Pharmacotherapy

A Pathophysiologic Approach

Eighth Edition

NOTICE

Medicine is an ever-changing science. As new research and clinical experience broaden our knowledge, changes in treatment and drug therapy are required. The authors and the publisher of this work have checked with sources believed to be reliable in their efforts to provide information that is complete and generally in accord with the standards accepted at the time of publication. However, in view of the possibility of human error or changes in medical sciences, neither the authors nor the publisher nor any other party who has been involved in the preparation or publication of this work warrants that the information contained herein is in every respect accurate or complete, and they disclaim all responsibility for any errors or omissions or for the results obtained from use of the information contained in this work. Readers are encouraged to confirm the information contained herein with other sources. For example and in particular, readers are advised to check the product information sheet included in the package of each drug they plan to administer to be certain that the information contained in this work is accurate and that changes have not been made in the recommended dose or in the contraindications for administration. This recommendation is of particular importance in connection with new or infrequently used drugs.

Laboratory	Conventional Units	Conversion Factor	SI Units
CD8 lymphocyte count	18–39% of total lymphocytes		
Cerebrospinal fluid (CSF)			
Pressure	75–175 mm H_2O		
Glucose	40–70 mg/dL	0.0555	2.2–3.9 mmol/L
Protein	15–45 mg/dL	0.01	0.15–0.45 g/L
WBC	Less than 10/mm³		
Ceruloplasmin	18–45 mg/dL	10	180–450 mg/L
		0.063	1.1–2.8 μmol/L
Chloride	97–110 mEq/L	1	97–110 mmol/L
Cholesterol			
Desirable	Less than 200 mg/dL	0.0259	Less than 5.18 mmol/L
Borderline high	200–239 mg/dL	0.0259	5.18–6.19 mmol/L
High	Greater than or equal to 240 mg/dL	0.0259	Greater than or equal to 6.2 mmol/L
Chorionic gonadotropin (β-hCG)	Less than 5 milliunits/mL	1	Less than 5 units/L
Clozapine	Minimum trough 300–350 ng/mL or mcg/L	3.06	918–1071 nmol/L
CO_2 content	22–30 mEq/L	1	22–30 mmol/L
Complement component 3 (C3)	70–160 mg/dL	0.01	0.7–1.6 g/L
Complement component 4 (C4)	20–40 mg/dL	0.01	0.2–0.4 g/L
Copper	70–150 mcg/dL	0.157	11–24 μmol/L
Cortisol (fasting, morning)	5–25 mcg/dL	27.6	138–690 nmol/L
Cortisol (free, urinary)	10–100 mcg/day	2.76	28–276 nmol/day
Creatine kinase			
Male	30–200 IU/L	0.01667	0.50–3.33 μkat/L
Female	20–170 IU/L	0.01667	0.33–2.83 μkat/L
MB fraction	0–7 IU/L	0.01667	0.0–0.12 μkat/L
Creatinine clearance (CrCl) (urine)	85–135 mL/minute/1.73 m²	0.00963	0.82–1.3 mL/s/m²
Creatinine			
Male 4–20 years	0.2–1.0 mg/dL	88.4	18–88 μmol/L
Female 4–20 years	0.2–1.0 mg/dL	88.4	18–88 μmol/L
Male (adults)	0.7–1.3 mg/dL	88.4	62–115 μmol/L
Female (adults)	0.6–1.1 mg/dL	88.4	53–97 μmol/L
Cyclosporin			
Renal transplant	100–300 ng/mL or mcg/L	0.832	83–250 nmol/L
Cardiac, liver, or pancreatic transplant	200–350 ng/mL or mcg/L	0.832	166–291 nmol/L
Cryptococcal antigen	Negative		
D-dimers	Less than 250 ng/mL	1	Less than 250 mcg/L
Desipramine	75–300 ng/mL or mcg/L	3.75	281–1125 mmol/L
Dexamethasone suppression test (DST) (overnight)	8:00 am cortisol less than 5 mcg/dL	0.0276	Less than 0.14 μmol/L
DHEAS			
Male	170–670 mcg/dL	0.0271	4.6–18.2 μmol/L
Female			
Premenopausal	50–540 mcg/dL	0.0271	1.4–14.7 μmol/L
Postmenopausal	30–260 mcg/dL	0.0271	0.8–7.1 μmol/L
Digoxin, therapeutic	0.5–1.0 ng/mL or mcg/L	1.28	0.6–1.3 nmol/L
Erythrocyte count (blood) See under Red blood cell count			
Erythrocyte sedimentation rate (ESR)			
Westergren			
Male	0–20 mm/hour		
Female	0–30 mm/hour		
Wintrobe			
Male	0–9 mm/hour		
Female	0–15 mm/hour		
Erythropoietin	2–25 mIU/mL	1	2–25 IU/L
Estradiol			
Male	10–36 pg/mL	3.67	37–132 pmol/L
Female	34–170 pg/mL	3.67	125–624 pmol/L
Ethanol, legal intoxication	Greater than or equal to 50–100 mg/dL	0.217	10.9–21.7 mmol/L
	Greater than or equal to 0.05–0.1%	217	
Ethosuccimide, therapeutic	40–100 mg/L or mcg/mL	7.08	283–708 μmol/L
Factor VIII or factor IX			
Severe hemophilia	Less than 1 IU/dL	0.01	Less than 0.01 units/mL
Moderate hemophilia	1–5 IU/dL	0.01	0.01–0.05 units/mL
Mild hemophilia	Greater than 5 IU/dL	0.01	Greater than 0.05 units/mL
Usual adult levels	60–140 IU/dL	0.01	0.60–1.40 units/mL
Ferritin			
Male	20–250 ng/mL	1	20–250 mcg/L
Female	10–150 ng/mL	1	10–150 mcg/L
Fibrin degradation products (FDP)	2–10 mg/L		
Fibrinogen	200–400 mg/dL	0.01	2.0–4.0 g/L
Folate (plasma)	3.1–12.4 ng/mL	2.266	7.0–28.1 nmol/L
Folic acid (RBC)	125–600 ng/mL	2.266	283–1360 nmol/L
Follicle-stimulating hormone (FSH)			
Male	1–7 mIU/mL	1	1–7 IU/L
Female			
Follicular phase	1–9 mIU/mL	1	1–9 IU/L
Midcycle	6–26 mIU/mL	1	6–26 IU/L
Luteal phase	1–9 mIU/mL	1	1–9 IU/L
Postmenopausal	30–118 mIU/mL	1	30–118 IU/L
Free thyroxine index (FT_4I)	6.5–12.5		
Gamma glutamyl transferase (GGT)	0–30 IU/L	0.01667	0–0.5 μkat/L
Gastrin (fasting)	0–130 pg/mL	1	0–130 ng/L
Gentamicin, therapeutic	4–10 mg/L peak	2.09	8.4–21 μmol/L peak
	Less than or equal to 2 mg/L trough		Less than or equal to 4.2 μmol/L trough
Globulin	2.3–3.5 g/dL	10	23–35 g/L
Glucose (fasting, plasma)	65–109 mg/dL	0.0555	3.6–6.00 mmol/L
Glucose, two hour postprandial blood (PPBG)	Less than 140 mg/dL	0.0555	Less than 7.8 mmol/L
Granulocyte count	1.8–6.6 × 10³/μL	10⁶	1.8–6.6 × 10⁹/L
Growth hormone (fasting)			
Male	Less than 5 ng/mL	1	Less than 5 mcg/L
Female	Less than 10 ng/mL	1	Less than 10 mcg/L

(continued on back inside cover)

Pharmacotherapy
A Pathophysiologic Approach
Eighth Edition

Joseph T. DiPiro, PharmD, FCCP

Executive Dean and Professor, South Carolina
College of Pharmacy, University of South Carolina, Columbia South Carolina
and Medical University of South Carolina, Charleston, South Carolina

Robert L. Talbert, PharmD, FCCP, BCPS, CLS

Professor, College of Pharmacy, University of Texas at Austin,
Pharmacotherapy Division, Professor, School of Medicine,
University of Texas Health Science Center at San Antonio,
Pharmacotherapy Education & Research Center
(PERC), UTHSCSA-PERC, San Antonio, Texas

Gary C. Yee, PharmD, FCCP, BCOP

Professor and Associate Dean for Academic Affairs, College of
Pharmacy, University of Nebraska Medical Center, Omaha, Nebraska

Gary R. Matzke, PharmD, FCP, FCCP, FASN

Professor and Associate Dean for Clinical Research and Public Policy,
School of Pharmacy, Professor of Internal Medicine, Nephrology Division,
School of Medicine, Virginia Commonwealth University, Richmond, Virginia

Barbara G. Wells, PharmD, FCCP, BCPP

Dean and Professor, Executive Director of the Research
Institute of Pharmaceutical Sciences, School of Pharmacy,
The University of Mississippi, Oxford, Mississippi

L. Michael Posey, BSPharm

Editorial Director, Periodicals Department,
American Pharmacists Association, Washington D.C.

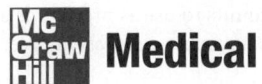

New York   Chicago   San Francisco   Lisbon   London   Madrid   Mexico City
Milan   New Delhi   San Juan   Seoul   Singapore   Sydney   Toronto

Pharmacotherapy: A Pathophysiologic Approach, Eighth Edition

1 2 3 4 5 6 7 8 9 0   CTP/CTP   14 13 12 11

ISBN 978-0-07-170354-3
MHID 0-07-170354-3

This book was set in Minion Pro by Thomson Digital.
The editors were Michael Weitz and Karen G. Edmonson.
The production supervisor was Sherri Souffrance.
Project management was provided by Aakriti Kathuria, Thomson Digital.
The interior designer is Alan Barnett; cover design by The Gazillion Group with
    photo by David Mack/Photo Researchers, Inc.
China Translation & Printing, Ltd. was printer and binder.

Library of Congress Cataloging-in-Publication Data

Pharmacotherapy: a pathophysiologic approach / editors, Joseph T. DiPiro ... [et al.]. — 8th ed.
    p. ; cm.
  Includes bibliographical references and index.
  Summary: "The most comprehensive, widely used, and evidence-based pharmacotherapy text available. Hailed by Doody's Review Service as "one of the best in pharmacy" Pharmacotherapy: A Pathophysiologic Approach is unmatched in its ability to help students develop a mastery of evidence-based medicine for optimum patient outcomes. The eighth edition will feature the addition of SI units throughout and an increased number of global examples and clinical questions. Features unparalleled guidance in the development of pharmaceutical care plans. Full-color presentation. Key Concepts in each chapter. Critical Presentation boxes summarize common disease signs and symptoms. Clinical Controversy boxes examine complicated issues you face when providing drug therapy. NEW material added to the online learning center. EXPANDED evidence-based recommendations. EXPANDED coverage of timely issues such as palliative care and pain medicine. Therapeutic recommendations in each disease-specific chapter"—Provided by publisher.
  ISBN-13: 978-0-07-170354-3 (pbk. : alk. paper)
  ISBN-10: 0-07-170354-3 (pbk. : alk. paper)
  1. Chemotherapy. 2. Physiology, Pathological. I. DiPiro, Joseph T.
  [DNLM: 1. Drug Therapy. WB 330]
  RM263.P56 2011
  615.5'8—dc22

                                                                                    2010039580

Please tell the authors and publisher what you think of this book by sending your comments to *pharmacotherapy@mcgraw-hill.com*. Please put the author and title of the book in the subject line.

DEDICATION

To our patients, who have challenged and inspired us
and given meaning to all our endeavors.

To practitioners who continue to improve patient health outcomes
and thereby serve as role models for their colleagues and students
while clinging tenaciously to the highest standards of practice.

To our mentors, whose vision provided educational and training
programs that encouraged our professional growth and challenged us
to be innovators in our patient care, research, and education.

To our faculty colleagues for their efforts and support for our mission
to provide a comprehensive and challenging educational
foundation for the pharmacists of the future.

And finally to our families for the time that they have sacrificed
so that this eighth edition would become a reality.

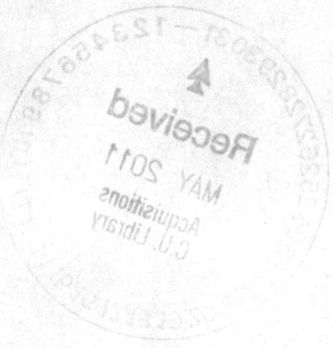

CONTENTS

The complete chapter, learning objectives, and other resources can be found at **www.pharmacotherapyonline.com**.

SECTION 3

Respiratory Disorders

Section Editor: Robert L. Talbert

SECTION 4

Gastrointestinal Disorders

Section Editor: Joseph T. DiPiro

SECTION 5

Renal Disorders

Section Editor: Gary R. Matzke

🖰 The complete chapter, learning objectives, and other resources can be found at **www.pharmacotherapyonline.com**.

SECTION 6

Neurologic Disorders

Section Editor: Barbara G. Wells

SECTION 7

Psychiatric Disorders

Section Editor: Barbara G. Wells

🖱 The complete chapter, learning objectives, and other resources can be found at **www.pharmacotherapyonline.com**.

The complete chapter, learning objectives, and other resources can be found at **www.pharmacotherapyonline.com**.

SECTION 15

Hematologic Disorders

Section Editor: Gary C. Yee

SECTION 16

Infectious Diseases

Section Editor: Joseph T. DiPiro

SECTION 17

Oncologic Disorders

Section Editor: Gary C. Yee

The complete chapter, learning objectives, and other resources can be found at **www.pharmacotherapyonline.com**.

SECTION 18
Nutritional Disorders

Section Editor: Gary R. Matzke

The complete chapter, learning objectives, and other resources can be found at **www.pharmacotherapyonline.com**.

CONTRIBUTORS

Val R. Adams, PharmD, FCCP, BCOP

Associate Professor, Department of Pharmacy Practice and Science, University of Kentucky, College of Pharmacy, Lexington, Kentucky

Chapter 137

Sarah E. Adkins, PharmD

The Ohio State University, College of Pharmacy, Columbus, Ohio

Chapter 5

Jeffrey R. Aeschlimann, PharmD

Associate Professor, University of Connecticut School of Pharmacy, Storrs, Connecticut

Chapter 113

Rondall E. Allen, B.S. PharmD

Associate Dean for Student Affairs and Curricular Assessment, Clinical Assistant Professor, Xavier University of Louisiana, College of Pharmacy, New Orleans, Louisiana

Chapter 45

J. V. Anandan, PharmD

Pharmacy Specialist, Center for Drug Use Analysis and Information, Henry Ford Hospital and Adjunct Associate Professor, Eugene Apppelbaum College of Pharmacy and Health Sciences, Wayne State University, Detroit, Michigan

Chapter 124

Peter L. Anderson, PharmD

Associate Professor, Department of Pharmoceutical Sciences, School of Pharmacy, University of Colorado - Denver, Aurora, Colorado

Chapter 134

Tami R. Argo, PharmD, MS, BCPP

Clinical Pharmacy Specialist-Psychiatry, Iowa City Veterans Affairs Medical Center, Iowa City, Iowa

Chapter 76

Edward P. Armstrong, PharmD

Professor, Department of Pharmacy Practice and Science, College of Pharmacy, University of Arizona, Tuscon, Arizona

Chapter 127

Jill Astolfi, PharmD

Client Relations Liaison, Hospice Pharmacia, a service of excelleRx, Inc., an Omnicare company

Chapter 12

Daniel H. Atchley, PhD, MS, MT-ASCP

Associate Professor and Director of Assessment, Harding University College of Pharmacy, Harding University, Searcy, Arkansas

Chapter 95

Rebecca L. Attridge, PharmD, MSC

Assistant Professor, Department of Pharmacy Practice, Feik School of Pharmacy, University of The Incarnate Word, San Antonio, Texas

Chapter 35

Jacquelyn L. Bainbridge PharmD, FCCI

Professor, Department of Clinical Pharmacy and Department of Neurology, University of Colorado - Denver, Aurora, Colorado

Chapter 64

Jeffrey F. Barletta, PharmD, FCCM

Associate Professor, Department of Pharmacy Practice, Midwestern University, College of Pharmacy, Glendale, Arizona

Chapter 18

Chad M. Barnett, PharmD, BCOP

Clinical Pharmacy Specialist, Breast Oncology, University of Texas M.D. Anderson Cancer Center, Houston, Texas

Chapter 136

Larry A. Bauer, PharmD, FCP, FCCP

Professor, Departments of Pharmacy and Laboratory Medicine, Schools of Pharmacy and Medicine, University of Washington, Seattle, Washington

Chapter 8

Jerry L. Bauman, PharmD, FCCP, FACC

Dean, University of Illinois at Chicago College of Pharmacy, Professor, Departments of Pharmacy Practice and Medicine, Section of Cardiology, University of Illinois at Chicago, Chicago, Illinois

Chapter 25

Terry J. Baumann, BS, PharmD

Clinical Manager and Clinical Pharmacist, Munson Medical Center, Traverse City, Michigan

Chapter 69

Oralia V. Bazaldua, PharmD, FCCP, BCPS

Associate Professor, Department of Family & Community Medicine, The University of Texas Health Science Center at San Antonio

Chapter 3

Rosemary R. Berardi, PharmD, FCCP, FASHP, FAPHA

Professor of Pharmacy, College of Pharmacy, University of Michigan, Ann Arbor, Michigan

Chapter 40

Martha G. Blackford, PharmD

Division of Clinical Pharmacology and Toxicology, Department of Pediatrics, Children's Hospital Medical Center, Akron Children's Hospital, Akron, Ohio

Chapter 116

Scott Bolesta, PharmD, BCPS

Assistant Professor, Department of Pharmacy Practice, Clinical Pharmacists, Mercy Hospital, Scranton, Pennsylvania

Chapter 46

Bradley A. Boucher, PharmD, FCCP, FCCM

Professor of Clinical Pharmacy, Department of Clinical Pharmacy, College of Pharmacy, and Associate Professor of Neurosurgery, Department of Neurosurgery, College of Medicine, University of Tennessee, Memphis, Tennessee

Chapter 67

Denise Boudreau, RPh, PhD

Scientific Investigator, Group Health Center for Health Studies, Seattle, Washington

Chapter 13

Sharya V. Bourdet, PharmD, BCPS

Critical Care Pharmacist/Clinical Inpatient Program Manager, Veterans Affairs Medical Center, Health Sciences Clinical Assistant Professor, School of Pharmacy, University of California, San Francisco, San Francisco, California

Chapter 34

Nancy Brahm, PharmD, MS, BCPP, CGP

Clinical Associate Professor, Department of Clinical and Administrative Sciences, College of Pharmacy, University of Oklahoma, Tulsa, Oklahoma

Chapter 82

Donald F. Brophy, PharmD, MSc, FCCP, FASN, BCPS

Professor and Chairman Department of Pharmacotherapy & Outcomes Science, School of Pharmacy and Professor of Internal Medicine, Virginia Commonwealth University Medical College of Virginia Campus, Richmond, Virginia

Chapter 60

Jason E. Brouillard, PharmD

Critical Care Pharmacist, Sacred Heart Medical Center, Spokane, WA, Adjunct Clinical Instructor, Department of Pharmacotherapy College of Pharmacy, Washington State University, Spokane, Washington

Chapter 15

Thomas E. R. Brown, PharmD

Associate Professor, Leslie Dan Faculty of Pharmacy, University of Toronto and Sunnybrook Health Science Center, Toronto, Ontario

Chapter 129

Dianne M. Brundage, PharmD, FCCP, BCPS, BCOP

Oncology Clinical Pharmacy Specialist, Park Nicollet Health Services Methodist Hospital, Assistant Professor, College of Pharmacy, University of Minnesota, Minneapolis, Minnesota

Chapter 142

Edward M. Buchanan, MD

Thomas Jefferson University, Jefferson Medical College, Philadelphia, Pennsylvania

Chapter 89

Peter F. Buckley, MD

Professor and Chairman, Psychiatry and Health Behavior, Senior Associate Dean for Leadership Development, Medical College of Georgia, Augusta, Georgia

Chapter 76

David S. Burgess, PharmD, FCCP

James T. Doluisio Regents Clinical Professor and Head, Pharmacotherapy, College of Pharmacy, The University of Texas at Austin, Clinical Professor, Department of Medicine, Division of Infectious Diseases, Director, Pharmacotherapy Education and Research Center School of Medicine, The University of Texas Health Science Center, San Antonio, Texas

Chapter 114

Julianna A. Burzynski, PharmD, BCPS, BCOP

Clinical Pharmacy Specialist, Hematology/Oncology, Mayo Clinic, Rochester, Minnesota

Chapter 145

Lucinda M. Buys, PharmD, BCPS

Associate Professor (Clinical), Department of Pharmacy Practice and Science, University of Iowa College of Pharmacy and the Siouxland Medical Education Foundation, Sioux City, Iowa

Chapter 101

Karim Anton Calis, PharmD, MPH, FASHP, FCCP

Adjunct Clinical Investigator, Program in Developmental Endocrinology and Genetics, *Eunice Kennedy Shriver* National Institute of Child Health and Human Development, National Institutes of Health; Clinical Professor, University of Maryland and Virginia Commonwealth University, Richmond, Virginia

Chapters 86, 91, and 154

Kimberly A. Cappuzzo, PharmD, MS, CGP

Senior Regional Medical Liason, Metabolic Bone Team, Scientific Affairs, Amgen, Richmond, Virginia

Chapter 96

Peggy L. Carver, PharmD, FCCP

Associate Professor, Department of Clinical, Social, and Administrative Sciences, The University of Michigan, College of Pharmacy, Clinical Pharmacist, The University of Michigan Health System

Chapter 130

Larisa H. Cavallari, PharmD, FCCP, BCPS

Associate Professor, Department of Pharmacy Practice, College of Pharmacy, University of Illinois at Chicago

Chapters 9 and 20

Jose E. Cavazos, MD, PhD

Associate Professor of Neurology, Pharmacology and Physiology, University of Texas Health Science Center, San Antonio, Texas

Chapter 65

Alexandre Chan, PharmD, BCPS, BCOP

Assistant Professor, Department of Pharmacy, Faculty of Science, National University of Singapore, Clinical Pharmacist, Department of Pharmacy, National Cancer Centre, Singapore, Singapore

Chapter 140

C. Y. Jennifer Chan, PharmD

Clinical Associate Professor of Pediatrics, University of Texas Health Science Center at San Antonio, Clinical Assistant Professor of Pharmacy, University of Texas in Austin, San Antonio, Texas
Chapter 111

Jack J. Chen, PharmD, BCPS, CGP

Associate Professor (Neurology), Movement Disorders Center, Schools of Medicine and Pharmacy, Loma Linda University, Loma Linda, California
Chapter 68

Judy T. Chen, PharmD, BCPS

Clinical Assistant Professor of Pharmacy Practice Purdue University - School of Pharmacy and Pharmaceutical Sciences West Lafayette, Indiana
Chapter 154

Katherine Hammond Chessman, PharmD, FCCP, BCPS, BCNSP

Professor, Department of Pharmacy and Clinical Sciences, South Carolina College of Pharmacy, MUSC Campus, Clinical Pharmacy Specialist, Pediatrics/Pediatric Surgery, Department of Pharmacy Services, Medical University of South Carolina Children's Hospital, Charleston, South Carolina
Chapters 149 and 152

Thomas W. F. Chin*, BScPhm, PharmD, FCSHP

Clinical Pharmacy Specialist/leader- Antimicrobials & Infectious Diseases, St. Michael's Hospital and Assistant Professor, Leslie Dan Faculty of Pharmacy, University of Toronto, Toronto, Ontario
Chapter 129

Elaine Chiquette, PharmD. BCPS

Director, Research & Development Strategic Relations, Amylin Pharmaceuticals, Inc., San Antonio, Texas
Chapter 6

Mariann D. Churchwell, PharmD, BCPS

Assistant Professor, University of Toledo College of Pharmacy, Toledo, Ohio
Chapter 54

Peter A. Chyka, PharmD, FAACT, DABAT

Professor, Department of Clinical Pharmacy; Associate Dean, Knoxville Campus, University of Tennessee College of Pharmacy, Knoxville, Tennessee
Chapter 14

Elizabeth C. Clark, MD, MPH

Assistant Professor, Department of Family Medicine, University of Medicine and Dentistry of New Jersey, Robert Wood Johnson Medical School, New Brunswick, New Jersey
Chapter 102

Kristen Cook, PharmD, BCPS

Assistant Professor, Department of Pharmacy Practice, University of Nebraska Medical Center College of Pharmacy, Clinical Pharmacist, Nebraska-Western Iowa VA Healthcare System, Omaha, Nebraska
Chapter 109

Stephen Joel Coons, PhD

Director, Patient-Reported Outcomes Consortium, Critical Path Institute, Tucson, Arizona
Chapter 2

John R. Corboy, MD

Professor, Neurology, University of Colorado School of Medicine, Co-Director, Rocky Mountain Multiple Sclerosis Center at Anschutz Medical Center, Staff Neurologist, Denver Veteran's Affairs Medical Center, Aurora, Colorado
Chapter 64

Lisa T. Costanigro, PharmD, BCPS

Staff Pharmacist, Paudre Valley Health System, Fort Collins, Colorado
Chapter 15

Elizabeth A. Coyle, PharmD, BCPS

Clinical Associate Professor, University of Houston College of Pharmacy, Houston, Texas
Chapter 125

James D. Coyle

Assistant Professor of Clinical Pharmacy, College of Pharmacy, The Ohio State University, Columbus, Ohio
Chapter 58

Catherine M. Crill, PharmD, BCPS, BCNSP

Associate Professor, Departments of Clinical Pharmacy and Pediatrics, The University of Tennessee Health Science Center, Memphis, Tennessee
Chapter 151

M. Lynn Crismon, PharmD

Dean, James T. Doluisio Regents Chair & Behren's Centennial Professor, College of Pharmacy, The University of Texas at Austin, Austin, Texas
Chapter 76

Michael A. Crouch, PharmD, FASHP, BCPS

Professor and Associate Dean, Gatton College of Pharmacy, East Tennessee State University, Johnson City, Tennessee
Chapter 120

William Dager, PharmD, BCPS, FCSHP, FCCP, FCCM

Pharmacist Specialist, UC Davis Medical Center, Clinical Professor of Pharmacy, UC San Francisco School of Pharmacy, Clinical Professor of Medicine, UC Davis School of Medicine, Clinical Professor of Pharmacy, Touro School of Pharmacy, Sacramento, California
Chapter 51

Devra K. Dang, PharmD, BCPS, CDE

Associate Clinical Professor, University of Connecticut School of Pharmacy, Storrs, Connecticut
Chapter 91

Larry H. Danziger, PharmD

Professor of Pharmacy, College of Pharmacy, University of Illinois at Chicago, Chicago, Illinois
Chapter 119

*Deceased

Joseph F. Dasta, MSc, FCCM, FCCP

Professor Emeritus, The Ohio State University, Columbus, Ohio, Adjunct Professor, University of Texas, Austin, Texas

Chapter 30

Lisa E. Davis, PharmD, BCPS, BCOP

Associate Professor of Clinical Pharmacy, Philadelphia College of Pharmacy, University of the Sciences in Philadelphia, Philadelphia, Pennsylvania

Chapter 138

Susan R. Davis, MBBS, FRACP, PhD

Department of Medicine, Monash University, Melbourne, Australia

Chapter 91

Jeffrey C. Delafuente, MS, FCCP, FASCP

Associate Dean for Professional Education and Professor of Pharmacotherapy and Outcomes Science, Virginia Commonwealth University School of Pharmacy, Richmond, Virginia

Chapter 96

Mark DeLegge, MD, FACG, CNSP, AGAF, FASGE

Professor of Medicine and Director Digestive Disease Center, Director of Nutrition, Medical University of South Carolina, Charleston, South Carolina

Chapter 153

Paulina Deming, PharmD

University of New Mexico College of Pharmacy, Project ECHO Hepatitis C Community Clinic, Alburquerque, New Mexico

Chapter 47

Simon De Denus, B.Pharm, MSC, PhD

Faculty of Pharmacy, University de Montreal, Montreal Heart Institute, Montreal, Quebec

Chapter 24

Vimal K. Derebail, MD

Clinical Assistant Professor UNC Kidney Center, Division of Nephrology and Hypertension, University of North Carolina at Chapel Hill

Chapter 52

John W. Devlin, PharmD, FCCP, FCCM, BCPS

Associate Professor, Northeastern University School of Pharmacy, Adjunct Associate Professor, Tufts University School of Medicine, Boston, Massachusetts

Chapter 61

Vanessa A. Diaz, MD, MS

Medical University of South Carolina, Department of Family Medicine, Charleston, South Carolina

Chapter 88

Roland N. Dickerson, PharmD, BCNSP, FACN, FCCP

Professor of Clinical Pharmacy, University of Tennessee Health Science Center, Memphis, Tennessee

Chapter 150

Cecily V. DiPiro, PharmD

Consultant Pharmacist, Mt. Pleasant, South Carolina

Chapter 42

Joseph T. DiPiro, PharmD, FCCP

Executive Dean and Professor, South Carolina College of Pharmacy, Medical University of South Carolina and the University of South Carolina

Chapters 97 and 123

Paul L. Doering, MS

Distinguished Service Professor of Pharmacy Practice, College of Pharmacy, University of Florida, Gainesville, Florida

Chapters 74 and 75

Julie A. Dopheide, PharmD, BCPP

Associate Professor, Clinical Pharmacy, Psychiatry and the Behavioral Sciences, University of Southern California Schools of Pharmacy and Medicine, Los Angeles, California

Chapter 72

John M. Dopp, PharmD

Assistant Professor, School of Pharmacy, University of Wisconsin, Madison, Wisconsin

Chapter 81

Thomas C. Dowling, PharmD, PhD, FCP

Associate Professor and Vice Chair, Department of Pharmacy Practice and Science, University of Maryland School of Pharmacy, Baltimore, Maryland

Chapter 50

Shannon J. Drayton, PharmD, BCPP

Assistant Professor, Department of Clinical Pharmacy and Outcomes Research, South Carolina College of Pharmacy, MUSC Campus, Charleston, South Carolina

Chapter 78

Linda D. Dresser, PharmD

Assistant Professor Leslie Dan Faculty of Pharmacy, University of Toronto and University Health Network, Toronto, Canada

Chapter 129

Deepak P. Edward, MD, FACS

Summa Health System and Northeastern Ohio Universities College of Medicine, Akron, Ohio

Chapter 103

Mary Elizabeth Elliott, PharmD, PhD

Associate Professor, Pharmacy Practice Division, University of Wisconsin-Madison School of Pharmacy, Madison, Wisconsin, Clinical Pharmacist, Osteoporosis Clinic, VA Medical Center, Madison, Wisconsin

Chapter 101

Michael E. Ernst, PharmD

Professor (Clinical), Department of Pharmacy Practice and Science, College of Pharmacy; and Department of Family Medicine, Carver College of Medicine, The University of Iowa, Iowa City, Iowa

Chapter 102

Brian L. Erstad, PharmD, FCCM, FCCP, FASHP

Professor, Department of Pharmacy Practice and Science, University of Arizona College of Pharmacy, Tucson Arizona

Chapter 31

Francisco J. Esteva, MD, PhD

Director, Breast Cancer Translational Research Laboratory, Professor, Departments of Breast Medical Oncology and Molecular and Cellular Oncology, University of Texas M.D. Anderson Cancer Center, Houston, Texas

Chapter 136

Susan C. Fagan, PharmD, BCPS, FCCP

Jowdy Professor, Associate Head, Assistant Dean, University of Georgia College of Pharmacy, Augusta, Georgia

Chapters 27 and 62

Christopher A. Fausel, PharmD, BCPS, BCOP

Clinical Director, Oncology Pharmacy Services, Indiana University Simon Cancer Center, Indianapolis, Indiana

Chapter 143

Richard G. Fiscella, PharmD, MPH

Clinical Professor, Department of Pharmacy Practice and Adjunct Assistant Professor, Department of Ophthalmology, University of Illinois at Chicago, Chicago, Illinois

Chapter 103

Douglas N. Fish, PharmD

Professor, Department of Clinical Pharmacy, University of Colorado Denver School of Pharmacy, Clinical Specialist in Infectious Diseases/Critical Care, University of Colorado Hospital, Aurora, Colorado

Chapters 119 and 131

Virginia H. Fleming, PharmD

Clinical Assistant Professor, Department of Clinical and Administrative Pharmacy, University of Georgia College of Pharmacy, Athens, Georgia

Chapter 43

Courtney V. Fletcher, PharmD

Dean and Professor, College of Pharmacy, University of Nebraska Medical Center, Omaha, Nebraska

Chapter 134

Bradi Frei, PharmD, BCPS, BCOP

Assistant Professor, Department of Pharmacy Practice, University of the Incarnate Word, San Antonio, Texas

Chapter 117

Christopher Frei, PharmD, MSc, BCPS

Assistant Professor, Pharmacotherapy Division, College of Pharmacy, The University of Texas at Austin; Clinical Assistant Professor, Department of Medicine, Division of Infectious Diseases and Pharmacotherapy Education & Research Center, School of Medicine, The University of Texas Health Science Center at San Antonio, Texas

Chapter 117

Allan D. Friedman, MD, MPH

Professor and Chair, Division of General Pediatrics, Department of Pediatrics, Virginia Commonwealth University, Richmond, Virginia

Chapter 127

Deborah A. Frieze, PharmD, BCOP

Inpatient Pharmacy Manager, University of Washington Medical Center, Clinical Assistant Professor, University of Washington School of Pharmacy, Seattle, Washington

Chapter 137

Jane Frumin, PharmD

Assistant Professor, Clinical and Administrative Sciences, College of Notre Dame of Maryland School of Pharmacy, Baltimore, Maryland

Chapter 60

Randolph V. Fugit, PharmD, BCPS

Internal Medicine Clinical Specialist, Denver Veterans Affairs Medical Center, Clinical Assistant Professor, Clinical Pharmacy Practice, University of Colorado Denver Health Sciences Center, Denver, Colorado

Chapter 40

Mark L. Glover, BS Pharm, PharmD

Associate Professor and Director, West Palm Beach program, Department of Pharmacy Practice, College of Pharmacy, Nova Southeastern University, Palm Beach Gardens, Florida

Chapter 116

Shelly L. Gray, PharmD, MS

Professor, School of Pharmacy, University of Washington, Seattle, Washington

Chapter 11

David R.P. Guay, PharmD

Professor, Department of Experimental and Clinical Pharmacology, College of Pharmacy, University of Minnesota, Division of Geriatrics, Health Partners Inc., Minneapolis, Minnesota

Chapters 11 and 94

Wayne P. Gulliver, MD, FRCP

Professor of Medicine and Dermatology, and Chair, Discipline of Medicine, Faculty of Medicine, Memorial University of Newfoundland, St. John's Newfoundland and Labrador, Canada

Chapter 107

John G. Gums, PharmD, FCCP

Professor of Pharmacy and Medicine, Associate Chair, Department of Pharmacotherapy and Translational Research, Director of Clinical Research in Family Medicine Departments of Pharmacotherapy and Translational Research and Community Health and Family Medicine, University of Florida

Chapter 85

Stuart T. Haines, PharmD, FCCP, FASHP, FAPHA

Professor, Department of Pharmacy Practice and Science, University of Maryland School of Pharmacy, Baltimore, Maryland and Clinical Pharmacy Specialist, Patient Care Services, West Palm Beach, Virginia Medical Center

Chapter 26

Emily R. Hajjar, PharmD, BCPS, CGP

Associate Professor, Jefferson School of Pharmacy, Thomas Jefferson University, Philadelphia, Pennsylvania

Chapter 11

Jenana Halilovic, PharmD, BCPS

Assistant Professor, Thomas J Long School of Pharmacy, University of the Pacific, Stockton, California and Clinical Pharmacist, UC Davis Medical Center, Sacramento, California

Chapter 51

Philip D. Hall, PharmD, FCCP, BCPS, BCOP

Professor, South Carolina College of Pharmacy, Medical University of South Carolina, Charleston, South Carolina

Chapter 95

Steven M. Handler, Md, PhD

Assistant Professor, University of Pittsburgh School of Medicine, Department of Biomedical Informatics and Division of Geriatric Medicine, Geriatric Research Education and Clinical Center (GRECC), Veterans Affairs Pittsburgh Healthcare Center (VAPHS), Pittsburgh, Pennsylvania

Chapter 11

Joseph T. Hanlon, PharmD, MS

Professor of Medicine, Pharmacy and Epidemiology, University of Pittsburgh and Health Scientist, CHERP/GRECC, Pittsburgh Veterans Affairs Pittsburgh Health System, Pittsburgh, Pennsylvania

Chapter 11

Christine N. Hansen, PharmD

Clinical Pharmacy Specialist, Department of Pharmacy, Lakeland Regional Medical Center, Lakeland, Florida

Chapter 112

Michelle Harkins, MD

Associate Professor of Medicine, Pulmonary and Critical Care, University of New Mexico Health Sciences Center, Albuquerque, New Mexico

Chapter 36

Mary S. Hayney, PharmD, MPH

Professor of Pharmacy (CHS), University of Wisconsin School of Pharmacy

Chapter 133

Thomas K. Hazlet, PharmD, DrPH

Associate Professor, Pharmaceutical Outcomes Research & Policy Program, School of Pharmacy, University of Washington, Seattle, Washington

Chapter 13

Brian A. Hemstreet, PharmD, BCPS

Associate Professor, Department of Clinical Pharmacy, University of Colorado, Denver School of Pharmacy, Aurora, Colorado

Chapter 41

Elizabeth D. Hermsen, PharmD, MBA, BCPS-ID

Antimicrobial Stewardship Program Coordinator, Pharmacy Relations & Clinical Decision Support, The Nebraska Medical Center; Adjunct Assistant Professor, Department of Pharmacy Practice, University of Nebraska Medical Center, College of Pharmacy; Adjunct Assistant Professor, Section of Infectious Diseases, Department of Internal Medicine, University of Nebraska Medical Center, College of Medicine, Omaha, Nebraska

Chapters 115 and 118

Chris M. Herndon, PharmD, BCPS, CPE

Assistant Professor, Department of Pharmacy Practice, Southern Illinois University, Edwardsville School of Pharmacy, Edwardsville, Illinois

Chapter 69

David C. Hess, MD

Professor and Chairman, Department of Neurology, Medical College of Georgia, Augusta, Georgia

Chapter 27

Angela Massey Hill, PharmD, BCPP

Florida A & M University, College of Pharmacy, Professor and Division Director of Pharmacy Practice, Tallahassee, Florida

Chapter 63

L. David Hillis, MD

Professor and Chair, Department of Medicine, University of Texas Health Science Center, San Antonio, Texas

Chapter 17

Jonathan Himmelfarb, MD

Professor of Medicine, Joseph W. Eschbach, MD, Endowed Chair for Kidney Research, Director, Kidney Research Institute, Department of Medicine, Division of Nephrology, University of Washington, Seattle, Washington

Chapter 55

Brian M. Hodges, PharmD, BCPS, BCNSP

Assistant Professor, Department of Clinical Pharmacy, West Virginia University School of Pharmacy, West Virginia

Chapter 153

Barbara J. Hoeben, PharmD, MSPharm, BCPS

Pharmacy Flight Commander, Davis-Monthan Air Force Base, Tucson, Arizona

Chapter 29

Collin A. Hovinga, PharmD

University of Tennessee Health Science Center, LeBonheur Children's Medical Center, Memphis, Tennessee

Chapter 66

Thomas R. Howdieshell, MD, FACS, FCCP

Professor of Surgery, Trauma/Surgical Critical Care, University of New Mexico HSC, Albuquerque, New Mexico

Chapter 123

Joanna Q. Hudson, PharmD, BCPS, FASN

Associate Professor, Departments of Clinical Pharmacy and Medicine (Nephrology), The University of Tennessee Health Science Center, Memphis, Tennessee

Chapter 53

Grant F. Hutchins, MD

Assistant Professor Gastroenterology/Hepatology, Director of Advanced Endoscopy, University of Nebraska Medical Center, Omaha, Nebraska

Chapter 38

Robert J. Ignoffo, PharmD

Touro University, Vallejo, California

Chapter 42

Beata A. Ineck, PharmD, BCPS, CDE

Home Based Primary Care, Clinical Pharmacist, Boise VA Medical Center, Boise, Idaho

Chapter 109

Arthur A. Islas, MD, MPH, CAQ–Sports Medicine, FAWM

Associate Professor, Department of Family & Community Medicine, Paul L. Foster School of Medicine, Texas Tech University Health Science Center, El Paso, Texas

Chapter 4

Heather J. Johnson, PharmD, BCPS, FASN

Assistant Professor, Department of Pharmacy and Therapeutics, University of Pittsburgh School of Pharmacy, Clinical Pharmacist, University of Pittsburgh Medical Center, Pittsburgh, Pennsylvania

Chapter 98

Jacqueline Jonklaas, MD, PhD

Associate Professor, Division of Endocrinology, Georgetown University Medical Center, Washington DC

Chapter 84

Melanie S. Joy, PharmD, PhD, FCCP, FASN

Associate Professor, School of Medicine, Division of Nephrology & Hypertension, UNC Kidney Center, and Associate Professor, School of Pharmacy, Division of Pharmacotherapy and Experimental Therapeutics, University of North Carolina at Chapel Hill, Chapel Hill, North Carolina

Chapter 52

Rose Jung, PharmD, MPH, BCPS

Visiting Associate Professor, Department of Pharmacy Practice, University of Toledo, College of Pharmacy, Toledo, Ohio

Chapter 122

Thomas N. Kakuda, PharmD

Director, Clinical Pharmacology, Tibotec, Inc., Titusville, New Jersey

Chapter 134

Sophia N. Kalantaridou, MD, PhD

Associate Professor, Department of Obstetrics and Gynecology, Division of Reproductive Endocrinology, University of Ioannina Medical School, Ioannina, Greece

Chapter 91

Judith C. Kando, PharmD, BCPP

Ortho-McNeil Janssen Scientific Affairs, LLC, Tewksbury, Massachusetts

Chapter 77

S. Lena Kang-Birken, PharmD, FCCP

Associate Professor, Department of Pharmacy Practice, Thomas J. Long School of Pharmacy and Health Sciences, University of The Pacific, Stockton, California

Chapter 128

Salmaan Kanji, PharmD

Clinical Pharmacy Specialist (ICU), Department of Pharmacy and Critical Care, The Ottawa Hospital, Associate Scientist, Clinical Epidemiology Program, Ottawa Hospital Institute, Ottawa, Ontario

Chapter 132

H. William Kelly, PharmD

Professor Emeritus Pediatrics, University of New Mexico Health Sciences Center, Albuquerque, New Mexico

Chapter 33

Patrick J. Kiel, PharmD, BCPS, BCOP

Clinical Pharmacy Specialist, Hematology/Stem Cell Transplant, Indiana University Simon Cancer Center, Indianapolis, Indiana

Chapter 143

Karla Killgore-Smith, PharmD, BCPS

Clinical Pharmacist, Santa Barbara Cottage Hospital, Adjunct Professor of Pharmacy, University of Pacific, Santa Barbara, California

Chapter 128

William R. Kirchain, PharmD, CDE

Wilbur and Mildred Robichaux Endowed Professor, Division of Clinical and Administrative Sciences, College of Pharmacy, Xavier University of Louisiana, New Orleans, Louisiana

Chapter 45

Cynthia K. Kirkwood, PharmD, BCPP

Associate Professor of Pharmacy, Vice Chair for Education, Department of Pharmacotherapy and Outcome Science, School of Pharmacy, Virginia Commonwealth University, Richmond, Virginia

Chapters 79 and 80

Leroy C. Knodel, PharmD

Associate Professor, Department of Surgery, The University of Texas Health Science Center, San Antonio, San Antonio, Texas, Clinical Associate Professor, College of Pharmacy, The University of Texas at Austin, Austin, Texas

Chapter 126

Jill M. Kolesar, PharmD, BCPS, FCCP

Professor of Pharmacy, University of Wisconsin, School of Pharmacy, University of Wisconsin Carbone Cancer Center, Madison, Wisconsin

Chapter 139

Sunil Kripalani, MD, MSc

Associate Professor and Chief, Section of Hospital Medicine, Vanderbilt University, Nashville, Tennessee

Chapter 3

Abhijit V. Kshirsagar, MD, MPH

Associate Professor of Medicine Division of Nephrology and Hypertension, UNC Kidney Center, University of North Carolina at Chapel Hill, Chapel Hill, North Carolina

Chapter 52

Vanessa J. Kumpf, PharmD, BCNSP

Clinical Specialist, Nutrition Support, Vanderbilt University Medical Center, Nashville, Tennessee

Chapters 149 and 152

Po Gin Kwa, MD, FRCP

Clinical Associate Professor, Faculty of Medicine, Memorial University of Newfoundland, St. John's Newfoundland, Canada

Chapter 108

Ninh M. La-Beck, PharmD

Assistant Professor, Center for Immunotherapeutic Research and Department of Pharmacy Practice, School of Pharmacy, Texas Tech University Health Sciences Center, Abilene, Texas

Chapter 146

Thomas Lackner, PharmD

Experimental and Clinical Pharmacology, College of Pharmacy, University of Minnesota, Minneapolis, Minnesota

Chapter 94

Y. W. Francis Lam, PharmD, FCCP

Professor of Pharmacology, University of Texas Health Science Center at San Antonio, Associate Professor of Medicine, University of Texas Health Science Centre at San Antonio, Clinical Associate Professor of Pharmacy, University of Texas at Austin, Austin, Texas

Chapters 9 and 48

Richard A. Lange, MD, MBA

Professor and Executive Vice Chairman, Department of Medicine, The University of Texas Health Science Center, San Antonio, Texas

Chapter 17

Kerry L. Laplante, PharmD

University of Rhode Island, Department of Pharmacy Practice, Infectious Diseases Research Laboratory, Providence Veterans Affairs Medical Center, Division of Infectious Diseases, Department of Medicine, Warren Alpert Medical School of Brown University, Providence, Rhode Island

Chapter 113

Alan H. Lau, PharmD, FCCP

Professor of Pharmacy Practice and Director, International Clinical Pharmacy Education College of Pharmacy University of Illinois at Chicago, Chicago, Illinois

Chapter 56

David T.S. Law, BSc, MD, PhD, CCFP

Assistant Professor, Department of Community and Family Medicine, University of Toronto, and Staff Physician, Department of Family Practice, The Scarborough Hospital and Rouge Valley Health System, Scarborough, Ontario, Canada

Chapter 105

Rebecca M. Law, PharmD

Associate Professor, School of Pharmacy and Discipline of Family Medicine, Faculty of Medicine, Memorial University of Newfoundland, St. John's, Newfoundland, Canada

Chapters 105, 107, and 108

Craig R. Lee, PharmD, PhD

Assistant Professor, Division of Pharmacotherapy and Experimental Therapeutics, UNC Eshelman School of Pharmacy, University of North Carolina at Chapel Hill, Chapel Hill, North Carolina

Chapter 22

Mary Lee, PharmD, BCPS, FCCP

Professor of Pharmacy Practice, Chicago College of Pharmacy, Vice President and Chief Academic Officer, Pharmacy and Health Sciences Education, Midwestern University, Downers Grove, Illinois

Chapters 92 and 93

Timothy S. Lesar, PharmD

Director of Clinical Pharmacy Service, Albany Medical Center, Albany, New York

Chapter 103

Deborah J. Levine

Associate Professor of Medicine, Division of Pulmonary and Critical Care, University of Texas, San Antonio, San Antonio, Texas

Chapter 35

Stephanie M. Levine, MD

Professor of Medicine, Division of Pulmonary Diseases and Critical Care Medicine, University of Texas Health Science Center, San Antonio, San Antonio, Texas

Chapter 32

Robin Moorman Li, PharmD

Assistant Professor Department of Pharmacotherapy and Translational Research, College of Pharmacy, University of Florida, Gainesville, Florida

Chapter 75

Jeffrey D. Little, PharmD, MPH

Pharmacy Manager, Finance and Ancillary Services, Children's Mercy Hospital and Clinics, Kansas City, Missouri

Chapter 5

Amanda M. Loya, PharmD

Clinical Assistant Professor, University of Texas at El Paso College of Health Sciences and University of Texas at Austin College of Pharmacy, El Paso, Texas

Chapter 4

William L. Lyons, MD

Associate Professor, Section of Geriatrics, Department of Internal Medicine, University of Nebraska Medical Center, Omaha, Nebraska

Chapter 109

George E. MacKinnon III, BS, MS, PhD, RPh, FASHP

Founding Dean and Professor, College of Pharmacy, Roosevelt University, Schaumburg, Illinois

Chapter 7

Neil J. MacKinnon, PhD, FCSHP

Associate Director for Research and Professor, College of Pharmacy, Dalhousie University, Halifax, Nova Scotia, Canada

Chapter 7

Robert MacLaren, BSc, PharmD, FCCM, FCCP

Associate Professor, Department of Clinical Pharmacy, School of Pharmacy, University of Colorado Denver, Aurora, Colorado

Chapter 30

Eric J. MacLaughlin, PharmD, FCCP, BCPS

Associate Professor and Head of Adult Medicine, Department of Pharmacy Practice, Texas Tech University Health Sciences Center School of Pharmacy, Amarillo, Texas

Chapter 19

Robert A. Mangione, EdD, RPh

Dean and Professor, St. John's University, College of Pharmacy and Allied Health Professions, Queens, New York

Chapter 49

Scott M. Mark, PharmD, MS, MEd, MPH, MBA, FASHP, FACHE, FABC

Director of Pharmacy, University of Pittsburgh Medical Center, Director, Pharmacy Practice Management Residency, Associate Professor and Vice Chair, University of Pittsburgh School of Pharmacy, Pittsburgh, Pennsylvania

Chapter 5

Patricia L. Marshik, PharmD

Associate Professor, Department of Pharmacy Practice, College of Pharmacy, University of New Mexico, Albuquerque, New Mexico

Chapter 36

Steven Martin, PharmD, BCPS, FCCP, FCCM

Professor and Chairman, Department of Pharmacy Practice, College of Pharmacy, The University of Toledo, Toledo, Ohio

Chapter 122

Todd W. Mattox, PharmD, BCNSP

Nutrition Support Team Lead, Moffitt Cancer Center and Research Institute, Tampa, Florida

Chapter 151

Gary R. Matzke, PharmD, FCP, FCCP, FASN, FNAP

Professor and Associate Dean for Clinical Research and Public Policy, School of Pharmacy, Virginia Commonwealth University-MCV Campus, Richmond, Virginia

Chapters 57, 58, and 61

J. Russell May, PharmD, FASHP

Clinical Professor, Department of Clinical and Administrative Pharmacy, University of Georgia, College of Pharmacy, Medical College of Georgia Campus, Augusta, Georgia

Chapter 104

Timothy R. McGuire, PharmD, FCCP, BCOP

Associate Professor, Department of Pharmacy Practice, College of Pharmacy, University of Nebraska Medical Center, Omaha, Nebraska

Chapter 144

Jerry McKee, PharmD, MS, BCPP

Pharmacy Clinical Practice Specialist, University of Texas Medical Branch, Correctional Managed Care, Huntsville, Texas

Chapter 82

Patrick J. Medina, PharmD, BCOP

Associate Professor, University of Oklahoma, College of Pharmacy, Oklahoma City, Oklahoma

Chapters 135 and 138

Sarah T. Melton, PharmD, BCPP, CGP

Director of Addiction Outreach, Associate Professor of Pharmacy Practice, Appalachian College of Pharmacy, Oakwood, Virginia

Chapter 79

Laura Boehnke Michaud, PharmD, BCOP, FASHP

Manager, Clinical Pharmacy Services, The University of Texas M. D. Anderson Cancer Center, Adjunct Assistant Professor of Pharmacy Practice, University of Houston, College of Pharmacy, Houston, Texas

Chapter 136

Deborah S. Minor, PharmD

Associate Professor, Department of Medicine, School of Medicine, University of Mississippi Medical Center, Assistant Professor, Department of Pharmacy Practice, University of Mississippi, Jackson, Mississippi

Chapter 70

Isaac F. Mitropoulos, PharmD

Ortho-McNeil Janssen Scientific Affairs, Cary, North Carolina

Chapter 115

Patricia A. Montgomery, PharmD

Clinical Pharmacy Specialist, Mercy General Hospital, Sacramento, California

Chapter 46

Reginald Moore, MD

Clinical Associate Professor, University of Texas Health Science Center, San Antonio, Texas, Director, Regional Sickle Cell Program, San Antonio, Texas

Chapter 111

Rebecca Moote, PharmD, MSc, BCPS

Assistant Professor, Department of Pharmacy Practice, Regis University School of Pharmacy, Denver, Colorado

Chapter 35

Stuart Munro, MD

Professor and Chair, Department of Psychiatry, School of Medicine, University of Missouri-Kansas City, Kansas City, Missouri

Chapter 71

Milap C. Nahata, PharmD, MS, FCCP

Professor of Pharmacy, Pediatrics and Internal Medicine, Division Chair, Pharmacy Practice and Administration, College of Pharmacy, Ohio State University, Associate Director of Pharmacy, Ohio State University Medical Center, Columbus, Ohio

Chapter 10

Rocsanna Namdar, PharmD, BCPS

Assistant Professor, University of Colorado, Aurora, Colorado

Chapter 121

Jean M. Nappi, BS, PharmD, FCCP, BCPS

Professor of Clinical Pharmacy and Outcome Sciences, South Carolina College of Pharmacy -MUSC Campus Professor of Medicine, Medical University of South Carolina, Charleston, South Carolina

Chapter 21

Leigh Anne Nelson, PharmD, BCPP

Assistant Professor, Division of Pharmacy Practice and Administration, University of Missouri-Kansas City School of Pharmacy, Kansas City, Missouri

Chapter 71

Merlin V. Nelson, PharmD, MD

Neurologist, Affiliated Community Medical Centers, Willmor, Minnesota

Chapter 68

Fenwick T. Nichols III, MD, FACP, FAAN, FAHA

Professor, Neurology; Professor, Radiology; Medical College of Georgia, Augusta, Georgia

Chapter 62

Jessica C. Njoku, PharmD, BCPS

Pharmacy Relations & Clinical Decision Suport, The Nebraska Medical Center, University of Nebraska Medical Center, College of Pharmacy, Department of Pharmacy Practice, Omaha, Nebraska

Chapter 118

Thomas D. Nolin, PharmD, PhD

Assistant Professor, Department of Pharmacy and Therapeutics, and Department of Medicine Renal Electrolyte Division, University of Pittsburgh Schools of Pharmacy and Medicine, Pittsburgh, Pennsylvania

Chapter 55

LeAnn B. Norris, PharmD, BCPS, BCOP

Assistant Professor, Department of Clinical Pharmacy and Outcomes Sciences, South Carolina College of Pharmacy, University of South Carolina Campus, Columbia, South Carolina

Chapter 139

Edith A. Nutescu, PharmD, FCCP

Clinical Professor, Department of Pharmacy Practice and Center for Pharmacoeconomic Research, Director, Antithrombosis Center, The University of Illinois at Chicago, College of Pharmacy & Medical Center, Chicago, Illinois

Chapter 26

Barbara M. O'Brien, MD

Assistant Professor Obstetrics and Gynecology, Warren Alpert School of Medicine at Brown University, Director of Maternal Fetal Medicine; Director of Perinatal Genetics, Providence Rhode Island

Chapter 87

Cindy L. O'Bryant, PharmD, FCCP, BCOP

Associate Professor, Department of Clinical Pharmacy, School of Pharmacy, University of Colorado Denver, Aurora, Colorado

Chapter 147

Mary Beth O'Connell, PharmD, BCPS, FASHP, FCCP

Associate Professor, Pharmacy Practice Department, Eugene Applebaum College of Pharmacy and Health Systems, Wayne State University, Detroit, Michigan

Chapter 99

Jessica S. Oftebro, PharmD, BA

Kelley-Ross Pharmacy, Seattle, Washington

Chapter 15

Keith M. Olsen, PharmD, FCCP, FCCM

Professor and Chair, Department of Pharmacy Practice, University of Nebraska Medical Center, Omaha, Nebraska

Chapter 38

Robert L. Page II, PharmD, MSPH, FCCP, FAHA, FASHP, BCPS, CGP

Associate Professor of Clinical Pharmacy and Physical Medicine, University of Colorado Denver Schools of Pharmacy and Medicine, Clinical Specialist, Division of Cardiology, University of Colorado Hospital, Aurora, Colorado

Chapter 21

Amy Barton Pai, PharmD, BCPS, FCCP, FASN

Associate Professor, Department of Pharmacy Practice, ANephRx-Albany Nephrology Pharmacy, Albany College of Pharmacy and Health Sciences, Albany, New York

Chapter 59

Robert B. Parker, PharmD, FCCP

Professor, University of Tennessee College of Pharmacy, Department of Clinical Pharmacy, Memphis, Tennessee

Chapter 20

Priti N. Patel, PharmD, BCPS

Assistant Clinical Professor, College of Pharmacy and Alliec Health Professions, St. John's University, Queens, New York

Chapter 49

Charles A. Peloquin

Professor and Director of Infectious Disease Pharmacokinetics Laboratory, College of Pharmacy, and Emerging Infectious Pathogens Institute, University of Florida, Gainesville, Florida

Chapter 121

Susan L. Pendland, MS, PharmD

St. Joseph Beren Hospital, Beren Kentucky, University of Illinois at Chicago, Department of Pharmacy Practice, Chicago, Illinois

Chapter 119

Janelle B. Perkins, PharmD, BCOP

Assistant Member, Blood and Marrow Transplantation, H. Lee Moffitt Cancer Center and Research Institute, Tampa, Florida

Chapter 148

Jay I. Peters, MD

Professor of Medicine, Division of Pulmonary and Critical Care, University of Texas Health Science Center at San Antonio, San Antonio, Texas

Chapter 32

Stephanie J. Phelps, PharmD, BCPS

Professor, Clinical Pharmacy and Pediatrics, University of Tennessee Health Science Center, College of Pharmacy, Memphis, Tennessee

Chapter 66

Bradley G. Phillips, PharmD, BCPS, FCCP

Millikan-Reeve Professor and Head, Department of Clinical and Administrative Pharmacy, University of Georgia College of Pharmacy, Athens, Georgia

Chapter 81

Lisa B. Phipps, PharmD, PhD

Assistant Professor, Department of Pharmacotherapy & Outcomes Science, Virginia Commonwealth University, Richmond, Virginia

Chapter 80

Nicole Weimert Pilch, PharmD, MSCR, BCPS

Clinical Specialist, Solid Organ Transplantation, Clinical Assistant Professor, Department of Pharmacy and Clinical Sciences, South Carolina College of Pharmacy, MUSC Campus, Medical University of South Carolina, Department of Pharmacy Services, Charleston, South Carolina

Chapter 95

Stephen R. Pliszka, MD

Professor and Vice Chair, Chief Division of Child and Adolescent Psychiatry, Department of Psychiatry, The University of Texas Health Science, Center at San Antonio, San Antonio, Texas

Chapter 72

Betsy Bickert Poon, PharmD, FCCP

Clinical Specialist, Pediatric Hematology/Oncology, Florida Hospital for Children, Clinical Assistant Professor, University of Florida College of Pharmacy, Orlando, Florida

Chapters 110 and 142

L. Michael Posey, BSPharm

Editorial Director, Periodicals Department, American Pharmacists Association, Washington, DC

Chapter 6

Jamie C. Poust, PharmD, BCOP

Oncology Clinical Specialist, Department of Pharmacy, University of Colorado Hospital, Aurora, Colorado

Chapter 147

Patricia H. Powell, PharmD, BCPS

Assistant Professor, Clinical Pharmacy and Outcomes Sciences, South Carolina College of Pharmacy, University of South Carolina Campus, Columbia, South Carolina

Chapter 43

Randall A. Prince, PharmD, PhD

Professor, University of Houston College of Pharmacy, Houston, Texas

Chapter 125

Jane Pruemer, PharmD, BCOP, FASHP

Professor of Pharmacy Practice, Oncology Clinical Pharmacy Specialist, James L. Winkle College of Pharmacy, University of Cincinnati, Cincinnati, Ohio

Chapter 110

Kelly R. Ragucci, PharmD, FCCP, BCPS, CDE

Associate Professor, Clinical Pharmacy and Outcomes Sciences, South Carolina College of Pharmacy, Medical University of South Carolina Campus, Charleston, South Carolina

Chapter 88

Hengameh H. Raissy, PharmD

Department of Pediatrics, School of Medicine, University of New Mexico, Alburquerque, Mew Mexico

Chapter 36

Charles A. Reasner, MD

Professor of Medicine/Diabetes, University of Texas Health Science Center at San Antonio and Medical Director at the Texas Diabetes Institute, San Antonio, Texas

Chapter 83

Michael D. Reed, PharmD, FCCP, FCP

Director, Division of Clinical Pharmacology and Toxicology, and the Rebecca D. Considine Research Institute, Children's Hospital Medical Center of Akron and Professor & Associate Chair, Department of Pediatrics NEOUCOM, Akron, Ohio

Chapter 116

José O. Rivera, PharmD

Clinical Professor, University of Texas at El Paso College of Health Sciences and University of Texas at Austin College of Pharmacy, El Paso, Texas

Chapter 4

Jo E. Rodgers, PharmD, FCCP, BCPS

Clinical Associate Professor, Department of Pharmacotherapy and Experimental Therapeutics, Eshelman School of Pharmacy, University of North Carolina at Chapel Hill, Chapel Hill, North Carolina

Chapter 22

Susan J. Rogers, PharmD, BCPS

Assistant Clinical Professor, University of Texas at Austin; Clinical Pharmacy Specialist Neurology, South Texas Healthcare System, Audie L. Murphy Veterans Hospital, San Antonio, Texas

Chapter 65

Amy F. Rosenberg, PharmD, BCPS

Clinical Pharmacy Specialist, Shands at the University of Florida, Gainesville, Florida

Chapter 112

John C. Rotschafer, PharmD, FCCP

Professor, Experimental and Clinical Pharmacology, College of Pharmacy, Minneapolis, Minnesota

Chapter 115

Eric S. Rovner, MD

Professor of Urology, Department of Urology, Medical University of South Carolina, Charleston, South Carolina

Chapter 94

Maria I. Rudis, PharmD, BScPharm

Clinical Pharmacy Specialist - Emergency Medicine, Program Director, Emergency Medicine Pharmacy Residency, Chair, Research Committee, Department of Pharmacy Services, St. Mary's Hospital, Mayo Clinic, Rochester, Minnesota

Chapter 30

Michael J. Rybak, PharmD, MPH

Associate Dean for Research, Professor of Pharmacy and Medicine, Director, Anti-Infective Research Laboratory Department of Pharmacy Practice, Eugene Applebaum College of Pharmacy, Wayne State University, Detroit, Michigan

Chapter 113

Gordon S. Sacks, PharmD, BCNSP

Professor and Head, Department of Pharmacy Practice, Harrison School of Pharmacy, Auburn University, Auburn, Alabama

Chapter 150

Cynthia A. Sanoski, PharmD, BCPS, FCCP

Chair, Department of Pharmacy Practice, Associate Professor, Jefferson School of Pharmacy, Thomas Jefferson University, Philadelphia, Pennsylvania

Chapter 25

Joseph J. Saseen, PharmD

Professor, Clinical Pharmacy and Family Medicine, Schools of Pharmacy and Medicine University of Colorado Denver, Aurora, Colorado

Chapter 19

Robert R. Schade, MD, FACP, AGAF, FACG, FASGE

Medical College of Georgia, Professor of Medicine, Chief, Section of Gastroenterology/Hepatology Medical College of Georgia, Augusta, Georgia

Chapter 39

Mark E. Schneiderhan, PharmD, BCPP

University of Minnesota College of Pharmacy, Duluth, Department of Pharmacy Practice and Pharmaceutical Sciences, Human Development Center, Duluth, Minnesota

Chapter 71

Kristine S. Schonder, PharmD

Assistant Professor, Pharmacy and Therapeutics, University of Pittsburgh School of Pharmacy; Clinical Pharmacist, Thomas E. Starzl Transplantation Institute, University of Pittsburgh Medical Center, Pittsburgh, Pennsylvania

Chapter 98

Arthur A. Schuna, MS, FASHP

Clinical Coordinator, William S. Middleton VA Medical Center, Clinical Professor, University of Wisconsin School of Pharmacy, Madison, Wisconsin

Chapter 100

Richard B. Schwartz, MD

Associate Professor, Department of Emergency Medicine, Medical College of Georgia, Augusta, Georgia

Chapter 16

Julie M. Sease, PharmD, BCPS, CDE

Associate Professor of Pharmacy Practice, Department of Pharmacy Practice, Presbyterian College School of Pharmacy, Clinton, South Carolina

Chapter 44

Amy Heck Sheehan, PharmD

Associate Professor, Department of Pharmacy Practice, Purdue University School of Pharmacy and Pharmaceutical Sciences, Indianapolis, Indiana

Chapters 86 and 154

Greene Shepherd, PharmD

Clinical Associate Professor, College of Pharmacy, University of Georgia, Augusta, Georgia

Chapter 16

Stacy S. Shord, PharmD, BCOP, FCCP

Reviewer, Office of Clinical Pharmacology, Office of Translational Science, Center for Drug Evaluation and Research, U.S. Food and Drug Administration, Silver Spring, Maryland

Chapter 135

Sarah P. Shrader PharmD, BCPS, CDE

Assistant Professor, Department of Clinical Pharmacy and Outcomes Sciences, South Carolina College of Pharmacy -MUSC Campus, Charleston, South Carolina

Chapter 88

Jeri J. Sias, PharmD, MPH

Clinical Associate Professor, University of Texas at El Paso/ UT Austin Cooperative Pharmacy Program, Adjunct Clinical Assistant Professor, Department of Family and Community Medicine, Texas Tech University Health Sciences Center - El Paso, El Paso, Texas

Chapter 4

Debra J. Sibbald, BScPhm, ACPR, MA, PhD

Senior Tutor, Division of Pharmacy Practice, Leslie Dan Faculty of Pharmacy, University of Toronto, Toronto, Ontario, Canada

Chapter 106

Patricia W. Slattum, PharmD, PhD

Associate Professor of Pharmacy, Geriatric Pharmacotherapy Program, Virginia Commonwealth University, School of Pharmacy, Richmond, Virginia

Chapter 63

Judith A. Smith, PharmD, BCOP, FCCP, FISOPP

Associate Professor and Director of Pharmacology Research, Department of Gynecologic Oncology, Division of Surgery, The University of Texas M.D. Anderson Cancer Center, Houston, Texas

Chapter 141

Philip H. Smith, MD

Assistant Professor of Medicine, Medical College of Georgia, Director of Allergy Services, Charlie Norwood VA Hospital, Augusta, Georgia

Chapter 104

Steven M. Smith, PharmD

Postdoctoral Fellow, Departments of Pharmacotherapy and Translational Research and Community Health and Family Medicine, Colleges of Pharmacy and Medicine, University of Florida, Gainesville, Florida

Chapter 85

Christine A. Sorkness, PharmD

Professor of Pharmacy and Medicine, University of Wisconsin, Madison, Wisconsin

Chapter 33

Kevin M. Sowinski, PharmD, FCCP

Professor, Department of Pharmacy Practice, School of Pharmacy and Pharmaceutical Sciences, Purdue University, West Lafayette and Indianapolis, Indiana, Adjunct Professor, Department of Medicine, School of Medicine, Indiana University, Indianapolis, Indiana

Chapter 54

Sarah A. Spinler, PharmD, FCCP, FAHA, FASHP, BCPS (AQ Cardiology)

Professor of Clinical Pharmacy, Residency Programs Coordinator, Philadelphia College of Pharmacy, University of the Sciences in Philadelphia, Philadelphia, Pennsylvania

Chapter 24

Catherine I. Starner, PharmD, BCPS, CGP

Senior Clinical Pharmacist, Prime Theapeutics, LLC. Eagan, Minnesota

Chapter 11

Andy Stergachis, PhD, RPh

Professor of Epidemiology and Global Health, Adjunct Professor of Pharmacy & Health Services, Director, Global Medicines Program, School of Public Health, University of Washington, Seattle, Washington

Chapter 13

Douglas Stewart, DO, MPH

Associate Professor, Department of Pediatrics, University of Oklahoma College of Medicine, Tulsa, Oklahoma

Chapter 82

Steven C. Stoner, PharmD, BCPP

Chair and Clinical Professor of Psychiatric Pharmacy, UMKC School of Pharmacy, Division of Pharmacy Practice and Administration, Kansas City, Missouri

Chapter 73

Jennifer M. Strickland, PharmD, BCPS

Co-Director, Center of Advancing Quality of Life, Director, Pharmacy, Pain & Palliative Care Specialist, Lakeland Regional Medical Center, Lakeland, Florida

Chapter 69

Deborah A. Sturpe, PharmD, BCPS

Associate Professor, Department of Pharmacy Practice and Science, University of Maryland School of Pharmacy, Baltimore, Maryland

Chapter 90

Weijing Sun, MD

Associate Professor of Medicine, Director, GI Medical Oncology Program, Abramson Cancer Center, University of Pennsylvania, Philadelphia, Pennsylvania

Chapter 138

Russell H. Swerdlow, MD

Professor, Neurology and Molecular & Integrative Physiology, University of Kansas School of Medicine, Kansas City, Kansas

Chapter 63

David M. Swope, MD

Associate Professor of Neurology, Loma Linda University, Loma Linda, California

Chapter 68

Lynne M. Sylvia, PharmD

Clinical Pharmacy Specialist, Tufts Medical Center, Adjunct Clinical Professor, Northeastern University, School of Pharmacy, Boston, Massachusetts

Chapter 97

Carol Taketomo, PharmD

Director of Pharmacy, Children's Hospital Los Angeles, Adjunct Assistant Professor of Pharmacy Practice, University of Southern California, School of Pharmacy, Los Angeles, California

Chapter 10

Robert L. Talbert, PharmD, FCCP, BCPS, FAHA

SmithKline Professor, College of Pharmacy, The University of Texas at Austin, Professor, School of Medicine, University of Texas Health Science Center at San Antonio, Texas

Chapters 23, 28, 29, and 84

Colleen M. Terriff, PharmD

Clinical Associate Professor, Washington State University, College of Pharmacy, Deaconess Medical Center Pharmacy Department, Spokane, Washington

Chapter 15

Christian J. Teter, PharmD, BCPP

Assistant Professor, Pharmacy Practice, School of Pharmacy, Northeastern University, Boston, Massachusetts, Clinician-Researcher, Alcohol and Drug Abuse Treatment Program, McLean Hospital, Belmont, Massachusetts

Chapter 77

Shelly D. Timmons, MD, PhD, FACS

Associate Professor and Chief of Neurotrauma Division, Department of Neurosurgery, University of Tennessee Health Science Center, Semmes-Murphey Neurologic and Spine Institute, Memphis, Tennessee

Chapter 67

Lisa Sanchez Trask, PharmD

Executive Manager, Clinical Science & Outcomes Manager, Takeda Pharmaceuticals America, Inc. Denver, Colorado

Chapter 1

Curtis L. Triplitt, PharmD, CDE

Clinical Assistant Professor, Department of Medicine, Division of Diabetes, University of Texas Health Science Center at San Antonio, Texas

Chapter 83

Elena M. Umland, PharmD

Associate Dean for Academic Affairs, Associate Professor of Pharmacy Practice Jefferson School of Pharmacy, Thomas Jefferson University, Philadelphia, Pennsylvania

Chapter 89

Ulysses J. Urquidi, MD, MS, FAAFP

Associate Professor and Chief, Division of Community Medicine, Texas Tech Health Sciences Center, Paul L. Foster School of Medicine, Department of Family and Community Medicine, El Paso, Texas

Chapter 4

Yolanda Y. Vera, PharmD

Pediatric Patient Care Pharmacist, Department of Pharmacy, The Children's Hospital at Scott & White, Temple, Texas

Chapter 37

Angie Veverka, PharmD

Associate Professor of Pharmacy, Wingate University School of Pharmacy, Wingate, North Carolina

Chapter 120

Sheryl F. Vondracek, PharmD

Associate Professor, Department of Clinical Pharmacy, School of Pharmacy, University of Colorado Denver, Aurora, Colorado

Chapter 99

Christine M. Walko, PharmD, BCOP

Clinical Assistant Professor, Division of Pharmacotherapy and Experimental Therapeutics, Institute of Pharmacogenomics and Individualized Therapy, University of North Carolina School of Pharmacy, Chapel Hill, North Carolina

Chapter 146

Mark D. Walsh, PharmD

Hematology/Oncology Fellow, Division of Pharmacotherapy and Experimental Therapeutics, UNC Eshelman School of Pharmacy, University of North Carolina, Chapel Hill, North Carolina

Chapter 146

Tracey Walsh-Chocolaad, PharmD, BCOP

Clinical Pharmacist, Outpatient Stem Cell Transplantation, National Heart, Lung and Blood Institute, National Institutes of Health, Bethesda, Maryland

Chapter 145

Kristina E. Ward, BS, PharmD, BCPS

Clinical Assistant Professor of Pharmacy Practice, Director, Drug Information Services, College of Pharmacy, University of Rhode Island, Kingston, Rhode Island

Chapter 87

Robert J. Weber, PharmD, MS, BCPS, FASHP

Senior Director, Pharmaceutical Services, and Assistant Dean for Medical Center Affairs, The Ohio State University Medical Center and College of Pharmacy, Columbus, Ohio

Chapter 5

Lara Carson Weinstein, MD

Assistant Professor, Department of Family and Community Medicine, Thomas Jefferson University, Philadelphia, Pennsylvania

Chapter 89

Barbara G. Wells, PharmD, FCCP, BCPP

Dean and Professor, Executive Director of the Research Institute of Pharmaceutical Sciences, School of Pharmacy, The University of Mississippi, Oxford, Mississippi

Chapters 77 and 80

James W. Wheless, MD

Professor and Chief of Pediatric Neurology, Le Bonheur Chair in Pediatric Neurology, University of Tennessee Health Science Center, Director, Le Bonheur Comprehensive Epilepsy Program, Director, Neuroscience Institute Le Bonheur Children's Medical Center, Clinical Chief & Director of Pediatric Neurology St Jude Children's Research Hospital, Memphis, Tennessee

Chapter 66

Casey B. Williams, PharmD, BCOP

Hematology/Oncology Clinical Coordinator and PGY-2 Residency Director, University of Kansas Hospital; Adjunct Clinical Assistant Professor, University of Kansas School of Pharmacy, Kansas City, Kansas

Chapter 144

Dennis M. Williams, PharmD, BCPS, AE-C

Associate Professor and Vice-Chair, Division of Pharmacotherapy and Experimental Therapeutics, University of North Carolina at Chapel Hill, Eshelman School of Pharmacy

Chapter 34

Dianne B. Williams, PharmD, BCPS

Clinical Associate Professor, Campus Director for Pharmacy Practice Experiences, Department of Clinical and Administrative Pharmacy Office of Experience Programs, University of Georgia College of Pharmacy, Augusta, Georgia

Chapter 39

Jeffrey L. Wilt, M.D. FACP, FCC

Associate Professor of Medicine, Michigan State University

Chapter 18

Char Witmer, MD

Assistant Professor, Pediatrics, The Children's Hospital of Philadelphia, Division of Hematology, Philadelphia, Pennsylvania

Chapter 110

Daniel M. Witt, PharmD, FCCP, BCPS, CACP

Senior Manager Clinical Pharmacy and Research, Kaiser Permanente Colorado, Aurora, Colorado

Chapter 26

Judith K. Wolf, MD

Professor, Department of Gynecologic Oncology, The University of Texas M.D. Anderson Cancer Center, Houston, Texas

Chapter 141

Chanin C. Wright, PharmD

Assistant Professor, Department of Pediatrics, Texas A&M College of Pharmacy, The Children's Hospital at Scott and White, Temple, Texas

Chapter 37

Jean Wyman, PhD, RN

Professor and Cora Meidl Siehl Chair in Nursing Research, Director, Minnesota Hartford Center of Geriatric Nursing Excellence, University of Minnesota School of Nursing, Minneapolis, Minnesota

Chapter 94

Jack A. Yanovski, MD, PhD

Head, Unit on Growth and Obesity, Program in Developmental Endocrinology and Genetics, Eunice Kennedy Shriver National Institute of Child Health and Human Development, National Institutes of Health, Bethesda, Maryland

Chapters 86 and 154

Gary C. Yee, PharmD, FCCP, BCOP

Professor and Associate Dean for Academic Affairs, College of Pharmacy, University of Nebraska Medical Center, Omaha, Nebraska

Chapters 140 and 148

George Zhanel, PharmD, PhD

Professor, Department of Medical Microbiology/Infectious Diseases, Faculty of Medicine, University of Manitoba, Winnipeg, Canada and Research Director-Canadian Antimicrobial Resistance Alliance (CARA) Winnipeg, Canada

Chapter 117

FOREWORD

The saying that "timing is everything" aptly describes the circumstances surrounding medication use in health care as this edition of *Pharmacotherapy: A Pathophysiologic Approach* goes to print. The U.S. Congress passed hallmark health reform legislation in March 2010 to expand access to health coverage, including pharmaceuticals and medication therapy management services, to millions of Americans. At the same time, many private sector efforts to make care safer and more affordable are moving forward. Massive movement is under way to enhance access to and coordinate electronic health records in health delivery in and between hospitals, physicians' offices and pharmacies.

What does this mean with respect to medication use? Perhaps the Patient-Centered Primary Care Collaborative[1] says it best.

Now is an important time in health care. Medications hold the promise to significantly improve the health of all Americans by effectively preventing and controlling many diseases, but they have fallen far short of this goal. Our current health care system rewards splintered, episodic care, which cripples our primary care system and silos medication use and costs from medical care and costs. As we truly coordinate care, we must also deliver on the promise of modern medications to prevent and control disease by directly linking their use to clinical goals and outcomes in a patient-centered fashion in a primary care team-based approach. Only with appropriate and optimal medication use will we see real quality of care improve and health care costs decrease in the patient-centered medical home (PCMH). Adherence to medications and recommended therapies is optimized when patients have a thorough understanding of all of their medications, including over-the-counter drugs, and how they impact their health when incentives are fairly aligned. Whole-person, patient-centered care—considering the mental and physical aspects of health—can be advanced by fully integrated care that includes clinically linked, comprehensive medication management.

When the first edition of *Pharmacotherapy: A Pathophysiologic Approach* was published in 1988 the role of the clinical pharmacist was in the midst of its evolution and most who were prepared for advanced clinical roles utilized their skills and expertise in acute care settings. US colleges and schools of pharmacy only graduated about 1,000 PharmD graduates annually and debates were still raging about whether the accreditation standards for pharmacy education should change to make the Doctor of Pharmacy degree the entry level for licensure and practice. With the exception of a few key products for distinct diagnoses, medications were not a covered benefit for Medicare beneficiaries. Prescriptions were an optional benefit for state Medicaid programs. The federal government had little 'skin in the game' so to speak with respect to medications and their proper use and federal health policy makers devoted very little

time to the pharmacotherapeutic elements of public or private sector health programs.

For so long pharmacy leaders seemed to be lone rangers when it came to identifying unmet needs for patient care related to the proactive management of patients' drug regimens. Justification for introducing clinical pharmacy services into hospitals and health systems, clinics, and other environments seemed to have to be made one unit, or one physician, or one chief financial officer at a time. For patients it would seem that the prevailing attitude was "if the FDA says this drug is approved and my physician prescribes it, it must be safe to take; and why would I need a pharmacist's services anyway?"

A glance back at the table of contents of the first edition of *Pharmacotherapy: A Pathophysiologic Approach* in comparison to the contents of the 8th edition is also revealing. With credit to the editors, the basic organizational structure of this world renowned text remains consistent. The first edition provided 111 chapters of essential information on pharmacotherapy for pharmacists and others who needed an essential reference on the pathophysiology and management of this array of diseases. The 8th edition has 154 chapters, almost a 50 percent increase in the coverage of specific conditions or areas of focus. This says nothing of the expansion of the depth of material in a given chapter.

It is also of interest to observe the transformation since 1988 of material the editors consider to be the "Foundational Issues" contained in Section 1 of the text. While important chapters such as geriatrics, pediatrics and pharmacokinetics remain at the core of the foundational pharmacotherapeutic content, these are accompanied by new chapters, including pharmacoeconomics and health outcomes, medication safety, health literacy and cultural competency. Biological, chemical and radiological terrorism also now appear in Section 1.

These simple but striking examples reveal the complexity of these times in health care and in pharmacy practice. As noted in the PCPCC treatise on MTM, "Medications hold the promise to significantly improve the health of all Americans by effectively preventing and controlling many diseases, but they have fallen far short of this goal." It is the growing recognition by health policy experts, health care delivery system leaders, patient safety advocates and others that a laisee faire approach to medication management is insufficient to advance contemporary care models.

As we enter the second decade of the 21st century a new recognition is dawning. Medication use is central to high quality, safe and effective patient care. This is true in prevention, acute care and chronic disease management. To use a term from the writing of Donald M. Berwick, MD, recently named the Administrator of the Centers for Medicare and Medicaid Services, medication management might well be an "integrator" in health care.[2] An integrator in Berwick's analysis enters a partnership with individuals and families, redesigns primary care, addresses population health management, financial management and macro system integration.

Well designed programs of pharmacotherapy management touch on each of these elements and call upon the knowledge, skills and abilities of medication use specialists. Colleges and schools of pharmacy and their faculty members offer curricula that provide the foundational abilities for pharmacists to enter practice across all settings of care and manage patients' drug therapy. Often with post-graduate training, pharmacists apply their unique insights into the care of patients with the broad array of conditions described in this text and especially those that are most challenging. That may be a patient with a newly transplanted and life-saving organ or an elderly woman with six chronic ailments and a pharmacotherapy regimen of 10 to 12 prescriptions, over the counter and nutritional products. Longitudinal care management for individuals with chronic conditions such as diabetes, asthma, congestive heart failure and depression that respond to well-designed pharmacotherapeutic regimens also shows consistent improvement when a medication use specialist is directly involved in the patient's care.

There are numerous stakeholders in the realm of effective medication use and the management of complex medical conditions. Fortunately, *Pharmacotherapy: A Pathophysiologic Approach* continues the fine tradition of organizing essential information in a systematic fashion to guide the evaluation, individualization, and rationalization of drug therapy for the entire array of patients and their medical conditions. The depth and breadth of information contained in this text long ago surpassed the ability of any one clinician to command it entirely. We have therefore seen specialists emerge in virtually each area while many clinicians continue to work to coordinate and optimize care plans that are more routine but require continuous patient education and monitoring. The time is now to make good on the promise of relief of suffering and compassionate care that can be achieved when medications are used properly and managed effectively. The 8th edition of *Pharmacotherapy: A Pathophysiologic Approach* will help assure the promise is realized.

Lucinda L. Maine, PhD, RPh
Executive Vice President and CEO
American Association of Colleges of Pharmacy

References

1. McInnis T, Strand LM, and Webb CE. The Patient Centered Medical Home: Integrating Comprehensive Medication Management to Optimize Patient Outcomes. Available from the Patient Centered Primary Care Collaborative at http://www.pcpcc.net/files/medmanagepub.pdf.

2. Berwick DM, Nolan TW, Whittington J. The Triple Aim: Care, Health, and Cost. Health Affairs 2008;27(3):759–769.

FOREWORD TO THE FIRST EDITION

Evidence of the maturity of a profession is not unlike that characterizing the maturity of an individual; a child's utterances and behavior typically reveal an unrealized potential for attainment, eventually, of those attributes characteristic of an appropriately confident, independently competent, socially responsible, sensitive, and productive member of society.

Within a period of perhaps 15 or 20 years, we have witnessed a profound maturation within the profession of pharmacy. The utterances of the profession, as projected in its literature, have evolved from mostly self-centered and self-serving issues of trade protection to a composite of expressed professional interests that prominently include responsible explorations of scientific/technological questions and ethical issues that promote the best interests of the clientele served by the profession. With the publication of *Pharmacotherapy: A Pathophysiologic Approach,* pharmacy's utterances bespeak a matured practitioner who is able to call upon unique knowledge and skills so as to function as an appropriately confident, independently competent pharmacotherapeutics expert.

In 1987, the Board of Pharmaceutical Specialties (BPS), in denying the petition filed by the American College of Clinical Pharmacy (ACCP) to recognize "clinical pharmacy" as a specialty, conceded nonetheless that the petitioning party had documented in its petition a specialist who does in fact exist within the practice of pharmacy and whose expertise clearly can be extricated from the performance characteristics of those in general practice. A refiled petition from ACCP requests recognition of "pharmacotherapy" as a Specialty Area of Pharmacy Practice. While the BPS had issued no decision when this book went to press, it is difficult to comprehend the basis for a rejection of the second petition.

Within this book one will find the scientific foundation for the essential knowledge required of one who may aspire to specialty practice as a pharmacotherapist. As is the case with any such publication, its usefulness to the practitioner or the future practitioner is limited to providing such a foundation. To be socially and professionally responsible in practice, the pharmacotherapist's foundation must be continually supplemented and complemented by the flow of information appearing in the primary literature. Of course this is not unique to the general or specialty practice of pharmacy; it is essential to the fulfillment of obligations to clients in any occupation operating under the code of professional ethics.

Because of the growing complexity of pharmacotherapeutic agents, their dosing regimens, and techniques for delivery, pharmacy is obligated to produce, recognize, and remunerate specialty practitioners who can fulfill the profession's responsibilities to society for service expertise where the competence required in a particular case exceeds that of the general practitioner. It simply is a component of our covenant with society and is as important as any other facet of that relationship existing between a profession and those it serves.

The recognition by BPS of pharmacotherapy as an area of specialty practice in pharmacy will serve as an important statement by the profession that we have matured sufficiently to be competent and willing to take unprecedented responsibilities in the collaborative, pharmacotherapeutic management of patient-specific problems. It commits pharmacy to an intention that will not be uniformly or rapidly accepted within the established health care community. Nonetheless, this formal action places us on the road to an avowed goal, and acceptance will be gained as the pharmacotherapists proliferate and establish their importance in the provision of optimal, cost-effective drug therapy.

Suspecting that other professions in other times must have faced similar quests for recognition of their unique knowledge and skills I once searched the literature for an example that might parallel pharmacy's modern-day aspirations. Writing in the *Philadelphia Medical Journal,* May 27, 1899, D. H. Galloway, MD, reflected on the need for specialty training and practice in a field of medicine lacking such expertise at that time. In an article entitled "The Anesthetizer as a Speciality," Galloway commented:

> *The anesthetizer will have to make his own place in medicine: the profession will not make a place for him, and not until he has demonstrated the value of his services will it concede him the position which the importance of his duties entitles him to occupy. He will be obliged to define his own rights, duties and privileges, and he must not expect that his own estimate of the importance of his position will be conceded without opposition. There are many surgeons who are unwilling to share either the credit or the emoluments of their work with anyone, and their opposition will be overcome only when they are shown that the importance of their work will not be lessened, but enhanced, by the increased safety and dispatch with which operations may be done. . . .*

It has been my experience that, given the opportunity for one-on-one, collaborative practice with physicians and other health professionals, pharmacy practitioners who have been educated and trained to perform at the level of pharmacotherapeutics specialists almost invariably have convinced the former that "the importance of their work will not be lessened, but enhanced, by the increased safety and dispatch with which" individualized problems of drug therapy could be managed in collaboration with clinical pharmacy practitioners.

It is fortuitous—the coinciding of the release of *Pharmacotherapy: A Pathophysiologic Approach* with ACCP's petitioning of BPS for recognition of the pharmacotherapy specialist. The utterances of a maturing profession as revealed in the contents of this book, and the intraprofessional recognition and acceptance of a higher level of responsibility in the safe, effective, and economical use of drugs and drug products, bode well for the future of the profession and for the improvement of patient care with drugs.

Charles A. Walton, PhD
San Antonio, Texas

PREFACE

Health care has entered an era of change more dramatic than any in the last few decades. While issues related to health care access and coverage, including payment for care, dominate the media, health care providers are challenged daily to meet the needs and demands for wellness services, primary care and chronic disease management, end-of-life care, and specialty care. Effective health care practitioners now must be able to manage the economic burdens of care, including psychosocial dimensions, and apply the latest advances in the health sciences. This is true just as much with the management of patient-centered pharmacotherapy as with any other aspect of health care. To remain relevant and effective, the pharmacotherapist must maintain a commitment to life-long learning in the interest of caring for patients.

The 8th edition of *Pharmacotherapy: A Pathophysiologic Approach* has six new chapters. The first section of the book includes new chapters on Palliative Care, Health Literacy, Cultural Competency, and Medication Safety. A new chapter on Celiac Disease addresses a condition that is now recognized as affecting as many as 1 of every 300 people in the United States. There is also a new chapter on Renal Cell Carcinoma, and the chapters on acutely decompensated heart failure and cystic fibrosis have been completely rewritten. Most importantly, each chapter of the book has been updated to reflect the latest in evidence-based information and recommendations. We have done our best to balance the need for accurate, thorough, and unbiased information about the treatment of diseases with the practical limitations of paper books.

With each edition, the editors recommit to our founding precepts:

- Advance the quality of patient care through evidence-based medication therapy management based on sound pharmacotherapeutic principles.
- Enhance the health of our communities by incorporating contemporary health promotion and disease-prevention strategies in our practice environments.
- Motivate young practitioners to enhance the breadth, depth, and quality of care they provide to their patients.
- Challenge established pharmacists and other primary-care providers to learn new concepts and refine their understanding of the pathophysiologic tenets that undergird the development of individualized therapeutic regimens.
- Present the pharmacy and health care communities with innovative patient assessment, triage, and pharmacotherapy management skills.

The eighth edition continues the emphasis on evidenced-based pharmacotherapy. Most of the disease-oriented chapters have incorporated updated evidence-based treatment guidelines that include, when available, ratings of the level of evidence to support the key therapeutic approaches. Also, in this edition key features have been retained, including:

- Key concepts listed at the beginning of each chapter are identified in the text with numbered icons so that the reader can easily jump to the material of interest.
- The most common signs and symptoms of diseases are presented in highlighted *Clinical Presentation* tables in disease-specific chapters.
- Clinical controversies in treatment or patient management are highlighted to assure that the reader is aware of these issues and how practitioners are responding to them.
- Each chapter has approximately 100 of the most important and current references relevant to each disease, with most published since 2005.
- The diagnostic flow diagrams, treatment algorithms, dosing guideline recommendations, and monitoring approaches that were present in the last edition have been refined.

We have made a special effort with this edition to have authors summarize concepts more succinctly or use tables to present details more concisely. This process continued as the book entered production, and even during the review of final proofs, we continued to make changes to ensure that this book is as current and complete as is possible.

To make room for new chapters and stay with a single volume of *Pharmacotherapy*, 21 chapters of this edition are being published in our Pharmacotherapy Online Learning Center, accessible at www.pharmacotherapyonline.com or http://highered.mcgraw-hill.com/sites/0071416137/information_center_view0/. The chapters chosen for Web publication include those of specialized application that may be predominantly used by practitioners, rather than being core elements of the pharmacotherapy sequences at colleges of pharmacy. The online chapters include those describing details about the diagnosis of organ system diseases. In addition, 14 chapters printed in the book also appear online to enhance student and instructor access.

As the world increasingly relies on electronic means of communication, we are committed to keeping *Pharmacotherapy* and its companion works, *Pharmacotherapy Casebook: A Patient-Focused Approach and Pharmacotherapy Handbook,* integral components of clinicians' toolboxes. The Online Learning Center continues to provide unique features designed to benefit students, practitioners, and faculty around the world. The site includes learning objectives and self-assessment questions for each chapter, and the full text of this book is now available on the publisher's AccessPharmacy site (www.accesspharmacy.com). In AccessPharmacy, each section of the book also has updates published periodically and editorial comment about the relevance of more recent information.

In closing, we acknowledge the many hours that *Pharmacotherapy's* more than 300 authors contributed to this labor of love. Without their devotion to the cause of improved pharmacotherapy and dedication in maintaining the accuracy, clarity, and relevance of their chapters, this text would unquestionably not be possible. In addition, we thank Michael Weitz, Karen Edmonson, and James Shanahan and their colleagues at McGraw-Hill for their consistent support of the *Pharmacotherapy* family of resources, insights into trends in publishing and higher education, and the critical attention to detail so necessary in pharmacotherapy.

The Editors
March 2011

SECTION 1
FOUNDATION ISSUES

CHAPTER

1

Pharmacoeconomics: Principles, Methods, and Applications

LISA SANCHEZ TRASK

KEY CONCEPTS

❶ Pharmacoeconomics identifies, measures, and compares the costs and consequences of drug therapy to healthcare systems and society.

❷ The perspective of a pharmacoeconomic evaluation is paramount because the study results will be highly dependent on the perspective selected.

❸ Healthcare costs can be categorized as direct medical, direct nonmedical, indirect nonmedical, intangible, opportunity, and incremental costs.

❹ Economic, humanistic, and clinical outcomes should be considered and valued using pharmacoeconomic methods, to inform local decision making whenever possible.

❺ To compare various healthcare choices, economic valuation methods are used, including cost-minimization, cost-benefit, cost-effectiveness, and cost-utility analyses. These methods all provide the means to compare competing treatment options and are similar in the way they measure costs (dollar units). They differ, however, in their measurement of outcomes and expression of results.

❻ In today's healthcare settings, pharmacoeconomic methods can be applied for effective formulary management, individual patient treatment, medication policy determination, and resource allocation.

❼ When evaluating published pharmacoeconomic studies, the following factors should be considered: study objective, study

perspective, pharmacoeconomic method, study design, choice of interventions, costs and consequences, discounting, study results, sensitivity analysis, study conclusions, and sponsorship.

❽ Both the use of economic models and conducting pharmacoeconomic analyses on a local level can be useful and relevant sources of pharmacoeconomic data when rigorous methods are employed, as outlined in this chapter.

Today's cost-sensitive healthcare environment has created a competitive and challenging workplace for clinicians. Competition for diminishing resources has necessitated that the appraisal of healthcare goods and services extends beyond evaluations of safety and efficacy and considers the economic impact of these goods and services on the cost of healthcare. A challenge for healthcare professionals is to provide quality patient care while assuring an efficient use of resources.

Defining the *value* of medicine is a common thread that unites today's healthcare practitioners. With serious concerns about rising medication costs and consistent pressure to decrease pharmacy expenditures and budgets, clinicians/prescribers, pharmacists, and other healthcare professionals must answer the question, "What is the value of the pharmaceutical goods and services I provide?" *Pharmacoeconomics*, or the discipline of placing a value on drug therapy,[1] has evolved to answer that question.

Challenged to provide high-quality patient care in the least expensive way, clinicians have developed strategies aimed at containing costs. However, most of these strategies focus solely on determining the least expensive alternative rather than the alternative that represents the best value for the money. The "cheapest" alternative—with respect to drug acquisition cost—is not always the best value for patients, departments, institutions, and healthcare systems.

Quality patient care must not be compromised while attempting to contain costs. The products and services delivered by today's healthcare professionals should demonstrate *pharmacoeconomic value*—that is, a balance of economic, humanistic, *and* clinical outcomes. Pharmacoeconomics can provide the systematic means for this quantification. This chapter discusses the principles and methods of pharmacoeconomics and how they can be applied to clinical pharmacy practice, and thereby how they can assist in the valuation of pharmacotherapy and other modalities of treatment in clinical practice.

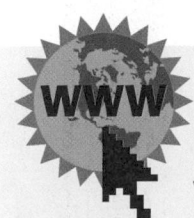

2

Health Outcomes and Health-Related Quality of Life

STEPHEN JOEL COONS

KEY CONCEPTS

❶ The evaluation of healthcare is increasingly focused on the assessment of the *outcomes* of medical interventions.

❷ An essential patient-reported outcome is self-assessed function and well-being, or health-related quality of life (HRQOL).

❸ In certain chronic conditions, HRQOL may be the most important health outcome to consider in assessing treatment impact.

❹ Information about the impact of pharmacotherapy on HRQOL can provide additional data for making decisions regarding medication use.

❺ HRQOL instruments can be categorized as generic/general or targeted/specific.

❻ In HRQOL research, the quality of the data collection tool is the major determinant of the overall quality of the results.

The medical care marketplace in the United States continues to experience change in both the financing and delivery of care.[1] This change is evidenced by a variety of developments, including an increase in investor-owned organizations, consolidation through mergers and acquisitions, increasingly sophisticated clinical and administrative information systems, and new financing and organizational structures. In this dynamic and increasingly complex environment, there is a concern that healthcare quality is being compromised in the push to contain costs.[2] ❶ As a consequence, there has been a growing movement to focus the evaluation of healthcare on the assessment of the end results, or *outcomes,* associated with medical care delivery systems as well as specific medical interventions. The primary objective of this effort is to maximize the net health benefit derived from the use of finite healthcare resources.[3] However, there is a profound lack of critical information as to what value is received for the tremendous amount of resources expended on medical care.[4] This lack of critical information as to

the outcomes produced is an obstacle to optimal healthcare decision making at all levels.

HEALTH OUTCOMES

Although the implicit objective of medical care is to improve health outcomes, until relatively recently, little attention was paid to the explicit measurement of them. An outcome is one of the three components of the conceptual framework articulated by Donabedian for assessing and ensuring the quality of healthcare: *structure, process,* and *outcome.*[4] For far too long, the approach to evaluating healthcare had emphasized the structure and processes involved in medical care delivery rather than the outcomes. However, healthcare regulators, payers, providers, manufacturers, and patients are placing increasing emphasis on the outcomes that medical care products and services produce.[5] As stated by Ellwood, outcomes research is "designed to help patients, payers, and providers make rational medical care choices based on better insight into the effect of these choices on the patient's life."[6]

TYPES OF OUTCOMES

The types of outcomes that result from medical care interventions can be described in a number of ways. One classic list, called the *five D's*—death, disease, disability, discomfort, and dissatisfaction—captures a limited range of outcomes for use in assessing the quality of medical care.[7] The *five D's* do not reflect any positive health outcomes and, as a result, have little value in contemporary outcomes research. A more comprehensive conceptual framework, the ECHO model, places outcomes into three categories: *economic, clinical,* and *humanistic outcomes.*[8] As described by Kozma et al.,[8] *economic outcomes* are the direct, indirect, and intangible costs compared with the consequences of a medical intervention. *Clinical outcomes* are the medical events that occur as a result of the condition and/or its treatment. ❷ *Humanistic outcomes,* which now are more commonly called *patient-reported outcomes,*[9] are the consequences of the disease and/or its treatment as perceived and reported by the patient.

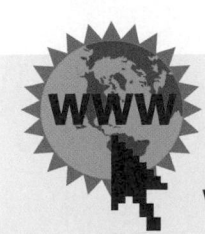

The complete chapter, learning objectives, and other resources can be found at **www.pharmacotherapyonline.com**.

CHAPTER 3

Health Literacy and Medication Use

ORALIA V. BAZALDUA AND SUNIL KRIPALANI

KEY CONCEPTS

❶ Limited health literacy is common and must be considered when providing medication management services.

❷ Some groups of people are at higher risk for having limited literacy skills, but in general, you cannot tell by looking.

❸ Patients with limited health literacy are more likely to misunderstand medication instructions and have difficulty demonstrating the correct dosing regimen.

❹ Limited health literacy is associated with increased healthcare costs and worse health outcomes, including increased mortality.

❺ Despite numerous efforts to improve safe medication practices, current strategies have been inadequate, and this may have a larger impact in patients with limited literacy.

❻ Most printed materials are written at higher comprehension levels than most adults can read.

❼ Health literacy experts are advocating standardization of prescription medication labels to minimize patient confusion.

❽ Several instruments exist to measure health literacy, but some experts advocate "universal precautions" under which all patients are assumed to benefit from plain language and clear communication.

❾ Obtaining a complete medication history and providing medication counseling are vital components in the medication management of patients with limited health literacy.

Every day, thousands of patients are not taking their medications correctly. Some take too much. Others take too little. Some use a tablespoon instead of a teaspoon. Parents pour an oral antibiotic suspension in their child's ear instead of giving it by mouth because it was prescribed for an ear infection. Others are in the emergency department because they did not know how to use their asthma inhaler. It is not a deliberate revolt against the doctor's orders but rather a likely and an unfortunate result of a hidden risk factor—limited health literacy.

❶ *Literacy*, at the basic level, is simply the ability to read and write. When these skills are applied to a health context, it is called *health literacy*, but health literacy is more than just reading and writing. *Health literacy*, as defined by the Institute of Medicine (IOM), is "the degree to which individuals have the capacity to obtain, process and understand basic health information and services needed to make appropriate health decisions." A growing body of evidence associates low health literacy with less understanding, worse outcomes, and increased cost, and these poor outcomes have led this topic to receive national attention. Health literacy has been made "a priority area for national action" by the IOM[1] and Healthy People 2010.[2] Likewise, the Agency for Healthcare Research and Quality (AHRQ) and the National Institutes of Health (NIH) have dedicated a website to this topic and have provided funding to support studies and interventions that are specifically relevant to health literacy.[3,4] Indeed, health literacy should be a national priority for the medical community as its consequences are far-reaching and crosscutting.

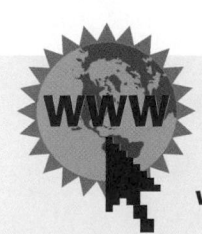

The complete chapter, learning objectives, and other resources can be found at **www.pharmacotherapyonline.com**.

JERI J. SIAS, AMANDA M. LOYA, JOSÉ O. RIVERA,
ARTHUR A. ISLAS, AND ULYSSES J. URQUIDI

CHAPTER

4

Cultural Competency

KEY CONCEPTS

❶ Healthcare providers should strive toward cultural competency to improve care to patients and communities from diverse cultures and backgrounds.

❷ Changes in demographics in the United States, health disparities, and patient safety are among the reasons that cultural competency needs to be emphasized in healthcare.

❸ Stages of cultural competency include cultural destructiveness, incapacity, blindness, pre-competency, competency, and proficiency.

❹ Legal and regulatory issues surrounding cultural competency include understanding and interpreting accreditation standards for healthcare organizations and Title VI of the Civil Rights Act.

❺ Patients may enter the healthcare setting with a different explanation of their illnesses than found in the Western biomedical model.

❻ Factors that can influence cultural values and beliefs toward healthcare include racial, ethnic, age, gender, sexual orientation, as well as religious backgrounds.

❼ Developing communication skills to interact with diverse populations includes recognizing personal styles of communication as well as barriers to patient understanding.

❽ Linguistic competency encompasses understanding issues related to working with patients with limited English proficiency and/or hearing impairments, such as learning basic terms and greetings, working with an interpreter or language-assistance lines, using non-English patient education/materials.

❾ Skills for working with patients from diverse cultures include being able to listen to the patient's perception of health, acknowledge difference, be respectful, and negotiate treatment options.

❿ Before they can understand other cultures, practitioners should understand personal and organizational values and beliefs.

CULTURE, COMMUNITY, AND SOCIAL DETERMINANTS OF HEALTH

Culture defines us.[1] Although our genetic make-up influences who we are, social determinants of health are also of great influence (Fig. 4–1). For example, our socioeconomic status, our race and ethnicity, our gender, our age, and our communities (environments), as part of our cultures, shape us.[2] Consider the following brief descriptions of three individuals. Patient 1 is a 30-year-old bilingual Vietnamese American Buddhist woman living on the West Coast whose family immigrated to the United States 5 years ago. Patient 2 is a 30-year-old African American Muslim upper-middle class man living in a major city in the Great Lakes region of the United States. Patient 3 is a 30-year-old trilingual European American Protestant middle class man living on the East Coast. Can healthcare professionals assume that because these patients are the same age that their healthcare beliefs and values as well as their approach to healthcare are the same? While each of the patients described above will have a unique health situation, their cultural backgrounds have likely influenced their health beliefs and behaviors.

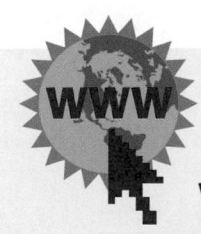

The complete chapter,
learning objectives, and other
resources can be found at
www.pharmacotherapyonline.com.

CHAPTER 5

Principles and Practices of Medication Safety

SCOTT M. MARK, JEFFREY D. LITTLE, SARAH E. ADKINS, AND ROBERT J. WEBER

KEY CONCEPTS

❶ Medication errors (MEs) are defined as *any* mistake at *any* stage of the medication use process; adverse drug events (ADEs) are the result of an injury to a drug-related intervention, regardless of whether an error has occurred.

❷ All MEs can be prevented, while ADEs can be categorized as preventable, nonpreventable, or potential.

❸ MEs occur at an alarmingly high rate, and some MEs and ADEs have fatal outcomes for patients.

❹ MEs can result from any step of the medication-use process: selection and procurement, storage, ordering and transcribing, preparing and dispensing, administration, or monitoring.

❺ MEs can be prevented by determining the actual and potential root causes in the medication-use system and correcting them.

❻ Quality improvement methods that prevent MEs and thereby minimize ADEs include identifying the ME/ADE, understanding the reasons for the ME/ADE, designing and implementing a change to prevent an ADE/ME, and checking the outcome of that change.

❼ A "Just Culture" of medication safety cultivates trust in the workplace that makes personnel feel comfortable sharing safety information (e.g., unsafe situations) and assuming personal responsibility for complying with safe medication practices.

Medical mistakes that cause harm have a devastating effect on patients in the healthcare system. In 1991, the Harvard Medical Practice Study showed that a significant number of people are victims of MEs. This landmark study reviewing safety in the state of New York showed that almost four percent of patients experienced an iatrogenic injury (one caused by healthcare practices or procedures), prolonging their hospital stays.[1] Importantly, nearly 14% of those mistakes were fatal. Examples of mistakes noted in the Harvard study included renal failure from angiographic dye, colon laceration during a therapeutic abortion, and a missed diagnosis of colon cancer. Drug complications were the most common type of outcome attributed to negligence, accounting for 19% of these preventable adverse events.[1]

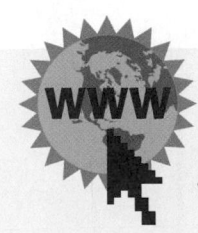

The complete chapter, learning objectives, and other resources can be found at **www.pharmacotherapyonline.com**.

CHAPTER 6

Evidence-Based Medicine

ELAINE CHIQUETTE AND L. MICHAEL POSEY

KEY CONCEPTS

❶ The best current evidence integrated into clinical expertise ensures optimal care for patients.

❷ The four steps in the process of applying evidence-based medicine (EBM) in practice are (a) formulate a clear question from a patient's problem, (b) identify relevant information, (c) critically appraise available evidence, and (d) implement the findings in clinical practice.

❸ The decision to implement results of a specific study, conclusions of a review article, or another piece of evidence in clinical practice depends on the quality (i.e., internal validity) of the evidence, its clinical importance, whether benefits outweigh risks and costs, and its relevance in the clinical setting and patient's circumstances.

❹ EBM strategies help keep one current in their field of expertise.

❺ EBM is realistic.

In the information age, clinicians are presented with a daunting number of diseases and possible treatments to consider as they care for patients each day. As knowledge increases and technology for accessing information becomes widely available, healthcare professionals are expected to stay current in their fields of expertise and to remain competent throughout their careers. In addition, the number of information sources for the typical practitioner has ballooned, and clinicians must sort out information from many sources, including college courses and continuing education (e.g., seminars and journals), pharmaceutical representatives, and colleagues, as well as guidelines from committees of healthcare facilities, government agencies, and expert committees and organizations.

❶ How does the healthcare professional find valid information from such a cacophony? Increasingly, clinicians are turning to the principles of EBM to identify the best course of action for each patient. EBM strategies help healthcare professionals to ferret out these gold nuggets, enabling them to integrate the best current evidence into their pharmacotherapeutic decision making. These strategies can help physicians, pharmacists, and other healthcare professionals to distinguish reliably beneficial pharmacotherapies from those that are ineffective or harmful. In addition, EBM approaches can be applied to keep up-to-date and to make an overwhelming task seem more manageable.

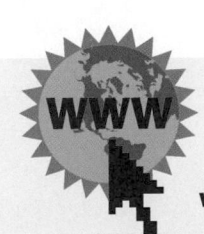

The complete chapter, learning objectives, and other resources can be found at **www.pharmacotherapyonline.com**.

CHAPTER

7

Documentation of Pharmacy Services

GEORGE E. MACKINNON III AND NEIL J. MACKINNON

KEY CONCEPTS

❶ Documentation of pharmacists' interventions, their actions and impact on patient outcomes is central to the process of pharmaceutical care.

❷ Unless pharmacists in all practice settings document their activities and communicate with other healthcare professionals, they may not be considered an essential and integral part of the healthcare team.

❸ Manual systems of documentation for pharmacists have been described in detail, but increasingly electronic systems are used to facilitate integration with other clinicians, payer records, and healthcare systems.

❹ Integrated electronic information systems can facilitate provision of seamless care as patients move among ambulatory, acute, and long-term care settings.

❺ Medication reconciliation, a process of ensuring documentation of the patient's correct medication profile, has become a central part of patient safety activities in recent years.

❻ Systems of pharmacy documentation are becoming increasingly important models in the United States as the Medicare Part D Prescription Drug Plan and accompanying medication therapy management services are further implemented.

❼ Electronic medical records and prescribing systems have several advantages over manual systems that will facilitate access by community pharmacists and their participation as fully participating and acknowledged members of the healthcare team.

As the opportunities to become more patient-focused increase and market pressures exert increased accountability for pharmacists' actions, the importance of documenting pharmacists' professional activities related to patient care will become paramount in the years to come. Processes to document the clinical activities and therapeutic interventions of pharmacists have been described extensively in the pharmacy literature, yet universal adoption of documentation throughout pharmacy practice remains inconsistent, incomplete, and misunderstood.

❶ Documentation is central to the provision of patient-centered care/pharmaceutical care.[1] Pharmaceutical care is provided through a "system" in which feedback loops are established for monitoring purposes. This has advantages compared with the traditional medication-use process because the system enhances communication among members of the healthcare team and the patient. Pharmaceutical care requires responsibility by the provider to identify drug-related problems (DRPs), provide a therapeutic monitoring plan, and ensure that patients receive the most appropriate medicines and ultimately achieve their desired level of health-related quality of life (HRQOL).

To provide pharmaceutical care, the pharmacist, patient, and other providers enter a covenantal relationship that is considered to be mutually beneficial to all parties. The patient grants the pharmacist the opportunity to provide care, and the pharmacist, in turn, must accept this and the responsibility it entails. Documentation enables the pharmaceutical care model of pharmacy practice to be maximized and communicated to vested parties. Communication among sites of patient care must be accurate and timely to facilitate pharmaceutical care. As discussed by Hepler,[1] documentation supports care that is coordinated, efficient, and cooperative.

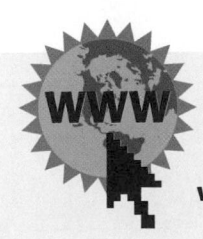

The complete chapter, learning objectives, and other resources can be found at **www.pharmacotherapyonline.com**.

CHAPTER 8

Clinical Pharmacokinetics and Pharmacodynamics

LARRY A. BAUER

KEY CONCEPTS

❶ Clinical pharmacokinetics is the discipline that describes the absorption, distribution, metabolism, and elimination of drugs in patients requiring drug therapy.

❷ Clearance is the most important pharmacokinetic parameter because it determines the steady-state concentration for a given dosage rate. Physiologically, clearance is determined by blood flow to the organ that metabolizes or eliminates the drug and the efficiency of the organ in extracting the drug from the bloodstream.

❸ The volume of distribution is a proportionality constant that relates the amount of drug in the body to the serum concentration. The volume of distribution is used to calculate the loading dose of a drug that will immediately achieve a desired steady-state concentration. The value of the volume of distribution is determined by the physiologic volume of blood and tissues and how the drug binds in blood and tissues.

❹ Half-life is the time required for serum concentrations to decrease by one-half after absorption and distribution are complete. It is important because it determines the time required to reach steady state and the dosage interval. Half-life is a dependent kinetic variable because its value depends on the values of clearance and volume of distribution.

❺ The fraction of drug absorbed into the systemic circulation after extravascular administration is defined as its bioavailability.

❻ Most drugs follow linear pharmacokinetics, whereby steady-state serum drug concentrations change proportionally with long-term daily dosing.

❼ Some drugs do not follow the rules of linear pharmacokinetics. Instead of steady-state drug concentration changing proportionally with the dose, serum concentration changes more or less than expected. These drugs follow nonlinear pharmacokinetics.

❽ Pharmacokinetic models are useful to describe data sets, to predict serum concentrations after several doses or different routes of administration, and to calculate pharmacokinetic constants such as clearance, volume of distribution, and half-life. The simplest case uses a single compartment to represent the entire body.

❾ Factors to be taken into consideration when deciding on the best drug dose for a patient include age, gender, weight, ethnic background, other concurrent disease states, and other drug therapy.

❿ Cytochrome P450 is a generic name for the group of enzymes that are responsible for most drug metabolism oxidation reactions. Several P450 isozymes have been identified, including CYP1A2, CYP2C9, CYP2C19, CYP2D6, CYP2E1, and CYP3A4.

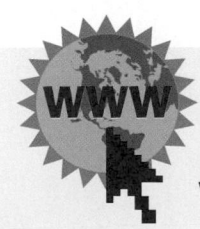

The complete chapter, learning objectives, and other resources can be found at **www.pharmacotherapyonline.com**.

CHAPTER 9

Pharmacogenetics

LARISA H. CAVALLARI AND Y. W. FRANCIS LAM

KEY CONCEPTS

❶ Genetic variation contributes to pharmacokinetic and pharmacodynamic drug properties.

❷ Genetic variation occurs for drug metabolism, drug transporter, and drug target proteins, as well as disease-associated proteins.

❸ Single-nucleotide polymorphisms are the most common gene variations associated with drug response.

❹ Genetic polymorphisms may influence drug efficacy or toxicity.

❺ Pharmacogenetics is the study of the impact of genetic polymorphisms on drug response.

❻ The goals of pharmacogenetics are to optimize drug efficacy and limit drug toxicity based on an individual's DNA.

❼ Gene therapy aims to cure disease caused by genetic defects by changing gene expression.

❽ Inadequate gene delivery and expression and serious adverse effects are obstacles to successful gene therapy.

Great variability exists among individuals in response to drug therapy, and it is difficult to predict how effective or safe a medication will be for a particular patient. For example, when treating a patient with hypertension, it may be necessary to try several agents or a combination of agents before achieving adequate blood pressure control with acceptable tolerability. A number of clinical factors are known to influence drug response, including age, body size, renal and hepatic function, and concomitant drug use. However, considering these factors alone is often insufficient in predicting the likelihood of drug efficacy or safety for a given patient. For instance, identical antihypertensive therapy in two patients of similar age, sex, race, and with similar medical histories and concomitant drug therapy may produce inadequate blood pressure reduction in one patient and symptomatic hypotension in the other.

❶ ❷ The observed interpatient variability in drug response may result largely from genetically determined differences in drug metabolism, drug distribution, and drug target proteins. The influence of heredity on drug response was demonstrated as early as 1956 with the discovery that an inherited deficiency of glucose-6-phosphate dehydrogenase (G6PD) was responsible for hemolytic reactions to the antimalarial drug primaquine.[1] Variations in genes encoding cytochrome P450 (CYP) and other drug-metabolizing enzymes are now well recognized as causes of interindividual differences in plasma concentrations of certain drugs. These variations may have serious implications for narrow-therapeutic-index drugs such as warfarin, phenytoin, and mercaptopurine.[2-4] Other variations associated with drug response occur in genes for drug transporters such as P-glycoprotein and drug targets such as receptors, enzymes, and proteins involved in intracellular signal transduction. Genetic variations for drug-metabolizing enzymes and drug transporter proteins may influence drug disposition, thus altering pharmacokinetic drug properties. Drug target genes may alter pharmacodynamic mechanisms by affecting sensitivity to a drug at its target site. Finally, genes associated with disease severity have been correlated with drug efficacy despite having no direct effect on pharmacokinetic or pharmacodynamic mechanisms.

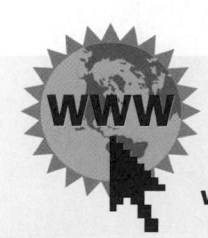

The complete chapter, learning objectives, and other resources can be found at **www.pharmacotherapyonline.com**.

CHAPTER 10

Pediatrics

MILAP C. NAHATA AND CAROL TAKETOMO

KEY CONCEPTS

1 Children are not just "little adults," and lack of data on important pharmacokinetic and pharmacodynamic differences has led to several disastrous situations in pediatric care.

2 Variations in absorption of medications from the gastrointestinal tract, intramuscular injection sites, and skin are important in pediatric patients, especially in premature and other newborn infants.

3 The rate and extent of organ function development and the distribution, metabolism, and elimination of drugs differ not only between pediatric versus adult patients but also among pediatric age groups.

4 The effectiveness and safety of drugs may vary among age groups and from one drug to another in pediatric versus adult patients.

5 Concomitant diseases may influence dosage requirements to achieve a targeted effect for a specific disease in children.

6 Use of weight-based dosing of medications for obese children may result in suboptimal drug therapy.

7 The myth that neonates and young infants do not experience pain has led to inadequate pain management in this pediatric population.

8 Special methods of drug administration are needed for infants and young children.

9 Many medicines needed for pediatric patients are not available in appropriate dosage forms; thus, the dosage forms of drugs marketed for adults may require modification for use in infants and children, necessitating assurance of potency and safety of drug use.

10 The pediatric medication-use process is complex and error-prone because of the multiple steps required in calculating, verifying, preparing, and administering doses.

Remarkable progress has been made in the clinical management of disease in pediatric patients. This chapter highlights important principles of pediatric pharmacotherapy that must be considered when the diseases discussed in other chapters of this book occur in pediatric patients, defined as those younger than 18 years. Newborn infants born before 37 weeks of gestational age are termed *premature*; those between 1 day and 1 month of age are *neonates*; 1 month to 1 year are *infants*; 1 to 11 years are *children*; and 12 to 16 years are *adolescents*. This chapter covers notable examples of problems in pediatrics, pharmacokinetic differences in pediatric patients, drug efficacy and toxicity in this patient group, and various factors affecting pediatric pharmacotherapy. Specific examples of problems and special considerations in pediatric patients are cited to enhance understanding.

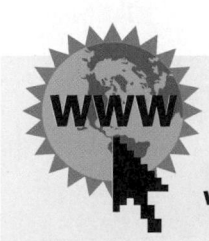

EMILY R. HAJJAR, SHELLY L. GRAY, DAVID R.P. GUAY, CATHERINE I. STARNER, STEVEN M. HANDLER, AND JOSEPH T. HANLON

CHAPTER 11

Geriatrics

KEY CONCEPTS

❶ The population of persons aged 65 years and older is increasing.

❷ Age-related changes in physiology can affect the pharmacokinetics and pharmacodynamics of numerous drugs.

❸ Improving and maintaining functional status is a cornerstone of care for older adults.

❹ Drug-related problems in older adults are common and cause considerable morbidity.

❺ Pharmacists can play a major role in optimizing drug therapy and preventing drug-related problems in older adults.

Pharmacotherapy for older adults can cure or palliate disease as well as enhance health-related quality of life (HRQOL). HRQOL considerations for older adults include focusing on improvements in physical functioning (e.g., activities of daily living), psychological functioning (e.g., cognition, depression), social functioning (e.g., social activities, support systems), and overall health (e.g., general health perception).[1] Despite the benefits of pharmacotherapy, HRQOL can be compromised by drug-related problems. The prevention of drug-related adverse consequences in older adults requires that health professionals become knowledgeable about a number of age-specific issues. To address these knowledge needs, this chapter discusses the epidemiology of aging; physiologic changes associated with aging, with emphasis on those changes that can affect the pharmacokinetics and pharmacodynamics of drugs; clinical conditions commonly seen in older adult patients; epidemiology of drug-related problems in older adults; and an approach to reducing drug-related problems through the provision of comprehensive geriatric assessment.

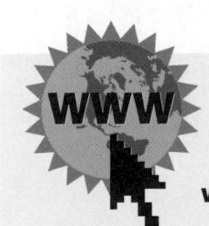

The complete chapter, learning objectives, and other resources can be found at **www.pharmacotherapyonline.com**.

CHAPTER 12

Palliative Care

JILL ASTOLFI

KEY CONCEPTS

❶ The goal of palliative care is to improve overall quality of life for patients, caregivers, and families while managing both general and disease-specific symptoms each patient may experience.

❷ Both palliative care and hospice use a team approach to address the total care of the patient and manage his or her symptoms.

❸ Palliative care should be instituted at the time of diagnosis and carried through to a patient's death; it can and should be administered simultaneously while a patient is receiving curative or life-prolonging therapies.

❹ It is important to address and manage each end-of-life symptom to improve the quality of life for the patient.

❺ Patients may experience different pain syndromes at the end of life. Knowledge of pain classification is important and necessary to determine the appropriate medication treatment for each patient.

❻ An interdisciplinary team approach is beneficial throughout the care of the patient. This is evident when addressing more psychologically based symptoms, such as delirium.

❼ Various symptoms will develop as death approaches. Anticipation, preparation, and access to appropriate treatment measures are necessary for a peaceful death.

❶ Approximately 2.4 million people die each year in the United States, most as a result of chronic illnesses.[1] For patients with advanced disease or life-limiting illness, access to appropriate symptom management is of great concern, as are access to social,

psychological, and spiritual support. A field of medicine known as palliative care focuses on reducing suffering and improving the quality of life for patients, their families, and caregivers. The purpose of palliative care is symptom assessment, prevention, and management. In addition, palliative care establishes goals of care with each patient and caregiver and extends support to the patient, family, and caregivers while addressing the individual patient's needs across all models of patient care settings (i.e., hospital, home, nursing home, and hospice).[2] Palliative care teams depend on the expertise of healthcare professionals from various disciplines; this helps to address the complex needs of seriously ill patients and their families. Typical members of a palliative care team are physicians, nurses, and social workers, with additional support from pharmacy, chaplaincy, nutrition, and other disciplines as needed.

Pharmacists serve an integral role in palliative care and hospice teams. They often participate in interdisciplinary team meetings, while others are employed by home health and hospital agencies and provide consultative services to interdisciplinary teams. Other pharmacists may work for an in-house hospice pharmacy or be employed by specialized hospice pharmacies throughout the country. Pharmacists typically provide appropriate medication recommendations and education for both staff and patients on appropriate use of medications. Some pharmacists are allowed to alter or initiate medications and dosages within a confined algorithm. Others provide recommendations to nurses and physicians regarding the medication therapy.

Overall, pharmacists can improve patient outcomes and symptom management by providing cost-effective medication recommendations, reviewing medication profiles, decreasing or eliminating duplicative medications, recommending alternative medication dosage forms (i.e., compounded medications) when appropriate, monitoring medications for both effectiveness and side effects, and educating staff, patients, and family on appropriate use of medication.

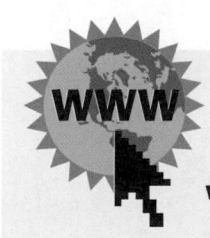

The complete chapter, learning objectives, and other resources can be found at **www.pharmacotherapyonline.com**.

CHAPTER 13

Pharmacoepidemiology

ANDY STERGACHIS, THOMAS K. HAZLET, AND DENISE BOUDREAU

KEY CONCEPTS

❶ Risks and benefits are commonly identified only after a drug is widely used by the general population.

❷ Observational study designs are essential for the study of risks and benefits associated with marketed drugs.

❸ Regulatory agencies are under pressure to identify and respond to postapproval drug safety issues and work with stakeholders on risk management and risk communication.

❹ Not all drug–disease associations represent cause–effect relationships.

❶ The practice of pharmacotherapy presents numerous challenges to clinicians as they apply knowledge of the benefits and risks of pharmaceuticals to the provision of individual and population-based care. A great deal of our understanding about the efficacy and short-term safety of drugs arises from well-controlled studies conducted during the drug development and approval process. However, many additional risks and, increasingly, additional benefits are only identified after the drug is used widely by the general population. Our gaps in knowledge of risks and benefits at the time a drug is marketed is due to numerous characteristics of premarketing studies, including limited sample size, relatively short study follow-up, restricted characteristics of persons studied, and differences in research settings from real-life conditions once a drug is marketed. Benefits and risks learned following a drug's approval may range from relatively minor to clinically important effects that seriously alter an individual drug's risk-benefit profile. The association between certain appetite-suppressant drugs and primary pulmonary hypertension/valvular heart disease and some cyclooxygenase-2 (COX-2) inhibitors and cardiovascular events are two examples where serious adverse effects were discovered only after these drugs had come into widespread use.[1-4] These examples highlight the inherent limitations of the drug development process, the limitations of contemporary medical product regulatory framework, and the need to study populations using medications, biologics, and medical devices obtained through real-world healthcare delivery. The liver toxicity seen with troglitazone and rosiglitazone is another example of the valuable contribution of close monitoring to drug safety. The first thiazolidinedione introduced for treatment of type 2 diabetes mellitus in 1997, troglitazone was withdrawn from the market based on reports of serious hepatocellular injury. In the mid-2007s, heart attacks and related deaths were observed in pooled clinical trials data for some patients receiving rosiglitazone, another thiazolidinedione subsequently approved for diabetes.[5] Medical products must be monitored closely following their introduction into the marketplace, and this information has value when applied to clinical practice. The purpose of this chapter is to describe the role of pharmacoepidemiology in drug development and therapeutics and to characterize the primary methods and contemporary issues in this field.

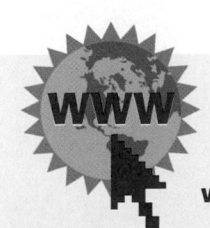

The complete chapter, learning objectives, and other resources can be found at **www.pharmacotherapyonline.com**.

CHAPTER 14

Clinical Toxicology

PETER A. CHYKA

KEY CONCEPTS

❶ Poisoning can result from exposure to excessive doses of any chemical, with medicines being responsible for most childhood and adult poisonings.

❷ The total number and rate of poisonings have been increasing, but preventive measures, such as child-resistant containers, have reduced mortality in young children.

❸ Immediate first aid may reduce the development of serious poisoning, and consultation with a poison control center may indicate the need for further therapy.

❹ The use of ipecac syrup, gastric lavage, and cathartics has fallen out of favor as routine therapies, whereas activated charcoal and whole-bowel irrigation still are useful for gastric decontamination of appropriate patients.

❺ Antidotes can prevent or reduce the toxicity of certain poisons, but symptomatic and supportive care is essential for all patients.

❻ Acute acetaminophen poisoning produces severe liver injury and occasionally kidney failure. A determination of serum acetaminophen concentration may indicate whether there is risk of hepatotoxicity and the need for acetylcysteine therapy.

❼ Anticholinesterase insecticides may produce life-threatening respiratory distress and paralysis by all routes of exposure and can be treated with symptomatic care, atropine, and pralidoxime.

❽ An overdose of calcium channel antagonists will produce severe hypotension and bradycardia and can be treated with supportive care, calcium, insulin with supplemental dextrose, and glucagon.

❾ Poisoning with iron-containing drugs produces vomiting, gross gastrointestinal bleeding, shock, metabolic acidosis, and coma and can be treated with supportive care and deferoxamine.

❿ Overdoses of tricyclic antidepressants can cause arrhythmias, such as prolonged QRS intervals and ventricular dysrhythmias, coma, respiratory depression, and seizures and are treated with symptomatic care and intravenous sodium bicarbonate.

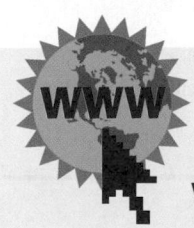

The complete chapter, learning objectives, and other resources can be found at **www.pharmacotherapyonline.com**.

Poisoning is an adverse effect from a chemical that has been taken in excessive amounts. The body is able to tolerate and, in some cases, detoxify a certain dose of a chemical; however, once a critical threshold is exceeded, toxicity results. Poisoning can produce minor local effects that can be treated readily in the outpatient setting or systemic life-threatening effects that require intensive medical intervention. This spectrum of toxicity is typical for many chemicals with which humans come in contact. Virtually any chemical can become a poison when taken in sufficient quantity, but the potency of some compounds leads to serious toxicity with small quantities (Table 14–1).[1] Poisoning by chemicals includes exposure to drugs, industrial chemicals, household products, plants, venomous animals, and agrochemicals. This chapter describes some examples of this spectrum of toxicity, outlines means to recognize poisoning risk, and presents principles of treatment.

EPIDEMIOLOGY

Each year poisonings account for approximately 37,000 deaths and at least 1.7 million emergency department visits in the United States.[2,3] Males have a nearly two-fold higher incidence of death than do females and 15% of adult poisoning deaths are attributed to suicide. Approximately 0.2% of poisoning deaths involve children younger than 5 years.[2] Of emergency department visits, typically 31% involve illicit drugs only, 28% involve pharmaceuticals only, 13% involve illicit drugs with alcohol, and 10% involve alcohol with pharmaceuticals.[2] Approximately 40% of emergency department visits for poisoning involve abuse of prescription and nonprescription drugs with one half of these patients taking multiple drugs. The number and rates of poisoning deaths from all circumstances have been increasing steadily, with a 90% overall increase from 1999 to 2006, representing 37,286 deaths in 2006.[3] This increasing mortality trend has placed poisoning as the second leading cause of injury death overall and the leading cause of injury death of people 35 to 54 years of age. Poisoning deaths were most frequently due to drugs. The number of deaths from opioid analgesics has nearly tripled from 1999 to 2006 and opioids were involved in nearly 40% of all poisoning deaths in 2006.[4]

TABLE 14-1	Serious Toxicity in a Child Associated with Ingestion of One Mouthful or One Dosage Unit	
Acids[a]		Cocaine
Anticholinesterase insecticides[a]		Colchicine
Caustics or alkalis[a]		Cyanide[a]
Cationic detergents[a]		Hydrocarbons[a]
Chloroquine		Methanol[a]
Clonidine		Phencyclidine or LSD

[a]Concentrated or undiluted form.

TABLE 14-2	Comparison of Various Poisoning Databases
Database (Abbreviation)	**Characteristics**
Death certificates from state health departments compiled by the National Center for Health Statistics (NCHS) www.cdc.gov/injury/wisqars/index.html	Compiles all death certificates whether the cause of death was by disease or external forces. Typically verified by laboratory and clinical observations
National Electronic Injury Surveillance System – All Injury Program of U.S. Consumer Product Safety Commission (NEISS) www.cdc.gov/injury/wisqars/index.html	Surveys electronically all injuries, including poisonings, treated daily at approximately 100 emergency departments. Used to identify product-related injuries
Drug Abuse Warning Network (DAWN) of the Federal Substance Abuse and Mental Health Services Administration (SAMHSA) www.dawninfo.samhsa.gov	Identifies substance abuse–related episodes and deaths as reported to approximately 1,100 hospitals and 600 medical examiners
The American Association of Poison Control Centers' National Poison Data System (AAPCC-NPDS) www.aapcc.org	Represents largest database of poisonings with high representation of children based on voluntary reporting to poison control centers

❶ Several databases in the United States provide different levels of insight into and documentation of the poisoning problem (Table 14–2). Poisonings documented by U.S. poison centers are compiled in the annual report of the American Association of Poison Control Centers' National Poison Data System (AAPCC-NPDS).[5] Although it represents the largest database on poisoning, it is not complete because it relies on individuals voluntarily contacting a poison control center. The AAPCC-NPDS dataset captures approximately 5% of the annual number of deaths from poisoning tabulated in death certificates.[5,6] Despite this shortcoming, AAPCC-NPDS provides valuable insight into the characteristics and frequency of poisonings. In the 2007 AAPCC-NPDS summary, 2,482,041 poisoning exposures were reported by 61 participating poison centers that served the entire United States.[5] Children younger than 6 years accounted for 51% of cases. The home was the site of exposure in 93% of the cases, and a single substance was involved in 91% of cases. An acute exposure accounted for 91% of cases, 83% of which were unintentional or accidental exposures. Only 13% were intentional. Fatalities accounted for 1,239 (0.05%) cases, of which 3% were children younger than 6 years. The distribution of substances most frequently involved in pediatric and adult exposures differed; however, medicines were the most frequently involved (52%) substances (Table 14–3).

TABLE 14-3	Poison Exposure by Age Group and Fatal Outcome, Ranked in Decreasing Order	
Pediatric	**Adult**	**Fatal Outcome**
Medicines	Medicines	Medicines
Cosmetics, personal care items	Cosmetics, personal care items	Alcohols
Cleaning substances	Cleaning substances	Gases, fumes
Pesticides	Pesticides	Chemicals
Arts and crafts, office supplies	Plants	Automotive products
Alcohols	Arts and crafts, office supplies	Pesticides
Food products	Alcohols	Cleaning substances

From reference Bronstein et al.[5]

Seventy-three percent of the poison exposures were treated at the scene, typically a home. In summary, children account for most of the reported poison exposures, but adults account for a greater proportion of life-threatening effects from poisoning.

ECONOMIC IMPACT OF POISONING

Poisoning accounted for a total lifetime cost of $12.6 billion annually in 2003 dollars.[7] Estimates of the lifetime cost of injury include related healthcare costs and lost lifetime earnings of the victim; however, they do not include the costs of suffering, reduced productivity of caregivers, or legal costs. The definition of poisoning for this economic estimate excluded poisoning from alcohol and illicit drugs.

POISON PREVENTION STRATEGIES

❷ The number of poisoning deaths in children has declined dramatically over the past four decades, due, in part, to the implementation of several poison prevention approaches.[7,8] These include the Poison Prevention Packaging Act (PPPA) of 1970, the evolution of regional poison control centers, the application of prompt first aid measures, improvements in overall critical care, development of less toxic product formulations, better clarity in the packaging and labeling of products, and public education on the risks and prevention of poisoning.[9] Although all these factors play a role in minimizing poisoning dangers, particularly in children, the PPPA has perhaps had the most significant influence.[8] The intent of the PPPA was to develop packaging that is difficult for children younger than 5 years to open or to obtain harmful amounts within a reasonable period of time. However, the packaging was not to be difficult for normal adults to use properly. Safety packaging is required for a number of products and product categories (Table 14–4). Child-resistant containers are not totally childproof and may be opened by children, which can result in poisoning. Despite the success of child-resistant containers, many adults disable the hardware or simply use no safety cap, thus placing children at risk. Fatigue of the packaging materials can occur, which underscores the need for new prescription ware for refills, as required in the PPPA.[10]

Poison prevention requires constant vigilance because of new generations of families in which parents and grandparents must be educated on poisoning risks and prevention strategies. New products and changes in product formulations present different poisoning dangers and must be studied to provide optimal management. Strategies to prevent poisonings should consider the various psychosocial circumstances of poisoning (Table 14–5), prioritize risk groups and behaviors, and customize an intervention for specific situations.[11,12]

TABLE 14-4	Examples of Products Requiring Child-resistant Closures	
Acetaminophen	Kerosene
Aspirin	Methanol
Diphenhydramine	Naproxen
Ethylene glycol	Oral prescription drugs[a]
Glue removers containing acetonitrile	Sodium hydroxide
Ibuprofen	Sulfuric acid
Iron pharmaceuticals	Turpentine

[a]With certain exceptions such as nitroglycerin and oral contraceptives.

TABLE 14-5	Psychosocial Characteristics of Poisoning Patients
Children	**Young Adults**	**Elderly**
Act purposefully or are poisoned by caretaker or sibling	Intentional abuse or suicidal intent is possible	Act with suicidal intent or unintentional misuse
Act with developmentally appropriate curiosity	Disregard or cannot read directions	Confuse product identity and directions for use
Attracted by product appearance	Do not recognize poisoning risk	Do not recognize poisoning risk
Ingest substances that adults find unpleasant	Reluctant to seek assistance until ill	Comorbid conditions complicate toxicity
React to stressful and disrupted household	Exaggerate or misrepresent situation	Unable or unwilling to describe situation
Imitate adult behaviors (e.g., taking medicine)	Peer pressure to experiment with drugs	Multiple drugs may lead to adverse reactions

RECOGNITION AND ASSESSMENT

The clinician's initial responsibility is to determine whether a poisoning has occurred or a potential for development of a poisoning exists. Some patients provide a clear account of an exposure that occurred with a known quantity of a specific agent. Other patients appear with an unexplained illness characterized by nonspecific signs and symptoms and no immediate history of ingestion. Exposure to folk remedies, dietary supplements, and environmental toxins also should be considered. Patients with suicide gestures can deliberately give an unclear history, and poisoning should be suspected routinely. Poisoning and drug overdoses should be suspected in any patient with a sudden, unexplained illness or with a puzzling combination of signs and symptoms, particularly in high-risk age groups. Nearly any symptom can be seen with poisoning, but some signs and symptoms are suggestive of a particular toxin exposure.[13] Compounds that produce characteristic clinical pictures (toxidromes), such as organophosphate poisoning with pinpoint pupils, rales,

bradycardia, central nervous system depression, sweating, excessive salivation, and diarrhea, are most readily recognizable.[14] The recognition of chemicals responsible for acute mass emergencies resulting from industrial disasters, hazardous materials accidents, or acts of terrorism may be aided by evaluating characteristic signs and symptoms.[15] Some drugs may be adulterated or counterfeit products and delay appropriate recognition of a possible toxin.[16] Assessment of the patient may be aided by consultation with a poison control center. A center can provide information on product composition, typical symptoms, range of toxicity, laboratory analysis, treatment options, and bibliographic references. Furthermore, a center will have specially trained physicians, pharmacists, nurses, and toxicologists on staff or available for consultation to assist with difficult cases. Consultation with a poison control center also may identify changes in recommended therapy. A nationwide toll-free poison center access number (1-800-222-1222) routes callers to a local poison control center.

When the circumstances of a poison exposure indicate that it is minimally toxic, many poisonings can be managed successfully at the scene of the poisoning.[5,17] Poison control centers typically monitor the victim by telephone during the first 2 to 6 hours of the exposure to assess the patient's status and outcome of first aid.

Once a poisoning is suspected and confirmation of the diagnosis is needed for medical or legal purposes, appropriate biologic material should be sent to the laboratory for analysis. Gastric contents may contain the greatest concentration of drug, but they are difficult to analyze. Blood or urine can be tested by qualitative screening in order to detect a drug's presence.[18,19] The results of a qualitative drug screen can be misleading because of interfering or low-level substances (Table 14–6); it rarely guides emergency therapy and thus has questionable value for nonspecific, general screening purposes.[18,19] Consultation with the laboratory technician and review of the assay package insert will help to determine the sensitivity and specificity of the assay. Quantitative determination of serum concentrations may be important for the assessment of some poisonings, such as those containing acetaminophen, ethanol, methanol, iron, theophylline, and digoxin.[20]

TABLE 14-6	Considerations in Evaluating the Results of Some Common Immunoassays Used for Urine Drug Screening
Drug	**Detection After Stopping Use**	**Comments**
Amphetamines	2–5 days	Many sympathomimetic amines, such as pseudoephedrine, ephedra, phenylephrine, fenfluramine, and phentermine, may cause positive results
	Up to 2 weeks with prolonged or heavy use	Other drugs, such as selegiline, chlorpromazine, trazodone, bupropion, and amantadine, may cause false-positive results depending on the assay
Benzodiazepines	Up to 2 weeks Up to 6 weeks with chronic use of some drugs	Ability to detect benzodiazepines varies by drug
Cannabinoid metabolite (marijuana)	7–10 days Up to 1–2 months with prolonged or heavy use	Extent and duration of use will affect detection time. Drugs such as ibuprofen and naproxen may cause false-positive results depending on the assay
Cocaine metabolite (benzoylecgonine)	12–72 hours Up to 1–3 weeks with prolonged or heavy use	Cocaine is metabolized rapidly and specific metabolites are typically the substance detected. False-positive results from "caine" anesthetics and other drugs are unlikely
Opioids	2–3 days Up to 6 days with sustained-release formulations Up to 1 week with prolonged or heavy use	Because the assay was made to detect morphine, detection of other opioids, such as codeine, oxycodone, hydrocodone, and other semisynthetic opioids, may be limited. Some synthetic opioids, such as fentanyl and meperidine, may not be detected. Drugs such as rifampin and some fluoroquinolones may cause false-positive results depending on the assay
Phencyclidine	2–10 days 1 month or more with prolonged or heavy use	Drugs such as ketamine, dextromethorphan, diphenhydramine, and sertraline may cause false-positive results depending on the assay

TABLE 14-7	Examples of the Influence of Drug Overdosage on Pharmacokinetic and Pharmacodynamic Characteristics
Effect of Overdosage[a]	**Examples**
Slowed absorption due to formation of poorly soluble concretions in the gastrointestinal tract	Aspirin, lithium, phenytoin, sustained-release theophylline
Slowed absorption due to slowed gastrointestinal motility	Benztropine, nortriptyline
Slowed absorption due to toxin-induced hypoperfusion	Procainamide
Decreased serum protein binding Increased volume of distribution associated with toxin-induced acidemia	Lidocaine, salicylates, valproic acid Salicylates
Slowed elimination due to saturation of biotransformation pathways	Ethanol, phenytoin, salicylates, theophylline
Slowed elimination due to toxin-induced hypothermia (<35°C)	Ethanol, propranolol
Prolonged toxicity due to formation of longer-acting metabolites	Carbamazepine, dapsone, glutethimide, meperidine

[a]Compared to characteristics following therapeutic doses or resolution of toxicity.

PHARMACOKINETICS OF OVERDOSE

The pharmacokinetic characteristics of drugs taken in overdose may differ from those observed following therapeutic doses (Table 14–7).[21,22] These differences are the result of dose-dependent changes in absorption, distribution, metabolism, or elimination; pharmacologic effects of the drug; or pathophysiologic consequences of the overdose. Dose-dependent changes may decrease the rate and extent of absorption, whereas the bioavailability of the agent may be increased due to saturation of first-pass metabolism. The distribution of a compound may be altered due to saturation of protein-binding sites. Metabolism and elimination of a compound may be retarded due to saturation of biotransformation pathways leading to nonlinear elimination kinetics. Delayed gastric emptying by anticholinergic drugs or as the result of general central nervous system depression caused by many drugs may alter the rate and extent of absorption. Patients with a drug overdose may inherently exhibit prolonged gastric emptying and gastric hypomotility.[23] The formation of concretions or bezoars of solid dosage forms may delay the onset, prolong the duration, or complicate the therapy for an acute overdose.[24] A combination of pharmacokinetic and pharmacodynamic factors may lead to delayed onset of toxicity of several toxins, such as thyroid hormones, oral anticoagulants, acetaminophen, and drugs in sustained-release dosage forms.[25] Drug-induced hypoperfusion may affect drug distribution and result in reduced hepatic or renal clearance. Changes in blood pH may alter the distribution of weak acids and bases. Drug-induced renal or hepatic injury also can decrease clearance significantly. Implications of these changes for poisoning management include delayed achievement of peak concentrations with a corresponding longer period of opportunity to remove the drug from the gastrointestinal tract. The expected duration of effects may be much greater than that observed with therapeutic doses because of continued absorption and impaired clearance. The application of pharmacokinetic variables, such as percentage protein binding and volume of distribution, from therapeutic doses may not be appropriate in poisoning cases.[21,22] Data on toxicokinetics often are difficult to interpret and compare because the doses and times of ingestion are uncertain, the duration of sampling is inadequate, active metabolites may not be measured, protein binding typically is not assessed, and the severity of toxicity may vary dramatically.

TREATMENT

Clinical Toxicology

GENERAL APPROACHES TO TREATMENT OF THE POISONED PATIENT

■ PREHOSPITAL CARE

First Aid

❸ The presence of adequate airway, breathing, and circulation should be assessed, and cardiopulmonary resuscitation should be started if needed. The most important step in preventing a minor exposure from progressing to a serious intoxication is early decontamination of the poison. Basic poisoning first aid and decontamination measures (Table 14–8) should be instituted immediately at the scene of the poisoning. If there is any question about the potential severity of the poison exposure, a poison control center should be consulted immediately (1-800-222-1222). While awaiting transport, placing the patient on the left side may afford easier clearance of the airway if emesis occurs and may slow absorption of drug from the gastrointestinal tract.[26]

Ipecac Syrup

❹ Ipecac syrup, a nonprescription drug, has been used in the United States for the past 50 years as a means to induce vomiting for treatment of ingested poisons. Despite its widespread use, concerns about its effectiveness and safety have been raised recently. An expert panel of North American and European toxicologists concluded that its routine use in the emergency department should be abandoned.[27] In 2003 the American Academy of Pediatrics issued a policy statement indicating that ipecac syrup was no longer to be used routinely to treat poisonings at home and that parents should discard any ipecac.[28] The key reason for the policy change was that research failed to show benefits in children who were treated with ipecac syrup. It likely will take several years for these recommendations to be adopted fully by parents and healthcare professionals, and rare exceptions may arise. In the 2007 AAPCC-NPDS report, 0.07% of 2.48 million cases received ipecac syrup, with or without poison center direction.[5]

There are several contraindications to the use of ipecac syrup or any form of induced emesis, such as gagging.[27] If the patient is without a gag reflex; is lethargic, comatose, or convulsing; or is expected to become unresponsive within the next 30 minutes, emesis should not be induced. If a fruitful emesis has occurred

TABLE 14-8	First Aid for Poison Exposures

Inhaled poison
Immediately get the person to fresh air. Avoid breathing fumes. Open doors and windows. If victim is not breathing, start artificial respiration.

Poison on the skin
Remove contaminated clothing and flood skin with water for 10 minutes. Wash gently with soap and water and rinse. Avoid further contamination of victim or first aid providers.

Poison in the eye
Flood the open eye with lukewarm or cool water poured from a glass 2 or 3 inches from the eye. Repeat for 10–15 continuous minutes. Remove contact lenses.

Swallowed poison
Unless the patient is unconscious, having convulsions, or cannot swallow, give 2–4 ounces of water immediately and then seek further help.

spontaneously shortly after ingestion, further emesis may not be necessary. Ingestions of caustics, corrosives, ammonia, and bleach are definite contraindications to induced emesis. Ingestion of aliphatic hydrocarbons (e.g., gasoline, kerosene, and charcoal lighter fluid) typically does not require emesis. When the agent is definitely known to be nontoxic, induction of emesis is purposeless and potentially dangerous. The rapid onset of coma or seizures or the potential to exaggerate the toxic effects of the poison may preclude further the induction of emesis. Some examples include poisonings with diphenoxylate, propoxyphene, clonidine, tricyclic antidepressants, hypoglycemic agents, nicotine, strychnine, β-blocking agents, and calcium channel blockers. Debilitated, pregnant, and elderly patients may be further compromised by induction of emesis.

■ HOSPITAL TREATMENT

General Care

Supportive and symptomatic care is the mainstay of treatment of a poisoned patient. In the search for specific antidotes and methods to increase excretion of the drug, attention to vital signs and organ functions should not be neglected. Establishment of adequate oxygenation and maintenance of adequate circulation are the highest priorities. Other components of the acute supportive care plan include the management of seizures, arrhythmias, hypotension, acid-base balance, fluid status, electrolyte balance, and hypoglycemia. Placement of intravenous and urinary catheters is typical to ensure delivery of fluids and drugs when necessary and to monitor urine production, respectively.[13,14]

Gastric Lavage

Gastric lavage involves the placement of an orogastric tube and washing out of the gastric contents through repetitive instillation and withdrawal of fluid. Gastric lavage may be considered only if a potentially toxic agent has been ingested within the past hour for most patients. If the patient is comatose or lacks a gag reflex, gastric lavage should be performed only after intubation with a cuffed or well-fitting endotracheal tube. The largest orogastric tube that can be passed (external diameter at least 12 mm in adults and 8 mm in children) should be used to ensure adequate evacuation, especially of undissolved tablets. Lavage should be performed with warm (37°C–38°C) normal saline or tap water until the gastric return is clear; this usually requires 2 to 4 L or more of fluid. Relative contraindications for gastric lavage include ingestion of a corrosive or hydrocarbon agent. Complications of gastric lavage include aspiration pneumonitis, laryngospasm, mechanical injury to the esophagus and stomach, hypothermia, and fluid and electrolyte imbalance.[29] Use of gastric lavage has declined in recent years as evidenced by the finding that only 1.5% of 588,262 cases treated at a healthcare facility received gastric lavage in the 2007 AAPCC-NCDS report.[5]

Single-Dose Activated Charcoal

Reduction of toxin absorption can be achieved by administration of activated charcoal. It is a highly purified, adsorbent form of carbon that prevents gastrointestinal absorption of a drug by chemically binding (adsorbing) the drug to the charcoal surface. There are no toxin-related contraindications to its use, but it is generally ineffective for iron, lead, lithium, simple alcohols, and corrosives. It is not indicated for aliphatic hydrocarbons because of the increased risk for emesis and pulmonary aspiration. Activated charcoal is most effective when given within the first few hours after ingestion, ideally within the first hour.[30] The recommended dose of activated charcoal for a child (1 to 12 years old) is 25 to 50 g; for an adolescent or adult the recommended dose is 25 to 100 g. Children younger than 1 year

can receive 1 g/kg.[9] Activated charcoal is mixed with water to make a slurry, shaken vigorously, and administered orally or via a nasogastric tube. Activated charcoal is contraindicated when the gastrointestinal tract is not intact. Activated charcoal is relatively nontoxic, but two identified risks are (a) emesis following administration and (b) pulmonary aspiration of charcoal and gastric contents leading to pneumonitis in patients with an unprotected airway or absent gag reflex.[30] Some activated charcoal products contain sorbitol, a cathartic that may be associated with an increased incidence of emesis following use.[31] Single-dose activated charcoal use has remained relatively steady during the past decade, with 4.1% of 2.48 million cases having received it according to the 2007 AAPCC-NPDS report.[5]

CLINICAL CONTROVERSY

Activated charcoal has been promoted for use at home as a replacement for ipecac syrup, but some have contended that little evidence indicates activated charcoal can be used safely and properly in this setting.

Cathartics

Cathartics, such as magnesium citrate and sorbitol, were thought to decrease the rate of absorption by increasing gastrointestinal elimination of the poison and the poison-activated charcoal complex, but their value is unproven. Poisoned patients do not routinely require a cathartic, and it is rarely, if ever, given without concurrent activated charcoal administration.[32] If used, a cathartic should be administered only once and only if bowel sounds are present. Infants, the elderly, and patients with renal failure should be given saline cathartics cautiously, if at all.[9,32]

Whole-Bowel Irrigation

Polyethylene glycol electrolyte solutions, such as GoLYTELY and Colyte, are used routinely as whole-bowel irrigants prior to colonoscopy and bowel surgery.[33] These solutions also can be used to decontaminate the gastrointestinal tract of ingested toxins.[9,13,34] Large volumes of these osmotically balanced solutions are administered continuously through a nasogastric or duodenal tube for 4 to 12 hours or more. They quickly cause gastrointestinal evacuation and are continued until the rectal discharge is relatively clear. This procedure may be indicated for certain patients in whom the ingestion occurred several hours prior to hospitalization and the drug still is suspected to be in the gastrointestinal tract, such as drug smugglers who swallow condoms filled with cocaine.[35] In addition, patients who have ingested delayed-release or enteric-coated drug formulations or have ingested substances such as iron that are not well adsorbed by activated charcoal may benefit from whole-bowel irrigation.[34] It should not be used in patients with a bowel perforation or obstruction, gastrointestinal hemorrhage, ileus, or intractable emesis. Emesis, abdominal cramps, and intestinal bloating have been reported with whole-bowel irrigation.[34] During 2007, whole-bowel irrigation was used in 0.5% of 588,262 cases managed at a healthcare facility.[5]

CLINICAL CONTROVERSY

Some clinicians believe that whole-bowel irrigation should be used more routinely as a rapid means to evacuate the gastrointestinal tract. Others recognize that it does have a quick onset but point out that little proof indicates whole-bowel irrigation makes a difference in patient outcome.

Perspectives on Gastric Decontamination

Although there are a variety of options for gastric decontamination, two clinical toxicology groups (the American Academy of Clinical Toxicology and the European Association of Poison Centers and Clinical Toxicologists) have concluded that no means of gastric decontamination should be used routinely for a poisoned patient without careful consideration.[27,29,30,32,34] They indicate that therapy is most effective within the first hour and that effectiveness beyond this time cannot be supported or refuted with the available data. A clinical policy statement by the American College of Emergency Physicians concludes that although no definitive recommendation can be made on the use of ipecac syrup, gastric lavage, cathartics, or whole-bowel irrigation, activated charcoal is advocated for most patients when appropriate.[36] The clinical policy also states that ipecac syrup is rarely of value in the emergency department and that the use of whole-bowel irrigation following ingestion of substances not well adsorbed by activated charcoal is not supported by evidence. The efficacy of activated charcoal has been demonstrated for many compounds,[30] but a randomized, controlled clinical trial of poisoned patients indicated that charcoal therapy did not reduce length of hospital stay or positively influence patient outcomes.[37] Although gastric lavage can reduce drug absorption if performed within 1 hour of ingestion, its use is not recommended routinely.[29,36,38] In recent years, the use of ipecac syrup has declined markedly in part because of its apparent lower efficacy compared with activated charcoal in minimizing drug absorption.[5,27,30] The American Academy of Pediatrics has recommended that ipecac syrup no longer be used for treatment of poisonings at home and has called for its removal from the home.[28] Recently, activated charcoal has been promoted for treatment of poisonings at home, but issues of safety, patient compliance, and effectiveness have not been proven in the home setting.[1,28,39] Poison control centers may be a source of guidance on the contemporary application of gastric decontamination techniques for a specific patient.

Enhanced Elimination Numerous methods have been used to increase the rate of excretion of poisons from the body. Of these, only diuresis, multiple-dose activated charcoal, and hemodialysis have demonstrated usefulness. These approaches should be considered only if the risks of the procedure are significantly outweighed by the expected benefits or if the recovery of the patient is seriously in doubt and the method has been shown to be helpful.

Diuresis Diuresis can be used for poisons excreted predominantly by the renal route; however, most drugs and poisons are metabolized, and only a good urine flow (e.g., 2–3 mL/kg/h) needs to be maintained for most patients. Fluid and electrolyte balance should be monitored closely. Ionized diuresis by altering urinary pH may increase excretion of certain chemicals that are weak acids or bases by trapping ionized drug in the renal tubule and minimizing reabsorption.[13] Alkalinization of the urine to achieve a urine pH of 7.5 or greater for poisoning by weak acids such as salicylates or phenobarbital can be achieved by intravenous administration of sodium bicarbonate 1 to 2 mEq/kg (1–2 mmol/kg) over a 1- to 2-hour period. Complications of urinary alkalinization include alkalosis, fluid and electrolyte disturbances, and inability to achieve target urinary pH values.[40] Acid diuresis may enhance the excretion of weak bases, such as amphetamines, but it is rarely, if ever, used because it risks worsening rhabdomyolysis commonly associated with amphetamine overdose.[13] Generally, diuresis or ionized diuresis is rarely indicated for poisoned patients because it is inefficient relative to other methods of enhancing elimination, it is associated with a risk of unacceptable adverse effects, and renal elimination of most drugs is not enhanced dramatically.

Multiple-Dose Activated Charcoal Multiple doses of activated charcoal can augment the body's clearance of certain drugs by enhanced passage from the bloodstream into the gastrointestinal tract and subsequent adsorption. This process, termed *charcoal intestinal dialysis* or *charcoal-enhanced intestinal exsorption,* describes the attraction of drug molecules across the capillary bed of the intestine by activated charcoal in the intestinal lumen and subsequent adsorption of the drug to the charcoal.[41] Furthermore, it may interrupt the enterohepatic recirculation of certain drugs.[13,41] Once the drug is adsorbed to the charcoal, it is eliminated with the charcoal in the stool. Systemic clearance of several drugs has been shown to be enhanced up to several-fold.[41,42] An international toxicology group's position statement on multiple-dose activated charcoal concluded that it should be considered only if a patient has ingested a life-threatening amount of carbamazepine, dapsone, phenobarbital, quinine, or theophylline.[42] Although a prospective, randomized study of the effects of multiple-dose activated charcoal on phenobarbital-overdosed patients demonstrated increased drug elimination, no demonstrable effect on patient outcome was observed.[43]

This approach provides a rapid onset of action that is limited by blood flow and a maximal "ceiling effect" related to the dose of charcoal present in the intestine. The response to multiple-dose activated charcoal is greatest for drugs with the following characteristics: good affinity for adsorption by activated charcoal, low intrinsic clearance, sufficient residence time in the body (long serum half-life), long distributive phase, and nonrestrictive protein binding. A small volume of distribution is desirable, but it has a marginal influence as an isolated characteristic,[44] particularly if multiple-dose activated charcoal is instituted during the toxin's distributive phase. A typical dosage schedule is 15 to 25 g of activated charcoal every 2 to 6 hours until serious symptoms abate or the serum concentration of the toxin is below the toxic range. This procedure has been used in premature and full-term infants in doses of 1 g/kg every 1 to 4 hours. Serious complications, such as pulmonary aspiration, occur in <1% of patients.[45] The risks of aspiration pneumonitis in obtunded or uncooperative patients and of intestinal obstruction in patients prone to ileus following a period of bowel ischemia (e.g., after cardiopulmonary arrest in the elderly) may be higher.[46] Contraindications are the same as those for single-dose charcoal.

Hemodialysis Hemodialysis may be necessary for certain severe cases of poisoning. Dialysis should be considered when the duration of symptoms is expected to be prolonged, normal pathways of excretion are compromised, clinical deterioration is present, the drug is dialyzable, and appropriate personnel and equipment are available. Drugs that are hemodialyzable usually have a low molecular weight, are not highly or tightly protein bound, and are not highly distributed to tissues. The principles of hemodialysis for acutely ill individuals are described in Chapter 54. Hemodialysis and charcoal hemoperfusion are efficient methods of dialysis, but both pose serious risks related to anticoagulation, blood transfusions, loss of blood elements, fluid and electrolyte disturbances, and infection.[47] Hemodialysis may be lifesaving for methanol and ethylene glycol poisoning and effective for other poisons, such as lithium, salicylates, ethanol, and theophylline.[13,36] Charcoal hemoperfusion was popular in the 1970s and 1980s as a means to remove toxins, but this approach has fallen out of favor because of poor clinical results, inappropriate use for drugs with large volumes of distribution, and limited availability of charcoal hemoperfusion columns.[48] Continuous hemofiltration transports drugs across a semipermeable membrane by convection in response to hydrostatic pressure gradients.[13,47] Limited experience is reported with the use of hemofiltration for poisonings, but it may be attractive

TABLE 14-9 Systemic Antidotes Available in the United States

Toxic Agent	Antidote
Acetaminophen	Acetylcysteine
Anticholinesterase insecticides	Atropine
Anticoagulants	Phytonadione
Benzodiazepines	Flumazenil
Botulism	Botulism antitoxin
Carbon monoxide	Oxygen
Cyanide	Cyanide antidote kit (amyl nitrite, sodium nitrate, and sodium thiosulfate)
Cyanide	Hydroxocobalamin
Digoxin	Digoxin immune Fab
Ethylene glycol, methanol	Ethanol
Ethylene glycol, methanol	Fomepizole
Heavy metals (copper, lead)	Dimercaprol
Heavy metals (copper, lead)	Penicillamine
Iron	Deferoxamine
Isoniazid	Pyridoxine
Lead	Calcium EDTA
Lead	Succimer
Methemoglobinemia	Methylene blue
Opioids	Nalmefene
Opioids	Naloxone
Organophosphate insecticides	Pralidoxime
Radioactive americium, curium, plutonium	Diethylenetriamene pentaacetate
Radioactive iodine	Potassium iodide
Snake, coral	*Micrurus fulvius* antivenin
Snakes (rattlesnakes, cottonmouth, copperhead)	*Crotalidae* polyvalent antivenin *Crotalidae* polyvalent immune Fab
Spider, black widow	*Lactrodectus mactans* antivenin
Thallium	Prussian blue

for the hemodynamically unstable patient who cannot tolerate hemodialysis.

Antidotes

5 The search for and use of an antidote should never replace good supportive care.[36] Specific systemic antidotes are available for many common poisonings (Table 14–9).[49,50] Inadequate availability of antidotes at acute care hospitals has been noted throughout the United States and can complicate the care of a poisoned patient. An evidenced-based consensus of experts has recommended minimum stocking requirements for 24 antidotes for acute care hospitals and that 12 be available for immediate administration upon patient arrival.[51] These recommendations may provide guidance to pharmacy and therapeutics committees in establishing a hospital's antidote needs. Drugs used conventionally for nonpoisoning situations may act as antidotes to reverse acute toxicity, such as insulin-dextrose or glucagon for β-adrenergic blocker or calcium channel antagonist overdose and octreotide for sulfonylurea-induced hypoglycemia.[52] As our understanding of drug toxicity increases, antidotes may have applications beyond contemporary indications, such as for acetylcysteine, which has shown promise for treating approximately 25 different poisonings and adverse drug reactions.[53] Commercially available intravenous lipid emulsions, e.g. Intralipid, have recently been used to reduce cardiac toxicity from several lipid-soluble drugs.[54] The use of toxin-specific antibodies (e.g., fragment antigen binding [Fab] antibody fragments for digoxin[55] or crotalid snake venom[56]) has offered a new approach to treatment of poisoning victims.

Assessing the Effectiveness of Therapies

Our knowledge of poisoning treatment is derived from case reports, clinical studies, human volunteer studies, animal investigations, and in vitro tests. Each of these approaches has limited applicability to the care of humans who have been poisoned. Case reports often are difficult to assess because they are uncontrolled, the histories are uncertain, and multiple therapies frequently are used. However, they can be useful to describe unique or new toxicities or characterize adverse effects associated with a therapy. Although clinical studies may describe tens to hundreds of patients, they can exhibit serious shortcomings, such as weak randomization procedures, no laboratory confirmation or correlation with history, insufficient number of severe cases, no control group, and no quantitative measure of outcome. Extrapolation of data from human volunteer studies to patients who overdose is difficult because of potential or unknown variations in pharmacokinetics (e.g., differing dissolution, gastric emptying, and absorption rates) seen with toxic as opposed to therapeutic doses,[21,22] differences in time to institute therapy in the emergency setting, and differences in absorption in fasted human volunteers compared with the full stomach of some patients who overdose. However, these studies provide the most controlled and objective measures of the efficacy of a treatment. Experiences from animal studies cannot be applied directly to humans because of interspecies differences in toxicity and metabolism. In vitro tests serve to screen the efficacy of some approaches, such as activated charcoal adsorption, but they do not mimic physiologic conditions sufficiently to allow direct clinical application of the findings. Despite their limitations, these data compose the basis for the therapy of poisoned patients and are tempered with the consideration of nonpoisoning-related factors such as a particular patient's underlying medical condition, age, and need for concurrent supportive measures.

CLINICAL SPECTRUM OF POISONING

Poisoning and drug overdose with acetaminophen, anticholinesterase insecticides, calcium channel blockers, iron, and tricyclic antidepressants are the focus of the remainder of this chapter because they represent commonly encountered poisonings for which pharmacotherapy is indicated. These agents also were chosen because they represent common examples with different mechanisms of toxicity, and they illustrate the application of general treatment approaches as well as some agent-specific interventions.

ACETAMINOPHEN

Clinical Presentation

6 Acute acetaminophen poisoning characteristically results in hepatotoxicity[57,58] and is the leading cause of acute liver failure in the United States.[59] Clinical presentation (see below) is dependent on the time since ingestion, presence of risk factors, and the ingestion of other drugs. During the first 12 to 24 hours after ingestion, nausea, vomiting, anorexia, and diaphoresis may be observed; however, many patients are asymptomatic. During the next 1 to 3 days, which is a latent phase of lessened symptoms, patients often have an asymptomatic rise in liver enzymes and bilirubin. Signs and symptoms of hepatic injury become manifest 3 to 5 days after ingestion and include right upper quadrant abdominal tenderness, jaundice, hypoglycemia, and encephalopathy. Prolongation of the international normalized ratio (INR) worsens as hepatic necrosis progresses and may lead to disseminated intravascular coagulopathy.

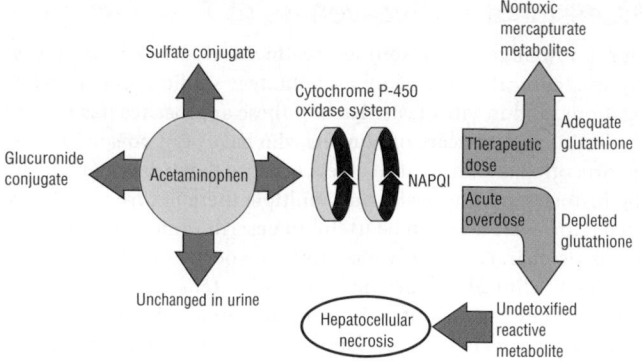

FIGURE 14-1. Pathway of acetaminophen metabolism and basis for hepatotoxicity. (NAPQI, *N-acetyl-p*-benzoquinoneimine, a reactive acetaminophen metabolite.)

Patients with hepatic damage may develop hepatic coma and hepatorenal syndrome, and death can occur.[57,58,60] Survivors of severe hepatotoxicity usually exhibit no residual functional or histologic abnormalities of the liver within 1 to 6 months of the incident.[58]

Mechanism of Toxicity

Acetaminophen is metabolized in the liver primarily to glucuronide or sulfate conjugates, which are excreted into the urine with small amounts (<5%) of unchanged drug. Approximately 5% of a therapeutic dose is metabolized by the cytochrome P450 mixed-function oxygenase system, primarily CYP2E1, to a reactive metabolite, *N*-acetyl-*p*-benzoquinoneimine (NAPQI). This metabolite normally is conjugated with glutathione, a sulfhydryl-containing compound, in the hepatocyte and excreted in the urine as a mercapturate conjugate (Fig. 14–1).[60]

In an acute overdose situation, sulfate stores are depleted, shifting more drug through the cytochrome system, thereby depleting the available glutathione used to detoxify the reactive metabolite. The reactive metabolite NAPQI then reacts with other hepatocellular sulfhydryl compounds such as those in the cytosol, cell wall, and endoplasmic reticulum. This results in centrilobular hepatic necrosis.[60] Several other mechanisms, such as cytokine release and oxidative stress, also may be initiated by the initial cellular injury.[60]

In many cases of severe hepatotoxicity, renal injury also is present and may range from oliguria to acute renal failure. The etiology of the renal injury may be a direct effect of the toxic metabolite of acetaminophen, NAPQI, generated by renal cytochrome oxidase, or a consequence of hepatic injury resulting in hepatorenal syndrome.[61]

Causative Agents

Acetaminophen, also known as paracetamol, is available widely without prescription as an analgesic and antipyretic. It is available in various oral dosage forms, including extended-release preparations. Acetaminophen may be combined with other drugs, such as antihistamines or opioid analgesics, and marketed in cough and cold preparations, menstrual remedies, and allergy products. Some patients may not recognize that they are consuming several products containing acetaminophen which can increase the total daily dose taken and the subsequent risk of hepatotoxicity.

Incidence

Acetaminophen is one of the drugs most commonly ingested by small children and is used commonly in suicide attempts by

adolescents and adults. The 2007 AAPCC-NPDS report documented 50,758 nonfatal single-drug product exposures and 74 deaths from acetaminophen alone or in combination products, with 27% of the exposures in children younger than 6 years.[5]

Age-based differences in the metabolism of acetaminophen appear to be responsible for major differences in the incidence of serious toxicity. Despite the common ingestion of acetaminophen by young children, few develop hepatotoxicity from acute overdosage.[5] In children younger than 9 to 12 years, acetaminophen undergoes more sulfation and less glucuronidation. The reduced fraction available for metabolism by the cytochrome system may explain the rare development of serious toxicity in young children who take large overdoses. Earlier treatment intervention and spontaneous emesis also may reduce the risk of toxicity in children.

Risk Assessment

There is a risk of developing hepatotoxicity when patients 6 years or older acutely ingest at least 10 g or 200 mg/kg, whichever is less, of acetaminophen or when children younger than 6 years acutely ingest 200 mg/kg or more.[62] Patients have survived much larger doses, particularly with early treatment. Initial symptoms, if present, do not predict how serious the toxicity eventually may become.

Chronic exposure to drugs that induce the cytochrome oxidase system—specifically isoenzyme CYP2E1, which is responsible for most of the formation of NAPQI—may increase the risk of acetaminophen hepatotoxicity. Poorer outcomes have been noted in patients who chronically ingest alcohol and those receiving anticonvulsants, both known to induce CYP2E1.[58,63] Patients with chronic alcoholism have a 3.5 greater odds of mortality with acute acetaminophen poisoning.[64] Concurrent acute ingestion of alcohol and acetaminophen may decrease the risk of acetaminophen-induced hepatotoxicity by ethanol acting as a competitive substrate for CYP2E1, thus reducing NAPQI formation.[65] Ethanol coingestion is not advocated as a preventive measure, and it is difficult to account for its specific impact on care.

Repeated ingestion of supratherapeutic doses of acetaminophen (defined for patients <6 years: ≥200 mg/kg over 8 to 24 hours, ≥150 mg/kg/day for 2 days, ≥100 mg/kg/day for 3 days or longer; for patients ≥6 years: ≥10 g or 200 mg/kg (whichever is less) over a single 24-hour period, ≥6 g or 150 mg/kg (whichever is less) per 24-hour period for ≥48 hours) has been associated with hepatotoxicity.[58,62] Patients who are fasting or have ingested alcohol in the preceding 5 days appear to be at greater risk.[66] Young children who receive repetitive supratherapeutic doses of acetaminophen have a higher risk of developing hepatotoxicity, particularly when they have been acutely fasting as the result of a febrile illness or gastroenteritis.[62,67] Patients with suspected risk factors, such as alcoholism, isoniazid therapy, or prolonged fasting, should be referred for medical evaluation if there is evidence that the ingestion exceeded 4 g/day or 100 mg/kg/day, whichever is less.[62]

The risk of developing hepatotoxicity may be predicted from a nomogram (Fig. 14–2) based on the acetaminophen serum concentration and time after ingestion.[57,59] The treatment line of the nomogram (150 mcg/mL [1,000 mmol/L] at 4 hours), which allows a margin of error in laboratory analysis and time of ingestion, should be used to make treatment decisions. The other lines on the nomogram indicate differing levels of risk for hepatotoxicity based on a multicenter study of 11,195 patients.[57,68]

If the plasma concentration plotted on the nomogram falls above the nomogram treatment line, indicating that hepatic damage is possible, a full course of treatment with acetylcysteine is indicated. When the results of the acetaminophen determination will be available later than 8 hours after the ingestion, acetylcysteine therapy should be initiated based on the history and later discontinued if the results indicate nontoxic concentrations. The nomogram has not been evaluated and thus is not useful for assessing chronic exposure to acetaminophen. Some have advocated that patients with chronic alcoholism should be treated with acetylcysteine regardless of the risk estimation.[64,68]

Management of Toxicity

Therapy of an acute acetaminophen overdose depends on the amount ingested, time after ingestion, and serum concentration of acetaminophen. When excessive amounts are ingested, the history is unclear, or an intentional ingestion is suspected, the patient should be evaluated at an emergency department and acetaminophen serum concentrations obtained.[62] No prehospital care generally is indicated, and ipecac syrup typically is not recommended.[62] If the patient presents to the emergency department within 4 hours of the ingestion or ingestion of other drugs is suspected, one dose of activated charcoal can be administered.

Acetylcysteine (also known as *N*-acetylcysteine), a sulfhydryl-containing compound, replenishes the hepatic stores of glutathione by serving as a glutathione surrogate that combines directly with reactive metabolites or by serving as a source of sulfate, thus preventing hepatic damage.[69] It should be started within 10 hours of the ingestion to be most effective.[57] Initiation of therapy 24 to 36 hours after the ingestion may be of value in some patients, particularly those with measurable serum acetaminophen concentrations.[69,70] Patients with fulminant hepatic failure may benefit through other mechanisms by the administration or initiation of acetylcysteine several days after ingestion.[69]

Therapy should be initiated with acetylcysteine within 10 hours of ingestion when indicated. The oral liquid was the only approved form of acetylcysteine in the United States until 2004, when the Food and Drug Administration (FDA) approved an intravenous formulation.[71] The dosage regimen for the intravenous form is based on one used in Europe for two decades, and outcomes similar to the 72-hour oral regimen have been reported.[53,71] A systematic review of the literature indicated that acetylcysteine is superior to supportive care, but there is no clear evidence of which regimen is better.[73] There are several notable differences between the oral and intravenous forms of acetylcysteine (Table 14–10),[53,57,71,72] most notable is the occurrence (approximately 10% of cases) of anaphylactoid reactions (see Chapter 97) following the intravenous infusion. An equal number of patients were treated with the intravenous or oral forms of acetylcysteine

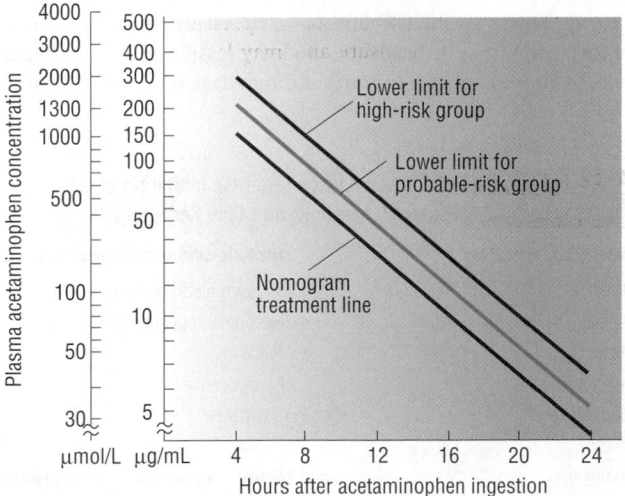

FIGURE 14-2. Nomogram for assessing hepatotoxic risk following acute ingestion of acetaminophen. (*Adapted from Smilkstein MJ, Knapp GL, Kulig KW, Rumack BH. Efficacy of oral N-acetylcysteine in the treatment of acetaminophen overdose: Analysis of the national multicenter study (1976–1985). N Engl J Med 1988;319:1557–1562. Copyright ©1988 Massachusetts Medical Society. All rights reserved.*)

TABLE 14-10	Comparison of Intravenous and Oral Regimens for Acetylcysteine in the Treatment of Acute Acetaminophen Poisoning	
Characteristic	**Intravenous**	**Oral**
Regimen	150 mg/kg in 200 mL D$_5$W infused over 1 hour, then 50 mg/kg in 500 mL D$_5$W over 4 hours, followed by 100 mg/kg in 1,000 mL D$_5$W over 16 hours[a]	140 mg/kg, followed 4 hours later by 70 mg/kg every 4 hours for 17 doses diluted to 5% with juice or soft drinks
Total dose (mg/kg)	300	1,330
Duration (h)	21	72
Adverse effects	Anaphylactoid reactions (rash, hypotension, wheezing, dyspnea); acute flushing and erythema in first hour of the infusion that typically resolves spontaneously	Nausea, vomiting
Ancillary therapy, if needed	Antihistamines and epinephrine for severe anaphylactic reactions	Antiemetics, e.g., metoclopramide, ondansetron, or droperidol
Trade name	Acetadote	Mucomyst
Available strength	20%	10%, 20%

[a]For patients <40 kg and those requiring fluid restriction, the total volume for dilution should be reduced as directed in the package insert.

D$_5$W, 5% dextrose in water for injection.

as reported in the 2007 AAPCC-NPDS.[5] When acetaminophen plasma concentrations are below the nomogram treatment line, there is little risk of toxicity, protective therapy with acetylcysteine is not necessary, and medical therapy likely is unnecessary.[57] The acetaminophen blood sample should be drawn no sooner than 4 hours after the ingestion to ensure that peak acetaminophen concentrations have been reached. If a concentration is obtained less than 4 hours after ingestion, it is not interpretable, and a second determination should be done at least 4 hours after ingestion. Serial determinations of a serum concentration, 4 to 6 hours apart, typically are unnecessary unless there is some evidence of slowed gastrointestinal motility as the result of the ingestion of certain drugs (e.g., opioids, antihistamines, or anticholinergics) or unless an extended-release product is involved. In these circumstances, therapy with acetylcysteine is continued if any concentration is above the treatment line of the nomogram, and provisional therapy is discontinued when both concentrations are below the treatment line.

Although young children have an inherently lower risk of acetaminophen-induced hepatotoxicity, these patients should be managed in the same manner as adults. When acetaminophen serum concentrations predict that toxicity is probable, young children should receive acetylcysteine in the dosing regimen described previously.[67] If fulminant hepatic failure develops, the approaches described in Chapter 44 should be considered. In unresponsive patients, liver transplantation is a lifesaving option.[58]

CLINICAL CONTROVERSY

The routine administration of acetylcysteine more than 24 hours after acetaminophen overdose has been proposed. Case reports and animal studies indicate that it is relatively safe and that its use may minimize hepatotoxicity. Although accepted criteria for its use are lacking, it may be considered for patients with fulminant hepatotoxicity, when acetaminophen is still measurable in the serum, or when the ingestion was not recognized within 24 hours and liver toxicity is apparent.

Monitoring and Prevention

Baseline liver function tests (AST, ALT, bilirubin, INR), serum creatinine determination, and urinalysis should be obtained on admission and repeated at 24-hour intervals until at least 96 hours have elapsed for patients at risk. Most patients with liver injury develop elevated transaminase concentrations within 24 hours of ingestion. AST or ALT concentrations >1,000 international units per liter (>16.7 mkat/L) commonly are associated with other signs of liver dysfunction and have been used as the threshold concentration in outcome studies to define severe liver toxicity.[57] The extent of transaminase elevation is not correlated directly with the severity of hepatic injury, with nonfatal cases demonstrating peak concentrations as high as 30,000 international units per liter (500 mkat/L) between 48 and 72 hours after ingestion.[58]

Prevention of acetaminophen poisoning is based on recognition of the maximum daily therapeutic doses (4 g in adults), observance of general poison prevention practices, and early intervention in cases of suspected overdose. The frequent involvement of acetaminophen in poisonings and overdoses, whether or not declared by the patient, has led to the routine determination of acetaminophen

concentrations in patients admitted to emergency departments for any overdose.[18]

ANTICHOLINESTERASE INSECTICIDES

Clinical Presentation

❼ The clinical manifestations of anticholinesterase insecticide poisoning include any or all of the following: pinpoint pupils, excessive lacrimation, excessive salivation, bronchorrhea, bronchospasm and expiratory wheezes, hyperperistalsis producing abdominal cramps and diarrhea, bradycardia, excessive sweating, fasciculations and weakness of skeletal muscles, paralysis of skeletal muscles (particularly those involved with respiration), convulsions, and coma.[74] Symptoms of anticholinesterase poisoning and their response to antidotal therapy depend on the action of excessive acetylcholinesterase at different receptor types (Table 14–11).

The time of onset and severity of symptoms depend on the route of exposure, potency of the agent, and total dose received (see presentation box below). Toxic signs and symptoms develop most rapidly after inhalation or intravenous injection and slowest after skin contact. Anticholinesterase insecticides are absorbed through the skin, lungs, conjunctivae, and gastrointestinal tract. Severe symptoms can occur from absorption by any route. Most patients are symptomatic within 6 hours, and death may occur within 24 hours without treatment. Death typically is caused by respiratory failure resulting from the combination of pulmonary and cardiovascular effects (Fig. 14–3).[74] Poisoning may be complicated by aspiration pneumonia, urinary tract infections, and sepsis.[74,75]

Organophosphate poisoning has been associated with several residual effects, such as intermediate syndrome, extrapyramidal symptoms, neuropsychiatric effects, and delayed chronic neuropathy. Intermediate syndrome becomes manifest in some patients approximately 1 to 3 days after exposure and generally resolves within weeks of onset without further treatment. It is characterized by muscle weakness of proximal limbs, cranial nerve innervated muscles, and muscles of respiration. The inability of the patient to raise his or her head is often an initial sign. Extrapyramidal symptoms, which may develop 1 to 7 days after exposure, usually resolve spontaneously within a few days of onset. Neuropsychiatric effects, such as confusion, lethargy, memory impairment, headache, and depression, typically begin weeks to months after exposure and may last for years. Chronic

TABLE 14-11	Effects of Acetylcholinesterase Inhibition at Muscarinic, Nicotinic, and CNS Receptors
Muscarinic receptors	**Nicotinic-sympathetic neurons**
Diarrhea	Increased blood pressure
Urination	Sweating and piloerection
Miosis[a]	Mydriasis[a]
Bronchorrhea	Hyperglycemia
Bradycardia[a]	Tachycardia[a]
Emesis	Priapism
Lacrimation	**Nicotinic-neuromuscular neurons**
Salivation	Muscular weakness
CNS receptors (mixed type)	Cramps
Coma	Fasciculations
Seizures	Muscular paralysis

[a]Generally muscarinic effects predominate, but nicotinic effects can be observed.

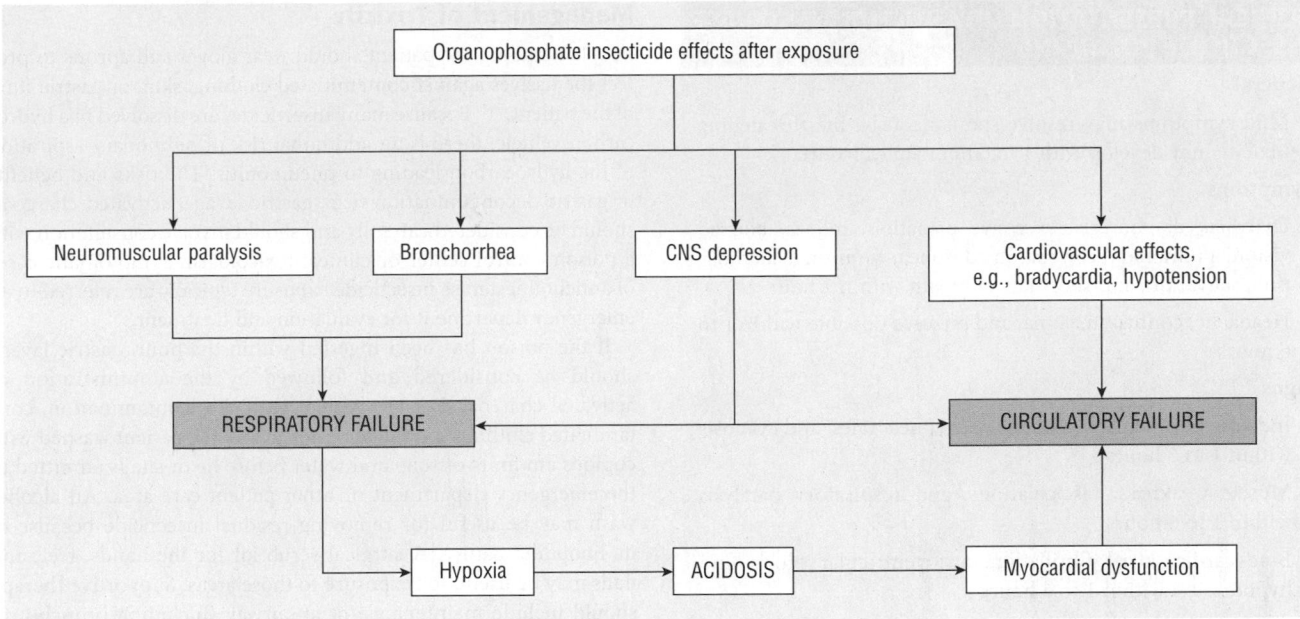

FIGURE 14-3. Pathogenesis of life-threatening effects of organophosphate poisoning. (CNS, central nervous system.)

neuropathy often presents as cramping muscle pain in the legs (upper extremities are sometimes involved), followed by rapidly progressive weakness and paralysis and develops 1 to 5 weeks after recovery from the acute poisoning exposure. Paresthesia and pain may be present. It is unresponsive to further atropine or pralidoxime therapy. Improvement may be delayed for months to years, and in some cases the patient develops permanent disability. It is not associated with all organophosphates.[74,76]

Mechanism of Toxicity

Anticholinesterase insecticides phosphorylate the active site of cholinesterase in all parts of the body.[74,77] Inhibition of this enzyme leads to accumulation of acetylcholine at affected receptors and results in widespread toxicity. Acetylcholine is the neurotransmitter responsible for physiologic transmission of nerve impulses from preganglionic and postganglionic neurons of the cholinergic (parasympathetic) nervous system, preganglionic adrenergic (sympathetic) neurons, neuromuscular junction in skeletal muscles, and multiple nerve endings in the central nervous system (Fig. 14–4).

Causative Agents

Anticholinesterase insecticides include organophosphate and carbamate insecticides. These insecticides are currently in widespread use throughout the world for eradication of insects in dwellings and crops. Carbamates typically are less potent and inactivate cholinesterase in a more reversible fashion through carbamylation compared with organophosphates.[74] The prototype anticholinesterase agent is the organophosphate, which is the focus of this discussion. A large number of organophosphates are used as pesticides (e.g., dichlorphos disulfoton, malathion, mevinphos, phosmet), and several were specifically developed for use as potent chemical warfare agents (see Chapter 16).[74,75,78,79] The chemical warfare agents act like organophosphate insecticides, but they are highly potent, are quickly absorbed, and can be deadly to humans within minutes.[79,80] An anticholinesterase insecticide typically is stored in a garage, chemical storage area, or living area. Anticholinesterase agents also can be found in occupational (e.g., pest exterminators) or agricultural (e.g., crop dusters or farm workers) settings. These agents also have been used as a means for suicide or homicide.

Incidence

Anticholinesterase insecticides are among the most poisonous substances commonly used for pest control and are a frequent source of serious poisoning in children and adults in rural and urban settings. The 2007 AAPCC-NPDS report documented 7,190 nonfatal single-product exposures and nine deaths from anticholinesterase insecticides alone or in combination with other pesticides, with 30% of exposures in children younger than 6 years.[5]

Risk Assessment

The triad of miosis, bronchial secretions, and muscle fasciculations should suggest the possibility of anticholinesterase insecticide poisoning and warrants a therapeutic trial of the antidote atropine. In cases of low-level exposure, failure to develop signs within 6 hours indicates a low likelihood of subsequent toxicity.[74] Ruling out other chemical exposures may be guided initially by symptoms at presentation.[15]

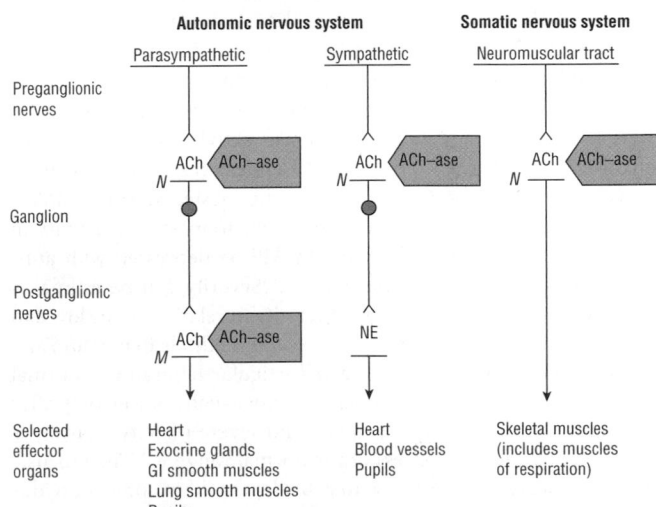

FIGURE 14-4. Organization of neurotransmitters of the peripheral nervous system and site of acetylcholinesterase action. (ACh, acetylcholine; ACh-ase, acetylcholinesterase; M, muscarinic receptor; N, nicotinic receptor; NE, norepinephrine.)

CLINICAL PRESENTATION OF ANTICHOLINESTERASE INSECTICIDE POISONING

General

- Mild symptoms may resolve spontaneously; life-threatening toxicity may develop with 1 to 6 hours of exposure

Symptoms

- Diarrhea, diaphoresis, excessive urination, miosis, blurred vision, pulmonary congestion, dyspnea, vomiting, lacrimation, salivation, and shortness of breath within 1 hour

- Headache, confusion, coma, and seizures possible within 1 to 6 hours

Signs

- Increased bronchial secretions, tachypnea, rales, and cyanosis within 1 to 6 hours

- Muscle weakness, fasciculations, and respiratory paralysis within 1 to 6 hours

- Bradycardia, atrial fibrillation, atrioventricular block, and hypotension within 1 to 6 hours

Laboratory Tests

- Markedly depressed serum pseudocholinesterase activity below normal range

- Altered arterial blood gases (acidosis), serum electrolytes, BUN, and serum creatinine in response to respiratory distress and shock within 1 to 6 hours

Other Diagnostic Tests

- Chest radiographs for progression of pulmonary edema or hydrocarbon pneumonitis in symptomatic patients

- Electrocardiogram (ECG) with continuous monitoring and pulse oximetry for complications from toxicity and hypoxia

Although the lethal dose for parathion is approximately 4 mg/kg, as little as 10 to 20 mg can be lethal to an adult and 2 mg (0.1 mg/kg) to a child. Small children may be more susceptible to toxicity because less pesticide is required per body weight to produce toxicity.[74,78] Estimation of an exact dose is impossible in most cases of acute poisoning; thus, tabulated "toxic" doses generally are not helpful in assessing risk of toxicity. Generally, ingestion of a small mouthful (~5 mL in adults) of the concentrated forms of an organophosphate intended to be diluted for commercial or agricultural use will produce serious, life-threatening toxicity, whereas a mouthful of an already diluted household product, such as an aerosol insecticide for household use, typically does not produce serious toxic effects.[78]

Measurement of acetylcholinesterase activity at the neuronal synapse is not feasible clinically. Cholinesterase activity can be measured in the blood as the pseudocholinesterase (butylcholinesterase) activity of the plasma and acetylcholinesterase activity in the erythrocyte. Both cholinesterases will be depressed with anticholinesterase insecticide poisoning.[74,78] Severity can be estimated roughly by the extent of depressed activity in relation to the low end of normal values. Because there are several methods to measure and report cholinesterase activity, each particular laboratory's normal range must be considered. Clinical toxicity usually is seen only after a 50% reduction in enzyme activity, and severe toxicity typically is observed at levels 20% or less of the normal range.[77,78] The intrinsic activity of acetylcholinesterase may be depressed in some individuals, but the absence of any manifestations in most people does not permit recognition of the relative deficiency in the general population. Therapy should not be delayed pending laboratory confirmation when insecticide poisoning is clinically suspected.

Management of Toxicity

People handling the patient should wear gloves and aprons to protect themselves against contaminated clothing, skin, or gastric fluid of the patient.[74,78] Because many insecticides are dissolved in a hydrocarbon vehicle, there is an additional risk of pulmonary aspiration of the hydrocarbon leading to pneumonitis. The risks and benefits of gastric decontamination (e.g., gastric lavage, activated charcoal) should be considered carefully and should involve consultation with a poison control center or clinical toxicologist. Symptomatic cases of anticholinesterase insecticide exposure typically are referred to an emergency department for evaluation and treatment.

If the poison has been ingested within the hour, gastric lavage should be considered and followed by the administration of activated charcoal. For the patient with skin contamination, contaminated clothing should be removed and the patient washed with copious amounts of soap and water before he or she is admitted to the emergency department or other patient care area. An alcohol wash may be useful for removing residual insecticide because of its lipophilic nature. A surgical scrub kit for the hands, feet, and nails may be useful for exposure to those areas. Supportive therapy should include maintenance of an airway (including bronchotracheal suctioning), provision of adequate ventilation, and establishment of an intravenous line. Based on a history of an exposure and presence of typical symptoms, the anticholinesterase syndrome should be recognized without difficulty.

Pharmacologic management of organophosphate intoxication relies on the administration of atropine and pralidoxime.[74,77,78] Atropine has no effect on inhibited cholinesterase, but it competitively blocks the actions of acetylcholine on cholinergic and some central nervous system receptors. It thereby alleviates bronchospasm and reduces bronchial secretions. Although atropine has little effect on the flaccid muscle paralysis or the central respiratory failure of severe poisoning, it is indicated in all symptomatic patients and can be used as a diagnostic aid. It should be given intravenously and in larger than conventional doses of 0.05 to 0.1 mg/kg in children younger than 12 years and 2 to 5 mg in adolescents and young adults.[78] It should be repeated at 5- to 10-minute intervals until bronchial secretions and pulmonary rales resolve. Therapy may require large doses over a period of several days until all absorbed organophosphate is metabolized, and acetylcholinesterase activity is restored.

Restoration of enzyme activity is necessary for severe poisoning, characterized by a reduction of cholinesterase activity to <20% of normal, profound weakness, and respiratory distress. Pralidoxime (Protopam), also called 2-PAM or 2-pyridine aldoxime methiodide, breaks the covalent bond between the cholinesterase and organophosphate and regenerates enzyme activity. Organophosphate-cholinesterase binding is reversible initially, but it gradually becomes irreversible. Therefore, therapy with pralidoxime should be initiated as soon as possible, preferably within 36 to 72 hours of exposure.[78] The drug should be given at a dose of 25 to 50 mg/kg up to 1 g intravenously over 5 to 20 minutes. If muscle weakness persists or recurs, the dose can be repeated after 1 hour and again if needed. A continuous infusion of pralidoxime has been shown to be effective in adults when administered at 2 to 4 mg/kg/h preceded by a loading dose of 4 to 5 mg/kg[81] and in children at 10 to 20 mg/kg/h with a loading dose of 15 to 50 mg/kg.[82] Both atropine and pralidoxime should be given together because they have complementary actions (Table 14–12). Systematic reviews of the literature indicate that the effectiveness of pralidoxime and similar oxime compounds in the treatment of organophosphate poisoning is inconclusive because of problems with study design.[83,84] Carbamate insecticide poisonings typically do not require the administration of pralidoxime.

One of the pitfalls of therapy is the delay in administering sufficient doses of atropine or pralidoxime.[74,78] The adverse effects of

TABLE 14-12	Comparative Characteristics of Atropine and Pralidoxime for Anticholinesterase Poisoning	
Characteristic	Atropine	Pralidoxime
Interaction	Synergy with pralidoxime	Reduces atropine dose requirement
Indication	Any anticholinesterase agent	Typically needed for organophosphates
Primary sites of action	Muscarinic, CNS	Nicotinic > muscarinic > CNS
Adverse effects	Coma, hallucinations, tachycardia	Dizziness, diplopia, tachycardia, headache
Daily dose[a]	2–1,600 mg	1–12 g
Total dose[a]	2–11,422 mg	1–92 g

[a]Range of reported cases; higher doses may be required in rare cases.

atropine and pralidoxime, predictable extensions of their anticholinergic actions, are minimally important compared with the life-threatening effects of severe anticholinesterase poisoning and can be minimized easily by decreasing the dose.

CLINICAL CONTROVERSY

Some references indicate that pralidoxime should be avoided in the treatment of carbamate (another type of anticholinesterase insecticide) poisoning because of reports of worsened toxicity in animals. Pralidoxime may be considered when exposure to carbamates is not known but an anticholinesterase is suspected based on symptoms or when respiratory paralysis due to nicotinic effects is not managed sufficiently by mechanical ventilation.

Monitoring and Prevention

Poisoned patients may require monitoring of vital signs, measurement of ventilatory adequacy such as blood gases and pulse oximetry, leukocyte count with differential to assess development of pneumonia, and chest radiographs to assess the degree of pulmonary edema or development of hydrocarbon pneumonitis. Workers involved in the formulation and application of pesticides should be monitored by periodic measurement of cholinesterase activity in their bloodstream. Untreated, anticholinesterase-depressed acetylcholinesterase activity returns to normal values in approximately 120 days. Long-term follow-up for severe cases of poisoning may be necessary to detect the presence of delayed or persistent neuropsychiatric effects.

Many anticholinesterase insecticide poisonings are unintentional as a result of misuse, improper storage, failure to follow instructions for mixing or application, or inability to read directions for use. Training and vigilant adherence to directions may minimize some poisonings. Storing pesticides in original or labeled containers can minimize the risk of unintentional ingestion. Keeping pesticides out of children's reach may decrease the risk of childhood poisoning.[85]

CALCIUM CHANNEL BLOCKERS

Clinical Presentation

❽ Overdosage with calcium channel blockers typically results in bradycardia and hypotension (Fig. 14–5). Many patients become lethargic and may develop agitation and coma. If the degree of hypotension becomes severe or is prolonged, the secondary effects of seizures, coma, and metabolic acidosis usually develop. Pulmonary edema, nausea and vomiting, and hyperglycemia are

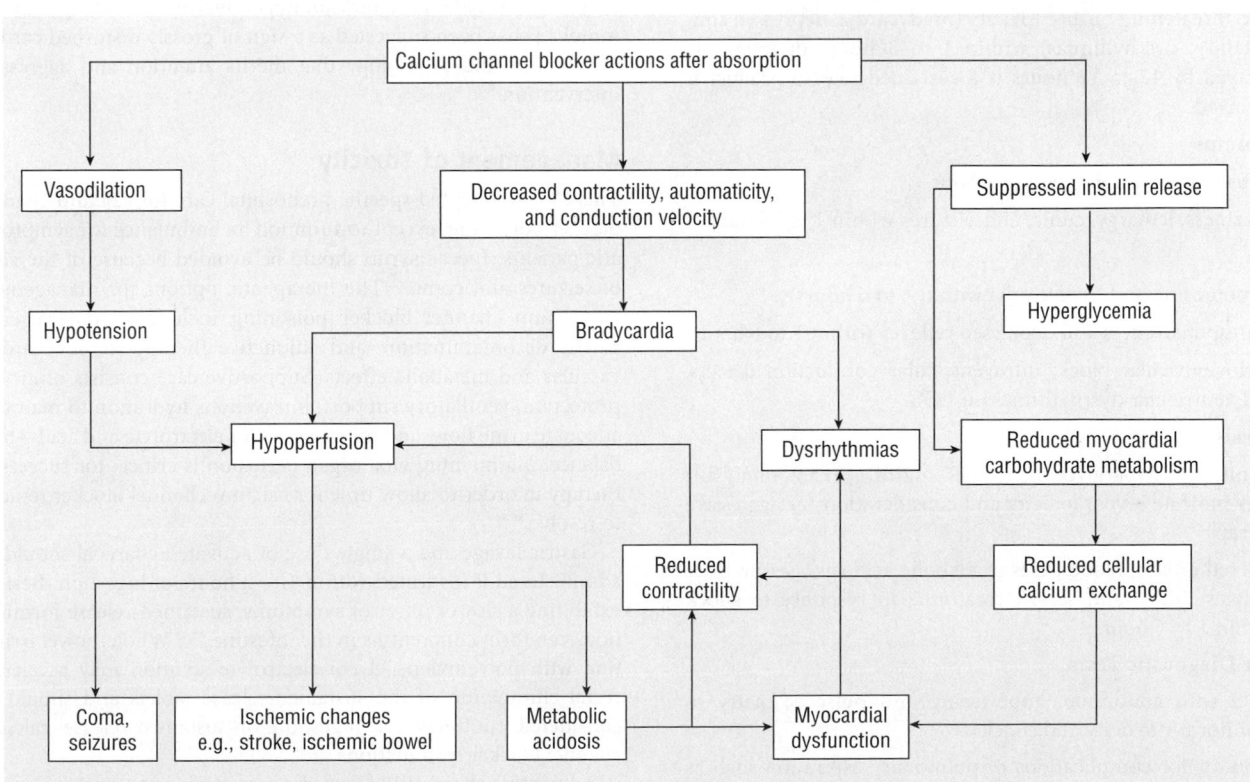

FIGURE 14-5. Pathophysiologic changes associated with calcium channel blocker poisoning.

frequent complications of calcium channel blocker overdoses. Paralytic ileus, mesenteric ischemia, and colonic infarction have been observed in patients with severe hypotension. Many symptoms become manifest within 1 to 2 hours of ingestion (see presentation box below). If a sustained-release formulation is involved, the onset of overt toxicity may be delayed by 6 to 18 hours from the time of ingestion. Severe poisoning can result in refractory shock and cardiac arrest. Death can occur within 3 to 4 hours of ingestion.[86–89]

Mechanism of Toxicity

Most toxic effects of calcium channel blockers are produced by three basic actions on the cardiovascular system: vasodilation through relaxation of smooth muscles, decreased contractility by action on cardiac tissue, and decreased automaticity and conduction velocity through slow recovery of calcium channels. Calcium channel blockers interfere with calcium entry by inhibiting one or more of the several types of calcium channels and binding at one or more cellular binding sites. Selectivity of these actions varies with the calcium channel blocker and provides some therapeutic distinctions, but these differences are less clear with overdosage.[89] Calcium channel blockers also inhibit insulin secretion, which results in hyperglycemia and changes in fatty acid oxidation in the myocardium that alter myocardial calcium flow and reduce contractility.[90] Current experiences suggest that the signs and symptoms of calcium channel blocker toxicity are similar among the drugs in this class.

CLINICAL PRESENTATION OF CALCIUM CHANNEL BLOCKER POISONING

General

- Life-threatening cardiac toxicity (bradycardia, depressed contractility, dysrhythmias) within 1 to 3 hours of ingestion, delayed by 12 to 18 hours if a sustained-release product is involved

Symptoms

- Nausea and vomiting within 1 hour
- Dizziness, lethargy, coma, and seizures within 1 to 3 hours

Signs

- Hypotension and bradycardia within 1 to 6 hours
- Unresponsiveness and depressed reflexes within 1 to 6 hours
- Atrioventricular block, intraventricular conduction defects, and ventricular dysrhythmias on ECG

Laboratory Tests

- Significant hyperglycemia (>250 mg/dL [>13.9 mmol/L]) may indicate severe toxicity and consideration for aggressive therapy
- Altered arterial blood gases (metabolic acidosis), serum electrolytes, BUN, and serum creatinine in response to shock within 1 to 6 hours

Other Diagnostic Tests

- ECG with continuous monitoring and pulse oximetry to monitor for toxicity and shock
- Monitor for complications of pulmonary aspiration such as hypoxia and pneumonia by physical findings and chest radiographs

Causative Agents

Approximately 10 calcium channel antagonists are marketed in the United States for treatment of hypertension, certain dysrhythmias, and some forms of angina. The calcium channel blockers are classified by their chemical structure (see Chapter 19) as phenylalkylamines (e.g., verapamil), benzothiapines (e.g., diltiazem), and dihydropyridines (e.g., amlodipine, felodipine, nicardipine, and nifedipine). Several of these agents, namely, diltiazem, nicardipine, nifedipine, and verapamil, are formulated as sustained-release oral dosage forms or have a slow onset of action and longer half-life (e.g., amlodipine[91]), allowing once-daily administration.

Incidence

In 2007, the AAPCC-NPDS report documented 4,759 single-product toxic exposures to a calcium channel blocker; 74 patients exhibited and survived major toxic effects, and 17 died.[5]

Risk Assessment

Ingestion of doses near or in excess of 1 g of diltiazem, nifedipine, or verapamil may result in life-threatening symptoms or death in an adult.[86] Ingestion of an amount that exceeds the usual maximum single therapeutic dose or a dose equal to or greater than the lowest reported toxic dose (whichever is less) warrants referral to a poison control center and/or an emergency department. The threshold doses of several agents and dosage forms vary (e.g., diltiazem: adults, >120 mg for immediate release and chewed sustained release, >360 mg for sustained release, >540 mg for extended release; children younger than 6 years: >1 mg/kg).[92] Patients on chronic therapy with these agents who acutely ingest an overdose may have a greater risk of serious toxicity. Elderly patients and those with underlying cardiac disease may not tolerate mild hypotension or bradycardia. Concurrent ingestion of β-adrenergic blocking drugs, digitalis, class I antiarrhythmics, and other vasodilators may worsen the cardiovascular effects of calcium channel blockers.[87,89,92] The presence of persistent and significant hyperglycemia (>250 mg/dL [13.9 mmol/L]) has been suggested as a sign of grossly disturbed cardiac metabolism and physiology that merits attention and aggressive intervention.[93]

Management of Toxicity

There is no accepted specific prehospital care for calcium channel blocker poisoning, except to summon an ambulance for symptomatic patients. Ipecac syrup should be avoided because of the risks of seizures and coma.[92] The therapeutic options for management of calcium channel blocker poisoning include supportive care, gastric decontamination, and adjunctive therapy for the cardiovascular and metabolic effects. Supportive care consists of airway protection, ventilatory support, intravenous hydration to maintain adequate urine flow, and maintenance of electrolyte and acid—base balance. Maintaining vital organ perfusion is critical for successful therapy in order to allow time for calcium channel blocker toxicity to resolve.[88,89]

Gastric lavage and a single dose of activated charcoal should be administered if instituted within 1 to 2 hours of ingestion. Besides exhibiting a slower onset of symptoms, sustained-release formulations can form concretions in the intestine.[88,89] Whole-bowel irrigation with polyethylene glycol electrolyte solution may accelerate rectal elimination of the sustained-release tablets and should be considered routinely for ingestion of sustained-release calcium channel blocker formulations.[34,94]

Adjunctive therapy is focused on treating hypotension, bradycardia, and resulting shock. Hypotension is treated primarily by correction of coexisting dysrhythmias (e.g., bradycardia, heart block) and implementation of conventional measures to treat decreased blood pressure. Infusion of normal saline and placement of the patient in the Trendelenburg position are initial therapies. Further fluid therapy should be guided by central venous pressure monitoring. Dopamine and epinephrine in conventional doses for cardiogenic shock should be considered next. If hypotension persists, dysrhythmias are present, or other signs of serious toxicity are present, calcium should be administered intravenously.[86,89]

A calcium chloride bolus test dose (10–20 mg/kg up to 1–3 g) is the preferred therapy for patients with serious toxicity. In adults, calcium chloride 10% can be diluted in 100 mL normal saline and infused over 5 minutes through a central venous line. If a positive cardiovascular response is achieved with this test dose, a continuous infusion of calcium chloride (20–50 mg/kg/h) should be started. Calcium gluconate is less desirable to use because it contains less elemental calcium per milligram of final dosage form. Intravenous calcium salts can produce vomiting and tissue necrosis on extravasation.[52,89] Atropine also may be considered for treatment of bradycardia, but it is seldom sufficient as a sole therapy.[88]

For severe cases of calcium channel blocker toxicity refractory to conventional therapy, an infusion of high-dose insulin with supplemental dextrose and potassium to produce a state of hyperinsulinemia and euglycemia should be considered.[52,86–90] Case reports suggest that an intravenous bolus of regular insulin (0.5–1 U/kg) with 50 mL dextrose 50% (0.25 mg/kg for children) followed by a continuous infusion of regular insulin (0.5 to 1 U/kg/h) may improve myocardial contractility. The effect of insulin is presently unclear, but it may improve myocardial metabolism that is adversely affected by calcium channel blocker overdoses, such as decreased cellular uptake of glucose and free fatty acids and a shift from fatty acid oxidation to carbohydrate metabolism.[86,88,90] This insulin regimen is titrated to improvement in systolic blood pressure over 100 mm Hg and heart rate over 50 beats/min. Serum glucose concentrations should be monitored closely to maintain euglycemia. Patients with serum potassium concentrations <2.5 mEq/L (<2.5 mmol/L) may need supplemental potassium (see Chapter 60). The insulin infusion rate can be reduced gradually as signs of toxicity resolve. Intravenous sodium bicarbonate may be also necessary to establish acid—base balance and correct the metabolic acidosis that is common with serious calcium channel blocker overdoses.

If the bradycardia and hypotension are refractory to the foregoing therapy, a bolus infusion of glucagon (0.05–0.20 mg/kg, initial adult dose is 3–5 mg over 1–2 min) should be considered. Benefit typically is observed within 5 minutes of administration and can be sustained with a continuous intravenous infusion (0.05–0.1 mg/kg/h) titrated to clinical response.[95] Glucagon possesses chronotropic and inotropic effects in part by stimulating adenylate cyclase and increasing cyclic adenosine monophosphate, which may promote intracellular entry of calcium through calcium channels. It thereby may improve hypotension and bradycardia.[52] Vomiting is not uncommon with these large doses of glucagon, and the airway should be protected to prevent pulmonary aspiration. Hyperglycemia may occur or be exacerbated in those patients receiving glucagon therapy.

Therapies with glucagon and insulin are based on animal studies and case reports; clinical trials demonstrating effectiveness have not been performed to date.[52,86–90]

Several lifesaving options may be warranted for patients with cardiogenic shock that is refractory to conventional therapy. Electrical cardiac pacing may restore an acceptable heart rate in patients with severe bradycardia.[89] Intraaortic balloon counterpulsation or cardiopulmonary bypass may improve shock in patients unresponsive to other therapies.[52,89,96,97] Animal studies and cases from the anesthesiology literature suggest that the emergent infusion of lipid emulsion, e.g., Intralipid, can dramatically "rescue" patients with severe cardiac toxicity from lipid soluble drugs such as calcium

channel blockers. Some current hypotheses on the actions responsible for this effect include serving as a "lipid sink" for lipophillic drugs and as an energy substrate for the myocardium. There are several dosing schemes and none are well studied to date. Better and more evidence is needed to know if it has a place in therapy.[54,98]

Measures to enhance elimination from the bloodstream by hemodialysis or multiple-dose activated charcoal have not been shown to be effective and are not indicated for calcium channel blocker poisoning.[42,87,89,99]

CLINICAL CONTROVERSY

Some clinicians believe that hyperinsulinemia/euglycemia or glucagon therapy for calcium channel blocker poisoning should be used early in the course of therapy. Others reserve it for life-threatening symptoms not responsive to other therapy. More safety and effectiveness data are needed to define the place of these two agents in therapy.

Monitoring and Prevention

Regular monitoring of vital signs and ECG is essential in suspected calcium channel blocker poisoning. Determinations of serum electrolytes, serum glucose, arterial blood gases, urine output, and renal function are indicated to assess and monitor symptomatic patients. If serious toxicity is likely to develop, overt symptoms will manifest within 6 hours of ingestion.[92] For ingestions of sustained-release products in toxic doses, observation for 24 hours in a critical care unit may be prudent because the onset of symptoms may be slow and delayed up to 12 to 18 hours after ingestion.[86,92,94,99,100] Serum concentrations of these agents in overdose patients do not correlate well with the ingested dose, degree of toxicity, or outcome.

Poisonings resulting from these agents may be the result of an intentional suicide or unintentional ingestion by young children. Prevention of calcium channel blocker poisonings in children rests with the education of patients receiving these agents, particularly of grandparents and those who have children visit their homes infrequently, of their dangers on overdosage. Safe storage and use of child-resistant closures may reduce the opportunities for unintentional poisonings by children.[87]

IRON

Clinical Presentation

❾ In the first few hours after ingestion of toxic amounts of iron, symptoms of gastrointestinal irritation (e.g., nausea, vomiting, and diarrhea) are common (see presentation box below). In certain severe cases, acidosis and shock can become manifest within 6 hours of ingestion. Some have observed a quiescent phase between 6 and 48 hours after ingestion when symptoms improve or abate, but this phenomenon is poorly characterized.[101] Continued gastrointestinal symptoms, poor perfusion, and oliguria should suggest the development of severe toxicity, with other effects still to become manifest. Generally, within 24 to 36 hours of the ingestion, central nervous system involvement with coma and seizures; hepatic injury characterized by jaundice, increased INR, increased bilirubin, and hypoglycemia; cardiovascular shock; and acidosis also develop.[101,102] Adult respiratory distress syndrome (ARDS) may develop in patients with severe cardiovascular shock and further compromise recovery.[103] Coagulopathy with decreased thrombin formation is one of the early direct effects of excessive iron concentrations, and later disturbances of coagulation (after 24 to 48 hours of ingestion) are a consequence of hepatotoxicity.[104] Mucosal injury, an iron-rich circulation, or deferoxamine therapy may promote septicemia with *Yersinia enterocolitica* during iron overdose; other bacteria or viruses also may cause septicemia.[101] Two to 4 weeks after the exposure, a small percentage of patients experience persistent vomiting from gastric outlet obstruction as the result of pyloric and duodenal stenosis from the earlier gastric mucosal necrosis. Autopsy findings in children indicate prominent iron deposition in intestinal mucosa and periportal necrosis of the liver that correlate with the primary symptoms of serious iron poisoning.[105]

Mechanism of Toxicity

The toxicity of acute iron poisoning includes local effects on the gastrointestinal mucosa and systemic effects induced by excessive iron in the body.[101,103] Iron is irritating to the gastric and duodenal mucosa, which may result in hemorrhage and occasional perforations. Once absorbed, iron is taken up by tissues, particularly the liver, and acts as a mitochondrial poison. It occasionally causes hepatic injury. Iron may inhibit aerobic glycolysis and perturb the electron transport system. Further, iron may shunt electrons away from the electron transport system, thereby reducing the efficiency of oxidative phosphorylation. These biochemical factors, along with the cardiovascular effects of iron, lead to metabolic acidosis. The pathogenesis of shock is not well understood but may include the development of hypovolemia and lactic acidosis, release of endogenous vasodilators, and the direct vasodepressant effects of iron and ferritin on the circulation (Fig. 14–6).

Causative Agents

Iron poisoning results from the ingestion and absorption of excessive amounts of iron from iron tablets, multiple vitamins with iron, and prenatal vitamins. Different iron salts and formulations contain varying amounts of elemental iron (see Chapter 109). Generally, children's chewable vitamins are less likely to produce systemic iron poisoning in part because of their lower iron content.[106]

Incidence

Acute iron poisoning can produce death in children and adults.[105,106] The 2007 AAPCC-NPDS report documented 3,196 single-agent iron ingestions, with 3.1% of the exposures exhibiting moderate to severe toxicity. Children younger than 6 years accounted for 60% of the exposures. Multiple vitamins with iron were involved in 23,535 cases, with 0.2% exhibiting moderate-severe toxicity. No deaths were associated with any iron product during this year.[5]

CLINICAL PRESENTATION OF ACUTE IRON POISONING

General

- Gastrointestinal symptoms shortly after ingestion with possible rapid progression to shock and coma

Symptoms

- Vomiting, abdominal pain, and diarrhea within 1 to 6 hours
- Lethargy, coma, seizures, bloody vomiting, bloody diarrhea, and shock within 6 to 24 hours

Signs

- Hypotension and tachycardia within 6 to 24 hours
- Liver dysfunction and failure possible in 2 to 5 days

Laboratory Tests

- Toxic serum iron concentrations >500 mcg/dL (>90 mmol/L)
- Altered arterial blood gases and serum electrolytes associated with a high anion gap metabolic acidosis within 3 to 24 hours
- Elevated BUN, serum creatinine, AST, ALT, and INR within 1 to 2 days

Other Diagnostic Tests

- Guaiac test of stools for the presence of blood
- Abdominal radiograph to detect solid iron tablets in gastrointestinal tract

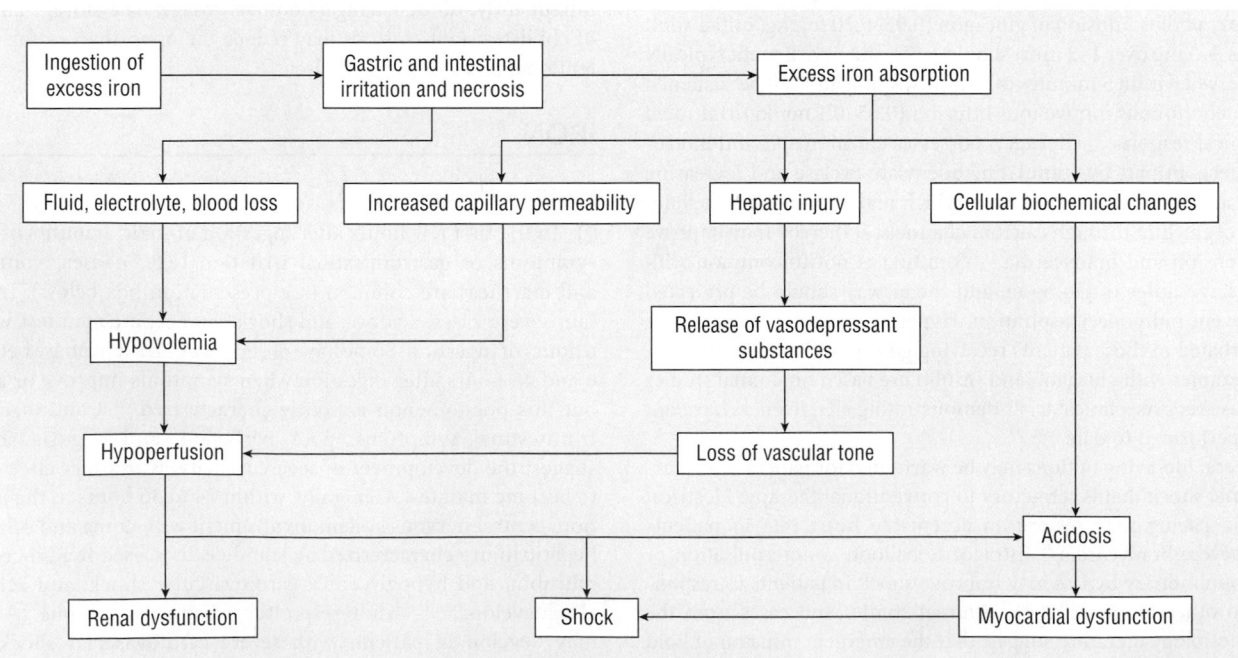

FIGURE 14-6. Pathophysiology of acute iron poisoning.

Risk Assessment

A patient who exhibits lethargy, paleness, persistent or bloody emesis, or diarrhea should be immediately referred to an emergency department.[106] Ingestion of 10 to 20 mg/kg elemental iron usually elicits mild gastrointestinal symptoms. Ingestion of 20 to 40 mg/kg is not likely to produce systemic toxicity, and typically these patients can be conservatively managed at home. Ingestions of 40 mg/kg or more of elemental iron are often associated with serious toxicity and require immediate medical attention.[106] Psychiatric as well as medical intervention is indicated for adults and adolescents who intentionally ingest iron as a suicide gesture.[101,103,106]

An abdominal radiograph may help to confirm the ingestion of iron tablets and indicate the need for aggressive gastrointestinal evacuation with whole-bowel irrigation. An abdominal radiograph is most useful within 2 hours of ingestion. The visualization of radiopaque iron tablets is confounded by the presence of other hard-coated tablets and some extended-release tablets that also are radiopaque. Furthermore, the radiopacity of iron tablets diminishes as the tablets disintegrate, and chewable and liquid formulations typically are not radiopaque.[107]

Iron poisoning causes vomiting and diarrhea, but these symptoms are poor indicators of later serious toxicity. The presence of a combination of findings such as coma, radiopacities, leukocytosis, and increased anion gap, however, is associated with dangerously high serum concentrations >500 mcg/dL (>90 mmol/L). The presence of single signs and symptoms, such as vomiting, leukocytosis, or hyperglycemia, is not a reliable indicator of the severity of iron poisoning in adults or children.[108,109]

Once iron is absorbed, it is eliminated only as the result of blood loss or sloughing of the intestinal and epidermal cells. Thus, iron kinetics essentially represent a closed system with multiple compartments. The serum iron concentration represents a small fraction of the total-body content of iron and is at its greatest concentration in the postabsorptive and distributive phases, typically 2 to 10 hours after ingestion.[110] Serum iron concentrations >500 mcg/dL (>90 mmol/L) have been associated with severe toxicity, whereas concentrations <350 mcg/dL (<62.7 mmol/L) typically are not associated with severe toxicity; however, exceptions have been reported for both thresholds.[110] Serious toxicity is best determined by assessing the development of gross gastrointestinal bleeding, metabolic acidosis, shock, and coma regardless of the serum iron concentration.[103] The serum iron concentration serves as a guide for further assessment and treatment options. The ratio of the serum iron concentration to the total iron-binding capacity is unreliable, insensitive, and has little relationship to acute toxicity.[109]

Management of Toxicity

Many patients vomit spontaneously, and ipecac syrup should be avoided.[106] At the emergency department, gastric lavage with normal saline can be considered. Lavage with normal saline may remove iron tablet fragments and dissolved iron, but because the lumen of the tube is often smaller than some whole tablets, effective removal is unlikely.[101] Activated charcoal administration is not warranted routinely because it adsorbs iron poorly. If abdominal radiographs reveal a large number of iron tablets, whole-bowel irrigation with polyethylene glycol electrolyte solution typically is necessary.[34] Although removal by gastrostomy has been used in a few cases,[103] early and aggressive decontamination and evacuation of the gastrointestinal tract usually will be adequate to minimize iron absorption and thereby reduce the risk of systemic toxicity. Lavage solutions of phosphate or deferoxamine have been proposed previously as a means to render iron insoluble, but they were found ineffective and dangerous.[103,106]

Patients with systemic symptoms (e.g., shock, coma, or gross gastrointestinal bleeding or metabolic acidosis) should receive parenteral deferoxamine as soon as possible. If the serum iron concentration is >500 mcg/dL (>90 mmol/L), deferoxamine is also indicated because serious systemic toxicity is likely.[101,103] Its use is less clear in patients with serum iron concentrations in the range from 350 to 500 mcg/dL (62.7–90 mmol/L) because many of these patients do not develop systemic symptoms.[110]

Deferoxamine is a highly selective chelator of iron that theoretically binds ferric (Fe^{3+}) iron in a 1:1 molar ratio (100 mg deferoxamine to 8.5 mg ferric iron) that is more stable than the binding of iron to transferrin. Deferoxamine removes excess iron from the circulation and some iron from transferrin by chelating ferric complexes in equilibrium with transferrin. The resulting iron—deferoxamine complex, ferrioxamine, is then excreted in the urine. Its action on intracellular iron is unclear, but it may have a protective intracellular effect or may chelate extramitochondrial iron.[103] The parenteral administration of deferoxamine produces an orange—red-colored urine within 3 to 6 hours because of the presence of ferrioxamine in the urine.[101] For mild-to-moderate cases of iron poisoning, where its use is unclear, the presence of discolored urine indicates the persistent presence of chelatable iron and the need to continue deferoxamine. The reliance on discolored urine as a therapeutic end point has been challenged because it is not sensitive and is difficult to detect.[111]

An initial intravenous infusion of 15 mg/kg/h generally is indicated, although some have used up to 30 mg/kg/h for life-threatening cases. In these situations, the dose must be titrated carefully to minimize deferoxamine-induced hypotension.[101,103,112] The rapid intravenous infusion of deferoxamine (>15 mg/kg/h) has been associated with tachycardia, hypotension, shock, generalized erythema, and urticaria.[101,113] Anaphylaxis has been reported rarely. The use of deferoxamine for more than 24 hours at doses used for treatment of acute poisoning has been associated with exacerbation or development of ARDS.[113–115] Although the manufacturer states that the total dose in 24 hours should not exceed 6 g, the basis for this recommendation is unclear, and daily doses as high as 37.1 g have been administered without incident.[112,114] Good hydration and urine output may moderate some of the secondary physiologic effects of iron toxicity and ensure urinary elimination of ferrioxamine. In the patient who develops renal failure, hemodialysis or hemofiltration does not remove excess iron but will remove ferrioxamine.[101]

The desired end point for deferoxamine therapy is not clear. Some have suggested that deferoxamine therapy should cease when the serum iron concentration falls below 150 mcg/dL (26.9 mmol/L).[103] The decline of serum iron concentrations, however, may not account for the potential cellular action of deferoxamine irrespective of its effect on iron elimination. The cessation of orange-red urine production that is indicative of ferrioxamine excretion is not reliable because many individuals cannot distinguish its presence in the urine.[111] Considering these shortcomings, deferoxamine therapy should be continued for 12 hours after the patient is asymptomatic and the urine returns to normal color or until the serum iron concentration falls below 350 mcg/dL (62.7 mmol/L) and approaches 150 mcg/dL (26.9 mmol/L).

CLINICAL CONTROVERSY

There is little evidence on how much deferoxamine should be given for iron poisoning or for how long it should be administered. The dosage regimen should balance the benefits of increased iron removal in patients with exceedingly high serum iron concentrations versus the risk of developing ARDS when therapy lasts for more than 1 to 3 days.

Monitoring and Prevention

Once a poisoning has occurred, acid—base balance (anion gap and arterial blood gases), fluid and electrolyte balance, and perfusion should be monitored. Other indicators of organ toxicity, such as

ALT, AST, bilirubin, INR, serum glucose and creatinine concentrations, as well as markers of physiologic stress or infection such as leukocytosis, also should be monitored.

Iron poisoning often is not recognized as a potentially serious problem by parents or victims until symptoms develop; thus, valuable time to institute treatment is lost. Parents should be made aware of the potential risks and asked to observe basic poison prevention measures. Some hard-coated iron tablets resemble candy-coated chocolates and are confused easily by children. Based on these considerations and the frequency of this poisoning, iron tablets are packaged in child-resistant containers.

TRICYCLIC ANTIDEPRESSANTS

Clinical Presentation

❿ Patients may deteriorate rapidly and progress from no symptoms to life-threatening cardiotoxicity or seizures within 1 hour.[116,117] Major symptoms of tricyclic antidepressant overdose typically are manifest within 6 hours of ingestion.[116] The principal effects of tricyclic antidepressant poisoning involve the cardiovascular system and the central nervous system and can result in arrhythmias, hypotension, coma, and seizures (see presentation box below).

Prolongation of the QRS complex on ECG indicating nonspecific intraventricular conduction delay or bundle-branch block is the most distinctive feature of tricyclic antidepressant overdose.[117] Sinus tachycardia with rates typically <160 beats/min is common and does not cause serious hemodynamic changes in most patients. Ventricular tachycardia is a common ventricular arrhythmia, but it may be difficult to distinguish from sinus tachycardia in the presence of QRS complex prolongation and the apparent absence of P waves. It often occurs in patients with marked QRS complex prolongation or hypotension and may be precipitated by seizures.[117,118] High rates of mortality are associated with ventricular tachycardia; ventricular fibrillation is the terminal rhythm. Torsade de pointes is observed infrequently with tricyclic antidepressant poisoning. With massive tricyclic antidepressant overdose, slow ventricular rhythms may be observed. Hypotension is a significant factor in most cases of tricyclic antidepressant poisoning. Refractory hypotension leading to death is due to vasodilation and impaired cardiac contractility.[117] Other factors, such as extreme heart rates, intravascular volume depletion, hypoxia, hyperthermia, seizures, and acidosis, may contribute to refractory hypotension.

Coma usually is present in patients with tricyclic antidepressant poisoning and may or may not be associated with QRS complex prolongation. In severe cases, coma is sufficient to depress respirations. Delirium, manifest as agitation or disorientation, may occur early in the course of severe poisoning or with poisoning of moderate severity. Seizures often occur within 2 hours of ingestion and usually are generalized, single, and brief. Seizures may result in acidosis, hyperthermia, or rhabdomyolysis, and 10% to 20% of patients may abruptly develop cardiovascular deterioration.[117] Myoclonus also may be observed with tricyclic antidepressant overdose. Hyperthermia often results from seizure and myoclonic activity in the presence of decreased sweating and is associated with a high incidence of neurologic sequelae and mortality. Anticholinergic symptoms, such as urinary retention, ileus, and dry mucous membranes, often are observed with tricyclic antidepressant overdose.[116,117] Pupil size is variable.

Tricyclic antidepressant overdose can be staged based on the patient's symptoms and recovery time. In stage 1, patients are responsive to pain, have sinus tachycardia, and recover within 24 hours. In stage 2, seizures, coma, and cardiac conduction problems are evident; respiratory support typically is needed. Patients recover within 24 to 48 hours of ingestion. Stage 3 is characterized by the features of stage 2 with the addition of respiratory arrest, hypotension, ventricular dysrhythmias, and asystole, which may occur within 1 to 24 hours

of ingestion. Typically symptoms appear within 2 hours, and more serious effects usually are not seen until 6 hours postingestion; rarely rapid clinical deterioration is observed within 1 to 2 hours.[119]

Amoxapine, bupropion, and maprotiline are atypical antidepressants associated with a higher incidence of seizures on overdose; amoxapine produces minimal cardiotoxicity,[117,120] but venlafaxine has been associated with greater mortality.[121] The selective serotonin reuptake inhibitors (SSRIs) generally produce a common toxicity profile on overdose despite their structural and pharmacologic distinctions.[122] The SSRIs inhibit presynaptic neuronal uptake of serotonin, resulting in increased synaptic serotonin levels. When ingested in excess, SSRIs rarely cause death and typically produce nausea, vomiting, diarrhea, tremor, and decreased level of consciousness.[122] Tachycardia and seizures are infrequent.[117,120,123]

Serotonin syndrome is a condition in which certain drugs (e.g., meperidine, nonselective monoamine oxidase inhibitors, dextromethorphan, linezolid, tricyclic antidepressants, SSRIs) acutely increase serotonin levels and develops within minutes to hours (typically within 6 hours) after starting a medication, increasing the dose of a medication, or overdosing. It is characterized by a collection of neurobehavioral (e.g., confusion, agitation, coma, seizures), autonomic (e.g., hyperthermia, diaphoresis, tachycardia, hypertension), and neuromuscular (e.g., myoclonus, rigidity, tremor, ataxia, shivering, nystagmus) signs and symptoms.[124] Most cases are mild and resolve spontaneously within 24 to 72 hours. Cardiac arrest, coma, and multiorgan system failure have been reported as consequences of serotonin syndrome.[124] Recognition of the syndrome is based on a high index of suspicion and identification of risk factors.

CLINICAL PRESENTATION OF TRICYCLIC ANTIDEPRESSANT POISONING

General

☐ Sedating and cardiovascular effects observed within 1 hour of ingestion, quickly leading to life-threatening symptoms; death is possible within 1 to 2 hours

Symptoms

☐ Lethargy, coma, and seizures occur within 1 to 6 hours

☐ Dry mouth, mydriasis, urinary retention, and hypoactive bowel sounds, develop within 1 to 6 hours

Signs

☐ Tachycardia within 1 to 3 hours

☐ Mild hypertension early will change to severe hypotension and shock within 1 to 6 hours

☐ Unresponsiveness and depressed reflexes within 1 to 3 hours

☐ Depressed respiratory rate and depth depending on the degree of coma

☐ Common arrhythmias, such as prolonged QRS and QT intervals to ventricular dysrhythmias, within 1 to 6 hours

Laboratory Tests

☐ Altered arterial blood gases associated with metabolic acidosis from hypoxia and seizures

☐ Altered serum electrolytes, BUN, and serum creatinine in response to seizures and shock within 3 to 12 hours

Other Diagnostic Tests

☐ ECG with continuous monitoring and pulse oximetry to monitor for toxicity and shock

☐ Monitor for complications of pulmonary aspiration, such as hypoxia and pneumonia, by physical findings and chest radiograph

Mechanism of Toxicity

Many of the toxic effects of tricyclic antidepressants are associated with an exaggeration of their pharmacologic action. The tricyclic antidepressants, such as type Ia antiarrhythmic drugs, inhibit the fast sodium channel so that phase 0 depolarization of the myocardium is slowed.[117] This action leads to QRS complex prolongation, atrioventricular block, ventricular tachycardia, and decreased myocardial contractility. Tricyclic antidepressants also block vascular *a*-adrenergic receptors, resulting in vasodilation, which contributes to hypotension. Sinus tachycardia is related to the inhibition of norepinephrine reuptake and anticholinergic effects. Other anticholinergic effects include urinary retention, ileus, dry mucous membranes, and impaired sweating. Inhibition of norepinephrine reuptake also may account for the early, transient, and self-limiting elevation of blood pressure observed in some patients. The central nervous system toxicity of tricyclic antidepressants is not well understood.

Causative Agents

Tricyclic antidepressants and SSRIs are used to treat a variety of behavioral conditions (see Chapters 77–79). The tricyclic antidepressants include drugs such as amitriptyline, desipramine, doxepin, imipramine, and nortriptyline. Atypical agents include amoxapine, bupropion, maprotiline, nefazodone, trazodone, and venlafaxine. The SSRIs include fluoxetine, paroxetine, and sertraline. The tricyclic antidepressants are generally highly protein bound, exhibit a large volume of distribution, and possess elimination half-lives of 8 to 24 hours or more. Virtually none of the drug is eliminated unchanged in the urine. Metabolism of the parent drug produces active metabolites in most cases (e.g., amitriptyline to nortriptyline) that may contribute to toxicity after the first 12 to 24 hours.[117] Genetic polymorphism at *CYP2D6* may lead to slower recovery in patients who are slow hydroxylators.[125]

Incidence

Tricyclic antidepressant poisoning is a common cause of death from drug overdose.[117,118] The 2007 AAPCC-NPDS report documented 43,198 patients with single-agent exposures to tricyclic antidepressants; 42% of these cases were considered to be intentional overdoses. A total of 922 people experienced a major effect, and 32 people died.[5] The SSRIs accounted for 19,407 nonfatal single-agent exposures with 84 people exhibiting severe toxicity but no deaths were reported this year.

Risk Assessment

Referral to an emergency department is warranted for ingestions >5 mg/kg of amitriptyline, clomipramine, doxepin, and imipramine; >2.5 mg/kg of desipramine, nortriptyline, and trimipramine; and >1 mg/kg of protriptyline.[119] Patients who exhibit weakness, drowsiness, dizziness, tremulousness, and palpitations after an ingestion of a tricyclic antidepressant and patients suspected of a suicide gesture or those who are suspected victims of malicious poisoning should be promptly referred to an emergency department.[119] A QRS complex >160 milliseconds or progressive prolongation of the QRS complex is an indicator of toxicity such as seizures or ventricular arrhythmias and often precedes the onset of serious symptoms.[116,118,126] The QRS complex duration should not be used as the sole indicator of risk for tricyclic antidepressant poisoning.[126] Although urine drug analyses routinely screen for tricyclic antidepressants, the qualitative result can only suggest or confirm a potential risk for the development of toxicity.

Patients with coexisting cardiovascular and pulmonary conditions (e.g., ARDS, pulmonary infection, pulmonary aspiration) may be more susceptible to the toxic effects or complications of tricyclic antidepressant poisoning.[119] Tricyclic antidepressants interact with other central nervous system depressant drugs, which together may lead to increased central nervous system and respiratory depression.

Consult a poison control center for current recommendations for doses of SSRIs that would warrant referral to an emergency department.[127] The risk of serotonin syndrome may be increased shortly after dosage increases of SSRIs or when drug interactions increase serotonin activity.[124] Concomitant or proximal use of SSRIs, tricyclic antidepressants, or nonselective monoamine oxidase inhibitors may cause serotonin syndrome. Furthermore, the addition of certain drugs, such as tryptophan, dextromethorphan, cocaine, or sympathomimetics, to SSRI therapy may increase the risk of developing serotonin syndrome.[124]

Management of Toxicity

Once the ingestion of an overdose of tricyclic antidepressant is suspected or for any intentional ingestions, medical evaluation and treatment should be sought promptly. If the patient is symptomatic, it may be prudent to call for an ambulance because of the rapid progression of some cases. At the emergency department, the patient should be monitored carefully, have vital signs assessed regularly, and have an intravenous line started. Supportive and symptomatic care includes oxygen, intravenous fluids, and other treatments as indicated. Prompt administration of activated charcoal may decrease the absorption of any remaining tricyclic antidepressant. It also may be useful beyond the first hour of ingestion because of decreased gastrointestinal motility from the anticholinergic action of tricyclic antidepressants. Gastric lavage may be considered if the time of the ingestion is unknown or if ingestion occurred within the past 1 to 2 hours. Some practitioners avoid gastric lavage altogether.[117] Ipecac syrup should be avoided in patients who ingest tricyclic antidepressants because the rapid onset of toxicity compromises its safety. Multiple-dose activated charcoal has been shown to increase the elimination of some tricyclic antidepressants in human volunteers[42] and has been used in poisoned patients.[116,117] It may be most useful during the first 12 hours of ingestion while the drug is distributing to tissue compartments. Because the tricyclic antidepressants possess a large volume of distribution, little of the drug is present in the bloodstream; thus hemodialysis is not useful for the extracorporeal removal of tricyclic antidepressants.

Intravenous sodium bicarbonate is part of the first-line treatment of QRS complex prolongation, ventricular arrhythmias, and hypotension caused by tricyclic antidepressant overdose.[52,117,128] Typically 1 to 2 mEq/kg (1–2 mmol/kg) sodium bicarbonate (1 mEq/mL [1 mmol/mL]) is administered as a bolus infusion (usually a 50-mEq [50-mmol] ampule in an adult) and repeated as necessary to achieve an arterial blood pH of 7.50 to 7.55 or abatement of toxicity.[116,117] A therapeutic effect usually is observed within minutes. Excessive use of sodium bicarbonate may produce dangerous alkalemia, which by itself is associated with ventricular arrhythmias.[117] The mechanism of action of sodium bicarbonate is unclear. Although some practitioners have proposed that sodium bicarbonate increases protein binding of tricyclic antidepressants, this theory has been discounted. Sodium may play an important role by stabilizing tricyclic antidepressant—induced changes to the sodium gradient of the myocardium.[117,129] Regardless of its action, it is effective and generally safe. Hyperventilation to produce a mild state of respiratory alkalosis has been used to treat some dysrhythmias, but it is used less widely than sodium bicarbonate.[116,117]

CLINICAL CONTROVERSY

Because intravenous sodium bicarbonate is used as therapy for certain arrhythmias and hypotension caused by tricyclic antidepressant poisoning, some practitioners have advocated its prophylactic use. Little evidence indicates which patients would benefit from prophylactic use. The risks of potentially producing alkalosis in a patient who is not seriously toxic should be considered.

Treatment of the complications of tricyclic antidepressant poisoning is outlined in Table 14–13 and includes pharmacologic and nonpharmacologic approaches.[116,117] Several agents generally should be avoided in the treatment of tricyclic antidepressant poisoning. Other drugs that inhibit the fast sodium channel, such as procainamide and quinidine, are contraindicated. Phenytoin has limited usefulness in treating tricyclic antidepressant seizures and has questionable efficacy in managing cardiotoxicity.[116] Physostigmine was used in the past as a treatment of tricyclic antidepressant-induced cardiotoxicity and seizures because it antagonizes anticholinergic actions. However, physostigmine has been associated with bradycardia and asystole[117,130] and has been avoided in the contemporary treatment of tricyclic antidepressant cardiovascular or central nervous system toxicity. Flumazenil is used to antagonize the effects of benzodiazepines, but its use in the presence of a tricyclic antidepressant has been associated with the development of seizures and should be avoided.[131]

Treatment of an overdose of the atypical antidepressants and SSRIs is directed primarily toward decontamination of the gastrointestinal tract with activated charcoal, symptomatic treatment, and general supportive care. Management of the serotonin syndrome involves discontinuation of the serotoninergic agent and supportive therapy. Benzodiazepines, propranolol, and cyproheptadine, a serotonin antagonist, have been used successfully.[124]

Monitoring and Prevention

Measurement of vital signs, electrolytes, and BUN and a urinalysis are indicated for initial assessment. Patients should be monitored continuously by ECG, and a 12-lead ECG should be obtained if QRS complex prolongation is noted. If patients start to show signs of cardiotoxicity, arterial blood gases should be determined. Patients who show no signs of toxicity during 6 hours of observation and have received activated charcoal promptly require no further medical monitoring. Psychiatric evaluation is indicated for adolescents and adults. When signs of tricyclic antidepressant toxicity are present in a patient, cardiac monitoring generally is recommended for at least 24 hours after the patient is without findings.[117]

Prevention of tricyclic antidepressant poisoning poses unique challenges. Many of the dosage forms are small in size, and adults and children can consume large numbers easily. In the course of treating depression, several antidepressant agents may be tried to achieve results. By not discarding unused medicines, a storehouse of potentially deadly drugs may be available for children to discover or for the despondent patient to use to attempt suicide. Although patients take tricyclic antidepressants for therapeutic relief of depression, they are also a group likely to contemplate suicide with tricyclic antidepressants. Strategies that would limit the amount of tricyclic antidepressant prescribed at one time also potentially would impair adherence to a dosage regimen and thereby compromise the therapeutic potential of these agents.[117,128] Patients with a history of suicidal gestures may be candidates for the atypical antidepressants or SSRIs, which possess less cardiotoxicity. General poison prevention measures may limit childhood poisonings; and monitoring depressed patients for suicidal ideation may identify patients at risk.[132]

ABBREVIATIONS

AAPCC-NPDS: American Association of Poison Control Centers' National Poison Data System

ALT: alanine aminotransferase

ARDS: adult respiratory distress syndrome

AST: aspartate aminotransferase

BUN: blood urea nitrogen

ECG: electrocardiogram

INR: international normalized ratio

NAPQI: N-acetyl-p-benzoquinoneimine

PPPA: Poison Prevention Packaging Act (of 1970)

TABLE 14-13	Treatment Options for Acute Tricyclic Antidepressant Toxicity
Toxicity	**Treatment**
Cardiovascular	
QRS prolongation, if progressive or >0.16 s	Intravenous sodium bicarbonate to a blood pH of 7.5 even in the absence of acidosis; generally avoid other antiarrhythmic drugs
Hypotension	Intravascular fluids; intravenous sodium bicarbonate; consider norepinephrine or dopamine
Ventricular tachycardia	Intravenous sodium bicarbonate; lidocaine, overdrive pacing
Ventricular bradycardia	Epinephrine drip; cardiac pacemaker
Atrioventricular block type II, second or third degree	Cardiac pacemaker
Cardiac arrest	Advanced cardiac life support, prolonged resuscitation may be needed
Neurologic	
Seizures, agitation	Benzodiazepines; neuromuscular blockade may be needed if hyperthermia or acidosis is present
Coma	Endotracheal intubation; mechanical ventilation if needed
Homeostatic	
Hyperthermia	Treat seizures and agitation; consider cooling blanket, ice water lavage, and cool water mist of body
Acidosis	Intravenous sodium bicarbonate

REFERENCES

1. Eldridge DL, Van Eyk J, Kornegay C. Pediatric toxicology. Emerg Med Clin North Am 2007;25:283–308.
2. Substance Abuse and Mental Health Services Administration, Office of Applied Studies. Drug Abuse Warning Network, 2006: National Estimates of Drug-Related Emergency Department Visits. DAWN Series D-30, DHHS Publication No. (SMA) 08–4339, Rockville, MD, 2008. http://dawninfo.samhsa.gov/files/ED2006/DAWN2k6ED.pdf.
3. Centers for Disease Control and Prevention. Web-based Injury Statistics Query and Reporting System (WISQARS) (online). Washington, DC: National Center for Injury Prevention and Control, Centers for Disease Control and Prevention; 2009. www.cdc.gov/injury/wisqars/index.html.
4. Warner M, Chen LH, Makuc DM. Increase in fatal poisonings involving opioid analgesics in the United States, 1999–2006. NCHS data brief, no 22. Hyattsville, MD: National Center for Health Statistics. 2009. http://cdc.gov/nchs/data/databriefs/db22.pdf.

5. Bronstein AC, Spyker DA, Cantilena LR, et al. 2007 Annual Report of the American Association of Poison Control Centers' National Poison Data System (NPDS): 25th Annual Report. Clin Toxicol (Phila) 2008;46:927–1057. *http://www.aapcc.org/DNN*.

6. Hoppe-Roberts JH, Lloyd LM, Chyka PA. Poisoning mortality in the United States: Comparison of national mortality statistics and poison control center reports. Ann Emerg Med 2000;35:440–448.

7. Institute of Medicine. Forging a Poison Prevention and Control System. Committee on Poison Prevention and Control. Board on Health Promotion and Disease Prevention. Washington, DC: National Academy Press, 2004.

8. Rodgers GB. The safety effects of child-resistant packaging for oral pre-scription drugs: Two decades of experience. JAMA 1996;275:1661–1665.

9. Shannon M. Ingestion of toxic substances by children. N Engl J Med 2000;342:186–191.

10. Poison Prevention Packaging: A Textbook for Pharmacists and Physicians. Publication number 384. Washington, DC: US Consumer Product Safety Commission, 2005. *http://www.cpsc.gov/cpscpub/pubs/384.pdf*.

11. Buckley NA, Whyte IM, Dawson AH, et al. Correlations between prescriptions and drugs taken in self-poisoning. Med J Aust 1995;162:194–197.

12. Haselberger MB, Kroner BA. Drug poisoning in older patients: Preventative and management strategies. Drugs Aging 1995;7:292–297.

13. Mokhlesi B, Leiken JB, Mirray P, Corbridge TC. Adult toxicology in critical care: I. General approach to the intoxicated patient. Chest 2003;123:577–592.

14. Erickson TB, Thompson TM, Lu JJ. The approach to the patient with an unknown overdose. Emerg Med Clin North Am 2007;25:249–281.

15. Kales SN, Christiani DC. Acute chemical emergencies. N Engl J Med 2004;350:800–808.

16. Hubbard WK. Can the Food and Drug Administration ensure that our pharmaceuticals are safely manufactured? [editorial]. Arch Intern Med 2009;169:1655–1656.

17. Kearney TE, Van Bebber SL, Hiatt PH, Olson KR. Protocols for pedi-atric poisonings from nontoxic substances: Are they valid? Pediatr Emerg Care 2006;22:215–221.

18. Chyka PA. Substance abuse and toxicological tests. In: Lee M, ed. Basic Skills in Interpreting Laboratory Data, 4th ed. Bethesda, MD: American Society of Health System Pharmacists; 2009:47–72.

19. Moeller KE, Lee KC, Kissack JC. Urine drug screening: practical guide for clinicians. Mayo Clin Proc 2008;83:66–76.

20. Wu AB, McKay C, Broussard LA, et al. National Academy of Clinical Biochemistry Laboratory Medicine Practice Guidelines: Recommendations for the use of laboratory tests to support poisoned patients who present to the emergency department. Clin Chem 2003;49:357–379.

21. Roberts DM, Buckley NA. Pharmacokinetic considerations in clinical toxicology. Clin Pharmacokinet 2007;46:897–939.

22. Young-Jin S, Shannon M. Pharmacokinetics of drugs in overdose. Clin Pharmacokinet 1992;23:93–105.

23. Adams BK, Mann MD, Aboo A, et al. Prolonged gastric emptying halftime and gastric hypomotility after drug overdose. Am J Emerg Med 2004;22:548–554.

24. Taylor JR, Streetman DS, Castle SS. Medication bezoars: A literature review and report of a case. Ann Pharmacother 1998;32:940–946.

25. Bosse GM, Matyunas NJ. Delayed toxidromes. J Emerg Med 1999;17:679–690.

26. Vance MV, Selden BS, Clark RF. Optimal patient position for trans-port and initial management of toxic ingestions. Ann Emerg Med 1992;21:243–246.

27. Krenzelok EP, McGuigan M, Lheur P. American Academy of Clinical Toxicology, European Association of Poison Centres and Clinical Toxicologists. Position statement: Ipecac syrup. J Toxicol Clin Toxicol 1997;35:699–709. *http://www.clintox.org/positionstatements.cfm*.

28. Committee on Injury, Violence, and Poison Prevention. American Academy of Pediatrics policy statement: Poison treatment in the home. Pediatrics 2003;112:1180–1181.

29. Vale JA. American Academy of Clinical Toxicology, European Association of Poison Centres and Clinical Toxicologists. Position statement: Gastric lavage. J Toxicol Clin Toxicol 1997;35:711–719. *http://www.clintox.org/positionstatements.cfm*.

30. Chyka PA, Seger D, Krenzelok EP, Vale JA; American Academy of Clinical Toxicology; European Association of Poisons Centres and Clinical Toxicologists. Position paper: Single-dose activated charcoal. Clin Toxicol (Phila) 2005;43:61–87. *http://www.clintox.org/positionstatements.cfm*.

31. McFarland AK III, Chyka PA. Selection of activated charcoal products for the treatment of poisonings. Ann Pharmacother 1993;27:358–361.

32. Barceloux D, McGuigan M, Hartigan-Go K. American Academy of Clinical Toxicology, European Association of Poisons Centres and Clinical Toxicologists. Position statement: Cathartics. J Toxicol Clin Toxicol 1997;35:743–752. *http://www.clintox.org/positionstatements.cfm*.

33. Oral electrolyte solutions for colonic lavage before colonoscopy or barium enema. Med Lett Drugs Ther 1985;27:39–40.

34. Tenenbein M. American Academy of Clinical Toxicology, European Association of Poison Centres and Clinical Toxicologists. Position statement: Whole bowel irrigation. Clin Toxicol 2004;42:843–854. *http://www.clintox.org/positionstatements.cfm*.

35. Traub SJ, Hoffman RS, Nelson LS. Body packing: The internal conceal-ment of illicit drugs. N Engl J Med 2003;349:2519–2526.

36. American College of Emergency Physicians. Clinical policy for the initial approach to patients presenting with acute toxic ingestion or dermal or inhalation exposure. Ann Emerg Med 1999;33:735–761.

37. Cooper GM, Le Couteur DG, Richardson D, Buckley NA. A random-ized clinical trial of activated charcoal for the routine management of oral drug overdose. QJM 2005;98:655–660.

38. Bond GR. The role of activated charcoal and gastric emptying in gas-trointestinal decontamination: A state-of-the-art review. Ann Emerg Med 2002;39:273–286.

39. McGuigan MA. Activated charcoal in the home. Clin Pediatr Emerg Med 2000;1:191–194.

40. Elenbaas RM. Critical review of forced alkaline diuresis in acute sali-cylism. Crit Care Q 1982;4:89–95.

41. Chyka PA. Multiple-dose activated charcoal and enhancement of systemic drug clearance: Summary of studies in animals and humans. J Toxicol Clin Toxicol 1995;33:399–405.

42. American Academy of Clinical Toxicology, European Association of Poison Centres and Clinical Toxicologists. Position statement and practice guidelines on the use of multidose activated charcoal in the treatment of acute poisoning. J Toxicol Clin Toxicol 1999;37:731–751. *http://www.clintox.org/positionstatements.cfm*.

43. Pond SM, Olson KR, Osterloh JD, et al. Randomized study of the treatment of phenobarbital overdose with repeated doses of activated charcoal. JAMA 1984;251:3104–3108.

44. Chyka PA, Holley JE, Mandrell TM, Sugathan P. Correlation of drug pharmacokinetics and effectiveness of multiple-dose activated char-coal therapy. Ann Emerg Med 1995;25:356–362.

45. Dorrington CL, Johnson DW, Brant R, et al. The frequency of com-plications associated with the use of multiple-dose activated charcoal. Ann Emerg Med 2003;42:370–377.

46. Tomaszewski C. Activated charcoal: Treatment or toxin? (editorial). Clin Toxicol 1999;37:17–18.

47. Zimmerman JL. Poisonings and overdoses in the intensive care unit: General and specific management issues. Crit Care Med 2003;31:2794–2801.

48. Tyagi PK, Winchester JF, Feinfeld DA. Extracorporeal removal of toxins. Kidney Int 2008;74:1231–1233.

49. Calello DP, Osterhoudt KC, Henretig FM. New and novel antidotes in pediatrics. Pediatr Emerg Care 2006;22:523–530.

50. Trujillo MH, Guerrero J, Fragachan C, Fernandez MA. Pharmacologic antidotes in critical care medicine: A practical guide for drug adminis-tration. Crit Care Med 1998;26:377–391.

51. Dart RC, Borron SW, Caravati EM et al. Expert consensus guidelines for stocking of antidotes in hospitals that provide emergency care. Ann Emerg Med 2009;54:386–394.

52. Albertson TE, Dawson A, de Latorre F, et al. Tox-ACLS: Toxicologic-oriented advanced cardiac life support. Ann Emerg Med 2001;37:S78–S90.

53. Chyka PA, Butler AY, Holliman BJ, Herman MI. Utility of *N*-acetylcysteine in treating poisonings and adverse drug reactions. Drug Saf 2000;22:123–148.

54. Turner-Lawrence DE, Kerns W. Intravenous fat emulsion: a potential novel antidote. J Med Toxicol 2008;4:109–114.

55. Antman EM, Wenger TL, Butler VP, et al. Treatment of 150 cases of life-threatening digitalis intoxication with digoxin-specific Fab antibody fragments. Circulation 1990;81:1744–1752.

56. Dart RC, Seifert SA, Boyer LV, et al. A randomized multicenter trial of Crotalidae polyvalent immune Fab (ovine) antivenom for the treatment for crotaline snakebite in the United States. Arch Intern Med 2001;161:2030–2036.

57. Smilkstein MJ, Knapp GL, Kulig KW, Rumack BH. Efficacy of oral N-acetylcysteine in the treatment of acetaminophen overdose: Analysis of the national multicenter study (1976–1985). N Engl J Med 1988;319:1557–1562.

58. Chun LJ, Tong MJ, Busuttil RW, Hiatt JR. Acetaminophen hepatotoxicity and acute liver failure. J Clin Gastroenterol 2009;43:342–349.

59. Larson AM, Polson J, Fontana RJ, et al. Acetaminophen-induced acute liver failure: Results of a United States multicenter, prospective study. Hepatology 2005;42:1364–1372.

60. James LP, Mayeux PR, Hinson JA. Acetaminophen-induced hepatotoxicity. Drug Metab Dispos 2003;31:1499–1506.

61. Mazer M, Perrone J. Acetaminophen-induced nephrotoxicity: pathophysiology, clinical manifestations, and management. J Med Toxicol 2008;4:2–6.

62. Dart RC, Erdman AR, Olson KR, et al. Acetaminophen poisoning: An evidence-based consensus guideline for out-of-hospital management. Clin Toxicol (Phila) 2006;44:1–18. http://www.clintox.org/guidelines.cfm.

63. Bray GP, Harrison PM, O'Grady JG, et al. Long-term anticonvulsant therapy worsens outcome in paracetamol-induced fulminant hepatic failure. Hum Exp Toxicol 1992;11:265–270.

64. Schmidt LE, Dalhoff K, Poulsen HE. Acute versus chronic alcohol consumption in acetaminophen-induced hepatoxicity. Hepatology 2002;35:876–882.

65. Lee WM. Drug-induced hepatotoxicity. N Engl J Med 2003;349:474–485.

66. Draganov P, Durrence H, Cox C, Reuben A. Alcohol-acetaminophen syndrome: Even moderate social drinkers are at risk. Postgrad Med 2000;107:189–195.

67. Kearns GL, Leeder JS, Wasserman GS. Acetaminophen intoxication during treatment: What you don't know can hurt you. Clin Pediatr 2000;39:133–144.

68. Wolf SJ, Heard K, Sloan EP, Jagoda AS; American College of Emergency Physicians. Clinical policy: critical issues in the management of patients presenting to the emergency department with acetaminophen overdose. Ann Emerg Med 2007;50:292–313.

69. Jones AL. Mechanism of action and value of N-acetylcysteine in the treatment of early and late acetaminophen poisoning: A critical review. J Toxicol Clin Toxicol 1998;36:277–285.

70. Heard KJ. Acetylcysteine for acetaminophen poisoning. N Engl J Med 2008;359:285–292.

71. Acetadote (acetylcysteine) Injection [package insert]. Nashville, TN: Cumberland Pharmaceuticals; 2006.

72. Sandilands EA, Bateman DN. Adverse reactions associated with acetylcysteine. Clin Toxicol (Phila) 2009;47:81–88.

73. Brok J, Buckley N, Gluud C. Interventions for paracetamol (acetaminophen) overdose. Cochrane Database Syst Rev 2006;(2):CD003328.

74. Reigart JR, Roberts JR. Recognition and Management of Pesticide Poisonings, 5th ed. Washington, DC: US Environmental Protection Agency; 1999. http://www.epa.gov/oppfead1/safety/healthcare/handbook/handbook.pdf.

75. Roberts DM, Aaron CK. Management of acute organophosphorus pesticide poisoning. BMJ 2007;334:629–634.

76. Abou-Donia MB. Organophosphorus ester-induced chronic neurotoxicity. Arch Environ Health 2003;58:484–497.

77. Kwong TC. Organophosphate pesticides: Biochemistry and clinical toxicology. Ther Drug Monit 2002;24:144–149.

78. Eddleston M, Buckley NA, Eyer P, Dawson AH. Management of acute organophosphorus pesticide poisoning. Lancet 2008;371:597–607.

79. Okumura T, Takasu N, Ishimatsu S, et al. Report on 640 victims of the Tokyo subway sarin attack. Ann Emerg Med 1996;28:129–135.

80. Evison D, Hinsley D, Rice P. Chemical weapons. Br Med J 2002;324:332–335.

81. Medicis JJ, Stork CM, Howland MA, et al. Pharmacokinetics following a loading dose plus a continuous infusion of pralidoxime compared with the traditional short infusion regimen in human volunteers. J Toxicol Clin Toxicol 1996;34:289–295.

82. Farrar HC, Wells TG, Kearns GL. Use of continuous infusion of pralidoxime for treatment of organophosphate poisoning in children. J Pediatr 1990;116:658–661.

83. Buckley NA, Eddleston M, Szinicz L. Oximes for acute organophosphate pesticide poisoning. Cochrane Database Syst Rev 2005;(1):CD005085.

84. Peter JV, Moran JL, Graham P. Oxime therapy and outcomes in human organophosphate poisoning: An evaluation using meta-analytic techniques. Crit Care Med 2006;34:502–510.

85. Pesticides: Health and Safety. Washington, DC: US Environmental Protection Agency. http://www.epa.gov/pesticides/health.

86. Salhanick SD, Shannon MW. Management of calcium channel antagonist overdose. Drug Saf 2003;26:65–79.

87. Kerns W 2nd. Management of beta-adrenergic blocker and calcium channel antagonist toxicity. Emerg Med Clin North Am 2007;25:309–331.

88. DeWitt CR, Waksman JC. Pharmacology, pathophysiology and management of calcium channel blocker and beta-blocker toxicity. Toxicol Rev 2004;23:223–238.

89. Harris NS. Case records of the Massachusetts General Hospital. Case 24–2006. A 40-year-old woman with hypotension after an overdose of amlodipine. N Engl J Med 2006;355:602–611.

90. Shepherd G. Treatment of poisoning caused by beta-adrenergic and calcium-channel blockers. Am J Health Syst Pharm 2006;63:1828–1835.

91. Adams BD, Browne WT. Amlodipine overdose causes prolonged calcium channel blocker toxicity. Am J Emerg Med 1998;16:527–528.

92. Olson KR, Erdman AR, Woolf AD, et al. Calcium channel blocker ingestion: An evidence-based consensus guideline for out-of-hospital management. Clin Toxicol (Phila) 2005;43:797–821. http://www.clintox.org/guidelines.cfm.

93. Levine M, Boyer EW, Pozner C, et.al. Assessment of hyperglycemia after calcium channel blocker overdoses involving diltiazem or verapamil. Crit Care Med 2007;35:2071–2075.

94. Buckley N, Dawson AH, Howarth D, Whyte IM. Slow-release verapamil poisoning: Use of polyethylene glycol whole-bowel lavage and high-dose calcium. Med J Aust 1993;158:202–204.

95. Papadopoulos J, O'Neil MG. Utilization of a glucagon infusion in the management of a massive nifedipine overdose. J Emerg Med 2000;18:453–455.

96. Holzer M, Sterz F, Schoerkhuber W, et al. Successful resuscitation of a verapamil-intoxicated patient with percutaneous cardiopulmonary bypass. Crit Care Med 1999;27:2818–2823.

97. Durward A, Guerguerian AM, Lefebvre M, Shemie SD. Massive diltiazem overdose treated with extracorporeal membrane oxygenation. Pediatr Crit Care Med 2003;4:372–376.

98. Corman SL, Skledar SJ. Use of lipid emulsion to reverse local anesthetic-induced toxicity. Ann Pharmacother 2007;41:1873–1877.

99. Luomanmaki K, Tiula E, Kivisto KT, Neuvonen PJ. Pharmacokinetics of diltiazem in massive overdose. Ther Drug Monit 1997;19:240–242.

100. Morimoto S, Sasaki S, Kiyama M, et al. Sustained-release diltiazem overdose. J Hum Hypertens 1999;13:643–644.

101. Fine JS. Iron poisoning. Curr Probl Pediatr 2000;30:71–90.

102. Robertson A, Tenenbein M. Hepatotoxicity in acute iron poisoning. Hum Exp Toxicol 2005;24:559–562.

103. Chyka PA, Banner W Jr. Hematopoietic agents. In: Dart RC, ed. Medical Toxicology, 3rd ed. Philadelphia: Lippincott Williams & Wilkins, 2004: 605–614.

104. Tenenbein M, Israels SJ. Early coagulopathy in severe iron poisoning. J Pediatr 1988;113:695–697.

105. Pestaner JP, Ishak KG, Mullick FG, Centeno JA. Ferrous sulfate toxicity: A review of autopsy findings. Biol Trace Element Res 1999;69:191–198.

106. Manoguerra AS, Erdman AR, Booze LL, et al. Iron ingestion: An evidence-based consensus guideline for out-of-hospital management. Clin Toxicol (Phila) 2005;43:553–570. http://www.clintox.org/guidelines.cfm.

107. Everson GW, Oukjhane K, Young LW, et al. Effectiveness of abdominal radiographs in visualizing chewable iron supplements following overdose. Am J Emerg Med 1989;7:459–463.

108. Palatnick W, Tenenbein M. Leukocytosis, hyperglycemia, vomiting, and positive x-rays are not indicators of severity of iron overdose in adults. Am J Emerg Med 1996;14:454–455.

109. Chyka PA, Butler AY. Assessment of acute iron poisoning by laboratory and clinical observations. Am J Emerg Med 1993;11:99–103.

110. Chyka PA, Butler AY, Holley JE. Serum iron concentrations and symptoms of acute iron poisoning in children. Pharmacotherapy 1996;16:1053–1058.

111. Eisen TF, Lacouture PG, Woolf A. Visual detection of ferrioxamine color changes in urine. Vet Hum Toxicol 1988;30:369–370.

112. Peck M, Rogers J, Riverbach J. Use of high doses of deferoxamine (Desferal) in an adult patient with acute iron overdosage. J Toxicol Clin Toxicol 1982;19:865–869.

113. Howland MA. Risks of parenteral deferoxamine for acute iron poisoning. J Toxicol Clin Toxicol 1996;34:491–497.

114. Shannon M. Desferrioxamine in acute iron poisoning [letter]. Lancet 1992;339:1601.

115. Tenenbein M, Kowalski S, Sienko A, et al. Pulmonary toxic effects of continuous desferrioxamine administration in acute iron poisoning. Lancet 1992;339:699–701.

116. Kerr GW, McGuffie AC, Wilkie S. Tricyclic antidepressant overdose: A review. Emerg Med J 2001:18:236–241.

117. Pentel PR, Keyler DE, Haddad LM. Tricyclic antidepressants and selective serotonin reuptake inhibitors. In: Haddad LM, Shannon MW, Winchester JI, eds. Clinical Management of Poisoning and Drug Overdose, 3rd ed. Philadelphia: WB Saunders, 1998: 437–451.

118. James LP, Kearns GL. Cyclic antidepressant toxicity in children and adolescents. J Clin Pharmacol 1995;35:343–350.

119. Woolf AD, Erdman AR, Nelson LS, et al. Tricyclic antidepressant poisoning: An evidence-based consensus guideline for out-of-hospital management. Clin Toxicol (Phila) 2007;45:203–233. *http://www.clintox.org/guidelines.cfm.*

120. Henry JA. Epidemiology and relative toxicity of antidepressant drugs in overdose. Drug Saf 1997;16:374–390.

121. Buckley NA, McManus PR. Fatal toxicity of serotoninergic and other antidepressant drugs: Analysis of United Kingdom mortality data. Br Med J 2002;325:1332–1333.

122. Reilly TH, Kirk MA. Atypical antipsychotics and newer antidepressants. Emerg Med Clin North Am 2007;25:477–497.

123. Borys DJ, Setzer SC, Ling LJ, et al. Acute fluoxetine overdose: A report of 234 cases. Am J Emerg Med 1992;10:115–120.

124. Boyer EW, Shannon M. The serotonin syndrome. N Engl J Med 2005; 352:1112–1120.

125. Spina E, Henthorn TK, Eleborg L, et al. Desmethylimipramine overdose: Nonlinear kinetics in a slow hydroxylator. Ther Drug Monit 1985;7:239–241.

126. Buckley NA, Chevalier S, Leditschke A, et al. The limited utility of electrocardiography variables used to predict arrhythmia in psychotropic drug overdose. Crit Care 2003;7:R102—R107. *http://ccforum.com/content/7/5/R101.*

127. Nelson LS, Erdman AR., Booze LL, et al. Selective serotonin reuptake inhibitor poisoning: An evidence-based consensus guideline for out-of-hospital management. Clin Toxicol (Phila) 2007;45:315–332. *http://www.clintox.org/guidelines.cfm.*

128. Smilkstein MJ. Reviewing cyclic antidepressant cardiotoxicity: Wheat and chaff. J Emerg Med 1990;8:645–648.

129. McCabe JL, Cobaugh DJ, Mengazzi JJ, Fata J. Experimental tricyclic antidepressant toxicity: A randomized, controlled comparison of hypertonic saline solution, sodium bicarbonate, and hyperventilation. Ann Emerg Med 1998;32:329–333.

130. Suchard JR. Assessing physostigmine's contraindication in cyclic antidepressant ingestions. J Emerg Med 2003;25:185–191.

131. Weinbroum AA, Flaishon R, Sorkine P. A risk-benefit assessment of flumazenil in the management of benzodiazepine overdose. Drug Saf 1997;17:181–196.

132. Friedman RA, Leon AC. Expanding the Black Box—depression, antidepressants, and the risk of suicide. N Engl Med 2007;356: 2343–2346.

15

Emergency Preparedness: Identification and Management of Biologic Exposures

COLLEEN M. TERRIFF, JASON E. BROUILLARD, LISA T. COSTANIGRO, AND JESSICA S. OFTEBRO

KEY CONCEPTS

❶ Bioterrorism agents are organisms or toxins that can cause disease and death in humans, animals, or plants and elicit terror.

❷ Category A bioterrorism agents include anthrax (*Bacillus anthracis*), tularemia (*Francisella tularensis*), smallpox (*variola major*), plague (*Yersinia pestis*), botulinum toxin (*Clostridium botulinum*), and viral hemorrhagic fevers.

❸ An important therapeutic concept surrounding prophylaxis involves prompt initiation of a regimen with the appropriate empiric antimicrobial.

❹ Anthrax is a highly virulent, lethal infection; human-to-human transmission, however, has not been documented.

❺ Rapid recognition of botulism based on clinical presentation is essential to ensure antitoxin therapy within 24 hours of presentation.

❻ Primary septicemic plague can lead to severe complications, such as multi-organ dysfunction and adult respiratory distress syndrome.

❼ Smallpox vaccine stockpiles are maintained for response to a smallpox emergency.

❽ Pharmacologic treatment of viral hemorrhagic fever, with the exception of infection caused by viruses from the *Filoviridae* or *Flaviviridae* family, includes oral or intravenous ribavirin.

❾ Infectious disease outbreaks following natural disasters, like bioterror agent exposures, can cause panic, social unrest, and tax any country's medical and public health system.

The fall of 2001 forever changed how many people throughout the world felt about flying, airport security, and even opening their mail. Terrorism, especially bioterrorism, became a common term used by the media, military analysts, government and public health officials, and the public at large. Anxiety caused by the 2001 intentional anthrax release through the United States mail system, and the ensuing exposures and deaths, was further escalated by numerous false alarms surrounding the delivery of parcels containing unidentified white powder.[1] Recent devastating natural disasters, such as tsunamis and hurricanes, have reawakened our appreciation of the power and destruction associated with natural disasters. In April 2009, a novel influenza A virus (swine-originated H1N1) caused outbreaks of respiratory illness in Mexico and the United States, leading to a declaration of a worldwide pandemic by June.[2] Later that month, the Secretary of the U.S. Department of Health and Human Services, determined that a nationwide public health emergency existed.[3] With goals of reducing transmission and illness severity, the CDC's Division of the Strategic National Stockpile (SNS) released antiviral drugs, respiratory protection devices, and personal protective equipment to state departments of health, who in turn allocated supplies to local health jurisdictions.[4] Vaccine development and distribution, as well as execution of immunization campaigns for recommended targeted groups, was tasked to health departments. Management of stockpiles of antibiotics, antivirals, or vaccines for bioterrorism attacks or pandemic influenza is becoming a crucial public health issue. Healthcare providers need to play an active role in awareness and preparedness for biological threats released by terrorists or nature, and the decision-making process regarding postexposure prophylaxis (PEP), mass vaccination, and treatment of biologic exposures to help protect the public.

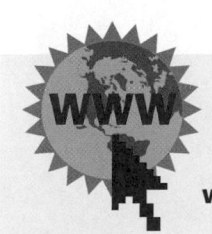

The complete chapter, learning objectives, and other resources can be found at **www.pharmacotherapyonline.com**.

CHAPTER

16

Emergency Preparedness: Identification and Management of Chemical and Radiologic Exposures

GREENE SHEPHERD AND RICHARD B. SCHWARTZ

KEY CONCEPTS

❶ In mass casualty events with chemical or radiologic exposure, the majority of victims can be managed with decontamination, observation, and supportive care. Antidotal therapies should be reserved for more critically injured victims.

❷ Nerve agent poisoning is similar to organophosphate insecticide poisoning, with atropine and pralidoxime being the primary antidotes.

❸ Cyanide gas exposure can be rapidly fatal but most victims that are conscious upon arrival to the hospital will not require antidote therapy.

❹ Respiratory problems caused by pulmonary agents with low water solubility may take several hours to develop, thus requiring extended observation.

❺ Vesicant chemical weapons are less lethal than other chemical weapons but cause significant morbidity, leaving many survivors who need extensive care.

❻ Therapeutic agents are available that can block the uptake or enhance the elimination of radioactive contamination.

❼ Clinicians, especially pharmacists, need to be prepared to take an active role in the design and operations of disaster plans for their workplace and community. Pharmacists may participate on established disaster response teams, which may be deployed to assist in the care of individuals outside of their local area.

Life-threatening hazardous material exposures may happen anywhere and at any time. The exposure may be due to an unintentional release or at the other extreme be the result of an intentional and catastrophic act of terrorism.[1-6] A hazardous material is defined as any substance that poses a substantial risk to the health or safety of individuals, or the environment when improperly handled, stored, transported, or disposed.[1] The specific risks are dependent on the quantity and concentration of the substance exposure and the physical, chemical, or infectious characteristics of the material. Many of these substances have the potential to be used as weapons. Small quantities of hazardous materials are used in many commercial products, such as pesticides. Larger and more concentrated quantities are found at industrial sites and in their waste byproducts. Injuries from hazardous materials are relatively common as evidenced by the tens of thousands of hazardous material incidents recorded by the U.S. Environmental Protection Agency during the last decade. The majority of these incidents occur during transport rather than at the site of manufacture or use and represent a complex and significant danger for emergency healthcare workers.[1] Violent acts of nature, such as hurricanes or earthquakes, can lead to environmental contamination due to the release of a wide variety of hazardous materials when pipelines or storage tanks rupture. At the other extreme, a hazardous material exposure may be the result of an intentional and catastrophic act of terrorism. Historically, acts of chemical or radiologic terrorism have been rare but have had very high visibility and marked psychological impact. Terrorism represents a profound threat to many countries around the world. Terrorists, whether representing foreign governments, organized religious sects, or individuals, have the capacity to endanger our communities with hazardous materials. Even a single patient contaminated with a hazardous material has the potential to overwhelm an unprepared healthcare facility.

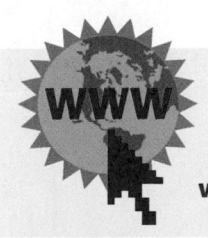

The complete chapter, learning objectives, and other resources can be found at **www.pharmacotherapyonline.com**.

CHAPTER

17

Cardiovascular Testing

RICHARD A. LANGE AND L. DAVID HILLIS

KEY CONCEPTS

❶ A careful patient history and physical examination are extremely important in diagnosing cardiovascular disease and should be done prior to any test.

❷ Heart sounds and heart murmurs are important in identifying heart valve abnormalities and other structural cardiac defects.

❸ Elevated jugular venous pressure is an important sign of heart failure and may be used to assess severity and response to therapy.

❹ Electrocardiography is useful for determining rhythm disturbances (tachy- or bradyarrhythmias).

❺ Exercise stress testing provides important information concerning the likelihood and severity of coronary artery disease; changes in the electrocardiogram, blood pressure, and heart rate are used to assess the response to exercise.

❻ Cardiac catheterization and angiography are used to assess coronary anatomy and ventricular performance.

❼ Echocardiography is used to assess valve structure and function as well as ventricular wall motion; transesophogeal echocardiography is more sensitive for detecting thrombus and vegetations than transthoracic echocardiography.

❽ Radionuclides such as technetium-99m and thallium-201 are used to assess ischemia and myocardial viability in patients with suspected coronary artery disease and heart failure.

❾ Pharmacologic stress testing is used when patients cannot perform physical exercise to assess the likelihood of coronary artery disease.

Learning objectives, review questions, and other resources can be found at
www.pharmacotherapyonline.com.

In the United States, cardiovascular disease (CVD) afflicts an estimated 80 million people (i.e., approximately 1 in 3 adults) and accounts for 35% of all deaths. In 2009, the estimated direct and indirect cost of CVD—which includes hypertension, coronary heart disease, heart failure, and stroke—was $475.3 billion.[1]

Atherosclerosis, the cause of most CVD events, is typically present for decades before symptoms appear. With a thorough history, comprehensive physical examination, and appropriate testing, the individual with subclinical CVD usually can be identified, and the subject with symptomatic CVD can be assessed for the risk of an adverse event and can be managed appropriately.

THE HISTORY

The elements of a comprehensive history include the chief complaint, current symptoms, past medical history, family history, social history, and review of systems.

The chief complaint is a brief statement describing the reason the patient is seeking medical attention. The patient is asked to describe his or her current symptoms, including their duration, quality, frequency, severity, progression, precipitating and relieving factors, associated symptoms, and impact on daily activities.

The past medical history may reveal previous cardiovascular problems, conditions that predispose the patient to develop CVD (i.e., hypertension, hyperlipidemia, or diabetes mellitus) (Table 17–1), or comorbid conditions that influence the identification or management of CVD. The patient should be asked about social habits that affect the cardiovascular system, including diet, amount of regular physical activity, tobacco use, alcohol intake, and illicit drug use. At present, family history is the best available screening tool to identify patients with a genetic predisposition for CVD.

CARDIOVASCULAR HISTORY

❶ Chest pain is a frequent symptom and may occur as a result of myocardial ischemia (angina pectoris) or infarction or a variety of noncardiac conditions, such as esophageal, pulmonary, or musculoskeletal disorders. The quality of chest pain, its location and duration, and the factors that provoke or relieve it are important in ascertaining its etiology.

TABLE 17-1	Risk Factors for Cardiovascular Disease

Non-Modifiable
Advancing age
Male
Family history of early onset CVD
Postmenopausal status
Modifiable
Hypertension
Diabetes mellitus
Dyslipidemia
Cigarette smoking
Obesity
Physical inactivity
Excessive alcohol
Stress
Chronic inflammation (i.e., gingivitis, arthritis, elevated C-reactive protein, etc.)
Illicit drug use (e.g., cocaine or methamphetamine)

Typically, patients with angina describe a sensation of heaviness or pressure in the retrosternal area that may radiate to the jaw, left shoulder, back, or left arm. It typically lasts only a few minutes. It is precipitated by exertion, emotional stress, eating, smoking a cigarette, or exposure to cold, and it is usually relieved with rest or a sublingual nitroglycerin, although the latter also is effective in relieving chest pain due to esophageal spasm. Angina that is increasing in severity, longer in duration, or occurring at rest is called unstable angina; it should prompt the patient to seek medical attention expeditiously.

The patient with congestive heart failure and pulmonary vascular congestion may complain of shortness of breath (dyspnea) with exertion or even at rest, orthopnea, paroxysmal nocturnal dyspnea, and nocturia. The patient with congestive heart failure and peripheral venous congestion may report abdominal swelling (from hepatic congestion or ascites), nausea, vomiting, lower extremity edema, fatigue, and dyspnea.

The New York Heart Association (NYHA) grading system is used to indicate whether a patient has angina or symptoms of congestive heart failure with vigorous (Class I), moderate (Class II), mild (Class III), or minimal/no (Class IV) exertion.

PHYSICAL EXAMINATION

The patient with suspected heart disease should undergo a comprehensive physical examination, with particular attention to the cardiovascular system. This should include an assessment of the jugular venous pulse, carotid and peripheral arterial pulses, examination of the heart and lungs (i.e., palpation, percussion, and auscultation), and inspection of the abdomen and extremities.

JUGULAR VENOUS PRESSURE

❸ The jugular venous pressure (JVP) is an indirect assessment of right atrial pressure. With the patient lying supine at 30 degrees and his/her head rotated slightly to the left, the height of the fluid wave in the right internal jugular vein is determined relative to the sternal angle. The normal JVP is 1 to 2 cm above the sternal angle. The JVP typically is elevated in the patient with heart failure. The extent of elevation can be used to assess the severity of peripheral venous congestion, and its diminution can be used to assess the response to therapy.

ARTERIAL PULSES

The carotid arterial pulse is examined for its intensity and, concurrently with the apical impulse, for concordance within the cardiac cycle. Diminished carotid arterial pulsations may be the result of a reduced stroke volume, atherosclerotic narrowing of the carotid artery, or obstruction to left ventricular outflow, as may occur with aortic valve stenosis or hypertrophic obstructive cardiomyopathy. Conversely, very forceful, hyperdynamic, "bounding" carotid arterial pulsations may be palpated in the patient with an increased stroke volume and suggests the presence of chronic aortic valve regurgitation or a high cardiac output due, for example, to hyperthyroidism, an arteriovenous shunt, or marked anemia.

The pulses in the arms and legs also are examined. Diminished peripheral pulses suggest the presence of a reduced stroke volume or atherosclerotic peripheral arterial disease (PAD). Concomitant pallor, skin atrophy, hair loss, or ulcerations is consistent with PAD, which often coexists with coronary artery disease. To quantify the severity of PAD, systolic arterial pressure is measured in all four extremities. Normally, the systolic arterial pressure in the feet should be similar or even slightly higher than the pressure in the arms. Thus, the ratio of the systolic arterial pressures in the foot and arm (the so-called ankle-brachial index [ABI]) is normally >1.0. An ABI <0.9 suggests PAD.[2]

CHEST

In the patient with chest pain, a thorough lung examination should be performed to exclude a pulmonary cause. The anterior chest wall is palpated to assess for the presence of tenderness in the sternal area, which may indicate that the patient has costochondritis. Percussion of the posterior chest is done to determine if a pleural effusion is present. Auscultation of the anterior and posterior lung fields is performed to assess for the presence of findings suggestive of pneumonia, airway obstruction, pleural effusion, or pulmonary edema.

HEART SOUNDS

❷ The typical "lub-dub" sound of the normal heart consists of the first heart sound (S_1), which precedes ventricular contraction and is due to closure of the mitral and tricuspid valves, and the second heart sound (S_2), which follows ventricular contraction and is due to closure of the aortic and pulmonic valves. Other heart sounds, which are normally not present (i.e., a third heart sound (S_3), fourth heart sound (S_4), or murmur), may indicate the presence of underlying heart disease (Fig. 17–1).

The S_3, a so-called ventricular gallop, is a low-pitched sound usually heard at the cardiac apex in early diastole (i.e., immediately after S_2). It is caused by the vibrations that occur when blood rapidly rushes from a "tense" atrium into a stiff, noncompliant ventricle. Thus, it is usually associated with decompensated congestive heart failure or intravascular volume overload. A so-called "physiologic" S_3 is heard commonly in healthy children and may persist into young adulthood.

The S_4 is a dull, low-pitched sound that is caused by the vibrations that occur when atrial contraction forces blood into a stiff, noncompliant ventricle. It is audible at the cardiac apex just before ventricular contraction (i.e., just before S_1); it is not present in the subject with a normal heart. An S_4 may be present in the patient with aortic stenosis, systemic arterial hypertension, hypertrophic cardiomyopathy, or coronary artery disease.

Murmurs are auditory vibrations resulting from turbulent blood flow within the heart chambers or across the valves. They are classified by their timing and duration within the cardiac cycle (systolic, diastolic, or continuous), location on the chest wall, intensity (grade 1 to 6, from softest to loudest), pitch (high or low frequency), and

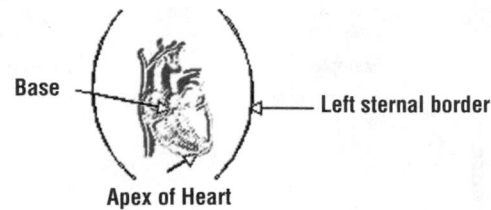

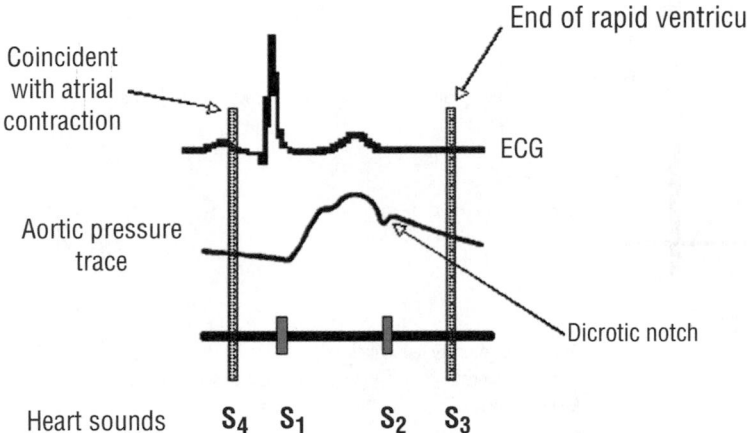

FIGURE 17-1. Correlation of the electrocardiogram (ECG) with an aortic pressure tracing and heart sounds. Normal heart sounds are S$_1$ (mitral and tricuspid valve closure) and S$_2$ (aortic and pulmonic valve closure). The S$_3$ and S$_4$ "gallops" are usually abnormal. The S$_3$ occurs in early diastole as blood rapidly rushes into a stiff, noncompliant ventricle (e.g., with decompensated congestive heart failure). The S$_4$ occurs in late diastole and is caused by atrial contraction into a hypertrophied ventricle (e.g., hypertension).

radiation (Fig. 17–2 and Table 17–2). Some murmurs are said to be "innocent" or "physiologic" and result from rapid, turbulent blood flow in the absence of cardiac disease. Fever, anxiety, anemia, hyperthyroidism, and pregnancy increase the intensity of a physiologic murmur.

Systolic murmurs occur during ventricular contraction. They begin with or after S$_1$ and end at or before S$_2$, depending on the origin of the murmur. They are classified based on time of onset and termination within systole: midsystolic or holosystolic (pansystolic). Examples of midsystolic murmurs include pulmonic stenosis, aortic stenosis, and hypertrophic obstructive cardiomyopathy. Holosystolic murmurs occur when blood flows from a chamber of higher pressure to one of lower pressure throughout systole, such as occurs with mitral or tricuspid valve regurgitation or a ventricular septal defect.

Diastolic murmurs occur during ventricular filling. They begin with or after S$_2$, depending on the origin of the murmur. Aortic

or pulmonic valve regurgitation causes a high-pitched diastolic murmur that begins with S$_2$, whereas stenosis of the mitral or tricuspid valves causes a low-pitched, "rumbling" diastolic murmur.

Continuous murmurs begin in systole and continue without interruption into all or part of diastole. Such murmurs are mainly a result of aortopulmonary connections (e.g., patent ductus arteriosus) or arteriovenous connections (e.g., arteriovenous fistula, coronary artery fistula, or arteriovenous malformation).

When a murmur is heard, the cardiac abnormality underlying it usually can be confirmed and assessed with echocardiography or other imaging modalities, such as cardiac angiography or magnetic resonance imaging (MRI) (see below).

PRACTICE GUIDELINES FOR DIAGNOSTIC AND PROGNOSTIC TESTING IN CARDIOVASCULAR DISEASE TESTING

The American Heart Association (AHA) and American College of Cardiology (ACC) Task Force on Practice Guidelines provide the indications and utility of various diagnostic cardiac tests (Fig. 17–3). Class I indications are those for which evidence or agreement that the specific procedure is useful and effective is unequivocal. Class II indications are those for which a divergence of opinion concerning the usefulness of the test is present: class IIa are those for which evidence or opinion in favor of the test exists, whereas class IIb are those for which less evidence favoring the test is present. Class III indications are those for which evidence or agreement exists that a diagnostic test is not useful.

For a specific clinical scenario, the guidelines also indicate the level of evidence for the recommendation. Level A evidence is said to be present if the recommendation is based on the results of multiple randomized clinical trials. Level B evidence is said to exist if only a single randomized trial or multiple nonrandomized trials exist. Level C evidence is said to be present if the recommendation is made based on expert opinion only.

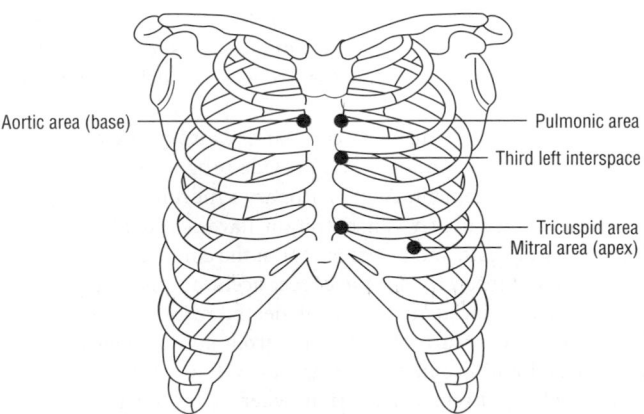

FIGURE 17-2. Schematic illustrations of topographic areas on the precordium for cardiac auscultation. Auscultatory areas do not correspond to anatomic locations of the valves but to the sites at which particular valves are heard best. *(Redrawn from Kinney MR, Packa DR, eds. Andreoli's Comprehensive Cardiac Care, 8th ed. St. Louis, MO: Mosby, 1996, with permission.)*

TABLE 17-2 Characteristic Murmurs

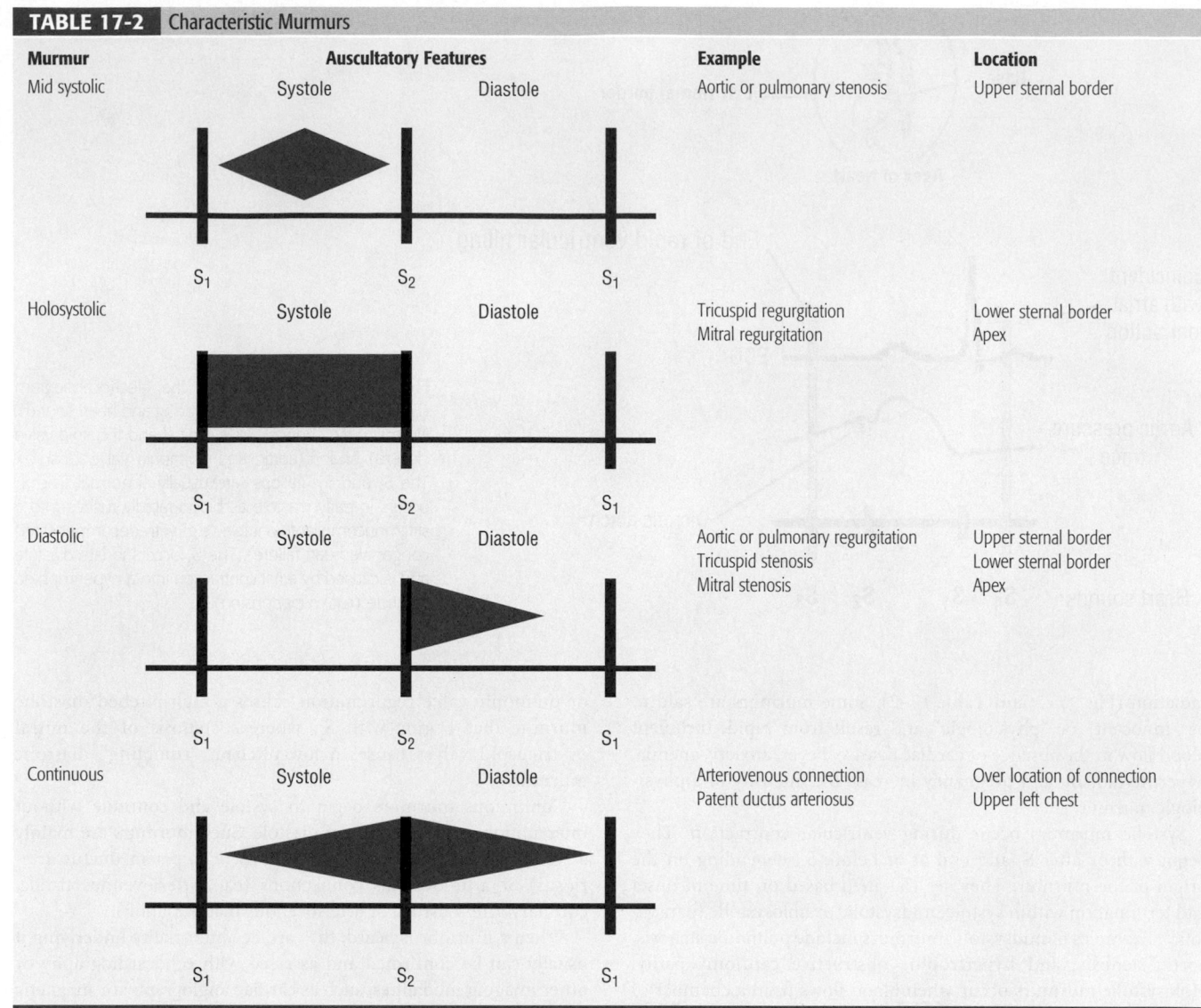

Murmur	Auscultatory Features			Example	Location
Mid systolic	Systole	Diastole		Aortic or pulmonary stenosis	Upper sternal border
Holosystolic	Systole	Diastole		Tricuspid regurgitation Mitral regurgitation	Lower sternal border Apex
Diastolic	Systole	Diastole		Aortic or pulmonary regurgitation Tricuspid stenosis Mitral stenosis	Upper sternal border Lower sternal border Apex
Continuous	Systole	Diastole		Arteriovenous connection Patent ductus arteriosus	Over location of connection Upper left chest

TESTING MODALITIES

BIOMARKERS

Blood tests are available for several substances that suggest the presence of myonecrosis (i.e., recent death of myocardial cells), inflammation, or hemodynamic stress (Fig. 17–4).[3–5]

Markers of Myonecrosis

When myocardial infarction (myonecrosis) occurs, proteins from the recently necrotic myocytes are released into the peripheral blood, where they can be detected using specific biochemical assays. These biomarkers of myonecrosis (a) aid in the diagnosis (or exclusion) of myocardial infarction as the cause of chest pain; (b) facilitate triage and risk stratification of patients with chest discomfort; and (c) identify patients who are appropriate candidates for specific therapeutic strategies or interventions. Cardiac troponin (cTn) is the preferred biomarker for the diagnosis of myonecrosis.[6] Other available biomarkers of necrosis include creatine kinase-MB (CK-MB) and myoglobin.

Troponin I and T are contractile proteins found only in cardiac myocytes. In the patient with myocardial infarction, cTn is detectable in the blood 2 to 4 hours after the onset of symptoms and remains detectable for 5 to 10 days (Fig. 17–5). cTn is the preferred marker for evaluating the patient suspected of having an acute myocardial infarction, since it is the most sensitive and tissue-specific biomarker available. In the patient with ischemic chest pain and electrocardiographic (e.g., ST segment) abnormalities, the presence of an elevated serum cTn concentration establishes the diagnosis of myocardial infarction, and the absence of such an elevation excludes it.

In the patient with an acute coronary syndrome, detection and quantitation of cTn in the blood provide prognostic information and guide management. Acute coronary syndrome patients with an elevated serum cTn concentration have a roughly four-fold higher risk of death and recurrent MI in the coming months when compared to those with normal cTn concentrations.[7] They benefit (i.e., have a reduced incidence of death, recurrent myocardial infarction, and recurrent ischemia) from more intensive antiplatelet and antithrombotic therapy as well as prompt coronary angiography and revascularization, whereas those with a normal serum cTn do not benefit from such intensive therapy.[8] Thus, serum cTn concentrations are used for diagnostic, prognostic, and therapeutic purposes in the patient with suspected or proven coronary artery disease.

On occasion, the serum cTn concentration may be elevated in a patient without coronary artery disease in whom myonecrosis

Size of treatment effect

Estimate of certainty (precision) of treatment effect		Class I	Class IIa	Class IIb	Class III
		Benefit >>> Risk Procedure/Treatment SHOULD be performed/administered	Benefit >>> Risk Additional studies with focused objectives needed **IT IS REASONABLE to perform procedure/administer treatment**	Benefit ≥ Risk Additional studies with broad objectives needed; Additional registry data would be helpful **IT IS NOT UNREASONABLE to perform procedure/administer treatment**	Risk ≥ Benefit No additional studies needed **Procedure/Treatment should NOT be performed/administered SINCE IT IS NOT HELPFUL AND MAY BE HARMFUL**
Level A Multiple (3–5) population risk strata evaluated General consistency of direction and magnitude of effect		• Recommendation that procedure or treatment is useful/effective • Sufficient evidence from multiple randomized trials or meta-analyses	• Recommendation in favor of treatment or procedure being useful/effective • Some conflicting evidence from multiple randomized trials or meta-analyses	• Recommendation's usefulness/efficacy less well established • Greater conflicting evidence from multiple randomized trials or meta-analyses	• Recommendation that procedure or treatment not useful/effective and may be harmful • Sufficient evidence from multiple randomized trials or meta-analyses
Level B Limited (2–3) population risk strata evaluated		• Recommendation that procedure or treatment is useful/effective • Limited evidence from single randomized trial or non-randomized studies	• Recommendation in favor of treatment or procedure being useful/effective • Some conflicting evidence from single randomized trial or non-randomized studies	• Recommendation's usefulness/efficacy less well established • Greater conflicting evidence from single randomized trial or non-randomized studies	• Recommendation that procedure or treatment not useful/effective and may be harmful • Limited evidence from single randomized trial or non-randomized studies
Level C Very limited (1–2) population risk strata evaluated		• Recommendation that procedure or treatment is useful/effective • Only expert opinion, case studies, or standard-of-care	• Recommendation in favor of treatment or procedure being useful/effective • Only diverging expert opinion, case studies, or standard-of-care	• Recommendation's usefulness/efficacy less well established • Only diverging expert opinion, case studies, or standard-of-care	• Recommendation that procedure or treatment not useful/effective and may be harmful • Only expert opinion, case studies, or standard-of-care

FIGURE 17-3. Classification of recommendations and level of evidence.

occurs because myocardial oxygen demands markedly exceed oxygen supply (i.e., severe systemic arterial hypertension) or nonischemic cardiac injury occurs (i.e., myocardial contusion caused by blunt trauma to the chest) (Table 17–3). In the patient with an elevated serum cTn concentration, the responsible physician must decide if the observed abnormal serum cTn concentration is the result of coronary artery disease or another condition.

When serum cTn measurements are not available, the best alternative is the MB isoenzyme of creatine kinase (CK-MB), which is a cytosolic carrier protein for high-energy phosphates that is released into the blood when myonecrosis occurs. Although it was initially thought to be cardiac specific, CK-MB is now known to be present in small amounts in skeletal muscle; as a result, it may be detectable in the blood of patients with massive muscle injury, as occurs with rhabdomyolysis or myositis.

In the patient with an acute myocardial infarction, CK-MB can be detected in the blood 2 to 4 hours after symptom onset; its serum concentration peaks within 24 hours, and it remains detectable in the blood for 48 to 72 hours. To document the characteristic rise and fall of CK-MB concentrations, blood samples should be obtained every 4 to 8 hours. Although CK-MB is not as sensitive or cardiac-specific a biomarker as cTn, its blood concentration declines more rapidly than cTn, which makes

Cardiac Biomarkers

Markers of myonecrosis
- Cardiac troponin (cTn)
- Creatine kinase MB (CK-MB)
- Myoglobin

Markers of inflammation
- C reactive protein (CRP)
- Myeloperoxidase
- P-selectin
- CD40 ligand
- Interleukin
- Fibrinogen

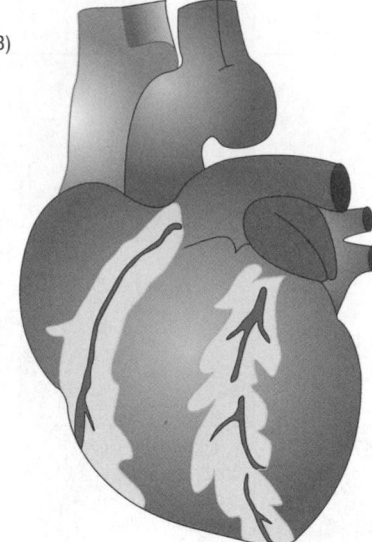

Markers of hemodynamic stress
- B-type natriuretic peptide (BNP)
- N-terminal pro BNP (NT-proBNP)

FIGURE 17-4. Cardiac biomarkers classified according to the different pathologic processes they indicate.

it the preferred biomarker for evaluating suspected recurrent infarction in the patient who experiences recurrent chest pain within several days of myocardial infarction. With recurrent infarction, the typical rise and fall of the serum CK-MB concentration is interrupted by a second elevation. Since serum cTn concentrations decline slowly following myocardial infarction, they are not as sensitive as CK-MB for diagnosing recurrent infarction.

The serum myoglobin concentration is elevated in the patient with myonecrosis, but it has a low specificity for myocardial infarction because of its high concentration in skeletal muscle. Because of its small molecular size and consequent rapid release (within 1 hour) following the onset of myonecrosis, it is valuable as a very early marker of myocardial infarction. When it is combined with a more specific marker of myonecrosis, such as cTn or CK-MB, myoglobin is useful for the early exclusion of myocardial infarction.

Markers of Inflammation

Inflammatory processes participate in the development of atherosclerosis and contribute to the destabilization of atherosclerotic plaques, which may ultimately lead to an acute coronary syndrome. Several mediators of the inflammatory response, including acute phase proteins, cytokines, and cellular adhesion molecules, have been evaluated as potential indicators of underlying atherosclerosis and as predictors of acute cardiovascular events.

C-reactive protein (CRP) is an acute-phase reactant protein produced by the liver.[9] Although a receptor for CRP is present on endotheial cells, controversy exists regarding whether CRP is simply a marker for systemic inflammation or participates actively in atheroma formation.[10,11] In the absence of acute illness or myocardial infarction, serum concentrations of CRP are relatively stable, although their concentrations are influenced by gender and ethnicity.

Epidemiologic studies have shown that the relative risk of future vascular events increases as the serum hs-CRP concentration increases.[9] Values >3 mg/L are associated with an increased risk for developing CVD; conversely, values <1 mg/L are associated with a low risk. Those between 1 and 3 mg/L are considered to be

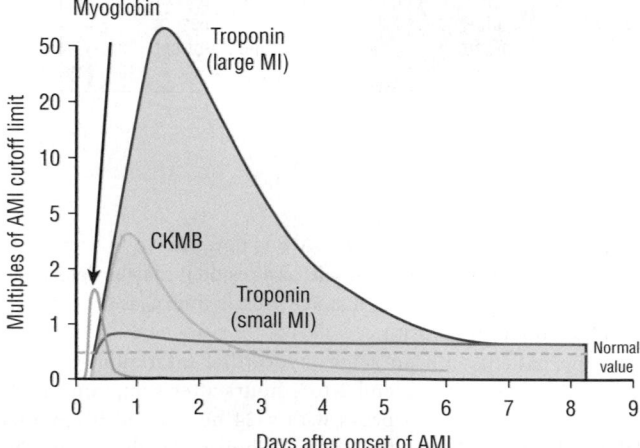

FIGURE 17-5. Time course of the appearance of various markers in the blood after acute myocardial infarction. *(Reprinted from JACC, Vol. 48, Jaffe et al, Biomarkers in Acute Cardiac Disease-The Present and the Future, page 4, Copyright © 2006, with permission from Elsevier.)*

TABLE 17-3	Conditions Associated With an Increased Serum Troponin Concentration
Myocardial infarction	Pulmonary embolism
Acute coronary syndrome	Strenuous exercise
Coronary intervention	Chemotherapy
Pericarditis	Severe asthma
Congestive heart failure	Respiratory distress
Cardiac defibrillation	Infiltrative disorders
Cardiac ablation	Acute limb ischemia
Cardiac contusion	Inflammatory disease
Tachycardia	Influenza
Aortic dissection	Hemodialysis
Stroke	Sepsis
Renal failure	Shock
Hyper- or hypotension	Rhabdomyolysis

at intermediate risk. To measure serum CRP concentrations accurately, a high-sensitive CRP (hs-CRP) assay is required. In an individual with an elevated serum CRP concentration, the measurement should be repeated several weeks later to exclude the possibility that an acute illness was responsible for the elevation. Measurements should not be taken when subjects are acutely ill (for example, with any acute febrile illness) or have a known autoimmune or rheumatologic disorder. Serum CRP concentrations above 10 mg/L are likely caused by an acute or chronic systemic illness.[12]

Although the relative risk of future vascular events increases as the serum concentration of hs-CRP increases, controversy continues as to whether hs-CRP concentrations provide sufficient incremental information above traditional risk factors to warrant routine testing in subjects without known CVD in an attempt to prevent an adverse event (so-called primary prevention).[9,13] Recent guidelines have suggested that CRP be used in patients who are considered (on the basis of traditional risk factors) to be at intermediate risk for coronary artery disease in an attempt to guide the intensity with which their risk factors are modified.[9] Only limited data have suggested that interventions that lower CRP concentrations (i.e., aspirin and statins) are beneficial.[14–16]

Multiple studies[17,18] of patients with acute coronary syndromes have demonstrated the capacity of hs-CRP concentrations—measured at the time of hospitalization or hospital discharge—to help to predict cardiovascular outcomes during the hospitalization or during long-term follow-up. This prognostic information appears to be independent of and complementary to data obtained from the history and electrocardiogram. Moreover, hs-CRP concentrations appear to provide additional prognostic information in patients with a normal cTn concentration,[19] and they may be useful for monitoring the response to statin therapy, in that those with low hs-CRP concentrations after statin therapy have better clinical outcomes than those in whom these concentrations are high.[14,16] Based on these data, the measurement of serum hs-CRP concentrations in patients with acute coronary syndromes is recommended as reasonable (class IIa) for risk stratification when additional prognostic information is desired.[5] In contrast, its routine use is not recommended in the absence of compelling data identifying its role in guiding specific therapy.

Other novel markers of inflammation that have been shown to provide prognostic information in patients with an acute coronary syndrome are myeloperoxidase, CD40 ligand, and P-selectin (a marker of platelet activation and a potential participant in plaque destabilization), interleukin 6, and fibrinogen.[3,5]

Markers of Hemodynamic Stress

B-type natriuretic peptide (BNP) and its precursor, N-terminal pro-brain natriuretic protein (NT-proBNP), are released from ventricular myocytes in response to increases in wall stress. As a result, their serum concentrations typically are increased in patients with congestive heart failure. They may also be elevated in patients with an acute coronary syndrome as a result of left ventricular systolic dysfunction, impairment of ventricular relaxation, and myocardial stunning.[5]

Since serum BNP and NT-proBNP concentrations manifest substantial biologic variability, their serum concentrations in an individual subject must increase or decrease at least 2-fold to provide assurance that a "real" change has occurred. In addition, when considering the normal range for an individual, one must be aware that considerable variation in serum concentrations exists according to age, gender, weight, and renal function. Women and older patients have a higher normal range, whereas obese patients have lower values than the nonobese. Patients with renal failure often have substantially higher values.

Elevated BNP and NT-proBNP concentrations support a suspected diagnosis of heart failure or lead to a suspicion of heart failure when a diagnosis is unclear. Conversely, a normal value (BNP <100 pg/mL or NT-proBNP <300 pg/mL) in an untreated patient strongly suggests that heart failure is not present.[20,21] In a study of 1,568 patients seeking medical attention because of acute dyspnea, plasma BNP was significantly higher in those with clinically diagnosed heart failure than in those without (mean value, 675 compared with 110 pg/mL, respectively), with intermediate values in those with known heart failure but with a noncardiac cause of dyspnea (mean, 346 pg/mL).[22]

Plasma BNP concentrations provide prognostic information in patients with acute decompensated heart failure: in-hospital mortality is 3-fold higher in those in the highest BNP quartile when compared to the lowest quartile.[23] Similarly, in patients with compensated CHF, plasma BNP concentrations provide valuable prognostic information, in that each 100 pg/mL increase in plasma BNP in these subjects is associated with a 35% increase in the relative risk of death.[24] Although the measurement of BNP can be used for prognostic purposes in patients with CHF, its role in assessing treatment efficacy and modifying drug therapy is not clearly established.

Elevated plasma concentrations of BNP and NT-pro BNP have been observed in subjects with heart failure with depressed left ventricular systolic function, heart failure with preserved left ventricular systolic function, elevated left ventricular filling pressures, left ventricular hypertrophy, atrial fibrillation, and myocardial ischemia. They may be elevated in certain noncardiac conditions, including pulmonary embolism, chronic obstructive pulmonary disease, hypoxemia, sepsis, cirrhosis, and renal failure. As a result, values of BNP or NT-pro BNP should not be used in isolation either to confirm or to refute a diagnosis of heart failure.

Elevated serum concentrations of BNP and NT-proBNP may be detected in patients with acute coronary syndrome. Data from at least 10 studies have indicated that BNP and NT-proBNP are among the most robust predictors of death and heart failure in patients hospitalized with acute coronary syndrome.[5,25–27] Nonetheless, data regarding the potential for these substances to guide specific therapeutic decisions, such as whether to perform coronary angiography and revascularization, have been mixed. At present, therefore, the use of BNP and NT-proBNP in patients with acute coronary syndrome is limited to risk stratification, for which they can be used to help in the assessment of prognosis.

CHEST RADIOGRAPHY

The chest radiograph provides supplemental information to the physical examination. Although it does not provide detailed information about internal cardiac structures, it can provide information about the position and size of the heart and its chambers as well as adjacent structures. The standard chest radiographs for evaluation of the lungs and heart are standing posteroanterior and lateral views taken with maximal inspiration; portable chest radiographs usually are less helpful. When possible, previous radiographs should be obtained for comparison.

The posteroanterior chest radiograph outlines the superior vena cava, right atrium, aortic knob, main pulmonary artery, left atrial appendage (especially if enlarged), and left ventricle. In the lateral view, the chest radiograph allows one to assess the right ventricle, inferior vena cava, and left ventricle. These structures are visualized as shadows of differing density rather than as discrete entities.

Cardiac enlargement is determined by the cardiothoracic ratio (CTR), which is the maximal transverse diameter of the heart divided by the maximal transverse diameter of the thorax on the posteroanterior view. The CTR normally is ≤0.45, but it may be higher (i.e., ≤0.55) in subjects with a large stroke volume (e.g., highly conditioned athletes). Certain cardiac conditions, such as heart failure and hypertension, may cause cardiac enlargement, with a resultant high CTR. Individual chamber enlargement can be seen on the chest radiograph. Right ventricular enlargement is best seen on the lateral film, on which the heart appears to occupy the retrosternal space. Left atrial enlargement is suspected if there is elevation of the left bronchus or an enlarged atrial appendage. Left ventricular enlargement is the most common feature identified on chest radiography and is seen as a lateral and downward displacement of the cardiac apex. A large pericardial effusion may appear as a large heart on a chest radiograph, but, in contrast to heart failure, pulmonary vascular congestion is not present (see below).

The pulmonary vessels are examined for size and filling. With diminished pulmonary blood flow, as would be present in the patient with tetralogy of Fallot or pulmonic valvular stenosis, the peripheral pulmonary vessels are small in caliber and under-filled. Increased pulmonary blood flow, as occurs with a high cardiac output or left-to-right intracardiac shunting, may lead to enlargement and tortuosity of the central and peripheral pulmonary vessels. Pulmonary arterial hypertension (increased pulmonary resistance) is identified by enlargement of the central pulmonary arteries and diminished peripheral perfusion. Elevated pulmonary venous pressure—usually as a result of an elevated left atrial pressure—is characterized by dilation of vessels in the upper lung zones (e.g., cephalization of flow), owing to recruitment of upper lung vessels when blood is diverted from the constricted vessels in the lower lung zones.

Congestive heart failure causes Kerley B lines (edema of interlobular septa), which appear as thin, horizontal reticular lines in the costophrenic angles. As pulmonary venous pressure increases, alveolar edema becomes evident, and pleural effusions may appear as blunting of the costophrenic angles.

ELECTROCARDIOGRAPHY

❹ The electrocardiogram (ECG) is a graphic recording of the electrical potentials generated by the heart. The signals are detected by using electrodes attached to the extremities and chest wall (Figs. 17–6 and 17–7), which are then amplified and recorded

(Fig. 17–8). The ECG leads display the instantaneous differences in potential between electrodes. As electrical activity approaches the positive electrode of the lead, it registers a positive (upright) deflection on the ECG, whereas electrical activity in the opposite direction of the positive electrode of the lead registers a negative (downward) deflection.

The ECG can be used to detect arrhythmias, conduction disturbances, myocardial ischemia or infarction, metabolic disturbances that may result in lethal arrhythmias (e.g., hyperkalemia), and increased susceptibility to sudden cardiac death (e.g., prolonged QT interval). It is simple to perform, noninvasive, and inexpensive.

Depolarization of the heart initiates cardiac contraction. The electrical current that depolarizes the heart originates in special cardiac pacemaker cells located in the sinoatrial (SA) node, or sinus node, which is located in the upper right atrium near the insertion of the superior vena cava (Fig. 17–9). The depolarization wave is transmitted through the atria, which initiates atrial contraction. Subsequently, the impulse is transmitted through specialized conduction tissues in (a) the atrioventricular (AV) node, which is located in the inferior right atrium near the tricuspid valve; (b) the bundle of His, which is located in the interventricular septum; and (c) the right and left bundles, which rapidly conduct the electrical impulse to the right and left ventricular myocardium via (d) the Purkinje fibers. The depolarization wavefront then spreads through the ventricular muscle, from endocardium to epicardium, triggering ventricular contraction.

The ECG waveforms (Fig. 17–10), which are recorded during electrical depolarization of the heart, are labeled alphabetically and are read from left to right, beginning with the P wave, which represents depolarization of the atria. The normal duration of the P wave is up to 0.12 second. The *PR segment,* created by passage of the impulse through the AV node and the bundle of His and its branches, has a duration of 0.12 to 0.20 second. The *QRS complex* represents electrical depolarization of the ventricles. Initially, a negative deflection (the Q wave) appears, followed by a positive deflection, the R wave, and finally a negative deflection, the S wave. The normal duration of the QRS complex is <0.12 second. Since the left ventricle is much thicker than the right ventricle, most of the electrical wavefront is directed toward the former. Accordingly, the precordial leads positioned over the left ventricle (leads V_5 and V_6) demonstrate a positive (upright) QRS complex, whereas those positioned over the right ventricle (V_1 and V_2) record a negative (downward) QRS complex.

Following the QRS complex is a plateau phase called the *ST segment,* which extends from the end of the QRS complex (called the *J point*) to the beginning of the T wave. When ischemia occurs, one may observe depression of the ST segment (Fig. 17–11A). When infarction from total obstruction of a coronary artery occurs, ST segment elevation may be observed (Fig. 17–11B). Repolarization of the ventricle leads to the T wave. The T wave usually goes in the same direction as the QRS complex.

The *QT interval*—measured from the beginning of the QRS complex to the end of the T wave—includes the time required for ventricular depolarization and repolarization, and it varies inversely with heart rate. A rate-related ("corrected") QT interval (QTc) can be calculated as QT√R-R interval; it should be <0.44 second. A prolonged QTc interval is caused by abnormalities in depolarization or repolarization that are associated with sudden cardiac death. QTc prolongation may be due to genetic defects in action potential ion channels (e.g., congenital long QT syndrome), drugs (Table 17–4), or electrolyte disturbances (i.e., hypokalemia, hypocalcemia, hypomagnesemia). Regardless of the cause, QT prolongation increases susceptibility to a potentially lethal arrhythmia, torsades de pointes (a type of ventricular tachycardia).

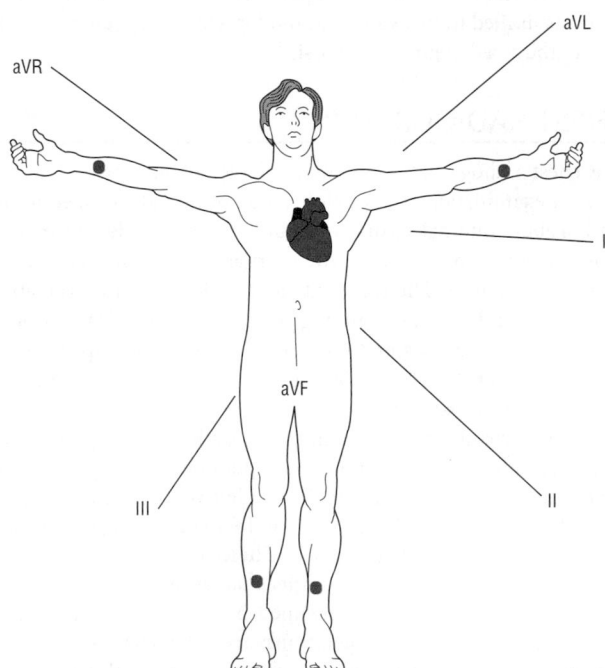

FIGURE 17-6. With electrodes (depicted as dots) attached to each arm and leg, electrical activity on the torso (i.e., frontal plane) is recorded from six different directions. These are known as the limb leads; leads I, II, III, aVF, aVL, and aVR.

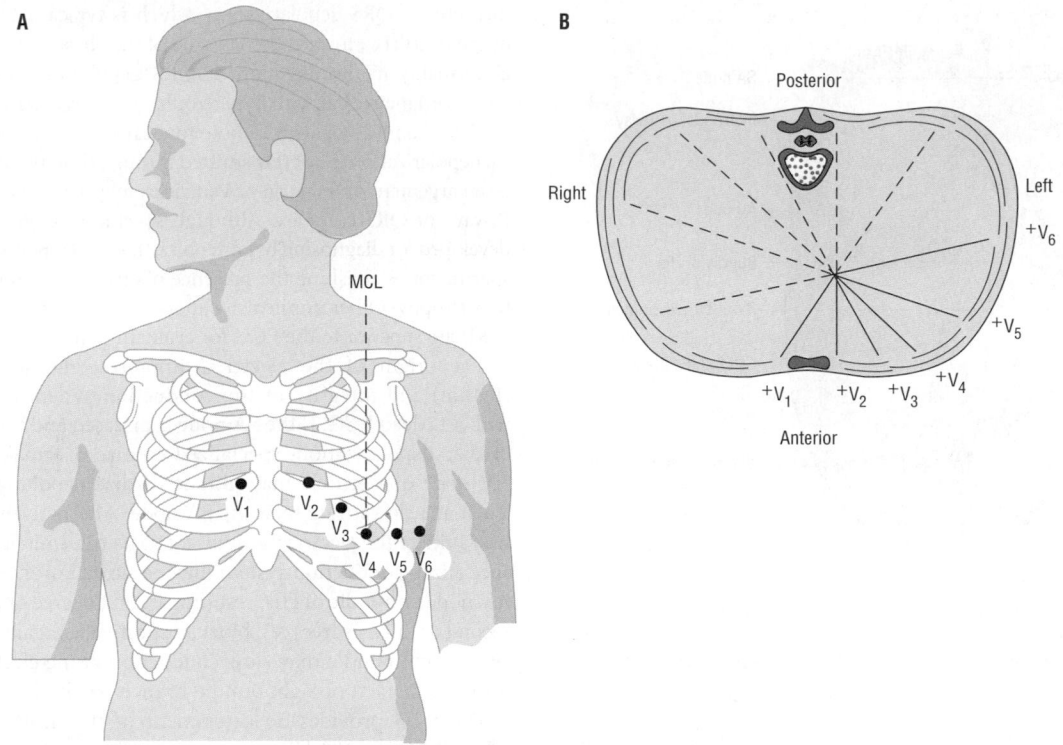

FIGURE 17-7. **A.** Electrode positions of the precordial leads. (MCL, midclavicular line; V1, fourth intercostal space at the right sternal border; V_2, fourth intercostal space at the left sternal border; V_3, halfway between V_2 and V_4; V_4, fifth intercostal space at the midclavicular line; V_5, anterior axillary line directly lateral to V_4; V_6, anterior axillary space directly lateral to V_5.). **B.** The precordial reference figure. Leads V_1 and V_2 are called right-sided precordial leads; leads V_3 and V_4, midprecordial leads; and leads V_5 and V_6, left-sided precordial leads. *(Redrawn from Kinney MR, Packa DR, eds. Andreoli's Comprehensive Cardiac Care, 8th ed. St. Louis: Mosby, 1996, with permission.)*

The 12 conventional ECG leads record the electrical potential difference between electrodes placed on the surface of the body (Fig. 17–9). The 6 frontal plane and the 6 horizontal plane leads provide a three-dimensional representation of cardiac electrical activity. Each lead provides the opportunity to view atrial and ventricular depolarization from a different angle, much the same way that multiple video cameras positioned in different locations can view an event from different perspectives.

The 6 frontal leads can be subdivided into those that view electrical potentials directed inferiorly (leads II, III, aVF), laterally

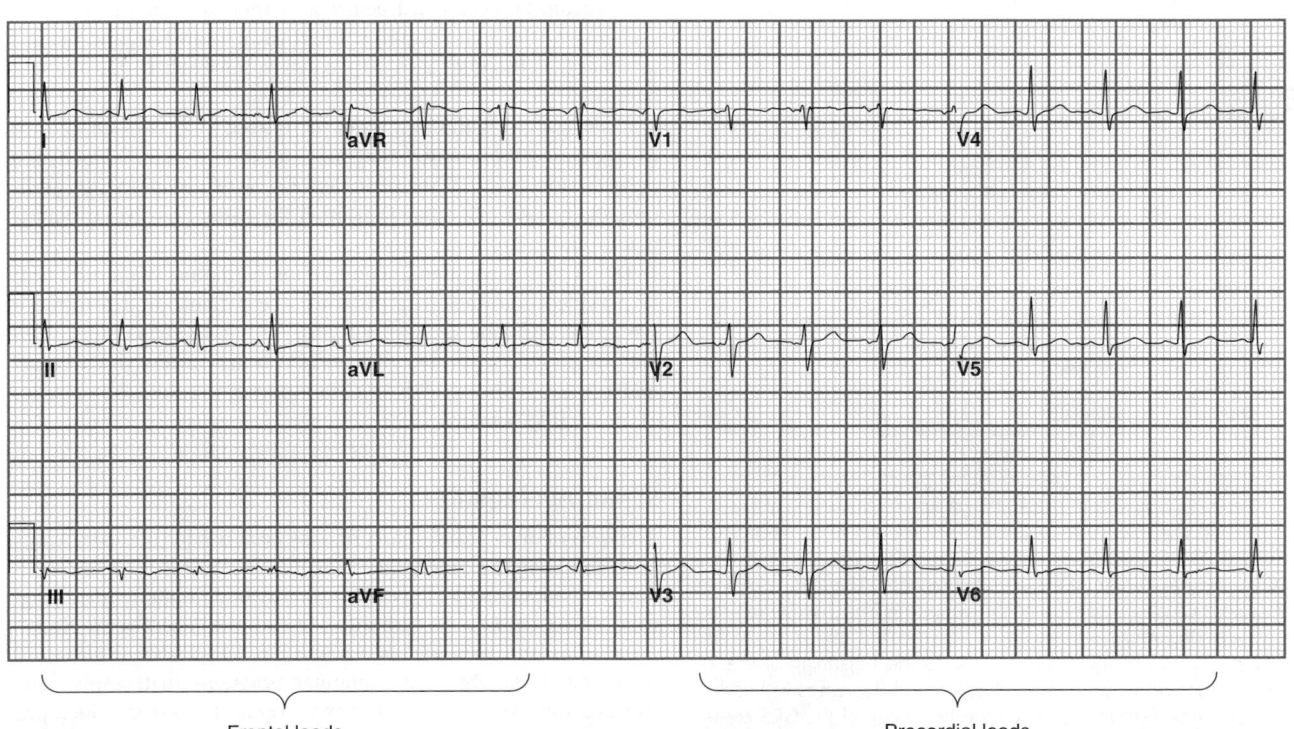

FIGURE 17-8. Standard 12-lead electrocardiogram, with 6 frontal and 6 precordial leads.

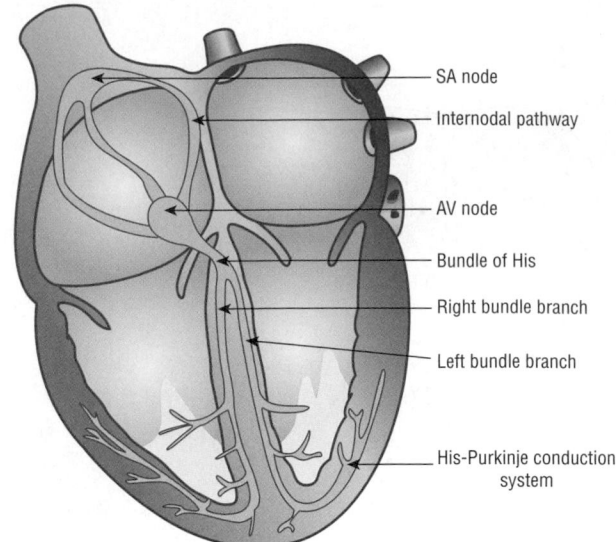

FIGURE 17-9. Schematic representation of the cardiac conduction system. (AV, atrioventricular; SA, sinoatrial.) *(From Vijayaraman P, Ellenbogen KA. Bradyarrhythmias and Pacemakers. In: Fuster V, O'Rourke RA, Walsh RA, Poole-Wilson P: Hurst's the Heart, 12th ed. New York: McGraw-Hill, 2004:1021.)*

(leads I, aVL), or rightward (aVR). Likewise, the 6 precordial leads can be subdivided into those that view electrical potentials directed toward the septal (leads V_1, V_2), apical (leads V_3, V_4), or lateral (leads V_5, V_6) regions of the heart. Thus, when ischemia or infarction-related ECG changes occur, the region of the heart affected can be localized by determining which leads manifest abnormalities.

The mean orientation of the QRS vector with reference to the 6 frontal plane leads is known as the QRS axis. It describes the "major"

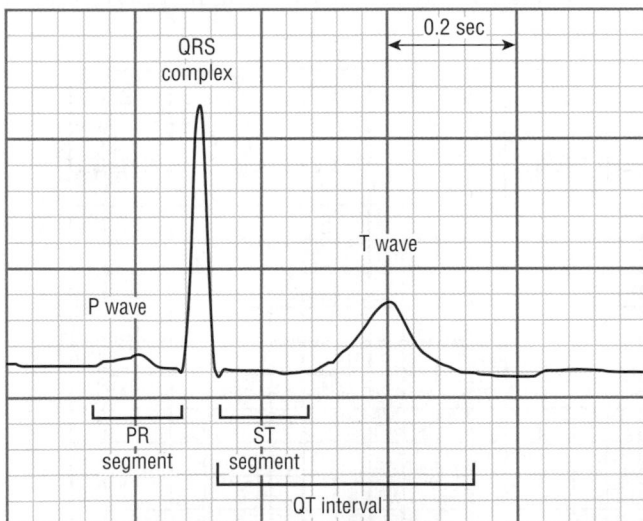

FIGURE 17-10. ECG waveforms are labeled alphabetically and are read from left to right. The *P wave* represents depolarization of the atria. The *PR segment* is created by passage of the impulse through the atrioventricular node and the bundle of His and its branches. The *QRS complex* represents electrical depolarization of the ventricles. The *T wave* results from ventricular depolarization. A plateau phase called the *ST segment* extends from the end of the QRS complex to the beginning of the T wave. The ST segment elevates with infarction and depresses with ischemia. The *QT interval*—measured from the beginning of the QRS complex to the end of the T wave—includes the time required for ventricular depolarization and repolarization.

direction of QRS depolarization, which is typically toward the apex of the heart (i.e., toward the left side of the chest and downward). An abnormality in the direction of QRS depolarization (so-called axis deviation) may occur with hypertrophy or enlargement of one or more cardiac chambers or with remote myocardial infarction, since electrical depolarization is not transmitted through dead tissue. Hypertrophy or enlargement of the atria or ventricles may also affect the size of the P wave or QRS complex. Although specific ECG criteria have been developed for diagnosing hypertrophy, the ECG is neither sensitive nor specific for establishing the presence of atrial dilatation or ventricular hypertrophy. Other noninvasive modalities (i.e., echocardiography or MRI) are superior to the ECG for evaluating these conditions.

The origin of the electrical impulses (the so-called cardiac rhythm) and integrity of the conduction system can be assessed with a 12-lead ECG. If the SA node is diseased and unable to initiate cardiac depolarization, specialized cardiac pacemaker cells in the AV node or ventricle may initiate cardiac depolarization instead, albeit at a slower rate than the SA node. Alternatively, the SA node may initiate the electrical impulse, but its transmission through the specialized conduction system may be slowed or interrupted in the AV node or bundle of His, resulting in first degree or advanced (i.e., second or third degree) AV block, respectively. Finally, disease in the left or right bundle may slow conduction of the electrical impulse, resulting in a left or right bundle-branch block, respectively.

The ECG provides an assessment of the heart rate, which is normally 60 to 100 beats per minute (bpm) at rest. Tachycardia is present when the heart rate exceeds 100 bpm, and bradycardia is present when it is <60 bpm. Tachycardia may originate in the SA node (sinus tachycardia), atrium (atrial flutter or fibrillation, ectopic atrial tachycardia, or multifocal atrial tachycardia), or AV node (junctional tachycardia or AV nodal reentry tachycardia). Collectively, these are termed supraventricular tachycardias. Alternatively, a tachycardia may have its origin in the right or left ventricle (ventricular tachycardia, ventricular fibrillation, and right ventricular outflow tract tachycardia).

Many drugs can affect the specialized cardiac pacemaker cells, causing tachycardia or bradycardia, or the conduction system, which may lead to AV block or sudden cardiac death. A resting ECG should be performed before and after the administration of such drugs, with examination of the rhythm, heart rate, and various intervals (i.e., PR, QRS, and QT) to determine if substantial changes have occurred.

In the patient with chest pain, the resting ECG is examined for ST segment abnormalities that may indicate myocardial ischemia or infarction (i.e., ST segment depression or elevation). In addition, the resting ECG may indicate if the patient has had a remote myocardial infarction.

The ECG is used often in conjunction with other diagnostic tests to provide additional data, monitor the patient, or determine if symptoms correlate with what is observed on the ECG. For example, the patient suspected of having coronary artery disease may undergo stress testing with ECG monitoring to assess the presence of provocable ischemia.

Signal-Averaged ECG

Survivors of myocardial infarction may be at risk for life-threatening arrhythmias. In these individuals, myocardial scar tissue creates zones of slow conduction that appear as low amplitude, high frequency signals that are continuous with the QRS complex. These small electrical currents (so-called late potentials) are not detectable on a routine, traditional ECG. By using computer programs that amplify and enhance the electrical signal, signal-averaged electrocardiography (SAECG) provides a high-resolution ECG that measures ventricular

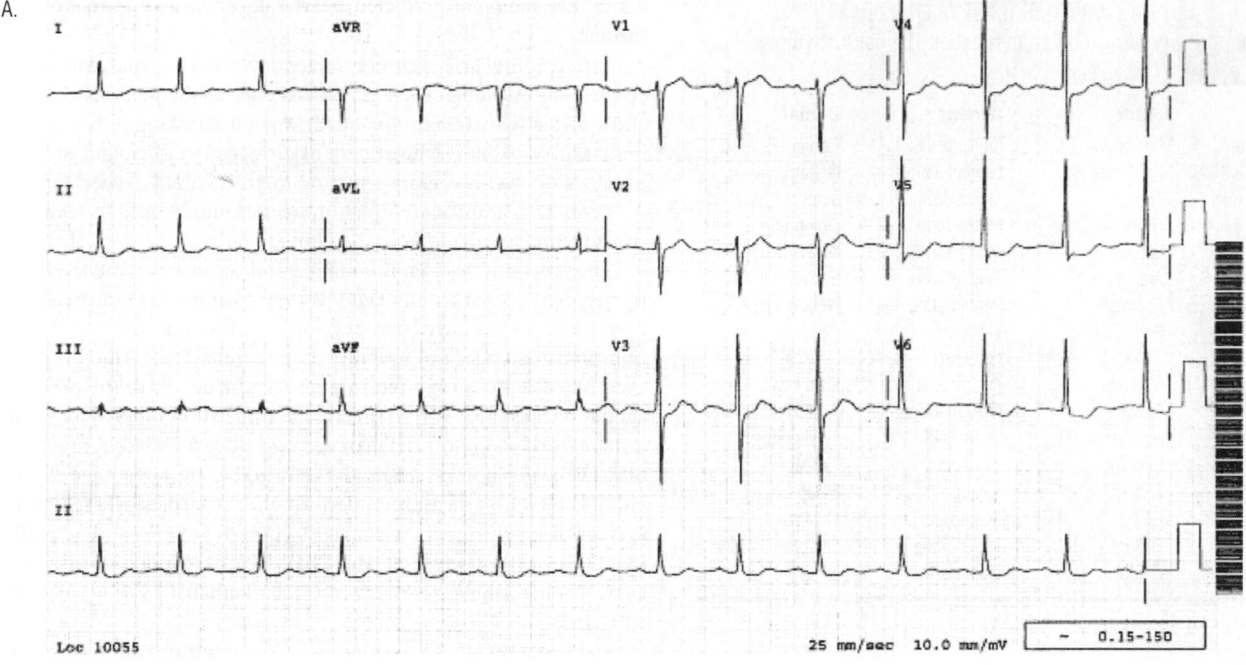

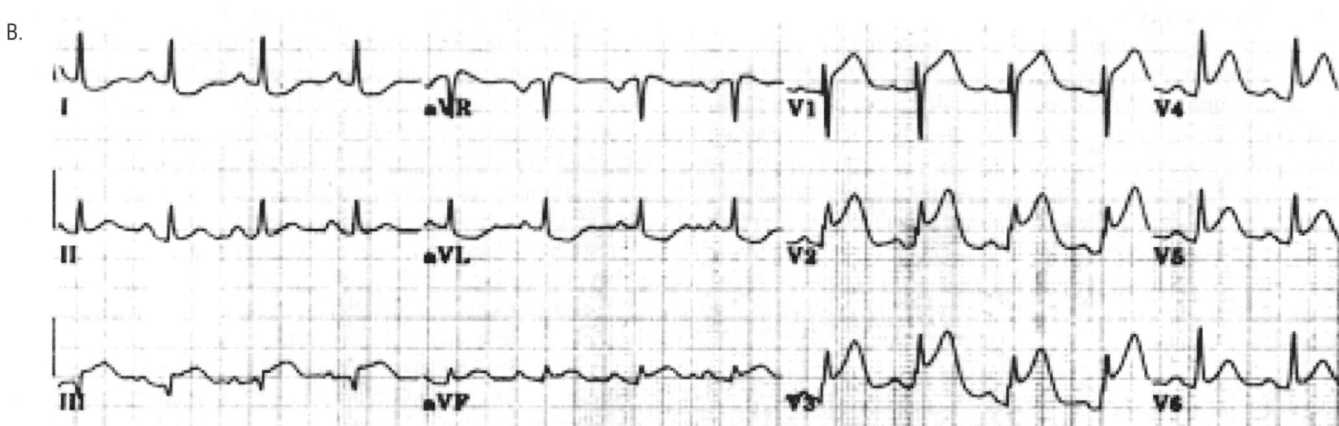

FIGURE 17-11. *A.* Electrocardiogram recorded during an episode of chest pain at rest in a patient with unstable angina. ST-segment depression >1 mm is present in leads V_4 to V_6. *B.* EKG from a patient with acute myocardial infarction. Note the ST segment elevation in the inferior (leads III and aVF) and precordial (leads V_1–V_6) leads, indicating that the inferior and anterior regions of the heart are affected. *(From Vijayaraman P, Ellenbogen KA. Bradyarrhythmias and Pacemakers. In: Fuster V, O'Rourke RA, Walsh RA, Poole-Wilson P: Hurst's the Heart, 12th ed. New York: McGraw-Hill, 2004:1046.)*

late potentials, thereby identifying patients at risk of sustained ventricular tachycardia after myocardial infarction.[28]

Patients with ischemic heart disease and unexplained syncope who are at risk for sustained ventricular tachycardia may be candidates for a SAECG. A SAECG may be useful in the patient with nonischemic cardiomyopathy and sustained ventricular tachycardia, detection of acute rejection following heart transplant, and assessment of the proarrhythmic potential of antiarrhythmic drugs.

AMBULATORY ELECTROCARDIOGRAPHIC MONITORING

Ambulatory electrocardiography (AECG), so-called Holter monitoring, can be used to detect, document, and characterize the cardiac rhythm or ECG abnormalities during ordinary daily activities. Current continuous AECG equipment is capable of providing an analysis of cardiac electrical activity, including arrhythmias, ST segment abnormalities, and heart rate variability. An AECG can be

obtained with continuous recorders (Holter monitors) or intermittent recorders.

During continuous Holter monitoring, the patient wears a portable ECG recorder (weighing 8 to 16 oz) that is attached to 2 to 4 leads placed on the chest wall. During monitoring, the patient maintains a diary, in which he/she records the occurrence, duration, and severity of symptoms (e.g., lightheadedness, chest pain, palpitations, etc). The device is typically worn for 24 to 48 hours, after which the continuous ECG recording is scanned by computer to detect arrhythmias or ST segment abnormalities.

Intermittent recorders (also known as event monitors or loop recorders) are worn for longer periods of time (weeks to months). Although they continuously monitor the ECG, only brief (minutes) segments of it are recorded when the patient activates the device (i.e., when symptoms occur) or a preprogrammed abnormal ECG event occurs. Some intermittent event recorders incorporate a memory loop that permits capture of a rhythm recording during fleeting symptoms, tachycardia onset, and, in some cases, syncope that occurs infrequently. When the patient activates a looping

TABLE 17-4 Drugs With Known Risk of QT interval Prolongation and Potentially Lethal Arrhythmia (Torsades de Pointes)

Generic	Brand	Generic	Brand
Amiodarone	Cordarone	Ibutilide	Corvert
Amiodarone	Pacerone	Levomethadyl	Orlaam
Arsenic trioxide	Trisenox	Mesoridazine	Serentil
Astemizole	Hismanal	Methadone	Dolophine
Bepridil	Vascor	Methadone	Methadose
Chloroquine	Aralen	Pentamidine	Pentam
Chlorpromazine	Thorazine	Pentamidine	NebuPent
Cisapride	Propulsid	Pimozide	Orap
Clarithromycin	Biaxin	Probucol	Lorelco
Disopyramide	Norpace	Procainamide	Pronestyl
Dofetilide	Tikosyn	Procainamide	Procan
Domperidone	Motilium	Quinidine	Cardioquin
Droperidol	Inapsine	Quinidine	Quinaglute
Erythromycin	Erythrocin	Sotalol	Betapace
Erythromycin	E.E.S.	Sparfloxacin	Zagam
Halofantrine	Halfan	Terfenadine	Seldane
Haloperidol	Haldol	Thioridazine	Mellaril

monitor, it records several minutes of the preceding rhythm as well as the subsequent rhythm.

When monitoring is performed to evaluate the cause of intermittent symptoms, the frequency of symptoms dictates the type of recording. Continuous recordings are indicated for the assessment of frequent (at least once a day) symptoms that may be related to disturbances of heart rhythm, for the assessment of syncope or near syncope, and for patients with recurrent unexplained palpitations. In contrast, for patients whose symptoms are infrequent, intermittent event recorders may be more cost-effective in attempting to determine the cause of symptoms. For patients receiving antiarrhythmic drug therapy, continuous monitoring is indicated to assess drug response and to exclude proarrhythmia.

EXERCISE STRESS TESTING

⑤ Exercise stress testing, a well-established, relatively low-cost procedure, has been in widespread use for decades. It may be performed (a) to evaluate an individual's exercise capacity; (b) to assess the presence of myocardial ischemia in the patient with symptoms suggestive of coronary artery disease; (c) to obtain prognostic information in the patient with known coronary artery disease or recent myocardial infarction; (d) to evaluate the severity of valvular abnormalities; or (e) to assess the presence of arrhythmias or conduction abnormalities in the patient with exercise-induced cardiac symptoms (i.e., palpitations, lightheadedness, or syncope).

The patient who is to undergo an exercise stress test should fast for several hours beforehand and dress appropriately for exercise. Before exercise begins, a limited cardiac examination is performed (i.e., auscultation of the lungs and heart); blood pressure and heart rate are measured and the values recorded; and a standard 12-lead ECG is recorded. Exercise is then initiated, and the ECG, heart rate, and blood pressure are monitored carefully and recorded as the intensity of exercise increases incrementally. The patient is monitored for the development of symptoms (i.e., chest pain, dyspnea, lightheadedness, etc.), transient rhythm disturbances, ST segment abnormalities, and other electrocardiographic manifestations of myocardial ischemia. Exercise is terminated with the onset of limiting symptoms, diagnostic electrocardiographic (e.g., ST segment) changes, arrhythmias, or a decrease in blood pressure >10 mm Hg. Otherwise, exercise is continued until the patient achieves 85% of

his or her maximal predicted heart rate or is unable to exercise further.

Both treadmill and cycle ergometer devices are available for exercise testing. Although cycle ergometers are less expensive, smaller, and quieter than treadmills, quadricep muscle fatigue is a major limitation in patients who are not experienced cyclists, and subjects usually stop cycling before reaching their maximal oxygen uptake. As a result, treadmills are much more commonly used for exercise stress testing, particularly in the United States.

With treadmill testing, the incline and/or speed of the treadmill is increased incrementally every 2 to 3 minutes. Several treadmill exercise protocols have been developed to accommodate the variations in fitness, age, and mobility of individuals. Accordingly, if the exercise capacity is reported in minutes, the details of the protocol should be specified. Alternatively, the translation of exercise duration or workload into METs (oxygen uptake expressed in multiples of basal oxygen uptake, 3.5 mLO$_2$/kg/min) has the advantage of providing a common measure of performance regardless of the type of exercise test or protocol used. Most domestic chores and activities require <5 METs, whereas participation in strenuous sports, such as swimming, singles tennis, football, basketball, or skiing, requires >10 METs.

Interpretation of the results of exercise testing should include exercise capacity as well as the clinical, hemodynamic, and electrocardiographic responses. The occurrence of chest pain consistent with angina is important, particularly if it results in termination of the test. Abnormalities in exercise capacity, the response of systolic blood pressure to exercise, and the response of heart rate to exercise and recovery may provide valuable information. The most important electrocardiographic findings are ST segment depression and elevation. A positive exercise test is said to have occurred if the ECG shows at least 1 mm of horizontal or downsloping ST segment depression or elevation for at least 60 to 80 milliseconds after the end of the QRS complex.

ST segment changes suggestive of myocardial ischemia that occur at a low level of exercise (<6 minutes of exercise or <5 METS) are associated with more severe coronary artery disease and a worse prognosis than those that occur at a higher workload. An estimate of myocardial oxygen demands can be obtained by calculating the so-called "rate-pressure product" (double product) (i.e., heart rate × systolic arterial pressure).

Most treadmill exercise testing is performed in adults with symptoms of known or suspected ischemic heart disease. In patients for whom the diagnosis of coronary artery disease is certain, stress testing is often used for risk stratification or prognostic assessment to determine the need for possible coronary angiography or revascularization. Patients who are candidates for exercise testing may (a) have stable chest pain; (b) be stabilized by medical therapy following an episode of unstable chest pain; or (c) be post-myocardial infarction or post-revascularization.

The ability of the exercise stress test to identify (or to exclude) individuals with coronary artery disease is influenced by (a) their exercise capacity (i.e., can the individual perform maximal or nearly maximal exercise?); (b) the presence of baseline electrocardiographic abnormalities (i.e., bundle-branch block or ST segment depression); (c) medications that affect the electrocardiogram or the hemodynamic response to exercise (i.e., digoxin and beta-adrenergic blocking agents, respectively); and (d) concomitant cardiac conditions that are associated with electrocardiographic abnormalities (i.e., left ventricular hypertrophy, paced rhythm, pre-excitation) (Table 17–5). Thus, patients who are unable to exercise or who have baseline ECG abnormalities require imaging (i.e., radionuclide or echocardiographic) stress testing to detect (or to exclude) coronary artery disease, since routine stress testing is unreliable in these individuals.

TABLE 17-5 Meta-Analyses of Exercise Testing

Grouping	Number of Studies	Total Number of Patients	Sens (%)	Spec (%)	Predictive Accuracy (%)
Meta-analysis of standard exercise test	147	24,047	68	77	73
Meta-analysis without MI	58	11,691	67	72	69
Meta-analysis without workup bias	3	>1000	50	90	69
Meta-analysis with ST depression	22	9153	69	70	69
Meta-analysis without ST depression	3	840	67	84	75
Meta-analysis with digoxin	15	6338	68	74	71
Meta-analysis without digoxin	9	3548	72	69	70
Meta-analysis with LVH	15	8016	68	69	68
Meta-analysis without LVH	10	1977	72	77	74

Sens indicates sensitivity; Spec, specificity; MI, myocardial infarction; and LVH, left ventricular hypertrophy.

From Gibbons RJ, Balady GJ, Bricker JT, et al. ACC/AHA 2002 guideline update for exercise testing: a report of the American College of Cardiology/American Heart Association Task Force on Practice Guidelines (Committee on Exercise Testing); 2002. American College of Cardiology Website. www.acc.org/clinical/guidelines/exercise/dirIndex.htm.

The ability of the exercise stress test to identify the presence of coronary artery disease is influenced by the pretest probability of coronary artery disease in the population tested. For example, exercise-induced ST segment depression in a 60-year-old man with typical anginal chest pain and multiple risk factors for atherosclerosis (i.e., a high pretest probability) is considered a "true positive" stress test, whereas the same findings in a 30-year-old woman with chest pain believed to be atypical for angina (i.e., a low pretest probability) is most likely to be a "false-positive" test. The relatively poor accuracy of the exercise ECG for diagnosing coronary artery disease in asymptomatic subjects has led to the recommendation that exercise testing not be used as a screening tool,[29] since false-positive tests are common among asymptomatic adults, especially women, and may lead to unnecessary testing and treatment.

The ACC and AHA have jointly developed guidelines describing the indications for exercise stress testing.[29,30]

Exercise stress testing is relatively safe, with an estimated risk of acute myocardial infarction or death of 1 per 2,500 tests. It should be supervised by a physician or a properly trained health professional working directly under the supervision of a physician, who should be in the immediate vicinity and available for emergencies. Exercise stress testing is contraindicated in subjects who are unable to exercise or who should not exercise because of physiologic or psychological limitations (Table 17–6). Although unstable angina is usually a contraindication to exercise stress testing, it can be performed safely once the patient has responded appropriately to intensive medical therapy. Exercise testing is contraindicated in patients with untreated life-threatening arrhythmias or congestive heart failure. Patients with comorbid diseases, such as chronic obstructive pulmonary disease or peripheral vascular disease, may be limited in their exercise capacity. For patients with disabilities or other medical conditions that limit their exercise capacity, pharmacologic stress testing (with dipyridamole, adenosine, or dobutamine) is an alternative (see Pharmacologic Stress Testing below).

Drug therapy is not routinely altered before exercise stress testing, since few data suggest that doing so improves its diagnostic accuracy. Although patients receiving a beta-adrenergic or calcium channel blocker may have a blunted increase in heart rate and blood pressure with exercise, exercise stress testing in such patients nonetheless provides information regarding exercise capacity and ischemic ECG alterations. Nitrates do not directly alter exercise capacity, but they may increase the patient's exercise capacity by preventing or relieving exercise-induced angina. Digoxin interferes with the interpretation of ST segment alterations, and patients taking it rarely manifest ST segment depression of more than 1 mm even in the face of substantial myocardial ischemia. Because of its long half-life, discontinuing digoxin immediately before the test does not ameliorate its effects.

ECHOCARDIOGRAPHY

❼ Using echocardiography, one can evaluate cardiac function and structure with images produced by ultrasound. High frequency sound waves transmitted from a hand-held transducer "bounce" off tissue and are reflected back to the transducer, where the waves are collected and used to construct a real-time image of the heart.

With the exception of the ECG, echocardiography is the most frequently performed cardiovascular test. It is noninvasive, relatively inexpensive, safe, devoid of ionizing radiation, and portable, so that it can be done at the patient's bedside, in the operating room, or in the physician's office. Serial echocardiograms can be performed, especially following a cardiac procedure or a change in clinical condition, as well as to follow the progression of the underlying cardiac disease over time. It is the procedure of choice for the diagnosis and evaluation of many cardiac conditions, including valvular abnormalities, intracardiac thrombi, pericardial effusions, and congenital abnormalities. Echocardiography often is used to assess chamber sizes, function, and wall thickness. In the patient suspected of having CAD, echocardiography can be performed before, during, and immediately after exercise or pharmacologic stress (e.g., dobutamine) to evaluate the presence of ischemia-induced ventricular wall motion abnormalities.

Two approaches to echocardiography are used in clinical practice. Transthoracic echocardiography (TTE) is performed with the transducer positioned on the anterior chest wall, whereas transesophageal echocardiography (TEE) is performed with the transducer

TABLE 17-6 Contraindications to Exercise Testing

Absolute
Acute myocardial infarction (within 2 days)
High-risk unstable angina
Uncontrolled cardiac arrhythmias causing symptoms or hemodynamic compromise
Symptomatic severe aortic stenosis
Uncontrolled symptomatic heart failure
Acute pulmonary embolus or pulmonary infarction
Acute myocarditis or pericarditis
Acute aortic dissection

Relative
Left main coronary stenosis
Moderate stenotic valvular heart disease
Electrolyte abnormalities
Severe arterial hypertension
Tachyarrhythmias or bradyarrhythmias
Hypertrophic cardiomyopathy and other forms of outflow tract obstruction
Mental or physical impairment leading to inability to exercise adequately
High-degree atrioventricular block

Adapted from AHA/ACC guidelines.

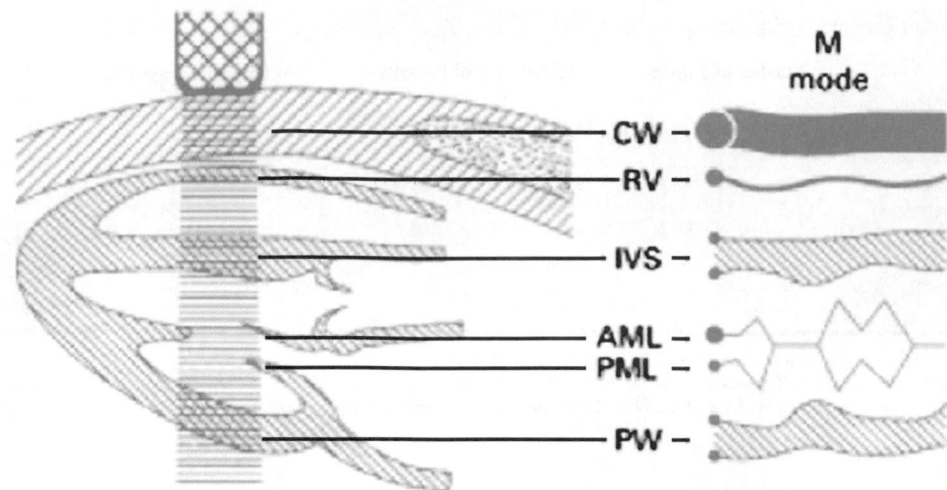

FIGURE 17-12. M-mode echocardiogram. The transducer emits an ultrasound beam, which reflects at each anatomic interface. The reflected wavefronts are detected by the probe, which records the images of cardiac structures in one plane, producing a static picture of a small region of the heart, a so-called "ice pick view." (AML, anterior mitral leaflet; CW, chest wall; IVS, interventricular septum; PML, posterior mitral leaflet; PW, posterior wall; RV, right ventricle.) *(Modified from Hagan AD, DeMaria AN. Clinical Applications of Two-Dimensional Echocardiography and Cardiac Doppler. Boston, MA: Little, Brown; 1989, with permission.) (From Fuster V. O'Rourke RA, Walsh RA, Poole-Wilson P: Hurst's The Heart, 12th ed. http://www.accessmedicine.com. Copyright © The McGraw-Hill Companies, Inc. All rights reserved.)*

positioned in the esophagus. Following transducer placement, several modes of operation are possible: M-mode (motion), two-dimensional (2D), three-dimensional (3D), and Doppler imaging.

With M-mode echocardiography, a transducer placed at a site on the anterior chest (usually along the sternal border) records the images of cardiac structures in one plane, producing a static picture of a small region of the heart, a so-called "ice pick view" (Fig. 17–12). Results depend on the exact placement of the transducer with respect to the underlying structures. Conventional M-mode echocardiography provides visualization of the right ventricle, left ventricle, and posterior left ventricular wall and pericardium. If the transducer is swept in an arc from the apex to the base of the heart, virtually the whole heart can be visualized, including the valves and left atrium.

Two-dimensional echocardiography employs multiple windows of the heart, and each view provides a wedge-shaped image (Figs. 17–13 and 17–14). These views are processed to produce a motion picture of the beating heart. When compared to M-mode echocardiography, two-dimensional echocardiography provides increased accuracy in calculating ventricular volumes, wall thickness, and the severity of valvular stenoses.

Three-dimensional echocardiography, which uses an ultrasound probe with an array of transducers and an appropriate processing system, enables a detailed assessment of cardiac anatomy and pathology, particularly valvular abnormalities as well as ventricular size and function (Fig. 17–15). The ability to "slice" the heart in an infinite number of planes in an anatomically appropriate manner and to reconstruct 3D images of anatomic structures makes this technique very powerful in understanding congenital cardiac conditions.[31]

Doppler echocardiography is used to detect the velocity and direction of blood flow by measuring the change in frequency produced when ultrasound waves are reflected from red blood cells. Color enhancement allows blood flow direction and velocity to be visualized, with different colors used for antegrade and retrograde flow. Blood flow moving toward the transducer is displayed in red, and flow moving away from the transducer is displayed in blue; increasing velocity is depicted in brighter shades of each color. Thus, with Doppler echocardiography, information

regarding the presence, direction, velocity, and turbulence of blood flow can be acquired. Cardiac hemodynamic variables (e.g., intracardiac pressures) and the presence and severity of valvular disease can be assessed noninvasively with Doppler echocardiography.

When TTE is performed, the transducer is placed on the anterior chest wall, and imaging is performed in three orthogonal planes: long axis (from aortic root to apex), short axis (perpendicular to the long axis), and four-chamber (visualizing both ventricles and atria through the mitral and tricuspid valves) (Figs. 17–13 and 17–14). Sound energy is poorly transmitted through air and bone, and the ability to record adequate images is dependent on a thoracic window that gives the ultrasound beam adequate access to cardiac structures. Accordingly, in approximately 15% of subjects, suboptimal TTE images are obtained, particularly those with large lung volumes (i.e., chronic lung disease or those being ventilated mechanically) or marked obesity. In addition, TTE may not provide adequate or complete images of the posterior cardiac structures (i.e., left atrium, left atrial appendage, mitral valve, interatrial septum, descending aorta, etc.) that are located far away from the transducer.

With TEE, a flexible transducer is advanced into the esophagus and rests just behind the heart, adjacent to the left atrium and descending aorta. When compared with TTE, TEE provides more detailed images of the mitral valve, left atrium, left atrial appendage, pulmonary veins, and descending thoracic aorta. Because of the transducer's proximity to the heart, TEE allows one to delineate small cardiac structures (i.e., vegetations and thrombi <3mm in diameter) that may not be seen with TTE. As a result, TEE often is used to assess the presence of (a) mitral valve vegetations, (b) endocarditis complications (e.g., myocardial abscess), (c) left atrial appendage thrombus in the patient with a stroke or under consideration for an elective cardioversion, and (d) aortic dissection.[32-38] In addition, the transducer can be advanced into the fundus of the stomach to obtain images of the ventricles. TEE is widely utilized intraoperatively to assess the success of valve repair or replacement and to delineate cardiac anatomy in subjects with congenital heart disease at the time of surgical repair.

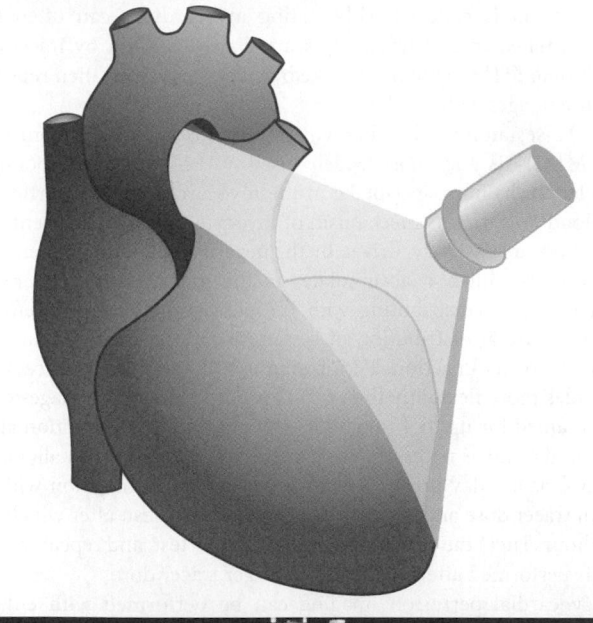

A

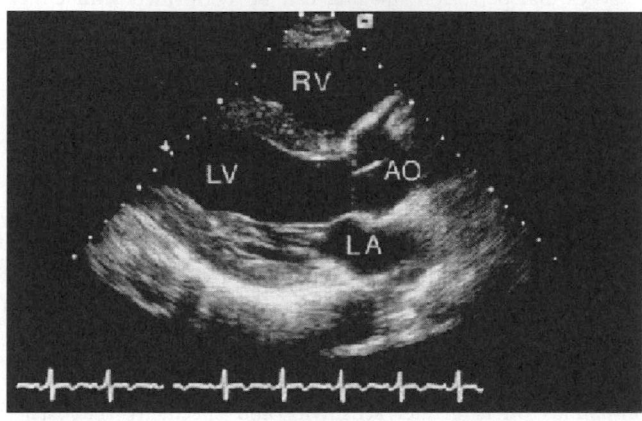

B

FIGURE 17-13. 2D transthoracic echocardiography. **A.** Orientation of the sector beam and transducer position for the parasternal long-axis view of the left ventricle. **B.** 2D image of the heart, parasternal long-axis view. (Ao, aorta; LA, left atrium; LV, left ventricle; RV, right ventricle.) *(From DeMaria AN, Daniel G. Blanchard DG. Echocardiography. In: Fuster V, O'Rourke RA, Walsh RA, Poole-Wilson P: Hurst's the Heart, 12th ed. New York: McGraw-Hill, 2004:369.)*

Although TEE is a low-risk invasive procedure, complications, such as tearing or perforation of the esophagus, esophageal burns, transient ventricular tachycardia, minor throat irritation, and transient vocal cord paralysis, occur rarely. In one series of 10,218 TEEs, 1 death (0.0098%) was reported.[39] TEE is contraindicated in patients with esophageal abnormalities, in whom passage of the transducer may be difficult or hazardous (e.g., esophageal strictures or varices).

The ACC/AHA task force has published guidelines for application of echocardiography and stress echocardiography.[35,40]

NUCLEAR CARDIOLOGY

❽ Myocardial perfusion imaging, the most commonly performed nuclear cardiology procedure, is used to assess the presence, location, and severity of ischemic or infarcted myocardium. It consists of a combination of (a) some form of stress (exercise or pharmacologic), (b) administration of a radiopharmaceutical, and (c) detection of the radiopharmaceutical in the myocardium via a nuclear camera positioned adjacent to the subject's chest wall.

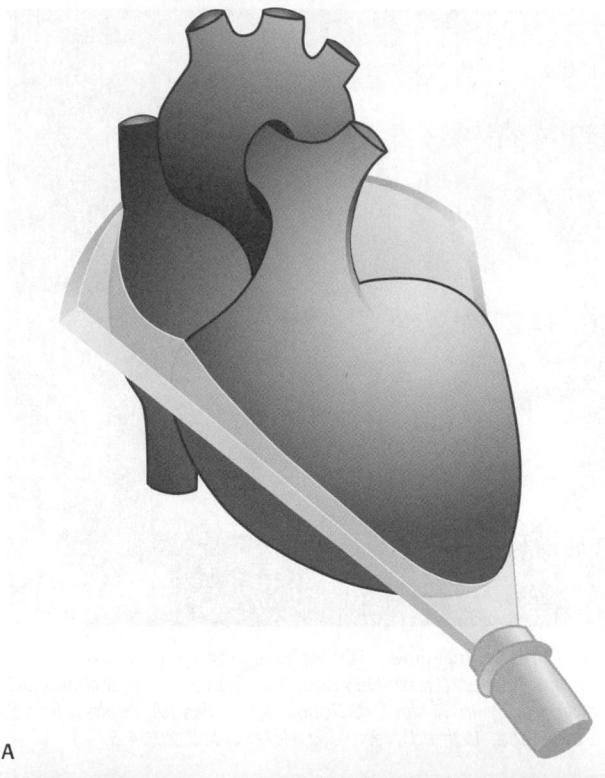

A

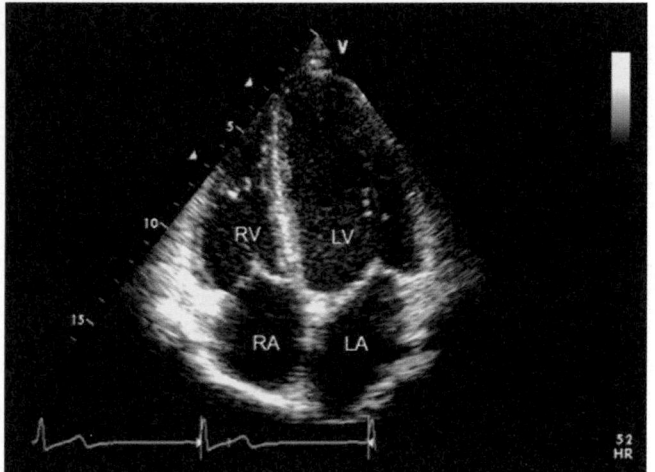

B

FIGURE 17-14. 2D transthoracic echocardiography. **A.** Orientation of the sector beam and transducer position for the apical four-chamber plane. **B.** 2D image of the apical four-chamber plane. (LA, left atrium; LV, left ventricle; RA, right atrium; RV, right ventricle.) *(From DeMaria AN, Daniel G. Blanchard DG. Echocardiography. In: Fuster V, O'Rourke RA, Walsh RA, Poole-Wilson P: Hurst's the Heart, 12th ed. New York: McGraw-Hill, 2004:372.)*

The most widely used radionuclides are technetium sestamibi or tetrofosmin-99m (^{99m}Tc-sestamibi or ^{99m}Tc-tetroforsmin) and thallium-201 (^{201}Tl). ^{99m}Tc is ideal for clinical imaging because it has a short half-life (about 6 hours) and can be generated in-house with a benchtop generator, thereby providing immediate availability. Because of its short half-life, repeat injections can be given to evaluate the efficacy of reperfusion therapy. ^{201}Tl has a much longer half-life (73 hours), which prevents the use of multiple doses in close temporal proximity but allows for delayed imaging following its administration. The production of ^{201}Tl requires a cyclotron. With both radiopharmaceuticals, myocardial perfusion images are obtained with a conventional gamma camera (see below).

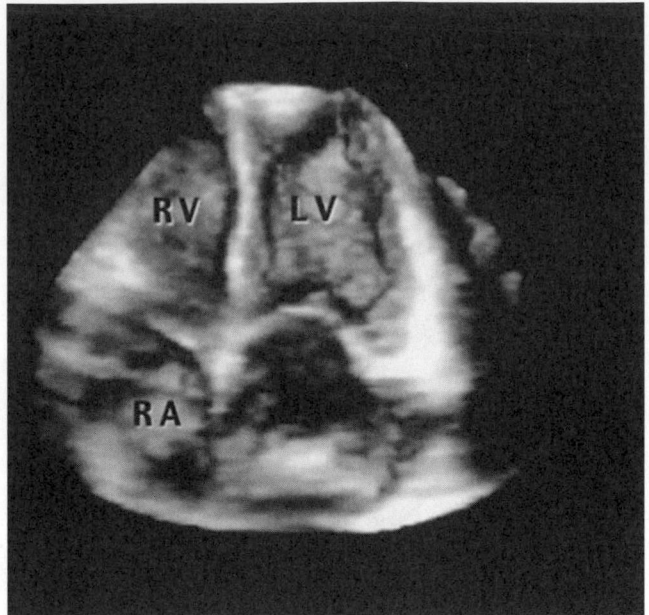

FIGURE 17-15. Real-time 3D echocardiography image, apical four-chamber plane. *(From DeMaria AN, Daniel G. Blanchard DG. Echocardiography. In: Fuster V, O'Rourke RA, Walsh RA, Poole-Wilson P: Hurst's the Heart, 12th ed. New York: McGraw-Hill, 2004:374.)*

Although both [99m]Tc- and ^{201}Tl-labeled compounds are useful for the detection of ischemic or infarcted myocardium, each offers certain advantages. [99m]Tc provides better image quality and is superior for detailed single photon emission computed tomography (SPECT) imaging (see below), whereas ^{201}Tl imaging provides superior detection of myocardial cellular viability.

With ^{201}Tl imaging, the radioisotope is injected intravenously as the patient is completing exercise or pharmacologic stress. Since thallium is a potassium analogue, it enters normal myocytes that have an active sodium-potassium ATPase pump (i.e., viable myocytes). The intracellular concentration of thallium depends on the perfusion of the tissue and its viability. In the normal heart, homogeneous distribution of thallium occurs in myocardial tissue. Conversely, regions that are scarred due to previous infarction or have stress-induced ischemia do not accumulate as much thallium as normal muscle; as a result, these areas appear as "cold" spots on the perfusion scan.

When evaluating for myocardial ischemia, an initial set of images is obtained immediately after stress and ^{201}Tl injection, and the images are examined for regions of decreased radioisotope uptake. Delayed images are obtained 3 to 4 hours later, since ^{201}Tl accumulation does not remain fixed in myocytes. Continuous redistribution of the isotope occurs across the cell membrane, with (a) differential washout rates between hypoperfused but viable myocardium and normal zones and (b) wash-in to previously hypoperfused zones. Thus, when additional images are obtained after 3 to 4 hours of redistribution, viable myocytes have similar concentrations of [201]Tl. Consequently, any uptake abnormalities that were caused by myocardial ischemia will have resolved (i.e., "filled in") on the delayed scan and are termed "reversible" defects, whereas those representing scarred or infarcted myocardium will persist as cold spots.

Myocardial segments that demonstrate persistent ^{201}Tl hypoperfusion with stress and redistribution imaging may represent so-called "hibernating myocardium." This markedly hypoperfused myocardium is chronically ischemic and noncontractile but metabolically active; as a result, it has the potential to regain function if perfusion is restored. Hibernating myocardium can often be differentiated from irreversibly scarred myocardium by injecting additional ^{201}Tl to enhance uptake by viable myocytes, then repeating the images 24 hours later.[41,42]

[99m]Tc-sestamibi—also known as methoxy-isobutyl isonitrile (Tc-MIBI)—is the most widely used ^{99m}Tc-labeled compound. Similar to thallium, its uptake in the myocardium is proportional to blood flow, but its mechanism of myocyte uptake is different, in that it occurs passively, driven by the negative membrane potential. Once intracellular, it accumulates in the mitochondria, where it remains, not redistributing with the passage of time. Therefore, the myocardial distribution of sestamibi reflects perfusion at the moment of its injection. Performing a ^{99m}Tc-sestamibi procedure provides more flexibility than a ^{201}Tl procedure, in that images can be obtained for up to 4 to 6 hours after radioisotope injection and acquired again as necessary. A ^{99m}Tc-sestamibi study is usually performed as a 1-day protocol, with which an initial injection with a small tracer dose and imaging are performed at rest, after which (a few hours later) the patient undergoes a stress test, and repeat imaging is performed after injection of a larger tracer dose.

Myocardial perfusion imaging can be performed with either planar or single photon emission computed tomographic (SPECT) approaches. The planar technique consists of three 2D image acquisitions, usually for 10 to 15 minutes each. With SPECT, the camera detectors rotate around the patient in a circular or elliptical fashion, collecting a series of planar projection images at regular angular intervals (Fig. 17-16). The 3D distribution of radioactivity in the myocardium is then "reconstructed" by computer from the 2D projections. Gated SPECT is a further refinement of the process, whereby the projection images are acquired in specific phases of the cardiac cycle based on ECG triggering (so-called "gating"). With gated SPECT, myocardial perfusion and function can be evaluated.

Although stress perfusion imaging with [99m]Tc- or ^{201}Tl-labeled compounds offers greater sensitivity and specificity than standard exercise electrocardiography for the detection of ischemia (Fig. 17-17),[42] they are considerably more expensive and expose the patient to ionizing radiation. As a result, they should be used judiciously. Stress perfusion scans are particularly useful in patients with an underlying ECG abnormality that precludes its accurate interpretation during conventional exercise stress testing, such as patients with a bundle branch block, previous myocardial infarction, baseline ST segment abnormalities, or taking medications that affect the ST segments (e.g., digoxin).[43] When compared with standard exercise testing, nuclear perfusion imaging also provides more accurate anatomic localization of ischemia and quantitation of the extent of ischemia.[44]

Technetium Scanning

Technetium scanning is used for the evaluation of cardiac function, myocardial perfusion, and the presence of infarcted myocardium.[42,45]

Radionuclide ventriculography—so-called MUGA (multigated acquisition) scanning—is a noninvasive method for determining right and left ventricular systolic function, detecting intracardiac shunting, estimating ventricular volumes, and assessing regional wall motion. For the most part, it has been replaced by other noninvasive techniques (i.e., echocardiography and MRI) that provide similar information without ionizing radiation. Nonetheless, it may be performed in the subject in whom suitable echocardiographic images cannot be obtained or who is unable to undergo an MRI study.

During radionuclide ventriculography, ^{99m}Tc-pertechnate is introduced into the blood stream and imaged as it circulates through the heart. The resulting images of the blood pool in the

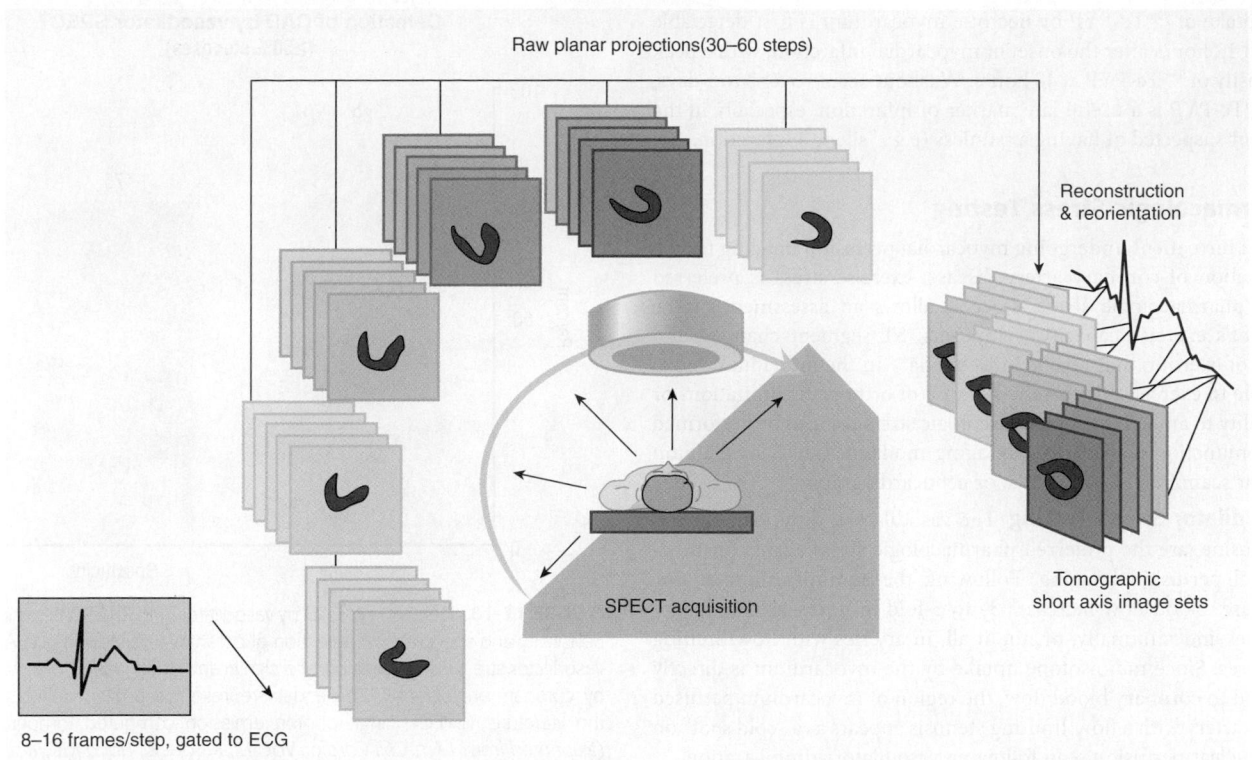

Raw planar projections(30–60 steps)

Reconstruction & reorientation

SPECT acquisition

Tomographic short axis image sets

8–16 frames/step, gated to ECG

FIGURE 17-16. Schematic representation of ECG-gated SPECT imaging and acquisition. *(From Berman DS, Hachamovitch R, Shaw LJ, et al. Nuclear Cardiology. In: Fuster V, O'Rourke RA, Walsh RA, Poole-Wilson P: Hurst's the Heart, 12th ed. New York: McGraw-Hill, 2004:545.)*

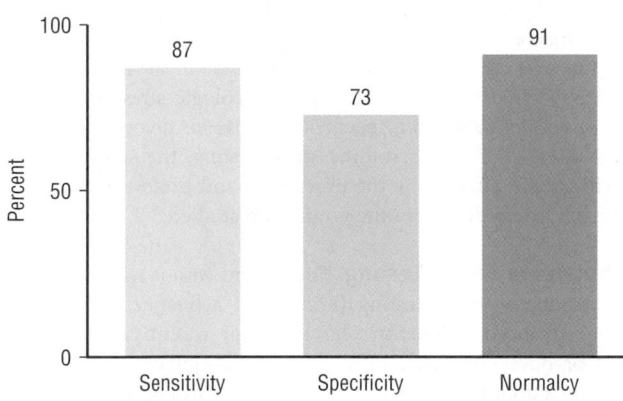

Detection of CAD by exercise SPECT:
Pooled analysis of 33 studies (≥50% stenoses)

FIGURE 17-17. Detection of CAD by exercise SPECT: pooled analysis of 33 studies (≥50% stenoses). Sensitivity, specificity, and normalcy rates from a pooled analysis of 33 studies in the literature using exercise single-photon emission computed tomography (SPECT) myocardial perfusion imaging for detection of coronary artery disease (CAD). Note that the normalcy rate, which is derived from the percentage of patients with normal scans who have <5% pretest likelihood of CAD is shown. This normalcy rate of 91% is significantly higher than specificity. *(Reprinted from J Am Coll Cardiol, Vol. 42, Klocke FJ, Baird MG, Bateman TM, et al, ACC/AHA/ASNC guidelines for the clinical use of cardiac radionuclide imaging—executive summary: a report of the American College of Cardiology/American Heart Association Task Force on Practice Guidelines (ACC/AHA/ASNC Committee to Revise the 1995 Guidelines for the Clinical Use of Radionuclide Imaging), pages 1318–1333, Copyright © 2003, with permission from Elsevier.)*

cardiac chambers are analyzed by computer to calculate right and left ventricular ejection fractions.

The radioactive marker can be introduced to the patient's blood in vivo or in vitro. With the in vivo method, stannous (tin) ions are injected intravenously, after which an intravenous injection of ^{99m}Tc-pertechnate labels the red blood cells in vivo. With the in vitro method, an aliquot of the patient's blood is withdrawn, to which the stannous ions and ^{99m}Tc-pertechnate are added, after which the labeled blood is reinfused into the patient. The stannous chloride is given to prevent the technetium from leaking from the red blood cells.

Once the radiolabeled red blood cells are circulating, the patient is placed under a gamma camera, which detects the radioactive ^{99m}Tc. As the images are acquired, the patient's heart beat is used to "gate" the acquisition, resulting in a series of images of the heart at various stages of the cardiac cycle.

Depending on the objectives of the test, the operator may decide to perform a resting or a stress MUGA. During the resting MUGA, the patient lies stationary, whereas during a stress MUGA, the patient is asked to exercise on a supine bicycle ergometer as images are acquired. The stress MUGA allows the operator to assess cardiac performance at rest and during exercise. It is usually performed to assess the presence of suspected coronary artery disease.

Infarct-avid radionuclides, such as technetium-pyrophosphate (^{99m}Tc-PYP), are used to assess the presence and extent of infarcted myocardium. Since ^{99m}Tc-PYP binds to calcium that is deposited in the infarcted area, it is known as *hot-spot scanning*. Hot spots appear where necrotic myocardial tissue is present, which may occur with recent myocardial infarction, myocarditis, myocardial abscesses, and myocardial trauma. Additionally, ^{99m}Tc-PYP uptake has been observed on occasion in patients with unstable angina, severe diabetes mellitus, and cardiac amyloidosis.

Uptake of ^{99m}Tc-PYP by necrotic myocardium is first detectable about 12 hours after the onset of myocardial infarction, with a peak intensity of ^{99m}Tc-PYP at 48 hours. Washout occurs over 5 to 7 days, so ^{99m}Tc-PYP is a useful late marker of infarction, especially in the patient suspected of having a painless (e.g., "silent") infarction.

Pharmacologic Stress Testing

❾ In the patient undergoing myocardial perfusion imaging for the evaluation of coronary artery disease, exercise stress is preferred over pharmacologic stress, since it allows an assessment of the patient's exercise capacity, symptoms, ST segment changes, and level of exertion that results in ischemia.[44] In the individual who is unable to exercise adequately (because of orthopedic limitations or inability to ambulate), a pharmacologic stress test can be performed in conjunction with various imaging modalities, such as thallium planar scanning, SPECT, MRI, or echocardiography.[42–44]

Vasodilator Stress Testing The vasodilators, dipyridamole and adenosine, are the preferred pharmacologic stress agents for myocardial perfusion imaging. Following the administration of one of these, blood flow increases 3- to 5-fold in undiseased coronary arteries and minimally, or not at all, in arteries with flow-limiting stenoses. Since radioisotope uptake by the myocardium is directly related to coronary blood flow, the region of myocardium perfused by an artery with a flow-limiting stenosis appears as a "cold spot" on the nuclear perfusion scan following vasodilator administration.

Adenosine dilates coronary arteries by binding to specific adenosine receptors on smooth muscle cells in the coronary arterial media. Dipyridamole causes coronary vasodilatation by blocking the cellular uptake of adenosine, thereby increasing the extracellular adenosine concentration. Currently, adenosine is used more often than dipyridamole because of its rapid onset and termination of action. Since methylxanthines (i.e., caffeine and theophylline) block adenosine binding and can interfere with the vasodilatory effects of these agents, foods and beverages containing caffeine should not be ingested during the 24 hours before their administration.

During a vasodilator stress test, the patient normally manifests a modest increase in heart rate, a fall in blood pressure, and no or minimal electrocardiographic changes. Chest pain, shortness of breath, flushing, and dizziness occur commonly during vasodilator administration. As a result, the hemodynamic, electrocardiographic, and symptomatic responses to vasodilator administration do not provide insight into the presence or absence of coronary artery disease.

Dipyridamole is administered intravenously at 0.142 mg/kg/min for 4 minutes, with the maximal effect occurring 3 to 4 minutes after the infusion has ended. Adenosine is administered intravenously at 0.140 mcg/kg/min for 6 minutes, with the maximum effect occurring 30 seconds after the infusion is completed. At the end of the dipyridamole infusion or 3 minutes after initiation of adenosine infusion, thallium is administered, after which nuclear imaging follows immediately and can be repeated 24 hours later to distinguish scarred from hibernating myocardium.

Since these agents may induce severe bronchospasm in subjects with a history of asthma, they should not be administered to such individuals. With adenosine, advanced atrioventricular block may occur. Fortunately, severe side effects are rare, occurring in only 1 in 10,000 patients receiving these agents, and are usually reversed with intravenous aminophylline 75 to 125 mg.

In the patient referred for stress testing to assess the presence of CAD, pharmacologic stress is indicated for those unable or with a contraindication to exercise. This includes patients with (a) a chronic debilitating illness, such as COPD, liver, or kidney disease; (b) older age and decreased functional capacity; (c) limited exercise capacity due to injury, arthritis, orthopedic problems, neurologic disorders,

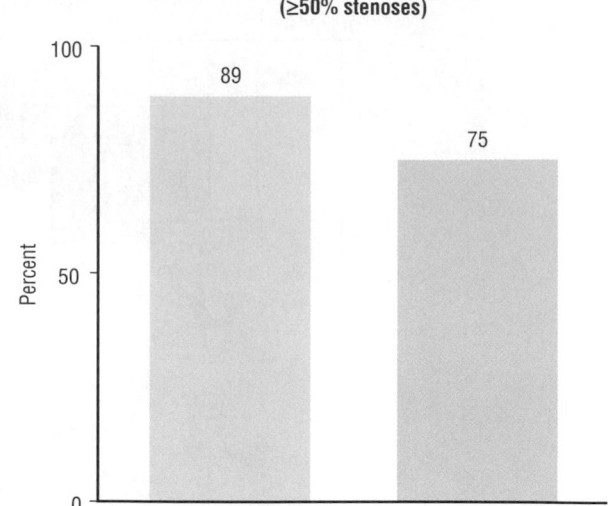

FIGURE 17-18. Detection of CAD by vasodilator SPECT (≥50% stenoses). Sensitivity and specificity for detection of coronary artery disease (CAD) by vasodilator stress. The definition of a significant lesion was ≥50% stenosis by coronary angiography. These data represent a pooled analysis from the literature. (SPECT, single-photon emission computed tomography.) *(Reprinted from J Am Coll Cardiol, Vol. 42, Klocke FJ, Baird MG, Bateman TM, et al, ACC/AHA/ASNC guidelines for the clinical use of cardiac radionuclide imaging—executive summary: a report of the American College of Cardiology/American Heart Association Task Force on Practice Guidelines (ACC/AHA/ASNC Committee to Revise the 1995 Guidelines for the Clinical Use of Radionuclide Imaging), pages 1318–1333, Copyright © 2003, with permission from Elsevier.)*

myopathic diseases, or peripheral vascular disease; (d) an acute coronary syndrome; (e) postoperative state; and (f) beta-blocker or other negative chronotropic agents that interfere with the subject's ability to achieve an adequate increase in heart rate in response to exercise.

Pharmacologic stress testing has a similar sensitivity and specificity to exercise stress testing (Fig. 17–18). In an analysis of 17 studies of almost 2000 patients, pharmacologic stress testing had a sensitivity of 89% and a specificity of 75% for detecting ischemic heart disease.[42] As with routine stress testing, the sensitivity and specificity are affected by the prevalence and pretest likelihood of coronary artery disease in the population studied.

Dobutamine Stress Testing The patient who is not a candidate for vasodilator stress testing (because of a history of bronchospasm, advanced atrioventricular block, or recent caffeine ingestion) or does not desire infusion of a radiopharmaceutical may undergo a dobutamine stress test with echocardiographic imaging. Dobutamine, a synthetic catecholamine, is an inotropic agent that increases heart rate and myocardial contractility, thereby increasing myocardial oxygen demands. In regions of the heart where myocardial oxygen supply is insufficient to meet the increase in demands (because of a flow-limiting stenosis in the coronary artery supplying that region), ischemia develops and causes regional abnormalities in contraction that may be observed with echocardiography.

When used for stress testing, dobutamine is infused intravenously at 10 mcg/kg/min, with the dose increased at 3-minute intervals in increments of 10 mcg/kg/min to a maximum of 40 mcg/kg/min. To achieve a further increase in myocardial oxygen demands, atropine (0.5 to 1 mg) may be injected to augment the dobutamine-induced increase in heart rate, and handgrip exercise may be performed concomitantly to achieve an increase in blood pressure. The ECG and blood pressure are monitored throughout the test, and echocardiographic images are

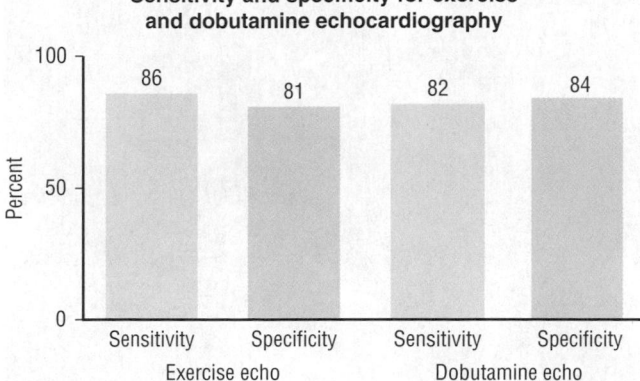

Sensitivity and specificity for exercise and dobutamine echocardiography

FIGURE 17-19. Sensitivity and specificity for exercise and dobutamine echocardiography. Note a slightly higher sensitivity for exercise echo compared to dobutamine echo. *(Reprinted from J Am Coll Cardiol, Vol. 42, Cheitlin MD, Armstrong WF, Aurigemma GP, et al. ACC/AHA/ASE 2003 guideline update for the clinical application of echocardiography–summary article: a report of the American College of Cardiology/American Heart Association Task Force on Practice Guidelines (ACC/AHA/ASE Committee to Update the 1997 Guidelines for the Clinical Application of Echocardiography), pages 954–970, Copyright © 2003, with permission from Elsevier.)*

obtained during the last minute of each dobutamine dose infusion and during recovery. For the patient with suboptimal echocardiographic images, dobutamine stress testing may be combined with radionuclide perfusion imaging, in which case, thallium is injected 2 to 3 minutes before completion of the dobutamine infusion.

Since beta-blocker and calcium channel blocker therapy may interfere with the heart rate response to dobutamine, it is recommended that they be discontinued before the test. Dobutamine stress testing is relatively well tolerated, with ventricular irritability occurring rarely (0.05%). The dobutamine infusion is discontinued with the appearance of severe chest pain, extensive new wall motion abnormalities, substantial ST segment changes suggestive of severe ischemia, tachyarrhythmias, or a symptomatic fall in systemic arterial pressure. Beta-blockers can be used to reverse most adverse effects if they persist. Dobutamine stress testing is contraindicated in patients with aortic stenosis, uncontrolled hypertension, and severe ventricular arrhythmias.

A review of 37 studies of 3,280 patients reported that dobutamine stress testing had a sensitivity of 82% and a specificity of 84% for detecting coronary artery disease (Fig. 17-19). The sensitivity was highest in subjects with three vessel coronary artery disease (92%).[46]

COMPUTED TOMOGRAPHY

Computed tomographic (CT) scanning is becoming increasingly popular as a primary screening procedure in the evaluation of individuals with suspected or known CVD, since it provides similar information as other diagnostic modalities, such as catheterization and echocardiography, yet it is less invasive than the former.[47–49] In recent years, technologic advances have enhanced CT's definition and spatial resolution of cardiac structures, such as coronary arteries, valves, pericardium, and cardiac masses. In addition, CT provides an accurate measurement of chamber volumes and sizes as well as wall thickness.

CT scanners produce images by rotating an x-ray beam around a circular gantry (e.g., opening), through which the patient advances on a moving couch. Two types of CT scanners are used for cardiac imaging: electron beam computed tomography (EBCT)

and mechanical CT.[49] With EBCT, the electron x-ray tube remains stationary, and the electron beam is swept electronically around the patient. With mechanical or conventional CT, the x-ray tube itself rotates around the patient, and the use of multirow detector systems rays (i.e., multislice CT) allows acquisition of up to 256 simultaneous images, each 0.5 mm in thickness. With either type of CT, the image acquisition is gated to the ECG to minimize radiation exposure, and cardiac images are obtained at end inspiration (i.e., during a breath hold) to minimize artifact caused by cardiac motion.

Since EBCT has no moving parts, it requires a shorter image acquisition time and exposes the patient to less radiation when compared with conventional CT (<1.0 rad vs 15 rads, respectively). With EBCT, image resolution is sufficient to assess global and regional ventricular function and coronary anatomy, but it is not sufficient to provide an accurate assessment of the presence and severity of coronary artery disease. However, it can reliably detect the presence and extent of coronary arterial calcification, which is expressed as a coronary artery calcium score in Agatston units (Fig. 17-20). Although the presence of coronary arterial calcification correlates with the total atherosclerotic plaque burden in epicardial coronary arteries, it does not predict the presence or location of flow-limiting (>50% luminal diameter narrowing) coronary arterial stenoses, nor does the lack of coronary calcium exclude the presence of atherosclerotic plaque.[47–49]

The distribution of calcification scores in populations of individuals without known heart disease has been studied extensively. These studies have shown that the amount of coronary arterial calcification increases with age, and men typically develop calcification 10 to 15 years earlier than women.[49] In the majority of asymptomatic men over 55 years of age and women over 65 years of age, coronary arterial calcification is detectable. The person who undergoes coronary calcium screening with EBCT receives a score in Agatston units as well as a calcium score percentile with which his/her score is compared to a population of subjects of similar age and gender.

Unlike EBCT, multislice CT has sufficient resolution to visualize the coronary arteries (Fig. 17-21). To accomplish this, radiographic contrast material is administered intravenously, and a beta-blocker is given to slow the heart rate to <70 beats/min to minimize motion artifact. Compared with conventional coronary angiography, cardiac CT has a sensitivity of 85%, a specificity of 90%, a positive predictive value of 91%, and a negative predictive value of 83% for detecting or excluding a coronary arterial stenosis of 50% or more luminal diameter narrowing.[50] It has limited diagnostic utility in patients with extensive coronary arterial calcification or a rapid heart rate, due to artifacts caused by high-density calcified coronary arterial stenoses or cardiac motion. Vessels with a luminal diameter <1.5mm cannot be assessed reliably with cardiac CT, since the resolution is insufficient.

Independent of its use in assessing coronary arteries, cardiac CT often is used in the subject with suspected aortic dissection, in whom its accuracy in detecting dissection is >90%. In the patient with possible constrictive pericarditis, the pericardium can be evaluated for thickening and calcification. In the patient with a possible cardiac mass, CT scanning allows one to assess the size and location of the mass, and tissue density differentiation may aid in its characterization. Cardiac CT can be used to calculate left ventricular volumes, ejection fraction, and mass, and these measurements obtained with CT scanning are superior in accuracy and reproducibility to those obtained with angiography or echocardiography. CT scans allow visualization of congenital heart defects. Although MRI may provide similar information without exposing the patient to ionizing radiation, many patients have contraindications to MRI (i.e., those with an implanted metallic device). In such patients, cardiac CT is an alternative method for visualizing cardiac anatomy.

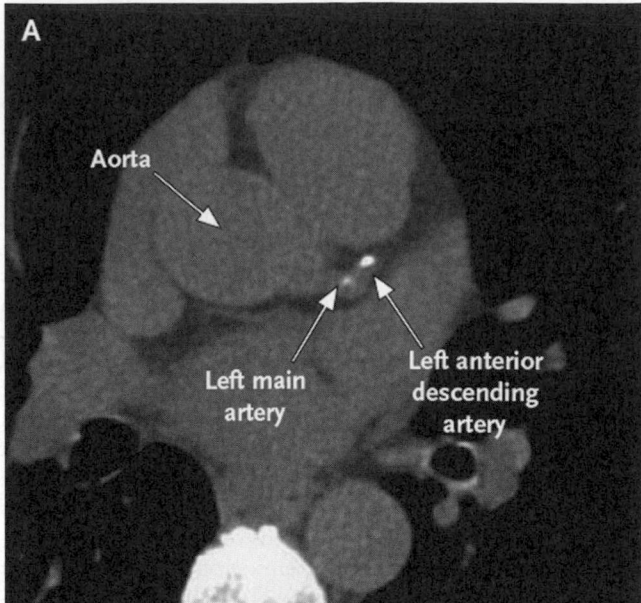

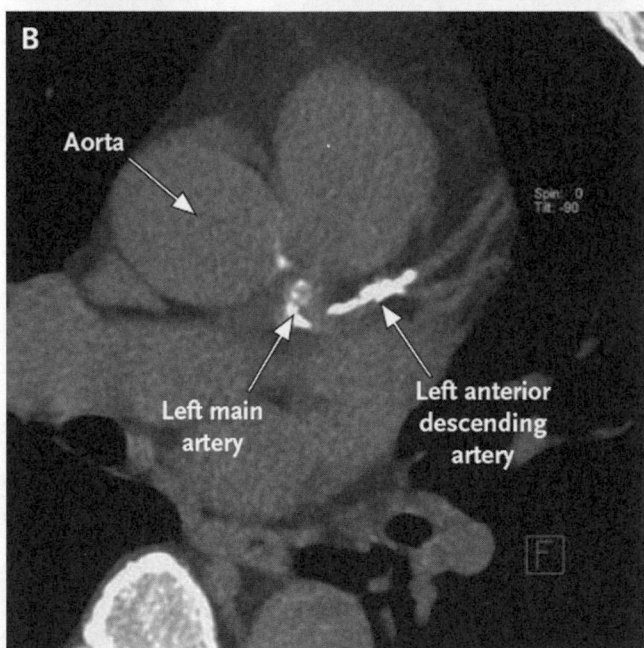

FIGURE 17-20. CT scans of the left coronary artery in two asymptomatic men. Two asymptomatic men, 51 years of age and 81 years of age, underwent coronary-artery calcium (CAC) imaging with multidetector CT. There is calcification of the left main and proximal left anterior descending coronary arteries in both the younger patient (*panel A*) and the older patient (*panel B*). The CAC score for the younger man, although relatively low at 80, places him in the 85th percentile for severity of CAC for men in his age group. The older man's CAC score is higher, at 1,054, but the severity of his CAC relative to that for men in his age group is lower—in the 70th percentile. (*Bonow RO. Should Coronary Calcium Screening Be Used in Cardiovascular Prevention Strategies? N Engl J Med 2009;361:990–997. Copyright © 2009 Massachusetts Medical Society. All rights reserved.*)

POSITRON EMISSION TOMOGRAPHY

Positron emission tomography (PET) is a relatively new modality for diagnostic imaging in patients with suspected or known CVD. Among imaging techniques, it is unique in its ability (a) to provide quantitative imaging with high temporal resolution; (b) to image a large number of physiologically active radiotracers; and (c) to apply tracer kinetic principles so that in vivo imaging can be performed. With PET, myocardial metabolic activity, perfusion, and viability

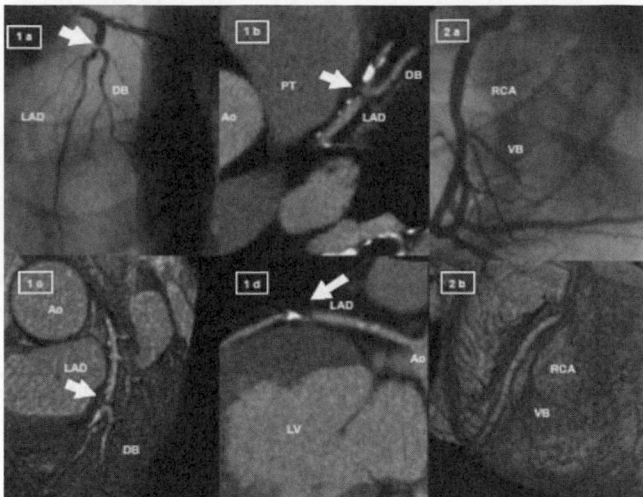

FIGURE 17-21. 16-slice MDCT in a 49-year-old male with chest pain. (*1a*) Coronary angiography showing severe lesion in LAD. (*1b*) MDCT axial slice visualizing high-grade lesion (arrow) and calcification. (*1c*) MDCT 3-dimensional volume-rendering technique showing the LAD stenosis. (*1d*) MDCT curved multiplanar reconstruction of the LAD. (*2a*) Coronary angiography of RCA, which is normal. (*2b*) MDCT volume-rendering technique of RCA. (Ao, aorta; DB, diagonal branch; LV, left ventricle; MDCT, multidetector computed tomography; PT, pulmonary trunk; VB, ventricular branch.) (*Reproduced with permission from Berman DS, Hachamovitch R, Shaw LJ, et al. Roles of Nuclear Cardiology, Cardiac Computed Tomography, and Cardiac Magnetic Resonance: Assessment of Patients with Suspected Coronary Artery Disease. J Nucl Med 2006;47:74–82.*)

can be assessed.[41,42] Using appropriate positron-emitting biologically active tracers, PET can measure regional myocardial uptake of exogenous glucose and fatty acids, quantitate free fatty acid metabolism, ascertain myocardial energy substrates, and evaluate myocardial chemoreceptor sites.

In the fasting state (i.e., low serum glucose and insulin concentrations), fatty acids are the preferred energy source of the myocardium. Following the ingestion of carbohydrate, serum glucose and insulin concentrations increase, and glucose becomes the preferred myocardial fuel. Glucose also is the major myocardial fuel during ischemia, since ischemia impairs mitochondrial fatty acid oxidation. Using positron-emitting isotopes, such as oxygen-15 (^{15}O-oxygen), carbon-11 (^{11}C-palmitate or ^{11}C acetate), and fluoride-18 (^{18}F-fluorodeoxyglucose), myocardial oxygen consumption and substrate utilization can be measured, from which ischemic and nonischemic regions of the heart can be identified.[41] PET usually is used in conjunction with pharmacologic stress testing to provoke ischemia, with images obtained before and after stress.

Tracers such as rubidium 82 (^{82}Rb) and nitrogen 13 (^{13}N) are retained in the myocardium in proportion to blood flow. PET imaging with these agents allows one to measure myocardial blood flow at rest and during pharmacologically induced hyperemia. Thus, PET can be used to assess the physiologic significance of coronary arterial stenoses, which is useful when attempting to determine if a luminal diameter narrowing of intermediate severity (50%–70%) is causing ischemia.

In the patient with noncontractile myocardium, PET is considered to be the "gold standard" technique for distinguishing infarcted myocardium from chronically ischemic, metabolically active myocardium that has the potential to regain function if perfusion is restored (hibernating myocardium).[41] Myocardial infarction and ischemia can be distinguished by analysis of PET images of the glucose analog ^{8}F-fluorodeoxyglucose (FDG), which is injected after glucose administration, and the perfusion

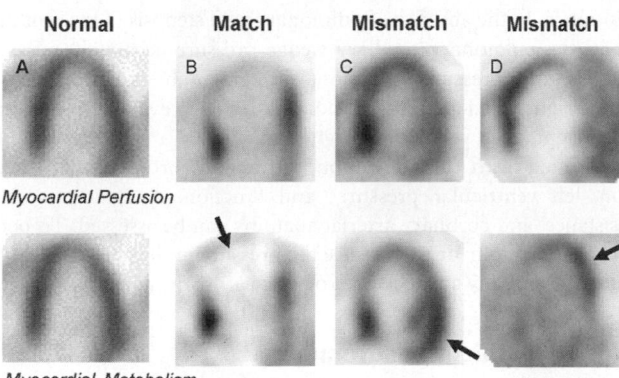

Normal	Match	Mismatch	Mismatch
A	B	C	D

Myocardial Perfusion

Myocardial Metabolism

FIGURE 17-22. Patterns of myocardial perfusion (*upper panel*) and metabolism (with ¹⁸F-FDG; *lower panel*). **A.** Normal myocardial perfusion and metabolism. **B.** Severely reduced myocardial perfusion in the anterior wall associated with a concordant reduction in ¹⁸F-FDG uptake (arrow), corresponding to a match. **C.** Mildly reduced perfusion in the lateral and posterior lateral wall associated with a segmental increase in glucose metabolism (mismatch). **D.** Severely reduced myocardial perfusion in the lateral wall with a segmental increase in ¹⁸F-FDG uptake (arrow), reflecting a perfusion metabolism mismatch. *(From Schelbert HR. Positron Emission Tomography for the Noninvasive Study and Quantitation of Myocardial Blood Flow and Metabolism in Cardiovascular Disease. In: Fuster V, O'Rourke RA, Walsh RA, Poole-Wilson P: Hurst's the Heart, 12th ed. New York: McGraw-Hill, 2004:675.)*

tracer ¹³N-ammonia. Regions that show a concordant reduction in myocardial blood flow and FDG uptake ("flow-metabolism match") are considered to be irreversibly injured, whereas regions in which FDG uptake is relatively preserved or increased despite a perfusion defect ("flow-metabolism mismatch") are considered to be ischemic (Fig. 17–22). This approach more accurately predicts recovery of regional function after revascularization than does SPECT imaging. The magnitude of improvement in heart failure symptoms after revascularization in patients with left ventricular dysfunction correlates with the preoperative extent of FDG "mismatch."[51]

The main strengths of PET compared with SPECT are its superior spatial resolution and ability to assess myocardial viability accurately.[41,42] The limited availability of PET scanners and the need for a cyclotron on site are its main limitations. Recently, the number of PET scanners has increased to approximately 1,200 in the United States and 400 in Europe. In the United States, more than 150,000 cardiac PET scans are performed annually, of which about 68,000 are viability and about 86,000 are perfusion scans.[41]

CARDIAC CATHETERIZATION AND ANGIOGRAPHY

❻ Cardiac catheterization plays a pivotal role in the evaluation of patients with suspected or known cardiac disease; in addition, it has become an important therapeutic alternative to cardiac surgery in many patients who require nonmedical therapy.

Indications

Diagnostic cardiac catheterization is appropriate under several conditions. First, it is often performed to confirm or to exclude the presence of a cardiac condition that is suspected from the patient's history, physical examination, or noninvasive evaluation. In such a circumstance, it allows an assessment of the presence and severity of cardiac disease. For example, in a subject with progressive angina

TABLE 17-7	Relative Contraindications to Cardiac Catheterization

Decompensated heart failure (e.g., pulmonary edema)
Uncontrolled ventricular irritability
Uncontrolled systemic arterial hypertension
Acute or severe renal insufficiency
Difficulty with vascular access
Electrolyte imbalance (i.e., hypo- or hyperkalemia)
Digitalis intoxication
Active infection or febrile illness
Uncorrected bleeding diathesis
Severe anemia
Active bleeding from internal organ
Severe allergy to radiographic contrast material
Mental incompetence

pectoris or a positive exercise stress test, coronary angiography allows the physician to visualize the coronary arteries sufficiently to assess the presence and extent of coronary artery disease. Second, catheterization is often helpful in the patient with a confusing or difficult clinical presentation in whom the noninvasive evaluation is inconclusive. For instance, a hemodynamic evaluation or coronary angiography may be useful in the patient with unexplained dyspnea. Third, data obtained at catheterization may provide prognostic information that is helpful in guiding therapy. Such is the case, for example, in the patient with cardiomyopathy, in whom the hemodynamic data obtained at catheterization are used to guide medical therapy and to assess the need for and timing of cardiac transplantation.

Contraindications

The only absolute contraindication to catheterization is the refusal of a mentally competent patient to provide informed consent. Relative contraindications (Table 17–7) mostly involve conditions in which the risks of the procedure are increased or the information obtained from it is potentially unreliable. In these circumstances, the benefits of having the data that are obtained at catheterization must be weighed against the procedure's increased risks. Catheterization usually is not performed in the patient who refuses therapy for the condition for which diagnostic catheterization is recommended.

Complications

Because catheterization is an invasive procedure, its performance is associated with major and minor risks. The incidence of a major complication (death, myocardial infarction, or cerebrovascular accident) during or within 24 hours of diagnostic catheterization is 0.2% to 0.3%. Deaths, which occur in 0.1 to 0.2% of patients, may be caused by perforation of the heart or great vessels, cardiac arrhythmias, acute myocardial infarction, or anaphylaxis to radiographic contrast material.

Numerous minor complications may cause morbidity but exert no effect on mortality. Local vascular complications occur in 0.5% to 1.5% of patients. The injection of radiographic contrast material occasionally is associated with allergic reactions of varying severity, and a rare individual has anaphylaxis. Of patients with a known allergy to contrast material, only about 15% have an adverse reaction with its repeat administration, and most of these reactions are minor (e.g., urticaria, nausea, vomiting). In most patients with a previous allergic reaction to radiographic contrast material, angiography can be performed safely, but premedication with glucocorticosteroids and antihistamines and the use of a different contrast material are usually recommended. Use of excessive quantities of radiographic contrast material may result in renal insufficiency, particularly in patients with preexisting renal dysfunction and diabetes mellitus.

Techniques

Cardiac catheterization is generally performed with the patient in the fasting state and mildly sedated. Anticoagulants are discontinued before the procedure (warfarin for several days, heparin for 4–6 hours). Cardiac catheterization requires vascular access, which is usually obtained percutaneously via the femoral, brachial, or radial vessels.

With the *percutaneous approach,* the area overlying the vessel is aseptically prepared and locally anesthetized. The vessel is punctured with a needle, through which a flexible metal wire is advanced into the vessel's lumen, over which a sheath with a sideport extension is advanced into the vessel. The sideport extension allows continuous monitoring of arterial pressure (through an arterial sheath) or infusion of fluids (through a venous sheath) as catheters are advanced through the sheath to the heart. When the procedure is completed, the catheters and sheaths are removed, after which local pressure is applied or a closure device is used to achieve hemostasis. If the femoral approach is used, the patient remains at bed rest for 2 to 8 hours to minimize the chance of hemorrhage. With the radial and brachial approach, bed rest following sheath removal is not necessary.

During routine right heart catheterization, measurements of pressures and blood oxygen saturations in the vena cavae, right atrium, right ventricle, pulmonary artery, and pulmonary capillary wedge position can be performed, and cardiac output can be quantified (Table 17–8 lists normal values). The measurement of right-sided pressures helps the physician to evaluate the severity of tricuspid or pulmonic stenosis, to assess the presence and severity of pulmonary hypertension, and to calculate pulmonary vascular resistance. In the absence of pulmonary vein stenosis (a rare condition), the pulmonary capillary wedge pressure accurately reflects the left atrial pressure. Occasionally angiography is performed to define right-sided anatomic abnormalities or to evaluate the severity of right-sided valvular regurgitation.

With left heart catheterization, mitral and aortic valvular function, left ventricular pressures and function, systemic vascular resistance, and coronary arterial anatomy can be assessed. To perform angiography or to measure the pressure in the left ventricle, a catheter is usually advanced retrograde across the aortic valve.

Hemodynamic Measurements

Cardiac Output The blood flow measurement most often performed during catheterization is the quantitation of cardiac output. This variable allows assessment of overall cardiovascular function, vascular resistances, valve orifice areas, and valvular regurgitation. In the catheterization laboratory, the three common methods of measuring cardiac output are the Fick principle, the indicator dilution technique, and angiography.

Fick Principle

The Fick principle is based on the fact that when a substance is consumed by an organ, its concentration is the product of blood flow to the organ and the substance's arteriovenous difference across the organ. Using the lungs as the organ of interest and oxygen as the substance, one can calculate pulmonary blood flow (e.g., cardiac output) using the formula:

$$\text{Cardiac output (L/min)} = \text{Oxygen consumption (mL/min)} / \text{Arteriovenous oxygen difference (mL/L)}$$

Oxygen consumption is measured by analyzing the patient's exhaled air, and the arteriovenous oxygen difference is calculated by measuring the oxygen content in a blood sample procured from the aorta and the pulmonary artery.

Dilution Method

With indicator dilution, a known amount of indicator is injected as a bolus into the circulation and allowed to mix completely in the blood, after which its concentration is measured. A time-concentration curve is generated, and a minicomputer calculates the cardiac output from the area of the inscribed curve. The most widely used indicator for the measurement of cardiac output is cold solution. A balloon-tipped, flow-directed, polyvinyl chloride catheter (a so-called Swan-Ganz catheter) with a thermistor at its tip and an opening 25 to 30 cm proximal to the tip is inserted into a vein and advanced to the pulmonary artery, so that the proximal opening is located in the vena cavae or right atrium and the thermistor is in the pulmonary artery. A known amount of cold fluid is injected through the proximal port; it mixes completely in the right ventricle and causes a change in blood temperature, which is detected by the thermistor. The thermodilution method is relatively inexpensive and easy to perform and does not require arterial sampling or blood withdrawal.

Angiographic Method

From the left ventriculogram, the volume of blood ejected with each heartbeat (stroke volume) can be determined. It is then multiplied by the heart rate, yielding the angiographic cardiac output. The measurement of cardiac output by the angiographic method is potentially erroneous in patients with extensive segmental wall motion abnormalities or misshapen ventricles, in whom the determination of stroke volume may be inaccurate.

TABLE 17-8	Normal Hemodynamic Values
Measurement	**Value**
Flows	
Cardiac index (L/min/m²)	2.6–4.2
Stroke volume index (mL/m²)	35–55
Pressures (mm Hg)	
Aorta/systemic artery	
Peak systolic/end-diastolic	100–140/60–90
Mean	70–105
Left ventricle	
Peak systolic/end-diastolic	100–140/3–12
Left atrium (PCW)	
Mean	1–10
a wave	3–15
v wave	3–15
Pulmonary artery	
Peak systolic/end-diastolic	16–30/4–12
Mean	10–16
Right ventricle	
Peak systolic/end-diastolic	16–30/0–8
Right atrium	
Mean	0–8
a wave	2–10
v wave	2–10
Resistances	
Systemic vascular resistance	
Wood units	10–20
dynes-sec-cm⁻⁵	770–1,500
Pulmonary vascular resistance	
Wood units	0.25–1.5
dynes-sec-cm⁻⁵	20–120
Oxygen Consumption	
(mL/min/m²)	110–150
AV O₂ Difference (mL/dL)	3.0–4.5

AV, arteriovenous; PCW, pulmonary capillary wedge.

Pressures

One of the most important functions of cardiac catheterization is to measure and to record intracardiac pressures. Once a catheter is positioned in a cardiac chamber, it is connected through fluid-filled, stiff, plastic tubing to a pressure transducer, which transforms the pressure signal into an electrical signal that is recorded. During catheterization, pressures are usually measured directly from each of the cardiac chambers: right atrium, right ventricle, pulmonary artery, ascending aorta, and left ventricle. Because the left atrial pressure is transmitted to the pulmonary capillaries, it can be recorded "indirectly" as the pulmonary capillary "wedge" pressure. In addition to measuring pressures from each cardiac chamber, pressures from certain chambers are examined simultaneously to identify or to exclude a gradient between them indicative of valvular stenosis.

Resistances

The resistance of a vascular bed is calculated by dividing the pressure gradient across the bed by the blood flow through it. Thus,

Systemic vascular resistance = (Mean systemic arterial pressure – mean right atrial pressure)/Sytemic blood flow

and

Pulmonary vascular resistance = (Mean Pulmonary arterial pressure – mean left atrial pressure)/Pulmonary blood flow

Because a properly obtained pulmonary capillary wedge pressure is similar to left atrial pressure, it can be substituted for it in the above equation. These formulae express resistances in arbitrary resistance units. Most often, these values are multiplied by 80 to express them in metric units of dynes-sec-cm^{-5}. Normal values are displayed in Table 17–8.

An elevated systemic vascular resistance is often present in the patient with systemic arterial hypertension. It may also be observed in patients with a reduced forward cardiac output and compensatory arteriolar vasoconstriction (often seen in patients with heart failure). Conversely, systemic vascular resistance may be reduced in patients with arteriolar vasodilation (due, for example, to sepsis) or those with an increased cardiac output (due, for example, to an arteriovenous fistula, severe anemia, fever, or thyrotoxicosis). An elevated pulmonary vascular resistance often is observed in patients with primary lung disease, pulmonary vascular disease, and a greatly elevated pulmonary venous pressure resulting from left-sided myocardial or valvular dysfunction.

ANGIOGRAPHY

During angiography, radiographic contrast material is injected into the cardiovascular structure of interest, and the images are digitally recorded and stored on a computer-accessible medium (i.e., CD-ROM, DVD, external memory drives, etc.). The resultant angiogram permits the study of cardiac structures in real time, in slow motion, or by single frame.

Left Ventriculography

With angiography of the left ventricle, global and segmental left ventricular function, left ventricular volumes and ejection fraction, and the presence and severity of mitral regurgitation can be assessed. A segment of the left ventricular wall with reduced systolic motion is said to be hypokinetic; a segment that does not move is akinetic; and a segment that moves paradoxically during systole is dyskinetic.

Coronary Angiography

Selective coronary angiography is usually performed to determine the presence and severity of fixed, atherosclerotic coronary artery disease and to guide subsequent percutaneous (e.g., angioplasty with or without stent placement) or surgical (e.g., bypass grafting) therapy. Under fluoroscopic guidance, the ostia of the native right and left coronary arteries or bypass grafts are engaged selectively with a catheter, and radiographic contrast material is injected manually during digital image recording. Because atherosclerotic coronary arterial stenoses are often eccentric and the coronary vessels often overlap one another, images are obtained in multiple obliquities, thereby ensuring a complete angiographic assessment of each arterial segment.

Coronary angiography provides radiographic images of the coronary lumina but does not visualize the actual arterial walls. A stenosis is present when a discrete reduction in luminal diameter is noted, and its severity is assessed by comparing it with presumably normal adjacent segments of the same artery. Thus, if atherosclerosis is diffuse and involves the entire artery, angiography may lead to an underestimation of the severity of disease.

Aortography

Aortography is accomplished with the rapid injection of radiographic contrast material into the aorta. With proximal aortography, the severity of aortic valve regurgitation, the location of saphenous vein bypass grafts, and the anatomy of the proximal aorta and its branches can be assessed. Distal aortography usually is performed to assess the presence of vascular abnormalities, such as aneurysm, dissection, intraluminal thrombus, or branch vessel stenosis.

Valvular Stenosis or Regurgitation

In patients with valvular stenosis, the effective valve orifice area can be calculated with data obtained during catheterization using principles of standard fluid dynamics. The pressures on either side of a stenotic valve are recorded simultaneously and the flow across it is measured, after which the valve area is calculated.

The presence and severity of valvular regurgitation may be evaluated qualitatively by observing the amount of radiographic contrast material that regurgitates in a retrograde direction across the valve. The magnitude of regurgitation is estimated as trivial (1+), mild (2+), moderate (3+), or severe (4+).

Endomyocardial Biopsy

Through a long sheath positioned across the tricuspid valve, a bioptome can be advanced to obtain small pieces (1–2 mm^2) of myocardial tissue from the right ventricular side of the interventricular septum. Endomyocardial biopsy is used most often to detect transplant rejection and to monitor immunosuppressive therapy in survivors of cardiac transplantation. Less commonly, it is undertaken in the patient with suspected infiltrative cardiomyopathy or active inflammation of the heart (e.g., myocarditis). In experienced hands, complications are uncommon: cardiac perforation occurs in only 0.3% to 0.5%, and the procedure-related mortality is only 0.05%.

INTRAVASCULAR ULTRASOUND

Intravascular ultrasound (IVUS) employs a small catheter-mounted ultrasound transducer to provide detailed images of the coronary arterial lumen. In contrast to coronary angiography, which does not visualize the actual arterial wall, IVUS provides quantitative information from within the vessel regarding vessel diameter, circumference, luminal diameter, plaque volume, and percent narrowing. Qualitative information regarding the amount of plaque stenosis, plaque composition (e.g., calcific, fibrous, or fatty plaque), and the presence of plaque versus thrombus, thrombus versus tumor, and aneurysm and hematoma can be provided by IVUS. IVUS is used as a therapeutic adjunct to PTCA, atherectomy, stent or graft placement, and fibrinolysis, although its routine use with these modalities may not be justified. These combination procedures may be monitored in real time as the procedure (e.g., atherectomy) is being performed. In recent studies, IVUS has been helpful in the evaluation of the progression or regression of atherosclerosis. Current trials are testing medications for atherosclerosis regression and changes in plaque morphology.

Intravascular optical coherence tomography provides high-resolution, cross-sectional images of tissue with an axial resolution of 10 microns and a lateral resolution of 20 microns.[63] Optical coherence tomographic images of human coronary atherosclerotic plaques are much more structurally detailed than those obtained with IVUS.[63] Clinically, the detection of thin fibrous caps (vulnerable atheromas) (<65 microns) is below the resolution of the current 40-MHz IVUS (100–200 microns).[60] A summary of testing modalities used in cardiovascular medicine is provided in Appendices 17–1 and 17–2.

ABBREVIATIONS

ABI=ankle-brachial index

ACC=American College of Cardiology

AECG=ambulatory electrocardiography

AHA=American Heart Association

AV=atrioventricular

BPM=beats per minute

BNP=B-type natriuretic protein

CAC=coronary artery calcium

CAD=coronary artery disease

CK-MB=creatine kinase-MB

CRP: C-reactive protein

CT: computed tomography

cTn: cardiac troponin

CTR: cardiothoracic ratio

CVD: cardiovascular disease

EBCT: electron beam computed tomography

ECG: electrocardiogram

FDG: flurodeoxyglucose

Hs-CRP: high sensitivity C-reactive protein

IVUS: intravascular ultrasound

JVP: jugular venous pressure

MDCT: multidetector computed tomography

MRI-magnetic resonance imaging

MUGA: multigated acquisition

NT-proBNP: N-terminal pro brain-type natriuretic protein

NYHA: New York Heart Association

PAD: peripheral arterial disease

PCW: pulmonary capillary wedge

PET: positron emission tomography

S_1: first heart sound

S_2: second heart sound

S_3: third heart sound

S_4: fourth heart sound

SA: sinoatrial

SAECG: signal-averaged electrocardiography

SPECT: single photon emission computed tomography

Tn: troponin

TEE: transesophageal echocardiography

TTE: transthoracic echocardiography

REFERENCES

1. Lloyd-Jones D, Adams R, Carnethon M, et al. Heart disease and stroke statistics–2009 update: a report from the American Heart Association Statistics Committee and Stroke Statistics Subcommittee. Circulation 2009;119:e21–e181.
2. White C. Clinical practice. Intermittent claudication. N Engl J Med 2007;356:1241–1250.
3. Jaffe AS, Babuin L, Apple FS. Biomarkers in acute cardiac disease: the present and the future. J Am Coll Cardiol 2006;48:1–11.
4. Maisel AS, Bhalla V, Braunwald E. Cardiac biomarkers: a contemporary status report. Nat Clin Pract Cardiovasc Med 2006;3:24–34.
5. Morrow DA, Cannon CP, Jesse RL, et al. National Academy of Clinical Biochemistry Laboratory Medicine Practice Guidelines: Clinical characteristics and utilization of biochemical markers in acute coronary syndromes. Circulation 2007;115:e356– e375.
6. Babuin L, Jaffe AS. Troponin: the biomarker of choice for the detection of cardiac injury. CMAJ 2005;173:1191–1202.
7. Heidenreich PA, Alloggiamento T, Melsop K, McDonald KM, Go AS, Hlatky MA. The prognostic value of troponin in patients with non-ST elevation acute coronary syndromes: a meta-analysis. J Am Coll Cardiol 2001;38:478–485.
8. Hillis LD, Lange RA. Optimal management of acute coronary syndromes. N Engl J Med 2009;360:2237–2240.
9. Musunuru K, Kral BG, Blumenthal RS, et al. The use of high-sensitivity assays for C-reactive protein in clinical practice. Nat Clin Pract Cardiovasc Med 2008;5:621–635.
10. Schunkert H, Samani NJ. Elevated C-reactive protein in atherosclerosis–chicken or egg? N Engl J Med 2008;359:1953–1955.
11. Zacho J, Tybjaerg-Hansen A, Jensen JS, Grande P, Sillesen H, Nordestgaard BG. Genetically elevated C-reactive protein and ischemic vascular disease. N Engl J Med 2008;359:1897–1908.
12. Rifai N, Ridker PM. Proposed cardiovascular risk assessment algorithm using high-sensitivity C-reactive protein and lipid screening. Clin Chem 2001;47:28–30.
13. Helfand M, Buckley DI, Freeman M, et al. Emerging risk factors for coronary heart disease: a summary of systematic reviews conducted for the U.S. Preventive Services Task Force. Ann Intern Med 2009;151:496–507.
14. Ridker PM, Danielson E, Fonseca FA, et al. Rosuvastatin to prevent vascular events in men and women with elevated C-reactive protein. N Engl J Med 2008;359:2195–2207.
15. Prasad K. C-reactive protein (CRP)-lowering agents. Cardiovasc Drug Rev 2006;24:33–50.
16. Ridker PM, Cannon CP, Morrow D, et al. C-reactive protein levels and outcomes after statin therapy. N Engl J Med 2005;352:20–28.
17. James SK, Armstrong P, Barnathan E, et al. Troponin and C-reactive protein have different relations to subsequent mortality and myocardial infarction after acute coronary syndrome: a GUSTO-IV substudy. J Am Coll Cardiol 2003;41:916–924.
18. Lindahl B, Toss H, Siegbahn A, Venge P, Wallentin L. Markers of myocardial damage and inflammation in relation to long-term mortality in unstable coronary artery disease. FRISC Study Group. Fragmin during Instability in Coronary Artery Disease. N Engl J Med 2000;343:1139–1147.
19. Rebuzzi AG, Quaranta G, Liuzzo G, et al. Incremental prognostic value of serum levels of troponin T and C-reactive protein on admission in patients with unstable angina pectoris. Am J Cardiol 1998;82:715–719.
20. Januzzi JL Jr, Camargo CA, Anwaruddin S, et al. The N-terminal Pro-BNP investigation of dyspnea in the emergency department (PRIDE) study. Am J Cardiol 2005;95:948–954.

21. Maisel A, Mueller C, Adams K Jr, et al. State of the art: using natriuretic peptide levels in clinical practice. Eur J Heart Fail 2008;10:824–839.

22. Maisel AS, Krishnaswamy P, Nowak RM, et al. Rapid measurement of B-type natriuretic peptide in the emergency diagnosis of heart failure. N Engl J Med 2002;347:161–167.

23. Fonarow GC, Peacock WF, Phillips CO, Givertz MM, Lopatin M. Admission B-type natriuretic peptide levels and in-hospital mortality in acute decompensated heart failure. J Am Coll Cardiol 2007;49: 1943–1950.

24. Doust JA, Pietrzak E, Dobson A, Glasziou P. How well does B-type natriuretic peptide predict death and cardiac events in patients with heart failure: systematic review. BMJ 2005;330:625.

25. de Lemos JA, Morrow DA, Bentley JH, et al. The prognostic value of B-type natriuretic peptide in patients with acute coronary syndromes. N Engl J Med 2001;345:1014–1021.

26. James SK, Lindback J, Tilly J, et al. Troponin-T and N-terminal pro-B-type natriuretic peptide predict mortality benefit from coronary revascularization in acute coronary syndromes: a GUSTO-IV substudy. J Am Coll Cardiol 2006;48:1146–1154.

27. Morrow DA, de Lemos JA, Sabatine MS, et al. Evaluation of B-type natriuretic peptide for risk assessment in unstable angina/non-ST-elevation myocardial infarction: B-type natriuretic peptide and prognosis in TACTICS-TIMI 18. J Am Coll Cardiol 2003;41:1264–1272.

28. Goldberger JJ, Cain ME, Hohnloser SH, et al. American Heart Association/American College of Cardiology Foundation/Heart Rhythm Society scientific statement on noninvasive risk stratification techniques for identifying patients at risk for sudden cardiac death: a scientific statement from the American Heart Association Council on Clinical Cardiology Committee on Electrocardiography and Arrhythmias and Council on Epidemiology and Prevention. Circulation 2008;118:1497–1518.

29. Lauer M, Froelicher ES, Williams M, Kligfield P. Exercise testing in asymptomatic adults: a statement for professionals from the American Heart Association Council on Clinical Cardiology, Subcommittee on Exercise, Cardiac Rehabilitation, and Prevention. Circulation 2005;112:771–776.

30. Gibbons RJ, Balady GJ, Bricker JT, et al. ACC/AHA 2002 guideline update for exercise testing: summary article: a report of the American College of Cardiology/American Heart Association Task Force on Practice Guidelines (Committee to Update the 1997 Exercise Testing Guidelines). Circulation 2002;106:1883–1892.

31. Marwick TH. The future of echocardiography. Eur J Echocardiogr 2009;10:594–601.

32. Ayres NA, Miller-Hance W, Fyfe DA, et al. Indications and guidelines for performance of transesophageal echocardiography in the patient with pediatric acquired or congenital heart disease: report from the task force of the Pediatric Council of the American Society of Echocardiography. J Am Soc Echocardiogr 2005;18:91–98.

33. Baddour LM, Wilson WR, Bayer AS, et al. Infective endocarditis: diagnosis, antimicrobial therapy, and management of complications: a statement for healthcare professionals from the Committee on Rheumatic Fever, Endocarditis, and Kawasaki Disease, Council on Cardiovascular Disease in the Young, and the Councils on Clinical Cardiology, Stroke, and Cardiovascular Surgery and Anesthesia, American Heart Association: endorsed by the Infectious Diseases Society of America. Circulation 2005;111:e394–e434.

34. Baumgartner H, Hung J, Bermejo J, et al. Echocardiographic assessment of valve stenosis: EAE/ASE recommendations for clinical practice. J Am Soc Echocardiogr 2009;22:1–23; quiz 101–102.

35. Douglas PS, Khandheria B, Stainback RF, et al. ACCF/ASE/ACEP/ASNC/SCAI/SCCT/SCMR 2007 appropriateness criteria for transthoracic and transesophageal echocardiography: a report of the American College of Cardiology Foundation Quality Strategic Directions Committee Appropriateness Criteria Working Group, American Society of Echocardiography, American College of Emergency Physicians, American Society of Nuclear Cardiology, Society for Cardiovascular Angiography and Interventions, Society of Cardiovascular Computed Tomography, and the Society for Cardiovascular Magnetic Resonance endorsed by the American College of Chest Physicians and the Society of Critical Care Medicine. J Am Coll Cardiol 2007;50:187–204.

36. Singer DE, Albers GW, Dalen JE, et al. Antithrombotic therapy in atrial fibrillation: American College of Chest Physicians Evidence-Based Clinical Practice Guidelines (8th Edition). Chest 2008;133:546S–592S.

37. Vahanian A, Baumgartner H, Bax J, et al. Guidelines on the management of valvular heart disease: The Task Force on the Management of Valvular Heart Disease of the European Society of Cardiology. Eur Heart J 2007;28:230–268.

38. Warnes CA, Williams RG, Bashore TM, et al. ACC/AHA 2008 Guidelines for the Management of Adults with Congenital Heart Disease: a report of the American College of Cardiology/American Heart Association Task Force on Practice Guidelines (writing committee to develop guidelines on the management of adults with congenital heart disease). Circulation 2008;118:e714–e833.

39. Daniel WG, Erbel R, Kasper W, et al. Safety of transesophageal echocardiography. A multicenter survey of 10,419 examinations. Circulation 1991;83:817–821.

40. Douglas PS, Khandheria B, Stainback RF, et al. ACCF/ASE/ACEP/AHA/ASNC/SCAI/SCCT/SCMR 2008 appropriateness criteria for stress echocardiography: a report of the American College of Cardiology Foundation Appropriateness Criteria Task Force, American Society of Echocardiography, American College of Emergency Physicians, American Heart Association, American Society of Nuclear Cardiology, Society for Cardiovascular Angiography and Interventions, Society of Cardiovascular Computed Tomography, and Society for Cardiovascular Magnetic Resonance: endorsed by the Heart Rhythm Society and the Society of Critical Care Medicine. Circulation 2008;117:1478–1497.

41. Camici PG, Prasad SK, Rimoldi OE. Stunning, hibernation, and assessment of myocardial viability. Circulation 2008;117:103–114.

42. Klocke FJ, Baird MG, Lorell BH, et al. ACC/AHA/ASNC guidelines for the clinical use of cardiac radionuclide imaging–executive summary: a report of the American College of Cardiology/American Heart Association Task Force on Practice Guidelines (ACC/AHA/ASNC Committee to Revise the 1995 Guidelines for the Clinical Use of Cardiac Radionuclide Imaging). Circulation 2003;108:1404–1418.

43. Hendel RC, Berman DS, Di Carli MF, et al. ACCF/ASNC/ACR/AHA/ASE/SCCT/SCMR/SNM 2009 appropriate use criteria for cardiac radionuclide imaging: a report of the American College of Cardiology Foundation Appropriate Use Criteria Task Force, the American Society of Nuclear Cardiology, the American College of Radiology, the American Heart Association, the American Society of Echocardiography, the Society of Cardiovascular Computed Tomography, the Society for Cardiovascular Magnetic Resonance, and the Society of Nuclear Medicine. Endorsed by the American College of Emergency Physicians. J Am Coll Cardiol 2009;53:2201–2229.

44. Sabharwal NK, Lahiri A. Role of myocardial perfusion imaging for risk stratification in suspected or known coronary artery disease. Heart 2003;89:1291–1297.

45. Somsen GA, Verberne HJ, Burri H, Ratib O, Righetti A. Ventricular mechanical dyssynchrony and resynchronization therapy in heart failure: a new indication for Fourier analysis of gated blood-pool radionuclide ventriculography. Nucl Med Commun 2006;27:105–112.

46. Cheitlin MD, Armstrong WF, Aurigemma GP, et al. ACC/AHA/ASE 2003 guideline update for the clinical application of echocardiography: summary article: a report of the American College of Cardiology/American Heart Association Task Force on Practice Guidelines (ACC/AHA/ASE Committee to Update the 1997 Guidelines for the Clinical Application of Echocardiography). Circulation 2003; 108:1146–1162.

47. Berman DS, Hachamovitch R, Shaw LJ, et al. Roles of nuclear cardiology, cardiac computed tomography, and cardiac magnetic resonance: assessment of patients with suspected coronary artery disease. J Nucl Med 2006;47:74–82.

48. Bluemke DA, Achenbach S, Budoff M, et al. Noninvasive coronary artery imaging: magnetic resonance angiography and multidetector computed tomography angiography: a scientific statement from the American Heart Association Committee on Cardiovascular Imaging and Intervention of the Council on Cardiovascular Radiology and Intervention, and the Councils on Clinical Cardiology and Cardiovascular Disease in the Young. Circulation 2008;118: 586–606.

49. Budoff MJ, Achenbach S, Fayad Z, et al. Task Force 12: training in advanced cardiovascular imaging (computed tomography): endorsed by the American Society of Nuclear Cardiology, Society for Cardiovascular Angiography and Interventions, Society of Atherosclerosis Imaging and Prevention, and Society of Cardiovascular Computed Tomography. J Am Coll Cardiol 2006;47:915–920.

50. Miller JM, Rochitte CE, Dewey M, et al. Diagnostic performance of coronary angiography by 64-row CT. N Engl J Med 2008;359: 2324–2336.

51. Slart RH, Bax JJ, van Veldhuisen DJ, et al. Prediction of functional recovery after revascularization in patients with coronary artery disease and left ventricular dysfunction by gated FDG-PET. J Nucl Cardiol 2006;13:210–219.

Appendix 17-1
Types of Tests Used to Evaluate the Cardiovascular System

	Cardiac Function[a]			
	Myocardial Perfusion	**Pump**	**Electrical Rhythm**	**Anatomy**
Types of tests	Stress tests	Angiography	ECG	Echocardiography
	Nuclear imaging	MUGA	Electrophysiologic studies	Angiography
	Angiography	Echocardiography	Holter monitoring	Intravascular ultrasound
	Echocardiography			
Parameters evaluated	Coronary anatomy and blood flow	Cardiac output	Rhythm	Chamber size
	Myocardial perfusion	Ejection fraction	Rate	Wall motion
		Valvular function	Conduction pathways	Valve function
		Shunts		Valve structure
				Pericardium
				Coronary anatomy

ECG, electrocardiogram; MUGA, multigated acquisition.
[a]Not all tests for any one cardiac function are used to evaluate all parameters listed.

Appendix 17-2
Types of Tests for Various Cardiac Diseases or Features

Feature/Disorder	CXR	Echo	Angiography	Nuclear Scan	CT	MRI	ET	ECG	PET
Ischemic	−	+++	++++	+++	++/++	++	++	++	+++
Valvular	+	++++	+++	+	+++	+++	++	+	+
Congenital	++	++++	+++	+	+++	++++	+	+	+
Anatomy	+	+++	++	+	+++	++++	−	+	+
Cardiomyopathy	+	++++	+++	++	+++	+++	−	−	++
Pericardial	+	++++	++	−	++++	++++	−	±	−
Endocarditis	−	++++[a]	+	−	++	+++	−	±	−
Masses	−	++++	+	−	+++	+++	−	−	+
Metabolism	−	−	−	+	−	−	−	−	++++
Graft patency	−	±	+++	++	+	++	++	+	+++
CA anatomy	−	−	++++	++	+	++	++	+	+
Ventricular function	−	++++	+++	++	+++	+++	+	−	++

CA, coronary artery; CT, computed tomography; CXR, chest radiograph; ECG, electrocardiogram; echo, echocardiography; ET, exercise testing; PET, positron emission.
[a] Transesophageal echocardiography is superior to transthoracic echocardiography.

18

Cardiac Arrest

JEFFREY F. BARLETTA AND JEFFREY L. WILT

KEY CONCEPTS

❶ High-quality cardiopulmonary resuscitation with minimal interruptions in chest compressions should be emphasized in all patients following cardiac arrest.

❷ Chest compressions prior to defibrillation [consistent with the cardiocerebral resuscitation (CCR) model] may lead to more successful outcomes especially with arrests that are not witnessed.

❸ The purpose of using vasopressor therapy following cardiac arrest is to augment low coronary and cerebral perfusion pressures encountered during cardiopulmonary resuscitation (CPR).

❹ Despite several theoretical advantages with vasopressin, clinical trials have not consistently demonstrated superior results over that achieved with epinephrine

❺ Amiodarone remains the preferred antiarrhythmic during cardiac arrest according to the 2005 American Heart Association Guidelines for Cardiopulmonary Resuscitation and Emergency Cardiovascular Care (or 2005 AHA guidelines) with lidocaine considered as an alternative.

❻ Successful treatment of both pulseless electrical activity (PEA) and asystole depends almost entirely on diagnosis of the underlying cause.

❼ Intraosseous administration is the preferred alternative route for administration if IV access can not be achieved.

Cardiac arrest is defined as the cessation of cardiac mechanical activity as confirmed by the absence of signs of circulation (e.g., a detectable pulse, unresponsiveness, and apnea).[1] While there is wide variation in the reported incidence of cardiac arrest, it is estimated that there are 294,851 emergency medical services (EMS)-treated out-of-hospital cardiac arrests annually in the United States.[2] Unfortunately, outcomes remain alarmingly poor with survival to hospital discharge ranging from 1.1% to 8.1% in patients who suffer out-of-hospital cardiac arrest.[3] In-hospital cardiac arrest, on the other hand, yields a survival of approximately 20%.[1]

EPIDEMIOLOGY

In adult patients, cardiac arrest usually results from the development of an arrhythmia.[4] Historically, ventricular fibrillation (VF) and pulseless ventricular tachycardia (PVT) have been the most common initial rhythm; however, this has changed markedly over time. In one study of out-of-hospital arrests, VF was the first identified rhythm in 61% of patients in 1980 compared to 41% of patients in 2000, a reduction of greater than 30%.[5] More recently, a second study identified VF/PVT as the first recorded rhythm in only 13% of patients.[3] The declining incidence of VF could potentially be due to its association with ischemia and other cardiac causes of arrest (vs noncardiac causes) and the improvements made in the treatment of coronary artery disease.[4,5]

In contrast to out-of-hospital cardiac arrest, VF is the initial rhythm in roughly 20% to 35% of in-hospital cardiac arrests.[1] As in-hospital cardiac arrest is typically preceded by hypoxia or hypotension, asystole, or pulseless electrical activity (PEA) occur more commonly. In fact, one study noticed an incidence of asystole and PEA of 35% and 32%, respectively, while the incidence of VF or PVT was only 23%.[6]

This declining incidence of VF or PVT is somewhat concerning as survival rates are substantially higher compared to asystole or PEA. Hospital survival for in-hospital cardiac arrest related to VF or PVT is approximately 36% (vs 11% with asystole/PEA) with most patients having a good neurologic outcome.[6] Survival for out-of-hospital cardiac arrest due to VF or PVT is approximately 25% to 40%, with higher survival rates being observed in communities that have an organized rapid response system.[3]

In contrast to adult patients, only 14% of pediatric patients with in-hospital arrest present with VF or PVT as the initial rhythm of which 29% survive to hospital discharge.[6] This is probably because most pediatric arrests are respiratory-related as opposed to the primary cardiac etiology seen in adult patients. Unfortunately, survival following pediatric out-of-hospital cardiopulmonary arrest is roughly 7% with most survivors having a poor neurologic status.[2]

ETIOLOGY

Coronary artery disease is the most common clinical finding in adult patients who suffer cardiac arrest and is the etiologic cause for roughly 80% of sudden cardiac deaths.[4] Approximately 10% to 15% of sudden cardiac deaths occur in patients with cardiomyopathies (e.g., hypertrophic cardiomyopathy, dilated cardiomyopathy), while the remaining 5% to 10% are composed of either structurally abnormal congenital cardiac conditions or patients with structurally normal but electrically abnormal heart. Unfortunately, in at least 67% of patients, cardiac arrest is the first clinical sign of coronary artery disease with no preceding signs or symptoms.[7]

In pediatric patients, cardiac arrest is often the terminal event of respiratory failure or progressive shock.[8] Out-of-hospital arrests frequently are associated with events such as trauma, sudden infant death syndrome, drowning, poisoning, choking, severe asthma, and pneumonia, while in-hospital arrests are associated with sepsis, respiratory failure, drug toxicity, metabolic disorders, and arrhythmias.

PATHOPHYSIOLOGY OF CARDIAC ARREST

There are two distinctly different pathophysiologic conditions associated with cardiac arrest. The first is primary cardiac arrest whereby arterial blood is typically fully oxygenated at the time of arrest. The second is cardiac arrest secondary to respiratory failure in which lack of ventilation leads to severe hypoxemia, hypotension, and secondary cardiac arrest. It is important to understand specific condition at hand as different treatment approaches are likely necessary.[9]

TREATMENT

Cardiopulmonary resuscitation (CPR) is an attempt to restore spontaneous circulation by performing chest compressions (to restore threshold blood flows, particularly to the heart and brain) with or without ventilations. There are two proposed theories describing the mechanism of blood flow during CPR.[10] The original theory is known as the cardiac pump theory and is based on the active compression of the heart between the sternum and vertebrae thereby creating forward flow. Echocardiography, however, has revealed that left ventricular size does not always change with compressions and the mitral valve may in fact be open.[10] The second, more recent theory is the thoracic pump theory. This theory is based on intrathoracic pressure alterations induced by chest compressions and the differential compressibility of the arteries and veins. In this model, the heart merely acts as a passive conduit for flow.

The concept of cough CPR supports the importance of changes in intrathoracic pressure as a means of generating forward blood.[11] During vigorous coughing, intrathoracic pressures increase secondary to contractions of the diaphragm, abdominal muscles, and intercostal muscles. These pressure changes occur without direct chest compression and are sufficient to maintain consciousness. The observation that coughing alone can maintain consciousness led many investigators to question the cardiac pump theory and accept the thoracic pump theory. It is likely that both models contribute to the mechanism of blood flow with CPR.

High-quality CPR as suggested in the 2005 AHA guidelines has continued to be evaluated. In one animal model, high-quality compressions compared to standard compressions led to an increase in restoration of spontaneous circulation and neurologically normal survival.[12] In addition, the use of an impedance threshold device, which harnesses the recoil energy of the chest wall decompression (thereby improving cardiac filling) seems to be of benefit and is under continued investigation.[13]

■ DESIRED OUTCOME

The goal of CPR is the return of spontaneous circulation (ROSC), with effective perfusion (and similarly, ventilation) as quickly as possible to minimize hypoxic damage to vital organs. It is not sufficient to restore spontaneous circulation if the patient is left neurologically devastated or incurs severe morbidity in the process. Factors proved to enhance survival to hospital discharge include the occurrence of a witnessed arrest, rapid implementation of bystander CPR, presence of VF as the initial rhythm, and early defibrillation therapy for

VF.[14] In fact, survival rates from witnessed cardiac arrest due to VF/PVT decrease by approximately 7% for every minute between collapse and defibrillation if no CPR is provided. If bystander CPR is provided, however, the decrease in survival is 3% to 4% per minute.[8] Investigators are now evaluating predictors of outcome depending on type of arrest, time to ROSC, and are even validating new tools to evaluate functional outcome after cardiac arrest.[15,16]

■ GENERAL APPROACH TO TREATMENT

Cardiopulmonary Resuscitation

National conferences and organized committees have played a major role in encouraging widespread competency in CPR technique. The most recent conference was held in 2005 which provides the latest set of recommendations for CPR and emergency cardiovascular care (ECC) (Table 18–1).[8] These guidelines continue to emphasize the "chain of survival" to highlight the treatment approach and illustrate the importance of a timely response.[8] The four links of the chain of survival are

1. Early recognition of the emergency and activation of EMS
2. Early bystander basic life support (BLS) and CPR
3. Early delivery of a shock with a defibrillator
4. Early advanced cardiac life support (ACLS) followed by postresuscitation care delivered by healthcare professionals

While all four links of the chain of survival are important, the most crucial may be the first three, particularly early CPR.[8] CRP provides critical blood flow to the heart and brain, prolongs the time VF is present (prior to the deterioration to asystole) and increases the likelihood that a shock will terminate VF resulting in a rhythm compatible with life.[8] In one study of out-of-hospital cardiac arrest, early recognition of cardiac arrest [odds ratio (OR) 4.4 {95% confidence interval (CI), 3.1-6.4}], early CPR [OR 3.7 (95% CI, 2.5-5.4)], and defibrillation within 8 minutes [OR 3.4 (95% CI, 1.4-8.4] were associated with an increase in survival to hospital discharge.[14] ACLS, on the other hand, did not improve survival [OR 1.1 (95% CI, 0.8-1.5)]. ❶ The 2005 AHA guidelines for CPR and ECC, therefore emphasize the provision of high-quality CPR with minimal interruptions in chest compressions.[8]

The use of drug therapy as part of ACLS has devolved to a minimal role since survival to hospital discharge does not appear to be impacted.

Basic Life Support Based on the 2005 AHA guidelines, the initial algorithm is BLS, and the first action is to determine responsiveness of the patient. If there is no response, the rescuer should immediately activate the emergency medical response team, and obtain an automated external defibrillator (AED) if one is available. Next, the victim's airway should be opened, with an assessment of effective breathing. If the victim is not breathing, then two rescue breaths should be administered. Subsequent to this, the rescuer should determine if there is an effective pulse. If there is an effective pulse, then rescue breathing with frequent assessments of effective circulation should be continued until help arrives. If there is no pulse, then chest compressions need to be immediately instituted. The recommended rate is 100 beats/minute, with cycles of 30 compressions followed by 2 rescue breaths. The 2005 AHA guidelines for CPR and ECC stress that there should be minimal interruptions in chest compressions. If there is no AED available, then cycles of compressions/breaths should continue, with pulse checks every 2 minutes (5 cycles) until help arrives or the patient regains spontaneous circulation. If there is an AED available, then the rhythm should be checked to determine if defibrillation is advised. If so, then one shock should be delivered with the immediate resumption

TABLE 18-1 Evidence-Based Treatment Recommendations

Recommendations	Recommendation Grades[b]
Immediate bystander CPR[a] High-quality CPR should be performed with minimal interruption in chest compressions and defibrillation as soon as it can be accomplished.	Class I
Epinephrine One milligram IV/IO should be administered every 3 to 5 minutes in patients with VF, PVT, PEA, or asystole	Class IIb
Vasopressin Forty units IV/IO may replace either the first or second dose of epinephrine in patients with VF, PVT, or asystole. There is insufficient evidence to recommend either for or against its use in PEA.	Class Indeterminate
Amiodarone Three hundred milligrams IV/IO can be followed by 150 mg IV/IO in patients with VF/PVT unresponsive to CPR, shock, and a vasopressor.	Class IIb
Lidocaine Lidocaine can be considered an alternative to amiodarone in patients with VF/PVT. The initial dose is 1 to 1.5 mg/kg IV. Additional doses of 0.5 to 0.75 mg/kg can be administered at 5- to 10-minute intervals to a maximum dose of 3 mg/kg if VF/PVT persists.	Class Indeterminate
Magnesium Magnesium is recommended for VF/PVT that is caused by torsades de pointes. One to 2 g diluted in 10 mL D5W should be administered IV/IO push over 5 to 20 minutes. Clinical studies have not demonstrated a benefit when magnesium was routinely administered during CPR when torsades de pointes was not present.	Class IIa
Fibrinolysis Thrombolytics should be considered on a case-by-case basis when pulmonary embolism is suspected.	Class IIa
Hypothermia Hypothermia should be implemented in unconscious adult patients with ROSC after out-of-hospital cardiac arrest when the initial rhythm was VF. These patients should be cooled to 32°C to 34°C for 12 to 24 hours. Hypothermia may be beneficial for patients with non-VF arrest out of hospital or for in-hospital cardiac arrest.	Class IIa Class IIb
Atropine Atropine 1 mg IV/IO every 3 to 5 minutes (maximum total of 3 doses or 3 mg) can be considered for patients with asystole or PEA.	Class Indeterminate

[a] CPR, cardiopulmonary resuscitation; IV, intravenous; IO, intraosseous; VF, ventricular fibrillation; PVT, pulseless ventricular tachycardia; PEA, pulseless electrical activity; D5W, dextrose 5% in water.

[b] Key for evidence-based classifications:[8]

Class I: High-level prospective studies support the action or therapy, and the benefit substantially outweighs the potential for harm. The treatment should be administered.

Class IIa: The weight of evidence supports the action or therapy, and the therapy is considered acceptable and useful. It is reasonable to administer the treatment.

Class IIb: The evidence documented only short-term benefits, or positive results were documented with lower levels of evidence. Class IIb recommendations can be considered either optional or recommended by experts despite the absence of high-level supporting evidence.

Class III: The risk outweighs the benefit for a particular treatment. The treatment should not be administered and may be harmful.

Class Indeterminate: This is either a continuing area of research or an area where research is just getting started. No recommendation (either for or against) can be made.

of chest compressions and rescue breaths. After 5 cycles, the rhythm should be reevaluated to determine the need for defibrillation. This algorithm should be repeated until help arrives, or the rhythm is no longer "shockable." If the rhythm is not shockable, then chest compressions—rescue breath cycles should be continued until help arrives, or the victim recovers spontaneous circulation. (Fig. 18–1)

Despite widespread dissemination of cardiac arrest guidelines, and the ongoing education even of health care providers, there is ample evidence that chest compression quality remains poor in general. This has led to further educational interventions in an attempt to increase quality of CPR. In one study, the combination of debriefing and feedback improved the effectiveness of chest compressions from 29% to 64%.[17]

Advanced Cardiac Life Support Once ACLS providers arrive, then further definitive therapy is given. If the rhythm is not shockable, then it is likely to be either asystole or PEA. (Fig. 18–2) The general management of these rhythms is CPR and pharmacologic therapy as listed below. For PEA, the rescuer must consider reversible causes. (Table 18–2) If the person is in VF or PVT, then one shock should be delivered (appropriate to the available electrical device), with the immediate resumption of 30 compressions and 2 breaths for 5 cycles prior to rechecking the rhythm or pulse. If there is still a shockable rhythm, then one shock should be delivered, and at this time pharmacologic intervention can be considered. After the first unsuccessful shock, vasopressors are the initially recommended pharmacologic intervention (before or after the second shock), and after the second unsuccessful shock, antiarrhythmics can be considered (before or after the third shock). Five cycles of chest compressions—breaths should be performed in between attempts at defibrillation. This algorithm will repeat until either a pulse is obtained with effective circulation, the rhythm changes, or the patient expires. For completeness, please refer to the guidelines published by the AHA.[8]

Cardiocerebral Resuscitation

The appropriateness of the 2005 AHA guidelines for ECC has recently been questioned in favor of a concept known as cardiocerebral resuscitation (CCR).[9] This "clarion call for change" was made in light of the suboptimal outcomes observed with the ECC guidelines as well as several limitations with the guideline process.[18] CCR is composed of three major components: (1) continuous chest compressions for bystander resuscitation, (2) a new ACLS algorithm for EMS, and (3) aggressive postresuscitation care including therapeutic hypothermia and early catheterization/intervention.

CCR advocates continuous chest compressions without mouth-to-mouth ventilations for witnessed cardiac arrests. Chest compressions deliver a small but critical amount of oxygen to the brain and myocardium. Cerebral and coronary perfusion pressures, however, build up slowly once chest compressions are begun. These perfusion pressures are lost if chest compressions are stopped to deliver mouth-to-mouth ventilation. In fact, approximately 16 seconds are required to deliver 2 breaths as recommended by the ECC guidelines.[19] The loss of perfusion during this time period is extremely detrimental as ROSC is closely related to perfusion pressures generated during chest compressions.[20] Several clinical trials have documented the benefit of continuous chest compressions (without ventilation) compared to conventional CPR.[21]

The second component of CCR is a new ACLS protocol for EMS. This protocol is based on the 3-phase time-sensitive model of cardiac arrest.[22] The first phase is the electrical phase (0 to 5 minutes), where prompt defibrillation is the most important intervention. The second phase is the hemodynamic phase (5 to 15 minutes), where adequate coronary and cerebral perfusion pressures, before and after defibrillation, are crucial. In fact, defibrillation prior to CPR in this phase commonly leads asystole or PEA. This is likely due to the presence of global tissue ischemia and the need for blood flow (via chest compressions) to "flush out" deleterious metabolic factors that have accumulated during ischemia. The third phase is the metabolic phase (beyond 15 minutes) in which survival is very low and hypothermia may be the most beneficial approach.

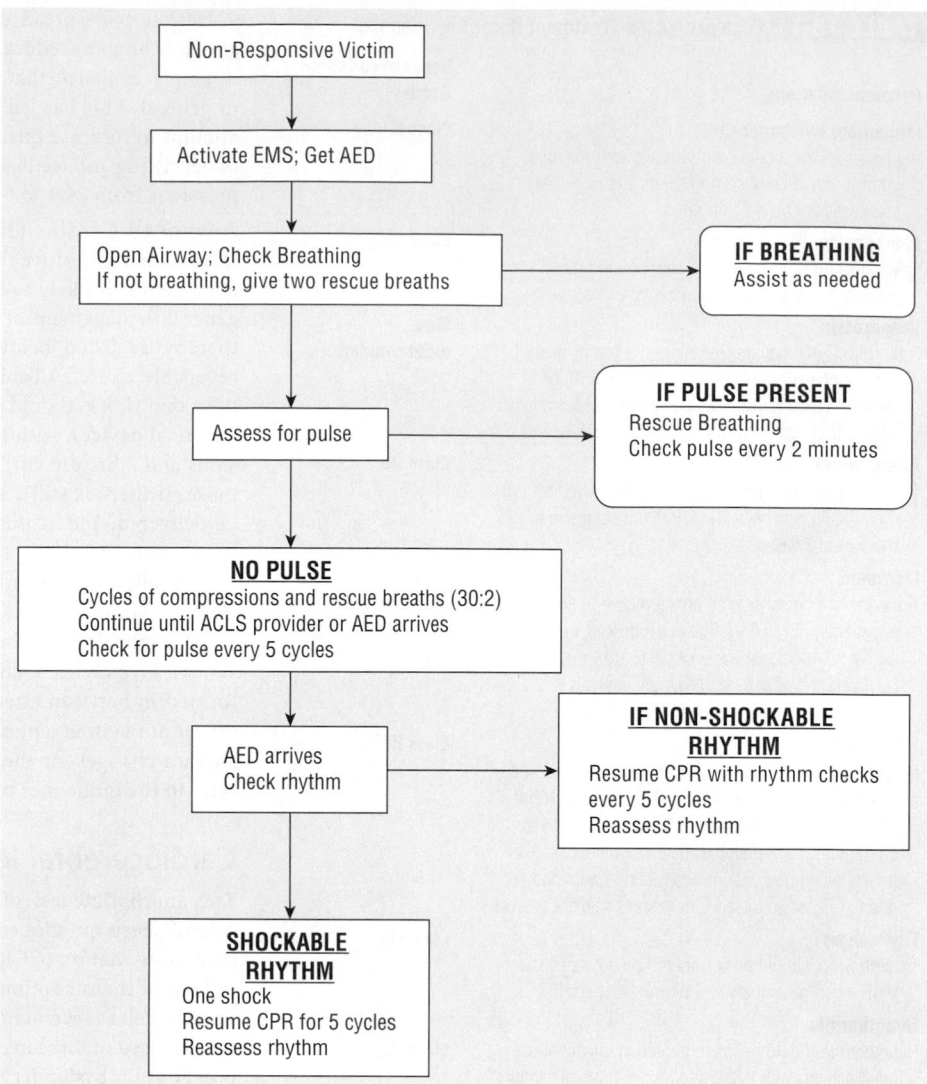

FIGURE 18-1. Treatment algorithm for adult cardiopulmonary arrest: basic life support (BLS)

The third component of CCR is aggressive postresuscitation care. This consists of the use of hypothermia for all comatose patients and emergent cardiac catheterization and percutaneous coronary intervention for patients with myocardial ischemia as a potential cause of their arrest. This and other differences between CCR and CPR are highlighted in Table 18–3. Since its conception in 2003, clinical studies evaluating CCR have demonstrated an improvement in survival of 250% to 300% compared to conventional CPR.[9]

■ VENTRICULAR FIBRILLATION AND VENTRICULAR TACHYCARDIA

Nonpharmacologic Therapy

Electrical defibrillation is the only effective method of restoring a perfusing cardiac rhythm in either VF or PVT; therefore, it is a crucial link in the "chain of survival," especially for a witnessed arrest.[8] The probability of successful defibrillation is directly related to the time interval between the onset of VF and the delivery of the first shock.[8] In one study, a 23% relative improvement in survival was observed with each 1 minute reduction in the time to defibrillation [OR 0.77 (95% CI, 0.73-0.81)].[23]

❷ Although early defibrillation is crucial for survival following cardiac arrest, several studies have suggested that CPR prior to defibrillation (consistent with the CCR model) may lead to more successful outcomes.[24–27]

In one trial, the provision of roughly 90 seconds of CPR prior to defibrillation was associated with an increased rate of hospital survival (compared with a historical control group) when response intervals were 4 minutes or longer (27% vs 17%; $P = 0.01$).[24] A second trial reported higher survival rates in patients with response intervals greater than 5 minutes when 3 minutes of CPR was administered prior to defibrillation (22% vs 4%; $P = 0.006$).[27] In a study where each defibrillation, including the first, was preceded by 200 uninterrupted chest compressions, an increase in total survival [57% (19/33) vs 20% (18/92), $P = 0.001$] and neurologically normal survival [48% (16/33) vs 15% (14/92), $P = 0.001$] was reported compared to standard CPR practices.[26] Finally, one study noted an improvement in hospital survival (from 22% to 44%, $P = 0.0024$) in patients with witnessed VF using a modified resuscitation protocol which included 200 pre-shock chest compressions.[25] In lieu of these results, the 2005 AHA guidelines offer that EMS personnel may give two minutes of chest compressions prior to attempting defibrillation. Recommendations are similar for victims in the metabolic phase recognizing the likelihood of achieving ROSC, however, is drastically lower.

As opposed to the previous guidelines, where "stacked," multiple shocks were initially given, persons in VF or PVT should receive electrical defibrillation with one shock.[8] This revision is largely due to the prolonged time noted (approximately 55 seconds) to deliver three stacked shocks without providing adequate chest compressions.[28] The defibrillation attempt should be with

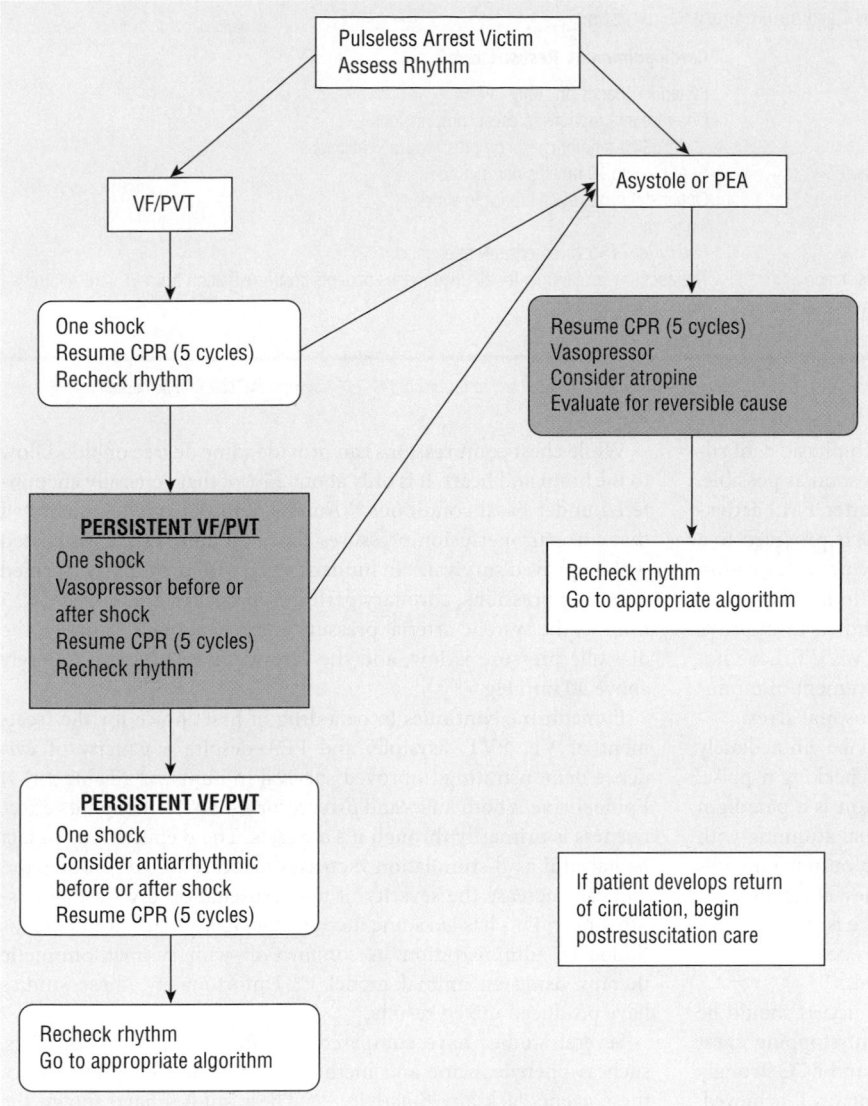

FIGURE 18-2. Treatment algorithm for adult cardiopulmonary arrest: advanced cardiac life support (ACLS)

TABLE 18-2	Potentially Reversible Causes of PEA and Asystole (Think: 6 H's; 6 T's)	
Condition	**Clues**	**Treatment**
Hypovolemia	History, flat neck veins	Intravenous fluids
Hypoxia	Cyanosis, blood gases, airway problems	Ventilation, oxygen
Hydrogen ion (acidosis)	History of bicarbonate-responsive preexisting acidosis	Sodium bicarbonate, hyperventilation
Hyper (Hypo) kalemia	History of renal failure, diabetes, recent dialysis, dialysis fistulas, medications	Calcium chloride, insulin, glucose, sodium bicarbonate, sodium polystyrene sulfonate, dialysis
Hypothermia	History of exposure to cold, central body temperature	Rewarming, oxygen, intravenous fluids
Hypoglycemia	History of diabetes	Glucose infusion
Toxin (Drug overdose)	Bradycardia, history of ingestion, empty bottles at the scene, pupils, neurologic exam	Drug screens, intubation, lavage, activated charcoal
Tamponade (Cardiac)	History (trauma, renal failure, thoracic malignancy), no pulse with CPR, vein distention, impending tamponade-tachycardia, hypotension, low pulse pressure changing to sudden bradycardia as terminal event	Pericardiocentesis
Tension pneumothorax	History (asthma, ventilator, chronic obstructive pulmonary disease, trauma), no pulse with CPR, neck vein distention, tracheal deviation	Needle decompression
Thrombosis, coronary	History, ECG, enzymes	PCI, thrombolytics, oxygen, nitroglycerin, heparin, aspirin, morphine
Thrombosis, pulmonary	History, no pulse with CPR, distended neck veins	Pulmonary arteriogram, surgical embolectomy, thrombolytics
Trauma	History, examination	Volume infusion, intracranial pressure monitoring, bleeding control, surgical intervention

Data from references (8, 126)

TABLE 18-3 Cardiocerebral Resuscitation Versus Cardiopulmonary Resuscitation

Cardiocerebral Resuscitation	Cardiopulmonary Resuscitation
Continuous chest compressions for bystanders	Bystander "hands-on" only CPR
Decrease rescue breathing	Decrease interruptions in chest compressions
BLS: No rescue breathing	BLS: 30:2 ratio of chest compressions to ventilations
ACLS: Passive oxygen insufflation or limited breaths per minute	ACLS: 8 to 10 breaths per minute
Two hundred chest compressions prior to shock	Optional 5 cycles of 30:2 prior to shock
Single shock	Single shock
Two hundred chest compressions immediately after shock	Five cycles of 30:2 immediately after shock
Therapeutic hypothermia for all unconscious patients postresuscitation	Therapeutic hypothermia for all unconscious patients postresuscitation from VF cardiac arrest
Early emergent catheterization and PCI for all resuscitated victims regardless of EKG findings	No official statement

Reprinted from J Am Coll Cardiol., Vol. 53(2), Ewy GA, Kern KB. Recent advances in cardiopulmonary resuscitation: cardiocerebral resuscitation, 149–157, Copyright © 2009, with permission from Elsevier.

360 J (monophasic defibrillator) or 150 to 200 J (biphasic defibrillator). If an AED is available, it should be used as soon as possible. However, CPR should be started immediately (after EMS activation), as the AED is being prepared. If early CPR is provided to a witnessed VF arrest, and defibrillation is able to be provided within 3 to 5 minutes, survival rates have been reported to be has high as 74%.[8,29] Interestingly, AEDs, which have been shown to improve survival in out-of-hospital cardiac arrest due to VF/VT, have not been shown to improve outcome following replacement of monophasic defibrillators with biphasic AEDs for in-hospital arrest.[30]

After defibrillation is attempted, CPR should be immediately restarted and continued for 2 minutes without checking a pulse. The omission of the pulse check after defibrillation is a paradigm shift in the algorithm that is related to myocardial stunning with resultant poor perfusion and diminished cardiac output immediately after electrical therapy.[8] After 2 minutes of chest compressions, the rhythm and pulse should be rechecked. If there is still evidence of VF or PVT, then pharmacologic therapy with repeat attempts at single-discharge defibrillation should be attempted.

Endotracheal intubation and intravenous (IV) access should be obtained when feasible, but not at the expense of stopping chest compressions. The 2005 AHA guidelines for CPR and ECC strongly stress the need for uninterrupted CPR.[8] Once an airway is achieved, patients should be ventilated with 100% oxygen. The recent guidelines suggest that lower tidal volumes and rates may be beneficial.[8] There are several airway adjuncts that are potentially available, such as laryngeal mask airways and esophageal-tracheal combination tubes. However, the definitive airway is an endotracheal tube placed with direct laryngoscopy.

Other interventions are also being evaluated as non-pharmacologic therapy. In a porcine model of VF arrest, a percutaneously placed left ventricular assist device (LVAD) was shown to sustain vital organ perfusion.[31] As well, the performance of angiography and percutaneous coronary intervention during suspected myocardial infarction has been studied in both animals and anecdotally in humans refractory to traditional ACLS protocol without ROSC. A review of this topic suggests that this intervention is feasible and that further investigation is warranted.[32] Extracorporeal membrane oxygenation (ECMO) has also been evaluated and has been shown to improve outcomes in some series, but the logistics of widespread implementation is daunting.[33] While there are no conclusive human data regarding these issues, it does raise interesting concepts to deliberate and research.

Pharmacologic Therapy

Sympathomimetics The use of sympathomimetics is a major part of drug therapy in CPR. ❸ The primary goal of sympathomimetic therapy is to augment low coronary and cerebral perfusion pressures encountered during CPR.

While chest compressions can provide some degree of blood flow to the brain and heart, it is only about 25% of that generally encountered under basal conditions.[34] Animal studies have demonstrated that coronary perfusion pressures above 30 mm Hg are associated with improved survival.[35] In humans, even with properly performed chest compressions, coronary perfusion pressures are only 10 to 15 mmHg, the systolic arterial pressure is rarely above 80 mmHg, the diastolic pressure is low, and the carotid mean pressure is rarely above 40 mm Hg.[8,36]

Epinephrine continues to be a drug of first choice for the treatment of VF, PVT, asystole, and PEA despite a paucity of evidence demonstrating improved survival in humans.[8] (Table 18–4) Epinephrine is both an α- and β-receptor agonist, although its effectiveness is primarily through it's α effects. The β effects may in fact be harmful as β-stimulation increases myocardial oxygen demand and can increase the severity of postresuscitation myocardial dysfunction.[37] This has led some investigators to evaluate simultaneous β-blocker administration in conjunction with sympathomimetic therapy using an animal model.[35,38] Unfortunately, these studies have produced mixed results.

Several studies have compared the effects of pure α_1-agonists, such as phenylephrine and methoxamine, with epinephrine since these agents lack any β-activity.[39,40] These studies have shown the use of α_1-agonists to have no long-term survival advantage over epinephrine. One reason that selective α_1-agonists are not superior to epinephrine is related to the α_2 effects. Agents that have potent α_2 effects (e.g., epinephrine and norepinephrine) may be more effective because the α_2-adrenergic receptors lie extrajunctionally in the intima of the blood vessels, making them more accessible to circulating catecholamines—even in low-flow states that occur during CPR.[40] Furthermore, during ischemia, the number of postsynaptic α_1-receptors decreases, which suggests a greater role for α_2-agonist activity during CPR.[41]

Several investigators have compared norepinephrine with epinephrine.[36,42,43] Norepinephrine is a potent α-agonist (both α_1 and α_2) but also has β_1-agonist effects. In the only large-scale randomized, double-blind, prospective trial that compared norepinephrine with epinephrine in the prehospital cardiac arrest setting, there were no significant differences in ROSC, hospital admission or discharge.[42] A second, smaller study demonstrated higher resuscitation rates with norepinephrine compared to epinephrine (64% vs 32%) but no significant difference in hospital discharge.[43] Consequently, epinephrine remains the first-line sympathomimetic for CPR.

The recommended dose for epinephrine is 1 mg administered by IV or intraosseous (IO) injection every 3 to 5 minutes.[8] This epinephrine dose was derived from animal studies (0.1 mg/kg in a 10 kg dog) and equates to approximately 0.015 mg/kg for a 70 kg human.[44] Both animal and human studies have demonstrated a positive dose—response relationship with epinephrine suggesting that higher doses might be necessary to improve hemodynamics and

TABLE 18-4 Summary of Adult High-Dose Epinephrine Studies

Author	Design	Epinephrine Dosing SDE versus HDE	N	Initial Resuscitation SDE versus HDE		Hospital Discharge SDE versus HDE		Discharge Neurologic Status SDE versus HDE	
Gueugniaud et al[50]	P, MC, R, DB	1 mg vs 5 mg, up to 15 doses	3327	601/1650 (36.4%)	678/1677* (40.4%)	46/1650 (2.8%)	38/1677 (2.3%)	26/46 (56.5%)	26/38 (68.4%)
								Discharged without neurologic impairment	
Sherman et al[52]	P, MC, R, DB	0.01 mg/kg versus 0.1 mg/kg, up to 4 doses	140	7/62 (11%)	15/78 (19%)	Not addressed		Not addressed	
Choux et al[49]	P, R, DB	1 mg versus 5 mg, up to 15 doses	536	85/265 (32%)	96/271 (35.5%)	20/54 (37%)	23/63† (35.4%)	GCS ≥ 9 (at day 3):	
								4/20	3/23
								EEG Normal (at day 3):	
								1/20	3/23
Lipman et al[51]	P, R, DB	1 mg versus 10 mg, up to 3 doses	35	11/16 (69%)	15/19 (79%)	1/16 (6.3%)	0/19 (0%)	Not addressed	
Stiell et al[53]	P, R, DB	1 mg versus 7 mg, up to 5 doses	650	76/333 (23%)	56/317 (18%)	16/333 (5%)	10/317 (3%)	94%	90%
								Remained in their best CPC on discharge	
Brown et al[47]	P, MC, R, DB	0.02 mg/kg versus 0.2 mg/kg for the first dose	1280	190/632 (30%)	217/648 (33%)	26/632 (4%)	31/648 (5%)	92%	94%
								Conscious at discharge (CPC = 1-3)	
Callaham et al[42]	P, R, DB	1 mg versus 15 mg, up to 3 doses	556	22/270 (8%)	37/286* (13%)	3/270 (1.2%)	5/286 (1.7%)	2.3	3.2
								Mean CPC score	
Lindner et al[43]	P, R, DB	1 mg versus 5 mg for the first dose	68	6/40 (15%)	16/28* (57%)	2/40 (5%)	4/28 (14%)	Not addressed	
Callaham et al[48]	Ret	HDE: ≥ 50 mcg/kg or total dose > 2.8 mcg/kg/min	68	Not addressed		11/35 (31%)	6/33 (18.2%)	Intact: 8/11 versus 4/6	
								Impaired: 2/11 versus 2/6	
								Vegetative: 1/11 versus 0/6	

*$p < 0.05$.

†Number of patients admitted to the hospital alive on day 3.

Abbreviations: SDE, standard dose epinephrine; HDE, high-dose epinephrine; P, prospective; MC, multicenter; R, randomized; DB, double-blind; Ret, retrospective; GCS, Glasgow Coma Scale; EEG, electroencephalogram; CPC, cerebral performance category.

Data from references (42, 47–54)

achieve successful resuscitation.[45,46] These results, however, have not been replicated in human studies[42,47-54] (Table 18–4). Collectively, these studies have shown that high-dose epinephrine may increase the initial resuscitation success rate but that overall survival is not significantly different. The discrepancy between animal and human studies may be due to the fact that most victims of cardiac arrest have coronary artery disease, a condition not present in an animal model. In a human model, however, atherosclerotic plaques can aggravate the balance between myocardial oxygen supply and demand. Moreover, the interval from arrest to treatment in animal studies is shorter than the interval frequently reported in human studies. Since time to CPR and defibrillation are crucial variables for success, prolonging this time period can lower resuscitation rates.

Vasopressin Vasopressin, also known as *antidiuretic hormone*, is a potent, nonadrenergic vasoconstrictor that increases blood pressure and systemic vascular resistance. Although it acts on various receptors throughout the body, its vasoconstrictive properties are due primarily to its effects on the V_1 receptor.[55] Measurement of vasopressin levels in patients undergoing CPR has shown a high correlation between the levels of endogenous vasopressin released and the potential for ROSC.[55] In fact, in one study, plasma vasopressin concentrations were approximately three times as high in survivors compared with nonsurvivors, suggesting that vasopressin is released as an adjunct vasopressor to epinephrine in life-threatening events such as cardiac arrest.[56]

Vasopressin may have several advantages over epinephrine. First, the metabolic acidosis that frequently accompanies cardiac arrest can blunt the vasoconstrictive effect of adrenergic agents such as epinephrine. This effect does not occur with vasopressin. Second, the stimulation of β-receptors caused by epinephrine can increase myocardial oxygen demand and complicate the postresuscitative phase of CPR. Because vasopressin does not act on β-receptors, this effect does not occur with its use. Vasopressin also may have a beneficial effect on renal blood flow by stimulating V_2-receptors in the kidney, causing vasodilation and increased water reabsorption. With regard to splanchnic blood flow, however, vasopressin has a detrimental effect when compared to epinephrine.[57]

❹ Despite several theoretical advantages with vasopressin, clinical trials have not consistently demonstrated superior results over that achieved with epinephrine. (Table 18–5) In one large trial of out-of-hospital arrest, no significant differences were noted in ROSC, hospital admission rate or discharge rate.[58] Although, when patients were stratified according to their initial rhythm, patients with asystole, had a significantly higher rate of hospital admission (29% vs 20%; $P = 0.02$) and discharge (4.7% vs 1.5%; $P = 0.04$) with vasopressin compared to epinephrine. In addition, a subgroup analysis of 732 patients who required additional epinephrine therapy despite the two doses of study drug revealed significant benefits in ROSC (37% vs 26%; $P = 0.002$), hospital admission rate (26% vs 16%; $P = 0.002$), and discharge rate (6.2% vs 1.7%; $P = 0.002$) with vasopressin. There was a trend, however, toward a poorer neurologic state or coma among the patients who survived to discharge and received vasopressin.

The favorable results from the subgroup analysis led to a prospective study evaluating the combination of vasopressin and

TABLE 18-5 Summary of Adult Vasopressin Comparative Trials[a]

Author	Design	Setting	Initial rhythm	Intervention[a]	N	Initial Resuscitation Vasopressin	Initial Resuscitation Epinephrine	Hospital Discharge Vasopressin	Hospital Discharge Epinephrine
Lindner et al[128]	P, R, DB	Out of hospital	VF: 100%	Vasopressin 40 units versus epinephrine 1 mg for initial drug treatment	40	16/20 (80%)	11/20 (55%)	8/20 (40%)	3/20 (15%)
Stiell et al[129]	P, R, TB, MC	In hospital	VF/PVT: 21% PEA: 48% Asystole: 31%	Vasopressin 40 units versus epinephrine 1 mg for initial drug treatment	200	62/104 (60%)	57/96 (59%)	12/104 (12%)	13/96 (14%)
Wenzel et al[58]	P, R, DB, MC	Out of hospital	VF/PVT: 40% PEA: 16% Asystole: 45%	Vasopressin 40 units versus epinephrine 1 mg for 2 doses as initial drug treatment	1186	145/589 (25%)	167/597 (28%)	57/578 (10%)	58/588 (10%)
Guyette et al[127]	Ret	Out of hospital	VF/PVT: 27% PEA: 17% Asystole: 51%	Epinephrine versus epinephrine + vasopressin	298	16/37[b] (43%)	58/231[b] (25%)	NR	NR
Grmec et al[130]	P, O with Ret control	Out of hospital	VF/PVT: 100%	Epinephrine 1 mg versus vasopressin 40 units initially versus vasopressin 40 units after 3 doses of epinephrine 1 mg	109	Initial therapy: 17/27 (63%)[b] Delayed therapy: 19/31 (61%)[b]	23/51 (45%)[b]	Initial therapy: 7/27 (26%) Delayed therapy: 8/31 (26%)	10/51 (20%)
Callaway et al[131]	P, R, DB	Out of hospital	VF: 15% PEA: 22% Asystole: 50%	Vasopressin 40 units or placebo as soon as possible after the first dose of epinephrine 1 mg	325	52/167 (31%)	48/158 (30%)	NR	NR
Gueugniaud et al[59]	P, R, DB, MC	Out of hospital	VF: 9% PEA: 8% Asystole: 83%	Epinephrine 1 mg followed by vasopressin 40 units (<10 seconds apart) versus epinephrine alone for 2 doses	2894	413/1442 (29%)	428/1452 (30%)	24/1439 (1.7%)	33/1448 (2.3%)
Mentzelopoulos et al[60]	P, R, DB	In hospital	VF/PVT: 14% PEA: 25% Asystole: 61%	Vasopressin 20 units + epinephrine 1 mg + methylprednisolone 40 mg (vasopressin + epinephrine were repeated during each of 4 subsequent CPR cycles versus epinephrine 1 mg)	100	39/48 (81%)[b]	27/52 (52%)	9/48 (19%)[b]	2/52 (4%)

[a]All study groups received epinephrine following the initial study drug.

[b]$p < 0.05$.

Abbreviations: P, prospective; MC, multicenter; R, randomized; DB, double-blind; TB, triple-blind; Ret, retrospective; O, observational; VF, ventricular fibrillation; PVT, pulseless ventricular tachycardia; PEA, pulseless electrical activity; NR, not reported. *Data from references (58-60, 127–131)*

epinephrine versus epinephrine alone.[59] In this study, patients were randomized to receive either 1 mg of epinephrine followed by 40 units of vasopressin (in less than 10 seconds) or 1 mg of epinephrine plus saline placebo. Unfortunately, there were no significant differences between the combination therapy group and epinephrine only group in any of the outcome measures studied (ROSC, survival to hospital admission, survival to hospital discharge, 1 year survival and good neurologic recovery at discharge). In contrast, a post-hoc subgroup analysis revealed a lower rate of survival (0% vs 5.8%, $P = 0.02$) with combination therapy when the initial rhythm was PEA.

A second study evaluated combination therapy for in-hospital cardiac arrest.[60] In this study, patients were randomized to receive either epinephrine alone or 20 units of vasopressin plus 1 mg of epinephrine and 40 mg of methylprednisolone (followed by

hydrocortisone in the post-resuscitative phase). Vasopressin 20 units plus epinephrine 1 mg were repeated during each of 4 subsequent CPR cycles. This study marks the first to include corticosteroids as part of drug-therapy during CPR. The rationale is based on the hemodynamic effects of steroids alone with their potential to impact the intensity of the postresuscitation systemic inflammatory response and organ dysfunction. Significant benefits were observed in ROSC (81% vs 52%, $P = 0.003$) and survival to hospital discharge (19% vs 4%, $P = 0.02$) with combination therapy including corticosteroids. Future studies are required to determine the role of vasopressin and corticosteroids for cardiac arrest.

Antiarrhythmics The purpose of antiarrhythmic drug therapy following unsuccessful defibrillation and vasopressor administration is to prevent the development or recurrence of VF and PVT by raising the fibrillation threshold. Clinical evidence demonstrating improved survival to hospital discharge however is lacking. As the role of antiarrhythmics during CPR remains limited, only two individual agents are currently recommended in the 2005 AHA guidelines for CPR and ECC: amiodarone and lidocaine.

The use of lidocaine has been beneficial in animal studies and in patients with arrhythmias following an acute myocardial infarction but its benefit in cardiac arrest remains questionable. In the only published case-control trial where patients were classified according to whether they received lidocaine, no significant difference was noted in ROSC, admission to the hospital, or survival to hospital discharge between groups.[61] Similarly, a prospective study comparing the effectiveness of lidocaine with that of standard-dose epinephrine showed not only a lack of benefit with lidocaine but also a higher tendency to promote asystole.[62] In contrast, a retrospective analysis in patients with VF indicated that lidocaine was associated with a higher rate of ROSC and hospitalization ($P<0.01$) but not an increase in the hospital discharge rate.[63]

Amiodarone is classified as a class III antiarrhythmic but possesses electrophysiologic characteristics of all four Vaughn Williams classifications. In a large, randomized, double-blind trial in out-of-hospital cardiac arrest secondary to VF or PVT (also known as the *ALIVE trial*), patients were randomized to receive either amiodarone 300 mg or placebo.[64] Recipients of amiodarone were more likely to be resuscitated and survive to hospital admission than were recipients of placebo (44% and 34%, respectively; $P = .03$). There was no difference in survival to hospital discharge (amiodarone, 13.4% vs placebo, 13.2%; $P = $ NS). This was the first trial to demonstrate the benefit of an antiarrhythmic agent over placebo in patients with out-of-hospital cardiac arrest.

A subsequent trial (known as the *ALIVE trial*) compared amiodarone 5 mg/kg with lidocaine 1.5 mg/kg in patients with out-of-hospital cardiac arrest due to VF.[65] In this trial, amiodarone was associated with a relative improvement of 90% in survival to hospital admission compared with lidocaine [22.8% vs 12%; OR 2.17 (95% CI 1.21-3.83); $P = 0.009$]. Similar to the ARREST trial, there was no difference in survival to hospital discharge (amiodarone, 5% vs lidocaine, 3%; $P = .34$).

Amiodarone and lidocaine have also been compared following in-hospital cardiac arrest secondary to VF or PVT. In a multicentered, retrospective review, 194 patients who received amiodarone ($n = 74$), lidocaine ($n = 79$), or both ($n = 41$) were evaluated.[66] The rate of survival at 24 hours was 55%, 63%, and 50% for patients receiving amiodarone, lidocaine, or both, respectively ($P = 0.39$). There was no difference in survival to hospital discharge (39% for amiodarone, 45% for lidocaine, and 42% for patients receiving both agents; $P = 0.72$). After adjusting for multiple covariates, Cox regression analysis revealed higher mortality for those patients who received amiodarone (as opposed to lidocaine) [survival to 24 hours: hazard ratio was 3.15 (95% CI, 1.68-5.92), $P<0.001$; survival to hospital discharge: hazard ratio was 3.25 (95% CI, 1.22-8.65), $P = 0.02$] and in those patients with VF/PVT as the initial rhythm (as opposed to bradycardia followed by VF/PVT) [survival to 24 hours: hazard ratio was 3.36 (95% CI, 1.98-5.71), $P<0.001$; survival to hospital discharge: hazard ratio was 3.6 (95% CI, 1.2-10.6), $P = 0.021$]. The mean initial dose of amiodarone, though, was 190 mg, and only 25% of patients received the recommended dose of 300 mg. Additionally, the time to first dose of antiarrhythmic was significantly longer in the amiodarone group than in the lidocaine group (14 minutes vs 6 minutes, $P<0.001$). While these differences could have biased the results in favor of lidocaine, they provide a real-world experience with the use of amiodarone. Further large-scale trials are needed to determine the preferred antiarrhythmic for both in-hospital and out-of-hospital cardiac arrest. ❺ In the meantime, amiodarone remains the preferred antiarrhythmic during cardiac arrest according to the 2005 AHA guidelines for CPR and ECC with lidocaine considered as an alternative.[8]

Thrombolytics Since most cardiac arrests are related to either MI or PE, several investigators have evaluated the role of thrombolytics during CPR. While these studies have demonstrated successful use of thrombolytics, few have shown improvements to hospital discharge[67-76] (Table 18–6). In the largest published randomized controlled trial to date, tenecteplase was compared with placebo for out-of-hospital cardiac arrest. Unfortunately, enrollment was stopped early due to futility in meeting their primary endpoint, 30 day survival.[74] Survival in the tenecteplase and placebo groups, respectively, was 15% and 17% ($P = 0.36$). Potential reasons for failure in this study include the lack of antiplatelet and antithrombin medications and decreased delivery of the thrombolytic to the coronary arteries (where the clots exist) due to impaired flow and perfusion. Of note, intracranial hemorrhage occurred with significantly greater frequency with tenecteplase versus placebo (2.7% vs 0.4%, $P = 0.006$). The role of thrombolytics as part of CPR will require further study.

Magnesium While severe hypomagnesemia has been associated with VF/PVT, clinical trials have not demonstrated any benefit with the routine administration of magnesium during a cardiac arrest. Two observation trials though have shown an improvement in ROSC in patients with arrests associated with torsades de pointes.[8] Therefore, magnesium administration should be limited to these patients.

Postresuscitative Care

Following the ROSC from a cardiac arrest, a complex phase of resuscitation begins which has been termed post-cardiac arrest syndrome.[77] There are four main components of post-cardiac arrest syndrome which highlight succinct pathophysiologic processes and potential areas for treatment (Table 18–7). They are post-cardiac arrest brain injury, myocardial dysfunction, systemic ischemia/reperfusion response and persistent precipitating pathology.[77] In general, many of the concepts within these 4 components surround the principles of basic ICU care (e.g., early hemodynamic optimization, circulatory support, sedation, etc). For a detailed description, the reader is referred either to the corresponding chapter in this text or to evidence-based consensus statements.[77] One particular area, however that is specific to cardiac arrest is the concept of therapeutic hypothermia.

Restoration of blood flow following cardiac arrest can lead to several chemical cascades and destructive enzymatic reactions that can result in cerebral injury. These reactions include free-radical production, excitatory amino acid release, and calcium shifts, leading to mitochondrial damage and apoptosis (programmed cell death).[78] Hypothermia can protect from cerebral injury by suppressing these chemical reactions, thereby reducing the production of free radicals. Various animal models have demonstrated improved functional recovery and reduced cerebral deficits with the induction of mild therapeutic hypothermia[78,79] Recent data has attempted to refine this concept, and even expand upon the organ systems protected. In a pig model of VF treated after 10 minutes, rapid head cooling led to more beneficial effects than surface cooling in terms of postresuscitation myocardial dysfunction.[80] In addition, a similar pig model of cardiac arrest showed that delayed surface cooling led to less favorable survival and neurologic outcome than early head cooling.[81]

Interestingly, hypothermia as a therapeutic endeavor in humans has been described since antiquity. It is reported that Hippocrates suggested packing bleeding patients in snow and ice for treatment, and also that a chief surgeon of Napoleon Bonaparte's noticed that wounded soldiers who were rewarmed survived less than those who were left in the cold.[82,83]

TABLE 18-6 Summary of Adult Thrombolytic Comparative Trials

Author	Design	Drug Studied	N	Initial Resuscitation		Hospital Discharge		Major Bleeding	
				Thrombolytic	No Thrombolytic	Thrombolytic	No Thrombolytic	Thrombolytic	No Thrombolytic
Kurkciyan, et al, 2000[71]	Ret	tPA 100 mg	42	17/21[a] (81%)	9/21[a] (43%)	2/21 (10%)	1/21 (5%)	5/21 (24%)	NA
Bottiger, et al, 2001[68]	P, NR, PC	tPA 50 mg, up to 2 doses	90	27/40[a] (68%)	22/50[a] (44%)	6/40 (15%)	4/50 (8%)	2/40 (5%)	0/50 (0%)
Ruiz-Bailen, et al, 2001[73]	Ret	SK (3%) tPA (94%) Other (3%)	303	22/67[a] (33%)	144/236[a] (61%)	12/67[a] (18%)	109/236[a] (46%)	5/67 (7%)	2/236 (1%)
Lederer, et al, 2001[72]	Ret	tPA	324	76/108[a] (70%)	110/214[a] (51%)	27/108[a] (25%)	33/214[a] (15%)	6/45 (13%)	7/46 (15%)
Abu-Laban, et al, 2002[67]	P, R, MC, PC	tPA 100 mg	233	25/117 (21%)	27/116 (23%)	1/117 (1%)	0/116 (0%)	2/117 (2%)	0/116 (0%)
Janata et al, 2003[70]	Ret	tPA 0.6-1 mg/kg (100mg max)	66	24/36 (67%)	13/30 (43%)	7/36 (19%)	2/30 (7%)	9/36 (25%)	3/30 (10%)
Fatovich, et al, 2004[69]	P, R, DB, PC	Tenecteplase 50 mg	35	8/19[a] (42%)	1/16[a] (6%)	1/19 (5%)	1/16 (6%)	0	0
Stadlbauer, et al, 2006[76]	Ret	Tenecteplase or reteplase	1186	44/99[a] (46%)	355/1087[a] (33%)	14/99 (14%)	101/1067 (10%)	0	NA
Bozeman, et al 2006[75]	P, NR, MC	Tenecteplase	163	13/50[a] (26%)	14/113[a] (12%)	2/50 (4%)	0/113 (0%)	1/50 (2%)	NA
Bottiger, et al 2008[74]	P, R, DB, MC, PC	Tenecteplase (30 mg – 50 mg)	1050	283/515 (55%)	279/511 (55%)	78/517 (15%)	90/514 (18%)	14/518 (2.7%)[a]	2/514 (0.4%)[a]

[a]p<0.05

Abbreviations: Ret, retrospective, tPA, tissue plasminogen activator, NA, not available, P, prospective, NR, non-randomized, PC, placebo controlled, SK, streptokinase, R, randomized, MC, multicentered, DB, double-blind.

Data from references (67–76)

These early human observations, as well as current animal model investigations, have been parlayed into the clinical bedside in human trials, and literature continues to accumulate. Early human success with hypothermia was described in two pivotal trials.[84,85]

The first trial was conducted in nine centers in five European countries.[84] In this study, patients who had been resuscitated after cardiac arrest due to VF but remained comatose were assigned randomly to undergo therapeutic hypothermia, targeting a temperature of 32° to 34°C, for 24 hours. The primary end point was neurologic outcome within 6 months of cardiac arrest. Secondary end points were mortality (within 6 months) and complication rate within 7 days. A favorable neurologic outcome was achieved in 55% of patients in the hypothermia group as opposed to 39% in the normothermia group ($P = 0.009$). Additionally, mortality rates were improved significantly in the hypothermia group (41% vs 55%; $P = 0.02$). Based on this difference, seven patients would need to be treated with hypothermia to prevent one death. The rate of complications (e.g., bleeding, pneumonia, sepsis, and renal failure) did not differ between the two groups (73% for the hypothermia group and 70% for the normothermia group; $P = 0.70$).

The second trial was conducted in four hospitals in Melbourne, Australia.[85] Entry criteria were similar to the previous trial, but the target temperature for hypothermia was 33°C, which was maintained for 12 hours. The primary outcome measure was survival to hospital discharge with good neurologic function. Forty-nine percent of patients in the hypothermia group had good neurologic function on discharge (to either home or a rehabilitation facility) compared with 26% of patients in the normothermia group ($P = 0.046$). Mortality rates were similar between the two

groups (51% for the hypothermia group and 68% for the normothermia group; $P = 0.145$). Hypothermia was associated with a lower cardiac index, higher systemic vascular resistance, and hyperglycemia. It is important to note that only 8% of patients with cardiac arrest were selected for therapeutic hypothermia in these two studies.

Since that time, further data has continued to accumulate. In one study therapeutic hypothermia (combined with percutaneous coronary intervention, tight glycemic control, and seizure control) doubled the one-year survival rate (reportedly with good brain function) from 26% to 56%.[86] The implementation of therapeutic hypothermia in clinical practice (i.e., outside of the context of a clinical trial) has also been evaluated. A review of this topic showed that there is a significant variation in reported protocols, but that survival and neurological outcomes benefit from post-arrest hypothermia "are robust when compared over a wide range of studies of actual implementation" [OR (95% CI) = 2.5 (1.8-3.3)].[87] Nevertheless, there is significant debate about hypothermia including when to consider limitation of care given predicted poor outcome.[88] Initially hypothermia was described with only VF without sustained circulatory shock. As part of the "cardiocerebral" concept described above, investigators are expanding the use to non VF arrests since similar benefit is being found.[15]

Methods of inducing hypothermia are also in evaluation. There is debate over how quickly to achieve a therapeutic temperature, and in at least one animal model, a novel immersion device showed an average time to reach target temperature of only 9 minutes.[89] As well, simple maneuvers, such as iced saline infusion, can be used even in the pre-hospital setting with subsequent cooling by other

TABLE 18–7 Post-Cardiac Arrest Syndrome

Syndrome	Pathophysiology	Potential Treatments
Post-cardiac arrest brain injury	Impaired cerebrovascular autoregulation Cerebral edema Postischemic neurodegeneration	Therapeutic hypothermia Early hemodynamic optimization Mechanical ventilation Seizure control Controlled reoxygenation Supportive care
Post-cardiac arrest myocardial dysfunction	Global hypokinesis ACS	Early revascularization Early hemodynamic optimization IV fluids Inotropes IABP LVAD ECMO
Systemic ischemia/reperfusion response	SIRS Impaired vasoregulation Increased coagulation Adrenal suppression Impaired tissue oxygen delivery and utilization Impaired resistance to infection	Early hemodynamic optimization IV fluids Vasopressors High-volume hemofiltration Temperature control Glucose control Antibiotics for documented infection
Persistent precipitating pathology	AMI/ACS COPD/asthma CVA PE Overdose/poisoning Sepsis Hypovolemia	Disease-specific interventions

Abbreviations: ACS, acute coronary syndrome; SIRS, systemic inflammatory response syndrome; AMI, acute myocardial infarction; COPD, chronic obstructive pulmonary disease; CVA, cerebrovascular accident; PE, pulmonary embolism; IABP, intra-aortic balloon pump; LVAD, left ventricular assist device; ECMO, extracorporeal membrane oxygenation.

Data from reference (77)

means.[90] This has led to editorials clamoring for ongoing studies regarding methodologies and outcomes.[91,92]

In light of these accumulating data, unconscious adult patients with spontaneous circulation after out-of-hospital cardiac arrest should be cooled to 32°C to 34°C for 12 to 24 hours when the initial rhythm was VF.[8,78,87] Such cooling also may be of benefit for other rhythms or in-hospital cardiac arrests. There is insufficient evidence to make a recommendation on the use of therapeutic hypothermia in children, however an evaluation in neonates with asphyxiation suggested that hypothermia in this select population may be beneficial.[93]

Hypothermia must be used with caution, however, as there are several complications that can develop. Coagulopathy, dysrhythmias, hyperglycemia, increased incidence of pneumonia, as well as sepsis have been described.[85,94] In addition, hypothermia can have profound effects on drug distribution and elimination.[95] Further research is proceeding in this area.

■ NON-VF/PVT RHYTHMS: PEA AND ASYSTOLE

Nonpharmacologic Therapy

Pulseless electrical activity is defined as the absence of a detectable pulse and the presence of some type of electrical activity other than VF or PVT. Several studies have documented that patients with PEA actually have mechanical cardiac contractions, but they are too weak to produce a palpable pulse or blood pressure. Asystole is defined as the presence of a flat line on the ECG monitor. Although PEA is still classified as a "rhythm of survival," the success rate of treatment is much lower than the rates seen with VF/PVT.[6] PEA is often caused by treatable conditions, and the resuscitation team needs to identify and correct these conditions emergently if the resuscitation is to be successful. The rate of survival among patients with out-of-hospital cardiac arrest secondary to asystole is 1% to 2% but may be up to 10% in patients with in-hospital arrest.[5,6,14] ❻ Successful treatment of both PEA and asystole depends almost entirely on diagnosis of the underlying cause (Table 18–2).

The algorithm for treatment of PEA is the same as the treatment of asystole. Both conditions require CPR, airway control, and IV access. Asystole should be reconfirmed by checking a second lead on the cardiac monitor. Defibrillation should be avoided in patients with asystole because the parasympathetic discharge that occurs with defibrillation may reduce the chance of ROSC and worsen the chance of survival. The emphasis in resuscitation is good quality CPR without interruption, and to try to identify a correctable cause. If available, transcutaneous pacing can be attempted. Asystole often represents confirmation of death rather than a rhythm to be treated; therefore, withdrawal of efforts must be strongly considered if there is not a rapid ROSC.[8]

Much like VF/PVT, there is an interest in hypothermia in these post-arrest patients. Metabolic parameters (e.g., lactate and O_2 extraction) have been shown to be improved when post-arrest comatose adults survived their arrest and were treated with hypothermia.[96] Further studies are warranted in this area.

Pharmacologic Therapy

The primary pharmacologic agents used in the treatment of asystole are vasopressors (i.e., epinephrine and vasopressin) and atropine. Studies comparing epinephrine and vasopressin in patients with PEA and asystole have not consistently demonstrated an advantage with one agent over the other. In one large trial of patients with out-of-hospital cardiac arrest, a post-hoc, subgroup analysis was conducted for those patients with asystole.[58] In these patients, survival to hospital admission (29% vs 20%, $P = 0.02$) and discharge (4.7% vs 1.5%, $P = 0.04$) were significantly higher with vasopressin compared to epinephrine. There was, however, a non-statistically significant increase in coma/vegetative state with vasopressin (40% vs 0%, $P = 0.014$). In contrast to these findings, a second study which evaluated combination therapy with vasopressin and epinephrine, did not report an advantage with vasopressin in patients with asystole.[59] In fact, a post-hoc subgroup analysis of patients with PEA as the initial rhythm, revealed a lower rate of survival (0% vs 5.8%, $P = 0.02$) with combination therapy compared to epinephrine alone.

Atropine is an antimuscarinic agent that blocks the depressant effect of acetylcholine on both the sinus and atrioventricular nodes, thus decreasing parasympathetic tone. During asystole, parasympathetic tone may increase because of the vagal stimulation that occurs secondary to intubation, the effects of hypoxia and acidosis, or alterations in the balance of parasympathetic and sympathetic control.[97] Unfortunately, there are no prospective controlled trials showing benefit from atropine for the treatment of asystole or PEA.

Earlier small observational reports found some response to atropine in asystole or pulseless idioventricular rhythm but little evidence to suggest that long-term outcomes were altered.[98] In one retrospective case-control study, a success rate of 14% (6 of 43) was noted with atropine compared with to a 0% (0 of 41) rate with a control but no patients survived to hospital discharge.[98] In a second retrospective study, asystole was terminated in only 4 of 22 patients (18%) when atropine was administered.[99] Once again, none survived to hospital discharge. Finally, a third retrospective review evaluated 101 patients who received atropine for asystole.[100]

Twenty-four patients (24%) survived 24 hours after resuscitation. It is unclear how many survived to hospital discharge. These results show that although atropine may achieve ROSC in some instances, asystolic arrest is almost always fatal. Given the relative safety of atropine, the ease of administration, low cost and theoretical advantages, atropine should be considered for asystole or PEA.[8] The beneficial effects however are limited.

■ ACID-BASE MANAGEMENT

Acidosis seen during cardiac arrest is the result of decreased blood flow (leading to anaerobic metabolism) or inadequate ventilation. Chest compressions generate only approximately 20% to 30% of normal cardiac output, leading to inadequate organ perfusion, tissue hypoxia, and metabolic acidosis. In addition, the lack of ventilation causes retention of carbon dioxide, leading to respiratory acidosis. This combined acidosis produces not only reduced myocardial contractility and negative inotropic effect, but also the appearance of arrhythmias because of a lower fibrillation threshold. In early cardiac arrest, adequate alveolar ventilation has been considered the mainstay of control to limit the accumulation of carbon dioxide and control the acid-base imbalance.[8] With the evolution to CCR, however, there are experts arguing against ventilation because of the negative effects it can have on the effectiveness of CPR. This has led to evidence showing no negative effects if compression-only CPR is used for out-of-hospital cardiac arrest (exceptions being pediatric arrest, drowning, trauma, airway obstruction, non-cardiac etiology, or due to acute respiratory disease).[101] With arrests of long duration, buffer therapy is often considered, however little data supports its use during cardiac arrest.

Although sodium bicarbonate was once given routinely to reduce the detrimental effects associated with acidosis (e.g., reduced myocardial contractility), enhance the effect of epinephrine, and improve the rate of defibrillation, there are few clinical data supporting its use.[102] In fact, sodium bicarbonate may have some detrimental effects.[102,103] The effect of sodium bicarbonate can be described by the following reaction:

$$[HCO_3^-] + [H^+] \leftrightarrow [H_2CO_3] \leftrightarrow [H_2O] + [CO_2]$$

When sodium bicarbonate is added to an acidic environment, this reaction will shift to the right, thereby increasing tissue and venous hypercarbia. The carbon dioxide generated by this reaction will diffuse into the cell and decrease intracellular pH. The accumulation of intracellular carbon dioxide, specifically within the myocardium, is inversely correlated with coronary perfusion pressure produced by CPR. Intracellular acidosis also will decrease myocardial contractility, further complicating the low-flow state associated with CPR.[102] Furthermore, treatment with sodium bicarbonate often overcorrects extracellular pH because sodium bicarbonate has a greater effect when the pH is closer to normal.[103] The induced alkalosis, causes an increase in the affinity of oxygen to hemoglobin ("left shift"), thus interfering with oxygen release into the tissues. More recently, the early administration of bicarbonate (1 mEq/kg) had no effect on survival in pre-hospital cardiac arrest. There was a slight trend toward improvement in prolonged arrest (>15 mins) with a twofold improvement in survival (32.8% vs 15.4%).[104]

Sodium bicarbonate can be used in special circumstances (i.e., underlying metabolic acidosis, hyperkalemia, salicylate overdose, or tricyclic antidepressant overdose), however the dosage should be guided by laboratory analysis if possible. There has been clinical interest in other buffering agents (Carbicarb, Tham, Tribonat) as they have shown less potential for the adverse effects seen with sodium bicarbonate.[8] However there is a dearth of clinical experience with these agents, and outcome studies are not available.

■ MODIFICATIONS FOR SPECIAL SITUATIONS

Drowning

Drowning is a process resulting in primary respiratory impairment from immersion in a liquid. It is a common, preventable cause of morbidity and mortality. The most important inciting event is the hypoxia induced by submersion. Thus, early care of the drowning patient includes immediate rescue breathing, even before they are removed from the water. Prompt initiation of this therapy increases chance of survival.[105] Once the victim is removed from the water, immediate chest compressions should be started if they are pulseless. Drowning victims can present with any of the pulseless rhythms; standard guidelines need to be followed for therapy of these rhythms.

Hypothermia

Unintentional hypothermia (as opposed to the therapeutic hypothermia used post-arrest, described above) is defined by a body temperature <30°C (86°F), and is associated with marked derangements in body function. Because it can depress virtually every body system, including pulse and respiration, the patient may appear to be dead upon the initial evaluation. Hypothermia may lead to benefit on brain recovery after cardiac arrest (discussed earlier), thus aggressive intervention is clearly indicated when there is a hypothermic arrest victim.

If the patient still has a perfusing rhythm, therapy is mainly based upon rewarming techniques. For mild hypothermia [i.e., >34°C (>93.2°F)], passive rewarming is recommended. For moderate hypothermia [i.e., 30°C to 34°C (86°F to 93.2°F)], active external rewarming is recommended, and for severe hypothermia [i.e., <30°C (<86°F)] active internal rewarming is recommended. These patients need to be manipulated very gently as VF is sometimes precipitated by movement.[106]

If the patient is in cardiac arrest, then the standard BLS algorithm should be followed. However, there are some modifications that the rescuer needs to consider. The rescuer should evaluate for respiration and pulse for a longer timeframe, since these may be slow or very difficult to realize. If there is no breathing, then rescue breaths should ensue. If there is any doubt about the presence of a pulse, then chest compressions should be started immediately. If the patient is in VF or PVT then electrical therapy should be given in a standard manner. However, the hypothermic heart may be less responsive to medications or defibrillation, and thus there have been worries about the optimal temperature at which to start defibrillation attempts.[8] There are no published consensus guidelines regarding this. Immediately after defibrillation, CPR should resume as in the standard manner. During CPR, continued attempts at rewarming are of paramount importance. Included in this concept is preventing further heat loss (i.e., removal of wet clothing, protection from the environment, etc). Patients often require significant volume challenges during the rewarming process. The use of steroids, antibiotics, and barbiturates has been proposed, but none of these agents have ever been shown to increase survival rates.[8]

It is debatable when to stop resuscitative efforts in the hypothermic patient. Many authors have proposed that a patient should not be pronounced until the core temperature has been restored to near normal.[8] Once the patient is in the hospital, it is still the judgment of the treating physician when efforts should be terminated.

Pregnancy

Pregnancy is a unique situation in that survival of both the fetus and the mother depend on CPR. The best hope for survival of the fetus is maternal survival. Because of the gravid uterus, resuscitation needs to be modified. Since the vena cava and aorta can be obstructed by a uterus of approximately 20 weeks gestation or later, it is appropriate to position the patient approximately 15 to 30 degrees back from the left lateral decubitus position, or to pull the uterus to the side.[107] The optimal angle has been cited to be 27 degrees, and has led to the development of the "Cardiff resuscitation wedge" which has been specifically designed for performing CPR on pregnant patients.[108]

Airway control is important in the pregnant patient. The airway may be smaller because of the hormonal changes and edema which accompany pregnancy.[108] Similarly, because of increased intra-abdominal pressure exerted by the uterus, as well as hormonal changes that change the resting state of the gastroesophageal sphincter, clinicians need to be acutely aware of the increased risk of aspiration. Because of this, cricoid pressure needs to be maintained continuously during airway manipulation. The rescuer may need to give smaller tidal volumes than normal because of the diaphragm elevation that accompanies the later stages of pregnancy. Because of the increased ventilatory needs in pregnancy as well as the anatomic changes, some authors have suggested that it is important to perform early intubation during cardiac arrest in pregnancy and cite this rapid intubation as a difference from non-pregnant patients.[108] Similarly, circulatory support also has to be adjusted. In particular, chest compressions need to be administered slightly above the center of the sternum to adjust for the anatomic changes of the pregnant uterus.[8]

In an arrest situation during pregnancy the ACLS provider needs to follow the standard guidelines, including the same use of defibrillation and medications. While it is true that vasoactive agents, such as epinephrine, can diminish uterine blood flow, safer alternatives do not exist.[8] Available literature, though scant, suggests that the energy requirements for defibrillation do not change in pregnancy.[109]

While etiologies of arrest in pregnancy are often the same as in the non-pregnant patient, there are several unique situations that need to be considered in the differential diagnosis of a pregnancy arrest. These include excess magnesium sulfate institution (i.e., iatrogenic from treating eclampsia) in which case the therapeutic administration of calcium gluconate can be lifesaving; amniotic embolism, which is associated with complete cardiovascular collapse during labor and delivery (cardiopulmonary bypass has been reportedly successful in salvaging this condition); pre-eclampsia/eclampsia developing after the 20th week of gestation producing hypertension and multiple organ dysfunction; as well as vascular events including acute coronary syndromes and acute pulmonary embolism.[108,110,111]

It is paramount to remember that unless circulation is restored to the mother, both the mother and the fetus will succumb, especially if standard therapy is not used correctly and promptly. Because of this the resuscitation leader should consider the need for emergent hysterotomy (i.e., Cesarean delivery) and delivery as soon as the arrest happens. The best survival reported for infants > 24 weeks gestation happens when delivery occurs no more than 5 minutes after the arrest of the mother.[8]

Trauma

Cardiac resuscitation of the trauma arrest patient is basically performed with the same guidelines as any other arrest. There are some specific etiologies to rapidly consider however, since the survival of an out-of-hospital cardiac arrest due to trauma is rare.[8] The rescuer needs to consider airway obstruction, pneumothorax, tracheobronchial injury, cardiac or large arterial injury, cardiac tamponade, severe head injury with secondary cardiac collapse, and other injuries specific to the particular trauma.[8] The best survival seems to be in young patients with treatable penetrating injuries.

Trauma patients often suffer head or cervical injuries; thus cervical spine precautions should be used in these patients. A jaw thrust maneuver is the preferred way to open the airway, with in-line stabilization during attempts at advanced airway placement.[8] The rescuer must be vigilant for the development of tension pneumothorax during ventilation. Inadequate ventilation of one side is usually due to tube malposition, tension pneumothorax, or hemothorax. These conditions are usually treated by medical personnel at the hospital after transport.

Chest compressions should be performed in a standard manner. Any visible hemorrhage should be controlled with direct pressure. Fluid resuscitation is done with a goal of adequate blood pressure and organ perfusion. The specific details of fluid resuscitation are highly controversial however, and the optimal volume infusion for trauma resuscitation is a subject of ongoing debate.

Open thoracotomy for trauma-induced arrest has been performed in many instances. For penetrating chest trauma patients who arrest immediately before arrival or in the emergency department, open thoracotomy can allow relief of tamponade, control of major vessel hemorrhage, or direct repair of cardiac insult.[8] In the case of blunt trauma however, open thoracotomy has not been shown to definitively improve outcome. However, there is some suggesting that a physician-led out-of-hospital thoracotomy for penetrating trauma may have a higher chance of survival.[112]

For definitive post-arrest care, trauma patients should be rapidly transferred to a facility with expertise in the provision of trauma care.

Electrical Shock

There are many etiologies of electrical shock injuries, from lightning strike (mortality estimated to be 30%, with 70% of survivors sustaining significant morbidity) to high-tension current, to household current.[8] The severity of injury depends on the site, type of current, duration of contact, pathway, and the magnitude of delivered electricity.

Cardiac arrest is common in electrical injury due to current passing through the heart during the "vulnerable period" of the cardiac cycle. In large-current events, such as lightning strike, the heart undergoes massive depolarization simultaneously.[113] Sometimes the intrinsic pacemaker can restore an organized cardiac electrical cycle, but because of injury to other muscles, specifically the thoracic musculature, the patient cannot retain or sustain viable circulation due to the lack of ventilation and oxygenation.[114]

When approaching a victim of electrocution, the rescuer must first be certain of his or her own safety. Thereafter, standard BLS, prompt CPR, and ACLS when available is indicated. Electric shock is often associated with multiple trauma, including spinal injury, multiple injuries to the skeletal muscles, as well as fractures. These factors need to be evaluated by the resuscitation team.

Airway control may be difficult due to the edema that often accompanies such injuries; thus an advanced airway early in the treatment process is recommended.[8] With soft tissue swelling, there is often a need for aggressive fluid resuscitation in these patients. The underlying tissue, or visceral organ damage, is often worse than the external appearance. It is usually recommended that these patients be transferred to centers with expertise in dealing with these types of injuries.

GUIDELINES FOR DRUG ADMINISTRATION

The routes of administration that are available for drug delivery during CPR include IV (both central and peripheral access), IO, and endotracheal. The chosen route represents a compromise between the availability of access and their apparent efficacy in introducing the drug into the central circulation. When selecting a route for drug administration, it is of utmost importance to minimize any interruptions in chest compressions during CPR.

Central venous access will result in a faster and higher peak drug concentration than peripheral access but central line access is not needed in most resuscitation attempts. If a central line is already present, however, it should be the access site of choice. Central lines located above the diaphragm are preferable to those located below the diaphragm because of poor blood flow during CPR.[115] If IV access (either central or peripheral) has not been established a large peripheral venous catheter should be inserted. It has been suggested that only one attempt at peripheral IV insertion be allowed.[116] If this is not successful, an IO device should be inserted. Of note, peripheral drug administration yields a peak concentration in the major systemic arteries in roughly 1.5 to 3 minutes but circulation time can be shortened by up to 40% if the drug is followed by a 20-mL fluid bolus with elevation of the extremity.[115]

❼ IO administration is the preferred alternative route for administration if IV access can not be achieved.[8] Drug administration using the IO route is as quick and effective as drug administration via central access and superior to that achieved with peripheral access. Several studies have documented the effectiveness and safety of this administration route in both adults and children.[8] Potential anatomic sites for insertion for an IO needle are the distal tibia, the proximal tibia and the distal femur.[117] IO infusion devices are available that allow for rapid insertion (i.e., within 60 seconds) and are easy to use.[118]

In the event that neither IV nor IO access can be established, then a few drugs can be administered endotracheally. These drugs are atropine, lidocaine, epinephrine, naloxone, and vasopressin.[8] Medications administered through the endotracheal route however, will have both a lower and delayed peak concentration than when they are administered by the IV or IO routes.[8] Furthermore, clinical trials have failed to demonstrate any benefit with using the endotracheal route.[119,120] In fact, one clinical trial noted lower rates of ROSC [15% vs 27%, $P \leq 0.01$], hospital admission [9% vs 20%, $P \leq 0.02$] and hospital discharge [0% vs 5%, $P \leq 0.02$] with endotracheal drug administration compared to IV.[120] Currently, the recommended endotracheal dose is 2 to 2.5 times larger than the IV/IO dose.[8] Given the unpredictable absorption and the lack of clinical effectiveness though, either the IV or IO routes are preferred.

ETHICAL AND ECONOMICAL CONSIDERATIONS

The primary endpoint of CPR is to survive to hospital discharge with good neurologic function. Simply surviving to hospital discharge, but in a vegetative or comatose state, can not be considered a favorable outcome and can impose a tremendous economic burden on the healthcare system. Additionally, most patients would choose not to continue living in this state and would have preferred withdrawal of support.[121] One difficulty in making these decisions is defining medical futility. The two major determinants of medical futility are length of life and quality of life.[8] An intervention that cannot increase length or quality of life is considered futile. Ethically, health care providers are obligated to respect patient autonomy, which is easiest in the arrest situation if the patient has an advance directive. If the patient loses the ability to make informed decisions regarding medical care, then a spouse or a designated healthcare advocate must act as a surrogate decision maker, invoking what has been termed substituted judgment: following the predetermined wishes of the patient.

Many health care professionals have attempted to identify patients unlikely to benefit from cardiac resuscitation. One study evaluated 2 termination rules for resuscitation following out-of-hospital arrest.[122] The first was the BLS rule which consisted of (1) the event was not witnessed by EMS personnel, (2) no AED was used or manual shock applied and (3) ROSC was not achieved in the out-of-hospital setting. The second rule was the advanced life support rule which consisted of the BLS criteria plus (1) the arrest was not witnessed by a bystander and (2) no bystander CPR administered. These rules accurately identified patients who were unlikely to benefit from rapid transport to a hospital with a positive predictive value of 0.998 (BLS rule) and 1.000 (ALS rule).

If the patient survives to hospital admission, guidelines from the American Academy of Neurology are available to aid in the decisions relative to outcome prediction for comatose survivors of cardiac arrest.[123] Collectively, these factors could improve the cost-effectiveness of CPR programs and decrease the economic burden of cardiac arrest to the healthcare system.

EVALUATION OF THERAPEUTIC OUTCOMES

To measure the success of resuscitation outcomes, therapeutic outcome monitoring should occur both during the resuscitation attempt and in the postresuscitation phase. The optimal outcome following CPR is an awake, responsive, spontaneously breathing patient. Patients must remain neurologically intact with minimal morbidity following the resuscitation if it is to be truly classified as a success.

Unfortunately, there are no reliable criteria for clinicians to use to gauge the efficacy of CPR. Nonetheless, heart rate, cardiac rhythm, and blood pressure should be assessed and documented throughout the resuscitation attempt and subsequent to each intervention. Coronary perfusion pressure (CPP = aortic diastolic pressure minus right atrial diastolic pressure) should be assessed in patients whom intra-arterial monitoring is in place. Determination of the presence or absence of a pulse is paramount to deciding which interventions may be appropriate. Palpating a pulse to determine the efficacy of blood flow during CPR has not been shown to be useful, however.

End-tidal carbon dioxide monitoring is a safe and effective method to assess cardiac output during CPR and has been associated with ROSC.[8] The main determinant for carbon dioxide excretion is the rate of delivery from the peripheral sites (where it is produced) to the lungs. Increasing cardiac output (through effective CPR) will yield higher end-tidal carbon dioxide levels as delivery of carbon dioxide to the lungs increases.

Clinicians should also consider the precipitating cause of the cardiac arrest, such as an MI, electrolyte imbalance, or primary arrhythmia. Pre-arrest status should be carefully reviewed, particularly if the patient was receiving drug therapy. Altered cardiac, hepatic, and renal function resulting from ischemic damage during the cardiopulmonary arrest warrant special attention and may require advanced care. Neurologic function should be assessed by means of the Cerebral Performance Category and the Glasgow Coma Scale.[124,125] Nonresponse to an array of suitable interventions may indicate that resuscitation is impossible.

CLINICAL CONTROVERSIES

1. The concept of CCR has led to an alternative treatment approach for cardiac arrest that some clinicians feel is superior to that proposed by the AHA.

2. Some clinicians feel that vasopressin offers substantial benefit to patients following cardiac arrest while others feel it has no advantage over epinephrine alone.

3. Although amiodarone is considered the preferred antiarrhythmic in patients with VF/PVT, there is conflicting data regarding its effect on outcome when compared to lidocaine.

4. Some clinicians support the use of therapeutic hypothermia for all comatose patients following cardiac arrest while others recommend its use only after arrests due to VF.

ABBREVIATIONS

ACLS: advanced cardiac life support

AED: automated external defibrillator

AHA: American Heart Association

BLS: basic life support

CCR: cardiocerebral resuscitation

CI: confidence interval

CPP: coronary perfusion pressure

CPR: cardiopulmonary resuscitation

ECC: emergency cardiovascular care

ECMO: extracorporeal membrane oxygenation

EMS: emergency medical services

IO: intraosseous

IV: intravenous

LVAD: left ventricular assist device

MI: myocardial infarction

OR: odds ratio

PCI: percutaneous coronary intervention

PEA: pulseless electrical activity

PE: pulmonary embolism

ROSC: return of spontaneous circulation

PVT: pulseless ventricular tachycardia

VF: ventricular fibrillation

CLINICAL PRESENTATION

Symptoms

Anxiety, change in mental status or unconscious

Cold, clammy extremities

Dyspnea, shortness of breath or no respiration

Chest pain

Diaphoresis

Nausea and vomiting

Signs

Hypotension

Tachycardia, bradycardia, irregular or no pulse

Cyanosis

Hypothermia

Distant or absent heart and lung sounds

REFERENCES

1. Sandroni C, Nolan J, Cavallaro F, Antonelli M. In-hospital cardiac arrest: Incidence, prognosis and possible measures to improve survival. Intensive Care Med 2007;33:237–245.

2. Lloyd-Jones D, Adams R, Carnethon M, et al. Heart disease and stroke statistics—2009 update: A report from the American Heart Association Statistics Committee and Stroke Statistics Subcommittee. Circulation 2009;119:e21–181.

3. Nichol G, Thomas E, Callaway CW, et al. Regional variation in out-of-hospital cardiac arrest incidence and outcome. JAMA 2008;300:1423–1431.

4. Chugh SS, Reinier K, Teodorescu C, et al. Epidemiology of sudden cardiac death: Clinical and research implications. Prog Cardiovasc Dis 2008;51:213–228.

5. Cobb LA, Fahrenbruch CE, Olsufka M, Copass MK. Changing incidence of out-of-hospital ventricular fibrillation, 1980–2000. JAMA 2002;288:3008–3013.

6. Nadkarni VM, Larkin GL, Peberdy MA, et al. First documented rhythm and clinical outcome from in-hospital cardiac arrest among children and adults. JAMA 2006;295:50–57.

7. Myerburg RJ, Castellanos A. Emerging paradigms of the epidemiology and demographics of sudden cardiac arrest. Heart Rhythm 2006;3:235–239.

8. 2005 American Heart Association Guidelines for Cardiopulmonary Resuscitation and Emergency Cardiovascular Care. Circulation 2005;112(suppl 24):IV1–203.

9. Ewy GA, Kern KB. Recent advances in cardiopulmonary resuscitation: Cardiocerebral resuscitation. J Am Coll Cardiol 2009;53:149–157.

10. Cooper JA, Cooper JD, Cooper JM. Cardiopulmonary resuscitation: History, current practice, and future direction. Circulation 2006;114:2839–2849.

11. Tucker KJ, Savitt MA, Idris A, Redberg RF. Cardiopulmonary resuscitation. Historical perspectives, physiology, and future directions. Arch Intern Med 1994;154:2141–2150.

12. Wu JY, Li CS, Liu ZX, et al. A comparison of 2 types of chest compressions in a porcine model of cardiac arrest. Am J Emerg Med 2009;27:823–829.

13. Aufderheide TP, Alexander C, Lick C, et al. From laboratory science to six emergency medical services systems: New understanding of the physiology of cardiopulmonary resuscitation increases survival rates after cardiac arrest. Crit Care Med 2008;36:S397–S404.

14. Stiell IG, Wells GA, Field B, et al. Advanced cardiac life support in out-of-hospital cardiac arrest. N Engl J Med 2004;351:647–656.

15. Oddo M, Ribordy V, Feihl F, et al. Early predictors of outcome in comatose survivors of ventricular fibrillation and non-ventricular fibrillation cardiac arrest treated with hypothermia: A prospective study. Crit Care Med 2008;36:2296–2301.

16. Stiell IG, Nesbitt LP, Nichol G, et al. Comparison of the Cerebral Performance Category score and the Health Utilities Index for survivors of cardiac arrest. Ann Emerg Med 2009;53:241–248.

17. Dine CJ, Gersh RE, Leary M, et al. Improving cardiopulmonary resuscitation quality and resuscitation training by combining audiovisual feedback and debriefing. Crit Care Med 2008;36:2817–2822.

18. Ewy GA. A clarion call for change. Curr Opin Crit Care 2009;15:181–184.

19. Assar D, Chamberlain D, Colquhoun M, et al. Randomised controlled trials of staged teaching for basic life support. 1. Skill acquisition at bronze stage. Resuscitation 2000;45:7–15.

20. Ewy GA. Cardiocerebral resuscitation: The new cardiopulmonary resuscitation. Circulation 2005;111:2134–2142.

21. Nagao K. Chest compression-only cardiocerebral resuscitation. Curr Opin Crit Care 2009;15:189–197.

22. Weisfeldt ML, Becker LB. Resuscitation after cardiac arrest: A 3-phase time-sensitive model. JAMA 2002;288:3035–3038.

23. De Maio VJ, Stiell IG, Wells GA, Spaite DW. Optimal defibrillation response intervals for maximum out-of-hospital cardiac arrest survival rates. Ann Emerg Med 2003;42:242–250.

24. Cobb LA, Fahrenbruch CE, Walsh TR, et al. Influence of cardiopulmonary resuscitation prior to defibrillation in patients with out-of-hospital ventricular fibrillation. JAMA 1999;281:1182–1188.

25. Garza AG, Gratton MC, Salomone JA, et al. Improved patient survival using a modified resuscitation protocol for out-of-hospital cardiac arrest. Circulation 2009;119:2597–2605.

26. Kellum MJ, Kennedy KW, Ewy GA. Cardiocerebral resuscitation improves survival of patients with out-of-hospital cardiac arrest. Am J Med 2006;119:335–340.

27. Wik L, Hansen TB, Fylling F, et al. Delaying defibrillation to give basic cardiopulmonary resuscitation to patients with out-of-hospital ventricular fibrillation: A randomized trial. JAMA 2003;289:1389–1395.

28. Nolan JP, Soar J. Defibrillation in clinical practice. Curr Opin Crit Care 2009;15:209–215.

29. Valenzuela TD, Roe DJ, Nichol G, et al. Outcomes of rapid defibrillation by security officers after cardiac arrest in casinos. N Engl J Med 2000;343:1206–1209.

30. Forcina MS, Farhat AY, O'Neil WW, Haines DE. Cardiac arrest survival after implementation of automated external defibrillator technology in the in-hospital setting. Crit Care Med 2009;37:1229–1236.

31. Tuseth V, Salem M, Pettersen R, et al. Percutaneous left ventricular assist in ischemic cardiac arrest. Crit Care Med 2009;37:1365–1372.

32. Sunde K. Experimental and clinical use of ongoing mechanical cardiopulmonary resuscitation during angiography and percutaneous coronary intervention. Crit Care Med 2008;36:S405–S408.

33. Varon J, Acosta P. Extracorporeal membrane oxygenation in cardiopulmonary resuscitation: Are we there yet? Crit Care Med 2008;36:2685–2686.

34. Chamberlain D, Frenneaux M, Fletcher D. The primacy of basics in advanced life support. Curr Opin Crit Care 2009;15:198–202.

35. Hilwig RW, Kern KB, Berg RA, et al. Catecholamines in cardiac arrest: Role of alpha agonists, beta-adrenergic blockers and high-dose epinephrine. Resuscitation 2000;47:203–208.

36. Robinson LA, Brown CG, Jenkins J, et al. The effect of norepinephrine versus epinephrine on myocardial hemodynamics during CPR. Ann Emerg Med 1989;18:336–340.

37. Zhong JQ, Dorian P. Epinephrine and vasopressin during cardiopulmonary resuscitation. Resuscitation 2005;66:263–269.

38. Cammarata G, Weil MH, Sun S, et al. Beta$_1$-adrenergic blockade during cardiopulmonary resuscitation improves survival. Crit Care Med 2004;32(suppl 9):S440–S443.

39. Holmes HR, Babbs CF, Voorhees WD, et al. Influence of adrenergic drugs upon vital organ perfusion during CPR. Crit Care Med 1980;8:137–140.

40. Ornato JP. Use of adrenergic agonists during CPR in adults. Ann Emerg Med 1993;22(2 Pt 2):411–416.

41. Brown C, Wiklund L, Bar-Joseph G, et al. Future directions for resuscitation research. IV. Innovative advanced life support pharmacology. Resuscitation 1996;33:163–177.

42. Callaham M, Madsen CD, Barton CW, et al. A randomized clinical trial of high-dose epinephrine and norepinephrine vs standard-dose epinephrine in prehospital cardiac arrest. JAMA 1992;268:2667–2672.

43. Lindner KH, Ahnefeld FW, Grunert A. Epinephrine versus norepinephrine in prehospital ventricular fibrillation. Am J Cardiol 1991;67:427–428.

44. Redding JS, Pearson JW. Evaluation of drugs for cardiac resuscitation. Anesthesiology 1963;24:203–207.

45. Brown CG, Werman HA, Davis EA, et al. Comparative effect of graded doses of epinephrine on regional brain blood flow during CPR in a swine model. Ann Emerg Med 1986;15:1138–1144.

46. Gonzalez ER, Ornato JP, Garnett AR, et al. Dose-dependent vasopressor response to epinephrine during CPR in human beings. Ann Emerg Med 1989;18:920–926.

47. Brown CG, Martin DR, Pepe PE, et al. A comparison of standard-dose and high-dose epinephrine in cardiac arrest outside the hospital. The Multicenter High-Dose Epinephrine Study Group. N Engl J Med 1992;327:1051–1055.

48. Callaham M, Barton CW, Kayser S. Potential complications of high-dose epinephrine therapy in patients resuscitated from cardiac arrest. JAMA 1991;265:1117–1122.

49. Choux C, Gueugniaud PY, Barbieux A, et al. Standard doses versus repeated high doses of epinephrine in cardiac arrest outside the hospital. Resuscitation 1995;29:3–9.

50. Gueugniaud PY, Mols P, Goldstein P, et al. A comparison of repeated high doses and repeated standard doses of epinephrine for cardiac arrest outside the hospital. European Epinephrine Study Group. N Engl J Med 1998;339:1595–1601.

51. Lipman J, Wilson W, Kobilski S, et al. High-dose adrenaline in adult in-hospital asystolic cardiopulmonary resuscitation: A double-blind randomised trial. Anaesth Intensive Care 1993;21:192–196.

52. Sherman BW, Munger MA, Foulke GE, et al. High-dose versus standard-dose epinephrine treatment of cardiac arrest after failure of standard therapy. Pharmacotherapy 1997;17:242–247.

53. Stiell IG, Hebert PC, Weitzman BN, et al. High-dose epinephrine in adult cardiac arrest. N Engl J Med 1992;327:1045–1050.

54. Lindner KH, Ahnefeld FW, Prengel AW. Comparison of standard and high-dose adrenaline in the resuscitation of asystole and electromechanical dissociation. Acta Anaesthesiol Scand 1991;35:253–256.

55. Miano TA, Crouch MA. Evolving role of vasopressin in the treatment of cardiac arrest. Pharmacotherapy 2006;26:828–839.

56. Lindner KH, Strohmenger HU, Ensinger H, et al. Stress hormone response during and after cardiopulmonary resuscitation. Anesthesiology 1992;77:662–668.

57. Voelckel WG, Lindner KH, Wenzel V, et al. Effects of vasopressin and epinephrine on splanchnic blood flow and renal function during and after cardiopulmonary resuscitation in pigs. Crit Care Med 2000;28:1083–1088.

58. Wenzel V, Krismer AC, Arntz HR, et al. A comparison of vasopressin and epinephrine for out-of-hospital cardiopulmonary resuscitation. N Engl J Med 2004;350:105–113.

59. Gueugniaud PY, David JS, Chanzy E, et al. Vasopressin and epinephrine vsersus epinephrine alone in cardiopulmonary resuscitation. N Engl J Med 2008;359:21–30.

60. Mentzelopoulos SD, Zakynthinos SG, Tzoufi M, et al. Vasopressin, epinephrine, and corticosteroids for in-hospital cardiac arrest. Arch Intern Med 2009;169:15–24.

61. Harrison EE. Lidocaine in prehospital countershock refractory ventricular fibrillation. Ann Emerg Med 1981;10:420–423.

62. Weaver WD, Fahrenbruch CE, Johnson DD, et al. Effect of epinephrine and lidocaine therapy on outcome after cardiac arrest due to ventricular fibrillation. Circulation 1990;82:2027–2034.

63. Herlitz J, Ekstrom L, Wennerblom B, et al. Lidocaine in out-of-hospital ventricular fibrillation. Does it improve survival? Resuscitation 1997;33:199–205.

64. Kudenchuk PJ, Cobb LA, Copass MK, et al. Amiodarone for resuscitation after out-of-hospital cardiac arrest due to ventricular fibrillation. N Engl J Med 1999;341:871–878.

65. Dorian P, Cass D, Schwartz B, et al. Amiodarone as compared with lidocaine for shock-resistant ventricular fibrillation. N Engl J Med 2002;346:884–890.

66. Rea RS, Kane-Gill SL, Rudis MI, et al. Comparing intravenous amiodarone or lidocaine, or both, outcomes for inpatients with pulseless ventricular arrhythmias. Crit Care Med 2006;34:1617–1623.

67. Abu-Laban RB, Christenson JM, Innes GD, et al. Tissue plasminogen activator in cardiac arrest with pulseless electrical activity. N Engl J Med 2002;346:1522–1528.

68. Bottiger BW, Bode C, Kern S, et al. Efficacy and safety of thrombolytic therapy after initially unsuccessful cardiopulmonary resuscitation: A prospective clinical trial. Lancet 2001;357(9268):1583–1585.

69. Fatovich DM, Dobb GJ, Clugston RA. A pilot randomised trial of thrombolysis in cardiac arrest (The TICA trial). Resuscitation 2004;61:309–313.

70. Janata K, Holzer M, Kurkciyan I, et al. Major bleeding complications in cardiopulmonary resuscitation: The place of thrombolytic therapy in cardiac arrest due to massive pulmonary embolism. Resuscitation 2003;57:49–55.

71. Kurkciyan I, Meron G, Sterz F, et al. Pulmonary embolism as a cause of cardiac arrest: Presentation and outcome. Arch Intern Med 2000;160:1529–1535.

72. Lederer W, Lichtenberger C, Pechlaner C, et al. Recombinant tissue plasminogen activator during cardiopulmonary resuscitation in 108 patients with out-of-hospital cardiac arrest. Resuscitation 2001;50: 71–76.

73. Ruiz-Bailen M, Aguayo de Hoyos E, Serrano-Corcoles MC, et al. Efficacy of thrombolysis in patients with acute myocardial infarction requiring cardiopulmonary resuscitation. Intensive Care Med 2001;27:1050–1057.

74. Bottiger BW, Arntz HR, Chamberlain DA, et al. Thrombolysis during resuscitation for out-of-hospital cardiac arrest. N Engl J Med 2008;359:2651–2662.

75. Bozeman WP, Kleiner DM, Ferguson KL. Empiric tenecteplase is associated with increased return of spontaneous circulation and short term survival in cardiac arrest patients unresponsive to standard interventions. Resuscitation 2006;69:399–406.

76. Stadlbauer KH, Krismer AC, Arntz HR, et al. Effects of thrombolysis during out-of-hospital cardiopulmonary resuscitation. Am J Cardiol 2006;97:305–308.

77. Neumar RW, Nolan JP, Adrie C, et al. Post-cardiac arrest syndrome: Eepidemiology, pathophysiology, treatment, and prognostication. A consensus statement from the International Liaison Committee on Resuscitation (American Heart Association, Australian and New Zealand Council on Resuscitation, European Resuscitation Council, Heart and Stroke Foundation of Canada, InterAmerican Heart Foundation, Resuscitation Council of Asia, and the Resuscitation Council of Southern Africa); the American Heart Association Emergency Cardiovascular Care Committee; the Council on Cardiovascular Surgery and Anesthesia; the Council on Cardiopulmonary, Perioperative, and Critical Care; the Council on Clinical Cardiology; and the Stroke Council. Circulation 2008;118:2452–2483.

78. Nolan JP, Morley PT, Vanden Hoek TL, et al. Therapeutic hypothermia after cardiac arrest: An advisory statement by the advanced life support task force of the International Liaison Committee on Resuscitation. Circulation 2003;108:118–121.

79. Safar P, Xiao F, Radovsky A, et al. Improved cerebral resuscitation from cardiac arrest in dogs with mild hypothermia plus blood flow promotion. Stroke 1996;27:105–113.

80. Tsai M, Barbut D, Wang H, et al. Intra-arrest rapid head cooling improves postresuscitation myocardial function in comparison with delayed postresuscitation surface cooling. Crit Care Med 2008;36:S434–S439.

81. Guan J, Barbut D, Wang H, et al. A comparison between head cooling begun during cardiopulmonary resuscitation and surface cooling after resuscitation in a pig model of cardiac arrest. Crit Care Med 2008;36:S428–S433.

82. Dine CJ, Abella BS. Therapeutic hypothermia for neuroprotection. Emerg Med Clin North Am 2009;27:137–149.

83. O'Sullivan ST, O'Shaughnessy M, O'Connor TP. Baron Larrey and cold injury during the campaigns of Napoleon. Ann Plast Surg 1995;34:446–449.

84. Mild therapeutic hypothermia to improve the neurologic outcome after cardiac arrest. N Engl J Med 2002;346:549–556.

85. Bernard SA, Gray TW, Buist MD, et al. Treatment of comatose survivors of out-of-hospital cardiac arrest with induced hypothermia. N Engl J Med 2002;346:557–563.

86. Sunde K, Pytte M, Jacobsen D, et al. Implementation of a standardised treatment protocol for post resuscitation care after out-of-hospital cardiac arrest. Resuscitation 2007;73:29–39.

87. Sagalyn E, Band RA, Gaieski DF, Abella BS. Therapeutic hypothermia after cardiac arrest in clinical practice: Review and compilation of recent experiences. Crit Care Med 2009;37(suppl 7):S223–S226.

88. Sunde K, Steen PA. Studies in hypothermia-treated cardiac arrest patients are needed to establish the accuracy of proposed outcome predictors. Crit Care Med 2009;37:2485–2486.

89. Janata A, Weihs W, Bayegan K, et al. Therapeutic hypothermia with a novel surface cooling device improves neurologic outcome after prolonged cardiac arrest in swine. Crit Care Med 2008;36: 895–902.

90. Kim F, Olsufka M, Carlbom D, et al. Pilot study of rapid infusion of 2 L of 4°C normal saline for induction of mild hypothermia in hospital-ized, comatose survivors of out-of-hospital cardiac arrest. Circulation 2005;112:715–719.

91. Drabek T, Kochanek PM. In quest of the optimal cooling device: Isn't faster "too fast"? Crit Care Med 2008;36:1018–1020.

92. Levine RL. Cardiocerebral resuscitation: Few answers, more questions. Crit Care Med 2009;37:747–748.

93. Shankaran S, Laptook AR, Ehrenkranz RA, et al. Whole-body hypothermia for neonates with hypoxic-ischemic encephalopathy. N Engl J Med 2005;353:1574–1584.

94. Bunch TJ, White RD, Gersh BJ, et al. Long-term outcomes of out-of-hospital cardiac arrest after successful early defibrillation. N Engl J Med 2003;348:2626–2633.

95. Arpino PA, Greer DM. Practical pharmacologic aspects of therapeutic hypothermia after cardiac arrest. Pharmacotherapy 2008;28:102–111.

96. Hachimi-Idrissi S, Corne L, Ebinger G, et al. Mild hypothermia induced by a helmet device: A clinical feasibility study. Resuscitation 2001;51:275–281.

97. Gonzalez ER. Pharmacologic controversies in CPR. Ann Emerg Med 1993;22(2 Pt 2):317–323.

98. Stueven HA, Tonsfeldt DJ, Thompson BM, et al. Atropine in asystole: Human studies. Ann Emerg Med 1984;13(9 Pt 2):815–817.

99. Ornato JP, Gonzales ER, Morkunas AR, et al. Treatment of presumed asystole during pre-hospital cardiac arrest: Superiority of electrical countershock. Am J Emerg Med 1985;3:395–399.

100. Tortolani AJ, Risucci DA, Powell SR, Dixon R. In-hospital cardiopulmonary resuscitation during asystole. Therapeutic factors associated with 24-hour survival. Chest 1989;96:622–626.

101. Bohm K, Rosenqvist M, Herlitz J, et al. Survival is similar after standard treatment and chest compression only in out-of-hospital bystander cardiopulmonary resuscitation. Circulation 2007;116:2908–2912.

102. Levy MM. An evidence-based evaluation of the use of sodium bicarbonate during cardiopulmonary resuscitation. Crit Care Clin 1998;14:457–483.

103. Bjerneroth G. Tribonat-a comprehensive summary of its properties. Crit Care Med 1999;27:1009–1013.

104. Vukmir RB, Katz L. Sodium Bicarbonate Study G. Sodium bicarbonate improves outcome in prolonged prehospital cardiac arrest. Am J Emerg Med 2006;24:156–161.

105. Kyriacou DN, Arcinue EL, Peek C, Kraus JF. Effect of immediate resuscitation on children with submersion injury. Pediatrics 1994;94(2 Pt 1):137–142.

106. Hanania NA, Zimmerman JL. Accidental hypothermia. Crit Care Clin 1999;15:235–149.

107. Goodwin AP, Pearce AJ. The human wedge. A manoeuvre to relieve aortocaval compression during resuscitation in late pregnancy. Anaesthesia 1992;47:433–434.

108. Atta E, Gardner M. Cardiopulmonary resuscitation in pregnancy. Obstet Gynecol Clin North Am 2007;34:585–597.

109. Nanson J, Elcock D, Williams M, Deakin CD. Do physiological changes in pregnancy change defibrillation energy requirements? Br J Anaesth 2001;87:237–239.

110. Munro PT. Management of eclampsia in the accident and emergency department. J Accid Emerg Med 2000;17:7–11.

111. Stanten RD, Iverson LI, Daugharty TM, et al. Amniotic fluid embolism causing catastrophic pulmonary vasoconstriction: Diagnosis by transesophageal echocardiogram and treatment by cardiopulmonary bypass. Obstet Gynecol 2003;102:496–498.

112. Lockey D, Crewdson K, Davies G. Traumatic cardiac arrest: Who are the survivors? Ann Emerg Med 2006;48:240–244.

113. Browne BJ, Gaasch WR. Electrical injuries and lightning. Emerg Med Clin North Am 1992;10:211–229.

114. Milzman DP, Moskowitz L, Hardel M. Lightning strikes at a mass gathering. South Med J 1999;92:708–710.

115. Vincent R. Drugs in modern resuscitation. Br J Anaesth 1997;79:188–197.

116. Kellum MJ. Improving performance of emergency medical services personnel during resuscitation of cardiac arrest patients: The McMAID approach. Curr Opin Crit Care 2009;15:216–220.

117. West VL. Alternate routes of administration. J Intraven Nurs 1998;21:221–231.

118. Brenner T, Bernhard M, Helm M, et al. Comparison of two intraosseous infusion systems for adult emergency medical use. Resuscitation 2008;78:314–319.

119. Niemann JT, Stratton SJ. Endotracheal versus intravenous epinephrine and atropine in out-of-hospital "primary" and postcountershock asystole. Crit Care Med 2000;28:1815–1819.

120. Niemann JT, Stratton SJ, Cruz B, Lewis RJ. Endotracheal drug administration during out-of-hospital resuscitation: Where are the survivors? Resuscitation 2002;53:153–157.

121. Young GB. Clinical practice. Neurologic prognosis after cardiac arrest. N Engl J Med 2009;361:605–611.

122. Sasson C, Hegg AJ, Macy M, et al. Prehospital termination of resuscitation in cases of refractory out-of-hospital cardiac arrest. JAMA 2008;300:1432–1438.

123. Wijdicks EF, Hijdra A, Young GB, et al. Practice parameter: Prediction of outcome in comatose survivors after cardiopulmonary resuscitation (an evidence-based review): Report of the Quality Standards Subcommittee of the American Academy of Neurology. Neurology 2006;67:203–210.

124. Jennett B, Bond M. Assessment of outcome after severe brain damage. Lancet 1975;1(7905):480–484.

125. Jennett B, Teasdale G. Aspects of coma after severe head injury. Lancet 1977;1(8017):878–881.

126. Ornato JP, Peberdy MA. Prehospital and emergency department care to preserve neurologic function during and following cardiopulmonary resuscitation. Neurol Clin 2006;24:23–39.

127. Guyette FX, Guimond GE, Hostler D, Callaway CW. Vasopressin administered with epinephrine is associated with a return of a pulse in out-of-hospital cardiac arrest. Resuscitation 2004;63:277–282.

128. Lindner KH, Dirks B, Strohmenger HU, et al. Randomised comparison of epinephrine and vasopressin in patients with out-of-hospital ventricular fibrillation. Lancet 1997;349(9051):535–537.

129. Stiell IG, Hebert PC, Wells GA, et al. Vasopressin versus epinephrine for inhospital cardiac arrest: A randomised controlled trial. Lancet 2001;358(9276):105–109.

130. Grmec S, Mally S. Vasopressin improves outcome in out-of-hospital cardiopulmonary resuscitation of ventricular fibrillation and pulseless ventricular tachycardia: A observational cohort study. Crit Care 2006;10:R13.

131. Callaway CW, Hostler D, Doshi AA, et al. Usefulness of vasopressin administered with epinephrine during out-of-hospital cardiac arrest. Am J Cardiol 2006;98:1316–1321.

CHAPTER

19

Hypertension

JOSEPH J. SASEEN AND ERIC J. MACLAUGHLIN

KEY CONCEPTS

❶ The risk of cardiovascular (CV) morbidity and mortality is directly correlated with blood pressure (BP).

❷ Outcome trials have shown that antihypertensive drug therapy substantially reduces the risks of CV events and death in patients with high BP.

❸ Essential hypertension is usually an asymptomatic disease. A diagnosis cannot be made based on one elevated BP measurement. An elevated value from the average of two or more measurements, present during two or more clinical encounters, is needed to diagnose hypertension.

❹ The overall goal of treating hypertension is to reduce hypertension-associated morbidity and mortality from CV events. These are considered hypertension-associated complications. The selection of specific drug therapy is based on evidence that demonstrates CV risk reduction.

❺ A goal BP of less than 140/90 mm Hg is appropriate for general prevention of CV events and CV risk reduction. A lower goal BP of less than 130/80 mm Hg is recommended for patients with diabetes and significant chronic kidney disease. However, recommendations from the American Heart Association also recommend this lower goal BP of less than 130/80 mm Hg for patients with known coronary artery disease [myocardial infarction (MI), stable angina, unstable angina], noncoronary atherosclerotic vascular disease (ischemic stroke, transient ischemic attack, peripheral arterial disease, abdominal aortic aneurysm) or a 10% or greater 10 year risk of fatal coronary heart disease or nonfatal MI based on Framingham risk scoring.

❻ Magnitude of BP elevation should be used to guide determination of the number of agents to start when implementing drug therapy. Most patients with Stage 1 hypertension should be started on one drug, with the option of starting two for some patients. However, most patients presenting with Stage 2 hypertension should be started on two drugs.

❼ Lifestyle modifications should be prescribed in all patients, especially those with prehypertension and hypertension. However, they should never be used as a replacement for antihypertensive drug therapy for patients with hypertension, especially in those with additional CV risk factors.

❽ Thiazide-type diuretics, angiotensin-converting enzyme (ACE) inhibitors, angiotensin II receptor blockers (ARB), and calcium channel blockers (CCB) are all considered first-line agents for most patients with hypertension for general prevention of CV events and CV risk reduction. These first-line options are for patients with hypertension that do not have any compelling indications for a specific antihypertensive drug class.

❾ For general prevention of CV events and CV risk reduction in most patients with hypertension, β-blockers do not reduce CV events to the extent as thiazide-type diuretics, ACE inhibitors, ARBs, or CCBs.

❿ Compelling indications are comorbid conditions where specific antihypertensive drug classes have been shown in outcome trials to provide unique long-term benefits (reducing the risk of CV events).

⓫ Patients with diabetes are at high risk for CV events. All patients with diabetes and hypertension should be managed with either an ACE inhibitor or an ARB. These are typically in combination with one or more other antihypertensive agents because multiple agents frequently are needed to control BP.

⓬ Older patients with isolated systolic hypertension are often at risk for orthostatic hypotension when antihypertensive drug therapy is started, particularly with diuretics, ACE inhibitors, and ARBs. Although overall antihypertensive drug therapy should be the same, low initial doses should be used and dosage titrations should be gradual to minimize risk of orthostatic hypotension.

⓭ Alternative antihypertensive agents have not been proven to reduce the risk of CV events compared with first-line antihypertensive agents. They should be used primarily in combination with first-line agents to provide additional BP lowering.

⓮ Initial therapy with the combination of two antihypertensive agents should be used in most patients presenting with stage 2 hypertension. This is also an option for patients presenting with stage 1 hypertension. Most patients require combination therapy to achieve goal BP values.

⓯ Patients are considered to have resistant hypertension when they fail to attain goal BP values while adherent to a regimen that includes at least three agents at maximum dose, one of which includes a diuretic.

⓰ Hypertensive urgency is ideally managed by adjusting maintenance therapy (adding a new antihypertensive and/or increasing the dose of a present medication). This provides a gradual reduction in BP, which is a safer treatment approach than rapid reductions in BP.

Learning objectives, review questions, and other resources can be found at **www.pharmacotherapyonline.com**.

Hypertension is a common disease that is simply defined as persistently elevated arterial blood pressure (BP). Although elevated BP was perceived to be "essential" for adequate perfusion of vital organs during the early and middle 1900s, it is now identified as one of the most significant risk factors for cardiovascular (CV) disease in the United States. Increasing awareness and diagnosis of hypertension, and improving control of BP with appropriate treatment, are considered critical public health initiatives to reduce CV morbidity and mortality.

The Seventh report of the Joint National Committee on the Detection, Evaluation, and Treatment of High Blood Pressure (JNC7) is the most prominent evidence-based clinical guideline in United States for the management of hypertension,[1] supplemented by the 2007 American Heart Association (AHA) Scientific Statement on the treatment of hypertension.[2] This chapter reviews relevant components of both these guidelines and additional evidence from clinical trials, with a focus on the pharmacotherapy of hypertension. The Eight report of the Joint National Committee (JNC8) will represent the most updated treatment guideline, although publication is not expected until 2011.

The National Health and Nutrition Examination Survey and the National Center for Health Statistics regularly assess hypertension in the United States.[3] Data from 2003 to 2006 indicate that of the population of Americans with hypertension, 77.6% are aware that they have hypertension, only 67.9% are on some form of antihypertensive treatment, and only 44.1% of all patients have controlled BP. This control rate is substantially higher than in the past. However, there remain many opportunities for clinicians to improve the care of patients with hypertension.

EPIDEMIOLOGY

Approximately 31% of Americans (74.5 million people) have elevated BP, defined as greater than or equal to 140/90 mm Hg.[3] The overall incidence is similar between men and women, but varies depending on age. The percentage of men with high BP is higher than for women before the age of 45 and is similar to that of women between the ages 45 and 64. However, after the age of 64, a much higher percentage of women have high BP than men.[3] Prevalence rates are highest in non-Hispanic blacks (45% in women, 44% in men), followed by non-Hispanic whites (31% in women, 34% in men), Mexican Americans (32% in women, 26% in men), American Indians/Alaska Natives (25% in women and men), and Asians (21% in women and men).[3]

BP values increase with age, and hypertension (persistently elevated BP values) is very common in the elderly. The lifetime risk of developing hypertension among those 55 years of age and older who are normotensive is 90%.[1] Most patients have prehypertension before they are diagnosed with hypertension, with most diagnoses occurring between the third and fifth decades of life.

ETIOLOGY

In most patients, hypertension results from unknown pathophysiological etiology (*essential* or *primary hypertension*). This form of hypertension cannot be cured, but it can be controlled. A small percentage of patients have a specific cause of their hypertension (*secondary hypertension*). There are many potential secondary causes that either are concurrent medical conditions or are endogenously induced. If the cause can be identified, hypertension in these patients can be mitigated or potentially be cured.

ESSENTIAL HYPERTENSION

Over 90% of individuals with high BP have essential hypertension.[1] Numerous mechanisms have been identified that may contribute to the pathogenesis of this form of hypertension, so identifying the exact underlying abnormality is not possible. Genetic factors may play an important role in the development of essential hypertension. There are monogenic and polygenic forms of BP dysregulation that may be responsible for essential hypertension.[4] Many of these genetic traits feature genes that affect sodium balance, but genetic mutations altering urinary kallikrein excretion, nitric oxide release, and excretion of aldosterone, other adrenal steroids, and angiotensinogen are also documented.[4] In the future, genetic testing for these traits could lead to alternative approaches to preventing or treating hypertension; however, this is not currently recommended.

SECONDARY HYPERTENSION

Fewer than 10% of patients have secondary hypertension where either a comorbid disease or drug (or other product) is responsible for elevating BP (see Table 19–1).[1,5] In most of these cases, renal dysfunction resulting from severe chronic kidney disease or renovascular disease is the most common secondary cause. Certain drugs (or other products), either directly or indirectly, can cause hypertension or exacerbate hypertension by increasing BP. The most common agents are listed in Table 19–1. When a secondary cause is identified, removing the offending agent (when feasible) or treating/correcting the underlying comorbid condition should be the first step in management.

PATHOPHYSIOLOGY[4,6]

Multiple factors that control BP are potential contributing components in the development of essential hypertension. These include malfunctions in either humoral [i.e., the renin-angiotensin-aldosterone system (RAAS)] or vasodepressor mechanisms, abnormal neuronal mechanisms, defects in peripheral autoregulation, and disturbances in sodium, calcium, and natriuretic hormone. Many of these factors are cumulatively affected by the multifaceted RAAS, which ultimately regulates arterial BP. It is probable that no one factor is solely responsible for essential hypertension.

ARTERIAL BP

Arterial BP is the pressure in the arterial wall measured in millimeters of mercury (mm Hg). The two typical arterial BP values are *systolic BP* (SBP) and *diastolic BP* (DBP). SBP represents the peak value, which is achieved during cardiac contraction. DBP is achieved after contraction when the cardiac chambers are filling, and represents the nadir value. The difference between SBP and DBP is called the pulse pressure and is a measure of arterial wall tension. Mean arterial pressure (MAP) is the average pressure throughout the cardiac cycle of contraction. It is sometimes used clinically to represent overall arterial BP, especially in hypertensive emergency. During a cardiac cycle, two-thirds of the time is spent in diastole and one-third in systole. Therefore, the MAP is calculated by using the following equation:

$$MAP = (SBP \times 1/3) + (DBP \times 2/3)$$

Arterial BP is hemodynamically generated by the interplay between blood flow and the resistance to blood flow. It is mathematically defined as the product of cardiac output (CO)

TABLE 19-1 Secondary Causes of Hypertension[1,5]

Disease	Drugs and Other Products Associated with Hypertension[a]
Chronic kidney disease	**Prescription drugs**
Cushing syndrome	• Amphetamines (amphetamine, dexmethylphenidate, dextroamphetamine, lisdexamfetamine, methylphenidate, phendimetrazine, phentermine) and anorexiants (sibutramine)
Coarctation of the aorta	
Obstructive sleep apnea	
Parathyroid disease	
Pheochromocytoma	• Anti-vascular endothelin growth factor agents (bevacizumab, sorafenib, sunitinib)
Primary aldosteronism	
Renovascular disease	• Corticosteroids (cortisone, dexamethasone, fludrocortisone, hydrocortisone, methylprednisolone, prednisolone, prednisone, triamcinolone)
Thyroid disease	

• Calcineurin inhibitors (cyclosporine, tacrolimus)
• Decongestants (pseudoephedrine, phenylephrine)
• Ergot alkaloids (ergonovine, methysergide)
• Erythropoiesis stimulating agents (erythropoetin, darbopoetin)
• Estrogen-containing oral contraceptives
• Nonsteroidal antiinflammatory drugs—Cyclooxygenase-2 selective (celecoxib) and nonselective (aspirin, choline magnesium trisalicylate, diclofenac, diflunisal, etodolac, fenoprofen, flurbiprofen, ibuprofen, indomethacin, ketoprofen, ketorolac, meclofenamate, mefenamic acid, meloxicam, nabumetone, naproxen, naproxen sodium, oxaprozin, piroxicam, salsalate, sulindac, tolmetin)
• Others: Desvenlafaxine, venlafaxine, bupropion

Situations: β-blocker or centrally acting α agonists (when abruptly discontinued); β-blocker without α-blocker first when treating pheochromocytoma; use of a monoamine oxidase inhibitor (isocarboxazid, phenelzine, tranylcypromine) with tryamine containing foods or certain drugs

Street drugs and other products
Cocaine and cocaine withdrawal
Ephedra alkaloids (e.g., Ma huang), "herbal ecstasy," other analogues
Nicotine and withdrawal, anabolic steroids, narcotic withdrawal, ergot-containing herbal products, St. John's wort

Food substances
Sodium
Ethanol
Licorice

[a]Agents of most clinical importance.

and total peripheral resistance (TPR) according to the following equation:

$$BP = CO \times TPR$$

CO is the major determinant of SBP, whereas TPR largely determines DBP. In turn, CO is a function of stroke volume, heart rate, and venous capacitance. Table 19–2 lists physiologic causes of increased CO and TPR and correlates them to potential mechanisms of pathogenesis.

Under normal physiologic conditions, arterial BP fluctuates throughout the day following a circadian rhythm. BP decreases to its lowest daily values during sleep followed by a sharp rise starting a few hours prior to awakening with the highest values occurring midmorning. BP is also increased acutely during physical activity or emotional stress.

TABLE 19-2 Potential Mechanisms of Pathogenesis

Blood pressure (BP) is the mathematical product of cardiac output and peripheral resistance. Elevated BP can result from increased cardiac output and/or increased total peripheral resistance.

Increased cardiac output	Increased cardiac preload:
	• Increased fluid volume from excess sodium intake or renal sodium retention (from reduced number of nephrons or decreased glomerular filtration)
	Venous constriction:
	• Excess stimulation of the renin-angiotensin aldosterone system (RAAS)
	• Sympathetic nervous system overactivity
Increased peripheral resistance	Functional vascular constriction:
	• Excess stimulation of the RAAS
	• Sympathetic nervous system overactivity
	• Genetic alterations of cell membranes
	• Endothelial-derived factors
	Structural vascular hypertrophy:
	• Excess stimulation of the RAAS
	• Sympathetic nervous system overactivity
	• Genetic alterations of cell membranes
	• Endothelial-derived factors
	• Hyperinsulinemia resulting from the metabolic syndrome

Classification

The JNC7 classification of BP in adults (age greater than or equal to 18) is based on the average of 2 or more properly measured BP values from 2 or more clinical encounters (Table 19–3).[1] It includes 4 categories: normal, prehypertension, Stage 1 hypertension, and Stage 2 hypertension. Prehypertension is not considered a disease category but identifies patients whose BP is likely to increase into the classification of hypertension in the future.

Hypertensive crises are clinical situations where BP values are very elevated, typically greater than 180/120 mm Hg.[6] They are categorized as either *hypertensive emergency* or *hypertensive urgency*. Hypertensive emergencies are extreme elevations in BP that are accompanied by acute or progressing target-organ damage. Hypertensive urgencies are high elevations in BP without acute or progressing target-organ injury.

Cardiovascular Risk and Blood Pressure

❶ Epidemiologic data clearly indicate a strong correlation between BP and CV morbidity and mortality.[7] Risk of stroke, myocardial infarction (MI), angina, heart failure, kidney failure, or early death from a CV cause are directly correlated with BP. Starting at a BP of 115/75, risk of CV disease doubles with every 20/10 mm Hg increase.[1] Even patients with prehypertension have an increased risk of CV disease.

TABLE 19-3 Classification of Blood Pressure in Adults (Age ≥18 Years)[a]

Classification	Systolic Blood Pressure (mm Hg)		Diastolic Blood Pressure (mm Hg)
Normal	Less than 120	and	Less than 80
Prehypertension[b]	120–139	or	80–89
Stage 1 hypertension	140–159	or	90–99
Stage 2 hypertension	≥160	or	≥100

[a]Classification determined based on the average of two or more properly measured seated BP values from two or more clinical encounters. If systolic and diastolic BP values yield different classifications, the highest category is used for the purpose of determining a classification.
[b]For certain patients, BP values within the prehypertension range are considered above goal (see Box 19–2).

❷ Treating patients with hypertension with antihypertensive drug therapy provides significant clinical benefits. Large-scale placebo-controlled outcome trials have shown that the increased risks of CV events and death associated with elevated BP are reduced substantially by antihypertensive therapy.[8-11] This is discussed in the Treatment Section.

SBP is a stronger predictor of CV disease than DBP in adults ≥50 years and is the most important clinical BP parameter for most patients.[1] Patients are considered to have *isolated systolic hypertension* when their SBP values are elevated (greater than or equal to 140 mm Hg) and DBP values are not (less than 90 mm Hg, but commonly less than 80 mm Hg). Isolated systolic hypertension is believed to result from pathophysiologic changes in the arterial vasculature consistent with aging. These changes decrease the compliance of the arterial wall and portend an increased risk of CV morbidity and mortality. The elevated pulse pressure (SBP minus DBP) is believed to reflect extent of atherosclerotic disease in the elderly and is a measure of increased arterial stiffness. Higher pulse pressure values seen in those with isolated systolic hypertension are correlated with an increased risk of CV mortality.

HUMORAL MECHANISMS

Several humoral abnormalities involving the RAAS, natriuretic hormone, and hyperinsulinemia may be involved in the development of essential hypertension.

The Renin-Angiotensin-Aldosterone System (RAAS)

The RAAS is a complex endogenous system that is involved with most regulatory components of arterial BP. Activation and regulation are primarily governed by the kidney (see Fig. 19-1). The RAAS regulates sodium, potassium, and blood volume. Therefore, this system significantly influences vascular tone and sympathetic nervous system activity and is the most influential contributor to the homeostatic regulation of BP.

Renin is an enzyme that is stored in the juxtaglomerular cells, which are located in the afferent arterioles of the kidney. The release of renin is modulated by several factors: intrarenal factors (e.g., renal perfusion pressure, catecholamines, angiotensin II), and extrarenal factors (e.g., sodium, chloride, and potassium).

Juxtaglomerular cells function as a baroreceptor-sensing device. Decreased renal artery pressure and kidney blood flow is sensed by these cells and stimulate secretion of renin. The juxtaglomerular apparatus also includes a group of specialized distal tubule cells referred to collectively as the *macula densa*. A decrease in sodium and chloride delivered to the distal tubule stimulates renin release. Catecholamines increase renin release probably by directly stimulating sympathetic nerves on the afferent arterioles that in turn activate the juxtaglomerular cells.

Renin catalyzes the conversion of angiotensinogen to angiotensin I in the blood. Angiotensin I is then converted to angiotensin II by angiotensin-converting enzyme (ACE). After binding to specific

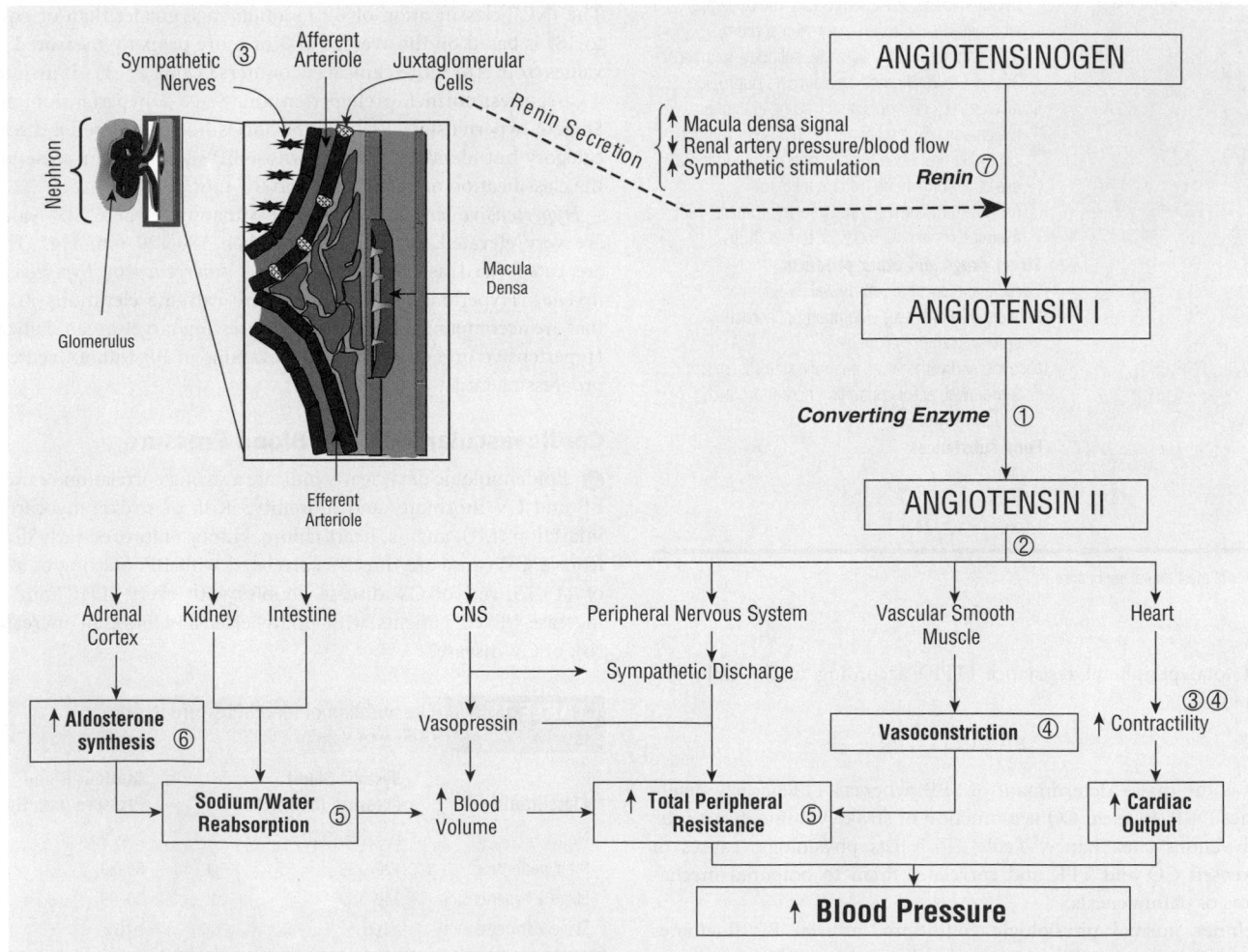

FIGURE 19-1. Diagram representing the renin-angiotensin-aldosterone system. The interrelationship between the kidney, angiotensin II, and regulation of blood pressure are depicted. Renin secretion from the juxtaglomerular cells in the afferent arterioles is regulated by three major factors to trigger conversion of angiotensinogen to angiotensin 1. The primary sites of action for major antihypertensive agents are included: ① ACE inhibitors; ② angiotensin II receptor blockers; ③ β-blockers; ④ calcium channel blockers; ⑤ diuretics; ⑥ aldosterone antagonists; ⑦ direct renin inhibitor.

receptors (classified as either AT_1 or AT_2 subtypes), angiotensin II exerts biologic effects in several tissues. The AT_1 receptor is located in brain, kidney, myocardium, peripheral vasculature, and the adrenal glands. These receptors mediate most responses that are critical to CV and kidney function. The AT_2 receptor is located in adrenal medullary tissue, uterus, and brain. Stimulation of the AT_2 receptor does not influence BP regulation.

Circulating angiotensin II can elevate BP through pressor and volume effects. Pressor effects include direct vasoconstriction, stimulation of catecholamine release from the adrenal medulla, and centrally mediated increases in sympathetic nervous system activity. Angiotensin II also stimulates aldosterone synthesis from the adrenal cortex. This leads to sodium and water reabsorption that increases plasma volume, TPR, and ultimately BP. Aldosterone also has a deleterious role in the pathophysiology of other CV diseases (heart failure, MI, and kidney disease) by promoting tissue remodeling leading to myocardial fibrosis and vascular dysfunction. Clearly, any disturbance in the body that leads to activation of the RAAS could explain chronic hypertension.

The heart and brain contain a local RAAS. In the heart, angiotensin II is also generated by angiotensin I convertase (human chymase). This enzyme is not blocked by ACE inhibition. Activation of the myocardial RAAS increases cardiac contractility and stimulates cardiac hypertrophy. In the brain, angiotensin II modulates the production and release of hypothalamic and pituitary hormones, and enhances sympathetic outflow from the medulla oblongata.

Natriuretic Hormone

Natriuretic hormone inhibits sodium and potassium-ATPase and thus interferes with sodium transport across cell membranes. Inherited defects in the kidney's ability to eliminate sodium can cause an increased blood volume. A compensatory increase in the concentration of circulating natriuretic hormone theoretically could increase urinary excretion of sodium and water. However, this hormone might block the active transport of sodium out of arteriolar smooth muscle cells. The increased intracellular sodium concentration ultimately would increase vascular tone and BP.

Insulin Resistance and Hyperinsulinemia

The development of hypertension and associated metabolic abnormalities is referred to as the metabolic syndrome.[12] Hypothetically, increased insulin concentrations may lead to hypertension because of increased renal sodium retention and enhanced sympathetic nervous system activity. Moreover, insulin has growth hormone–like actions that can induce hypertrophy of vascular smooth muscle cells. Insulin also may elevate BP by increasing intracellular calcium, which leads to increased vascular resistance. The exact mechanism by which insulin resistance and hyperinsulinemia occur in hypertension is unknown. However, this association is strong because many of the criteria used to define this population (i.e., elevated BP, abdominal obesity, dyslipidemia, and elevated fasting glucose) are often present in patients with hypertension.[12]

NEURONAL REGULATION

Central and autonomic nervous systems are intricately involved in the regulation of arterial BP. Many receptors that either enhance or inhibit norepinephrine release are located on the presynaptic surface of sympathetic terminals. The alpha (α) and beta (β) presynaptic receptors play a role in negative and positive feedback to the norepinephrine-containing vesicles. Stimulation of presynaptic α-receptors (α_2) exerts a negative inhibition on norepinephrine release. Stimulation of presynaptic β-receptors facilitates norepinephrine release.

Sympathetic neuronal fibers located on the surface of effector cells innervate the α- and β-receptors. Stimulation of postsynaptic α-receptors (α_1) on arterioles and venules results in vasoconstriction. There are two types of postsynaptic β-receptors, β_1 and β_2. Both are present in all tissue innervated by the sympathetic nervous system. However, in some tissues β_1-receptors predominate, and in other tissues β_2-receptors predominate. Stimulation of β_1-receptors in the heart results in an increase in heart rate and contractility, whereas stimulation of β_2-receptors in the arterioles and venules causes vasodilatation.

The baroreceptor reflex system is the major negative-feedback mechanism that controls sympathetic activity. Baroreceptors are nerve endings lying in the walls of large arteries, especially in the carotid arteries and aortic arch. Changes in arterial BP rapidly activate baroreceptors that then transmit impulses to the brain stem through the ninth cranial nerve and vagus nerves. In this reflex system, a decrease in arterial BP stimulates baroreceptors, causing reflex vasoconstriction and increased heart rate and force of cardiac contraction. These baroreceptor reflex mechanisms may be less responsive in the elderly and those with diabetes.

Stimulation of certain areas within the central nervous system (nucleus tractus solitarius, vagal nuclei, vasomotor center, and the area postrema) can either increase or decrease BP. For example, α_2-adrenergic stimulation within the central nervous system decreases BP through an inhibitory effect on the vasomotor center. However, angiotensin II increases sympathetic outflow from the vasomotor center, which increases BP.

The purpose of these neuronal mechanisms is to regulate BP and maintain homeostasis. Pathologic disturbances in any of the four major components (autonomic nerve fibers, adrenergic receptors, baroreceptors, central nervous system) could chronically elevate BP. These systems are physiologically interrelated. A defect in one component may alter normal function in another. Therefore, cumulative abnormalities may explain the development of essential hypertension.

PERIPHERAL AUTOREGULATORY COMPONENTS

Abnormalities in renal or tissue autoregulatory systems could cause hypertension. It is possible that a renal defect in sodium excretion may develop, which can then cause resetting of tissue autoregulatory processes resulting in a higher BP. The kidney usually maintains a normal BP through a volume-pressure adaptive mechanism. When BP drops, the kidneys respond by increasing retention of sodium and water, which leads to plasma volume expansion that increases BP. Conversely, when BP rises above normal, renal sodium and water excretion are increased to reduce plasma volume and CO.

Local autoregulatory processes maintain adequate tissue oxygenation. When tissue oxygen demand is normal to low, the local arteriolar bed remains relatively vasoconstricted. However, increases in metabolic demand triggers arteriolar vasodilation that lowers peripheral vascular resistance and increases blood flow and oxygen delivery through autoregulation.

Intrinsic defects in these renal adaptive mechanisms could lead to plasma volume expansion and increased blood flow to peripheral tissues, even when BP is normal. Local tissue autoregulatory processes that vasoconstrict would then be activated to offset the increased blood flow. This effect would result in increased peripheral vascular resistance and, if sustained, would also result in thickening of the arteriolar walls. This pathophysiological component is plausible because increased TPR is a common underlying finding in patients with essential hypertension.

VASCULAR ENDOTHELIAL MECHANISMS

Vascular endothelium and smooth muscle play important roles in regulating blood vessel tone and BP. These regulating functions are mediated by vasoactive substances that are synthesized by endothelial cells. It has been postulated that a deficiency in the local synthesis of vasodilating substances (prostacyclin and bradykinin) or excess vasoconstricting substances (angiotensin II and endothelin I) contribute to essential hypertension, atherosclerosis, and other CV diseases.

Nitric oxide is produced in the endothelium, relaxes the vascular epithelium, and is a very potent vasodilator. The nitric oxide system is an important regulator of arterial BP. Patients with hypertension may have an intrinsic nitric oxide deficiency, resulting in inadequate vasodilatation.

ELECTROLYTES

Epidemiologic and clinical data have associated excess sodium intake with hypertension. Population-based studies indicate that high sodium diets are associated with a high prevalence of stroke and hypertension. Conversely, low sodium diets are associated with a low prevalence of hypertension. Clinical studies have consistently shown that dietary sodium restriction lowers BP in many (but not all) patients with elevated BP. The exact mechanisms by which excess sodium leads to hypertension are not known.

Altered calcium homeostasis also may play an important role in the pathogenesis of hypertension. A lack of dietary calcium hypothetically can disturb the balance between intracellular and extracellular calcium, resulting in an increased intracellular calcium concentration. This imbalance can alter vascular smooth muscle function by increasing peripheral vascular resistance. Some studies have shown that dietary calcium supplementation results in a modest BP reduction for patients with hypertension.

The role of potassium fluctuations is also inadequately understood. Potassium depletion may increase peripheral vascular resistance, but the clinical significance of small serum potassium concentration changes is unclear. Furthermore, data demonstrating reduced CV risk with dietary potassium supplementation are very limited.

CLINICAL PRESENTATION

The clinical presentation of hypertension is described in Box 19–1.

DIAGNOSTIC CONSIDERATIONS

❸ Hypertension is termed the *silent killer* because most patients do not have symptoms. The primary physical finding is elevated BP. The diagnosis of hypertension cannot be made based on one elevated BP measurement. The average of two or more measurements taken during two or more clinical encounters should be used to diagnose hypertension.[1] This BP average should be used to establish a diagnosis, and then classify the stage of hypertension using Table 19–3.

Measuring BP

The measurement of BP is a common routine medical screening tool that should be conducted at every healthcare encounter.[1]

Cuff Measurement Using Sphygmomanometry[13] The most common procedure to measure BP in clinical practice is the indirect measurement of BP using sphygmomanometry. The appropriate procedure to indirectly measure BP using sphygmomanometry has been described by the AHA.[13] It is imperative that the measurement equipment (inflation cuff, stethoscope, and manometer) meet

---

BOX 19-1 CLINICAL PRESENTATION OF HYPERTENSION

General: the patient may appear healthy or may have the presence of additional CV risk factors:

- Age (greater than or equal to 55 for men, greater than or equal to 65 for women)
- Diabetes mellitus
- Dyslipidemia
- Microalbuminuria
- Family history of premature CV disease
- Obesity (body mass index greater than or equal to 30 kg/m²)
- Physical inactivity
- Tobacco use

Symptoms: Usually none related to elevated BP.

Signs: Previous BP values in either the prehypertension or the hypertension category.

Laboratory Tests: BUN/serum creatinine, fasting lipid panel, fasting blood glucose, serum electrolytes (sodium, potassium), spot urine albumin-to-creatinine ratio. The patient may have normal values and still have hypertension. However, some may have abnormal values that are consistent with either additional CV risk factors or hypertension-related damage.

Other Diagnostic Tests: 12-lead electrocardiogram, estimated glomerular filtration rate [using modification of diet in renal disease (MDRD) equation].

Hypertension-Related Target-Organ Damage: The patient may have a previous medical history or diagnostic findings that indicate the presence of hypertension-related target-organ damage:

- Brain (stroke, transient ischemic attack, dementia)
- Eyes (retinopathy)
- Heart (left ventricular hypertrophy, angina, prior MI, prior coronary revascularization, heart failure)
- Kidney (chronic kidney disease)
- Peripheral vasculature (peripheral arterial disease)

---

certain national standards to ensure maximum quality and precision with measurement.

The AHA stepwise technique is recommended:

- Patients should ideally refrain from nicotine and caffeine ingestion for 30 minutes and sit with lower back supported in a chair. Bare arm should be supported and resting near heart level. Feet should be flat on the floor (with legs not crossed). The measurement environment should be relatively quiet and provide privacy. Measuring BP in a position other than seated (supine or standing position) may be required under special circumstances (suspected orthostatic hypotension, or dehydration).

- Measurement should begin only after a 5-minute period of rest.

- A properly sized cuff (pediatric, small, regular, large, or extra large) should be used. The inflatable rubber bladder inside the cuff should cover at least 80% of the arm of the upper arm circumference and 40% of the upper arm width.

- The palpatory method should be used to estimate the SBP:

  - Place the cuff on the upper arm 2 to 3 cm above the antecubital fossa and attach it to the manometer (either a mercury or aneroid).

- Close the inflation valve and inflate the cuff to 70 mm Hg.

- Palpate the radial pulse with the index and middle fingers of the opposite hand.

- Inflate further in increments of 10 mm Hg until the radial pulse is no longer palpated.

- Note the pressure at which the radial pulse is no longer palpated; this is the estimated SBP.

- Release the pressure in the cuff by opening the value.

- The bell (not the diaphragm) of the stethoscope should be placed on the skin of the antecubital fossa, directly over where the brachial artery is palpated. The stethoscope earpieces should be inserted appropriately. The valve should be closed with the cuff then inflated to 30 mm Hg above the estimated SBP from the palpatory method. The value should be slightly opened to slowly release pressure at a rate of 2 to 3 mm Hg/second.

- The clinician should listen for Korotkoff sounds with the stethoscope. The first phase of Korotkoff sounds are the initial presence of clear tapping sounds. Note the pressure at the first recognition of these sounds. This is the SBP. As pressure deflates, note the pressure when all sounds disappear, right at the last sound. This is the DBP.

- Measurements should be rounded to the nearest 2 mm Hg.

- A second measurement should be obtained after at least 1 minute. If these values differ by more than 5 mm Hg, additional measurements should be obtained.

- Neither the patient nor the observer should talk during measurement.

- When first establishing care with a patient, BP should be measured in both arms. If consistent inter-arm differences exist, the arm with the higher value should be used.

Inaccuracies with indirect measurements result from inherent biological variability of BP, inaccuracies related to suboptimal technique, and the white coat effect.[13] Variations in BP occur with environmental temperature, the time of day and year, meals, physical activity, posture, alcohol, nicotine, and emotions. In the clinic setting, standard BP measurement procedures (e.g., appropriate rest period, poor technique, minimal number of measurements) are often not followed, which results in poor estimation of true BP. It is recommended that the stethoscope bell, rather than the diaphragm, be used for measurement, though some studies suggest little difference between two.[13]

Approximately 15% to 20% of patients have *white coat hypertension,* where BP values rise in a clinical setting but return to normal in nonclinical environments using home or ambulatory BP measurements.[13] Interestingly, the rise in BP dissipates gradually over several hours after leaving the clinical setting. It may or may not be precipitated by other stresses in the patient's daily life. This is in contrast to *masked hypertension,* where a decrease in BP occurs in the clinical setting.[14] With masked hypertension, home BP is hypertensive, while the in-office BP is normotensive or substantially lower than at home. This situation may lead to under treatment or lack of treatment for hypertension. Moreover, patients with either white coat or masked hypertension have a high risk of progressing to develop sustained hypertension, which can result in a higher risk of CV events compared with normotensive patients.[15]

Pseudohypertension is a falsely elevated BP measurement. It may be seen in the elderly, those with long-standing diabetes, or those with chronic kidney disease due to rigid, calcified brachial arteries.[13] In these patients, the true arterial BP when measured directly with intraarterial measurement (the most accurate measurement of BP) is much lower than that measured using the indirect cuff method.

The Osler maneuver can be used to test for pseudohypertension. In this maneuver, the BP cuff is inflated above peak SBP. If the radial artery remains palpable, the patient has a positive Osler sign (rigid artery), which may indicate pseudohypertension.

Elderly patients with a wide pulse pressure may have an auscultatory gap that can lead to underestimated SBP or overestimated DBP measurements.[13] In this situation, as the cuff pressure falls from the true SBP value, the Korotkoff sound may disappear (indicating a false DBP measurement), reappear (a false SBP measurement), and then disappear again at the true DBP value. When an auscultatory gap is present, Korotkoff sounds are usually heard when pressure in the cuff first starts to decrease after inflation. This may be eliminated by raising the arm overhead by 30 seconds before bringing it to the proper position and inflating the cuff. This maneuver decreases the intravascular volume and improves inflow thereby allowing Korotkoff sounds to be heard.[13]

Ambulatory and Self-BP Monitoring Ambulatory BP (ABP) monitoring using an automated device can document BP at frequent time intervals (e.g., every 15 to 30 minutes) throughout a 24-hour period.[13] ABP values are usually lower than clinic-measured values. The upper limit for normal ABP is 140/90 mm Hg during the day, 125/75 mm Hg at night, and 135/85 mm Hg during 24 hours. Self-BP measurements are collected by patients, preferably in the morning, using home monitoring devices.

Neither ABP nor self-BP monitoring are needed for the routine diagnosis of hypertension; however, these modalities can enhance the ability to identify patients with white coat and masked hypertension.[14] ABP and self-BP measurements may also be useful in evaluating BP control for patients on antihypertensive drug therapy.[14] ABP monitoring may be helpful for patients with apparent drug resistance, hypotensive symptoms while on antihypertensive therapy, episodic hypertension (e.g., white coat hypertension), and autonomic dysfunction and in identifying "non-dippers" whose BP does not decrease by >10% during sleep and who may portend increased risk of BP-related complications.[1,13]

Limitations of ABP and self-BP measurements may prohibit routine use of such technology. These include complexity of use, costs, and lack of prospective outcome data describing normal ranges for these measurements. Although self-monitoring of BP at home is less complicated and less costly than ambulatory monitoring, patients may omit or fabricate readings.

CLINICAL EVALUATION

Frequently, the only sign of essential hypertension is elevated BP. The rest of the physical examination may be completely normal. However, a complete medical evaluation (a comprehensive medical history, physical examination, and laboratory and/or diagnostic tests) is recommended after diagnosis to (1) identify secondary causes, (2) identify other CV risk factors or comorbid conditions that may define prognosis and/or guide therapy, and (3) assess for the presence or absence of hypertension-associated target-organ damage.[1] All patients with hypertension should have the tests described in Box 19–1 measured prior to initiating therapy.[1] For patients without a history of coronary artery disease, noncoronary atherosclerotic vascular disease, left ventricular dysfunction, or diabetes it is also important to estimate a 10-year risk of fatal coronary heart disease or nonfatal MI using Framingham risk scoring. (*http://www.nhlbi.nih.gov/guidelines/cholesterol/risk_tbl.htm*).[2]

Secondary Causes

The most common secondary causes of hypertension are listed in Table 19–1. A complete medical evaluation should provide clues for identifying secondary hypertension.

Patients with secondary hypertension might have signs or symptoms suggestive of the underlying disorder. Patients with pheochromocytoma may have a history of paroxysmal headaches, sweating, tachycardia, and palpitations. Over half of these patients suffer from episodes of orthostatic hypotension. In primary hyperaldosteronism symptoms related to hypokalemia usually include muscle cramps and muscle weakness. Patients with Cushing syndrome may complain of weight gain, polyuria, edema, menstrual irregularities, recurrent acne, or muscular weakness and have several classic physical features (e.g., moon face, buffalo hump, hirsutism). Patients with coarctation of the aorta may have higher BP in the arms than legs and diminished or even absent femoral pulses. Patients with renal artery stenosis may have an abdominal systolic-diastolic bruit.

Routine laboratory tests may also help identify secondary hypertension. Baseline hypokalemia may suggest mineralocorticoid-induced hypertension. Protein, red blood cells, and casts in the urine may indicate renovascular disease. Some laboratory tests are used specifically to diagnose secondary hypertension. These include plasma norepinephrine and urinary metanephrine for pheochromocytoma, plasma and urinary aldosterone concentrations for primary hyperaldosteronism, plasma renin activity, captopril stimulation test, renal vein renin, and renal artery angiography for renovascular disease.

Certain drugs and other products can result in drug-induced hypertension (see Table 19-1). For some patients, the addition of these agents can be the cause of hypertension or can exacerbate underlying hypertension. Identifying a temporal relationship between starting the suspected agent and developing elevated BP is most suggestive of drug-induced BP elevation.

NATURAL COURSE OF DISEASE

Essential hypertension is usually preceded by elevated BP values that are in the prehypertension category. BP values may fluctuate between elevated and normal levels for an extended period of time. During this stage, many patients have a hyperdynamic circulation with increased CO and normal or even low peripheral vascular resistance. As the disease progresses, peripheral vascular resistance increases, and BP elevation becomes chronic.

Hypertension-Associated Target-Organ Damage

Target-organ damage (see Box 19-1) can develop as a complication of hypertension. CV events (e.g., MI, cerebrovascular accidents, kidney failure) are clinical end points of hypertension-associated target-organ damage and are the primary causes of CV morbidity and mortality for patients with hypertension. The probability of CV events and CV morbidity and mortality in patients with hypertension is directly correlated with the severity of BP elevation.

Hypertension accelerates atherosclerosis and stimulates left ventricular and vascular dysfunction. These pathologic changes are thought to be secondary to both a chronic pressure overload and a variety of nonhemodynamic stimuli. Several nonhemodynamic disturbances have been implicated in these effects (e.g., the adrenergic system, RAAS, increased synthesis and secretion of endothelin I, and a decreased production of prostacyclin and nitric oxide). Atherosclerosis in hypertension is accompanied by proliferation of smooth muscle cells, lipid infiltration into the vascular endothelium, and an enhancement of vascular calcium accumulation.

Cerebrovascular disease is a consequence of hypertension. A neurologic assessment can detect either gross neurologic deficits or a slight hemiparesis with some incoordination and hyperreflexia that are indicative of cerebrovascular disease. Stroke can result from lacunar infarcts caused by thrombotic occlusion of small vessels or intracerebral hemorrhage resulting from ruptured microaneurysms. Transient ischemic attacks secondary to atherosclerotic disease in the carotid arteries are common for patients with hypertension.

Retinopathies can occur in hypertension and may manifest as a variety of different findings. A funduscopic examination can detect hypertensive retinopathy, and the result can be categorized according to the Keith-Wagener-Barker retinopathy classification. Retinopathy manifests as arteriolar narrowing, focal arteriolar constrictions, arteriovenous crossing changes (nicking), retinal hemorrhages and exudates, and disk edema. Accelerated arteriosclerosis, a long-term consequence of essential hypertension, can cause nonspecific changes such as increased light reflex, increased tortuosity of vessels, and arteriovenous nicking. Focal arteriolar narrowing, retinal infarcts, and flame-shaped hemorrhages usually are suggestive of accelerated or malignant phase of hypertension. Papilledema is swelling of the optic disk caused by a breakdown in autoregulation of capillary blood flow in the presence of high pressure. It is usually only present in hypertensive emergencies.

Heart disease is the most well-identified form of target-organ damage. A thorough cardiac and pulmonary examination can identify cardiopulmonary abnormalities. Clinical manifestations include left ventricular hypertrophy, coronary heart disease (angina, prior MI, and prior coronary revascularization), and heart failure. These complications may lead to cardiac arrhythmias, angina, MI, and sudden death. Coronary disease (also called *coronary heart disease*) and associated CV events are the most common causes of death in patients with hypertension.

The kidney damage caused by hypertension is characterized pathologically by hyaline arteriosclerosis, hyperplastic arteriosclerosis, arteriolar hypertrophy, fibrinoid necrosis, and atheroma of the major renal arteries. Glomerular hyperfiltration and intraglomerular hypertension are early stages of hypertensive nephropathy. Microalbuminuria is followed by a gradual decline in renal function. The primary renal complication in hypertension is nephrosclerosis, which is secondary to arteriosclerosis. Atheromatous disease of a major renal artery may give rise to renal artery stenosis. Although overt kidney failure is an uncommon complication of essential hypertension, it is an important cause of end-stage kidney disease, especially in African-Americans, Hispanics, and Native Americans.

The peripheral vasculature is a target organ. Physical examination of the vascular system can detect evidence of atherosclerosis, which may present as arterial bruits (aortic, abdominal, or peripheral), distended veins, diminished or absent peripheral arterial pulses, or lower extremity edema. Peripheral arterial disease is a clinical condition that can result from atherosclerosis, which is accelerated in hypertension. Other CV risk factors (e.g., smoking) can increase the likelihood of peripheral arterial disease as well as all other forms of target-organ damage.

TREATMENT

■ DESIRED OUTCOMES

Overall Goal of Treatment

❹ The overall goal of treating hypertension is to reduce hypertension-associated morbidity and mortality.[1] This morbidity and mortality is related to hypertension-associated target-organ damage (e.g., CV events, cerebrovascular events, heart failure, kidney disease). Reducing CV risk remains the primary purpose of hypertension therapy and the specific choice of drug therapy is significantly influenced by evidence demonstrating such CV risk reduction.

Surrogate Targets—Blood Pressure Goals

❺ Treating patients with hypertension to achieve a desired target BP value is simply a surrogate goal of therapy. Reducing BP to goal does not guarantee prevention of hypertension-associated target-organ damage, but is associated with a lower risk of hypertension-associated target-organ damage.[1] Targeting a goal BP value is a tool that clinicians use to evaluate response to therapy. It is the primary method used to determine the need for titration and regimen modification.

The JNC7 and AHA 2007 guidelines each recommend BP goals (Box 19–2) for the management of hypertension. Both guidelines recommend a goal BP of less than 140/90 mm Hg for most patients for the general prevention of CV events or CV disease (e.g., coronary artery disease).[1,2] A lower BP goal of less than 130/80 mm Hg is recommended by both of these guidelines for patients with diabetes or significant chronic kidney disease, although data supporting that this goal provides better reductions in CV events than less than 140/90 mm Hg is not definitive.[1,2] Moreover, the AHA 2007 guidelines also recommend the goal of less than 130/80 mm Hg for patients with known coronary artery disease (MI, stable angina, unstable angina), noncoronary atherosclerotic vascular disease (ischemic stroke, transient ischemic attack, peripheral arterial disease, abdominal aortic aneurysm) or a 10% or greater 10-year risk of fatal coronary heart disease or non-fatal MI based on Framingham risk scoring (*http://www.nhlbi.nih.gov/guidelines/cholesterol/risk_tbl.htm*).[2] The AHA 2007 guidelines also recommend BP goal of less than 120/80 mm Hg for patients with left ventricular dysfunction (heart failure).[2] Similar to diabetes or chronic kidney disease, data supporting that these lower BP goal provides better reductions in CV events than less than 140/90 mm Hg are not definitive.

The BP goals recommended by the JNC7 should be considered standard, or minimum, BP goals. The expanded, lower BP goals

BOX 19-2 GOAL BP VALUES RECOMMENDED BY THE JNC 7 IN 2003[1] AND AHA IN 2007[2]

	JNC7	AHA
Most Patients for General Prevention:	<140/90 mm Hg	<140/90 mm Hg
Patients with Diabetes	<130/80 mm Hg	<130/80 mm Hg
Significant chronic kidney disease		
Patients with Known coronary artery disease (MI, stable angina, unstable angina)	No specific recommendation	<130/80 mm Hg
Noncoronary atherosclerotic vascular disease (ischemic stroke, transient ischemic attack, peripheral arterial disease, abdominal aortic aneurysm)		
Framingham risk score of 10% or greater		
Patients with left ventricular dysfunction (heart failure)	No specific recommendation	120/80 mm Hg

Significant chronic kidney disease is considered to be moderate-to-severe chronic kidney disease, defined as estimated glomerular filtration rate (GFR) <60 mL/minute/1.73 m² (correlating to a serum creatinine >1.3 mg/dL in women or >1.5 in men); or albuminuria (>300 mg/day or >200 mg/g creatinine).

Framingham risk score calculated using the risk calculator available at *http://www.nhlbi.nih.gov/guidelines/cholesterol/risk_tbl.htm*

recommended by the AHA 2007 guidelines for patients with known coronary artery disease, noncoronary atherosclerotic vascular disease, a Framingham risk score of 10% or greater, or left ventricular dysfunction should be considered optional goals for more aggressive management of hypertension. The determination of which approach to follow has been widely debated.[16] Definitive evidence proving that the lower optional BP goals recommended by the AHA reduce risk of hypertension-associated target organ damage greater than the standard JNC7 goals is not available. When available, the BP goals recommended in the JNC8 will represent the most updated expert consensus. Until that time, clinicians should at minimum target the JNC7 BP goals, and then target the extended, more aggressive AHA 2007 guideline BP goals based on clinical judgment.

Evidence Supporting <140/90 mm Hg in Most Patients Lower goal DBP values have been evaluated prospectively in the Hypertension Optimal Treatment (HOT) study.[17] In this study, over 18,700 patients were randomized to target DBP values of ≤90 mm Hg, ≤85 mm Hg, ≤ or 80 mm Hg. Although the actual DBP values achieved were 85.2, 83.2, and 81.1 mm Hg, respectively, there were no significant differences in risk of major CV events when the three treatment groups were compared to each other among the total population. This lack of a benefit in reducing risk of CV events is consistent with findings from a 2009 Cochrane Collaboration systematic review that included 7 clinical trials which evaluated different goal DBP values in hypertension.[18] When the relationship between actual BP values and risk of CV events was evaluated there was trend that lower was better. The risk of major CV events was the lowest with a BP of 139/83 mm Hg, and lowest risk of stroke was with a BP of 142/80 mm Hg.

A major limitation of the HOT study and the 2009 Cochrane Collaboration review is the use of DBP goal values. SBP is more directly correlated to CV risk than DBP in most patients with hypertension, especially those above the age of 50. Therefore, data from the HOT study can not answer this question. It is important to note that no J-curve relationship was seen. The *J-curve hypothesis* suggests that lowering BP too much might increase the risk of CV events.[19] This theoretical hypothesis was described many years ago and was originally suggested in observational studies. Therefore, it remains an unproven hypothesis.

Limited data suggests lower is better when SBP goal values are targeted. The Cardio-Sys trial was a small open-label study in 1,111 patients with hypertension and without a history of diabetes.[20] These patients had additional CV risk factors and roughly reflect a population with a Framingham risk score of 10% or greater. Patients were randomized to SBP goals of less than 140 mm Hg or less than 130 mm Hg. After a median of 2 years, the incidence of left ventricular hypertrophy was lower in the group randomized to a SBP goal of less than 130 mm Hg. Interestingly, the incidence of CV events, which was a secondary end point, was also significantly lower in the less than 130 mm Hg group. These data suggest that the optional lower BP goals may be better. Left ventricular hypertrophy is only a surrogate end point for CV events, and the open-label nature of this study limits broad application to patient care.

CLINICAL CONTROVERSY

How low to go in most patients?

A standard BP goal of less than 140/90 mm Hg is recommended by both the JNC7 and AHA guidelines for most patients, while less than 130/80 mm Hg is recommended in other higher risk patient populations (e.g., diabetes, significant chronic kidney disease, coronary artery disease, ischemic stroke).[1,2] However, some clinicians believe that lower BP goals are better, even for patients that do not have one of the aforementioned higher risk conditions. One ongoing trial that is sponsored by National Heart, Lung, and Blood Institute (NHLBI), the Systolic Pressure Intervention Trial (SPRINT), is a prospective randomized trial that is evaluating standard BP goals with lower BP goals for patients without a history of diabetes or a history of stroke. Once this trial is completed, hopefully the controversy of how low to go in most patients will be resolved.

Evidence Supporting <130/80 mm Hg in Diabetes A BP goal of <130/80 mm Hg has been recommended for patients with diabetes for many years, by multiple organizations.[1,2,21,22] The primary evidence supporting this recommendation was from the HOT study, where the only subgroup to show a lower risk of major CV events in the less than 80 mm Hg group versus the less than 90 mm Hg group was in patient with diabetes (n = 1,501). There was a trend that lower was better in the 3,080 patients with ischemic heart disease [e.g., previous MI, other forms of coronary heart disease (CHD)], but this failed to meet statistical significance.

In 2010, results of the NHLBI-sponsored Action to Control Cardiovascular Risk in Diabetes Blood Pressure (ACCORD-BP) study further questioned the benefit of lower BP goals for patients with diabetes.[23] The ACCORD-BP was an open-label study that randomized 4,733 patients with type 2 diabetes to intensive therapy targeting a SBP of less than 120 mm Hg, or to standard therapy to targeting a SBP less than 140 mm Hg for a mean follow up of 4.7 years. After 1 year, a mean number of medications of 3.4 was needed in the intensive therapy group to attain a mean SBP of 119.3 mm Hg, compared with a mean number of medications of 2.1 in the standard therapy group to attain a mean SBP of 133.5 mm Hg. This difference was generally maintained throughout the study duration. However, there was no significant difference in the annual rate of the primary end point (nonfatal MI, nonfatal stroke, or CV death) between the two groups. The annual incidence of the secondary end point of stroke was lower with the intensive therapy group versus the standard therapy group, and this was the only prespecified end point that was different between the two groups.

Despite consensus guidelines recommending a BP goal of less than 130/80 mm Hg for patients with diabetes, evidence supporting this approach over a standard goal of less than 140/90 mm Hg is marginal. If there are additional clinical benefits of this lower BP goal, they may be limited to certain types of CV events (e.g., stroke). While the ACCORD-BP provided additional evidence regarding BP goals for patients with diabetes, these data do not provide all of the clinical answers that are needed. The ACCORD-BP was open-label, and those in the standard group (SBP less than 140 mm Hg) actually had SBP values that were closer to 130 mm Hg than 140 mm Hg. Clinicians should acknowledge that the best available evidence suggests that a BP goal of less than 130/80 mm Hg is possibly only marginally better than a standard goal BP of less than 140/90 mm Hg for patients with diabetes.

■ AVOIDING CLINICAL INERTIA

Although hypertension is one of the most common medical conditions, BP control rates are poor. *Clinical inertia* in hypertension has been defined as an office visit at which no therapeutic move was made to lower BP in a patient with uncontrolled hypertension.[24] Clinical inertia is not the entire reason why many patients with hypertension do not achieve goal BP values. However, it is certainly a major reason that can be remedied simply through more aggressive treatment with drug therapy. This can involve initiating, titrating, or changing drug therapy.

■ GENERAL APPROACH TO TREATMENT

After a diagnosis of hypertension is made, most patients should be placed on both lifestyle modifications and drug therapy concurrently. Lifestyle modification alone is appropriate therapy for most patients with prehypertension. However, lifestyle modifications alone are not considered adequate for patients with hypertension and additional CV risk factors or hypertension-associated target organ damage.

❻ The choice of initial drug therapy depends on the degree of BP elevation and presence of compelling indications (discussed in the Pharmacotherapy section). Most patients with stage 1 hypertension should be initially treated with a first-line antihypertensive drug, or the combination of two agents. Combination drug therapy is recommended for patients with more severe BP elevation (stage 2 hypertension), using preferably two first-line antihypertensive drugs. This general approach is outlined in Figure 19–2. There are six compelling indications where specific

FIGURE 19-2. Algorithm for treatment of hypertension. Drug therapy recommendations are graded with strength of recommendation and quality of evidence in brackets. Strength of recommendations: A, B, and C are good, moderate, and poor evidence to support recommendation, respectively. Quality of evidence: (1) Evidence from more than 1 properly randomized, controlled trial. (2) Evidence from at least one well-designed clinical trial with randomization, from cohort or case-controlled studies, or dramatic results from uncontrolled experiments or subgroup analyses. (3) Evidence from opinions of respected authorities, based on clinical experience, descriptive studies, or reports of expert communities. *(Adapted from the JNC7 and the AHA.[1,2])*

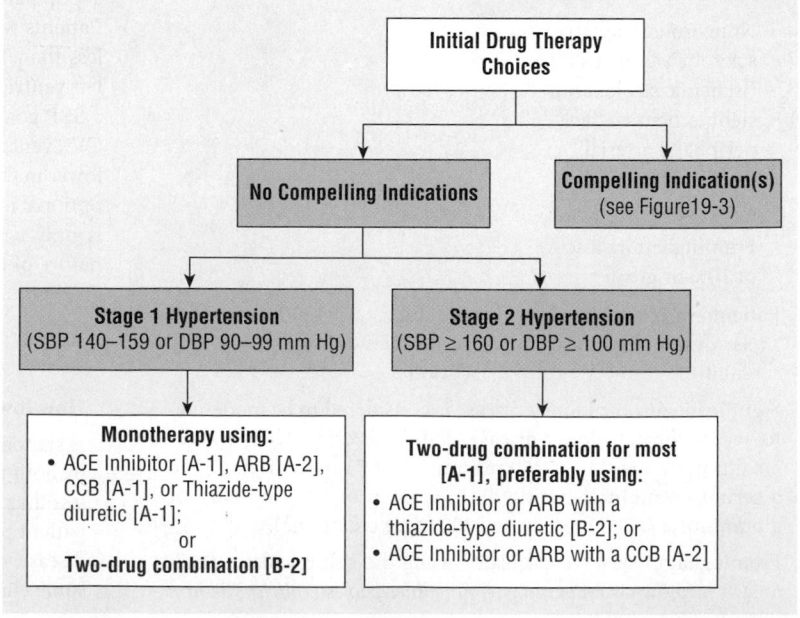

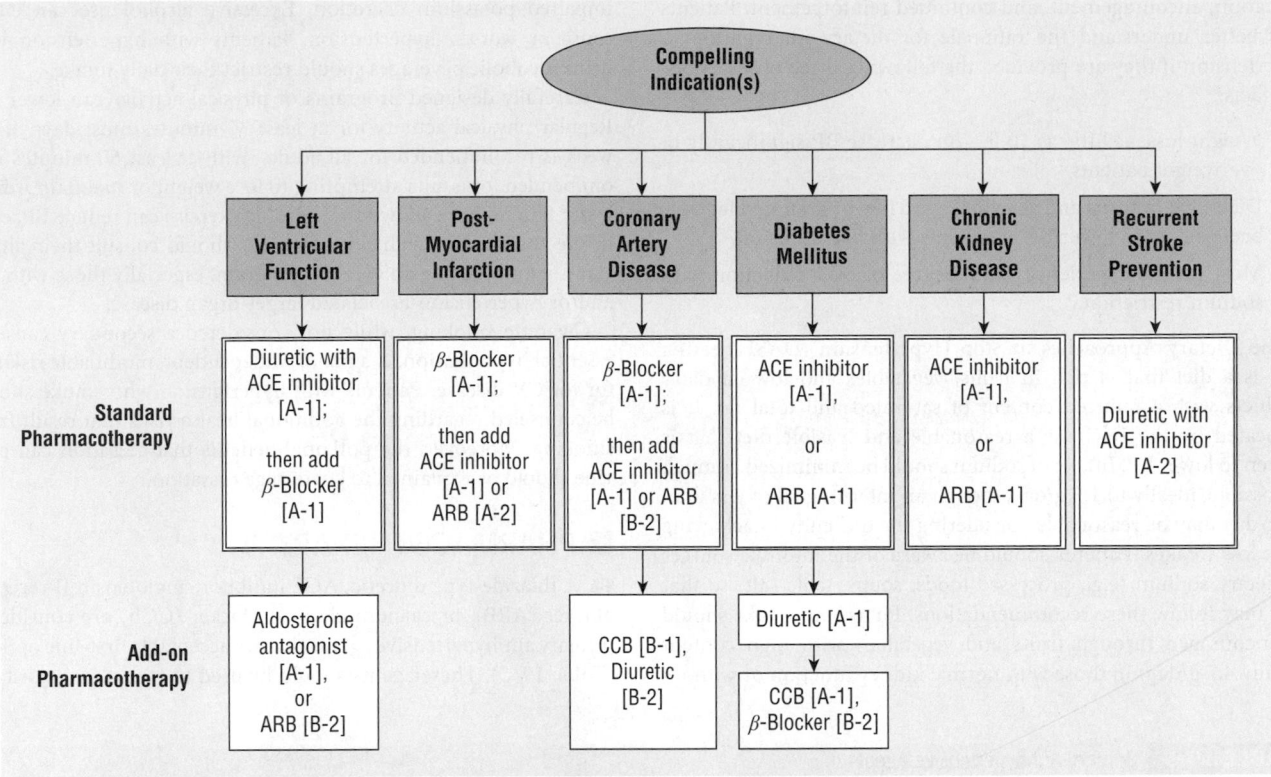

FIGURE 19-3. Compelling indications for individual drug classes (adapted from the JNC7,[1] AHA,[2] and other evidence[58]). Compelling indications for specific drugs are evidenced-based recommendations from outcome studies or existing clinical guidelines. The order of drug therapies serves as a general guidance that should be balanced with clinical judgment and patient response; however, standard pharmacotherapy should be considered first-line recommendations, preferably in the order depicted. Then add-on pharmacotherapy recommendations are intended to further reduce risk of cardiovascular events when additional pharmacotherapy is needed to lower blood pressure to goal values. Blood pressure control should be managed concurrently with the compelling indication. Drug therapy recommendations are graded with strength of recommendation and quality of evidence in brackets. Strength of recommendations: A, B, and, C are good, moderate, and poor evidence to support recommendation, respectively. Quality of evidence: (1) Evidence from more than one properly randomized, controlled trial. (2) Evidence from at least one well-designed clinical trial with randomization, from cohort or case-controlled analytic studies or multiple time series, or dramatic results from uncontrolled experiments or subgroup analyses. (3) Evidence from opinions of respected authorities, based on clinical experience, descriptive studies, or reports of expert communities.

antihypertensive drug classes have evidence showing unique benefits in patients with hypertension and the listed compelling indication (Fig. 19–3).

■ NONPHARMACOLOGIC THERAPY

❼ All patients with prehypertension and hypertension should be prescribed lifestyle modifications. Recommended modifications that have been shown to lower BP are listed in Table 19–4.[1,25] They

can provide small to moderate reductions in SBP. Aside from lowering BP in patients with known hypertension, lifestyle modification can decrease the progression to hypertension in patients with prehypertension BP values.[25]

A sensible dietary program is one that is designed to reduce weight gradually (for overweight and obese patients) and one that restricts sodium intake with only moderate alcohol consumption. Successful implementation of dietary lifestyle modifications by clinicians requires aggressive promotion through reasonable patient

TABLE 19-4	Lifestyle Modifications to Prevent and Manage Hypertension	
Modification	**Recommendation**	**Approximate Systolic Blood Pressure Reduction (mm Hg)[a]**
Weight loss	Maintain normal body weight (body mass index, 18.5–24.9 kg/m²)	5–20 per 10-kg weight loss
DASH-type dietary patterns	Consume a diet rich in fruits, vegetables, and low-fat dairy products with a reduced content of saturated and total fat	8–14
Reduced salt intake	Reduce daily dietary sodium intake as much as possible, ideally to ≈65 mmol/day (1.5 g/day sodium, or 3.8 g/day sodium chloride)	2–8
Physical activity	Regular aerobic physical activity (at least 30 minutes/day, most days of the week)	4–9
Moderation of alcohol intake	Limit consumption to less than or equal to 2 drink equivalents per day in men and less than or equal to 1 drink equivalent per day in women and lighter weight persons[b]	2–4

[a]Effects of implementing these modifications are time- and dose-dependent and could be greater for some patients.
[b]One drink equivalent is equal to 1.5 oz of 80-proof distilled spirits (e.g., whiskey), a 5 oz glass of wine (12%), or 12 oz of beer.
Data from references (1, 24)

education, encouragement, and continued reinforcement. Patients may better understand the rationale for dietary intervention in hypertension if they are provided the following three observations and facts:[25]

1. Weight loss, as little as 10 lb, can decrease BP significantly in overweight patients.

2. Diets rich in fruits and vegetables and low in saturated fat have been shown to lower BP in patients with hypertension.

3. Most people experience some degree of SBP reduction with sodium restriction.

The Dietary Approaches to Stop Hypertension (DASH) eating plan is a diet that is rich in fruits, vegetables and low-fat dairy products with a reduced content of saturated and total fat. It is advocated by the JNC7 as a reasonable and feasible diet that is proven to lower BP. Intake of sodium should be minimized as much as possible, ideally to 1.5 g/day, though an interim goal of less than 2.3 g/day may be reasonable considering the difficulty in achieving these low intakes. Patients should be aware of the multiple sources of dietary sodium (e.g., processed foods, soups, table salt) so that they may follow these recommendations. Potassium intake should be encouraged through fruits and vegetables with high content (ideally 4.7 g/day) in those with normal kidney function or without

impaired potassium excretion. Excessive alcohol use can either cause or worsen hypertension. Patients with hypertension who drink alcoholic beverages should restrict their daily intake.

Carefully designed programs of physical activity can lower BP. Regular physical activity for at least 30 minutes most days of the week is recommended for all adults, with at least 60 minutes recommended for adults attempting to lose weight or maintain weight loss.[26] Studies have shown that aerobic exercise can reduce BP, even in the absence of weight loss. Patients should consult their physicians before starting an exercise program, especially those with CV and/or hypertension-associated target-organ disease.

Cigarette smoking, while not considered a secondary cause of essential hypertension, is a major, independent, modifiable risk factor for CV disease. Patients with hypertension who smoke should be counseled regarding the additional health risks that result from smoking. Moreover, the potential benefits that cessation can provide should be explained to encourage cessation.

■ PHARMACOTHERAPY

8 A thiazide-type diuretic, ACE inhibitor, angiotensin II receptor blocker (ARB), or calcium channel blocker (CCB) are considered primary antihypertensive agents that are acceptable first-line options (Table 19–5). These agents should be used to treat the majority of

TABLE 19-5	Primary Antihypertensive Agents				
Class	Subclass	Drug (Brand Name)	Usual Dose Range, mg/day	Daily Frequency	Comments
Diuretics	Thiazides	Chlorthalidone (Hygroton)	6.25–25	1	Dose in the morning to avoid nocturnal diuresis; thiazides are more effective antihypertensives than loop diuretics in most patients; use usual doses to avoid adverse metabolic effects; hydrochlorothiazide and chlorthalidone are preferred; chlorthalidone is approximately 1.5 times as potent as hydrochlorothiazide; have additional benefits in osteoporosis; may require additional monitoring in patients with a history of gout or hyponatremia
		Hydrochlorothiazide (Esidrix, HydroDiuril, Microzide, Oretic)	12.5–25	1	
		Indapamide (Lozol)	1.25–2.5	1	
		Metolazone (Mykrox)	0.5–1	1	
		Metolazone (Zaroxolyn)	2.5–10	1	
	Loops	Bumetanide (Bumex)	0.5–4	2	Dose in the morning and late afternoon (when twice daily) to avoid nocturnal diuresis; higher doses may be needed for patients with severely decreased glomerular filtration rate or heart failure
		Furosemide (Lasix)	20–80	2	
		Torsemide (Demadex)	5–10	1	
	Potassium sparing	Amiloride (Midamor)	5–10	1 or 2	Dose in the morning and late afternoon (when twice daily) to avoid nocturnal diuresis; weak diuretics that are generally used in combination with thiazide-type diuretics to minimize hypokalemia; do not significantly lower BP unless used with a thiazide-type diuretic; should generally be reserved for patients experiencing diuretic-induced hypokalemia; avoid in patients with chronic kidney disease (estimated creatinine clearance <30 mL/min); may cause hyperkalemia, especially in combination with an ACE inhibitor, ARB, direct renin inhibitor, or potassium supplements
		Amiloride/ hydrochlorothiazide (Moduretic)	5–10/50–100	1	
		Triamterene (Dyrenium)	50–100	1 or 2	
		Triamterene/ hydrochlorothiazide (Dyazide)	37.5–75/25–50	1	
	Aldosterone Antagonists	Eplerenone (Inspra)	50–100	1 or 2	Dose in the morning and late afternoon (when twice daily) to avoid nocturnal diuresis; eplerenone contraindicated in patients with an estimated creatinine clearance <50 mL/min, elevated serum creatinine (>1.8 mg/dL in women, >2 mg/dL in men), and type 2 diabetes with microalbuminuria; sprionolactone often used as add-on therapy in resistant hypertension; avoid spironolactone in patients with chronic kidney disease (estimated creatinine clearance <30 mL/min); may cause hyperkalemia, especially in combination with an ACE inhibitor, ARB, direct renin inhibitor or potassium supplements
		Spironolactone (Aldactone)	25–50	1 or 2	
		Spironolactone/ hydrochlorothiazide (Aldactazide)	25–50/25–50	1	

(continued)

TABLE 19-5 Primary Antihypertensive Agents (continued)

Class	Subclass	Drug (Brand Name)	Usual Dose Range, mg/day	Daily Frequency	Comments
ACE inhibitors		Benazepril (Lotensin)	10–40	1 or 2	May cause hyperkalemia in patients with chronic kidney disease or in those receiving potassium-sparing diuretic, aldosterone antagonist, ARB, or direct renin inhibitor; can cause acute kidney failure in patients with severe bilateral renal artery stenosis or severe stenosis in artery to solitary kidney; do not use in pregnancy or in patients with a history of angioedema; starting dose should be reduced 50% in patients who are on a diuretic, are volume depleted, or are very elderly due to risks of hypotension.
		Captopril (Capoten)	12.5–150	2 or 3	
		Enalapril (Vasotec)	5–40	1 or 2	
		Fosinopril (Monopril)	10–40	1	
		Lisinopril (Prinivil, Zestril)	10–40	1	
		Moexipril (Univasc)	7.5–30	1 or 2	
		Perindopril (Aceon)	4–16	1	
		Quinapril (Accupril)	10–80	1 or 2	
		Ramipril (Altace)	2.5–10	1 or 2	
		Trandolapril (Mavik)	1–4	1	
ARBs		Candesartan (Atacand)	8–32	1 or 2	May cause hyperkalemia in patients with chronic kidney disease or in those receiving potassium-sparing diuretic, aldosterone antagonist, ACE inhibitor, or direct renin inhibitor; can cause acute kidney failure in patients with severe bilateral renal artery stenosis or severe stenosis in artery to solitary kidney; do not cause a dry cough like ACE inhibitors may; do not use in pregnancy; starting dose should be reduced 50% in patients who are on a diuretic, are volume depleted, or are very elderly due to risks of hypotension.
		Eprosartan (Teveten)	600–800	1 or 2	
		Irbesartan (Avapro)	150–300	1	
		Losartan (Cozaar)	50–100	1 or 2	
		Olmesartan (Benicar)	20–40	1	
		Telmisartan (Micardis)	20–80	1	
		Valsartan (Diovan)	80–320	1	
Calcium channel blockers	Dihydropyridines	Amlodipine (Norvasc)	2.5–10	1	Short-acting dihydropyridines should be avoided, especially immediate-release nifedipine and nicardipine; dihydropyridines are more potent peripheral vasodilators than nondihydropyridines and may cause more reflex sympathetic discharge (tachycardia), dizziness, headache, flushing, and peripheral edema; have additional benefits in Raynaud's syndrome
		Felodipine (Plendil)	5–20	1	
		Isradipine (DynaCirc)	5–10	2	
		Isradipine SR (DynaCirc SR)	5–20	1	
		Nicardipine sustained release (Cardene SR)	60–120	2	
		Nifedipine long-acting (Adalat CC, Nifedical XL, Procardia XL)	30–90	1	
		Nisoldipine (Sular)	10–40	1	
	Non-dihydropyridines	Diltiazem sustained-release (Cardizem SR)	180–360	2	Extended-release products are preferred for hypertension; these agents reduce heart rate; may produce heart block, especially in combination with β-blockers; these products are not AB rated as interchangeable on a equipotent mg-per-mg basis due to different release mechanisms and different bioavailability parameters; Cardizem LA, Covera HS, and Verelan PM have delayed drug release for several hours after dosing, when dosed in the evening can provide chronotherapeutic drug delivery starting shortly before patients awake from sleep; non-dihydropyridines have additional benefits in patients with atrial tachyarrhythmia
		Diltiazem sustained-release (Cardizem CD, Cartia XT, Dilacor XR, Diltia XT, Tiazac, Taztia XT)	120–480	1	
		Diltiazem extended-release (Cardizem LA)	120–540	1 (morning or evening)	
		Verapamil sustained-release (Calan SR, Isoptin SR, Verelan)	180–480	1 or 2	
		Verapamil controlled-onset extended-release (Covera HS)	180–420	1 (in the evening)	
		Verapamil chronotherapeutic oral drug absorption system (Verelan PM)	100–400	1 (in the evening)	
β-blockers	Cardioselective	Atenolol (Tenormin)	25–100	1	Abrupt discontinuation may cause rebound hypertension; inhibit β_1 receptors at low to moderate dose, higher doses also block β_2 receptors; may exacerbate asthma when selectivity is lost; have additional benefits in patients with atrial tachyarrhythmia or preoperative hypertension
		Betaxolol (Kerlone)	5–20	1	
		Bisoprolol (Zebeta)	2.5–10	1	
		Metoprolol tartrate (Lopressor)	100–400	2	
		Metoprolol succinate extended release (Toprol XL)	50–200	1	
	Nonselective	Nadolol (Corgard)	40–120	1	Abrupt discontinuation may cause rebound hypertension; inhibit β_1 and β_2 receptors at all doses; can exacerbate asthma; have additional benefits in patients with essential tremor, migraine headache, thyrotoxicosis
		Propranolol (Inderal)	160–480	2	
		Propranolol long-acting (Inderal LA, InnoPran XL)	80–320	1	
		Timolol (Blocadren)	10–40	1	

(continued)

TABLE 19-5 Primary Antihypertensive Agents (continued)

Class	Subclass	Drug (Brand Name)	Usual Dose Range, mg/day	Daily Frequency	Comments
	Intrinsic sympathomimetic activity	Acebutolol (Sectral)	200–800	2	Abrupt discontinuation may cause rebound hypertension; partially stimulate β-receptors while blocking against additional stimulation; no clear advantage for these agents; contraindicated in patients post-myocardial infarction
		Carteolol (Cartrol)	2.5–10	1	
		Penbutolol (Levatol)	10–40	1	
		Pindolol (Visken)	10–60	2	
	Mixed α- and β-blockers	Carvedilol (Coreg)	12.5–50	2	Abrupt discontinuation may cause rebound hypertension; additional α blockade produces vasodilation and more orthostatic hypotension
		Carvedilol phosphate (Coreg CR)	20–80	1	
		Labetalol (Normodyne, Trandate)	200–800	2	
	Cardioselective and vasodilatory	Nebivolol (Bystolic)	5–20	1	Abrupt discontinuation may cause rebound hypertension; additional vasodilation does not result in more orthostatic hypotension

patients with hypertension because evidence from outcome data has demonstrated CV risk-reduction benefits with these classes. Several have subclasses where significant differences in mechanism of action, clinical use, side effects, or evidence from outcome studies exist. β-blockers are effective antihypertensive agents that previously were considered primary agents. They are now preferred either to treat a specific compelling indication, or in combination with one or more of the aforementioned primary antihypertensive agents for patients without a compelling indication. Other antihypertensive drug classes are considered alternative drug classes that may be used in select patients after first-line agents (Table 19–6).

Thiazide-Type Diuretics as First-Line Agents

JNC7 guidelines (from 2003) recommend thiazide-type diuretics whenever possible, as first-line therapy for most patients, and is consistent with the traditional pharmacotherapy of hypertension.[1] However, the AHA 2007 guidelines do not identify thiazide-type diuretics as preferred over an ACE inhibitor, ARB, or CCB for first-line therapy. Figure 19–2 displays the algorithm for the treatment of hypertension. This recommendation is specifically for patients without compelling indications and is based on best available evidence demonstrating reductions in CV morbidity and mortality.

Landmark placebo-controlled clinical trials demonstrate that thiazide-type diuretic therapy irrefutably reduces risk of CV morbidity and mortality.[27] The Systolic Hypertension in the Elderly Program (SHEP),[8] Swedish Trial in Old Patients with Hypertension (STOP-Hypertension),[9] and Medical Research Council (MRC)[10] studies showed significant reductions in stroke, MI, all cause CV disease, and mortality with thiazide-type diuretic-based therapy versus placebo. These trials allowed for β-blockers as add on therapy for BP control. Newer agents (ACE inhibitors, ARBs, and CCBs) were not available at the time of these studies. However, subsequent clinical trials have compared these newer antihypertensive agents to thiazide-type diuretics.[28–33] These data show similar effects, but most trials used a prospective open-label, blinded end point (PROBE) study methodology that is not double-blinded and limited their ability to prove equivalence of newer drugs to diuretics. Other prospective trials have compared different primary antihypertensive agents to each other.[30,34,35] Although these studies used head-to-head comparisons, they did not use a thiazide-type diuretic as their comparator treatment.

The Antihypertensive and Lipid Lowering Treatment to Prevent Heart Attack Trial (ALLHAT)[31] The results of the ALLHAT was the deciding evidence that the JNC7 used to justify thiazide-type diuretics as first-line therapy.[31] It was designed to test the hypothesis that newer antihypertensive agents (an α-blocker, ACE inhibitor, or dihydropyridine CCB) would be superior to thiazide-type diuretic-based therapy. The primary objective was to compare the combined end point of fatal CHD and nonfatal MI. Other hypertension-related complications (e.g., heart failure, stroke)

TABLE 19-6 Alternative Antihypertensive Agents

Class	Drug (Brand Name)	Usual Dose Range in mg/day	Daily Frequency	Comments
α₁-Blockers	Doxazosin (Cardura)	1–8	1	Give first dose at bedtime; patients should rise from sitting or laying down slowly to minimize risk of orthostatic hypotension; additional benefits in men with benign prostatic hyperplasia
	Prazosin (Minipress)	2–20	2 or 3	
	Terazosin (Hytrin)	1–20	1 or 2	
Direct renin inhibitor	Aliskiren (Tekturna)	150–300	1	May cause hyperkalemia in patients with chronic kidney disease and diabetes or in those receiving a potassium-sparing diuretic, aldosterone antagonist, ACE inhibitor, or ARB; may cause acute kidney failure in patients with severe bilateral renal artery stenosis or severe stenosis in artery to solitary kidney; do not use in pregnancy
Central α₂-agonists	Clonidine (Catapress)	0.1–0.8	2	Abrupt discontinuation may cause rebound hypertension; most effective if used with a diuretic to diminish fluid retention; clonidine patch is replaced once per week
	Clonidine patch (Catapress- TTS)	0.1–0.3	1 weekly	
	Methyldopa (Aldomet)	250–1000	2	
Peripheral adrenergic antagonist	Reserpine (generic only)	0.05–0.25		Used in many of the landmark clinical trials; should be used with a diuretic to diminish fluid retention
Direct arterial vasodilators	Minoxidil (Loniten)	10–40	1 or 2	Should be used with diuretic and β-blocker to diminish fluid retention and reflex tachycardia
	Hydralazine (Apresoline)	20–100	2 to 4	

were evaluated as secondary end points. This was the largest prospective hypertension trial ever conducted and included 42,418 patients age 55 and older with hypertension and one additional CV risk factor. This double-blind trial randomized patients to chlorthalidone, amlodipine, doxazosin, or lisinopril-based therapy for a mean of 4.9 years.

The doxazosin arm was terminated early when a significantly higher risk of heart failure versus chlorthalidone was observed.[36] The other arms were continued as scheduled and no significant differences in the primary end point were seen between the chlorthalidone and lisinopril or amlodipine treatment groups. However, chlorthalidone had statistically fewer secondary end points than amlodipine (heart failure) and lisinopril (combined CV disease, heart failure, and stroke). The study conclusions were that chlorthalidone-based therapy was superior in preventing one or more major forms of CV disease and was less expensive than amlodipine or lisinopril-based therapy.

ALLHAT was designed as a superiority study with the hypothesis that amlodipine, doxazosin, and lisinopril would be better than chlorthalidone.[37] It did not prove this hypothesis because the primary end point was no different between chlorthalidone, amlodipine and lisinopril. Many subgroup analyses of specific populations (e.g., black patients, chronic kidney disease, diabetes) from the ALLHAT have been conducted to assess response in certain unique patient populations.[38–40] Surprisingly, none of these analyses demonstrated superior CV event reductions with lisinopril or amlodipine versus chlorthalidone. Overall, thiazide-type diuretics remain unsurpassed in their ability to reduce CV morbidity and mortality in most patients.

The preponderance of evidence supports the JNC7 recommendation of using a thiazide-type diuretic as a first-line antihypertensive agent, unless there are contraindications or if a compelling indication for another agent is present, for most patients.

CLINICAL CONTROVERSY

Is chlorthalidone superior to hydrochlorothiazide?

Chlorthalidone undisputedly reduces CV morbidity and mortality. It was used in the most influential landmark long-term placebo-controlled trials in hypertension, and is almost twice more potent in lowering BP on a milligram-per-milligram basis than hydrochlorothiazide, which has not been as extensively studied in major long term hypertension clinical trials. In clinical practice, it is well accepted that CV benefits in hypertension apply to all thiazide-type diuretics, and benefits are considered a class effect.[2] However, it is not definitively known if the clinical benefits of reducing CV morbidity and mortality that have been proven with chlorthalidone can be extrapolated to hydrochlorothiazide.

ACE Inhibitors, ARBs, and CCBs as First-Line Agents

Clinical trials data cumulatively demonstrate that ACE inhibitor, CCB, or ARB-based antihypertensive therapy reduces CV events. These agents may be used for patients without compelling indications as a first-line therapy. The Blood Pressure Lowering Treatment Trialists' Collaboration has evaluated the incidence of major CV events and death among different antihypertensive drug classes from 29 major randomized trials in 162,341 patients.[41] In placebo-controlled trials, the incidences of major CV events were significantly lower with ACE inhibitor and CCB-based regimens versus placebo. Although there were differences in the incidences of certain CV events in some comparisons (e.g., stroke was lower with diuretic or CCB-based regiments versus ACE inhibitor-based regimens), there were no differences in total major CV events when

ACE inhibitors, CCBs, or diuretics were compared to each other. In studies evaluating ARB-based therapy to control regimens, the incidence of major CV events was lower with ARB-based therapy. However, the control regimens used in these comparisons included both active antihypertensive drug therapies and placebo.

Data from meta-analyses may not be as influential as data from well-designed, prospective, randomized controlled trials (e.g., the ALLHAT). However, they provide clinically useful data that support using ACE inhibitor, CCB, or ARB-based treatment for hypertension as first-line antihypertensive agents. Clinicians can use meta-analyses data as supporting evidence when selecting a first-line antihypertensive regimen for hypertension in most patients.

Other major consensus guidelines recommend multiple first-line options for treating hypertension in most patients. The 2007 European Society of Hypertension-European Society of Cardiology guidelines and the 2006 United Kingdom's National Institute for Health and the Clinical Excellence guidelines list more than one drug therapy option as an acceptable first-line treatment approach.[42,43] The European Society of Hypertension–European Society of Cardiology guidelines are founded on the principle that CV risk reduction is a function of BP control that is largely independent of specific antihypertensives.[42] The United Kingdom guidelines stratify patients based on age and race; they recommend an ACE inhibitor first-line for patients under the age of 55, and either a CCB or thiazide-type diuretic first-line for patients age 55 or older or for black patients.[43]

❾ β-Blockers Versus First-Line Agents Clinical trials data cumulatively suggests that β-blockers may not reduce CV events to the extent that ACE inhibitors, CCB, or ARB do. These data are from three meta-analyses of clinical trials evaluating β-blocker-based therapy for hypertension.[44–47] Overall, these analyses demonstrated fewer reductions in CV events with β-blocker-based antihypertensive therapy compared mostly with ACE inhibitor and CCB based therapy. Although comparative data with ARB based therapy are more limited, a similar trend was observed.

Meta-analyses data evaluating β-blockers and their ability to reduce CV events have limitations. Most studies that were included used atenolol as the β-blocker studied. Therefore, it is possible that atenolol is the only β-blocker that reduces CV events less than the other primary antihypertensive drug classes. However, consensus guidelines do extrapolate these findings to the β-blocker drug class in general.[2] The 2006 United Kingdom guidelines recommend a β-blocker only after other primary antihypertensive agents (e.g., thiazide-type diuretics, CCBs, ACE inhibitors, or ARBs) have been used.[43] These findings also call in question the validity of results from prominent prospective, controlled clinical trials evaluating antihypertensive drug therapy that use β-blocker-based therapy, especially atenolol, as the primary comparator.[30,35,47] Of note, these studies used once daily atenolol, which may be inadequate based on the shorter half-life of this agent.

CLINICAL CONTROVERSY

Is atenolol the reason that β-blockers should not be used first-line?

Many of the clinical trials included in the meta-analyses data that suggest β-blocker-based therapy may not reduce CV events as well as these other agents used atenolol dosed once daily.[44–47] Atenolol has a half-life of 6 to 7 hours and is nearly always dosed once daily, while immediate release forms of carvedilol and metoprolol have half-lives 6 to 10 hours and 3 to 7 hours, respectively, and are always dosed at least twice daily. Therefore, it is possible that these findings might only apply to atenolol and also that these findings may be a result of using atenolol once daily instead of twice daily.

β-Blocker therapy for patients without compelling indications still has a role in the management of hypertension. It is important for clinicians to remember that β-blocker-based antihypertensive therapy does not increase risk of CV events; β-blocker-based therapy reduces risk of CV events compared to no antihypertensive therapy. Using a β-blocker as a primary antihypertensive agent is optimal when a thiazide-type diuretic, ACE inhibitor, ARB, or CCB cannot be used as the primary agent. β-blockers still have an important add-on role after first-line agents to reduce BP in patients with hypertension but without compelling indications.

Patients with Compelling Indications[1]

🔟 The JNC7 report identifies six compelling indications. Compelling indications represent specific comorbid conditions where evidence from clinical trials supports using specific antihypertensive classes to treat both the compelling indication and hypertension. Drug therapy recommendations typically consist of combination drug therapies (see Fig. 19–3). Data from these clinical trials have demonstrated reduction in CV morbidity and/or mortality that justify use for patients with hypertension and with such a compelling indication. Some compelling indications include recommendations that are provided by other national treatment guidelines, or from newer clinical trials, which are complementary to the JNC7 guidelines.

Left Ventricular Dysfunction (Systolic Heart Failure)[48] Five drug classes are listed as compelling indications for left ventricular dysfunction [also known as (aka) systolic heart failure]. The primary physiologic abnormality in this compelling indication is decreased CO. Standard pharmacotherapy for left ventricular dysfunction, sometimes called *standard pharmacotherapy*, consists of three drugs: an ACE inhibitor plus diuretic therapy, followed by the addition of an appropriate β-blocker.

Evidence from clinical trials shows that ACE inhibitors significantly modify disease progression by reducing morbidity and mortality. Although left ventricular dysfunction was the primary disease in these studies, ACE inhibitor therapy will also control BP in patients with systolic heart failure and hypertension. ACE inhibitors should be started with low-doses for patients with systolic heart failure, especially those in acute exacerbation. Heart failure induces a compensatory high-renin condition, and starting ACE inhibitors under these conditions can cause a pronounced first-dose effect and possible orthostatic hypotension.

Diuretics are also a part of standard pharmacotherapy primarily to control symptoms. They provide symptomatic relief of edema by inducing diuresis. Loop diuretics are often needed, especially for patients with more advanced heart failure. However, some patients with well-controlled heart failure and without significant chronic kidney disease may be managed with a thiazide-type diuretic.

β-Blocker therapy is appropriate to further modify disease in left ventricular dysfunction and is a component of standard therapy for these patients. For patients on an initial regimen of diuretics and ACE inhibitors, β-blockers have been shown to reduce CV morbidity and mortality.[49,50] It is of paramount importance that β-blockers be dosed appropriately due to the risk of inducing an acute exacerbation of heart failure. They must be started in very low doses, doses much lower than that used to treat hypertension, and titrated slowly to high doses based on tolerability. Bisoprolol, carvedilol, and sustained release metoprolol succinate are the only β-blockers proven to be beneficial in left ventricular dysfunction.[48]

After implementation of a standard three-drug regimen, other agents may be added to further reduce CV morbidity and mortality, and reduce BP if needed. The addition of an aldosterone antagonist can reduce CV morbidity and mortality in left ventricular dysfunction.[51,52] Spironolactone has been studied in severe

left ventricular dysfunction and has shown benefit in addition to diuretic and ACE inhibitor therapy.[51] Eplerenone has been studied in patients with symptomatic left ventricular dysfunction within 3 to 14 days after an acute MI in addition to a standard three-drug regimen.[52] An aldosterone antagonist may be considered in addition to a diuretic, ACE inhibitor or ARB, and β-blocker. It is not currently recommended to use both an aldosterone inhibitor and an ARB as add-on therapy to a standard three-drug regimen because of the potential increase in risk of severe hyperkalemia.[48]

Early data suggested that ARBs may be better than ACE inhibitors in left ventricular dysfunction.[53] However, when directly compared in a well-designed prospective trial, ACE inhibitors were found to be better.[54] ARBs are acceptable as an alternative therapy for patients who cannot tolerate ACE inhibitors and possibly as add-on therapy to those already on a standard three-drug regimen based on data from the Candesartan in Heart Failure-Assessment of Reduction in Mortality and Morbidity (CHARM) studies.[55,56] However, the clinical benefit of adding an ARB to a regimen that already includes an ACE inhibitor seems to be limited to reducing the incidence of hospitalization for heart failure. Therefore, if a fourth agent needs to be added, many clinicians will select an aldosterone antagonist. For patients self-described as African-Americans, the combination of a fixed dose of isosorbide dinitrate and hydralazine to standard three drug regimen is recommended as an option to improve CV outcomes.[48]

Post-MI[57] β-Blocker [those without intrinsic sympathomimetic activity (ISA)] and ACE inhibitor therapy are recommended in the AHA/American College of Cardiology and JNC7 guidelines.[1,2,57] β-blockers decrease cardiac adrenergic stimulation and have been shown in clinical trials to reduce the risk of a subsequent MI or sudden cardiac death. ACE inhibitors have been shown to improve cardiac remodeling and cardiac function and to reduce CV events post-MI. These two drug classes, with β-blockers first, are considered the first drugs of choice for patients who have experienced an MI. One study, the Valsartan in acute MI (VALIANT) trial, demonstrated that ARB therapy is similar to ACE inhibitor therapy for patients post-MI with left ventricular dysfunction.[58] However, ARBs are considered alternatives to ACE inhibitors in post-MI patients with left ventricular dysfunction.

Eplerenone reduces CV morbidity and mortality in patients soon after an acute MI (within 3 to 14 days).[52] However, this supporting evidence was specifically for patients with symptoms of acute left ventricular dysfunction. Considering that this drug has the propensity to cause significant hyperkalemia, eplerenone should only be used in selected patients following an MI and left ventricular dysfunction with very diligent monitoring of potassium.

Coronary Artery Disease[57,59] Chronic stable angina and acute coronary syndrome (unstable angina and acute MI) are forms of coronary artery disease (aka ischemic heart disease). These are the most common forms of hypertension-associated target-organ disease. This compelling indication is also referred to as high coronary disease risk and high CV disease risk in the JNC7 report.[1] This compelling indication does not refer to patients without established CV disease (primary prevention patients) even if they have very high Framingham risk score (e.g., greater than 20%). β-Blocker therapy has the most evidence demonstrating benefits in these patients. β-blockers are first-line therapy in chronic stable angina and have the ability to reduce BP and improve ischemic symptoms by decreasing myocardial oxygen consumption and demand.

Long-acting CCBs are either alternatives (the nondihydropyridine CCBs diltiazem and verapamil) or add-on therapy (dihydropyridine CCBs) to β-blockers in chronic stable angina for patients with ischemic symptoms.[59] The International Verapamil-Trandolapril Study (INVEST) demonstrated no difference in CV risk reduction when β-blocker-based therapy was compared to nondihydropyridine CCB-based therapy in this population.[60] Nonetheless, the preponderance of data are with β-blockers and they remain the therapy of choice.[1,57,59]

For acute coronary syndromes (ST-elevation MI and unstable angina/non-ST-segment MI), first-line therapy should consist of a β-blocker and ACE inhibitor.[61,62] This regimen will lower BP, control acute ischemia, and reduce CV risk.

CCBs (especially nondihydropyridine CCBs) and β-blockers provide anti-ischemic effects; they lower BP and reduce myocardial oxygen demand in patients with hypertension and coronary artery disease. However, cardiac stimulation may occur with dihydropyridine CCBs or β-blockers with ISA, making these agents less desirable. Therefore, β-blockers with ISA should be avoided. Nondihydropyridines CCBs should be used as alternatives to β-blockers, and dihydropyridines should be add-on therapy to β-blockers.

Once ischemic symptoms are controlled with β-blocker and/or CCB therapy, other antihypertensive drugs can be added to provide additional CV risk reduction. Clinical trials have demonstrated that the addition of an ACE inhibitor further reduces risk CV events in patients with chronic stable angina.[63] ARBs may provide similar benefits but have not been as extensively studied as ACE inhibitors have in clinical trials.[63] Therefore, in coronary artery disease, ARBs are generally considered an alternative to ACE inhibitor therapy. Thiazide-type diuretics can be added thereafter to provide additional BP lowering and to further reduce CV risk; they do not provide anti-ischemic effects.

Diabetes Mellitus[1,21] The primary cause of mortality in diabetes is CV disease, and hypertension management is a very important risk-reduction strategy. Five antihypertensive agents have evidence supporting their compelling indications in diabetes (see Fig. 19–3). All of these agents have been shown to reduce CV events in patients with diabetes. However, risk reduction may not be equal when comparing these agents.

❶ All patients with diabetes and hypertension should be treated with an ACE inhibitor or an ARB.[21] Pharmacologically, both of these agents should provide nephro protection due to vasodilatation in the efferent arteriole of the kidney. Moreover, ACE inhibitors have overwhelming data demonstrating CV risk reduction in patients with established forms of heart disease. Evidence from outcome studies have demonstrated reductions in both CV risk (mostly with ACE inhibitors) and reduction in risk of progressive kidney dysfunction (mostly with ARBs) in patients with diabetes.[21] There is debate surrounding which agent is better because data support both drug classes. Nonetheless, either drug class should be used to control BP as one of the drugs in the antihypertensive regimen for patients with diabetes because multiple agents are often needed to attain goal BP values.

A thiazide-type diuretic is recommended as the second agent to lower BP and provide additional CV risk-reduction. A subgroup analysis of patients with diabetes from the ALLHAT trial showed no difference in long-term risk of CV events in the chlorthalidone and lisinopril treatment groups.[39] Therefore, some argue that thiazide-type diuretics, used in low-doses, are equally effective for patients with hypertension and diabetes. Nonetheless, the entire body of evidence evaluating pharmacotherapy for patients with hypertension and diabetes and consensus guidelines support an ACE inhibitor or ARB first-line, with a thiazide-type diuretic as add-on therapy.[1,21,64]

CCBs are useful add-on agents for BP control for patients with diabetes. Several studies have compared an ACE inhibitor with either a dihydropyridine CCB or a β-blocker. In the studies comparing a dihydropyridine with an ACE inhibitor, the ACE inhibitor group had significantly lower rates of CV end points, including

MIs and all CV events.[65] These data do not suggest that CCBs are harmful in patients with diabetes, but indicate that they are not as protective as ACE inhibitors. While data are limited, nondihydropyridine CCBs (diltiazem and verapamil) appear to have more renal protective effects than the dihydropyridines.[64]

β-blockers, similar to CCBs, are useful add-on agents for BP control for patients with diabetes. These agents should also be used to treat another compelling indication (e.g., post-MI). β-blockers (especially non-selective agents) can possibly mask the signs and symptoms of hypoglycemia in patients with tightly controlled diabetes because most of the symptoms of hypoglycemia (i.e., tremor, tachycardia, and palpitations) are mediated through the sympathetic nervous system. Sweating, a cholinergically mediated symptom of hypoglycemia, should still occur during a hypoglycemic episode despite β-blocker therapy. Patients may also have a delay in hypoglycemia recovery time because compensatory recovery mechanisms need the catecholamine inputs that are antagonized by β-blocker therapy. Finally, unopposed α-receptor stimulation during the acute hypoglycemic recovery phase (due to endogenous epinephrine release intended to reverse hypoglycemia) may result in acutely elevated BP due to vasoconstriction. Despite these potential problems, β-blockers can be safely used for patients with diabetes.

Based on the weight of all evidence, ACE inhibitors or ARBs are preferred first-line agents for controlling hypertension in diabetes. The need for combination therapy should be anticipated, and thiazide-type diuretics should the second agent added. Based on scientific evidence, CCBs and even β-blockers are useful evidenced-based agents in this population, but are considered add-on therapies to the aforementioned agents.

Chronic Kidney Disease[66] Patients with hypertension may develop damage to either the renal tissue (parenchyma) or the renal arteries. Chronic kidney disease initially presents as microalbuminuria (30 to 299 mcg/mg albumin/creatinine ratio on a spot urine sample or greater than or equal 30 mg albumin in a 24 hour urine collection) that can progress to overt kidney failure. The rate of kidney function deterioration is accelerated when both hypertension and diabetes are present. Once patients have an estimated GFR less than 60 mL/min/1.73 m² or albuminuria they have significant chronic kidney disease and risk of CV disease and progression to severe chronic kidney disease increases.[1]

BP control to a goal of less than 130/80 mm Hg can slow the decline in kidney function. Although this BP goal is recommended in significant chronic kidney disease, long term benefits of this BP goal have mostly been demonstrated for patients with both significant chronic kidney disease and diabetes.[67]

In addition to lowering BP, ACE inhibitors and ARBs reduce intraglomerular pressure, which can theoretically provide additional benefits by further reducing the decline in kidney function. ACE inhibitors and ARBs have been shown to reduce progression of chronic kidney disease in diabetes[21] and in those without diabetes.[64,68] It is difficult to differentiate whether the kidney protection benefits are from RAAS blockade versus BP lowering. A meta-analysis failed to demonstrate any unique long term kidney protective effects of RAAS blocking drugs compared with other antihypertensive drugs.[69] Moreover, a subgroup analysis of patients from the ALLHAT stratified by different baseline GFR values also did not show a difference in long term outcomes with chlorthalidone versus lisinopril.[38] Nonetheless, consensus guidelines recommend either an ACE inhibitor or ARB as first-line therapy to control BP and preserve kidney function in chronic kidney disease.

Patients may experience a rapid and profound drop in BP or acute kidney failure when given an ACE inhibitor or ARB. The potential to produce acute kidney failure is particularly problematic in patients with bilateral renal artery stenosis or a solitary functioning kidney with stenosis. Patients with renal artery stenosis are usually older, and the condition is more common in patients with diabetes or those who smoke. Patients with renal artery stenosis do not always have evidence of kidney disease unless sophisticated tests are performed. Starting with low dosages and evaluating serum creatinine soon after starting the drug can minimize this risk.

Recurrent Stroke Prevention Stroke (specifically ischemic stroke, not hemorrhagic stroke) is considered a form of hypertension-associated target organ damage. Attaining goal BP values in patients who have experienced an ischemic stroke is considered a primary modality to reduce risk of a second stroke. However, BP lowering should only be attempted after patients have stabilized following an acute cerebrovascular event. One clinical trial, the Protection Against Recurrent Stroke Study (PROGRESS), showed that the incidence of recurrent stroke in patients with a history of ischemic stroke can be reduced when a thiazide-type diuretic is added to an ACE inhibitor.[32] Reduction in recurrent stroke was seen with this combination therapy, even in those who had BP values less than 140/90 mm Hg. Recurrent stroke was not reduced with ACE inhibitor monotherapy in the PROGRESS; it was only reduced when the thiazide-type diuretic was added.

An ACE inhibitor with a thiazide-type diuretic is an evidence-based antihypertensive regimen for patients with a history of cerebrovascular disease.[1,70] This recommendation does not apply to patients with a history of hemorrhagic stroke. However, it does apply to patients with a history of transient ischemic attack, which is considered a form of this compelling indication.

CLINICAL CONTROVERSY

Does ARB-based therapy reduce recurrent stroke risk?

Two large, prospective clinical trials have evaluated whether ARB-based therapy reduces the risk of recurrent stroke in patients with established cerebrovascular disease. In the Morbidity and Mortality after Stroke- Eprosartan Compared With Nitrendipine for Secondary Prevention (MOSES) study, patients with a history of cerebrovascular disease (ischemic stroke or transient ischemic attack) had a lower risk of a recurrent stoke when treated with ARB-based therapy compared to dihydropyridine CCB-based therapy.[71] However, in the PROFESS trial, there was no difference in the incidence of recurrent stroke with ARB-based treatment versus placebo.[72] Therefore, the exact role of ARB-based therapy for patients with a history of ischemic stroke is unknown.

Alternative Drug Treatments

It is necessary to use other agents such as a direct renin inhibitor, α-blockers, central α₂-agonists, adrenergic inhibitors, and arterial vasodilators in some patients. Although these agents are effective in lowering BP, they do not have compelling outcome data showing reduced morbidity and mortality in hypertension. Moreover, there is a much greater incidence of adverse effects with some of these agents (i.e., α-blockers, central α₂-agonists, and arterial vasodilators) than with first-line agents. They are generally reserved for patients with resistant hypertension or as add-on therapy with multiple other primary antihypertensive agents.

Special Populations[1] Selection of drug therapy should follow the guidelines provided by the JNC7 and AHA 2007 recommendations, which are summarized in Figures 19–2 and 19–3. These should be maintained as the guiding principles of drug therapy. However, there are some patient populations where the approach to drug therapy may be slightly different or utilize recommended agents using

tailored dosing strategies. In some cases, this is because other agents have unique properties that benefit a coexisting condition, but may not be based on evidence from outcome studies in hypertension.

Hypertension in Older People Hypertension often presents as isolated systolic hypertension in the elderly. Epidemiologic data indicate that CV morbidity and mortality are more directly correlated to SBP than to DBP for patients age 50 and older, so this population is at high risk for hypertension related target-organ damage.[1] Although several placebo-controlled trials have specifically demonstrated risk reduction in this form of hypertension, many older people with hypertension are either not treated, or treated yet not controlled.[73]

The SHEP was a landmark double-blind, placebo-controlled trial that evaluated chlorthalidone-based treatment (with atenolol or reserpine as add-on therapy) for isolated systolic hypertension.[8] A 36% reduction in total stroke, a 27% reduction in coronary artery disease, and 55% reduction in heart failure were demonstrated versus placebo. The Systolic Hypertension in Europe (Syst-Eur) trial was another placebo-controlled trial that evaluated treatment with a long acting dihydropyridine CCB.[11] Treatment resulted in a 42% reduction in stroke, 26% reduction in coronary artery disease, and 29% reduction in heart failure. These data clearly demonstrate reductions in CV morbidity and mortality in older patients with isolated systolic hypertension, especially with thiazide-type diuretics and long-acting dihydropyridine CCBs.

The very elderly population, greater than or equal 80 years, were underrepresented in the SHEP and Syst-Eur studies. Historically, this population often is not treated to goal either because of a fear of side effects or because of limited data demonstrating benefit. However, the Hypertension in the Very Elderly Trial (HYVET) in 2008 provided definitive proof that antihypertensive drug therapy provides significant clinical benefits in the very elderly.[74] The HYVET was a prospective controlled clinical trial that randomized patients 80 years and older with hypertension to placebo or antihypertensive drug therapy. It was stopped early after a median of only 1.8 years because the incidence of death was 21% higher in placebo-treated patients. Based on these results, hypertension should be treated in the very elderly.

CLINICAL CONTROVERSY

How aggressively should BP be lowered in the very elderly?

It has been advocated for several years to target standard BP goals in the elderly population, regardless of age. This is a well-accepted standard of care for patients with hypertension that continue to have hypertension as they age, meaning that a patient with a history of hypertension should not have their BP goal adjusted just because they have become older. However, for patients that initially develop hypertension when they are very elderly, it is less clear what their BP goal should be. The HYVET trial established that treating hypertension in patients age 80 years or older reduces mortality, but the treatment goal in that population was less than 150/80 mm Hg with a mean SBP and DBP achieved of 145 mm Hg and 79 mm Hg, respectively at 2 years.

Thiazide-type diuretics or β-blockers have been compared with either ACE inhibitors or CCBs in elderly patients with either systolic or diastolic hypertension or both in the Swedish Trial in Old Patients with Hypertension-2 (STOP-2) study.[75] In this trial no significant differences were seen between conventional drugs and either ACE inhibitors or CCBs. However, there were significantly fewer MIs and cases of heart failure in the ACE inhibitor group compared with the CCB group. These data suggest that overall treatment may be more important than specific antihypertensive agents in this population.

Elderly patients are more sensitive to volume depletion and sympathetic inhibition than younger patients. This may lead to orthostatic hypotension (see next section). In the elderly, this can increase the risk of falls due to the associated dizziness. Centrally acting agents and α-blockers should generally be avoided or used with caution in the elderly because they are frequently associated with dizziness and orthostatic hypotension. Diuretics, ACE inhibitors, and ARBs provide significant benefits and can safely be used in the elderly, but smaller-than-usual initial doses must be used for initial therapy.

The JNC7 and AHA goal BP recommendations are independent of age.[1,2] Age adjusted goals are currently not appropriate. Moreover, treatment of hypertension in older patients should follow the same principles that are outlined for general care of hypertension. However, initial drug doses may be lower, and dosage titrations over a longer period of time to minimize the risk of hypotension are usually needed.

⑫ **Patients at Risk for Orthostatic Hypotension** *Orthostatic hypotension* is a significant drop in BP when standing and can be associated with dizziness and/or fainting. It is defined as an SBP decrease of greater than 20 mm Hg or DBP decrease of greater than 10 mm Hg when changing from supine to standing.[1] Older patients (especially those with isolated systolic hypotension) and patients with diabetes, severe volume depletion, baroreflex dysfunction, autonomic insufficiency, and use of venodilators (α-blockers, mixed α-/β-blockers, nitrates, and phosphodiesterase inhibitors) all increase risk of orthostatic hypotension. For patients with these risks, antihypertensive agents should be started in low doses, especially diuretics, ACE inhibitors, and ARBs.

Hypertension in Children and Adolescents[76] Detecting hypertension in children requires special attention to BP measurement, which is defined as SBP and/or DBP that is greater than 95th percentile for sex, age, and height on at least three occasions.[76] Blood pressure between the 90th and 95th percentile, or greater than 120/80 mmHg in adolescents, is considered prehypertension. Hypertensive children often have a family history of high BP, and many are overweight predisposing them to insulin resistance and associated CV disease. Unlike hypertension in adults, secondary hypertension is more common in children and adolescents. An appropriate workup for secondary causes is required if elevated BP is identified. Kidney disease (e.g., pyelonephritis, glomerulonephritis) is the most common cause of secondary hypertension in children. Coarctation of the aorta can also produce secondary hypertension. Medical or surgical management of the underlying disorder usually normalizes BP.

Non-pharmacologic treatment, particularly weight loss in those overweight, is the cornerstone of therapy for essential hypertension in children.[76] The goal is to reduce the BP to below the 95th percentile for sex, age, and height, or below the 90th percentile if concurrent conditions such as chronic kidney disease, diabetes, or target organ damage are present. ACE inhibitors, ARBs, β-blockers, CCBs, and thiazide-type diuretics are all acceptable choices in children and have data supporting their use. ACE inhibitors and ARBs are contraindicated in sexually active girls due to potential teratogenic effect. As with adults, selection of initial agents should be based on the presence of compelling indications or concurrent conditions that may warrant their use (e.g., ACE inhibitor or ARB for those with diabetes or microalbuminuria).

Pregnancy[1,77] Hypertension during pregnancy is a major cause of maternal and neonatal morbidity and mortality. Hypertension during pregnancy is categorized as preeclampsia, eclampsia, gestational, chronic, and superimposition of preeclampsia on chronic hypertension. *Preeclampsia*, defined as an elevated BP greater than 140/90 that appears after 20 weeks gestation accompanied by new-onset proteinuria (greater than or equal to 300 mg/24 hours), can lead to life-threatening complications for both mother and fetus. Eclampsia, the onset of convulsions in preeclampsia, is a medical emergency. *Gestational hypertension* is defined as new onset hypertension arising after mid-pregnancy in the absence of proteinuria, and chronic hypertension is elevated BP that is noted before the pregnancy began. It is controversial whether treating elevated BP for patients with chronic hypertension in pregnancy is beneficial. However, women with chronic hypertension prior to pregnancy are at increased risk of a number of complications including superimposed preeclampsia, preterm delivery, fetal growth restriction or demise, placental abruption, heart failure, and acute kidney failure.[77]

Definitive treatment of preeclampsia is delivery. Delivery is indicated if pending or frank eclampsia is present. Otherwise, management consists of restricting activity, bed rest, and close monitoring. Salt restriction, or any other measures that contract blood volume, should not be employed. Antihypertensive agents are used prior to induction of labor if DBP is greater than 105 mm Hg with a target DBP of 95 to 105 mm Hg. Intravenous hydralazine is most commonly used, and intravenous labetalol is also effective. Immediate-release oral nifedipine has been used in the past, but it is not approved by the Food and Drug Administration (FDA) for hypertension, and untoward fetal and maternal effects (hypotension with fetal distress) have been reported.

Many agents can be used to treat chronic hypertension in pregnancy (Table 19–7). Unfortunately, there is little consensus and few data regarding the most appropriate therapy in pregnancy. Methyldopa is still considered the drug of choice.[1] It is viewed as very safe based on long-term follow-up data (7.5 years) that has not demonstrated adverse effects on childhood development. β-blockers (other than atenolol), labetalol and CCBs are also reasonable alternatives. ACE inhibitors and ARBs are known teratogens and are absolutely contraindicated.[78]

African-Americans[1,79] Hypertension affects African-American patients at a disproportionately higher rate, and hypertension-related target-organ damage is more prevalent than in other populations. Reasons for these differences are not fully understood, but may be related to differences in electrolyte homeostasis, GFR, sodium excretion and transport mechanisms, plasma renin activity, and BP response to plasma volume expansion.

African-Americans have an increased need for combination therapy to attain and maintain BP goals.[79] The Hypertension in African American Working Group of the International Society on

TABLE 19-7	Treatment of Chronic Hypertension in Pregnancy
Drug/Class	**Comments**
Methyldopa	Preferred agent based on long-term follow-up data supporting safety; traditional drug of choice
β-blockers	Generally safe, but intrauterine growth retardation reported (mostly with atenolol)
Labetalol	Increasingly preferred over methyldopa because of fewer side effects
Clonidine	Limited data available; used mainly in third trimester
CCBs	Limited data available; no increase in major teratogenicity with exposure (except immediate-release oral nifedipine should not be used)
Diuretics	Not first-line agents but probably safe in low doses if started prior to conception for essential hypertension
ACE inhibitors, ARBs, direct renin inhibitors	Contraindicated; major teratogenicity reported with exposure (fetal toxicity and death)

Hypertension in Blacks published treatment guidelines that are similar to the JNC7.[79] Lifestyle modifications are recommended to augment drug therapy. They support thiazide-type diuretics as first-line for most patients and selecting specific drug therapy to treat compelling indications, if present. These guidelines aggressively promote combination therapy. They recommend starting with two drugs for patients with SBP values greater than or equal to 15 mm Hg from goal. This aggressive approach is reasonable considering that overall goal BP attainment rates are low in African-Americans.

BP lowering effects of antihypertensive classes varies in African-Americans, primarily when used as monotherapy. Thiazide diuretics and CCBs are most effective at lowering BP in African-Americans. When either of these two classes (especially thiazide-type diuretics) are used in combination with a β-blocker, ACE inhibitor, or ARB (which are three classes known to be less effective at lowering BP in African-Americans), antihypertensive response is significantly increased. This may be due to the low-renin pattern of hypertension in African Americans, which can result in less BP lowering with β-blockers, ACE inhibitors, or ARBs when used as monotherapy compared to Caucasian patients. Interestingly, African-Americans have a higher risk of angioedema and cough from ACE inhibitors compared with Caucasians.[79]

Despite potential differences in antihypertensive effects, drug therapy selection should be based upon evidence, no different from what is recommended for the hypertensive population in general. Drug therapies should be used if a compelling indication is present, even if antihypertensive effect may not be as great as with another drug class (e.g., a β-blocker is first line for BP control in a African-American patient who is post-MI).

Other Concomitant Conditions

Most patients with hypertension have some other coexisting conditions that may influence selection or utilization of drug therapy. The influence of concomitant conditions should only be complementary to, and never in replacement of, drug therapy choices indicated by compelling indications. Under some circumstances, these considerations are helpful in deciding on a particular antihypertensive agent when more than one antihypertensive class is recommended to treat a compelling indication. In some cases, an agent should be avoided because it may aggravate a concomitant disorder. In other cases, an antihypertensive can be used to treat hypertension, a compelling indication, and another concomitant condition. These are briefly summarized in Table 19–5.

Pulmonary Disease and Peripheral Arterial Disease[80]
β-blockers, especially non-selective agents, have been generally avoided for patients with hypertension and reactive airway disease (asthma or chronic obstructive pulmonary disease [COPD] with a reversible obstructive component) due to a fear of inducing bronchospasm. This precaution is more of a myth than a fact. Data suggests that cardioselective β-blockers can safely be used in patients with asthma or COPD.[81] Therefore cardioselective β-blockers should be used to treat a compelling indication (i.e., post-MI, coronary disease, or heart failure) for patients with reactive airway disease.

Peripheral arterial disease (PAD) is considered a noncoronary form of atherosclerotic vascular disease and is a coronary artery disease risk equivalent. ACE inhibitors may be ideal for patients with symptomatic lower extremity PAD who also have hypertension, as they have been shown to decrease CV events in these patients.[80] β-blockers can theoretically be problematic for patients with PAD due to possible decreased peripheral blood flow secondary to unopposed stimulation of α-receptors that results in vasoconstriction. If problematic, this can be mitigated by using a β-blocker that also has α-blocking properties (e.g., carvedilol). However, β-blockers are not contraindicated in PAD and have not been shown to adversely affect walking capacity.[80]

Metabolic Syndrome[12]
Metabolic syndrome is a cluster of multiple cardiometabolic risk factors. It has been most recently defined as the presence of 3 of the following 5 criteria: abdominal obesity (based on waist circumference measurements), elevated triglycerides, low HDL cholesterol, elevated BP (≥130/≥85 mm Hg or receiving drug treatment for high BP), and elevated fasting blood glucose.[12]

Despite the debate regarding whether or not metabolic syndrome is a true "disease" or rather simply a cluster of risk factors, it is widely accepted that patients with metabolic syndrome have increased risk of developing CV disease and/or type 2 diabetes. Using an ACE inhibitor or ARB is associated with the lowest rate of developing new onset diabetes in patients with hypertension.[82] However, studies specifically evaluating the most effective antihypertensive regimen for patients with metabolic syndrome have not been done. In addition, an ALLHAT subgroup analysis of patients with impaired fasting glucose showed that CV events were reduced more with chlorthalidone compared to lisinopril.[39] Thus, thiazide-type diuretics can be used first line for patients with metabolic syndrome, similar to ACE inhibitors, ARBs, or CCBs, but treated patients will have a higher risk of developing elevated fasting glucose.

Erectile Dysfunction[83]
Most antihypertensive agents have been associated with erectile dysfunction in men. However, it is not clear if erectile dysfunction associated with antihypertensive treatment is solely a result of drug therapy or rather a symptom of underlying CV disease. β-blockers have traditionally been labeled as agents that significantly cause sexual dysfunction, and many practitioners have avoided prescribing them as a result. However, data supporting this notion are limited. A systematic review of 15 studies involving 35,000 patients assessing β-blocker use for MI, heart failure, and hypertension found only a very slight increased risk for erectile dysfunction.[84] In addition, prospective long-term data from the Treatment of Mild Hypertension Study (TOMHS) and the Veterans Administration Cooperative trial show no difference in the incidence of erectile dysfunction between diuretics and β-blockers versus ACE inhibitors and CCBs.[85,86] Centrally acting agents are associated with higher rates of sexual dysfunction and should be avoided in men with erectile dysfunction.

Hypertensive men frequently have atherosclerotic vascular disease, which frequently results in erectile dysfunction. Therefore, erectile dysfunction is associated with chronic arterial changes resulting from elevated BP, and lack of control may increase the risk of erectile dysfunction. These changes are even more pronounced in hypertensive men with diabetes.

Individual Antihypertensive Agents[1,6]

Diuretics[87] There are four subclasses of diuretics that are used in the treatment of hypertension: thiazide-type diuretics, loops, potassium-sparing agents, and aldosterone antagonists (see Table 19–5). Thiazide-type diuretics are the preferred type of diuretic for most patients with hypertension.[1,2] The best available evidence justifying this recommendation is from ALLHAT.[31] Moreover, when combination therapy is needed in hypertension to control BP, a thiazide-type diuretic as the second agent is very effective in lowering BP.[1,88]

Loops are more potent agents for inducing a diuresis, but they are not ideal antihypertensive agents unless relief of edema is also needed. In general, loops are often preferred over a thiazide-type diuretic for hypertension in patients with chronic kidney disease when estimated GFR is less than 30 mL/min/1.73 m[2].[87]

Are loop diuretics always preferred over thiazide-type diuretics in chronic kidney disease?

Thiazide-type diuretics have been traditionally viewed as less effective compared with loop diuretics for patients with severe chronic kidney disease. Some clinicians routinely replace thiazide-type diuretics with a loop diuretic for patients that have estimated creatinine clearances below 30 mL/min. However, limited data demonstrate that hydrochlorothiazide is equally effective for BP lowering when compared with furosemide for patients with severe renal failure and hypertension.[89]

Potassium-sparing diuretics are very weak antihypertensive agents when used alone but provide minimal additive effect when used in combination with a thiazide or loop diuretic. Their primary use in combination with another diuretic is to counteract the potassium-wasting properties of the other diuretic agents. Aldosterone antagonists (spironolactone and eplerenone) may be technically considered potassium-sparing agents but are more potent as antihypertensives. However, they are viewed by the JNC7 as an independent class due to evidence supporting compelling indications.

The exact hypotensive mechanism of action of diuretics is not known, but has been well hypothesized. The drop in BP seen when diuretics are first started is caused by an initial diuresis. Diuresis causes reductions in plasma and stroke volume, which decreases CO and BP. This initial drop in CO causes a compensatory increase in peripheral vascular resistance. With chronic diuretic therapy, extracellular fluid and plasma volume return to near pretreatment values. However, peripheral vascular resistance decreases to values that are lower than the pretreatment baseline. This reduction in peripheral vascular resistance is responsible for chronic antihypertensive effects.

Thiazide-type diuretics have additional actions that may further explain their antihypertensive effects. Thiazide-type diuretics mobilize sodium and water from arteriolar walls. This effect would lessen the amount of physical encroachment on the lumen of the vessel created by excessive accumulation of intracellular fluid. As the diameter of the lumen relaxes and increases, there is less resistance to the flow of blood and peripheral vascular resistance further drops. High dietary sodium intake can blunt this effect and a low salt intake can enhance this effect. Thiazide-type diuretics are also postulated to cause direct relaxation of vascular smooth muscle.

Diuretics should ideally be dosed in the morning if given once daily and in the morning and late afternoon when dosed twice daily to minimize risk of nocturnal diuresis. However, with chronic use, thiazide-type diuretics, potassium sparing diuretics, and aldosterone antagonists rarely cause a pronounced diuresis.

The major pharmacokinetic differences between the various thiazide-type diuretics are serum half-life and duration of diuretic effect. The clinical relevance of these differences is unknown because the serum half-life of most antihypertensive agents does not correlate with the hypotensive duration of action. Moreover, diuretics lower BP primarily through extrarenal mechanisms. Hydrochlorothiazide and particularly chlorthalidone are the two most frequently used thiazide diuretics in landmark clinical trials that have demonstrated reduced morbidity and mortality. These agents are not equipotent on a milligram-per-milligram basis; chlorthalidone is 1.5 to 2.0 times more potent than hydrochlorothiazide.[87,90] This has been attributed to a longer half-life (45 to 60 hours vs 8 to 15 hours) and longer duration of effect (48 to 72 hours vs 16 to 24 hours) with chlorthalidone.

Diuretics are very effective in lowering BP when used in combination with most other antihypertensives.[88] This additive response is explained by two independent pharmacodynamic effects. First, when two drugs cause the same overall pharmacologic effect (BP lowering) through different mechanisms of action, their combination usually results in an additive or synergistic effect. This is especially relevant when a β-blocker or ACE inhibitor is indicated in an African-American, but does not elicit sufficient antihypertensive effect. Adding a diuretic in this situation can often significantly lower BP. Second, a compensatory increase in sodium and fluid retention may be seen with antihypertensive agents. This problem is counteracted with the concurrent use of a diuretic.

The side effects of thiazide-type diuretics include hypokalemia, hypomagnesemia, hypercalcemia, hyperuricemia, hyperglycemia, dyslipidemia, and sexual dysfunction. Many of these side effects were identified when high-doses of thiazides were used in the past (e.g., hydrochlorothiazide 100 mg/day). Current guidelines recommend limiting the dose of hydrochlorothiazide or chlorthalidone to 12.5 to 25 mg/day, which markedly reduces the risk for most metabolic side effects. Loop diuretics may cause the same side effects, although the effect on serum lipids and glucose is not as significant, hypokalemia is more pronounced and hypocalcemia may occur.

Hypokalemia and hypomagnesemia may cause muscle fatigue or cramps. However, serious cardiac arrhythmias can occur in patients with severe hypokalemia and hypomagnesemia. Patients at greatest risk for this are patients with LVH, coronary disease, post-MI, a history of arrhythmia, or those concurrently receiving digoxin. Low-dose therapy (i.e., 25 mg hydrochlorothiazide or 12.5 mg chlorthalidone daily) causes small electrolyte disturbances. Efforts should be made to keep potassium in the therapeutic range by careful monitoring.

Diuretic-induced hyperuricemia can precipitate gout. This side effect may be especially problematic for patients with a previous history of gout and is more common with thiazide-type diuretics. However, acute gout is unlikely in patients with no previous history of gout. If gout does occur in a patient who requires diuretic therapy, allopurinol can be given to prevent gout and will not compromise the antihypertensive effects of the diuretic. High doses of thiazide-type and loop diuretics may increase fasting glucose and serum cholesterol values. These effects, however, usually are transient and often inconsequential.[91]

Potassium-sparing diuretics can cause hyperkalemia, especially in patients with chronic kidney disease or diabetes and in patients receiving concurrent treatment with an ACE inhibitor, ARB, direct renin inhibitor, or potassium supplements. Hyperkalemia is especially problematic for the newest aldosterone antagonist eplerenone. This agent is a very selective aldosterone antagonist, and its propensity to cause hyperkalemia is greater than with the other potassium sparing agents and even spironolactone. Due to this increased risk of hyperkalemia, eplerenone is contraindicated for patients with impaired kidney function or type 2 diabetes with proteinuria (see Table 19–5). While spironolactone may cause gynecomastia in up to 10% of patients, this occurs rarely with eplerenone.

Diuretics can be used safely with most other agents. However, concurrent administration with lithium may result in increased lithium serum concentrations and can predispose patients to lithium toxicity.

Minimizing Hyperglycemia with Thiazide-type Diuretic Therapy

Patients treated with thiazide-type diuretic therapy have a higher incidence of developing type 2 diabetes than patients treated with other antihypertensive therapies.[82] There is a plausible theory that insulin utilization is linked to intracellular potassium. This increase in risk has been associated with potassium concentrations and hypokalemia.[92] Patients that are treated with a thiazide-type diuretic and have the lowest serum potassium concentrations have the largest increases in glucose concentrations. The potassium cut point at which this relationship appears is when serum potassium is less than 4.0 mEq/L.

Despite the increased risk of hyperglycemia, and possibly development of type 2 diabetes, thiazide-type diuretics must still be used as a first-line drug therapy option for many patients with hypertension. However, clinicians should be proactive in trying to minimize potential hyperglycemia. Three strategies might be considered as modalities to minimize thiazide induced hyperglycemia: (1) use the lowest effective dose (e.g., hydrochlorothiazide 12.5 or 25 mg daily), (2) maintain serum potassium values between 4.0 and 5.0 mEq/L during treatment with a thiazide type diuretic, and (3) lifestyle modification.[93] While these strategies are not definitively proven to reduce risk of hyperglycemia and progression to type 2 diabetes, they are considered reasonable in the overall care of patients with hypertension. Moreover, other than potassium supplementation, the other strategies that would maintain serum potassium between 4.0 and 5.0 mEq/L could be accomplished by adding an ACE inhibitor, ARB, or potassium sparing drug. These additional drug therapies are easily available in fixed dose combination products and may aid in achieving BP goals for patients with hypertension.

ACE Inhibitors ACE inhibitors are a first-line therapy option in most patients with hypertension.[1,2] The ALLHAT demonstrated less heart failure and stroke with chlorthalidone versus lisinopril.[31] However, another outcome study has demonstrated similar, if not better outcomes with ACE inhibitors versus hydrochlorothiazide.[33] It is possible that the different thiazide-type diuretics have different abilities to reduce hypertension associated target organ damage. Nonetheless, most clinicians will agree that if ACE inhibitors are not the first agent used in most patients with hypertension, they should be the second agent used.

ACE facilitates production of angiotensin II that has a major role in arterial BP regulation as depicted in Figure 19–1. ACE is distributed in many tissues and is present in several different cell types, but its principal location is in endothelial cells. Therefore, the major site for angiotensin II production is in the blood vessels, not the kidney. ACE inhibitors block the ACE, thus inhibiting conversion of angiotensin I to angiotensin II. Angiotensin II is a potent vasoconstrictor that stimulates aldosterone secretion, causing an increase in sodium and water reabsorption with accompanying potassium loss. By blocking the ACE, vasodilatation and a decrease in aldosterone occur.

ACE inhibitors also block degradation of bradykinin and stimulate the synthesis of other vasodilating substances (prostaglandin E$_2$ and prostacyclin). The observation that ACE inhibitors lower BP in patients with normal plasma renin activity suggests that bradykinin and perhaps tissue production of ACE are important in hypertension. Increased bradykinin enhances the BP lowering effects of ACE inhibitors, but also is responsible for the side effect of dry cough. ACE inhibitors effectively prevent or regress LVH by reducing direct stimulation by angiotensin II on myocardial cells.

There are many evidence-based uses for ACE inhibitors (see Fig. 19–3). ACE inhibitors reduce CV morbidity and mortality in patients with left ventricular dysfunction,[48] and decrease progression of chronic kidney disease.[64] They should be first-line as disease modifying therapy in all of these patients unless absolutely contraindicated. ACE inhibitors (or ARBs in certain patients), are first-line for patients with diabetes and hypertension because of demonstrated CV disease and kidney benefits. A regimen including an ACE inhibitor with a thiazide-type diuretic is considered first-line in recurrent stroke prevention base on proven benefits from the PROGRESS trial showing reduced risk of secondary stroke.[32] In combination with β-blocker therapy, evidence shows that ACE inhibitors further reduce CV risk in coronary disease and in patients post-MI.[57,59,61,62] These benefits of ACE inhibitors occur in patients with atherosclerotic vascular disease even in the absence of left ventricular dysfunction and have the potential to reduce the development of new-onset type 2 diabetes.[94]

Most ACE inhibitors can be dosed once daily in hypertension (Table 19–5). In some patients, especially when higher doses are used, twice daily dosing is needed to maintain 24-hour effects with enalapril, benazepril, moexipril, quinapril and ramipril.

ACE inhibitors are well tolerated,[95] but are not absent of side effects. ACE inhibitors decrease aldosterone and can increase potassium serum concentrations. While this increase is usually small, hyperkalemia is possible. Patients with chronic kidney disease or those on concomitant potassium supplements, potassium-sparing diuretics, ARBs, or a direct renin inhibitor are at risk for hyperkalemia. Judicious monitoring of serum potassium and creatinine values within 4 weeks of starting or increasing the dose of an ACE inhibitor can often identify these abnormalities early before they evolve into serious adverse events.

The most worrisome adverse effect of ACE inhibitor is acute kidney failure. This serious adverse effect is rare, occurring in less than 1% of patients. Preexisting kidney disease increases the risk of this side effect. Bilateral renal artery stenosis or unilateral stenosis of a solitary functioning kidney render patients dependent on the vasoconstrictive effect of angiotensin II on the efferent arteriole of the kidney, thus explaining why these patients are particularly susceptible to acute kidney failure from ACE inhibitors. Slow titration of the ACE inhibitor dose and judicious kidney function monitoring can minimize risk and allow for early detection of those with renal artery stenosis.

It is important to note that GFR does decrease somewhat in patients when started on ACE inhibitors or ARBs.[64] This is attributed to the inhibition of angiotensin II vasoconstriction on the efferent arteriole. This decrease in GFR often increases serum creatinine, and small increases should be anticipated when monitoring patients on ACE inhibitors. Modest elevations of either ≤35% (for baseline creatinine values less than or equal to 3 mg/dL) or absolute increases less than 1 mg/dL do not warrant changes.[64] If larger increases occur, ACE inhibitor therapy should be stopped or the dose reduced.

Angioedema is a serious potential complication of ACE inhibitor therapy. It occurs in less than 1% of the population, and it is more likely in African-Americans and smokers. Symptoms include lip and tongue swelling and possibly difficulty breathing. Drug withdrawal is appropriate for treating patients with angioedema. However, angioedema associated with laryngeal edema and/or pulmonary symptoms occasionally occurs and requires additional treatment with epinephrine, corticosteroids, antihistamines, and/or emergent intubations to support respiration. A history of angioedema, even if not from an ACE inhibitor, precludes use of another ACE inhibitor (it is a contraindication). Cross-reactivity between ACE inhibitors and ARBs does not appear to be a significant concern. The Telmisartan randomized assessment study in ACE intolerant subjects with cardiovascular disease (TRANSCEND) trial enrolled 75 patients with a history of ACE-inhibitor–induced angioedema, and randomized these patients to either placebo or ARB therapy.[96] There were no cases of repeat angioedema among these patients. These data suggest the cross-reactivity is very low. Hence, an ARB can be used in a patient with a history of ACE-inhibitor–induced angioedema when it is needed. However, clinicians should monitor for repeat occurrences, since idiopathic angioedema may still occur.

A persistent dry cough develops in up to 20% of patients treated with an ACE inhibitor. It is pharmacologically explained by the inhibition of bradykinin breakdown. This cough does not cause respiratory illness but is annoying to patients and can compromise adherence. It should be clearly differentiated from a wet cough due to pulmonary edema, which may be a sign of uncontrolled heart failure versus an ACE-inhibitor–induced cough.

ACE inhibitors, as well as ARBs, are absolutely contraindicated in pregnancy.[1,78] Female patients of child-bearing age should be counseled regarding effective forms of birth control as ACE inhibitors have been associated with major congenital malformations when exposed in the first trimester and fetopathy (group of conditions that includes renal failure, renal dysplasia, hypotension, oligohydramnios, pulmonary hypotension, hypocalvaria, and death) has occurred when exposed in the second and third trimester.[78] Similar to diuretics, ACE inhibitors can increase lithium serum concentrations in patients on lithium therapy. Concurrent use of an ACE with a potassium sparing diuretic (including aldosterone antagonists), potassium supplements, an ARB, or a direct renin inhibitor may result in hyperkalemia.

Starting doses of ACE inhibitors should be low, with even lower doses for patients at risk for orthostatic hypotension or severe renal dysfunction (e.g., elderly, chronic kidney disease). Acute hypotension may occur at the onset of ACE inhibitor therapy. Patients who are sodium or volume depleted, in heart failure exacerbation, very elderly, or on concurrent vasodilators or diuretics are at high risk for this effect. It is important to start with half the normal dose of an ACE inhibitor for all patients with these risk factors and to use slow dose titration.

ARBs Angiotensin II is generated by two enzymatic pathways: the RAAS, which involves ACE, and an alternative pathway that uses other enzymes such as chymase (aka "tissue ACE"). ACE inhibitors inhibit only the effects of angiotensin II produced through the RAAS, whereas ARBs inhibit angiotensin II from all pathways. It is unclear how these differences affect tissue concentrations of ACE. ACE inhibitors only partially block the effects of angiotensin II, though the clinical significance of this is not known.

ARBs directly block the angiotensin II type 1 (AT_1) receptor that mediates the known effects of angiotensin II in humans: vasoconstriction, aldosterone release, sympathetic activation, antidiuretic hormone release, and constriction of the efferent arterioles of the glomerulus. They do not block the angiotensin II type 2 (AT_2) receptor. Therefore, beneficial effects of AT_2 receptor stimulation (vasodilatation, tissue repair, and inhibition of cell growth) remain intact when ARBs are used. Unlike ACE inhibitors, ARBs do not block the breakdown of bradykinin. Therefore, some of the beneficial effects of bradykinin, such as vasodilation, regression of myocyte hypertrophy and fibrosis, and increased levels of tissue plasminogen activator, are not present with ARB therapy.

ARB therapy has been directly compared to ACE inhibitor therapy in the management of hypertension.[97] The Ongoing Telmisartan Alone and in Combination with Ramipril Global End point Trial (ON-TARGET) was a double-blind trial that randomized 25,620 patients with hypertension to either ACE-inhibitor–based therapy, ARB-based therapy, or the combination of an ACE inhibitor with an ARB. The primary end point was a composite end point of CV death or hospitalization for heart failure. After a median follow-up of 56 months, there was no difference in the primary end point between any of the three treatment groups. Therefore, these data establish that the CV event lowering benefits of ARB therapy are similar to ACE inhibitor therapy in hypertension. Moreover, the combination of an ACE inhibitor with an ARB had no additional CV event lowering but was associated with a higher risk of side effects (renal dysfunction, hypotension). Therefore, there is no reason to use an ACE inhibitor with an ARB for the management of hypertension.

For patients with certain compelling indications, ARBs have outcome data showing long-term reductions in progression of target-organ damage. For patients with type 2 diabetes and nephropathy,

progression of nephropathy has been shown to be significantly reduced with ARB therapy.[21] Some benefits appear to be independent of BP lowering, suggesting that the pharmacologic effects of ARBs on the efferent arteriole may result in attenuated progression of kidney disease. For patients with left ventricular dysfunction, the CHARM studies showed that ARB therapy reduces risk of hospitalization for heart failure when added to a stable regimen of a diuretic, ACE inhibitor, and β-blocker or as an alternative therapy in ACE intolerant patients.[55,56] Importantly, the Evaluation of Losartan in the Elderly (ELITE) studies have shown that losartan is not superior to captopril in left ventricular dysfunction when compared head-to-head.[53,54]

ARBs have been compared head-to-head with CCBs. The MOSES demonstrated that eprosartan reduced the occurrence of recurrent stroke greater than nitrendipine in patients with a past medical history of cerebrovascular disease.[71] Using nitrendipine was a reasonable comparator because the Syst-Eur had already demonstrated that nitrendipine reduces the occurrence of CV events, particularly stroke, in older patients with isolated systolic hypertension compared to placebo.[11] These data support the common notion that ARBs may have cerebroprotective effects that may explain CV event reductions.[98] Another outcome study, the Valsartan Antihypertensive Long-term Use Evaluation (VALUE) trial, showed that valsartan-based therapy is equivalent to amlodipine-based therapy for the primary composite outcome of first CV event in patients with hypertension and additional CV risk factors.[34] However, occurrence of certain components of the primary end point (stroke and MI) and new onset type 2 diabetes was lower in the valsartan group. Although patients treated with amlodipine had slightly lower mean BP values than valsartan treated patients, there was no difference in the primary end point.

The addition of low doses of a thiazide-type diuretic to an ARB or a CCB to an ARB significantly increases antihypertensive efficacy. Similar to ACE inhibitors, most ARBs have long enough half-lives to allow for once daily dosing. However, candesartan, eprosartan, losartan, and valsartan have the shortest half-lives and may require twice daily dosing for sustained BP lowering.

ARBs have the lowest incidence of side effects compared to other antihypertensive agents.[95] Because they do not affect bradykinin, they do not illicit a dry cough like ACE inhibitors. While these drugs have been referred to as "ACE inhibitors without the cough," pharmacologic differences highlight that they could have very different effects on vascular smooth muscle and myocardial tissue that can correlate to different effects on target-organ damage and CV risk reduction when compared with ACE inhibitors. It is possible that their effects may be superior to ACE inhibitors for patients with type 2 diabetic nephropathy but may be inferior to ACE inhibitors in patients with more advanced heart disease (e.g., heart failure, post-MI). Regardless, their role for patients with type 2 diabetic nephropathy is well established, and they also are very reasonable alternatives for patients requiring an ACE inhibitor but who experience an intolerable cough.

Like ACE inhibitors, ARBs may cause renal insufficiency, hyperkalemia, and orthostatic hypotension. The same precautions that apply to ACE inhibitors for patients with suspected bilateral renal artery stenosis, those on drugs that can raise potassium and those on drugs that increase risk of hypotension apply to ARBs. As discussed in the section "ACE Inhibitors, ARBs, and CCBs as First-Line Agents", patients with a history of ACE inhibitor angioedema can be treated with an ARB when needed.[96] ARBs should not be used in pregnancy.[78]

CCBs CCBs, both dihydropyridine CCBs and non-dihydropyridine CCBs, are first-line therapy options and are very effective antihypertensive agents.[1,2] They also have compelling indications in coronary artery disease and in diabetes. However, with these compelling indications, they are in addition to, or in instead of, other first-line antihypertensive drug classes.

Contraction of cardiac and smooth muscle cells requires an increase in free intracellular calcium concentrations from the extracellular fluid. When cardiac or vascular smooth muscle is stimulated, voltage-sensitive channels in the cell membrane are opened, allowing calcium to enter the cells. The influx of extracellular calcium into the cell releases stored calcium from the sarcoplasmic reticulum. As intracellular free calcium concentration increases, it binds to a protein, calmodulin, which then activates myosin kinase enabling myosin to interact with actin to induce contraction. CCBs work by inhibiting influx of calcium across the cell membrane. There are two types of voltage-gated calcium channels: a high-voltage channel (L-type) and a low-voltage channel (T-type). Currently available CCBs only block the L-type channel, which leads to coronary and peripheral vasodilatation.

The two subclasses of CCBs, dihydropyridines and non-dihydropyridines (see Table 19–5), are pharmacologically very different from each other. Antihypertensive effectiveness is similar with both subclasses, but they differ somewhat in other pharmacodynamic effects. Non-dihydropyridines (verapamil and diltiazem) decrease heart rate and slow atrioventricular nodal conduction. Similar to β-blockers these drugs may also treat supraventricular tachyarrhythmias (e.g., atrial fibrillation). Verapamil produces negative inotropic and chronotropic effects that are responsible for its propensity to precipitate or cause systolic heart failure in high risk patients. Diltiazem also has these effects but to a lesser extent than verapamil. All CCBs (except amlodipine and felodipine) have negative inotropic effects. Dihydropyridines may cause a baroreceptor-mediated reflex tachycardia because of their potent peripheral vasodilating effects. This effect appears to be more pronounced with the first-generation dihydropyridines (e.g., nifedipine) and is significantly diminished with the newer agents (e.g., amlodipine) and when given in sustained release dosage forms. Dihydropyridines do not alter conduction through the atrioventricular node and thus are not effective agents in supraventricular tachyarrhythmias.

Dihydropyridine CCBs

CCBs, both dihydropyridines and non-dihydropyridines, are as effective at lowering CV events as other first-line agents in most patients with hypertension. The dihydropyridine CCBs have been extensively studied. In ALLHAT there was no difference in the primary outcome between chlorthalidone and amlodipine, and only the secondary outcome of heart failure was higher with amlodipine.[31] A subgroup analysis of ALLHAT directly compared amlodipine to lisinopril and demonstrated that there was no difference in the primary outcome.[99] However, amlodipine was superior to lisinopril for BP control in blacks, and for stroke reduction in blacks and in women. There was a lower risk of heart failure in the lisinopril group. As discussed previously, the VALUE study also showed no difference between valsartan and amlodipine in the primary outcome of first CV event in high-risk patients.[34]

Dihydropyridine CCBs are very effective in older patients with isolated systolic hypertension. The Syst-Eur, a placebo-controlled trial, demonstrated that a long-acting dihydropyridine CCB reduced the risk of CV events markedly in isolated systolic hypertension.[11] A long-acting dihydropyridine CCB should be strongly considered as preferred add-on therapy when a thiazide-type diuretic is not controlling BP in a patient with isolated systolic hypertension and no other compelling indications.

Among dihydropyridines, short-acting nifedipine may rarely cause an increase in the frequency, intensity, and duration of angina in association with acute hypotension. This effect is most likely due to a reflex sympathetic stimulation and is likely obviated by using sustained-release formulations of nifedipine. For this reason, all other dihydropyridines have an intrinsically long half-life or are sustained-release formulations. Immediate-release nifedipine has been associated with an increased incidence of adverse CV effects, is not approved for treatment of hypertension, and should not be used to treat hypertension. Other side effects with dihydropyridines include dizziness, flushing, headache, gingival hyperplasia, peripheral edema, mood changes, and various gastrointestinal complaints. Side effects due to vasodilatation such as dizziness, flushing, headache, and peripheral edema occur more frequently with all dihydropyridines than with the non-dihydropyridines (i.e., verapamil, diltiazem) because they are less potent vasodilators.

Non-Dihydropyridine CCBs

Diltiazem and verapamil can cause cardiac conduction abnormalities such as bradycardia or atrioventricular block. These problems occur mostly with high doses or when used for patients with preexisting abnormalities in the cardiac conduction system. Heart failure has been reported in otherwise healthy patients due to negative inotropic effects. Both drugs can cause anorexia, nausea, peripheral edema, and hypotension. Verapamil causes constipation in about 7% of patients. This side effect also occurs with diltiazem, but to a lesser extent.

Verapamil and to a lesser extent diltiazem, can cause drug interactions due to their ability to inhibit the cytochrome P450 3A4 isoenzyme system. This inhibition can increase serum concentrations of other drugs that are metabolized by this isoenzyme system (e.g., cyclosporine, digoxin, lovastatin, simvastatin, tacrolimus, theophylline). Verapamil and diltiazem should be given very cautiously with a β-blocker because there is an increased risk of heart block with these combinations. When a CCB is needed in combination with a β-blocker for BP lowering, a dihydropyridine should be selected because it will not increase risk of heart block. The hepatic metabolism of CCBs, especially felodipine, nicardipine, nifedipine, and nisoldipine may be inhibited by ingesting large quantities of grapefruit juice (greater than or equal to 1 qt daily).

Many different formulations of verapamil and diltiazem are currently available (see Table 19–5). Although certain sustained release verapamil and diltiazem products contain the same active drug (e.g., Calan SR and Verelan), they are usually not AB rated by the FDA as interchangeable on a milligram-per-milligram basis due to different biopharmaceutical release mechanisms. However, the clinical significance of these differences is likely negligible.

Two sustained-release verapamil products (Covera HS and Verelan PM) and one diltiazem product (Cardizem LA) are chronotherapeutically designed to target the circadian BP rhythm. These agents are primarily dosed in the evening (with the exception of Cardizem LA, which may be dosed in the morning or evening) so that drug is released during the early morning hours when BP first starts to increase. The rationale behind chronotherapy in hypertension is that blunting the early morning BP surge may result in greater reductions in CV events than conventional dosing of regular antihypertensive products in the morning. However, evidence from the Controlled ONset Verapamil Investigation of Cardiovascular End-points (CONVINCE) trial showed that chronotherapeutic verapamil was similar, but not better than, a thiazide-type diuretic–β-blocker-based regimen with respect to CV events.[29]

β-Blockers

β-blockers have been used in several large outcome trials in hypertension. However, in most of these trials, a thiazide-type diuretic was the primary agent with a β-blocker added on for additional BP lowering. Moreover, as previously discussed, for patients with hypertension but without compelling indications, other primary agents (thiazide-type diuretics, ACE inhibitors, ARBs, and CCBs) should be used as the initial first-line agent before β-blockers. While this may be surprising to experienced clinicians, this recommendation is consistent with the 2007 AHA guidelines and the 2006 United Kingdom's National Institute for Health and the Clinical Excellence guidelines.[2,43] It is based on meta-analyses that suggest β-blocker-based therapy may not reduce CV events as well as these other agents when used as the initial drug to treat patients with hypertension and without a compelling indication for a β-blocker.[44–47]

β-blockers are only considered appropriate first-line agents to treat specific compelling indications (post-MI, coronary artery disease). β-blockers are also evidenced-based as additional therapy for other compelling indications (left ventricular dysfunction and diabetes). Numerous trials have shown reduced CV risk when β-blockers are used following an MI, during an acute coronary syndrome, or in chronic stable angina. Although once contraindicated in heart failure, studies have shown that bisoprolol, carvedilol, and metoprolol succinate reduce mortality in patients with left ventricular dysfunction who are treated with a diuretic and ACE inhibitor.

Several mechanisms of action have been proposed for β-blockers, but none of them alone has been shown to be consistently associated with a reduction in arterial BP. β-blockers have negative chronotropic and inotropic cardiac effects that reduce CO, which explains some of the antihypertensive effect. However, CO falls equally for patients treated with β-blockers regardless of BP lowering. Additionally, β-blockers with ISA do not reduce CO, yet they lower BP and decrease peripheral resistance.

β-Adrenoceptors are also located on the surface membranes of juxtaglomerular cells, and β-blockers inhibit these receptors and thus the release of renin. However, there is a weak association between plasma renin and antihypertensive efficacy of β-blocker therapy. Some patients with low plasma renin concentrations do respond to β-blockers. Therefore, additional mechanisms must also account for the antihypertensive effect of β-blockers. However, the ability of β-blockers to reduce plasma renin and thus angiotensin II concentrations may play a major role in their ability to reduce CV risk.

There are important pharmacodynamic and pharmacokinetic differences among β-blockers, but all agents provide a similar degree of BP lowering. There are three pharmacodynamic properties of the β-blockers that differentiate this class: cardioselectivity, ISA, and membrane-stabilizing effects. β-blockers that possess a greater affinity for β_1-receptors than β_2-receptors are *cardioselective*.

β_1-Adrenoceptors and β_2-adrenoceptors are distributed throughout the body, but they concentrate differently in certain organs and tissues. There is a preponderance of β_1-receptors in the heart and kidney, and a preponderance of β_2-receptors in the lungs, liver, pancreas, and arteriolar smooth muscle. β_1-Receptor stimulation increases heart rate, contractility, and renin release. β_2-Receptor stimulation results in bronchodilation and vasodilation. Cardioselective β-blockers are not likely to provoke bronchospasm and vasoconstriction. Insulin secretion and glycogenolysis are mediated by β_2-receptors. Blocking β_2-receptors may reduce these processes and cause hyperglycemia or blunt recovery from hypoglycemia.

Cardioselective β-blockers (e.g., atenolol, metoprolol, nebivolol) have clinically significant advantages over nonselective β-blockers (e.g., propranolol, nadolol), and are preferred when using a β-blocker to treat hypertension. Cardioselective agents are safer than nonselective agents for patients with asthma or diabetes that have a compelling indication for a β-blocker. However, cardioselectivity is a dose-dependent phenomenon; at higher doses, cardioselective agents lose their relative selectivity for β_1-receptors and block β_2-receptors as effectively as they block β_1-receptors. The dose at which cardioselectivity is lost varies from patient to patient.

Some β-blockers (e.g., acebutolol, pindolol) have ISA and act as partial β-receptor agonists. When they bind to the β-receptor, they stimulate it, but far less than a pure β-agonist. If sympathetic tone is low, as it is during resting states, β-receptors are partially stimulated by ISA β-blockers. Therefore, resting heart rate, CO, and peripheral

blood flow are not reduced when these type of β-blockers are used. Theoretically, ISA agents would appear to have advantages over β-blockers in certain patients with heart failure or sinus bradycardia. Unfortunately, they do not appear to reduce CV events as well as other β-blockers. In fact, they may increase risk post-MI or in those with coronary artery disease. Thus, agents with ISA are rarely needed.

All β-blockers exert a *membrane-stabilizing action* on cardiac cells when large doses are given. This activity is needed when β-blockers are used as an antiarrhythmic agent.

Pharmacokinetic differences among β-blockers relate to first-pass metabolism, route of elimination, degree of being lipophilic, and serum half-lives. Propranolol and metoprolol undergo extensive first-pass metabolism, so the dose needed to attain β-blockade with either drug varies from patient to patient. Atenolol and nadolol are renally excreted. The dose of these agents may need to be reduced for patients with moderate to severe chronic kidney disease.

β-blockers, especially those with high lipophilic properties, penetrate the central nervous system and may cause other effects. Propranolol is the most lipophilic drug and atenolol is the least lipophilic. Therefore, higher brain concentrations of propranolol compared to atenolol are seen after equivalent doses are given. It is thought that higher lipophilicity is associated with more central nervous system side effects (dizziness, drowsiness). However, the lipophilic properties can provide better effects for non-CV conditions such as migraine headache prevention, essential tremor, and thyrotoxicosis. BP lowering is equal among β-blockers regardless of lipophilicity.

Most side effects of β-blockers are an extension of their ability to antagonize β-adrenoceptors. β-blockade in the myocardium can be associated with bradycardia, atrioventricular conduction abnormalities (e.g. second- or third-degree heart block), and the development of acute heart failure. The decreases in heart rate may actually benefit certain patients with atrial arrhythmias (atrial fibrillation, atrial flutter) and hypertension by both providing rate control and BP lowering. β-blockers usually only produce heart failure if they are used in high initial doses for patients with preexisting left ventricular dysfunction or if started in these patients during an acute heart failure exacerbation. Blocking β_2-receptors in arteriolar smooth muscle may cause cold extremities and may aggravate intermittent claudication or Raynaud phenomenon as a result of decreased peripheral blood flow. In addition, there is an increase of sympathetic tone during periods of hypoglycemia in patients with diabetes that may result in a significant increase in BP because of unopposed α-receptor-mediated vasoconstriction.

Abrupt cessation of β-blocker therapy can produce unstable angina, MI, or even death in patients with coronary disease. Abrupt cessation may also lead to rebound hypertension (a sudden increase in BP to or above pretreatment values). To avoid this, β-blockers should always be tapered gradually over 1 to 2 weeks before eventually discontinuing the drug. This acute withdrawal syndrome is believed to be secondary to progression of underlying coronary disease, hypersensitivity of β-adrenergic receptors due to up regulation, and increased physical activity after withdrawal of a drug that decreases myocardial oxygen requirements. For patients without coronary disease, abrupt discontinuation may present as tachycardia, sweating, and generalized malaise in addition to increased BP.

Like diuretics, β-blockers have been shown to increase serum cholesterol and glucose values, but these effects are transient and of little clinical significance. For patients with diabetes, the reduction in CV events was as great with β-blockers as with an ACE inhibitor in the United Kingdom Prospective Diabetes Study (UKPDS)[100] and far superior to placebo in the SHEP trial.[8] In the Glycemic Effects in Diabetes Mellitus: Carvedilol-Metoprolol Comparison in Hypertensives (GEMINI) trial, patients with diabetes and hypertension who were randomized to metoprolol had an increase in hemoglobin A1C values, while patients randomized to carvedilol did not.[101] This suggests that mixed α and β-blocking effects of carvedilol may be preferential to metoprolol for patients with uncontrolled diabetes. However, differences in hemoglobin A1C values were too small to make this application clinically relevant in all patients with diabetes that need treatment with a β-blocker. Nebivolol is considered a third-generation β-blocker. Similar to carvedilol and labetalol, this β-blocker results in vasodilatation. However, carvedilol and labetalol cause vasodilatation because of their ability to block α-receptors, while nebivolol causes vasodilatation through release of nitric oxide. The long-term clinical benefits of the nitric oxide effects seen with nebivolol are currently unknown, but this might explain a lower risk of β-blocker associated fatigue, erectile dysfunction, and metabolic side effects (e.g., hyperglycemia) with this agent.

⑬ Alternative Agents The primary role of an alternative antihypertensive agent is to provide additional BP lowering in patients that are already treated with antihypertensive agents from a drug class proven to reduce hypertension associated CV events (diuretics, ACE inhibitors, ARBs, CCBs, and/or β-blockers).

α_1-Blockers[36] Prazosin, terazosin, and doxazosin are selective α_1-receptor blockers. They work in the peripheral vasculature and inhibit the uptake of catecholamines in smooth muscle cells resulting in vasodilatation and BP lowering.

Doxazosin was one of the original treatment arms of the ALLHAT. However, it was stopped prematurely when statistically more secondary end points of stroke, heart failure, and CV events were seen with doxazosin compared with chlorthalidone.[36] There were no differences in the primary end point of fatal coronary heart disease and nonfatal MI. These data suggest that thiazide-type diuretics are superior to α_1-blockers in preventing CV events in patients with hypertension. Therefore, α_1-blockers are alternative agents that should be used in combination with first-line antihypertensive agents.

α_1-Blockers can provide symptomatic benefits in men with benign prostatic hypertrophy. These agents block postsynaptic α_1-adrenergic receptors located on the prostate capsule, causing relaxation and decreased resistance to urinary outflow. However, when used to lower BP, they should only be in addition to other first-line antihypertensive agents.

A potentially severe side effect of α_1-blockers is a "first-dose" phenomenon that is characterized by transient dizziness or faintness, palpitations, and even syncope within 1 to 3 hours of the first dose. This adverse reaction can also happen after dose increases. These episodes are accompanied by orthostatic hypotension and can be obviated by taking the first dose and subsequent first increased doses at bedtime. Because orthostatic hypotension and dizziness may persist with chronic administration, these agents should be used very cautiously in elderly patients. Even though antihypertensive effects are achieved through a peripheral α_1-receptor antagonism, these agents cross the blood–brain barrier and may cause central nervous system side effects such as lassitude, vivid dreams, and depression. α_1-Blockers also may cause priapism. Sodium and water retention can occur with higher doses, and sometimes even with chronic administration of low doses. Therefore, these agents are most effective when given in combination with a diuretic to maintain antihypertensive efficacy and minimize potential edema.

Aliskiren[102,103] Aliskiren is the first oral agent within a new antihypertensive drug class that directly inhibits renin.[102] This drug blocks the RAAS at its point of activation, which results in reduced plasma renin activity and BP lowering. It has a 24-hour half-life, is primarily eliminated through biliary excretion unchanged, and provides 24-hour antihypertensive effects with once daily dosing.

The exact role of this drug class in the management of hypertension is unclear. Aliskiren is approved as monotherapy or in combination therapy. However, because of the lack of long-term studies evaluating CV event reduction and significant drug cost compared to older generic agents with outcome data; it should clearly be used as an alternative therapy for the treatment of hypertension. The Aliskiren in the Evaluation of Proteinuria in Diabetes (AVOID) trial demonstrated that the combination of aliskiren with losartan resulted in a reduction in proteinuria compared to losartan alone in patients with type 2 diabetes.[104] This may be a future role for this particular drug class after more clinical trials have been completed. Aliskiren is effective in lowering BP when used in combination with thiazide-type diuretics, ACE inhibitors, ARBs, or a CCB; however, its effectiveness in combination with maximum doses of ACE inhibitor, ARB, or other CCBs has not been adequately studied.

Many of the cautions and adverse effects seen with ACE inhibitors and ARBs apply to direct renin inhibitors (e.g., aliskiren). Aliskiren should never be used in pregnancy due to the known teratogenic effects of using other drugs that block the RAAS system. Angioedema has also been reported for patients treated with aliskiren. Increases in serum creatinine and serum potassium values have been observed. The mechanisms of these adverse effects are likely similar to those with ACE inhibitors and ARBs. It is reasonable to utilize similar monitoring strategies by measuring serum creatinine and serum potassium in patients treated with aliskiren. This is particularly important for patients treated with the combination of aliskiren and an ACE inhibitor or an ARB who are at higher risk for hyperkalemia (e.g., patients with diabetes and chronic kidney disease).

Central α_2-Agonists Clonidine, guanabenz, guanfacine, and methyldopa lower BP primarily by stimulating α_2-adrenergic receptors in the brain. This stimulation reduces sympathetic outflow from the vasomotor center in the brain and increases vagal tone. It is also believed that peripheral stimulation of presynaptic α_2-receptors may further reduce sympathetic tone. Reduced sympathetic activity together with enhanced parasympathetic activity can decrease heart rate, CO, TPR, plasma renin activity, and baroreceptor reflexes. Clonidine is often used in resistant hypertension, and methyldopa is a first-line agent for pregnancy-induced hypertension.

Chronic use of centrally acting α_2-agonists results in sodium and water retention, which is most prominent with methyldopa. Low doses of clonidine (and guanfacine or guanabenz) can be used to treat hypertension without the addition of a diuretic. However, methyldopa should be given in combination with a diuretic to avoid the blunting of antihypertensive effect that happens with prolonged use when used to treat chronic hypertension (not necessary in pregnancy induced hypertension). Sedation and dry mouth are common anticholinergic side effects that typically improve with chronic use of low doses, but they are more troublesome in the elderly. As with other centrally acting antihypertensives, depression can occur, especially with high doses. The incidence of orthostatic hypotension and dizziness is higher than with other antihypertensive agents, so they should be used very cautiously in the elderly. Lastly, clonidine has a relatively high incidence of anticholinergic side effects (sedation, dry mouth, constipation, urinary retention and blurred vision). Thus, it should generally be avoided for chronic antihypertensive therapy in the elderly.

Abrupt cessation of central α_2-agonists may lead to rebound hypertension. This effect is thought to be secondary to a compensatory increase in norepinephrine release after abrupt discontinuation. In addition, other effects such as nervousness, agitation, headache, and tremor can also occur, which may be exacerbated by concomitant β-blocker use, particularly with clonidine. Thus, if clonidine is to be discontinued it should be tapered. For patients who are receiving concomitant β-blocker therapy, the β-blocker should be gradually discontinued first several days before gradual discontinuation of clonidine.

Methyldopa can cause hepatitis or hemolytic anemia, although this is rare. Transient elevations in serum hepatic transaminases are occasionally seen with methyldopa therapy but are clinically irrelevant unless they are greater than 3 times the upper limit or normal. Methyldopa should be quickly discontinued if persistent increases in serum hepatic transaminases or alkaline phosphatase are detected because this may indicate the onset of fulminant life threatening hepatitis. A Coombs-positive hemolytic anemia occurs in less than 1% of patients receiving methyldopa, although 20% exhibit a positive direct Coombs test without anemia. For these reasons, methyldopa has limited use in routine management of hypertension, except in pregnancy.

Reserpine Reserpine lowers BP by depleting norepinephrine from sympathetic nerve endings and blocking transport of norepinephrine into its storage granules. Norepinephrine release into the synapse following nerve stimulation is reduced and results in reduced sympathetic tone, peripheral vascular resistance, and BP. Reserpine also depletes catecholamines in the brain and the myocardium, which may lead to sedation, depression, and decreased CO.

Reserpine has a slow onset of action and long half-life that allows for once daily dosing. However, it may take 2 to 6 weeks before the maximal antihypertensive effect is seen. Because reserpine can cause significant sodium and water retention, it should be given in combination with a diuretic (preferably a thiazide). Reserpine's strong inhibition of sympathetic activity results in increased parasympathetic activity. This effect explains why side effects such as nasal stuffiness, increased gastric acid secretion, diarrhea, and bradycardia can occur. Depression has been reported, which is a consequence of central nervous system depletion of catecholamines and serotonin. The initial reports of depression with reserpine were in the 1950s and are not consistent with current definitions of depression. Regardless, reserpine-induced depression is dose related. Moreover, very high doses (above 1 mg daily) were frequently used in the 1950s, resulting in more depression. When reserpine is dosed between 0.05 and 0.25 mg daily (recommended doses), the rate of depression is equal to that seen with β-blockers, diuretics, or placebo.[8]

Reserpine was used as a third-line agent in many of the landmark clinical trials that have documented the benefit in treating hypertension, including the Veterans Administration Cooperative trials and the SHEP trial.[8] An analysis of the SHEP data found that reserpine was very well tolerated and that the combination of a thiazide-type diuretic and reserpine is very effective at lowering BP.

Direct Arterial Vasodilators Hydralazine and minoxidil directly relax arteriolar smooth muscle resulting in vasodilatation and BP lowering. They exert little to no venous vasodilatation. Both agents cause potent reductions in perfusion pressure that activates the baroreceptor reflexes. Activation of baroreceptors results in a compensatory increase in sympathetic outflow, which leads to an increase in heart rate, CO, and renin release. Consequently, tachyphylaxis can develop resulting in a loss of hypotensive effect with continued use. This compensatory baroreceptor response can be counteracted by concurrent use of a β-blocker.

All patients receiving hydralazine or minoxidil long-term for hypertension should first receive both a diuretic and a β-blocker. Direct arterial vasodilators can precipitate angina in patients with underlying coronary disease unless the baroreceptor reflex mechanism is completely blocked with a β-blocker. Non-dihydropyridine CCBs can be used as an alternative to β-blockers in these patients, but a β-blocker is preferred. The side effect of sodium and water retention is significant but is minimized by using a diuretic concomitantly.

One side effect unique to hydralazine is a dose-dependent drug-induced lupus-like syndrome. Hydralazine is eliminated by hepatic N-acetyltransferase. This enzyme displays genetic polymorphism, and "slow acetylators" are especially prone to develop drug-induced lupus with hydralazine. This syndrome is more common in women and is reversible upon discontinuation. Drug-induced lupus may be avoided by using less than 200 mg of hydralazine daily. Because of side effects, hydralazine has limited clinical use for chronic management of hypertension. However, it is especially useful for patients with severe chronic kidney disease and in kidney failure on hemodialysis.

Minoxidil is a more potent vasodilator than hydralazine. Therefore, the compensatory increases in heart rate, CO, renin release, and sodium retention are even more dramatic. Sodium and water retention can be so severe with minoxidil that heart failure can be precipitated. It is even more important to co-administer a β-blocker and a diuretic with minoxidil. A loop diuretic is often more effective than a thiazide in patients treated with minoxidil. A troublesome side effect of minoxidil is hypertrichosis (hirsutism), presenting as increased hair growth on the face, arms, back, and chest. This usually ceases when the drug is discontinued. Other minoxidil side effects include pericardial effusion and a nonspecific T-wave change on the electrocardiogram. Minoxidil is reserved for very difficult to control hypertension and for patients requiring hydralazine that experience drug-induced lupus.

PHARMACOECONOMIC CONSIDERATIONS

The cost of effectively treating hypertension is substantial. However, these costs are offset by savings that would be realized by reducing CV morbidity and mortality. Cost related to treating target-organ damage (e.g., MI, end-stage kidney failure) can drastically increase healthcare costs. The cost per life-year saved from treating hypertension has been estimated to be $40,000 for younger adults and even less for older adults.[105] Treatments that cost less than $50,000 per life-year saved generally are considered favorable by health economists.

Antihypertensive drug costs are a major portion of the total cost of hypertensive care. First-line drug classes recommended by the JNC7 and AHA guidelines, such as diuretics, ACE-inhibitors, and CCBs, are predominantly generic.[1,2] Using these agents to treat hypertension result in lower drug acquisition costs. There are even multiple generic fixed-dose combinations of these agents. A comparative analysis of 133,624 patients with hypertension aged 65 and older from a state prescription drug assistance program demonstrated that 40% of patients were prescribed pharmacotherapy that was not necessarily according to JNC7 guidelines recommendations.[106] If these 40% had drug therapy modifications made to follow evidence-based treatment, a reduction in costs of $11.6 million would have been realized in the 2001 calendar year based on discounted prices. This was projected to increase to $20.5 million using usual Medicaid pricing limits.

Other factors contribute to the overall cost of treating hypertension. Supplemental drugs, laboratory tests, clinic visits, and costs to treat complications of hypertension (e.g., CV events) can be staggering. A cost-minimization analysis found that 86 middle-aged or 29 elderly patients with hypertension would need to be treated to prevent one MI, stroke, or death.[107]

It is crucial to identify ways to control the cost of care without increasing the morbidity and mortality associated with uncontrolled hypertension. Using evidence-based pharmacotherapy will save costs. Thiazide-type diuretics, ACE inhibitors, and CCBs are first-line treatment options in most patients without compelling indications and are very inexpensive. Even the ARBs have one generic option (losartan, although more are expected in 2012). Just utilizing generic agents, either as monotherapy or in combination, is appropriate under most circumstances in hypertension management. Brand name drugs should also be used when needed. However, considerations to implement once daily options, and even fixed-dose combination options that are economical should be considered.

Team-Based Collaborative Care

Team-based care for patients with hypertension is a proven strategy that improves goal BP attainment rates.[108] These patient care models are intraprofessional models of disease state management that utilize physicians, pharmacists, nurses, and other healthcare professionals. With the advent of healthcare reform, such approaches to chronic diseases are being viewed as high-quality and cost-effective improvement modalities. Within these models, pharmacists have been proven to be an effective component of these team-based models both in ambulatory clinic settings[109] and in community pharmacist settings.[110] In addition to optimizing selection and implementation of antihypertensive drug therapy, clinical interventions by pharmacists have been proven to reduce risk of adverse drug events and medication errors in ambulatory patients with CV disease.[111]

EVALUATION OF THERAPEUTIC OUTCOMES

MONITORING THE PHARMACOTHERAPY PLAN

Routine ongoing monitoring to assess disease progression, the desired effects of antihypertensive therapy (efficacy, including BP goal attainment), and undesired adverse side effects (toxicity) is needed in all patients treated with antihypertensive drug therapy.

Disease Progression

Patients should be monitored for signs and symptoms of progressive hypertension-associated target-organ disease. A careful history for ischemic chest pain (or pressure), palpitations, dizziness, dyspnea, orthopnea, headache, sudden change in vision, one-sided weakness, slurred speech, and loss of balance should be taken to assess the presence of CV and cerebrovascular hypertensive complications. Other clinical monitoring parameters that may be used to assess target-organ disease include funduscopic changes on eye exam, left ventricular hypertrophy on electrocardiogram, proteinuria, and changes in kidney function. These parameters should be monitored periodically because any sign of deterioration requires immediate assessment and follow-up.

Efficacy

The most important strategy to prevent CV morbidity and mortality in hypertension is BP control to goal values (see Box 19–2). Routine goal BP values should be attained in elderly patients and in those with isolated systolic hypertension, but actual BP lowering can occur at a very gradual pace over a period of several months to avoid orthostatic hypotension. Modifying other CV risk factors (e.g., smoking, dyslipidemia, and diabetes) is also important.

Clinic-based BP monitoring remains the standard for managing hypertension. BP response should be evaluated 2 to 4 weeks after initiating or making changes in therapy. With some agents, monitoring BP 4 to 6 weeks later may better represent steady state BP values (e.g., thiazide-type diuretics, reserpine). Once goal BP values are attained, assuming no signs or symptoms of acute target-organ disease are present, BP monitoring can be done every 3 to 6 months. More frequent evaluations are required for patients with a history of poor control, nonadherence, progressive target-organ damage, or symptoms of adverse drug effects.

TABLE 19-8	Select Monitoring for Antihypertensive Pharmacotherapy
Class	**Parameters**
Diuretics	Blood pressure; BUN/serum creatinine; serum electrolytes (potassium, magnesium, sodium); uric acid (for thiazides)
Aldosterone antagonists	Blood pressure; BUN/serum creatinine; serum potassium
ACE inhibitors	Blood pressure; BUN/serum creatinine; serum potassium
ARBs	Blood pressure; BUN/serum creatinine; serum potassium
Calcium channel blockers	Blood pressure; heart rate
β-blockers	Blood pressure; heart rate

Self-measurements of BP or automated ambulatory BP monitoring can be useful clinically to establish effective 24-hour control. This type of monitoring may become the standard of care in the future, but currently, ambulatory BP monitoring is used in select situations such as suspected white coat hypertension.[14] If patients are measuring their BP at home, it is important that they measure during the early morning hours for most days and then at different times of the day on alternative days of the week.

Toxicity

Patients should be monitored routinely for adverse drug effects. The most common side effects associated with each class of antihypertensive agents were discussed in the Individual Antihypertensive Agents section, and laboratory parameters for primary agents are listed in Table 19–8. Laboratory monitoring should typically occur 2 to 4 weeks after starting a new agent or dose increase, and then every 6 to 12 months in stable patients. Additional monitoring may be needed for other concomitant diseases if present (e.g., diabetes, dyslipidemia, gout). Moreover, patients treated with an aldosterone antagonist (eplerenone or spironolactone) should have potassium concentrations and kidney function assessed within 3 days of initiation and again at 1 week to detect potential hyperkalemia.[48] The occurrence of an adverse drug event may require dosage reduction or substitution with an alternative antihypertensive agent.

Adherence

Lack of persistence with hypertension treatment is a major problem in the United States and is associated with significant increases in costs due to development of complications. Since hypertension is a relatively asymptomatic disease, poor adherence is frequent, particularly in patients newly treated. It has been estimated that up to 50% of patients with newly diagnosed hypertension are continuing treatment at 1 year.[112] It has also been demonstrated that long-term risk of CV events is significantly reduced when newly diagnosed patients are adherent with their antihypertensive drug therapy.[113] Therefore, it is imperative to assess patient adherence on a regular basis.

Identification of nonadherence should be followed up with appropriate patient education, counseling, and intervention. Once-daily regimens are preferred in most patients to improve adherence. Although some may believe that aggressive treatment may negatively impact quality of life and thus adherence, several studies have found that most patients actually feel better once their BP is controlled. Patients on antihypertensive therapy should be questioned periodically about changes in their general health perception, energy level, physical functioning, and overall satisfaction with treatment. Lifestyle modifications should always be recommended to provide additional BP lowering and other potential health benefits. Persistence with lifestyle modifications should be continually encouraged for patients engaging in such endeavors.

COMBINATION THERAPY

🟦 Initial therapy with a combination of two drugs is highly recommended for patients with Stage 2 hypertension and is an option for treating patients with Stage 1 hypertension where goal achievement may be difficult (e.g., those with BP goals of less than 130/80 mm Hg, African-Americans). Using a fixed-dose combination product is an option for these types of patients and has been shown to improve adherence.[114] Initial two-drug combination therapy may also be appropriate for patients with multiple compelling indications for different antihypertensive agents. Moreover, combination therapy is often needed to control BP in patients that are already on drug therapy and most patients require two or more agents.[1,42,64,73]

The Avoiding Cardiovascular Events Through Combination Therapy for Patients Living with Systolic Hypertension (ACCOMPLISH) Trial

Long-term safety and efficacy of initial two drug therapy for hypertension has been evaluated in the ACCOMPLISH trial.[115] This was a prospective, randomized, double-blind trial in 11,506 patients with hypertension and other CV risk factors. All of these patients either had stage 2 hypertension or were on antihypertensive drug therapy upon enrollment. Patients were randomized to receive either benazepril-with-hydrochlorothiazide or benazepril-with-amlodipine as initial drug therapy. Treatment was titrated to a goal BP of less than 140/90 mm Hg for most patients and less than 130/80 mm Hg for patients with diabetes or chronic kidney disease.

The trial was terminated early after a mean of only 36 months because the incidence of CV events was 20% lower in the benazepril-with-amlodipine group compared with the benazepril-with-hydrochlorothiazide group. What is most important for clinical practice is that this trial established that initial therapy, as is recommended in the JNC7 and AHA guidelines, was safe and highly effective in lowering BP. Mean BP measurements were 132/73 mm Hg and 133/74 mm Hg in the benazepril-with-amlodipine and the benazepril-with-hydrochlorothiazide groups, respectively. However, rates of attaining a BP of less than 140/90 mm Hg were 75.4% and 72.4% (benazepril with amlodipine and benazepril with hydrochlorothiazide, respectively). These goal attainment rates are higher than in any other long-term prospective study and are higher than what is seen in clinical practice.

The ACCOMPLISH trial established initial two-drug antihypertensive therapy as an evidence-based strategy to treat hypertension. Clinicians should consider this study as positive justification for implementing initial two-drug therapy antihypertensive regimens in appropriate patients.

CLINICAL CONTROVERSY

What is the most effective two-drug combination for reducing CV events?

The ACCOMPLISH trial demonstrated that the combination of an ACE inhibitor with a dihydropyridine CCB was more effective in reducing risk of CV events than the combination of an ACE inhibitor with a thiazide-type diuretic.[115] However, thiazide-type diuretics are very effective at lowering BP, especially when used in combination with other agents, and have been traditionally viewed as the most appropriate second drug (if not used as the first drug) to treat hypertension.[88] Therefore, the most ideal two-drug combination for the treatment of hypertension is debatable.

Optimal Use of Combination Therapy

Clinicians should anticipate the need for three drugs to control BP in most patients when an aggressive BP goal of less than 130/80 mm Hg is targeted.[64] Using low-dose combinations also provides greater reductions in BP compared to high doses of single agents, with fewer drug-related side effects.[95] Contrary to popular myth, appropriately increasing the number of antihypertensive medications to attain goal BP values does not increase the risk of adverse effects.[116] Ideal combinations include two drugs with discretely different mechanisms of action that are supported by evidence demonstrating the ability to lower CV events.

Combination regimens for hypertension that include a diuretic, preferably a thiazide-type, are inexpensive and effective in lowering BP.[87,88] Diuretics, when combined with several agents (especially an ACE inhibitor, ARB, or β-blocker), can result in additive antihypertensive effects that are independent of reversing fluid retention. These fixed dose products are also readily available. BP lowering from certain antihypertensive agents can activate the RAAS as a compensatory mechanism to counteract BP changes and can regulate fluid loss. Most alternative antihypertensive agents (i.e., reserpine, arterial vasodilators, and centrally acting agents) need to be given with a diuretic to avoid sodium and water retention.

Some combinations either are less effective in lowering BP or are not effective long term in treating hypertension. As previously discussed, the ON-TARGET trial demonstrated that the use of an ACE inhibitor with an ARB in the management of hypertension results in no additional reduction in incidence of CV events.[97] Moreover, this combination results in a higher risk of adverse events. This combination should not be used for the purpose of managing hypertension. Other combinations such as a thiazide-diuretic with a potassium sparing agent, both of which appear to have overlapping mechanisms of action, should be implemented primarily to minimize side effects. The combination of two CCBs, a dihydropyridine with a non-dihydropyridine, might provide additional BP lowering[117,118] but has limited use in the routine management of patients with hypertension, perhaps for patient with diabetes.[64] Under no circumstance should two drugs from the same exact class of medications (e.g., two β-blockers, two ACE inhibitors) be used to treat hypertension.

Fixed-Dose Combination Products Many fixed-dose combination products are commercially available, and some are generic (see Table 19–9). Most of these products contain a thiazide-type diuretic and have multiple dose strengths available. Individual dose titration is more complicated with fixed-dose combination products, but this strategy can reduce the number of daily tablets/capsules and can simplify regimens to improve adherence by decreasing pill burden.[114] This alone may increase the likelihood of achieving or maintaining goal BP values. Depending on the product, some may be less expensive to patients and to health systems. Nonadherence rates are 24% lower when fixed-dose combination products are used to treat hypertension compared to using free drug components (separate pills) to treat hypertension.[119]

RESISTANT HYPERTENSION

🟦 Resistant hypertension is defined as patients who are uncontrolled (failure to achieve goal BP of <140/90 mm Hg, or lower when indicated) with the use of three or more drugs.[120] Ideally, these should be patients who are adhering to full doses of an appropriate three-drug regimen that includes a diuretic.[1] This also includes patients who are controlled but require the use of four or more mediations.[120] Patients with newly diagnosed hypertension or who are not receiving drug therapy should not be considered to have resistant hypertension.[121] Difficult-to-control hypertension is

TABLE 19-9 Fixed-Dose Combination Products

Combination	Drugs (Brand Name)	Strengths (mg/mg)	Daily Frequency
ACE inhibitor with a thiazide-type diuretic	Benazepril/hydrochlorothiazide (Lotensin HCT)	5/6.25, 10/12.5, 20/12.5, 20/25	1
	Captopril/hydrochlorothiazide (Capozide)	25/15, 25/25, 50/15, 50/25	1 to 3
	Enalapril/hydrochlorothiazide (Vaseretic)	5/12.5, 10/25	1
	Lisinopril/hydrochlorothiazide (Prinizide, Zestoretic)	10/12.5, 20/12.5, 20/25	1
	Moexipril/hydrochlorothiazide (Uniretic)	7.5/12.5, 15/25	1 or 2
	Quinapril/hydrochlorothiazide (Accuretic)	10/12.5, 20/12.5, 20/25	1
ARB with a thiazide-type diuretic	Candesartan/hydrochlorothiazide (Atacand HCT)	16/12.5, 32/12.5	1
	Eprosartan/hydrochlorothiazide (Teveten HCT)	600/12.5, 600/25	1
	Irbesartan/hydrochlorothiazide (Avalide)	75/12.5, 150/12.5, 300/12.5	1
	Losartan/hydrochlorothiazide (Hyzaar)	50/12.5, 100/25	1
	Olmesartan/hydrochlorothiazide (Benicar HCT)	20/12.5, 40/12.5, 40/25	1
	Telmisartan/hydrochlorothiazide (Micardis HCT)	40/12.5, 80/12.5	1
	Valsartan/hydrochlorothiazide (Diovan HCT)	80/12.5, 160/12.5	1
β-blocker with a thiazide-type diuretic	Atenolol/chlorthalidone (Tenoretic)	50/25, 100/25	1
	Bisoprolol/hydrochlorothiazide (Ziac)	2.5/6.25, 5/6.25, 10/6.25	1
	Propranolol/hydrochlorothiazide (Inderide)	40/25, 80/25	2
	Propranolol LA/hydrochlorothiazide (Inderide LA)	80/50, 120/50, 160/50	1
	Metoprolol/hydrochlorothiazide (Lopressor HCT)	50/25, 100/25	1 or 2
	Nadolol/bendroflumethazide (Corzide)	40/5, 80/5	1
	Timolol/hydrochlorothiazide (Timolide)	10/25	1 or 2
ACE inhibitor with CCB	Amlodipine/benazepril (Lotrel)	2.5/10, 5/10, 10/20	1
	Enalapril/felodipine (Lexxel)	5/5	1
	Trandolapril/verapamil (Tarka)	2/180, 1/240, 2/240, 4/240	1 or 2
ARB with CCB	Amlodipine/olmesartan (AZOR)	5/20, 10/20, 5/40, 10/40	1
	Telmisartan/amlodipine (Twynsta)	40/5, 40/10, 80/5, 80/10	1
	Valsartan/amlodipine (Exforge)	5/160, 10/160, 5/320,10/320	1
ARB with direct renin inhibitor	Aliskiren/valsartan (Valturna)	150/160, 300/320	1
Direct renin inhibitor with thiazide-type diuretic	Aliskiren/hydrochlorothiazide (Tekturna HCT)	150/12.5, 150/25, 300/12.5, 300/25	1
ARB with CCB with a thiazide-type diuretic	Amlodipine/valsartan/hydrochlorothiazide (Exforge HCT)	5/160/12.5, 5/160/25, 10/160/12.5, 10/160/25, 10/320/25	1
	Olmesartan, amlodipine, hydrochlorothiazide (Tribenzor)	20/5/12.5, 40/5/12.5, 40/5/25, 40/10/12.5, 40/10/25	1

persistently elevated BP despite treatment with two or three drugs that does not meet the criteria for resistant hypertension (e.g., maximum doses that include a diuretic).

Several causes of resistant hypertension are listed in Table 19–10. Volume overload is a common cause, thus highlighting the importance of diuretic therapy in the management of hypertension. Pseudoresistance should also be ruled out by assuring adherence with prescribed therapy and possibly use of home BP measurements (by using a self-monitoring device or 24-hour ABP monitor).[120] Patients should be closely evaluated to see if any of these causes can be reversed.

Treatment of patients with resistant hypertension should ultimately follow the principle of drug therapy selection from the JNC7 and AHA guidelines. Compelling indications, if present, should guide selection assuming these patients are on a diuretic.

TABLE 19-10 Causes of Resistant Hypertension

Improper BP measurement
Volume overload:
• Excess sodium intake
• Volume retention from kidney disease
• Inadequate diuretic therapy
Drug-induced or other causes:
• Nonadherence
• Inadequate doses
• Agents listed in Table 19–1
Associated conditions:
• Obesity, excess alcohol intake
Secondary hypertension

However, there are treatment philosophies that are germane to the management of resistant hypertension: (1) assuring adequate diuretic therapy, (2) appropriate use of combination therapies, and (3) using alternative antihypertensive agents when needed.[120]

Assuring Appropriate Diuretic Therapy

Diuretics have a large role in the pharmacotherapy of resistant hypertension. Thiazide-type diuretics are the mainstay of treatment, but chlorthalidone should be preferentially used instead of hydrochlorothiazide for patients with resistant hypertension because it is more potent on a milligram-per-milligram basis.[87,120] Clinicians should identify that chlorthalidone therapy, like all thiazide-type diuretics, has dose-dependent metabolic side effects (hypokalemia and hyperglycemia) and that appropriate monitoring should be implemented. An aldosterone antagonist (e.g., spironolactone) is also very effective as an add-on agent.[120] Evolving data indicate that many patients with resistant hypertension have some degree of underlying hyperaldosteronism, emphasizing the role of adding an aldosterone antagonist. Clinicians should consider using a loop diuretic, even in place of a thiazide-type diuretic, for patients with resistant hypertension that have very compromised kidney function (estimated GFR less than 30 mL/min/1.73 m²). Torsemide can be dosed once daily while furosemide must be dosed twice daily or three times daily.

HYPERTENSIVE URGENCIES AND EMERGENCIES[1,6]

Hypertensive urgencies and emergencies both are characterized by the presence of very elevated BP, typically greater than 180/120 mm Hg. However, the need for urgent or emergent antihypertensive therapy must be determined based on the presence of acute or immediately progressing target-organ injury, not elevated BP alone. Urgencies are not associated with acute or immediately progressing target-organ injury, while emergencies are. Examples of acute target-organ injury include encephalopathy, intracranial hemorrhage, acute left ventricular failure with pulmonary edema, dissecting aortic aneurysm, unstable angina, and eclampsia or severe hypertension during pregnancy.

Hypertensive Urgency

🔞 A common error with hypertensive urgency is overly aggressive antihypertensive therapy. This treatment has likely been perpetrated by the classification terminology "urgency." Hypertensive urgencies are ideally managed by adjusting maintenance therapy, by adding a new antihypertensive, and/or by increasing the dose of a present medication. This is the preferred approach to these patients as it provides a more gradual reduction in BP. Very rapid reductions in BP to goal values should be discouraged due to potential risks. Because autoregulation of blood flow in patients with hypertension occurs at a much higher range of pressure than in normotensive persons, the inherent risks of reducing BP too precipitously include cerebrovascular accidents, MI, and acute kidney failure. Hypertensive urgency requires BP reductions with oral antihypertensive agents to stage 1 values over a period of several hours to several days. All patients with hypertensive urgency should be reevaluated within and no later than 7 days (preferably after 1 to 3 days).

Acute administration of a short-acting oral antihypertensive (e.g., captopril, clonidine, or labetalol) followed by careful observation for several hours to assure a gradual reduction in BP is an option for hypertensive urgency. However, there are no data supporting this approach as being absolutely needed. Oral captopril is one of the agents of choice and can be used in doses of 25 to 50 mg at 1- to 2-hour intervals. The onset of action of oral captopril is 15 to 30 minutes, and a marked fall in BP is unlikely to occur if no hypotensive response is observed within 30 to 60 minutes. For patients with hypertensive rebound following withdrawal of clonidine, 0.2 mg can be given initially, followed by 0.2 mg hourly until the DBP falls below 110 mm Hg or a total of 0.7 mg clonidine has been administered. A single dose may be all that is necessary. Labetalol can be given in a dose of 200 to 400 mg, followed by additional doses every 2 to 3 hours.

Oral or sublingual immediate-release nifedipine has been used for acute BP lowering in the past but is potentially dangerous. This approach produces a rapid reduction in BP. Immediate-release nifedipine should never be used for hypertensive urgencies due risk of causing of severe adverse events such as MIs and strokes.[122]

Hypertensive Emergency

Hypertensive emergencies are those rare situations that require immediate BP reduction to limit new or progressing target-organ damage (see "Classification" under the Arterial Blood Pressure section). Hypertensive emergencies require parenteral therapy, at least initially, with one of the agents listed in Table 19–11. The goal in

TABLE 19-11	Parenteral Antihypertensive Agents for Hypertensive Emergency				
Drug	**Dose**	**Onset (minutes)**	**Duration (minutes)**	**Adverse Effects**	**Special Indications**
Clevidipine	1–2 mg/h (32 mg/h max)	2–4	5–15	Headache, nausea, tachycardia, hypertriglyceridemia	Most hypertensive emergencies except acute heart failure; caution with coronary ischemia; contraindicated in soy or egg allergy or if defective lipid metabolism
Enalaprilat	1.25–5 mg intravenous every 6 h	15–30	360–720	Precipitous fall in pressure in high-renin states; variable response	Acute left ventricular failure; avoid in acute myocardial infarction
Esmolol hydrochloride	250–500 mcg/kg/min intravenous bolus, then 50–100 mcg/kg/min intravenous infusion; may repeat bolus after 5 minutes or increase infusion to 300 mcg/min	1–2	10–20	Hypotension, nausea, asthma, first-degree heart block, heart failure	Aortic dissection; perioperative
Fenoldopam mesylate	0.1–0.3 mcg/kg/min intravenous infusion	<5	30	Tachycardia, headache, nausea, flushing	Most hypertensive emergencies; caution with glaucoma
Hydralazine hydrochloride	12–20 mg intravenous 10–50 mg intramuscular	10–20 20–30	60–240 240–360	Tachycardia, flushing, headache vomiting, aggravation of angina	Eclampsia
Labetalol hydrochloride	20–80 mg intravenous bolus every 10 min; 0.5–2.0 mg/min intravenous infusion	5–10	180–360	Vomiting, scalp tingling, bronchoconstriction, dizziness, nausea, heart block, orthostatic hypotension	Most hypertensive emergencies except acute heart failure
Nicardipine hydrochloride	5–15 mg/h intravenous	5–10	15–30, may exceed 240	Tachycardia, headache, flushing, local phlebitis	Most hypertensive emergencies except acute heart failure; caution with coronary ischemia
Nitroglycerin	5–100 mcg/min intravenous infusion	2–5	5–10	Headache, vomiting, methemoglobinemia, tolerance with prolonged use	Coronary ischemia
Sodium nitroprusside	0.25–10 mcg/kg/min intravenous infusion (requires special delivery system)	Immediate	1–2	Nausea, vomiting, muscle twitching, sweating, thiocynate and cyanide intoxication	Most hypertensive emergencies; caution with high intracranial pressure, azotemia, or in chronic kidney disease

hypertensive emergencies is not to lower BP to less than 140/90 mm Hg; rather, the initial target is a reduction in MAP of up to 25% within minutes to hours. If the patient is then stable, BP can be reduced toward 160/100 mm Hg to 160/110 mm Hg within the next 2 to 6 hours. Precipitous drops in BP may lead to end-organ ischemia or infarction. If patients tolerate this reduction well, additional gradual reductions toward goal BP values can be attempted after 24 to 48 hours. The exception to this guideline is for patients with an acute ischemic stroke where maintaining an elevated BP is needed for a much longer period of time.

The clinical situation should dictate which intravenous medication is used to treat hypertensive emergencies. Regardless, therapy should be provided in a hospital or emergency room setting with intraarticular BP monitoring. Table 19–11 lists special indications for agents that can be used.

Nitroprusside is widely considered the agent of choice for most cases, but it can be problematic for patients with chronic kidney disease. It is a direct-acting vasodilator that decreases peripheral vascular resistance but does not increase CO unless left ventricular failure is present. Nitroprusside can be given to treat most hypertensive emergencies, but in aortic dissection, propranolol should be given first to prevent reflex sympathetic activation. Nitroprusside is metabolized to cyanide and then to thiocyanate, which is eliminated by the kidneys. Therefore, serum thiocyanate levels should be monitored when infusions are continued longer than 72 hours. Nitroprusside should be discontinued if the concentration exceeds 12 mg/dL. The risk of thiocyanate accumulation and toxicity is increased for patients with impaired kidney function.

Intravenous nitroglycerin dilates both arterioles and venous capacitance vessels, thereby reducing both cardiac afterload and cardiac preload, which can decrease myocardial oxygen demand. It also dilates collateral coronary blood vessels and improves perfusion to ischemic myocardium. These properties make intravenous nitroglycerin ideal for the management of hypertensive emergency in the presence of myocardial ischemia. Intravenous nitroglycerin is associated with tolerance when used over 24 to 48 hours and can cause severe headache.

Fenoldopam, nicardipine, and clevidipine are newer and more expensive agents. Fenoldopam is a dopamine-1 agonist. It can improve renal blood flow and may be especially useful for patients with kidney insufficiency. Nicardipine and clevidipine are dihydropyridine CCBs that provides arterial vasodilatation and can treat cardiac ischemia similar to nitroglycerin, but they may provide more predictable reductions in BP.

The hypotensive response of hydralazine is less predictable than with other parenteral agents. Therefore, its major role is in the treatment of eclampsia or hypertensive encephalopathy associated with renal insufficiency.

CONCLUSIONS

Hypertension is a very common medical condition in the United States. Treatment of patients with hypertension should include both lifestyle modifications and pharmacotherapy. Outcome-based studies have definitively demonstrated that treating hypertension reduces the risk of CV events and subsequently reduces morbidity and mortality. Moreover, evidence evaluating individual drug classes has resulted in an evidence-based approach to selecting pharmacotherapy in an individual patient, which is outlined in the JNC7 and 2007 AHA guidelines. Thiazide-type diuretics, ACE inhibitors, ARBs, and CCBs are all first-line agents. Data suggests that using a β-blocker as the primary agent to treat patients with hypertension, without the presence of a compelling indication, may not be as beneficial in reducing risk of CV events

compared to thiazide-type diuretic, ACE inhibitor, ARB, or CCB-based therapy. Therefore, they are not first-line therapy options unless an appropriate compelling indication is present.

An often overlooked concept in managing hypertension is to treat patients to a goal BP value. In addition to selecting the most appropriate agent, attaining a goal BP is also of paramount importance to ensure maximum reduction in risk for CV events is provided. A BP goal of at least less than 140/90 mm Hg is recommended for most patients with hypertension and some patients are candidates for lower goal values. Most patients with hypertension require more than one pharmacologic agent to attain goal BP values; therefore, combination therapy is often needed.

Optimizing hypertension management can be achieved many ways. Team-based approaches to implement care and attain goal BP values are effective. Judicious use of cost effective treatments and fixed-dose combination products should always be considered to improve sustainability of treatment. Lastly, interventions to reinforce adherence and lifestyle modifications also are highly recommended in the comprehensive management of hypertension.

ABBREVIATIONS

ACE: angiotensin converting enzyme

ARB: angiotensin II receptor blocker

AHA: American Heart Association

BP: blood pressure

BUN: blood urea nitrogen

CCB: calcium channel blocker

COPD: chronic obstructive pulmonary disease

CV: cardiovascular

DBP: diastolic blood pressure

GFR: glomerular filtration rate

JNC7: Seventh report of the Joint National Committee on Prevention, Detection, Evaluation, and Treatment of High Blood Pressure

MI: myocardial infarction

ISA: intrinsic sympathomimetic activity

LVH: left ventricular hypertrophy

RAAS: renin-angiotensin-aldosterone system

SBP: systolic blood pressure

REFERENCES

1. Chobanian AV, Bakris GL, Black HR, et al. Seventh Report of the Joint National Committee on Prevention, Detection, Evaluation, and Treatment of High Blood Pressure. Hypertension 2003;42:1206–1252.

2. Rosendorff C, Black HR, Cannon CP, et al. Treatment of hypertension in the prevention and management of ischemic heart disease: A scientific statement from the American Heart Association Council for High Blood Pressure Research and the Councils on Clinical Cardiology and Epidemiology and Prevention. Circulation 2007;115:2761–2788.

3. Lloyd-Jones D, Adams RJ, Brown TM, et al. Heart Disease and Stroke Statistics—2010 Update. A Report from the American Heart Association. Circulation 2009.

4. Staessen JA, Wang J, Bianchi G, Birkenhager WH. Essential hypertension. Lancet 2003;361:1629–1641.

5. Saseen JJ. Hypertension. In: Tisdale JE, Miller DA, eds. Drug-Induced Diseases: Prevention, Detection, and Management. Bethesda; American Society of Health-Systems Pharmacists, Inc.; 2010.

6. Kaplan NM. Kaplan's Clinical Hypertension. 9th ed. Philadelphia: Lipincott Williams & Wilkins; 2006:1–518.

7. MacMahon S, Peto R, Cutler J, et al. Blood pressure, stroke, and coronary heart disease. Part 1: Prolonged differences in blood pressure: Prospective observational studies corrected for the regression dilution bias. Lancet 1990;335:765–774.

8. SHEP Cooperative Research Group. Prevention of stroke by antihypertensive drug treatment in older persons with isolated systolic hypertension. Final results of the Systolic Hypertension in the Elderly Program (SHEP). JAMA 1991;265:3255–3264.

9. Dahlof B, Lindholm LH, Hansson L, Schersten B, Ekbom T, Wester PO. Morbidity and mortality in the Swedish trial in old patients with hypertension (STOP-hypertension). Lancet 1991;338:1281–1285.

10. MRC Working Party. Medical Research Council trial of treatment of hypertension in older adults: Principal results. BMJ 1992;304:405–412.

11. Staessen JA, Fagard R, Thijs L, et al. Randomised double-blind comparison of placebo and active treatment for older patients with isolated systolic hypertension. The Systolic Hypertension in Europe (Syst-Eur) Trial Investigators. Lancet 1997;350:757–764.

12. Alberti KG, Eckel RH, Grundy SM, et al. Harmonizing the metabolic syndrome: A joint interim statement of the International Diabetes Federation Task Force on Epidemiology and Prevention; National Heart, Lung, and Blood Institute; American Heart Association; World Heart Federation; International Atherosclerosis Society; and international association for the Study of Obesity. Circulation 2009;120:1640–1645.

13. Pickering TG, Hall JE, Appel LJ, et al. Recommendations for blood pressure measurement in humans and experimental animals: Part 1: Blood pressure measurement in humans: A statement for professionals from the Subcommittee of Professional and Public Education of the American Heart Association Council on High Blood Pressure Research. Circulation 2005;111:697–716.

14. Pickering TG, White WB. ASH Position Paper: Home and ambulatory blood pressure monitoring. When and how to use self (home) and ambulatory blood pressure monitoring. J Clin Hypertens (Greenwich) 2008;10:850–855.

15. Mancia G, Bombelli M, Facchetti R, et al. Long-term risk of sustained hypertension in white-coat or masked hypertension. Hypertension 2009;54:226–232.

16. Mitka M. Aggressively treating hypertension remains strategy of uncertain benefit. JAMA 2009;302:1047–1048.

17. Hansson L, Zanchetti A, Carruthers SG, et al. Effects of intensive blood-pressure lowering and low-dose aspirin in patients with hypertension: Principal results of the Hypertension Optimal Treatment (HOT) randomised trial. HOT Study Group. Lancet 1998;351:1755–1762.

18. Arguedas JA, Perez MI, Wright JM. Treatment blood pressure targets for hypertension. Cochrane Database Syst Rev 2009:CD004349.

19. Farnett L, Mulrow CD, Linn WD, Lucey CR, Tuley MR. The J-curve phenomenon and the treatment of hypertension. Is there a point beyond which pressure reduction is dangerous? JAMA 1991;265:489–495.

20. Verdecchia P, Staessen JA, Angeli F, et al. Usual versus tight control of systolic blood pressure in non-diabetic patients with hypertension (Cardio-Sis): An open-label randomised trial. Lancet 2009;374:525–533.

21. American Diabetes Association. Standards of medical care in diabetes—2010. Diabetes Care 2010;33(suppl 1):S11–S61.

22. National Kidney Foundation. K/DOQI clinical practice guidelines on hypertension and antihypertensive agents in chronic kidney disease. Am J Kidney Dis 2004;43(5 suppl 1):S1–S290.

23. The ACCORD Study Group. Effects of intensive blood-pressure control in type 2 diabetes mellitus. N Engl J Med 2010;362(17):1575–1585.

24. O'Connor PJ. Overcome clinical inertia to control systolic blood pressure. Arch Intern Med 2003;163:2677–2678.

25. Appel LJ, Brands MW, Daniels SR, Karanja N, Elmer PJ, Sacks FM. Dietary approaches to prevent and treat hypertension: A scientific statement from the American Heart Association. Hypertension 2006;47:296–308.

26. Lichtenstein AH, Appel LJ, Brands M, et al. Diet and lifestyle recommendations revision 2006: A scientific statement from the American Heart Association Nutrition Committee. Circulation 2006;114:82–96.

27. Moser M, Feig PU. Fifty years of thiazide diuretic therapy for hypertension. Arch Intern Med 2009;169:1851–1856.

28. Saseen JJ, MacLaughlin EJ, Westfall JM. Treatment of uncomplicated hypertension: Are ACE inhibitors and calcium channel blockers as effective as diuretics and beta-blockers? J Am Board Fam Pract 2003;16:156–164.

29. Black HR, Elliott WJ, Grandits G, et al. Principal results of the Controlled Onset Verapamil Investigation of Cardiovascular End Points (CONVINCE) trial. JAMA 2003;289:2073–2082.

30. Dahlof B, Devereux RB, Kjeldsen SE, et al. Cardiovascular morbidity and mortality in the Losartan Intervention For Endpoint reduction in hypertension study (LIFE): A randomised trial against atenolol. Lancet 2002;359:995–1003.

31. ALLHAT Officers and Coordinators for the ALLHAT Collaborative Research Group. Major outcomes in high-risk hypertensive patients randomized to angiotensin-converting enzyme inhibitor or calcium channel blocker vs diuretic: The Antihypertensive and Lipid-Lowering Treatment to Prevent Heart Attack Trial (ALLHAT). JAMA 2002;288:2981–2997.

32. PROGRESS Collaborative Group. Randomised trial of a perindopril-based blood-pressure-lowering regimen among 6,105 individuals with previous stroke or transient ischaemic attack. Lancet 2001;358:1033–1041.

33. Wing LM, Reid CM, Ryan P, et al. A comparison of outcomes with angiotensin-converting enzyme inhibitors and diuretics for hypertension in the elderly. N Engl J Med 2003;348:583–592.

34. Julius S, Kjeldsen SE, Weber M, et al. Outcomes in hypertensive patients at high cardiovascular risk treated with regimens based on valsartan or amlodipine: The VALUE randomised trial. Lancet 2004;363:2022–2031.

35. Dahlof B, Sever PS, Poulter NR, et al. Prevention of cardiovascular events with an antihypertensive regimen of amlodipine adding perindopril as required versus atenolol adding bendroflumethiazide as required, in the Anglo–Scandinavian Cardiac Outcomes Trial–Blood Pressure Lowering Arm (ASCOT–BPLA): A multicentre randomised controlled trial. Lancet 2005;366:895–906.

36. Diuretic versus alpha-blocker as first-step antihypertensive therapy: Final results from the Antihypertensive and Lipid-Lowering Treatment to Prevent Heart Attack Trial (ALLHAT). Hypertension 2003;42:239–246.

37. Davis BR, Cutler JA, Gordon DJ, et al. Rationale and design for the Antihypertensive and Lipid Lowering Treatment to Prevent Heart Attack Trial (ALLHAT). ALLHAT Research Group. Am J Hypertens 1996;9:342–360.

38. Rahman M, Pressel S, Davis BR, et al. Renal outcomes in high-risk hypertensive patients treated with an angiotensin-converting enzyme inhibitor or a calcium channel blocker vs a diuretic: A report from the Antihypertensive and Lipid-Lowering Treatment to Prevent Heart Attack Trial (ALLHAT). Arch Intern Med 2005;165:936–946.

39. Whelton PK, Barzilay J, Cushman WC, et al. Clinical outcomes in antihypertensive treatment of type 2 diabetes, impaired fasting glucose concentration, and normoglycemia: Antihypertensive and Lipid-Lowering Treatment to Prevent Heart Attack Trial (ALLHAT). Arch Intern Med 2005;165:1401–1409.

40. Wright JT, Jr., Dunn JK, Cutler JA, et al. Outcomes in hypertensive black and nonblack patients treated with chlorthalidone, amlodipine, and lisinopril. JAMA 2005;293:1595–1608.

41. Turnbull F. Effects of different blood-pressure-lowering regimens on major cardiovascular events: Results of prospectively-designed overviews of randomised trials. Lancet 2003;362:1527–1535.

42. Mancia G, De Backer G, Dominiczak A, et al. 2007 Guidelines for the Management of arterial hypertension. The Task for Management of the European Society of Cardiology (ESC). Eur Heart J 2007;28:1462–1536.

43. National Collaborating Centre for Chronic Conditions. Hypertension: Management of hypertension in adults in primary care: Partial update. London: Royal College of Physicians, 2006.

44. Carlberg B, Samuelsson O, Lindholm LH. Atenolol in hypertension: Is it a wise choice? Lancet 2004;364:1684–1689.

45. Lindholm LH, Carlberg B, Samuelsson O. Should beta-blockers remain first choice in the treatment of primary hypertension? A meta-analysis. Lancet 2005;366:1545–1553.

46. Khan N, McAlister FA. Re-examining the efficacy of beta-blockers for the treatment of hypertension: A meta-analysis. CMAJ 2006;174:1737–1742.

47. Wiysonge C, Bradley H, Mayosi B, et al. Beta-blockers for hypertension. Cochrane Database Syst Rev 2007:CD002003.

48. Hunt SA, Abraham WT, Chin MH, et al. 2009 Focused update incorporated into the ACC/AHA 2005 Guidelines for the Diagnosis and Management of Heart Failure in Adults A Report of the American College of Cardiology Foundation/American Heart Association Task Force on Practice Guidelines Developed in Collaboration With the International Society for Heart and Lung Transplantation. J Am Coll Cardiol 2009;53:e1–e90.

49. Effect of metoprolol CR/XL in chronic heart failure: Metoprolol CR/XL randomised intervention trial in congestive heart failure (MERIT–HF). Lancet 1999;353:2001–2007.

50. Packer M, Coats AJ, Fowler MB, et al. Effect of carvedilol on survival in severe chronic heart failure. N Engl J Med 2001;344:1651–1658.

51. Pitt B, Zannad F, Remme WJ, et al. The effect of spironolactone on morbidity and mortality in patients with severe heart failure. Randomized Aldactone Evaluation Study Investigators. N Engl J Med 1999;341:709–717.

52. Pitt B, Remme W, Zannad F, et al. Eplerenone, a selective aldosterone blocker, in patients with left ventricular dysfunction after myocardial infarction. N Engl J Med 2003;348:1309–1321.

53. Pitt B, Segal R, Martinez FA, et al. Randomised trial of losartan versus captopril in patients over 65 with heart failure (Evaluation of Losartan in the Elderly Study, ELITE). Lancet 1997;349:747–752.

54. Pitt B, Poole-Wilson PA, Segal R, et al. Effect of losartan compared with captopril on mortality in patients with symptomatic heart failure: Randomised trial—The Losartan Heart Failure Survival Study ELITE II. Lancet 2000;355:1582–1587.

55. Granger CB, McMurray JJ, Yusuf S, et al. Effects of candesartan in patients with chronic heart failure and reduced left-ventricular systolic function intolerant to angiotensin-converting-enzyme inhibitors: The CHARM–Alternative trial. Lancet 2003;362:772–776.

56. McMurray JJ, Ostergren J, Swedberg K, et al. Effects of candesartan in patients with chronic heart failure and reduced left-ventricular systolic function taking angiotensin-converting-enzyme inhibitors: The CHARM–Added trial. Lancet 2003;362:767–771.

57. Smith SC, Jr., Allen J, Blair SN, et al. AHA/ACC guidelines for secondary prevention for patients with coronary and other atherosclerotic vascular disease: 2006 update endorsed by the National Heart, Lung, and Blood Institute. J Am Coll Cardiol 2006;47:2130–2139.

58. Pfeffer MA, McMurray JJ, Velazquez EJ, et al. Valsartan, captopril, or both in myocardial infarction complicated by heart failure, left ventricular dysfunction, or both. N Engl J Med 2003;349:1893–1906.

59. Fraker TD, Jr., Fihn SD, Gibbons RJ, et al. 2007 chronic angina focused update of the ACC/AHA 2002 Guidelines for the management of patients with chronic stable angina: A report of the American College of Cardiology/American Heart Association Task Force on Practice Guidelines Writing Group to develop the focused update of the 2002 Guidelines for the management of patients with chronic stable angina. Circulation 2007;116:2762–2772.

60. Pepine CJ, Handberg EM, Cooper-DeHoff RM, et al. A calcium antagonist vs a non-calcium antagonist hypertension treatment strategy for patients with coronary artery disease. The International Verapamil–Trandolapril Study (INVEST): A randomized controlled trial. JAMA 2003;290:2805–2816.

61. Anderson JL, Adams CD, Antman EM, et al. ACC/AHA 2007 guidelines for the management of patients with unstable angina/non-ST-Elevation myocardial infarction: A report of the American College of Cardiology/American Heart Association Task Force on Practice Guidelines (Writing Committee to Revise the 2002 Guidelines for the Management of Patients With Unstable Angina/Non-ST-Elevation Myocardial Infarction) developed in collaboration with the American College of Emergency Physicians, the Society for Cardiovascular Angiography and Interventions, and the Society of Thoracic Surgeons endorsed by the American Association of Cardiovascular and Pulmonary Rehabilitation and the Society for Academic Emergency Medicine. J Am Coll Cardiol 2007;50:e1–e157.

62. Antman EM, Hand M, Armstrong PW, et al. 2007 Focused Update of the ACC/AHA 2004 Guidelines for the Management of Patients With ST-Elevation Myocardial Infarction: A report of the American College of Cardiology/American Heart Association Task Force on Practice Guidelines: Developed in collaboration With the Canadian Cardiovascular Society endorsed by the American Academy of Family Physicians: 2007 Writing Group to Review New Evidence and Update the ACC/AHA 2004 Guidelines for the Management of Patients With ST-Elevation Myocardial Infarction, Writing on Behalf of the 2004 Writing Committee. Circulation 2008;117:296–329.

63. Baker WL, Coleman CI, Kluger J, et al. Systematic review: Comparative effectiveness of angiotensin-converting enzyme inhibitors or angiotensin II-receptor blockers for ischemic heart disease. Ann Intern Med 2009;151:861–871.

64. Bakris GL, Williams M, Dworkin L, et al. Preserving renal function in adults with hypertension and diabetes: A consensus approach. National Kidney Foundation Hypertension and Diabetes Executive Committees Working Group. Am J Kidney Dis 2000;36:646–661.

65. Pahor M, Psaty BM, Alderman MH, Applegate WB, Williamson JD, Furberg CD. Therapeutic benefits of ACE inhibitors and other antihypertensive drugs in patients with type 2 diabetes. Diabetes Care 2000;23:888–892.

66. National Kidney Foundation. K/DOQI clinical practice guidelines on hypertension and antihypertensive agents in chronic kidney disease. Am J Kidney Dis 2004;43:S1–S290.

67. Ruggenenti P, Perna A, Loriga G, et al. Blood-pressure control for renoprotection in patients with non-diabetic chronic renal disease (REIN-2): Multicentre, randomised controlled trial. Lancet 2005;365:939–946.

68. Wright JT, Jr., Bakris G, Greene T, et al. Effect of blood pressure lowering and antihypertensive drug class on progression of hypertensive kidney disease: Results from the AASK trial. JAMA 2002;288:2421–2431.

69. Casas JP, Chua W, Loukogeorgakis S, et al. Effect of inhibitors of the renin-angiotensin system and other antihypertensive drugs on renal outcomes: Systematic review and meta-analysis. Lancet 2005;366:2026–2033.

70. Sacco RL, Adams R, Albers G, et al. Guidelines for prevention of stroke in patients with ischemic stroke or transient ischemic attack: A statement for healthcare professionals from the American Heart Association/American Stroke Association Council on Stroke: Co-sponsored by the Council on Cardiovascular Radiology and Intervention: The American Academy of Neurology affirms the value of this guideline. Stroke 2006;37:577–617.

71. Schrader J, Luders S, Kulschewski A, et al. Morbidity and Mortality After Stroke, Eprosartan Compared with Nitrendipine for Secondary Prevention: Principal results of a prospective randomized controlled study (MOSES). Stroke 2005;36:1218–1226.

72. Yusuf S, Diener HC, Sacco RL, et al. Telmisartan to prevent recurrent stroke and cardiovascular events. N Engl J Med 2008;359:1225–1237.

73. Hyman DJ, Pavlik VN. Characteristics of patients with uncontrolled hypertension in the United States. N Engl J Med 2001;345:479–486.

74. Beckett NS, Peters R, Fletcher AE, et al. Treatment of hypertension in patients 80 years of age or older. N Engl J Med 2008;358:1887–1898.

75. Hansson L, Lindholm LH, Ekbom T, et al. Randomised trial of old and new antihypertensive drugs in elderly patients: Cardiovascular mortality and morbidity the Swedish Trial in Old Patients with Hypertension-2 study. Lancet 1999;354:1751–1756.

76. The fourth report on the diagnosis, evaluation, and treatment of high blood pressure in children and adolescents. Pediatrics 2004;114:555–576.

77. Roberts JM, Pearson G, Cutler J, Lindheimer M. Summary of the NHLBI Working Group on Research on Hypertension During Pregnancy. Hypertension 2003;41:437–445.

78. Cooper WO, Hernandez-Diaz S, Arbogast PG, et al. Major congenital malformations after first-trimester exposure to ACE inhibitors. N Engl J Med 2006;354:2443–2451.

79. Douglas JG, Bakris GL, Epstein M, et al. Management of high blood pressure in African Americans: Consensus statement of the Hypertension in African Americans Working Group of the International Society on Hypertension in Blacks. Arch Intern Med 2003;163:525–541.

80. Hirsch AT, Haskal ZJ, Hertzer NR, et al. ACC/AHA 2005 Practice Guidelines for the management of patients with peripheral arterial disease (lower extremity, renal, mesenteric, and abdominal aortic): A collaborative report from the American Association for Vascular Surgery/Society for Vascular Surgery, Society for Cardiovascular

Angiography and Interventions, Society for Vascular Medicine and Biology, Society of Interventional Radiology, and the ACC/AHA Task Force on Practice Guidelines (Writing Committee to Develop Guidelines for the Management of Patients With Peripheral Arterial Disease): Endorsed by the American Association of Cardiovascular and Pulmonary Rehabilitation; National Heart, Lung, and Blood Institute; Society for Vascular Nursing; TransAtlantic Inter-Society Consensus; and Vascular Disease Foundation. Circulation 2006;113:e463–e654.

81. Salpeter SR, Ormiston TM, Salpeter EE. Cardioselective beta-blockers in patients with reactive airway disease: A meta-analysis. Ann Intern Med 2002;137:715–725.

82. Elliott WJ, Meyer PM. Incident diabetes in clinical trials of antihypertensive drugs: A network meta-analysis. Lancet 2007;369:201–207.

83. Barksdale JD, Gardner SF. The impact of first-line antihypertensive drugs on erectile dysfunction. Pharmacotherapy 1999;19:573–581.

84. Ko DT, Hebert PR, Coffey CS, Sedrakyan A, Curtis JP, Krumholz HM. Beta-blocker therapy and symptoms of depression, fatigue, and sexual dysfunction. JAMA 2002;288:351–357.

85. Materson BJ, Reda DJ, Cushman WC, et al. Single-drug therapy for hypertension in men. A comparison of six antihypertensive agents with placebo. The Department of Veterans Affairs Cooperative Study Group on Antihypertensive Agents. N Engl J Med 1993;328:914–921.

86. Grimm RH, Jr., Grandits GA, Prineas RJ, et al. Long-term effects on sexual function of five antihypertensive drugs and nutritional hygienic treatment in hypertensive men and women. Treatment of Mild Hypertension Study (TOMHS). Hypertension 1997;29:8–14.

87. Ernst ME, Moser M. Use of diuretics in patients with hypertension. N Engl J Med 2009;361:2153–2164.

88. Chen JM, Heran BS, Wright JM. Blood pressure lowering efficacy of diuretics as second-line therapy for primary hypertension. Cochrane Database Syst Rev 2009:CD007187.

89. Dussol B, Moussi-Frances J, Morange S, Somma-Delpero C, Mundler O, Berland Y. A randomized trial of furosemide versus hydrochlorothiazide in patients with chronic renal failure and hypertension. Nephrol Dial Transplant 2005;20:349–353.

90. Carter BL, Ernst ME, Cohen JD. Hydrochlorothiazide versus chlorthalidone: Evidence supporting their interchangeability. Hypertension 2004;43:4–9.

91. Grimm RH, Jr., Flack JM, Grandits GA, et al. Long-term effects on plasma lipids of diet and drugs to treat hypertension. Treatment of Mild Hypertension Study (TOMHS) Research Group. JAMA 1996;275:1549–1556.

92. Zillich AJ, Garg J, Basu S, Bakris GL, Carter BL. Thiazide diuretics, potassium, and the development of diabetes: A quantitative review. Hypertension 2006;48:219–224.

93. Carter BL, Ernst ME. Thiazide-induced hyperglycemia: Can it be prevented? Am J Hypertens 2009;22:473.

94. Dagenais GR, Pogue J, Fox K, Simoons ML, Yusuf S. Angiotensin-converting-enzyme inhibitors in stable vascular disease without left ventricular systolic dysfunction or heart failure: A combined analysis of three trials. Lancet 2006;368:581–588.

95. Law MR, Wald NJ, Morris JK, Jordan RE. Value of low dose combination treatment with blood pressure lowering drugs: Analysis of 354 randomised trials. BMJ 2003;326:1427.

96. Yusuf S, Teo K, Anderson C, et al. Effects of the angiotensin-receptor blocker telmisartan on cardiovascular events in high-risk patients intolerant to angiotensin-converting enzyme inhibitors: A randomised controlled trial. Lancet 2008;372:1174–1183.

97. Yusuf S, Teo KK, Pogue J, et al. Telmisartan, ramipril, or both in patients at high risk for vascular events. N Engl J Med 2008;358:1547–1559.

98. Fournier A, Messerli FH, Achard JM, Fernandez L. Cerebroprotection mediated by angiotensin II: A hypothesis supported by recent randomized clinical trials. J Am Coll Cardiol 2004;43:1343–1347.

99. Leenen FH, Nwachuku CE, Black HR, et al. Clinical events in high-risk hypertensive patients randomly assigned to calcium channel blocker versus angiotensin-converting enzyme inhibitor in the antihypertensive and lipid-lowering treatment to prevent heart attack trial. Hypertension 2006;48:374–384.

100. UK Prospective Diabetes Study Group. Efficacy of atenolol and captopril in reducing risk of macrovascular and microvascular complications in type 2 diabetes: UKPDS 39. BMJ 1998;317:713–720.

101. Bakris GL, Fonseca V, Katholi RE, et al. Metabolic effects of carvedilol vs metoprolol in patients with type 2 diabetes mellitus and hypertension: A randomized controlled trial. JAMA 2004;292:2227–2236.

102. Staessen JA, Li Y, Richart T. Oral renin inhibitors. Lancet 2006;368:1449–1456.

103. Gradman AH, Vivas Y. New drugs for hypertension: What do they offer? Curr Hypertens Rep 2006;8:425–432.

104. Parving HH, Persson F, Lewis JB, Lewis EJ, Hollenberg NK. Aliskiren combined with losartan in type 2 diabetes and nephropathy. N Engl J Med 2008;358:2433–2446.

105. Edelson JT, Weinstein MC, Tosteson AN, Williams L, Lee TH, Goldman L. Long-term cost-effectiveness of various initial monotherapies for mild to moderate hypertension. JAMA 1990;263:407–413.

106. Fischer MA, Avorn J. Economic implications of evidence-based prescribing on hypertension: Can better care cost less? JAMA 2004;291:1850–1856.

107. Pearce KA, Furberg CD, Psaty BM, Kirk J. Cost-minimization and the number needed to treat in uncomplicated hypertension. Am J Hypertens 1998;11:618–629.

108. Carter BL, Rogers M, Daly J, Zheng S, James PA. The potency of team-based care interventions for hypertension: A meta-analysis. Arch Intern Med 2009;169:1748–1755.

109. Carter BL, Ardery G, Dawson JD, et al. Physician and pharmacist collaboration to improve blood pressure control. Arch Intern Med 2009;169:1996–2002.

110. McLean DL, McAlister FA, Johnson JA, et al. A randomized trial of the effect of community pharmacist and nurse care on improving blood pressure management in patients with diabetes mellitus: Study of cardiovascular risk intervention by pharmacists-hypertension (SCRIP-HTN). Arch Intern Med 2008;168:2355–2361.

111. Murray MD, Ritchey ME, Wu J, Tu W. Effect of a pharmacist on adverse drug events and medication errors in outpatients with cardiovascular disease. Arch Intern Med 2009;169:757–763.

112. Degli Esposti L, Valpiani G. Pharmacoeconomic burden of undertreating hypertension. Pharmacoeconomics 2004;22:907–928.

113. Mazzaglia G, Ambrosioni E, Alacqua M, et al. Adherence to antihypertensive medications and cardiovascular morbidity among newly diagnosed hypertensive patients. Circulation 2009;120:1598–1605.

114. Bangalore S, Shahane A, Parkar S, Messerli FH. Compliance and fixed-dose combination therapy. Curr Hypertens Rep 2007;9:184–189.

115. Jamerson K, Weber MA, Bakris GL, et al. Benazepril plus amlodipine or hydrochlorothiazide for hypertension in high-risk patients. N Engl J Med 2008;359:2417–2428.

116. Weber CA, Leloux MR, Carter BL, Farris KB, Xu Y. Reduction in adverse symptoms as blood pressure becomes controlled. Pharmacotherapy 2008;28:1104–1114.

117. Saseen JJ, Carter BL. Dual calcium-channel blocker therapy in the treatment of hypertension. Ann Pharmacother 1996;30:802–810.

118. Saseen JJ, Carter BL, Brown TE, Elliott WJ, Black HR. Comparison of nifedipine alone and with diltiazem or verapamil in hypertension. Hypertension 1996;28:109–114.

119. Bangalore S, Kamalakkannan G, Parkar S, Messerli FH. Fixed-dose combinations improve medication compliance: A meta-analysis. Am J Med 2007;120:713–719.

120. Calhoun DA, Jones D, Textor S, et al. Resistant hypertension: Diagnosis, evaluation, and treatment: A scientific statement from the American Heart Association Professional Education Committee of the Council for High Blood Pressure Research. Circulation 2008;117:e510–e526.

121. Moser M, Setaro JF. Clinical practice. Resistant or difficult-to-control hypertension. N Engl J Med 2006;355:385–392.

122. Grossman E, Messerli FH, Grodzicki T, Kowey P. Should a moratorium be placed on sublingual nifedipine capsules given for hypertensive emergencies and pseudoemergencies? JAMA 1996;276:1328–1331.

20

Systolic Heart Failure

ROBERT B. PARKER AND LARISA H. CAVALLARI

KEY CONCEPTS

❶ Heart failure is a clinical syndrome caused by the inability of the heart to pump sufficient blood to meet the metabolic needs of the body. It can result from any disorder that reduces ventricular filling (diastolic dysfunction) and/or myocardial contractility (systolic dysfunction). The leading causes of heart failure are coronary artery disease and hypertension. The primary manifestations of the syndrome are dyspnea, fatigue, and fluid retention.

❷ Heart failure is a progressive disorder that begins with myocardial injury. In response to the injury, several compensatory responses are activated in an attempt to maintain adequate cardiac output, including activation of the sympathetic nervous system (SNS) and the renin—angiotensin—aldosterone system (RAAS), resulting in vasoconstriction and sodium and water retention, as well as ventricular hypertrophy/remodeling. These compensatory mechanisms are responsible for the symptoms of heart failure and contribute to disease progression.

❸ Our current understanding of heart failure pathophysiology is best described by the neurohormonal model. Activation of endogenous neurohormones, including norepinephrine, angiotensin II, aldosterone, vasopressin, and numerous proinflammatory cytokines, plays an important role in ventricular remodeling and the subsequent progression of heart failure. Pharmacotherapy targeted at antagonizing this neurohormonal activation has slowed the progression of heart failure and improved survival.

❹ Most patients with symptomatic heart failure should be routinely treated with an angiotensin-converting enzyme (ACE) inhibitor, a β-blocker, and a diuretic. The benefits of these medications on slowing heart failure progression, reducing morbidity and mortality, and improving symptoms are clearly established. Patients should be treated with a diuretic if there is evidence of fluid retention. Treatment with digoxin may also be considered to improve symptoms and reduce hospitalizations.

❺ In patients with heart failure, ACE inhibitors improve survival, slow disease progression, reduce hospitalizations, and improve quality of life. The doses for these agents should be targeted at those shown in clinical trials to improve survival.

Learning objectives, review questions, and other resources can be found at **www.pharmacotherapyonline.com**.

When ACE inhibitors are contraindicated or not tolerated, an angiotensin II receptor blocker and the combination of hydralazine and isosorbide dinitrate are reasonable alternatives. Patients with asymptomatic left ventricular dysfunction and/or a previous myocardial infarction (MI; stage B of the American College of Cardiology/American Heart Association [ACC/AHA] classification scheme) should also receive ACE inhibitors, with the goal of preventing symptomatic heart failure and reducing mortality.

❻ The β-blockers carvedilol, metoprolol controlled release/extended release (CR/XL), and bisoprolol have been shown to prolong survival, decrease hospitalizations and the need for transplantation, and cause "reverse remodeling" of the left ventricle. These agents are recommended for all patients with a reduced left ventricular ejection fraction. Therapy must be instituted at low doses, with slow upward titration to the target dose.

❼ Although chronic diuretic therapy frequently is used in patients with heart failure, it is not mandatory. Diuretic therapy, along with sodium restriction, is required only in those patients with peripheral edema and/or pulmonary congestion. Many patients will need continued diuretic therapy to maintain euvolemia after fluid overload is resolved.

❽ Digoxin does not improve survival in patients with heart failure but does provide symptomatic benefits. Digoxin doses should be adjusted to achieve plasma concentrations of 0.5 to 1.0 ng/mL; higher plasma concentrations are not associated with additional benefits but may be associated with increased risk of toxicity.

❾ Aldosterone antagonism with low-dose spironolactone has been shown to reduce mortality in patients with New York Heart Association (NYHA) class III and IV heart failure and thus should be strongly considered in these patients provided that potassium levels and renal function can be carefully monitored. Aldosterone antagonists should also be considered soon after MI in patients with left ventricular dysfunction and either heart failure or diabetes.

❿ The combination of hydralazine and nitrates has been shown to improve the composite endpoint of mortality, hospitalizations for heart failure, and quality of life in African Americans receiving standard therapy. Current guidelines recommend the addition of hydralazine and nitrates to self-described African Americans with moderate to severe symptoms despite therapy with ACE inhibitors, diuretics, and β-blockers. This combination is also reasonable to consider in all patients who continue to have symptoms despite optimized therapy with an ACE inhibitor (or angiotensin receptor blocker [ARB]) and β-blocker. Hydralazine and a nitrate might be reasonable in patients unable to tolerate either an ACE inhibitor or an ARB because of renal insufficiency, hyperkalemia, or hypotension.

⓫ Pharmacists should play an important role as part of a multidisciplinary team to optimize therapy in heart failure. They should be responsible for such activities as optimizing regimens for heart failure drug therapy (namely, ensuring that appropriate drugs at appropriate doses are used), educating patients about the importance of adherence to their heart failure regimen (including pharmacologic and dietary interventions), screening for drugs that may exacerbate or worsen heart failure, and monitoring for adverse drug effects and drug interactions.

❶ ❷ Heart failure is a progressive clinical syndrome that can result from any abnormality in cardiac structure or function that impairs the ability of the ventricle to fill with or eject blood, thus rendering the heart unable to pump blood at a rate sufficient to meet the metabolic demands of the body.[1] It is the final common pathway for numerous cardiac disorders, including those affecting the pericardium, heart valves, and myocardium. Diseases that adversely affect ventricular diastole (filling), ventricular systole (contraction), or both can lead to heart failure. For many years it was believed that reduced myocardial contractility, or systolic dysfunction (i.e., reduced left ventricular ejection fraction [LVEF]), was the sole disturbance in cardiac function responsible for heart failure. However, it is now recognized that large numbers of patients with the heart failure syndrome have relatively normal systolic function (i.e., normal LVEF). This is now referred to as heart failure with preserved LVEF and is believed to be primarily due to diastolic dysfunction of the heart.[1] Recent estimates suggest approximately 50% of patients with heart failure have preserved LVEF with disturbances in relaxation (lusitropic) properties of the heart, or diastolic dysfunction.[2] However, regardless of the etiology of heart failure, the underlying pathophysiologic process and principal clinical manifestations (fatigue, dyspnea, and volume overload) are similar and appear to be independent of the initial cause. Historically, this disorder was commonly referred to as *congestive heart failure*; the preferred nomenclature is now *heart failure*, because a patient may have the clinical syndrome of heart failure without having symptoms of congestion. This chapter will focus on treatment of patients with systolic heart failure due to systolic dysfunction (with or without concurrent diastolic dysfunction). Chapters 21 and 22 discuss the treatment of heart failure with preserved LVEF (diastolic dysfunction) and acute decompensated heart failure, respectively.

EPIDEMIOLOGY

Heart failure is an epidemic public health problem in the United States. Nearly 6 million Americans have heart failure, with an additional 670,000 cases diagnosed each year.[3] Unlike most other cardiovascular diseases, the incidence, prevalence, and hospitalization rates associated with heart failure are increasing and are expected to continue to increase over the next few decades as the population ages. A large majority of patients with heart failure are elderly, with multiple comorbid conditions that influence morbidity and mortality.[3,4] The incidence of heart failure doubles with each decade of life and affects nearly 10% of individuals over age 75. Improved survival after myocardial infarction (MI) is thought to be a likely contributor to the increased incidence and prevalence of

heart failure.[4] Heart failure is the most common hospital discharge diagnosis in individuals over age 65. Annual hospital discharges for heart failure now total over 1 million, a 174% increase over the last 2 decades.[3] Heart failure also has a tremendous economic impact, with this expected to increase markedly as the baby boom generation ages. Current estimates suggest annual expenditures for heart failure of approximately $37 billion, with the majority of these costs spent on hospitalized patients.[3] In the United States, over $3 billion is spent annually on drug therapy for heart failure.[3] Thus, heart failure is a major medical problem, with a substantial economic impact that is expected to become even more significant as the population ages.

Despite prodigious advances in our understanding of the etiology, pathophysiology, and pharmacotherapy of heart failure, the prognosis for patients with this disorder remains grim. Although the mortality rates have declined over the past 50 years, the overall 5-year survival remains approximately 50% for all patients with a diagnosis of heart failure, with mortality increasing with symptom severity.[5] For patients under age 65, 80% of men and 70% of women will die within 8 years. Death is classified as sudden in about 40% of patients, implicating serious ventricular arrhythmias as the underlying cause in many patients.[1,5] Factors affecting the prognosis of patients with heart failure include, but are not limited to, age, gender, LVEF, renal function, diabetes, anemia, extent of underlying coronary artery disease, blood pressure, heart failure etiology, and drug or device therapy. Recent models incorporating these and other factors enable clinicians to develop reliable estimates of an individual patient's prognosis.[6,7]

ETIOLOGY

❶ ❷ Heart failure can result from any disorder that affects the ability of the heart to contract (systolic function) and/or relax (diastolic dysfunction); common causes of heart failure are shown in Table 20-1.[8] Heart failure with impaired systolic function (i.e., reduced LVEF) is the classic, more familiar form of the disorder, but current estimates suggest up to 50% of patients with heart failure have preserved left ventricular systolic function with presumed diastolic dysfunction.[2] In contrast to systolic heart failure that is usually caused by previous MI, patients with preserved LVEF typically are elderly, female, obese, and have hypertension, atrial fibrillation, or diabetes.[2] Recent data indicate that survival is similar in patients with impaired or preserved LVEF.[2] Common cardiovascular diseases such as MI and hypertension can cause both

TABLE 20-1	Causes of Heart Failure

Systolic dysfunction (decreased contractility)
- Reduction in muscle mass (e.g., myocardial infarction)
- Dilated cardiomyopathies
- Ventricular hypertrophy
  - Pressure overload (e.g., systemic or pulmonary hypertension, and aortic or pulmonic valve stenosis)
  - Volume overload (e.g., valvular regurgitation, shunts, and high-output states)

Diastolic dysfunction (restriction in ventricular filling)
- Increased ventricular stiffness
  - Ventricular hypertrophy (e.g., hypertrophic cardiomyopathy; other examples above)
  - Infiltrative myocardial diseases (e.g., amyloidosis, sarcoidosis, and endomyocardial fibrosis)
  - Myocardial ischemia and infarction
- Mitral or tricuspid valve stenosis
- Pericardial disease (e.g., pericarditis and pericardial tamponade)

systolic and diastolic dysfunction; thus, many patients have heart failure as a result of reduced myocardial contractility and abnormal ventricular filling. Heart failure with preserved LVEF is discussed in Chapter 21.

❶ Coronary artery disease is the most common cause of systolic heart failure, accounting for nearly 70% of cases.[4] MI leads to reduction in muscle mass due to the death of affected myocardial cells. The degree to which contractility is impaired will depend on the size of the infarction. In an attempt to maintain cardiac output, the surviving myocardium undergoes a compensatory remodeling, thus beginning the maladaptive process that initiates heart failure syndrome and leads to further injury to the heart. This is discussed in greater detail in the Pathophysiology section. Myocardial ischemia and infarction also affect the diastolic properties of the heart by increasing ventricular stiffness and slowing ventricular relaxation. Thus, MI frequently results in systolic and diastolic dysfunction.

Impaired systolic function is a cardinal feature of dilated cardiomyopathies. Although the cause of reduced contractility frequently is unknown, abnormalities such as interstitial fibrosis, cellular infiltrates, cellular hypertrophy, and myocardial cell degeneration are seen commonly on histologic examination. Genetic causes of dilated cardiomyopathies may also occur.[9]

Pressure or volume overload causes ventricular hypertrophy, which attempts to return contractility to a near-normal state. If the pressure or volume overload persists, the remodeling process results in alterations in the geometry of the hypertrophied myocardial cells and is accompanied by increased collagen deposition in the extracellular matrix. Thus, both systolic and diastolic function may be impaired.[8] Examples of pressure overload include systemic or pulmonary hypertension and aortic or pulmonic valve stenosis.

Hypertension remains an important cause and/or contributor to heart failure in many patients, particularly women, the elderly, and African Americans.[1] The role of hypertension should not be underestimated because hypertension is an important risk factor for ischemic heart disease and thus is also present in a high percentage of patients with this disorder. A recent analysis emphasized that heart failure is a largely preventable disorder. Modifiable risk factors such as uncontrolled hypertension, coronary heart disease, smoking, and chronic kidney disease are strongly associated with increased risk of heart failure.[10] Thus, appropriate management of cardiovascular risk is key to minimizing the risk of heart failure development.

the Frank-Starling mechanism, the ability of the heart to alter the force of contraction depends on changes in preload. As myocardial sarcomere length is stretched, the number of cross-bridges between thick and thin myofilaments increases, resulting in an increase in the force of contraction. The length of the sarcomere is determined primarily by the volume of blood in the ventricle; therefore, left ventricular end-diastolic volume (LVEDV) is the primary determinant of preload. In normal hearts, the preload response is the primary compensatory mechanism such that a small increase in end-diastolic volume results in a large increase in cardiac output. Because of the relationship between pressure and volume in the heart, left ventricular end-diastolic pressure (LVEDP) is often used in the clinical setting to estimate preload. The hemodynamic measurement used to estimate LVEDP is the pulmonary artery occlusion pressure (PAOP). Afterload is a more complex physiologic concept that can be viewed pragmatically as the sum of forces preventing active forward ejection of blood by the ventricle. Major components of global ventricular afterload are ejection impedance, wall tension, and regional wall geometry. In patients with left ventricular systolic dysfunction, an inverse relationship exists between afterload (or SVR) and stroke volume such that increasing afterload causes a decrease in stroke volume (Fig. 20–1). Contractility is the intrinsic property of cardiac muscle describing fiber shortening and tension development.

COMPENSATORY MECHANISMS IN HEART FAILURE

❷ Heart failure is a progressive disorder initiated by an event that impairs the ability of the heart to contract and/or relax, resulting in a decrease in cardiac output. The index event may have an acute onset, as with MI, or the onset may be slow, as with long-standing hypertension. Regardless of the index event, the decrease in the heart's pumping capacity results in the heart having to rely on compensatory responses to maintain an adequate cardiac output.[11] These compensatory responses include (a) tachycardia and increased contractility through sympathetic nervous system (SNS) activation; (b) the Frank-Starling mechanism, whereby an increase in preload results in an increase in stroke volume; (c) vasoconstriction; and (d) ventricular hypertrophy and remodeling. Compensatory responses are intended to provide short-term support to maintain circulatory homeostasis after acute reductions in blood pressure or renal perfusion. However, the persistent decline in cardiac output in heart failure leads to long-term activation of these compensatory

PATHOPHYSIOLOGY

NORMAL CARDIAC FUNCTION

To understand the pathophysiologic processes in heart failure, a basic understanding of normal cardiac function is necessary. *Cardiac output* (CO) is defined as the volume of blood ejected per unit time (L/min) and is the product of heart rate (HR) and stroke volume (SV):

$$CO = HR \times SV$$

The relationship between CO and mean arterial pressure (MAP) is

$$MAP = CO \times \text{systemic vascular resistance (SVR)}$$

Heart rate is controlled by the autonomic nervous system. Stroke volume, or the volume of blood ejected during systole, depends on preload, afterload, and contractility.[8] As defined by

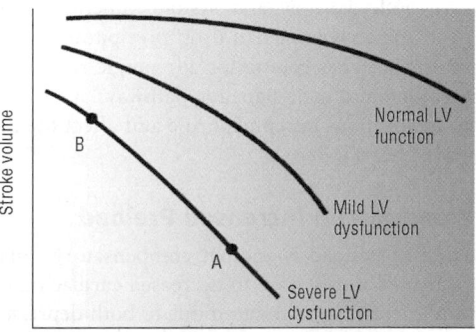

FIGURE 20-1. Relationship between stroke volume and systemic vascular resistance. In an individual with normal left ventricular (LV) function, increasing systemic vascular resistance has little effect on stroke volume. As the extent of LV dysfunction increases, the negative, inverse relationship between stroke volume and systemic vascular resistance becomes more important (*B* to *A*).

TABLE 20-2 Beneficial and Detrimental Effects of the Compensatory Responses in Heart Failure

Compensatory Response	Beneficial Effects of Compensation	Detrimental Effects of Compensation
Increased preload (through Na+ and water retention)	Optimize stroke volume via Frank-Starling mechanism	Pulmonary and systemic congestion and edema formation Increased MVO_2
Vasoconstriction	Maintain BP in face of reduced CO Shunt blood from nonessential organs to brain and heart	Increased MVO_2 Increased afterload decreases stroke volume and further activates the compensatory responses
Tachycardia and increased contractility (due to SNS activation)	Helps maintain CO	Increased MVO_2 Shortened diastolic filling time β_1-receptor downregulation, decreased receptor sensitivity Precipitation of ventricular arrhythmias Increased risk of myocardial cell
Ventricular hypertrophy and remodeling	Helps maintain CO Reduces myocardial wall stress Decreases MVO_2	Diastolic dysfunction Systolic dysfunction Increased risk of myocardial cell death Increased risk of myocardial ischemia Increased arrhythmia risk Fibrosis

Abbreviations: BP, blood pressure; CO, cardiac output; MVO_2, myocardial oxygen demand; SNS, sympathetic nervous system.

responses, resulting in the complex functional, structural, biochemical, and molecular changes important for the development and progression of heart failure. The beneficial and detrimental effects of these compensatory responses are described later in this chapter and are summarized in Table 20–2.

Tachycardia and Increased Contractility

The change in heart rate and contractility that rapidly occurs in response to a drop in cardiac output is primarily due to the release of norepinephrine from adrenergic nerve terminals, although parasympathetic nervous system activity is also diminished. Cardiac output increases with heart rate until diastolic filling becomes compromised, which in the normal heart is at 170 to 200 beats per minute. Loss of atrial contribution to ventricular filling also can occur (atrial fibrillation, ventricular tachycardia), reducing ventricular performance even more. Because ionized calcium is sequestered into the sarcoplasmic reticulum and pumped out of the cell during diastole, shortened diastolic time also results in a higher average intracellular calcium concentration during diastole, increasing actin—myosin interaction, augmenting the active resistance to fibril stretch, and reducing lusitropy. Conversely, the higher average calcium concentration translates into greater filament interaction during systole, generating more tension.[8] Increasing heart rate greatly increases myocardial oxygen demand. If ischemia is induced or worsened, both diastolic and systolic function may become impaired, and stroke volume can drop precipitously. In addition, polymorphisms in genes coding for adrenergic receptors (e.g., β_1 and α_{2c} receptors) and their signaling pathways appear to alter the response to endogenous norepinephrine and affect the risk for the development of heart failure.[12,13]

Fluid Retention and Increased Preload

Augmentation of preload is another compensatory response that is rapidly activated in response to decreased cardiac output. Renal perfusion in heart failure is reduced due to both depressed cardiac output and redistribution of blood away from nonvital organs. The kidney interprets the reduced perfusion as an ineffective blood volume, resulting in activation of the renin—angiotensin—aldosterone system (RAAS) in an attempt to maintain blood pressure and increase renal sodium and water retention. Reduced renal perfusion and increased sympathetic tone also stimulate renin release from juxtaglomerular cells in the kidney. As shown in Figure 20–2, renin

is responsible for conversion of angiotensinogen to angiotensin I. Angiotensin I is converted to angiotensin II by angiotensin-converting enzyme (ACE). Angiotensin II may also be generated via non-ACE-dependent pathways. Angiotensin II stimulates aldosterone release from the adrenal gland, thereby providing an additional mechanism for renal sodium and water retention. As intravascular volume increases secondary to sodium and water retention, left ventricular volume and pressure (preload) increase, sarcomeres are stretched, and the force of contraction is enhanced.[8] Although the preload response is the primary compensatory mechanism in normal hearts, the chronically failing heart usually has exhausted its preload reserve.[8] As shown in Figure 20–3, increases in preload will increase stroke volume only to a certain point. Once the flat portion of the curve is reached, further increases in preload will only lead to pulmonary or systemic congestion, a detrimental result.[8] Figure 20–3 also shows that the curve is flatter in patients with left ventricular dysfunction. Consequently, a given increase in preload in a patient with heart failure will produce a smaller increment in stroke volume than in an individual with normal ventricular function.

Vasoconstriction and Increased Afterload

Vasoconstriction occurs in patients with heart failure to help redistribute blood flow away from nonessential organs to coronary and cerebral circulations to support blood pressure, which may be reduced secondary to a decrease in cardiac output (MAP = CO × SVR).[8] A number of neurohormones likely contribute to the vasoconstriction, including norepinephrine, angiotensin II, endothelin-1, neuropeptide Y, and arginine vasopressin (AVP).[8,14] Vasoconstriction impedes forward ejection of blood from the ventricle, further depressing cardiac output and heightening the compensatory responses. Because the failing ventricle usually has exhausted its preload reserve (unless the patient is intravascularly depleted), its performance is exquisitely sensitive to changes in afterload (Fig. 20–1). Thus, increases in afterload often potentiate a vicious cycle of continued worsening and downward spiraling of the heart failure state.

Ventricular Hypertrophy and Remodeling

❸ Although the signs and symptoms of heart failure are closely associated with the items described above, the progression of heart failure appears to be independent of the patient's hemodynamic

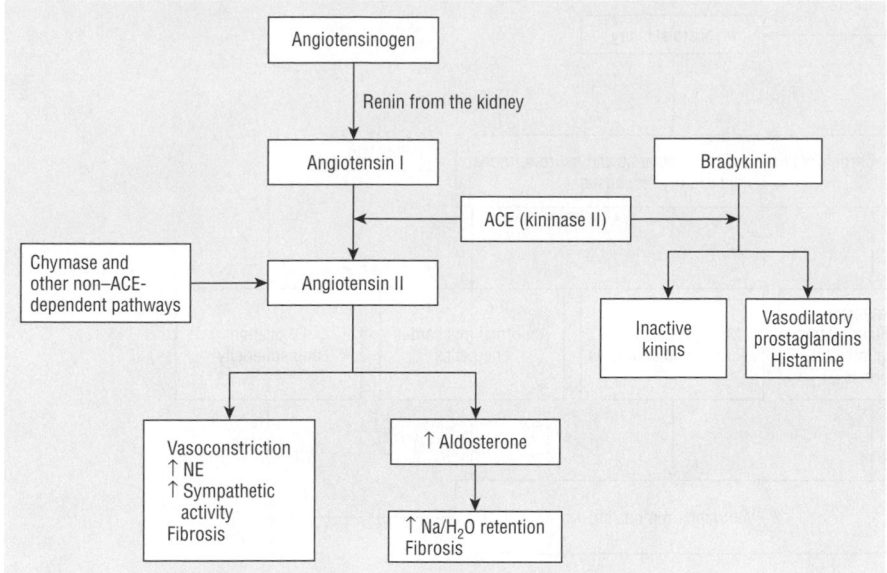

FIGURE 20-2. Physiology of the renin-angiotensin-aldosterone system. Renin produces angiotensin I from angiotensinogen. Angiotensin I is cleaved to angiotensin II by angiotensin-converting enzyme (ACE). Angiotensin II has a number of physiologic actions that are detrimental in heart failure. Note that angiotensin II can be produced in a number of tissues, including the heart, independent of ACE activity. ACE is also responsible for the breakdown of bradykinin. Inhibition of ACE results in accumulation of bradykinin that, in turn, enhances the production of vasodilatory prostaglandins. (NE, norepinephrine.)

status. It is now recognized that ventricular hypertrophy and remodeling are key components in the pathogenesis of progressive myocardial failure.[8,11] *Ventricular hypertrophy* is a term used to describe an increase in ventricular muscle mass. *Cardiac or ventricular remodeling* is a broader term describing changes in both myocardial cells and extracellular matrix that result in changes in the size, shape, structure, and function of the heart. These progressive changes in ventricular structure and function ultimately result in a change in the shape of the left ventricle from an ellipse to a sphere. This change in ventricular size and shape serves to further depress the mechanical performance of the heart, increases regurgitant flow through the mitral valve, and, in turn, fuels the continued progression of remodeling. Ventricular hypertrophy and remodeling can occur in association with any condition that causes myocardial injury, including MI, cardiomyopathy, hypertension, and valvular heart disease. The onset of the remodeling process precedes the development of heart failure symptoms.

Cardiac remodeling is a complex process that affects the heart at the molecular and cellular level. Key elements in the process are shown in Figure 20–4. Collectively, these events result in

progressive changes in myocardial structure and function, such as cardiac hypertrophy, myocyte loss, and alterations in the extracellular matrix. The progression of the remodeling process leads to reductions in myocardial systolic and/or diastolic function that, in turn, result in further myocardial injury, perpetuating the remodeling process and the decline in ventricular dysfunction. Angiotensin II, norepinephrine, endothelin, aldosterone, vasopressin, and numerous inflammatory cytokines, as well as substances under investigation that are activated both systemically and locally in the heart and vasculature, play an important role in initiating the signal-transduction cascade responsible for ventricular remodeling. Although these mediators produce deleterious effects on the heart, their increased circulating and tissue concentrations play important roles in other organs, such as the brain, that serve to sustain the heart failure syndrome.[15] This serves as an important reminder that heart failure is a systemic as well as a cardiac disorder.

Pressure overload (and probably hormonal activation) associated with hypertension produces a concentric hypertrophy (increase in the ventricular wall thickness without chamber enlargement). Conversely, eccentric left ventricular hypertrophy (myocyte lengthening with increased chamber size with minimal increase in wall thickness) characterizes the hypertrophy seen in patients with systolic dysfunction or previous MI. As the myocytes undergo change, so do various components of the extracellular matrix. For example, there is evidence for collagen degradation, which may lead to slippage of myocytes, fibroblast proliferation, and increased fibrillar collagen synthesis, resulting in fibrosis and stiffening of the entire myocardium. Thus, a number of important ventricular changes that occur with remodeling include changes in the geometry of the heart from an elliptical to spherical shape, increases in ventricular mass (from myocyte hypertrophy), and changes in ventricular composition (especially the extracellar matrix) and volumes, all of which likely contribute to the impairment of cardiac function. If the event that produces cardiac injury is acute (e.g., MI), the ventricular remodeling process begins immediately. However, it is the progressive nature of this process that results in continual worsening of the heart failure state, and thus is now the major focus for identification of therapeutic targets. In fact, it is believed that all the heart failure therapies that have been associated with decreased mortality and/or slowing of the progression of the disease produce this effect largely through their ability to slow or reverse the ventricular remodeling

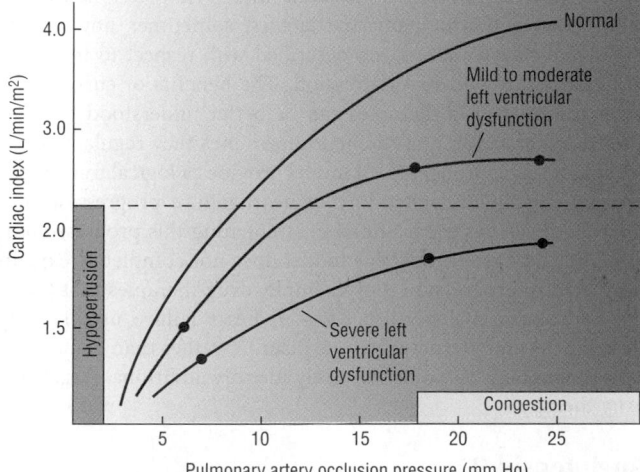

FIGURE 20-3. Relationship between cardiac output (shown as cardiac index, which is cardiac output [CO]/body surface area [BSA]) and preload (shown as pulmonary artery occlusion pressure).

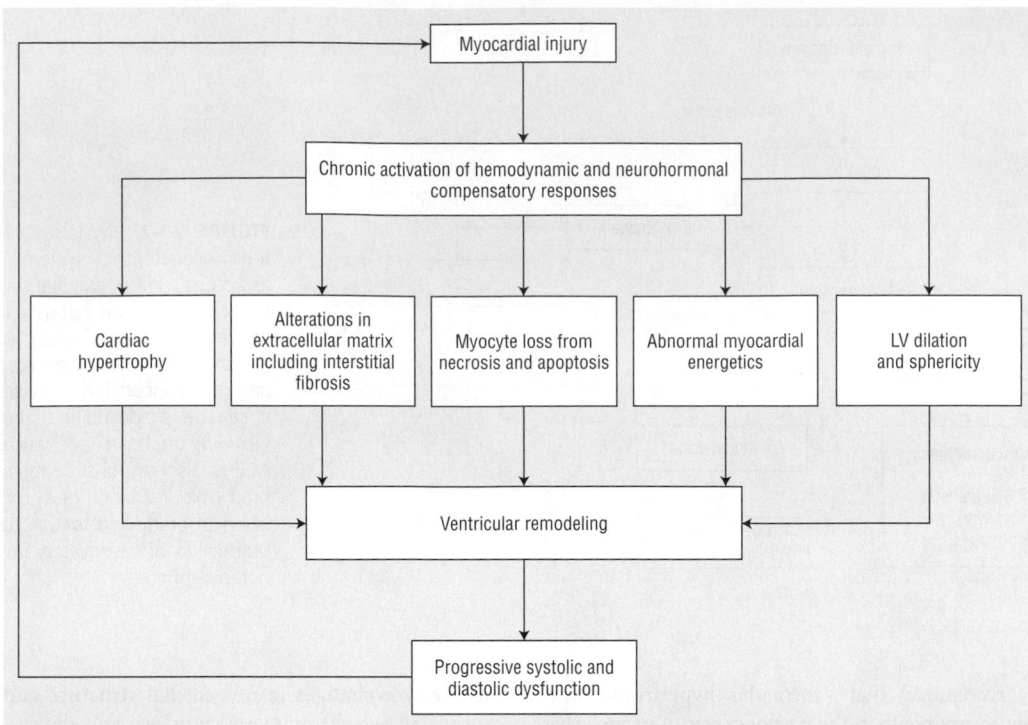

FIGURE 20-4. Key components of the pathophysiology of cardiac remodeling. Myocardial injury (e.g., myocardial infarction) results in the activation of a number of hemodynamic and neurohormonal compensatory responses in an attempt to maintain circulatory homeostasis. Chronic activation of the neurohormonal systems results in a cascade of events that affect the myocardium at the molecular and cellular levels. These events lead to the changes in ventricular size, shape, structure, and function known as ventricular remodeling. The alterations in ventricular function result in further deterioration in cardiac systolic and diastolic function, which further promotes the remodeling process. (LV, left ventricular.)

process, a process often referred to as *reverse remodeling.* Thus, while ventricular hypertrophy and remodeling may have some beneficial effects by helping maintain cardiac output, they also are believed to play an essential role in the progressive nature of heart failure.

THE NEUROHORMONAL MODEL OF HEART FAILURE AND THE THERAPEUTIC INSIGHTS IT PROVIDES

❷ ❸ Over the years, several different paradigms have guided our understanding of the pathophysiology and treatment of heart failure.[8,11,16] The early paradigm, often called the *cardiorenal model,* viewed the problem as excess sodium and water retention, and diuretic therapy was the main therapeutic approach. The next paradigm, the *cardiocirculatory model,* focused on impaired cardiac output (viewed as being due to both the reduced pumping capacity of the heart and systemic vasoconstriction). This paradigm focused on positive inotropes and, later, vasodilators as the primary therapies to overcome reductions in cardiac output. Although the therapeutic approaches associated with these paradigms provided some symptomatic benefits to patients with heart failure, they did little to slow progression of the disease. In fact, the detrimental effects of positive inotropic drugs on survival highlighted the inadequacy of the cardiocirculatory model to explain the progressive nature of heart failure. Initial studies with ACE inhibitors were conducted with the thought that they might be effective due to their balanced (arterial and venous) vasodilation. Subsequent realization that ACE inhibitors were providing benefit beyond their vasodilating effects, followed by the positive results with β-adrenergic receptor blockers and aldosterone antagonists, has led to the current paradigm used to describe heart

failure: the *neurohormonal model.* This model recognizes that there is an initiating event (e.g., MI, long-standing hypertension) that leads to decreased cardiac output and begins the "heart failure state." Subsequently, the problem moves beyond the heart, and it becomes a systemic disease whose progression is mediated largely by neurohormones and autocrine/paracrine factors that drive myocyte injury, oxidative stress, inflammation, and extracellular-matrix remodeling. Although the former paradigms still guide us to some extent in the symptomatic management of the disease (e.g., diuretics and digoxin), it is the latter paradigm that helps us understand disease progression, in particular, the ways to slow disease progression. In the sections that follow, key neurohormones and autocrine/paracrine factors, sometimes now collectively termed *biomarkers,* are described with respect to their role in heart failure and its progression. The benefits of current and investigational drug therapies can be better understood through a solid understanding of the neurohormones they regulate/affect. Although the neurohormonal model provides a logical framework for our current understanding of heart failure progression and the role of various medications in attenuating this progression, it must be emphasized that this model does not completely explain heart failure progression. For example, drug therapies that target the neurohormonal perturbations in heart failure usually only slow the progressive nature of the disorder rather than completely stop it. Ongoing research will likely identify additional targets for drug therapy.

Angiotensin II

Of the neurohormones and autocrine/paracrine factors that play an important role in the pathophysiology of heart failure, angiotensin II is probably the best understood.[8,11] Although circulating angiotensin II produced from ACE activity is the most familiar route for generation of angiotensin II, recent evidence indicates that this hormone is synthesized directly in the myocardium through non-ACE-dependent pathways. This tissue production of angiotensin II also plays an important role in heart failure pathophysiology. Angiotensin II has multiple actions that contribute to its detrimental effects in heart failure. It increases systemic vascular resistance directly by binding to the angiotensin I receptor in the vasculature and promoting potent vasoconstriction and indirectly by causing release of AVP and endothelin-1. Angiotensin II also facilitates the release of norepinephrine from adrenergic nerve terminals, heightening SNS activation. It promotes sodium retention through direct effects on the renal tubules and by stimulating aldosterone release. Its vasoconstriction of the efferent glomerular arteriole helps to maintain perfusion pressure in patients with severe heart failure or impaired renal function. Thus, in patients dependent on angiotensin II for maintenance of perfusion pressure, initiation of an ACE inhibitor or a type I angiotensin receptor blocker (ARB) causes efferent arteriole vasodilation, decreased perfusion pressure, and decreased glomerular filtration. This explains the risk of transient impairment in renal function associated with initiation of ACE inhibitor or ARB therapy. Finally, angiotensin II and many of the neurohormones released in response to angiotensin II play a central role in stimulating ventricular hypertrophy, remodeling, myocyte apoptosis (programmed cell death), oxidative stress, inflammation, and alterations in the extracellular matrix. Clinical data suggest that blocking angiotensin II-mediated effects contributes substantially to the prolonged survival of patients treated with ACE inhibitors and ARBs.[17,18] The favorable effects of ACE inhibitors and ARBs on hemodynamics, symptoms, quality of life, and survival in heart failure highlight the importance of angiotensin II in the pathophysiology of heart failure.

Norepinephrine

Many of the detrimental effects of norepinephrine in heart failure are described earlier in this chapter. Norepinephrine plays a central role in the tachycardia, vasoconstriction, and increased contractility observed in heart failure. It also plays a role in the increased plasma renin activity seen in heart failure. Plasma norepinephrine concentrations are elevated in correlation with the degree of heart failure, and patients with the highest concentrations have the poorest prognosis.[8,11,14] In addition to the detrimental effects described, excessive SNS activation causes downregulation of β_1-receptors, with a subsequent loss of sensitivity to receptor stimulation. Evidence suggests that genetic variations in the β_1- and α_{2c}-receptors, which are targets for norepinephrine's actions, may modify the extent of receptor downregulation and increase the risk of heart failure.[12,13] Excess catecholamines increase the risk of arrhythmias and can cause myocardial cell loss by stimulating both necrosis and apoptosis. Finally, norepinephrine contributes to ventricular hypertrophy and remodeling. The detrimental effects of SNS activation are further highlighted by the clinical trials of chronic therapy with β-agonists, phosphodiesterase inhibitors, or other drugs that cause SNS activation, as they have been shown uniformly to increase mortality in heart failure. Conversely, β-blockers, ACE inhibitors, and digoxin all help to decrease SNS activation, through various mechanisms, and are beneficial in heart failure. Thus, it is clear that norepinephrine plays a critical role in the pathophysiology of the heart failure state.

Aldosterone

Aldosterone-mediated sodium retention and its key role in volume overload and edema have long been recognized as important components of the heart failure syndrome.[19,20] Circulating aldosterone is increased in heart failure due to stimulation of its synthesis and release from the adrenal cortex by angiotensin II and to decreased hepatic clearance secondary to reduced hepatic perfusion. Although its enhancement of sodium retention is an important component of heart failure symptoms, recent studies indicate the direct effects of aldosterone on the heart that may be even more important in heart failure pathophysiology. Chief among these is the ability of aldosterone to produce interstitial cardiac fibrosis through increased collagen deposition in the extracellular matrix of the heart. This cardiac fibrosis may decrease systolic function and impair diastolic function by increasing the stiffness of the myocardium. Current research shows that extra-adrenal production of aldosterone in the heart, kidneys, and vascular smooth muscle also contributes to the progressive nature of heart failure through target organ fibrosis and vascular remodeling. Induction of a systemic proinflammatory state, increased oxidative stress, wasting of soft tissues and bone, secondary hyperparathyroidism, and mineral/micronutrient dyshomeostasis are other important pathological actions of aldosterone that directly contribute to ventricular remodeling and heart failure progression.[21] Aldosterone also may increase the risk of ventricular arrhythmias through a number of mechanisms, including creation of reentrant circuits as a result of fibrosis, inhibition of cardiac norepinephrine reuptake, depletion of intracellular potassium and magnesium, and impairment of parasympathetic traffic. Other recently identified detrimental effects of aldosterone are insulin resistance and endothelial and baroreceptor dysfunction. Recent studies demonstrate that the aldosterone antagonists spironolactone[22] and eplerenone[23] produce significant reductions in mortality in patients with heart failure, without appreciable effects on diuresis or hemodynamics, providing substantial evidence that the direct cardiac effects of aldosterone play an important role in heart failure pathophysiology.

Natriuretic Peptides

The natriuretic peptide family has three members: atrial natriuretic peptide (ANP), B-type natriuretic peptide (BNP), and C-type natriuretic peptide (CNP).[24–26] ANP is stored mainly in the right atrium, whereas BNP is found primarily in the ventricles. Both are released in response to pressure or volume overload. CNP is found mainly in the brain and has very low plasma concentrations. ANP and BNP plasma concentrations are elevated in patients with heart failure and are thought to balance the effects of the RAAS by causing natriuresis, diuresis, vasodilation, decreased aldosterone release, decreased hypertrophy, and inhibition of the SNS and RAAS.

The development of easily performed commercial assays for BNP and the related biologically inactive peptide, NT-proBNP, resulted in significant attention to the role of these peptides as a biomarker for prognostic, diagnostic, and therapeutic use. In patients with systolic heart failure, the degree of elevation in BNP levels is closely associated with increased mortality, risk of sudden death, symptoms, and hospital readmission. Current data indicate BNP is more sensitive than norepinephrine for predicting morbidity and mortality in patients with heart failure. Accurate diagnosis of acute decompensated heart failure in acute care settings is often difficult, as many of the symptoms (e.g., dyspnea) mimic those of other disorders, such as pulmonary disease and obesity. The most well established clinical application of BNP testing is in the urgent care setting, where the BNP assay is useful when combined with clinical evaluation for discriminating dyspnea secondary to heart failure from other causes. Much interest has focused on the benefits of serial measurement of BNP as a target to guide the titration of drug doses. Recent studies evaluating this approach have not shown consistent improvement in long-term outcomes compared with standard medical therapy.[27] As a result, current guidelines do not support the routine use of serial measurement of BNP in the management of systolic heart failure.

Arginine Vasopressin

AVP is a pituitary peptide hormone that plays an important role in the regulation of renal water and solute excretion.[16,28] AVP secretion is directly linked to changes in plasma osmolality, thus attempting to maintain body fluid homeostasis. The physiologic effects of AVP are mediated through the V_{1a} and V_2 receptors. V_{1a} receptors are located in vascular smooth muscle and in myocytes, where AVP stimulation results in vasoconstriction and increased cardiac contractility, respectively. V_2 receptors are located in the collecting duct of the kidney, where AVP stimulation causes reabsorption of free water.

Plasma concentrations of AVP are elevated in patients with heart failure, supporting current research that indicates AVP plays a role in the pathophysiology of heart failure. Important effects associated with increased circulating AVP concentrations include (a) increased renal free water reabsorption in the face of plasma hypo-osmolality, resulting in volume overload and hyponatremia; (b) increased arterial vasoconstriction, which contributes to reduced cardiac output; and (c) stimulation of remodeling by cardiac hypertrophy and extracellular matrix collagen deposition.

Given the importance of AVP in heart failure, recent efforts have focused on the development of AVP antagonist drugs for treatment of acute and systolic heart failure. By blocking the AVP receptor, these agents primarily increase free water excretion (i.e., an "aquaretic" effect). Clinical trials with the oral V_2 receptor antagonist tolvaptan indicate it improves acute symptoms and increases serum sodium and urine output without affecting heart rate, blood pressure, renal function, or other electrolytes. However, neither overall mortality nor morbidity from heart failure was improved by tolvaptan treatment.[29] Therefore, the role of chronic therapy with vasopressin antagonists remains uncertain.

Endothelin

The endothelin peptides are potent vasoconstrictors that may be involved in heart failure pathophysiology through a number of mechanisms.[16] Endothelin-1, the best characterized of these peptides, is synthesized by endothelial and vascular smooth muscle cells, with its release enhanced by norepinephrine, angiotensin II, and inflammatory cytokines. Like other peptides and hormones described earlier, endothelin-1 plasma concentrations are elevated in heart failure and have been correlated directly with the severity of hemodynamic abnormality, symptoms, and mortality. Its arterial and venous constrictive effects increase preload and afterload, and its vasoconstriction of both efferent and afferent renal arterioles may decrease renal plasma flow and induce sodium retention. Endothelin-1 has direct cardiotoxic and arrhythmogenic effects and is a potent stimulator of cardiac myocyte hypertrophy. The putative role of endothelin in heart failure led to the development of a number of endothelin-receptor antagonists. Although these agents improved hemodynamics, no benefit on morbidity or mortality has been demonstrated, and further clinical development is unlikely.

Other Circulating Biomarkers

In addition to neurohormones, a number of other biomarkers may play a role in heart failure pathogenesis, risk stratification, and identification of patients at risk for developing heart failure.[16] Inflammation is a key component of the systemic heart failure state, resulting in significant interest in associated biomarkers.[30] Elevated plasma concentrations of the acute phase reactant C-reactive protein are associated with poor outcomes in patients with heart failure. The proinflammatory cytokines tumor necrosis factor-α (TNF-α) and interleukins-1, -6, and -18 have all been shown to be elevated in heart failure, with a direct relationship between the degree of elevation and the severity of heart failure. These cytokines produce multiple deleterious actions, including negative inotropic effects, uncoupling β-adrenergic receptors from adenylyl cyclase (thus reducing β-receptor-mediated responses), increasing myocardial cell apoptosis/necrosis, and stimulating remodeling via several mechanisms.

The role of inflammation and endothelial dysfunction has generated significant interest in the use of a number of antiinflammatory therapies in patients with heart failure. Clinical trials evaluating anti-TNF-α therapies (e.g., etanercept and infliximab) have been disappointing, with no improvement in outcomes demonstrated. In addition to the ability of statins to lower cholesterol and reduce the risk of death and other atherosclerotic vascular diseases, their pleiotropic effects (e.g., antiinflammatory, improved endothelial function, and promotion of angiogenesis) were thought to be beneficial in heart failure. However, two recent major trials with statins failed to show any benefit on important clinical outcomes.[31,32] At this time, statins cannot be recommended for routine use specifically for their benefits in heart failure. Although it is uncertain if reductions are due to antiinflammatory effects, fish oil supplementation reduced total mortality and hospitalizations for cardiovascular disease in patients with heart failure.[33]

Numerous other biomarkers are under investigation for their role in heart failure, including those associated with inflammation, oxidative stress, extracellular matrix remodeling, and myocyte injury and stress. It is hoped that data from investigations will lead to improved understanding of disease pathophysiology, prognosis, and targets for therapy.

FACTORS PRECIPITATING/ EXACERBATING HEART FAILURE

Although significant advancements have been made in treatment, symptom exacerbation, to the point that hospitalization is required, is a common and growing problem in patients with systolic heart failure. Hospitalization for heart failure exacerbation consumes large amounts of healthcare dollars and significantly impairs the patient's quality of life; thus, there is great interest in identifying and then remedying factors that increase the risk of decompensation. Appropriate therapy can often maintain patients in a "compensated" state, indicating that they are relatively symptom-free. However, there are many aggravating or precipitating factors that may cause a previously compensated patient to develop worsened symptoms, necessitating hospitalization. Often, these precipitating factors are reversible or treatable, such that a thorough evaluation for their presence in hospitalized patients is imperative.

Cardiac events are a frequent cause of worsening heart failure.[1,34] Myocardial ischemia and infarction are potentially reversible causes that must be carefully considered, as nearly 70% of patients with heart failure have coronary artery disease. Revascularization should be considered in appropriate patients. Atrial fibrillation occurs in 10% to 50% of patients with heart failure and is associated with increased morbidity and mortality.[35] Atrial fibrillation can exacerbate heart failure through rapid ventricular response and loss of atrial contribution to ventricular filling. Conversely, heart failure can precipitate atrial fibrillation by worsening atrial distention, resulting from ventricular volume overload. Control of ventricular response, maintenance of sinus rhythm in appropriate patients, and prevention of thromboembolism are important elements in the treatment of heart failure patients with atrial fibrillation. Uncontrolled hypertension is also an important contributing factor and should be treated according to current guidelines.[36]

A number of noncardiac events may also be associated with heart failure decompensation. Pulmonary infections frequently cause worsening of heart failure. Many of these events would be preventable with more widespread use of the pneumococcal and influenza vaccines. Pulmonary embolus, diabetes, worsening renal function, hypothyroidism, and hyperthyroidism should also be considered.

Nonadherence with prescribed heart failure medications or with dietary recommendations (e.g., sodium intake and fluid restriction) are also common causes of heart failure exacerbation.[1,34] Recent estimates indicate that nonadherence accounts for between 3% and 64% of hospital admissions for heart failure and that socioeconomically disadvantaged patients appear to be disproportionately affected.

A number of drugs are associated with the ability to precipitate or exacerbate heart failure by one or more of the following mechanisms: negative inotropic effects, direct cardiotoxicity, or increased sodium and/or water retention (Table 20–3). The resulting symptoms are typically those associated with volume overload, but in more severe cases, hypoperfusion may also be present. Nonsteroidal antiinflammatory drugs (NSAIDs) are increasingly recognized for their ability to exacerbate heart failure through a number of mechanisms, including volume retention, decreased renal function, and increased blood pressure. A recent analysis demonstrated that NSAIDs are associated with increased mortality and hospitalization risk in patients with heart failure.[37]

⑫ What should be evident is that many of the precipitating factors are preventable, particularly through appropriate pharmacist intervention. Specifically, patient education and counseling by a pharmacist should help to decrease a common reason for heart failure exacerbation: noncompliance with dietary sodium and water restrictions, drug therapy, or both. Pharmacists also should be able to identify and address inadequate heart failure therapy, poorly controlled hypertension, and administration of drugs that may worsen heart failure (Table 20–3). A careful medication history is an important aspect of evaluating the cause(s) of heart failure exacerbation. Discontinuation of medications that may exacerbate heart failure may help prevent hospitalizations. Use of medications such as antiarrhythmic agents and non—dihydropyridine calcium channel blockers are important precipitants of exacerbations. The widespread use of NSAIDs, particularly those obtained over-the-counter that are perceived by many patients as having a low risk of adverse effects, is also problematic, and their use should be discouraged in patients with heart failure. The thiazolidinedione hypoglycemic drugs rosiglitazone and pioglitazone are associated with the development of fluid retention and weight gain that may exacerbate heart failure. Current guidelines indicate these agents should not be used in patients with New York Heart Association (NYHA) class III or IV heart failure.[1,38] Thus, many of the factors precipitating heart failure exacerbations (nonadherence, inadequate/inappropriate drug therapy, uncontrolled hypertension, etc.) are amenable to pharmacist intervention. The value of the pharmacist's role in careful and repeated education of patients and monitoring of the drug regimen should not be underestimated.[39,40] Attention to these factors may make an important contribution to reducing the risk of hospitalization and improving the patient's quality of life.

CLINICAL PRESENTATION

SIGNS AND SYMPTOMS

❷ The primary manifestations of heart failure are dyspnea and fatigue, which lead to exercise intolerance, and fluid overload, which can result in pulmonary congestion and peripheral edema.[41] The presence of these signs and symptoms may vary considerably from patient to patient, such that some patients have dyspnea but no signs of fluid retention, whereas others may have marked volume overload with few complaints of dyspnea or fatigue. However, many patients may have both dyspnea and volume overload. Clinicians should remember that symptom severity often does not correlate with the degree of left ventricular dysfunction. Patients with a low LVEF (less than 20–25%) may be asymptomatic, whereas those with preserved LVEF may have significant symptoms. It is also important to note that symptoms can vary considerably over time in a given patient even in the absence of changes in ventricular function or medications.

Historically, signs and symptoms are classified as being due to left ventricular failure (pulmonary congestion) or right ventricular failure (systemic congestion). Because of the complex nature of this syndrome, it has become exceedingly more difficult to attribute a specific sign or symptom as caused by either right or left ventricular failure. Therefore, the numerous signs and symptoms associated with this disorder are collectively attributed to heart failure, rather than due to dysfunction of a specific ventricle.

Pulmonary congestion arises as the left ventricle fails and is unable to accept and eject the increased blood volume that is delivered to it. Consequently, pulmonary venous and capillary pressures rise, leading to interstitial and bronchial edema, increased airway resistance, and dyspnea. The associated signs and symptoms may include (a) dyspnea (with or without exertion), (b) orthopnea, (c) paroxysmal nocturnal dyspnea (PND), and (d) pulmonary edema. Exertional dyspnea occurs when there is a reduction in the level of exertion that causes breathlessness. This is typically described as more breathlessness than was associated previously with a specific activity (e.g., vacuuming, stair climbing). As heart failure progresses, many patients eventually have dyspnea at rest.

TABLE 20-3	Drugs that May Precipitate or Exacerbate Heart Failure

Negative inotropic effect
- Antiarrhythmics (e.g., disopyramide, flecainide, and propafenone)
- Beta-blockers (e.g., propranolol, metoprolol, and atenolol)
- Calcium channel blockers (e.g., verapamil and diltiazem)
- Itraconazole
- Terbinafine

Cardiotoxic
- Doxorubicin
- Daunomycin
- Cyclophosphamide
- Trastuzumab
- Ethanol
- Amphetamines (e.g., cocaine and methamphetamine)

Sodium and water retention
- NSAIDs
- COX-2 inhibitors
- Rosiglitazone and pioglitazone
- Glucocorticoids
- Androgens and estrogens
- Salicylates (high-dose)
- Sodium-containing drugs (e.g., carbenicillin disodium and ticarcillin disodium)
- Imatinib

Abbreviations: COX-2, cyclooxygenase-2; NSAIDs, nonsteroidal antiinflammatory drugs.

Orthopnea is dyspnea that occurs with assumption of the supine position. It occurs within minutes of recumbency and is due to reduced pooling of blood in the lower extremities and abdomen. Orthopnea is relieved almost immediately by sitting upright and typically is prevented by elevating the head with pillows. An increase in the number of pillows required to prevent orthopnea (e.g., a change from "two-pillow" to "three-pillow" orthopnea) suggests worsening heart failure.

Attacks of paroxysmal nocturnal dyspnea or PND typically occur after 2 to 4 hours of sleep; the patient awakens from sleep with a sense of suffocation. The attacks are due to severe pulmonary and bronchial congestion, leading to shortness of breath, cough, and wheezing. The reasons these attacks occur at night are unclear but may include (a) reduced pooling of blood in the lower extremities and abdomen (as with orthopnea), (b) slow resorption of interstitial fluid from sites of dependent edema, (c) normal reduction in sympathetic activity that occurs with sleep (e.g., less support for the failing ventricle), and (d) normal depression in respiratory drive that occurs with sleep.

Rales (crackling sounds heard on auscultation) are present in the lung bases due to transudation of fluid into alveoli. The rales typically are bibasilar, but if heard unilaterally, they are usually right-sided. Rales are not present in most patients with systolic heart failure even though there is volume overload. This is thought to be due to a compensatory increase in lymphatic drainage. Detection of rales is usually indicative of a rapid onset of worsening heart failure rather than the amount of excess fluid volume. A third heart sound, or S_3 gallop, is heard frequently in patients with left ventricular failure and may be due to elevated atrial pressure and altered distensibility of the ventricle.

Pulmonary edema is the most severe form of pulmonary congestion and is caused by accumulation of fluid in the interstitial spaces and alveoli. In patients with heart failure, it is the result of increased pulmonary venous pressure. The patient experiences extreme breathlessness and anxiety and may cough pink, frothy sputum. Pulmonary edema can be terrifying for the patient, causing a feeling of suffocation or drowning. Patients with pulmonary edema may also report any of the above-mentioned signs or symptoms of pulmonary congestion.

Systemic congestion is associated with a number of signs and symptoms. Jugular venous distention (JVD) is the simplest and most reliable sign of fluid overload. Examination of the right internal jugular vein with the patient at a 45-degree angle is the preferred method for assessing JVD. The presence of JVD >4 cm above the sternal angle suggests systemic venous congestion. In patients with mild systemic congestion, JVD may be absent at rest, but application of pressure to the abdomen will cause an elevation of JVD (hepatojugular reflux).

Peripheral edema is a cardinal finding in heart failure. Edema usually occurs in dependent parts of the body, and thus is seen as ankle or pedal edema in ambulatory patients, although it may be manifested as sacral edema in bedridden patients. Adults typically have a 10 lb fluid weight gain before trace peripheral edema is evident; therefore, patients with acute decompensated heart failure may have no clinical evidence of systemic congestion except weight gain. Body weight is thus the best short-term end point for evaluating fluid status. Nonfluid weight gain and loss of muscle mass due to cardiac cachexia are potential confounders for long-term use of weight as a marker for fluid status. Hepatomegaly and ascites are other signs of systemic congestion.

Patients with heart failure may exhibit signs and symptoms of low cardiac output alone or in addition to volume overload. The primary complaint associated with such poor perfusion is fatigue. Patients may also complain of poor appetite or early satiety due to limited perfusion of the gastrointestinal (GI) tract.

Conversely, patients with such GI complaints may simply be experiencing gut edema. More subjective measures of low cardiac output include worsening renal function, cool extremities, change in mental status, resting tachycardia, and narrow pulse pressure.

CLINICAL PRESENTATION OF HEART FAILURE

General

- Patient presentation may range from asymptomatic to cardiogenic shock.

Symptoms

- Dyspnea, particularly on exertion
- Orthopnea
- Paroxysmal nocturnal dyspnea
- Exercise intolerance
- Tachypnea
- Cough
- Fatigue
- Nocturia
- Hemoptysis
- Abdominal pain
- Anorexia
- Nausea
- Bloating
- Poor appetite, early satiety
- Ascites
- Mental status changes

Signs

- Pulmonary rales
- Pulmonary edema
- S_3 gallop
- Cool extremities
- Pleural effusion
- Cheyne-Stokes respiration
- Tachycardia
- Narrow pulse pressure
- Cardiomegaly
- Peripheral edema
- JVD
- Hepatojugular reflux
- Hepatomegaly

Laboratory Tests

- BNP >100 pg/mL
- Electrocardiogram may be normal, or it could show numerous abnormalities, including acute ST-T wave changes from myocardial ischemia, atrial fibrillation, bradycardia, and left ventricular hypertrophy.
- Serum creatinine may be increased due to hypoperfusion. Preexisting renal dysfunction can contribute to volume overload.
- Complete blood count (CBC) can be useful in determining if heart failure is due to a reduced oxygen-carrying capacity.

- Chest x-ray: useful for detecting cardiac enlargement, pulmonary edema, and pleural effusions
- Echocardiogram: used to assess the size of the left ventricle, valve function, pericardial effusion, wall motion abnormalities, and ejection fraction
- Hyponatremia: serum sodium <130 mEq/L is associated with reduced survival and may indicate worsening volume overload and/or disease progression.

DIAGNOSIS

No single test is available to confirm the diagnosis of heart failure—it is a clinical syndrome associated with specific signs and symptoms.[1,41] Because heart failure can be caused or worsened by multiple cardiac and noncardiac disorders, many of which may be treatable or reversible, accurate diagnosis is essential for development of therapeutic strategies. Heart failure is often initially suspected in a patient based on symptoms. These often include dyspnea, exercise intolerance, fatigue, and/or fluid retention. However, it must be emphasized that signs and symptoms lack sensitivity for diagnosing heart failure, as these symptoms are frequently found with many other disorders. Even in patients with known heart failure, there is a poor correlation between the presence or severity of symptoms and the hemodynamic abnormality.

A complete history and physical examination targeted at identifying cardiac or noncardiac disorders or behaviors that may cause or hasten heart failure development or progression are essential in the initial evaluation of a symptomatic patient. A careful medication history should also be obtained with a focus on use of ethanol, tobacco, illicit drugs (e.g., cocaine or methamphetamine), vitamins and supplements (including herbal or "natural" supplements), NSAIDs, and antineoplastic agents (anthracyclines, cyclophosphamide, trastuzumab, and imatinib).

Particular attention should be paid to cardiovascular risk factors and to other disorders that can cause or exacerbate heart failure, such as hypertension, diabetes, dyslipidemia, tobacco use, sleep-disordered breathing, and thyroid disease. Because coronary artery disease is the cause of heart failure in many patients, careful attention and evaluation of the possibility of coronary disease is essential, especially in men. If coronary artery disease is detected, appropriate revascularization procedures may then be considered. The patient's volume status should be documented by assessing the body weight, JVD, and presence or absence of pulmonary congestion and peripheral edema. Laboratory testing may assist in identification of disorders that cause or worsen heart failure. The initial evaluation should include a complete blood count, serum electrolytes (including calcium and magnesium), tests of renal and hepatic function, urinalysis, lipid profile, hemoglobin A1C, thyroid function tests, chest x-ray, and 12-lead electrocardiogram (ECG). There are no specific ECG findings associated with heart failure, but findings may help detect coronary artery disease or conduction abnormalities that could affect prognosis and guide treatment decisions. Measurement of BNP may also assist in differentiating dyspnea caused by heart failure from other causes.[25,26]

Although the history, physical examination, and laboratory tests provide important insight into the underlying cause of heart failure, the echocardiogram is the single most useful test in the evaluation of the patient. The echocardiogram is used to assess abnormalities in cardiac structure and function, including evaluation of the pericardium, myocardium, and heart valves, and to quantify the LVEF to determine if systolic or diastolic dysfunction is present.

TREATMENT OF SYSTOLIC HEART FAILURE

DESIRED OUTCOMES

The goals of therapy in the management of systolic heart failure are to improve the patient's quality of life, relieve or reduce symptoms, prevent or minimize hospitalizations for exacerbations of heart failure, slow progression of the disease process, and prolong survival. Although these goals are still important, identification of risk factors for heart failure development and recognition of its progressive nature have led to increased emphasis on preventing the development of this disorder. With this in mind, the American College of Cardiology/American Heart Association (ACC/AHA) guidelines for the evaluation and management of systolic heart failure utilize a staging system that not only recognizes the evolution and progression of the disorder, but also emphasizes risk factor modification and preventive treatment strategies.[1] The system is composed of four stages (Fig. 20–5). This staging system differs from the New York Heart Association (NYHA) functional classification (Table 20–4) with which most clinicians are familiar. The NYHA system is primarily intended to classify symptomatic heart failure according to the clinician's subjective evaluation and does not recognize preventive measures or the progression of the disorder. A patient's symptoms can change frequently over a short period of time due to changes in medications, diet, intercurrent illnesses, and so on. For example, a patient with ACC/AHA stage C heart failure with NYHA class IV symptoms such as marked volume overload could rapidly improve to class I or II with aggressive diuretic therapy. Despite these limitations, this system can be useful for monitoring patients and is widely used in heart failure studies. In contrast, and consistent with the progressive nature of heart failure, a patient's ACC/AHA heart failure stage could not improve (e.g., go from stage C to stage B) even though the patient's symptoms could fluctuate from NYHA class IV to I. In addition, the ACC/AHA staging system provides a more comprehensive framework for evaluation, prevention, and treatment of heart failure.

GENERAL MEASURES

The complexity of the heart failure syndrome necessitates a comprehensive approach to management that includes accurate diagnosis, identification, and treatment of risk factors, elimination or minimization of precipitating factors, appropriate pharmacologic and nonpharmacologic therapy, and close monitoring and follow-up.

The first step in management of systolic heart failure is to determine the etiology (see Table 20–1) and/or any precipitating factors. Treatment of underlying disorders such as hyperthyroidism may obviate the need for treatment of heart failure. Patients with valvular diseases may derive significant benefit from valve replacement or repair. Revascularization or anti-ischemic therapy in patients with coronary disease may reduce heart failure symptoms. Drugs that aggravate heart failure (see Table 20–3) should be discontinued if possible.

Restriction of physical activity reduces cardiac workload and is recommended for virtually all patients with acute congestive symptoms. However, once the patient's symptoms have stabilized, and excess fluid is removed, restrictions on physical activity are discouraged. Current guidelines support exercise training programs in stable patients with heart failure to improve clinical status.[1] More recently, exercise training in patients with left ventricular systolic dysfunction produced nonsignificant reductions in total mortality or hospitalization.[42]

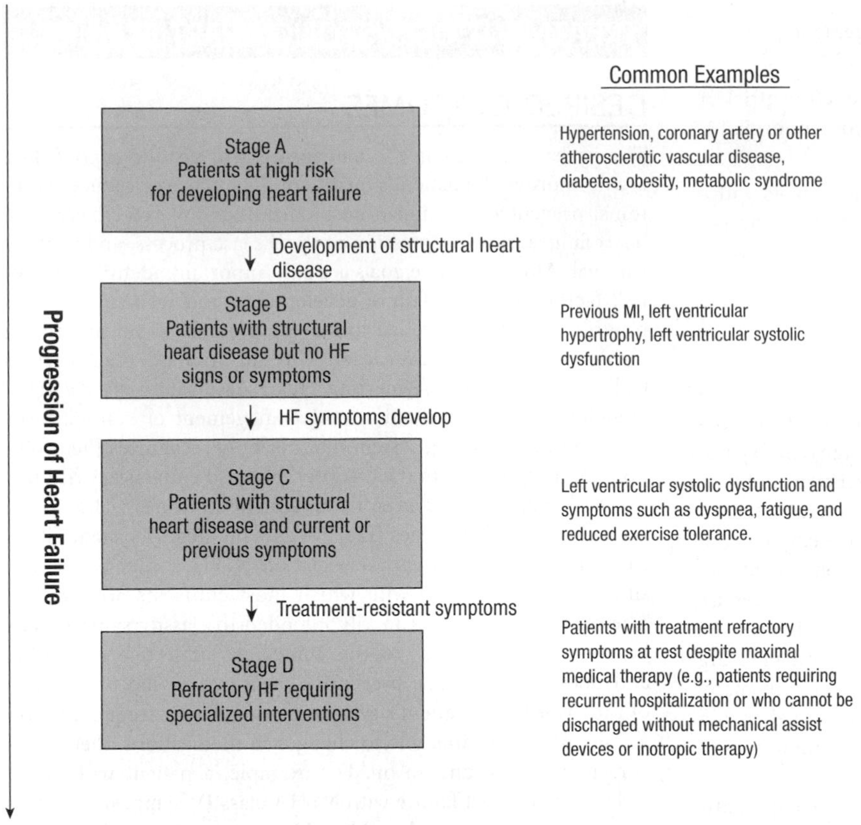

Common Examples

Progression of Heart Failure

Stage A
Patients at high risk
for developing heart failure

Hypertension, coronary artery or other
atherosclerotic vascular disease,
diabetes, obesity, metabolic syndrome

↓ Development of structural heart
disease

Stage B
Patients with structural
heart disease but no HF
signs or symptoms

Previous MI, left ventricular
hypertrophy, left ventricular systolic
dysfunction

↓ HF symptoms develop

Stage C
Patients with structural
heart disease and current or
previous symptoms

Left ventricular systolic dysfunction and
symptoms such as dyspnea, fatigue, and
reduced exercise tolerance.

↓ Treatment-resistant symptoms

Stage D
Refractory HF requiring
specialized interventions

Patients with treatment refractory
symptoms at rest despite maximal
medical therapy (e.g., patients requiring
recurrent hospitalization or who cannot be
discharged without mechanical assist
devices or inotropic therapy)

FIGURE 20-5. American College of Cardiology/ American Heart Association (ACC/AHA) heart failure staging system. (HF, heart failure; MI, myocardial infarction.) *(Source: Hunt SA, Abraham WT, Chin MH, et al. 2009 focused update incorporated into the ACC/AHA 2005 Guidelines for the Diagnosis and Management of Heart Failure in Adults: a report of the American College of Cardiology Foundation/American Heart Association Task Force on Practice Guidelines: developed in collaboration with the International Society for Heart and Lung Transplantation. Circulation 2009;119:e391–e479.)*

Because a major compensatory response in heart failure is sodium and water retention, restriction of dietary sodium and fluid intake are important lifestyle interventions. Mild (<3 g per day) to moderate (<2 g per day) sodium restriction, in conjunction with daily measurement of weight, should be implemented to minimize volume retention and allow use of lower and safer diuretic doses. The typical American diet contains 8 to 10 g of sodium per day, so most patients would need to reduce their intake by approximately 50%. This can often be accomplished by not adding salt to prepared foods and eliminating foods high in sodium (e.g., salt-cured meats, salted snack foods, pickles, soups, delicatessen meats, and processed foods). In patients with hyponatremia (serum Na <130 mEq/L) or those with persistent volume retention despite high diuretic doses and sodium restriction, daily fluid intake should be limited to 2 L per day from all sources.

Other important general measures include patient and family counseling on the signs and symptoms of heart failure, detailed written instructions on the importance of appropriate medication use and compliance, activity level, diet, discharge medications, weight monitoring, and the need for close monitoring and follow-up to reinforce compliance and minimize the risk of heart failure exacerbations and subsequent hospitalization. These activities are now referred to as self-care and constitute an important means to improve such important outcomes as hospitalization and quality of life.[43]

GENERAL APPROACH TO TREATMENT

❹ Current ACC/AHA treatment guidelines are organized around the four identified stages of heart failure, and the treatment recommendations are summarized in Figures 20–6 and 20–7.[1] Clinicians are reminded that, in addition to the ACC/AHA, other cardiology professional societies have developed guidelines for evaluation and treatment of heart failure. The Heart Failure Society of America (HFSA) issued practice guidelines in 2006.[44] The HFSA and ACC/AHA guidelines are very similar with regard to care and treatment of patients with systolic heart failure. In addition, the HFSA guidelines provide a thorough discussion of other areas, including acute decompensated heart failure, heart failure with preserved LVEF, and management of patients with heart failure and a number of comorbid diseases. The HFSA guidelines will be periodically updated on the HFSA website (www.hfsa.org). Finally, the European Society of Cardiology (ESC) published guidelines for the management of both acute and systolic heart failure.[45] Although minor differences exist between the recommendations in the American and European guidelines, they are in general agreement in their overall approach. Clinicians caring for patients with heart failure should be familiar with these guidelines but should also remember that these indeed are only guidelines and that evaluation and treatment should be individualized for each patient.

Treatment of Stage A Heart Failure

Patients in stage A do not have structural heart disease or heart failure symptoms but are at high risk for developing heart failure because of the presence of risk factors (Fig. 20–6). The emphasis

TABLE 20-4	New York Heart Association Functional Classification

Functional class

I. Patients with cardiac disease but without limitations of physical activity. Ordinary physical activity does not cause undue fatigue, dyspnea, or palpitation.

II. Patients with cardiac disease that results in slight limitations of physical activity. Ordinary physical activity results in fatigue, palpitation, dyspnea, or angina.

III. Patients with cardiac disease that results in marked limitation of physical activity. Although patients are comfortable at rest, less than ordinary activity will lead to symptoms.

IV. Patients with cardiac disease that results in an inability to carry on physical activity without discomfort. Symptoms of congestive heart failure are present even at rest. With any physical activity, increased discomfort is experienced.

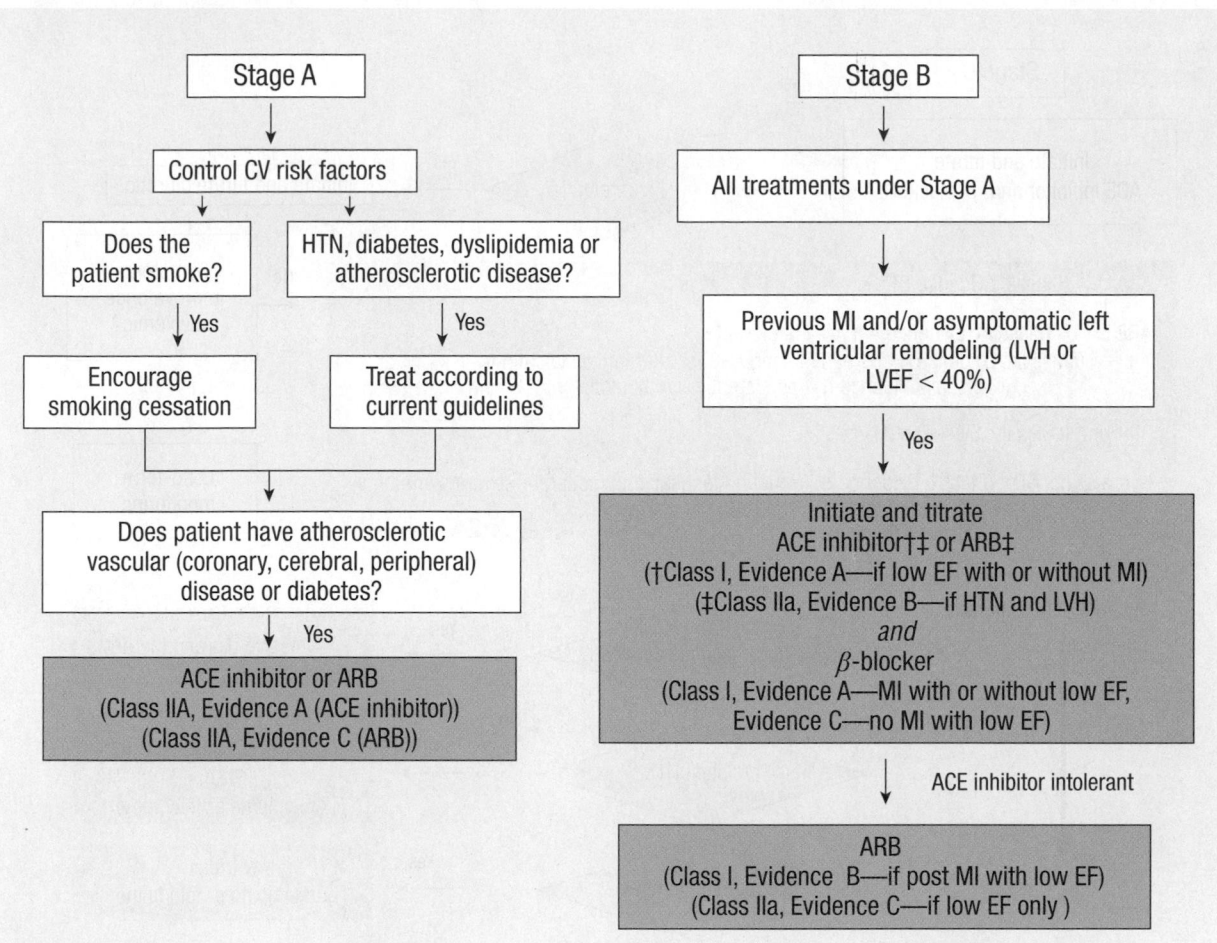

FIGURE 20-6. Treatment algorithm for patients with ACC/AHA stages A and B heart failure. (ACE, angiotensin-converting enzyme; ARB, angiotensin receptor blocker; CV, cardiovascular; EF, ejection fraction; HTN, hypertension; LVEF, left ventricular ejection fraction; LVH, left ventricular hypertrophy; MI, myocardial infarction.) *(Source: Hunt SA, Abraham WT, Chin MH, et al. 2009 focused update incorporated into the ACC/AHA 2005 Guidelines for the Diagnosis and Management of Heart Failure in Adults: a report of the American College of Cardiology Foundation/American Heart Association Task Force on Practice Guidelines: developed in collaboration with the International Society for Heart and Lung Transplantation. Circulation 2009;119:e391–e479.)*

here is on identification and modification of these risk factors to prevent the development of structural heart disease and subsequent heart failure. Commonly encountered risk factors include hypertension, dyslipidemia, diabetes, obesity, metabolic syndrome, smoking, and coronary artery disease. Although each of these disorders individually increases risk, they frequently coexist in many patients and act synergistically to foster the development of heart failure. Effective control of both systolic and diastolic blood pressure reduces the risk of developing heart failure by approximately 50%; thus, current hypertension treatment guidelines should be followed.[36] Diabetes dramatically increases the risk of developing heart failure and adversely affects the prognosis of patients with known heart failure. Appropriate diabetic control is important to minimize the risk of end-organ damage but has not been shown to affect the risk of developing heart failure. Appropriate management of coronary disease and its associated risk factors is also important, including treatment of dyslipidemia and smoking cessation.[46] Although treatment must be individualized, ACE inhibitors or ARBs can be useful for antihypertensive therapy in patients with multiple vascular risk factors.[1] Adding further evidence that heart failure is a preventable disorder, a recent study found that such modifiable risk factors as body weight, smoking, exercise, alcohol intake, and consumption of fruits and vegetables reduced the lifetime risk of developing heart failure.[47]

Treatment of Stage B Heart Failure

Patients in stage B have structural heart disease but do not have heart failure symptoms (Fig. 20–6). This group includes patients with left ventricular hypertrophy, recent or remote MI, valvular disease, or reduced LVEF (less than 40%). These individuals are at risk for developing heart failure, and treatment is targeted at minimizing additional injury and preventing or slowing the remodeling process. In addition to the treatment measures outlined in stage A, ACE inhibitors and β-blockers are important components of therapy. Patients with a previous MI should receive both ACE inhibitors and β-blockers, regardless of the LVEF.[1] Similarly, patients with a reduced LVEF should also receive both of these agents, whether or not they have had an MI.[1] ARBs are an effective alternative in patients intolerant to ACE inhibitors.[1]

Treatment of Stage C Heart Failure

❹ ❺ ❻ ❼ ❽ ❾ ❿ Patients with structural heart disease and previous or current heart failure symptoms are classified as stage C (Fig. 20–7). In addition to treatments in stages A and B, most patients in stage C should be routinely treated with three medications: a diuretic, an ACE inhibitor, and a β-blocker (see Drug Therapies for Routine Use in Patients with Stage C Heart Failure).

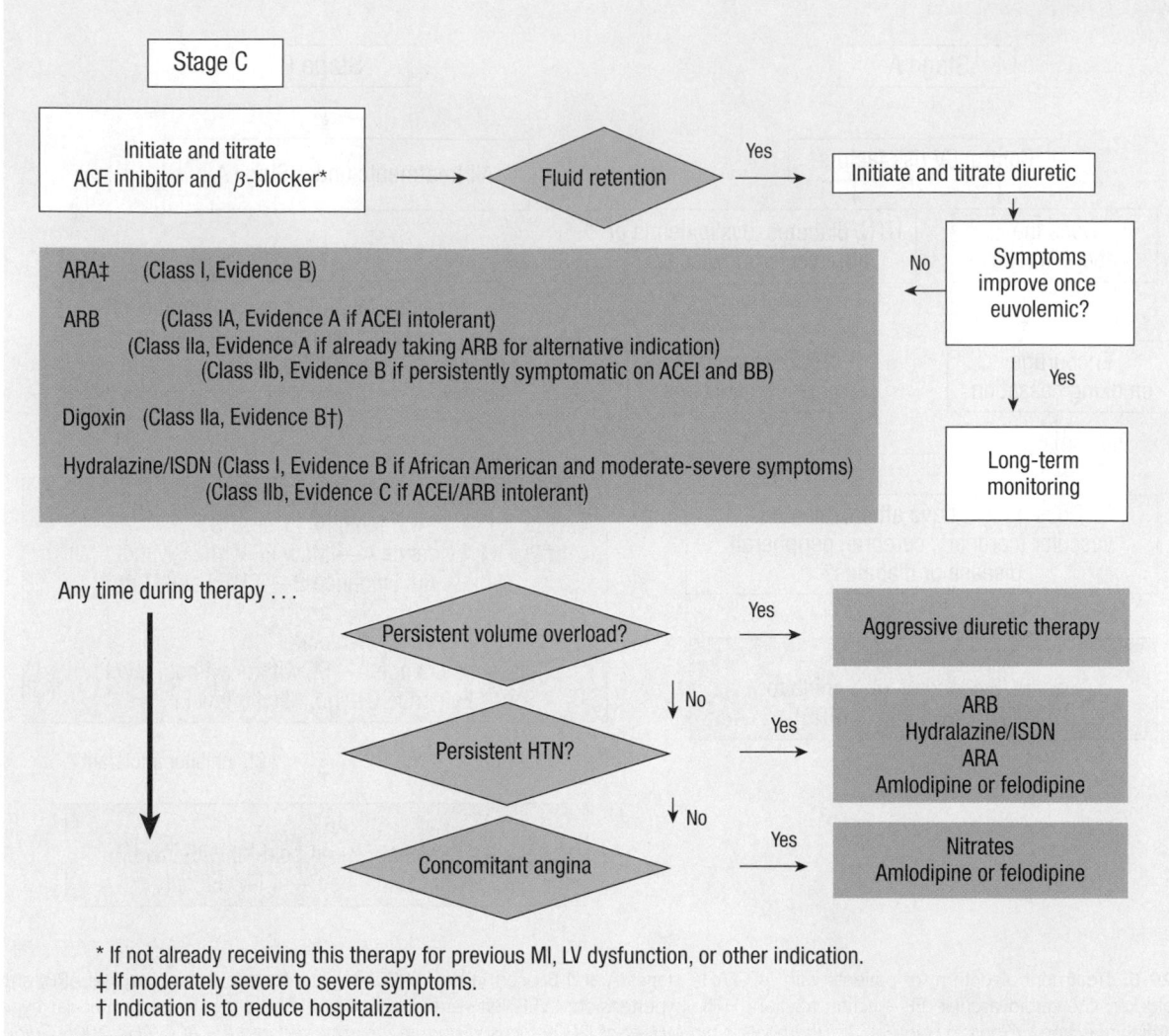

FIGURE 20-7. Treatment algorithm for patients with ACC/AHA stage C heart failure. (ACEI, angiotensin-converting enzyme I; ARA, aldosterone receptor antagonist; ARB, angiotensin receptor blocker; BB, β-blocker; HTN, hypertension; ISDN, isosorbide dinitrate; LV, left ventricular; MI, myocardial infarction.) *(Source: Hunt SA, Abraham WT, Chin MH, et al. 2009 focused update incorporated into the ACC/AHA 2005 Guidelines for the Diagnosis and Management of Heart Failure in Adults: a report of the American College of Cardiology Foundation/American Heart Association Task Force on Practice Guidelines: developed in collaboration with the International Society for Heart and Lung Transplantation. Circulation 2009;119:e391–e479.)*

The benefits of these medications on slowing heart failure progression, reducing morbidity and mortality, and improving symptoms are clearly established. Aldosterone receptor antagonists, ARBs, digoxin, and hydralazine-isosorbide dinitrate are also useful in selected patients. Nonpharmacologic therapy with devices such as an implantable cardiac defibrillator (ICD) or cardiac resynchronization therapy (CRT) with a biventricular pacemaker is also indicated in certain patients in stage C (see Nonpharmacologic Therapy). Other general measures are also important, including moderate sodium restriction, daily weight measurement, immunization against influenza and pneumococcus, modest physical activity, and avoidance of medications that can exacerbate heart failure. Recent evidence suggests that careful follow-up and patient education that reinforces dietary and medication compliance can prevent clinical deterioration and reduce hospitalization.[1,43]

Treatment of Stage D Heart Failure

Stage D heart failure includes patients with symptoms at rest that are refractory despite maximal medical therapy and those patients who undergo recurrent hospitalizations or cannot be discharged from the hospital without special interventions. These individuals have the most advanced form of heart failure and should be referred to heart failure management programs so that specialized therapies, including mechanical circulatory support, continuous intravenous (IV) positive inotropic therapy, and cardiac transplantation, can be considered in addition to standard treatments outlined in stages A, B, and C. A new continuous-flow left ventricular assist device was shown to improve outcomes with fewer adverse events compared with the traditional pulsatile-flow devices.[48] When no additional treatments are appropriate, discussions about prognosis and end of life care should be initiated.[1,49]

Management of volume status can be challenging in these patients. Restriction of sodium and fluid intake may be beneficial. High doses of diuretics, combination therapy with a loop and thiazide diuretic, or mechanical methods of fluid removal such as ultrafiltration may be required. Patients in stage D may be less tolerant to ACE inhibitors (hypotension, worsening renal insufficiency) and β-blockers (worsening heart failure), as circulatory homeostasis is maintained by high levels of neurohormonal activation. Initiation of therapy with low doses, slow upward dose titration, and close monitoring for signs and symptoms of intolerance are essential in this group of patients. The approach to the treatment of patients with stage D heart failure is discussed in more detail in Chapter 22.

NONPHARMACOLOGIC THERAPY

Sudden cardiac death, primarily due to ventricular tachycardia and fibrillation, is responsible for 40% to 50% of the mortality in patients with heart failure. In general, patients in the earlier stages of heart failure with milder symptoms are more likely to experience sudden death, whereas death from pump failure is more frequent in those with advanced heart failure. Many of these patients have complex and frequent ventricular ectopy, although it remains unknown whether these ectopic beats contribute to the risk of malignant arrhythmias or merely serve as markers for individuals at higher risk for sudden death. Drugs that attenuate disease progression such as β-blockers and aldosterone antagonists reduce the risk of sudden death. However, empiric treatment with class I antiarrhythmic agents, although they can suppress ventricular ectopy, adversely affects survival.[50]

Amiodarone is reported to have a neutral effect on survival in patients with heart failure and low LVEF. The role of the ICD compared with amiodarone for primary prevention of sudden death was evaluated in Sudden Cardiac Death in Heart Failure Trial (SCD-HeFT). The ICD was superior to amiodarone or placebo for reducing mortality in patients with NYHA class II or III symptoms and LVEF ≤35%, regardless of the etiology of heart failure.[51] Importantly, this study also found that amiodarone had no benefit compared with placebo; thus, this drug, because of its multiple adverse effects, drug interactions, and lack of effect on mortality, should not be used for primary prevention of sudden death. However, because of the neutral effects of amiodarone on survival, it is often used in patients with symptomatic atrial fibrillation to maintain sinus rhythm and/or to prevent ICD discharges. Thus, the ACC/AHA guidelines recommend the ICD for both primary and secondary prevention to improve survival in patients with current or previous heart failure symptoms and reduced LVEF.[1] A thorough review of ICD therapy can be found in Chapter 25.

Recent studies demonstrate that CRT offers a promising approach to select patients with systolic heart failure.[52,53] Delayed electrical activation of the left ventricle, characterized on the ECG by a QRS duration that exceeds 120 msec, occurs in approximately one third of patients with moderate to severe systolic heart failure. Because the left and right ventricles normally activate simultaneously, this delay results in asynchronous contraction of the ventricles, which contributes to the hemodynamic abnormalities of heart failure. Implantation of a specialized biventricular pacemaker to restore synchronous activation of the ventricles can improve ventricular contraction and hemodynamics. Use of CRT is associated with improvements in exercise capacity, NYHA classification, quality of life, hemodynamic function, hospitalizations, and mortality.[52,53] Current guidelines indicate CRT should be used only in NYHA class III and IV patients receiving optimal medical therapy and with a QRS duration ≥120 msec and LVEF ≤35%. However, the recently published Multicenter Automatic Defibrillator Implantation Trial with Cardiac Resynchronization Therapy (MADIT-CRT) trial found that the combination of CRT plus an ICD reduced death or heart failure events by 34% compared with an ICD alone in patients with an LVEF ≤30% and a QRS duration ≥130 msec and less severe symptoms (NYHA class I or II).[54] This earlier use of CRT is also associated with reverse remodeling.[55] It remains to be determined if these new data will result in changes to the guidelines. Combined CRT and ICD devices are available and can be used if the patient meets the indications for both devices.

PHARMACOLOGIC THERAPY

Drug Therapies for Routine Use in Patients with Stage C Heart Failure

4 5 6 7 A treatment algorithm for management of patients with stage C heart failure is shown in Figure 20–7. In general, these patients should receive combined therapy with an ACE inhibitor or ARB and a β-blocker, plus a diuretic if there is evidence of fluid retention. Initiation of digoxin therapy can be considered at any time for symptom reduction, to decrease hospitalizations, or to slow ventricular response in patients with concomitant atrial fibrillation.[1] An aldosterone receptor antagonist should also be considered in select patients.[1]

Diuretics 7 The compensatory mechanisms in heart failure stimulate excessive sodium and water retention, often leading to pulmonary and systemic congestion.[56,57] Diuretic therapy, in addition to sodium restriction, is recommended in all patients with clinical evidence of fluid retention. Once fluid overload has been resolved, many patients require chronic diuretic therapy to maintain euvolemia. Among the drugs used to manage heart failure, diuretics are the most rapid in producing symptomatic benefits. However, diuretics do not prolong survival or (with the possible exception of torsemide) alter disease progression, and therefore are not considered mandatory therapy. Thus, patients who do not have fluid retention would not require diuretic therapy.

The primary goal of diuretic therapy is to reduce symptoms associated with fluid retention, improve exercise tolerance and quality of life, and reduce hospitalizations from heart failure. They accomplish this by decreasing pulmonary and peripheral edema through reduction of preload. Although preload is a determinant of cardiac output, the Frank-Starling curve (see Fig. 20–3) shows that patients with congestive symptoms have reached the flat portion of the curve. A reduction in preload improves symptoms but has little effect on the patient's stroke volume or cardiac output until the steep portion of the curve is reached. However, diuretic therapy must be used judiciously because overdiuresis can lead to a reduction in cardiac output, renal perfusion, and symptoms of dehydration.

Diuretic therapy is usually initiated in low doses in the outpatient setting, with dosage adjustments based on symptom assessment and daily body weight. Change in body weight is a sensitive marker of fluid retention or loss, and it is recommended that patients monitor their status by taking daily morning body weights. Patients who gain 1 lb per day for several consecutive days or 3 to 5 lb in a week should contact their healthcare provider for instructions (which often will be to increase the diuretic dose temporarily). Such action often will allow patients to prevent a decompensation that requires hospitalization. One study demonstrated a significant reduction in emergency department visits with a protocol that directed patients to self-adjust their diuretic dose based on changes in heart failure symptoms and daily body weight.[58] Hypotension or worsening renal function (e.g., increases in serum creatinine) may be indicative of volume depletion and necessitate a reduction in the diuretic dose. Assessing volume status is particularly important before ACE inhibitor or β-blocker initiation or dose uptitration, as overdiuresis may predispose patients to hypotension and other adverse effects with increases in ACE inhibitor or β-blocker doses.

Thiazide diuretics Thiazide diuretics such as hydrochlorothiazide block sodium reabsorption in the distal convoluted tubule (~5–8% of filtered sodium). The thiazides therefore are relatively weak diuretics and infrequently are used alone in heart failure. However, thiazides or the thiazide-like diuretic metolazone can be used in combination with loop diuretics to promote a very effective diuresis. In addition, thiazide diuretics may be preferred in patients with only mild fluid

TABLE 20-5 Loop Diuretics: Use in Heart Failure

	Furosemide	Bumetanide	Torsemide
Usual daily dose (po)	20–160 mg/d	0.5–4 mg/d	10–80 mg/d
Ceiling dose[a]			
Normal renal function	80-160 mg	1–2 mg	20–40 mg
CL_{CR} 20–50 mL/min	160 mg	2 mg	40 mg
CL_{CR} <20 mL/min	400 mg	8–10	100 mg
Bioavailability	10–100%	80–90%	80–100%
	Average: 50%		
Affected by food	Yes	Yes	No
Half-life	0.3–3.4 h	0.3–1.5 h	3–4 h

[a] Ceiling dose: single dose above which additional response is unlikely to be observed.
Adapted from Brater DC. Pharmacology of Diuretics. Am J Med Sci 2000;319:38–50.

retention and elevated blood pressure because of their more persistent antihypertensive effects compared with loop diuretics.

Loop diuretics Loop diuretics are usually necessary to restore and maintain euvolemia in heart failure. They act by inhibiting a Na-K-2Cl transporter in the thick ascending limb of the loop of Henle, where 20% to 25% of filtered sodium normally is reabsorbed. Because loop diuretics are highly bound to plasma proteins, they are not highly filtered at the glomerulus. They reach the tubular lumen by active transport via the organic acid transport pathway. Competitors for this pathway (probenecid or organic by-products of uremia) can inhibit delivery of loop diuretics to their site of action and decrease effectiveness. Loop diuretics also induce a prostaglandin-mediated increase in renal blood flow, which contributes to their natriuretic effect. Coadministration of NSAIDs blocks this prostaglandin-mediated effect and can diminish diuretic efficacy. Excessive dietary sodium intake may also reduce the efficacy of loop diuretics. Unlike thiazides, loop diuretics maintain their effectiveness in the presence of impaired renal function, although higher doses may be necessary to obtain adequate delivery of the drug to the site of action.

Heart failure is one of the disease states in which the maximal response to loop diuretics is reduced. This is believed to result from a decrease in the rate of diuretic absorption and/or increased proximal or distal tubule reabsorption of sodium, possibly due to increased activity of the Na-K-2Cl transporter.[56] As a consequence, doses above the recommended ceiling produce no additional diuresis. Thus, once the ceiling dose is reached, it is recommended that more frequent doses be given for additional effect rather than progressively higher doses. The appropriate chronic dose of a loop diuretic is that which maintains the patient at a stable dry weight without symptoms of dyspnea. Ranges of doses of loop diuretics and recommended ceiling doses are shown in Table 20–5.

ACE Inhibitors ❺ ACE inhibitors are the cornerstone of pharmacotherapy for patients with heart failure. By blocking the conversion of angiotensin I to angiotensin II by ACE, the production of angiotensin II and, in turn, aldosterone is decreased, but not completely eliminated.[17] This decrease in angiotensin II and aldosterone attenuates many of the deleterious effects of these neurohormones, including ventricular remodeling, myocardial fibrosis, myocyte apoptosis, cardiac hypertrophy, norepinephrine release, vasoconstriction, and sodium and water retention.[17] Thus, ACE inhibitor therapy plays an important role in preventing RAAS-mediated progressive worsening of myocardial function. The endogenous vasodilator bradykinin, which is inactivated by ACE, is also increased by ACE inhibitors, along with the release of vasodilatory prostaglandins and histamine.[17] The precise contribution of the effects of ACE inhibitors on bradykinin and vasodilatory prostaglandins is unclear. However, the persistence of clinical benefits with ACE inhibitors despite the fact that angiotensin II and aldosterone levels return to

pretreatment levels in some patients suggests this is a potentially important effect.[17]

Numerous placebo-controlled clinical trials involving over 7,000 patients with reduced LVEF have documented the favorable effects of ACE inhibitor therapy on symptoms, NYHA functional classification, clinical status, exercise tolerance, and quality of life.[17] When compared with placebo, patients treated with ACE inhibitors have fewer treatment failures, hospitalizations, and increases in diuretic dosages.[17]

More importantly, these trials show that ACE inhibitors improve survival by 20% to 30% compared with placebo and that these benefits are maintained for years after therapy is initiated.[17] In addition to improving survival, ACE inhibitors reduce the combined risk of death or hospitalization, slow the progression of heart failure, and reduce the rates of reinfarction.[17] The benefits of ACE inhibitor therapy are independent of the etiology of heart failure (ischemic vs nonischemic) and are observed in patients with mild, moderate, or severe symptoms.

ACE inhibitors also are effective for preventing the development of heart failure and reducing cardiovascular risk. Enalapril decreases the risk of hospitalization for worsening heart failure and reduces the composite end point of death and heart failure hospitalization in patients with asymptomatic left ventricular dysfunction.[59] In patients with established atherosclerotic vascular disease (e.g., coronary, cerebral, or peripheral circulations) and normal LVEF, ACE inhibitors reduce the development of new-onset heart failure and diabetes, cardiovascular death, overall mortality, MI, and stroke.[60]

The most common cause of heart failure is ischemic heart disease, where MI results in loss of myocytes, followed by ventricular dilation and remodeling. Captopril, ramipril, and trandolapril have all been shown to benefit patients following MI whether they are initiated early (within 36 hours) and continued for 4 to 6 weeks or started later and administered for several years.[17] Collectively, these studies indicate that ACE inhibitors after MI improve overall survival, decrease development of severe heart failure, and reduce reinfarction and heart failure hospitalization rates.[17] The effects are most pronounced in higher-risk patients, such as those with symptomatic heart failure or reduced LVEF, with 20% to 30% reductions in mortality reported in these patients.[17] Post-MI patients without heart failure symptoms or decreases in LVEF (stage B) should also receive ACE inhibitors to prevent the development of heart failure and to reduce mortality.[1,17]

The clear benefit of ACE inhibitors is evident in the Joint Commission for Accreditation of Healthcare Organizations (JCAHO) and Centers for Medicare and Medicaid Services (CMS) selection of ACE inhibitor use in patients with heart failure and decreased LVEF as a key performance measure. This measure states that patients with left ventricular systolic dysfunction discharged from the hospital should receive ACE inhibitors unless there is documentation in the medical record of an absolute contraindication or drug intolerance. Despite the overwhelming benefit demonstrated with these agents, they remain underused and underdosed.[61] Also, for patients receiving an ACE inhibitor at hospital discharge, use significantly decreases over time, and patients not prescribed ACE inhibitors at discharge were unlikely to have therapy initiated in the outpatient setting.[61] Common reasons cited for underuse or underdosing are concerns about safety and adverse reactions to ACE inhibitors, especially in patients with underlying renal dysfunction or hypotension.

The use of ACE inhibitors in patients with renal insufficiency is particularly relevant, as it is present in 25% to 50% of patients with heart failure and is associated with an increased risk of mortality.[62] Despite the perceived risks, recent data indicate that ACE inhibitors may be more effective in those patients with renal insufficiency.[63,64] Because many patients with heart failure have concomitant disorders (e.g., diabetes, hypertension, and previous MI) that also may be favorably affected by ACE inhibitors, renal dysfunction should not be an absolute contraindication to ACE inhibitor use in patients with left ventricular dysfunction. However, these patients should be monitored carefully for the development of worsening renal function and/or hyperkalemia with special attention to risk factors associated with this complication of ACE inhibitor therapy.[1]

An important practical consideration is determining the proper dose of an ACE inhibitor. The ability to achieve target doses shown to be effective in clinical trials may be limited by hypotension and/or a decline in renal function. Clinical trials establishing the efficacy of these agents titrated drug doses to a predetermined target rather than according to therapeutic response. Although data on the dose-dependent effects of ACE inhibitors in patients with heart failure are limited, higher doses may reduce the risk of hospitalization compared with lower doses, but there do not appear to be significant differences in mortality.[65] In many positive trials of other heart failure therapies (e.g., β-blockers and aldosterone antagonists), intermediate ACE inhibitor doses were generally used as background therapy. These results emphasize that clinicians should attempt to use ACE inhibitor doses proven beneficial in clinical trials, but if these doses are not tolerated, lower doses can be used with the knowledge that there are likely only small differences in mortality outcomes between the high and low doses. Also, initiation of β-blocker therapy should not be delayed until target ACE inhibitor doses are achieved, because the addition of a β-blocker is proven to reduce mortality, whereas that is not the case with increasing ACE inhibitor doses.

In summary, the evidence that ACE inhibitors improve symptoms, slow disease progression, and decrease mortality in patients with heart failure and reduced LVEF (stage C) is unequivocal. Current guidelines indicate these patients should receive ACE inhibitors, unless contraindications are present.[1]

Beta-Blockers ❻

There is overwhelming evidence from multiple randomized, placebo-controlled clinical trials that β-blockers reduce morbidity and mortality in patients with heart failure. As such, the ACC/AHA guidelines on the management of heart failure recommend that β-blockers should be used in all stable patients with heart failure and a reduced LVEF in the absence of contraindications or a clear history of β-blocker intolerance.[1] Patients should receive a β-blocker even if their symptoms are mild or well controlled with diuretic and ACE inhibitor therapy. Importantly, it is not essential that ACE inhibitor doses are optimized before a β-blocker is started because the addition of a β-blocker is likely to be of greater benefit than an increase in ACE inhibitor dose.[1] Beta-blockers are also recommended for asymptomatic patients with a reduced LVEF (stage B) to decrease the risk of progression to heart failure.

Beta-blockers have been studied in over 20,000 patients with heart failure in placebo-controlled trials. Three β-blockers have been shown to significantly reduce mortality compared with placebo: carvedilol, metoprolol CR/XL, and bisoprolol. Each was studied in a large population with the primary end point of mortality. Carvedilol was the first β-blocker shown to improve survival in heart failure. In the U.S. Carvedilol Heart Failure Study, 1,094 patients were randomized to carvedilol or placebo in addition to standard therapy, including an ACE inhibitor, digoxin, and diuretic.[66] The study was stopped early because of a 65% reduction in the risk of death with carvedilol. Nearly 4,000 patients were randomized to metoprolol CR/XL (Toprol XL) or placebo in the Metoprolol CR/XL Randomised Intervention Trial in Congestive Heart Failure (MERIT-HF), the largest β-blocker mortality trial to date.[67] This trial was also stopped early because of a significant survival benefit with β-blockade. Specifically, metoprolol was associated with a 34% reduction in total mortality, a 41% reduction in sudden death, and a 49% reduction in death from worsening heart failure. Bisoprolol was studied in over 2,600 patients enrolled in the Cardiac Insufficiency Bisoprolol Study II (CIBIS II).[68] This study

was also stopped prematurely because of a 34% reduction in total mortality with bisoprolol compared with placebo. Bisoprolol was associated with a 44% reduction in sudden death and a 26% reduction in death due to worsening heart failure. Multiple post hoc subgroup analyses of data from the MERIT-HF and CIBIS II trials suggest that the benefits of β-blockade occur regardless of heart failure etiology or disease severity.

The majority of participants in MERIT-HF and CIBIS II had either NYHA class II or class III heart failure, and β-blockers became standard therapy in patients with class II or III disease after these trials were published. However, the efficacy and safety of β-blockers in patients with class IV heart failure were unclear until publication of the Carvedilol, Prospective, Randomized, Cumulative Survival (COPERNICUS) trial.[69] This trial randomized nearly 2,300 clinically stable patients who had symptoms at rest or with minimal exertion to carvedilol or placebo. Like the other studies, COPERNICUS was stopped prematurely after carvedilol produced a 35% relative reduction in mortality. Carvedilol was well tolerated in this population, with fewer participants receiving carvedilol compared with placebo requiring permanent discontinuation of study medication.

Data supporting the use of β-blockers in asymptomatic patients with left ventricular systolic dysfunction (stage B) come from a study of carvedilol in post-MI patients with a decreased LVEF.[70] Although the primary end point of all-cause mortality or hospital admission for cardiovascular problems was similar in the carvedilol and placebo groups, carvedilol significantly reduced all-cause mortality alone compared with placebo. Cardiovascular mortality and nonfatal MI were also lower among carvedilol-treated patients.

In addition to improving survival, β-blockers have been shown to improve multiple other end points. All the large clinical trials demonstrated 15% to 20% reductions in all-cause hospitalization and 25% to 35% reductions in hospitalizations for worsening heart failure with β-blocker therapy.[68,71,72] Studies have also shown consistent improvements in left ventricular systolic function with β-blockers, with increases in LVEF of 5 to 10 units (e.g., from an EF of 20% to 25% or 30%) after several weeks to months of therapy. Beta-blockers have also been shown to decrease ventricular mass, improve the sphericity of the ventricle, and reduce systolic and diastolic volumes (left ventricular end-systolic volume and left ventricular end-diastolic volume).[73,74] These effects are often collectively called *reverse remodeling*, referring to the fact that they return the heart toward more normal size, shape, and function.

The effects of β-blockers on symptoms and exercise tolerance varied among studies. Many studies showed improvements in NYHA functional class, patient symptom scores or quality-of-life assessments (e.g., the Minnesota Living with Heart Failure Questionnaire), and exercise performance, as assessed by the 6-minute walk test.[71–73] Other investigators found significant reductions in mortality with β-blockers but no significant improvement in symptoms.[75] As such, it is important to educate patients that β-blocker therapy is expected to positively influence disease progression and survival even if there is little to no symptomatic improvement.

The majority of participants in β-blocker trials were on ACE inhibitors at baseline because the benefits of ACE inhibitors were proven prior to β-blocker trials. Whether the strategy of starting a β-blocker prior to an ACE inhibitor is safe and effective has been debated. This issue was addressed in CIBIS III, in which patients with mild to moderate symptoms were randomized to initial therapy with either bisoprolol or enalapril.[76] Rates of death or hospitalization were similar with the two strategies. However, the trial failed to satisfy the prespecified statistical criterion for noninferiority of initial therapy with a β-blocker compared with an ACE inhibitor. In the absence of more compelling evidence, ACE inhibitors should be started first in most patients. Initiating a β-blocker first may be advantageous for patients with evidence of excessive SNS activity (e.g., tachycardia) and may also be appropriate for patients whose renal function or potassium concentrations preclude starting an ACE inhibitor (or ARB) at that time. However, the risk for decompensation during β-blocker initiation may be greater in the absence of preexisting ACE inhibitor therapy, and careful monitoring is essential.

Beta-blockers antagonize the detrimental effects of the SNS described earlier in the chapter. To this end, potential mechanisms to explain the favorable effects of β-blockers in heart failure include antiarrhythmic effects, attenuating or reversing ventricular remodeling, decreasing myocyte death from catecholamine-induced necrosis or apoptosis, preventing fetal gene expression, improving left ventricular systolic function, decreasing heart rate and ventricular wall stress, thereby reducing myocardial oxygen demand, and inhibiting plasma renin release.[1]

Components that are critical for successful β-blocker therapy include appropriate patient selection, drug initiation and titration, and patient education. Beta-blockers should be initiated in stable patients who have no or minimal evidence of fluid overload.[1] Although β-blockers are typically started in the outpatient setting, there are data indicating that initiation of a β-blocker prior to discharge in patients who are hospitalized for decompensated heart failure increases β-blocker usage compared with outpatient initiation without increasing the risk of serious adverse effects.[77] However, β-blockers should not be started in patients who are hospitalized in the intensive care unit or recently required IV inotropic support. In unstable patients, other heart failure therapy should be optimized and then β-blocker therapy reevaluated once stability is achieved.

Initiation of a β-blocker at normal doses in patients with heart failure may to lead to symptomatic worsening or acute decompensation owing to the drug's negative inotropic effect. For this reason, β-blockers are listed as drugs that may exacerbate or worsen heart failure (see Table 20–3). To minimize the likelihood of acute decompensation, β-blockers should be started in very low doses with slow upward dose titration. The starting doses and target doses achieved in clinical trials are described in Table 20–6. Of note, the smallest commercially available tablet of bisoprolol is a scored 5 mg tablet. Because the recommended starting dose of 1.25 mg/day is not readily available, bisoprolol is the least commonly used of the three agents and, in fact, is not approved by the FDA for use in heart failure. Thus, therapy is generally limited to either carvedilol or metoprolol CR/XL, and there is no compelling evidence that one drug is superior to the other. A controlled-release formulation of carvedilol (carvedilol CR) that allows once-daily dosing is available, and pharmacokinetic studies demonstrate similar degrees of drug exposure with the controlled- and immediate-release formations of the drug.[78] There are data showing similar adherence rates with the once- and twice-daily formulations of carvedilol.[79] Nonetheless, carvedilol CR may be considered in patients with difficulty maintaining adherence to the immediate-release formulation.

Beta-blocker doses should be doubled no more often than every 2 weeks, as tolerated, until the target or maximally tolerated dose is reached. According to current guidelines, target doses are those associated with reductions in mortality in placebo-controlled clinical trials.[1] Data with both metoprolol and carvedilol suggest that heart rate may serve as a guide to the degree of β-blockade and that lower β-blocker doses might be considered reasonable if the reduction in heart rate indicates a good response to β-blocker therapy.[80] In fact, it remains uncertain whether β-blocker dose or the degree of heart rate reduction is the optimal end point to guide dose—titration and predict survival.

A recent meta-analysis of 23 randomized trials involving over 19,000 patients receiving β-blockers for heart failure compared heart rate reduction and β-blocker dose as predictors of survival.[80] Overall, β-blocker treatment was associated with a 24% mortality reduction. However, trials with the largest decrease in heart rate (median 15 beats/min) reported a 36% reduction in mortality, whereas trials with the smallest heart rate reduction (median 8 beats/min) showed only a 9% mortality reduction. Greater magnitude of heart rate reduction was significantly associated with greater improvement in survival. On the other hand, no relationship between β-blocker dose and magnitude of mortality decrease was found. The results from this study suggest that the degree of β-blocker-mediated reduction in resting heart rate, but not β-blocker dose, is associated with the magnitude of improved survival. However, the analysis is limited by its retrospective design, inability to account for other factors affecting heart rate (e.g., vagal activity, β-receptor pharmacogenomics) and reliance on resting heart rate as a surrogate marker for the extent of β-blockade. Although resting heart rate is routinely used clinically to evaluate the extent of β-blockade, it is not as accurate as inhibition of exercise heart rate. Whether magnitude of resting heart rate reduction or achievement of clinical trial doses is the optimal surrogate marker for improved outcomes with β-blockers in heart failure remains uncertain and may only be definitively determined by prospective trials.

Good communication between the patient and healthcare provider(s) is particularly important for successful therapy. Patients should understand that dose uptitration is a long, gradual process and that achieving the target dose is important to maximize the benefits of therapy. Patients should also be aware that response to therapy may be delayed and that heart failure symptoms may actually worsen during the initiation period. In the event of worsening symptoms, patients who understand the potential benefits of long-term β-blocker therapy may be more likely to continue treatment.

In summary, the data provide clear evidence that β-blockers slow disease progression, decrease hospitalizations, and improve survival in heart failure. Beta-blockers have also been shown to improve quality of life in many patients with heart failure, although this is not a universal finding. Based on these data, β-blockers are recommended as standard therapy for all patients with systolic dysfunction, regardless of the severity of their symptoms. Clinical trial experience shows that target β-blocker doses can be achieved in the majority of patients provided that appropriate initiation, titration, and education are implemented.

Drug Therapies to Consider for Select Patients

Angiotensin II Receptor Blockers ❺ The crucial role of the RAAS in heart failure development and progression is well established, as are the benefits of inhibiting this system with ACE inhibitors. Despite the efficacy of ACE inhibitors, heart failure still progresses in many patients. ACE inhibitors decrease angiotensin II production in the short term, but these agents do not completely suppress generation of this hormone. With chronic administration of ACE inhibitors, ACE escape, characterized by increases

TABLE 20–6	Initial and Target Doses for β-blockers Used in Treatment of Heart Failure	
Drug	**Initial Dose**[b]	**Target Dose**
Bisoprolol[a]	1.25 mg once daily	10 mg once daily
Carvedilol[a]	3.125 mg bid	25 mg bid[c]
Carvedilol CR	10 mg once daily	80 mg once daily
Metoprolol succinate CR/XL[a]	12.5–25 mg once daily[d]	200 mg once daily

[a]Regimens proven in large trials to reduce mortality.
[b]Doses should be doubled approximately every 2 weeks, or as tolerated by the patient, until the highest tolerated or target dose is reached.
[c]Target dose for patients >85 kg is 50 mg bid.
[d]In MERIT-HF, the majority of NYHA class II patients were given 25 mg once daily, while the majority of class III patients were given 12.5 mg once daily as their starting dose.

in circulating angiotensin II and aldosterone, often occurs.[81] In addition, angiotensin II can be formed in a number of tissues, including the heart, through non-ACE-dependent pathways (e.g., chymase, cathepsin, and kallikrein).[17,81] Therefore, blockade of the detrimental effects of angiotensin II by ACE inhibition is incomplete. In addition, troublesome adverse effects of ACE inhibitors such as cough are linked to accumulation of bradykinin.[17] The ARBs block the angiotensin II receptor subtype, AT_1, preventing the deleterious effects of angiotensin II, regardless of its origin. Because ARBs do not inhibit the ACE enzyme, these agents do not appear to affect bradykinin.[81] By inhibiting both the formation of angiotensin II and its effects on the AT_1 receptor, combination therapy with an ACE inhibitor plus an ARB offers a theoretical advantage over either agent used alone through more complete blockade of the deleterious effects of angiotensin II. Also, by directly blocking AT_1 receptors, ARBs would allow unopposed stimulation of AT_2 receptors, causing vasodilation and inhibition of ventricular remodeling.[81] Because bradykinin-related adverse effects of ACE inhibitors such as angioedema and cough lead to drug discontinuation in some patients, the potential for an ARB to produce similar clinical benefits with fewer side effects is of great interest. Whether ARBs add incremental benefit to current established therapies or are superior (or equivalent) to ACE inhibitors is the focus of several clinical trials.[81]

Although a number of ARBs are currently available, the primary clinical trials supporting the use of these agents in heart failure used either valsartan or candesartan.[81] The Valsartan Heart Failure Trial (Val-HeFT) evaluated whether the addition of valsartan to standard background heart failure therapy (which included an ACE inhibitor in 93% and a β-blocker in 35% of patients) improved survival.[82] The addition of valsartan had no effect on all-cause mortality but produced a 13% reduction in morbidity and mortality (principally due to reductions in heart failure hospitalizations). Based on these results, valsartan is now approved for use in patients with NYHA class II to IV heart failure. The Valsartan in Acute Myocardial Infarction (VALIANT) trial compared the effect of valsartan, captopril, and the combination of the two agents in post-MI patients with symptomatic heart failure, reduced left ventricular systolic function, or both in a noninferiority trial design.[83] There were no differences in the primary end point of total mortality between patients receiving valsartan and captopril, captopril alone, or valsartan alone. Thus, in this high-risk post-MI population, valsartan was as effective as captopril in reducing the risk of death, but combination therapy only increased the risk of adverse effects and did not improve survival compared to monotherapy with either agent. Based on these findings, valsartan is now approved for use in post-MI patients with left ventricular failure or left ventricular dysfunction.

The Candesartan in Heart Failure: Assessment of Reduction in Mortality and Morbidity (CHARM) trials were designed as three studies to evaluate candesartan in patients with symptomatic heart failure.[84] Both the CHARM-Added (patients receiving background ACE inhibitor therapy)[85] and CHARM-Alternative (patients intolerant of ACE inhibitor therapy)[86] trials found significant reductions in the primary end point of cardiovascular death or hospitalization for heart failure in patients receiving candesartan, although the benefit was modest in CHARM-Added (17% reduction). No significant benefit of candesartan was observed in CHARM-Preserved (patients with LVEF >40%).[87] Overall, candesartan was well tolerated, but its use was associated with an increased risk of hypotension, hyperkalemia, and renal dysfunction. On the basis of these results, candesartan is now approved for use in symptomatic heart failure in patients with LVEF ≤40% to reduce cardiovascular death and reduce heart failure hospitalizations. These benefits are present when candesartan is used alone or with an ACE inhibitor.

The effect of high-dose compared with low-dose losartan treatment was evaluated in the Heart Failure Endpoint Evaluation of Angiotensin II Antagonist Losartan (HEAAL) study.[88] Over 3,800 patients who were intolerant to ACE inhibitors with an LVEF ≤40% and NYHA class II to IV symptoms were randomly assigned to losartan 50 or 150 mg daily. The primary end point was a composite of death or heart failure admission, and all patients received standard background heart failure pharmacotherapy. The higher losartan dose was associated with significant reductions (~10%) in the primary end point. Significant increases in renal insufficiency, hyperkalemia, and hypotension were also associated with the higher dose, but the development of these adverse effects did not result in increased rates of drug discontinuation. Although losartan is not approved for the treatment of heart failure, these results suggest that incremental benefit can be achieved by increasing doses of ARBs and ACE inhibitors[65] to achieve higher degrees of RAAS inhibition.

Although ACE inhibitors remain first-line therapy in patients with stage C heart failure and reduced LVEF, the current ACC/AHA guidelines recommend the use of ARBs in patients who are unable to tolerate ACE inhibitors.[1] Similarly, ARBs are alternatives to ACE inhibitors in patients with stage A or B heart failure.[1] Cough and angioedema are the most common causes of ACE inhibitor intolerance. Caution should be exercised when ARBs are used in patients with angioedema from ACE inhibitors, as some cross-reactivity has been reported.[89,90] ARBs are not an alternative in patients with hypotension, hyperkalemia, or renal insufficiency secondary to ACE inhibitors because they are as likely to cause these adverse effects. Also, the combined use of ACE inhibitors, ARBs, and aldosterone antagonists is not recommended because of the increased risk of renal dysfunction and hyperkalemia.[1] The specific drugs and doses proven to be effective in clinical trials should be used.

The role of combination therapy with an ACE inhibitor and an ARB remains controversial. The CHARM-Added trial found the addition of candesartan to ACE inhibitor and β-blocker therapy produced incremental reductions in cardiovascular death and hospitalizations for heart failure but did not improve overall survival.[85] In contrast, neither the VALIANT nor the Val-HeFT trials found additional benefit from the addition of valsartan to ACE inhibitor treatment.[82,83] Moreover, a recent meta-analysis showed that combination therapy is associated with increased risk of medication discontinuation due to adverse effects, hyperkalemia, renal insufficiency, and hypotension.[91] Collectively, these results suggest the addition of an ARB to optimal heart failure therapy (ACE inhibitors, β-blockers, diuretics, etc.) offers, at best, marginal benefits with increased risk of adverse effects. The current guidelines indicate that the addition of an ARB can be considered in patients who remain symptomatic despite receiving conventional heart failure pharmacotherapy. Some clinicians suggest that the addition of an aldosterone antagonist to ACE inhibitor and β-blocker therapy is preferred over that of an ARB. The proven survival benefit of aldosterone antagonists in patients with NYHA class III or IV heart failure (RALES trial) and in post-MI patients with left ventricular systolic dysfunction (EPHESUS trial), as discussed in the following section, supports this approach.[22,23]

Aldosterone Antagonists ❾ Spironolactone and eplerenone are aldosterone antagonists that work by blocking the mineralocorticoid receptor, the target site for aldosterone. In the kidney, aldosterone antagonists inhibit sodium reabsorption and potassium excretion. Although the diuretic effects with low doses of aldosterone antagonists are minimal, the potassium-sparing effects can have significant consequences, as discussed later in the chapter. In the heart, aldosterone antagonists inhibit cardiac extracellular matrix and collagen deposition, thereby attenuating cardiac fibrosis and ventricular remodeling.[92] Spironolactone also interacts with androgen and progesterone receptors, which may lead to gynecomastia

and other sexual side effects in some patients. Such adverse effects are less frequent with eplerenone owing to its low affinity for the progesterone and androgen receptors.

Evidence that ACE inhibitors incompletely suppress aldosterone provided the impetus for examining the benefits of adding an aldosterone antagonist to ACE inhibitor therapy.[93] The Randomized Aldactone Evaluation Study (RALES) randomized over 1,600 patients with current or recent NYHA class IV heart failure to aldosterone blockade with spironolactone 25 mg daily or placebo.[22] Patients were also treated with standard therapy, usually including an ACE inhibitor, loop diuretic, and digoxin. Those with a serum creatinine concentration >2.5 mg/dL or a serum potassium concentration >5 mEq/L were excluded. The study was stopped prematurely after an average follow-up of 24 months because of a significant 30% reduction in the primary end point of total mortality with spironolactone. Spironolactone reduced mortality due to both progressive heart failure and sudden cardiac death. It also produced a 35% reduction in hospitalizations for worsening heart failure and significant symptomatic improvement, as assessed by changes in NYHA functional class. The low dose of spironolactone was well tolerated in RALES. The most common adverse effect was gynecomastia, which occurred in 10% of men on spironolactone compared with 1% of men on placebo, and led to treatment discontinuation in 2% of patients. There were statistically (but not clinically) significant increases in serum creatinine (by 0.05–0.10 mg/dL) and potassium concentrations (by 0.30 mEq/L) with spironolactone. The incidence of serious hyperkalemia (>6 mEq/L) was minimal and did not differ between spironolactone- and placebo-treated groups.

More recently, the EPHESUS trial evaluated the effect of selective antagonism of the mineralocorticoid receptor with eplerenone in patients with left ventricular dysfunction after MI.[23] To be eligible for study participation, patients had to have evidence of either heart failure or diabetes. Over 6,600 patients were randomized within 3 to 14 days of MI to eplerenone, titrated to 50 mg daily, or placebo in addition to standard therapy, which usually included an ACE inhibitor, β-blocker, aspirin, and diuretics. Similar to the RALES trial, patients with serum creatinine concentrations greater than 2.5 mg/dL or serum potassium concentrations greater than 5 mEq/L were excluded. Treatment with eplerenone was associated with a significant 15% relative reduction in the risk for death from any cause and a 15% reduction in the risk of hospitalization from heart failure. Serious hyperkalemia occurred in 5.5% of eplerenone-treated patients and 3.9% of placebo-treated patients. Eplerenone was not associated with gynecomastia.

The benefits of aldosterone antagonists in heart failure are not just due to the inhibition of aldosterone's actions in the heart resulting in inhibition of aldosterone-mediated cardiac fibrosis and ventricular remodeling. Recent evidence points to an important role of aldosterone antagonists in attenuating the systemic proinflammatory state and oxidative stress caused by aldosterone.[94,95] In addition, there is evidence that aldosterone antagonists may attenuate aldosterone-induced calcium excretion and reductions in bone mineral density and protect against fractures in heart failure.[96,97] And although spironolactone historically has been viewed as a diuretic, this is believed to contribute little to its benefits in heart failure, in part because the doses used have minimal diuretic effect.[22] Thus, as with ACE inhibitors and β-blockers, the data on aldosterone antagonists also support the neurohormonal model of heart failure.

Current guidelines recommend adding a low-dose aldosterone antagonist to standard therapy in select patients provided that potassium and renal function can be carefully monitored.[1] Based on data from RALES and EPHESUS, low-dose aldosterone antagonists are appropriate for two groups of patients: those with moderately severe to severe heart failure and reduced LVEF who are receiving

standard therapy and those with left ventricular dysfunction early after MI.[1] For patients who fall outside the populations studied in these clinical trials, there are no clear guidelines on aldosterone antagonist use. Trials to address the efficacy of aldosterone antagonism in patients with mild to moderate heart failure symptoms and in patients with preserved left ventricular systolic function are ongoing. In the interim, guidelines state that it might be reasonable to consider use of aldosterone antagonists for some patients with mild to moderate symptoms. Such patients might include those who require potassium supplementation. The premise for use in this setting would be that it might be possible to reduce or eliminate potassium supplementation while potentially providing additional benefit with respect to altering the disease course.

Despite the clear benefits of aldosterone antagonists in patients with moderately severe to severe heart failure and left ventricular systolic dysfunction, registry data show that only one third of patients meeting guideline criteria for an aldosterone antagonist actually receive one.[98,99] The low use of aldosterone antagonists is likely due in large part to safety concerns. The clinical trial data suggest that aldosterone antagonists in heart failure are associated with minimal risk when used appropriately (e.g., in those with adequate renal function and with close laboratory monitoring). However, shortly after publication of RALES, an observational study of approximately 1.3 million elderly patients in the Ontario Drug Benefit Program found that the increase in the spironolactone prescription rate following the publication of RALES was accompanied by nearly threefold increases in the rate of hospital admissions and the rate of death related to hyperkalemia.[100] In addition, small case series showed that 25% to 35% of patients treated outside the controlled clinical trial setting developed hyperkalemia (>5 mEq/L) and that 10% to 12% developed serious hyperkalemia.[101,102]

Potential factors contributing to the high incidence of hyperkalemia in clinical practice include the initiation of aldosterone antagonists in patients with impaired renal function or high potassium concentrations and the failure to decrease or stop potassium supplements when starting aldosterone antagonists. Other risk factors for hyperkalemia include diabetes, inadequate laboratory monitoring, and concomitant use of both ACE inhibitors and ARBs or NSAIDs. ACC/AHA recently recommended strategies to minimize the risk for hyperkalemia with aldosterone antagonists in heart failure.[1] These strategies are summarized in Table 20–7. Chief among these recommendations is to avoid aldosterone antagonists in patients with renal dysfunction or elevated serum potassium. It is important to emphasize here that serum creatinine may overestimate renal function in the elderly and in patients with decreased muscle mass, in whom creatinine clearance should serve as a guide for the appropriateness of aldosterone antagonist therapy. The risk for hyperkalemia is dose dependent, and the morbidity and mortality reductions with aldosterone antagonists in clinical trials occurred at low doses (i.e., spironolactone 25 mg/day and eplerenone 50 mg/day). Therefore, the doses of aldosterone antagonists should be limited to those associated with beneficial effects in order to decrease the risk for hyperkalemia.

Only 10% of RALES participants were taking β-blockers at baseline because the benefits of β-blockers in heart failure were not appreciated fully at the time the trial began.[22] Beta-blockers inhibit plasma renin release and may provide additional suppression of the RAAS when used with ACE inhibitors. Thus, there has been some speculation about whether spironolactone will provide further benefit in patients receiving both ACE inhibitors and β-blockers. However, data from EPHESUS provide some clarity to this issue, as the majority of EPHESUS participants were on β-blockers at baseline, and the trial still demonstrated significant reductions in mortality with the addition of eplerenone.[23]

TABLE 20-7	Recommended Strategies for Reducing the Risk of Hyperkalemia with Aldosterone Antagonists

1. Avoid starting aldosterone antagonists in patients with any of the following:
   - Serum creatinine concentration >2 mg/dL in women or >2.5 mg/dL in men or a creatinine clearance <30 mL/min
   - Recent worsening of renal function
   - Serum potassium concentration ≥5 mEq/L
   - History of severe hyperkalemia
2. Start with low doses (12.5 mg/d for spironolactone and 25 mg/d for eplerenone), especially in the elderly and in those with diabetes or a creatinine clearance <50 mL/min.
3. Decrease or discontinue potassium supplements when starting an aldosterone antagonist.
4. Avoid concomitant use of NSAIDs or COX-2 inhibitors.
5. Avoid concomitant use of high-dose ACE inhibitors or ARBs.
6. Avoid triple therapy with an ACE inhibitor, ARB, and aldosterone antagonist.
7. Monitor serum potassium concentrations and renal function within 3 days and 1 week after the initiation or dose titration of an aldosterone antagonist or any other medication that could affect potassium homeostasis. Thereafter, potassium concentrations and renal function should be monitored monthly for the first 3 months, then every 3 months.
8. If potassium exceeds 5.5 mg/dL* at any point during therapy, discontinue any potassium supplementation, or, in the absence of potassium supplements, reduce or stop aldosterone antagonist therapy.
9. Counsel patients to
   - Limit intake of high potassium-containing foods and salt substitutes.
   - Avoid the use of nonprescription NSAIDs.
   - Temporarily discontinue aldosterone antagonist therapy if diarrhea develops or diuretic therapy is interrupted.

Abbreviations: ACE, angiotensin-converting enzyme; ARB, angiotensin receptor blocker; COX-2, cyclooxygenase-2; NSAID, nonsteroidal antiinflammatory drug.
Source: Adapted from Hunt SA, Abraham WT, Chin MH, et al. 2009 focused update incorporated into the ACC/AHA 2005 guidelines for the diagnosis and management of heart failure in adults: A report of the American College of Cardiology Foundation/American Heart Association Task Force on Practice Guidelines. Circulation 2009;119:e391–e479.

Digoxin ⑧ In 1785, William Withering was the first to report extensively on the use of foxglove or *Digitalis purpurea* for the treatment of dropsy (i.e., edema). Although digitalis glycosides have been in clinical use for more than 200 years, not until the 1920s were they clearly demonstrated to have a positive inotropic effect on the heart. Furthermore, it was not until the late 1980s that clinical trials were conducted to critically evaluate the role of digoxin in the therapy of systolic heart failure. The results of the Digitalis Investigation Group (DIG) trial helped clarify the role of digoxin in this setting.[103] The view of digoxin has also shifted over the past decade. Although it was historically considered useful in heart failure because of its positive inotropic effects, it now seems clear that its real benefits in heart failure are related to its neurohormonal modulating activity.[104,105]

The efficacy of digoxin in patients with heart failure and supraventricular tachyarrhythmias such as atrial fibrillation is well established and widely accepted. Its role in patients with normal sinus rhythm has been considerably more controversial. Until the 1980s, most data supporting the efficacy of digoxin in these patients came from anecdotal evidence and seriously flawed or uncontrolled studies. Since then, a number of clinical trials have shown that digoxin improves cardiac function, quality of life, exercise tolerance, and heart failure symptoms.[105,106] However, these studies involved small numbers of patients followed for short time periods. Although these trials demonstrated hemodynamic and symptomatic improvement in patients with heart failure receiving digoxin, an unresolved issue was the unknown effect of digoxin on mortality. This was of particular concern, given the increased mortality seen with other positive inotropic drugs, and finally led to organization

and performance of the DIG trial to determine the effects of digoxin on survival in patients with heart failure in sinus rhythm.[103]

The DIG trial was a double-blind, randomized, placebo-controlled trial with the primary end point of all-cause mortality.[103] Patients ($n = 6,800$) with heart failure symptoms and an EF ≤45% were eligible for the main DIG trial and were randomized to received digoxin or placebo for a mean follow-up period of 37 months. Most patients received background therapy with diuretics and ACE inhibitors. Digoxin serum concentrations of 0.5 to 2 ng/mL were targeted, with a mean serum digoxin concentration of 0.8 ng/mL achieved after 12 months of therapy. No significant differences in all-cause mortality were found between patients receiving digoxin and placebo. A trend toward lower mortality due to worsening heart failure was observed in the digoxin group, although this was offset by a trend toward an increased mortality from other cardiovascular causes (presumably arrhythmias) in patients receiving digoxin. Importantly, digoxin reduced hospitalizations for worsening heart failure by 28% compared with placebo ($P < 0.001$). Therefore, DIG is the first trial to show that a positive inotropic agent does not increase mortality and actually decreases morbidity in patients with heart failure and reduced systolic function. On the other hand, among an additional 988 patients with an EF greater than 45% (diastolic dysfunction) who were enrolled in an ancillary DIG trial, there was no apparent benefit of digoxin on hospitalizations or mortality during the 37-month follow-up period.[107]

The Prospective Randomized Study of Ventricular Failure and the Efficacy of Digoxin (PROVED) and Randomized Assessment of Digoxin and Inhibitors of Angiotensin-Converting Enzyme (RADIANCE) trials investigated the effect of digoxin withdrawal in patients with systolic heart failure and normal sinus rhythm and further defined the role of digoxin in this setting.[108,109] Both of these trials were short-term (12-week), prospective, randomized, and placebo-controlled and were conducted prior to the use of β-blockers. Together, data from these trials suggested that digoxin produces important symptomatic benefits and that digoxin withdrawal results in worsening heart failure, decreased exercise capacity, and a reduction in EF. A post hoc analysis of the DIG trial data supports previous findings that discontinuation of digoxin may be detrimental. Specifically, among patients treated with digoxin prior to enrollment in the DIG trial, those assigned to the placebo arm (i.e., those discontinuing digoxin therapy) had an increased risk of all-cause hospitalization and heart failure—related hospitalization compared with patients assigned to the digoxin arm (i.e., those continuing digoxin therapy).[110]

Retrospective analyses of the combined PROVED/RADIANCE database[111] and the DIG trial database[112] suggest that the clinical benefits of digoxin are achieved at lower serum digoxin concentrations (SDCs), with no additional benefit with higher concentrations. In particular, analysis of digoxin-treated patients in the PROVED and RADIANCE trials showed similar clinical outcomes among those with an SDC between 0.5 and 0.9 ng/mL as those with higher serum concentrations.[111] Although the DIG trial showed no reduction in mortality in the study population overall, a comprehensive analysis of the DIG trial database found that lower SDCs were associated with decreased mortality, whereas higher concentrations were not.[112] Specifically, compared with placebo, SDCs of 0.5 to 0.9 ng/mL 1 month after digoxin initiation were associated with lower mortality, all-cause hospitalizations, and heart failure hospitalizations. Serum concentrations greater than or equal 1 ng/mL were associated with lower heart failure hospitalizations with no effect on mortality. A digoxin dose of ≤0.125 mg daily was predictive of SDCs of 0.4 to 0.9 ng/mL. Although an initial, well-publicized study suggested that digoxin might be harmful in women,[113] subsequent analyses show no increased risks with digoxin in women, particularly with SDCs less than 1 ng/mL.[112,114]

Another post hoc analysis of DIG trial data evaluated the effect of digoxin on mortality at 1 year.[115] In contrast to the original DIG data, the investigators observed a reduction in all-cause mortality in addition to reductions in heart failure—related mortality and all-cause hospitalizations with digoxin compared with placebo. The investigators postulated that increased use of open-label digoxin in the placebo group and worsening renal function over time leading to increased SDCs in the digoxin group may explain the lack of sustained effects of digoxin on mortality. Because this analysis was retrospective and nonprespecified, the results should be interpreted with caution. However, it provides reassurance of the safety of digoxin early after initiation.

Based on the available data, for most patients, the target SDC should be 0.5 to 1 ng/mL. This more conservative target would also be expected to decrease the risk of adverse effects from digoxin toxicity. In fact, recent assessment of the rate of digoxin toxicity has suggested a significant decline in the overall incidence.[116] In most patients with normal renal function, this serum concentration range can be achieved with a daily dose of 0.125 mg. Patients with decreased renal function, the elderly, or those receiving interacting drugs (e.g., amiodarone) should receive 0.125 mg daily or every other day. Routine measuring of SDCs is not necessary in the absence of suspected digoxin toxicity, worsening renal function, institution of an interacting drug, or other conditions that may significantly affect SDC. In patients with atrial fibrillation and a rapid ventricular response, the historic practice of increasing digoxin doses (and concentrations) until rate control is achieved is no longer recommended. Digoxin alone is often ineffective in controlling ventricular response in patients with atrial fibrillation, and increasing the dose only increases the risk of toxicity. Digoxin combined with a β-blocker or amiodarone is superior to either agent alone for controlling ventricular response in patients with atrial fibrillation and heart failure.[1] Therefore, target SDCs are the same regardless of whether the patient is in sinus rhythm or atrial fibrillation. Several equations and nomograms have been proposed to estimate digoxin maintenance doses based on estimated renal function for a particular patient and population pharmacokinetic parameters. These methods are extensively reviewed elsewhere.[117] More recently, based on post hoc analyses from the DIG, PROVED, and RADIANCE trials, investigators developed a digoxin-dosing nomogram that targets a lower digoxin plasma concentration.[118] In the absence of supraventricular tachyarrhythmias, a loading dose is not indicated because digoxin is a mild inotropic agent that will produce gradual effects over several hours, even after loading.

Digoxin's place in the pharmacotherapy of systolic heart failure can therefore be summarized for two patient groups. In patients with heart failure and supraventricular tachyarrhythmias such as atrial fibrillation, it should be considered early in therapy to help control the ventricular response rate. For patients in normal sinus rhythm, although digoxin does not improve survival, its effects on symptom reduction and clinical outcomes are evident in patients with mild to severe heart failure with reduced systolic function. Thus, it should be used in conjunction with other standard heart failure therapies, including diuretics, ACE inhibitors, and β-blockers, in patients with symptomatic heart failure to reduce hospitalizations. In the absence of digoxin toxicity or serious adverse effects, digoxin should be continued in most patients. Digoxin withdrawal may be considered for asymptomatic patients who have significant improvement in systolic function with optimal ACE inhibitor and β-blocker treatment.[106]

Nitrates and Hydralazine ⑩ Nitrates and hydralazine were combined originally in the treatment of heart failure because of their complementary hemodynamic actions. Nitrates, by serving as nitric oxide donors, activate guanylate cyclase to increase cyclic guanosine monophosphate (cGMP) in vascular smooth muscle. This results in venodilation and reductions in preload. Hydralazine is a direct-acting vasodilator that acts predominantly on arterial smooth muscle to reduce SVR and increase stroke volume and cardiac output (see Fig. 20–1). Hydralazine also has antioxidant properties and appears to prevent nitrate tolerance.[119] Evidence also suggests that the combination of hydralazine and nitrates may exert beneficial effects beyond their hemodynamic actions by interfering with the biochemical processes associated with heart failure progression.[1,120]

The efficacy of the combination of hydralazine and isosorbide dinitrate (ISDN) has been evaluated in three large, randomized heart failure trials. The first trial predated the use of ACE inhibitors and β-blockers in heart failure and found that the combination of hydralazine 75 mg and ISDN 40 mg, each given four times daily, reduced mortality compared with placebo in patients receiving diuretics and digoxin.[121] However, a subsequent trial comparing the combination with an ACE inhibitor demonstrated greater mortality reduction with the ACE inhibitor.[122] Post hoc analysis of these trials suggested that the combination of hydralazine and ISDN was particularly effective in African Americans and led to examining the efficacy of adding the combination to standard therapy in this group.[123]

The African-American Heart Failure Trial (A-HeFT) randomized 1,050 self-identified African Americans with NYHA class III or IV heart failure to hydralazine plus ISDN or placebo, each in addition to standard therapy, usually including an ACE inhibitor (or ARB), β-blocker, and diuretic, with or without digoxin and spironolactone.[120] The trial used a fixed-dose combination product, BiDil, that contains hydralazine 37.5 mg and ISDN 20 mg. Therapy was initiated as a single tablet given three times daily, then titrated to two tablets three times daily if tolerated. The trial was terminated early after a mean follow-up of 10 months because of a significant 43% reduction in all-cause mortality in patients receiving hydralazine/ISDN compared with placebo. The primary composite end point of mortality, hospitalizations for heart failure, and quality of life was also significantly improved with the combination product. Based on these results, BiDil was approved by the FDA to treat heart failure exclusively in African Americans.

The mechanism for the beneficial effects of hydralazine/ISDN is believed to relate to an increase in nitric oxide bioavailability secondary to nitric oxide donation from ISDN and a hydralazine-mediated reduction in oxidative stress.[119] Nitric oxide has been shown to attenuate myocardial remodeling and may play a protective role in heart failure. It is suggested that African Americans have less nitric oxide availability compared with non—African Americans, and thus may derive particular benefit from therapy that enhances nitric oxide bioavailability. Whether the benefits of adding hydralazine/ISDN to standard therapy extend to non—African Americans remains to be prospectively evaluated. However, a recent nonrandomized trial found that the addition of ISDN and hydralazine improved hemodynamics and clinical outcomes (all-cause mortality and the combined end point of mortality and heart failure hospitalization) in patients of any race with advanced systolic heart failure receiving ACE inhibitors and/or ARBs who were discharged from the hospital after an episode of acute decompensated heart failure.[124]

Approximately 350 A-HeFT participants were enrolled in a genetic substudy to examine whether genotype influenced response to hydralazine/ISDN. Separate analyses examined the associations between the endothelial nitric oxide synthase-3 (NOS3) Glu298Asp and corin Gln568Pro variants and treatment outcomes.[125,126] The NOS3 study showed that hydralazine/ISDN improved the composite end point of survival, hospitalization, and quality of life in those with the Glu/Glu genotype, but not in those with the Asp allele.[125] The corin study suggested that hydralazine/ISDN abolishes adverse consequences of the 568Pro allele. Corin is a protein expressed in cardiomyocytes that cleaves pro-ANP and pro-BNP into active natriuretic peptides. The corin 568Pro variant leads to a dysfunctional protein and lower BNP levels.[126] Among A-HeFT participants in the placebo group, the 568Pro allele was associated with an increased risk for death or heart failure hospitalization.[126] However, no detrimental effect of the 568Pro variant was observed in the hydralazine/ISDN treatment group. Both the *NOS3* Glu/Glu genotype and corin 568Pro variant occur predominantly in persons of African descent, potentially explaining why hydralazine/ISDN is especially effective in African Americans.

In the future, treatment with hydralazine and nitrates could be guided by genotype. Until then, current guidelines recommend the addition of hydralazine and nitrates to self-described African Americans with moderate to severe symptoms despite therapy with ACE inhibitors, diuretics, and β-blockers.[1] This combination is also reasonable to consider in all patients who continue to have symptoms despite optimized therapy with an ACE inhibitor (or ARB) and β-blocker.[1] For patients unable to tolerate an ACE inhibitor because of cough or angioedema, an ARB is recommended as the first-line alternative.[1] Hydralazine and a nitrate might be reasonable in patients unable to tolerate either an ACE inhibitor or an ARB because of renal insufficiency, hyperkalemia, or possibly hypotension.[1]

There are several potential obstacles to successful therapy with hydralazine and nitrates in heart failure. The first is the need for frequent dosing, with the fixed-dose combination dosed three times daily and the individual drugs dosed four times daily in clinical trials. Second, adverse effects are common with hydralazine/nitrates, with headache, dizziness, and GI distress occurring more frequently with hydralazine/nitrates compared with placebo in clinical trials.[120,121] A third potential obstacle is the high cost of the brand-name fixed-dose combination product compared with the individual generic drugs purchased separately. Because of the high cost of the combination product, many clinicians use generic hydralazine and isosorbide as separate agents rather than the combination product, although this approach has not been evaluated in clinical trials.

Treatment of Concomitant Disorders

Heart failure is often accompanied by other disorders whose natural history or therapy may affect morbidity and mortality. In select patients, optimal management of these concomitant disorders may have a profound impact on heart failure symptoms and outcomes.

Hypertension Although ischemic heart disease has replaced hypertension as the most common cause of heart failure, still nearly two thirds of heart failure patients have current hypertension or a previous history of hypertension.[1] Hypertension can contribute directly to the development of left ventricular systolic and/or diastolic dysfunction and heart failure. It can also contribute indirectly by increasing the risk of coronary artery disease. Effective treatment of hypertension reduces the risk of developing heart failure, especially in patients with diabetes.[1]

Pharmacotherapy of hypertension in patients with heart failure should initially involve agents that can treat both disorders, such as ACE inhibitors, β-blockers, and diuretics. Target levels of blood pressure should be consistent with current guidelines.[1,46] If control of hypertension is not achieved after optimizing treatment with these agents, the addition of an ARB, aldosterone antagonist, isosorbide dinitrate/hydralazine, or a second-generation calcium channel blocker such as amlodipine (or possibly felodipine) should be considered. Medications that should be avoided include the calcium channel blockers with negative inotropic effects (e.g., verapamil, diltiazem, and most dihydropyridines) and direct-acting vasodilators (e.g., minoxidil) that cause sodium retention.

Angina Coronary artery disease is the most common heart failure etiology. Appropriate management of coronary disease and its risk factors is thus an important strategy for the prevention and treatment of heart failure. Coronary revascularization should be strongly considered in patients with both heart failure and angina.[1] Pharmacotherapy of angina in patients with heart failure should utilize drugs that can successfully treat both disorders. Nitrates and β-blockers are effective antianginals and are the preferred agents for patients with both disorders, as they may improve hemodynamics and clinical outcomes.[1] It should be noted that the antianginal effectiveness of these agents may be significantly limited if fluid retention is not controlled with diuretics. Similar to their use in hypertension, both amlodipine and felodipine appear to be safe to use in this setting. Optimization of other treatments for secondary prevention of coronary and other atherosclerotic vascular disease should also be considered.[46] Two large trials found that despite significant reductions in low-density lipoprotein (LDL) cholesterol, rosuvastatin did not improve outcomes including mortality, nonfatal MI, nonfatal stroke, or hospital admission for cardiovascular causes in patients with heart failure and reduced LVEF.[31,32] Therefore, the current data do not support the routine use of statins in systolic heart failure, although the precise role of statins in these patients remains controversial.

Atrial Fibrillation Atrial fibrillation is the most frequently encountered arrhythmia. It is commonly found in patients with heart failure, affecting 10% to 50% of patients, with the prevalence increasing in parallel to the severity of heart failure.[35] The high incidence of atrial fibrillation in the heart failure population is not surprising, as each of these two disorders predisposes to the other, and they share many risk factors, including coronary artery disease, diabetes, obesity, and hypertension. The presence of atrial fibrillation in patients with heart failure is associated with a worse long-term prognosis.[1,35] The combination of atrial fibrillation and heart failure may exert a number of detrimental effects, which include increased risk of thromboembolism secondary to stasis of blood in the atria, a reduction in cardiac output due to loss of the atrial contribution to ventricular filling, and hemodynamic compromise from the rapid ventricular response.[35] Moreover, heart failure exacerbations and atrial fibrillation are closely linked, and it is often difficult to determine which disorder caused the other. For example, worsening heart failure results in volume overload, which in turn causes atrial distention and increases the risk of atrial fibrillation. Similarly, atrial fibrillation with a rapid ventricular response can reduce cardiac output and lead to heart failure exacerbation. Thus, optimal management according to established guidelines is required, with careful attention paid to control of ventricular response and anticoagulation for stroke prevention (see Chapter 25).[127]

Recent studies suggest that ACE inhibitors, ARBs, and β-blockers decrease the incidence of atrial fibrillation in patients with heart failure, providing further support for their use in these patients.[128,129] Digoxin is frequently used to slow ventricular response in patients with heart failure and atrial fibrillation. However, it is more effective at rest than with exercise, and it does not affect the progression of heart failure. Beta-blockers are more effective than digoxin and have the added benefits of improving heart failure—related morbidity and mortality. Combination therapy with digoxin and a β-blocker may be more effective for rate control than either agent used alone. Calcium channel blockers with negative inotropic effects such as verapamil and diltiazem should be avoided. Amiodarone is a reasonable alternative for rate control in those patients not responding to digoxin and/or β-blockers or with contraindications to these agents.[127] Appropriate selection of antithrombotic therapy for stroke prevention that takes into consideration the presence of risk factors for thromboembolism in an individual patient is also required.[127]

Because of the close association between atrial fibrillation, heart failure exacerbations, and hospitalizations, restoration and maintenance of sinus rhythm (i.e., rhythm control) is often attempted instead of the rate control approach. Although initial trials such as

AFFIRM showed no difference in outcomes between the rhythm control and rate control approaches, less than 10% of the patients in this study had significant left ventricular dysfunction.[130] The Atrial Fibrillation and Congestive Heart Failure (AF-CHF) trial prospectively compared the rhythm and rate control approaches in nearly 1,400 patients with symptomatic heart failure and LVEF ≤35%.[131] Rhythm control was primarily achieved with amiodarone, whereas a β-blocker and digoxin were used for rate control. Compared with rate control, there were no improvements in mortality, stroke, death from cardiovascular causes, or heart failure hospitalizations in the rhythm control arm. Therefore, overall rhythm control appears to offer no specific advantages over rate control in this population and can be reserved for patients in whom the rate cannot be controlled or who remain symptomatic. In general, amiodarone is the preferred agent if the rhythm control approach is taken. Although it has many noncardiac toxicities, amiodarone does not have cardiodepressant or significant proarrhythmic effects and appears to be safe in heart failure. Dofetilide also appears to be safe and effective in this population.[35,127] Class I antiarrhythmics should be avoided.[35,127]

Diabetes Diabetes is highly prevalent in the heart failure population, with current estimates indicating it is present in approximately one third of patients with heart failure.[38,132] As an important risk factor for coronary artery disease, diabetes directly contributes to the development of heart failure. Importantly, though, diabetes is a risk factor for heart failure independent of coronary artery disease or hypertension, is associated with hastened heart failure progression, and is a significant predictor of mortality in patients with heart failure.[132]

Pharmacotherapy of diabetes in patient with heart failure is complicated by concerns about adverse effects associated with metformin and the thiazolidinedione (TZD) drugs (rosiglitazone and pioglitazone). The beneficial effects of these agents on glucose control and cardiovascular risk factors lead to their widespread use in patients with heart failure despite the warnings in the product labeling against their use.[132] Use of metformin in patients with heart failure has been contraindicated because of the purported risk of lactic acidosis. However, the product labeling was recently revised removing this contraindication, although a warning still remains specifically in patients with hypoperfusion and hypoxemia. Data from observational studies and a systematic review suggest that metformin is safe (no reports of lactic acidosis or hospital admissions) and is associated with decreased mortality in patients with heart failure.[133,134] Therefore, some clinicians suggest that the concerns about metformin use in hemodynamically stable patients with normal renal function should be reexamined. However, the lack of prospective data about the safety and efficacy of metformin in this population suggests that if metformin is used, it should be used cautiously with careful monitoring of volume status and renal function.[132]

Although the mechanisms are presently unclear, TZDs are associated with weight gain, peripheral edema, and heart failure. The TZD package inserts indicate these agents should not be used in patients with NYHA class III or IV heart failure because they may cause intravascular volume expansion and heart failure exacerbation. Most clinical trials with these drugs excluded patients with moderate to severe heart failure; thus, there is a lack of prospective data to guide clinical decision making. A systematic review and an observational study both suggest TZDs do not increase mortality but do increase the risk of hospital admission for heart failure.[133,134] Because of the potential risk, a recent consensus statement indicates TZDs should not be used in patients with NYHA class III or IV heart failure.[38] TZDs should be used cautiously in patients with class I or II symptoms, with close observation needed to detect weight gain, edema formation, or heart failure exacerbation.[38]

Anemia Anemia occurs frequently in patients with heart failure and is associated with worse clinical outcomes, including increased risk of death, hospitalization for heart failure, reduced exercise capacity, and worse quality of life.[135] The exact cause of anemia in patients with heart failure is uncertain but likely involves reduced response to erythropoietin, the presence of inhibitors to hematopoiesis, renal dysfunction, proinflammatory state, bone marrow suppression, and/or iron deficiency.[135] As a result, there is widespread interest in the correction of anemia as a therapeutic target in heart failure. A recent meta-analyis suggests erythropoiesis-stimulating agents improve symptoms and exercise capacity and decrease plasma natriuretic peptide levels in patients with heart failure and anemia.[136] A recently completed trial using darbepoetin in patients with type 2 diabetes, chronic kidney disease, and anemia (~30% of the patients had heart failure) did not improve cardiovascular outcomes and increased the risk of stroke.[137] Administration of IV iron to patients with NYHA class II or III symptoms, an LVEF ≤45%, and iron deficiency was associated with improvements in exercise capacity and quality of life with no increased risk of adverse events.[138] The results of ongoing prospective trials are needed to characterize the risks and benefits of treating anemia in this population.

Drug Class Information

Diuretics ❼ Loop diuretics, as described earlier, represent the typical diuretic therapy for patients with heart failure due to their potency and, as such, are the only diuretics discussed here.[57] There are currently three loop diuretics available that are used routinely: furosemide, bumetanide, and torsemide. They share many similarities in their pharmacodynamics, with their differences being largely pharmacokinetic in nature. Relevant information on the loop diuretics is shown in Table 20–5. Following oral administration, the peak effect with all the agents occurs in 30 to 90 minutes, with duration of 2 to 3 hours (slightly longer for torsemide). Following IV administration, the diuretic effect begins within minutes. All three drugs are highly (>95%) bound to serum albumin and enter the nephron by active secretion in the proximal tubule. The magnitude of effect is determined by the peak concentration achieved in the nephron, and there is a threshold concentration that must be achieved before any diuresis is seen.

The biggest difference between the agents is bioavailability. Bioavailability of bumetanide and torsemide is essentially complete (80–100%), whereas furosemide bioavailability exhibits marked intra- and interpatient variability. Furosemide bioavailability ranges from 10% to 100%, with an average of 50%. Thus, if bioequivalent IV and oral doses are desired, oral furosemide doses should be approximately double that of the IV dose, whereas IV and oral doses are the same for torsemide and bumetanide. Coadministration of furosemide and bumetanide with food can decrease bioavailability significantly, whereas food has no effect on the bioavailability of torsemide. The intra-abdominal congestion that can occur in heart failure also may slow the rate (and thus decrease the peak concentration) of furosemide, which can reduce the diuretic's efficacy. Thus, furosemide is most problematic with respect to rate and extent of absorption and the factors that influence it, whereas torsemide has the least variable bioavailability.

Recent data suggest that these differences in bioavailability and variability may have clinical implications. For example, several studies have suggested that torsemide is absorbed reliably and is associated with better outcomes than the more variably absorbed furosemide.[139,140] Torsemide is preferred in patients with persistent fluid retention despite high doses of other loop diuretics. Although the costs of torsemide exceed those of furosemide, pharmacoeconomic analyses suggest that the costs of care are similar or less with torsemide.[140] These data require confirmation in double-blind, controlled clinical trials but provide preliminary evidence that the more reliably absorbed loop diuretics may be superior to furosemide.

The loop diuretics exhibit a ceiling effect in heart failure, meaning that once the ceiling dose is reached, no additional response is achieved by increasing the dose. Thus, when this dose is reached, additional diuresis is achieved by giving the drug more often (twice daily or occasionally three times daily) or by giving combination diuretic therapy. The ceiling doses are listed in Table 20–5. Multiple daily dosing achieves a more sustained diuresis throughout the day. When dosed two or three times daily, the first dose is usually given first thing in the morning and the final dose in late afternoon/early evening.

Diuretics cause a variety of metabolic abnormalities, with severity related to the potency of the diuretic. The reader is referred to Chapter 19 for a detailed discussion of the adverse effects of diuretic therapy. Hypokalemia is the most common metabolic disturbances with thiazide and loop diuretics, which in patients with heart failure may be exacerbated by hyperaldosteronism. Hypokalemia increases the risk for ventricular arrhythmias in heart failure and is especially worrisome in patients receiving digoxin. Hypokalemia is often accompanied by hypomagnesemia. Because adequate magnesium is necessary for entry of potassium into the cell, cosupplementation with both magnesium and potassium may be necessary to correct the hypokalemia. Concomitant ACE inhibitor (or ARB) and/or aldosterone antagonist therapy may help to minimize diuretic-induced hypokalemia because these drugs tend to increase serum potassium concentration through their inhibitory effect on aldosterone secretion. Nonetheless, the serum potassium concentration should be monitored closely in patients with heart failure and supplemented appropriately when needed. In addition to metabolic abnormalities, a recent post hoc analysis of the DIG trial suggested that chronic diuretic use was associated with increased risk of mortality and hospitalization.[141] These findings must be interpreted with caution because this trial was not designed to evaluate outcomes associated with diuretic therapy. However, they do serve to remind clinicians of the importance of appropriate patient selection and monitoring when using diuretic therapy.

ACE Inhibitors ⑤ A number of ACE inhibitors are currently available; those commonly used in the treatment of patients with heart failure are summarized in Table 20–8. Although ACE inhibitors vary in their chemical structure (e.g., sulfhydryl- vs nonsulfhydryl-containing agents) and tissue affinity, the major differences in the ACE inhibitors are not in these pharmacologic properties but in their pharmacokinetic properties.[17] To date all ACE inhibitors studied have shown improvement in heart failure symptoms or mortality.[17] However, it seems most prudent to use those agents

documented to reduce morbidity and mortality because the dose required for these end points has been determined.[1]

To minimize the risk of hypotension and renal insufficiency, ACE inhibitor therapy should be started with low doses followed by gradual titration as tolerated to the target doses.[1] Asymptomatic hypotension should not be considered a contraindication to initiation of an ACE inhibitor, although initiation or dose increases in patients with systolic blood pressures less than 90 to 100 mm Hg should be done cautiously. Renal function and serum potassium should be evaluated within 1 to 2 weeks after therapy is started with subsequent periodic assessments, especially after dose increases. Careful attention to appropriate doses of diuretics is important, as fluid overload may blunt the beneficial effects of ACE inhibitors, and overdiuresis increases the risk of hypotension and renal insufficiency. After titration of the drug to the target dose, most patients tolerate chronic therapy with few complications. Although symptoms may improve within a few days of initiating therapy, it may take weeks to months before the full benefits are apparent. Even if symptoms do not improve, long-term ACE inhibitor therapy should be continued to reduce the risk of mortality and hospitalization.

Because ACE inhibitors were the first agents to show improvements in heart failure survival and were frequently used as background therapy in clinical trials of other medications, they are often used as the initial therapy in patients with heart failure. Traditionally, after titration of the ACE inhibitor dose, the addition of β-blockers was then considered. The expected ACE inhibitor—mediated decrease in blood pressure made some clinicians reluctant to initiate β-blocker therapy. Because of the impressive benefits of β-blockers, initiation of β-blocker therapy should not be delayed in patients who fail to reach target ACE inhibitor doses, as low-intermediate ACE inhibitor doses are as effective as higher doses for improving symptoms and survival.[1,65] Also, in β-blocker clinical trials, most patients were receiving background therapy with low-intermediate ACE inhibitor doses. Thus, in most patients, ACE inhibitors should be the initial therapy, but it is important to remember that the greatest benefit is seen when both an ACE inhibitor and a β-blocker are used.

Because of the high prevalence of coronary artery disease in patients with heart failure, aspirin is frequently coadministered with ACE inhibitors. Whether aspirin may attenuate the hemodynamic and mortality benefits of ACE inhibitors remains controversial.[142,143] The postulated mechanism of this interaction involves opposing effects on synthesis of vasodilatory prostaglandins. The ACE inhibitor—mediated increase in bradykinin increases the synthesis of vasodilatory prostaglandins that have favorable hemodynamic benefits in heart failure. Because of aspirin's effect on prostaglandin synthesis, this potentially beneficial action of ACE

TABLE 20-8	ACE Inhibitors Routinely Used for the Treatment of Heart Failure			
Generic Name	Brand Name	Initial Dose	Target Dosing: Survival Benefit[a]	Elimination[b]
Captopril	Capoten	6.25 mg tid	50 mg tid	Renal
Enalapril	Vasotec	2.5–5 mg bid	10–20 mg bid	Renal
Lisinopril	Zestril, Prinivil	2.5–5 mg once daily	20–40 mg once daily[c]	Renal
Quinapril	Accupril	5 mg bid	20–40 mg bid[d]	Renal
Ramipril	Altace	1.25–2.5 mg bid	5 mg bid	Renal
Fosinopril	Monopril	5–10 mg once daily	40 mg once daily[d]	Renal/hepatic
Trandolapril	Mavik	0.5–1 mg once daily	4 mg once daily	Renal/hepatic
Perindopril	Aceon	2 mg once daily	8–16 mg once daily[d]	Renal/hepatic

Abbreviations: bid, twice daily; tid, three times daily.
[a]Target doses associated with survival benefits in clinical trials.
[b]Primary route of elimination.
[c]Note that in the ATLAS trial (Circulation 1999;100:2312–2318), no significant difference in mortality was found between low-dose (~5 mg/d) and high-dose (~35 mg/d) lisinopril therapy.
[d]Effects on mortality have not been evaluated.

inhibitors may be attenuated. However, in contrast with studies that showed an ACE inhibitor—aspirin interaction, other investigators have found no interaction, even in patients without coronary artery disease or with impaired renal function.[143,144] It is currently recommended that the decision to use each of these medications be made based on whether an individual patient has indications for each drug. Use of aspirin doses of 160 mg per day or less should be considered.

Adverse Effects The primary adverse effects of ACE inhibitors are secondary to their major pharmacologic effects of suppressing angiotensin II and increasing bradykinin. The reductions in angiotensin II are associated with hypotension and functional renal insufficiency, which are the most adverse effects observed with these agents. ACE inhibitors reduced blood pressure in nearly all patients with hypotension, becoming problematic when symptoms such as dizziness, lightheadedness, blurred vision, presyncope, and syncope are observed. Hypotension occurs most commonly early in therapy or after an increase in dose, although it may occur at any time during treatment. Risk factors for hypotension include hyponatremia (serum sodium <130 mEq/L), hypovolemia, and overdiuresis.[1] The occurrence of hypotension may be minimized by initiating therapy with lower ACE inhibitor doses and/or temporarily withholding or reducing the dose of diuretic and liberalizing salt and fluid intake.[1] An often overlooked solution to hypotension is to space the administration times of vasoactive medications (e.g., diuretics and β-blockers) throughout the day so that these medications are not all administered at or near the same time. Many patients who experience symptomatic hypotension early in therapy are still good candidates for long-term treatment if risk factors for low blood pressure are addressed.

Functional renal insufficiency is manifested as increases in serum creatinine and blood urea nitrogen (BUN). As cardiac output and renal blood flow decline, renal perfusion is maintained by the vasoconstrictor effect of angiotensin II on the efferent arteriole. Patients most dependent on this system for maintenance of renal perfusion (and therefore most likely to develop functional renal insufficiency with ACE inhibitors) are those with severe heart failure, hypotension, hyponatremia, volume depletion, bilateral renal artery stenosis, and concomitant use of NSAIDs.[145] Sodium depletion, usually secondary to diuretic therapy, is the most important factor in the development of functional renal insufficiency with ACE inhibitor therapy. Renal insufficiency therefore can be minimized in many cases by reduction of diuretic dosage or liberalization of sodium intake. Increases in serum creatinine of 10% to 20% from baseline are commonly observed after initiation of ACE inhibitor therapy. In some patients, the serum creatinine will return to baseline levels without a reduction in ACE inhibitor dose.[145] Increases in serum creatinine of >0.5 mg/dL if the baseline creatinine is <2 mg/dL or >1 mg/dL if the creatinine is >2 mg/dL should prompt clinicians to reconsider ACE therapy and evaluate potential causes for the abrupt decline in renal function.[145] The safety and efficacy of ACE inhibitors in patients with baseline serum creatinine >2.5 mg/dL are uncertain, as these patients were usually excluded from clinical trials. Caution should also be exercised when using ACE inhibitors in such patients. Because renal dysfunction with ACE inhibitors is secondary to alterations in renal hemodynamics, it is almost always reversible upon discontinuation of the drug.[145]

Careful dose titration can minimize the risks of hypotension and transient worsening of renal function. Thus, usual initial doses should be about one fourth the final target dose, with slow upward dose titration based on blood pressure and serum creatinine. In certain patients, especially those hospitalized patients who seem at high risk for hypotension or worsening of renal function, it may be advisable to initiate therapy with a short-acting agent such as

captopril. This will help minimize the duration of adverse effects should they occur. Once stabilized on captopril, the patient can then be switched to an ACE inhibitor given once daily.

Retention of potassium with ACE inhibitor therapy can occur and is due to the reduced feedback of angiotensin II to stimulate aldosterone release. Hyperkalemia is most likely to occur in patients with renal insufficiency and in those taking concomitant potassium supplements, potassium-containing salt substitutes, or potassium-sparing diuretic therapy (including an aldosterone antagonist), especially if they have diabetes.[145] The more widespread use of aldosterone antagonists (e.g., spironolactone) in patients with heart failure may increase the risk of hyperkalemia.[100]

ACE inhibitors are associated with other important adverse effects. A dry, hacking cough occurs with a similar frequency (5–15% of patients) with all the agents and is related to bradykinin accumulation. The cough is usually nonproductive, occurs within the first few months of therapy, resolves within 1 to 2 weeks of drug discontinuation, and reappears with rechallenge. Cough occurs in up to 40% of patients with heart failure, independent of ACE inhibitor use; therefore, it is important to rule out other potential causes of cough, such as pulmonary congestion. Because cough is a bradykinin-mediated effect, replacement of ACE inhibitor therapy with an ARB would be reasonable in those patients who cannot tolerate the cough. Angioedema is a rare but potentially life-threatening complication that is also believed to be related to bradykinin accumulation. It may occur more frequently in African Americans than in other populations.[1] Use of ACE inhibitors is contraindicated in patients with a history of angioedema. ARBs may be an alternative therapy in patients with ACE inhibitor—induced angioedema, although caution is advised, as rare cross-reactivity is reported.[1,86,90] ACE inhibitors are contraindicated during the second and third trimesters of pregnancy due to the increased risk of fetal renal failure, intrauterine growth retardation, and other congenital defects. A recent analysis using a Medicaid database of nearly 30,000 patients suggests that first trimester use of ACE inhibitors should also be avoided, as the risk of major congenital defects was increased 2.7-fold in infants exposed to these agents during the first trimester.[146]

Angiotensin II Receptor Blockers ❺ Although ACE inhibitors remain the agents of first choice to treat stage C heart failure with reduced LVEF, ARBs approved for the treatment of heart failure are now the recommended alternatives in patients who are unable to tolerate an ACE inhibitor.[1] Although numerous ARBs are currently available, only two, candesartan and valsartan, are approved for the treatment of heart failure. The efficacy of these two agents is supported by clinical trial data that document a target dose associated with improved survival and other important outcomes in patients with decreased LVEF.[82–84,86] Thus, candesartan and valsartan are the preferred agents in patients with heart failure, whether used alone or in combination with ACE inhibitors. ARBs are also alternatives to ACE inhibitors in patients with stage A or B heart failure.[1]

The clinical use of ARBs is similar to that of ACE inhibitors. Therapy should be initiated at low doses (candesartan 4–8 mg once daily, valsartan 20–40 mg twice daily) and then titrated to target doses (candesartan 32 mg once daily, valsartan 160 mg twice daily).[1] Blood pressure, renal function, and serum potassium should be evaluated within 1 to 2 weeks after initiation of therapy and after increases in dose, and these end points should be used to guide subsequent dose changes. It is not necessary to reach target doses before adding a β-blocker, although incremental benefits may be associated with higher doses of ARBs.[88]

Adverse Effects ARBs have a low incidence of adverse effects. Because they do not affect bradykinin, they are not associated with cough and have a lower risk of angioedema than ACE inhibitors. However, because of reports of recurrences of ACE inhibitor—related angioedema after ARB administration, ARBs should be used cautiously in any patient with a history of angioedema, as a recent meta-analysis suggests that from 2% to 17% of patients experiencing angioedema with an ACE inhibitor will cross-react with an ARB.[86,90,147] The major adverse effects are related to suppression of the RAAS. The incidence and risk factors for developing hypotension, decreases in renal function, and hyperkalemia with the ARBs are similar to that of ACE inhibitors.[81] Thus, ARBs are not alternatives in patients who develop these complications from ACE inhibitors. Careful monitoring is required when an ARB is used with another inhibitor of the RAAS (e.g., ACE inhibitor or aldosterone antagonist), as this combination increases the risk of these adverse effects. As with ACE inhibitors, ARBs are contraindicated in the second and third trimesters of pregnancy and should be avoided in the first trimester because of increased risk of fetal/neonatal morbidity and mortality. Neither candesartan nor valsartan is metabolized by the cytochrome P450 system, so no pharmacokinetic drug—drug interactions with these agents are expected.

β-Blockers ⑥

Metoprolol CR/XL, carvedilol, and bisoprolol are the only β-blockers shown to reduce mortality in large heart failure trials. Metoprolol and bisoprolol selectively block the β_1-receptor, whereas carvedilol blocks the β_1-, β_2-, and α_1-receptors and also possesses antioxidant effects. Although there is no clear evidence that these pharmacologic differences result in differences in efficacy among agents, they may aid in selection of a specific agent. For example, carvedilol is expected to have greater antihypertensive effects than the other agents because of its α-receptor-blocking properties and may be preferred in patients with poorly controlled blood pressure. Conversely, metoprolol or bisoprolol may be preferred in patients with low blood pressure or dizziness and in patients with significant airway disease.

Bisoprolol is eliminated approximately 50% by the kidneys, whereas metoprolol and carvedilol are essentially completely metabolized and undergo extensive hepatic first-pass metabolism. Both metoprolol and carvedilol are also substrates for the cytochrome P450 2D6, which is known to be polymorphic. The 7% of the white population and 1% to 2% of the Asian American and African American populations who are CYP2D6 poor metabolizers would be expected to have more pronounced plasma concentrations than anticipated at the usual doses of carvedilol and metoprolol. However, given that β-blockers have a wide therapeutic index, it is unclear whether CYP2D6 phenotype significantly impacts hemodynamic and clinical effects.

There is fairly strong evidence that benefits of β-blockers in heart failure are not a class effect. Specifically, in a study powered for mortality reduction, there was no difference in survival between the nonselective β-blocker bucindolol and placebo.[148] Although there has been considerable debate over why bucindolol failed to provide a survival benefit, it may be related to the drug's ancillary properties or differences among β-blocker trials in the characteristics of study participants. Additional data suggest that bucindolol's effects on survival might be genotype specific, with a potential survival benefit in patients with the β_1-adrenergic receptor Arg389Arg genotype, but not in those with the Gly389 allele.[149] However, in the absence of bucindolol approval for heart failure, β-blocker use should be confined to one of the agents with proven survival benefits, especially given the diversity among β-blockers in their receptor sensitivities and ancillary properties.

There has been much debate over whether one β-blocker is superior to another. Specifically, it has been hypothesized that nonselective blockade with carvedilol might produce greater benefits than β_1-selective blockade. This hypothesis is based on observations that the β_1-receptor is downregulated, and the β_2-

and α_1-receptors account for a larger proportion of total cardiac adrenergic receptors in the failing heart. Only one trial with a mortality end point has provided a head-to-head comparison of carvedilol and a β_1-selective blocker. The Carvedilol or Metropolol European Trial (COMET) compared carvedilol 25 mg twice daily and immediate-release metoprolol 50 mg twice daily and found a significant 17% lower mortality rate in patients treated with carvedilol.[150] However, concerns regarding the formulation and dose of metoprolol used in COMET limit the conclusions that can be drawn from these findings. Specifically, the study used the immediate-release formulation of metoprolol (metoprolol tartrate), not the sustained-release formulation (metoprolol succinate) shown to reduce mortality. The efficacy of the immediate-release formulation in reducing mortality in heart failure has not been proven. Metoprolol CR/XL provides more consistent plasma concentrations over a 24-hour period and appears to provide more favorable effects on heart rate variability, autonomic balance, and blood pressure, suggesting that this formulation might be superior to immediate-release metoprolol.[151] The target dose of metoprolol also differed between COMET and MERIT-HF. The target dose in COMET was 100 mg/day (50 mg twice daily), whereas the target dose of metoprolol in MERIT-HF was 200 mg/day. Many question whether the degree of β-blockade achieved in COMET with immediate-release metoprolol 50 mg twice daily is comparable to that achieved with metoprolol CR/XL 200 mg/day in MERIT-HF or carvedilol 25 mg twice daily in COMET. Thus, the debate over β-blocker superiority continues, and although some clinicians would argue the superiority of carvedilol, it seems clear that what is most important is that one of the three β-blockers proven to reduce mortality is used.

Adverse Effects

Possible adverse effects with β-blocker use in heart failure include bradycardia or heart block, hypotension, fatigue, impaired glycemic control in diabetic patients, bronchospasm in patients with asthma, and worsening heart failure. Clinicians should monitor vital signs and carefully assess for signs and symptoms of worsening heart failure during β-blocker initiation and uptitration. Hypotension is more common with carvedilol due to its α_1-receptor-blocking properties. Bradycardia and hypotension generally are asymptomatic and require no intervention; however, β-blocker dose reduction is warranted in symptomatic patients. Fatigue usually resolves after several weeks of therapy but sometimes requires dose reduction. In diabetic patients, β-blockers may worsen glucose tolerance and can mask the tachycardia and tremor (but not sweating) that accompany hypoglycemia. In addition, nonselective agents such as carvedilol may prolong insulin-induced hypoglycemia and slow recovery from a hypoglycemic episode. Despite this, there is evidence that carvedilol produces better glycemic control in diabetic patients compared with immediate-release metoprolol and may improve insulin sensitivity.[152] Furthermore, carvedilol and metoprolol provide similar survival benefits in patients with concomitant heart failure and diabetes.[153] Diabetic patients should be warned of these potential adverse effects, and blood glucose should be monitored with initiation, adjustment, and discontinuation of β-blocker therapy. Adjustment of hypoglycemic therapy may be necessary with concomitant β-blocker use in diabetics.

Uptitration should be avoided if the patient experiences signs of worsening heart failure, including volume overload and poor perfusion. Fluid overload may be asymptomatic and manifest solely as an increase in body weight. Mild fluid overload may be managed by intensifying diuretic therapy. The treatment of moderate to severe congestion is discussed in Chapter 22. Once the patient has been stabilized, dose titration may continue as tolerated until the target or highest tolerated dose is reached. Despite their negative inotropic effects, continuing β-blocker therapy during hospitalization for acute heart failure appears to neither worsen symptoms nor delay clinical improvement. In fact, β-blocker withdrawal may increase the risk for mortality after hospital discharge.[154,155] Furthermore, stopping β-blocker therapy during acute decompensation may lead to lower chronic β-blocker use due to failure to reinstitute β-blocker therapy once the patient has stabilized.[155,156] Guidelines recommend continuing β-blocker therapy during hospitalization for heart failure whenever possible.

Absolute contraindications to β-blocker use include uncontrolled bronchospastic disease, symptomatic bradycardia, advanced heart block without a pacemaker, and acute decompensated heart failure. However, β-blockers may be tried with caution in patients with asymptomatic bradycardia or well-controlled asthma. Particular caution is warranted in patients with marked bradycardia (<55 bpm) or hypotension (systolic blood pressure <80 mm Hg). Importantly, concerns of masking symptoms of hypoglycemia or worsening glycemic control should not preclude β-blocker use in patients with diabetes. Indeed, post hoc analysis of heart failure trials shows that β-blockers are well tolerated and significantly reduce morbidity and mortality in patients with diabetes and heart failure.[157] Beta-blockers should be used cautiously in patients with diabetes and recurrent hypoglycemia.

Digoxin Digoxin exerts its positive inotropic effect by binding to sodium- and potassium-activated adenosine triphosphatase (Na,K-ATPase or sodium pump). Inhibition of Na,K-ATPase decreases outward transport of sodium and leads to increased intracellular sodium concentrations. Higher intracellular sodium concentrations favor calcium entry and reduce calcium extrusion from the cell through effects on the sodium—calcium exchanger. The result is increased storage of intracellular calcium in the sarcoplasmic reticulum and, with each action potential, a greater release of calcium to activate contractile elements. Digoxin also has beneficial neurohormonal actions. These effects occur at low plasma concentrations, where little inotropic effect is seen, and are independent of inotropic activity. Unlike other positive inotropes that increase intracellular cyclic adenosine monophosphate (cAMP), digoxin attenuates the excessive SNS activation present in patients with heart failure. Although the precise mechanism is unknown, a digoxin-mediated reduction in central sympathetic outflow and improvement in impaired baroreceptor function appear to play an important role. Because mortality and progression of heart failure are linked to the extent of SNS activation, these sympathoinhibitory effects may be an important component of the clinical response to the drug. Systolic heart failure is also marked by autonomic dysfunction, most notably suppression of the parasympathetic (vagal) system. Digoxin increases parasympathetic activity in patients with heart failure and leads to a decrease in heart rate, thus enhancing diastolic filling. The vagal effects also result in slowed conduction and prolongation of atrioventricular node refractoriness, thus slowing the ventricular response in patients with atrial fibrillation. Because atrial fibrillation is a common complication of heart failure, the combined positive inotropic, neurohormonal, and negative chronotropic effects of digoxin can be particularly beneficial for such patients. The overall response to digoxin is usually an increase in cardiac index and a decrease in PAOP with relatively little change in arterial blood pressure.[105,106,158]

Pharmacokinetics Numerous studies of digoxin pharmacokinetics have been published and are summarized in Table 20–9. Digoxin has a large volume of distribution and is extensively bound to various tissues, most notably to Na,K-ATPase in skeletal and cardiac muscles. Because it does not distribute appreciably to body fat, loading doses of digoxin (when necessary) should be calculated based on estimates of lean body weight. There is a long "distribution

TABLE 20-9 Clinical Pharmacokinetics of Digoxin

Oral bioavailability	
Tablets	0.5–0.9 (0.65)[a]
Elixir	0.75–0.85 (0.80)
Capsules	0.9–1.0 (0.95)
Onset of action	
Oral	1.5–6 h
Intravenous	15–30 min
Peak effect	
Oral	4–6 h
Intravenous	1.5–4 h
Terminal half-life	
Normal renal function	36 h
Anuric patients	5 d
Volume of distribution at steady state	7.3 L/kg
Fraction unbound in plasma	0.75–0.80
Fraction excreted unchanged in urine	0.65–0.70

[a]Range and mean value in parentheses.

Source: Data from Schentag JJ, Bang AJ, Kozinski-Tober JL. Digoxin. In: Burton ME, Shaw LM, Schentag JJ, Evans WE, eds. Applied Pharmacokinetics and Pharmacodynamics: Principles of Therapeutic Drug Monitoring. 4th ed. Baltimore, MD: Lippincott Williams & Wilkins; 2006:410–439.

phase" after administration of oral or IV digoxin, resulting in a lag time before maximum pharmacologic response is observed (see Table 20–9). Transiently elevated SDCs during the distribution phase are not associated with increased therapeutic or adverse effects, although they can mislead the clinician who is unaware of the timing of blood sampling relative to the previous digoxin dose. Consequently, blood samples for measurement of SDCs should be collected at least 6 hours and preferably 12 hours or more after the last dose.

In patients with normal renal function, 60% to 80% of a dose of digoxin is eliminated unchanged in urine via glomerular filtration and tubular secretion. The terminal half-life of digoxin is approximately 1.5 days in subjects with normal renal function but approximately 5 days in anuric patients (see Table 20–9). Recent evidence indicates that the drug efflux transporter P-glycoprotein (P-gp) plays an important role in the bioavailability, renal and nonrenal clearance, and drug interactions with digoxin. Clinically important pharmacokinetic/pharmacodynamic drug interactions are summarized in Table 20–10. An extensive review of the pharmacokinetics and pharmacodynamics of digoxin is available.[158]

Adverse Effects Digoxin can produce a variety of cardiac and noncardiac adverse effects, but it is usually well tolerated by most patients (Table 20–11).[105,106] Noncardiac adverse effects frequently involve the CNS or GI system but also may be nonspecific (e.g., fatigue or weakness). Cardiac manifestations include numerous different arrhythmias that are believed to be caused by multiple electrophysiologic effects (Table 20–11). Cardiac arrhythmias may be the first evidence of toxicity in a patient (before any noncardiac symptoms occur). Rhythm disturbances are of particular concern because patients with systolic heart failure are already at increased risk of sudden cardiac death, presumably due to ventricular arrhythmias. Patients at increased risk of toxicity include those with impaired renal function and/or decreased lean body mass, the elderly, and those taking interacting drugs. Hypokalemia, hypomagnesemia, and hypercalcemia will predispose patients to cardiac manifestations of digoxin toxicity. Thus, concomitant therapy with diuretics may lead to electrolyte abnormalities and increase the likelihood of cardiac arrhythmias. Similarly, hypothyroidism, myocardial ischemia, and acidosis will increase the risk of cardiac adverse effects. Although digoxin toxicity is commonly associated with plasma concentrations greater than 2 ng/mL, clinicians should remember that digoxin

TABLE 20-10 Selected Digoxin Drug Interactions

Drug	Mechanism/Effecy	Suggested Clinical Management
Amiodarone, dronedarone	Inhibits P-glycoprotein, resulting in decrease in renal and nonrenal clearance; can increase SDC by 70–100%	Monitor SDC and adverse effects; anticipate the need to reduce the dose by 50%
Antacids	Concurrent administration may decrease digoxin bioavailability by 20-35%	Space doses at least 2 h apart or avoid concurrent use if possible
Cholestyramine, colestipol	Bind digoxin in gut and decrease bioavailability 20-35%; may also decrease enterohepatic recycling	Space doses at least 2 h apart or avoid concurrent use if possible
Diuretics	Thiazides or loop diuretics may cause hypokalemia and hypomagnesemia, thereby increasing the risk of digitalis toxicity	Monitor and replace electrolytes if necessary
Erythromycin, clarithromycin, tetracycline	Alter gut bacterial flora; bioavailability and SDC increase 40–100% in about 10% of patients who extensively metabolize digoxin in the gut, may also be due to inhibition of P-glycoprotein by macrolides	Monitor SDC and anticipate the need to reduce the dose; avoid concurrent use if possible
Ketoconazole, itraconazole	Decrease in renal and nonrenal clearance by inhibition of P-glycoprotein; SDC may increase by 50–100%	Monitor SDC and anticipate the need to reduce the dose by 50%
Kaolin-pectin	Large dose (30–60 mL) may decrease digoxin bioavailability by ~60%	Space doses at least 2 h apart or avoid concurrent use if possible
Metoclopramide	Increase in gut mobility may decrease bioavailability of slow-dissolving tablets; unknown significance	Effect is minimized by administration of digoxin capsules
Neomycin, sulfasalazine	Decrease in bioavailability by 20–25%	Space doses at least 2 h apart or avoid concurrent use if possible
Propafenone	Decrease in renal clearance; SDC may increase 30–40%	Monitor SDC and anticipate the need to reduce the dose
Quinidine	Inhibits P-glycoprotein, resulting in decrease in renal and nonrenal clearance; also, displacement of digoxin from tissue-binding sites, with decrease in the volume of distribution; SDC generally increases about twofold	Monitor SDC and adverse effects; anticipate the need to reduce dose by 50%
Spironolactone	Decrease in renal and nonrenal clearance; also, interference with some digoxin assays, thus increasing apparent SDC	Monitor SDC and anticipate the need to reduce dose; check assay for interference
Verapamil	Inhibits P-glycoprotein, resulting in decrease in renal and nonrenal clearance, SDC may increase 70–100%	Monitor SDC and anticipate the need to reduce the dose by 50%; consider using another calcium channel blocker

Abbreviation: SDC, serum digoxin concentration.

toxicity is based on the presence of symptoms rather than a specific plasma concentration.[158] Usual treatment of digoxin toxicity includes drug withdrawal or dose reduction and treatment of cardiac arrhythmias and electrolyte abnormalities. In patients with life-threatening digoxin toxicity, purified digoxin-specific Fab antibody fragments should be administered. Serum digoxin concentrations will not be reliable until the antidote has been eliminated from the body.[106]

TABLE 20-11 Signs and Symptoms of Digoxin Toxicity

Noncardiac (mostly CNS) adverse effects
Anorexia, nausea, vomiting, and abdominal pain
Visual disturbances:
Halos, photophobia, problems with color perception (i.e., red-green or yellow-green vision), and scotomata
Fatigue, weakness, dizziness, headache, neuralgia, confusion, delirium, and psychosis
Cardiac adverse effects[a,b]
Ventricular arrhythmias
Premature ventricular depolarizations, bigeminy, trigeminy, ventricular tachycardia, ventricular fibrillation
AV block
First-degree, second-degree (Mobitz type I), or third-degree
AV junctional escape rhythms, junctional tachycardia
Atrial arrhythmias with slowed AV conduction or AV block
Particularly paroxysmal atrial tachycardia with AV block
Sinus bradycardia

[a]Some adverse effects may be difficult to distinguish from the signs/symptoms of heart failure.
[b] Digoxin toxicity has been associated with almost every known rhythm abnormality (only the more common manifestations are listed).
Abbreviation: AV, atrioventricular.
Source: Data from Eichorn EJ, Gheorghiade M. Digoxin. Prog Cardiovasc Dis 2002;44:251–66.

Pharmacoeconomic Considerations

Heart failure imposes a tremendous economic burden on the healthcare system. In patients over age 65, it is the most common reason for hospitalization, with hospital admission rates for this disorder continuing to increase. Heart failure is also associated with unacceptably high readmission rates during the 3 to 6 months after initial discharge. Current estimates of costs of heart failure treatment in the United States approach $40 billion, with most of the costs associated with hospitalization.[1,3] The prevalence of heart failure and the costs associated with patient care are expected to increase as the population ages and as survival from ischemic heart disease improves. Thus, approaches to improve the quality and cost-effectiveness of care for these patients may have a significant impact on healthcare costs.

Studies to assess the cost-effectiveness of drug therapy for heart failure have been recently reviewed.[159] Many studies provide direct cost estimates demonstrating an economic value when employing standard heart failure therapies, specifically ACE inhibitors, β-blockers, and digoxin. Much of the economic benefit of these therapies is due to a reduction in hospitalization. Although the clinical and economic benefits of these therapies are well recognized, standard heart failure therapies are often underprescribed or underdosed, which may increase the risk of poor clinical outcomes.[61] For example, a recent observational analysis of a heart failure quality improvement initiative found that only 32.5% of over 12,000 patients who were admitted to the hospital for heart failure and met guidelines for aldosterone antagonist therapy received these agents at discharge.[98]

More recent pharmacoeconomic studies have focused on the impact of newer heart failure therapies or those used as alternatives to standard therapy. ARBs have been shown to be cost-effective in patients not receiving ACE inhibitors.[160] Eplerenone has been shown to be a cost-effective therapy in patients with post-MI heart failure.[161] Fixed-dose combination hydralazine and ISDN is cost-effective in African American patients with severe heart failure.[162] Other cost-effective studies have focused on device therapy. Both prophylactic ICD implantation in patients with systolic dysfunction and CRT therapy appear to be cost-effective.[163,164] However, cost-effectiveness is limited if devices are implanted in patients with any comorbid illnesses that may shorten life expectancy.

As the management of heart failure has become increasingly complex, the development of disease management programs approaches that use multidisciplinary teams has been studied extensively. These programs utilize several broad approaches, including heart failure specialty clinics, home-based interventions, and close patient follow-up. Most are multidisciplinary and may include physicians, advanced practice nurses, dietitians, and pharmacists. In general, the programs focus on optimization of drug and no-drug therapy, patient and family education and counseling, exercise and dietary advice, intense follow-up by telephone or home visits, encouragement of self-care, and monitoring and management of signs and symptoms of decompensation.[1] Such programs have typically focused on patients with more severe heart failure who are at high risk of hospital admission. In general, multidisciplinary disease management programs improve quality of life and reduce heart failure and all-cause hospitalizations and costs, although these benefits are not consistently demonstrated in all studies.[165,166]

⓫ Pharmacists can play an important role in the multidisciplinary team management of heart failure.[39,167,168] Compared with conventional treatment, pharmacist interventions, which included medication evaluation and therapeutic recommendations, patient education, and follow-up telephone monitoring, reduced hospitalizations for heart failure, adverse drug events, and medication errors. Adherence to guideline-recommended therapy was also improved by pharmacist intervention. A recent study found that pharmacist intervention improved medication adherence and reduced emergency department visits and hospitalizations in low-income patients with heart failure.[168] Thus, the role and cost benefits of pharmacist involvement in the multidisciplinary care of patients with heart failure are now apparent and should include optimizing doses of heart failure drug therapy, screening for drugs that exacerbate heart failure, monitoring for adverse drug effects and drug interactions, educating patients, and patient follow-up. The role of pharmacists in optimizing pharmacotherapy is underscored by the finding that heart failure is associated with an increased risk of experiencing adverse drug reactions.[169]

CURRENT CONTROVERSIES

Diabetes is a frequently occurring comorbidity in patients with heart failure. Metformin is effective for reducing the microvascular and macrovascular complications of diabetes. The use of metformin in patients with heart failure is controversial because of the potential risk for lactic acidosis. However, recent observational studies show that metformin is commonly used by many clinicians and that it may be safe and effective in this population. Prospective data are needed to determine the benefits and risks of metformin in patients with heart failure.

Inflammation plays a key role in the pathophysiology of heart failure. Because of their pleiotropic actions, there is great interest in the use of statins in patients with heart failure. Despite significant decreases in LDL cholesterol, two recent well-designed clinical trials failed to demonstrate that statins improved clinical outcomes.[31,32] Because coronary artery disease is a frequent cause of heart failure, many clinicians still use statins in patients with both disorders in the belief that these agents reduce cardiovascular risk.

EVALUATION OF THERAPEUTIC OUTCOMES

Although mortality is an important end point, it does not give a complete measure of the overall impact of heart failure because many patients are hospitalized repeatedly for heart failure exacerbations and continue to survive, albeit with a significantly reduced quality of life. Thus, some of the more important therapeutic outcomes in heart failure management, such as prolonged survival or prevention or slowing of the progression of heart failure, cannot be quantified in an individual patient. However, after appropriate diagnostic evaluation to determine the etiology of heart failure, ongoing clinical assessment of patients typically focuses on three general areas: (a) evaluation of functional capacity, (b) evaluation of volume status, and (c) laboratory evaluation.

The evaluation of functional capacity should focus on the presence and severity of symptoms the patient experiences during activities of daily living and how his or her symptoms affect these activities. Questions directed toward the patient's ability to perform specific activities may be more informative than general questions about the symptoms the patient may be experiencing. For example, patients should be asked if they can exercise, climb stairs, get dressed without stopping, check the mail, go shopping, or clean the house. Another important component of assessment of functional capacity is to ask patients what activities they would like to do but are now unable to perform.

Assessment of volume status is a vital component of the ongoing care of patients with heart failure. This evaluation provides the clinician important information about the adequacy of diuretic therapy. Because the cardinal signs and symptoms of heart failure are caused by excess fluid retention, the efficacy of diuretic treatment is readily evaluated by the disappearance of these signs and symptoms. The physical examination is the primary method for the evaluation of fluid retention, and specific attention should be focused on the patient's body weight, extent of JVD, presence of hepatojugular reflux, presence and severity of pulmonary congestion, and peripheral edema. Specifically, in a patient with pulmonary congestion, monitoring is indicated for resolution of rales and pulmonary edema and improvement or resolution of dyspnea on exertion, orthopnea, and PND. For patients with systemic congestion, a decrease or disappearance of peripheral edema, JVD, and hepatojugular reflux is sought. Other therapeutic outcomes include an improvement in exercise tolerance and fatigue and a decrease in nocturia and heart rate. Clinicians also will want to monitor blood pressure and ensure that the patient does not develop symptomatic hypotension as a result of drug therapy. Body weight is a sensitive marker of fluid loss or retention, and patients should be counseled to weigh themselves daily, reporting changes to their healthcare provider so that adjustments can be made in diuretic doses. It should be noted that, particularly with β-blocker therapy, symptoms may worsen initially and that it may take weeks to months of treatment before patients notice improvement in symptoms. Also, patients and healthcare providers should be aware that heart failure progression may be slowed even though symptoms have not resolved.

Routine monitoring of serum electrolytes and renal function is required in patients with heart failure. Assessment of serum potassium is especially important because hypokalemia is a common adverse effect of diuretic therapy and is associated with an increased risk of arrhythmias and digoxin toxicity. Serum potassium monitoring is also required because of the risk of hyperkalemia associated with ACE inhibitors, ARBs, and aldosterone antagonists. A serum potassium ≥4 mEq/L should be maintained, with some evidence suggesting it should be ≥4.5 mEq/L.[170] Assessment of renal function (BUN and serum creatinine) is also an important end point for monitoring diuretic and ACE inhibitor therapy. Common causes

TABLE 20-12 ACC/AHA Clinical Performance Measures for Adults with Systolic Heart Failure

Performance Measure	Recommendation
Inpatient measures	
Evaluation of left ventricular systolic function[a]	Echocardiogram with Doppler flow studies is the most useful test, as it enables clinicians to determine the presence of pericardial, myocardial, or valvular abnormalities. Patients with LVEF <40% should be considered for specific therapy (e.g., ACE inhibitors, β-blockers). Class I recommendation, Level of Evidence C.
ACE inhibitors or ARBs for patients with left ventricular systolic dysfunction[a]	Patients with LVEF <40% or moderate or severe systolic dysfunction should receive an ACE inhibitor or ARB unless contrainidcations are present or there is a history ot intolerance to both drugs. ACE inhibitors: Class I recommendation, Level of Evidence A. ARBs: Class 1, Level of Evidence A.
Anticoagulant therapy with warfarin for patients with atrial fibrillation	Patients without contraindications should receive warfarin to reduce the risk of a thromboembolic event. Class I recommendation, Level of Evidence A.
Discharge instructions[a]	Patients discharged home should receive written instructions that address activity levels, diet, discharge medications, follow-up appointments, weight monitoring, and what to do if symptoms worsen. Education of both patients and families is important.
Smoking cessation counseling[a]	All current or recent smokers should receive counseling on smoking cessation and offered smoking cessation pharmacotherapy. Class I recommendation, Level of Evidence C.
Outpatient measures	
Initial laboratory evaluation	Laboratory tests may identify the cause of or factors that may exacerbate heart failure. Recommended tests include complete blood count, urinalysis, serum electrolytes, BUN, serum creatinine, blood glucose, liver function, TSH. Class I, Level of Evidence C.
Evaluation of left ventricular systolic function	Echocardiogram with Doppler flow studies is the most useful test, as it enables clinicians to determine the presence of pericardial, myocardial, or valvular abnormalities. Patients with LVEF <40% should be considered for specific therapy (e.g., ACE inhibitors, β-blockers). Class I recommendation, Level of Evidence C.
Weight measurement	Important measure for assessment and follow-up of patient's volume status. Helps determine the need for adjustment of diuretic therapy. Class I recommendation, Level of Evidence C.
Blood pressure measurement	Hypertension is an important risk factor for heart failure development and progression. Class I recommendation, Level of Evidence C.
Assessment of clinical symptoms of volume overload	Along with weight, plays an important role in determining the need for adjustment of diuretic therapy. Assess for the presence of orthopnea and dyspnea. Orthostatic blood pressure evaluation should also be performed. Class I recommendation, Level of Evidence C.
Assessement of clinical signs of volume overload	Assessment of the presence of the following signs should be performed: peripheral edema, rales, hepatomegaly, ascites, jugular venous pressure, S_3 and S_4 gallop. Class I recommendation, Level of Evidence C.
Assessment of activity level	Longitudinal assessment of functional capacity allows for determination of whether symptoms are improving and serve as basis for additional treatment decisions. Class I recommendation, Level of Evidence C.
Patient education	Patients should be provided with written and/or verbal instructions at one or more visits on the following: weight monitoring, diet (sodium restriction), symptom management, physical activity, smoking cessation, medication instruction, minimizing or avoiding NSAIDs, referral to educational/disease management programs, prognosis/end-of-life issues. Class I recommendation, Level of Evidence C.
Beta-blocker therapy	All patients with stable heart failure and LVEF <40% should receive treatment with one of the three β-blockers proven to reduce mortality unless contraindicated. Class I recommendation, Level of Evidence A.
ACE inhibitors or ARBs for patients with left ventricular systolic dysfunction	Patients with LVEF <40% or moderate or severe systolic dysfunction should receive an ACE inhibitor or ARB unless contraindications are present or there is a history ot intolerance to both drugs. ACE inhibitors: Class I recommendation, Level of Evidence A. ARBs: Class I recommendation, Level of Evidence A.
Warfarin therapy for patients with atrial fibrillation	Patients without contraindications should receive warfarin to reduce the risk of a thromboembolic event. Class I recommendation, Level of Evidence A.

[a]Also Center for Medicare and Medicaid Services and the Joint Commission Core Measures.

Abbreviations: ACE, angiotensin-converting enzyme; ARB, angiotensin receptor blocker; BUN, blood urea nitrogen; LVEF, left ventricular ejection fraction; NSAID, nonsteroidal antiinflammatory drug; TSH, thyroid-stimulating hormone.

Source: Adapted from Bonow RW, Bennett S, Casey DE, et al. ACC/AHA clinical performance measures for adults with systolic heart failure: A report of the American College of Cardiology/American Heart Association Task Force on Performance Measures (Writing Committee to Develop Heart Failure Clinical Performance Measures). J Am Coll Cardiol 2005;46:1144–1178.

of worsening renal function in patients with heart failure include overdiuresis, adverse effects of ACE inhibitor or ARB therapy, and hypoperfusion.

Most of these therapeutic end points are incorporated into the ACC/AHA performance measures outlined in Table 20–12.

ABBREVIATIONS

ACC: American College of Cardiology
ACE: angiotensin-converting enzyme
AHA: American Heart Association
ANP: atrial natriuretic peptide
ARB: angiotensin receptor blocker
AVP: arginine vasopressin
BNP: B-type natriuretic peptide
cAMP: cyclic adenosine monophosphate
CNP: C-type natriuretic peptide
CO: cardiac output
COX-2: cyclooxygenase-2
CRT: cardiac resynchronization therapy
ESC: European Society of Cardiology
HFSA: Heart Failure Society of America
IABP: intra-aortic balloon pump
ICD: implantable cardioverter-defibrillator
JVD: jugular venous distention

LVAD: left ventricular assist device

LVEDP: left ventricular end-diastolic pressure

LVEDV: left ventricular end-diastolic volume

LVEF: left ventricular ejection fraction

MI: myocardial infarction

NSAID: nonsteroidal antiinflammatory drug

NYHA: New York Heart Association

PAOP: pulmonary artery occlusion pressure

P-gp: P-glycoprotein

RAAS: renin—angiotensin—aldosterone system

SDC: serum digoxin concentration

SNS: sympathetic nervous system

SVR: systemic vascular resistance

TNF-α: tumor necrosis factor-α

TZD: thiazolidinedione

REFERENCES

1. Hunt SA, Abraham WT, Chin MH, et al. 2009 focused update incorporated into the ACC/AHA 2005 Guidelines for the Diagnosis and Management of Heart Failure in Adults: A report of the American College of Cardiology Foundation/American Heart Association Task Force on Practice Guidelines developed in collaboration with the International Society for Heart and Lung Transplantation. Circulation 2009;119:e391–479.

2. Maeder MT, Kaye DM. Heart failure with normal left ventricular ejection fraction. J Am Coll Cardiol 2009;53:905–918.

3. Lloyd-Jones D, Adams R, Carnethon M, et al. Heart disease and stroke statistics—2009 update: A report from the American Heart Association Statistics Committee and Stroke Statistics Subcommittee. Circulation 2009;119:480–486.

4. Gheorghiade M, Sopko G, De Luca L, et al. Navigating the crossroads of coronary artery disease and heart failure. Circulation 2006;114:1202–1213.

5. Roger VL, Weston SA, Redfield MM, et al. Trends in heart failure incidence and survival in a community-based population. JAMA 2004;292:344–350.

6. Levy WC, Mozaffarian D, Linker DT et al. The Seattle Heart Failure Model: Prediction of survival in heart failure. Circulation 2006;113:1424–133.

7. Kalogeropoulos AP, Georgiopoulou VV, Giamouzis G, et al. Utility of the Seattle Heart Failure Model in patients with advanced heart failure. J Am Coll Cardiol 2009;53:334–342.

8. Mann D. Pathophysiology of heart failure. In: Libby P, Bonow RO, Mann DL, Zipes DP, eds. Braunwald's Heart Disease: A Textbook of Cardiovascular Medicine. 8th ed. Philadelphia, PA: Elsevier; 2007:541–560.

9. Richard P, Villard E, Charron P, Isnard R. The genetic bases of cardiomyopathies. J Am Coll Cardiol 2006;48:A79–89.

10. Kalogeropoulos A, Georgiopoulou V, Kritchevsky SB, et al. Epidemiology of incident heart failure in a contemporary elderly cohort: The health, aging, and body composition study. Arch Intern Med 2009;169:708–715.

11. Mann DL, Bristow MR. Mechanisms and models in heart failure: The biomechanical model and beyond. Circulation 2005;111:2837–2849.

12. Small KM, Wagoner LE, Levin AM, et al. Synergistic polymorphisms of beta$_1$- and alpha$_{2C}$-adrenergic receptors and the risk of congestive heart failure. N Engl J Med 2002;347:1135–1142.

13. Liggett SB, Cresci S, Kelly RJ, et al. A GRK5 polymorphism that inhibits beta-adrenergic receptor signaling is protective in heart failure. Nat Med 2008;14:510–517.

14. Triposkiadis F, Karayannis G, Giamouzis G, et al. The sympathetic nervous system in heart failure physiology, pathophysiology, and clinical implications. J Am Coll Cardiol 2009;54:1747–1762.

15. Felder RB, Yu Y, Zhang ZH, Wei SG. Pharmacological treatment for heart failure: A view from the brain. Clin Pharmacol Ther 2009;86:216–220.

16. Braunwald E. Biomarkers in heart failure. N Engl J Med 2008;358:2148–2159.

17. Wong J, Patel RA, Kowey PR. The clinical use of angiotensin-converting enzyme inhibitors. Prog Cardiovasc Dis 2004;47:116–130.

18. Lee VC, Rhew DC, Dylan M et al. Meta-analysis: angiotensin-receptor blockers in systolic heart failure and high-risk acute myocardial infarction. Ann Intern Med 2004;141:693–704.

19. Weber KT. The proinflammatory heart failure phenotype: A case of integrative physiology. Am J Med Sci 2005;330:219–226.

20. Selektor Y, Weber KT. The salt-avid state of congestive heart failure revisited. Am J Med Sci 2008;335:209–218.

21. Weber KT, Weglicki WB, Simpson RU. Macro- and micronutrient dyshomeostasis in the adverse structural remodelling of myocardium. Cardiovasc Res 2009;81:500–508.

22. Pitt B, Zannad F, Remme WJ, et al. The effect of spironolactone on morbidity and mortality in patients with severe heart failure. Randomized Aldactone Evaluation Study Investigators. N Engl J Med 1999;341:709–717.

23. Pitt B, Remme W, Zannad F, et al. Eplerenone, a selective aldosterone blocker, in patients with left ventricular dysfunction after myocardial infarction. N Engl J Med 2003;348:1309–1321.

24. Gallegos PJ, Maclaughlin EJ, Haase KK. Serial monitoring of brain natriuretic peptide concentrations for drug therapy management in patients with systolic heart failure. Pharmacotherapy 2008;28:343–355.

25. Tang WH, Francis GS, Morrow DA, et al. National Academy of Clinical Biochemistry Laboratory Medicine practice guidelines: Clinical utilization of cardiac biomarker testing in heart failure. Circulation 2007;116:e99–109.

26. Daniels LB, Maisel AS. Natriuretic peptides. J Am Coll Cardiol 2007;50:2357–2368.

27. Pfisterer M, Buser P, Rickli H, et al. BNP-guided vs symptom-guided heart failure therapy: The Trial of Intensified vs Standard Medical Therapy in Elderly Patients with Congestive Heart Failure (TIME-CHF) randomized trial. JAMA 2009;301:383–392.

28. Greenberg A, Verbalis JG. Vasopressin receptor antagonists. Kidney Int 2006;69:2124–2130.

29. Konstam MA, Gheorghiade M, Burnett JC Jr, et al. Effects of oral tolvaptan in patients hospitalized for worsening heart failure: The EVEREST Outcome Trial. JAMA 2007;297:1319–1331.

30. Fildes JE, Shaw SM, Yonan N, Williams SG. The immune system and systolic heart failure: is the heart in control? J Am Coll Cardiol 2009;53:1013–1020.

31. Kjekshus J, Apetrei E, Barrios V, et al. Rosuvastatin in older patients with systolic heart failure. N Engl J Med 2007;357:2248–2261.

32. Tavazzi L, Maggioni AP, Marchioli R, et al. Effect of rosuvastatin in patients with systolic heart failure (the GISSI-HF trial): A randomised, double-blind, placebo-controlled trial. Lancet 2008;372:1231–1239.

33. Tavazzi L, Maggioni AP, Marchioli R, et al. Effect of n-3 polyunsaturated fatty acids in patients with systolic heart failure (the GISSI-HF trial): A randomised, double-blind, placebo-controlled trial. Lancet 2008;372:1223–1230.

34. Fonarow GC, Abraham WT, Albert NM, et al. Factors identified as precipitating hospital admissions for heart failure and clinical outcomes: Findings from OPTIMIZE-HF. Arch Intern Med 2008;168:847–854.

35. Anter E, Jessup M, Callans DJ. Atrial fibrillation and heart failure: Treatment considerations for a dual epidemic. Circulation 2009;119:2516–2525.

36. Chobanian AV, Bakris GL, Black HR, et al. The Seventh Report of the Joint National Committee on Prevention, Detection, Evaluation, and Treatment of High Blood Pressure: the JNC 7 report. JAMA 2003;289:2560–2572.

37. Gislason GH, Rasmussen JN, Abildstrom SZ, et al. Increased mortality and cardiovascular morbidity associated with use of nonsteroidal anti-inflammatory drugs in systolic heart failure. Arch Intern Med 2009;169:141–149.

38. Nesto RW, Bell D, Bonow RO, et al. Thiazolidinedione use, fluid retention, and congestive heart failure: A consensus statement from

the American Heart Association and American Diabetes Association. Circulation 2003;108:2941–2948.

39. Koshman SL, Charrois TL, Simpson SH, et al. Pharmacist care of patients with heart failure: A systematic review of randomized trials. Arch Intern Med 2008;168:687–694.

40. Murray MD, Young J, Hoke S, et al. Pharmacist intervention to improve medication adherence in heart failure: A randomized trial. Ann Intern Med 2007;146:714–725.

41. Hess O, Carroll J. Clinical assessment of heart failure. In: Libby P, Bonow RO, Mann DL, Zipes DP, eds. Braunwald's Heart Disease: A Textbook of Cardiovascular Medicine. 8th ed. Philadelphia, PA: Elsevier; 2007:561–582.

42. O'Connor CM, Whellan DJ, Lee KL, et al. Efficacy and safety of exercise training in patients with systolic heart failure: HF-ACTION randomized controlled trial. JAMA 2009;301:1439–1450.

43. Riegel B, Moser DK, Anker SD, et al. State of the science: promoting self-care in persons with heart failure: A scientific statement from the American Heart Association. Circulation 2009;120:1141–1163.

44. Adams K, Lindenfeld J, Arnold J, et al. Executive summary: HFSA 2006 Comprehensive Heart Failure Practice Guideline. J Card Fail 2006;12:10–38.

45. Dickstein K, Cohen-Solal A, Filippatos G, et al. ESC guidelines for the diagnosis and treatment of acute and systolic heart failure 2008: The Task Force for the Diagnosis and Treatment of Acute and Systolic heart failure 2008 of the European Society of Cardiology, developed in collaboration with the Heart Failure Association of the ESC (HFA) and endorsed by the European Society of Intensive Care Medicine (ESICM). Eur Heart J 2008;29:2388–2442.

46. Smith SC Jr, Allen J, Blair SN, et al. AHA/ACC guidelines for secondary prevention for patients with coronary and other atherosclerotic vascular disease: 2006 update. Endorsed by the National Heart, Lung, and Blood Institute. Circulation 2006;113:2363–2372.

47. Djousse L, Driver JA, Gaziano JM. Relation between modifiable lifestyle factors and lifetime risk of heart failure. JAMA 2009;302:394–400.

48. Slaughter MS, Rogers JG, Milano CA, et al. Advanced heart failure treated with continuous-flow left ventricular assist device. N Engl J Med 2009;361:2241–2251.

49. Goodlin SJ. Palliative care in congestive heart failure. J Am Coll Cardiol 2009;54:386–396.

50. Echt DS, Liebson PR, Mitchell LB, et al. Mortality and morbidity in patients receiving encainide, flecainide, or placebo: The Cardiac Arrhythmia Suppression Trial. N Engl J Med 1991;324:781–788.

51. Bardy GH, Lee KL, Mark DB, et al. Amiodarone or an implantable cardioverter-defibrillator for congestive heart failure. N Engl J Med 2005;352:225–237.

52. Cleland JG, Daubert JC, Erdmann E, et al. The effect of cardiac resynchronization on morbidity and mortality in heart failure. N Engl J Med 2005;352:1539–1549.

53. Abraham WT. Cardiac resynchronization therapy. Prog Cardiovasc Dis 2006;48:232–238.

54. Moss AJ, Hall WJ, Cannom DS, et al. Cardiac-resynchronization therapy for the prevention of heart-failure events. N Engl J Med 2009;361:1329–1338.

55. St John Sutton M, Ghio S, Plappert T, et al. Cardiac resynchronization induces major structural and functional reverse remodeling in patients with New York Heart Association class I/II heart failure. Circulation 2009;120:1858–1865.

56. Shankar SS, Brater DC. Loop diuretics: from the Na-K-2Cl transporter to clinical use. Am J Physiol Renal Physiol 2003;284:F11–21.

57. Brater DC. Pharmacology of diuretics. Am J Med Sci 2000;319:38–50.

58. Prasun MA, Kocheril AG, Klass PH, et al. The effects of a sliding scale diuretic titration protocol in patients with heart failure. J Cardiovasc Nurs 2005;20:62–70.

59. Dries DL, Strong MH, Cooper RS, Drazner MH. Efficacy of angiotensin-converting enzyme inhibition in reducing progression from asymptomatic left ventricular dysfunction to symptomatic heart failure in black and white patients. J Am Coll Cardiol 2002;40:311–317.

60. Dagenais GR, Pogue J, Fox K, et al. Angiotensin-converting-enzyme inhibitors in stable vascular disease without left ventricular systolic dysfunction or heart failure: A combined analysis of three trials. Lancet 2006;368:581–588.

61. Rodgers JE, Stough WG. Underutilization of evidence-based therapies in heart failure: the pharmacist's role. Pharmacotherapy 2007;27:18S–28S.

62. Smith GL, Lichtman JH, Bracken MB, et al. Renal impairment and outcomes in heart failure: Systematic review and meta-analysis. J Am Coll Cardiol 2006;47:1987–1996.

63. Frances CD, Noguchi H, Massie BM, et al. Are we inhibited? Renal insufficiency should not preclude the use of ACE inhibitors for patients with myocardial infarction and depressed left ventricular function. Arch Intern Med 2000;160:2645–2650.

64. Solomon SD, Rice MM, K AJ, et al. Renal function and effectiveness of angiotensin-converting enzyme inhibitor therapy in patients with chronic stable coronary disease in the Prevention of Events with ACE inhibition (PEACE) trial. Circulation 2006;114:26–31.

65. Packer M, Poole-Wilson PA, Armstrong PW, et al. Comparative effects of low and high doses of the angiotensin-converting enzyme inhibitor, lisinopril, on morbidity and mortality in systolic heart failure. ATLAS Study Group. Circulation 1999;100:2312–2318.

66. Packer M, Bristow MR, Cohn JN, et al. The effect of carvedilol on morbidity and mortality in patients with systolic heart failure. U.S. Carvedilol Heart Failure Study Group. N Engl J Med 1996;334:1349–1355.

67. Effect of metoprolol CR/XL in systolic heart failure: Metoprolol CR/XL Randomised Intervention Trial in Congestive Heart Failure (MERIT-HF). Lancet 1999;353:2001–2007.

68. The Cardiac Insufficiency Bisoprolol Study II (CIBIS-II): A randomised trial. Lancet 1999;353:9–13.

69. Packer M, Coats AJ, Fowler MB, et al. Effect of carvedilol on survival in severe systolic heart failure. N Engl J Med 2001;344:1651–1658.

70. Dargie HJ. Effect of carvedilol on outcome after myocardial infarction in patients with left-ventricular dysfunction: The CAPRICORN randomised trial. Lancet 2001;357:1385–1390.

71. Packer M, Fowler MB, Roecker EB, et al. Effect of carvedilol on the morbidity of patients with severe systolic heart failure: Results of the carvedilol prospective randomized cumulative survival (COPERNICUS) study. Circulation 2002;106:2194–2199.

72. Hjalmarson A, Goldstein S, Fagerberg B, et al. Effects of controlled-release metoprolol on total mortality, hospitalizations, and well-being in patients with heart failure: The Metoprolol CR/XL Randomized Intervention Trial in congestive heart failure (MERIT-HF). MERIT-HF Study Group. JAMA 2000;283:1295–1302.

73. Kukin ML, Kalman J, Charney RH, et al. Prospective, randomized comparison of effect of long-term treatment with metoprolol or carvedilol on symptoms, exercise, ejection fraction, and oxidative stress in heart failure. Circulation 1999;99:2645–2651.

74. Metra M, Nodari S, Parrinello G, et al. Marked improvement in left ventricular ejection fraction during long-term beta-blockade in patients with systolic heart failure: Clinical correlates and prognostic significance. Am Heart J 2003;145:292–299.

75. Bristow MR, Gilbert EM, Abraham WT, et al. Carvedilol produces dose-related improvements in left ventricular function and survival in subjects with systolic heart failure. MOCHA Investigators. Circulation 1996;94:2807–2816.

76. Willenheimer R, van Veldhuisen DJ, Silke B, et al. Effect on survival and hospitalization of initiating treatment for systolic heart failure with bisoprolol followed by enalapril, as compared with the opposite sequence: results of the randomized Cardiac Insufficiency Bisoprolol Study (CIBIS) III. Circulation 2005;112:2426–2435.

77. Gattis WA, O'Connor CM, Gallup DS, et al. Predischarge initiation of carvedilol in patients hospitalized for decompensated heart failure: results of the Initiation Management Predischarge: Process for Assessment of Carvedilol Therapy in Heart Failure (IMPACT-HF) trial. J Am Coll Cardiol 2004;43:1534–1541.

78. Packer M. Controlled-release carvedilol: A concluding perspective. Am J Cardiol 2006;98:67–69.

79. Udelson JE, Pressler SJ, Sackner-Bernstein J, et al. Adherence with once daily versus twice daily carvedilol in patients with heart failure: The Compliance And Quality of Life Study Comparing Once-Daily Controlled-Release Carvedilol CR and Twice-Daily Immediate-Release Carvedilol IR in Patients with Heart Failure (CASPER) Trial. J Card Fail 2009;15:385–393.

80. McAlister FA, Wiebe N, Ezekowitz JA, et al. Meta-analysis: beta-blocker dose, heart rate reduction, and death in patients with heart failure. Ann Intern Med 2009;150:784–794.

81. Bhatia V, Bhatia R, Mathew B. Angiotensin receptor blockers in congestive heart failure: evidence, concerns, and controversies. Cardiol Rev 2005;13:297–303.

82. Cohn JN, Tognoni G. A randomized trial of the angiotensin-receptor blocker valsartan in systolic heart failure. N Engl J Med 2001;345:1667–1675.

83. Pfeffer MA, McMurray JJ, Velazquez EJ, et al. Valsartan, captopril, or both in myocardial infarction complicated by heart failure, left ventricular dysfunction, or both. N Engl J Med 2003;349:1893–1906.

84. Pfeffer MA, Swedberg K, Granger CB, et al. Effects of candesartan on mortality and morbidity in patients with systolic heart failure: The CHARM-Overall programme. Lancet 2003;362:759–766.

85. McMurray JJ, Ostergren J, Swedberg K, et al. Effects of candesartan in patients with systolic heart failure and reduced left-ventricular systolic function taking angiotensin-converting-enzyme inhibitors: The CHARM-Added trial. Lancet 2003;362:767–771.

86. Granger CB, McMurray JJ, Yusuf S, et al. Effects of candesartan in patients with systolic heart failure and reduced left-ventricular systolic function intolerant to angiotensin-converting-enzyme inhibitors: The CHARM-Alternative trial. Lancet 2003;362:772–776.

87. Yusuf S, Pfeffer MA, Swedberg K, et al. Effects of candesartan in patients with systolic heart failure and preserved left-ventricular ejection fraction: The CHARM-Preserved Trial. Lancet 2003;362: 777–781.

88. Konstam MA, Neaton JD, Dickstein K, et al. Effects of high-dose versus low-dose losartan on clinical outcomes in patients with heart failure (HEAAL study): A randomised, double-blind trial. Lancet 2009;374:1840–1848.

89. Haymore BR, Yoon J, Mikita CP, et al. Risk of angioedema with angiotensin receptor blockers in patients with prior angioedema associated with angiotensin-converting enzyme inhibitors: A meta-analysis. Ann Allergy Asthma Immunol 2008;101:495–499.

90. Cicardi M, Zingale LC, Bergamaschini L, Agostoni A. Angioedema associated with angiotensin-converting enzyme inhibitor use: Outcome after switching to a different treatment. Arch Intern Med 2004;164:910–913.

91. Phillips CO, Kashani A, Ko DK, et al. Adverse effects of combination angiotensin II receptor blockers plus angiotensin-converting enzyme inhibitors for left ventricular dysfunction: A quantitative review of data from randomized clinical trials. Arch Intern Med 2007;167:1930–1936.

92. Zannad F, Dousset B, Alla F. Treatment of congestive heart failure: interfering the aldosterone-cardiac extracellular matrix relationship. Hypertension 2001;38:1227–1232.

93. Struthers AD. The clinical implications of aldosterone escape in congestive heart failure. Eur J Heart Fail 2004;6:539–545.

94. Sun Y, Ahokas RA, Bhattacharya SK, et al. Oxidative stress in aldosteronism. Cardiovasc Res 2006;71:300–309.

95. Farquharson CA, Struthers AD. Spironolactone increases nitric oxide bioactivity, improves endothelial vasodilator dysfunction, and suppresses vascular angiotensin I/angiotensin II conversion in patients with systolic heart failure. Circulation 2000;101:594–597.

96. Chhokar VS, Sun Y, Bhattacharya SK, et al. Hyperparathyroidism and the calcium paradox of aldosteronism. Circulation 2005;111: 871–878.

97. Carbone LD, Cross JD, Raza SH, et al. Fracture risk in men with congestive heart failure risk reduction with spironolactone. J Am Coll Cardiol 2008;52:135–138.

98. Albert NM, Yancy CW, Liang L, et al. Use of aldosterone antagonists in heart failure. JAMA 2009;302:1658–1665.

99. Fonarow GC, Yancy CW, Albert NM, et al. Heart failure care in the outpatient cardiology practice setting: findings from IMPROVE HF. Circ Heart Fail 2008;1:98–106.

100. Juurlink DN, Mamdani MM, Lee DS, et al. Rates of hyperkalemia after publication of the Randomized Aldactone Evaluation Study. N Engl J Med 2004;351:543–551.

101. Bozkurt B, Agoston I, Knowlton AA. Complications of inappropriate use of spironolactone in heart failure: When an old medicine spirals out of new guidelines. J Am Coll Cardiol 2003;41:211–214.

102. Svensson M, Gustafsson F, Galatius S, et al. How prevalent is hyperkalemia and renal dysfunction during treatment with spironolactone in patients with congestive heart failure? J Card Fail 2004;10:297–303.

103. The effect of digoxin on mortality and morbidity in patients with heart failure: The Digitalis Investigation Group. N Engl J Med 1997;336:525–533.

104. Terra SG, Washam JB, Dunham GD, Gattis WA. Therapeutic range of digoxin's efficacy in heart failure: What is the evidence? Pharmacotherapy 1999;19:1123–1126.

105. Eichhorn EJ, Gheorghiade M. Digoxin. Prog Cardiovasc Dis 2002;44:251–266.

106. Gheorghiade M, van Veldhuisen DJ, Colucci WS. Contemporary use of digoxin in the management of cardiovascular disorders. Circulation 2006;113:2556–2564.

107. Ahmed A, Rich MW, Fleg JL, et al. Effects of digoxin on morbidity and mortality in diastolic heart failure: the ancillary digitalis investigation group trial. Circulation 2006;114:397–403.

108. Uretsky BF, Young JB, Shahidi FE, et al. Randomized study assessing the effect of digoxin withdrawal in patients with mild to moderate chronic congestive heart failure: Results of the PROVED trial. PROVED Investigative Group. J Am Coll Cardiol 1993;22:955–962.

109. Packer M, Gheorghiade M, Young JB, et al. Withdrawal of digoxin from patients with systolic heart failure treated with angiotensin-converting-enzyme inhibitors. RADIANCE Study. N Engl J Med 1993;329:1–7.

110. Ahmed A, Gambassi G, Weaver MT, et al. Effects of discontinuation of digoxin versus continuation at low serum digoxin concentrations in systolic heart failure. Am J Cardiol 2007;100:280–284.

111. Adams KF Jr, Gheorghiade M, Uretsky BF, et al. Clinical benefits of low serum digoxin concentrations in heart failure. J Am Coll Cardiol 2002;39:946–953.

112. Ahmed A, Rich MW, Love TE, et al. Digoxin and reduction in mortality and hospitalization in heart failure: A comprehensive post hoc analysis of the DIG trial. Eur Heart J 2006;27:178–186.

113. Rathore SS, Wang Y, Krumholz HM. Sex-based differences in the effect of digoxin for the treatment of heart failure. N Engl J Med 2002;347:1403–1411.

114. Adams KF Jr, Patterson JH, Gattis WA, et al. Relationship of serum digoxin concentration to mortality and morbidity in women in the digitalis investigation group trial: A retrospective analysis. J Am Coll Cardiol 2005;46:497–504.

115. Ahmed A, Waagstein F, Pitt B, et al. Effectiveness of digoxin in reducing one-year mortality in systolic heart failure in the Digitalis Investigation Group trial. Am J Cardiol 2009;103:82–87.

116. Bauman JL, Didomenico RJ, Galanter WL. Mechanisms, manifestations, and management of digoxin toxicity in the modern era. Am J Cardiovasc Drugs 2006;6:77–86.

117. Schentag JJ, Bang AJ, Kozinski-Tober JL. In: Burton ME, Shaw LM, Schentag JJ, Evans WE, eds. Applied Pharmacokinetics and Pharmacodynamics: Principles of Therapeutic Drug Monitoring, 4th edition. Baltimore, MD, Lippincott Williams and Wilkins, 2006:410–439.

118. Bauman JL, DiDomenico RJ, Viana M, Fitch M. A method of determining the dose of digoxin for heart failure in the modern era. Arch Intern Med 2006;166:2539–2545.

119. Daiber A, Mulsch A, Hink U, et al. The oxidative stress concept of nitrate tolerance and the antioxidant properties of hydralazine. Am J Cardiol 2005;96:25i–36i.

120. Taylor AL, Ziesche S, Yancy C, et al. Combination of isosorbide dinitrate and hydralazine in blacks with heart failure. N Engl J Med 2004;351:2049–2057.

121. Cohn JN, Archibald DG, Ziesche S, et al. Effect of vasodilator therapy on mortality in chronic congestive heart failure: Results of a Veterans Administration Cooperative Study. N Engl J Med 1986;314: 1547–1552.

122. Cohn JN, Johnson G, Ziesche S, et al. A comparison of enalapril with hydralazine-isosorbide dinitrate in the treatment of chronic congestive heart failure. N Engl J Med 1991;325:303–310.

123. Carson P, Ziesche S, Johnson G, Cohn JN. Racial differences in response to therapy for heart failure: Analysis of the vasodilator-heart failure trials. Vasodilator-Heart Failure Trial Study Group. J Card Fail 1999;5:178–187.

124. Mullens W, Abrahams Z, Francis GS, et al. Usefulness of isosorbide dinitrate and hydralazine as add-on therapy in patients discharged for advanced decompensated heart failure. Am J Cardiol 2009;103:1113–1119.

125. McNamara DM, Tam SW, Sabolinski ML, et al. Endothelial nitric oxide synthase (NOS3) polymorphisms in African Americans with heart failure: results from the A-HeFT trial. J Card Fail 2009;15:191–198.

126. Rame JE, Tam SW, McNamara D, et al. Dysfunctional corin i555(p568) allele is associated with impaired brain natriuretic peptide processing and adverse outcomes in blacks with systolic heart failure: Results from the genetic risk assessment in heart failure substudy. Circ Heart Fail 2009;2:541–548.

127. Fuster V, Ryden LE, Cannom DS, et al. ACC/AHA/ESC 2006 guidelines for the management of patients with atrial fibrillation: A report of the American College of Cardiology/American Heart Association Task Force on Practice Guidelines and the European Society of Cardiology Committee for Practice Guidelines (Writing Committee to Revise the 2001 Guidelines for the Management of Patients with Atrial Fibrillation), developed in collaboration with the European Heart Rhythm Association and the Heart Rhythm Society. Circulation 2006;114:e257–354.

128. Anand K, Mooss AN, Hee TT, Mohiuddin SM. Meta-analysis: Inhibition of renin-angiotensin system prevents new-onset atrial fibrillation. Am Heart J 2006;152:217–222.

129. Nasr IA, Bouzamondo A, Hulot JS, et al. Prevention of atrial fibrillation onset by beta-blocker treatment in heart failure: a meta-analysis. Eur Heart J 2007;28:457–462.

130. Wyse DG, Waldo AL, DiMarco JP, et al. A comparison of rate control and rhythm control in patients with atrial fibrillation. N Engl J Med 2002;347:1825–1833.

131. Roy D, Talajic M, Nattel S, et al. Rhythm control versus rate control for atrial fibrillation and heart failure. N Engl J Med 2008;358:2667–2677.

132. Choy CK, Rodgers JE, Nappi JM, Haines ST. Type 2 diabetes mellitus and heart failure. Pharmacotherapy 2008;28:170–192.

133. Masoudi FA, Inzucchi SE, Wang Y, et al. Thiazolidinediones, metformin, and outcomes in older patients with diabetes and heart failure: an observational study. Circulation 2005;111:583–590.

134. Eurich DT, McAlister FA, Blackburn DF, et al. Benefits and harms of antidiabetic agents in patients with diabetes and heart failure: Systematic review. BMJ 2007;335:497.

135. Anand IS. Anemia and systolic heart failure implications and treatment options. J Am Coll Cardiol 2008;52:501–511.

136. Tehrani F, Dhesi P, Daneshvar D, et al. Erythropoiesis stimulating agents in heart failure patients with anemia: A meta-analysis. Cardiovasc Drugs Ther 2009;23:511–518.

137. Pfeffer MA, Burdmann EA, Chen CY, et al. A trial of darbepoetin alfa in type 2 diabetes and chronic kidney disease. N Engl J Med 2009;361:2019–2032.

138. Anker SD, Comin Colet J, Filippatos G, et al. Ferric carboxymaltose in patients with heart failure and iron deficiency. N Engl J Med 2009;361:2436–2448.

139. Murray MD, Deer MM, Ferguson JA, et al. Open-label randomized trial of torsemide compared with furosemide therapy for patients with heart failure. Am J Med 2001;111:513–520.

140. Young M, Plosker GL. Torasemide: A pharmacoeconomic review of its use in systolic heart failure. Pharmacoeconomics 2001;19:679–703.

141. Ahmed A, Husain A, Love TE, et al. Heart failure, chronic diuretic use, and increase in mortality and hospitalization: An observational study using propensity score methods. Eur Heart J 2006;27:1431–1439.

142. Massie BM. Aspirin use in systolic heart failure: What should we recommend to the practitioner? J Am Coll Cardiol 2005;46:963–966.

143. Masoudi FA, Wolfe P, Havranek EP, et al. Aspirin use in older patients with heart failure and coronary artery disease: National prescription patterns and relationship with outcomes. J Am Coll Cardiol 2005;46:955–962.

144. McAlister FA, Ghali WA, Gong Y, et al. Aspirin use and outcomes in a community-based cohort of 7352 patients discharged after first hospitalization for heart failure. Circulation 2006;113:2572–2578.

145. Schoolwerth AC, Sica DA, Ballermann BJ, Wilcox CS. Renal considerations in angiotensin converting enzyme inhibitor therapy: a statement for healthcare professionals from the Council on the Kidney in Cardiovascular Disease and the Council for High Blood Pressure Research of the American Heart Association. Circulation 2001;104:1985–1991.

146. Cooper WO, Hernandez-Diaz S, Arbogast PG, et al. Major congenital malformations after first-trimester exposure to ACE inhibitors. N Engl J Med 2006;354:2443–2451.

147. Haymore BR, DeZee KJ. Use of angiotensin receptor blockers after angioedema with an angiotensin-converting enzyme inhibitor. Ann Allergy Asthma Immunol 2009;103:83–84.

148. A trial of the beta-blocker bucindolol in patients with advanced systolic heart failure. N Engl J Med 2001;344:1659–1667.

149. Liggett SB, Mialet-Perez J, Thaneemit-Chen S, et al. A polymorphism within a conserved beta(1)-adrenergic receptor motif alters cardiac function and beta-blocker response in human heart failure. Proc Natl Acad Sci U S A 2006;103:11288–11293.

150. Poole-Wilson PA, Swedberg K, Cleland JG, et al. Comparison of carvedilol and metoprolol on clinical outcomes in patients with systolic heart failure in the Carvedilol or Metoprolol European Trial (COMET): randomised controlled trial. Lancet 2003;362:7–13.

151. Aquilante CL, Terra SG, Schofield RS et al. Sustained restoration of autonomic balance with long- but not short-acting metoprolol in patients with heart failure. J Card Fail 2006;12:171–176.

152. Bakris GL, Fonseca V, Katholi RE et al. Metabolic effects of carvedilol vs metoprolol in patients with type 2 diabetes mellitus and hypertension: A randomized controlled trial. JAMA 2004;292:2227–2236.

153. Torp-Pedersen C, Metra M, Charlesworth A, et al. Effects of metoprolol and carvedilol on pre-existing and new onset diabetes in patients with systolic heart failure: Data from the Carvedilol or Metoprolol European Trial (COMET). Heart 2007;93:968–973.

154. Metra M, Torp-Pedersen C, Cleland JG, et al. Should beta-blocker therapy be reduced or withdrawn after an episode of decompensated heart failure? Results from COMET. Eur J Heart Fail 2007;9:901–909.

155. Fonarow GC, Abraham WT, Albert NM, et al. Influence of beta-blocker continuation or withdrawal on outcomes in patients hospitalized with heart failure: findings from the OPTIMIZE-HF program. J Am Coll Cardiol 2008;52:190–199.

156. Jondeau G, Neuder Y, Eicher JC, et al. B-CONVINCED: Beta-blocker CONtinuation vs. INterruption in patients with Congestive heart failure hospitalizED for a decompensation episode. Eur Heart J 2009;30:2186–2192.

157. Deedwania PC, Giles TD, Klibaner M, et al. Efficacy, safety and tolerability of metoprolol CR/XL in patients with diabetes and systolic heart failure: Experiences from MERIT-HF. Am Heart J 2005;149:159–167.

158. Schentag J, Bang A, Kozinski-Tober J. Digoxin. In: Burton M, Shaw L, Schentag J, Evans W, eds. Applied Pharmacokinetics and Pharmacodynamics. 4th ed. Baltimore, MD: Lippincott Williams & Wilkins; 2006:411–439.

159. Lee WC, Chavez YE, Baker T, Luce BR. Economic burden of heart failure: A summary of recent literature. Heart Lung 2004;33:362–371.

160. Smith DG, Cerulli A, Frech FH. Use of valsartan for the treatment of heart-failure patients not receiving ACE inhibitors: a budget impact analysis. Clin Ther 2005;27:951–959.

161. Croom KF, Plosker GL. Eplerenone: A pharmacoeconomic review of its use in patients with post-myocardial infarction heart failure. Pharmacoeconomics 2005;23:1057–1072.

162. Angus DC, Linde-Zwirble WT, Tam SW et al. Cost-effectiveness of fixed-dose combination of isosorbide dinitrate and hydralazine therapy for blacks with heart failure. Circulation 2005;112:3745–3753.

163. Sanders GD, Hlatky MA, Owens DK. Cost-effectiveness of implantable cardioverter-defibrillators. N Engl J Med 2005;353:1471–1480.

164. Yao G, Freemantle N, Calvert MJ, et al. The long-term cost-effectiveness of cardiac resynchronization therapy with or without an implantable cardioverter-defibrillator. Eur Heart J 2007;28:42–51.

165. Holland R, Battersby J, Harvey I et al. Systematic review of multidisciplinary interventions in heart failure. Heart 2005;91:899–906.

166. Clark AM, Savard LA, Thompson DR. What is the strength of evidence for heart failure disease-management programs? J Am Coll Cardiol 2009;54:397–401.

167. Murray MD, Ritchey ME, Wu J, Tu W. Effect of a pharmacist on adverse drug events and medication errors in outpatients with cardiovascular disease. Arch Intern Med 2009;169:757–763.

168. Murray M, Young J, Hoke S et al. Pharmacist intervention to improve medication adherence in heart failure: A randomized trial. Ann Intern Med 2007;146:714–725.

169. Catananti C, Liperoti R, Settanni S et al. Heart failure and adverse drug reactions among hospitalized older adults. Clin Pharmacol Ther 2009;86:307–310.

170. MacDonald JE, Struthers AD. What is the optimal serum potassium level in cardiovascular patients? J Am Coll Cardiol 2004;43:155–161.

21

Diastolic Heart Failure and the Cardiomyopathies

JEAN M. NAPPI AND ROBERT L. PAGE II

KEY CONCEPTS

❶ Diastolic heart failure is a frequent cause of heart failure (35–50% prevalence) and has a significant effect on mortality (25–35% 5-year mortality rate) and morbidity (50% 1-year readmission rate).

❷ Hypertension is a common cause of diastolic heart failure.

❸ The diagnosis of diastolic heart failure can be made when a patient has both symptoms and signs of congestive heart failure on physical examination and preserved left ventricular (LV) function.

❹ Treatment should be targeted at symptom reduction, causal clinical disease, and underlying basic mechanisms. Patients with diastolic heart failure may be treated differently than those with systolic dysfunction.

❺ Nonpharmacologic treatment measures include weight loss, smoking cessation, dietary changes, and exercise.

❻ Symptom-targeted therapy includes decreasing pulmonary venous pressure, maintaining atrial contraction and atrioventricular synchrony, and reducing heart rate. Exercise tolerance is increased by reducing exercise-induced increases in blood pressure and heart rate.

❼ Disease-targeted therapy includes preventing or treating myocardial ischemia and preventing or regressing LV hypertrophy.

❽ Treatment strategies for patients with hypertrophic cardiomyopathy (HCM) are aimed at improving symptoms and preventing sudden cardiac death.

❾ Patients with HCM who are at high risk for sudden cardiac death should receive an implantable cardioverter-defibrillator.

❿ Patients with HCM who are symptomatic may benefit from β-blockade or verapamil.

DIASTOLIC HEART FAILURE

Heart failure (HF) may be caused by a primary abnormality in systolic function, diastolic function, or both. Making the distinction is important because the prevalence, prognosis, and treatment of

Learning objectives, review questions, and other resources can be found at **www.pharmacotherapyonline.com**.

HF may be quite different depending on whether the predominant mechanism causing the symptoms is systolic or diastolic dysfunction. Clinical studies have reported that up to 74% of patients with HF have preserved left ventricular ejection fraction (LVEF), variably defined as exceeding 40%, 45%, or 50%.[1-3] When patients with preserved EF exhibit symptoms consistent with effort intolerance and dyspnea, especially in the presence of venous congestion and edema, the term *diastolic heart failure* (DHF) is often used.[4] Despite recognition of its importance, no strong consensus exists regarding appropriate terminology for this syndrome; therefore, the terms DHF, HF with preserved EF, and HF with normal EF are often used synonymously.

DHF can be defined as a condition in which myocardial relaxation and filling are impaired and incomplete. The ventricle is unable to accept an adequate volume of blood from the venous system, does not fill at low pressure, and/or is unable to maintain normal stroke volume. In its most severe form, DHF results in overt symptoms of HF. In modest DHF, symptoms of dyspnea and fatigue occur only during stress or activity, when heart rate and end-diastolic volume increase. In its mildest form, DHF can be manifested as a slow or delayed pattern of relaxation and filling with little or no elevation in diastolic pressure and few or no cardiac symptoms. The congestive symptoms that occur with DHF are a manifestation of increased pulmonary venous pressures. DHF is caused by impaired myocardial relaxation and/or increased diastolic stiffness. When HF is caused by a predominant abnormality in diastolic function, the ventricular chamber is not enlarged, and EF may be normal or even elevated.[5] Figure 21–1 shows the pressure—volume relationship in a patient with normal versus abnormal diastolic function. Changes in the myocardium are associated with a shift upward and to the left of the pressure—volume curve, so that for any increase in LV volume, diastolic pressure rises to a much greater level than normally would occur. Clinically, patients present with reduced exercise tolerance and dyspnea when they have elevated LV diastolic

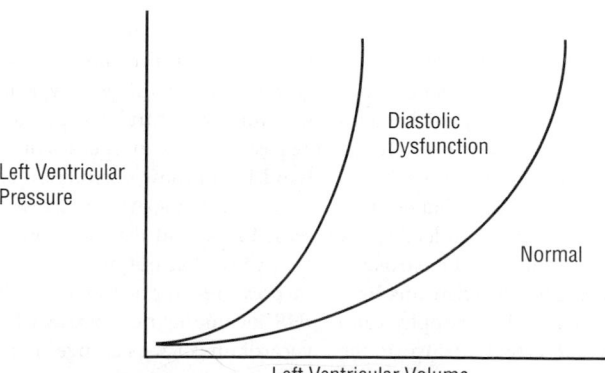

FIGURE 21-1. Diastolic pressure—volume relationship in a normal patient (*right trace*) and a patient with diastolic dysfunction (*left trace*).

pressures. Patients with DHF have a predominant abnormality in diastolic function, whereas patients with systolic heart failure (SHF) have a predominant abnormality in systolic function of the LV. Furthermore, patients with DHF are more likely to be female, obese, have diabetes, and be hypertensive.[1]

EPIDEMIOLOGY

❶ Recent studies suggest that as many as half of all patients presenting with overt HF have preserved EF.[7,8] The prevalence of DHF depends on a number of determinants: patient age, patient gender, study design, particular population under consideration, and EF. It is important to recognize that these determinants are not independent but interdependent. The most important determinant appears to be patient age. DHF is relatively uncommon in young and middle-aged patients. The prevalence of DHF increases with age, approximating 15% in patients younger than 60 years, 35% in patients between 60 and 70 years, and 50% in patients older than 70 years. Prospective community-based studies showed that in patients older than 70 years, the prevalence of DHF approaches 50%.[9,10] As the proportion of the population older than 65 years continues to grow, it has been estimated that DHF may eventually become the most common form of HF.[11]

ETIOLOGY

❷ Several disorders can impair ventricular function and play a role in the development of DHF. DHF is seen often in patients with hypertension, coronary artery disease (CAD), valvular heart disease, atrial fibrillation, diabetes, and hypertrophic cardiomyopathy (HCM).[12,13] Hypertension and valvular heart disease are common underlying cardiovascular disorders in patients with DHF.[14] There are several proposed mechanisms by which hypertension may impair diastolic function. Hypertension can alter diastolic function through its effects on wall tension, myocardial hypertrophy and fibrosis, and small-vessel structure and function, as well as by predisposing to epicardial CAD. An association between impaired LV filling and subnormal high-energy phosphate metabolism has been shown in hypertensive patients, even in the absence of left ventricular hypertrophy (LVH).[15]

LVH plays a central role in the adaptation of the myocardium to pressure overload. Severe and long-standing pressure overload has been associated with phenotypic alterations at the myocyte level, which differs from the physiologic hypertrophy seen in athletes.[16] Long-term chronic pressure overload stimulates cardiac growth and collagen production, which lead to an increase in myocardial mass and structural remodeling. The results of these changes are an increase in myocardial stiffness and a decrease in diastolic filling.

PATHOPHYSIOLOGY

The pathologic disease processes that cause DHF include myocardial ischemia with or without epicardial CAD, pressure overload hypertrophy, and genetic hypertrophy. HCM is a prototype for DHF. The grossly thickened myocardium, structural changes, and interstitial fibrosis severely alter the passive elastic properties of the myocardium. Patients with HCM and LV outflow obstruction are sensitive to small changes in volume, such that a small decrease in filling pressure can lead to a decrease in LV end-diastolic volume and a dramatic fall in stroke volume and cardiac output.

The basic mechanisms by which pressure-overload hypertrophy and genetic hypertrophy cause DHF include extramyocardial factors and factors intrinsic to the myocardium, such as changes in the cardiac muscle cell and in the extracellular matrix that surrounds the cardiomyocyte (Table 21–1).[17–19] Intracellular processes, such as changes in calcium homeostasis, contractile and noncontractile

TABLE 21-1 Potential Pathologic Mechanisms of Diastolic Heart Failure

Mechanisms directly affecting myocardial tissue	
Cardiomyocyte	Increased intracellular calcium, producing calcium overload
	Myofilaments
	Increased troponin C calcium binding and increased myofilament calcium sensitivity
	Cytoskeleton
	Changes in cytoskeletal proteins
	Energetics
	Decrease in ATP availability, leading to decreased rate or extent of actomyosin dissociation
Extracellular matrix	Increased content of fibrillar collagen
	Thickening of existing fibrillar collagen
	Decreased MMP and/or increased TIMP
Neurohormones	Increased renin–angiotensin–aldosterone
	Increased endothelin
Extramyocardial mechanisms	
Increased hemodynamic load: preload or afterload	
Increased heterogeneity	
Systemic neurohormones	Increased levels of angiotensin II
Pericardium	Pericardium may have a constraining effect as LV filling pressure and end-diastolic volume increase

ATP = adenosine triphosphate, LV = left ventricular, MMP = matrix metalloproteinase, TIMP = tissue inhibitor of MMP

proteins, energetics, and the cytoskeleton, contribute to abnormalities in myocardial relaxation and stiffness. Changes in the extracellular matrix, particularly changes in fibrillar collagen, alter relaxation and stiffness. In addition to the cardiomyocyte and the extracellular matrix, local myocardial neuroendocrine activation can impair relaxation and increase stiffness. Activation of neurohormones such as the renin—angiotensin—aldosterone system (RAAS) may act directly to alter diastolic properties or act indirectly by altering calcium homeostasis. Finally, extramyocardial changes in loading conditions and changes in heterogeneity occur in hypertrophied ventricles and contribute to changes in relaxation and stiffness, so that even when the myocardium itself is normal, changes in these extramyocardial factors can cause abnormalities in diastolic function.[19]

Myocardial ischemia, particularly in the subendocardial region, is common when ventricular hypertrophy is present. Slow or delayed myocardial relaxation and perivascular fibrosis can adversely affect coronary blood flow and coronary blood flow reserve. This may contribute to the development of myocardial ischemia and sudden death.[20,21] Therefore, myocardial ischemia may be part of the clinical syndrome of DHF even if no epicardial CAD is present.

An association between diabetes and diastolic dysfunction leading to heart failure has been identified.[22] This may occur even in the absence of atherosclerotic heart disease. Hyperinsulinemia is thought to trigger cardiac hypertrophy, and hyperglycemia alters the expression and function of the intracellular receptors, ultimately leading to systolic and diastolic dysfunction.

CLINICAL PRESENTATION OF DIASTOLIC DYSFUNCTION

General

▪ The majority of patients do not show symptoms at rest but in response to stress conditions. Symptoms may be induced or worsened by physical exercise but also by events such as anemia, fever, tachycardia, and systemic pathologies.

Symptoms

- The patient may complain of exertional dyspnea, orthopnea, paroxysmal dyspnea, and exercise intolerance.

Signs

- Pulmonary congestion (rales)
- Exaggerated rise in blood pressure and heart rate in response to exercise
- Presence of an S4 gallop

Laboratory Tests

- B-type natriuretic peptide and N-terminal pro–B-type natriuretic peptide will be elevated.

Other Diagnostic Tests

- Two-dimensional echocardiography will show a normal or elevated EF, normal or decreased cardiac output, and LVH and/or concentric remodeling.
- Doppler echocardiography will show elevated pulmonary venous pressures.
- Chest radiography will show pulmonary congestion.
- Electrocardiography may reflect LVH.

DIAGNOSIS

❸ The criteria used to make the diagnosis of DHF remain controversial. However, making an accurate diagnosis is extremely important. Guidelines from the European Society of Cardiology (ESC) propose that three requirements must be present to make the diagnosis of DHF: (a) symptoms or signs of HF; (b) normal or only mildly abnormal systolic function (EF exceeding 45–50%); and (c) abnormal diastolic function (e.g., abnormal relaxation, filling, distensibility, or stiffness).[23] The first two requirements appear to be well justified; the third requirement may not be.[6]

Three clinical factors have been proposed to categorize patients with DHF: the presence/absence of elevated blood pressure or history of hypertension, the presence/absence of LVH, and the presence/absence of increased LV volume.[22] Based on these factors, patients are divided into four subgroups according to the underlying pathophysiology: HCM, infiltrative or restrictive cardiomyopathy, increased preload, and abnormal ventricular-arterial coupling.

With few exceptions, DHF cannot be distinguished from SHF on the basis of the history, physical examination, chest x-ray, and electrocardiogram (ECG) alone. The frequency with which patients have symptoms and signs of HF on physical examination or chest x-ray is not dependent on whether they have SHF or DHF.[21] Patients with DHF are often elderly, hypertensive women.[1,22]

The data from a number of studies demonstrate that signs and symptoms of HF do not predict EF. In contrast, they do predict the presence of increased LV diastolic pressure. The question then becomes whether the increase in LV diastolic pressure occurs in association with normal LV volume and EF, as would occur in DHF, or whether the increase in LV diastolic pressure occurs in association with an increased LV volume and decreased EF, as would occur with SHF. Therefore, determining whether HF is caused by systolic or diastolic dysfunction requires some estimate of LV size and EF. These measurements can be made using echocardiography, radionuclide ventriculography, or contrast ventriculography. When a patient presents with dyspnea, pulmonary rales, and radiographic evidence of pulmonary venous hypertension, the detection of normal LV end-diastolic volume and normal EF supports the diagnosis of DHF. Conditions such as mitral stenosis, pulmonary disease, sleep apnea, anemia, cirrhosis, hypothyroidism, and drug-induced

fluid retention must be ruled out because they can cause similar symptoms.[24]

B-type natriuretic peptide (BNP) and its biologically inactive fragment, N-terminal proBNP (NT-proBNP), are cardiac neurohormones secreted from the myocardium in response to increases in ventricular volume and pressure. Both are used as an aid in the differential diagnosis of dyspnea. The Breathing Not Properly study evaluated 452 patients with echocardiography within 30 days of an emergency department visit. Of the 452 patients, 165 (36.5%) had EF >45% (mean EF 59%).[25] In these patients with preserved EF who had been admitted to the hospital for dyspnea, BNP levels were significantly lower than those found in patients with SHF (413 vs 821 pg/mL). However, there was considerable overlap in the BNP levels in patients with DHF compared with those without HF, making BNP levels less useful. Furthermore, the sensitivity, specificity, and predictive accuracy of BNP levels in DHF are limited in part because BNP is altered by age, adiposity, gender, and other factors. Similar findings have been documented with NT-proBNP. In a study of 68 symptomatic patients with isolated DHF (EF >50%), NT-proBNP was significantly increased in patients with isolated DHF and correlated with disease severity. Compared with conventional echocardiography, Doppler imaging, and heart catheterization, NT-proBNP exhibited the best negative predictive value for detection of DHF.[26]

PROGNOSIS

The prognosis in patients with DHF, although less ominous than in those with SHF, is worse than that of age-matched control patients. The 5-year mortality rate of these patients approximates 25%, although mortality rates as high as 13% over a 6-month period have been reported.[1,7] In comparison, the annual mortality rate of patients with SHF approximates 10% to 15%, whereas age-matched control mortality approaches 1%. However, in a population-based cohort study of 2,802 patients with HF, no significant difference was demonstrated in the adjusted 1-year mortality rate for patients with EF <40% compared with those with EF >50%.[27] Unfortunately, compared with SHF, little improvement in the survival rate among patients with DHF has been seen.[11]

In patients with DHF, the prognosis is also affected by the clinical pathologic etiology causing the disease. When patients with CAD are excluded, the annual mortality rate for DHF is 2% to 3%. In addition to the clinical pathologic etiology causing HF, other predictors of mortality are impaired renal function ≤60 mL/min/m², worse functional class (New York Heart Association [NYHA] class III—IV), male gender, and older age (>74 years).[28,29]

The mode of death appears similar in patients with systolic versus diastolic HF. Sudden death and death from progressive pump failure occurred with equal frequency in patients with SHF as those with DHF. Morbidity also is similar between patients with SHF and DHF. The 1-year hospital readmission rate can approach 50%, thereby placing significant pressure on healthcare resources. However, patients with DHF appear to have a higher risk of nonfatal myocardial infarction (MI) and stroke.[12,27]

TREATMENT

Diastolic Heart Failure

The general principles used to guide the treatment of SHF are based on numerous large, randomized, double-blind, multicenter trials. Until recently, no such randomized trials had been performed in patients with DHF. Consequently, the guidelines for the management of DHF are based primarily on clinical investigations in relatively small groups of patients, clinical experience, and concepts

TABLE 21-2 Targeted Approach to Treatment of Diastolic Heart Failure

Symptom-targeted treatment	Rationale	Agent
Decrease pulmonary venous pressure	Reduce left ventricular volume	Diuretics, nitrates, salt restriction
	Reduce heart rate	
Decrease myocardial oxygen consumption	Control blood pressure	β-blockers, diltiazem, verapamil
		ACE inhibitors, angiotensin receptor blockers, calcium channel blockers
Maintain atrial contraction	Restore and/or maintain sinus rhythm	Cardioversion of atrial fibrillation
Improve exercise tolerance	As above	Use positive inotropic agents with caution
Disease-targeted treatment		
Prevent/treat myocardial ischemia		β-blockers, diltiazem, verapamil, nitrates
Prevent/regress ventricular hypertrophy		Antihypertensive therapy
Mechanism-targeted treatment		
Modify myocardial and extramyocardial mechanisms		Possibly ACE inhibitors or angiotensin receptor blockers, diuretics, spironolactone
Modify intracellular and extracellular mechanisms		Possibly ACE inhibitors or angiotensin receptor blockers, spironolactone

ACE = angiotensin-converting enzyme

based on the knowledge and understanding of the pathophysiology of the disease process. The treatment regimen outlined in Table 21–2 applies to patients with DHF who have clear manifestations of congestion either at rest or with exertion. Whether treatment of asymptomatic diastolic dysfunction confers any benefit has not been demonstrated.

DESIRED OUTCOME

④ Treatment should be targeted at reducing symptoms, principally those of increased pulmonary venous pressure. It should include decreasing diastolic pressure by decreasing LV volume, maintaining atrial contraction, and reducing heart rate without reducing cardiac output. Also, treatment should be targeted at the pathologic diseases that cause DHF. For example, CAD, hypertensive heart disease, and aortic stenosis have relatively specific therapeutic targets, such as lowering blood pressure, inducing LVH regression, performing aortic valve replacement, and treating ischemia by increasing myocardial blood flow and reducing myocardial oxygen demand. Finally, treatment should be targeted at the underlying mechanisms that are altered by the disease processes just mentioned.[30]

NONPHARMACOLOGIC THERAPY

Diet and Lifestyle

⑤ The initial effort in the treatment of DHF is aimed at decreasing symptoms. The first step in this effort is to decrease pulmonary congestion by decreasing LV volume using sodium and fluid restriction. A low-sodium diet (≤2 g/day) and moderate fluid restriction will help to prevent volume overload. Both sodium and fluid restriction must be done with care. Excessive restriction can lead to hypotension, low-output state, and/or renal insufficiency. Daily weights may help to assess volume status. Dietary and lifestyle factors that decrease the risk of development of epicardial CAD and high blood pressure should be encouraged.[23,31]

Moderate aerobic exercise to improve cardiovascular conditioning is beneficial to maintain a slower heart rate, improve cardiac reserve, and maintain skeletal muscle function. Isometric exercise should be avoided.[32]

Interventional/Surgical Procedures

An important step in symptom-targeted therapy that acts to decrease pulmonary venous pressures is to maintain atrial contraction and atrioventricular (AV) synchrony. Maintaining atrial contraction and AV synchrony is important both in preserving normal cardiac output and in keeping LV diastolic pressure low. Chemical or electrical cardioversion of persistent atrial tachyarrhythmias will decrease diastolic pressure, increase cardiac output, and resolve pulmonary edema. An AV sequential pacemaker should be used to treat bradyarrhythmias in patients requiring pacing.

Therapy also should be aimed at preventing or treating the underlying pathologic cause of DHF. Aortic valve replacement should be performed in symptomatic patients with pressure-overload hypertrophy caused by aortic stenosis. Revascularization should be performed in selected patients with DHF caused by CAD-induced myocardial ischemia. In addition, myocardial oxygen consumption and myocardial blood flow should be increased using medical treatment, including nitrates, β-blockers, and calcium channel blockers.[33]

Indications for Hospitalization

Patients with DHF may present with an acute onset of pulmonary edema. Potential causes for the acute decompensation of these patients include volume overload, uncontrolled hypertension, acute myocardial ischemia, progressive valvular disease (aortic stenosis), and new-onset or uncontrolled tachyarrhythmias. Treatment strategies for these patients eventually may include the need for surgery, as in the case of valvular disease.

The initial management focuses on relieving pulmonary congestion and maintaining oxygenation. IV diuretic agents and nesiritide for patients are effective for volume overload. Caution must be exercised to avoid overdiuresis or excessive lowering of LV end-diastolic volume, which can lead to a decrease in stroke volume. Morphine and nitroglycerin also are effective in reducing LV end-diastolic pressure.[34]

PHARMACOLOGIC TREATMENT

Drug Treatments of First Choice

With a few notable exceptions, many of the drugs used to treat SHF are the same as those used to treat DHF. However, the rationale for their use, the pathophysiologic process that is being altered by the drug, and the dosing regimen may be entirely different depending on whether the patient has SHF or DHF. For example, β-blockers are recommended for the treatment of both SHF and DHF. In DHF, however, β-blockers are used to decrease heart rate, increase diastolic duration, and modify the hemodynamic response to exercise. In SHF, β-blockers are used in the long run to increase the inotropic state and modify LV remodeling. Diuretics also are used in the treatment of both SHF and DHF. However, the doses of diuretics used to treat DHF are, in general, much smaller than the doses used to treat SHF. Antagonists of the

TABLE 21-3 Evidence-Based Pharmacotherapy for Diastolic Heart Failure

Recommendations	Recommendation Grade[a]
Diuretics	
• A loop or a thiazide diuretic should be considered for patients with volume overload. However, with more severe volume overload or inadequate response to a thiazide, a loop diuretic should be implemented. Caution is warranted not to lower preload excessively, which may reduce stroke volume and cardiac output.	C
ACE inhibitors	
• ACE inhibitors may be considered in all patients.	C
• ACE inhibitors should be considered in all patients who have symptomatic atherosclerotic cardiovascular disease or diabetes and one additional risk factor.	C
Angiotensin receptor blockers	
• Angiotensin receptor blockers may be considered in all patients.	C
• In patients who are intolerant of ACE inhibitors, an angiotensin receptor blocker can be considered an alternative.	C
β-Blockers	
• β-blockers should be considered in patients with one or more of the following conditions:	
Myocardial infarction	A
Hypertension	B
Atrial fibrillation requiring ventricular rate control	B
Calcium channel blockers	
• In patients with atrial fibrillation warranting ventricular rate control who either are intolerant to or have not responded to a β-blocker, diltiazem or verapamil should be considered.	C
• A nondihydropyridine or dihydropyridine calcium channel blocker can be considered for symptom-limiting angina.	A
• A nondihydropyridine or dihydropyridine calcium channel blocker can be considered for hypertension.	C

[a]Strength of recommendations: A, randomized controlled clinical trials; B, cohort and case control studies based on observations from observational studies or registries, post hoc, subgroup, and meta-analysis; C, expert opinion, epidemiologic findings from observational studies, and safety findings from large-scale use.
ACE = angiotensin-converting enzyme
Data from Heart Failure Society of America. Evaluation and management of patients with heart failure and preserved left ventricular ejection fraction. J Card Fail 2010;16:e126–133.

RAAS are useful in lowering blood pressure and reducing LVH. Some drugs, however, are used to treat either SHF or DHF but not both. Calcium channel blockers such as diltiazem, nifedipine, and verapamil have little utility in the treatment of SHF. In contrast, each of these drugs has been proposed as being useful in the treatment of DHF.

Published Guidelines

Much less objective information on the treatment of DHF is available. This relative paucity of objective information is reflected in guidelines for the diagnosis and management of HF published by the American College of Cardiology (ACC)/American Heart Association (AHA), the ESC, and the Heart Failure Society of America (HFSA).[23,31,36] In general, all three guidelines recommend treating comorbid conditions by controlling heart rate and blood pressure, alleviating causes of myocardial ischemia, reducing volume, and restoring and maintaining sinus rhythm. Table 21–3 summarizes the therapeutic recommendations from the HFSA.

General Information

Although dozens of trials evaluating pharmacologic therapy have been conducted in patients with SHF, few trials have focused on patients with DHF. In fact, most published HF trials have specifically excluded patients with preserved EF. A few published large clinical studies and several trials examining various agents in the treatment of DHF are under way (Table 21–4). With these studies and others that are currently under way, an evidence-based treatment for DHF will be defined.

Alternative Drug Treatment

As a result of the controversy regarding the diagnosis of DHF, the development and design of large clinical trials have been hindered. At this time, most antihypertensive agents would be acceptable forms of therapy for hypertensive heart disease, with the exception of α-blockers (e.g., doxazosin). In the Antihypertensive and Lipid-Lowering Treatment to Prevent Heart Attack Trial (ALLHAT), the doxazosin treatment arm was dropped because patients randomized to doxazosin had an increased risk for developing HF and stroke compared with the chlorthalidone arm.[37]

Special Populations

DHF is associated with hypertension and aging, making it a common diagnosis in elderly white women. Because these women often are frail and have low muscle mass, their creatinine clearance and renal function may be compromised. Special care must be taken when selecting and titrating doses of drugs, monitoring levels of serum creatinine and electrolytes, and using diuretics, angiotensin-converting enzyme (ACE) inhibitors, and angiotensin receptor blockers.[38]

Diabetes is often a comorbid condition in patients with HF. Because the thiazolidinediones (pioglitazone and rosiglitazone) are associated with fluid retention, caution is warranted when initiating these drugs in patients with a history of DHF. Thiazolidinediones should be discontinued in patients with symptoms related to volume overload.[3,36]

■ DRUG CLASS INFORMATION

Diuretics

6 Diuretics can provide symptom-targeted therapy by decreasing systemic and LV volume. By decreasing LV diastolic volumes, LV pressures slide down the curvilinear diastolic pressure—volume relationship toward a lower, less steep portion of the curve. As pressure throughout diastole falls, mean diastolic pressure, pulmonary capillary wedge pressure, and pulmonary venous pressure fall. These agents effectively reduce the central blood volume and lower diastolic pressures, thus alleviating the symptoms of the congestive state. Diuretics can provide disease-targeted therapy by decreasing blood pressure and favorably affecting the myocardial oxygen supply versus demand ratio. Lower LV diastolic pressures may increase subendocardial blood flow, preventing or alleviating the imbalance

TABLE 21-4 Completed and Ongoing Large Clinical Trials for Diastolic Heart Failure

Trial (No. of Patients)	Treatment	Inclusion Criteria	Primary End Point	Results
DIG Ancillary Study[53] (n = 988)	Digoxin vs placebo for a mean of 37 months. Patients received ACE inhibitor (86%) and diuretics (85%).	EF >45%, NYHA II–IV, normal sinus rhythm	Composite of HF hospitalization or HF mortality	No significant difference was found in the primary end point between treatment groups (HR = 0.82, P = 0.136). Digoxin had no effect on all-cause mortality or cause-specific mortality or on all-cause or CV hospitalization. Compared with placebo, digoxin use was associated with a trend toward a reduction in HF hospitalizations (HR = 0.79, P = 0.094) and an increase in unstable angina admissions (HR = 1.37, P = 0.061).
CHARM-Preserved[13] (n = 3,023)	Candesartan vs placebo for a mean of 36.6 months. Patients continued their background HF medications: ACE inhibitor (19%), β-blocker (55%), diuretics (75%), spironolactone (11%).	EF >40%, NYHA II–IV, ≥1 hospitalization for CV reason	Composite of CV mortality or HF hospitalization	No significant difference was found in the primary end point between treatment groups (adjusted HR = 0.86, P = 0.051) or in CV deaths (adjusted HR = 0.95, P = 0.635). Compared with placebo, candesartan use was associated with fewer HF admissions (P = 0.047), lower incidence of new diabetes (HR = 0.60, P = 0.005), and a reduction in the composite of CV death, hospitalization for HF, MI, and stroke (adjusted HR = 0.86, P = 0.037).
PEP-CHF[47] (n = 850)	Perindopril vs placebo for a mean of 2.1 years	Clinical criteria for HF, EF ≥40%, age ≥70 years	Composite of total mortality and HF hospitalization	At 1 year and at study completion, no significant difference was found in the primary end point between treatment groups (HR = 0.69, P = 0.055; HR = 0.70, P = 0.545). In a subgroup analysis, patients ≤75 years of age (HR = 0.29, P = 0.035) and with a history of MI (HR = 0.38, P = 0.004) showed a reduction in the primary end point. Compared with placebo, perindopril use at 1 year was associated with fewer unplanned hospital admissions (HR = 0.63, P = 0.033), greater improvements in exercise tolerance (P = 0.011), and improvement in NYHA class (P = 0.030).
I-Preserve[49] (n = 4,128)	Irbesartan vs placebo for 2 years. ACE inhibitor can be used for any indication other than HTN.	Clinical criteria for HF or hospitalized within 6 months for HF, age ≥60 years, NYHA II–IV, EF ≥45%	Composite of all-cause mortality or CV hospitalization	No significant difference was found in the primary end point between treatment groups (HR = 0.95, P = 0.35), overall death rates (HR = 1.00, P = 0.98), or CV hospitalization rate (HR = 0.95, P = 0.44).
J-DHF[73] (n = 800)	Carvedilol vs placebo for 2 years	Clinical criteria for HF, EF >40%	Composite of CV mortality and unplanned HF hospitalization	Expected to be completed in 2010
SENIORS[43] (n = 2,111)	Nebivolol vs placebo for 21 months	Clinical criteria for HF with either documented heart failure hospitalization with 1 year or documented EF ≤35% within 6 months, age ≥70 years	All-cause mortality or cardiovascular hospitalization	In the study, 1,359 patients (64%) had an EF ≤35% (mean 28.7%), and 752 (36%) had an EF >35% (mean 49.2%). In patients with EF >35%, the HR for nebivolol vs placebo for the primary end point was 0.81 (P = 0.104). No significant difference existed between groups (EF ≤35% vs EF >35%, P = 0.720).
TOPCAT[74] (n = 4,500)	Spironolactone vs placebo for 2 years	Clinical criteria for HF, age ≥50 years, EF ≥45%, ≥1 hospitalization for HF, controlled SBP	CV mortality, aborted cardiac arrest, HF hospitalization	Expected to be completed in 2011

ACE = angiotensin-converting enzyme; CHARM = Candesartan in Heart Failure: Assessment of Reduction in Mortality and Morbidity; CV = cardiovascular; DIG, Digitalis Investigational Group; EF = ejection fraction; HF, heart failure; HR, hazard ratio; HTN, hypertension; I-Preserve = Irbesartan in Heart Failure with Preserved EF; J-DHF: Japanese Diastolic Heart Failure Study; MI, myocardial infarction; NYHA, New York Heart Association; PEP-CHF = Perindopril for Elderly Persons with Chronic Heart Failure; SBP, systolic blood pressure; SENIORS, Study of Effects of Nebivolol Intervention on Outcomes and Rehospitalization in Seniors with Heart Failure; TOPCAT = Trial of Aldosterone Antagonist Therapy in Adults with Preserved Ejection Fraction Congestive Heart Failure

between myocardial oxygen supply and demand (see Fig. 21–1). Diuretics alone and especially in combination with other antihypertensive drugs are an effective approach to therapy.

In a small subpopulation of ALLHAT, admissions for 1,367 patients hospitalized for heart failure were adjudicated in a centrally blinded manner.[39] In this study, signs and symptoms of HF were similar between patients with reduced and preserved EF. Treatment with chlorthalidone significantly reduced the risk for hospitalization in patients with preserved EF when compared with amlodipine, lisinopril, or doxazosin (hazard ratio 0.69, 0.74, and

0.53, respectively). After the onset of HF symptoms, patients with a preserved EF had a better prognosis when compared with patients with a reduced EF; however, the long-term outcome is still poor.

Treatment with diuretics should be initiated at low doses in order to avoid hypotension and fatigue. Hypotension can be a significant problem in the treatment of DHF because these patients have a very steep LV diastolic pressure—volume curve such that a small change in volume causes a large change in filling pressure and cardiac output. After the acute treatment of DHF has been completed, long-term treatment should include small to moderate oral doses of diuretics (furosemide 20 to 40 mg/day, chlorthalidone 25 to 100 mg or hydrochlorothiazide 12.5 to 25 mg/day). If prompt and sustained diuresis is not achieved, the dosage of a single diuretic should be increased, or a loop and thiazide or thiazide-like diuretic should be used in combination. Aldosterone antagonists such as spironolactone and eplerenone may be especially effective for long-term use because of their potassium-sparing effects and because their antagonism of RAAS activation may alter intramyocardial and extramyocardial mechanisms, causing abnormalities in diastolic function.[40] Because aldosterone is profibrotic and stimulates hypertrophy, aldosterone blockade may be of benefit in patients with DHF and is under investigation in TOPCAT (Trial of Aldosterone Antagonist Therapy in Adults with Preserved Ejection Fraction Congestive Heart Failure).[41]

Torsemide may also offer a benefit beyond diuresis. In a small, open-label trial in patients with diastolic and systolic heart failure, torsemide in comparison to furosemide was shown to decrease two different indices of fibrillar collagen turnover and myocardial fibrosis.[42] These findings are interesting, but clinical importance remains to be established.

Excessive diuresis may result in hypotension, low-output syndrome, and worsening renal insufficiency. Electrolyte imbalances, including hypokalemia and hypomagnesemia, are common with diuretics. Carbohydrate intolerance and hyperuricemia are dose-related adverse drug reactions seen with thiazide diuretics. Thiazide diuretics generally are ineffective in patients with a creatinine clearance <30 mL/min. Spironolactone can cause hyperkalemia and gynecomastia. Eplerenone may be used as an alternative to spironolactone in patients who complain of gynecomastia. In general, diuretic agents are very cost-effective in the management of DHF.

Nitrates

❼ Similar to diuretics, nitrates can provide symptom-targeted therapy by acting to decrease LV volume by increasing venous capacitance. In addition, nitrates can provide disease-targeted therapy by providing antiischemic effects in patients with DHF due to CAD.

Like diuretics, therapy should be initiated at low doses to avoid hypotension. Isosorbide dinitrate 10 mg three or four times daily, isosorbide mononitrate (Imdur) 30 mg daily, nitroglycerin paste 0.5 to 1 inch every 4 to 6 hours, and nitroglycerin patch 0.1 to 0.2 mg/h applied each day are common initial doses. Doses can be increased during long-term therapy and titrated against symptoms. Nitrate tolerance has not been studied in this patient population but probably occurs. Like diuretics, nitrates can cause hypotension and a low-output syndrome. Headaches are common but may be less frequent with continued use.

Sublingual nitroglycerin tablets or nitroglycerin spray may be used for patients who develop shortness of breath with mild exercise, and they can be used much in the same way as in patients with ischemic symptoms. Nitroglycerin will decrease LV end-diastolic volume, resulting in relief of breathlessness.

Beta-Adrenergic Blockers

Beta-blockers can provide symptom-targeted therapy by decreasing heart rate and can provide disease-targeted therapy by treating high blood pressure and CAD. By decreasing heart rate and increasing the duration of diastole, β-blockers can help to lower and maintain low pulmonary venous pressures. Tachycardia is poorly tolerated in patients with DHF for several reasons. First, rapid heart rates cause an increase in myocardial oxygen demand and a decrease in coronary perfusion time. This rapid rate can promote ischemic diastolic dysfunction even in the absence of epicardial CAD, especially in patients with LVH. Second, incomplete relaxation between cardiac cycles may result in an increase in diastolic pressure relative to volume. Thus, LV distensibility is reduced. Third, a rapid rate reduces diastolic filling time and ventricular filling. Fourth, hearts with diastolic dysfunction exhibit a flat or even negative relaxation rate versus frequency relationship. Thus, as heart rate increases in these hearts, relaxation does not become augmented and may become slower and incomplete, causing diastolic pressures, especially early in diastole, to increase.[9] For these and other reasons, most clinicians use β-blockers (and calcium channel blockers) to prevent excessive tachycardia and produce a relative bradycardia in patients with diastolic dysfunction. However, excessive bradycardia can result in a fall of cardiac output despite an increase in LV filling. Such considerations underscore the need for individualizing therapeutic interventions that affect heart rate. Although the optimal heart rate must be individualized, an initial goal might be a resting heart rate of approximately 60 beats/min, with a blunted exercise-induced increase in heart rate not to exceed 110 beats/min.[9]

No evidence suggests a specific therapeutic advantage of one β-blocker over another. Selective and nonselective β-blockers appear equally effective in DHF. Interestingly, a subanalysis of the SENIORS (Study of Effects of Nebivolol Intervention on Outcomes and Rehospitalization in Seniors with Heart Failure) trial showed a similar response to nebivolol in patients with preserved and reduced EF.[43]

In a small prospective cohort analysis, patients with DHF prescribed β-blockers had improved survival compared with those not receiving β-blocker therapy at hospital discharge.[44] Furthermore, in a community-based registry, carvedilol use had similar 1-year mortality rates in patients with preserved and reduced EF but less reduction in hospitalizations for patients with a reduced EF.[45]

In general, it is not necessary to start the drug at an extremely low dose and titrate the β-blocker in a slow, progressive fashion in DHF as it is in SHF. However, because patients tend to be older, have numerous comorbidities, and take concomitant medications, it is prudent to start with a moderate dose of β-blockers. Doses such as metoprolol tartrate 25 mg twice daily, metoprolol succinate 25 mg daily, atenolol 25 mg daily, carvedilol 3.125 mg twice daily, and nebivolol 1.25 mg daily titrated to a higher dose with a treatment target of a heart rate of approximately 60 beats/min can be considered.

Prinzmetal vasospastic angina, occlusive peripheral vascular disease, diabetes mellitus type 1 that is prone to hypoglycemia, severe heart block, and excessive bradycardia are contraindications to β-blockers. Beta-blockers may be considered in patients with reactive airway disease or asymptomatic bradycardia but should be used with extreme caution. The main side effects of β-blockers are depression, fatigue, bradycardia, bronchospasm, and impotence. Many of the β-blockers are eliminated via hepatic metabolism and may be affected by other drugs that either inhibit (e.g., cimetidine and verapamil) or enhance (e.g., barbiturates) hepatic enzymes. Because the doses are titrated to patient response, these interactions are managed easily.

Calcium Channel Blockers

Calcium channel blockers can provide symptom-targeted treatment by decreasing heart rate and increasing exercise tolerance. They can provide disease-targeted treatment by treating high blood pressure and CAD. However, the beneficial effect of these agents on exercise tolerance is not always paralleled by improved LV diastolic function or increased relaxation rate. Nonetheless, a number of small clinical trials have shown that the use of these agents results in both short- and long-term improvement in exercise capacity in patients with DHF.[30,35]

Of the calcium channel blockers, the nondihydropyridines (verapamil and diltiazem) are the most effective because they lower heart rate in addition to lowering blood pressure.[22] Sustained-release nifedipine, because of its strong vasodilator properties, tends to cause hypotension and reflex tachycardia. In addition, nifedipine causes peripheral edema. These characteristics make it less useful in DHF. Amlodipine may be effective because it reduces blood pressure. Initial doses are verapamil 120 to 240 mg/day, diltiazem 90 to 120 mg/day, and amlodipine 2.5 mg/day.

Heart block is a contraindication for the nondihydropyridines. The most common side effects are bradycardia and heart block (for the nondihydropyridines). Peripheral edema and headache also are common. Nondihydropyridines exacerbate the bradycardic effects of β-blockers, and verapamil raises digoxin serum concentrations by 70%. Diltiazem raises cyclosporine, tacrolimus, and sirolimus serum concentrations. IV calcium salts inhibit the pharmacologic effect of calcium channel blockers. Generic formulations or similar products, but not necessarily generic equivalents to the original brand names, are available for some of the calcium channel blockers.

Neurohormonal Antagonists

Both basic and clinical studies suggest that DHF is associated with activation of systemic and local cardiac neuroendocrine systems such as the RAAS. One mechanism causing fluid retention and the increases in central and systemic volume in patients with DHF is activation of these neuroendocrine systems. Therefore, treatment of DHF could include agents such as angiotensin-converting enzyme (ACE) inhibitors, angiotensin receptor blockers, and aldosterone antagonists that attenuate the fluid retention caused by neuroendocrine activation. In addition to promoting fluid retention, neuroendocrine activation can have direct effects on cellular and extracellular mechanisms that contribute to the development of DHF. Modulation of neuroendocrine activation may provide mechanism-targeted treatment by decreasing fibroblast activity and interstitial fibrosis, improving intracellular calcium handling, and decreasing myocardial stiffness. Finally, the RAAS antagonists provide disease-targeted treatment by treating hypertension.[18,46]

The mechanisms that evoke activation of the neuroendocrine system remain incompletely understood in patients with DHF. A number of factors have been suggested. Myocardial ischemia, uncontrolled hypertension, and excessive dietary sodium or sodium-retaining medications may contribute to neuroendocrine activation. Limited distensibility of the atria may attenuate the secretion of atrial natriuretic factor and thereby reduce its diuretic effect. In others, low systemic vascular resistance and/or low arterial pressure may contribute to an increase in RAAS activation and salt and water retention. Elevated venous pressure may cause renal sodium retention directly. The reduction in blood volume that follows the use of diuretics triggers an increase in sympathetic tone and further activation of the RAAS. Such neurohormonal activation can lead to vasoconstriction and a worsening of the congestive state. Some vasodilators, particularly nitrates and pure arteriolar vasodilators, evoke a similar response. By contrast, ACE inhibitors, aldosterone antagonists, and β-blockers blunt neurohormonal activation and decrease the salt and water retention that complicates the treatment of HF.

Angiotensin-Converting Enzyme Inhibitors

ACE inhibitors can provide symptom-targeted treatment by decreasing LV volume and directly improving relaxation. They can provide disease-targeted treatment by treating high blood pressure, preventing LVH, promoting regression, and preventing fibrosis. Treatment of high blood pressure with ACE inhibitors has been shown to normalize load, prevent and/or regress LVH, correct the

abnormality in intracellular processes, and modify the extracellular matrix response.[46]

The largest study with an ACE inhibitor, the Perindopril for Elderly Persons with Chronic Heart Failure (PEP-CHF) trial, failed to find a significant effect on clinical outcomes at 1 year in patients with DHF who received perindopril (see Table 21–4). Based on these limited data, it appears that ACE inhibitors may improve HF symptomatology and exercise capacity while not impacting mortality.[47]

At this time, no evidence suggests an advantage of one ACE inhibitor over another. Their effects appear to be a class effect. Initial doses should be small to moderate to avoid hypotension, especially if the patient examination does not indicate volume overload. Examples of initial starting doses are captopril 6.25 mg three times daily, enalapril 2.5 mg/day, and lisinopril 2.5 mg/day.

A history of angioedema and pregnancy are contraindications to ACE inhibitors. Hyperkalemia, persistent cough, hypotension, taste disturbances, and worsening renal function are common side effects but are managed by decreasing the dose or discontinuing the drug.

Angiotensin Receptor Blockers

Angiotensin receptor blockers can provide symptom-targeted treatment by decreasing LV pressure, decreasing LV volume, and increasing exercise tolerance. They can provide disease-targeted treatment by lowering blood pressure. The Candesartan in Heart Failure: Assessment of Reduction in Mortality and Morbidity (CHARM)-Preserved trial (see Table 21–4) was the first large prospective study to demonstrate some benefit of an angiotensin receptor blocker in patients with preserved EF currently receiving the usual treatment.[13] However, in a cost analysis study of the CHARM program using European data, there was a net increase in the daily cost of care in the CHARM-Preserved trial.[48] In addition, 22% of candesartan-treated patients discontinued therapy because of hypotension ($P = 0.009$), increased serum creatinine ($P = 0.0005$), and hyperkalemia ($P = 0.029$).

In the I-PRESERVE (Irbesartan in Heart Failure with Preserved EF) trial, irbesartan was compared with placebo in over 4,000 patients with symptoms of heart failure and an EF of at least 45%.[49] There was no significant difference between irbesartan and placebo with regard to death or hospitalization for cardiovascular causes. No benefit was seen in quality-of-life measures. There was a high discontinuation rate of the study drug in this trial (33%), as well as a high rate of postrandomization initiation of ACE inhibitors (20%) and spironolactone (10%), that may have contributed to the outcome in this trial.

Angiotensin receptor blockers may be used as antihypertensive agents in patients with DHF. Initial doses of candesartan start at 4 mg/day, irbesartan 150 mg/day, losartan 25 mg/day, telmisartan 40 mg/day, and valsartan 80 mg/day. As with the ACE inhibitors, angiotensin receptor blockers are contraindicated in pregnancy. The side effects of angiotensin receptor blockers are similar to those of ACE inhibitors, but they are not associated with persistent cough.

Aldosterone Antagonists

Aldosterone antagonists can provide improved myocardial functioning by decreasing LV volume and chamber stiffness.[50,51] They can provide disease-targeted treatment by decreasing the fibrosis that accompanies LVH. An analysis of the Randomized Aldactone Evaluation Study (RALES) found that spironolactone significantly decreased the levels of serum markers for cardiac collagen turnover. The benefit from spironolactone was seen in patients with higher levels of collagen synthesis markers. This was the first study to show that serum levels of markers of cardiac collagen synthesis were associated with a poor clinical outcome and could be decreased with spironolactone. This property distinguishes spironolactone from other diuretics that have no effect on myocardial necrosis or collagen turnover.

Like other diuretics, spironolactone should be initiated at a low dose and increased to treat symptoms. Spironolactone may be initiated at doses of 12.5 to 25 mg/day. It should be avoided in patients with severe renal failure. Hyperkalemia and gynecomastia are the most common side effects. Eplerenone is a viable alternative to spironolactone in patients complaining of sex hormone—related side effects and may be initiated at 25 mg/day.[40]

Positive Inotropic Agents

Positive inotropic agents, such as β-agonists and phosphodiesterase inhibitors, are generally not used in the treatment of patients with isolated DHF because LVEF is preserved, and there appears to be little potential for a beneficial effect. Such agents have the potential to worsen DHF by adversely affecting energetics, inducing ischemia, raising heart rate, and inducing arrhythmias.[9] In contrast to long-term use, positive inotropic drugs may be beneficial in the short-term treatment of pulmonary edema associated with DHF. These agents can enhance sarcoplasmic reticular function, promote more rapid and complete relaxation, increase splanchnic blood flow, increase venous capacitance, and facilitate diuresis.[9] However, they should be used with caution, if they are used at all, because the risk-to-benefit ratio is not clearly established.

Istaroxime is an investigational agent with inotropic and lusitropic properties. It was evaluated in acutely hospitalized patients with systolic heart failure (mean EF 27%).[52] In addition to lowering pulmonary capillary wedge pressure, istaroxime was found to decrease diastolic stiffness. Whether this property would be useful in patients with a preserved EF presenting with acute decompensation is unknown at this time.

Digitalis Derivatives

Digoxin, by inhibiting the Na^+,K^+-adenosine triphosphatase (ATPase) pump, augments intracellular calcium and thereby augments contractile state. In this manner, digoxin produces an increase in systolic energy demands while adding to a relative calcium overload in diastole. These effects may not be apparent clinically under many circumstances, but during hemodynamic stress or ischemia, digoxin may promote or contribute to diastolic dysfunction.[9] However, based on the data from the Digitalis Investigational Group (DIG) Ancillary Study (see Table 21–4), it appears that digoxin has, at most, a very limited role in the management of patients with DHF in normal sinus rhythm.[53]

PHARMACOECONOMIC CONSIDERATIONS

Frequent admission to the hospital is common in patients with DHF. Five-year cost estimates associated with HF are similar in patients with a preserved EF and those with a reduced EF.[54] Because DHF is primarily a disease of the elderly, comorbid conditions will create challenges in any trial design. When developing a pharmacotherapeutic plan, cost to the patient should be carefully considered because adherence to an antihypertensive regimen is paramount to a beneficial outcome.

CLINICAL CONTROVERSIES

- Digoxin may increase hospitalizations for unstable angina in patients with DHF and normal sinus rhythm.
- Antihypertensive drugs that antagonize the RAAS may be preferred for patients with DHF.

EVALUATION OF THERAPEUTIC OUTCOMES

The end points used in assessing effective therapies for DHF include mortality, hospitalization for worsening HF, functional status or quality-of-life indicators, and cost. Other end points may target underlying mechanisms of disease, such as calcium homeostasis and regression of fibrosis. A paucity of data exits regarding the most effective regimen for DHF.

CARDIOMYOPATHIES

Diastolic dysfunction plays a role in the presentation of some types of cardiomyopathy. Over the past decade, the terminology and classification used for the cardiomyopathies have been confusing because of overlap among the diseases and/or classification schemes. In 2006, the ACC/AHA suggested a broader definition for the cardiomyopathies. The expert panel defined the cardiomyopathies as

> a heterogeneous group of diseases of the myocardium associated with mechanical and/or electrical dysfunction that usually (but not invariably) exhibit inappropriate ventricular hypertrophy or dilation and are due to a variety of causes that frequently are genetic. Cardiomyopathies either are confined to the heart (primary cardiomyopathy) or are part of generalized systemic disorders (secondary cardiomyopathy), often leading to cardiovascular death or progressive HF-related disability.[55]

The primary cardiomyopathies are further divided into genetic, mixed (genetic and nongenetic), and acquired. Endocrine conditions, inflammation, metabolic disorders, infiltrative diseases, and toxins are a few of the causative factors of secondary cardiomyopathy.[55] It is important to note that this new contemporary classification does not include pathologic myocardial processes that are a direct result of other cardiovascular conditions, such as valvular heart disease, hypertension, and CAD. Therefore, ischemic cardiomyopathy is not considered a "true" cardiomyopathy.

Frequently, a specific etiology is not evident. Therefore, another commonly used categorization of the cardiomyopathies is based on the structural and/or functional abnormalities present. The three groups of primary cardiomyopathies usually are described as dilated, hypertrophic, or restrictive. An understanding of the pathophysiologic basis for each type of cardiomyopathy leads to a rational selection of drug therapy or other treatment modality. The characteristics for each of the types of cardiomyopathy are listed in Table 21–5. The distinction among the cardiomyopathies is not absolute, and there is some overlap in their functional abnormalities.

In dilated cardiomyopathy, the cardinal feature is ventricular chamber enlargement. Systolic function is abnormal with normal LV wall thickness, leading to a decreased cardiac output. In patients with hypertrophic cardiomyopathy (HCM), the ventricular cavity is not dilated, but the ventricular muscle mass is increased, existing in the absence of known causes of LVH. Ventricular cavity size is normal or decreased, and systolic function often is preserved. Patients with HCM may have an obstructive or nonobstructive form. Patients with restrictive cardiomyopathy have inadequate ventricular compliance, causing diastolic dysfunction as a result of endocardial and/or myocardial disease. The clinical presentation is similar to that of constrictive pericarditis.

HYPERTROPHIC CARDIOMYOPATHY

HCM is a primary, genetic cardiomyopathy that is inherited as an autosomal dominant trait caused by mutations in any of 12 genes. The distribution of the hypertrophy usually is asymmetric, meaning that segments of the LV are thickened to varying degrees. There also may be enlargement of the atria, thickening of the mitral valve leaflets, and fibrotic areas within the ventricular wall. In the past, the terms *idiopathic hypertrophic subaortic stenosis* and *hypertrophic*

TABLE 21-5 Characteristics of the Cardiomyopathies

	Dilated	Hypertrophic	Restrictive
Myocardial mass	$\uparrow \rightarrow \uparrow\uparrow$	$\uparrow\uparrow\uparrow$	$nl \rightarrow \uparrow$
Ventricular cavity size	$\uparrow\uparrow\uparrow\uparrow\uparrow$	$\downarrow\downarrow \rightarrow nl$	$nl \rightarrow \downarrow$
Contractile function	$\downarrow\downarrow\downarrow$	$\uparrow\uparrow \rightarrow$	$nl \rightarrow \downarrow$
LV filling pressure	$\uparrow\uparrow$	$nl \rightarrow \uparrow$	$\uparrow$
Chest x-ray film	Moderate to marked cardiac enlargement	Mild to moderate cardiac enlargement	Mild cardiac enlargement
Electrocardiogram	ST-segment and T-wave abnormalities	ST-segment and T-wave abnormalities, LV hypertrophy	Low voltage, conduction defects
Echocardiogram	LV dilation and dysfunction	Asymmetric septal hypertrophy, systolic anterior motion of the mitral valve	Increased LV wall thickness possible
Radionuclide studies	LV dilation and dysfunction	Vigorous systolic function	Normal systolic function

$\uparrow$ = increased, $\downarrow$ = decreased, LV = left ventricular, nl = normal

obstructive cardiomyopathy were used to describe patients with HCM and outflow obstruction.

Epidemiology

Recent epidemiologic investigations estimate the prevalence of phenotypically expressed HCM in the general adult population to be approximately 0.2% (1:500), making it the most frequently occurring cardiomyopathy. HCM is the most common genetic cardiovascular disease and the most common cause of sudden death in young athletes.[56] More than 430 mutations in 12 genes have been identified to date; however, many individuals with a mutant gene go undetected.[57]

Etiology

The genetic predisposition to HCM is thought to be an autosomal dominant trait with variable penetrance. Because of the wide variability of presentation, not all cases in a family may be detected. HCM usually is caused by mutations in the genes for β-myosin heavy chain, myosin-binding protein C, and cardiac troponin T.[58]

Pathophysiology

HCM appears to have several different pathophysiologic mechanisms leading to similar clinical manifestations, although the prognoses for patients will vary. The pathophysiology of HCM is a complex relationship among several factors, including (a) asymmetric LVH, (b) diastolic dysfunction, (c) dynamic obstruction of the outflow tract, and (d) myocardial ischemia. Each of these components contributes to the overall presentation of the patient to a varying degree.[56,58]

Left Ventricular Hypertrophy The hypertrophy seen in HCM usually is diffuse and involves the septum and LV anterolateral free wall to a greater degree than the posterior segment. Asymmetric septal hypertrophy is a sensitive marker for HCM but is not specific for this disorder. In patients with outflow obstruction, the basal septum usually is markedly thickened at the level of the mitral valve. In patients with nonobstructive HCM, the outflow tract is larger, and the septal hypertrophy that occurs has a more distal or apical distribution.[59]

Cellular disorganization is a common histologic finding in HCM. Morphologic abnormalities are found at the gross, microscopic, and ultrastructural levels. The disarray of myocytes may contribute to diastolic and systolic dysfunction, as well as serving as a nidus for ventricular arrhythmias. The degree of LVH is associated with a worse clinical course. The presence of hypertrophy correlates directly with myocardial infarction, HF, stroke, and ventricular arrhythmias. Spirito and Autore found that the magnitude of LVH was directly related to the risk of sudden cardiac death.[56]

Diastolic Dysfunction Diastolic dysfunction is the most common abnormality found in patients with HCM. Approximately 80% of patients exhibit symptoms associated with diastolic dysfunction.

Studies of the LV led to the realization that diastolic dysfunction is the result of abnormalities in relaxation, distensibility (compliance), and filling. The abnormalities of diastolic function can be both regional and global and lead to an incoordination of contraction and relaxation. Beta-adrenergic stimulation can aggravate these abnormalities, whereas β-receptor blockade may diminish them.[58]

Abnormalities in filling are also associated with changes in chamber stiffness that occur in HCM. This stiffness may be the result of myocardial fibrosis, cellular disorganization, or increased myocardial mass. The decreased distensibility leads to an abnormally steep slope of the diastolic pressure—volume curve, such that an increase in LV volume results in a disproportionate increase in diastolic pressure.

Myocardial relaxation is an energy-dependent process that is sensitive to episodes of ischemia. Diastolic resequestration of calcium ions by the sarcoplasmic reticulum is an energy-dependent process. In the event of ischemia, the sequestration of calcium is inhibited, allowing the calcium to continue its interaction with the myofibrillar contractile proteins. Calcium channel blockers have been used with some success in patients with diastolic dysfunction.[57]

Systolic Function and Outflow Tract Obstruction Abnormalities of systolic function also occur in patients with HCM. The hypertrophied LV may cause a powerful but sometimes uncoordinated contraction presumably as a result of the abnormal architecture of the myocardium. The increase in LV wall thickness results in decreased wall stress during systole. Therefore, the LV contracts against a decreased afterload so that the LV is described as being hyperdynamic. EF often is increased.

Over the past 5 decades, controversy has surrounded the issue of the importance of outflow tract obstruction in conjunction with HCM. The presence of a gradient (the systolic pressure difference between the body and the outflow tract of the LV) is indicative of a dynamic obstruction of the LV outflow tract. Outflow tract gradients occur in approximately 30% to 50% of patients with HCM.[57] The obstruction that occurs usually shows spontaneous variability and may be reduced by interventions that decrease myocardial contractility. The gradient can be augmented by factors that increase contractility (Table 21–6). LV outflow tract obstruction at rest has been found to be a predictor of progression to severe HF symptoms, stroke, and death. It is important to identify and treat these gradients aggressively with medications, surgery, or alcohol septal ablation procedures.[60]

Myocardial Ischemia Chest pain in the absence of CAD is a common symptom of patients with HCM. However, it is appropriate to consider typical CAD in patients with HCM if they have the usual risk factors for atherosclerosis.[61,62] Several mechanisms are proposed for the myocardial ischemia seen in this patient population. There may be inadequate capillary density in relation to the increased LV muscle mass. The small intramural coronary arteries may be abnormally narrowed or excessively compressed during

TABLE 21-6 Factors Known to Affect Outflow Gradients in Hypertrophic Cardiomyopathy

Factors that diminish gradients
Decreasing myocardial contractility
   β-blocking drugs
   Verapamil
Increasing ventricular volume
Increasing arterial pressure

Factors that enhance gradients
Increasing myocardial contractility
   Exercise
   Inotropic agents
Decreasing ventricular volume
Decreasing arterial pressure

systole. Impaired relaxation during diastole may inhibit blood flow to the subendocardium. Once myocardial ischemia develops, further increases in LV filling pressure may occur, which, in turn, lead to more ischemia. Repeated episodes of ischemia may be responsible for progressive myocyte loss and fibrosis. The subendocardium is at greatest risk for ischemic damage because of the lower capillary density and higher oxygen demand secondary to wall tension.

CLINICAL PRESENTATION OF HYPERTROPHIC CARDIOMYOPATHY

General

- The clinical presentation varies widely, ranging from no symptoms to severe symptoms of angina, HF, and sudden death. The severity of symptoms corresponds to the degree of LVH, but this relationship is not absolute.

Symptoms

- The patient may complain of dyspnea, chest pain, fatigue, palpitations, presyncope, and syncope.

Signs

- Systolic murmur

Other Diagnostic Tests

- Echocardiography will show increased myocardial mass.
- Electrocardiography will reveal LVH with or without ST-segment and T-wave abnormalities.

Diagnosis

Making the diagnosis of HCM may be difficult because the disorder may be confused with CAD, aortic stenosis, or mitral regurgitation. Patients with HCM can be young and physically active. The physical signs of the cardiac examination depend on the presence of a systolic pressure gradient within the LV. If a gradient is present, a late-onset systolic murmur is often heard. The murmur is intensified by standing and the Valsalva maneuver and lessened with squatting or hand grip. Very rarely, some patients develop an end-stage LV dilation and a declining LVEF, which often are confused with idiopathic dilated cardiomyopathy. HCM should be considered in the differential diagnosis in patients with HF and unexplained LVH, significant heart murmurs, unexplained syncope, abnormal electrocardiogram patterns (pseudoinfarction or giant negative T waves), or a positive family history.[57]

Echocardiography is used to confirm the diagnosis. The diagnosis of HCM is made with two-dimensional echocardiography, with the usual criterion of LV wall thickness ≥15 mm. Magnetic resonance imaging of the entire LV may add valuable information, especially if the echocardiogram is of suboptimal quality.[55,61]

The development of or increase in a murmur suggests progression of disease, but disappearance of a murmur does not imply improvement. In fact, disappearance of a murmur may herald further impairment of systolic function. Some patients will progress to congestive heart failure (CHF) as a result of atrial fibrillation, mitral regurgitation, or myocardial infarction. If SHF develops, the patient has a poor prognosis.

Contemporary methods of diagnosis consist of genotype assessment. Genetic testing allows for a definitive diagnosis and precise identification of mutations in myocardial sarcomere proteins. Unfortunately, screening for more than 200 mutations in multiple genes is complex, time consuming, and costly. Although becoming more common, therapeutic decisions based on genetic testing are not recommended. Genetic testing is useful in identifying at-risk relatives for potential follow-up and treatment.[63]

Prognosis

The clinical course for a patient with HCM should be viewed in terms of the specific subtypes of the disease spectrum. Patients fall into one of several relatively discrete pathways: (a) high risk for sudden death; (b) symptoms of DHF, including syncope; (c) progression toward advanced end-stage HF; and (d) atrial fibrillation and its sequelae. Of major concern is the incidence of sudden cardiac death among patients with HCM. Approximately 10% to 20% of patients with HCM are at increased risk for sudden death. The mechanism responsible for sudden cardiac death is thought to be related to an electrically unstable myocardium leading to complex ventricular arrhythmias. Less often, sudden death may be the result of hemodynamic changes. The onset of atrial fibrillation in the face of severe LV diastolic dysfunction may result in a significant decrease in stroke volume. This decrease in cardiac output could lead to acute LV failure, MI, or sudden death. Sudden death can be a complication, especially in young athletes with HCM. It is recommended that young patients with HCM refrain from competitive athletics.[55,61]

Quantification of the risk of sudden death remains elusive for patients with HCM. The clinical markers associated with an increased risk for sudden death (Table 21–7) have a high negative predictive value. The absence of all these markers can be used to develop a profile for a patient at low risk for sudden death. The magnitude of hypertrophy appears to be a strong predictor, with the cumulative risk nearly zero for patients with a wall thickness ≤19 mm. Young patients with severe hypertrophy (wall thickness

TABLE 21-7 Risk Factors Associated with Sudden Cardiac Death in Hypertrophic Cardiomyopathy

Major risk factors
Prior cardiac arrest
Spontaneous sustained ventricular tachycardia
Positive family history of premature death
Multiple syncopal or near-syncopal episodes, especially if associated with exertion
Multiple and repetitive or prolonged episodes of nonsustained ventricular tachycardia
Marked left ventricular hypertrophy ≥30 mm
Hypotensive blood pressure response to exercise

Potential individual risk factors
Atrial fibrillation
Myocardial ischemia
Left ventricular outflow obstruction
Identification of a malignant genotype
Intense (competitive) physical exertion

Reprinted with permission Circulation. 2006;114:e385–e484, © 2006 American Heart Association, Inc.

>30 mm) are at high risk for sudden death even if they are asymptomatic. A high LV outflow tract pressure gradient ≥30 mm Hg is a strong predictor for older patients.[64] Presentation of HCM in the later decades of life is common. Patients who present with HCM at an advanced age of 65 years or older usually have a prognosis that is no different from that of age- and gender-matched controls. Elderly patients with HCM tend to have mild degrees of LVH, and their symptoms are not severe.[65] Because systolic hypertension and diastolic HF are common in the elderly, the diagnosis of HCM may be challenging. However, marked LVH out of proportion to blood pressure, unusual patterns of LVH, or an outflow obstruction at rest strongly suggests HCM.[55]

TREATMENT

Hypertrophic Cardiomyopathy

■ DESIRED OUTCOMES

Because no known means are available for preventing HCM, the focus must be on methods to minimize the consequences of the disorder.

■ GENERAL APPROACH TO TREATMENT

❽ The treatment of HCM is designed to reduce symptoms, improve exercise tolerance, retard disease progression, and improve prognosis. Agents that decrease contractility, improve diastolic

dysfunction, reduce ischemia, and suppress arrhythmias have been used with some success (Fig. 21–2). In 2003, the ACC in conjunction with the ESC published a consensus document on HCM.[66]

■ NONPHARMACOLOGIC THERAPY

In the past, surgical treatment was reserved for patients who were refractory to medical management and had an outflow gradient ≥50 mm Hg, a very thick ventricular septum, and high LV pressures. Surgical intervention relieves the outflow obstruction and the elevated LV pressures. The surgeon accomplishes this by performing a myectomy (i.e., removal of excess tissue). The procedure results in a reduction in LV filling pressures and a long-term improvement in symptoms. Myectomy has demonstrated a long-term survival benefit in severely symptomatic patients with obstruction by altering the course of the disease.[60]

Ablation of the myocardium using alcohol is an alternative to surgery. Septal ablation with alcohol results in the same type of outcomes as seen with myectomy. Long-term follow-up is limited because this procedure has been used for less than a decade. Because it is a percutaneous procedure (similar to cardiac catheterizations), it is being performed more frequently than myectomy. There is some concern that the risk for arrhythmia-related cardiac events may increase following alcohol ablation. Long-term follow-up is needed to assess this risk. Complete heart block is a common complication of septal ablation (14% in one case series) and requires a permanent pacemaker if it occurs.[58,60]

The results of uncontrolled studies suggested that dual-chamber pacing decreased LV outflow gradients and improved symptoms.

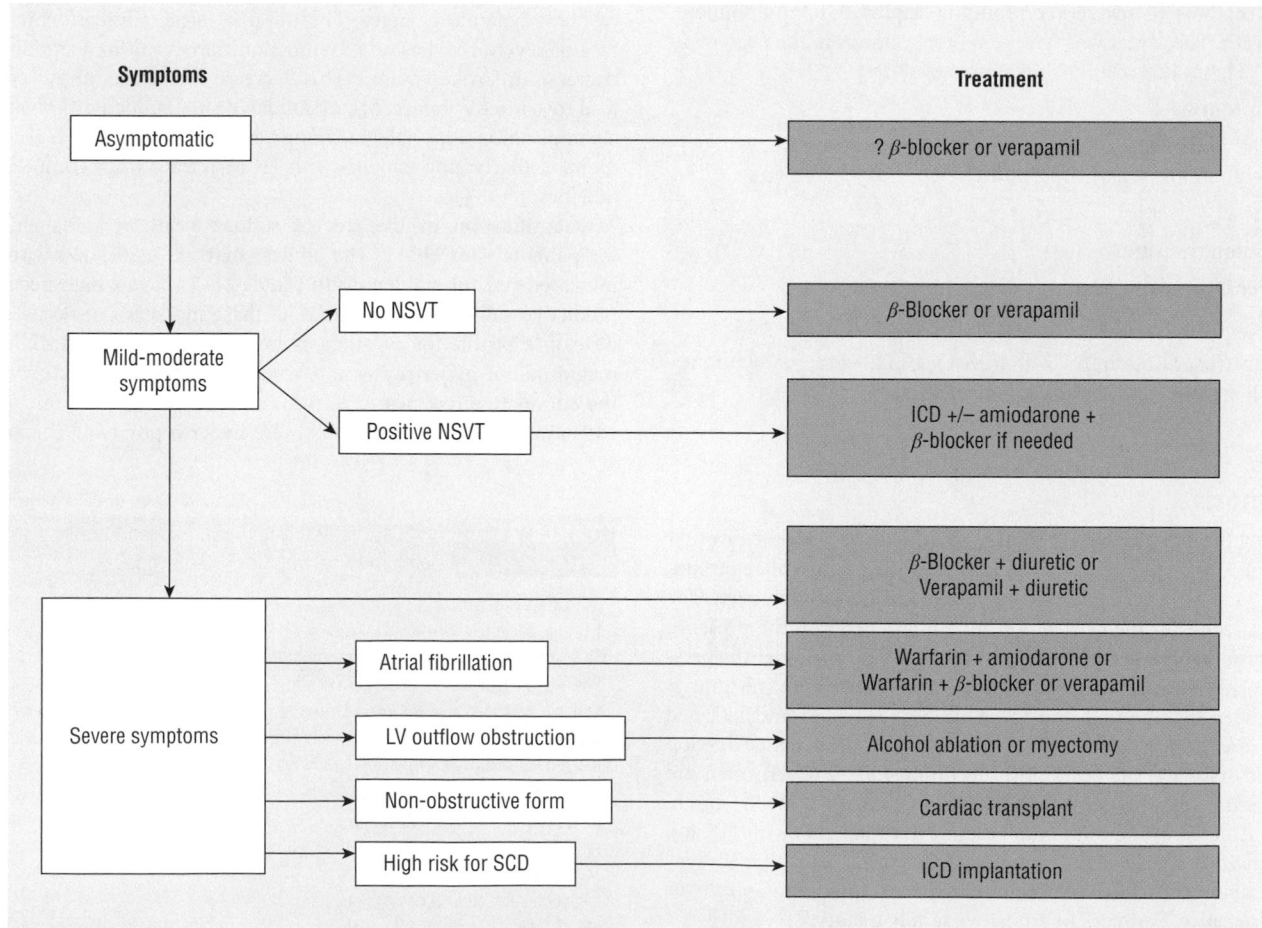

FIGURE 21-2. Treatment algorithm for hypertrophic cardiomyopathy (ICD = implantable cardioverter-defibrillator; LV = left ventricular; NSVT = nonsustained ventricular tachycardia; SCD = sudden cardiac death; ? = questionable role).

Subsequent controlled trials were not able to replicate the initial findings and demonstrated more modest improvement. Consequently, the ACC/AHA/HRS issued guidelines suggesting pacing for severely symptomatic patients who have not responded to medical management (class IIb recommendation, or one in which the efficacy is less well established by evidence).[67] The Canadian Cardiovascular Society recommends following the guidelines for LV systolic dysfunction regarding dual chamber pacing.[57]

■ IMPLANTABLE CARDIOVERTER-DEFIBRILLATOR

❾ Sudden death is the most worrisome outcome of HCM, and the implantable cardioverter-defibrillator (ICD) is the most effective therapy for prevention of sudden death. It is difficult to know when to implant an ICD, especially in a young patient diagnosed with HCM. Patients who are candidates for an ICD for primary prevention will be young and relatively asymptomatic. In 2006, the ACC/AHA with the ESC published updated guidelines designating the ICD for prevention of sudden death (class IIa recommendation or one in which the weight of the evidence or opinion favors efficacy). These guidelines stipulate that patients should exhibit one or more major risk factors for sudden death (see Table 21-7), are currently be receiving chronic medical therapy, and have a reasonable survival with good functional status at 1 year. For secondary prevention following cardiac arrest, ICD placement is considered a class I recommendation, where there is evidence or general agreement that the procedure is beneficial.[68] Conducting a clinical trial to provide evidence for a higher-level recommendation for primary prevention is unlikely to occur.

■ PHARMACOLOGIC THERAPY

Beta-Adrenergic Blockers

❿ Beta-blocking agents have been used in obstructive and nonobstructive forms of HCM since the 1960s and are recommended as first-line drug therapy to control symptoms.[57] Doses up to 480 mg/day of propranolol or its equivalent are used. Resting heart rate should be 60 beats/min, and the maximum exercise heart rate should be <120 beats/min. The mechanism by which β-blockade is beneficial is by inhibiting sympathetic stimulation of the heart. Myocardial oxygen demand is reduced by decreasing heart rate, LV contractility, and myocardial wall stress during systole. Outflow tract obstruction may be minimized with β-blockade, especially under conditions of stress or exercise, when sympathetic stimulation is high.

Calcium Channel Blockers

Patients who have an inadequate response to β-blockade may respond to verapamil.[56] Doses of verapamil up to 480 mg/day have beneficial effects on symptoms.[66] Calcium channel blockers may be of benefit to patients with HCM for several reasons. Increased calcium concentrations have been shown to play a role in prolonging ventricular depolarization, as well as the duration of isometric contraction and relaxation. Patients with HCM have a hyperdynamic ventricle in systole and delayed relaxation and decreased compliance during diastole. Calcium channel blockers decrease the myocardial oxygen demand, resulting in an improved balance between oxygen supply and demand; therefore, diastolic function may be improved.

Most patients with HCM who have been treated with a calcium channel blocker have received verapamil, although others also have been used. IV verapamil has been noted to acutely reduce the outflow tract gradient in patients with obstructive HCM. The mechanism may be a decrease in systolic function as well as an increase in LV volumes as a result of enhanced LV diastolic filling.

The adverse effects associated with use of verapamil include constipation, sinus nodal blockade, prolongation of the PR interval, AV dissociation, hypotension, and pulmonary congestion. The risks may outweigh the benefits in patients with (a) a markedly elevated pulmonary capillary wedge pressure or pulmonary artery occlusion pressure, (b) a history of paroxysmal nocturnal dyspnea or orthopnea, (c) sick sinus syndrome or significant AV nodal disease in the absence of a permanent pacemaker, (d) low systolic blood pressure, and (e) a substantial outflow gradient. Verapamil should be avoided in patients with HF as a result of systolic dysfunction.[66] There is no evidence that either β-blockade or verapamil protects the patient from sudden cardiac death.

Studies using other calcium channel blockers are limited. Improvement in diastolic dysfunction may occur, but the dihydropyridines may cause a reflex increase in heart rate or hypotension or worsen the outflow tract gradient.

Antiarrhythmic Agents

Disopyramide has been used for treating both the supraventricular and ventricular arrhythmias occurring in patients with HCM. In addition, the negative inotropic effect and the ability to increase peripheral vascular resistance attributed to disopyramide have been used to reduce outflow tract obstruction. The anticholinergic side effects (blurred vision, dry mouth, and urinary retention) make disopyramide a problematic agent for long-term therapy in some patients. The QT interval on the ECG should be monitored in patients on disopyramide.[66]

The role of amiodarone for the prevention of sudden death in patients with HCM has been questionable. A few nonrandomized studies have suggested a protective effect, whereas others demonstrate only symptomatic improvement. Nonetheless, the 2006 ACC/AHA/ESC guidelines give amiodarone a class IIb recommendation for primary prophylaxis against sudden death in patients with HCM when ICD placement is not feasible and who demonstrate one or more major risk factors for sudden death (see Table 21-7). Furthermore, in patients with HCM who are not candidates for ICD placement and have suffered a cardiac arrest, amiodarone therapy is considered the preferred treatment (class I recommendation).[68]

A significant number of patients with HCM develop atrial fibrillation. Amiodarone is one of the most effective agents available to maintain normal sinus rhythm in these patients. For patients in chronic atrial fibrillation requiring rate control, a β-blocker or verapamil may be used. Anticoagulation should be considered because these patients are at risk for systemic embolization and stroke. If amiodarone is added to the therapy of a patient already receiving warfarin, the prothrombin time or international normalized ratio will be increased and should be monitored closely.[56]

Other Drugs

There is a small risk for bacterial endocarditis in patients with LV outflow obstruction under resting conditions and in those with intrinsic mitral valve disease. Patients undergoing dental or selected surgical procedures that cause bloodborne bacteremia should receive appropriate antibiotic therapy. The administration of nitroglycerin and digoxin generally is discouraged in the presence of LV outflow obstruction.[66]

CLINICAL CONTROVERSY

Some clinicians believe that ACE inhibitors have no role in the management of HCM with LV outflow obstruction. Others believe that ACE inhibitors may be beneficial by limiting hypertrophy.

Evaluation of Therapeutic Outcomes

The goal of treatment of patients with HCM is primarily to reduce their symptoms of dyspnea and exercise intolerance. Either β-blocker or calcium channel blockers can be used. If a β-blocker is chosen, it is best to use an agent that does not have intrinsic sympathomimetic activity. The dose should be maximized. If the patient does not tolerate a β-blocker or has a contraindication to use of a β-blocker, then verapamil can be tried. Patients should be monitored for resolution of symptoms and an increase in exercise tolerance. Resolution of symptoms may take months to occur. In addition, both β-blockers and calcium channel blockers may cause hypotension and conduction abnormalities. Beta-blockers may worsen pulmonary function. If dyspnea continues with maximal doses of a β-blocker or calcium channel blocker, a diuretic agent or a nitrate may be added with caution. Patients who are at high risk for sudden cardiac death should be considered candidates for an ICD.

For patients with significant obstruction to LV outflow who do not respond to medical management, a surgical approach may be necessary. Septal myectomy and alcohol ablation have been used. These approaches generally are reserved for patients who have an exercise outflow gradient >50 mm Hg or resting outflow gradient >30 mm Hg and/or severe symptoms and who have not responded to an adequate trial of medical therapy.

RESTRICTIVE CARDIOMYOPATHY

Restrictive cardiomyopathy is primarily an abnormality of diastolic function that results in impaired filling and increases in ventricular end-diastolic pressures with normal or decreased diastolic volume. It is associated with normal systolic function early in the course of the disease but a decrease in systolic function later in the disease process. Either one or both of the ventricles may be affected; therefore, restrictive cardiomyopathy may present as either left- or right-sided HF.[55]

Epidemiology and Etiology

Restrictive cardiomyopathy is encountered less frequently in Western countries. Because restrictive cardiomyopathy is rare, the natural course of the disease is not well characterized, and reports on prognosis have been highly variable. Restrictive cardiomyopathies may be classified as either myocardial or endomyocardial. The myocardial types may be noninfiltrative, infiltrative, or storage diseases. The endomyocardial types are due to endomyocardial fibrosis, hypereosinophilic syndrome, carcinoid heart disease, metastatic cancers, radiation, and anthracycline toxicity or secondary to drugs known to cause fibrosis.[57]

Restrictive myocardial disease may result from several local or systemic disorders. Amyloidosis, hemochromatosis, scleroderma, carcinoid, sarcoidosis, diabetes, pseudoxanthoma elasticum, and endomyocardial fibrosis have been known to cause restrictive cardiomyopathy. The most common cause of restrictive cardiomyopathy in the industrialized world is amyloidosis, whereas endomyocardial fibrosis is a common cause in tropical areas of the world. There may be a genetic predisposition to idiopathic restrictive cardiomyopathy.[57]

Pathophysiology

The major hemodynamic abnormality in restrictive cardiomyopathy is a limitation in ventricular filling leading to reduced diastolic volumes of one or both ventricles.[57] The cavity size and wall thickness of the ventricles usually are normal. Atrial dimensions often are increased. Thrombi are found frequently in the cardiac chambers. Patients may have signs and symptoms consistent with HF. The abnormality is similar to that seen in pericardial disease causing constriction or tamponade.

Diagnosis

The diagnosis of restrictive cardiomyopathy should be considered in any patient who presents with signs and symptoms of HF but has only mild cardiomegaly. A positive Kussmaul sign is common when symptoms of HF are present.[57] Differentiation from constrictive pericarditis is important because pericardectomy is an effective form of treatment of constrictive pericarditis. Recent studies have focused on using BNP as a potential noninvasive marker for differentiation of the two conditions.[69] Other laboratory tests or endomyocardial biopsy can be performed to look for diseases such as amyloidosis and hemachromatosis.

TREATMENT

Restrictive Cardiomyopathy

The treatment of restrictive cardiomyopathy is complex because of the heterogeneity of the pathophysiologic abnormalities.[57] Diuretics are used for the symptoms of venous congestion in the presence of restrictive cardiomyopathy, but caution is advised because these patients require high filling pressures to maintain an adequate stroke volume and cardiac output. Hypotension and hypoperfusion may occur as a result of excessive use of diuretics. Because systolic function often is normal, digoxin is of little benefit and may be proarrhythmic. Amiodarone can be used to maintain normal sinus rhythm in patients who have episodes of atrial fibrillation. Anticoagulation is needed to decrease the risk of systemic embolization, particularly in patients with atrial fibrillation, valvular regurgitation, and low cardiac output. In the case of hemochromatosis, chelation therapy and/or repeated phlebotomy may be of benefit. Treatment with corticosteroids and cytotoxic drugs has been used with some success in the early phase of endomyocardial fibrosis and eosinophilic cardiomyopathy.

Evaluation of Therapeutic Outcomes

The first step in assessing and treating a patient with restrictive cardiomyopathy is to rule out constrictive pericarditis because the two conditions have a similar presentation. Patients with constrictive pericarditis are treated easily with surgery, whereas patients with restrictive cardiomyopathy undergo a varied approach to therapy depending on the etiology of their disorder. The treatment is aimed at relieving the symptoms associated with high filling pressures. This is achieved generally through the use of diuretics. Diuretic therapy should be initiated with low doses. Normalization of filling pressures is not possible or desirable. Patients' symptoms should be monitored for improvement. Excessive diuresis will result in inadequate cardiac output. Chelation therapy has been advocated for patients with hemochromatosis. Prednisone has been suggested for patients with sarcoidosis. There is no curative treatment for restrictive cardiomyopathy.

OTHER CARDIOMYOPATHIES

Tachycardia-induced cardiomyopathy (TIC) is a reversible form of HF. The incidence of TIC is unknown but generally thought to be uncommon. It is associated with persistent supraventricular or ventricular arrhythmias and may occur in patients of all ages.[57,70] With prolonged tachycardia, the heart dilates, LVEF decreases, but hypertrophy does not occur. Recovery of EF and resolution of symptoms may occur within 1 month after treatment. However, if tachycardia recurs, a precipitous decline in EF may occur, along with possible sudden cardiac death.[70] The sinus node inhibitor ivabradine has been reported to improve symptoms and systolic function and may warrant further evaluation.[71]

There are also a number of endocrine disorders associated with cardiomyopathy, including acromegaly, adrenal insufficiency, Cushing disease, hyperthyroidism, myxedema, and pheochromocytoma.[57] Treatment is targeted at the underlying endocrine disease.

When patients present with dilated cardiomyopathy, alcohol consumption should be investigated. Alcohol consumption is associated with myocardial fibrosis, impaired sarcoplasmic reticulum uptake of calcium, inhibition of myosin ATPase, and diastolic dysfunction. Generally, excessive alcohol intake for a prolonged period (10 or more years) is likely to occur before symptoms develop. Treatment is abstinence from alcohol.[57] Patients receiving other known cardiotoxic agents, such as anthracyclines, should follow established dosing guidelines and be monitored closely. Chronic cocaine use can cause cardiomyopathy through direct toxicity to the myocardium as well as promoting atherosclerosis- and vasospasm-induced ischemia. As with alcohol, abstinence is critical for patients with cocaine-induced cardiomyopathy. Standard HF therapies should be initiated; however, use of β-blockers is discouraged if the patient is likely to continue the use of cocaine.[72]

ABBREVIATIONS

ACC: American College of Cardiology

ACE: Angiotensin-converting enzyme

AHA: American Heart Association

ALLHAT: Antihypertensive and lipid-lowering treatment to prevent heart attack trial

AV: Atrioventricular

BNP: B-type natriuretic peptide

CAD: Coronary artery disease

CHARM: Candesartan in Heart Failure: Assessment of Reduction in Mortality and Morbidity

DHF: Diastolic heart failure

DIG: Digitalis Investigational Group

ECG: Electrocardiogram

EF: Ejection fraction

ESC: European Society of Cardiology

HCM: Hypertrophic cardiomyopathy

HF: Heart failure

HFSA: Heart Failure Society of America

HR: Hazard ratio

ICD: Implantable cardioverter-defibrillator

I-Preserve: Irbesartan in Heart Failure with Preserved Ejection Fraction

LV: Left Ventricular

LVH: Left Ventricular Hypertrophy

MI: Myocardial infarction

MMP: Matrix metalloproteinase

NT-proBNP: N-terminal proBNP

NYHA: New York Heart Association

PEP-CHF: Perindopril for Elderly Persons with Chronic Heart Failure

RALES: Randomized aldactone evaluation study

SBP: Systolic blood pressure

SENIORS: Study of Effects of Nebivolol Intervention on Outcomes and Rehospitalization in Seniors with Heart Failure

SHF: Systolic heart failure

TIC: Tachycardia-induced cardiomyopathy

REFERENCES

1. Owan TE, Redfield MM. Epidemiology of diastolic heart failure. Prog Cardiovasc Dis 2005;47:320–332.
2. Brutsaert DL, De Keulenaer GW. Diastolic heart failure: A myth. Curr Opin Cardiol 2006;21:240–248.
3. Executive summary: HFSA 2006 Comprehensive Heart Failure Practice Guideline. J Card Fail 2006;12:10–38.
4. Sanderson JE, Yip GWK. Heart failure with a normal ejection fraction. BMJ 2009;338:367–368.
5. Leite-Moreira AF. Current perspectives in diastolic dysfunction and diastolic heart failure. Heart 2006;92:712–718.
6. Zile MR. Heart failure with preserved ejection fraction: Is this diastolic heart failure? J Am Coll Cardiol 2003;41:1519–1522.
7. Smith GL, Masoudi FA, Vaccarino V, et al. Outcomes in heart failure patients with preserved ejection fraction: Mortality, readmission, and functional decline. J Am Coll Cardiol 2003;41:1510–1518.
8. Fonarow GC, Adams KF Jr, Abraham WT, et al. Risk stratification for in-hospital mortality in acutely decompensated heart failure: Classification and regression tree analysis. JAMA 2005;293:572–580.
9. Zile MR. Diastolic heart failure. Diagnosis, prognosis, treatment. Minerva Cardioangiol 2003;51:131–142.
10. Redfield MM, Jacobsen SJ, Burnett JC Jr, et al. Burden of systolic and diastolic ventricular dysfunction in the community: Appreciating the scope of the heart failure epidemic. JAMA 2003;289:194–202.
11. Owan TE, Hodge DO, Herges RM, et al. Trends in prevalence and outcome of heart failure with preserved ejection fraction. N Engl J Med 2006;355:251–259.
12. Franklin KM, Aurigemma GP. Prognosis in diastolic heart failure. Prog Cardiovasc Dis 2005;47:333–339.
13. Yusuf S, Pfeffer MA, Swedberg K, et al. Effects of candesartan in patients with chronic heart failure and preserved left-ventricular ejection fraction: The CHARM-Preserved Trial. Lancet 2003;362:777–781.
14. Lee DS, Gona P, Vasan RS, et al. Relation of disease pathogenesis and risk factors to heart failure with preserved or reduced ejection fraction: insights from the Framingham heart study of the National Heart, Lung and Blood Institute. Circulation 2009;119:3070–3077.
15. Galderisi M. Diastolic dysfunction and diastolic heart failure: Diagnostic, prognostic and therapeutic aspects. Cardiovasc Ultrasound 2005;3:1–14.
16. Neilan TG, Yoerger DM, Douglas PS, et al. Persistent and reversible cardiac dysfunction among amateur marathon runners. Eur Heart J 2006;27:1079–1084.
17. Ahmed SH, Clark LL, Pennington WR, et al. Matrix metalloproteinases/tissue inhibitors of metalloproteinases: Relationship between changes in proteolytic determinants of matrix composition and structural, functional, and clinical manifestations of hypertensive heart disease. Circulation 2006;113:2089–2096.
18. Gaddam KK, Oparil S. Diastolic dysfunction and heart failure with preserved ejection fraction: rationale for RAAS antagonist/CCB combination therapy. J Am Soc Hypertens 2009;3:52–68.
19. Zile MR, Baicu CF, Gaasch WH. Diastolic heart failure—Abnormalities in active relaxation and passive stiffness of the left ventricle. New Engl J Med 2004;350:1953–1959.
20. Cecchi F, Olivotto I, Gistri R, et al. Coronary microvascular dysfunction and prognosis in hypertrophic cardiomyopathy. N Engl J Med 2003;349:1027–1035.
21. Torosoff M, Philbin EF. Improving outcomes in diastolic heart failure: Techniques to evaluate underlying causes and target therapy. Postgrad Med 2003;113:51–58.
22. Chinnaiyan KM, Alexander D, Maddens M, McCullough PA. Curriculum in cardiology: Integrated diagnosis and management of diastolic heart failure. Am Heart J 2007;153:189–200.
23. Swedberg K, Cleland J, Dargie H, et al. Guidelines for the diagnosis and treatment of chronic heart failure: Executive summary (update 2005): The Task Force for the Diagnosis and Treatment of Chronic Heart Failure of the European Society of Cardiology. Eur Heart J 2005;26:1115–1140.
24. Massie BM. Natriuretic peptide measurements for the diagnosis of "nonsystolic" heart failure: Good news and bad. J Am Coll Cardiol 2003;41:2018–2021.

25. Maisel AS, McCord J, Nowak RM, et al. Bedside B-type natriuretic peptide in the emergency diagnosis of heart failure with reduced or preserved ejection fraction: Results from the Breathing Not Properly Multinational Study. J Am Coll Cardiol 2003;41:2010–2017.

26. Tschope C, Kasner M, Westermann D, et al. The role of NT-proBNP in the diagnostics of isolated diastolic dysfunction: Correlation with echocardiographic and invasive measurements. Eur Heart J 2005;26:2277–2284.

27. Bhatia RS, Tu JV, Lee DS, et al. Outcome of heart failure with preserved ejection fraction in a population-based study. N Engl J Med 2006;355:260–269.

28. Deswal A, Bozkurt B. Comparison of morbidity in women versus men with heart failure and preserved ejection fraction. Am J Cardiol 2006;97:1228–1231.

29. Jones RC, Francis GS, Lauer MS. Predictors of mortality in patients with heart failure and preserved systolic function in the Digitalis Investigation Group trial. J Am Coll Cardiol 2004;44:1025–1029.

30. Little WC, Brucks S. Therapy for diastolic heart failure. Prog Cardiovasc Dis 2005;47:380–388.

31. Hunt SA, Abraham WT, Chin MH, et al. 2009 Focused update incorporated into the ACC/AHA 2005 Guidelines for the Diagnosis and Management of Heart Failure in Adults: A report of the American College of Cardiology Foundation/American Heart Association Task Force on Practice Guidelines Developed in Collaboration with the International Society for Heart and Lung Transplantation. J Am Coll Cardiol 2009;53:e1–e90.

32. Pina IL, Apstein CS, Balady GJ, et al. Exercise and heart failure: A statement from the American Heart Association Committee on exercise, rehabilitation, and prevention. Circulation 2003;107:1210–1225.

33. Colucci WS, Braunwald E. Pathophysiology of heart failure. In: Zipes DP, Libby P, Bonow RO, Braunwald E, eds. Braunwald's Heart Disease. 7th ed. Philadelphia, PA: Elsevier Saunders; 2005:509–538.

34. Gaasch WH, Zile MR. Left ventricular diastolic dysfunction and diastolic heart failure. Annu Rev Med 2004;55:373–394.

35. Heart Failure Society of America. Evaluation and management of patients with heart failure and preserved left ventricular ejection fraction. J Card Fail 2010;16:e126–133.

36. Hunt SA. ACC/AHA 2005 guideline update for the diagnosis and management of chronic heart failure in the adult: A report of the American College of Cardiology/American Heart Association Task Force on Practice Guidelines (Writing Committee to Update the 2001 Guidelines for the Evaluation and Management of Heart Failure). J Am Coll Cardiol 2005;46:e1–e82.

37. Major cardiovascular events in hypertensive patients randomized to doxazosin vs chlorthalidone: The Antihypertensive and Lipid-Lowering Treatment to Prevent Heart Attack Trial (ALLHAT). ALLHAT Collaborative Research Group. JAMA 2000;283:1967–1975.

38. Banerjee P, Clark AL, Cleland JG. Diastolic heart failure: A difficult problem in the elderly. Am J Geriatr Cardiol 2004;13:16–21.

39. Davis BR, Kostis JB, Simpson LM, et al for the ALLHAT Collaborative Research Group. Heart failure with preserved and reduced left ventricular ejection fraction in the antihypertensive and lipid-lowering treatment to prevent heart attack trial. Circulation 2008;118:2259–2267.

40. Davis KL, Nappi JM. The cardiovascular effects of eplerenone, a selective aldosterone-receptor antagonist. Clin Ther 2003;25:2647–2668.

41. Krum H, Abraham WT. Heart failure. Lancet 2009;373:941–955.

42. Lopez B, Querejeta R, Gonzalez A, et al. Effects of loop diuretics on myocardial fibrosis and collagen type I turnover in chronic heart failure. J Am Coll Cardiol 2004:43:2028–2035.

43. van Veldhuisen DJ, Cohen-Solal A, Bohm M, et al on behalf of the SENIORS Investigators. Beta-blockade with nebivolol in elderly heart failure patients with impaired and preserved left ventricular ejection fraction. J Am Coll Cardiol 2009;53:2150–2158.

44. Dobre D, van Veldhuisen DJ, DeJongste MJ, et al. Prescription of beta-blockers in patients with advanced heart failure and preserved left ventricular ejection fraction: Clinical implications and survival. Eur J Heart Fail 2007; 9:280–286.

45. Massie BM, Nelson JJ, Lukas MA, et al. Comparison of outcomes and usefulness of carvedilol across a spectrum of left ventricular ejection fractions in patients with heart failure in clinical practice. Am J Cardiol 2007;99:1263–1268.

46. Hogg K, McMurray J. Neurohumoral pathways in heart failure with preserved systolic function. Prog Cardiovasc Dis 2005;47:357–366.

47. Cleland J, Tendera M, Adamus J, et al. The perindopril in elderly people with chronic heart failure (PEP-CHF) study. Eur Heart J 2006;27:2338–2345.

48. McMurray JJV, Andersson FL, Stewart S, et al, for the CHARM Investigators and Committees. Resource utilization and costs in the candesartan in heart failure: Assessment of reduction in mortality and morbidity (CHARM) programme. Eur Heart J 2006;27:1447–1458.

49. Massie, BM, Carson PE, McMurray JJ, et al, for the I-PRESERVE Investigators. Irbesartan in patients with heart failure and preserved ejection fraction. New Engl J Med 2008;359:2456–2467.

50. Mottram PM, Haluska B, Leano R, et al. Effect of aldosterone antagonism on myocardial dysfunction in hypertensive patients with diastolic heart failure. Circulation 2004;110:558–565.

51. Roongsritong C, Sutthiwan P, Bradley J, et al. Spironolactone improves diastolic function in the elderly. Clin Cardiol 2005;28:484–487.

52. Shah SJ, Blair JEA, Filippatos GS, et al, for the HORIZON-HF Investigators. Effects of istaroxime on diastolic stiffness in acute heart failure syndromes: Results from the Hemodynamic, Echocardiographic, and Neurohormonal Effects of Istaroxime, a Novel Intravenous Inotropic and Lusitropic Agent: A Randomized Controlled Trial in Patients Hospitalized with Heart Failure (HORIZON-HF) trial. Am Heart J 2009;1035–1041.

53. Ahmed A, Rich MW, Fleg JL, et al. Effects of digoxin on morbidity and mortality in diastolic heart failure: The ancillary digitalis investigation group trial. Circulation 2006;114:397–403.

54. Liao L, Jollis JG, Anstrom KJ, et al. Costs for heart failure with normal vs reduced ejection fraction. Arch Int Med 2006;166:112–118.

55. Maron BJ, Towbin JA, Thiene G, et al. Contemporary definitions and classification of the cardiomyopathies: An American Heart Association Scientific Statement from the Council on Clinical Cardiology, Heart Failure and Transplantation Committee; Quality of Care and Outcomes Research and Functional Genomics and Translational Biology Interdisciplinary Working Groups; and Council on Epidemiology and Prevention. Circulation 2006;113:1807–1816.

56. Spirito P, Autore C. Management of hypertrophic cardiomyopathy. BMJ 2006;332:1251–1255.

57. Arnold JMO, Howlett JG, Ducharme A, et al. Canadian Cardiovascular Society Consensus Conference guidelines on heart failure—2008 update: Best practices for the transition of care of heart failure patients, and the recognition, investigation and treatment of cardiomyopathies. Can J Cardiol 2008;24:21–40.

58. Roberts R, Sigwart U. Current concepts of the pathogenesis and treatment of hypertrophic cardiomyopathy. Circulation 2005;112:293–296.

59. Poliac LC, Barron ME, Maron BJ. Hypertrophic cardiomyopathy. Anesthesiology 2006;104:183–192.

60. Maron BJ, Maron MM, Wigle ED, Braunwald E. The 50-year history, controversy, and clinical implications of left ventricular outflow tract obstruction in hypertrophic cardiomyopathy. J Am Coll Cardiol 2009;54:191–200.

61. Ho CY, Seidman CE. A contemporary approach to hypertrophic cardiomyopathy. Circulation 2006;113:e858–e862.

62. Maron MS, Olivotto I, Maron BJ, et al. The case for myocardial ischemia in hypertrophic cardiomyopathy. J Am Coll Cardiol 2009;54:866–875.

63. Bos JM, Towbin JA, Ackerman MJ. Diagnostic, prognostic, and therapeutic implications of genetic testing for hypertrophic cardiomyopathy. J Am Coll Cardiol 2009;54:201–211.

64. Klein GJ, Krahn AD, Skanes AC, et al. Primary prophylaxis of sudden death in hypertrophic cardiomyopathy, arrhythmogenic right ventricular cardiomyopathy, and dilated cardiomyopathy. J Cardiovasc Electrophysiol 2005;16(Suppl 1):S28–S34.

65. Maron BJ, Casey SA, Hauser RG, Aeppli DM. Clinical course of hypertrophic cardiomyopathy with survival to advanced age. J Am Coll Cardiol 2003;42:882–888.

66. Maron BJ, McKenna WJ, Danielson GK, et al. American College of Cardiology/European Society of Cardiology clinical expert consensus document on hypertrophic cardiomyopathy: A report of the American College of Cardiology Foundation Task Force on Clinical Expert Consensus Documents and the European Society of Cardiology Committee for Practice Guidelines. J Am Coll Cardiol 2003;42:1687–1713.

67. ACC/AHA/HRS 2008 guidelines for device-based therapy of cardiac rhythm abnormalities: A report of the American College of Cardiology/American Heart Association Task Force on Practice Guidelines (Writing Committee to Revise the ACC/AHA/NASPE 2002 Guideline Update for Implantation of Cardiac Pacemakers and Antiarrhythmia Devices) developed in collaboration with the American Association for Thoracic Surgery and Society of Thoracic Surgeons. J Am Coll Cardiol. 2008; 27;51:e1–e62.

68. Zipes DP, Camm AJ, Borggrefe M, et al. ACC/AHA/ESC 2006 guidelines for management of patients with ventricular arrhythmias and the prevention of sudden cardiac death: A report of the American College of Cardiology/American Heart Association Task Force and the European Society of Cardiology Committee for Practice Guidelines (Writing Committee to Develop Guidelines for Management of Patients with Ventricular Arrhythmias and the Prevention of Sudden Cardiac Death): Developed in collaboration with the European Heart Rhythm Association and the Heart Rhythm Society. Circulation 2006;114:e385–e484.

69. Leya FS, Arab D, Joyal D, et al. The efficacy of brain natriuretic peptide levels in differentiating constrictive pericarditis from restrictive cardiomyopathy. J Am Coll Cardiol 2005;45:1900–1902.

70. Nerheim P, Birger-BotkinS, Piracha L, Olshansky B. Heart failure and sudden death in patients with tachycardia-induced cardiomyopathy and recurrent tachycardia. Circulation 2004;110:247–252.

71. Winum PF, Cayla G, Rubini M, et al. A case of cardiomyopathy induced by inappropriate sinus tachycardia and cured by ivabradine. Pacing Clin Electrophysiol 2009;32:942–944.

72. Phillips K, Luk A, Soor GS, Abraham JR, et al Cocaine cardiotoxicity: A review of the pathophysiology, pathology, and treatment options. Am J Cardiovasc Drugs 2009;9:177–196.

73. Hori M, Kitabatake A, Tsutsui H, et al. Rationale and design of a randomized trial to assess the effects of beta-blocker in diastolic heart failure; Japanese Diastolic Heart Failure Study (J-DHF). J Card Failure 2005;7:542–547.

74. Massie BM, Fabi MR. Clinical trials in diastolic heart failure. Prog Cardiovasc Dis 2005;47:389–395.

22

Acute Decompensated Heart Failure

JO E. RODGERS AND CRAIG R. LEE

KEY CONCEPTS

❶ Unlike chronic heart failure therapies whose primary benefit is an improvement in survival, treatment goals of acute decompensated heart failure (ADHF) are directed toward relief of symptoms of pulmonary edema, restoration of systemic oxygen transport and tissue perfusion, and limitation of further cardiac damage and other adverse effects.

❷ Maximizing oral chronic heart failure therapy and using combinations of short-acting intravenous medications with different cardiovascular actions are often needed to optimize cardiac output, relieve pulmonary edema, and limit myocardial ischemia.

❸ Patients presenting to the hospital with ADHF can be categorized into four subsets based upon fluid status (euvolemic or "dry" vs fluid overload or "wet") and cardiac output (adequate cardiac output or "warm" vs hypoperfusion or "cold"). Thus, patients are warm and dry, warm and wet, cold and dry, or cold and wet.

❹ While invasive hemodynamic monitoring using a pulmonary artery or Swan Ganz catheter has been shown to not alter outcomes in a broad population of ADHF patients not requiring such monitoring, it is indicated for patients who are refractory to initial therapy, whose volume status is unclear, or who have clinically significant hypotension such as a systolic blood pressure less than 80 mm Hg or worsening renal function despite therapy. In addition, pulmonary artery catheter monitoring may also be necessary to provide immediate feedback on treatment efficacy and adverse effects.

❺ Key hemodynamic parameters to assess with pulmonary artery catheter monitoring include pulmonary capillary wedge pressure, which reflects fluid status or preload; cardiac output, which reflects the innate contractility of the heart; and systemic vascular resistance, which reflects vascular tone or afterload. While a normal pulmonary capillary wedge pressure (6 to 12 mm Hg) is desirable in most healthy patients, higher filling pressures (15 to 18 mm Hg) are necessary in patients with heart failure.

❻ Three major therapeutic categories exist for managing ADHF: diuretics, inotropes, and vasodilators. No therapy for ADHF studied to date has been shown conclusively to decrease mortality. Inotropic therapy consistently has been associated with increased mortality and adverse effects in multiple studies.

❼ Intravenous loop diuretics are considered first-line therapy for management of ADHF associated with fluid overload. A variety of therapeutic options are recommended for managing refractory fluid overload, including increasing loop diuretic intravenous bolus dose, adding a diuretic with a different mechanism of action, and transitioning to a continuous infusion of loop diuretic. Ultrafiltration is also an option for patients refractory to diuretics. If patients continue to be refractory to and experience worsening renal function with diuretic therapy, vasodilator and inotropic therapy may be indicated. Placement of a pulmonary artery catheter may be helpful in guiding therapy in such patients.

❽ Intravenous inotropes are recommended for symptom relief or end-organ dysfunction for patients with left ventricular dysfunction and low cardiac output syndrome. Such therapy may be especially useful for patients with low systolic blood pressure (less than 90 mm Hg) or symptomatic hypotension in the setting of adequate filling pressures. Inotropic therapy may also be considered for patients who do not tolerate or respond to intravenous vasodilators or who present worsening renal function. These agents should be avoided in patients with reduced left heart filling pressures, and patients should be monitored continuously for arrhythmias.

❾ Given the potential risks associated with inotropic therapy, vasodilators should be considered prior to using inotropes.

❿ Intravenous vasodilators may be considered in addition to diuretics for rapid symptom resolution and may be especially useful for patients with acute pulmonary edema or severe hypertension as well as for patients who fail to respond to aggressive treatment with diuretics. It is essential to avoid use of vasodilators for patients with symptomatic hypotension, and frequent blood pressure monitoring is essential for the safe use of these agents. In addition, these agents should not be used for patients with reduced left heart filling pressures. If patients fail to respond to the above therapies or experience worsening renal function, intravenous inotropic therapy should be considered.

⓫ Vasopressin antagonists provide a new therapeutic option for managing hyponatremia in patients with euvolemic or hypervolemic hyponatremia. Tolvaptan is the only vasopressin antagonist indicated for managing hyponatremia associated with heart failure. Despite tolvaptan being an oral agent, it should only be initiated in the hospital setting to allow for

Learning objectives, review questions, and other resources can be found at **www.pharmacotherapyonline.com**.

close monitoring of rapidity of serum sodium correction and volume status. Over-rapid correction of serum sodium may result in adverse neurological sequelae.

⓬ Given extended wait times for patients on the cardiac transplant list, insertion of a ventricular assist device may be considered for patients in whom extended time to identify a suitable donor is likely to occur (i.e., "bridge" to transplant) or in whom transplantation is not an option (i.e., "destination" therapy).

As discussed in Chap. 20 (Systolic Heart Failure), the number of patients with heart failure is substantial and continues to increase. Although survival from heart failure, has improved, the growing number of patients with the disorder and the progressive nature of the syndrome have lead to substantial increases in hospitalizations for heart failure.[1] Recent data indicate approximately 1 million patients are hospitalized annually for heart failure resulting in significant morbidity, mortality, and consumption of large quantities of healthcare resources.[1,2] Inpatient admission for heart failure is associated with an increased risk of subsequent hospitalization and decreased survival.[3] In fact, recent data suggest that the mortality rate following hospitalization for heart failure is 10.4%, 22%, and 42.3% at 30 days, 1 year, and 5 years, respectively. Additional data suggest an in-hospital mortality rate of 5.1%.[2] The economic impact of heart failure is considerable, with cost driven primarily by inpatient care.[1,2]

A number of descriptive terms have been used to characterize patients with worsening heart failure requiring hospitalization. Patients with persistent symptoms or *refractory* heart failure requiring specialized interventions despite optimal standard therapy such as angiotensin-converting enzyme (ACE) inhibitors and β-blockers are classified as stage D in the American College of Cardiology/ American Heart Association (ACC/AHA) classification scheme.[4,5] These patients typically fall into the category of New York Heart Association (NYHA) class III or IV heart failure with symptoms upon minimal exertion or at rest. The terms *decompensated heart failure* or *exacerbation of heart failure* refer to those patients with new or worsening signs or symptoms that are usually caused by volume overload and/or hypoperfusion and lead to additional medical care such as emergency room visits and hospitalizations. The term *acute* heart failure may be misleading as it more often refers to the patient with a sudden onset of signs or symptoms of heart failure in the setting of previously normal cardiac function. This chapter will focus on the management of patients with acute decompensated heart failure (ADHF). Clinical syndromes within decompensated heart failure include pulmonary or systemic volume overload, low cardiac output, and acute pulmonary edema. It is important to recognize that such patients may present with impaired (left ventricular ejection fraction less than 40%) or preserved (left ventricular ejection fraction greater than or equal to 40%) left ventricular systolic function and a variety of etiologies may be responsible for the primary disease process. The clinical course of heart failure manifests as periods of relative stability with an increasing frequency in episodes of decompensation as the underlying disease progresses.[6]

Despite the considerable morbidity and mortality associated with decompensated heart failure, the first randomized placebo-controlled trials in this patient population were published in 2002.[7,8] In addition, it was not until 2005 that guidelines specifically focused on managing decompensated heart failure were generated. The Heart Failure Society of America (HFSA) and the European Society of Cardiology have published separate guidelines for evaluating and treating decompensated heart failure.[9,10] The 2005 ACC/AHA guidelines had previously focused a portion of their recommendations for chronic heart failure on the decompensated patient.[4] However, the 2009 update has also provided specific recommendations for the

hospitalized patient.[5] Since available drug therapies differ between Europe and the United States, the HFSA and ACC/AHA guidelines will be the focus of the remainder of this chapter.

PATHOPHYSIOLOGY AND CLINICAL PRESENTATION

Patients requiring intensive therapy for decompensated heart failure may have a variety of underlying etiologies and clinical presentations.[5,9] Patients with worsening chronic heart failure comprise approximately 70% of heart failure hospital admissions. These patients can become refractory to available oral therapy and decompensate following a relatively mild insult (e.g., dietary indiscretion, nonsteroidal antiinflammatory drug use), cardiac medication noncompliance, or a noncardiac concurrent illness (e.g., infection). A new cardiac event, such as recurrent myocardial infarction, atrial fibrillation, hypertensive urgency/emergency, myocarditis, or acute valvular insufficiency also can cause a stable patient to decompensate. Secondly, de novo heart failure may occur following a large myocardial infarction or sudden increase in blood pressure in the setting of left ventricular dysfunction and represents approximately 25% of admissions. A third group of patients with severe left ventricular systolic dysfunction associated with progressive worsening of cardiac output and refractoriness to therapy represents about 5% of heart failure admissions.[11] Additional insight into the clinical characteristics of decompensated heart failure patients unexpectedly indicates that a high percentage of patients present with hypertension and preserved left ventricular systolic function.[12]

Several studies have also provided a better understanding of the prognostic factors associated with decompensated heart failure. Data from the Acute Decompensated Heart Failure Registry (ADHERE), a registry of hospitalized patients with a primary diagnosis of decompensated heart failure, found BUN greater than or equal to 43 mg/dL to be the best individual predictor of in-hospital mortality, followed by systolic blood pressure less than 115 mm Hg, and then serum creatinine greater than or equal to 2.75 mg/dL. Using these three parameters, patients were identified as low, intermediate, high, and very high risk with in-hospital mortality of 2%, 6%, 13%, and 20%, respectively.[13] Additional studies have confirmed an increase in in-hospital mortality for patients with low systolic blood pressure and worsening renal function on admission.[14,15] Hyponatremia, elevations in troponin I, ischemic etiology, and poor functional capacity are additional negative prognostic factors.[11] Importantly, patients who survive a hospitalization for ADHF remain at high risk for rehospitalization or death.[5] Data from the Organized Program to Initiate Lifesaving Treatment in Hospitalized Patients with Heart Failure (OPTIMIZE-HF), another registry of hospitalized patients with a primary diagnosis of ADHF, have reported overall mortality and rehospitalization rates of 8.6% and 29.6%, respectively, 60 to 90 days postdischarge.[16] Similarly, low blood pressure and poor renal function are negative prognostic factors.[16] However, use of a β-blocker, ACE inhibitor, angiotensin receptor blocker, or lipid-lowering therapy at discharge, and coronary angiography or implantable cardioverter–defibrillator placement during hospitalization were associated with improved prognosis,[16] suggesting that optimal management of these patients in the hospital can yield beneficial effects on prognosis.

GENERAL APPROACH TO TREATMENT

❶ ❷ The overall goals of therapy for the patient with decompensated heart failure are to relieve congestive symptoms or optimize volume status, as well as treat symptoms of low cardiac output, so that the patient can be discharged in a compensated state on oral drug therapy. Although diuretic, vasodilator, and positive inotrope therapy can be very effective at achieving these goals, their efficacy must be balanced against the potential for serious toxicity. Thus, another important goal is to minimize the risks of pharmacologic therapy. Maintenance of vital organ perfusion to preserve renal function and prevention of additional myocardial injury, diuretic-induced electrolyte depletion, hypotension from vasodilators, and myocardial ischemia and arrhythmias from positive inotropes are all important goals.

In addition, all patients should be evaluated for potential etiologies and precipitating factors, including atrial fibrillation and other arrhythmias, worsening hypertension, myocardial ischemia or infarction, anemia, hypothyroidism or hyperthyroidism, or other causes. Medications, including noncardiac medications, which may worsen cardiac function, should also be considered as precipitating or contributing factors. Patients who may benefit from revascularization should also be identified. Prior to discharge, optimization of chronic oral therapy and patient education are critical to preventing future hospitalizations. When available and appropriate, patients should be referred to a heart failure disease management program.[9] A careful history and physical examination are key components in the diagnosis of decompensated heart failure. The history should focus on the potential etiologies of heart failure; the presence of any precipitating factors, onset, duration, and severity of symptoms; and a careful medication history. Current guidelines recommend making the diagnosis of decompensated heart failure based primarily on signs and symptoms.[9] With congestion representing the more common presentation of heart failure, orthopnea is the main symptom of fluid overload that best correlates with elevated pulmonary pressures.[15] Important elements of the physical examination include assessment of vital signs and weight, cardiac auscultation for heart sounds and murmurs, pulmonary exam for the presence of rales, and evaluation for the presence of peripheral edema. The jugular venous pressure is the most reliable indicator of the patient's volume status and should be carefully evaluated on admission and closely followed during hospitalization as an indicator of the efficacy of diuretic therapy.[15] An S3 gallop also represents ventricular filling and has high diagnostic specificity for heart failure decompensation. Other physical findings such as pulmonary crackles and lower extremity edema have low specificity and sensitivity for the diagnosis of decompensated heart failure.[9] The development of a bedside assay for plasma b-type natriuretic peptide (BNP) has focused considerable attention on the use of natriuretic peptide levels as an aid in the diagnosis of suspected heart failure.[17] Plasma BNP and N-terminal pro-BNP levels are positively correlated with the degree of left ventricular dysfunction and heart failure, and these assays are now frequently used in acute care settings to assist in the differential diagnosis of dyspnea (heart failure vs asthma, COPD, or infection). A low BNP concentration has a 96% predictive value for excluding heart failure as an etiology when evaluating patients presenting with dyspnea. In addition, an elevated pre-hospital discharge BNP concentration is associated with an increased risk of worse long-term outcome. It is important to note that any disease process that increases right heart pressures will elevate BNP, including pulmonary emboli, chronic obstructive lung disease, and primary pulmonary hypertension. Also, BNP levels may be mildly increased with increasing age, female gender, and renal dysfunction while concentrations may be lower with obesity.[15] Additional research will better characterize the role of BNP measurement in the diagnosis and treatment of heart failure. When the diagnosis of decompensated heart failure is uncertain, current guidelines recommend obtaining a BNP concentration in conjunction with assessing signs and symptoms.[5,9]

TABLE 22-1	Recommendations for Hospitalizing Patients Presenting with ADHF
Recommendation	**Clinical Circumstances**
Hospitalization recommended	Evidence of severely decompensated HF, including • Hypotension • Worsening renal function • Altered mentation Dyspnea at rest • Typically reflected by resting tachypnea • Less commonly reflected by oxygen saturation <90% Hemodynamically significant arrhythmia • Including new onset of rapid atrial fibrillation Acute coronary syndromes
Hospitalization should be considered	Worsened congestion • Even without dyspnea • Typically reflected by a weight gain of ≥5 kg Signs and symptoms of pulmonary or systemic congestion • Even in the absence of weight gain Major electrolyte disturbance Associated comorbid conditions • Pneumonia • Pulmonary embolus • Diabetic ketoacidosis • Symptoms suggestive of transient ischemic accident or stroke Repeated implantable cardioverter-defibrillator firings Previously undiagnosed HF with signs and symptoms of systemic or pulmonary congestion

Data from Adams KF, Lindenfeld J, Arnold JMO, et al. HFSA 2006 Comprehensive Heart Failure Practice Guidelines. J Cardiac Fail 2006;12:e1–e122.

Hospitalization *is recommended* or *should be considered*, depending on each patient's presenting symptoms and physical exam. Table 22–1 describes the clinical presentation of patients in whom hospitalization should occur or should be considered. Most patients do not require admission to an intensive care unit and are admitted to a monitored unit or general medical floor. Admission to an intensive care unit may be required if the patient experiences hemodynamic instability requiring frequent monitoring of vital signs, invasive hemodynamic monitoring, or rapid titration of intravenous medications with concurrent monitoring to assure safe and effective outcomes.

The first step in the management of decompensated heart failure is to ascertain that optimal treatment with oral medications has been achieved.[5,9] If fluid retention is evident on physical examination, aggressive diuresis should be accomplished. Although increasing the dose of oral diuretic may be effective in some cases, the use of intravenous diuretics frequently is necessary. Every effort should be made to optimally treat the patient with an ACE inhibitor. β-blocker therapy should generally be continued during the hospital admission unless recent dose initiation or uptitration was responsible for the decompensated state. In such cases, β-blocker therapy may need to be temporarily held or dose reduced. Appropriateness of initiating this therapy prior to hospital discharge will be discussed later in this chapter. Discontinuation of ACE inhibitor or β-blocker therapy occasionally may be necessary in the setting of cardiogenic shock or symptomatic hypotension. Certain therapies may also need to be temporarily held in the setting of renal dysfunction especially in the setting of oliguria or hyperkalemia (e.g., ACE inhibitor, angiotensin receptor blocker, and/or aldosterone antagonist) or elevated serum digoxin concentrations. Most patients should be receiving digoxin at a low dose prescribed to achieve a trough serum concentration of 0.5 to 1.0 ng/mL.[18]

There are two general approaches to maximize therapy in the decompensated heart failure patient. One is to use simple clinical

TABLE 22-2 Monitoring Recommendations for Patients Hospitalized with ADHF

Value	Frequency	Specifics
Weight	At least daily	Determine after voiding in the morning Account for possible increased food intake due to improved appetite
Fluid intake/ output	At least daily	Strict documentation necessary
Vital signs	More than daily	Including orthostatic blood pressure
Signs	At least daily	Edema, ascites, pulmonary rales, hepatomegaly, increased jugular venous pressure, hepatojugular reflux, liver tenderness
Symptoms	At least daily	Orthopnea, paroxysmal nocturnal dyspnea, nocturnal cough, dyspnea, fatigue
Electrolytes	At least daily	Potassium, magnesium, sodium
Renal function	At least daily	blood urea nitrogen, serum creatinine

Data from Adams KF, Lindenfeld J, Arnold JMO, et al. HFSA 2006 Comprehensive Heart Failure Practice Guidelines. J Cardiac Fail 2006;12:e1–e122.

parameters (e.g., signs and symptoms, blood pressure, renal function), and the other is to use invasive hemodynamic monitoring in addition to these clinical parameters. In all decompensated heart failure patients, close monitoring is essential for assuring optimal response to therapy while avoiding adverse effects. Daily monitoring should include weight, strict fluid intake and output, and heart failure signs and symptoms to assess clinical efficacy of drug therapy. Foley catheter placement is not recommended unless close monitoring of urine output is needed. As safety end points, monitoring for electrolyte depletion, symptomatic hypotension, and renal dysfunction should be assessed frequently. While many of the above parameters may be monitored daily, some will need to be monitored more frequently as dictated by the patient's clinical status. Vital signs should be assessed multiple times throughout the day at a frequency that is appropriate for a given patient's level of stability. Orthostatic blood pressure should be assessed at least once daily.[9] Recommendations for monitoring are summarized in Table 22–2.

PRINCIPLES OF THERAPY BASED ON CLINICAL PRESENTATION

3 Appropriate medical management of the patient presenting with decompensated heart failure is aided by determination of whether the patient has signs and symptoms of fluid overload ("wet" heart failure) or low cardiac output ("cold" heart failure).[15,19] As previously discussed, most patients present with *fluid overload* (or the "wet" profile). Symptoms consistent with pulmonary congestion include orthopnea and dyspnea with minimal exertion and those of systemic congestion include gastrointestinal discomfort, ascites, and peripheral edema. Patients with no or minimal fluid overload (or the "dry" category of decompensated heart failure) may have symptoms that are more difficult to distinguish. Such patients may present with a syndrome of *low cardiac output* ("cold" heart failure), which is characterized principally by extreme fatigue and tiredness as well as other symptoms not commonly attributed to cardiac causes such as poor appetite, nausea, and early satiety. It is important to recognize that gastrointestinal symptoms may be associated with congestion rather than low cardiac output to the gastrointestinal tract. Moreover, these patients frequently exhibit worsening renal function and a decline in serum sodium level, which, as previously discussed, are each associated with poor prognosis. Many patients will present with signs and symptoms of both wet and cold types of

ADHF. In these patients, low-output symptoms may not be obvious until congestion is optimally treated. Figure 22–1 outlines a suggested treatment approach based on whether the patient has signs and symptoms of fluid overload and/or low cardiac output.

PRINCIPLES OF THERAPY BASED ON HEMODYNAMIC SUBSETS

Patients with decompensated heart failure may have critically reduced cardiac output, usually with low arterial blood pressure and systemic hypoperfusion resulting in organ system dysfunction (i.e., cardiogenic shock). They also may have pulmonary edema with hypoxemia, respiratory acidosis, and markedly increased work of breathing. With cardiopulmonary support, response to interventions should be assessed promptly to allow for timely adjustments in treatment. Since cardiopulmonary support must be instituted and adjusted rapidly, immediate assessment of the results of an intervention limits risks and makes adjustments in therapy more prompt. ECG monitoring, continuous pulse oximetry, urine flow monitoring, and automated blood pressure recording are now the minimal noninvasive standard of care for critically ill patients with cardiopulmonary decompensation. Peripheral or femoral arterial catheters may be utilized for continuous and accurate assessment of arterial pressure.

HEMODYNAMIC MONITORING

4 **5** The role of invasive hemodynamic monitoring for improving outcomes for patients with decompensated heart failure remains controversial. The Evaluation Study of Congestive Heart Failure and Pulmonary Artery Catheterization Effectiveness (ESCAPE) trial assessed the role of invasive hemodynamic monitoring in the management of patients hospitalized for heart failure.[20] The use of a pulmonary artery catheter had no impact on survival after hospital discharge. It is important to note that patients with a clear indication for pulmonary artery catheter placement were excluded from this trial. Based upon these study results, the routine use of invasive monitoring is not recommended. However, invasive hemodynamic monitoring often provides essential information to achieve optimal drug therapy for patients with a confusing or complicated clinical picture and during dose titration of rapidly acting medications. Such invasive monitoring should be considered for patients who are refractory to initial therapy, whose volume status is unclear, or who have clinically significant hypotension such as a systolic blood pressure less than 80 mmHg or worsening renal function despite therapy. In addition, documentation of adequate hemodynamic response to inotropic therapy is often necessary prior to committing to chronic outpatient inotropic therapy.[9] Finally, assessment of hemodynamic parameters is required to document adequate reversal of pulmonary hypertension prior to cardiac transplantation.[15]

Invasive hemodynamic monitoring is usually performed with a flow-directed pulmonary artery (PA) or Swan-Ganz catheter placed percutaneously through a central vein and advanced through the right side of the heart and into the PA. Inflation of a balloon proximal to the end port allows the catheter to "wedge," yielding the pulmonary artery occlusion pressure, which estimates the pulmonary venous (left atrial) pressure and, in the absence of intracardiac shunt, mitral valve disease, or pulmonary disease, the left ventricular end diastolic pressure. While the term pulmonary artery occlusion pressure has been utilized in the distant past to describe the filling pressure of the heart, the term *pulmonary capillary wedge pressure* (PCWP) is used more commonly in clinical practice and thus will be used henceforth throughout this chapter. The PCWP is a useful marker of volume status with an elevated

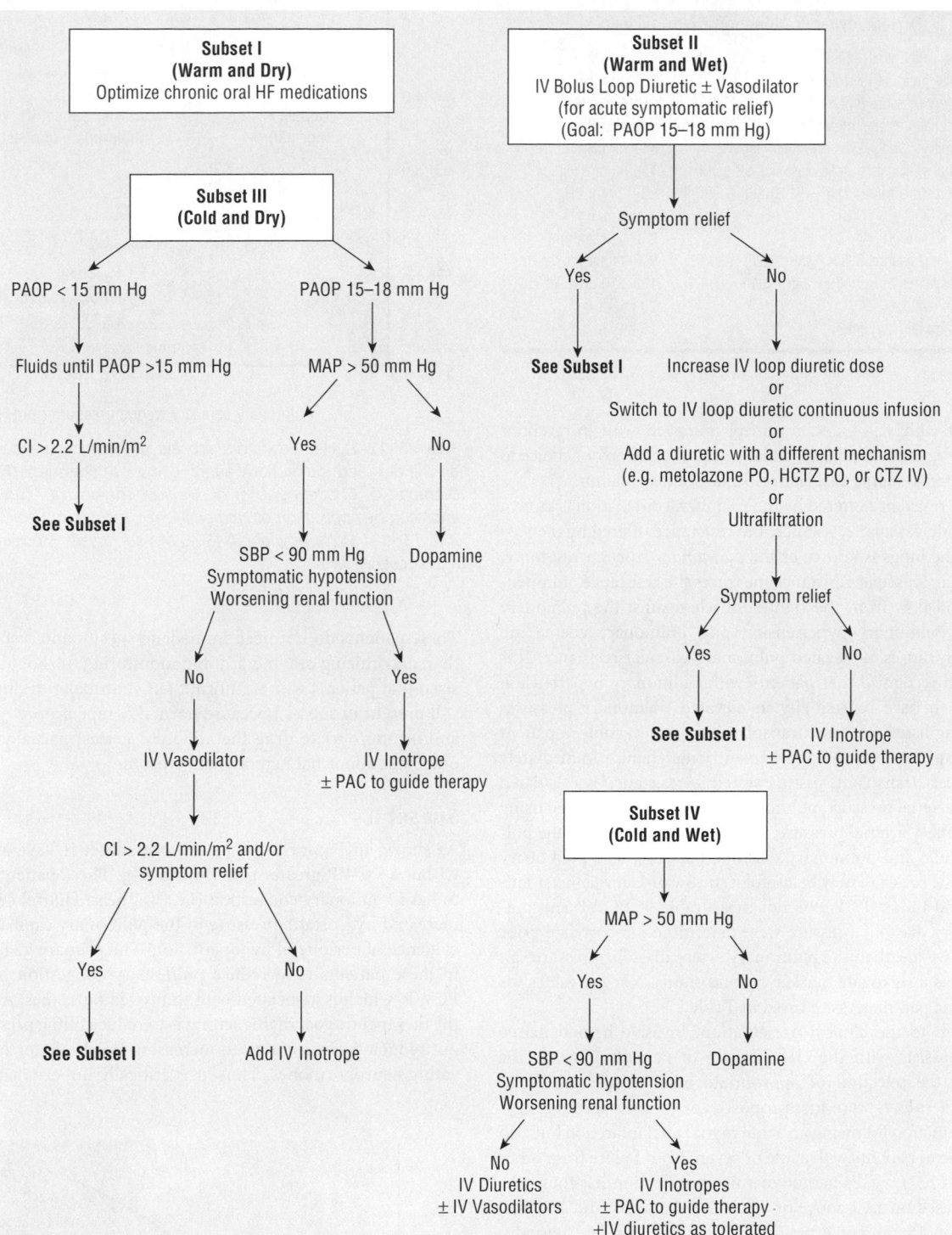

FIGURE 22-1. General treatment algorithm for ADHF based on clinical presentation. IV vasodilators that may be used include nitroglycerin, nesiritide, or nitroprusside. Metolazone or spironolactone may be added if the patient fails to respond to loop diuretics and a second diuretic is required. IV inotropes that may be used include dobutamine or milrinone. *(Reprinted from J Cardiac Fail, Vol 12(1), Heart Failure Society of America, HFSA 2006 Comprehensive Heart Failure Practice Guideline, e120–e122, Copyright © 2006, with permission from Elsevier.)*

PCWP in fluid overload and a reduced PCWP in dehydration. Cardiac output may be measured and represents the volume of blood being pumped by the heart, in particular by the left ventricle, in a minute. Cardiac index (CI) relates the cardiac output to body surface area, thus relating heart performance to the size of the individual. Systemic vascular resistance is calculated using cardiac output and thus is inversely related to cardiac output. Mixed venous oxygen saturation represents the end result of both oxygen delivery and consumption at the tissue level.

The systemic vascular resistance measures the afterload or resistance applied to the left ventricle and is the force impeding the ejection of blood from the left ventricle. The systemic vascular resistance may also be referred to as the *total peripheral resistance*. Vasoconstriction (i.e., decrease in blood vessel diameter) increases vascular resistance, whereas vasodilation (i.e., increase in diameter) decreases resistance. An elevated systemic vascular resistance is common with untreated or decompensated heart failure and is generally responsive to oral or intravenous arterial vasodilators, while reduction in resistance

TABLE 22-3	Hemodynamic Monitoring: Normal Values
Central venous (right atrial) pressure, mean, CVP	<5 mm Hg
Right ventricular pressure (systolic/diastolic)	25/0 mm Hg
Pulmonary artery pressure (systolic/diastolic), PAS/PAD	25/10 mm Hg
Pulmonary arterial pressure, mean, PAP	<18 mm Hg
Pulmonary capillary wedge pressure, mean, PCWP	<12 mm Hg
Systemic arterial pressure (systolic/diastolic), SBP/DBP	120/80 mm Hg
Mean arterial pressure, MAP = DBP + [(1/3)(SBP − DBP)]	90–110 mm Hg
Cardiac output, CO	4–6 L/min
Cardiac index, CI = CO/BSA	2.8–4.2 L/min/m²
Systemic vascular resistance, SVR = (MAP − CVP) × 80/CO	900–1400 dyne.sec/cm⁵
Pulmonary vascular resistance, PVR = (PAP − CVP) × 80/CO	150–250 dyne.sec/cm⁵
Arterial oxygen content	20 mL/dL
Mixed venous oxygen content	15 mL/dL

BSA, body surface area

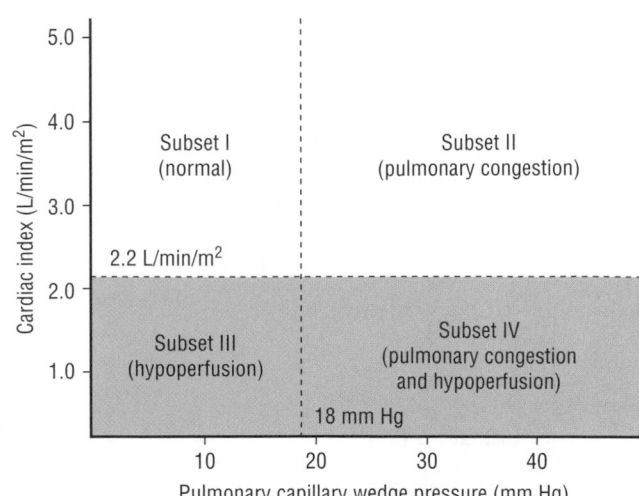

FIGURE 22-2. Hemodynamic subsets of heart failure based on cardiac index and pulmonary artery occlusion pressure. (*Forrester, JS, Diamond G, Chatterjee K, et al. Medical Therapy of Acute Myocardial Infarction by Application of Hemodynamic Subsets. N Engl J Med 1976; 295:1356–1362. Copyright ©1976 Massachusetts Medical Society. All rights reserverd.*)

is consistent with sepsis and routinely managed with intravenous vasopressive agents. Arterial vasodilators are the therapy of choice to reduce elevated systemic vascular resistance in heart failure.

While the resistance offered by the peripheral circulation is known as the systemic vascular resistance, the resistance offered by the vasculature of the lungs is known as the *pulmonary vascular resistance*. The pulmonary vascular resistance measures the resistance or impedance of blood flow from the right ventricle against the pulmonary circulation. Pulmonary hypertension and pulmonary edema are two common causes of elevated pulmonary vascular resistance. It is important to recognize that patients with pulmonary hypertension must prove to have reversibility in elevated pulmonary pressures prior to being listed for heart transplant. If not reversible, a patient will likely experience isolated right ventricular failure immediately following heart transplant. Just as systemic resistance is calculated using mean arterial pressure, pulmonary resistance is calculated using mean pulmonary arterial pressure, which is calculated using the pulmonary systolic and pulmonary diastolic pressure. The pulmonary artery diastolic pressure may be useful if the Swan-Ganz catheter fails to wedge, and thus a PCWP is not measurable. If PCWP and pulmonary artery diastolic pressure were determined to correlate prior to failure to wedge, then the pulmonary artery diastolic pressure can be followed as a surrogate marker of fluid status. Normal values for hemodynamic parameters are listed in Table 22–3.

In addition to the clinical presentation, invasive hemodynamic monitoring assists with the classification of patients into specific subsets and the selection of appropriate medical therapy. These *hemodynamic subsets* were first proposed for patients with left ventricular dysfunction following an acute myocardial infarction but also are applicable to patients with acute or severe heart failure from other causes (Fig. 22–2).[21] This hemodynamic classification has four subsets and is based on a CI above or below 2.2 L/min/m² and a PCWP above or below 18 mm Hg. A treatment algorithm, based on hemodynamic subsets, is provided in Figure 22–1. In addition to utilizing the above profiles or categories to stratify patients with decompensated heart failure, these four hemodynamic profiles are predictive for outcome with patients in the wet-warm profile having a twofold greater risk of death and those in the wet-cold profile having a 2.5-fold increased risk of death at 1 year compared to dry-warm patients.[15] It is important to note that patients may experience compromised cardiac index in the setting of significant fluid overload and cardiac index may improve as diuresis occurs. The underlying mechanism for how increasing fluid overload further worsens cardiac function is not clearly understood and is depicted in Figure 22–3.

Subset I

Patients in hemodynamic subset I have a CI and PCWP within generally acceptable ranges and have the lowest mortality of any subset.

These patients do not need immediate specific interventions other than maximizing oral therapy and monitoring. It should be emphasized that patients with significant left ventricular dysfunction may still present in subset I because normal compensatory mechanisms and/or appropriate drug therapy may at least partially correct an otherwise abnormal hemodynamic profile.

Subset II

As shown in Figure 22–2, patients in subset II have an adequate CI but a PCWP greater than 18 mm Hg. These patients are likely to have pulmonary congestion (i.e., wet heart failure) secondary to increased hydrostatic pressure in the pulmonary capillaries but no evidence of peripheral hypoperfusion. The primary goal of therapy in these patients is to reduce pulmonary congestion by lowering PCWP, which is associated with improved outcomes. Accordingly, the therapeutic goal in this setting is to reduce filling pressures without reducing cardiac output, increasing heart rate, or further activating neurohormones. Thus, it is critically important that PCWP

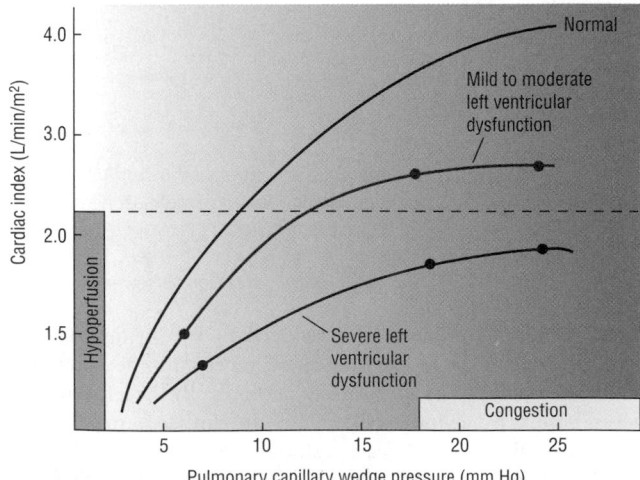

FIGURE 22-3. Relationship between cardiac output (shown as cardiac index, which is CO/BSA) and preload (shown as pulmonary capillary wedge pressure).

not be decreased excessively so as to cause a significant decline in cardiac output. Although the normal range of PCWP is 5 to 12 mm Hg for individuals without cardiac dysfunction, higher pressures of 15 to 18 mm Hg commonly are necessary for heart failure patients to optimize CI. Generally, the PCWP can be lowered to the range of 15 to 18 mm Hg with relatively little decrease in cardiac output because the Frank–Starling curve is flatter at higher PCWP values for patients with heart failure. The Frank–Starling curve in normal and heart failure patients is depicted in Figure 22–3. It is important to note that cardiac output also declines when the PCWP desired in a heart failure patient (i.e., PCWP 15 to 18 mm Hg) is exceeded. This phenomenon may explain why patients may experience enhanced diuresis and improved renal function when the PCWP range of 15 to 18 mm Hg is achieved in a heart failure patient with fluid overload. Intravenous administration of agents that reduce preload (i.e., loop diuretics, nitroglycerin, or nesiritide) are the most appropriate acute therapy to achieve the therapeutic goal for patients in subset II. Despite a very rapid onset with diuretic therapy, the time required for adequate enough diuresis to allow for significant improvement in oxygenation with intravenous loop diuretics may take several hours in select patients. Thus, intravenous nitroglycerin and nesiritide may be utilized for rapid venodilation, which can acutely aid in improving hypoxia.[8]

Current guidelines recommend loop diuretics as first-line therapy for management of heart failure patients admitted with fluid overload and that such agents should typically be administered intravenously.[5,9] The rate of diuresis should achieve a desirable volume status without causing a rapid reduction in intravascular volume resulting in symptomatic hypotension or renal dysfunction. Electrolyte depletion should be monitored for closely, especially when high dose or diuretic combination therapy is utilized. In addition to sodium restriction (less than 2 g daily), supplemental oxygen should be administered as needed for hypoxemia. For patients with moderate hyponatremia (less than 130 mEq/L), fluid restriction (less than 2 L daily) should be considered, and for patients with worsening or severe hyponatremia (less than 125 mEq/L), stricter fluid restriction may be necessary.[5,9] The arginine vasopressin (AVP) antagonists are a new class of agents indicated for the management of euvolemic or hypervolemic hyponatremia in a variety of disease states including heart failure.[22] The currently available vasopressin antagonists are discussed in greater detail later in this chapter.

Intravenous vasodilators may be considered in addition to diuretics for rapid symptom resolution and may be especially useful for patients with acute pulmonary edema or severe hypertension as well as for patients who fail to respond to aggressive treatment with diuretics. It is essential to avoid use of vasodilators for patients with symptomatic hypotension, and frequent blood pressure monitoring is essential for the safe use of these agents. In addition, these agents should not be used for patients with reduced left heart filling pressures. If symptomatic hypotension occurs with vasodilator therapy, the dose should be reduced or the agent discontinued. If patients fail to respond to the above therapies or experience worsening renal function, intravenous inotropic therapy should be considered.[9]

Subset III

Patients in hemodynamic subset III have a CI of less than 2.2 L/min/m² but without an abnormally elevated PCWP (Fig. 22–2). These patients usually will present without evidence of pulmonary congestion, but low cardiac output will result in signs and symptoms of peripheral hypoperfusion (i.e., decreased urine output, weakness, peripheral vasoconstriction, weak pulses). The mortality rate of subset III patients is reported to be higher than that of patients without hypoperfusion.[21] Although the treatment goal is to alleviate signs

and symptoms of hypoperfusion by increasing CI and perfusion to essential organs, therapy will differ among patients. If the PCWP is significantly below 15 mm Hg, initial therapy will be to administer intravenous fluids to provide a more optimal left ventricular filling pressure of 15 to 18 mm Hg and consequently improve CI. When there is only mild left ventricular dysfunction, intravenous fluid administration may be all that is necessary to achieve a CI above 2.2 L/min/m². However, many patients will have significant left ventricular dysfunction and a depressed Frank–Starling relationship despite adequate preload (i.e., PCWP of 15 to 18 mm Hg). In these patients, intravenous administration of positive inotropic agents (e.g., dobutamine, milrinone) and/or arterial vasodilators (e.g., nitroprusside or nitroglycerin) is often necessary to achieve an adequate CI. It is noteworthy that some positive inotropic medications also will have arterial vasodilating activity (see specific drug classes that follow).

Current guidelines recommend intravenous inotropes for symptom relief or end-organ dysfunction for patients with left ventricular dysfunction and low cardiac output syndrome.[5,9] Such therapy may be especially useful for patients with low systolic blood pressure (less than 90 mm Hg) or symptomatic hypotension in the setting of adequate filling pressures. As previously discussed (see Subset II), inotropic therapy may be considered for patients who do not tolerate or respond to intravenous vasodilators or patients with worsening renal function. As with vasodilators, inotrope administration requires frequent blood pressure monitoring as well as continuous monitoring for arrhythmias. If arrhythmias arise, dose reduction or discontinuation of inotropic therapy should occur. As with vasodilators, these agents should be avoided for patients with low left heart filling pressures. Given the potential risks associated with inotropic therapy, vasodilators should be considered prior to using inotropes.[9]

In general, inotropic therapy should not be used widely in the decompensated heart failure population. They are useful to increase cardiac output in the specific patients described above. These agents may be used to "bridge" patients to heart transplantation or left ventricular assist device. Inotropes may also be utilized as palliative therapy to improve functional status and quality of life for patients who are not considered optimal candidates for these definitive therapies.[9]

Subset IV

Patients with a CI of less than 2.2 L/min/m² and a PCWP higher than 18 mm Hg are in hemodynamic subset IV. These patients have the worst prognosis of any subset and illustrate the typical hemodynamic profile for the patient hospitalized for end-stage heart failure. Because of severe pump failure, these patients cannot maintain an adequate CI despite the elevated left ventricular filling pressure and increased myocardial fiber stretch. These patients will present with signs and symptoms of both congestion and hypoperfusion. The treatment goals are to alleviate these signs and symptoms by increasing CI above 2.2 L/min/m² and reducing PCWP to 15 to 18 mm Hg while maintaining an adequate mean arterial pressure. Thus, therapy will involve a combination of agents used for subset II and subset III patients to achieve these goals (i.e., combination of diuretic plus positive inotrope). These targets may be difficult to achieve and will necessitate careful monitoring and individualization of drug therapy. Nitroprusside may be a particularly useful agent in this setting because of its mixed arterial–venous vasodilating effects. In the presence of significant hypotension and low mean arterial pressures, inotropic agents with vasopressor activity (e.g., dopamine) may be required initially to achieve an adequate perfusion pressure to essential organs and can then be combined, if necessary, with diuretics and/or therapies to obtain the desired hemodynamic effects and clinical response.

TABLE 22-4 Usual Hemodynamic Effects of Intravenous Agents Commonly Used for Treatment of Advanced or Decompensated Heart Failure[a]

Drug	Dose	HR	MAP	PCWP	CO	SVR
Dopamine	0.5–3 mcg/kg/min	0	0	0	0/+	–
Dopamine	3–10 mcg/kg/min	+	+	0	+	0
Dopamine	10–20 mcg/kg/min	+	+	+	+	+
Dobutamine	2.5–20 mcg/kg/min	0/+	0	–	+	–
Milrinone	0.1–0.75 mcg/kg/min	0/+	0/–	–	+	–
Nitroprusside	0.25–3 mcg/kg/min	0/+	0/–	–	+	–
Nitroglycerin	5–200 mcg/min	0/+	0/–	–	0/+	0/–
Furosemide	20–80 mg IVB (<4 mg/min)[b] 2–3 times/day or 0.1 mg/kg/h CI	0	0/–	–	0	0
Enalaprilat	1.25–2.5 mg every 6–8 h	0	0/–	–	+	–
Nesiritide	2 mcg/kg IVB; 0.01 mcg/kg/min	0	0/–	–	+	–

[a]See text for a more detailed description of the interpatient variability in response.
[b]Intravenous bolus administered <4 mg/min.
Abbreviations: +, increase; –, decrease; 0, no change; HR, heart rate; MAP, mean arterial pressure; PCWP, pulmonary capillary wedge pressure; CI, continuous infusion; CO, cardiac output; IVB, intravenous bolus; SVR, systemic vascular resistance.

PHARMACOLOGIC THERAPY OF ACUTE DECOMPENSATED HEART FAILURE

6 Unfortunately, the treatment of decompensated heart failure has not improved substantially in the past decade due in large part to the lack of clinical trial data in this population. The pharmacotherapeutic agents used to treat patients with decompensated heart failure rarely, if ever, produce a single cardiovascular action. Even when intended for a single purpose (e.g., a positive inotrope), other drug effects (tachycardia, vasodilation, or vasoconstriction) may either add to the therapeutic effect or cause adverse events that negate or even outweigh the intended therapeutic benefit. It often can be difficult to anticipate how an individual patient will respond to a given intervention. For this reason, hemodynamic monitoring can be useful, and many drugs are considered first-line therapy due in part to their short half-lives and ease of titration. The description of expected drug actions outlined below should be viewed as a general guide to the clinician, who must continuously reassess the patient for desired outcomes. Table 22–4 contains a summary of the expected hemodynamic effects of the various drugs discussed in the following sections.

DIURETICS[23-26]

7 Intravenous loop diuretics, including furosemide, bumetanide, and torsemide, are used in the management of decompensated heart failure, with furosemide being the most widely studied and used agent in this setting. Bolus administration of diuretics reduces preload within 5 to 15 minutes by functional venodilation and later (>20 minutes) via sodium and water excretion, thereby improving pulmonary congestion. However, the acute reduction in venous return may severely compromise effective preload for patients with significant diastolic dysfunction or intravascular depletion or for those whose CI are significantly dependent on adequate filling pressure (i.e., preload dependent). This reduction in preload may result in a reflex elevation in renin, norepinephrine, and AVP and the expected consequences of arteriolar and coronary constriction, tachycardia, and increased myocardial oxygen consumption. Unlike arterial dilators and positive inotropic agents, diuretics do

not cause an upward shift in the Frank–Starling curve or increase CI significantly in most patients (Table 22–4 and Fig. 22–3). In contrast, excessive preload reduction with diuretics, specifically diuresis to PCWP less than 15 mm Hg, can lead to a decline in cardiac output (Fig. 22–3). Furthermore, intravascular depletion may occur in the setting of rapid diuresis despite continued relative total body fluid overload, and thus, daily diuresis goals must be highly individualized. Most patients tolerate a 2 L/day net negative diuresis. However, some end-stage patients, especially those who are malnourished due to early satiety, will only tolerate a 1 L/day net negative diuresis. Thus, diuretics must be used judiciously to obtain the desired improvement in symptoms of congestion while avoiding a reduction in cardiac output, symptomatic hypotension, or worsening renal function. Although counter intuitive, patients with excessive fluid overload may experience compromised cardiac output, and this may improve with diuresis once PCWP reach more near normal ranges. This concept was described earlier in the chapter (Fig. 22–3) and may explain why renal function occasionally improves in the setting of diuresis.

Diuretic Resistance

Occasionally, patients respond poorly to large doses of loop diuretics, and heart failure is the most common clinical setting in which diuretic resistance is observed. Multiple retrospective analyses suggest that diuretics, especially aggressive diuretic administration, may be harmful. The use of diuretics is associated with a dose-dependent increase in mortality.[27] Recent evidence also suggests that high diuretic doses are associated with a decline in renal function in decompensated heart failure,[25,28] which further exacerbates diuretic resistance. Thus, the need for increased exposure to diuretics in the setting of diuretic resistance is concerning.

The mechanisms responsible for diuretic resistance in heart failure patients appear to be both pharmacokinetic and pharmacodynamic.[29] The bioavailability of furosemide is relatively normal in heart failure patients, but the rate of absorption is prolonged approximately twofold, and peak concentrations are reduced approximately 50%. Because loop diuretics have a sigmoidal-shaped urine concentration-response curve, prolonged absorption may result in concentrations that fail to reach the steep portion of this curve, resulting in diminished responsiveness. Despite normal pharmacokinetics following intravenous administration, diuretic resistance is also observed with this route, suggesting an important pharmacodynamic component to diuretic resistance. The decreased responsiveness in heart failure patients is explained in part by the high concentrations of sodium reaching the distal tubule as a result of the blockade of sodium reabsorption in the loop of Henle. As a consequence, the distal tubule hypertrophies, increasing its ability to reabsorb sodium. In addition, neurohormonal activation, low cardiac output, reduced renal perfusion, and subsequent decreased delivery of drug to the kidney may also contribute to resistance.

Several maneuvers can be attempted to overcome diuretic resistance. Current guidelines support one of three options for managing patients who do not initially respond to diuretic therapy.[5,9] First, larger intravenous bolus doses of loop diuretics may achieve concentrations closer to the top of the concentration-response curve. Second a continuous intravenous infusion may be used to maintain more constant concentrations in the steep portion of this curve. Initial studies of continuous-infusion furosemide suggest a greater natriuretic effect and no difference in metabolic adverse effects when compared with the same total daily dose given by intravenous bolus.[9,26,30] More recently, Thomson et al conducted a prospective, randomized, parallel-group study comparing continuous intravenous with intermittent intravenous infusion of furosemide in 56 patients with decompensated heart failure.[31] The primary end point of the study was net urine output (nUOP) per 24 hours, which was 2098 ± 1132 mL with continuous dosing of intravenous furosemide versus 1575 ± 1100 mL with intermittent dosing ($P = 0.086$). The continuous dosing group had significantly greater total urine output ($P = 0.019$), although mean weight loss was not significantly different between the groups. The continuous dosing group did experience a shorter length of hospital stay ($P = 0.006$). A larger study, the DOSE-AHF Trial, is ongoing and will compare four study arms: low dose and high dose intermittent dosing and low dose and high dose continuous infusion.

Third, a second diuretic with a different mechanism of action can be administered. Combining a loop diuretic with a distal tubule blocker such as oral metolazone, oral hydrochlorothiazide, or intravenous chlorothiazide can produce a synergistic diuretic effect. The synergism is not a pharmacokinetic interaction but is related to the increased delivery of sodium to the distal convoluted tubule. Enhanced sodium delivery to (and reabsorption in) the distal tubule can then be blocked by the thiazide-type diuretic. Thus, when thiazide-type diuretics are added to a loop diuretic, they block more than their normal 5% to 8% of filtered sodium, and the combination results in synergistic natriuresis. The loop diuretic–thiazide combination generally should be reserved for the inpatient setting, where the patient can be monitored closely given the increased likelihood of a more profound diuresis with severe electrolyte and volume depletion. When used in the outpatient setting, very low doses or only occasional doses of the thiazide-type diuretic should be used along with close follow-up (e.g., weight, vital signs, serum potassium, dizziness) to avoid serious adverse events.

Current guidelines support each of the three options described above for managing patients who do not initially respond to diuretic therapy. Further restricting sodium and fluid (e.g., less than 1 g and less than 1 L per day, respectively) beyond that which is routine may also prove useful in managing diuretic refractory patients. Such severe fluid restrictions will also be helpful in managing moderate to severe hyponatremia. Ultrafiltration is an additional therapeutic option in the diuretic refractory patient. This topic is discussed within the section of Mechanical Circulatory Support.

Treatment of heart failure with other agents (e.g., positive inotropes or arterial vasodilators) may improve diuresis by increasing cardiac output and renal perfusion. As previously discussed, given the adverse effects of inotropic therapy, this option is generally reserved for patients not responding to all other therapies or those with apparent low cardiac output. Administration of low doses of dopamine with the hope of enhancing diuresis was previously common practice. However, data suggest that addition of dopamine to furosemide provides no additional diuresis.[32]

POSITIVE INOTROPIC AGENTS[33,34]

8 Drugs that increase intracellular cyclic adenosine monophosphate (cAMP) are the only positive inotropic agents currently approved for the treatment of acute heart failure. β-agonists activate adenylate cyclase through stimulation of β-adrenergic receptors, with the enzyme then catalyzing the conversion of adenosine triphosphate to cAMP. Phosphodiesterase inhibitors raise cAMP concentrations by reducing its degradation. Thus, both drug classes increase intracellular cAMP, which enhances phospholipase (and subsequently phosphorylase) activity, increasing the rate and extent of calcium influx during systole and enhancing contractility. Additionally, cAMP enhances reuptake of calcium by the sarcoplasmic reticulum during diastole, improving active relaxation. The receptor activities of the β-agonists are summarized in Table 22–5. Although rarely used in management of heart failure, the receptor effects of epinephrine, norepinephrine, and isoproterenol are provided for reference.

TABLE 22-5	Relative Effects of Adrenergic Drugs on Receptors			
Drug	α_1	β_1	β_2	**Dopamine₁**
Dopamine[a]	++++	++++	++	++
Epinephrine	++++	++++	++	0
Norepinephrine	++++	++++	0	0
Phenylephrine	++++	0	0	0
Dobutamine	+	++++	++	0
Isoproterenol	0	++++	++++	0

[a]See text for a more detailed description of the dose-dependent hemodynamic effects.

Digoxin has little, if any, place in the acute treatment of patients with decompensated heart failure who are hemodynamically unstable. The delay in peak inotropic effect, limited inotropic effect, long duration of action, and potential toxicity (arrhythmic, neurologic) are disadvantages in the acute setting. However, for patients with acute decompensation who are taking digoxin as part of their chronic therapy, it is generally unnecessary to adjust the dose or discontinue its use unless changes in renal function increase the risk of toxicity.

Although a number of parenteral agents have been used for the treatment of patients with decompensated heart failure, dobutamine and milrinone have emerged as the two drugs most commonly administered. These drugs differ in their mechanism of action and resulting pharmacologic effects and provide advantages and disadvantages in any given patient.

Dobutamine

Dobutamine, a synthetic catecholamine, is a β_1- and β_2-receptor agonist with some α_1-agonist effects (Table 22–5). Unlike dopamine, dobutamine does not cause release of norepinephrine from nerve terminals. The positive inotropy is primarily a β_1-receptor mediated effect. Cardiac β_1-receptor stimulation by dobutamine causes an increase in contractility but generally no significant change in heart rate and may provide an explanation for the apparently more modest chronotropic actions of dobutamine compared with dopamine. The overall hemodynamic effects of dobutamine are the result of its effects on adrenergic receptors and reflex-mediated actions. Modest peripheral β_2-receptor-mediated vasodilation will tend to offset minor α_1-receptor-mediated vasoconstriction with dobutamine. In addition, the increase in cardiac output will often cause a reflexive decline in systemic vascular resistance. Thus the net vascular effect is usually vasodilation.

The overall hemodynamic effects of dobutamine are those of a potent inotropic agent with vasodilating action. Initial doses of 2.5 to 5 mcg/kg per minute can be increased progressively to 20 mcg/kg/min based on clinical and hemodynamic responses. The onset of action is within minutes; however, peak effects may take 10 minutes to become evident. Dobutamine has a half-life of 2 minutes. Cardiac index is increased because of inotropic stimulation, arterial vasodilation, and a variable increase in heart rate. Because of the offsetting changes in arteriolar resistance and CI, dobutamine usually will cause relatively little change in mean arterial pressure, although these effects may be variable. This is compared with the more consistent increase observed with dopamine. Dobutamine's vasodilating action usually reduces PCWP, making it particularly useful in the presence of low CI and an elevated left ventricular filling pressure, or detrimental in the presence of a reduced filling pressure. Unfortunately, an increase in oxygen consumption with dobutamine has been demonstrated for patients with both ischemic and nonischemic cardiomyopathy. The major adverse effect of dobutamine is tachycardia. While concern over attenuation of dobutamine's hemodynamic effects has been raised with prolonged administration, some effect is likely still retained. Thus, dobutamine dose should be tapered rather than abruptly discontinued.

For some patients, dobutamine (or milrinone) dose reduction or discontinuation results in acute decompensation, and these patients may then require placement of an indwelling intravenous catheter for continuous therapy. This approach may be used to "bridge" patients awaiting cardiac transplantation or left ventricular assist device and may also be used to facilitate the discharge of patients who are not transplant candidates but who cannot be weaned from inotrope therapy. In this latter group, the use of continuous outpatient dobutamine therapy is for palliative use and should only be considered after multiple unsuccessful attempts to maximize oral therapy and discontinue inotrope therapy. Although effective for symptom palliation, it should be realized that the risk of mortality is likely increased. In contrast, the use of regularly scheduled intermittent dobutamine infusions is not recommended in the current guidelines.[5,9]

Milrinone

Milrinone is a bipyridine derivative that inhibits phosphodiesterase III, an enzyme responsible for the breakdown of cAMP to AMP. Milrinone has supplanted the use of amrinone, the prototype drug for milrinone, given the more frequent occurrence of thrombocytopenia with amrinone. Milrinone's positive inotropic, arterial vasodilating, and venous vasodilating effects contribute to the therapeutic response in heart failure patients; hence, milrinone has been referred to as an *inodilator*. The relative balance of these pharmacologic effects may vary with dose and underlying cardiovascular pathology.

During intravenous administration, there is an increase in stroke volume (and, therefore, cardiac output) with little change in heart rate (Table 22–4). Despite the increase in CI, mean arterial pressure may remain constant due to a concomitant decrease in arteriolar resistance. In contrast, the vasodilating effects may predominate and lead to a decrease in blood pressure and a reflex tachycardia. Like dobutamine, milrinone lowers PCWP by venodilation and thus is particularly useful for patients with a low CI and an elevated left ventricular filling pressure. Such a reduction in preload, however, can be hazardous for patients without excessive filling pressure (especially those with subset III heart failure), leading to further decline in CI. Such an effect would blunt the improvement in cardiac output that would otherwise be produced by the positive inotropic and arterial dilating actions. Milrinone should be used cautiously as a single agent in severely hypotensive heart failure patients because it will not increase, and may even decrease, arterial blood pressure. The results of controlled studies comparing dobutamine with milrinone indicate that these agents produce generally similar hemodynamic effects. A clinically insignificant but greater increase in heart rate with dobutamine is the most consistent difference in these studies.

Milrinone has a longer terminal elimination half-life than other adrenergic agonists. The average milrinone half-life in healthy subjects is about 1 hour and approximately 3 hours for patients with heart failure. This long elimination half-life may be a disadvantage in this patient population because a loading dose may be necessary to obtain a prompt initial response, minute-to-minute titrations in dose cannot be made based on response, and adverse effects (arrhythmias or hypotension) will persist longer after drug discontinuation. The usual loading dose for milrinone is 50 mcg/kg administered over 10 minutes. However, if rapid hemodynamic changes are not necessary, the loading dose should be eliminated given an increased risk of hypotension. Thus, most patients are simply started on the maintenance infusion without a preceding

bolus dose. Lower initial doses, such as 0.1 mcg/kg/min, may be considered. The maintenance infusion for milrinone is commonly 0.1 to 0.3 mcg/kg/min (up to 0.75 mcg/kg/min). Milrinone is excreted unchanged in urine, and thus, its infusion rate should be decreased by 50% to 70% for patients with significant renal impairment.

The most notable adverse events associated with milrinone are arrhythmia, hypotension, and thrombocytopenia. While the incidence of thrombocytopenia associated with milrinone therapy is rare, patients should still have platelet counts determined before and during therapy.

The combination of dobutamine and milrinone would be expected to produce additive effects on CI and PCWP reduction, suggesting this regimen as an option for patients who have dose-limiting adverse effects with either drug class. It is unclear, however, if this combination provides a therapeutic advantage over the combination of a positive inotrope and a traditional pure vasodilator such as nitroprusside.

One study with milrinone points out the risk associated with routine administration of inotropic therapy to a broad population of patients admitted to the hospital for decompensated heart failure. Although this approach is not supported by clinical trial data, many patients without signs or symptoms of hypoperfusion receive milrinone or other inotropic therapy with the belief that the hemodynamic effects may shorten hospitalization and improve clinical outcomes. Designed to evaluate this strategy, the Outcomes of a Prospective Trial of Intravenous Milrinone for Exacerbations of Chronic Heart Failure (OPTIME-CHF) trial was a randomized, double-blind trial comparing the effects of milrinone and placebo for patients hospitalized with an acute exacerbation of chronic heart failure who, in the investigator's opinion, did not require inotropic therapy.[7] The 949 patients received a 48-hour infusion of milrinone 0.5 mcg/kg/min with no loading dose or placebo. No difference between milrinone and placebo was found in the primary end point, the number of days patients were hospitalized for cardiovascular causes within 60 days of randomization. However, adverse events were more common in the milrinone group. Sustained hypotension requiring intervention (10.7% vs 3.2%; $P < 0.001$) and new onset of atrial fibrillation or flutter (4.6% vs 1.5%; $P = 0.004$) occurred more frequently for patients receiving milrinone.

Recently, data from the ADHERE Registry ($n = 15,230$) was used to compare in-hospital mortality with intravenous nitroglycerin, nesiritide, milrinone, or dobutamine. After adjusting for baseline parameters that predict in-hospital mortality, both dobutamine- and milrinone-treated patients had a higher in-hospital mortality when compared to patients receiving either nitroglycerin or nesiritide ($P < 0.005$). There was no difference in in-hospital mortality between nitroglycerin- and nesiritide-treated patients ($P = 0.58$). In-hospital mortality was higher for patients receiving dobutamine compared to milrinone ($P = 0.027$).[35]

These results add to the growing concern regarding the use of inotropic drugs for patients with decompensated heart failure and strongly suggest that milrinone, and probably other inotropes, should not be routinely used for the treatment of acute heart failure exacerbations. Although the routine use of milrinone should be discouraged, clinicians should be aware that inotropic therapy may be needed in selected patients such as those with low cardiac output states with organ hypoperfusion or with cardiogenic shock.[5,9] Generally, milrinone should be considered for patients who are receiving chronic β-blocker therapy because its positive inotropic effect does not involve stimulation of β-receptors. In contrast to dobutamine, milrinone's positive hemodynamic effects persist despite concomitant β-blocker therapy.

Dopamine

Although dopamine generally should be avoided in the treatment of decompensated heart failure, the only clinical scenario where its pharmacologic actions may be preferable to dobutamine or milrinone is for the patient with marked systemic hypotension or cardiogenic shock in the face of elevated ventricular filling pressures, where dopamine in doses greater than 5 mcg/kg/min may be necessary to raise central aortic pressure. However, there are no data to support this commonly employed practice.

Dopamine, the endogenous precursor of NE, exerts its effects by directly stimulating adrenergic receptors as well as causing release of NE from adrenergic nerve terminals. Dopamine produces dose-dependent hemodynamic effects because of its relative affinity for α_1-, β_1-, β_2-, and D1- (vascular dopaminergic) receptors (see Table 22–5). The following dose-dependent actions are intended as a general guide to the clinician.

Positive inotropic effects mediated primarily by β_1-receptors become more prominent with dopamine doses of 2 to 5 mcg/kg/min. Cardiac index is increased because of an increase in stroke volume and a variable increase in heart rate, which is partially dose dependent. There is usually little change in systemic vascular resistance, presumably because neither vasodilation (D1- and β_2-receptor-mediated) nor vasoconstriction (α_1-receptor-mediated) predominates. At doses between 5 to 10 mcg/kg/min, chronotropic and α_1-receptor-mediated vasoconstricting effects become more prominent. Mean arterial pressure usually increases due to an increase in both CI and systemic vascular resistance (Table 22–4). The vasoconstricting effects of higher doses could indirectly limit the increase in CI by increasing afterload and PCWP, thus complicating the management of patients with preexisting high afterload. For such patients, alternative agents (dobutamine, milrinone) or the addition of diuretics and/or vasodilators may be necessary.

Dopamine, particularly at higher doses, may alter several parameters that increase myocardial oxygen demand (increased heart rate, contractility, and systolic pressure) and potentially decrease myocardial blood flow (coronary vasoconstriction and increased wall tension), worsening ischemia in some patients with coronary disease. As with dobutamine and milrinone, arrhythmogenesis is also more common at higher doses.

VASODILATORS[25,36]

9 **10** As previously discussed, activation of the sympathetic nervous system, renin angiotensin system, and other mediators results in vasoconstriction and increased systemic vascular resistance as well as fluid retention and increased PCWP. The influence of individual vasodilators on these hemodynamic parameters varies depending on the unique properties of each agent (Fig. 22–4). Agent selection should be based upon individual patient presentation and, if available, hemodynamic parameters.

Vasodilators typically are described by their prominent site of action (arterial or venous). Arterial vasodilators act as impedance-reducing agents, reducing afterload and causing a reflexive increase in cardiac output. Venodilators act as preload reducers by increasing venous capacitance, reducing symptoms of pulmonary congestion for patients with high cardiac filling pressures. Mixed vasodilators act on both resistance and capacitance vessels, reducing congestive symptoms while increasing cardiac output. Nitroprusside, nitroglycerin, and nesiritide are the most commonly used intravenous vasodilating agents in decompensated heart failure.

Nitroprusside

Sodium nitroprusside, a mixed arterial–venous vasodilator, acts on vascular smooth muscle, increasing synthesis of nitric oxide

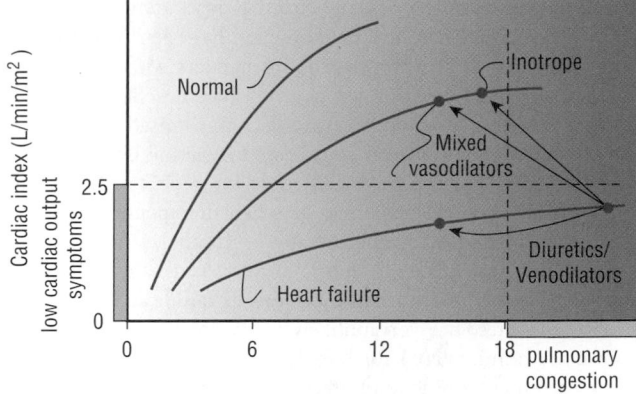

FIGURE 22-4. Relationship between cardiac output and pulmonary capillary wedge pressure. See text for more detailed description of how various vasodilators and inotropes influence these hemodynamic parameters.

to produce its balanced vasodilating action. As such, it increases CI and decreases venous pressure. Nitroprusside's effects on these parameters are qualitatively similar to those produced by dobutamine and phosphodiesterase inhibitors, despite the fact that it has no direct inotropic activity (Table 22–4). However, nitroprusside generally causes a greater decrease in PCWP, systemic vascular resistance, and blood pressure than these agents do. Mean arterial pressure may remain fairly constant but often decreases, depending on the relative increase in cardiac output and reduction in arteriolar tone. Hypotension is an important dose-limiting adverse effect of nitroprusside and other vasodilators. Therefore, this drug is used primarily for patients who have a significantly elevated systemic vascular resistance and often requires invasive hemodynamic monitoring.

Patients with normal left ventricular function will not experience an increase in stroke volume when systemic vascular resistance falls because the normal ventricle is fairly insensitive to small changes in afterload. Consequently, these patients experience a significant decrease in blood pressure after administration of arterial vasodilators. This explains why nitroprusside is a potent antihypertensive agent for patients without heart failure but causes less hypotension and reflex tachycardia for patients with left ventricular dysfunction. Nonetheless, even a modest increase in heart rate could have adverse consequences for patients with underlying ischemic heart disease and/or resting tachycardia, and close monitoring is necessary during therapy.

Nitroprusside has been studied extensively and shown to be effective in the short-term management of patients with severe heart failure in a variety of settings (i.e., acute MI, valvular regurgitation, after coronary bypass surgery, decompensated chronic heart failure). Generally, nitroprusside will not worsen, and may improve, the balance between myocardial oxygen demand and supply. This is mainly due to a decrease in oxygen demand caused by the lowering of left ventricular wall tension and a possible increase in subendocardial blood flow resulting from decreased left ventricular end-diastolic pressure. However, an excessive decrease in systemic arterial pressure can reduce coronary perfusion and worsen ischemia, leading to an increased risk of coronary steal.

Nitroprusside has a rapid onset of action and duration of action of less than 10 minutes, necessitating its administration by continuous intravenous infusion. This allows for precise dose titration based on measured clinical and hemodynamic parameters. It, like other vasodilators used in heart failure, should be initiated at a low dose (0.1 to 0.2 mcg/kg/min) to avoid excessive hypotension and then increased by small increments (0.1 to 0.2 mcg/kg/min) every 5 to 10 minutes as needed and tolerated. Usually effective doses range from 0.5 to 3.0 mcg/kg/min. A rebound phenomenon has been reported after abrupt withdrawal of nitroprusside for patients with heart failure and is apparently due to reflex neurohormonal activation during therapy. If renal perfusion pressure is compromised by the drug, salt and water retention can contribute to volume expansion and tachyphylaxis; this is seen typically only for patients with chronic hypertension, baseline azotemia, or when therapeutic augmentation of cardiac output during therapy is minimal. When stopping nitroprusside and switching to oral drugs, it is usually advisable to taper doses slowly. Nitroprusside can cause cyanide and thiocyanate toxicity, but these are very unlikely when doses less than 3 mcg/kg/min are administered for less than 3 days, except for patients with a serum creatinine level greater than 3 mg/dL. Nitroprusside should not be used in the presence of elevated intracranial pressure because it may worsen cerebral edema in this setting. Given the potent pulmonary vasodilator effects of nitroprusside as well as its short half-life, this agent is frequently used to determine reversibility of pulmonary hypertension for patients being assessed for heart transplantation. This is the most common use of nitroprusside for the management of decompensated heart failure.

Nitroglycerin

Intravenous nitroglycerin is often considered the preferred agent for preload reduction for patients with severe heart failure. Because of its short half-life, intravenous nitroglycerin is administered by continuous infusion. Its major hemodynamic actions are reductions in preload and PCWP via functional venodilation and mild arterial vasodilation that is particularly evident in patients with heart failure and elevated systemic vascular resistance or when given in doses approaching 200 mcg/min (Table 22–4). Intravenous nitroglycerin is used primarily as a preload reducer for patients with pulmonary congestion. In higher doses, nitroglycerin displays potent coronary vasodilating properties and beneficial effects on myocardial oxygen demand and supply, making it the vasodilator of choice for patients with severe heart failure and ischemic heart disease.

Nitroglycerin should be initiated at a dose of 5 to 10 mcg/min (0.1 mcg/kg/min) and increased every 5 to 10 minutes as necessary and tolerated. Hypotension and an excessive decrease in PCWP are important dose-limiting side effects. Maintenance doses usually vary from 35 to 200 mcg/min (0.5 to 3.0 mcg/kg/min). While tolerance to the hemodynamic effects of nitroglycerin may develop over 12 to 72 hours of continuous administration, some patients experience a sustained response. Like nitroprusside, nitroglycerin should not be used in the presence of elevated intracranial pressure because it may worsen cerebral edema in this setting.

Nesiritide

Nesiritide is the first new drug approved for the treatment of decompensated heart failure since milrinone. Manufactured by recombinant techniques, it is identical to the endogenous human BNP secreted by the ventricular myocardium in response to volume overload. Exogenous administration of nesiritide mimics the vasodilator and natriuretic actions of the endogenous peptide by stimulating the natriuretic peptide receptor A, which leads to increased levels of cGMP in target tissues. Nesiritide produces dose-dependent venous and arterial vasodilation, increases cardiac output, natriuresis, and diuresis, and decreases cardiac filling pressures, sympathetic nervous system, and renin–angiotensin–aldosterone system activity. Unlike nitroglycerin or dobutamine, tolerance does not develop to nesiritide's pharmacologic actions. It does not affect cAMP or stimulate β-receptors, mechanisms that are thought to contribute to the myocardial toxicity associated with the positive inotropic agents. Thus, nesiritide does not have the proarrhythmic

effects related with inotropic therapy. Nesiritide is eliminated by several pathways including the natriuretic peptide receptor C on target tissues, proteolytic cleavage by neutral endopeptidase, and renal filtration. Its elimination half-life of 18 minutes is considerably longer than that of other intravenous vasoactive agents.

The Vasodilation in the Management of Acute CHF (VMAC) trial was a randomized, double-blind trial that compared the effects of nesiritide, IV nitroglycerin, or placebo for patients with decompensated heart failure and dyspnea receiving standard background therapy.[8] Patients received pulmonary artery catheterization at the discretion of the investigators. The primary study end points were the patient's self-assessment of dyspnea (all patients) and the change in PCWP at 3 hours after the start of the study drug infusion (only for patients with a pulmonary artery catheter) compared to placebo. Nesiritide significantly reduced PCWP at 3 hours compared to placebo and nitroglycerin. Although nesiritide reduced dyspnea at 3 hours compared to placebo, no difference between nesiritide and nitroglycerin was found.

The precise role of nesiritide in the pharmacotherapy of decompensated heart failure remains controversial. Some of this controversy centers on the marginal lack of improvement in mortality or other clinical outcomes with nesiritide compared to nitroglycerin (or nitroprusside) balanced against nesiritide's significantly greater costs (~$450 for a 24-hour nesiritide infusion compared to $10 to $15 for nitroglycerin). In addition, two metaanalyses suggested an increased risk of negative outcomes with nesiritide: the first, an increased risk of worsening renal function and the second, an increased risk in mortality.[37,38] The authors of these studies concluded that these finding are hypothesis generating and should be further investigated. To clarify these issues about the safety and efficacy of nesiritide, its manufacturer is conducting an additional prospective randomized controlled trial, the Double-Blind, Placebo-Controlled, Multicenter Acute Study of Clinical Effectiveness of Nesiritide in Subjects With Decompensated Heart Failure (ASCEND-HF) trial.

VASOPRESSIN RECEPTOR ANTAGONISTS

⑪ Fluid balance depends on the relative concentrations of sodium and water. Abnormally low sodium concentrations or hyponatremia, commonly defined as a serum sodium less than 125 mmol/L, can arise from a variety of causes. Diuretic administration can cause hypovolemic hyponatremia or excessive water consumption or result in euvolemic hyponatremia (urine sodium less than 30 mmol/L), and heart failure can be associated with hypervolemic hyponatremia (urine sodium greater than 30 mmol/L). There are many other causes of hyponatremia including, but not limited to, syndrome of inappropriate diuretic hormone (SIADH), cirrhosis with ascites and certain medications.[39]

Hyponatremia is commonly characterized by inappropriately elevated concentrations of AVP, which is also known as *antidiuretic hormone*. In the setting of heart failure, excess total body volume exceeds excess total body sodium. Arterial baroreceptors stimulate increased AVP release and net water retention. While the prevalence of hyponatremia in heart failure varies with definition, the Acute and Chronic Therapeutic Impact of Vasopressin Antagonists in Heart Failure (ACTIV-HF) trial found that approximately 20% of patients admitted to the hospital for acute heart failure had hyponatremia, defined as a serum sodium less than 136 mmol/L.[40] Importantly, the presence of hyponatremia is associated with increased mortality in heart failure patients.[41]

While the majority of cases of hyponatremia are mild, asymptomatic, and self-limited, the primary concern is the less common but life-threatening presentation that may include lethargy, confusion, respiratory arrest, cerebral edema, seizures, and coma, which may result in death. Thus, prompt diagnosis and management is critical. Treatment is specific to the underlying etiology, duration of symptoms, and severity of symptoms. Treatment may include removal of the underlying cause, fluid restriction, isotonic or hypertonic saline administration, and/or administration of diuretics, vasopressin antagonists, or other therapies. Importantly, while neurological sequelae may occur if treatment is not initiated promptly, overly rapid correction of hyponatremia (greater than 12 mmol/L per 24 hours) results in the same.[42]

Currently available vasopressin receptor antagonists affect one or two AVP receptors, V_{1A} or V_2.[43] Present in the vascular smooth muscle cells and myocardium, stimulation of V_{1A} results in vasoconstriction as well as myocyte hypertrophy, coronary vasoconstriction, and positive inotropic effects. The V_2 receptors are present in the renal tubules where they regulate water reabsorption. Tolvaptan selectively binds to and inhibits the V_2 receptor, whereas conivaptan nonselectively inhibits both the V_{1A} and V_2 receptor. Tolvaptan is an oral agent indicated for hypervolemic and euvolemic hyponatremia for patients with SIADH, cirrhosis, and heart failure. Importantly, tolvaptan is a substrate of cytochrome P450-3A4 and contraindicated with potent inhibitors of this enzyme. Tolvaptan is typically initiated at 15 mg orally daily and then titrated to 30 or 60 mg as needed to resolve hyponatremia. Conivaptan is an intravenous agent indicated for hypervolemic and euvolemic hyponatremia due to a variety of causes; however, it is not indicated for hyponatremia associated with heart failure, and thus it will not be further discussed. Patients receiving either agent must be monitored closely to avoid an overly rapid rise in serum sodium. If serum sodium rises too rapidly, hypotension or hypovolemia can occur, and the vasopressin antagonist should be discontinued. Therapy may be restarted at a lower dose if hyponatremia recurs or persists and/or these side effects resolve.[44]

In the Studies of Ascending Levels of Tolvaptan in Hyponatremia 1 and 2 (SALT-1 and SALT-2) trials, tolvaptan effectively increased serum sodium at 4 and 30 days in euvolemic or hypervolemic patients; approximately one third of the patients had heart failure as the etiology of hyponatremia.[45] The Efficacy of Vasopressin Antagonism in Heart Failure Outcome Study With Tolvaptan (EVEREST) trial was conducted in 4,133 patients hospitalized with NYHA class III-IV heart failure who experienced significant improvement in hyponatremia with tolvaptan compared with placebo.[46,47] In addition, patients experienced an improvement in diuresis, as well as signs and symptoms of congestion. Unfortunately, this study failed to demonstrate an improvement in global clinical status at discharge or a reduction in 2-year all-cause mortality, cardiovascular mortality, and heart failure rehospitalization. Thus, the role of vasopressin antagonists in the long-term management of heart failure remains unclear.

Overall, tolvaptan was very well tolerated in these trials with the most common side effects being dry mouth, thirst, urinary frequency, constipation, and hyperglycemia. It is important to recognize that while tolvaptan is an oral agent, it was initiated in clinical trials in the inpatient setting where serum sodium and volume status were closely monitored. This is an important safety aspect of this therapy that cannot be over emphasized. Two other vasopressin antagonists are currently being investigated: lixivaptan and satavaptan.

MECHANICAL CIRCULATORY SUPPORT[48]

INTRAAORTIC BALLOON PUMP

The intraaortic balloon pump (IABP) is a form of mechanical circulatory assistance occasionally employed for patients with advanced heart failure who do not respond adequately to drug therapy such as those with intractable myocardial ischemia or patients in cardiogenic shock. The IABP consists of a polyethylene balloon mounted on a catheter that is usually inserted percutaneously into the femoral artery, and the balloon is then advanced into the descending thoracic aorta. During counterpulsation, the balloon is synchronized with the ECG so that it inflates during diastole and displaces aortic blood, thus increasing aortic diastolic pressure and coronary perfusion. The balloon deflates just prior to the opening of the aortic valve during systole and causes a sudden decrease in aortic pressure, allowing the left ventricle to pump against reduced arterial impedance. IABP support results in increased CI, coronary artery perfusion, and myocardial oxygen supply accompanied by decreased myocardial oxygen demand. Thus, it is particularly useful for short-term use for patients with decompensated heart failure in the setting of myocardial ischemia (evolving infarction, patients awaiting emergency coronary bypass surgery). It is also used in hemodynamically unstable patients who are unresponsive to inotropic therapy. In the latter circumstance, the IABP may serve as a bridge to a surgical device or transplantation. Intravenous vasodilators and inotropic agents generally are used in conjunction with the IABP to maximize hemodynamic and clinical benefits.

VENTRICULAR ASSIST DEVICES[49]

⑫ A number of ventricular assist devices (VAD) are available or under investigation. These pumps are surgically implanted and assist, or in some cases replace, the pumping functions of the right and/or left ventricles. A left VAD (LVAD) removes blood directly from the left ventricle or the left atrium and pumps it to the aorta. The right VAD works similar to the LVAD and may be used alone or in conjunction with the LVAD.

LVADs can be used in the short-term (days to a couple of weeks) for temporary stabilization of a patient awaiting an intervention that would correct the underlying cardiac dysfunction. Alternatively, these devices can be used in the long term (several months to a couple of years) as a bridge to heart transplantation. More recently, permanent device implantation has become an option for patients who are not heart transplant candidates.

The Randomized Evaluation of Mechanical Assistance for the Treatment of Congestive Heart Failure (REMATCH) trial randomized 129 patients with decompensated heart failure who were ineligible for transplant to the HeartMate VE LVAD (Thoratec Corp., Pleasanton, CA) or optimal medical therapy. LVAD patients experienced improved 1- and 2-year survival (52% vs 25% at 1 year and 23% vs 8% at 2 years, $P = 0.009$); however, the overall survival was admittedly low in both groups.[50] The REMATCH trial was responsible for the approval of the use of these devices as "destination" therapy—destination being the last therapeutic option for a patient who is not a transplant candidate. More recently, the Investigation of Non-Transplant Eligible Patients who are Inotrope Dependent (INTrEPID) trial evaluated the Novacor LVAD (WorldHeart, Ottawa, Canada) in an inotrope-dependent heart failure population. Although the 1-year survival was improved in the LVAD arm (21% vs 11% in medically treated patients, $P = 0.02$), overall outcomes in the LVAD arm were inferior to those of the HeartMate VE in the REMATCH trial. Some of the patients in the INTrEPID trial were much sicker and thus would have been considered too high risk for surgery in the REMATCH trial.[51] Despite modifications leading to the HeartMate XVE design to improve safety and reliability of the device, long-term survival in the post-REMATCH era did not appreciably change (56% vs 51% 1-year survival).[52] In the post-REMATCH era, complications were unrelated to device malfunction and thus the role of operative candidate selection and the critical need to identify the "optimal" window for LVAD implantation was emphasized. Ongoing studies are assessing the next generation axial flow device, the HeartMate II LVAD (Thoratec Corporation), as well as making direct comparisons of various devices. These studies have also raised awareness regarding some of the limitations of these devices. Complications with LVADs include bleeding, air embolism, right ventricular failure, as well as those associated with a major surgical procedure including infection. In addition, these pumps can cause hemolysis, thrombosis, renal and hepatic dysfunction, and arrhythmias. Finally, device malfunction may occur. Controversy exists regarding the cost of such procedures given the already significant economic impact of this disease state on the healthcare system.[53] Although only a small number of patients were studied, recent research suggests that prolonged unloading of the left ventricle with an LVAD in combination with drug therapy to induce reverse remodeling can produce sustained recovery in LV function and amelioration of symptoms.[54] Furthermore, data that are more recent suggest that patients referred for LVAD prior to major complications of heart failure developing experience improved survival.[52]

For complete heart replacement therapy, the total artificial heart systems continue to be investigated; however, embolic complications as well as the large size of the currently available systems are limiting their use. Inserted percutaneously, catheter-based LVADs are a more recent advancement. These small pumps may offer an advantage as they avoid the need for open-heart surgery; however, this technology is still in developmental stages.

ULTRAFILTRATION

Renal dysfunction often occurs in the setting of decompensated heart failure, and thus, renal replacement therapy may be necessary. Ultrafiltration provides an additional modality for fluid removal by rapidly removing salt and water (up to 500 mL/hr) in a predictable manner. It has been shown to reduce PCWP and increases diuresis without adversely affecting blood pressure, heart rate, or renal function. In addition, ultrafiltration has been proposed to be safer than diuretics because removal of sodium and water is isotonic. Potential candidates for ultrafiltration include patients with diuretic resistance, renal impairment with diuretic administration, or renal impairment despite inotropic therapy. Complications of ultrafiltration include those associated with central venous access such as infection as well as those associated with rapid volume removal and intravascular depletion. Electrolyte depletion is less significant but still requires close monitoring.

Small studies suggest that ultrafiltration is an effective method to remove fluid in heart failure patients and that early initiation prior to intravenous diuretics was effective and safe in reducing hospital length of stay and readmission in diuretic resistant patients. Recently, the Ultrafiltration versus Intravenous Diuretics for Patients Hospitalized for Acute Decompensated Congestive Heart Failure (UNLOAD) trial investigated the effects of early ultrafiltration alone compared to intravenous diuretics alone in 200 patients hospitalized for decompensated heart failure and evidence of fluid overload. The primary end point of weight loss after 48 hours was significantly greater in the ultrafiltration group (5.0 kg) than in the diuretic group (3.1 kg). There was no significant difference between the two treatment groups in the dyspnea score at 48 hours, another primary end point. Compared with the diuretic group, the net fluid loss was significantly greater in the ultrafiltration group (4.6 L vs 3.3 L) after 48 hours. After 90 days, the incidence and duration of rehospitalization and the incidence of unscheduled office or emergency department visits were significantly lower for patients treated using ultrafiltration than for patients treated with intravenous diuretics.[55] Larger studies are ongoing to determine the role of ultrafiltration in managing decompensated heart failure.

SURGICAL THERAPY

Orthotopic cardiac transplantation remains the best therapeutic option for patients with chronic, irreversible NYHA class IV heart failure, with a 10-year survival of approximately 50% in well-selected patients.[56] Unfortunately, the shortage of acceptable donor hearts has resulted in long waiting times for transplantation with many patients succumbing to their disease prior to transplantation. Another large percentage of patients is rejected from consideration for transplant because of age, concurrent illnesses, psychosocial factors, and other reasons. The shortage of donor hearts has prompted development of new surgical techniques, including ventricular aneurysm resection, mitral valve repair, and myocardial cell transplantation, which have resulted in variable degrees of symptomatic improvement. Further development of these and other techniques may offer additional options for patients who are not candidates for transplantation.

PREPARATION FOR HOSPITAL DISCHARGE

For patients hospitalized with decompensated heart failure, all factors contributing to decompensation should be addressed. Patients should be near if not at optimal fluid status and transitioned from intravenous to oral diuretic therapy. Both the patient and family should receive appropriate education (see details in the following paragraphs). Chronic drug therapy should be optimized and appropriate follow-up clinic appointments scheduled. Typically, patients should be seen in the clinic within 7 to 10 days of hospital discharge. For patients with recurrent hospital admissions, additional discharge criteria should be considered (Table 22–6).[5,9]

Patient education is essential in the discharge process and should be multidisciplinary involving input from dietitians, pharmacists, and other healthcare providers. Teaching should promote self-care by incorporating identification of specific positive and negative behaviors. By having a better understanding of the key concepts of the disease and its management, patient self-care should improve and future hospitalizations may be avoided.[9]

While all patients would benefit from education, those with more severe symptoms (NYHA class III or IV) will require the most

TABLE 22-6	Discharge Criteria for Patients with HF
Recommended for all HF patients	• Exacerbating factors addressed • At least near optimal volume status achieved • Transition from intravenous to oral diuretic successfully completed • Patient and family education completed. • At least near optimal pharmacologic therapy achieved • Follow-up clinic visit scheduled, usually for 7–10 days
Should be considered for patients with advanced HF or recurrent admissions for HF	• Oral medication regimen stable for 24 hours • No intravenous vasodilator or inotropic agent for 24 hours • Ambulation before discharge to assess functional capacity after therapy • Plans for postdischarge management (scale present in home, visiting nurse or telephone follow-up generally no longer than 3 days after discharge) • Referral for disease management

Data from Adams KF, Lindenfeld J, Arnold JMO, et al. HFSA 2006 Comprehensive Heart Failure Practice Guidelines. J Cardiac Fail 2006;12:e1–e122.

intensive counseling. During a hospitalization, only essential education is recommended and should be supplemented within a couple of weeks after discharge in the clinic setting. Patients recently hospitalized for heart failure should be considered for referral to a disease management program.

For patients with end-stage disease, quality of life and prognosis should be discussed with the patient and caregivers. If possible, this discussion should occur while the patient is still able to participate in the decision-making process. End-of-life care should be considered for patients with persistent symptoms at rest despite multiple attempts to optimize therapy as evidenced by: frequent hospitalizations, ongoing limited quality of life, requiring intermittent or continuous intravenous therapy, or consideration of assist devices as destination therapy. In such cases, inactivation of an implantable cardioverter–defibrillator should be discussed and patients may be considered for hospice services.[9] Integration of a palliative care approach may be necessary. As clinical status deteriorates and medical therapies become ineffective, healthcare providers should transition from focusing on mortality reduction to palliative care.[57]

PHARMACOECONOMIC CONSIDERATIONS

Heart failure imposes a tremendous economic burden on the healthcare system. For patients over age 65, it is the most common reason for hospitalization, with hospital admission rates for this disorder continuing to increase. Heart failure is also associated with unacceptably high readmission rates during the 3 to 6 months after initial discharge. Current estimates of costs of heart failure treatment in the United States approach $37 billion with most of the costs associated with hospitalization.[1] The prevalence of heart failure and the costs associated with patient care are expected to increase as the population ages and as survival from ischemic heart disease is improved. Thus, approaches to improve the quality and cost-effectiveness of care for these patients may have a significant impact on healthcare costs. Finally, LVADs as a bridge to heart transplantation were found to be cost-ineffective unless costs associated with their implantation decrease or their clinical benefits increase.[58]

As the management of heart failure has become increasingly complex, the development of disease management programs that use multidisciplinary teams has been studied extensively. These programs utilize several broad approaches, including heart failure specialty clinics and/or home-based interventions. Most are multidisciplinary and may include physicians, advanced practice nurses, dieticians, and pharmacists. In general, programs focus on optimization of drug and nondrug therapy, patient and family education and counseling, exercise and dietary advice, intense follow-up by telephone or home visits, and monitoring and management of signs and symptoms of decompensation. In general, multidisciplinary disease management programs reduce mortality, heart failure and all-cause hospitalizations, and costs.[59]

Pharmacists can play an important role in the multidisciplinary team management of heart failure.[60,61] Compared with conventional treatment, pharmacist interventions that included medication evaluation and therapeutic recommendations, patient education and follow-up telephone monitoring reduced hospitalizations for heart failure. Adherence to guideline-recommended therapy also improved with pharmacist intervention. A recent study found that pharmacist intervention improved medication adherence and reduced emergency department visits and hospitalizations in low-income patients with heart failure.[62] Thus, the role and cost benefits of pharmacist involvement in the

multidisciplinary care of heart failure patients are now apparent and should include optimizing doses of heart failure drug therapy, screening for drugs that exacerbate heart failure, monitoring for adverse drug effects and drug interactions, educating patients, and patient follow-up.

CURRENT CONTROVERSIES

1. The optimal pharmacotherapy for patients with acute decompensated heart failure that are refractory to diuretic therapy is controversial. The following questions remain unaddressed by the current literature: change to continuous infusion loop diuretic versus addition of thiazide diuretic, which thiazide diuretic should be added (metolazone, HCTZ, other) and at what dose, high dose versus low dose continuous infusion, and the role of ultrafiltration. Ongoing studies such as the DOSE-AHF trial should address these questions.

2. The role of nesiritide remains highly controversial. After two metaanalyses suggested that nesiritide use is associated with worsening renal function and increased mortality, prescribing of nesiritide has declined considerably. However, the safety of other vasodilators such as nitroglycerin or nitroprusside is not well established, and the use of positive inotropes is associated with poor outcomes. The results of the ongoing ASCEND trials will address both the efficacy and safety of this agent.

3. The role of vasopressin antagonists beyond managing hypervolemic or euvolemic hyponatremia in heart failure patients remains unclear. Future trials addressing impact on long-term outcomes in heart failure patients including morbidity and mortality are warranted.

4. Evolving data regarding the role of LVADs as a bridge to transplant or destination therapy provide further support for the use of these therapeutic modalities. Additional data are warranted to further define the most optimal candidates, timelines for insertion, and how to best minimize complications associated with these mechanical devices.

EVALUATION OF THERAPEUTIC OUTCOMES

Assessment of adequacy of therapy in the acute decompensated HF patient can be separated into two general categories: initial improvement of physiologic parameters and safe discharge from the intensive care unit following conversion to a chronic oral therapeutic regimen. Both goals are equally important because hemodynamic improvement alone has not been correlated with prolonged symptom improvement or enhanced survival.

Initial stabilization requires achievement of adequate arterial oxygen saturation and content. Cardiac index and blood pressure must be sufficient to ensure adequate organ perfusion, as assessed by alert mental status, creatinine clearance sufficient to prevent metabolic azotemic complications, hepatic function adequate to maintain synthetic and excretory functions, a stable heart rate and rhythm (predominately sinus rhythm, rate-stabilized atrial fibrillation or flutter, or paced rhythm), absence of ongoing myocardial ischemia or infarction, skeletal muscle and skin blood flow sufficient to prevent ischemic injury, and normal arterial pH (7.34 to 7.47) with a normal serum lactate concentration. Although these goals are achieved most often with a CI greater than 2.2 L/min/m², a mean arterial blood pressure greater than 60 mm Hg, and a PCWP of 15 mm Hg or greater, the absolute values are highly variable and depend on chronicity of illness, efficacy of chronic compensatory mechanisms, previous chronic therapy, and concurrent illnesses.

Discharge from the intensive care unit requires maintenance of the preceding parameters in the absence of ongoing intravenous infusion therapy, mechanical circulatory support, or positive-pressure ventilation. Some patients may achieve this goal with markedly lower blood pressure or higher filling pressure than suggested earlier; hence, numerical goals cannot always be substituted for clinical status. Nonpharmacologic treatments aimed at the precipitants of a patient's HF exacerbation include permanent pacing, chronic resynchronization therapy (also know as *biventricular pacing*) with or without an implantable cardioverter–defibrillator, coronary angioplasty or valvuloplasty, pericardial drainage, cardiac surgery (coronary bypass, valve replacement or reconstruction, closure of intracardiac shunts), or even cardiac transplantation, to achieve initial stabilization, definitive therapy, or both.

ABBREVIATIONS

ACC: American College of Cardiology

ACE: angiotensin-converting enzyme

ADHF: acute decompensated heart failure

AHA: American Heart Association

ANP: atrial natriuretic peptide

AVP: arginine vasopressin

BNP: B-type natriuretic peptide

cAMP: cyclic adenosine monophosphate

CI: cardiac index

CO: cardiac output

HFSA: Heart Failure Society of America

IABP: intraaortic balloon pump

LVAD: left ventricular assist device

NYHA: New York Heart Association

PCWP: pulmonary capillary wedge pressure

VAD: ventricular assist device

REFERENCES

1. Rosamond W, Flegal K, Furie K, et al. Heart disease and stroke statistics—2008 update: A Report from the American Heart Association Statistics Committee and Stroke Statistics Subcommittee. Circulation 2008;117:e25–146.
2. Lloyd-Jones D, Adams RJ, Brown TM, et al. Heart Disease and Stroke Statistics—2010 Update. A Report from the American Heart Association. Circulation. 2010;121:e46–e215.
3. Mehra MR. Optimizing outcomes in the patient with acute decompensated heart failure. Am Heart J 2006;151:571–579.
4. Hunt SA, Abraham WT, Chin MH, et al. ACC/AHA 2005 Guideline Update for the Diagnosis and Management of Chronic Heart Failure in the Adult: A Report of the American College of Cardiology/American Heart Association Task Force on Practice Guidelines (Writing Committee to Update the 2001 Guidelines for the Evaluation and Management of Heart Failure): Developed in collaboration with the American College of Chest Physicians and the International Society for Heart and Lung Transplantation: endorsed by the Heart Rhythm Society. Circulation 2005;112:e154–235.
5. Jessup M, Abraham WT, Casey DE, et al. 2009 focused update: ACCF/AHA Guidelines for the Diagnosis and Management of Heart Failure in Adults: A Report of the American College of Cardiology Foundation/American Heart Association Task Force on Practice Guidelines: developed in collaboration with the International Society for Heart and Lung Transplantation. Circulation 2009;119:1977–2016.
6. Felker GM, Adams KF, Jr., Konstam MA, O'Connor CM, Gheorghiade M. The problem of decompensated heart failure: nomenclature, classification, and risk stratification. Am Heart J 2003;145:S18–S25.
7. Cuffe MS, Califf RM, Adams KF, et al. Short-term intravenous milrinone for acute exacerbation of chronic heart failure: A randomized controlled trial. JAMA 2002;287:1541–1547.
8. The VMAC Investigators. Intravenous nesiritide vs nitroglycerin for treatment of decompensated congestive heart failure: A randomized controlled trial. JAMA 2002;287:1531–1540.
9. Adams KF, Lindenfeld J, Arnold JMO, et al. HFSA 2006 Comprehensive Heart Failure Practice Guideline: Section 12: Evaluation and management of patients with acute decompensated heart failure. J Card Fail 2006;12:e86–e103.
10. Nieminen MS, Bohm M, Cowie MR, et al. Executive summary of the guidelines on the diagnosis and treatment of acute heart failure: The Task Force on Acute Heart Failure of the European Society of Cardiology. Eur Heart J 2005;26:384–416.
11. Gheorghiade M, Zannad F, Sopko G, et al. Acute heart failure syndromes: Current state and framework for future research. Circulation 2005;112:3958–3968.
12. Adams KF, Jr., Fonarow GC, Emerman CL, et al. Characteristics and outcomes of patients hospitalized for heart failure in the United States: Rationale, design, and preliminary observations from the first 100,000 cases in the Acute Decompensated Heart Failure National Registry (ADHERE). Am Heart J 2005;149:209–216.
13. Fonarow GC, Adams KF, Jr., Abraham WT, Yancy CW, Boscardin WJ. Risk stratification for in-hospital mortality in acutely decompensated heart failure: Classification and regression tree analysis. JAMA 2005;293:572–580.
14. Gheorghiade M, Abraham WT, Albert NM, et al. Systolic blood pressure at admission, clinical characteristics, and outcomes in patients hospitalized with acute heart failure. JAMA 2006;296:2217–2226.
15. Nohria A, Mielniczuk LM, Stevenson LW. Evaluation and monitoring of patients with acute heart failure syndromes. Am J Cardiol 2005;96:32G–40G.
16. O'Connor CM, Abraham WT, Albert NM, et al. Predictors of mortality after discharge in patients hospitalized with heart failure: An analysis from the Organized Program to Initiate Lifesaving Treatment in Hospitalized Patients with Heart Failure (OPTIMIZE-HF). Am Heart J 2008;156:662–673.
17. Maisel A, Mueller C, Adams K, Jr., et al. State of the art: using natriuretic peptide levels in clinical practice. Eur J Heart Fail 2008;10:824–839.
18. Adams KF, Lindenfeld J, Arnold JMO, et al. HFSA 2006 Comprehensive Heart Failure Practice Guideline: Section 7: Heart failure in patients with left ventricular systolic dysfunction. J Card Fail 2006;12:e38–e57.
19. Nohria A, Lewis E, Stevenson LW. Medical management of advanced heart failure. Jama 2002;287:628–640.
20. Binanay C, Califf RM, Hasselblad V, et al. Evaluation study of congestive heart failure and pulmonary artery catheterization effectiveness: the ESCAPE trial. JAMA 2005;294:1625–1633.
21. Forrester JS, Diamond G, Chatterjee K, Swan HJC. Medical therapy of acute myocardial infarction by application of hemodynamic subsets. N Engl J Med 1976;295:1356–1362.
22. Finley JJt, Konstam MA, Udelson JE. Arginine vasopressin antagonists for the treatment of heart failure and hyponatremia. Circulation 2008;118:410–421.
23. Brater DC. Pharmacology of diuretics. Am J Med Sci 2000;319:38–50.
24. Brater DC. Diuretic therapy in congestive heart failure. CHF 2000;6:197–210.
25. Stough WG, O'Connor CM, Gheorghiade M. Overview of current noninodilator therapies for acute heart failure syndromes. Am J Cardiol 2005;96:41G–46G.
26. Iyengar S, Abraham WT. Diuretics for the treatment of acute decompensated heart failure. Heart Fail Rev 2007;12:125–130.
27. Eshaghian S, Horwich TB, Fonarow GC. Relation of loop diuretic dose to mortality in advanced heart failure. Am J Cardiol 2006;97:1759–1764.
28. Butler J, Forman DE, Abraham WT, et al. Relationship between heart failure treatment and development of worsening renal function among hospitalized patients. Am Heart J 2004;147:331–338.

29. Cleland JG, Coletta A, Witte K. Practical applications of intravenous diuretic therapy in decompensated heart failure. Am J Med 2006;119:S26–S36.

30. Dormans TP, van Meyel JJ, Gerlag PG, Tan Y, Russel FG, Smits P. Diuretic efficacy of high dose furosemide in severe heart failure: Bolus injection versus continuous infusion. J Am Coll Cardiol 1996;28: 376–382.

31. Thomson MR, Nappi JM, Dunn SP, Hollis IB, Rodgers JE, VanBakel A. Continuous versus intermittent infusion furosemide in acute decompensated heart failure. J Card Fail 2010;(in press).

32. Vargo DL, Brater DC, Rudy DW, Swan SK. Dopamine does not enhance furosemide-induced natriuresis in patients with congestive heart failure. J Am Soc Nephrol 1996;7:1032–1037.

33. Bayram M, De Luca L, Massie MB, Gheorghiade M. Reassessment of dobutamine, dopamine, and milrinone in the management of acute heart failure syndromes. Am J Cardiol 2005;96:47G–58G.

34. Lehtonen LA, Antila S, Pentikainen PJ. Pharmacokinetics and pharmacodynamics of intravenous inotropic agents. Clin Pharmacokinet 2004;43:187–203.

35. Abraham WT, Adams KF, Fonarow GC, et al. In-hospital mortality in patients with acute decompensated heart failure requiring intravenous vasoactive medications: an analysis from the Acute Decompensated Heart Failure National Registry (ADHERE). J Am Coll Cardiol 2005;46:57–64.

36. Dorsch MP, Rodgers JE. Nesiritide: harmful or harmless? Pharmacotherapy 2006;26:1465–1478.

37. Sackner-Bernstein JD, Skopicki HA, Aaronson KD. Risk of worsening renal function with nesiritide in patients with acutely decompensated heart failure. Circulation 2005;111:1487–1491.

38. Sackner-Bernstein JD, Kowalski M, Fox M, Aaronson K. Short-term risk of death after treatment with nesiritide for decompensated heart failure: A pooled analysis of randomized controlled trials. JAMA 2005;293:1900–1905.

39. Reynolds RM, Padfield PL, Seckl JR. Disorders of sodium balance. BMJ 2006;332:702–705.

40. Gheorghiade M, Gattis WA, O'Connor CM, et al. Effects of tolvaptan, a vasopressin antagonist, in patients hospitalized with worsening heart failure: A randomized controlled trial. JAMA 2004;291: 1963–1971.

41. Lee WH, Packer M. Prognostic importance of serum sodium concentration and its modification by converting-enzyme inhibition in patients with severe chronic heart failure. Circulation 1986;73:257–267.

42. Adrogue HJ, Madias NE. Hyponatremia. N Engl J Med 2000;342: 1581–1589.

43. Lee CR, Watkins ML, Patterson JH, et al. Vasopressin: a new target for the treatment of heart failure. Am Heart J 2003;146:9–18.

44. Tolvaptan (Samsca) package insert. Rockville, MD: Otsuka America Pharmaceutical, Inc.; May 2009.

45. Schrier RW, Gross P, Gheorghiade M, et al. Tolvaptan, a selective oral vasopressin V2-receptor antagonist, for hyponatremia. N Engl J Med 2006;355:2099–2112.

46. Gheorghiade M, Konstam MA, Burnett JC, Jr., et al. Short-term clinical effects of tolvaptan, an oral vasopressin antagonist, in patients hospitalized for heart failure: The EVEREST Clinical Status Trials. JAMA 2007;297:1332–1343.

47. Konstam MA, Gheorghiade M, Burnett JC, Jr., et al. Effects of oral tolvaptan in patients hospitalized for worsening heart failure: The EVEREST Outcome Trial. JAMA 2007;297:1319–1331.

48. Boehmer JP, Popjes E. Cardiac failure: Mechanical support strategies. Crit Care Med 2006;34:S268–S277.

49. Lietz K, Miller LW. Destination therapy: Current results and future promise. Semin Thorac Cardiovasc Surg 2008;20:225–233.

50. Rose EA, Gelijns AC, Moskowitz AJ, et al. Long-term mechanical left ventricular assistance for end-stage heart failure. N Engl J Med 2001;345:1435–1443.

51. Rogers JG, Butler J, Lansman SL, et al. Chronic mechanical circulatory support for inotrope-dependent heart failure patients who are not transplant candidates: results of the INTrEPID Trial. J Am Coll Cardiol 2007;50:741–747.

52. Lietz K, Long JW, Kfoury AG, et al. Outcomes of left ventricular assist device implantation as destination therapy in the post-REMATCH era: implications for patient selection. Circulation 2007;116: 497–505.

53. Russo MJ, Gelijns AC, Stevenson LW, et al. The cost of medical management in advanced heart failure during the final two years of life. J Card Fail 2008;14:651–658.

54. Birks EJ, Tansley PD, Hardy J, et al. Left ventricular assist device and drug therapy for the reversal of heart failure. N Engl J Med 2006;355:1873–1884.

55. Costanzo MR, Guglin ME, Saltzberg MT, et al. Ultrafiltration versus intravenous diuretics for patients hospitalized for acute decompensated heart failure. J Am Coll Cardiol 2007;49:675–683.

56. Taylor DO, Edwards LB, Boucek MM, et al. Registry of the International Society for Heart and Lung Transplantation: Twenty-third official adult heart transplantation report—2006. J Heart Lung Transplant 2006;25:869–879.

57. Hauptman PJ, Havranek EP. Integrating palliative care into heart failure care. Arch Intern Med 2005;165:374–378.

58. Clegg AJ, Scott DA, Loveman E, Colquitt JL, Royle P, Bryant J. Clinical and cost-effectiveness of left ventricular assist devices as a bridge to heart transplantation for people with end-stage heart failure: A systematic review and economic evaluation. Eur Heart J 2006;27:2929–2938.

59. Holland R, Battersby J, Harvey I, Lenaghan E, Smith J, Hay L. Systematic review of multidisciplinary interventions in heart failure. Heart 2005;91:899–906.

60. Gattis WA, Hasselblad V, Whellan DJ, O'Connor CM. Reduction in heart failure events by the addition of a clinical pharmacist to the heart failure management team. Arch Int Med 1999;159: 1939–1945.

61. Whellan DJ, Gaulden L, Gattis WA, et al. The benefit of implementing a heart failure disease management program. Arch Intern Med 2001;161:2223–2228.

62. Murray M, Young J, Hoke S, et al. Pharmacist intervention to improve medication adherence in heart failure. A randomized trial. Ann Intern Med 2007;146:714–725.

Appendix

This chapter was prepared prior to the publication of the 2010 Heart Failure Society of America Guidelines (Lindenfeld J, Albert NM, Boehmer JP, et al. HFSA 2010 Comprehensive Heart Failure Practice Guideline. J Card Fail. 2010;16:e1–194). The 2010 updated guideline does not differ from the content referenced within this chapter.

CHAPTER

23

Ischemic Heart Disease

ROBERT L. TALBERT

KEY CONCEPTS

❶ Ischemic heart disease (IHD) is primarily caused by coronary atherosclerotic plaque formation that leads to an imbalance between oxygen supply and demand resulting in myocardial ischemia.

❷ Chest pain is the cardinal symptom of myocardial ischemia due to coronary artery disease (CAD).

❸ Risk factor identification and modification are important interventions for individual patients with known or suspected IHD and as a population-based policy to reduce the impact of this disease.

❹ Major risk factors that can be altered include dyslipidemia (high total and LDL cholesterol, low HDL cholesterol, and high triglycerides), smoking, glycemic control in diabetes mellitus, hypertension, and adoption of therapeutic lifestyle changes (exercise, weight reduction, and reduced cholesterol and fat in the diet). Reduction in inflammation may also play an important role.

❺ Most patients with CAD should receive antiplatelet therapy. Chronic stable angina should be managed initially with β-blockers because they provide better symptomatic control at least as well as nitrates or calcium channel blockers and decrease the risk of recurrent myocardial infarction (MI) and CAD mortality.

❻ Nitroglycerin and other nitrate products are useful for prophylaxis of angina when patients are undertaking activities known to provoke angina; however, when angina is occurring on a regular, routine basis, chronic prophylactic therapy should be instituted.

❼ Although calcium channel blockers are effective as monotherapy, they are generally used in combination with β-blockers or as monotherapy if patients are intolerant of β-blockers; most patients with moderate to severe angina will require two drugs to control their symptoms. Ranolazine is a second-line drug to be used with β-blockers and certain calcium channel blockers.

❽ Pharmacologic management is as effective as revascularization (e.g., percutaneous transluminal coronary angioplasty [PTCA], coronary artery bypass grafting [CABG]) if one or two vessels are involved and there are no differences in survival, recurrent MI, or other measures of effectiveness.

❾ Multivessel involvement, especially if the patient has left main CAD, left main equivalent disease, or two- to three-vessel involvement with significant left ventricular dysfunction, is best managed with revascularization. With improvements in stent technology, more patients are eligible for this approach compared to CABG.

❿ PTCA and CABG produce similar results overall, but certain patient subsets (e.g., diabetics) should have CABG done.

⓫ The clinical performance measures for chronic stable CAD recommended by the American College of Cardiology and the American Heart Association include blood pressure measurement, lipid profile, symptom and activity assessment, smoking cessation, antiplatelet therapy, drug therapy for lowering LDL cholesterol, β-blocker therapy for prior MI, angiotensin-converting enzyme (ACE) inhibitor therapy, and screening for diabetes.

Learning objectives, review questions, and other resources can be found at **www.pharmacotherapyonline.com**.

Ischemic heart disease (IHD) due to atherosclerosis of the epicardial vessels leading to coronary heart disease (CHD) is the main etiology of IHD. This process begins early in life, often not being clinically manifest until the middle-aged years and beyond. IHD may present as an acute coronary syndrome (ACS), which includes unstable angina, non–ST-segment elevation MI, or ST-segment elevation MI (see Chap. 24), chronic stable exertional angina pectoris, and ischemia without clinical symptoms. Coronary artery vasospasm (variant of Prinzmetal angina) produces similar symptoms but is not due to atherosclerosis. Microvascular angina, which is myocardial ischemia without occlusive CHD, is seen more commonly in women than men. Other manifestations of atherosclerosis include heart failure, arrhythmias, cerebrovascular disease (stroke), and peripheral vascular disease. The American Heart Association, the American College of Cardiology, and the European Society of Cardiology have published management guidelines for stable and unstable angina.[1-3]

EPIDEMIOLOGY

The American Heart Association (AHA) estimates that 81,100,000 American adults have one or more types of cardiovascular disease (CVD) based on data from 2003 through 2006.[4] Nearly 2,300 Americans die of CVD each day, or an average of 1 death every 38 seconds. In 2006, the death rates from CVD were 422.8 (per 100,000) for black males, 306.6 for white males, 298.2 for black females, and 215.5 for white females.[4] Mortality data for 2006 show that CVD accounted for 34.3% of 2,426,264 deaths in 2006 or 1 of every 2.9 deaths in the United States. Men die earlier from IHD and acute myocardial infarction (AMI) than women, and aging of both sexes is associated with a higher incidence of these afflictions. The disparity in mortality from IHD between men and women decreases with aging, being about four to five times more common in men from the age of the mid-30s to a preponderance of female deaths in the very elderly.

The syndrome of angina pectoris is reported to occur with an average annual incidence rate (number of new cases per time period divided by the total number of persons in the population for the same time period) of about 1.5% (range 0.1 to 5/1000) depending on the patient's age, gender, and risk factor profile.[5] The presenting manifestation in women is more commonly angina, whereas men more frequently have MI as the initial event. Estimates of the incidence and prevalence of angina are not entirely accurate due to waxing and waning of symptoms; angina may disappear in up to 30% of patients with angina that is less severe and of recent onset.

Data from the Framingham study show that the prevalence in a 1970 cohort followed for 10 years was about 1.5% for women and 4.3% for men aged 50 to 59 years at inception.[5] The annual rate of new episodes of angina range from 28.3 to 33 per 1,000 population for nonblack men, 22.4 to 39.5 for black men, 14.1 to 22.9 for nonblack women, and 15.3 to 35.9 for black women in the age range of 65 to 84 years or older.[4] AHA estimates that the prevalence of angina was 10.2 million in 2006.[4] Between 1980 and 2002, death rates due to CHD among men and women ≥65 years of age fell by 52% in men and 49% in women.[4] The risk of developing IHD is not the same worldwide. Countries such as Japan and France are on the low end of the spectrum whereas Finland, Northern Ireland, Scotland, and South Africa have very high rates of IHD.[6,7]

Angina may be classified according to symptom severity, disability induced, or a specific activity scale (Tables 23–1 and 23–2). The specific activity scale developed by Goldman and coworkers[8] may be preferable because it has been shown to be equal to or better than the New York Heart Association or Canadian Cardiovascular Society functional classifications for reproducibility and provides better agreement with exercise treadmill testing.

An important determinate of outcome for the angina patient is the number of vessels obstructed. Twelve-year survival from the Coronary Artery Surgery Study (CASS) for patients with zero-, one-, two-, and three-vessel disease was 88%, 74%, 59%, and 40%, respectively.[9] Other factors that increase the risk of death in medically managed patients include the presence of heart failure (or markers such as poor ventricular wall motion and low ejection fraction), smoking, left main or left main–equivalent coronary artery disease (CAD), diabetes, or prior MI. Twelve-year survival for patients with at least one diseased vessel and ejection fractions in the ranges of ≥50%, 35% to 49%, and 0% to 34% is 73%, 54%, and 21%, respectively. Of particular note, patients with left main (or left main–equivalent) CAD are at extremely high risk and constitute a unique group for therapeutic consideration.[10] In the CASS, at 15 years of follow-up, 37% of the surgery group and 27% of the medical group are surviving; median survival is 13.3 years versus 6.7 years, respectively ($P<0.0001$). It is important to realize that these surgery studies are 15 years old and event rates are now likely lower. Technology advances in coronary artery stent development may now allow more patients to be treated with primary percutaneous intervention rather than coronary artery bypass grafting (CABG).[11] If systolic function was normal, then median survival and percent surviving were not different between the surgery and medical groups (median survival of about 15 years). Patients screened but not randomized to Coronary Artery Surgery Study (CASS) had similar survival rates, suggesting that results from randomized patients may be applicable to more generalized populations as a measure of external reliability.

TABLE 23-1	Criteria for Determination of the Specific Activity Scale Functional Class		
		Any Yes	**No**
1. Can you walk down a flight of steps without stopping (4.5–5.2 MET[a])?		Go to 2	Go to 4
2. Can you carry anything up a flight of 8 steps without stopping (5–5.5 MET)? Or can you		Go to 3	Class III
a. Have sexual intercourse without stopping (5–5.2 MET)			
b. Garden, rake, weed (5.6 MET)			
c. Roller skate, dance foxtrot (5–6 MET)			
d. Walk at a 4 miles/h rate on level ground (5–6 MET)			
3. Can you carry at least 24 lb up 8 steps (10 MET)? Or can you		Class I	Class II
a. Carry objects that weigh at least 80 lb (18 MET)			
b. Do outdoor work, shovel snow, spade soil (7 MET)			
c. Do recreational activities such as skiing, basketball, touch football, squash, handball (7–10 MET)			
d. Jog/walk 5 miles/h (9 MET)			
4. Can you shower without stopping (3.6–4.2 MET)? Or can you		Class III	Go to 5
a. Strip and make bed (3.9–5 MET)			
b. Mop floors (4.2 MET)			
c. Hang washed clothes (4.4 MET)			
d. Clean windows (3.7 MET)			
e. Walk 2.5 miles/h (3–3.5 MET)			
f. Bowl (3–4.4 MET)			
g. Play golf, walk and carry clubs (4.5 MET)			
h. Push a power lawnmower (4 MET)			
5. Can you dress without stopping because of symptoms (2–2.3 MET)?		Class III	Class IV

[a]MET, metabolic equivalents of activity.
From reference 8, with permission.

ETIOLOGY AND PATHOPHYSIOLOGY

The pathophysiology that underlies this disease process is dynamic, evolutionary, and complex. An understanding of the determinants of myocardial oxygen demand (MVO_2), regulation of coronary blood flow, the effects of ischemia on the mechanical and metabolic function of the myocardium, and how ischemia is recognized are

TABLE 23-2	Grading of Angina Pectoris by the Canadian Cardiovascular Society Classification System
Class	**Description of Stage**
Class I	Ordinary physical activity does not cause angina, such as walking, climbing stairs. Angina occurs with strenuous, rapid, or prolonged exertion at work or recreation.
Class II	Slight limitation or ordinary activity. Angina occurs on walking or climbing stairs rapidly, walking uphill, walking or stair climbing after meals, or in cold, or in wind, or under emotional stress, or only during the few hours after wakening. Walking more than 2 blocks on the level and climbing more than 1 flight of ordinary stairs at a normal pace and in normal condition.
Class III	Marked limitations of ordinary physical activity. Angina occurs on walking 1 to 2 blocks on the level and climbing 1 flight of stairs in normal conditions and at a normal pace.
Class IV	Inability to carry on any physical activity without discomfort–anginal symptoms may be present at rest.

From Campeau L. Grading of angina [letter]. Circulation 1976;54:522–523, with permission.

important in understanding the rationale for the selection and use of pharmacotherapy for IHD.

1 Ischemia may be defined as lack of oxygen and decreased or no blood flow in the myocardium. In contrast, anoxia, defined as the absence of oxygen to the myocardium, results in continued perfusion with washout of acid by-products of glycolysis, thereby preserving the mechanical and metabolic status of the heart to a greater extent than does ischemia for short periods of time.

DETERMINANTS OF OXYGEN DEMAND (MVO₂)

The major determinants of MVO_2 are (1) heart rate, (2) contractility, and (3) intramyocardial wall tension during systole. Overall, intramyocardial wall tension is thought to be the most important among these three factors. As the consequences of IHD are a result of increased demand in the face of a fixed supply of oxygen in most situations, alterations in MVO_2 are critically important in producing ischemia and for interventions intended to alleviate ischemia. MVO_2 can not be directly measured in patients; however, an indirect assessment that correlates reasonably well with MVO_2 as determined in experimental animal models is the tension–time index (TTI). This is a measure of the area under the curve of the left ventricular (LV) pressure curve. Tension in the ventricle wall is a function of the radius of the LV and intraventricular pressure. These factors are related through Laplace law, which states that wall stress is related directly to the product of intraventricular pressure and internal radius and inversely to wall thickness multiplied by a factor of 2. Increasing systemic blood pressure or ventricular dilation would increase wall tension and oxygen demand, whereas ventricular hypertrophy would tend to minimize increasing MVO_2. Clinical application of these principles has led to the use of the double product (DP), which is heart rate (HR) multiplied by systolic blood pressure (SBP) (DP = HR × SBP). Although this is a clinically useful indirect estimate of MVO_2, it does not consider changes in contractility (an independent variable), and because only changes in pressure are considered with the double product, volume loading of the LV and increased MVO_2 related to ventricular dilation are underestimated.

REGULATION OF CORONARY BLOOD FLOW

Coronary blood flow is influenced by multiple factors; however, the caliber of the resistance vessels delivering blood to the myocardium and MVO_2 are the prime determinants in the occurrence of ischemia. The anatomy of the vascular bed will affect oxygen supply and, subsequently, myocardial metabolism and mechanical function.

Anatomic Factors

The normal coronary system (see Fig. 23–1 for normal anatomy) consists of large epicardial or surface vessels (R1) that normally offer little intrinsic resistance to myocardial flow and intramyocardial arteries and arterioles (R2), which branch into a dense capillary network (about 4,000 capillaries/mm²) to supply basal blood flow of 60 to 90 mL/min per 100 g of myocardium. R1 and R2 are in series and total resistance is the algebraic sum; however, under normal circumstances, the resistance in R2 is much greater. Myocardial blood flow is inversely related to arteriolar resistance and directly related to the coronary driving pressure. The arterioles dynamically alter their intrinsic tone in response to demands for oxygen and other factors, and as a result, myocardial oxygen delivery and myocardial oxygen demand are tightly coupled in a rapidly responsive system.

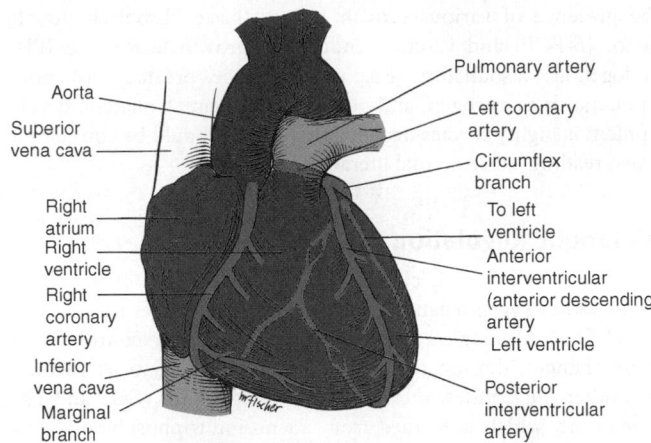

FIGURE 23-1. Coronary anatomy. *(From Tintinalli JE, Kelen GD, Stapczynski JR. Tintinalli's Emergency Medicine: A Comprehensive Study Guide, 6th ed. Copyright The McGraw Hill Companies, Inc. with permission. http://www.accessemergencymedicine.com.)*

Atherosclerotic lesions encroaching on the luminal cross-sectional area of the larger epicardial vessels (R1) transform the relationships among R1, R2, and blood flow. As resistance increases in R1 owing to occlusion, R2 can vasodilate to maintain coronary blood flow. This response is inadequate with greater degrees of obstruction, and the coronary flow reserve afforded by R2 vasodilation is insufficient to meet oxygen demand (also referred to as *autoregulation*). The extent of functional obstruction is important in the limitation of coronary blood flow, and the presence of relatively severe stenosis (>70%) may provoke ischemia and symptoms at rest, whereas less severe stenosis may allow a reserve of coronary blood flow for exertion.[12]

The diameter of the lesion impeding blood flow through a vessel is important, but other factors such as length of the lesion and the influence of pressure drop across an area of stenosis also affect coronary blood flow and function of the collateral circulation. Resistance to flow in a vessel is directly related to length of the obstructing lesion, but resistance is inversely related to the diameter of the vessel to the fourth power. Diameter is, therefore, much more important. As blood flows across a stenotic lesion, the pressure drops (energy losses) due to friction between blood and the lesion and to the abrupt turbulent expansion as blood emerges from the stenosis. This pressure drop is dynamic and directly related to flow giving rise to a resistance that is not fixed, but rather fluctuates, as flow is changed. This relationship can dramatically affect collateral blood flow and its response to exercise, resulting in what has been called *coronary steal*. A similar situation may also occur when the epicardial or subepicardial vessels "steal" blood flow from the endocardium in the presence of a stenotic lesion.

Large and small coronary arteries may undergo dynamic changes in coronary vascular resistance and coronary blood flow. Dynamic coronary obstruction can occur in normal vessels and vessels with stenosis in which vasomotion or spasm may be superimposed on a fixed stenosis. Although it is possible that these changes may be "active" in small coronary arteries, it is also possible that the observed changes may reflect collapse owing to poststenotic intraluminal pressure drop or increased intramyocardial compressive forces associated with inadequate ventricular relaxation.

Collateral blood flow exists to a certain extent from birth as native collaterals, but persisting ischemia may promote collateral growth as developed collaterals. These two types of collaterals differ in anatomy and in their ability to regulate coronary blood flow. Collateral development is dependent on the severity of obstruction, the presence of various growth factors (basic fibroblast growth factor [β-FGF] and vascular endothelial growth factor [VEGF]), endogenous vasodilators (e.g., nitrous oxide, prostacyclin), hormones such as estrogen, and potentially exercise. Collateral development is highly species dependent, and this should be considered when reading experimental literature.

Metabolic Regulation

Coronary blood flow is closely tied to oxygen needs of the heart. Changes in oxygen balance lead to very rapid changes in coronary blood flow. Although a number of mediators may contribute to these changes, the most important ones are likely to be adenosine, other nucleotides, nitric oxide, prostaglandins, CO_2, and H^+. Adenosine, which is formed from adenosine triphosphate (ATP) and adenosine monophosphate (AMP) under conditions of ischemia and stress, is a potent vasodilator that links decreased perfusion to metabolically induced vasodilation or "reactive hyperemia." The synthesis and release of adenosine into coronary sinus venous effluent occurs within seconds after coronary artery occlusion, and about 30% of the hyperemic response can be blocked by metabolic blockers of adenosine. Coronary reactivity can be used to detect individuals at risk for future events.[13]

Endothelial Control of Coronary Vascular Tone

The vascular endothelium, a single-cell tissue with an enormous surface area separating the blood from vascular smooth muscle of the artery wall, is capable of a broad range of metabolic functions. The endothelium functions as a protective surface for the artery wall, and as long as it remains intact and functional, it promotes vascular smooth muscle relaxation and inhibits thrombogenesis and atherosclerotic plaque formation; damaged endothelium reacts to numerous stimuli with vasoconstriction, thrombosis, and plaque formation. The vascular endothelium of the coronary arteries synthesizes large molecules such as fibronectin, interleukin-1, tissue plasminogen activator, and various growth factors. Small molecules that are also produced include prostacyclin, platelet-activating factor, endothelin-1, and endothelium-derived relaxing factor (EDRF) that is now characterized as nitric oxide. EDRF is synthesized from 1-arginine via nitric oxide synthase and released by shear force on the endothelium as well as through interaction with many biochemical stimuli such as acetylcholine, histamine, arginine, catecholamines, arachidonic acid, adenosine diphosphate (ADP), endothelin-1, bradykinin, serotonin, and thrombin. Nitric oxide then causes relaxation of the underlying smooth muscle and may be thought of as a paracrine homeopathic defense mechanism against noxious stimuli. Denudation or loss of the vascular endothelium results in loss of EDRF and this protective mechanism. Loss of the endothelial cell layer and function may occur secondary to physical disruption (percutaneous transluminal angioplasty [PTCA]), factors impinging from the vascular side (cyanide from smoke), or disruption of the intimal-medial layers (oxidized low-density lipoprotein). Impaired endothelial function may be related to the development of premature atherosclerosis based on recent family studies. Endothelial function may be improved with ACE inhibitors, statins, and exercise.[14]

Factors Extrinsic to the Vascular Bed

Blood flow to the coronary arteries arises from orifices located immediately distal to the aorta valve. Perfusion pressure is equal to the difference between the aortic pressure at an instantaneous point in time and the intramyocardial pressure. Coronary vascular resistance is influenced by phasic systolic compression of the vascular bed. The driving force for perfusion is, therefore, not constant throughout the cardiac cycle. Opening of the aortic valve may also lead to a Venturi effect, which can slightly decrease perfusion pressure. If perfusion pressure is elevated for a period of time, coronary vascular resistance declines and blood flow increases; however, continued perfusion pressure increases lead, within limits, to a return of coronary blood flow back toward baseline levels through autoregulation.

Alterations in intramyocardial wall tension throughout the cardiac cycle will also impose significant changes in coronary blood flow. Diastole is the period during which coronary artery filling can occur due to these pressure differences and little or no coronary blood flow occurs to the left ventricle during systole. The extent of pressure development in the ventricle and heart rate have a major effect on the development of wall tension, time for diastolic coronary artery filling, and myocardial oxygen demand.

Under normal conditions, the average global distribution of blood flow between the epicardial and endocardial layer is about 1:1 at rest and remains approximately even during exercise secondary to autoregulatory changes. Regional disparity of blood flow distribution does exist normally, and these disparities are magnified in the presence of diseased coronary arteries and with increased cardiac work as the vasodilator reserve in the resistance vessels of the subendocardial layers is exhausted. Factors that favor a reduction in subendocardial blood flow include decreased perfusion pressure due to decreased diastolic blood pressure or coronary artery obstruction by atherosclerotic plaques with or without vasomotion, abbreviation of diastole (increased heart rate), and increased intraventricular diastolic pressure (e.g., valvular obstruction to flow).

Extravascular resistance may decrease coronary blood flow, primarily during systole. This effect is much more pronounced in the left ventricle compared with the right ventricle (RV). When the effect of increased contractility is separated from the effect of ventricular pressure, about 75% of extravascular resistance is accounted for by passive stretch in equilibrium with ventricular pressure whereas only 25% results from active myocardial contraction.

Factors Intrinsic to the Vascular Bed

Metabolic factors, myogenic responses, neural reflexes, and humoral substances within the vascular bed of the coronary circulation function in an orchestrated fashion to maintain relative consistency in blood flow to the myocardium in the face of imposed changes in perfusion pressures. Autoregulation, mediated primarily through the effects of myogenic responses and metabolic factors, is thought to be responsible for maintaining regional blood flow in a narrow range while systemic pressure varies over a range of approximately 50 to 150 mm Hg.

Myogenic control (also known as the *Bayliss effect*) of coronary artery tone occurs when the vessel is stretched secondary to an increase in pressure and contracts to return blood flow to normal. It is thought that the myogenic response to stretching in coronary arteries is a modest one and that metabolic factors such as nitric oxide play a much larger role in autoregulation.

There are three well-studied metabolic factors that have the ability to modify coronary artery resistance and blood flow at the local level. Basal coronary blood flow meets oxygen demands of 8 to 10 mL/min per 100 g of myocardium with essentially complete extraction of oxygen from the blood. As cardiac output or mean arterial blood pressure increases, the increased demand for oxygen is met by increasing blood flow because little additional oxygen is available from hemoglobin. Decreased oxygen availability causes vasodilation of vascular smooth muscle and relaxation of precapillary sphincters, which increase tissue oxygen and help maintain blood flow on a regional basis.

At perfusion pressures below 60 mm Hg, as the coronary arteries are maximally dilated and the buffering effect of autoregulation has reached its capacity, further reduction in coronary blood flow will decrease perfusion pressure and tissue oxygenation. It is thought that autoregulation works more efficiently in the epicardial layers than in subendocardial layers, and this may contribute to coronary steal.

Neural components that participate in the regulation of coronary blood flow include the sympathetic nervous system, the parasympathetic nervous system, coronary reflexes, and possibly central control of coronary blood flow. Within the sympathetic system, stimulation of the stellate ganglion elicits coronary vasodilation, which is associated with tachycardia and enhanced contractility. This indirect coronary vasodilation is secondary to increased MVO_2 related to increased heart rate, contractility, and aortic pressure and occurs following stellate stimulation. The direct effect of the sympathetic system is α_1-mediated vasoconstriction at rest and during exercise. Other receptor types, α_2 and β_1, have little influence on tone, whereas β_2 stimulation produces a modest vasodilating effect. Although coronary atherosclerosis may decrease blood flow secondary to obstruction, severe coronary atherosclerosis and obstruction may also increase the sensitivity of coronary arteries to the effects of $\beta1$ stimulation and vasoconstriction.

Vagal stimulation within the parasympathetic system produces a small to moderate increase in coronary blood flow, which involves the coronary efferent and afferent parasympathetic components (Bezold–Jarish reflex). Indirectly, vasoconstriction may result, with vagal stimulation as the result of bradycardia and decreased contractility reducing myocardial oxygen demand.

Coronary reflexes have an undetermined role in the regulation of coronary blood flow. Based on experimental data, coronary reflexes that may be important include the baroreceptor, the chemoreceptor, Bezold–Jarish reflex, and the pulmonary inhalation reflex.

FACTORS LIMITING CORONARY PERFUSION

During exercise and pacing, as MVO_2 increases, coronary vascular resistance can be reduced to about 25% of basal values, which results in a fourfold to fivefold increase in coronary blood flow. The cross-sectional area can be reduced by about 80% prior to any mechanical or biochemical changes in the myocardium, reflecting a margin of safety for coronary blood flow. The extent of cross-sectional obstruction, the length of the lesion, lesion composition, and the geometry of the obstructing lesion can each affect flow across coronary arteries with atherosclerosis. Bernoulli's theorem states that the pressure drop across a lesion is directly related to the length of the lesion and inversely related to the radius of the lesion to the fourth power; critical stenosis occurs when the obstructing lesion encroaches on the luminal diameter and exceeds 70%. Lesions creating obstruction of 50% to 70% may reduce blood flow; however, these obstructions are not consistent and vasospasm and thrombosis superimposed on a "noncritical" lesion may lead to clinical events such as MI.[14] If the lesion enlarges from 80% to 90%, resistance in that vessel is tripled. Coronary reserve is diminished at about 85% obstruction owing to vasoconstriction. Exaggerated responsiveness can be seen when coronary stenosis reaches this critical level, and the role of vasoactive substances such as prostaglandins, thromboxanes, and serotonin may play more of a role in the regulation of coronary vascular tone and thrombosis.

Little reserve exists for coronary blood flow, and a relatively small reduction of 10% to 20% results in decreased myocardial fiber shortening as the first evidence for abnormal function. The subendocardial layers are affected to a greater extent than the epicardium by ischemia, considering changes in fiber shortening, arteriovenous (AV) difference in oxygen saturation, and lactate production. A reduction of 80% gives rise to akinesis and a 95% reduction of coronary blood flow produces dyskinesis during contraction of the ventricles. Although these abnormalities of contraction are associated with transient impaired function, depletion of high-energy phosphate compounds and ultrastructural changes may last for days even after transient ischemia; this has been referred to as *stunned myocardium*. Chronic hypoperfusion may lead to "hibernation," in which ventricular function is impaired over longer time intervals. Hibernating myocardium can be differentiated from necrosis with various techniques (see Chap. 17) and revascularization of hibernating myocardium is useful in improving ventricular function. Regional loss of contractility may impose a burden on the remaining myocardial tissue, resulting in heart failure, increased MVO_2, and rapid depletion of blood flow reserve. Consequently, zones of tissue with marginal blood flow may develop in a lateral or transmural fashion; such development puts this tissue at risk for more severe damage if the ischemic episode persists or becomes more severe. Nonischemic areas of myocardium may compensate for the severely ischemic and border zones of ischemia by developing more tension than usual in an attempt to maintain cardiac output. At the cellular level, ischemia and the attendant acidosis are thought to alter calcium release from storage sites such as the sarcolemma and the sarcoplasmic reticulum as well as inhibiting the binding of calcium to troponin, thereby impairing the association of actin and myosin. The clinical correlates of these cellular biochemical events leading to the development of LV or RV dysfunction include an S3, dyspnea, orthopnea, tachycardia, fluctuating blood pressure, transient murmurs, and mitral or tricuspid regurgitation.

Calcium accumulation and overload secondary to ischemia impairs ventricular relaxation as well as contraction. This is apparently a result of impaired calcium uptake after systole from the myofilaments, leading to a less negative decline of the pressure in the ventricle over time. Impaired relaxation is associated with enhanced diastolic stiffness, decreased rate of wall thinning, and slowed pressure decay, producing an upward shift in the ventricular pressure–volume relationship; put more simply, MVO_2 is likely to be increased secondary to increased wall tension. Impairment of both diastolic and systolic function leads to elevation of the filling pressure of the left ventricle.

CLINICAL PRESENTATION AND DIAGNOSIS OF ANGINA

General

- Many episodes of ischemia do not cause symptoms of angina (silent ischemia).
- Patients often have a reproducible pattern of pain or other symptoms that appear after a specific amount of exertion.
- Increased frequency, severity, duration, or symptoms at rest suggest an unstable angina pattern, and the patient should seek help immediately.

Symptoms

- ❷ Sensation of pressure or burning over the sternum or near it, often but not always radiating to the left jaw, shoulder, and arm; also chest tightness and shortness of breath.
- Pain usually lasts from 0.5 to 30 minutes often with a visceral quality (deep location).
- Precipitating factors include exercise, cold environment, walking after a meal, emotional upset, fright, anger, and coitus.
- Relief occurs with rest and nitroglycerin.

Signs

- Abnormal precordial (over the heart) systolic bulge
- Abnormal heart sounds

Laboratory Tests

- Typically no laboratory tests are abnormal; however, if the patient has intermediate- to high-risk features for unstable angina, electrocardiographic changes and serum troponin, or creatine kinase, they may become abnormal (see Table 23-3).
- Patients are likely to have laboratory test abnormalities for the risk factors for IHD such as elevated total and LDL cholesterol, low HDL cholesterol, impaired fasting glucose or elevated glucose, high blood pressure, elevated C-reactive protein, and abnormal renal function. Hemoglobin should be checked to make sure the patient is not anemic.

Other Diagnostic Tests (See Chap. 17)

- A resting electrocardiogram and then an exercise tolerance test are usually the first tests done in stable patients. A chest x-ray should be done if the patient has heart failure symptoms. Cardiac imaging using radioisotopes to detect ischemic myocardium and to measure ventricular function are commonly done when revascularization is being considered. Echocardiography may also be used to assess ventricular wall motion at rest or during stress. Cardiac catheterization and coronary arteriography are used to determine coronary artery anatomy and whether the patient would benefit from angioplasty, coronary artery bypass surgery, or other revascularization procedures. Coronary artery calcium (CAC) may be useful in detecting early disease.

Important aspects of the clinical history for chest pain for patients with angina include the nature or quality of the pain, precipitating factors, duration, pain radiation, and the response to nitroglycerin or rest. Because there can be considerable variation in the manifestations of angina, it is more accurate to refer to these symptoms as an anginal syndrome. For some patients with significant coronary disease, their presenting symptoms may differ from the classical symptoms; yet the symptoms are due to ischemic pain, and these are often referred to as *anginal equivalents*. Obtaining an accurate and detailed family history is useful in placing symptoms in perspective. Significant positive information includes

premature CHD (<55 years in men and <65 years in women) as manifested as fatal and nonfatal MI, stroke, peripheral vascular disease as well as other risk factors such as hypertension, smoking, familial lipid disorders, and diabetes mellitus (considered to be a risk equivalent). Typical pain radiation patterns include anterior chest pain (96%), left upper arm pain (83.7%), left lower arm pain (29.3%), and neck pain at some time (22%). Pain from other areas is less common. Ischemia detected by ECG monitoring is more likely to be detected in the morning hours (6 am to 12 noon) than other periods throughout the day. Patients suffering from variant or Prinzmetal angina secondary to coronary spasm are more likely to experience pain at rest and in the early morning hours. Prinzmetal anginal pain is not usually brought on by exertion or emotional stress nor relieved by rest; and the ECG pattern is that of current injury with ST elevation rather than depression. Typical pain that occurs in nonocclusive CAD is referred to as *microvascular angina*.

It is also important to differentiate the pattern of pain for stable angina from that of unstable angina. Unstable angina may be stratified into categories of risk ranging from high to low (Table 23–3).[15] Ischemia may also be painless, or "silent," in 60% to 100% of patients depending on the series cited and the patient population.[16] In patients with myocardial ischemia, approximately 70% of the episodes of documented ischemia are painless as determined by ambulatory ECG monitoring, and the ST segment changes associated with these episodes can be ST elevation or depression. The mechanism of silent ischemia is unclear, but studies have shown that patients not experiencing pain have altered pain perception, with the threshold and tolerance for pain being higher than that of patients who have pain more frequently. Although patients with diabetes tend to have more extensive and microvascular coronary disease than those without diabetes and may suffer from autonomic neuropathy, asymptomatic ischemia is not more prevalent based on the Asymptomatic Cardiac Ischemia Pilot (ACIP) study.[17]

Lastly, it should be recognized that the threshold for pain due to exertion is fixed for some patients and variable for others and that the amount of exercise or stress necessary to provoke symptoms can change over time. A fixed threshold for the induction of pain or ECG evidence of ischemia means these indicators of ischemia occur at the same, or nearly so, double rate–pressure product (systolic blood pressure × heart rate). This is apparently due to at least two factors. Over long periods of time atherosclerosis may progress, leading to more severe stenosis, reduced oxygen supply, and less

TABLE 23-3	Short-Term Risk of Death or Nonfatal Myocardial Infarction in Patients with Unstable Angina		
Feature	High Risk (At Least 1 of the Following Features must be Present)	Intermediate Risk (No High-Risk Feature but must have 1 of the Following)	Low Risk (No High- or Intermediate-Risk Feature but may have any of the Following)
History	Accelerating tempo of ischemic symptoms in preceding 48 hours	Prior MI, peripheral or cerebrovascular disease, or CABG, prior aspirin use	New-onset CCS class III or IV angina in the past 2 weeks without prolonged (>20 minutes) rest pain but with moderate or high likelihood of CAD
Character of pain	Prolonged ongoing (>20 minutes), rest pain	Prolonged (>20 minutes), rest angina, now resolved, with moderate or high likelihood of CAD	
Clinical findings	Pulmonary edema, most likely caused by ischemia New or worsening MR murmur S₃ or new/worsening rales Hypotension, bradycardia, tachycardia Age >75 years		
ECG	Angina at rest with transient ST-segment changes >0.05 mV Bundle-branch block, new or presumed new	T-wave inversions >0.2 mV Pathologic Q waves	Normal or unchanged ECG during an episode of chest discomfort
Cardiac markers	Markedly elevated (e.g., TnT or TnI > 0.1 ng/mL)	Slightly elevated (e.g., TnT > 0.01 but <0.1 ng/mL)	Normal

CABG, coronary artery bypass grafting; CAD, coronary artery disease; CCS, Canadian Cardiovascular Society; ECG, electrocardiogram; MI, myocardial infarction; MR, mitral regurgitation; TnI, troponin I; TnT, troponin T.

TABLE 23-4 Differential Diagnosis of Episodic Chest Pain Resembling Angina Pectoris

	Duration	Quality	Provocation	Relief	Location	Comment
Effort angina	5–15 minutes	Visceral (pressure)	During effort or emotion	Rest, NTG	Substernal, radiates	First episode vivid
Rest angina	5–15 minutes	Visceral (pressure)	Spontaneous (with exercise?)	NTG	Substernal, radiates	Often nocturnal
Mitral prolapse	Minutes to hours	Superficial (rarely visceral)	Spontaneous (no pattern)	Time	Left anterior	No pattern, variable
Esophageal reflux	10 minutes to 1 hour	Visceral	Spontaneous, cold liquids, exercise, lying down	Foods, antacids, H₂ blockers, proton pump inhibitors, NTG	Substernal, radiates	Mimics angina
Peptic ulcer	Hours	Visceral, burning	Lack of food, "acid" foods	Foods, antacids, H₂ blockers, proton pump inhibitors	Epigastric, substernal	
Biliary disease	Hours	Visceral (wax and wane)	Spontaneous, food	Time, analgesia	Epigastric, radiates	Colic
Cervical disk	Variable (gradually subsides)	Superficial	Spontaneous, food	Time, analgesia	Arm, neck	Not relieved by rest
Hyperventilation	2–3 minutes	Visceral	Emotion, tachypnea	Stimulus removed	Substernal	Facial paraesthesia
Musculoskeletal	Variable	Superficial	Movement, palpation	Time, analgesia	Multiple	Tenderness
Pulmonary	30 minutes	Visceral (pressure)	Often spontaneous	Rest, time bronchodilator	Substernal	Dyspneic

NTG, nitroglycerin.

of an increase in demand to precipitate ischemic symptoms. Once stenotic lesions reach a critical level of about 80% or greater, vasomotion, vasospasm, and thrombotic occlusion become significant factors impairing blood flow to the myocardium. Consequently, anatomic considerations and vasoactive substances may interact to provide an environment amenable to changing thresholds for the production of angina.

There appears to be little relationship between the historical features of angina and the severity or extent of coronary artery vessel involvement. Therefore, one may speculate that severe symptoms might be associated with multivessel disease, but no predictive markers exist on a routine basis.

Chest pain may resemble pain arising from a variety of noncardiac sources, and the differential diagnosis of anginal pain from other etiologies may be quite difficult based on history alone. Table 23–4 outlines other common problems that may present with episodic chest pain. Although much less common, nonatherosclerotic etiologies of CAD do exist and should be excluded with appropriate tests. The clinical classification of chest pain encompasses typical angina including (1) substernal chest pain with a characteristic quality and duration that is (2) provoked by exertion or emotional stress and (3) relieved by rest or nitroglycerin; atypical angina meets 2 of the characteristics for typical angina, and noncardiac chest pain meets ≤1 of the typical angina characteristics.[1,2]

There are few signs apparent on physical examination to indicate the presence of CAD and usually only the cardiovascular system reveals any useful information. Elevated heart rate or blood pressure can yield an increased double product and may be associated with angina, and it would be important to correct extreme tachycardia or hypertension if present. Other noncardiac physical findings that suggest that significant CVD may be associated with angina include abdominal aortic aneurysms or peripheral vascular disease. Cardiac examination findings in CAD are noted in Table 23–5. During an angina attack, these findings may appear or become more prominent, making them more valuable if present.

In addition to screening for CVD risk factors (Table 28–7), other recommended tests include hemoglobin, fasting glucose, fasting lipoprotein panel, resting ECG, and chest x-ray in patients with signs or symptoms of heart failure, valvular heart disease, pericardial disease or aortic dissection/aneurysm.[2] Hemoglobin is assessed to insure adequate oxygen carrying capacity. Fasting glucose determinations to exclude diabetes and glucose monitoring for concurrent diabetes should be performed routinely. Lipids are assessed

total, LDL, and HDL cholesterol and triglycerides (see Chap. 28).[18] Other risk factors that may be important for some patients include C-reactive protein, homocysteine level, evidence of chlamydia infection, and elevations in lipoprotein(a), fibrinogen, and plasminogen

TABLE 23-5 Cardiac Findings for Patients with Coronary Artery Disease

Sign	Clinical Significance	Frequency
Abnormal precordial systolic bulge	Left ventricular wall motion abnormality	Not usually present unless patient has sustained a prior MI (especially anterior wall) or is experiencing angina at time of examination
Decreased intensity of S₁	Decrease in left ventricular contractility	Difficult to evaluate in resting state, but can be commonly demonstrated during angina
Paradoxical splitting of S₂	Left ventricular wall motion abnormality	Very uncommon but occasionally noted during angina
S₃ (ventricular gallop)	Increased left ventricular diastolic pressure, with or without clinical CHF	Not usually present unless patient sustained extensive MI; may occasionally be present during angina
S₄ (atrial gallop)	Reduced ventricular compliance ("stiff heart")	Common; very common in patients who have sustained a prior MI as well as during angina
Apical systolic murmur (in absence of rheumatic mitral regurgitation or Barlow syndrome)	Papillary muscle dysfunction	Not usually present unless patient has sustained prior MI
Diastolic murmur (in absence of aortic regurgitation)	Coronary artery stenosis	Rare

CHF, congestive heart failure; MI, myocardial infarction; S₁, first heart sound; S₂, second heart sound; S₃, third heart sound; S₄, fourth heart sound.

From Cohn PF, ed. Diagnosis and Therapy of Coronary Artery Disease, 2d ed. Boston: Martinus Nijhoff; 1985:101, with permission.

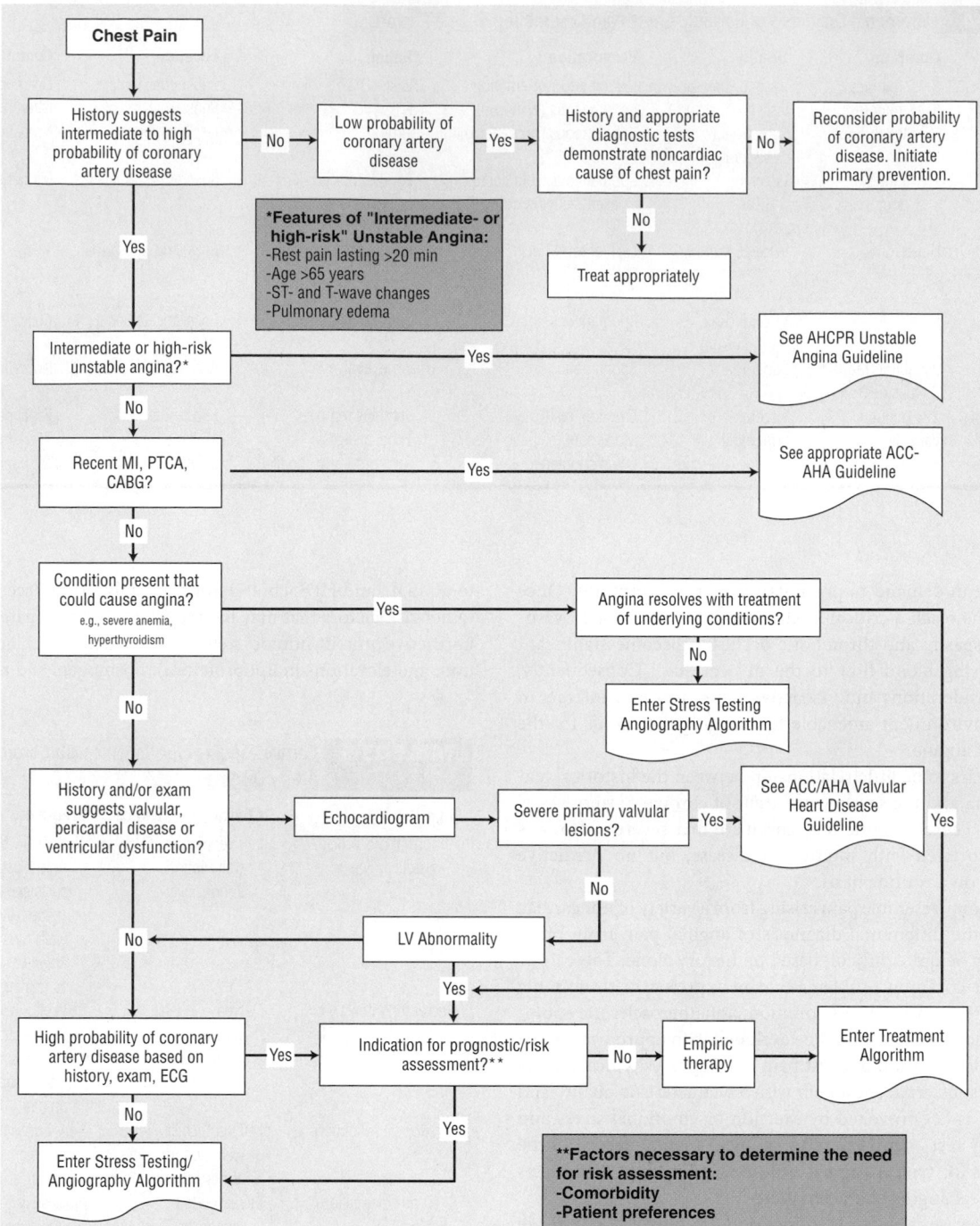

FIGURE 23-2. Clinical assessment (ACC/AHA, American College of Cardiologists/American Heart Association; AHCPR, Agency for Health Care Policy and Research; CABG, coronary artery bypass graft; ECG, electrocardiogram; LV, left ventricular; MI, myocardial infarction; PTCA, percutaneous transluminal coronary angioplasty).

activator inhibitor.[19] Cardiac enzymes should all be normal in stable angina. Troponin T or I, myoglobin or creatinine phosphokinase-MB isoform may be elevated in patients with unstable angina, and interventions such as anticoagulation or antiplatelet therapy have been shown to reduce cardiac end points when these markers for injury are elevated (Table 23–3).[20]

Patients presenting with chest pain are stratified into chronic stable angina or having features of intermediate or high-risk unstable angina (Fig. 23–2 and Table 23–3). These features include rest pain lasting >20 minutes, age >65 years, ST and T wave changes, and pulmonary edema. Patients with ACS (unstable angina, non-ST-segment

elevation AMI and ST-segment elevation AMI) are managed differently than chronic stable angina.

DIAGNOSTIC TESTS

See also Chap. 17.

Electrocardiogram

The ECG is normal in about one half of patients with angina who are not experiencing an acute attack. Typical ST-T-wave changes include depression, T-wave inversion, and ST-segment elevation.

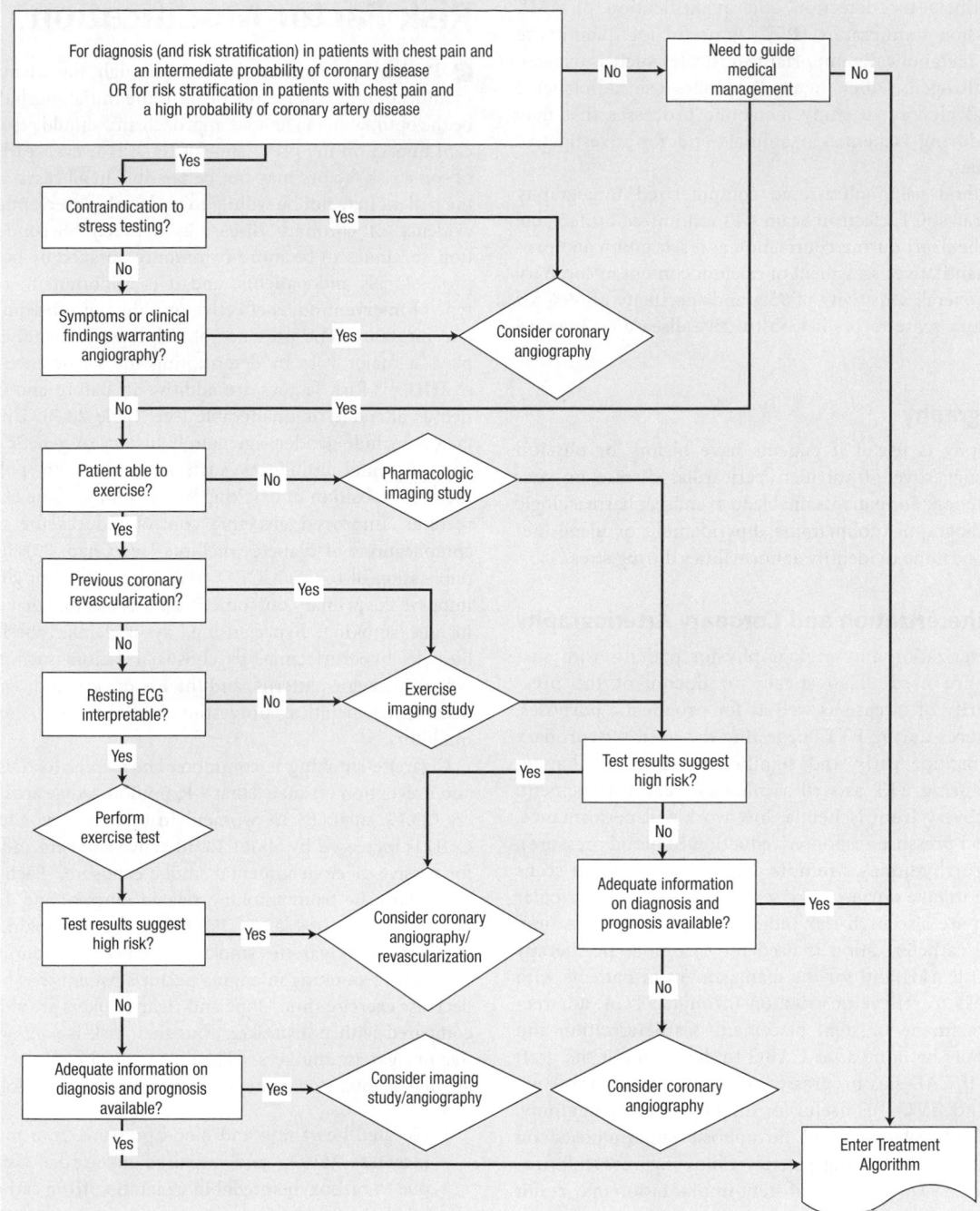

FIGURE 23-3. Stress testing/angiography algorithm. (ECG, electrocardiogram.)

Forms of ischemia other than exertional angina may have ECG manifestations that are different; variant angina is associated with ST-segment elevation, whereas silent ischemia may produce elevation or depression. Significant ischemia is associated with ST-segment depression of greater than 2 mm, exertional hypotension, and reduced exercise tolerance.

Exercise Tolerance Testing[21]

Exercise tolerance (stress) testing (ETT) is recommended for patients with intermediate pretest probability of CAD based on age, gender, and symptoms, including those with complete right bundle branch block or <1 mm of rest ST depression (Fig. 23–3). Although ETT is insensitive for predicting coronary artery anatomy, it does correlate well with outcomes such as the likelihood

of progressing to angina, the occurrence of acute MI, and cardiovascular death. Ischemic ST depression that occurs during ETT is an independent risk factor for cardiac events and cardiovascular mortality. Thallium (^{201}Tl) myocardial perfusion scintigraphy may be used in conjunction with ETT to detect reversible and irreversible defects in blood flow to the myocardium because it is more sensitive than ETT.

Cardiac Imaging

Radionuclide angiocardiography (performed with technetium-99m, a radioisotope) is used to measure ejection fraction, regional ventricular performance, cardiac output, ventricular volumes, valvular regurgitation, asynchrony or wall motion abnormalities, and intracardiac shunts.[22–24] Technetium pyrophosphate scans are used routinely for detection and quantification of AMI. Positron emission tomography (PET) is useful for quantifying ischemia with metabolically important substrates such as oxygen, carbon, and nitrogen. Other metabolic probes use radiolabeled fatty acids and glucose to study metabolic processes that may be deranged during ischemia in animals and for investigative purposes in man.

A new method using ultra-rapid computerized tomography (spiral CT, ultrafast CT, electron beam CT) minimized artifact due to motion of the heart during contraction and relaxation and provides a semiquantitative assessment of calcium content in coronary arteries.[22] The overall sensitivity of 95% and specificity of 66% for coronary calcium score to predict obstructive disease on invasive angiography.

Echocardiography

Echocardiography is useful if patients have history or physical examination suggestive of valvular, pericardial disease or ventricular dysfunction. For patients unable to exercise, pharmacologic stress echocardiography (dobutamine, dipyridamole, or adenosine) or pacing may be done to identify abnormalities during stress.

Cardiac Catheterization and Coronary Arteriography

Cardiac catheterization and angiography for patients with suspected CAD are used diagnostically to document the presence and severity of disease as well as for prognostic purposes. High-risk features during ETT suggesting the need for coronary angiography include early and significant (≥ 2 mm) changes on the ECG during ETT as well as multiple lead involvement, prolonged recovery from ischemia, low workload performance, abnormal blood pressure response (reduction in blood pressure), or ventricular arrhythmias. Multiple defects with thallium scans as well as lung uptake during exercise or postexercise ventricular cavity dilation are also high-risk indications for catheterization. Interventional catheterization is used for thrombolytic therapy for patients with AMI and for the management of patients with significant CAD to relieve obstruction through PTCA, atherectomy, laser treatment, or stent placement. Catheterization and angiography may be done after CABG to determine if the graft has closed or if CAD has progressed. Coronary artery intravascular ultrasound (IVUS) is useful for directly imaging anatomy, calcified and fatty plaques, and thrombosis superimposed on plaque as well as determining patency following revascularization procedures. IVUS guidance of stent implantation may result in more effective stent expansion compared with angiographic guidance alone.[23]

TREATMENT

Desired Outcome

The short-term goals of therapy for IHD are to reduce or prevent the symptoms of angina that limit exercise capability and impair quality of life. Long-term goals of therapy are to prevent CHD events such as MI, arrhythmias, and heart failure and extend the patient's life. Since there is little evidence that revascularization procedures such as angioplasty and coronary artery bypass surgery extend life, the primary focus should be on altering the underlying and ongoing process of atherosclerosis through risk factor modification while providing symptomatic relief through the use of nitrates, β-blockers, calcium channel blockers and ranolazine for anginal symptoms.

Risk Factor Modification

❸ Primary prevention of IHD through the identification and modification of risk factors prior to the initial morbid event would be the optimal management approach and should result in a significant impact on the prevalence of IHD. However, early recognition of some risk factors may not be possible in all cases, and in others, the patient may not be willing to undertake intervention until overt evidence of coronary disease is apparent. Secondary intervention continues to be more commonly pursued by both healthcare professionals and patients, and it is important to recognize this type of intervention as effective in reducing subsequent morbidity and mortality. The presence of risk factors in individual patients plays a major role in determining the occurrence and severity of IHD.[24,25] Risk factors are additive in nature and can be classified as alterable or unalterable (see Table 28-7). Unalterable risk factors include gender; age; family history or genetic composition; environmental influences such as climate, air pollution, trace metal composition of drinking water; and, to some extent, diabetes mellitus. Improved glycemic control reduces the microvascular complications of diabetes mellitus (see Chap. 83); however, with publication of the ACCORD trial strict control of glucose did not improve the primary outcome.[26] ❹ Risk factors that can be altered include smoking, hypertension, dyslipidemia, obesity, sedentary lifestyle, hyperuricemia, psychosocial factors such as stress and type A behavior patterns, and the use of certain drugs that may be detrimental including progestins, corticosteroids, and calcineurin inhibitors.

Cigarette smoking is common. The Center for Disease Control and Prevention estimates that ~46 million people are current smokers (23.1% men; 18.3% women) in this country, and the risk for CHD is increased by about 1.8 in active smokers and by about 1.3 for passive or environmental smoke exposure.[4] Each year 443,000 Americans die from smoking-related illnesses and 142,000 of the deaths are attributable to CVD.[4] Risk due to smoking is related to the number of cigarettes smoked per day and the duration of smoking. Passive smoking in angina pectoris patients has been shown to decrease exercise time.[6] Pipe and cigar smokers are at increased risk compared with nonsmokers, but their risk is somewhat less than that of cigarette smokers.[27] The direct effects of cigarette smoke that are detrimental to patients with angina include the following:

1. Elevated heart rate and blood pressure from nicotine, which increases MVO_2, and impaired myocardial oxygen delivery due to carboxyhemoglobin generation from carbon monoxide inhalation in smoke

2. The negative inotropic effect of carboxyhemoglobin

3. Increased platelet adhesiveness and promotion of aggregation resulting in thrombotic tendencies due to nicotine and carboxyhemoglobin

4. Lowered threshold for ventricular fibrillation during ischemia due to carboxyhemoglobin

5. Impaired endothelial function owing to smoking[28-31]

Similar changes have been noted for marijuana smoking as well. Smoking also accelerates the risk for MI, sudden death, cerebrovascular disease, peripheral vascular disease, and hypertension, and it reduces high-density lipoprotein concentrations. Clearly, primary prevention is needed for this risk factor and much of the education effort to discourage initiation of smoking should be targeted for teenagers. Techniques for cessation of smoking that may be useful include aversive conditioning, group programs, self-help programs, hypnosis, "cold turkey," and the use of nicotine substitutes (lobeline) or other sources of nicotine replacement products for short-term substitution during withdrawal syndrome. The antidepressant sustained-release bupropion has been shown to be more effective than placebo and best used with smoking cessation counseling. Varenicline, a partial agonist selective for the $\alpha_4\beta_2$ nicotinic acetylcholine receptor subtype has been shown to improve cessation rates as well.[28,29] Cessation of smoking reduces the incidence of coronary events to about 15% to 25% of that associated with continued smoking and these benefits are noted within 2 years of cessation.[30] A public ordinance reducing exposure to secondhand smoke was associated with a decrease in AMI hospitalizations in Pueblo, Colorado by 27% in 2 years.[31]

Hypertension, whether labile or fixed, borderline or definite, casual or basal, systolic or diastolic, at any age regardless of gender, is the most common and a powerful contributor to atherosclerotic coronary vascular disease.[32] Morbidity and mortality increase progressively with the degree of blood pressure elevation of either systolic or diastolic pressure and pulse pressure, and no discernible critical value exists (see Chap. 19). Numerous trials have documented the reduction in risk associated with blood pressure lowering; however, most of these studies show that mortality and morbidity reduction is a result of fewer strokes and less renal failure and heart failure. The reduction in CHD end points is significant but not as dramatic. The reasons for this are unclear but perhaps relate to the multifactorial etiology of IHD. Recent guideline changes from the AHA recommend goal blood pressure of <130/80 mmHg for patients with stable angina, unstable angina, non–ST-segment MI, and ST-segment MI and <120/80 mmHg for patients with LV dysfunction.[32]

Hypercholesterolemia is a significant cardiovascular risk factor, and risk is directly related to the degree of cholesterol elevation.[24,33] As with hypertension, there is no critical value that defines risk, but rather, risk is incrementally related to the degree of elevation and the presence of other risk factors (see Chap. 28 for a detailed discussion). A fasting lipoprotein panel should be obtained in all patients with known CAD. The goals for total, LDL, and HDL cholesterol and triglycerides are discussed in Chap. 28. All patients should undertake therapeutic lifestyle changes. Reductions in LDL cholesterol for primary prevention and secondary intervention have been shown to reduce total and CAD mortality and stroke as well as the need for interventions such as PTCA and CABG. Supplemental vitamin E or other antioxidants reduce the susceptibility of LDL cholesterol to oxidation, but clinical trial data have failed to show any benefit with supplementation.[34]

The prevalence of overweightness and obesity, defined as a body mass index (BMI)—weight in kg divided by height in meters squared—of ≥25 kg/m² and ≥30 kg/m², respectively, are estimated to occur in 66.3% and 34.3% of the U.S. population. BMI is associated with an increased mortality ratio compared with individuals of normal body weight, and the objective for patients with IHD is to maintain or reduce to a normal body weight.[4] This may be accomplished through dietary modification, exercise, pharmacologic therapy, or surgical therapy. Frequently associated with obesity is a sedentary lifestyle, and inactivity may contribute to higher blood pressure, elevated blood lipid levels, and insulin resistance associated with glucose intolerance in diabetics (insulin resistance or metabolic syndrome). Exercise to the level of about 300 kcal 3 times/week is useful in improving maximal oxygen uptake, improving cardiorespiratory efficiency, promoting collateral artery formation, and promoting potential alterations in the risk of ventricular fibrillation, coronary thrombosis, and improved tolerance to stress. Epidemiologic studies have found that mortality is directly related to resting heart rate and a low heart rate difference between resting and maximal exercise heart rate and inversely related to exercise heart rate. A regular exercise program has been shown to reduce all-cause and cardiac mortality.[35,36]

Competitiveness, intense striving for achievement, easily provoked hostility, a sense of urgency about doing things quickly and being punctual, impatience, abrupt and rapid speech and gestures, and concentration on self-selected goals to the point of not perceiving and attending to other aspects of the environment are traits that characterize the behavioral pattern known as the type A or coronary prone personality. Although the issue is somewhat controversial, type A individuals may have increased cardiovascular risk with risk ratios ranging from insignificant to 3 times that of a matched population. Psychological stress and type D personality have been associated with adverse cardiac prognosis, but little is known about their relative effect on the pathogenesis of CHD. Type D refers to the tendency to experience negative emotions and to inhibit the expression of these emotions in social interactions. The mechanism by which personality affects the cardiovascular system is not understood but may reflect the activity of the sympathetic system and enhanced responsiveness of other stress hormones when compared with non-type A personalities.

Alcohol ingestion in small to moderate amounts (<40 g/d of pure ethanol) reduces the risk of CHD; however, consumption of large amounts (>50 g/d) or binge drinking of alcohol is associated with increased mortality from stroke, cancer, vehicular accidents, and cirrhosis.[37,38] There appears to be a differential effect depending on race with an inverse relationship between ethanol consumption in whites and CAD risk but a direct relationship in blacks between consumption and CAD risk. The mechanisms for the presumed protective effects of alcohol are not known but the effects may be related to increased high-density lipoprotein levels, impaired platelet function, or associations between the amount of alcohol ingested and personality type. Whatever the relationship, it is well to remember that alcohol drinking is implicated in over 40% of all fatal automobile accidents and consumption of alcohol predisposes to hepatic cirrhosis, the sixth to seventh most common cause of death of the middle aged in the United States. With this in mind, it seems illogical to suggest alcohol ingestion as a prophylactic measure for coronary disease but rather advise moderation of alcohol consumption, if it is the preference of the individual.

Thiazide diuretics have been shown to elevate serum cholesterol and triglyceride levels, whereas β-blockers tend to lower HDL and raise LDL slightly; however, a direct association between these drugs and cardiovascular risk is tenuous and based on aggregating results rather than randomized clinical trials. Conjugated equine estrogen alone or in combination with progestin lowers LDL and raises HDL; unfortunately, the Heart and estrogen/progestin replacement study (HERS) trial showed no benefit of hormone replacement therapy for secondary intervention and increased risk for thromboembolism.[39] In secondary intervention, hormone replacement therapy (HRT) or estrogen alone in women after hysterectomy found that hormonal therapy health risks exceeded benefits as well.[40] Unopposed estrogen is the optimal regimen for elevation of HDL, but the high rate of endometrial hyperplasia restricts use to women without a uterus. In women with a uterus, estrogen with cyclic medroxyprogesterone has the most favorable effect on HDL and no excess risk of endometrial hyperplasia. Use of oral contraceptives in women who smoke and are over the age of 35 years increases the risk of MI, stroke, and venous thromboembolism by threefold or higher. Alternative forms of contraception and cessation of smoking should be promoted for these patients. The risk for nonsmoking oral contraceptive users under the age of 35 is very small. The relative risk of breast cancer is increased, but in the absence of risk factors for breast cancer, the relative risk is approximately 1.3 (30% increase). Coffee consumption has also been linked to CHD and caffeine does transiently elevate blood pressure; however, the overall risk, if any, appears to be low and may be related to genetic makeup (cytochrome P450 (CYP)

| TABLE 23-6 | The American College of Cardiology and American Heart Association Evidence Grading System |

Recommendation Class		Level of Evidence	
I	Conditions for which there is evidence or general agreement that a given procedure or treatment is useful and effective	A	Data derived from multiple randomized clinical trials with large numbers of patients
II	Conditions for which there is conflicting evidence or a divergence of opinion that the usefulness/efficacy of a given procedure or treatment is useful and effective	B	Data derived from a limited number of randomized trials with small numbers of patients, careful analyses of nonrandomized studies, or observational registries
IIa	Weight of evidence/opinion is in favor or usefulness/efficacy	C	Expert consensus was the primary basis for the recommendation
IIb	Usefulness/efficacy is less well established by evidence/opinion		
III	Conditions for which there is evidence or general agreement that a given procedure or treatment is not useful/effective and in some cases may be harmful		

1A2 mutation).[41] Although thiazide diuretics and β-blockers (nonselective without intrinsic sympathomimetic activity) may elevate both cholesterol and triglycerides by some 10% to 20%, and these effects may be detrimental, no objective evidence exists from prospective well-controlled studies to support avoiding these drugs at this time. This controversy is most pertinent in the treatment of mild hypertension, and it is discussed in greater detail in Chap. 19.

TREATMENT

Stable Exertional Angina Pectoris

(Table 23–6 contains evidence grading recommendations.)

The current national guidelines recommend that all patients be given the following unless contraindications exist:

1. Aspirin (Class I, Level A);

2. β-blockers with prior MI (Class I, Level A)

3. ACE inhibitor to patients with CAD and diabetes or LF systolic dysfunction (Class I, Level A)

4. LDL-lowering therapy with CAD and LDL >130 mg/dL (Class I, Level A) (target LDL <100 mg/dL; <70 mg/dL for patients with CHD and multiple risk factors is reasonable)[33]

5. SL nitroglycerin or immediate relief of angina (Class I, Level B)

6. Calcium antagonists or long-acting nitrates for reduction of symptoms when β-blockers are contraindicated (Class I, Level B)

7. Calcium antagonists or long-acting nitrates in combination with β-blockers when initial treatment with β-blockers is not successful (Class I, Level C)

8. Calcium antagonists or long-acting nitrates are recommended as a substitute for β-blockers if initial treatment with β-blockers leads to unacceptable side effects (Class I, Level A).

Clopidogrel may be substituted when aspirin is absolutely contraindicated (Class IIa, Level B) and long-acting non-dihydropyridine calcium antagonists instead of β-blockers as initial therapy (Class IIa, Level B). ACE inhibitors are recommended for patients with CAD or other vascular disease (Class IIa, Level B). Angiotensin receptor antagonists are not mentioned in these guidelines, but substitution for ACE inhibitor intolerance is reasonable. Low-intensity anticoagulation with warfarin, in addition to aspirin, is recommended, but bleeding would be increased (Class IIb, Level B).[1,42]

Therapies to be avoided include dipyridamole (Class III, Level B) and chelation therapy (Class III, Level B). Ranolazine is not addressed in these guidelines because it was released after their

publication. The European Society of Cardiology guidelines have a Class IIb, Level B recommendation.[3]

After assessing and manipulating the alterable risk factors as discussed previously, the next intervention that could be undertaken is the institution of a regular exercise program. Training is possible in many patients with angina and the observed benefits include decreased heart rate and systolic blood pressure as well as increased ejection fraction and duration of exercise. Although the mechanism of these effects has been debated, improved overall cardiovascular and muscular condition is probably most important. Improved production of nitric oxide and coronary vasomotion may account partially for the beneficial effects of exercise. The intensity of exercise influences training and more vigorous programs provide better overall results.[35,36] Obviously, an exercise program should be undertaken with caution and in a graded fashion with adequate supervision.

❺ Chronic prophylactic therapy for patients with more than one angina episode per day may also be instituted with β-adrenergic blocking agents, and in many instances β-blockers may be preferable because of less frequent dosing and other properties inherent in β-blockade (e.g., potential cardioprotective effects, antiarrhythmic effects, lack of tolerance, and antihypertensive effects), as well as their antianginal effects and documented protective effects in post-MI patients.[1,42] β-Blockers may also slow the progression of plaque volume.[43] Patients who continue to smoke have reduced antianginal efficacy of β-blockers. This may be due to enhanced hepatic metabolism of drugs that are eliminated through this route or related to the effects of smoking on MVO_2 and oxygenation.[44] The one characteristic that is relevant is the duration of effect on the double product. β-Blockers with longer half-lives (e.g., nadolol) are more likely to affect the double product for a longer period of time and require fewer doses per day. The choice of β-blocker for angina rests on choosing the appropriate dose to achieve the goals outlined for heart rate and double product and choosing an agent that is well tolerated by individual patients and cost. Selective use may incorporate ancillary properties, but these are secondary considerations in overall drug product selection. Patients most likely to respond well to β-blockade are those who have a high resting heart rate and those having a relatively fixed anginal threshold. In other words, their symptoms appear at the same level of exercise or workload on a consistent basis. Symptoms appearing with variable workloads suggest fluctuations in myocardial oxygen supply, perhaps due to coronary artery vasomotion, and these patients are more likely to respond to calcium channel antagonists.

❻ Nitrate therapy should be the first step in managing acute attacks for patients with chronic stable angina if the attacks are infrequent (i.e., a few times per month) or for prophylaxis of symptoms when undertaking activities known to precipitate attacks. In general, if angina occurs no more often than once every few days, then sublingual (SL) nitroglycerin tablets or spray or buccal products may be sufficient to allow the patient to maintain an

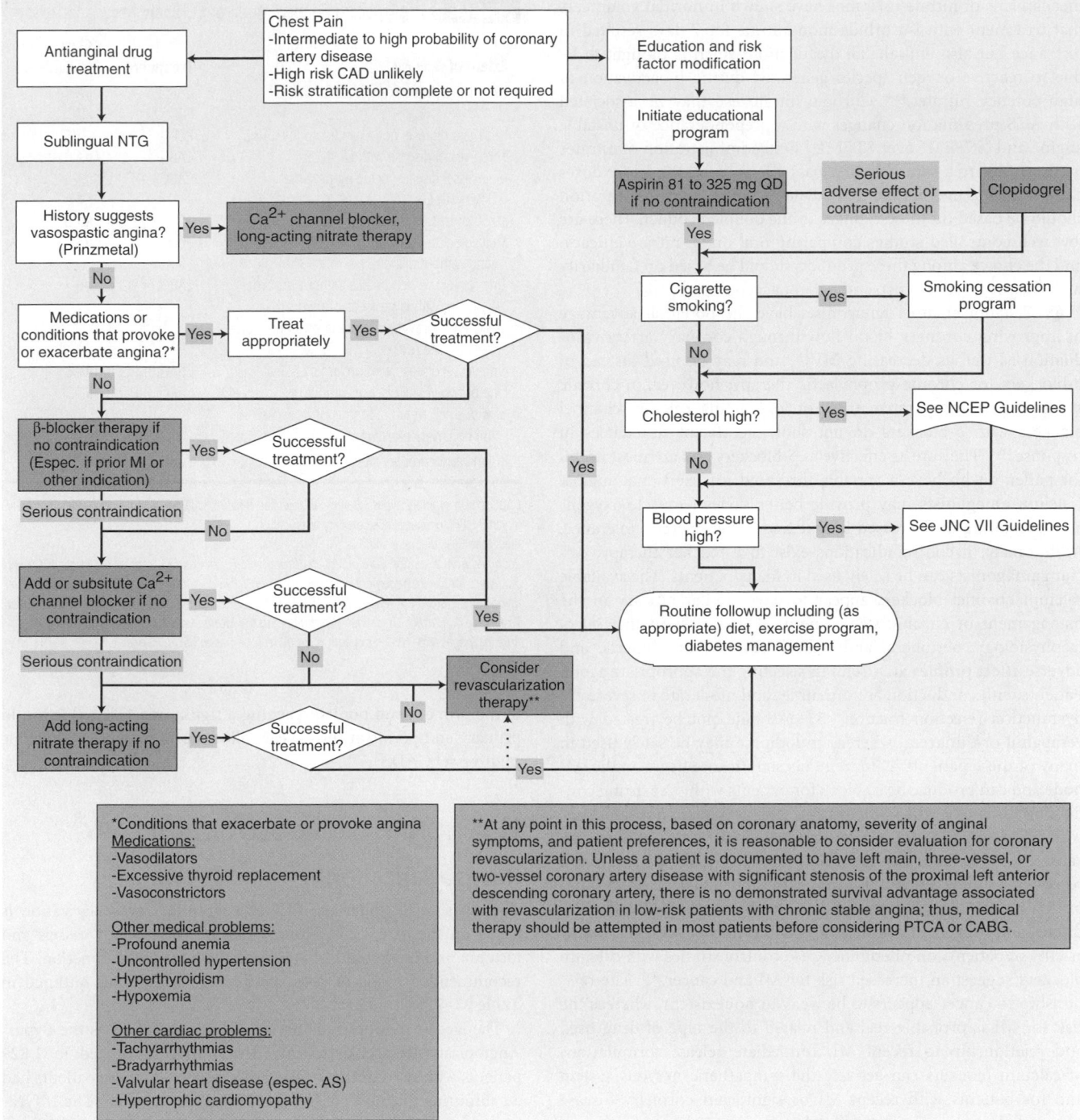

FIGURE 23-4. Treatment algorithm (AS, aortic stenosis; CABG, coronary artery bypass grafting; CAD, coronary artery disease; JNC VII, Seventh Report of the Joint National Committee on Prevention, Detection, Evaluation, and Treatment of High Blood Pressure; MI, myocardial infarction; NCEP, National Cholesterol Education Program; NTG, nitroglycerin; PTCA, percutaneous transluminal coronary angioplasty; QD, every day.)

adequate lifestyle. For episodes of "first-effort" angina occurring in a predictable fashion, nitroglycerin may be used in a prophylactic manner with the patient taking 0.3 to 0.4 mg sublingually about 5 minutes prior to the anticipated time of activity. Nitroglycerin spray may be useful when inadequate saliva is produced to rapidly dissolve SL nitroglycerin or if a patient has difficulty opening the container. Most patients have a response that lasts about 30 minutes or so, but this is subject to interindividual variability. When angina occurs more frequently than once a day, a chronic prophylactic regimen using β-blockers as the first line of therapy should be considered (see Fig. 23–4 for the stable angina algorithm).

Chronic prophylactic therapy with long-acting forms of nitroglycerin (oral or transdermal), isosorbide dinitrate, 5-mononitrate, and pentaerythritol trinitrate may be effective; however, the development of tolerance is a major limiting step in their continued effectiveness. Since long-acting nitrates are not as effective as β-blockers and do not have beneficial effects, monotherapy with nitrates should not be first-line therapy unless β-blockers and calcium channel blockers are contraindicated or not tolerated. As described previously, providing a nitrate-free interval of 8 hours per day or longer appears to be the most promising approach to maintaining the efficacy of chronic nitrate therapy. Recent investigations into the mechanisms of nitrate tolerance have shown in normal volunteers that treatment with isosorbide mononitrate for 7 days resulted in tolerance but also endothelial dysfunction which is thought to be due to reactive oxygen species generated during bioactivation of high-potency nitrates.[45,46] Chronic nitrate use may be associated with ACS presentation changes with a preponderance of unstable angina and NSTEMI over STEMI.[47] Oral administration of nitrates is susceptible to a saturable first-pass effect; therefore, larger doses can produce a measurable hemodynamic effect and dose titration should be based on these changes in the double product. There are few well-controlled studies comparing oral or SL nitrate efficacy, and the choice among these products should be based on familiarity with the preparation, cost, and patient acceptance.

❼ Calcium channel antagonists have the potential advantage of improving coronary blood flow through coronary artery vasodilation as well as decreasing MVO_2 and may be used instead of β-blockers for chronic prophylactic therapy; however, in chronic stable angina comparative trials of long-acting calcium channel blockers with β-blockers do not show significant differences in response.[48,49] They are as effective as β-blockers and are most useful for patients who have a variable threshold for exertional angina. Calcium antagonists may provide better skeletal muscle oxygenation, resulting in decreased fatigue and better exercise tolerance. Additionally, if contraindications exist to β-blocker therapy, calcium antagonists can be safely used in many patients. The available calcium channel blockers appear to have similar efficacy in the management of chronic stable angina. Differences in their electrophysiology, peripheral and central hemodynamic effects, and adverse effect profiles are useful in selecting the appropriate agent. Patients with conduction abnormalities and moderate to severe LV dysfunction (ejection fraction <35%) should not be treated with verapamil or diltiazem, whereas amlodipine may be safely used in many of these patients. Diltiazem has significant effects on the AV node and can produce heart block for patients with preexisting conduction disease or when other drugs, such as digoxin or β-blockers, with effects on conduction are used concurrently. Nifedipine may cause excessive heart rate elevation, especially if the patient is not receiving a β-blocker, and this may offset the beneficial effect it has on MVO_2. Gingival hyperplasia has also been reported with nifedipine, and some dental authorities say this may be seen in as many as 20% of patients on nifedipine. Case control studies with calcium blockers suggest an increased risk for MI and cancer.[50,51] The relationship to cancer appears to be weak to nonexistent, whereas the risk for MI is probably real and related to the type of drug used and relationship to recent MI. Immediate release formulations of calcium blockers can activate the sympathetic nervous system and for patients with recent MI or significant coronary disease may induce ischemia. This effect has not been shown for longer acting products. The hemodynamic effect of calcium antagonists is complementary to β-blockade, and consequently, combination therapy is rational, but clinical trial data do not support the notion that combination therapy is always more effective.[48,52]

While revascularization (see the following section) would seem to provide better symptomatic relief and improved survival rates, recent randomized trials have shown no advantage of angioplasty or surgery over medical therapy for patients with stable CAD. In the Clinical Outcomes Utilizing Revascularization and Aggressive Drug Evaluation (COURAGE) trial the 4.6-year cumulative primary-event rates (death from any cause and nonfatal MI) were 19.0% in the PCI group and 18.5% in the medical-therapy group (hazard ratio for the PCI group, 1.05; 95% confidence interval [CI], 0.87 to 1.27; P = 0.62).[53,54] Medicine, Angioplasty, or Surgery Study (MASS II) found medical therapy was associated with an incidence of long-term events and rate of additional revascularization similar to those for PCI. CABG was superior to medical therapy in terms

TABLE 23-7 Recommended Mode of Coronary Revascularization

Extent of Disease	Treatment	Class/Level of Evidence
Left main disease,[a] candidate for CABG	CABG	I/A
	PCI	III/C
Left main disease, not a candidate for CABG	PCI	IIb/C
Three-vessel disease with EF <0.50	CABG	I/A
Multivessel disease including proximal LAD with EF	CABG	I/A
<0.50 or treated diabetes	PCI	IIb/B
Multivessel disease with EF >0.50 and without diabetes	PCI	I/A
One- or two-vessel disease without proximal LAD but with large areas of myocardial ischemia or high-risk criteria on noninvasive testing (see text)	CABG or PCI	I/B
One-vessel disease with proximal LAD	CBAG or PCI	IIa/B
One-or two-vessel disease without proximal LAD with small area of ischemia or no ischemia on noninvasive testing	CABG or PCI	III/C
Insignificant coronary stenosis	CABG or PCI	III/C

CABG, coronary artery bypass grafting; EF, ejection fraction; LAD, left anterior descending coronary artery; PCI, percutaneous coronary intervention.
[a]Less than 50% diameter stenosis.
Reprinted from J Am Coll Cardiol, Vol. 36, Braunwald E, Antman EM, Beasley JW, et al., ACC/AHA guidelines for the management of patients with unstable angina and non–ST-segment elevation myocardial infarction: A report of the American College of Cardiology/American Heart Association Task Force on Practice Guidelines (Committee on the Management of Patients with Unstable Angina), pages 970–1062, Copyright © 2000 with permission from Elsevier.

of the primary end points, reaching a significant 44% reduction in primary end points at the 5-year follow-up of patients with stable multivessel CAD.[55]

■ ❽ NONPHARMACOLOGIC THERAPY

Revascularization

The decision to undertake PCI or CABG for revascularization is based on the extent of coronary disease (number of vessels and location and/or amount of stenosis) and ventricular function. The recommended mode of coronary revascularization is outlined in Table 23-7.[56,57]

The largest randomized trial of PCI versus CABG is the Bypass Angioplasty Revascularization (BARI) trial conducted in 1,829 patients with two- or three-vessel disease; 64% of these patients had an admitting diagnosis of UA and 19% were diabetic.[58] The 10-year survival was 71.0% for PTCA and 73.5% for CABG (P = 0.18). At 10 years, the PTCA group had substantially higher subsequent revascularization rates than the CABG group (76.8% vs 20.3%, P<0.001), but angina rates for the two groups were similar. In the subgroup of patients with no treated diabetes, survival rates were nearly identical by randomization (PTCA 77.0% vs CABG 77.3%, P = 0.59).[59] Insulin-requiring diabetics and chronic kidney disease seem to be at the highest risk, and CABG is the revascularization procedure of choice for this population.[54] In a large observational study by Hannan et al., patients with proximal LAD lesions and multivessel disease had higher survival rates with CABG than with PTCA.[58,60,61] High-risk patients who should be considered for CABG over PCI are those with LV systolic dysfunction, patients with diabetes, and those with two-vessel disease with severe proximal LAD involvement or severe three-vessel or left main disease[56] (Table 23-7). Angina with Extremely Serious Operative Mortality (AWESOME) found that patients who were older than 70 years of age support the trial conclusions that either bypass or percutaneous intervention effectively relieves medically refractory ischemia among high-risk unstable angina patients whose age was >70 years.[62]

PCI has been used successfully in the management of unstable angina.[63] PTCA involves the insertion of a guidewire and inflatable balloon into the affected coronary artery and enlarging the lumen of the artery by stretching the vessel wall. This frequently causes atheroma plaque fracture by stretching inelastic components and denudation of the endothelium resulting in loss of nitric oxide and other vasodilators and exposure of plaque contents to the vascular compartment. Consequently, immediate vascular recoil, platelet adhesion and aggregation, mural thrombus formation, smooth muscle proliferation, and synthesis of extracellular matrix may give rise to acute occlusion and early or late restenosis.[64–66] The presence of coronary artery spasm and intraluminal thrombus, common occurrences in unstable angina, increases the hazard of these complications. The advent of combination therapy with Aspirin (ASA), Unfractonated Heparin (UFH), or Low Molecular Weight Heparin LMWH) and IIb/IIIa receptor antagonists and coronary artery stents has dramatically reduced the occurrence of early reocclusion and late restenosis.[67,68] Patients best suited for PTCA are those with recent onset of worsening of angina without a long history of symptoms. Angiographic characteristics associated with these clinical findings that allow the greatest probability of success for PTCA are severe, discrete, proximal lesions found in a large epicardial vessel subtending a moderate or large area of viable myocardium and have high risk. Patients with focal saphenous-vein-graft lesions who are poor candidates for reoperation have a Class IIa recommendation for PCI. Class IIb indications include patients with one or more lesions to be dilated in vessels subtending a less than moderate area of viable myocardium and patients with multivessel disease and proximal LAD lesions, diabetes, or abnormal LV function.[57] Previously, candidates for PTCA must also be suited for CABG because a small percentage of procedures results in emergency CABG. Improvements in PCI and stent technology have lead to some institutions performing procedures without surgical backup.[69] Success of PCI may be defined as angiographic success (TIMI 3 flow and <20% residual stenosis), procedural success (lack of in-hospital clinical complications), and clinical success (anatomic and procedural success with relief of ischemic pain for at least 6 months). In trials of invasive versus conservative strategies (medical management) using PCI, death or MI is less frequent in some trials but not all.[53,70,71] Numerous studies support the use of IIb/IIIa receptor antagonists in addition to ASA and UFH or LMWH and as described previously, abciximab was superior to tirofiban in the only comparative study available.[72,73] The initial success rate for PTCA in unstable angina is ~80% to 90%, but these patients are at risk for more complications than are those with stable angina because of the underlying pathophysiology.

In the event of prolonged chest pain and ischemic ECG changes unrelieved by nitrate therapy or calcium channel antagonists, one may assume total occlusion of a coronary vessel and steps should be taken to restore blood flow with either PCI or CABG.

Coronary Artery Bypass Grafting[74]

Following the introduction of saphenous-vein-graft replacement for the severely occluded coronary arteries by Favorolo and Garrett in 1967, CABG became an accepted and commonly used approach for the management of IHD. The objectives in performing CABG are twofold: (1) reduce the number of symptomatic anginal attacks not controlled with medical management or PCI and improve the lifestyle of the patient and (2) reduce the mortality associated with CAD. Surgery is effective in providing pain relief in large numbers of patients, with about 70% to 95% being pain free at 1 year and

46% to 55% being pain free at 5 years. This compares favorably with medical management, for which only about 30% are free of symptoms at 5 years. Mortality at 10 years from the largest published studies is 26.4% with CABG and 30.5% with medical management ($P = 0.03$), but there are significant differences based on subgroup analysis (e.g., left main disease vs one-vessel without a proximal LAD lesion).[74] The second objective is met for certain patients and this has been addressed in three large, well-controlled trials of bypass surgery. These three studies, the Veterans Administration (VA), European Cooperative Surgery Study (ECSS), and the CASS, are not directly comparable because the inclusion and exclusion criteria for entry into each study were different and patients were followed for different periods of time. They have also been criticized for not being representative of the population that may be candidates for surgery, lacking women or late-middle-aged or elderly patients, and for crossover of medically managed patients to the surgical group. A major change in medical practice that influences the interpretation of these older studies is the common procedure of stent placement at the time of angioplasty.[11,75] There are about 20 different types of stents available, and their use is associated with greater luminal diameter after angioplasty, fewer acute reocclusions, and less restenosis after stent placement.[76] Consequently, the validity of generalizing the results from these studies to routine practice has been questioned, but these studies are useful for providing a basis for decisions concerning surgery. Current class I recommendations for CABG in asymptomatic or mild angina patient includes significant (>50%) left main coronary artery stenosis, left main equivalent (≥70% stenosis of the proximal LAD and proximal left circumflex artery), and three-vessel disease, especially for patients with LV ejection fraction <0.50.[74] Class IIa recommendations for CABG are proximal LAD stenosis with one- or two-vessel disease and Class IIb one- or two-vessel disease not involving the proximal LAD. In stable angina, Class I recommendations are the same as for mild angina with the following additions: one- or two-vessel disease without significant proximal LAD stenosis, but with a large area of viable myocardium and high-risk criteria in noninvasive testing; disabling angina despite maximal medical therapy, when surgery can be performed with acceptable risk. Class IIb recommendations in stable angina include proximal LAD stenosis with one-vessel disease and one- or two-vessel disease without significant proximal LAD stenosis but with a moderate area of viable myocardium and ischemia on noninvasive testing. The indications for CABG in UA/NSTEMI are described previously. In ST-segment MI CABG is indicated for ongoing ischemia/infarction not responsive to maximal medical therapy (Class IIb).

For patients with poor LV function CABG is indicated for the same indications as in mild angina for Class I. Class IIa recommendations include poor LV function with significant viable, noncontracting, revascularizable myocardium without any of the aforementioned anatomic patterns (e.g., left main disease). CABG is useful for patients with life-threatening ventricular arrhythmia in the presence of left main disease, three-vessel disease (Class I) and in bypassable one- or two-vessel disease causing life-threatening ventricular arrhythmias and proximal LAD disease with one- or two-vessel disease (Class IIa).

CABG may also be used for patients who have failed PTCA if there is ongoing ischemia or threatened occlusion with significant myocardium at risk and for patients with hemodynamic compromise (Class I). Class IIa recommendations for failed PTCA include a foreign body in a crucial anatomic position and hemodynamic compromise for patient with impairment of the coagulation system and without a previous sternotomy. CABG may be repeated for patients with a previous CABG if disabling angina exists despite maximal noninvasive therapy (Class I) and if a large area of myocardium is threatened and is subtended by bypassable distal vessels (Class IIa).

The need for nitrates and β-blockers is clearly reduced by surgery, with only 30% of CABG patients requiring chronic medication, whereas 70% of their medical counterparts received anginal drugs. Employment status after surgery has been shown in CASS to be more dependent on the pretreatment status than an effect induced by the treatment arm, and about 70% of patients are employed before and after surgery. Recent follow-up analyses of these studies suggest that patients who have diabetes or peripheral vascular disease, who are African American, or who continued to smoke are at high risk for CAD events, and diabetics, in particular, are more likely to have a better outcome with CABG than PTCA.[58,70] The overall benefit noted after CABG is similar in men and women, and elderly patients appear to have outcomes similar to younger patients.

Operative mortality is reported to range from 1% to 3% and is related to the number of vessels involved and preoperative ventricular function. Patients in CASS with one-, two-, or three-vessel disease had operative mortalities of 1.4%, 2.1%, and 2.8%, respectively. The relationship to LV ejection fraction follows a similar trend with ejection fractions of >50%, 20% to 40%, and <20% having operative mortality rates of 1.9%, 4.4%, and 6.7%, respectively. Perioperative infarction averages 5% depending on the sensitivity of the method for assessment, and the occurrence of an infarct reduces long-term survival. Neurologic dysfunction is relatively common postoperatively in CABG patients (~6%), but many of the deficits are clinically insignificant and resolve with time. Fatal brain damage occurs in 0.3% to 0.7%, stroke in about 5%, and ophthalmologic defects occur in 25%, but only 3% have clinically apparent field defects. Peripheral nerve lesions (12%) and brachial plexopathy (7%) are also reported to occur. Other complications include constrictive pericarditis (0.2%), cellulitis at the site of vein graft, and mediastinal infections (1% to 4%).

Graft patency influences the success for symptom control, and survival and the mechanism for early graft occlusion are probably different from that associated with late closure. Early occlusion is related to platelet adhesion and aggregation, whereas late occlusion may be related to endothelial proliferation and progression of atherosclerosis. Patency of grafts early on after the CABG is reported to range from 88% to 97% in at least one graft and 58% to 81% in all grafts at 1 year. Long-term patency based on the CASS Montreal Heart Institute experience suggests that 60% to 67% of all grafts remain patent at 5 to 11 years. Antiplatelet therapy has been demonstrated to improve early and late patency rates and should probably be used for all patients who do not have any contraindications.[72,73,77] Aspirin with or without other antiplatelet agents reduces the late development of vein-graft occlusions. At the current time, prasugrel, a new antiplatelet drug is only indicated for patients with ACS who are going to undergo PCI.[78] Late graft closure is related to elevated lipid levels and the progression of atherosclerosis in the grafted vessels as well as the native circulation. Elevation of very low density lipoprotein (VLDL), low-density lipoprotein (LDL), and LDL apolipoprotein B is correlated to disease progression and graft closure. Aggressive lipid lowering can stabilize the progression of CAD and may induce regression in selected coronary artery segments within a patient following CABG. Cessation of smoking is an important preoperative and postoperative objective as well as in the management of other coronary risk factors (e.g., hypertension), and institution of a supervised, daily exercise program is recommended. Internal mammary artery grafts should be used for revascularizing the left anterior descending artery system when possible due to better graft survival and clinical outcomes.

Valvular heart disease can coexist with CHD, although this is relatively uncommon with rheumatic valve disease, usually the mitral valve, and more common with aortic stenosis and regurgitation. Angina may occur in 35% to 65% of patients with aortic stenosis or regurgitation and, if severe, may be the cause of angina in the absence of CAD. Patients being evaluated for possible CABG should also be evaluated for valvular disease to determine if valve replacement needs to be performed along with bypass grafting.

Percutaneous Transluminal Coronary Angioplasty[63]

Since the introduction into clinical cardiology of PTCA by Gruentzig in 1977, this procedure has gained rapid acceptance as a safe and effective means of managing CAD. It is estimated that more than 750,000 PCI procedures are done each year in this country and 525,000 of them are PTCA. The proposed mechanisms of reduced stenosis with PTCA include (1) compression and redistribution of the atherosclerotic plaque, (2) embolization of plaque contents, (3) aneurysm formation, and (4) disruption of the plaque and arterial wall with distortion and tearing of the intima and media, which leads to denudation of the endothelium, platelet adhesion and aggregation, thrombus formation, and smooth muscle proliferation. Of these mechanisms, mechanism (4) is felt to be the most important, but the others may contribute to opening of the lesions in some situations.

9 The indications for PTCA have been provided by the ACC/AHA and now span single- or multivessel disease as well as asymptomatic and symptomatic patients (see Table 23–8).[63] In addition to providing recommendations for which type of patients are appropriate for PTCA, the guidelines also provide recommendations for the volume of procedures, the use of IVUS and surgery backup when PTCA is being considered. **10** PTCA generally is not useful if only a small area of viable myocardium is at risk, when ischemia cannot be demonstrated, when borderline (<50%) stenosis or lesions are difficult to dilate, or when patients are at high risk for morbidity or mortality or both (e.g., left main or equivalent disease or three-vessel disease). PTCA alone or when used sequentially or in conjunction with thrombolysis for AMI is discussed in Chap. 18. Stent placement accompanies balloon angioplasty in about 80% of cases in the United States. The current recommendations for PCI are provided in Table 23–8 based on class of angina.

Assessment of outcome with PCI can be based on several angiographic, procedural and clinical outcomes as discussed previously. The success of PCI is dependent on the experience of the operator (high volume, better outcome), complicating factors for the patient (including the number of vessels to be dilated), and technical advances in the equipment used (e.g., steerable and low-profile catheters). The acute success rate for opening of uncomplicated stenotic lesions ranges from 96% to 99% with the combined balloon–device–pharmacologic approach in experienced hands, and angina is decreased or eliminated in about 80% of cases. The success rate for totally occluded lesions is somewhat less (~65%). Mortality at 1 year is 1% and 2.5% for single-vessel disease and multiple-vessel involvement, respectively, reflecting the good prognosis associated with this degree of CAD. At 10 years, survival is 95% and 81% for single and multiple disease, respectively.[63] Most patients remain event free (no death, MI, or CABG) for an extended period. Symptomatic status, as measured by the New York Heart Association (NYHA) classification, is improved in many patients. Restenosis is noted in 32% to 40% after balloon angioplasty at 6 months, and half of these patients will have symptoms associated with restenosis.[63] A few late restenotic events occur, but most restenosis occurs within the first 6 months. Anatomic factors that predict restenosis include lesions >20 mm in length, excessive tortuosity of the proximal segment, extremely angulated segments (>90°), total occlusions >3 months old and and/or bridging collaterals, and the inability to protect

TABLE 23-8 Percutaneous Coronary Intervention Based on Angina Class

Patients with Asymptomatic Ischemia or Canadian Cardiovascular Society (CCS) Class I or II Angina

Class I	**Class IIa**	Phrasing has been changed to reflect current terminology. The recommendation and all of those that follow in Section 5 have been reworded to be consistent with the CCS classification system of angina. This recommendation has been changed to class IIa to reflect the published data and Writing Committee consensus that not all patients in this clinical category must have PCI performed.
Patients who do not have treated diabetes with asymptomatic ischemia or mild angina with 1 or more significant lesions in 1 or 2 coronary arteries suitable for PCI with a high likelihood of success and low risk of morbidity and mortality. The vessels to be dilated must subtend a large area of viable myocardium. (Level of Evidence: B)	1. PCI is reasonable in patients with asymptomatic ischemia or CCS class I or II angina and with 1 or more significant lesions in 1 or 2 coronary arteries suitable for PCI with a high likelihood of success and a low risk of morbidity and mortality. The vessels to be dilated must subtend a moderate to large area of viable myocardium or be associated with a moderate to severe degree of ischemia on noninvasive testing. (Level of Evidence: B)	
Class IIa		This recommendation has been merged with other class IIa recommendations of this section, and the phrasing has been changed to reflect current terminology.
1. The same clinical and anatomic requirements as for class I, except the myocardial area at risk is of moderate size or the patient has treated diabetes. (Level of Evidence: B)	2. PCI is reasonable for patients with asymptomatic ischemia or CCS class I or II angina, and recurrent stenosis after PCI with a large area of viable myocardium or high-risk criteria on noninvasive testing. (Level of Evidence: C)	This is a new recommendation dealing with the management of recurrent stenosis after PCI among patients with asymptomatic ischemia or class I or II angina.
	3. Use of PCI is reasonable for patients with symptomatic ischemia or CCS class I or II angina with significant left main CAD (>50% diameter stenosis) who are candidates for revascularization but are not eligible for CABG. (Level of Evidence: B)	This recommendation for PCI among patients who are eligible for CABG who have significant left main disease has been added to reflect the favorable results noted by several trials with PCI.
Class IIb		This recommendation has been eliminated and replaced by the following 2 recommendations. For each, the phrasing has been constructed to reflect current terminology.
Patients with asymptomatic ischemia or mild angina with greater than or equal to 3 coronary arteries suitable for PCI with a high likelihood of success and a low risk of morbidity and mortality. The vessels to be dilated must subtend at least a moderate area of viable myocardium. In the physician's judgment, there should be evidence of myocardial ischemia by ECG exercise testing, stress nuclear imaging, stress echocardiography or ambulatory ECG monitoring, or intracoronary physiologic measurements. (Level of Evidence: B)		
	Class IIb	Phrasing has been changed to reflect current terminology. Among patients who are eligible, CABG with 1 arterial conduit is generally preferred for treatment of multivessel disease with significant proximal LAD obstruction in patients with treated diabetes and/or abnormal OV function.
	1. The effectiveness of PCI for patients with asymptomatic ischemia or CCS class I or II angina who have two- or three- vessel disease with significant proximal LAD CAD who are otherwise eligible for CABG with 1 arterial conduit and who have treated diabetes or abnormal LV function is not well established. (Level of Evidence: B)	
	2. PCI might be considered for patients with asymptomatic ischemia or CCS class I or II angina with nonproximal LAD CAD that subtends a moderate area of viable myocardium and demonstrates ischemia on noninvasive testing. (Level of Evidence: C)	Phrasing has been changed to reflect current terminology. PCI might be considered in this clinical setting.
Class III	**Class III**	
Patients with asymptomatic ischemia or mild angina who do not meet the criteria as listed under class I or class II and who have	PCI is not recommended for patients with asymptomatic ischemia or CCS class I or II angina who do not meet the criteria as listed under the class II recommendations or who have 1 or more of the following:	
a. Only a small area of viable myocardium at risk	a. Only a small area of viable myocardium at risk (Level of Evidence: C)	
b. No objective evidence of ischemia	b. No objective evidence of ischemia (Level of Evidence: C)	
c. Lesions that have a low likelihood of successful dilation	c. Lesions that have a low likelihood of successful dilation (Level of Evidence: C)	
d. Mild symptoms that are unlikely to be due to myocardial ischemia	d. Mild symptoms that are unlikely to be due to myocardial ischemia (Level of Evidence: C)	
e. Factors associated with increased risk of morbidity or mortality	e. Factors associated with increased risk of morbidity or mortality (Level of Evidence: C)	
f. Left main disease	f. Left main disease and eligibility for CABG (Level of Evidence: C)	
g. Insignificant disease <50% (Level of Evidence: C)	g. Insignificant disease (<50% coronary stenosis) (Level of Evidence: C)	

(continued)

TABLE 23-8 Percutaneous Coronary Intervention Based on Angina Class (continued)

Patients with CCS Class III Angina

Class I	Class IIa	
Patient with 1 or more significant lesions in 1 or more coronary arteries suitable for PCI with a high likelihood of success and low risk of morbidity or mortality. The vessel(s) to be dilated must subtend a moderate or large area of viable myocardium and high risk. (Level of Evidence: B)	1. It is reasonable that PCI be performed in patients with CCS class III angina and single-vessel or multivessel CAD who are undergoing medical therapy and who have 1 or more significant lesions in 1 or more coronary arteries suitable for PCI with a high likelihood of success and low risk of morbidity or mortality. (Level of Evidence: B)	Phrasing has been changed to reflect current terminology. Recommendation has been reworded to be consistent with CCS classification system for angina. The recommendation class has been changed to IIa to reflect published data and Writing Committee consensus. Criteria regarding viable and high-risk myocardium have been deleted from this commendation.
Class IIa Patients with focal saphenous vein graft lesions or multiple stenoses that are poor candidates for reoperative surgery. (Level of Evidence: C)	2. It is reasonable that PCI be performed in patients with CCS class III angina with single-vessel or multivessel CAD who are undergoing medical therapy with focal saphenous vein graft lesions or multiple stenoses who are poor candidates for reoperative surgery. (Level of Evidence: C)	Phrasing has been changed to reflect current terminology.
	3. Use of PCI is reasonable in patients with CCS class III angina with significant left main CAD (>50% diameter stenosis) who are candidates for revascularization but are not eligible for CABG. (Level of Evidence: B)	This recommendation for PCI among patients with significant left main disease who are not eligible for CABG has been added to reflect the favorable results noted by several trials with PCI.
Class IIb Patient has 1 or more lesions to be dilated with reduced likelihood of success of the vessel(s) subtend a less than moderate area of viable myocardium. Patients with two- or three-vessel disease, with significant proximal LAD CAD and treated diabetes or abnormal LV function. (Level of Evidence: B)	**Class IIb** 1. PCI may be considered in patients with CCS class III angina with single-vessel or multivessel CAD who are undergoing medical therapy and who have 1 or more lesions to be dilated with a reduced likelihood of success. (Level of Evidence: B)	Phrasing has been changed to reflect current terminology. The 2001 recommendation has been split into 2 separate recommendations.
	2. PCI may be considered in patients with CCS class III angina and no evidence of ischemia on noninvasive testing or who are undergoing medical therapy and have two- or three-vessel CAD with significant proximal LAD CAD and treated diabetes or abnormal LV function. (Level of Evidence: B)	Phrasing has been changed to reflect current terminology. The use of noninvasive testing to evaluate for evidence of ischemia has been added.
Class III Patient has no evidence of myocardial injury or ischemia on objective testing and has not had a trial of medical therapy, or has a. Only a small area of myocardium at risk b. All lesions or the culprit lesion to be dilated with morphology with a low likelihood of success c. A high risk of procedure-related morbidity or mortality. (Level of Evidence: C)	**Class III** PCI is not recommended for patients with CCS class III angina with single-vessel or multivessel CAD, no evidence of myocardial injury or ischemia on objective testing, and no trial of medical therapy, or who have 1 of the following: a. Only a small area of myocardium at risk (Level of Evidence: C) b. All lesions or the culprit lesion to be dilated with morphology that conveys a low likelihood of success (Level of Evidence: C) c. A high risk of procedure-related morbidity or mortality (Level of Evidence: C) d. Insignificant disease (<50% coronary stenosis) (Level of Evidence: C) e. Significant left main CAD and candidacy for CABG (Level of Evidence: C)	Phrasing has been changed to reflect current terminology. Class II recommendations two and three from the 2001 guidelines have been merged into this recommendation.
2. Patients with insignificant coronary stenosis (e.g., <50% diameter). (Level of Evidence: C) 3. Patients with significant left main CAD who are candidates for CABG. (Level of Evidence: B)		

CAEBG, coronary artery bypass graft; CAD, coronary artery disease; ECG, electrocardiography; LAD, left anterior descending; LV, left ventricle; OV, outflow volume; PCI, percutaneous coronary intervention.
Reprinted with permission, Circulation. 2006;113:156–175, © 2006 American Heart Association, Inc.

major side branches and degenerated vein grafts with friable lesions. Clinical factors that predict worse outcome include diabetes, advanced age, female gender, unstable angina, heart failure, and multivessel disease. A 4-variable scoring system that predicts cardiovascular collapse for failed PTCA includes percentage of myocardium at risk (e.g., >50% viable myocardium at risk and LV ejection fraction <25%), preangioplasty percent diameter stenosis, multivessel CAD, and diffuse disease in the dilated segment or a high myocardial jeopardy score.[63] Strut thickness of the stent influences restenosis as well, and thicker struts are associated with angiographic and clinical restenosis.[76,79] With the development of drug-eluting stents (DES), early reocclusion has been reduced dramatically, but late in-stent thrombosis has been a problem. As stent technology has evolved better polymers, better strut design, and better antiproliferative agents (e.g., everolimus), stent thrombosis has dropped to as low as 0.3%, MI to 1.9%, and target-lesion revascularization to 2.5%.[76]

The overall complication rate ranges from 2% to 21% depending on the lesion type. Coronary occlusion, dissection, or spasm occurs in 4% to 8% of patients, whereas ST-segment-elevation MI occurs in 1.6% to 4.8%.[63] Prolonged angina and ventricular tachycardia or fibrillation occurs in 6.9% and 2.3%, respectively. In-hospital mortality ranges from 0.7% to 2.5% overall, and high-risk events for mortality included ventricular arrhythmias and MI. The frequency of urgent CABG because of complications ranges from 0.4% to 5.8%.[63]

Current AHA/ACC recommendations for antithrombotic therapy in PCI are outlined in Table 23–9.[63,77] Antiplatelet therapy with ASA 80 to 325 mg/day given at least 2 hours prior to angioplasty is currently recommended. If patients are sensitive to ASA, clopidogrel or prasugrel are acceptable alternatives. In elective settings, clopidogrel should be started at least 72 hours in advance of the procedure to allow for maximal antiplatelet effects. Alternatively, a loading dose of clopidogrel (300 to 600 mg) or

prasugrel 60 mg may be given to achieve a more rapid antiplatelet effect.[80-82] The combination of ASA plus clopidogrel or prasugrel is currently recommended for patients undergoing angioplasty and stenting, and this combination is safer and superior to antiplatelet therapy plus anticoagulation with warfarin-like drugs.[77] Follow-up for up to 4 years from the Intracoronary Stenting and Antithrombotic Regimen (ISAR) trial shows that the benefit of combined antiplatelet therapy evident after 30 days is maintained after 4 years.[83] Aspirin is an incomplete inhibitor of platelet aggregation and combination therapy of ASA plus a GP IIb/IIIa receptor antagonist for PCI has shown a relative risk reduction of 37.5% for death and nonfatal MI at 30 days favoring GP IIb/IIIa receptor antagonists over placebo (absolute rates of 5.5% vs 8.9% based on PCI trials of EPIC, IMPACT-II, EPILOG, CAPTURE,

---

TABLE 23-9 Pharmacologic Management of Percutaneous Coronary Intervention

Antiplatelet and antithrombotic adjunctive therapies for PCI—oral antiplatelet therapy

Class I

1. Patients already taking daily chronic aspirin therapy should take 75 to 325 mg of aspirin before the PCI procedure is performed. (Level of Evidence: A)

2. Patients not already taking daily chronic aspirin therapy should be given 300–325 mg of aspirin at least 2 hours and preferably 24 hours before the PCI procedure is performed. (Level of Evidence: C)

3. After the PCI procedure, in patients with neither aspirin resistance, allergy, nor increased risk of bleeding, aspirin 325 mg daily should be given for at least 1 month after bare-metal stent implantation, 3 months after sirolimus-eluting stent implantation, and 6 months after paclitaxel-eluting stent implantation, after which daily chronic aspirin use should be continued indefinitely at a dose of 75 to 162 mg. (Level of Evidence: B)

4. A loading dose of clopidogrel should be administered before PCI is performed. (Level of Evidence: A) An oral loading dose of 300 mg, administered at least 6 hours before the procedure, has the best established evidence of efficacy. (Level of Evidence: B)

5. In patients who have undergone PCI, clopidogrel 75 mg daily should be given for at least 1 month after bare-metal stent implantation (unless the patient is at increased risk for bleeding; then it should be given for a minimum of 2 weeks), 3 months after sirolimus stent implantation, and 6 months after paclitaxel stent implantation, and ideally up to 12 months for patients who are not at high risk of bleeding. (Level of Evidence: B)

Class IIa

1. If clopidogrel is given at the time of procedure, supplementation with GP IIb/IIIa receptor antagonists can be beneficial to facilitate earlier platelet inhibition than with clopidogrel alone. (Level of Evidence: B)

2. For patients with an absolute contraindication to aspirin, it is reasonable to give a 300 mg loading dose of clopidogrel, administered at least 6 hours before PCI, and/or GP IIb/IIIa antagonists, administered at the time of PCI. (Level of Evidence: C)

3. When a loading dose of clopidogrel is administered, a regimen of greater than 300 mg is reasonable to achieve higher levels of antiplatelet activity more rapidly, but the efficacy and safety compared with a 300-mg loading dose are less established. (Level of Evidence: C)

4. It is reasonable that patients undergoing brachytherapy be given daily clopidogrel 75 mg indefinitely and daily aspirin 75 to 325 mg indefinitely unless there is significant risk for bleeding. (Level of Evidence: C)

Class IIb

For patients in whom subacute thrombosis may be catastrophic or lethal (unprotected left main, bifurcating left main, or last patent coronary vessel), platelet aggregation studies may be considered and the dose of clopidogrel increased to 150 mg/day if less than 505 inhibition of platelet aggregation is demonstrated. (Level of Evidence: C)

Glycoprotein IIb/IIIa inhibitors

Class I

For patients with UA/NSTEMI undergoing PCI without clopidogrel administration, a C IIb/IIIa inhibitor (abciximab, eptifibatide, or tirofiban) should be administered. (Level of Evidence: A) It is acceptable to administer the GP IIb/IIIa inhibitor before performance of the diagnostic angiogram ("upstream treatment") or just before PCI ("in-lab treatment").

A daily dose of 75 mg of aspirin has been shown to result in improved cardiovascular outcomes similar to daily doses of 325 mg but with fewer bleeding complications.

Higher doses of aspirin are recommended for patients not already taking aspirin therapy immediately before PCI procedures.

The doses and duration of aspirin therapy recommended herein and derived from those used for US Food and Drug Administration approval of the specific stent types noted in the recommendation. Daily chronic aspirin therapy is based on recommendations in the ACC/AHA Guidelines for the Management of Patents with ST-Elevation Myocardial Infarction and evidence indicating that aspiring therapy in dosages as low as 75 mg per day yields outcomes similar to those achieved with 325 mg per day but with fewer side effects.

Clopidogrel is an important adjunctive therapy for patients undergoing PCI with stent placement. The best evidence of efficacy exists for 300 mg given at lest 6 hours before PCI is performed.

Clopidogrel therapy in the dosage of 75 mg daily should be given after stent placement to all patients. The duration of therapy varies for each stent and is based on data from clinical trails used for U.S. Food and Drug Administration approval of that stent.

When clopidogrel is given at the time of a PCI procedure, supplementation with glycoprotein IIb/IIIa receptor antagonists can be beneficial, especially among high-risk patients.

A significant number of patients will have resistance to aspirin. The strongest evidence for clopidogrel benefit exists for doses of 300 mg given at least 6 hours before the procedure.

Many patients receive clopidogrel therapy at the time of PCI in dosages greater than 600 mg. Although more pronounced inhibition of platelet function has been demonstrated for doses of clopidogrel greater than 300 mg, the safety of these higher doses and their benefits on clinical outcome are not fully established.

Subacute or later thrombosis has been observed for patients undergoing brachytherapy, and for this reason long-term antiplatelet therapy is recommended.

Clopidogrel resistance is a significant problem, and owing to its contribution to catastrophic clinical outcomes, the Writing Committee recommends studies be performed with increases in clopidogrel dose being recommended for use in those with higher risk lesions.

This recommendation and phrasing are compatible with the ACC/AHA 2002 Guideline Update for the Management of Patients with Unstable Angina and Non–ST-Segment Myocardial Infarction and current evidence from randomized clinical trials. The benefits of GP IIb/IIa inhibition are especially efficacious when clopidogrel is not given.

(continued)

TABLE 23-9 Pharmacologic Management of Percutaneous Coronary Intervention (continued)

Class IIa

1. For patients with UA/NSTEMI undergoing PCI with clopidogrel administration, it is reasonable to administer a GP IIb/IIIa inhibitor (abciximab, eptifibatide, or tirofiban). (Level of Evidence: B)

It is acceptable to administer the GP IIb/IIIa inhibitor before performance of the diagnostic angiogram ("upstream treatment") or just before PCI ("in-lab treatment").

2. In patients with STEMI undergoing PCI, it is reasonable to administer abciximab as early as possible. (Level of Evidence: B)

3. In patients undergoing elective PCI with stent placement, it is reasonable to administer a GP IIb/IIIa inhibitor (abciximab, epitifibatide, or tirofiban). (Level of Evidence: B)

Recommendation has been added for consistency with the ACC/AHA Guidelines for the Management of Patients With ST-Elevation Myocardial Infarction.

Phrasing has been changed to reflect current terminology, especially in a high-risk patient.

Class IIb

In patients with STEMI undergoing PCI, treatment with eptifibatide or tirofiban may be considered. (Level of Evidence: C)

Recommendation has been added for consistency with the ACC/AHA Guidelines for the Management of Patients with ST-Elevation Myocardial Infarction.

Antithrombotic therapy

Unfractionated heparin, low-molecular-weight heparin, and bivalirudin

Class I

1. Unfractionated heparin should be administered to patients undergoing PCI. (Level of Evidence: C)

Phrasing has been changed to reflect current terminology.

2. For patients with heparin-induced thrombocytopenia, it is recommended that bivalirudin or argatroban be used to replace heparin. (Level of Evidence: B)

Bivalirudin and argatroban are established therapies in place of heparin among patients with heparin-induced thrombocytopenia.

Class IIa

1. It is reasonable to use bivalirudin as an alternative to unfractionated heparin and glycoprotein IIb/IIIa antagonists in low-risk patients undergoing elective PCI. (Level of Evidence: B)

2. Low-molecular-weight heparin is a reasonable alternative to unfractionated heparin in patients with UA/NSTEMI undergoing PCI. (Level of Evidence: B)

New recommendation is based on data from a clinical trial (REPLACE-2) indicating bivalirudin is an acceptable alternative to heparin and GP IIb/IIIa antagonists in low-risk patients undergoing PCI.

Recommendation from the ACC/AHA 2002 Guideline Update for the Management of Patients with Unstable Angina and Non–ST-Segment Myocardial Infarction has been approved by this Writing Committee and included in these guidelines for consistency.

Class IIb

Low-molecular-weight heparin may be considered as an alternative to unfractionated heparin in patients with STEMI undergoing PCI. (Level of Evidence: B)

Recommendation from the ACC/AHA Guidelines for the Management of Patients with ST-Elevation Myocardial Infarction has been approved by this Writing Committee and included in these guidelines for consistency.

GP, glycoprotein; NSTEMI, non–ST-segment elevation myocardial infarction; PCU, percutaneous coronary intervention; STEMI, ST-segment elevation myocardial infarction; UA, unstable angina.
Reprinted with permission, Circulation. 2006;113:156–175, © 2006 American Heart Association, Inc.

RESTORE, and EPISTENT).[63] As discussed under unstable angina, high risk patients and those having a stent placed are most likely to benefit from GP IIb/IIIa receptor antagonist use. Patients presenting with elevated cardiac biomarkers are also more likely to receive benefit from GP IIb/IIIa receptor antagonists than patients with normal levels of biomarkers.[84] In the only comparative trial (TARGET), abciximab was superior to tirofiban.[85]

During PTCA, patients are usually heparinized to prevent immediate thrombus formation at the site of arterial injury and on coronary guidewires and catheters; anticoagulation is continued for up to 24 hours. The intensity of anticoagulation is monitored using the activated clotting time (ACT), and the targeted range for ACT is 250 to 300 seconds (HemoTec device) in the absence of GP IIb/IIIa receptor antagonist use.[63] When GP IIb/IIIa receptor antagonists are not used, UFH is given as an IV bolus of 70 to 100 international units/kg to achieve a target ACT of 200 seconds. The loading dose is lowered 50 to 70 international units/kg when GP IIb/IIIa receptor antagonists are given. Target ACT for eptifibatide and tirofiban is <300 seconds during angioplasty; postprocedural UFH infusions are not recommended during GP IIb/IIIa receptor antagonist therapy. Mechanisms that result in restenosis include acute lumen loss owing to "recoil," mural thrombosis formation, and smooth muscle cell proliferation with synthesis of extracellular matrix.[65] Approaches to prevent restenosis may be aimed at altering the underlying mechanisms. Recoil and loss of luminal diameter may

be reduced by the use of stent placement; however, this beneficial effect is offset by an increased number of vascular complications. Cracking of the plaque leads to severe damage to the arterial wall, exposure of collagen, and endothelial dysfunction. These factors promote mural thrombi, and the propensity for thrombus formation is related, in part, to the composition of the plaque as well as the depth of injury. Combination therapy with ASA, heparin, and IIb/IIIa receptor antagonists is recommended to minimize acute occlusion and numerous clinical trials document the efficacy of this combined approach.[63,73,86] Bivalirudin is a specific and reversible direct thrombin inhibitor that is indicated for use as an anticoagulant for patients with unstable angina undergoing PTCA. Based on the REPLACE-2 and ACUITY studies, bivalirudin is comparable to heparin in preventing thrombosis and may be associated with less bleeding.[87,88] A more complete discussion of antithrombotic therapy can be found in Chap. 24.

When medical therapy, PTCA, and CABG have been compared, low-risk patients with single-vessel CAD and normal LV function had greater alleviation of symptoms with PTCA than those with medical treatment; mortality rates and rates of MI were unchanged. In high-risk patients (risk was defined by severity of ischemia, number of diseased vessels, and presence of LV dysfunction), improvement of survival was greater with CABG than with medical therapy. In moderate-risk patients with multivessel CAD (most had two-vessel disease and normal LV function), PTCA and CABG produced equivalent mortality rates and rates of MI.

The development of DES has changed the natural course of stent thrombosis when compared to bare metal stents (BMS) that have existed for a longer period of time. Currently there are three types of DES available: sirolimus (Cypher), paclitaxel (Taxus), and everolimus (Zortress). Soon after the introduction of BMS, it became apparent that early stent thrombosis (≤30 days) was an uncommon but serious complication of therapy.[65,76,79,89] Stent thrombosis is an infrequent but severe complication of both BMS and DES; while there is no apparent difference in overall stent thrombosis frequency at 4 years of follow-up, the time course appears to be different. There is a relative numeric excess of stent thrombosis late after DES implantation; however, no differences in death or death and infarction have been observed. Target lesion revascularization is needed less often with DES compared with BMS. Implantation of DES stents outside of approved indications and lack of proper positioning of the stent are related to the occurrence of late stent thrombosis. Longer-term follow-up with larger subsets of patients (i.e., lesion number, type and location, and patient comorbidities) is needed to fully understand this issue and the evolution of newer platforms for drug delivery will likely alter the natural history of DES stent thrombosis.[90] A very important consideration is the use of combination antiplatelet therapy (aspirin plus clopidogrel or prasugrel) for at least a year following implantation.[72,73,77,91] Patients who are unable to activate clopidogrel due to a reduced function allele for CYP2C19 may be treated with 150 mg/day rather than 75 mg/day or switched to prasugrel.[92] Drugs which inhibit CYP2C19 should probably be avoided although there is conflicting evidence in the literature.[93-95]

■ PHARMACOLOGIC THERAPY

Historically, about 30% of anginal syndrome symptoms have responded regardless of which therapy was instituted. These observations stem from two problems inherent in clinical trials undertaken to assess the efficacy of any therapy for angina: (1) adequate trial design incorporating appropriate controls and washout periods, and (2) assessment of treatment effects using objective measures of efficacy including improvement in exercise performance, resting and ambulatory ECG improvement in ischemic changes, or other objective tests to address other aspects of myocardial function or metabolism. The use of pain episode frequency and nitroglycerin consumption is subjective, and their use as sole measures of efficacy should be avoided. Objective assessment using ETT has shown that placebo does not provide improvement for patients with exertional angina, substantiating this as a valid means to assess efficacy.

β-Adrenergic Blocking Agents[96,97]

Decreased heart rate, decreased contractility, and a slight to moderate decrease in blood pressure with β-adrenergic receptor antagonism reduce MVO_2. The predominant receptor type in the heart is the β1-receptor, and competitive blockade minimizes the influence of endogenous catecholamines on the chronotropic and inotropic state of the myocardium. These beneficial effects may be countered to some degree with increased ventricular volume and ejection time seen with β-blockade; however, the overall effect of β-blockers for patients with effort-induced angina is a reduction in oxygen demand (Table 23–10). The β-blockers do not improve oxygen supply, and in certain instances, unopposed α-adrenergic stimulation following the use of β-blockers may lead to coronary vasoconstriction. For patients with chronic exertional stable angina, β-blockers improve symptoms about 80% of the

TABLE 23–10 Effect of Drug Therapy on Myocardial Oxygen Demand[a]

| | Heart Rate | Myocardial Contractility | LV Wall Tension | | |
			Systolic Pressure	LV Volume	
Nitrates	⇑	0	⇓	⇓⇓	
β-Blockers	⇓⇓	⇓	⇓	⇑	
Nifedipine	⇓	0 or ⇓	0 or ⇓	0 or ⇓	
Verapamil	⇓	⇓	⇓	0 or ⇓	
Diltiazem	⇓⇓	0 or ⇓	⇓	0 or ⇓	

LV, left ventricular.
[a]Calcium channel antagonists and nitrates also may increase myocardial oxygen supply through coronary vasodilation. Diastolic function also may be improved with verapamil, nifedipine, and perhaps diltiazem. These effects may vary from those indicated in the table depending on individual patient baseline hemodynamics.

time, and objective measures of efficacy demonstrate improved exercise duration and delay in the time at which ST-segment changes and initial or limiting symptoms occur. β-Blockers do not alter the rate-to-pressure product (double product) for maximal exercise, therefore substantiating reduced demand rather than improved supply as the major consequence of their actions. Reflex tachycardia from nitrate therapy can be blunted with β-blocker therapy, making this a common and useful combination. Although β-blockade may decrease exercise capacity in healthy individuals or for patients with hypertension, it may allow angina patients previously limited by symptoms to perform more exercise and ultimately improve overall cardiovascular performance through a training effect. Ideal candidates for β-blockers include patients in whom physical activity figures prominently in their anginal attacks, those who have coexistent hypertension, those with a history of supraventricular arrhythmias or post-MI angina, and those who have a component of anxiety associated with angina.[3] β-Blockers may also be safely used in angina and heart failure as described in Chap. 20. Pertinent pharmacokinetics for the β-blockers include half-life and route elimination, which are reviewed in Chap. 19. Drugs with longer half-lives need to be dosed less frequently than ones with shorter half-lives; however, disparity exists between half-life and duration of action for several β-blockers (e.g., metoprolol), and this may reflect attenuation of the central nervous system–mediated effects on the sympathetic system as well as the direct effects of this category on heart rate and contractility. Renal and hepatic dysfunction can affect the disposition of β-blockers, but these agents are dosed to effect, either hemodynamic or symptomatic, and route of elimination is not a major consideration in drug selection.

Guidelines for the use of β-blockers in treating angina include the objective of lowering resting heart rate to 50 to 60 beats per minute and limiting maximal exercise heart rate to about 100 beats per minute or less. It has also been suggested that exercise heart rate should be no more than about 20 beats per minute or a 10% increment over resting heart rate with modest exercise. Because β-blockade is competitive and circulating catecholamine concentrations vary depending on the intensity of exercise and other factors and cholinergic tone may be important in controlling heart rate in some patients, these guidelines are general in nature. These effects are generally dose and plasma concentration related, and for propranolol, plasma concentrations of 30 ng/mL are needed for a 25% reduction of anginal frequency. Initial doses of β-blockers should be at the lower end of the usual dosing range and titrated to response as indicated above.

There is little evidence to suggest superiority of any β-blocker; however, the duration of β-blockade is dependent partially on the half-life of the agent used, and those with longer half-lives may be dosed less frequently. Of note, propranolol may be dosed twice a day in most patients with angina, and the efficacy is similar to that seen with more frequent dosing. The ancillary property of membrane stabilizing activity is irrelevant in the treatment of angina, and intrinsic sympathomimetic activity appears to be detrimental in rest or severe angina because the reduction in heart rate would be minimized, therefore limiting a reduction in MVO_2. Cardioselective β-blockers may be used in some patients to minimize adverse effects such as bronchospasm in asthma, intermittent claudication, and sexual dysfunction. A common misunderstanding is that β-blockers are not well tolerated in peripheral arterial disease, but in fact, their use is associated with a reduction in death and improved quality of life.[98] It should be remembered that cardioselectivity is a relative property and that the use of larger doses (e.g., metoprolol 200 mg/day) is associated with the loss of selectivity and with adverse effects. Post-acute-MI patients with angina are particularly good candidates for β-blockade both because anginal symptoms may be treated as well as reducing the risk of post-MI reinfarction and because mortality has been demonstrated with timolol, propranolol, and metoprolol (see Chap. 24). Combined β- (nonselective) and α-blockade with labetalol may be useful in some patients with marginal LV reserve, and fewer deleterious effects on coronary blood flow are seen when compared with other β-blockers.

Extension of pharmacologic effect is the underlying reason for many of the adverse effects seen with β-blockade. Hypotension, decompensated heart failure, bradycardia and heart block, bronchospasm, and altered glucose metabolism are directly related to β-adrenoreceptor antagonism. Patients with preexisting LV systolic decompensated and heart failure and the use of other negative inotropic agents are most prone to developing overt heart failure, and in the absence of these, heart failure is uncommon (less than 5%). Other drugs that depress conduction are additive to β-blockade, and intrinsic conduction system disease predisposes the patient to conduction abnormalities. Altered glucose metabolism is most likely to be seen in insulin-dependent diabetics, and β-blockade obscures the symptoms of hypoglycemia except for sweating. β-Blockers may also aggravate the lipid abnormalities seen in patients with diabetes; however, these changes are dose related, are more common with normal baseline lipids than dyslipidemia, and may be of short-term significance only. One of the more common reasons for discontinuation of β-blocker therapy is related to central nervous system adverse effects of fatigue, malaise, and depression. Cognition changes seen with β-blockers are usually minimal and comparable to other categories of drugs based on studies done in hypertension.[99] Abrupt withdrawal of β-blocker therapy for patients with angina has been associated with increased severity and number of pain episodes and MI. The mechanism of this effect is unknown but may be related to increased receptor sensitivity or disease progression during therapy, which becomes apparent following discontinuation of β-blockade. In any event, tapering of β-blocker therapy over about 2 days should minimize the risk of withdrawal reactions for those patients in whom therapy is being discontinued.

β-adrenoreceptor blockade is effective in chronic exertional angina as monotherapy and in combination with nitrates and/or calcium channel antagonists. β-blockers should be the first-line drug in chronic angina requiring daily maintenance therapy because β-blockers are more effective in reducing episodes of silent ischemia, reducing early morning peak of ischemic activity, and improving mortality after Q-wave MI than nitrates or calcium channel blockers (Fig. 23–4).[3] If β-blockers are ineffective or not tolerated, then monotherapy with a calcium channel blocker may be instituted or, if monotherapy is ineffective for either alone, combination therapy may be instituted. Patients with severe angina, rest angina, or variant angina (i.e., a component of coronary artery spasm) may be better treated with calcium channel blockers or long-acting nitrates.

Nitrates[100]

Nitroglycerin has a well-documented role in the alleviation of acute anginal attacks when used as rapidly absorbed and readily available preparations by the oral and intravenous routes (see Table 23–10 and Table 23–11)). SL, buccal, or spray products are the products of choice for this indication. Prevention of symptoms may be accomplished by the prophylactic use of oral or transdermal products; however, recent concern has been expressed over the long-term efficacy of many of these preparations and the development of tolerance.[101–103]

Nitrates have multiple potential mechanisms of action, and for a given patient it is not always clear which of these is most important. In general, the major action appears to be indirectly mediated through a reduction of myocardial oxygen demand secondary to venodilation and arterial-to-arteriolar dilation, leading to a reduction in wall stress from reduced ventricular volume and pressure (see Table 23–10). Systemic venodilation also promotes increased flow to deep myocardial muscle by reducing the gradient between intraventricular pressure and coronary arteriolar (R2) pressure. Direct actions on coronary circulation include dilation of large and small intramural coronary arteries, collateral dilation, coronary artery stenosis dilation, abolition of normal tone in narrowed vessels, and relief of spasm; these actions occur even if the endothelium is denuded or dysfunctional. It is likely that depending on the underlying pathophysiology, different mechanisms become operative. For example, in the presence of a 60% to 70% stenosis, venodilation with MVO_2 reduction is most important; however, with higher grade lesions, direct effects on the coronary circulation and vessel tone are the predominant effects. Nitroglycerin and pentaerythritol tetranitrate (PETN) in low doses are bioactivated by mitochondrial aldehyde dehydrogenase (ALDH-2) to nitrite or dinitrated metabolites that require further activation by cytochrome oxidase or acidic disproportionation in the inner membrane space finally yielding nitric oxide. Nitric oxide activates soluble guanylate cyclase to increase intracellular concentrations of cyclic GMP resulting in vasorelaxation.[103] In contrast, isosorbide dinitrate (ISDN) and isosorbide mononitrate (ISMN) are bioactivated via CYP enzymes to nitric oxide. At higher concentrations, nitroglycerin and PETN may also be bioactivated to nitric oxide via CYP enzymes. Increased cyclic GMP induces a sequence of protein phosphorylation associated with reduced intracellular

TABLE 23–11	Nitrate Products		
Product	**Onset (minutes)**	**Duration**	**Initial Dose**
Nitroglycerin			
IV	1–2	3–5 minutes	5 mcg/min
Sublingual/lingual	1–3	30–60 minutes	0.3 mg
Oral	40	3–6 hours	2.5–9 mg 3 times a day
Ointment	20–60	2–8 hours	0.5–1 in
Patch	40–60	>8 hours	1 patch
Erythritol tetranitrate	5–30	4–6 hours	5–10 mg 3 times a day
Pentaerythritol tetranitrate	30	4–8 hours	10–20 mg 3 times a day
Isosorbide dinitrate			
Sublingual/chewable	2–5	1–2 hours	2.5–5 mg 3 times a day
Oral	20–40	4–6 hours	5–20 mg 3 times a day
Isosorbide mononitrate	30–60	6–8 hours	20 mg daily, twice a day[a]

[a]Product dependent.

calcium release from the sarcoplasmic reticulum or reduced permeability to extracellular calcium and, consequently, smooth muscle relaxation. Oxidative stress within the mitochondria causes inactivation of ALDH-2 leading to impaired bioactivation of nitroglycerin during prolonged treatment.[104] Thomas et al.[101] performed a study in normal volunteers to evaluate the effect of ISMN 120 mg/day given for 7 days on endothelial function. They found that ISMN impaired endothelial function suggesting a role for oxygen free radicals and nitrate induced abnormalities in endothelial-dependent vasomotor responses that were reversed with a vitamin C infusion of 24 mg/min given for 15 minutes.[101] Furthermore, ISDN has been shown to impair flow mediated dilation and carotid intimal-media thickness after three months of treatment.[105] These deleterious changes in endothelial function, intima-media thickness and the occurrence of tolerance suggest that the role of nitrates in IHD may be changing.

Pharmacokinetic characteristics common to the organic nitrates used for angina include a large first-pass effect of hepatic metabolism, short to very short half-lives (except for ISMN), large volumes of distribution, high clearance rates, and large interindividual variations in plasma or blood concentrations. Pharmacodynamic-pharmacokinetic relationships for the entire class remain poorly defined, presumably due to methodological difficulty in characterizing the parent drug and metabolite concentrations at or within vascular smooth muscle and secondary to counterregulatory or adaptive mechanisms from the drug's effects as well as the occurrence of tolerance. Nitroglycerin is extracted by a variety of tissues and metabolized locally; differential extraction and metabolite generation occur depending on the tissue site. There are also numerous technical problems limiting the generation of reliable pharmacokinetic parameter estimates including the following: assay sensitivity; arteriovenous extraction gradients and therefore extrahepatic metabolism; in vitro degradation; drug adsorption to polyvinyl chloride tubing and syringes; potentially saturable metabolism; accumulation of metabolites (some of which are active) with multiple doses; postural and exercise-induced changes in pharmacokinetics; a variety of variables associated with transdermal delivery including the delivery system (matrix, membrane-limited, ointment); vehicle used; the surface area and thickness of application; the site application; and other skin variables (temperature, moisture content).

Nitroglycerin concentrations are affected by the route of administration, with the highest concentrations usually obtained with intravenous administration, the lowest seen with lower oral doses. Peak concentrations with SL nitroglycerin appear within 2 to 4 minutes, with the oral route producing peaks at about 15 to 30 minutes and by the transdermal route at 1 to 2 hours. The half-life of nitroglycerin is 1 to 5 minutes regardless of route; hence the potential advantage of sustained-release and transdermal products. Transdermal nitroglycerin does produce sufficient concentrations for acute hemodynamic effects to occur and these concentrations are maintained for long intervals; however, the hemodynamic and antianginal effects are minimal after 1 week or less with chronic, continuous (24 h/day) therapy.

ISDN is metabolized to isosorbide 2-mono- and 5-mononitrate ISMN. ISMN is well absorbed and has a half-life of about 5 hours and may be given once or twice daily depending on the product chosen. Multiple, larger doses of ISDN lead to disproportionate increases in the area under the plasma time profile, suggesting that metabolic pathways are being saturated or that metabolite accumulation may influence the disposition of ISDN. Little pharmacokinetic information is available for other nitrate compounds.

Nitrate therapy may be used to terminate an acute anginal attack, to prevent effort or stress-induced attacks, or for long-term prophylaxis, usually in combination with β-blockers or calcium channel blockers. SL nitroglycerin 0.3 to 0.4 mg will relieve pain in about 75% of patients within 3 minutes, with another 15% becoming pain free in 5 to 15 minutes. Pain persisting beyond about 20 to 30 minutes following the use of two or three nitroglycerin tablets is suggestive of ACS, and the patient should be instructed to seek emergency aid. Patients should be instructed to keep nitroglycerin in the original, tightly closed glass container and to avoid mixing with other medication, because mixing may reduce nitroglycerin adsorption and vaporization. Additional counseling should include the facts that nitroglycerin is not an analgesic but rather it partially corrects the underlying problem and that repeated use is not harmful or addicting. Patients should also be aware that enhanced venous pooling in the sitting or standing positions may improve the effect as well as the symptoms of postural hypotension and that inadequate saliva may slow or prevent tablet disintegration and dissolution. An acceptable albeit expensive alternative is lingual spray, which may be more convenient and has a shelf life of 3 years compared with 6 months or so for some forms of nitroglycerin tablets.

Chewable, oral, and transdermal products are acceptable for the long-term prophylaxis of angina; however, considerable controversy surrounds their use and it appears that the development of tolerance or adaptive mechanisms limits the efficacy of all chronic nitrate therapies regardless of route. Dosing of the longer acting preparations should be adjusted to provide a hemodynamic response, and as an example, this may require doses of oral ISDN ranging from 10 to 60 mg as often as every 3 to 4 hours owing to tolerance or first-pass metabolism, and similar large doses are required for other products. Nitroglycerin ointment has a duration of up to 6 hours, but it is difficult to apply in a cosmetically acceptable fashion over a consistent surface area, and its response varies depending on the epidermal thickness, vascularity, and amount of hair. Percutaneous adsorption of nitroglycerin ointment may occur unintentionally if someone other than the patient applies the ointment, and limiting exposure through the use of gloves or some other means is advisable.

Peripheral edema may also impair the response to nitroglycerin because venodilation cannot increase capacitance to a maximum and pooling may be reduced. Transdermal patch delivery systems were approved on the basis of sustained and equivalent plasma concentrations to other forms of therapy. Trials required by the Food and Drug Administration using transdermal patches as a continuous 24-hour delivery system revealed a lack of efficacy for improved exercise tolerance. Subsequently, large, randomized, double-blind, placebo-controlled trials of intermittent (10 to 12 hours on, 12 to 14 hours off) transdermal nitroglycerin therapy in chronic stable angina demonstrated modest but significant improvement in exercise time after 4 weeks for the highest doses at 8 to 12 hours after patch placement.[106] Subjective assessment methods for nitrate effects include reduction in the number of painful episodes and the amount of nitroglycerin consumed. Objective assessment includes the resolution of ECG changes at rest, during exercise, or with ambulatory ECG monitoring. Because nitrates work primarily through a reduction in MVO_2, the double product can be used to optimize the dose of SL and oral nitrate products. It is important to realize that reflex tachycardia may offset the beneficial reduction in systolic blood pressure and calculation of the observed changes is necessary. The double product is best assessed in the sitting position and at intervals of 5 to 10 minutes and 30 to 60 minutes following SL and oral therapy, respectively. Owing to the placebo effect, unpredictable and variable course of angina, numerous pharmacologic effects of nitroglycerin, diurnal variation in pain patterns, stringent investigative protocols, and interindividual sensitivity to nitroglycerin, assessment with transdermal and sustained-release products is difficult. ETT provides valuable information concerning efficacy and mechanism of action for nitrates but its use is usually reserved for clinical investigation rather than routine patient care. Most ETT studies have shown nitrates to delay the onset of ischemia (ST-segment changes or initial chest discomfort) at submaximal exercise, but the threshold for maximal exercise is unaltered, suggesting a reduction in oxygen demand rather than an improved oxygen supply. More sophisticated studies of myocardial function such as wall motion abnormalities and myocardial metabolism could be used to document efficacy; however, these studies are generally only for investigative purposes.

Adverse effects of nitrates are related most commonly to an extension of their pharmacologic effects and include postural hypotension with associated central nervous system symptoms, headaches and flushing secondary to vasodilation, and occasional nausea from smooth muscle relaxation. If hypotension is excessive, coronary and cerebral filling may be compromised leading to MI and stroke. While reflex tachycardia is most common, bradycardia with nitroglycerin has been reported. Other noncardiovascular adverse effects include rash with all products but particularly with transdermal nitroglycerin, the production of methemoglobinemia with high doses given for extended periods, and measurable concentrations of ethanol (intoxication has been reported) and propylene glycol (found in the diluent) with intravenous nitroglycerin.

Tolerance with nitrate therapy was first described in 1867 with the initial experience using amyl nitrate for angina and later widely recognized in munitions workers who underwent withdrawal reactions during periods of absence from exposure. Tolerance to nitrates is associated with a reduction in tissue cyclic Guanyl Mono Phosphate (GMP), which results from decreased production (guanylate cyclase) and increased breakdown via cyclic GMP-phosphodiesterase and increased superoxide levels. One proposed mechanism for the lack of cyclic GMP is lack of conversion of organic nitrates to nitric oxide as described previously.[100]

Most of the published information from controlled trials examining nitrate tolerance have been done with either ISDN or transdermal nitroglycerin, and these studies demonstrate the development of tolerance within as little as 24 hours of therapy. While the onset of tolerance is rapid, the offset may be just as rapid, and one alternative dosing strategy to circumvent or minimize tolerance is to provide a daily nitrate-free interval of 6 to 8 hours. Studies with a variety of nitrate preparations and dosing schedules demonstrate that this approach is useful and the nitrate-free interval should be a minimum of 8 hours and perhaps 12 hours for even better effects.[100] Another concern for intermittent transdermal nitrate therapy is the occurrence of rebound ischemia during the nitrate-free interval. Freedman et al. found more silent ischemia during the patch-free interval during a randomized, double-blind, placebo-controlled trial than during the placebo patch phase, although others have not noted this effect.[107] ISDN, for example, should not be used more often than three times per day if tolerance is to be avoided. Interestingly, hemodynamic tolerance does not always coincide with antianginal efficacy, but this is not well studied.

Nitrates may be combined with other drugs for anginal therapy including β-adrenergic blocking agents and calcium channel antagonists. These combinations are usually instituted for chronic prophylactic therapy based on complimentary or offsetting mechanisms of action (Table 23–10). Combination therapy is generally used for patients with more frequent or symptoms not responding to β-blockers alone (nitrates plus β-blockers or calcium blockers), for patients intolerant of β-blockers or calcium channel blockers, and for patients having an element of vasospasm leading to decreased supply (nitrates plus calcium blockers).[108]

Calcium Channel Blockers

Modulation of calcium entry into vascular smooth muscle and myocardium as well as a variety of other tissues is the principle action of the calcium antagonists. The cellular mechanism of these drugs is not completely understood, and it differs among the available classes of the phenylalkylamines (verapamil-like), dihydropyridines (nifedipine-like), benzothiazepines (diltiazem-like), bepridil, and a recent class referred to as *T-channel blockers*. Receptor-operated channels stimulated by norepinephrine and other neurotransmitters, and potential-dependent channels activated by membrane depolarization, control the entry of calcium, and consequently the cytosolic concentration of calcium responsible for activation of actin–myosin complex leading to contraction of vascular smooth muscle and myocardium. In the myocardium, calcium entry triggers the release of intracellular stores of calcium to increase cytosolic calcium, whereas in smooth muscle calcium derived from the extracellular fluid may do this directly. Binding proteins within the cell, calmodulin and troponin, after binding with calcium, participate in phosphorylation reactions leading to contraction. Decreased calcium availability, through the actions of calcium antagonists, inhibits these reactions. Direct actions of the calcium antagonists include vasodilation of systemic arterioles and coronary arteries, leading to a reduction of arterial pressure and coronary vascular resistance as well as depression of the myocardial contractility and conduction velocity of the sinoatrial and atrioventricular nodes (see Chap. 25). Reflex β-adrenergic stimulation overcomes much of the negative inotropic effect, and depression of contractility becomes clinically apparent only in the presence of LV dysfunction and when other negative inotropic drugs are used concurrently. Verapamil and diltiazem cause less peripheral vasodilation than nifedipine, and, consequently, the risk of myocardial depression is greater with these two agents. Conduction through the AV node is predictably depressed with verapamil and diltiazem, and they must be used with caution for patients with preexisting conduction abnormalities or in the presence of other drugs with negative chronotropic properties. MVO_2 is reduced with all of the calcium channel antagonists because of reduced wall tension secondary to reduced arterial pressure and, to a minor extent, depressed contractility (Table 23–10). Heart rate changes are dependent on the drug used and the state of the conduction system. Nifedipine generally increases heart rate or causes no change whereas either no change or decreased heart rate is seen with verapamil and diltiazem because of the interaction of these direct and indirect effects. In contrast to the β-blockers, calcium channel antagonists have the potential to improve coronary blood flow through areas of fixed coronary obstruction and by inhibiting coronary artery vasomotion and vasospasm. Beneficial redistribution of blood flow from well-perfused myocardium to ischemic areas and from epicardium to endocardium may also contribute to improvement in ischemic symptoms. Overall, the benefit provided by calcium channel antagonists is related to reduced MVO_2 rather than improved oxygen supply based on lack of alteration in the rate pressure product at maximal exercise in most studies performed to date. However, as CAD progresses and vasospasm becomes superimposed on critical stenotic lesions, improved oxygen supply through coronary vasodilation may become more important.

Absorption of the calcium channel antagonists is characterized by excellent absorption and large, variable first-pass metabolism resulting in oral bioavailability ranging from about 20% to 50% or greater for diltiazem, nicardipine, nifedipine, verapamil, felodipine, and isradipine. Amlodipine has a range of bioavailability of ~60% to 80%. Saturation of this effect may occur with verapamil and diltiazem, resulting in greater amounts of drug being absorbed with chronic dosing. Nifedipine may have slow or fast absorption patterns, and the ingestion of food delays and impairs its absorption as well as potential enhanced absorption in elderly patients. This variability in absorption produces fluctuation in the hemodynamic response with nifedipine. SL nifedipine is frequently used to provide a more rapid response; however, the rationale for this application is suspect because little nifedipine is absorbed from the buccal mucosa and the swallowed drug is responsible for the observed plasma concentrations. Absorption of verapamil in sustained-release products may be influenced by food, and when used in the fasted state, dose dumping may occur, resulting in high peak concentrations with some products. The approved sustained-release products for nifedipine, verapamil, and diltiazem are approved primarily for the treatment of hypertension (see Chapter 19). The presence of severe liver disease (e.g., alcoholic liver disease with cirrhosis) has been shown to reduce the first-pass metabolism of verapamil, and this shunting of drug around the liver gives rise to higher plasma concentrations and lower dose requirements in these patients. Interestingly, this effect appears to be stereoselective for the more active isomer of verapamil. Verapamil may also reduce liver blood flow; however, evidence for this reduction is based primarily on animal experiments. Few data are available regarding the influence of liver disease on the kinetics of calcium blockers; however, these drugs undergo extensive hepatic metabolism with little unchanged drug being renally excreted, and liver disease can be expected to alter the pharmacokinetics. Nifedipine has no active metabolites whereas norverapamil possesses 20% or less activity of the parent compound. Desacetyldiltiazem has not been studied in man, but canine studies suggest its potency ranges from 100% to 40% of the parent compound for various cardiovascular effects; the clinical importance of these observations remains to be determined. With chronic dosing of verapamil and diltiazem, apparent saturation of metabolism occurs, producing higher plasma concentrations of each drug than those seen with single-dose administration. Consequently, the elimination half-life for verapamil is prolonged, and less frequent dosing intervals may be used in some patients. The elimination half-life for diltiazem is also somewhat prolonged and the half-life of desacetyldiltiazem is longer than that of the parent drug, but it is not clear if less frequent dosing may be used. Bepridil also undergoes hepatic elimination and an active metabolite, 4-hydroxyphenyl bepridil, is produced; the parent compound has a long half-life of 30 to 40 hours. Nifedipine does not accumulate with chronic dosing; however, it is eliminated via oxidative pathways that may be polymorphic, and slow and fast metabolizers have been described for nifedipine. Most of the calcium channel blockers are eliminated via cytochrome (CYP) 3A4 and other CYP isoenzymes and many inhibit CYP 3A4 activity as well. Renal insufficiency has little or no effect on the pharmacokinetics of these three drugs. Although disease alterations in kinetics have been described, the most important quantitative alteration is the influence of liver disease on bioavailability and elimination that reduce the clearance of verapamil and diltiazem, and dosing in this population should be done with caution. Altered protein binding due to renal disease, decreased protein concentration, or increased α1-acid glycoprotein has been noted, but the clinical import of these changes is unknown.

Good candidates for calcium channel blockers in angina include patients with contraindications or intolerance of β-blockers, coexisting conduction system disease (except for verapamil and diltiazem), patients with Prinzmetal angina (vasospastic or variable threshold angina), the presence of peripheral vascular disease, severe ventricular dysfunction (amlodipine is probably calcium channel blocker of choice and others need to be used with caution if the ejection fraction is <40%), and concurrent hypertension.

Ranolazine

Ranolazine is a new drug for angina that has a unique mechanism of action unlike any other drugs used to alter the relationship between oxygen supply and demand. Ranolazine reduces calcium overload in the ischemic myocyte through inhibition of the late sodium current (I_{Na}). Myocardial ischemia produces a cascade of complex ionic exchanges that can result in intracellular acidosis, excess cytosolic Ca^{2+}, myocardial cellular dysfunction, and, if sustained, cell injury and death. Activation of the adenosine triphosphate–dependent K^+ current during ischemia results in a strong efflux of K^+ ions from myocytes. Sodium channels are activated on depolarization, leading to a rapid influx of sodium into the cells. The inactivation of I_{Na} has a fast component lasting a few milliseconds and a slowly inactivating component that can last hundreds of milliseconds.[109] Ranolazine is a relatively selective inhibitor for late I_{Na}. In isolated ventricular myocytes in which the late I_{Na} was pathologically augmented, ranolazine prevented or reversed the induced mechanical dysfunction, as well as ameliorated abnormalities of ventricular repolarization. Ranolazine does not affect heart rate, inotropic state, or hemodynamic state or increase coronary blood flow.

Ranolazine is extensively metabolized via CYP 450 3A and potent inhibitors of 3A increase the plasma concentration by a factor of about three. Ketoconazole, diltiazem, and verapamil should not be coadministered with ranolazine. Absorption from the gut is quite variable and the apparent half-life is 7 hours. Steady state is reached after 3 days of twice daily dosing. Ranolazine is indicated for the treatment of chronic angina, and because it prolongs the QT interval, it should be reserved for patients who have not achieved an adequate response with other antianginal agents. Contraindications include preexisting QT interval prolongation, hepatic impairment, concurrent QT interval prolonging drugs and moderately potent to potent concurrent 3A inhibitors. QT prolongation occurs in a dose-dependent fashion with ranolazine with an average increase of 6 milliseconds, but 5% of the population has QTc prolongation of 15 milliseconds. Baseline and follow-up ECGs should be obtained to evaluate effects of the QT interval. In controlled trials, the most common adverse reactions are dizziness, headache, constipation, and nausea. Ranolazine should be started at 500 mg twice daily and increased to 1000 mg twice daily as needed based on symptoms.[110]

Based on randomized, placebo-controlled trials, the improvement in exercise time is a modest increase of 15 to about 45 seconds compared with placebo.[111-113] In a large ACS trial, ranolazine reduced recurrent ischemia but did not improve the primary efficacy end point of the composite of cardiovascular death, MI, or recurrent ischemia.[114] Ranolazine may have antiarrhythmic effects as assessed by continuous ECG monitoring of patients in the first week after admission for ACS.[115]

Coronary Artery Spasm and Variant Angina Pectoris (Prinzmetal Angina)

Prinzmetal, in his original description of variant angina pectoris, noted the waxing and waning course of this syndrome associated with ST-segment elevation and most commonly resolves without progression to MI. Patients who develop variant angina are usually younger, have fewer coronary risk factors, but more commonly smoke than patients with chronic stable angina. Hyperventilation, exercise, exposure to cold may precipitate variant angina attacks or there may be no apparent precipitating cause. The onset of chest discomfort is usually in the early morning hours. The exact cause of variant angina is not well understood, but may be an imbalance between endothelium-produced vasodilator factors (prostacyclin, nitric oxide) and vasoconstrictor factors (e.g., endothelin, angiotensin II) as well as an imbalance of autonomic control characterized by parasympathetic dominance, or inflammation may also play a role.[116,117] More recently there have been a number potential common adrenoreceptor polymorphisms that may predispose patients to developing vasospasm.[118-121] Another possible explanation is a recently discovered genetic mutation. The eNOS T-786C mutation appears to be a reversible etiology of Prinzmetal variant angina in white Americans whose angina might be ameliorated by L-arginine.[119]

The diagnosis of variant angina is based on ST-segment elevation during transient chest discomfort (usually at rest) that resolves when the chest discomfort diminishes for patients who have normal or nonobstructive coronary lesions. In the absence of ST-segment elevation, a provocative test using ergonovine, acetylcholine, or methacholine may be used to precipitate coronary artery spasm, ST-segment elevation, and typical symptoms. Nitrates and calcium antagonists should be withdrawn prior to provocative testing. Provocative testing should not be used for patients with high-grade lesions. Hyperventilation may also be used to provoke spasm, and patients who have positive a hyperventilation test are more likely to have higher frequency of attacks, multivessel disease, and a high degree of AV block or ventricular tachycardia.

Optimization of therapy includes dose titration using sufficiently high doses to obtain clinical efficacy without unacceptable adverse effects in individual patients. All patients should be treated for acute attacks and maintained on prophylactic treatment for 6 to 12 months following the initial episode. The occurrence of serious arrhythmias during attacks is associated with a greater risk of sudden death, and these patients should be treated more aggressively and for prolonged periods. For patients without arrhythmias who become asymptomatic and remain so for several months after treatment has been instituted, withdrawal of therapy may be safe after first ascertaining that disease activity is quiescent. Aggravating factors such as alcohol or cocaine use or cigarette smoking should be eliminated when instituting treatment.

Nitrates have been the mainstay of therapy for the acute attacks of variant angina and coronary artery spasm for many years. Most patients respond rapidly to SL nitroglycerin or ISDN; however, intravenous and intracoronary nitroglycerin may be very useful for patients not responding to SL preparations. In particular, vasospasm provoked by ergonovine may require intracoronary nitroglycerin. Although studies with nitrates generally show them to be efficacious, high does are often required, and it is unclear if they reduce mortality. Because calcium antagonists may be more effective, have few serious adverse effects in effective doses, and can be given less frequently than nitrates, some consider them the agents of choice for variant angina.

Nifedipine, verapamil, and diltiazem are all equally effective as single agents for the initial management of variant angina and coronary artery spasm. Dose titration is important to maximize the response with calcium antagonists. Comparative trials, which are few number and do not reveal significant differences among these three drugs for variant angina. Patients unresponsive to calcium antagonists alone may have nitrates added. Combination therapy with nifedipine–diltiazem or nifedipine–verapamil has been reported useful for patients unresponsive to single-drug regimens. This is probably rational because, at the cellular level, the drugs have different receptors, but the combination of verapamil–diltiazem should be used cautiously owing to their potential additive effects on contractility and conduction.

β-adrenergic blockade has little or no role in the management of variant angina according to most authorities.[120] Although not all studies report increased painful episodes of variant angina with the addition of β-blockers, they may induce coronary vasoconstriction and prolong ischemia, as documented by continuous ECG monitoring. Other approaches to therapy attempting to modify sympathetic/parasympathetic tone include α-antagonists, anticholinergics, plexectomy, surgical interruption of the sympathetic innervation of the heart, thromboxane receptor antagonism, prostacyclin, lipoxygenase inhibition, and ticlopidine but these drugs or procedures do not occupy a major place in therapy at the present time. One interesting case report found that the likely cause of MI was coronary artery spasm in a woman with migraine headaches because of the possible increased serotonergic activity secondary to concomitant use of zolmitriptan and citalopram.[121]

Silent Ischemia[16]

The objective in the treatment of silent myocardial ischemia is to reduce the total number of ischemic episodes, both symptomatic and asymptomatic, regardless of the direction of ST-segment shift. The incidence of silent ischemia in the general, asymptomatic population is not known. Significant day-to-day variability in the number of episodes, the duration of ischemia, and the amount of ST-segment deviation complicates both the understanding of this process and the utility of various therapeutic interventions. Silent ischemia for patients with known CAD is common (~80% of all ischemic episodes) and associated with the extent of disease as well as a high risk for MI and sudden death when compared with symptomatic episodes of ischemia. Although the underlying mechanisms for silent ischemia are continuing to be defined, increased physical activity, activation of the sympathetic nervous system, increased cortisol secretion, increased coronary artery tone, and enhanced platelet aggregation due to endothelia dysfunction leading to intermittent coronary obstruction may be additive in lowering the threshold for ischemia. Platelet aggregability is increased in the morning hours (7 AM to 11 AM), corresponding to circadian rhythms noted for the peak frequency of ischemia, AMI, and sudden death. Silent ischemia is associated with ST-segment elevation or depression and frequently occurs without antecedent changes in heart rate or blood pressure, suggesting that this form of ischemia is a result of primary reduction in oxygen supply. Silent ischemia is classified into Class I, patients who do not experience angina at any time, and Class II, patients who have both asymptomatic and symptomatic ischemia. Patients with silent ischemia have a defective warning system for angina pain that may encourage excessive myocardial demand. Regardless of the exact mechanism, there is increasing concern that painless ischemia carries considerable risk for myocardial perfusion defects, detrimental hemodynamic changes, arrhythmogenesis, and sudden death.[122] Silent ischemia is associated with reduced survival and increased need for PTCA and CABG as well as increased risk of AMI.[123,124] Because it is apparently very common in some settings, major emphasis should be placed on its management. A consensus has not been reached for the most appropriate method of detecting and quantifying the magnitude of silent ischemia; however, ambulatory electrocardiogram monitoring is felt by many to be the most useful tool at the present time.

The initial step in management is to modify the major risk factors for IHD, hypertension, hypercholesterolemia, and smoking, and data from the Multiple Risk Factor Intervention Trial (MRFIT) show these interventions to be useful for patients with silent ischemia. In a subset of the study population who had abnormal baseline exercise ECG responses, the special intervention group had a 57% reduction in CHD death (22.2/1000 vs 51.8/1000) and a reduction in sudden death resulting from cessation of smoking and lowering of blood pressure and cholesterol when compared with the usual-care group.

Asymptomatic Cardiac Ischemia Pilot (ACIP), a randomized trial of medical therapy versus revascularization (PTCA or CABG), at the 2-year follow-up demonstrates that total mortality was 6.6% in the angina-guided strategy (i.e., therapy based on symptoms), 4.4% in the ischemia-guided strategy (based on ECG changes), and 1.1% in the revascularization strategy (P<0.02). The rate of death or MI was 12.1% in the angina-guided strategy, 8.8% in the ischemia-guided strategy, and 4.7% in the revascularization strategy (P<0.04).[124] The rate of death, MI, or recurrent cardiac hospitalization was 41.8% in the angina-guided strategy, 38.5% in the ischemia-guided strategy, and 23.1% in the revascularization strategy (P<0.001). Post-MI patients and those with a high level of sympathetic nervous system activity are perhaps the best candidates for β-blocker therapy.

Calcium channel antagonists alone and in combination have been shown to be effective in reducing symptomatic and asymptomatic ischemia; however, they do not interrupt the diurnal surge in ischemia observed on ambulatory monitoring and, in general, they are somewhat less effective than β-blockers for silent ischemia.[125,126] Nifedipine in particular seems to provide less protection and provides wide fluctuations in response with approximate reductions in the number of episodes ranging from 0% to 93% and in duration from 23% to 65% unless combined with β-blockers. Fewer studies are available with other calcium blockers and comparative trials are uncommon. Earlier studies have shown that combination therapy with calcium and β-blockers provides a better response than calcium blockers and nitrates or monotherapy.[124,127]

A randomized, unblinded, controlled trial Swiss Interventional Study on Silent Ischemia Type II (SWISSI II) of PCI for patients with silent ischemia after AMI found that PCI compared with antiischemic drug therapy reduced the long-term risk of major cardiac events with better preservation of ventricular function than with medical therapy.[128,129]

PHARMACOECONOMIC CONSIDERATIONS

Pharmacoeconomic studies have been performed primarily for patients with ACSs and only with low molecular weight heparins, glycoprotein IIb/IIIa receptor antagonists and statins.[130] Most of the studies on LMWHs have been cost-minimization analyses and have focused on enoxaparin sodium, because this is the only LMWH proven to be superior to UFH. Several analyses show that, compared with UFH plus aspirin, enoxaparin sodium provides cost savings both during hospitalization (30 days) and 1-year follow-up. These cost savings are mainly attributable to fewer cardiac interventions, shorter hospital stays, and lower administrative costs. Indeed, the clinical and economic advantages of enoxaparin sodium have led to its recommendation in recent guidelines as the antithrombotic agent of choice for CAD. Most of the economic analyses of GP IIb/IIIa inhibitors have been cost-effectiveness analyses.[131] Such analyses indicate that the high acquisition costs of these drugs may be at least partially offset by reductions in other costs if a noninvasive approach to risk stratification is used. Furthermore, use of GP IIb/IIIa inhibitors appears to give favorable cost-effectiveness ratios compared with other accepted therapies, such as fibrin-specific thrombolytic therapy, in the cardiovascular field, particularly in high-risk patients and those undergoing percutaneous coronary intervention. However, more comprehensive economic data on the GP IIb/IIIa inhibitors are needed. Bivalirudin combined with provisional glycoprotein IIb/IIIa inhibitors appears to be an acceptable alternative to the standard of care, is superior to UFH alone in PCI, and is considered to be cost effective.[132]

Atorvastatin when used in ACS has been shown to reduce events and this offsets the upfront acquisition costs.[133] The total expected cost was £784.05 (British) per patient in the placebo cohort and £851.59 per patient in the atorvastatin cohort, resulting in an incremental cost of £67.54 per patient in the atorvastatin group. The cost per event avoided was £1762.04. A third of the cost of atorvastatin treatment was offset within 16 weeks by the cost savings resulting from the reduction in the number of events in the atorvastatin cohort compared with the placebo cohort. Other analyses of statins have found this class to be cost-effective especially for patients at higher risk.[133]

Aspirin and clopidogrel have been evaluated for secondary prevention of CHD, and while aspirin is very cost effective, clopidogrel is only cost effective or patients who cannot take aspirin.[134]

CLINICAL CONTROVERSIES

Once patients with angina develop symptoms sufficient for pharmacologic therapy on a daily basis, the initial prophylactic therapy recommended is a β-blocker. There is a paucity of comparative, long-term clinical trials of β-blockade versus calcium channel blockers to determine which is superior for survival benefit. β-blockers are recommended first-line therapy because of their efficacy in post-MI patients and favorable adverse effect profile.

Recent developments in the understanding of bioactivation of organic nitrates have given rise to concern over endothelial dysfunction induced by nitrates when administered long term. Not all nitrate products are activated via the same mechanisms, and this may impact how effective individual drugs are in long-term treatment.

In stable CAD, medical management has been reported for outcomes similar to revascularization, and these findings may have a significant impact on how healthcare resources are utilized in the future.

EVALUATION OF THERAPEUTIC OUTCOMES

Improved symptoms of angina, improved cardiac performance and improvement in risk factors may all be used to assess the outcome of treatment of IHD and angina. Symptomatic improvement in exercise capacity (longer duration) or fewer symptoms at the same level of exercise is subjective evidence that therapy is working. Once patients have been optimized on medical therapy, symptoms should improve over 2 to 4 weeks and remain stable until their disease progresses. There are several instruments (e.g., Seattle angina questionnaire, specific activity scale [Table 23–1], Canadian classification system [Table 23–2]) that could be used improve the reproducibility of symptom assessment.[2] If the patient is doing well, then no other assessment may be necessary. Objective assessment is obtained through increase exercise duration on ETT and the absence of ischemic changes on ECG or deleterious hemodynamic changes. Echocardiography and cardiac imaging may also be used, however, due to their expense, they are only used if a patient is not doing well to determine if revascularization or other measures should be undertaken. Coronary angiography may be used to assess the extent of stenosis or re-stenosis after angioplasty or CABG. ⓫ The performance measurement set recommended by the ACC/AHA is provided in Table 23–12.

TABLE 23-12 American College of Cardiology, American Heart Association, and Physician Consortium for Performance Improvement Chronic Stable Coronary Artery Disease Core Physician Performance Measurement Set[a]

	Clinical Recommendations
Blood pressure measurement	A blood pressure ready is recommended at every visit. Recommended blood pressure management targets are ≤130 mm Hg systolic (Class I Recommendation, Level A Evidence) and ≤85 mm Hg diastolic for patients with CAD coexisting condition (e.g., diabetes, heart failure, or renal failure) and <140/90 mm Hg for patients with CAD and no coexisting condition.
Lipid profile	A lipid profile is recommended and should include total cholesterol, high-density lipoprotein cholesterol (HDL-C), low-density lipoprotein cholesterol (LDL-C), and triglycerides. (*Class I Recommendation, Level C Evidence*)
Symptom and activity assessment	Regular assessment of patients' anginal symptoms and levels of activity is recommended. (Serves as a basis for treatment modification.)
Smoking cessation	Smoking status should be determined and smoking cessation counseling and interventions are recommended. (*Class I Recommendation, Level B Evidence*)
Antiplatelet therapy[d] *Denominator exclusion* Documentation of medical reason(s)[b] for not prescribing antiplatelet therapy; documentation of patient reason(s)[c] for not prescribing antiplatelet therapy	Routine use of aspirin is recommended in the absence of contraindications. If contraindications exist, other antiplatelet therapies may be substituted. (*Class I Recommendation, Level A Evidence*)
Drug therapy for lowering LCL-cholesterol *Denominator exclusion* Documentation that a statin was not indicated;[e] documentation of medical reason(s)[b] for not prescribing a statin; documentation of patient reason(s)[c] for not prescribing statin	The LCL-C treatment goal is <100 mg/dL. Persons with established coronary heart disease (CHD) who have a baseline LCL-C ≥130 mg/dL should be started on a cholesterol-lowering drug simultaneously with therapeutic lifestyle changes and control of nonlipid risk factors. (*Class I Recommendation, Level A Evidence*)
β-blocker therapy–prior myocardial infarction (MI) *Denominator inclusion* Prior MI *Denominator exclusion* Documentation that a β-blocker was not indicated; documentation of medical reason(s)[b] for not prescribing a β-blocker; documentation of patient reason(s)[c] for not prescribing a β-blocker	β-Blocker therapy is recommended for all patients with prior MI in the absence of contraindications. (*Class I Recommendation, Level A Evidence*)
ACE inhibitor therapy *Denominator inclusion* Patient with CAD who also has diabetes and/or left ventricular systolic dysfunction (LVSD) (left ventricular ejection fraction [LVEF] <40% or moderately or severely depressed left ventricular systolic function) *Denominator exclusion* Documentation that ACE inhibitor was not indicated (e.g., patients on angiotensin receptor blockers [ARB]); documentation of medical reason(s)[b] for not prescribing ACE inhibitor; documentation of patient reason(s)[c] for not prescribing ACE inhibitor	ACE inhibitor use is recommended in all patients with CAD who also have diabetes and/or LVSD (*Class I Recommendation, Level A Evidence*) ACE inhibitor use is also recommended in patients with CAD or other vascular disease (*Class IIa Recommendation, Level B Evidence*)
Screening for diabetes[f,g] *Denominator exclusion* Patients with documented diabetes	Screening for diabetes is recommended in patients who are considered high risk (e.g., CAD) (*Class I Recommendation, Level A Evidence*)

ACE, angiotensin-converting enzyme; CAD, coronary artery disease; MI, myocardial infarction.

[a]Refers to all patients diagnosed with CAD

[b]Medical reasons for not prescribing *antiplatelet therapy* (aspirin, clopidogrel, or combination of aspirin and dipyridamole): active bleeding in the previous 6 months with required hospitalization and/or transfusion(s), patient on other antiplatelet therapy, etc. Medical reasons for not prescribing a *statin*: clinical judgement, documented LCL-C <130 mg/dL, etc. Medical reasons for not prescribing a *β-blocker*: bradycardia (defined as heart rate <50 beats/min without β-blocker therapy), history of class IV (congestive) heart failure, history of secondor third-degree atrioventricular block without permanent pacemaker, etc. Medical reasons for not prescribing *ACE inhibitor* (ACEI): allergy, angioedema caused by ACEI, anuric rental failure caused by ACEI, pregnancy, moderate or severe aortic stenosis, etc.

[c]Patient reasons for not prescribing antiplatelet therapy, statin, β-blocker, or ACEI: economic, social, and/or religious, etc.

[d]Antiplatelet therapy may include aspirin, clopidogrel, or combination of aspirin and dipyridamole.

[e]Not indicated for a stat refers to LCL-C <100 mg/dL.

[f]Test measure.

[g]Screening for diabetes is usually done by fasting blood glucose or 2-hour glucose tolerance testing. Clinical recommendations indicate screening should be considered at 3-year intervals.

REFERENCES

1. Fraker TD, Jr., Fihn SD, Gibbons RJ, et al. 2007 chronic angina focused update of the ACC/AHA 2002 guidelines for the management of patients with chronic stable angina: a report of the American College of Cardiology/American Heart Association Task Force on Practice Guidelines Writing Group to develop the focused update of the 2002 guidelines for the management of patients with chronic stable angina. J Am Coll Cardiol 2007;50:2264–2274.

2. Gibbons RJ, Abrams J, Chatterjee K, et al. ACC/AHA 2002 guideline update for the management of patients with chronic stable angina—Summary article: A report of the American College of Cardiology/American Heart Association Task Force on practice guidelines (Committee on the Management of Patients With Chronic Stable Angina). J Am Coll Cardiol 2003;41:159–168.

3. Fox K, Garcia MA, Ardissino D, et al. Guidelines on the management of stable angina pectoris: executive summary: The Task Force on the Management of Stable Angina Pectoris of the European Society of Cardiology. Eur Heart J 2006;27:1341–1381.

4. Lloyd-Jones D, Adams RJ, Brown TM, et al. Heart disease and stroke statistics—2010 update: a report from the American Heart Association. Circulation 2010;121:e46–e215.

5. Sytkowski PA, D'Agostino RB, Belanger A, Kannel WB. Sex and time trends in cardiovascular disease incidence and mortality: The Framingham Heart Study, 1950–1989. Am J Epidemiol 1996;143: 338–350.

6. Menotti A, Keys A, Blackburn H, et al. Comparison of multivariate predictive power of major risk factors for coronary heart diseases in different countries: results from eight nations of the Seven Countries Study, 25-year follow-up. J Cardiovasc Risk 1996;3:69–75.

7. Keys A. Mediterranean diet and public health: personal reflections. Am J Clin Nutr 1995;61:1321S–1323S.

8. Goldman L, Hashimoto B, Cook EF, Loscalzo A. Comparative reproducibility and validity of systems for assessing cardiovascular functional class: Advantages of a new specific activity scale. Circulation 1981;64:1227–1234.

9. Emond M, Mock MB, Davis KB, et al. Long-term survival of medically treated patients in the Coronary Artery Surgery Study (CASS) Registry. Circulation 1994;90:2645–2657.

10. Caracciolo EA, Davis KB, Sopko G, et al. Comparison of surgical and medical group survival in patients with left main coronary artery disease. Long-term CASS experience. Circulation 1995;91: 2325–2334.

11. Park SJ, Park DW. Percutaneous coronary intervention with stent implantation versus coronary artery bypass surgery for treatment of left main coronary artery disease: Is it time to change guidelines? Circ Cardiovasc Interv 2009;2:59–68.

12. Epstein SE, Cannon RO, 3rd, Talbot TL. Hemodynamic principles in the control of coronary blood flow. Am J Cardiol 1985;56:4E–10E.

13. von Mering GO, Arant CB, Wessel TR, et al. Abnormal coronary vasomotion as a prognostic indicator of cardiovascular events in women: Results from the National Heart, Lung, and Blood Institute-Sponsored Women's Ischemia Syndrome Evaluation (WISE). Circulation 2004;109:722–725.

14. Ferrari R, Fox K. Insight into the mode of action of ACE inhibition in coronary artery disease: the ultimate 'EUROPA' story. Drugs 2009;69:265–277.

15. Anderson JL, Adams CD, Antman EM, et al. ACC/AHA 2007 guidelines for the management of patients with unstable angina/non ST-elevation myocardial infarction: A report of the American College of Cardiology/American Heart Association Task Force on Practice Guidelines (Writing Committee to Revise the 2002 Guidelines for the Management of Patients With Unstable Angina/Non ST-Elevation Myocardial Infarction): Developed in collaboration with the American College of Emergency Physicians, the Society for Cardiovascular Angiography and Interventions, and the Society of Thoracic Surgeons: Endorsed by the American Association of Cardiovascular and Pulmonary Rehabilitation and the Society for Academic Emergency Medicine. Circulation 2007;116:e148–e304.

16. Cohn PF. A new look at benefits of drug therapy in silent myocardial ischaemia. Eur Heart J 2007;28:2053–2054.

17. Caracciolo EA, Chaitman BR, Forman SA, et al. Diabetics with coronary disease have a prevalence of asymptomatic ischemia during exercise treadmill testing and ambulatory ischemia monitoring similar to that of nondiabetic patients. An ACIP database study. ACIP Investigators. Asymptomatic Cardiac Ischemia Pilot Investigators. Circulation 1996;93:2097–2105.

18. Panel E. Summary of the second report of the National Cholesterol Education Program (NCEP) Expert Panel on Detection, Evaluation, and Treatment of High Blood Cholesterol in Adults (Adult Treatment Panel II). JAMA 1993;269:3015–3023.

19. Glynn RJ, Koenig W, Nordestgaard BG, Shepherd J, Ridker PM. Rosuvastatin for primary prevention in older persons with elevated C-reactive protein and low to average low-density lipoprotein cholesterol levels: Exploratory analysis of a randomized trial. Ann Intern Med 2010;152:488–496, W174.

20. Crowe E, Lovibond K, Gray H, Henderson R, Krause T, Camm J. Early management of unstable angina and non-ST segment elevation myocardial infarction: Summary of NICE guidance. BMJ 2010;340:c1134.

21. Gibbons RJ, Balady GJ, Bricker JT, et al. ACC/AHA 2002 guideline update for exercise testing: summary article. A report of the American College of Cardiology/American Heart Association Task Force on Practice Guidelines (Committee to Update the 1997 Exercise Testing Guidelines). J Am Coll Cardiol 2002;40:1531–1540.

22. Greenland P, Bonow RO, Brundage BH, et al. ACCF/AHA 2007 clinical expert consensus document on coronary artery calcium scoring by computed tomography in global cardiovascular risk assessment and in evaluation of patients with chest pain: A report of the American College of Cardiology Foundation Clinical Expert Consensus Task Force (ACCF/AHA Writing Committee to Update the 2000 Expert Consensus Document on Electron Beam Computed Tomography). Circulation 2007;115:402–426.

23. Fitzgerald PJ, Oshima A, Hayase M, et al. Final results of the Can Routine Ultrasound Influence Stent Expansion (CRUISE) study. Circulation 2000;102:523–530.

24. Panel E. Executive Summary of The Third Report of The National Cholesterol Education Program (NCEP) Expert Panel on Detection, Evaluation, And Treatment of High Blood Cholesterol In Adults (Adult Treatment Panel III). JAMA 2001;285:2486–2497.

25. Grundy SM, Cleeman JI, Merz CN, et al. Implications of recent clinical trials for the National Cholesterol Education Program Adult Treatment Panel III Guidelines. J Am Coll Cardiol 2004;44:720–732.

26. Skyler JS, Bergenstal R, Bonow RO, et al. Intensive glycemic control and the prevention of cardiovascular events: Implications of the ACCORD, ADVANCE, and VA diabetes trials: A position statement of the American Diabetes Association and a scientific statement of the American College of Cardiology Foundation and the American Heart Association. Circulation 2009;119:351–357.

27. Wald NJ, Watt HC. Prospective study of effect of switching from cigarettes to pipes or cigars on mortality from three smoking related diseases. BMJ 1997;314:1860–1863.

28. Rigotti NA, Pipe AL, Benowitz NL, Arteaga C, Garza D, Tonstad S. Efficacy and safety of varenicline for smoking cessation in patients with cardiovascular disease: A randomized trial. Circulation 2010;121: 221–229.

29. Swan GE, McClure JB, Jack LM, et al. Behavioral counseling and varenicline treatment for smoking cessation. Am J Prev Med 2010;38:482–490.

30. Russell LB, Carson JL, Taylor WC, Milan E, Dey A, Jagannathan R. Modeling all-cause mortality: projections of the impact of smoking cessation based on the NHEFS. NHANES I Epidemiologic Follow-up Study. Am J Public Health 1998;88:630–636.

31. Bartecchi C, Alsever RN, Nevin-Woods C, et al. Reduction in the incidence of acute myocardial infarction associated with a citywide smoking ordinance. Circulation 2006;114:1490–1496.

32. Rosendorff C. Hypertension and coronary artery disease: a summary of the American Heart Association scientific statement. J Clin Hypertens (Greenwich) 2007;9:790–795.

33. Grundy SM, Cleeman JI, Merz CN, et al. Implications of recent clinical trials for the National Cholesterol Education Program Adult Treatment Panel III guidelines. Circulation 2004;110:227–239.

34. Bleys J, Miller ER, 3rd, Pastor-Barriuso R, Appel LJ, Guallar E. Vitamin-mineral supplementation and the progression of atherosclerosis: A meta-analysis of randomized controlled trials. Am J Clin Nutr 2006;84:880–887; quiz 954–955.

35. Haskell WL, Lee IM, Pate RR, et al. Physical activity and public health: updated recommendation for adults from the American College of Sports Medicine and the American Heart Association. Circulation 2007;116:1081–1093.

36. Williams MA, Haskell WL, Ades PA, et al. Resistance exercise in individuals with and without cardiovascular disease: 2007 update: A scientific statement from the American Heart Association Council on Clinical Cardiology and Council on Nutrition, Physical Activity, and Metabolism. Circulation 2007;116:572–584.

37. Fuchs FD, Chambless LE, Folsom AR, et al. Association between alcoholic beverage consumption and incidence of coronary heart disease in whites and blacks: The Atherosclerosis Risk in Communities Study. Am J Epidemiol 2004;160:466–474.

38. Britton A, Marmot MG, Shipley MJ. How does variability in alcohol consumption over time affect the relationship with mortality and coronary heart disease? Addiction 2010;105:639–645.

39. Hulley S, Grady D, Bush T, et al. Randomized trial of estrogen plus progestin for secondary prevention of coronary heart disease in postmenopausal women. Heart and Estrogen/progestin Replacement Study (HERS) Research Group. JAMA 1998;280:605–613.

40. Rossouw JE, Cushman M, Greenland P, et al. Inflammatory, lipid, thrombotic, and genetic markers of coronary heart disease risk in the women's health initiative trials of hormone therapy. Arch Intern Med 2008;168:2245–2253.

41. El-Sohemy A, Cornelis MC, Kabagambe EK, Campos H. Coffee, CYP1A2 genotype and risk of myocardial infarction. Genes Nutr 2007;2:155–156.

42. Gibbons RJ, Abrams J, Chatterjee K, et al. ACC/AHA 2002 guideline update for the management of patients with chronic stable angina— summary article: a report of the American College of Cardiology/ American Heart Association Task Force on Practice Guidelines (Committee on the Management of Patients With Chronic Stable Angina). Circulation 2003;107:149–158.

43. Sipahi I, Tuzcu EM, Wolski KE, et al. Beta-blockers and progression of coronary atherosclerosis: pooled analysis of 4 intravascular ultrasonography trials. Ann Intern Med 2007;147:10–18.

44. Kroon LA. Drug interactions with smoking. Am J Health Syst Pharm 2007;64:1917–1921.

45. Munzel T, Daiber A, Mulsch A. Explaining the phenomenon of nitrate tolerance. Circ Res 2005;97:618–628.

46. Daiber A, Munzel T. Characterization of the antioxidant properties of pentaerythrityl tetranitrate (PETN)-induction of the intrinsic antioxidative system heme oxygenase-1 (HO-1). Methods Mol Biol 2010;594:311–326.

47. Ambrosio G, Del Pinto M, Tritto I, et al. Chronic nitrate therapy is associated with different presentation and evolution of acute coronary syndromes: insights from 52,693 patients in the Global Registry of Acute Coronary Events. Eur Heart J 2009;31:430–438.

48. Pehrsson SK, Ringqvist I, Ekdahl S, Karlson BW, Ulvenstam G, Persson S. Monotherapy with amlodipine or atenolol versus their combination in stable angina pectoris. Clin Cardiol 2000;23:763–770.

49. Verdecchia P, Reboldi G, Angeli F, et al. Angiotensin-converting enzyme inhibitors and calcium channel blockers for coronary heart disease and stroke prevention. Hypertension 2005;46:386–392.

50. Opie LH, Yusuf S, Kubler W. Current status of safety and efficacy of calcium channel blockers in cardiovascular diseases: a critical analysis based on 100 studies. Prog Cardiovasc Dis 2000;43:171–196.

51. Howes LG, Edwards CT. Calcium antagonists and cancer. Is there really a link? Drug Saf 1998;18:1–7.

52. Knight CJ, Fox KM. Amlodipine versus diltiazem as additional antianginal treatment to atenolol. Centralised European Studies in Angina Research (CESAR) Investigators. Am J Cardiol 1998;81:133–136.

53. Boden WE, O'Rourke RA, Teo KK, et al. Optimal medical therapy with or without PCI for stable coronary disease. N Engl J Med 2007;356:1503–1516.

54. Maron DJ, Boden WE, O'Rourke RA, et al. Intensive multifactorial intervention for stable coronary artery disease: Optimal medical therapy in the COURAGE (Clinical Outcomes Utilizing Revascularization and Aggressive Drug Evaluation) trial. J Am Coll Cardiol 2010;55:1348–1358.

55. Hueb W, Lopes NH, Gersh BJ, et al. Five-year follow-up of the Medicine, Angioplasty, or Surgery Study (MASS II): A randomized controlled clinical trial of 3 therapeutic strategies for multivessel coronary artery disease. Circulation 2007;115:1082–1089.

56. Braunwald E, Antman EM, Beasley JW, et al. ACC/AHA guideline update for the management of patients with unstable angina and non-ST-segment elevation myocardial infarction—2002: Summary article: A report of the American College of Cardiology/American Heart Association Task Force on Practice Guidelines (Committee on the Management of Patients With Unstable Angina). Circulation 2002;106:1893–1900.

57. King SB, 3rd, Smith SC, Jr., Hirshfeld JW, Jr., et al. 2007 Focused Update of the ACC/AHA/SCAI 2005 Guideline Update for Percutaneous Coronary Intervention: a report of the American College of Cardiology/American Heart Association Task Force on Practice Guidelines: 2007 Writing Group to Review New Evidence and Update the ACC/AHA/SCAI 2005 Guideline Update for Percutaneous Coronary Intervention, Writing on Behalf of the 2005 Writing Committee. Circulation 2008;117:261–295.

58. Sobel BE. Coronary revascularization in patients with type 2 diabetes and results of the BARI 2D trial. Coron Artery Dis 2010;21:189–198.

59. The final 10-year follow-up results from the BARI randomized trial. J Am Coll Cardiol 2007;49:1600–1606.

60. Hannan EL, Racz MJ, Gold J, et al. Adherence of catheterization laboratory cardiologists to American College of Cardiology/American Heart Association guidelines for percutaneous coronary interventions and coronary artery bypass graft surgery: What happens in actual practice? Circulation 2010;121:267–275.

61. Simoons ML, Windecker S. Controversies in cardiovascular medicine: Chronic stable coronary artery disease: Drugs vs. revascularization. Eur Heart J 2010;31:530–541.

62. Ramanathan KB, Weiman DS, Sacks J, et al. Percutaneous intervention versus coronary bypass surgery for patients older than 70 years of age with high-risk unstable angina. Ann Thorac Surg 2005;80:1340–1346.

63. Smith SC, Jr., Feldman TE, Hirshfeld JW, Jr., et al. ACC/AHA/SCAI 2005 guideline update for percutaneous coronary intervention: A report of the American College of Cardiology/American Heart Association Task Force on Practice Guidelines (ACC/AHA/SCAI Writing Committee to Update 2001 Guidelines for Percutaneous Coronary Intervention). Circulation 2006;113:e166–e286.

64. Rathore S, Kinoshita Y, Terashima M, et al. A comparison of clinical presentations, angiographic patterns, and outcomes of in-stent restenosis between bare metal stents and drug eluting stents. EuroIntervention 2010;5:841–846.

65. Lemesle G, Maluenda G, Collins SD, Waksman R. Drug-eluting stents: Issues of late stent thrombosis. Cardiol Clin 2010;28:97–105.

66. Onuma Y, Serruys PW, Kukreja N, et al. Randomized comparison of everolimus- and paclitaxel-eluting stents: Pooled analysis of the 2-year clinical follow-up from the SPIRIT II and III trials. Eur Heart J 2010;31:1071–1078.

67. Coons JC, Battistone S. 2007 Guideline update for unstable angina/ non-ST-segment elevation myocardial infarction: Focus on antiplatelet and anticoagulant therapies. Ann Pharmacother 2008;42:989–1001.

68. Vermeer NS, Bajorek BV. Utilization of evidence-based therapy for the secondary prevention of acute coronary syndromes in Australian practice. J Clin Pharm Ther 2008;33:591–601.

69. Tebbe U, Hochadel M, Bramlage P, et al. In-hospital outcomes after elective and non-elective percutaneous coronary interventions in hospitals with and without on-site cardiac surgery backup. Clin Res Cardiol 2009;98:701–707.

70. Chaitman BR, Hardison RM, Adler D, et al. The Bypass Angioplasty Revascularization Investigation 2 Diabetes randomized trial of different treatment strategies in type 2 diabetes mellitus with stable ischemic heart disease: Impact of treatment strategy on cardiac mortality and myocardial infarction. Circulation 2009;120:2529–2540.

71. Curzen NP. Is there evidence for prognostic benefit following PCI in stable patients? COURAGE and its implications: An interventionalist's view. Heart 2009;96:103–105.

72. Bottorff MB, Nutescu EA, Spinler S. Antiplatelet therapy in patients with unstable angina and non-ST-segment-elevation myocardial infarction: Findings from the CRUSADE national quality improvement initiative. Pharmacotherapy 2007;27:1145–1162.

73. Levine GN, Berger PB, Cohen DJ, et al. Newer pharmacotherapy in patients undergoing percutaneous coronary interventions: A guide for pharmacists and other health care professionals. Pharmacotherapy 2006;26:1537–1556.

74. Eagle KA, Guyton RA, Davidoff R, et al. ACC/AHA 2004 guideline update for coronary artery bypass graft surgery: A report of the American College of Cardiology/American Heart Association Task Force on Practice Guidelines (Committee to Update the 1999 Guidelines for Coronary Artery Bypass Graft Surgery). Circulation 2004;110:e340–e437.

75. King SB, 3rd, Marshall JJ, Tummala PE. Revascularization for coronary artery disease: stents versus bypass surgery. Annu Rev Med 2009;61:199–213.

76. Lange RA, Hillis LD. Second-generation drug-eluting coronary stents. N Engl J Med 2010;362:1728–1730.

77. Spinler SA. Managing acute coronary syndrome: evidence-based approaches. Am J Health Syst Pharm 2007;64:S14–S24.

78. Toth PP. The potential role of prasugrel in secondary prevention of ischemic events in patients with acute coronary syndromes. Postgrad Med 2009;121:59–72.

79. Doostzadeh J, Clark LN, Bezenek S, Pierson W, Sood PR, Sudhir K. Recent progress in percutaneous coronary intervention: Evolution of the drug-eluting stents, focus on the XIENCE V drug-eluting stent. Coron Artery Dis 2010;21:46–56.

80. Bertrand ME, Rupprecht HJ, Urban P, Gershlick AH. Double-blind study of the safety of clopidogrel with and without a loading dose in combination with aspirin compared with ticlopidine in combination with aspirin after coronary stenting: The clopidogrel aspirin stent international cooperative study (CLASSICS). Circulation 2000;102:624–629.

81. Wiviott SD, Braunwald E, McCabe CH, et al. Prasugrel versus clopidogrel in patients with acute coronary syndromes. N Engl J Med 2007;357:2001–2015.

82. Mahoney EM, Wang K, Arnold SV, et al. Cost-effectiveness of prasugrel versus clopidogrel in patients with acute coronary syndromes and planned percutaneous coronary intervention: Results from the trial to assess improvement in therapeutic outcomes by optimizing platelet inhibition with Prasugrel-Thrombolysis in Myocardial Infarction TRITON-TIMI 38. Circulation 2010;121:71–79.

83. Schuhlen H, Kastrati A, Pache J, Dirschinger J, Schomig A. Sustained benefit over four years from an initial combined antiplatelet regimen after coronary stent placement in the ISAR trial. Intracoronary Stenting and Antithrombotic Regimen. Am J Cardiol 2001;87:397–400.

84. Takakuwa KM, Ou FS, Peterson ED, et al. The usage patterns of cardiac bedside markers employing point-of-care testing for troponin in non-ST-segment elevation acute coronary syndrome: results from CRUSADE. Clin Cardiol 2009;32:498–505.

85. Topol EJ, Moliterno DJ, Herrmann HC, et al. Comparison of two platelet glycoprotein IIb/IIIa inhibitors, tirofiban and abciximab, for the prevention of ischemic events with percutaneous coronary revascularization. N Engl J Med 2001;344:1888–1894.

86. Spinler SA, Rees C. Review of prasugrel for the secondary prevention of atherothrombosis. J Manag Care Pharm 2009;15:383–395.

87. Stone GW, Ware JH, Bertrand ME, et al. Antithrombotic strategies in patients with acute coronary syndromes undergoing early invasive management: One-year results from the ACUITY trial. JAMA 2007;298:2497–2506.

88. Lincoff AM, Kleiman NS, Kereiakes DJ, et al. Long-term efficacy of bivalirudin and provisional glycoprotein IIb/IIIa blockade vs heparin and planned glycoprotein IIb/IIIa blockade during percutaneous coronary revascularization: REPLACE-2 randomized trial. JAMA 2004;292:696–703.

89. Canan T, Lee MS. Drug-eluting stent fracture: incidence, contributing factors, and clinical implications. Catheter Cardiovasc Interv 2010;75:237–245.

90. Stone GW, Rizvi A, Newman W, et al. Everolimus-eluting versus paclitaxel-eluting stents in coronary artery disease. N Engl J Med 2010;362:1663–1674.

91. Grines CL, Bonow RO, Casey DE, Jr., et al. Prevention of premature discontinuation of dual antiplatelet therapy in patients with coronary artery stents: A science advisory from the American Heart Association, American College of Cardiology, Society for Cardiovascular Angiography and Interventions, American College of Surgeons, and American Dental Association, with representation from the American College of Physicians. J Am Coll Cardiol 2007;49:734–739.

92. Mega JL, Close SL, Wiviott SD, et al. Cytochrome p-450 polymorphisms and response to clopidogrel. N Engl J Med 2009;360:354–362.

93. Ray WA, Murray KT, Griffin MR, et al. Outcomes with concurrent use of clopidogrel and proton-pump inhibitors: A cohort study. Ann Intern Med 2010;152:337–345.

94. Zairis MN, Tsiaousis GZ, Patsourakos NG, et al. The impact of treatment with omeprazole on the effectiveness of clopidogrel drug therapy during the first year after successful coronary stenting. Can J Cardiol 2010;26:e54–e57.

95. Juurlink DN, Gomes T, Ko DT, et al. A population-based study of the drug interaction between proton pump inhibitors and clopidogrel. CMAJ 2009;180:713–718.

96. Hall SL, Lorenc T. Secondary prevention of coronary artery disease. Am Fam Physician 2010;81:289–296.

97. Messerli FH, Bangalore S, Yao SS, Steinberg JS. Cardioprotection with beta-blockers: Myths, facts and Pascal's wager. J Intern Med 2009;266:232–241.

98. Feringa HH, van Waning VH, Bax JJ, et al. Cardioprotective medication is associated with improved survival in patients with peripheral arterial disease. J Am Coll Cardiol 2006;47:1182–1187.

99. Prince MJ, Bird AS, Blizard RA, Mann AH. Is the cognitive function of older patients affected by antihypertensive treatment? Results from 54 months of the Medical Research Council's trial of hypertension in older adults. BMJ 1996;312:801–805.

100. Abrams J, Thadani U. Therapy of stable angina pectoris: the uncomplicated patient. Circulation 2005;112:e255–e259.

101. Thomas GR, DiFabio JM, Gori T, Parker JD. Once daily therapy with isosorbide-5-mononitrate causes endothelial dysfunction in humans: Evidence of a free-radical-mediated mechanism. J Am Coll Cardiol 2007;49:1289–1295.

102. Schuhmacher S, Wenzel P, Schulz E, et al. Pentaerythritol tetranitrate improves angiotensin II-induced vascular dysfunction via induction of heme oxygenase-1. Hypertension 2010;55:897–904.

103. Daiber A, Oelze M, Wenzel P, et al. Nitrate tolerance as a model of vascular dysfunction: Roles for mitochondrial aldehyde dehydrogenase and mitochondrial oxidative stress. Pharmacol Rep 2009;61:33–48.

104. Gori T, Daiber A, Di Stolfo G, et al. Nitroglycerine causes mitochondrial reactive oxygen species production: In vitro mechanistic insights. Can J Cardiol 2007;23:990–992.

105. Sekiya M, Sato M, Funada J, Ohtani T, Akutsu H, Watanabe K. Effects of the long-term administration of nicorandil on vascular endothelial function and the progression of arteriosclerosis. J Cardiovasc Pharmacol 2005;46:63–67.

106. Parker JO, Amies MH, Hawkinson RW, et al. Intermittent transdermal nitroglycerin therapy in angina pectoris. Clinically effective without tolerance or rebound. Minitran Efficacy Study Group. Circulation 1995;91:1368–1374.

107. Freedman SB, Daxini BV, Noyce D, Kelly DT. Intermittent transdermal nitrates do not improve ischemia in patients taking beta-blockers or calcium antagonists: Potential role of rebound ischemia during the nitrate-free period. J Am Coll Cardiol 1995;25:349–355.

108. Ajani AE, Yan BP. The mystery of coronary artery spasm. Heart Lung Circ 2007;16:10–15.

109. Reffelmann T, Kloner RA. Ranolazine: An anti-anginal drug with further therapeutic potential. Expert Rev Cardiovasc Ther 2010;8:319–329.

110. Fernandez SF, Tandar A, Boden WE. Emerging medical treatment for angina pectoris. Expert Opin Emerg Drugs 2010;15(2):283–98

111. Chaitman BR. Efficacy and safety of a metabolic modulator drug in chronic stable angina: Review of evidence from clinical trials. J Cardiovasc Pharmacol Ther 2004;9 (suppl 1):S47–S64.

112. Chaitman BR, Skettino SL, Parker JO, et al. Anti-ischemic effects and long-term survival during ranolazine monotherapy in patients with chronic severe angina. J Am Coll Cardiol 2004;43:1375–1382.

113. Chaitman BR, Pepine CJ, Parker JO, et al. Effects of ranolazine with atenolol, amlodipine, or diltiazem on exercise tolerance and angina frequency in patients with severe chronic angina: a randomized controlled trial. JAMA 2004;291:309–316.

114. Morrow DA, Scirica BM, Karwatowska-Prokopczuk E, et al. Effects of ranolazine on recurrent cardiovascular events in patients with non-ST-elevation acute coronary syndromes: the MERLIN-TIMI 36 randomized trial. JAMA 2007;297:1775–1783.

115. Scirica BM, Morrow DA, Hod H, et al. Effect of ranolazine, an antianginal agent with novel electrophysiological properties, on the incidence of arrhythmias in patients with non ST-segment elevation acute coronary syndrome: Results from the Metabolic Efficiency with Ranolazine for Less Ischemia in Non ST-Elevation Acute Coronary Syndrome Thrombolysis in Myocardial Infarction 36 (MERLIN-TIMI 36) randomized controlled trial. Circulation 2007;116:1647–1652.

116. Sakata K, Miura F, Sugino H, et al. Assessment of regional sympathetic nerve activity in vasospastic angina: analysis of iodine 123-labeled metaiodobenzylguanidine scintigraphy. Am Heart J 1997;133: 484–489.

117. Hung MJ, Cherng WJ, Yang NI, Cheng CW, Li LF. Relation of high-sensitivity C-reactive protein level with coronary vasospastic angina pectoris in patients without hemodynamically significant coronary artery disease. Am J Cardiol 2005;96:1484–1490.

118. Park JS, Zhang SY, Jo SH, et al. Common adrenergic receptor polymorphisms as novel risk factors for vasospastic angina. Am Heart J 2006;151:864–869.

119. Glueck CJ, Munjal J, Khan A, Umar M, Wang P. Endothelial nitric oxide synthase T-786C mutation, a reversible etiology of Prinzmetal's angina pectoris. Am J Cardiol 2010;105:792–796.

120. Lanza GA, Pedrotti P, Pasceri V, Lucente M, Crea F, Maseri A. Autonomic changes associated with spontaneous coronary spasm in patients with variant angina. J Am Coll Cardiol 1996;28:1249–1256.

121. Acikel S, Dogan M, Sari M, Kilic H, Akdemir R. Prinzmetal-variant angina in a patient using zolmitriptan and citalopram. Am J Emerg Med 2010;28:257 e3–e6.

122. Schoenenberger AW, Kobza R, Jamshidi P, et al. Sudden cardiac death in patients with silent myocardial ischemia after myocardial infarction (from the Swiss Interventional Study on Silent Ischemia Type II [SWISSI II]). Am J Cardiol 2009;104:158–163.

123. Conti CR, Geller NL, Knatterud GL, et al. Anginal status and prediction of cardiac events in patients enrolled in the asymptomatic cardiac ischemia pilot (ACIP) study. ACIP investigators. Am J Cardiol 1997;79:889–892.

124. Davies RF, Goldberg AD, Forman S, et al. Asymptomatic Cardiac Ischemia Pilot (ACIP) study two-year follow-up: Outcomes of patients randomized to initial strategies of medical therapy versus revascularization. Circulation 1997;95:2037–2043.

125. Singh N, Mironov D, Goodman S, Morgan CD, Langer A. Treatment of silent ischemia in unstable angina: A randomized comparison of sustained-release verapamil versus metoprolol. Clin Cardiol 1995;18:653–658.

126. Dwivedi SK, Saran RK, Mittal S, Gupta R, Narain VS, Puri VK. Silent ischemic interval on exercise test is a predictor of response to drug therapy: A randomized crossover trial of metoprolol versus diltiazem in stable angina. Clin Cardiol 2001;24:45–49.

127. Pratt CM, McMahon RP, Goldstein S, et al. Comparison of subgroups assigned to medical regimens used to suppress cardiac ischemia (the Asymptomatic Cardiac Ischemia Pilot [ACIP] Study). Am J Cardiol 1996;77:1302–1309.

128. Erne P, Schoenenberger AW, Burckhardt D, et al. Effects of percutaneous coronary interventions in silent ischemia after myocardial infarction: The SWISSI II randomized controlled trial. JAMA 2007;297:1985–1991.

129. Erne P, Schoenenberger AW, Zuber M, et al. Effects of anti-ischaemic drug therapy in silent myocardial ischaemia type I: The Swiss Interventional Study on Silent Ischaemia type I (SWISSI I): A randomized, controlled pilot study. Eur Heart J 2007;28:2110–2117.

130. Bosanquet N, Jonsson B, Fox KA. Costs and cost effectiveness of low molecular weight heparins and platelet glycoprotein IIb/IIIa inhibitors: In the management of acute coronary syndromes. Pharmacoeconomics 2003;21:1135–1152.

131. Plosker GL, Ibbotson T. Eptifibatide: A pharmacoeconomic review of its use in percutaneous coronary intervention and acute coronary syndromes. Pharmacoeconomics 2003;21:885–912.

132. Caron MF, McKendall GR. Bivalirudin in percutaneous coronary intervention. Am J Health Syst Pharm 2003;60:1841–1849.

133. Hay JW, Yu WM, Ashraf T. Pharmacoeconomics of lipid-lowering agents for primary and secondary prevention of coronary artery disease. Pharmacoeconomics 1999;15:47–74.

134. Yang F, Cho SW, Son SM, et al. Genetic engineering of human stem cells for enhanced angiogenesis using biodegradable polymeric nanoparticles. Proc Natl Acad Sci USA 2010;107:3317–3322.

SARAH A. SPINLER AND SIMON DE DENUS

CHAPTER 24

Acute Coronary Syndromes

KEY CONCEPTS

❶ The cause of an acute coronary syndrome (ACS) is the erosion or rupture of an atherosclerotic plaque with subsequent platelet adherence, activation, aggregation, and activation of the clotting cascade. Ultimately, a clot forms and is composed of fibrin and platelets.

❷ The American Heart Association (AHA) and the American College of Cardiology (ACC) recommend strategies or guidelines for ACS patient care for ST-segment elevation (STE) myocardial infarction (MI) and unstable angina, non-ST-segment elevation (NSTE) MI, also termed NSTE ACS.

❸ Patients with ischemic chest discomfort and suspected ACS are risk stratified based on a 12-lead electrocardiogram (ECG), past medical history, signs and symptoms, and results of creatine kinase myocardial band (CK-MB) and troponin biochemical marker tests.

❹ The diagnosis of MI is confirmed based on the results of the CK-MB and troponin tests.

❺ Early reperfusion therapy with either primary percutaneous coronary intervention (PCI) or administration of a fibrinolytic agent is the recommended therapy for patients presenting with STE MI.

❻ High-risk patients with NSTE ACS should undergo early coronary angiography and revascularization with either PCI or coronary artery bypass graft (CABG) surgery.

❼ In addition to reperfusion therapy, additional pharmacotherapy that all patients with STE MI and without contraindications should receive within the first day of hospitalization and preferably in the emergency department are intranasal oxygen (if oxygen saturation is low), aspirin, a thienopyridine (agent and timing dependent on reperfusion strategy), sublingual (SL) nitroglycerin (NTG), and anticoagulation with either bivalirudin, unfractionated heparin (UFH), or enoxaparin (agent dependent on reperfusion strategy). A glycoprotein IIb/IIIa inhibitor should be administered with UFH for patients undergoing primary PCI. Intravenous (IV) β-blockers and NTG should be given to select patients.

❽ In the absence of contraindications, all patients with NSTE ACS should be treated in the emergency department with intranasal oxygen (if oxygen saturation is low), aspirin, SL NTG, and an anticoagulant, either UFH, enoxaparin, fondaparinux, or bivalirudin. High-risk patients should proceed to early coronary angiography and may additionally receive a glycoprotein IIb/IIIa inhibitor. Clopidogrel or prasugrel [agent and timing dependent on selection of an interventional (PCI) or medical management strategy] should be administered to all patients. Intravenous β-blockers and nitroglycerin should be given to select patients.

❾ Following MI, all patients, in the absence of contraindications, should receive indefinite therapy with aspirin, a β-blocker (started within 24 hours of hospital arrival), and an angiotensin-converting enzyme (ACE) inhibitor for secondary prevention of death, stroke, and recurrent infarction. Most patients will receive a statin to reduce low-density lipoprotein cholesterol to less than 100 mg/dL and ideally less than 70 mg/dL. Clopidogrel or prasugrel should be continued for at least 12 months for patients undergoing PCI, and clopidogrel should be continued for at least 14 days in patients with STE MI who either did not receive reperfusion therapy or received fibrinolytic therapy without PCI and who are at low risk of bleeding. Anticoagulation with warfarin should be considered for patients at high risk of death, reinfarction, or stroke.

Learning objectives, review questions, and other resources can be found at **www.pharmacotherapyonline.com**.

Since the early 1900s, cardiovascular disease (CVD) has been the leading cause of death. Acute coronary syndromes (ACSs), including unstable angina (UA) and myocardial infarction (MI), are forms of coronary heart disease (CHD) that constitute the most common cause of CVD death.[1] ❶ The cause of an ACS is the erosion or rupture of an atherosclerotic plaque with subsequent platelet adherence, activation, aggregation, and activation of the clotting cascade. Ultimately, a clot forms in the culprit coronary artery and is composed of fibrin and platelets. Correspondingly, pharmacotherapy of ACS has advanced to include combinations of fibrinolytics, antiplatelets, and anticoagulants with more traditional therapies such as nitrates and β-adrenergic blockers. Pharmacotherapy is integrated with reperfusion therapy and revascularization of the culprit coronary artery through interventional means such as percutaneous coronary intervention (PCI) and coronary artery bypass graft (CABG) surgery. ❷ The American Heart Association (AHA) and the American College of Cardiology (ACC) recommend strategies or guidelines for ACS patient care for ST-segment elevation (STE) myocardial infarction (MI) and non-ST-segment elevation (NSTE) ACS. These joint practice guidelines are based on a review of available clinical evidence, have graded recommendations based on the weight and quality of evidence, and are updated periodically. The guidelines form the cornerstone for quality patient care of the ACS patient.[2-6]

EPIDEMIOLOGY

Each year more than 1.2 million Americans will experience an ACS, and 220,000 will die of an MI.[1] In the United States, more than 17.6 million, or 7.9% of living persons age 20 years and older, have CHD, and 3.6% have survived an MI.[1] Chest discomfort is the most frequent specific reason for patient presentation to emergency departments with up to 6.3 million emergency department visits, or approximately 5.4% of all emergency department visits, linked to chest discomfort and possible ACS.[7] CHD is the leading cause of premature, chronic disability in the United States. The cost of CHD is high, with direct and indirect costs estimated at $177.1 billion for 2010.[1] The median length of hospital stay for MI in 2001 was 4 days but had decreased to a median of 3 days in 2006.[1]

Much of the epidemiologic data regarding ACS treatment and survival come from the ACC's National Cardiovascular Data Registry (NCDR) Acute Coronary Treatment and Interventions Network (ACTION)—Get with the Guidelines (GWTG), the Global Registry of Acute Coronary Events (GRACE), and statistical summaries of U.S. hospital discharges prepared by the AHA. In patients with STE ACS, in-hospital death rates are approximately 4.6%, while it is lower, 2.2%, for patients with NSTE ACS.[8] Patients with STE MI who are treated with reperfusion therapy, either fibrinolytics or primary PCI, have lower mortality rates than patients treated without reperfusion. Reperfusion rates and mortality rates are higher in the elderly and women. For example, the mortality rate is 19% in elderly patients who were eligible for reperfusion therapy but did not receive it compared with 10.5% in those that did.[8-10] In women, the mortality rate is 18% in those eligible for but who did not receive reperfusion therapy compared with 9.3% in those who did.[8-10] In the first year following MI, 23% of women and 18% of men will die, most from recurrent infarction.[1] At 1 year, rates of mortality and reinfarction are similar between STE and NSTE MI.[10]

The rate of developing heart failure during hospitalization for ACS is declining rapidly. Compared with data from 1999, the 2006 incidence of in-hospital heart failure in patients with STE MI declined from 19.5% to 11% and that for patients with NSTE ACS declined from 13% to 6.1%.[9] In-hospital death rates for patients who present with or develop heart failure are more than threefold higher than for those who do not.[8]

Because reinfarction and death are major outcomes following ACS, therapeutic strategies to reduce morbidity and mortality, particularly use of coronary angiography, revascularization, and pharmacotherapy, will have a significant impact on the social and economic burden of CHD in the United States.

ETIOLOGY

In this section we will discuss the formation of atherosclerotic plaques, the underlying cause of coronary artery disease (CAD) and ACS in most patients. The process of atherosclerosis starts early in life. Although atherosclerosis was once considered only a disease of cholesterol excess, it is now clear that inflammation also plays a central role in the genesis, progression, and complication of this disease.[11] In its earliest stage, endothelial dysfunction, the induction and/or repression of several genes, occurs in response to sheer stress of the blood flowing over the atherosclerotic plaque on the endothelial lining of the artery. In response to gene induction and repression, the endothelial cells decrease the synthesis of nitric oxide, increase the oxidation of lipoproteins and facilitate their

entry into the arterial wall, promote the adherence of monocytes to the vessel wall and deposition of extracellular matrix, cause smooth muscle cell proliferation, and release local vasoconstrictor and prothrombotic substances into the blood, each with subsequent inflammatory response.[11] Taken together, all these factors contribute to the evolution of endothelial dysfunction to the formation of fatty streaks in the coronary arteries and eventually to atherosclerotic plaques. Therefore, the endothelium serves as an important autocrine and paracrine organ in the development of atherosclerosis.

A number of factors are directly responsible for the development and progression of endothelial dysfunction and atherosclerosis, including hypertension, age, male gender, tobacco use, diabetes mellitus, obesity, and dyslipidemias.[1]

PATHOPHYSIOLOGY

SPECTRUM OF ACS

Acute coronary syndromes is a term that includes all clinical syndromes compatible with acute myocardial ischemia resulting from an imbalance between myocardial oxygen demand and supply. In contrast to stable angina, an ACS results primarily from diminished myocardial blood flow secondary to an occlusive or partially occlusive coronary artery thrombus. ACSs are classified according to electrocardiographic changes into STE MI and NSTE ACS, which includes NSTE MI and UA (Fig. 24–1).[2-6,12,13] For patients presenting with suspected ACS, the percentage of patients diagnosed with STE MI varies by registry or database but is approximately 30%, while 31% are diagnosed with NSTE MI, 26% with UA, and 12% with another cardiac or noncardiac condition.[14] NSTE MI differs from UA in that ischemia is severe enough to produce myocardial necrosis, resulting in the release of a detectable amount of biochemical markers, mainly troponins I or T, and creatine kinase (CK) myocardial band (MB) from the necrotic myocytes, into the bloodstream.[6] The clinical significance of serum biochemical markers is discussed in more detail in the section entitled "Biochemical Markers" of this chapter. Following an STE MI, pathologic Q waves are seen frequently on the electrocardiogram (ECG), whereas such an ECG manifestation is seen less commonly in patients with NSTE MI.[2,6] The presence of Q waves usually indicates transmural MI.

PLAQUE RUPTURE AND CLOT FORMATION

❶ The predominant cause of ACS in more than 90% of patients is atheromatous plaque rupture, fissuring, or erosion of an unstable atherosclerotic plaque. Plaques that encompass less than 50% of the coronary lumen are more likely to rupture than those that occlude 70% to 90% of the coronary artery.[6] Such stable 70% to 90% stenoses of the coronary artery are characteristic of stable angina and tend to have a small lipid core, a thick fibrous cap, more calcification and less compensatory enlargement.[15] Plaques that are more susceptible to rupture are characterized by an eccentric shape, a thin fibrous cap (particularly in the shoulder region of the plaque), large fatty core, a high content in inflammatory cells, such as macrophages and lymphocytes, limited amounts of smooth muscle, and significant compensatory enlargement. Compensatory enlargement is the growth of the lesion pushing the vessel outward rather than the growth of plaque inward. Therefore, compensatory enlargement may result in an underestimation of the atherosclerotic stenosis as measured by coronary angiography. Inflammatory cells promote the thinning of the fibrous cap through the release of proteolytic enzymes, particularly matrix metalloproteinases.[11]

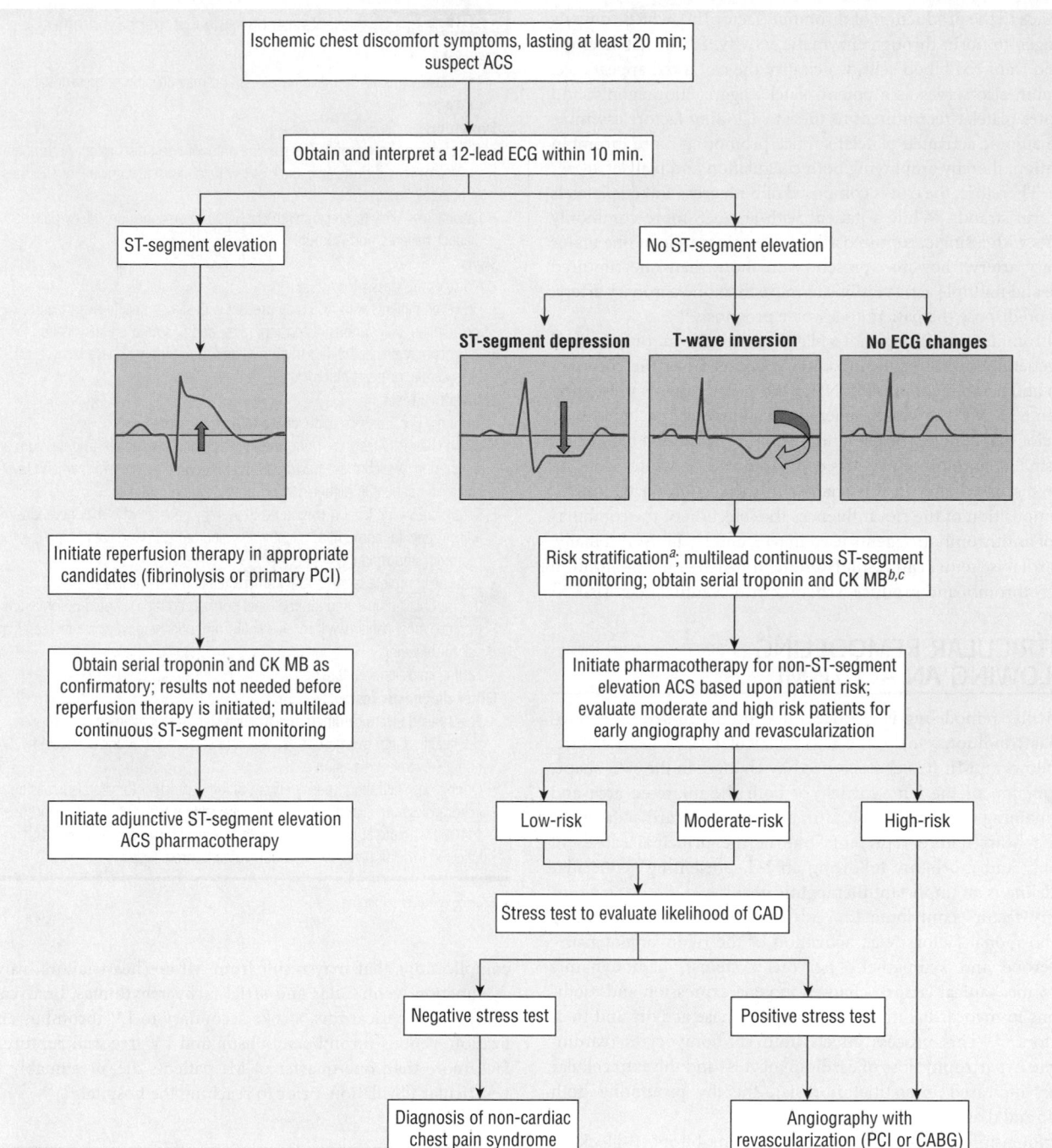

FIGURE 24-1. Evaluation of the Acute Coronary Syndrome Patient. (ACS, acute coronary syndrome; CABG, coronary artery bypass graft surgery; CAD, coronary artery disease; CK, creatine kinase; ECG, electrocardiogram; PCI, percutaneous coronary intervention.) [a]As described in Table 24–2. [b]Positive means above the MI decision limit. [c]Negative means below the MI decision limit. *(Reproduced with permission from: Spinler SA. Acute coronary syndromes. In: Dunsworth TS, Richardson MM, Cheng JWM, Chessman KH, Hume AL, Hutchison LC, Jackson AB, Karpiuk EL, Martin LG, Semla TP, Wittbrodt ET, editors. Pharmacotherapy self-assessment program Book 1, 6th ed., Cardiology. Kansas City: American College of Clinical Pharmacy; 2007. p. 59–83.)*

Following plaque rupture, a partially occlusive or completely occlusive thrombus, a clot, forms on top of the ruptured plaque. The thrombogenic contents of the plaque are exposed to blood elements. Exposure of exposed subendothelial collagen and tissue factor via shear forces promote platelet adhesion to the site of injury via binding of platelet glycoprotein (GP) Ib to von Willebrand factor. This binding interaction integrates signals that cause platelets to become activated—undergoing a shape change, as well as synthesizing and releasing thromboxane A_2 (TXA_2), adenosine diphosphate (ADP), and vasoactive and other prothrombotic substances from dense α-granules. Furthermore, during platelet activation, ADP binds to the platelet $P2Y_1$ and $P2Y_{12}$ receptors, and $P2Y_{12}$ bind-

ing promotes a conformational change in the GP IIb/IIIa surface receptors of platelets, increasing their affinity for fibrinogen that results in cross-linking of platelets to each other through fibrinogen bridges. This is considered the final common pathway of platelet aggregation. Additionally, ADP binding to the $P2Y_{12}$ receptor promotes amplification of platelet aggregation and recruitment of other platelets to the site of injury by promoting release of other platelet aggregation agonists such as serotonin, thrombin, TXA_2, and epinephrine. Inclusion of platelets gives the clot a white appearance.

Simultaneously, the extrinsic coagulation cascade pathway is activated as a result of exposure of blood components to the thrombogenic lipid core and endothelium, which are rich in tissue factor.

This leads to the production of thrombin (factor IIa), which converts fibrinogen to fibrin through enzymatic activity. Fibrin stabilizes the clot and traps red blood cells, which give the clot a red appearance. Thrombin also serves as a potent platelet aggregation agonist and promotes platelet recruitment to the site. Clotting factors assemble on the anionic activated platelet surface promoting more thrombin generation, thereby amplifying both coagulation and platelet aggregation. Therefore, the clot is composed of both cross-linked platelets and fibrin strands. While a patient with an ACS more commonly presents with a single, ruptured atherosclerotic plaque in one major coronary artery, they may present with more than one ruptured plaque and multiple active lesions in more than one coronary artery, which predispose the patient to a worse prognosis.[11]

A thrombus containing more platelets than fibrin, or a "white" clot, generally produces an incomplete occlusion of the coronary lumen and is more common in NSTE ACS. For patients presenting with an STE MI, the vessel generally is completely occluded by a "red" clot that contains larger amounts of fibrin and red blood cells but a smaller amount of platelets compared with a "white" clot.[2] As will be discussed later in this chapter in the section on treatment, the composition of the clot influences the selection of the combinations of antithrombotic agents used in STE and NSTE ACS. Finally, myocardial ischemia can result from the downstream embolization of microthrombi and produce ischemia with eventual necrosis.[2]

VENTRICULAR REMODELING FOLLOWING AN ACUTE MI

Ventricular remodeling is a process that occurs in several cardiovascular conditions, including left ventricular (LV) heart failure, and follows an MI. It is characterized by changes in the size, shape, and function of the left ventricle of both the infarcted area and the remaining ventricle, and it ultimately leads to cardiac failure.[16] Because heart failure represents one of the principal causes of mortality and morbidity following an MI, preventing ventricular remodeling is an important therapeutic goal.[16]

Many factors contribute to ventricular remodeling, including neurohormonal factors (e.g., activation of the renin–angiotensin–aldosterone and sympathetic nervous systems), hemodynamic factors, mechanical factors, changes in gene expression and modifications in myocardial matrix metalloproteinase activity and their inhibitors.[17,18] This process affects both cardiomyocytes (cardiomyocyte hypertrophy, loss of cardiomyocytes) and the extracellular matrix (increased interstitial fibrosis), thereby promoting both systolic and diastolic dysfunction.[18]

Angiotensin-converting enzyme (ACE) inhibitors, β-blockers, and aldosterone antagonists are all agents that slow down or reverse ventricular remodeling through neurohormonal blockage and/or through improvement in hemodynamics (decreasing preload or afterload).[16] These agents also improve survival and will be discussed in more detail in subsequent sections of this chapter describing treatment and secondary prevention. This underlines the importance of the remodeling process and the urgency of preventing, halting, or reversing it for patients who have experienced an MI.

COMPLICATIONS

This chapter will focus on management of the uncomplicated ACS patient. However, it is important for clinicians to recognize complications of MI because such patients have increased mortality. The most serious complication is cardiogenic shock, occurring in approximately 5% to 6% of patients presenting with STE MI and less than 2% of those presenting with NSTE ACS.[14] Mortality in cardiogenic shock patients with MI is high, approaching 60%.[8] Other

TABLE 24-1	Presentation of Acute Coronary Syndromes

General
- The patient typically is in acute distress and may develop or present with cardiogenic shock.

Symptoms
- The classic symptom of ACS is midline anterior chest discomfort. Accompanying symptoms may include arm, back or jaw pain, nausea, vomiting, or shortness of breath.
- Patients less likely to present with classic symptoms include elderly patients, diabetic patients, and women.

Signs
- No signs are classic for ACS.
- However, patients with ACS may present with signs of acute heart failure, including jugular venous distension, rales, and S_3 sound on auscultation.
- Patients may present with arrhythmias and therefore may have tachycardia, bradycardia, or heart block.

Laboratory tests
- Troponin I or T and creatine kinase MB are measured.
- Blood chemistry tests are performed with particular attention to potassium and magnesium, which may affect heart rhythm, and glucose, which when elevated places the patient at higher risk for morbidity and mortality.
- Serum creatinine level is measured to identify patients who may need dosing adjustments for some pharmacotherapy and patients who are at high risk for morbidity and mortality.
- Baseline complete blood count and coagulation tests (activated partial thromboplastin time and international normalized ratio) should be obtained because most patients will receive antithrombotic therapy, which increases the risk for bleeding.
- Fasting lipid panel is obtained.

Other diagnostic tests
- The 12-lead electrocardiogram is the first step in management. Patients are risk stratified into two groups: ST-segment elevation ACS and suspected non–ST-segment elevation ACS.
- During hospitalization, measurement of left ventricular function, such as an echocardiogram, is performed to identify patients with low ejection fractions (<40%) who are at high risk for death following hospital discharge.
- Selected low-risk patients may undergo early stress testing.

ACS, acute coronary syndrome.

complications that may result from MI are heart failure, valvular dysfunction, ventricular and atrial tachyarrhythmias, bradycardia, heart block, pericarditis, stroke secondary to LV thrombus embolization, venous thromboembolism, and LV free wall rupture.[19] In fact, more than one-quarter of MI patients die, presumably from ventricular fibrillation, prior to reaching the hospital.[20]

CLINICAL PRESENTATION

The key points in clinical presentation of the patient with ACS are described in Table 24–1.

SYMPTOMS AND PHYSICAL EXAMINATION FINDINGS

The classic symptom of an ACS is midline anterior anginal chest discomfort, most often either at rest, severe new-onset, or increasing angina that is at least 20 minutes in duration. The chest discomfort may radiate to the shoulder, down the left arm, to the back, or to the jaw. Associated symptoms that may accompany the chest discomfort include nausea, vomiting, diaphoresis, or shortness of breath. Typically, patients with STE MI present with unremitting chest discomfort. Patients with NSTE ACS may present with either (1) rest angina, (2) new onset (less than 2 months) angina, or (3) angina that is increasing in either frequency, duration, or intensity. All healthcare professionals should review these warning symptoms

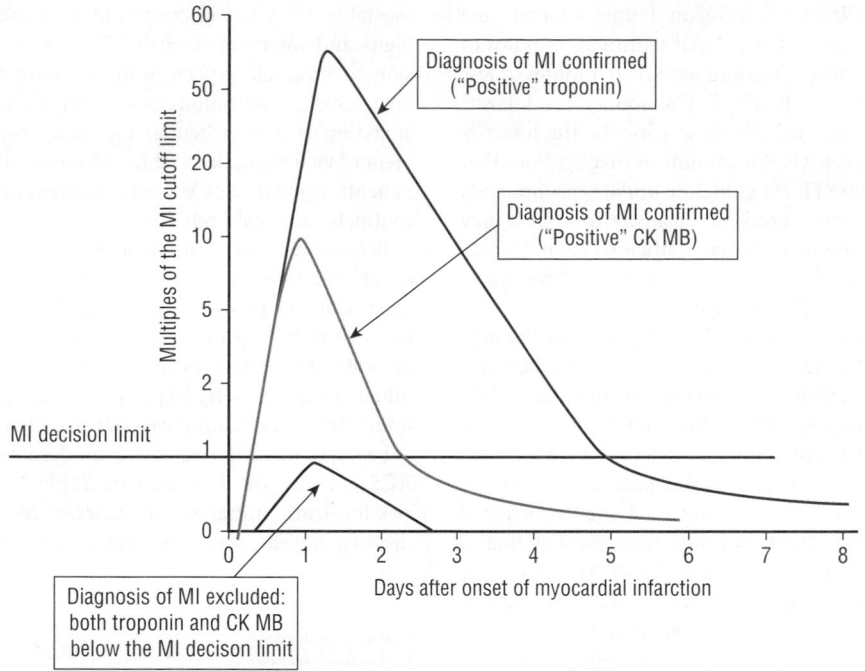

FIGURE 24-2. Biochemical markers in suspected acute coronary syndrome.

with patients at high risk for CHD. On physical examination, no specific features are indicative of ACS.

TWELVE-LEAD ELECTROCARDIOGRAM (ECG)

❸ There are key features of a 12-lead ECG that identify and risk stratify a patient with an ACS. Within 10 minutes of presentation to an emergency department with symptoms of ischemic chest discomfort (or preferably prehospital), a 12-lead ECG should be obtained and interpreted. If available, a prior 12-lead ECG should be reviewed to identify whether the findings on the current ECG are new or old, with new findings being more indicative of an ACS. Key findings on review of a 12-lead ECG that indicate myocardial ischemia or MI are ST-segment elevation, ST-segment depression, and T-wave inversion (Fig. 24–1).[13] ST-segment and/or T-wave changes in contiguous leads help to identify the location of the coronary artery that is the cause of the ischemia or infarction. In addition, the appearance of a new left bundle branch block accompanied by chest discomfort is highly specific for acute MI. About 40% of patients diagnosed with MI present with ST-segment elevation on their ECG, with the remainder having ST-segment depression, T-wave inversion, or in some instances, no ECG changes.[21] Some parts of the heart are more "electrically silent" than others, and myocardial ischemia may not be detected on a surface ECG. Therefore, it is important to review findings from the ECG in conjunction with biochemical markers of myocardial necrosis, such as troponin I or T, and other risk factors for CHD to determine the patient's risk for experiencing a new MI or having other complications.

BIOCHEMICAL MARKERS

❹ Biochemical markers of myocardial cell death are important for confirming the diagnosis of MI. *Evolving MI* is defined by the ACC as "typical rise and gradual fall (troponin) or more rapid rise and fall (CK-MB) of biochemical markers of myocardial necrosis."[22] Troponin and CK-MB rise in the blood following the onset of complete coronary artery occlusion subsequent myocardial cell death. Their time course is depicted in Figure 24–2. Typically, blood is

obtained from the patient at least two times, once in the emergency department and again in 6 to 9 hours, in order to measure troponin and CK-MB.[23] A single measurement of a biochemical marker is not adequate to exclude a diagnosis of MI because up to 15% of the values that were below the level of detection initially (a negative test) are above the level of detection (a positive test) in the subsequent hours. An MI is identified if at least one troponin value is greater than the MI decision limit, defined as above the 99th percentile of a reference population (set by the hospital laboratory and dependent upon the assay used) with a typical rise or fall.[23] If a troponin test is not available, an increase CK-MB (above the 99th percentile of a reference population with a cut-off value dependent upon assay), may also be used to make the diagnosis of MI. These are termed *positive* biochemical markers for MI. While troponins and CK-MB appear in the blood within 6 hours of infarction, troponins stay elevated in the blood for 7 to 14 days, whereas CK-MB returns to normal values within 48 hours. If early reinfarction is suspected, blood should be drawn and troponin and CK-MB repeated. Reinfarction is diagnosed when the CK-MB or troponin are elevated at least 20% above the previous value (as well as above the 99th percentile of the reference population).[23] Biochemical markers, such as troponin measurements, that are below the hospital laboratories reference range are termed *negative* and the diagnosis of MI is excluded.

RISK STRATIFICATION

Patient signs and symptoms, past medical history, ECG, and troponin or CK-MB determinations are used to stratify patients into low, medium, or high risk of death, initial MI, reinfarction, or likelihood of failing pharmacotherapy and needing urgent coronary angiography and PCI (Fig. 24–1). Patients with STE MI are at the highest risk of death. In a report from the Global Registry of Acute Coronary Events (GRACE) of almost 30,000 patients from 2001 to 2007, in-hospital mortality rates were 6.2% for STE MI, 2.9% for NSTE MI, and 1.7% for UA.[14] Initial treatment of STE MI should proceed without evaluation of the troponin or CK-MB levels because these patients have a greater than 97% chance of having an MI subsequently diagnosed with biochemical markers. The

ACC/AHA as well as The Joint Commission defines a target time to initiate reperfusion treatment for STE MI within 30 minutes of hospital presentation for fibrinolytics and within 90 minutes or less from presentation for primary PCI.[6,23,24] The sooner the infarct-related coronary artery is opened for these patients, the lower is their mortality, and the greater is the amount of myocardium that is preserved.[14,25,26] The 2009 STE MI guideline update recommends that patients be evaluated for interhospital transfer for PCI if they present to a hospital without a cardiac catheterization laboratory and primary PCI capability as an alternative to fibrinolysis.[5] Regionalized systems of STE MI care are encouraged.[5,27]

While all patients should be evaluated for reperfusion therapy, not all patients may be eligible. Indications and contraindications for fibrinolytic therapy as well as eligibility criteria for primary PCI are described in the treatment section of this chapter. In the United States in 2006, 66% of patients presenting with STE MI met eligibility for reperfusion therapy. Among all eligible patients, only 70.8% received reperfusion therapy in 2006.[14] Since 2004, the frequency of primary PCI has exceeded the frequency of fibrinolysis such that in 2006, 43.2% of eligible patients presenting with STE MI underwent primary PCI, while 27.6% received fibrinolysis.[14] Most of those not eligible for reperfusion therapy present more than 12 hours after the onset of symptoms, outside of the eligibility window.[14,28,29] In addition, fewer than 50% of patients with MI in the United States present to hospitals that are equipped to perform primary PCI, and approximately 5% to 6% of patients present with at least one contraindication to fibrinolysis.[21,28,29] Unfortunately, 28% of patients *eligible* for reperfusion therapy with either fibrinolysis or primary PCI do not receive it, suggesting there is still a need for more thorough patient evaluation and treatment triage.[14]

If patients are not eligible for reperfusion therapy or interhospital transfer, additional pharmacotherapy for STE patients should be initiated in the emergency department, and the patient should be transferred to a coronary intensive care unit (Fig. 24–1).[30]

Risk stratification of the patient with NSTE ACS is more complex because in-hospital outcomes for this group of patients vary, with reported rates of death of 0% to 12%, reinfarction of 0% to 3%, and recurrent severe ischemia of 5% to 20%.[31] Not all patients presenting with suspected NSTE ACS will even have CAD. Some will be diagnosed eventually with nonischemic chest discomfort. Additional information regarding risk stratification of NSTE ACS is presented in the section general approach to treatment.

TREATMENT

Acute Coronary Syndromes

■ DESIRED OUTCOMES

The short-term goals of treatment for the ACS patient are

1. Early restoration of blood flow to the infarct-related artery to prevent infarct expansion (in the case of MI) or prevent complete occlusion and MI (in UA)

2. Prevention of death and other MI complications

3. Prevention of coronary artery reocclusion with reinfarction

4. Relief of ischemic chest discomfort

5. Resolution of ST-segment and T-wave changes on ECG

■ GENERAL APPROACH TO TREATMENT

❷ Selecting evidence-based therapies described in the ACC/AHA guidelines for patients without contraindications results in lower

mortality.[32-34] General treatment measures for all STE MIs and high- and intermediate-risk NSTE ACS patients include admission to hospital, oxygen administration (if oxygen saturation is low, <90%), continuous multilead ST-segment monitoring for arrhythmias and ischemia, glycemic control, frequent measurement of vital signs, bed rest for 12 hours in hemodynamically stable patients, avoidance of Valsalva maneuver (prescribe stool softeners routinely), and pain relief.

Because risk varies and resources are limited, it is important to triage and treat patients according to their risk category. Initial approaches to treatment of the STE and NSTE ACS patient are outlined in Figure 24–1.[2-6,12] Patients with STE MI are at high risk of death, and efforts to reestablish coronary perfusion should be initiated immediately. Reperfusion therapy should be considered immediately and adjunctive pharmacotherapy initiated.[6]

Features identifying low-, moderate-, and high-risk NSTE ACS patients are described in Table 24–2.[2,35-37] Patients at low risk for death, initial MI or recurrent MI or for refractory angina needing urgent coronary artery revascularization typically are

---

TABLE 24-2 Risk Stratification for ACS[35-37]

TIMI risk score for NSTE ACS

One point is assigned for each of the seven medical history and clinical presentation findings. The point total is calculated and the patient is assigned a risk for experiencing the composite endpoint of death, myocardial infarction, or urgent need for revascularization as follows:

- Age ≥ 65 years
- 3 or more CHD risk factors: smoking, hypercholesterolemia, hypertension, diabetes mellitus, family history of premature CHD death/events
- Known CAD (≥50% stenosis of at least one major coronary artery on coronary angiogram)
- Aspirin use within the past 7 days
- 2 or more episodes of chest discomfort within the past 24 hrs
- ST-segment depression ≥0.5 mm
- Positive biochemical marker for infarction

High-risk	**Medium-risk**	**Low-risk**
TIMI risk score 5–7 points	TIMI risk Score 3–4 points	TIMI risk score 0–2 points

TIMI risk score	**Mortality, MI, or severe recurrent ischemic requiring urgent target vessel revascularization**
0/1	4.7%
2	8.3%
3	13.2%
4	19.9%
5	26.2%
6/7	40.9%

GRACE risk factors for increased mortality and the composite of death or MI in ACS

- Signs and symptoms of heart failure
- Low systolic blood pressure
- Elevated heart rate
- Older age
- Elevated serum creatinine
- Baseline risk factors on clinical evaluation: cardiac arrest at admission, ST-segment deviation, elevated troponin
- A high-risk patient is defined as a GRACE risk score of >140 points

TIMI = Thrombolysis in Myocardial Infarction; CAD = coronary artery disease; MI = myocardial infarction; GRACE = Global Registry of Acute Coronary Events.

An online calculator for the GRACE Risk Model is available at http://www.outcomes-umassmed.org/externalwindow.cfm?URL=http://www.outcomes.org/grace/acs_risk/acs_risk.html&Link=http://www.outcomes-umassmed.org/grace/acs_risk.cfm&DeptName=Center%20for%20Outcomes%20Research (Accessed March 22, 2010).

Reprinted with permission from Spinler SA. Evolution of antithrombotic therapy used in acute coronary syndromes. In: Richardson MM, Chessman KH, Chant C, Cheng JWM, Hemstreet BA, Hume AL, et al, eds. Pharmacotherapy Assessment Program, 7th ed. Cardiology. Lenexa, KS: American College of Clinical Pharmacy; 2010, 97–124.

evaluated in the emergency department, where serial biochemical marker tests are obtained, and if they are negative, the patient may be admitted to a general medical floor with ECG telemetry monitoring for ischemic changes and arrhythmias, undergo a noninvasive stress test, or be discharged from the emergency department. Moderate- and high-risk patients are admitted to a coronary intensive care unit, an intensive care step-down unit, or a general medical floor in the hospital depending on the patient's symptoms and perceived level of risk. High-risk patients should undergo early coronary angiography (within 12 to 24 hours) and revascularization (with PCI or CABG) if a significant coronary artery stenosis is found[5] (Fig. 24–1 and Table 24–2). Moderate-risk patients with positive biochemical markers for infarction typically also will undergo angiography and revascularization during hospital admission. Moderate-risk patients with negative biochemical markers for infarction also may undergo angiography and revascularization or first undergo a noninvasive stress test, with only select patients with a positive stress test proceeding to angiography. Following risk stratification, pharmacotherapy for NSTE ACS is initiated.

■ NONPHARMACOLOGIC THERAPY

Primary PCI for STE ACS

❺ Either fibrinolysis or immediate primary PCI is the treatment of choice for reestablishing coronary artery blood flow for patients with STE ACS when the patient presents within 3 hours of symptom onset and both options are available at the institution. For primary PCI, the patient is taken from the emergency department to the cardiac catheterization laboratory and undergoes coronary angiography with either balloon angioplasty or placement of a bare-metal or drug-eluting intracoronary stent. Additional details regarding angioplasty and intracoronary stenting are provided in Chap. 23. Results from a meta-analysis of trials comparing fibrinolysis with primary PCI indicate a lower mortality rate with primary PCI.[38] One reason for the superiority of primary PCI compared with fibrinolysis is that more than 90% of occluded infarct-related coronary arteries are opened with primary PCI compared with less than 60% of coronary arteries with currently available fibrinolytics.[4,6] In addition, the stroke [including intracranial hemorrhage (ICH)] and major bleeding risks from primary PCI are lower than following fibrinolysis.[4,6] An invasive strategy of primary PCI is generally preferred for patients presenting to institutions with skilled interventional cardiologists and a catheterization laboratory immediately available, for patients with cardiogenic shock, for patients with contraindications to fibrinolytics, and for patients presenting with symptom onset greater than 3 hours.[6] Patients presenting to a facility that is not capable of performing primary PCI may receive fibrinolysis or be immediately transferred to another hospital for primary PCI.[5] Patients best suited for transfer are those presenting more than 4 hours after symptom onset and those at high-risk for bleeding with fibrinolysis. The ACC/AHA guidelines encourage the formation of systems of care for rapid STE MI reperfusion treatment.[5] A quality performance measure in the care of patients with STE MI is the time from hospital presentation to the time that the occluded artery is opened with PCI. This "door-to-primary PCI time" should be ≤90 minutes (Table 24–3).[6,12,23] In 2006, the median time to primary PCI in the United States was 79 min for nontransferred patients and 139 minutes for transferred patients.[10] In 2006, only 54% of patients met the performance measure target of ≤90 minutes.[10] However more recent data from 2008 suggested that more than 75% of nontransferred patients had door-to-primary PCI times of ≤90 minutes, suggesting that efforts such as the Door to Balloon (D2B) Time Alliance educational materials and tools available on line have been successful.[39] Unfortunately, most hospitals do not have interventional cardiology services capable of performing primary PCI 24 hours a day.

Patients in whom fibrinolysis is not successful (as determined by persistent rest ischemic symptoms), as well as those receiving fibrinolysis but at continued high risk for death (including patients in cardiogenic shock patients with life-threatening ventricular arrhythmias or signs of ischemia on stress testing following MI), should be transferred to a hospital capable of cardiac catheterization and undergo angiography and PCI as early as possible (Fig. 24–1).[3-6] A randomized study established that "rescue" PCI for failed fibrinolysis was superior to repeated fibrinolytic administration or conservative management, resulting in lower cardiac and cerebrovascular events.[40] The strategy of routine angiography and revascularization in all STE patients later during hospitalization was controversial for more than a decade, but data from the Occluded Artery Trial (OAT) demonstrated that routine angiography followed by PCI in stable patients 3 to 28 days post-MI, without recurrent unprovoked ischemia or ischemia induced by stress testing, is not beneficial in reducing mortality or heart failure

---

TABLE 24-3 ACC/AHA 2008 Quality Performance Measures and Test Measures for Acute Coronary Syndrome[12]

Quality Performance Measure	Test Measure
Aspirin at arrival	LDL-C Assessment
Aspirin prescribed at discharge	Excessive initial heparin dose
β-blocker prescribed at hospital discharge	Excessive initial LMWH dose
Statin prescribed at hospital discharge	Excessive initial abciximab dose
ACE inhibitor or ARB for LVD prescribed at discharge	Excessive initial eptifibatide dose
Evaluation of LV function	Excessive initial tirofiban dose
Time to fibrinolytic therapy for patients with STE MI or LBBB	Presence of an anticoagulation dosing protocol for ACS (structural measure)
Time to PCI for patient with STE MI	Presence of an anticoagulant medication error tracking system
Time from ED arrival to ED discharge when transferring for STE MI PCI to another hospital	
Time from ED arrival at STE MI referral facility to PCI at receiving facility	
Percent of eligible patients with STE MI or LBBB receiving reperfusion therapy	
Smoking cessation counseling	
Cardiac rehabilitation referral	

ACE = angiotensin converting enzyme; ACS = acute coronary syndrome; ARB = angiotensin receptor blocker; ED = emergency department; LBBB = left bundle branch block; LDL-C = low-density lipoprotein cholesterol; LMWH = low-molecular weight heparin; LVD = left ventricular dysfunction; PCI = percutaneous coronary intervention; STE MI = ST-segment elevation myocardial infarction.

Reprinted with permission from Spinler SA. Evolution of antithrombotic therapy used in acute coronary syndromes. In: Richardson MM, Chessman KH, Chant C, Cheng JWM, Hemstreet BA, Hume AL, et al, eds. Pharmacotherapy Assessment Program, 7th ed. Cardiology. Lenexa, KS: American College of Clinical Pharmacy; 2010, 97–124.

and may increase the risk of recurrent MI.[41] Therefore, routine *late* restoration of antegrade coronary artery blood flow in patients not at high risk should not be performed.[5]

Percutaneous Coronary Intervention in Non-ST-Segment Elevation ACS

❻ The most recent ACC/AHA PCI and STEMI practice guideline update recommends early coronary angiography within 12 hours following hospital presentation and subsequent revascularization for patients with suitable coronary anatomy with either PCI and bare-metal or drug-eluting stent placement or CABG as an early treatment for high-risk NSTE ACS patients, and that such an approach be considered for patients not at high risk.[5] Several clinical trials support an "early invasive strategy" with PCI or CABG versus a "medical stabilization management strategy" whereby coronary angiography with revascularization is reserved for patients with symptoms refractory to pharmacotherapy and patients with signs of ischemia on stress testing (Fig. 24–1).[5,12] An early invasive approach results in a lower rate of refractory angina during hospital admission and over the first year, as well as a lower frequency of MI at 5 years, but an increased frequency of minor bleeding related to the procedure.[42] An early invasive strategy is also less costly than the conservative medical stabilization approach.[43]

Additional Testing and Risk Stratification

At some point during hospitalization but prior to discharge, patients with MI should have their LV function evaluated for risk stratification.[1,6,23] The most common way LV function is measured is using an echocardiogram to calculate the patient's LV ejection fraction (LVEF). LV function is the single best predictor of mortality following MI. Patients with LVEFs of less than 40% are at highest risk of death. Patients with an estimated survival of more than 1 year who are receiving medical therapy for secondary MI prevention and are in New York Heart Association (NYHA) functional Class II or III who have an LVEF <35% or those in NYHA functional class I who have an LVEF of <30% at 40 days following MI should receive an implantable cardioverter defibrillator (ICD) for primary prevention of sudden cardiac death.[44] The Multicenter Automatic Defibrillator Implantation II trial (MADIT) demonstrated a 29% reduction in mortality for patients with a history of MI, low LVEFs, and no history of symptomatic ventricular arrhythmias who received prophylactic implantation of an ICD.[45] Additional discussion of the role of ICDs in the management of high-risk patients and those with ventricular arrhythmias may be found in Chap. 25.

Predischarge stress testing may be performed in moderate- or low-risk patients in order to determine which patients would benefit from coronary angiography to establish the diagnosis of CAD and also for patients following MI to predict intermediate and long-term risk of recurrent MI and death[2,46] (Fig. 24–1). In most cases, patients with a positive stress test indicating coronary ischemia will then undergo coronary angiography and subsequent revascularization of significantly occluded coronary arteries. Exercise stress testing, most often with the addition of a radionuclide imaging agent, is preferred over nonpharmacologic stress testing because it evaluates the workload achieved with exercise as well as the occurrence of ischemia. If a patient has a negative exercise stress test for ischemia, the patient is at low risk for subsequent CHD events. Therefore, exercise stress testing has high negative predictive value. Additional discussion of the types of stress testing may be found in Chap. 23.

Patients admitted for ACS should have a fasting lipid panel drawn within the first 24 hours of hospitalization with statins the preferred agents to achieve a target low-density lipoprotein (LDL) cholesterol of less than 100 mg/dL and ideally <70 mg/dL.[3]

◼ EARLY PHARMACOTHERPY FOR ST-SEGMENT ELEVATION ACS

Pharmacotherapy for early treatment of STE MI is outlined in Figure 24–3.[3–6] **❼** According to the ACC/AHA STE MI practice guidelines and updates, early pharmacotherapy of STE MI should include intranasal oxygen (if oxygen saturation is <90%), sublingual (SL) nitroglycerin (NTG), aspirin, an anticoagulant, and fibrinolysis in eligible candidates. Morphine is administered to patients with refractory angina as an analgesic and a venodilator that lowers preload, but it does not reduce mortality.[47] These agents should be administered early, while the patient is still in the emergency department. A thienopyridine, either prasugrel or clopidogrel, should be administered for patients undergoing PCI, while only clopidogrel is recommended for patients receiving fibrinolytics and those not undergoing reperfusion therapy.[5] An ACE inhibitor should be started within 24 hours of presentation, particularly for patients with an LVEF ≤40%, signs of heart failure (HF) or an anterior wall MI, in the absence of contraindications. Intravenous (IV) NTG, β-blockers, and an aldosterone antagonist should be administered in select patients. A statin should be initiated prior to hospital discharge for patients with an LDL cholesterol of >100 mg/dL.[3,6] Dosing and contraindications for SL and IV NTG, aspirin, β-blockers, anticoagulants, ACE inhibitors, aldosterone antagonists, and fibrinolytics are listed in Table 24–4.[3–6,12]

Fibrinolytic Therapy

Administration of a fibrinolytic agent is indicated for patients with STE MI presenting to hospital within 12 hours of the onset of chest discomfort (that has persisted for at least 20 minutes) who have at least 1 mm of ST-segment elevation in two or more contiguous ECG leads (suggestive of infarct location) or a new left bundle branch block.[6] Fibrinolytic therapy should also be considered for patients presenting within 12–24 hours who have persistent symptoms of ischemia and at least 1 mm of STE in two or more contiguous leads.[6] The mortality benefit of fibrinolysis is highest with early administration and diminishes after 12 hours. Fibrinolytic therapy is preferred over primary PCI for patients presenting within 3 hours of symptom onset where there is a delay to primary PCI because of a delay in access to a cardiac catheterization laboratory or a delay in obtaining patient vascular access that would result in a "door-to-primary PCI" delay that would be greater than 90 minutes.[3] Contraindications to fibrinolysis include a history of hemorrhagic stroke (at any time), history of ischemic stroke within the 3 months, active internal bleeding, known intracranial neoplasm, suspected aortic dissection.[6] It is not necessary to obtain the results of biochemical markers before initiating fibrinolytic therapy. Because administration of fibrinolytics results in clot lysis, patients at high risk for major bleeding, including ICH, have either relative or absolute contraindications. Patients presenting with an absolute contraindication likely will not receive fibrinolytic therapy, and primary PCI is preferred. Patients with a relative contraindication may receive fibrinolytic therapy if the perceived risk of death from the MI is higher than the risk of major hemorrhage. For every 1,000 patients with anterior wall MI, treatment with fibrinolysis saves 37 lives compared with placebo. For patients with inferior wall MI, who generally have smaller MIs and are at lower risk of death, treatment with fibrinolysis saves 8 lives per 1,000 patients treated.[25]

Fibrinolytic therapy is controversial for patients older than 75 years of age. More than 60% of all MI deaths occur in this group. Benefit, in terms of absolute mortality reduction compared with placebo, varies from approximately 1% to 9%, with some observational studies suggesting higher mortality in the very elderly treated with fibrinolysis compared with no fibrinolysis. Stroke rates also

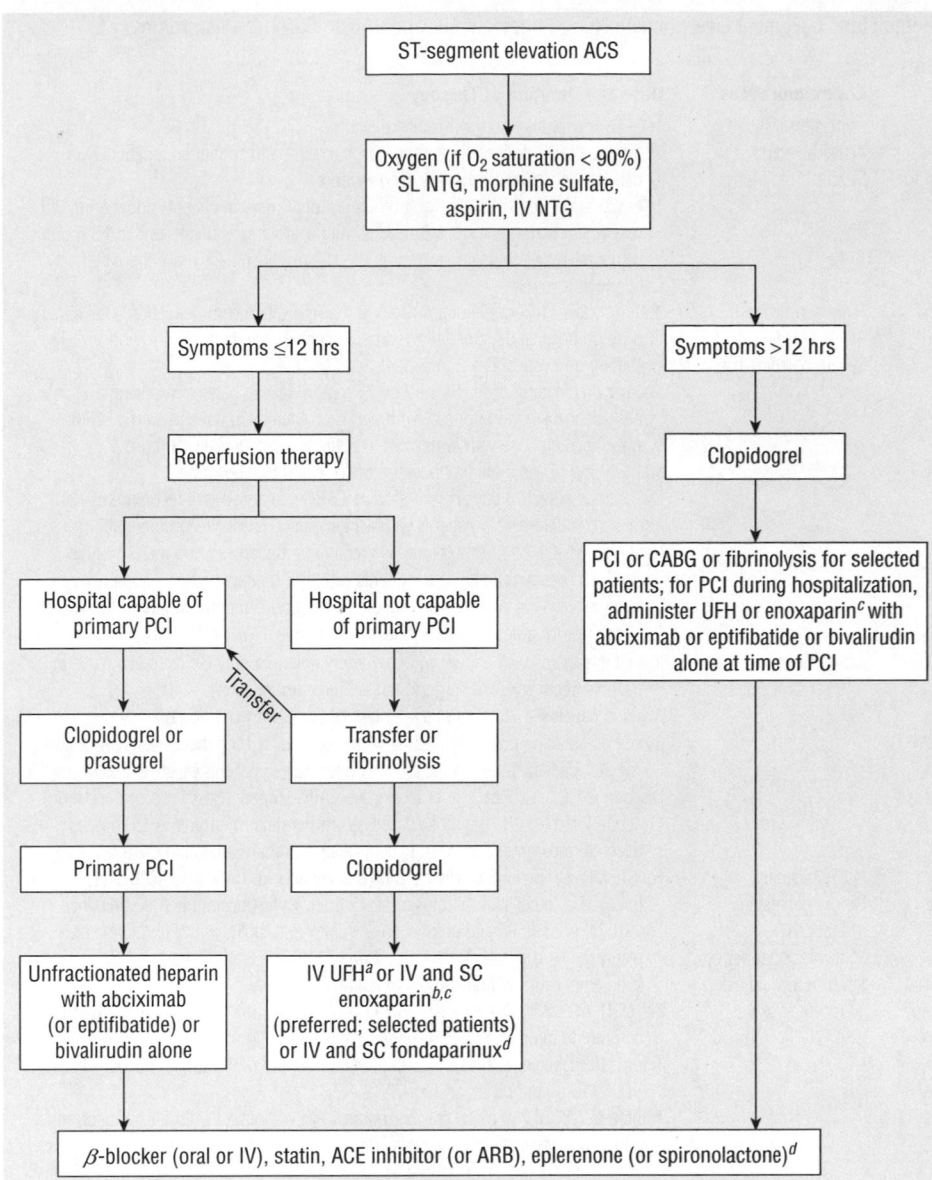

FIGURE 24-3. Initial pharmacotherapy for ST-segment elevation myocardial infarction. (ACS, acute coronary syndromes; CABG, coronary artery bypass graft surgery; IV, intravenous; NTG, nitroglycerin; PCI, percutaneous coronary intervention; SL, sublingual; UFH, unfractionated heparin.) [a]For at least 48 hours. [b]See Table 24–4 for dosing and specific types of patients who should not receive enoxaparin. [c]For the duration of hospitalization, up to 8 days. [d]For select patients, see Table 24–4. *(Reprinted with permission from Spinler SA. Evolution of antithrombotic therapy used in acute coronary syndromes. In: Richardson MM, Chessman KH, Chant C, Cheng JWM, Hemstreet BA, Hume AL, et al, eds. Pharmacotherapy Assessment Program, 7th ed. Cardiology. Lenexa, KS: American College of Clinical Pharmacy; 2010, 97–124.)*

grow in number with increasing patient age. While the ICH rate is approximately 1% in younger patients, it is 2% to 3% in older patients. There is no excess risk of stroke for patients younger than 55 years of age, whereas patients older than 75 years of age experience an excess of 8 strokes per 1,000 patients treated.[25] However, the ACC/AHA practice guidelines recommend the use of fibrinolytics for this age group, provided that the patient has no contraindications.[6] A 1% absolute mortality benefit is felt to be clinically significant, and the benefit in terms of lives saved per 1,000 patients treated has been reported to range from 10 to 80 for patients older than age of 75 years.[25] An AHA Scientific Statement concluded that a mortality benefit with fibrinolysis compared with no reperfusion has been demonstrated in patients up to age 85 years and includes deaths related to ICH, stroke, and shock which are all higher in the elderly compared with younger patients.[48] Careful attention to correct dosing of unfractionated heparin (UFH) and enoxaparin can reduce ICH and bleeding rates.[48] Because older patients may have cognitive impairment, careful history taking and assessment weighing the bleeding risk versus the benefit must be performed prior to administration of fibrinolysis.

According to the ACC/AHA STE ACS practice guideline, a more fibrin-specific agent, such as alteplase, reteplase, or tenecteplase, is preferred over a non-fibrin-specific agent, such as streptokinase.[6]

Early administration of more fibrin-specific fibrinolytics opens a greater percentage of infarct arteries. Because an early open artery results in smaller infarcts, administration of fibrin-specific agents should result in lower mortality. This concept has been termed the *open-artery hypothesis.* In a large clinical trial, administration of alteplase reduced mortality by 1% (absolute reduction) and costs about $30,000 per year of life saved compared with streptokinase.[49] Two other trials compared alteplase with reteplase and alteplase with tenecteplase and found similar mortality between agents.[50,51] Therefore, either alteplase, reteplase, or tenecteplase is acceptable as a first-line agent. Most hospitals have at least two agents on their formulary. Most often, formulary decisions are based on frequency of use of fibrinolytics for other approved indications, such as ischemic stroke or pulmonary embolism, with alteplase having the most indications of the fibrin-specific agents. Administration considerations also guide formulary decision making and choice for patient treatment with alteplase being the most complex to administer as a weight-based bolus dose and a series of two sequential infusions over 90 minutes, whereas tenecteplase is given as a single, weight-based dose, and reteplase is given as two fixed doses administered 30 minutes apart without weight adjustment (Table 24–4). Therefore, both tenecteplase and reteplase are easier to administer than alteplase.

TABLE 24-4 Evidence-Based Pharmacotherapy for ST-segment Elevation and Non-ST-segment Elevation Acute Coronary Syndromes

Drug	Clinical Condition and ACC/AHA Guideline Recommendation[a]	Contraindications[b]	Dose and Duration of Therapy
Aspirin	STEMI, class I recommendation for all patients NSTE ACS, class I recommendation for all patients	Hypersensitivity, Active bleeding, Severe bleeding risk	160–325 mg orally once on hospital day 1 75–162 mg once daily orally starting hospital day 2 and continued indefinitely in patients not receiving an intracoronary stent 162–325 mg once daily orally for a minimum of 30 days in patients undergoing PCI receiving a bare metal stent, 3 months with a sirolimus-eluting stent and 6 months with a paclitaxel-eluting, followed by 75–162 mg once daily orally thereafter Continue indefinitely
Clopidogrel	NSTE ACS, class I recommendation added to aspirin STE MI, class I recommendation added to aspirin PCI in STE and NSTE ACS, class I recommendation In patients with aspirin allergy, class I recommendation	Hypersensitivity, Active bleeding, Severe bleeding risk	300 mg (class I recommendation) to 600 mg (class IIa recommendation) oral loading dose on hospital day one followed by a maintenance dose of 75 mg once daily starting on hospital day 2 in patients with NSTE ACS 300 mg oral loading dose followed by 75 mg po daily in patients receiving a fibrinolytic or that do not receive reperfusion therapy in patients with a STEMI Avoid loading dose with fibrinolytic in patients aged 75 years or more 300–600 mg (Class I) loading dose before or when PCI performed Discontinue at least 5 days before elective CABG surgery (class I recommendation) Administer indefinitely in patients with aspirin allergy (class I recommendation) Continue for at least 12 months (class I recommendation) and up to 15 months (class IIb recommendation) in patients with ACS managed with PCI/stent In patients receiving a fibrinolytic or that do not receive reperfusion therapy, administer for at least 14 days (Class I) and up to 1 year (Class IIa)
Prasugrel	PCI in STE and NSTE ACS, added to aspirin, class I recommendation	Active bleeding, Prior stroke or TIA	Initiate in patients with known coronary artery anatomy only (so as to avoid use in patients needing CABG surgery) (class I recommendation) Avoid in patients ≥ 75 years of age unless DM or history of prior MI 60 mg oral loading dose followed by 10 mg once daily for patients weighing ≥ 60 kg 60 mg oral loading dose followed by 5 mg once daily in patients weighing < 60 kg Discontinue at least 7 days prior to elective CABG surgery (class I recommendation) Continue for at least 12 months (class I recommendation) and up to 15 months (class IIb recommendation) in patients with ACS managed with PCI/stent
Unfractionated heparin	STE MI, class I recommendation in patients undergoing PCI, and for those patients treated with fibrinolytics, class IIa recommendation for patients not treated with fibrinolytic therapy. NSTE ACS, Class I recommendation in combination with antiplatelet therapy for conservative or invasive approach PCI, class I recommendation (NSTE ACS and STE MI)	Active bleeding, History of heparin-induced thrombocytopenia, Severe bleeding risk, recent stroke	For STE MI with fibrinolytics, administer 60 units/kg IV bolus (maximum 4000 units) heparin followed by a constant IV infusion at 12 units/kg/hr (maximum 1000 units/hr) For STE MI primary PCI, administer 50–70 units/kg IV bolus if a GPIIb/IIIa inhibitor planned; 70–100 units/kg IV bolus if no GPIIb/IIIa inhibitor planned and supplement with IV bolus doses to maintain target ACT For NSTE ACS, administer 60 Units/kg IV bolus (maximum 4000 Units) followed by a constant IV infusion at 12 Units/kg/hr (maximum 1000 Units/hr) Titrated to maintain an aPTT of 1.5 to 2.0 times control (approximately 50 to 70 sec) for STE MI with fibrinolytics and for NSTE ACS Titrated to ACT of 250 to 350 sec for primary PCI without a GP IIb/IIIa inhibitor and 200 to 250 sec in patients given a concomitant GP IIb/IIIa inhibitor The first aPTT should be measured at 4 to 6 hours for NSTE ACS and STE ACS in patients *not* treated with fibrinolytics or undergoing primary PCI The first aPTT should be measured at 3 hours in patients with STE ACS who are treated with fibrinolytics Continue for 48 hrs or until the end of PCI
Enoxaparin	STE MI class I recommendation in patients receiving fibrinolytics and class IIa for patients not undergoing reperfusion therapy NSTE ACS, class I recommendation in combination with aspirin for conservative or invasive approach For PCI, class IIa recommendation as an alternative to UFH in patients with NSTE ACS For primary PCI in STE MI, class IIb recommendation as an alternative to UFH	Active bleeding, History of heparin-induced thrombocytopenia Severe bleeding risk, Recent stroke, Avoid enoxaparin if CrCl < 15 mL/min, Avoid if CABG surgery	Enoxaparin 1 mg/kg SC every 12 hrs for patients with NSTE ACS (CrCl ≥ 30 mL/min) Enoxaparin 1 mg/kg SC every 24 hrs (CrCl 15–29 mL/min) for NSTE or STE MI For all patients undergoing PCI following initiation of SC enoxaparin for NSTE ACS, a supplemental 0.3 mg/kg IV dose of enoxaparin should be administered at the time of PCI if the last dose of SC enoxaparin was given 8–12 hrs prior to PCI For patients with STE MI receiving fibrinolytics: Age <75 yrs: administer enoxaparin 30 mg IV bolus followed immediately by 1 mg/kg SC every 12 hours (first two doses administer maximum of 100 mg for patients for weighing more than 100 kg) For patients with STE MI ≥ 75 yrs old: administer enoxaparin 0.75 mg/kg SC every 12 hours (first two doses administer maximum of 75 mg for patients weighing more than 75 kg) Continue throughout hospitalization or up to 8 days for STE MI Continue for 24–48 hours for NSTE ACS or until the end of PCI for NSTE MI
Bivalirudin	NSTE ACS class I recommendation for invasive strategy	Active bleeding, Severe bleeding risk	For NSTE ACS, administer 0.1 mg/kg IV bolus followed by 0.25 mg/kg/hr infusion For PCI in NSTE ACS, administer a second bolus of 0.5 mg/kg IV and increase infusion rate to 1.75 mg/kg/hr For PCI in STEMI administer 0.75 mg/kg IV bolus followed by 1.75 mg/kg/hr infusion If prior UHF given, discontinue UHF and wait 30 mins before initiating bivalirudin Dosage adjustment for renal failure: none required in the HORIZONS-AMI trial Discontinue at end of PCI or continue at 0.25 mg/kg/hr if prolonged anticoagulation necessary

(continued)

| TABLE 24-4 | Evidence-Based Pharmacotherapy for ST-segment Elevation and Non-ST-segment Elevation Acute Coronary Syndromes (continued) |

Drug	Clinical Condition and ACC/AHA Guideline Recommendation[a]	Contraindications[b]	Dose and Duration of Therapy
Fondaparinux	STE MI class I recommendation receiving fibrinolytics and IIa for patients not undergoing reperfusion therapy NSTE ACS class I recommendation for invasive or conservative approach	Active bleeding, Severe bleeding risk SCr ≥ 3.0 mg/dL or Clcr < 30 mL/min	For STE MI, 2.5 mg IV bolus followed by 2.5 mg SC once daily starting on hospital day 2 For NSTE ACS, 2.5 mg SC once daily For PCI, give 50 to 60 units/kg IV bolus of UFH (regimen not rigorously studied) Continue until hospital discharge or up to 8 days

Fibrinolytic therapy	STE MI, class I recommendation for patients presenting within 12 hrs following the onset of symptoms, class IIa in patients presenting between 12 and 24 hrs, following the onset of symptoms with continuing signs of ischemia
	NSTE ACS, class III recommendation
		Any prior intracranial hemorrhage
		Known structural cerebrovascular lesions, such as an arterial venous malformation
		Known intracranial malignant neoplasm
		Ischemic stroke within 3 months
		Active bleeding (excluding menses),
		Significant closed head or facial trauma within 3 months
			Streptokinase: 1.5 MU IV over 60 min
			Alteplase: 15 mg IV bolus followed by 0.75 mg/kg IV over 30 min (max 50 mg) followed by 0.5 mg/kg (max 35 mg) over 60 min (maximum dose = 100 mg)
			Reteplase: 10 units IV x 2, 30 min apart
			Tenecteplase:
			  <60 kg (<132 lbs) = 30 mg IV bolus
			  60–69.9 kg (132–153 lbs) = 35 mg IV bolus
			  70–79.9 kg (154–176 lbs) = 40 mg IV bolus

Drug	Clinical Condition and ACC/AHA Guideline Recommendation[a]	Contraindications[b]	Drug	Dose for STE MI PCI and NSTE ACS	Dose for NSTE ACS without PCI	Dose adjustment for renal insufficiency
Glycoprotein IIb/IIIa receptor inhibitors	NSTE ACS, class IIa recommendation for either tirofiban or eptifibatide for patients with either continuing ischemia, elevated troponin or other high-risk features, class I recommendation for patients undergoing PCI, class IIb recommendation for patients without high-risk features who are not undergoing PCI STE MI, class IIa for abciximab for primary PCI and class IIb for either tirofiban or eptifibatide for primary PCI	Active bleeding Thrombocytopenia Prior stroke Renal dialysis (eptifibatide)	Abciximab	0.25 mg/kg IV bolus followed by 0.125 mcg/kg/min (maximum 10 mcg/min) for 12 hrs	Not recommended	None
			Eptifibatide	180 μ/kg IV bolus X 2, 10 min apart with an infusion of 2 mcg/kg/min for 18–24 hrs after PCI	180 μ/kg IV bolus followed by an infusion of 2 mcg/kg/min for 12–72 hrs	Reduce maintenance infusion to 1 mcg/kg/min for patients with CrCl <50 mL/min; not studied in patients with serum creatinine >4.0 mg/dL; Patients weighing 121 kg (266 lbs) or more should receive a maximum infusion rate of 22.6 mg per bolus and a maximum infusion rate of 15 mg/hour
			Tirofiban	25 μ/kg IV bolus Followed by an Infusion of 0.15 mcg/kg/minute for up to 18 hours	0.4 mg/kg IV bolus administered over 30 min followed by an infusion of 0.1 mcg/kg/min for 18 to 72 hours	Reduce maintenance infusion to 0.05 mcg/kg/min for patients with CrCl < 30 mL/min

(continued)

TABLE 24-4 Evidence-Based Pharmacotherapy for ST-segment Elevation and Non-ST-segment Elevation Acute Coronary Syndromes (continued)

Drug	Clinical Condition and ACC/AHA Guideline Recommendation[a]	Contraindications[b]	Dose and Duration of Therapy
Nitroglycerin	STE MI and NSTE ACS, class I indication in patients with ongoing ischemic discomfort, control of hypertension or management of pulmonary congestion	Hypotension Sildenafil or vardenafil within 24 hrs or tadalafil within 48 hours	0.4 mg SL, repeated every 5 minutes x 3 doses 5 to 10 mcg/min IV infusion titrated up to 75 to 100 mcg/min until relief of symptoms or limiting side-effects (headache) with a systolic blood pressure < 90 mm Hg or more than 30 percent below starting mean arterial pressure levels if significant hypertension is present Topical patches or oral nitrates are acceptable alternatives for patients without ongoing or refractory symptoms. Continue IV infusion for 24 to 48 hours
β-blockers[c]	STE MI and NSTE ACS, class I recommendation for oral beta-blockers in all patients without contraindications in the first 24 hrs, class IIa for IV beta-blockers in hypertensive patients	PR ECG segment >0.24 sec, 2nd degree or 3rd degree atrioventricular heart block Heart rate < 60 beats per min Systolic blood pressure < 90 mm Hg Shock Left ventricular failure with congestive heart failure Severe reactive airway disease	Target resting heart rate of 50–60 beats/min Metoprolol 5 mg slow IV push (over 1 to 2 min), repeated every 5 min for a total of 15 mg followed in 1 to 2 hours by 25 to 50 mg by mouth every 6 hours; if a very conservative regimen is desired, initial doses can be reduced to 1 to 2 mg Propranolol 0.5 to 1 mg IV dose followed in 1–2 hours by 40–80 mg by mouth every 6 to 8 hours Atenolol 5 mg IV dose followed in 5 min by a second 5 mg IV dose for a total of 10 mg, followed in 1 to 2 hours by 50 to 100 mg by mouth once daily Alternatively, initial intravenous therapy can be omitted Continue oral β-blocker indefinitely
Calcium channel blockers	STE MI class IIa recommendation and NSTE ACS class I recommendation for patients with ongoing ischemia who are already taking adequate doses of nitrates and β-blockers or in patients with contraindications to or intolerance to β-blockers (diltiazem or verapamil preferred during initial presentation) NSTE ACS, class IIb recommendation for diltiazem for patients with AMI	Pulmonary edema Evidence of left ventricular dysfunction Systolic blood pressure < 100 mm Hg PR ECG segment >0.24 sec 2nd or 3rd degree atrio-ventricular heart block for verapamil and diltiazem, pulse rate < 60 beats per min for diltiazem or verapamil	Diltiazem 120–360 mg sustained release orally once daily Verapamil 180–480 mg sustained release orally once daily Nifedipine 30–90 mg sustained release orally once daily Amlodipine 5–10 mg orally once daily Continue indefinitely if contraindication to oral β-blocker persists

ACE inhibitors — NSTE ACS and STE MI, class I recommendation for patients with heart failure, left ventricular dysfunction and EF ≤ 40%, type 2 diabetes mellitus or chronic kidney disease in the absence of contraindications. Consider in all patients with CAD (class I recommendation, class IIa in low risk patients). Indicated indefinitely for all patients with EF <40% (class I recommendation)

Contraindications: Systolic blood pressure < 100 mm Hg; History of intolerance to an ACE inhibitor; Bilateral renal artery stenosis; Serum potassium > 5.5 mEq/L (> 5.5 mmol/L); Acute renal failure; Pregnancy

Drug	Initial dose (mg)	Target dose (mg)
Captopril	6.25–12.5	50 twice daily orally to 50 three times daily
Enalapril	2.5–5.0	10 twice daily orally
Lisinopril	2.5–5.0	10–20 once daily orally
Ramipril	1.25–2.5	5 twice daily or 10 mg once daily orally
Trandolapril	1.0	4 mg once daily orally

Angiotensin receptor blockers — NSTE MI and STE MI, class I recommendation in patients with clinical signs of heart failure or left ventricular EF < 40% and intolerant of an ACE inhibitor, class IIa recommendation in patients with clinical signs of heart failure or EF < 40% and no documentation of ACE inhibitor intolerance, class I in other ACE inhibitor intolerant patients with hypertension

Contraindications: Systolic blood pressure < 100 mm Hg; Bilateral renal artery stenosis; Serum potassium > 5.5 mEq/L; Acute renal failure; Pregnancy

Drug	Initial dose (mg)	Target dose (mg)
Candesartan	4–8 mg	32 mg once daily orally
Valsartan	40 mg	160 mg twice daily orally
Continue indefinitely		

(continued)

TABLE 24-4 Evidence-Based Pharmacotherapy for ST-segment Elevation and Non-ST-segment Elevation Acute Coronary Syndromes (continued)

Drug	Clinical Condition and ACC/AHA Guideline Recommendation[a]	Contraindications[b]	Dose and Duration of Therapy		
Aldosterone antagonists	NSTE MI and STE MI class I recommendation with ejection fraction ≤40% and either DM or heart failure symptoms who are already receiving an ACE inhibitor	Hypotension Hyperkalemia, serum potassium >5.0 mEq/L SCr >2.5 mg/dL and/or CrCl <30 mL/min	**Drug**	**Initial dose (mg)**	**Maximum dose (mg)**
			Eplerenone	25 mg	50 mg once daily orally
			Spironolactone	12.5 mg	25–50 mg once daily orally
			Continue indefinitely		
Morphine sulfate	STE and NSTE ACS, class I recommendation for patients whose symptoms are not relieved after three serial SL nitroglycerin tablets or whose symptoms recur with adequate anti- ischemic therapy	Hypotension Respiratory depression Confusion Obtundation	2 to 4 mg IV bolus dose May be repeated every 5 to 15 minutes as needed to relieve symptoms and maintain patient comfort		

[a]Class I recommendations are conditions for which there is evidence and/or general agreement that a given procedure or treatment is useful and effective. Class II recommendations are those conditions for which there is conflicting evidence and/or divergence of opinion about the usefulness/efficacy of a procedure or treatment. For Class IIa recommendations, the weight of the evidence/opinion is in favor of usefulness/efficacy. Class IIb recommendations are those for which usefulness/efficacy is less well established by evidence/opinion. Class III recommendations are those where the procedure or treatment is not useful and may be harmful.

[b]Allergy or prior intolerance contraindication for all categories of drugs listed in this chart.

[c]Choice of the specific agent is not as important as ensuring that appropriate candidates receive this therapy. If there are concerns about patient intolerance due to existing pulmonary disease, especially asthma, selection should favor a short-acting agent, such as metoprolol or the ultra short-acting agent, esmolol. Mild wheezing or a history of chronic obstructive pulmonary disease should prompt a trial of a short-acting agent at a reduced dose (e.g., 2.5 mg intravenous metoprolol, 12.5 mg oral metoprolol, or 25 mcg/kg/min esmolol as initial doses) rather than complete avoidance of beta-blocker therapy.

ACC = American College of Cardiology; ACE = angiotensin converting enzyme inhibitor; AHA = American Heart Association; ACS = acute coronary syndrome; ACT = activated clotting time; ACUITY = Acute Catheterization and Urgent Intervention Triage Strategy; CABG = coronary artery bypass graft; CAD = coronary artery disease; CrCl = creatinine clearance; DM = diabetes mellitus; ECG = electrocardiogram; IV = intravenous; MI = myocardial infarction; NSTE = non-ST-segment elevation; OASIS = Organization to Assess Strategies in Acute Ischemic Syndromes; PCI = percutaneous coronary intervention; SC = subcutaneous; SCr = serum creatinine; SL = sublingual; STE = ST-segment elevation; TIA = transient ischemic attack

Reprinted with permission from Spinler SA. Evolution of antithrombotic therapy used in acute coronary syndromes. In: Richardson MM, Chessman KH, Chant C, Cheng JWM, Hemstreet BA, Hume AL, et al, eds. Pharmacotherapy Assessment Program, 7th ed. Cardiology. Lenexa, KS: American College of Clinical Pharmacy; 2010; 97–124.

ICH and major bleeding are the most serious side effects of fibrinolytic agents. The risk of ICH is higher with fibrin-specific agents than with streptokinase. Models are available for use in clinical practice to predict an individual patient's risk of ICH following administration of a fibrinolytic.[6] The risk of systemic bleeding other than ICH is higher with streptokinase than with other, more fibrin-specific agents.[49]

The percentage of eligible patients who receive reperfusion therapy is another quality performance measure of care for patients with STE MI.[23] (see Table 24–3). The "door-to-needle time," the time from hospital arrival to start of fibrinolytic therapy, is also a quality performance measure.[23] (Table 24–3) While the ACC/AHA guidelines recommend a door-to-needle time of less than 30 minutes, the median administration time in the United States in 2006 was 29 minutes with only 50% of patients meeting the quality performance measure target of <30 minutes.[10] Therefore, healthcare professionals can work to shorten fibrinolytic administration times.

Aspirin

Based on several randomized trials, aspirin is the preferred antiplatelet agent in the treatment of all ACSs.[2–6] Early aspirin administration to all patients without contraindications within the first 24 hours of hospital admission is a quality care indicator[23] (Table 24–3). The antiplatelet effects of aspirin are mediated by inhibiting the synthesis of TXA_2 through an irreversible inhibition of platelet cyclooxygenase-1.[52] Following the administration of a non-enteric-coated formulation, aspirin rapidly (<10 minutes) inhibits TXA_2 production in the platelets. Aspirin also has antiinflammatory actions, which decrease C-reactive protein and also may contribute to its effectiveness in ACS.[52] For patients undergoing PCI, aspirin prevents acute thrombotic occlusion during the procedure and likely stent thrombosis following PCI.

The Second International Study of Infarct Survival (ISIS-2), which studied the impact of streptokinase and aspirin (162.5 mg/day) either alone or in combination, is a landmark clinical trial that convincingly demonstrated the value of aspirin for patients with STE ACS.[53] In this trial ($n = 17,187$), patients receiving aspirin demonstrated a lower risk of 35-day vascular mortality compared with placebo (9.4% vs 11.8%; $P<0.0001$). The use of aspirin was not associated with any increase in major bleeding, although the incidence of minor bleeding was increased. Furthermore, the combination of aspirin plus streptokinase reduced mortality compared with placebo, as well as compared with either agent alone, thereby highlighting the additive effects of combination antithrombotic therapy.

For patients experiencing an ACS, an initial dose equal to greater than 160 mg nonenteric aspirin is necessary to achieve a rapid platelet inhibition[52,53] (Table 24–4). This first dose can be chewed in order to achieve high blood concentrations and platelet inhibition rapidly.[6] The notion of chewing aspirin came from the use of an enteric-coated formulation of aspirin in the ISIS-2 trial in order to break the enteric coating to ensure more rapid effect.[53] Current data suggest that although an initial dose 160 to 325 mg is required, long-term therapy with doses of 75 to 150 mg daily are as effective as higher doses, and therefore,[54,55] a daily maintenance dose of 75 to 162 mg is recommended in most patients to inhibit the 10% of the total platelet pool that is regenerated daily.[2–6,55] Whether these lower doses are as effective as a dose of 325 mg daily for patients undergoing intracoronary stent placement remains uncertain and current AHA/ACC guidelines recommend the use of 162 mg to 325 mg daily for one month after the placement of a bare-metal stent, 3 months after the placement of a sirolimus coated stent and 6 months after the placement of a paclitaxel coated stent, following which a daily aspirin dose of 75 mg to 162 mg should be used indefinitely.[4]

TABLE 24-5 Pharmacokinetics of Clopidogrel and Prasugrel[58,59]

	Prasugrel	Clopidogrel
Absorption and Metabolism	Prodrug Active metabolite R-138727 Metabolism to R-138727 is primarily by CYP3A4 and CYP2B6 Exposure to the active metabolite is not affected by CYP2C19 and CYP2C9 polymorphism Rapid conversion of the parent drug to active metabolite (median time to peak plasma concentration of active metabolite ≈30 minutes)	Prodrug Inactive metabolite SR266334 Active metabolite R-130946 Metabolism to R-130946 is primarily via CYP2C19, CYP3A4, CYP2B6 and CYP1A2, with lesser contribution from CYP2C9 Exposure to the active metabolite is affected by CYP2C19 genotype polymorphisms (e.g CYP2C19*2 or CYP2C19*3) Rapid conversion of the parent drug to active metabolite (mean time to peak plasma concentration of active metabolite ≈1 hour)
Food effect	Fasting administration preferred; C_{max} is reduced by 49% and t_{max} delayed 0.5–1.5 hours when administered with high-fat high-calorie meal, although AUC is unaffected	One report in healthy volunteers of bioavailability of inactive metabolite concentrations unaffected by food; one report in healthy volunteers of clopidogrel t_{max} delayed by 1.5 hrs, C_{max} increased 6-fold and bioavailability increased 9-fold
Disposition	Linear pharmacokinetics at doses up to 75 mg	Linear pharmacokinetics at doses of 50 to 150 mg
Elimination	Median elimination half-life of the active metabolite ≈7.4 hours Excretion is primarily urinary (≈70%); fecal excretion <30%	Elimination half-life of active metabolite not properly characterized, but reported to be a mean of 1.9 hours in one analysis Excretion is 50% urinary and 46% fecal
Labeled drug-drug interactions and management strategy	Enhanced bleeding with warfarin: monitor carefully for bleeding and target INR of 2.0 to 2.5 NSAIDs: avoid use if possible	Enhanced bleeding with warfarin: monitor carefully for bleeding and target INR of 2.0 to 2.5 NSAIDs: Avoid use if possible Reduced active metabolite and antiplatelet effect with inhibitors of CYP2C19: Administration of clopidogrel with agents known to inhibit CYP2C19 should be avoided. (e.g., omeprazole, esomeprazole, cimetidine, fluconazole, ketoconazole, voriconazole, etravirine, felbamate, fluoxetine, fluvoxamine)

AUC = area under the curve; CYP = cytochrome P450; INR = international normalized ratio; NSAIDs = nonsteroidal antiinflammatory drugs

Reprinted with permission from Spinler SA. Evolution of antithrombotic therapy used in acute coronary syndromes. In: Richardson MM, Chessman KH, Chant C, Cheng JWM, Hemstreet BA, Hume AL, et al, eds. Pharmacotherapy Assessment Program, 7th ed. Cardiology. Lenexa, KS: American College of Clinical Pharmacy; 2010, 97–124.

Therefore, although the risk of major bleeding, particularly gastrointestinal bleeding appears to be reduced by using lower doses of aspirin, low-dose aspirin, taken chronically, is not free of adverse effects.[55,56] Patients should be counseled on the potential risk of bleeding.

Nonselective nonsteroidal antiinflammatory agents (except aspirin) as well as cyclooxygenase-2 (COX-2) selective antiinflammatory agents should be discontinued at the time of STE MI secondary to increased risk of mortality, reinfarction, HF, and myocardial rupture.[3] Finally, although some concern has been voiced regarding the possible increased risk of hemorrhagic stroke in patients taking aspirin, this risk appears to be very small and is outweighed by the benefit in reducing the risk of ischemic stroke and other vascular events.[54] The risk of hemorrhagic stroke appears to be minimal for patients with adequate blood pressure control,[25] and there are no specific contraindications to antiplatelet therapy in a hypertensive patient presenting with ACS. Aspirin therapy should be continued indefinitely.[2–6]

Thienopyridines

Although aspirin is effective in the setting of ACS, it is a relatively weak platelet inhibitor that blocks platelet aggregation through only one pathway. The thienopyridines, ticlopidine, clopidogrel, and prasugrel, are antiplatelet agents that mediate their antiplatelet effects through a blockade of ADP $P2Y_{12}$ receptors on platelets. Because ticlopidine is associated with the occurrence of neutropenia that requires frequent monitoring of the complete blood count (CBC) during the first 3 months of use,[57] either clopidogrel or prasugrel are the preferred thienopyridines for ACS and PCI patients.[5] (Table 24–4)

Clopidogrel is currently recommended by the AHA/ACC guidelines as an alternative to aspirin for patients who have an allergy to

aspirin.[2,6] For STE MI, either clopidogrel or prasugrel, in addition to aspirin 325 mg, should be administered to patients undergoing primary PCI.[5] Both clopidogrel and prasugrel are prodrugs that are converted to an active metabolite by a variety of CYP isoenzymes (Table 24–5).[12,58,59] Prasugrel is a third-generation thienopyridine that is a more potent antiplatelet agent, resulting in a higher percentage of platelet aggregation inhibition and is less dependent on CYP 2C19 to produce its active metabolite and therefore has fewer drug–drug interactions.[59,60]

For primary PCI, clopidogrel is administered as a 300 mg to 600 mg loading dose followed by 75 mg once daily, to prevent subacute stent thrombosis and long-term CV events.[5,61] Prasugrel is administered as a loading dose of 60 mg followed by a maintenance dose of 10 mg daily. A large randomized, double-blind study, Trial to Assess Improvement in Therapeutic Outcomes by Optimizing Platelet Inhibition with Prasugrel (TRITON)-Thrombolysis in Myocardial Infarction (TIMI) 38, compared the 15-month efficacy and safety of prasugrel versus clopidogrel added to aspirin for patients undergoing PCI in the setting of STE MI or NSTE ACS.[62] Prasugrel significantly reduced the frequency of the primary composite end point of CV death, stroke or MI by 19% (9.9% vs 12.1%), as well as MI and stent thrombosis, but increased the risk of major bleeding (not ICH), by 32% (2.4% vs 1.8%). Patients with a history of prior stroke or transient ischemic attack had an increased risk of ICH and no net clinical benefit from prasugrel and thus the product label lists prior stroke or transient ischemic attack (TIA) as a contraindication to prasugrel.[59,62] Patients over the age of 75 years and those weighing less than 60 kg are at increased risk of bleeding with prasugrel compared with clopidogrel.[59] Two subgroups of patients *do not* have an increased bleeding risk with prasugrel compared with clopidogrel and have even greater benefit, namely patients undergoing primary PCI for STE MI and those patients with a history of diabetes mellitus.[63,64] While some have suggested that prasugrel is preferred in those two groups of patients, the most recent ACC/AHA STE MI and PCI practice guideline update does not favor one agent over another.[5,65]

Pharmacogenetic differences in thienopyridine metabolism, namely poor metabolism of CYP2C19, also can result in some patients being less responsive and thus displaying lower antiplatelet aggregation inhibition effects.[66] Lower rates of platelet aggregation inhibition [also known as (aka) responsiveness] to clopidogrel have been associated with higher rates of CV events, especially stent thrombosis and periprocedural MI in clinical trials.[67] While clopidogrel product labeling currently suggests that genetic testing and alternative therapy should be sought for patients that are CYP2C19 poor metabolizers, the cost of testing is estimated to be between $275 and $500 per patient; no prospective studies on using such a strategy to direct therapy have been published to assess the cost-effectiveness of such an approach.[58] In addition, poor responsiveness of antiplatelet effect to clopidogrel is but one predictor of increased risk of recurrent CV events following PCI. While functional platelet aggregation testing is available, there is no one gold-standard test. Prasugrel is not as dependent on CYP2C19 genotype for its conversion to the active metabolite and has a lower frequency of poor antiplatelet responsiveness.[68] Higher maintenance doses of clopidogrel of 150 mg daily have been studied for short-term administration and appear to have a lower frequency of poor antiplatelet responsiveness, but prasugrel's antiplatelet effects at 10 mg daily are still greater than clopidogrel at 150 mg daily.[60,69] Therefore, at the time of this writing, practitioners have no clear direction on how to incorporate pharmacogenetic testing of patients taking clopidogrel into practice.

The recommended duration of thienopyridine therapy for a patient undergoing PCI for ACS, either STE MI or NSTE ACS, is at least 12 months for patients receiving either a bare-metal or a drug-eluting stent, and up to 15 months for patients receiving a drug-eluting stent for patients at low risk of bleeding (Table 24–4).[5]

While prasugrel has been studied in the setting of PCI, no studies have evaluated its use when added to both aspirin and a fibrinolytics. Therefore, clopidogrel is the preferred thienopyridine for patients receiving fibrinolysis reperfusion therapy.[3] A large trial of more than 45,000 Chinese patients with STE MI showed that early therapy with clopidogrel 75 mg once daily (started within 24 hours of hospital presentation), added to aspirin for the duration of hospitalization (average 15 days) or up to 28 days, reduced mortality and reinfarction compared with placebo for patients treated with medical therapy, including fibrinolytics, without increasing the risk of major bleeding.[70] Another smaller study showed that clopidogrel added to aspirin reduced the composite rate of 30-day death, MI, or stroke by 20% for patients ages 18 to 75 years with STE MI treated with fibrinolytics.[71] Clopidogrel or placebo was administered as an initial dose of 300 mg orally on day one followed by 75 mg daily. Angiography was encouraged as early as hospital day 2 and patients undergoing PCI at the time of angiography continued on open-label, clopidogrel, a 300 mg loading dose followed by 75 mg once daily, for the duration of the study. Patients who did not undergo revascularization received clopidogrel up to the time of discharge or hospital day 8. At the time of angiography, there were more open infarct arteries in the clopidogrel-treated patients. Based on current data, therefore, clopidogrel (either 75 mg or 300 mg on day 1 followed by 75 mg once daily) should be given for at least 14 to 28 days in addition to aspirin for patients treated by fibrinolytics and in those receiving no revascularization therapy with either PCI or CABG surgery.[3] The safety of a 300 mg loading dose has not been evaluated in patients over the age of 75 years receiving a fibrinolytic.

The most frequent side effects of clopidogrel and prasugrel are nausea, vomiting, and diarrhea, which occur in approximately 2% to 5% of patients.[58,59] Rarely, thrombotic thrombocytopenic purpura has been reported with clopidogrel and is a precaution in the prasugrel product labeling.[58,59] The most serious side effect of thienopyridines is bleeding, and patients should be counseled on self-monitoring for signs of gastrointestinal bleeding and intolerable bruising. Abrupt discontinuation of thienopyridines for patients with intracoronary stents has resulted in abrupt stent closure which carries a high mortality risk.[72] Therefore, pharmacists play an integral role in reinforcing adherence to dual antiplatelet therapy.

Glycoprotein IIb/IIIa Receptor Inhibitors

GP IIb/IIIa receptor inhibitors block the final common pathway of platelet aggregation, namely, cross-linking of platelets by fibrinogen bridges between the GP IIb and IIIa receptors on the platelet surface. If UFH is selected for primary PCI in STE MI, a GP IIb/IIIa inhibitor, most commonly eptifibatide or abciximab, should be added to UFH (in addition to clopidogrel or prasugrel and aspirin) to reduce the likelihood of reinfarction for patients who have not received fibrinolytics.[4,6,73] GP IIb/IIIa inhibitors should not be administered for medical management of the patient with STE MI who will not be undergoing PCI. Abciximab is the most common GP IIb/IIIa receptor inhibitor studied in primary PCI trials.[3,4,73] Abciximab, in combination with aspirin, a thienopyridine, and UFH (administered as an infusion for the duration of the procedure) reduced mortality and reinfarction without increasing the risk of major bleeding in a meta-analysis of primary PCI clinical trials.[73] Administration of a GP IIb/IIIa inhibitor with bivalirudin, an alternative anticoagulant to UFH for PCI, is associated with increased risk of bleeding and should be avoided if possible.[74]

Dosing and contraindications for GP IIb/IIIa inhibitors are described in Table 24–4.[12] Abciximab typically is initiated as an IV bolus followed by an IV infusion at the time of PCI, and the infusion is continued for 12 hours while eptifibatide is administered as a double IV bolus followed by an infusion and continued for 12 to 18 hours. Administration of a GP IIb/IIIa receptor inhibitor may increase the risk of bleeding, especially if it is given in the setting of recent (<4 hours) administration of fibrinolytic therapy.[73,75] An immune-mediated thrombocytopenia occurs in approximately 5% of patients with abciximab and less than 1% of patients receiving eptifibatide or tirofiban.[76]

Anticoagulants

Options for anticoagulant therapy for patients with STE ACS are outlined in Figure 24–3 and Table 24–4.[2–6,12] For patients undergoing primary PCI, either UFH or bivalirudin is preferred whereas for fibrinolysis, enoxaparin is preferred.[3,6,77–79]

Unfractionated heparin has been the traditional anticoagulant administered to patients with STE MI to prevent reocclusion of an infarct artery for more than 40 years. A meta-analysis of small randomized studies from the 1970s and 1980s suggests that UFH reduces mortality by approximately 17% compared with no anticoagulant therapy.[6] In studies of patients receiving fibrinolytics, both fondaparinux, an indirect-acting factor Xa inhibitor, and reviparin, an investigational low-molecular-weight heparin (LMWH), have shown mortality reductions compared with placebo (no anticoagulant therapy).[80,81] Other beneficial effects of anticoagulation are prevention of cardioembolic stroke, as well as venous thromboembolism in MI patients.[6] Because randomized controlled clinical trials comparing UFH with placebo are lacking, no conclusive data exist supporting a benefit of UFH over placebo in reducing mortality or reinfarction in STE MI.[82] On the contrary, the results of a meta-analysis of more than 7,500 patients suggests that LMWHs reduce both mortality and reinfarction compared with placebo.[82]

Limitations of UFH anticoagulation include the need for intravenous infusion therapy, frequent aPTT monitoring, and the risk of heparin-induced thrombocytopenia. Bivalirudin is a direct thrombin inhibitor that has been associated with similar outcomes and reduced bleeding rates in primary PCI compared with UFH. In the Harmonizing Outcomes with Revascularization and Stents in Acute Myocardial Infarction (HORIZONS-AMI) open-label trial, patients treated with bivalirudin as a bolus and short-term infusion continued only through the PCI procedure, reduced the frequency of CV and all-cause mortality at 1 year, and lowered the risk of in-hospital major bleeding events compared with UFH.[77]

Enoxaparin, administered for a median of 7 days, has shown a reduction in the risk of death or nonfatal MI compared with UFH administered for a median of 2 days in the large, randomized Enoxaparin and Thrombolysis Reperfusion for Acute Myocardial Infarction Treatment (ExTRACT)-TIMI 25 trial.[78] (See Table 24–4 for enoxaparin dosing for STE MI.) The benefit, although modest, was already apparent after 48 hours of treatment. Enoxaparin use was associated with a small (2.1% vs 1.4%) but significant increased risk of major bleeding. Whether the observed benefits and increase in bleeding observed in this trial can be solely attributed to the pharmacokinetic and pharmacodynamic differences between UFH and enoxaparin or the longer duration of treatment in the enoxaparin group is uncertain. Although the bleeding rates were increased for patients over the age of 75 years compared with younger patients, the rates of major bleeding were similar between enoxaparin and UFH.[79] Therefore, enoxaparin can be considered a valuable anticoagulant when fibrinolysis reperfusion therapy is select for STE MI. Insufficient data are available studying IV enoxaparin in the setting of primary PCI.[83]

Fondaparinux has recently been studied in the setting of STE MI. In the Organization for the Assessment of Strategies for Ischemic Syndromes (OASIS) 6 trial, fondaparinux, administered for a median of 8 days, had similar efficacy and safety as UFH, administered for a median of 2 days, for patients receiving fibrinolytic therapy with either alteplase, reteplase, or tenecteplase[84] (see Table 24–4 for dosing). A small reduction in mortality was observed for patients treated with fondaparinux versus placebo for patients treated with streptokinase or receiving no fibrinolytic therapy. No benefit of fondaparinux was observed in the subgroup of patients undergoing PCI during hospitalization.[84] Because of the lack of benefit of fondaparinux compared with UFH as well as in the subgroup of patients undergoing PCI, coupled with the relatively long duration of administration, it is unlikely fondaparinux will be used widely in practice in the United States for STE MI.

Anticoagulant therapy should be initiated in the emergency department and continued for 48 hours or longer in select patients who will be bridged over to receive chronic warfarin anticoagulation following acute MI.[5] If a patient undergoes a PCI, UFH or bivalirudin is discontinued immediately after the procedure. The dose of the UFH infusion is adjusted frequently to a target activated partial thromboplastin time (aPTT) (see Table 24–4). When coadministered with a fibrinolytic, aPTTs above the target range are associated with an increased rate of bleeding, whereas aPTTs below the target range are associated with increased mortality and reinfarction.[85] Enoxaparin dosing is adjusted for body weight and renal function and, when administered in combination with fibrinolysis, has special dosing requirements for older patients and those weighing more than 100 kg. Fondaparinux is administered as a comparatively low, fixed dose of 2.5 mg subcutaneously daily and is contraindicated for patients with creatinine clearance less than

30 mL/min. For patients who do not undergo reperfusion therapy, it is reasonable to administer anticoagulant therapy for the duration of hospitalization, up to 8 days. Besides bleeding, the most frequent adverse effect of UFH is an immune-mediated clotting disorder, heparin-induced thrombocytopenia (see Chap. 26), which occurs in up to 5% of patients treated with UFH. Heparin-induced thrombocytopenia is less common for patients receiving LMWHs.[6]

Nitrates

Nitrates promote the release of nitric oxide from the endothelium, which results in venous and arterial vasodilation at higher doses. Venodilation lowers preload and myocardial oxygen demand. Arterial vasodilatation may lower blood pressure, thus reducing myocardial oxygen demand. Arterial vasodilatation also relieves coronary artery vasospasm, dilating coronary arteries to improve myocardial blood flow and oxygenation. One SL NTG tablet (0.4 mg) should be administered every 5 minutes for up to 3 doses to relieve myocardial ischemia. If patients have previously been prescribed SL NTG and ischemic chest discomfort persists for more than 5 minutes after the first dose, the patient should be instructed to contact emergency medical services before self-administering subsequent doses in order to activate emergency care sooner. IV NTG is indicated for patients with an ACS who do not have a contraindication and who have persistent ischemic symptoms, HF, or uncontrolled high blood pressure in the absence of contraindications (see Table 24–4). IV NTG should be continued for approximately 24 hours after ischemia is relieved.[6] Importantly, other life-saving therapies, such as ACE inhibitors or β-blockers, should not be withheld to use nitrates because the mortality benefit of nitrates is unproven. Nitrates play a limited role in the treatment of ACS patients because two large, randomized clinical trials failed to show a mortality benefit for IV followed by oral nitrate therapy in acute MI.[86,87] The most significant adverse effects of nitrates are tachycardia, flushing, headache, and hypotension. Nitrate administration is contraindicated for patients who have received oral phosphodiesterase-5 inhibitors, such as sildenafil and vardenafil within the past 24 hours and tadalafil within the past 48 hours. Because PCI or CABG restores coronary artery blood flow, NTG is typically not continued following revascularization.

β-Blockers

A β-blocker should be administered early in the care of patients with STE ACS and continued indefinitely. In ACS, the benefit of β-blockers results mainly from the competitive blockade of $β_1$-adrenergic receptors located on the myocardium. $β_1$-Blockade produces a reduction in heart rate, myocardial contractility, and blood pressure, decreasing myocardial oxygen demand. In addition, the reduction in heart rate increases diastolic time, thus improving ventricular filling and coronary artery perfusion.[88] As a result of these effects, β-blockers reduce the risk for recurrent ischemic, infarct size, risk of reinfarction, and occurrence of ventricular arrhythmias in the hours and days following MI.[88]

Landmark clinical trials have established the role of early β-blocker therapy in reducing MI mortality. Most of these trials were performed in the 1970s and 1980s before routine use of early reperfusion therapy.[89–92] However, data regarding the acute benefit of β-blockers in MI in the reperfusion era are derived mainly from a more recent large clinical trial that suggests that although initiating IV followed by oral β-blockers early in the course of STE MI was associated with a lower risk of reinfarction or ventricular fibrillation, there may be an early risk of cardiogenic shock, especially for patients presenting with pulmonary congestion or systolic blood pressure >120 mm Hg.[93] Therefore, initiation of β-blockers, particularly when administered intravenously, should be limited to patients who are hemodynamically stable and who do not demonstrate any signs or symptoms of acute HF.[3] Careful assessment for signs of hypotension and HF should be performed following β-blocker initiation and prior to any dose titration. Patients already taking β-blockers can continue taking them. STEMI 2007 The Joint Commission has retired the "Beta Blocker at Hospital Arrival" Core Measure and is no longer requiring hospital reporting of this measure.

The most serious side effects of β-blocker administration early in ACS are hypotension, acute HF, bradycardia, and heart block. While initial acute administration of β-blockers is not appropriate for patients who present with acute HF, initiation of β-blockers may be attempted before hospital discharge for most patients following treatment of acute HF. β-Blockers are continued indefinitely.[6]

Calcium Channel Blockers

Administration of calcium channel blockers in the setting of STE MI is reserved for patients who have contraindications to β-blockers and is used for relief of ischemic symptoms.[6] Patients prescribed calcium channel blockers for treatment of hypertension who are not receiving β-blockers and who do not have a contraindication to β-blockers should have the calcium channel blocker discontinued and a β-blocker initiated. Calcium channel blockers inhibit calcium influx into myocardial and vascular smooth muscle cells, causing vasodilation. Although all calcium channel blockers produce coronary vasodilatation and decrease blood pressure, other effects are more heterogeneous between agents. Dihydropyridine calcium channel blockers (e.g., amlodipine, felodipine, and nifedipine) primarily produce their antiischemic effects through peripheral vasodilatation with no clinical effects on atrioventricular (AV) node conduction and heart rate. Diltiazem and verapamil, on the other hand, have additional antiischemic effects by reducing contractility and AV nodal conduction and slowing heart rate.[94]

Current data suggest little benefit on clinical outcomes beyond symptom relief for calcium channel blockers in the setting of ACS.[94,95] Moreover, the use of first-generation short-acting dihydropyridines, such as nifedipine, should be avoided because they appear to worsen outcomes through their negative inotropic effects, induction of reflex sympathetic activation, tachycardia, and increased myocardial ischemia.[94] Therefore, the role of verapamil or diltiazem appears to be limited to relief of ischemia-related symptoms or control of heart rate in patients with supraventricular arrhythmias for whom β-blockers are contraindicated or ineffective.[6]

Adverse effects and contraindications of calcium channel blockers are described in Table 24–4. Verapamil, diltiazem, and first-generation dihydropyridines also should be avoided for patients with acute HF or LV systolic dysfunction because they can worsen HF and potentially increase mortality secondary to their negative inotropic effects. For patients with HF requiring treatment with a calcium channel blocker, amlodipine is the preferred agent.[96,97]

Two groups of patients may benefit from calcium channel blockers as opposed to β-blockers as initial therapy. Cocaine-induced ACS and variant (or Prinzmetal) angina are two conditions in which coronary vasospasm plays an important role.[6,98] Calcium channel blockers and/or NTG generally are considered the agents of choice in these patients because they can reverse the coronary spasm by inducing smooth muscle relaxation in the coronary arteries. In contrast, β-blockers generally should be avoided in these patients unless there is uncontrolled sinus tachycardia (>100 beats per minute) or severe uncontrolled hypertension following cocaine use because β-blockers actually may worsen vasospasm through an unopposed β_2-blocking effect on the smooth muscle cells.[98]

■ EARLY PHARMACOTHERAPY FOR NON-ST-SEGMENT ELEVATION ACS

In general, early pharmacotherapy for NSTE ACS (see Fig. 24–4)[12] is similar to that for STE. ❽ According to the 2007 ACC/AHA NSTE ACS practice guidelines, early pharmacotherapy includes intranasal oxygen (if oxygen saturation is low), aspirin, SL NTG, and an anticoagulant, either UFH, enoxaparin, fondaparinux, or bivalirudin. High-risk patients should proceed to early coronary angiography and may additionally receive a glycoprotein IIb/IIIa receptor inhibitor. Clopidogrel or prasugrel [agent and timing dependent on selection of an interventional (PCI) or medical management strategy] should be administered to all patients. Intravenous β-blockers and nitroglycerin should be given to select patients. Morphine is also administered to patients with refractory angina, as described previously. Intravenous NTG should be administered in select patients. Aspirin, SL NTG, and anticoagulation should be initiated early, while the patient is still in the emergency department. Fibrinolytic therapy is never administered. Dosing and contraindications for SL and IV NTG, aspirin, β-blockers, thienopyridines, and anticoagulants are listed in Table 24–4.[2–6,12]

Fibrinolytic Therapy

Fibrinolytic therapy is not indicated in any patient with NSTE ACS, even those who have positive biochemical markers (e.g., troponin) that indicate infarction. Because the risk of death from MI is lower for patients with NSTE ACS, whereas the risk for life-threatening adverse effects, such as ICH, with fibrinolytics is similar between patients with STE and NSTE ACS, the risks of fibrinolytic therapy outweigh the benefit for NSTE ACS patients. In fact, increased mortality has been reported with fibrinolytics compared with controls in clinical trials where fibrinolytics have been administered to patients with NSTE ACS (patients with normal or ST-segment-depression ECGs).[25]

Aspirin

Aspirin reduces the risk of death or developing MI by about 50% (compared with no antiplatelet therapy) for patients with non-STE ACS.[55] Therefore, aspirin remains the cornerstone of early treatment for all ACSs. Dosing of aspirin for NSTE ACS is the same as that for STE ACS (see Table 24–4).[2] Aspirin is continued indefinitely.

Thienopyridines

For patients with NSTE ACS, either clopidogrel or prasugrel is indicated for patients managed invasively with early coronary angiography and revascularization, while clopidogrel is indicated in those early conservatively managed patients. Clopidogrel is recommended for low- to moderate-risk patients, in addition to aspirin, who are managed with early conservative therapy, while clopidogrel or prasugrel may be selected in addition to aspirin and anticoagulation, in high-risk patients.[2,5] Clopidogrel is initiated as either a 300 mg or 600 mg loading dose followed by 75 mg daily, while prasugrel is initiated as a 60 mg loading dose followed by 10 mg daily.[5] Efficacy and safety of dual oral antiplatelet therapy were demonstrated in the Clopidogrel in Unstable Angina to Prevent Recurrent Events (CURE) trial.[99,100] In CURE, 12,562 patients with UA or an NSTEMI and new ECG changes consistent with ischemia or positive cardiac markers were randomized to a loading dose of 300 mg clopidogrel followed by a daily dose of 75 mg or placebo in addition to aspirin for a mean duration of 9 months and up to 12 months.[99] Clopidogrel reduced the combined risk of death from cardiovascular causes, nonfatal MI, or stroke from 11.4% to 9.4% compared with placebo, mainly through a reduction in the risk of MI. Cardiovascular mortality was similar between groups. In the subgroup of patients undergoing PCI, clopidogrel reduced the rate

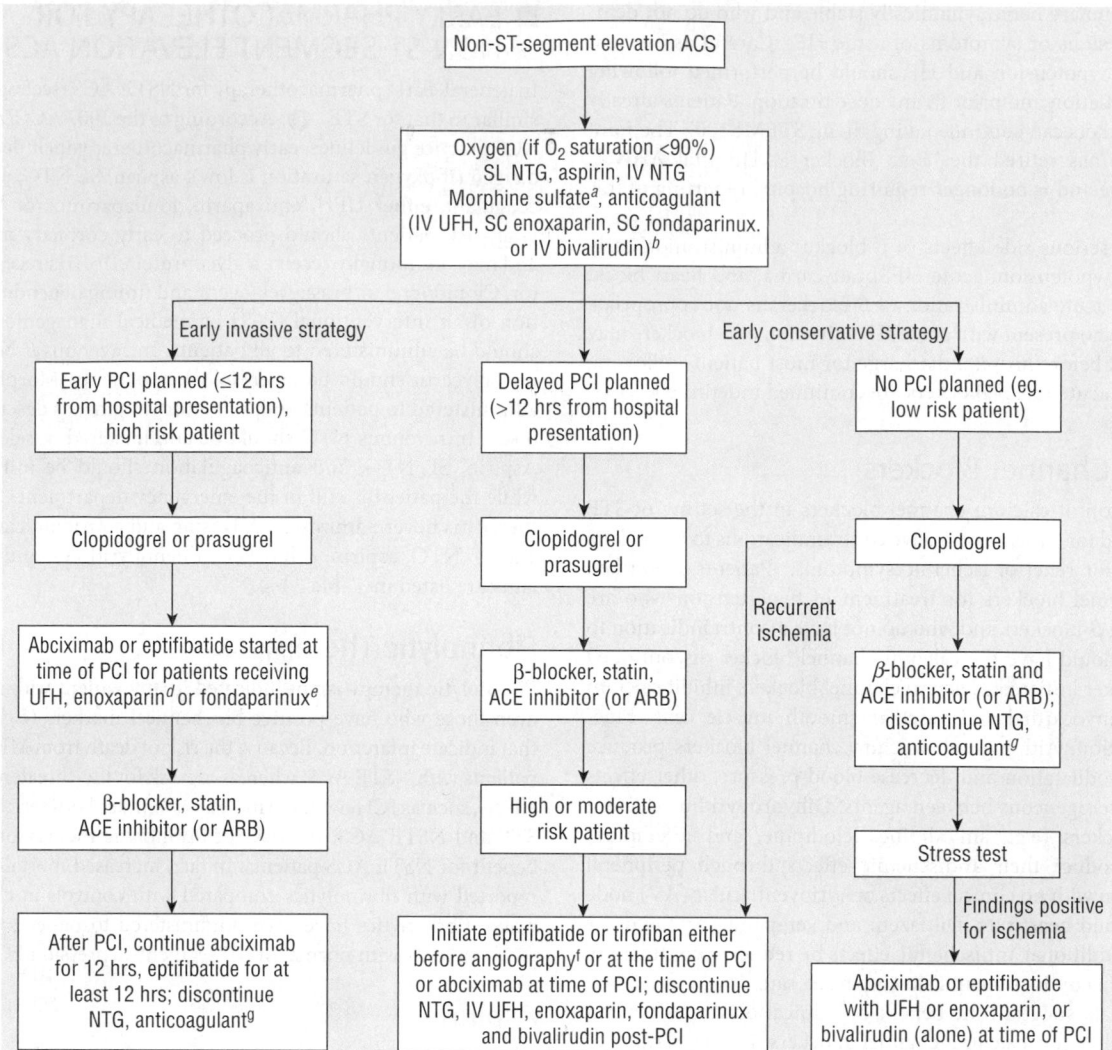

FIGURE 24-4. Initial pharmacotherapy for non-ST-segment elevation acute coronary syndrome. (ACE, angiotensin-converting enzyme; ARB, angiotensin receptor blocker; ACS, acute coronary syndrome; CABG, coronary artery bypass graft surgery; IV, intravenous; NTG, nitroglycerin; PCI, percutaneous coronary intervention; SC, subcutaneous; SL, sublingual; UFH, unfractionated heparin.) [a]For select patients, see Table 24–4. [b]Enoxaparin, UFH, fondaparinux plus UFH, or bivalirudin for early invasive strategy; enoxaparin or fondaparinux if no angiography/PCI planned; fondaparinux or bivalirudin preferred if high risk of bleeding; UFH preferred if patients going for CABG. [c]For patients unlikely to undergo CABG. [d]May require an IV supplemental dose of enoxaparin, see Table 24–4. [e]May require an IV supplemental dose of UFH, see Table 24–4. [f]For signs and symptoms of recurrent ischemia. [g]SC enoxaparin or UFH can be continued at a lower dose for venous thromboembolism prophylaxis. *(Reprinted with permission from Spinler SA. Evolution of antithrombotic therapy used in acute coronary syndromes. In: Richardson MM, Chessman KH, Chant C, Cheng JWM, Hemstreet BA, Hume AL, et al, eds. Pharmacotherapy Assessment Program, 7th ed. Cardiology. Lenexa, KS: American College of Clinical Pharmacy; 2010, 97–124.)*

of CV death or MI by 28% compared with placebo.[100] Results from a second trial in PCI patients, the Clopidogrel for the Reduction of Events During Observation (CREDO) trial, in which patients treated with long-term clopidogrel (1 year), demonstrated a lower risk of death, MI, or stroke compared with patients receiving only 28 days of clopidogrel added to aspirin compared with placebo (8.5% vs 11.5%; P = .02).[101] However, the interpretation of this study is limited in that the control group did not receive a loading dose of clopidogrel on the first day.

Prasugrel, a thienopyridine with greater antiplatelet effects than clopidogrel, reduced the risk of CV death, MI, and stroke in the TRITON-TIMI 38 trial as described in the section Early Pharmacotherapy for STE MI.[62] In TRITON-TIMI 38, 74% of patients enrolled had NSTE ACS. As described previously, prasugrel-treated patients had a higher rate of major bleeding. As part of the study design, the thienopyridine was initiated following coronary angiography at the time of PCI rather than initiated in

the emergency department. Therefore, the 2009 ACC/AHA STEMI and PCI guideline update provides an option for these agents to be initiated at the time of angiography/PCI in high-risk patients and also reserve prasugrel for patients in the early intervention strategy.[5] Clopidogrel remains the thienopyridine of choice for patients not undergoing revascularization (also termed *medical therapy alone*).[2] In CURE, the subgroup of patients not undergoing revascularization had a significant 20% reduction in CV events.[99]

Based upon the duration of thienopyridine administration in CURE and TRITON-TIMI 38, current guidelines for patients with NSTE ACS recommend that clopidogrel or prasugrel be administered for at least 12 months for patients undergoing PCI with placement of either a bare-metal or drug-eluting stent and up to 15 months for patients with a drug-eluting stent, where the risk of thrombotic occlusion may be greater.[5] For medical therapy of NSTE ACS, clopidogrel should be administered for up to 12 months for patients not at high risk of bleeding[2] (see Table 24–4).

The major concern when combining two antiplatelet agents is the increased risk of bleeding. In CURE, the risk of major bleeding was increased for patients receiving clopidogrel plus aspirin compared with aspirin alone (3.7% vs 2.7%; $P = 0.001$).[99] A post hoc analysis of CURE revealed that the rate of major bleeding depends on the dose of aspirin and showed that doses equal to or less than 100 mg daily reduced the risk of bleeding with similar efficacy when compared with higher doses.[102] The recommendation to use a lower dose of aspirin with clopidogrel is also supported by the results of a recent systematic review of clinical trials that found no benefit to aspirin as a sole antiplatelet agent for chronic treatment in doses greater than 75 to 81 mg.[54] However, a dose of 162 to 325 mg of aspirin is recommended to be administered with clopidogrel to patients with recent intracoronary stent placement, as described in the section on STE MI Pharmacotherapy, to prevent stent thrombosis[5] (see Table 24–4).

For patients undergoing CABG, major bleeding was increased in patients having the procedure within 5 days of clopidogrel discontinuation (9.6% vs 6.3%; $P = 0.06$) but not in patients for which clopidogrel was discontinued more than 5 days before the procedure.[99] Aspirin was continued up to and after CABG. Therefore, for patients scheduled for CABG, clopidogrel should be withheld at least 5 days and preferably 7 days before the procedure.[2,3,5]

In TRITON-TIMI 38, the frequency of major bleeding was higher in prasugrel- versus clopidogrel-treated patients (2.4% vs 1.8%, hazard ratio 1.32; 95% CI, 1.03–1.68; $P = 0.03$).[62] Prasugrel is contraindicated for patients with a prior history of stroke or TIA as the ICH rate was numerically higher without a net clinical benefit.[59,62] Patients older than 75 years of age have a greater risk of bleeding with prasugrel compared with clopidogrel as do patients weighing less than 60 kg.[59] For patients weighing less than 60 kg, a lower maintenance dose of 5 mg is recommended.[59] No outcome information from clinical trials evaluating safety of this dose has been reported. Hence, clopidogrel may be preferred for patients older than 75 years of age and in those weighing less than 60 kg.

Glycoprotein IIb/IIIa Receptor Inhibitors

Administration of abciximab or eptifibatide (alternatively tirofiban) with aspirin and UFH or enoxaparin is recommended for high-risk NSTE ACS patients undergoing PCI.[2,3] Administration of tirofiban or eptifibatide is also indicated for patients with continued or recurrent ischemia despite treatment with aspirin, clopidogrel, and an anticoagulant.[2] The pharmacologic similarities and differences between GP IIb/IIIa receptor inhibitors are reviewed in Chap. 23. As discussed in Chap. 23, the benefits of GP IIb/IIIa receptor inhibitors in PCI is well established, and they are considered a first-line agent to reduce the risk of reinfarction and the need for repeat PCI when added to aspirin and either UFH or enoxaparin.[2,3] A limitation of such studies is that they were conducted at a time when thienopyridines were not routinely administered prior to angiography and the practice was not standardized during the GP IIb/IIIa receptor inhibitor trials, and so such use was inconsistent between studies. A meta-analysis of five contemporary trials where clopidogrel pretreatment was required demonstrated no additional benefit for GP IIb/IIIa inhibitors over placebo, in terms of reduction in mortality, MI, or need for coronary artery revascularization with PCI, for either elective PCI for patients with stable angina or PCI in the setting of ACS.[103] In another 2008 meta-analysis of all studies published at the time, the beneficial reduction in the frequency of death or MI was greater for the patients with highest-risk such as those with positive troponins or those with a history of diabetes mellitus.[104] A third meta-analysis estimated that 30 adverse outcomes (either death or MI) are prevented for every 1,000 patients treated with a GP IIb/IIIa inhibitor before PCI, whereas only 4 events are prevented for medical management of patients with NSTE ACS using GP IIb/IIIa

inhibitors without PCI.[104] Major and minor bleeding rates were increased in all of these reports.[103–105] A study of routine use of these agents in high-risk patients prior to angiography, termed *upstream* administration, compared with initiation at the time of coronary angiograph, termed *downstream administration*, showed that upstream administration does not reduce ischemic events but does increase risk of bleeding.[106] Therefore, the use of GP IIb/IIIa receptor inhibitors in NSTE ACS is restricted to high-risk patients undergoing PCI and those lower-risk patients with unremitting or recurrent ischemic symptoms after initial medical therapy who will eventually undergo coronary angiography and PCI[2,5] (Table 24–4).

Doses and contraindications to GP IIb/IIIa inhibitors are described in Table 24–4, and common adverse effects are described in the preceding section on STEMI Pharmacotherapy. Administration of an IV GP IIb/IIIa receptor inhibitor in combination with aspirin and either UFH or enoxaparin results in major bleeding rates of 0.4% to 10.6% but no increased risk of ICH in the absence of concomitant fibrinolytic treatment.[107,108] Risk factors that increase the chance of bleeding with a GP IIb/IIIa inhibitor include female gender, older age, and reduced renal function.[109] In fact, older patients, especially women, are more likely to receive an excessive dose of a GP IIb/IIIa inhibitor, which can result in bleeding.[110] Since both eptifibatide and tirofiban require dose reductions for patients with renal insufficiency (see Table 24–4), careful attention to calculating creatinine clearance and dose adjustment is required for these agents. The risk of thrombocytopenia with tirofiban and eptifibatide appears to be lower than that with abciximab. Bleeding risks appear similar among agents.

Anticoagulants

The choice of anticoagulant for a patient with NSTE ACS is guided by risk stratification, treatment strategy, and the results of recent clinical trials.[2,74] For patients undergoing an early invasive strategy with early coronary angiography and PCI, either UFH, LMWH, low-dose fondaparinux, or bivalirudin should be administered.[3] If fondaparinux is chosen for a patient who undergoes PCI, it should be administered in combination with UFH as the dose of fondaparinux studied appears too low to prevent thrombotic events during PCI. UFH is the preferred anticoagulant following angiography for patients subsequently undergoing CABG during the same hospitalization.[2] For patients receiving an early conservative strategy, either enoxaparin or fondaparinux is preferred.[2] Therapy should be continued for up to at least 48 hours for UFH, until the patient is discharged from the hospital for either enoxaparin or fondaparinux and until the end of PCI or angiography procedure (or up to 72 hours following PCI) for bivalirudin.[2] UFH is the preferred anticoagulant following angiography for patients subsequently undergoing CABG during the same hospitalization as it has a short duration of action following discontinuation when the patient is proceeding to surgery.[2] For patients presenting with NSTE ACS in whom clinicians suspect a high risk for bleeding while receiving an anticoagulant, fondaparinux is the preferred anticoagulant recommended by the ACC/AHA NSTE ACS guidelines.[2] Neither fondaparinux or bivalirudin are Food and Drug Administration (FDA) approved for NSTE ACS despite being recommended by the ACC/AHA NSTE ACS guidelines. For patients initiating warfarin therapy, UFH or LMWHs should be continued until the international normalization ratio (INR) with warfarin is in the therapeutic range.

Data supporting the addition of UFH to aspirin stem from a meta-analysis of six randomized trials demonstrating a 33% reduction in the risk of death or MI at 6 weeks with UFH plus aspirin compared with aspirin alone.[111] One trial compared the LMWH dalteparin plus aspirin with aspirin alone and found a 60% reduction in death or MI at 6 days.[112] Three clinical trials have compared

UFH with LMWHs using an early conservative strategy in NSTE ACS.[113-115] One large clinical trial of enoxaparin compared with UFH in more than 10,000 patients using an early interventional approach found similar efficacy with a higher risk of major bleeding with enoxaparin (9.1% vs 7.6%; $P = 0.008$).[116] The risk of major bleeding with UFH or LMWHs is higher in patients undergoing angiography because there is an associated risk of hematoma at the femoral access site. The risk of heparin-induced thrombocytopenia is lower in some, but not all, clinical trials with LMWHs compared with UFH.

A low-dose of fondaparinux, 2.5 mg administered once daily subcutaneously, was compared with the usual NSTE ACS dose of enoxaparin, 1 mg/kg administered every 12 hours, in OASIS-5, the largest NSTE ACS trial performed to date (N = 20,000).[117] Fondaparinux was found to be non-inferior to enoxaparin with respect to the clinical end point of 9-day death, MI or refractory ischemia (5.8% vs 5.7%, hazard ratio 1.01, 95% CI, 0.90–1.13). Fondaparinux also reduced the rate of major bleeding compared with enoxaparin (2.2% vs 4.1%, $P < 0.001$). At 30 days, mortality was lower in fondaparinux-treated patients (8.0 vs 8.6%, hazard ratio 0.83, 95% CI, 0.71–0.97), and the investigators suggested that the excess mortality observed in enoxaparin-treated patients was related to bleeding events. The major limitation of OASIS-5 is that only 30% of patients underwent PCI. In addition, the duration of study drug administration, (median of about 5 days) was longer than usual in the United States, which may have increased bleeding events. Supplemental doses of UFH were administered to patients randomized to enoxaparin who underwent PCI. For patients randomized to fondaparinux who underwent PCI, the protocol was changed. The original protocol specified that intravenous fondaparinux be administered to patients undergoing PCI. When this practice was associated with catheter thrombosis, the protocol was changed to recommend supplemental UFH be given (see Table 24-4 for recommendations) to fondaparinux-treated patients undergoing PCI. As a result, interventional cardiologists may be reluctant to use low-dose fondaparinux for patients undergoing PCI.

Bivalirudin is an IV direct thrombin inhibitor that has a short duration of action. When administered as a bolus and short infusion that is continued during the PCI procedure only, bivalirudin has been shown to lower bleeding risk compared with UFH and enoxaparin.

In the Acute Catheterization and Urgent Intervention Triage Strategy (ACUITY) trial 13,819 patients with NSTE ACS at moderate- to high-risk of death or MI (expected to undergo coronary angiography within the first 48 to 72 hours of hospital admission) were randomized to one of three antithrombotic treatment strategies: (1) heparin (UFH or enoxaparin) plus a glycoprotein (GP) IIb/IIIa inhibitor, (2) bivalirudin plus GP IIb/IIIa inhibitor, or (3) bivalirudin alone in a noninferiority trial (see Table 24-4 for dosing).[74] The primary end point was "net clinical outcome" at 30 days, which was a quadruple end point consisting of the composite ischemic end point (death, MI, or unplanned revascularization for ischemia) plus non-CABG major bleeding. The results of the quadruple end point were that bivalirudin alone was noninferior to bivalirudin plus a GP IIb/IIIa inhibitor and superior to heparin plus a GP IIb/IIIa inhibitor. The benefit of bivalirudin alone was that it reduced the rate of major bleeding by 47% compared with heparin plus a GP IIb/IIIa receptor inhibitor. Although numerically higher in the bivalirudin group, the ischemic end points were not statistically different between the groups.[74]

With similar efficacy and a lower bleeding rate, on the surface bivalirudin alone appears the preferred therapy. However, several issues surround the study design and application to practice. The main issue surrounds the noninferiority margin of 25% used in the trial. This means that bivalirudin could be 25% "worse" than heparin plus GPI treated and still be called noninferior. In fact, the upper boundary of the 95% CI for the ischemic composite end point comparing bivalirudin alone with heparin plus a GP IIb/IIIa inhibitor was 1.24.[74] Other contemporary NSTE ACS trials, have used lower margins. More than 60% of patients received on average more than 14 hours of prerandomized treatment prior to study enrollment and were "crossed over" to study medications. Study medications were administered for a median duration of less than 6 hours before coronary angiography and PCI, and the overall duration of study drug administration was less than 18 hours since most study drugs were discontinued after angiography. Therefore although patients were randomized, there was potential for the prerandomization therapy to impact study outcomes, and some could question whether the short duration of treatment was long enough to impact outcomes. So while bivalirudin is a choice for higher-risk patients with NSTE ACS anticipated to undergo angiography and PCI, it was not given a "preferred" recommendation in the 2007 NSTE ACS guidelines.[2,3]

Because LMWHs are eliminated renally and patients with renal insufficiency generally have been excluded from clinical trials, some practice protocols recommend UFH for patients with creatinine clearance rates of less than 30 mL/min. (Creatinine clearance is calculated based on total patient body weight using the Cockroft-Gault equation estimated using total body weight.[2,3]) However, while recommendations for dosing adjustment of enoxaparin for patients with creatinine clearance between 10 and 30 mL/min are listed in the product manufacturer's label, the safety and efficacy of LMWH in this patient population remain vastly understudied. Administration of LMWHs should be avoided in dialysis patients with ACS. It is unclear whether bivalirudin requires dose adjustment for patients with significant renal dysfunction. While bivalirudin is eliminated renally, the duration of infusion in recent trials has been short (several hours only), and therefore the actual need for dosing adjustment is unlikely.[74] Patients with serum creatinine greater than 3.0 mg/dL were excluded from ACS trials with fondaparinux, and the product label states that fondaparinux is contraindicated for patients with creatinine clearance <30 mL/min and for patients weighing less than 50 kg.

UFH is monitored and the dose adjusted to a target aPTT, whereas LMWHs are administered by a fixed, actual body weight-based dose without routine monitoring of antifactor Xa levels. Some experts recommend antifactor Xa monitoring for LMWHs for patients with renal impairment during prolonged courses of administration of more than several days.[118] No monitoring of coagulation is recommended for bivalirudin and fondaparinux.

Since there is a variety of anticoagulants recommended by the guidelines, practitioners should be familiar with the study designs, patient demographics, and results for recent NSTE ACS studies and develop protocols for dosing each agent that is on the hospital formulary. Dosing information and contraindications are described in Table 24-4.

Nitrates

For patients with ischemic chest discomfort, SL NTG, 0.4 mg every 5 minutes for a total of 3 doses should be administered. IV NTG should be administered to all patients with NSTE ACS with persistent ischemia, HF symptoms or hypertension in the absence of contraindications (see Table 24-4).[2] The mechanism of action, dosing, contraindications, and adverse effects are the same as described in the section Early Pharmacotherapy for STE MI. IV NTG typically is continued for approximately 24 hours following ischemia relief. The mechanism of action, dosing, contraindications, and adverse effects are the same as described in the section Early Pharmacotherapy for STE MI.

β-Blockers

Oral β-blockers should be administered to all patients with NSTE ACS prior to hospital discharge in the absence of contraindications.[2] IV β-blockers should be considered in hemodynamically stable patients who present with persistent ischemia, hypertension, or tachycardia. The mechanism of action, dosing, contraindications, and adverse effects are the same as described in the section Early Pharmacotherapy for ST-Segment Elevation ACS. β-Blockers are continued indefinitely.

Calcium Channel Blockers

As previously described, calcium channel blockers should not be administered to most patients with ACS.[2] Their role is a second-line treatment for patients with certain contraindications to β-blockers and those with continued ischemia despite β-blocker and nitrate therapy. They are a first-line therapy for patients with Prinzmetal vasospastic angina and those with cocaine-associated ACS. Administration of amlodipine, diltiazem, or verapamil is preferred.[2] Agent selection based on heart rate and LV dysfunction (diltiazem and verapamil contraindicated for patients with bradycardia, heart block, or systolic HF) is described in more detail in the section Early Pharmacotherapy for ST-Segment Elevation ACS. Dosing and contraindications are described in Table 24–4.

Glycemic Control

While there are numerous guidelines and standards addressing the management of diabetes mellitus in the outpatient setting, only recently has there been sufficient evidence to warrant the development of standards of care to optimize inpatient glycemic control for hospitalized individuals with diabetes or illness-induced hyperglycemia. In 2004, a joint practice guideline from the American Diabetes Association and the American College of Endocrinology recommend that the blood glucose level in critically ill patients, such as those with ACS, be kept as close to 110 mg/dL (6.1 mmol/L) as possible.[119] This was supported by the 2004 ACC/AHA STE MI guidelines that recommend normalization of blood glucose during the first 24 to 48 hours of care.[6] Elevated blood glucose levels are associated with higher mortality rates and larger infarct size in patients with acute MI.[119] Beneficial outcomes that have been associated with "tight" glucose control in some trials of critically ill patients include reductions in the development of renal dysfunction, infections, and length of mechanical ventilation.[6,119] For patients with MI, glucose control has been associated with a reduction in inflammatory markers and improvement in LVEF.[5] More recently, results from a large international trial of more than 6,000 patients in either medical or surgical intensive care units, Normoglycemia in Intensive Care Evaluation—Survival Using Glucose Algorithm Regulation (NICE-SUGAR), revealed increased mortality in patients randomized to tight glucose control targeted to 80 to 108 mg/dL (mean achieved was 115 mg/dL) versus less than 180 mg/dL (mean achieved 144 mg/dL) thought secondary to an increased number of hypoglycemic events in the intensive-control group.[120] Therefore, in 2009, the ACC/AHA revised the practice guidelines to recommend a less intensive target of <180 mg/dL for patients with STEMI, often achieved using an insulin-based regimen while avoiding episodes of hypoglycemia.[5]

■ SECONDARY PREVENTION FOLLOWING MI

The long-term goals following MI are to

1. Control modifiable CHD risk factors
2. Prevent the development of systolic HF
3. Prevent recurrent MI and stroke
4. Prevent death, including sudden cardiac death

❾ Pharmacotherapy that has been proven to decrease mortality, HF, reinfarction, or stroke should be initiated prior to hospital discharge for secondary prevention. Guidelines from the ACC/AHA suggest that following MI from either STE or NSTE ACS patients should receive indefinite treatment with aspirin, a β-blocker, and an ACE inhibitor (or alternatively and ARB).[2,3,6] All patients should receive SL NTG or lingual spray and instructions for use in case of recurrent ischemic chest discomfort.[2,6] Clopidogrel or prasugrel should be considered for most patients, but the duration of therapy is individualized according to the type of ACS and whether the patient is treated medically or with PCI and whether a drug-eluting versus a bare-metal stent is placed.[2,5] All patients should receive annual influenza vaccination.[121,122] Select patients, such as those with atrial fibrillation, also will be treated with long-term warfarin anticoagulation, in addition to aspirin and a thienopyridine.[6] Eplerenone should be added to therapy with a β-blocker and an ACE inhibitor for patients with an LVEF less than 40%.[2,6,112] For all patients with ACS, treatment and control of modifiable risk factors such as hypertension, dyslipidemia, and diabetes mellitus are essential. Most patients with CHD will require drug therapy for dyslipidemia, usually with a statin (hydroxymethylglutaryl coenzyme A reductase inhibitor).[2,3] Benefits and adverse effects of long-term treatment with these medications are discussed in more detail in the following sections.

Aspirin

Aspirin decreases the risk of death, recurrent MI, and stroke following MI. An aspirin prescription at hospital discharge is a quality care indicator in MI patients[23] (see Table 24–3). The clinical value of aspirin in secondary prevention of ACS and other vascular diseases was demonstrated in a large number of clinical trials. Following an MI, aspirin is expected to prevent 36 vascular events per 1,000 patients treated for 2 years.[52,55] Because the benefit of antiplatelet agents appears to be sustained for at least 2 years following an MI,[55] all patients should receive aspirin indefinitely, or clopidogrel for patients with a contraindication to aspirin.[2–6]

Thienopyridines

For patients with ACS, clopidogrel and prasugrel decrease the risk of developing either death, MI, or stroke in patients post-PCI.[62,99] The benefit is primarily in reducing the rate of MI.[99] For patients with an STEMI treated medically without revascularization including PCI or CABG, clopidogrel can be given for 14 days and up to 1 year.[3] For patients in which an intracoronary stent was placed, clopidogrel and prasugrel should be continued for up to 12 months for patients at low risk of bleeding, with an option for up to 15 months of therapy for patients with a drug-eluting stent.[5]

The most common adverse effects for patients receiving clopidogrel and prasugrel are rash (approximately 5%) and diarrhea or gastrointestinal upset (approximately 3%).[58,59]

Anticoagulation

Warfarin should be considered in select patients following an ACS, including patients with a LV thrombus, patients demonstrating extensive ventricular wall motion abnormalities on cardiac echocardiogram, and patients with a history of thromboembolic disease or chronic atrial fibrillation.[3] An INR of 2.0 to 2.5 is recommended when warfarin is added to dual antiplatelet therapy with a thienopyridine.[3] Clopidogrel is preferred in such patients because the risk of bleeding with prasugrel is increased compared with clopidogrel and the risk of bleeding with warfarin added to dual antiplatelet therapy is even greater. A more detailed discussion regarding the use of warfarin is available in Chap. 26.

β-Blockers, Nitrates, and Calcium Channel Blockers

Current treatment guidelines recommend that following an ACS, patients should receive a β-blocker indefinitely[2,3] whether they have residual symptoms of angina or not.[123] β-Blocker prescription at hospital discharge in the absence of contraindications is a quality performance measure (see Table 24–3).[23] Overwhelming data support the use of β-blockers for patients with a previous MI. Data from a systematic review of long-term trials of patients with recent MI demonstrate that the NNT for 1 year with a β-blocker to prevent one death is only 84 patients.[123] Because the benefit from β-blockers appears to be maintained for at least 6 years following an MI,[124] it is recommended that all patients receive β-blockers indefinitely in the absence of contraindications or intolerance.[2,3] Currently, there are no data to support the superiority of one β-blocker over another, although the only β-blocker with intrinsic sympathomimetic activity that has been shown to be beneficial following MI is acebutolol in one study of modest size.[125]

Although β-blockers should be avoided for patients with HF from LV systolic dysfunction complicating an MI, clinical trial data suggest that it is safe to initiate β-blockers prior to hospital discharge in these patients once HF symptoms have resolved.[126] These patients actually may benefit more than those without LV dysfunction.[127]

For patients who cannot tolerate or have a contraindication to a β-blocker, a calcium channel blocker can be used to prevent anginal symptoms but should not be used routinely in the absence of such symptoms.[2,3,128] Finally, all patients should be prescribed short-acting SL NTG or lingual NTG spray to relieve any anginal symptoms when necessary and should be instructed on its use.[2,3] Chronic long-acting nitrate therapy has not been shown to reduce CHD events following MI. Therefore, IV NTG is not followed routinely by chronic, long-acting oral nitrate therapy in ACS patients who have undergone revascularization unless the patient has chronic stable angina or significant coronary stenoses that were not revascularized.[128]

ACE Inhibitors and Angiotensin Receptor Blockers

ACE inhibitors should be initiated in all patients following MI to reduce mortality, decrease reinfarction, and prevent the development of HF.[2,3,121] Dosing and contraindications are described in Table 24–4. The benefit of ACE inhibitors and angiotensin receptor blockers (ARBs) for patients with MI most likely comes from their ability to prevent cardiac remodeling. Other proposed mechanisms include improvement in endothelial function, a reduction in atrial and ventricular arrhythmias, and promotion of angiogenesis, leading to a reduction in ischemic events. The largest reduction in mortality with ACE inhibitors is observed for patients with LV dysfunction (low LVEF) or HF symptoms.[129] Long-term studies in patients with LV systolic dysfunction with or without HF symptoms demonstrate greater benefit because mortality reductions are larger (23.4% vs 29.1%; $P<0.0001$) such that only 17 patients need treatment to prevent 1 death, with 57 lives saved for every 1,000 patients treated.[130] The use of ACE inhibitors in a wide range of patient types without a contraindication to ACE inhibitors may be expected to save 5 lives per 1,000 patients treated for 30 days.[129] ACE inhibitor prescription at hospital discharge following MI, in the absence of contraindications, to patients with depressed LV function (LVEF <40%) is currently a quality care indicator[23] (see Table 24–3).

Early initiation (within 24 hours) of an *oral* ACE inhibitor appears to be crucial during an acute MI because 40% of the 30-day survival benefit is observed during the first day, 45% from days 2 to 7, and approximately 15% from days 8 to 30.[129] However, data do not support the early administration of *intravenous* ACE inhibitors for patients experiencing an MI because mortality may be increased.[131] Hypotension should be avoided because coronary artery filling may be compromised. Because the benefits of ACE inhibitor administration have been documented out to 12 years following therapy for 2 to 4 years following MI for patients with LV dysfunction,[130,132] administration should continue indefinitely.

Additional data suggest that even patients with preserved LV function benefit from ACE inhibitors for secondary prevention as ACE inhibitors have demonstrated reductions in mortality, reinfarction, stroke, and development of HF.[133] Therefore all patients, and not just those with reduced LVEFs, should be considered for ACE inhibitor therapy prior to hospital discharge. However, ACE inhibitor prescription (or alternatively an ARB) at hospital discharge following MI, in the absence of contraindications, to patients with depressed LV function (LVEF less than 40%) is currently the only quality performance measure reported.[23] Similar outcomes have been demonstrated with both valsartan and candesartan for patients following myocardial infarction or with chronic HF compared with ACE inhibitors.[134,135]

Besides hypotension, the most frequent adverse reaction to an ACE inhibitor is cough, which may occur in up to 30% of patients. Patients with ACE inhibitor cough and either clinical signs of HF or LVEF less than 40% may be prescribed an ARB.[3] Other less common but more serious adverse effects of ACE inhibitors and ARBs include acute renal failure and hyperkalemia. While the incidence of angioedema appears higher for patients receiving ACE inhibitors (0.1% to 1.0% with an ACE inhibitor), ARBs have also been associated with angioedema, including recurrent angioedema in patients with a prior history of angioedema while receiving an ACE inhibitor.[136] Therefore, while ARBs are not contraindicated, the severity of angioedema while receiving an ACE inhibitor, for example, tongue or laryngeal edema necessitating intubation and mechanical ventilation, should be considered before starting an ARB for a patient with prior ACE inhibitor-associated angioedema.

Aldosterone Antagonists

Administration of an aldosterone antagonist, either eplerenone or spironolactone, should be considered within the first 2 weeks following MI in all patients already receiving an ACE inhibitor who experienced HF symptoms during hospitalization for MI and have an LVEF of 40% or less to reduce mortality.[3,121] Aldosterone plays an important role in HF and MI because it promotes vascular and myocardial fibrosis, endothelial dysfunction, hypertension, LV hypertrophy, sodium retention, potassium and magnesium loss, and arrhythmias. Aldosterone blockers have been shown in experimental and human studies to attenuate these adverse effects.[137] As discussed in Chap. 20, the benefit of aldosterone blockade for patients with stable, severe HF was highlighted in the Randomized Aldactone Evaluation Study (RALES), where spironolactone decreased the risk of all-cause mortality.[138]

Eplerenone, like spironolactone, is an aldosterone blocker that blocks the mineralocorticoid receptor. In contrast to spironolactone, eplerenone has no effect on the progesterone or androgen receptor, thereby minimizing the risk of gynecomastia, sexual dysfunction, and menstrual irregularities.[139] The Eplerenone Post-Acute Myocardial Infarction Heart Failure Efficacy and Survival Study (EPHESUS) evaluated the effect of aldosterone antagonism for patients with an MI complicated by HF or LV dysfunction. Patients ($n = 6,642$) were randomized 3 to 14 days following the MI to eplerenone or placebo.[139] Eplerenone significantly reduced the risk of mortality (14.4% vs 16.7%; $P = 0.008$). Data from EPHESUS suggest that eplerenone reduced mortality from sudden death, HF, and MI. Eplerenone also reduced the risk of hospitalizations for HF. Most patients in EPHESUS also were being treated with aspirin, a β-blocker, and an ACE inhibitor. Approximately half the patients also were receiving a statin. Therefore, the mortality reduction observed was in addition to that of standard therapy for secondary CHD prevention. These benefits were obtained at the expense of an increased risk of severe hyperkalemia (5.5% vs 3.9%; $P = 0.002$), defined as a potassium concentration equal or greater than 6 mEq/L. Patients with a serum creatinine concentration of greater than 2.5 mg/dL or a serum potassium concentration of greater than 5 mEq/L at baseline were excluded. The risk of hyperkalemia was particularly alarming for patients with a creatinine clearance of less than 50 mL/min. This highlights the importance of close monitoring of potassium level and renal function for patients being treated with eplerenone. There was no increase in gynecomastia, breast pain, or impotence.

The results from EPHESUS have raised the question of which aldosterone blocker, spironolactone or eplerenone, should be used preferentially. Currently, there are no data to support that the more selective, but more expensive eplerenone is superior to or should be preferred to the less expensive generic spironolactone unless a patient has experienced gynecomastia, breast pain, or impotence while receiving spironolactone. Finally, it should be noted that hyperkalemia is just as likely to appear with both these agents.

Lipid-Lowering Agents

There are now overwhelming data supporting the benefits of statins for patients with CAD in the prevention of total mortality, cardiovascular mortality, and stroke. According to the National Cholesterol Education Program (NCEP) Adult Treatment Panel recommendations, all patients with CAD should receive dietary counseling and pharmacologic therapy in order to reach an LDL cholesterol concentration of less than 100 mg/dL, with statins being the preferred agents to lower LDL cholesterol.[121,140,141] Although the primary effect of statins is to decrease LDL cholesterol, statins are believed to produce many non-lipid-lowering or "pleiotropic" effects. These effects, which include improvement in endothelial dysfunction, antiinflammatory and antithrombotic properties, and a decrease in matrix metalloproteinase activity, may be relevant for patients experiencing an ACS and result in short-term (<1 year) benefit. A meta-analysis of randomized, controlled clinical trials in almost 18,000 patients with recent ACS (<14 days) indicated that statin therapy reduces mortality by 19% with benefits observed after approximately 4 months of treatment.[142]

Recommendations from the NCEP give an optional goal of an LDL cholesterol of less than 70 mg/dL for secondary prevention.[2,141] This recommendation is based upon a large clinical trial evaluating recurrence of major cardiovascular events in patients with a history of an ACS occurring within the past 10 days. This trial documented the benefit of lowering LDL cholesterol to, on average, 62 mg/dL, with 80 mg of atorvastatin compared with 95 mg/dL for patients treated with pravastatin 40 mg daily.[143] Whether a statin should be used routinely in all patients irrespective of their baseline LDL cholesterol level is currently being investigated, but preliminary data from the Heart Protection Study suggest that patients benefit from statin therapy irrespective of their baseline LDL cholesterol level.[144] The 2007 ACC/AHA NSTE ACS guidelines recommended statin therapy, in addition to diet, for all ACS patients, regardless of LDL cholesterol level, although the exact target LDL, if the patient's LDL cholesterol at hospital presentation is already less than 70 mg/dL, is not stated.[2]

A fibrate or niacin may be considered in select patients with a low high-density lipoprotein (HDL) cholesterol concentration (<40 mg/dL) and/or a high triglyceride level (>200 mg/dL).[2,121,141] In a large, randomized trial in men with established CAD and low levels of HDL cholesterol, the use of gemfibrozil (600 mg twice daily) significantly decreased the risk of nonfatal MI or death from coronary causes.[145] No such benefit was observed with fenofibrate in two large multicenter primary and secondary prevention studies for patients with diabetes mellitus.[146,147] However, due to the increased risk of myopathy, gemfibrozil is not recommended for patients receiving a statin.

Additional discussion, dosing, monitoring, and adverse effects of using lipid-lowering drugs for secondary prevention may be found in Chap. 28.

Fish Oils (Marine-Derived Omega-3 Fatty Acids)

Eicosapentaenoic acid (EPA) and docosahexaenoic acid (DHA) are omega-3 polyunsaturated fatty acids that are most abundant in fatty fish such as sardines, salmon, and mackerel. Epidemiologic and randomized trials have demonstrated that a diet high in EPA plus DHA or supplementation with these fish oils reduces the risk of cardiovascular mortality, reinfarction, and stroke in patients who have experienced an MI.[148] Although the exact mechanism responsible for the beneficial effects of omega-3 fatty acids has not been clearly elucidated, potential mechanisms include triglyceride-lowering effects, antithrombotic effects, retardation in the progression of atherosclerosis, endothelial relaxation, mild antihypertensive effects, and reduction in ventricular arrhythmias.[148]

The GISSI-Prevenzione trial, the largest randomized trial of fish oils published to date, evaluated the effects of open-label EPA plus DHA (LOVAZA) in 11,324 patients with recent MI who were randomized to receive 850 to 882 mg/day of n-3 polyunsaturated fatty acid (EPA plus DHA) in a ratio of EPA:DHA of 1.2:1, 300 mg vitamin E, both, or neither.[149,150] The use of EPA plus DHA reduced the risk of death, nonfatal acute MI, or nonfatal stroke, whereas the use of vitamin E had no significant impact on this combined clinical end point. Therefore, based on current data, the AHA recommends that CHD patients consume approximately 1 g EPA plus DHA per day, preferably from oily fish.[121,148] Because oil content in fish varies, the number of 6-oz servings of fish that would need to be consumed to provide 7 g EPA plus DHA per week varies from approximately 4 to more than 14 for secondary prevention. The average diet only contains one-tenth to one-fifth the recommended amount.[148] Supplements could be considered for select patients who do not eat fish, have limited access to fish, or who cannot afford to purchase fish. Approximately three 1 g fish oil capsules per day should be consumed to provide 1 g omega-3 fatty acids depending on the brand of supplement.[148] Alternatively, the prescription drug, LOVAZA may be used in a dose of 1 g/day. Finally, current guidelines suggest that higher doses of EPA plus DHA (2 to 4 g/day) also can be considered for the management of hypertriglyceridemia.[2,121,148] Adverse effects from fish oils include fishy aftertaste, nausea, and diarrhea.[148]

Other Modifiable Risk Factors

Smoking cessation, control of hypertension, weight loss, and tight glucose control for patients with diabetes mellitus, in addition to treatment of dyslipidemia, are important treatments for secondary prevention of CHD events.[3,121] All patients with CAD should receive annual influenza vaccination.[121,122] Influenza-related deaths are highest among patients with CVD compared with patients with other medical conditions.[122] Annual influenza vaccination has been shown in randomized controlled clinical trials to reduce

CV mortality and MI.[122] Smoking cessation is accompanied by a significant reduction in all-cause mortality in patients with CAD.[151] Smoking cessation counseling at the time of discharge following MI is a quality care indicator[23] (see Table 24–3). The use of nicotine patches or gum, bupropion alone or in combination with nicotine patches, or varenicline should be considered in appropriate patients.[3] Following MI, hypertension should be strictly controlled to a target blood pressure of <140/90 according to the Joint National Committee on Prevention, Detection, Evaluation, and Treatment of High Blood Pressure guidelines.[152] Patients who are overweight should be educated on the importance of regular exercise, healthy eating habits, and of reaching and maintaining an ideal weight.[153] Finally, because diabetics have up to a fourfold increased risk of mortality compared with nondiabetics, the importance of glucose control, as well as other CHD risk factor modification, cannot be understated.

■ MEDICATION ADHERENCE AND PERSISTENCE

It is becoming increasingly clear that medication nonadherence poses a problem for patients following ACS. Indeed, it is estimated that almost 7% of patients do not fill prescriptions for thienopyridines following hospitalization for PCI and stent placement.[154] Approximately 15% do not fill prescriptions for β-blockers following discharge following MI, and persistence is only 60% at 6 months.[155] Primary nonadherence at 120 days following discharge for MI was 26% in one large study of 4,591 patients >65 years of age.[156] Medication discontinuation has been associated with an increased risk of CV events and mortality in patients with various types of CVD.[156-159] In clinical trials, poor adherence is associated with poor outcome, regardless of treatment assignment,[159] highlighting that this behavior may be related with other health-related behaviors in patients. Increased adherence to statins and β-blockers has been associated with lower long-term mortality.[160]

The discontinuation of thienopyridines may be particularly problematic for patients treated with a drug-eluting stent,[161] because this places the patient at an increased risk for stent thrombosis and increased mortality.[72,154] Current data suggest that long-term adherence and persistence to statins for patients with an ACS and for patients with chronic CAD is variable.[162-165] Persistence to statins is associated with lower risk of MI.[166] Early initiation of statins for patients with ACS appears to increase long-term persistence with statin therapy, which should result in clinical benefit.[142] Therefore, for patients with an ACS, statin therapy initiation should not be delayed, and statins should be prescribed at or prior to discharge in most patients.

Several clinical trials have documented the value of a pharmacist in the management in improving adherence and persistence to medication, which in turn can significantly improve the treatment of risk factors such as hypertension, HF, and dyslipidemia.[167,168]

PHARMACOECONOMIC CONSIDERATIONS

The risks of CHD events, such as death, recurrent MI, and stroke, are higher for patients with established CHD and a history of MI than for patients with no known CHD. Because the costs for chronic preventative pharmacotherapy are the same for primary and secondary prevention, while the risk of events is higher with secondary prevention, secondary prevention is more cost-effective than primary prevention of CHD.[169] Pharmacotherapy that has demonstrated cost-effectiveness to prevent death in the ACS and post-MI patient includes fibrinolytics ($2,000 to $33,000 cost per

year of life saved),[169,170] aspirin[171], glycoprotein IIb/IIIa receptor blockers ($ 13,700 to $16,500 per year of life added),[172] β-blockers (less than $5,000 to $15,000 cost per year of life saved),[173] ACE inhibitors ($3,000 to $5,000 cost per year of life saved),[174,175] eplerenone ($15,300 to $32,400 per life year gained),[176] statins ($4,500 to $9,500 per year of life saved),[177] gemfibrozil ($17,000 per year of life saved),[178] and fish oil.[179] The cost-effectiveness of prasugrel compared with clopidogrel is $9,727 per year of life gained based upon data from the TRITON-TIMI 28 trial.[180] Because cost-effectiveness ratios of less than $50,000 per added life-year are considered economically attractive from a societal perspective,[169] pharmacotherapy above for ACS and secondary prevention are standards of care because of their efficacy and cost-attractiveness to payers.

EVALUATION OF THERAPEUTIC OUTCOMES

The monitoring parameters for *efficacy* of nonpharmacologic and pharmacotherapy for both STE MI and NSTE ACS are similar:

- Relief of ischemic discomfort
- Return of ECG changes to baseline
- Absence or resolution of HF signs

Monitoring parameters for recognition and prevention of *adverse effects* from ACS pharmacotherapy are described in Table 24–6. In general, the most common adverse reactions from ACS therapies are hypotension and bleeding. Treatment for bleeding and hypotension involves discontinuation of the offending agent(s) until symptoms resolve. Severe bleeding resulting in hypotension secondary to hypovolemia may require blood transfusion.

CONCLUSIONS

The AHA and ACC published evidence-based practice guidelines for the treatment of patients with STE and NSTE ACS. Mainstays of therapy include risk stratification, primary PCI for STE MI, early angiography and revascularization with either PCI or CABG for patients with NSTE ACS at high risk of MI and death. Pharmacotherapy for acute treatment includes sublingual NTG, antiplatelets, and anticoagulants. Routine pharmacotherapy for secondary prevention of recurrent ACS, MI, and CHD death includes aspirin, a thienopyridine, statin, β-blocker and either an ACE inhibitor or an ARB. Ensuring selection of evidence-based therapies for all patients without contraindications results in lower mortality. Encouraging adherence and persistence of pharmacotherapy is also important role for pharmacists.

ABBREVIATIONS

ACC: American College of Cardiology

ACE: angiotensin-converting enzyme

ACS: acute coronary syndrome

ACT: activated clotting time

ACTION: Acute Coronary Treatment and Interventions Network

ACUITY: Acute Catheterization and Urgent Intervention Triage Strategy

ADP: adenosine diphosphate

AHA: American Heart Association

aPTT: activated partial thromboplastin time

ARB: angiotensin receptor blocker

TABLE 24-6 Therapeutic Drug Monitoring for Adverse Effects of Pharmacotherapy for Acute Coronary Syndromes

Drug	Adverse Effects	Monitoring
Aspirin	Dyspepsia, bleeding, gastritis	Clinical signs of bleeding,[a] gastrointestinal upset; baseline CBC and platelet count; CBC platelet count every 6 months
Clopidogrel and prasugrel	Bleeding, diarrhea, rash, TTP (rare)	Clinical signs of bleeding[a]; baseline CBC and platelet count; CBC and platelet count every 6 months following hospital discharge
Unfractionated heparin	Bleeding, heparin-induced thrombocytopenia	Clinical signs of bleeding[a]; baseline aPTT, INR, CBC and platelet count; aPTT every 6 hours until target then every 24 hours; daily CBC; platelet count every 2–3 days from day 4 to 14 until heparin is stopped (minimum, preferably every day)
Enoxaparin	Bleeding, heparin- induced thrombocytopenia	Clinical signs of bleeding[a]; baseline SCr, aPTT, INR, CBC and platelet count; daily CBC, no routine platelet count monitoring unless recent UFH (less than 100 days) then baseline and within 24 hours; daily CBC and SCr
Fondaparinux	Bleeding	Clinical signs of bleeding[a]; baseline SCr, aPTT, INR, CBC and platelet count; daily CBC and SCr
Bivalirudin	Bleeding	Clinical signs of bleeding[a]; baseline SCr, aPTT, INR, CBC and platelet count; daily CBC and SCr
Fibrinolytics	Bleeding, especially intracranial hemorrhage	Clinical signs of bleeding[a]; baseline aPTT, INR, CBC and platelet count; mental status every 2 hours for signs of intracranial hemorrhage; daily CBC
Glycoprotein IIb/IIIa receptor blockers	Bleeding, acute profound thrombocytopenia	Clinical signs of bleeding[a]; baseline SCr (for eptifibatide and tirofiban), CBC, and platelet count; platelet count at 4 hours after initiation; daily CBC (and SCr for eptifibatide and tirofiban)
Intravenous nitrates	Hypotension, flushing, headache, tachycardia	BP and HR every 2 hours
β-Blockers	Hypotension, bradycardia, heart block, bronchospasm, acute heart failure, fatigue, depression, sexual dysfunction	BP, RR, HR, 12-lead ECG and clinical signs of heart failure every 5 minutes during bolus intravenous dosing; BP, RR, HR, and clinical signs of heart failure every shift during oral administration during hospitalization, then BP and HR every 6 months following hospital discharge
Diltiazem and verapamil	Hypotension, bradycardia, heart block, heart failure, gingival hyperplasia	BP and HR every shift during oral administration during hospitalization then every 6 months following hospital discharge; dental exam and teeth cleaning every 6 months
Amlodipine	Hypotension, dependent peripheral edema, gingival hyperplasia	BP every shift during oral administration during hospitalization, then every 6 months following hospital discharge; dental exam and teeth cleaning every 6 months
Angiotensin-converting enzyme (ACE) inhibitors and angiotensin receptor blockers (ARBs)	Hypotension, cough (with ACE inhibitors), hyperkalemia, prerenal azotemia, acute renal failure, angioedema (ACE inhibitors more so than ARBs)	BP every 2 hours × 3 for first dose, then every shift during oral administration during hospitalization, then once every 6 months following hospital discharge; baseline SCr and potassium; daily SCr and potassium while hospitalized then every 6 months (or 1–2 weeks after each outpatient dose titration); closer monitoring required in selected patients using spironolactone or eplerenone or if renal insufficiency; counsel patient on throat, tongue, and facial swelling
Aldosterone antagonists	Hypotension, hyperkalemia	BP and HR every shift during oral administration during hospitalization, then once every 6 months; baseline SCr and serum potassium concentration; SCr and potassium at 48 hours, at 7 days, then monthly for 3 months, then every 3 months thereafter following hospital discharge
Warfarin	Bleeding, skin necrosis	Clinical signs of bleeding[a]; baseline CBC and platelet count; CBC and platelet count every 6 months following hospital discharge; baseline aPTT and INR; daily INR until two consecutive INRs are within the target range then once weekly × 2 weeks, then every month; See Chapter 26 for patient counseling points
Morphine	Hypotension, respiratory depression	BP and RR 5 minutes after each bolus dose
Statins	Gastrointestinal upset, myopathy, hepatotoxicity	Liver function tests at baseline, at 6 weeks following initiation, and after titration to highest dose, then annually thereafter; counsel patient on myalgia; consider creatinine kinase at baseline if adding a fibrate or niacin

[a]Clinical signs of bleeding include bloody stools, melena, hematuria, hematemesis, bruising, and oozing from arterial or venous puncture sites.

ACE, angiotensin-converting enzyme; aPTT, activated partial thromboplastin time; ARB, angiotensin receptor blocker; BP, blood pressure; CBC, complete blood count; ECG, electrocardiogram; HR, heart rate; INR, International Normalized Ratio; RR, respiratory rate; SCr, serum creatinine, TTP, thrombotic thrombocytopenic purpura.

AV: atrioventricular

CABG: coronary artery bypass graft

CAD: coronary artery disease

CBC: complete blood count

CHD: coronary heart disease

CK: creatine kinase

CK-MB: creatine kinase myocardial band

CREDO: Clopidogrel for the Reduction of Events During Observation

CURE: Clopidogrel in Unstable Angina to Prevent Recurrent Events

CVD: cardiovascular disease

DHA: docosahexaenoic acid

ECG: electrocardiogram

EPA: eicosapentaenoic acid

EPHESUS: Eplerenone Post-Acute Myocardial Infarction Heart Failure Efficacy and Survival Study

ExTRACT: Enoxaparin and Thrombolysis Reperfusion for Acute Myocardial Infarction Treatment

GP: glycoprotein

GRACE: Global Registry of Acute Coronary Events

GWTG: Get with the Guidelines

HORIZONS-AMI: Harmonizing Outcomes with Revascularization and Stents in Acute Myocardial Infarction

ICD: implantable cardioverter defibrillator

ICH: intracranial hemorrhage

INR: international normalized ratio

ISIS-2: Second International Study of Infarct Survival

IV: intravenous

LDL: low-density lipoprotein

LMWH: low-molecular-weight heparin

LV: left ventricular

LVEF: left ventricular ejection fraction

MADIT: Multicenter Automatic Defibrillator Implantation Trial

MB: myocardial band

MI: myocardial infarction

NCDR: National Cardiovascular Data Registry

NCEP: National Cholesterol Education Program

NICE-SUGAR: Normoglycemia in Intensive Care Evaluation—Survival Using Glucose Algorithm Regulation

NNH: number need to harm

NNT: number needed to treat

NSTE: non-ST-segment elevation

NTG: nitroglycerin

NYHA: New York Heart Association

OASIS: Organization for the Assessment of Strategies for Ischemic Syndromes

OAT: Occluded Artery Trial

PCI: percutaneous coronary intervention

RALES: Randomized Aldactone Evaluation Study

SL: sublingual

STE: ST-segment elevation

TIMI: Thrombolysis in Myocardial Infarction

TRITON: Trial to Assess Improvement in Therapeutic Outcomes by Optimizing Platelet Inhibition with Prasugrel

TXA_2: thromboxane A_2

UA: unstable angina

UFH: unfractionated heparin

REFERENCES

1. Lloyd-Jones D, Adams RJ, Brown TM, et al. Executive summary: Heart disease and stroke statistics—2010 update: A report from the American Heart Association. Circulation 2010;121:948–954.

2. Anderson JL, Adams CD, Antman EM, et al. ACC/AHA 2007 guidelines for the management of patients with unstable angina/non ST-elevation myocardial infarction: A report of the American College of Cardiology/American Heart Association Task Force on Practice Guidelines (Writing Committee to Revise the 2002 Guidelines for the Management of Patients With Unstable Angina/Non ST-Elevation Myocardial Infarction). Developed in collaboration with the American College of Emergency Physicians, the Society for Cardiovascular Angiography and Interventions, and the Society of Thoracic Surgeons. Endorsed by the American Association of Cardiovascular and Pulmonary Rehabilitation and the Society for Academic Emergency Medicine. Circulation 2007;116:803–877.

3. Antman EM, Hand M, Armstrong PW, et al. 2007 Focused Update of the ACC/AHA 2004 Guidelines for the Management of Patients with ST-Elevation Myocardial Infarction: A report of the American College of Cardiology/American Heart Association Task Force on Practice Guidelines. Circulation. 2008;117:296–329.

4. King SB 3rd, Smith SC Jr, Hirshfeld JW Jr, et al. 2007 Focused Update of the ACC/AHA/SCAI 2005 guideline Update for Percutaneous Coronary Intervention: A report of the American College of Cardiology/American Heart Association Task Force on Practice Guidelines: 2007 Writing Group to Review New Evidence and Update the ACC/AHA/SCAI 2005 Guideline Update for Percutaneous Coronary Intervention, Writing on Behalf of the 2005 Writing Committee. Circulation 2008;117:261–295.

5. Kushner FG, Hand M, Smith SC Jr, et al. 2009 Focused Updates: ACC/AHA Guidelines for the Management of Patients with ST-Elevation Myocardial Infarction (updating the 2004 Guideline and 2007 Focused Update) and ACC/AHA/SCAI Guidelines on Percutaneous Coronary Intervention (updating the 2005 Guideline and 2007 Focused Update): A report of the American College of Cardiology Foundation/American Heart Association Task Force on Practice Guidelines. Circulation 2009;120:2271–2306.

6. Antman EM, Anbe DT, Armstrong PW, et al. ACC/AHA Guidelines for the Management of Patients with ST-Elevation Myocardial Infarction: Executive summary. A report of the American College of Cardiology/American Heart Association Task Force on Practice Guidelines (Committee to revise the 1999 Guidelines for the Management of Patients with Acute Myocardial Infarction). Circulation 2004;110:588–636.

7. Centers for Disease Control: National Health Statistics Report: National Hospital Ambulatory Medical Care Survey: 2006 Emergency Department Summary, http://www.cdc.gov/nchs/data/nhsr/nhsr007.pdf.

8. Fox KAA, Steg PG, Eagle KA, et la. Decline in rates of death and heart failure in acute coronary syndromes, 1999–2006. JAMA 2007;297:1892–1900.

9. Gibson CM, Pride YB, Frederick PD, et al. Trends in reperfusion strategies, door-to-needle and door-to-balloon times, and in-hospital mortality among patients with ST-segment elevation myocardial infarction enrolled in the National Registry of Myocardial Infarction from 1990 to 2006. Am Heart J 2008;156:1035–1044.

10. Gibson CM. NRMI and current treatment patterns for ST-elevation myocardial infarction. Am Heart J 2004;148(5 suppl):S29–S33.

11. Fuster V, Moreno PR, Fayad ZA, et al. Atherothrombosis and high-risk plaque: Part I: Evolving concepts. J Am Coll Cardiol. 2005;46:937–954.

12. Spinler SA. Evolution of antithrombotic therapy used in acute coronary syndromes. In: Richardson MM, Chessman KH, Chant C, et al, eds. Pharmacotherapy self-assessment program, Book 1 Cardiology, 7th ed. Lenexa, KS: American College of Clinical Pharmacy; 2010:97–124.

13. Spinler SA. Acute coronary syndromes. In: Dunsworth TS, Richardson MM, Cheng JWM, et al, eds. Pharmacotherapy self-assessment program Book 1 Cardiology, 6th ed. Kansas City, KS: American College of Clinical Pharmacy; 2007:59–83.

14. Goodman SG, Huang W, Yan AT, et al. The expanded Global Registry of Acute Coronary Events: Baseline characteristics, management practices and outcomes of patients with acute coronary syndromes. Am Heart J 2009;158:193–205.e5.

15. Ruberg FL, Leopold JA, Loscalzo J. Atherothrombosis: Plaque instability and thrombogenesis. Prog Cardiovasc Dis 2003;44:381–394.

16. St John Sutton M, Ferrari VA. Prevention of left ventricular remodeling after myocardial infarction. Curr Treat Options Cardiovasc Med 2002;4:97–108.

17. Opie LH, Commerford PJ, Gersh BJ, Pfeffer MA. Controversies in ventricular remodeling. Lancet 2006;367:356–67.

18. Mann DL. Mechanisms and models in heart failure: A combinatorial approach. Circulation 1999;100:999–1008.

19. Lavie CJ, Gersh BJ. Mechanical and electrical complications of acute myocardial infarction. Mayo Clin Proc 1990;65:709–730. Erratum in Mayo Clin Proc 1990;65:1032.

20. Zheng ZJ, Croft JB, Giles WH, et al. Sudden cardiac death in the United States, 1989 to 1998. Circulation 2001;104:2158–63.

21. Rogers WJ, Frederick PD, Stoehr E, et al. Trends in presenting characteristics and hospital mortality among patients with ST elevation and non-ST-elevation myocardial infarction in the National

Registry of Myocardial Infarction from 1990–2006. Am Heart J 2008;156:1026–1034.

22. Thygesen K, Alpert JS, White HD, et al. Universal definition of myocardial infarction. Circulation 2007;116:2634–2653.

23. Krumholz HM, Anderson JL, Brooks NH, et al. ACC/AHA clinical performance measures for adults with ST-elevation and non-ST-elevation myocardial infarction: A report of the American College of Cardiology/American Heart Association Task Force on Performance Measures (Writing Committee to Develop Performance Measures on ST-Elevation and Non-ST-Elevation Myocardial Infarction). J Am Coll Cardiol 2006;47(1):236–265.

24. Acute myocardial infarction core measure set. The Joint Commission, *http://www.jointcommission.org/PerformanceMeasurement/ PerformanceMeasurement/Acute+Myocardial+Infarction+Core+Meas ure+Set.htm.*

25. Fibrinolytic Therapy Trialists' (FTT) Collaborative Group. Indications for fibrinolytic therapy in suspected myocardial infarction: Collaborative overview of early mortality and major morbidity results from all randomized trials of more than 1000 patients. Lancet 1994;343:311–322.

26. Rathore SS, Curtis JP, Chen J, et al. Association of door-to-balloon time and mortality in patients admitted to hospital with ST elevation myocardial infarction : national cohort study. BMJ 2009;338:b1807. doi: 10.1136/bmj.b1807.

27. Jacobs A. Regionalized care for patients with ST-elevation myocardial infarction: It's closer than you think. Circulation 2006;113:1159–1161.

28. Cohen M, Gensini GF, Maritz F, et al. TETAMI Investigators. Prospective evaluation of clinical outcomes after acute ST-elevation myocardial infarction in patients who are ineligible for reperfusion therapy: preliminary results from the TETAMI registry and randomized trial. Circulation 2003;108 (16 suppl I): III14–21.

29. Eagle KA, Goodman, SG, Avezum A, et al. Practice variation and missed opportunities for reperfusion in ST-segment-elevation myocardial infarction: findings from the Global Registry of Acute Coronary Events (GRACE). Lancet 2002;359:373–377.

30. Svilaas T, Zijlstra F. The benefit of an invasive approach in thrombolysis-ineligible patients with acute myocardial infarction. Am J Med 2005;118:123–125.

31. Steg PG, Goldberg RJ, Gore JM, et al. Baseline characteristics, management practices, and in-hospital outcomes of patients hospitalized with acute coronary syndromes in the Global Registry of Acute Coronary Events (GRACE). Am J Cardiol 2002;90:358–363.

32. Peterson ED, Roe MT, Muglund J, et al. Association between hospital process performance and outcomes among patients with acute coronary syndromes. JAMA 2006;295:1912–1920.

33. Eagle KA, Montoye CK, Riba AL, et al. Guideline-based standardized care is associated with substantially lower mortality in Medicare patients with acute myocardial infarction: the American College of Cardiology's Guidelines Applied in Practice (GAP) Projects in Michigan. J Am Coll Cardiol 2005;46:1242–1248.

34. Heidenreich PA, Lewis WR, LaBresh KA, et al. Hospital performance recognition with the Get with the Guidelines Program and mortality for acute myocardial infarction and heart failure. Am Heart J 2009;158:546–553.

35. Antman EM, Cohen M, Bernink PJ, et al. The TIMI risk score for unstable angina/non-ST-segment-elevation MI: A method for prognostication and therapeutic decision-making. JAMA 2000;284:835–842.

36. Pieper KS, Gore JM, FitzGerald G, et al. Validity of a risk-prediction tool for hospital mortality: the Global Registry of Acute Coronary Events. Am Heart J 2009;157:1097–1105.

37. Grace Risk Model Calculator, *http://www.outcomes-umassmed.org/ externalwindow.cfm?URL=http://www.outcomes.org/grace/acs_risk/ acs_risk.html&Link=http://www.outcomes-umassmed.org/grace/acs_ risk.cfm&DeptName=Center%20for%20Outcomes%20Research.*

38. Huynh T, Perron S, O'Loughlin J, et al. Comparison of primary percutaneous coronary intervention and fibrinolytic therapy in ST-segment-elevation myocardial infarction: Bayesian hierarchical meta-analyses of randomized controlled trials and observational studies. Circulation 2009;119:3101–3109.

39. Bradley EH, Nallamothu BK, Herrin J, et al. National efforts to improve door-to-balloon time. J Am Coll Cardiol 2009;54:2423–2429.

40. Gershlick AH, Stephens-Lloyd A, Hughes S, et al. Rescue angioplasty after failed thrombolytic therapy for acute myocardial infarction. N Engl J Med 2005;353:2758–2768.

41. Hochman JS, Lamas GA, Buller CE et al. Coronary intervention for persistent occlusion after myocardial infarction. N Engl J Med 2006;355:2395–2407.

42. Hoenig MR, Aroney CN, Scott IA. Early invasive versus conservative strategies for unstable angina and non-ST elevation myocardial infarction in the stent era. Corchrane Database Syst rev 2010;Mar 17;3:CD004815.

43. Mahoney M, Jurkovitz CT, Chu H, et al. Cost and cost-effectiveness of an early invasive vs conservative strategy for the treatment of unstable angina and non-ST-segment elevation myocardial infarction. JAMA 2002;288:1851–8185.

44. Epstein AE, DiMarco JP, Ellenbogen KA, et al. ACC/AHA/HRS 2008 Guidelines for Device-Based Therapy of Cardiac Rhythm Abnormalities: A report of the American College of Cardiology/ American Heart Association Task Force on Practice Guidelines (Writing Committee to Revise the ACC/AHA/NASPE 2002 Guideline Update for Implantation of Cardiac Pacemakers and Antiarrhythmia Devices) developed in collaboration with the American Association for Thoracic Surgery and Society of Thoracic Surgeons. J Am Coll Cardiol 2008;51:e1–e62.

45. Moss AJ, Zareba W, Hall WJ. Prophylactic implantation of a defibrillator in patients with myocardial infarction and reduced ejection fraction. N Engl J Med 2002;346:877–883.

46. Bertrand ME, Simoons ML, Fox KAA. Management of acute coronary syndromes in patients presenting without persistent ST-segment elevation. The Task Force on the Management of Acute Coronary Syndromes of the European Society of Cardiology. Eur Heart J 2002;23:1809–1840.

47. Meine TJ, Roe MT, Chen AY, et al. Association of intravenous morphine use and outcomes in acute coronary syndromes: results from the CRUSADE Quality Improvement Initiative. Am Heart J. 2005;149:1043–1049.

48. Alexander KP, Newby K, Armstrong PW, et al. Acute coronary syndromes in the elderly, Part II: ST-segment-elevation myocardial infarction. A scientific statement for healthcare professionals from the American Heart Association Council on Clinical Cardiology. Circulation 2007;115:2570–2589.

49. The Global Use of Strategies to Open Occluded Coronary Arteries (GUSTO) Investigators. An international randomized trial comparing four thrombolytic strategies for acute myocardial infarction. N Engl J Med 1993;329:673–682.

50. The Global Use of Strategies to Open Occluded Coronary Arteries (GUSTO III) Investigators. A comparison of reteplase with alteplase for acute myocardial infarction. N Engl J Med 1997;337:1118–1123.

51. Assessment of the Safety and Efficacy of a New Thrombolytic (ASSENT-2) Investigators. Single-bolus tenecteplase compared with front-loaded alteplase in acute myocardial infarction: The ASSENT-2 double-blind, randomized trial. Lancet 2001;354:716–722.

52. Awtry EH, Loscalzo J. Aspirin. Circulation 2000;101:1206–1218.

53. ISIS-2 (Second International Study of Infarct Survival) Collaborative Group. Randomised trial of intravenous streptokinase, oral aspirin, both, or neither among 17,187 cases of suspected acute myocardial infarction: ISIS-2. Lancet 1988;2:349–360.

54. Campbell CL, Smyth S, Montalescot G, Steinhubl SR. Aspirin dose for the prevention of cardiovascular disease. JAMA 2007;297:2018–2024.

55. Antiplatelet Trialists' Collaboration. Collaborative meta-analysis of randomised trials of antiplatelet therapy for prevention of death, myocardial infarction, and stroke in high risk patients. Br Med J 2002;324:71–86.

56. Serebruany VL, Steinhubl SR, Berger PB, et al. Analysis of risk of bleeding complications after different doses of aspirin in 193,036 patients enrolled in 31 randomized controlled trials. Am J Cardiol 2005;95:1218–1222.

57. Bertrand ME, Rupprecht HJ, Urban P, et al. Double-blind study of the safety of clopidogrel with and without a loading dose in combination with aspirin compared with ticlopidine in combination with aspirin

after coronary stenting: the clopidogrel aspirin stent international cooperative study (CLASSICS). Circulation 2000;102:624–629.

58. Plavix (clopidogrel) prescribing information, *http://products.sanofi-aventis.us/PLAVIX/PLAVIX.html.*

59. Effient (prasugrel) prescribing information, *http://pi.lilly.com/us/effient.pdf.*

60. Wiviott SD, Trenk D, Frelinger AL, et al. Prasugrel compared with high loading- and maintenance-dose clopidogrel in patients with planned percutaneous coronary intervention: the Prasugrel in Comparison to Clopidogrel for Inhibition of Platelet Activation and Aggregation-Thrombolysis in Myocardial Infarction 44 trial. Circulation 2007;116:2923–2932.

61. Einstein EL, Anstrom KJ, Kong DF, et al. Clopidogrel use and long-term clinical outcomes after drug-eluting stent implantation. JAMA 2007;297:159–168.

62. Wiviott SD, Braunwald E, McCabe CH, et al. Prasugrel versus clopidogrel in patients with acute coronary syndromes. N Engl J Med 2007;357;2001–2015.

63. Montalescot G, Wiviott SD, Braunwald E, et al. Prasugrel compared with clopidogrel in patients undergoing percutaneous coronary intervention for ST-elevation myocardial infarction (TRITON-TIMI 38): Double-blind, randomised controlled trial. Lancet 2009;373:723–731.

64. Wiviott SD, Braunwald E, Angiolillo DJ, et al. Greater clinical benefit of more intensive oral antiplatelet therapy with prasugrel in patients with diabetes mellitus in the trial to assess improvement in therapeutic outcomes by optimizing platelet inhibition with prasugrel-Thrombolysis in Myocardial Infarction 38. Circulation 2008;118:1626–1636.

65. Dobesh P. Clopidogrel versus prasugrel: Times are changing, but not for everyone. Pharmacotherapy 2009;29:1393–1396.

66. Mega JL Close SL, Wiviott SD, et al. Cytochrome p-450 polymorphisms and response to clopidogrel. N Engl J Med 2009;360:354–362.

67. Ferreiro JL, Angiolillo DJ. Clopidogrel response variability: current status and future directions. Thromb Haemost. 2009;102:7–14.

68. Mega JL, Close SL, Wiviott SD, et al. Cytochrome P450 genetic polymorphisms and the response to prasugrel: Relationship to pharmacokinetic, pharmacodynamic, and clinical outcomes. Circulation 2008; Circulation 2009;119:2553–2560.

69. Pena A, Collet JP, Hulot JS, et al. Can we override clopidogrel resistance? Circulation 2009;119:2854–2857.

70. Chen ZM, Jiang XL, Chen YP, et al. Addition of clopidogrel to aspirin in 45,852 patients with acute myocardial infarction: randomised placebo-controlled trial. Lancet 2005;366:1607–1621.

71. Sabatine MS, Cannon CP, Gibson CM, et al. Addition of clopidogrel to aspirin and fibrinolytic therapy for myocardial infarction with ST-segment elevation. N Engl J Med 2005;352:1179–1189.

72. Grines CL, Bonow RO, Casey DE, et al. Prevention of premature discontinuation of dual antiplatelet therapy in patients with coronary artery stents: A science advisory from the American Heart Association, American College of Cardiology, Society for Cardiovascular Angiography and Interventions, American College of Surgeons, and American Dental Association, with representation from the American College of Physicians. J Am Dent Assoc 2007;138:652–655.

73. De Luca G, Suryapranata H, Stone GW, et al. Abciximab as adjunctive therapy to reperfusion in acute ST-segment elevation myocardial infarction: A meta-analysis of randomized trials. JAMA 2005;293:1759–1765.

74. Stone GW, McLaurin BT, Cox DA, et al. Bivalirudin for patients with acute coronary syndromes. N Engl J Med 2006;355:2203–2216.

75. The Assessment of the Safety and Efficacy of a New Thrombolytic Regimen (ASSENT) 3 Investigators. Efficacy and safety of tenecteplase in combination with enoxaparin, abciximab, or unfractionated heparin: The ASSENT-3 randomised trial in acute myocardial infarction. Lancet 2001;358:605–613.

76. Dasgupta H, Blankenship JC, Wood C, et al. Thrombocytopenia complicating treatment with intravenous glycoprotein IIb/IIIa receptor inhibitors: A pooled analysis. Am Heart J 2000;140:206–211.

77. Mehran R, Lansky AJ, Witzenbichler B, et al. Bivalirudin in patients undergoing primary angioplasty for acute myocardial infarction (HORIZONS-AMI): 1-year results of a randomized controlled trial. Lancet 2009;374:1149–1159.

78. Antman EM, Morrow DA, McCabe CH, et al. Enoxaparin versus unfractionated heparin with fibrinolysis for ST-elevation myocardial infarction. N Engl J Med 2006;354:1477–1488.

79. White HD, Braunwald E, Murphy SA, et al. Enoxaparin vs unfractionated heparin with fibrinolysis for ST-elevation myocardial infarction in elderly and younger patients: results from ExTRACT-TIMI 25. Eur Heart J 2007;28:1066–1071.

80. Peters RJ, Joyner C, Bassand JP et al. The role of fondaparinux as an adjunct to thrombolytic therapy in acute myocardial infarction: A subgroup analysis of the OASIS-6 trial. Eur Heart J 2008;29(3):324–331.

81. Yusuf S, Mehta SR, Xie C, et al. Effects of reviparin, a low-molecular-weight heparin, on mortality, reinfarction, and strokes in patients with acute myocardial infarction presenting with ST-segment elevation JAMA 2005;293(4):427–435.

82. Eikelboom JW, Quinlan DJ, Mehta SR, et al. Unfractionated and low-molecular-weight heparin as adjuncts to Thrombolysis in aspirin-treated patients with ST-Elevation acute myocardial infarction: A meta-analysis of the randomized trials. Circulation 2005;112:3855–3867.

83. Montalescot G, Ellis SG, de Belder MA, et al. Enoxaparin in primary and facilitated percutaneous coronary intervention A formal prospective nonrandomized substudy of the FINESSE trial (Facilitated INtervention with Enhanced Reperfusion Speed to Stop Events). JACC Cardiovasc Interv 2010;3:203–212.

84. Yusuf S, Mehta SR, Chrolavicius S, et al. Effects of fondaparinux on mortality and reinfarction in patients with acute ST-segment elevation myocardial infarction: the OASIS-6 randomized trial. JAMA 2006;295:1519–1530.

85. Granger CB, Hirsh J, Califf RM, et al. Activated partial thromboplastin time and outcome after thrombolytic therapy for acute myocardial infarction. Circulation 1996;93:870–878.

86. Gruppo Italioano per Lo Studio della Sopravvivenza Nell'infarcto Myiocardio. GISSI-3: Effects of lisinopril and transdermal glyceryl trinitrate singly and together on 6-week mortality and ventricular function after acute myocardial infarction. Lancet 1994;343:1115–1122.

87. ISIS-4 (Fourth International Study of Infarct Survival Collaborative Group). ISIS-4: A randomised factorial trial assessing early oral captopril, oral mononitrate, and intravenous magnesium sulphate in 58,050 patients with suspected acute myocardial infarction. Lancet 1995;345:669–685.

88. Gheorghiade M, Goldstein S. β-Blockers in the post-myocardial infarction patient. Circulation 2002;106:394–398.

89. First International Study of Infarct Survival Collaborative Group. Randomised trial of intravenous atenolol among 16,027 cases of suspected acute myocardial infarction: ISIS-1. Lancet 1986;2:57–661.

90. Metoprolol in acute myocardial infarction (MIAMI). A randomised, placebo-controlled international trial. Eur Heart J 1985;6:199–226.

91. Hjalmarson A, Herlitz J, Homberg S, et al. The Goteborg metoprolol trial. Effects on mortality and morbidity in acute myocardial infarction. Circulation. 1983 Jun;67(6 Pt 2):I26-I32.

92. Goldstein S. Propranolol therapy in patients with acute myocardial infarction: The Beta-Blocker Heart Attack Trial. Circulation 1983;67:I53-I57.

93. Chen Z, Pan HC, Chen YP, et al. Early intravenous then oral metoprolol in 45,852 patients with acute myocardial infarction: Randomised placebo-controlled trial. Lancet 2005;366:1622–1632.

94. Abernethy DR, Schwartz JB. Calcium-antagonist drugs. N Engl J Med 1999;341:1447–1457.

95. Boden WE, van Gilst WH, Scheldewaert RG, et al. Diltiazem in acute myocardial infarction treated with thrombolytic agents: A randomised, placebo-controlled trial. Incomplete Infarction Trial of European Research Collaborators Evaluating Prognosis post-Thrombolysis (INTERCEPT). Lancet 2000;355:1751–1756.

96. Pitt B, Byington RP, Furberg CD, et al. Effect of amlodipine on the progression of atherosclerosis and the occurrence of clinical events. PREVENT Investigators. Circulation 2000;102:1503–1510.

97. Packer M, O'Connor CM, Ghali JK, et al. Effect of amlodipine on morbidity and mortality in severe chronic heart failure: Prospective Randomized Amlodipine Survival Evaluation Study Group. N Engl J Med 1996;335:1107–1114.

98. McCord J, Jneid H, Hollander JE, Management of cocaine-associated chest pain and myocardial infarction: A scientific statement from

the American Heart Association Acute Cardiac Care Committee of the Council on Clinical Cardiology. Circulation. 2008;117:1897–907

99. Yusuf S, Zhao F, Meta SR, et al. Effects of clopidogrel in addition to aspirin in patients with acute coronary syndromes without ST-segment elevation. N Engl J Med 2001;345:494–502.

100. Mehta SR, Yusuf S, Peters RJ, et al. Effects of pretreatment with clopidogrel and aspirin followed by long-term therapy in patients undergoing percutaneous coronary intervention: The PCI-CURE study. Lancet 2001;358:527–533.

101. Steinhubl SR, Berger PB, Mann JT 3d, et al: Early and sustained dual oral antiplatelet therapy following percutaneous coronary intervention: A randomized, controlled trial. JAMA 2002;288:2411–2420.

102. Peters RJ, Mehta SR, Fox KA, et al. Effects of aspirin dose when used alone or in combination with clopidogrel in patients with acute coronary syndromes: Observations from the clopidogrel in unstable angina to prevent recurrent events (CURE) study. Circulation 2003;108:1682–1687.

103. Pannu R, Andraws R. Effects of glycoprotein IIb/IIIa inhibitors in patients undergoing percutaneous coronary intervention after pretreatment with clopidogrel: A meta-analysis of randomized trials. Crit Pathw Cardiol 2008;7:5–10.

104. Boersma E, Harrington RA, Moliterno DJ et al. Platelet glycoprotein IIb/IIIa inhibitors in acute coronary syndromes: A meta-analysis of all major randomised clinical trials. Lancet 2002;359:189–198. Erratum in: Lancet 2002;359:2120.

105. Roffi M, Chew DP, Mukherjee D, et al. Platelet glycoprotein IIb/IIIa inhibitors in acute coronary syndromes: A meta-analysis of all major randomised clinical trials. Eur Heart J 2002;23:1408–1411.

106. Giugliano RP, White JA, Bode C, et al. Early versus delayed, provisional eptifibatide in acute coronary syndromes. N Engl J Med. 2009 May 21;360:2176–2190.

107. The PURSUIT Trial Investigators. Inhibition of platelet glycoprotein IIb/IIIa with eptifibatide in patients with acute coronary syndromes. N Engl J Med 1998;339:436–443.

108. Platelet Receptor Inhibition in Ischemic Syndrome Management in Patients Limited by Unstable Signs and Symptoms (PRISM-PLUS) Study Investigators. Inhibition of the platelet glycoprotein IIb/IIIa receptor with tirofiban in unstable angina and non-Q-wave myocardial infarction. N Engl J Med 1998;338:1488–1497.

109. Alexander KP, Chen AY, Newby K, et al. Sex differences in major bleeding with GP IIb/IIIa inhibitors: Results from the CRUSADE (Can Rapid Risk Stratification of Unstable Angina Patients Suppress Adverse Outcomes with Early Implementation of the ACC/AHA Guidelines) Initiative. Circulation 2006;114:1380–1387.

110. Alexander KP, Chen AY, Roe MT, et al. Excess dosing of antiplatelet and antithrombin agents in the treatment of non-ST-segment elevation acute coronary syndromes. JAMA 2005;294:3108–3116.

111. Oler A, Whooley MA, Oler J. Grady D. Adding heparin to aspirin reduces the incidence of myocardial infarction and death in patients with unstable angina: A meta-analysis. JAMA 1996;276:811–815.

112. Fragmin During Instability in Coronary Artery Disease Study Group. Low-molecular-weight heparin during instability in coronary artery disease. Lancet 1996;347:561–568.

113. Klein W, Buchwald A, Hillis SE, et al. Comparison of low-molecular-weight heparin with unfractionated heparin acutely and with placebo for 6 weeks in the management of unstable coronary artery disease: Fragmin in Unstable Coronary Artery Disease Study (FRIC). Circulation 1997;96:61–68.

114. Antman EM, McCabe CH, Gurfinkle EP, et al. Enoxaparin prevents deaths and cardiac ischemic events in unstable angina/non-Q-wave myocardial infarction: Results of the Thrombolysis in Myocardial Infarction (TIMI 11B) trial. Circulation 1999;100:1593–1601.

115. Cohen M, Demers C, Gurfinkle EP, et al. A comparison of low-molecular-weight heparin with unfractionated heparin for unstable coronary artery disease. N Engl J Med 1997;337:447–452.

116. Ferguson JJ, Califf RM, Antman EM, et al. The Synergy Trial Investigators. Enoxaparin versus unfractionated heparin in high-risk patients with non-ST-segment elevation acute coronary syndromes managed with an intended early invasive strategy. JAMA 2004;292:45–54.

117. Yusuf S, Mehta SR, Chrolavicius S, et al. Comparison of fondaparinux and enoxaparin in acute coronary syndromes. N Engl J Med. 2006 Apr 6;354(14):1464–1476.

118. Nutescu EA, Spinler SA, Wittkowsky A, et al. Low-molecular-weight heparins in renal impairment and obesity: Available evidence and clinical practice recommendations across medical and surgical settings. Ann Pharmacother. 2009;43:1064–1083.

119. ACE/ADA Task Force on Inpatient diabetes. American College of Endocrinology and American Diabetes Association Consensus statement on inpatient diabetes and glycemic control: A call to action. Diabetes Care 2006;29:1955–1962.

120. Finfer S, Chittock DR, Su SY, et al. Intensive versus conventional glucose control in critically ill patients. N Engl J Med. 2009;360:1283–1297.

121. Smith SC, Allen J, Blair SN, et al. AHA/ACC Guidelines for secondary prevention for patients with coronary and other atherosclerotic vascular disease: 2006 update. Endorsed by the National Heart Lung and Blood Institute. J Am Coll Cardiol 2006;47:2130–2139.

122. Davis MM, Taubert K, Benin AL, et al. Influenza vaccination as secondary prevention for cardiovascular disease: A science advisory from the American Heart Association/American College of Cardiology. J Am Coll Cardiol 2006;48:1498–1502.

123. Freemantle N, Cleland J, Young P, et al. β-Blockade after myocardial infarction: Systematic review and meta regression analysis. Br Med J 1999;318:1730–1737.

124. Pedersen TR. Six-year follow-up of the Norwegian Multicenter Study on Timolol after Acute Myocardial Infarction. N Engl J Med 1985;313:1055–1058.

125. Cucherat M, Boissel JP, Leizorovicz A. Persistent reduction of mortality for five years after one year of acebutolol treatment initiated during acute myocardial infarction. The APSI Investigators. Acebutolol et Prevention Secondaire de l'Infarctus. Am J Cardiol 1997;79:587–589.

126. Dargie HJ. Effect of carvedilol on outcome after myocardial infarction in patients with left-ventricular dysfunction: The CAPRICORN randomised trial. Lancet 2001;357:1385–1390.

127. Houghton T, Freemantle N, Cleland JG, et al. Are beta-blockers effective in patients who develop heart failure soon after myocardial infarction? A meta-regression analysis of randomised trials. Eur J Heart Fail 2000;2:333–340.

128. Gibbons RJ, Abrams J, Chatterjee K, et al. ACC/AHA 2002 guideline update for the management of patients with chronic stable angina: Summary article. A report of the American College of Cardiology/American Heart Association Task Force on Practice Guidelines (Committee on the Management of Patients With Chronic Stable Angina). J Am Coll Cardiol 2003;41:159–168.

129. ACE Inhibitor Myocardial Infarction Collaborative Group. Indications for ACE inhibitors in the early treatment of acute myocardial infarction: Systematic overview of individual data from 100,000 patients in randomized trials. Circulation 1998; 97:2202–2212.

130. Flather MD, Yusuf S, Kober L, et al. Long-term ACE inhibitor therapy in patients with heart failure or left ventricular dysfunction: A systematic overview of data from individual patients. ACE Inhibitor Myocardial Infarction Collaborative Group. Lancet 2000;355:1575–1581.

131. Swedberg K, Held P, Kjekshus J, et al. Effects of the early administration of enalapril on mortality in patients with acute myocardial infarction: Results of the Cooperative New Scandinavian Enalapril Survival Study II (CONSENSUS II). N Engl J Med 1992;327:678–684.

132. Buch P, Rasmussen PS, Abildstrom AZ, et al. The long-term impact of the angiotensin-converting enzyme inhibitor trandolapril on mortality and hospital admissions in patients with left ventricular dysfunction after a myocardial infarction: Follow-up to 12 years. Eur Heart J 2005;26:145–152.

133. Saha, SA, Molnar J, Arora RR. Tissue ACE inhibitors for secondary prevention of cardiovascular disease in patients with preserved left ventricular function: A pooled meta-analysis of randomized placebo-controlled trials. J Cardiovasc Pharmacol 2007;12:192–204.

134. Pfeffer MA, McMurray JJV, Velazquez EJ, et al. Valsartan, captopril, or both in myocardial infarction complicated by heart failure, left ventricular dysfunction, or both. N Engl J Med 2003;349:1893–1906.

135. Granger CB, McMurray JV, Yusuf S, et al., eds. CHARM Investigators and Committees. Effects of candesartan in patients with chronic heart failure and reduced left-ventricular systolic function intolerant to

angiotensin-converting-enzyme inhibitors: CHARM Alternative trial. Lancet 2004;362:772–776.

136. Warner KK, Visconti JA, Tschampel MM. Angiotensin II receptor blockers in patients with ACE inhibitor-induced angioedema. Ann Pharmacother 2000;34:526–528.

137. Zillich AJ, Carter BL. Eplerenone: A novel selective aldosterone blocker. Ann Pharmacother 2002;36:1567–1576.

138. Pitt B, Zannad F, Remme WJ, et al. The effect of spironolactone on morbidity and mortality in patients with severe heart failure. Randomized Aldactone Evaluation Study Investigators. N Engl J Med 1999;341:709–717.

139. Pitt B, Remme W, Zannad F, et al. Eplerenone, a selective aldosterone blocker in patients with left ventricular dysfunction after myocardial infarction. N Engl J Med 2003;348:1309–1321.

140. Executive Summary of the Third Report of the National Cholesterol Education Program (NCEP) Expert Panel on Detection, Evaluation, and Treatment of High Blood Cholesterol in Adults (Adult Treatment Panel III). JAMA 2001;285:2486–2497.

141. Grundy SM, Cleeman JI, Bairey Merz, CN, et al., eds. Coordinating Committee of the National Cholesterol Education Program, Endorsed by the National Heart, Lung, and Blood Institute, American College of Cardiology Foundation, and American Heart Association. Implications of Recent Clinical Trials for the National Cholesterol Education Program Adult Treatment Panel III Guidelines. Circulation 2004;110:227–239.

142. Hulten E, Jackson JL, Douglas K, et al. The effect of early, intensive statin therapy on acute coronary syndrome: A meta-analysis of randomized controlled trials. Arch Intern Med 2006;166:1814–1821.

143. Cannon CP, Braunwald E, McCabe CH, et al. Pravastatin or Atorvastatin Evaluation and Infection Therapy: Thrombolysis in Myocardial Infarction 22 Investigators. Intensive versus moderate lipid lowering with statins after acute coronary syndromes. N Engl J Med 2004;350:1495–1504.

144. Anonymous. MRC/BHF Heart Protection Study of cholesterol lowering with simvastatin in 20,536 high-risk individuals: A randomised placebo-controlled trial. Lancet 2002;360:7–22.

145. Rubins HB, Robins SJ, Collins D, et al. Gemfibrozil for the secondary prevention of coronary heart disease in men with low levels of high-density lipoprotein cholesterol. Veterans Affairs High-Density Lipoprotein Cholesterol Intervention Trial Study Group. N Engl J Med 1999;341:410–418.

146. Keech A, Simes RJ, Barter P, et al. Effects of long-term fenofibrate therapy on cardiovascular events in 9795 people with type 2 diabetes mellitus (the FIELD study): Randomised controlled trial. Lancet 2005;366:1849–1861.

147. The ACCORD Study Group. Effects of combination lipid therapy in type 2 diabetes mellitus. N Engl J Med. 2010 Mar 18. [Epub ahead of print].

148. Kris-Etherton PM, Harris WS, Appel LJ. Fish consumption, fish oil, omega-3 fatty acids, and cardiovascular disease. Circulation 2002;106:2747–2757.

149. Gruppo Italiano per lo Studio della Sopravvivenza nell'infarcto miocardio. Dietary supplementation with n-3 fatty acids and vitamin E after myocardial infarction: Results of GISSI-Prevenzione trial. Lancet 1999;354:447–455.

150. Bays H. Fish oil composition of Omacor and the GISSI trial. Am J Cardiol 2007;99:1483–1484.

151. Critchley JA, Capewell S. Mortality risk reduction associated with smoking cessation in patients with coronary heart disease: A systematic review. JAMA 2003;290:86–97.

152. Chobanian AV, Bakris GL, Black HR, et al. The seventh report of the Joint National Committee on Prevention, Detection, Evaluation, and Treatment of High Blood Pressure: The JNC 7 report. JAMA 2003;289:2560–2572.

153. Thompson PD, Bucner D, Pina IL, et al. Exercise and physical activity in the prevention and treatment of atherosclerotic cardiovascular disease: A statement from the Council on Clinical Cardiology (Subcommittee on Exercise, Rehabilitation and Prevention) and the Council on Nutrition, Physical Activity, and Metabolism (Subcommittee on Physical Activity). Circulation 2003;107: 3109–3116.

154. Ko DT, Chiu M, Guo H, et al. Patterns of thienopyridine drug therapy after percutaneous coronary interventions with drug-eluting and bare-metal stents. Am Heart J 2009;158:592–598.e1.

155. Jackevicius CA, Li P, Tu JV. Prevalence, predictors, and outcomes of primary nonadherence after myocardial infarction. Circulation 2008;117:1028–1036.

156. Butler J, Arbogast PG, BeLue R, et al. Outpatient adherence to beta-blocker therapy after acute myocardial infarction. J Am Coll Cardiol 2002;6:40:1589–1595.

157. Ho PM, Spertus JA, Masoudi FA, et al. Impact of medication therapy discontinuation on mortality after myocardial infarction. Arch Intern Med 2006;166:1842–1847.

158. Biondi-Zoccai GG, Lotrionte M, Agostoni P, et al. A systematic review and meta-analysis on the hazards of discontinuing or not adhering to aspirin among 50,279 patients at risk for coronary artery disease. Eur Heart J 2006;27:2667–2674.

159. Granger BB, Swedberg K, Ekman I, et al. Adherence to candesartan and placebo and outcomes in chronic heart failure in the CHARM programme: Double-blind, randomised, controlled clinical trial. Lancet 2005;366:1989–1991.

160. Rasmussen JN, Chong A, Alter DA. Relationship between adherence to evidence-based pharmacotherapy and long-term mortality after acute myocardial infarction. JAMA 2007;297:177–186.

161. Spertus JA, Kettelkamp R, Vance C, et al. Prevalence, predictors, and outcomes of premature discontinuation of thienopyridine therapy after drug-eluting stent placement: Results from the PREMIER registry. Circulation 2006;113:2803–2809.

162. Muhlestein JB, Horne BD, Bair TL, et al. Usefulness of in-hospital prescription of statin agents after angiographic diagnosis of coronary artery disease in improving continued compliance and reduced mortality. Am J Cardiol 2001;87:257–261.

163. Jackevicius CA, Mamdani M, Tu JV. Adherence with statin therapy in elderly patients with and without acute coronary syndromes. JAMA 2002;288:462–467.

164. Lachaine J, Rinfret S, Merikle EP, Terride JE. Persistence and adherence to cholesterol lowering agents: Evidence from Regie de l'Assurance Maladie du Quebec data. Am Heart J 2006;152: 164–169.

165. Kulkarni SP, Alexander KP, Lytle B, et al. Long-term adherence with cardiovascular drug regimens. Am Heart J 2006;151:185–191.

166. Blackburn DF, Dobson RT, Blackburn JL, et al. Cardiovascular morbidity associated with nonadherence to statin therapy. Pharmacotherapy 2005;25:1035–1043.

167. Murray MD, Young J, Hoke S, et al. Pharmacist intervention to improve medication adherence in heart failure: A randomized trial. Ann Intern Med 2007;146:714–725.

168. Lee JK, Grace KA, Taylor AJ. Effect of a pharmacy care program on medication adherence and persistence, blood pressure, and low-density lipoprotein cholesterol: A randomized controlled trial. JAMA 2006;296:2563–2571.

169. Mark DB. Medical economics in cardiovascular medicine. In: Topol EJ, Califf RM, Isner J, et al, eds. Textbook of Cardiovascular Medicine. Philadelphia, Lippincott Williams & Wilkins, 2003:957–979.

170. Hlatky MA, Califf RM, Naylor CD, et al. Cost-effectiveness of thrombolytic therapy with tissue plasminogen activator as compared with streptokinase for acute myocardial infarction. N Engl J Med 1996;332:1418–1424.

171. Eccles M, Freemantle N, Mason J, et al. North of England evidence based guideline development project: Guideline on the use of aspirin as secondary prophylaxis for vascular disease in primary care. Br Med J 1998;316:1303–1309.

172. Mark DB, Harrington RA, Lincoff AM, et al. Cost effectiveness of platelet glycoprotein IIb/IIIa inhibition with eptifibatide in patients with non-ST-segment-elevation acute coronary syndromes. Circulation 2000;101:366–371.

173. Phillips KA, Shlipak MG, Coxson P, et al. Health and economic benefits of increased beta-blocker use following myocardial infarction. JAMA 2001;284:2748–2754.

174. McMurray JJ, McGuire A, Davie AP, Hughs D. Cost-effectiveness of different ACE inhibitor treatment scenarios post-myocardial infarction. Eur Heart J 1997;18:1411–1415.

175. Franzosi MG, Maggioni AP, Santoro E. Cost-effective analysis of early lisinopril use with acute myocardial infarction: Results from GISSI-3 trial. Pharmacoeconomics 1998;13:337–346.

176. Weintraub WS, Zhang Z, Mahoney EM, et al. Cost-effectiveness of eplerenone compared with placebo in patients with myocardial infarction complicated by left ventricular dysfunction and heart failure. Circulation 2005;11:1106–1113.

177. Grover SA, Coupal L, Paquet S, Zowall H. Cost-effectiveness of 3-hydroxy-3-methylglutaryl-coenzyme A reductase inhibitors in the secondary prevention of cardiovascular disease: Forecasting the incremental benefits of preventing coronary and cerebrovascular events. Arch Intern Med 1999;159:593–600.

178. Nyman JA, Martinson MS, Nelson D, et al. Cost-effectiveness of gemfibrozil for coronary heart disease patients with low levels of high-density lipoprotein cholesterol: The Department of Veterans Affairs High-Density Lipoprotein Cholesterol Intervention Trial. Arch Intern Med 2002;162:177–182.

179. Franzosi MG, Brunetti M, Marchioli R, et al. Cost-effectiveness analysis of n-3 polyunsaturated fatty acids (PUFA) after myocardial infarction: Results from Gruppo Italiano per lo Studio della Sopravvivenza nell'Infarcto (GISSI)-Prevenzione Trial. Pharmacoeconomics 2001:19:411–420.

180. Mahoney EM, Wang K, Arnold SV, et al. Cost-effectiveness of prasugrel versus clopidogrel in patients with acute coronary syndromes and planned percutaneous coronary intervention: Results from the trial to assess improvement in therapeutic outcomes by optimizing platelet inhibition with Prasugrel-Thrombolysis in Myocardial Infarction TRITON-TIMI 38. Circulation 2010;121:71–79.

CHAPTER

25

The Arrhythmias

CYNTHIA A. SANOSKI AND JERRY L. BAUMAN

KEY CONCEPTS

❶ The use of antiarrhythmic drugs (AADs) in the United States has declined because of major trials that show increased mortality with their use in several clinical situations, the realization of proarrhythmia as a significant side effect, and the advancing technology of nonpharmacologic therapies such as ablation and the implantable cardioverter-defibrillator (ICD).

❷ AADs frequently cause side effects and are complex in their pharmacokinetic characteristics. Close monitoring is required of all of these drugs to assess for adverse effects as well as potential drug interactions.

❸ The most commonly prescribed AAD is now amiodarone. This drug is effective in terminating and preventing a wide variety of symptomatic supraventricular and ventricular arrhythmias. However, because this AAD is plagued by frequent side effects, it requires close monitoring. The most concerning toxicity is pulmonary fibrosis; side effect profiles of the intravenous (IV) (acute, short-term) and oral (chronic, long-term) forms of amiodarone differ substantially.

❹ In patients with artial fibrillation (AF), therapy is traditionally aimed at controlling ventricular rate (digoxin, nondihydropyridine [non-DHP] calcium channel blockers [CCBs], β-blockers), preventing thromboembolic complications (warfarin, aspirin), and restoring and maintaining sinus rhythm (SR) (AADs, direct-current cardioversion [DCC]). Studies show there is no need to aggressively pursue strategies to maintain SR (i.e., long-term AAD therapy); rate control alone (leaving the patient in AF) is often sufficient in patients who can tolerate it. Nonetheless, chronic AAD therapy may still be needed in patients who continue to have symptoms despite adequate ventricular rate control.

❺ Paroxysmal supraventricular tachycardia (PSVT) is usually a result of reentry in or proximal to the atrioventricular (AV) node or AV reentry incorporating an extranodal pathway; common tachycardias can be terminated acutely with AV nodal-blocking drugs such as adenosine, and recurrences can be prevented by ablation with radiofrequency current.

❻ Patients with Wolff-Parkinson-White (WPW) syndrome may have several different tachycardias that are acutely treated by different strategies: orthodromic reentry (adenosine), antidromic reentry (adenosine or procainamide), and AF

Learning objectives, review questions,
and other resources can be found at
www.pharmacotherapyonline.com.

(procainamide or amiodarone). AV nodal-blocking drugs are contraindicated in patients with WPW and AF.

❼ Because of the results of the Cardiac Arrhythmia Suppression Trial (CAST) and other trials, AADs (with the exception of β-blockers) should not be routinely used in patients with prior myocardial infarction (MI) or left ventricular (LV) dysfunction and minor ventricular rhythm disturbances (e.g., premature ventricular complexes [PVCs]).

❽ Patients with hemodynamically significant ventricular tachycardia (VT) or ventricular fibrillation (VF) not associated with an acute MI who are successfully resuscitated (electrical cardioversion, vasopressors, amiodarone) are at high risk for sudden cardiac death (SCD) and should receive an ICD ("secondary prevention").

❾ Implantation of an ICD should be considered for the primary prevention of SCD in certain high-risk patient populations. High-risk patients include those with a history of MI and LV dysfunction (regardless of whether they have inducible sustained ventricular arrhythmias), as well as those with New York Heart Association (NYHA) class II or III heart failure (HF) as a result of either ischemic or nonischemic causes.

❿ Life-threatening ventricular proarrhythmia generally takes two forms: sinusoidal or incessant monomorphic VT (class Ic AADs) and torsades de pointes (TdP) (class Ia or III AADs and many other noncardiac drugs).

The heart has two basic properties, namely an electrical property and a mechanical property. The synchronous interaction between these two properties is complex, precise, and relatively enduring. The study of the electrical properties of the heart has grown at a steady rate, interrupted by periodic salvos of scientific breakthroughs. Einthoven's pioneering work allowed graphic electrical tracings of cardiac rhythm and probably represents the first of these breakthroughs. This discovery of the surface electrocardiogram (ECG) has remained the cornerstone of diagnostic tools for cardiac rhythm disturbances. Since then, intracardiac recordings and programmed cardiac stimulation have advanced our understanding of arrhythmias, and microelectrode, voltage-clamping, and patch-clamping techniques have allowed considerable insight into the electrophysiologic actions and mechanisms of AADs. Certainly, the new era of molecular biology and mapping of the human genome promises even greater insights into mechanisms (and potential therapies) of arrhythmias. Noteworthy in this regard is the discovery of genetic abnormalities in the ion channels that control electrical repolarization (heritable long QT syndrome) or depolarization (Brugada syndrome).

The clinical use of drug therapy started with the use of digitalis and then quinidine. A surge of new agents followed somewhat later in the 1980s. A theme of drug discovery during this decade was initially to find orally absorbed lidocaine congeners (such as mexiletine and tocainide); later, the emphasis was on drugs with extremely potent effects on conduction (i.e., flecainide-like agents). The most recent focus of investigational AADs are the potassium channel blockers, with dronedarone being the most recently approved AAD in the United States in nearly a decade. Previously, there was some expectation that advances in AAD discovery would lead to a highly effective and nontoxic agent that would be effective for a majority of patients (i.e., the so-called magic bullet). Instead, significant problems with drug toxicity and proarrhythmia have resulted in a decline in the overall volume of AAD usage in the United States since 1989. ❶ The other phenomenon that has significantly contributed to the decline in AAD utilization is the development of extremely effective nonpharmacologic therapies. Technical advances have made it possible to permanently interrupt reentry circuits with radiofrequency ablation, which renders long-term AAD use unnecessary in certain arrhythmias. Furthermore, the impressive survival data associated with the use of ICDs for the primary and secondary prevention of SCD has led most clinicians to choose "device" therapy as the first-line treatment for patients who are at high risk for life-threatening ventricular arrhythmias. Both of these nonpharmacologic therapies have become increasingly popular for the management of arrhythmias so that the potential proarrhythmic effects and organ toxicities associated with AADs can be avoided.

This chapter reviews the principles involved in both normal and abnormal cardiac conduction and addresses the pathophysiology and treatment of the more commonly encountered arrhythmias. Certainly, many volumes of complete text could be (and have been) devoted to basic and clinical electrophysiology. Consequently, this chapter briefly addresses those principles necessary for clinicians.

ARRHYTHMOGENESIS

NORMAL CONDUCTION

Electrical activity is initiated by the sinoatrial (SA) node and moves through cardiac tissue by a treelike conduction network. The SA node initiates cardiac rhythm under normal circumstances because this tissue possesses the highest degree of automaticity or rate of spontaneous impulse generation. The degree of automaticity of the SA node is largely influenced by the autonomic nervous system in that both cholinergic and sympathetic innervations control the sinus rate. Most tissues within the conduction system also possess varying degrees of inherent automatic properties. However, the rates of spontaneous impulse generation of these tissues are less than that of the SA node. Thus these latent automatic pacemakers are continuously overdriven by impulses arising from the SA node (primary pacemaker) and do not become clinically apparent.

From the SA node, electrical activity moves in a wave front through an atrial specialized conducting system and eventually gains entrance to the ventricle via the AV node and a large bundle of conducting tissue referred to as the bundle of His. Aside from this AV node–bundle of His pathway, a fibrous AV ring that will not permit electrical stimulation separates the atria and ventricles. The conducting tissues bridging the atria and ventricles are referred to as the junctional areas. Again, this area of tissue (junction) is largely influenced by autonomic input and possesses a relatively high degree of inherent automaticity (about 40 beats/min, less than that of the SA node). From the bundle of His, the cardiac conduction system bifurcates into several (usually three) bundle branches: one right bundle and two left bundles. These bundle branches further arborize into a conduction network referred to as the Purkinje system. The conduction system as a whole innervates the mechanical myocardium and serves to initiate excitation–contraction coupling and the contractile process. After a cell or group of cells within the heart is electrically stimulated, a brief period of time follows in which those cells cannot again be excited. This time period is referred to as the refractory period. As the electrical wavefront moves down the conduction system, the impulse eventually encounters tissue refractory to stimulation (recently excited) and subsequently dies out. The SA node subsequently recovers, fires spontaneously, and begins the process again.

Prior to cellular excitation, an electrical gradient exists between the inside and the outside of the cell membrane. At this time, the cell is polarized. In atrial and ventricular conducting tissue, the intracellular space is approximately 80 to 90 mV negative with respect to the extracellular environment. The electrical gradient just prior to excitation is referred to as the resting membrane potential (RMP) and is the result of differences in ion concentrations between the inside and the outside of the cell. At RMP, the cell is polarized primarily by the action of active membrane ion pumps, the most notable of these being the sodium-potassium pump. For example, this specific pump (in addition to other systems) attempts to maintain the intracellular sodium concentration at 5 to 15 mEq/L and the extracellular sodium concentration at 135 to 142 mEq/L; the intracellular potassium concentration at 135 to 140 mEq/L and the extracellular potassium concentration at 3 to 5 mEq/L. The RMP can be calculated by using the Nernst equation:

$$RMP = 61.5 \log\left(\frac{[K^+] \text{ outside}}{[K^+] \text{ inside}}\right)$$

Electrical stimulation (or depolarization) of the cell will result in changes in membrane potential over time or a characteristic action potential curve (Fig. 25–1). The action potential curve results from the transmembrane movement of specific ions and is divided into different phases. Phase 0 or initial, rapid depolarization of atrial and ventricular tissues is caused by an abrupt increase in the permeability of the membrane to sodium influx. This rapid depolarization more than equilibrates (overshoots) the electrical potential, resulting in a brief initial repolarization or phase 1. Phase 1 (initial depolarization) is caused by a transient and active potassium efflux (i.e., the I_{Kto} current). Calcium begins to move into the intracellular space at about –60 mV (during phase 0), causing a slower depolarization. Calcium influx continues throughout phase 2 of the action potential (plateau phase) and is balanced to some degree by potassium efflux. Calcium entrance (only through L channels in myocardial tissue) distinguishes cardiac conducting cells from nerve tissue and provides the critical ionic link to excitation–contraction coupling and the mechanical properties of the heart as a pump. The membrane remains permeable to potassium efflux during phase 3, resulting in cellular repolarization. Phase 4 of the action potential is the gradual depolarization of the cell and is related to a constant sodium leak into the intracellular space balanced by a decreasing (over time) efflux of potassium. The slope of phase 4 depolarization determines, in large part, the automatic properties of the cell. As the cell is slowly depolarized during phase 4, an abrupt increase in sodium permeability occurs, allowing the rapid cellular depolarization of phase 0. The juncture of phase 4 and phase 0 where rapid sodium influx is initiated is referred to as the threshold potential of the cell. The level of threshold potential also regulates the degree of cellular automaticity.

Not all cells in the cardiac conduction system rely on sodium influx for initial depolarization. Some tissues depolarize in response to a slower inward ionic current caused by calcium influx. These "calcium-dependent" tissues are found primarily in the SA and AV nodes (both L and T channels) and possess distinct conduction properties in comparison to "sodium-dependent" fibers.

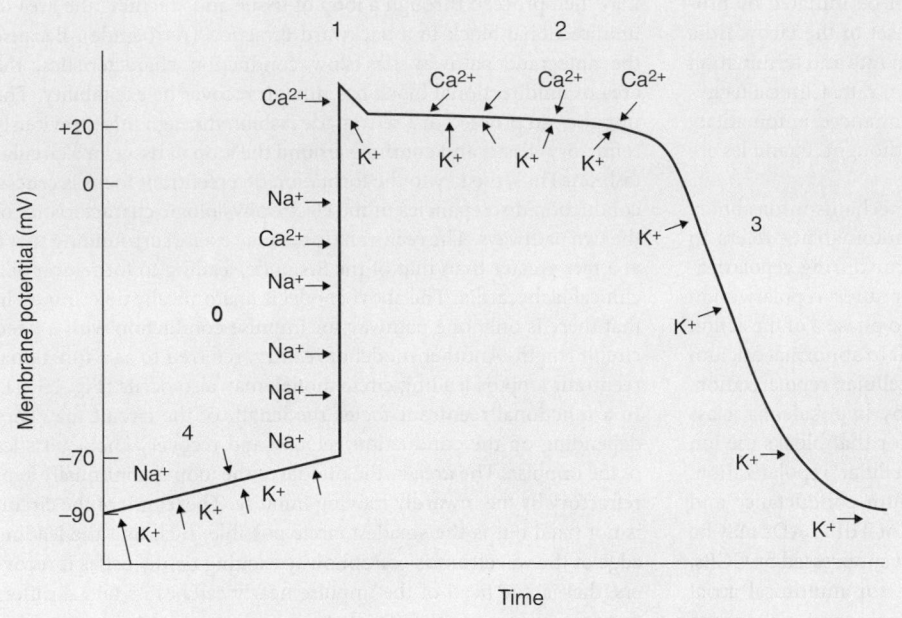

FIGURE 25-1. Purkinje fiber action potential showing specific ion flux responsible for the change in membrane potential. Ions outside of the line (e.g., sodium) move from the extracellular space to the intracellular space and ions on the inside of the line (e.g., potassium) move from the inside of the cell to the outside. Below the line is the corresponding ventricular excitation and recovery from the surface electrocardiogram. One can see that excessive sodium channel blockade from drugs may lead to QRS prolongation and excessive potassium channel blockade from drugs may lead to QT interval prolongation.

Calcium-dependent cells generally have a less negative RMP (–40 to –60 mV) and a slower conduction velocity. Furthermore, in calcium-dependent tissues, recovery of excitability outlasts full repolarization, whereas in sodium-dependent tissue, recovery is prompt after repolarization. These two types of electrical fibers also differ dramatically in how drugs modify their conduction properties.

Ion conductance across the lipid bilayer of the cell membrane occurs via the formation of membrane pores or "channels" (Fig. 25–2). Selective ion channels probably form in response to specific electrical potential differences between the inside and the outside of the cell (voltage dependence). The membrane itself is composed of both organized and disorganized lipids and phospholipids in a dynamic sol-gel matrix. During ion flux and electrical excitation, changes in this sol-gel equilibrium occur and permit the formation of activated ion channels. Besides channel formation and membrane composition, intrachannel proteins or phospholipids,

referred to as gates, also regulate the transmembrane movement of ions. These gates are thought to be positioned strategically within the channel to modulate ion flow (Fig. 25–2). Each ion channel conceptually has two types of gates: an activation gate and an inactivation gate. The activation gate opens during depolarization to allow the ion current to enter or exit from the cell, and the inactivation gate later closes to stop ion movement. When the cell is in a rested state, the activation gates are closed and the inactivation gates are open. The activation gates then open to allow ion movement through the channel, and the inactivation gates later close to stop ion conductance. Thus the cell cycles between three states: resting, activated or open, and inactivated or closed. Activation of SA and AV nodal tissue is dependent on a slow depolarizing current through calcium channels and gates, whereas the activation of atrial and ventricular tissue is dependent on a rapid depolarizing current through sodium channels and gates.

ABNORMAL CONDUCTION

The mechanisms of tachyarrhythmias have been classically divided into two general categories: those resulting from an abnormality in impulse generation or "automatic" tachycardias and those resulting from an abnormality in impulse conduction or "reentrant" tachycardias.

Automatic tachycardias depend upon spontaneous impulse generation in latent pacemakers and may be a result of several different mechanisms. Drugs, such as digoxin or catecholamines, and conditions, such as hypoxia, electrolyte abnormalities (e.g., hypokalemia), and fiber stretch (cardiac dilation), may lead to an increased slope of phase 4 depolarization in cardiac tissues other than the SA node. These factors that experimentally lead to abnormal automaticity are also known to be arrhythmogenic in clinical situations. The increased slope of phase 4 causes heightened automaticity of these tissues and competition with the SA node for dominance of cardiac rhythm. If the rate of spontaneous impulse generation of the abnormally automatic tissue exceeds that of the SA node, then an automatic tachycardia may result. Automatic tachycardias have the following characteristics: (a) the onset of the tachycardia is unrelated to an initiating event such as a premature beat; (b) the initiating beat is usually identical to subsequent beats

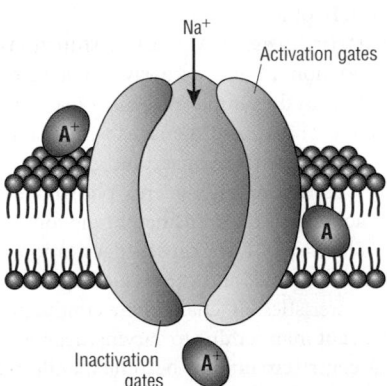

FIGURE 25-2. Lipid bilayer, sodium channel, and possible sites of action of the class I AADs (A). Class I AADs may theoretically inhibit sodium influx at an extracellular, intramembrane, or intracellular receptor site. However, all approved agents appear to block sodium conductance at a single receptor site by gaining entrance to the interior of the channel from an intracellular route. Active ionized drugs block the channel predominantly during the activated or inactivated state and bind and unbind with specific time constants (described as fast on-off, slow on-off, and intermediate) (AADs, antiarrhythmic drugs).

of the tachycardia; (c) the tachycardia cannot be initiated by programmed cardiac stimulation; and (d) the onset of the tachycardia is usually preceded by a gradual acceleration in rate and termination is usually preceded by a gradual deceleration in rate. Clinical tachycardias resulting from the classic forms of enhanced automaticity already described are not as common as once thought. Examples are sinus tachycardia and junctional tachycardia.

Triggered automaticity is also a possible mechanism for abnormal impulse generation. Briefly, triggered automaticity refers to transient membrane depolarizations that occur during repolarization (early after-depolarizations [EADs]) or after repolarization (late after-depolarizations [LADs]) but prior to phase 4 of the action potential. After-depolarizations may be related to abnormal calcium and sodium influx during or just after full cellular repolarization. Experimentally, EADs may be precipitated by hypokalemia, class Ia AADs, or slow stimulation rates—any factor that blocks the ion channels (e.g., potassium) responsible for cellular repolarization. EADs provoked by drugs that block potassium conductance and delay repolarization are the underlying cause of TdP. LADs may be precipitated by digoxin or catecholamines and suppressed by CCBs, and have been suggested as the mechanism for multifocal atrial tachycardia, digoxin-induced tachycardias and exercise-provoked VT. Triggered automatic rhythms possess some of the characteristics of automatic tachycardias and some of the characteristics of reentrant tachycardias (description follows).

As previously mentioned, the impulse originating from the SA node in an individual with SR eventually meets previously excited and thus refractory tissue. Reentry is a concept that involves indefinite propagation of the impulse and continued activation of previously refractory tissue. There are three conduction requirements for the formation of a viable reentrant focus: two pathways for impulse conduction, an area of unidirectional block (prolonged refractoriness) in one of these pathways, and slow conduction in the other pathway (Fig. 25–3). Usually a critically timed premature beat initiates reentry. This premature impulse enters both conduction pathways but encounters refractory tissue in one of the pathways at the area of unidirectional block. The impulse dies out because the tissue is still refractory from the previous (sinus) impulse. Although it fails to propagate in one pathway, the impulse may still proceed in a forward direction (antegrade) through the other pathway because of this pathway's relatively shorter refractory period. The impulse

may then proceed through a loop of tissue and "reenter" the area of unidirectional block in a backward direction (retrograde). Because the antegrade pathway has slow conduction characteristics, the area of unidirectional block has time to recover its excitability. The impulse can proceed in a retrograde fashion through this (previously refractory) tissue and continue around the loop of tissue in a circular fashion. Thus, the key to the formation of a reentrant focus is crucial conduction discrepancies in the electrophysiologic characteristics of the two pathways. The reentrant focus may excite surrounding tissue at a rate greater than that of the SA node, leading to formation of a clinical tachycardia. The above model is anatomically determined in that there is only one pathway for impulse conduction with a fixed circuit length. Another model of reentry, referred to as a functional reentrant loop or leading circle model, may also occur (Fig. 25–4).[1] In a functional reentrant focus, the length of the circuit may vary depending on the conduction velocity and recovery characteristics of the impulse. The area in the middle of the loop is continually kept refractory by the inwardly moving impulse. The length of the circuit is not fixed but is the smallest circle possible, such that the leading edge of the wavefront is continuously exciting tissue just as it recovers; that is, the head of the impulse nearly catches its tail. It differs from the anatomic model in that the leading edge of the impulse is not preceded by an excitable gap of tissue, and it does not have an obstacle in the middle or a fixed anatomic circuit. Clinically, many reentrant foci probably have both anatomic and functional characteristics. In the figure 8 model, a zone of unidirectional block is present, allowing for two impulse loops that join and reenter the area of block in a retrograde fashion to form a pretzel-shaped reentrant circuit. This model combines functional characteristics with an excitable gap. All of these theoretical models require a critical balance of refractoriness and conduction velocity within the circuit and as such have helped to explain the effects of drugs on terminating, modifying, and causing cardiac rhythm disturbances.

What causes reentry to become clinically manifest? Reentrant foci may occur at any level of the conduction system: within the branches of the specialized atrial conduction system, within the Purkinje network, and even within portions of the SA and AV nodes. The anatomy of the Purkinje system appears to provide a suitable substrate for the formation of microreentrant loops and is often used as a model to facilitate the understanding of reentry concepts (see Fig. 25–4). Of course, because reentry does not usually occur in normal, healthy conduction tissue, various forms of heart disease or conduction abnormalities must usually be present before reentry becomes manifest. In other words, the various forms of heart disease (e.g., coronary artery disease [CAD], LV dysfunction) can result in changes in conduction in the pathways of a suitable reentrant substrate. An often-used example is reentry occurring as a consequence of ischemic or hypoxic damage: with inadequate cellular oxygen, cardiac tissue resorts to anaerobic glycolysis for adenosine triphosphate production. As high-energy phosphate concentration diminishes, the activity of the transmembrane ion pumps declines and RMP rises. This rise in RMP causes inactivation in the voltage-dependent sodium channel, and the tissue begins to assume slow conduction characteristics. If changes in conduction parameters occur in a discordant manner due to varying degrees of ischemia or hypoxia, then a reentry circuit may become manifest. Furthermore, an ischemic, dying cell liberates intracellular potassium, which also causes a rise in RMP. In other cases, reentry may occur as a consequence of anatomic or functional variants in the normal conduction system. For instance, patients may possess two (instead of one) conduction pathways near or within the AV node, or have an anomalous extranodal AV pathway that possesses different electrophysiologic characteristics from the normal AV nodal pathway. Reentry in these cases may occur within the AV node or encompass both atrial and ventricular tissue. Reentrant tachycardias have the

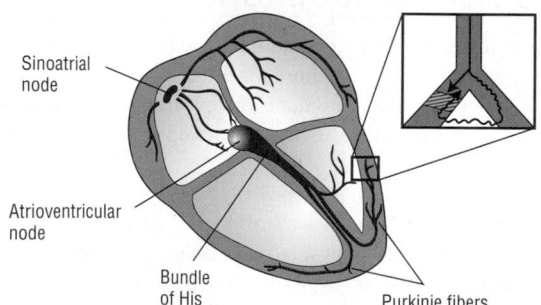

Sinoatrial node

Atrioventricular node

Bundle of His

Purkinje fibers

FIGURE 25-3. Conduction system of the heart. The magnified portion shows a bifurcation of a Purkinje fiber traditionally explained as the etiology of reentrant VT. A premature impulse travels to the fiber, damaged by heart disease or ischemia. It encounters a zone of prolonged refractoriness (area of unidirectional block; *cross-hatched area*) but fails to propagate because it remains refractory to stimulation from the previous impulse. However, the impulse may slowly travel *(squiggly line)* through the other portion of the Purkinje twig and will "reenter" the cross-hatched area if the refractory period is concluded and it is now excitable. Thus, the premature impulse never meets refractory tissue; circus movement ensues. If this site stimulates the surrounding ventricle repetitively, clinical reentrant VT results (VT, ventricular tachycardia).

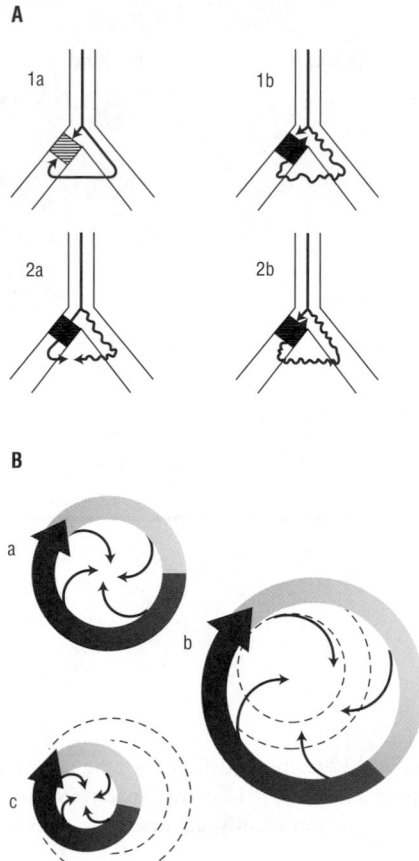

A

B

FIGURE 25-4. *A.* Possible mechanism of proarrhythmia in the anatomic model of reentry. *(1a)* Nonviable reentrant loop due to bidirectional block *(shaded area)*. *(1b)* Instance where a drug slows conduction velocity without significantly prolonging the refractory period. The impulse is now able to reenter the area of unidirectional block *(shaded area)* because slowed conduction through the contralateral limb allows recovery of the block. A new reentrant tachycardia may result. *(2a)* Nonviable reentrant loop due to a lack of a unidirectional block. *(2b)* Instance where a drug prolongs the refractory period without significantly slowing conduction velocity. The impulse moving antegrade meets refractory tissue *(shaded area)* allowing for unidirectional block. A new reentrant tachycardia may result. *B.* Mechanism of reentry and proarrhythmia. *(a)* Functionally determined *(leading circle)* reentrant circuit. This model should be contrasted with anatomic reentry; here the circuit is not fixed (it does not necessarily move around an anatomic obstacle) and there is no excitable gap. All tissue inside is held continuously refractory. *(b)* Instance where a drug prolongs the refractory period without significantly slowing conduction velocity. The tachycardia may terminate or slow in rate as shown as a consequence of a greater circuit length. The *dashed lines* represent the original reentrant circuit prior to drug treatment. *(c)* Instance where a drug slows conduction velocity without significantly prolonging the refractory period (i.e., class Ic antiarrhythmic drugs) and accelerates the tachycardia. The tachycardia rate may increase (proarrhythmia) as shown as a consequence of a shorter circuit length. The dashed lines represent the original reentrant circuit prior to drug treatment. *(From McCollam PL, Parker RB, Beckman KJ, et al. Proarrhythmia: A paradoxic response to antiarrhythmic agents. Pharmacotherapy 1989;9:146, with permission.)*

following characteristics: (a) the onset of the tachycardia is usually related to an initiating event (i.e., premature beat); (b) the initiating beat is usually different in morphology from subsequent beats of the tachycardia; (c) the initiation of the tachycardia is usually possible with programmed cardiac stimulation; and (d) the initiation and termination of the tachycardia is usually abrupt without an acceleration or deceleration phase. There are many examples of reentrant tachycardias, including AF, atrial flutter, AV nodal or AV reentrant tachycardia, and recurrent VT.

ANTIARRHYTHMIC DRUGS

In a theoretical sense, drugs may have antiarrhythmic activity by directly altering conduction in several ways. First, a drug may depress the automatic properties of abnormal pacemaker cells. A drug may do this by decreasing the slope of phase 4 depolarization and/or by elevating threshold potential. If the rate of spontaneous impulse generation of the abnormally automatic foci becomes less than that of the SA node, normal cardiac rhythm can be restored. Second, drugs may alter the conduction characteristics of the pathways of a reentrant loop.[1,2] A drug may facilitate conduction (shorten refractoriness) in the area of unidirectional block, allowing antegrade conduction to proceed. On the other hand, a drug may further depress conduction (prolong refractoriness) either in the area of unidirectional block or in the pathway with slowed conduction and a relatively shorter refractory period. If refractoriness is prolonged in the area of unidirectional block, retrograde propagation of the impulse is not permitted, causing a "bidirectional" block. In the anatomic model, if refractoriness is prolonged in the pathway with slow conduction, antegrade conduction of the impulse is not permitted. In either case, drugs that reduce the discordance and cause uniformity in conduction properties of the two pathways may suppress the reentrant substrate. In the functionally determined model, if refractoriness is prolonged without significantly slowing conduction velocity, the tachycardia may terminate or slow in rate as a consequence of a greater circuit length (see Fig. 25–4). There are other theoretical ways to stop reentry: a drug may eliminate the critically timed premature impulse that triggers reentry; a drug may slow conduction velocity to such an extent that conduction is extinguished; or a drug may reverse the underlying form of heart disease that was responsible for the conduction abnormalities that led to the arrhythmia (i.e., "reverse remodeling").

AADs have specific electrophysiologic actions that alter cardiac conduction in patients with or without heart disease. These actions form the basis of grouping AADs into specific categories based upon their electrophysiologic actions *in vitro*. Vaughan Williams proposed the most frequently used classification system (Table 25–1).[2] This classification has been criticized for the following reasons: (a) it is incomplete and does not allow for the classification of drugs such as digoxin or adenosine; (b) it is not pure, and many agents have properties of more than one class of drugs; (c) it does not incorporate drug characteristics such as mechanisms of tachycardia termination/prevention, clinical indications, or side effects; and (d) drugs become "labeled" within a class, although they may be distinct in many regards.[3] These criticisms formed the basis for an attempt to reclassify AADs based upon a variety of basic and clinical characteristics (called the Sicilian Gambit[3]). Nonetheless, the Vaughan Williams classification remains the most frequently used despite many proposed modifications and alternative systems.

The class Ia AADs, quinidine, procainamide, and disopyramide, slow conduction velocity, prolong refractoriness, and decrease the automatic properties of sodium-dependent (normal and diseased) conduction tissue. Although class Ia AADs are primarily considered sodium channel blockers, their electrophysiologic actions can also be attributed to blockade of potassium channels. In reentrant tachycardias, these drugs generally depress conduction and prolong refractoriness, theoretically transforming the area of unidirectional block into a bidirectional block. Clinically, class Ia drugs are broad-spectrum AADs that are effective for both supraventricular and ventricular arrhythmias. Procainamide is only available in the IV formulation as all of its oral formulations have been discontinued.

The class Ib AADs, lidocaine, mexiletine, and phenytoin, were historically categorized separately from quinidine-like drugs. This was a result of early work demonstrating that lidocaine had distinctly different electrophysiologic actions. In normal tissue models,

TABLE 25-1 Classification of Antiarrhythmic Drugs

Class	Drug	Conduction Velocity[a]	Refractory Period	Automaticity	Ion Block
Ia	Quinidine Procainamide Disopyramide	↓	↑	↓	Sodium (intermediate) Potassium
Ib	Lidocaine Mexiletine	0/↓	↓	↓	Sodium (fast on-off)
Ic	Flecainide Propafenone[b]	↓↓	0	↓	Sodium (slow on-off)
II[c]	β-blockers	↓	↑	↓	Calcium (indirect)
III	Amiodarone[d] Dofetilide Dronedarone[d] Sotalol[b] Ibutilide	0	↑↑	0	Potassium
IV[c]	Verapamil Diltiazem	↓	↑	↓	Calcium

AV, atrioventricular; SA, sinoatrial.

[a]Variables for normal tissue models in ventricular tissue.

[b]Also has β-blocking actions.

[c]Variables for SA and AV nodal tissue only.

[d]Also has sodium, calcium, and β-blocking actions; see Table 25–2 (for amiodarone).

lidocaine generally facilitates actions on cardiac conduction by shortening refractoriness and having little effect on conduction velocity. Thus, it was postulated that these agents could improve antegrade conduction, eliminating the area of unidirectional block. Of course, arrhythmias do not usually arise from normal tissue, leading investigators to study the actions of lidocaine and phenytoin in ischemic and hypoxic tissue models. Interestingly, studies have shown these drugs to possess class Ia quinidine-like properties in diseased tissues. Therefore, it is probable that lidocaine acts in a similar fashion to the class Ia AADs (i.e., prolong refractoriness in diseased ischemic tissues leading to bidirectional block in a reentrant circuit). Lidocaine and similar agents have accentuated effects in ischemic tissue caused by the local acidosis and potassium shifts that occur during cellular hypoxia. Changes in pH alter the time that local anesthetics occupy the sodium channel receptor, thereby affecting the agent's electrophysiologic actions. In addition, the intracellular acidosis that ensues as a consequence of ischemia could cause lidocaine to become "trapped" within the cell, allowing increased access to the receptor. The class Ib AADs are considerably more effective in ventricular arrhythmias than supraventricular arrhythmias. As a group these drugs are relatively weak sodium channel antagonists (at normal stimulation rates).

The class Ic AADs, propafenone and flecainide, are extremely potent sodium channel blockers, profoundly slowing conduction velocity while leaving refractoriness relatively unaltered. The class Ic AADs theoretically eliminate reentry by slowing conduction to a point where the impulse is extinguished and cannot propagate further. Although the class Ic AADs are effective for both ventricular and supraventricular arrhythmias, their use for ventricular arrhythmias has been limited by the risk of proarrhythmia.

Class I AADs are grouped together because of their common action in blocking sodium conductance. The receptor site for these AADs is probably inside the sodium channel so that, in effect, the drug plugs the pore. The agent may gain access to the receptor either via the intracellular space through the membrane lipid bilayer or directly through the channel. Several principles are inherent in antiarrhythmic sodium channel receptor theories:[4]

1. Class I AADs have predominant affinity for a particular state of the channel (e.g., during activation or inactivation).

For example, lidocaine and flecainide block sodium current primarily when the cell is in the inactivated state, whereas quinidine is predominantly an open (or activated)-channel blocker.

2. Class I AADs have specific binding and unbinding characteristics to the receptor. For example, lidocaine binds to and dissociates from the channel receptor quickly ("fast on-off") but flecainide has very "slow on-off" properties. This explains why flecainide has such potent effects on slowing ventricular conduction, whereas lidocaine has little effect on normal tissue (at normal heart rates). In general, the class Ic AADs are "slow on-off", the class Ib AADs are "fast on-off", and the class Ia AADs are intermediate in their binding kinetics.

3. Class I AADs possess rate dependence (i.e., sodium channel blockade and slowed conduction are greatest at fast heart rates and least during bradycardia). For "slow on-off" drugs, sodium channel blockade is evident at normal rates (60 to 100 beats/min) but for "fast on-off" agents, slowed conduction is only apparent at fast heart rates.

4. Class I AADs (except phenytoin) are weak bases with a $pK_a > 7.0$ and block the sodium channel in their ionized form. Consequently, pH will alter these actions: acidosis accentuates and alkalosis diminishes sodium channel blockade.

5. Class I AADs appear to share a single receptor site in the sodium channel. It should be noted, however, that a number of class I AADs have other electrophysiologic properties. For instance, quinidine has potent potassium channel blocking activity (manifest predominantly at low concentrations) as does N-acetylprocainamide (manifest predominantly at high concentrations), the primary metabolite of procainamide. Additionally propafenone has β-blocking actions.

These principles are important in understanding additive drug combinations (e.g., quinidine and mexiletine), antagonistic combinations (e.g., flecainide and lidocaine), and potential antidotes to excess sodium channel blockade (sodium bicarbonate). They also explain a number of clinical observations, such as why lidocaine-like drugs are relatively ineffective for supraventricular tachycardia. The class Ib AADs are "fast on-off", inactivated sodium channel blockers; atrial cells, however, have a very brief inactivated phase relative to ventricular tissue.

The β-blockers are classified as class II AADs. For the most part, the clinically relevant acute antiarrhythmic mechanisms of the β-blockers result from their antiadrenergic actions. Because the SA and AV nodes are heavily influenced by adrenergic innervation, β-blockers would be most useful in tachycardias in which these nodal tissues are abnormally automatic or are a portion of a reentrant loop. These drugs are also helpful in slowing ventricular response in atrial arrhythmias (e.g., AF) by their effects on the AV node. Furthermore, some tachycardias are exercise-related or precipitated by states of high sympathetic tone (perhaps through triggered activity), and β-blockers may be useful in these instances. β-adrenergic stimulation results in increased conduction velocity, shortened refractoriness, and increased automaticity of the nodal tissues; β-blockers will antagonize these effects. In the nodal tissues, β-blockers interfere with calcium entry into the cell by altering catecholamine-dependent channel integrity and gating kinetics. In sodium-dependent atrial and ventricular tissue, β-blockers shorten repolarization somewhat but otherwise have little direct effect. The antiarrhythmic properties of β-blockers observed with long-term, chronic therapy in patients with heart disease are less well understood. Although it is clear that β-blockers decrease the likelihood of SCD (presumably arrhythmic death) after MI, the mechanism for this benefit remains unclear but may relate to the complex interplay of changes in sympathetic tone, damaged myocardium, and ventricular conduction. In patients with HF, drugs such as β-blockers, angiotensin-converting enzyme inhibitors, and angiotensin II receptor blockers may prevent arrhythmias such as AF by attenuating the structural and/or electrical remodeling process in the myocardium.[5,6]

The class III AADs include those agents that specifically prolong refractoriness in atrial and ventricular tissue. This class includes very different drugs: amiodarone, dronedarone, sotalol, ibutilide, and dofetilide; they share the common effect of delaying repolarization by blocking potassium channels. Amiodarone and sotalol are effective in most supraventricular and ventricular arrhythmias. Amiodarone displays electrophysiologic characteristics of all four Vaughan Williams classes; it is a sodium channel blocker with relatively "fast on-off" kinetics, has nonselective β-blocking actions, blocks potassium channels, and also has a small degree of calcium channel blocking activity (Table 25–2). At normal heart rates and with chronic use, its predominant effect is to prolong repolarization. Upon IV administration, its onset is relatively quick (unlike the oral form) and β-blockade predominates initially. Theoretically, amiodarone, like class I AADs, may interrupt the reentrant substrate by transforming an area of unidirectional block into an area of bidirectional block. However, electrophysiologic studies using programmed cardiac stimulation imply that amiodarone may leave the reentrant loop intact. The impressive effectiveness of amiodarone

coupled with its low proarrhythmic potential has challenged the notion that selective ion channel blockade by AADs is preferable. Sotalol is a potent inhibitor of outward potassium movement during repolarization and also possesses nonselective β-blocking actions. Unlike amiodarone and sotalol, dronedarone, ibutilide and dofetilide are only approved for the treatment of supraventricular arrhythmias. Both ibutilide (only available IV) and dofetilide (only available orally) can be used for the acute conversion of AF or atrial flutter to SR. Dofetilide can also be used to maintain SR in patients with AF or atrial flutter of longer than 1 week's duration who have been converted to SR. Dronedarone is approved to reduce the risk of cardiovascular hospitalization in patients with paroxysmal or persistent AF or atrial flutter who experienced a recent episode of this arrhythmia, have cardiovascular risk factors (at least 70 years of age, hypertension, diabetes, prior stroke, left atrial diameter ≥50 mm, or left ventricular ejection fraction [LVEF] <40%), and are in or will be cardioverted to SR. Although structurally related to amiodarone, dronedarone's structure has been modified through the addition of a methylsulfonyl group and the removal of iodine. Dronedarone is also similar to amiodarone in exhibiting electrophysiologic characteristics of all four Vaughan Williams classes (sodium channel blocker with relatively "fast on-off" kinetics, nonselective β-blocker, potassium channel blocker, and calcium channel antagonist).

There are a number of different potassium channels that function during normal conduction; all approved class III AADs inhibit the delayed rectifier current (I_K) responsible for phases 2 and 3 repolarization. Subcurrents make up I_K; an ultrarapid component (I_{Kur}), a rapid component (I_{Kr}), and the slow component (I_{Ks}). N-acetylprocainamide, sotalol, ibutilide, and dofetilide selectively block I_{Kr}, whereas amiodarone and dronedarone block both I_{Kr} and I_{Ks}. New drugs that selectively block I_{Kur} (found predominantly in the atrium but not ventricle) are being investigated for supraventricular arrhythmias. The clinical relevance of selectively blocking components of the delayed rectifier current remains to be determined. Potassium channel blockers (particularly those with selective I_{Kr} blocking properties) display "reverse use dependence" (i.e., their effects on repolarization are greatest at low heart rates). Sotalol and drugs like it also appear to be much more effective in preventing VF (in dog models) than the traditional sodium channel blockers. They also decrease defibrillation threshold in contrast to class I AADs, which tend to increase this parameter. This feature could be important in patients with ICDs, as concurrent therapy with class I AADs may require more energy for successful cardioversion or may render the ICD ineffective in terminating the ventricular arrhythmia. The Achilles' heel of all class III AADs is an extension of their underlying ionic mechanism (i.e., by blocking potassium channels and delaying repolarization, they may also cause proarrhythmia in the form of TdP by provoking EADs).

The non-DHP CCBs, verapamil and diltiazem, are categorized as class IV AADs. At least two types of calcium channels are operative

TABLE 25-2	Time Course and Electrophysiologic Effects of Amiodarone						
				IV		Oral	
Class	Mechanism	EP	ECG	*Minutes–Hours*	*Hours–Days*	*Days–Weeks*	*Weeks–Months*
Class I	Na⁺ block	↑ HV	↑ QRS	0	+	+	++
Class II	β-block	↑ AH	↑ PR ↓ HR	++	++	++	++
Class III	K⁺ block	↑ VERP ↑ AERP	↑ QT	0	+	++	++++
Class IV	Ca²⁺ block[a]	↑ AH	↑ PR	+	+	+	+

[a]Rate-dependent.

AERP, atrial effective refractory period; AH, atria–His interval; ECG, electrocardiographic effects; EP, electrophysiologic actions; HR, heart rate; HV, His–ventricle interval; VERP, ventricular effective refractory period.

in SA and AV nodal tissues: an L-type channel and a T-type channel. Both L-type channel blockers (verapamil and diltiazem) and selective T-type channel blockers (mibefradil was previously approved but withdrawn from the market) will slow conduction, prolong refractoriness, and decrease automaticity (e.g., due to EADs or LADs) of the calcium-dependent tissue in the SA and AV nodes. Therefore, these agents are effective in automatic or reentrant tachycardias, which arise from or use the SA or AV nodes. In supraventricular arrhythmias (e.g., AF), these drugs can slow ventricular response by slowing AV nodal conduction. Furthermore, because calcium entry seems to be integral to exercise-related tachycardias and/or tachycardias caused by some forms of triggered automaticity, these agents may be effective in the treatment of these types of arrhythmias. The DHP CCBs (e.g., nifedipine) do not have significant antiarrhythmic activity because a reflex increase in sympathetic tone caused by vasodilation counteracts their direct negative dromotropic action.

All AADs currently available have an impressive side effect profile (Table 25–3). A considerable percentage of patients cannot tolerate long-term therapy with these drugs and will have to discontinue therapy because of side effects. ❷ In one trial,[7] more than 50% of patients had to discontinue long-term procainamide (mostly because of a lupus-like syndrome) after MI. In another study,[8] disopyramide caused anticholinergic side effects in approximately 70% of patients. Flecainide, propafenone, and disopyramide may precipitate congestive HF in a significant number of patients with underlying LV systolic dysfunction; consequently, these drugs should be avoided in this patient population.[9] The class Ib AAD,

mexiletine, causes neurologic and/or gastrointestinal toxicity in a high percentage of patients. One of the most frightening side effects related to AADs is the aggravation of underlying ventricular arrhythmias or the precipitation of new (and life-threatening) ventricular arrhythmias.[10]

Amiodarone has assumed a prominent place in the treatment of both chronic and acute supraventricular and ventricular arrhythmias and is now the most commonly prescribed AAD.[11] Once considered a drug of last resort, it is now the first AAD considered in many arrhythmias. Yet amiodarone is a peculiar and complex drug, displaying unusual pharmacologic effects, pharmacokinetics, dosing regimens, and multiorgan side effects. Amiodarone has an extremely long elimination half-life (greater than 50 days) and large volume of distribution; consequently, its onset of action with the oral form is delayed (days to weeks) despite the use of a loading regimen, and its effects persist for a long period (months) after discontinuation. Amiodarone is a substrate of the cytochrome P450 (CYP) 3A4 isoenzyme, a moderate inhibitor of many CYP isoenzymes (e.g., CYP2C9, CYP2D6, CYP3A4), and a P-glycoprotein inhibitor, all of which can result in the potential for numerous drug interactions. Amiodarone interacts with digoxin and warfarin and can significantly increase plasma concentrations of both drugs. By inhibiting P-glycoprotein, amiodarone can increase digoxin concentrations by approximately twofold; therefore, the digoxin dose should be empirically reduced by 50% when amiodarone is initiated. When amiodarone and warfarin are initiated concurrently, warfarin should be started at a dose of 2.5 mg daily. When amiodarone is initiated in a patient already receiving warfarin, the warfarin dose should be reduced by approximately 30%.[12] Acute administration of amiodarone is usually well tolerated by patients, but severe organ toxicities may result with chronic use. Severe bradycardia (sometimes requiring pacing to allow the patient to remain on amiodarone), hyper- and hypothyroidism, peripheral neuropathy, gastrointestinal discomfort, photosensitivity, and a blue-gray skin discoloration on exposed areas are common. Fulminant hepatitis (uncommon) and pulmonary fibrosis (5% to 10% of patients) have caused death.[13,14] Although amiodarone can cause corneal microdeposits (which usually do not affect vision) in virtually every patient, it has also been associated with the development of optic neuropathy/neuritis, which can lead to blindness. All of these side effects mandate close and continued monitoring (liver enzymes, thyroid function tests, eye exams, chest radiographs, pulmonary function tests) and have led to a proliferation of "amiodarone clinics" designed just for patients receiving this drug on a chronic basis (Table 25–4). ❸[15]

The modifications to dronedarone's chemical structure may confer an improved safety profile when compared with amiodarone. With the addition of a methylsulfonyl group and the deletion of the iodine moiety, dronedarone is less lipophilic than amiodarone; consequently, dronedarone is much less likely to accumulate in tissues and to cause various organ toxicities. Dronedarone also has a considerably shorter half-life (~24 hours) when compared with amiodarone, which allows for steady-state to be achieved in 5 to 7 days, without the need for using loading doses. Like amiodarone, dronedarone is a substrate of the CYP3A isoenzyme and a moderate inhibitor of the CYP2D6 and CYP3A isoenzymes. Its use with potent CYP3A4 inhibitors or inducers should be avoided. No significant interaction has been observed when dronedarone was used concomitantly with warfarin. Dronedarone also inhibits P-glycoprotein and can increase digoxin concentrations by about 2.5-fold. Consequently, when concomitantly using dronedarone and digoxin, the digoxin dose should be empirically reduced by 50%.

Table 25–5 summarizes the pharmacokinetics of the AADs and Table 25–6 lists recommended dosages of the oral dosage forms. Table 25–7 lists the dosing recommendations for the IV forms of various AADs.

TABLE 25-3	Side Effects of Antiarrhythmic Drugs
Disopyramide	Anticholinergic symptoms (dry mouth, urinary retention, constipation, blurred vision), nausea, anorexia, TdP, HF, conduction disturbances, ventricular arrhythmias
Procainamide[a]	Hypotension, TdP, worsening HF, conduction disturbances, ventricular arrhythmias
Quinidine	Cinchonism, diarrhea, abdominal cramps, nausea, vomiting, hypotension, TdP, worsening HF, conduction disturbances, ventricular arrhythmias, fever, hepatitis, thrombocytopenia, hemolytic anemia
Lidocaine	Dizziness, sedation, slurred speech, blurred vision, paresthesia, muscle twitching, confusion, nausea, vomiting, seizures, psychosis, sinus arrest, conduction disturbances
Mexiletine	Dizziness, sedation, anxiety, confusion, paresthesia, tremor, ataxia, blurred vision, nausea, vomiting, anorexia, conduction disturbances, ventricular arrhythmias
Flecainide	Blurred vision, dizziness, dyspnea, headache, tremor, nausea, worsening HF, conduction disturbances, ventricular arrhythmias
Propafenone	Dizziness, fatigue, bronchospasm, headache, taste disturbances, nausea, vomiting, bradycardia or AV block, worsening HF, ventricular arrhythmias
Amiodarone	Tremor, ataxia, paresthesia, insomnia, corneal microdeposits, optic neuropathy/neuritis, nausea, vomiting, anorexia, constipation, TdP (<1%), bradycardia or AV block (IV and oral use), pulmonary fibrosis, liver function test abnormalities, hepatitis, hypothyroidism, hyperthyroidism, photosensitivity, blue-gray skin discoloration, hypotension (IV use), phlebitis (IV use)
Dofetilide	Headache, dizziness, TdP
Dronedarone	Nausea, vomiting, diarrhea, serum creatinine elevations, bradycardia, TdP (<1%)
Ibutilide	Headache, TdP, hypotension
Sotalol	Dizziness, weakness, fatigue, nausea, vomiting, diarrhea, bradycardia or AV block, TdP, bronchospasm, worsening HF

[a]Side effects listed are for the IV formulation only; oral formulations are no longer available.
AV, atrioventricular; HF, heart failure; IV, intravenous; TdP, torsade de pointes.

TABLE 25-4 Amiodarone Monitoring

Side Effect	Monitoring Recommendations	Management of Side Effect
Pulmonary fibrosis	Chest radiograph (baseline, then every 12 months) Pulmonary function tests (if symptoms develop)	Discontinue amiodarone immediately; initiate corticosteroid therapy
Hypothyroidism	TFTs (baseline, then every 6 months)	Thyroid hormone supplementation (e.g., levothyroxine)
Hyperthyroidism	TFTs (baseline, then every 6 months)	Antithyroid drugs (e.g., methimazole)
Optic neuritis/neuropathy	Ophthalmologic examination (baseline [only if significant visual abnormalities present], then if symptoms develop)	Discontinue amiodarone immediately
Corneal microdeposits	Slit-lamp examination (routine monitoring not necessary)	No treatment necessary
Hepatotoxicity	LFTs (baseline, then every 6 months)	Lower the dose or discontinue amiodarone if LFTs >3× the upper limit of normal
Bradycardia/heart block	ECG (baseline, then every 3 to 6 months)	Lower the dose, if possible, or discontinue amiodarone if severe
Tremor, ataxia, peripheral neuropathy	History/physical examination (each office visit)	Lower the dose, if possible, or discontinue amiodarone if severe
Photosensitivity/blue-gray skin discoloration	History/physical examination (each office visit)	Advise patients to wear sunblock while outdoors

ECG, electrocardiogram; LFTs, liver function tests, TFTs, thyroid function tests.

TABLE 25-5 Pharmacokinetics of Antiarrhythmic Drugs

Drug	Oral Bioavailability (%)	Primary Route of Elimination[a]	Substrate[b]	Inhibitor[b]	V_{Dss} (L/kg)	Protein Binding (%)	$t_{1/2}$[c]	Therapeutic Range (mg/L)
Disopyramide	70–95	H/R	CYP3A4 (M)	–	0.8–2.0	50–80	4–8 h	2–6
Procainamide	75–95	H/R	NAT CYP2D6 (M)	–	1.5–3.0	10–20	5–6 h (SAs) 2–3 h (FAs)	4–15
Quinidine	70–80	H	CYP3A4 (M) CYP2C9	CYP2D6 (S) CYP3A4 (S) CYP2C9 P-GP	2.0–3.5	80–90	5–9 h	2–6
Lidocaine	–	H	CYP3A4 (M) CYP2D6 (M) CYP1A2 CYP2C9	CYP1A2 (S) CYP2D6 CYP3A4	1–2	65–75	1–3 h	1.5–5.0
Mexiletine	80–95	H	CYP2D6 (M) CYP1A2 (M)	CYP1A2 (S)	5–12	60–75	12–20 h (PMs) 7–11 h (EMs)	0.8–2.0
Flecainide	90–95	H/R	CYP2D6 (M) CYP1A2	CYP2D6	8–10	35–45	14–20 h (PMs) 10–14 h (EMs)	0.2–1.0
Propafenone[d]	11–39	H	CYP2D6 (M) CYP1A2 CYP2D6	CYP1A2 CYP2D6	2.5–4.0	85–95	10–25 h (PMs) 3–7 h (EMs)	–
Amiodarone	22–88	H	CYP3A4 (M) CYP1A2 CYP2C19 CYP2D6	CYP2C9 CYP2D6 CYP3A4 CYP1A2 CYP2C19 P-GP	70–150	95–99	15–100 d	1.0–2.5
Dofetilide	85–95	R/H	CYP3A4	–	2.5–3.5	60–70	6–10 h	–
Dronedarone	4 (fasting) 15 (with food)	H	CYP3A4	CYP2D6 CYP3A4	20	>98	13–19	–
Ibutilide	–	H	–	–	6–12	40–50	3–6 h	–
Sotalol	90–95	R	–	–	1.2–2.4	30–40	10–20 h	–
Diltiazem	35–50	H	CYP3A4 (M) CYP2C9 CYP2D6	CYP3A4 CYP2C9 CYP2D6 P-GP	3–5	70–85	4–10 h	–
Verapamil	20–40	H	CYP3A4 (M) CYP1A2 CYP2C9	CYP3A4 CYP1A2 CYP2C9 CYP2D6 P-GP	1.5–5.0	95–99	4–12 h	–

[a]H, hepatic; R, renal.
[b]CYP, cytochrome P450 isoenzyme; M, major; NAT, N-acetyltransferase; P-GP, P-glycoprotein; S, strong.
[c]EMs, extensive metabolizers; FAs, fast acetylators; PMs, poor metabolizers; SAs, slow acetylators.
[d]Variables for parent compound (not 5-OH-propafenone).

TABLE 25-6 Typical Maintenance Doses of Oral Antiarrhythmic Drugs

Drug	Dose	Dose Adjusted
Disopyramide	100–150 mg q 6 h 200–300 mg q 12 h (SR form)	HEP, REN
Quinidine	200–300 mg sulfate salt q 6 h 324–648 gluconate salt q 8–12 h	HEP
Mexiletine	200–300 mg q 8 h	HEP
Flecainide	50–200 mg q 12 h	HEP, REN
Propafenone	150–300 mg q 8 h 225-425 mg q 12 h (SR form)	HEP
Amiodarone	400 mg two to three times daily until 10 g total, then 200–400 mg daily[a]	
Dofetilide	500 mcg q 12 h	REN[b]
Dronedarone	400 mg twice daily (with meals)[c]	
Sotalol	80–160 mg q 12 h	REN[d]

HEP, hepatic disease; REN, renal dysfunction; SR, sustained release.

[a]Usual maintenance dose for atrial fibrillation is 200 mg/day (may further decrease dose to 100 mg/day with long-term use if patient clinically stable in order to decrease risk of toxicity); usual maintenance dose for ventricular arrhythmias is 300–400 mg/day.

[b]Dose should be based upon creatinine clearance; should not be used when creatinine clearance <20 mL/min.

[c]Should not be used in severe hepatic impairment.

[d]Should not be used for atrial fibrillation when creatinine clearance <40 mL/min.

TABLE 25-7 Intravenous Antiarrhythmic Dosing

Drug	Clinical Situation	Dose
Amiodarone	Pulseless VT/VF	300 mg IV/IO push (can give additional 150 mg IV/IO push if persistent VT/VF), followed by infusion of 1 mg/min for 6 h, then 0.5 mg/min
	Stable VT (with a pulse)	150 mg IV over 10 min, followed by infusion of 1 mg/min for 6 h, then 0.5 mg/min
	AF (termination)	5 mg/kg IV over 30 min, followed by infusion of 1 mg/min for 6 h, then 0.5 mg/min
Diltiazem	PSVT; AF (rate control)	0.25 mg/kg IV over 2 min (may repeat with 0.35 mg/kg IV over 2 min), followed by infusion of 5–15 mg/h
Ibutilide	AF (termination)	1 mg IV over 10 min (may repeat if needed)
Lidocaine	Pulseless VT/VF	1–1.5 mg/kg IV/IO push (can give additional 0.5–0.75 mg/kg IV/IO push every 5–10 min if persistent VT/VF [maximum cumulative dose = 3 mg/kg], followed by infusion of 1–4 mg/min (1–2 mg/min if liver disease or HF)
	Stable VT (with a pulse)	1–1.5 mg/kg IV push (can give additional 0.5–0.75 mg/kg IV push every 5–10 min if persistent VT [maximum cumulative dose = 3 mg/kg]), followed by infusion of 1–4 mg/min (1–2 mg/min if liver disease or HF)
Procainamide	AF (termination); stable VT (with a pulse)	15–18 mg/kg IV over 60 min, followed by infusion of 1–4 mg/min
Sotalol[a]	AF/AFl (SR maintenance) Ventricular arrhythmias	75–150 mg IV once or twice daily (infused over 5 h)[b]
Verapamil	PSVT; AF (rate control)	2.5–5 mg IV over 2 min (may repeat up to maximum cumulative dose of 20 mg); can follow with infusion of 2.5–10 mg/h

AF, atrial fibrillation; AFl, atrial flutter; HF, heart failure; IO, intraosseous; IV, intravenous; PSVT, paroxysmal supraventricular tachycardia; VF, ventricular fibrillation; VT, ventricular tachycardia.

[a]Should be used only when patients are unable to take sotalol orally.

[b]IV sotalol should be administered at the same frequency as oral sotalol (based on creatinine clearance). Oral sotalol may be converted to IV sotalol as follows: 80 mg oral = 75 mg IV; 120 mg oral = 112.5 mg IV; 160 mg oral = 150 mg IV.

SUPRAVENTRICULAR ARRHYTHMIAS

The common supraventricular tachycardias that often require drug treatment are (a) AF or atrial flutter; (b) PSVT; and (c) automatic atrial tachycardias. Other common supraventricular arrhythmias that usually do not require drug therapy include premature atrial complexes, wandering atrial pacemaker, sinus arrhythmia, and sinus tachycardia. As an example, premature atrial complexes rarely cause symptoms, never cause hemodynamic compromise, and therefore drug therapy is usually not indicated. Likewise, sinus tachycardia is usually the result of underlying metabolic or hemodynamic disorders (e.g., infection, dehydration, hypotension), and therapy should be directed at the underlying cause, not the tachycardia per se. Of course, there are exceptions to these suggestions. For example, sinus tachycardia may be deleterious in patients after cardiac surgery or MI. Therefore, AADs, such as β-blockers, may be indicated in these situations. Stated in another way, although many arrhythmias generally do not require therapy, clinical judgment and patient-specific variables play an important role in this decision. Nevertheless, for the purpose of this discussion, only the tachycardias usually requiring AAD therapy, as listed earlier, are addressed.

ATRIAL FIBRILLATION AND ATRIAL FLUTTER

Mechanisms and Background

AF and atrial flutter are common supraventricular tachycardias. AF continues to be the most common sustained arrhythmia encountered in clinical practice, affecting approximately 2.2 million Americans.[16] In the general population, the overall prevalence of AF is 0.4% to 1%, and this increases with age (e.g., approximately an 8% prevalence in patients >80 years old).[17] The prevalence of AF also appears to increase as patients develop more severe HF, increasing from 4% in asymptomatic NYHA class I patients to 50% in patients with NYHA class IV HF.[17] With the aging population; improved survival in patients with HF, CAD, and hypertension; and the increased frequency of surgical procedures being performed,

it is expected that the prevalence of AF will dramatically increase to an estimated 12 to 15 million by the year 2050.[18] Based on data derived from the Framingham study cohort, the general lifetime risk for AF in men and women at least 40 years of age is estimated to be 1 in 4.[19]

AF and atrial flutter may present as a chronic, established tachycardia; an acute tachycardia; or a self-terminating, paroxysmal form. The following semantics and definitions are sometimes used specifically for AF:[17,20] acute AF (onset within 48 hours); paroxysmal AF (terminates spontaneously in <7 days); recurrent AF (two or more episodes); persistent AF (duration >7 days and does not terminate spontaneously); and permanent AF (does not terminate with attempts at pharmacologic or electrical cardioversion). AF is characterized by extremely rapid (atrial rate of 400 to 600 beats/min) and disorganized atrial activation. With this disorganized atrial activity, there is a loss of the contribution of synchronized atrial contraction (atrial kick) to forward cardiac output. Supraventricular impulses penetrate the AV conduction system in

CLINICAL PRESENTATION: SUPRAVENTRICULAR TACHYCARDIAS

Atrial Fibrillation/Flutter
General

☐ These rhythms are usually not directly life threatening and do not generally cause hemodynamic collapse or syncope; 1:1 atrial flutter (ventricular response ~300 beats/min) is an exception. Also, patients with underlying forms of heart disease that are heavily reliant on atrial contraction to maintain adequate cardiac output (e.g., mitral stenosis, obstructive cardiomyopathy) display more severe symptoms of AF or atrial flutter.

Symptoms

☐ Most often, patients complain of rapid heart rate/palpitations and/or worsening symptoms of HF (shortness of breath, fatigue). Medical emergencies are severe HF (i.e., pulmonary edema, hypotension) or AF occurring in the setting of acute MI.

Diagnostic Tests/Signs (ECG; See Text for Details)

☐ AF is an irregularly irregular supraventricular rhythm with no discernible, consistent atrial activity (P waves). Ventricular response is usually 120 to 180 beats/min and the pulse is irregular. Atrial flutter is (usually) a regular supraventricular rhythm with characteristic flutter waves (or sawtooth pattern) reflecting more organized atrial activity. Commonly, the ventricular rate is in factors of 300 beats/min (e.g., 150, 100, or 75 beats/min).

Paroxysmal Supraventricular Tachycardia Caused by Reentry
General

☐ These rhythms can be transient, resulting in little, if any, symptoms.

Symptoms

☐ Patients frequently complain of intermittent episodes of rapid heart rate/palpitations that abruptly start and stop, usually without provocation (but occasionally as a result of exercise). Severe symptoms include syncope. Often (in particular, those with AV nodal reentry), patients complain of a chest pressure or neck sensation. This is caused by simultaneous AV contraction with the right atrium contracting against a closed tricuspid valve. Life-threatening symptoms (syncope, hemodynamic collapse) are associated with an extremely rapid heart rate (e.g., >200 beats/min) and AF associated with an accessory AV pathway.

Diagnostic Tests/Signs (ECG; See Text for Details)

☐ Most commonly, PSVT is a rapid, narrow QRS tachycardia (regular in rhythm) that starts and stops abruptly. Atrial activity, although present, is difficult to ascertain on surface ECG because P waves are "buried" on the QRS or T wave.

variable degrees resulting in an irregular activation of the ventricles and an irregularly, irregular pulse. The AV junction will not conduct most of the supraventricular impulses, causing ventricular response to be considerably slower (120 to 180 beats/min) than the atrial rate. It is sometimes stated that "AF begets AF"; that is, the arrhythmia tends to perpetuate itself. Long episodes are more difficult to terminate perhaps because of tachycardia-induced changes in atrial function (mechanical and/or electrical "remodeling").

Atrial flutter occurs less frequently than AF but is similar in its precipitating factors, consequences, and drug therapy approach. This arrhythmia is characterized by rapid (270 to 330 atrial beats/min) but regular atrial activation. The slower and regular electrical activity results in a regular ventricular response that is in approximate factors of 300 beats/min (i.e., 1:1 AV conduction = ventricular rate of 300 beats/min; 2:1 AV conduction = ventricular rate of 150 beats/min; 3:1 AV conduction = ventricular rate of 100 beats/min). Atrial flutter may occur in two distinct forms (type I and type II). Type I flutter is the more common classic form with atrial rates of approximately 300 beats/min and the typical "sawtooth" pattern of atrial activation as shown by the surface ECG. Type II flutter tends to be faster, being somewhat of a hybrid between classic atrial flutter and AF. Although the ventricular response usually has a regular pattern, atrial flutter with varying degrees of AV block or that occur with episodes of AF ("fib-flutter") can cause an irregular ventricular rate.

It is generally accepted that the predominant mechanism of AF and atrial flutter is reentry. AF appears to result from multiple atrial reentrant loops (or wavelets), whereas atrial flutter is caused by a single, dominant, reentrant substrate (counterclockwise circus movement in the right atrium around the tricuspid annulus). AF or atrial flutter usually occurs in association with various forms of structural heart disease (SHD) that cause atrial distension, including myocardial ischemia or infarction, hypertensive heart disease, valvular disorders such as mitral stenosis or mitral insufficiency, congenital abnormalities such as septal defects, dilated or hypertrophic cardiomyopathy, and obesity. Disorders that cause right atrial stretch and are associated with AF or atrial flutter include acute pulmonary embolus and chronic lung disease resulting in pulmonary hypertension and cor pulmonale. AF may also occur in association with states of high adrenergic tone such as thyrotoxicosis, surgery, alcohol withdrawal, sepsis, and excessive physical exertion. AF that develops in the absence of clinical, electrocardiographic, radiographic, and echocardiographic evidence of SHD is defined as lone AF. Other states in which patients are predisposed to episodes of AF are the presence of an anomalous AV pathway (i.e., Kent bundle) and sinus node dysfunction (i.e., sick sinus syndrome).

Patients with AF or atrial flutter may experience the entire range of symptoms associated with other supraventricular tachycardias, although syncope as a presenting symptom is uncommon. Because atrial kick is lost with the onset of AF, patients with LV systolic or diastolic dysfunction may develop worsening signs and symptoms of HF as they often depend on the contribution of their atrial kick to maintain an adequate cardiac output. Thromboembolic events, resulting from atrial stasis and poorly adherent mural thrombi, are an additional complication of AF. Of course, the most devastating complication in this regard is the occurrence of an embolic stroke. Approximately 15% of all strokes in the United States can be attributed to AF.[21] The average rate of ischemic stroke in patients with AF who are not receiving antithrombotic therapy is approximately 5% per year.[21,22] Stroke can precede the onset of documented AF, probably as a result of undetected paroxysms prior to the onset of established AF. The risk of stroke significantly increases with age, with the annual attributable risk increasing from 1.5% in individuals 50 to 59 years of age to almost 24% in those 80 to 89 years of age.[21] Patients with concomitant AF and rheumatic heart disease are at particularly high risk for stroke, with their risk being increased 17-fold compared to patients in SR.[21] Other risk factors for stroke identified from recent trials are previous ischemic stroke, transient ischemic attack, or other systemic embolic event; age >75 years; moderate or severe LV systolic dysfunction and/or congestive HF; hypertension; and diabetes.[21] The risk of stroke in patients with only atrial flutter has been traditionally believed to be low, prompting some to recommend only aspirin for prevention of thromboembolism in this particular patient population. However, because patients with atrial flutter may also intermittently have episodes of AF, this patient population also may be at risk for a thromboembolic event. Although the role of antithrombotic therapy

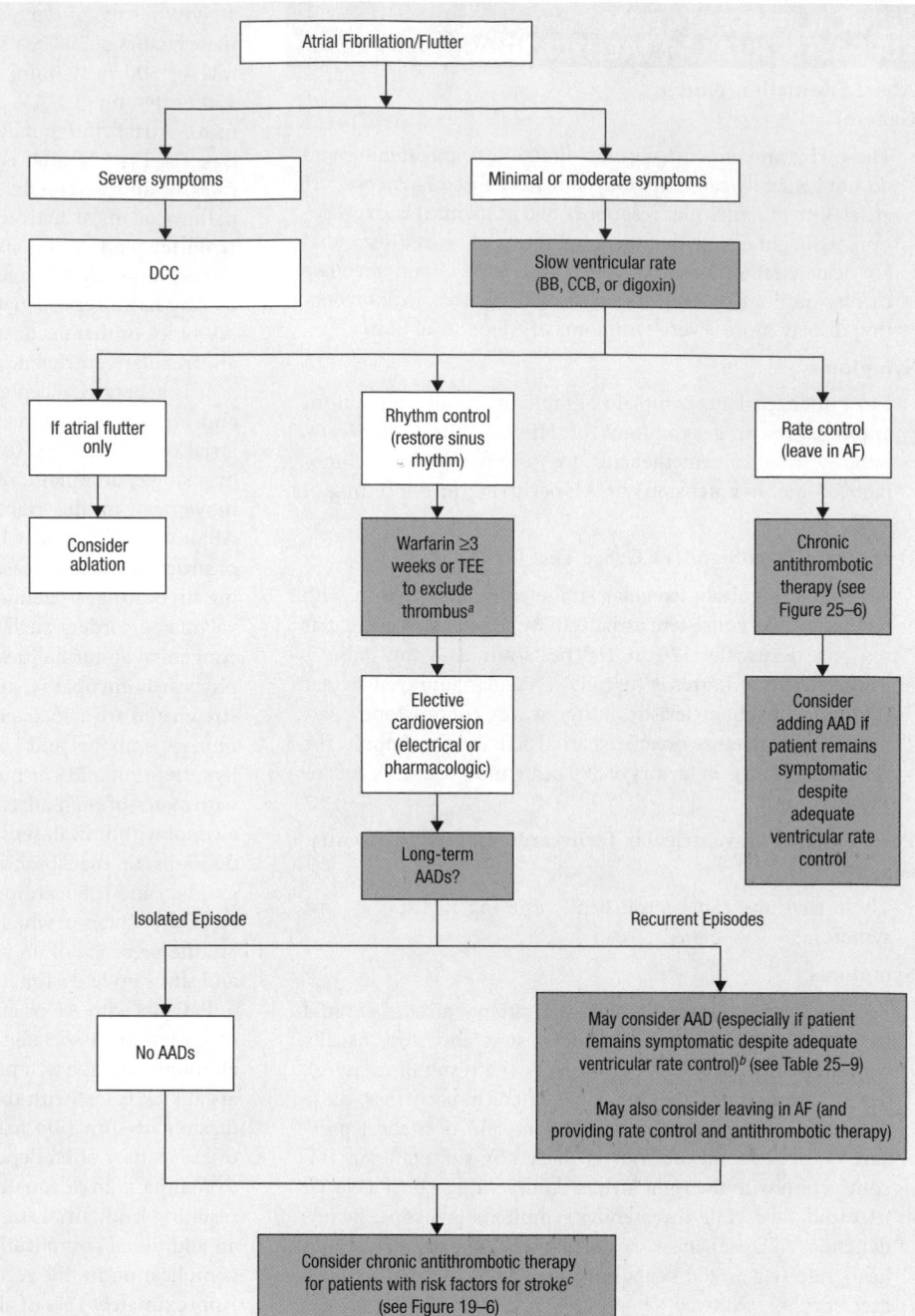

FIGURE 25-5. Algorithm for the treatment of AF and atrial flutter. [a]If AF <48 hours, anticoagulation prior to cardioversion is unnecessary; may consider TEE if patient has risk factors for stroke. [b]Ablation may be considered for patients who fail or do not tolerate ≥1 AAD. [c]Chronic antithrombotic therapy should be considered in all patients with AF and risk factors for stroke regardless of whether or not they remain in sinus rhythm. (AAD, antiarrhythmic drug; AF, atrial fibrillation; BB, β-blocker; CCB, calcium channel blocker [i.e., verapamil or diltiazem]; DCC, direct-current cardioversion; TEE, transesophageal echocardiogram)

in patients with atrial flutter has not been adequately studied in clinical trials, the most recent guidelines suggest that the same risk stratification scheme and antithrombotic recommendations used in patients with AF should also be applied to those with atrial flutter.[21]

Management

The traditional approach to the treatment of AF can be organized into several sequential goals. First, evaluate the need for acute treatment (usually administering drugs that slow ventricular rate). Next, contemplate methods to restore SR, taking into consideration the risks (e.g., thromboembolism). Lastly, consider ways to prevent the long-term complications of AF such as arrhythmia recurrence and thromboembolism. ❹ One of the biggest controversies in the management of AF is whether restoring and maintaining SR is a desirable goal for all patients. A review of the management of AF and atrial flutter, including a discussion of

this controversy, follows, organized according to the goals already outlined. Figure 25–5 shows an algorithm for the management of AF and atrial flutter. In addition, Table 25–8 summarizes the recommendations for pharmacologically controlling ventricular rate and restoring and maintaining SR from the most recent AF guidelines developed by the American College of Cardiology (ACC)/American Heart Association (AHA)/European Society of Cardiology (ESC).[17]

Acute Treatment First, consider the patient with new-onset, symptomatic AF or atrial flutter. Although uncommon, patients may present with signs and/or symptoms of hemodynamic instability (e.g., severe hypotension, angina, or pulmonary edema), which qualifies as a medical emergency. In these situations, DCC is indicated as first-line therapy in an attempt to immediately restore SR (without regard to the risk of thromboembolism). Atrial flutter often requires relatively low energy levels of countershock

TABLE 25-8 Evidence-Based Pharmacologic Treatment Recommendations for Controlling Ventricular Rate, Restoring Sinus Rhythm, and Maintaining Sinus Rhythm in Patients with Atrial Fibrillation

Treatment Recommendations	ACC/AHA/ESC Guideline Recommendation
Ventricular rate control (acute setting)	
In the absence of an accessory pathway, IV β-blockers or IV non-DHP CCBs are recommended for patients without hypotension or HF.	Class I
In the absence of an accessory pathway, IV digoxin or IV amiodarone is recommended for patients with HF.	Class I
IV amiodarone can be used to control the ventricular rate in patients who are refractory to or have contraindications to IV β-blockers, non-DHP CCBs, or digoxin.	Class IIa
IV procainamide or ibutilide is a reasonable alternative in patients with an accessory pathway when DCC is not necessary.	Class IIa
IV procainamide, ibutilide, or amiodarone may be considered for hemodynamically stable patients with an accessory pathway.	Class IIb
IV non-DHP CCBs are not recommended in patients with decompensated HF.	Class III
Ventricular rate control (chronic setting)	
Oral digoxin is effective for controlling the ventricular rate at rest in patients with HF or LV dysfunction, and in those who are sedentary.	Class I
Combination therapy with oral digoxin and either an oral β-blocker or non-DHP CCB is reasonable to control the ventricular rate both at rest and during exercise.	Class IIa
Oral amiodarone can be used when the ventricular rate cannot be adequately controlled at rest and during exercise with an oral β-blocker, non-DHP CCB, and/or digoxin.	Class IIb
Digoxin should not be used as the only agent for controlling the ventricular rate in patients with paroxysmal AF.	Class III
Restoration of sinus rhythm	
Flecainide, dofetilide, propafenone, or ibutilide is recommended for pharmacologic cardioversion of AF.	Class I
Amiodarone is a reasonable option for pharmacologic cardioversion of AF.	Class IIa
The "pill-in-the-pocket" approach (see text) can be used to terminate persistent AF on an outpatient basis once the treatment has been used safely in the hospital, in patients without sinus or AV node dysfunction, bundle-branch block, QT interval prolongation, Brugada syndrome, or SHD. (Note: AV node must be adequately blocked before initiating this therapy.)	Class IIa
Amiodarone can be used on an outpatient basis in patients with paroxysmal or persistent AF when rapid restoration of sinus rhythm is not necessary.	Class IIa
Quinidine or procainamide might be considered for pharmacologic cardioversion of AF, but their efficacy is not well established.	Class IIb
Digoxin and sotalol should not be used for pharmacologic cardioversion of AF (may be harmful).	Class III
Quinidine, procainamide, disopyramide, and dofetilide should not be initiated on an outpatient basis.	Class III
Maintenance of sinus rhythm	
Antiarrhythmic therapy can be useful for maintaining sinus rhythm and preventing tachycardia-induced cardiomyopathy.	Class IIa
Outpatient initiation of antiarrhythmic therapy is reasonable in patients without SHD.	Class IIa
Propafenone or flecainide may be initiated on an outpatient basis in patients with paroxysmal AF who have no SHD and are in sinus rhythm at the time therapy is initiated.	Class IIa
Sotalol may be initiated on an outpatient basis in patients without SHD, QT interval prolongation, electrolyte abnormalities, or other risk factors for proarrhythmia.	Class IIa
An antiarrhythmic drug should not be used when patients have risk factors for proarrhythmia with that particular agent.	Class III
Antiarrhythmic therapy is not recommended in patients with sinus or AV node dysfunction unless a pacemaker is present.	Class III

ACC, American College of Cardiology; AF, atrial fibrillation; AHA, American Heart Association; AV, atrioventricular; CCB, calcium channel blocker; DCC, direct-current cardioversion; DHP, dihydropyridine; ESC, European Society of Cardiology; HF, heart failure; IV, intravenous; LV, left ventricular; SHD, structural heart disease.
Adapted from Fuster et al.[17]

(i.e., 50 joules), whereas AF often requires higher energy levels (i.e., greater than 200 joules).

If patients are hemodynamically stable, there is no emergent need to restore SR. Instead, the focus should be directed toward controlling the patient's ventricular rate. Achieving adequate ventricular rate control should be a treatment goal for all patients with AF. To achieve this goal, drugs that slow conduction and increase refractoriness in the AV node (e.g., β-blockers, non-DHP CCBs, or digoxin) should be used as initial therapy. Although loading doses of digoxin have been historically recommended as first-line treatment to slow ventricular rate, use of this drug for this purpose, especially in patients with normal LV systolic function (LVEF >40%) has declined.[11] In this patient population, IV β-blockers (propranolol, metoprolol, esmolol), diltiazem, or verapamil are preferred. A few of the potential reasons for the declining use of digoxin in this patient population are its relatively slow onset and its inability to control the heart rate during exercise. Although an initial decrease in the ventricular rate can sometimes be observed within 1 hour of IV administration of digoxin, full control (heart rate <80 beats/min at rest and <100 beats/min during exercise) is usually not achieved for 24 to 48 hours. In addition, digoxin tends to be ineffective for controlling ventricular rate under conditions of increased sympathetic tone (i.e., surgery, thyrotoxicosis) because it slows AV nodal conduction primarily through vagotonic mechanisms. In contrast, IV β-blockers and non-DHP CCBs have a relatively quick onset and can effectively control the ventricular rate at rest and during exercise. β-blockers are also effective for controlling ventricular rate under conditions of increased sympathetic tone.

Based on the most recent guidelines for the treatment of AF, the selection of a drug to control ventricular rate in the acute setting should be primarily based on the patient's LV function.[17] In patients with normal LV function (LVEF >40%), IV β-blockers, diltiazem or verapamil is recommended as first-line therapy to control ventricular rate.[17] All of these drugs have proven efficacy in controlling the ventricular rate in patients with AF. Propranolol and metoprolol can be administered as intermittent IV boluses, whereas esmolol (because of its very short half-life of 5 to 10 minutes) must be administered as a series of loading doses followed by a continuous infusion. Likewise, because control of ventricular rate can be transient with a single bolus, verapamil or diltiazem can be given as an initial IV bolus followed by a continuous infusion.[23] These continuous infusions can be adjusted in monitored settings to the desired ventricular response (e.g., acutely <100 beats/min). In situations where AF or atrial flutter is precipitated by states of increased sympathetic tone, IV β-blockers can be highly effective and should be considered first.

In patients with LV dysfunction (LVEF ≤40%), both IV diltiazem and verapamil should be avoided because of their potent negative inotropic effects. IV β-blockers should be used with caution in this patient population and should be avoided if patients are in the midst of an episode of decompensated HF. In those patients who are having an exacerbation of HF symptoms, IV administration of either digoxin or amiodarone should be used as first-line therapy to achieve ventricular rate control.[17] IV amiodarone can also be used in patients who are refractory to or have contraindications to β-blockers, non-DHP CCBs, and digoxin.[17] However, clinicians should be aware that the use of amiodarone for controlling ventricular rate may also stimulate the conversion of AF to SR, and place the patient at risk for a thromboembolic event, especially if the AF has persisted at least 48 hours or is of unknown duration.

Patients may present with a slow ventricular response (in the absence of AV nodal-blocking drugs) and thus do not require therapy with β-blockers, non-DHP CCBs, or digoxin. This type of presentation should alert the clinician to the possibility of preexisting SA or AV nodal conduction disease such as sick sinus syndrome. In these patients, DCC should not be attempted without a temporary pacemaker in place.

Restoration of Sinus Rhythm? After treatment with AV nodal-blocking drugs and a subsequent decrease in the ventricular rate, the patient should be evaluated for the possibility of restoring SR if AF persists. Within the context of this evaluation, several factors should be considered. First, many patients spontaneously convert to SR without intervention, obviating the need for therapy to achieve this goal. For instance, AF occurs frequently as a complication of cardiac surgery and often spontaneously reverts to SR without therapy. Second, restoring SR is not a necessary or realistic goal in some patients. The results of six landmark clinical trials (Pharmacological Intervention in Atrial Fibrillation [PIAF], Rate Control versus Electrical Cardioversion for Persistent Atrial Fibrillation [RACE], Atrial Fibrillation Follow-up Investigation of Rhythm Management trial [AFFIRM], Strategies of Treatment of Atrial Fibrillation [STAF], How to Treat Chronic Atrial Fibrillation [HOT-CAFE], and Atrial Fibrillation and Congestive Heart Failure [AF-CHF]), have shed significant light on the comparative efficacy of rate-control (controlling ventricular rate; patient remains in AF) and rhythm-control (restoring and maintaining SR) treatment strategies in patients with AF.[24-29] The AFFIRM trial is the largest rate- versus rhythm-control study to be conducted to date in patients with AF.[26] In this trial, patients with AF and at least one risk factor for stroke were randomized to either a rate-control or rhythm-control group. Rate-control treatment involved AV nodal-blocking drugs (digoxin, β-blockers, and/or non-DHP CCBs) first, then nonpharmacologic treatment (AV nodal ablation with pacemaker implantation), if necessary. All patients in this group were anticoagulated with warfarin to achieve an international normalized ratio (INR) of 2.0 to 3.0. In the rhythm-control group, class I or III AADs were used to maintain SR. The choice of AAD therapy was left up to each patient's physician; however, by the end of the trial, more than 60% of patients had received at least one trial of amiodarone and approximately 40% of patients had received at least one trial of sotalol. In this group, anticoagulation was encouraged but could be discontinued if SR had been maintained for at least 4 weeks. After a mean follow-up period of 3.5 years, overall mortality was not statistically different between the two strategies but tended ($P = 0.08$) to be higher in the rhythm-control group. The results of the PIAF, RACE, STAF, and HOT-CAFE trials were consistent with those of the AFFIRM trial.[24,25,27,28] In addition, meta-analysis of the data from all of these trials demonstrated no significant

difference in overall mortality between rate-control and rhythm-control strategies, which persisted even when the results from the AFFIRM trial were excluded from this analysis.[30]

Even though the results of the PIAF, RACE, STAF, HOT-CAFE, and AFFIRM trials collectively demonstrate that a rate-control strategy is a viable alternative to a rhythm-control strategy in patients with persistent AF, a significant limitation of these results is that they cannot be applied to patients with HF because only a small proportion of patients enrolled in these trials had LV systolic dysfunction. The AF-CHF trial was conducted to specifically evaluate the safety and efficacy of rate-control and rhythm-control strategies in patients with systolic HF.[29] In this trial, patients with an LVEF ≤35%, a history of congestive HF (defined as NYHA class II–IV HF within the past 6 months, NYHA class I HF with a hospitalization for HF during the previous 6 months, or an LVEF ≤25%), and a history of AF were randomized to either a rate-control or rhythm-control group. Rate-control treatment involved concomitant therapy with a β-blocker and digoxin first, then nonpharmacologic treatment (AV nodal ablation with pacemaker implantation), if necessary. In the rhythm-control group, amiodarone was the preferred AAD, whereas sotalol and dofetilide were considered alternatives (most of the patients ultimately received amiodarone). If patients in this group did not convert to SR within 6 weeks, electrical cardioversion was performed. Anticoagulation was recommended for all patients in both treatment groups. After a mean follow-up period of 37 months, no significant difference was observed between the treatment groups with regard to the primary end point of death from cardiovascular causes. Patients in the rhythm-control group tended to have more hospitalizations, primarily due to repeated cardioversions and adjustment of AAD therapy, compared with patients in the rate-control group, although this difference was not statistically significant ($P = 0.06$). It is important to note that the results of this trial should not be applied to patients with HF and preserved LV function (i.e., diastolic HF). Nevertheless, the results of this trial are generally consistent with those of the PIAF, RACE, AFFIRM, STAF, and HOT-CAFE trials and suggest that a rhythm-control strategy does not confer any advantage over a rate-control strategy in patients with AF and systolic HF.

Clearly, these important findings temper the old approach of aggressively attempting to maintain SR. Because a rhythm-control strategy does not offer any significant advantage over a rate-control strategy in the management of patients with persistent or recurrent AF (including those with concomitant HF), it is acceptable to allow patients to remain in AF, while being chronically treated not only with AV nodal-blocking drugs to achieve adequate ventricular rate control (e.g., heart rate <80 beats/min at rest and <100 beats/min during exercise) but also with appropriate antithrombotic therapy to prevent thromboembolic complications. ❹ As in the acute setting, the selection of an AV nodal-blocking drug to control ventricular rate in the chronic setting should be primarily based on the patient's LV function.[17] In patients with normal LV function (LVEF >40%), oral β-blockers, diltiazem, or verapamil is preferred over digoxin because of their relatively quick onset and maintained efficacy during exercise. When adequate ventricular rate control cannot be achieved with one of these drugs, the addition of digoxin may provide an additive lowering of the heart rate. Verapamil and diltiazem should not be used in patients with LV dysfunction (LVEF ≤40%). Instead, β-blockers (i.e., metoprolol succinate, carvedilol, or bisoprolol) and digoxin are preferred in these patients, as these drugs are also concomitantly used to treat chronic HF. Specifically, in patients with NYHA class II or III HF, β-blockers should be considered over digoxin because of their survival benefits in patients with LV systolic dysfunction. If patients are having an episode of decompensated HF (NYHA class IV), digoxin is preferred as first-line therapy to achieve ventricular rate control because of the potential for worsening HF symptoms with the initiation and subsequent titration of β-blocker therapy. If adequate ventricular rate control during rest and exercise cannot be achieved with β-blockers, non-DHP CCBs, and/or digoxin in patients with normal or depressed LV function, oral amiodarone can be used as alternative therapy to control the heart rate.[17]

Because a rate-control strategy is now considered a reasonable initial approach for the chronic management of AF, the question that remains to be answered is, "In which patients should restoration of SR be considered?" Electrical or pharmacologic cardioversion should be considered for those patients with AF who remain symptomatic despite having adequate ventricular rate control or for those patients in whom adequate ventricular rate control cannot be achieved. In addition, a rhythm-control strategy may be considered in patients who are experiencing their first episode of AF if they are likely to convert to and remain in SR. Chronic AAD therapy is usually not needed in this latter population since the AF is often self-limiting.

In those patients in whom it is decided to restore SR, one must consider that this very act (regardless of whether an electrical or pharmacologic method is chosen) places the patient at risk for a thromboembolic event. The reason for this is that the return of SR restores effective contraction in the atria, which may dislodge poorly adherent thrombi. Administering antithrombotic therapy prior to cardioversion not only prevents clot growth and the formation of new thrombi but also allows existing thrombi to become organized and well-adherent to the atrial wall. It is a generally accepted principle that patients become at increased risk of thrombus formation and a subsequent embolic event if the duration of the AF exceeds 48 hours. Therefore, it is vital for clinicians to estimate the duration of the patient's AF, so that appropriate antithrombotic therapy can be administered prior to cardioversion if needed.

According to the most recent guidelines on antithrombotic and thrombolytic therapy developed by the American College of Chest Physicians (ACCP), patients with AF lasting at least 48 hours or an unknown duration should receive warfarin treatment (target INR 2.5; range: 2.0 to 3.0) for at least 3 weeks prior to elective cardioversion.[21] After restoration of SR, full atrial contraction does not occur immediately. Rather, it returns gradually to a maximum contractile force over a 3- to 4-week period. Consequently, warfarin should be continued for at least 4 weeks after successful cardioversion and return of SR.[21] Patients with risk factors for thromboembolism should be continued on warfarin therapy for longer than 4 weeks unless it is definitively known that they are remaining in SR. If the 3 weeks of therapeutic warfarin therapy prior to cardioversion is not feasible, patients may alternatively undergo transesophageal echocardiography (TEE) to provide guidance regarding the need for antithrombotic therapy prior to cardioversion. If no thrombus is noted on TEE, then these patients can be cardioverted without the mandatory 3 weeks of warfarin pretreatment. However, IV unfractionated heparin should still be administered during the TEE and cardioversion procedure to prevent the formation of thrombi during the peri- and postcardioversion periods. After successful cardioversion and return of SR, these patients should receive 4 weeks of warfarin therapy, as their atria may still be mechanically stunned during this period. Patients with risk factors for thromboembolism should be continued on warfarin for longer than 4 weeks unless it is definitively known that they are remaining in SR. If the TEE performed prior to cardioversion reveals a thrombus, patients should then be anticoagulated indefinitely, and cardioversion should not be attempted until there is absence of thrombus on repeat TEE. Overall, the use of TEE in this manner has been compared to the conventional 3 weeks of anticoagulation before cardioversion in patients with AF.[31] In this large, multicenter, randomized trial, the incidence of thromboembolic events was not

different between the two strategies, but bleeding episodes were higher in the group that received 3 weeks of warfarin therapy before cardioversion. Patients in the TEE strategy group had a higher success rate of achieving SR, probably because it is more difficult to terminate AF the longer a patient remains in this arrhythmia.

In patients with AF that is less than 48 hours in duration, anticoagulation prior to cardioversion is unnecessary because there has not been sufficient time to form atrial thrombi.[21] However, it is recommended that these patients should receive either IV unfractionated heparin or a low-molecular-weight heparin (subcutaneously at treatment doses) at presentation prior to cardioversion. If these patients have risk factors for stroke, a TEE could alternatively be performed prior to cardioversion to exclude the presence of thrombus. Patients with AF less than 48 hours in duration do not require the 4 weeks of postcardioversion anticoagulation therapy unless they have risk factors for stroke or the AF recurs.

After prior anticoagulation or TEE, the process of restoring SR can be considered. There are two methods of restoring SR in patients with AF or atrial flutter: pharmacologic cardioversion and DCC. The decision to use either of these methods is generally a matter of clinical preference. The disadvantages of pharmacologic cardioversion are the risk of significant side effects (e.g., drug-induced TdP),[32] the potential for drug–drug interactions (e.g., digoxin–amiodarone), and the lower efficacy of AADs when compared with DCC. The advantages of DCC are that it is quick and more often successful (80% to 90% success rate). The disadvantages of DCC are the need for prior sedation/anesthesia and a risk (albeit small) of serious complications such as sinus arrest or ventricular arrhythmias. Contrary to past beliefs, DCC carries very little risk in patients who are receiving digoxin and have no evidence of digoxin toxicity.

Nonetheless, despite the relatively high success rate associated with DCC, clinicians often elect to use AADs first, then resort to DCC in the event that these drugs fail. Pharmacologic cardioversion appears to be most effective when initiated within 7 days after the onset of AF.[17] According to the most recent treatment guidelines for AF, there is relatively strong evidence for efficacy of the class III pure I_K blockers (ibutilide and dofetilide), the class Ic AADs (e.g., flecainide and propafenone), and amiodarone (oral or IV) within this time frame.[17] Class Ia AADs have limited efficacy or have not been adequately studied in this setting. Sotalol is not effective for cardioversion of paroxysmal or persistent AF. Single, oral loading doses of propafenone (600 mg) and flecainide (300 mg) are effective compared with placebo for conversion of recent-onset AF and have been incorporated into the "pill-in-the-pocket" approach endorsed by the treatment guidelines.[17,33] With this method, outpatient, patient-controlled self-administration of a single, oral loading dose of either flecainide or propafenone can be a relatively safe and effective approach for the termination of recent-onset AF in a selected patient population that does not have sinus or AV node dysfunction, bundle-branch block, QT interval prolongation, Brugada syndrome, or SHD.[34] In addition, this treatment regimen should only be considered in patients who have previously been successfully cardioverted with these drugs on an inpatient basis. In patients with AF that is longer than 7 days in duration, only dofetilide, amiodarone, and ibutilide have proven efficacy for cardioversion.[17] The class Ia and Ic AADs have limited efficacy or have been inadequately studied in this setting.

Overall, when considering pharmacologic cardioversion, the selection of an AAD should be based on whether the patient has SHD (e.g., LV dysfunction, CAD, valvular heart disease, LV hypertrophy).[17] In the absence of any type of SHD, the use of a single, oral loading dose of flecainide or propafenone is a reasonable approach for cardioversion. Ibutilide can also be used as an alternative in this patient population; however, use of this agent is restricted to a monitored setting in the hospital because it requires QT interval monitoring. In patients with underlying SHD, flecainide, propafenone, and ibutilide should be avoided because of the increased risk of proarrhythmia; amiodarone or dofetilide should be used instead. Although amiodarone can be administered safely on an outpatient basis because of its low proarrhythmic potential, dofetilide therapy can only be initiated in the hospital (for QT interval monitoring). Additionally, it should be remembered that a patient's ventricular rate should be adequately controlled with AV nodal-blocking drugs prior to administering a class Ic (or Ia) AAD for cardioversion. The class Ia and Ic AADs may paradoxically increase ventricular response. Traditionally, this observation has been attributed to the vagolytic action of these drugs despite the fact that only disopyramide displays significant anticholinergic side effects. Therefore, a more likely alternative explanation exists: all of these drugs slow atrial conduction, decreasing the number of impulses reaching the AV node; as a result, the AV node paradoxically allows more impulses to gain entrance to the ventricular conduction system, thereby increasing ventricular rate.

Long-Term Complications There are two forms of therapy that the clinician must consider in each patient with AF: long-term antithrombotic therapy to prevent stroke, and long-term AADs to prevent recurrences of AF. Consider the issue of antithrombotic therapy first. In the past, patients with AF were not routinely anticoagulated (unless there was a history of stroke or concurrent mitral valve disease) because it was believed that the risk of warfarin exceeded its potential (though unknown) benefit. In the past several years, numerous randomized, placebo-controlled trials

have demonstrated that warfarin is the most effective agent for preventing stroke in patients with AF. The results of these studies have been incorporated into the most recent ACCP guidelines for antithrombotic therapy in patients with AF.[21] When initiating chronic antithrombotic therapy in patients with AF, assessing the patient's risk for stroke becomes important for selecting the most appropriate regimen. Based on the most recent ACCP guidelines, the CHADS2 index is now recommended for stroke risk stratification in patients with AF.[21] With this risk index, patients with AF are given two points if they have a history of a previous stroke or transient ischemic attack, and one point each for being ≥75 years old, having hypertension, having diabetes, or having congestive HF (CHADS2 is an acronym for each of these risk factors). The points are added up and the total score is then used to determine the most appropriate antithrombotic therapy for the patient (Fig. 25-6). Patients with a CHADS2 score of ≥2 are considered to be at high risk for stroke and should receive warfarin (target INR: 2.5; range: 2.0 to 3.0). Patients with a CHADS2 score of 1 are considered to be at intermediate risk for stroke and should receive either warfarin (target INR: 2.5; range: 2.0 to 3.0) or aspirin (75 to 325 mg/day). However, because of its superior efficacy in preventing stroke, the use of warfarin is suggested over that of aspirin in this particular group of patients. Patients with a CHADS2 score of 0 are considered to be at low risk for stroke and should receive aspirin (75 to 325 mg/day).

The safety and efficacy of combination antithrombotic therapy with aspirin and clopidogrel in patients with AF has been recently investigated in the Atrial Fibrillation Clopidogrel Trial with

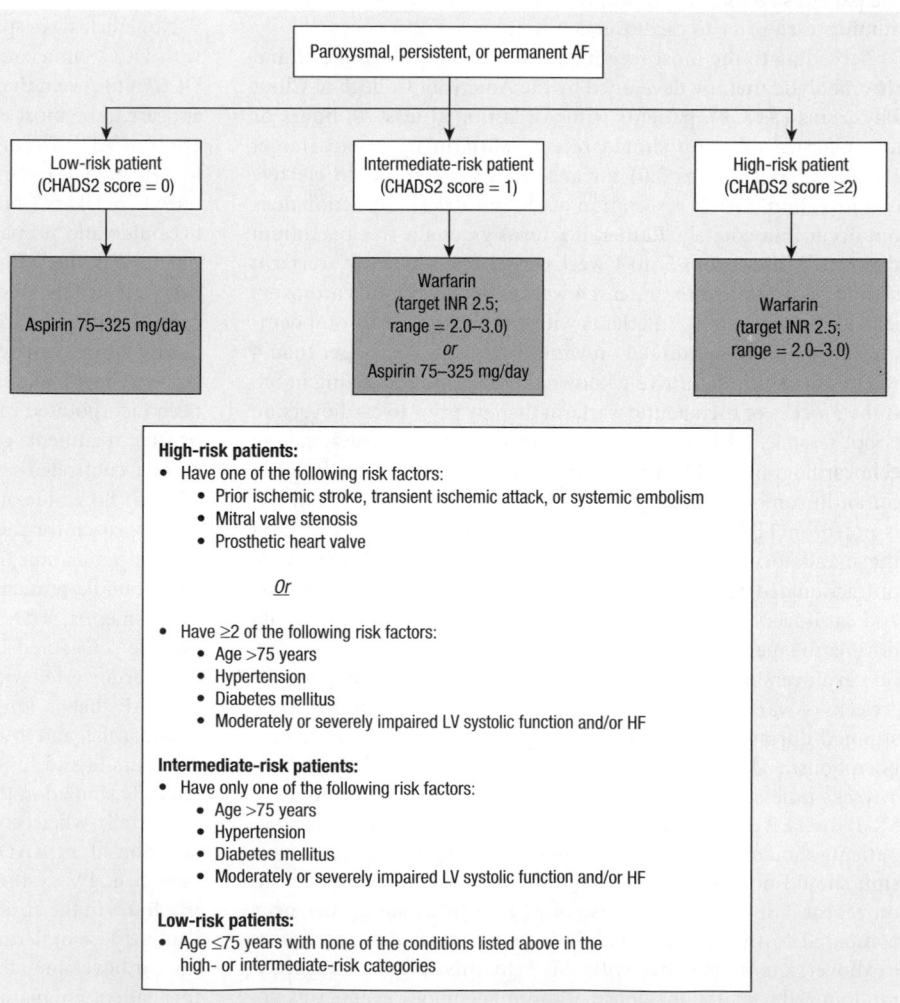

FIGURE 25-6. Algorithm for the prevention of thromboembolism in paroxysmal, persistent, or permanent AF.[a] The target INR for patients with prosthetic heart valves should be based upon the type of valve that is present. (AF, atrial fibrillation; INR, international normalized ratio; HF, heart failure; LV, left ventricular)

Irbesartan for Prevention of Vascular Events (ACTIVE) research program. Both the ACTIVE W and ACTIVE A evaluated the efficacy and safety of this combination therapy in patients with AF and at least one risk factor for stroke.[35,36] In the ACTIVE W, patients were randomized to receive oral anticoagulation therapy (with the vitamin K antagonist used in the investigator's country) titrated to achieve a target INR of 2.0 to 3.0 or clopidogrel 75 mg/day plus aspirin 75 to 100 mg/day.[35] After a median follow-up of 1.3 years, this trial was prematurely discontinued when the oral anticoagulation therapy was found to be superior to the combination antiplatelet regimen in reducing the occurrence of stroke, non–central nervous system systemic embolism, MI, or vascular death. While major bleeding events were similar between the two groups, significantly more minor bleeding episodes occurred in the clopidogrel plus aspirin group than in the oral anticoagulation group.

Patients who had a contraindication to or were unwilling to take oral anticoagulant therapy were enrolled in the ACTIVE A.[36] In this trial, patients were randomly assigned to receive clopidogrel 75 mg/day plus aspirin 75 to 100 mg/day or aspirin monotherapy (75 to 100 mg/day). After a median follow-up of 3.6 years, the incidence of stroke, non–central nervous system systemic embolism, MI, or vascular death was significantly reduced in the clopidogrel plus aspirin group when compared with the aspirin group. However, significantly more patients in the clopidogrel plus aspirin group experienced major bleeding than in the aspirin group. While the results of ACTIVE W were evaluated when the most recent ACCP guidelines were developed, the ACTIVE A was published after this time period. Although no official recommendations regarding the use of clopidogrel and aspirin therapy in patients with AF have been published, based on the results of ACTIVE A, this combination regimen may be considered in patients who are deemed to be unsuitable candidates for warfarin therapy (e.g., unable to comply with monitoring or dosing regimen requirements). If these patients are considered to be at high risk for bleeding, aspirin monotherapy can then be used.

Although it was previously an acceptable practice to continue antithrombotic therapy for only 4 weeks after successful cardioversion (with the belief that a patient's risk for thromboembolism had abated since they were in SR), data from the RACE and AFFIRM trials, in particular, strongly suggest that patients with AF and other risk factors for stroke continue to be at risk for stroke even when maintained in SR.[25,26] It is possible that these patients may be having undetected episodes of paroxysmal AF, placing them at risk for stroke. Consequently, the most recent ACCP guidelines recommend that chronic antithrombotic therapy be considered for all patients with AF and risk factors for stroke regardless of whether or not they remain in SR.[21]

The second form of chronic therapy to be considered is AADs to prevent recurrences of AF. Historically, many clinicians have aggressively attempted to maintain SR by prescribing oral AADs (usually quinidine) to prevent AF recurrences despite the fact that only small studies with conflicting results existed evaluating this approach. To evaluate the efficacy of quinidine in preventing AF, a well-known meta-analysis of the existing literature was completed.[37] This meta-analysis demonstrated that indeed more patients remain in SR with quinidine therapy (compared to placebo); however, approximately 50% have recurrences of AF within a year despite quinidine. This reported effectiveness was at the cost of an associated increase in mortality (presumably due, in part, to proarrhythmia) in the quinidine-treated patients. These disturbing results (published soon after the CAST[38]) became widely quoted and highly visible, making clinicians question the wisdom of long-term prevention of recurrences of AF with AADs. These results coupled with the more recent findings of the PIAF, RACE, AFFIRM, STAF, HOT-CAFE, and AF-CHF trials question the need to use AADs to prevent AF recurrences.[20-24] In fact, based on

TABLE 25-9	Guidelines for Selecting Antiarrhythmic Drug Therapy for Maintenance of Sinus Rhythm in Patients with Recurrent Paroxysmal or Recurrent Persistent Atrial Fibrillation

No structural heart disease[a]
First line: flecainide, propafenone, or sotalol
Second line: amiodarone, dofetilide, or dronedarone (catheter ablation could also be considered as an alternative to antiarrhythmic therapy)

Heart failure[a]
First line: amiodarone or dofetilide
Second line: catheter ablation

Coronary artery disease[a]
First line: sotalol (to be used only if patients have normal LV systolic function)
Second line: amiodarone, dofetilide, or dronedarone[b] (catheter ablation could also be considered as an alternative to antiarrhythmic therapy)

Hypertension[a]
Presence of significant LVH
    First line: amiodarone
    Second line: catheter ablation
Absence of significant LVH:
    First line: flecainide, propafenone, or sotalol
    Second line: amiodarone, dofetilide, or dronedarone (catheter ablation could also be considered as an alternative to antiarrhythmic therapy)

LV, left ventricular; LVH, left ventricular hypertrophy.
[a]Drugs are listed alphabetically and not in order of suggested use.
[b]Dronedarone should only be used in this situation if the patient has normal LV systolic function.

the results of these landmark trials, the use of AADs to maintain SR may be more reasonable to consider in patients who remain symptomatic despite having adequate ventricular rate control or for those patients in whom adequate ventricular rate control cannot be achieved.

According to the most recent treatment guidelines for AF, the class Ic or III AADs are reasonable to consider to maintain patients in SR (Table 25–9).[17] The role of the class Ia AADs for maintenance of SR has been deemphasized throughout these guidelines as they are considered less effective or incompletely studied compared to the class Ic and III AADs. Realistically, however, these drugs can still be considered as last-line therapy in select patients. Interestingly, a recent systematic review of AADs for the maintenance of SR after cardioversion in patients with AF demonstrated that AF recurrences were significantly reduced with the use of class Ia, Ic, and III AADs; however, mortality was significantly increased with the class Ia drugs, in particular.[39]

The class Ic AADs, flecainide and propafenone, are effective for maintaining SR. However, because of the increased risk for proarrhythmia, these drugs should be avoided in patients with SHD.

Although all of the oral class III AADs have demonstrated efficacy in preventing AF recurrences, amiodarone is clearly the most effective agent and is now the most frequently used AAD despite its potential for causing significant organ toxicity.[11] The superiority of amiodarone over other AADs for maintaining patients in SR has been demonstrated in a number of clinical trials. In the Canadian Trial of Atrial Fibrillation, amiodarone was significantly more effective than sotalol or propafenone in maintaining SR in patients with persistent or paroxysmal AF.[40] Furthermore, in a substudy of the AFFIRM trial, amiodarone appeared to be the most effective AAD of those used in the study.[41] In the Sotalol Amiodarone Atrial Fibrillation Efficacy Trial, amiodarone and sotalol were equally effective at converting AF to SR.[42] However, amiodarone was significantly more effective than sotalol at maintaining SR in all patient subgroups, except for those with CAD where the efficacy of these two drugs was comparable.

Although sotalol is not effective for conversion of AF, it is an effective drug for maintaining SR. Sotalol has been shown to be at least as effective as quinidine or propafenone in preventing recurrences of AF.[40,43] However, treatment with either quinidine or sotalol is associated with a similar incidence of TdP. Because this form of proarrhythmia primarily occurs with higher doses of sotalol (quinidine usually causes TdP at low or therapeutic concentrations), it may be more easily predicted and therefore avoided. Nonetheless, sotalol may increase mortality in patients with AF similar to quinidine; however, this requires further study.[44]

Dofetilide is effective in preventing recurrences of AF[45] but has not been directly compared with either amiodarone or sotalol. In a large, multicenter trial,[46] dofetilide (dose adjusted for renal function and QT interval) was more effective than placebo in maintaining SR (approximately 35% to 50% at 1 year). The efficacy of dofetilide for the maintenance of SR has also specifically been demonstrated in patients with LV dysfunction.[47] Like sotalol and quinidine, dofetilide also has significant potential to cause TdP (in a dose-related fashion).

The safety and efficacy of dronedarone for the treatment of AF and atrial flutter have been evaluated in several clinical trials. In the European Trial in Atrial Fibrillation or Flutter Patients Receiving Dronedarone for the Maintenance of Sinus Rhythm and the American-Australian-African Trial with Dronedarone in Atrial Fibrillation or Flutter Patients for the Maintenance of Sinus Rhythm, which were similar in design, dronedarone was more effective than placebo in maintaining SR in patients with paroxysmal or persistent AF or atrial flutter.[48] In another trial, the use of dronedarone in patients with persistent or paroxysmal AF or atrial flutter was associated with significantly fewer hospitalizations due to cardiovascular events or death when compared to placebo.[49] The safety and efficacy of dronedarone were also evaluated in a trial that included patients with NYHA class III or IV HF and an LVEF of 35% or less.[50] This trial was prematurely terminated because all-cause mortality (primarily due to worsening HF) was significantly higher in the dronedarone group when compared with the placebo group. Consequently, based on these findings, dronedarone is contraindicated in and has received a black-box warning for patients with advanced HF (NYHA class IV or NYHA class II or III with a recent hospitalization for decompensated HF).

Overall, the selection of an AAD to maintain SR should be primarily based on whether the patient has SHD.[17] However, other factors, including renal and hepatic function, concomitant disease states and drugs, and the AAD's side effect profile, also need to be considered. For those patients with no underlying SHD, flecainide, propafenone, or sotalol should be considered initially because these drugs have the most optimal long-term safety profile in this setting. However, amiodarone, dofetilide, or dronedarone could be used as alternative therapy if the patient fails or does not tolerate one of these initial AADs. In the presence of SHD, flecainide and propafenone should be avoided because of the risk of proarrhythmia. If LV dysfunction is present (LVEF ≤40%), amiodarone should be considered the AAD of choice. Dofetilide can be used as an alternative if patients develop intolerable side effects with amiodarone. At this time, only amiodarone and dofetilide have been shown to be mortality-neutral in patients with AF and HF. Both dronedarone and sotalol should be avoided in patients with LV dysfunction because of the risk for increased mortality (dronedarone) or worsening HF (sotalol). In patients with CAD, sotalol can be used initially, provided that the patient's LV function is normal. Amiodarone, dofetilide, or dronedarone could be used as an alternative therapy if the patient fails or does not tolerate sotalol. The presence of LV hypertrophy may predispose the myocardium to proarrhythmic events. Because of its low proarrhythmic potential, amiodarone should be considered first-line therapy in these patients.

Nonpharmacologic forms of therapy, designed to maintain SR are becoming increasingly popular treatment options for patients with AF or atrial flutter. For patients who have "pure" (i.e., not associated with concurrent AF) type I atrial flutter, ablation of the

reentrant substrate with radiofrequency current is highly effective (~90%)[51] and can be considered first-line treatment of atrial flutter to prevent recurrences.[52] Catheter ablation for patients with AF is much more technically difficult for a variety of reasons, including the lack of a single, identifiable, and ablatable reentrant focus (as in atrial flutter). Nonetheless, progress has been made in this area. Patients with AF have been found to have arrhythmogenic foci that occur in atrial tissue near and within the pulmonary veins. During the ablation procedure, radiofrequency energy can be delivered to these areas in an attempt to abolish the foci. Historically, this procedure was often considered last-line therapy for patients who had failed all AADs, including amiodarone. However, in some of the recent trials, the use of catheter ablation in patients with AF has been associated with a significant reduction in recurrent episodes of AF and an improvement in quality of life when compared with AAD therapy.[53,54] There is even some evidence[55,56] to suggest that this procedure may be superior to AADs as first-line therapy of symptomatic AF; however, these results will have to be validated in larger trials. Based on these recent data, the guidelines now recommend that catheter ablation be considered as a reasonable treatment alternative for patients with symptomatic episodes of recurrent AF who fail or do not tolerate at least one class I or III AAD.[57] This procedure is not without its risks, as major complications, such as pulmonary vein stenosis, thromboembolic events, cardiac tamponade, and new atrial flutter, have been reported in up to 6% of patients.[58]

PAROXYSMAL SUPRAVENTRICULAR TACHYCARDIA CAUSED BY REENTRY

PSVT arising by reentrant mechanisms includes those arrhythmias caused by AV nodal reentry, AV reentry incorporating an anomalous AV pathway, SA nodal reentry, and intraatrial reentry. AV nodal reentry and AV reentry are by far the most common of these tachycardias. **5**

Mechanisms

The underlying substrate of AV nodal reentry is the functional division of the AV node into two (or more) longitudinal conduction pathways or "dual" AV nodal pathways.[59] It is now clear that there are not two distinct anatomic pathways inside the AV node itself; rather, it is likely that a fanlike network of perinodal fibers inserts into the AV node and represents the second pathway. The pathways possess key differences in conduction characteristics: one is a fast-conducting pathway with a relatively long refractory period (fast pathway), and the other is a slower-conducting pathway with a shorter refractory period (slow pathway). The presence of dual pathways does not necessarily imply that the patient will have clinical PSVT. In fact, it is estimated that between 10% and 50% of patients have discernible dual pathways, but the incidence of PSVT is considerably lower.[59] Sustenance of the tachycardia depends on the critical electrophysiologic discrepancies and the ability of one pathway (usually the slow) to allow repetitive antegrade conduction, and the ability of the other pathway (usually the fast) to allow repetitive retrograde conduction. During SR, a patient with dual pathways conducts supraventricular impulses antegrade through both pathways. Electrical activity reaches the distal common pathway at the level of or above the His bundle and continues to depolarize the ventricles in an antegrade direction. Conduction proceeds via the two pathways but reaches the distal common pathway first through the fast AV nodal route (Fig. 25–7). For this reason, a short PR interval is sometimes observed during SR.

PSVT caused by AV nodal reentry may occur by the following sequence of events. The occurrence of an appropriately timed premature impulse penetrates the AV node but is blocked in the fast pathway that is still refractory from the previous beat. However,

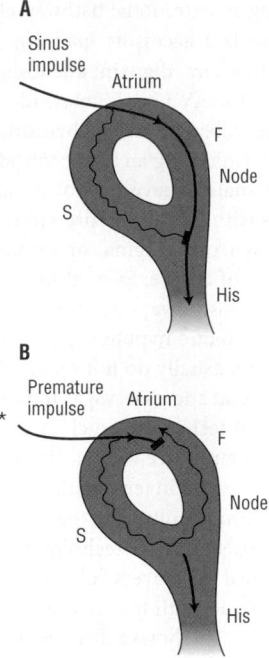

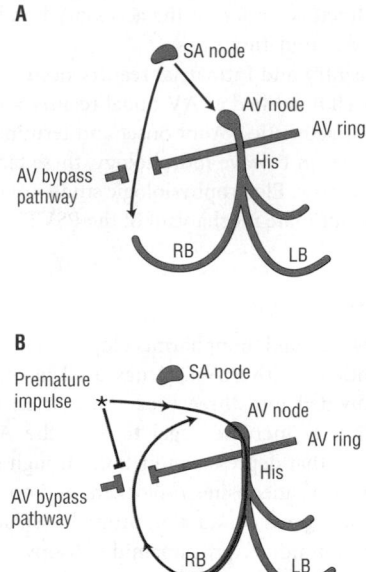

FIGURE 25-7. Reentry mechanism of dual AV nodal pathway PSVT. *A.* Sinus rhythm: The impulse travels from the atrium through the fast pathway *(F)* and then to the His-Purkinje system *(His)*. The impulse also travels through the slow pathway *(S)* but is stopped when refractory tissue is encountered. *B.* Dual AV nodal reentry: A critically timed premature impulse (*) is stopped in the fast pathway (because of prolonged refractoriness) but is able to travel antegrade down the slow pathway and retrograde through the fast pathway. (AV, atrioventricular; PSVT, paroxysmal supraventricular tachycardia)

FIGURE 25-8. Reentry mechanism for AV accessory pathway PSVT in Wolff-Parkinson-White syndrome. *A.* Sinus rhythm: The impulse travels from the atrium to the ventricle by two pathways—the AV node and an accessory bypass pathway. *B.* AV reentry: A critically timed premature impulse (*) is stopped in the Kent bundle (because of prolonged refractoriness) but travels antegrade through the AV node and retrograde through the Kent bundle. (AV, atrioventricular; His, His-Purkinje system; LB, left bundle-branch; PSVT, paroxysmal supraventricular tachycardia; RB, right bundle-branch; SA, sinoatrial)

the slow pathway, which has a shorter refractory period, permits antegrade conduction of the premature impulse. By the time the impulse has reached the distal common pathway, the fast pathway has recovered its excitability and now will permit retrograde conduction. The impulse reaches the common proximal pathway, preceded by an excitable gap of tissue, and reenters the slow pathway. A reentrant circuit that does not require atrial or ventricular tissue is completed within the AV node, and a tachycardia is thereby initiated (see Fig. 25-7). The common form of this tachycardia uses the slow pathway for antegrade conduction and the fast pathway for retrograde conduction; an uncommon form exists in which the reentrant impulse travels in the opposite direction.

AV reentrant tachycardia depends upon the presence of an anomalous, or accessory, extranodal pathway that bypasses the normal AV conduction pathway. Several different types of accessory pathways have been described, depending on the specific anatomic areas they connect (e.g., AV bundles or nodoventricular tracts); some are also referred to as eponyms, such as the Kent bundle. A Kent bundle is an extranodal AV connection that is associated with WPW syndrome. During SR (Fig. 25-8), patients with WPW syndrome depolarize the ventricles simultaneously through both AV pathways (AV nodal pathway and the Kent bundle), creating a fusion pattern on the early portion of the QRS complex (delta wave). The degree of ventricular "preexcitation" depends on the contribution of antegrade ventricular activation through the accessory pathway. Patients may have an accessory pathway that is not evident on ECG, which is referred to as a "concealed" Kent bundle. These concealed accessory pathways are often incapable of antegrade conduction and can only accept electrical stimulation in a retrograde fashion. The electrocardiographic expression of preexcitation (delta wave) depends on the location of the accessory pathway, the distance from the wavefront of sinus activation, and

the conduction characteristics of the various structures involved. It should be noted that (similar to patients with dual AV nodal pathways) not all patients with preexcitation with an accessory AV pathway are capable of having clinical PSVT.

Patients with an accessory AV pathway may have three forms of supraventricular tachycardia: orthodromic reentry, antidromic reentry, and/or AF or atrial flutter. AV reentrant PSVT usually occurs by the following sequence of events. Analogous to AV nodal reentry, two pathways (the normal AV nodal pathway and the accessory AV pathway) exist that have different electrophysiologic characteristics. The AV nodal pathway usually has a relatively slower conduction velocity and shorter refractory period, and the accessory pathway has a faster conduction velocity and a longer refractory period. A critically timed premature impulse may be blocked in the accessory pathway because this area is still refractory from the previous sinus beat. However, the AV nodal pathway, with a relatively shorter refractory period, may accept antegrade conduction of the premature impulse. Meanwhile, the accessory pathway may recover its excitability and now allow retrograde conduction. A macroreentrant tachycardia is thereby initiated in which the antegrade pathway is the AV nodal pathway; the distal common pathway is the ventricle; the retrograde pathway is the accessory pathway; and the proximal common pathway is the atrium (see Fig. 25-8). This sequence of events (down the AV node, up the Kent bundle), termed *orthodromic PSVT*, is the common variety of reentry in patients with an accessory AV pathway, resulting in a narrow QRS tachycardia. In the uncommon variety, conduction proceeds in the opposite direction (down the Kent bundle, up the AV node), resulting in a wide QRS tachycardia, which is termed *antidromic PSVT*. Patients with WPW syndrome can have a third type of tachycardia, namely AF. The occurrence of AF in the setting of an accessory AV pathway (i.e., WPW syndrome) can be extremely serious. As AF is an extremely rapid atrial tachycardia, conduction can proceed down the accessory AV pathway, resulting in a very fast ventricular response or even VF. Unlike the AV nodal pathway, the refractory period of the accessory bundle shortens in response to rapid stimulation rates.

Sinus node reentry and intraatrial reentry occur less commonly and are not as well described as AV nodal reentry and AV reentry. Aside from a characteristic abrupt onset and termination, coupled with subtle changes in P-wave morphology, these tachycardias can be difficult to diagnose. Electrophysiologic studies may be necessary to determine the ultimate mechanism of the PSVT.

Management

Both pharmacologic and nonpharmacologic methods have been used to treat patients with PSVT. Drugs used in the treatment of PSVT can be divided into three broad categories: (a) those that directly or indirectly increase vagal tone to the AV node (e.g., digoxin); (b) those that depress conduction through slow, calcium-dependent tissue (e.g., adenosine, β-blockers, and non-DHP CCBs); and (c) those that depress conduction through fast, sodium-dependent tissue (e.g., quinidine, procainamide, disopyramide, and flecainide). Drugs within these categories alter the electrophysiologic characteristics of the reentrant substrate so that PSVT cannot be sustained. In PSVT caused by AV nodal reentry, class I AADs, such as flecainide, act primarily on the retrograde fast pathway. Digoxin and β-blockers may work on either the retrograde fast or the antegrade slow pathway. Verapamil, diltiazem, and adenosine prolong conduction time and increase refractoriness, primarily in the slow antegrade pathway of the reentrant loop. In PSVT caused by AV

reentry incorporating an extranodal pathway, class I AADs increase refractoriness in the fast accessory pathway or within the His-Purkinje system. β-blockers, digoxin, adenosine, and verapamil all act by their effects on the AV nodal (antegrade, slow) portion of the reentrant circuit. Regardless of the mechanism, treatment measures are directed first at terminating an acute episode of PSVT and then at preventing symptomatic recurrences of the arrhythmia.

For those patients with PSVT who present with severe symptoms (i.e., syncope, near syncope, angina, or severe HF), synchronized DCC is the treatment of choice. Even at low energy levels (such as 25 joules), DCC is almost always effective in quickly restoring SR and correcting symptomatic hypotension. Patients with only mild to moderate symptoms usually do not require DCC, and nonpharmacologic measures that increase vagal tone to the AV node can be used initially. Vagal techniques, such as unilateral carotid sinus massage, Valsalva maneuver, ice water facial immersion, or induced retching, are often successful in terminating PSVT, although carotid massage and Valsalva maneuver are the simplest, least obtrusive, and most frequently used of these techniques.

In the event that vagal maneuvers fail (approximately 80% of acute episodes) in those patients with tolerable symptoms, drug therapy is the next option. Figure 25–9 shows a therapeutic approach to the acute treatment of the different forms of reentrant PSVT. ❻ This approach is based on analysis of the electrocardiographic characteristics of the rhythm because PSVT is not always discernible from other arrhythmias, and some forms of PSVT require different treatment. In patients with a narrow QRS, regular arrhythmia (AV nodal reentry

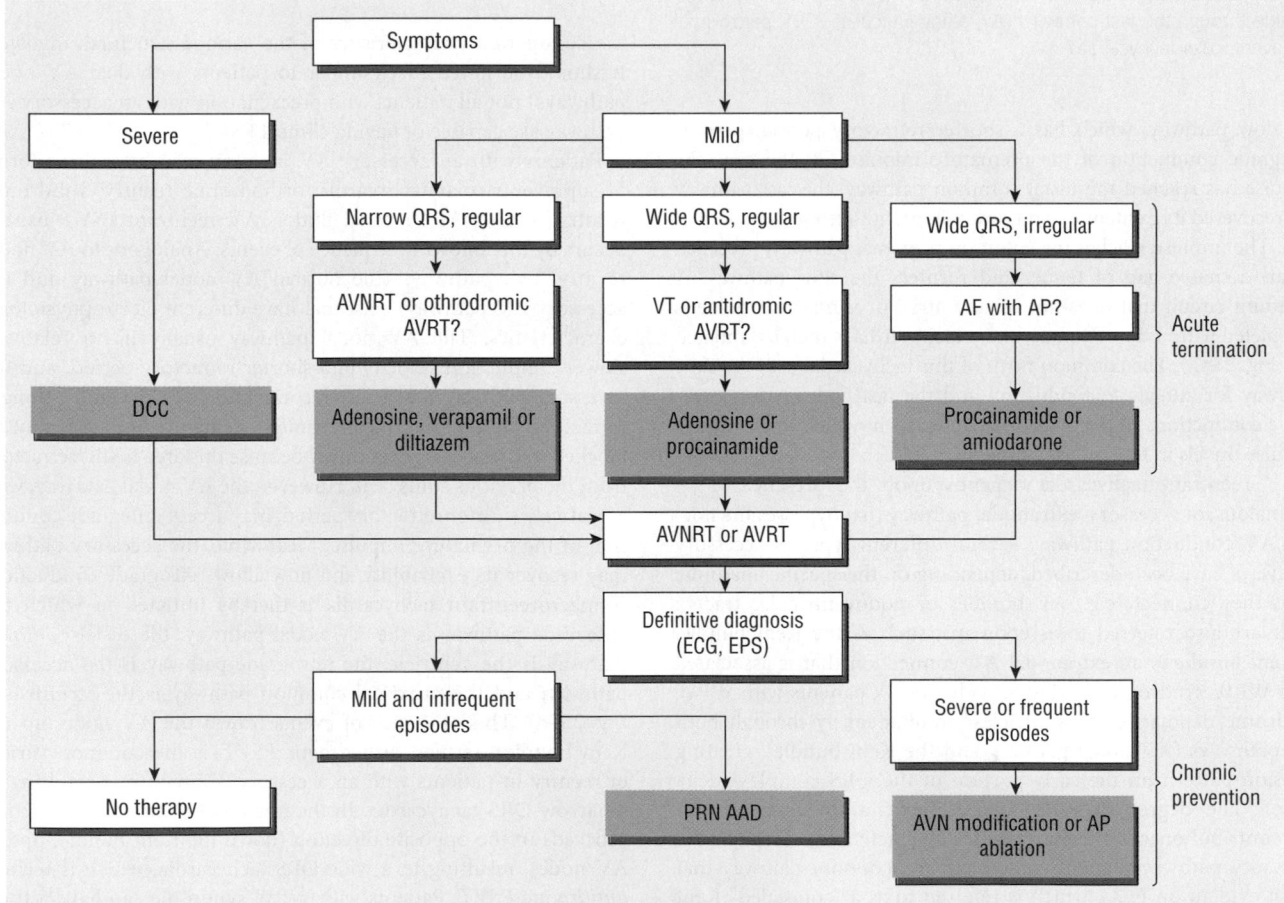

FIGURE 25-9. Algorithm for the treatment of acute *(top portion)* PSVT and chronic prevention of recurrences *(bottom portion)*. *Note:* For empiric bridge therapy prior to radiofrequency ablation procedures, CCBs (or other AV nodal blockers) should not be used if the patient has AV reentry with an accessory pathway. (AAD, antiarrhythmic drugs; AF, atrial fibrillation; AP, accessory pathway; AV, atrioventricular; AVN, atrioventricular nodal; AVNRT, atrioventricular nodal reentrant tachycardia; AVRT, atrioventricular reentrant tachycardia; CCBs, calcium channel blockers; DCC, direct-current cardioversion; ECG, electrocardiogram; EPS, electrophysiologic studies; PRN, as needed; PSVT, paroxysmal supraventricular tachycardia; VT, ventricular tachycardia.)

or orthodromic AV reentry), IV verapamil (5 to 10 mg), IV diltiazem (15 to 25 mg), and adenosine (6 to 12 mg) are all equally efficacious. Approximately 80% to 90% of PSVT episodes will revert to SR within 5 minutes of these drug therapies.[60] The most recent guidelines for cardiopulmonary resuscitation (CPR) and emergency cardiovascular care (ECC) from the AHA,[61] and practice guidelines from the ACC/AHA/ESC,[52] promote adenosine as the drug of first choice in patients with PSVT. ❺ These recommendations are particularly important when treating a patient who presents with a wide QRS, regular tachycardia that may be VT or PSVT (antidromic AV reentry or as a result of aberrancy). Because of its ultrashort duration of action (seconds), adenosine will not cause the severe and prolonged hemodynamic compromise seen in patients with VT who were mistakenly treated with verapamil and suffered from its negative inotropic effects and vasodilator properties.[62] If, in fact, the arrhythmia is PSVT, adenosine will likely terminate it. An alternative treatment for this type of patient is IV procainamide, which works on the fast, sodium-dependent extranodal pathway and is also effective for VT. Likewise, IV procainamide, or perhaps IV amiodarone (particularly in patients with LV dysfunction), or IV sotalol should be used for the patient who presents with a wide QRS, irregular arrhythmia that is hemodynamically stable.[61] This rhythm could represent AF with rapid ventricular activation occurring primarily through an extranodal pathway. Administration of IV verapamil, diltiazem, digoxin, or adenosine to these patients may result in a paradoxical increase in ventricular response, causing severe symptoms requiring cardioversion. Consequently, these drugs are considered contraindicated in this specific setting.

Once the acute episode of PSVT is terminated, a decision on long-term preventive therapy must follow. Most patients require long-term therapy; preventive treatment is indicated if (a) frequent episodes occur that necessitate therapeutic intervention (i.e., emergency department visits or interference with the patient's lifestyle), or (b) infrequent but severely symptomatic symptoms occur. For those patients in whom a preventive treatment is deemed necessary, two methods of management have been used: preventive drug therapy and ablation.

AADs are no longer the treatment of choice to prevent recurrences of reentrant PSVT for the following reasons: (a) lifelong treatment is necessary in these generally young, but otherwise healthy, individuals; (b) there are few, if any, large controlled or comparative trials to assist the clinician in rationally choosing effective agents; and (c) most importantly, other nonpharmacologic treatments are clearly more effective. Nevertheless, drug therapy may occasionally be necessary in some patients, particularly those with mild symptoms and infrequent recurrences. A trial-and-error approach may be used, complemented by the use of ambulatory electrocardiographic recordings (Holter) or telephonic transmissions of cardiac rhythm (event monitors) to objectively document the efficacy or failure of the chosen drug regimen. Drugs known to be effective in preventing recurrences of PSVT are the AV nodal-blocking drugs (digoxin, β-blockers, non-DHP CCBs, and combinations of these agents) and the class Ic AADs (flecainide, propafenone). Drugs such as quinidine, disopyramide, amiodarone, and dofetilide, although effective in some patients, should be discouraged because of the risk of toxicity with long-term treatment.

One concept that can serve as an aid to arriving at an effective regimen is that there are patterns of drug response in patients with PSVT; in other words, the tachycardia behaves as if it has a "weak link." Patients who respond to agents that act on one limb of the reentrant loop are less likely to respond to drugs that block conduction in the other limb. For instance, in a patient with AV nodal reentry, one may first choose a non-DHP CCB or β-blocker (to affect the antegrade, slow pathway). If symptomatic recurrences are subsequently documented, it may be prudent to switch to a class Ic AAD (to affect the retrograde, fast pathway) in an attempt to find the weak link or susceptible pathway. Patients with evidence of pre-excitation (delta waves during SR) should not be treated with only AV nodal-blocking drugs. If AF were to occur, these drugs would facilitate rapid conduction over the accessory pathway. The trial-and-error method for determining drug effectiveness in this setting has inherent shortcomings. If the PSVT episodes are infrequent, a considerable time period may be consumed before an effective regimen is realized, or in the case of moderate to severe symptoms associated with PSVT, the patient may experience several troublesome episodes before the correct drug is identified. Alternatively, self-administered, single-dose oral therapy (i.e., the "pill-in-the-pocket" strategy) has been shown effective. Specifically, 120 mg of oral diltiazem coupled with 80 mg of oral propranolol has been shown to be superior to single-dose flecainide in terminating PSVT, decreasing the need to visit the emergency department for treatment.[63] Nonetheless, *all* forms of drug treatment designed to prevent or terminate the arrhythmia by self-administered therapy should probably be avoided in most patients because of the superior efficacy of nonpharmacologic treatment strategies.

Transcutaneous catheter ablation using radiofrequency current on the PSVT substrate has dramatically altered the traditional treatment of these patients (Fig. 25-10). ❺ Radiofrequency energy delivered through a transvenous or arterial catheter causes small, discrete lesions through thermal energy. During invasive electrophysiologic studies, portions of the reentrant circuit can be located (or mapped) by the use of a number of catheters. Once this is completed, radiofrequency energy is applied, creating thermal injury in the tissue necessary for reentry. In this way, the substrate for reentry is destroyed, "curing" the patient of recurrent episodes of PSVT and obviating the need for chronic drug therapy. Historically, ablation procedures were reserved for drug-refractory patients because they necessitated open-heart surgery. However, breakthroughs in technology initially included transvenous catheter approaches, followed by the use of radiofrequency (rather than direct current) energy. Complications, although unusual, include tamponade, pericarditis, valvular insufficiency, and AV block. Radiofrequency ablation is highly effective, preventing the recurrences of PSVT in 85% to 98% of patients.[64,65] The procedure was originally used in patients with WPW syndrome.[64] In these patients, the extranodal pathway is most often located at the left lateral free wall of the left ventricle (Fig. 25-10). After the pathway is located, the catheter is put as close to the site as possible, and radiofrequency current is applied to make small burns in the tissue. Ablation of the extranodal connection occurs promptly, and evidence of preexcitation (delta waves) disappears. Thereafter, a similar approach was developed for patients with AV nodal reentry, placing the catheter in the coronary sinus, proximal to the AV node.[65] The preferred method in these individuals is to apply small amounts of radiofrequency current to the slow pathway of the reentrant circuit in order to modify its properties enough so that PSVT cannot recur.

It has been suggested that *all* patients with symptomatic PSVT undergo radiofrequency catheter ablation.[66] This is because the procedure is highly effective and curative, rarely results in complications, and obviates the need for chronic AAD therapy. In other words, radiofrequency catheter ablation should be considered in *any* patient who would previously be considered for chronic AAD treatment. Radiofrequency ablation is also a cost-effective approach (in the long term) because, if effective, the costs of drugs and repeated hospital visits are avoided. In one cost-effectiveness analysis, radiofrequency ablation improved quality of life and reduced lifetime medical expenditures by nearly $30,000 compared with chronic drug treatment.[67]

AUTOMATIC ATRIAL TACHYCARDIAS

Automatic atrial tachycardias, such as multifocal atrial tachycardia, appear to arise from supraventricular foci that have enhanced automatic properties.[68] It is presumed that multifocal atrial

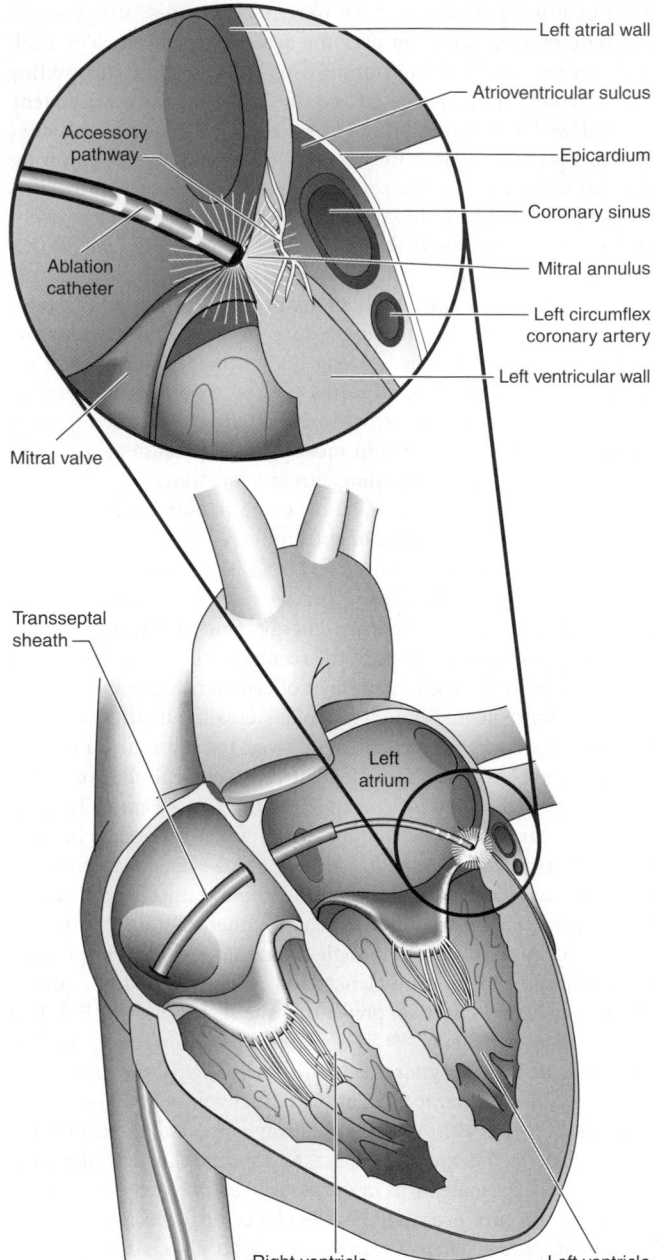

FIGURE 25-10. Drawing showing catheter placement for radiofrequency ablation of a left lateral free wall accessory pathway. Here, a venous (atrial) transseptal puncture to gain access to the Kent bundle is shown; a retrograde arterial approach has also been used. *(Lerman BB, Basson CT. High risk patients with ventricular preexcitation: A pendulum in motion. N Engl J Med 2003;349:1787–1789. Copyright © 2003 Massachusetts Medical Society. All rights reserved.)*

tachycardia is the result of multiple ectopic atrial pacemakers, which account for the variable P-wave morphologies. In unifocal atrial tachycardia (more often referred to as ectopic atrial tachycardia), a single P-wave morphology, different from that of SR, is recorded. In either case, the underlying, precipitating disorder present in the majority (60% to 80%) of these patients is severe pulmonary disease. Other disease states associated with these arrhythmias include acute infection (pneumonia and sepsis) and dilated cardiomyopathy. It should be noted that young patients without associated precipitating factors might rarely present with rapid atrial tachycardias from unknown etiologies. In these cases, long-standing tachycardias cause the cardiomyopathic state. Effective treatment of the tachycardia may result in reversal of the LV dysfunction. Traditionally, many

factors (i.e., electrolyte disturbances, hypoxia, catecholamines, and tissue stretch) may cause an elevated slope of phase 4 depolarization and theoretically result in abnormal heightened automaticity. It is noteworthy that many of these factors are often clinically present in patients with concurrent pulmonary disease and automatic atrial tachycardia. However, it appears that triggered activity (i.e., LADs) is a more likely mechanism in the genesis of these tachycardias. Atrial tachycardias with AV block or a slow ventricular response should alert the clinician to the possibility of digoxin toxicity.

The first step in the treatment of automatic atrial tachycardias is to correct the underlying, precipitating factors.[68] One should ensure proper oxygenation and ventilation and correct acid–base or electrolyte disturbances. These measures alone may result in the return of SR, but in some cases, the tachycardia will persist. Patients with an asymptomatic atrial tachycardia and a relatively slow ventricular rate usually require no drug therapy. In symptomatic patients, medical therapy can be tailored either to control ventricular rate or to restore SR. Class I AADs, such as procainamide and quinidine, are only occasionally effective in restoring SR and are usually not considered first-line therapy. DCC is also ineffective in restoring SR. The use of IV β-blockers to slow ventricular rate is usually contraindicated because of the frequent coexistence of bronchospastic pulmonary disease or decompensated HF. Digoxin has been used but is controversial because of its ability to increase the automatic properties of atrial tissue, and the high sympathetic state of these patients frequently overrides the vagotonic effects of digoxin, rendering it ineffective. Non-DHP CCBs, such as verapamil, are most effective and are now considered first-line drug therapy.[52,69] Interestingly, verapamil seems to decrease ventricular rate by altering atrial automaticity, not by slowing AV nodal conduction.[69]

VENTRICULAR ARRHYTHMIAS

The common ventricular arrhythmias include (a) PVCs, (b) VT, and (c) VF. These arrhythmias may result in a wide variety of symptoms. PVCs often cause no symptoms or only mild palpitations. VT may be a life-threatening situation associated with hemodynamic collapse or may be totally asymptomatic. VF, by definition, is an acute medical emergency necessitating CPR.

CLINICAL PRESENTATION: VENTRICULAR ARRHYTHMIAS

Premature Ventricular Contractions

■ PVCs are non-life-threatening and usually asymptomatic. Occasionally, patients will complain of palpitations or uncomfortable heartbeats. Since the PVC, by definition, occurs early and the ventricle contracts when it is incompletely filled, patients do not feel the PVC. Rather, the next beat (after the PVC and a compensatory pause) is usually responsible for the patient's symptoms.

Ventricular Tachycardia

■ The symptoms of VT (monomorphic VT or TdP), if prolonged (i.e., sustained), can vary from nearly completely asymptomatic to pulseless, hemodynamic collapse. Fast heart rates and underlying poor LV function will result in more severe symptoms. Symptoms of nonsustained, self-terminating VT also correlate with duration of episodes (e.g., patients with 15-second episodes will be more symptomatic than those with three-beat episodes).

Ventricular Fibrillation

■ By definition, VF results in hemodynamic collapse, syncope, and cardiac arrest. Cardiac output and blood pressure are not recordable.

PREMATURE VENTRICULAR COMPLEXES AND PREVENTION OF SUDDEN CARDIAC DEATH

PVCs are very common ventricular rhythm disturbances that occur in patients with or without SHD. Experimental models show that PVCs may be elicited by abnormal automaticity, triggered activity, or reentrant mechanisms. It is well known that PVCs are commonly observed in apparently healthy individuals; in these patients, the PVCs seem to have little if any prognostic significance. PVCs occur more frequently and in more complex forms in patients with SHD than in healthy individuals. The prognostic meaning of PVCs has been well studied in patients with MI (acute or remote) with several consistent themes. Patients with some forms of PVCs are at higher risk for sudden death than if they did not have these minor rhythm disturbances. SCD can be defined as unexpected death occurring in a patient within 1 hour of experiencing symptoms. Studies of patients who experienced SCD (and happened to be wearing an electrocardiographic monitor at the time) often demonstrate the cause to be VF preceded by a short run of VT and frequent PVCs.[70]

Significance

Historically, investigators promoted the concept that patients in the acute phase of MI may have types of PVCs that are predictive of VF and SCD. These types of PVCs were referred to as "warning arrhythmias" and included frequent ventricular ectopy (more than 5 beats/min), multiform configuration (different morphology), couplets (two in a row), and R-on-T phenomenon (PVCs occurring during the repolarization phase of the preceding sinus beat in the vulnerable period of ventricular recovery). However, as a result of using continuous electrocardiographic monitoring techniques, it has become apparent that almost all patients have warning arrhythmias in the acute MI setting. In those patients who experience VF, warning arrhythmias are no more common than in those without VF. Consequently, warning arrhythmias observed during acute MI are neither sensitive nor specific for determining which patients will have VF. Thus there is little need to direct drug therapy specifically at PVC suppression in these particular patients. Studies show that effective prevention of VF in the acute MI setting may be achieved without the abolition of PVCs.

Conversely, data strongly imply that PVCs documented in the convalescence period of MI do carry important long-term prognostic significance.[71] PVCs occurring after an MI seem to be a risk factor for patient death that is independent of the degree of LV dysfunction or the extent of coronary atherosclerosis. Ruberman et al.[71] employed a simple classification of PVCs: simple or benign (infrequent and monomorphic) versus "complex" (≥5 PVCs/min, couplets, R-on-T beats, and multiform). These investigators found that the presence of complex (but not simple) ventricular ectopy in the setting of CAD was associated with a higher incidence of overall mortality and cardiac death. One can see that within the controversy of the significance of PVCs is a basic question: Are complex forms of PVCs simply an unimportant marker of underlying SHD or are PVCs an important electrical disorder that should be addressed independently?

Because PVCs without associated SHD, in apparently healthy individuals, carry little or no risk, drug therapy is unnecessary. However, because of the prognostic significance of complex PVCs in patients with SHD, the use of AAD therapy to suppress them has been controversial. Historically, many supported the aggressive use of AAD therapy to suppress PVCs, based on the underlying premise of eliminating a risk factor for SCD in patients with CAD (namely the presence of complex PVCs). However, others favored a more conservative approach and disregarded the use of AAD therapy in the absence of significant symptoms. An important study, the CAST,[38] abruptly put an end to this debate in noteworthy fashion; its results are reviewed in the following section because of its great historical significance and lingering impact.

The Cardiac Arrhythmia Suppression Trial

The CAST[38,72] was initiated by the National Institutes of Health in 1987 to determine if suppression of ventricular ectopy with encainide, flecainide, or moricizine could decrease the incidence of death from arrhythmia in patients who had suffered an MI. **❼** Entrance criteria included documented MI between 6 days and 2 years prior to enrollment, and ≥6 PVCs/hour (associated with no or minimal symptoms) without runs of VT >15 beats in length. Also, patients were required to have an LVEF ≤55% if recruited within 90 days of the MI or an LVEF ≤40% if recruited ≥90 days after the MI. Patients with an LVEF <30% were randomized only to encainide or moricizine. Patients were randomized to receive AAD therapy or placebo after demonstrating PVC suppression with one of the agents.

In April 1989, a routine, preliminary review of the study by the Safety and Monitoring Board revealed alarming results, and the study was interrupted. The results showed that when compared with placebo, treatment with encainide or flecainide was associated with a significantly higher rate of total mortality and death due to arrhythmia, presumably caused by proarrhythmia (Fig. 25–11). Analysis of the moricizine arm indicated neither harm nor benefit from this therapy; therefore, only this portion of the study was allowed to continue as CAST II.[72] However, in July 1991, CAST II was also prematurely discontinued because there was a trend toward an increase in mortality in moricizine-treated patients. This increase in mortality was primarily observed during the initiation of moricizine (dose-titration phase) but not during the chronic treatment phase. The overall results of the two CASTs conclusively prove that the use of AAD therapy (beyond the general use of β-blockers) to suppress PVCs in patients after an MI does not improve survival and is most likely detrimental. These studies also put into perspective the risk associated with the use of AAD therapy and the need to carefully select only those patients who would derive a defined therapeutic benefit from this therapy.

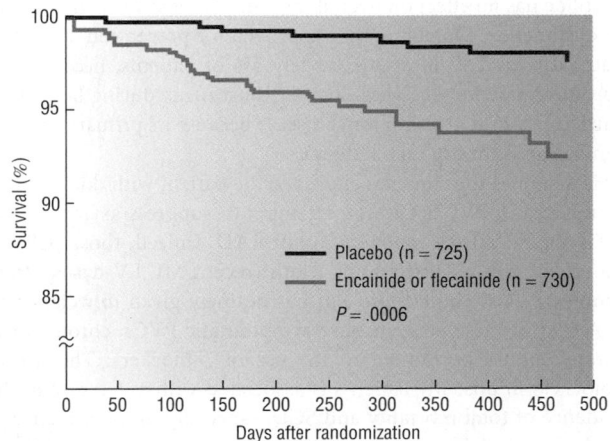

FIGURE 25-11. Life table curves from the Cardiac Arrhythmia Suppression Trial (CAST), specifically for patients receiving encainide or flecainide *(lighter line)* and matching placebo *(darker line)*. Note the divergent slopes of each line, implying a sustained risk of death (presumed proarrhythmia). *(The CAST Investigators. Preliminary report: Effect of encainide and flecainide on mortality in a randomized trial of arrhythmia suppression after myocardial infarction. N Engl J Med 1989;321:406–412. Copyright © 1989 Massachusetts Medical Society. All rights reserved.)*

Even though the CAST was conducted more than 2 decades ago, it is considered one of the most important trials ever undertaken and has had a tremendous influence on the overall approach to the treatment of arrhythmias, as well as a far-reaching impact on AAD development. The results of the CAST have clearly had a negative influence on the long-term use of all AADs, causing a broad skepticism in the risk-versus-benefit analysis of this class of drugs. Consequently, pharmaceutical companies have shifted their drug discovery and investigative efforts away from potent sodium channel blockers. The findings of the CAST have also provided additional fuel for the pursuit of nonpharmacologic therapies for arrhythmias, such as ablation and implantable devices.

Despite the discouraging results of the CAST, post-MI patients with complex ventricular ectopy remain at risk for death. Other drugs, besides the class Ic AADs, have been studied in this patient population, including sotalol. Sotalol is marketed as a racemic mixture of a *d* and *l* isomer: both are class III potassium channel blockers but the *l* isomer has β-blocking actions. Chronic therapy with *d*-sotalol was studied in patients with a remote MI complicated by complex ectopy in the Survival With Oral *d*-Sotalol trial.[73] In this trial, *d*-sotalol treatment was not designed to cause PVC suppression (unlike the CAST), yet (like the CAST) the trial was halted prematurely because of excessive mortality in the treatment arm. Again, the presumed reason for this observation was *d*-sotalol–related proarrhythmia. Currently, only two AADs have been shown *not* to increase mortality in post-MI patients with long-term use: amiodarone and dofetilide. A number of trials[74,75] have shown amiodarone to decrease the incidence of sudden (or arrhythmic) death, but not total mortality, in post-MI patients with complex ventricular ectopy. A meta-analysis of all trials (6,553 combined patients) demonstrated a reduction in total mortality (by 13%) with long-term amiodarone therapy.[76] It is unclear if these findings can be attributed to one of amiodarone's electrophysiologic properties (e.g., β-blocking) or a combination of its complex pharmacologic effects on conduction. It is noteworthy to mention that in two major studies, patients treated with amiodarone and a β-blocker generally did better than when no β-blocker was used.[74,75] Clearly, because of its impressive side effect profile and its inability to improve survival, amiodarone should not routinely be recommended in patients with heart disease such as remote MI and complex PVCs. Two randomized, controlled trials[77,78] have also shown that chronic therapy with dofetilide has no effect on overall mortality in post-MI patients with LV dysfunction. Dofetilide (not approved for prevention of sudden death) caused TdP in approximately 5% of patients, necessitating a protocol amendment with dosage adjustments during both trials (particularly in those with renal disease because its primary route of elimination is through the kidney).

How should the clinician approach the patient with documented asymptomatic PVCs? Clearly, attempts to suppress asymptomatic PVCs should *not* be made with any AAD. Indeed, those patients who are at risk for arrhythmic death (recent MI, LV dysfunction, complex PVCs) should also *not* be routinely given *any* class I or III AAD.[79] If these patients have symptomatic PVCs, chronic drug therapy should be limited to the use of β-blockers. The use of β-blockers in post-MI patients is associated with a decrease in the incidence of total mortality and SCD, especially in the presence of LV dysfunction. These drugs can also be used in patients without underlying SHD to suppress symptomatic PVCs. ❼

VENTRICULAR TACHYCARDIA

Mechanisms and Types of VT

VT is a wide QRS tachycardia that may acutely occur as a result of metabolic abnormalities, ischemia, or drug toxicity, or chronically

recur as a paroxysmal form. On ECG, VT may appear as either repetitive monomorphic or polymorphic ventricular complexes. The definition of VT is three or more consecutive PVCs occurring at a rate >100 beats/min. An acute episode of VT may be precipitated by severe electrolyte abnormalities (hypokalemia or hypomagnesemia), hypoxia, or digoxin toxicity, or (most commonly) may occur during an acute MI or ischemia complicated by HF. In these cases, correction of the underlying precipitating factors will usually prevent further recurrences of VT. As an example, if VT occurs during the first 24 hours of an acute MI, it will probably not reappear on a chronic basis after the infarcted area has been reperfused or healed with scar formation. This form of acute VT may be caused by a transient reentrant mechanism within temporarily ischemic or dying ventricular tissue. In contrast, some patients have a chronic recurrent form of VT that is almost always associated with some type of underlying SHD. Common examples are paroxysmal VT associated with idiopathic dilated cardiomyopathy or remote MI with an LV aneurysm. In chronic, recurrent VT, microreentry within the distal Purkinje network is presumed to be responsible for the underlying substrate in a large majority of patients (see Fig. 25–3). Theoretically, electrophysiologic discrepancies occur as a result of structural damage and heart disease within the ventricular conducting system. The reentrant circuit may possess both anatomically determined and functional properties coursing through normal tissue, damaged (but not dead) tissue, and islands of necrosed tissue. In a minority of patients, macroreentrant circuits may be responsible for recurrent VT, including reentry incorporating the bundle branches.

Patients with acute VT associated with a precipitating factor often suffer severe symptoms, requiring immediate treatment measures. Chronic recurrent VT may also cause severe hemodynamic compromise but may also be associated with only mild symptoms that are generally well tolerated. Sustained VT is that which requires therapeutic intervention to restore a stable rhythm or persists for a relatively long time (usually >30 seconds). Nonsustained VT is that which self-terminates after a brief duration (usually <30 seconds). If the patient has VT more frequently than SR (i.e., VT is the dominant rhythm), this is referred to as incessant VT. In monomorphic VT, the QRS complexes are similar in morphologic characteristics from beat to beat. In polymorphic VT, the QRS complexes vary in shape and/or size between beats. A characteristic type of polymorphic VT, in which the QRS complexes appear to undulate around a central axis and that is associated with evidence of delayed ventricular repolarization (long QT interval or prominent U waves), is referred to as TdP.

Most but not all forms of recurrent VT occur in patients with extensive SHD. VT occurring in a patient without SHD is sometimes referred to as idiopathic VT and may take several forms.[80–82] Fascicular tachycardia arises from a fascicle of the left bundle branch (usually posterior) and is usually not associated with severe underlying SHD. In distinct contrast to the common form of recurrent VT associated with extensive SHD, non-DHP CCBs (but not adenosine) are effective in terminating an acute episode of fascicular VT. Ventricular outflow tract tachycardia (usually originating from the right ventricular outflow tract) originates from near the pulmonic valve (or uncommonly the aortic valve or LV outflow tract) and also occurs in patients with normal LV function without discernible SHD.[82] Unlike other forms of VT, right ventricular outflow tract tachycardia often terminates with adenosine and may be prevented with β-blockers and/or non-DHP CCBs.

Some unusual forms of VT are congenital or heritable (Table 25–10). TdP can be associated with heritable defects in the flux of ions that govern ventricular repolarization. Although multiple syndromes and genetic mutations have been described, the more common examples are long QT syndrome 1 (depressed I_{Ks}), long QT syndrome 2 (depressed I_{Kr}), and long QT syndrome 3

TABLE 25-10 Heritable Polymorphic Ventricular Tachycardia

Syndrome	Channel Defect	Mutant Gene	Characteristics	Treatment
LQTS$_1$	↓ I$_{Ks}$	KVLQT1	SCD/TdP with exercise	BB/ICD
LQTS$_2$	↓ I$_{Kr}$	HERG	SCD/TdP with arousal	BB/ICD
LQTS$_3$	↑ I$_{Na}^+$ during plateau/repolarization	SCN5A	SCD/TdP at rest/sleep	Flecainide/mexiletine/ICD
Brugada	↓ I$_{Na}^+$	SCN5A	SCD/PMVT or VF at rest/sleep in Asian males	ICD/quinidine

BB, β-blocker; ICD, implantable cardioverter-defibrillator; LQTS, long QT syndrome; PMVT, polymorphic ventricular tachycardia; SCD, sudden death; TdP, torsade de pointes; VF, ventricular fibrillation.

Note: LQTS can be provoked by potassium channel blockers (e.g., quinidine, sotalol), and Brugada syndrome can be provoked by potent sodium channel blockers (e.g., cocaine, flecainide). LQTS$_3$ and Brugada syndrome may coexist.

(enhanced inward sodium ion flux during repolarization).[83,84] Polymorphic VT (without a long QT interval) or VF may also occur as a result of a heritable defect in the sodium channel. This is the case in Brugada syndrome, which is described as a typical ECG pattern (ST-segment elevation in leads V$_1$ to V$_3$) in SR that is associated with SCD, and commonly occurs in males of Asian descent.[85] It is estimated that Brugada syndrome accounts for approximately 40% of all cases of VF in patients without heart disease.

Management

Consider the patient with the more common form of sustained monomorphic VT (i.e., those with SHD, usually ischemic in nature). Like other rapid tachycardias, the initial management of an acute episode of VT (with a pulse) requires a quick assessment of the patient's status and symptoms. If severe symptoms are present (i.e., severe hypotension, angina, pulmonary edema), synchronized DCC should be delivered immediately to attempt to restore SR. An investigation should be made into possible precipitating factors, and these should be corrected if possible. The diagnosis of acute MI should always be entertained. If the episode of VT is thought to be an isolated electrical event associated with a transient initiating factor (such as acute myocardial ischemia or digoxin toxicity), there is no need for long-term AAD therapy once the precipitating factors are corrected (e.g., an MI has been reperfused and healed and the patient is stable). Nevertheless, the patient should be monitored closely for possible recurrences of VT.

Patients presenting with an acute episode of VT (with a pulse) associated with only mild symptoms can be initially treated with AADs. The reader is referred to the most recent AHA guidelines for CPR and ECC.[61] IV procainamide amiodarone, or sotalol can be considered in this situation. Lidocaine can be considered as an alternative. In one small study, procainamide was shown to be superior to lidocaine in terminating VT.[86] Synchronized DCC should be delivered if the patient's status deteriorates, VT degenerates to VF (would be unsynchronized in this situation), or drug therapy fails.

Once an acute episode of sustained VT has been successfully terminated by electrical or pharmacologic means and an acute MI has been ruled out, the possibility of a patient having recurrent episodes of VT should be considered. Evidence for the possibility of VT recurrence can often be gleaned from invasive electrophysiologic studies using programmed ventricular stimulation. The management of the patient with chronic, recurrent, sustained VT deserves considerable attention. Because these patients are at extremely high risk for death, trial-and-error attempts to find effective therapy are unwarranted. To gain some objective evidence of a response to a specific AAD regimen, serial testing of these drugs using the following two surrogate end points has been used: (a) inability to induce sustained VT with programmed extrastimuli by invasive electrophysiologic studies and (b) suppression of ventricular ectopic beats by serial 24-hour continuous electrocardiographic (Holter) monitoring. These two strategies have been compared[87,88] but largely abandoned for several reasons. First, the yield for finding an effective AAD is low. For instance, sustained monomorphic VT can be rendered noninducible or nonsustained by programmed stimulation protocols in only 20% to 25% of patients. Therefore, the clinician frequently must search for other therapeutic options or settle for other treatment end points such as slower and more tolerable inducible VT. Second, amiodarone is clearly the most effective (approximately 50% effective after 2 years) AAD in patients with recurrent VT; however, electrophysiologic drug testing does not necessarily predict the clinical efficacy of amiodarone. Patients may have continued inducibility of VT on amiodarone despite long-term success. Indeed, empiric amiodarone has been compared to therapy (with other AADs) guided by electrophysiologic testing in patients at high risk for recurrent VT.[89] In this trial, amiodarone therapy without invasive testing was superior in preventing SCD and recurrences of severe ventricular arrhythmias at all time points. Third, the recurrence rate of life-threatening VT is high (20% to 50% per year depending on the AAD chosen), regardless of the method of acute drug testing. Fourth, as referred to previously, there is a substantial side-effect profile of the class I and III AADs. Lastly, and perhaps most importantly, is the impressive demonstrated effectiveness of nonpharmacologic approaches to the treatment of recurrent VT/VF.[90] For instance, some forms of recurrent VT are amenable to catheter ablation therapy using radiofrequency current. This approach is highly effective (approximately 90%) in idiopathic VT (right ventricular outflow tract or fascicular VT), but less so in recurrent VT associated with a cardiomyopathic process or remote MI with LV aneurysm. In the latter patients, ablation is usually regarded as second-line therapy after other methods have failed. Additionally, numerous trials have established the ICD as a superior treatment over AAD therapy not only for the prevention of SCD in patients who have been resuscitated from an episode of cardiac arrest or had sustained VT ("secondary prevention") but also for the prevention of an initial episode of SCD in certain high-risk patient populations ("primary prevention").

The Implantable Cardioverter-Defibrillator The introduction of and advances in the ICD (Fig. 25–12) have obviated the need to rely solely on the use of AADs to prevent episodes of life-threatening ventricular arrhythmias.[91] ❽ Numerous advancements in device technology have allowed the ICD to become smaller, less invasive to implant, and programmable with advanced functions. Early ICDs required a thoracotomy to place the generator in the abdomen, whereas with the newer, smaller models, the leads are implanted transvenously with the generator placed into the pectoral region in a manner similar to cardiac pacemakers. Modern ICDs now employ a "tiered-therapy approach" meaning that overdrive pacing (i.e., antitachycardia pacing) can be

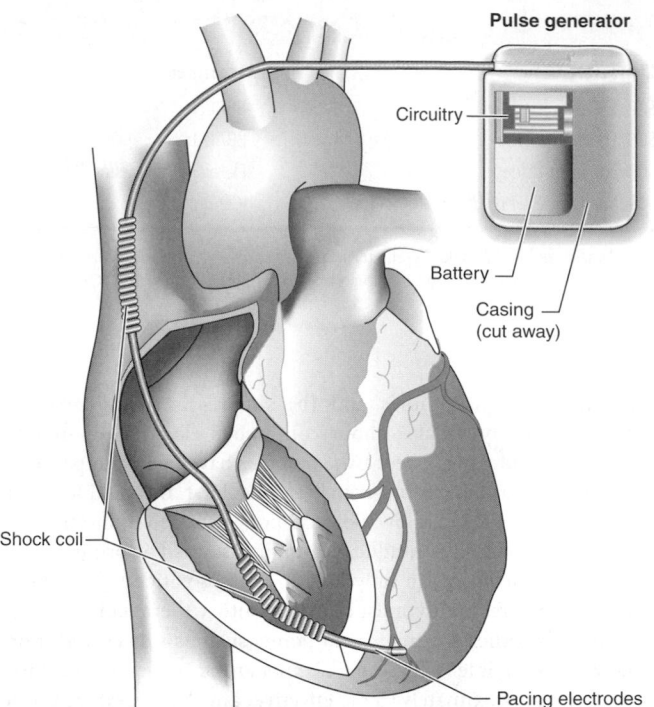

Pulse generator

Circuitry

Battery

Casing
(cut away)

Shock coil

Pacing electrodes

FIGURE 25-12. Drawing showing ICD. *(DiMarco JP. Implantable Cardioverter-defibrillators. N Engl J Med 2003;349:1836–1847. Copyright © 2003 Massachusetts Medical Society. All rights reserved.)*

attempted first to terminate the tachyarrhythmia (no painful shock delivered), followed by low-energy cardioversion, and, finally, by high-energy defibrillation shocks. In addition, backup antibrady-cardia pacing and extended battery lives have made these newer devices much more attractive. All models store recordings during delivery of pacing shocks, which is extremely important in discerning appropriate shocks (i.e., delivers shock for serious ventricular arrhythmia) from inappropriate shocks (i.e., delivers shock for AF with rapid ventricular rate) and in documenting true recurrences of the patient's tachycardia.

Although the ICD is a highly effective method for preventing SCD due to recurrent VT or VF, several problems remain. First, the device itself, the implantation procedure, electrophysiologic studies, hospitalization, and physician fees are costly. Given that the indications for receiving an ICD have significantly expanded over the past several years, the total cost associated with the implantation of this device is likely to place a great burden on the healthcare system. Second, many patients (as high as 70% of patients) with ICDs end up receiving concomitant AAD therapy (usually amiodarone or sotalol).[92,93] AADs can be initiated in these patients for a number of reasons, including (a) decreasing the frequency of VT/VF episodes to subsequently reduce the frequency of appropriate shocks; (b) reducing the rate of VT so that it can be terminated with antitachycardia pacing; and (c) decreasing episodes of concomitant supraventricular arrhythmias (e.g., AF, atrial flutter) that may trigger inappropriate shocks. As a result of these potential benefits, the concomitant use of AADs can minimize patient discomfort and prolong the battery life of the ICD. The decision to initiate concomitant AAD therapy should be individualized, with treatment usually being reserved for those with frequent shocks because of VT or AF. If AADs are added to ICD therapy, one should note that many of these drugs alter defibrillation thresholds; consequently, the device should be reprogrammed to account for this alteration.[94]

Secondary Prevention of Sudden Cardiac Death
The results of three trials, the Antiarrhythmics Versus Implantable

Defibrillators (AVID), Cardiac Arrest Study Hamburg (CASH), and Canadian Implantable Defibrillator Study (CIDS), definitively support the ICD as first-line therapy for the secondary prevention of SCD.[95-97] Of these, the AVID trial was the largest, randomizing more than 1,000 patients with resuscitated VF, sustained VT with syncope, or hemodynamically significant sustained VT (with LVEF ≤40%) to either an ICD or AADs (~95% receiving amiodarone at discharge).[95] The trial was stopped early because of a demonstrated superiority of the ICD; patients in the ICD group had a better overall survival when compared with those in the AAD group (75% vs. 64%, respectively, at 3 years). Although they were smaller trials, both CASH and CIDS demonstrated the efficacy of an ICD compared with amiodarone in patients with a history of sustained VT or VF, with the ICD reducing overall mortality by 20% to 25%.[96,97] Overall, the results of these three trials provide strong support for the aggressive use of the ICD in patients who are at high risk for recurrent, life-threatening ventricular arrhythmias. Implantation of an ICD can be cost-effective, particularly in patients with poor LV function. Although nearly all clinicians now consider the ICD as first-line treatment for secondary prevention of SCD, there is at least one possible patient group that may do as well with AAD therapy alone. In the AVID trial, there was no differences in survival between ICD and AAD treatment in patients with mild LV dysfunction (LVEF >35%), which suggests that long-term amiodarone therapy may be appropriate to use in this lower-risk patient population.[95] However, because these data were obtained from a post hoc analysis, additional trials are needed to confirm these findings.

Primary Prevention of Sudden Cardiac Death Over the past decade, the AVID, CASH, and CIDS trials have established the ICD as an effective treatment for the secondary prevention of SCD in patients who have previously suffered a documented episode of VT or VF. Most of the studies that have been performed in the past several years have focused on the efficacy of the ICD for primary prevention in patients deemed to be at high risk for SCD.[98-101]

One of the patient populations that appears to be at high risk for a first episode of SCD includes those with a prior MI, LV dysfunction, and nonsustained VT. The use of AADs to prevent SCD in this high-risk group has been significantly limited by the results of the CAST and other similar trials that have collectively demonstrated that these drugs may actually increase the risk of mortality in these patients. As a result of these trials, clinicians have sought a more clearly defined strategy for risk stratification in these patients before initiating drug therapy.

Traditionally, there are three strategies to approach the treatment of nonsustained VT: (a) conservative (i.e., no AAD treatment beyond β-blockers); (b) empiric amiodarone; and (c) aggressive (i.e., electrophysiologic studies with possible insertion of an ICD) (Fig. 25–13). ❾ A number of early studies[102,103] suggested that tests such as electrophysiologic studies could be used to determine long-term risk in patients with nonsustained VT. For instance, Wilber et al.[102] demonstrated that post-MI patients with nonsustained VT and inducible *sustained* VT after programmed stimulation were at increased risk for subsequent VT/VF or SCD compared with those in whom sustained VT could not be induced. These data provided the basis for the Multi-center Automatic Defibrillator Implantation Trial (MADIT) and the Multicenter Unsustained Tachycardia Trial (MUSTT).[98,99] The MADIT was the first of these trials to be conducted to evaluate the efficacy of ICD therapy in this high-risk patient population. Specifically, this trial randomized patients with a previous MI, LVEF ≤36%, asymptomatic nonsustained VT, and inducible VT that was not suppressed with the use of IV procainamide to receive an ICD or conventional medical therapy (74% of patients in this particular group received amiodarone).[98] This trial was terminated prematurely after a significant survival benefit

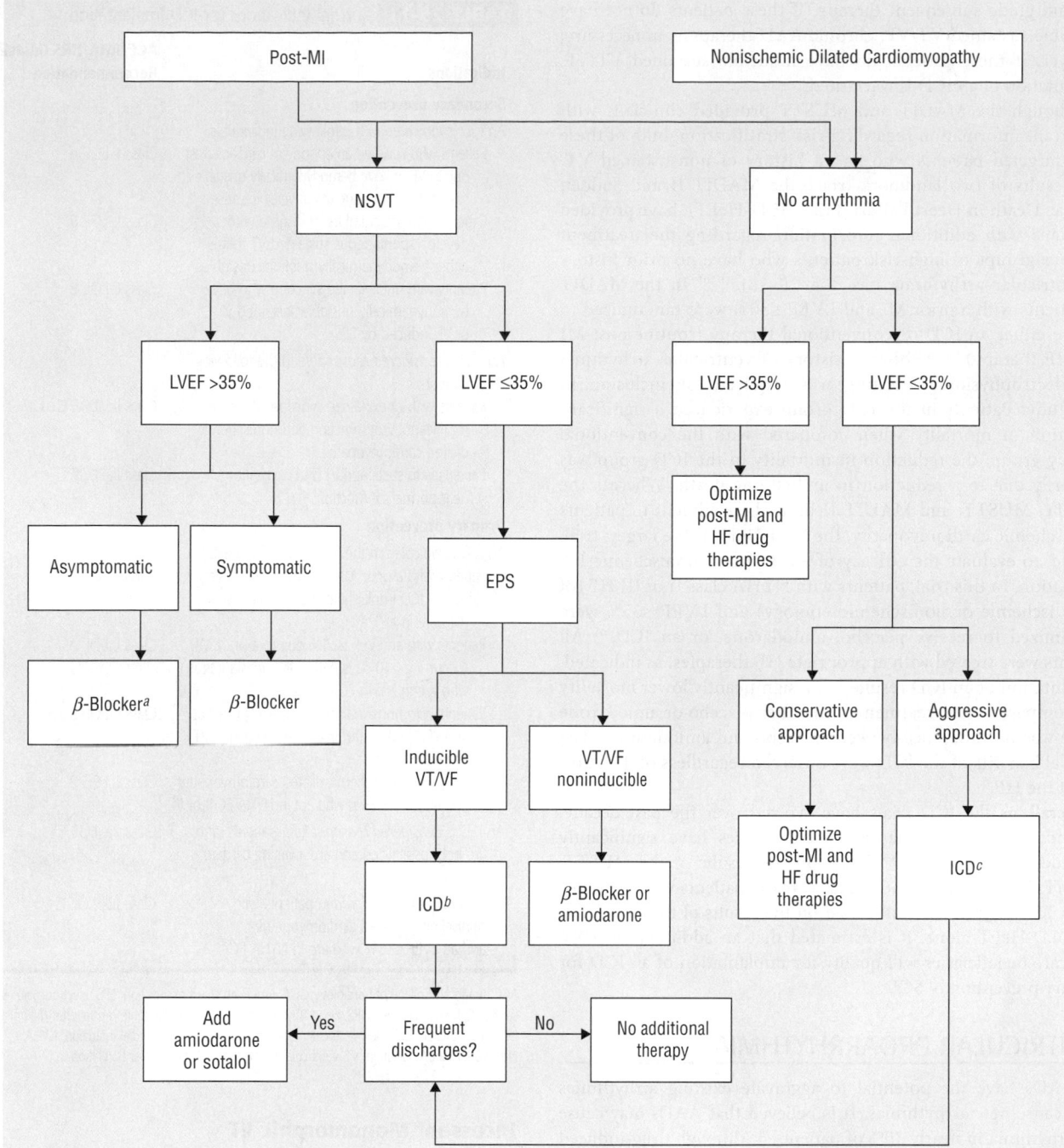

FIGURE 25-13. Algorithm for the primary prevention of SCD in patients with a history of MI or with a nonischemic dilated cardiomyopathy. [a]In these patients, the β-blocker is being used to reduce post-MI mortality. [b]Patients should be >40 days post-MI prior to insertion of the ICD. [c]Patients with an ischemic cardiomyopathy should be >40 days post-MI prior to insertion of the ICD. (EPS, electrophysiologic study; HF, heart failure; ICD, implantable cardioverter-defibrillator; LVEF, left ventricular ejection fraction; MI, myocardial infarction; NSVT, nonsustained VT; SCD, sudden cardiac death; VF, ventricular fibrillation; VT, ventricular tachycardia.)

was detected in the ICD group. The findings of the MADIT were subsequently supported by those of the MUSTT. In the MUSTT, patients with a history of MI, LVEF ≤40%, asymptomatic nonsustained VT, and inducible sustained VT were randomized to a conservative approach (no AAD therapy beyond β-blockers) or electrophysiologically guided therapy (AADs and/or ICD).[99] The results showed that the conservative approach had a significantly higher event rate (cardiac arrest or death from arrhythmia). However, when the results of the electrophysiologically guided group were further stratified, those receiving only AADs (no ICD) were no different in terms of outcomes than those who received no

treatment. In other words, only those treated with an ICD had a significantly lower event rate and greater survival. One problem with the MUSTT, however, is that, because the trial was initiated in 1989, nearly 50% of patients received class I AADs or drugs that are now known not to improve survival in patients with CAD, LV dysfunction, and ventricular arrhythmias; only 10% of patients received the most effective agent in this setting, amiodarone. Based on the results of the MADIT and MUSTT, it is reasonable for patients with CAD, LV dysfunction, and nonsustained VT to undergo electrophysiologic testing;[104] that is, invasive electrophysiologic studies with programmed stimulation are used to determine risk and guide subsequent therapy. If these patients do not have inducible sustained VT/VF, chronic AAD therapy is unnecessary; however, if these patients do have inducible sustained VT/VF, implantation of an ICD is warranted.

Although the MADIT and MUSTT provided clinicians with important information regarding risk stratification, both of these trials targeted patients who had a history of nonsustained VT. The results of two landmark trials, the MADIT II and Sudden Cardiac Death in Heart Failure Trial (SCD-HeFT), have provided clinicians with additional information regarding the treatment of other groups of high-risk patients who have no prior history of ventricular arrhythmia (see Fig. 25–13).[100,101] In the MADIT II, patients with a prior MI and LVEF ≤30% were randomized to receive either an ICD or conventional therapy (routine post-MI and HF therapy).[100] Neither a history of ventricular arrhythmia nor electrophysiologic testing was required for inclusion in this study. Patients in the ICD group experienced a significant reduction in mortality when compared with the conventional therapy group; the reduction in mortality in the ICD group was primarily due to a reduction in arrhythmic death. Whereas the MADIT, MUSTT, and MADIT II limited enrollment to patients with ischemic cardiomyopathy, the SCD-HeFT is the largest trial, to date, to evaluate the efficacy of an ICD in a nonischemic HF population. In this trial, patients with NYHA class II or III HF (of either ischemic or nonischemic etiology) and LVEF ≤35% were randomized to receive placebo, amiodarone, or an ICD.[101] All patients were treated with appropriate HF therapies, as indicated. Implantation of an ICD resulted in a significantly lower mortality rate compared with treatment with either placebo or amiodarone (there was no difference between placebo and amiodarone). The survival benefits of the ICD were observed regardless of the etiology of the HF.

Overall, as the ICD trials have evolved over the past decade, the indications for implanting these devices have significantly expanded (Table 25–11).[105] Based on the results of the MUSTT, MADIT, MADIT II, and SCD-HeFT, many patients will be eligible for an ICD. ❾ In fact, just based on the results of the MADIT II and SCD-HeFT alone, it is estimated that an additional 500,000 Medicare beneficiaries will qualify for implantation of an ICD for primary prevention of SCD.

VENTRICULAR PROARRHYTHMIA

All AADs have the potential to aggravate existing arrhythmias or to cause new arrhythmias. It is believed that AADs may cause proarrhythmia in nearly 30% of patients.[10] Although drug-induced arrhythmias have been recognized for several years, only recently has this adverse effect gained widespread attention. Many definitions for proarrhythmia have been proposed; however, in the simplest terms, it indicates the development of a significant new arrhythmia (such as VT, VF, or TdP) or worsening of an existing arrhythmia (episodes are longer, faster, or more frequent). As with all arrhythmias, the consequences of proarrhythmia are varied. Some patients who develop proarrhythmia may be totally asymptomatic, others may notice a worsening of symptoms, and some may die suddenly. The development of proarrhythmia results from the same mechanisms that cause arrhythmias in general (e.g., quinidine-induced TdP due to EADs) or from an alteration in the underlying substrate due to the AAD (e.g., development of an accelerated tachycardia caused by flecainide, which decreases conduction velocity without significantly altering the refractory period) (see Fig. 25–4).[10] The diagnosis of proarrhythmia is sometimes difficult to make because of the variable nature of the underlying arrhythmias. However, in all cases, the drug should be discontinued if proarrhythmia is detected or suspected.

TABLE 25-11 Current Indications for ICD Implantation

Indications	ACC/AHA/HRS Guideline Recommendation
Secondary prevention	
An ICD is *indicated* in the following individuals:	
Patients who survived an episode of cardiac arrest due to VF or have hemodynamically unstable sustained VT, not due to a reversible cause.	Class I, LOE A
Patients with structural heart disease who develop spontaneous sustained VT that is either hemodynamically stable or unstable.	Class I, LOE B
Patients with unexplained syncope who have hemodynamically unstable sustained VT or VF induced by EPS.	Class I, LOE B
An ICD is *considered reasonable* in the following individuals:	
Patients with unexplained syncope who have significant LV dysfunction and nonischemic dilated cardiomyopathy.	Class IIa, LOE C
Patients with sustained VT and normal or near-normal LV function.	Class IIa, LOE C
Primary prevention	
An ICD is *indicated* in the following individuals:	
Patients with a prior MI (occurring >40 days before ICD implantation) and LVEF ≤30% who are in NYHA FC I.	Class I, LOE A
Patients with an LVEF ≤35% due to a prior MI (occurring >40 days before ICD implantation) who are in NYHA FC II or III.	Class I, LOE A
Patients with nonsustained VT due to prior MI, an LVEF ≤40%, and inducible, sustained VT or VF at EPS.	Class I, LOE B
Patients with nonischemic dilated cardiomyopathy and an LVEF ≤35% who are in NYHA FC II or III	Class I, LOE B
An ICD is *considered reasonable* in patients who are not hospitalized and are awaiting cardiac transplantation.	Class IIa, LOE C
An ICD *may be considered* in patients with nonischemic dilated cardiomyopathy and an LVEF ≤35% who are in NYHA FC I	Class IIb, LOE C

ACC, American College of Cardiology; AHA, American Heart Association; EPS, electrophysiological study; FC, functional class; HRS, Heart Rhythm Society; ICD, implantable cardioverter-defibrillator; LV, left ventricular; LVEF, left ventricular ejection fraction; MI, myocardial infarction; NYHA, New York Heart Association; VT, ventricular tachycardia; VF, ventricular fibrillation.

Incessant Monomorphic VT

The prototypical form of proarrhythmia caused by the class Ic AADs is a rapid, sustained, monomorphic VT with a characteristic sinusoidal QRS pattern that is often resistant to resuscitation with cardioversion or overdrive pacing. ❿ It is sometimes referred to as sinusoidal or incessant VT and is the result of excessive sodium channel blockade and slowed conduction. Sinusoidal VT caused by the class Ic AADs was thought to occur within the first several days of drug initiation; however, the results of the CAST indicate that the risk for this type of proarrhythmia may exist as long as the drug is continued. Factors that definitely predispose a patient to this form of proarrhythmia include: (a) the presence of underlying ventricular arrhythmias; (b) CAD; and (c) LV dysfunction. Provocation of proarrhythmia by the class Ic AADs is sometimes reported during exercise, which is most likely a result of augmented slowed conduction at rapid heart rates (i.e., rate-dependent sodium blockade). The incidence of proarrhythmia caused by class Ic AADs is greatest in patients with all three risk factors (approximately 10% to 20%) and extremely uncommon in those without risks, such as patients with supraventricular tachycardias and normal LV function. In one

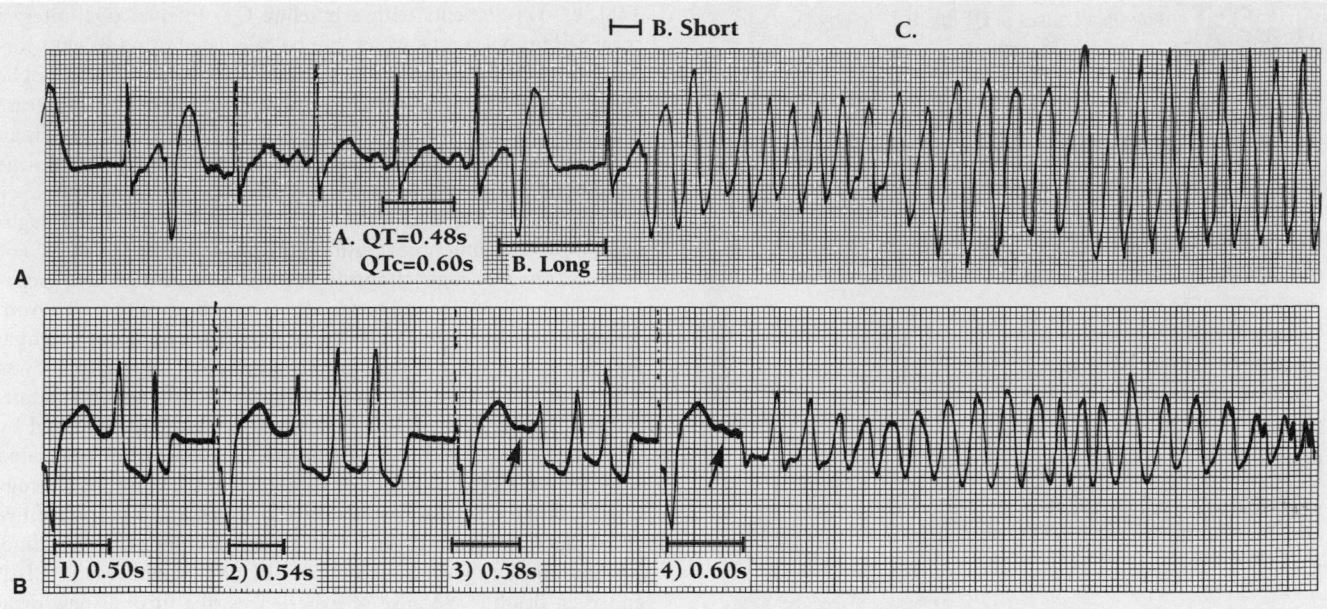

FIGURE 25-14. Torsade de pointes caused by quinidine. Note the presence of a couplet and two triplets following each extra systolic pause. The pause gets progressively longer until it is long enough to result in an episode of sustained torsade de pointes. Also, as the pause lengthens, discernible U waves (labeled ↑) (EADs?) begin to appear. The amplitude of the U wave is somewhat greater with the longest pause. *(From Bauman JL. Drug safety: Cardiac arrhythmias. Antihistamine update symposium. Hosp Med 1995;31:24, with permission.)*

study, in patients with risk factors, the incidence of death due to proarrhythmia from encainide and flecainide was approximately the same as the chance of long-term effectiveness.[106] Other factors that have a less well-defined association with proarrhythmia are elevated AAD serum concentrations and rapid dosage escalation. It has been proposed that the presence of underlying ventricular conduction delays may also pose a risk for proarrhythmia. As mentioned earlier, this arrhythmia is often resistant to resuscitation; however, some have had success with lidocaine ("fast on-off" AAD, which successfully competes with a "slow on-off" agent such as flecainide for sodium channel receptor) or sodium bicarbonate (reverses the excessive sodium channel blockade).

Torsade de Pointes

As defined previously, TdP is a rapid form of polymorphic VT (Fig. 25–14) that is associated with evidence of delayed ventricular repolarization (long QT interval or prominent U waves) on ECG. It is important to note that most forms of polymorphic VT occurring in the setting of a normal QT interval are similar to monomorphic VT in terms of etiology and treatment strategies (thus, a long QT interval is crucial to the diagnosis of TdP). Much has been learned about the underlying etiology of TdP. Basic defects (genetic, drugs, or diseases) that delay repolarization by influencing ion movement (usually by blocking potassium efflux) provoke EADs, preferentially in cells deep in the heart muscle (termed *M cells*), which, in turn, trigger reentry and TdP. Drugs that cause TdP usually delay ventricular repolarization in an inhomogeneous way (termed *dispersion of refractoriness*), which facilitates the formation of multiple reentrant loops in the ventricle.[107] TdP may occur in association with hereditary syndromes or as an acquired form (i.e., a result of drugs or diseases). The underlying etiology in both cases is delayed ventricular repolarization due to blockade of potassium conductance. It is possible, however, that some individuals have a partially expressed form of these congenital syndromes but never suffer TdP unless some other external factor (e.g., drugs, diseases, electrolyte disturbances, abrupt heart rate changes) further delays ventricular repolarization. Specifically, acquired forms of TdP are associated

with electrolyte disturbances (hypokalemia or hypomagnesemia), subarachnoid hemorrhage, myocarditis, liquid protein diets, arsenic poisoning, severe hypothyroidism, or, most commonly, drug therapy (notably phenothiazines, antibiotics, antihistamines, antidepressants, and AADs) (Table 25–12). **❿**

The class Ia AADs (especially quinidine) and class III I_{Kr} blockers are most notorious for precipitating TdP; the class Ib and Ic AADs rarely, if ever, cause TdP (they do not appreciably delay repolarization). Most AADs with I_{Kr} blocking activity cause TdP in approximately 2% to 4% of patients, with the exceptions being amiodarone and dronedarone (<1%). Risk factors and associated features of drug-induced TdP have been identified and can be summarized as follows:[32,108] (a) high dosages or plasma concentrations of the offending drug ("dose-related") (except for quinidine-induced TdP, which tends to occur more frequently at low-to-therapeutic concentrations); (b) concurrent SHD (e.g., CAD, HF, and/or LV hypertrophy); (c) evidence of mild delayed repolarization (prolonged QT interval) at baseline; (d) evidence of a prolonged QT interval shortly after initiation of the offending drug; (e) concomitant electrolyte disturbances such as hypokalemia or hypomagnesemia; (f) female gender; and (g) a characteristic long–short initiating sequence (so-called "pause dependence") of the episode of TdP (see Fig. 25–14). However, none of these associations are absolute prerequisites to the development of drug-induced TdP. For instance, although TdP is usually documented early in the course of quinidine therapy, patients may develop this arrhythmia during chronic treatment.[109] The reason for quinidine's relatively unique propensity for causing TdP at relatively low dosages and concentrations requires explanation. Quinidine's ability to block I_{Kr} is clinically manifest at low concentrations; at higher concentrations, its sodium-channel blocking properties predominate. Other drugs that block I_{Kr} usually do so in a concentration-dependent fashion. The observation that most patients who suffer drug-induced TdP have evidence of mildly delayed repolarization (long QT intervals) even before they are prescribed the offending drug has stimulated a search for a potential genetically linked risk. Indeed, it appears that at least some patients with acquired drug-induced TdP appear to possess mutations of genes that encode for I_{Kr} or I_{Ks}.[108]

TABLE 25-12 Potential Causes of QT Interval Prolongation and Torsade de Pointes

Conditions

Congenital long QT syndromes

Myocarditis

Myocardial ischemia/infarction

Heart failure

Severe bradycardia (<50 beats/min)

Hypokalemia

Severe hypothermia

Hypomagnesemia

Severe starvation/liquid-protein diets

Subarachnoid hemorrhage

Drugs

Antiarrhythmic drugs

   Quinidine

   Procainamide (also *N*-acetylprocainamide)

   Disopyramide

   Amiodarone (<1%)

   Dofetilide

   Dronedarone (<1%)

   Sotalol

   Ibutilide

Psychotropics

   Phenothiazines (e.g., thioridazine, chlorpromazine)

   Tricyclic and tetracyclic antidepressants

   Haloperidol/droperidol

   Pimozide

   Atypical antipsychotics (e.g., quetiapine, ziprasidone)

Toxins

   Organophosphate insecticides

   Arsenic

Antibiotics

   Pentamidine

   Macrolides (erythromycin and clarithromycin)

   Trimethoprim-sulfamethoxazole

   Fluoroquinolones (levofloxacin, moxifloxacin, gemifloxacin)

   Voriconazole

Pain

   Methadone

Miscellaneous

   Liquid-protein diets[a]

   Corticosteroids[a]

   Diuretics[a]

   Quinine

   Chloroquine

   Chloral hydrate

   Tacrolimus

[a]More than likely a result of severe electrolyte imbalance.

Note: For a complete list, see *www.qtdrugs.org.*

The common underlying electrophysiologic cause of TdP is a delay in ventricular repolarization (provoking EADs), which usually results from inhibition (drug-induced or genetic) of I_K current and manifests as QT interval prolongation on the ECG. Therefore, the extent of QT interval prolongation has been used as a measurement of risk of TdP; however, considerable controversy exists. Amiodarone, for example, commonly causes significant QT prolongation but is a relatively infrequent cause of TdP. Nonetheless, the QT interval should be measured and monitored in all patients prescribed drugs that have a high potential for causing TdP (see

Table 25–12). Patients with a baseline QT_c interval (QT interval corrected for heart rate, which can be calculated using Bazett's formula: $QT_c = QT$ measured$/\sqrt{R\text{-}R \text{ interval}}$) >450 msec should not be given drugs that have a high potential for causing TdP; an increase in the QT_c interval to ≥ 560 msec after the initiation of the drug is an indication to discontinue the agent or, at least, to reduce its dosage and carefully observe and monitor.

Drug-induced TdP has become an extremely visible hazard plaguing new drugs, sometimes resulting in public health disasters. For instance, several drugs (cisapride, astemizole, levomethadyl, grepafloxacin, sparfloxacin, and terfenadine) have been withdrawn from the market in the United States because of their significant potential for causing TdP. One of the most visible and striking examples was with regard to the popular nonsedating antihistamine, terfenadine. Terfenadine is a potent I_{Kr} blocker but is rapidly metabolized by CYP3A4 to an active moiety (fexofenadine) that is not associated with delayed repolarization. Consequently, in the presence of drugs that block the CYP3A4 isoenzyme (e.g., ketoconazole, erythromycin, diltiazem), accumulation of the parent compound, terfenadine, causes clinically significant blockade of I_{Kr} that could result in TdP and even death.[110] Because of experiences like this, all new drug entities under investigation are screened for their ability to block I_K and cause significant QT prolongation.

Acute treatment of TdP is different than treatment for the more common acute monomorphic VT. For an acute episode of TdP, most patients will require and respond to DCC. However, TdP tends to be paroxysmal in nature and often will rapidly recur after DCC. Therefore, after the initial restoration of a stable rhythm, therapy designed to prevent recurrences of TdP should be instituted. AADs that further prolong repolarization such as IV procainamide are absolutely contraindicated. Lidocaine is usually ineffective. Although there are no true efficacy trials, IV magnesium sulfate, by suppressing EADs, is now considered the drug of choice in preventing recurrences of TdP.[111] If IV magnesium sulfate is ineffective, treatment strategies designed to increase heart rate, shorten ventricular repolarization, and prevent the pause dependency should be initiated. Either temporary transvenous pacing (105 to 120 beats/min) or pharmacologic pacing (isoproterenol or epinephrine infusion) can be initiated for this purpose. All drugs that prolong the QT interval should be discontinued, and exacerbating factors (e.g., hypokalemia or hypomagnesemia) should be corrected.

VENTRICULAR FIBRILLATION

Background and Prevention

VF is electrical anarchy of the ventricle resulting in no cardiac output and cardiovascular collapse. Death will ensue rapidly if effective treatment measures are not taken. Patients who die abruptly (within 1 hour of initial symptoms) and unexpectedly (i.e., "sudden death") usually have VF recorded at the time of death.[112] SCD accounts for about 310,000 deaths per year in the United States.[16] SCD occurs most commonly in patients with CAD and those with LV dysfunction; it occurs less commonly in those with WPW syndrome or mitral valve prolapse, and occasionally in those without associated heart disease (e.g., Brugada syndrome). Patients who have SCD (not associated with acute MI) but survive because of appropriate CPR and defibrillation (where warranted), often have inducible sustained VT and/or VF during electrophysiologic studies. These individuals are at high risk for the recurrence of VT and/or VF.

In contrast, patients who have VF associated with acute MI (i.e., within the first 24 hours after symptoms) usually have little risk of recurrence. Of all patients who die as a result of an acute MI, approximately 50% die suddenly prior to hospitalization.

VF associated with acute MI can be subdivided into two types: primary VF and complicated or secondary VF. Primary VF occurs in an uncomplicated MI not associated with HF; secondary VF occurs in an MI complicated by HF. The time course, incidence, mechanisms, treatment, and complications of these two forms of VF are different. For example, approximately 2% to 6% of patients with acute MI suffer primary VF within 24 hours of chest pain, but the risk of VF declines rapidly over time and is nearly zero after the initial 24-hour period. Complicated or secondary VF does not follow such a predictable time course and may occur in the late infarction period. The premise of prophylactic AADs administered to all patients with uncomplicated MI is based on (a) the inability to predict which patients are at risk for primary VF and (b) the predictable time course of primary VF (in contrast to complicated VF). Of the prophylactic therapies used, lidocaine has been the most widely debated and studied. Lie et al.[113] performed the classic study showing the effectiveness of lidocaine in preventing primary VF. Although lidocaine significantly reduced the incidence of VF compared with placebo, there was no significant difference in mortality due to VF between the groups. These results, along with the effectiveness of rapidly instituted defibrillation in modern coronary care units with sophisticated monitoring techniques, have caused most to reject the notion of prophylactic lidocaine administration for all patients with uncomplicated MI. In support of this, two meta-analyses[114,115] concluded against the routine use of prophylactic lidocaine because of a possible increase in mortality in lidocaine-treated patients[114] as well as the declining incidence of primary VF documented in recent years (probably a result of the more aggressive and rapid use of β-blockers, thrombolytics, and percutaneous intervention for the treatment of acute coronary syndromes).[115]

The use of IV magnesium sulfate has also been entertained for the prevention of VF during the acute infarction period. Small trials implying its effectiveness were subsequently incorporated into a meta-analysis.[116] This meta-analysis found a decrease in the incidence of VT/VF and a reduction in total mortality with IV magnesium therapy. A subsequent large multicenter trial[117] found similar results, although most of the reduction in mortality with IV magnesium was (surprisingly) attributed to HF deaths rather than to deaths caused by ventricular arrhythmia. These results would lead one to conclude that magnesium sulfate should be routinely administered to patients with suspected MI because of its ease of administration and safety. However, data from another large trial apparently have verified no such effectiveness of magnesium therapy in this setting.[118] Hence, prophylactic magnesium cannot be recommended for this purpose. In addition, AADs have not shown any conclusive benefit in preventing VF in the acute infarction period; as such, these drugs also cannot be recommended in this setting.

Acute Management

A patient with pulseless VT or VF should be managed according to the most recent AHA guidelines for CPR and ECC.[61] A detailed discussion regarding the acute management of pulseless VT/VF can be found in Chapter 18 (Cardiopulmonary Resuscitation).

BRADYARRHYTHMIAS

SINUS NODE DYSFUNCTION

The previous sections reviewed the pathophysiology and treatment of tachyarrhythmias, and this section serves to briefly consider the bradyarrhythmias. For the most part, the symptoms of bradyrrhythmias result from a decline in cardiac output. Because cardiac output decreases as heart rate decreases (to a point), patients with bradyarrhythmias may experience symptoms in association with hypotension, such as dizziness, syncope, fatigue, and confusion. If LV dysfunction exists, patients may experience worsening HF symptoms. Except in the case of recurrent syncope, symptoms associated with bradyarrhythmias are often subtle and nonspecific.

SINUS BRADYCARDIA

Sinus bradyarrhythmias (heart rate <60 beats/min) are a common finding, especially in young, athletically active individuals, and usually are neither symptomatic nor in need of therapeutic intervention. On the other hand, some patients, particularly the elderly, have sinus node dysfunction. This may be the result of underlying SHD and the normal aging process that attenuate SA nodal function over time. Sick sinus syndrome refers to this process resulting in symptomatic sinus bradycardia and/or periods of sinus arrest.[119,120] Sinus node dysfunction is usually reflective of diffuse conduction disease, and accompanying AV block is relatively common. Furthermore, symptomatic bradyarrhythmias may be accompanied by alternating periods of paroxysmal tachycardias such as AF. In this instance, AF sometimes presents with a rather slow ventricular response (in the absence of AV nodal blocking drugs) because of diffuse conduction disease. The occurrence of alternating bradyarrhythmias and tachyarrhythmias is referred to as the tachy-brady syndrome. The occurrence of paroxysmal AF in a patient with sinus node dysfunction may be a result of underlying SHD with atrial dysfunction or atrial escape in response to reduced sinus node automaticity. In fact, because the rate of impulse generation by the sinus node is generally depressed or may fail altogether, other automatic pacemakers within the conduction system may "rescue" the sinus node. These rescue rhythms often present as paroxysmal atrial rhythms (e.g., AF) or as a junctional escape rhythm.

The treatment of sinus node dysfunction involves the elimination of symptomatic bradycardia and potentially managing alternating tachycardias such as AF. In general, the long-term therapy of choice is a permanent ventricular pacemaker. Dual-chamber, rate-adaptive chronic pacing clearly improves symptoms and overall quality of life and decreases the incidence of paroxysmal AF and systemic embolism.[119] Drugs commonly employed to treat supraventricular tachycardias should be used with caution, if at all, in the absence of a functioning pacemaker. AADs prescribed to prevent AF recurrences may also suppress the escape or rescue rhythms that appear in severe sinus bradycardia or sinus arrest. Consequently, these drugs may transform an asymptomatic patient with bradycardia into a symptomatic one. The addition of class I AADs can also affect pacemaker threshold and result in loss of capture if the pacemaker is not appropriately interrogated and adjusted. Other drugs that depress SA or AV nodal function, such as β-blockers and non-DHP CCBs, may also significantly exacerbate bradycardia. Even drugs with indirect sympatholytic actions, such as methyldopa and clonidine, may worsen sinus node dysfunction. The use of digoxin in these patients is controversial; however, in most cases, it can be used safely.

Other Causes

Another reason for paroxysmal bradycardia and sinus arrest that is not directly due to sinus node dysfunction is carotid-sinus hypersensitivity.[121,122] Again, this syndrome occurs commonly in the elderly with underlying SHD, and may precipitate falls and hip fractures. Symptoms occur when the carotid sinus is stimulated, resulting in an accentuated baroreceptor reflex. Often, however, symptoms are not well correlated with the obvious physical manipulation of the carotid sinus (in the lateral neck region). Patients may experience intermittent episodes of dizziness or syncope because of sinus arrest caused by increased vagal tone and sympathetic withdrawal (the cardioinhibitory type), a drop in systemic blood pressure caused by sympathetic withdrawal (the vasodepressor type), or both (mixed cardioinhibitory and vasodepressor types). The diagnosis can be confirmed by performing carotid-sinus massage with ECG and blood pressure monitoring in controlled conditions. Symptomatic carotid-sinus hypersensitivity should also be treated with permanent pacemaker therapy.[121] However, some patients, particularly those with a significant vasodepressor component, still experience syncope or dizziness. The choice of definitive drug therapy in this situation is marred by the lack of controlled trials, although α-adrenergic stimulants such as midodrine are often tried in addition to the pacemaker.[122]

Vasovagal syndrome, by causing bradycardia, sinus arrest, and/or hypotension, is the cause of syncope in many patients who present with recurrent fainting of unknown origin.[123-125] By history, many individuals can recount rare instances of fainting spells at times of duress or fear. These are most often caused by vasovagal syncope. However, some have extremely frequent, unexpected syncopal episodes that interfere with the patient's quality of life and cause physical danger (sometimes referred to as neurocardiogenic syncope syndrome or malignant vasovagal syndrome). Vasovagal syncope is presumed to be a neurally mediated, paradoxical reaction involving stimulation of cardiac mechanoreceptors (i.e., Bezold-Jarisch reflex). Forceful contraction of the ventricle (e.g., as with adrenergic stimulation) coupled with low ventricular volumes (e.g., with upright posture or dehydration) provides a powerful stimulus for cardiac mechanoreceptors. Syncope results from the spontaneous development of transient hypotension (sympathetic withdrawal) and bradycardia (vagotonia). However, the true mechanism of vasovagal syncope remains to be definitively determined. For instance, patients with denervated hearts (e.g., heart transplant recipients) can still experience this form of syncope. This observation has led some to question the ultimate role of the Bezold-Jarisch reflex in these patients. Regardless, patients believed to have frequent episodes of vasovagal syncope have been evaluated and diagnosed using the upright body-tilt test,[126] a potent stimulus for the development of vasovagal symptoms. Although commonly used, the sensitivity and reproducibility of this test have been questioned.[127]

Traditionally, β-blockers, such as metoprolol, were frequently chosen as the drugs of choice in preventing episodes of vasovagal syncope. Although these drugs may seem inappropriate to treat a syndrome resulting from vasodilation and bradycardia, the therapeutic approach is designed to block an inappropriate vasovagal reaction (i.e., they inhibit the sympathetic surge that causes forceful ventricular contraction and precedes the onset of hypotension and bradycardia). To most clinicians' surprise, most controlled trials of the use of β-blockers in patients with severe vasovagal syncope have shown no effect compared with placebo in preventing syncopal episodes.[128] Some trials have suggested that β-blockers are more effective and should be used in older patients (>40 years of age) with vasovagal syncope rather than the relatively young.[129] Other drugs that have been used successfully (with or without β-blockers) include mineralocorticoids as volume expanders (fludrocortisone), anticholinergic drugs (scopolamine patches, disopyramide), α-adrenergic agonists (midodrine), adenosine analogs (theophylline, dipyridamole), and selective serotonin receptor antagonists (sertraline, paroxetine).[130] Permanent pacing has been used with some success but should be reserved for drug-refractory patients.[124,125] Because of the questionable effectiveness of β-blockers and the paucity of controlled or comparative trials, there is not a true drug of choice for severe vasovagal syncope, and clinicians are left with choosing agents and judging clinical effectiveness in individual patients on a case-by-case basis.

ATRIOVENTRICULAR BLOCK

Conduction delay or block may occur in any area of the AV conduction system: the AV node, the His bundle, or the bundle branches.

TABLE 25-13	Forms of Atrioventricular Block	
Type	**Criteria**	**Site of Block**
First-degree block	Prolonged PR interval (>0.2 s); 1:1 AV conduction	Usually AVN
Second-degree block		
Mobitz I	Progressive PR prolongation until QRS is dropped; <1:1 AV conduction	AVN
Mobitz II	Random nonconducted beats (absence of QRS); <1:1 AV conduction	Below AVN
Third-degree block	AV dissociation; absence of AV conduction	AVN or below

AV, atrioventricular; AVN, atrioventricular node.

AV block is usually categorized into three different types based on ECG findings (Table 25-13). First-degree AV block is 1:1 AV conduction with a prolonged PR interval. Second-degree AV block is divided into two forms: Mobitz I AV block (Wenckebach periodicity) is less than 1:1 AV conduction with progressively lengthening PR intervals until a ventricular complex is dropped; Mobitz II AV block is intermittently dropped ventricular beats in a random fashion without progressive PR lengthening. Third-degree AV block is complete heart block where AV conduction is totally absent (AV dissociation). By using intracardiac His bundle ECGs, the actual site of conduction delay/block can be determined and correlated to the type of AV block. First-degree AV block usually represents prolonged conduction in the AV node. Mobitz I, second-degree AV block is also usually caused by prolonged conduction in the AV node. Indeed, Wenckebach periodicity is a normal AV nodal response to rapid supraventricular stimulation or high vagal tone. In contrast, Mobitz II, second-degree AV block is usually caused by conduction disease below the AV node (i.e., His bundle). Third-degree AV block may be caused by disease at any level of the AV conduction system: complete AV nodal block, His bundle block, or trifascicular block. In this situation, the ventricle beats independently of the atria (AV dissociation), and the rate of ventricular activation and QRS configuration are determined by the site of the AV block. The usual degree of automaticity of ventricular pacemakers progressively declines as the site of impulse generation moves down the ventricular conduction system. Therefore, the ventricular escape rate in cases of trifascicular block will be significantly less than complete AV nodal block. Consequently, trifascicular block is a much more dangerous form of AV block. For instance, complete AV block at the level of the AV node usually results in the ventricular rhythm being controlled by the stable AV junctional pacemaker (rate ~40 beats/min). In contrast, in complete AV block due to trifascicular or His bundle block, a much less reliable pacemaker with slower rates below the site of block controls ventricular rhythm.

AV block may be found in patients without underlying SHD such as trained athletes or during sleep when vagal tone is high. Also, AV block may be transient where the underlying etiology is reversible such as in myocarditis, myocardial ischemia, after cardiovascular surgery, or during drug therapy. β-blockers, digoxin, or non-DHP CCBs may cause AV block, primarily in the AV nodal area. Class I AADs may exacerbate conduction delays below the level of the AV node (sodium-dependent tissue). In other cases, AV block may be irreversible, such as that caused by acute MI, rare degenerative diseases, primary myocardial disease, or congenital heart disease.

If patients with Mobitz II AV block or third-degree AV block develop signs or symptoms of poor perfusion (e.g., altered mental status, chest pain, hypotension, shock), IV atropine (0.5 mg given every 3 to 5 minutes, up to 3 mg total dose) should be administered.[61] If these patients do not respond to atropine, transcutaneous pacing can be initiated. Sympathomimetic infusions such as epinephrine (2 to 10 mcg/min) or dopamine (2 to 10 mcg/kg/min) can also be used in the event of atropine failure and are particularly effective in sinus bradycardia/arrest and AV nodal block. An isoproterenol infusion (2 to 10 mcg/min) may be considered if the patient does not respond to dopamine or epinephrine however, this drug should be used with caution because of its vasodilating properties and ability to increase myocardial oxygen consumption (particularly during active MI). As would be expected, these drugs usually do not help when the site of AV block is below the AV node (e.g., Mobitz II or trifascicular AV block) because their primary mechanism is to accelerate conduction through the AV node. If patients with bradycardia or AV block present with signs and symptoms of adequate perfusion, no acute therapy other than close observation is recommended.

Patients with chronic symptomatic AV block should be treated with the insertion of a permanent pacemaker. Patients without symptoms can sometimes be followed closely without the need for a pacemaker. The reader is referred for more detail to the national consensus guidelines for pacemaker implantation, which were last updated in 2008.[105] Patients with acute MI and evidence of new AV block or conduction disturbances will often require the insertion of a temporary transvenous pacemaker. AV block more commonly occurs as a complication of inferior wall MIs because of high vagal innervation at this site, and the coronary blood flow to the nodal areas usually supplies the inferior wall. However, the AV block may only be transient, obviating the need for permanent pacing. In patients with chronic AV conduction disturbances, intracardiac recordings (His bundle ECGs) are sometimes used to document the actual site of block and define the potential need for and specific type of pacemaker therapy.

EVALUATION OF THERAPEUTIC AND ECONOMIC OUTCOMES

Generally, patients who suffer from tachyarrhythmias can be monitored for one or several possible therapeutic outcomes. Obviously, the presence or recurrence of any arrhythmia can be documented by electrocardiographic means (e.g., surface ECG, Holter monitor, or event monitor). Furthermore, patients may experience a decrease in blood pressure that may result in symptoms ranging from lightheadedness to abrupt syncope, depending on the rate of the arrhythmia and the status of the underlying heart disease. For some patients, the potential alteration in hemodynamics may result in death if the arrhythmia is not detected and treated immediately. Besides these clinical outcomes, many patients with tachyarrhythmias experience alterations in quality of life as a result of recurrent symptoms of the arrhythmia or from side effects of therapy. And, finally, there are the economic considerations of medical or surgical intervention, continued medical care, and chronic drug or nonpharmacologic treatment.[131,132] Most of the studies are limited to the use of nonpharmacologic therapies such as the ICD or radiofrequency ablation.[50,104] Because that technology is rapidly evolving, what is not very cost-effective now may indeed be cost-effective in the next several years. For example, original cost-effectiveness analysis of the ICD showed it to be highly sensitive to the life of the generator, yet newer-generation devices have made significant advances not only in the size but also in battery life. More recent data on the effect of the ICD on mortality coupled with the declining costs of an ICD imply that the device is indeed cost-effective in certain subsets of patients, which is similar to well-proven drug therapies used for other disorders.[104,133] Other

TABLE 25-14 Arrhythmia Outcomes

Mortality
  Total, all-cause
  Arrhythmic death (i.e., sudden cardiac death)
Recurrences documented by electrocardiogram
  Time to recurrence
  Frequency of recurrences
Tolerance
  Symptoms
  Blood pressure
  Rate of tachycardia
Surrogate markers of efficacy such as:
  Number of premature ventricular complexes/day
  Inducibility of tachycardia with programmed stimulation
Necessity of nondrug interventions (e.g., ICD)
ICD shocks
Side effects of drugs/treatment complications
Quality of life
Economics
Outcomes specific to tachycardia (e.g., systemic embolism in atrial fibrillation)

ICD, implantable cardioverter-defibrillator.

nonpharmacologic treatments, such as radiofrequency ablation, for PSVT not only improve quality of life but also save money on medical expenditures compared with chronic drug therapy.[52]

There are some therapeutic outcomes that are unique to certain arrhythmias. For instance, patients with AF or atrial flutter need to be monitored for thromboembolism and for complications of antithrombotic therapy (bleeding, drug interactions). However, the most important monitoring parameters for most patients fall into the following categories: (a) mortality (total and arrhythmic); (b) arrhythmia recurrence (duration, frequency, symptoms); (c) hemodynamic consequences (heart rate, blood pressure, symptoms); and (d) treatment complications (side effects or need for alternative or additional drugs, devices, surgery) (Table 25-14). When evaluating the arrhythmia literature, care should be taken to consider real outcomes. For example, total mortality is more meaningful than only SCD rates; it is possible an intervention prevents arrhythmic death but patients die from other causes, leaving all-cause mortality unaltered. Likewise, surrogate markers of drug efficacy (e.g., noninducible tachycardia, suppression of minor arrhythmias) should be judged with a degree of skepticism. One should ask: Did the treatment make patients live longer (reduce mortality)? Did the treatment make them feel better (improve humanistic outcomes or quality of life)? Was the treatment economically worth it (cost-effective)?

ABBREVIATIONS

AAD: antiarrhythmic drug

ACC: American College of Cardiology

ACCP: American College of Chest Physicians

ACTIVE: Atrial Fibrillation Clopidogrel Trial with Irbesartan for Prevention of Vascular Events

AF: atrial fibrillation

AFFIRM: Atrial Fibrillation Follow-up Investigation of Rhythm Management trial

AHA: American Heart Association

AV: atrioventricular

AVID: Antiarrhythmics Versus Implantable Defibrillators trial

CAD: coronary artery disease

CASH: Cardiac Arrest Study Hamburg

CAST: Cardiac Arrhythmia Suppression Trial

CCB: calcium channel blocker

CIDS: Canadian Implantable Defibrillator Study

CPR: cardiopulmonary resuscitation

CYP: cytochrome P450

DCC: direct-current cardioversion

DHP: dihydropyridine

EAD: early after-depolarization

ECC: emergency cardiovascular care

ECG: electrocardiogram

ESC: European Society of Cardiology

HF: heart failure

HOT-CAFE: How to Treat Chronic Atrial Fibrillation trial

ICD: implantable cardioverter-defibrillator

INR: international normalized ratio

IV: intravenous

LAD: late after-depolarization

LV: left ventricular

LVEF: left ventricular ejection fraction

MADIT: Multicenter Automatic Defibrillator Implantation Trial

MI: myocardial infarction

MUSTT: Multicenter Unsustained Tachycardia Trial

NYHA: New York Heart Association

PIAF: Pharmacological Intervention in Atrial Fibrillation trial

PSVT: paroxysmal supraventricular tachycardia

PVC: premature ventricular complex

RACE: Rate Control versus Electrical Cardioversion for Persistent Atrial Fibrillation trial

RMP: resting membrane potential

SA: sinoatrial

SCD: sudden cardiac death

SCD-HeFT: Sudden Cardiac Death in Heart Failure Trial

SHD: structural heart disease

SR: sinus rhythm

STAF: Strategies of Treatment of Atrial Fibrillation trial

TdP: torsade de pointes

TEE: transesophageal echocardiography

VF: ventricular fibrillation

VT: ventricular tachycardia

WPW: Wolff-Parkinson-White syndrome

REFERENCES

1. Alice MA, Bonke FIM, Schopman FJG. Circus movement in rabbit atrial muscle as a mechanism of tachycardia III. The "leading circle" concept: A new model of circus movement in cardiac tissue without the involvement of an anatomic obstacle. Circ Res 1977;41:9–18.

2. Vaughan Williams EM. A classification of antiarrhythmic actions reassessed after a decade of new drugs. J Clin Pharmacol 1984;24:129–147.

3. Working Group on Arrhythmias of the European Society of Cardiology. The Sicilian Gambit: A new approach to the classification of antiarrhythmic drugs based upon their actions on arrhythmogenic mechanisms. Circulation 1991;84:1831–1851.

4. Hondeghem LM, Katzung BG. Antiarrhythmic agents: The modulated receptor mechanism of action of sodium and calcium channel-blocking drugs. Annu Rev Pharmacol Toxicol 1984;24:387–423.

5. Nasr IR, Bouzamondo A, Hulot JS, et al. Prevention of atrial fibrillation onset by beta-blocker treatment in heart failure: A meta-analysis. Eur Heart J 2007;28:457–462.

6. Makkar KM, Sanoski CA, Spinler SA. Role of angiotensin-converting enzyme inhibitors, angiotensin II receptor blockers, and aldosterone antagonists in the prevention of atrial and ventricular arrhythmias. Pharmacotherapy 2009;29:31–48.

7. Kosowsky BD, Taylor J, Lown B, et al. Long-term procaine amide following acute myocardial infarction. Circulation 1973;47:1204–1210.

8. Bauman JL, Gallastegui J, Strasberg B, et al. Long-term therapy with disopyramide phosphate: Side effects and effectiveness. Am Heart J 1986;111:654–660.

9. Podrid PJ, Schoeneburger A, Lown B. Congestive heart failure caused by oral disopyramide. N Engl J Med 1980;302:614–617.

10. Podrid PJ. Proarrhythmia, a serious complication of antiarrhythmic drugs. Curr Cardiol Rep 1999;1:289–296.

11. Fang MC, Stafford RS, Ruskin JN, et al. National trends in antiarrhythmic and antithrombotic medication use in atrial fibrillation. Arch Intern Med 2004;164:55–60.

12. Sanoski CA, Bauman JL. Clinical observations with the amiodarone/warfarin interaction: Dosing relationships with long-term therapy. Chest 2002;121:19–23.

13. Camus P, Martin WJ, Rosenow EC. Amiodarone pulmonary toxicity. Clin Chest Med 2004;25:65–75.

14. Babatin M, Lee SS, Pollak PT. Amiodarone hepatotoxicity. Curr Vasc Pharmacol 2008;6:228–236.

15. Sanoski C, Schoen MD, Gonzalez RD, et al. Rational, development and outcomes of a multidisciplinary clinic for patients receiving chronic oral amiodarone. Pharmacotherapy 1998;18:1465–1515.

16. Lloyd-Jones D, Adams R, Brown TM, et al. Heart disease and stroke statistics 2010 update: A report from the American Heart Association. Circulation 2010;121:e1–e170.

17. Fuster V, Rydén LE, Cannom DS, et al. ACC/AHA/ESC 2006 guidelines for the management of patients with atrial fibrillation: A report of the American College of Cardiology/American Heart Association Task Force on Practice Guidelines and the European Society of Cardiology Committee for Practice Guidelines (Writing Committee to Revise the 2001 Guidelines for the Management of Patients with Atrial Fibrillation). J Am Coll Cardiol 2006;48:e149–e246.

18. Lloyd-Jones DM, Wang TJ, Leip EP, et al. Lifetime risk for developing atrial fibrillation: the Framingham Heart Study. Circulation 2004;110:1042–1046.

19. Miyasaka Y, Barnes ME, Gersh BJ, et al. Secular trends in incidence of atrial fibrillation in Olmsted County, Minnesota, 1980 to 2000, and implications on the projections for future prevalence. Circulation 2006;114:119–125.

20. Levy S, Camm AJ, Saksena S, et al. International consensus on nomenclature and classification of atrial fibrillation. A collaborative project of the Working Group on Arrhythmias and the Working Group on Cardiac Pacing of the European Society of Cardiology and the North American Society of Pacing and Electrophysiology. Europace 2003;5:119–122.

21. Singer DE, Albers GW, Dalen JE, et al. Antithrombotic therapy in atrial fibrillation: American College of Chest Physicians Evidence-Based Clinical Practice Guidelines (8th edition). Chest 2008;133:546S–592S.

22. Atrial Fibrillation Investigators. Risk factors for stroke and efficacy of antithrombotic therapy in atrial fibrillation: Analysis of pooled data from five randomized controlled trials. Arch Intern Med 1994;154:1449–1457.

23. Phillips BG, Gandhi AJ, Sanoski CA, et al. Comparison of intravenous diltiazem and verapamil for the acute treatment of atrial fibrillation and flutter. Pharmacotherapy 1997;17:1238–1245.

24. Hohnloser SH, Kuck KH, Lilienthal J. Rhythm or rate control in atrial fibrillation—Pharmacological Intervention in Atrial Fibrillation (PIAF): A randomised trial. Lancet 2000;356:1789–1794.

25. Van Gelder IC, Hagens VE, Bosker HA, et al. The Rate Control Versus Electrical Cardioversion for Persistent Atrial Fibrillation Study Group.

A comparison of rate control and rhythm control in patients with recurrent persistent atrial fibrillation. N Engl J Med 2002;347:1834–1840.

26. The Atrial Fibrillation Follow-up Investigation of Rhythm Management (AFFIRM) Investigators. A comparison of rate control and rhythm control in patients with atrial fibrillation. N Engl J Med 2002;347:1825–1833.

27. Carlsson J, Miketic S, Windeler J, et al. Randomized trial of rate-control versus rhythm-control in persistent atrial fibrillation: The Strategies of Treatment of Atrial Fibrillation (STAF) study. J Am Coll Cardiol 2003;41:1690–1696.

28. Opolski G, Torbicki A, Kosior DA, et al. Rate control vs rhythm control in patients with nonvalvular persistent atrial fibrillation: The results of the Polish How to Treat Chronic Atrial Fibrillation (HOT CAFE) Study. Chest 2004;126:476–486.

29. Roy D, Talajic M, Nattel S, et al. Rhythm control versus rate control for atrial fibrillation and heart failure. N Engl J Med 2008;358:2667–2677.

30. de Denus S, Sanoski CA, Carlsson J, Opolski G, Spinler SA. Rate vs rhythm control in patients with atrial fibrillation: A meta-analysis. Arch Intern Med 2005;165:258–262.

31. Klein AL, Grimm RA, Murray D, et al. Use of transesophageal echocardiography to guide cardioversion in patients with atrial fibrillation. N Engl J Med 2001;344:1411–1420.

32. Bauman JL, Bauernfeind RA, Hoff JV, et al. Torsade de pointes due to quinidine: Observations in 31 patients. Am Heart J 1984;107:425–430.

33. Slavik RS, Tisdale JE, Borzak S. Pharmacologic conversion of atrial fibrillation: A systematic review of available evidence. Prog Cardiovasc Dis 2001;44:121–152.

34. Alboni P, Botto GL, Baldi N, et al. Outpatient treatment of recent-onset atrial fibrillation with the "pill-in-the-pocket" approach. N Engl J Med 2004;351:2384–2391.

35. Connolly SJ, Pogue J, Hart R, et al. Clopidogrel plus aspirin versus oral anticoagulation for atrial fibrillation in the Atrial fibrillation Clopidogrel Trial with Irbesartan for prevention of Vascular Events (ACTIVE W): A randomised controlled trial. Lancet 2006;367:1903–1912.

36. The ACTIVE Investigators. Effect of clopidogrel added to aspirin in patients with atrial fibrillation. N Engl J Med 2009;360:2066–2078.

37. Coplen SE, Antman EM, Berlin JA, et al. Efficacy and safety of quinidine therapy for maintenance of sinus rhythm after cardioversion: A meta-analysis of randomized control trials. Circulation 1990;82:1106–1116.

38. Echt DS, Liebson PR, Mitchell B, et al. Mortality and morbidity in patients receiving encainide, flecainide, or placebo. The Cardiac Arrhythmia Suppression Trial. N Engl J Med 1991;324:781–788.

39. Lafuente-LaFuente C, Mouly S, Longás-Tejero MA, Mahé I, Bergmann JF. Antiarrhythmic drugs for maintaining sinus rhythm after cardioversion of atrial fibrillation. Arch Intern Med 2006;166:719–728.

40. Roy D, Talajic M, Dorian P, et al. Amiodarone to prevent recurrence of atrial fibrillation. Canadian Trial of Atrial Fibrillation Investigators. N Engl J Med 2000;324:913–920.

41. AFFIRM First Antiarrhythmic Drug Substudy Investigators. Maintenance of sinus rhythm in patients with atrial fibrillation: An AFFIRM substudy of the first antiarrhythmic drug. J Am Coll Cardiol 2003;42:20–29.

42. Singh BN, Singh SN, Reda DJ, et al. Amiodarone versus sotalol for atrial fibrillation. N Engl J Med 2005;352:1861–1872.

43. Juul-Moller S, Edvardsson N, Rehnqvist-Ahlberg N. Sotalol versus quinidine for the maintenance of sinus rhythm after direct current conversion of atrial fibrillation. Circulation 1990;82:1932–1939.

44. Southworth MR, Zarembski D, Viana M, Bauman JL. Comparison of sotalol versus quinidine for maintenance of normal sinus rhythm in patients with chronic atrial fibrillation. Am J Cardiol 1999;83:1629–1632.

45. Pedersen OD, Bagger H, Keller N, et al. Efficacy of dofetilide in the treatment of atrial fibrillation-flutter in patients with reduced left ventricular function, A Danish Investigation of Arrhythmia and Mortality ON Dofetilide (DIAMOND) Substudy. Circulation 2001;104:292–296.

46. Singh S, Zoble RG, Yellen L, et al. Efficacy and safety of oral dofetilide in converting and maintaining sinus rhythm in patients with chronic atrial fibrillation or atrial flutter. The Symptomatic Atrial Fibrillation Investigative Research on Dofetilide (SAFIRE-D) Study. Circulation 2000;102:2385–2390.

47. Pedersen OD, Bagger H, Keller N, et al. Efficacy of dofetilide in the treatment of atrial fibrillation-flutter in patients with reduced left ventricular function: A Danish investigations of arrhythmia and mortality on dofetilide (DIAMOND) substudy. Circulation 2001;104:292–296.

48. Singh BN, Connolly SJ, Crijns HJGM, et al. Dronedarone for maintenance of sinus rhythm in atrial fibrillation or flutter. N Engl J Med 2007;357:987–999.

49. Hohnloser SH, Crijns HJGM, van Eickels M, et al. Effect of dronedarone on cardiovascular events in atrial fibrillation. N Engl J Med 2009;360:668–678.

50. Køber L, Torp-Pedersen C, McMurray JJV, et al. Increased mortality after dronedarone therapy for severe heart failure. N Engl J Med 2008;358:2678–2687.

51. Spector P, Reynolds MR, Calkins H, et al. Meta-analysis of ablation of atrial flutter and supraventricular tachycardia. Am J Cardiol 2009;104:671–677.

52. Blomstrom-Lundgrist C, Scheimanman MM, Aliot EM, et al. ACC/AHA/ESC Guidelines for the management of patients with supraventricular arrhythmias. A report of the American College of Cardiology/American Heart Association Task Force and the European Society of Cardiology Committee for Practice Guidelines. J Am Coll Cardiol 2003;42:1493–1531.

53. Pappone C, Augello G, Sala S, et al. A randomized trial of circumferential pulmonary vein ablation versus antiarrhythmic drug therapy in paroxysmal atrial fibrillation: The APAF Study. J Am Coll Cardiol 2006;48:2340 –2347.

54. Oral H, Pappone C, Chugh A, et al. Circumferential pulmonary-vein ablation for chronic atrial fibrillation. N Engl J Med 2006;354:934–941.

55. Wazni OM, Marrouche NF, Martin DO, et al. Radiofrequency ablation vs antiarrhythmic drugs as first-line treatment of symptomatic atrial fibrillation: A randomized trial. JAMA 2005;293:2634–2640.

56. Jaïs P, Cauchemez B, Macle L, et al. Catheter ablation versus antiarrhythmic drugs for atrial fibrillation: the A4 study. Circulation 2008;118:2498–2505.

57. Calkins H, Brugada J, Packer DL, et al. HRS/EHRA/ECAS expert consensus statement on catheter and surgical ablation of atrial fibrillation: recommendations for personnel, policy, and follow-up. Heart Rhythm 2007;4:816–861.

58. Cappato R, Calkins H, Chen SA, et al. Worldwide survey on the methods, efficacy, and safety of catheter ablation for human atrial fibrillation. Circulation 2005;111:1100–1105.

59. Sung RJ, Lauer MR, Chun H. Atrioventricular Node Reentry: Current concepts and new perspectives. Pacing Clin Electrophysiol 1994;17:1413–1430.

60. DiMarco JP, Miles W, Akhtar M, et al. Adenosine for paroxysmal supraventricular tachycardia: Dose ranging and comparison with verapamil. Assessment in placebo-controlled, multicenter trials. Ann Intern Med 1990;1113:104–110.

61. 2010 American Heart Association guidelines for cardiopulmonary resuscitation and emergency cardiovascular care science. Circulation 2010;122:5640–5933.

62. Rankin AC, McGovern BA. Adenosine or verapamil for the acute treatment of supraventricular tachycardia? Ann Intern Med 1991;114:513–515.

63. Alboni P, Tomasi C, Menozzi C, et al. Efficacy and safety of out-of-hospital self-administered single-dose oral drug treatment in the management of infrequent, well-tolerated paroxysmal supraventricular tachycardia. J Am Coll Cardiol 2001;37:548–553.

64. Jackman WM, Wang Z, Friday KJ, et al. Catheter ablation of accessory atrioventricular pathways (Wolff-Parkinson-White syndrome) by radiofrequency current. N Engl J Med 1991;324:1605–1611.

65. Jackman WM, Beckman KJ, McClelland JH, et al. Treatment of supraventricular tachycardia due to atrioventricular nodal reentry by radiofrequency catheter ablation of slow pathway conduction. N Engl J Med 1992;327:313–318.

66. Scheinman MM. Radiofrequency catheter ablation for patients with supraventricular tachycardia. Pacing Clin Electrophysiol 1993;16:671–679.

67. Cheng CH, Sanders GD, Hlatky MA, et al. Cost effectiveness of radiofrequency ablation for supraventricular tachycardia. Ann Intern Med 2000;133:864–876.

68. McCord J, Borzak S. Multifocal atrial tachycardia. Chest 1998;113: 203–209.

69. Levine JH, Michael JR, Guarnier T. Treatment of multifocal atrial tachycardia with verapamil. N Engl J Med 1985;312:21–25.

70. Bayes deLuna A, Coumel P, LeClercq IF. Ambulatory sudden cardiac death: Mechanisms of production of fatal arrhythmia on the basis of data from 157 cases. Am Heart J 1989;117:151–159.

71. Ruberman W, Weinblatt E, Goldberg JD, et al. Ventricular premature beats and mortality after myocardial infarction. N Engl J Med 1977;297:750–757.

72. The Cardiac Arrhythmia Suppression Trial II Investigators. Effect of the antiarrhythmic agent moricizine on survival after myocardial infarction. N Engl J Med 1992;327:227–233.

73. Waldo AL, Camm AJ, deRuyter H, et al. Effect of d-sotalol on mortality in patients with left ventricular dysfunction and remote myocardial infarction. Lancet 1996;348:7–12.

74. Julian DG, Camm AJ, Frangin G, et al. Randomized trial of effect of amiodarone on mortality in patients with left ventricular dysfunction after recent myocardial infarction: EMIAT. Lancet 1997;349:667–674.

75. Cairns JA, Connolly SJ, Roberts R, et al. Randomized trial of outcome after myocardial infarction in patients with frequent or repetitive ventricular premature depolarizations: CAMIAT. Lancet 1997;349:675–682.

76. Amiodarone Trials Meta-Analysis Investigators. Effect of prophylactic amiodarone on mortality after acute myocardial infarction and in congestive heart failure: Meta-analysis of individual data from 6,500 patients in randomized trials. Lancet 1997;350:1417–1424.

77. Torp-Pederson C, Moller M, Bloch-Thomsen PE, et al. Dofetilide in patients with congestive heart failure and left ventricular dysfunction. N Engl J Med 1999;341:857–865.

78. Kober L, Block-Thomsen PE, Moller M, et al. Effect of dofetilide in patients with recent myocardial infarction and left ventricular dysfunction: A randomized trial. Lancet 2000;356:2052–2058.

79. Hilleman DE, Bauman JL. Role of antiarrhythmic therapy in patients at risk for sudden cardiac death: An evidence-based review. Pharmacotherapy 2001;21:556–575.

80. Edhouse J, Morris F. Broad complex tachycardia—Part I. BMJ 2002;312:719–722.

81. Edhouse J, Morris F. Broad complex tachycardia—Part II. BMJ 2002;324:776–779.

82. Cole CR, Marrouche NF, Natale A. Evaluation and management of ventricular outflow tract tachycardias. Card Electrophysiol Rev 2002;6: 442–447.

83. Modell SM, Lehmann MH. The long QT syndrome family of cardiac ion channelopathies: A HuGE review. Genet Med 2006;8:143–155.

84. Keating MT, Sanguinetti MC, Molecular and cellular mechanisms of cardiac arrhythmias. Cell 2001;104:569–580.

85. Antzelevitch C, Brugada P, Brugada J, et al. Brugada syndrome: 1992–2002: A historical perspective. J Am Coll Cardiol 2003;41:1665–1671.

86. Gorgels A, van den Dool A, Hofs A, et al. Comparison of procainamide and lidocaine in terminating sustained monomorphic ventricular tachycardia. Am J Cardiol 1996;78:43–46.

87. Mason JW and the Electrophysiologic Study versus Electrocardiographic Monitoring Investigators. A comparison of electrophysiologic testing with Holter monitoring to predict antiarrhythmic drug efficacy for ventricular tachyarrhythmias. N Engl J Med 1993;329:445–451.

88. Mason JW and the Electrophysiologic Study versus Electrocardiographic Monitoring Investigators. A comparison of seven antiarrhythmic drugs in patients with ventricular tachyarrhythmias. N Engl J Med 1993;329:452–458.

89. The Cascade Investigators. Randomized antiarrhythmic drug therapy in survivors of cardiac arrest (the CASCADE Study). Am J Cardiol 1993;72:280–287.

90. Aliot EM, Stevenson WG, Almendral-Garrote JM, et al. EHRA/HRS Expert Consensus on Catheter Ablation of Ventricular Arrhythmias: Developed in a partnership with the European Heart Rhythm Association (EHRA), a Registered Branch of the European Society of Cardiology (ESC), and the Heart Rhythm Society (HRS); in collaboration with the American College of Cardiology (ACC) and the American Heart Association (AHA). Europace 2009;11:771–817.

91. DiMarco JP. Implantable cardioverter-defibrillators. N Engl J Med 2003;349:1836–1847.

92. Pacifico A, Hohnloser SH, Williams JH, et al. Prevention of implantable-defibrillator shocks by treatment with sotalol. N Engl J Med 1999;340:1855–1862.

93. Connolly SJ, Dorian P, Roberts RS, et al. Comparison of beta-blockers, amiodarone plus beta-blockers, or sotalol for prevention of shocks from implantable defibrillators: The OPTIC Study: A randomized trial. JAMA 2006;295:165–171.

94. Dopp AL, Miller JM, Tisdale JE. Effects of drugs on defibrillation capacity. Drugs 2008;68:607–630.

95. The AVID Investigators. A comparison of antiarrhythmic-drug therapy with implantable defibrillators in patients resuscitated from near-fatal ventricular arrhythmias. N Engl J Med. 1997;337:1576–1583.

96. Connolly SJ, Gene M, Roberts TS, et al. Cardiac Implantable Defibrillator Study (CIDS): A randomized trial of the implantable cardioverter-defibrillator against amiodarone. Circulation 2000;101:1297–1302.

97. Kuck KH, Cappato R, Siebels J, et al. Randomized comparison of antiarrhythmic drug therapy with implantable defibrillators in patients resuscitated from cardiac arrest: The Cardiac Arrest Study Hamburg (CASH). Circulation 2000;102:748–754.

98. Moss AJ, Hall WJ, Cannom DS, et al. Improved survival with an implanted defibrillator in patients with coronary disease at high risk for ventricular arrhythmia. N Engl J Med 1996;335:1933–1940.

99. Buxton AE, Lee KL, Fisher JD, et al. A randomized study of the prevention of sudden death in patients with coronary artery disease. N Engl J Med 1999;341:1882–1890.

100. Moss AJ, Zareba W, Hall WJ, et al. Prophylactic implantation of a defibrillator in patients with myocardial infarction and reduced ejection fraction. N Engl J Med 2002;346:877–883.

101. Bardy GH, Lee KL, Mark DB, et al. Amiodarone or an implantable cardioverter-defibrillator for congestive heart failure. N Engl J Med 2005;352:225–237.

102. Wilber DJ, Olshansky B, Moran JF, et al. Electrophysiological testing and nonsustained VT. Use and limitations in patients with coronary artery disease and impaired ventricular function. Circulation 1990;82:350–358.

103. Buxton AE, Leek KL, DiCarlo L, et al. Electrophysiologic testing to identify patients with coronary artery disease who are at risk for sudden death. Multicenter Unsustained Tachycardia trial. N Engl J Med 2000;342:1937–1945.

104. Zipes DP, Camm AJ, Borggrefe M, et al. ACC/AHA/ESC 2006 guidelines for management of patients with ventricular arrhythmias and the prevention of sudden cardiac death—Executive summary: A report of the American College of Cardiology/American Heart Association Task Force and the European Society of Cardiology Committee for Practice Guidelines (Writing Committee to Develop Guidelines for Management of Patients with Ventricular Arrhythmias and the Prevention of Sudden Cardiac Death). Circulation 2006;114:1–45.

105. Epstein AE, DiMarco JP, Ellenbogen KA, et al. ACC/AHA/HRS 2008 guidelines for device-based therapy of cardiac rhythm abnormalities: A report of the American College of Cardiology/American Heart Association Task Force on Practice Guidelines (Writing Committee to Revise the ACC/AHA/NASPE 2002 Guideline Update for Implantation of Cardiac Pacemakers and Antiarrhythmia Devices). J Am Coll Cardiol 2008;51:e1–e62.

106. Herre JM, Titus C, Oeff M, et al. Inefficacy and proarrhythmic effects of flecainide and encainide for sustained ventricular tachycardia and ventricular fibrillation. Ann Intern Med 1990;113:671–676.

107. Antzelevitch C. Heterogeneity of cellular repolarization in LQTS: The role of M cells. Eur Heart J 2001;3:K2–K16.

108. Roden DM. Long QT syndrome: Reduced repolarization reserve and the genetic link. J Intern Med 2006;259:59–69.

109. Oberg KC, O'Toole MF, Gallastegui JL, Bauman JL. "Late" proarrhythmia due to quinidine. Am J Cardiol 1994;74:192–194.

110. Bauman JL. The role of pharmacokinetics, drug interactions and pharmacogenetics in the acquired long QT syndrome. Eur Heart J 2001;3:K93–K100.

111. Tzivoni D, Banai S, Schuger C, et al. Treatment of torsade de pointes with magnesium sulfate. Circulation 1987;77:392–397.

112. Koplan BA, Stevenson WG. Ventricular tachycardia and sudden cardiac death. Mayo Clin Proc 2009;84:289–297.

113. Lie KI, Wellens HJJ, Van Capelle FJ. Lidocaine in the prevention of primary ventricular fibrillation. N Engl J Med 1974;291:1324–1326.

114. MacMahon S, Collin R, Peto R, et al. Effects of prophylactic lidocaine in suspected acute myocardial infarction: An overview of results from the randomized controlled trials. JAMA 1988;260:1910–1916.

115. Antman EM, Berlin JA. Declining incidence of ventricular fibrillation in myocardial infarction: Implications for the prophylactic use of lidocaine. Circulation 1992;86:764–773.

116. Horner SM. Efficacy of intravenous magnesium in acute myocardial infarction in reducing arrhythmias and mortality: Meta-analysis of magnesium in acute myocardial infarction. Circulation 1992;86:774–779.

117. Woods KL, Fletcher S, Roffe C, Haider Y. A randomized trial of intravenous magnesium sulfate in suspected acute myocardial infarction: Results of the second Leicester Intravenous Magnesium Intervention Trial (LIMIT-2). Lancet 1992;339:1553–1558.

118. Sleight P. Vasodilators after myocardial infarction—ISIS IV. Am J Hypertens 1994;7:1025–1055.

119. Task Force on Syncope, European Society of Cardiology. Guidelines on the management (diagnosis and treatment) of syncope—Update 2004. Europace 2004;6:467–537.

120. Sneddon JF, Camm AJ. Sinus node disease: Current concepts in diagnosis and therapy. Drugs 1992;44:728–737.

121. Sugrue DD, Gersh BJ, Holmes DR, et al. Symptomatic "isolated" carotid sinus hypersensitivity: Natural history and results of treatment with anticholinergic drugs or pacemaker. J Am Coll Cardiol 1986;7:158–162.

122. Strasberg B, Sagie A, Erdman S, et al. Carotid sinus hypersensitivity and the carotid sinus syndrome. Prog Cardiovasc Dis 1989;31:379–391.

123. Zagga M, Massumi A. Neurally mediated syncope. Tex Heart Inst J 2000;27:268–272.

124. Grubb BP. Neurocardiogenic syncope and related disorders of orthostatic intolerance. Circulation 2005;111:2997–3006.

125. Grubb BP. Neurocardiogenic syncope. N Engl J Med 2005;352: 1004–1010.

126. Milstein S, Reyes WJ, Benditt DG. Upright body tilt for evaluation of patients with recurrent, unexplained syncope. Pacing Clin Electrophysiol 1989;12:117–124.

127. Almquist A, Goldenberg I, Milstein S. Provocation of bradycardia and hypotension by isoproterenol and upright posture in patients with unexplained syncope. N Engl J Med 1990;320:346–351.

128. Brignole M. Randomized clinical trials of neurally mediated syncope. J Cardiovasc Electrophysiol 2003;14(suppl):S64–S69.

129. Sheldon R, Connolly S, Rose S, for the POST Investigators. Prevention of Syncope Trial (POST). A randomized, placebo-controlled study of metoprolol in the prevention of vasovagal syncope. Circulation 2006; 113:1164–1170.

130. Bloomfield DM. Strategy for the management of vasovagal syncope. Drugs Aging 2002;19:179–202.

131. Kupersmith J, Holmes-Novner M, Hogan A, et al. Cost-effectiveness analysis in heart disease, I: General principles. Prog Cardiovasc Dis 1994;37:161–184.

132. Kupersmith J, Holmes-Novner M, Hogan A, et al. Cost-effectiveness analysis in heart disease, III: Ischemia, congestive heart failure, and arrhythmias. Prog Cardiovasc Dis 1995;37:307–346.

133. Sanders GD, Hlatky MA, Owens DK. Cost-effectiveness of implantable cardioverter-defibrillators. N Engl J Med 2005;353:1471–1480.

26 Venous Thromboembolism

DANIEL M. WITT, EDITH A. NUTESCU, AND STUART T. HAINES

KEY CONCEPTS

❶ The risk of venous thromboembolism (VTE) is related to several easily identifiable factors, including age, major surgery (particularly orthopedic procedures of the lower extremities), previous VTE, trauma, malignancy, prolonged immobility or limb paralysis, and hypercoagulable states. These risks are additive.

❷ The diagnosis of VTE should be confirmed by objective testing.

❸ Antithrombotic therapies require meticulous and systematic monitoring as well as ongoing patient education. Well-organized anticoagulation management services improve the quality of patient care and reduce overall cost.

❹ Bleeding is the most common adverse effect associated with anticoagulant drugs. A patient's risk of major hemorrhage is related to the intensity and stability of therapy, concurrent drug use, history of gastrointestinal bleeding, history of prior noncadioembolic stroke, renal or hepatic impairment, thrombocytopenia, recent surgery or trauma, and increasing age.

❺ At the time of hospital admission, all patients should receive prophylaxis against venous thromboembolism that corresponds to their level of risk. Prophylaxis should be continued throughout the period of risk.

❻ In the absence of contraindications, the treatment of VTE should initially include a rapid-acting anticoagulant (e.g., unfractionated heparin, low-molecular-weight heparin, or fondaparinux). If the patient is transitioned to warfarin therapy, the rapid-acting anticoagulant should be overlapped with warfarin for at least 5 days and until the patient's international normalized ratio is greater than 2.0. Anticoagulation therapy should be continued for a minimum of 3 months. The duration of anticoagulation therapy should be based on the patient's risks of VTE recurrence and major bleeding, and preference regarding continued treatment.

❼ Most patients with an uncomplicated deep vein thrombosis, with or without pulmonary embolism, can be safely treated as an outpatient.

Learning objectives, review questions, and other resources can be found at **www.pharmacotherapyonline.com**.

Venous thromboembolism (VTE) is a potentially fatal disorder and a significant health problem in our aging society.[1,2] Although it can strike young, otherwise healthy adults, it most frequently occurs in patients who sustain multiple trauma, undergo major surgery, are immobile for a lengthy period of time, or have a hypercoagulable disorder. Resulting from clot formation within the venous circulation (Fig. 26–1), VTE is manifested as deep vein thrombosis (DVT) and pulmonary embolism (PE). Death from PE can occur within minutes after the onset of symptoms, before effective treatment can be given.

Unfortunately, the disease is often clinically silent, and the first manifestation may be sudden death. In some case series, 80% of patients who died suddenly had some evidence of PE at the time of autopsy.[2] Beyond the symptoms produced by the acute event, the complications of VTE, such as the postthrombotic syndrome and chronic thromboembolic pulmonary hypertension (CTPH), also cause substantial disability and suffering.[1]

The treatment of VTE is fraught with substantial risks.[3] Antithrombotic drugs require precise dosing and meticulous monitoring.[4,5] Systematic approaches to drug therapy management substantially reduce the risks, but bleeding remains an all too common and serious complication of administering antithrombotic drugs. Consequently, the prevention of VTE in at-risk patients is paramount to improving outcomes.[2] When there is a suspicion of VTE, the rapid and accurate diagnosis of the disorder is critical to making appropriate treatment decisions.[6,7] The optimal use of antithrombotic drugs requires not only an in-depth knowledge of their pharmacology and pharmacokinetic properties, but also a comprehensive approach to patient management.[4,5]

EPIDEMIOLOGY

The true incidence of VTE in the general population is unknown, because a substantial portion of patients, perhaps more than 50%, have clinically silent disease. An estimated 350,00 to 600,00 people in the United States develop VTE each year and more than 100,000 die.[8] The estimated annual direct medical costs of managing the disease are well over $1 billion and growing. The estimated age-adjusted annual incidence of symptomatic VTE in whites is 100 per 100,000.[9] The incidence of VTE nearly doubles in each decade of life over the age of 50 years and is slightly higher in men. African Americans appear to be at somewhat higher risk of VTE than are Americans of predominantly European ancestry, whereas Hispanic Americans may be at slightly lower risk. Asian Americans and Pacific Islanders appear to have a strikingly low incidence of VTE. While the age-adjusted incidence of PE has declined slightly in recent years, the total number of cases of DVT and PE continues to climb as the population ages.

The incidence of VTE in specific high-risk patient populations has been extensively studied.[2] Patients who sustain multiple traumas

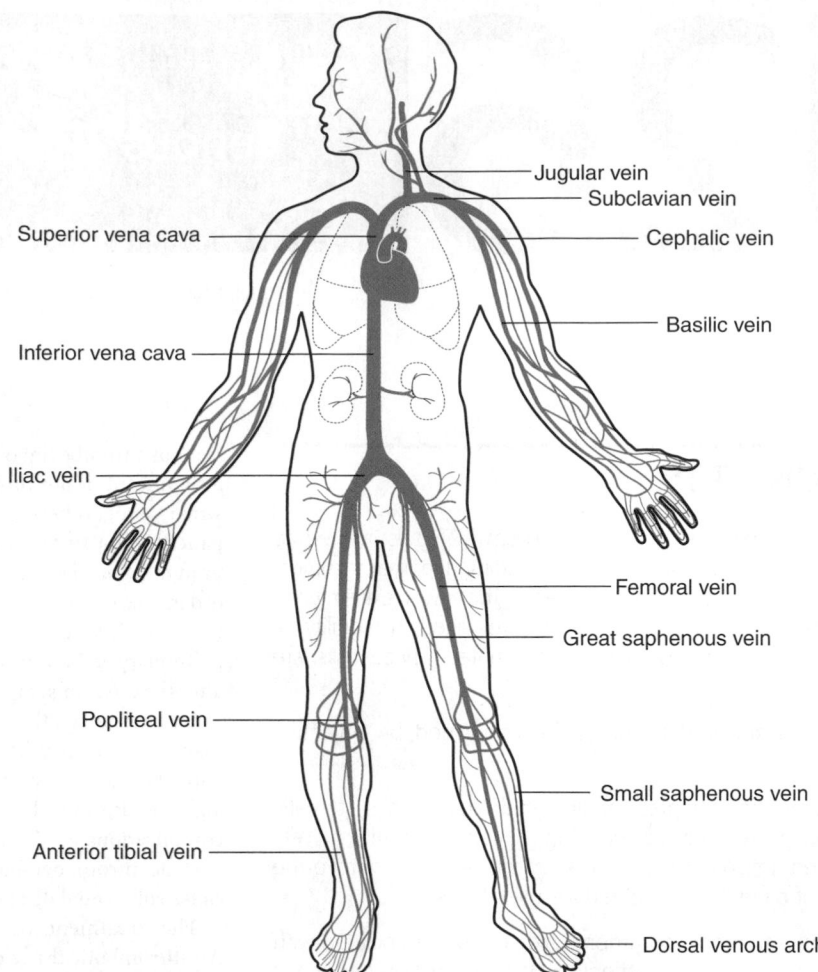

FIGURE 26-1. Venous circulation.

Jugular vein
Subclavian vein
Superior vena cava
Cephalic vein
Basilic vein
Inferior vena cava
Iliac vein
Femoral vein
Great saphenous vein
Popliteal vein
Small saphenous vein
Anterior tibial vein
Dorsal venous arch

or undergo an orthopedic procedure involving a lower extremity are at particularly high risk, with the incidence of VTE often exceeding 50% in the absence of effective prophylaxis. Among those undergoing major surgeries other than procedures involving the lower extremities, the incidence of VTE is 20% to 40% when one or more other risk factors are present, such as age older than 60 years. The long-term incidence of VTE among patients who have a prior history of VTE and who have metastatic cancer is extremely high. Likewise, the incidence of VTE after a myocardial infarction, stroke, and spinal cord injury is high. Several disorders of hypercoagulability have also been linked to a high lifetime incidence of VTE.[10]

ETIOLOGY

❶ A number of factors increase the risk of developing VTE (Table 26-1). These additive risk factors can be easily identified in clinical practice. Stasis of blood favors thrombogenesis in part through reduced clearance of activated clotting factors from sites of thrombus formation. The rate of blood flow in the venous circulation, particularly in the deep veins of the lower extremities, is relatively slow. Valves in the deep veins of the legs, as well as contraction of the calf and thigh muscles, facilitate the flow of blood back to the heart and lungs; thus, damage to the venous valves and periods of prolonged immobility result in venous stasis. Vessel obstruction, either from external compression or a thrombus, also promotes clot propagation. Reduced venous blood flow explains, at least in part, why numerous medical conditions and surgical procedures are associated with an increased risk of VTE

(Table 26–1). Increased blood viscosity, seen in myeloproliferative disorders like polycythemia vera, for example, may also contribute to slowed blood flow and thrombus formation.

A growing list of hereditary deficiencies, gene mutations, and acquired diseases has been linked to hypercoagulability (see Table 26–1).[11] Activated protein C resistance is the most common genetic disorder of hypercoagulability, with a prevalence rate of about 5% in healthy people of Northern European ancestry, and a rate as high as 20% among patients with a first VTE.[11] About 90% of activated protein C resistance results from a mutation on factor V that renders it resistant to degradation by activated protein C.[12] This mutation is known as factor V Leiden, named after the city of Leiden, Holland, where the defect was first described in 1994. The prothrombin G20210A mutation is another common defect, occurring in about 4% of the general population and in about 6% of those with an initial VTE.[11] This mutation increases VTE risk by increasing the basal level of functionally normal prothrombin.[11] Although the rarity (present in <1% of the population) of inherited deficiencies of the natural anticoagulants protein C, protein S, and antithrombin, precludes accurate quantification of their effect on the risk of initial VTE, many experts believe the lifetime risk is high.[13] Conversely, excessively high concentrations of factors VIII, IX, and XI or fibrinogen also increase the risk of VTE.[11] Given the prevalence of these inherited abnormalities in the general population, some patients have multiple genetic defects that have additive effects in terms of increasing the lifetime thrombotic risk.[11]

Acquired disorders of hypercoagulability may result from malignancy, the presence of antiphospholipid antibodies, and

TABLE 26-1 Risk Factors for Venous Thromboembolism

Risk Factor	Comments/Examples
Age	Annual incidence increases from 1 per 100,000 in childhood to 1 per 100 in old age
History of VTE	Strongest known risk factor for recurrence, risk is highest during the first 6 months after VTE
Venous stasis	Acute medical illness requiring hospitalization
	Surgery (especially general anesthesia >30 minutes)
	Paralysis (e.g., status post-stroke, spinal cord injury) Immobility (e.g., plaster casts, status post-stroke, or spinal cord injury)
	Polycythemia vera
	Obesity
	Varicose veins
Vascular injury	Major orthopedic surgery (e.g., knee and hip replacement)
	Trauma (especially fractures of the pelvis, hip, or leg)
	Indwelling venous catheters
	Hypercoagulable states
	Malignancy, diagnosed or occult
	Activated protein C resistance/factor V Leiden
	Prothrombin (G20210A) gene mutation
	Protein C deficiency
	Protein S deficiency
	Antithrombin deficiency
	Factor VIII excess (>90th percentile)
	Factor XI excess (>90th percentile)
	Antiphospholipid antibodies
	Lupus anticoagulant
	Anticardiolipin antibodies
	Anti-β_2-glycoprotein I antibodies
	Dysfibrinogenemia
	Hyperhomocysteinemia
	Plasminogen activator inhibitor-1 excess
	Inflammatory bowel disease
	Nephrotic syndrome
	Paroxysmal nocturnal hemoglobinuria
	Pregnancy/postpartum
Drug therapy	Estrogen-containing contraception
	Estrogen replacement therapy
	Selective estrogen receptor modulators (e.g., tamoxifen, raloxifene)
	Cancer therapy
	Heparin-induced thrombocytopenia

VTE, venous thromboembolism.
Data from Rosendaal et al.,[17] Geerts et al.,[2] Giannakopoulos et al.[15]

estrogen use.[11] The strong link between cancer and thrombosis has been recognized since the late 1800s.[14] Tumor cells secrete a number of procoagulant substances that activate the coagulation cascade. Furthermore, patients with cancer often have suppressed levels of protein C, protein S, and antithrombin. It has been postulated that cancer cells use thrombotic mechanisms to recruit a blood supply (angiogenesis), metastasize, and create a barrier against host defense mechanisms.[14] Antiphospholipid antibodies, most commonly found in patients with autoimmune disorders such as systemic lupus erythematosus and inflammatory bowel disease, can cause venous and arterial thrombosis.[15] These antibodies are also associated with repeated pregnancy loss presumably caused by placental thrombosis.[16] The precise mechanism by which the antiphospholipid antibodies provoke thrombosis is unclear, but they appear to activate complement, the coagulation cascade and platelets, as well as to inhibit the anticoagulant activity of proteins C and S and fibrinolysis.[15] Estrogen-containing contraception, estrogen replacement therapy, and the selective estrogen receptor modulators are all linked to venous thrombosis.[17] Women with an underlying disorder of hypercoagulability are at particularly high risk of developing venous thrombosis while taking estrogens.

Although the mechanisms are not clearly understood, estrogens increase serum clotting factor concentrations and induce activated protein C resistance. Increased serum estrogen concentrations may explain, in part, the increased risk of VTE observed during pregnancy and the immediate postpartum period.[16]

In many cases, VTE is the result of converging combinations of inherited and acquired thrombotic risk factors. Thus, many individuals with congenital hypercoagulable conditions experience a first VTE only after being placed in situations of high risk for thrombosis such as orthopedic surgery, immobilization, the use of estrogen-containing oral contraceptives, or pregnancy.[12]

PATHOPHYSIOLOGY

The arrest of bleeding following vascular injury (hemostasis) is an amazingly complex process that is essential to life. Within the vascular system, blood remains in a fluid state, transporting oxygen, nutrients, plasma proteins, and waste. With vascular injury, a dynamic series of reactions involving a complex interplay of thrombogenic and antithrombotic stimuli result in the local formation of a hemostatic plug that seals the vessel wall and prevents further blood loss but does not spread to other areas of the vasculature (Figs. 26–2, 26–3, 26–4).[18] A disruption of this delicate system of checks and balances may lead to inappropriate clot formation within the blood vessel that subsequently obstructs blood flow or embolizes to a distant vascular bed. In the late 1800s, Dr. Rudolf Virchow, a German pathologist, recognized the role played by blood vessels, circulating elements in the blood, and the speed of blood flow in the regulation of clot formation (Table 26–2).[10] Alterations in any one of these elements, known today as the Virchow triad, may lead to pathologic clot formation.

Hemostasis occurs in three distinct but overlapping steps: initiation, amplification, and propagation (see Fig. 26–4).[18] Under normal circumstances, the endothelial cells that form the intima of vessels maintain blood flow by physically separating extravascular collagen and tissue factor from platelets and by producing substances that inhibit platelet adherence and prevent the activation of the coagulation cascade. Vascular injury allows key components of the coagulation process, namely platelets and factor VIII complexed to von Willebrand factor to come into contact with collagen and tissue factor bearing cells in the extravascular space initiating the hemostatic process (see Fig. 26–3). During initiation, tissue factor bearing cells produce small (picomolar) amounts of thrombin via what has traditionally been termed the "extrinsic" coagulation pathway (namely the factor VIIa/tissue factor complex and the factor Xa/Va complex).[19] A major function of this thrombin is amplification of the hemostatic process by inducing platelets partially activated during adherence to collagen at the site of vascular injury to higher levels of procoagulant activity. This dual activation by collagen and thrombin is a mechanism by which the most procoagulant form of activated platelets are produced at the site of vascular injury.[18] In addition, the thrombin formed during initiation activates cofactors V and VIII and factor XI on platelet surfaces in preparation for large-scale thrombin production. This so-called propagation phase involves much of what has traditionally been termed the "intrinsic" coagulation pathway (namely factor XIa, the factor IXa/VIIIa complex and the factor Xa/Va complex) occurring on the negatively charged phospholipid surfaces of activated platelets (see Fig. 26–4). Thus while the coagulation cascade has historically been divided into distinct parts: the intrinsic, extrinsic, and common pathways, this artificial division is somewhat misleading, as the intrinsic and extrinsic pathways cannot function as independent, redundant pathways in vivo, but are both required for physiologic hemostasis operating on different cell surfaces and playing unique roles.[18]

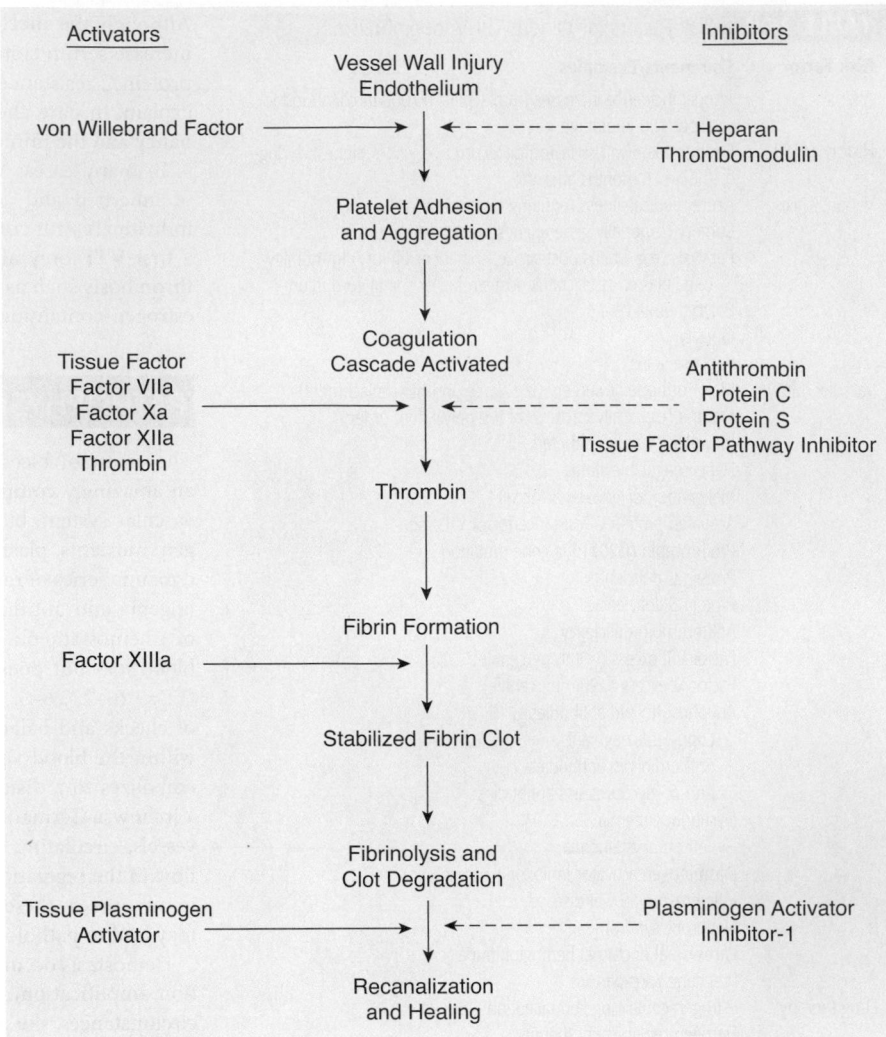

Activators

Inhibitors

Vessel Wall Injury
Endothelium

von Willebrand Factor → ← Heparan
Thrombomodulin

Platelet Adhesion
and Aggregation

Coagulation
Cascade Activated

Tissue Factor
Factor VIIa
Factor Xa
Factor XIIa
Thrombin

Antithrombin
Protein C
Protein S
Tissue Factor Pathway Inhibitor

Thrombin

Fibrin Formation

Factor XIIIa →

Stabilized Fibrin Clot

Fibrinolysis and
Clot Degradation

Tissue Plasminogen
Activator

Plasminogen Activator
Inhibitor-1

Recanalization
and Healing

FIGURE 26-2. Hemostasis and thrombosis.

The final step in hemostasis is the thrombin-mediated conversion of fibrinogen to form fibrin monomers. As fibrin monomers reach a critical concentration, they begin to precipitate and polymerize to form fibrin strands. Factor XIIIa covalently bonds these strands to one another. Local deposition of fibrin forms an extensive meshwork that surrounds and encases aggregated platelets to form a stabilized clot that seals the site of vascular injury and prevents blood loss.[20] Coagulation reactions are eventually terminated when this expanding meshwork of platelets and fibrin "paves over" the initiation site and activated factors are unable to diffuse through the overlying layer of clot.[18]

Normally, a number of tempering mechanisms control coagulation (see Table 26–2 and Fig. 26–2).[18] Without effective self-regulation, the coagulation cascade would proceed unabated causing vascular occlusion at the site of injury. The intact endothelium adjacent to the damaged tissue actively secretes several antithrombotic substances. As its name implies, thrombomodulin modulates thrombin activity by converting protein C to its active form (activated protein C [aPC]). When joined with its cofactor protein S, aPC enzymatically inactivates factors Va and VIIIa. The physiologic role of aPC is to prevent coagulation reactions from spreading to healthy, uninjured vessel walls. Antithrombin is a circulating protein that inhibits thrombin and factor Xa. Heparan sulfate, a heparin-like compound secreted by endothelial cells, exponentially accelerates antithrombin activity. By a similar mechanism, heparin cofactor II also inhibits thrombin. Tissue factor pathway inhibitor plays an important role by

regulating the initiation of the coagulation cascade. When these self-regulatory mechanisms are intact, the formation of the fibrin clot is limited to the zone of tissue injury. However, disruptions in the system, so-called hypercoagulable states, often result in pathologic thrombosis.

The fibrinolytic system is responsible for the dissolution of formed blood clots.[21] An inactive proenzyme, plasminogen, is converted to an active enzyme, plasmin, that degrades the fibrin mesh into soluble end products collectively known as fibrin split products or fibrin degradation products.[21] The fibrinolytic system is also under the control of a series of stimulatory and inhibitory substances. Tissue plasminogen activator and urokinase plasminogen activator convert plasminogen to plasmin. Plasminogen activator inhibitor-1 inhibits the plasminogen activators, and α_2-antiplasmin inhibits plasmin activity. Impaired activation of the fibrinolytic system has also been linked to hypercoagulability and thrombotic complications.[21]

CLINICAL PRESENTATION AND DIAGNOSIS

Although a thrombus can form in any part of the venous circulation, the majority begin in the lower extremities. Once formed, a venous thrombus may either (a) remain asymptomatic, (b) spontaneously lyse, (c) obstruct the venous circulation, (d) propagate into more proximal veins, (e) embolize, or (f) act in any combination of these ways.[22] Many patients with VTE never develop symptoms

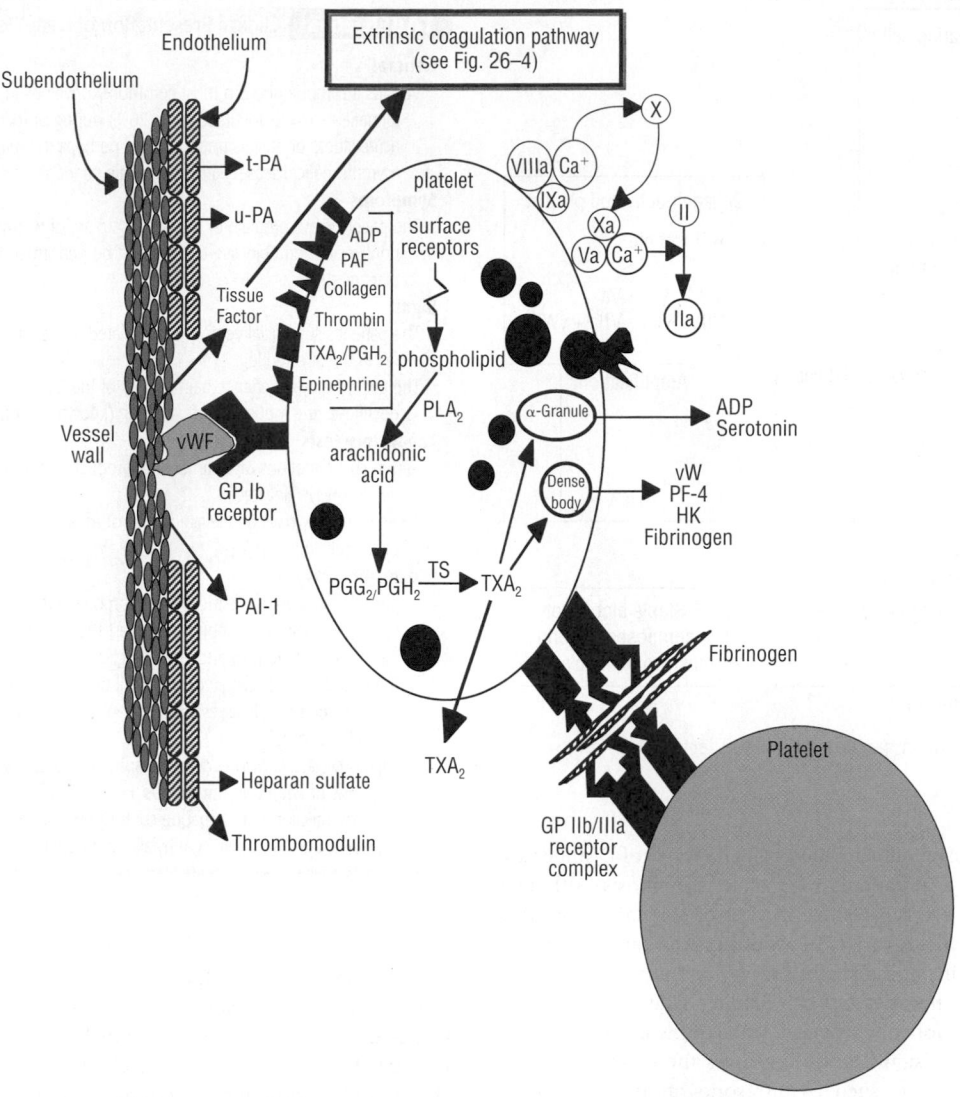

FIGURE 26-3. Vascular injury and thrombosis. (ADP, adenosine diphosphate; CO, cyclooxygenase; GP Ib, glycoprotein Ib; GP IIb/IIa, glycoprotein IIb/IIa; HK, high-molecular-weight kininogen; PAF, platelet-activating factor; PAI-1, plasminogen activator inhibitor; PF4, platelet factor 4; PGG/PGH, prostaglandins; PGI, prostacyclin; PLA, phospholipase A; TS, thromboxane synthetase; TXA$_2$, thromboxane A$_2$; t-PA, tissue plasmogen activator; u-PA, urokinase plasmogen activator; vWF, von Willebrand factor.)

from the acute event. However, even in the absence of symptoms, patients may develop long-term consequences, such as the post-thrombotic syndrome, CTPH, and recurrent VTE. The symptoms of DVT or PE (Tables 26-3, 26-4), are nonspecific and objective tests are required to confirm or exclude the diagnosis.[23] Patients with DVT frequently present with unilateral leg pain and swelling. The postthrombotic syndrome, a long-term complication of DVT caused by damage to the venous valves, also produces similar symptoms including chronic lower extremity swelling, pain, tenderness, skin discoloration, and ulceration. Symptomatic PE often produces dyspnea, tachypnea, and tachycardia.[24] Hemoptysis, while distressing, occurs in less than one third of patients. Cardiovascular collapse, characterized by cyanosis, shock, and oliguria, is an ominous sign.

❷ Given that VTE can be debilitating or fatal, it is important to treat it quickly and aggressively.[6] Conversely, because major bleeding induced by antithrombotic drugs can be equally harmful, it is important to avoid treatment when the diagnosis is not a reasonable certainty.[25] Assessment of the patient's status should focus on the search for risk factors in the patient's medical history (see Table 26-1). Venous thrombosis is uncommon in the absence of

risk factors, and the effects of these risks are additive. Even in the presence of mild, seemingly inconsequential symptoms, VTE should be strongly suspected in those with multiple risk factors.

Because radiographic contrast studies are the most accurate and reliable methods for the diagnosis of VTE, they are considered the gold standards in clinical trials.[26] Contrast venography allows visualization of the entire venous system in the lower extremity and abdomen. Pulmonary angiography allows the visualization of the pulmonary arteries. The diagnosis of VTE can be made if there is a persistent intraluminal filling defect observed on multiple radiographic films. Contrast studies are expensive, invasive procedures that are technically difficult to perform and evaluate. Severely ill patients often are unable to tolerate the procedure, and many develop hypotension and cardiac arrhythmias. Furthermore, the contrast medium is irritating to vessel walls and toxic to the kidneys. For these reasons, noninvasive tests, such as ultrasonography, computed tomography scans, and the ventilation–perfusion scan, are frequently used in clinical practice for the initial evaluation of patients with suspected VTE.

D-dimer is a simple blood test frequently used in the diagnostic evaluation of patients suspected to have VTE.[25] D-dimer is a

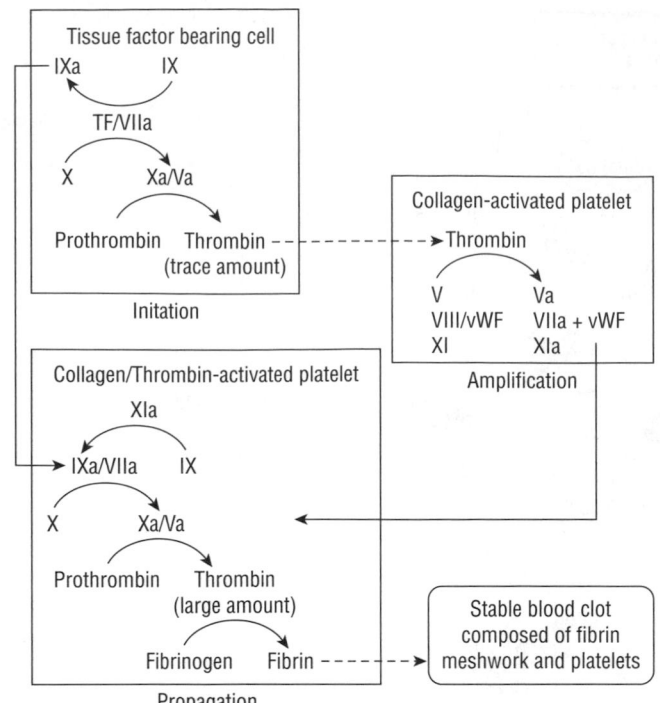

FIGURE 26-4. Coagulation cascade. (TF, tissue factor; vWF, von Willebrand factor.)

degradation product of a fibrin blood clot and levels of D-dimer are significantly elevated in patients with acute thrombosis. Although the D-dimer test is a very sensitive marker of clot formation, it is not sufficiently specific. A variety of conditions can cause elevations of serum D-dimer, including recent surgery or trauma, pregnancy, and cancer. While a negative test can help to "rule out" a DVT or PE, a positive test is not conclusive evidence of the diagnosis.

Clinical assessment significantly improves the diagnostic accuracy of noninvasive tests such as ultrasonography, ventilation–perfusion scanning, and D-dimer.[27] Simple assessment checklists can be used to determine if a patient has a high, moderate, or low probability of a DVT or PE (Table 26–5). Patients with a high pretest probability of VTE have a greater than 60% chance of having VTE, compared with only 5% for the low pretest probability group. Clinical assessment can rule in or out the diagnosis of VTE with reasonable certainty when the results are consistent with those of a noninvasive test.[25] For example, in patients with a high or moderate

TABLE 26-3 Clinical Presentation of Deep Vein Thrombosis

General

Venous thromboembolism most commonly develops in patients with identifiable risk factors (see Table 26-1) during or following a period of acute illness or hospitalization. Many, perhaps the majority, of patients have asymptomatic disease. Patients may die suddenly of pulmonary embolism.

Symptoms

The patient may complain of leg swelling, pain, or warmth. Symptoms are nonspecific and objective testing must be performed to establish the diagnosis.

Signs

The patient's superficial veins may be dilated and a "palpable cord" may be felt in the affected leg.

The patient may experience pain in back of the knee when the examiner dorsiflexes the foot of the affected leg (known as Homans sign).

Laboratory tests

Serum concentrations of D-dimer, a byproduct of thrombin generation, is nearly always elevated.

The patient may have an elevated erythrocyte sedimentation rate and white blood cell count.

Diagnostic tests

Duplex ultrasonography is the most commonly used test to diagnosis deep vein thrombosis. It is a noninvasive test that can measure the rate and direction of blood flow and visualize clot formation in proximal veins of the legs. It cannot reliably detect small blood clots in distal veins. Coupled with a careful clinical assessment, it can rule in or out the diagnosis in the majority of cases.

Venography (also known as phlebography) is the gold standard for the diagnosis of deep vein thrombosis. However, it is an invasive test that involves injection of radiopaque contrast dye into a foot vein. It is expensive and can cause anaphylaxis and nephrotoxicity.

pretest probability of VTE and an abnormal lower-extremity ultrasonogram, the diagnosis of VTE can be reasonably concluded. In patients with a low pretest probability of VTE and a negative D-dimer test (≤500 ng/mL), the diagnosis of VTE can be reasonably excluded without radiographic testing. However, if the results of the clinical assessment and the ultrasonogram are discordant, additional tests should be performed to confirm the diagnosis.

PHARMACOLOGIC AGENTS USED IN THE MANAGEMENT OF VENOUS THROMBOEMBOLISM

The following agents are most commonly used in the prevention and treatment of VTE. A brief overview of selected investigational agents is also provided.

UNFRACTIONATED HEPARIN

Unfractionated heparin (UFH) has been used for the prevention and treatment of thrombosis for decades.[5] Commercially available UFH preparations are derived from bovine lung or porcine intestinal mucosa. Although some differences exist between the two sources, no differences in antithrombotic activity have been demonstrated. Today, UFH and the low-molecular-weight heparins (LMWHs) are the most commonly used therapies for the acute treatment of venous thrombosis.[6]

Pharmacology

Unfractionated heparin is a heterogeneous mixture of sulfated mucopolysaccharides of variable lengths and pharmacologic properties (Table 26–6).[5] Each heparin molecule is composed of

TABLE 26-2 Factors Regulating Hemostasis and Thrombosis

	Thrombogenic	Antithrombotic
Vessel wall	Exposed subendothelium	Preserved endothelial integrity
	Tissue factor	Heparan sulfate
	Plasminogen activator inhibitor-1	Dermatan sulfate
		Thrombomodulin
		Tissue plasminogen activator
		Urokinase plasminogen activator
Circulating elements	Platelets	Antithrombin
	Platelet activating factor	Heparin cofactor II
	The clotting factors	Protein C
	Prothrombin (factor II)	Protein S
	Fibrinogen (factor I)	Plasminogen
	von Willebrand factor	Tissue factor pathway inhibitor
	β_2-Antiplasmin	Proteolytic enzymes
Blood flow	Slow rate of flow	Fast rate of flow
	Turbulent flow	Laminar flow

TABLE 26-4	Clinical Presentation of Pulmonary Embolism

General

Pulmonary embolism (PE) most commonly develops in patients with risk factors for venous thromboembolism (see Table 26–1) during or following a hospitalization. Although many patients develop a symptomatic deep vein thrombosis prior to developing a PE, many do not. Patients may die suddenly before effective treatment can be initiated.

Symptoms

The patient may complain of cough, chest pain, chest tightness, shortness of breath, or palpitation. The patient may spit or cough up blood (hemoptysis). When PE is massive, the patient may complain of dizziness or lightheadedness. Symptoms may be confused for a myocardial infarction, requiring objective testing to establish the diagnosis.

Signs

The patient may have tachypnea (increased respiratory rate) and tachycardia (increased heart rate). The patient may appear diaphoretic (sweaty). The patient's neck veins may be distended. In massive PE, the patient may appear cyanotic and become hypotensive. In such cases, oxygen saturation by pulse oximetry or arterial blood gas will likely indicate that the patient is hypoxic. In the worse cases, the patient may go into circulatory shock and die within minutes.

Laboratory tests

Serum concentrations of D-dimer, a byproduct of thrombin generation, are nearly always elevated.

The patient may have an elevated erythrocyte sedimentation rate and white blood cell count.

Diagnostic tests

Computerized tomography (CT) scan is the most commonly used test to diagnose PE but some centers still use the ventilation-perfusion (V/Q) scan. Spiral CT scans can detect emboli in the pulmonary arteries. A V/Q scan measures the distribution of blood and air flow in the lungs. When there is a large mismatch between blood and air flow in one area of the lung, there is a high probability that the patient has a PE.

Pulmonary angiography is the gold standard for the diagnosis of PE. However, it is an invasive test that involves injection of radiopaque contrast dye into the pulmonary artery. The test is expensive and associated with a significant risk of mortality.

TABLE 26-5	Clinical Assessment Models for Deep Vein Thrombosis and Pulmonary Embolism

Pretest Probability of Deep Vein Thrombosis

Clinical feature	Score
Tenderness along entire deep vein system	1.0
Swelling of the entire leg	1.0
Greater than 3 cm difference in calf circumference	1.0
Pitting edema	1.0
Collateral superficial veins	1.0
Risk factors present:	
Active cancer	1.0
Prolonged immobility or paralysis	1.0
Recent surgery or major medical illness	1.0
Alternative diagnosis likely (ruptured Baker cyst, rheumatoid arthritis, superficial thrombophlebitis, or infective cellulitis)	−2.0

Score ≥3 = high probability; 1–2 = moderate probability; ≤0 = low probability

Pretest Probability of Pulmonary Embolism

Clinical feature	Score
Deep vein thrombosis suspected	
Clinical features of deep vein thrombosis	3.0
Recent prolonged immobility or surgery	1.5
Active cancer	1.0
History of deep vein thrombosis or pulmonary embolism	1.5
Hemoptysis	1.0
Resting heart rate >100 beats/min	1.5
No alternative explanation for acute shortness of breath or chest pain	3.0

Score ≥6 = high probability; 2–6 = moderate probability; ≤1.5 = low probability

Adapted from Hunt.[27]

repetitive units of D-glycosamine and uronic acid. The molecular weight of UFH molecules ranges from 3,000 to 30,000 daltons, with a mean of 15,000 daltons. The anticoagulant profile and clearance of each UFH molecule varies based on its length. The smaller chains are cleared less rapidly than their longer counterparts.[5]

The anticoagulant effect of UFH is mediated through a specific pentasaccharide sequence on the heparin molecule that binds to antithrombin, provoking a conformational change (Fig. 26–5). Only one third of the UFH molecules possess the unique pentasaccharide sequence with affinity for antithrombin. The UFH–antithrombin complex is 100 to 1,000 times more potent as an anticoagulant compared to antithrombin alone. Antithrombin inhibits the activity of several clotting factors including IXa, Xa, XIIa, and thrombin. Through its action on thrombin, the UFH–antithrombin complex also inhibits the thrombin-induced activation of factors V and VIII.[5] UFH prevents the growth and propagation of a formed thrombus and allows the patient's own thrombolytic system to degrade the clot.

Factors IIa (thrombin) and Xa are the most sensitive to inhibition by the UFH–antithrombin complex. To inactivate thrombin, the heparin molecule must form a ternary complex bridging between antithrombin and thrombin (see Fig. 26–5). Only molecules that contain more than 18 saccharides are able to bind to both antithrombin and thrombin simultaneously. Smaller heparin molecules cannot facilitate the interaction between antithrombin and thrombin. In contrast, the inactivation of factor Xa does not require UFH to form a bridge with antithrombin. It only requires that UFH bind to antithrombin using the specific pentasaccharide sequence. Heparin molecules with as few as 5 saccharide units are able to catalyze the inhibition of factor Xa. Heparin uncouples from antithrombin after it has produced its effect and quickly recouples with another antithrombin molecule. Because of its relatively large size, the UFH–antithrombin complex is incapable of inactivating thrombin or factor Xa within a formed clot or bound to surfaces. At high doses, UFH also binds to heparin cofactor II, further inhibiting the activity of thrombin. UFH increases the release of tissue factor pathway inhibitor from vascular endothelium, augmenting its inhibitory effect on factor Xa. UFH, especially high-molecular-weight heparin fractions, also binds to platelets and inhibits platelet aggregation.[5]

Pharmacokinetics

Unfractionated heparin is not reliably absorbed when taken orally as a result of its large molecular size and anionic structure. The bioavailability and biologic activity of UFH is limited by its propensity to bind to plasma proteins, platelet factor 4 (PF4), macrophages, fibrinogen, lipoproteins, and endothelial cells.[5] This may explain the substantial inter- and intra-patient variability observed in the anticoagulation response to UFH.[5]

The subcutaneous bioavailability of UFH is dose dependent and ranges from 30% at low doses to as much as 70% at high doses. Higher doses presumably saturate protein-binding sites, thereby permitting a larger proportion to reach the systemic circulation. The onset of anticoagulant effect is usually evident 1 to 2 hours after subcutaneous injection and peaks at 3 hours.[28] When UFH is administered via the IV route, a continuous infusion is preferable. Intermittent IV boluses produce relatively high peaks in anticoagulation activity and have been associated with a greater risk of major bleeding.[6] Intramuscular administration is discouraged because of erratic absorption and risk of large hematoma formation.

Unfractionated heparin has a dose-dependent half-life of approximately 30 to 90 minutes, but may be prolonged to as much as 150 minutes when given in high doses to some patients.[5] There are two primary mechanisms for the elimination of UFH. The relative contribution of each mechanism to the total clearance of heparin is related

TABLE 26-6 Comparison of the Chemical and Pharmacokinetic Properties of Antithrombotic Drugs Used for Venous Thrombosis

Agent	FDA Approved	Method of Preparation	Mean Molecular Weight (Daltons)	Plasma Half-Life	Anti-Xa: Anti-IIa Activity	Bioavailability
Unfractionated heparin	Yes	Extracted from porcine gut mucosa or beef lung	≈15,000	30–90 min (dose dependent)	1:1	SC: 30–70% (dose dependent)
Low-molecular-weight heparins						
Dalteparin (Fragmin)	Yes	Nitrous acid depolymerization	≈6,000	119–139 min	2.7:1	SC: 87%
Enoxaparin (Lovenox)	Yes	Benzoylation and alkaline depolymerization	≈4,200	129–180 min	3.8:1	SC: 92%
Tinzaparin (Innohep)	Yes	Heparinase digestion	≈4,500	111–234 min	2.8:1	SC: 90%
Heparinoid						
Danaparoid (Orgaran)	Yes (no longer marketed in U.S.)	Extracted from porcine gut mucosa	≈6,500	22–24 h	20:1	SC: 95%
Anti-factor Xa inhibitors						
Fondaparinux (Arixtra)	Yes	Synthetic	1,728	15–18 h	100% anti-Xa	SC: 100%
Idraparinux and biotinylated idraparinux	No	Synthetic	≈1,700	≈80 h	100% anti-Xa	SC: 100%
Rivaroxaban (Xarelto)	No (Available in EU and Canada)	Synthetic	NA	7–11 h	100% anti-Xa	PO: 80%-100%
Abipxaban	No	Synthetic	460	9-14 h	100% anti-Xa	PO: 50%
Direct thrombin inhibitors						
Argatroban (Argatroban)	Yes	Synthetic	509	30–50 min	100% anti-IIa	
Bivalirudin (Angiomax)	Yes	Semisynthetic	2,180	25 min	100% anti-IIa	
Desirudin (Iprivask)	Yes	Recombinant DNA technology	6,964	120 min	100% anti-IIa	SC: >90%
Lepirudin (Refludan)	Yes	Recombinant DNA technology	6,980	80 min	100% anti-IIa	SC: 70%
Dabigatran	Yes (for stroke prevention in atrial fibrillation)	Synthetic	471	14 h	100% anti-IIa	Oral: 7%
Vitamin K antagonists						
Warfarin (Coumadin)	Yes	Synthetic	330	40 h	1:1	Oral: 90–100%

SC, subcutaneous; NA, not available.
Data from Nutescu et al.,[53] Abrams et al.,[97] and Karthikeyan et al.[40]

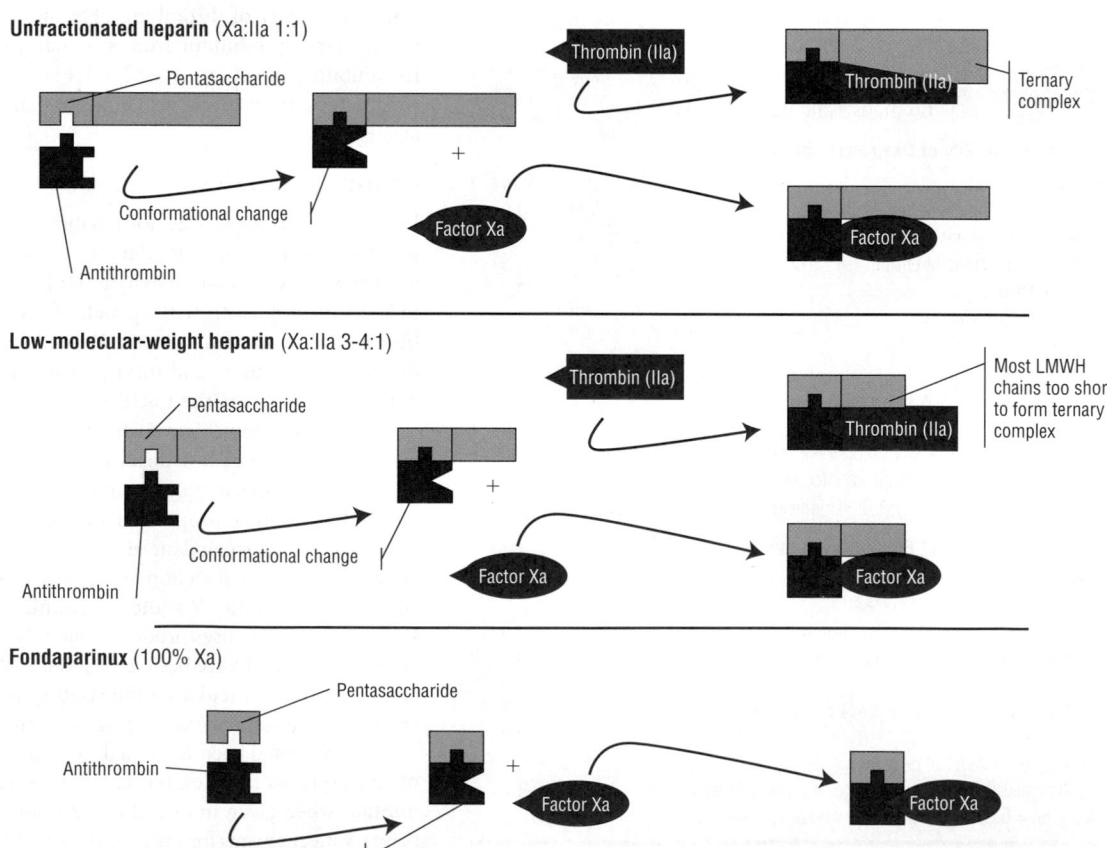

Unfractionated heparin (Xa:IIa 1:1)

Pentasaccharide
Conformational change
Antithrombin
Thrombin (IIa)
Thrombin (IIa) — Ternary complex
Factor Xa
Factor Xa

Low-molecular-weight heparin (Xa:IIa 3-4:1)

Pentasaccharide
Conformational change
Antithrombin
Thrombin (IIa)
Thrombin (IIa) — Most LMWH chains too short to form ternary complex
Factor Xa
Factor Xa

Fondaparinux (100% Xa)

Pentasaccharide
Antithrombin
Factor Xa
Factor Xa
Conformational change

FIGURE 26-5. Pharmacologic activity of unfractionated heparin, low-molecular-weight heparins (LMWHs), and fondaparinux.

to the dose and size of the UFH molecules. One mechanism is a rapid, but saturable zero-order process. Heparinases and desulfatases enzymatically inactivate heparin molecules bound to endothelial cells and macrophages, reducing them to smaller and less sulfated molecules.[5] Heparin is also eliminated renally. This first-order process is slower and nonsaturable. Low doses of UFH are cleared principally by the saturable, rapid, zero-order mechanism, whereas the renal route predominates at very high doses. With typical therapeutic regimens, a combination of the two mechanisms are used to eliminate UFH with the saturable mechanism predominating. Renal and hepatic dysfunction reduces the rate of clearance of UFH. Patients with active thrombosis may eliminate UFH more rapidly, possibly because of increased binding to acute phase reactants.[28]

Dose and Administration

The dose and route of administration for UFH are based on the indication, the therapeutic goals, and the patient's individual response to therapy. The dose of UFH is expressed in units of activity. The number of units per milligram is variable and depends on the manufacturing process. For the prevention of VTE, UFH is given by subcutaneous injection in the abdominal fat layer over the iliac crest. The typical dose for prophylaxis is 5,000 units every 8 to 12 hours. When immediate and full anticoagulation is required, a weight-based IV bolus dose followed by a continuous infusion is preferred (Table 26–7).[5] Subcutaneous UFH (initial dose of 333 units/kg followed by 250 units/kg every 12 hours) also provides adequate therapeutic anticoagulation for the treatment of acute VTE.[29]

Therapeutic Monitoring

❸ Administration of UFH has traditionally required close monitoring because of the unpredictable anticoagulant patient response.[5] Several tests are available to monitor UFH therapy including whole blood clotting time, activated partial thromboplastin time (aPTT), activated clotting time (ACT), antifactor Xa activity, and plasma heparin concentrations. The aPTT is the most widely used test to determine the degree of therapeutic anticoagulation. The therapeutic range of aPTT has traditionally been considered to be 1.5 to 2.5 times the mean normal control value.[5] Many currently available aPTT reagents do not accurately measure the response to heparin

within this fixed therapeutic range; thus, the use of a fixed aPTT therapeutic range of 1.5 to 2.5 times the control represents a subtherapeutic dose of UFH in many instances.[5] Because of substantial interlaboratory variability in the aPTT, an institution-specific aPTT therapeutic range that correlates with a plasma heparin concentration of 0.3 to 0.7 units/mL by an amidolytic antifactor Xa assay should be established.[5]

Although most experts advocate using the aPTT to monitor UFH provided that institution-specific therapeutic ranges are defined, the use of aPTT has several limitations. First, preanalytical variables such as reagent sensitivity, temperature, phlebotomy methods, and hemodilution may result in aPTT results that do not correlate with the in vivo level of heparin anticoagulation present.[28] Second, the aPTT response exhibits diurnal variation, with a peak response occurring around 3 AM during continuous IV infusion. Adjusting infusion rates in response to this diurnal variation could lead to subsequent over- or underdosing.[30] Third, the aPTT is prolonged beyond measurable limits when the heparin concentration exceeds 1 unit/mL; consequently, the aPTT is unsuitable for monitoring heparin therapy in patients who require doses of heparin that will produce serum concentrations >1 unit/mL. The ACT is the most suitable assay when high doses of heparin are used, especially during coronary angioplasty or coronary bypass surgery.[5] Fourth, the lower-weight heparin fragments accumulate but have little effect on the aPTT in vivo.[28] Lastly, the data supporting the currently recommended heparin concentration therapeutic range is not derived from scientifically rigorous research.[5]

The aPTT should be measured prior to the initiation of therapy to determine the patient's baseline. When administered by IV infusion, the response to therapy should be measured 6 hours after the initiation of therapy or a dose change. This is usually sufficient time for heparin to reach steady state. The dose of heparin should be promptly adjusted based on the patient's response and the institution-specific therapeutic range (see Table 26–7).[28]

Some patients with acute VTE and myocardial infarction have a diminished response to UFH (so-called heparin resistance), presumably because of variations in the plasma concentrations of heparin-binding proteins. Some patients are reported to have acute elevations in factor VIII, preventing the prolongation of the aPTT by UFH. In some cases, antithrombin deficiency might be the culprit. The possibility of this phenomenon should be suspected in patients who require more than 35,000 units of UFH per 24-hour period. The recommended management of patients with "heparin resistance" is to adjust the UFH dose based on antifactor Xa concentrations.[5]

Adverse Effects

❹ Bleeding is the primary adverse effect associated with all anticoagulant drugs (Table 26–8).[3] There is not solid evidence linking supratherapeutic aPTT values and the risk for bleeding in patients receiving UFH. The risk for bleeding is more closely related to underlying risk factors than to high aPTT values.[30] Therefore, UFH should not be administered to patients with contraindications to anticoagulation therapy (Table 26–9). Low-dose subcutaneous UFH is associated with a minimal risk of major bleeding. The rates of major bleeding for patients receiving full therapeutic doses of UFH range from 0% to 2%.[3] The presence of concomitant bleeding risks such as thrombocytopenia, the use other antithrombotic therapy, and a preexisting source of bleeding increase the risk of UFH-induced hemorrhage. The risk of bleeding also increases with age. Recent surgery, hemostatic defects, heavy alcohol consumption, renal failure, peptic ulcers, and neoplasms also increase the risk of major bleeding while receiving UFH.[3]

TABLE 26–7	Weight-Based[a] Dosing for Unfractionated Heparin Administered by Continuous Intravenous Infusion	
Indication	**Initial Loading Dose**	**Initial Infusion Rate**
Deep venous thrombosis/pulmonary embolism	80–100 units/kg Maximum = 10,000 units	17–20 units/kg/h Maximum = 2,300 units/h
Activated Partial Thromboplastin Time (seconds)	**Maintenance Infusion Rate** *Dose adjustment*	
<37 (or >12 s below institution-specific therapeutic range)	80 units/kg bolus then increase infusion by 4 units/kg/h	
37–47 (or 1–12 s below institution-specific therapeutic range)	40 units/kg bolus then increase infusion by 2 units/kg/h	
48–71 (or within institution-specific therapeutic range)	No change	
72–93 (or 1–22 s above institution-specific therapeutic range)	Decrease infusion by 2 units/kg/h	
>93 (or <22 s above institution-specific therapeutic range)	Hold infusion for 1 h then decrease by 3 units/kg/h	

[a]Use actual body weight for all calculations. Adjusted body weight may be used for obese patients (>130% of ideal body weight).
From Hirsh et al.[5]

TABLE 26-8	Risk Factors for Major Bleeding While Taking Anticoagulation Therapy

Anticoagulation intensity (e.g., international normalized ratio >4.0)
Initiation of therapy (first few days and weeks)
Unstable anticoagulation response
Age >65 years
Concurrent antiplatelet drug use
Concurrent nonsteroidal antiinflammatory drug use
History of gastrointestinal bleeding
Recent surgery or trauma
High risk for fall/trauma
Heavy alcohol use
Renal failure
Cerebrovascular disease
Malignancy

From Schulman et al.[3]

Anatomic sites commonly associated with UFH-related bleeding include the gastrointestinal and urinary tracts, as well as soft tissues. Minor bleeding, such as epistaxis, gingival bleeding, and prolonged bleeding from cuts, is frequently reported. Bruising from minor trauma and at the sites of subcutaneous injections and venous access is also common. Local irritation, mild pain, erythema, histamine-like reactions, and hematoma can occur during UFH administration. Even small amounts of bleeding into critical sites

TABLE 26-9	Contraindications to Anticoagulation Therapy

General
Active major bleeding
Hemophilia or other hemorrhagic tendencies
Severe liver disease with elevated baseline PT
Severe thrombocytopenia (platelet count <20,000 mm^3)
Malignant hypertension
Inability to meticulously supervise and monitor treatment
Product-specific contraindications
  Argatroban
    Hypersensitivity to argatroban
  Bivalirudin
    Hypersensitivity to bivalirubin
  Fondaparinux
    Hypersensitivity to fondaparinux
    Severe renal insufficiency (creatinine clearance <30 mL/min)
    Body weight <50 kg (prophylaxis only)
    Bacterial endocarditis
    Thrombocytopenia with a positive in vitro test for anti-platelet antibodies in the presence of fondaparinux
  Lepirudin
    Hypersensitivity to hirudins
  LMWHs
    Hypersensitivity to LMWH, UFH, pork products, methylparaben, or propylparaben
    Thrombocytopenia associated with a positive in vitro test for anti-platelet antibody in the presence of LMWH
  UFH
    Hypersensitivity to UFH
    Thrombocytopenia associated with a positive in vitro test for anti-platelet antibody in the presence of UFH
  Warfarin
    Hypersensitivity to warfarin
    Pregnancy
    History of warfarin-induced skin necrosis
    Inability to obtain regular PT/INR measurements
    Inappropriate medication use or lifestyle behaviors

HIT, heparin-induced thrombocytopenia; INR, international normalized ratio; LMWH, low-molecularweight heparin; PT, prothrombin time; UFH, unfractionated heparin.

such as the central nervous system (CNS) or the structures of the eye can cause catastrophic consequences.

Heparin-induced thrombocytopenia (HIT) is a serious drug-induced problem requiring immediate intervention (see Heparin-Induced Thrombocytopenia below).[31] A baseline platelet count should be obtained before UFH therapy is initiated. If the patient has received UFH within the previous 100 days, or if previous UFH exposure is uncertain, a repeat platelet count should be performed within 24 hours.[31] Monitoring platelet counts every other day for 14 days or until UFH therapy is stopped, whichever occurs first, is recommended for patients who are receiving therapeutic doses of UFH.[31]

Long-term UFH has been reported to cause alopecia, priapism, and suppressed aldosterone synthesis with subsequent hyperkalemia. The use of UFH in doses ≥20,000 units/day for more than 6 months, especially during pregnancy, is associated with significant bone loss and may lead to osteoporosis.[30] Few drug interactions are reported with UFH. Concurrent use with other antithrombotic drugs, thrombolytics, and antiplatelet agents increases the risk of bleeding, however.

Management of Bleeding and Excessive Anticoagulation

Hemorrhage can occur at any site in patients receiving UFH and close monitoring for signs and symptoms of bleeding is crucial.[3,5] In addition to an appropriate coagulation study to measure the response to UFH, it is necessary to regularly monitor hemoglobin, hematocrit, and blood pressure. Bleeding can produce a wide variety of symptoms, depending on the site of hemorrhage. Symptoms can include severe headache, joint pain, chest pain, abdominal pain, swelling, tarry stools, frank hematuria, or the passage of bright red blood through the rectum. Life-threatening bleeding, either as a consequence of a significant volume loss or because of the location (e.g., bleeding into a critical space), must be recognized swiftly and immediately treated. Critical areas include intracranial, pericardial, and intraocular sites, as well as the adrenal glands.

When major bleeding occurs, UFH should be immediately discontinued and the underlying source of bleeding should be identified and treated. Intravenous protamine sulfate, given in a dose of 1 mg per 100 units of UFH up to a maximum of 50 mg, can be administered to reverse the anticoagulant effects of UFH.[5] Protamine sulfate has intrinsic anticoagulation activity, but when administered with UFH, it forms a stable salt that results in the loss of anticoagulation activity of both drugs. Protamine sulfate neutralizes UFH in 5 minutes, and its activity persists for 2 hours. It should be given by slow IV infusion.[5] In cases of large heparin overdoses or in patients with renal failure, a "rebound" effect may occur with a return of some anticoagulant activity several hours after the administration of protamine sulfate. Therefore, the patient's aPTT should be closely monitored. Multiple doses or prolonged infusion of protamine sulfate may be necessary if hemorrhage continues.[5]

Use in Special Populations

Heparin-related compounds such as UFH or LMWH are the anticoagulants of choice during pregnancy.[16] Because UFH does not cross the placenta, it is not associated with teratogenicity or fetal bleeding complications.[16] UFH should be used cautiously during the last trimester of pregnancy and the peripartum period because of the risk of maternal hemorrhage. Induction of labor is advisable so that UFH can be discontinued prior to delivery to minimize the risk for excessive bleeding during delivery. Long-term use of UFH during pregnancy may result in bone loss and increased risk for

TABLE 26-10 FDA-Approved Indications and Doses for Low-Molecular-Weight Heparins

Indications	Enoxaparin	Dalteparin	Tinzaparin
Hip-replacement surgery (prophylaxis)	30 mg SC q 12 h initiated 12–24 h after surgery *or* 40 mg SC q 24 h initiated 12 h prior to surgery Extended prophylaxis may be given for up to 3 wk	Postoperative start: 2,500 units SC given 4-8 h after surgery then 5,000 international units SC q 24 h *or* Preoperative start (evening before surgery): 5,000 units SC 10–14 h before surgery then 5,000 units given 4–8 h after surgery then 5,000 units SC q 24 h *or* Preoperative start (day of surgery): 2,500 units SC within 2 h of surgery, then 2,500 units given 4–8 h after surgery then 5,000 units SC q 24 h	
Knee-replacement surgery (prophylaxis)	30 mg SC q 12 h initiated 12–24 h after surgery		
Abdominal surgery (prophylaxis)	40 mg SC q 24 h initiated 2 h prior to surgery	2,500 units SC q 24 h initiated 1–2 h prior to surgery Patients with malignancy: 5,000 units SC the evening prior surgery then 5,000 units SC q 24 h *or* 2,500 units SC 1–2 h prior to surgery then 2,500 units 12 h after surgery followed by 5,000 units SC q 24 h	
Acute medical illness (prophylaxis)	40 mg SC q 24 h	5,000 units SC q 24 h	
Deep vein thrombosis treatment (with or without pulmonary embolism)	1 mg/kg SC q 12 h *or* 1.5 mg/kg SC q 24 h		175 units/kg SC q 24 h
Venous thromboembolism treatment in patients with cancer		200 units/kg SC q 24 h for 30 days, followed by 150 units SC q 24 h (total daily dose should not exceed 18,000 units)	

osteoporosis-related fractures.[16] However, UFH has been successfully in pregnant patients without evidence of osteoporosis.[32] Unfractionated heparin is not excreted in breast milk and is considered safe to use by women who are breastfeeding.[16]

Advances in tertiary care for pediatric patients have resulted in increasing numbers of children requiring antithrombotic therapy, and UFH is commonly used in this setting (see General Approach to the Treatment of Venous Thromboembolism below).[33]

LOW-MOLECULAR-WEIGHT HEPARIN

Produced by either chemical or enzymatic depolymerization (see Table 26–6), LMWHs are fragments of UFH.[5] They are heterogeneous mixtures of sulfated glycosaminoglycans with approximately one-third the molecular weight of UFH. Although all the LMWHs share similarities in their mechanisms of action with UFH, their molecular weight distributions vary, resulting in differences in their activity against factor Xa and thrombin, affinity for plasma proteins, propensity to release tissue factor pathway inhibitor, and duration of activity.[28] The mean molecular weight of the LMWHs is product specific. These agents have several advantages over UFH, including (a) predictable anticoagulation dose response, (b) improved subcutaneous bioavailability, (c) dose-independent clearance, (d) longer biologic half-life, (e) lower incidence of thrombocytopenia, and (f) a reduced need for routine laboratory monitoring.[5]

Currently, there are three LMWH products available in the United States. The usefulness of LMWHs has been extensively evaluated for a wide array of indications, including the treatment of acute coronary syndromes, DVT, and PE, as well as for the prevention of VTE in several high-risk populations. The FDA-approved indications and doses for the LMWHs are product specific (Table 26–10). The LMWHs have largely replaced UFH for the prevention and treatment of VTE in some hospitals. However, institutional resources and individual patient needs should determine their precise role in the management of VTE.

Pharmacology

The LMWHs prevent the growth and propagation of formed thrombi. Like UFH, the LMWHs enhance and accelerate the activity of antithrombin through binding to a specific pentasaccharide sequence. Fewer than one third of LMWH molecules contain the specific sequence necessary to interact with antithrombin.[5] The principal difference in the pharmacologic activity of the LMWHs and UFH is their relative inhibition of factor Xa and thrombin. Because of their smaller chain length, the LMWHs have limited activity against thrombin (see Fig. 26–5). Fewer than 50% of the LMWH molecules have the requisite chain length to simultaneously bind antithrombin and thrombin. For this reason, the LMWHs have proportionally greater antifactor Xa activity. The ratio of antifactor Xa-to-IIa activity varies between 4:1 and 2:1.[5] By comparison, UFH has an antifactor Xa-to-IIa activity ratio of 1:1. Like UFH, the LMWHs cause the endothelium to release tissue factor pathway inhibitor, which is believed to enhance the inhibition of factor Xa and to inactivate factor VIIa.[28]

Pharmacokinetics

Compared with UFH, the LMWHs have a more predictable anticoagulation response. The improved pharmacokinetic profile of LMWHs is the result of reduced binding to proteins and cells.[5] The bioavailability of LMWHs is about 90% when administered subcutaneously, whereas the absorption of UFH is relatively poor and erratic. The subcutaneous bioavailability of the available LMWH products differs only slightly. The peak anticoagulation effect is seen in 3 to 5 hours.[5]

The renal route is the predominant mode of elimination for the LMWHs. Consequently, their biologic half-life may be prolonged in patients with renal impairment. Longer heparin chains bind to macrophages and are rapidly degraded. Therefore, antifactor Xa activity, which is mediated by smaller heparin molecules, persists longer than antithrombin activity. The plasma half-life of the LMWH preparations is two to four times longer than UFH. The clearance of LMWHs is independent of dose.[5]

Dosing and Administration

The LMWHs are given in fixed or weight-based doses based on the product and indication (see Table 26–10). Doses should be based on actual body weight and studies in obese patients indicate that full weight-based doses do not lead to elevated LMWH concentrations when compared with normal subjects; consequently, capping of the dose is not recommended.[30] The dose for enoxaparin is expressed in milligrams, whereas dalteparin and tinzaparin are expressed in units of antifactor Xa activity. Although they can be given by continuous intravenous infusion, the LMWHs are generally given by subcutaneous injection in the abdominal area or the upper outer part of the thigh while the patient is in a supine position. The clinician or patient pinches a layer of skin between the thumb and forefinger, and then introduces the entire length of the needle into a skin fold at a 90° angle. Injection sites should be alternated between right and left sides. Following subcutaneous administration, the drug is absorbed slowly, resulting in sustained antithrombotic activity over several hours.

The dosing interval for the LMWHs is every 12 or 24 hours depending on the indication and product. Larger doses are given once daily and produce significantly higher peak plasma concentrations. Given that the elimination half-life of the LMWHs is prolonged in patients with severe renal impairment, high doses may lead to a significant accumulation in these patients.[5] The enoxaparin dose should be reduced and the dosing interval extended to once daily in patients with creatinine clearance <30 mL/min.[34] The pharmacokinetics of dalteparin and tinzaparin are less-well characterized in patients with renal insufficiency, but some studies suggest that there is a lower degree of accumulation with tinzaparin.[5] Data on the use of LMWH in patients with end-stage renal disease receiving hemodialysis is very limited, thus UFH is preferred for these patients.[5] Given that few published data are available regarding the use of LMWHs in the setting of renal insufficiency, some experts recommend measuring antifactor Xa activity if therapy is continued for more than a few days.[5]

For the prevention of VTE, the LMWHs have been studied in a variety of high-risk circumstances, including orthopedic surgery, abdominal surgery, acute spinal cord injury, neurosurgery, multiple trauma, and critical illness.[2] The effectiveness of the LMWHs has been extensively evaluated for the treatment of VTE in hospitalized patients and used in the outpatient management of DVT.[6] They are also a reasonable alternative to warfarin therapy in circumstances when a prothrombin time (PT)/international normalized ratio (INR) can not be routinely obtained.

Therapeutic Monitoring

Because the LMWHs achieve predictable anticoagulant response when given subcutaneously, routine laboratory monitoring is unnecessary to guide the dosing of these agents.[5] The PT, the ACT, and the aPTT are minimally affected by LMWHs.[28] Prior to initiation of LMWH, a baseline complete blood cell count with platelet count, and serum creatinine should be obtained. The complete blood cell count should be checked every 5 to 10 days during the first 2 weeks of LMWH therapy and every 2 to 4 weeks thereafter to monitor for occult bleeding.

Although several methods to monitor LMWHs have been explored, measurement of antifactor Xa activity has been the most widely used method in clinical practice. Routine antifactor Xa activity measurement is unnecessary in patients whose condition is stable and uncomplicated.[5] Although very limited data support the use of laboratory monitoring to guide LMWH therapy, measuring antifactor Xa activity may be helpful in patients who have significant renal impairment (e.g., creatinine clearance <30 mL/min), weigh less than 50 kg, are morbidly obese, or require prolonged therapy (e.g., longer than 14 days). Periodic antifactor Xa activity monitoring may also be useful in women treated with a LMWH during pregnancy because of changing pharmacokinetic variables (e.g., volume of distribution and renal function).[5] Patients who are at very high risk of bleeding or thrombotic recurrence may also benefit from antifactor Xa monitoring to avoid periods of over-or underanticoagulation. Because newborns and pediatric patients have unpredictable pharmacokinetic profiles, they may require monitoring to ensure adequate therapy.[33]

When anti-factor Xa activity is used to monitor LMWH therapy, the sample should be drawn after steady state has been achieved (after the second or third dose) and approximately 4 hours after the subcutaneous injection, during the peak period of antifactor Xa activity.[28] A calibrated LMWH heparin should be used to establish the standard curve for the assay. The therapeutic range for antifactor Xa activity is not well defined and not been clearly correlated with efficacy or the risk of bleeding.[5] For the treatment of VTE, an acceptable target range for the peak level is 0.6 to 1.0 units/mL with twice daily enoxaparin or nadroparin dosing. For once daily dosing likely peak targets are >1 units/mL for enoxaparin, 0.85 units/mL for tinzaparin, 1.3 units/mL for nadroparin, and 1.05 units/mL for dalteparin.[5] For the prevention of VTE an acceptable target range for the peak level is 0.2 to 0.4 units/mL.

Adverse Effects

As with UFH, bleeding is the most common adverse effect of the LMWHs.[3] Although not consistently demonstrated in clinical trials, the frequency of major bleeding is purported to be less with the LMWHs than with UFH.[3] This difference may be partly a result of their reduced effects on platelet function, endothelial cells, and microvascular permeability. The incidence of major bleeding reported in clinical trials is less than 3% and varies among the LMWH preparations, their indication for use, patient population, and dose administered. Minor bleeding, particularly at the site of injection, occurs frequently with LMWH use. Epidural and spinal hematoma resulting in long-term or permanent paralysis have been reported with the use of LMWH during spinal and epidural anesthesia or spinal puncture.[34] The risk of these events is higher with the use of indwelling epidural catheters and concomitant use of drugs that affect hemostasis. Patients should be frequently monitored for signs and symptoms of neurological impairment. If neurological compromise is noted, urgent treatment is necessary.[34]

Although there is no proven method for reversing LMWH, if major bleeding does occur in a patient receiving an LMWH, it is recommended that IV protamine sulfate be administered.[5] However, because of its limited binding to the shorter LMWH chains, protamine sulfate cannot completely neutralize the anticoagulant effects of LMWH. When given in equimolar concentrations, protamine sulfate neutralizes an estimated 60% to 75% of the antithrombotic activity of LMWH. The recommended dose of protamine sulfate is 1 mg/1 mg of enoxaparin or 1 mg/100 anti-factor Xa units of dalteparin or tinzaparin administered in the previous 8 hours. A second protamine sulfate dose of 0.5 mg/100 anti-factor Xa can be given if bleeding continues. Smaller doses of protamine sulfate can be used if the LMWH dose was given in the previous 8 to 12 hours. The use of protamine sulfate is not recommended if the LMWH was administered more than 12 hours earlier.[5]

Although thrombocytopenia can occur with the use of a LMWH, the incidence of HIT is substantially lower than that observed with the use of UFH.[5,31] The explanation may lie in the reduced propensity of the LMWHs to bind to platelets and PF-4.[5] Because the LMWHs exhibit nearly 100% cross-reactivity with heparin antibodies in vitro, the LMWHs should be avoided in patients with an established diagnosis or history of HIT.[31] Platelet counts should be periodically monitored in all patients who are receiving LMWH, and thrombocytopenia of any degree should be promptly evaluated. The risk of osteoporosis appears to be lower with the LMWHs than with UFH, but both agents have the potential to produce osteopenia.[5]

Use in Special Populations

There is growing experience with the use of LMWHs during pregnancy.[16] The LMWHs do not cross the placenta. According to the results of a few large case series, the LMWH appear to be relatively safe to use during pregnancy and are an attractive alternative to UFH when long-term anticoagulation therapy is required. Furthermore, the LMWHs may have less effect on bone formation.[16] Dalteparin, enoxaparin, and tinzaparin are classified as FDA pregnancy category B.

The LMWHs are becoming the preferred agents in pediatric populations despite the fact that the safety and effectiveness of the LMWHs to treat VTE in children and infants has not been extensively studied. The reduced need for routine monitoring associated with LMWH is especially attractive as many pediatric patients have limited venous access.[33] Weight-based LMWH doses provide a less-predictable anticoagulant response in children compared to adults. For enoxaparin, suggested therapeutic doses are 1.5 mg/kg every 12 hours for infants <2 months old and 1.0 mg/kg every 12 hours for those >2 months old. The suggested dose for dalteparin is 86 to 172 units/kg every 24 hours, keeping in mind that neonates appear to require higher doses/kg than older children or adults.[33] Until more data are available, it is prudent to periodically monitor anti-factor Xa activity in these special populations during long-term use.[33]

FONDAPARINUX

Fondaparinux, also known as pentasaccharide, is a synthetic molecule consisting of the five critical saccharide units that bind specifically, but reversibly, to antithrombin (see Fig. 26–5).[5] Fondaparinux is the first in a class of anticoagulants that selectively inhibits factor Xa activity.[35]

Pharmacology

Similar to UFH and the LMWHs, fondaparinux prevents thrombus generation and clot formation by indirectly inhibiting factor Xa activity through its interaction with antithrombin. When fondaparinux binds to antithrombin it causes a permanent conformational change in antithrombin's active site and catalyzes antifactor Xa activity by about 300-fold.[36] Fondaparinux is not destroyed during this process and is released to bind many other antithrombin molecules.[5] Unlike UFH and LMWH, fondaparinux has no direct effect on thrombin activity at therapeutic plasma concentrations.[5]

Selective inhibition of factor Xa may provide more efficient control over fibrin generation while preserving thrombin's regulatory functions in the control of hemostasis. Fondaparinux has no known effect on platelet function.[36]

Pharmacokinetics

Fondaparinux is rapidly and completely absorbed following subcutaneous administration (absolute bioavailability 100%). Peak plasma concentrations are achieved in approximately 2 hours after a single dose and 3 hours with repeated once-daily dosing. It is distributed primarily in blood. At therapeutic concentrations, fondaparinux is highly and specifically bound to antithrombin. It does not bind to red blood cells or other plasma proteins including albumin, glycoprotein, platelets, or PF4.[5] Fondaparinux is primarily eliminated unchanged in the urine. It is contraindicated in patients with severe renal function impairment (creatinine clearance <30 mL/min). The terminal elimination half-life is 17 to 21 hours and is independent of the patient's age or sex.[5] The anticoagulant effect of fondaparinux persists for 2 to 4 days following discontinuation of the drug in patients with normal renal function. Fondaparinux has no known pharmacokinetic drug interactions. However, concurrent use with other drugs with antithrombotic activity increases the risk of hemorrhage.[37]

Dose and Administration

Fondaparinux is FDA-approved for the prevention of VTE following orthopedic (hip fracture, hip replacement, and knee replacement) or abdominal surgery and for the treatment of DVT and PE (in conjunction with warfarin).[37] In the setting of VTE prevention, the dose of fondaparinux is 2.5 mg injected subcutaneously once daily starting 6 to 8 hours following surgery providing hemostasis has been established. It is important to avoid initiating fondaparinux too soon because there is a significant relationship between the timing of the first dose and the risk of major bleeding complications. Patients who weigh less than 50 kg should not be given fondaparinux for VTE prophylaxis. The usual duration of therapy is 5 to 9 days, but may be given as extended prophylaxis following hospital discharge for up to 21 days.[37] For the treatment of DVT or PE, the dose of fondaparinux is 7.5 mg given subcutaneously once daily. Patients who weight more than 100 kg should be given 10 mg once daily and those who weigh less than 50 kg should receive only 5 mg daily.[37]

Similar to the LMWHs, fondaparinux is administered into the fatty tissue of the abdominal wall. Patients should be instructed to pinch a fold of skin at the injection site and hold it throughout the injection. The needle should be inserted at a 90° angle. Injection sites should be alternated from side to side.[37]

CLINICAL CONTROVERSY

The ACCP Clinical Practice Guidelines recommend against the use of aspirin as the primary method of VTE prophylaxis. However, the American Academy of Orthopedic Surgeons continues to advocate for the use of aspirin 325 mg daily for the prevention of PE following hip and knee replacement surgery. While antiplatelet drugs clearly reduce the risk of coronary artery and cerebrovascular events in patients with arterial disease, aspirin produces a very modest reduction in VTE following orthopedic surgeries of the lower extremities. The relative contribution of platelets in the pathogenesis of venous thrombosis compared with that of arterial thrombosis can explain the reason for this difference.

Therapeutic Monitoring

A complete blood cell count should be measured at baseline and monitored periodically to detect the possibility of occult bleeding.[37] Baseline kidney function should be determined and monitored closely in patients at risk of developing renal failure. Fondaparinux should be discontinued if the creatinine clearance drops below 30 mL/min. Signs and symptoms of bleeding should be monitored daily, particularly in patients with a baseline creatinine clearance between 30 and 50 mL/min. If neuraxial anesthesia has been used, patients should be closely monitored for signs and symptoms of neurologic impairment.

Fondaparinux does not alter coagulation tests such as the aPTT and PT. The role of antifactor Xa monitoring during fondaparinux is not well defined. Patients receiving fondaparinux therapy do not require routine coagulation testing. The anticoagulant activity can be measured with using anti-Xa assays provided fondaparinux is used as a reference standard.[5]

Adverse Effects

The primary adverse effect associated with fondaparinux therapy is bleeding.[37] The rate of major bleeding in the VTE prophylaxis trials was approximately 2% to 3%. Because the risk of major bleeding appears to be related to weight, in patients who weigh less than 50 kg, fondaparinux is contraindicated for VTE prophylaxis and the treatment dose is only 5 mg every 24 hours. Similar to UFH and the LMWHs, fondaparinux should be used with extreme caution in patients with neuraxial anesthesia or following a spinal puncture because of the risk for spinal or epidural hematoma formation. Some case reports have documented successful treatment of HIT with fondaparinux, while others have implicated fondaparinux as a cause of HIT.[38] A specific antidote to reverse the antithrombotic activity of fondaparinux is not currently available, if uncontrollable bleeding occurs during fondaparinux therapy, factor VIIa may be effective.[5]

Use in Special Populations

Fondaparinux has been used safely in elderly patients but the risk of major bleeding increases with age.[37] This is an important consideration because many patients who undergo orthopedic surgery are elderly. Elderly patients are also more likely to have decreased renal function and careful assessment of renal status should be conducted prior to initiating therapy.

Fondaparinux is a pregnancy category B drug.[37] However, there is very limited information regarding fondaparinux use during pregnancy. The drug is excreted in the milk of lactating rats, but excretion in human milk is unknown. Until more data becomes available, UFH and LMWH should remain the agents of choice during pregnancy. Fondaparinux use in pediatric populations has not been studied. Because the dose of fondaparinux is 10 mg for all patients >100 kg, some prefer fondaparinux for VTE treatment in obese patients.

IDRAPARINUX

Idraparinux is an experimental analog of fondaparinux that has very long duration of effect (see Table 26–6) and was developed to be administered once weekly by subcutaneous injection.[35] Idraparinux has shown similar efficacy and safety as warfarin in the treatment of DVT but was less effective than warfarin in patients with PE.[6] A drug that increases bleeding risk with duration of effect persisting for a week is concerning. A novel biotinylated formulation of idraparinux (SSR 126517) has been developed that can be rapidly reversed with injection of avidin an egg white protein.[35] Avidin binds biotin with high affinity to form a stable complex that is renally cleared within minutes terminating the anticoagulant

effect of SSR 126517.[39] Further development of idraparinux has been halted with focus turning to SSR 126517. Whether biotinylation of idraparinux will improve results in the treatment of VTE remains to be defined.[39]

EMERGING ANTI-XA INHIBITORS

The introduction of LMWH and fondaparinux transformed the initial treatment of VTE from a purely inpatient endeavor to one where the majority of patients can be treated as outpatients. However, the need for daily subcutaneous injections is a significant barrier for some patients.[39] Warfarin therapy poses even greater challenges as discussed previously and the required monitoring is labor intensive and stressful for patients and anticoagulation providers.[40] These shortcomings in available anticoagulants have driven the search for replacements with rapid onset of effect that can be administered orally without the need for anticoagulant monitoring. Two such agents that target factor Xa, rivaroxaban and apixaban are in advanced stages of clinical development. Rivaroxaban has been approved in Europe and Canada for prevention of VTE following orthopedic surgery.[40]

Pharmacology and Pharmacokinetics

Rivaroxaban and apixaban are potent and selective inhibitors of factor Xa that do not require antithrombin to exert their anticoagulant effect.[39] Both drugs have good oral bioavailability (80% and 50% for rivaroxaban and abixaban, respectively) and reach peak plasma concentrations in about 3 hours.[39] The terminal half-life of rivaroxaban is 5 to 9 hours and 9 to 14 hours for abixaban.[39] Both drugs are excreted in the urine and feces and are metabolized by CYP 3A4 (among others) and CYP-independent mechanisms.[39] Inhibitors of CYP3A4 and P-glycoprotein may increase plasma concentrations of either drug.[40]

Monitoring

Rivaroxaban and abixaban prolong the PT and the aPTT. For rivaroxaban, the effect on PT and aPTT is short-lived and only appreciable at peak concentrations. Apixiban's effect on PT and aPTT is minimal at therapeutic concentrations. Both drugs can be monitored using factor Xa inhibition assay; however, clinical trials have demonstrated that routine coagulation monitoring is unnecessary for either.[39]

Opportunities and Limitations

Rivaroxaban and apixaban represent a potential advancement in the prevention and treatment of VTE. The rapid onset of effect of these new agents could eliminate the need for injectable anticoagulants in the initial management of VTE. Fixed dosing without the need for routine coagulation monitoring and less drug interaction potential would also offer advantages over warfarin for long-term VTE management.[39]

The lack of a safe, rapidly acting antidote for either of these agents may complicate the management of patients who develop bleeding during treatment.[39] While the lack of routine coagulation monitoring is generally regarded as beneficial, there are instances when monitoring is helpful. Examples include patients with renal or hepatic impairment or in those taking drugs that could affect the metabolism of rivaroxaban or abixaban. Without knowledge of the degree of coagulation inhibition in these circumstances, it will be difficult to know if dose adjustments are necessary to prevent the risk of adverse events.[39] The routine coagulation monitoring associated with warfarin provides a method to assess compliance with therapy. Compliance with new anticoagulants may be more challenging to assess and will require careful patient supervision.[39] The cost of rivaroxaban and abixaban may limit use, particularly if no

TABLE 26-11 Pharmacologic and Clinical Properties of Direct Thrombin Inhibitors

	Lepirudin	Desirudin	Bivalirudin	Argatroban	Dabigatran[a]
Route of administration	IV or SC	IV or SC	IV	IV	PO
Indication	Treatment of thrombosis in patients with HIT	DVT prevention after THA (not available in the U.S.)	Patients with UA undergoing PTCA; PCI with provisional use of GPI Patients with or at risk for HIT undergoing PCI	Treatment of thrombosis in patients with HIT; patients at risk for HIT undergoing PCI	Investigational for VTE prevention and treatment, and stroke prevention in AF
Binding to thrombin	Irreversible catalytic site and exosite-1	Irreversible catalytic site and exosite-1	Partially Reversible catalytic site and exosite-1	Reversible catalytic site	Reversible catalytic site
Monitoring	aPTT (IV) S_{cr}/Cl_{cr}	aPTT (IV) S_{cr}/Cl_{cr}	aPTT/ACT S_{cr}/Cl_{cr}	aPTT/ACT Liver function	S_{cr}/Cl_{cr} Effect on liver function unclear at this time[b]
Clearance	Renal	Renal	Enzymatic (80)% and Renal (20%)	Hepatic	Renal
Antibody development	Antihirudin antibodies in up to 60% of patients	Possible; lower incidence than with lepirudin	May cross-react with antihirudin antibodies	No	Unknown
Effect on INR	Slight increase	Slight increase	Slight increase	Increase	Unpredictable and variable

ACT, activated clotting time; AF, atrial fibrillation; aPTT, activated partial thromboplastin time; Cl_{cr}, creatinine clearance; DVT, deep vein thrombosis; HIT, heparin induced thrombocytopenia; INR, international normalized ratio; IV, intravenous; PCI, percutaneous coronary intervention; PO, oral; SC, subcutaneous; S_{cr}, serum creatinine; THA, total hip arthroplasty; VTE, venous thromboembolism.

[a] Investigational.
[b] Routine monitoring of anticoagulant effect may not be necessary.
From Nutescu et al.[42]

efficacy and/or safety advantage can be demonstrated in comparison to existing anticoagulants. As many patients with VTE will require indefinite anticoagulation therapy, the long-term safety of these new agents will need to be established.[40] Until providers become comfortable with new anticoagulants and the cost differential with existing agents narrows, these drugs may initially be second-line choices for patients who cannot be adequately controlled on warfarin or for those in whom routine coagulation testing cannot be readily performed (e.g., geographic inaccessibility, poor venous access).[39]

DIRECT THROMBIN INHIBITORS

In recent years, research has focused on the development of direct thrombin inhibitors (DTIs) that may offer benefits over traditional agents in the treatment and prevention of various thrombotic disorders. The DTIs have been studied for many indications such as HIT, prophylaxis and treatment of VTE, acute coronary syndromes with and without percutaneous transluminal coronary angioplasty, and nonvalvular atrial fibrillation. Currently four parenteral agents—lepirudin, desirudin, bivalirudin, and argatroban—are approved for use in the United States, and several oral compounds are in various phases of clinical development (Table 26–11).[41,42]

Pharmacology and Pharmacokinetics

The direct thrombin inhibitors, as their name implies, directly interact with the thrombin molecule (see Fig. 26–6). The agents in this class differ in terms of their molecular weight, chemical structure, and binding to the thrombin molecule. Unlike UFH, LMWH, and fondaparinux, DTIs do not require a cofactor (antithrombin) to exert their antithrombotic activity. They are capable of inhibiting both circulating and clot-bound thrombin, a potential advantage over UFH and LMWH. Furthermore, DTIs do not induce immune mediated thrombocytopenia and are widely used for the treatment of HIT.[41,42]

Hirudin, the prototype of this class, is a 65-amino-acid polypeptide that was originally isolated from the salivary secretions of the medicinal leech (*Hirudo medicinalis*). Although not commercially available, the discovery of hirudin led to the development of deriva-

tives such as lepirudin and desirudin via recombinant DNA technology. The hirudins (lepirudin, desirudin, and bivalirudin) form a stoichiometric and very slowly reversible complex by binding to both the active site and exosite-1 of the thrombin molecule (see Fig. 26–6). Because of this bivalent bond, hirudins are considered the most potent inhibitors of thrombin.[41,42]

Lepirudin, a recombinant analogue of hirudin, is a 65-amino acid polypeptide that is administered parenterally, either by continuous IV infusion or subcutaneous injection.[43] It is indicated for anticoagulation in patients with HIT and associated thrombosis to prevent further thromboembolic complications. Research is also being conducted on the use of lepirudin for other indications, such as acute coronary syndromes and VTE. Because of the strong, almost irreversible bond between lepirudin and thrombin, lepirudin is associated with bleeding complications.[43] The primary route of elimination for lepirudin is through renal excretion, and systemic clearance is directly proportional to the glomerular filtration rate. Lepirudin has a terminal half-life of 1.3 hours in young healthy volunteers. In patients with marked renal insufficiency (ClCr <15 mL/min) and on hemodialysis, elimination half-lives are prolonged up to 2 days.[41,42] Thus, dose adjustment is required in the setting of impaired renal function, a potential disadvantage of this agent (Table 26–12). Many patients develop antibodies to lepirudin. Up to 60% of patients treated with lepirudin for 10 days or more will develop antibodies. This may increase the anticoagulant effect of lepirudin, possibly as a result of delayed renal elimination of active lepirudin–antihirudin complexes. Consequently, strict monitoring of aPTT is necessary during prolonged therapy.[41,42] Because fatal anaphylaxis has been reported in patients who developed antibodies, patients should not be treated with lepirudin more than once.[44]

Desirudin, also a recombinant hirudin analogue, is administered by subcutaneous injection and approved by the FDA in 2003 for the prevention of venous thrombosis in patients undergoing elective hip surgery. Although approved for use, the agent is not currently commercially available in the United States. Studies are evaluating the use of subcutaneous desirudin for the treatment of HIT. For acute myocardial infarction and unstable angina, desirudin has

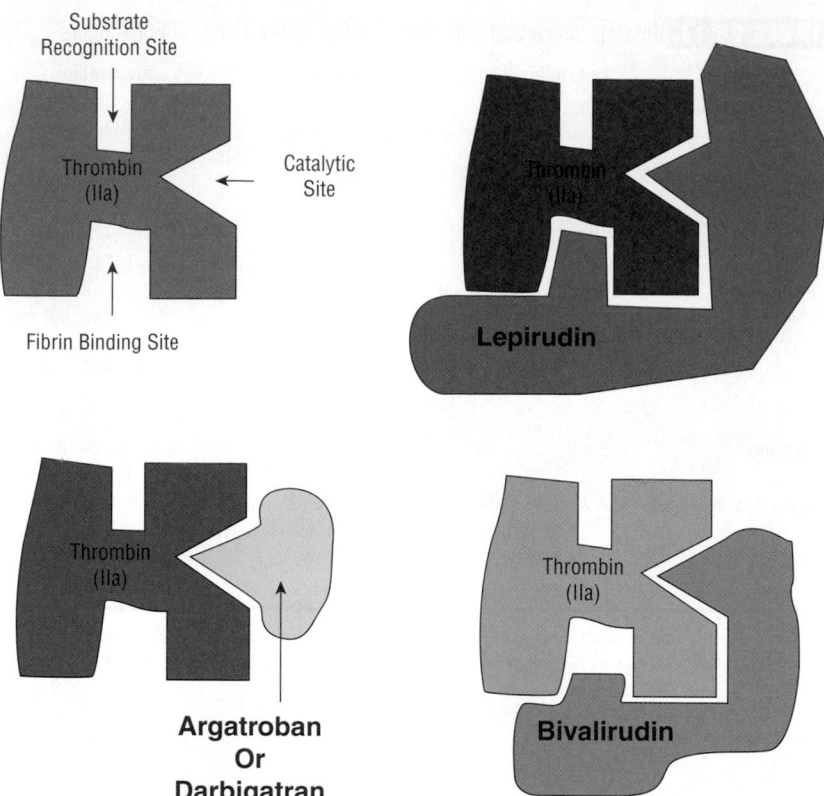

FIGURE 26-6. Pharmacologic activity of lepirudin, bivalirudin, argatroban, and dabigatran.

TABLE 26-12	Dosing Considerations for Direct Thrombin Inhibitors in Patients with Renal and Hepatic Dysfunction	
	Renal Impairment	**Hepatic Impairment**
Lepirudin	Bolus: 0.2 mg/kg (bolus dose is should be avoided in patients with renal impairment) Infusion: Cl_{cr} 45–60 mL/min: 0.075 mg/kg/h Cl_{cr} 30–44 mL/min: 0.045 mg/kg/h Cl_{cr} 15–29 mL/min: 0.0225 mg/kg/h Cl_{cr} <15 mL/min: no bolus; avoid or stop infusion HD: stop infusion & additional IV bolus doses of 0.1 mg/kg every other day should be considered if the aPTT ratio falls below 1.5	Dose adjustment not required
Desirudin	Cl_{cr} 31–60 mL/min: 5mg SC q 12 h Cl_{cr} <30 mL/min: 1.7 mg SC q 12 h	Dose adjustment not required
Bivalirudin	Bolus: no dose adjustment Infusion: Cl_{cr} <30: 1 mg/kg/h HD: 0.25 mg/kg/h	Dose adjustment not required
Argatroban	Dose adjustment not required	Initiate at 0.5 mcg/kg/min then titrate to aPTT 1.5–3.0 × baseline
Dabigatran	Dose adjustment will be required; degree of dose decrease not defined at this time.	Unclear at this time

aPTT, activated partial thromboplastin time; Cl_{cr}, creatinine clearance; HD, hemodialysis; SC, subcutaneous.
From Nutescu et al.[42]

been given via continuous IV infusion.[42,45] Desirudin has a terminal elimination half-life after subcutaneous dosing of approximately 2 hours, and 80% to 90% of the elimination is by renal clearance and metabolism. The total urinary excretion of unchanged drug amounts to 40% to 50% of the administered dose. Similar to lepirudin, in patients with moderate to severe renal impairment, the dosage should be reduced (see Table 26–12). Although antihirudin antibodies also have been documented with desirudin, the incidence appears to be lower than with lepirudin.[42,46]

Bivalirudin, formerly known as Hirulog, is a semisynthetic 20-amino-acid polypeptide analogue of recombinant hirudin that is FDA approved for use in patients with unstable angina who are undergoing percutaneous transluminal coronary angioplasty and with provisional use of glycoprotein IIb/IIIa inhibitor for use as an anticoagulant in patients undergoing percutaneous coronary intervention.[47] Recent reports also support the use of bivalirudin in patients with acute ST elevation myocardial infarction and in patients with HIT, although the agent is not currently FDA approved for these indications. Unlike lepirudin, bivalirudin is a reversible inhibitor of thrombin and provides transient antithrombotic activity with an estimated 20 to 30 minute half-life. This difference may reduce the risk of bleeding and antibody production.[42,48] The ACT can be used to monitor the anticoagulant effect of bivalirudin. Therapeutic ACT levels are achieved within 5 minutes after initiating bivalirudin therapy, and ACT levels return to subtherapeutic levels within 1 hour of discontinuing the infusion. The aPTT test has also been used to monitor the anticoagulant effect of bivalirudin in patients with HIT. Bivalirudin is mostly cleared by proteolytic cleavage and by hepatic metabolism, with approximately 20% eliminated renally. The manufacturer recommends reducing the dose by 20% to 60% in patients with renal impairment and monitoring the ACT closely (see Table 26–12).[42,48]

Argatroban differs from the hirudins in that it is a small, synthetic molecule derived from arginine that reversibly binds only to the active catalytic site of thrombin. Its small size relative to other DTIs enables it to inhibit both clot-bound and soluble thrombin, offering a potential therapeutic advantage over other agents in its class.[42,49] Argatroban is primarily eliminated by hydroxylation and aromatization in the liver to inactive metabolites. A small percentage is excreted unchanged in the bile. The elimination half-life is 39 to 51 minutes, but extends to approximately 181 minutes in hepatic impairment. Dose adjustment is required in patients with hepatic impairment (see Table 26–12). The aPTT and ACT can be used to monitor the anticoagulant effect of argatroban. It is FDA approved for the prophylaxis or treatment of thrombosis in patients with HIT, and also as an anticoagulant in patients with HIT, or at risk of HIT, who are undergoing percutaneous coronary intervention.[42,50]

Oral Direct Thrombin Inhibitors

Recent progress has also been made in the development of oral DTIs. These agents appear promising and offer various advantages such as oral administration, predictable pharmacokinetics and pharmacodynamics, a broader therapeutic window, no need for routine laboratory monitoring, no significant drug interactions, and fixed dose administration without the need of dosing adjustments.[42] Several of these compounds are being investigated with dabigatran etexilate being in most advanced phases of clinical development. A previous oral DTI (ximelagatran) was denied FDA approval because of concerns of drug-induced liver toxicity. Dabigatran is being investigated in the prevention and treatment of venous thrombosis and for stroke prevention in atrial fibrillation. Available data suggest that dabigatran is at least as effective and safe as LMWH in the prevention of VTE after major orthopedic surgery and at least as effective and safe as warfarin in patients with atrial fibrillation.[51,52] Dabigatran has been approved in Canada and Europe for VTE prevention after hip and knee replacement surgery, but it is not yet approved by the FDA. Dabigatran shows promise as an effective and convenient oral anticoagulant. The first safe, oral DTI to make it to the U.S. market has the potential to revolutionize the provision of antithrombotic therapy.

Therapeutic Monitoring

Although the DTIs produce changes in the prothrombin time, the aPTT is used to monitor the patient's response to lepirudin, desirudin, and argatroban.[42,45] After obtaining baseline coagulation studies, doses of lepirudin and argatroban should be titrated to achieve the institution-specific therapeutic range or an aPTT 1.5 to 3.0 times the mean normal control. Daily aPTT monitoring is also recommended for patients on desirudin, particularly those with impaired renal function.[46] Although bivalirudin doses should be adjusted based on the ACT, some experience is also available using the aPTT.[47,48] The ecarin clotting time is a potentially more suitable test to measure the antithrombotic activity of the DTIs, but it is not readily available in most clinical labs in the United States. Oral DTIs appear to produce a predictable antithrombotic response in fixed doses and have a relatively large therapeutic window.[42] Consequently, routine anticoagulation monitoring may not be required for these agents. A CBC should be obtained at baseline and periodically thereafter to detect potential bleeding.

Adverse Effects

Contraindications for use of the DTIs and risk factors for bleeding are similar to other antithrombotic drugs (see Tables 26–8, 26–9). Hemorrhage is the most serious and common adverse effect related to the DTIs.[42,45] In studies evaluating the use of lepirudin for the treatment of patients with HIT, the incidence of major bleeding was relatively high (13%–17%).[43] However, no fatal or intracranial bleeding events occurred. A slightly lower rate of major hemorrhage

was reported in HIT trials using argatroban (approximately 5%) and, similarly, there were no reports of fatal or intracranial bleeding.[50] Bleeding complications with desirudin were similar to enoxaparin in a trial of patients undergoing elective hip surgery. Serious bleeding occurred in less than 1% of all patients in the trial.[46] Minor bleeding and small reductions in red blood cell counts occurred relatively frequently but typically did not require drug discontinuation. There are no known agents that reverse the activity of the DTIs. Nonhemorrhagic effects such as fever, nausea, vomiting, and allergic reactions occur infrequently.

Drug–Drug and Drug–Food Interactions

The concurrent use of DTIs and thrombolytic agents substantially increases bleeding risk, particularly intracranial hemorrhage, and should be undertaken with great caution. Warfarin and antiplatelet agents can be concurrently initiated with DTIs. Because the DTIs prolong the PT and INR, close monitoring for bleeding complications is required. Few pharmacokinetic drug interactions with this class of agents are known. Drugs that alter renal function could prolong lepirudin, desirudin, and bivalirudin activity. Drugs that inhibit liver enzymes have the potential to interact with argatroban.[43,47,50,53]

Use in Special Populations

Lepirudin, bivalirudin, and argatroban are classified by the FDA as pregnancy category B drugs but they should be used cautiously in women of child bearing age because experience is very limited.[43,47,50] Desirudin is classified as pregnancy category C with no controlled trials in pregnant women. Lepirudin and argatroban have been evaluated in a very small number of children. Dosing requirements can vary widely in pediatric patients, thus product-specific dosing guidelines and monitoring should be followed.[54] Critically ill patients and patients with renal or hepatic impairment will require dosage adjustments according to the specific DTI used, and lower initiation doses are recommended (see Table 26–12).[55]

WARFARIN

The most widely prescribed anticoagulant worldwide is warfarin sodium.[4] It was serendipitously discovered in the early 1940s at the University of Wisconsin after hemorrhagic deaths occurred in cattle eating spoiled sweet clover. Warfarin is currently the anticoagulant of choice when long-term or extended anticoagulation is indicated. Warfarin is FDA approved for the prevention and treatment of VTE, as well as for the prevention of thromboembolic complications associated with atrial fibrillation, heart valve replacement, and myocardial infarction.[56] Because of its narrow therapeutic index, predisposition to drug and food interactions, and propensity to cause hemorrhage, warfarin requires continuous patient monitoring and education to achieve optimal outcomes.[4]

Pharmacology

Warfarin exerts its anticoagulation effect by inhibiting the enzymes responsible for the cyclic interconversion of vitamin K in the liver (Fig. 26–7).[4] Reduced vitamin K is a cofactor required for the carboxylation of the vitamin K-dependent coagulation proteins, namely factors II (prothrombin), VII, IX, and X, as well as the endogenous anticoagulant proteins C and S. Carboxylation of the N-terminal region of these proteins in the liver is required for biologic activity. By inhibiting the supply of vitamin K to serve as a cofactor in the production of these proteins, warfarin results in the production of partially carboxylated and decarboxylated coagulation proteins with reduced activity.[4] Warfarin has no direct effect on previously circulating clotting factors or previously formed thrombus. The time required for warfarin to achieve its pharmacologic

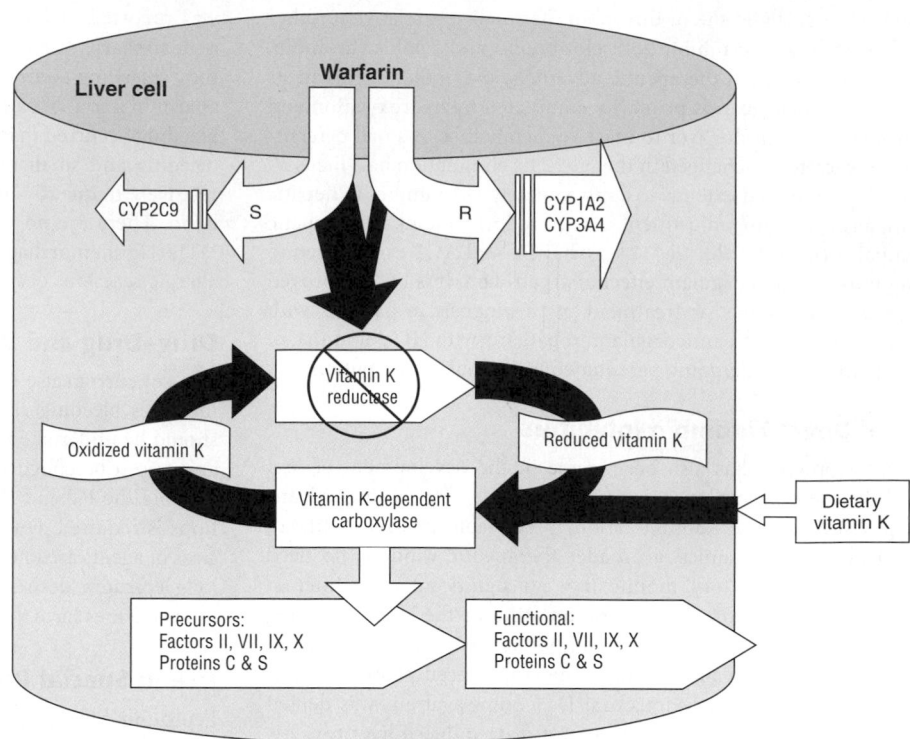

FIGURE 26-7. Pharmacologic activity and metabolism of warfarin.

effect is dependant on the elimination half-lives of the coagulation proteins (Table 26–13). Given that prothrombin has a 2- to 3-day half-life, warfarin's full antithrombotic effect is not achieved for 8 to 15 days after the initiation of therapy. By suppressing the production of clotting factors, warfarin prevents the initial formation and propagation of thrombus.[4]

Pharmacokinetics

Commercially available warfarin is a racemic mixture of *R* and *S* isomers. The *S* isomer is 2.7 to 3.8 times more potent that the *R* isomer.[4] Warfarin is rapidly and extensively absorbed from the gastrointestinal tract and reaches peak plasma concentration within 4 hours with a bioavailability of greater than 90% following oral administration. Warfarin is 99% bound to plasma proteins.[56] Warfarin undergoes stereoselective metabolism via cytochrome P450 (CYP) 1A2, 2C9, 2C19, 2C8, 2C18, and 3A4 isoenzymes in the liver (see Fig. 26–7), with 2C9 being the main enzyme to modulate *in vivo* anticoagulant activity.[56] The pharmacokinetic parameters of warfarin, particularly hepatic metabolism, vary substantially between individuals leading to large interpatient differences in dose requirements. Genetic variations in the 2C9 isoenzyme and vitamin K epoxide reductase (VKOR) have been shown to correlate with warfarin dose requirements.[4] Given the relatively greater potency of *S*-warfarin, coadministration of drugs that induce or inhibit the

CYP2C isoenzymes are more likely to cause clinically significant interactions.[4] These and other pharmacokinetic variations in warfarin metabolism likely explain the large interpatient dose-response seen with warfarin in clinical practice.

Dosing and Administration

The dose of warfarin is patient-specific based on the desired intensity of anticoagulation and the patient's individual response.[4] There is tremendous interpatient variability with regard to the pharmacodynamic response and pharmacokinetic disposition of warfarin. In addition, there is significant intrapatient variability in these parameters over time. Therefore, the dose of warfarin must be based on continual clinical and laboratory monitoring.[4] At the initiation of therapy, it is difficult to predict the specific dose that an individual will require. Warfarin dosing algorithms that incorporate pharmacogenetic information regarding CYP2C9 and VKOR polymorphisms are currently being evaluated. However, the clinical utility and cost-effectiveness of using pharmacogenetic information to guide warfarin initiation remains unproven.[4,57]

Although the average weekly dose of warfarin is between 25 mg and 55 mg, some patient-related variables are associated with lower than usual dose requirement, including advanced age (>65 years old), elevated baseline INR, poor nutritional status, liver disease, hyperthyroidism, genetic polymorphisms in CYP2C9 and VKOR, and concurrent use of medications known to enhance the effect of warfarin (Table 26–14).[4] Prior to initiating therapy, the clinician should screen for the presence of contraindications to anticoagulation therapy and risk factors for major bleeding (see Tables 26–8, 26–9). It is essential to collect a complete medication history, including the use of herbal and nutritional products (Tables 26–15, 26–16).

For most patients, initiating therapy with 5 mg to 10 mg daily and adjusting the dose based on the INR response will produce therapeutic INRs in 4 to 5 days (Fig. 26–8). Lower starting doses may be acceptable based on patient-related factors such as advanced age, malnutrition, liver disease, or heart failure. Starting doses >10 mg should be avoided.[4] Warfarin therapy can be safely initiated on an outpatient basis; the response to therapy should be measured

TABLE 26-13	Biologic Half-Life of Vitamin K–Dependent Coagulation Proteins
Protein	**Half-Life (hours)**
Prothrombin (factor II)	42–72
Factor VII	4–6
Factor IX	21–30
Factor X	27–48
Protein C	9
Protein S	60

From Wittkowsky.[98]

TABLE 26-14	Clinically Important Warfarin Drug Interactions

Increase Anticoagulation Effect (↑INR)	Decrease Anticoagulation Effect (↓INR)	Increase Bleeding Risk
Acetaminophen	Amobarbital	Argatroban
Alcohol binge	Butabarbital	Aspirin
Allopurinol	Carbamazepine	Clopidogrel
Amiodarone	Cholestyramine	Danaparoid
Cephalosporins (with NMTT side chain)	Dicloxacillin Griseofulvin	Dipyridamole
Chloral hydrate	Nafcillin	Unfractionated/low-molecular-weight heparin
Cimetidine	Phenobarbital	Nonsteroidal antiinflammatory drugs
Ciprofloxacin	Phenytoin	Ticlopidine
Clofibrate	Primidone	
Chloramphenicol	Rifampin	
Danazol	Rifabutin	
Disulfuram	Secobarbital	
Doxycycline	Sucralfate	
Erythromycin	Vitamin K	
Fenofibrate		
Fluconazole		
Fluorouracil		
Fluoxetine		
Fluvoxamine		
Gemfibrozil		
Influenza vaccine		
Isoniazid		
Itraconazole		
Lovastatin		
Moxalactam		
Metronidazole		
Miconazole		
Neomycin		
Norfloxacin		
Ofloxacin		
Omeprazole		
Phenylbutazone		
Piroxicam		
Propafenone		
Propoxyphene		
Quinidine		
Sertraline		
Sulfamethoxazole		
Sulfinpyrazone		
Tamoxifen		
Testosterone		
Vitamin E		
Zafirlukast		

INR, international normalized ratio; NMTT, *N*-methylthiotetrazole.
From Coumadin Prescribing Information.[56]

TABLE 26-15	Warfarin Dietary Supplements Interactions Involving Cytochrome P450 Metabolism

Dietary Supplement	Mechanism
Bergamottin (component of grapefruit juice)	2C9 inhibitor
Bishop's weed (Bergapten)	3A4 inhibitor
Bitter orange	3A4 Inhibitor
Cat's claw	3A4 inhibitor
Chrysin	1A2 inhibitor
Cranberry	2C9 inhibitor
Devil's claw	2C9 Inhibitor
Dehydroepiandrosterone (DHEA)	3A4 inhibitor
Diindolymethane	1A2 inducer
Echinacea	3A4 inhibitor
Eucalyptus	3A4, 2C9, 2C19, 1A2 inhibitor
Feverfew	1A2, 2C9, 2C19, 3A4 inhibitor
Fo-ti	1A2, 2C9, 2C19, 3A4 inhibitor
Garlic	2C9, 2C19, and 3A4 inhibitor
Ginseng	CYP P450 inducer
Goldenseal	3A4 inhibitor
Guggul	3A4 inducer
Grape	1A2 inducer
Grapefruit juice	1A2, 2A6, and 3A4 inhibitor
Indole-3-carbinol	1A2 Inducer
Ipriflavone	2C9, 1A2 inhibitor
Kava	1A2, 2C9, 2C19, 2D6, 3A4 inhibitor
Licorice	3A4 inhibitor
Lime	3A4 inhibitor
Limonene	2C9, 2C19 substrate, and 2C9 inducer
Lycium (Chinese wolfberry)	2C9 inhibitor
Milk thistle	2C9 and 3A4 inhibitor
Peppermint	1A2, 2C9, 2C19, 3A4 inhibitor
Red clover	1A2, 2C9, 2C19, 3A4 inhibitor
Resveratrol	1A, 2E1 3A4 inhibitor
St. John's wort	1A2, 2C9, 3A4 inducer
Sulforaphane	1A2 inhibitor
Valerian	3A4 inhibitor
Wild cherry	3A4 inhibitor

From Nutescu et al.[63]

Therapeutic Monitoring

Warfarin requires frequent laboratory monitoring to ensure optimal therapeutic outcomes and minimize bleeding complications. The prothrombin time has been used for decades to monitor the anticoagulation effects of warfarin. The PT measures the biologic activity of factors II, VII, and X activity and correlates well to warfarin's anticoagulation effect. The test is performed by measuring the time required for clot formation after adding calcium and thromboplastin to citrated plasma.[4] Several thromboplastins, varying in responsiveness to reductions in vitamin K-dependent clotting factors are commercially available. The PT is problematic to interpret because the variable sensitivity of thromboplastin reagents. With a given blood sample, thromboplastins of differing sensitivity will produce substantially different results some of which could lead to inappropriate dosing decisions. The World Health Organization (WHO) addressed the need for standardization in the late 1970s by developing a reference thromboplastin and recommending the use of the INR to monitor warfarin therapy. The INR corrects for differences in thromboplastin reagents through the following formula:

$$INR = \left(\frac{PT^{Patient}}{PT^{Control}} \right)^{ISI}$$

every 1 to 3 days until stabilized. For patients with acute venous thrombosis, UFH, LMWH, or fondaparinux should be overlapped with warfarin therapy for at least 5 days regardless of whether the target INR has been achieved earlier.[6]

When adjusting the dose of warfarin, the clinician should allow sufficient time for changes in the INR to occur. In general, maintenance dose changes should not be made more frequently than every 3 days. Doses should be adjusted by calculating the weekly dose and reducing or increasing the weekly dose by 5% to 25%. The effect of dose changes may not become evident for 5 to 7 days. During maintenance therapy, patients should not have follow-up INR tests sooner than anticipated changes are likely to occur.[4]

TABLE 26-16 Dietary Supplements That Can Affect Platelet Function and Anticoagulation Status

Agent	Mechanism	Comments
Bladderwrack	Has anticoagulant effects	Increased risk of bleeding or bruising
Boldo	Constituents may have antiplatelet effects	Increased risk of bleeding or bruising
Bromelain	Decreased platelet aggregation	Increased risk of bleeding or bruising
Burdock	Decreased platelet aggregation by inhibiting platelet activation factor	Increased risk of bleeding or bruising
Caffeine	May have antiplatelet activity; not reported in humans	Increased risk of bleeding or bruising; found in black tea, green tea, guarana, mate, oolong tea
Clove	Eugenol has antiplatelet activity	Increased risk of bleeding or bruising
Cod liver oil	May inhibit platelet aggregation	Increased risk of bleeding or bruising; avoid concomitant use
Coltsfoot	May inhibit platelet aggregation	Increased risk of bleeding or bruising; avoid concomitant use
Danshen	Decreased platelet aggregation; may also have antithrombotic effects	Increased risk of bleeding or bruising; avoid concomitant use
Dong quai	May inhibit platelet aggregation	Increased risk of bleeding or bruising
Fenugreek	Constituents may have antiplatelet effects; concentration may not be clinically significant	Increased risk of bleeding or bruising
Fish oil	Has antiplatelet effects	Increased risk of bleeding or bruising
Flax seed	Decreased platelet aggregation and increased bleeding time	Increased risk of bleeding or bruising
Gamma linolenic acid (GLA)	Has anticoagulant effects	Increased risk of bleeding or bruising; found in borage and evening primrose oil
Garlic	Has anticoagulant effects and may inhibit platelet aggregation	Increased risk of bleeding or bruising
Ginger	Inhibit thromboxane synthetase and decrease platelet aggregation	Increased risk of bleeding or bruising
Ginkgo	Decreased platelet aggregation; ginkgolide B, a component of ginkgo, is a potent inhibitor of PAF	Increased risk of bleeding or bruising
Ginseng, panax	Components may decrease platelet aggregation through PAF antagonism; not shown in humans	Increased risk of bleeding or bruising; use with caution until more is known.
Ginseng, Siberian	A component, dihydroxybenzoic acid, may inhibit platelet aggregation	Increased risk of bleeding or bruising
Melatonin	Unknown; might increase the anticoagulant or antiplatelet effect; decreased prothrombin activity observed	Increased risk of bleeding or bruising
Nattokinase	Has thrombolytic activity	Increased risk of bleeding or bruising
Onion	Decreased platelet aggregation	Increased risk of bleeding or bruising
Pantethine	Decreased platelet aggregation	Increased risk of bleeding or bruising
Policosanol	Inhibits platelet aggregation	Increased risk of bleeding or bruising
Poplar	Contains salicylates and may cause decreased platelet aggregation	Increased risk of bleeding or bruising
Resveratrol	Has antiplatelet effects	Increased risk of bleeding or bruising
Sea buckthorn	Inhibits platelet aggregation	Increased risk of bleeding or bruising
Turmeric	Decreased platelet aggregation; has antiplatelet effects	Increased risk of bleeding or bruising
Vinpocetine	Has antiplatelet effects	Increased risk of bleeding or bruising
Vitamin E	Inhibits platelet aggregation and antagonizes the effects of vitamin K–dependent clotting factors	Dose dependent and significant with doses greater than 800 units per day; advise patients to avoid high doses of vitamin E; increased risk of bleeding or bruising
Willow bark	Decreased platelet aggregation; has antiplatelet effects but less than aspirin	Increased risk of bleeding or bruising

PAF, platelet-activating factor.
From Nutescu et al.[63]

The International Sensitivity Index (ISI) is a measure of the thromboplastin's responsiveness compared to the WHO reference standard.[4] Each thromboplastin reagent manufactured has an ISI value that should be used to calculate the INR. Although the INR system has a number of potential problems, it is currently the best means available to interpret the PT and the preferred method for monitoring oral anticoagulation therapy.

The recommended target INR and associated goal range is based on the therapeutic indication.[4] For most indications, the target INR is 2.5 with an acceptable range of 2.0 to 3.0. The target INR is higher for some patients with mechanical prosthetic heart valves (target INR, 3.0; range, 2.5–3.5).[4] A baseline PT and complete blood cell count should be obtained prior to initiating warfarin therapy. In patients with an acute thromboembolic event, an INR should be measured minimally every 3 days during the first week of therapy (daily INRs are common in hospitalized patients). Once the patient's dose-response is established, an INR should be determined every 7 to 14 days until it stabilizes and optimally every 4 to 8 weeks thereafter.[4,58]

At each encounter, patients should be meticulously questioned regarding their medication use and symptoms related to bleeding and thromboembolic complications. Any changes in medications, including changes in dose as well as non-prescription drug and dietary supplement use, should be carefully explored (see Tables 26–14, 26–15, 26–16). Dietary intake of vitamin K rich foods should also be evaluated (Table 26–17).

Anticoagulation therapy management services can improve the care of patients who take warfarin therapy by providing structured, comprehensive patient education and evaluation.[4] When staffed by experienced and knowledgeable practitioners, anticoagulation management services improve the safety and effectiveness of warfarin therapy compared to "usual" medical care.[59] Anticoagulation patient management services lower the overall cost of care by reducing the frequency of major bleeding and recurrent thromboembolic events.[59]

Portable finger stick INR devices are available for monitoring warfarin therapy. These devices permit clinicians to do "real-time" therapeutic drug monitoring, and enable patients to engage in self-testing at home.[60] Self-monitoring, in its simplest form, requires the patient to report their test results to a healthcare professional. In such arrangements, the clinician continues to make warfarin dosing decisions. Highly motivated and sophisticated patients can be trained to manage themselves, independently altering the dose of

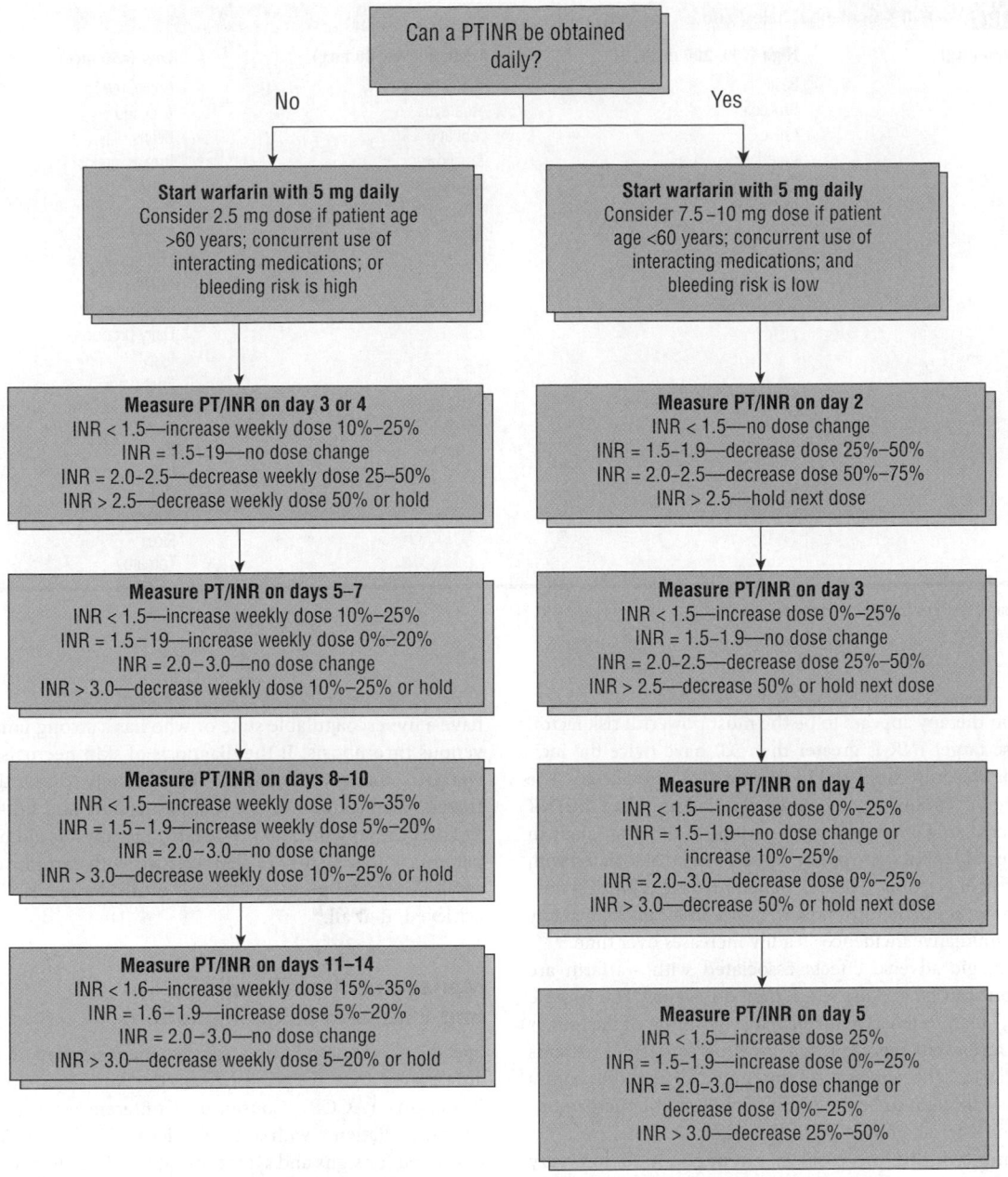

FIGURE 26-8. Initiation of warfarin therapy. (INR, international normalized ratio; PT, prothrombin time.)

warfarin therapy based on their INR results. Patients who engage in INR self-monitoring and warfarin self-management report high levels of satisfaction with care and maintain the INR within the therapeutic range more frequently than those managed by "usual care."[60] Home INR testing and self management are clearly not for everyone, however. These modalities require careful patient selection and considerable education. Finger stick INR devices are relatively expensive, but some Medicare patients may qualify for limited coverage of the monitor and testing strips.

Adverse Effects

Warfarin's primary adverse effect is bleeding.[3] Hemorrhagic complications, ranging from mild to life-threatening, can occur at any site in the body. Although warfarin is not believed to cause bleeding per se, it can "unmask" bleeding from an existing lesion or enable massive bleeding from an ordinarily minor source. The gastrointestinal tract and the nose are the most frequent sites of bleeding. Intracranial hemorrhage is the most serious and feared complication

related to warfarin therapy, often resulting in permanent disability or death.[3]

The annual incidence of major bleeding ranges from 1% in highly selected patient populations who are carefully managed, to greater than 10% in patients managed in less-structured environments.[3,4] There are no universally accepted criteria for defining a bleeding event as major or minor. Most studies have defined major bleeding as any bleeding into a critical anatomic space (e.g., intracranial bleeding, hemarthrosis, or intraocular bleeding), bleeding that requires transfusion of 2 or more units of blood or plasma, or that leads to a greater than 2 g/dL drop in hemoglobin concentration. Bleeding that does not meet the criteria for a major hemorrhage is generally considered to be a minor. Minor bleeding is common during warfarin therapy. Few studies have prospectively evaluated the incidence of minor bleeding but it is likely to be greater than 15% annually even in the most expertly managed patients.[3,4]

Several risk factors for bleeding while taking anticoagulation therapy have been identified (see Table 26-8).[3,4] Intensity of

TABLE 26-17 Vitamin K Content of Select Foods[a]

Very High (>200 mcg)	High (100–200 mcg)	Medium (50–100 mcg)	Low (<50 mcg)
Brussel sprouts	Basil	Apple, green	Apple, red
Chickpea	Broccoli	Asparagus	Avocado
Collard greens	Chive	Cabbage	Beans
Coriander	Coleslaw	Cauliflower	Breads, grains
Endive	Cucumber (with peel)	Mayonnaise	Carrot
Kale	Canola oil	Nuts, pistachio	Cereal
Lettuce, red leaf	Green onion/scallion	Squash, summer	Celery
Parsley	Lettuce, butterhead		Coffee
Spinach	Mustard greens		Corn
Swiss chard	Soybean oil		Cucumber (without peel)
Tea, green			Dairy products
Tea, black			Eggs
Turnip greens			Fruit (varies)
Watercress			Lettuce, iceberg
			Meats, fish, poultry
			Pasta
			Peanuts
			Peas
			Potato
			Rice
			Tomato

[a]Approximate amount of vitamin K per 100 g (3.5 oz) serving.
From Booth and Centurelli.[99]

anticoagulation therapy appears to be the most powerful risk factor. Patients whose target INR is greater than 3.0 have twice the incidence of major bleeding compared to those with a target of 2.5. The risk of intracranial hemorrhage increases significantly when the INR remains greater than 4.0 for prolonged periods of time especially in the elderly. Unstable INR control also appears to be associated with an increased risk of bleeding. The risk of hemorrhage is greatest during the first few weeks of therapy; however, bleeding can occur at any time and the cumulative incidence steadily increases over time.[3,4]

Nonhemorrhagic adverse effects associated with warfarin are uncommon, but can be serious when they do occur.[4] The "purple toe syndrome," manifested as a purplish discoloration of the toes, is an extremely rare event reported in a small percentage of patients receiving warfarin. The etiology of this unusual phenomenon is unknown, but is thought to be the result of cholesterol microembolization into the arterial circulation of the toes.[56]

Warfarin-induced skin necrosis is an uncommon but very serious dermatologic reaction that is manifested by a painful maculopapular rash and ecchymosis or purpura that subsequently progresses to necrotic gangrene. It most frequently appears in areas of the body rich in subcutaneous fat, such as the breasts, thighs, buttocks, and abdomen. The incidence of warfarin-induced skin necrosis is less than 0.1%.[61] It occurs most commonly in middle-aged women who are being treated for acute venous thrombosis. Although symptoms generally appear during the first week of therapy, it has been reported in a small number of patients who had taken warfarin for months and even years. The pathogenesis of warfarin-induced skin necrosis is not clearly understood. Many believe imbalances between procoagulant and anticoagulant proteins that occur early in the course of warfarin therapy resulting in capillary thrombosis and secondary hemorrhages. The observation that patients with proteins C or S deficiency appear to be at greater risk for warfarin-induced skin necrosis supports this theory. Warfarin-induced skin necrosis has also been reported in patients with other disorders of hypercoagulability, such as antithrombin deficiency and antiphospholipid antibodies. Patients who receive large "loading" doses of warfarin may also be at greater risk.[61] Overlapping warfarin and injectable anticoagulants is especially important in any patient suspected to

have a hypercoagulable state or who has a strong family history of venous thrombosis. If the diagnosis of skin necrosis is suspected, warfarin therapy should be immediately discontinued, fresh-frozen plasma and vitamin K administered, and full-dose UFH or LMWH therapy initiated. Warfarin therapy should be restarted in patients with a history of skin necrosis with extreme caution using small doses and gradual titration until therapeutic INR has been achieved, if at all.[61]

Management of Bleeding and Excessive Anticoagulation

Specific recommendations for the management of patients with an elevated INR are published by the American College of Chest Physicians (ACCP) Consensus Conference on Antithrombotic Therapy.[4] Patients with a mildly elevated INR (3.5–5.0) should be examined for signs and symptoms of bleeding, as well as factors that increase bleeding risk. In this circumstance, either reducing the dose of warfarin or holding one or two doses will safely manage most patients. When a swift reduction in an elevated INR is required, oral or intravenous vitamin K_1 (phytonadione) can be given. In the absence of major bleeding, the oral route of administration is preferred. While the IV route produces a more rapid reversal, previous parenteral formulations have been associated with rare but serious anaphylactoid reactions. The risk of this reaction can be reduced with slow infusion of diluted vitamin K solution. If the INR is between 5 and 9 and no bleeding is present, doses of warfarin should be withheld and may be combined with a low dose of oral vitamin K (≤2.5 mg). Administering vitamin K in this situation will increase both the rate of INR decline and the potential for INR overcorrection; however, neither of these outcomes has been shown to affect the risk of developing subsequent bleeding or thromboembolism compared to simply withholding warfarin alone.[62] Therefore, the decision to administer vitamin K should be individualized based on the patient's bleeding risk and the underlying indication for anticoagulation therapy (see Fig. 26–9). Vitamin K should be used with caution in patients at high risk of recurrent thromboembolism because of the possibility of INR overcorrection. Conversely, simply withholding warfarin therapy may not lower a high INR quickly

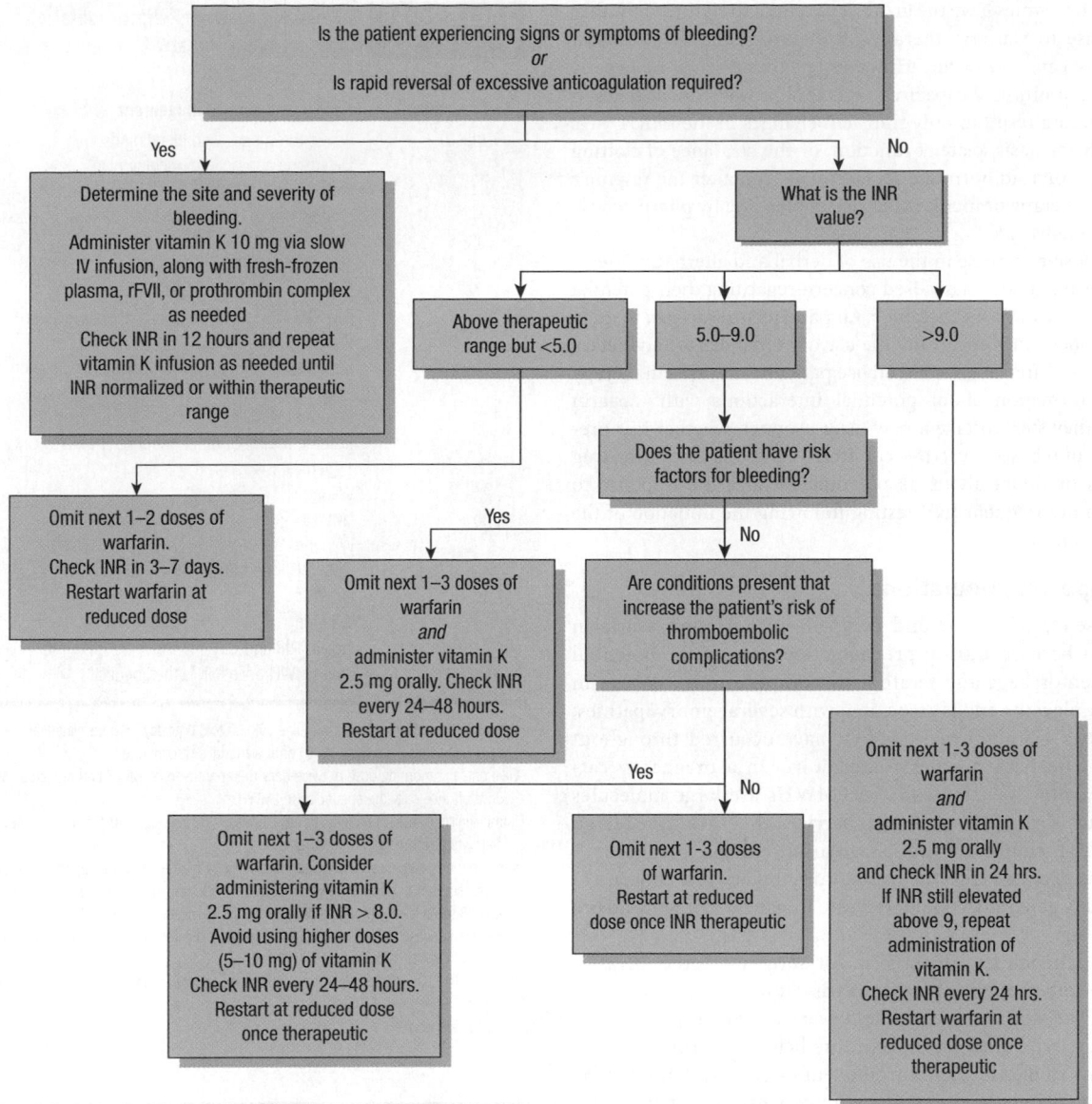

FIGURE 26-9. Management of an elevated international normalized ratio (INR) in patients taking warfarin. Dose reductions should be made by determining the weekly warfarin dose and reducing the weekly dose by 10% to 25% based on degree of INR elevation. Conditions that increase the risk of thromboembolic complications include history of hypercoagulability disorders (e.g., protein C or S deficiency, presence of antiphospholipid antibodies, antithrombin deficiency, activated protein C resistance), arterial or venous thrombosis within the previous month, thromboembolism associated with malignancy, and mechanical mitral valve in conjunction with atrial fibrillation, previous stroke, poor ventricular function, or coexisting mechanical aortic valve. (INR, international normalized ratio; rFVII, recombinant factor VII.)

enough in patients at high risk for developing bleeding complications. Most patients with asymptomatic INR elevations can be safely managed by withholding warfarin alone. If the INR is greater than 9, 2.5 mg to 5mg of oral vitamin K is recommended.[4] High doses of vitamin K (e.g., 10 mg) are associated with prolonged resistance to warfarin and the occurrence of thromboembolic complications and should only be administered to patients with serious bleeding. In the event of a serious or life-threatening bleeding, intravenous vitamin K should be administered as well as fresh-frozen plasma, clotting factor concentrates, or recombinant FVII.[4]

Drug–Drug and Drug–Food Interactions

The pharmacokinetic and pharmacodynamic properties of warfarin, coupled with its narrow therapeutic index, predispose this agent to numerous clinically important food and drug interactions (see Tables 26–14, 26–15, 26–16, 26–17).[4,56] Vitamin K can reverse warfarin's pharmacologic activity, and many foods contain sufficient vitamin K to reduce the anticoagulation effect of warfarin if a patient consumes them in large portions or repetitively within a short period of time.[63] Patients should be given a list of vitamin K-rich foods and instructed to maintain a relatively consistent intake. It is important to stress consistency and moderation rather than absolute abstinence. Abrupt changes in vitamin K intake should be considered when unexplained changes in the INR occur.[64] Alternative sources of vitamin K, such as multivitamins and nutritional supplements (e.g., Sustacal and Ensure) should also be considered. Patients who require parenteral nutrition should not receive a weekly bolus dose of vitamin K if they are taking warfarin therapy.

Pharmacokinetic drug interactions with warfarin are primarily a result of alterations in hepatic metabolism or binding to plasma proteins. Drugs that inhibit or induce the CYP2C9, CYP1A2, and

CYP3A4 isoenzymes have the greatest potential to significantly alter the response to warfarin therapy.[4] Protein-binding displacement interactions can also occur. However, in the absence of hepatic disease or a diminished capacity to metabolize warfarin, changes in protein binding result in only transient changes in the INR. Drugs that alter hemostasis, platelet function, or the clearance of clotting factors (e.g., thyroid hormone replacement) can alter the response to warfarin therapy or increase the risk of bleeding by pharmacodynamic mechanisms.[4]

The explosive increase in the use of herbal and alternative therapies in North America has raised concern regarding their potential to interact with warfarin therapy.[63] All patients on warfarin therapy should be questioned regarding the use of herbal drugs and dietary supplements. Clinicians should advise patients on warfarin therapy to seek information about potential interactions with warfarin whenever they start to take a new drug product, whether it is prescribed or purchased over the counter. If there is a known drug interaction or doubt about its potential to alter the response to warfarin, more frequent INR testing following the initiation of the new agent is prudent.[4]

Use in Special Populations

In the absence of a clear and compelling indication, warfarin should not be used during pregnancy because of the potential for fetal hemorrhage and teratogenic complications.[16] Warfarin crosses the placenta and is associated with several embryopathies, particularly CNS abnormalities that have occurred throughout gestation. The FDA has designated warfarin a pregnancy category X agent.[56] As UFH and the LMWHs are large molecules that do not cross the placental barrier, they are considered the drugs of choice for anticoagulation during pregnancy.[16] Warfarin is excreted into the breast milk in very low concentrations[56] and is generally considered safe to use by women who are breastfeeding.

Patients scheduled to undergo major surgery or other invasive procedures often require temporary discontinuation of warfarin therapy.[65] The decision to withhold warfarin therapy should be based on the type of surgical procedure being performed and the patient's risk of bleeding and thromboembolism. Warfarin therapy should generally not be discontinued in patients undergoing minimally invasive procedures such as dental work.[65] If the bleeding risk from the procedure is considerable, warfarin should be stopped 4 to 5 days prior to the procedure in order to allow the INR to return to near-normal values. Alternatively, warfarin can be stopped and a low dose (1–2 mg) of oral vitamin K may be given 1 to 2 days prior to the procedure.[65] Patients at high risk of thromboembolism (i.e., DVT or PE in the previous month) should be given so-called bridge therapy with UFH or a LMWH before and/or after the procedure (Table 26–18).

Warfarin use among elderly patients is increasingly common. Although the drug has been extensively studied in this population, some debate still remains regarding the relative risks of warfarin therapy in the elderly.[4] Accumulating evidence indicates that increasing age is an independent risk factor for major bleeding during anticoagulation therapy.[3] Age >75 years is associated with an increased risk of intracranial hemorrhage, especially when the INR is supratherapeutic.[3] Elderly patients may be more prone to excessive anticoagulation as a consequence of nutritional deficiencies, comorbidities, and multiple drug interactions. However, age >70 has also been associated with an increased likelihood of achieving stable INR control.[58] The elderly are often at greater risk of falls. Although they often derive the greatest benefit from anticoagulation therapy, elderly patients should be monitored with greater vigilance, and warfarin dose changes should be made more cautiously.

TABLE 26-18	General Approach to Periprocedural Anticoagulation Therapy Management
Days Relative to Procedure	**Anticoagulation Management**
−7 to −10	Assess thrombosis and bleeding risk
	Determine appropriate bridging plan
	Obtain baseline INR
−7	Stop aspirin or other antiplatelet therapy if necessary
−6 or −5	Stop warfarin[a]
−4 or −3	Start LMWH[b]
−2	LMWH
−1	Give last dose of LMWH 24 h before procedure[c]
	Obtain INR
0 = Procedure	Resume warfarin[d] at usual maintenance dose on evening after procedure
+1	Resume LMWH[e]
	Resume aspirin or other antiplatelet therapy once hemostasis secured
	Warfarin
+2 to +3	LMWH[e]
	Warfarin
	Obtain INR and CBC
+4 to +5	LMWH
	Warfarin
	Obtain INR and CBC
<+6	Stop LMWH once INR is therapeutic

[a] Warfarin stopped on day −5 if baseline INR 2.0 to 3.0 or day −6 if baseline INR is 2.5 to 3.5.
[b] LMWH is initiated 2 days (36–48 h) after warfarin is discontinued.
[c] Give only the morning dose of twice-daily therapeutic-dose LMWH and reduce by 50% the total dose of once-daily therapeutic-dose LMWH.
[d] Some clinicians instruct patients to take "booster" doses (e.g., 150% of usual dose) for 1 to 2 days when resuming warfarin therapy.
[e] Resume therapeutic-dose LMWH approximately 24 h after (e.g., the day after) the procedure for minor surgical or other invasive procedures; for major surgery or high bleeding risk procedures wait 48 to 72 h after the procedure and when hemostasis is secured before resuming therapeutic-dose LMWH, or administer prophylactic-dose LMWH when hemostasis is secured, or avoid LMWH completely.

CBC, complete blood count; INR, international normalized ratio; LMWH, low-molecular-weight heparin.

From Douketis et al.[65]

GENERAL APPROACH TO THE PREVENTION OF VENOUS THROMBOEMBOLISM

Given that VTE is potentially fatal and costly to treat, strategies to prevent DVT in at-risk populations will have the greatest impact on patient outcomes.[2,8,66] To rely on the early diagnosis and treatment of VTE is unacceptable because many patients will die before treatment can be initiated. Despite an immense body of literature that overwhelmingly supports the widespread use of pharmacologic and mechanical strategies to prevent VTE, prophylaxis is underused in many hospitals. Even when prophylaxis is given, many patients receive prophylaxis that is less than optimal. Educational programs and clinical decision support systems have been shown to improve the appropriate use of VTE prevention methods.

❺ The goal of an effective VTE prophylaxis program is to identify all patients at risk, determine each patient's level of risk, select and implement regimens that provide sufficient protection for the level of risk, and avoid or limit complications from the selected regimens. As hospitalized patients are frequently at high risk for VTE, screening all patients prior to or at the time of admission to determine their level of risk is the first step in an effective VTE prevention program.[2] The risk classification criteria and suggested prophylaxis strategies published by the ACCP Clinical Practice Guidelines and the Surgical Care Improvement Project

(SCIP) are widely used (Table 26–19). Several pharmacologic and mechanical methods are effective for preventing VTE, and these can be used alone or in combination. Mechanical methods improve venous blood flow, whereas drug therapy counteracts the propensity for thrombus formation by inhibiting the coagulation cascade.

MECHANICAL STRATEGIES

Resumption of ambulation as soon as possible following surgery reduces the incidence of VTE in low-risk patients.[2] Walking increases venous blood flow and promotes the flow of natural antithrombotic factors into the lower extremities. During prolonged surgeries, venous foot pumps that mimic the pumping action produced during ambulation can be beneficial.

Graduated compression stockings reduce the incidence of VTE by approximately 60% following general surgery, neurosurgery, and stroke.[2] Compression stockings work by increasing the velocity of venous blood flow through the application of graded pressure, with the greatest amount applied at the ankle. This treatment option is inexpensive and safe, and an excellent choice when pharmacologic intervention is either contraindicated or difficult to adequately monitor. When combined with pharmacologic interventions, graduated compression stockings have an additive effect. However, compression stockings can be uncomfortable and some patients are unable to wear them because of the size or shape of their legs.

Intermittent pneumatic compression (IPC) devices increase the velocity of blood flow in the lower extremities.[2] The technique involves the sequential inflation of a series of cuffs wrapped around the patient's legs. The cuffs use graded pressure and inflate in 1- to 2-minute continuous cycles from the ankles to the thighs. IPC reduces the risk of VTE by more than 60% following general surgery, neurosurgery, and orthopedic surgery.[2] There is some theoretical concern that external compression may dislodge a previously formed clot. Although IPC is well tolerated and safe to use in patients who have contraindications to pharmacologic therapies, it does have drawbacks. It is more expensive than the use of graduated compression stockings; it is a relatively cumbersome technique; and some patients have difficulty sleeping while using it. Compliance with IPC use throughout the day is relatively poor in many hospitals, leaving patients without effective thromboprophylaxis. Like graduated compression hose, IPC can be used in combination with pharmacologic strategies.

Inferior vena cava (IVC) filters can provide short-term protection against PE in very high-risk patients by preventing the embolization of a thrombus formed in the lower extremities into the pulmonary circulation.[2] Percutaneous insertion of a filter into the IVC is a minimally invasive procedure performed via fluoroscopy. Despite the widespread use of IVC filters, there are limited data regarding their effectiveness and long-term safety. The evidence suggests that IVC filters, particularly in the absence of effective antithrombotic therapy, increase the long-term risk of recurrent DVT.[67] Although IVC filters can reduce the short-term risk of PE in patients who are at highest risk, they should be reserved for patients in whom other prophylactic strategies cannot be used. To reduce the long-term risk of DVT associated with IVC filter use, pharmacologic prophylaxis is needed. Anticoagulation therapy should begin as soon as the patient is able to tolerate it.

PHARMACOLOGIC STRATEGIES

Numerous pharmacologic options have been extensively evaluated in randomized clinical trials (see Table 26–19).[2,68] Appropriately selected drug therapies can significantly reduce the incidence of VTE following hip and knee replacement, hip fracture repair, general surgery, myocardial infarction, and ischemic stroke. The choice of agent and dose to use for VTE prevention must be based on the patient's level of risk for thrombosis and bleeding complications, as well as cost and availability.

The most extensively studied agents for the prevention of VTE are UFH, the LMWHs, and fondaparinux.[2,68] The LMWHs and fondaparinux provide superior protection against VTE when compared with low-dose UFH. Their more predictable absorption when given by subcutaneous injection may be the explanation. Even so, UFH remains an effective, cost-conscious choice for many patient populations, provided that it is given in the appropriate dose. Low-dose UFH (5,000 units every 12 hours or every 8 hours) given subcutaneously reduces the risk of VTE by 55% to 70% in patients undergoing a wide range of general surgical procedures and following myocardial infarction or stroke. For the prevention of VTE following hip and knee replacement surgery, the effectiveness of low-dose UFH is considerably lower. The LMWHs and fondaparinux appear to provide a high degree of protection against VTE

TABLE 26-19	DVT Risk Classification and Suggested Prevention Strategies		
Level of Risk		**Risk of DVT without Thromboprophylaxis**	**Suggested Prevention Strategies**
Low			
Patients undergoing minor surgery and fully ambulatory		<10%	Early and aggressive ambulation
Patients who are medically ill and fully ambulatory			
Moderate			
Most patients undergoing general, gynecological, or urological surgeries		10–40%	UFH 5,000 units SC q 8 or 12 h
Most patients who are hospitalized for an acute medical illness (e.g., MI, ischemic stroke, CHF exacerbation, acute respiratory illness)			LMWH (at recommended dose) Fondaparinux
Patients who are at moderate DVT risk and high risk for bleeding			Mechanical thromboprophylaxis[a]
High			
Patients undergoing major lower-extremity orthopedic surgery (hip or knee arthroplasty, hip fracture repair)		40–80%	LMWH (at recommended dose) Fondaparinux
Spinal cord injury			Warfarin (INR goal = 2.0–3.0)
Major trauma			Oral factor Xa inhibitors[b] Oral direct thrombin inhibitors[b]
Patients who are at high DVT risk and high risk for bleeding			Mechanical thromboprophylaxis[a]

[a] Mechanical thromboprophylaxis includes intermittent pneumatic compression (IPC), graduated compression stockings (GCS), and venous foot pumps (VFP)

[b] Oral factor Xa inhibitors and oral direct thrombin inhibitors are investigational agents. These agents have not yet been formally endorsed as appropriate VTE prevention strategies in clinical practice guidelines.

DVT, deep vein thrombosis; CHF, congestive heart failure; INR, international normalized ratio; MI, myocardial infarction; UFH, unfractionated heparin.

Adapted from Geerts et al.[2]

in most high-risk populations. The appropriate prophylactic dose for each LMWH product is indication specific (see Table 26–10). There is no evidence that one LMWH is superior to another for the prevention of VTE. Fondaparinux was significantly more effective than enoxaparin at preventing venographically detected DVT and proximal DVT in several clinical trials that enrolled patients undergoing high risk orthopedic procedures but has not shown superiority in reducing the incidence of symptomatic PE or mortality. Fondaparinux has also been show to cause more bleeding than enoxaparin when administered within 6 hours of orthopedic surgery.[2] To provide optimal protection, some experts believe that the LMWHs should be initiated prior to surgery.[2]

Warfarin is a commonly used option for the prevention of VTE following orthopedic surgeries of the lower extremities.[2] The evidence is equivocal regarding the relative effectiveness of warfarin compared to the LMWHs for the prevention of clinically important VTE events in the highest risk populations. When used to prevent VTE, the dose of warfarin should be adjusted to maintain an INR between 2.0 and 3.0; however, some orthopedic surgeons favor lower initial INR goal ranges (e.g., 1.5–2.5) because of fear of bleeding at the surgical site. Oral administration and low drug cost give warfarin some advantages over LMWHs and fondaparinux. However, warfarin does not achieve its full antithrombotic effect for several days, requires frequent monitoring and periodic dosage adjustments, and carries a substantial risk of major bleeding. Furthermore, warfarin should be recommended only when a well-coordinated monitoring system is available.[4]

The optimal duration for VTE prophylaxis following surgery is not well established.[2] Prophylaxis should be given throughout the period of risk. For general surgical procedures and medical conditions, once the patient is able to ambulate regularly and other risk factors are no longer present, prophylaxis can be discontinued. Because of the relatively high incidence of VTE in the first month following hospital discharge among patients who have undergone a lower extremity orthopedic procedure, extended prophylaxis following hospital discharge with either LMWH, fondaparinux, or warfarin appears to be beneficial. Most clinical trials support the use of antithrombotic therapy for 21 to 35 days following total hip replacement and hip fracture repair surgeries.[2,68]

Given the limitations of warfarin, there has been considerable interest in alternative medications and several new oral agents are in various stages of development.[69] New oral anticoagulants hold the promise of fixed dosing, rapid onset, fewer drug–drug interactions, and simplified monitoring requirements.[70] A few of these agents, specifically rivaroxaban, apixaban, and dabigatran, have been evaluated in phase 3 clinical trials for use in high-risk populations for the prevention of VTE. In patients who have undergone elective knee or hip replacement placement, these new agents appear to be comparable or superior to enoxaparin in terms of efficacy and safety. To date, none of these agents have been compared with warfarin in the setting of VTE prevention. While the results of initial clinical trials have been favorable, they should be viewed with caution until postmarketing studies are completed, providing a greater sense of the potential value of these new agents in a variety of patient populations.

PHARMACOECONOMIC CONSIDERATIONS

Only a handful of studies have formally evaluated the cost-effectiveness of VTE prevention strategies. The acquisition costs of graduated compression stockings, UFH, and warfarin are considerably less than those of LMWH and fondaparinux. However, the acquisition cost for drug therapy is relatively small when compared with the overall cost of care.[66] Economic analyses must take into account the efficacy of the strategy, duration of use, complications, and monitoring costs.[71,72]

The determination of the cost-effectiveness of VTE prophylaxis is based on the premise that a reduction in future VTE events will reduce overall healthcare costs.[71] Furthermore, the incremental cost per patient will decrease proportionally with increasing frequency of VTE in the population. Stated another way, the cost of providing prophylaxis to 1,000 patients will decline as the incidence of VTE in the given population increases. Consequently, more expensive and effective strategies become more cost-effective in higher-risk populations. In populations at low risk for VTE, early ambulation appears to be the most cost-effective strategy. Although LMWH provides slightly greater reductions in the risk of VTE in patients who are at moderate risk of VTE, the additional cost is estimated to be $107 (in 1999 dollars) per patient when compared to low-dose UFH.[73] Whether universal use of LMWH in moderate-risk patients is a cost-effective strategy is controversial.

In high-risk patients, the cost-effectiveness of prevention is far greater because the incidence of VTE is higher.[71] Following hip replacement surgery, regardless of the strategy selected, prophylaxis saves money when compared with no prophylaxis. LMWHs and fondaparinux slightly increase the total mean cost of care after total hip and knee replacement when compared with low-dose UFH and warfarin.[74] However, because of their superior effectiveness, LMWH and fondaparinux have a significantly lower cost per DVT and PE avoided. Based on typical drug-acquisition costs, LMWH and fondaparinux are generally considered cost-effective choices in the highest-risk patient populations.

GENERAL APPROACH TO THE TREATMENT OF VENOUS THROMBOEMBOLISM

6 Before initiating anticoagulation therapy for the treatment of VTE, it is imperative to establish an accurate diagnosis; thus preventing unnecessary risk and expense to the patient. Anticoagulation therapy remains the mainstay of treatment for VTE. DVT and PE are manifestations of the same disease process and are treated similarly.[6] Full "therapeutic" doses of antithrombotic drugs prevent thrombus extension and embolization as well as reduce the risk of long-term sequelae such as the postthrombotic syndrome, chronic thromboembolic pulmonary hypertension, and recurrent thromboembolism.[6] The standard approach is to initiate therapy with an injectable anticoagulant and to make the transition to warfarin for maintenance therapy (Table 26–20 and Fig. 26–10). Determining the optimal duration of anticoagulation involves weighing the risk of recurrent VTE against the risk of bleeding associated with anticoagulation therapy and determining patient preference regarding treatment duration. When bleeding risk outweighs VTE recurrence risk or if the informed patient's preference is to stop treatment, anticoagulation should be stopped.[6] In some circumstances, elimination of the obstructing thrombus is warranted and the use of venous thrombectomy or thrombolysis can be considered.[6] Inferior vena cava interruption with a filter is also an option in those with contraindications to anticoagulation therapy or in whom anticoagulant therapy has failed.[6]

Once the diagnosis of VTE has been objectively confirmed (see Clinical Presentation and Diagnosis below), anticoagulant therapy with UFH, LMWH, or fondaparinux should be instituted as soon as possible. Evidence indicates that currently available injectable anticoagulants can be administered in the outpatient setting in most patients with DVT and some patients with PE. The decision to initiate therapy on an outpatient basis should be based on institutional resources and patient specific variables (Table 26–21).[75] **7**

For the treatment of an acute VTE, LMWHs should be dosed based on the patient's actual (or total) body weight. Some clinicians believe that dose adjustments or dosing "caps" are not recommended in obese patients. However, some clinicians continue to "cap" LMWH doses for patients weighing more than 150 kg.

UNFRACTIONATED HEPARIN

The parenteral administration of UFH followed by warfarin has been the conventional treatment of patients with VTE for decades and is still preferred in patients with severe renal insufficiency.[6] For acute treatment of VTE, UFH has traditionally be administered by continuous IV infusion (see Table 26–7). When UFH is administered by IV infusion, the aPTT or a suitable coagulation study is generally used to monitor the anticoagulant effect. The infusion rate should be adjusted to maintain an appropriate range corresponding to a heparin concentration of 0.3 to 0.7 international units/mL anti-Xa activity by the amidolytic assay.[6] Weight-based dosing of UFH achieves a therapeutic aPTT in the vast majority of patients in the first 24 hours (see Table 26–7).[5] Failure to give a sufficient dose of IV UFH has been shown to increase the risk of VTE recurrence not only during the initial treatment but also during long-term therapy.[6] Intravenous UFH requires hospitalization with frequent monitoring and dose adjustment. Well-organized inpatient anticoagulation management services have been shown to improve patient care by increasing the proportion of aPTT values in the therapeutic range, reducing the length of hospital stay, and lowering total hospital costs when compared with usual care.[76] However, despite the widespread use of weight-based dosing protocols, some patients still fail to achieve an adequate response to UFH therapy. There is also evidence that UFH does not prevent thrombus progression in some patients with DVT, and rebound thrombin generation has been observed when UFH is discontinued abruptly.[30] These limitations of traditional IV UFH in the acute treatment of VTE have led to the investigation of alternative approaches.

Evidence suggests that if a sufficient dose of UFH is administered, aPTT-guided dose titration may not be necessary. Weight-based LMWH compared to weight-based UFH (initial dose 333 units/kg subcutaneously followed by 250 units/kg twice daily) without coagulation monitoring for the treatment of acute VTE revealed no difference in recurrent VTE, major bleeding or death during follow-up. Both groups received warfarin therapy overlapped for at least 5 days and continued after LMWH or UFH was discontinued.[29] UFH administered in this manner may be a less costly option for treatment of acute VTE in appropriately selected patients. For patients weighing more than 80 kg, injection volume may be problematic since 20,000 unit/mL is the most concentrated commercially available preparation of UFH.

LOW-MOLECULAR-WEIGHT HEPARIN

Because of their improved pharmacokinetic and pharmacodynamic profile as well as ease of use, the LMWHs have largely replaced UFH for the treatment of VTE. The LMWHs given subcutaneously in fixed, weight-based doses (see Table 26–10) are at least as effective as UFH given IV for the treatment of VTE.[6] There appears to be similar efficacy and safety with inpatient or outpatient LMWH administration, once- or twice-daily dosing regimens, and use of different LMWH preparations.[6] However, a subgroup analysis in one study suggested that patients with cancer and obese patients have higher VTE recurrence rates with once-daily enoxaparin.[77]

TABLE 26-20	Consensus Guidelines for Venous Thromboembolism Treatment	
	Recommendation	**Grade**[a]
Acute anticoagulation	Acute treatment of objectively confirmed DVT or PE should be with subcutaneous LMWH, subcutaneous fondaparinux, subcutaneous fixed-dose UFH, intravenous UFH, or adjusted-dose subcutaneous UFH	1A
	The dose of monitored UFH (subcutaneous or intravenous) should be sufficient to prolong the aPTT to a range that corresponds to a plasma heparin level of 0.3 to 0.7 international units/mL anti-Xa activity	1C
	LMWH (as an outpatient if possible) is recommended rather than intravenous UFH for patients with acute DVT	1C (outpatient); 1A (inpatient)
	UFH is suggested over LMWH for patients with severe renal failure	2C
Duration of acute treatment	Treatment with UFH, LMWH, or fondaparinux should be overlapped with warfarin for at least 5 d and until the INR is ≥2.0 for 24 h	1C
	Warfarin should initiated together with UFH, LMWH, or fondaparinux on the first treatment day	1A
	Patients with cancer should be treated with a LMWH for the first 3 to 6 mo	1A
Long-term anticoagulation	Warfarin (target INR 2.5, range: 2.0 to 3.0) should be continued for at least 3 mo *in all patients*	1A
	All patients with unprovoked VTE should be evaluated for the risk-benefit ratio of long-term anticoagulation	1C
	Patients with a first unprovoked proximal DVT or PE who are at low risk for bleeding and for whom good anticoagulant monitoring is achievable should receive long-term anticoagulation	1A
	Patients with recurrent unprovoked VTE should receive long-term anticoagulation	1A
	Patients receiving long-term anticoagulation should receive periodic reassessment of the risk-benefit ratio of continuing anticoagulation	1C
	In patients with cancer, following 3 to 6 mo of LMWH, subsequent anticoagulation with either warfarin or LMWH should continue indefinitely or until the cancer is resolved	1C

[a] Refers to grade of recommendation (1A, strong recommendation applying to most patients in most circumstances; 1C, strong recommendation applying to most patients in many circumstances; higher quality research likely to impact confidence in the estimate of effect and may well change the estimate; 2B, weak recommendation where alternative approaches likely to be better for some patients under some circumstances).

aPTT, activated partial thromboplastin time; DVT, deep vein thrombosis; INR, international normalized ratio; LMWH, low-molecular-weight heparin; PE, pulmonary embolism; UFH, unfractionated heparin; VTE, venous thromboembolism.
From Kearon et al.[6]

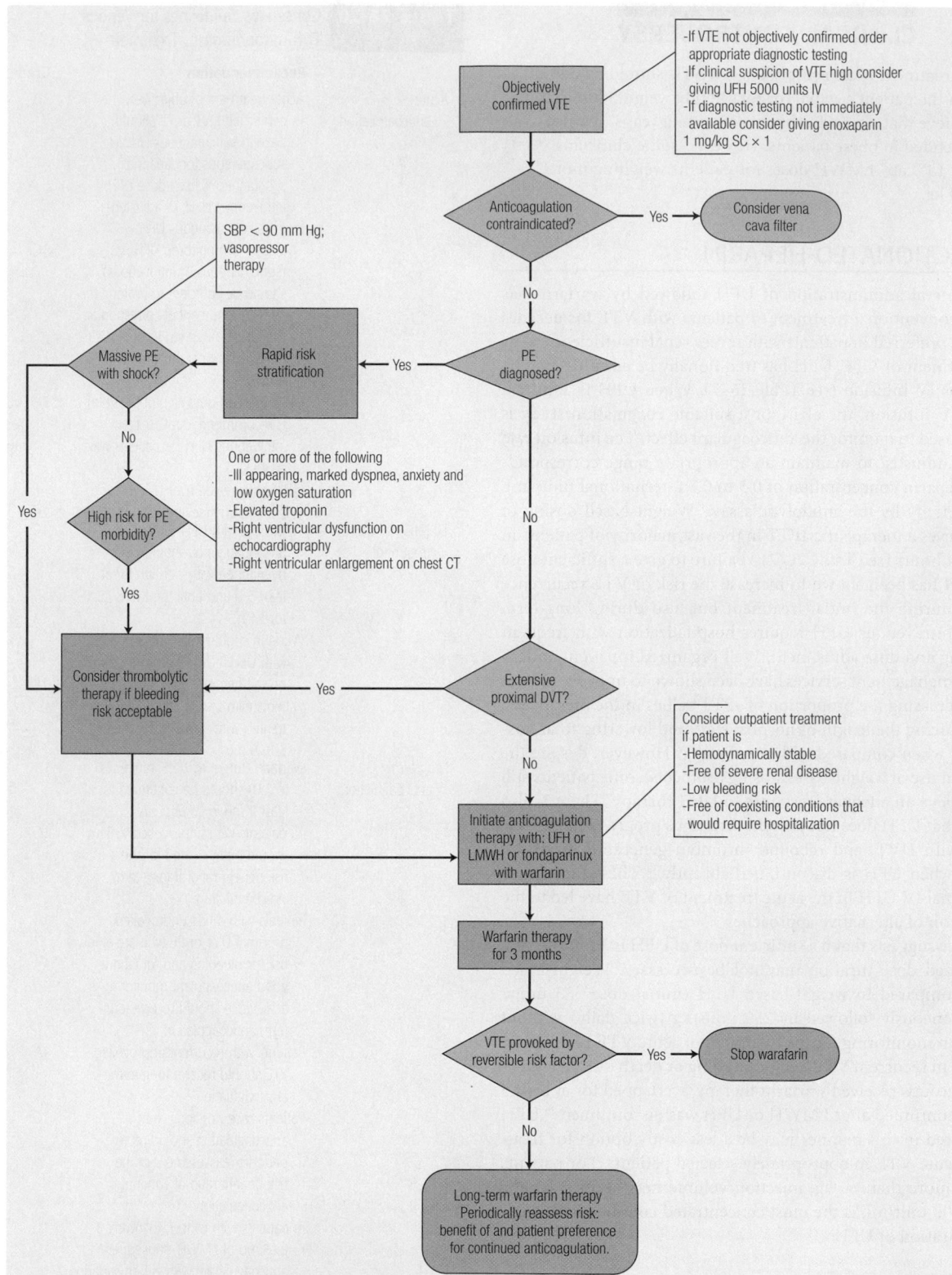

FIGURE 26-10. Treatment of venous thromboembolism (VTE). (IV, intravenous; SC, subcutaneous; DVT, deep vein thrombosis; LMWH, low-molecular-weight heparin; PE, pulmonary embolism; SBP, systolic blood pressure; UFH, unfractionated heparin.)

Given the predictable response and the reduced need for laboratory monitoring with LMWH, stable patients with DVT who have normal vital signs, low bleeding risk and no other comorbid conditions requiring hospitalization can be discharged early or treated entirely on an outpatient basis (see Table 26–21).[75] The efficacy and safety of LMWH in the home-based treatment of proximal DVT was initially established in large clinical studies. The results

of randomized controlled clinical trials, as well as the experience of several successful outpatient DVT treatment programs in a variety of healthcare settings, have led to an increased acceptance for outpatient management. Indeed, surveys of patients who received outpatient DVT treatment indicate a high degree of satisfaction and comfort, with 91% expressing satisfaction with home treatment.[75]

TABLE 26-21 Outpatient Treatment Protocol for Deep Venous Thrombosis

Target population: Inclusion/exclusion criteria for outpatient venous thromboembolism (VTE) treatment

Inclusion: Patients with objectively diagnosed VTE

Relative exclusion: Patients with clinical evidence of pulmonary embolus or suspected embolism who are hemodynamically stable

Exclusion: Arterial thromboembolism or patients who are currently receiving dialysis, actively bleeding, have had recent (within 2 weeks) major surgery/trauma, or have other severe uncompensated comorbid conditions

Recommended procedure: May vary depending on the patient's clinical condition

A. Confirm diagnosis of VTE by objective testing
1. Venous ultrasonogram
2. Ventilation–perfusion (V/Q) scan
3. Computed tomography (CT) scan

B. Day 1
1. Baseline laboratory evaluation
  a. Prothrombin time (PT) and calculated international normalized ration (INR)
  b. Activated partial thromboplastin time (aPTT)
  c. Serum creatinine (Scr)
  d. Complete blood count (CBC) with platelets
2. Medication
  a. Low-molecular-weight heparin (LMWH) or fondaparinux injections
    i. Enoxaparin 1 mg/kg subcutaneously (SC) q 12 h or
    ii. Enoxaparin 1.5 mg/kg SC q 24 h (not recommended for patients with cancer or for obese patients)
    iii. Dalteparin 100 units/kg SC q 12 h or
    iv. Dalteparin 200 units/kg SC q 24 h or
    v. Tinzaparin 175 units/kg SC q 24 h or
    vi. Fondaparinux 7.5 mg SC q 24 h (5 mg if <50 kg and 10 mg if >100 kg)
  b. Warfarin sodium 5–10 mg orally every evening
  c. Pain medication if necessary (avoid nonsteroidal antiinflammatory drugs [NSAIDs])
3. Patient education
  a. Clinical pharmacy/nursing
    i. Educate patient regarding the importance of proper monitoring of anticoagulation therapy and indications for additional medical evaluation; document activities in the medical record
    ii. Teach patient how to self-administer LMWH (if patient or family member unwilling or unable to self-administer LMWH injection, visiting nurse services should be arranged); initial LMWH injection should be administered in the medical office or hospital
    iii. Instruct patient regarding local therapy: elevation of affected extremity; localized heat, antiembolic exercises (flexion–extension of ankle for lower-extremity VTE, or hand squeezing–relaxation for upper-extremity VTE)
  b. Pharmacy operations
    i. Provide backup for clinical pharmacy/nursing; reinforce patient education regarding indication, use, monitoring, side effects, and drug interactions with antithrombotic therapy
    ii. Repackage LMWH syringes (if indicated) in patient-specific doses and dispense 5 to 7 days of therapy
    iii. Screen patient's pharmacy profile for potential drug–drug interactions with anticoagulation therapy
  c. Anticoagulation service enrollment
    i. The physician should forward outpatient VTE treatment orders to the anticoagulation service

C. Day 2
1. Laboratory evaluation: not required on day 2 of therapy
2. Medications: continue LMWH and warfarin as directed
3. Anticoagulation service
  a. Contact patient and evaluate for symptoms of pulmonary embolism (PE), clot extension, and/or bleeding
  b. Arrange for visiting nursing service if family or family member is having difficulty with outpatient therapy
  c. Continue reduced activity as long as pain persists (when possible, elevate extremity); increase activity as tolerated
  d. Document activities in medical record

D. Day 3
1. Laboratory evaluation: check INR
2. Medications: continue LMWH and warfarin directed
3. Anticoagulation service
  a. Contact patient and evaluate for symptoms of PE, clot extension, and/or bleeding
  b. Interpret results of INR and adjust dose of warfarin to achieve a target INR of 2.5
  c. Patient activity: continue reduced activity as long as pain persists (when possible, elevate extremity); increase activity as tolerated
  d. Document activities in medical record

E. Day 4
1. Laboratory evaluation: check INR
2. Medications: continue LMWH and warfarin as directed
3. Anticoagulation service
  a. Contact patient and evaluate for symptoms of PE, clot extensions, and/or bleeding
  b. Interpret results of INR and adjust dose of warfarin to achieve a target INR of 2.5
  c. Patient activity: no restrictions; if pain increases, contact anticoagulation service or provider
  d. Document activities in medical record

(continued)

TABLE 26-21 Outpatient Treatment Protocol for Deep Venous Thrombosis (continued)

F. Day 5
1. Laboratory evaluation: check INR and CBC with platelets
2. Medications: continue LMWH if indicated and warfarin as directed
3. Anticoagulation service
   a. Contact patient and evaluate for symptoms of PE, clot extension, and/or bleeding
   b. Interpret results of INR and adjust does of warfarin to achieve a target INR of 2.5
   c. Patient activity: no restriction; if pain increases, contact primary care provider
   d. Document activities in medical record

Patients presenting with PE and no evidence of hemodynamic instability are at low risk of subsequent morbidity and mortality. Evidence exists suggesting that patients with submassive PE who are hemodynamically stable can be managed safely as outpatients with LMWH or fondaparinux.[30] However, hemodynamically unstable patients with PE should generally be admitted for initiation of anticoagulation therapy. If thrombolytic therapy or embolectomy is anticipated, UFH, which can be rapidly reversed, is preferred.[78]

Not all patients are appropriate candidates for outpatient DVT treatment. At a minimum, patients with objectively diagnosed DVT must be reliable or have adequate caregiver support.[75] Patients and their caregivers must be willing and active participants in the outpatient management of DVT (Table 26–22). Patients who are unable to manage or who decline at-home treatment should be admitted to the hospital. These patients may subsequently opt for early discharge on LMWH. Daily patient contact either in person or via telephone is essential to identify potential complications and to address questions and concerns promptly. During daily contacts patients must be asked about symptoms that may indicate bleeding, thrombus extension, and PE.[75] Once acute treatment with LMWH has been transitioned to long-term warfarin therapy (usually after about 5 to 10 days), patient contact can occur less frequently.

FONDAPARINUX

Fondaparinux has been shown to be a safe and effective alternative to LMWH for the treatment of VTE.[6] Fondaparinux is dosed once daily via subcutaneous injection based on weight in the following doses: 5 mg if <50 kg, 7.5 mg if 50 kg to 100 kg, and 10 mg if >100 kg.[37] Careful attention should be paid to renal function when fondaparinux is used to treat VTE.

WARFARIN

Warfarin monotherapy is an unacceptable choice for the acute treatment of VTE because it does not produce a rapid anticoagulation effect and is associated high incidence of recurrent thromboembolism. However, warfarin is very effective in the long-term management of VTE and should be started concurrently with rapid acting injectable anticoagulant therapy.[6] The rapid-acting injectable anticoagulant should overlap with warfarin therapy for at least 5 days and until INR ≥2.0 has been achieved for at least 24 hours.[6] The initial dose of warfarin should be 5 to 10 mg (see Fig. 26–8) and periodically adjusted to achieve and maintain an INR between 2.0 and 3.0.

The appropriate initial duration of warfarin therapy to effectively treat an acute first episode of VTE for all patients is 3 months. The one exception to this rule is that isolated distal DVT provoked by a major transient risk factor can safely be treated with only 6 weeks of warfarin therapy.[6] Three months of warfarin therapy reduces the risk of recurrent VTE to as low a value as can be achieved by a time-limited duration of therapy. To prevent new episodes of VTE that are not directly related to the preceding episode, continued warfarin therapy is required.[79] Individually tailoring

warfarin maintenance duration therapy for 3 months requires careful consideration of the circumstances surrounding the initial thromboembolic event, the presence of ongoing thromboembolic risk factors, and the risk of bleeding and patient preference.[6] The most important consideration in determining the risk of recurrent VTE once anticoagulation therapy is stopped is whether the initial thrombotic event was associated with a major transient or reversible risk factor (e.g., surgery, plaster cast immobilization of a leg, or hospitalization in the month prior to VTE). For patients in this situation, the risk of recurrence is relatively small, approximately 3% in the first year and approximately 10% over 5 years, and only 3 months of oral anticoagulation treatment is warranted.[79] For VTE associated with a minor transient or reversible risk factor (e.g., within 6 weeks of initiation of estrogen therapy, air travel lasting >8 hours, pregnancy, less marked leg injuries or immobilization, or the aforementioned major risk factors when they have occurred 1 to 3 months prior to VTE), 3 months of oral anticoagulation therapy is also reasonable.[79]

Patients with a first unprovoked (idiopathic) VTE have a recurrence risk of approximately 10% in the first year and approximately 30% and 50% over 5 and 10 years, respectively. These patients should be considered for indefinite warfarin therapy when feasible.[6] Indefinite in this context refers to warfarin that is continued without a scheduled stop date, but which may be stopped because of a subsequent increase in the risk of bleeding or change in patient preference for anticoagulation.[6] Indefinite warfarin therapy targeted to an INR of 2.0 to 3.0 reduces recurrent VTE by about 90% with the trade off of a doubled frequency of major bleeding rate to about 1% to 2% per year.[79] Factors that may lead to the decision to stop warfarin therapy after 3 months include noncompliance with warfarin therapy, initial clot although idiopathic was isolated in calf veins, or a moderate to high risk of bleeding.[6] Clinically important risk factors for bleeding include age >75 years, previous non-cardioembolic stroke, history of gastrointestinal bleeding, renal or hepatic impairment, anemia, thrombocytopenia, concurrent antiplatelet use (avoid if possible), noncompliance, poor anticoagulant control, serious acute or chronic illness, and the presence of a structural lesion (e.g., tumor, recent surgery) expected to be associated with bleeding. Presence of one to two bleeding risk factors suggests moderate bleeding risk while three or more risk factors suggest a high bleeding risk.[79] For patients with second episode of idiopathic VTE, indefinite anticoagulation is recommended.[6]

Various strategies aimed at identifying patients at very low risk of recurrence after a first idiopathic VTE are being evaluated in clinical trials. Safe withdrawal of warfarin therapy may be possible if reliable identification of these patients proves possible. Estimating an individual patient's risk of recurrent VTE using a variety of interacting clinical, laboratory, and radiologic findings can be accomplished with increasing precision.[80] Some factors that may predict lower risk of recurrence include female gender, low D-dimer levels 1 month after stopping warfarin therapy, absence of residual clot on ultrasound, absence of hereditary and acquired thrombophilia, and absence of the postthrombotic syndrome.[79]

TABLE 26-22 Patient Education for Outpatient Deep Vein Thrombosis Therapy

General information regarding DVT and the goals of treatment
- Anticoagulant medications (injections and warfarin tablets) have been prescribed to prevent the blood clot from growing larger so that the body can begin to dissolve the clot
- Your body may be able to completely dissolve the clot, but in some cases the clot never goes completely away; even with adequate anticoagulation therapy, some people will have chronic pain and swelling in the affected extremity; people who have had one clot are at increased risk of having future clots
- Warfarin tablets take several days to begin to work; LMWH injections work right away so at first LMWH injections and warfarin tablets are used together
- When the warfarin has become effective, you will be able to stop the LMWH injections; you will continue to take warfarin tablets for 3 to 6 months or longer to prevent blood clots from returning
- It is important for you to administer your LMWH or fondaparinux and warfarin exactly as directed

Subcutaneous injection technique
- You must learn to give yourself a subcutaneous injection of LMWH or fondaparinux; alternatively, you may have a family member or visiting nurse give it to you
- If your LMWH or fondaparinux syringes were filled by the manufacturer, they can be stored at room temperature; if your syringes were filled by the pharmacy, they should be stored in the refrigerator; if you were instructed to fill your own syringes, you should prepare the syringe immediately prior to injecting its contents
- If you see a bubble in the syringe, do not try to get it out, you may accidentally squirt out part of your dose
- Choose an injection site on your abdomen; clean the area with alcohol, then position an uncapped syringe at a 90-degree angle; pinch the skin, stick the needle in as far as it will go and gently but firmly push the plunger down; this will inject the medicine into the skin; when all the medication has been injected, remove the needle and dispose of it in an appropriate container
- You will likely experience a burning sensation when the medication is injected; this will go away after a few minutes
- Rotate injection sites from side to side, do not inject into the same site more than once; avoid the area around your navel; do not inject into any bruises

Blood test monitoring
- Regular blood tests are required to make sure your medication is working properly
- The prothrombin time tells how quickly your blood forms a clot; it is used to tell how well warfarin is working
- The INR is a way to standardize the prothrombin time between laboratories; your goal INR range is between 2.0–3.0; if your INR is <2.0, you are at higher risk for clotting, if your INR is >3.0, you are at higher risk for bleeding; your dose of warfarin will be adjusted based on the results of this test
- You need to have a complete blood count test both before you begin therapy and after you have been on LMWH or fondaparinux for about 5 days; this will help detect internal bleeding and the occurrence of a rare side effect of heparin therapy that can decrease a component of your blood called platelets

Warfarin information
- Each strength of warfarin has a unique color; each time you refill your prescription, make sure your new tablets are the same color you have been taking; if they are not the same color, ask your pharmacist why
- Warfarin should be taken at approximately the same time each day
- The most common and serious side effect of warfarin is bleeding; you should be careful to avoid situations or activities that increase your risk of injury; apply direct pressure to control bleeding from superficial cuts
- Warfarin has many drug interactions; always check with your provider before taking any new medications (including over-the-counter medications and dietary supplements)
- Foods rich in vitamin K (green leafy vegetables, etc.) may interfere with warfarin; you do not need to avoid foods rich in vitamin K, but you should try to maintain consistent dietary habits
- Alcohol can increase your risk for bleeding and interfere with warfarin therapy; drink alcohol in moderation (1–2 drinks per day); avoid binge drinking

Contact your provider if you experience
- Persistent bleeding from a cut or scrape
- Blood in your urine
- Blood in your stool
- Persistent nose bleeding
- Increased swelling or pain in your affected extremity

Go to the emergency department if you experience
- Shortness of breath
- Chest pain
- Coughing up blood
- Black tarry-appearing stool
- Severe headache of sudden onset
- Slurred speech

DVT, deep vein thrombosis; INR, international normalized ratio; LMWH, low-molecular-weight heparin.

Risk assessment tools derived from combining several independent risk factors for recurrence has also been investigated.[81] While low D-dimer level one month after stopping warfarin therapy currently appears to hold the greatest promise as a method for identifying patients who could possibly stop warfarin therapy due to low risk of recurrence, further validation is needed before any one factor or prediction rule using a combination of factors can justify routinely stopping warfarin after 3 months of therapy.[79] The decision to continue anticoagulation therapy indefinitely should be reassessed periodically.[6] Patients should be involved in any decision to continue anticoagulation therapy with consideration given to the patient's long-term prognosis, risk of bleeding, ability to adhere to anticoagulation therapy instructions, financial resources, lifestyle, and quality of life.[6]

Increasingly, patients with VTE are being tested for hereditary and acquired hypercoagulable states (thrombophilia). The available evidence does not support an association between genetically transmitted thrombophilias and a higher chance of recurrent VTE.[11] Despite a lack of convincing evidence, most experts recommend indefinite anticoagulation for individuals with the antiphospholipid antibody syndrome, homozygotes for the factor V Leiden mutation, and heterozygotes with both the factor V Leiden and prothrombin 20210 gene mutations.

THROMBOLYSIS AND THROMBECTOMY

Most cases of VTE require only anticoagulation therapy. In rare cases, however, removal of the occluding thrombus by either pharmacologic or surgical means may be warranted.[6] Consensus panel recommendations regarding either thrombolysis or thrombectomy in the management of VTE are based on low-quality evidence, and more study is clearly needed to clarify their precise role.

Thrombolytic agents are proteolytic enzymes that enhance the conversion of plasminogen to plasmin which subsequently degrades the fibrin matrix. Thrombolytic therapy for DVT should theoretically improve long-term outcomes and reduce the risk of recurrent VTE. Indeed, thrombolytic therapy improves venous patency.[6] There is some evidence from pooled study analyses suggesting that thrombolytic therapy is superior to anticoagulation therapy alone in preventing postthrombotic morbidity.[6] Catheter-directed instillation of a thrombolytic agent directly into the clot is increasingly being used. The risk of bleeding associated with catheter-directed drug administration appears to be less than systemic administration.[6] Patients who present within 14 days of symptom onset with extensive proximal DVT, with good functional status, low bleeding risk and a life expectancy of a year or more are candidates for thrombolysis (Table 26–23). Catheter-directed thrombolysis is preferred provided appropriate expertise and resources are available. Catheter-based fragmentation of thrombus, with or without aspiration of the thrombus fragments, can be combined with catheter-directed thrombolysis and the combination has been associated with shorter treatment times and reduced cost.[6] The same duration and intensity of anticoagulation therapy is recommended as for DVT patients who do not receive thrombolysis.[6]

In the management of acute PE, successful dissolution of fibrin with thrombolytic therapy reduces elevated pulmonary artery pressure and normalizes right ventricular dysfunction. However, the risk of death from PE should outweigh the risk of serious bleeding associated with thrombolytic therapy. Patients being considered for thrombolytic therapy should be screened carefully for contraindications relating to bleeding risk (e.g., intracranial disease, uncontrolled hypertension at presentation, and recent major surgery or trauma).[6]

Thrombolytic therapy is considered the standard of care for patients with massive PE manifested by shock and cardiovascular collapse (about 5% of patients diagnosed with PE).[6] These patients have the highest risk of mortality and require aggressive interventions such as volume expansion, vasopressor therapy, intubation, and mechanical ventilation in addition to antithrombotic therapy.[78] Thrombolytic therapy in these patients should be administered without delay to reduce the risk of progression to multisystem organ failure and death. While life-saving in the acute phase of massive PE with hypotension, the hemodynamic benefit of thrombolysis is comparable to that of heparin after a few days.[80]

The benefit of thrombolytic therapy in patients with severe PE without hemodynamic compromise is less clear and rapid risk stratification is required to determine whether the patient will benefit from thrombolysis or embolectomy in addition to anticoagulation therapy.[78] Risk stratification helps inform the intensity of initial treatment, low risk patients being discharged early or managed as outpatients and high risk patients receiving intensive surveillance in the intensive care unit and/or advanced therapies such as thrombolysis.[82] Three key components of risk stratification are clinical evaluation, determination of cardiac biomarker levels such as troponin, and assessment of right ventricular size and function.[6,78] The Pulmonary Embolism Severity Index (PESI) is a prognostic tool utilizing 11 routinely available clinical parameters namely demographics (age and gender), comorbid illnesses (cancer, heart failure, and chronic lung disease) and clinical findings (pulse, systolic blood pressure, respiratory rate, temperature, mental status, and arterial oxygen saturation) that accurately stratifies patients into five risk classes with classes I and II considered low risk.[82] Poor

---

TABLE 26-23 Thrombolysis for the Treatment of Venous Thromboembolism

- The majority of patients with VTE do not require thrombolytic therapy
- Thrombolytic therapy for DVT should be reserved for patients who present with extensive proximal DVT (e.g., ileofemoral) within 14 days of symptom onset, have good functional status, and are at low risk of bleeding
- Thrombolytic therapy should be administered to patients with massive PE with evidence of hemodynamic compromise (hypotension or shock) unless contraindicated by bleeding risk
- Thrombolytic therapy should be considered for selected high-risk patients without hypotension provided the risk of bleeding is acceptable
- Factors associated with high risk for adverse PE outcomes include
  - Ill-appearing patients with marked dyspnea, anxiety, and low oxygen saturation
  - Elevated troponin levels
  - Right ventricular dysfunction on echocardiography
  - Right ventricular enlargement on chest CT
- Factors that increase the risk of bleeding must be evaluated before thrombolytic therapy is initiated (i.e., recent surgery, trauma or internal bleeding, uncontrolled hypertension, recent stroke or intracranial hemorrhage)
- Baseline labs should include CBC and blood typing in case transfusion is needed
- Alteplase 100 mg infused via peripheral vein over 2 hours is the most commonly used thrombolytic for patients with PE
- Before thrombolytic therapy for PE, intravenous UFH should be administered in full therapeutic doses
- During thrombolytic thereapy it is acceptable to either continue or suspend intravenous UFH (suspending UFH is the most common practice in the U.S.)
- aPTT should be measured following the completion of thrombolytic therapy
  - If aPTT is <80 seconds, UFH infusion should be started and adjusted to maintain aPTT in therapeutic range
  - If aPTT is >80 seconds, remeasure every 2–4 hours and start UFH infusion when aPTT is <80 seconds
- Avoid phlebotomy, arterial puncture, and other invasive procedures during thrombolytic therapy to minimize the risk of bleeding

aPTT, activated partial thromboplastin time; CBC, complete blood cell count; DVT, deep vein thrombosis; PE, pulmonary embolism; UFH, unfractionated heparin.
From Kearon et al.[6] and Goldhaber.[78]

---

prognostic indicators include patients who appear ill, with marked dyspnea, anxiety, and low oxygen saturation; elevated troponin levels; right ventricular dysfunction on echocardiography; and right ventricular enlargement on chest CT. Patients with one or more of these clinical features are at high risk for PE-related morbidity and mortality and may benefit from thrombolytic therapy, provided bleeding risk is acceptable, even in the absence of hemodynamic compromise (see Table 26–23).[6] The optimal role of thrombolysis in the management of PE requires further study and it is important to note that current data has not shown a benefit of thrombolytic therapy in submassive PE despite recruitment of over 800 patients in several studies.[80,82]

In high-risk patients, whose clinical status may rapidly deteriorate necessitating the need for thrombolysis or thrombectomy, initial anticoagulation with short-acting intravenous UFH may be preferred.[78] The most common thrombolytic agent for PE is alteplase at a dose of 100 mg via a peripheral vein over 2 hours with or without concomitant intravenous UFH (suspending UFH during alteplase administration is the more common practice in the United States).[6]

Actual removal of clot can be achieved by catheter-directed interventions or surgery and is usually reserved for the patient who is either not a candidate for or has not responded to thrombolysis.[6,78] For DVT, catheter-based interventions are not recommended unless combined with catheter-directed thrombolysis.[6] In rare circumstances surgical thrombectomy for extensive ileofemoral DVT may be necessary, but catheter-directed thrombolysis is preferred if bleeding risk is acceptable.[6] For treatment of acute PE, catheter-based embolectomy might be particularly suitable for patients too frail for surgery (surgical pulmonary embolectomy requires cardiopulmonary bypass).[78] Catheter-based embolectomy in PE can be combined with catheter-directed thrombolysis although catheter embolectomy is usually attempted first with combined therapy reserved for those not responding to mechanical intervention alone.[78] Surgical embolectomy is effective for massive PE and hemodynamic instability when thrombolysis is contraindicated and for when thrombolysis has failed clinically.[78] In cases of chronic PE—where persistent emboli produce CTPH, hypoxemia, and right-sided heart failure—surgical pulmonary thromboendarterectomy offers greater benefit than anticoagulants and may be the treatment of choice if performed by an experienced surgical team. A permanent vena cava filter is usually inserted before or during the procedure and these patients need indefinite oral anticoagulation therapy targeted to an INR of 2.5 (range, 2.0–3.0).[6]

VENA CAVA INTERRUPTION

Anticoagulation therapy is the accepted standard for treating DVT and PE. However, an IVC filter may be indicated in special situations when anticoagulants are ineffective or unsafe, including in (a) patients with an absolute contraindication to anticoagulation therapy because of active bleeding or anticipated bleeding from a predisposing lesion; (b) patients with a massive PE who survive but in whom recurrent embolism might be fatal; (c) patients who have recurrent VTE despite adequate anticoagulation therapy; and (d) demonstration of large free-floating clot loosely attached to the wall of the IVC.[67] There is little evidence to support the widespread use of vena cava filters. Vena cava filters reduce the risk of PE in the short-term, but also appear to increase the long-term risk for recurrent DVT presumably as a consequence of the accumulation of thrombus on the filter, which may partially occlude the vena cava, resulting in venous stasis.[67] Patients with permanent IVC filters should probably receive anticoagulant therapy as soon as possible and continue it indefinitely.[67] Given these concerns, retrievable filters that can be removed after the period of greatest risk for PE or after a transient bleeding risk has resolved have been developed and have been suggested for use in patients with transient contraindications to anticoagulation therapy. In reality most (65% in one report) "retrievable" filters are not removed.[67]

ANCILLARY THERAPY

In addition to anticoagulant therapy for patients with proximal DVT, wearing graduated compression stockings can reduce the risk of developing the postthrombotic syndrome by 50%.[80] To be effective, graduated compression stockings must fit properly and provide adequate pressure at the ankle (30–40 mm Hg). While the use of elastic compression stockings should be recommended for all patients with symptomatic DVT, in reality the discomfort associated with wearing properly fitted stockings along with the expense and unflattering cosmetic appeal makes routine use of compression stockings undesirable for many patients.

Strict bedrest was traditionally recommended following acute DVT based on the assumption that leg movement would dislodge the clot, resulting in PE. However, the evidence contradicts this assumption. Ambulation in conjunction with graduated compression stockings results in faster reduction in pain and swelling with no apparent increase in the rate of clot embolization.[6] Early ambulation and continued high activity level also reduce the likelihood of postthrombotic syndrome.[80] Patients should be encouraged to ambulate as much as their symptoms permit. If pain and swelling increase with ambulation, the patient should be instructed to lie down and elevate the affected leg until symptoms subside.

TREATMENT OF VENOUS THROMBOEMBOLISM IN SPECIAL POPULATIONS

Certain patient populations require unique considerations as outlined in the following sections.

Pregnancy

The use of anticoagulation therapy for the treatment of DVT or PE in pregnant women is common.[16] UFH and LMWH are the preferred anticoagulants for use during pregnancy (Table 26–24). They do not cross the placenta and evidence suggests they are safe for the fetus.[16] Warfarin should be avoided because it crosses the placenta and can produce fetal bleeding, central nervous system abnormalities, and embryopathy. The direct thrombin inhibitors also cross the placenta. To date, fondaparinux has not been formally evaluated in pregnant patients.[5]

Long-term UFH therapy has been linked to significant bone loss and osteoporosis, requires multiple daily injections, and must be monitored frequently (every 1–2 weeks) throughout pregnancy. Because of these limitations, many experts suggest the use of LMWH over UFH throughout pregnancy.[16] The evidence supporting this preference is weak however and UFH has been successfully used to prevent and treat VTE during pregnancy.[32] Anticoagulation for acute DVT during pregnancy should continue for at least 6 months postpartum (minimum total duration of therapy of 6 months).[16]

Pediatric Patients

Although seen far more frequently in adults, VTE in pediatric patients has become increasingly common secondary to prematurity, cancer, trauma, surgery, congenital heart disease, and systemic lupus erythematosus. Pediatric patients often develop DVTs associated with an indwelling central venous catheter. In contrast to adults, pediatric patients rarely develop idiopathic VTE.[33] While recommendations for antithrombotic therapy in pediatric patients are largely extrapolated from recommendations in adults, there are likely important pharmacokinetic and pharmacodynamic differences when antithrombotic medications are given to pediatric patients. The majority of literature supporting pediatric recommendations is derived from uncontrolled studies, case reports, or in vitro experiments. When possible, a pediatric hematologist with experience managing VTE should manage pediatric patients.[33]

Anticoagulation with UFH and warfarin remains the most frequently used approach for the treatment of VTE in pediatric patients. The recommended target aPTT and INR ranges as well as the duration of therapy are extrapolated from clinical trials in adults. Recent data suggest that extrapolating aPTT range from adults to pediatric patients is unlikely to be valid. However, in the absence of supporting clinical data, extrapolation of the adult aPTT range to pediatric patients remains necessary.[33] The recommended initial bolus dose of UFH is 75 to 100 units/kg given intravenously over 10 minutes followed by a maintenance infusion of 28 units/kg/h for infants 2 to 12 months of age and 20 unit/kg/h for children age 1 year or older.[33] Subsequent adjustments should be made every 4 to 6 hours to maintain the aPTT within the institution-specific therapeutic range. The usual warfarin starting dose is 0.2 mg/kg with a maximum of 10 mg. Infants require higher doses of warfarin per kg to maintain a target INR of 2.0 to 3.0 compared to teenagers and adults (mean dose 0.33 mg/

TABLE 26-24	Unfractionated and Low-Molecular-Weight Heparin Use During Pregnancy
Acute treatment	LMWH • Enoxaparin 1 mg/kg SC q 12 h or 1.5 mg/kg q 24 h or • Dalteparin 100 U/kg SC q 12 h or • Tinzaparin 175 U/kg SC q 24 h or UFH • Initiate using weight-based intravenous therapy and adjust dose to achieve therapeutic anti-Xa level for at least 5 days • Transition to SC adjusted-dose UFH administered q 8–12 h with midinterval anti-Xa activity in the therapeutic range[a]
Long-term treatment[b]	LMWH Maintain initial LMWH dose regimen throughout pregnancy or Alter LMWH dose in proportion to any weight change (usually gain) or Obtain monthly anti-Xa level measurements 4–6 hours after morning dose and adjust LMWH dose based on anti-Xa level (target = 0.5–1.2 units/mL if twice daily dosing; 1.0 to 2.0 units/mL if once-daily dosing) or UFH Obtain anti-Xa level at the midpoint of the dosing interval and adjust UFH dose to achieve an anti-Xa level of 0.3–0.7 units/mL
Issues at time of delivery	Elective induction of labor • Discontinue UFH or LMWH 24 hours prior to induction • Initiate therapeutic doses of UFH by IV infusion and discontinue 4–6 hours prior to expected time of delivery if risk of recurrent VTE is deemed high Spontaneous labor • For LMWH, if there is a reasonable expectation that significant anticoagulant effect will be present at time of delivery (a) epidural should be avoided, and (b) reversal with protamine sulfate may be considered • For UFH, monitor the aPTT and reverse with protamine sulfate if aPTT is prolonged near the time of delivery Postpartum • Commence UFH or LMWH as soon as safely possible (usually 12 hours following delivery) • Concurrently initiate warfarin therapy and discontinue UFH or LMWH when the INR is ≥2.0 • Continue anticoagulants for at least 4 weeks following delivery • Warfarin can be safely used by women who are breastfeeding

[a] Anti-Xa monitoring preferred as the relationship between aPTT and heparin levels differs in pregnant compared to nonpregnant patients.

[b] As pregnancy progresses the volume of distribution of LMWH changes, glomerular filtration rate increases, and most women gain weight.

aPTT, activated partial thromboplastin time; INR, international normalized ratio; IV, intravenous; LMWH, low-molecular-weight heparin; SC, subcutaneously; UFH, unfractionated heparin; VTE, venous thromboembolism.

From Bates et al.[16] and Ginsberg and Bates.[100]

kg, 0.09 mg/kg, and 0.04 to 0.08 mg/kg, respectively). The INR target range is 2.0 to 3.0. Frequent INR monitoring and warfarin dose adjustments are typically required. When compared to adults, only 10% to 20% of pediatric patients can be safely monitored once monthly. Obtaining coagulation monitoring tests in pediatric patients is problematic because many have poor or nonexistent

venous access. To address this problem, many clinicians recommend using fingerstick blood samples with a portable point-of-care monitor.[33] Because LMWHs have low drug-interaction potential, are less likely to cause HIT or osteoporosis, and require less frequent laboratory testing, they are an attractive alternative in pediatric patients. Enoxaparin, dalteparin, tinzaparin, and reviparin have been evaluated in pediatric patients. Most experts recommend that anti-Xa activity be monitored and the dose adjusted to maintain antifactor Xa levels between 0.5 and 1.0 units/mL 4 to 6 hours following subcutaneous injection. Compared to adults, children younger than 2 to 3 months of age or who weigh less than 5 kg have higher per-kilogram dose requirements to achieve a "therapeutic" response. The doses of LMWH for older children are generally similar to the weight-adjusted doses used in adults.[33] Warfarin can be initiated concurrently with UFH or LMWH therapy. Therapy should be overlapped for a minimum of 5 days and until the INR is therapeutic. Warfarin should be continued for at least 3 months for provoked VTE and 6 months for idiopathic VTE.[33] Thrombolysis and thrombectomy have been successfully employed in pediatric patients but published data are very limited—routine use is not recommended.[33]

Patients with Cancer

VTE is a frequent complication of malignancy. Furthermore, compared to patients without cancer, the rate of recurrent VTE in patients with cancer is threefold higher.[14] Warfarin therapy in cancer patients is often complicated by drug interactions (e.g., chemotherapy and antibiotics) and the need to frequently interrupt therapy for invasive procedures (e.g., thoracentesis, percutaneous biopsies, and abdominal paracentesis). Maintaining stable INR control is more difficult in this patient population because of nausea, anorexia, and vomiting.

CLINICAL CONTROVERSY

Evidence suggests that LMWH administered for 3 to 6 months after a DVT or PE is more effective than warfarin in preventing recurrent VTE events in patients with cancer. Despite the fact that current consensus guidelines recommend the use of a LMWH over warfarin for the long-term treatment of VTE in cancer patients, many practitioners still prefer the use of warfarin in these patients.

Randomized trials provide evidence that long-term LMWH monotherapy for VTE in cancer patients significantly decrease the rate of recurrent VTE without increasing bleeding risks compared to traditional therapy with warfarin.[6] Despite compelling data that cancer patients should be given LMWH instead of warfarin for the long-term treatment of VTE, the economic implications of this strategy have not yet been evaluated. In the absence of insurance coverage to offset the relatively high cost of long-term LMWH therapy, most patients are unable to afford it. Meta-analysis of 6 randomized, controlled clinical trials demonstrated no survival advantage of LMWH monotherapy compared to traditional therapy with warfarin.[83]

For patients with VTE and cancer who do receive LMWH, therapy should continue for at least the first 3 to 6 months of long-term treatment, at which time further LMWH can be considered or warfarin therapy can be substituted.[6] Anticoagulation therapy should continue for as long as the cancer is "active" and while the patient is receiving antitumor therapy.[6] A risk-to-benefit assessment should be performed on a regular basis and the overall clinical status of the patient should be considered, along with the risk for bleeding, quality of life, and life expectancy.[6] Many patients with terminal cancer receiving palliative care prefer LMWH over warfarin.[84] Consideration should be given to stopping anticoagulant therapy even in the presence of active cancer for patients who are at very high risk of bleeding complications.[85]

PHARMACOECONOMIC CONSIDERATIONS

Hospitalization is the main cost driver in the management of VTE.[86] Although the drug acquisition cost for the LMWHs and fondaparinux are substantially higher than UFH, avoiding hospitalization dramatically decreases the overall costs of DVT treatment. Cost-effectiveness analyses using decision modeling suggests that the treatment of DVT with LMWHs is more cost effective than the treatment with UFH in both inpatient and outpatient settings.[87] Based on this decision model, the LMWHs will reduce overall healthcare cost if as few as 8% of patients are treated entirely on an outpatients basis or 13% of patients are discharged from hospital early.

Despite the substantial cost savings stemming from outpatient DVT treatment from the perspective of the insurer, the reality is that some patients are unable to afford LMWH or fondaparinux prescriptions and are therefore denied outpatient treatment. Fixed dose UFH as described previously may provide a lower cost option for the outpatient treatment of VTE for selected patients who otherwise would not have been able to afford it.[29]

HEPARIN-INDUCED THROMBOCYTOPENIA

HIT is an uncommon but extremely serious adverse effect associated with heparin use.[31] The immune-mediated platelet activation and thrombin generation seen during HIT can lead to severe and unusual thrombotic complications. Morbidity and mortality associated with HIT is disturbingly high—up to 50% of patients who develop the disorder will suffer a thrombotic complication or die within 30 days in the absence of treatment. The diagnosis of HIT is based on laboratory findings that confirm heparin antibody formation and platelet activation (Table 26–25). To prevent the thrombotic complications associated with HIT, prompt discontinuation of heparin and initiation of an alternative anticoagulant therapy is imperative.[31]

ETIOLOGY AND PATHOPHYSIOLOGY OF HIT

Two types of thrombocytopenia associated with heparin use have been described.[88] As many as 25% of patients receiving heparin therapy develop a benign, mild reduction in platelet counts referred to as non–immune-mediated heparin-associated thrombocytopenia (HAT; previously called HIT type 1). HAT produces a transient fall in platelet count that occurs early, typically between days 2 and 4 of heparin therapy. The degree of thrombocytopenia is usually mild, with platelet counts rarely going below 100,000 mm³. It is not necessary to discontinue heparin therapy in these patients as platelet counts generally rebound to baseline values despite continued use. The exact mechanism of HAT is unknown; however, it may be the result of platelet aggregation, a dilutional effect, or diminished platelet production often seen in acutely ill patients. No clinical sequelae are associated with this benign phenomenon.

The second type of thrombocytopenia associated with heparin use is known as immune-mediated HIT (formally known as HIT type 2).[44,88] HIT is a severe pathologic adverse effect of heparin with a significant potential to cause thrombotic complications (see Table 26–25). The time course and magnitude of thrombo-

TABLE 26-25 Presentation of Heparin-Induced Thrombocytopenia

General

Venous thromboembolism is the most common presentation of heparin-induced thrombocytopenia (HIT), although arterial events (e.g., myocardial infarction, stroke) can occur. HIT should be suspected if a patient develops a deep vein thrombosis or pulmonary embolism while or soon after receiving unfractionated heparin.

Symptoms and signs

Thromboembolic events secondary to HIT produce the same signs and symptoms as those of other etiologies (see Clinical Presentation and Diagnosis).

Laboratory tests

The patient's platelet- count will typically be below 150,000/mm³ or drop more than 50% from baseline. The platelet count usually drops after 5 to 10 days of unfractionated heparin therapy, but may drop sooner if the patient has received heparin in the past 3 months.

Other diagnostic tests

An enzyme-linked immunoabsorbent assay (ELISA) for the presence of antibodies to the heparin–PF4 complex should be performed to confirm the diagnosis. Functional assays, including the heparin-induced platelet activation assay (HIPAA), the serotonin release assay (SRA), or the platelet-aggregation assay (PAA), may also be performed to confirm the diagnosis.

cytopenia associated with HIT differs from that of HAT. Platelet counts typically begin to fall 5 to 10 days following initiation of heparin and reach a nadir by days 7 to 14. The development of thrombocytopenia can be delayed (delayed-onset HIT) up to 20 days, and begin several days after heparin has been stopped in patients naive to heparin therapy. Conversely, so-called rapid-onset HIT can occur rapidly and abruptly (within 24 hours following heparin initiation) in patients with a recent exposure to heparin (i.e., previous 3 months).[31] Platelet counts commonly fall below 150,000 mm³ but rarely nadir as low as 20,000 mm³. In some cases, overt thrombocytopenia may not occur, but a drop in platelet count greater than 50% from baseline is considered indicative of HIT.[31]

The frequency of immune-mediated HIT is most powerfully related to the duration and type of heparin used and to a lesser extent the dose and route of administration.[31,44] The incidence of HIT associated with intravenous full dose UFH given for prolonged periods is significantly higher than that of low-dose subcutaneous UFH or LMWHs. The estimated overall incidence of HIT after 5 days of UFH use is 1% to 3% but the cumulative incidence may be as high as 6% after 14 days of continuous intravenous use. The incidence of HIT with low dose subcutaneous UFH in medical patients has been reported to be approximately 1%.[89] Low-molecular-weight heparins are associated with a significantly lower risk of HIT (<1%).[31] The incidence of HIT is higher with bovine UFH versus porcine UFH. In addition, the HIT risk varies with the exposed patient population: surgical patients > medical patients > pregnant patients.[31]

The pathogenesis of HIT involves an immunoglobulin mediated response to the heparin molecule leading to platelet activation and thrombin generation (Fig. 26–11).[44,88] With platelet activation there is release of PF4 from platelet granules. Heparin binds to PF4 forming a negatively charged polysaccharide molecule that is highly antigenic and stimulates the production of immunoglobulin (Ig) G antibodies. Although heparin-induced antibody formation occurs in 10% to 20% of patients treated with heparin, the vast majority never develop HIT. In patients who develop HIT, the heparin–PF4–IgG complexes bind to the Fc receptor on platelets, leading to further platelet activation and the release of PF4 and procoagulant microparticles from platelet granules. In addition, PF4 and heparin-like molecules bind to the surface of endothelial cells resulting in antibody-induced endothelial cell damage and the

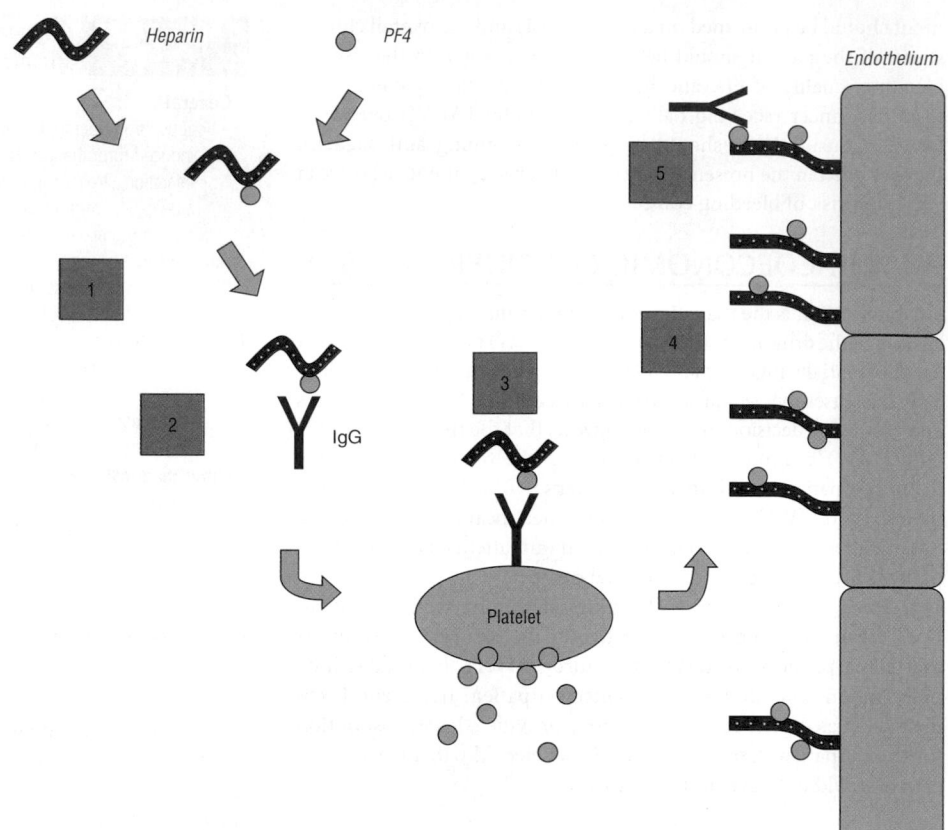

FIGURE 26-11. Pathogenesis of heparin-induced thrombocytopenia. (IgG, immunoglobulin G; PF4, platelet factor 4.)

release of tissue factor. The net result of this cascade of events is an increased risk of thrombotic events secondary to platelet activation, endothelial damage, and thrombin generation despite moderate to severe thrombocytopenia. Antibodies to the heparin/PF4 complex are transient, and they have been reported to disappear from the circulation within a median of 85 days.[31,44]

CLINICAL PRESENTATION AND DIAGNOSIS OF HIT

Thrombotic complications are the most common clinical sequelae of HIT (see Table 26–25).[31,44] The incidence of thrombosis can be as high as 50% in those patients with laboratory-confirmed immune mediated thrombocytopenia. Thrombosis may occur in patients with seemingly mild thrombocytopenia but platelet counts invariably have dropped more than 50% from baseline. This syndrome is poorly recognized and many, perhaps most, patients diagnosed with HIT initially present with thrombosis. Even among those diagnosed prior to the development of thrombosis, the prognosis is poor. In patients diagnosed with HIT without thrombosis and managed only by discontinuation of UFH, the risk of symptomatic thrombosis is 25% to 50%, and fatal thrombosis is 5%.[31,44]

Thrombotic risk is 30 times higher in patients with HIT compared with control populations.[89] Venous thrombosis is the most common thrombotic complication associated with HIT and most patients develop proximal DVT. PE occurs in 25% of patients with thrombotic complications and contributes significantly to mortality. Arterial thrombosis occurs less commonly.[31,88] Limb artery occlusion, stroke, and myocardial infarction are the most commonly reported arterial events. HIT has also been linked with atypical manifestations such as skin necrosis, venous limb gangrene, and anaphylactic-type reactions after intravenous bolus of UFH. Heparin-induced skin lesions occur in 10% to 20% of patients with HIT. Lesions range from painful, localized ery-

thematous plaques to widespread dermal necrosis. Amputation in such cases is frequently required. Mortality from HIT may be as high as 50% in patients with acute thrombosis. The relatively high frequency of thrombotic complications and poor outcomes associated with HIT emphasize the need for prompt recognition and diagnosis.[31,44]

The diagnosis of immune-mediated HIT is made based on clinical findings supplemented by laboratory tests confirming the presence of antibodies to heparin or platelet activation induced by heparin.[31,44] Thrombocytopenia is the most common initial event suggesting the diagnosis of HIT. New thrombosis shortly after the development of thrombocytopenia is a distinguishing feature in nearly half of all patients with HIT. The time course and magnitude of thrombocytopenia distinguish immune-mediated HIT from HAT. Acute thrombosis and skin lesions may also occur prior to the development of overt thrombocytopenia. HIT should immediately be suspected when these events occur in any patient on UFH or LMWH therapy.

Laboratory testing must be performed to confirm the diagnosis of HIT.[31,88] Laboratory testing is very helpful in patients with only mild to moderate thrombocytopenia in whom HIT is suspected. Two types of assays are available to detect the presence of heparin antibodies. Platelet activation assays, also known as functional assays, confirm in vitro platelet activation in the presence of therapeutic heparin levels. Functional assays include the heparin-induced platelet-activation assay, the serotonin release assay, and the platelet-aggregation assay. The heparin-induced platelet-activation assay and serotonin release assay tests have higher sensitivity and specificity than the platelet-aggregation assay but are technically more difficult to perform. Antigen assays that detect the presence of specific antibodies against the heparin–PF4 complex using enzyme-linked immunosorbent assays are also available. These tests have reasonably high sensitivity and specificity. The optimal test for laboratory confirmation of immune-mediated HIT is

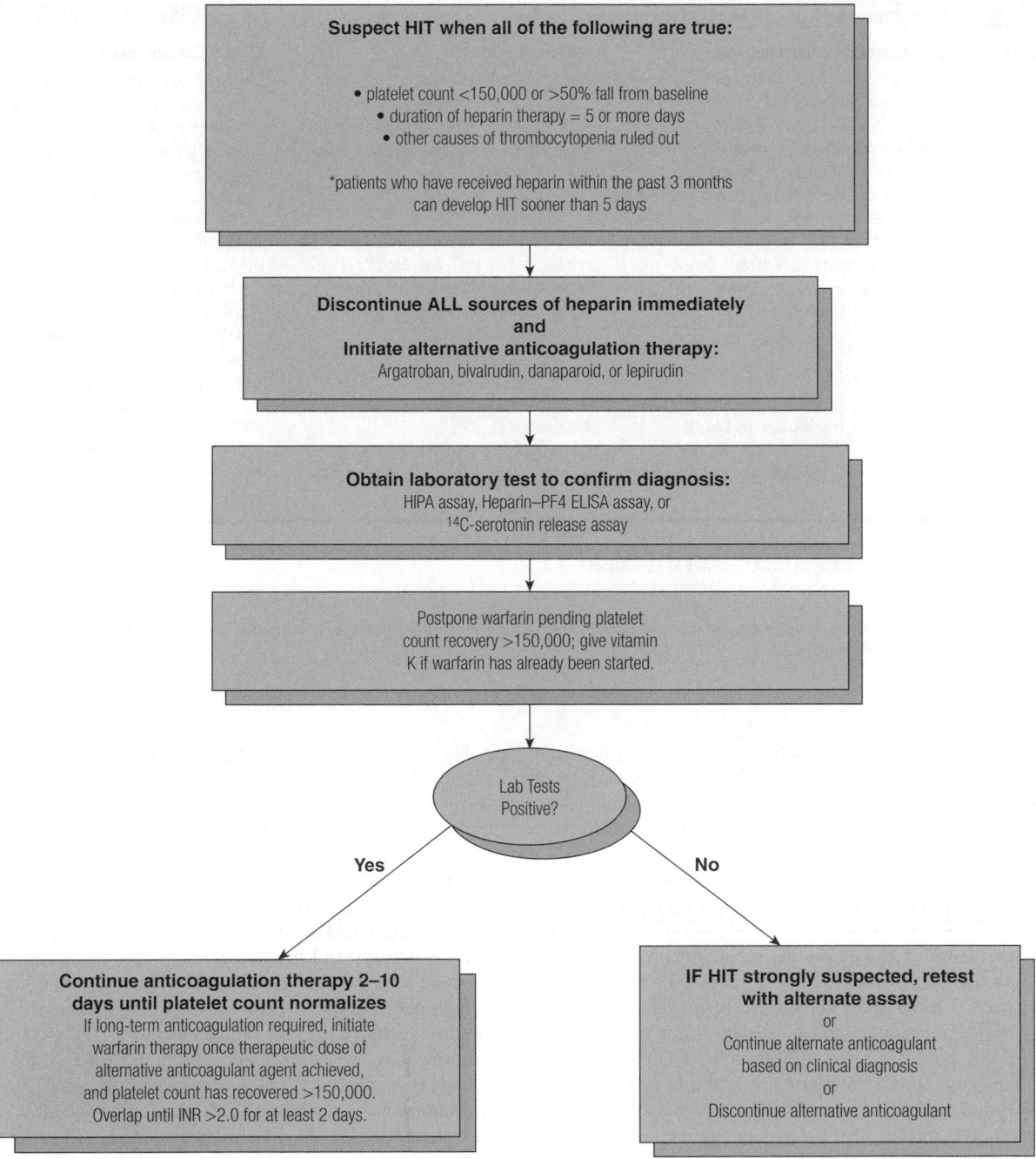

FIGURE 26-12. Treatment of heparin-induced thrombocytopenia (HIT). (HIPA assay, heparin-induced platelet activation assay; ELISA, enzyme-linked immunosorbent assay; INR, international normalized ratio.)

unclear. The most readily available test with the greatest sensitivity and specificity should be used. The combined use of functional and enzyme-linked immunosorbent assays may reduce false-negative results. When results of one test are negative or indeterminate in patients suspected of HIT, another test should be considered.

GENERAL APPROACHES TO THE TREATMENT OF HIT

The goal of therapy in patients with HIT is to reduce the thrombosis risk by decreasing thrombin generation and platelet activation. The 8th ACCP Consensus Conference on Antithrombotic Therapy has established recommendations for the treatment of HIT.[31] Once the diagnosis of HIT is established or strongly suspected, all sources of heparin, including heparin flushes, should

be discontinued and an alternative anticoagulant agent should be initiated (Fig. 26–12).[31,44] Even in the absence of thrombosis, patients with HIT are at extremely high risk for subsequently developing serious thrombotic complications without treatment. Because the time required for diagnostic laboratory results to be reported can be prolonged, it is crucial that alternate anticoagulant agents be initiated in a timely fashion to prevent new thrombosis. Anticoagulant agents that rapidly inhibit thrombin activity and are devoid of significant cross-reactivity with heparin–PF4 antibodies are the drugs of choice for the management of HIT (Table 26–26). In cases of severe or life-threatening thrombosis, surgical extraction of thrombi may be required. Limited data exists regarding the use of thrombolytic therapy in severe HIT with thrombosis. The use of warfarin for long-term anticoagulation in patients with HIT and thrombosis is recommended, but warfarin should

TABLE 26-26	Recommended Dose and Monitoring Parameters for Direct Thrombin Inhibitors to Treat Heparin-Induced Thrombocytopenia		
Agent Dose	**Manufacturer Recommended Dose**	**Monitoring Parameters**	**Clinical Considerations**
Lepirudin	0.4 mg/kg (up to 110 kg) slow IV bolus[a] (can also be given without bolus), followed by 0.15 mg/kg/h (up to 110 g) IV infusion[b] **Guidelines recommended dose[c]** Omit initial IV bolus or give at reduced dose of 0.2mg/kg if life-threatening thrombosis; The highest starting infusion rate should not exceed 0.1mg/kg/h	Obtain baseline PT, aPTT, CBC, Scr Check aPTT 2 hours after initiation and each dose change and adjust dose to achieve aPTT 1.5–2.5 times control. Once stable, monitor aPTT every 12 h	Dose must be reduced in patients with renal impairment; avoiding the bolus dose may reduce the risk of accumulation and may reduce the risk of anaphylaxis; antihirudin antibodies can occur in 40–60% of patients and can lead to reduced clearance. Concomitant warfarin requires dose adjustment
Argatroban	2 mcg/kg/min continuous IV infusion (no bolus); maximum infusion 10 mcg/kg/min	Obtain baseline PT, aPTT, CBC. Monitor aPTT 2 hours after initiation and each dose change and adjust dose to achieve aPTT of 1.5–3 times control (max. 100 s)	Dose reduction is necessary for those patients with hepatic impairment and in critically ill; will cause significant elevation in PT/INR; concurrent warfarin therapy requires special management (when INR >4, argatroban therapy should be withheld and the INR rechecked to determine if it is therapeutic)
Bivalirudin	0.15–0.20 mg/kg/h IV infusion (no bolus); approved dose for PCI: 0.75 mg IV bolus, followed by 1.75 mg/kg/h infusion up to 4 hours	Obtain baseline PT, aPTT, CBC, Scr Check aPTT 2 hours after initiation and adjust dose to achieve aPTT 1.5–2.5 times control	Not FDA approved for treatment of HIT

[a] Bolus dose is not advised in patients with renal impairement.

[b] Dose in isolated HIT: no bolus, 0.1 mg/kg/h infusion with aPTT adjusted to 1.5–2.0 times control.

[c] Clinical guidelines and more current data[31] suggest lower dose requirements for lepirudin compared to manufacturer recommended doses due to concern of heightened bleeding complications with the higher manufacturer recommended doses.

aPTT, activated partial thromboplastin time; CBC, complete blood cell count; HIT, heparin-induced thrombocytopenia; INR, international normalized ratio; IV, intravenous; PCI, percutaneous coronary intervention; PT, prothrombin time; Scr, serum creatinine.

only be initiated after substantial platelet count recovery has been documented (e.g., >150,000/mm³). In addition, great care must be taken when initiating warfarin in these patients as the risk of inducing further thrombosis secondary to inhibition of proteins C and S is possible.[31,44]

PHARMACOLOGIC TREATMENT OPTIONS

DTIs are the drugs of choice for the treatment of HIT with or without thrombosis (see Table 26–26).[31] Three DTIs are currently available in the United States for the treatment of patients with HIT—lepirudin, argatroban, and bivalirudin—but only the first two are FDA approved for this indication.[43,50] For the treatment of HIT, lepirudin and argatroban are administered by intravenous infusion and should be titrated based on aPTT testing. The comparative efficacy of these agents has not been formally evaluated, and they are considered equally suitable for the initial treatment of HIT. Some clinicians prefer argatroban because it has a shorter half-life, modest bleeding risk, and lower cost when compared to lepirudin.[90] Because of a short half-life, low immunogenicity, minimal effect on INR, and enzymatic metabolism, bivalirudin appears to be a promising alternative for treatment of HIT. However, to date, efficacy data is based only on case series.[48] Given fondaparinux is devoid of in vitro cross-reactivity to HIT antibodies, does not interfere with PT/INR measurement, and has enjoyed favorable experience in a few HIT case reports, it is a promising alternative for the management of HIT.[91] Further study is required, however, as fondaparinux has also been associated with HIT in rare cases.[38] Patient-related factors, such as the presence of renal or hepatic dysfunction, drug-specific features such as prior exposure to lepirudin, as well as institutional preference, availability, and cost should be used to determine the most appropriate agent. LMWHs are not recommended for use in HIT because they have nearly 100% cross-reactivity with heparin antibodies by in vitro testing.[31]

The use of warfarin during the initial treatment of HIT is potentially dangerous.[31,44] The rapid reduction in protein C concentrations induced early in the course of warfarin therapy further increases the risk thrombosis in patients with HIT. This concern is supported by the observation that several patients with HIT have developed venous limb gangrene and warfarin-induced skin necrosis when treated with warfarin. Patients with venous limb gangrene had relatively high INRs after the initiation of warfarin therapy and presumably had rapid depletion of protein C but persisting thrombin generation. Therefore, warfarin is contraindicated as monotherapy for the initial treatment of patients diagnosed with HIT. However, patients with HIT and thrombosis requiring long-term anticoagulation can be treated with warfarin if therapy is appropriately timed and carefully initiated. A conservative approach is to withhold warfarin until the patient is stabilized and platelet counts have substantially recovered at least above 100,000 mm³, and preferably above 150,000 mm³. If warfarin has already been initiated when HIT is diagnosed, reversing therapy with vitamin K (5–10 mg either IV or oral) is recommended. This may prevent the development of further thrombotic adverse events caused by protein C depletion. Warfarin can be reinitiated once platelet counts have been recovered (>150,000 mm³) but it should be overlapped with a DTI for a minimum of 5 days and until the full anticoagulant effect of warfarin has been achieved (i.e., INR within the therapeutic range for at least 2 consecutive days). Initial doses of warfarin greater than 5 mg should be strictly avoided in these patients.[31,44]

The management of pregnant patients with a history of HIT requiring anticoagulation therapy presents a challenge. Both UFH and LMWH are the anticoagulants of choice for pregnant patients requiring anticoagulation therapy. Women who develop HIT during pregnancy or who have a recent history of HIT (e.g., < 3 months) cannot use UFH or LMWH safely. Limited evidence exists for the use of DTIs in pregnancy. Lepirudin is known to cross the placenta; however, case reports suggest it may be safe for the management of HIT with thrombosis in pregnancy.[92] Danaparoid, a low-molecular-weight heparinoid not available in the United States that does not cross the placenta has also been investigated as a potential anticoagulant option in pregnant patients with HIT.[16] Limited case reports suggest that fondaparinux may also be a future potential alternative in pregnant patients.[93]

EVALUATION OF THERAPEUTIC OUTCOMES

The appropriate duration of therapy in patients with HIT will depend on whether the patient had a thrombotic event. HIT patients without thrombosis should continue therapeutic doses of alternative anticoagulant agents until platelet counts have normalized. Platelet counts should be monitored frequently, and patients should be watched closely for the development of new thrombosis after starting an alternate anticoagulant. Patients with thrombosis, either at the time of presentation or following the diagnosis of HIT, should receive therapy with an alternative anticoagulant such as lepirudin or argatroban followed by a transition to warfarin after the platelet count has recovered to >150,000 mm³. Warfarin therapy is usually continued for at least 6 months, or longer if indicated. The initial anticoagulant used should be continued until the INR is stable and therapeutic for more than two consecutive days. In addition, it is important to clearly document the occurrence of immune-mediated HIT in the patient's medical record and educate the patient regarding this adverse effect. Future use of UFH, particularly in the next 3 to 6 months, should be strictly avoided. As PF4–heparin antibodies are transient and usually cleared within 3 months, patients with a history of HIT should be tested for HIT antibodies prior to any future use of UFH. Although there are few data regarding the use if UFH in patients with a remote history of HIT, these patients should receive alternative anticoagulant agents for most indications until more rigorous data are available.[31,44]

NATIONAL QUALITY INITIATIVES

Despite the fact that several clinical interventions are known to be effective in preventing and treating VTE, adherence with various consensus guidelines regarding thrombophrophylaxis remains alarmingly low.[2] Although preventing VTE is a significant patient safety issue, there is little public awareness of the life-threatening nature of DVT and PE. A survey conducted on behalf of the American Public Health Association suggests that 75% of Americans have little or no awareness of DVT, and less than one half of respondents could identify any risk factors associated with its development.[94] Recognizing the lack of public awareness, several organizations have focused on increasing consumer knowledge of the risks, signs, and symptoms of VTE through increased media visibility.

Given the number and variety of clinical conditions or circumstances that place individuals at risk for VTE, improvements in VTE prevention and care have the potential to benefit many patients. Over the past decade, the focus on quality healthcare has been emphasized by the call to accountability through the Joint Commission's Agenda for Change, the Institute of Medicine's report on medical errors, the National Quality Forum's endorsed safe practices, the Leapfrog Group, and the demand for value by healthcare consumers (Table 26–27).[95,96] The National Quality Forum (NQF) has developed national consensus standards for VTE prevention and treatment that will be applicable to a variety of healthcare settings.[96] The outcomes of this effort will provide a

---

TABLE 26-27 Organizations Monitoring Quality Care

The Joint Commission
  www.jointcommission.org
  A not-for-profit healthcare accreditation organization that issues performance-based standards and assesses organizational compliance to improve patient safety and quality of care.
Leapfrog Group
  www.leapfroggroup.org
  An initiative of healthcare purchasing organizations seeking improvements in safety, quality, and affordability of healthcare, with funding from the Business Roundtable, Robert Wood Johnson Foundation, and member organizations.
National Quality Forum
  www.qualityforum.org
  A not-for-profit that develops and implements national strategies for healthcare quality measurement and reporting.

---

framework for measuring the effective screening, prevention, and treatment of VTE. NQF's recommendations include developing organizational policies that address staff education, treatment protocols, and adherence measurements to improve VTE prevention in the hospital. The ultimate goal of the NQF consensus standards is to facilitate early promulgation of VTE policies, risk assessment, prophylaxis, diagnosis and treatment services as well as patient education and organizational accountability. To that end, the Joint Commission has developed performance measures to enforce the NQF's recommendations.[95] Four major domains have been identified: risk assessment, prevention, diagnosis, and treatment. Six measures have been selected for implementation as core VTE quality measures. It is expected that compliance and reporting on these measures eventually will be tied to payment from governmental entities like Medicare and Medicaid (Table 26–28).

Hopefully, through the concerted efforts of government and accrediting agencies working with hospitals and other healthcare institutions, the incidence of DVT and PE will begin to fall. Systematic approaches to this problem are needed at every level, starting with increased public and health practitioner awareness, continuing with the uniform use of effective prophylactic strategies in patients at risk, and concluding with greater accountability with precise quality measurements.

TABLE 26-28 The Joint Commission's Proposed Performance Measures for the Prevention and Treatment of Venous Thrombosis

Number	Description of Proposed Performance Measure
1	Documentation of Venous Thromboembolism Risk Assessment/Prophylaxis within 24 Hours of Hospital Admission
2	Documentation of Venous Thromboembolism Risk Assessment/Prophylaxis within 24 Hours of Transfer to ICU
3	Venous Thromboembolism Patients with Overlap of Parenteral and Warfarin Anticoagulation Therapy
4	Venous Thromboembolism Patients Receiving Unfractionated Heparin by Nomogram/Protocol and with Platelet Count Monitoring
5	Venous Thromboembolism Discharge Instructions
6	Incidence of Potentially Preventable Hospital-Acquired Venous Thromboembolism

From The Joint Commission.[95]

ABBREVIATIONS

ACCP: American College of Chest Physicians

ACT: activated clotting time

aPC: activated protein C

aPTT: activated partial thromboplastin time

CNS: central nervous system

CTPH: chronic thromboembolic pulmonary hypertension

CYP: cytochrome p450

DTI: direct thrombin inhibitor

DVT: deep vein thrombosis

FDA: Food and Drug Administration

HAT: heparin-associated thrombocytopenia

HIT: heparin-induced thrombocytopenia

Ig: immunoglobin

INR: international normalized ratio

IPC: Intermittent Pneumatic Compression

ISI: International Sensitivity Index

IV: intravenous

IVC: inferior vena cava

LMWH: low-molecular-weight heparin

NQF: National Quality Forum

PE: pulmonary embolism

PESI: Pulmonary Embolism Severity Index

PF4: platelet factor 4

PT: prothrombin time

SC: subcutaneous

SCIP: Surgical Care Improvement Project

UFH: unfractionated heparin

VKOR: vitamin K epoxide reductase

VTE: venous thromboembolism

WHO: World Health Organization

REFERENCES

1. Blann AD, Lip GY. Venous thromboembolism. BMJ 2006;332: 215–219.

2. Geerts WH, Bergqvist D, Pineo GF et al. Prevention of venous thromboembolism: American College of Chest Physicians Evidence-Based Clinical Practice Guidelines (8th Edition). Chest 2008;133:381S-453S.

3. Schulman S, Beyth RJ, Kearon C, Levine MN. Hemorrhagic complications of anticoagulant and thrombolytic treatment: American College of Chest Physicians Evidence-Based Clinical Practice Guidelines (8th Edition). Chest 2008;133:257S-298S.

4. Ansell J, Hirsh J, Hylek E et al. Pharmacology and management of the vitamin K antagonists: American College of Chest Physicians Evidence-Based Clinical Practice Guidelines (8th Edition). Chest 2008;133:160S-198S.

5. Hirsh J, Bauer KA, Donati MB et al. Parenteral anticoagulants: American College of Chest Physicians Evidence-Based Clinical Practice Guidelines (8th Edition). Chest 2008;133:141S-159S.

6. Kearon C, Kahn SR, Agnelli G et al. Antithrombotic therapy for venous thromboembolic disease: American College of Chest Physicians Evidence-Based Clinical Practice Guidelines (8th Edition). Chest 2008;133:454S-545S.

7. Merli G. Diagnostic assessment of deep vein thrombosis and pulmonary embolism. Am J Med 2005;118(Suppl 8A):3S-12S.

8. The Surgeon General's call to action to prevent deep vein thrombosis and pulmonary embolism. 2008. Washington, DC: US Department of Health and Human Services.

9. White RH. The epidemiology of venous thromboembolism. Circulation 2003;107:I4-I8.

10. Dahlback B. Advances in understanding pathogenic mechanisms of thrombophilic disorders. Blood 2008;112:19–27.

11. Rosendaal FR, Reitsma PH. Genetics of venous thrombosis. J Thromb Haemost 2009;7(Suppl 1):301–304.

12. Crowther MA, Kelton JG. Congenital thrombophilic states associated with venous thrombosis: a qualitative overview and proposed classification system. Ann Intern Med 2003;138:128–134.

13. Dalen JE. Should patients with venous thromboembolism be screened for thrombophilia? Am J Med 2008;121:458–463.

14. Buller HR, van Doormaal FF, van Sluis GL, Kamphuisen PW. Cancer and thrombosis: from molecular mechanisms to clinical presentations. J Thromb Haemost 2007;5(Suppl 1):246–254.

15. Giannakopoulos B, Passam F, Rahgozar S, Krilis SA. Current concepts on the pathogenesis of the antiphospholipid syndrome. Blood 2007;109:422–430.

16. Bates SM, Greer IA, Pabinger I, Sofaer S, Hirsh J. Venous thromboembolism, thrombophilia, antithrombotic therapy, and pregnancy: American College of Chest Physicians Evidence-Based Clinical Practice Guidelines (8th Edition). Chest 2008;133:844S-886S.

17. Rosendaal FR, Helmerhorst FM, Vandenbroucke JP. Female hormones and thrombosis. Arterioscler Thromb Vasc Biol 2002;22:201–210.

18. Monroe DM, Hoffman M. What does it take to make the perfect clot? Arterioscler Thromb Vasc Biol 2006;26:41–48.

19. Mann KG, Brummel-Ziedins K, Orfeo T, Butenas S. Models of blood coagulation. Blood Cells Mol Dis 2006;36:108–117.

20. Crawley JT, Zanardelli S, Chion CK, Lane DA. The central role of thrombin in hemostasis. J Thromb Haemost 2007;5(Suppl 1):95–101.

21. Rijken DC, Lijnen HR. New insights into the molecular mechanisms of the fibrinolytic system. J Thromb Haemost 2009;7:4–13.

22. Kearon C. Natural history of venous thromboembolism. Circulation 2003;107:I22-I30.

23. McRae SJ, Ginsberg JS. Update in the diagnosis of deep-vein thrombosis and pulmonary embolism. Curr Opin Anaesthesiol 2006;19:44–51.

24. Tapson VF. Acute pulmonary embolism. N Engl J Med 2008;358:1037–1052.

25. Fancher TL, White RH, Kravitz RL. Combined use of rapid D-dimer testing and estimation of clinical probability in the diagnosis of deep vein thrombosis: systematic review. BMJ 2004;329:821.

26. Haines ST, Bussey HI. Diagnosis of deep vein thrombosis. Am J Health Syst Pharm 1997;54:66–74.

27. Hunt D. Determining the clinical probability of deep venous thrombosis and pulmonary embolism. South Med J 2007;100:1015–1021.

28. Hirsh J, Raschke R. Heparin and low-molecular-weight heparin: the Seventh ACCP Conference on Antithrombotic and Thrombolytic Therapy. Chest 2004;126:188S-203S.

29. Kearon C, Ginsberg JS, Julian JA et al. Comparison of fixed-dose weight-adjusted unfractionated heparin and low-molecular-weight heparin for acute treatment of venous thromboembolism. JAMA 2006;296:935–942.

30. Hull RD, Pineo GF. Heparin and low-molecular-weight heparin therapy for venous thromboembolism: will unfractionated heparin survive? Semin Thromb Hemost 2004;30(Suppl 1):11–23.

31. Warkentin TE, Greinacher A, Koster A, Lincoff AM. Treatment and prevention of heparin-induced thrombocytopenia: American College of Chest Physicians Evidence-Based Clinical Practice Guidelines (8th Edition). Chest 2008;133:340S-380S.

32. Clark NP, Delate T, Witt DM, Parker S, McDuffie R. A descriptive evaluation of unfractionated heparin use during pregnancy. J Thromb Thrombolysis 2009;27:267–273.

33. Monagle P, Chalmers E, Chan A et al. Antithrombotic therapy in neonates and children: American College of Chest Physicians Evidence-Based Clinical Practice Guidelines (8th Edition). Chest 2008;133:887S-968S.

34. Lovenox [package insert]. Sanofi-Aventis Pharmaceuticals, Bridgewater, NJ; December 2009. http://products.sanofi-aventis.us/lovenox/lovenox.html

35. Savi P, Herault JP, Duchaussoy P et al. Reversible biotinylated oligo-saccharides: a new approach for a better management of anticoagulant therapy. J Thromb Haemost 2008;6:1697–1706.

36. Bauer KA. New anticoagulants. Hematology Am Soc Hematol Educ Program 2006;450–456.

37. Arixtra [package insert]. GlaxoSmithKline, Reaserch Triangle Park, NC; January 2010. http://us.gsk.com/products/assets/us_arixtra.pdf

38. Blackmer AB, Oertel MD, Valgus JM. Fondaparinux and the management of heparin-induced thrombocytopenia: the journey continues. Ann Pharmacother 2009;43:1636–1646.

39. Gross PL, Weitz JI. New anticoagulants for treatment of venous thromboembolism. Arterioscler Thromb Vasc Biol 2008;28:380–386.

40. Karthikeyan G, Eikelboom JW, Hirsh J. New oral anticoagulants: not quite there yet. Pol Arch Med Wewn 2009;119:53–58.

41. Nutescu EA, Wittkowsky AK. Direct thrombin inhibitors for anticoagulation. Ann Pharmacother 2004;38:99–109.

42. Nutescu EA, Shapiro NL, Chevalier A. New anticoagulant agents: direct thrombin inhibitors. Cardiol Clin 2008;26:169–187.

43. Refludan [package insert]. Berlex Laboratories, Montville, NJ; 31 July, 2007. http://www.rxlist.com/refludan-drug.htm.

44. Arepally GM, Ortel TL. Clinical practice. Heparin-induced thrombocytopenia. N Engl J Med 2006;355:809–817.

45. Frenkel EP, Shen YM, Haley BB. The direct thrombin inhibitors: their role and use for rational anticoagulation. Hematol Oncol Clin North Am 2005;19:119–145.

46. Matheson AJ, Goa KL. Desirudin: a review of its use in the management of thrombotic disorders. Drugs 2000;60:679–700.

47. Angiomax [package insert]. The Medicines Company, Parssipany, NJ; December 2005. http://www.angiomax.com/Files/SalesAidRef/PI.pdf

48. Seybert AL, Coons JC, Zerumsky K. Treatment of heparin-induced thrombocytopenia: is there a role for bivalirudin? Pharmacotherapy 2006;26:229–241.

49. Serebruany MV, Malinin AI, Serebruany VL. Argatroban, a direct thrombin inhibitor for heparin-induced thrombocytopaenia: present and future perspectives. Expert Opin Pharmacother 2006;7:81–89.

50. Argatroban [package insert]. GlaxoSmithKline, Reaserch Triangle Park, NC; March 2009. http://us.gsk.com/products/assets/us_argatroban.pdf

51. Connolly SJ, Ezekowitz MD, Yusuf S et al. Dabigatran versus warfarin in patients with atrial fibrillation. N Engl J Med 2009;361:1139–1151.

52. Wolowacz SE, Roskell NS, Plumb JM, Caprini JA, Eriksson BI. Efficacy and safety of dabigatran etexilate for the prevention of venous thromboembolism following total hip or knee arthroplasty. A meta-analysis. Thromb Haemost 2009;101:77–85.

53. Nutescu EA, Shapiro NL, Chevalier A, Amin AN. A pharmacologic overview of current and emerging anticoagulants. Cleve Clin J Med 2005;72(Suppl 1):S2-S6.

54. Hursting MJ, Dubb J, Verme-Gibboney CN. Argatroban anticoagulation in pediatric patients: a literature analysis. J Pediatr Hematol Oncol 2006;28:4–10.

55. Kiser TH, Fish DN. Evaluation of bivalirudin treatment for heparin-induced thrombocytopenia in critically ill patients with hepatic and/or renal dysfunction. Pharmacotherapy 2006;26:452–460.

56. Coumadin [package insert]. Bristol-Myers Squibb, Princeton, NJ; January 2010. http://packageinserts.bms.com/pi/pi_coumadin.pdf

57. Eckman MH, Rosand J, Greenberg SM, Gage BF. Cost-effectiveness of using pharmacogenetic information in warfarin dosing for patients with nonvalvular atrial fibrillation. Ann Intern Med 2009;150:73–83.

58. Witt DM, Delate T, Clark NP et al. Outcomes and predictors of very stable INR control during chronic anticoagulation therapy. Blood 2009;114:952–956.

59. Witt DM, Sadler MA, Shanahan RL, Mazzoli G, Tillman DJ. Effect of a centralized clinical pharmacy anticoagulation service on the outcomes of anticoagulation therapy. Chest 2005;127:1515–1522.

60. Nutescu EA. Point of care monitors for oral anticoagulant therapy. Semin Thromb Hemost 2004;30:697–702.

61. Nazarian RM, Van Cott EM, Zembowicz A, Duncan LM. Warfarin-induced skin necrosis. J Am Acad Dermatol 2009;61:325–332.

62. Crowther MA, Ageno W, Garcia D et al. Oral vitamin K versus placebo to correct excessive anticoagulation in patients receiving warfarin: a randomized trial. Ann Intern Med 2009;150:293–300.

63. Nutescu EA, Shapiro NL, Ibrahim S, West P. Warfarin and its interactions with foods, herbs and other dietary supplements. Expert Opin Drug Saf 2006;5:433–451.

64. de Assis MC, Rabelo ER, Avila CW, Polanczyk CA, Rohde LE. Improved oral anticoagulation after a dietary vitamin k-guided strategy: a randomized controlled trial. Circulation 2009;120:1115–1122.

65. Douketis JD, Berger PB, Dunn AS et al. The perioperative management of antithrombotic therapy: American College of Chest Physicians Evidence-Based Clinical Practice Guidelines (8th Edition). Chest 2008;133:299S-339S.

66. Dobesh PP. Economic burden of venous thromboembolism in hospitalized patients. Pharmacotherapy 2009;29:943–953.

67. Anderson RC, Bussey HI. Retrievable and permanent inferior vena cava filters: selected considerations. Pharmacotherapy 2006;26: 1595–1600.

68. Dobesh PP, Wittkowsky AK, Stacy Z et al. Key articles and guidelines for the prevention of venous thromboembolism. Pharmacotherapy 2009;29:410–458.

69. Weitz JI, Hirsh J, Samama MM. New antithrombotic drugs: American College of Chest Physicians Evidence-Based Clinical Practice Guidelines (8th Edition). Chest 2008;133:234S-256S.

70. Merli G, Spyropoulos AC, Caprini JA. Use of emerging oral anticoagulants in clinical practice: translating results from clinical trials to orthopedic and general surgical patient populations. Ann Surg 2009;250:219–228.

71. Davidson BL, Sullivan SD, Kahn SR et al. The economics of venous thromboembolism prophylaxis: a primer for clinicians. Chest 2003;124:393S-396S.

72. Matchar DB, Mark DB. Strategies for incorporating resource allocation and economic considerations: American College of Chest Physicians Evidence-Based Clinical Practice Guidelines (8th Edition). Chest 2008;133:132S-140S.

73. Etchells E, McLeod RS, Geerts W, Barton P, Detsky AS. Economic analysis of low-dose heparin vs the low-molecular-weight heparin enoxaparin for prevention of venous thromboembolism after colorectal surgery. Arch Intern Med 1999;159:1221–1228.

74. Gordois A, Posnett J, Borris L et al. The cost-effectiveness of fondaparinux compared with enoxaparin as prophylaxis against thromboembolism following major orthopedic surgery. J Thromb Haemost 2003;1:2167–2174.

75. ASHP Therapeutic Position Statement on the Use of Low-Molecular-Weight Heparins for Adult Outpatient Treatment of Acute Deep-Vein Thrombosis. Am J Health Syst Pharm 2004;61:1950–1955.

76. Mamdani MM, Racine E, McCreadie S et al. Clinical and economic effectiveness of an inpatient anticoagulation service. Pharmacotherapy 1999;19:1064–1074.

77. Merli G, Spiro TE, Olsson CG et al. Subcutaneous enoxaparin once or twice daily compared with intravenous unfractionated heparin for treatment of venous thromboembolic disease. Ann Intern Med 2001;134:191–202.

78. Goldhaber SZ. Advanced treatment strategies for acute pulmonary embolism, including thrombolysis and embolectomy. J Thromb Haemost 2009;7(Suppl 1):322–327.

79. Kearon C. Balancing risks and benefits of extended anticoagulant therapy for idiopathic venous thrombosis. J Thromb Haemost 2009;7(Suppl 1):296–300.

80. Baglin T. What happens after venous thromboembolism? J Thromb Haemost 2009;7(Suppl 1):287–290.

81. Rodger MA, Kahn SR, Wells PS et al. Identifying unprovoked thromboembolism patients at low risk for recurrence who can discontinue anticoagulant therapy. CMAJ 2008;179:417–426.

82. Aujesky D, Hughes R, Jimenez D. Short-term prognosis of pulmonary embolism. J Thromb Haemost 2009;7(Suppl 1):318–321.

83. Akl EA, Muti P, Schunemann HJ. Anticoagulation in patients with cancer: an overview of reviews. Pol Arch Med Wewn 2008;118:183–193.

84. Noble SI, Finlay IG. Is long-term low-molecular-weight heparin acceptable to palliative care patients in the treatment of cancer related venous thromboembolism? A qualitative study. Palliat Med 2005;19:197–201.

85. Kearon C. Long-term management of patients after venous thromboembolism. Circulation 2004;110:I10-I18.

86. Tillman DJ, Charland SL, Witt DM. Effectiveness and economic impact associated with a program for outpatient management of acute deep vein thrombosis in a group model health maintenance organization. Arch Intern Med 2000;160:2926–2932.

87. Gould MK, Dembitzer AD, Sanders GD, Garber AM. Low-molecular-weight heparins compared with unfractionated heparin for treatment of acute deep venous thrombosis. A cost-effectiveness analysis. Ann Intern Med 1999;130:789–799.

88. Kelton JG. The pathophysiology of heparin-induced thrombocytopenia: biological basis for treatment. Chest 2005;127:9S-20S.

89. Girolami B, Prandoni P, Stefani PM et al. The incidence of heparin-induced thrombocytopenia in hospitalized medical patients treated with subcutaneous unfractionated heparin: a prospective cohort study. Blood 2003;101:2955–2959.

90. Lewis BE, Wallis DE, Hursting MJ, Levine RL, Leya F. Effects of argatroban therapy, demographic variables, and platelet count on thrombotic risks in heparin-induced thrombocytopenia. Chest 2006;129:1407–1416.

91. Efird LE, Kockler DR. Fondaparinux for thromboembolic treatment and prophylaxis of heparin-induced thrombocytopenia. Ann Pharmacother 2006;40:1383–1387.

92. Messmore H, Jeske W, Wehrmacher W, Walenga J. Benefit-risk assessment of treatments for heparin-induced thrombocytopenia. Drug Saf 2003;26:625–641.

93. Mazzolai L, Hohlfeld P, Spertini F et al. Fondaparinux is a safe alternative in case of heparin intolerance during pregnancy. Blood 2006;108:1569–1570.

94. American Public Health Association. Deep-Vein Thrombosis: Advancing Awareness to Protect Patient Lives. Public Health Leadership Conference on Deep-Vein Thrombosis. White paper; February 26, 2003. http://www.apha.org/NR/rdonlyres/A209F84A-7C0E-4761-9ECF-61D22E1E11F7/0/DVT_White_Paper.pdf

95. The Joint Commission. National Consensus Standards on the Prevention and Care of Venous Thromboembolism; April 2009. http://www.jointcommission.org/PerformanceMeasurement/PerformanceMeasurement/VTE.htm

96. The National Quality Forum. Establishing a patient-centered national action plan for deep vein thrombosis prevention, treatment, and research. Conference Proceedings; 2007.

97. Abrams PJ, Emerson CR. Rivaroxaban: a novel, oral, direct factor Xa inhibitor. Pharmacotherapy 2009;29:167–181.

98. Wittkowsky AK. Pharmacology of warfarin and related anticoagulants. In: Ansell JE, Oertel LB, Wittkowsky AK, eds. Managing Oral Anticoagulation Therapy. St. Louis, MO: Wolters Kluwer Health, 2009:149–160.

99. Booth SL, Centurelli MA. Vitamin K: a practical guide to the dietary management of patients on warfarin. Nutr Rev 1999;57:288–296.

100. Ginsberg JS, Bates SM. Management of venous thromboembolism during pregnancy. J Thromb Haemost 2003;1:1435–1442.

CHAPTER 27

Stroke

SUSAN C. FAGAN AND DAVID C. HESS

KEY CONCEPTS

❶ Stroke is one of the leading killers of individuals worldwide.

❷ Stroke can be either ischemic (87%) or hemorrhagic (13%).

❸ Transient ischemic attacks (TIAs) require urgent intervention to reduce the risk of stroke, which is known to be highest in the first few days after TIA.

❹ Carotid endarterectomy should be performed in ischemic stroke patients with 70% to 99% stenosis of the ipsilateral carotid artery, provided that it is done in an experienced center.

❺ Early reperfusion (<4.5 hours from onset) with tissue plasminogen activator (t-PA) has been shown to reduce the ultimate disability caused by ischemic stroke.

❻ Antiplatelet therapy is the cornerstone of antithrombotic therapy for the secondary prevention of ischemic stroke.

❼ Warfarin is the drug of choice for secondary prevention of cardioembolic stroke.

❽ Blood pressure lowering is effective in both the primary and secondary prevention of both ischemic and hemorrhagic stroke regardless of blood pressure.

❾ Blood pressure lowering in the acute stroke period (first 7 days) can result in decreased cerebral blood flow and worsened symptoms.

❿ Statin therapy is recommended for all ischemic stroke patients, regardless of baseline cholesterol, to reduce recurrent vascular events.

❶ Stroke is the leading cause of disability among adults and the third leading cause of death in the United States, behind cardiovascular disease and all cancers. Despite a 30% reduction in stroke mortality between 1995 and 2005, stroke occurs in the United States at a rate of almost 800,000 per year and results in 150,000 deaths.[1] Aggressive efforts to organize stroke care at the local and regional levels and increased utilization of evidence-based recommendations and national guidelines may have contributed to the improved outcomes.

Learning objectives, review questions, and other resources can be found at **www.pharmacotherapyonline.com**.

EPIDEMIOLOGY

There are currently 6.5 million stroke survivors in the United States, and stroke is the leading cause of adult disability.[1] Of those free of the diagnosis of stroke or TIA, however, almost 20% of individuals over the age of 45 years reported at least one stroke symptom,[2] suggesting rampant underdiagnosing. Owing in part to the need for expensive posthospitalization rehabilitation and nursing home care, the annual cost of stroke in the United States is estimated to be $69 billion.[1] Current projections are that death caused by stroke will increase exponentially in the next 30 years owing to aging of the population and our inability to control risk factors.[3]

African Americans have stroke rates that are twice those of whites, and the difference is exaggerated at younger ages.[1] In addition, geographic disparity in stroke incidence exists, such that many states in the southeastern United States have stroke mortality rates more than twice that of the national average.[1]

ETIOLOGY AND CLASSIFICATION

❷ Stroke can be either ischemic or hemorrhagic (87% and 13%, respectively, of all strokes in the 2009 American Heart Association report).[1,4] A classification of stroke by mechanism is given in Figure 27–1. Hemorrhagic strokes include subarachnoid hemorrhage, intracerebral hemorrhage, and subdural hematomas. Subarachnoid hemorrhage occurs when blood enters the subarachnoid space (where cerebrospinal fluid is housed) owing to either trauma, rupture of an intracranial aneurysm, or rupture of an arteriovenous malformation (AVM). By contrast, intracerebral hemorrhage occurs when a blood vessel ruptures within the brain parenchyma itself, resulting in the formation of a hematoma. These types of hemorrhages very often are associated with uncontrolled high blood pressure and sometimes antithrombotic or thrombolytic therapy. Subdural hematomas refer to collections of blood below the dura (covering of the brain), and they are caused most often by trauma. Hemorrhagic stroke, although less common, is significantly more lethal than ischemic stroke, with 30-day case-fatality rates that are two to six times higher.[5,6]

Ischemic strokes are caused either by local thrombus formation or by embolic phenomena, resulting in occlusion of a cerebral artery. Atherosclerosis, particularly of the cerebral vasculature, is a causative factor in most cases of ischemic stroke, although 30% are cryptogenic. Emboli can arise from either intra- or extracranial arteries (including the aortic arch) or, as is the case in 20% of all ischemic strokes, the heart. Cardiogenic embolism is presumed to have occurred if the patient has concomitant atrial fibrillation, valvular heart disease, or any other condition of the heart that can lead to clot formation.[7] Distinguishing between cardiogenic embolism and other causes of ischemic stroke is important in determining long-term pharmacotherapy in a given patient.

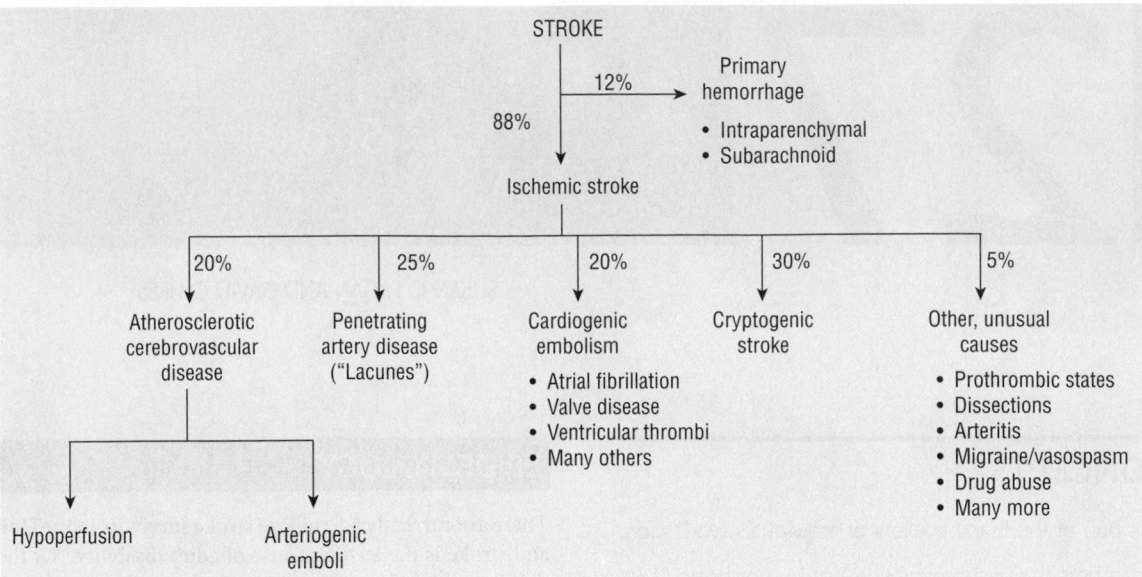

FIGURE 27-1. A classification of stroke by mechanism with estimates of the frequency of various categories of abnormalities. Approximately 30% of ischemic strokes are cryptogenic.

RISK FACTORS

Risk factors for stroke can be subdivided into nonmodifiable, modifiable, and potentially modifiable. In addition, risk factors can be either well documented or less well documented.[8] The main risk factors of stroke are listed in Table 27–1. Recommendations for risk factor reduction aggressively target the modifiable, well-documented risk factors, even in individuals with nonmodifiable risk.[8] The nonmodifiable risk factors are age, race, sex, low birth weight, and family history. An individual's risk of having a stroke increases substantially as he or she ages, with a doubling of risk for each decade older than 55 years of age. African Americans, Asian-Pacific Islanders, and Hispanics experience higher death rates than their Caucasian counterparts.[1,4] Men are at a higher risk of stroke than women when matched for age, but women who suffer from a stroke are more likely to die from it.[1]

The most common modifiable, well-documented risk factors for stroke include hypertension, cigarette smoking, diabetes, atrial fibrillation, and dyslipidemia. The treatment of hypertension, beginning in the mid-20th century, is thought to be primarily responsible for the drastic reduction in stroke death rates between 1950 and 1980 in the United States.[4] A second very important risk factor for stroke is cardiac disease. Patients with coronary artery disease, congestive heart failure, left ventricular hypertrophy, and especially atrial fibrillation are at increased risk of stroke.[8,9] In fact, the presence of atrial fibrillation is one of the most potent risk factors for ischemic stroke, with stroke rates from 5% to 20% per year depending on the patient's comorbid conditions.[10,11] Other known risk factors for atherosclerosis are also known to place patients at risk of stroke. Diabetes mellitus, dyslipidemia, and cigarette smoking are known atherogenic states that lead to cerebrovascular disease and ischemic stroke.[8,9,12]

TABLE 27-1	Risk Factors for Ischemic Stroke

Nonmodifiable risk factors or risk markers
Age
Gender
Race
Family history of stroke
Low birth weight

Modifiable, well documented
Hypertension–single most important risk factor for ischemic stroke
Atrial fibrillation–most important and treatable cardiac cause of stroke
Other cardiac diseases
Diabetes–independent risk factor
Dyslipidemia
Cigarette smoking
Alcohol
Sickle cell disease
Asymptomatic carotid stenosis
Postmenopausal hormone therapy
Lifestyle factors–associated with stroke risk
    Obesity
    Physical inactivity
    Diet

Potentially modifiable, less well documented
Oral contraceptives
Migraine
Drug and alcohol abuse
Hemostatic and inflammatory factors–fibrinogen linked to increased risk
Homocysteine
Sleep-disordered breathing

Goldstein LB, Adams R, Alberts MJ, et al. Primary prevention of ischemic stroke: A guideline from the American Heart Association/American Stroke Association Stroke Council: Cosponsored by the Atherosclerotic Peripheral Vascular Disease Interdisciplinary Working Group; Cardiovascular Nursing Council; Clinical Cardiology Council; Nutrition, Physical Activity, and Metabolism Council; and the Quality of Care and Outcomes Research Interdisciplinary Working Group. Stroke 2006;37:1583–1633. Source: American Heart Association, Inc.

PATHOPHYSIOLOGY

ISCHEMIC STROKE

In carotid atherosclerosis, progressive accumulation of lipids and inflammatory cells in the intima of the affected arteries, combined with hypertrophy of arterial smooth muscle cells, results in plaque formation. Eventually, sheer stress may result in plaque rupture, collagen exposure, platelet aggregation, and clot formation. The clot can remain in the vessel, causing local occlusion, or travel distally as an embolism, eventually lodging downstream in a cerebral vessel. In the case of cardiogenic embolism, stasis of blood in the atria or ventricles of the heart leads to the formation of local clots that can become dislodged and travel directly through the aorta to the cerebral circulation. The final result of both thrombus formation

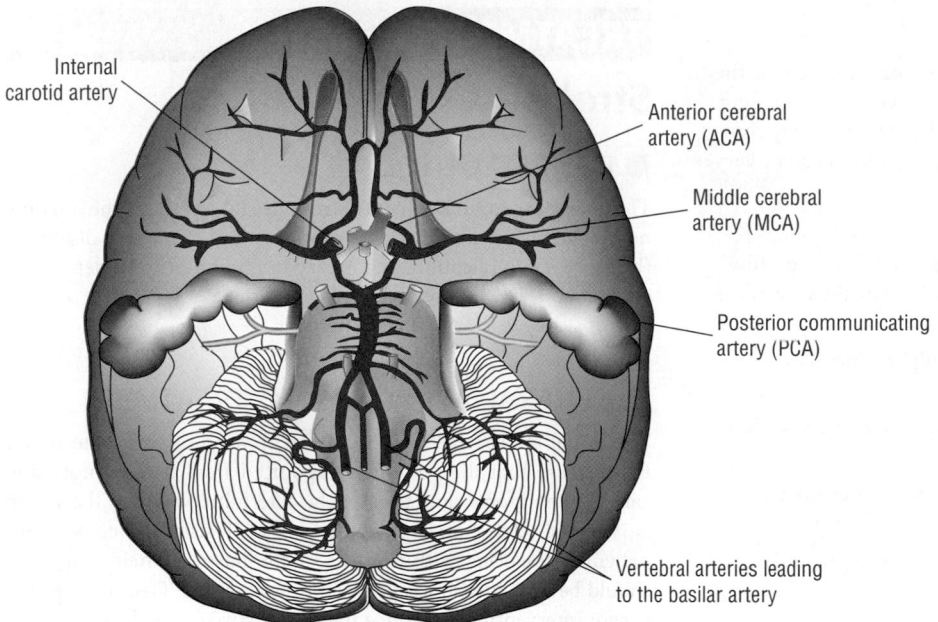

Internal carotid artery

Anterior cerebral artery (ACA)

Middle cerebral artery (MCA)

Posterior communicating artery (PCA)

Vertebral arteries leading to the basilar artery

FIGURE 27-2. Main arterial blood supply to the brain.

and embolism is an arterial occlusion, decreasing cerebral blood flow and causing ischemia distal to the occlusion.[13]

Normal cerebral blood flow averages 50 mL/100 g per minute, and this is maintained over a wide range of blood pressures (mean arterial pressures of 50 to 150 mm Hg) by a process called *cerebral autoregulation.* Cerebral blood vessels dilate and constrict in response to changes in blood pressure, but this process can be impaired by atherosclerosis, chronic hypertension, and acute injury, such as stroke. When local cerebral blood flow decreases below 20 mL/100 g per minute, ischemia ensues, and when further reductions below 12 mL/100 g per minute persist, irreversible damage to the brain occurs, which is called *infarction.* Tissue that is ischemic but maintains membrane integrity is referred to as the ischemic *penumbra* because it usually surrounds the infarct core. This penumbra is potentially salvageable through therapeutic intervention.

Reduction in the provision of nutrients to the ischemic cell eventually leads to depletion of the high-energy phosphates (e.g., adenosine triphosphate [ATP]), accumulation of extracellular potassium, intracellular sodium, and water, leading to cell swelling and eventual lysis. The increase in intracellular calcium that follows results in the activation of lipases, proteases, and endonucleases and the release of free fatty acids from membrane phospholipids. The critical step is damage to the mitochondria. In addition, there is a release of excitatory amino acids, such as glutamate and aspartate, that perpetuates the neuronal damage and the accumulation of free fatty acids, including arachidonic acid, and results in the formation of prostaglandins, leukotrienes, and free radicals. In ischemia, the magnitude of free-radical production overwhelms normal scavenging systems, leaving these reactive molecules to attack cell membranes and contribute to the mounting intracellular acidosis. All these events occur within 2 to 3 hours of the onset of ischemia and contribute to the ultimate cell death.[13]

Later targets for intervention in the pathophysiologic process involved after cerebral ischemia include the influx of activated inflammatory cells, starting from 2 hours after the onset of ischemia and lasting for several days. Also, the initiation of apoptosis, or programmed cell death, is thought to occur many hours after the acute insult and can interfere with recovery and repair of brain tissue.[14]

HEMORRHAGIC STROKE

The pathophysiology of hemorrhagic stroke is not as well studied as that of ischemic stroke. However, it is known that the presence of blood in the brain parenchyma causes damage to the surrounding tissue through the mechanical effect it produces (mass effect) and the neurotoxicity of the blood components and their degradation products.[5,6] Approximately 30% of intracerebral hemorrhages continue to enlarge over the first 24 hours, most within 4 hours, and clot volume is the most important predictor of outcome, regardless of location.[15] Hemorrhage volumes >60 mL are associated with 71% to 93% mortality at 30 days.[5,6] Much of the early mortality of hemorrhagic stroke (up to 50% at 30 days) is caused by the abrupt increase in intracranial pressure that can lead to herniation and death.[1] There is also evidence to support that both early and late edema contributes to worsened outcome after intracerebral hemorrhage.[6]

CLINICAL PRESENTATION (INCLUDING DIAGNOSTIC CONSIDERATIONS)

Stroke is a term used to describe an abrupt-onset focal neurologic deficit that lasts at least 24 hours and is of presumed vascular origin. A transient ischemic attack (TIA) is the same but lasts less than 24 hours and usually less than 30 minutes. The abrupt onset and the duration of the symptoms are determined through the history. The use of sensitive imaging techniques (magnetic resonance imaging [MRI] with diffusion-weighted imaging [DWI]) has revealed that symptoms lasting more than 1 hour and less than 24 hours, are associated with infarction, making TIA and minor stroke clinically indistinguishable. The location of the central nervous system injury and its reference to a specific arterial distribution in the brain are determined through the neurologic examination and confirmed by imaging studies such as computed tomography (CT) scanning and MRI. The main arterial supply to the brain is illustrated in Figure 27–2. Further diagnostic tests are performed to identify the cause of the patient's stroke and to design appropriate therapeutic strategies to prevent further events.[16]

CLINICAL PRESENTATION OF STROKE

General

☐ The patient may not be able to reliably report the history owing to cognitive or language deficits. A reliable history may have to come from a family member or another witness.

Symptoms

- The patient may complain of weakness on one side of the body, inability to speak, loss of vision, vertigo, or falling. Ischemic stroke is not usually painful, but patients may complain of headache, and with hemorrhagic stroke, it can be very severe.

Signs

- Patients usually have multiple signs of neurologic dysfunction, and the specific deficits are determined by the area of the brain involved.

- Hemi- or monoparesis occurs commonly, as does a hemisensory deficit.

- Patients with vertigo and double vision are likely to have posterior circulation involvement.

- Aphasia is seen commonly in patients with anterior circulation strokes.

- Patients may also suffer from dysarthria, visual field defects, and altered levels of consciousness.

Laboratory Tests

- Tests for hypercoagulable states (protein C deficiency, antiphospholipid antibody) should be done only when the cause of the stroke cannot be determined based on the presence of well-known risk factors for stroke. Protein C, protein S, and antithrombin III are best measured in the "steady state," not in the acute stage. Antiphospholipid antibodies as measured by anticardiolipin antibodies, β_2-glycoprotein I, and lupus anticoagulant screen are of higher yield than protein C, protein S, and antithrombin III but should be reserved for patients who are young (<50 years of age), have had multiple venous/arterial thrombotic events, or have livedo reticularis (a skin rash).

Other Diagnostic Tests

- CT scan of the head will reveal an area of hyperintensity (white) in the area of hemorrhage and will be normal or hypointense (dark) in the area of infarction. The CT scan may take 24 hours (and rarely longer) to reveal the area of infarction.

- MRI of the head will reveal areas of ischemia with higher resolution and earlier than the CT scan. Diffusion-weighted imaging (DWI) will reveal an evolving infarct within minutes.

- Carotid Doppler (CD) studies will determine whether the patient has a high degree of stenosis in the carotid arteries supplying blood to the brain (extracranial disease).

- An electrocardiogram (ECG) will determine whether the patient has atrial fibrillation, a potent etiologic factor for stroke.

- Transthoracic echocardiography (TTE) will determine whether valve abnormalities or wall-motion abnormalities are sources of emboli to the brain. A "bubble test" can be done to look for an intraatrial shunt indicating an atrial septal defect or a patent foramen ovale.

- Transesophageal echocardiography (TEE) is a more sensitive test for thrombus in the left atrium. It is effective at examining the aortic arch for atheroma, a potential source of emboli.

- Transcranial Doppler (TCD) will determine whether the patient is likely to have intracranial stenosis (e.g., middle cerebral artery stenosis).

TREATMENT

Stroke

■ DESIRED OUTCOME

The goals of treatment of acute stroke are (a) to reduce the ongoing neurologic injury and decrease mortality and long-term disability, (b) prevent complications secondary to immobility and neurologic dysfunction, and (c) prevent stroke recurrence.[17–19] Primary prevention of stroke is reviewed elsewhere.[8]

■ GENERAL APPROACH TO TREATMENT

The initial approach to the patient with a presumed acute stroke is to ensure that the patient is supported from a respiratory and cardiac standpoint and to quickly determine whether the lesion is ischemic or hemorrhagic, based on a CT scan. Ischemic stroke patients presenting within hours of the onset of their symptoms should be evaluated for reperfusion therapy. ❸ TIAs also require urgent intervention to reduce the risk of stroke, which is known to be highest in the first few days after TIA.[20] According to the ASA Guidelines, patients with elevated blood pressure should remain untreated unless their blood pressure exceeds 220/120 mm Hg, or they have evidence of aortic dissection, acute myocardial infarction (AMI), pulmonary edema, or hypertensive encephalopathy. However, this level of blood pressure may be too high, and a number of clinical trials are currently testing more aggressive treatment of hypertension in the acute setting. If blood pressure is treated, short-acting parenteral agents, such as labetalol and nicardipine, or nitroprusside, are favored. Current recommendations regarding management of arterial hypertension in stroke patients is given in Table 27–2.[17–19] In patients with subarachnoid hemorrhage, if an aneurysm is found by angiography, endovascular coiling or clipping via a craniotomy should be performed to reduce the risk of rebleeding. In intracerebral hemorrhage, patients may require external ventricular drainage (EVD) if there is intraventricular blood and evolving hydrocephalus (enlargement of the ventricles). Once the patient is out of the hyperacute phase, attention is placed on preventing worsening, minimizing complications, and instituting appropriate secondary prevention strategies. The acute phase of the stroke includes the first week after the event.[17]

■ NONPHARMACOLOGIC THERAPY

Ischemic Stroke

Surgical interventions in the acute ischemic stroke patient are limited. In certain cases of ischemic cerebral edema owing to a large

TABLE 27-2	Blood Pressure Treatment Guidelines in Acute Ischemic Stroke Patients	
Treatment	**Received t-PA**	**Did Not Receive t-PA**
None	<180/105	<220/120
Labetalol IV[a] or Nicardipine IV[b]	180–230/105–120	>220/121–140
Nitroprusside[c]	Diastolic >140	Diastolic >140

t-PA, tissue plasminogen activator.
[a]Labetalol IV = 10–20 mg, doubled every 10–20 minutes, to a maximum of 300 mg. Also can use an infusion of 2–8 mg/min.
[b]Nicardipine IV = infusion starting at 5 mg/h up to 15 mg/h.
[c]Nitroprusside IV = infusion starting at 0.5 mcg/kg/min, with continuous arterial blood pressure monitoring.
Adams HP, del Zoppo G, Alberts MJ, et al. Stroke 2007;38:1655–1711. Source: American Heart Association, Inc.

infarction, craniectomy to release some of the rising pressure has been tried. In cases of significant swelling associated with a cerebellar infarction, surgical decompression can be lifesaving. Beyond surgical intervention, however, the use of an organized, multidisciplinary approach to stroke care that includes early rehabilitation has been shown to be very effective in reducing the ultimate disability owing to ischemic stroke. In fact, the use of "stroke units" has been associated with outcomes similar to those achieved with early thrombolysis when compared with usual care.[17]

❹ In secondary prevention, carotid endarterectomy of an ulcerated and/or stenotic carotid artery is a very effective way to reduce stroke incidence and recurrence in appropriate patients and in centers where the operative morbidity and mortality are low. In fact, in ischemic stroke patients with 70% to 99% stenosis of an ipsilateral internal carotid artery, recurrent stroke risk can be reduced by up to 48% compared with medical therapy alone when combined with aspirin 325 mg daily.[21] In patients in whom the risk of endarterectomy is thought to be excessive, carotid stenting can be effective in reducing recurrent stroke risk.[22] Carotid endarterectomy remains preferred in elderly patients.[22]

Hemorrhagic Stroke

As in patients with subarachnoid hemorrhage owing to a ruptured intracranial aneurysm, in arteriovenous malformations (AVMs), surgical intervention to either clip or ablate the offending vascular abnormality substantially reduces mortality owing to rebleeding.[23] In the case of primary intracerebral hemorrhage, however, the benefits of surgery are less well documented. Although some patients undergo surgical evacuation of intracerebral hematomas, recommendations are limited to lobar (near the surface) and cerebellar hemorrhages.[6,15] Insertion of an external ventricular drain (EVD) for hydrocephalus and subsequent monitoring of intracranial pressure are done commonly and are the least invasive of the procedures done in these patients.

■ PHARMACOLOGIC THERAPY

Ischemic Stroke

Drug Treatments of First Choice: Published Guidelines The Stroke Council of the American Stroke Association has created and published guidelines that address the management of acute ischemic stroke.[17] In general, the only two pharmacologic agents with class I recommendations are intravenous t-PA within 4.5 hours of onset and aspirin within 48 hours of onset.

❺ Early reperfusion (<4.5 hours from onset) with intravenous t-PA has been shown to reduce the ultimate disability caused by ischemic stroke.[24,25] Caution must be exercised when using this therapy, and adherence to a strict protocol is essential to achieving positive outcomes.[17] The essentials of the treatment protocol can be summarized as (a) stroke team activation, (b) treat as early as possible within 4.5 hours of onset, (c) CT scan to rule out hemorrhage, (d) meet inclusion and exclusion criteria (Table 27–3), (e) administer t-PA 0.9 mg/kg over 1 hour, with 10% given as initial bolus over 1 minute, (f) avoid antithrombotic (anticoagulant or antiplatelet) therapy for 24 hours, and (g) monitor the patient closely for elevated blood pressure, response, and hemorrhage.[17]

Early aspirin therapy has also been shown to reduce long-term death and disability[26,27] but should never be given within 24 hours of the administration of t-PA because it can increase the risk of bleeding in such patients.[17]

The American Heart Association/American Stroke Association (AHA/ASA) guidelines address all pharmacotherapy used in the secondary prevention of ischemic stroke and are updated every 3 years.[28] It is clear that antiplatelet therapy is the cornerstone

TABLE 27-3 Inclusion and Exclusion Criteria for Alteplase Use in Acute Ischemic Stroke[17,25,29]

Inclusion criteria (all YES boxes must be checked before treatment)

YES
- ☐ Age 18 years or older
- ☐ Clinical diagnosis of ischemic stroke causing a measurable neurologic deficit
- ☐ Time of symptom onset well established to be less than 4.5 hours before treatment would begin

Exclusion criteria (all NO boxes must be checked before treatment)

NO
- ☐ Evidence of intracranial hemorrhage on noncontrast head CT
- ☐ Only minor or rapidly improving stroke symptoms
- ☐ High clinical suspicion of subarachnoid hemorrhage even with normal CT
- ☐ Active internal bleeding (e.g., GI/GU bleeding within 21 days)
- ☐ Known bleeding diathesis, including but not limited to platelet count <100,000/mm³
- ☐ Patient has received heparin within 48 hours and had an elevated APTT
- ☐ Recent use of anticoagulant (e.g., warfarin) and elevated PT (>15 second)/INR
- ☐ Intracranial surgery, serious head trauma, or previous stroke within 3 months
- ☐ Major surgery or serious trauma within 14 days
- ☐ Recent arterial puncture at noncompressible site
- ☐ Lumbar puncture within 7 days
- ☐ History of intracranial hemorrhage, arteriovenous malformation, or aneurysm
- ☐ Witnessed seizure at stroke onset
- ☐ Recent acute myocardial infarction
- ☐ SBP >185 mm Hg or DBP >110 mm Hg at time of treatment

Additional exclusion criteria if within 3-4.5 hours of onset:[29]
- ☐ Age greater than 80 years
- ☐ Current treatment with oral anticoagulants
- ☐ NIH Stroke Scale Score >25 (severe stroke)
- ☐ History of both stroke and diabetes

APTT, activated partial thromboplastin time; CT, computed tomography; DBP, diastolic blood pressure; GI, gastrointestinal; GU, genitourinary; INR, international normalized ratio; PT, prothrombin time; SBP, systolic blood pressure.

of antithrombotic therapy for the secondary prevention of ischemic stroke and should be used in noncardioembolic strokes. All three currently used agents, aspirin, clopidogrel, and extended-release dipyridamole plus aspirin (ERDP-ASA), are considered first-line antiplatelet agents.

In patients with atrial fibrillation and a presumed cardiac source of embolism, warfarin is the antithrombotic agent of first choice. Other pharmacotherapy recommended for secondary prevention of stroke includes blood pressure lowering and statin therapy. Current recommendations regarding the acute treatment and secondary prevention of stroke are given in Table 27–4.

■ GENERAL INFORMATION REGARDING SAFETY AND EFFICACY (INCLUDING PIVOTAL CLINICAL TRIALS)

t-PA

The effectiveness of IV t-PA in the treatment of ischemic stroke was first demonstrated in the National Institutes of Neurologic Disorders and Stroke (NINDS) Recombinant Tissue-Type Plasminogen Activator (rt-PA) Stroke Trial, published in 1995.[24] In 624 patients treated in equal numbers with either t-PA 0.9 mg/kg IV or placebo within 3 hours of the onset of their neurologic symptoms, 39% of the treated patients achieved an "excellent outcome" at 3 months compared with 26% of the placebo patients. An "excellent outcome" was defined as minimal or no disability by several different neurologic scales. This beneficial effect was reported despite a 10-fold increase in the risk of symptomatic intracerebral hemorrhage in the t-PA-treated patients (0.6% vs. 6.4%). Overall

TABLE 27-4	Recommendations for Pharmacotherapy of Ischemic Stroke	
	Recommendation	**Evidence**[a]
Acute treatment	t-PA 0.9 mg/kg IV[7–17] (maximum 90 mg) over 1 hour in selected patients within 3 hours of onset	IA
	t-PA 0.9 mg/kg IV[25,29] (maximum 90 mg) over 1 hour between 3 and 4.5 hours of onset	IB
	ASA 160–325 mg daily[7,17] started within 48 hours of onset	IA
Secondary prevention		
Noncardioembolic	Antiplatelet therapy	IA
	Aspirin 50–325 mg daily[7,28]	IIa A (all three as initial options)
	Clopidogrel 75 mg daily[7,28]	IIb B (over aspirin)
	Aspirin 25 mg + extended-release dipyridamole 200 mg twice daily[7,28]	IIa A (over aspirin)
Cardioembolic (esp. atrial fibrillation)	Warfarin (INR = 2.5)[7,28]	IA
All	Antihypertensive treatment[28]	IA
Previously hypertensive	ACE inhibitor + diuretic[28]	IA
Previously normotensive	ACE inhibitor + diuretic[28]	IIa B
Dyslipidemic	Statin[28]	IA
Normal lipids	Statin[48]	IB

ACE, angiotensin-converting enzymes; ASA, aspirin; INR, international normalized ratio; t-PA, tissue plasminogen activator.

[a]Classes and levels of evidence: I, evidence or general agreement that useful and effective; II, conflicting evidence about the usefulness; IIa, weight of evidence in favor of the treatment; IIb, usefulness less well established; III, not useful and maybe harmful. Levels of evidence: A, multiple randomized clinical trials; B, a single randomized trial or nonrandomized studies; C, expert opinion or case studies.[28] (Level A in reference 7–t-PA recommendation–does not require multiple trials, just randomized, well-controlled clinical trial.)

Data from Albers et al.,[7] Adams et al.,[17] Sacco et al.,[28] and Adams et al.[48]

mortality was not significantly different between the two groups (17% with t-PA and 21% with placebo). Patients with very severe symptoms at baseline (National Institutes of Health Stroke Scale [NIHSS] >20) and early ischemic changes on CT scan were shown to be at highest risk for the development of symptomatic intracranial hemorrhage. Even in patients at highest risk for bleeding, however, those receiving t-PA had better outcomes at 90 days than those who received placebo.[24]

Thirteen years after the NINDS trial, the European Cooperative Acute Stroke Study (ECASS) III demonstrated that, even when administered between 3 and 4.5 hours after the onset of symptoms, ischemic stroke patients benefit from t-PA when compared with placebo (52.4% vs. 45.2% excellent outcome; $P = 0.04$).[25] The benefit was less than reported with earlier treatment but the rate of excess hemorrhage was similar, leading to a change in AHA guidelines to recommend extension of the window.[29] An important caveat was that the exclusion criteria for later treatment are more strict and are given in Table 27–3.

Aspirin

The use of early aspirin to reduce long-term death and disability owing to ischemic stroke is supported by two large, randomized clinical trials. In the International Stroke Trial (IST),[27] aspirin 300 mg/day significantly reduced stroke recurrence within the first 2 weeks without effect on early mortality, resulting in a significant decrease in death and dependency at 6 months. In the Chinese Acute Stroke Trial (CAST),[26] aspirin 160 mg/day reduced the risk

of recurrence and death in the first 28 days, but long-term death and disability were not different than with placebo. In both trials, a small but significant increase in hemorrhagic transformation of the infarction was demonstrated. Overall, the beneficial effects of early aspirin have been embraced and adopted into clinical guidelines.

Antiplatelet Agents

All patients who have had an acute ischemic stroke or TIA should receive long-term antithrombotic therapy for secondary prevention.[28] ❻ In patients with noncardioembolic stroke, this will be some form of antiplatelet therapy. In a recent meta-analysis, the overall benefit of antiplatelet therapy in patients with atherothrombotic disorders was estimated to be 22%.[30] Aspirin is the best-studied of the available agents and, until recently, was considered the sole first-line agent. However, published literature has supported the use of clopidogrel and the combination product ERDP-ASA as additional first-line agents in secondary stroke prevention.

The efficacy of clopidogrel as an antiplatelet agent in atherothrombotic disorders was demonstrated in the Clopidogrel versus Aspirin in Patients at Risk of Ischemic Events (CAPRIE) trial.[31] In this study of more than 19,000 patients with a history of either myocardial infarction (MI), stroke, or peripheral arterial disease (PAD), clopidogrel 75 mg/day was compared with aspirin 325 mg/day for its ability to decrease MI, stroke, or cardiovascular death. In the final analysis, clopidogrel was slightly (8% relative risk reduction [RRR]) more effective than aspirin ($P = 0.043$) and had a similar incidence of adverse effects. It is not associated with the blood dyscrasias (neutropenia) common with its congener, ticlopidine, and is used widely in patients with atherosclerosis.

In the European Stroke Prevention Study 2 (ESPS-2), aspirin 25 mg and ERDP 200 mg twice daily were compared alone and in combination with placebo for their ability to reduce recurrent stroke over a 2-year period.[32] In a total of more than 6,600 patients, all three treatment groups were shown to be superior to placebo—aspirin alone (18% RRR), ERDP alone (16% RRR), and the combination (37% RRR). In addition, the combination demonstrated a significant advantage over the aspirin-alone group (23% RRR; $P = 0.006$) and the ERDP-alone group (24% RRR; $P = 0.002$). Headache resulting in discontinuation occurred in approximately 15% of the ERDP groups (four times more common than in the placebo group), and the aspirin-treated patients, even at the low dose of 50 mg/day, experienced significantly more bleeding than the other groups. The European/Australasian Stroke Prevention in Reversible Ischemia Trial (ESPRIT) confirmed the results of ESPS-2, in that the combination of dipyridamole (83% extended release) and aspirin (30–325 mg daily) was more effective than aspirin alone in reducing recurrent stroke.[33] Headache was again an important cause of discontinuation in the ESPRIT trial.

Lastly, in a large, multinational trial (PRoFESS—Prevention Regimen for Effectively Avoiding Second Strokes) comparing ERDP-ASA to clopidogrel, the risk of recurrent stroke was similar for the two antiplatelet agents, but clopidogrel was better tolerated with less bleeding and headache.[34]

Warfarin

❼ Warfarin is the treatment of choice for the prevention of stroke in patients with atrial fibrillation.[10,11,35] In patients with atrial fibrillation and a recent history of stroke or TIA, the risk of recurrence places these patients in one of the highest risk categories known. In the European Atrial Fibrillation Trial (EAFT), 669 patients with nonvalvular atrial fibrillation (NVAF) and a prior stroke or TIA were randomized to either warfarin (international normalized ratio [INR] = 2.5–4), aspirin 300 mg/day, or placebo. Patients in the placebo group experienced stroke, MI, or vascular death at a rate of

17% per year compared with 8% per year in the warfarin group and 15% per year in the aspirin group. This represents a 53% reduction in risk with anticoagulation.[10] Subsequent studies in the primary prevention of stroke in patients with NVAF have demonstrated that targeting an international normalization ratio (INR) of 2.5 prevents stroke with the lowest bleeding risk (Stroke Prevention in Atrial Fibrillation [SPAF III]); therefore, a target INR of 2.5 is recommended in the secondary prevention of stroke.[11,35] The emergence of orally active direct thrombin inhibitors (dabigatran) may challenge the favored position of warfarin for stroke prevention in atrial fibrillation.[36]

Use of warfarin in the secondary prevention of noncardioembolic stroke was addressed in the Warfarin Aspirin Recurrent Stroke Study.[37] In 2,206 patients with recent stroke, warfarin (INR = 1.4–2.8) was not superior to aspirin 325 mg/day in the prevention of recurrent events. Further data from the Warfarin-Aspirin in Intracranial Disease (WASID) trial demonstrated that aspirin therapy was as effective and safer than warfarin in patients with intracranial stenosis.[38] These studies led most clinicians to abandon the practice of using warfarin in all but patients with cardioembolic sources of emboli, mainly atrial fibrillation.

Blood Pressure Lowering

8 Elevated blood pressure is very common in ischemic stroke patients, and treatment of hypertension in these patients is associated with a decreased risk of stroke recurrence.[39] In the Perindopril pROtection aGainst REcurrent Stroke Study (PROGRESS), a multinational stroke population (40% Asian) was randomized to receive either blood pressure lowering with the angiotensin-converting enzyme (ACE) inhibitor perindopril (with or without the thiazide diuretic indapamide) or placebo.[40] Treated patients achieved an overall 9 mm Hg systolic and 4 mm Hg diastolic blood pressure reduction, and this was associated with a 28% reduction in stroke recurrence. In the patients who received the combination treatment (clinician's discretion), the average blood pressure lowering achieved was 12 systolic and 5 diastolic mm Hg, and this was associated with an even larger reduction in stroke recurrence (43%). Similar results were achieved in patients with and without hypertension. Based on the results of this study and other evidence of the tolerability and vascular protective properties of the ACE inhibitors, the Seventh Report of the Joint National Committee on Prevention, Detection, Evaluation, and Treatment of High Blood Pressure (JNC7) and the AHA/ASA guidelines recommend an ACE inhibitor and a diuretic for the reduction of blood pressure in patients with stroke or TIA.[28,41] **9** Early blood pressure lowering can worsen symptoms; therefore, recommendations are limited to patients outside of the acute stroke period (first 7 days).[28] Despite this, there is support for carefully restarting antihypertensive therapy after 24 hours in the acute stroke patient.[17]

Statins

10 The statins have been shown to reduce the risk of stroke by approximately 30% in patients with coronary artery disease and elevated plasma lipids.[42–44] The National Cholesterol Education Program (NCEP) considers ischemic stroke or TIA to be a coronary "equivalent" and has recommended the use of statins to achieve a low-density lipoprotein (LDL) concentration of less than 100 mg/dL.[45] When the Heart Protection Study was published, it provided evidence that simvastatin 40 mg/day reduced stroke risk in high-risk individuals (including patients with prior stroke) by 25% ($P < 0.0001$), even in patients with LDL concentrations of less than 116 mg/dL.[46] The investigators also showed that this practice is extremely safe, with an excess incidence of myopathy of 0.01%. The Stroke Prevention by Aggressive Reduction in Cholesterol (SPARCL) study went one step further by demonstrating, in stroke

patients, that atorvastatin 80 mg daily reduced the risk of recurrent stroke by 16% and coronary events by 42% while causing an increase in liver enzymes, but no increase in myopathy.[47] It is now recommended that ischemic stroke patients, regardless of baseline cholesterol, be treated with high-dose statin therapy for secondary stroke prevention.[48]

Heparin for Prophylaxis of Deep-Vein Thrombosis (DVT)

The use of low-molecular-weight heparins or low-dose subcutaneous unfractionated heparin (5,000 units three times daily) can be recommended for the prevention of DVT in hospitalized patients with decreased mobility owing to their stroke and should be used in all but the most minor strokes.[7,17]

■ ALTERNATIVE DRUG TREATMENTS

Aspirin Plus Clopidogrel

In the Management of ATherothrombosis with Clopidogrel in High-risk patients (MATCH) study, clopidogrel in combination with aspirin 75 mg daily was no better than clopidogrel alone in secondary stroke prevention.[49] However, the combination has been studied in patients with acute coronary syndromes and patients undergoing percutaneous coronary interventions and shown to be significantly more effective than aspirin alone in reducing MI, stroke, and cardiovascular death.[50,51] Also, when clopidogrel was used with aspirin, the risk of life-threatening bleeding increased from 1.3% to 2.6%.[49] In the Clopidogrel for High Atherothrombotic Risk and Ischemic Stabilization, Management and Avoidance (CHARISMA) trial, the combination was again found to significantly increase serious bleeding in a high-risk atherosclerosis population (clinically evident disease or multiple risk factors) with no consistent benefit in terms of preventing vascular events, when compared with aspirin alone.[52] This combination can only be recommended in patients with a recent history of MI or coronary stent placement and only with ultra–low-dose aspirin to minimize bleeding risk.[53]

Angiotensin II Receptor Blockers

Angiotensin II receptor blockers (ARBs) have also been shown to reduce the risk of stroke. In the Losartan Intervention For Endpoint Reduction in Hypertension (LIFE) study, losartan and metoprolol were compared for their ability to reduce blood pressure and prevent cardiovascular events in a group of severely hypertensive patients.[54] Despite similar reductions in blood pressure of approximately 30/16 mm Hg, the losartan group experienced a 24% reduction in the risk of stroke. In a similar study comparing eprosartan to nitrendipine, the ARB eprosartan was superior to the calcium channel blocker in reducing recurrent stroke risk, when equal blood pressure lowering was achieved.[55] Although the use of telmisartan failed to add additional benefit to adequately treated stroke patients in the PRoFESS trial,[34] the ARBs should be considered in patients unable to tolerate ACE inhibitors for blood pressure lowering after acute ischemic stroke.

Heparins

The use of full-dose unfractionated heparin in the acute stroke period has never been proven to positively affect stroke outcome, and it significantly increases the risk of intracerebral hemorrhage.[7,17] Trials of low-molecular-weight heparins or heparinoids have been largely negative and do not support their routine use in stroke patients.[56–58] Other potential but unproven uses for treatment doses of either unfractionated or low-molecular-weight heparins include bridge therapy in patients being initiated on warfarin, carotid dissection, or continuous worsening of ischemia despite adequate antiplatelet therapy.[7]

■ DRUG CLASS INFORMATION

Aspirin

Aspirin exerts its antiplatelet effect by irreversibly inhibiting cyclooxygenase, which, in platelets, prevents conversion of arachidonic acid to thromboxane A_2 (TXA_2), which is a powerful vasoconstrictor and stimulator of platelet aggregation. Platelets remain impaired for their life span (5 to 7 days) after exposure to aspirin. Aspirin also inhibits prostacyclin (PGI_2) activity in the smooth muscle of vascular walls. PGI_2 inhibits platelet aggregation, and the vascular endothelium can synthesize prostacyclin such that the platelet antiaggregating effect is maintained. The suppression of PGI_2 production by aspirin has been found to be dose and duration related; the higher the dose, the longer the cyclooxygenase production is suppressed. Therefore, the lower the aspirin dose, the less effect on PGI_2.[7] The optimal dose of aspirin should be the dose that inhibits TXA_2 with the least amount of PGI_2 inhibition. It has been shown that an aspirin dose of 325 mg/day will inhibit TXA_2 but will not significantly inhibit PGI_2 production. There is probably a point at which lower doses of aspirin do not completely block TXA_2, and recent studies indicate that the lowest effective dose may be in the range of 50 mg/day.[59] Upper GI discomfort and bleeding are the most common adverse effects of aspirin and have been shown to be dose related. The highest rates of GI bleeding (5%) have been reported in patients receiving 1,200 mg/day as compared with rates of 2% in patients taking the more commonly prescribed 300 mg/day. Upper GI symptoms are much more common than frank bleeding, however, with 40% of patients affected at 1,200 mg/day and 25% at 300 mg/day.[60] In the ESPS-2 study, even 50 mg/day of aspirin was associated with a twofold increase in bleeding over the placebo group.[32]

Low doses (<100 mg) of aspirin quickly inhibit cyclooxygenase in all the platelets in the circulation. Therefore, the onset of the antiplatelet effect of aspirin is less than 60 minutes.[61] It has been reported, however, that some patients either have or develop "aspirin resistance" and can require higher doses to achieve the desired antiplatelet effect.[62] Despite this, routine testing for aspirin resistance is not recommended. It was observed recently that administration of ibuprofen prior to the administration of a daily aspirin dose inhibits the aspirin from binding irreversibly to the cyclooxygenase and can decrease its antiplatelet effect.[63] Current recommendations are to administer aspirin at least 2 hours before ibuprofen or to wait at least 4 hours after an ibuprofen dose.

Aspirin also has an antiinflammatory effect as it reduces levels of C-reactive protein (CRP), and this may partially explain its mechanism of action at reducing vascular events.[64]

Extended-Release Dipyridamole Plus Aspirin

Early studies of the role of dipyridamole in stroke prevention failed to show a benefit over that realized by aspirin alone. Dipyridamole in high doses is thought to inhibit platelet aggregation by inhibiting phosphodiesterase, leading to accumulation of cyclic adenosine monophosphate (cAMP) and cyclic guanosine monophosphate (cGMP) intracellularly, which prevent platelet activation. In addition, dipyridamole also enhances the antithrombotic potential of the vascular wall.[65] The ESPS-2 demonstrated the efficacy of high-dose ERDP alone and in combination with aspirin in secondary stroke prevention.[32] The extended-release formulation of dipyridamole is important in that it allows twice-daily administration and higher doses to be tolerated in patients. The use of immediate-release generic dipyridamole in combination with regular aspirin, in order to reduce costs, is unproven and should be discouraged.

In the ESPS-2, 25% of the patients who received combination dipyridamole and aspirin discontinued the therapy early, and the rate of discontinuation owing to headache was more than three times as common (10%) as in the aspirin-alone group (3%).[32] Even when patients were carefully educated and coached in the PRoFESS trial, discontinuation due to headache was six times higher in the ERDP-aspirin group (5.9% vs. 0.9%).[34] The headache caused by ERDP-ASA is mostly self-limiting and decreases after several days.[66]

Clopidogrel

Clopidogrel has a unique platelet antiaggregatory effect in that it is an inhibitor of the adenosine diphosphate (ADP) pathway of platelet aggregation and inhibits known stimuli to platelet aggregation.[7,31] This effect causes an alteration of the platelet membrane and interference with the membrane–fibrinogenic interaction leading to a blocking of the platelet glycoprotein IIb/IIIa receptor. A time lag of 3 to 7 days before the antiplatelet effect is maximal should be expected. The tolerability of clopidogrel 75 mg/day is at least as good as medium-dose (325 mg/day) aspirin, and there is less GI bleeding.[31] Clopidogrel is associated with an increased risk of diarrhea and rash, but discontinuation rates owing to adverse effects are similar to those with aspirin 325 mg/day (5.3% to 6%, respectively).[31] There is no excess neutropenia in patients taking clopidogrel, and rates of thrombotic thrombocytopenic purpura probably are no greater than background rates.[67]

Clopidogrel is a thienopyridine prodrug and needs to be biotransformed by the liver to an active metabolite. Evidence suggests that the antiplatelet effects of clopidogrel can be diminished in patients with reduced function CYP2C19[68] or in those receiving agents that inhibit hepatic metabolism.[69] Although high doses of the lipophilic statins atorvastatin and simvastatin can diminish the effectiveness of clopidogrel to inhibit platelet aggregation in vitro, there does not appear to be any adverse effect on atherothrombotic event rates.[70] In contrast, in a retrospective analysis of 8,205 patients, concomitant proton pump inhibitor and clopidogrel treatment was associated with increased adverse vascular outcomes after acute coronary syndromes.[69] Careful consideration should be given to using clopidogrel in patients with reduced ability to biotransform the agent to its active metabolite.

■ INVESTIGATIONAL STRATEGIES

Reperfusion

Various investigations aimed at opening the occluded cerebral artery and preserving its patency are under way in acute ischemic stroke patients.[71] Strategies being tried include longer-acting fibrinolytic agents, intraarterial fibrinolysis with t-PA and other agents, and endovascular clot removal using mechanical and laser-guided approaches. In addition, investigators are trying to identify, using sensitive MRI techniques, which patients benefit from reperfusion at time points outside the approved time window. Undoubtedly, efforts to reperfuse the ischemic brain will continue to be explored, so more patients will be eligible for this therapy.

Neuroprotection and Neurorestoration

Although many different neuroprotective agents have been studied in clinical trials of acute ischemic stroke, most have been unsuccessful.[72] Some of the most promising are agents with multiple proposed mechanisms of protection (e.g., albumin infusions, and minocycline).[72] In addition, hope exists that clinicians will be able to enhance the reparative process of the brain (neurorestoration) through targeted neurorehabilitation, membrane stabilization (citicoline),[73] and the use of neural and cell transplantation.[74]

A promising nonpharmacologic strategy that has been shown to provide neuroprotection in patients has been hypothermia.[72]

Clinical trials are under way to optimize the mechanism of cooling the ischemic brain (intravascular coils vs. surface cooling) and rewarming the patient after hypothermia.

HEMORRHAGIC STROKE

There are currently no standard pharmacologic strategies for treating intracerebral hemorrhage (ICH).[6] Medical guidelines for the management of blood pressure, raised intracranial pressure, and other medical complications of ICH are those required for the management of any acutely ill patient in a neurointensive care unit.[15] When ICH occurs in a patient on warfarin (INR >1.3), rapid reversal of anticoagulation to prevent expansion and allow surgical intervention is recommended. The methods recommended to achieve reversal include intravenous vitamin K, fresh frozen plasma (FFP), and hemostatic agents (factor VIIa and prothrombin-complex concentrate (PCC).[15,75] The optimal approach is yet to be determined.

Subarachnoid hemorrhage (SAH) owing to aneurysm rupture is associated with a high incidence of delayed cerebral ischemia (DCI) in the 2 weeks following the bleeding episode. Vasospasm of the cerebral vasculature is thought to be responsible for DCI and occurs between 4 and 21 days after the bleed, peaking at days 5 through 9.[23] The calcium channel blocker nimodipine (60 mg every 4 hours for 21 days), along with maintenance of intravascular volume with pressor therapy, is recommended to reduce the incidence and severity of neurologic deficits owing to DCI.[23]

PHARMACOECONOMIC CONSIDERATIONS

Although t-PA is expensive, when the total healthcare costs are factored in, savings can accrue to the healthcare system as a direct result of appropriate t-PA therapy.[76] It has been estimated that, at a rate of $600 per patient treated, annual cost savings of $15 and $22 million could be realized by increasing national t-PA use to 4% and 6%, respectively (from the current 2%).[77]

In antithrombotic prophylaxis for atrial fibrillation, warfarin therapy was evaluated using quality-adjusted life-years (QALYs) saved.[78] It was found that in patients with atrial fibrillation and one additional risk factor, warfarin therapy cost $8,000 per QALY saved. In higher-risk patients, those with atrial fibrillation and two or more risk factors, warfarin use is cost saving. The cost-effectiveness of the various other secondary prevention strategies have been determined as well.[79,80] Without a doubt, aspirin, owing to its extremely low acquisition cost (pennies daily), is cost saving. In other words, it reduces costs at the same time as saving QALYs. The use of clopidogrel or ERDP-ASA is associated with higher efficacy but significantly greater costs as well (up to $3 daily). In fact ERDP-ASA was associated with $5,000 to $15,000 per QALY (adjusted for the acquisition cost) and clopidogrel was $26,580 per QALY. In addition, high-dose atorvastatin, as administered to stroke patients in the SPARCL trial, was estimated to result in an additional cost of $6,500 to $21,000 per QALY gained.[80] Any cost per QALY less than $50,000 is thought to be "cost-effective."[79] These estimates are extremely dependent on the assumptions made in the model. Cost-effectiveness in an individual patient is much more difficult to discern.

Primary prevention strategies that address the risk factors for ischemic stroke can be powerful in reducing the costs of stroke. Many of the stroke risk factors can be modified and some eliminated at very low costs (lifestyle changes), therefore developing risk-factor-reduction strategies can be the most cost-effective measure of all. More research is needed in identifying the cost-effectiveness of other forms of acute stroke treatment.

CLINICAL CONTROVERSIES

The use of full-dose unfractionated heparin in the management of acute ischemic stroke remains controversial despite years of debate and a lack of evidence supporting its use. Proponents of the therapy cite strong anecdotal evidence of positive responses in selected patients who have never been studied in clinical trials.

The use of intracranial angioplasty and stenting is strongly supported in the few institutions where the technology exists. Whether these procedures should be attempted in patients outside clinical trials remains controversial.

The use of surgical evacuation of intracranial hemorrhage with and without instillation of fibrinolytic agents is controversial. Although fervently pursued in select centers and countries, indications and outcomes are not known. Results of ongoing clinical trials can assist in settling this controversy.

EVALUATION OF THERAPEUTIC OUTCOMES

MONITORING OF THE PHARMACEUTICAL CARE PLAN

Patients with acute stroke should be monitored intensely for the development of neurologic worsening (recurrence or extension), complications (thromboembolism or infection), or adverse effects from pharmacologic or nonpharmacologic interventions. The most common reasons for deterioration in a stroke patient are (a) extension of the original lesion—ischemic or hemorrhagic—in the brain, (b) development of cerebral edema and raised intracranial pressure, (c) hypertensive emergency, (d) infection (urinary and respiratory most common), (e) venous thromboembolism (DVT and pulmonary embolism), (f) electrolyte abnormalities and cardiac rhythm disturbances (can be associated with brain injury), and (g) recurrent stroke.

The approach to monitoring the stroke patient is summarized in Table 27–5. The plan should be customized for individual patients based on their comorbidities and ongoing disease processes.

ABBREVIATIONS

ACE: angiotensin-converting enzyme

AMI: acute myocardial infarction

ADP: adenosine diphosphate

AHA: American Heart Association

ARB: angiotensin II receptor blocker

ATP: adenosine triphosphate

AVM: arteriovenous malformation

cAMP: cyclic adenosine monophosphate

CD: carotid Doppler

cGMP: cyclic guanosine monophosphate

CRP: C-reactive protein

CT scan: computed tomographic scan

CYP2C19: cytochrome P450 2C19

DCI: delayed cerebral ischemia

DVT: deep vein thrombosis

DWI: diffusion-weighted imaging

TABLE 27-5 Monitoring the Hospitalized Acute Stroke Patient

	Treatment	Parameter(s)	Frequency	Comments
Ischemic stroke	t-PA	BP, neurologic function, bleeding	Every 15 minutes × 1 hour; every 0.5 h × 6 h; every 1 h × 17 h; every shift after	
	Aspirin	Bleeding	Daily	
	Clopidogrel	Bleeding	Daily	
	ERDP-ASA	Headache, bleeding	Daily	Headache usually transient (2–3 days) and may respond to simple analgesics
	Warfarin	Bleeding, INR, Hb/Hct	INR daily × 3 days; weekly until stable; monthly	
Hemorrhagic stroke		BP, neurologic function, ICP	Every 2 hours in ICU	Many patients require intervention with short-acting agents to reduce BP to <180 mm Hg systolic
All	Nimodipine (for SAH)	BP, neurologic function, fluid status	Every 2 hours in ICU	For infectious complications such as UTI or pneumonia
		Temperature, CBC	Temp. every 8 hours; CBC daily	
		Pain (calf or chest)	Every 8 hours	For DVT, MI, acute headache
		Electrolytes and ECG	Up to daily	For fluid and electrolyte imbalances, cardiac rhythm abnormalities
	Heparins for DVT prophylaxis	Bleeding, platelets	Bleeding daily, platelets if suspected thrombocytopenia	

BP, blood pressure; CBC, complete blood count; DVT, deep-vein thrombosis; ECG, electrocardiography, ERDP-ASA, extended-release dipyridamole plus aspirin; Hb/Hct, hemoglobin/hematocrit; ICP, intracranial pressure; ICU, intensive care unit; MI, myocardial infarction; SAH, subarachnoid hemorrhage.

ECG: electrocardiogram

ERDP: extended-release dipyridamole

ESPRIT: European/Australasian Stroke Prevention in Reversible Ischemia Trial

ESPS-2: European Stroke Prevention Study 2

EVD: external ventricular drainage

FFP: fresh frozen plasma

GI: gastrointestinal

ICH: intracerebral hemorrhage

INR: international normalized ratio

JNC: Joint National Committee

LDL: low-density lipoprotein

MI: myocardial infarction

MRI: magnetic resonance imaging

NCEP: National Cholesterol Education Program

NIHSS: National Institutes of Health Stroke Scale

NINDS: National Institute of Neurologic Disorders and Stroke

NVAF: nonvalvular atrial fibrillation

PAD: peripheral arterial disease

PCC: prothrombin-complex concentrate

PGI_2: prostacyclin

PRoFESS: Prevention Regimen for Effectively Avoiding Second Strokes

QALY: quality-adjusted life-year

RRR: relative risk reduction

SAH: subarachnoid hemorrhage

TCD: transcranial Doppler

TEE: transesophageal echocardiography

TIA: transient ischemic attack

TTE: transthoracic echocardiography

TXA_2: thromboxane A_2

t-PA: tissue plasminogen activator

REFERENCES

1. Lloyd-Jones D, Adams R, Carnethon M, et al. Heart disease and stroke statistics—2009 update: A report from the American Heart Association Statistics Committee and Stroke Statistics Subcommittee. Circulation 2009;119:e21–e181.

2. Howard VJ, McClure LA, Meschia JF, Pulley L, Orr SC, Friday GH. High prevalence of stroke symptoms among persons without a diagnosis of stroke or transient ischemic attack in a general population: The Reasons for Geographic and Racial Differences in Stroke (REGARDS) Study. Arch Int Med 2006;166:1952–1958.

3. Elkins JS, Johnston SC. Thirty-year projections for deaths from ischemic stroke in the United States. Stroke 2003;34:2109–2113.

4. Cooper R, Cutler J, Desvigne-Nickens P, et al. Trends and disparities in coronary heart disease, stroke, and other cardiovascular diseases in the United States: Findings of the National Conference on Cardiovascular Disease Prevention. Circulation 2000;102:3137–3147.

5. Juvela S, Kase CS. Advances in intracerebral hemorrhage management. Stroke 2006;37:301–304.

6. Qureshi AI, Mendelow AD, Hanley DF. Intracerebral hemorrhage. Lancet 2009;373:1632–1644.

7. Albers GW, Amerenco P, Easton JD, Sacco RL, Teal P. Antithrombotic and thrombolytic therapy for ischemic stroke. American College of Chest Physicians Evidence-Based Clinical Practice Guidelines (8th Edition). Chest 2008;133:630S–669S.

8. Goldstein LB, Adams R, Alberts MJ, et al. Primary prevention of ischemic stroke. A Guideline from the American Heart Association/American Stroke Association Stroke Council: Cosponsored by the Atherosclerotic Peripheral Vascular Disease Interdisciplinary Working Group; Cardiovascular Nursing Council; Clinical Cardiology Council; Nutrition, Physical Activity, and Metabolism Council; and the Quality of Care and Outcomes Research Interdisciplinary Working Group. Stroke 2006;37:1583–1633.

9. Helgason CM, Wolf PA. American Heart Association Prevention Conference IV. Prevention and rehabilitation of stroke. Circulation 1997;96:701–707.

10. European Atrial Fibrillation Trial Study Group. Secondary prevention in nonrheumatic atrial fibrillation after transient ischaemic attack or minor stroke. Lancet 1993;342:1255–1262.

11. Hart RG, Halperin JL, Pearce LA, et al. Lessons from the stroke prevention in atrial fibrillation trials. Ann Intern Med 2003;138:831–838.

12. Wolf PA. Fifty years at Framingham: Contributions to stroke epidemiology. Adv Neurol 2003;92:165–172.

13. Dirnagl U, Iadecola C, Moskowitz MA. Pathobiology of ischemic stroke: An integrated view. Trends Neurosci 1999;22:391–397.

14. Feuerstein GZ, Wang X. New opportunities for stroke prevention and therapeutics: A hope from anti-inflammatory drugs? In: Feuerstein GZ, ed. Inflammation and Stroke. Basel: Birkhauser-Verlag; 2001:3–10.

15. Broderick J, Connelly S, Feldman E, et al. Guidelines for the management of spontaneous intracerebral hemorrhage in adults: 2007 Update. Stroke 2007;38:2001–2023.

16. Greenberg DA, Aminoff MJ, Simon RP, eds. Stroke. In: Clinical Neurology, 5th ed. New York: McGraw-Hill; 2002:282–316.

17. Adams HP Jr, del Zoppo G, Alberts MJ, et al. Guidelines for the early management of adults with ischemic stroke: A guideline from the American Heart Association. Stroke 2007;38:1655–1711.

18. Khaja AM, Grotta JC. Established treatments for acute ischemic stroke. Lancet 2007;369:319–330.

19. Goldstein LB. Acute ischemic stroke treatment in 2007. Circulation 2007;116:1504–1514.

20. Johnston SC, Nguyen-Huynh MN, Schwartz ME, et al. National Stroke Association guidelines for the management of transient ischemic attacks. Ann Neurol 2006;60(3):301–313.

21. Cina CA, Clase CM, Haynes RB. Carotid endarterectomy for symptomatic carotid stenosis (Cochrane Review on CD-ROM). Oxford: Cochrane Library Update Software; 2001: issue 1.

22. Brott TG, Hobson RW, Howard G et al. Stenting versus endarterectomy for treatment of carotid artery stenosis. N Engl J Med 2010; [10.1056/NEJMoa0912321] May 26, 2010.

23. Miller J, Diringer M. Management of aneurysmal subarachnoid hemorrhage. Neurol Clin 1995;13:451–478.

24. The National Institute of Neurological Disorders and Stroke rt-PA Stroke Study Group. Tissue plasminogen activator for acute ischemic stroke. N Engl J Med 1995;333:1581–1587.

25. Hacke W, Kaste M, Bluhmki E, et al. Thrombolysis with alteplase 3 to 4.5 hours after acute ischemic stroke. N Engl J Med 2008;359:1317–1329.

26. Chinese Acute Stroke Trial (CAST) Collaborative Group. CAST: A randomized, placebo-controlled trial of early aspirin use in 20,000 patients with acute ischemic stroke. Lancet 1997;349:1641–1649.

27. International Stroke Trial Collaborative Group. The International Stroke Trial (IST): A randomized trial of aspirin, subcutaneous heparin, both, or neither among 19,435 patients with acute ischemic stroke. Lancet 1997;349:1560–1581.

28. Sacco RL, Adams R, Albers G, et al. Guidelines for prevention of stroke in patients with ischemic stroke or transient ischemic attack. A statement for health care professionals from the American Heart Association/American Stroke Association Council on Stroke. Stroke 2006;37:577–617.

29. del Zoppo GJ, Saver JL, Jauch EC, Adams HP on behalf of the American Heart Association Stroke Council. Expansion of the time window for treatment of acute ischemic stroke with intravenous tissue plasminogen activator. A science advisory for the American Heart Association/American Stroke Association. Stroke 2009;40:2945–2948.

30. Antithrombotic Trialists' Collaboration. Collaborative meta-analysis of randomized trials of antiplatelet therapy for prevention of death, myocardial infarction, and stroke in high risk patients. BMJ 2002;324:71–86.

31. CAPRIE Steering Committee. A randomized, blinded trial of clopidogrel versus aspirin in patients at risk of ischaemic events (CAPRIE). Lancet 1995;348:1329–1339.

32. Diener HC, Cunha L, Forbes C, et al. European Stroke Prevention Study 2: Dipyridamole and acetylsalicylic acid in the secondary prevention of stroke. J Neurol Sci 1996;143:1–13.

33. ESPRIT Study Group. Aspirin plus dipyridamole versus aspirin alone after cerebral ischaemia of arterial origin (ESPRIT): Randomized controlled trial. Lancet 2006;367:1665–1673.

34. Sacco RL, Diener HC, Yusuf S, et al. Aspirin and extended-release dipyridamole versus clopidogrel for recurrent stroke. N Engl J Med 2008;359:1238–1251.

35. American Society of Health-System Pharmacists. ASHP therapeutics position statement on antithrombotic therapy in chronic atrial fibrillation. Am J Health Syst Pharm 1998;55:376–381.

36. Connolly SJ, Ezekowitz MD, Yusuf S, et al. Dabigatran versus warfarin in patients with atrial fibrillation. N Engl J Med 2009;361(12):1139–1151.

37. Mohr JP, Thompson JLP, Lazar RM, et al. A comparison of warfarin and aspirin for the prevention of recurrent ischemic stroke. N Engl J Med 2001;345:1444–1451.

38. Chimowitz MI, Lynn MJ, Howlett-Smith H, et al. Comparison of warfarin and aspirin for symptomatic intracranial arterial stenosis. N Engl J Med 2005;352:1305–1316.

39. Gueyffer F, Boissel JP, Bouttie F, et al. for the INDANA Project Collaborators. Effect of antihypertensive treatment in patients having already suffered from stroke: Gathering of the evidence. Stroke 1997;28:2557–2562.

40. PROGRESS Collaborative Group. Randomized trial of perindopril-based blood-pressure-lowering regimen among 6105 individuals with previous stroke or transient ischaemic attack. Lancet 2001;358:1033–1041.

41. Chobanian AV, Bakris GL, Black HR, et al. The Seventh Report of the Joint National Committee on Prevention, Detection, Evaluation, and Treatment of High Blood Pressure. The JNC7 Report. JAMA 2003;289(19):2560–2572.

42. Hebert PR, Gaziano JM, Chan KS, Hennekens CH. Cholesterol lowering with statin drugs, risk of stroke, and total mortality: An overview of randomized trials. JAMA 1997;278:313–321.

43. Scandinavian Simvastatin Survival Study Group. Randomized trial of cholesterol lowering in 4444 patients with coronary heart disease: The Scandinavian Simvastatin Survival Study (4S). Lancet 1994;344:1383–1389.

44. Byrington RP, Davis BR, Plehn JF, et al. Reduction of stroke events with pravastatin: The Prospective Pravastatin Pooling (PPP) Project. Circulation 2001;103:387–392.

45. Executive Summary of the Third Report of the National Cholesterol Education Program (NCEP) Expert Panel on Detection, Evaluation, and Treatment of High Blood Cholesterol in Adults (Adult Treatment Panel III). JAMA 2001;285:2486–2497.

46. Heart Protection Study Collaborative Group. MRC/BHF Heart Protection Study of cholesterol lowering with simvastatin in 20,536 high-risk individuals: A randomized, placebo-control trial. Lancet 2002;360:7–22.

47. The Stroke Prevention by Aggressive Reduction in Cholesterol Levels (SPARCL) Investigators. High-dose atorvastatin after stroke or transient ischemic attack. N Engl J Med 2006;355:549–559.

48. Adams RJ, Albers G, Alberts MJ, et al. Update to the AHA/ASA recommendations for the prevention of stroke in patients with stroke and transient ischemic attack. Stroke 2008;39:1647–1652.

49. Diener HC, Bogousslavsky J, Brass LM, et al. Aspirin and clopidogrel compared with clopidogrel alone after recent ischemic stroke or transient ischaemic attack in high-risk patients (MATCH): Randomized, double-blind, placebo-controlled trial. Lancet 2004;364:331–337.

50. Yusuf S, Zhao F, Mehta SR, et al. Effects of clopidogrel in addition to aspirin in patients with acute coronary syndromes without ST-segment elevation. N Engl J Med 2001;54:1022–1028.

51. Steinhubl SR, Berger PB, Mann JT, et al. Early and sustained dual oral antiplatelet therapy following percutaneous coronary intervention: A randomized, controlled trial. JAMA 2002;288:2411–2420.

52. Bhatt DL, Fox KAA, Hacke W, et al. Clopidogrel and aspirin versus aspirin alone for the prevention of atherothrombotic events. N Engl J Med 2006;354:1706–1717.

53. Peters RJG, Mehta SR, Fox KAA, et al. Effects of aspirin dose when used alone or in combination with clopidogrel in patients with acute coronary syndromes: Observations from the clopidogrel in unstable angina to prevent recurrent events (CURE) study. Circulation 2003;108:1682–1687.

54. Dahlof B, Devereux RB, Kjeldsen SE, et al. Cardiovascular morbidity and mortality in the Losartan Intervention for Endpoint Reduction in Hypertension Study (LIFE). Lancet 2002;359:995–1003.

55. Schrader J, Luders S, Kulschewski A, et al. Morbidity and mortality after stroke, eprosartan compared with nitrendipine for secondary prevention. Principal results of a prospective randomized controlled study (MOSES). Stroke 2005;36:1218–1226.

56. The Publications Committee for the Trial of ORG 10172 in Acute Stroke Treatment (TOAST) Investigators. Low-molecular-weight heparinoid,

ORG 10172 (danaparoid), and outcome after acute ischemic stroke: A randomized, controlled trial. JAMA 1998;279:1265–1272.

57. Bath PM, Lidenstrom E, Boysen G, et al. Tinzaparin in acute ischaemic stroke (TAIST): A randomized, aspirin-controlled trial. Lancet 2001;358:702–710.

58. Berge E, Abdelnoor M, Nakstad PH, et al. Low-molecular-weight heparin versus aspirin in patients with acute ischaemic stroke and atrial fibrillation: A double-blind, randomised study. HAEST Study Group. Heparin in Acute Embolic Stroke Trial. Lancet 2000;355:1205–1210.

59. Food and Drug Administration. FDA Approves New Prescribed Uses for Aspirin. FDA Talk Paper. 1998;T98–76, *www.fda.gov/bbs/topics/ANSWERS/ANS00919.html.*

60. Farrell B, Godwin J, Richards S, Warlow C. The United Kingdom transient ischaemic attack (UK-TIA) aspirin trial: Final results. J Neurol Neurosurg Psychiatry 1991;54:1044–1054.

61. Serebruany VL, Malinin AI, Sane DC. Rapid platelet inhibition after a single capsule of Aggrenox: Challenging a conventional full-dose aspirin antiplatelet advantage? Am J Hematol 2003;72:280–281.

62. Eikelboom JW, Hankey GJ. Aspirin resistance: A new independent predictor of vascular events? J Am Coll Cardiol 2003;41:966–968.

63. Catella-Lawson F, Reilly MP, Kapoor SC, et al. Cyclooxygenase inhibitors and the antiplatelet effects of aspirin. N Engl J Med 2001;345:1809–1817.

64. Ridker PM, Cushman M, Stampfer MJ et al. Inflammation, aspirin, and the risk of cardiovascular disease in apparently healthy men. N Engl J Med 1997;336:973–979. Erratum in: N Engl J Med 1997;337:356.

65. Eisert WG. Near-field amplification of antithrombotic effects of dipyridamole through vessel wall cells. Neurology 2001;57(suppl 2):S20–S23.

66. Theis JG, Deichsel G, Marshall S. Rapid development of tolerance to dipyridamole-associated headaches. Br J Clin Pharm 1999;48:750–755.

67. Bennett CL, Connors JM, Carwile JM, et al. Thrombotic thrombocytopenic purpura associated with clopidogrel. N Engl J Med 2000;342:1773–1777.

68. Mega JL, Close SL, Wiviott SD, et al. Cytochrome P-450 polymorphisms and response to clopidogrel. N Engl J Med 2009;360:354–362.

69. Ho PM, Maddox TM, Wang L, Fihn SD, Jesse RL, Peterson ED, Rumsfeld JS. Risk of adverse outcomes associated with concomitant use of clopidogrel and proton pump inhibitors following acute coronary syndrome. JAMA 2009;301:937–944.

70. Saw J, Steinhubl SR, Berger PB, et al. Lack of adverse clopidogrel atorvastatin clinical interaction from secondary analysis of a randomized, placebo-controlled clopidogrel trial. Circulation 2003;108:921–924.

71. Broderick JP, Hacke W. Treatment of acute ischemic stroke, I: Recanalization strategies. Circulation 2002;106:1563–1569.

72. Ginsberg MD. Current status of neuroprotection for cerebral ischemia: Synoptic overview. Stroke 2009;40(suppl 1);S111–S11473.

73. Saver JL. Citicoline: Update on a promising and widely available agent for neuroprotection and neurorepair. Rev Neurol Dis 2008;5(4):167–177.

74. Garber K. Stroke treatment—light at the end of the tunnel? Nature Biotech 2007;25(8):838–840.

75. Freeman WD, Aguilar MI. Management of warfarin-related intracerebral hemorrhage. Expert Rev Neurotherapeutics 2008;8(2):271–290.

76. Fagan SC, Morgenstein LB, Peitta A, et al. Cost effectiveness of tissue plasminogen activate for acute ischemic stroke. Neurology 1998;50:883–890.

77. Demaerschalk BM, Yip TR. Economic benefit of increasing utilization of intravenous tissue plasminogen activator for acute ischemic stroke in the United States. Stroke 2005;36:2500–2503.

78. Gage BF, Cardinalli AB, Albers GW, Owens DK. Cost-effectiveness of warfarin and aspirin for prophylaxis of stroke in patients with nonvalvular atrial fibrillation. JAMA 1995;274:1839–1845.

79. Sarasin FP, Gaspoz JM, Bournameaux H. Cost-effectiveness of new antiplatelet regimens used as secondary prevention of stroke or transient ischemic attack. Arch Intern Med 2000;160:2773–2778.

80. Kongnakorn T, Ward A, Roberts CS, O'Brien JA, Proskorovsky I, Caro JJ. Economic evaluation of atorvastatin for prevention of recurrent stroke based on the SPARCL trial. Val Health 2009;12(6):880–887.

28

Dyslipidemia

ROBERT L. TALBERT

KEY CONCEPTS

❶ Hypercholesterolemia, elevated low-density lipoprotein (LDL), and low high-density lipoprotein (HDL) are unequivocally linked to increased risk for coronary heart disease and cerebrovascular morbidity and mortality; LDL is the primary target.

❷ Multiple genetic abnormalities and environmental factors are involved in clinical lipid abnormalities and routinely used clinical laboratory measurements do not define the underlying abnormalities.

❸ Initial therapy for any lipoprotein disorder is therapeutic lifestyle changes with restricted intake of total and saturated fat and cholesterol and a modest increase in polyunsaturated fat intake, along with a program of regular exercise and weight reduction, if needed.

❹ If pharmacologic therapy is insufficient after therapeutic lifestyle changes, lipid-lowering agents should be chosen based on the specific lipoprotein disorder presentation and the severity of the lipid abnormality.

❺ Considering compliance, adverse effects, and effectiveness, statins are the drugs of choice for patients with hypercholesterolemia because they are the most potent form of monotherapy and are cost effective in patients with known CAD or multiple risk factors and in high risk primary prevention patients.

❻ Patients not responding to statin monotherapy may be treated with combination therapy for hypercholesterolemia, but should be monitored closely because of an increased risk for adverse effects and drug interactions.

❼ Hypertriglyceridemia usually responds well to niacin, gemfibrozil, and fenofibrate; high dose niacin should be used cautiously in diabetics because of worsening glycemic control. Statins lower triglycerides to a variable extent, depending on baseline triglyceride concentration and statin potency.

❽ Low HDL-C is addressed with lifestyle modifications such as smoking cessation and increased exercise; niacin and gemfibrozil and fenofibrate can significantly increase HDL-C as well.

❾ Reductions in elevated total cholesterol and LDL-C reduce CHD mortality and total mortality; increasing HDL reduces CHD events as well. Aggressive treatment of hypercholesterolemia results in fewer patients progressing to myocardial infarction, angina, and stroke, and reduces the need for interventions such as coronary artery bypass graft and percutaneous transluminal coronary angioplasty.

❿ Lipid-lowering therapy is generally considered to be cost effective, particularly in secondary intervention and high risk patients.

Cholesterol, triglycerides, and phospholipids are the major lipids in the body and they are transported as complexes of lipids and proteins known as lipoproteins. Plasma lipoproteins are spherical particles with surfaces that consist largely of phospholipid, free cholesterol, and protein, and cores that consist mostly of triglyceride and cholesterol ester (Fig. 28–1). The three major classes of lipoproteins found in serum are low density lipoproteins (LDL), high density lipoproteins (HDL), and very low density lipoproteins (VLDL). VLDL is carried in the circulation as triglyceride and VLDL can be estimated by dividing the triglyceride concentration by five if the triglyceride concentration is below 250 mg/dL. Intermediate density lipoprotein resides between VLDL and LDL and is included in the LDL measurement in routine clinical measurement. Abnormalities of plasma lipoproteins can result in a predisposition to coronary, cerebrovascular, and peripheral vascular arterial disease and constitutes one of the major risk factors for coronary heart disease (CHD). Accumulating evidence over the last decades had linked elevated total and LDL cholesterol and reduced HDL to the development of CHD. Premature coronary atherosclerosis, leading to the manifestations of ischemic heart disease (see Chapter 23), is the most common and significant consequence of dyslipidemia. The National Cholesterol Education Program (NCEP) Adult Treatment Panel III (ATP III) published its third report summarizing these data and giving recommendations for the management of hypercholesterolemia in adults.[1,2] This report and the later update modify earlier recommendations and provide a new way of risk-stratifying patients based on multiple risk factors, the presence of diabetes, and the metabolic syndrome. The American Heart Association (AHA) also provides guidelines for primary and secondary prevention of CHD.[3,4,5]

Total cholesterol and LDL-C increase throughout life in men and women, representing an atherogenic pattern characteristic of Westernized society diets.[6] Based on estimates from the American Heart Association (AHA), 46.8% or 10.2 million American adults over age 20 years have total cholesterol levels of 200 mg/dL or higher.[7] More than half of individuals at borderline-high risk remain unaware that they have hypercholesterolemia and fewer than half of highest risk persons (those with symptomatic CHD) are receiving

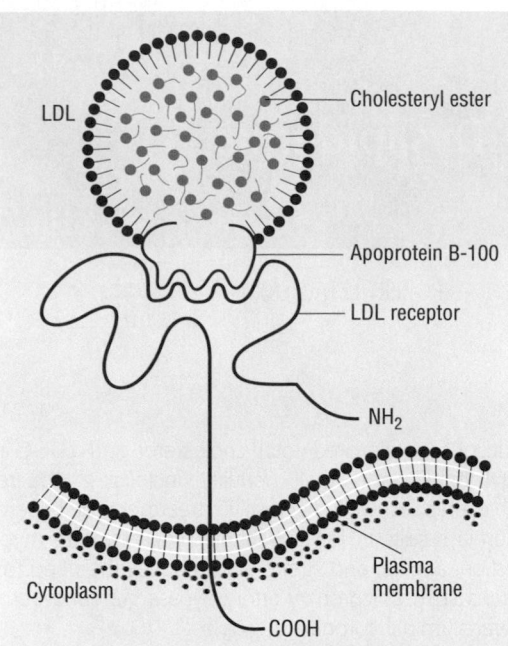

FIGURE 28-1. Diagrammatic representation of the structure of low-density lipoprotein (LDL), the LDL receptor, and the binding of LDL to the receptor via apolipoprotein B-100. *(From Ganong WF. Review of Medical Physiology, 22nd ed. New York: McGraw-Hill, 2005:303.)*

lipid-lowering treatment. About one-third of treated patients are achieving their LDL goal; fewer than 20% of CHD patients are at their LDL goal.[8,9] Changes in the NCEP guidelines have increased the number of persons eligible for therapeutic lifestyle changes (TLC) or lipid-lowering therapy by millions. NCEP estimates that only 26% of patients have an optimal LDL-C (<100 mg/dL) and that large numbers of patients are either untreated or under-treated.[1] Unfortunately, those patients at highest risk are less likely to be treated to desirable levels of LDL.[10] Although these numbers seem staggering in their enormity, substantial progress has been made, and the number of Americans with a desirable blood cholesterol level (<200 mg/dL) has risen to 49% from 45% from the earlier survey (1976 to 1980), while the average total cholesterol in this country has fallen from 220 mg/dL in 1960 to 1962, to 203 mg/dL in 2002.[11] Patients who are at risk but who have not yet experienced their first cardiovascular or cerebrovascular event [e.g., myocardial infarction (MI)] are termed primary prevention; whereas those with manifest vascular disease are termed secondary intervention.

❶ Data from the Framingham and other studies demonstrate that the risk for developing cardiovascular disease is related to the degree of total cholesterol and LDL elevation in a graded, continuous fashion.[12] Hypercholesterolemia is additive to the other non-lipid risk factors for CHD, including cigarette smoking, hypertension, diabetes, low HDL levels, and electrocardiographic abnormalities. The presence of established CHD or prior MI increases the risk of MI five to seven times that seen in men or women without CHD, and LDL is a significant predictor of subsequent morbidity and mortality. About 50% of all MIs and at least 70% of CHD deaths occur in patients with known CHD, and these patients should therefore be a target for screening, identification, and treatment. Unfortunately, the identification of patients at high risk because of hypercholesterolemia or other lipid disorders is too frequently overlooked, because blood lipid levels are not always evaluated in this population, even after an event such as MI.

A comparison of the United States to other countries shows similar relationships between total cholesterol, LDL, and an inverse relationship with HDL to coronary artery disease (CAD) mortality.[12] On a positive note, the U.S. mortality rate is midway among the countries studied, and this country has had the greatest decline in CAD mortality (35% to 40%) in men and women over the last 10 years as compared to other countries. A decline in the prevalence of hypercholesterolemia in certain segments of the U.S. population parallels these trends in mortality.[1] LDL and the ratio of LDL to HDL have also been used to assess risk, but their use adds little information to total cholesterol alone, unless HDL is abnormally high or low. McQueen, et al., found that the ratio of apolipoprotein (Apo) B to ApoA1 was more predictive and consistent across gender and ethnic groups.[13] HDL transports cholesterol from lipid-laden foam cells to the liver. HDL has been shown to be protective for the occurrence of CHD, and an inverse relationship exists between CHD and HDL levels.[14]

VLDL, the major lipoprotein associated with triglycerides, is enriched with cholesterol esters, is smaller, denser, and more atherogenic than less-dense VLDL. Routine measurement of triglycerides cannot distinguish between the types of VLDL present in plasma. Elevation of triglyceride-rich lipoproteins is associated with low HDL, and this ratio predicts increased risk. The eight-year follow-up of the Copenhagen male study found a clear gradient of risk of ischemic heart disease (IHD) with increasing triglyceride levels within each level of HDL cholesterol. When compared to the lowest tertile of triglyceride concentrations, the highest tertile had 2.2 relative risk for IHD and the relationship extended across all concentrations of HDL.[15] The Helsinki heart study shows that hypertriglyceridemia and low HDL are associated with obesity (body mass index [BMI] >26 kg/m²), smoking, sedentary life-style, blood pressure of ≥140/90 mm Hg, and blood glucose above 4.4 mmol/L, and that the benefit of gemfibrozil (risk reduction 68%, $P < 0.03$) was largely confined to overweight subjects.[16] Hypertriglyceridemia in certain instances—for example, diabetes mellitus, nephrotic syndrome, and chronic renal disease, and perhaps in women—is associated with increased cardiovascular risk. This is thought to be a consequence of the presence of atherogenic lipoproteins and of hypertriglyceridemia being a marker for them, as triglycerides are usually not independently predictive for CHD.[17]

LIPOPROTEIN METABOLISM AND TRANSPORT

Cholesterol and triglycerides, as the major plasma lipids, are essential substrates for cell membrane formation and hormone synthesis, and provide a source of free fatty acids.[18] Dyslipidemia may be defined as an elevation of total cholesterol, elevation in LDL cholesterol, elevation in triglycerides or low HDL cholesterol concentration, or some combination of these abnormalities. Lipids, being water immiscible, are not present in free form in the plasma, but rather circulate as lipoproteins. *Hyperlipoproteinemia* describes an increased concentration of the lipoprotein macromolecules that transport lipids in the plasma. The density of plasma lipoproteins is determined by their relative content of protein and lipid. Density, composition, size, and electrophoretic mobility divide lipoproteins into four classes (Table 28-1).

LDL has been further divided into LDL$_1$, or intermediate-density lipoprotein (density 1.006–1.019 g/mL), and LDL$_2$ (1.019–1.063 g/mL). LDL$_2$ is the major LDL component in plasma and it carries 60% to 70% of the total serum cholesterol. HDL has been subfractionated into HDL$_2$ (density 1.063–1.125 g/mL) and HDL$_3$ (1.125–1.21 g/mL). Fluctuations in HDL are usually caused by alterations in the levels of HDL$_2$. HDL normally carries about 20% to 30% of the total cholesterol. VLDL has also been subdivided

TABLE 28-1 Composition of Lipoprotein Isolated from Normal Subjects

Lipoprotein Class[a]	Density Range (g/mL)	Diameter (nm)	Protein	Triglyceride	Cholesterol Free	Cholesterol Ester	Phospholipid
Chylomicrons	<0.94	75–1200	1–2	80–95	1–3	2–4	3–9
VLDL	0.94–1.006	30–80	6–10	55–80	4–8	16–22	10–20
LDL	1.006–1.063	18–25	18–22	5–15	6–8	45–50	18–24
HDL	1.063–1.21	5–12	45–55	5–10	3–5	15–20	20–30

[a]VLDL denotes very-low-density lipoprotein, LDL low-density lipoprotein, and HDL high-density lipoprotein.

into three classes, and it carries about 10% to 15% of serum cholesterol and most of the triglyceride in the fasting state. VLDL is the precursor for LDL, and VLDL remnants may also be atherogenic. Table 28–2 shows the characteristics of the protein constituent of lipoproteins known as apolipoproteins. The structure of LDL, the LDL receptor, and the binding of the LDL to the receptor via apolipoprotein (Apo) B-100 is shown in Figure 28–1.

Chylomicrons, large triglyceride-rich particles containing apolipoprotein B-48, B-100, and E, are formed from dietary fat solubilized by bile salts in intestinal mucosal cells. Chylomicrons are normally not present in the plasma after a fast of 12 to 14 hours and are catabolized by lipoprotein lipase (LPL), which is activated by apolipoprotein C-II and in the vascular endothelium and hepatic lipase to form chylomicron remnants. The remnants that contain apolipoprotein E (Fig. 28–2) are taken up by the "remnant receptor," which may be an LDL receptor-related protein in the liver. Free cholesterol is liberated intracellularly after attachment to the remnant receptor. Chylomicrons also function to deliver dietary triglyceride to skeletal muscle and adipose tissue. During the catabolism of nascent chylomicrons to remnants, triglyceride is converted to free fatty acids and apolipoproteins A-I, A-II, A-IV (free in plasma), C-I, C-II, and C-III, and phospholipids are transferred to HDL. Apolipoprotein E and apolipoprotein C-II are transferred to chylomicrons from HDL and eventually back through these metabolic events. Hepatic VLDL synthesis is regulated in part by diet and hormones, and is inhibited by uptake of

chylomicron remnants in the liver. VLDL is secreted from the liver and serially converted via LPL to intermediate-density lipoprotein (IDL), and finally, to LDL. VLDL receptors are found in adipose tissue and muscle, and bear close homology to the structure of LDL receptors.

LDL, the major cholesterol transport lipoprotein and having virtually only apolipoprotein B-100, is mostly derived from VLDL catabolism and cellular synthesis. When fasting and on low-fat intake in normal subjects, most cholesterol is synthesized and used in the extrahepatic organs, while most of the cholesterol carried by LDL is taken up by the liver for catabolism. In patients with homozygous familial hypercholesterolemia, enhanced synthesis of LDL may occur, because LDL clearance is reduced as a consequence of the lack of LDL receptors. LDL is catabolized through interaction of cell surface receptors found on liver, adrenal, and peripheral cells (including fibroblasts and smooth muscle cells). These cells recognize apolipoprotein B-100 on LDL, and after binding to a receptor on the cell membrane, LDL is internalized and degraded. In the normal fasting state, approximately 70% of LDL is cleared through a receptor-dependent mechanism, although this is highly dependent on the availability and type of saturated and mono- or polyunsaturated fat from dietary sources. Ingestion of cholesterol and saturated fatty acids such as C12:0, C14:0, and C16:0 are associated with reduction in LDL receptor activity, increased LDL production rate, and elevation in LDL plasma concentration. Receptor-independent mechanisms are

TABLE 28-2 Characteristics and Functions of Apolipoproteins

Apolipoprotein	Lipoprotein Density Class	Approximate Plasma Concentration (mg/dL)	Approximate Molecular Weight (kd)	Reported Functions	Major Site of Synthesis
A-I	Chylomicrons, HDL	120	28	Cofactor with LCAT, structural protein on HDL, ligand for HDL receptor	Liver, intestine
A-II	Chylomicrons, HDL	35	17	Structural protein for HDL, ligand for HDL receptor	Liver
A-IV	Chylomicrons, 1.21B	15	46	Possibly facilitates transfer of other apos between HDL and chylomicrons	Intestine
ApoLp(a)	LDL, HDL	10	500±	Bound to B-100, high homology with plasminogen, may prevent LDL uptake by B, E receptor	Liver
B-100	VLDL, LDL, IDL	100	540	Necessary for assembly and secretion of VLDL from the liver, structural protein of VLDL, IDL, LDL, ligand for LDL receptor	Liver
B-48	Chylomicrons	Trace	264	Necessary for assembly and secretion of chylomicrons from the small intestine	Intestine
C-I	Chylomicrons, VLDL, HDL	7	6.6	Cofactor with LCAT; may inhibit hepatic uptake of chylomicron and VLDL remnants	Liver
C-II	Chylomicrons, VLDL, HDL	4	8.9	Activator of LPL	Liver
C-III	Chylomicrons, VLDL, HDL	13	8.8	Inhibitor with LPL; may inhibit hepatic uptake of chylomicron and VLDL remnants	Liver
D	HDL	6	32	?	?
E2-E4	Chylomicrons, VLDL, HDL	5	34	Ligand for several lipoproteins to LDL receptor, LRP and possibly to a separate hepatic apo E receptor	Liver

LCAT, lecithin-cholesterol acyltransferase; HL, hepatic lipase; IDL, intermediate density lipoprotein; LRP, LDL receptor-related protein. Other abbreviations are in Table 28-1.

FIGURE 28-2. Simplified diagram of lipoprotein systems for transporting lipids in humans. In the exogenous system, chylomicrons rich in triglycerides of dietary origin are converted to chylomicron remnants rich in cholesteryl esters by the action of lipoprotein lipase (LPL). In the endogenous system, very-low-density lipoproteins (VLDL) rich in triglycerides are secreted by the liver and converted to intermediate-density lipoproteins (LDL) and then to low-density lipoproteins (LDL) rich in cholesteryl esters. Some of the LDLs enter the subendothelial space of arteries, are oxidized, and then are taken up by macrophages, wchich become foam cells. The letters on the chylomicrons, chylomicron remnants, VLDL, IDL, and LDL identify the primary apoproteins (ApoB, ApoC, ApoE) found in them. (LDLR, low-density lipoprotein receptor.) *(From Kasper DL, Braunwald E, Fauci AS, et al., eds. Harrison's Principles of Internal Medicine, 16th ed. New York, McGrawHill, 2005, p. 2289.)*

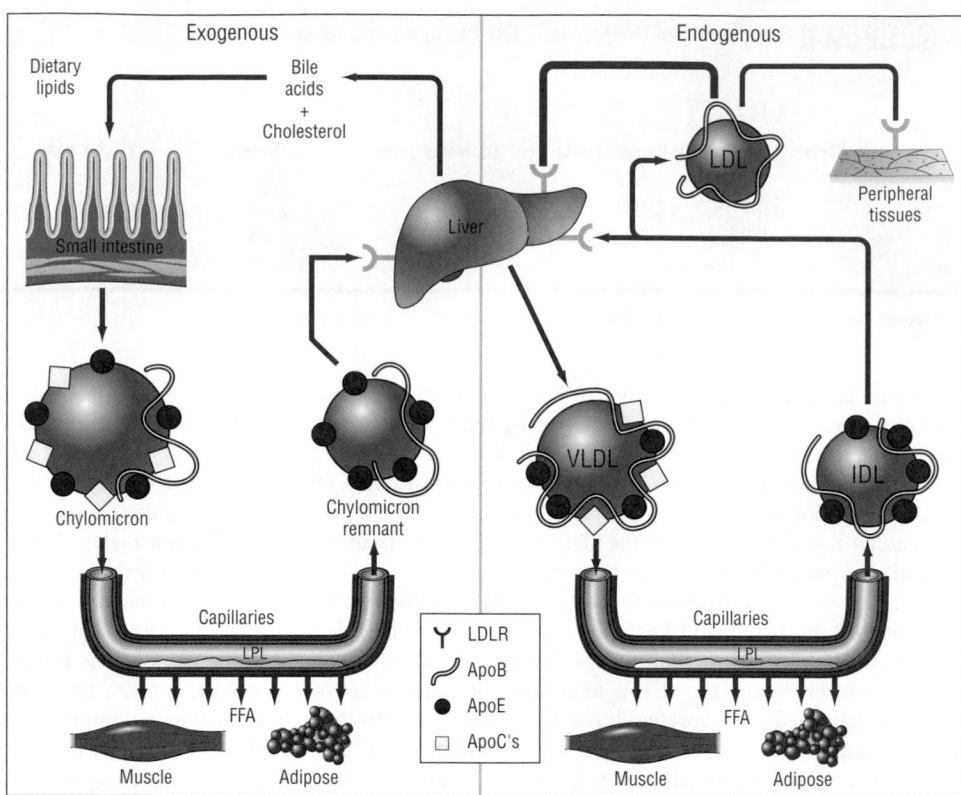

also involved to a lesser extent in the catabolism of LDL, and these receptors are present in many tissues, but are most active in animals in the adrenals and ovary. Increased intracellular cholesterol resulting from LDL catabolism inhibits the activity of 3-hydroxy-3-methylglutaryl coenzyme A reductase (HMG-CoA reductase), the rate-limiting enzyme for intracellular cholesterol biosynthesis (Fig. 28–3). Additional consequences of increased intracellular cholesterol include reduced synthesis of LDL receptors, which limits subsequent cholesterol uptake from the plasma, and accelerated activity of acyl coenzyme-A:cholesterol acyltransferase to facilitate cholesterol storage within cells. LDL cholesterol may also be excreted into bile and become part of the enterohepatic pool or may be lost in the stool. Lp(a) is a cholesterol-rich lipoprotein similar to LDL in composition and density and with close homology to fibrinogen. It is reported to be an important independent risk factor for the development of premature cardiovascular disease.

Nascent HDL is derived from liver and gut synthesis, primarily in the form of apolipoprotein A-I phospholipid discs.[14] Esterification of free cholesterol in nascent HDL and from peripheral tissues to cholesteryl esters by lecithin-cholesterol acyltransferase (LCAT) results in the production of HDL$_3$. Further addition of tissue cholesterol to HDL$_3$ results in the formation of HDL$_2$. HDL$_2$ can also be formed from remodeling of chylomicrons and VLDL catabolism. HDL$_2$ may be converted back to HDL$_3$ by the action of hepatic lipase and by the transfer of cholesteryl esters to the liver, LDL, and VLDL. Apolipoprotein A-I production is increased by estrogens, leading to higher HDL levels in women and in individuals receiving estrogen. Transfer of excess cholesterol from peripheral tissues by HDL is called *reverse cholesterol transport.* Putative HDL receptors in peripheral cells facilitate the uptake of cholesterol by HDL, which transfers cholesterol to either VLDL and LDL, or to the liver for secretion into bile or conversion into bile acids. These processes serve to rid peripheral tissue (e.g., coronary arteries) of excessive amounts of cholesterol, and account for some of the protective effects noted with increasing HDL in women and other

factors that elevate HDL levels. Variants of the cholesterol ester transfer protein (CETP) have been demonstrated in humans, and the B1B1 genotype is associated with lower HDL and progression of coronary atherosclerosis. Inhibition of CETP leads to elevations in HDL. Unfortunately, when CETP inhibitors have been tested in clinical trials, they did not induce regression of atherosclerotic plaque and were associated with higher blood pressure and CHD events.[19–21] The effect of CETP inhibition on blood pressure and HDL are disconcordant.[22]

The "response-to-injury" hypothesis states that risk factors such as oxidized LDL, mechanical injury to the endothelium (e.g., percutaneous transluminal angioplasty), excessive homocysteine, immunologic attack, or infection-induced (e.g., *Chlamydia*, herpes simplex virus-1) changes in endothelial and intimal function lead to endothelial dysfunction and a series of cellular interactions that culminate in atherosclerosis. *C-reactive protein* (CRP) is an acute phase reactant and a marker for inflammation; it may be useful in identifying patients at risk for developing CAD.[23] The eventual outcomes of this atherogenic cascade are clinical events such as angina, MI, arrhythmias, stroke, peripheral arterial disease, abdominal aortic aneurysm, and sudden death. Atherosclerotic lesions are thought to arise from transport and retention of plasma LDL-cholesterol through the endothelial cell layer into the extracellular matrix of the subendothelial space. Once in the artery wall, LDL is chemically modified through oxidation and non-enzymatic glycation. Mildly oxidized LDL then recruits monocytes into the artery wall, which become transformed into macrophages. Macrophages have tremendous potential for accelerating LDL oxidation and apolipoprotein B accumulation, and altering the receptor-mediated uptake of LDL into the artery wall from the usual LDL-receptor to a "scavenger receptor" not regulated by cell content of cholesterol. Oxidized LDL increases plasminogen inhibitor levels (promotion of coagulation), induces the expression of endothelin (vasoconstrictive substance), inhibits the expression of nitric oxide (a vasodilator and platelet inhibitor), and is toxic to macrophages if highly oxidized. As oxidation of biologically

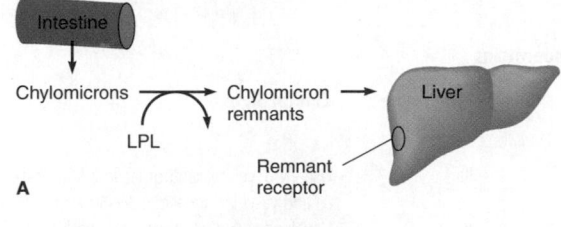

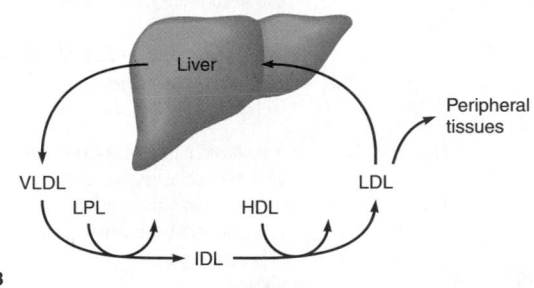

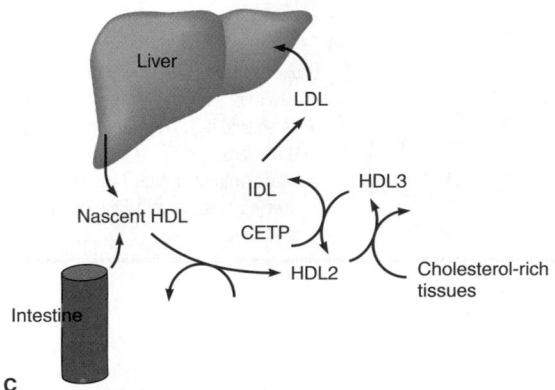

FIGURE 28-3. Biosynthetic pathway for cholesterol. The rate-limiting enzyme in this pathway is 3-hydroxy-3-methylglutaryl coenzyme A reductase (HMG-CoA reductase). (CETP, cholesterol ester transfer protein; HDL, high-density lipoprotein; IDL, intermediate-density lipoprotein; LDL, low-density lipoprotein; LPL, lipoprotein lipase; VLDL, very-low-density lipoprotein.) *(Modified from Breslow JL. Genetic basis of lipoprotein disorders. J Clin Invest 1989;84:373.).* A. Exogenous pathway; B. Endogenous pathway; C. Reverse cholesterol transport.

active lipids proceeds, other lipids such as lysophosphatidylcholine, hydroperoxides, and aldehydic breakdown products of fatty acids and oxysterol are formed, which continue the reaction within the tissue. These events lead to a massive accumulation of cholesterol. The cholesterol-laden macrophages become foam cells; *foam cells* are the earliest recognized cells of the arterial fatty streak.

Oxidized LDL provokes an inflammatory response, which is mediated by a number of chemoattractants and cytokines. Examples of each that appear to be involved at different stages of lesion development include monocyte chemoattractant protein 1 (MCP-1); monocyte colony stimulating factor (M-CSF); *gro;* vascular cell adhesion molecule (VCAM-1); E-selectin (ELAM-1); intercellular adhesion molecule (ICAM-1); platelet-derived growth factor (PDGF); vascular endothelial growth factor (VEGF); transforming growth factors (TGFα and TGFβ); interleukin-1 and interleukin-6 (IL-1, IL-6); and the ratio of interleukin-10 and interleukin-12 (IL-10, IL-12). It appears that some of these factors (e.g., MCP-1 and M-CSF) participate early in the process of monocyte-macrophage attachment and transmigration across the endothelium, whereas others (PDGF and VCAM-1) promote later lesion growth.[24] The extent of oxidation and the inflammatory response is under genetic control of a major gene termed *Ath*-1 based on murine model studies. The process of aging may lead to lipoproteins that are more

TABLE 28-3 Fredrickson-Levy-Lees Classification of Hyperlipoproteinemia

Type	Lipoprotein Elevation
I	Chylomicrons
IIa	LDL
IIb	LDL + VLDL
III	IDL (LDL₁)
IV	VLDL
V	VLDL + Chylomicrons

LDL indicates low-density lipoprotein; VLDL indicates very low-density lipoprotien; IDL indicates intermediate-density lipoprotein.

susceptible to oxidation and have longer resident time in the vascular compartment. Two proteins associated with HDL—apolipoprotein J (apoJ) and paraxonase (PON) appear to play an important role in minimizing the oxidation of LDL-C.[25] Increased recognition of the role of these growth-regulatory molecules provides the possibility of future directions for antagonists to regulatory molecules such as PDGF, TGFβ, and the interleukins. Repeated injury and repair within an atherosclerotic plaque eventually leads to a fibrous cap protecting the underlying core of lipids, collagen, calcium, and inflammatory cells such as T-lymphocytes. Maintenance of the fibrous plaque is critical to prevent plaque rupture and subsequent coronary thrombosis.[26] An imbalance between plaque synthesis and degradation may lead to a weakened or vulnerable plaque prone to rupture. The fibrous cap may become weakened through decreased synthesis of the extracellular matrix or increased degradation of the matrix. The cytokine interferon-γ, produced by T-lymphocytes, inhibits the ability of smooth muscle cells to synthesize collagen, a structurally important component of the fibrous cap. A family of enzymes known as matrix metalloproteinases can degrade all major constituents of the vascular extracellular matrix: collagen, elastin, and proteoglycans.[27]

❷ Lipoprotein disorders are classified into six categories, which are commonly used for phenotypical description of dyslipidemia (Table 28–3). Specific genetic defects with disrupted protein, cell, and organ function give rise to several disorders within each family of lipoproteins (Table 28–4). In other words, an elevated cholesterol level does not necessarily equate with familial hypercholesterolemia or type IIa, as cholesterol may also be elevated in other lipoprotein disorders and the lipoprotein pattern does not describe the underlying genetic defect. The preceding discussion has focused on primary or genetic dyslipoproteinemia. It should be remembered that secondary forms exist and that several drugs may also elevate lipid levels (Table 28–5). These secondary forms of hyperlipidemia should be initially managed by correcting the underlying abnormality, including modification of drug therapy when appropriate.

Familial hypercholesterolemia is characterized by (a) a selective elevation in the plasma level of LDL; (b) deposition of LDL-derived cholesterol in tendons (xanthomas) and arteries (atheromas); and (c) inheritance as an autosomal dominant trait with homozygotes more severely affected than heterozygotes. Homozygotes (prevalence 1 in 1,000,000) have severe hypercholesterolemia (650–1000 mg/dL), with the early appearance of cutaneous xanthomas and fatal CHD generally before the age of 20. The primary defect in familial hypercholesterolemia is the inability to bind LDL to the LDL receptor (LDL-R) or, rarely, a defect of internalizing the LDL-R complex into the cell after normal binding. Homozygotes have essentially no functional LDL receptors. This leads to lack of LDL degradation by cells and unregulated biosynthesis of cholesterol, with total cholesterol and LDL-C being inversely proportional to the deficit in LDL receptors. Heterozygotes have only about one-half of the normal

TABLE 28-4 Lipoprotein Disorders

Lipid Phenotype	Plasma Lipid Levels, mmol/L (mg/dL)L	Lipoproteins Elevated	Phenotype	Clinical Signs
Isolated hypercholesterolemia				
Familial hypercholesterolemia	Heterozygotes TC = 7–13 (275–500)	LDL	IIa	Usually develops xanthomas in adulthood and vascular disease at 30–50 years
	Homozygotes TC >13 (>500)	LDL	IIa	Usually develops xanthomas in adulthood and vascular disease in childhood
Familial defective apo B100	Heterozygotes TC = 7–13 (275–500)	LDL	IIa	
Polygenic hypercholesterolemia	TC = 6.5–9 (250–350)	LDL	IIa	Usually asymptomatic until vascular disease develops; no xanthomas
Isolated hypertriglyceridemia				
Familial hypertriglyceridemia	TG = 2.8–8.5 (250–750)	VLDL	IV	Asymptomatic; may be associated with increased risk of vascular disease
Familial LPL deficiency	TG >8.5 (750)	Chylomicrons, VLDL	I, V	May be asymptomatic; may be associated with pancreatitits, abdominal pain, hepatosplenoggaly
Familial apo CII deficiency	TG >8.5 (>750)	Chylomicrons, VLDL	I, V	As above
Hypertriglyceridemia and hypercholesterolemia				
Combined hyperlipidemia	TG = 2.8–8.5 (250–750); TC = 6.5–13 (250–500)	VLDL, LDL	IIb	Usually asymptomatic until vascular disease develops; familial form may also present as isolated high TG or an isolated high LDL cholesterol
Dysbetalipoproteinemia	TG = 2.8–8.5 (250–750); TC = 6.5–13 (250–500)	VLDL, IDL; LDL normal	III	Usually asymptomatic until vascular disease develops; may have palmar or tuboeruptive xanthomas

Abbreviations: TC, total cholesterol; TG, triglycerides, LPL, lipoprotein lipase. Other abbreviations as in Table 28–1.

TABLE 28-5 Secondary Causes of Lipoprotein Abnormalities

Hypercholesterolemia	Hypothyroidism
	Obstructive liver disease
	Nephrotic syndrome
	Anorexia nervosa
	Acute intermittent porphyria
	Drugs: Progestins, thiazide diuretics, glucocorticoids, β-blockers, isotretinoin, protease inhibitors, cyclosporine, mirtazapine, sirolimus
Hypertriglyceridemia	Obesity
	Diabetes mellitus
	Lipodystrophy
	Glycogen storage disease
	Ileal bypass surgery
	Sepsis
	Pregnancy
	Acute hepatitis
	Systemic lupus erythematous
	Monoclonal gammopathy: multiple myeloma, lymphoma
	Drugs: Alcohol, estrogens, isotretinoin, β-blockers, glucocorticoids, bile-acid resins, thiazides; asparaginase, interferons, azole antifungals, mirtazapine, anabolic steroids, sirolimus, bexarotene
Hypocholesterolemia	Malnutrition
	Malabsorption
	Myeloproliferative diseases
	Chronic infectious diseases: AIDS, tuberculosis
	Monoclonal gammopathy
	Chronic liver disease
Low HDL	Malnutrition
	Obesity
	Drugs: Non-ISA β-blockers, anabolic steroids, probucol, isotretinoin, progestins

number of LDL receptors, total cholesterol levels in the range of 300–600 mg/dL, and cardiovascular events beginning in the third and fourth decades of life.

Familial LPL deficiency is a rare, autosomal recessive trait characterized by a massive accumulation of chylomicrons and corresponding increase in plasma triglycerides or a type I lipoprotein pattern. VLDL concentration is normal. The presenting manifestations include repeated attacks of pancreatitis and abdominal pain, eruptive cutaneous xanthomatosis, and hepatosplenomegaly beginning in childhood. Symptom severity is proportional to dietary fat intake, and consequently to the elevation of chylomicrons. LPL is normally released from vascular endothelium or by heparin and hydrolyzes chylomicrons and VLDL (see Fig. 28–2). Diagnosis is based on low or absent enzyme activity with normal human plasma or apolipoprotein C-II, a cofactor of the enzyme. Accelerated atherosclerosis is not associated with this disease. Abdominal pain, pancreatitis, eruptive xanthomas, and peripheral polyneuropathy characterize type V (VLDL and chylomicrons). Symptoms may occur in childhood, but usually the disorder is expressed at a later age. The risk of atherosclerosis is increased with this disorder. These patients are commonly obese, hyperuricemic, and diabetic, and alcohol intake, exogenous estrogens, and renal insufficiency tend to be exacerbating factors.

Patients with familial type III hyperlipoproteinemia (also called dysbetalipoproteinemia, broad-band or β-VLDL) develop these clinical features after 20 years of age: xanthoma striata palmaris (yellow discolorations of the palmar and digital creases); tuberous or tuberoeruptive xanthomas (bulbous cutaneous xanthomas); and severe atherosclerosis involving the coronary arteries, internal carotids, and abdominal aorta. A defective structure of apolipoprotein E does not allow normal hepatic surface receptor binding of remnant particles derived from chylomicrons and VLDL (known as IDL). Aggravating factors such as obesity, diabetes, or pregnancy may promote overproduction of apo-B-containing lipoproteins. Although homozygosity for the defective allele (E_2/E_2) is common (1 in 100), only 1 in 10,000 express the full-blown picture, and interaction with other genetic or environmental factors, or both, is needed to produce clinical disease.

Familial combined hyperlipidemia is characterized by elevations in total cholesterol, triglycerides, decreased HDL, increased apolipoprotein B and small, dense LDL.[28] It is associated with premature CHD and may be difficult to diagnose since the lipid levels do not consistently display the same pattern.

Type IV hyperlipoproteinemia is common and occurs in adulthood, primarily in patients who are obese, diabetic, and hyperuricemic and do not have xanthomas. It may be secondary to alcohol ingestion and can be aggravated by stress, progestins, oral contraceptives, thiazides, or β-blockers. Two genetic patterns occur in type IV hyperlipoproteinemia: familial hypertriglyceridemia, which does not carry a great risk for premature CAD, and familial combined hyperlipidemia, which is associated with increased risk of cardiovascular disease.

Rare forms of lipoprotein disorders may include hypobetalipoproteinemia, abetalipoproteinemia, Tangier disease, LCAT deficiency (fish-eye disease), cerebrotendinous xanthomatosis, and sitosterolemia. Most of these rare lipoprotein disorders do not result in premature atherosclerosis, with the exceptions of familial LCAT deficiency, cerebrotendinous xanthomatosis (CTX), and sitosterolemia with xanthomatosis. Their treatment consists of dietary restriction of plant sterols (sitosterolemia with xanthomatosis), chenodeoxycholic acid (CTX), or, potentially, blood transfusion (LCAT deficiency).

CLINICAL PRESENTATION

General

- Most patients are asymptomatic for many years prior to clinically evident disease.
- Patients with the metabolic syndrome may have three or more of the following: abdominal obesity, atherogenic dyslipidemia, raised blood pressure, insulin resistance ± glucose intolerance, prothrombotic state, or proinflammatory state.

Symptoms

- None to chest pain, palpitations, sweating, anxiety, shortness of breath, loss of consciousness or difficulty with speech or movement, abdominal pain, sudden death.

Signs

- None to abdominal pain, pancreatitis, eruptive xanthomas, peripheral polyneuropathy, high blood pressure, body mass index >30 kg/m² or waist size >40 inches in men (35 inches in women).

Laboratory Tests

- Elevations in total cholesterol, LDL, triglycerides, apolipoprotein B, C-reactive protein (CRP).
- Low HDL

Other Diagnostic Tests

- Lipoprotein (a), and small, dense LDL (pattern B), HDL subclassification, apolipoprotein E isoforms, apolipoprotein A-1, fibrinogen, folate, lipoprotein-associated phospholipase A_2.
- Various screening tests for manifestations of vascular disease (ankle-brachial index, exercise testing, magnetic resonance imaging) and diabetes (fasting glucose, oral glucose tolerance test, hemoglobin A_{1c}).

TABLE 28-6 Classification of Total-, LDL-, HDL-Cholesterol and Triglycerides

Total cholesterol	
<200 mg/dL	Desirable
200–239 mg/dL	Borderline high
≥240 mg/dL	High
LDL cholesterol	
<100 mg/dL	Optimal
100–129 mg/dL	Near or above optimal
130–159 mg/dL	Borderline high
160–189 mg/dL	High
≥190 mg/dL	Very high
HDL cholesterol	
<40 mg/dL	Low
≥60 mg/dL	High
Triglycerides	
<150 mg/dL	Normal
150–199 mg/dL	Borderline high
200–499 mg/dL	High
≥500 mg/dL	Very high

HDL indicates high-density lipoproteins
LDL indicates low-density lipoproteins

PATIENT EVALUATION

A fasting lipoprotein profile including total cholesterol, LDL-C, HDL-C, and triglycerides should be measured in all adults 20 years of age or older at least once every five years.[1] If the profile is obtained in the nonfasted state, only total cholesterol and HDL-C will be usable because LDL-C is usually a calculated value. If total cholesterol is ≥200 mg/dL, or if HDL-C is <40 mg/dL, a follow-up fasting lipoprotein profile should be obtained. After a lipid abnormality is confirmed (Table 28–6), major components of the evaluation are the history (including age, gender, and, if female, menstrual and hormone replacement status), physical examination, and laboratory investigations. A complete history and physical exam should assess (a) presence or absence of cardiovascular risk factors (Table 28–7) or definite cardiovascular disease in the individual; (b) family history of premature cardiovascular disease or lipid disorders; (c) presence or absence of secondary causes of lipid abnormalities, including concurrent medications (see Table 28–5); and (d) presence or absence of xanthomas or abdominal pain, or history of pancreatitis, renal or liver disease, peripheral vascular disease, abdominal aortic aneurysm, or cerebral vascular disease (carotid bruits, stroke, or transient ischemic attack). An important change in the ATP III guidelines is that diabetes mellitus is regarded

TABLE 28-7 Major Risk Factors (Exlusive of LDL Cholesterol) That Modify LDL Goals[a]

Age
  Men: ≥45 years
  Women: ≥55 years or premature menopause without estrogen replacement therapy
Family history of premature CHD (definite myocardial infarction or sudden death before 55 years of age in father or other male first-degree relative, or before 65 years of age in mother or other female first-degree relative)
Cigarette smoking
Hypertension (≥140/90 mm Hg or on antihypertensive medication)
Low HDL cholesterol (<40 mg/dL)[b]

[a]Diabetes is regarded as a coronary heart disease (CHD) risk equivalent, LDL indicates low-density lipoprotein, HDL indicates high-density lipoprotein.
[b]HDL cholesterol (≥60 mg/dL counts as a "negative" risk factor; its presence removes 1 risk factor from the total count).

TABLE 28-8 LDL Cholesterol Goals and Cutpoints for Therapeutic Lifestyle Changes (TLC) and Drug Therapy in Different Risk Categories[a]

Risk Category	LDL Goal (mg/dL)	LDL Level at Which to Initiate TLC (mg/dL)	LDL Level at Which to Consider Drug Therapy (mg/dL)
High risk: CHD or CHD risk equivalents (10-year risk >20%)	<100 mg/dL (optional goal: <70)	≥100	≥100 (<100 mg/dL; consider drug options)[b]
Moderately high risk: 2+ risk factors (10-year risk >10–20%)	<130	≥130	≥130 (100–129: consider drug options)
Moderate risk: 2+ risk factors (10-year risk <10%)	<130	≥130	≥160
Lower risk: 0–1 Risk factor[c]	<160	≥160	≥190 (160–189: LDL-lowering drug optional)

[a]LDL indicates low-density lipoprotein; CHD, coronary heart disease.
[b]Some authorities recommend use of LDL-lowering drugs in this category if an LDL cholesterol level of <100 mg/dL cannot be achieved by TLC. Others prefer use of drugs that primarily modify triglycerides and HDL, (e.g., nicotinic acid or fibrates). Clinical judgment also may call for deferring drug therapy in this subcategory.
[c]Almost all people with 0–1 risk factor have a 10-year risk <10%; thus, 10-year risk assessment in people with 0–1 risk factor is not necessary.

as a CHD risk equivalent.[1] The presence of diabetes in patients without known CHD is associated with the same level of risk as patients without diabetes but having confirmed CHD.[29,30] ATP III identifies four categories of risk that modify the goals and modalities of LDL-lowering therapy (Table 28–8).[2] The highest category is known CHD or CHD risk equivalents, which is defined as the risk for major coronary events equal to or greater than established CHD, that is, >20% per 10 years (2% per year). The next category is moderately high risk consisting of patients with multiple (2+) risk factors in which 10-year risk for CHD is 10–20%. Moderate risk is defined as ≥2 risk factors and a 10-year risk of ≤10%. The lowest risk category consists of persons with 0 to 1 risk factor. Risk is estimated from Framingham risk scores.[31] Risk is estimated based on the patient's age, LDL-C or total cholesterol level, blood pressure, the presence of diabetes, and smoking status (Table 28–7). This approach for a single patient is referred to as case finding or patient-based, whereas large-scale screening and recommendations for the general populace, health care providers, and the food industry are called a population-based approach.

Measurement of plasma cholesterol (which is about 3% lower than serum determinations), triglyceride, and HDL-C levels after a 12-hour or longer fast is important, as triglycerides may be elevated in nonfasted individuals. Total cholesterol is only modestly affected by fasting. Analytic and biologic variability can have a major impact on the measurement and interpretation of cholesterol (or any other laboratory test). Analytic variability can be minimized through the use of adequate quality control procedures, including internal training, routine calibration and monitoring, and external proficiency testing. Even with these measures, the coefficient of variability in the best procedures can acceptably be up to 5%, and when combined with average biologic variability, total variability may be as high as about 22%. Analytic variability with desktop equipment generally is greater in the fingerstick capillary blood methods, usually yielding measurements less than those from a clinical laboratory, and this technology should be considered for use only as a screening method. Reliance on desktop methods can result in misclassification of 7% to 14% of patients if capillary blood is used. Two determinations, one to eight weeks apart, with the patient on a stable diet and weight, and in the absence of acute illness, are recommended to minimize variability and to obtain a reliable baseline.[1] If the total cholesterol is greater than 200 mg/dL, a second determination is recommended, and if the values are more than 30 mg/dL apart, the average of three values should be used. Familiarity with the method and quality control procedures employed by local laboratories is essential for interpretation of reported values. If the physical examination and history are insufficient to diagnose a familial disorder, then agarose-gel lipoprotein electrophoresis is useful to determine which class of lipoproteins is affected. If the triglyceride levels are below 400 mg/dL and neither type III hyperlipidemia nor

chylomicrons are detected by electrophoresis, then one can calculate VLDL and LDL concentrations: VLDL = triglyceride/5; LDL = total cholesterol – (VLDL + HDL).

Because total cholesterol is comprised of cholesterol derived from LDL, VLDL, and HDL, determination of HDL is useful when total plasma cholesterol is elevated. HDL may be elevated by moderate alcohol ingestion (less than two drinks per day), physical exercise, smoking cessation, weight loss, oral contraceptives, phenytoin, and terbutaline. Smoking, obesity, a sedentary lifestyle and drugs such as β-blockers lower HDL. Only exercise and smoking cessation could be recommended as interventions for low HDL concentrations. Niacin and gemfibrozil also increase HDL concentrations.

The range of lipid concentrations represents a population mean plus or minus two standard deviations and does not define the risk of disease. Reference values for plasma total, LDL, and HDL cholesterol concentrations for men and women, as well as various ethnic groups, are available from the NHANES III.[6] Cholesterol and triglycerides increase throughout life until about the fifth decade for men and the sixth decade for women. Past these ages, total cholesterol and LDL plateau and fall slightly. HDL tends to fall slightly with time and more rapidly after menopause in women. Institution of a population-based approach for cholesterol reduction should shift the entire curve to the left, and the potential reduction in cardiovascular mortality would be proportional to mean reductions at any cholesterol concentration.

Based on a careful review of the experimental pathologic, genetic, and epidemiologic evidence relating to the relationship between blood cholesterol levels and CHD, the adult treatment panel III of the NCEP recommends that a fasting lipoprotein profile and risk factor assessment be used in the initial classification of adults.[1,32] If total cholesterol is less than 200 mg/dL, then the patient has a *desirable blood cholesterol level* (Table 28–6). Cholesterol levels between 200 and 239 mg/dL are classified as *borderline-high blood cholesterol levels*, and assessment of risk factors (Table 28–7) is needed to more clearly define disease risk. Blood cholesterol levels of 240 mg/dL and above are classified as *high blood cholesterol levels*. If the total cholesterol is below 200 mg/dL and the HDL is above 40 mg/dL, no further follow-up is recommended for patients without known CHD and who have fewer than two risk factors. In patients with evidence of CHD or other clinical atherosclerotic disease, the LDL goal is less than 100 mg/dL and most patients will require diet and/or drug intervention. For patients with very high risk (known CHD and multiple risk factors) the LDL goal may be set <70 mg/dL, based on evidence from newer studies.[32] Decisions regarding classification and management are based on the LDL-C levels as outlined in Table 28–8. An increasing number of persons have the metabolic syndrome that is characterized by abdominal obesity, atherogenic dyslipidemia (elevated triglycerides, small LDL particles, low HDL-C), raised blood pressure, insulin resistance (with or without glucose intolerance), and prothrombotic and proinflammatory states. ATP III recognizes the metabolic syndrome as a secondary target of risk-reduction therapy after LDL-C has been addressed and if the metabolic syndrome is present, the patient is considered to have a CHD risk equivalent. Other lipid targets include non-HDL goals for patients with triglycerides >200 mg/dL. Non-HDL is calculated by subtracting HDL from total cholesterol, and the targets are 30 mg/dL greater than LDL for each risk stratum. Non-HDL takes into consideration atherogenic particles such as remnant lipoproteins and intermediate-density lipoproteins that are not measured in routine clinical laboratory testing.[33] HDL-raising has potential benefit, but no specific goals are set in the current guidelines and the evidence is modest to support aggressively increasing HDL levels.[34]

The Expert Panel on Children and Adolescents of the NCEP recommends screening in higher-risk children (positive family history or parental high blood cholesterol, ≥240 mg/dL).[35] The American Academy of Pediatrics categorizes total and LDL cholesterol into Acceptable (<75th percentile; total cholesterol <170 mg/dL), Borderline (75th–95th percentile; total cholesterol 170–199 mg/dL, LDL cholesterol 11–129 mg/dL) and Elevated (>95th percentile; total cholesterol >200 mg/dL, LDL cholesterol >130 mg/dl).[35] The rationale, in part, for this approach is based on the recognition that atherosclerosis begins in the childhood and adolescent years as documented in the pathobiologic determinants of atherosclerosis in youth (PDAY) and the Bogalusa studies.[36] Similarly, if children with high blood lipids or lipoprotein levels are identified, and the levels in the parents are unknown, the parents should be screened as well, as they are likely to be at high risk. Racial and gender differences do exist in the determination of lipoprotein fractions, and these factors should be considered in screening. Use of the serum cholesterol level alone may be of insufficient specificity or sensitivity, depending on the cut points used in screening, and other discretionary factors, such as hypertension, smoking, obesity, high-fat diet, and use of cholesterol-raising medication, may be needed to correctly identify children at risk. Presently, children over the age of 10 years are candidates for drug therapy if a trial of diet (6 months to 1 year) proves to be inadequate and LDL-C remains above 190 mg/dL, or above 160 mg/dL, if two or more risk factors or CHD are present in the child or adolescent, or if there is a history of premature CHD. In children with diabetes mellitus, pharmacologic treatment should be considered when LDL cholesterol is ≥130 mg/dL.[35] The Dietary Intervention Study in Children (DISC) in pubertal children found that a fat-restricted diet modestly lowered LDL-C and maintained psychologic well-being, and dietary changes are acceptable to children.[37,38] Although bile acid sequestrants have been the recommended drugs for this population, clinical trials demonstrate that statin therapy is effective and well tolerated in pediatric populations.[39,40] The long-term consequences of drug therapy in this population are unknown. In special instances, familial hypercholesterolemia (particularly the homozygous form), or the existence of CHD or two or more risk factors in the child, would prompt the earlier institution of drug therapy after a trial of dietary intervention.

TREATMENT

■ DESIRED OUTCOMES

The goals of therapy expressed as LDL-C levels and the level of initiation of therapeutic lifestyle change (TLC) and drug therapy are provided in Table 28–8 for adults and children, respectively. While these goals are surrogate endpoints, the primary reason to institute TLC and drug therapy is to reduce the risk first or recurrent events such as MI, angina, heart failure, or ischemic stroke or other forms of peripheral arterial disease such as carotid stenosis or abdominal aortic aneurysm.

■ GENERAL APPROACH[1]

Establishing targeted changes and outcomes with consistent reinforcement of goals and measures at follow-up visits to attain goals are important to reduce barriers for optimizing TLC and pharmacologic therapy. ❸ TLC should be implemented in all patients prior to considering drug therapy. The components of TLC include reduced intakes of saturated fats and cholesterol, dietary options to reduce LDL such as plant stanols and sterols and increased soluble fiber intake, weight reduction, and increased physical activity. In general, physical activity of moderate intensity 30 minutes per day for most days of the week should be encouraged.[41,42] Patients with known CAD or at high risk should be evaluated before undertaking vigorous exercise. Weight and body mass index (BMI) should be determined at each visit and lifestyle patterns to induce a weight loss of 10% should be discussed in persons who are overweight. All patients should also be counseled to stop smoking and to meet the Joint National Committee VII guidelines for control of hypertension.

■ NONPHARMACOLOGIC THERAPY

Individualized diet counseling that provides acceptable substitutions for unhealthy foods and ongoing reinforcement by a registered dietitian are necessary for maximal effect. The objectives of dietary therapy are to progressively decrease the intake of total fat, saturated fatty acids (i.e., saturated fat), and cholesterol, and to achieve a desirable body weight. Typical American diets now include 13% to 20% of total calories from saturated fat and a cholesterol intake of 350–450 mg/d, both in excess of a "heart healthy" diet for normal Americans, let alone patients with a lipid disorder. Excessive dietary intake of cholesterol and saturated fatty acids leads to decreased hepatic clearance of LDL and deposition of LDL and oxidized LDL in peripheral tissues. The targeted saturated fatty acids have carbon chain lengths of 12 (lauric acid), 14 (myristic acid), and 16 (palmitic acid). The rationale for using a nutritionally balanced low-fat, low-cholesterol diet for the treatment of hypercholesterolemia is based on these principles: (a) it represents a reasonable extension of the diet recommended for the general public; (b) it progressively decreases the major cholesterol-raising constituent of the diet; (c) it precludes large intakes of polyunsaturated fats; and (d) it facilitates weight reduction by removing foods of high caloric density.[43–46]

Dietary expertise in providing a wide range of options and suggestions in preparation of food can make the difference between a good and an inadequate response to diet. Information concerning eating out in a healthy fashion and advice for shopping are also important factors for success in diet therapy. An example is being aware of products with misleading labels such as coffee creamers that state they contain "no cholesterol," when they may contain hydrogenated (saturated) fats or oils (e.g., palmitic acid, palm kernel oil, or coconut oil), which makes them undesirable because of their saturated fat content. Variations in polyunsaturated and saturated fat and cholesterol intake influence the LDL concentration, but the amount of cholesterol has been found to have a greater effect than the proportion of polyunsaturated or saturated fat. There were also racial differences in elevation of LDL with high saturated fat diets being greater in whites than in other racial groups. The isomeric form of fatty acids is also important.[43] Fatty acids with the *cis* configuration are the preferred substrate for the ACAT reaction and significantly increase hepatic LDL receptor clearance while

TABLE 28-9 Macronutrient Recommendations for the TLC Diet

Component[a]	Recommended Intake
Total fat	25–35% of total calories
Saturated fat	Less than 7% of total calories
Polyunsaturated fat	Up to 10% of total calories
Monounsaturated fat	Up to 20% of total calories
Carbohydrates[b]	50–60% of total calories
Cholesterol	<200 mg per day
Dietary Fiber	20–30 grams per day
Plant sterols	2 grams per day
Protein	Approximately 15% of total calories
Total calories	To achieve and maintain desirable body weight

[a]Calories from alcohol not included.
[b]Carbohydrates should derive from foods rich in complex carbohydrates such as whole grains, fruits, and vegetables.

reducing LDL cholesterol production rate. The *trans* isomeric form cannot be used by ACAT and is biologically inactive with no effect on LDL concentration.

Ideally, therapeutic TLC including reduced intake of saturated fats and cholesterol, increased stanol/sterol and fiber intake, weight reduction, and increased physical activity should be used to attain lower LDL-C and to achieve reductions in CHD risk (Table 28–9). TLC may obviate the need for drug therapy, augment LDL-lowering drug therapy, and allow for lower doses. Weight control plus increased physical activity reduces risk beyond LDL-cholesterol lowering, is the primary management approach for the metabolic syndrome, raises HDL, and reduces non-HDL cholesterol.[47,48] Many persons should be given a three-month trial (two visits spaced 6 weeks apart) of dietary therapy and TLC before advancing to drug therapy unless patients are at very high risk (severe hypercholesterolemia, known CHD, CHD risk equivalents, multiple risk factors, strong family history). Although changes in blood lipid levels may change before three months, adoption of a different eating pattern may require a longer period of time. It is important to involve all family members, especially if the patient is not the primary person preparing food. The NCEP and AHA both have excellent Internet-based resources to aid patients in altering their diet in a culturally sensitive manner (*http://www.americanheart. org/presenter.jhtml?identifier=1200009*; *http://www.nhlbi.nih.gov/ health/index.htm*). If all of the recommended dietary changes from NCEP are made, the estimated reduction, on average, in LDL would range from 20–30%.[1] Adherence to diet and inter-individual variability in macronutrient intake would obviously influence the eventual LDL level achieved. Based on the NHANES data, less than one-half of the patients who should be instructed on a heart healthy diet receive any dietary instructions.

Other dietary interventions or diet supplements may be useful in certain patients with lipid disorders. Increased intake of soluble fiber in the form of oat bran, pectins, certain gums, and psyllium products can result in useful adjunctive reductions in total and LDL cholesterol, but these dietary alterations or supplements should not be substituted for more active forms of treatment. Total daily fiber intake should be about 20–30 g/d, with about 25% or 6 g/d, being soluble fiber.[1] Studies with psyllium seed in doses of 10–15 g/d show reductions in total and LDL cholesterol ranging from about 5% to 20%.[49,50] They have little or no effect on HDL-C or triglyceride concentrations. These products may also be useful in managing constipation associated with the bile acid sequestrants. Psyllium binds cholesterol in the gut but also reduces hepatic production and clearance. Fish oil supplementation provides an increased amount of the omega-3 polyunsaturated fatty acids such as eicosapentaenoic acid and docosahexaenoic acid. In epidemiologic studies, ingestion of large amounts of cold water,

oily fish is associated with a reduction in CHD risk, but it is unclear whether the same advantage is conferred with commercially prepared fish oil products. Each 20 gm per day ingestion of fish lowers CHD risk by 7% and eating fish once weekly or more should reduce CHD mortality.[51] Fish oil supplementation has a fairly large effect in reducing triglycerides and VLDL-C, but it either has no effect on total and LDL cholesterol or may cause elevations in these fractions. Other actions of fish oil may account for their protective effects. These effects include quantitative and qualitative alterations in the synthesis of prostanoid substances, changes in immune function and cellular proliferation, and potential antioxidative actions.[52] Responses noted with fish oil are further discussed under drug therapy.[53]

Fat substitutes such as Olestra (Olean, sucrose polyester, Procter and Gamble), a mixture of hexa-, hepta-, and octa-esters formed from the reaction of sucrose with long-chain fatty acids, are approved by the FDA as a nondigestible, nonabsorbable, noncaloric fat substitute for snack foods. Olestra is heat stable, an advantage over several other fat substitutes, enabling it to be used in the preparation of fried and baked foods. It is similar in composition to triglycerides, but Olestra is not hydrolyzed in the gastrointestinal tract by pancreatic lipase, and, consequently, is not taken up by the intestinal mucosa. The principal adverse effects associated with Olestra use are bloating, flatulence, diarrhea, and "anal leakage." Because of the ability of Olestra to solubilize lipophilic substances, there has been concern over potential drug interactions in which lipophilic drugs (e.g., cyclosporin or colchicine) or vitamins (vitamins A, D, E, and K) are solubilized in Olestra and excreted in the feces.

Recent studies have demonstrated the LDL-lowering effect of plant sterols, which are isolated from soybean and tall pine tree oils. Ingestion of 2–3 grams per day will reduce LDL by 6–15%.[1] Plant sterols can be esterified to unsaturated fatty acids (creating sterol esters) to increase lipid solubility. Hydrogenating sterols produces plant stanols and, with esterification, stanol esters. The efficacy of plant sterols and plant stanols is considered to be comparable. Because lipids are needed to solubilize stanol/sterol esters, they are usually available in commercial margarines. The presence of plant stanols/sterols is listed on the food label. When margarine products are used, persons must be advised to adjust caloric intake to account for the calories contained in the products. Benecol® (McNeil), as an example, is a butter-like spread that contains a plant stanol ester, an ingredient that can lower cholesterol and which is derived from plant stanols found naturally in small amounts in foods like wheat, rye, and corn.[54] In August 2007, the Food and Drug Administration issued a warning about the consumption of red yeast rice and red yeast rice/policosonal containing products. These products contained lovastatin that could interact with other drugs and would have the same toxicity of statins but would not be recognized by the consumer and the reduction in LDL is minimal.[55]

Drug therapy is indicated following an adequate trial of TLC changes as outlined in Table 28–8.

PHARMACOLOGIC THERAPY

There are now numerous randomized, double-blinded clinical trials demonstrating that reduction of LDL reduces CHD event rates in primary prevention, secondary intervention, and in angiographic trials.[56] Generally speaking, for every 1% reduction in LDL, there is a 1% reduction in CHD event rates.[1] However, if treatment extends beyond the typical duration of a clinical trial (2–5 years), the accumulated benefit could be greater. Elevations of HDL of 1% result in approximately a 2% reduction in CHD events.[14,57] Of interest, angiographic trials, which typically cause small changes in luminal diameter (e.g., about a 0.04-mm difference in change between

TABLE 28-10 Effects of Drug Therapy on Lipids and Lipoproteins

Drug	Mechanism of Action	Effects on Lipids	Effects on Lipoproteins	Comment
Cholestyramine, colestipol, and colesevelam	↑ LDL catabolism ↓ Cholesterol absorption	↓ Cholesterol	↓ LDL ↑ VLDL	Problem with compliance; binds many co-administered acidic drugs
Niacin	↓ LDL and VLDL synthesis	↓ Triglyceride and ↓ Cholesterol	↓ VLDL, ↓ LDL, ↑ HDL	Problems with patient acceptance; good in combination with bile acid resins; extended release niacin causes less flushing and is less hepatotoxic than sustained release
Gemfibrozil, fenofibrate, clofibrate	↑ VLDL clearance ↓ VLDL synthesis	↓ Triglyceride and ↓ cholesterol	↓ VLDL, ↓ LDL, ↑ HDL	Clofibrate causes cholesterol gall stones; modest LDL lowering; raises HDL; gemfibrozil inhibits glucuronidation of simvastatin, lovastatin, and atorvastatin
Lovastatin, pravastatin, simvastatin, fluvastatin, atorvastatin, rosuvastatin	↑ LDL catabolism; inhibit LDL synthesis	↓ Cholesterol	↓ LDL	Highly effective in heterozygous familial hypercholesterolemia and in combination with other agents
Ezetimibe	Blocks cholesterol absorption across the intestinal border	↓ Cholesterol	↓ LDL	Few adverse effects; effects additive to other drugs

placebo and active treatment), result in fewer clinical events such as MI or the need for revascularization. This unexpected finding suggests that plaque size and luminal encroachment by plaque may be less important than the effects that cholesterol lowering may have on the activity in the plaque and endothelial dysfunction. These studies provide a strong rationale for attempting to lower plasma cholesterol and LDL in patients with hypercholesterolemia.

❹ Although many efficacious lipid-lowering drugs exist, none is effective in all lipoprotein disorders, and all such agents are associated with some adverse effects.[58] Lipid-lowering drugs can be broadly divided into agents that decrease the synthesis of VLDL and LDL, agents that enhance VLDL clearance, agents that enhance LDL catabolism, agents that decrease cholesterol absorption, agents that elevate HDL, or some combination of these characteristics (Table 28–10). Table 28–11 lists recommended drugs of choice for each lipoprotein phenotype and alternate agents. Table 28–12 lists available products and their doses.

Treatment of type I hyperlipoproteinemia is directed toward reduction of chylomicrons derived from dietary fat with the subsequent reduction in plasma triglycerides. Total daily fat intake should be no more than 10–25 g/d, or approximately 15% of total calories. Secondary causes of hypertriglyceridemia (see Table 28–5) should be excluded or, if present, the underlying disorder should be treated appropriately. Type V hyperlipoproteinemia also requires a stringent restriction of the fat component of dietary intake. In addition, drug therapy is indicated, as outlined in Table 28–11, if the response to diet alone is inadequate. Medium-chain triglycerides, which are absorbed without chylomicron formation, may be used as a dietary supplement for caloric intake if needed for types I and V. Hepatic fibrosis has been reported with medium-chain triglycerides. Omega-3 fatty acids may be useful in lipoprotein lipase deficiency in some patients. In patients with apolipoprotein C-II deficiency, infusion of plasma may normalize plasma triglyceride levels.

Primary hypercholesterolemia (familial hypercholesterolemia, familial combined hyperlipidemia, type IIa hyperlipoproteinemia) is treated with the bile acid resins or sequestrants (BAR, colestipol, cholestyramine, and colesevelam), HMG Co-A reductase inhibitors (statins), niacin, or eztimibe. ❺ Of these choices, statins are first choice because they are the most potent LDL lowering agents. Statins interrupt the conversion of HMG-CoA to mevalonate, the rate-limiting step in de novo cholesterol biosynthesis, by inhibiting HMG-CoA reductase (see Fig. 28–3). Currently available products include lovastatin, pravastatin, simvastatin, fluvastatin, atorvastatin, and pitvastatin.[59] Rosuvastatin is currently the most potent statin on the market. Table 28–13 lists the pharmacokinetic properties of the statins.[60] The plasma half-lives for all the statins are reported to be short except for atorvastatin and rosuvastatin, and this may account for their potency. In CURVES, the largest head-to-head comparison of statins, atorvastatin was found to be the most potent drug for lowering total cholesterol and LDL-C, with reductions in LDL-C of 38%, 46%, 51%, and 54% for the 10-, 20-, 40-, and 80-mg doses, respectively.[61] Metabolic studies with statins in normal volunteers and patients with hypercholesterolemia suggest reduced synthesis of LDL-C, as well as enhanced catabolism of LDL mediated through LDL receptors, as the principal mechanisms for lipid-lowering effects. Total and LDL cholesterol are reduced in a dose-related fashion by 30% or more on average when added to dietary therapy, with the effects being more pronounced in nonfamilial than in familial hypercholesterolemia. ❻ Combination therapy with bile acid sequestrants and lovastatin is rational as LDL receptor numbers are increased, leading to greater degradation of LDL-C; intracellular synthesis of cholesterol is inhibited, and

TABLE 28-11 Lipoprotein Phenotype and Recommended Drug Treatment

Lipoprotein Type	Drug of Choice	Combination therapy
I	Not indicated	–
IIa	Statins	Niacin or BAR
	Cholestyramine or colestipol	Statins or niacin
	Niacin	Statins or BAR
	Ezetimibe	
IIb	Statins	BAR or fibrates or niacin
	Fibrates	Statins or niacin or BAR[a]
	Niacin	Statins or fibrates
	Ezetimibe	
III	Fibrates	Statins or niacin
	Niacin	Statins or fibrates
	Ezetimibe	
IV	Fibrates	Niacin
	Niacin	Fibrates
V	Fibrates	Niacin
	Niacin	Fish oils

BAR, bile acid resins; fibrates include gemfibrozil or fenofibrate
[a]BAR are not used as first-line therapy if triglycerides are elevated at baseline, since hypertriglyceridemia may worsen with BAR alone.

TABLE 28-12 Comparison of Drugs Used in the Treatment of Hyperlipidemia

Drug	Manufacturer	Dosage Forms	Usual Daily Dose	Maximum Daily Dose
Cholestyramine(Questran)	BMS	Bulk powder/4-g packets	8 g tid	32 g
Cholestyramine(Questran Light)	BMS	Bulk powder/4-g packets		
Cholestyramine Cholybar)	Parke-Davis	4-g resin per bar		
Colestipol hydrochloride (Colestid)	Upjohn	Bulk powder/5-g packets	10 g bid	30 g
Colesevelam (Welchol)	Sankyo	625 mg tablets	1,875 mg bid	4,375 mg
Niacin	Various	50-, 100-, 250-, and 500-mg tablets; 125-, 250-, and 500-mg capsules	0.5–1 g tid	6 g/day
Extended release niacin (Niaspan)	Kos	500, 750, and 1000 mg tablets	1–2 g/day	2,000 mg
Extended release niacin + lovastatin (Advicor)[a]	Kos	Niacin/lovastatin 500 mg/20 mg tablets Niacin/lovastatin 750 mg/20 mg tablets Niacin/lovastatin 1000 mg/20 mg tablets	Niacin/lovastatin 500 mg/ 20 mg	Niacin/lovastatin 1000 mg/ 20 mg
Fenofibrate (Tricor and others)	Abbott, various	67, 134, and 200 mg capsules (micronized); 54 and160 mg tablets; 40, 120 mg tablets; 50, 160 mg tablets	54 mg or 67 mg	201 mg
Gemfibrozil (Lopid)	Parke-Davis	300-mg capsules	600 mg bid	1.5 g
Lovastatin (Mevacor)	MSD	20- and 40-mg tablets	20–40 mg	80 mg
Pravastatin (Pravachol)	Bristol-Myers Squibb	10- and 20-mg tablets	10–20 mg	40 mg
Simvastatin (Zocor)	MSD	5, 10, 20, 40 and 80-mg tablets	10–20 mg	80 mg
Atorvastatin (Lipitor)	Pfizer	10 mg tablets	10 mg	80 mg
Rosuvastatin (Crestor)	Astra-Zeneca	5- and 10-mg tablets	5 mg	40 mg
Pitavastatin (Livalo)	Kowa	1, 2, and 4 mg tablets	2 mg	4 mg
Ezetimibe (Zetia)	MSD	10 mg tablet	10 mg	10 mg
Atorvastatin/amlodipine (Caduet)	Pfizer	Atorvastatin/amlodipine 10 mg/5 mg Atorvastatin/amlodipine 20 mg/5 mg Atorvastatin/amlodipine 40 mg/5 mg Atorvastatin/amlodipine 80 mg/5 mg Atorvastatin/amlodipine 10 mg/10 mg Atorvastatin/amlodipine 20 mg/10 mg Atorvastatin/amlodipine 40 mg/10 mg Atorvastatin/amlodipine 80 mg/10 mg	Atovastatin/amlodipine 10 mg/5 mg	Atovastatin/amlodipine 80 mg/10 mg
Pravastatin/aspirin (Pravigard PAC)	BMS	Pravastatin/aspirin 20 mg/81 mg Pravastatin/aspirin 20 mg/325 mg Pravastatin/aspirin 40 mg/81 mg Pravastatin/aspirin 40 mg/325 mg Pravastatin/aspirin 80 mg/81 mg Pravastatin/aspirin 80 mg/325 mg		
Simvastatin/ezetimibe (Vytorin)	Merck/Schering-Plough	Simvastatin/ezetimibe 10 mg/ 10 mg Simvastatin/ezetimibe 20 mg/ 10 mg Simvastatin/ezetimibe 40 mg/ 10 mg	Simvastatin/ezetimibe 20 mg/10 mg	Simvastatin/ezetimibe 40 mg/10 mg
Omega-3 acid ethyl esters (Lovaza)	Reliant	Eicosapentaenoic acid (EPA) 465 mg, docosahexaenoic acid (DHA) 375 mg	4 1 gram capsules QD or 2 1 gram capsules BID	4 1 gram capsules QD or 2 1 gram capsules BID

Legend: bid indicates twice daily; probucol is no longer on the market in the U.S.; gemfibrozil, fenofibrate, and lovastatin are available as generic products. BMS, Bristol-Myers Squibb; MSD, Merck Sharp & Dohme.

[a]The manufacturer does not recommend use of the fixed combination as initial therapy of primary hypercholesterolemia or mixed dyslipidemia. It is specifically indicated in patients receiving lovastatin alone plus diet who require an additional reduction in triglyceride levels or increase in HDL-cholesterol levels; it is also indicated in those treated with niacin alone who require additional decreases in LDL cholesterol.

enterohepatic recycling of bile acids is interrupted. Combination therapy with a statin plus eztimibe is also rational, since eztimibe inhibits cholesterol absorption across the gut border and adds 12–20% further reduction when combined to a statin or other drugs.[62] However, the combination of a statin and eztimibe has not been shown to affect surrogate endpoints such as carotid intimal medial thickness (CIMT), even with further reduction in LDL cho-

lesterol.[63] Elevation of serum transaminase levels (primarily alanine aminotransferase) to greater than three times the upper limit of normal occurs in approximately 1.3% of patients on moderate to high doses of statins, and serious muscle toxicity occurs in <0.6% of patients.[64] Meta-analysis of placebo-controlled studies with statins demonstrate a low risk of abnormal ALT or CK and a low risk of myopathy without or with rhadomyolysis.[65] Lens opacities have been

TABLE 28-13 Pharmacokinetics of the Statins

Parameter	Lovastatin	Simvastatin	Pravastatin	Fluvastatin	Atorvastatin	Rosuvastatin	Pitavastatin
Isoenzyme	3A4	3A4	None	2C9	3A4	2C9/2C19	UGT1A3/UGT2B7
Lipophilic	Yes	Yes	No	Yes	Yes	No	Yes
Protein binding (%)	>95	95–98	~50	>90	96	88	99
Active metabolites	Yes	Yes	No	No	Yes	Yes	No
Elimination half-life (hr.)	3	2	1.8	1.2	7–14	13–20	12

Isoenzyme refers to the specific isoenzyme in the cytochrom P450 system which is responsible for the metabolism of each drug. Pharmacokinetic parameters in this table are based on studies and reviews presented in the literature.

reported with lovastatin. However, in the age groups studied, these abnormalities are common and tend to wax and wane with time irrespective of drug therapy, and no statistical association is known to exist. As a category of monotherapy, the HMG-CoA reductase inhibitors are the most potent total and LDL cholesterol-lowering agents and among the best tolerated.[64,65] In an analysis of more than 75,000 patients allocated to statins in clinical trials, Alsheikh-Ali et al. found that risk of statin-associated elevated liver enzymes or rhabdomyolysis is not related to the magnitude of LDL-C lowering. A highly significant inverse relationship between achieved LDL-C levels and rates of newly diagnosed cancer was observed (R^2 = 0.43, p = 0.009).[66] The WHO Foundation Collaborating Centre for International Drug Monitoring has issued a report suggesting that a rare relationship may exist between statin use and the onset of upper motor neuron diseases such as amyotrophic lateral sclerosis but this association remains uncertain.[67] Statin use is associated with a small risk of diabetes (9%).[68] There are numerous pharmacokinetic and pharmacodynamic differences among statins and patients that give rise to variable response to therapy.[69]

The primary action of BAR is to bind bile acids in the intestinal lumen, with a concurrent interruption of enterohepatic circulation of bile acids and a markedly increased excretion of acidic steroids in the feces. This decreases the bile acid pool size and stimulates hepatic synthesis of bile acids from cholesterol. Depletion of the hepatic pool of cholesterol results in an increase in cholesterol biosynthesis and an increase in the number of LDL receptors on the hepatocyte membrane. The increased number of receptors stimulates an enhanced rate of catabolism from plasma and lowers LDL levels. CETP, which is correlated with total and LDL cholesterol concentrations, is also reduced by BAR, perhaps by interfering with hepatic microsomal cholesterol content, but this effect is not as great as with statins.[70] Patients with homozygous familial hypercholesterolemia genetically lack the ability to increase synthesis of LDL receptors and bile acid resins are generally ineffective. The increase in hepatic cholesterol biosynthesis may be paralleled by increased hepatic VLDL production and consequently, bile acid resins may aggravate hypertriglyceridemia in patients with combined hyperlipidemia. Gastrointestinal complaints of constipation, bloating, epigastric fullness, nausea, and flatulence are most commonly reported.[1] With intensive education, patients can learn to tolerate resins on a long-term basis as evidenced by adherence in clinical trials to active drug regimens. However, in routine clinical practice 40% or more of patients will discontinue therapy within one year but with pharmacists' interventions, adherence rates can be improved.[71,72] These adverse effects can be managed by increasing the fluid intake, modifying the diet to increase bulk, and using stool softeners. The other major limiting complaint is the gritty texture and bulk; these problems may be minimized by mixing the powder with orange drink or juice. Tablet forms of bile acid sequestrants should help in improving compliance with this form of therapy, whereas resin does not improve compliance.[73] Other potential adverse effects include impaired absorption of fat-soluble vitamins A, D, E, and K; hypernatremia and hyperchloremia; gastrointestinal obstruction; and reduced bioavailability of acidic drugs such as coumarin anticoagulants, nicotinic acid, thyroxine, acetaminophen, hydrocortisone, hydrochlorothiazide, loperamide, and possibly iron. Hyperchloremic metabolic acidosis, hypernatremia, and gastrointestinal obstruction have been reported almost exclusively in children, and malabsorption of fat-soluble vitamins is probably most common with high doses (e.g., 30 g/d of cholestyramine) of the bile acid resins. Drug interactions may be avoided by alternating administration times with an interval of six hours or greater between the bile acid resin and other drugs. Colestipol and cholestyramine have comparable side effects; however, colestipol may have better palatability because it is odorless and tasteless. Colesevelam is the

newest BAR and total and LDL-C reduction is dose related. The adverse effects are qualitatively similar to the older BAR but may occur less often. Because of adverse effects occurring commonly with BAR at higher doses, BARs are increasingly used in combination with other drugs, as low doses are tolerated well and they work in a complementary fashion with other agents.

Niacin (nicotinic acid) may also be used in primary hypercholesterolemia in combination with bile acid sequestrants or as monotherapy for this disorder and others (Table 28–11). Niacin reduces the hepatic synthesis of VLDL, which in turn leads to a reduction in the synthesis of LDL. Factors responsible for decreased production of VLDL include inhibition of lipolysis with a decrease in free fatty acids in plasma, decreased hepatic esterification of triglycerides, and a possible direct effect on the hepatic production of apolipoprotein B.[74] The complementary action of niacin and bile acid sequestrants to increase catabolism and decrease synthesis of LDL may account for the additive effects of this combination in hyperlipidemia. Niacin also increases HDL by reducing its catabolism. Niacin selectively decreases hepatic removal of HDL apoA-I but not removal of cholesterol esters, thereby increasing the capacity of retained apoA-I to augment reverse cholesterol transport in isolated hepatic cells. The principal use of niacin is for mixed hyperlipemia or as a second-line agent in combination therapy for hypercholesterolemia. It is also considered to be the first-line agent or an alternative for the treatment of hypertriglyceridemia and diabetic dyslipidemia.[75,76] There are numerous smaller trials suggesting that lower doses of niacin may be combined with statins or gemfibrozil to minimize adverse effects and maximize response. One meta-analysis showed that combination therapy was no more effective than high dose statin therapy.[77] These combinations require careful monitoring because interactions do occur.

Niacin has many adverse drug reactions that occur commonly; fortunately, most of the symptoms and biochemical abnormalities seen do not require discontinuation of therapy. Cutaneous flushing and itching appear to be prostaglandin-mediated and can be reduced by aspirin 325 mg given shortly before niacin ingestion.[1,78] Flushing seems to be related to rising plasma concentrations of niacin; taking the dose with meals and slowly titrating the dose upward may minimize these effects. Laropiprant is a selective antagonist of the prostaglandin D(2) receptor subtype 1 (DP1), which may mediate niacin-induced vasodilation. Coadministration of laropiprant 30, 100, and 300 mg with extended-release (ER) niacin significantly lowered flushing symptom scores (by approximately 50% or more) and also significantly reduced malar skin blood flow measured by laser Doppler perfusion imaging.[79,80] Gastrointestinal intolerance and flushing are common problems. Acanthosis nigricans, a darkening of the skin in skinfold areas and an external marker of insulin resistance, may be seen with high doses of niacin. Sustained-release products may minimize these complaints in some patients, but controlled trials with regular-release products do not demonstrate much of a difference between sustained- and regular-release products. The only legend form of niacin, Niaspan® (Abbott), is an extended release form of niacin with pharmacokinetics intermediate between instant and sustained-release products which are sold as food supplements rather than legend products. In controlled trials, Niaspan® is reported to have fewer dermatologic reactions and has a low risk for hepatoxicity. When combined with statins, this combination produces large reductions in LDL and increases in HDL.[81] Potentially important laboratory abnormalities occurring with niacin therapy include elevated liver function tests, hyperuricemia, and hyperglycemia. Recent experience with niacin in diabetes suggests that some diabetic patients do not have worsened glycemic control with dose-titration and sustained-release products.[82] Body mass index and fasting plasma glucose predict loss of blood glucose control.[83] With less than 3 grams per day, the degree of liver function test elevation is generally not marked and often transient, and a temporary reduction in dosage frequently corrects the problem. Niacin-associated hepatitis is more common with sustained-release preparations, and their use should be restricted to patients intolerant of regular-release products.[82,84] Sustained-release products are often more expensive and given the lack of data for reduced adverse effects and increased incidence of hepatitis, regular-release products should always be used first. Preexisting gout and diabetes may be exacerbated by niacin; these patients should be monitored more closely and their medication titrated appropriately. Patients with well-controlled Type 2 diabetes mellitus do not have significant changes in glycemic control with niacin at doses of 2 grams per day or less.[84] Niacin is contraindicated in patients with active liver disease. Dry eyes and other ophthalmologic complaints are also occasionally noted. Concomitant alcohol and hot drinks may magnify flushing and pruritus with niacin and they should be avoided at the time of ingestion. Nicotinamide should not be used in the treatment of hyperlipidemia, as it does not effectively lower cholesterol or triglyceride levels.

Combined hyperlipoproteinemia (type IIb) may be treated with statins, niacin, or gemfibrozil combinations to lower LDL cholesterol without elevating VLDL and triglycerides. Niacin is the most effective agent and may be combined with a bile acid sequestrant. Bile acid resins alone in this disorder may elevate VLDL and triglycerides, and their use as single agents for treating combined hyperlipoproteinemia should be avoided. Fibric acid (gemfibrozil, fenofibrate) monotherapy is effective in reducing VLDL, but a reciprocal rise in LDL may occur, and total cholesterol values may remain relatively unchanged. Gemfibrozil reduces the synthesis of VLDL and to a lesser extent, apolipoprotein B, with a concurrent increase in the rate of removal of triglyceride-rich lipoproteins from plasma. Plasma HDL concentrations may rise 10% to 15% or more with fibrates. Fenofibrate may have fewer drug interactions than gemfibrozil but fenofibrate has been reported to worsen renal function.[85] Ezetimibe could also be used in combination therapy in Type IIb. Gastrointestinal complaints with fibric acid derivatives occur in 3% to 5% of patients; rash in 2% of patients; dizziness in 2.4% of patients; and transient elevations in transaminase levels and alkaline phosphatase in 4.5% and 1.3% of patients, respectively.[86] Gemfibrozil and probably fenofibrate may enhance the formation of gallstones associated with an increase in the lithogenic index; however, the rate is low (0.5–7%) and similar to that seen with placebo in the Helsinki heart study.[86] Fibric acid derivatives may potentiate the effects of oral anticoagulants and international normalized ratio (INR) should be monitored very closely with this combination.

Type III hyperlipoproteinemia may be treated with fibric acid derivatives or niacin. Although fibric acid derivatives have been suggested as the drugs of choice for this disorder, given the lack of data supporting its efficacy in altering cardiovascular mortality in the major studies on hypercholesterolemia, and numerous, well-documented, and serious adverse effects, it is reasonable to consider niacin. Gemfibrozil increases the activity of lipoprotein lipase and reduces to a lesser extent the synthesis or secretion of VLDL from the liver into the plasma. A myositis syndrome of myalgia, weakness, stiffness, malaise, and elevations in creatinine phosphokinase and aspartate aminotransaminase is seen with the fibric acid derivatives, and it seems to be more common in patients with renal insufficiency.[86] Enhanced hypoglycemic effects are reported to occur when fibric acid derivatives are given to patients on sulfonylurea compounds, but the mechanisms for these interactions are not well understood.

Two fibric acid derivatives (gemfibrozil and fenofibrate) are approved in the United States. Both reduce LDL-C by 20% to 25% in heterozygous familial hypercholesterolemia. The response of LDL-C, HDL-C, and triglycerides to this category of drug is very dependent on the specific lipoprotein type (e.g., type IIa versus IIb) and the baseline triglyceride concentration.[87]

As a potential alternative therapy, for this phenotype, numerous epidemiologic and normal volunteer studies have found that diets high in omega-3 polyunsaturated fatty acids (from fish oil), mostly commonly eicosapentaenoic acid, reduce cholesterol, triglycerides, LDL-C, and VLDL-C, and may elevate HDL-C.[53] The effects of fish oil on lipoprotein metabolism are mediated through a reduction in VLDL production and suppression of VLDL apolipoprotein B. In patients with hypertriglyceridemia, either phenotypes type IIb or type V, a diet high in omega-3 fatty acids given for 4 weeks reduced cholesterol 27% and 45%, and triglyceride 64% and 79%, in the type IIb and type V patients, respectively.[51] A diet high in eicosapentaenoic acid given to hyperlipidemic hemodialysis patients resulted in significant decreases in cholesterol and triglycerides for as long as 13 weeks. Fish oil supplementation may be most useful in patients with hypertriglyceridemia; however, its role in treatment is not well defined. Potential complications of fish oil supplementation, such as thrombocytopenia and bleeding disorders, have been noted, especially with high doses (eicosapentaenoic acid 15–30 g/d); and well-controlled trials are needed to determine if fish oils are safe and effective before their use may be broadly recommended. Based on a recent meta-analysis, fish consumption lowers the risk of CHD but nutricueticals have not been adequately tested.[51] Recently, a prescription form of concentrated fish oil, Lovaza®, has become available.[53] This product lowers triglycerides by 14% to 30% and raises HDL by about 10%, depending on baseline values.

Combination drug therapy may be considered after adequate trials of monotherapy and for patients documented compliant to the prescribed regimen. Two or three lipoprotein profiles at 6-week intervals should confirm lack of response prior to initiation of combination therapy. Cholestyramine may be added in patients with fasting hypertriglyceridemia, but it should not be used as the initial drug, because triglycerides are likely to increase. Contraindications to and drug interactions with combined therapy should be carefully screened, as well as consideration of the extra cost of drug product and monitoring that may be required. In general, a statin and a BAR or niacin with a BAR provide the greatest reduction in total and LDL cholesterol. Regimens intended to increase HDL levels should include either gemfibrozil or niacin, and it should be remembered that statins combined with either of these drugs may result in a greater incidence of hepatotoxicity or myositis. This is particularly important for statins that are eliminated via cytochrome 3A4 or through glucuronidation.[60] Familial combined hyperlipidemia may respond better to a fibric acid and a statin than to a fibric acid and a BAR.[88]

Severe forms of hypercholesterolemia, such as familial hypercholesterolemia, familial defective apolipoprotein B-100, severe polygenic hypercholesterolemia, familial combined hyperlipidemia, and familial dysbetalipoproteinemia (type III)—may require more intensive therapy. In particular, familial hypercholesterolemia patients often require combination therapy (two or three drugs) and are managed with surgical therapy (partial ileal bypass), plasmapheresis (LDL-apheresis), and liver transplantation (to replace LDL receptors).

■ HYPERTRIGLYCERIDEMIA

It is important to remember that lipoprotein pattern types I, III, IV, and V are associated with hypertriglyceridemia, and that these primary lipoprotein disorders and underlying diseases should be excluded prior to implementing therapy (see Table 28–5). In a national survey, approximately one third of participants tested had a triglyceride concentration exceeding 150 mg/dL.[89] A positive family history of CHD is important in identifying patients at risk for premature atherosclerosis.[17,90] If a patient with CHD has elevated triglycerides, the associated abnormality is probably a contributing factor to CHD and should be treated.[32]

High serum triglycerides (see Tables 28–6 and 28–11) should be treated by achieving desirable body weight, consumption of a low saturated fat and cholesterol diet, regular exercise, smoking cessation, and restriction of alcohol (in selected patients). ATP III identifies the sum of LDL + VLDL (termed *non-HDL* [total cholesterol - HDL]) as a secondary target of therapy in persons with high triglycerides (≥200 mg/dL).[1,32] This approach is used when triglycerides exceed 200 mg/dL and accounts for atherogenic particles carried in VLDL and remnant particles. The goal for non-HDL in persons with high serum triglycerides can be set at 30 mg/dL higher than that for LDL on the premise that a VLDL level ≤30 mg/dL is normal. ❼ In patients with borderline-high triglycerides but with accompanying risk factors of established CHD disease, family history of premature CHD, concomitant LDL elevation or low HDL, and genetic forms of hypertriglyceridemia associated with CHD (familial dysbetalipoproteinemia, familial combined hyperlipidemia), drug therapy with niacin should be considered. Niacin may be used cautiously in diabetics based on the results of the ADMIT trial, which found that triglycerides were reduced by 23%, HDL-C increased by 29%, there was only a slight increase in glucose (mean 8.7 mg/dL), and no change in hemoglobin A$_{1c}$.[91] Elevated body mass index and plasma glucose predict loss of glycemic control.[83] Alternative therapies include gemfibrozil or fenofibrate, statins, and fish oil.[17,92,93] Fibrates may increase LDL, and their use in borderline-high triglyceridemia requires careful monitoring to detect this deleterious change in lipid profile. Statins may also be used, because they provide modest reductions in triglycerides and modest elevations in HDL. Higher doses of statins may reduce HDL as well as LDL and triglycerides with the amount of reduction related to the baseline concentration and dose.[17,93] The goal of therapy in this situation is to lower triglycerides and VLDL particles that may be atherogenic, increase HDL, and reduce LDL.

Very high triglycerides are associated with pancreatitis and other consequences of the chylomicron syndrome. At this level of elevation of triglycerides, a genetic form of hypertriglyceridemia often coexists with other causes of elevated triglycerides such as diabetes. Dietary fat restriction (10% to 20% of calories as fat), weight loss, alcohol restriction, and treatment of the coexisting disorder are the basic elements of management. Drugs useful in hypertriglyceridemia include gemfibrozil or fenofibrate, niacin, and higher potency statins (atorvastatin, rosuvastatin, pitavastatin, and simvastatin). Gemfibrozil or fenofibrate are the preferred drugs in diabetics because of the effect of niacin on glycemic control unless the newer extended-release forms are used. Fenofibrate may be preferred in combination with statin therapy since it does not impair glucuronidation and minimizes potential drug interactions. Success in treatment is defined as a reduction in triglycerides below 500 mg/dL.[1]

■ LOW HDL CHOLESTEROL

Low HDL is a strong independent risk predictor of CHD. ATP III redefined low HDL-C as <40 mg/dL, but specified no goal for HDL-C raising.[1] Low HDL may be a consequence of insulin resistance, physical inactivity, Type 2 diabetes, cigarette smoking, very high carbohydrate intake, and certain drugs (see Table 28–5). ❽ In low HDL, the primary target remains LDL according to ATP III, but emphasis shifts to weight reduction, increased physical activity, and smoking cessation, and if drug therapy is required, to fibric acid derivatives and niacin. Niacin has the potential for the greatest increase in HDL and the effect is more pronounced with regular or immediate-release forms than with sustained-release forms.[94]

■ DIABETIC DYSLIPIDEMIA

Diabetic dyslipidemia is characterized by hypertriglyceridemia, low HDL, and LDL that is minimally elevated. Small, dense LDL (pattern B) in diabetes is more atherogenic than larger, more buoyant forms of LDL (pattern A); routine lipoprotein profiles do not differentiate between pattern A and pattern B.[95–97] Diabetes in ATP III is a CHD risk equivalent and the primary target is LDL with a goal of treatment being to lower LDL-C <100 mg/dL.[1] When LDL is >130 mg/dL, most patients will require simultaneous therapeutic lifestyle changes and drug therapy. When LDL-C is between 100 and 129 mg/dL, intensifying glycemic control, adding drugs for the atherogenic dyslipidemia (fibric acid derivatives, niacin) and intensifying LDL-C-lowering therapy are options. Because the primary target is LDL-C in diabetic dyslipidemia, statins are considered by many to be initial drugs of choice.[1,32] The relative risk reduction for CHD in diabetics versus nondiabetics is greater in the West of Scotland, (37% versus 20%)[98] AFCAPS/TexCAPS (43% versus 36%),[99] CARE (25% versus 23%),[100] and 4S (55% versus 32%) trials.[101] All statins are fairly comparable in triglyceride lowering and because statins differ in potency for LDL reduction, a ratio of LDL reduction to triglyceride reduction can be applied. Statin therapy may protect against the development of diabetes.[29] The most recent trial LDL-lowering in Type 2 diabetes mellitus is the Collaborative Atorvastatin Diabetes Study (CARDS).[102] This was a randomized, double-blind placebo comparison of atorvastatin 10 mg per day versus placebo in 2,838 diabetes patients to reduce first CHD events. Baseline LDL was 118 mg/dL and with atorvastatin LDL fell by 46 mg/dL. The primary end point, a composite of acute CHD death, nonfatal MI, hospitalized unstable angina, resuscitated cardiac arrest, and coronary revascularization or stroke, was reduced by 37%. This study suggests that all diabetics should have a LDL much lower than 100 mg/dL and these results are consistent with the Heart Protection Study analysis of diabetic patients.[103]

Fenofibrate, according to the DIAS trial, reduced the angiographic progression of CAD in type 2 diabetes.[104] Fewer CHD events were seen with fenofibrate compared with placebo but the difference was not significant. Fibric acids principally lower VLDL and triglycerides while increasing HDL with only modest lowering of total and LDL cholesterol. On occasion, fibric acid derivatives may increase LDL levels. Fibric acid derivatives tend to improve glucose tolerance, in contrast to niacin; the greatest effect has been seen with bezafibrate. The Helsinki Heart Study found gemfibrozil to be most effective in diabetic dyslipidemia.[105] Although the effect of statins on triglycerides and HDL abnormalities commonly seen in diabetes is less than with fibric acids, the subgroup analyses cited earlier suggest that they reduce CHD risk significantly. In the Action to Control Cardiovascular Risk in Diabetes (ACCORD) the combination of a statin and fenofibrate in patients with type 2 diabetes did not reduce the rate of fatal cardiovascular events, nonfatal myocardial infarction, or nonfatal stroke compared to simvastatin alone.[106] Cholestyramine in diabetic patients may result in lower LDL levels, but VLDL and triglyceride levels, which are commonly elevated in diabetes, may be further increased in this population. Resins may aggravate constipation, which is common in diabetics. As demonstrated in the ADMIT and ADVENT trials, immediate-release and extended-release niacin are very effective in raising HDL and lowering triglycerides and LDL.[91,107]

■ SPECIAL CONSIDERATIONS

Elderly

Hypercholesterolemia is an independent risk factor for CHD in the elderly (>65 years old), as it is in the younger patient. The attributable risk, which is the difference in absolute rates of CHD between segments of the population with higher or lower serum cholesterol levels, increases with age. Older patients potentially benefit to a greater extent from cholesterol lowering than younger populations. Data from studies of elderly men in a variety of settings are consistent with a relative risk of at least 1.5 in the highest quartile compared to the lowest quartile of cholesterol levels and a relative risk reduction of 22% for heart-related mortality.[108,109,110] Treatment of hypercholesterolemia in the elderly may bring about a comparable reduction in absolute risk to that obtained in younger persons.[1] Subgroup analyses of the West of Scotland (primary) and 4S (secondary) intervention studies show that elderly patients have lower CHD risk reduction (relative risk reduction of 27% and 29%, respectively) as compared to younger patients (relative risk reduction of 40% and 39%, respectively).[98,111] The Framingham study suggests that elderly women are at higher risk because of high blood cholesterol levels, but no other large studies included women; and their risks or benefits from cholesterol reduction are not well defined. Primary prevention in younger patients requires about two years before reduction in CHD risk is apparent, and this lag time should be taken into consideration in patient selection for therapy. Non-lipid CHD risk factors do not decline in relative risk with aging, and aggressive management of the modifiable non-lipid risk factors is important in the older patient. High-risk elderly patients are less likely to be prescribed statins and their potent benefits are not realized.[112] Because most women with CHD are elderly and also at risk for osteoporosis, they are logical candidates for diet therapy with consideration of calcium intake consistent with osteoporosis prevention, exercise, and perhaps estrogen replacement therapy. Recent evidence suggests that statins may reduce the risk of osteoporosis; however, there are conflicting data from various studies.[113]

Drug therapy in principle differs little from younger patients, and older patients respond to lipid-lowering drugs as well as younger patients.[114,115] Based on the Heart Protection Study with more elderly patients than any other trial, simvastatin 40 mg per day produced the same CHD event rate reduction in patients over 70 years of age as in younger patients.[116] The gain in life expectancy may be small depending on the age at the start of treatment and the magnitude of cholesterol reduction. Changes in body composition, renal function, and other physiologic changes of aging may make older patients more susceptible to adverse effects of lipid-lowering drug therapy. In particular, older patients are more likely to have constipation (bile acid resins), skin and eye changes (niacin), gout (niacin), gallstones (fibric acid derivatives), and bone/joint disorders (fibric acid derivatives, statins). Therapy should be started with lower doses and titrated up slowly to minimize adverse effects.

Women

Cholesterol is an important determinant of CHD in women, but the relationship is not as strong as that seen in men. HDL may be a more important predictor of disease in women.[4] LDL and HDL genetic regulation in women and men does not appear to be different. Based on the Nurses' Health Study, obesity is an important determinant of CHD in women, with the relative risk being 3.3 in the highest Quetelet index (weight in kilograms divided by the square of the height in meters) as compared to the lowest category (i.e., <21 vs ≥29); low HDL levels usually accompany obesity.[117] No major differences exist in the influence of exercise, alcohol ingestion, and smoking on lipid levels between men and women. Women

in the highest tertile of cholesterol appear to be more responsive to dietary therapy than those in the lower tertiles, and more responsive than formulas based on men predict.

Based on the HERS[118] and WHI trials[119–121], recently published national guidelines recommended similar types of lifestyle and risk factor goals and interventions as recommended by NCEP for the entire population.[4] Hormone therapy may continue to have a role for postmenopausal symptoms, however, a notable exception is hormone replacement therapy and heart protection. Combined estrogen plus progestin hormone therapy should not be initiated to prevent CVD in postmenopausal women. Combined estrogen plus progestin hormone therapy should not be continued to prevent CVD in postmenopausal women. Other forms of menopausal hormone therapy (e.g., unopposed estrogen) should not be initiated or continued to prevent CVD in postmenopausal women pending the results of ongoing trials. Results of the WISDOM trial confirm a lack of benefit as seen in HERS and WHI.[122] In a recent, post-hoc analysis of the WHI, women who initiated hormone therapy closer to menopause tended to have reduced CHD risk compared with the increase in CHD risk among women more distant from menopause, but this trend did not meet statistical signifance.[119] Based on the Justification for the Use of Statins in Prevention: An Intervention Trial Evaluating Rosuvastatin (JUPITER) trial, women experience the same benefit of LDL cholesterol lowering as men with rosuvastatin.[123]

Cholesterol and triglyceride levels rise progressively throughout pregnancy, with an average increment in cholesterol of 30–40 mg/dL occurring around the 36th to 39th weeks. Triglyceride levels may go up by as much as 150 mg/dL. Drug therapy is not instituted nor is it usually continued during pregnancy. If the patient is very high risk, a bar acid resin may considered since there is no systemic drug exposure.[1] Statins are category X and are contraindicated. Ezetimibe might be an alternative, since it is a Category C drug (animal studies have shown that the drug exerts teratogenic or embryocidal effects, and there are no adequate, well-controlled studies in pregnant women, or no studies are available in either animals or pregnant women) but no data are available in humans. Dietary therapy is the mainstay of treatment, with emphasis on maintaining a nutritionally balanced diet as per the needs of pregnancy.

Children

Drug therapy in children is not recommended until the age of 8 years or older, and the guidelines for institution of therapy and the goals of therapy are different from those in adults.[124] Younger children are generally managed with therapeutic lifestyle changes until after the age of 2 years.[1,46] Although bile acid sequestrants have been recommended in the past as first line therapy, there is now evidence that statins are safe and effective in children and provide greater lipid lowering than BAR.[125–127,128] Severe forms of hypercholesterolemia (e.g., familial hypercholesterolemia) may require more aggressive treatment.

■ CONCURRENT DISEASE STATES

Nephrotic syndrome, end-stage renal disease and nephrotic syndrome, and hypertension compound the risk of dyslipidemia and may present difficult-to-treat lipid abnormalities. Abnormalities of lipoprotein metabolism in the nephrotic syndrome include elevated total and LDL cholesterol, Lp(a), VLDL, and triglycerides. The apolipoprotein C-III to C-II ratio is elevated, consistent with greater lipoprotein lipase inhibitor activity, and the extent of hypoalbuminemia is correlated with dyslipidemia. The basic abnormality appears to be one of overproduction of LDL-apoB from VLDL, rather than reduced clearance of LDL-C and related proteins. Protein restriction and a "vegan" diet corrects lipid abnormalities to some extent. Statins have been shown to be effective in reducing elevated total and LDL cholesterol in the nephrotic syndrome, although the levels do not usually return to normal.[129] Fibric acid derivatives and statins reduce small, dense LDL-C by different mechanisms, suggesting a potential role for combination therapy to optimize lowering of small, dense LDL-C and remnant lipoproteins. Statins appear to safe and effective for lowering LDL cholesterol in renal insufficiency but they may not affect CHD endpoints.[130,131]

Renal insufficiency without proteinuria leads to hypertriglyceridemia, slightly elevated total and LDL cholesterol (particularly with chronic ambulatory peritoneal dialysis), and low HDL levels (especially during hemodialysis). These abnormalities are thought to be caused by a deficiency in apolipoprotein C-II, perhaps as a result of sustained use of heparin during hemodialysis and depletion of lipoprotein lipase, carbohydrate-induced obesity and hypertriglyceridemia, loss of carnitine during hemodialysis, use of acetate buffer (acetate is a precursor to fatty acid synthesis) during hemodialysis, and decreased LCAT activity during hemodialysis. Dialysis does not correct the lipid abnormalities. Renal transplantation may correct lipid abnormalities in some patients. However, in others, the use of transplantation-related medications such as corticosteroids, cyclosporine, and certain antihypertensive agents (see Chapters 19 and 98) may aggravate the lipid abnormalities. Cyclosporine interferes with the metabolism of statins metabolized by cytochrome P450 3A4 (Table 28–13), and patients need to be observed closely for myositis and worsening renal function. Of interest, correction of lipid abnormalities may improve renal hemodynamics. Pravastatin and fluvastatin may be safer than other statins, but this needs to be validated in larger, long-term trials. Diet will modify lipoprotein levels and polyunsaturated fatty acids may have a role in impeding the progression of renal disease as well as the cardiovascular complications. Bile acid sequestrants do not correct the lipid abnormalities seen in renal insufficiency. Lovastatin or its active metabolite may accumulate in renal insufficiency, and lower doses of reductase inhibitors should be used to avoid adverse effects. Gemfibrozil may be used with caution as its pharmacokinetics are unchanged and it lowers triglycerides and increases HDL.[132] Statins (simvastatin, lovastatin, and atorvastatin) and fibric acid derivatives may increase the risk of severe myopathy, and attention to symptoms of myositis is needed. Niacin may also be useful in nondiabetic patients with renal insufficiency.

Hypertensive patients have a greater-than-expected prevalence of high blood-cholesterol levels and, conversely, patients with hypercholesterolemia have a higher than expected prevalence of hypertension caused by the metabolic syndrome. Recommendations for the management of hypertension in patients with hypercholesterolemia include avoiding the use of drugs that elevate cholesterol such as diuretics and β-blockers and using agents that are either lipid-neutral or that may reduce cholesterol slightly (see Chapter 19).[1] Bile acid sequestrants may bind to thiazide diuretics and some β-blockers, and may interfere with their absorption; reaction may be avoided by giving the antihypertensive 1 hour before or 4 hours after the resin. Niacin may magnify the hypotensive effects of vasodilators.

■ PHARMACOECONOMIC CONSIDERATIONS

🔟 The clinical benefits of lipid-lowering therapy for primary and secondary intervention are now well established, based on the results of studies showing a reduction in CHD morbidity and mortality.[133,134,135] The balance of benefits and costs has been examined in a few studies. The cost per year of life saved has been estimated to range from less than $10,000 to over $1 million dollars, depending on the presence or absence of CHD, age of the patient, baseline total or LDL-C level and reduction in cholesterol, and number of risk factors present. In general, intervention in patients with known CHD, those who have CHD risk equivalents, or those with a 10-year risk of 10% to 20%, are cost-effective with statin therapy, while other types of therapy may be cost-effective if certain assumptions concerning compliance, efficacy, and so forth, are met. The range for secondary intervention based on the 4S study is $3,800 for a 70-year-old man with a high cholesterol level to $27,400 per year of life gained for a middle-aged woman with an average cholesterol level.[136] In contrast, primary prevention in men based on the West of Scotland trial averages about $35,000 per year of life gained.[137] These studies demonstrate that primary and secondary interventions are well within the accepted boundary of less than $50,000 for a medical intervention to be considered cost-effective. Based on the specific lipoprotein phenotype, fibric acid derivatives, niacin, or combination therapy of statins plus BAR may be cost-effective. Cost-effectiveness is maximized by treating high-risk patients and those with established CHD.

Specialty lipid clinics have become increasingly popular and many use pharmacists to provide direct patient care in this setting. An interesting recent analysis shows that a specialty clinic may be more expensive ($659 ± $43 versus $477 ± $42 per patient, $P < .001$) than usual care. However, the overall cost-effectiveness is improved when expressed as program costs per unit (mmol/L) reduction in the LDL-C, a measure of cost-effectiveness that was significantly lower for specialized care ($758 ± $58 versus $1,058 ± $70, $P = .002$)because more patients achieve their targeted goal.[138] Project ImPACT demonstrated that pharmacists, working collaboratively with patients and physicians can improve persistence and compliance and that nearly two-thirds of patients achieved their NCEP lipid goal.[139] Other programs show similar trends.[72,140,141]

■ OTHER THERAPIES

Partial ileal bypass has been used in severe heterozygous and homozygous familial hypercholesterolemia; however, it is ineffective in the latter case. Ileal bypass removes the site of bile acid reabsorption, depleting the bile acid pool and increasing the catabolism of cholesterol. A randomized trial of diet versus surgery program on the surgical control of the hyperlipidemias (POSCH), reported that total and LDL cholesterol were decreased (23.3% and 37.7%, respectively) and HDL increased (4.3%) in patients who had undergone ileal bypass for hypercholesterolemia.[142] Overall death was delayed by nearly 3 years ($P = .032$) and CHD mortality was delayed by nearly 4 years ($P = .046$) by surgery, as compared to the control group. Revascularization procedures were delayed by an average of 7 years ($P < .001$). Post-surgery diarrhea was more common in the surgical group, as was the rate of kidney stones (4% versus 0.4%), gallstones (10% versus 2%), and bowel obstruction (13.5% versus 3.6%).

Portacaval shunts have been used to decrease the formation of LDL-C and reductions of 10% to 20% have been reported. Plasma exchange combined with niacin was found to reduce plasma cholesterol levels by about 50% in homozygous familial hypercholesterolemia over 5 years, and coronary atherosclerosis did not progress as documented by angiography. LDL-apheresis, selective removal of LDL-C via a filtering system, plus statin therapy is effective in LDL-C and appears to affect the progression of vascular disease. LDL-apheresis may be combined with statin therapy for greater effect. Combined liver and heart transplantation in homozygous familial hypercholesterolemia reduces total and LDL cholesterol concentrations from about 1100 and 900 mg/dL to about 300 and 185 mg/dL, prior to and after surgery, respectively. Liver transplantation replaced the missing LDL receptors, enhanced catabolism, and reduced lipoprotein synthesis in this patient.

TABLE 28-14 Primary Prevention Trials with Lipid-Lowering Drugs

Trial	F/U (yr)	N	Treatment	Control Events	Treatment Events	P Value	RRR	ARR	NNT
AFCAPS/TexCAPS	5	6,605	Lovastatin 20–40 mg	5.5%	3.5%	<0.001	36.4%	2.0%	50
Helsinki	5	4,081	Gemfibrozil 1200 mg	4.1%	2.7%	<0.02	34.0%	1.4%	71
LRC-CPPT	7.4	3,806	Cholestyramine 24 g	9.8%	8.1%	<0.05	17.3%	1.7%	59
Oslo	5	1,232	Diet + smoking cessation	4.2%	2.5%	0.03	40.5%	1.7%	59
WOSCOPS	4.9	6,595	Pravastatin 40 mg	7.8%	5.5%	<0.001	29.5%	2.3%	43
ALLHAT	4.8	10,355	Usual care Pravastatin 40 mg	10.4%	9.3%	0.16	9%	1.1%	91
WHI	5.2	16,608	Usual care Diet, CEE 0.625 mg + MPA 2.5 mg	1.5%	1.9%	0.05	1.29[a]	0.4%	200[b]
WHI	5.2	16,608	Usual care Diet, CEE 0.625 mg	3.7%	3.3%	NS	9%	0.4%	250
CARDS	4	2,838	Atorvastatin 10 mg	9.0%	5.8%	0.001	37%	3.2%	32
JUPITER	1.9	17,802	Rosuvastatin 20 mg	2.82%	1.59%	0.00001	44%	1.2%	82

Legend: AFCAPS/TexCAPS, Air Force/Texas Coronary Atherosclerosis Prevention Study (Downs et al, 1998); Helsinki, The Helsinki Heart Study (Frick et al., 1987); LRC-CPPT, The Lipid Research Clinics Coronary Primary Prevention Trial (Insull et al., 1984); Oslo, The Oslo Study (Hjermann et al., 1988); WOSCOPS, The West of Scotland Coronary Prevention Study (Shepherd et al., 1995); ALLHAT, Antihypertensive and Lipid-Lowering Treatment to Prevent Heart Attack Trial; approximately 13–15% of patients had a history of coronary heart disease (CHD); events are CHD events only; JUPITER, Justification for the Use of Statins in Prevention (Ridker, 2008); WHI, Women's Health Initiative; RRR, Relative Risk Reduction; ARR, Absolute Risk Reduction; NNT, Number Needed to Treat; NA, Not available; CEE, conjugated equine estrogen; MPA medtroxyprogesterone acetate; CARDS, Collaborative Atorvastatin Diabetes Study (presented at the 2004 American Diabetes Association meeting).
[a]HR, hazard ratio. The risk of CHD was increased by 29%.
[b]Number needed to harm since CEE + MPA was worse than placebo.

■ SUMMARY OF MAJOR STUDIES

⑨ Primary and secondary prevention diet and drug trials have been performed to determine whether lowering of cholesterol will prevent CHD. Table 28–14 and Table 28–15 summarize these trials. A number of earlier angiographic studies demonstrated that cholesterol reduction leads to regression of atherosclerosis and plaque stabilization. Most of the primary and secondary studies were double blinded, randomized, and placebo controlled, lasting for 5 years or longer, and most had sufficient patient numbers to be meaningful. Exceptions to these qualifications were seen in the early studies such as the Newcastle and Edinburgh trials, which were small and generally did not show much benefit; and the Coronary Drug Project (CDP) using dextrothyroxine, which was terminated early due to adverse effects on CHD mortality. The Helsinki heart

study, using gemfibrozil, resulted in a reduction in nonfatal MI, which was the primary contributor to reduced CHD incidence (Table 28–14).[16]

Total and LDL cholesterol were reduced an average of 13.4% and 20.3%, respectively, by cholestyramine in the LRC-CPPT, and the reduction of lipid levels was related to the amount of drug ingested (e.g., 1 to 2 packets, 5.4% reduction in total cholesterol, versus 5 or more packets, 19.0% reduction).[143] The prescribed dose of cholestyramine was 24 g, or 6 packets, per day. The cholestyramine group experienced a 19% reduction in risk ($P < .05$) of the primary end point: Definite CHD death and/or definite nonfatal MI, reflecting a 24% reduction in definite CHD death and a 19% reduction in nonfatal MI. Other end points were reduced by 25%, 20%, and 21% for new positive exercise tests, angina, and coronary bypass

TABLE 28-15 Secondary Prevention Trials with Lipid-Lowering Drugs

Trial	F/U (yr)	N	Treatment	Control Events	Treatment Events	P Value	RRR	ARR	NNT
VA-HIT	5.1	2,531	Gemfibrozil 1200 mg	23.7%	17.3%	0.006	22%	4.4%	23
AVERT	1.5	341	Atorvastatin 80 mg	21%	13%	0.048	38%	8%	12
CARE	5	4,159	Pravastatin 40 mg	13.2%	10.2%	0.003	22.7%	3.0%	33
CDP	5	8,341	Niacin 3 g + Clofibrate 1.8 g	20.9%	20.6%	NS	1.4%	0.3%	333
HERS	4.1	2,673	Estrogen 0.625 mg + Progestin 2.5 mg	12.7%	12.5%	0.91	1.6%	0.2%	500
LIPID	7.4	3,806	Pravastatin 40 mg	9.8%	8.1%	<0.05	17.3%	1.7%	59
4S	5	4,444	Simvastatin 20 mg	11.5%	8.2%	0.0003	28.7%	3.3%	30
WHO	5.3	15,745	Clofibrate 1.6 g	3.9%	3.1%	<0.005	20.5%	0.8%	125
BIP	6.2	3,090	Placebo Bezafibrate 400 mg	15.0%	13.6%	0.26	9.3%	1.4%	72
TIMI-22	2	4,162	Pravastatin 40 mg Atorvastatin 80 mg	26.3% (P)	22.4% (A)	0.005	16%	3.9%	26
HPS	5	20,536	Simvastatin 40 mg	14.7%	12.9%	0.003	13%	1.8%	56
MIRACL		3,086	Atorvastatin 80 mg	17.4%	14.8%	0.048	16%	2.6%	39
PROSPER	3	5,804	Pravastatin 40 mg	16.2%	14.1%	0.014	24%	2.1%	48
SPARCL	4.0	4,731	Atorvastatin 80 mg	13.1%	11.2%	0.03	16%	2.2%	46
TNT	4.9	10,001	Atorvastatin 10 mg vs. 80 mg	10.9%	8.7%	<0.001	22%	2.2%	46
ACCORD	4.7	5,518	Fenofibrate 160 mg	2.4%	2.2%	0.32	8%	0.2%	500

Legend: VA-HIT, Veterans Administration-High-Density Lipoprotein Cholestol (HDL-C) Intervention Trial; AVERT, The Atorvastatin Versus Revascularization Treatments; CARE, Cholesterol and Recurrent Events (Melendez et al., 1996); CDP, Coronary Drug Project (Berge et al., 1975); HERS, Heart and Estrogen Replacement Study (Hulley et al., 1998); LIPID, Long-Term Intervention with Pravastatin in Ischaemic Disease Study (MacMahon et al., 1995); 4S, Scandinavian Simvastatin Survival Study (Pederson et al., 1994); WHO, World Health Organization (Committee of Principal Investigators, 1978); BIP, Bezafibrate Infarction Prevention; TIMI-22, Thrombolysis in Myocardial Infarction study 22; also known as the PROVE-IT trial (Cannon, et al., 2004); HPS, Heart Protection Study; results expressed as all cause mortality (HPS Collaborative Group, 2002); MIRACL, Myocardial Ischemia Reduction with Aggressive Cholesterol Lowering (Schwartz, et al., 2001); PROSPER, PROspective Study of Pravastatin in the Elderly at Risk (Shepher, 2002); SPARCL, Stroke Prevention by Aggressive Reduction in Cholesterol Levels (SPARCL investigators, 2006); TNT, Treatment to New Targets (LaRosa, 2005); ACCORD, Action to Control Cardiovascular Risk in Diabetes (Accord Study Group, 2010); RRR, Relative Risk Reduction; ARR, Absolute Risk Reduction; NNT, Number Needed to Treat.

surgery, respectively. Death from all causes was not significantly reduced by cholestyramine secondary to more accidents and violence in this group. The mean falls in total and LDL cholesterol in the cholestyramine group were 8% and 12% relative to levels in placebo-treated men, providing evidence that for every 1% reduction in cholesterol, a 2% decline in CHD mortality can be realized.

AFCAPS/TexCAPS, a primary prevention trial conducted in 6,605 men and women aged 57 to 63 years with average total cholesterol and LDL (<221 mg/dL and <150 mg/dL, respectively) who were treated with lovastatin 20–40 mg/d for 5.2 years, a 37% reduction (P < .001) was shown in the risk for first acute major coronary event (fatal or nonfatal MI, unstable angina, or sudden cardiac death).[99] The need for revascularization procedures was also reduced by 33% (P < .001). The implications of this trial are enormous. Potentially millions of "normal" people could benefit from lipid-lowering with statins based on these results. The number of patients that need to be treated (NNT, Table 28–14) for primary prevention ranges from 43 in the West of Scotland trial to 71 in the Helsinki Heart Study. This range is within the typical boundary used for treatment decisions and described previously; cost-effectiveness is achieved routinely in patients with moderate to high risk. The Antihypertensive and Lipid-Lowering Treatment to Prevent Heart Attack Trial (ALLHAT-LLT) tested pravastatin 40 mg per day versus placebo in hypertensive patients with at least one CHD risk factor. Pravastatin did not reduce either all-cause mortality or CHD significantly when compared with usual care in older participants with well-controlled hypertension and moderately elevated LDL-C. The results may be due to the modest differential in total cholesterol (9.6%) and LDL-C (16.7%) between pravastatin and usual care compared with prior statin trials supporting cardiovascular disease prevention.[144] The Women's Health Initiative trial proved to be disappointing, with no beneficial effects on CHD event reduction in the hormone replacement arm (conjugated equine estrogens (CEE) + medroxyprogesterone) or the CEE alone arm compared to placebo.[118,120] Women did experience greater risk for thromboembolism and a slight increase in breast cancer and a reduced risk of hip fracture. Consequently, hormone replacement therapy can no longer be recommended for cardiovascular protection.[4] Publication of the recent WISDOM trial found that when combined hormone therapy (n = 2196) was compared with placebo (n = 2189), there was a significant increase in the number of major cardiovascular events (7 vs 0, P = 0.016) and venous thromboembolism (22 vs 3, hazard ratio 7.36 [95% CI 2.20 to 24.60]) confirming the findings of HERS and WHI. There were no statistically significant differences in numbers of breast or other cancers, cerebrovascular events, fractures, and overall death.[122]

Niacin in the CDP significantly reduced definite, nonfatal MI as compared to placebo (10.1% versus 13.9%), whereas clofibrate did not reduce death from any cause or nonfatal or fatal MI at the 5-year follow-up period.[145]

One of the most important studies published in the last few years is the 4S trial, a secondary intervention trial in a large number of patients.[146] Simvastatin, 20–40 mg/d, reduced LDL cholesterol by 35% and reduced the risk of death from any cause by 30%. Coronary deaths were also reduced with simvastatin (relative risk, 0.58; confidence interval, 0.46–0.73). Therapy was also shown to be effective in women (18% to 19% of patients enrolled) and in the elderly (≥60 years). Indeed, the relative risk of death or major coronary event was reduced to a greater extent in the elderly than in younger patients. Death from noncardiovascular causes was similar for simvastatin and placebo (2.1% and 2.2%, respectively). The survival curves for simvastatin and placebo began to separate at 1 year and became more divergent with additional follow-up. The 4S study clearly demonstrates the benefit in cholesterol lowering and placates long-held fears of death from non-CHD causes. The long-term intervention with pravastatin in ischemic disease (LIPID) study (N = 7498 men and 1516 women) has investigated the effect of pravastatin on CHD mortality in patients with prior MI or unstable angina and mean cholesterol level of 219 mg/dL over 6 years.[147] Pravastatin reduced the risk of CHD mortality by 24% (8.3% versus 6.4%, P = .0004) and total mortality by 23% (14.1% versus 11.0%, P = .00002); stroke was also reduced by 20% (4.3% versus 3.5%, P = .22) as well as a reduction in the need for coronary artery bypass graft (11.3% versus 8.9%, P = .0001) or percutaneous transluminal coronary angioplasty (5.3% versus 4.4%, P = .04).

The Veterans Administration High-Density Lipoprotein intervention trial (VA-HIT) was a double-blind trial that compared gemfibrozil (1200 mg/d) with placebo in 2,531 men with CHD, an HDL cholesterol level of ≤40 mg/dL, and an LDL cholesterol level of ≤140 mg/dL.[148] The primary study outcome was nonfatal MI or death from coronary causes. The median follow-up was 5.1 years. At 1 year, the mean HDL cholesterol level was 6% higher, the mean triglyceride level was 31% lower, and the mean total cholesterol level was 4% lower in the gemfibrozil group than in the placebo group. LDL cholesterol levels did not differ significantly between the groups. A primary event occurred in 21.7% of the patients assigned to placebo and in 17.3% of the patients assigned to gemfibrozil. The overall reduction in the risk of an event was 4.4 percentage points, and the reduction in relative risk was 22% (P = 0.006). This trial presents the strongest evidence to date that raising HDL-C and lowering triglycerides reduces risk for CHD.

The Atorvastatin Versus Revascularization Treatments (AVERT) study compared atorvastatin 80 mg/d with percutaneous transluminal coronary angioplasty.[149] The follow-up period was 18 months. Of the patients who received aggressive lipid-lowering treatment with atorvastatin, 13% had ischemic events, as compared to 21% of the patients who underwent angioplasty. The incidence of ischemic events was thus 36% lower in the atorvastatin group over an 18-month period (P = 0.048, which was not statistically significant after adjustment for interim analyses). This reduction in events was because of a smaller number of angioplasty procedures, coronary-artery bypass operations, and hospitalizations for worsening angina (the most common end point). As compared to the patients who were treated with angioplasty and usual care, the patients who received atorvastatin had a significantly longer time to the first ischemic event (P = 0.03). In low-risk patients with stable CAD, aggressive lipid-lowering therapy is at least as effective as angioplasty and usual care in reducing the incidence of ischemic events.

Pravastatin in the elderly individuals at risk for vascular disease (PROSPER) studied men and women in the age range of 70–82 years and found that pravastatin 40 mg per day reduced CHD events by 24% with no affect on cognitive function.[150] A more recent trial, TIMI-22 (also known as PROVE-IT, Pravastatin or Atorvastatin Evaluation and Infection Therapy) enrolled 4,162 patients who had been hospitalized for an acute coronary syndrome within the preceding 10 days and compared 40 mg of pravastatin daily (standard therapy) with 80 mg of atorvastatin daily (intensive therapy).[151] An intensive lipid lowering statin regimen with atorvastatin 80 mg per day provided greater protection against death or major cardiovascular events than did a standard regimen. This study clearly points to "lower is better" for LDL concentration and will likely lead to revision in guideline goals to lower LDL levels. The Treatment to New Targets (TNT) assessed the efficacy and safety of lowering LDL cholesterol levels below 100 mg per deciliter (2.6 mmol per liter) in patients with stable coronary heart disease (CHD).[152,153] Intensive lipid-lowering therapy with 80 mg of atorvastatin per day in patients with stable CHD provides significant clinical benefit beyond that afforded by treatment with 10 mg of atorvastatin per day, providing further evidence that intensive lipid lowering brings greater benefits.

Statins reduce the incidence of strokes among patients at increased risk for cardiovascular disease. Whether they reduce the risk of stroke after a recent stroke or transient ischemic attack (TIA) was addressed by Stroke Prevention by Aggressive Reduction in Cholesterol Levels (SPARCL). During a median follow-up of 4.9 years, 265 patients (11.2 percent) receiving atorvastatin 80 mg/day and 311 patients (13.1 percent) receiving placebo had a fatal or nonfatal stroke (5-year absolute reduction in risk, 2.2 percent; adjusted hazard ratio, 0.84; 95 percent confidence interval, 0.71 to 0.99; P = 0.03; unadjusted P = 0.05).[154] JUPITER randomized healthy patients to rosuvastatin on placebo on the basis of elevated CRP and found a 55% reduction in vascular events (event rate 1.11 vs. 0.51 per 100 person-years; hazard ratio 0.45, p <0.0001).[23]

CLINICAL CONTROVERSIES

The CETP inhibitor torcetrapib was associated with a substantial increase in HDL cholesterol and decrease in LDL cholesterol. It was also associated with an increase in blood pressure, and there was no significant decrease in the progression of coronary atherosclerosis. The lack of efficacy may be related to the mechanism of action of this drug class or to molecule-specific adverse effects. Other means of raising HDL cholesterol (HDL mimetics, which include ApoA1 mutants and peptide mimetics of ApoA1 and HDL Milano A, a synthetic form of HDL) still hold hope of HDL modification leading a reduction in clinical events.

The enzyme acyl-coenzyme A:cholesterol acyltransferase (ACAT) esterifies cholesterol in a variety of tissues. In some animal models, ACAT inhibitors have antiatherosclerotic effects. Unfortunately, when tested in clinical trials, ACAT inhibition is not an effective strategy for limiting atherosclerosis and may promote atherogenesis.[155]

Statins differ in their pharmacokinetic properties and in pleotropic effects (i.e., non-lipid lowering). The contribution of lipid lowering alone (a class effect) versus other effects (anti-inflammatory, antithombotic, etc.) continues to create controversy.

Proteinuria has been associated with high dose rosuvastatin therapy (40 mg/day), but a review of a clinical trial database revealed an increase in eGFR for rosuvastatin-treated patients was consistent across all major demographic and clinical subgroups of interest, including patients with baseline proteinuria, baseline eGFR <60 ml/min/1.73 m2, and in patients with hypertension and/or diabetes.[156]

Mipomersen, an investigational apoliprotein B synthesis inhibitor, reduced LDL cholesterol in patients with homozygous hypercholesterolemia by nearly 25% with the most common adverse events being injection site pain.[157]

The role of non-traditional risk factors (hsCRP, homocysteine, etc.) continues to be clarified and may lead to recommendations for the use of these tests in patient evaluation.

EVALUATION OF THERAPEUTIC OUTCOMES

Short-term evaluation of therapy for hyperlipidemia is based on response to diet and drug treatment as measured in the clinical laboratory by total cholesterol, LDL cholesterol, HDL cholesterol, and triglycerides for patients being treated for primary intervention, as well as on response to secondary intervention. The interval for follow-up is dependent on the severity of illness, and patients with known CAD or multiple risk factors should be monitored

more closely. Less commonly used laboratory measurements include C-reactive protein, homocysteine, apolipoprotein B, and Lp(a) levels. Because many patients being treated for primary hyperlipidemia have no symptoms and may not have any clinical manifestations of a genetic lipid disorder such as xanthomas or eruptions, monitoring and outcome are solely laboratory based. In patients treated for secondary intervention, symptoms of atherosclerotic cardiovascular disease, such as angina or intermittent claudication, may improve over months to years. If patients have xanthomas or other external manifestations of hyperlipidemia, these lesions should regress with therapy. Lipid measurements should be obtained in the fasted state to minimize interference from chylomicrons, and once the patient is stable, monitoring is needed at intervals of 6 months to 1 year. The goals for LDL and HDL cholesterol are provided in Table 28–8.

Patients with multiple risk factors and established CHD should also be monitored and evaluated for progress in managing their other risk factors such as hypertension, smoking cessation, exercise and weight control, and glycemic control if diabetic. The goals are to maintain a blood pressure of below 130/80 mm Hg or less (presence of diabetes or renal insufficiency), stop smoking, maintain an ideal body weight, exercise for at least 20 minutes three or more times per week, and keep plasma glucose below 100 mg/dL (threshold for glucose intolerance). Invasive evaluation, such as cardiac catheterization, is useful in patients with established CHD and is typically used for planning revascularization rather than monitoring of lipid-lowering therapy.

Evaluation of dietary therapy is part of the outcome evaluation for treating hyperlipidemia and the assistance of a dietitian is recommended. Use of diet diaries and recall survey instruments enable information about diet to be collected in a systematic fashion and may improve patient adherence to dietary recommendations. Patients on resin therapy should have a FLP panel checked every 4–8 weeks until a stable dose is reached; triglycerides should be checked at the stable dose to ensure they have not increased. Niacin requires baseline liver function tests, uric acid and glucose; repeat tests are appropriate at doses of 1,000–1,500 mg per day. Symptoms of myopathy or diabetes-like symptoms should be investigated and may require CK or glucose determinations; more frequent monitoring in diabetics may be necessary. A FLP 4–8 weeks after the initial dose or dose changes with statins is appropriate. Liver function tests should be obtained at baseline and periodically thereafter based on package insert information. Recognized experts believe that monitoring for hepatotoxicity and myopathy should be symptom-triggered.[58,65] Ezetimibe requires little specific monitoring. However, with the publication of the SEAS trial, there is concern over the increased risk of cancer.[158] Other studies underway will clarify this issue.

REFERENCES

1. Expert Panel on Detection E, and Treatment of High Blood Cholesterol in Adults. Executive summary of the third report of the National Cholesterol Education Program (NCEP) Expert Panel on Detection, Evaluation and Treatment of High Blood Cholesterol in Adults (Adult Treatment Panel III). Jama 2001;285:2486–2497.
2. Grundy SM, Cleeman JI, Merz CN, et al. Implications of recent clinical trials for the National Cholesterol Education Program Adult Treatment Panel III guidelines [erratum appears in Circulation. 2004 Aug 10;110(6):763]. Circulation 2004;110:227–239.
3. Smith SC, Jr., Allen J, Blair SN, et al. AHA/ACC guidelines for secondary prevention for patients with coronary and other atherosclerotic vascular disease: 2006 update: endorsed by the National Heart, Lung, and Blood Institute [erratum appears in Circulation. 2006 Jun 6;113(22):e847]. Circulation 2006;113:2363–2372.

4. Mosca L, Banka CL, Benjamin EJ, et al. Evidence-based guidelines for cardiovascular disease prevention in women: 2007 update. Circulation 2007;115:1481–1501.

5. Fletcher B, Berra K, Ades P, et al. Managing abnormal blood lipids: a collaborative approach. Circulation 2005;112:3184–3209.

6. Ford ES, Mokdad AH, Giles WH, Mensah GA. Serum total cholesterol concentrations and awareness, treatment, and control of hypercholesterolemia among US adults: findings from the National Health and Nutrition Examination Survey, 1999 to 2000. Circulation 2003;107:2185–2189.

7. Lloyd-Jones D, Adams RJ, Brown TM, et al. Heart disease and stroke statistics-2010 update: a report from the American Heart Association. Circulation 2010;121:e46–e215.

8. Arnett DK, Jacobs DR, Jr., Luepker RV, Blackburn H, Armstrong C, Claas SA. Twenty-year trends in serum cholesterol, hypercholesterolemia, and cholesterol medication use: the Minnesota Heart Survey, 1980–1982 to 2000–2002. Circulation 2005;112:3884–3891.

9. Lloyd-Jones D, Adams RJ, Brown TM, et al. Executive Summary: Heart Disease and Stroke Statistics-2010 Update A Report From the American Heart Association. Circulation 2010;121:948–954.

10. Foley KA, Denke MA, Kamal-Bahl S, et al. The impact of physician attitudes and beliefs on treatment decisions: lipid therapy in high-risk patients. Medical Care 2006;44:421–428.

11. Carroll MD, Lacher DA, Sorlie PD, et al. Trends in serum lipids and lipoproteins of adults, 1960–2002. Jama 2005;294:1773–1781.

12. Menotti A, Lanti M, Nedeljkovic S, Nissinen A, Kafatos A, Kromhout D. The relationship of age, blood pressure, serum cholesterol and smoking habits with the risk of typical and atypical coronary heart disease death in the European cohorts of the Seven Countries Study. International Journal of Cardiology 2006;106:157–163.

13. McQueen MJ, Hawken S, Wang X, et al. Lipids, lipoproteins, and apolipoproteins as risk markers of myocardial infarction in 52 countries (the INTERHEART study): a case-control study. Lancet 2008;372: 224–233.

14. Rader DJ. Mechanisms of disease: HDL metabolism as a target for novel therapies. Nature Clinical Practice Cardiovascular Medicine 2007;4:102–109.

15. Jeppesen J, Hein HO, Suadicani P, Gyntelberg F. Triglyceride concentration and ischemic heart disease: an eight-year follow-up in the Copenhagen Male Study. Circulation 1998;97:1029–1036.

16. Huttunen JK, Manninen V, Manttari M, et al. The Helsinki Heart Study: central findings and clinical implications. Annals of Medicine 1991;23:155–159.

17. Yuan G, Al-Shali KZ, Hegele RA. Hypertriglyceridemia: its etiology, effects and treatment. CMAJ Canadian Medical Association Journal 2007;176:1113–1120.

18. Ganong WF. Pathophysiology of Disease: An Introduction to Clinical Medicine, 5th Edition. New York: McGraw Hill; 2006.

19. Nissen SE, Tardif JC, Nicholls SJ, et al. Effect of torcetrapib on the progression of coronary atherosclerosis. New England Journal of Medicine 2007;356:1304–1316.

20. Libby P, Aikawa M, Jain MK. Vascular endothelium and atherosclerosis. Handbook of Experimental Pharmacology 2006;176:285–306.

21. Miller DT, Ridker PM, Libby P, Kwiatkowski DJ. Atherosclerosis: the path from genomics to therapeutics. Journal of the American College of Cardiology 2007;49:1589–1599.

22. Sofat R, Hingorani AD, Smeeth L, et al. Separating the mechanism-based and off-target actions of cholesteryl ester transfer protein inhibitors with CETP gene polymorphisms. Circulation 2010;121: 52–62.

23. Ridker PM, Danielson E, Fonseca FA, et al. Reduction in C-reactive protein and LDL cholesterol and cardiovascular event rates after initiation of rosuvastatin: a prospective study of the JUPITER trial. Lancet 2009;373:1175–1182.

24. Eagle KA, Ginsburg GS, Musunuru K, et al. Identifying patients at high risk of a cardiovascular event in the near future: current status and future directions: report of a national heart, lung, and blood institute working group. Circulation 2010;121:1447–1454.

25. Kujiraoka T, Hattori H, Miwa Y, et al. Serum apolipoprotein in health, coronary heart disease and type 2 diabetes mellitus. Journal of Atherosclerosis & Thrombosis 2006;13:314–322.

26. Libby P. How our growing understanding of inflammation has reshaped the way we think of disease and drug development. Clin Pharmacol Ther 2010;87:389–391.

27. Huang CY, Wu TC, Lin WT, et al. Effects of simvastatin withdrawal on serum matrix metalloproteinases in hypercholesterolaemic patients. European Journal of Clinical Investigation 2006;36:76–84.

28. Suviolahti E, Lilja HE, Pajukanta P. Unraveling the complex genetics of familial combined hyperlipidemia. Annals of Medicine 2006;38: 337–351.

29. Buse JB, Ginsberg HN, Bakris GL, et al. Primary prevention of cardiovascular diseases in people with diabetes mellitus: a scientific statement from the American Heart Association and the American Diabetes Association. Diabetes Care 2007;30:162–172.

30. Grundy SM, Cleeman JI, Daniels SR, et al. Diagnosis and management of the metabolic syndrome: an American Heart Association/National Heart, Lung, and Blood Institute Scientific Statement [erratum appears in Circulation. 2005 Oct 25;112(17):e297]. Circulation 2005;112: 2735–2752.

31. Grundy SM, Pasternak R, Greenland P, Smith S, Jr., Fuster V. AHA/ACC scientific statement: Assessment of cardiovascular risk by use of multiple-risk-factor assessment equations: a statement for healthcare professionals from the American Heart Association and the American College of Cardiology. Journal of the American College of Cardiology 1999;34:1348–1359.

32. Grundy SM, Cleeman JI, Merz CN, et al. A summary of implications of recent clinical trials for the National Cholesterol Education Program Adult Treatment Panel III guidelines. Arteriosclerosis, Thrombosis & Vascular Biology 2004;24:1329–1330.

33. Grundy SM, Cleeman JI, Merz CN, et al. Implications of recent clinical trials for the National Cholesterol Education Program Adult Treatment Panel III Guidelines. Journal of the American College of Cardiology 2004;44:720–732.

34. Singh IM, Shishehbor MH, Ansell BJ. High density lipoprotein as a therapeutic target. A systematic review. JAMA 2007;298:786–798.

35. Daniels SR, Greer FR. Lipid screening and cardiovascular health in childhood. Pediatrics 2008;122:198–208.

36. Strong JP, Malcom GT, Oalmann MC, Wissler RW. The PDAY Study: natural history, risk factors, and pathobiology. Pathobiological Determinants of Atherosclerosis in Youth. Annals of the New York Academy of Sciences 1997;811:226–35; discussion 35–37.

37. Lauer RM, Obarzanek E, Hunsberger SA, et al. Efficacy and safety of lowering dietary intake of total fat, saturated fat, and cholesterol in children with elevated LDL cholesterol: the Dietary Intervention Study in Children. American Journal of Clinical Nutrition 2000;72:1332S–1342S.

38. Van Horn L, Obarzanek E, Friedman LA, Gernhofer N, Barton B. Children's adaptations to a fat-reduced diet: the Dietary Intervention Study in Children (DISC). Pediatrics 2005;115:1723–1733.

39. Iughetti L, Predieri B, Balli F, Calandra S. Rational approach to the treatment for heterozygous familial hypercholesterolemia in childhood and adolescence: a review. J Endocrinol Invest 2007;30:700–719.

40. Wierzbicki AS, Viljoen A. Hyperlipidaemia in paediatric patients: the role of lipid-lowering therapy in clinical practice. Drug Saf 2010;33: 115–125.

41. Trejo-Gutierrez JF, Fletcher G. Impact of exercise on blood lipids and lipoproteins. Journal of Clinical Lipidology 2007;1:175–181.

42. Williams MA, Haskell WL, Ades PA, et al. Resistance exercise in individuals with and without cardiovascular disease: 2007 update: a scientific statement from the American Heart Association Council on Clinical Cardiology and Council on Nutrition, Physical Activity, and Metabolism. Circulation 2007;116:572–584.

43. Eckel RH, Borra S, Lichtenstein AH, Yin-Piazza SY. Trans Fat Conference Planning G. Understanding the complexity of trans fatty acid reduction in the American diet: American Heart Association Trans Fat Conference 2006: report of the Trans Fat Conference Planning Group. Circulation 2007;115:2231–2246.

44. American Heart Association Nutrition Committee, Lichtenstein AH, Appel LJ, et al. Diet and lifestyle recommendations revision 2006: a scientific statement from the American Heart Association Nutrition Committee [erratum appears in Circulation. 2006 Jul 4;114(1):e27]. Circulation 2006;114:82–96.

45. Sacks FM, Lichtenstein A, Van Horn L, et al. Soy protein, isoflavones, and cardiovascular health: an American Heart Association Science Advisory for professionals from the Nutrition Committee. Circulation 2006;113:1034–1044.

46. Gidding SS, Dennison BA, Birch LL, et al. Dietary recommendations for children and adolescents: a guide for practitioners: consensus statement from the American Heart Association [erratum appears in Circulation. 2005 Oct 11;112(15):2375]. Circulation 2005;112: 2061–2075.

47. Grundy SM, Cleeman JI, Daniels SR, et al. Diagnosis and management of the metabolic syndrome: an American Heart Association/National Heart, Lung, and Blood Institute scientific statement. Current Opinion in Cardiology 2006;21:1–6.

48. Assmann G, Guerra R, Fox G, et al. Harmonizing the definition of the metabolic syndrome: comparison of the criteria of the Adult Treatment Panel III and the International Diabetes Federation in United States American and European populations. American Journal of Cardiology 2007;99:541–548.

49. Shrestha S, Volek JS, Udani J, et al. A combination therapy including psyllium and plant sterols lowers LDL cholesterol by modifying lipoprotein metabolism in hypercholesterolemic individuals. Journal of Nutrition 2006;136:2492–2497.

50. Petchetti L, Frishman WH, Petrillo R, Raju K. Nutriceuticals in cardiovascular disease: psyllium. Cardiology in Review 2007;15:116–122.

51. He K, Song Y, Davigius ML, et al. Accumulated evidence on fish consumption and coronary heart disease mortality: a meta-analysis of cohort studies. Circulation 2004;109:2705–2711.

52. von Schacky C, Harris WS. Cardiovascular benefits of omega-3 fatty acids. Cardiovascular Research 2007;73:310–315.

53. McKenney JM, Sica D. Role of prescription omega-3 fatty acids in the treatment of hypertriglyceridemia. Pharmacotherapy 2007;27:715–728.

54. Bhattacharya S. Therapy and clinical trials: plant sterols and stanols in management of hypercholesterolemia: where are we now? Current Opinion in Lipidology 2006;17:98–100.

55. Berthold HK, Unverdorben S, Degenhardt R, Bulitta M, Gouni-Berthold I. Effect of policosanol on lipid levels among patients with hypercholesterolemia or combined hyperlipidemia: a randomized controlled trial. Jama 2006;295:2262–2269.

56. Baigent C, Keech A, Kearney PM, et al. Efficacy and safety of cholesterol-lowering treatment: prospective meta-analysis of data from 90,056 participants in 14 randomised trials of statins. Lancet 2005;366:1267–1278.

57. Link JJ, Rohatgi A, de Lemos JA. HDL cholesterol: physiology, pathophysiology, and management. Current Problems in Cardiology 2007;32:268–314.

58. McKenney JM. Introduction. Report of the National Lipid Association's Safety Task Force: The nonstatins. American Journal of Cardiology 2007;99:1C–58C.

59. Wensel TM, Waldrop BA, Wensel B. Pitavastatin: a new HMG-CoA reductase inhibitor. Ann Pharmacother 2010;44:507–514.

60. Shitara Y, Sugiyama Y. Pharmacokinetic and pharmacodynamic alterations of 3-hydroxy-3-methylglutaryl coenzyme A (HMG-CoA) reductase inhibitors: drug-drug interactions and interindividual differences in transporter and metabolic enzyme functions. Pharmacology & Therapeutics 2006;112:71–105.

61. Jones P, Kafonek S, Laurora I, Hunninghake D, Investigators C. Comparative dose efficacy study of atorvastatin versus simvastatin, pravastatin, lovastatin, and fluvastatin in patients with hypercholesterolemia. (The CURVES Study). American Journal of Cardiology 1998;81:582–587.

62. Robinson JG, Davidson MH. Combination therapy with ezetimibe and simvastatin to achieve aggressive LDL reduction. Expert Review of Cardiovascular Therapy 2006;4:461–476.

63. Nissen SE. ENHANCE and ACCORD: controversy over surrogate end points. Curr Cardiol Rep 2008;10:159–161.

64. Davidson MH, Robinson JG. Safety of aggressive lipid management. Journal of the American College of Cardiology 2007;49:1753–1762.

65. McKenney JM, Davidson MH, Jacobson TA, Guyton JR, National Lipid Association Statin Safety Assessment Task F. Final conclusions and recommendations of the National Lipid Association Statin Safety Assessment Task Force. American Journal of Cardiology 2006;97:17.

66. Alsheikh-Ali AA, Maddukuri PV, Han H, Karas RH. Effect of the Magnitude of Lipid Lowering on Risk of Elevated Liver Enzymes, Rhabdomyolysis, and Cancer: Insights From Large Randomized Statin Trials. Journal of the American College of Cardiology 2007;50:409–418.

67. Edwards IR, Star K, Kiuru A. Statins, neuromuscular degenerative disease and an amyotrophic lateral sclerosis-like syndrome: an analysis of individual case safety reports from vigibase. Drug Safety 2007;30: 515–525.

68. Sattar N, Preiss D, Murray HM, et al. Statins and risk of incident diabetes: a collaborative meta-analysis of randomised statin trials. Lancet 2010;375:735–742.

69. Mangravite LM, Thorn CF, Krauss RM. Clinical implications of pharmacogenomics of statin treatment. Pharmacogenomics Journal 2006;6:360–374.

70. McPherson R. Comparative effects of simvastatin and cholestyramine on plasma lipoproteins and CETP in humans. Canadian Journal of Clinical Pharmacology 1999;6:85–90.

71. Tsuyuki RT, Bungard RJ. Poor adherence with hypolipidemic drugs: a lost opportunity. Pharmacotherapy 2001;21.

72. Tsuyuki RT, Olson KL, Dubyk AM, Schindel TJ, Johnson JA. Effect of community pharmacist intervention on cholesterol levels in patients at high risk of cardiovascular events: the Second Study of Cardiovascular Risk Intervention by Pharmacists (SCRIP-plus). American Journal of Medicine 2004;116:130–133.

73. McCrindle BW, O'Neill MB, Cullen-Dean G, Helden E. Acceptability and compliance with two forms of cholestyramine in the treatment of hypercholesterolemia in children: a randomized, crossover trial. Journal of Pediatrics 1997;130:266–273.

74. Zhang Y, Schmidt RJ, Foxworthy P, et al. Niacin mediates lipolysis in adipose tissue through its G-protein coupled receptor HM74A. Biochemical & Biophysical Research Communications 2005;334: 729–732.

75. Carlson LA. Nicotinic acid: the broad-spectrum lipid drug. A 50th anniversary review. Journal of Internal Medicine 2005;258:94–114.

76. Shepherd J, Betteridge J, Van Gaal L, European Consensus P. Nicotinic acid in the management of dyslipidaemia associated with diabetes and metabolic syndrome: a position paper developed by a European Consensus Panel. Current Medical Research & Opinion 2005;21: 665–682.

77. Sharma M, Ansari MT, Abou-Setta AM, et al. Systematic review: comparative effectiveness and harms of combination therapy and monotherapy for dyslipidemia. Ann Intern Med 2009;151:622–630.

78. Stern RH. The role of nicotinic acid metabolites in flushing and hepatoxicity. Journal of Clinical Lipidology 2007;1:191–193.

79. Lai E, De Lepeleire I, Crumley TM, et al. Suppression of niacin-induced vasodilation with an antagonist to prostaglandin D2 receptor subtype 1. Clinical Pharmacology & Therapeutics 2007;81:849–857.

80. Maccubbin D, Koren MJ, Davidson M, et al. Flushing profile of extended-release niacin/laropiprant versus gradually titrated niacin extended-release in patients with dyslipidemia with and without ischemic cardiovascular disease. Am J Cardiol 2009;104:74–81.

81. McKenney JM, Jones PH, Bays HE, et al. Comparative effects on lipid levels of combination therapy with a statin and extended-release niacin or ezetimibe versus a statin alone (the COMPELL study). Atherosclerosis 2007;192:432–437.

82. McKenney J. Niacin for dyslipidemia: considerations in product selection. American Journal of Health System Pharmacy 2003;60: 995–1005.

83. Libby A, Meier J, Lopez J, Swislocki AL, Siegel D. The effect of body mass index on fasting blood glucose and development of diabetes mellitus after initiation of extended-release niacin. Metab Syndr Relat Disord 2010;8:79–84.

84. Guyton JR, Bays HE. Safety considerations with niacin therapy. American Journal of Cardiology 2007;99:19.

85. Forsblom C, Hiukka A, Leinonen ES, Sundvall J, Groop PH, Taskinen MR. Effects of long-term fenofibrate treatment on markers of renal function in type 2 diabetes: the FIELD Helsinki substudy. Diabetes Care 2010;33:215–220.

86. Davidson MH, Armani A, McKenney JM, Jacobson TA. Safety considerations with fibrate therapy. American Journal of Cardiology 2007;99:19.

87. Sveger T, Flodmark CE, Nordborg K, Nilsson-Ehle P, Borgfors N. Hereditary dyslipidaemias and combined risk factors in children with a family history of premature coronary artery disease. Archives of Disease in Childhood April 2000;82:292–296.

88. Grundy SM, Vega GL, Yuan Z, Battisti WP, Brady WE, Palmisano J. Effectiveness and tolerability of simvastatin plus fenofibrate for combined hyperlipidemia (the SAFARI trial) [erratum appears in Am J Cardiol. 2006 Aug 1;98(3):427–8]. American Journal of Cardiology 2005;95:462–468.

89. Ford ES, Li C, Zhao G, Pearson WS, Mokdad AH. Hypertriglyceridemia and its pharmacologic treatment among US adults. Arch Intern Med 2009;169:572–578.

90. Capell WH, Eckel RH. Treatment of hypertriglyceridemia. Current Diabetes Reports 2006;6:230–240.

91. Elam MB, Hunninghake DB, Davis KB, et al. Effect of niacin on lipid and lipoprotein levels and glycemic control in patients with diabetes and peripheral arterial disease: the ADMIT study: A randomized trial. Arterial Disease Multiple Intervention Trial. Jama 2000;284:1263–1270.

92. McKenney JM, Sica D. Prescription omega-3 fatty acids for the treatment of hypertriglyceridemia. American Journal of Health System Pharmacy 2007;64:595–605.

93. Oh RC, Lanier JB. Management of hypertriglyceridemia. American Family Physician 2007;75:1365–1371.

94. McKenney J. New perspectives on the use of niacin in the treatment of lipid disorders. Archives of Internal Medicine 2004;164:697–705.

95. Gadi R, Samaha FF. Dyslipidemia in type 2 diabetes mellitus. Current Diabetes Reports 2007;7:228–234.

96. Tan KC. Management of dyslipidemia in the metabolic syndrome. Cardiovascular & Hematological Disorders Drug Targets 2007;7:99–108.

97. Garg A, Simha V. Update on dyslipidemia. Journal of Clinical Endocrinology & Metabolism 2007;92:1581–1589.

98. Shepherd J, Cobbe SM, Ford I, et al. Prevention of coronary heart disease with pravastatin in men with hypercholesterolemia. West of Scotland Coronary Prevention Study Group. New England Journal of Medicine 1995;333:1301–1307.

99. Downs JRMD, Clearfield MDO, Weis SDO, et al. Primary prevention of acute coronary events with lovastatin in men and women with average cholesterol levels: results of AFCAPS/TexCAPS. JAMA May 1998;279:1615–1622.

100. Sacks FM, Pfeffer MA, Moye LA, et al. The effect of pravastatin on coronary events after myocardial infarction in patients with average cholesterol levels. New England Journal of Medicine October 1996;335:1001–1009.

101. Anonymous. Design and baseline results of the Scandinavian Simvastatin Survival Study of patients with stable angina and/or previous myocardial infarction. American Journal of Cardiology 1993;71:393–400.

102. Colhoun HM, Betteridge DJ, Durrington PN, et al. Primary prevention of cardiovascular disease with atorvastatin in type 2 diabetes in the Collaborative Atorvastatin Diabetes Study (CARDS): multicentre randomised placebo-controlled trial. Lancet 2004;364:685–696.

103. Collins R, Armitage J, Parish S, Sleight P, Peto R, Heart Protection Study Collaborative G. Effects of cholesterol-lowering with simvastatin on stroke and other major vascular events in 20536 people with cerebrovascular disease or other high-risk conditions. Lancet 2004;363:757–767.

104. Anonymous. Effect of fenofibrate on progression of coronary-artery disease in type 2 diabetes: the Diabetes Atherosclerosis Intervention Study, a randomised study. Lancet 2001;357:905–90.

105. Backes JM, Gibson CA, Ruisinger JF, Moriarty PM. Fibrates: what have we learned in the past 40 years? Pharmacotherapy 2007;27:412–424.

106. Effects of combination lipid therapy in type 2 diabetes mellitus. N Engl J Med 2010.

107. Grundy SM, Vega GL, McGovern ME, et al. Efficacy, safety, and tolerability of once-daily niacin for the treatment of dyslipidemia associated with type 2 diabetes: results of the assessment of diabetes control and evaluation of the efficacy of niaspan trial. Archives of Internal Medicine 2002;162:1568–1576.

108. Davidson MH, Kurlandsky SB, Kleinpell RM, Maki KC. Lipid management and the elderly. Preventive Cardiology 2003;6:128–133.

109. Mazza A, Tikhonoff V, Schiavon L, Casiglia E. Triglycerides + high-density-lipoprotein-cholesterol dyslipidaemia, a coronary risk factor in elderly women: the CArdiovascular STudy in the ELderly. Internal Medicine Journal 2005;35:604–610.

110. Afilalo J, Duque G, Steele R, Jukema JW, de Craen AJ, Eisenberg MJ. Statins for secondary prevention in elderly patients: a hierarchical bayesian meta-analysis. J Am Coll Cardiol 2008;51:37–45.

111. Anonymous. Randomised trial of cholesterol lowering in 4444 patients with coronary heart disease: the Scandinavian Simvastatin Survival Study (4S). Lancet 1994;344:1383–1389.

112. Berger AK, Duval SJ, Armstrong C, Jacobs DR, Jr., Luepker RV. Contemporary diagnosis and management of hypercholesterolemia in elderly acute myocardial infarction patients: a population-based study. American Journal of Geriatric Cardiology 2007;16:15–23.

113. Hatzigeorgiou C, Jackson JL. Hydroxymethylglutaryl-coenzyme A reductase inhibitors and osteoporosis: a meta-analysis. Osteoporosis International 2005;16:990–998.

114. Blue Cross Blue Shield A, Technology Evaluation C. Special report: the efficacy and safety of statins in the elderly. Technology Evaluation Center Assessment Program Executive Summary 2007;21:1–3.

115. Anonymous. Pravastatin benefits elderly patients: results of PROSPER study. Cardiovascular Journal of Southern Africa 2003;14: Jan-Feb.

116. Heart Protection Study Collaborative G. MRC/BHF Heart Protection Study of cholesterol lowering with simvastatin in 20,536 high-risk individuals: a randomised placebo-controlled trial [summary for patients in Curr Cardiol Rep. 2002 Nov;4(6):486–7; PMID: 12379169]. Lancet 2002;360:7–22.

117. Abate N. Obesity and cardiovascular disease. Pathogenetic role of the metabolic syndrome and therapeutic implications. Journal of Diabetes & its Complications 2000;14:154–174.

118. Hulley S, Grady D, Bush T, et al. Randomized trial of estrogen plus progestin for secondary prevention of coronary heart disease in postmenopausal women. Heart and Estrogen/progestin Replacement Study (HERS) Research Group. Jama 1998;280:605–613.

119. Rossouw JE, Prentice RL, Manson JE, et al. Postmenopausal hormone therapy and risk of cardiovascular disease by age and years since menopause. Jama 2007;297:1465–1477.

120. Anderson GL, Limacher M, Assaf AR, et al. Effects of conjugated equine estrogen in postmenopausal women with hysterectomy: the Women's Health Initiative randomized controlled trial. Jama 2004;291:1701–1712.

121. Wassertheil-Smoller S, Hendrix SL, Limacher M, et al. Effect of estrogen plus progestin on stroke in postmenopausal women: the Women's Health Initiative: a randomized trial. Jama 2003;289:2673–2684.

122. Vickers MR, MacLennan AH, Lawton B, et al. Main morbidities recorded in the women's international study of long duration oestrogen after menopause (WISDOM): a randomised controlled trial of hormone replacement therapy in postmenopausal women. BMJ 2007;335:doi:10.1136/bmj.39266.425069.AD.

123. Mora S, Glynn RJ, Hsia J, MacFadyen JG, Genest J, Ridker PM. Statins for the primary prevention of cardiovascular events in women with elevated high-sensitivity C-reactive protein or dyslipidemia: results from the Justification for the Use of Statins in Prevention: An Intervention Trial Evaluating Rosuvastatin (JUPITER) and meta-analysis of women from primary prevention trials. Circulation 2010;121:1069–1077.

124. Davis V, Schatz D, Winter W. Pediatric lipid disorders in clinical practice. eMedicine 2006;http://www.emedicine.com/ped/topic2787.htm#section~pictures.

125. Clauss SB, Holmes KW, Hopkins P, et al. Efficacy and safety of lovastatin therapy in adolescent girls with heterozygous familial hypercholesterolemia. Pediatrics 2005;116:682–688.

126. Wiegman A, Hutten BA, de Groot E, et al. Efficacy and safety of statin therapy in children with familial hypercholesterolemia: a randomized controlled trial. Jama 2004;292:331–337.

127. de Jongh S, Ose L, Szamosi T, et al. Efficacy and safety of statin therapy in children with familial hypercholesterolemia: a randomized, double-blind, placebo-controlled trial with simvastatin. Circulation 2002;106:2231–2237.

128. O'Gorman CS, Higgins MF, O'Neill MB. Systematic review and metaanalysis of statins for heterozygous familial hypercholesterolemia in children: evaluation of cholesterol changes and side effects. Pediatr Cardiol 2009;30:482–489.

129. Toto RD, Grundy SM, Vega GL. Pravastatin treatment of very low density, intermediate density and low density lipoproteins in hypercholesterolemia and combined hyperlipidemia secondary to the nephrotic syndrome. American Journal of Nephrology 2000;20: 12–17.

130. Fellstrom BC, Jardine AG, Schmieder RE, et al. Rosuvastatin and cardiovascular events in patients undergoing hemodialysis. N Engl J Med 2009;360:1395–1407.

131. Baber U, Toto RD, de Lemos JA. Statins and cardiovascular risk reduction in patients with chronic kidney disease and end-stage renal failure. American Heart Journal 2007;153:471–477.

132. Samuelsson O, Attman PO, Knight-Gibson C, et al. Effect of gemfibrozil on lipoprotein abnormalities in chronic renal insufficiency: a controlled study in human chronic renal disease. Nephron 1997;75:286–294.

133. Peterson AM, McGhan WF. Pharmacoeconomic impact of noncompliance with statins. Pharmacoeconomics 2005;23:13–25.

134. Tarraga-Lopez PJ, Celada-Rodriguez A, Cerdan-Oliver M, et al. A pharmacoeconomic evaluation of statins in the treatment of hypercholesterolaemia in the primary care setting in Spain [erratum appears in Pharmacoeconomics. 2006;24(1):106]. Pharmacoeconomics 2005;23:275–287.

135. Cziraky MJ, Watson KE, Talbert RL. Targeting low HDL-Cholesterol to decrease residual cardiovascular risk in the managed care setting. Journal of Managed Care Pharmacy 2009;14:S3–S28.

136. Johannesson M, Jonsson B, Kjekshus J, Olsson AG, Pedersen TR, Wedel H. Cost effectiveness of simvastatin treatment to lower cholesterol levels in patients with coronary heart disease. Scandinavian Simvastatin Survival Study Group. New England Journal of Medicine 1997;336:332–336.

137. Caro J, Klittich W, McGuire A, et al. The West of Scotland coronary prevention study: economic benefit analysis of primary prevention with pravastatin. Bmj 1997;315:1577–1582.

138. Schectman G, Wolff N, Byrd JC, Hiatt JG, Hartz A. Physician extenders for cost-effective management of hypercholesterolemia. Journal of General Internal Medicine 1996;11:277–286.

139. Bluml BM, McKenney JM, Cziraky MJ. Pharmaceutical care services and results in project ImPACT: hyperlipidemia. Journal of the American Pharmaceutical Association 2000;40:157–165.

140. Charrois TL, Johnson JA, Blitz S, Tsuyuki RT. Relationship between number, timing, and type of pharmacist interventions and patient outcomes. American Journal of Health System Pharmacy 2005;62: 1798–1801.

141. Yamada C, Johnson JA, Robertson P, Pearson G, Tsuyuki RT. Long-term impact of a community pharmacist intervention on cholesterol levels in patients at high risk for cardiovascular events: extended follow-up of the second study of cardiovascular risk intervention by pharmacists (SCRIP-plus). Pharmacotherapy 2005;25: 110–115.

142. Buchwald H, Campos CT, Boen JR, Nguyen PA, Williams SE. Disease-free intervals after partial ileal bypass in patients with coronary heart disease and hypercholesterolemia: report from the Program on the Surgical Control of the Hyperlipidemias (POSCH). Journal of the American College of Cardiology 1995;26:351–357.

143. Anonymous. The Lipid Research Clinics Coronary Primary Prevention Trial results. I. Reduction in incidence of coronary heart disease. Jama 1984;251:351–364.

144. Officers A, Coordinators for the ACRGTA, Lipid-Lowering Treatment to Prevent Heart Attack T. Major outcomes in moderately hypercholesterolemic, hypertensive patients randomized to pravastatin vs usual care: The Antihypertensive and Lipid-Lowering Treatment to Prevent Heart Attack Trial (ALLHAT-LLT). Jama 2002;288:2998–3007.

145. Canner PL, Berge KG, Wenger NK, et al. Fifteen year mortality in Coronary Drug Project patients: long-term benefit with niacin. Journal of the American College of Cardiology 1986;8:1245–1255.

146. Strandberg TE, Pyorala K, Cook TJ, et al. Mortality and incidence of cancer during 10-year follow-up of the Scandinavian Simvastatin Survival Study (4S). Lancet 2004;364:771–777.

147. Tonkin AM, Colquhoun D, Emberson J, et al. Effects of pravastatin in 3260 patients with unstable angina: results from the LIPID study. Lancet 2000;356:1871–1875.

148. Rubins HB, Robins SJ, Collins D. The Veterans Affairs High-Density Lipoprotein Intervention Trial: baseline characteristics of normocholesterolemic men with coronary artery disease and low levels of high-density lipoprotein cholesterol. Veterans Affairs Cooperative Studies Program High-Density Lipoprotein Intervention Trial Study Group. American Journal of Cardiology 1996;78:572–575.

149. Pitt B, Waters D, Brown WV, et al. Aggressive lipid-lowering therapy compared with angioplasty in stable coronary artery disease. Atorvastatin versus Revascularization Treatment Investigators. New England Journal of Medicine 1999;341:70–76.

150. Shepherd J, Blauw GJ, Murphy MB, et al. Pravastatin in elderly individuals at risk of vascular disease (PROSPER): a randomised controlled trial. Lancet 2002;360:1623–1630.

151. Cannon CP, Braunwald E, McCabe CH, et al. Intensive versus moderate lipid lowering with statins after acute coronary syndromes [erratum appears in N Engl J Med. 2006 Feb 16;354(7):778]. New England Journal of Medicine 2004;350:1495–1504.

152. LaRosa JC, Grundy SM, Waters DD, et al. Intensive lipid lowering with atorvastatin in patients with stable coronary disease. New England Journal of Medicine 2005;352:1425–1435.

153. Waters DD, LaRosa JC, Barter P, et al. Effects of high-dose atorvastatin on cerebrovascular events in patients with stable coronary disease in the TNT (treating to new targets) study. Journal of the American College of Cardiology 2006;48:1793–1799.

154. Amarenco P, Bogousslavsky J, Callahan A, 3rd, et al. High-dose atorvastatin after stroke or transient ischemic attack. New England Journal of Medicine 2006;355:549–559.

155. Nissen SE, Tuzcu EM, Brewer HB, et al. Effect of ACAT inhibition on the progression of coronary atherosclerosis [erratum appears in N Engl J Med. 2006 Aug 10;355(6):638]. New England Journal of Medicine 2006;354:1253–1263.

156. Vidt DG, Harris S, McTaggart F, Ditmarsch M, Sager PT, Sorof JM. Effect of short-term rosuvastatin treatment on estimated glomerular filtration rate. American Journal of Cardiology 2006;97:1602–1606.

157. Raal FJ, Santos RD, Blom DJ, et al. Mipomersen, an apolipoprotein B synthesis inhibitor, for lowering of LDL cholesterol concentrations in patients with homozygous familial hypercholesterolaemia: a randomised, double-blind, placebo-controlled trial. Lancet 2010;375: 998–1006.

158. Pedersen TR. Lipid-lowering drugs and risk for cancer. Curr Atheroscler Rep 2009;11:350–357.

CHAPTER

29

Peripheral Arterial Disease

BARBARA J. HOEBEN AND ROBERT L. TALBERT

KEY CONCEPTS

❶ The prevalence of peripheral arterial disease is dependent upon age and the presence of traditional risk factors for cardiovascular disease, and many patients are undiagnosed; undiagnosed patients have substantial risk for coronary and cerebrovascular events.

❷ The clinical presentation of peripheral arterial disease is variable and includes a range of symptoms. The two most common characteristics of peripheral arterial disease are intermittent claudication and pain at rest in the lower extremities.

❸ The ankle-brachial index (ABI) is a simple, noninvasive, quantitative test that has been proven to be a highly sensitive and specific tool in the diagnosis of peripheral arterial disease.

❹ As with any atherosclerotic condition, several risk factors play an important role in the morbidity and mortality of peripheral vascular disease. Many of these risk factors are modifiable with the help of various nonpharmacologic and pharmacologic interventions.

❺ Nonpharmacologic interventions such as smoking cessation and walking exercise programs have the ability to positively impact several of the pathophysiologic abnormalities present for patients with peripheral arterial disease.

❻ Data proving that antiplatelet therapies can prevent or delay the progression of peripheral arterial disease are currently unavailable. However, aspirin therapy has repeatedly been proven to significantly reduce serious vascular events in these "high-risk" patients and, in the absence of contraindications, is highly recommended.

❼ After appropriate exercise therapy and therapeutic lifestyle changes have been implemented, patients who continue to experience severe intermittent claudication may benefit from additional pharmacologic therapy with cilostazol.

Peripheral arterial disease (PAD), the most common form of peripheral vascular disease, is a manifestation of progressive narrowing of arteries due to atherosclerosis.[1] PAD is associated with elevated risk of cardiovascular disease (CVD) morbidity and mortality, even in the absence of prior history of acute myocardial infarction (AMI),

Learning objectives, review questions, and other resources can be found at
www.pharmacotherapyonline.com.

stroke, or other manifestations of CVD.[1-3] Patients with PAD have approximately the same relative risk of death from CVD as do patients with a history of coronary or cerebrovascular disease, and PAD should be considered a surrogate marker of subclinical coronary artery disease (CAD) and other vascular territories.[1,4-5] The treatment of PAD focuses on decreasing the functional impairment caused by symptoms of intermittent claudication through nonpharmacologic and pharmacologic therapy and by minimizing the impact of other cardiovascular risk factors.[6]

EPIDEMIOLOGY

❶ Using the definition of an ankle-brachial index (ABI) of less than 0.9 in either leg, the National Health and Nutrition Examination Survey (NHANES) found a 4.3% prevalence of PAD among adults age 40 years and older in the United States.[2] The prevalence of PAD is highly dependent on age, being infrequent in younger individuals and common in older individuals (Fig. 29–1). In age- and gender-adjusted logistic regression analyses, black race/ethnicity [odds ratio (OR) 2.83] current smoking (OR 4.46), diabetes (OR 2.71), hypertension (OR 1.75), hypercholesterolemia (OR 1.68), and impaired renal function (estimated glomerular filtration rate less than 60 mL/min/1.73 m²) (OR 2.00) were associated with more prevalent PAD.[2,7] Individuals with PAD are also more likely to have a self-reported history of any CAD or CVD but, interestingly, no association with elevated body mass index. The reported relative risk of death from CVD for patients with PAD is reported to range from 2 to 5.1 for patients with or without CVD and 2.9 to 5.7 for patients with known CVD.[8] CVD accounts for 75% of all deaths in patients with PAD.[9] The risk of death is approximately the same in men and women and is elevated even in asymptomatic patients. Annual mortality is 25% for patients with critical leg ischemia who have the lowest ABI values.[10]

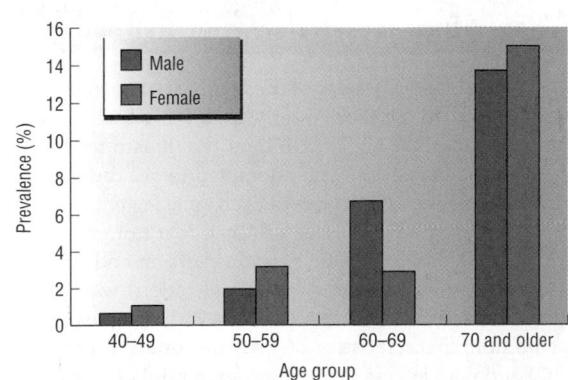

FIGURE 29-1. Prevalence of peripheral arterial disease by age and gender.

More than 5 million (estimated range 4 to 7 million) adults age 40 years or more have PAD. Ninety-five percent of individuals with PAD have at least one cardiovascular risk factor; the majority of patients have multiple risk factors for CVD.[2] Based on the PAD Awareness, Risk, and Treatment: New Resources for Survival (PARTNERS) program, the prevalence of PAD in primary care practices is high, yet physician awareness of the PAD diagnosis is relatively low.[11] In this cross-sectional study, PAD was detected in 29% of 6,979 patients. Eighty-three percent of the patients were aware of their diagnosis but only 49% of their patients' physicians were aware. The reason for this observation is that patient self-report of symptoms and the use of questionnaires to detect PAD are not sufficiently sensitive and specific to reproducibly diagnose PAD and the cardinal symptom of PAD—intermittent claudication—is present in the minority of patients (1 to 27%).[8,12,13] A simple ABI measurement will identify a large number of patients with previously unrecognized PAD. Atherosclerosis risk factors were very prevalent for PAD patients, but these patients received less intensive treatment for lipid disorders and hypertension and were prescribed antiplatelet therapy less frequently than were patients with CVD. These results demonstrate that underdiagnosed PAD in primary care practice may be a barrier to effective secondary prevention of the high ischemic cardiovascular risk associated with PAD.[11] Because of the systemic nature of atherosclerosis and the high risk of ischemic events, patients with PAD should be considered for secondary prevention strategies including aggressive risk-factor modification and antiplatelet drug therapy.[8,12-16]

ETIOLOGY AND PATHOPHYSIOLOGY

PAD is most commonly a manifestation of systemic atherosclerosis in which the arterial lumen of the lower extremities becomes progressively occluded by atherosclerotic plaque.[9] The major risk factors for the development of atherosclerosis are older age (greater than 40 years), cigarette smoking, diabetes mellitus, hypercholesterolemia, hypertension, and hyperhomocysteinemia.[8,9,12] The arteries most commonly involved, in order of occurrence, are the femoropopliteal-tibial, aortoiliac, carotid and vertebral, splenic and renal, and brachiocephalic.[15] Familial hypercholesterolemia (FH) leading to hypercholesterolemia and elevated low-density lipoprotein (LDL) levels are associated with accelerated development of atherosclerosis earlier and with more severe symptoms (e.g., intermittent claudication) and abnormal blood flow studies compared with controls.[16,17] Intima-media thickness can be used as a surrogate phenotype for cardiovascular risk in FH and carotid and/or femoral artery atherosclerosis results in increased intima-media thickness, and it is correlated to cardiovascular risk in FH patients compared with normolipidemic individuals.

CLINICAL PRESENTATION AND DIAGNOSIS

❷ The clinical presentation of PAD is variable, ranging from no symptoms at all (typically early in the disease) to pain and discomfort (Table 29–1). This finding was illustrated in a study by Wang and colleagues,[18] who attempted to aid the diagnosis of PAD by using defined categories of exertional leg pain for patients with and without PAD. They determined that not one of the five categories of leg pain (no pain, pain on exertion and rest, noncalf pain, atypical calf pain, and classic claudication) was sufficiently sensitive or specific to enable a link to a PAD diagnosis. The two most common characteristics of PAD are intermittent claudication (IC) and pain at rest in the lower extremities.[17-19] IC is generally regarded as the primary indicator of PAD. It is described as

| TABLE 29-1 | Clinical Presentation of PAD |

General
- Patients with peripheral arterial disease (PAD) are likely to be ≥ 40 years of age with hypertension, hypercholesterolemia, diabetes, impaired renal function, a history of coronary artery disease or cardiovascular disease, and/or a history of smoking.

Signs and symptoms
- The clinical presentation of PAD is variable and includes symptoms ranging from no symptoms at all (typically early in the disease) to pain and discomfort.
- The two most common characteristics of PAD are intermittent claudication and pain at rest in the lower extremities.
- Intermittent claudication is generally regarded as the primary indicator in PAD. It has been described as fatigue, discomfort, cramping, pain, or numbness in the affected extremities (typically the buttock, thigh, or calf) during exercise that resolves within a few minutes with rest.
- Physical examination may reveal nonspecific signs of decreased blood flow to the extremities (e.g., cool skin temperature, thickened toenails, lack of hair on the calf, feet, and/or toes).

Laboratory tests
- None specific to PAD.

Other diagnostic tests
- The ankle-brachial index (ABI) is a simple, noninvasive, quantitative test that has been proven to be a highly sensitive and specific (≥90%) tool in the diagnosis of PAD.

Data from references 2, 7, 12, 18, 20–22, 24–27, 29, 31, 85, and 86.

reproducible fatigue, discomfort, cramping, pain, or numbness in the affected extremities (typically the buttock, thigh or calf) during exercise and is resolved within a few minutes with rest.[17,19-23] Symptoms of IC occur during exercise as the increase in blood flow is limited by occlusive atherosclerotic lesions in the peripheral arteries leading to an inability for oxygen supply to meet the demands of increased metabolic demand by the muscles.[23] Resting pain typically occurs later in the disease when the blood supply is not adequate to perfuse the extremity (critical limb ischemia). This can be felt most often at night in the feet (typically the toes or heel) while the patient is lying in bed.[17-19] Although IC is the primary indicator of PAD, it alone cannot be used to diagnose PAD. As explained by the Inter-Society Consensus for the Management of Peripheral Arterial Disease (TASC II),[23] patients with PAD may not have symptoms of IC because they may have a sedentary lifestyle or some other condition that may be limiting the ability to exercise.

As with any good medical encounter, a detailed patient history of symptoms and atherosclerosis risk factors (e.g., smoking, hypertension, hyperlipidemia, and diabetes) can be helpful in the diagnosis of PAD. Unfortunately, as illustrated by the PARTNERS program, providers who rely on a history alone will miss approximately 85% to 90% of patients with PAD.[24] Therefore, examination of the patient is vital to proper diagnosis. Requesting that the patient remove socks and shoes may reveal nonspecific signs of decreased blood flow to the extremities (e.g., cool skin temperature, shiny skin, thickened toenails, lack of hair on the calf, feet, and/or toes) or, in severe cases, visible sores or ulcers that are slow to heal and may even be black in appearance.[17-19,24-25]

An important criterion for the accurate diagnosis of PAD is the exclusion of other conditions that possess similar signs and symptoms. Differential diagnosis should rule out other neurologic conditions (e.g., peripheral neuropathy), inflammatory conditions (e.g., arthritis), and vascular conditions (e.g., deep venous thrombosis or venous congestion) that may mimic PAD.[17,22,26]

❸ The ABI is a simple, noninvasive, quantitative test that has been proven to be a highly sensitive and specific (≥90%) tool in the diagnosis of PAD.[20,27,28] For measurement of the ABI, the patient lies in the supine position as the systolic blood pressure is measured at the brachial arteries on both arms and the dorsalis pedis and posterior tibial arteries of the legs with a standard sphygmomanometer and a continuous-wave Doppler device. The pressures obtained at the dorsalis pedis and posterior tibial arteries are averaged and divided by the mean measurement taken at the left and right brachial arteries.[8,23,24,29,30] An ABI of 1 is considered normal, while a measurement under 0.9 is consistent with PAD. ABI from 0.7 to 0.9 correlates with mild PAD, 0.4 to 0.7 indicates moderate disease, and under 0.4 denotes severe PAD.[9,21,29] In addition to providing diagnostic information, the ABI measurement has been shown to be a strong predictor of future cardiovascular events associated with PAD.[31,32] The ABI can also be useful after a test of exercise tolerance (e.g., 5 minutes on a treadmill or 30 to 50 repetitions of heel raises). Patients with PAD will demonstrate a significant drop in the ABI after exercise, but their pain will be normal or unchanged. ABI can rule out PAD and suggest alternate diagnoses.[9,21,23,24] ABI can be considered as a useful tool in diagnosing both symptomatic and nonsymptomatic patients at high risk of PAD.[11,33]

Other noninvasive tools are available for the diagnosis of PAD. One study has suggested a calculation that takes into consideration the patient's history of AMI and the number of auscultated and palpated posterior tibial arteries.[34,35] Magnetic resonance angiography (MRA) can be used to examine the presence and location of significant stenosis, or lack thereof, and is a reasonable option for patients who are being considered for surgical revascularization.[36] Similarly, computed tomographic angiography (CTA) can be used to determine the presence of significant stenosis and soft tissue diagnostic information that may be associated with PAD (e.g., aneurysms).[36,37] However, as ABI is a sufficient means of diagnosis, arteriography is not necessary or encouraged.[19,22,28]

TREATMENT

Peripheral Arterial Disease

■ GOALS OF TREATMENT

PAD is the result of atherosclerotic plaque formation in the arteries that results in decreased blood flow to the legs. Several of the treatment goals for these patients involve the reduction of confounding variables that attribute to the disease process, progress, and eventual outcome. Specific goals should include increasing maximal walking distance, increasing duration of pain-free walking, improving control of comorbid conditions contributing to the morbidity of the condition (e.g., hypertension, hyperlipidemia, and diabetes), improving overall quality of life and reducing cardiovascular complications and death.

■ GENERAL APPROACH TO TREATMENT

❹ As with any atherosclerotic condition, several risk factors play an important role in the morbidity and mortality of PAD. Many of these risk factors are modifiable with the help of various nonpharmacologic and pharmacologic interventions.

■ NONPHARMACOLOGIC THERAPY

Smoking Cessation

❺ Cigarette smoking not only increases the risk of developing PAD and other cardiovascular disorders, but the quantity smoked and the duration can negatively impact disease progression (e.g., increase the risk of amputation) and increase mortality.[8,23,26,31,32,38–41] As a result, providers must advise patients to quit and should offer nonpharmacologic and pharmacologic means to aid the patient in that goal. Individual or group behavior modification therapy with or without the addition of certain antidepressants (e.g., bupropion), varenicline, or nicotine replacement therapies (e.g., gum or patches) has been proven effective in numerous studies. Reassessment of smoking status and progress encouragement at each encounter can help to reemphasize to the patient the vital importance of this lifestyle change.

Exercise

❺ Walking exercise programs for patients with PAD have been proven to result in an increase in walking duration and distance, an increase in pain-free walking, and a delayed onset of claudication by 179%.[12,25,26,38,39,42–51] Walking, or any aerobic exercise program conducted under the supervision of a healthcare provider, has the ability to positively impact several of the pathophysiologic abnormalities present in patients with PAD. Benefits of exercise programs include improving diabetes and lipid management, reducing weight, improving blood viscosity and flow, and reducing blood pressure.[6] Walking distance can also be used as a prognostic tool for future outcomes for patients with normal and impaired ABIs. A recent study by de Liefde and colleagues[52] examined patients with normal ABI (≥0.90) and impaired ABI (<0.90) in relation to walking distance. It was demonstrated that walking impairment in conjunction with impaired ABI was associated with higher cardiovascular events, including death. Other studies have likewise observed a link between impaired exercise/walking distance and negative long-term outcomes for patients with PAD.[53,54]

The American College of Cardiology/American Heart Association (ACC/AHA) Guidelines for the Management of PAD recommends supervised exercise training for patients with IC, for a minimum of 30 to 45 minutes, to be performed at least 3 times per week for a minimum of 12 weeks.[36] During exercise sessions, walking should be performed with at a speed and grade of incline to produce the symptoms of IC within 3 to 5 minutes. The patient should stop walking when the symptoms become moderate in intensity, wait for the symptoms to resolve, and then resume walking thus repeating the cycle for the duration of the session.[23] A prospective, observational study performed by Gardner and colleagues concluded that PAD patients with higher physical activity (as measured with a vertical accelerometer) have reduced mortality and cardiovascular events compared with those with low physical activity, regardless of confounders.[48] Exercise treadmill walking testing should be repeated at regular intervals (e.g., quarterly to biannually) to assess improvement or decline in walking duration and distance, as well as the time to pain onset while performing this activity. The type of aerobic activity recommended, as well as the duration and frequency of the activity, should be individually designed on a patient-to-patient basis.

Surgical Interventions

Various surgical procedures are available for patients with severe, debilitating claudication who have attempted, and failed, other means of nonpharmacologic and pharmacologic therapy. The TransAtlantic Inter-Society Consensus (TASC) document on PAD provides clear recommendations for invasive therapy.[28] First, there must be a lack of adequate response to exercise therapy and risk factor modification. Second, the patient must have severe disability from IC resulting in impairment of daily activities. Third, there must be a thorough evaluation of the risks versus benefits of an invasive intervention including probability of success, the anticipated future course of the disease if an intervention is not performed, as well as an evaluation of concomitant disease states.[28] The decision to attempt percutaneous revascularization is often made with the guidance of diagnostic angiography. Angiography can help to identify the location and size of lesions and provide valuable information as to the likelihood of success with surgical revascularization.[28]

Percutaneous transluminal angioplasty (PTA) is an example of an invasive treatment for PAD. A randomized controlled clinical trial performed by Whyman and colleagues[55] determined that in a 2-year postintervention, PTA outcomes on maximum walking distance and ABI were not significantly different than for patients that had only received daily low-dose ASA ($P>0.05$). Nevertheless, patients who had received PTA had significantly fewer occluded arteries ($P = 0.003$), but the true clinical significance of this finding could not be realized in the time allotted for the study. PTA typically is reserved for patients whose lifestyle and/or job performance are compromised secondary to claudication despite adequate pharmacologic interventions and exercise.[12,40]

Stent placement for PAD patients has also been an area of study and controversy. A metaanalysis examining the use of stent placement versus PTA for the treatment of aortoiliac occlusive disease determined that although stent placement and PTA yielded similar complication and mortality rates, posttreatment ABI was more improved with stents (0.87 with PTA and 0.76 with stents, P<0.03), and the risk of long-term failure was 39% less with stent placement.[56] However, other studies have not demonstrated improvement in patency rates in peripheral arteries versus PTA alone.[20] The TASC document provides specific recommendations for PTA, with or without stenting, depending on how diffuse the disease process is, the number and size of the lesions, and the location of the lesions.[28]

For patients with severe IC resulting in critical leg ischemia, physicians may need to discuss alternate surgical interventions including aortofemoral bypass, femoropopliteal bypass, or even amputation.[20,21,42]

■ PHARMACOLOGIC THERAPY

Hypertension

Hypertension (HTN) is a major risk factor for PAD and can lead to AMI, stroke, heart failure (HF), and death.[14] Current guidelines recommend the treatment goal for blood pressure in patients with PAD to mirror those in patients with documented CVD, 130/85 mm Hg.[14,41] Although the Heart Outcomes Prevention Evaluation study (HOPE trial)[57] demonstrated that angiotensin-converting enzyme (ACE) inhibitors reduced not only blood pressure but other cardiovascular events (e.g., AMI, stroke, and death) in high-risk patients, including those with PAD, no specific class of antihypertensives are recommended over another for the treatment of hypertension for patients with PAD. Therefore, selection of drug therapy for hypertension should be made in accordance with the Joint National Committee on Prevention, Detection, Evaluation, and Treatment of High Blood Pressure (JNC VII)[14] guidelines on the basis of comorbid disease states, drug costs and availability, drug allergies, or other possible limiting factors. For example, patients with concomitant Raynaud phenomenon may benefit from calcium channel blockers, while patients with documented CAD may receive a dual benefit by the selection of a β-blocker whereas patients with.[14,41,58] Hesitation to use β-blockers in patients with PAD without harm was recently supported with the publication of a review of six randomized controlled trials by Paravastu and colleagues.[59] The review concluded that there was no evidence of harm in the use of these agents for patients with PAD; however, β-blockers should be used with caution for patients with critical leg ischemia where acute lowering of blood pressure is

contraindicated.[59] Dosing, monitoring guidelines and contraindications for specific agents used in the treatment of hypertension may be found in Chapter 19, Hypertension.

Hyperlipidemia

Although it has been shown that a reduction in lipid levels can reduce the progression of PAD and the severity of claudication, the current recommendations for the management of hyperlipidemia in PAD are based on only a few small studies and sub-hoc analyses from larger trials.[8,41,60–62] The Expert Panel on Detection, Evaluation, and Treatment of High Blood Cholesterol in Adults (Adult Treatment Panel III, or ATP III) considers PAD to be in the category of highest risk, or a coronary heart disease (CHD) risk equivalent. Therefore, it was recommended by the Expert Panel that levels of LDL be maintained at <100 mg/dL and non-high-density lipoprotein levels [total cholesterol minus high-density lipoprotein (HDL) cholesterol] at <130 mg/dL.[60] Results of clinical trials conducted since the time of this recommendation, specifically the Heart Protection Study (HPS)[62] and the Pravastatin or Atorvastatin Evaluation and Infection—Thrombolysis in Myocardial Infarction (PROVE IT)[63] trial, have lead many clinical experts to now recommend an LDL goal of <70 mg/dL for additional retardation of atherosclerotic plaque formation in persons considered to be at very high risk, including patients with PAD.[20] Regardless of the goal LDL chosen, initiation of patient therapeutic lifestyle changes (e.g., reduction in saturated fat, weight reduction, and increased physical activity) are vital to achieving these recommendations.[16,60] Unfortunately, in many cases, therapeutic lifestyle changes alone will not achieve the desired goals.

Several options are available for the initiation of drug therapy for LDL lowering for patients with PAD. Statins, bile acid sequestrants, and nicotinic acid are all effective treatment options. However, in most cases, statins are the preferred starting agent in this patient population.[24,42,60,62] As proven in the HPS, simvastatin demonstrated potent action not only in reducing LDL but also in providing a significant reduction in cardiovascular events overall as well (e.g., AMI, stroke, and death).[62] If an increase in HDL levels is also necessary, niacin should be considered alone or in combination with a statin without the fear of worsening glucose metabolism, as previously believed.[8,21,30,58,64] Dosing, monitoring guidelines, and contraindications for specific agents may be found in Chapter 28, Dyslipidemia.

Diabetes Mellitus

A metaanalysis of over 95,000 diabetic patients provided additional support for the accepted premise that glycemic control serves as a risk factor for CVD.[65] The analysis demonstrated an increasing risk of death from cardiovascular events as blood glucose concentrations increased, with the same relationship observed even at levels below the threshold of clinically defined diabetes mellitus. This relationship is just one illustration of the criticality of good glycemic control. Due to the high prevalence of PAD among diabetic patients, the American Diabetes Association recommends ABI screening for PAD in all diabetics older than 50 years.[66] Due to the presence of peripheral neuropathy, patients with diabetes may be less likely to experience or report symptoms of PAD, and the first sign may be as drastic as the appearance of a gangrenous foot ulcer. Therefore, although there is currently a lack of randomized controlled studies illustrating that the degree of glycemic control is predictive of the extent of PAD present, it is widely recommended that all patients with concomitant diabetes and PAD maintain good glycemic control, as evidenced by a hemoglobin A-1c level of <7%.[8,28,30,41,43,66,67] This recommendation was later supported by a prospective cohort study of 1,894 diabetic patients which demonstrated that patients with poor glucose control (A-1c>7.5%) were 5 times more likely to develop IC and also to be hospitalized for PAD compared with those with a hemoglobin A-1c<6%.[68] Despite this, a study by Rehring and colleagues[69] of 365 patients with known PAD and concomitant diabetes showed that only 45.8% of these patients had a hemoglobin A-1c<7%. Oral antidiabetic agents, insulin regimens, as well as other pharmacologic and nonpharmacologic strategies to reduce the risk of complications associated with diabetes mellitus are discussed at length in Chapter 83, Diabetes Mellitus.

■ ANTIPLATELET DRUG THERAPY (TABLE 29–2)

Aspirin

❻ By far, the most compelling evidence for the use of any pharmacologic agent in PAD can be found for aspirin (acetylsalicylic acid [ASA]). The Antithrombotic Trialists' Collaboration (ATC) conducted a metaanalysis of 195 randomized trials, composed of over 135,000 patients at high risk for occlusive arterial disease, and concluded that low-dose ASA (75 to 160 mg) and medium-dose ASA (160 to 325 mg/day) lead to a significant reduction in serious vascular events (12%) in "high-risk" patients, such as those with PAD.[70] The ATC also noted in this analysis that the risk of major extracranial bleed was similar between the low-dose and medium-dose regimens.

Tran and Anand[71] conducted a systematic review of the literature in an effort to summarize the best evidence for oral antiplatelet therapy for patients with cerebrovascular disease, CAD, and PAD. This review included 111 trials (42 of which included patients with PAD, n = 9,214) and concluded that patients with PAD should use ASA (160 to 325 mg/day) or clopidogrel (75 mg/day) when ASA is not tolerated or contraindicated.[71] This is in concordance with the recommendations of the Seventh American College of Chest Physicians (ACCP) Conference on Antithrombotic and Thrombolytic Therapy, which recommends lifelong ASA (75 to 325 mg/day) over clopidogrel, ticlopidine, and no antithrombotic therapy for patients with PAD.[72] Unfortunately, no data are currently available from large, clinical, randomized trials that ASA, or any other antiplatelet therapies, can actually prevent or delay the progression of PAD.[72]

Aspirin plus Dipyridamole Extended Release (Aggrenox)

The ATC also examined the use of dipyridamole extended release (Aggrenox) in combination with ASA in high-risk patients, such as those with PAD. The metaanalysis of 25 trials (which included more than 10,000 patients) concluded that the addition of dipyridamole to aspirin led to an additional reduction in serious vascular events over ASA alone (6%); however, this reduction was unable to reach statistical significance ($P = 0.32$).[70,71] It should also be taken into consideration that most of the reduction in nonfatal stroke in this analysis came from one trial, and these data are not replicated in the other studies.[70,73] The addition of dipyridamole to ASA may cause an increased risk of bleeding and gastrointestinal side effects when compared with placebo and should not be used with CAD.[73]

Clopidogrel (Plavix)

The ATC metaanalysis also reviewed the effectiveness of clopidogrel (Plavix) 75 mg/day in high risk patients, including those with PAD. The ATC concluded that although clopidogrel was able to reduce serious vascular events by 10%, this was significantly less than the reduction seen with ASA (12%, $P = 0.03$) described previously.[70] Included in this metaanalysis was the report from the Clopidogrel

---

TABLE 29-2 Pharmacotherapy Options for Patients with Peripheral Arterial Disease

Agent	Daily Dose (Oral)	Mechanism of Action (MOA)	Side Effects	Contraindications	Level of Evidence[b]
Aspirin	81–325 mg	Irreversibly inhibits prostaglandin cyclooxygenase in platelets, prevents formation of thromboxane A₂	Gastrointestinal upset and/or bleeding	Active bleeding; hemophilia; thrombocytopenia	With coronary or cerebrovascular (Grade 1A), without (Grade 1C+)
Dipyridamole ER (Aggrenox)	400 mg (+ aspirin 50 mg)	May act by inhibiting platelet aggregation (complete MOA unknown)	Angina; dyspnea; hypotension; headache; dizziness	Active bleeding; CAD ("coronary steal syndrome")	Recommendation for use not specified in report
Cilostazol (Pletal)[a]	100 mg BID	Phosphodiesterase inhibitor, suppresses platelet aggregation; direct artery vasodilator	Fever: infection; tachycardia	All CHF patients (decreased survival)	With IC (Grade 2A)
Clopidogrel (Plavix)	75 mg	Inhibits binding of ADP analogues to its platelet receptor causing irreversible inhibition of platelets	Chest pain; purpura generalized pain; rash	Active pathological bleeding (e.g., peptic ulcer, intracranial hemorrhage)	Recommend clopidogrel over no antiplatelet therapy (Grade 1C+)
Pentoxifylline (Trental)	1.2 g	Alters RBC flexibility; decreases platelet adhesion; reduces blood viscosity; decreases fibrinogen concentration	Dyspnea; nausea; vomiting; headache; dizziness	Recent retinal or cerebral hemorrhage; active bleeding	Not recommended in patients with IC (Grade 1B)
Ticlopidine (Ticlid)	500 mg	Inhibits binding of ADP analogues to its platelet receptor causing irreversible inhibition of platelets	Leukopenia; rash; thrombocytopenia; neutropenia; agranulocytosis; aplastic anemia	Active bleeding; hemophilia; thrombocytopenia	Clopidogrel recommended over ticlopidine (Grade 1C+)

Abbreviations: ER, extended-release; mg, milligrams; g, grams; BID, twice daily; ADP, adenosine 5'-diphosphate; RBC, red blood cell; CAD, coronary artery disease; CHF, congestive heart failure; IC, intermittent claudication.

[a]Cilostazol should be used in combination with antiplatelet therapy.

[b]Grades of recommendation for antithrombotic and thrombolytic therapy are part of the Seventh ACCP Conference on Antithrombotic and Thrombolytic Therapy.[87]

Data from references 5, 22, 30, 31, 70, 72, 76, 79, 88–91.

versus ASA in Patients at Risk of Ischemic Events (CAPRIE)5 trial, which had concluded that clopidogrel (75 mg daily) was more effective than ASA (325 mg daily) in preventing vascular events in high-risk patients. In comparison to the ASA therapy, the clopidogrel regimen resulted in an overall reduction in ischemic stroke, MI, or vascular death from 5.83% to 5.32% ($P = 0.043$). This difference was even more pronounced in the subgroup analysis of PAD patients, in which clopidogrel therapy led to a significant reduction of 4.86% versus 3.71% in the ASA group ($P = 0.0028$).[5,31,36] Although a generic clopidogrel product is now available, it not only remains significantly more expensive than ASA therapy, in drug costs, but clopidogrel also remains a by-prescription-only medication and thus requires a physician visit to obtain a prescription for the medication. For all these reasons, the current recommendations list clopidogrel as a first-line agent, but only in cases where ASA therapy is either not tolerated or contraindicated.[70]

Ticlopidine (Ticlid)

Although ticlopidine has the same mechanism of action as clopidogrel and possesses a similar molecular structure, the results of clinical trials among the two agents are strikingly different.[22] The Swedish Ticlopidine Multicenter Study (STIMS)[74] had determined that ticlopidine therapy (500 mg/day) was able to reduce total mortality in comparison with placebo for patients with IC ($P = 0.015$).[22,74,75] However, the once promising results seen with ticlopidine therapy have now been overshadowed by the severe hematologic side effects unique to this agent. Ticlopidine has a "black box" warning from the Food and Drug Administration (FDA) warning providers that use of this agent can cause neutropenia/agranulocytosis, thrombotic thrombocytopenic purpura, and aplastic anemia.[76] Other agents, namely clopidogrel, are now used instead of ticlopidine.[8,30,43]

■ INTERMITTENT CLAUDICATION (TABLE 29–2)

Cilostazol (Pletal)

❼ In a head-to-head, randomized, placebo-controlled study in 698 patients with moderate-to-severe claudication, Dawson and colleagues[77] assigned patients to cilostazol (100 mg twice a day), pentoxifylline (400 mg 3 times a day), or placebo in an effort to improve maximal walking distance. After 24 weeks, the cilostazol group demonstrated a 54% mean increase in distance versus pentoxifylline, which demonstrated only a 30% mean increase ($P <0.001$).[77] Similarly, a metaanalysis of 8 randomized, double-blind, placebo-controlled, parallel-design trials supported this conclusion with a reported increase in maximal walking distance and pain-free walking distance with cilostazol at doses of 50 mg and 100 mg twice-daily ($P <0.05$ for all) over placebo.[78] Regrettably, improvement in walking distance has appeared to come with a price (in addition to the high drug cost); cilostazol has a "black box" warning from the FDA warning providers not to use this medication for patients with PAD and coexisting heart failure.[79] However, the Seventh ACCP Conference on Antithrombotic and Thrombolytic Therapy does suggest the use of this agent for patients with PAD are not candidates for surgical interventions to improve severe IC that persists even after implementation of appropriate exercise therapy and therapeutic lifestyle changes.[72]

Pentoxifylline (Trental)

Unlike cilostazol, pentoxifylline has produced results in clinical trials that are less promising, as illustrated by the randomized, placebo-controlled trial by Dawson and colleagues.[77] Not only did cilostazol outperform pentoxifylline in improvement in walking distance, the improvement seen with pentoxifylline was no different from placebo ($P = 0.82$).[77] This nonsignificant improvement in walking distance has been observed in other studies as well.[8,80] Meanwhile, other metaanalyses of pentoxifylline in comparison with placebo for the improvement of maximal walking distance have shown some minimal improvement over placebo, but the average effects were relatively small.[8,81–91] For these reasons, the Seventh ACCP Conference on Antithrombotic and Thrombolytic Therapy does not recommend the use of this agent.[72,87]

EVALUATION OF THERAPEUTIC OUTCOMES

It is vital that the patient be counseled on the evaluation measures that will be used to monitor the outcomes of therapeutic interventions for PAD. Various laboratory measurements will assess patient progress in glycemic control (e.g., hemoglobin A-1c) and lipid management (e.g., total cholesterol, LDL, HDL, and non-HDL cholesterol), while blood pressure checks in the clinic and patient home blood pressure monitoring can assess the effectiveness of antihypertensive therapy. Repeat exercise treadmill walking testing should be repeated at regular intervals (e.g., quarterly to biannually) to assess improvement or decline in walking duration and distance, as well as the time to pain onset while performing this activity. Repeat ABI measurements should be assessed at each patient visit to determine if there has been stabilization or progression of the disease process. Most importantly to many patients, simple concern and questioning about improvements to their daily quality of life will highlight your concern for their well-being and aid in an overall picture of the patient's general state of health.

ABBREVIATIONS

ABI: ankle-brachial index

ACCP: American College of Chest Physicians

ACE: angiotensin-converting enzyme

AMI: acute myocardial infarction

ASA: aspirin (acetylsalicylic acid)

ATC: Antithrombotic Trialists' Collaboration

ATP III: adult treatment panel III (Expert Panel on Detection, Evaluation, and Treatment of High Blood Cholesterol in Adults)

CAD: coronary artery disease

CHD: coronary heart disease

CVD: cardiovascular disease

FDA: Food and Drug Administration

HF: heart failure

HOPE: Heart Outcomes Prevention Evaluation

HPS: Heart Protection Study

HTN: hypertension

IC: intermittent claudication

JNC VII: Seventh Report of the Joint National Committee on Prevention, Detection, Evaluation, and Treatment of High Blood Pressure

NHANES: National Health and Nutrition Examination Survey

OR: odds ratio

PAD: peripheral arterial disease

PARTNERS: PAD Awareness, Risk, and Treatment: New Resources for Survival

PTA: percutaneous transluminal angioplasty

STIMS: Swedish Ticlopidine Multicenter Study

TASC: TransAtlantic Inter-Society Consensus

TLC: therapeutic lifestyle changes

REFERENCES

1. Hiatt WR. Sounding the PAD alarm. GPs can diagnose peripheral artery disease with a simple ankle-and-arm blood pressure test. Health News 2004;10:4.

2. Selvin E, Erlinger TP. Prevalence of and risk factors for peripheral arterial disease in the United States. Results from the National Health and Nutrition Examination Survey, 1999–2000. Circulation 2004;110:738–743.

3. Golomb BA, Dang TT, Criqui MH. Peripheral arterial disease: Morbidity and mortality implications. Circulation 2006;114:688–699.

4. Newman AB, Shemanski L, Manolio TA, et al. Ankle-arm index as a predictor of cardiovascular disease and mortality in the Cardiovascular Health Study. The Cardiovascular Health Study Group. Arterioscl Thromb Vascular Biol 1999;19:538–545.

5. CAPRIE Steering Committee. A randomised, blinded, trial of clopidogrel versus aspirin in patients at risk of ischaemic events (CAPRIE). CAPRIE Steering Committee. Lancet 1996;348:1329–1339.

6. Stewart KJ, Hiatt WR, Regensteiner JG, Hirsch AT. Exercise training for claudication. N Engl J Med 2002;347:1941–1951.

7. O'Hare AM, Glidden DV, Fox CS, Hsu CY. High prevalence of peripheral arterial disease in persons with renal insufficiency: Results from the National Health and Nutrition Examination Survey 1999–2000. Circulation 2004;109:320–323.

8. Hiatt WR. Medical treatment of peripheral arterial disease and claudication. N Engl J Med 2001;344:1608–1621.

9. Mohler ER, 3rd. Peripheral arterial disease. Identification and implications. Arch Intern Med 2003;163:2306–2314.

10. Dormandy JA, Murray GD. The fate of the claudicant—A prospective study of 1969 claudicants. Eur J Vascular Surg 1991;5:131–133.

11. Hirsch AT, Hiatt WR, Committee PS. PAD awareness, risk, and treatment: New resources for survival—The USA PARTNERS program. Vascular Med 2001;6(3 suppl):9–12.

12. White C. Intermittent claudication. N Engl J Med 2007;356:1241–1250.

13. McDermott MM, Kerwin DR, Liu K, et al. Prevalence and significance of unrecognized lower extremity peripheral arterial disease in general medicine practice. J Gen Intern Med 2001;16:384–390.

14. Chobanian AV, Bakris GL, Black HR, et al. The Seventh Report of the Joint National Committee on Prevention, Detection, Evaluation, and Treatment of High Blood Pressure: The JNC 7 Report. JAMA 2003;289:2560–2571.

15. National Cholesterol Education Program Expert Panel on Detection Evaluation and Treatment of High Blood Cholesterol in Adults. Third Report of the National Cholesterol Education Program (NCEP) Expert Panel on Detection, Evaluation, and Treatment of High Blood Cholesterol in Adults (Adult Treatment Panel III) final report. Circulation 2002;106:3143–3421.

16. Grundy S, Cleeman J, Merz CB, et al. Implications of Recent Clinical Trials for the National Cholesterol Education Program Adult Treatment Panel III Guidelines. Circulation 2004;110:227–239.

17. Hutter C, Austin M, Humphries S. Familial hypercholesterolemia, peripheral arterial disease, and stroke: A HuGE minireview. Am J Epidemiol 2004;160:430–435.

18. Wang JC, Criqui MH, Denenberg JO, McDermott MM, Golomb BA, Fronek A. Exertional leg pain in patients with and without peripheral arterial disease. Circulation 2005;112:3501–3508.

19. Jackson M, Clagett G. Antithrombotic therapy in peripheral arterial occlusive disease. Chest 2001;119(suppl):283S–299S.

20. Hirsch AT, Haskal ZJ, Hertzer NR, et al. ACC/AHA 2005 Practice guidelines for the management of patients with peripheral artieral disease (lower extremity, renal, mesenteric, and abdominal aortic): A collaborative report from the American Association for Vascular Surgery/Society for Vascular Surgery, Society for Cardiovascular Angiography and Interventions, Society for Vascular Medicine and Biology, Societyof Interventional Radiology, and the ACC/AHA Task Force on Practice Guidelines (Writing Committee to Develop Guidelines for the Management of Patients with Peripheral Arterial Disease). Endorsed by the American Association of Cardiovascular and Pulmonary Rehabilitation; National Heart, Lung, and Blood Institute; Society for Vascular Nursing; TransAtlantic Inter-Society Consensus; and Vascular Disease Foundation. Circulation 2006;113:e463–e654.

21. Hiatt W, Nehler MR, eds. Peripheral arterial disease. 4th ed. New York: Spring-Verlag; 2003.

22. Hiatt WR. Preventing atherothrombotic events in peripheral arterial disease: The use of antiplatelet therapy. J Intern Med 2002;251:193–206.

23. Norgren L, Hiatt W, Dormandy J, Nehler MR, Harris KA, Fowkes FG. Inter-Society Consensus for the Management of Peripheral Arterial Disease (TASC II). J Vasc Surg 2007;45 (suppl S):S5–S67.

24. Hirsch AT, Criqui MH, Treat-Jacobson D, et al. Peripheral arterial disease detection, awareness, and treatment in primary care. JAMA 2001;286:1317–1324.

25. Dormandy JA, Rutherford RB. Management of peripheral arterial disease (PAD). TASC Working Group. TransAtlantic Inter-Society Concensus (TASC). J Vascular Surg 2000;31(1 Pt 2):S1–S296.

26. Carman TL, Fernandez BB, Jr. A primary care approach to the patient with claudication. Am Fam Physician 2000;61:1027–1032, 1034.

27. Schmieder FA, Comerota AJ. Intermittent claudication: Magnitude of the problem, patient evaluation, and therapeutic strategies. Am J Cardiol 2001;87(12A):3D-13D.

28. TransAtlantic Inter-Society Consensus (TASC) Working Group. Management of peripheral arterial disease (PAD). TransAtlantic Inter-Society Consensus (TASC). Section B: Intermittent claudication. Eur J Vascular Endovascular Surg 2000;19(suppl A):S47–S114.

29. Sontheimer DL. Peripheral vascular disease: Diagnosis and treatment. Am Fam Physician 2006;73:1971–1976.

30. Gey DC, Lesho EP, Manngold J. Management of peripheral arterial disease. Am Fam Physician 2004;69:525–532.

31. Aronow WS. Management of peripheral arterial disease of the lower extremities in elderly patients. J Gerontol Ser A—Biolog Sci Med Sci 2004;59:172–177.

32. Doobay AV, Anand SS. Sensitivity and specificity of the ankle-brachial index to predict future cardiovascular outcomes: A systematic review. Arterioscl Thromb Vasc Biol 2005;25:1463–1469.

33. Mourad JJ, Cacoub PP, Collet JP, et al. Screening of unrecognized peripheral arterial disease (PAD) using ankle-brachial index in high cardiovascular risk patients free from symptomatic PAD. J Vascular Surg 2009;doi:10.1016/j.jvs.2009.04.055.

34. McDermott MM, Greenland P, Liu K, et al. The ankle brachial index is associated with leg function and physical activity: The Walking and Leg Circulation Study. Ann Intern Med 2002;136:873–883.

35. McDermott MM, Criqui MH, Liu K, et al. Lower ankle/brachial index, as calculated by averaging the dorsalis pedis and posterior tibial arterial pressures, and association with leg functioning in peripheral arterial disease. J Vascular Surg 2000;32:1164–1171.

36. Belch JJ, Topol EJ, Agnelli G, et al. Critical issues in peripheral arterial disease detection and management: A call to action. Arch Intern Med 2003;163:884–892.

37. Met R, Bipat S, Legemate DA, Reekers JA, Koelemay MJW. Diagnostic Performance of Computed Tomography Angiography in Peripheral Arterial Disease: A Systematic Review and Meta-analysis. JAMA 2009;301:415–424.

38. Farkouh ME. Improving the clinical examination for a low ankle-brachial index. International J Angiol 2002;11:41–45.

39. Khan NA, Rahim SA, Anand SS, Simel DL, Panju A. Does the clinical examination predict lower extremity peripheral arterial disease? JAMA 2006;295:536–546.

40. Hirsch AT, Haskal ZJ, Hertzer NR, et al. ACC/AHA guidelines for the management of patients with peripheral arterial disease (lower extremity, renal, mesenteric, and abdominal aortic): Executive summary: A collaborative report from the Am Association for Vascular Surgery/ Society for Vascular Surgery, Society for Vascular Medicine and Biology, Society of Interventional Radiology, and the ACC/AHA Task Force on Practice Guidelines (Writing Committee to

Develop Guidelines for the Management of Patients With Peripheral Arterial Disease [Lower Extremity, Renal, Mesenteric, and Abdominal Aortic]). J the Am College of Cardiology 2006;46:1239–1312.

41. Hiatt WR. Pharmacologic therapy for peripheral arterial disease and claudication. J Vascular Surg 2002;36:1283–1291.

42. Burns P, Gough S, Bradbury AW. Management of peripheral arterial disease in primary care. Br Med J 2003;326(7389):584–588.

43. Regensteiner JG, Hiatt WR. Current medical therapies for patients with peripheral arterial disease: A critical review. Am J Med 2002;112:49–57.

44. Kannel WB, Shurtleff D. National Heart and Lung Institute, National Institutes of Health. The Framingham Study: Cigarettes and the development of intermittent claudication. Geriatr 1973;28:61–68.

45. Tierney S, Fennessy F, Hayes DB. ABC of arterial and vascular disease: Secondary prevention of peripheral vascular disease. BMJ 2000;320:1262–1265.

46. Gardner AW, Katzel LI, Sorkin JD, Goldberg AP. Effects of long-term exercise rehabilitation on claudication distances in patients with peripheral arterial disease: A randomized controlled trial. J Cardiopulmonary Rehabil 2002;22:192–198.

47. Langbein WE, Collins EG, Orebaugh C, et al. Increasing exercise tolerance of persons limited by claudication pain using polestriding. J Vascular Surg 2002;35:887–893.

48. Gardner AW, Katzel LI, Sorkin JD, et al. Exercise rehabilitation improves functional outcomes and peripheral circulation in patients with intermittent claudication: A randomized controlled trial. J Am Geriatr Soc 2001;49:755–762.

49. Falcone RA, Hirsch AT, Regensteiner JG, et al. Peripheral arterial disease rehabilitation: A review. J Cardiopulmonary Rehabilitation 2003;23:170–175.

50. Tan KH, De Cossart L, Edwards PR. Exercise training and peripheral vascular disease. Br J Surg 2000;87:553–562.

51. Garg PK, Tian L, Criqui MH, et al. Physical activity during daily life and mortality in patients with peripheral arterial disease. Circulation 2006;114:242–248.

52. de Liefde II, Hoeks SE, van Gestel YRBM, et al. The prognostic value of impaired walking distance on long-term outcome in patients with known or suspected peripheral arterial disease. Eur J Vasc Endovasc Surg 2009;doi:10.1016/j.ejvs.2009.02.022.

53. McDermott MM, Tian L, Liu K, Guralnik JM, Ferrucci L, Tan J. Prognostic value of functional performance for mortality in patients with peripheral artery disease. J Am Coll Cardiol 2008;51:1482–1489.

54. Schiano V, Brevetti G, Sirico G, Silvestro A, Giugliano G, Chiariello M. Functional status measured by walking impairment questionnaire and cardiovascular risk prediction in peripheral arterial disease: Results of the peripheral arteriopathy and cardiovascular events (PACE) study. Vasc Med 2006;11:147–154.

55. Whyman MR, Fowkes FG, Kerracher EM, et al. Is intermittent claudication improved by percutaneous transluminal angioplasty? A randomized controlled trial. J Vascular Surg 1997;26:551–557.

56. Bosch J, Hunink M. Meta-analysis of the results of percutaneous transluminal angioplasty and stent placement for aortoiliac occlusive disease [published erratum appears in Radiology 1997 Nov;205:584]. Radiol 1997;204:87–96.

57. The Heart Outcomes Prevention Evaluation Study Investigators. Effects of an Angiotensin-Converting-Enzyme Inhibitor, Ramipril, on Cardiovascular Events in High-Risk Patients. N Engl J Med 2000;342:145–153.

58. McDermott MM. Peripheral arterial disease: Epidemiology and drug therapy. Am J Geriatr Cardiol 2002;11:258–266.

59. Paravastu SCV, Mendonca DA, de Silva A. Beta Blockers for Peripheral Arterial Disease. Eur J Endovascular Surg 2009;38:66–70.

60. Expert Panel on Detection Evaluation and Treatment of High Blood Cholesterol in Adults. Executive Summary of the Third Report of the National Cholesterol Education Program (NCEP) Expert Panel on Detection, Evaluation, and Treatment of High Blood Cholesterol in Adults (Adult Treatment Panel III). JAMA 2001;285:2486–2497.

61. Leng GC, Price JF, Jepson RG. Lipid-lowering for lower limb atherosclerosis. Cochrane Database Syst Rev 2000;2(CD000123).

62. MRC/BHF Heart Protection Study of cholesterol lowering with simvastatin in 20536 high-risk individuals: A randomised placebo-controlled trial. Lancet 2002;360(9326):7–22.

63. Cannon CP, Braunwald E, McCabe CH, et al. Intensive versus Moderate Lipid Lowering with Statins after Acute Coronary Syndromes. N Engl J Med 2004;350:1495–1504.

64. Elam MB, Hunninghake DB, Davis KB, et al. Effect of niacin on lipid and lipoprotein levels and glycemic control in patients with diabetes and peripheral arterial disease: The ADMIT study: A randomized trial. JAMA 2000;284:1263–1270.

65. Coutinho M, Gerstein H, Wang Y, Yusuf S. The relationship between glucose and incident cardiovascular events. A metaregression analysis of published data from 20 studies of 95,783 individuals followed for 12.4 years. Diabetes Care 1999;22:233–240.

66. Am Diabetes Association. Peripheral arterial disease in people with diabetes. Diabetes Care 2003;26:3333–3341.

67. Creager MA, Luscher TF, Cosentino F, Beckman JA. Diabetes and vascular disease: Pathophysiology, clinical consequences, and medical therapy: Part I. Circulation 2003;108:1527–1532.

68. Selvin E, Wattanakit K, Steffes MW, Coresh J, Sharrett AR. HbA1c and peripheral arterial disease in diabetes: The atherosclerosis risk in communities study. Diabetes Care 2006;29:877–882.

69. Rehring TF, Sandhoff BG, Stolcpart RS, Merenich JA, Hollis Jr HW. Atherosclerotic risk factor control in patients with peripheral arterial disease. J Vasc Surg 2005;41:816–822.

70. Antithrombotic Trialists' Collaboration. Collaborative meta-analysis of randomised trials of antiplatelet therapy for prevention of death, myocardial infarction, and stroke in high risk patients. BMJ 2002;324:71–86.

71. Tran H, Anand SS. Oral antiplatelet therapy in cerebrovascular disease, coronary artery disease, and peripheral arterial disease. JAMA 2004;292:1867–1874.

72. Clagett GP, Sobel M, Jackson MR, Lip GYH, Tangelder M, Verhaeghe R. Antithrombotic therapy in peripheral arterial occlusive disease: The Seventh ACCP Conference on Antithrombotic and Thrombolytic Therapy. Chest 2004;126(3 suppl):609S–626S.

73. Diener HC, Cunha L, Forbes C, Sivenius J, Smets P, Lowenthal A. European Stroke Prevention Study 2. Dipyridamole and acetylsalicylic acid in the secondary prevention of stroke. J Neurol Sci 1996;143:1–13.

74. Janzon L. The STIMS trial: The ticlopidine experience and its clinical applications. Swedish Ticlopidine Multicenter Study. Vascular Med 1996;1:141–143.

75. Janzon L, Bergqvist D, Boberg J, et al. Prevention of myocardial infarction and stroke in patients with intermittent claudication; effects of ticlopidine. Results from STIMS, the Swedish Ticlopidine Multicentre Study [erratum appears in J Intern Med 1990 Dec;228:659]. J Intern Med 1990;227:301–308.

76. Ticlid—Ticlopidine hydrochloride. In: Roche Laboratories Inc; 2005.

77. Dawson DL, Cutler BS, Hiatt WR, et al. A comparison of cilostazol and pentoxifylline for treating intermittent claudication. Am J Med 2000;109:523–530.

78. Thompson PD, Zimet R, Forbes WP, Zhang P. Meta-analysis of results from eight randomized, placebo-controlled trials on the effect of cilostazol on patients with intermittent claudication. Am J Cardio 2002;90:1314–1319.

79. Cilostazol—"C" Monographs. In: DrugPoints. Thomson Healthcare; 2009.

80. Lindgarde F, Jelnes R, Bjorkman H, et al. Conservative drug treatment in patients with moderately severe chronic occlusive peripheral arterial disease. Scandinavian Study Group. Circulation 1989;80:1549–1556.

81. Girolami B, Bernardi E, Prins MH, et al. Treatment of intermittent claudication with physical training, smoking cessation, pentoxifylline, or nafronyl: A meta-analysis.[see comment]. Arch Intern Med 1999;159:337–345.

82. Radack K, Wyderski RJ. Conservative management of intermittent claudication. Ann Intern Med 1990;113:135–146.

83. Ernst E. Pentoxifylline for intermittent claudication. A critical review. Angiol 1994;45:339–345.

84. Hood SC, Moher D, Barber GG. Management of intermittent claudication with pentoxifylline: Meta-analysis of randomized controlled trials. CMAJ 1996;155:1053–1059.

85. Criqui MH. Systemic atherosclerosis risk and the mandate for intervention in atherosclerotic peripheral arterial disease. Am J Cardio 2001;88(7B):43J–47J.

86. Mannava K, Money SR. Current management of peripheral arterial occlusive disease: A review of pahrmacologic agents and other interventions. Am J Cardio Drugs 2007;7:59–66.

87. Guyatt G, Schunemann HJ, Cook D, Jaeschke R, Pauker S. Applying the Grades of Recommendation for Antithrombotic and Thrombolytic Therapy. The Seventh ACCP Conference on Antithrombotic and Thrombolytic Therapy. Chest 2004;126(3 suppl):179S-187S.

88. Plavix—Clopidogrel bisulfate. In: Bristol-Myers Squibb/Sanofi Pharmaceuticals Partnership; May 2009.

89. Aspirin—"A" Monographs. In: DrugPoints. Thomson Healthcare; 2009.

90. Dipyridamole—"D" Monographs. In: DrugPoints. Thomson Healthcare; 2009.

91. Pentoxifylline—"P" Monographs. In: DrugPoints. Thomson Healthcare; 2009.

30

Use of Vasopressors and Inotropes in the Pharmacotherapy of Shock

ROBERT MACLAREN, MARIA I. RUDIS, AND JOSEPH F. DASTA

KEY CONCEPTS

❶ Continuous hemodynamic monitoring with an arterial catheter or a central venous catheter capable of measuring mixed venous oxygen saturation (Svo_2) or central venous oxygen saturation ($Scvo_2$) should be used early and throughout the course of septic shock to assess intravascular fluid status and ventricular filling pressures, determine cardiac output (CO), and monitor arterial and venous oxygenation. They can be used for monitoring the response to drug therapy and guiding dosage titration.

❷ Early goal-directed therapy with aggressive fluid resuscitation in the emergency department within the first 6 hours of presentation improves survival of patients with sepsis and septic shock.

❸ Lactate production is increased under anaerobic conditions. Elevated serum lactate concentrations represent global perfusion abnormalities. Lactate may be used to assess repayment of oxygen to the tissues. Gastrointestinal tonometry and sublingual capnometry represent methods of assessing regional perfusion but are used infrequently.

❹ Derangements in adrenergic receptor sensitivity or activity frequently result in resistance to catecholamine vasopressor and inotropic therapy in critically ill patients. These changes may be a function of endogenous catecholamine concentrations, dosage/duration of exposure to and type of exogenously administered vasopressors, stage of septic shock, preexisting illness, and other factors.

❺ In refractory septic shock, rational use of vasopressor or inotropic agents should be guided by receptor activity, pharmacologic and pharmacokinetic characteristics, and regional and systemic hemodynamic effects of the drug and should be tailored to the patient's physiologic needs. Pharmacologically sound combinations of vasopressor and/or inotrope agents should be initiated early to optimize and facilitate rapid response.

❻ Goals of therapy with vasopressors and inotropes should be predetermined and should optimize global and regional perfusion parameters (e.g., cardiac, renal, mesenteric, and periphery). This can be accomplished by continuous or intermittent measurements. Targeted goals should be central venous pressure (CVP) of 8–12 mm Hg (up to 15 mm Hg in mechanically ventilated patients, patients with preexisting left ventricular

dysfunction, or patients with abdominal distension), mean arterial pressure (MAP) ≥65 mm Hg, and $Svo_2/Scvo_2$ ≥70%.

❼ Dose titration and monitoring of vasopressor and inotropic therapy should be guided by the "best clinical response" while observing for and minimizing evidence of myocardial ischemia (e.g., tachydysrhythmias, electrocardiographic changes), renal (decreased glomerular filtration rate and/or urine production), splanchnic/gastric [low intramucosal pH, bowel ischemia], or peripheral (cold extremities) hypoperfusion, and worsening of partial pressure of arterial oxygen (Pao_2), pulmonary artery occlusive pressure, and other hemodynamic variables.

❽ Much higher dosages of all vasopressors and inotropes than traditionally recommended are required to improve hemodynamic and oxygen-transport variables in patients with septic shock. Arbitrarily targeting vasopressor and inotrope therapy to supranormal values of global oxygen-transport variables cannot be recommended because of the lack of clear benefit and possible increased morbidity.

❾ First-line therapy of septic shock is aggressive volume resuscitation with crystalloid or colloid types of fluids. Dopamine or norepinephrine typically is used as the initial vasopressor agent for hemodynamic support. Dopamine is limited by its ability to increase CO and complications of tachycardia, tachydysrhythmias, increase in pulmonary artery occlusive pressure, and decrease in splanchnic oxygen use. Low-dose dopamine should not be used to prevent renal failure. Norepinephrine may achieve greater hemodynamic response than dopamine and is less likely to cause tachydysrhythmias and a decrease in splanchnic oxygen utilization.

❿ Phenylephrine may be a particularly useful alternative in patients who cannot tolerate tachycardia or tachydysrhythmia associated with the use of other agents. Its effects on cardiac performance and splanchnic oxygen utilization are variable.

⓫ Epinephrine appears to be effective as a single agent and as an add-on agent. It is particularly useful in the young, in patients with otherwise healthy myocardium, and potentially in patients when used early in the course of treatment. However, because epinephrine causes a significant increase in lactate and worsening of splanchnic oxygen utilization, it is not the agent of first choice in patients with septic shock. It should be used cautiously in patients with a history of coronary artery disease or underlying cardiac disturbances.

⓬ Dobutamine may be used as adjunctive therapy for its inotropic effect. It enhances CO and may increase $Svo_2/Scvo_2$. Concurrent vasopressor therapy is needed because dobutamine causes vasodilation. Dobutamine therapy may be limited by tachycardia and dysrhythmias.

⑬ Therapy with vasopressors and inotropes is continued until the myocardial depression and vascular hyporesponsiveness of septic shock improve, usually measured in hours to days. Discontinuation of vasopressor or inotropic therapy should be executed slowly; therapy should be "weaned" to avoid a precipitous worsening in regional and systemic hemodynamics.

⑭ Vasopressin produces vasoconstriction independent of adrenergic receptors and reduces the dosages of catecholamine vasopressors. Replacement dosages of vasopressin (0.01–0.04 units/min) can be considered in patients with septic shock refractory to catecholamine vasopressors despite adequate fluid resuscitation. Dosage rates should not be titrated upward. Vasopressin may enhance urine production but it may worsen splanchnic and peripheral perfusion. Given the current data, corticosteroids can be administered to patients with septic shock refractory to vasopressors or when adrenal insufficiency is present. Side effects of short-term corticosteroids are minimal.

Shock is an acute, generalized state of inadequate perfusion of critical organs that can produce serious pathophysiologic consequences, including death, when therapy is not optimal. Shock is defined as systolic blood pressure <90 mm Hg or reduction of at least 40 mm Hg from baseline with perfusion abnormalities despite adequate fluid resuscitation.[1] Previously, mortality from septic or cardiogenic shock exceeded 70% but now ranges between 30% to 50%.[2-5] This chapter reviews the theory and current status of hemodynamic monitoring and presents an update on the optimal use of inotropes and vasopressor drugs in shock states, specifically septic shock.[6-19]

Hemodynamic and perfusion monitoring can be categorized into two broad areas: global and regional monitoring. Global parameters, such as systemic blood pressure and pulse oximetry, assess perfusion and oxygen utilization of the entire body. Regional monitoring techniques, such as tonometry, focus on oxygen delivery and subsequent changes in metabolism of individual organs and tissues. Normal values for commonly monitored parameters are listed in Table 30–1. Evidence-based goals of therapy are listed in Table 30–2.[6-19] The adequacy of regional perfusion can be assessed

TABLE 30-1	Hemodynamic and Oxygen-Transport Monitoring Parameters
Parameter	**Normal Value**[a]
Blood pressure (systolic/diastolic)	100–130/70–85 mm Hg
Mean arterial pressure (MAP)	80–100 mm Hg
Pulmonary artery pressure (PAP)	25/10 mm Hg
Mean pulmonary artery pressure (MPAP)	12–15 mm Hg
Central venous pressure (CVP)	8–12 mm Hg
Pulmonary artery occlusive pressure (PAOP)	12–15 mm Hg
Heart rate (HR)	60–80 beats/min
Cardiac output (CO)	4–7 L/min
Cardiac index (CI)	2.8–3.6 L/min/m²
Stroke volume index (SVI)	30–50 mL/m²
Systemic vascular resistance index (SVRI)	1,300–2,100 dyne • s/m² • cm⁵
Pulmonary vascular resistance index (PVRI)	45–225 dyne • s/m² • cm⁵
Arterial oxygen saturation (Sao_2)	97% (range, 95%–100%)
Mixed venous oxygen saturation (Svo_2)	70%–75%
Arterial oxygen content (Cao_2)	20.1 vol% (range, 19–21)
Venous oxygen content (Cvo_2)	15.5 vol% (range, 11.5–16.5)
Oxygen content difference ($C[a–v]O_2$)	5 vol% (range, 4–6)
Oxygen consumption index (VO_2)	131 mL/min/m² (range, 100–180)
Oxygen delivery index (Do_2)	578 mL/min/m² (range, 370–730)
Oxygen extraction ratio (O_2ER)	25% (range, 22–30)
Intramucosal pH (pHi)	7.40 (range, 7.35–7.45)
Index (I)	Parameter indexed to body surface area

[a]Normal values may not be the same as values needed to optimize the management of a critically ill patient.

TABLE 30-2	Evidence-Based Treatment Recommendations for Management of Severe Sepsis or Septic Shock	
Recommendations		**Grade**
In patients requiring vasopressors, an arterial catheter should be placed as soon as practical to monitor blood pressure.		1D
Begin resuscitation immediately in patients with hypotension or elevated serum lactate.		1C
Goals of resuscitation should include (1) CVP 8–12 mm Hg,[a] (2) MAP ≥65 mm Hg, (3) urine production ≥0.5 mL/kg/h, and (4) Svo_2 or $Scvo_2$ ≥70%.		1C
If Svo_2 or $Scvo_2$ ≥70% not achieved, consider the following: (1) further fluid administration, (2) transfuse packed red blood cells to hematocrit ≥30%, or (3) dobutamine infusion ≤20 mcg/kg/min.		2C
Fluid resuscitate using crystalloids or colloids.		1B
Use a fluid challenge technique to determine associated hemodynamic improvement. Administer 1000 mL of crystalloid or 300–500 mL of colloid over 30 minutes. More rapid and larger volumes may be required. Rate of fluid administration should be reduced if cardiac filling pressures increase without concurrent improvement.		1D
Use vasopressors to maintain MAP ≥65 mm Hg.		1C
Either dopamine or norepinephrine centrally administered are the initial vasopressors of choice.		1C
Epinephrine, phenylephrine, or vasopressin should not be administered as the initial vasopressor. Vasopressin 0.03 units/min may be subsequently added to norepinephrine with an anticipation of an effect equivalent to norepinephrine alone.		2C
Use epinephrine as the first alternative agent when blood pressure is poorly responsive to dopamine or norepinephrine.		2B
Do not use low-dose dopamine for renal protection.		1A
Use dobutamine in patients with myocardial dysfunction as supported by elevated cardiac filling pressures and low CO.		1C
Do not increase cardiac output to predetermined supranormal indices.		1B
Consider intravenous hydrocortisone when hypotension remains poorly responsive to adequate fluid resuscitation and vasopressors.		2C
ACTH stimulation test is not recommended to identify the subset of patients who should receive hydrocortisone.		2B
Hydrocortisone is the preferred corticosteroid.		2B
Hydrocortisone dose should be ≤300 mg/day.		1A
Corticosteroid therapy may be weaned once vasopressors are no longer required.		2D
Do not use corticosteroids to treat sepsis in the absence of shock unless the patient's endocrine or corticosteroid history warrants it.		1D

[a]A higher target CVP of 12–15 mm Hg may be required in the presence of mechanical ventilation or preexisting left ventricular dysfunction or abdominal distension.
ACTH, adrenocorticotropic hormone; CO, cardiac output; CVP, central venous pressure; Do_2, oxygen delivery; MAP, mean arterial pressure; $Scvo_2$, central-venous oxygen saturation; Svo_2, mixed venous oxygen saturation. Level of recommendations: 1, a strong recommendation indicating that the intervention's desirable effects clearly outweigh its undesirable effects; 2, a weak recommendation indicating that the tradeoff between desirable and undesirable effects is less clear. Quality of evidence: A, supported by a randomized control trial; B, supported by a downgraded randomized control trial or upgraded observational studies; C, supported by observational studies; D, supported by case series or expert opinion.
Based on data from references 6–19.

by indices of specific organ perfusion.[7,16–21] These measurements include coagulation abnormalities (disseminated intravascular coagulation), altered renal function with reduced urine production or increased serum concentrations of blood urea nitrogen and creatinine, altered hepatic parenchymal function with increased serum concentrations of transaminases and bilirubin, altered gastrointestinal perfusion manifested by ileus and diminished bowel sounds, cardiac ischemia with elevated troponin levels and electrocardiographic changes, and altered sensorium. Although none of these indices alone is a reliable indicator of adequate resuscitation, they offer immediate detection and may be prognostic of recovery when combined and defined at the level of organ function. As a result, these indices are frequently used as surrogate endpoints for the goals of resuscitation.[22] While it is assumed that normalization of these parameters infers benefit, the clinician must first treat the patient rather than relying solely on data from continuous monitoring to guide therapy.[22]

GLOBAL PERFUSION MONITORING

ARTERIAL BLOOD PRESSURE MEASUREMENT

Mean arterial blood pressure (MAP) is the product of cardiac output (CO) and systemic vascular resistance (SVR). Conditions that may lower blood pressure in critically ill patients include cardiac failure (etiology may be myocardial infarction, arrhythmia, acute heart failure, or valvular disease) and hypovolemia (etiology may be hemorrhage, intractable diarrhea, or heat stroke) by lowering CO and vasodilation (etiology may be sepsis, drugs, anaphylaxis, acute hepatic failure, or neurotrauma) by lowering SVR. Arterial blood pressure is the end point of therapy; however, restoration of adequate perfusion pressure is the primary criterion of effectiveness.[6–21] Profound hypotension (MAP <50 mm Hg) is associated with a pressure-dependent decrease in coronary and cerebral blood flow and may rapidly produce myocardial and cerebral ischemia. Arterial blood pressure can be determined by noninvasive and invasive methods. All noninvasive blood pressure monitoring techniques depend on the use of an occluding cuff. Systolic and diastolic blood pressures are further determined by auscultation, palpation (systolic pressure only), oscillometry, or Doppler technique (systolic pressures are most reliable). Auscultation is the most commonly used method outside the intensive care unit (ICU). Its use, however, is limited in patients with hypovolemia, hypothermia, or cardiogenic shock when pulses or Korotkoff sounds may be difficult to hear. Similar constraints exist for the palpation and oscillometric methods. However, oscillometry is preferred in edematous patients. Oscillometry measures blood pressure by sensing arterial blood pressure changes, or oscillations, against an inflated cuff. Rapid changes in oscillation amplitude correspond to systolic and diastolic pressure. It is the only noninvasive method to measure MAP even in low-flow states and lends itself to automatic cycling and serial measurements (every 1–3 minutes) that do not require operator intervention, a key component in ICU monitoring. The use of narrow cuffs or cuffs applied too loosely can result in falsely high readings, whereas wide cuffs may produce falsely low readings. Fingertip devices offer another avenue for continuous indirect blood pressure measurement, but their accuracy in ICU patients may be significantly diminished by concurrent administration of vasoactive drugs.

❶ The use of invasive arterial catheters makes possible the continuous measurement of MAP as well as procurement of blood samples for blood gas monitoring. The radial artery is the most commonly used vessel, but the dorsalis pedis, femoral, brachial, and axillary arteries and the umbilical artery in the newborn also can be accessed. This method of blood pressure monitoring is the standard technique used in the ICU against which all other methods are compared. Major complications of peripheral artery catheterization include infection and distal ischemia. Acute distal ischemia and catheter-related bacteremia occur in <1% of catheter insertions. This translates to 2.9% of bloodstream infections per 1,000 catheter-days.[23] Ischemia is most common in patients with multiple or prolonged arterial cannulations, hypertension, or vasopressor therapy.[8] Invasive techniques are labor intensive, require aseptic techniques, and offer potential sources of equipment errors, such as length and quality of tubing, air bubbles, stopcocks, thrombus formation, tube kinking, and transducer placement. Hypertension, advanced age, and atherosclerosis also may affect the accuracy of invasive blood pressure readings.[19]

CENTRAL VENOUS CATHETER

❶ The central venous catheter is used to measure the central venous pressure (CVP), to obtain venous blood gas samples, and to administer drugs or fluids directly to the central circulation. A triple-lumen catheter frequently is used, whereby drugs with known incompatibility can be administered. Blood volume, venous wall compliance, right-sided cardiac function, intraabdominal and intrathoracic pressures, and vasopressor therapy affect CVP. The CVP is not a reliable estimate of blood volume but can be used to qualitatively assess blood volume changes in patients during the early phases of fluid resuscitation.[6–8] The goal of fluid administration is to maintain the CVP at 8 to 12 mm Hg, but values of 15 mm Hg may be targeted in mechanically ventilated patients or patients with abdominal distension or preexisting ventricular dysfunction.[6–8] Sustained elevated pressures may be indicative of fluid overloading. Few data support the use of continuous CVP monitoring in the ICU. However, CVP monitoring of fluid therapy during resuscitation of septic shock is associated with reduced mortality.[9]

PULMONARY ARTERY CATHETER

❶ Pulmonary artery catheterization provides multiple cardiovascular parameters, including CVP, pulmonary artery pressure, pulmonary artery occlusive pressures (PAOP), CO, SVR, and the mixed-venous oxygen saturation (Svo_2).[24] Ideally, the pulmonary artery catheter should be positioned fluoroscopically; however, satisfactory placement also may be obtained by observing pulmonary artery pressure readings and electrocardiographic waveforms during catheter advancement. Proper positioning in the lower lung (zone 3) is essential to measure PAOP and to prevent distal pulmonary artery collapse. Inflation of the balloon at the catheter tip occludes the pulmonary artery, isolates the distal catheter tip from the right side of the heart, and allows the user to measure the PAOP, an approximate measure of the left ventricular end-diastolic volume and a major determinant of left ventricular preload. Poor wedging may be caused by catheter migration, patient movement, mechanical ventilation, or eccentric balloon inflation. Pulmonary artery catheters equipped with a distal thermistor also allow measurement of CO by thermodilution. Rapid injection of saline or dextrose solutions via the right atrial port allows complete mixing of blood with the injectate, and the resulting change in blood temperature is measured in the pulmonary artery. From the temperature change, the patient's CO can be calculated. Newer pulmonary artery catheters contain a temperature coil that intermittently warms the blood in the right ventricle for near-continuous CO measurement. Significant tricuspid regurgitation, an intracardiac shunt, and significant positive end-expiratory pressure decrease the validity of CO measurements. The most common complications of pulmonary artery catheterization include mural thrombus formation (14%–91%), transient ventricular tachydysrhythmias (11%–63%), pulmonary infarction (1%–7%), pulmonary artery rupture (0.06%–2.0%), and sepsis (0.3%–0.5%).[25]

Most pulmonary artery catheters are heparin bonded, and the relative risk (RR) of infection is 2.6 per 1,000 patient-days, similar to the risk with central venous catheters of 2.3 per 1,000 patient-days.[23] Controversy surrounds the utility and safety of the pulmonary artery catheter, including issues surrounding correct placement and impact of the device on patient outcome. Recent studies failed to demonstrate beneficial outcomes with the use of the pulmonary artery catheter.[26] The most recent guidelines suggest careful evaluation of the indications and the risk of placing a pulmonary artery catheter for resuscitation of critically ill patients.[27]

❶ The optimal PAOP needs to be individualized for each patient. Administering a fluid bolus followed by simultaneous PAOP and CO measurements with the goal of increasing the PAOP until CO does not change can be accomplished and is based on Starling's law of the heart. However, clinical experience suggests that most patients have an optimal response to PAOP values in the range from 12 to 15 mm Hg.

CLINICAL CONTROVERSY: CVP VS PAOP

Limited data are available comparing the use of CVP and PAOP for guiding therapy in patients with shock. The results of recent studies of critically ill patients suggest CVP and PAOP are equivalent in terms of clinical outcomes, including mortality.[28] Therefore, a pulmonary artery catheter should be inserted when hemodynamic data are needed that cannot be obtained from a central venous catheter or when the validity of measurements from the central venous catheter is questionable.

---

❶ Other methods used to assess CO include carbon dioxide (CO_2) partial rebreathing and esophageal Doppler.[22,29] The CO_2 partial rebreathing technique compares end-tidal CO_2 partial pressure obtained during a nonrebreathing period with that obtained during a subsequent rebreathing period. The ratio of change in end-tidal CO_2 and CO_2 elimination estimates CO but must be corrected for blood shunting. Poor to acceptable agreement exists between this method and the thermodilution method of assessing CO in critically ill patients. Also, low minute ventilation, a high shunt fraction, or a high cardiac output produce inaccurate results. The esophageal Doppler technique measures flow velocity in the descending aorta by means of a Doppler transducer. CO is calculated based on the diameter of the aorta, the distribution of CO to the aorta, and the flow velocity of blood in the aorta. The CO reported by this method correlates with therapeutic interventions and demonstrates excellent agreement with the pulmonary artery catheter. Unfortunately, this method is technologically difficult and may not produce reliable measurements over time.

OXYGEN TENSION AND SATURATION MONITORING

Partial pressure of arterial oxygen (Pao_2) and arterial oxygen saturation (Sao_2) can be measured subjectively by assessing capillary refill or invasively by obtaining an arterial blood sample. Arterial blood gases measured by conventional arterial sampling are considered standard, but their accuracy and usefulness are affected by poor sampling techniques, transportation and analysis delays, analyzer accuracy, sample cellular metabolism, and inability to trend results. Indwelling fiberoptic and electrochemical systems that allow continuous monitoring and trend analyses of blood pH, Pao_2, and partial pressure of arterial carbon dioxide ($Paco_2$) while decreasing patient blood loss from less frequent sampling are in development.

❶ Mixed venous oxygen saturation (Svo_2) depends on CO, oxygen demand, hemoglobin, and Sao_2. It can be measured in patients using a pulmonary artery catheter. Initially, critically ill septic patients may present with a low Svo_2 value (<70%), indicating high extraction of oxygen by tissues and lack of adequate oxygen delivery (Do_2, or Do_2I, indexed to body surface area) to tissues. In patients with sepsis and other conditions who present with a low Svo_2 value, rapid intervention should be undertaken to increase Do_2 to tissues, with the goal of obtaining Svo_2 ≥70%.[30,31] The length of time Svo_2 is <70% is associated with mortality.[32] As sepsis worsens, however, Svo_2 may be ≥70%. This occurs because extraction of oxygen in the arteriolar beds is hampered and is indicative of poor outcome.

❶ Central venous oxygen saturation ($Scvo_2$) is a less invasive measure of venous oxygen saturation because the catheter is placed at the junction of the inferior and superior venae cavae rather than at the pulmonary artery.[17-21] It is as accurate as Svo_2 but provides slightly higher normal values. Although controversial, many clinicians use these measurements interchangeably. Concentrations of $Scvo_2$ <70% reliably indicate inadequate oxygenation in shock states and detect subclinical ("cryptic") shock much earlier than hypotension. Targeting fluid and hemodynamic resuscitation to achieve $Scvo_2$ ≥70% is a sensitive indicator and measure of the extent of global tissue hypoxia, a determinant of the adequacy of hemodynamic resuscitation, and is associated with improved survival in patients with sepsis and septic shock.[17-21]

OXYGEN DELIVERY AND CONSUMPTION

Tissue oxygen debt is indicative of organ damage in critical illness. In normal individuals, oxygen consumption (Vo_2 or Vo_2I, indexed to body surface area) depends on Do_2 (or Do_2I) up to a certain critical level (Vo_2 flow dependency). At this point, tissue oxygen requirements apparently are satisfied, and further increases in Do_2 will not alter Vo_2 (Vo_2 flow independency). Although animal models of sepsis substantiate this relationship, studies in critically ill humans show a continuous, pathologic dependence relationship of Vo_2 with Do_2.[17-21,31] The Vo_2/Do_2 ratio, or oxygen extraction ratio (O_2ER), can be used to assess adequacy of perfusion and metabolic response.[17-21,31] Maintaining the oxygen extraction ratio (O_2ER) at <25% without a changing Vo_2 may be helpful in maintaining or improving the body's reserve in meeting the oxygen demands.[17-21,31] However, low Vo_2 and O_2ER values are indicative of poor oxygen utilization and lead to greater mortality. Patients who are able to increase Vo_2 when Do_2 is increased show improved survival. This finding became the basis for targeting supranormal Do_2 and Vo_2 values in the treatment of ICU patients.[9] However, a meta-analysis of randomized clinical trials involving 1,016 adult ICU patients failed to show that achievement of this goal improved mortality.[33] This may have been due in part to the heterogeneous nature of the ICU patients studied and therapies provided, lack of study blinding, crossover patients (control patients who achieve supranormal Do_2 and Vo_2 values by themselves), or lack of adequate control of cointerventions. The debate continues in more homogeneous patient populations. For example, in high-risk surgical patients, supranormal DO_2 values decrease mortality except in the subgroup of patients exceeding 75 years of age in whom achieving Do_2I >600 mL/m^2/min show mixed mortality results.[31,33]

A review of alternative potential mechanisms of beneficial effect of supranormal Do_2 suggests that catecholamines exert antiinflammatory actions by modulating cytokine response.[34] In general, catecholamines inhibit the production of inflammatory cytokines (e.g., interleukin [IL]-6, tumor necrosis factor [TNF]-α) and may enhance synthesis of antiinflammatory cytokine (e.g., IL-4 and IL-10). The actions of epinephrine on these cytokines are blocked by propranolol and thus are mediated by adrenergic β-receptors.

Another problem with therapy directed to achieve supranormal oxygen transport values is that the apparent linear relationship between DO_2 and VO_2 has been questioned because both share variables, and this *mathematical coupling* can produce artifactual relationships between variables.[17-21] The DO_2 and VO_2 indexed parameters are calculated as follows:

$$DO_2 = CI \times CaO_2$$

$$VO_2 = CI \times (CaO_2 - CvO_2),$$

where CI = cardiac index, CaO_2 = arterial oxygen content determined by hemoglobin concentration and SaO_2, and CvO_2 = mixed venous oxygen content determined by hemoglobin concentration and SvO_2.

However, variable relationships between DO_2 and VO_2 are observed when VO_2 is measured independently by indirect calorimetry. Therefore, a linear relationship between DO_2 and VO_2 may be the result of mathematical coupling or flow-dependent VO_2. Currently available data do not support the concept that patient outcome or survival is improved by treatment measures directed toward achieving supranormal DO_2 and VO_2 values.[33] In fact, a consensus conference concluded that although pulmonary artery catheterization is useful for guiding therapy, routinely increasing cardiac index to predetermined supranormal values does not improve outcome.[6] Furthermore, achievement of a supranormal DO_2 does not ensure parallel improvements in regional organ blood flow and oxygenation. One approach that may decrease the effect of mathematical coupling and provide individualized therapy may lie in titrated therapy, with sequential measurements of DO_2 and VO_2 to achieve VO_2 flow independency along with normalization of blood lactate and hemodynamic parameters.

❷ The most recent data regarding goal-directed therapy in the hemodynamic support of sepsis relates to the importance of achieving predetermined parameters early in the management of sepsis.[35] In a meta-analysis of early (defined as 8–12 hours postoperatively or before the development of organ failure) versus late (defined as after the onset of organ failure) resuscitative efforts in patients stratified according to severity of illness (determined by control group mortality >20% [12 studies] or <15% [9 studies]) and targeting supranormal oxygen-transport variables, the data suggest that timing of resuscitation matters.[35] Early goal-directed therapy reduced mortality and the development of organ failure in patients who were more severely ill and when therapeutic interventions produced differences in DO_2. Moreover, outcome was not improved significantly in less severely ill patients (control group mortality <15% and normal DO_2 values as goals) or when therapy did not improve DO_2.

❷ ❻ More important than achieving supranormal DO_2 is the rapid initiation of therapy. In a prospective, randomized controlled trial, Rivers et al. demonstrated a significant reduction in mortality (30.5% vs 46.5%; P <0.001) in patients with severe sepsis and septic shock randomized to receive therapy based on goal-directed hemodynamic end points that were achieved within 6 hours of hospital presentation.[30] They used a strategy of serial administering (1) fluids rapidly to achieve CVP 8–12 mm Hg, (2) vasopressor agents to achieve MAP at least 65 mm Hg, (3) red blood cell transfusion to maintain hematocrit ≥30%, and (4) dobutamine to achieve $ScvO_2$ ≥70%. This approach demonstrates the benefits of initiating therapy early in the course of sepsis and directs therapy toward clearly defined goals in a consistent manner. The results of several evaluations of protocols or order sets designed to achieve the hemodynamic end points of early goal-directed therapy show that implementation is easily accomplished, cost is reduced, and patient outcomes, including survival, are improved.[36-41] A recent meta-analysis of nine studies showed reduced mortality when quantitative resuscitation goals are used to guide therapy (odds ratio [OR] 0.64; 95% confidence interval [CI] 0.43–0.96; P = 0.03).[42] Therefore,

healthcare facilities should implement strategies to achieve early goal-directed therapy using the predefined hemodynamic variables of the study by Rivers et al.[30]

CLINICAL CONTROVERSY: GOALS OF EARLY GOAL-DIRECTED THERAPY

The results of studies cannot delineate which end point or combination of end points was most beneficial with respect to early goal-directed therapy. These studies also offer limited information about specific interventions to achieve the predefined goals. In addition, whether these goals must be maintained after resuscitation is unknown. Several studies are ongoing to address some of these issues.

BLOOD LACTATE

❸ Lactate is a metabolic product of pyruvate. Its production is increased under anaerobic conditions, such as may occur during shock. Blood lactate concentrations are used as a diagnostic and prognostic tool in sepsis; they also are used to measure the repayment of oxygen debt to tissues.[17-21,31] It is a useful tool in combination with DO_2 and VO_2 because these measures change independently of one another. Serial lactate concentrations may show better correlation with outcome than oxygen transport parameters and may be superior to hemodynamic markers in determining adequacy of restoration of systemic oxygenation.[17-21,31] However, several caveats guide the use of lactate concentrations in septic patients. First, lactate may accumulate in patients with other conditions, such as significant hepatic dysfunction or acute respiratory distress syndrome, who are not in shock. Second, both well-perfused and poorly perfused tissues contribute to arterial and mixed venous lactate concentrations and therefore are not reflective of regional perfusion. Third, although increased lactate concentrations have been correlated with increased mortality, the utility of blood lactate measurements in guiding therapy has not been clearly demonstrated. Fourth, elevated lactate concentrations may result from cellular metabolic failure rather than global hypoperfusion in shock. Serial blood lactate measurements are more useful than single isolated measurements and continuously elevated concentrations are predictive of morbidity and mortality.

REGIONAL PERFUSION MONITORING

GASTROINTESTINAL TONOMETRY

Blood pressures, CO, blood lactate, and global oxygen homeostasis parameters do not offer information about the function of individual organs. Organ-specific hypoxia may be evident by coagulopathy as indicated by thrombocytopenia (platelet count <100,000/L and/or prolonged clotting times [international normalized ratio >1.5 or activated partial thromboplastin time at least 1.5-fold the upper limit of normal]), impaired renal function with urine production <0.5 mL/kg/h and/or increased serum concentrations of blood urea nitrogen and creatinine, altered hepatic function with substantially increased serum concentrations of transaminases and bilirubin, altered gastrointestinal perfusion manifested by ileus and diminished bowel sounds, cardiac ischemia with elevated troponin levels and electrocardiogram changes, and altered sensorium.[7,22] Objective measurement of regional perfusion to detect inadequate tissue oxygenation has focused on the mesenteric/splanchnic circulation, which is sensitive to changes in blood flow and oxygenation for several reasons.[17–21,43,44] First, the normally large majority of blood flow to the gut mucosa is redistributed toward the serosa and muscularis. Second, the gut may have a higher critical Do_2 threshold than other organs. Third, the tip of the villus has a countercurrent oxygen-exchange mechanism, rendering it highly sensitive to alterations in regional blood flow and oxygenation.

❸ Gastric tonometry measures gut luminal partial pressure of carbon dioxide (Pco_2) at equilibrium by placing a saline- or air-filled gas-permeable balloon in the gastric lumen. Assuming that carbon dioxide (Co_2) permeates freely among tissues and that the arterial bicarbonate (Hco_3^-) concentration is equal to that of the gut mucosa, the intramucosal pH (pHi) may be calculated using the Henderson-Hasselbalch equation:

$$pHi = 6.1 \log (HCO_3^-)\ 0.03 \times Pco_2$$

Increases in mucosal Pco_2 and calculated decreases in pHi are associated with mucosal hypoperfusion and perhaps increased mortality.[17–21,43,44] Calculation of pHi can be confounded by increases in luminal Pco_2, such as may occur when buffering antacids are used. Histamine$_2$-receptor antagonists or proton pump inhibitors can be used instead. The presence of respiratory acid–base disorders; systemic bicarbonate administration; arterial blood gas measurement errors; or enteral feeding products, blood, or stool in the gut may confound pHi determinations. As a result, the change in gastric mucosal Pco_2 may be more accurate than pHi. Furthermore, because mucosal Pco_2 is influenced by arterial Pco_2, the mucosal–arterial Pco_2 difference (Pco_2 gap) likely is the optimal measurement.[17–21,43,44] Gastric tonometry can be performed using either a saline- or air-filled balloon. The time delay (30 minutes) associated with equilibration of saline inside the balloon makes this method impractical for monitoring of resuscitation and inconvenient for routine bedside monitoring. An air-filled balloon requires a shorter equilibrium time, is simpler to use, and is equally accurate. However, the clinical utility of gastric tonometry remains uncertain. Clinical trials of pHi-directed therapy do not show that it aids resuscitation when other goals are concomitantly targeted. Gastric tonometry, in general, inconsistently predicts mortality.

❸ Evidence suggests that the most proximal part of the gastrointestinal tract, the sublingual mucosa, may be an acceptable location for monitoring regional perfusion and Pco_2.[17–21,43,44] Unlike gastrointestinal circulation, limited intra- and interpatient variability exists in the microvasculature and only few arterioles are available for assessment. Sublingual capnometry is noninvasive, is not technically complex, and provides results within minutes. The device consists of a disposable sublingual carbon dioxide pressure ($Pslco_2$) sensor, a fiberoptic cable that connects the disposable sensor to a blood gas analyzer, and a blood gas monitoring instrument. Small studies of critically ill patients with and without sepsis and septic shock show that the $Pslco_2$ and the sublingual-to-arterial Pco_2 gap correlate better with the enhancement of Do_2 with dobutamine than the mucosal Pco_2 and the mucosal-to-arterial Pco_2 gap.[17–21,43,44] The initial sublingual-to-arterial Pco_2 gap is a better predictor of mortality. These pilot studies must be expanded before this technology becomes part of routine practice, but it offers the possibility of noninvasive measurement of regional perfusion. Of note, some institutions have incorporated the $Pslco_2$ into their algorithms of early goal-directed therapy in an effort to provide additional information about the effectiveness of therapies during resuscitation.

MYOCARDIAL DYSFUNCTION

❶ Although loss of vascular tone is the hallmark of septic shock, myocardial dysfunction characterized by transient impairment of contractility is a recognized complication.[45,46] The range of left ventricular ejection fraction (LVEF) upon presentation is wide, but approximately 35% of patients with septic shock have left ventricular hypokinesis (mean ejection fraction 38% ± 17%) and low CO.[45,46] Because LVEF also is affected by preload and afterload, the low SVR of septic shock may mask depressed myocardial contractility that may be revealed upon restoration of MAP by administration of fluid and vasopressors. Therefore, CO may not reflect the extent of myocardial dysfunction. While it requires technical and interpretive training, echocardiography is a relatively simple method of assessing cardiac function.[47,48] It can assess chamber size, ventricular contractility, valve function, and blood flow. Patients with tissue hypoxia or a hyper-contractile left ventricle may benefit from fluid administration or vasopressor therapy; whereas, patients with poor left ventricular function may require inotropic intervention. Like sublingual capnometry, some institutions use echocardiography to direct resuscitation therapies.[48]

Cardiac troponin release in septic patients occurs in the absence of flow-limiting disease, likely due to a loss in membrane integrity with subsequent leakage or microvascular thrombosis. Elevation of cardiac troponin concentrations in patients with sepsis indicates left ventricular dysfunction and portends a poor prognosis.[45,46] Troponin concentrations also correlate with the duration of hypotension and the intensity of vasopressor therapy. Early recognition of myocardial dysfunction is crucial for administration of appropriate therapy. In the absence of other mechanisms for assessing cardiac function, echocardiographic findings and troponin concentrations may help guide and monitor therapy. Whereas cardiac troponins may be integrated into the monitoring of myocardial dysfunction to identify patients requiring aggressive therapy, natriuretic peptides show variable correlation with LVEF and should not be routinely monitored.[45,46]

VASOPRESSORS AND INOTROPES

❻ Vasopressors and inotropes in patients with septic shock are required when volume resuscitation fails to maintain adequate blood pressure (MAP ≥65 mm Hg) and organs and tissues remain hypoperfused despite optimizing CVP to 8 to 12 mm Hg or PAOP to 12 to 15 mm Hg.[7] However, vasopressors may be needed temporarily to treat life-threatening hypotension when filling pressures are inadequate despite aggressive fluid resuscitation. Inotropes are frequently used to optimize cardiac function in cases of cardiogenic shock. The clinician must decide on the choice of agent, therapeutic end points, and safe and effective doses of vasopressors and inotropes to be used. This section reviews adrenergic receptor pharmacology, exogenous catecholamine use, and alterations in receptor function in critically ill patients. It also provides guidelines for the clinical use of adrenergic agents, optimization of pharmacotherapeutic outcomes, and minimization of adverse effects in critically ill patients with septic shock. Therapies of hypovolemic shock and cardiogenic shock are discussed in other chapters.

Of note, agents other than catecholamines have been used as inotropes and vasopressors in shock states. They include phosphodiesterase III inhibitors, naloxone, nitric oxide (NO) synthase (NOS) inhibitors, and calcium sensitizers. This chapter focuses on catecholamines. Vasopressin and corticosteroids, as they relate to septic shock, also are emphasized because they have pharmacologic interactions with catecholamines, possess hemodynamic effects, and are frequently used.

CATECHOLAMINE RECEPTOR PHARMACOLOGY

❺ Comparative receptor activities of endogenous and exogenously administered catecholamines is summarized in Table 30–3.[6–19,49–53] Endogenous catecholamines are responsible for regulation of

TABLE 30-3 Adrenergic, Dopaminergic, and Vasopressin Receptor Pharmacology and Organ Distribution

Effector Organ	Receptor Subtype	Physiologic Response
Heart		
Sinoatrial node	β_1, β_2	Increased heart rate
Atria	β_1, β_2	Increased contractility
		Increased conduction velocity
Atrioventricular node	β_1, β_2	Increased automaticity
		Increased conduction velocity
His-Purkinje system	β_1, β_2	Increased automaticity
		Increased conduction velocity
Ventricles	β_1, β_2	Increased contractility
		Increased conduction velocity
		Increased automaticity
		Increased rate idioventricular pacemaker cells
Arterioles		
Coronary	$\alpha_1, \alpha_2, V_1; \beta_2, D_1, V_2$ (via NO)	Constriction; dilation
Skin and mucosa	α_1, α_2, V_1	Constriction
Skeletal muscle	$\alpha_1, V_1; \beta_2$	Constriction; dilation
Cerebral	$\alpha_1, V_1; V_2$ (via NO)	Constriction (slight); dilation
Pulmonary	$\alpha_1; \beta_2, V_2$ (via NO)	Constriction; dilation
Abdominal viscera (mesentery)	$\alpha_1, V_1; \beta_2, D_1$	Constriction; dilation
Renal	$\alpha_1, \alpha_2, V_1; \beta_1, \beta_2, D_1$	Constriction; dilation
Veins (systemic)	$\alpha_1, \alpha_2; \beta_2$	Constriction; dilation
Lungs		
Tracheal/bronchial smooth muscle	β_2	Relaxation
Bronchial glands	$\alpha_1; \beta_2$	Decreased; increased secretion
Stomach		
Motility and tone	$\alpha_1, \alpha_2, \beta_1, \beta_2$	Decreased (usually)
Sphincter	α_1	Contraction (usually)
Secretions	α_2	Inhibition
Intestine		
Motility and tone	$\alpha_1, \alpha_2, \beta_1, \beta_2; V_1$	Decreased (usually); increased?
Sphincters	α_1	Contraction
Secretions	α_2	Inhibition
Kidney		
Renin secretion	$\alpha_1; \beta_1$	Decreased; increased
Reabsorption of water	V_2	Increased
Skeletal muscle	β_2	Increased contractility, glyconeogenesis, K+ uptake
Liver	α_1, β_2	Glycogenolysis and gluconeogenesis
Fat cells	$\alpha_1, \beta_1, \beta_2$	Lipolysis (thermogenesis)

D, dopamine; NO, nitric oxide; V, vasopressin.
Based on data from references 6–19, 49–53.

vascular and bronchiolar smooth muscle tone and myocardial contractility. These effects are mediated by sympathetic adrenergic receptors of the autonomic nervous system located in the vasculature, myocardium, and bronchioles. Postsynaptic adrenoceptors are located at or near the synaptic junction. These receptors can be activated by naturally circulating or exogenous catecholamines (e.g., norepinephrine, epinephrine, and phenylephrine), whereas presynaptic adrenoceptors are stimulated by locally released neurotransmitters (e.g., norepinephrine) and are controlled by a negative feedback mechanism.

The signal transduction pathways associated with catecholamine and vasopressin-induced effects in the heart and blood vessels are illustrated in Figure 30–1. [6–19,49–53] Agonists of β-adrenoceptors

and dopamine (D_1) receptors stimulate adenylate cyclase by a G-protein (G_s)–dependent mechanism (Fig. 30–1, top). Adenylate cyclase generates cyclic adenosine monophosphate (cAMP) from adenosine triphosphate (ATP). cAMP-dependent protein kinase A, which is activated by elevations in intracellular cAMP, phosphorylates target proteins to modify cellular function. Through these mechanisms, β_1-adrenoceptor activation exerts positive inotropic and chronotropic effects in the heart, and β_2-adrenoceptor and D_1-receptor activation induces vascular smooth muscle relaxation. Agonists of α_1-adrenoceptors stimulate phospholipase C-β (PLC-β) through a G-protein (G_q)–dependent process (Fig. 30–1, bottom). PLC-β produces inositol trisphosphate and diacylglycerol from cell membrane phosphatidylinositol bisphosphate. Diacylglycerol activates protein kinase C, an enzyme that phosphorylates several key proteins (e.g., extracellular signal-regulated kinases, c-Jun NH2-terminal kinases, and mitogen-activated protein kinases) that modify cellular function (e.g., hypertrophy). Inositol trisphosphate elicits the release of calcium from intracellular stores, such as the sarcoplasmic reticulum. Calcium forms a complex with calmodulin, which then activates calcium–calmodulin-dependent protein kinases (CaMK). CaMKs phosphorylate target proteins to alter cellular function. Myosin light-chain kinase is an example of a CaMK. Its action of phosphorylating myosin light chain leads to vascular smooth muscle contraction.

The normal heart contains primarily postsynaptic β_1-receptors, which when stimulated cause increased rate and force of contraction. This effect is mediated by activation of adenylate cyclase and subsequent generation and accumulation of cAMP. Stimulation of postsynaptic cardiac α_1-receptors causes a significant increase in contractility without an increase in rate, an effect mediated by PLC rather than adenylate cyclase. The increased contractility is more pronounced at lower heart rates and has a slower onset and longer duration in comparison with β_1-mediated inotropic response. Presynaptic α_2-adrenoceptors also are found in the heart and appear to be activated by norepinephrine released by the sympathetic nerve itself. Their activation inhibits further norepinephrine release from the nerve terminal.

Both presynaptic and postsynaptic adrenoceptors are present in the vasculature. Postsynaptic α_1- and α_2-receptors mediate vasoconstriction, whereas postsynaptic β_2-receptors induce vasodilation. Presynaptic α_2-receptors inhibit norepinephrine release in the vasculature, also promoting vasodilation. Presynaptic β_1-adrenoceptors promote neurotransmitter release. Stimulation of peripheral D_1-receptors produces renal, coronary, and mesenteric vasodilation and a natriuretic response. Stimulation of D_2-receptors inhibits norepinephrine release from sympathetic nerve endings, sequesters prolactin and aldosterone, and may induce nausea and vomiting. D_1- and D_2-receptor stimulation also suppresses peristalsis and may precipitate ileus.

❺ Vasopressin-induced vasoconstriction occurs through a variety of direct and indirect mechanisms. [51–53] Stimulation of vascular vasopressin $(V)_1$ receptors causes vasoconstriction by receptor-coupled activation of PLC and calcium release from intracellular stores via secondary messengers similar to α_1-adrenergic stimulation (Fig. 30–1, bottom). Vasopressin also directly inhibits vascular potassium-sensitive ATP channels to produce vasoconstriction (Fig. 30–1, bottom). V_1-receptor stimulation inhibits the actions of IL-1β and thereby facilitates vasoconstriction. Vasopressin also increases the activity of adrenergic receptors. The greatest vasoconstriction occurs in the skin and soft tissue, skeletal muscle, fat tissue, pancreas, and thyroid gland. In contrast, vasopressin causes vasodilation in the cerebral, pulmonary, coronary, and selected renal vascular beds by enhancing endothelial NO release through V_1-receptor stimulation in these tissues. [51–53] Vasopressin has minimal to no inotropic or chronotropic effects.

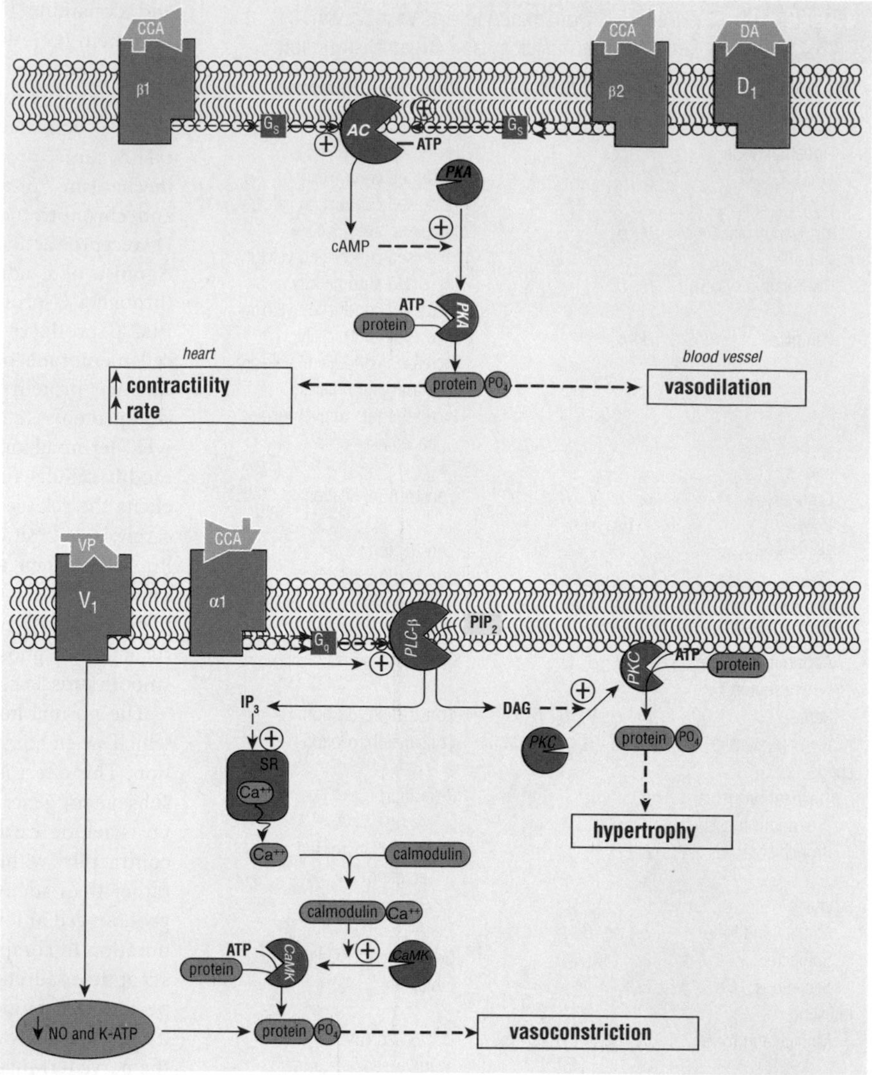

FIGURE 30-1. Signal transduction pathways in heart and blood vessels. Top: Catecholamine (CCA)-induced effects mediated in heart (β_1) or vascular smooth muscle (β_2, D_1). (AC, adenylate cyclase; ATP, adenosine triphosphate; cAMP, cyclic adenosine monophosphate; PKA, cAMP-dependent protein kinase; +, stimulation.) Bottom: CCA (α_1) and vasopressin (VP)-induced actions in vascular smooth muscle. (Ca++, calcium ion; CaMK, calcium/calmodulin-dependent protein kinase; DAG, diacylglycerol; IP3, inositol trisphosphate; NO, nitric oxide; PIP2, phosphatidylinositol bisphosphate; PKC, protein kinase C; PLC-β, phospholipase C-β; SR, sarcoplasmic reticulum.) These pathways have been extensively simplified, and denoted cellular effects represent one of many produced. (Figure based on data from references 6–19, 49–53.)

V_2 receptors located in the kidneys are responsible for the antidiuretic properties of vasopressin.[51-53] Stimulation of V_2 receptors facilitates integration of aquaporins into the luminal cell membrane of distal tubules and collecting duct capillaries to increase permeability and thus retain intravascular volume. However, vasopressin stimulation of V_1 receptors causes vasoconstriction of efferent arterioles and relative vasodilation of afferent arterioles to increase glomerular perfusion pressure and filtration rate to enhance urine production.

Vasopressin rapidly increases serum cortisol concentration by stimulating V_3 receptors in the pituitary gland to enhance the release of adrenocorticotropic hormone (ACTH).[51-53] Cortisol helps regulate the proinflammatory state associated with sepsis and increases blood pressure through several mechanisms, including inhibition of inducible NOS (iNOS) to reduce NO production, reversal of adrenergic receptor desensitization, and increased intravascular volume through retention of sodium and water.

ALTERED ADRENOCEPTOR FUNCTION: IMPLICATIONS FOR CRITICALLY ILL PATIENTS

❹ Most of the work describing receptor function and associated clinical pharmacology has been performed in either animal models or human volunteers. In critically ill septic patients, derangements in adrenergic receptor activity may result in resistance to exogenously administered catecholamine.[6-19,49,50] This "desensitization" frequently is characterized by myocardial and vascular hyporesponsiveness to high dosages of inotropes and vasopressor agents. Prolonged exposure of vascular endothelial tissue to vasopressor drugs (α-adrenergic agonists) or endogenous catecholamines may promote additional receptor downregulation. Increased endogenous catecholamine concentrations have been reported in endotoxemic and other critically ill patients, suggesting an acquired adrenergic receptor defect and desensitization of adrenergic receptors and alteration in voltage-sensitive calcium channels. The problem in critically ill patients may be related to decreased receptor activity or density. However, in patients with septic shock, catecholamine concentrations are even higher, so abnormalities in adrenergic receptor function are greater, with associated reductions in the concentrations of intracellular signal transduction mediators. The worsened receptor abnormality may be explained by defects distal to the receptor site, such as uncoupling of adrenergic receptors from adenylate cyclase or PLC, or dysfunction in the regulatory G-protein unit of signal transduction pathways.

In addition to catecholamines, circulating inflammatory cytokines may be partly responsible for distal alterations.[34] Macrophage-derived IL-1 and TNF-α produce impaired coupling of β-adrenoceptors to adenylate cyclase. Patients with septic shock exhibit impaired β-adrenergic receptor stimulation of cAMP associated with myocardial hyporesponsiveness to various vasopressors and inotropes. However, increased chronotropic sensitivity to β-adrenergic stimulation with hypersensitivity of the adenylate cyclase system to isoproterenol stimulation also has been reported in animal models of bacteremia and endotoxemia. In the presence of intrinsic myocardial dysfunction and increased metabolic demands, this dysfunctional adrenergic system is incapable of mobilizing functional cardiac reserve to maintain adequate myocardial performance.[45,46]

IL-1 and TNF-α suppress gene expression of α_1-adrenoceptors, resulting in fewer receptor proteins. Overproduction of NO by iNOS directly contributes to vasodilation by cyclic guanosine monophosphate–mediated smooth muscle relaxation. NO indirectly produces vasodilation by combining with superoxide to form peroxynitrite, a highly toxic reactive species that causes endothelial dysfunction, uncoupling of α_1-adrenoceptors to PLC, and deactivation of catecholamines. The result of sepsis-induced inflammation is a system that promotes adrenergic receptor dysfunction to accentuate vasodilation and shock.[6–19,49,50]

⑤ Functional α_1-adrenergic receptor changes occur at various stages of sepsis; thus, adrenoceptor sensitivity may be time dependent during progression of sepsis to septic shock. The findings are not always consistent in various animal models of sepsis and in critically ill septic patients. Time-dependent alterations in the production of NO, a potent vasodilator, may explain the apparent differences in vascular reactivity to phenylephrine during the phases of endotoxemia. This finding suggests that the clinical response to vasopressors and possibly inotropic agents is variable during the stages of hemodynamic, myocardial, and peripheral vascular derangements of septic shock. β-adrenergic receptor changes are present within 24 to 48 hours of septic shock. In summary, α- and β-adrenergic receptor derangements may vary among patients and during each bacteremic insult; therefore, doses of catecholamines vary among patients and during the insult.[6–19,49,50] For these reasons, these drugs should be dosed to clinical end points and not to arbitrary maximal doses. High dosages are frequently required.

RELATIVE DEFICIENCIES OF VASOPRESSIN AND CORTISOL

⑭ Endogenous arginine vasopressin, a peptide hormone also known as antidiuretic hormone, is important for osmoregulation under normal physiologic conditions. Vasopressin is produced in the hypothalamus, stored in the posterior pituitary, and released from magnocellular neurons of the hypothalamus.[51–53] Increased serum osmolality and hypovolemia are the major stimuli for vasopressin release.[51–53] Other stimuli commonly associated with shock are dopamine, histamine, angiotensin II, prostaglandins, pain, hypoxia, acidosis, hypotension, hypercarbia, and α_1-adrenergic receptor stimulation. Vasopressin release is inhibited by NO, natriuretic peptides, γ-aminobutyric acid, β-adrenergic receptor stimulation, and α_2-adrenergic receptor stimulation.[51–53]

Normal serum vasopressin concentrations are <4 pg/mL.[51–53] Serum vasopressin concentrations are elevated with hypotension. Vasopressin response in septic shock is biphasic. During the first 8 hours of septic shock requiring catecholamine adrenergic therapy, serum concentrations of vasopressin are appropriately high to help maintain blood pressure and organ perfusion. Thereafter, serum vasopressin concentrations decline dramatically over the next 96 hours to physiologically normal but inappropriately low values, resulting in a state of "relative deficiency." In contrast, serum vasopressin concentrations remain elevated in patients with cardiogenic shock. Administration of vasopressin at 0.01 to 0.06 units/min produces concentrations similar to those observed in early septic shock and other hypotensive states; however, vasopressin concentrations do not correlate with blood pressure.[51–53] Administration of vasopressin improves arterial pressure while minimizing the dose of catecholamine vasopressors.[51–53]

The mechanism of vasopressin insufficiency in septic shock is not well understood. Neurohypophyseal stores in the posterior lobe of the pituitary gland are depleted during septic shock, likely as a result of excessive and continuous baroreceptor stimulation that eventually exhausts the limited vasopressin secretory stores. In addition, secretion of vasopressin is inhibited by enhanced endothelial production of NO, high circulating concentrations of adrenergic agonists (both endogenous and exogenous), and tonic inhibition by stretch receptors in response to volume replacement and mechanical ventilation.[51–53]

⑭ As with vasopressin, during sepsis a state of "relative adrenal insufficiency" is produced by continuous activation of the hypothalamic–pituitary–adrenal axis by IL-1, IL-6, and TNF-α that causes depletion of cortisol in the adrenal glands.[54] Administration of corticosteroids improves arterial pressure while minimizing the dose of catecholamine vasopressors.[55,56] Current proposed mechanisms of the vasoconstrictor effect of corticosteroids include increasing the number and stimulating the function of α_1- and β-adrenergic receptors and attenuating the production of inflammatory mediators responsible for vasodilation.

The use of corticosteroids for treatment of septic shock has been a topic of controversy for many years. Meta-analyses of early studies of steroids in patients with sepsis demonstrated a lack of benefit and potential harm in sepsis and septic shock.[57,58] Interest in corticosteroid use is renewed because of the increased awareness of adrenocortical insufficiency in critically ill patients with septic shock.[54] Relative adrenal insufficiency has been defined as a random cortisol concentration <10 mcg/dL (278 nmol/L) or an increase of <9 mcg/dL (250 nmol/L) to a dose of synthetic ACTH irrespective of the initial serum cortisol level.[59] Although absolute insufficiency is rare, relative adrenocortical insufficiency is present in 50% to 70% of patients with septic shock and is associated with a poor outcome.[54–62]

An elevated random cortisol concentration (>34 mcg/dL) is an independent predictor of mortality.[59] Mortality is further increased if ACTH response is <9 mcg/dL, suggesting that the risk of mortality is greatest in situations of adrenal gland "fatigue" (i.e., degree of stress is not matched by sufficient cortisol production by the adrenal glands despite operating at maximal functional capacity).

CLINICAL PHARMACOLOGY OF VASOPRESSORS AND INOTROPES

⑤ ⑭ The receptor selectivity of clinically used, catecholamine-based vasopressors and inotropes and hemodynamic effects are listed in Table 30–4.[6–19,49–53] In general, these drugs are fast acting, with short durations of action. As such, these drugs are given as continuous infusions and titrated rapidly to predetermined effects.[7] Vasopressin is administered as a replacement dosage of 0.01 to 0.04 units/min and should not be titrated.[51–53] Careful monitoring and calculation of infusion rates are advised for all vasopressors because dosing adjustments are made frequently, and varying admixtures and concentrations are used in volume-restricted patients.

⑨ Dopamine has been described as having dose-related receptor activity at D_1-, D_2-, β_1-, and α_1-receptors (Table 30–4).[6–19,49,50] Unfortunately, this dose–response relationship has not been confirmed in critically ill patients. In patients with septic shock, great overlap of hemodynamic effects occurs, even at dosages as low as 3 mcg/kg/min.[63] Tachydysrhythmias are common due to the release of endogenous norepinephrine by dopamine entering the sympathetic nerve terminal. Dopamine may increase PAOP through pulmonary vasoconstriction. This drug also may depress ventilation and worsen hypoxemia in patients dependent on the hypoxic ventilatory drive. However, it is a first-line option for the initial therapy in patients with septic shock because it increases blood pressure by increasing myocardial contractility and vasoconstriction.[7]

⑨ Norepinephrine is a combined α- and β-agonist that produces vasoconstriction primarily via its more prominent α-effects on all

TABLE 30-4 Receptor Pharmacology and Adverse Events of Selected Inotropic and Vasopressor Agents Used in Septic Shock[a]

Agent (Adverse Events)	α_1	α_2	β_1	β_2	D	V_1	V_2
Dobutamine (0.5–4 mg/mL D₅W or NS)	Tachycardia, dysrhythmias, hypotension						
2–10 mcg/kg/min	+	0	++++	++	0	0	0
>10–20 mcg/kg/min	++	0	++++	+++	0	0	0
Dopamine (0.8–3.2 mg/mL D₅W or NS)	Tachycardia, dysrhythmias, decreased Pao₂, mesenteric hypoperfusion, gastrointestinal motility inhibition, T-cell inhibition						
1–3 mcg/kg/min	0	0	+	0	++++	0	0
3–10 mcg/kg/min	0/+	0	++++	+	++++	0	0
>10–20 mcg/kg/min	+++	0	++++	+	0	0	0
Epinephrine (0.008–0.016 mg/mL D₅W or NS)	Tachycardia, dysrhythmias, decreased Pao₂, mesenteric hypoperfusion, increased lactate, hyperglycemia, immunomodulation						
0.01–0.05 mcg/kg/min	++	++	++++	+++	0	0	0
0.05–3 mcg/kg/min	++++	++++	+++	+	0	0	0
Norepinephrine (0.016–0.064 mg/mL D₅W)	Mixed effects on myocardial performance and mesenteric perfusion, peripheral ischemia						
0.02–3 mcg/kg/min	+++	+++	+++	+/++	0	0	0
Phenylephrine (0.1–0.4 mg/mL D₅W or NS)	Mixed effects on myocardial performance, peripheral ischemia						
0.5–9 mcg/kg/min	+++	+	+	0	0	0	0
Vasopressin (0.8 units/mL D₅W or NS)	Mixed effects on myocardial performance, mesenteric hypoperfusion, peripheral ischemia, hyponatremia, thrombocytopenia						
0.01–0.04 units/min	0	0	0	0	0	+++	+++

[a]Activity ranges from no activity (0) to maximal (++++) activity.
D, dopamine; D₅W, dextrose 5% in water; NS, normal saline; Pao₂, arterial oxygen pressure; V, vasopressin.
Based on data from references 6–19, 49–53.

vascular beds, thus increasing SVR.[6–19,49,50] Norepinephrine administration generally produces either no change or some increase in CO. In addition to dopamine, norepinephrine is considered an option for initial vasopressor therapy for septic shock.[7,63]

❿ Phenylephrine is a pure α_1-agonist and increases blood pressure through vasoconstriction.[6–19,49,50] Given the presence of cardiac α_1-receptors, phenylephrine also may increase contractility and CO. It is a therapeutic option in hypotensive patients experiencing a tachyarrhythmia when a vasopressor with minimal to no β_1-agonist activity is indicated.[7]

⓫ Epinephrine exerts combined α- and β-agonist effects.[6–19,49,50] At the high epinephrine infusion rates used for patients with septic shock, predominantly α-adrenergic effects are observed, and SVR and MAP are increased. While epinephrine traditionally has been reserved as the vasopressor of last resort due to peripheral vasoconstriction, particularly in the splanchnic and renal beds, it is considered second-line therapy according to the current guidelines.[7] It is widely used in other countries where other agents may not be readily available or are relatively expensive.

⓬ Dobutamine, a synthetic catecholamine, is primarily a selective β_1-agonist with mild β_2- and vascular α_1-activity, resulting in strong positive inotropic activity without concomitant vasoconstriction.[6–19,49,50] In comparison with dopamine, dobutamine produces a larger increase in CO and is less arrhythmogenic. α_1-Adrenoceptors in the heart are directly stimulated by the (−) isomer of dobutamine, but β_1 and β_2 activity resides in the (+) isomer. The strong inotropic action of dobutamine is a function of its structure, the additive effect of cardiac α_1- and β_1-agonist activity, and a relatively weak chronotropic effect limited to the (+) isomer action on the β-receptors. Clinically, β_2-induced vasodilation and the increased myocardial contractility with subsequent reflex reduction in sympathetic tone lead to a decrease in SVR. Dobutamine is used optimally for patients in low CO states with high filling pressures (e.g., CI <3 L/min/m², left ventricular dysfunction demonstrated with echogardiography, or Scvo₂ <70%) or in those in cardiogenic shock; however, vasopressors may be needed to counteract arterial vasodilation.[7,30]

⓮ Unlike adrenergic receptor agonists, the vasoconstrictive effects of vasopressin are preserved during hypoxia and severe acidosis. Initiating vasopressin at ≤0.04 units/min in patients with

septic shock increases SVR and arterial blood pressure to reduce the dose requirements of catecholamine adrenergic agents.[51–53,64] These effects are rapid and sustained. Organ-specific vasodilation reduces pulmonary artery pressure and may preserve cardiac and renal function. It may enhance urine production, likely due to increased glomerular filtration rate.[51–53] At dosages exceeding 0.04 units/min, however, vasopressin is associated with ischemia of the mesenteric mucosa, skin, and myocardium. Limiting the dosage to a maximum of 0.04 units/min may minimize the development of these adverse effects. At present, vasopressin is not recommended as a replacement for norepinephrine or dopamine in patients with septic shock but may be considered as adjunctive therapy in patients who are refractory to catecholamine vasopressors despite adequate fluid resuscitation.[7] If used, vasopressin should be administered at dosages not exceeding 0.04 units/min.[7,51–53,64]

CLINICAL APPLICATION

Resuscitation of Septic Shock

❻ ❼ ❾ Initial hemodynamic therapy for septic shock is the administration of intravenous fluid (20–40 mL/kg of crystalloid fluid), with the goal of attaining CVP of 8 to 12 mm Hg or 15 mm Hg in mechanically ventilated patients or patients with abdominal distension or preexisting ventricular dysfunction.[6–19,30] Crystalloid fluids (e.g., normal saline, Ringer lactate) and colloid fluids (e.g., albumin, hydroxyethyl starch, blood products) are considered equivalent for shock resuscitation.[65] Crystalloid fluids are generally preferred unless patients are at risk for adverse events from redistribution of intravenous fluids to extravascular tissues and/or are fluid restricted (e.g., patients with renal dysfunction, decompensated heart failure, ascites compromising diaphragmatic function).[7] Recent data suggest hydroxyethyl starch may increase the risk of acute renal dysfunction in a dose-dependent manner and possibly enhance mortality.[66] Its use warrants caution.

❽ Traditional vasopressors and inotropes used for hemodynamic support of patients with hypotension refractory to fluid administration include dopamine, norepinephrine, phenylephrine epinephrine, and dobutamine. Optimizing MAP to 65 mm Hg as the goal of vasopressor therapy does not uniformly correlate with decreased mortality in patients with septic shock but global perfusion may be improved.[17-21] Historically, significant concerns about the adverse effects of vasopressors limited their use. The past focus of achieving supranormal oxygen-transport variables also yielded poor results in patients with septic shock.[33] In fact, normalization of systemic Do_2 and Vo_2, whether spontaneously or with intervention, is associated with improved outcome and is not dependent on administration of vasopressor agents.[33] Part of the inability to detect an improvement with vasopressor or inotropic therapies may result from the limited ability to quantify regional tissue perfusion. However, use of early goal-directed therapy to MAP $\geq$65 mm Hg and $Scvo_2$ $\geq$70% reduces mortality in patients with sepsis and septic shock.[30]

❻ ❼ ❽ ❾ Dosage titration and monitoring of vasopressor and inotropic therapy should be guided by the "best clinical response" and the goals of early goal-directed therapy.[6-19,30] Dopamine or norepinephrine is considered the agent of choice as initial vasopressor therapy.[7] Norepinephrine may be added in cases where suboptimal response is obtained from dopamine but adding dopamine to norepinephrine does not provide a hemodynamic benefit.[7] Phenylephrine may be tried as the initial vasopressor in cases of severe tachydysrhythmias.[7] The results of a recent survey of critical care pharmacists showed norepinephrine is the preferred initial agent (57%), followed by dopamine (28.6%) and phenylephrine (9.3%).[67] Norepinephrine is the most common second-line agent when used to augment dopamine or phenylephrine, whereas vasopressin is most frequently added to norepinephrine. Regardless of which vasopressor is chosen, low dosage rates are initiated and titrated rapidly (usually every 5-15 minutes) to clinical response. Clinically effective dosing of vasopressors and inotropes in septic shock often requires doses much larger than recommended by most references.[6-19] These large infusion rates must be tempered with the development of adverse effects. The goal is to use the minimally effective infusion rate while minimizing evidence of myocardial ischemia (e.g., tachydysrhythmias, electrocardiographic changes), renal (decreased glomerular filtration rate and/or urine output), splanchnic/gastric (low pHi, bowel ischemia), or peripheral (cold extremities) hypoperfusion, and worsening PaO_2, PAOP, and other hemodynamic variables.

⓭ Therapy with catecholamine vasopressors and inotropes is continued until myocardial depression and vascular hyporesponsiveness (i.e., blood pressure) of septic shock improve, usually measured in hours to days.[7] Discontinuation of vasopressor or inotropic therapy should be executed slowly; therapy should be "weaned" to avoid a precipitous worsening in regional and systemic hemodynamics. Careful monitoring of global and regional end points also should be geared toward discontinuation of vasopressors and inotropes as soon as the patient is hemodynamically stable. This requires constant observation. Because vasopressors and inotropes often are started while the patient is not yet optimally volume resuscitated, clinicians should reevaluate intravascular volume status continuously so that the patient can be weaned from the vasopressor as soon as possible. Dosage rates should be titrated carefully downward approximately every 10 minutes to determine if the patient can tolerate gradual withdrawal and eventual discontinuation of the vasopressor and/or inotrope. Discontinuation of agents may occur only minutes to hours after their initiation, or it may take days to weeks. Septic shock requiring vasopressor and/or inotropic support usually resolves within 1 week.

Comparative Studies of Catecholamine Vasopressors

❼ ❾ In a randomized study of 32 septic shock patients unresponsive to volume resuscitation, norepinephrine alone was superior to dopamine in achieving and maintaining preset hemodynamic

(MAP of at least 80 mm Hg) and oxygen-transport variables for at least 6 hours (93% vs 31% of patients; P <0.001).[68] Of the 11 patients who did not respond to dopamine, 10 achieved the desired hemodynamic goal when norepinephrine was added. The authors suggested that differences between the two agents resulted from norepinephrine's combined increase in Vo_2 and decrease in lactate concentrations due to reversal of splanchnic ischemia and efficient hepatic clearance of lactate or a preferential increase in Do_2 to areas of greatest oxygen demand, thus optimizing O_2ER. The same investigators showed in a prospective, observational cohort study of 97 adult patients with septic shock that use of norepinephrine to provide hemodynamic support was associated with a significant decrease in mortality (day 7: 28% vs 40%; P <0.005; day 28: 55% vs 82%; P <0.001; at hospital discharge: 62% vs 84%; P <0.001).[69] Using stepwise logistic regression analysis, norepinephrine was found to be the only factor associated with significantly improved survival (P = 0.03). Despite the drawback of the lack of randomization, this study is the first to demonstrate a survival benefit with any vasopressor. The results of another observational study found dopamine was an independent factor associated with ICU mortality in all 1,058 patients with shock (OR, 1.67; 95% CI, 1.19-2.35; P = 0.003) and the subgroup of 462 patients with septic shock (OR, 2.05; 95% CI, 1.25-3.37; P = 0.005).[70] Yet another observational study of 277 patients with septic shock found dopamine to be associated with 28-day mortality (OR, 6.2; 95% CI, 1.5-25; P = 0.01).[71] In contrast, a fourth observational study of 458 patients with community-acquired sepsis found norepinephrine was independently associated with 28-day mortality (OR, 2.5; 95% CI, 1.41-4.43; P = 0.002), whereas dopamine had no effect.[72] The results of a recent randomized study of norepinephrine and dopamine in 1,679 patients with shock unresponsive to volume resuscitation found similar 28-day mortality rates (48.5% vs 52.5% of patients; P = 0.10) although death from refractory shock tended to occur less frequently with norepinephrine (41% vs 46%; P = 0.05).[73] Mortality rate was significantly lower in the subgroup of 280 patients with cardiogenic shock that received norepinephrine (P = 0.03). Overall, patients receiving norepinephrine had fewer arrhythmic events (12.4% vs 24.2%; P <0.001) despite using dobutamine more frequently, had more vasopressor-free days, and were less likely to require open-label vasopressor support (20% vs 26%; P <0.001). Limitations of this landmark study include combining heterogeneous shock etiologies (cardiogenic, septic, hypovolemic, and other), the use of a relatively conservative definition of "shock unresponsive to fluid administration" (only 1 L of crystalloid or 0.5 L of colloid), the use of open-label norepinephrine in patients with inadequate hemodynamic response to study drug regimens, and the lack of standardization of other shock therapies that affect hemodynamic variables (e.g., corticosteroids, vasopressin, dobutamine, additional fluid administration). Another recent study randomized 252 septic shock patients found statistically similar 28-day mortality rates between norepinephrine and dopamine (43% vs 50%; P = 0.282).[74] Similar to the aforementioned study, arrhythmic events were less likely to occur with norepinephrine (5.3% vs 23.3%; P <0.0001).

❼ ❾ ⓫ Two randomized, double blind studies compared epinephrine with norepinephrine in 330 and 280 patients with septic shock, respectively.[75,76] Both studies found similar 28-day mortality rates with epinephrine and norepinephrine (40% vs 31%; P = 0.31; and 22.5% vs 26.1%; P = 0.48). Time to hemodynamic recovery and vasopressor withdrawal were also similar between agents in both studies. One study found more events of tachydysrhythmias with epinephrine leading to study discontinuation.[75] Both studies also showed that epinephrine was associated with lower arterial pH values and higher serum lactate concentrations over the first days of therapy, possibly demonstrating deleterious circulation, exaggerated glycolysis, or mobilization of lactate with epinephrine.

Low ("Renal") Dose Dopamine

❼ ❾ Historically, acute kidney injury from sepsis was believed to be due to renal ischemia.[77] In the critical care setting, low dosages (1–3 mcg/kg/min) of dopamine once were advocated for use in patients with septic shock receiving vasopressors with or without oliguria.[78] The goal of this therapy is to minimize or reverse renal vasoconstriction caused by other pressors, to prevent oliguric renal failure, or to convert oliguric to nonoliguric renal failure. At low dosages, dopamine has been shown to increase urine production as a result of enhanced renal blood flow from its D_1-receptor–mediated vasodilation, its D_2-receptor–mediated natriuretic effects (inhibition of Na^+/K^+ ATP of renal tubular cells), or its β_1-receptor–mediated increase in cardiac index.[49,50] In healthy subjects, the addition of dopamine to incremental doses of norepinephrine may blunt norepinephrine-induced renal vasoconstriction, thereby maintaining renal blood flow, natriuresis, urine production, and glomerular filtration. These effects also have been observed during the course of dopamine administration in oliguric and nonoliguric patients with septic shock. For this reason, low doses of dopamine sometimes are added to other vasopressors (e.g., norepinephrine). Tolerance to the vasodilatory effects of dopamine after 24 to 48 hours is evident in nonoliguric patients with sepsis syndrome.

Two studies have settled the debate surrounding low-dose dopamine. Friedrich et al. performed a meta-analysis to determine if low-dose dopamine reduces mortality or the need for dialysis in patients with critical illness.[78] Among 61 clinical trials (N = 3,359), low-dose dopamine had no effect on mortality (RR, 0.96; 95% CI, 0.78–1.19), need for dialysis (RR, 0.93; 95% CI, 0.76–1.15), or occurrence of adverse events (RR, 1.13; 95% CI, 0.90–1.41). Low-dose dopamine improved urine production by 24% (95% CI, 14%–35%) on the first day of therapy but failed to maintain this effect on days 2 and 3. No improvements in serum creatinine concentration (4% relative increase; 95% CI, 1%–7%) and measured creatinine clearance (6% relative increase; 95% CI, 1%–11%) occurred within 24 hours of initiating dopamine. One adequately designed prospective, controlled trial has been conducted with low-dose dopamine in critically ill patients.[79] Bellomo et al. randomized 328 critically ill patients with early renal dysfunction to either low-dose dopamine (2 mcg/kg/min) or placebo and found no differences in peak serum creatinine concentration (2.77 ± 1.63 mg/dL vs 2.82 ± 1.66 mg/dL), increase in serum creatinine concentration (0.7 ± 1.21 mg/dL vs 0.75 ± 1.22 mg/dL), need for renal replacement therapies (27.7% vs 24.5%), and urine production at any time point.[79] On the basis of available evidence, low-dose dopamine for treatment or prevention of acute renal failure cannot be justified and should be eliminated from routine clinical use in the ICU.[7]

Evidence now suggests that the etiology of acute renal failure from sepsis is due to efferent arteriole vasodilation.[76] Enhanced urine production has been shown to occur in hyperdynamic shock with use of agents that constrict the efferent arteriole such as vasopressin and norepinephrine.[49,50] In the randomized study of norepinephrine and dopamine by Martin et al.,[68] urine production increased with norepinephrine but not with dopamine (22 ± 7 mL/h to 189 ± 52 mL/h vs 24 ± 6 mL/h to 8.2 ± 10 mL/h; P <0.001). Adding norepinephrine to the dopamine group increased urine production to 107 ± 125 mL/h. An increase in urine production may be due to the localized vasoconstrictive effect of norepinephrine in the kidney (greater vasoconstriction of the efferent arteriole than the afferent arteriole) or enhanced glomerular filtration rate from increased renal perfusion pressure secondary to elevated CO and SVR. Delineating these differential effects of improved arterial blood pressure and CO from regional renal effects is difficult.

Vasopressin

⓮ Small studies of septic shock patients demonstrate that initial therapy with vasopressin achieves blood pressure control as effectively as traditional catecholamine vasopressors but the response is delayed.[51–53] Therefore, vasopressin therapy should not be initiated as first-line therapy. Several small studies showed that adjunctive vasopressin therapy reduces the dose requirements of catecholamine vasopressors and maintains blood pressure to expedite the discontinuation of catecholamine vasopressors.[51–53] Some studies document enhancement of urine production.[51–53] The results of a randomized, double-blind study of 776 patients with septic shock requiring catecholamine vasopressors showed that 28-day mortality rates were similar when vasopressin 0.01 to 0.03 units/min or norepinephrine 5 to 15 mcg/min was added to traditional catecholamine therapy (35.4% vs 39.3%; P = 0.26).[64] A trend toward reduced 28-day mortality favored vasopressin in the subset of patients categorized as having less severe septic shock defined by a baseline norepinephrine requirement of <15 mcg/min (26.5% vs 35.7%; P = 0.05). This trend was evident when sepsis severity was defined by lactate quartiles or number of organ failures, suggesting that adjunctive vasopressin may be most beneficial when it is started prior to escalation of therapy with catecholamine vasopressors. Posthoc analyses demonstrated greatest benefit with early vasopressin treatment relative to the onset of shock. The adverse event profiles were similar between groups. Of note, vasopressin therapy expedited the discontinuation of catecholamine vasopressors in all patients and helped preserve renal function in patients with acutely declining urine production.[64] Whereas V_2 stimulation promotes water retention from the distal tubules and collecting ducts, V_1 receptors cause vasoconstriction of efferent arterioles and relative vasodilation of afferent arterioles to increase glomerular perfusion pressure and filtration rate, enhancing urine production. In the studies reporting benefit on renal function, the maximum dosage used was 0.08 units/min.[51–53,64] Use of vasopressin for preventing dose escalation of adrenergic agents should be considered, but the risks must be considered prior to initiating therapy. At present, vasopressin should not be used for the sole purpose of improving or maintaining renal function.[7]

CLINICAL CONTROVERSY: VASOPRESSIN

Adding vasopressin reduces the dose of traditional catecholamine therapies and may improve renal function. However, the occurrence of ischemic events to digits and splanchnic circulation may be increased with vasopressin. Therefore, the lowest possible dose should be implemented if vasopressin is used.

Corticosteroids

⓮ Since two meta-analyses reported in 1995,[57,58] several randomized controlled trials of low-dose corticosteroids in vasopressor-dependent septic shock patients have been published.[54–56,60,61] These studies use moderate physiologic dosages (200–300 mg/day) of hydrocortisone. A meta-analysis of five studies (N = 465) showed that steroid therapy was associated with an overall improvement in survival rate (RR, 1.23; 95% CI, 1.01–1.50; P = 0.036) and shock reversal (RR, 1.71; 95% CI, 1.29–2.26; P <0.001).[55] These effects were beneficial in both responders and nonresponders to ACTH stimulation testing. These studies also showed that low-dose corticosteroid administration improves hemodynamics and reduces the duration of vasopressor support. All of these studies differ from earlier studies in that steroids were administered at lower total doses (hydrocortisone equivalents: 1,209 mg vs 23,975 mg; $P = 0.01$) starting later in septic shock (23 hours vs <2 hours; $P = 0.02$) for longer courses (6 days vs 1 day; $P = 0.01$) to patients with higher control group mortality rates (mean, 57% vs 34%; $P = 0.06$) who were more likely to be vasopressor dependent (100% vs 65%; $P = 0.03$). The relationship between corticosteroid dose and survival was linear, with survival benefit at low doses ($P = 0.02$). Another meta-analysis of 17 trials (N = 2,138) found similar results with long-term administration of corticosteroids associated with lower mortality in hospital (RR, 0.83; 95% CI, 0.68–1; $P = 0.05$) and at 28 days (RR, 0.84; 95% CI, 0.71–1; $P = 0.05$), reduced ICU stay by 4.49 days (95% CI, −7.04 to −1.95; $P < 0.001$), and greater shock reversal at 28 days (RR, 1.12; 95% CI, 1.02–1.23; $P = 0.02$).[56]

14 The results of these meta-analyses are heavily driven by data supplied by two, somewhat discordant, studies.[60,61] The first randomized 300 patients with septic shock within 8 hours of hypotension to placebo or a daily combination of hydrocortisone 50 mg IV every 6 hours and fludrocortisone 0.05 mg enterally for 7 days.[60] Similar to the meta-analyses, use of hydrocortisone reduced 28-day mortality (OR, 0.65; 95% CI, 0.39–1.07; $P = 0.09$), but all the benefit was seen in patients with adrenal insufficiency (OR, 0.54; 95% CI, 0.31–0.97; $P = 0.04$). The placebo group was more likely to continually require vasopressor therapy (hazard ratio [HR], 1.54; 95% CI, 1.10–12.16; $P = 0.01$), but differences between groups were exhibited only in patients with adrenal insufficiency (HR, 1.91; 95% CI, 1.29–2.84; $P = 0.001$). Approximately 77% of patients were deemed adrenally insufficient. The second study randomized 499 of 800 intended subjects with severe sepsis or shock within 72 hours of presentation to placebo or hydrocortisone 50 mg IV every 6 hours for 5 days followed by a 6-day taper.[61] Mortality rates were similar between groups (32% vs 34%), irrespective of adrenal function. Median time to shock reversal was shorter in patients receiving corticosteroid therapy (3.3 vs 5.8 days; $P < 0.001$), again irrespective of adrenal function. Unlike the previous study, however, only 47% of patients demonstrated adrenal insufficiency likely reflective of the entry criteria and lower overall mortality rate of the study population.

CLINICAL CONTROVERSY: CORTICOSTEROID THERAPY

Current guidelines do not suggest assessing adrenal function to determine the need for corticosteroid therapy.[7] Instead, they recommend initiating corticosteroids when hypotension is poorly responsive to vasopressor therapy. This is controversial given the limitations and differences between studies and the undefined term of "poorly responsive." Therefore, corticosteroid therapy may be considered in septic shock patients with adrenal insufficiency or when shock is refractory to other therapies.[54,62] Several questions surround the application of corticosteroid therapy in septic patients, including use in patients taking corticosteroids prior to ICU admission, most effective dosage regimen and duration, use of corticosteroids other than hydrocortisone, and the need for coadministration of fludrocortisone.

14 A post hoc analysis of the large vasopressin study revealed a significant interaction between vasopressin and corticosteroids.[80] In patients receiving vasopressin therapy, concurrent corticosteroid administration increased vasopressin concentrations by 33% to 67% over the initial 24 hours compared with patients only receiving vasopressin. The addition of corticosteroids to vasopressin was associated with reduced mortality compared with concurrent administration of corticosteroids and norepinephrine (35.9% vs 44.7%; $P = 0.03$). In the absence of corticosteroid therapy, however, mortality was greater with vasopressin therapy compared with norepinephrine (33.7% vs 21.3%; $P = 0.06$). Similar results were reported in a retrospective, matched assessment that found lower 7-day mortality was associated with combination therapy compared with vasopressin alone (19.1% vs 52.4%; $P = 0.02$).[81] This interaction warrants further investigation in studies.

Adverse Effects

5 7 9 10 11 Catecholamine vasopressors may result in adverse peripheral vasoconstrictive, metabolic, and dysrhythmogenic effects that limit or outweigh their positive effects on the central circulation.[6-19,49,50] Table 30–4 lists potential adverse effects of commonly used vasopressors and inotropes.[6-19,49-53] Norepinephrine, phenylephrine, and epinephrine can produce lactic acidosis secondary to excessive constriction in peripheral arterioles or enhanced glycogenolysis, or as a result of mobilization of lactate from peripheral tissues as a result of improved oxygenation. Additionally, excessive peripheral vasoconstriction may cause ischemia or necrosis of already poorly perfused tissues such as the skin and the mesenteric and splanchnic circulations. Some of these profound vasoconstrictive effects have been compounded by the concurrent use of other vasopressor agents in patients with septic shock who are significantly hypovolemic. These agents may be used in the context of late septic shock, where hypotension is refractory to less selective vasoconstrictors (e.g., dopamine) such that very large doses of norepinephrine or epinephrine or phenylephrine are required but provide little or no benefit. Myocardial ischemia and dysrhythmias may occur in patients with coronary artery disease, atherosclerosis, cardiomyopathies, left ventricular hypertrophy, congestive heart failure, or underlying dysrhythmias because of their inability to tolerate β_1 cardiac stimulation that mediates increases in CO. However, the effect usually is opposite in healthy myocardium and in young patients. β_1 Cardiac stimulation is well tolerated, ventricular filling pressures decrease, and CO and Do_2 increase, with a resulting increase in peripheral perfusion. The dysrhythmogenic potential of the catecholamine vasopressors includes a variety of resulting atrial and ventricular arrhythmias. Sympathomimetic vasopressors also have been found to possess immunomodulatory actions, primarily mediated by β_2-adrenergic actions (e.g., epinephrine) because almost all immune cells express this receptor.[34] The actions include downregulating expression of proinflammatory cytokines such as TNF-α by neutrophils, suppression of oxygen free radical production from neutrophils, and direct proapoptotic effects. Dopamine suppresses prolactin secretion from the anterior pituitary gland, which may lead to reduced T-cell responsiveness.[34] These effects may be either beneficial or deleterious by dampening harmful effects of oxygen free radical–mediated tissue injury or by reducing neutrophilic defense against bacteria.

Vasopressor catecholamines have the potential to cause extravasation-associated tissue damage if infusions infiltrate during peripheral administration. In the event of infiltration, an α-receptor antagonist such as phentolamine (10 mg in 10 mL saline) should be injected intradermally to reverse local vasoconstriction, with administration of vasopressor drugs into a large central vein.

Dopamine

7 8 9 13 Dopamine frequently is the initial vasopressor used for patients with septic shock.[6-19,67] Dosages of 5 to 10 mcg/kg/min are initiated to improve MAP. Most studies of patients with septic shock have shown that dopamine at these doses increases the cardiac index by improving contractility and heart rate, primarily from its β_1 effects. It increases MAP and SVR as a result of both increased CO and, at higher doses (>10 mcg/kg/min), its α_1 effects.

The clinical utility of dopamine as a vasopressor in the setting of septic shock is limited because large dosage rates frequently are necessary to maintain CO and MAP. At dosages exceeding 20 mcg/kg/min, further improvement in cardiac performance and regional hemodynamics is limited. Its clinical use frequently is hampered by tachycardia and tachydysrhythmias, which may lead to myocardial ischemia. Although tachydysrhythmias theoretically should not be expected to occur until administration of dopamine 5 to 10 mcg/kg/min, these β_1 effects are observed with dosages as low as 3 mcg/kg/min. They seem to be more prevalent in patients who are inadequately resuscitated (hypovolemic), in the elderly, in those with preexisting or concurrent cardiac ischemia or dysrhythmias, and in patients currently receiving other dysrhythmogenic agents, including vasopressors and inotropes.

Dopamine increases PAOP and pulmonary shunting to decrease Pao_2. The increase in PAOP may be due to changes in diastolic volumes from decreased cardiac compliance or increased venous return to the heart by α-adrenergic receptor–mediated venoconstriction. This may affect gas exchange and decrease Pao_2. The increase in pulmonary shunting also may result from acute enhancement of pulmonary blood flow to nonhomogeneous lung regions. Thus, dopamine should be used with caution in patients with elevated preload because the drug may worsen pulmonary edema. In the instance of high filling pressures, tachycardia, or tachydysrhythmias, dopamine should be replaced by another vasopressor and/or inotrope such as norepinephrine, dobutamine, phenylephrine, or epinephrine, depending on the desired effect.

The effect of dopamine on global oxygen-transport variables parallels the hemodynamic effects. Although dopamine improves global Do_2 in septic patients, it may compromise O_2ER in the splanchnic and mesenteric circulations by α_1-mediated vasoconstriction. Splanchnic blood flow and Do_2 increase with dopamine, but with no preferential increase in splanchnic perfusion as a fraction of CO and systemic increases in Do_2. Large doses of dopamine worsen pHi and the Pco_2 gap. This is reflected by a decrease or lack of change in regional Vo_2 and a decrease in tissue O_2ER. Dopamine at low or vasopressor dosages directly impedes gastric motility in critical illness and may aggravate gut ischemia in septic shock. Similar to high-dose administration, low-dose dopamine increases splanchnic blood flow but lowers splanchnic Vo_2 in sepsis. Therefore, dopamine at all dosages impairs hepatosplanchnic metabolism despite an increase in regional perfusion.

The use of dopamine as a first-line agent for septic shock may be questionable because regional hemodynamics, oxygen-transport variables, and functional parameters of improved organ perfusion are not consistently enhanced in a sustained manner and may be negatively impaired.[7,63] The negative findings of low-dose dopamine use (see Low ("Renal") Dose Dopamine above) and the deleterious effects of inotropic and vasopressor dosages of dopamine on regional hemodynamics and oxygen transport raise concern over whether dopamine should be considered the first-line vasopressor agent in patients with severe sepsis or septic shock.[7,7,79] Until dopamine is found to have definitive deleterious clinical outcomes compared to other vasopressors, empirical use of dopamine in a hypotensive patient in whom a pulmonary arterial catheter has not been inserted and in whom the cause of hypotension—low CO or vasodilation—is yet undetermined still may be reasonable. In addition, unlike other vasopressor agents, dopamine is available as premixed ready-to-use solutions of various concentrations that can be stored in automated dispensing systems for rapid initiation.

Norepinephrine

❼ ❾ ❽ ⓭ Use of norepinephrine as first-line therapy may be more rational than dopamine because norepinephrine is more potent and is more effective in increasing MAP.[7,67,68] It has combined strong α_1-activity and less potent β_1-agonist effects while maintaining weak vasodilatory effects of β_2-receptor stimulation.[6-19,49,50,68-76] Several retrospective analyses have demonstrated improved MAP and mortality in ICU patients with severe hypotension treated with norepinephrine either as first-line therapy or after therapeutic failure with fluid resuscitation and dopamine treatment.

Norepinephrine infusions can be titrated to preset goals of MAP (usually at least 65 mm Hg), improvement in peripheral perfusion (to restore urine production or decrease blood lactate), and/or achievement of desired oxygen-transport variables while not compromising the cardiac index. Norepinephrine 0.01 to 2 mcg/kg/min reliably and predictably improves hemodynamic parameters to "normal" or "supranormal" values in most patients with septic shock. As with other vasopressors, norepinephrine dosages exceeding those recommended by most references frequently are needed in critically ill patients with septic shock to achieve predetermined goals. A significant increase in MAP generally is caused by an increase in SVR. In contrast to dopamine, heart rate generally does not increase significantly with norepinephrine because of diminished stimulation of cardiac β_1-receptors in septic shock and reflex bradycardia from increased SVR.[68-76] Increasing norepinephrine doses to maintain higher MAPs may increase heart rates, cardiac index, DO_2, and cutaneous blood flow but these results are inconsistent. Older patients may benefit from the combined α- and β-adrenergic effects of norepinephrine given the higher incidence of coronary disease and compromised ventricles in this patient population. By virtue of restored MAP and hence coronary perfusion, cardiac index is increased in older patients, whereas in younger patients with less coronary artery disease and a higher cardiac index at baseline, norepinephrine acts primarily as a vasopressor. In contrast to dopamine, norepinephrine does not influence PAOP.

The effect of norepinephrine on oxygen transport parameters is variable and depends on baseline values and concurrently administered vasoactive agents. In most studies of norepinephrine alone, either an increase or no change in Do_2 is seen with no change in O_2ER, particularly when Do_2 values were "supranormal" prior to therapy. Norepinephrine demonstrates either no effect or improvement in Pco_2 gap, pHi, or serum lactate concentrations. Splanchnic blood flow and fractional blood flow are higher with norepinephrine than either dopamine or epinephrine despite higher CO with the two latter agents.

Taken together, these data suggest that norepinephrine should be the primary vasopressor of choice in patients in septic shock because of its multiple benefits: (1) norepinephrine may decrease mortality in septic shock; (2) it reverses inappropriate vasodilation and low global oxygen extraction; (3) it attenuates myocardial depression at unchanged or increased CO and increased coronary blood flow; (4) it improves renal perfusion pressure and renal filtration; (5) it enhances splanchnic perfusion; and (6) it is less likely than other vasopressors to cause tachycardias and tachydysrhythmias.[6-19,49,50,68-76]

Phenylephrine

❼ ❽ ❿ ⓭ Despite its purported use in refractory septic shock, little information is available regarding the clinical efficacy of phenylephrine. Nevertheless, it is an attractive agent for use in sepsis because of its selective α-agonism with primarily vascular effects.[6-19,49,50] It is generally initiated at dosages of 0.5 mcg/kg/min and can be titrated every 5 to 15 minutes to desired effects. As with other vasopressors, phenylephrine dosages required to achieve goals of therapy are significantly higher than dosages traditionally recommended for use.

Phenylephrine 0.5 to 9 mcg/kg/min, used alone or in combination with dobutamine or low doses of dopamine, improves blood pressure and myocardial performance in fluid-resuscitated septic patients. Incremental doses of phenylephrine result in linear dose-related increases in MAP, SVR, heart rate, and stroke index when administered alone as a single agent in stable, nonhypotensive but hyperdynamic, volume-resuscitated surgical ICU patients. In septic shock, phenylephrine does not impair the cardiac index, PAOP, or peripheral perfusion. In sepsis, phenylephrine improves MAP by increasing the cardiac index through enhanced venous return to the heart (increase in CVP and stroke index) and by acting as a positive inotrope. It improves myocardial performance in hyperdynamic, normotensive septic patients but worsens myocardial performance in cardiac controls. In cardiac patients, however, myocardial performance worsens as a result of a decrease in the cardiac index and an increase in SVR. Therefore, phenylephrine use warrants caution in septic shock patients with impaired myocardial performance.

In septic shock, phenylephrine appears to increase global tissue oxygen use, although information regarding the relationship of the oxygen-transport variables with increases in MAP and cardiac index is conflicting. Increases in Vo_2 appear to be dissociated from Do_2, representing an increase in O_2ER as the cardiac index remains unchanged. Increases in Vo_2 may result from redistribution of blood flow to previously underperfused areas, improving oxygen use as a result of changes in MAP and SVR. Evidence of globally improved peripheral tissue perfusion is observed as lactic acid concentration declines or remains unchanged and urine production increases significantly at increased or maximal Vo_2. An increased O_2ER may contribute to improved tissue response.

Few data regarding the effect of phenylephrine on regional hemodynamics and oxygen-transport variables are available. When phenylephrine replaced norepinephrine in patients with septic shock, phenylephrine selectively reduced splanchnic blood flow and thus splanchnic Do_2 and splanchnic lactate uptake rate without changing the overall splanchnic Vo_2. Concomitantly, pHi decreased and arterial lactate concentrations increased. Because all of these parameters normalized when norepinephrine was reinstated, these data suggest that exogenous β-adrenergic stimulation (norepinephrine) may determine hepatosplanchnic perfusion and oxygen availability but not utilization in septic shock. A small study comparing phenylephrine and norepinephrine for initial vasopressor therapy did not demonstrate significant differences between agents with respect to hemodynamic profiles or indices of global and regional perfusion.

The available data on hemodynamics, oxygen-transport variables, and mortality with phenylephrine in septic shock patients may not be generalizable because of the small numbers of patients evaluated. Adverse effects, such as tachydysrhythmias, are notably infrequent with phenylephrine, particularly when it is used as a single agent or at higher doses, because phenylephrine does not exert any activity on β_1-adrenergic receptors. Whether the beneficial effects can be sustained with longer administrations of phenylephrine is unclear. Phenylephrine may be a particularly useful alternative in patients who cannot tolerate tachycardia or tachydysrhythmias with use of dopamine or norepinephrine and in patients who are refractory to dopamine or norepinephrine (because of β-adrenergic receptor desensitization).[7] As with other vasopressors, phenylephrine is continued until resolution of the hemodynamic instability associated with the septic episode and is weaned when patients are clinically stable. Its use in patients with myocardial dysfunction warrants further investigation.

Epinephrine

❼ ❽ ⓫ ⓭ By convention, epinephrine has been reserved as a last-line agent for hemodynamic support of sepsis. Epinephrine, however, may be an acceptable choice as a single agent because of its combined vasoconstrictor and inotropic effects.[7] It is as effective

as norepinephrine for blood pressure control. Epinephrine infusion rates of 0.04 to 1 mcg/kg/min alone increase hemodynamic and oxygen-transport variables to "supranormal" values without adverse effects in septic patients without coronary artery disease. Large dosages (0.5–1 mcg/kg/min) often are required. Smaller dosages (0.10–0.50 mcg/kg/min) are effective when epinephrine is added to other vasopressors and inotropes. In addition, younger patients appear to respond better to epinephrine, possibly due to greater β-adrenergic stimulation.

Despite a linear dose–response curve with rapid improvement of hemodynamic variables and Do_2 epinephrine has deleterious effects on regional hemodynamics and oxygen utilization. Although Do_2 increases mainly as a function of increases in the cardiac index and a more variable increase in SVR, Vo_2 may not increase, and O_2ER may fall. A fall in pHi may be seen during epinephrine administration but the impairment in gastric mucosal perfusion can be counteracted in part by dobutamine. This may be explained by the vasodilatory effect of dobutamine on gastric mucosal microcirculation resulting in a redistribution of blood flow toward the mucosa. In contrast to other vasopressors, lactate concentrations frequently rise during epinephrine therapy resulting in variable arterial pH values. When compared with a combination of norepinephrine and dobutamine, epinephrine preferentially decreases splanchnic Do_2, worsens pHi, and increases systemic lactate concentration without increasing Vo_2. The effects of epinephrine on absolute and fractional splanchnic blood flow are more pronounced during severe shock. The increase in lactate may be a result of worsened Do_2 to the liver (and subsequent anaerobic metabolism) or to the hepatosplanchnic circulation, direct increase in calorigenesis and breakdown of glycogen, or lactate mobilization. However, evidence suggests that epinephrine, in contrast to dopamine, increases the proportion of total CO delivered to the splanchnic circulation, although Vo_2 is not increased sufficiently. As a result, O_2ER values are usually lower with epinephrine than with other vasopressors but the concomitant administration of dobutamine helps maintain O_2ER. Of all the vasopressors, epinephrine exhibits the most pronounced capacity to induce hyperglycemia by increased gluconeogenesis and glycogenolysis with α-mediated suppression of insulin secretion.[49,50]

Despite the administration of high doses, epinephrine-associated clinically important dysrhythmias or cardiac ischemia occur at variable rates irrespective of age or underlying cardiac status.[6–19,49,50,75,76] Nevertheless, caution must be exercised before considering epinephrine for managing hypoperfusion in hypodynamic patients with coronary artery disease, in whom ischemia, chest pain, or myocardial infarction may result. Based on the current evidence, epinephrine should not be used as initial therapy in patients with septic shock refractory to fluid administration.[7] Although it effectively increases CO and Do_2, it has deleterious effects on the splanchnic circulation. If it is used as a second-line agent in septic shock, factors that may influence successful therapy with epinephrine include the time from onset of septic shock to effective therapy and the age of the population.

Dobutamine

❻ ❼ ⓬ ⓭ Dobutamine is an inotrope with vasodilatory properties (an "inodilator").[6–19,49,50] It is used for treatment of septic and cardiogenic shock to increase the cardiac index, typically by 25% to 50%.[7] In septic shock, LVEF and right ventricular function are depressed despite a high cardiac index, whereas ventricular volumes and compliance are increased. Stroke index is maintained by an increased heart rate and ventricular dilation. In survivors, myocardial depression is reversible and normalizes 5 to 10 days after the onset of sepsis. Dobutamine increases stroke index, left ventricular stroke work index, and thus cardiac index and Do_2 without increasing

PAOP.[7] The ability of dobutamine to enhance cardiac index and Do_2 during septic shock appears to be related to its chronotropic effect. However, dosage increments of dobutamine beyond 20 mcg/kg/min are limited by complications of tachycardia, ischemic changes on electrocardiogram, hypertension, and tachydysrhythmias despite the absence of preexisting cardiac abnormalities. Of note, the combination of dobutamine and norepinephrine results in a lower increase in heart rate compared with use of other vasopressors alone.

Increased cardiac performance measures in response to adjunctive dobutamine therapy are predictive of survival during sepsis. However, the achievement of supranormal oxygen transport values with dobutamine is of little value compared with treatment to normal values. In addition, administration of dobutamine to achieve these high values may increase mortality rate and/or the incidence of adverse effects. Dobutamine increases Do_2 without affecting Vo_2, resulting in decreased O_2ER. Arterial lactate concentrations decrease significantly with norepinephrine and dobutamine compared with dopamine and epinephrine infusions.

Studies have focused on the effects of dobutamine on gastric mucosal flow and the splanchnic circulation. The addition of dobutamine to other vasopressors improves gastric mucosal perfusion without increasing the cardiac index. This is consistent with findings that dobutamine may improve pHi and mucosal perfusion in septic patients. The addition of dobutamine to norepinephrine or epinephrine treatment improves gastric mucosal perfusion as measured by improvements in pHi, and Pco_2 gap. This effect may relate to blood flow redistribution toward gastric mucosa, due to either an increase in the fraction of CO distributed to the global hepatosplanchnic blood flow and/or a redistribution of blood flow within gastric wall layers toward the mucosa by "stealing" blood away from the muscularis potentially as a result of greater β_2-mediated vasodilation. Sublingual microcirculation improves after dobutamine is added to vasopressor-dependent septic shock patients in a manner unrelated to arterial pressure or cardiac index, suggesting that enhanced perfusion is the result of the "steal" phenomenon. Of note, gastric mucosal perfusion and tissue oxygen utilization are most improved with concurrent norepinephrine and dobutamine therapies compared with other vasopressor combinations at the same level of MAP.

Dobutamine should be started at dosages ranging from 2.5 to 5 mcg/kg/min. In the study of early goal-directed therapy, dobutamine was administered to 13.7% of patients within 6 hours of resuscitation to achieve $Scvo_2 \geq 70\%$.[30] Although a dose response may be seen, evidence now suggests that dosages >5 mcg/kg/min may provide limited beneficial effects on oxygen transport values and hemodynamics and may increase adverse cardiac effects. If given to patients who are intravascularly depleted, dobutamine will result in hypotension and a reflexive tachycardia. Pathophysiologic factors influence dosing requirements and pharmacokinetic parameters over the time course of the illness and the duration of the infusion. Decreases in Pao_2, as well as myocardial adverse effects such as tachycardia, ischemic changes on electrocardiogram, tachydysrhythmias, and hypotension are seen. Thus, infusion rates should be guided by clinical end points and $Svo_2/Scvo_2$. Dobutamine, like other inotropes, usually is given until improvement in myocardial function with resolution of the septic episode or dose-limiting side effects are observed.

Vasopressin

14 Studies involving vasopressin infusion for management of septic shock show rapid and sustained improvement in hemodynamic parameters.[51-53,64] These effects are evident with administration of dosages not exceeding 0.04 units/min. Administration of dosages >0.04 units/min and 0.05 units/min are associated with negative changes in CO and mesenteric mucosal perfusion, respectively. The reduction in CO likely is the result of lowered stroke volume.[51-53] The

studies that reported cardiac function indicate patients had adequate CO prior to initiating vasopressin therapy. Therefore, vasopressin use in septic shock patients with cardiac dysfunction warrants extreme caution. Cardiac ischemia appears to be a rare occurrence and may be related to administration of dosages ≥ 0.05 units/min.

Mesenteric ischemia associated with vasopressin may be clinically relevant. Increased hepatic transaminases and total bilirubin concentrations may occur with vasopressin therapy, suggesting impaired hepatic blood flow or a direct effect on excretory hepatic function.[51-53] Most studies have found that vasopressin at dosages of 0.04 to 1.8 units/min worsen pHi or Pco_2 gap when it is added to low or high doses of catecholamine vasopressors.[51-53] Mesenteric mucosal hypoperfusion may be expected with vasopressin because mesenteric vasoconstriction occurs at vasopressin serum concentrations as low as 10 pg/dL, and the effect is dose dependent. Of concern is the additive effective with norepinephrine despite substantially reduced dosages of norepinephrine when vasopressin is initiated. Although controversial, the degree of hypoperfusion with vasopressin may be greater than with norepinephrine alone unless the dose of norepinephrine is markedly increased to maintain adequate arterial blood pressure.

Vasopressin's strongest vasoconstrictive action occurs in the skin and soft tissues, skeletal muscles, and fat tissues.[51-53] As a result, ischemic skin lesions have been observed in several studies, with an occurrence rate as high as 30% after vasopressin was added to norepinephrine-resistant shock. Although vasopressin may have deleterious effects on mesenteric and skin perfusion, studies report vasodilation of cerebral, pulmonary, coronary, and some renal vasculature beds. The clinical outcomes associated with selective vasodilation are not yet determined except for the possibility of enhanced urine production in patients not anuric at baseline.

In order to minimize the potential for adverse events and maximize the beneficial effects, vasopressin should be used as add-on therapy to one or two catecholamine adrenergic agents rather than as first-line therapy or salvage therapy and dosages should be limited to 0.04 units/min.[7,51-53] The results of studies showed that vasopressin markedly reduced the requirements for adrenergic agents, but few studies demonstrated complete discontinuation of these therapies.[51-53,64] Therefore, vasopressin should be used only if response to one or two adrenergic agents is inadequate or as a method for reducing the dosage of these therapies. Increased arterial pressure should be evident within the first hour of vasopressin therapy, at which time the dose(s) of adrenergic agent(s) should be reduced while maintaining blood pressure. This method should help limit the degree of ischemia.

Most studies evaluated vasopressin use for <48 hours, and several studies reported difficulty discontinuing vasopressin therapy. Whether additional benefits, deleterious effects, or tolerance is observed with longer infusions remains unclear. Long-term administration of vasopressin is associated with hyponatremia and thrombocytopenia. Because vasopressin is being used to replace a physiologic deficiency, it stands to reason that the requirement for vasopressin will subside with reversal of the septic process. Attempts to discontinue vasopressin should occur when the dosage(s) of adrenergic agent(s) has been minimized (e.g., dopamine ≤ 5 mcg/kg/min, norepinephrine ≤ 0.1 mcg/kg/min, phenylephrine ≤ 1 mcg/kg/min, epinephrine ≤ 0.15 mcg/kg/min). At present, vasopressin should not be initiated as first-line therapy or added to existing therapy solely because a patient is septic.

Corticosteroids

14 Corticosteroids can be initiated in cases of septic shock when adrenal insufficiency is present or when weaning of vasopressor therapy proves futile.[54,62] Adverse events are few because corticosteroids are administered for a finite period of time, usually 7 days.

Acutely, elevated serum concentrations of blood urea nitrogen, white blood cell count, and glucose occur. Although long-term administration of corticosteroids is associated with several chronic disease states, meta-analyses do not show an increase in adverse events, including gastrointestinal hemorrhage (RR, 1.12; 95% CI, 0.81–1.53; $P = 0.5$), superinfections (RR, 1.01; 95% CI, 0.82–1.25; $P = 0.92$), and neuromuscular weakness (RR, 0.63; 95% CI, 0.12–3.35; $P = 0.58$).[55,56] Hyperglycemia (RR, 1.16; 95% CI, 1.07–1.25; $P <0.001$) and hypernatremia (RR, 1.61; 95% CI, 1.26–2.06; $P < 0.001$) are associated with corticosteroid therapy.[55,56] Therefore, therapy of septic shock with corticosteroids improves hemodynamic variables and lowers catecholamine vasopressor dosages with minimal to no effect on patient safety.[7]

EXPERIMENTAL THERAPIES

NITRIC OXIDE INHIBITORS

NO is a short-acting, potent vasodilator derived from enzymatic oxidation of arginine. Its production is under control of NOS. This enzyme is present (expressed) in two forms: a constitutive form (ecNOS) and an inducible form (iNOS). Small amounts of NO normally are produced by the vascular endothelium under the control of ecNOS for physiologic control of vascular tone and blood flow distribution. Under pathophysiologic conditions such as stimulation by lipopolysaccharide or cytokines, iNOS becomes diffusely expressed, producing large amounts of NO. The latter has been implicated in the cardiovascular failure of septic shock.

Pharmacologic inhibition of NO production has been investigated as an adjunct to standard therapies of septic shock. L-Arginine analogs such as monomethyl-L-arginine (L-NMMA) and L-arginine-methylester (L-NAME) are competitive inhibitors of NOS and have been shown to increase blood pressure, partially restore vascular reactivity, and reduce vasopressor use.[7,11,12] However, because these arginine analogs nonselectively block ecNOS and iNOS, their use has been associated with extensive vasoconstriction, decreased CO, and regional hypoperfusion, thus promoting organ failure and mortality. Some S-substituted thiourea derivatives have demonstrated, both in vitro and in vivo (rodent), dose-dependent selectivity for iNOS inhibition, but the clinical application must be evaluated. A phase I/IIa clinical trial of septic shock patients is underway (see www.medinox.com).

Pyridoxalated hemoglobin polyoxyethylene is a scavenger of NO. A phase II study of 62 patients with vasodilatory shock requiring vasopressors showed that an infusion of 20 mg/kg/h for up to 100 hours rapidly increases blood pressure and shortens the duration of vasopressor therapy.[82] Additional studies are needed.

METHYLENE BLUE

Methylene blue counteracts ecNOS, iNOS, and soluble guanylate cyclase to reduce serum concentrations of NO and cyclic guanosine monophosphate.[83] Despite these effects, methylene blue does not alter the expression of inflammatory cytokines. Clinically, methylene blue at dosages of 0.25 to 3 mg/kg/h increases SVR, MAP, myocardial contractility, and DO_2 in septic shock patients refractory to vasopressors.[83] It may increase pulmonary vascular resistance, potentially worsening oxygenation. Additional studies are needed before methylene blue can be recommended; at present, it has been used only for salvage therapy.

TERLIPRESSIN

Terlipressin, a prodrug that is converted into lysine vasopressin, has been used in septic shock patients and is available in other countries.[84] This drug has a half-life of 6 hours and acts via vascular V_1 receptors and renal tubular V_2 receptors. Terlipressin increases MAP to a greater extent than norepinephrine when it is used as the initial vasopressor in septic shock. Despite a decrease in CO, heart rate, and Do_2I, terlipressin increases gastric mesenteric perfusion, urine production, and creatinine clearance while reducing lactate concentration. Both terlipressin and vasopressin increase blood pressure and decrease heart rate to the same extent but terlipressin is associated with less supplemental norepinephrine usage and improved mesenteric perfusion.[85,86] These preliminary findings suggest that a clinical trial evaluating mortality as well as hemodynamic effects should be conducted.

LEVOSIMENDAN

Levosimendan is a novel inotropic and vasodilator calcium-sensitizing drug.[87] In acute decompensated heart failure, it improves cardiac contractility by sensitizing troponin C to calcium. In septic shock patients with and without left ventricular dysfunction, levosimendan 0.1 to 0.2 mcg/kg/min decreases PAOP, increases LVEF and cardiac index, improves mesenteric perfusion, and enhances urine production.[87] Levosimendan improves $Scvo_2$ to the same extent as dobutamine when it is used in early goal-directed therapy. Levosimendan is associated with declining serum lactate concentration. While additional clinical trials of levosimendan in septic shock are needed, increased mortality was demonstrated in studies of acute decompensated heart failure.

DOPEXAMINE AND ISOPROTERENOL

Dopexamine is a structural and synthetic analog of dopamine that exerts systemic vasodilation through stimulation of β_2-adrenoceptors and peripheral D_1 and D_2 receptors and weak inotropic properties through stimulation of β_1-adrenoceptors.[49,50] It has been used in patients with acute heart failure and septic shock. Similar to dobutamine, dopexamine is administered in combination with a vasopressor in septic shock. In small studies of septic shock, dopexamine produced a dose-related (range, 2–6 mcg/kg/min) increase in cardiac index, stroke volume, and heart rate, as well as a decrease in SVR over the course of 0.5 to 1 hour while the dosages of other vasopressors were kept constant. The increase in myocardial oxygen demand is less than with dopamine, but tachycardia and tachydysrhythmia may lead to myocardial ischemia, especially when ischemic heart disease is present. Global oxygen-transport variables are similar to those of dopamine: Do_2 increases but Vo_2 increases insufficiently, resulting in impaired O_2ER. The combined β_2-adrenoceptors and peripheral D_1 agonistic effects of dopexamine should improve distribution of blood flow. However, the results of studies of dopexamine use in septic shock failed to show preferential increase in splanchnic blood flow. In fact, gastric pHi was lowered. When administered over 7 days, dopexamine had no impact on renal function. Therefore, initial data do not support a role for dopexamine in improving regional hemodynamics and blood flow, but studies continue to investigate dopexamine as an alternative therapy for septic shock.

Isoproterenol is a synthetic catecholamine that stimulates only β_1- and β_2-adrenoceptors to produce vasodilatory and inotropic effects.[88] Although not thought of as a traditional agent for managing septic shock, isoproterenol has received attention because of the concepts of early goal-directed therapy.[30] The strong β-adrenergic effects of isoproterenol make it a potential alternative to dobutamine for optimizing Do_2 in patients with low Svo_2 despite use of other therapies (e.g., fluid resuscitation, vasopressors, red blood cell transfusion). In patients with septic shock and Svo_2 <70% despite volume administration, norepinephrine, and red blood cell transfusion, adding isoproterenol increases Svo_2, cardiac index, and stroke

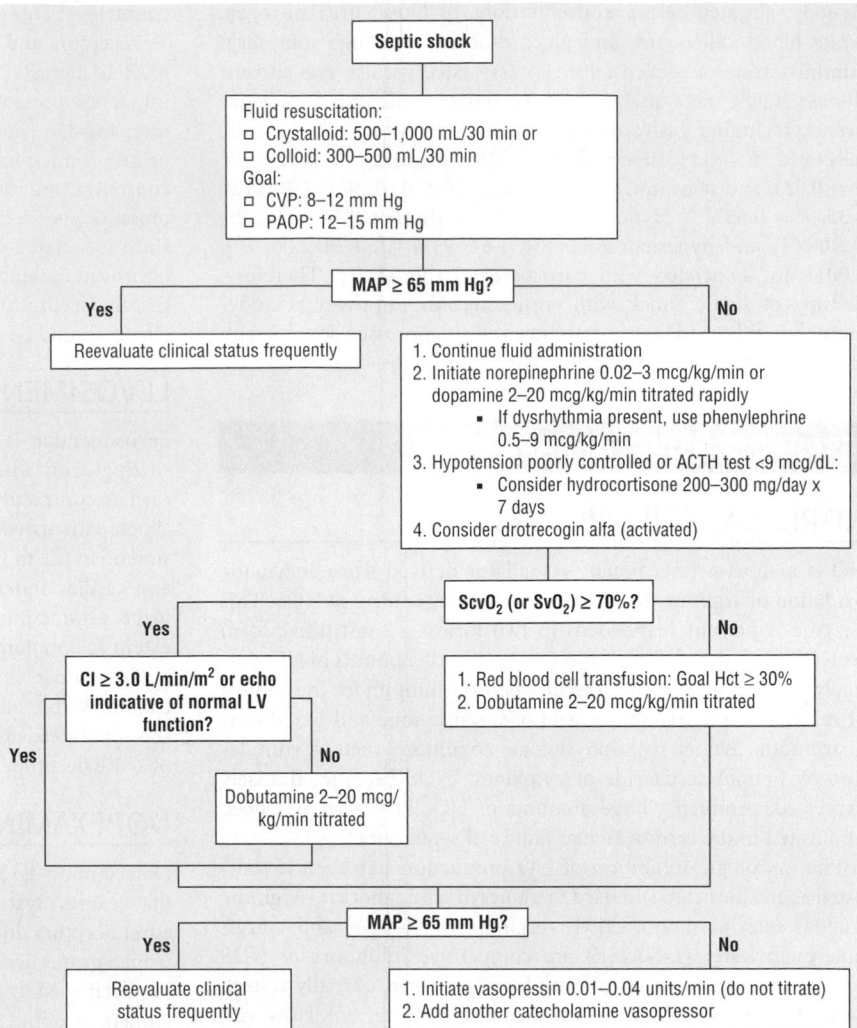

FIGURE 30-2. Algorithmic approach to resuscitative management of septic shock. Algorithmic approach is intended to be used in conjunction with clinical judgment, hemodynamic monitoring parameters, and therapy end points, as discussed in the text. (ACTH, adrenocorticotropic hormone; CI, cardiac index; CVP, central venous pressure; echo, echocardiography; Hct, hematocrit; MAP, mean arterial pressure; PAOP, pulmonary artery occlusive pressure; $Scvo_2$, central venous oxygen saturation; Svo_2, mixed venous oxygen saturation.) (*Figure based on data from references 6–19, 49–65.*)

index while decreasing lactate concentration without increasing heart rate or causing myocardial ischemia. Although these results are intriguing, additional studies are needed to define the role of isoproterenol, especially considering that dobutamine has become standard therapy for early goal-directed therapy. At present, isoproterenol is an agent of last resort.

OTHER THERAPIES

As with vasopressin and cortisol, critical illness impairs hypothalamic–pituitary function, producing relative deficiencies of triiodothyronine (T_3) and thyroxine (T_4). This condition, referred to as *euthyroid sick syndrome*, may contribute to hypotension.[89] Concentrations of thyrotropin-releasing hormone and thyroid-stimulating hormone are inappropriately low. Measured concentrations of free T_3 and T_4 may be low or normal, but synthesis is consistently impaired. Only scant data regarding the replacement of these hormones in critically ill patients are available, and the results are variable, depending on the extent of additional hormone replacement (growth hormone, gonadotropin-releasing hormone, leptin, insulin, thyrotropin-releasing hormone, and thyroid-stimulating hormone). Given the data for replacing vasopressin and cortisol in septic shock, it is reasonable to assume that one day a "thyroid replacement" regimen will be offered as an adjunctive treatment to vasopressors.

Drotrecogin alfa (activated) or recombinant activated protein C has been established as a treatment of severe sepsis because it reduces mortality when used early in patients with at least two

organ dysfunctions or an Acute Physiology and Chronic Health Evaluation (APACHE) II score of 25.[90] Drotrecogin alfa (activated) promotes fibrinolysis, inhibits coagulation, and modulates inflammation. It inhibits inflammation, possibly preventing endotoxin-induced hypotension. A study of 22 septic shock patients treated with drotrecogin alfa (activated) showed that the norepinephrine dosage rate decreased 33% over 24 hours.[91] In contrast, the norepinephrine dosage increased 38% in the matched control group despite MAP values similar to the drotrecogin alfa (activated) group. Although these results deserve further investigation, drotrecogin alfa (activated) likely will never be administered solely for hemodynamic support of septic shock patients because it is an expensive agent with concerns of hemorrhage as a side effect. Ultimately, patients who "qualify" for drotrecogin alfa (activated) will receive it irrespective of hemodynamic effect.

GENERAL CONCLUSIONS AND RECOMMENDATIONS

The choice of vasopressor or inotropic agent in septic shock should be made according to the needs of the patient. Figure 30–2 presents an algorithm for the management of septic shock.[6–19,49–65] This algorithm suggests a stepwise approach, first using dopamine or norepinephrine. Dobutamine is added for low CO states or to optimize $Svo_2/Scvo_2$. Occasionally, epinephrine and phenylephrine are used when necessary. Although this approach is empirical, it is used broadly in clinical practice and has been justified by the desire to avoid strong vasoconstriction. However, observations of improved outcomes with norepinephrine and decreased regional perfusion with dopamine are calling into question the use of dopamine as a first-line agent. Most clinicians now prefer norepinephrine as the initial vasopressor agent. Developing a strategy to titrate therapy early in the course of illness to predetermined values reduces mortality. Goals of initial resuscitation should include fluids to achieve CVP 8 to 12 mm Hg, vasopressor agents to achieve MAP at least 65 mm Hg, red blood cell transfusion to maintain hematocrit $\geq 30\%$, and inotropic therapy to achieve $Scvo_2 \geq 70\%$.[7,30] For all catecholamine vasopressors, doses higher than recommended traditionally are required for goal-directed therapy to MAP and for normalization of oxygen-transport variables, Do_2, and Vo_2. Patients who develop supranormal Do_2 and Vo_2 values have lower mortality, but whether this effect is achieved intrinsically or with exogenous administration of vasopressors/inotropes appears inconsequential. Therefore, goal-directed therapy to supranormal oxygen-transport variables cannot be recommended because little or no benefit has been demonstrated. Further work is required to better elucidate the differential effects of vasopressors on regional hemodynamic and oxygen-transport values as measures of local tissue perfusion.

The algorithmic approach (Fig. 30-2) we recommend for use of vasopressors and inotropes in the hemodynamic support of critically ill septic patients is consistent with the recommendations made in the Surviving Sepsis Campaign[7] and the American College of Critical Care Medicine's guidelines to the hemodynamic support of adult patients with sepsis (Table 30-2).[6,8] Although difficult to demonstrate, true differences in clinical outcomes as a result of differences in the pharmacologic activity of vasopressors and inotropes may exist. For example, evidence suggests that norepinephrine, when used appropriately with fluid replenishment, is safe and effective in treating septic shock; it decreases mortality, particularly when started early in the course of septic shock. It is effective in optimizing hemodynamic variables and improving systemic and regional (e.g., renal, gastric mucosal, and splanchnic) perfusion. Epinephrine causes a greater increase in the cardiac index and Do_2 and increases gastric mucosal flow but may not preserve splanchnic circulation adequately. It may cause increases in lactic acid. Epinephrine may be particularly useful when used earlier in the course of septic shock in young patients. Unlike epinephrine, dopamine does not increase the proportion of CO that preferentially goes to the splanchnic circulation. The ability of dopamine to increase CO by no more than 35% accompanied by a tachycardia or tachydysrhythmias limits its utility. Dopamine, as opposed to norepinephrine, has been shown to worsen splanchnic Vo_2 and O_2ER and is of limited value in improving urine production. Low-dose dopamine has not been shown consistently to increase the glomerular filtration rate, does not prevent renal failure, and actually worsens splanchnic tissue oxygen utilization. Low-dose dopamine should not be used. Phenylephrine should be used when a pure vasoconstrictor is desired in patients who may not require or cannot tolerate the β-effects of dopamine or norepinephrine with or without dobutamine. In patients with a high filling pressure and hypotension, the combination of phenylephrine and dobutamine may be useful.

Shortcomings of study methodology prevent the establishment of definitive conclusions. As a consequence, published guidelines for the management of severe sepsis and septic shock have many inconclusive recommendations (Table 30-2). Short infusions during studies may show differences that are not clinically significant after 24 hours, as demonstrated for epinephrine and dobutamine. Clinically, vasopressors and inotropes are used for hours to days. Possible confounding factors are the variable times at which studies are initiated with respect to the stage of sepsis or septic shock, the inherent differences in circulating catecholamine concentrations, changes in receptor activity, as well as differences in prestudy duration and type of exogenous catecholamine administration.

Initial studies with vasopressin suggest a potential role in the management of vasopressor-dependent septic shock patients. Vasopressin appears to reduce the requirements of adrenergic agents while maintaining hemodynamic function. While it may enhance urine production, it is associated with mesenteric and peripheral ischemia. Therefore, vasopressin should be used only if response to one or two adrenergic agents is inadequate or as a method for reducing the dosage of these therapies. Close monitoring of ischemic events is needed. Data indicate that moderate doses of hydrocortisone (200–300 mg/day) administered over several days may reverse septic shock and dependency on vasopressor agents, particularly in patients with relative adrenal insufficiency. As a result of a recent multicenter study, the presence of adrenal insufficiency to indicate therapy with corticosteroids is controversial. Given the discrepancy of the current data, corticosteroids may be administered to patients with septic shock refractory to vasopressors or when adrenal insufficiency is present. Data on optimal dosage regimens and definitive outcomes still are needed.

Further pharmacotherapeutic and outcomes studies are required to elucidate the place in therapy of individual vasopressors and inotropes or their combinations in the supportive care of patients with bacteremia or septic shock. As supportive therapy, it is imperative that primary therapy aimed at the source of (antimicrobials) and consequences of (anticytokines) infection be initiated quickly to afford the patient the best chance of survival. Once this goal is accomplished, we will need to direct our efforts to pharmacoeconomics and the cost effectiveness of these therapies.

ABBREVIATIONS

ACTH: adrenocorticotropic hormone

APACHE: Acute Physiology and Chronic Health Evaluation

ATP: adenosine triphosphate

CaMK: calcium-calmodulin-dependent protein kinase

cAMP: cyclic adenosine monophosphate

Cao_2: arterial oxygen content

CI: confidence interval

CO: cardiac output

CO_2: carbon dioxide

Cvo_2: venous oxygen content

CVP: central venous pressure

Do_2: oxygen delivery

DO_2I: oxygen delivery index

ecNOS: constitutive nitric oxide synthase

HR: hazard ratio

ICU: intensive care unit

IL: interleukin

iNOS: inducible nitric oxide synthase

L-NAME: L-arginine-methylester

L-NMMA: monomethyl-L-arginine

LVEF: left ventricular ejection fraction

MAP: mean arterial pressure

NO: nitric oxide

NOS: nitric oxide synthase

O$_2$ER: oxygen extraction ratio

OR: odds ratio

Paco$_2$: arterial carbon dioxide pressure (tension)

Pao$_2$: arterial oxygen pressure (tension)

PAOP: pulmonary artery occlusion pressure

Pco$_2$: gut luminal partial pressure of carbon dioxide

pHi: intramucosal pH

PLC: phospholipase

Pslco$_2$: sublingual carbon dioxide pressure

RR: relative risk

Sao$_2$: arterial oxygen saturation

Scvo$_2$: central venous oxygen saturation

Svo$_2$: mixed venous oxygen saturation

SVR: systemic vascular resistance

T$_3$: triiodothyronine

T$_4$: thyroxine

TNF: tumor necrosis factor

Vo$_2$: oxygen consumption

Vo$_2$I: oxygen consumption index

REFERENCES

1. Marik PE, Lipman J. The definition of septic shock: implications for treatment. Crit Care Resusc 2007;9:101–103.
2. Vincent JL, Sakr Y, Sprung CL, et al. Sepsis in European intensive care unit: Results of the SOAP study. Crit Care Med 2006;34:344–353.
3. Sakr Y, Vincent JL, Roukonen E, et al. Sepsis and organ failure are major determinants of post-intensive care unit mortality. J Crit Care 2008;23:475–483.
4. Blanco J, Muriel-Bombin A, Sagredo V, et al. Incidence, organ dysfunction and mortality in severe sepsis: a Spanish multicentre study. Crit Care 2008;12:R158.
5. Mann HJ, Nolan PE Jr. Update on the management of cardiogenic shock. Curr Opin Crit Care 2006;12:431–436.
6. Hollenberg SM, Ahrens TS, Annane D, et al. Practice parameters for hemodynamic support of sepsis in adult patients in sepsis. Crit Care Med 2004;32:1928–1948.
7. Dellinger RP, Levy MM, Carlet JM, et al. Surviving sepsis campaign: International guidelines for management of severe sepsis and septic shock: 2008. Crit Care Med 2008;36:296–327.
8. Beale RJ, Hollenberg SM, Vincent JL, et al. Vasopressor and inotropic support in septic shock: An evidence-based review. Crit Care Med 2004;32(Suppl):S455–S465.
9. Rudis MI, Rowland KL. Current concepts in severe sepsis and septic shock. J Pharm Practice 2005;18:351–362.
10. Holmes CL. Vasoactive drugs in the intensive care unit. Curr Opin Crit Care 2005;11:413–417.
11. Cinel I, Dellinger RP. Advances in the pathogenesis and management of sepsis. Curr Opin Infect Dis 2007;20:345–352.
12. Rivers EP, Coba V, Visbal A, et al. Management of sepsis: early resuscitation. Clin Chest Med 2008;29:689–704.
13. Holmes CL, Walley KR. Vasoactive drugs for vasodilatory shock in ICU. Curr Opin Crit Care 2009;15:398–402.
14. Gullo A, Bianco N, Berlot G. Management of severe sepsis and septic shock: challenges and recommendations. Crit Care Clin 2006;22: 489–501.
15. Leone M, Martin C. Vasopressor use in septic shock: an update. Curr Opin Anesthesiol 2008;21:141–147.
16. Bassi G, Radermacher P, Calzia E. Catecholamines and vasopressin during critical illness. Endocrinol Metab Clin N Am 2006;35: 839–857.
17. Zanotti-Cavazzoni SL, Dellinger RP. Hemodynamic optimization of sepsis-induced tissue hypoperfusion. Crit Care 2006;10(Suppl 3):S2.
18. Sevransky J. Clinical assessment of hemodynamically unstable patients. Curr Opin Crit Care 2009;15:234–238.
19. Dellinger RP. Cardiovascular management of septic shock. Crit Care Med 2003;32:946–955.
20. Pinsky MR. Hemodynamic evaluation and monitoring in the ICU. Chest 2007;132:2020–2029.
21. Marik PE, Baram M. Noninvasive hemodynamic monitoring in the intensive care unit. Crit Care Clin 2007;23:383–400.
22. Levy MM, Macias WL, Vincent JL, et al. Early changes in organ function predict eventual survival in severe sepsis. Crit Care Med 2005;33:2194–2201.
23. O'Grady N, Alexander M, Dellinger E, et al. Guidelines for the prevention of intravascular catheter-related infections. Clin Infect Dis 2002;35:1281–1307.
24. Greenberg SB, Murphy GS, Vender JS. Current use of the pulmonary artery catheter. Curr Opin Crit Care 2009;15:249–253.
25. Bernard GR, Sopko G, Cerra F, et al. Pulmonary artery catheterization and clinical outcomes: National Heart, Lung, and Blood Institute and Food and Drug Administration Workshop Report. Consensus Statement. JAMA 2000;283:2568–2572.
26. Harvey S, Young D, Brampton W, et al. Pulmonary artery catheter for adult patients in intensive care. Cochrane Database Syst Rev 2006;19:CD003408.
27. Practice guidelines for pulmonary artery catheterization: An updated report by the American Society of Anesthesiologists Task Force on Pulmonary Artery Catheterization. Anesthesiology 2003;99:988–1014.
28. The National Heart, Lung, and Blood Institute Acute Respiratory Distress Syndrome (ARDS) Clinical Trials Network. Pulmonary-artery central venous catheter to guide treatment of acute lung injury. N Engl J Med 2006;354:2213–2224.
29. Singer M. Oesophageal Doppler. Curr Opin Crit Care 2009;15: 244–248.
30. Rivers E, Nguyen B, Havstad S, et al. Early goal-directed therapy in the treatment of severe sepsis and septic shock. N Engl J Med 2001;345:1368–1377.
31. Caille V, Squara P. Oxygen uptake-to-delivery relationship: a way to assess adequate flow. Crit Care 2006;10(Suppl 3):S4.
32. Varpula M, Tallgren M, Saukkonen K, et al. Hemodynamic variables related to outcome in septic shock. Intensive Care Med 2005;31: 1066–1071.
33. Heyland DK, Cook DJ, King D, et al. Maximizing oxygen delivery in critically ill patients: A methodologic appraisal of the evidence. Crit Care Med 1996;24:517–524.
34. Oberbeck R. Catecholamines: physiological immunomodulators during health and illness. Curr Med Chem 2006;13:1979–1989.
35. Kern JW, Shoemaker WC. Meta-analysis of hemodynamic optimization in high-risk patients. Crit Care Med 2002;30:1686–1692.
36. Kortgen A, Neiderprum P, Bauer M. Implementation of an evidence-based standard operating procedure and outcome in septic shock. Crit Care Med 2006;34:943–949.
37. Micek ST, Roubinian N, Heuring T, et al. Before–after study of a standardized hospital order set for the management of septic shock. Crit Care Med 2006;34:2707–2713.
38. Shorr AF, Micek ST, Jackson WL, et al. Economic implications of an evidence-based sepsis protocol: can we improve outcomes and lower costs? Crit Care Med 2007;35:1257–1262.
39. Girardis P, Rinaldi L, Donno L, et al. Effects on management and outcome of severe sepsis and septic shock patients admitted to the intensive care unit after implementation of a sepsis program: a pilot study. Crit Care 2009;13:R143.
40. Shapiro NI, Howell MD, Talmor D, et al. Implementation and outcomes of the multiple urgent sepsis therapies (MUST) protocol. Crit Care Med 2006;34:1025–1032.
41. Talmor D, Greenberg D, Howell MD, et al. The costs and cost-effectiveness of an integrated sepsis treatment protocol. Crit Care Med 2008;36:1168–1174.
42. Jones AE, Brown MD, Trzeciak S. The effect of a quantatative resuscitation strategy on mortality in the patients with sepsis: a meta-analysis. Crit Care Med 2008;36:2734–2739.
43. Klijn E, Uil D, Bakker J, et al. The heterogeneity of the microcirculation in critical illness. Clin Chest Med 2008;29:643–654.

44. Boerma EC. The microcirculation as a clinical concept: work in progress. Curr Opin Crit Care 2009;15:261–265.

45. Zanotti-Cavazzoni SL, Hollenberg SM. Cardiac dysfunction in severe sepsis and septic shock. Curr Opin Crit Care 2009;15:392–397.

46. Fernandes CJ Jr, Akamine N, Knobel E. Myocardial depression in sepsis. Shock 2008;30(Suppl 1):14–17.

47. Price S, Nicol E, Gibson DG, et al. Echocardiography in the critically ill: Current and potential roles. Intensive Care Med 2006;32:48–59.

48. Boyd JH, Walley KR. The role of echocardiography in hemodynamic monitoring. Curr Opin Crit Care 2009;15:239–243.

49. Asfar P, Hauser B, Radermacher P, et al. Catecholamines and vasopressin during critical illness. Crit Care Clin 2006;22:131–149.

50. Senz A, Nunnink L. Review article: inotrope and vasopressor use in the emergency department. Emerg Med Australas 2009;21:342–351.

51. Obritsch M, Bestul D, Jung R, et al. The role of vasopressin in vasodilatory septic shock. Pharmacotherapy 2004;24:1050–1063.

52. Vincent JL. Vasopressin in hypotensive and shock states. Crit Care Clin 2006;22:187–197.

53. Russell JA. Vasopressin in septic shock. Crit Care Med 2007;35(Suppl):S609–S615.

54. MacLaren R, Jung R. Stress-dose corticosteroid therapy for sepsis and acute lung injury or acute respiratory distress syndrome in critically ill adults. Pharmacotherapy 2002;22:1140–1156.

55. Minneci PC, Deans KJ, Banks SM, et al. Meta-analysis: The effect of steroids on survival and shock during sepsis depends on the dose. Ann Intern Med 2004;141:47–56.

56. Annane D, Bellissant E, Bollaert PE, et al. Corticosteroids in the treatment of severe sepsis and septic shock in adults. JAMA 2009;301:2362–2375.

57. Lefering LR, Neugebauer EAM. Steroids controversy in sepsis and septic shock: A meta-analysis. Crit Care Med 1995;23:1294–1303.

58. Cronin L, Cook DJ, Carlet J, et al. Corticosteroid treatment for sepsis: A critical appraisal and meta-analysis. Crit Care Med 1995;23:1430–1439.

59. Annane D, Sebille V, Troche G, et al. A 3-level prognostic classification in septic shock based on cortisol levels and cortisol response to corticotropin. JAMA 2000;283:1038–1045.

60. Annane D, Sébille V, Charpentier C, et al. Effect of treatment with low doses of hydrocortisone and fludrocortisone on mortality in patients with septic shock. JAMA 2002;288:862–871.

61. Sprung CL, Annane D, Keh D, et al. Hydrocortisone therapy for patients with septic shock. N Engl J Med 2008;358:111–124.

62. Marik PE, Pastores SM, Annane D, et al. Recommendations for the diagnosis and management of corticosteroid insufficiency in critically ill adult patients: consensus statements from an international task force by the American College of Critical Care Medicine. Crit Care Med 2008;36:1937–1949.

63. Vincent JL, Biston P, Devriendt J, et al. Dopamine versus norepinephrine: is one better? Minerva Anestesiol 2009;75:533–537.

64. Russell JA, Walley KR, Singer J, et al. Vasopressin versus norepinephrine in patients with septic shock. N Engl J Med 2008;358:877–887.

65. Finfer S, Bellomo R, McEvoy S, et al. A comparison of albumin and saline for fluid resuscitation in the intensive care unit. N Engl J Med 2004;350:2247–2256.

66. Brunkhorst FM, Engel C, Bloos F, et al. Intensive insulin therapy and pentastarch resuscitation in severe sepsis. N Engl J Med 2008;358:125–139.

67. LeBlanc JM, Dasta JF, Hollenberg SM. North American survey of vasopressor and inotrope use in severe sepsis and septic shock. Crit Care Shock 2008;11:137–148.

68. Martin C, Papazian L, Perrin G, et al. Norepinephrine or dopamine for the treatment of hyperdynamic septic shock? Chest 1993;103:1826–1831.

69. Martin C, Viviand X, Leone M, Thirion X. Effect of norepinephrine on the outcome of septic shock. Crit Care Med 2000;28:2758–2765.

70. Sakr Y, Reinhart K, Vincent JL, et al. Does dopamine administration in shock influence outcome? Results of the sepsis occurrence in acutely ill patients (SOAP) study. Crit Care Med 2006;34:589–597.

71. Boulain T, Runge I, Bercault N, Benzekri-Lefevre D, Wolf M, Fleury C. Dopamine therapy in septic shock: detrimental effect on survival. J Crit Care 2009;24:575–582.

72. Povoa PR, Carneiro AH, Ribeiro OS, et al. Influence of vasopressor agent in septic shock mortality. Results from the Portuguese community-acquired sepsis study (SACiUCI study). Crit Care Med 2009;37:410–416.

73. De Backer D, Biston P, Devriendt J, et al. Comparison of dopamine and norepinephrine in the treatment of shock. N Engl J Med 2010;362:779–789.

74. Patel GP, Grahe JS, Sperry M, et al. Efficacy and safety of dopamine versus norepinephrine in the management of septic shock. Shock 2010;33:375–380.

75. Myburgh JA, Higgins A, Jovanovska A, et al. A comparison of epinephrine and norepinephrine in critically ill patients. Intensive Care Med 2008;34:2226–2234.

76. Annane D, Vignon P, Renault A, et al. Norepinephrine plus dobutamine versus epinephrine alone for the management of septic shock: a randomised trial. Lancet 2007;370:678–684.

77. Schrier RW, Wang W. Acute renal failure and sepsis. N Engl J Med 2004;351:159–169.

78. Friedrich JO, Adhikari N, Herridge MS, et al. Meta-analysis: Low-dose dopamine increases urine output but does not prevent renal dysfunction or death. Ann Intern Med 2005;142:510–524.

79. Bellomo R, Chapman M, Finfer S, et al. Low-dose dopamine in patients with early renal dysfunction: A placebo-controlled randomized trial. Australian and New Zealand Intensive Care Society (ANZICS) Clinical Trials Group. Lancet 2000;356:2139–2143.

80. Russell JA, Walley KR, Gordon AC, et al. Interaction of vasopressin infusion, corticosteroid treatment, and mortality of septic shock. Crit Care Med 2009;37:811–818.

81. Bauer SR, Lam SW, Cha SS, et al. Effect of corticosteroids on arginine vasopressin-containing vasopressor therapy for septic shock: a case control study. J Crit Care 2008;23:500–506.

82. Kinasewitz GT. Privalle CT, Imm A, et al. Multicenter, randomized, placebo-controlled study of the nitric oxide scavenger pyridoxalated hemoglobin polyoxyethylene in distributive shock. Crit Care Med 2008;36:1999–2007.

83. Kwok ES, Howes D. Use of methylene blue in sepsis: a systematic review. J Intensive Care Med 2006;21:359–363.

84. Morelli A, Ertmer C, Peitropaoli P, et al. Terlipressin: a promising vasoactive agent in hemodynamic support of septic shock. Expert Opin Pharmacother 2009;10:2569–2575.

85. Singer M. Arginine vasopressin vs. terlipressin in the treatment of shock states. Best Pract Res Clin Anaesthesiol 2008;22:359–368.

86. Lange M, Ertmer C, Westphal M. Vasopressin vs. terlipressin in the treatment of cardiovascular failure in sepsis. Intensive Care Med 2008;34:821–832.

87. Pinto BB, Rehberg S, Ertmer C, et al. Role of levosimendan in sepsis and septic shock. Curr Opin Anesthesiol 2008;21:168–177.

88. Leone M, Boyadjiev I, Boulos E, et al. A reappraisal of isoproterenol in goal-directed therapy of septic shock. Shock 2006;26:353–357.

89. De Groot LJ. Non-thyroidal illness syndrome is a manifestation of hypothalamic-pituitary dysfunction, and in view of current evidence, should be treated with appropriate replacement therapies. Crit Care Clin 2006;22:57–86.

90. Bernard GR, Vincent JL, Laterre PF, et al. Efficacy and safety of recombinant human activated protein C for severe sepsis. N Engl J Med 2001;344:699–709.

91. Monnet X, Lamia B, Anguel N, et al. Rapid and beneficial hemodynamic effects of activated protein C in septic shock patients. Intensive Care Med 2005;31:1573–1576.

CHAPTER

31

Hypovolemic Shock

BRIAN L. ERSTAD

KEY CONCEPTS

❶ Plasma does not have to be lost from the body for hypovolemic shock to occur.

❷ Patients may die of hypovolemic shock despite having normal serum electrolyte concentrations.

❸ Although the Starling equation of fluid transport is useful for understanding the factors involved in fluid shifting between compartments, it is not a practical tool for use in the clinical setting.

❹ Patients may have complications and death as a result of reperfusion injury as well as the initial insult.

❺ The clinical presentation of patients with hypovolemic shock can vary substantially, depending on concomitant disease states, medications, and cause of hypovolemia.

❻ The initial monitoring of a patient with suspected intravascular depletion always should include vital signs, urine output, mental status, and physical examination.

❼ The need for intravenous (versus oral) rehydration in children often is overestimated.

❽ Crystalloid (sodium-containing) solutions should be used for most forms of circulatory insufficiency that are associated with hemodynamic instability.

❾ Neither crystalloids nor colloids have the oxygen-carrying properties of red blood cells.

❿ Vasoactive medications should not be considered for hypovolemic shock until fluid resuscitation has been optimized.

This chapter discusses the assessment and management of hypovolemic shock. Neurogenic shock resulting from loss of sympathetic activity and anaphylactic shock resulting from increased vascular permeability often are considered separately from hypovolemic shock because fluid loss from the body is not necessary for their occurrence. Although these forms of shock are not discussed in detail, it is important to note that intravenous fluid administration (in conjunction with vasoactive medications) is a mainstay of therapy because circulating volume is decreased. In this regard,

Learning objectives, review questions, and other resources can be found at **www.pharmacotherapyonline.com**.

adequate fluid resuscitation to maintain circulating blood volume is a common principle in managing all forms of shock.

EPIDEMIOLOGY

Because shock is not a reportable category by state and federal agencies that track causes of death, the incidence is unknown. Estimates of deaths due to shock are complicated by differences in definitions and classification systems. Part of the problem is defining when progressive circulatory insufficiency results in the loss of normal compensatory responses by the body, which could reverse the processes leading to irreversible organ dysfunction. This loss of appropriate compensation varies from patient to patient and is not always readily apparent during the initial patient presentation. Therefore, forms of hypovolemic shock, such as hemorrhagic shock, are subsumed by more readily identifiable categories of death, such as accidental injuries and homicides. Crude and conservative estimates of death due to hypovolemic shock are available for some of its forms. More than 100,000 deaths each year in the United States are due to unintentional injuries that frequently involve bleeding,[1] and approximately 5,000 deaths are due to hyperthermia and dehydration associated with heat exposure.[2] The figures are much higher when considered on a global basis. For example, electrolyte depletion and dehydration due to diarrheal disease result in approximately 2 million deaths each year in children younger than 5 years.[3] The most liberal estimates of death include all causes of circulatory failure (i.e., the last stage of shock).

ETIOLOGY

❶ Hypovolemic shock may result from blood loss (plasma and red blood cells) due to trauma, surgery, or internal hemorrhage or from plasma loss due to fluid sequestered within the body or lost from the body (Table 31–1). In some cases, such as in

TABLE 31-1 Causes of Hypovolemic Shock[a]

Decreased blood (plasma + red blood cells) volume
  External: Surgery or trauma
  Internal (e.g., cerebral, chest, gastrointestinal and other abdominal sources, long bone fractures, retroperitoneum)
Decreased plasma volume
  External: Losses from urine, gastrointestinal tract (e.g., vomiting, nasogastric suctioning, fistula, diarrhea), lungs, or skin (including thermal injury)
  Internal (decreased oncotic pressure or increased capillary permeability): fluid accumulation in bowel, peritoneal or pleural cavities

[a]Shock may result from various combinations of blood and plasma volume losses listed (i.e., causes are not mutually exclusive).

postoperative patients, a number of these problems occur at the same time. For example, a patient may have blood loss secondary to trauma or surgery, with additional fluid being third spaced (e.g., as tissue edema in the gastrointestinal tract with a concomitant ileus) and lost through a high-output gastrointestinal fistula postoperatively. As this example of third-spaced fluid indicates, fluid (i.e., plasma) does not have to be lost from the body for a person to develop hypovolemic shock, although the fistula output would clearly aggravate the situation. Approximately 20 L of fluid is secreted and reabsorbed daily in the gastrointestinal tract, so it is not surprising that volume loss could be substantial, depending on the location of the fistula and function of the tract preceding the fistula.

Dehydration may result from primary water deficiency, usually because of decreased intake, but in some instances (e.g., diabetes insipidus) may result from increased losses of water. With most forms of dehydration, such as those caused by diarrheal disease and heat-related illness, a combination of inadequate intake and higher than normal losses occurs. In general, the term *dehydration* implies primary intracellular water depletion, in contrast to *volume depletion*, which implies extracellular, and particularly intravascular, sodium and water loss. However, there is substantial overlap in the definitions and use of terms such as *dehydration* and *volume depletion* in the medical literature, so the reader must be cognizant of the intended meaning. In the case of primary water deficit, cell dehydration occurs. Initially, the patient may be thirsty and possibly have some mental status changes, such as confusion. If cellular dehydration occurs slowly, intracellular substances, referred to as *idiogenic osmols*, develop that limit progressive complications (e.g., cerebral edema or coma). Death due to primary water deficit, if it occurs, is usually a result of delayed circulatory failure. With combined water and salt deficiencies, such as might occur with gastrointestinal (e.g., diarrhea) and skin losses (e.g., heat stroke), interstitial and intravascular depletion is an early occurrence. Fortunately, dehydration is relatively easy to prevent with routine vigilance and water replacement compared with some of the other causes of shock.

PATHOPHYSIOLOGY

❷ Hypovolemic shock often is described in terms of monitoring parameters such as lowered blood pressure, but patients with shock may die despite normal surrogate markers of circulatory insufficiency. Therefore, an appropriate definition should mention the underlying problem, which is inadequate tissue perfusion resulting from circulatory failure. In the case of hypovolemic shock, the cause of the altered perfusion is fluid (or volume) depletion resulting from trauma, surgery, thermal injury, or some form of dehydration. Figure 31–1 provides a simplified view of the pathophysiology of circulatory insufficiency assuming the acute insult causing the plasma volume depletion did not result in immediate patient death. Cell damage and death may occur from the primary insult or from reperfusion injury. The latter problem is associated most frequently with trauma and blood loss that cause a systemic inflammatory response syndrome (SIRS) with the release of a multitude of mediators of inflammation and injury that have complex interactions. Cells have varying responses to hypoxia, ranging from astrocytes that quit functioning almost immediately to hepatic cells that may function for several hours after injury to skin, muscle, and bone cells that may tolerate prolonged periods of hypoperfusion.[4,5] Left unmitigated, cell death occurs with prolonged injury and is usually heralded by acidosis, hypothermia, and coagulopathy—referred to as the lethal triad.[5]

The body attempts to compensate for volume depletion beginning with autoregulatory changes involving smaller blood vessels. When the cause of circulatory insufficiency continues unabated, local mechanisms eventually fail to provide adequate compensation, and macrocirculatory changes ensue. Approximately 75% of blood volume is contained in venous capacitance vessels, with gravity being the major impedance to flow back to the heart.[4] With increasing volume depletion, blood flow to the heart (preload) is decreased, with subsequent activation of baroreceptors and chemoreceptors leading to sympathetic discharge. Also, fluid shifting from the interstitial space to the intravascular space occurs through a phenomenon known as *transcapillary refill*, and hormones (e.g., adrenocorticotropic hormone, angiotensin, catecholamines, and vasopressin) that cause sodium and water retention by the kidneys are released. The phenomenon of transcapillary refill means that the body can have fluid losses exceeding normal plasma volume. These responses cause alterations in stroke volume, heart rate, and peripheral vascular resistance so that blood pressure and hence tissue perfusion can be maintained.

The microcirculatory changes associated with shock are complex and difficult to study. Although some mediators such as catecholamines, angiotensin II, arginine vasopressin, and endothelin-1 cause vasoconstriction, other mediators, such as adenosine and nitric oxide, yield vasodilation. These changes result in hypoperfusion or hyperperfusion, depending on the organs involved. As these microcirculatory changes fail to maintain adequate organ

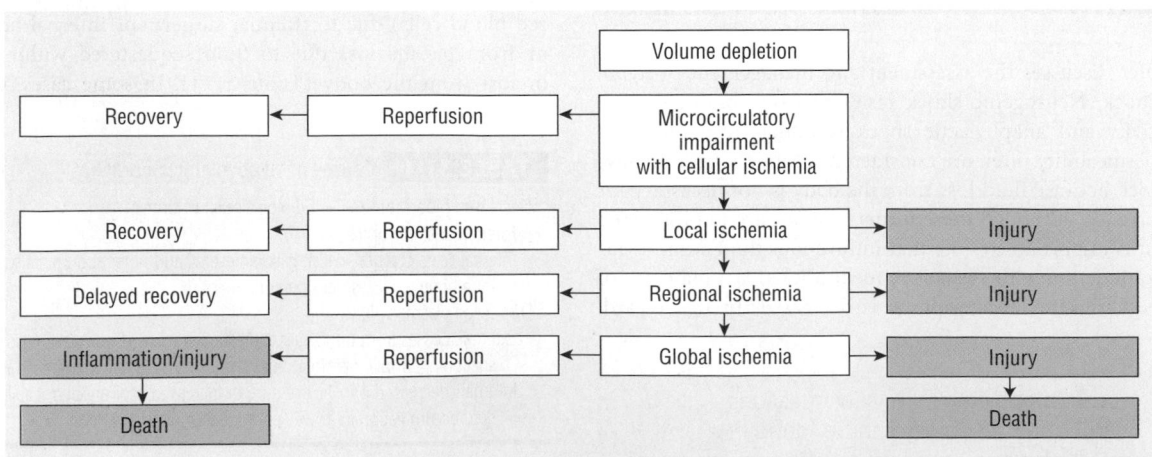

FIGURE 31-1. Pathophysiology of circulatory insufficiency.

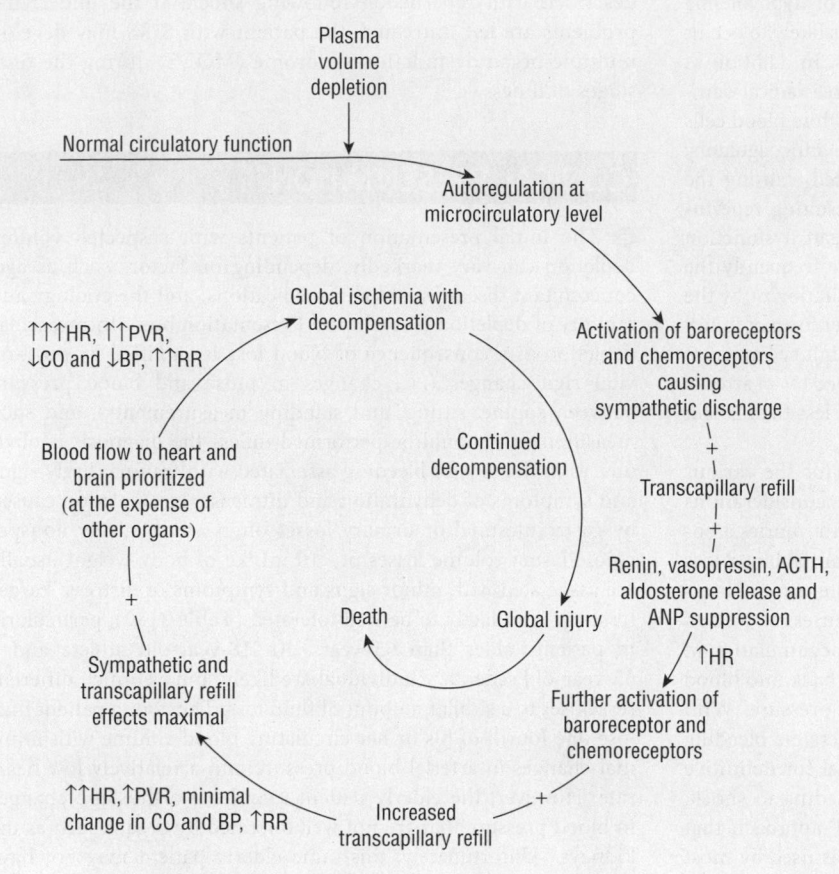

FIGURE 31-2. Activation of compensatory mechanisms with loss of circulatory volume. Certain stages may be absent, depending on a number of factors, such as age, preexisting disease states, and cause of circulatory insufficiency. (ACTH, adrenocorticotropin; BP, blood pressure; CO, cardiac output; HR, heart rate; PVR, peripheral vascular resistance; RR, respiratory rate.)

perfusion, more widespread sympathetic nervous system activation and vasoconstriction ensue. Even assuming general circulation is restored, capillaries may not function properly due to ongoing edema and ischemia. Failure to respond to sympathetic stimulation and fluid administration is indicative of the vasodilation that occurs in the final phase of circulatory failure leading to death.

The factors involved in fluid shifting between the intravascular and interstitial spaces are described by the modified Starling equation:

$$J_v = K_{f,c}[(P_c - P_t) - [\sigma(\pi_c - \pi_t)]$$

where J_v = net transvascular flow rate (cannot be measured in the clinical setting)

$K_{f,c}$ = capillary filtration coefficient for fluids (cannot be measured in the clinical setting)

P_c = capillary hydrostatic pressure (indirectly estimated in the clinical setting, e.g., pulmonary artery occlusive pressure)

P_t = tissue hydrostatic pressure (cannot be measured in the clinical setting)

σ = reflection coefficient for proteins (cannot be measured in the clinical setting)

π_c = plasma colloid osmotic pressure (not usually measured in the clinical setting, but technology is available)

π_t = tissue colloid osmotic pressure (cannot be measured in the clinical setting)

Proteins act as oncotic agents in each of these spaces to attract fluid, whereas hydrostatic forces push fluid into or out of the vessels. The equation has distinct permeability values for water and protein because each crosses the vascular membrane at a different rate. The values for the variables listed in the equation are not the same for capillaries in all parts of the body. For example, on a scale from 0 to 1 with 0 being free passage of protein and 1 being impermeable to protein, the typical value for the reflection coefficient in most capillaries is >0.9. However, in the pulmonary capillaries the value is closer to 0.7 and approaches 0 in inflammatory states associated with increased capillary permeability.[6] As the value approaches 0, the capillaries are freely permeable not only to the usual fluid and electrolytes but to plasma proteins such as albumin. Because albumin accounts for approximately 80% of the plasma oncotic pressure, its free passage into the interstitial space effectively negates its intravascular oncotic benefit. ❸ Although the Starling equation is useful to practitioners in terms of understanding the factors involved in fluid shifting between compartments, the rate and direction of transvascular flow cannot be calculated accurately in the clinical setting because most factors cannot be measured directly and the values for the factors vary in different capillaries in the body.

The body's compensatory mechanisms may have beneficial and harmful consequences. For example, cardiac output can be increased substantially by increases in stroke volume or heart rate. Although this may be useful for providing blood flow to inadequately perfused tissues, it may cause large increases in oxygen consumption by the heart that could aggravate preexisting ischemia in patients with underlying coronary artery disease (CAD). Another example is the sympathetic nervous system–mediated vasoconstriction that causes blood to shift from the skin, skeletal muscle, and some internal organs such as the kidneys and gastrointestinal tract to organs (e.g., heart and brain) that are less tolerant of inadequate flow. If the vasoconstriction continues unabated, the hypoperfused organs eventually become damaged. Figure 31–2 provides an overview of the compensatory changes that occur with a loss of circulating blood volume.

4 In addition to the more acute implications of hypovolemia and attendant complications, reperfusion damage is likely to occur, particularly after prolonged resuscitation attempts. In addition to edematous obstruction of capillaries and oxygen-free radical damage of cell membranes, a number of cellular (e.g., white blood cells and platelets) and humoral (e.g., procoagulants, anticoagulants, complement, and kinins) components are activated, causing the release of other inflammatory mediators.[6] The resulting reperfusion injury may range from readily reversible organ dysfunction to multiple-organ failure and death. The lungs are frequently the first system affected either by excessive fluid resuscitation or by the mediators of secondary reperfusion injury. The latter form of injury often results in the most severe form of acute lung injury known as the acute respiratory distress syndrome that is defined by an arterial oxygen tension: fraction of inspired oxygen ratio of less than 200 in the absence of hypervolemia.

Although the basic pathophysiology is similar for the various causes of hypovolemic shock, there are unique considerations relative to each. For example, whereas isolated head injuries associated with trauma typically do not result in substantial blood loss or shock, long bone or pelvic fractures may sequester several liters of blood. Patients with traumatic or thermal injuries, as well as postoperative patients, may have substantial fluid accumulation in sites where the fluid cannot be readily transferred back into blood vessels (i.e., third-spaced fluid) for maintaining pressure. With these types of injuries, prompt control of compressible bleeding sources with rapid patient transfer to the hospital for definitive treatment may preclude the cascade of events leading to shock. Indeed, with trauma patients, a "scoop and run" approach that places a priority on rapid transport to a hospital is used by most urban hospitals.

In the case of hemorrhagic shock, prompt attention must be given to cell as well as plasma losses. Red blood cells lost during the bleeding episode may lead to ischemic damage in vital organs. Packed red blood cell transfusions may be needed to increase the oxygen-carrying capacity of the blood because oxygen transport is a function not only of cardiac output but also of hemoglobin concentration and saturation and of hemoglobin affinity for oxygen. Once hemostasis has been achieved, a more restrictive transfusion strategy (i.e., transfusion if hemoglobin <7 g/dL) is indicated for the majority of patients without severe cardiovascular disease (see section on Trauma/Perioperative Patients).

Clotting factors and platelets are also lost in hemorrhage. The resulting bleeding problems may be aggravated by the dilutional effect of fluid resuscitation on clotting factor activity. Fresh-frozen plasma that contains necessary clotting factors and platelets are needed in massive blood loss to restore adequate coagulation. On the other hand, trauma patients are at increased risk for deep vein thrombosis and pulmonary embolism caused by multiple factors, including vessel damage, abnormal blood flow patterns, and the hypercoagulable state associated with injury. Therefore, some form of venous thromboembolism prophylaxis usually is indicated in multiple-trauma patients or patients with severe single-system injuries (e.g., spinal cord damage) once hemostasis of major injury-related bleeding has been achieved.

The pathophysiology becomes more complicated if the severity of shock is sufficient to require patient admission to the intensive care unit (ICU) after initial resuscitation or surgery. Most patients admitted to the ICU have SIRS, which is the body's response to injury. This syndrome is defined by a number of hypermetabolic changes reflected in the patient's temperature, white blood cell count and differential, and respiratory and heart rates. The stress response involves complex interactions between the nervous system and immunomodulating substances and has similar (if not the same) harmful and helpful consequences

described with reperfusion following shock. If the underlying problems are left untreated, the patient with SIRS may develop multiple-organ dysfunction syndrome (MODS) during the final stages of illness.

CLINICAL PRESENTATION

5 The initial presentation of patients with suspected volume depletion can vary markedly, depending on factors such as age, concomitant disease states and medications, and the etiology and rapidity of depletion (see Clinical Presentation box). Intravascular depletion as a consequence of blood loss is signified by postural vital sign changes (i.e., changes in pulse and blood pressure between supine, sitting, and standing measurements), and such measurements should be performed unless the diagnosis is obvious, as in the case of bleeding associated with trauma. Early signs and symptoms of dehydration and intravascular depletion caused by gastrointestinal or urinary losses often are relatively nonspecific. Plasma volume losses of <10 mL/kg of body weight usually are associated with minor signs and symptoms of distress. Larger losses are not likely to be well tolerated (Table 31–2), particularly in patients older than 65 years. An 18-year-old athlete and a 65-year-old sedentary individual are likely to have much different responses to a similar amount of fluid loss. The young patient may lose one fourth of his or her circulating blood volume with minimal changes in arterial blood pressure and a relatively low heart rate. However, the elderly patient may have orthostatic changes in blood pressure that are not well tolerated by organs such as the kidneys.[4] Unfortunately, this same elderly patient may not have common signs and symptoms of volume depletion, such as skin turgor changes or thirst, but instead may have more subtle changes (e.g., mental status alterations).

CLINICAL PRESENTATION OF HYPOVOLEMIC SHOCK

General

☐ The initial presentation of adult patients with suspected volume depletion could vary markedly, depending on factors such as age, concomitant disease states and medications, and the etiology and rapidity of depletion.

☐ Plasma volume losses of <10 mL/kg of body weight usually are associated with minor signs and symptoms of distress.

Symptoms

☐ Patients may present with thirst, nausea, anxiousness, weakness, light-headedness, and dizziness.

☐ Patients may report scanty urine output and dark-yellow urine.

Signs

With more severe volume loss:

☐ Patients would have marked increases in heart rate (e.g., >120 beats/min) and respiratory rate (e.g., >30 breaths/min).

☐ Blood pressure would be decreased (e.g., systolic blood pressure <90 mm Hg).

☐ Mental status changes or unconsciousness may occur.

☐ Agitation may be present if the patient is conscious.

☐ Body temperature would be low or normal [e.g., 36°–37°C (96.8°–98.6°F)] in the absence of concomitant infection with cold extremities and decreased capillary refill on physical examination.

Laboratory Tests

- Sodium and chloride concentrations usually are high with acute depletion but may be low or normal depending on type of fluid intake.

- The ratio of blood urea nitrogen (BUN) to creatinine is likely to be elevated initially, but the creatinine level would increase as renal dysfunction occurs.

- Elevated base deficit and lactate concentrations in conjunction with decreased bicarbonate concentrations and pH due to metabolic acidosis.

- The complete blood count should be normal in the absence of concomitant disease states such as infection; in hemorrhagic shock, the red cell count, hemoglobin, and hematocrit would decrease over time, while the prothrombin time and international normalized ratio would increase.

- With more severe volume depletion, other organs may become dysfunctional, which may be reflected in laboratory testing (e.g., elevated transaminase levels with hepatic dysfunction).

Other Diagnostic Tests

- Urine output would be decreased to <0.5 to 1 mL/h.

The diagnosis of dehydration and intravascular depletion in children is complicated by difficulties in obtaining an accurate history. However, some excellent resources are available for healthcare providers, such as the Centers for Disease Control and Prevention (CDC) guidelines (*www.cdc.gov*), which discuss the evaluation and management of diarrhea in patients of all ages. In younger children, parental observations are important for estimating fluid deficits and deciding whether hospitalization is necessary. Fortunately, prospective data suggest that parental histories are predictive of acidosis and the need for hospitalization.[7] ❻ Regardless of patient age or preexisting conditions, the initial monitoring of a patient with suspected volume depletion should include the following noninvasive

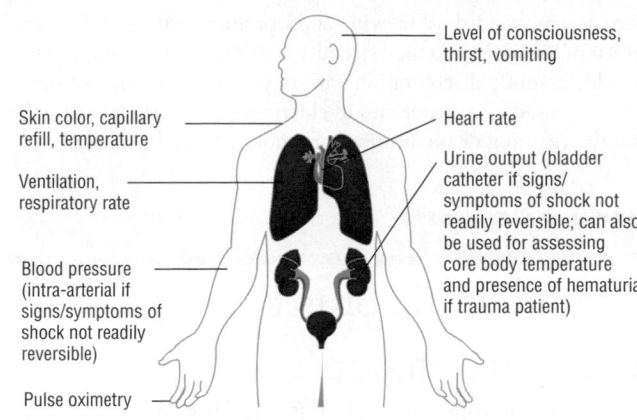

FIGURE 31-3. Noninvasive assessment of circulatory insufficiency.

parameters: vital signs, urine output, mental status, and physical examination (Fig. 31–3).

Although the presenting signs and symptoms of circulatory insufficiency are variable, patients usually have decreased blood pressure, increased heart and respiratory rates, and a normal or low–normal temperature (e.g., 36°–37°C [96.8°–98.6°F]) in the absence of infection, exposure to extremes of temperature, and medications that impair thermoregulation. As mentioned earlier, recordings of vital signs must be interpreted in light of known or suspected baseline conditions. For example, alcohol, β-blockers, butyrophenones such as haloperidol, diuretics, and medications with anticholinergic effects may impair thermoregulation.[8] Medications such as β-blockers and calcium channel blockers may alter resting blood pressure and heart rate, as well as the subsequent response to therapeutic interventions.

Although a blood pressure reading of 110/70 mm Hg (systolic/diastolic) may be acceptable in many patients, it may be inadequate in a patient with preexisting hypertension who normally has a blood pressure of 170/105 mm Hg. At the other extreme, patients with very low blood pressure may have inaudible or inaccurate determinations with cuff (sphygmomanometric) measurements. Chapter 19 details blood pressure measurement (e.g., cuff size, position). In this case, intraarterial monitoring is indicated. As a noninvasive tool, the respiratory rate may correlate better than the heart rate with volume loss, but respiratory rate often is not used.[4] The respiratory rate may be elevated because of anxiety or as a compensatory mechanism for the metabolic acidosis caused by lactic acidosis associated with poor tissue perfusion.

Although the kidneys continually produce urine, the bladder stores the urine for intermittent elimination. For the initial diagnosis and management of acute circulatory insufficiency, a catheter can be inserted into the bladder for measuring urine output. In contrast to thirst, which is a relatively insensitive indicator of volume depletion, urine output is generally diminished with inadequate fluid administration and increases with appropriate resuscitation. This presumes, of course, that acute renal failure or medications such as diuretics are not altering the expected response. Adults should produce at least 0.5 to 1 mL/kg/h of urine, whereas children up to 12 years of age should produce at least 1 mL/kg/h (2 mL/kg/h if younger than 1 year).

Mental status changes associated with volume depletion, if present, may range from subtle fluctuations in mood to unconsciousness. Although the latter finding typically is indicative of more severe depletion, less dramatic findings should not be interpreted as indicating mild fluid deficits. Losses of 4 L of plasma volume may be associated only with lassitude in an otherwise healthy adult patient.[4] Similar interpretation difficulties must be considered when performing the initial physical examination. An orderly progression

TABLE 31-2	Acute Circulatory Insufficiency: Initial Presentation and Therapy[a]	
	Mild	**Severe**
Plasma/blood loss	10 mL/kg adult 20 mL/kg child	30 mL/kg adult 35 mL/kg child
Mental status/level of consciousness	None–small changes (e.g., anxious, irritable)	Marked changes (e.g., confusion to unconsciousness)
Vital signs/orthostatic changes	Minor changes	Marked changes
Therapy	20 mL/kg lactated Ringer or normal saline IV[a] over 10–15 min Unlikely to need blood cell replacement even if hemorrhagic loss	Lactated Ringer or normal saline IV as rapidly as possible until response in adult, then decrease rate of infusion 20 mL/kg lactated Ringer or normal saline IV in child (repeat quickly if minimal response); likely to need blood cell replacement and surgery if hemorrhagic

[a]Patients may have intermediate degrees of volume loss in addition to those listed, but the amount of loss often is difficult to quantify. The presentations may also vary greatly in patients with similar amounts of loss (young athlete vs sedentary, elderly person). In patients particularly prone to complications associated with fluid overload, the fluid can be administered in multiple smaller boluses titrated to clinical response. See text for a more in-depth discussion of some of the guidelines in this table.

from warm, reddish skin with appropriate capillary refill (rapid return of blood flow to the extremity after removal of compression) to cold, cyanotic discoloration with impaired refill may not occur. Also, dry mucous membranes in elderly patients may be caused by mouth breathing or medications and not by fluid depletion.

TREATMENT

Hypovolemic Shock

■ DESIRED OUTCOME

The desired outcomes of therapy for patients with hypovolemic shock are to prevent further progression of the disease with subsequent organ damage and, to the extent possible, to reverse organ dysfunction that has already taken place.

■ GENERAL APPROACH TO TREATMENT

Milder forms of volume depletion may be managed in outpatient settings. For example, supplemental fluids can be added to the usual estimated daily requirements of 30 to 35 mL/kg in patients older than 12 years with dehydration. Commercially available carbohydrate/electrolyte drinks generally are more palatable than water and may promote earlier recovery. The rationale for combining carbohydrates with sodium is based on the cotransport absorption mechanism in the intestinal tract. With diarrheal states in particular, sodium absorption is impaired. Because water follows sodium, the diarrhea is likely to continue despite oral crystalloid fluid administration until the intestinal pathology resolves. However, when dextrose and sodium are combined in 1:1 equimolar amounts, both are absorbed via the cotransport mechanism, which also allows for absorption of water. This concept forms the basis for the World Health Organization's (WHO) oral rehydration solution, which contains 75 mmol/L of dextrose, 75 mmol/L of sodium, 20 mmol/L of potassium, 65 mmol/L of chloride, and 10 mmol/L of citrate for a total osmolarity of 245 mOsm/L.[3] Commercially available over-the-counter rehydration drinks for children in the United States also have an osmolarity of approximately 250 mOsm/L but typically contain 50 mmol/L or less of sodium, and the dextrose-to-sodium ratio often is 3:1. How these differences between commercially available formulations and the WHO rehydration formula might affect hospitalization rates is unclear, but ad hoc attempts to alter the commercially available products to make them more consistent with the WHO formula are not recommended.[3] Improper home mixing of a previous WHO formulation led to cases of hypernatremia.[9] Outpatient rehydration of children usually is recommended for those with uncomplicated (e.g., vomiting less than 48 hours) acute gastroenteritis and relatively mild dehydration after the exclusion of more severe illnesses such as bowel obstruction. ❼ The need for intravenous (IV) rehydration often is overestimated. Randomized studies conducted in pediatric emergency departments have found oral rehydration to be at least as effective as IV rehydration.[10] In one study, children receiving oral rehydration for acute gastroenteritis had shorter lengths of stay than those receiving IV rehydration (225 vs 358 minutes; $P < 0.01$). Furthermore, there was a trend toward decreased hospital admissions in the oral compared with the IV rehydration group (11% vs 25%; $P = 0.2$).[11]

Hospitalization is indicated for more severe forms of circulatory insufficiency. If access to the circulatory system for administration of fluids and medication was not obtained prior to hospitalization, this should be a priority. Venous access generally is obtained during the preliminary examination process that includes the ABCs of life support (i.e., airway, breathing, and circulation), assessment of vital signs and mental status, and determination of urine output after catheterization. Whenever large-volume fluid resuscitation is expected, as in hemorrhagic shock, at least two IV catheters are desirable. Because flow is a function of tubing length and catheter diameter, large-bore peripheral IV lines are preferred over longer central lines. Unfortunately, vascular access in some patients may be problematic, and other routes (e.g., intraosseous infusion in children) may be necessary. One interesting method of fluid administration that has been investigated in elderly patients is subcutaneous infusion, or hypodermoclysis. With hypodermoclysis, common dextrose and sodium-containing fluids typically given by the intravenous route are given by subcutaneous infusion at sites such as the upper arm, chest, abdomen, or thigh, depending on factors such as patient or provider preference. Hyaluronidase has been used as a spreading agent to facilitate fluid absorption by this route, but its benefit versus risk profile has yet to be clearly elucidated; in particular, allergic reactions with this agent have been a concern, although a recombinant form is now available that has the potential for fewer reactions compared to the older bovine-derived products. Hypodermoclysis is not used commonly in the United States, probably because of concerns of adverse effects that were found in early studies that used excessively hypotonic or hypertonic solutions, as well as issues related to reimbursement when considered in ambulatory, home, or palliative care settings. Although relatively high fluid administration rates have been achieved in some studies involving hypodermoclysis, this method of infusion should not be used in patients with more severe forms of dehydration or hypovolemia until additional supportive information from clinical trials is available. Although alternative methods of fluid administration, such as hypodermoclysis, are desirable, well-conducted trials are needed before such methods can be recommended for routine use.

■ PHARMACOLOGIC THERAPY

❽ Dextrose-in-water solutions may be appropriate for uncomplicated dehydration caused by water deprivation, but crystalloid (sodium-containing) solutions should be used for forms of circulatory insufficiency that are associated with hemodynamic instability. In the latter situation, IV solutions with sodium concentrations approximating normal serum sodium values usually are indicated because they cause more expansion of the intravascular and interstitial spaces compared with dextrose solutions (Table 31–3). Lactated Ringer's and normal saline solutions are examples of such crystalloid solutions that frequently need to be administered in large volumes when given to patients with more severe forms of hypovolemia (Table 31–4). A "large" amount of fluid does not mean a single bolus volume typically used as fluid challenge in a critically ill patient. An isolated bolus (e.g., 250–500 mL) in a young adult trauma patient is unlikely to cause a substantial change in blood pressure or acid–base balance.[12] Therefore, multiple fluid boluses usually are often needed in such patients to achieve hemodynamic stability in the perioperative period. On the other hand, overly aggressive fluid administration should be avoided, especially in patients with heart failure or impending pulmonary edema. In a randomized trial involving patients with acute lung injury and radiographic presence of pulmonary edema, a more conservative fluid management strategy led to significantly fewer ventilator-free days and days not spent in an ICU ($P < 0.001$).[13]

The choice between normal saline and lactated Ringer's solutions for hypovolemia is largely based on clinician preference. Traditionally, lactated Ringer's solution has been recommended for patients with hemorrhage because it is unlikely to cause the hyperchloremic metabolic acidosis that is seen with infusions of large volumes of normal saline. More recently, concerns have been raised relative to the proinflammatory effects (e.g., neutrophil

TABLE 31-3 Fluid Distribution and Major Indications[a]

Fluid	Intracellular	Interstitial	Intravascular	Major Indication
Normal saline or lactated Ringer	None	750 mL	250 mL	Intravascular repletion in symptomatic patients
3% sodium chloride	→	750 mL+	250 mL+	Small amounts (e.g., 250 mL) by intermittent infusion have been used in conjunction with normal saline or lactated Ringer for intravascular depletion in patients with head trauma
5% dextrose/0.45% sodium chloride	333 mL	500 mL	167 mL	Maintenance fluid in euvolemic or dehydrated (sodium and water loss) patients with mild signs/symptoms of volume depletion
5% dextrose	667 mL	250 mL	83 mL	Dehydration (primarily water loss) in patients with mild signs/symptoms of volume depletion
5% albumin	None	None	1,000 mL[b]	Intravascular repletion in symptomatic patients
25% albumin	→	→	1,000 mL+++[b]	Usually given by intermittent infusion of small volumes (e.g., 50–100 mL) or by continuous infusion titrated to response in hypovolemic patients with excess interstitial fluid accumulation

[a]Based on administration of 1 L of each solution *for comparative purposes only*. This amount of fluid, particularly for 3% saline and 25% albumin, would be inappropriate and likely harmful if given over a short period of time. Numbers are approximations; arrows indicate direction of fluid shift and plus signs indicate fluid pulled from other compartments.

[b]After distribution and attainment of steady-state conditions, 60% of albumin (and associated fluid) is in interstitial compartment and 40% is in intravascular compartment.

activation) of the L-isomer form of lactate that is contained along with the D-isomer in commercially available racemic isomer solutions. There are advocates for the use of lactated Ringer's solution containing only L-isomer lactate, particularly for more severe forms of hemorrhagic shock, since it avoids the proinflammatory effects of the racemic solution, while avoiding the hyperchloremia associated with normal saline.[14] Additionally, other substitutes for racemic lactate such as ketone or pyruvate have shown beneficial effects on neutrophil activation and gene expression in vitro and are the subject of ongoing studies.

Although lactated Ringer's solution does contain lactate, it does not cause substantial elevations in circulating lactate concentrations when used as a resuscitation solution.[15] Once adequate plasma volume has been restored by fluid administration, the body can readily clear the blood of the excess lactate that has accumulated from both anaerobic metabolism and from lactated Ringer's solution. However, blood samples for lactate determinations drawn through catheters (arterial and venous) that have not been cleared appropriately may have spurious increases or decreases in lactate concentrations because of retained lactated Ringer's and nonlactated solutions (e.g., varying concentrations of dextrose-in-water or sodium chloride), respectively.[16] Therefore, blood samples for lactate concentration determinations should be drawn from a catheter that has been cleared adequately (e.g., 5 mL) of infusate after temporarily stopping the fluid infusion.

A number of pharmacologic therapies show promise in animal models of shock, but few demonstrate success in subsequent trials involving patients with shock. In large part this is a result of the lack of acceptable animal models of shock that mimic the pathophysiology of patients.[17] In cases in which a relevant animal model is available, care must be taken when extrapolating the information to forms of shock other than the one under study. This may be the problem with naloxone, which has been shown to raise blood pressure in some studies of shock but not in others. While research continues on medications or fluids that improve oxygen transport, optimize oxygen utilization, reduce reactive oxygen species and reperfusion injuries, fluids remain the mainstay of therapy, although their use is not devoid of controversy.

Larger-molecular-weight solutions (i.e., >30,000) known as *colloids* have been recommended in conjunction with or as replacements for crystalloid solutions. Examples of colloids used as plasma expanders in the United States include albumin, hydroxyethyl starch, and dextran. Albumin is known as a *monodisperse colloid* because all its molecules are of the same molecular size and weight (~67,000), whereas hydroxyethyl starch and dextran solutions are *polydisperse compounds* with molecules of varying molecular size that are roughly proportional to molecular weight [weight *averaged* molecular weights of 600,000 (range 450,000–800,000) for 6% hetastarch in normal saline 450/0.75, 670,000 (range 450,000–800,000) for 6% hetastarch in lactated electrolyte 670/0.75, 130,000 (range 110,000–150,000) for 6% tetrastarch in normal saline 130/0.4, 40,000 (range 10,000–90,000) for dextran 40, or 70,000 to 75,000 (range 20,000–200,000) for dextran 70 or dextran 75, respectively]. In light of these differences, colloid comparisons are based on weight-averaged [(number of molecules at each weight × particle weight)/total weight of all molecules] or number-averaged (arithmetic mean of all particles' weights) molecular weight.[18] The size and weight differences of the colloids have important implications for the distribution of the products because lower-molecular-weight substances are retained in the intravascular space for a shorter period of time as a result of more rapid leakage across the vessel membrane. The theoretical benefit common to all colloids is based on their increased molecular weight (average molecular weight in the case of hydroxyethyl starch and dextran) that corresponds to increased intravascular retention time in the absence of increased capillary permeability compared with crystalloids. Even in patients with intact capillary permeability, the colloid molecules eventually will leak through the membrane. In the case of albumin with a distribution half-life of 15 hours in normal subjects, approximately 60% of administered albumin molecules (and associated fluid) would be shifted to the interstitial space within 3 to 5 days of exogenous administration. In patients with altered permeability (e.g., acute respiratory distress syndrome), the leakage of albumin from the intravascular to the

TABLE 31-4 Adverse Effects of Plasma Expanders: Crystalloids

Normal saline
  Primarily extensions of pharmacologic actions (e.g., fluid overload, dilutional coagulopathy)
  Hyperchloremic metabolic acidosis (has 154 mEq/L of chloride)
  Hypernatremia (has 154 mEq/L of sodium)
Lactated ringer
  Primarily extensions of pharmacologic actions (e.g., fluid overload, dilutional coagulopathy)
  Hyponatremia (has 130 mEq/L of sodium)
  Aggravation of preexisting hyperkalemia (has 4 mEq/L of potassium)
Hypertonic saline
  Primarily extensions of pharmacologic actions (e.g., fluid overload, dilutional coagulopathy; intracellular volume depletion)
  Hypernatremia (has 513 mEq/L of sodium)
  Hyperchloremia (has 513 mEq/L of chloride)

interstitial space may occur within hours, not days. The primary adverse effect concern of all colloids is fluid overload, which is an extension of their pharmacological action. Another adverse effect of increasing concern is renal dysfunction that seems to be related to hyperoncotic (e.g., 25%) albumin and other starch and dextran products. The mechanism of this adverse effect may be related to alteration of normal glomerular oncotic pressure differences or formation of lesions in the kidney.[19]

Albumin is available in 5% and 25% concentrations. Plasma protein fraction has oncotic actions similar to a 5% albumin solution, which is not surprising because albumin is the predominant protein in this product. When given in equipotent amounts, albumin is much more costly than crystalloid solutions. Additionally, the 5% and 25% albumin solutions typically are priced such that no cost-savings is associated with dilution of the 25% product to make a 5% concentration. In general, dilution should be avoided because of the possibility of preparation errors; cases of hemolysis and death have occurred when 25% albumin was inappropriately diluted with sterile water for injection, causing a dramatic lowering of effective osmolarity. The 5% albumin solution is relatively *isooncotic,* which means that it does not pull fluid into the compartment in which it is contained. In contrast, 25% albumin is referred to as *hyperoncotic* albumin because it tends to pull fluid into the compartment containing the albumin molecules. In general, the 5% albumin solution is used for hypovolemic states. The 25% solution should not be used for acute circulatory insufficiency unless it is used in combination with other fluids or it is being used in patients with excess total body water but intravascular depletion as a means of pulling fluid into the intravascular space. An example of the latter condition is cirrhosis with ascites in which total body water is substantially increased, but the patient is hypotensive as a consequence of lack of intravascular volume. To justify this use of hyperoncotic albumin from a cost-effectiveness standpoint presumes that there is evidence of adverse effects associated with the excess water (e.g., interstitial fluid accumulation in the lungs) and that the albumin remains in the intravascular space long enough to be of benefit. Albumin has a variety of functions beyond plasma expansion, such as binding properties, inflammatory gene modification, and antioxidant and free radical scavenging effects, which have been used to justify its administration instead of less expensive crystalloid or other colloid products. Although appealing theoretically, improved patient outcomes related to these properties have not been documented in adequately powered, randomized, controlled trials. Additionally, the clinician must realize that the properties of commercially available albumin products are not biologically identical to those of native albumin. For example, denaturation of the products may lead to inefficient binding and decreased oncotic activity.

Hydroxyethyl starch products have been developed as synthetic alternatives to albumin that is derived through the fractionation of donated human blood. The various products are differentiated by two numbers, one for the average mean molecular weight and one for the degree of hydroxyethyl substitution of glucose. For example, hetastarch is expressed as 450/0.7 based on weight and substitution, respectively. Most of the trials comparing albumin with hydroxyethyl starch products for volume expansion have found no significant differences in clinically important outcomes (e.g., mortality). Few trials have directly compared hydroxyethyl starch products with crystalloid solutions for intravascular expansion. Although hydroxyethyl starch products often are stated as being contraindicated in bleeding disorders, they have been most studied in patients with blood loss (e.g., trauma and perioperative patients). Hydroxyethyl starch should be avoided in situations where short-term impairments in hemostasis could have dire consequences, such as in patients undergoing cardiopulmonary bypass surgery and patients with intracranial bleeding. Hydroxyethyl starch may aggravate bleeding

through mechanisms specific to this colloid (e.g., decreased factor VIII/von Willebrand factor). These mechanisms have not been well elucidated and often are difficult to distinguish from the dilutional effects on clotting factors caused by all plasma expanders; however, the risk of coagulopathy appears to be related to increasing starch substitution (greater than 0.4), and increasing doses and durations of administration.[20] Renal dysfunction associated with hydroxyethyl starch products may also be a function of starch substitution and high doses. In a study comparing a pentastarch (200/0.5) to a crystalloid solution for severe sepsis, the cumulative dose of the starch product was associated with an increased need for renal replacement therapy ($P < 0.001$) and a higher 90-day mortality ($P = 0.001$).[21] Hydroxyethyl starch may cause elevations in serum amylase concentrations but does not cause pancreatitis.

Dextran 40, dextran 70, and dextran 75 are available for use as plasma expanders in the United States. The numbers refer to the average molecular weight of the solutions. In general, dextran solutions are not used as often as albumin or hydroxyethyl starch products for plasma expansion, possibly because of concerns related to aggravation of bleeding (i.e., anticoagulant actions related to inhibiting stasis of microcirculation) and anaphylaxis that is more likely to occur with the higher-molecular-weight solutions. However, both of these concerns can be reduced if proper attention is paid to patient selection and, in the case of bleeding, published dosing guidelines with regard to the amounts of these products that should be infused. There are few comparative trials involving the dextran solutions, but the intravascular expansion within hours after infusion is approximately equal to the amount of dextran infused.

The crystalloid versus colloid debate was intensified when a meta-analysis by the well-respected Cochrane group found an overall increase in mortality associated with albumin using pooled results of randomized investigations.[22] The meta-analysis involved 30 randomized trials with 1,419 patients (relative risk of death with albumin vs no administration or crystalloid administration, 1.68; 95% confidence interval [CI], 1.26–2.23). For hypovolemia (caused by blood loss in the majority of studies), the risk of death associated with albumin administration was not quite statistically significant (relative risk, 1.46; 95% CI, 0.97–2.22). With the notable exception of trauma patients, a subsequent and more comprehensive systematic review did not find increased mortality attributable to albumin.[23] Furthermore, a landmark investigation involving almost 7,000 critically ill patients (conducted after the previously mentioned meta-analyses) did not find statistically significant differences in 28-day mortality between patients resuscitated with either normal saline or 4% albumin.[24] As in the previous meta-analysis, there was a trend toward increased mortality in patients with trauma, which became statistically significant ($P = 0.003$) when analyzed at 24 months in a subset of patients with traumatic brain injury.[25] This multicenter, randomized, double-blind investigation, referred to as the Saline versus Albumin Fluid Evaluation (SAFE) study, involved a heterogeneous group of ICU patients and was not sufficiently powered to look at various subsets, so clinicians must be cautious when extrapolating the results to more specific patient populations. With this caution in mind, this trial provides strong evidence that crystalloid solutions should be considered first-line therapy in patients with hypovolemic shock, particularly in the United States where cost differences between crystalloids and colloids are substantial.

■ SPECIAL POPULATIONS

Trauma/Perioperative Patients

The need for immediate treatment of hemorrhagic circulatory insufficiency with plasma expanders (i.e., crystalloids or colloids) seems obvious, but no large, well-controlled trials conducted in humans have supported this practice. To the contrary, evidence suggests that fluid resuscitation beyond minimal levels (i.e., mean arterial pressure >40–60 mm Hg) is harmful in patients with penetrating abdominal trauma due to hemodilution and clot destabilization. One prospective study involving 598 adult patients with gunshot or stab wound injuries to the torso and systolic blood pressure measurements of 90 mm Hg or less found that delayed fluid resuscitation until operation was associated with increased survival and discharge from the hospital ($P = 0.04$).[26] Since concerns were expressed about the comparability of the immediate and delayed resuscitation groups, particularly because true randomization did not take place, a follow-up randomized trial was conducted to verify the findings. There were no differences in survival (four deaths in each group) in the second trial regardless of whether systolic blood pressure was titrated to >100 mm Hg or to 70 mm Hg.[27] Both studies were conducted in populated urban areas with approximately 2 hours from the time of injury to operation. Therefore, the results may not be applicable to rural areas with extended transport times. There also is a concern in applying the results of these investigations to patients with certain kinds of single-system injuries, particularly head trauma, where cerebral perfusion pressure is of primary importance. Although the applicability of these studies to other populations and settings is debatable, the *presumption* of benefits from immediate plasma expansion in all preoperative patients with circulatory insufficiency caused by hemorrhage is no longer valid. Instead, the initial priority should be surgical control of the bleeding source; until this is possible, fluids should be given in small aliquots to yield a palpable pulse and to maintain mean pressures no more than 60 mm Hg and systolic pressures no more than 90 mm Hg based on accurate measurements (e.g., arterial monitoring).

CLINICAL CONTROVERSY

Some clinicians believe that hypertonic solutions should be used to lower intracranial pressure in patients with head injuries.

By causing redistribution (i.e., pulling fluid) from the intracellular space, hypertonic solutions cause rapid expansion of the intravascular compartment, which is essential for vital organ perfusion. In head-injured patients, it has been postulated that this redistribution should decrease intracranial pressure because the vessels of the brain are more impermeable to sodium ions than are vessels in other areas of the body. Additionally, hypertonic saline solutions have beneficial immunomodulating actions when compared with more isotonic solutions in experiments with animals, although these actions have not always translated into similar beneficial effects in patients.[28]

Potential dosing and administration errors and related adverse events can occur when hypertonic saline is ordered and administered by clinicians relatively unfamiliar with its use. Potential adverse events include cellular crenation and damage caused by the dramatic fluid shifts associated with hypernatremia, hyperchloremic metabolic acidosis from hyperchloremia, and peripheral vein destruction from high osmolality. In the limited number of studies conducted in humans to date, such adverse effects have been uncommon and apparently of little clinical importance.[29,30]

Unfortunately, beneficial outcome data attributable to administration of these hypertonic solutions are lacking. Most of these studies were conducted in prehospital and emergency department settings using 250 mL of 7.5% sodium chloride with or without 6% dextran 70. A meta-analysis of randomized, controlled trials found no statistical difference between the survival rates of patients

receiving the hypertonic saline solutions and those receiving standard isotonic crystalloid solutions.[31] Additionally, a subsequent double-blind, randomized controlled trial involving 229 patients with hypotension and severe brain injury demonstrated no significant differences in neurologic function at 6 months when 250 mL of 7.5% saline or lactated Ringer's solution was administered as part of a prehospital resuscitation regimen.[32] Part of the explanation for this finding may be related to supplemental crystalloid fluids that were given routinely to patients in both the treatment and control groups, which probably would increase the number of patients needed to demonstrate a statistically significant difference in mortality. It is interesting to note that the hypertonic saline solutions in such prehospital trials appear to have been administered by peripheral veins, despite their very high osmolality. This is deserving of further investigation since intravenous solutions with osmolality values above 600 to 1,200 mOsm/kg (the high end for some peripheral parenteral nutrition solutions) are usually administered through central catheters. For example, the osmolality of 3% sodium chloride is 1,026 mOsm/kg and it is typically recommended for central line administration.

In order to address ongoing questions of efficacy, the National Heart, Lung, and Blood Institute evaluated hypertonic saline for traumo patients with shock and severe traumatic brain injury. These two trials were conducted by a network of sites known as the Resuscitation Outcomes Consortium (ROC). The parallel trials were both stopped when it was determined that hypertonic saline was no better than normal saline and further enrollment would not change the 33 outcomes.[33] Therefore, normal saline is the fluid of choice when a hypertonic solution is desirable because it contains 154 mmol/L of both sodium and chloride. Given their relatively poor intravascular expansion and association with poor outcome in animal models of closed head injury, hypotonic solutions should be avoided in this population.[34]

In addition to crystalloid solutions, colloids have been used for plasma expansion in patients with perioperative circulatory insufficiency. In the United States, albumin and starch (i.e., hydroxyethyl starch) derivatives are used most commonly, although dextran solutions also are available commercially.

CLINICAL CONTROVERSY

Some clinicians believe that colloid solutions have advantages beyond crystalloid solutions that justify their use for patients with hypovolemic shock.

The major theoretical advantage of these compounds is their prolonged intravascular retention time compared with crystalloid solutions. In contrast to isotonic crystalloid solutions that have substantial interstitial distribution within minutes of IV administration, colloids remain in the intravascular space for hours or days, depending on factors such as capillary permeability.

The colloids, particularly albumin, are expensive solutions. Therefore, it is difficult to justify the additional cost of colloidal products unless the benefit-to-risk ratio is substantially greater than that associated with inexpensive crystalloid solutions. This does not appear to be the case based on randomized, controlled studies and meta-analyses comparing colloid and crystalloid solutions for acute circulatory insufficiency. Because other colloids, such as hydroxyethyl starch, almost always have been compared with albumin and not with crystalloid solutions in published clinical studies (with no clinically important differences found), there is no reason to suspect that these other colloids have any unique advantages as volume expanders. Adverse effects associated with colloids appear to be

TABLE 31-5 Adverse Effects of Plasma Expanders: Colloids

Albumin
  Primarily extensions of pharmacologic actions (e.g., fluid overload; dilutional coagulopathy)
  Amino acid profile and catabolism alterations (clinical significance?); potential protein overload if given with exogenous protein (e.g., parenteral nutrition)
  Anaphylactoid/anaphylaxis reactions (life-threatening reactions rare; higher in patients with immunoglobulin A deficiency)
  Infectious complications (all reported cases have been associated with improper handling by manufacturer or institution; no reported cases of human immunodeficiency virus or hepatitis transmission)
  Interactions with medications and nutrients (clinical significance varies)
  Metal loading, particularly aluminum (long-term administration in patients with renal failure)
  Negative inotropic effect; reductions in ionized calcium concentrations (not well documented)
  Pyrogenic reactions (not well documented)
  Renal dysfunction with hyperoncotic albumin
Hydroxyethylstarch
  Primarily extensions of pharmacologic actions (e.g., fluid overload, dilutional coagulopathy)
  Bleeding (decreases factor VIII/C activity; not recommended in patients at high risk for bleeding or in patients with severe bleeding conditions such as subarachnoid hemorrhage)
  Macroamylase formation may cause elevation in blood amylase that leads to inaccurate diagnosis of pancreatitis
  Anaphylactoid/anaphylaxis reactions
  Pruritus (particularly when large amounts are given; may take months to resolve)
  Renal dysfunction
Dextrans
  Primarily extensions of pharmacologic actions (e.g., fluid overload, dilutional coagulopathy)
  Anaphylactoid/anaphylaxis reactions (increased incidence of anaphylaxis with increased molecular weight)
  Bleeding (sometimes used for anticoagulant activity, so not recommended for patients with severe bleeding)
  Renal dysfunction

TABLE 31-6 General Indications for Blood Products in Acute Circulatory Insufficiency Due to Hemorrhage[a]

Packed red blood cells
  Increase oxygen-carrying capacity of blood: Usually indicated in patients with continued deterioration after volume replacement or obvious exsanguination; must be warmed, particularly when used in children
Fresh-frozen plasma
  Replacement of clotting factors: Generally overused; indicated if ongoing hemorrhage in patients with PT/PTT >1.5 times normal, severe hepatic disease, or other bleeding diathesis
Platelets
Used for bleeding due to severe thrombocytopenia (i.e., platelet count <10,000 mcL) or rapidly dropping platelet counts as would occur with massive bleeding
Other products
  With the exception of recombinant activated factor VII, which is currently undergoing trials for use in life-threatening hemorrhage unresponsive to traditional blood product administration, components such as cryoprecipitate and factor VIII are generally not indicated in acute hemorrhage but rather are used after specific deficiencies are identified

[a]Although whole blood can be used for large-volume blood loss, most hospitals use component therapy, and use crystalloids or colloids for plasma expansion. PT, prothrombin time; PTT, partial thromboplastin time.

uncommon and generally are extensions of their pharmacologic activity (Table 31–5), but this is also true of crystalloids. The benefit-to-risk ratio appears to be similar for colloids and crystalloids; thus, based on cost, crystalloids are preferred for initial treatment of circulatory insufficiency in patients with hemorrhagic shock.

The preceding discussion dealt primarily with acute circulatory insufficiency, but there are other considerations with regard to fluid replacement in elective surgical procedures. Preoperative fluid deficits in patients undergoing minor procedures may be associated with increased perioperative morbidity, some of which (e.g., drowsiness, dizziness) may be reduced by appropriate fluid administration prior to surgery.[35] However, care must be taken to avoid overhydration in the perioperative period because excess fluid will lead to weight gain and decreased pulmonary function. Some evidence suggests that fluid restriction on the day of surgery may reduce postoperative morbidity in patients undergoing major surgical procedures. In one randomized, multicenter trial, use of a restricted intraoperative and postoperative IV fluid protocol led to significantly fewer cardiopulmonary (7% vs 24%; $P = 0.007$) and wound (16% vs 31%; $P = 0.04$) complications.[36] As the preceding discussion indicates, the benefits and risks of fluid administration in the perioperative period are not just a function of too little or too much fluid but involve other patient- and procedure-related issues.

Another consideration in the patient with penetrating injuries or surgery is the potential need for blood product administration (Table 31–6) to replace oxygen-carrying and clotting functions. Although a small group of trauma patients respond to the initial fluid bolus and remain stable, most patients respond initially and then deteriorate. The latter patients, as well as patients undergoing blood loss associated with surgery, frequently need blood components such as packed red blood cells. ❾ In the case of the latter component, red blood cells contain hemoglobin that delivers oxygen to tissues. Neither crystalloids nor colloids perform this function.

Administration of excessive blood products may be counterproductive. In the case of red blood cells, attempts to raise the hematocrit to high–normal or supranormal concentrations may decrease oxygen delivery by increasing blood viscosity. Additionally, there are immunomodulatory concerns with red blood cell administration. Although there is no optimal hematocrit value for all patients, a minimum hematocrit concentration of 30% (equivalent to a hemoglobin concentration of 10 gm/dL) traditionally has been used as the threshold for transfusion, particularly in patients at risk for ischemia, such as those with CAD. Use of a more liberal transfusion strategy has been curtailed in many institutions with the publication of a randomized, multicenter trial involving critically ill patients that found 30-day mortality to be similar whether patients were transfused at a hemoglobin concentration less than 7 or 10 g/dL (18.7% vs 23.3%, respectively; $P = 0.11$).[37] The mortality during hospitalization was significantly lower in the restrictive group (22.2% vs 28.1%; $P = 0.05$). Although the investigators were cautious about extrapolating the results of this investigation to patients with myocardial ischemia, the study does question the use of a liberal transfusion strategy for critically ill patients.

Blood products have risks beyond immunomodulation. There is the rare but important risk of virus transmission [e.g., human immunodeficiency virus (HIV), hepatitis]. Citrate that is added to stored blood to prevent coagulation may bind to calcium, resulting in hypocalcemia, although potassium and phosphate concentrations often are elevated in stored blood, particularly when hemolysis has occurred during storage. In patients receiving large amounts of blood, prophylactic calcium administration may be warranted until levels are available. Other issues that must be considered with blood product administration include monitoring for transfusion-related reactions and attention to appropriate warming, particularly when large volumes are given to pediatric patients, because hypothermia is associated with increased fluid requirements and mortality.

Since its commercial release in the United States, recombinant factor VIIa has been used for a variety of off-label uses related to trauma and bleeding. For example, in patients with massive blood loss a cocktail of cryoprecipitate, platelets, and recombinant factor

VIIa has been suggested to rapidly attain hemostasis.[38] These more severe forms of blood loss are not only a function of the type of injury but also factors such as medications (e.g., aspirin, coumadin, clopidogrel, enoxaparin) and disease states that impair normal coagulation. Large well-controlled trials are needed to define the role of recombinant factor VIIa in clinical practice given its high cost and potential thromboembolic complications. There are specific concerns with its use in trauma patients related to subpopulations most likely to see benefit since there are issues related to appropriate dose, timing, and diminished effectiveness in patients with acidosis and severe hypothermia. A large randomized controlled trial involving patients with penetrating and blunt trauma is currently underway that should help to resolve many of these concerns.[39]

The periodic shortages, high costs, and adverse effect concerns related to blood products have prompted investigations of alternative "bloodless" strategies. In addition to the use of more restrictive transfusion thresholds, as mentioned previously, these strategies have included hemoglobin-based oxygen carriers and perfluorocarbon compounds to deliver oxygen to tissues. Other strategies have aimed at reducing blood loss through the use of improved procedural and surgical techniques, as well as the administration of hemostatic medications.

Patients with Thermal Injuries

There are a number of formulas for estimating fluid requirements in thermally injured patients, but there is little reason to choose one over another based on well-controlled studies. In general, the amount of loss corresponds to the size of the thermal injury. Guidelines recommend approximately 2 to 4 mL/kg of isotonic fluid (lactated Ringer's solution) for each percent burn can be used for calculating the expected fluid requirements for the first 24 hours after the burn.[40] For example, a 60-kg person with 30% body surface area (BSA) burns is expected to require 5,400 to 7,200 mL of fluid over the initial 24 hours. Regardless of the calculated deficit, fluids should be administered until adequate tissue perfusion has been documented (e.g., maintenance of urine output of 0.5–1 mL/kg in adults) or adverse effects (e.g., pulmonary edema) occur. Crystalloids are preferred as initial therapy for burn victims because there is no substantial evidence that colloids mobilize edematous fluid, and there is a theoretical concern that extravascular fluid accumulation might be prolonged by the oncotic actions of albumin and other colloid products that have leaked through vessel walls.[41] Additionally, there is no evidence that colloids reduce mortality in patients with thermal injuries. Some novel therapies for thermal resuscitation have been studied, although larger confirmatory trials are needed prior to use apart from research protocols. For example, in a prospective study involving patients with >30% BSA burns, antioxidant therapy with extremely high doses on IV vitamin C (66 mg/kg/h for 24 hours) reduced resuscitation fluid requirements and wound edema.[42] The proposed mechanism is reduction in free radical–induced increases in capillary permeability.

CLINICAL CONTROVERSY

The appropriate use of invasive hemodynamic monitoring tools, such as right-sided heart catheterization in patients with hypovolemic shock, is controversial.

◼ ONGOING MONITORING

One form of monitoring that may take place in the emergency and operating rooms, as well as in the ICU, requires placement of a central venous pressure (CVP) line. Monitoring of CVP provides the clinician with a somewhat insensitive yet useful estimate of the relationship between increased right atrial pressure and cardiac output. A protocol that used a particular type of central catheter to perform continuous monitoring of central venous oxygen saturation in conjunction with so-called goal-directed therapy in the first 6 hours of patient arrival in an urban emergency department resulted in decreased mortality compared with standard monitoring (30.5% vs 46.5%; $P = 0.009$).[43] However, the patients in this study had severe sepsis and septic shock, so the results might not be applicable to other forms of shock with different pathophysiologic considerations. For example, in hemorrhagic shock due to trauma, the most important intervention is surgical control of bleeding, and anything that delays this control is likely to increase, not decrease, mortality. Until additional studies have been performed, it would be premature to mandate goal-directed therapy with the associated central venous monitoring in patients with nonseptic forms of shock, particularly shock due to blood loss. In fact, so-called "upstream" measurements of perfusion such as CVP are not a useful guide for fluid management in hospitalized patients,[44] and are being replaced by "downstream" markers such as urine output and lactate levels that are more likely to reflect end-organ dysfunction.[45] A more complete discussion of invasive and noninvasive hemodynamic monitoring is given in Chapter 30.

A number of laboratory tests are indicated for subacute monitoring of shock in the ICU setting. These include a renal battery for assessing possible electrolyte alterations and kidney perfusion (e.g., BUN and creatinine). Among other things, a complete blood count will enable assessment of possible infection (white blood cell count), oxygen-carrying capacity of the blood (hemoglobin, hematocrit), and ongoing bleeding (hemoglobin, hematocrit, and platelet count). The prothrombin time or international normalized ratio and partial thromboplastin time will give an indication of the ability of the blood to clot because, in the case of hemorrhagic shock, clotting factors are lost and diluted. An increasing lactate concentration (arterial, mixed venous, or central venous), an increasing arterial base deficit, or a decreasing bicarbonate concentration are global markers indicative of inadequate perfusion leading to anaerobic metabolism with accumulation of lactic acid. Although the value of these surrogate markers for improving patient outcomes is more controversial, they are considered traditional end points of resuscitation in certain populations such as trauma patients.[46] Other tests may be indicated if organ dysfunction is likely. For example, when blood flow to the liver is interrupted because of sustained hypotension, a condition known as *shock liver* may occur. In this condition, the levels of transaminases on a liver panel may be markedly elevated in the first couple of days after marked hypotension, although the concentrations should decrease over time.[4] Along with laboratory testing, a more extensive history can be obtained during the subacute monitoring period.

The value of pulmonary artery catheters (also known as right-sided heart or Swan-Ganz catheters) has been debated hotly since their introduction. Such catheters are placed to obtain various oxygen-transport variables, some of which cannot be determined reliably from peripheral or other central vessels. The debate was intensified when early studies suggested improved outcomes when cardiac output and other oxygen-transport variables were raised to supranormal levels, the monitoring of which required placement of a pulmonary artery catheter. Subsequent studies using similar monitoring parameters associated with pulmonary artery catheterization gave conflicting results.[47]

The controversy led to consensus conferences and workshops, the development of organizational guidelines, and the publication of a meta-analysis (which found a statistically significant reduction in *morbidity* using pulmonary artery catheters to guide therapy).[48] Ultimately, a large randomized, controlled trial involving pulmonary artery catheters was conducted in high-risk surgical patients.[49]

The trial involved 1,994 patients. The mortality was almost identical for the catheter and control groups (7.8% vs 7.7%; 95% CI, 2.3–2.5). There were no episodes of pulmonary embolism in the catheter group and eight episodes in the control group (P = 0.004). This trial is important not only because of the implications for high-risk surgical patients but also because it allows for the conduct of future trials in other patient populations without some of the ethical issues raised about such trials in the past.

Part of the concern regarding pulmonary artery catheterization relates to interpretation of its results by inexperienced practitioners. Studies in Europe and the United States found that one of two physicians incorrectly interpreted a tracing from a pulmonary artery catheter.[50] This could explain some of the results of studies finding no benefits to pulmonary artery catheterization or, in some cases, worse outcomes in the pulmonary artery catheterization group by actions taken as a result of inaccurate measurements or misinterpretation of information obtained from the monitoring process.

Complications related to pulmonary artery catheter insertion, maintenance, and removal include damage to vessels and organs during insertion, arrhythmias, infections, and thromboembolic damage. To avoid the complications associated with pulmonary artery catheterization, other less invasive tools were developed to obtain similar information. For example, cardiac output determinations have been made by Doppler, bioimpedance, dye, and ionic dilution techniques, although such measurements would not provide other data that are obtained routinely with pulmonary artery catheters (e.g., left-sided heart filling pressure). Additionally, advances in pulmonary artery catheter technology that expand the information obtained from such monitoring (e.g., mixed venous oxyhemoglobin) are under investigation. However, given the lack of well-defined outcome data associated with pulmonary artery catheterization, its use is best reserved for complicated cases of shock not responding to conventional fluid and medication therapies.

Commonly measured and calculated hemodynamic and oxygen-transport indices associated with invasive monitoring are primarily global indicators of tissue perfusion. Attempts have been made to find regional and local indicators of hypoperfusion so that circulatory insufficiency could be treated before overt shock occurs. One focus of recent research has been monitoring modalities involving the gastrointestinal tract.

Although the literature is fairly consistent concerning low gastric intramucosal pH (pHi) values being predictive of death, pHi-guided therapy to decrease mortality has not been demonstrated.[51] Additionally, a number of technical considerations remain to be resolved when using pHi or, more recently, capnometry (luminal P_{CO_2} tonometry) for monitoring and therapy. Despite these concerns, measures of regional tissue oxygenation continue to be investigated through a variety of novel monitoring techniques.

In addition to regional monitoring of tissue perfusion, local methods of monitoring are being studied. For example, subcutaneous measurement of tissue oxygen pressure shows promise in preliminary investigations. Regional and local measurements likely will not replace more global indicators of perfusion; rather, the methods will complement each other.

■ ONGOING MANAGEMENT

Proper attention to plasma expansion must be continued into the intraoperative and postoperative periods. A number of neurohormonal changes take place that affect urine output, and patients may have substantial third spacing of fluid depending on the operation and preexisting conditions. Furthermore, postoperative patients are prone to hyponatremia from renal generation of electrolyte-free water and from antidiuretic hormone release.[52] As in acute resuscitation, the administration of hypotonic solutions in the

perioperative period does not prevent the decrease in extracellular volume that often occurs. Therefore, although excess fluid administration is to be avoided in the perioperative setting, isotonic crystalloid solutions should be used when fluids are indicated to prevent intravascular depletion and circulatory insufficiency. There is general agreement that the choice of crystalloid solution in the perioperative period should be either normal saline or a lactated Ringer's (or equivalent) solution. However, there is substantial debate as to which of these two solutions is preferable since comparative studies have involved small numbers of patients.[53]

Of the randomized studies comparing albumin with crystalloid solutions in the perioperative period, the majority found no statistically significant differences between groups.[54] Any significant differences found involved isolated hemodynamic or respiratory variables with no obvious clinical correlates (e.g., duration of mechanical ventilation). Therefore, albumin and other colloids cannot be recommended for the prevention or initial treatment of circulatory insufficiency, although their use may be appropriate in patients who are not responding to crystalloids and are developing problems such as interstitial fluid accumulation. Practice guidelines published by a consortium of academic medical centers reflect this recommendation, but colloids continue to be used widely.[55]

In contrast to many other forms of shock, medications are not indicated in the initial therapy of hypovolemic shock but rather play an adjunctive role in patients who continue to have circulatory insufficiency after fluids have been maximized and volume overload concerns exist.[56] In a multicenter cohort study of blunt-injured patients with hemorrhagic shock, the use of vasopressors within 12 hours of injury was associated with significantly higher mortality at 24 hours (P = 0.001).[57] With hypovolemia, the body's natural response is to increase cardiac output and to constrict blood vessels to maintain blood pressure. There is no evidence that vasoactive medications improve outcome in patients with hypovolemic shock assuming that fluid therapy is adequate. ❿ However, once the cause of acute circulatory insufficiency has been stopped or treated and fluids have been optimized, some patients continue to have signs and symptoms of inadequate tissue perfusion. This may be caused by reperfusion injury. Although the search for a cryptogenic source (e.g., intraabdominal bleeding in a trauma patient) should continue, the clinician may need to administer vasoactive medications to improve perfusion.

Pressor agents such as norepinephrine and high-dose dopamine are to be avoided, if possible, because they may increase blood pressure at the expense of peripheral tissue ischemia. Some sources use stronger language and state that vasopressors are contraindicated in certain forms of shock (e.g., hemorrhagic). This does not help the clinician who is treating a patient with unstable blood pressure despite massive fluid replacement and increasing interstitial fluid accumulation. In such situations, inotropic agents such as dobutamine are preferred if blood pressure is adequate (e.g., systolic blood pressure ≥80–90 mm Hg) because they should not aggravate the existing vasoconstriction. The inotropic agents are justified by presumed inadequate cardiac output for the specific situation, although the measured values may be in the normal range.

When pressure cannot be maintained with inotropic agents or when inotropic agents with vasodilatory properties cannot be used because of inadequate blood pressure concerns, pressors may be required as a last resort. In general, the need for pressors is predictive of the development of MODS and increased length of hospital stay.[58] Although the response to pressor agents may be variable in hypovolemic shock, there does not appear to be resistance as a consequence of altered receptor response, as is sometimes seen in patients with septic shock.[4] Potent vasoconstrictors such as norepinephrine and phenylephrine should be given through central veins because of the possibility of extravasation and necrosis with peripheral administration.

In managing patients with hypovolemic shock, the clinician must be aware of potential adverse effects of medications being used for supportive care purposes. For example, some patients are particularly susceptible to the histamine release associated with morphine and may have substantial decreases in blood pressure. Sodium bicarbonate would seem to be a logical therapy in patients with shock who typically have a metabolic acidosis, but bicarbonate administration has not been shown to improve surrogate hemodynamic markers or patient outcomes and has known disadvantages such as the associated increase in arterial carbon dioxide levels and decrease in serum ionized calcium levels.[59] Propofol is commonly used for sedation in the ICU, but it may cause substantial decreases in blood pressure. The initial dose of propofol probably should be decreased by at least 50% in patients with hemorrhagic shock who have recently been resuscitated and by at least 80% (if it is given at all) in patients who may not be fully resuscitated.[60]

A number of interesting treatments for shock are under investigation, including autotransfusion for removing harmful cytokines from the body. Various alternatives to conventional blood components also are being studied, such as stroma-free hemoglobin and perfluorocarbon compounds, as virus-free alternatives to red blood cell transfusion. Hopefully, these methods will be useful adjuncts to adequate volume replacement, which is the primary therapeutic intervention in managing acute circulatory insufficiency as a result of volume depletion.

PHARMACOECONOMIC CONSIDERATIONS

The primary therapy for hypovolemic shock is fluid replacement. The institutional cost of 1 L of most crystalloid solutions is less than $1. Assuming that such fluids are used, the associated costs of personnel and equipment then become the primary economic considerations in the resuscitation of patients with hypovolemic shock. However, as mentioned, many clinicians recommend that colloid plasma expanders (e.g., albumin, hydroxyethyl starch, or dextrans) be used to replace some or all of the standard crystalloid solutions. Although the costs of these solutions vary, depending on contractual arrangements, as might occur with purchasing groups, in general, albumin solutions are more expensive than hydroxyethyl starch and dextran products. All these solutions are markedly more costly than crystalloid solutions; in some cases, the differences are 50- to 100-fold, even when used in equipotent amounts.

The only trial that investigated albumin use on a large-scale basis was an observational study involving 15 academic medical centers in the United States. Based on previously published guidelines, 62%

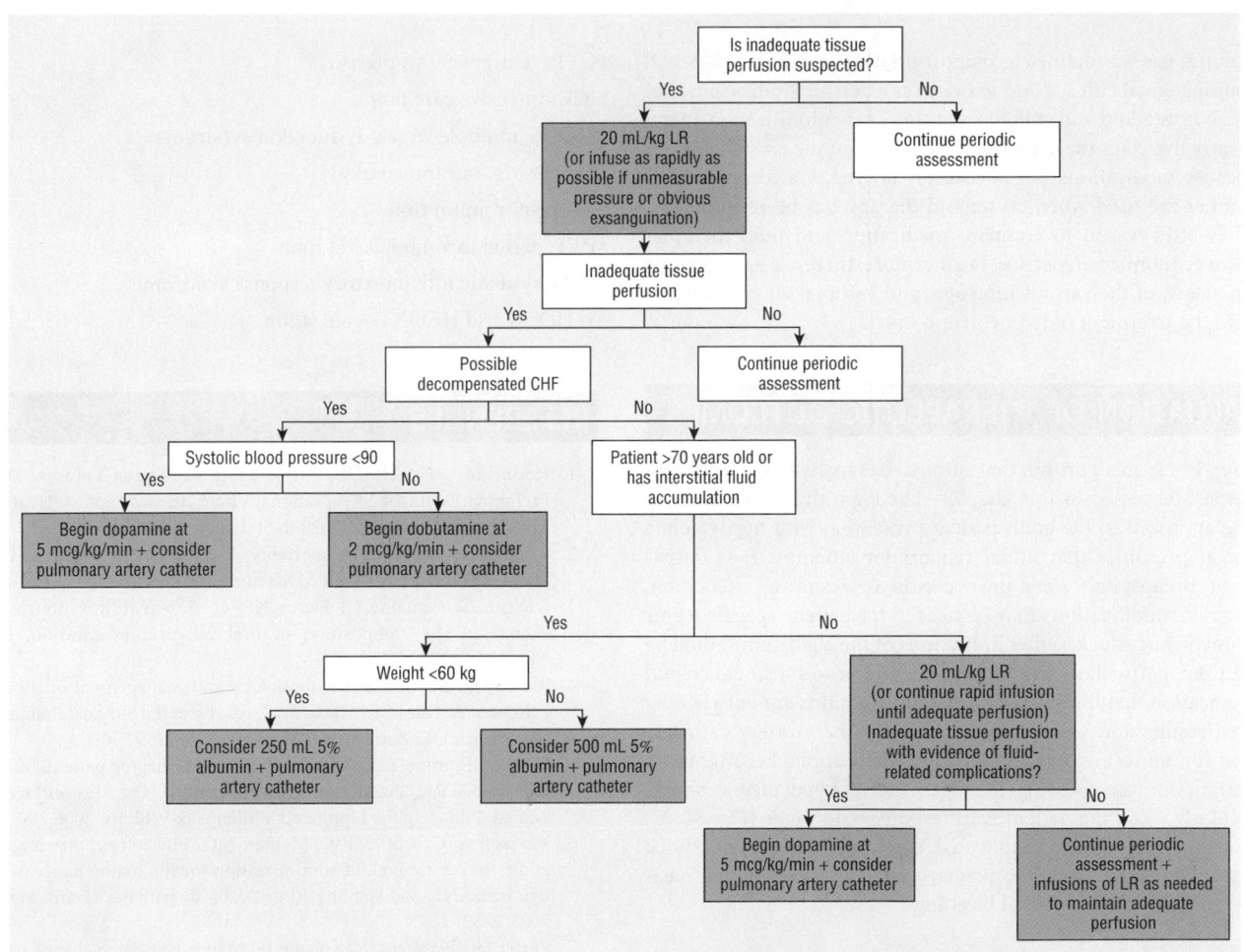

FIGURE 31-4. Hypovolemia protocol for adults. This protocol is not intended to replace or delay therapies such as surgical intervention or blood products for restoring oxygen-carrying capacity or hemostasis. If available, some measurements can be used in addition to those listed in the algorithm, such as mean arterial pressure or pulmonary artery catheter recordings. The latter can be used to assist in medication choices (e.g., agents with primary pressor effects may be desirable in patients with normal cardiac outputs, whereas dopamine or dobutamine may be indicated in patients with suboptimal cardiac outputs). Lower maximal doses of the medications in this algorithm should be considered when pulmonary artery catheterization is not available. Colloids that can be substituted for albumin are hydroxyethyl starch 6% and dextran 40. See text for an in-depth discussion of these and other issues involved in this protocol. (CHF, congestive heart failure; LR, lactated Ringer's solution.)

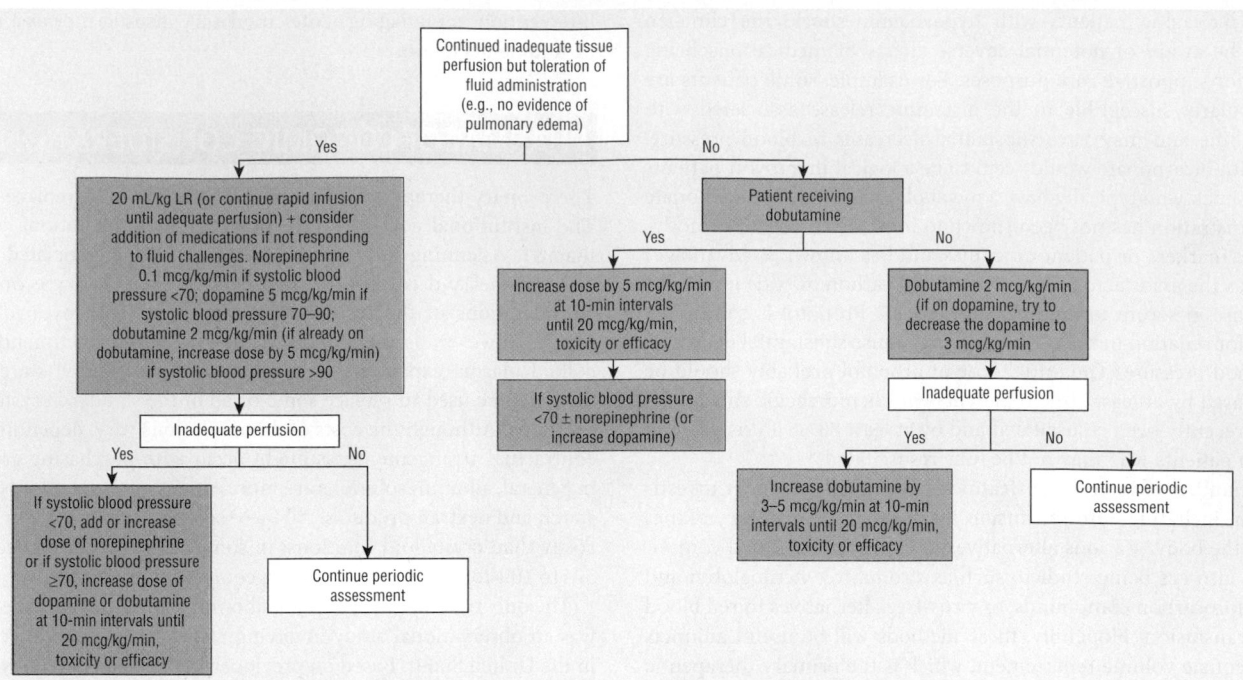

FIGURE 31-5. Ongoing management of inadequate tissue perfusion. (LR, lactated Ringer's solution.)

of albumin use was defined as inappropriate, at a cost of $124,939.[61] Presuming equal efficacy and toxicity (as available studies indicate) between crystalloid and colloid solutions, cost-minimization analysis clearly indicates the economic advantages of the crystalloids.

Because medications are not simply alternatives to crystalloids but rather are used when crystalloid therapy has been optimized, there is little reason to compare medication and fluid therapies from an economic perspective. Furthermore, there are no economic comparisons of the various inotropic and vasopressor medications used in the treatment of hypovolemic shock.

EVALUATION OF THERAPEUTIC OUTCOMES

Figure 31–4 is an algorithm that summarizes many of the treatment principles discussed in this chapter. The algorithm is an example of one approach to the adult patient presenting with hypovolemic shock. It presumes that initial rehydration attempts (i.e., outpatient or prehospital) were unsuccessful in restoring circulation. Obviously, modifications may be needed for patient-specific forms of hypovolemic shock. Other limitations of the algorithm should be recognized, particularly the decisions to add or to substitute colloid or medication therapies when crystalloid solutions are not yielding desired results and when to perform pulmonary artery catheterization for more invasive monitoring. Medications become more important for the ongoing management of hypovolemic shock, particularly when the patient is unresponsive to fluids (Fig. 31–5). Medications for more complicated cases of hemorrhagic shock should not detract from the primary effective resuscitative measure—surgical stabilization of bleeding.

ABBREVIATIONS

BSA: body surface area

CAD: coronary artery disease

CDC: Centers for Disease Control and Prevention

CVP: central venous pressure

ICU: intensive care unit

MODS: multiple-organ dysfunction syndrome

pHi: gastric intramucosal pH

PT: prothrombin time

PTT: partial thromboplastin time

SIRS: systemic inflammatory response syndrome

WHO: World Health Organization

REFERENCES

1. Heron MP, Hoyert DL, Xu J, Scott C, Tejada-Vera B. Deaths: Preliminary data for 2006. National Vital Statistics Reports. Hyattsville, MD: National Center for Health Statistics, 2008;56(16).
2. Anonymous. Heat-related mortality—Arizona, 1993–2002, and United States, 1979–2002. MMWR Morb Mortal Wkly Rep. 2005;54:628–630.
3. Duggan C, Fontaine O, Pierce NF, et al. Scientific rationale for a change in the composition of oral rehydration solution. JAMA 2004;291:2628–2635.
4. Ramsay G, Boom S. Pathophysiology and management of shock. In: Cuschieri A, Giles GR, Moossa AR, eds. Essential Surgical Practice, 3rd ed. Oxford, UK: Butterworth-Heinemann, 1995:72–89.
5. Dutton RP. Initial resuscitation of the hemorrhaging patient. In: Spiess BD, Spence RK, Shander A, eds. Perioperative Transfusion Medicine, 2nd ed. Philadelphia: Lippincott Williams & Wilkins, 2006:289–299.
6. Vercueil A, Grocott MPW, Mythen MG. Physiology, pharmacology, and rationale for colloid administration for the maintenance of effective hemodynamic stability in critically ill patients. Trans Med Rev 2005;19:93–109.
7. Porter SC, Fleisher GR, Kohane IS, Mandl KD. The value of parental report for diagnosis and management of dehydration in the emergency department. Ann Emerg Med 2003;41:196–205.
8. Anonymous. Prevention and treatment of heat injury. Med Lett 2003;45:58–60.
9. Nalin DR, Hirschhorn N, Greenough W, et al. Clinical concerns about reduced-osmolarity oral rehydration solution. JAMA 2004:291: 2632–2635.

10. Spandorfer PR, Alessandrini EA, Joffe MD, et al. Oral versus intravenous rehydration of moderately dehydrated children: a randomized, controlled trial. Pediatrics 2005;115:295–301.

11. Atherly-John YC, Cunningham SJ, Crain EF. A randomized trial of oral vs intravenous rehydration in a pediatric emergency department. Arch Pediatr Adolesc Med 2002;156:1240–1243.

12. Axler OA, Tousignant C, Thompson CR, et al. Small hemodynamic effect of typical rapid volume infusions in critically ill patients. Crit Care Med 1997;25:965–970.

13. The National Heart, Lung, and Blood Institute Acute Respiratory Distress Syndrome (ARDS) Clinical Trials Network. Comparison of two fluid-management strategies in acute lung injury. N Engl J Med 2006;354:2564–2575.

14. Alam HB, Rhee P. New developments in fluid resuscitation. Surg Clin N Am 2007;87:55–72.

15. Didwania A, Miller J, Kassel D, et al. Effect of intravenous lactated Ringer's solution infusion on the circulating lactate concentration: Results of a prospective, randomized, double-blind, placebo-controlled trial. Crit Care Med 1997;25:1851–1854.

16. Jackson EV, Wiese J, Sigal B, et al. Effects of crystalloid solutions on circulating lactate concentrations: 1. Implications for the proper handling of blood specimens obtained in critically ill patients. Crit Care Med 1996;24:1840–1846.

17. Deitch EA. Animal models of sepsis and shock: A review and lessons learned. Shock 1998;9:1–11.

18. Grocott MPW, Mythen MG, Gan TJ. Perioperative fluid management and clinical outcomes in adults. Anesth Analg 2005;100:1093–1106.

19. Schortgen F, Giron E, Deye N, Brochard L. The risk associated with hyperoncotic colloids in patients with shock. Intensive Care Med 2008;34:2157–2168.

20. Jungheinrich C, Neff TA. Pharmacokinetics of hydroxyethyl starch. Clin Pharmacokinet 2005;44:681–699.

21. Brunkhorst FM, Engel C, Bloos F, et al. Intensive insulin therapy and pentastarch resuscitation in severe sepsis. N Engl J Med 2008;358:125–139.

22. Cochrane Injuries Group Albumin Reviewers. Human albumin administration in critically ill patients: Systematic review of randomized controlled trials. BMJ 1998;317:235–240.

23. Choi PTL, Yip G, Quinonez LG, Cook DJ. Crystalloids vs. colloids in fluid resuscitation: A systematic review. Crit Care Med 1999;27:200–210.

24. The SAFE Study Investigators. A comparison of albumin and saline for fluid resuscitation in the intensive care unit. N Engl J Med 2004;350:2247–2256.

25. The SAFE Study Investigators. Saline or albumin for fluid resuscitation in patients with traumatic brain injury. N Engl J Med 2007;357:874–884.

26. Bickell WH, Wall MJ, Pepe PE, et al. Immediate versus delayed fluid resuscitation for hypotensive patients with penetrating torso injuries. N Engl J Med 1994;331:1105–1109.

27. Dutton RP, Mackenzie CF, Scalea TM. Hypotensive resuscitation during active hemorrhage: Impact on in-hospital mortality. J Trauma 2002;52:1141–1146.

28. Kolsen-Petersen JA, Nielsen JD, Tonnesen EM. Effect of hypertonic saline infusion on postoperative cellular outcome. Anesthesiology 2004;100:1108–1118.

29. Vassar MJ, Fischer RP, O'Brien PE, et al. A multicenter trial for resuscitation of injured patients with 7.5% sodium chloride: The effect of added dextran 70. Arch Surg 1993;128:1003–1013.

30. Suarez JI, Qureshi AI, Bhardwa A, et al. Treatment of refractory intracranial hypertension with 23.4% saline. Crit Care Med 1998;26:1118–1122.

31. Wade CE, Kramer GC, Grady JJ, et al. Efficacy of hypertonic 7.5% saline and 6% dextran-70 in treating trauma: A meta-analysis of controlled studies. Surgery 1997;122:609–616.

32. Cooper DJ, Myles PS, McDermott FT, et al. Prehospital hypertonic saline resuscitation of patients with hypotension and severe traumatic brain injury. JAMA 2004;291:1350–1357.

33. Anonymous. NHLBI stops enrollment in study of concentrated saline for patients with traumatic brain injury. http://www.nih.gov/news/health/may2009/nhlbi-12.htm(accessed 2010 July 1).

34. Gurevich B, Talmore D, Artru AA, et al. Brain edema, hemorrhagic necrosis volume, and neurological status with rapid infusion of 0.45% saline or 5% dextrose in 0.9% saline after closed head trauma in rats. Anesth Analg 1997;84:554–559.

35. Holte K, Klarskov B, Christensen DS, et al. Liberal versus restrictive fluid administration to improve recovery after laparoscopic cholecystectomy. Ann Surg 2004;240:892–899.

36. Brandstrup B, Tonnesen H, Beier-Holgersen R, et al. Effects of intravenous fluid restriction on postoperative complications: Comparison of two perioperative fluid regimens. Ann Surg 2003;238:641–648.

37. Hebert PC, Wells G, Blajchman MA, et al. A multicenter, randomized, controlled clinical trial of transfusion requirements in critical care. N Engl J Med 1999;340:409–417.

38. Dutton RP. Current concepts in hemorrhagic shock. Anesthesiol Clin 2007;25:23–34.

39. Patanawala AE. Factor VIIa (recombinant) for acute traumatic hemorrhage. Am J Health Syst Pharm 2008;65:1616–1623.

40. Pham TN, Cancio LC, Gibran NS. American Burn Association Practice Guidelines Burn Shock Resuscitation. J Burn Care Res 2008;29:257–266.

41. Zdolsek HJ, Lisander B, Jones AW, Sjoberg F. Albumin supplementation during the first week after a burn does not mobilise tissue oedema in humans. Intensive Care Med 2001;27:844–852.

42. Tanaka J, Matsuda T, Miyagantani Y, et al. Reduction of resuscitation fluid volumes in severely burned patients using ascorbic acid administration. Arch Surg 2000;135:326–331.

43. Rivers E, Nguyen B, Havstad S, et al. Early goal-directed therapy in the treatment of severe sepsis and septic-shock. N Engl J Med 2001;345:1368–1377.

44. Marik PE, Baram M, Vahid B. Does central venous pressure predict fluid responsiveness? Chest 2008;134:172–178.

45. Marik PE, Baram M. Noninvasive hemodynamic monitoring in the intensive care unit. Crit Care Clin 2007;25:383–400.

46. Bilkovski RN, Rivers EP, Horst HM. Targeted resuscitation strategies after injury. Curr Opin Crit Care 2004;10:529–538.

47. Yu M. Oxygen transport optimization. New Horiz 1999;7:46–53.

48. Ivanov R, Allen J, Calvin JE. The incidence of major morbidity in critically ill patients managed with pulmonary artery catheters: A meta-analysis. Crit Care Med 2000;28:615–619.

49. Sandham JD, Hull RD, Brant RF, et al. A randomized, controlled trial of the use of pulmonary-artery catheters in high-risk surgical patients. N Engl J Med 2003;348:5–14.

50. Ginosar Y, Thijs LG, Sprung CL. Raising the standard of hemodynamic monitoring: Targeting the practice or the practitioner? Crit Care Med 1997;25:209–211.

51. Gomersall CD, Joynt GM, Freebairn RC, et al. Resuscitation of critically ill patients based on the results of gastric tonometry: A prospective, randomized, controlled trial. Crit Care Med 2000;28:607–614.

52. Steele A, Gowrishankar M, Abrahamson S, et al. Postoperative hyponatremia despite near-isotonic saline infusion: A phenomenon of desalination. Ann Intern Med 1997;126:20–25.

53. Soni N. British consensus guidelines on intravenous fluid therapy for adult surgical patients – Cassandra's view. Anesthesia 2009;64:235–238.

54. Erstad BL. Concerns with defining appropriate uses of albumin by meta-analysis. Am J Health Syst Pharm 1999;56:1451–1454.

55. Fox DL, Vermeulen LC. UHC Technology Assessment: Albumin, Nonprotein Colloid, and Crystalloid Solutions. Oak Brook, IL: University Health System Consortium, 2000.

56. Ellender TJ, Skinner JC. The use of vasopressors and inotropes in the emergency medical treatment of shock. Emerg Med Clin N Am 2008;26:759–786.

57. Sperry JL, Minei JP, Frankel HL, et al. Early use of vasopressors after injury: caution before constriction. J Trauma 2008;64:9–14.

58. Goncalves JA, Hydo LJ, Barie PS. Factors influencing outcome of prolonged norepinephrine therapy for shock in critical surgical illness. Shock 1998;10:231–236.

59. Boyd JH, Walley KR. Is there a role for sodium bicarbonate in treating lactic acidosis from shock? Curr Opin Crit Care 2008;14:379–383.

60. Shafer SL. Shock values. Anesthesiology 2004;101:567–568.

61. Yim JM, Vermeulen LC, Erstad BL, et al. Albumin and nonprotein colloid solution use in US academic health centers. Arch Intern Med 1995;155:2450–2455.

CHAPTER 32

Introduction to Pulmonary Function Testing

JAY I. PETERS AND STEPHANIE M. LEVINE

KEY CONCEPTS

❶ Normal ventilation—perfusion ratio. The function of the lungs is to maintain Pao_2 and $Paco_2$ within normal ranges. This goal is accomplished by matching 1 mL mixed venous blood with 1 mL fresh air ($\dot{V}/\dot{Q} = 1$). Normally, ventilation ($\dot{V}$) is less than perfusion ($\dot{Q}$), and $\dot{V}/\dot{Q}$ ratio is 0.8.

❷ The air in the lung is divided into four compartments: tidal volume—air exhaled during quiet breathing; inspiratory reserve volume—maximal air inhaled above tidal volume; expiratory reserve volume—maximum air exhaled below tidal volume; and residual volume—air remaining in the lung after maximal exhalation. The sum of all four components is the total lung capacity.

❸ Obstructive lung disease is defined as an inability to get air out of the lung. It is identified on spirometry when FEV_1/FVC (force expiratory volume in the first second of expiration/forced vital capacity [total amount of air that can be exhaled during a forced exhalation]) is <70% to 75%.

❹ Reversible airway obstruction is common in asthma and chronic obstructive pulmonary disease. An increase in FEV_1 of 12% (and >0.2 L in adults) after an inhaled β-agonist suggests an acute bronchodilator response.

❺ Restrictive lung disease is defined as an inability to get air into the lung and is best defined as a reduction in total lung capacity. It is suspected when FVC is low and FEV_1/FVC is normal.

❻ Restrictive lung disease can be produced by a number of defects, such as increased elastic recoil (interstitial lung disease), respiratory muscle weakness (myasthenia gravis), mechanical restrictions (pleural effusion or kyphoscoliosis), and poor effort.

The primary function of the respiratory system is to maintain normality of arterial blood gases, that is, arterial pressure of oxygen (Pao_2) and arterial pressure of carbon dioxide ($Paco_2$). To achieve this goal, several processes must be accomplished, including alveolar ventilation, pulmonary perfusion, ventilation—perfusion matching, and gas transfer across the alveolar—capillary membrane. Alveolar ventilation is achieved by the cyclic process of air movement in and out of the lung. During inspiration, the inspiratory muscle contracts and generates negative pressure in the pleural space. This pressure gradient between the mouth and the alveoli draws fresh air (tidal volume) into the lung. Approximately one third of the inspired gas stays in the conducting airways (dead space), and two thirds reaches the alveoli.

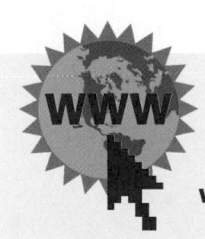

The complete chapter, learning objectives, and other resources can be found at **www.pharmacotherapyonline.com**.

CHAPTER 33

Asthma

H. WILLIAM KELLY AND CHRISTINE A. SORKNESS

KEY CONCEPTS

❶ Asthma is a disease of increasing prevalence that is a result of genetic predisposition and environmental interactions; it is one of the most common chronic diseases of childhood.

❷ Asthma is primarily a chronic inflammatory disease of the airways of the lung for which there is no known cure or primary prevention; the immunohistopathologic features include cell infiltration by neutrophils, eosinophils, T-helper type 2 lymphocytes, mast cells, and epithelial cells.

❸ Asthma is characterized by either the intermittent or persistent presence of highly variable degrees of airflow obstruction from airway wall inflammation and bronchial smooth muscle constriction; in some patients, persistent changes in airway structure occur.

❹ The inflammatory process in asthma is treated most effectively with corticosteroids, with the inhaled corticosteroids having the greatest efficacy and safety profile for long-term management.

❺ Bronchial smooth muscle constriction is prevented or treated most effectively with inhaled β_2-adrenergic receptor agonists.

❻ Variability in response to medications requires individualization of therapy within existing evidence-based guidelines for management. This is most evident in patients with severe asthma phenotypes.

❼ Ongoing patient education, for a partnership in asthma care, is essential for optimal patient outcomes and includes trigger avoidance and self-management techniques.

Asthma has been known since antiquity, yet it is a disease that still defies precise definition. The word *asthma* is of Greek origin and means "panting." More than 2,000 years ago, Hippocrates used the word *asthma* to describe episodic shortness of breath; however, the first detailed clinical description of the asthmatic patient was made by Aretaeus in the second century.[1] The National Institutes of Health, National Asthma Education and Prevention Program

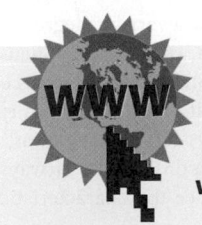

The complete chapter, learning objectives, and other resources can be found at **www.pharmacotherapyonline.com**.

Expert Panel Report 3 (EPR3), has provided the following working definition of asthma:[2]

> Asthma is a chronic inflammatory disorder of the airways in which many cells and cellular elements play a role: in particular, mast cells, eosinophils, T-lymphocytes, macrophages, neutrophils, and epithelial cells. In susceptible individuals, this inflammation causes recurrent episodes of wheezing, breathlessness, chest tightness, and coughing, particularly at night or in the early morning. These episodes are usually associated with widespread but variable airflow obstruction that is often reversible either spontaneously or with treatment. The inflammation also causes an associated increase in the existing bronchial hyperresponsiveness (BHR) to a variety of stimuli. Reversibility of airflow limitation may be incomplete in some patients with asthma.

This definition encompasses the important heterogeneity of the clinical presentation of asthma by describing the scientific and clinically accepted characteristics of asthma.

EPIDEMIOLOGY

❶ An estimated 22.9 million persons in the United States have asthma (about 7.7% of the population).[3] Asthma is the most common chronic disease among children in the United States, with approximately 6.7 million children affected. The prevalence rate is highest in children 5 to 17 years of age at 10.0%.[3] In the United States, as in other industrialized countries, the prevalence of asthma increased through the 1980s and 1990s but appears to be leveling off. Asthma accounts for 1.6% of all ambulatory care visits (10.6 million physician office visits and 1.2 million hospital outpatient visits) and resulted in 440,000 hospitalizations and 1.7 million emergency department (ED) visits in 2006 (both declined from peaks in the 1990s).[3] Asthma is the third leading cause of preventable hospitalization in the United States; however, hospitalizations have decreased over the past 10 years to 14.9 per 10,000 population with 33% reported in children less than 15 years of age. Asthma accounts for more than 12.8 million missed school days per year.[3] In young children (0–10 years of age), the risk of asthma is greater in boys than in girls, becomes about equal during puberty, and then is greater in women than in men.[3]

Ethnic minorities continue to share the burden of asthma disproportionately. African Americans have a 39% higher prevalence than whites.[3] African Americans are 3 times as likely to be hospitalized and approximately 3 times more likely to die from asthma than whites.[3] In addition, African Americans and Puerto Ricans living in inner cities are four times more likely to experience ED visits than whites.[3] However, Hispanics in general have lower prevalence and hospitalization rates than African Americans or whites.

The estimated direct medical cost of asthma in the United States in 2007 was $14.7 billion.[3] The societal burden of asthma (indirect medical expenditures: loss of productivity and death) in the United States was $5.0 billion. Prescription drugs were the largest single direct medical expenditure at $6.2 billion; however, the combined costs of emergency care of acute asthma exacerbations makes up 36% of direct medical costs.[3]

The natural history of asthma is still not well defined. Although asthma can occur at any time, it is principally a pediatric disease, with most patients being diagnosed by 5 years of age and up to 50% of children having symptoms by 2 years of age.[2] Between 30% and 70% of children with asthma will improve markedly or become symptom-free by early adulthood; chronic disease persists in about 30% to 40% of patients, and generally 20% or less develop severe chronic disease.[2] Predictors of persistent adult asthma include atopy, onset during school age, and presence of BHR.[4] Diminished lung growth may occur in some children (approximately 10%) with asthma.[2]

In adults, most longitudinal studies have suggested a more rapid rate of decline in lung function in asthmatics than in nonasthmatic normals, primarily reflected in forced expiratory volume in 1 second (FEV_1).[4] However, the annual decline in FEV_1 is less than in smokers or in patients with a diagnosis of emphysema. In general, individuals with less frequent asthma attacks and normal lung function on initial assessment have higher remission rates, whereas smokers have the lowest remission and highest relapse rates.[4] The level of BHR tends to predict the rate of decline in FEV_1, with a greater decline with high levels of BHR.[2] Thus airways obstruction in asthma not only may become irreversible but also may worsen over time owing to airway remodeling (see below).[2,4] However, most patients do not die from long-term progression of their disease and their life-span is not different from the general population.[4]

As with prevalence and morbidity, mortality from acute exacerbations of asthma has been decreasing over the past 10 years, with 3,565 deaths reported in 2007.[3] Despite the relatively low number of asthma deaths, 80% to 90% are preventable.[2] Most deaths from asthma occur outside the hospital, and death is rare after hospitalization. The most common cause of death from asthma is inadequate assessment of the severity of airways obstruction by the patient or physician and inadequate therapy. The most common cause of death in hospitalized patients is also inadequate or inappropriate therapy. Thus the key to prevention of death from asthma, as advocated by the U.S. National Asthma Education and Prevention Program (NAEPP), is education.[2]

ETIOLOGY

❶ Epidemiologic studies strongly support the concept of a genetic predisposition plus environmental interaction to the development of asthma, yet the picture remains complex and incomplete.[5] Genetic factors account for 60% to 80% of the susceptibility. Asthma represents a complex genetic disorder in that the asthma phenotype is likely a result of polygenic inheritance or different combinations of genes. Initial searches focused on establishing links between atopy (genetically determined state of hypersensitivity to environmental allergens) and asthma, but more recent genome-wide searches have found linkages with genes for metalloproteinases (e.g., *ADAM33*) and handling bacteria (*CHI3L1*).[5] Although genetic predisposition to atopy is a significant risk factor for developing asthma, not all atopic individuals develop asthma, nor do all patients with asthma exhibit atopy. Disparate phenotypes of asthma (progressive or remodelled versus non-progressive) are likely genetically determined.[5]

❶ Environmental risk factors for the development of asthma include socioeconomic status, family size, exposure to secondhand tobacco smoke in infancy and in utero, allergen exposure, urbanization, respiratory syncytial virus infection, and decreased exposure to common childhood infectious agents.[6,7] The "hygiene

TABLE 33-1	List of Agents and Events Triggering Asthma

Respiratory infection
  Respiratory syncytial virus (RSV), rhinovirus, influenza, parainfluenza, *Mycoplasma pneumonia*, *Chlamydia*
Allergens
  Airborne pollens (grass, trees, weeds), house-dust mites, animal danders, cockroaches, fungal spores
Environment
  Cold air, fog, ozone, sulfur dioxide, nitrogen dioxide, tobacco smoke, wood smoke
Emotions
  Anxiety, stress, laughter
Exercise
  Particularly in cold, dry climate
Drugs/preservatives
  Aspirin, NSAIDs (cyclooxygenase inhibitors), sulfites, benzalkonium chloride, nonselective β-blockers
Occupational stimuli
  Bakers (flour dust); farmers (hay mold); spice and enzyme workers; printers (arabic gum); chemical workers (azo dyes, anthraquinone, ethylenediamine, toluene diisocyanates, polyvinyl chloride); plastics, rubber, and wood workers (formaldehyde, western cedar, dimethylethanolamine, anhydrides)

hypothesis" proposes that genetically susceptible individuals develop allergies and asthma by allowing the allergic immunologic system (Th_2 lymphocytes) to develop instead of the system to fight infections (Th_1 lymphocytes) and may explain the increase of asthma in developed countries.[6,7] The first 2 years of life appear to be most important for the exposures to produce an alteration in the immune response system.[6] The hygiene hypothesis is supported by studies demonstrating a lower risk for asthma in children who are exposed to high levels of bacteria or endotoxin, in those with a large number of older siblings, in those with early enrollment into child care, in those with exposure to cats and dogs early in life, or in those with exposure to fewer antibiotics.[5–7]

Risk factors for early (<3 years of age) recurrent wheezing associated with viral infections include low birth weight, male gender, and parental smoking. However, this early pattern is due to smaller airways, and these risk factors are not necessarily risk factors for asthma in later life.[6] Atopy is the predominant risk factor for children to have continued asthma.[6,7] Asthma can begin in adults later in life. Occupational asthma in previously healthy individuals emphasizes the effect of environment on the development of asthma.[8] The heterogeneity of the asthma phenotype appears most obvious when listing the diverse triggers of bronchospasm[2,6] (Table 33–1). The various triggers have relative degrees of importance from patient to patient. Environmental exposures are the most important precipitants of severe asthma exacerbations[9] (see Table 33–1). Epidemics of severe asthma in cities have followed exposures to high concentrations of aeroallergens.[9] Viral respiratory tract infections remain the single most significant precipitant of severe asthma in children and are an important trigger in adults as well.[9] Other possible factors include air pollution, sinusitis, food preservatives, and drugs.

PATHOPHYSIOLOGY

❷ The major characteristics of asthma include a variable degree of airflow obstruction (related to bronchospasm, edema, and mucus hypersecretion), BHR, and airways inflammation (Fig. 33–1). To understand the pathogenetic mechanisms that underlie the many phenotypes of asthma, it is critical to identify factors that initiate, intensify, and modulate the inflammatory response of the airways and to determine how these processes produce the characteristic airway abnormalities.

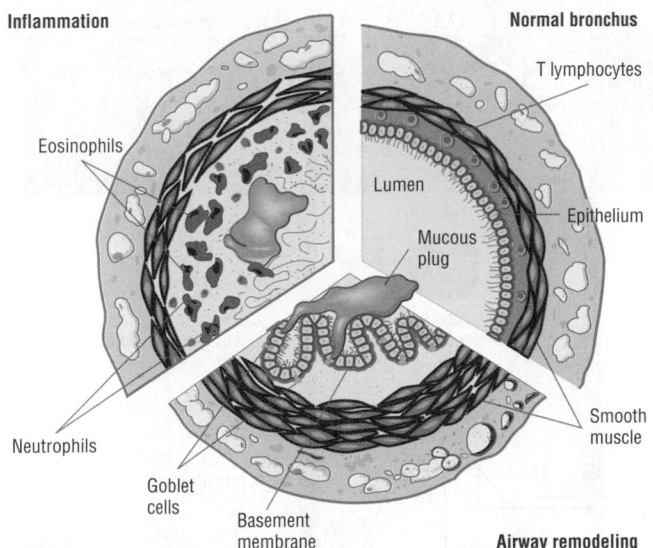

FIGURE 33-1. Representative illustration of the pathology found in the asthmatic bronchus compared with a normal bronchus (*upper right*). Each section demonstrates how the lumen is narrowed. Hypertrophy of the basement membrane, mucus plugging, smooth muscle hypertrophy, and constriction contribute (*lower section*). Inflammatory cells infiltrate, producing submucosal edema, and epithelial desquamation fills the airway lumen with cellular debris and exposes the airway smooth muscle to other mediators (*upper left*).

ACUTE INFLAMMATION

Inhaled allergen challenge models contribute most to our understanding of acute inflammation in asthma.[7] Inhaled allergen challenge in allergic patients leads to an early-phase reaction that, in some cases, may be followed by a late-phase reaction. The activation of cells bearing allergen-specific IgE initiates the early-phase reaction. It is characterized by the rapid activation of airway mast cells and macrophages leading to the rapid release of proinflammatory mediators such as histamine, eicosanoids, and reactive oxygen species that induce contraction of airway smooth muscle, mucus secretion, and vasodilatation.[7] The bronchial microcirculation has an essential role in this inflammatory process. Inflammatory mediators induce microvascular leakage with exudation of plasma in the airways.[7] Acute plasma protein leakage induces a thickened, engorged, and edematous airway wall and a consequent narrowing of the airway lumen. Plasma exudation may compromise epithelial integrity, and the presence of plasma in the lumen may reduce mucus clearance.[7] Plasma proteins also may promote the formation of exudative plugs mixed with mucus and inflammatory and epithelial cells. Together these effects contribute to airflow obstruction (Fig. 33–1).

The late-phase inflammatory reaction occurs 6 to 9 hours after allergen provocation and involves the recruitment and activation of eosinophils, CD4+ T cells, basophils, neutrophils, and macrophages.[7] There is selective retention of airway T cells, the expression of adhesion molecules, and the release of selected proinflammatory mediators and cytokines involved in the recruitment and activation of inflammatory cells.[7] The activation of T cells after allergen challenge leads to the release of T-helper cell type 2 (Th$_2$)–like cytokines that may modulate the late-phase response.[7] The release of preformed cytokines by mast cells is the likely initial trigger for the early recruitment of inflammatory cells that then recruit and induce the more persistent involvement by T cells.[7] The enhancement of nonspecific BHR usually can be demonstrated after the late-phase reaction but not after the early-phase reaction following allergen or occupational challenge.

CHRONIC INFLAMMATION

Airways inflammation has been demonstrated in all forms of asthma, and an association between the extent of inflammation and the clinical severity of asthma has been demonstrated in selected studies.[7] It is accepted that both central and peripheral airways are inflamed.

In asthma, all cells of the airways are involved and become activated (Fig. 33–2). Included are eosinophils, T cells, mast cells, macrophages, epithelial cells, fibroblasts, and bronchial smooth muscle cells. These cells also regulate airway inflammation and initiate the process of remodeling by the release of cytokines and growth factors.[7,10]

Epithelial Cells

Bronchial epithelial cells participate in mucociliary clearance and removal of noxious agents; however, they also enhance inflammation by releasing eicosanoids, peptidases, matrix proteins, cytokines, and nitric oxide (NO).[7,10] Epithelial cells can be activated by IgE-dependent mechanisms, viruses, pollutants, or histamine. In asthma, especially fatal asthma, extensive epithelial shedding occurs. The functional consequences of epithelial shedding may include heightened airways responsiveness, altered permeability of the airway mucosa, depletion of epithelial-derived relaxant factors, and loss of enzymes responsible for degrading proinflammatory neuropeptides. The integrity of airway epithelium may influence the sensitivity of the airways to various provocative stimuli. Epithelial cells also may be important in the regulation of airway remodeling and fibrosis.[7,10]

Eosinophils

Eosinophils play an effector role in asthma by releasing proinflammatory mediators, cytotoxic mediators, and cytokines.[7] Circulating eosinophils migrate to the airways by cell rolling, through interactions with selectins, and eventually adhere to the endothelium through the binding of integrins to adhesion proteins (vascular cell adhesion molecule 1 [VCAM-1] and intercellular adhesion molecule 1 [ICAM-1]). As eosinophils enter the matrix of the membrane, their survival is prolonged by interleukin 5 (IL-5) and granulocyte-macrophage colony-stimulating factor (GM-CSF). On activation, eosinophils release inflammatory mediators such as leukotrienes and granule proteins to injure airway tissue.[7]

Lymphocytes

Mucosal biopsy specimens from patients with asthma contain lymphocytes, many of which express surface markers of inflammation. There are two types of T-helper CD4+ cells. Type 1 T-helper (Th$_1$) cells produce IL-2 and interferon-γ (IFN-γ), both essential for cellular defense mechanisms. Th$_2$ cells produce cytokines (IL-4, -5, and -13) that mediate allergic inflammation. It is known that Th$_1$ cytokines inhibit the production of Th$_2$ cytokines, and vice versa. It is hypothesized that allergic asthmatic inflammation results from a Th$_2$-mediated mechanism (an imbalance between Th$_1$ and Th$_2$ cells).[7] However, more recently it has been observed that there exists a low Th$_2$ cytokine phenotype of asthma in adults that appears more resistant to usual therapies for asthma.[11]

Th$_1$ and Th$_2$ Cell Imbalance

The T-cell population in the cord blood of newborn infants is skewed toward a Th$_2$ phenotype.[6,7] The extent of the imbalance between Th$_1$ and Th$_2$ cells (as indicated by diminished IFN-γ production) during the neonatal phase may predict the subsequent development of allergic disease, asthma, or both. It has been

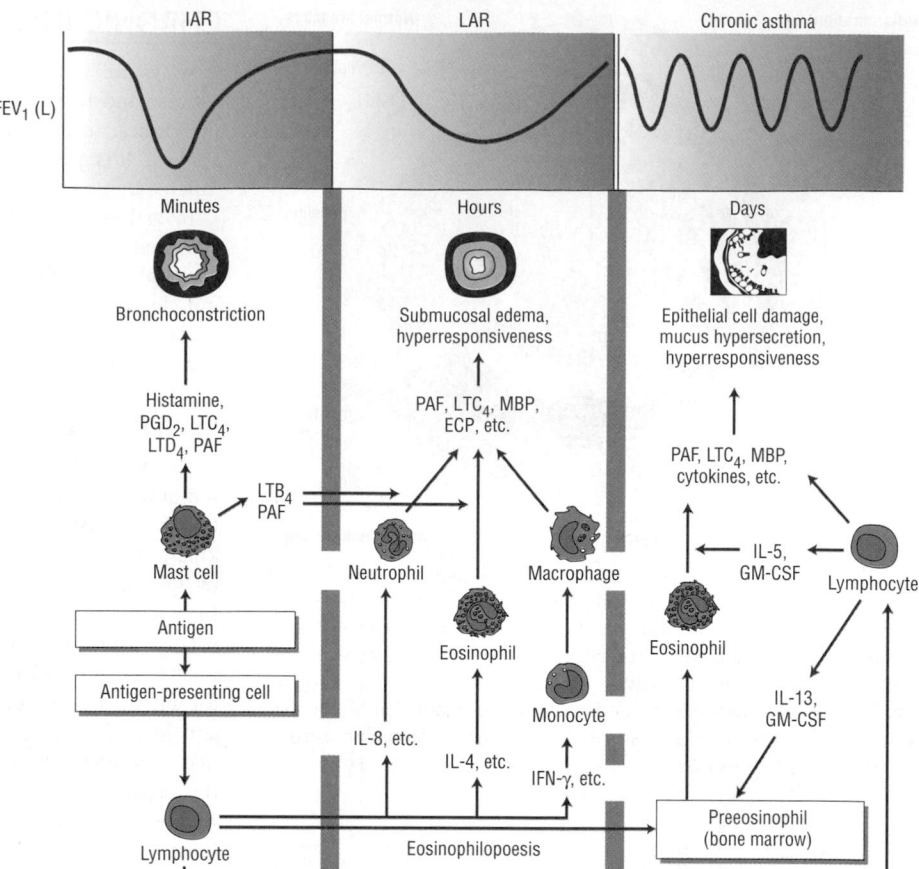

FIGURE 33-2. Diagrammatic presentation of the relationship between inflammatory cells, lipid and preformed mediators, inflammatory cytokines, and proposed pathogenesis and clinical presentation in asthma. See text for details. PG, prostaglandin; LT, leukotriene; PAF, platelet-activating factor; IL, interleukin; MBP, major basic protein; GM-CSF, granulocyte-macrophage colony-stimulating factor.

suggested that infants at high risk of asthma and allergies should be exposed to stimuli that upregulate Th$_1$-mediated responses in order to restore the balance during a critical time in the development of the immune system and the lungs.[6]

The basic premise of the hygiene hypothesis is that the newborn's immune system needs timely and appropriate environmental stimuli to create a balanced immune response. Factors that enhance Th$_1$-mediated responses include: infection with *Mycobacterium tuberculosis*, measles virus, and hepatitis A virus; increased exposure to infections through contact with older siblings; and day care attendance during the first 6 months of life. Restoration of the balance between Th$_1$ and Th$_2$ cells may be impeded by frequent administration of oral antibiotics, with concomitant alterations in gastrointestinal flora. Other factors favoring the Th$_2$ phenotype include residence in an industrialized country, urban environment exposure, diet, and sensitization to house dust mites and cockroaches.[6] Immune "imprinting" may begin in utero by transplacental transfer of allergens and cytokines.

Mast Cells

Mast cell degranulation is important in the initiation of immediate responses following exposure to allergens.[2] Mast cells reside throughout the walls of the respiratory tract, and increased numbers of these cells (3- to 5-fold) have been described in the airways of allergic asthmatics.[7] Once binding of allergen to cell-bound IgE occurs, mediators such as histamine; eosinophil and neutrophil chemotactic factors; leukotrienes (LTs) C$_4$, D$_4$, and E$_4$; prostaglandins; platelet-activating factor (PAF); and others are released from mast cells (see Fig. 33–2). Histologic examination has revealed decreased numbers of granulated mast cells in the airways of patients who have died from acute asthma attacks, suggesting that mast cell degranulation is a contributing factor. Sensitized mast

cells are also activated by osmotic stimuli to account for exercise-induced bronchospasm (EIB).[12]

Alveolar Macrophages

The primary function of alveolar macrophages in the normal airway is to serve as "scavengers," engulfing and digesting bacteria and other foreign materials. Macrophages are found in large and small airways, ideally located for affecting the asthmatic response. A number of mediators produced and released by macrophages have been identified, including PAF, LTB$_4$, LTC$_4$, and LTD$_4$.[7] Additionally, alveolar macrophages are able to produce neutrophil chemotactic factor and eosinophil chemotactic factor, which in turn amplify the inflammatory process.

Neutrophils

The role of neutrophils in the pathogenesis of asthma remains somewhat unclear because they normally may be present in the airways and usually do not infiltrate tissues showing chronic allergic inflammation despite the potential to participate in late-phase inflammatory reactions. However, high numbers of neutrophils have been observed in the airways of patients who died from sudden-onset fatal asthma and in those with severe disease.[13] This suggests that neutrophils may play a pivotal role in the disease process, at least in some patients with long-standing or corticosteroid-resistant asthma.[13] The neutrophil also can be a source for a variety of mediators, including PAF, prostaglandins, thromboxanes, and leukotrienes, that contribute to BHR and airway inflammation.[13]

Fibroblasts and Myofibroblasts

Fibroblasts are found frequently in connective tissue. Human lung fibroblasts may behave as inflammatory cells on activation by IL-4 and IL-13. The myofibroblast may contribute to the regulation of inflammation via the release of cytokines and to tissue remodeling. In asthma, myofibroblasts are increased in numbers beneath the reticular basement membrane, and there is an association between their numbers and the thickness of the reticular basement membrane.[7,10]

Inflammatory Mediators

Associated with asthma for many years, histamine is capable of inducing smooth muscle constriction and bronchospasm and is thought to play a role in mucosal edema and mucus secretion.[2] Lung mast cells are an important source of histamine. The release of histamine can be stimulated by exposure of the airways to a variety of factors, including physical stimuli (airway drying with exercise) and relevant allergens.[7] Histamine is involved in acute bronchospasm following allergen exposure; however, other mediators such as leukotrienes are also involved.

Besides histamine release, mast cell degranulation releases interleukins, proteases, and other enzymes that activate the production of other mediators of inflammation. Several classes of important mediators, including arachidonic acid and its metabolites (i.e., prostaglandins, leukotrienes, and PAF), are derived from cell membrane phospholipids.

Once arachidonic acid is released, it can be metabolized by the enzyme cyclooxygenase to form prostaglandins. Prostaglandin D_2 is a potent bronchoconstricting agent, however it is unlikely to produce sustained effects and its role in asthma remains to be determined. Similarly, prostaglandin $F_{2\alpha}$ is a potent bronchoconstrictor in patients with asthma and can enhance the effects of histamine.[2,7] However, its pathophysiologic role in asthma is unclear. Another cyclooxygenase product, prostacyclin (prostaglandin I_2), is known to be produced in the lung and may contribute to inflammation and edema owing to its effects as a vasodilator.

Thromboxane A_2 is produced by alveolar macrophages, fibroblasts, epithelial cells, neutrophils, and platelets within the lung.[7] Thromboxane A_2 may have several effects, including bronchoconstriction, involvement in the late asthmatic response, and involvement in the development of airway inflammation and BHR.

The 5-lipoxygenase pathway of arachidonic acid metabolism is responsible for the production of the *cysteinyl leukotrienes*.[7] Leukotriene C_4, LTD_4, and LTE_4 are released during inflammatory processes in the lung. Leukotrienes D_4 and E_4 share a common receptor (LTD_4 receptor) that, when stimulated, produces bronchospasm, mucus secretion, microvascular permeability, and airway edema, whereas LTB_4 is involved with granulocyte chemotaxis.

Thought to be produced by macrophages, eosinophils, and neutrophils within the lung, PAF is involved in the mediation of bronchospasm, sustained induction of BHR, edema formation, and chemotaxis of eosinophils.[7]

Adhesion Molecules

Adhesion molecules are glycoproteins that facilitate infiltration and migration of inflammatory cells to the site of inflammation. Adhesion molecules have additional functions involved in the inflammatory process aside from promoting cell adhesion, including activation of cells and cell–cell communication, and promoting cellular migration and infiltration.[2] The many adhesion molecules are divided into families on the basis of their chemical structure. These families are the integrins, cadherins, immunoglobulin supergene family, selectins, vascular adressins, and carbohydrate ligands.[7] Those thought to be important in inflammation include the integrins, immunoglobulin supergene family, selectins, and carbohydrate ligands, including ICAM-1 and

VCAM-1.[7] Adhesion molecules are found on a variety of cells, such as neutrophils, monocytes, lymphocytes, basophils, eosinophils, granulocytes, platelets, endothelial cells, and epithelial cells, and can be expressed or activated by the many inflammatory mediators present in asthma.[7]

CLINICAL CONSEQUENCES OF CHRONIC INFLAMMATION

Chronic inflammation is associated with nonspecific BHR and increases the risk of asthma exacerbations. Exacerbations are characterized by increased symptoms and worsening airways obstruction over a period of days or even weeks, and rarely hours. Hyperresponsiveness of the airways to physical, chemical, and pharmacologic stimuli is a hallmark of asthma.[2] BHR also occurs in some patients with chronic bronchitis and allergic rhinitis.[2] Normal healthy subjects also may develop a transient BHR after viral respiratory infections or ozone exposure. However, the degree of BHR in patients with asthma is quantitatively greater than in other populations. Bronchial responsiveness of the general population fits a unimodal distribution that is skewed toward increased reactivity; individuals with clinical asthma represent the extreme end of this distribution. The degree of BHR within asthma correlates with its clinical course and medication requirement necessary to control symptoms.[2] Patients with mild symptoms or in remission demonstrate lower levels of BHR.

The current understanding is that the BHR seen in asthma is at least in part due to and correlative with the extent of airways inflammation.[2] Airways remodeling also correlates somewhat with BHR.[10]

REMODELING OF THE AIRWAYS

Acute inflammation is a beneficial, nonspecific response of tissues to injury and generally leads to repair and restoration of the normal structure and function. In contrast, asthma represents a chronic inflammatory process of the airways followed by healing that in some may result in altered structure referred to as *remodeling*.[10] Repair involves replacement of injured tissue by parenchymal cells of the same type and replacement by connective tissue and its maturation into scar tissue. In asthma, remodeling presents as extracellular matrix fibrosis, an increase in smooth muscle and mucus gland mass, and angiogenesis.[10]

The precise mechanisms of remodeling of the airways are under intense study. Airways remodeling is of concern because it may represent an irreversible process that can have more serious sequelae such as the development of chronic obstructive pulmonary disease (COPD).[2,10] Observations in children with asthma indicate that some loss of lung function may occur during the first 5 years of life.[6] Importantly, no current therapies have been shown to alter either early decreased lung growth or later progressive loss of lung function.

MUCUS PRODUCTION

The mucociliary system is the lung's primary defense mechanism against irritants and infectious agents. Mucus, composed of 95% water and 5% glycoproteins, is produced by bronchial epithelial glands and goblet cells.[7] The lining of the airways consists of a continuous aqueous layer controlled by active ion transport across the epithelium in which water moves toward the lumen along the concentration gradient. Catecholamines and vagal stimulation enhance the ion transport and fluid movement. Mucus transport depends on its viscoelastic properties. Mucus that is either too watery or too viscous will not be transported optimally. The exudative inflammatory process and sloughing of epithelial cells into the airway lumen impair mucociliary transport. The bronchial glands are increased in size and the goblet cells are increased in size and number in asthma. Expectorated mucus from patients with asthma tends to have a high viscosity. The mucus plugs in the airways of patients who died in status asthmaticus are tenacious and tend to be connected by mucous strands to the goblet cells. Asthmatic airways also may become plugged with casts consisting of epithelial and inflammatory cells. Although it is tempting to speculate that death from asthma attacks is a result of the mucus plugging resulting in irreversible obstruction, there is no direct evidence for this. Autopsies of asthmatics who died from other causes have shown similar pathology. In addition, some patients who have died of sudden severe asthma did not show the characteristic mucus plugging on necropsy.[7]

AIRWAY SMOOTH MUSCLE

The smooth muscle of the airways does not form a uniform coat around the airways but is wrapped around in a connecting network best described as a spiral arrangement.[14] The muscle contraction displays a sphincteric action that is capable of completely occluding the airway lumen. The airway smooth muscle extends from the trachea through the respiratory bronchioles. When expressed as a percentage of wall thickness, the smooth muscle represents 5% of the large central airways and up to 20% of the wall thickness in the bronchioles. Total smooth muscle mass decreases rapidly past the terminal bronchioles to the alveoli, so the contribution of smooth muscle tone to airway diameter in this region is relatively small. In the large airways of asthmatics, smooth muscle may account for 11% of the wall thickness. It is possible that the increased smooth muscle mass of the asthmatic airways is important in magnifying and maintaining BHR in persistent disease. However, it appears that the hypertrophy and hyperplasia are secondary processes caused by chronic inflammation and are not the primary cause of BHR.[14]

NEURAL CONTROL/NEUROGENIC INFLAMMATION

The airway is innervated by parasympathetic, sympathetic, and nonadrenergic inhibitory nerves.[2] Parasympathetic innervation of the smooth muscle consists of efferent motor fibers in the vagus nerves and sensory afferent fibers in the vagus and other nerves.[14] The normal resting tone of human airway smooth muscle is maintained by vagal efferent activity. Maximum bronchoconstriction mediated by vagal stimulation occurs in the small bronchi and is absent in the small bronchioles. The nonmyelinated C fibers of the afferent system lie immediately beneath the tight junctions between epithelial cells lining the airway lumen.[14] These endings probably represent the irritant receptors of the airways. Stimulation of these irritant receptors by mechanical stimulation, chemical and particulate irritants, and pharmacologic agents such as histamine produces reflex bronchoconstriction.[7]

The nonadrenergic, noncholinergic (NANC) nervous system has been described in the trachea and bronchi. Substance P, neurokinin A, neurokinin B, and vasoactive intestinal peptide (VIP) are the best characterized neurotransmitters in the NANC nervous system.[7] VIP is an inhibitory neurotransmitter. Inflammatory cells in asthma can release peptidases that can degrade VIP, producing exaggerated reflex cholinergic bronchoconstriction. NANC excitatory neuropeptides such as substance P and neurokinin A are released by stimulation of C-fiber sensory nerve endings. The NANC system may play an important role in amplifying inflammation in asthma by releasing NO.

NITRIC OXIDE

NO is produced by cells within the respiratory tract. It has been thought to be a neurotransmitter of the NANC nervous system.[15] Endogenous NO is generated from the amino acid L-arginine by the enzyme NO synthase.[15] There are three isoforms of NO synthase. One isoform is induced in response to proinflammatory cytokines, inducible NO synthase (iNOS), in airway epithelial cells and inflammatory cells of asthmatic airways.[15] NO produces smooth muscle relaxation in the vasculature and bronchials; however, it appears to amplify the inflammatory process and is unlikely to be of therapeutic benefit. Investigations measuring the fraction of exhaled NO (FeNO) concentrations have suggested that it may be a useful measure of ongoing lower airways inflammation in patients with asthma and for guiding asthma therapy.[15]

CLINICAL PRESENTATION

CHRONIC ASTHMA

❸ Classic asthma is characterized by episodic dyspnea associated with wheezing; however, the clinical presentation of asthma is as diverse as the number of triggering events (see Clinical Presentation: Chronic Ambulatory Asthma). Although wheezing is the characteristic symptom of asthma, the medical literature is replete with the warning that "not all that wheezes is asthma." A wheeze is a high-pitched, whistling sound created by turbulent airflow through an obstructed airway, so any condition that produces significant obstruction can result in wheezing as a symptom. In addition, "all of asthma does not wheeze" is an equally justifiable warning. Patients may present with a chronic persistent cough as their only symptom.[2]

CLINICAL PRESENTATION: CHRONIC AMBULATORY ASTHMA

General

- Asthma is a disease of exacerbation and remission, so the patient may not have any signs or symptoms at the time of exam.

Symptoms

- The patient may complain of episodes of dyspnea, chest tightness, coughing (particularly at night), wheezing, or a whistling sound when breathing. These often occur in association with exercise, but also occur spontaneously or in association with known allergens.

Signs

- Expiratory wheezing on auscultation, dry hacking cough, or signs of atopy (allergic rhinitis and/or eczema) may occur.

Laboratory

- Spirometry demonstrates obstruction (reduced FEV_1/FVC) with reversibility following inhaled β_2-agonist administration (at least a 12% improvement in FEV_1).

Other Diagnostic Tests

- A fall in FEV_1 of at least 15% following 6 minutes of near maximal exercise. Elevated eosinophil count and IgE concentration in blood. Elevated FeNO (greater than 20 ppb in children less than 12 years of age and greater than 25 ppb in adults). Positive methacholine challenge (PC_{20} FEV_1 less than 12.5 mg/mL) or mannitol challenge (FEV_1 decrease of at least 15% from baseline after 635 mg or less).

A "yes" answer to any question suggests that an asthma diagnosis is likely. In the past 12 months....

- Have you had a sudden severe episode or recurrent episodes of coughing, wheezing (high-pitched whistling sounds when breathing out), chest tightness, or shortness of breath?
- Have you had colds that "go to the chest" or take more than 10 days to get over?
- Have you had coughing, wheezing, or shortness of breath during a particular season or time of the year?
- Have you had coughing, wheezing, or shortness of breath in certain places or when exposed to certain things (e.g., animals, tobacco smoke, perfumes)?
- Have you used any medications that help you breathe better? How often?
- Are your symptoms relieved when the medications are used?

In the past 4 weeks, have you had coughing, wheezing, or shortness of breath....

- At night that has awakened you?
- Upon awakening?
- After running, moderate exercise, or other physical activity?

[a]These questions are recommended by the NAEPP but have not been formally validated.

There is no single diagnostic test for asthma. The diagnosis is based primarily on a good history[2] (Table 33–2). The patient may have a family history of allergy or asthma or have symptoms of allergic rhinitis.[2] Reversibility of airways obstruction following administration of a short-acting inhaled β_2-agonist provides confirmation but is not by itself diagnostic. Patients with normal values of spirometry can be challenged by exercise or substances that produce bronchoconstriction, such as methacholine, to determine if they have BHR, but again, positive challenges are not diagnostic. Newer tests of inflammation in the airways such as induced sputum eosinophil counts and FeNO measurements are consistent with but not diagnostic of asthma.

Asthma has a widely variable presentation from chronic daily symptoms to only intermittent symptoms. The intervals between symptoms can be days, weeks, months, or years. Asthma also can vary as to its severity, the intrinsic intensity of the disease process. Severity is most easily and directly measured in a patient who is not currently receiving asthma treatment. The NAEPP has provided a means of classifying asthma severity that is broken down into two domains: impairment and risk.[2] This classification system is individualized for 3 age groups (0–4 years, 5–11 years, and ≥12 years) and summarized in Table 33–3. The intermittent and/or chronic nature of symptoms does not necessarily determine the severity of symptoms during exacerbations. Asthma severity is determined by lung function, symptoms, nighttime awakenings, and interference with normal activity prior to therapy. Patients can present with a range from intermittent symptoms that require no medications or only occasional use of short-acting inhaled β_2-agonists to severe persistent asthma symptoms despite treatment with multiple medications.

ACUTE SEVERE ASTHMA

Uncontrolled asthma, with its inherent variability, can progress to an acute state where inflammation, airways edema, excessive mucus accumulation, and severe bronchospasm result in a profound airways narrowing that is poorly responsive to usual bronchodilator therapy[2,9] (see Clinical Presentation: Acute Severe

TABLE 33-3 Classifying Asthma Severity for Patients who are not Currently Taking Long-Term Control Medications

Children 0–4 Years and 5–11 Years of Age

			Persistent		
Components	**Intermittent**	**Mild**	**Moderate**	**Severe**	
Symptoms	≤2 days/wk	>2 days/wk but not daily	Daily	Throughout the Day	
Nighttime Awakenings (0–4 y)	0	1–2 × mo	3–4 × mo	>1 × wk	
(5–11 y)	≤2 × mo	3–4 × mo	>1 × wk, but not nightly	Often 7 × wk	
SABA Use for Sx control	≤2 days/wk	>2 days/wk but not daily	Daily	Several times per day	
Interference with normal activity	None	Minor limitation	Some limitation	Extremely limited	
Lung function	FEV$_1$ >80%	FEV$_1$ >80%	FEV$_1$ 60%–80%	FEV$_1$ <60%	
(5–11 y)	FEV$_1$/FVC >85%	FEV$_1$/FVC >80%	FEV$_1$/FVC 75%–80%	FEV$_1$/FVC <75%	

Exacerbations	**Intermittent**	**Persistent**		
(0–4 y)	0–1/y	≥2 in 6 mo or ≥4 wheezing episodes/1 y lasting >1 day		
(5–11 y)	0–2/y	>2 in 1 y		
Recommended step for initiating Treatment	Step 1	Step 2	Step 3 and consider short course of oral corticosteroids	

Youths ≥12 Years of Age and Adults

			Persistent		
Components	**Intermittent**	**Mild**	**Moderate**	**Severe**	
Symptoms	≤2 days/wk	>2 days/wk but not daily	Daily	Throughout the day	
Nighttime Awakenings	≤2 × mo	3–4 × mo	>1 × wk, but not nightly	Often 7 × wk	
SABA Use for Sx control	≤2 days/wk	>2 days/wk, but not >1 × day	Daily	Several times per day	
Interference with normal activity	None	Minor limitation	Some limitation	Extremely limited	
Lung function*	FEV$_1$ >80%	FEV$_1$ >80%	FEV$_1$ 60%–80%	FEV$_1$ <60%	
*Normal FEV$_1$ / FVC: 8–19 y 85%; 20–39 y 80%; 40–59 y 75%; 60–80 y 70%.	FEV$_1$/FVC normal	FEV$_1$/FVC normal	FEV$_1$/FVC reduced 5%	FEV$_1$/FVC reduced >5%	

Exacerbations	**Intermittent**	**Persistent**		
	0–2/y	>2 in 1 y		
Recommended step for initiating Treatment	Step 1	Step 2	Step 3 and consider short course of oral corticosteroids	Step 4 or 5 course of oral corticosteroids

Asthma). Although this progression is the most common scenario, some patients experience rapid onset or hyper-acute attacks.[2,9] Hyperacute attacks are associated with neutrophilic as opposed to eosinophilic infiltration and resolve rapidly with bronchodilator therapy, suggesting that smooth muscle spasm is the major pathogenic mechanism.[9,13] In most cases, ED visits for acute severe asthma represent the failure of an adequate therapeutic regimen for persistent asthma. Underutilization of antiinflammatory drugs and excessive reliance on short-acting inhaled β_2-agonists are the major risk factors for severe exacerbations.[2] However, frequent exacerbations may represent a specific phenotype of asthma.[9] A blunted perception of airways obstruction may predispose certain individuals to fatal asthma attacks.[2]

CLINICAL PRESENTATION: ACUTE SEVERE ASTHMA

General

- An episode can progress over several days or hours (usual scenario) or progresses rapidly over 1 to 2 hours.

Symptoms

- The patient is anxious in acute distress and complains of severe dyspnea, shortness of breath, chest tightness, or burning. The patient is only able to say a few words with each breath. Symptoms are unresponsive to usual measures (short-acting inhaled β_2-agonist administration).

Signs

- Signs include expiratory and inspiratory wheezing on auscultation (breath sounds may be diminished with very severe obstruction), dry hacking cough, tachypnea, tachycardia, pale or cyanotic skin, hyperinflated chest with intercostal and supraclavicular retractions, and hypoxic seizures if very severe.

Laboratory

- PEF and/or FEV_1 less than 40% of normal predicted values. Decreased arterial oxygen (PaO_2), and O_2 saturations by pulse oximetry (SaO_2 less than 90% on room air is severe). Decreased arterial or capillary CO_2 if mild, but in the normal range or increased in moderate to severe obstruction.

Other Diagnostic Tests

- Blood gases to assess metabolic acidosis (lactic acidosis) in severe obstruction. Complete blood count if there are signs of infection (fever and purulent sputum). Serum electrolytes as therapy with β_2-agonist and corticosteroids can lower serum potassium, magnesium, and phosphate, and increase glucose. Chest radiograph if signs of consolidation on auscultation.

EXERCISE-INDUCED BRONCHOSPASM

During vigorous exercise, pulmonary function measurements (FEV_1 and peak expiratory flow [PEF]) in patients with asthma increase during the first few minutes but then begin to decrease after 6 to 8 minutes (Fig. 33–3).[2] Exercise-induced bronchospasm (EIB) is defined as a drop in FEV_1 of 15% or greater from baseline (pre-exercise value).[2] Most studies suggest that many patients with persistent asthma experience EIB.[2] The exact pathogenesis of EIB is unknown, but heat loss and/or water loss from the central airways appears to play an important role.[12] EIB is provoked more easily in cold, dry air; alternatively, warm, humid air can blunt or block it.[12] Studies have demonstrated increased plasma histamine, cysteinyl leukotrienes, prostaglandins and tryptase concentrations during EIB, suggesting a role for mast cell degranulation.[12] These findings have led to the development of inhaled mannitol, an osmotic agent

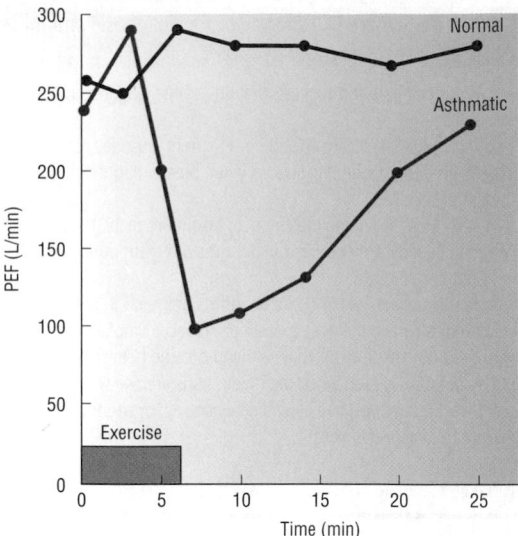

FIGURE 33-3. Typical responses to exercise in a normal subject and an asthmatic subject. Note the initial bronchodilation. PEF, peak expiratory flow.

as an indirect pharmacologic bronchoprovocation test to assist in the diagnosis of asthma.[16]

A refractory period following EIB lasts up to 3 hours after exercise in some patients. During this period, repeat exercise of the same intensity produces either no decrease in pulmonary function or a drop of less than 50% of the initial response.[12] This refractory period is thought to be caused by an acute depletion of mast cell mediators and time required for their repletion. Patients with known refractoriness to exercise will still respond to histamine, so acute hyporesponsiveness of airway smooth muscle does not appear to be a factor.[12]

EIB is believed to be a reflection of the increased BHR of asthmatics. A correlation, though not perfect, exists between EIB and reactivity to histamine, methacholine, and mannitol.[12,16] Other patient groups with BHR (e.g., after viral infection, cystic fibrosis, or allergic rhinitis) show bronchoconstriction after exercise to a lesser degree (5%–10% drops) than patients with asthma (15%–40% drops).[12] Patients will not always demonstrate the same sensitivity. During periods of remission, a decreased sensitivity to the same degree of exercise is often observed. Finally, a number of children and adults with EIB are otherwise normal, without symptoms or abnormal pulmonary function except in association with exercise.[2] Elite athletes have a higher prevalence of EIB than the general population.[12]

NOCTURNAL ASTHMA

❸ Worsening of asthma during sleep is referred to as *nocturnal asthma*. Patients with nocturnal asthma exhibit significant falls in pulmonary function between bedtime and awakening.[2] Typically, their lung function reaches a nadir at 3 to 4 AM. Although the pathogenesis of this phenomenon is unknown, it has been associated with diurnal patterns of endogenous cortisol secretion and circulating epinephrine.[2] Direct evidence for an inflammatory component to nocturnal asthma includes increased circulating histamine and activated eosinophils and leukotriene excretion at night associated with increased BHR to methacholine.[2]

Numerous other factors that may affect nocturnal worsening of asthma, including allergies and improper environmental control, gastroesophageal reflux, obstructive sleep apnea, and sinusitis, also must be considered when evaluating these patients.[2] Most experts consider nocturnal symptoms to be a sign of inadequately treated persistent asthma.[2] Awakening from nocturnal asthma is a sensitive indicator of both severity and asthma control.[2]

FACTORS CONTRIBUTING TO ASTHMA SEVERITY

VIRAL RESPIRATORY INFECTIONS

Viral respiratory infections are primarily responsible for exacerbations of asthma, particularly in children under age 10.[9] Infants are particularly susceptible to airways obstruction and wheezing with viral infections because of their small airways. The most common cause of exacerbations in both children and adults is the common rhinovirus.[9] Other viruses isolated include respiratory syncytial virus (RSV), parainfluenza virus, coronavirus, and influenza viruses. Certain viruses (RSV and parainfluenza virus) are capable of inducing specific IgE antibodies, and rhinovirus can activate eosinophils directly in asthmatics.[7] The increase in asthma symptoms and BHR that occurs may last for days or weeks following resolution of the symptoms of the viral infection. Evidence does not support a beneficial effect of influenza vaccine for preventing asthma exacerbations from subsequent influenza infections.[17]

ENVIRONMENTAL AND OCCUPATIONAL FACTORS

Agents and events and the mechanisms that are known to trigger asthma are listed in Table 33–1.[2] The general mechanisms are unknown but presumably are the result of epithelial damage and inflammation in the airway mucosa. Ozone and sulfur dioxide, common components of air pollution, have been used to induce BHR in animals. Exposure to 0.2 ppm ozone for 2 to 3 hours can induce bronchoconstriction and increase BHR in asthmatics.[2,8] Sulfur dioxide in the ambient atmosphere is highly irritating and presumably induces bronchoconstriction through mast cell or irritant-receptor involvement.[2] Asthma produced by repeated prolonged exposure to industrial inhalants is a significant health problem. It has been estimated that occupational asthma accounts for 2% of all asthmatic persons.[8] Persons with occupational asthma have the typical symptoms of asthma with cough, dyspnea, and wheeze. Typically, the symptoms are related to work place exposure and improve on days off and during vacations.[8] In some instances, symptoms may persist even after termination of exposure.[8]

STRESS, DEPRESSION, AND PSYCHOSOCIAL FACTORS IN ASTHMA

Observational studies demonstrate an association between increased stress and worsening asthma, but the role is not clearly defined.[2] Bronchoconstriction from psychological factors appears to be mediated primarily through excess parasympathetic input. Atropine has been shown to block experimental psychogenic bronchoconstriction. It is most important to emphasize to both patients and parents that asthma is not an emotional disease; however, coping skills may benefit the patient who becomes emotionally distraught during an asthma attack.

RHINITIS/SINUSITIS

Disorders of the upper respiratory tract, particularly rhinitis and sinusitis, have been linked with asthma for many years. As many as 40% to 50% of asthmatics have abnormal sinus radiographs.[2] However, chronic sinusitis may just represent a nonbacterial coexisting condition with allergic asthmatics because the histologic changes in the paranasal sinuses are similar to those seen in the lung and nose.[2] Treatment of upper airway disease may optimize overall asthma control. The mechanism by which sinusitis aggravates asthma is unknown. The treatment of allergic rhinitis with intranasal corticosteroids and cromolyn but not antihistamines will reduce BHR in asthmatic patients.[2] It has been postulated that transport of mucus chemotactic factors and inflammatory mediators from nasal passages during allergic rhinitis into the lung may accentuate BHR.

GASTROESOPHAGEAL REFLUX DISEASE

Symptoms of gastroesophageal reflux disease (GERD) as well as asymptomatic reflux are common in both children and adults who have asthma.[2] Nocturnal asthma may be associated with nighttime reflux.[2] Reflux of acidic gastric contents into the esophagus is thought to initiate a vagally mediated reflex bronchoconstriction.[2] Also of concern is that most medications that decrease airways smooth muscle tone may have a relaxant effect on gastroesophageal sphincter tone. However, treatment of reflux in asthma patients has produced inconsistent results on asthma control.[2,18] The current recommendation is to initiate standard antireflux therapy in those patients exhibiting symptoms of reflux.[2]

FEMALE HORMONES AND ASTHMA

Premenstrual worsening of asthma has been reported in as many as 30% to 40% of women in some studies, whereas worsening of pulmonary functions has been reported even in women not aware of worsening symptoms.[19] The pathophysiology is uncertain because estrogen replacement in postmenopausal women has been shown to worsen asthma, whereas estradiol and progesterone administration have been variably reported to improve or have no effect on asthma in women with premenstrual asthma.[19,20] The clinical significance of menstruation-related asthma is still unclear because some studies have reported that up to 50% of ED visits by women were premenstrual, whereas others have reported no association with menstrual phase.[19,20] In general, BHR and symptoms improve in asthmatic women during pregnancy.[2,19]

FOODS, DRUGS, AND ADDITIVES

Documentation in the literature of food allergens as triggers for asthma is not available.[2] However, additives, specifically sulfites used as preservatives, can trigger life-threatening asthma exacerbations. Beer, wine, dried fruit, and open salad bars in particular have high concentrations of metabisulfites.[2] Severe oral corticosteroid-dependent patients should be warned about ingesting foods processed with sulfites. Another additive producing bronchospasm is benzalkonium chloride, which is found as a preservative in some nebulizer solutions of antiasthmatic drugs.[21]

Aspirin and other nonsteroidal antiinflammatory drugs can precipitate an attack in up to 20% of adults and 5% of children with asthma.[22] The mechanism is related to cyclooxygenase inhibition, and 5-lipoxygenase inhibition can alter dose-response but not completely block the symptoms.[22] The prevalence increases with age and severity of asthma.[2] The greatest frequency occurs in severe corticosteroid-resistant asthmatics in their fourth and fifth decades who also have perennial rhinitis and nasal polyposis (presence of several polyps).[22] Other drugs that do not precipitate bronchospasm but which prevent its reversal are the nonselective β-blocking agents.[2]

NUTRITIONAL FACTORS

Epidemiologic data suggest that obesity increases the prevalence of asthma and may reduce asthma control.[23] Lung volume and tidal volume are reduced in obesity promoting airway narrowing. Obesity also produces low-grade systemic inflammation that may act on the lung to worsen asthma.[23] The mechanism is likely the release of adipose-derived pro-inflammatory mediators such as IL-6, IL-10, eotaxin, tumor necrosis factor-α, transforming growth factors-β_1, C-reactive protein, leptin, and adiponectin or a result of common predisposing dietary factors. Although not all studies find relationship between body mass index and asthma control, management of asthma in obese patients should include weight loss measures.[24]

More recently it has been shown that children with vitamin D insufficiency are at greater risk of uncontrolled asthma (increased hospitalizations, BHR and eosinophil counts).[25] Vitamin D helps regulate T-cells and improves their secretion of antiinflammatory cytokines in response to corticosteroids.[25]

TREATMENT

Asthma

■ AEROSOL THERAPY FOR ASTHMA

4 5 Aerosol delivery of drugs for asthma has the advantage of being site-specific and thus enhancing the therapeutic ratio.[2,26] Inhalation of short-acting β_2-agonists provides more rapid bronchodilation than either parenteral or oral administration, as well as the greatest degree of protection against EIB and other challenges.[2] Inhaled corticosteroids have been developed with rapid oral and systemic clearance to enhance lung activity and reduce systemic activity. Specific agents (e.g., cromolyn, formoterol, salmeterol, and ipratropium bromide) are only effective by inhalation.[26] Therefore, an understanding of aerosol drug delivery is essential to optimal asthma therapy. Table 33–4 lists the factors determining lung deposition of therapeutic aerosols.

TABLE 33-4	Factors Determining Lung Deposition of Aerosols	
Device	**Device Factors**	**Patient Factors**
Metered-dose inhaler (MDI)	Canister held inverted	Inspiratory flow (slow, deep)
	Formulation (CFC, HFA, solution, suspension)	Breath-holding
	Actuator cleanliness	Coordinating actuation with inhalation
	Addition of a spacer device	Priming and shaking the device
Dry-powder inhaler (DPI)	Device cleanliness	Inspiratory flow (deep, forceful)
	Resistance to inhalation	Tilting head back
	Humidity	Maintaining parallel to ground once activated
Jet nebulizer (small volume)	Volume fill (3–6 mL)	Inspiratory flow (slow, deep)
	Gas flow (6–12 L/min)	Breath-holding
	Dead-space volume	Tapping nebulizer
	Open vs closed system	
	Thumb-activating valve	
	Mouthpiece vs facemask	
Ultrasonic nebulizer	Volume fill	Inspiratory flow (slow, deep)
	Not effective for suspensions	Breath-holding
	Mouthpiece vs facemask	Tapping nebulizer
Spacer device	Volume (≥650 mL)	Inspiratory flow (slow, deep)
	One-way valves	Time between actuation and inhalation (<5 s)
	Holding chamber vs open-ended	Cleaning with detergent to reduce static
	Anti-static linning	Multiple actuations decrease delivery
	Mouthpiece vs facemask	Coordination of actuation and inhalation for the simple open-tube spacers

Device Determinants of Delivery

Devices used to generate therapeutic aerosols include jet nebulizers, ultrasonic nebulizers, metered-dose inhalers (MDIs), and dry-powder inhalers (DPIs). The single most important device factor determining the site of aerosol deposition is particle size.[26] Devices for delivering therapeutic aerosols generate particles with aerodynamic diameters from 0.5 to 35 microns.[26] Particles larger than 10 microns deposit in the oropharynx, particles between 5 and 10 microns deposit in the trachea and large bronchi, particles 1 to 5 microns in size reach the lower airways, and particles smaller than 0.5 microns act as a gas and are exhaled. In asthma, the airways, not the alveoli, are the target for delivery. Respirable particles are deposited in the airways by three mechanisms: (1) inertial impaction, (2) gravitational sedimentation, and (3) Brownian diffusion.[26] The first two mechanisms are the most important for therapeutic aerosols and probably are the only factors that can be manipulated by patients.

Each delivery device within a classification generates specific aerosol characteristics, so extrapolation of delivery data from one device cannot be applied to the other devices in the class. For instance, MDIs can deliver 15% to 50% of the actuated dose; DPIs, 10% to 30% of the labeled dose; and nebulizers, 2% to 15% of the starting dose.[26] MDIs and DPIs are portable and convenient, unlike jet nebulizers. Small portable ultrasonic nebulizers have also been developed. MDIs consist of a pressurized canister with a metering valve; the canister contains active drug, low-vapor-pressure propellants such as chlorofluorocarbon (CFC) or hydrofluoroalkane (HFA), cosolvents, and/or surfactants.[26] The international ban on the production and use of CFCs (due to their ozone layer–depleting properties) will result in no CFC propelled MDIs available in the United States by December 31, 2011. With any change in the components of an MDI, the Food and Drug Administration (FDA) considers it to be a new drug that requires stability, safety, and efficacy studies prior to approval. The drug is either in solution or a suspended micronized powder. In order to disperse the suspension for accurate delivery, the canister must be shaken. The metering chamber measures a liquid volume, and therefore, the device must be held with the valve stem downward so that the chamber is covered with liquid[26] (Fig. 33–4). When the canister is actuated, the device releases the propellant and drug in a forceful spray whose particles are large (mass median aerodynamic diameter [MMAD] = 45 microns) [26] (see Fig. 33–4). As evaporation occurs, the particle size is reduced to a final MMAD of 0.5 to 5.5 microns depending on the MDI. The aerosol cloud extends about 6 inches beyond the MDI at the lowest MMAD.[26] Each MDI has different conditions for storage and durations to expiration so the pharmacist must become familiar with and counsel the patient on these factors.

The breath-actuated MDI Autohaler is cocked with a lever to "load" the dose of medication, a baffle is opened by inspiratory

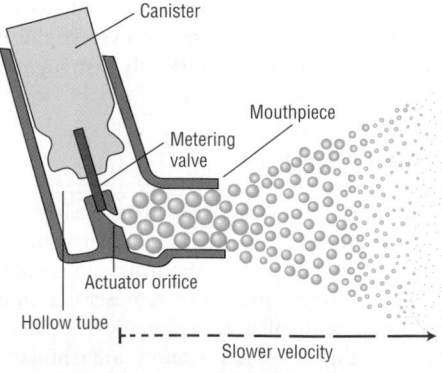

FIGURE 33-4. Illustration of a metered-dose inhaler demonstrating the particle size difference as the aerosol cloud extends outward.

TABLE 33-5 Characteristics of Various Inhalation Devices

Device	Drugs	Breath Activated	Dose Counter	Other Excipients	Disadvantages
CFC MDI	All classes	No	No	Propellants, surfactants	Requires coordination of actuation and inhalation Large pharyngeal deposition Difficult to teach
HFA-MDI	Albuterol	No	No/Yes	Propellants, surfactants, cosolvents	Same as CFC MDI
	Levalbuterol	No	No		
	Corticosteroids	No	No		
	ICS/LABA combinations	No	No		
Autohaler MDI	Pirbuterol	Yes	No	CFC propellant, surfactant	Requires rapid inhalation to activate
MDI plus valved holding chamber	All classes	No	No		More expensive than MDI alone; less portable; some payers will not pay; inconsistent effect on delivery; nonstatic preferred
Jet nebulizers	All classes	No	–	Preservatives in some solutions	Significant interbrand variability; expensive and time consuming; less efficient than MDIs; contamination possible; preparations may be light and temperature sensitive (short shelf-life)
Ulrasonic nebulizer	Cromolyn solution, short acting β_2-agonist solutions	No	–	Preservatives in some solutions	Same as for jet nebulizers plus cannot be used for suspensions
Flexhaler	Budesonide	Yes	Yes	Lactose filler	Requires high inspiratory flow (60 L/min). Pharyngeal deposition. Not approved for <6 years of age
Diskus	Fluticasone Salmeterol Fluticasone/salmeterol	Yes	Yes	Lactose filler	Not approved for <4 years of age Requires inspiratory flow of 30–60 L/min
Aerolizer	Formoterol	Yes	–	Lactose filler	Single-dose capsules. Not approved for <5 years of age Requires flow of 30–60 L/min
Twisthaler	Mometasone	Yes	Yes	Lactose filler	Not approved for <4 years of age

pressure, and the dose is expelled from the canister metering chamber.[26] While the need for hand-lung coordination for proper actuation is reduced significantly with breath-actuated MDIs, these devices do not allow the use of a spacer device.

Spacer devices are used frequently with an MDI to decrease oropharyngeal deposition and enhance lung delivery.[2] However, not all spacer devices produce similar effects. The design of spacers varies from simple open-ended tubes that separate the MDI from the mouth to valved holding chambers (VHCs) with one-way valves that open during inhalation (the preferred system). A VHC allows evaporation of the propellant prior to inhalation permitting a greater number of drug particles to achieve a respirable droplet size. VHC use also allows inhalation after actuation of the MDI, obviating the need for good hand-lung coordination.[26] Additionally, the large particles that normally would deposit in the oropharynx "rain out" in the spacer.[26] All the available spacers significantly reduce oropharyngeal deposition from MDIs, with the VHCs being superior to the open-ended tubes.[26] This reduction in oropharyngeal deposition is an important factor in reducing local adverse effects (e.g., hoarseness and thrush) from inhaled corticosteroids.[26] The change in lung delivery depends on both the MDI and the drug, where one spacer device may enhance delivery with one MDI preparation and decrease delivery with others.[26] The use of VHCs is less likely to enhance delivery from HFA propelled MDIs. Finally, over time, holding chambers can build up static electricity that attracts small particles to the sides of the chamber, significantly reducing aerosol availability. Some spacers should be washed weekly with household detergent with a single rinse and allowed to drip dry.[26] Other VHCs have been developed with antistatic lining.

Dry micronized powders can be inhaled directly into the lung. A number of DPIs are now available for use in the United States.[26] Currently, there are no generic DPIs as each drug plus device has

its own patent. Each DPI has unique characteristics with advantages and disadvantages (Table 33–5). The primary advantage of DPIs is that they are breath actuated and require minimal hand-lung coordination and are thus easier to teach patients proper technique.[26] Some DPIs are more flow-dependent than others.[26] Thus, similar to MDIs and spacers, delivery data from one DPI cannot be extrapolated to another.

Nebulizers come in two basic types, the jet nebulizer and the ultrasonic nebulizer. Jet nebulizers produce an aerosol from a liquid solution or suspension placed in a cup. A tube connected to a stream of compressed air or oxygen flows up through the bottom and draws the liquid up an adjacent open-ended tube.[26] The air and liquid strike a baffle, creating a droplet cloud that is then inhaled.[26] Ultrasonic nebulizers produce an aerosol by vibrating liquid lying above a transducer at speeds of about 1 mHz.[26] Both produce similar degrees of lung deposition, with the exception that ultrasonic nebulizers are ineffective for nebulizing currently available micronized suspensions.[26] The aerosol output and lung delivery vary significantly among the commercially available jet nebulizers even when operated in the same manner.[26] Increasing fill volume will increase the total amount of drug delivered; however, it also will take longer for the patient to nebulize the dose.[26] The MMAD of the droplets is related directly to the gas flow, with flows of 5 to 12 L/min providing an aerosol cloud with an MMAD of 4 to 8 microns for most jet nebulizers.[26] Each jet nebulizer comes with its optimal operating instructions.

Patient Determinants of Delivery (See Table 33–4)

6 7 The most important patient factor determining aerosol deposition is inspiratory flow.[2,26] High inspiratory flows increase the degree of deposition owing to impaction of particles of any size, thereby increasing deposition centrally (i.e., throat and large airways) and decreasing peripheral deposition. Optimal inspiratory flow for most MDIs is slow and deep (approximately 30 L/min or 5 seconds for a full inhalation).[2] In general, DPIs require higher inspiratory flows (≥60 L/min) and a change in inhalation technique (i.e., deep, forceful inspiration) for optimal dispersion of the powder, which, in turn, increases the amount of drug delivered to the larger central airways.[26] However, this difference in delivery may not produce clinically significant differences.[26] Patients should be cautioned not to exhale into DPIs because this causes loss of dose and moistens the dry powder, causing aggregation into larger particles. Patient factors that cannot be controlled include interpatient variability in airway geometry (particularly the differences between children and adults)[26] and the effects of bronchospasm, edema, and mucus hypersecretion. Mild obstruction increases aerosol deposition; however, severe obstruction probably leads to increased central deposition from impaction.[26] The absolute delivery to the lung is not as important as consistency of delivery, assuming that a sufficient dose to produce the desired therapeutic effect is achieved. No single inhalation device is the best for all patients. Table 33–5 lists the differing characteristics of inhalation devices.

Appropriate inhalation technique is essential to achieve optimal drug delivery and therapeutic effect.[2] The components are illustrated in Figure 33–5. Approximately 50% to 80% of a dose from MDIs and DPIs impacts on the oropharynx and is then swallowed; the rest is either left in the device or exhaled.[26] It is important that actuation occurs during inhalation, although the time during inspiration is unimportant.[2,26] Although radiolabeled studies with MDIs indicate improved delivery by holding the actuator 2 to 3 cm in front of an open mouth to allow more evaporation and less impaction, physiologic studies with bronchodilators have failed to document an advantage for this method.[2,26] Many patients do not use their MDIs optimally, and patient instruction with demonstration is the most effective means of improving inhaler technique.[2,26] Even with instruction, up to 30% of patients, particularly young children and the elderly, cannot master the use of an MDI. For these patients, attachment of a VHC to the MDI or use of a breath-actuated MDI can improve efficacy significantly.[2,26] However addition of a VHC offers no advantage in patients who can use an MDI optimally alone.[26] Mouth rinsing following treatment with MDI- and DPI-inhaled corticosteroids is important to minimize local effects and oral absorption.[2,26]

Delivery from high-resistance DPIs is more flow-dependent than from low-resistance DPIs. Thus, younger children and possibly elderly adults will have more variability in delivery from high resistance devices.[26] Most children younger than 4 years of age cannot generate a sufficient inspiratory flow to use DPIs. Young children (<4 years) and infants generally require the use of a facemask attached to either an MDI plus VHC or nebulizer. The use of a facemask results in a reduction in lung delivery due to the portion of the aerosol inhaled nasally so the doses of drugs used in these patients is often not decreased.

Steps for Using Your Inhaler

Please demonstrate your inhaler technique at every visit.

1. Remove the cap and hold inhaler upright.
2. Shake the inhaler.
3. Tilt your head back slightly and breathe out slowly.
4. Position the inhaler in one of the following ways (B is acceptable for those who have difficulty with A or C. C is required for breath-activated inhalers):

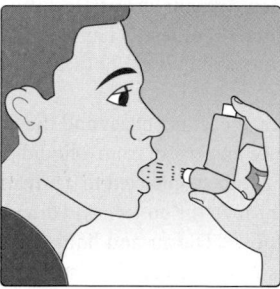 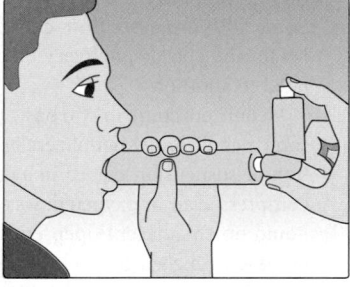 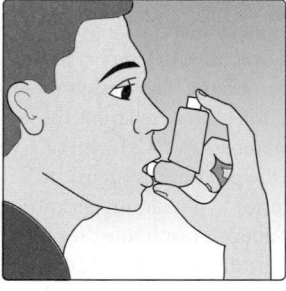 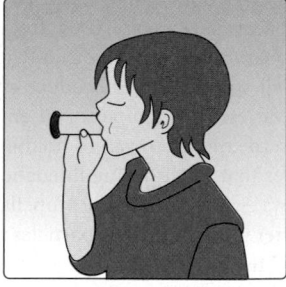

A Open mouth with inhaler 1 to 2 inches away.

B Use spacer/holding chamber (that is recommended especially for young children and for people using corticosteroids).

C In the mouth.

D NOTE: Inhaled dry powder capsules require a different inhalation technique. To use a dry powder inhaler, it is important to close the mouth tightly around the mouthpiece of the inhaler and to inhale rapidly.

5. Press down on the inhaler to release medication as you start to breathe in slowly.
6. Breathe in slowly (3 to 5 seconds).
7. Hold your breath for 10 seconds to allow the medicine to reach deeply into your lungs.
8. Repeat puff as directed. Waiting 1 minute between puffs may permit second puff to penetrate your lungs better.
9. Spacers/holding chambers are useful for all patients. They are particularly recommended for young children and older adults and for use with corticosteroids.

Avoid common inhaler mistakes. Follow these inhaler tips:

- Breathe out *before* pressing your inhaler.
- Inhale *slowly*.
- Breathe in through your mouth, not your nose.
- Press down on your inhaler at the *start* of inhalation (or within the first second of inhalation).
- Keep inhaling as you press down on inhaler.
- Press your inhaler only *once* while you are inhaling (one breath for each puff).
- Make sure you breathe in evenly and deeply.

NOTE: Other inhalers are becoming available in addition to those illustrated above. Different types of inhalers require different techniques.

FIGURE 33-5. Instructions for inhaler use from the adapted NAEPP Expert Panel Report 2. *http://www.nhlbi.nih.gov/guidelines/archives/epr-2/index.htm.*

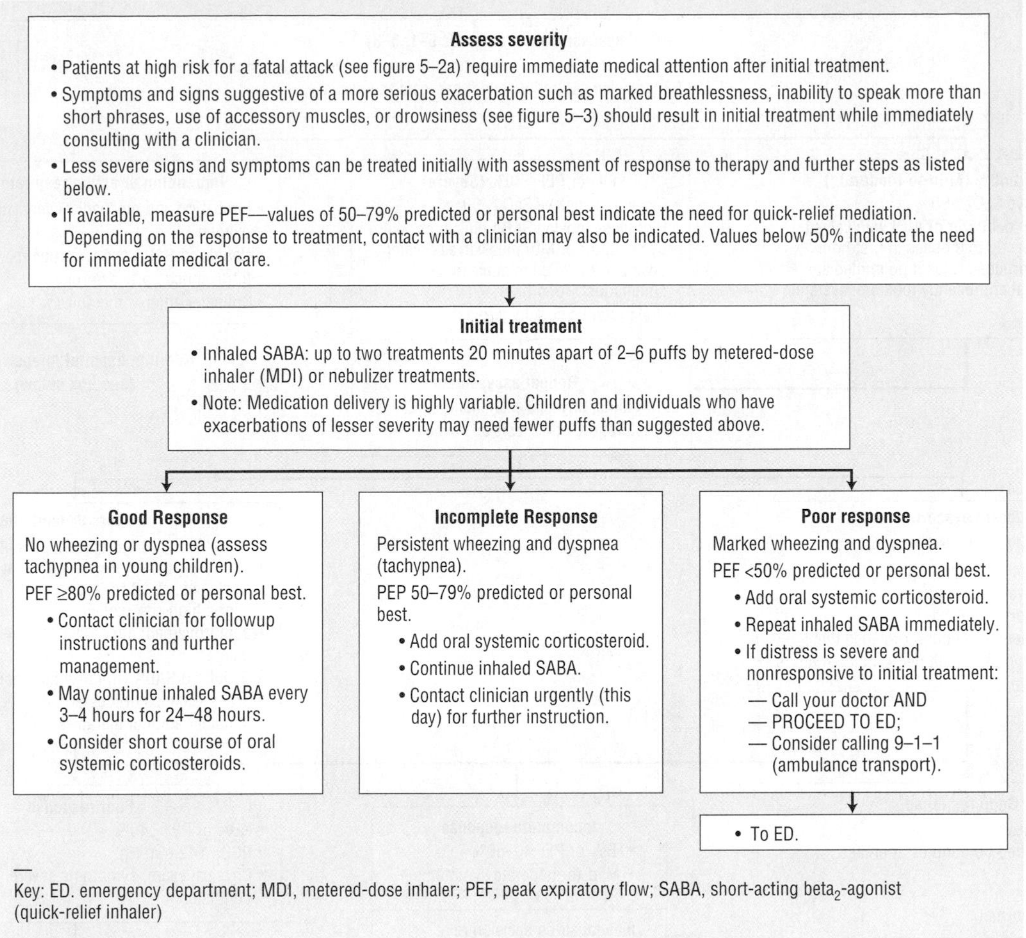

Assess severity
- Patients at high risk for a fatal attack (see figure 5–2a) require immediate medical attention after initial treatment.
- Symptoms and signs suggestive of a more serious exacerbation such as marked breathlessness, inability to speak more than short phrases, use of accessory muscles, or drowsiness (see figure 5–3) should result in initial treatment while immediately consulting with a clinician.
- Less severe signs and symptoms can be treated initially with assessment of response to therapy and further steps as listed below.
- If available, measure PEF—values of 50–79% predicted or personal best indicate the need for quick-relief mediation. Depending on the response to treatment, contact with a clinician may also be indicated. Values below 50% indicate the need for immediate medical care.

Initial treatment
- Inhaled SABA: up to two treatments 20 minutes apart of 2–6 puffs by metered-dose inhaler (MDI) or nebulizer treatments.
- Note: Medication delivery is highly variable. Children and individuals who have exacerbations of lesser severity may need fewer puffs than suggested above.

Good Response
No wheezing or dyspnea (assess tachypnea in young children).
PEF ≥80% predicted or personal best.
- Contact clinician for followup instructions and further management.
- May continue inhaled SABA every 3–4 hours for 24–48 hours.
- Consider short course of oral systemic corticosteroids.

Incomplete Response
Persistent wheezing and dyspnea (tachypnea).
PEP 50–79% predicted or personal best.
- Add oral systemic corticosteroid.
- Continue inhaled SABA.
- Contact clinician urgently (this day) for further instruction.

Poor response
Marked wheezing and dyspnea.
PEF <50% predicted or personal best.
- Add oral systemic corticosteroid.
- Repeat inhaled SABA immediately.
- If distress is severe and nonresponsive to initial treatment:
  — Call your doctor AND
  — PROCEED TO ED;
  — Consider calling 9–1–1 (ambulance transport).

- To ED.

Key: ED. emergency department; MDI, metered-dose inhaler; PEF, peak expiratory flow; SABA, short-acting beta₂-agonist (quick-relief inhaler)

FIGURE 33-6. Home management of acute asthma exacerbation. Patients at risk for asthma-related death should receive immediate clinical attention after initial treatment. Additional therapy may be required. *(From reference 2.)*

TREATMENT

Acute Severe Asthma

The primary goal is prevention of life-threatening asthma by early recognition of signs of deterioration and early intervention. As such, the principal goals of treatment include:[2]

- Correction of significant hypoxemia
- Rapid reversal of airflow obstruction
- Reduction of the likelihood of relapse of the exacerbation or future recurrence of severe airflow obstruction
- Development of a written asthma action plan in case of a further exacerbation

These goals are best achieved by early initiation or intensification of treatment and close monitoring of objective measures of oxygenation and lung function.[2] Early response to treatment as measured by the improvement in FEV_1 at 30 minutes following inhaled β_2-agonists is the best predictor of outcome.[2,27] Providing adequate oxygen supplementation to maintain oxygen (O_2) saturations above 90% (or >95% in pregnant women and those who have coexistent heart disease) is essential. In children younger than 6 years of age, in whom lung function measures are difficult to obtain, a combination of objective (e.g., oxygen saturation, capillary CO_2, respiratory rate, and heart rate) and subjective measures may be used to assess severity.[2]

The primary therapy of acute exacerbations is pharmacologic, which includes short-acting inhaled β_2-agonists and, depending on

the severity, systemic corticosteroids, inhaled ipratropium and O_2 (Figs. 33–6 and 33–7).[2] It is important that therapy not be delayed, so the history and physical examination should be obtained while initial therapy is being provided. Patients at risk for life-threatening exacerbations require special attention. Risk factors include: a history of previous severe asthma exacerbations (e.g., hospitalizations, intubations, or hypoxic seizures); difficulty perceiving asthma symptoms or severity of exacerbations; comorbidities (e.g., cardiac disease, other chronic lung disease, illicit drug use, or major psychosocial/psychiatric history); use of more than two canisters per month of short-acting inhaled β_2-agonists; and current intake of oral corticosteroids or recent withdrawal from oral corticosteroids.[2]

A complete blood count may be appropriate for patients with fever or purulent sputum, but modest leukocytosis is common in asthma exacerbations due to viral infection or secondary to corticosteroid administration. Chest radiography is not recommended for routine assessment but should be obtained for patients suspected of a complicating cardiopulmonary process or another pulmonary process (pneumothorax or pulmonary consolidation).[2] Serum electrolytes should be monitored if high-dose continuous inhaled or systemic β_2-agonists are to be used because they can produce transient decreases in potassium, magnesium, and phosphate.[2] Measurement of serum electrolytes is also prudent in patients who take diuretics regularly and in patients with coexistent cardiovascular disease. The combination of high-dose β_2-agonists and systemic corticosteroids occasionally may result in excessive elevations of glucose and lactic acid.[2]

Initial response should be achieved within minutes, and most patients experience significant improvement within the first 30 to

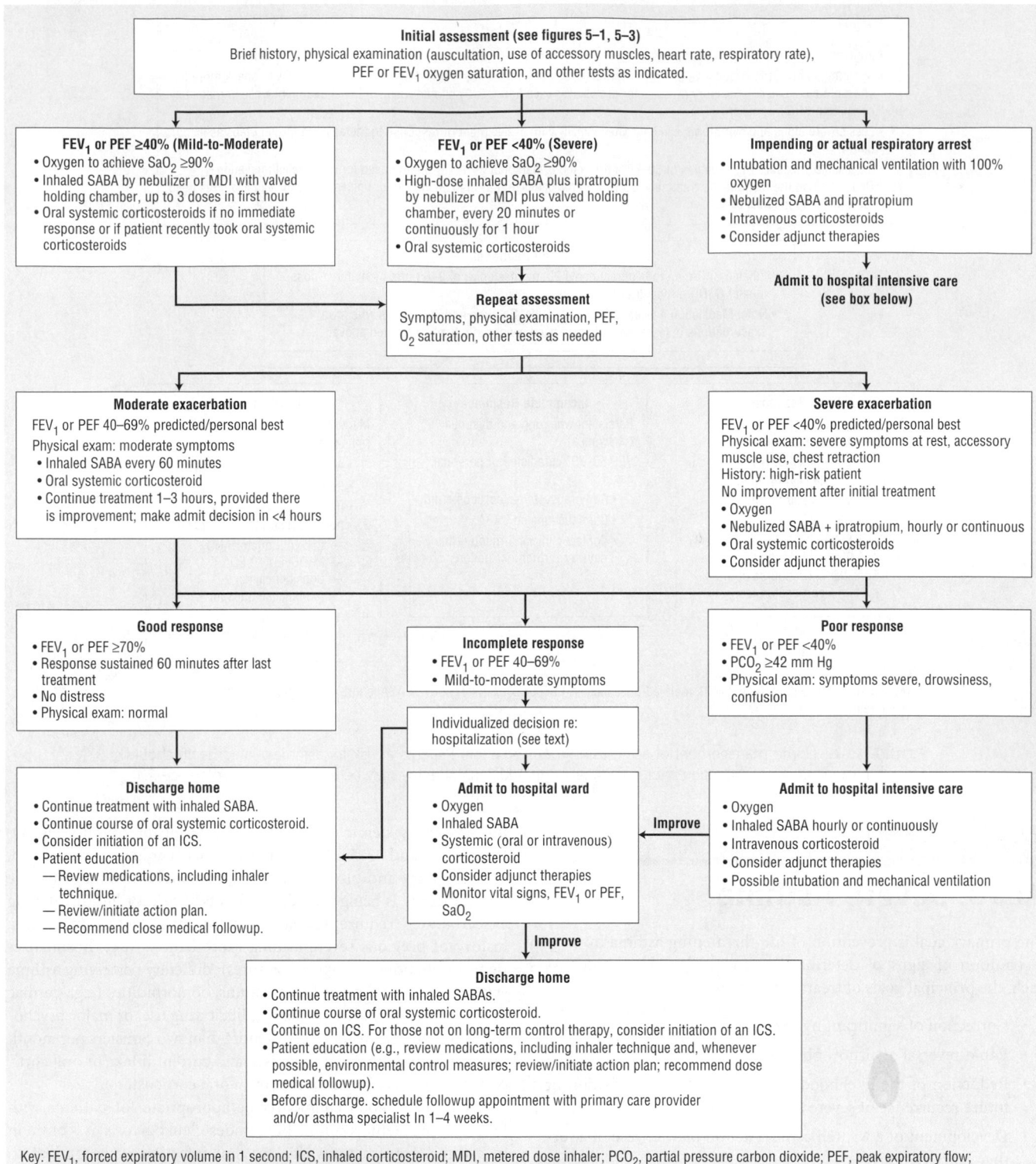

Initial assessment (see figures 5–1, 5–3)
Brief history, physical examination (auscultation, use of accessory muscles, heart rate, respiratory rate), PEF or FEV₁ oxygen saturation, and other tests as indicated.

FEV₁ or PEF ≥40% (Mild-to-Moderate)
- Oxygen to achieve SaO₂ ≥90%
- Inhaled SABA by nebulizer or MDI with valved holding chamber, up to 3 doses in first hour
- Oral systemic corticosteroids if no immediate response or if patient recently took oral systemic corticosteroids

FEV₁ or PEF <40% (Severe)
- Oxygen to achieve SaO₂ ≥90%
- High-dose inhaled SABA plus ipratropium by nebulizer or MDI plus valved holding chamber, every 20 minutes or continuously for 1 hour
- Oral systemic corticosteroids

Impending or actual respiratory arrest
- Intubation and mechanical ventilation with 100% oxygen
- Nebulized SABA and ipratropium
- Intravenous corticosteroids
- Consider adjunct therapies

Admit to hospital intensive care (see box below)

Repeat assessment
Symptoms, physical examination, PEF, O₂ saturation, other tests as needed

Moderate exacerbation
FEV₁ or PEF 40–69% predicted/personal best
Physical exam: moderate symptoms
- Inhaled SABA every 60 minutes
- Oral systemic corticosteroid
- Continue treatment 1–3 hours, provided there is improvement; make admit decision in <4 hours

Severe exacerbation
FEV₁ or PEF <40% predicted/personal best
Physical exam: severe symptoms at rest, accessory muscle use, chest retraction
History: high-risk patient
No improvement after initial treatment
- Oxygen
- Nebulized SABA + ipratropium, hourly or continuous
- Oral systemic corticosteroids
- Consider adjunct therapies

Good response
- FEV₁ or PEF ≥70%
- Response sustained 60 minutes after last treatment
- No distress
- Physical exam: normal

Incomplete response
- FEV₁ or PEF 40–69%
- Mild-to-moderate symptoms

Poor response
- FEV₁ or PEF <40%
- PCO₂ ≥42 mm Hg
- Physical exam: symptoms severe, drowsiness, confusion

Individualized decision re: hospitalization (see text)

Discharge home
- Continue treatment with inhaled SABA.
- Continue course of oral systemic corticosteroid.
- Consider initiation of an ICS.
- Patient education
  — Review medications, including inhaler technique.
  — Review/initiate action plan.
  — Recommend close medical followup.

Admit to hospital ward
- Oxygen
- Inhaled SABA
- Systemic (oral or intravenous) corticosteroid
- Consider adjunct therapies
- Monitor vital signs, FEV₁ or PEF, SaO₂

Improve

Admit to hospital intensive care
- Oxygen
- Inhaled SABA hourly or continuously
- Intravenous corticosteroid
- Consider adjunct therapies
- Possible intubation and mechanical ventilation

Improve

Discharge home
- Continue treatment with inhaled SABAs.
- Continue course of oral systemic corticosteroid.
- Continue on ICS. For those not on long-term control therapy, consider initiation of an ICS.
- Patient education (e.g., review medications, including inhaler technique and, whenever possible, environmental control measures; review/initiate action plan; recommend dose medical followup).
- Before discharge. schedule followup appointment with primary care provider and/or asthma specialist In 1–4 weeks.

Key: FEV₁, forced expiratory volume in 1 second; ICS, inhaled corticosteroid; MDI, metered dose inhaler; PCO₂, partial pressure carbon dioxide; PEF, peak expiratory flow; SABA, short-acting beta₂-agonist; SaO₂, oxygen saturation

FIGURE 33-7. Emergency department and hospital care of acute asthma exacerbations. *(From reference 2.)*

60 minutes of therapy, with most patients doubling their FEV₁ or PEF.[2] In patients ultimately admitted to the hospital, only a 10% to 20% improvement is seen within the first 2 hours. Hypoxemia, primarily a result of ventilation-perfusion mismatch, is immediately correctable by low-flow oxygen.[2] While reversal of lung function into the normal range may take 12 to 24 hours, complete restoration takes much longer—up to 3 to 7 days.[2] A strategy to prevent recurrence includes systemic corticosteroids and symptom or PEF monitoring.[2] It is essential to provide the patient with a written self-management action plan for dealing with exacerbations.

Patients at risk for severe exacerbations should be taught how to use a peak-flow meter and monitor morning peak flows at home.[2] In young children, an increased respiratory rate, increased heart rate, and inability to speak more than one or two words between breaths are signs of severe obstruction.[2] Oxygen saturations by pulse oximetry and peak flows should be measured in all patients not completely responding to initial intensive inhaled β₂-agonist therapy. Initially, on admission, the peak flows or clinical symptoms should be monitored every 2 to 4 hours. Prior to discharge from the ED or hospital, the patient should be given a sufficient supply

TABLE 33-6 Dosages of Drugs of Acute Severe Exacerbations of Asthma in the Emergency Department or Hospital

Medications	Dosages ≥12 Years Old	Dosages <12 Years Old	Comments
Inhaled β-agonists			
Albuterol nebulizer soln. (5 mg/mL, 0.63 mg/3 mL, 1.25 mg/3 mL, 2.5 mg/3 mL)	2.5–5 mg every 20 min for 3 doses, then 2.5–10 mg every 1–4 h as needed, or 10–15 mg/h continuously	0.15 mg/kg (minimum dose 2.5 mg) every 20 min for 3 doses, then 0.15–0.3 mg/kg up to 10 mg every 1–4 h as needed, or 0.5 mg/kg/h by continuous nebulization	Only selective β_2-agonists are recommended. For optimal delivery, dilute aerosols to minimum of 4 mL at gas flow of 6–8 L/min. Use face mask if <4 years.
Albuterol MDI (90 mcg/puff)	4–8 puffs every 30 min up to 4 h, then every 1–4 h as needed	4–8 puffs every 20 min for 3 doses, then every 1–4 h as needed	In patients in severe distress, nebulization is preferred; use VHC type spacer with facemask if <4 years old
Levalbuterol nebulizer soln. 0.31 mg/3 mL 0.63 mg/3 mL 2.5 mg/1 mL 1.25 mg/3 mL	Give at one-half the mg dose of albuterol above	Give at one-half the mg dose of albuterol above	The single isomer of albuterol is twice as potent on a mg basis
Levalbuterol MDI (45 mcg/puff)	See albuterol dose MOI dose	See albuterol dose MOI dose above	See albuterol MOI dose one-half as potent as albuterol on a microgram basis
Pirbuterol MDI (200 mcg/puff)	See albuterol MOI dose above		Has not been studied in acute severe asthma
Systemic β-agonists			
Epinephrine 1:1,000 (1 mg/mL)	0.3–0.5 mg every 20 min for 3 doses SQ	0.01 mg/kg up to 0.5 mg every 20 min for 3 doses SQ	No proven advantage of systemic therapy over aerosol
Terbutaline (1 mg/mL)	0.25 mg every 20 min for 3 doses SQ	0.01 mg/kg every 20 min for 3 doses, then every 2–6 h as needed SQ	Not recommended
Anticholinergics			
Ipratropium Br. nebulizer soln. (0.25 mg/mL)	500 mcg every 30 min for 3 doses, then every 2–4 h as needed	250 mcg every 20 min for 3 doses, then 250 mcg every 2–4 h	May mix in same nebulizer with albuterol; do not use as first-line therapy; only add to β_2-agonist therapy
Ipratropium Br. MDI (18 mcg/puff)	8 puffs every 20 min as needed for up to 3 h	4–8 puffs as needed every 2–4 h	
Corticosteroids			
Prednisone, methylprednisolone, prednisolone	40–80 mg in 1 or 2 divided doses until PEF reaches 70% of personal best	1 mg/kg (max. 60 mg/d) in 2 divided doses until PEF is 70% of normal predicted	For outpatient "burst" use 1–2 mg/kg/day, max. 60 mg, for 3–10 days in children and 40–60 mg/day in 1 or 2 divided doses for 5–10 days in adults

Note: No advantage has been found for very-high-dose corticosteroids in acute severe asthma, nor is there any advantage for intravenous administration over oral therapy. The usual regimen is to continue the oral corticosteroid for duration of hospitalization. The final duration of therapy following a hospitalization or emergency department visit may be from 3–10 days. If patients are then started on ICSs, there is no need to taper the systemic corticosteroid dose. ICSs can be started at any time during the exacerbation. (*From reference 2.*)

of prednisone, taught the purpose of the medications and proper inhaler technique, and referred to follow-up asthma care within 1 to 4 weeks; initiation of inhaled corticosteroids (ICSs) should also be considered.[2]

❼ Early recognition of deterioration and aggressive treatment are the keys to successful treatment of acute asthma exacerbations. Thus patient and/or parent education teaching self-management skills and written action plans for early institution of therapy for acute exacerbations improve outcomes.[2] For more moderate to severe patients, this therapeutic plan also may include the availability of oral prednisone to begin at home.[2] Easy access by telephone to healthcare providers is also needed. Because of the rapid progression to severe asthma that can occur, patients and parents should be encouraged to communicate promptly with their asthma care provider during an exacerbation.

Figures 33–6 and 33–7 illustrate the recommended therapies for the treatment of acute asthma of mild, moderate, and severe exacerbations in home and emergency department/hospital settings, respectively.[2] The dosages of the drugs for acute severe exacerbations are provided in Table 33–6.[2,6] Institutions should strongly consider developing critical-pathways/treatment algorithms for their EDs because their implementation has been shown to improve

outcomes and decrease the cost of care.[28] Finally, it is strongly recommended that an appointment with the patient's primary care provider be made within 1 week of the ED visit.[27]

■ NONPHARMACOLOGIC AND ANCILLARY THERAPY

Infants and young children may be mildly dehydrated owing to increased insensible loss, vomiting, and decreased intake.[2] Unless dehydration has occurred, increased fluid therapy is not indicated in acute asthma management because the capillary leak from cytokines and increased negative intrathoracic pressures may promote edema in the airways.[2] Correction of significant dehydration is always indicated, and the urine specific gravity may help to guide therapy in young children, in whom the state of hydration may be difficult to determine.[2] Chest physical therapy and mucolytics are not recommended in the therapy of acute asthma.[2] Sedatives should not be given because anxiety may be a sign of hypoxemia, which could be worsened by central nervous system depressants.[2] Antibiotics also are not indicated routinely because viral respiratory tract infections are the primary cause of asthma exacerbations.[2] Antibiotics should be reserved for patients who have signs and symptoms of pneumonia (e.g., fever, pulmonary consolidation, and purulent sputum from polymorphonuclear leukocytes). *Mycoplasma* and *Chlamydia* are infrequent causes of severe asthma exacerbations but should be considered in patients with high oxygen requirements.[2]

Respiratory failure or impending respiratory failure as measured by rising $PaCO_2$ (≥ 45 mm Hg) or failure to correct hypoxemia with supplemental oxygen therapy is treated with intubation and mechanical ventilation.[27] In order to prevent barotrauma and pneumothoraces from excess positive pressure, it is recommended that controlled hypoventilation or permissive hypercapnia be used (correcting the hypoxemia, $PaO_2 > 60$ mm Hg, but allowing the $PaCO_2$ to rise to the high 60 mm Hg range).[27]

■ PHARMACOTHERAPY

β_2-Agonists

❹ The short-acting inhaled β_2-agonists are the most effective bronchodilators and the treatment of first choice for the management of acute severe asthma.[2,27] Up to 66% of adults presenting to an ED require only three doses of 2.5 mg nebulized albuterol to be discharged.[27] Most well-controlled clinical trials have demonstrated equal to greater efficacy and greater safety of aerosolized β_2-agonists over systemic administration regardless of the severity of obstruction.[2,27] Systemic adverse effects, hypokalemia, hyperglycemia, tachycardia, and cardiac dysrhythmias are more pronounced in patients receiving systemic β_2-agonist therapy. Children younger than 2 years of age achieve clinically significant responses from nebulized albuterol.[2,29] Effective doses of aerosolized β_2-agonists can be delivered successfully through mechanical ventilator circuits to infants, children, and adults in respiratory failure secondary to severe airways obstruction.[29]

Frequent administration of inhaled β_2-agonists (every 20 minutes or continuous nebulization) has been found to be superior to the same dosage administered at 1-hour intervals.[30] In the subset of more severely obstructed patients, continuous nebulization decreases the hospital admission rate, provides greater improvement in the FEV_1 and PEF, and reduces duration of hospitalization when compared with intermittent (hourly) nebulized albuterol in the same total dose.[30] Thus continuous nebulization is recommended for patients having an unsatisfactory response (achieving less than 50% of normal FEV_1 or PEF) following the initial three doses (every 20 minutes) of aerosolized β_2-agonists and potentially for patients presenting initially with PEF or FEV_1 values of less than 30% of predicted normal.[2,30]

The doses of inhaled β_2-agonists for acute severe asthma exacerbations (see Table 33–6) have been derived empirically. The β_2-agonists follow a log-linear dose-response curve.[31] In addition, the dose-response curve is shifted to the right by more severe bronchospasm or by increased concentrations of bronchospastic mediators, which is characteristic of functional antagonists.[31] The ability to increase the dose of the short-acting aerosolized β_2-agonists by as much as 5- to 10-fold over doses producing adequate bronchodilation in chronic stable asthma is what contributes to their efficacy in reversing the bronchospasm of acute severe exacerbations. The nebulizer dose of inhaled β_2-agonists for children often is listed on a weight basis (milligrams per kilogram). However, a fixed minimal dose (2.5 mg albuterol or equivalent), as opposed to a weight-adjusted dose, is more appropriate in younger children because children younger than 5 years of age receive a lower lung dose.[2] Adults dosed on a weight basis demonstrate excessive cardiac stimulation, so they have fixed maximal doses[2] (see Table 33–6). Initial doses of inhaled β_2-agonists can produce vasodilation, worsening ventilation-perfusion mismatch, slightly lowering oxygen saturation or PaO_2.[27] High-doses of inhaled β_2-agonists can produce a decrease in serum potassium concentration, an increase in heart rate, and an increase in serum glucose and lactic acid concentration.[31] However, both children and adults receiving continuously nebulized β_2-agonists have demonstrated decreased heart rates as their lung function improves.[30] Thus, an elevated heart rate is not an indication to use lower doses or to avoid using inhaled β_2-agonists.

Some controversy exists concerning the most cost-effective delivery system (MDI plus VHC vs nebulization) to be used in treating acute severe exacerbations in the ED and hospital (see below).[2,29] The DPIs are currently not indicated for the treatment of acute severe asthma exacerbations due to the higher inspiratory flows required for adequate drug delivery.[2,29]

Corticosteroids

Systemic corticosteroids are indicated in all patients with acute severe asthma exacerbations not responding completely to initial inhaled β_2-agonist administration (every 20 minutes for three to four doses).[2] Intravenous therapy offers no therapeutic advantage over oral administration.[2,32] This therapy usually is continued until hospital discharge. Tapering the systemic corticosteroid dose following discharge from the hospital appears unnecessary, provided that patients are prescribed inhaled corticosteroids for outpatient therapy.[2] Most patients achieve 70% of predicted normal FEV_1 within 48 hours and 80% of predicted by 6 days after plateauing by day 3. Thus, maintaining systemic corticosteroid courses for 10 to 14 days may be unnecessarily long in some patients. Indeed, many patients not admitted to the hospital respond to 3- to 5-day courses of systemic corticosteroids. Short courses of oral prednisone (3–10 day "bursts") have been effective in preventing hospitalizations in infants and young children.[2] It is recommended that a full dose of the corticosteroid be continued until the patient's peak flow reaches 70% of predicted normal or personal best.[2]

Multiple daily dosing of systemic corticosteroids for the initial therapy of acute asthma exacerbations appears warranted because receptor-binding affinities of lung corticosteroid receptors are decreased in the face of airways inflammation.[32] However, patients with less severe exacerbations may be treated adequately with once-daily administration. High-dose and very-high-pulse-dose corticosteroid regimens have not been shown to enhance the outcomes in severe acute asthma but are associated with a higher likelihood of side effects.[32]

Studies of ICSs in acute exacerbations of asthma have provided conflicting results. Studies have demonstrated both greater and lesser efficacy than standard doses of oral corticosteroids.[32] Currently, there is insufficient evidence supporting efficacy in the ED setting, although continued research appears warranted.[2] There is evidence that prescribing ICSs on discharge from the ED reduces the risk of relapse.[32] This policy is reasonable because inflammation is the underlying cause of deterioration in most cases.[2]

Anticholinergics

Inhaled ipratropium bromide produces a further improvement in lung function of 10% to 15% over inhaled β_2-agonists alone. In children and adults, multiple-dose ipratropium bromide added to initial therapy reduces hospitalization rate in the subset of patients with a baseline FEV_1 of less than 30% of predicted.[33] Ipratropium bromide, a quaternary amine, is poorly absorbed and produces minimal or no systemic effects. Care should be used when administering ipratropium bromide by nebulizer. If a tight mask or mouthpiece is not used, the ipratropium bromide that deposits in the eyes may produce pupillary dilatation and difficulty in accommodation. Ipratropium bromide is not a vasodilator, so unlike β_2-agonists it will not worsen ventilation-perfusion mismatch.[33]

Alternative Therapies

The ED use of aminophylline, a moderate bronchodilator, for acute asthma has not been recommended for a number of years.[2] Aminophylline in adults and children hospitalized with acute asthma does not enhance improvement in lung function or reduce length of hospitalization but has increased the risk of adverse effects.[34] Adverse effects of theophylline include nausea and vomiting and potentiation of the cardiac effects of the inhaled β_2-agonists.

Magnesium sulfate is a moderately potent bronchodilator, producing relaxation of smooth muscle and central nervous system depression.[35] The use of intravenous magnesium sulfate in patients presenting to the ED is controversial (see below).[35,36] The adverse effects of magnesium sulfate include hypotension, facial flushing, sweating, nausea, loss of deep tendon reflexes, and respiratory depression.[35] Helium is an inert gas of low density with no pharmacologic properties that can lower resistance to gas flow and increase ventilation because the low density decreases the pressure gradient needed to achieve a given level of turbulent flow, converting turbulent flow to laminar flow.[2] Helium is given as a mixture of helium and oxygen (heliox), usually 60% to 70% helium with 30% to 40% oxygen.[37] Heliox has been effective in some but not all clinical trials. Although heliox is free of adverse effects, its use is limited to patients with a low inspired oxygen requirement because the decrease in density generally is insignificant clinically with less than 60% helium.[37]

The inhalational anesthetics halothane, isoflurane, and enflurane all have been reported to have a positive effect in children and adults with acute severe asthma that is unresponsive to standard medical therapy.[2] The proposed mechanisms for inhalational anesthetics include direct action on bronchial smooth muscle, inhibition of airway reflexes, attenuation of histamine-induced bronchospasm, and interaction with β_2-adrenergic receptors.[2] Well-controlled trials with these agents have not been completed.[27] Potential adverse effects include myocardial depression, vasodilation, arrhythmias, and depression of mucociliary function.[27] In addition, the practical problem of delivery and scavenging these agents in the intensive care environment as opposed to the operating room is a concern. The use of volatile anesthetics cannot be recommended based on insufficient evidence of efficacy.

Ketamine has been recommended for rapid induction of anesthesia in patients with asthma who require intubation and mechanical ventilation.[2] Although anecdotal reports have suggested that ketamine is useful as a short-term adjunct in acute severe asthma; controlled trials have not provided evidence of efficacy. Ketamine has several significant adverse effects, including the anesthesia emergence reaction, which can alter mood and cause delirium. These emergence phenomena occur in at least 25% of patients over 16 years of age; the incidence seems to be much lower in younger patients.[2] Other risks include an increase in heart rate, arterial blood pressure, and cerebral blood flow because of its sympathetic effects.[27]

■ SPECIAL POPULATIONS

❻ Infants and children younger than 4 years of age may be at greater risk of respiratory failure than older children and adults. Although treated with the same drugs, these younger children require the use of a facemask as opposed to a mouthpiece for delivery of aerosolized medication. Use of the facemask reduces delivery of drug to the lung by one-half so that a minimal dose is recommended as opposed to a weight-adjusted dose.[26,29] The facemask should be sized appropriately and should fit snugly over the nose and mouth. Use of the "blow by" method, where the respiratory therapist or parent places the mask or extension tubing near the

child's nose and mouth, should be discouraged because holding the mask as few as 2 cm from the patient's face reduces lung delivery of the aerosol by 80%.[2,26]

■ DRUG CLASS INFORMATION

Short-Acting β_2-Agonists

❺ ❻ The β_2-agonists are the most effective bronchodilators available. The β_2-adrenergic receptors are transmembrane proteins consisting of clusters of seven helices of amino acids that form the ligand-binding core.[31] The human β_2-adrenergic receptors are polymorphic in structure, with the most common polymorphisms in the amino terminus of the receptor at amino acid positions 16 (encoding either arginine [Arg] or glycine [Gly]) and 27 (encoding either glutamine [Gln] or glutamic acid [Glu]).[38] Some of the polymorphisms determine responsiveness to β_2-agonists, whereas others may act as disease modifiers (see below).[39] Stimulation of β_2-adrenergic receptor activates cytoplasmic G proteins, which in turn activate adenylyl cyclase to produce cyclic adenosine monophosphate (cAMP), generally thought to be responsible for the bulk of activity through activation of various proteins by cAMP-dependent protein kinase A (PKA).[31] This activation, in turn, decreases unbound intracellular calcium, producing smooth muscle relaxation, mast cell membrane stabilization, and skeletal muscle stimulation.[31] Despite the fact that β_2-agonists are potent inhibitors of mast cell degranulation in vitro, they do not inhibit the late asthmatic response to allergen challenge or the subsequent bronchial hyperresponsiveness.[2,31] Long-term administration of β_2-agonists does not reduce BHR, confirming a lack of significant antiinflammatory activity.[38] β_2-Adrenergic stimulation also activates Na^+-K^+-ATPase, produces gluconeogenesis, and enhances insulin secretion, resulting in a mild to moderate decrease in serum potassium concentration by driving potassium intracellularly.[31] The chronotropic response to β_2-agonists is mediated in part by baroreceptor reflex mechanisms as a result of the drop in blood pressure from vascular smooth muscle relaxation, as well as by direct stimulation of cardiac β_2-receptors and some β_1 stimulation at high concentrations.[31] Table 33-7 lists the pharmacologic effects of adrenergic receptor stimulation. Because β_1-receptor stimulation produces excessive cardiac stimulation, resulting in cardiac arrhythmias, and because the inotropic effect enhancing myocardial oxygen consumption leads to myocardial necrosis, there is no rationale for using non–β_2-selective agonists in the treatment of asthma.[31]

TABLE 33-7	Pharmacologic Responses to Sympathomimetic Agonists	
Tissue	**Receptor Type**	**Response**
Airways	β_2	Smooth muscle relaxation (bronchodilation), increased ciliary beat, increased serous secretion, and inhibition of mast cell degranulation
	α	Smooth muscle contraction (bronchoconstriction?)
Heart	β_1	Inotropic and chronotropic
	β_2	Chronotropic
Vasculature	β_2	Vasodilation, decreased microvascular leakage
	α	Vasoconstriction
Skeletal	β_2	Increased neuromuscular transmission (tremor and increased strength of contraction)
Uterus	β_2	Relaxation (tocolysis)
Metabolic	α, β_1	Glycogenolysis, lipolysis
	β_2	Gluconeogenesis, hypokalemia, increased lactate production

TABLE 33-8 Relative Selectivity, Potency, and Duration of Action of the β-Adrenergic Agonists

Agent	Selectivity β_1	Selectivity β_2	Potency, β_2[a]	Duration of Action[b] Bronchodilation (h)	Protection (h)[c]	Oral Activity
Isoproterenol	++++	++++	1	0.5–2	0.5–1	No
Albuterol	+	++++	2	4–8	2–4	Yes
Pirbuterol	+	++++	5	4–8	2–4	Yes
Terbutaline	+	++++	4	4–8	2–4	Yes
Formoterol	+	++++	0.12	≥12	6–12	Yes
Salmeterol	+	++++	0.5	≥12	6–12	No

[a]Relative molar potency to isoproterenol: 15 = lowest potency.
[b]Median durations with the highest value after a single dose and lowest after chronic administration.
[c]Protection refers to the prevention of bronchoconstriction induced by exercise or nonspecific bronchial challenges.

Table 33–8 compares the various β-adrenergic agonists used in asthma in terms of selectivity, potency, oral activity, and duration of action. The β_2-agonists are functional or physiologic antagonists in that they relax airway smooth muscle regardless of the mechanism for constriction.[31] When administered in equipotent doses, all the short-acting drugs produce the same intensity of response; the only differences are in duration of action and cardiac toxicity.[2,31] The catecholamine derivatives all have the disadvantage of rapid inactivation of their 3,4-hydroxyl catechol group from catechol-O-methyltransferase found in the gastrointestinal tract, rendering them orally inactive. In addition, catecholamines are taken up rapidly into tissues by secondary uptake mechanisms that limit their receptor occupancy and thus have a shorter duration of action.[31] All the β_2-agonists are more bronchoselective when administered by the aerosol route. Aerosol administration of the short-acting β_2-agonists provides more rapid response and greater protection against provocations that induce bronchospasm such as exercise and allergen challenges than does systemic administration.[2,31] Differences in myocardial effects are discernible between selective and nonselective agents even when administered as aerosols, particularly at the higher doses used for acute severe asthma. The β_2-agonists also differ in efficacy or ability to activate the β_2-adrenergic receptors. Full agonists include the catecholamines while the synthetic β_2-agonists all exhibit various levels of partial agonism in the following order of fuller agonism: formoterol > albuterol = terbutaline = pirbuterol > salmeterol.[31] Although partial agonists by definition cannot produce maximum dilation or protection as full agonists and can potentially block the effect of a full agonist, these differences have not been proven to be clinically significant.

All synthetic β_2-agonists are 1:1 racemic mixtures of two mirror images (enantiomers) owing to an asymmetric or chiral carbon.[31] Since most physiologic functions (receptor occupancy and activation and enzymatic metabolism) are stereoselective, the (R)-enantiomers of the β_2-agonists are the most pharmacologically active isomer.[31] While it was felt initially that the (S)-enantiomers were essentially inactive owing to the 100 to 1,000-fold potency difference between the enantiomers, studies in animal models and isolated in vitro tissue preparations have suggested that the (S)-enantiomer of albuterol may be proinflammatory and could induce BHR.[31] However, evidence that this occurs consistently in humans or is clinically relevant is lacking (see below).[31] The pharmacokinetics are stereoselective as well, although not predictable. (R)-Albuterol is metabolized more rapidly than (S)-albuterol, which could lead to accumulation of (S)-albuterol with continued dosing.[31] On the other hand, (S)-terbutaline is eliminated more rapidly than (R)-terbutaline.[38]

Both the intensity and duration of response are dose dependent, and more important, the dose-response relationship is dynamic.[31]

At increasing levels of baseline bronchoconstriction (irrespective of the stimulus), the dose-response curve is shifted to the right, and the duration of bronchodilation is decreased.[31] This shift is reflected in the need for higher, more frequent doses in acute asthma exacerbations; the duration of protection against significant provocation is much less than the duration of bronchodilation in chronic stable asthma (see Table 33–8).[31,38]

Chronic administration of β_2-agonists leads to downregulation (decreased number of β_2-receptors) and a decreased binding affinity (desensitization) for these receptors.[31] Systemic corticosteroid therapy can both prevent and partially reverse this phenomenon.[2,31] However, the use of inhaled corticosteroids appears to have minimal ability to prevent tolerance to β_2-agonists.[31] Although in vitro differences in downregulation of the β_2-receptors exist (Gly-16 homozygotes > Arg-16 homozygotes), clinical desensitization is seen in all polymorphisms.[38] Tolerance primarily reduces duration of bronchodilation as opposed to peak response, although that can occur as well. A significantly greater tolerance develops in other tissues (e.g., lymphocytes and cardiac and skeletal muscle) compared with the lung, primarily as a result of the surplus β_2-receptors found in respiratory smooth muscle.[31] Tolerance to the extrapulmonary effects (cardiac stimulation and hypokalemia) may account for a lack of significant cardiac effects with retention of the bronchodilator response despite chronic inhaled β_2-agonist therapy, whereas tolerance to mast cell stabilization may be a drawback to chronic use.[31] Thus, chronic β_2-agonist administration produces a tolerance of minimal clinical significance that is overcome easily by increasing the dose or by administering corticosteroids.[2,31,38] Most of the tolerance occurs within a week of regular administration and does not worsen with continued administration. As would be expected from a receptor phenomenon, tolerance is a cross-tolerance to all β_2-agonists.[31] Whether or not regular use of short-acting inhaled β_2-agonists produces worsening of asthma in a subset of patients remains controversial (see below), but it does not appear to occur in the entire population.[38] Regular treatment with short-acting β_2-agonists can increase BHR and in homozygous Arg-16 patients reduces morning PEF and increases exacerbations.[39] Regular treatment (4 times daily) does not improve symptom control over as-needed use and is not indicated.[2]

In conclusion, the short-acting inhaled selective β_2-agonists are indicated for the as needed treatment of intermittent episodes of bronchospasm. They are the first treatment of choice for acute severe asthma and exercise-induced bronchospasm.[2,31] They inhibit EIB in a dose-dependent fashion and provide complete protection for a 2-hour period following inhalation with varying levels of patient-dependent protection over 4 hours.[31] Although the regular administration of β_2-agonists slightly decreases the effect, two inhalations prior to exercise still

TABLE 33-9 Pharmacodynamic/Pharmacokinetic Comparison of the Corticosteroids

Systemic	Antiinflammatory potency	Mineralcorticoid potency	Duration of biologic activity (h)	Elimination half-life (h)
Hydrocortisone	1	1.0	8–12	1.5–2.0
Prednisone	4	0.8	12–36	2.5–3.5
Methylprednisolone	5	0.5	12–36	3.3
Dexamethasone	25	0	36–54	3.4–4.0

ICS	Receptor binding affinity	Oral bioavailability (%)	Systemic clearance (L/h)	Half-life (h) IV/inhaled
BDP/BMP[a]	0.4/13.5	20/40	150/120	(0.5/2.7)/(UK/2.7)
BUD	9.4	11	84	2.8/2.0
CIC/des-CIC[a]	0.12/12.0	<1/<1	152/228	(0.36/3.4)/(0.5/4.8)
FLU	1.8	20	58	1.6/1.6
FP	18	≤1	66	7.8/14.4
MF	23[b]	<1	53	5.8/UK
TAA	3.6	23	45–69	2.0/3.6

Note: Receptor binding affinities are relative to dexamethasone equal to 1. UK = unknown.
[a]BDP and CIC are prodrugs that are activated in the lung to their active metabolites BMP and des-CIC, respectively.
[b]MF studied in a different receptor system. Value estimated from relative values of BDP, TAA, and FP in that system.
BUD, budesonide; CIC, ciclesonide; des-CIC, des-ciclesonide; FLU, flunisolide; FP, fluticasone propionate; MF, mometasone furoate; TAA, triamcinolone acetonide; BDP, beclomethasone dipropionate; BMP, beclomethasone 17-monopropionate.

essentially blocks exercise-induced bronchospasm completely (1% vs 5% drop in FEV$_1$).[31]

Systemic Corticosteroids

❹ The corticosteroids are the most effective antiinflammatories available to treat asthma.[2] Actions useful in treating asthma include (1) increasing the number of β_2-adrenergic receptors and improving the receptor responsiveness to β_2-adrenergic stimulation, (2) reducing mucus production and hypersecretion, (3) reducing BHR, and (4) reducing airway edema and exudation.[2,40] The glucocorticoid receptor is found in the cytoplasm of most body cells, explaining the multiple effects of systemic corticosteroids. There is no difference between glucocorticoid receptors found throughout the body; however, genetic differences between glucocorticoid receptors from different individuals may determine some of the variations in response.[39] The corticosteroids are lipophilic, readily cross the cell membrane, and combine with the glucocorticoid receptor. The activated complex then enters the nucleus, where it acts as a transcription factor leading to gene activation or suppression.[40] This leads to specific mRNA production, resulting in increased production of antiinflammatory mediators; supression of several proinflammatory cytokines such as IL-1, GM-CSF, IL-4, IL-5, IL-6, and IL-8, reducing inflammatory cell activation, recruitment, and infiltration; and decreasing vascular permeability.[40] In addition, the activated glucocorticoid receptor complex can act directly with cytoplasmic transcription factors, nuclear factor κB, and activating protein 1 to prevent the action of proinflammatory cytokines on the cell.[40]

Owing to the mechanism that modifies gene expression, the time required to see the particular effect depends on the time required for new protein synthesis, decreased formation of the particular mediator, and resolution of the inflammatory response.[40] Generally, the cellular and biochemical effects are immediate, but varying amounts of time are required to produce a clinical response. β_2-Receptor density increases within 4 hours of corticosteroid administration.[40] Improved responsiveness to β_2-agonists occurs within 2 hours.[40] In acute severe asthma, 4 to 12 hours may be required before any clinical response is noted.[32,40] Reversal of seasonally increased BHR requires at least 1 week of therapy.[40] The chronic use of corticosteroids does not induce a state of corticosteroid dependence. Nor is there evidence of tolerance produced by chronic administration.

The corticosteroids used in asthma are compared in Table 33–9.[40,41] Besides acute severe asthma, systemic corticosteroids are also recommended for the treatment of impending episodes of severe asthma unresponsive to bronchodilator therapy.[2,32] The effects of corticosteroids in asthma are dose and duration dependent. This pattern is true for the adverse effects as well (Table 33–10). The clinician must continually balance the toxicity of chronic systemic corticosteroid therapy with control of asthma symptoms. Because short-term (1–2 weeks) high-dose corticosteroids (1–2 mg/kg per day of prednisone) do not produce serious toxicities, the ideal use is to administer the systemic corticosteroids in a short "burst" and then to maintain the patient on appropriate long-term control therapy with ICSs (discussed below).[2,32] In general, therapy for more than 5 days at doses that exceed the usual physiologic endogenous cortisol production will cause temporary aberration in adrenal cortisol release.[40] However, this hypothalamic-pituitary-adrenal (HPA) axis suppression is short-lived (1–3 days) and readily reversible following short bursts (≤10 days) of pharmacologic doses.[40] A maximum number of short bursts that a patient can receive probably exists, after which chronic corticosteroid side effects occur. Adult patients receiving at least eight bursts (≥10 days each) have a similar decrease in trabecular bone density as patients on daily or alternate-day corticosteroids over 1 year.[40] Children who received four or more bursts of prednisone exhibited a subnormal response to hypoglycemic stress or adrenocorticotropic hormone (ACTH) administration and two or more bursts/year increase the risk for osteopenia in

TABLE 33-10 Adverse Effects of Chronic Systemic Glucocorticoid Administration

Hypothalamic–pituitary-adrenal suppression	Hypertension
	Skin striae
Growth retardation	Impaired wound healing
Skeletal muscle myopathy	Inhibition of leukocyte and monocyte
Osteoporosis/fractures	function
Aseptic necrosis of bone	Subcutaneous tissue atrophy
Pancreatitis	Glaucoma
Pseudotumor cerebri	Posterior subcapsular cataracts
Psychiatric disturbances	Moon facies
Sodium and water retention	Central redistribution of fat
Hypokalemia/hyperglycemia	

children.[40,42] Very short courses (3–5 days) have been effective in reducing hospitalization from acute exacerbations.[2] Use of the shorter-acting corticosteroids such as prednisone will produce less adrenal suppression than the longer-acting dexamethasone.[40]

Anticholinergics

The anticholinergic agents have a long history of use for asthma, but they do not have a FDA labeled indication for asthma.[2] Anticholinergics are competitive inhibitors of muscarinic receptors.[43] Unlike β_2-agonists, they are not functional antagonists; they only reverse cholinergic-mediated bronchoconstriction. Normal bronchial tone is maintained through parasympathetic innervation of the airways via the vagus nerve.[40] A number of the triggers and mediators of asthma (i.e., histamine, prostaglandins, sulfur dioxide, exercise, and allergens) produce bronchoconstriction in part through vagal reflex mechanisms.[40] Studies consistently demonstrate that anticholinergics are effective bronchodilators in asthma, although not as effective as β_2-agonists. Anticholinergics attenuate but do not block allergen-induced asthma in a dose-dependent fashion and have no effect on BHR.[43] Anticholinergics attenuate but do not block EIB.[44]

Ipratropium bromide is a nonselective muscarinic receptor blocker, and blockade of inhibitory muscarinic receptors theoretically could result in an increased release of acetylcholine and overcome the block on the smooth muscle receptors (M_3).[43] Only the quaternary ammonium derivatives such as ipratropium bromide should be used because they have the advantage of poor absorption across mucosae and the blood–brain barrier. This attribute contributes to negligible systemic effects with a prolonged local effect (i.e., bronchodilation). In addition, the quaternary compounds do not appear to produce a decrease in mucociliary clearance.[43] Ipratropium bromide has a duration of action of 4 to 8 hours. Both intensity and duration of action are dose dependent. Tiotropium bromide, a long-acting inhaled anticholinergic with duration of 24 hours, is more selective for M_1 and M_3 receptors and less likely to affect the inhibitory M_2 receptors.[43] Time to reach maximum bronchodilation for ipratropium is considerably slower than from aerosolized short-acting β_2-agonists (30–60 minutes vs 5–10 minutes). However, this difference is of little clinical consequence because some bronchodilation is seen within 30 seconds; 50% of maximum response occurs within 3 minutes.[43] Ipratropium bromide is only indicated as adjunctive therapy in acute severe asthma not completely responsive to β_2-agonists alone because it does not improve outcomes in chronic asthma.[2,33] Tiotropium studies in chronic asthma are ongoing.

PHARMACOECONOMICS

Emergency department visits for asthma exceed the number of hospitalizations by approximately 4 times, yet the annual expenditures for ED visits remain significantly less than that spent on in-patient hospital services for patients with acute severe asthma.[3,27] Thus, reducing the number of patients requiring hospitalizations is a primary goal of therapy. Since the primary drugs used to treat acute severe asthma are available generically, drug costs account for only a small portion of the overall costs of care. Few of these therapies have been evaluated formally for their pharmacoeconomic impact. One evaluation based on a meta-analysis of inhaled anticholinergics added to short-acting inhaled β_2-agonists in children with acute severe asthma suggested that this approach was cost-effective and would reduce overall costs by reducing hospitalizations.[26,29] In children with acute severe asthma admitted to an intensive care unit, the use of continuously nebulized albuterol resulted in a decreased cost of care compared with intermittent nebulization.[26]

CLINICAL CONTROVERSIES

Some clinicians believe that intravenous magnesium sulfate is effective for the treatment of acute severe asthma exacerbations unresponsive to standard doses of inhaled β_2-agonists in the ED. This belief is based on subset analyses of two studies showing that patients with the most severe obstruction following initial inhaled β_2-agonists demonstrated a reduction in hospitalizations with magnesium treatment compared with placebo.[35] However, the subset with severe obstruction is the one demonstrating an improved response to the addition of ipratropium bromide and continuous nebulization of inhaled β_2-agonists. In addition, a large, randomized trial failed to confirm a decrease in hospitalization even in the severe group.[36] The 2007 NAEPP guidelines state that magnesium can be considered for use in patients with severe episodes with a poor response to initial inhaled β_2-agonists.[2]

Numerous studies have shown that the inhaled β_2-agonists administered by MDI plus VHC provide a similar outcome in acute severe asthma as drug administration by jet nebulizers.[29] Proponents of administration by MDI plus VHC argue that it is more cost-effective and so should replace nebulizer therapy. However, appropriate cost analyses have yet to be performed.[26] Comparisons in the most severe subsets with combination therapy and continuous nebulization have not been done.[2,26] Current practice should be based on the comfort level of the clinical staff until sufficient data are available to warrant a wholesale recommendation of one method.[2]

EVALUATION OF THERAPEUTIC OUTCOMES

Figures 33–6 and 33–7 provide the monitoring parameters for acute severe asthma. Lung function, either spirometric or peak flow measurements, should be monitored 5 to 10 minutes after each treatment.[2] Oxygen saturations can be easily monitored continuously with pulse oximetry. For young children and infants, pulse oximetry, lung auscultation, and observation of the presence of supraclavicular retractions are useful.[2,27] The majority of patients will respond within the first hour of initial inhaled β_2-agonists regardless of history of home administration of drug.[27] Patients not achieving an initial response should be monitored every half hour to 1 hour. Depending on whether there is a standard ED or a special unit for acute severe asthma, the decision to admit to the hospital should be made within 4 to 6 hours of entry to the emergency department.[27] The mean duration of hospitalization following admission is 2 to 3 days. Frequency of monitoring depends on the severity of the exacerbation. With mild exacerbations, monitor lung function every 2 to 3 hours and severe exacerbations every half hour to 1 hour.

TREATMENT

Chronic Asthma

The diagnosis of chronic asthma is made primarily by history and confirmatory spirometry (see Clinical Presentation above).[2] The NAEPP has provided a list of questions that would lead to the diagnosis of asthma[2] (see Table 33–2). In the older child and adult patient in whom spirometric evaluations can be performed, failure of pulmonary functions to improve acutely does not necessarily rule out asthma. Patients with long-standing disease or substantial inflammation may require an intensive, prolonged course of bronchodilators and glucocorticoids before reversibility is detected.[2] If baseline spirometry is normal, challenge testing with exercise, histamine, methacholine, or mannitol can be used to elicit BHR.[2] Patients with significant symptoms and/or an FEV_1 of less than 70% of predicted normal should not be challenged. Vocal cord dysfunction, particularly with exercise, may mimic asthma symptoms.[2] Studies for atopy such as serum IgE and sputum and blood eosinophil determinations are not necessary to make the diagnosis of asthma, but they may help differentiate asthma from chronic bronchitis in adults. Clinically, this distinction is often difficult to make. Some patients with chronic bronchitis may have a reversible component, and some patients with long-standing severe chronic asthma may have significant irreversible damage and obstruction. Very high peripheral blood eosinophil counts may point to the diagnosis of allergic bronchopulmonary aspergillosis (ABPA) or other hypereosinophilic syndromes.[2] Skin testing is of no value in diagnosing asthma but is useful in identifying triggers.[2] In small infants unable to perform spirometry, the diagnosis is more difficult. Hyperinflation may be demonstrated on the chest roentgenogram.[2] Radiologic examination is helpful in ruling out other causes of wheezing (e.g., foreign-body aspiration, parenchymal lung disease, cardiac disease, and congenital anomalies).[2] In place of pulmonary function measures, the parents should be given a diary card to record symptoms and precipitating events.

■ GOALS FOR MANAGING ASTHMA LONG-TERM

The NAEPP has provided key points for managing asthma long term.[2] The goal for therapy is to control asthma by:

Reducing impairment

1. Prevent chronic and troublesome symptoms (e.g. coughing or breathlessness in the daytime, in the night, or after exertion)

2. Require infrequent use (≤2 days a week) of short-acting inhaled β_2-agonist for quick relief of symptoms[2] (not including prevention of EIB)

3. Maintain (near) normal pulmonary function

4. Maintain normal activity levels (including exercise and other physical activity and attendance at work or school)

5. Meet patients' and families' expectations of and satisfaction with asthma care

Reducing risk

1. Prevent recurrent exacerbations of asthma and minimize the need for ED visits or hospitalizations

2. Prevent loss of lung function; for children, prevent reduced lung growth

3. Minimal or no adverse effects of therapy

■ NONPHARMACOLOGIC THERAPY

Although the mainstay of the management of asthma is pharmacologic therapy, it is likely to fail without concurrent attention to relevant environmental control and management of comorbid conditions. Figure 33–8 depicts the stepwise approach for managing asthma recommended in the newest update by the NAEPP.[2] Nonpharmacologic aspects of therapy are incorporated into the steps. The guidelines were designed to give primary healthcare providers a framework with which to develop the proper approach to the individualized therapy of patients. The heterogeneity of asthma demands an individualized approach to therapy with the basic goals of therapy as primary outcome measures.[2] The focus of therapy is the prevention and suppression of the underlying inflammation.[2] Thus current therapeutic options in asthma consist of acute reliever medications used for acute symptoms and exacerbations and long-term control medications used for the prevention

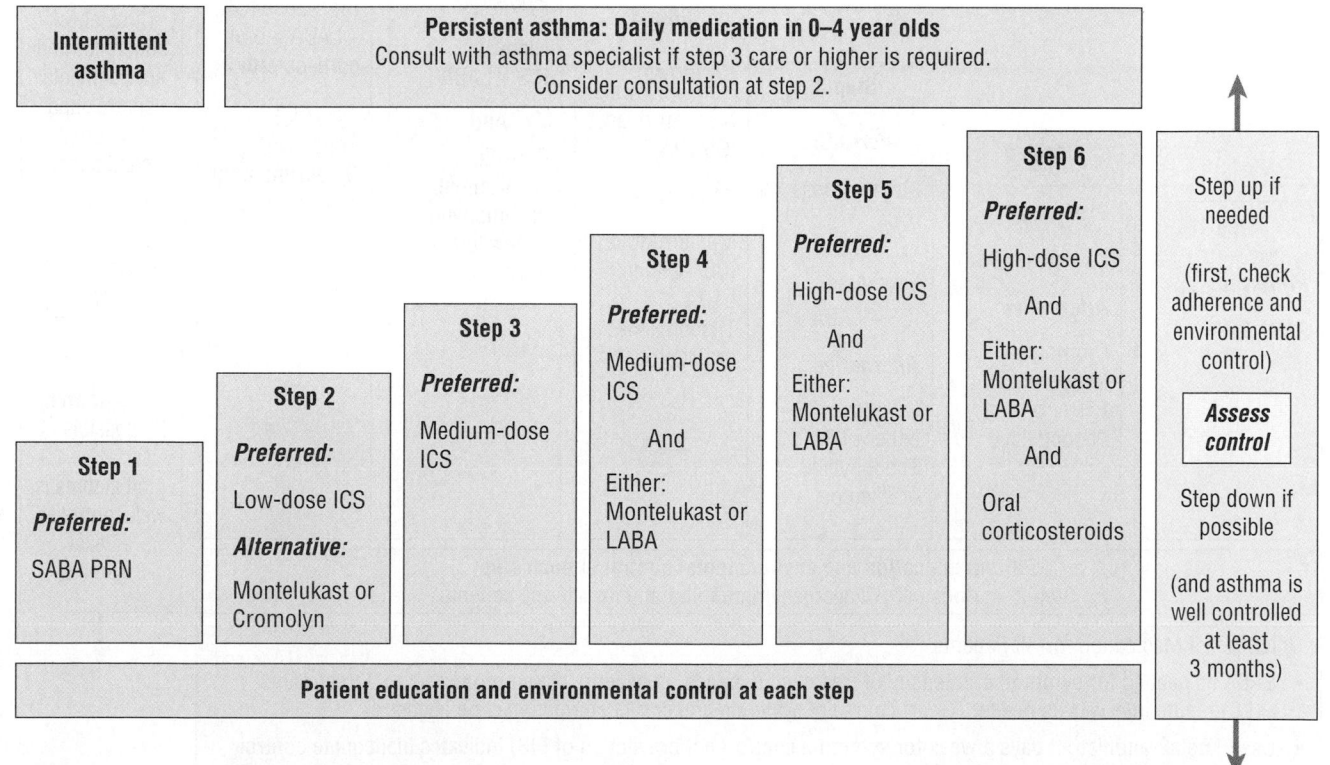

FIGURE 33-8. Stepwise approach for managing asthma in adults and children 0 to 4 years old and 5 to 11 years old. *(From reference 2.)*

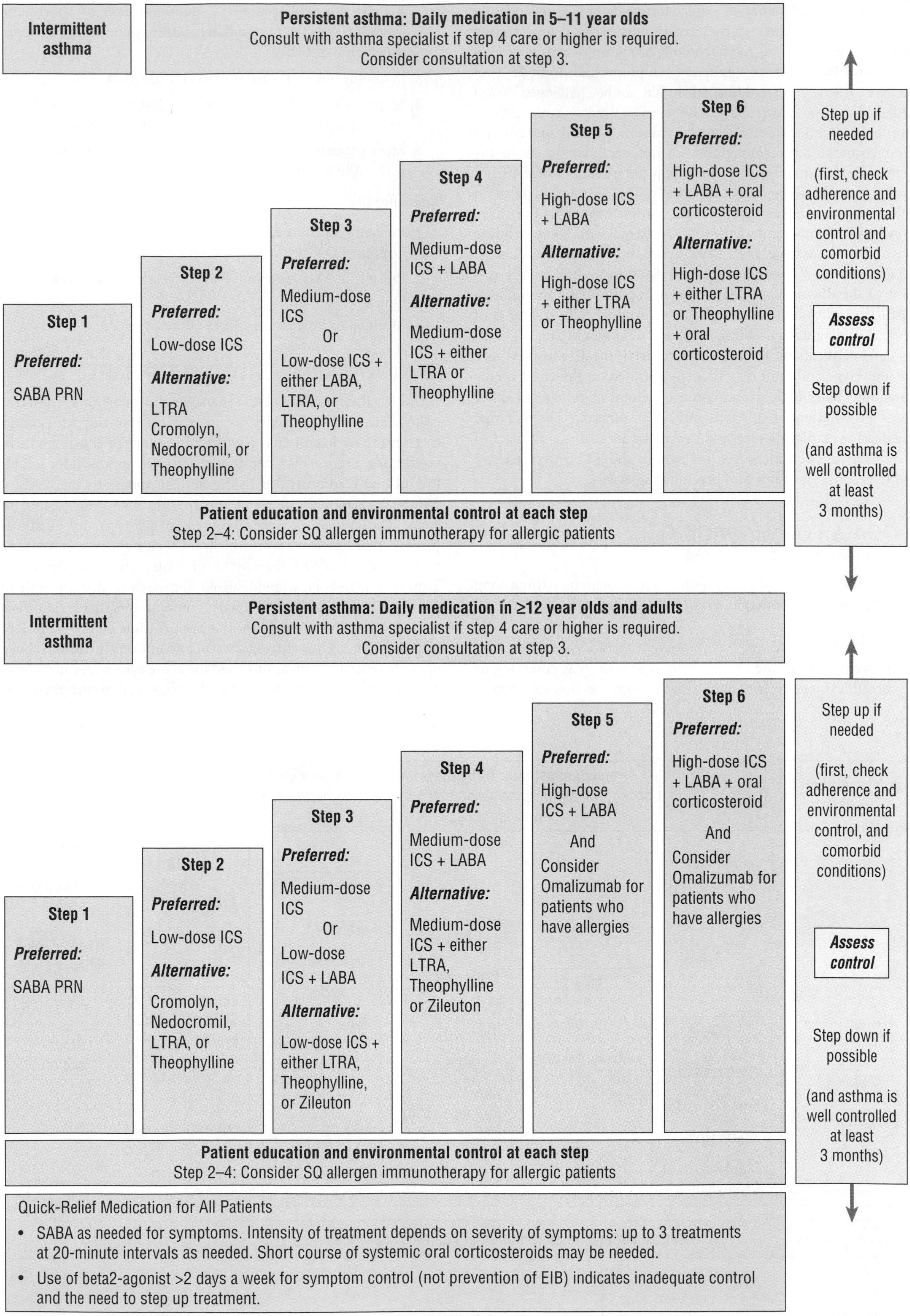

| Intermittent asthma | **Persistent asthma: Daily medication in 5–11 year olds**
Consult with asthma specialist if step 4 care or higher is required.
Consider consultation at step 3. |

Step 1

Preferred:

SABA PRN

Step 2

Preferred:

Low-dose ICS

Alternative:

LTRA
Cromolyn,
Nedocromil, or
Theophylline

Step 3

Preferred:

Medium-dose
ICS

Or

Low-dose ICS +
either LABA,
LTRA, or
Theophylline

Step 4

Preferred:

Medium-dose
ICS + LABA

Alternative:

Medium-dose
ICS + either
LTRA or
Theophylline

Step 5

Preferred:

High-dose ICS
+ LABA

Alternative:

High-dose ICS
+ either LTRA
or Theophylline

Step 6

Preferred:

High-dose ICS
+ LABA + oral
corticosteroid

Alternative:

High-dose ICS
+ either LTRA
or Theophylline
+ oral
corticosteroid

Step up if
needed

(first, check
adherence and
environmental
control and
comorbid
conditions)

*Assess
control*

Step down if
possible

(and asthma is
well controlled
at least
3 months)

Patient education and environmental control at each step
Step 2–4: Consider SQ allergen immunotherapy for allergic patients

| Intermittent asthma | **Persistent asthma: Daily medication in ≥12 year olds and adults**
Consult with asthma specialist if step 4 care or higher is required.
Consider consultation at step 3. |

Step 1

Preferred:

SABA PRN

Step 2

Preferred:

Low-dose ICS

Alternative:

Cromolyn,
Nedocromil,
LTRA, or
Theophylline

Step 3

Preferred:

Medium-dose
ICS

Or

Low-dose
ICS + LABA

Alternative:

Low-dose ICS +
either LTRA,
Theophylline,
or Zileuton

Step 4

Preferred:

Medium-dose
ICS + LABA

Alternative:

Medium-dose
ICS + either
LTRA,
Theophylline
or Zileuton

Step 5

Preferred:

High-dose
ICS + LABA

And

Consider
Omalizumab for
patients who
have allergies

Step 6

Preferred:

High-dose ICS
+ LABA + oral
corticosteroid

And

Consider
Omalizumab
for patients who
have allergies

Step up if
needed

(first, check
adherence and
environmental
control, and
comorbid
conditions)

*Assess
control*

Step down if
possible

(and asthma is
well controlled
at least
3 months)

Patient education and environmental control at each step
Step 2–4: Consider SQ allergen immunotherapy for allergic patients

Quick-Relief Medication for All Patients

- SABA as needed for symptoms. Intensity of treatment depends on severity of symptoms: up to 3 treatments at 20-minute intervals as needed. Short course of systemic oral corticosteroids may be needed.

- Use of beta2-agonist >2 days a week for symptom control (not prevention of EIB) indicates inadequate control and the need to step up treatment.

FIGURE 33-8. *(continued)*

TABLE 33-11 Key Educational Messages for Patients

Basic facts about asthma
- The contrast between asthmatic and normal airways
- What happens to the airways in an asthma attack

Roles of medications
- How medications work
- Long-term control: medications that prevent symptoms, often by reducing inflammation
- Quick relief: short-acting bronchodilator relaxes muscles around airways
- Stress importance of long-term-control medications and not to expect quick relief from them

Skills
- Inhaler use (patient demonstrate)
- Spacer and holding chamber use
- Use of the nebulizer
- Symptom monitoring, peak flow monitoring, and recognizing early signs of deterioration
- How to assess asthma control after therapy has begun

Environmental control measures
- Identifying and avoiding environmental precipitants or exposures, including tobacco smoke

When and how to adjust treatment
- Using written action plan
- Responding to changes in asthma control

of symptoms and exacerbations and the suppression of inflammation and reduction of BHR.[2]

❼ The development of a partnership in care through patient education and the teaching of patient self-management skills should be the cornerstone of any treatment program.[2] There are a number of published self-management programs for children and adults available through local American Lung Association chapters, as well as asthma treatment centers, and nationally through the NAEPP and the Asthma and Allergy Foundation of America.[2] Asthma self-management programs have been shown to improve patient adherence to medication regimens, improve self-management skills, and improve use of healthcare services.[2,46,47] Table 33–11 lists the key educational messages recommended by the NAEPP.[2]

Self-management programs instruct patients in the pathogenesis of asthma and the appropriate use of their medications but focus principally on teaching patients to recognize triggers for their asthma and how to recognize early signs of deterioration.[46] Home PEF monitoring is part of some programs.[2] However, routine PEF monitoring in and of itself does not improve patient outcomes.[2]

The NAEPP advocates the use of PEF monitoring only for patients with severe persistent asthma who have difficulty perceiving airway obstruction.[2] The NAEPP also has recommended a system based on a traffic light scenario (based on percentage of normal predicted values or personal best values): The green zone is equal to 80% to 100%, the yellow zone is equal to 50% to 79%, and the red zone is less than 50%. The yellow zone is cautionary and requires increasing as-needed bronchodilator use and possibly beginning prednisone if not improved, whereas the red zone warrants contacting the patient's healthcare provider.[2]

Patient education is essential before monitoring can be effective. Patient education has proved successful regardless of the health professional who provided the information (physician, nurse, or pharmacist). The NAEPP advocates significant involvement of all points of patient care in the educational process.[2] The provision of written action plans enhances the success of education and is considered an essential component of care.[2] Samples of clinically tested written action plans are available from NAEPP guidelines and other sources.[2]

In patients with known allergic triggers for their asthma, allergen avoidance has resulted in an improvement in symptoms, a reduction in medication use, and a decrease in BHR.[2] A comprehensive approach to environmental control is advocated. For example, for patients with house dust mite allergy removing carpeting from bedrooms, washing sheets in hot water (>130°F), and using special dust-proof pillow and mattress covers can reduce symptoms and need for medications.[2] Obvious environmental triggers (e.g., animal dander, cockroaches), if the patient is sensitive, should be avoided. Evidence for home air-filtering systems and chemicals for killing house dust mites is limited.[2] Immunotherapy (allergy shots) with single antigens particularly, has been beneficial and may be considered in patients with persistent asthma with documented sensitivity.[2] Immunotherapy with multiple antigens has been less effective.

Patients who smoke should be encouraged to stop. Parents of children with asthma should stop or at least not smoke around their children.[2]

■ PHARMACOLOGIC THERAPY

The current NAEPP recommendations for therapy of persistent asthma are illustrated in Figure 33–8.[2] Therapy should be adjusted based on control status of the patient (refer to later section). Regardless of the long-term therapy, all patients need to have quick-relief medication in the form of short-acting inhaled β_2-agonists available for acute symptoms. The ICSs are considered the preferred long-term control therapy for persistent asthma in all patients due to their potency and consistent effectiveness.[2] Low- to medium-dose ICSs reduce BHR, improve lung function, and reduce severe exacerbations leading to emergency department visits and hospitalizations. They are more effective than cromolyn, theophylline, or the leukotriene receptor antagonists.[2] In addition, the ICSs are the only therapy that reduces the risk of dying from asthma.[48] In the low to medium doses recommended by NAEPP guidelines (Table 33–12), ICSs are safe for long-term administration (see below).[2,41] The ICSs do not appear to reduce airway remodeling and loss of lung function found in some patients with persistent asthma. The ICSs do not enhance lung growth in children with asthma, prevent the development of asthma in high risk infants, nor do they induce remission of asthma as BHR and other measures of inflammation return to pretreatment levels upon discontinuation of therapy.[49,50] The sensitivity and consequent clinical response to ICSs can vary among patients.[2]

Although studies of the alternative long-term control therapies (e.g., cromolyn, leukotriene receptor antagonists, and theophylline) demonstrate improvement in symptoms, lung function, and as-needed, short-acting inhaled β_2-agonist use, they do not reduce BHR, suggesting minimal antiinflammatory activity.[2] The evidence suggests minimal to no differences in efficacy between these alternatives. Therefore, NAEPP lists them in alphabetical order to show no preference of one over the other.[2]

For those patients inadequately controlled on low dose ICSs either an increased dose of the ICS or the combination of ICS and long-acting inhaled β_2-agonist (LABA) is the next step to gain control of more moderate persistent asthma.[2] Alternatives could be the addition of leukotriene modifiers or theophylline to ICSs.[2] The addition of theophylline or leukotriene modifiers to ICSs is no more effective than doubling the dose of the ICS.[2] The combination of ICS/LABA is more effective at reducing severe asthma exacerbations than doubling the dose of ICS in moderate persistent asthma; increasing the dose of ICSs 4-fold also will result in a significant reduction in exacerbations.[51,52] However, doses of ICSs in the high range significantly enhance the risk of toxicity.[41,49] Thus, high doses of ICSs plus LABA are reserved for patients with severe persistent asthma.[2]

TABLE 33-12 Available Inhaled Corticosteroid Products, Lung Delivery, and Comparative Daily Dosages

ICS	Product	Lung Delivery[a]
Beclomethasone dipropionate (BDP)	40 and 80 mcg/actuation HFA MDI, 120 actuations	55%–60%
Budesonide (BUD)	90 or 180 mcg/dose DPI, Flexhaler, 200 doses	32% (15–30%)
	200 and 500 mcg ampules, 2 mL each	5%–8%
Ciclesonide (CIC)	80 or 160 mcg/actuation HFA MDI	50%
Flunisolide (FLU)	250 mcg/actuation CFC MDI, 100 actuations	20%
	80 mcg/actuation HFA MDI, 120 actuations	68%
Fluticasone propionate (FP)	44, 110, and 220 mcg/actuation HFA MDI, 120 actuations	20%
	50, 100 and 250 mcg/dose DPI, Diskus, 60 doses	15%
Mometasone furoate (MF)	110 and 220 mcg/dose DPI, Twisthaler, 14, 30, 60, and 120 doses	11%

	Comparative Daily Dosages (mcg) of Inhaled Corticosteroids		
	Low Daily Dose Child[a]/Adult	*Medium Daily Dose Child[a]/Adult*	*High Daily Dose Child[a]/Adult*
BDP			
HFA MDI	80–160/80–240	>160–320/>240–480	>320/>480
BUD			
DPI	180–360/180–540	>360720/>540–1,080	>720/>1,080
Nebules	500/UK	1,000/UK	2,000/UK
CIC	80–160/160–320	>160–320/>320–640	>320/>640
FLU			
CFC MDI	500–750/500–1,000	1,000–1,250/1,000–2,000	>1,250/>2,000
HFA MDI	160/320	320/320–640	≥640/>640
FP			
HFA MDI	88–176/88–264	176–352/264–440	>352/>440
DPIs	100–200/100–300	200–400/300–500	>400/>500
MF, DPI	110/220	220–440/440	>440/>440

[a]5 to 11 years of age, except for BUD Nebules which is 2 to 11 years of age.

Although the addition of a third controller medication is often used clinically in patients with severe persistent asthma uncontrolled on high dose ICS/LABA, there are few studies evaluating this practice.[2] Leukotriene receptor antagonists or theophylline added to high-dose combination ICS/LABA do not improve outcomes.[2] Omalizumab, a recombinant anti-IgE has demonstrated significant activity in these severe uncontrolled atopic patients.[2,53]

■ SPECIAL POPULATIONS

❻ Children younger than 5 years of age have not been studied adequately. Thus, many of the recommendations in this age group are extrapolated from older children and adults.[2] The studies of ICSs in this younger group demonstrate improvement in symptoms, as needed bronchodilator use, and exacerbations. The nebulized suspension of budesonide gained FDA approval from three pivotal efficacy and safety trials.[2] The FDA approval for montelukast in children younger than age 6 was based on safety and pharmacokinetic studies establishing doses but not on efficacy although improvement in symptoms and as needed bronchodilators was noted.[2] Cromolyn nebulizer solution was approved down to age 2 years based on efficacy.[2] Theophylline has not been evaluated adequately, except for pharmacokinetics.[2] Combination therapy of any kind has not been studied except for a small number of patients down to 4 years of age on ICS/LABA.[2]

The FDA approval of the fluticasone/salmeterol DPI 100/50 in patients 4 to 11 years of age was largely based on extrapolation of efficacy data from patients older than 12 years of age and by a single safety and efficacy study in children with asthma aged 4 to 11 years. In children 5 to 11 years old, the ICS/LABA combination has not yet been definitively shown to decrease exacerbations compared with medium dose ICS, although impairment domains improved.[2] The only study of the addition of montelukast to ICS showed minimal improvement in PEF and as needed albuterol use.[2] Thus, combination therapy has been inadequately studied to date in this population.

Owing to the increased risk of osteoporosis and cataracts in the elderly, patients requiring high doses of ICSs should have routine bone mineral density determinations and ophthalmic exams.[2,54] Appropriate therapies for prevention of osteoporosis should be instituted.[2,54]

Asthma affects 7% of pregnant women, making it potentially the most common serious medical condition to complicate pregnancy.[19] Maternal asthma has been reported to increase the risk of perinatal mortality, preeclampsia, preterm birth, and low-birth-weight infants.[19] More severe asthma is associated with increased risks, whereas better-controlled asthma is associated with decreased risks. A systematic review of the evidence on the safety of asthma medications has concluded that it is safer for pregnant women with asthma to be treated with effective medications than for them to have exacerbations.[19] Proper monitoring and control of asthma should enable a woman with asthma to maintain a normal pregnancy with little or no risk to mother or her fetus.

A stepwise approach to managing asthma during pregnancy and lactation has been published, with low-dose ICSs recommended as preferred treatment for mild persistent asthma with the addition of a LABA if not adequately controlled.[19] Budesonide is considered the preferred ICS to initiate because it has the greatest amount of safety data.[19] Albuterol is considered the preferred rescue therapy.[19]

■ DRUG CLASS INFORMATION

Inhaled Corticosteroids

The mechanism of action of the corticosteroids has been reviewed (see above). The principal advantage of the ICSs is their high topical potency to reduce inflammation in the lung and low systemic activity.[41,49] The ICSs have high antiinflammatory potency, approximately 1,000-fold greater than endogenous cortisol, and differ from each other by as much as 4- to 6-fold.[41] However, potency differences, which are simply a measure of binding affinity to the receptor, can be overcome simply by giving different microgram dosages of drug. Aerosol delivery of the preparations is remarkably variable, ranging from 10% to 60% of the nominal dose (i.e., that dose which leaves an actuator for an MDI or, in the case of a DPI, that which is released on actuation of the inhaler).[26,41] Different devices for the same chemical entity may result in 2-fold differences in delivery, so that delivery method can make a significant difference in the relative comparable dose or therapeutic index.[2,41]

The ICSs, beclomethasone dipropionate, budesonide, ciclesonide, flunisolide, fluticasone propionate, and mometasone furoate, that are currently available for use are compared and listed in Table 33–12. The ICSs have pharmacokinetic differences that result in different topical/systemic activity.[41] Most evidence is consistent with log-linear dose-response curves for both indirect and direct responses.[49] The log-linear nature of the dose-response curve for ICS activity raises the issue of how much of a difference in dose (or lung delivery) or potency is detectable. The measures used to assess efficacy (lung function, BHR, symptoms, and as-needed short-acting inhaled β_2-agonist use) are downstream events from the antiinflammatory activity.[49] It takes a 4-fold difference in potency or dose to detect clinically significant differences in efficacy. The table of comparable ICS doses (see Table 33–12) is based on extensive clinical trial data.[2,41] Clinically comparable doses take into consideration drug potency differences as well as device delivery differences but not the potential for systemic activity.

Since the glucocorticoid receptors within the various tissues are the same, differences in the pharmacokinetic profile are required to produce differences in the topical/systemic effect ratio (therapeutic index).[41] Pharmacokinetic properties that enhance topical selectivity include rapid systemic clearance, poor oral bioavailability, and prolonged residence time in the lung.[41] Owing to their high lipophilicity, systemic clearance of the available ICSs is very rapid, approaching the rate of liver blood flow with the exception of ciclesonide which is inactivated by blood esterases as well.[41] However, the ICSs differ markedly in their oral bioavailability, although they all undergo rather extensive first-pass metabolism to less active substances when absorbed[41] (see Table 33–9). The ICSs produce dose-dependent systemic effects, contributed by the orally absorbed fraction and the fraction absorbed from the lung[2,41,49] (Table 33–13). Essentially all the drug that reaches the lung is absorbed systemically; thus, a slow absorption from the lung results in an apparent long elimination half-life and enhances topical selectivity by lowering the systemic concentration.[41] Ciclesonide and beclomethasone dipropionate differ from the other ICSs in that the parent compounds are prodrugs that are metabolized in the lung to the active compounds des-ciclesonide and beclomethasone monopropionate.[41] The potential advantage of the drugs with low

oral bioavailability is obviated by using a spacer device with the MDI for the drugs with higher oral bioavailability because appropriate spacers reduce the oral dose by 80%.[41] The use of VHCs also can increase systemic activity by increasing lung delivery of drugs not absorbed significantly orally.[41] If this increase in lung deposition is 2-fold or less, it will increase systemic activity without producing a clinically important increase in efficacy, thus decreasing the therapeutic index.[41] Mouth rinsing and spitting will also reduce the oral availability and are particularly useful for DPI devices.[2,41] Although ciclesonide and its active metabolite have rapid systemic clearance suggesting an improved therapeutic index it has not yet been clearly established in clinical trials.[41]

The response to ICSs is somewhat delayed. Most patients' symptoms will improve in the first 1 to 2 weeks of therapy and will reach maximum improvement in 4 to 8 weeks.[49] Improvement in baseline FEV_1 and PEF may require 3 to 6 weeks for maximum improvement, whereas improvement in BHR requires 2 to 3 weeks and approaches maximum in 1 to 3 months but may continue to improve over 1 year.[49] Most of the improvement in these parameters occurs at low to medium doses, and there is a large variability in response, with 10% of patients not demonstrating an improvement in either parameter.[49] Whether these nonresponders also show no improvement in rates of exacerbations is unknown. Maximum decrease in FeNO occurs within 2 to 3 weeks.[15,49] Sensitivity to exercise challenge decreases after 4 weeks of therapy.[49] Although single doses do not inhibit the immediate asthmatic response to antigen challenge, continued therapy for 1 week partially suppresses the response. These two latter effects are likely due to a reduction in mucosal mast cells.[49]

Local adverse effects from ICSs include oropharyngeal candidiasis and dysphonia that are dose-dependent. The dysphonia (reported in 5%–20% of patients) appears to be due to a local corticosteroid-induced myopathy of the vocal cords.[2] The use of a spacer device with MDIs can decrease oropharyngeal deposition and thus decrease the incidence and severity of local side effects.[2,49] In infants who require ICS delivery through a facemask, the parent should clean the nasal-perioral area with a damp cloth following each treatment to prevent topical candidal infections.

Systemic adverse effects can occur with any of the ICSs given in a sufficiently high dose.[49] Long-term adverse effects of greatest concern include growth suppression in children, osteoporosis, cataracts, dermal thinning, and adrenal insufficiency and crisis.[49] Of these, only growth retardation occurs in low to medium doses. However, the growth reduction appears to be transient in that growth velocity is reduced in the first 6 months to 1 year of therapy and then returns to normal.[2,49] The effect is small (1–2 cm total) and not cumulative, and current studies suggest that attainment of predicted adult height is not affected.[2,49] The suppression of the hypothalamic-pituitary-adrenal axis and decreased bone mineralization are dose dependent and do not appear to be significant clinically except at high doses.[49] The risks therefore depend on the therapeutic index of each ICS and its delivery device. The effect of delivery device is illustrated by fluticasone propionate, which has both the greatest therapeutic index when administered by DPI and the lowest therapeutic index when administered by MDI plus VHC.[41] Many of the ICSs, including fluticasone propionate, budesonide, ciclesonide, and mometasone furoate, are metabolized in the gastrointestinal tract and liver by CYP3A4 isoenzymes. Potent inhibitors of CYP3A4 such as ritonavir and ketoconazole have the potential for increasing systemic concentrations of these ICSs by increasing oral availability and decreasing systemic clearance.[41] Some cases of clinically significant Cushing syndrome and secondary adrenal insufficiency have been reported.[41]

Most patients with moderate disease can be controlled with twice-daily dosing of most ICSs.[2,41] Twice-daily dosing produces less

---

TABLE 33-13 Effects of Inhaled Corticosteroids

Beneficial Effects	Potential Adverse Effects
Decrease eosinophil numbers	Growth retardation, skeletal muscle myopathy
Decrease mast cell numbers	Osteoporosis, fractures and aseptic necrosis of hip
Decrease T-lymphocyte cytokine production	Posterior subcapsular cataract formation and glaucoma
Inhibit transcription of inflammatory genes in airway epithelium	Adrenal axis suppression, immunosuppression
Reduce endothelial cell leak	Impaired wound healing, easy bruising, skin striae
Upregulate β_2-receptor production	Hyperglycemia/hypokalemia, hypertension
Reduce airway epithelial subbasement membrane thickening	Psychiatric disturbances

thrush than 3- to 4-times-daily dosing regimens. In milder asthma, once-daily dosing is often sufficient to maintain control.[41] Some of the newer products have gained once-daily dosing indications, particularly in mild asthma once initial control is established.[41] There does not appear to be any specific pharmacologic or pharmacokinetic aspect of the ICSs that allows for once-daily dosing because all the agents studied (both the older low-potency and newer high-potency ICSs) have been effective, provided that patients had relatively mild to moderate asthma.[41] More severe patients require multiple daily dosing. The inflammatory response of asthma has been shown to inhibit corticosteroid-receptor binding.[41] This provides strong theoretical evidence for initially beginning patients on higher and more frequent doses and then tapering down once control has been achieved. Once asthma is controlled many patients are able to reduce the ICS dose and maintain control.[49]

Long-Acting Inhaled β_2-Agonists

The two LABAs, formoterol and salmeterol, provide long-lasting bronchodilation ($\geq$12 hours) when administered as aerosols[38] (see Table 33–8). Unlike the more water-soluble short-acting β_2-agonists, the long-acting agents are lipid soluble, readily partitioning into the outer phospholipid layer of the cell membrane.[38] The LABA, are more β_2-selective than albuterol and more bronchoselective by virtue of its property of remaining in the lung tissue cell membrane, which produces its longer duration.[31] However, both formoterol and salmeterol will produce dose-dependent systemic β_2-agonist effects.[31]

The principal differences between formoterol and salmeterol are that formoterol has a more rapid onset of action and formoterol has greater agonist activty. These differences are unlikely to produce clinically significant differences because both are recommended for chronic therapy only in combination with ICSs.[6] LABAs are available singly and as fixed-dose combinations with ICSs (see below). Neither has approved FDA labeling for acute relief of asthma, although formoterol has an onset of activity similar to albuterol. Patients need to be counseled to continue to use their short-acting inhaled β_2-agonists for acute exacerbations while receiving the LABAs.

The LABAs are preferred adjunctive therapy to ICSs in children 12 years and older and adults for step 3 and children 5 to 11 years of age for steps 4 and 5.[2] Combination treatment with ICS/LABA provides greater asthma control than increasing the dose of ICS alone, while at the same time reducing the frequency of mild and severe exacerbations.[51,52] Since they are devoid of antiinflammatory activity, LABAs should not be used as monotherapy for asthma. Patients treated with LABA monotherapy added to usual therapy are at an increased risk for severe, life-threatening exacerbations and asthma-related death.[55,56] This risk may be greater in African American patients. Whether this risk is obviated by concomitant ICS use is unknown at this time but current evidence does not support an increased risk of severe, life-threatening exacerbations in patients receiving LABAs in combination with ICSs.[55–57] A recent controlled study failed to detect lung function deterioration or increased exacebations in Arg-16 homozygotes receiving a LABA plus ICS.[58]

As with short-acting β_2-agonists, tolerance is produced with chronic administration of LABAs. Long-term trials have shown no diminution in bronchodilator response but a partial loss of the bronchoprotective effect against methacholine, histamine, and exercise challenge.[31] In particular, the duration of protection against EIB following a single dose of salmeterol is up to 9 hours but is reduced to less than 4 hours following regular treatment.[31] Following regular treatment with LABAs, decreased protection against nonspecific bronchoprovocation with methacholine also occurs, although they continue to provide greater protection than placebo.[31] Responsiveness to short-acting β_2-agonists has been reported to be slightly decreased but easily overcome by increasing the dose (by approximately one puff) following chronic therapy with LABAs.[31]

There is ample evidence that the use of a LABA in combination with ICS therapy does not mask inflammation.[31] In children 4 to 11 years of age, LABAs added to ICS reduce impairment but have yet to be adequately studied for reducing the risk domain of exacerbations over ICS alone.[31,56] In children 0 to 4 years, the LABA/ICS combination has not been studied.[2]

Methylxanthines

Methylxanthines have been used for asthma therapy for more than 50 years, but their use in recent years has declined markedly owing to the high risk of severe life-threatening toxicity and numerous drug interactions, as well as decreased efficacy compared with ICSs and LABAs. Theophylline, the primary methylxanthine of interest, is a moderately potent bronchodilator with mild antiinflammatory properties.[2] Like the β_2-agonists, the methylxanthines are functional antagonists of bronchospasm; however, their clinical utility is limited by their low therapeutic index.[2] Theophylline as a sustained-release product is the preferred oral preparation, whereas its complex with ethylenediamine (aminophylline) is the preferred injectable product owing to increased solubility.[2]

The mechanism by which theophylline produces bronchodilation appears to be through nonselective phosphodiesterase inhibition–producing increased cAMP and cyclic guanosine monophosphate (cGMP) concentrations.[2] The phosphodiesterase (PDE) isoenzymes currently thought to be important for theophylline's clinical effects are isoenzymes III, predominant in airway smooth muscle, and IV, important in inflammatory cell regulation such as mast cells, neutrophils, eosinophils, and T-lymphocytes.[2] Selective PDE isoenzyme IV inhibitors, however, have no significant effects in clinical asthma. Theophylline also activates histone deacetylase that is involved in the corticosteroid-induced decrease in proinflammatory gene expression.[59] Theophylline is a competitive antagonist of adenosine and stimulates endogenous catecholamine release which are important determinants of toxic symptoms of excess theophylline.[2]

Theophylline has a log-linear dose-response curve.[60] Most chronic stable patients with asthma will obtain significant bronchodilation when the serum theophylline concentration reaches 5 mcg/mL, and most patients will have no toxic symptoms with serum concentrations of less than 15 mcg/mL.[2,60] The percentage of patients experiencing adverse effects increases sharply as concentrations exceed 15 mcg/mL. As with the β_2-agonists, the dose-response curves for smooth muscle relaxation by theophylline are dynamic and shifted to the right in the face of increasing contractile stimuli.[60] This property probably explains theophylline's relative lack of bronchodilatory effect in acute severe asthma.[2,60] The severity of theophylline's toxicity precludes even doubling the usual dosage. Toxicities include caffeine-like effects of nausea, vomiting, tachycardia, jitteriness, and difficulty sleeping to more severe toxicities such as cardiac tachyarrythmias and seizures. Death has occurred in children receiving their usual doses of theophylline during acute systemic viral illnesses.[60]

Routine monitoring of serum concentrations is essential for the safe and effective use of theophylline.[2] Theophylline is eliminated primarily by metabolism via the hepatic cytochrome P450 mixed-function oxidase microsomal enzymes (primarily the CYP1A2 and CYP3A3 isozymes), with 10% or less excreted unchanged in the kidney.[2] Theophylline clearance is age-dependent, with 1- to 9-year-olds having the highest systemic clearances and therefore

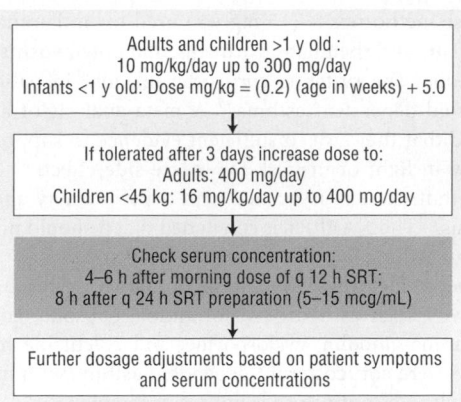

Adults and children >1 y old :
10 mg/kg/day up to 300 mg/day
Infants <1 y old: Dose mg/kg = (0.2) (age in weeks) + 5.0

↓

If tolerated after 3 days increase dose to:
Adults: 400 mg/day
Children <45 kg: 16 mg/kg/day up to 400 mg/day

↓

Check serum concentration:
4–6 h after morning dose of q 12 h SRT;
8 h after q 24 h SRT preparation (5–15 mcg/mL)

↓

Further dosage adjustments based on patient symptoms
and serum concentrations

FIGURE 33-9. Algorithm for slow titration of theophylline dosage and guide for final dosage adjusment based on serum theophylline concentration measurement. For infants younger than 1 year of age, the initial daily dosage can be calculated by the following regression equation: Dose (mg/kg) = (0.2) (age in weeks) + 5.0. Whenever side effects occur, dosage should be reduced to a previously tolerated lower dose.

requiring the largest dosages (on a weight basis). However, even within the same age groups, theophylline clearance can vary 2- to 3-fold.[2] Figure 33–9 outlines a dosing and monitoring schedule for theophylline. Factors affecting theophylline's hepatic metabolism are listed in Table 33–14.[2] Only drugs or diseases that produce a ≥20% inhibition or a ≥50% induction of theophylline metabolism are likely to result in clinically significant interactions.[60]

Sustained-release theophylline is less effective than ICSs and no more effective than oral sustained-release β_2-agonists, cromolyn, or leukotriene antagonists.[2] The addition of theophylline to ICSs is similar to doubling the dose of the ICS and is overall less effective than the LABAs as adjunctive therapy.[2] The addition of theophylline to patients with poorly controlled asthma receiving ICS/LABA combination does not improve outcomes.[61]

Cromolyn Sodium

Cromolyn is classified as a mast cell stabilizer and inhibits the early and late asthmatic response to allergen challenge, as well as inhibiting exercise-induced bronchospasm.[44,62] Treatment prevents the usual rise in BHR with specific pollen seasons, but long-term treatment produces minimal to no change in baseline BHR.[2] Cromolyn inhibits neurally mediated bronchoconstriction through C-fiber sensory nerve stimulation in the airways, although it does not have a bronchodilatory effect.[62]

Cromolyn is only effective by inhalation.[62] It is not bioavailable orally, but the portion of the dose that reaches the lung is absorbed completely.[62] Absorption from the airway is significantly slower than elimination (hours vs minutes). The short duration in the lung likely limits its efficacy. Both the intensity and duration of protection against various challenges are dose dependent.[62]

Cromolyn is remarkably nontoxic. No evidence of mutagenesis or teratogenesis has been found. Cough and wheeze have been reported following inhalation.[2] Tolerance to cromolyn has not been demonstrated. It is not considered to be an ICS-sparing agent.

Cromolyn is no more or less effective than theophylline or the leukotriene antagonists for persistent asthma.[2,60] Cromolyn is not as effective as the ICSs for controlling persistent asthma.[60] Cromolyn is not as effective as the inhaled β_2-agonists for preventing EIB but can be used in conjunction for patients not responding completely to the inhaled β_2-agonists.[44]

Most patients will experience an improvement in 1 to 2 weeks, but it may take longer to achieve maximum benefit. Patients initially should receive cromolyn 4 times daily, and then only after stabilization of symptoms may the frequency be reduced to 3 times daily.

Leukotriene Modifiers

Two cysteinyl leukotriene receptor antagonists (zafirlukast and montelukast) and one 5-lipoxygenase inhibitor (zileuton) are available in the United States.[63] In challenge studies, they reduce allergen-, exercise-, cold-air hyperventilation-, irritant-, and aspirin-induced asthma.[63] Clinical use of zileuton is limited due to the potential for elevated liver enzymes (especially in the first 3 months of therapy), and the potential inhibition of drugs metabolized by the CYP3A4 isoenzymes.[60,63] They are not preferred alternatives in mild persistent asthma nor as alternative add-on therapy for moderate persistent asthma (Fig. 33–8).[2]

These drugs improve pulmonary function tests (FEV$_1$ and PEF), decrease nocturnal awakenings and β_2-agonist use, and improve asthma symptoms.[63] A major advantage is that they are effective orally, and can be administered once or twice a day.[63] However, they are less effective in asthma than low doses of ICSs.[60,63] Although montelukast is approved for EIB in adults, it is significantly less effective than short-acting inhaled β_2-agonists. In adults with severe uncontrolled asthma they do not improve outcomes.[61] They are not as effective as LABAs when added to ICSs for moderate persistent asthma.[63] It is not yet possible to predict which patients respond best to leukotriene modifiers, although there is some evidence that patients with aspirin-sensitive asthma do well, as predicted by studies showing increased cysteinyl leukotriene production in these patients.[63] It is possible that genetic polymorphisms in the 5-lipoxygenase or LTC$_4$ synthase pathways or in cys-LT$_1$ receptors might predict better responders in the future.[63] Antileukotrienes also have modest efficacy in allergic rhinitis.

In general, the LTD$_4$ receptor antagonists are well tolerated and do not appear to have serious class-specific effects.[2] An idiosyncratic syndrome similar to the Churg-Strauss syndrome, with marked circulating eosinophilia, heart failure, and associated eosinophilic vasculitis, has been reported in a small number of patients treated with zafirlukast and montelukast.[60] The majority of these patients had been receiving high-dose ICS or oral corticosteroids and were able to reduce the dose as a consequence of the LTD$_4$ receptor antagonists. It is unclear whether the increased reports are due to increased

TABLE 33-14	Factors Affecting Theophylline Clearance		
Decreased Clearance	**% Decrease**	**Increased Clearance**	**% Increase**
Cimetidine	−25 to −60	Rifampin	+53
Macrolides: erythromycin, TAO, clarithromycin	−25 to −50	Carbamazepine	+50
		Phenobarbital	+34
		Phenytoin	+70
Allopurinol	−20	Charcoal-broiled meat	+30
Propranolol	−30		
Quinolones ciprofloxacin, enoxacin, perfloxacin	−20 to −50	High-protein diet	+25
		Smoking	+40
Interferon	−50	Sulfinpyrazone	+22
Thiabendazole	−65	Moricizine	+50
Ticlopidine	−25	Aminoglutethimide	+50
Zileuton	−35		
Systemic viral illness	−10 to −50		

case findings among patients with asthma prescribed a new drug or whether the syndrome is related to corticosteroid dose reduction or an idiosyncratic effect of leukotriene modifiers in general. Whatever the cause, it appears to be a rare syndrome, with an estimated incidence of fewer than 1 case per 15,000 to 20,000 patient-years of treatment.[60]

Reports of adverse neuropsychiatric events have caused the manufacturers of the leukotriene inhibitors to revise their labeling. However, evidence for causality of suicidal thoughts and suicide is lacking.[64] Reports of fatal hepatic failure associated with zafirlukast have prompted a warning for patients to be made aware of signs and symptoms of hepatic dysfunction.[2]

Zileuton can be administered twice daily as controlled release tablets.[2] Efficacy data is more limited, liver function monitoring is recommended, and drug interactions are reported with warfarin and theophylline.

Anti-IgE (Omalizumab)

Omalizumab is a recombinant anti-IgE antibody approved for the treatment of allergic asthma not well controlled on oral corticosteroids or ICSs.[65] Omalizumab is a composite of 95% human and 5% antihuman murine IgE sequences. Omalizumab binds to the Fc portion of the IgE antibody preventing the binding of IgE to its high-affinity receptor (FcεRI) on mast cells and basophils. The decreased binding of IgE on the surface of mast cells leads to a decrease in the release of mediators in response to allergen exposure. Omalizumab also decreases FcεRI expression on basophils and airway submucosal mast cells over 8 to 12 weeks.[65]

Omalizumab is administered subcutaneously and has a slow absorption rate; peak serum concentration is achieved in 3 to 14 days.[65] It is eliminated primarily through the reticuloendothelial system and has an elimination half-life of 17 to 22 days; serum free IgE levels return to baseline in about 3 weeks.[65] It should be administered under medical observation with drugs for treating anaphylaxis available.

The dosage of omalizumab is determined by the patient's baseline total serum IgE level (international units per milliliter) and body weight (kilograms).[65] Doses range from 150 to 375 mg and are given at either 2- or 4-week intervals. No further adjustments for variations in total serum IgE are required, and patients receive a consistent dose for the duration of treatment.[65] Omalizumab is approved for patients greater than 12 years with allergic asthma.[65] Clinical trials in 5- to 12-year-olds are ongoing. Due to its significant cost, it is only indicated as step 5 or 6 care for patients who have allergies and severe persistent asthma that are inadequately controlled with the combination of high dose ICS/LABA and at risk for severe exacerbations.[2,66] It is the only adjunctive therapy that has demonstrated improved outcomes in patients uncontrolled on ICS/LABA and has allowed oral corticosteroid reduction in a number of studies.[2,65] Omalizumab therapy is associated with a 0.2% rate of anaphylaxis prompting an FDA warning that patients should remain in the healthcare provider's office for a reasonable period of time past the injection as 70% of reactions occur within 2 hours. In addition, patients should be counseled on the signs and symptoms of anaphylaxis because some reactions have occurred up to 24 hours following an injection.[2,65]

■ MISCELLANEOUS THERAPIES (IMMUNOMODULATORS)

The following therapies have been loosely categorized by the NAEPP with omalizumab as immunomodulators because they either affect the immune system or have antiinflammatory properties. Many have been used experimentally in severe persistent uncontrolled asthma for years to try to avoid or lower oral corticosteroid dosages.

Low-dose methotrexate (15 mg/wk) used for inflammatory diseases, psoriatic and rheumatoid arthritis, and polymyositis has been used to reduce the systemic corticosteroid dose in patients with severe steroid-dependent asthma.[67] A meta-analysis of all studies determined that there was insufficient evidence to support its use, particularly in light of the risk for severe side effects.[67] Low-dose weekly methotrexate is associated with hepatotoxicity and pulmonary fibrosis.[67] The NAEPP has concluded that it should not be used in persistent asthma.[2]

A number of the drugs with antiinflammatory or immunomodulatory activity such as hydroxychloroquine, dapsone, gold, intravenous gamma-globulin, cyclosporine, and colchicine have been studied in severe corticosteroid-dependent asthma with mixed and limited results.[2,68] Routine use is not recommended.[2]

■ FUTURE THERAPIES

Agents that are now in development for asthma focus on the treatment of allergic inflammation.[69] Examples include inhibitors of eosinophilic inflammation, drugs that may inhibit allergen presentation, and inhibitors of Th$_2$ cells. Multiple cytokines have been implicated in allergic inflammation, and several possible inhibiting approaches are being explored. These range from drugs that inhibit cytokine synthesis (cyclosporin A and tacrolimus), humanized blocking antibodies to cytokines or their receptors, soluble receptors to mop up secreted cytokines, receptor antagonists, and drugs that block the signal-transduction pathways activated by cytokines.[69] Unfortunately specific anticytokine therapy against IL-5 and IL-4 have been disappointing to date.[69]

A FDA has approved Asthmatx Inc.'s Alair Bronchial Thermoplasty System to treat severe asthma in adult patients. This is the first nondrug treatment for asthma. The Alair treatment (3 sessions of 30 minutes each) is performed via a bronchoscope that is inserted into the lungs. A tip of a small catheter then expands to deliver thermal energy to reduce the presence of airway smooth muscle that narrows the airways.[70]

PHARMACOECONOMIC CONSIDERATIONS

Of the estimated $19.7 billion cost of asthma in the United States in 2004, direct medical expenditure accounted for $14.7 billion of the total, with emergency care (ED and in-patient hospital care) reaching $4.7 billion.[3] A cost-of-illness approach takes in all measurable costs; both indirect costs or costs to society and direct medical costs are considered.[71,72] Using this approach, indirect costs such as lost work and death accounted for 25% of total expenditures per patient. Although prescription drugs were the largest single direct medical expenditure at $6.7 billion,[3] an increase in these costs secondary to improved patient adherence could significantly reduce other costs due to missed school days and lost productivity secondary to asthma morbidity and mortality.

The medication cost increase over the past years resulted from an increase in prescribed medications, as well as an increase in unit cost per medication. Asthma severity affects cost of care as studies from health-maintenance organizations suggest that up to 45% of the cost of asthma is accrued by 10% of the patients, primarily as a result of emergency care.[72]

Numerous studies have demonstrated the cost-effectiveness of patient education programs for asthma, particularly those providing guided self-management.[2] Several studies have reported positive results from pharmacist interventions reducing overall cost of care.[2] Similar studies have demonstrated the cost-effectiveness of specialist care compared with generalist care. However, the results of these trials may be confounded by changes in prescribing as part of the overall program.[71] Indeed, use of ICSs reduces both morbidity, particularly hospitalizations, and mortality in asthma patients.[2,71]

The NAEPP recommendations provide numerous alternatives for long-term controllers in mild to moderate persistent asthma, and few studies have compared their relative cost-effectiveness. This comparison is important because outside the realm of randomized clinical trials that evaluate efficacy, other factors such as concern about adverse effects and adherence to therapy may alter the overall clinical effectiveness. Use of ICSs in children has produced a cost of $9.45 per symptom-free day gained and in adults $5.00 per symptom-free day.[2] Retrospective analyses of large managed-care-linked pharmacy claims and healthcare utilization databases has allowed direct comparisons of the various long-term controllers in a general population to assess clinical effectiveness and cost-effectiveness. While these studies have confirmed comparative randomized clinical trials showing ICSs to be significantly more cost-effective than leukotriene antagonists, many have flaws, including the short duration of followup for a chronic illness such as asthma.[71]

CLINICAL CONTROVERSY

The potential for chronic use of inhaled β_2-agonists to worsen asthma has been a concern for more than 30 years. Large multicenter, double-blind, placebo-controlled trials with both mild and moderate persistent asthma have not shown that regular administration with short-acting inhaled β_2-agonists worsened asthma. However, studies that have genotyped patients at the β-receptor suggest that homozygous Arg-16 patients (who make up about 16% of the population) are predisposed to worsening asthma with regular administration as measured by lower morning PEFs.[31,39] This phenomenon does not appear to occur with as-needed therapy with short-acting β_2-agonists. Regular treatment with LABAs does not produce similar effects.[58] The Arg-16 patients still respond acutely to the β_2-agonists without diminished response. Since the regular use of short-acting inhaled β_2-agonists does not improve control of symptoms, they should be used only for relief of symptoms.[2] The LABAs should be used only in combination with ICSs where the risk of severe life-threatening exacerbations has not been demonstrated.[56,57]

EVALUATION OF ASTHMA CONTROL

Control of asthma is defined as reducing both impairment and risk domains.[71] The stepwise approach to therapy should be used to achieve and maintain this control. The steps of care appropriate to the three age ranges of asthma have been outlined in Figure 33–8.[2] Depending on the severity of the patient's asthma, compromises from the ideal control are made, and the best possible outcome balancing disease control and possible adverse effects from the drugs is attempted. Regular follow-up contact is essential (at 1–6 month intervals, depending on control). A step-down in therapy can be considered, if well-controlled status has been achieved for at least 3 months.[2]

Components of control classification include symptoms, nighttime awakenings, interference with normal activities, pulmonary function, quality of life, exacerbations, medication adherence, treatment-related adverse effects, and satisfaction with care.[71] The categories of well controlled, not well controlled, and very poorly controlled are recommended.[6] Validated questionnaires such as the Asthma Therapy Assessment Questionnaire (ATAQ), the Asthma Control Questionnaire (ACQ), and the Asthma Control Test (ACT) can be regularly administered.[71] The NAEPP minimally recommends spirometric tests at initial assessment, after treatment is initiated, and then every 1 to 2 years.[2] In moderate to severe persistent asthma, PEF monitoring is recommended. PEF monitoring should also be considered in patients who are poor symptom perceivers or those with a history of severe exacerbations.[2] Patients should also be asked about exercise tolerance. All patients on inhaled drugs should have their inhalation delivery technique evaluated periodically—monthly initially and then every 3 to 6 months, before step-up in therapy, adherence, environmental control, and comorbid conditions should be reviewed.[2]

Following initiation of antiinflammatory therapy or an increase in dosage, most patients should begin experiencing a decrease in symptoms in 1 to 2 weeks and achieve maximum symptomatic improvement within 4 to 8 weeks. The use of higher ICS doses or more potent agents may accelerate the process. Improvement in FEV$_1$ and PEF should follow a similar time frame; however, a decrease in BHR, as measured by morning PEF, PEF variability, and exercise tolerance, may take longer and improve over 1 to 3 months.[2] Patients should be informed that following a viral respiratory infection, they may experience decreased exercise tolerance for up to 4 weeks.

Initial visits with the patient should focus on the patient's concerns, expectations, and goals of treatment. Basic education should focus on asthma as a chronic lung disease, the types of medications, and how they are to be used. Inhaler technique is taught, as is when to seek medical advice. Written action plans should be provided. Either peak flow-based or symptom-based self-monitoring can be effective, if taught and followed correctly.[2] The first follow-up visit should be in 2 to 6 weeks, to evaluate control. At that time, the educational messages of the first visit should be repeated, as well as review of the patient's current medications, adherence, and any difficulties related to the therapy.

CONCLUSION

Asthma is a complicated disease with a multitude of clinical presentations. The exact defect in asthma has not been defined, and it may be that asthma is a common presentation of a heterogeneous group of diseases. Asthma is defined and characterized by excessive reactivity of the bronchial tree to a wide variety of noxious stimuli. The reaction is characterized by bronchospasm, excessive mucus production, and inflammation. The central role of inflammation in inducing and maintaining BHR is now becoming widely appreciated. The goal of asthma therapy is to normalize, as much as possible, the patient's life and prevent chronic irreversible lung changes. Drugs are the mainstay of asthma management. The goal of drug therapy is to use the minimum amount of medications possible to completely control the disease. In persistent asthma, therapy should be aimed at both bronchospasm and inflammation in order to produce the best results. Patients should be followed and monitored diligently for toxicities. Although death from asthma is an uncommon event, the most common cause of death is under assessment of the severity of obstruction either by the patient or by the clinician; the next common cause is undertreatment. A cornerstone of any therapy is education and the realization that most asthma deaths are avoidable.

ABBREVIATIONS

ACTH: adrenocorticotropic hormone

Arg: arginine

BAL: bronchoalveolar lavage

BHR: bronchial hyperresponsiveness

CFC: chlorofluorocarbon

cAMP: cyclic adenosine monophosphate

CYP: cytochrome P450

DPI: dry powder inhaler

ED: emergency department

EIB: exercise-induced bronchospasm

FDA: Food and Drug Administration

FeNO: fraction of exhaled nitric oxide

FEV_1: forced expiratory volume in 1 second

FVC: forced vital capacity

GINA: Global Initiative for Asthma

Gln: glutamine

Glu: glutamic acid

Gly: glycine

GM-CSF: granulocyte-macrophage colony-stimulating factor

HFA: hydrofluoroalkane

ICAM-1: intercellular adhesion molecule 1

ICS: inhaled corticosteroids

IgE: immunoglobulin E

IL: interleukin

iNOS: inducible nitric oxide synthase

LABA: long-acting β-agonists

LT: leukotriene

MDI: metered-dose inhaler

MMAD: mass median aerodynamic diameter

NAEPP: National Asthma Education and Prevention Program

NANC: nonadrenergic, noncholinergic

NO: nitric oxide

PAF: platelet-activating factor

PEF: peak expiratory flow

PKA: protein kinase

RSV: respiratory syncytial virus

SABA: short-acting β-agonists

T-cells: thymically derived lymphocytes

VCAM-1: vascular cell adhesion molecule 1

VHC: valved holding chamber

VIP: vasoactive intestinal peptide

REFERENCES

1. Rosenblatt MB. History of bronchial asthma. In: Weiss EB, Segal MS, Stein M, eds. Bronchial Asthma: Mechanisms and Therapeutics, 2d ed. Boston: Little, Brown, 1976:5–17.
2. National Institutes of Health, National Heart, Lung, and Blood Institute. National Asthma Education and Prevention Program. Full Report of the Expert Panel: Guidelines for the Diagnosis and Management of Asthma (EPR-3); July 2007. *http://www.nhlbi.nih.gov/guidelines/asthma*.
3. American Lung Association. Trends in asthma morbidity and mortality. American Lung Association Epidemiology & Statistics Unit Research and Program Services; January 2009. *http://www.lungusa.org*.
4. Reed CE. The natural history of asthma. J Allergy Clin Immunol 2006;118:543–548.
5. Postma DS, Koppelman GH. Genetics of asthma: Where are we and where do we go? Proc Am Thorac Soc 2009;6:283–287.
6. Gelfand EW. Pediatric asthma: a different disease. Proc Am Thorac Soc 2009;6:278–282.
7. Busse WW, Lemanske RF Jr. Asthma. N Engl J Med 2001;344:350–362.
8. Dykewicz MS. Occupational asthma: current concepts in pathogenesis, diagnosis, and management. J Allergy Clin Immunol 2009;123:519–528.
9. Sears MR. Epidemiology of asthma exacerbations. J Allergy Clin Immunol 2008;122:662–668.
10. Fixman ED, Stewart A, Martin JG. Basic mechanisms of development of airway structural changes in asthma. Eur Respir J 2007;29:379–389.
11. Woodruff PG, Modrek B, Choy DF, et al. T-helper type 2-driven inflammation defines major subphenotypes of asthma. Am J Respir Crit Care Med 2009;180:388–395.
12. Anderson SD. How does exercise cause asthma attacks? Curr Opin Allergy Clin Immunol 2006;6:37–42.
13. Fahy JV. Eosinophilic and neutrophilic inflammation in asthma: insights from clinical studies. Proc Am Thorac Soc 2009;6:256–259.
14. An SS, Bai TR, Bates JHT, et al. Airway smooth muscle dynamics: a common pathway of airway obstruction in asthma. Eur Respir J 2007;29:834–860.
15. Kharitonov SA, Barnes PJ. Exhaled biomarkers. Chest 2006;130:1541–1546.
16. Anderson SD, Charlton B, Weiler JM, Nichols S, Spector SL, Pearlman DS; A305 Study Group. Comparison of mannitol and methacholine to predict exercise-induced bronchoconstriction and a clinical diagnosis of asthma. Respir Res 2009;10:4.
17. Cates CJ, Jefferson TO, Bara AI, Rowe BH. Vaccines for preventing influenza in people with asthma. Cochrane Database Syst Rev 2004;2:CD000364.
18. The American Lung Association Clinical Research Centers. Efficacy of esomeprazole for treatment of poorly controlled asthma. N Engl J Med 2009;360:1487–1499.
19. National Institutes of Health, National Heart, Lung and Blood Institute. NAEPP Expert Panel Report Managing Asthma During Pregnancy: Recommendations for Pharmacologic Treatment—Update 2004. NIH Publication No. 04–5246, March 2004.
20. Brenner BE, Holmes T M, Mazal B, Camargo CA Jr. Relation between phase of the menstrual cycle and asthma presentations in the emergency department. Thorax 2005;60:806–809.
21. Beasley R, Burgess C, Holt S. Call for a worldwide withdrawal of benzalkonium chloride from nebulizer solutions. J Allergy Clin Immunol 2001;107:222–223.
22. Jenkins C, Costello J, Hodge L. Systematic review of the prevalence of aspirin induced asthma and its implications for clinical practice. BMJ 2004;328(7437):434.
23. Shore SA. Obesity and asthma possible mechanisms. J Allergy Clin Immunol 2008;121:1087–1093.
24. Marcon A, Corsico A, Cazzoletti L, et al. Body mass index, weight gain, and other determinants of lung function decline in adult asthma. J Allergy Clin Immunol 2009;123:1069–1074.
25. Brehm JM, Celedon JC, Soto-Quiros ME, et al. Serum vitamin D levels and markers of severity of childhood asthma in Costa Rica. Am J Respir Crit Care Med 2009;179:765–771.
26. Dolovich MA, MacIntyre NR, Dhand R, et al. Consensus conference on aerosols and delivery devices. Respir Care 2000;45:589–596.
27. Schatz M, Kazzi AAN, Brenner B, et al. American Thoracic Society Documents: joint task force report: supplemental recommendations for the management and follow-up of asthma exacerbations. Proc Am Thor Soc 2009;6:353–393.
28. McFadden Jr ER, Elsanadi N, Dixon L, et al. Protocol therapy for acute asthma: therapeutic benefits and cost savings. Am J Med 1995;99:651–661.
29. Dolovich MB, Ahrens RC, Hess DR, et al. Device selection and outcomes of aerosol therapy: evidence-based guidelines. Chest 2005;127:335–371.
30. Camargo CA Jr, Spooner CH, Rowe BH. Continuous versus intermittent beta-agonists in the treatment of acute asthma. Cochrane Database Syst Rev 2003;4:CD001115.

31. Kelly HW. Risk versus benefit considerations for the beta(2)-agonists. Pharmacotherapy 2006;26:164S–174S.

32. Rowe BH, Edmonds ML, Spooner CH, Diner B, Camargo CA Jr. Corticosteroid therapy for acute asthma. Respir Med 2004;98:275–284.

33. Rodrigo GJ, Castro-Rodriguez JA. Anticholinergics in the treatment of children and adults with acute asthma: a systematic review with meta-analysis. Thorax 2005;60:740–746.

34. Parameswaran K, Belda J, Rowe BH. Addition of intravenous aminophylline to beta2-agonists in adults with acute asthma. Cochrane Database Syst Rev 2000;4:CD002742.

35. Rowe BH, Bretzlaff JA, Bourdon C, et al. Intravenous magnesium sulfate treatment for acute asthma in the emergency department: A systematic review of the literature. Ann Emerg Med 2000;36:181–190.

36. Silverman RA, Osborn H, Runge J, et al. IV magnesium sulfate in the treatment of acute severe asthma: a multicenter randomized controlled trial. Chest 2002;122:489–497.

37. Rodrigo G, Pollack C, Rodrigo C, Rowe BH. Heliox for non-intubated acute asthma patients. Cochrane Database Syst Rev 2006;4:CD002884.

38. Kelly HW. What is new with the β_2 agonists: issues in the management of asthma. Ann Pharmacother 2005;39:931–938.

39. Weiss ST, Litonja AA, Lange C, Lazarus R, Liggett SB, Bleecker ER, Tantisira KG. Overview of the pharmacogenetics of asthma treatment. Pharmacogenomics J 2006;6:311–326.

40. Green RH, Wardlaw AJ. Systemic corticosteroids in asthma. In: Pharmacotherapy of Asthma. Li JT ed. Taylor and Francis, New York, NY, 2006:233–262.

41. Kelly HW. Comparison of inhaled corticosteroids: an update. Ann Pharmacother 2009; 43:519–527.

42. Kelly HW, Van Natta ML, Covar RA, Tonascia J, Green RP, Strunk RC, CAMP Research Group. Effect of long-term corticosteroid use on bone mineral density in children: A prospective longitudinal assessment in the Childhood Asthma Management Program (CAMP) study. Pediatrics 2008; 122:e53–e61.

43. Gross NJ. Anticholinergic bronchodilators. In: Pharmacotherapy of Asthma. Li JT ed. Taylor and Francis, New York, NY, 2006:65–82.

44. Spooner CH, Spooner GR, Rowe BH. Mast-cell stabilising agents to prevent exercise-induced bronchoconstriction. Cochrane Database Syst Rev 2003;4:CD002307.

45. Weiss KB, Sullivan SD. The health economics of asthma and rhinitis. I. Assessing the economic impact. J Allergy Clin Immunol 2001; 107:3–8.

46. Boyd M, Lasserson TJ, McKean MC, Gibson PG, Ducharme FM, Haby M. Interventions for educating children who are at risk of asthma-related emergency department attendance. Cochrane Database Syst Rev 2009;2:CD001290.

47. Janson SL, McGrath KW, Covington JK, Cheng SC, Boushey HA. Individualized asthma self-management improves medication adherence and markers of asthma control. J Allergy Clin Immunol 2009;123:840–846.

48. Suissa S, Ernst P, Benayoun S, et al. Low-dose inhaled corticosteroids and the prevention of death from asthma. N Engl J Med 2000;343:332–336.

49. Masoli M, Shirtcliffe P, Weatherall M, Holt S, Beasley R. Inhaled corticosteroid therapy in the management of asthma in adults. In: Pharmacotherapy of Asthma. Li JT, ed. New York: Taylor & Francis, 2006:83–115.

50. Strunk RC, Sternberg AL, Szefler SJ, Zeiger RS, Bender B, Tonascia J; Childhood Asthma Management Program (CAMP) Research Group. Long-term budesonide or nedocromil treatment, once discontinued, does not alter the course of mild to moderate asthma in children and adolescents. J Pediatr 2009;154:682–687.

51. Greenstone I, Ni CM, Masse V, Danish A, Magdalinos H, Zhang X, Ducharme F. Combination of inhaled long-acting beta$_2$-agonists and inhaled steroids versus higher dose of inhaled steroids in children and adults with persistent asthma. Cochrane Database Syst Rev 2005;4:CD005533.

52. Masoli M, Weatherall M, Holt S, Beasley R. Moderate dose inhaled corticosteroids plus salmeterol versus higher doses of inhaled corticosteroids in symptomatic asthma. Thorax 2005;60:730–734.

53. Casale TB, Stokes JR. Immunomodulators for allergic respiratory disorders. J Allergy Clin Immunol 2008;121:288–296.

54. Weldon D. The effects of corticosteroids on bone growth and bone density. Ann Allergy Asthma Immunol 2009;103:3–11.

55. Nelson HS, Weiss ST, Bleecker ER, Yancey SW, Dorinsky PM. The Salmeterol Multicenter Asthma Research Trial: a comparison of usual pharmacotherapy for asthma or usual pharmacotherapy plus salmeterol. Chest 2006;129:15–26.

56. Levenson M. Long-acting β-agonist and adverse asthma events meta-analysis: statistical briefing package for joint meeting of the Pulmonary-Allergy Advisory Committee, Drug Safety and Risk Management Advisory Committee and Pediatric Advisory Committee; December 10–11, 2008. http://www.fda.gov/ohrms/dockets/ac/cder08.html#PulmonaryAllergy.

57. Jaeschke R, O'Byrne PM, Mejza F, et al. The safety of long-acting beta-agonists among patients with asthma using inhaled corticosteroids: systematic review and meta-analysis. Am J Respir Crit Care Med 2008;178:1009–1016.

58. Wechsler ME, Kunselman SJ, Chinchilli VM, et al. Effect of β_2-Adrenergic receptor polymorphism on response to longacting β_2 agonist in asthma (LARGE trial): a genotype-stratified, randomized, placebo-controlled, crossover trial. Lancet 2009;374: 1754–1764.

59. Adcock IM, Barnes PJ. Molecular mechanisms of corticosteroid resistance. Chest 2008;134:394–401.

60. Kelly HW. Non-corticosteroid therapy for the long-term control of asthma. Expert Opin Pharmacother 2007;8:2077–2087.

61. The American Lung Association Asthma Clinical Research Centers. Clinical trial of low-dose theophylline and montelukast in patients with poorly controlled asthma. Am J Respir Crit Care Med 2007;175: 235–242.

62. Lowery M, Kelly KJ. Cromolyn and nedocromil. In: Li JT, ed. Pharmacotherapy of Asthma. New York: Taylor & Francis, 2006: 195–231.

63. O'Byrne PM, Gauvreau GM, Murphy DM. Efficacy of leukotriene receptor antagonists and synthesis inhibitors in asthma. J Allergy Clin Immunol 2009;124:397–403.

64. Manalai P, Woo JM, Postolache TT. Suicidality and montelukast. Expert Opin Drug Saf 2009;8:273–282.

65. Ledford DK. Omalizumab: overview of pharmacology and efficacy in asthma. Expert Opin Biol Ther 2009;9:933–943.

66. Wu AC, Paltiel AD, Kuntz KM, et al. Cost-effectiveness of omalizumab in adults with severe asthma: results from the Asthma Policy Model. J Allergy Clin Immunol 2007;120:1146–1152.

67. Davies H, Olson L, Gibson P. Methotrexate as a steroid sparing agent for asthma in adults. Cochrane Database Syst Rev 2000;2:CD000391.

68. Dykewicz MS. Immunosuppressive and other alternate treatments for asthma. In: Pharmacotherapy of Asthma. Li JT, ed. New York: Taylor & Francis, 2006:299–317.

69. Barnes PJ. Drugs for asthma. Br J Pharmacol 2006;147(Suppl 1):S297–S303.

70. Castro M, Rubin AS, Laviolette M, et al. Effectiveness and safety of bronchial thermoplasty in the treatment of severe asthma: a multicenter, randomized, double-blind, sham-controlled clinical trial. Am J Respir Crit Care Med 2010;181:116–124.

71. Reddel HK, Taylor DR, Bateman ED, et al. An official American Thoracic Society/European Respiratory Society statement: asthma control and exacerbations: standardizing endpoints for clinical asthma trials and clinical practice. Am J Respir Crit Care Med 2009;180: 59–99.

72. Campbell JD, Spackman DE, Sullivan SD. Health economics of asthma: assessing the value of asthma interventions. Allergy 2008;63: 1581–1592.

34

Chronic Obstructive Pulmonary Disease

DENNIS M. WILLIAMS AND SHARYA V. BOURDET

KEY CONCEPTS

❶ Chronic obstructive pulmonary disease (COPD) is a treatable and preventable disease characterized by progressive airflow limitation that is not fully reversible and is associated with an abnormal inflammatory response of the lungs to noxious particles or gases.

❷ COPD is historically described as either *chronic bronchitis* or *emphysema*. Chronic bronchitis is defined in clinical terms, whereas emphysema is defined in terms of anatomic pathology. Because most patients exhibit some features of each disease, the appropriate emphasis of COPD pathophysiology is on small airway disease and parenchymal damage that contributes to chronic airflow limitation.

❸ Mortality from COPD has increased steadily over the past three decades; it currently is the fourth leading cause of death in the United States.

❹ The primary cause of COPD is cigarette smoking, implicated in 85% of diagnosed cases. Other risks include a genetic predisposition, environmental exposures (including occupational dusts and chemicals), and air pollution.

❺ Smoking cessation is the only management strategy proven to slow progression of COPD.

❻ Oxygen therapy has been shown to reduce mortality in selected patients with COPD. Oxygen therapy is indicated for patients with a resting Pao_2 of less than 55 mm Hg or a Pao_2 of less than 60 mm Hg and evidence of right-sided heart failure, polycythemia, or impaired neurologic function.

❼ Bronchodilators represent the mainstay of drug therapy for COPD. Pharmacotherapy is used to relieve patient symptoms and improve quality of life. Guidelines recommend short-acting bronchodilators as initial therapy for patients with mild or intermittent symptoms.

❽ For the patient who experiences chronic symptoms, long-acting bronchodilators are appropriate. Either a β_2-agonist or an anticholinergic offers significant benefits. Combining long-acting bronchodilators is recommended if necessary, despite limited data.

❾ The role of inhaled corticosteroid therapy in COPD is controversial. International guidelines suggest that patients with severe COPD and frequent exacerbations may benefit from inhaled corticosteroids.

❿ Acute exacerbations of COPD have a significant impact on disease progression and mortality. Treatment of acute exacerbations includes intensification of bronchodilator therapy and a short course of systemic corticosteroids.

⓫ Antimicrobial therapy should be used during acute exacerbations of COPD if the patient exhibits at least two of the following: increased dyspnea, increased sputum volume, and increased sputum purulence.

❶ Chronic obstructive pulmonary disease (COPD) is a common lung disease characterized by airflow limitation that is not fully reversible and is both chronic and progressive. COPD is preventable and treatable and causes significant extrapulmonary effects that contribute to disease severity in a subset of patients. The prevalence and mortality of COPD have increased substantially over the past two decades. Currently, COPD is the fourth leading cause of death in the United States. By 2020, it is estimated that COPD will rank fifth in burden of disease and third as a cause of death throughout the world.

There has been a renewed interest in research and in improving clinical management recommendations for patients with COPD in recent years. Although national guidelines for management have been available for over two decades, questions were raised concerning their quality and supporting evidence. In order to standardize the care of patients with COPD and present evidence-based recommendations, the National Heart, Lung, and Blood Institute (NHLBI) and the World Health Organization (WHO) launched the Global Initiative for Chronic Obstructive Lung Disease (GOLD) in 2001.[1] This report has been updated most recently in 2009, and a full revision is expected in 2011. The goals of the GOLD organization are to increase awareness of COPD and reduce morbidity and mortality associated with the disease. International guidelines have also been developed through a collaborative effort of the American Thoracic Society (ATS) and the European Respiratory Society (ERS) and are widely available.[2] These two guidelines are generally concordant in their recommendations.

COPD is differentiated from asthma in that the airflow limitation that is present is not fully reversible. In a subset of patients, it is fixed with minimal improvement in response to a bronchodilator or with optimal treatment. However, the natural course of the disease is quite variable among patients. The chronic and progressive nature of COPD is associated with an abnormal inflammatory response of the lungs to noxious particles or gases.[2] Nonetheless, COPD is preventable and treatable. In recent years, there has been an increased appreciation for the impact of the systemic consequences of chronic inflammatory diseases, including COPD, and for the impact of comorbidities in individual patients that can complicate COPD management.

Until recently, clinicians and researchers have exhibited a nihilistic attitude toward the value of treatments for COPD. This was based on the paucity of effective therapies, the destructive nature of the condition, and the fact that the common etiology is cigarette smoking, a modifiable health risk. There is now a renewed interest in evaluating the value of treatments and prevention based on the availability of new therapeutic options for pharmacotherapy and guidelines based on evidence.[3] The international guidelines emphasize the terms *preventable* and *treatable* to support a positive approach to managing the patient with COPD. Support is also reflected in the availability of research funding to improve understanding about this disease and its management. This includes NHLBI funding of Specialized Centers of Clinically Oriented Research (SCCOR) programs in COPD that have an objective to promote multidisciplinary research on clinically relevant questions enabling basic science findings to be more rapidly applied to clinical problems.[4]

❷ The term *chronic obstructive pulmonary disease* has historically been used to describe various pulmonary diseases with a fixed component of airflow limitation. The two principal conditions are chronic bronchitis and emphysema. Chronic bronchitis is associated with chronic or recurrent excessive mucus secretion into the bronchial tree with cough that is present on most days for at least 3 months of the year for at least 2 consecutive years in a patient in whom other causes of chronic cough have been excluded.[2] While chronic bronchitis is defined in clinical terms, emphysema is defined in terms of anatomic pathology. Emphysema historically was defined on histologic examination at autopsy. Because this histologic definition is of limited clinical value, emphysema also has been defined as abnormal permanent enlargement of the airspaces distal to the terminal bronchioles accompanied by destruction of their walls yet without obvious fibrosis.[2]

Differentiating COPD as either chronic bronchitis or emphysema as descriptive subsets of COPD is no longer considered relevant. This is based on the observation that the majority of COPD is caused by a common risk factor (cigarette smoking) and most patients exhibit features of both chronic bronchitis and emphysema. Currently, emphasis is placed on the pathophysiologic features of small airways disease and parenchymal destruction as contributors to chronic airflow limitation. Most patients with COPD demonstrate features of both chronic bronchitis and emphysema. Chronic inflammation affects the integrity of the airways and causes damage and destruction of the parenchymal structures. The underlying problem is persistent exposure to noxious particles or gases that sustain the inflammatory response. The airways of both the lung and the parenchyma are susceptible to inflammation, and the result is the chronic airflow limitation that characterizes COPD (see Fig. 34–1).

EPIDEMIOLOGY

The true prevalence of COPD is likely underreported in the United States. Data from the National Health Interview Survey in 2001 indicate that 12.1 million people over age 25 years have COPD.[5] Over 9 million of these individuals have chronic bronchitis; the remaining number have emphysema or a combination of both diseases. According to national surveys, the true prevalence of people with symptoms of chronic airflow obstruction may exceed 24 million.[6] The burden may be even greater because more than one-third of adults in the United States reported respiratory complaints compatible with symptomatic COPD in some surveys.[7]

❸ COPD is the fourth leading cause of death in the United States, exceeded only by cancer, heart disease, and cerebrovascular

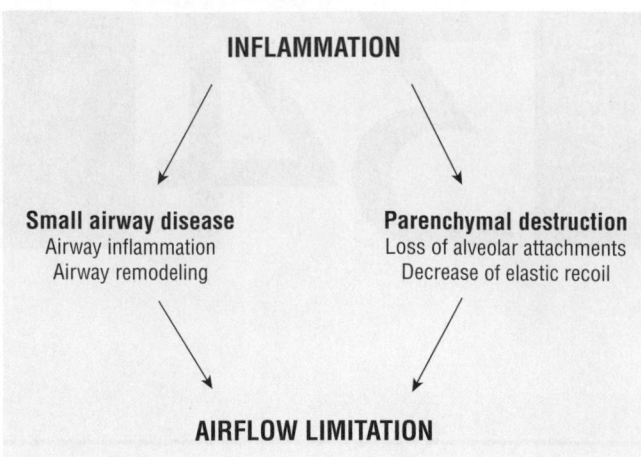

FIGURE 34-1. Mechanisms for developing chronic airflow limitation in COPD. *(From reference 1.)*

accidents. In 2005, COPD accounted for 126,005 deaths in the United States, representing one in every 20 deaths. Deaths attributed to COPD increased 8% from 2000 to 2005.[8] It is the only leading cause of death to increase over the last 30 years and is projected to be the third leading cause by 2020.[9] Overall, the mortality rate is higher in males; however, the female death rate has doubled over the last 25 years, and the number of female deaths exceeded male deaths in each year since 2000. The mortality rate is higher in whites compared with blacks.[9]

Cigarette smoking is the primary cause of COPD and, although the prevalence of cigarette smoking has declined compared with 1965, approximately 25% of individuals in the United States currently smoke. The trend of increasing COPD mortality likely reflects the long latency period between smoking exposure and complications associated with COPD.

The mortality of COPD is significant; however, morbidity associated with the disease also has a significant impact on patients, their families, and the healthcare system. COPD represents the second leading cause of disability in the United States. In the last 20 years, COPD has been responsible for nearly 50 million hospital visits nationwide.[10] In recent years, a diagnosis of COPD accounts for over 15 million physician office visits, 1.5 million emergency room visits, and 700,000 hospitalizations annually. A survey by the American Lung Association revealed that among COPD patients, 51% reported that their condition limits their ability to work, 70% were limited in normal physical activity, 56% were limited in performing household chores, and 50% reported that sleep was affected adversely.[11]

The economic impact of COPD continues to increase as well. It was estimated at $23 billion in 2000 and rose to $37.2 billion in 2004, including $20.9 billion in direct costs and $16.3 billion in indirect morbidity and mortality costs.[9,12] By 2020, COPD will be the fifth most burdensome disease, as measured by disability-adjusted life years lost due to illness. The cost of care for COPD patients is high compared with patients without the disease. There is a relationship among the severity of COPD, resources consumed, and the costs of care.[13]

ETIOLOGY

❹ Cigarette smoking is the most common risk factor and accounts for 85% to 90% of cases of COPD.[1] Components of tobacco smoke activate inflammatory cells, which produce and release the inflammatory mediators characteristic of COPD. Smokers are

TABLE 34-1	Risk Factors for Development of Chronic Obstructive Pulmonary Disease (COPD)
Exposures	**Host Factors**
Environmental tobacco smoke	Genetic predisposition (AAT deficiency)
Occupational dusts and chemicals	Airway hyperresponsiveness
Air pollution	Impaired lung growth

12 to 13 times more likely to die from COPD than nonsmokers.[14] Although the risk is lower in pipe and cigar smokers, it is still higher than in nonsmokers. Age of starting, total pack-years, and current smoking status are predictive of COPD mortality.

However, only 15% to 20% of all smokers go on to develop COPD, and not all smokers who have equivalent smoking histories develop the same degree of pulmonary impairment, suggesting that other host and environmental factors contribute to the degree of lung dysfunction. Nevertheless, the rate of loss of lung function is determined primarily by smoking status and history.[2] Children and spouses of smokers have increased risk of developing significant pulmonary dysfunction through passive smoking, also known as *environmental tobacco smoke* or *secondhand smoke.*

In addition to cigarette smoking, COPD is attributed to a combination of risk factors that results in lung injury and tissue destruction. Risk factors can be divided into host factors and environmental factors (Table 34–1), and commonly, the interaction between these risks leads to expression of the disease. Host factors, such as genetic predisposition, may not be modifiable but are important for identifying patients at high risk of developing the disease.

Environmental factors, such as tobacco smoke and occupational dust and chemicals, are modifiable factors that, if avoided, may reduce the risk of disease development. Environmental exposures associated with COPD are particles that are inhaled by the individual, which result in inflammation and cell injury. Exposure to multiple environmental toxins increases the risk of COPD. Thus, the total burden of inhaled particles (e.g., cigarette smoke as well as occupational and environmental particles and pollutants) can play a significant role in the development of COPD. In such cases, it is helpful to assess an individual's total burden of inhaled particles. For example, an individual who smokes and works in a textile factory has a higher total burden of inhaled particles than an individual who smokes and has no occupational exposure.

In nonindustrialized countries, occupational exposures may be a more common risk than cigarette smoking. These exposures include dust and chemicals such as vapors, irritants, and fumes. Reduced lung function and deaths from COPD are higher for individuals who work in gold and coal mining, in the glass or ceramic industries with exposure to silica dust, and in jobs that expose them to cotton dust or grain dust, toluene diisocyanate, or asbestos. Other occupational risk factors include chronic exposure to open cooking or heating fires.

It is unclear whether air pollution alone is a significant risk factor for the development of COPD in smokers and nonsmokers with normal lung function. However, in individuals with existing pulmonary dysfunction, significant air pollution worsens symptoms. As evidence for this, emergency department visits are increased during higher-intensity periods of air pollution.

Individuals exposed to the same environmental risk factors do not have the same chance of developing COPD, suggesting that host factors play an important role in pathogenesis.[1,2] While many not-yet-identified genes may influence the risk of developing COPD, the best documented genetic factor is a hereditary deficiency of α_1-antitrypsin (AAT). AAT-associated emphysema is an example of a pure genetic disorder inherited in an autosomal recessive pattern.

Inheritance is sometimes described as autosomal codominant by some researchers, because heterozygotes can also have decreased concentrations of AAT enzyme as well.[15] The consequences of AAT deficiency are discussed in the following section as protease-antiprotease imbalance. True AAT deficiency accounts for less than 1% of COPD cases.[2]

AAT is a 42 kDa plasma protein that is synthesized in hepatocytes. A primary role of AAT is to protect cells, especially those in the lung, from destruction by elastase released by neutrophils. In fact, AAT may be responsible for 90% of the inhibition of this destructive enzyme.[16] In individuals with the most common allele (M), plasma levels of AAT are approximately 20 to 50 µmol (100 to 350 mg/dL). The protective effect of AAT in the lungs is significantly diminished when plasma levels are less than 11 µmol (80 mg/dL).[16] AAT is an acute-phase reactant, and the serum concentration can be quite variable.

Several types of AAT deficiency have been identified and are due to mutations in the AAT gene. Two main gene variants, S and Z, have been identified. For patients who are homozygous with the S variant, AAT levels are at least 60% of those of normal individuals. These patients usually do not have an increased risk of COPD compared with normal individuals. Patients with homozygous Z deficiency (ZZ), represent 95% of clinical cases[15] and have AAT levels that are 10% of those of normal individuals, while patients with heterozygous Z variant (SZ) have levels closer to 40% of those of normal individuals. Homozygous Z patients have a higher risk of developing COPD compared with heterozygous Z patients. A history of cigarette smoking increases this risk. A small number of patients have a null phenotype and are at high risk for developing emphysema because they produce virtually no AAT.

Patients with AAT deficiency develop COPD at an early age (20 to 50 years) primarily owing to an accelerated decline in lung function. Compared with an average annual decline in forced expiratory volume in 1 second (FEV_1) of 25 mL/year in healthy nonsmokers, patients with homozygous Z deficiency have been reported to have declines of 54 mL/year for nonsmokers and 108 mL/year for current smokers. Effective diagnosis is dependent on clinical suspicion, diagnostic testing of serum concentrations, and genotype confirmation.[15] Patients developing COPD at an early age or those with a strong family history of COPD should be screened for AAT deficiency. If the concentration is low, genotype testing (DNA) should be performed.

Other genes have been implicated with increased risk of developing COPD, including chromosome 2q, transforming growth factor β_1, microsomal epoxide hydrolase 1, and tumor necrosis factor α. However, there are no definite conclusions about an association other than AAT. One genetic factor that may reduce the risk of developing COPD is a polymorphism in the gene encoding for matrix metalloproteinase 12 (MMP12). A cohort of smokers with the polymorphism exhibited a lower risk for developing COPD (0.63).[17]

Two additional host factors that may influence the risk of COPD include airway hyperresponsiveness and lung growth. Individuals with airway hyperresponsiveness to various inhaled particles may have an accelerated decline in lung function compared with those without airway hyperresponsiveness. Additionally, individuals who do not attain maximal lung growth owing to low birth weight, prematurity at birth, or childhood illnesses may be at risk for COPD in the future.[1]

PATHOPHYSIOLOGY

COPD is characterized by chronic inflammatory changes that lead to destructive changes and the development of chronic airflow limitation. The inflammatory process is widespread and not only

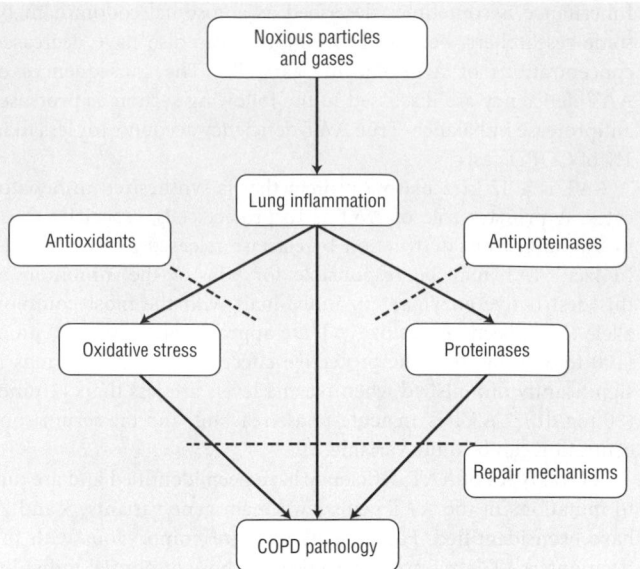

FIGURE 34-2. Pathogenesis of COPD. *(From reference 1.)*

TABLE 34-2	Features of Inflammation in COPD Compared with Asthma	
	COPD	**Asthma**
Cells	Neutrophils	Eosinophils
	Large increase in macrophages	Small increase in macrophages
	Increase in CD8+ T lymphocytes	Increase in CD4+ Th2 lymphocytes
		Activation of mast cells
Mediators	LTB$_4$	LTD$_4$
	IL-8	IL-4, IL-5
	TNF-α	(Plus many others)
Consequences	Squamous metaplasia of epithelium	Fragile epithelium
	Parenchymal destruction	Thickening of basement membrane
	Mucus metaplasia	Mucus metaplasia
	Glandular enlargement	Glandular enlargement
Response to treatment	Glucocorticosteroids have variable effect.	Glucocorticosteroids inhibit inflammation.

From reference 1.

involves the airways but also extends to the pulmonary vasculature and lung parenchyma. The inflammation of COPD is often referred to as *neutrophilic* in nature, but macrophages and CD8+ lymphocytes also play major roles.[18-20] The inflammatory cells release a variety of chemical mediators, of which tumor necrosis factor α (TNF-α), interleukin 8 (IL-8), and leukotriene B$_4$ (LTB$_4$) play major roles.[1,21] The actions of these cells and mediators are complementary and redundant, leading to the widespread destructive changes. The stimulus for activation of inflammatory cells and mediators is an exposure to noxious particles and gas through inhalation. The most common etiologic factor is exposure to environmental tobacco smoke, although other chronic inhalational exposures can lead to similar inflammatory changes.

Other processes that have been proposed to play a major role in the pathogenesis of COPD include oxidative stress and an imbalance between aggressive and protective defense systems in the lungs (proteases and antiproteases).[18] These processes may be the result of ongoing inflammation or occur as a result of environmental pressures and exposures (Fig. 34–2).

An altered interaction between oxidants and antioxidants present in the airways is responsible for the increased oxidative stress present in COPD. Increases in markers (e.g., hydrogen peroxide and nitric oxide) of oxidants are seen in the epithelial lining fluid.[1] The increased oxidants generated by cigarette smoke react with and damage various proteins and lipids, leading to cell and tissue damage. Oxidants also promote inflammation directly and exacerbate the protease-antiprotease imbalance by inhibiting antiprotease activity.

The consequences of an imbalance between proteases and antiproteases in the lungs were described over 40 years ago when the hereditary deficiency of the protective antiprotease AAT was discovered to result in an increased risk of developing emphysema prematurely. This enzyme (AAT) is responsible for inhibiting several protease enzymes, including neutrophil elastase. In the presence of unopposed activity, elastase attacks elastin, a major component of alveolar walls.[1]

In the inherited form of emphysema, there is an absolute deficiency of AAT. In cigarette smoking-associated emphysema, the imbalance is likely associated with increased protease activity or reduced activity of antiproteases. Activated inflammatory cells release several proteases other than AAT, including cathepsins and

metalloproteinases (MMPs). In addition, oxidative stress reduces antiprotease (or protective) activity.

It is helpful to differentiate inflammation occurring in COPD from that present in asthma because the response to antiinflammatory therapy differs. The inflammatory cells that predominate differ between the two conditions, with neutrophils playing a major role in COPD and eosinophils and mast cells in asthma. Mediators of inflammation also differ with LTB$_4$, IL-8, and TNF-α predominating in COPD, compared with LTD$_4$, IL-4, and IL-5 among the numerous mediators modulating inflammation in asthma.[1] Characteristics of inflammation for the two diseases are summarized in Table 34–2.

Pathologic changes of COPD are widespread, affecting large and small airways, lung parenchyma, and the pulmonary vasculature.[1] An inflammatory exudate is often present that leads to an increase in the number and size of goblet cells and mucus glands. Mucus secretion is increased, and ciliary motility is impaired. There is also a thickening of smooth muscle and connective tissue in the airways. Inflammation is present in central and peripheral airways. The chronic inflammation results in a repeated injury and repair process that leads to scarring and fibrosis. Diffuse airway narrowing is present and is more prominent in smaller peripheral airways. The decrease in FEV$_1$ is attributed to the presence of inflammation in the airways, while the blood gas abnormalities result from impaired gas transfer due to parenchymal damage.

Parenchymal changes affect the gas-exchanging units of the lungs, including the alveoli and pulmonary capillaries. The distribution of destructive changes varies depending on the etiology. Most commonly, smoking-related disease results in centrilobular emphysema that primarily affects respiratory bronchioles. Panlobular emphysema is seen in AAT deficiency and extends to the alveolar ducts and sacs.

The vascular changes of COPD include a thickening of pulmonary vessels and often are present early in the disease. Increased pulmonary pressures early in the disease are due to hypoxic vasoconstriction of pulmonary arteries. If persistent, the presence of chronic inflammation may lead to endothelial dysfunction of the pulmonary arteries. Later, structural changes lead to an increase in pulmonary pressures, especially during exercise. In severe COPD, secondary pulmonary hypertension leads to the development of right-sided heart failure.

TABLE 34-3 Etiology of Airflow Limitation in COPD
Reversible
Presence of mucus and inflammatory cells and mediators in bronchial secretions
Bronchial smooth muscle contraction in peripheral and central airways
Dynamic hyperinflation during exercise
Irreversible
Fibrosis and narrowing of airways
Reduced elastic recoil with loss of alveolar surface area
Destruction of alveolar support with reduced patency of small airways

Mucus hypersecretion is present early in the course of the disease and is associated with an increased number and size of mucus-producing cells. The presence of chronic inflammation perpetuates the process, although the resulting airflow obstruction and chronic airflow limitation may be reversible or irreversible. The various causes of airflow obstruction are summarized in Table 34–3.

Recently, there has been interest in the role of thoracic overinflation as it relates to the pathophysiology of COPD. Chronic airflow obstruction leads to air trapping, which results in thoracic hyperinflation that can be detected on chest radiograph. This problem results in several dynamic changes in the chest, including flattening of diaphragmatic muscles. Under normal circumstances, the diaphragms are dome-shaped muscles tethered at the base of the lungs. When the diaphragm contracts, the muscle becomes shorter and flatter, which creates the negative inspiratory force through which air flows into the lung during inspiration. In the presence of thoracic hyperinflation, the diaphragmatic muscle is placed at a disadvantage and is a less efficient muscle of ventilation. The increased work required by diaphragmatic contractions predisposes the patient to muscle fatigue, especially during periods of exacerbations.

The other consequence of thoracic hyperinflation is a change in lung volumes. For patients with COPD who exhibit thoracic hyperinflation, there is an increase in the functional residual capacity (FRC), which is the amount of air left in the lung after exhalation at rest. Therefore, these patients are breathing at higher lung volumes, which perturbs gas exchange. In addition, the increased FRC limits the inspiratory reserve capacity, which is the amount of air that the patient can inhale to fill the lungs. The increased FRC also limits the duration of inhalation time, and this has been associated with an increase in dyspnea complaints by patients.[22] Drug therapy for COPD, especially bronchodilators, can reduce thoracic hyperinflation by reducing airflow obstruction. This may partially explain the improvement in symptoms reported by patients with COPD despite minimal improvements in lung function with drug therapy.

Airflow limitation is assessed through spirometry, which represents the "gold standard" for diagnosing and monitoring COPD. The hallmark of COPD is a reduction in the ratio of FEV_1 to forced vital capacity (FVC) to less than 70%.[1,2] The FEV_1 generally is reduced, except in very mild disease, and the rate of FEV_1 decline is greater in COPD patients compared with normal subjects.

The impact of the numerous pathologic changes in the lung perturbs the normal gas-exchange and protective functions of the lung. Ultimately, these are exhibited through the common symptoms of COPD, including dyspnea and a chronic cough productive of sputum. As the disease progresses, abnormalities in gas exchange lead to hypoxemia and/or hypercapnia, although there often is not a strong relationship between pulmonary function and arterial blood gas (ABG) results.

Significant changes in ABGs usually are not present until the FEV_1 is less than 1 L.[1] In these patients, hypoxemia and hypercapnia can become chronic problems. Initially, when hypoxemia is present, it usually is associated with exercise. However, as the disease progresses, hypoxemia at rest develops. Patients with severe COPD can have a low arterial oxygen tension (Pao_2 = 45 to 60 mm Hg) and an elevated arterial carbon dioxide tension ($Paco_2$ = 50 to 60 mm Hg). The hypoxemia is attributed to hypoventilation ($\dot{V}$) of lung tissue relative to perfusion ($\dot{Q}$) of the area. This low $\dot{V}/\dot{Q}$ ratio will progress over a period of several years, resulting in a consistent decline in the Pao_2. Some COPD patients lose the ability to increase the rate or depth of respiration in response to persistent hypoxemia. Although this is not completely understood, the decreased ventilatory drive may be due to abnormal peripheral or central respiratory receptor responses. This relative hypoventilation subsequently leads to hypercapnia. In this case, the central respiratory response to a chronically increased $Paco_2$ can be blunted. These changes in Pao_2 and $Paco_2$ are subtle and progress over a period of many years. As a result, the pH usually is nearly normal because the kidneys compensate by retaining bicarbonate. If acute respiratory distress develops, such as might be seen in pneumonia or a COPD exacerbation with impending respiratory failure, the $Paco_2$ may rise sharply, and the patient presents with an uncompensated respiratory acidosis.

The consequences of long-standing COPD and chronic hypoxemia include the development of secondary pulmonary hypertension that progresses slowly if appropriate treatment of COPD is not initiated. Pulmonary hypertension is the most common cardiovascular complication of COPD and can result in cor pulmonale, or right-sided heart failure.[23]

The elevated pulmonary artery pressures are attributed to vasoconstriction (in response to chronic hypoxemia), vascular remodeling, and loss of pulmonary capillary beds. If elevated pulmonary pressures are sustained, cor pulmonale can develop, characterized by hypertrophy of the right ventricle in response to increases in pulmonary vascular resistance.

The risks of cor pulmonale include venous stasis with the potential for thrombosis and pulmonary embolism. Another important systemic consequence of COPD is a loss of skeletal muscle mass and general decline in the overall health status.

While airway inflammation is prominent for patients with COPD, there is also evidence of systemic inflammation.[24] A consequence is widespread skeletal muscle dysfunction, especially in the leg muscles involved with ambulation.[25] The systemic manifestations can have devastating effects on overall health status and comorbidities. These include cardiovascular events associated with ischemia, cachexia, osteoporosis, anemia, and muscle wasting. There is some interest in the role of measuring C-reactive protein as a parameter to assess systemic inflammation and its impact on COPD severity; however, it is premature to recommend this strategy currently.[26]

PATHOPHYSIOLOGY OF EXACERBATION

The natural history of COPD is characterized by recurrent exacerbations associated with increased symptoms and a decline in overall health status. An exacerbation is defined as a change in the patient's baseline symptoms (dyspnea, cough, or sputum production) beyond day-to-day variability sufficient to warrant a change in management.[1,2] Exacerbations have a significant impact on the natural course of COPD and occur more frequently for patients with more severe chronic disease. Because many patients experience chronic symptoms, the diagnosis of an exacerbation is based, in part, on subjective measures and clinical judgment. Repeated exacerbations, especially those requiring hospitalization, are associated with an increased mortality risk.

There are limited data about pathology during exacerbations owing to the nature of the disease and the condition of patients. However, inflammatory mediators including neutrophils and eosinophils are increased in the sputum. Chronic airflow limitation is a feature of COPD and may not change remarkably even during an exacerbation.[1] The lung hyperinflation present in chronic COPD is worsened during an exacerbation, which contributes to worsening dyspnea and poor gas exchange.

The primary physiologic change is often a worsening of ABG results owing to poor gas exchange and increased muscle fatigue. For a patient experiencing a severe exacerbation, profound hypoxemia and hypercapnia can be accompanied by respiratory acidosis and respiratory failure.

CLINICAL PRESENTATION

The diagnosis of COPD is made based on the patient's symptoms, including cough, sputum production, and dyspnea, and a history of exposure to risk factors such as tobacco smoke and occupational exposures. Patients may have these symptoms for several years before dyspnea develops and often will not seek medical attention until dyspnea is significant. A diagnosis of COPD should be considered for any patient, age 40 years or older, with persistent or progressive dyspnea, with chronic cough productive of sputum, and who exhibits an unusual or abnormal decline in activity, especially in the presence of positive cigarette smoke exposure. In addition, the presence of genetic factors, including AAT deficiency, and occupational exposures should be evaluated because approximately 15% of patients with COPD do not have a history of cigarette smoking.

The presence of airflow limitation should be confirmed with spirometry. Spirometry represents a comprehensive assessment of lung volumes and capacities. The hallmark of COPD is an $FEV_1:FVC$ ratio of less than 70%, which indicates airway obstruction, and a postbronchodilator FEV_1 of less than 80% of predicted confirms the presence of airflow limitation that is not fully reversible.[1] There is an increased awareness that the use of a fixed ratio of less than 70% may be problematic because normal aging may affect this result; however, it continues to be the current standard. An improvement in FEV_1 of less than 12% following inhalation of a rapid-acting bronchodilator is considered to be evidence of irreversible airflow obstruction. Reversibility of airflow limitation is measured by a bronchodilator challenge, which is described in Table 34–4. The use of peak expiratory flow measurements is not adequate for the diagnosis of COPD owing to low specificity and the high degree of effort dependence; however, a low peak expiratory flow is consistent with COPD. A comprehensive discussion about spirometry can be found in Chapter 33.

TABLE 34-4   Procedures for Reversibility Testing

Preparation
Tests should be performed when patients are clinically stable and free from respiratory infection.
Patients should not have taken inhaled short-acting bronchodilators in the previous 6 hours, long-acting β-agonists in the previous 12 hours, or sustained-release theophylline in the previous 24 hours.

Spirometry
FEV_1 should be measured before bronchodilator is given.
Bronchodilators can be given by either metered-dose inhaler or nebulization. Usual doses are 400 mcg of β-agonist, 80 mcg of anticholinergic, or the two combined.
FEV_1 should be measured again 30–45 minutes after bronchodilator is given.

Results
An increase in FEV_1 that is both greater than 200 mL and 12% above the prebronchodilator FEV_1 is considered significant.

From reference 1.

TABLE 34-5   Classification of COPD Severity

Stage I: mild
FEV_1/FVC <70%
$FEV_1 \geq 80\%$
With or without symptoms

Stage II: moderate
FEV_1/FVC <70%
50% <FEV_1 <80%
With or without symptoms

Stage III: severe
FEV_1/FVC <70%
30% <FEV_1 <50%
With or without symptoms

Stage IV: very severe
FEV_1/FVC <70%
FEV_1 <30% or <50% with presence of chronic respiratory failure or right-sided heart failure

From reference 1.

Spirometry combined with a physical examination improves the diagnostic accuracy of COPD.[7] Spirometry is also used to determine the severity of the disease, along with an assessment of symptoms and the presence of complications. A primary benefit of spirometry is to identify individuals who might benefit from pharmacotherapy to reduce exacerbations. Currently, the GOLD consensus guidelines suggest a 4-stage classification system (see Table 34–5).

Previously, guidelines have defined patients at risk for COPD who exhibit normal spirometry but experience chronic symptoms of cough or sputum production in the presence of risk factors. However, this category has been removed because there is not a reliable way to determine which patients might progress to COPD. This change was made because of inadequate evidence to identify patients who might progress to stage 1 disease. Patients with all levels of severity of COPD exhibit the hallmark finding of airflow obstruction, i.e., a reduction in the $FEV_1:FVC$ ratio to less than 70%. FVC is the total amount of air exhaled after a maximal inhalation. The extent of reduction in FEV_1 further defines the patient with mild, moderate, severe, or very severe disease.[1]

Spirometry is the primary tool in classifying COPD according to severity. The severity of symptoms also impacts the patient dramatically. Often symptoms do not correlate well with the degree of airflow limitation. Two important factors that influence disease severity, survival, and health-related quality of life are body mass index (BMI) and dyspnea.[2] A low BMI is a systemic consequence of chronic COPD, and a BMI of less than 21 kg/m² is associated with increased mortality.[27]

Dyspnea is often the most troublesome complaint for the patient with COPD and often is the stimulus for the patient seeking medical attention. Dyspnea can impair exercise performance and functional capacity and is frequently associated with depression and anxiety. Together, these have a significant effect on health-related quality of life.[22] As a subjective symptom, dyspnea is often difficult for the clinician to assess. Various tools are available to evaluate the severity of dyspnea. A version of the Medical Research Council (MRC) scale, modified by the ATS, is commonly employed and categorizes dyspnea grades from 0 to 4 (see Table 34–6).[28]

While a physical examination is appropriate in the diagnosis and assessment of COPD, most patients who present in the milder stages of COPD will have a normal physical examination. In later stages of the disease, when airflow limitation is severe, patients may have cyanosis of mucosal membranes, development of "barrel chest" due to hyperinflation of the lungs, an increased respiratory rate and shallow breathing, and changes in breathing mechanics such as pursing of the lips to help with expiration or use of accessory respiratory muscles.

TABLE 34-6	Modified Medical Research Council (MRC) Dyspnea Scale	
Grade 0	No dyspnea	Not troubled by breathlessness except with strenuous exercise
Grade 1	Slight dyspnea	Troubled by shortness of breath when hurrying on a level surface or walking up a slight hill
Grade 2	Moderate dyspnea	Walks slower than normal based on age on a level surface due to breathlessness or has to stop for breath when walking on level surface at own pace
Grade 3	Severe dyspnea	Stops for breath after walking 100 yards or after a few minutes on a level surface
Grade 4	Very severe dyspnea	Too breathless to leave the house or becomes breathless while dressing or undressing

From reference 2.

CLINICAL PRESENTATION

Symptoms

- Chronic cough
- Sputum production
- Dyspnea

Exposure to Risk Factors

- Tobacco smoke
- α_1-Antitrypsin deficiency
- Occupational hazards

Physical Examination

- Cyanosis of mucosal membranes
- Barrel chest
- Increased resting respiratory rate
- Shallow breathing
- Pursed lips during expiration
- Use of accessory respiratory muscles

Diagnostic Tests

- Spirometry with reversibility testing
- Radiograph of chest
- Arterial blood gas (not routine)

FEATURES OF COPD EXACERBATION

Symptoms

- Increased sputum volume
- Acutely worsening dyspnea
- Chest tightness
- Presence of purulent sputum
- Increased need for bronchodilators
- Malaise, fatigue
- Decreased exercise tolerance

Physical Examination

- Fever
- Wheezing, decreased breath sounds

Diagnostic Tests

- Sputum sample for Gram stain and culture
- Chest radiograph to evaluate for new infiltrates

PROGNOSIS

For the patient with COPD, the combination of impaired lung function and recurrent exacerbations promote a clinical scenario characterized by dyspnea, reduced exercise tolerance and physical activity, and deconditioning. These factors lead to disease progression, poor quality of life, possible disability, and premature mortality.[29] COPD is ultimately a fatal disease if it progresses and advanced directives and end-of-life care options are appropriate to consider. The primary causes of death of patients with COPD include respiratory failure, cardiovascular events or diseases, and lung cancer.[30]

The FEV_1 is the most important prognostic indicator for a patient with COPD. The average rate of decline of FEV_1 is the most useful objective measure to assess the course of COPD. The average rate of decline in FEV_1 for healthy, nonsmoking patients owing to age alone is 25 to 30 mL/year. The rate of decline for smokers is steeper, especially for heavy smokers compared with light smokers. The decline in pulmonary function is a steady curvilinear path. The more severely diminished the FEV_1 at diagnosis, the steeper is the rate of decline. Greater numbers of years of smoking and number of cigarettes smoked also correlate with a steeper decline in pulmonary function.[27] Conversely, the rate of decline of blood gases has not been shown to be a useful parameter to assess progression of the disease. Patients with COPD should have spirometry performed at least annually to assess disease progression.[31]

The survival rate of patients with COPD is highly correlated to the initial level of impairment in the FEV_1 and age. Other less important factors include degree of reversibility with bronchodilators, resting pulse, perceived physical disability, diffusing capacity (D_LCO), cor pulmonale, and blood gas abnormalities. A rapid decline in pulmonary function tests indicates a poor prognosis. Median survival is approximately 10 years when the FEV_1 is 1.4 L, 4 years when the FEV_1 is 1.0 L, and about 2 years when the FEV_1 is 0.5 L.

While ABG measurements are important, they do not carry the prognostic value of pulmonary function tests. Measurement of ABGs is more useful for patients with severe disease and is recommended for all patients with an FEV_1 of less than 40% of predicted or those with signs of respiratory failure or right-sided heart failure.[1]

Asthma is usually differentiated from COPD based on the patient's medical history, risk factors, and improvements on postbronchodilator spirometry; however, in some cases, asthma patients exhibit COPD-like features and COPD patients exhibit asthma-like features. It is also possible for the two conditions to coexist.

CLINICAL PRESENTATION OF COPD EXACERBATION

Because of the subjective nature of defining an exacerbation of COPD, the criteria used among clinicians varies widely; however, most rely on a change in one or more of the following clinical findings: worsening symptoms of dyspnea, increase in sputum volume, or increase in sputum purulence. Acute exacerbations have a significant impact of the economics of treating COPD as well, estimated at 35% to 45% of the total costs of the disease in some settings.[32]

A widely accepted definition of an exacerbation is that it is an event in the natural course of COPD that is characterized by a worsening in baseline dyspnea, cough, and/or sputum that is beyond the normal day-to-day variation, is acute in onset, and may warrant a change in regular medication. With an exacerbation, patients using rapid-acting bronchodilators may report an increase in the frequency of use. Exacerbations are commonly staged as mild, moderate, or severe according to the criteria summarized in Table 34–7.[33]

TABLE 34-7	Staging Acute Exacerbations of COPD[a]
Mild (type 1)	One cardinal symptom[a] plus at least one of the following: URTI[b] within 5 days, fever without other explanation, increased wheezing, increased cough, increase in respiratory or heart rate >20% above baseline
Moderate (type 2)	Two cardinal symptoms[a]
Severe (type 3)	Three cardinal symptoms[a]

[a]Cardinal symptoms include worsening of dyspnea, increase in sputum volume, and increase in sputum purulence.
[b]URTI, upper respiratory tract infection.

TABLE 34-8	Goals of COPD Management
Prevent disease progression
Relieve symptoms
Improve exercise tolerance
Improve overall health status
Prevent and treat exacerbations
Prevent and treat complications
Reduce morbidity and mortality

An important complication of a severe exacerbation is acute respiratory failure. In the emergency department or hospital, an ABG usually is obtained to assess the severity of an exacerbation. The diagnosis of acute respiratory failure in COPD is made based on an acute change in the ABGs. Defining acute respiratory failure as a Pao_2 of less than 50 mm Hg or a $Paco_2$ of greater than 50 mm Hg often may be incorrect and inadequate because these values may not represent a significant change from a patient's baseline values. A more precise definition is an acute drop in Pao_2 of 10 to 15 mm Hg or any acute increase in $Paco_2$ that decreases the serum pH to 7.3 or less. Additional acute clinical manifestations of respiratory failure include restlessness, confusion, tachycardia, diaphoresis, cyanosis, hypotension, irregular breathing, miosis, and unconsciousness.

PROGNOSIS

COPD exacerbations are associated with significant morbidity and mortality. While mild exacerbations may be managed at home, mortality rates are higher for patients admitted to the hospital. In one study of patients hospitalized with COPD exacerbations, in-hospital mortality was 6% to 8%.[34] Many patients experiencing an exacerbation do not have a return to their baseline clinical status for several weeks, significantly affecting their quality of life. Additionally, as many as half the patients originally hospitalized for an exacerbation are readmitted within 6 months.[35]

It is now evident that acute exacerbations of COPD have a tremendous impact on disease progression and ultimate mortality. For exacerbations requiring hospitalizations, mortality rates range from 22% to 43% after 1 year, and 36% to 49% in 2 years.[34,36,37]

TREATMENT

Chronic Obstructive Pulmonary Disease

■ DESIRED OUTCOME

Given the nature of COPD, a major focus in healthcare should be on prevention. However, for patients with a diagnosis of COPD, the primary goal is to prevent or minimize progression. Specific goals of management are listed in Table 34–8. The primary goal of pharmacotherapy has been relief of symptoms, including dyspnea. However, more recently there has been increased interest in the value of therapeutic interventions that reduce exacerbation frequency and severity, as well as reduce mortality.

Optimally, these goals can be accomplished with minimal risks or side effects. The therapy of the patient with COPD is multifaceted and includes pharmacologic and nonpharmacologic strategies. Appropriate measures of effectiveness of the management plan

include continued smoking cessation, symptom improvement, reduction in FEV_1 decline, reduction in the number of exacerbations, improvements in physical and psychological well-being, and reduction in mortality, hospitalizations, and days lost from work.

Unfortunately, most treatments for COPD have not been shown to improve survival or to slow the progressive decline in lung function. However, many therapies do improve pulmonary function and quality of life and reduce exacerbations and duration of hospitalization. Several disease-specific quality-of-life measures are available to assess the overall efficacies of therapies for COPD, including the Chronic Respiratory Questionnaire (CRQ) and the St. George's Respiratory Questionnaire (SGRQ). These questionnaires measure the impact of various therapies on such disease variables as severity of dyspnea and level of activity. They do not measure impact of therapies on survival. While early studies of COPD therapies focused primarily on improvements in pulmonary function measurements such as FEV_1, there is a trend toward greater use of these disease-specific quality-of-life measures to evaluate the benefits of therapy on larger clinical outcomes.

■ GENERAL APPROACH TO TREATMENT

To be effective, the clinician should address four primary components of management: Assess and monitor the condition, avoidance of or reduced exposure to risk factors, manage stable disease, and treat exacerbations. These components are addressed through a variety of nonpharmacologic and pharmacologic approaches.

■ NONPHARMACOLOGIC THERAPY

Patients with COPD should receive education about their disease, treatment plans, and strategies to slow progression and prevent complications.[1] Advice and counseling about smoking cessation are essential, if applicable. Because the natural course of the disease leads to respiratory failure, the clinician should address end-of-life decisions and advanced directives prospectively with the patient and family.[38]

Smoking Cessation

❺ Smoking cessation represents the single most important intervention in preventing the development, as well as the progression of COPD. A primary component of COPD management is avoidance of or reduced exposure to risk factors. Exposure to environmental tobacco smoke is a major risk factor, and smoking cessation is the most effective strategy to reduce the risk of developing COPD and to slow or stop disease progression. The cost-effectiveness of smoking-cessation interventions compares favorably with interventions made for other major chronic diseases.[39] The importance of smoking cessation cannot be overemphasized. Smoking cessation leads to decreased symptomatology and slows the rate of decline of pulmonary function even after significant abnormalities in pulmonary function tests have been detected (FEV_1:FVC <60%).[31] As confirmed by the Lung Health Study, smoking cessation is the only intervention proven at this time to affect long-term decline in

FEV$_1$ and slow the progression of COPD.[40] In this 5-year prospective trial, smokers with early COPD were randomly assigned to one of three groups: smoking-cessation intervention plus inhaled ipratropium 3 times a day, smoking-cessation intervention alone, or no intervention. During an 11-year follow-up, the rate of decline in FEV$_1$ among subjects who continued to smoke was more than twice the rate in sustained quitters. Smokers who underwent smoking-cessation intervention had fewer respiratory symptoms and a smaller annual decline in FEV$_1$ compared with smokers who had no intervention. However, this study also demonstrated the difficulty in achieving and sustaining successful smoking cessation.

Tobacco cessation has mortality benefits beyond those related to COPD. A follow-up analysis of the Lung Health Study data conducted more than 14 years later demonstrated an 18% reduction in all-cause mortality in patients that received the intervention compared with usual care.[41] Intervention patients had lower death rates due to coronary artery disease (the leading cause of mortality), cardiovascular diseases, and lung cancer, although all categories did not reach clinical significance.

Every clinician has a responsibility to assist smokers in smoking-cessation efforts. A clinical practice guideline for treating tobacco dependence from the U.S. Public Health Service (PHS) was updated in 2008.[42] The major findings and recommendations of that report are summarized in Table 34–9. An earlier report from the Surgeon General in 2004 on the health consequences of smoking broadened the scope of the detrimental effects of cigarette smoking, indicating that "Smoking harms nearly every organ of the body, causing many diseases and reducing the health of smokers in general."[14]

TABLE 34-9   **Key Guideline Recommendations Regarding Tobacco Use and Dependence[42]**

Tobacco dependence is a chronic disease that often requires repeated intervention and multiple attempts to quit. Effective treatments are available that can significantly improve rates of long-term abstinence.

Clinicians and healthcare delivery systems should consistently identify and document tobacco use status and treat every tobacco user.

Tobacco-dependence treatments are effective over a broad range of populations. Clinicians should encourage every patient willing to make a quit attempt to use counseling treatments and medications recommended in the guideline.

Brief tobacco-dependence treatments are effective. Clinicians should offer every patient who uses tobacco at least these brief treatments.

Individual, group, and telephone counseling are effective, and their effectiveness increases with treatment intensity. Practical counseling (problem-solving and/or skills training) and social support are especially effective and should be employed as a part of treatment.

There are numerous effective medications for tobacco dependence, and clinicians should encourage their use by patients during a quit attempt, except when medically contraindicated or with populations in which the evidence of effectiveness is insufficient (pregnancy, smokeless tobacco users, light smokers, and adolescents). Seven first-line medications (5 nicotine and 2 non-nicotine) consistently increase long-term abstinence rates. Clinicians should also consider the use of combinations as identified in the guideline.

Counseling and medication are effective when used by themselves for treating tobacco dependence. The combination of the two is more effective than either alone. Patients should be encouraged to use both counseling and medication.

Telephone quitline counseling is effective for diverse populations and offers the advantage of broad reach. Clinicians should ensure patient access to quitlines and promote quitline use.

For a tobacco user who is currently unwilling to make a quit attempt, clinicians should use motivational treatments that have been shown to be effective in increasing future quit attempts.

Tobacco-dependence treatments are both clinically effective and highly cost-effective relative to interventions for other clinical disorders. Providing coverage for these treatments increases quit rates. Insurers and purchasers should ensure that all insurance plans include the counseling and medications identified as effective in the guideline as covered benefits.

TABLE 34-10   **Five-Step Strategy for Smoking-Cessation Program (5 A's)**

Ask	Use systematic approach to identify all tobacco users.
Advise	Urge all tobacco users to quit.
Assess	Determine willingness to make a cessation attempt.
Assist	Provide support for the patient to quit smoking.
Arrange	Schedule follow-up and monitor for continued abstinence.

All clinicians should take an active role in assisting patients with tobacco dependence in order to reduce the burden on the individual, his or her family, and the healthcare system. It is estimated that over 75% of smokers want to quit and that one-third have made a serious effort. Yet complete and permanent tobacco cessation is difficult.[40] Counseling that is provided by clinicians is associated with greater success rates than self-initiated efforts.[42]

The PHS guidelines recommend that clinicians take a comprehensive approach to smoking-cessation counseling. Advice should be given to smokers even if they have no symptoms of smoking-related disease or if they are receiving care for reasons unrelated to smoking. Clinicians should be persistent in their efforts because relapse is common among smokers owing to the chronic nature of dependence. Brief interventions (3 minutes) of counseling are proven effective. However, it must be recognized that the patient must be ready to stop smoking because there are several stages of decision-making. Based on this, a 5-step intervention program is proposed (Table 34–10).

There is strong evidence to support the use of pharmacotherapy to assist in smoking cessation. In fact, it should be offered to most patients as part of a cessation attempt. In general, available therapies will double the effectiveness of a cessation effort. Agents that are considered first line are listed in Table 34–11. The usual duration of therapy is 8 to 12 weeks, although some individuals may require longer courses of treatment. Precautions to consider before using bupropion include a history of seizures or an eating disorder. Nicotine-replacement therapies are contraindicated for patients with unstable coronary artery disease, active peptic ulcers, or recent myocardial infarction or stroke. Nicotine patch, bupropion, and the combination of bupropion and the nicotine patch were compared with placebo in a controlled trial.[43] The treatment groups that received bupropion had higher rates of smoking cessation than the groups that received placebo or the nicotine patch. The addition of the nicotine patch to bupropion slightly improved the smoking-cessation rate compared with bupropion monotherapy. Recently, a new agent became available to assist in tobacco cessation attempts. Varenicline is a nicotine acetylcholine receptor partial agonist that has shown benefit in tobacco cessation.[44] Varenicline relieves physical withdrawal symptoms and reduces the rewarding properties of nicotine. Nausea and headache are the most frequent complaints associated with varenicline. Currently, varenicline has not been studied in combination with other tobacco-cessation therapies. Second-line agents are less effective or associated with greater side effects; however, they may be useful in selected clinical situations. These therapies include clonidine and nortriptyline, a tricyclic antidepressant.

Behavioral modification techniques or other forms of psychotherapy also may be helpful in assisting in smoking cessation. Programs that address the many issues associated with smoking (i.e., learned behaviors, environmental influences, and chemical dependence) using a team approach are more likely to be successful. The role of alternative-medicine therapies in smoking cessation is controversial. Hypnosis may aid in improving abstinence rates when added to a smoking-cessation program but appears to give little benefit when used alone. Acupuncture has not been shown to contribute to smoking cessation and is not recommended.[2]

TABLE 34-11	First-Line Pharmacotherapies for Smoking Cessation			
Agent	**Usual Dose**	**Duration**	**Common Complaints**
Bupropion SR	150 mg orally daily for 3 days, then twice daily	12 weeks, up to 6 months	Insomnia, dry mouth
Nicotine gum	2–4 mg gum prn, up to 24 pieces daily	12 weeks	Sore mouth, dyspepsia
Nicotine inhaler	6–16 cartridges daily	Up to 6 months	Sore mouth and throat
Nicotine nasal spray	8–40 doses daily	3–6 months	Nasal irritation
Nicotine patches	Various, 7–21 mg every 24 hours	Up to 8 weeks	Skin reaction, insomnia
Varenicline	0.5 mg daily for 3 days, then 0.5 mg twice daily for 4 days, then 1 mg twice daily	12 weeks	Nausea, sleep disturbances

Other Environmental Triggers

Although cigarette smoke represents the overwhelming majority of risk for developing COPD, exposure to other environmental toxins also confer risks. Exposures to occupational dusts and fumes have been implicated as a cause of COPD in 19% of smokers and 31% of nonsmokers with COPD in the United States. In the case of known environmental hazards, primary prevention is appropriate. Policies to limit airborne exposures in the workplace and outdoors, as well as education efforts of workers and policy makers are recommended.

Pulmonary Rehabilitation

Exercise training is beneficial in the treatment of COPD to improve exercise tolerance and to reduce symptoms of dyspnea and fatigue.[1] Pulmonary rehabilitation programs are an integral component in the management of COPD and should include exercise training along with smoking cessation, breathing exercises, optimal medical treatment, psychosocial support, and health education. Pulmonary rehabilitation has no direct effect on lung function or gas exchange. Instead, it optimizes other body systems so that the impact of poor lung function is minimized. Exercise training reduces the CNS response to dyspnea, ameliorates anxiety and depression, reduces thoracic hyperinflation, and improves skeletal muscle function.[47] High-intensity training (70% maximal workload) is possible even in advanced COPD patients, and the level of intensity improves peripheral muscle and ventilatory function. Studies have demonstrated that pulmonary rehabilitation with exercise 3 to 7 times per week can produce long-term improvement in activities of daily living, quality of life, exercise tolerance, and dyspnea for patients with moderate to severe COPD.[48] Improvements in dyspnea can be achieved without concomitant improvements in spirometry. Programs using less intensive exercise regimens (2 times per week) have not been shown to be of benefit.[49]

Immunizations

Vaccines can be considered as pharmacologic agents; however, their role is described here in reducing risk factors for COPD exacerbations. Because influenza is a common complication in COPD that can lead to exacerbations and respiratory failure, an annual vaccination with the inactivated intramuscular influenza vaccine is recommended. Immunization against influenza can reduce serious illness and death by 50% in COPD patients.[50] Influenza vaccine should be administered in the fall of each year (October and November) during regular medical visits or at vaccination clinics. There are few contraindications to influenza vaccine except for a patient with a serious allergy to eggs. An oral antiinfluenza agent (oseltamivir) can be considered for patients with COPD during an outbreak for patients who have not been immunized; however, this therapy is less effective and causes more side effects.[51]

The polyvalent pneumococcal vaccine, usually administered 1 time, is widely recommended for people from 2 to 64 years of age who have chronic lung disease and for all people older than 65 years. Thus, COPD patients at any age are candidates for vaccination. Although evidence for the benefit of the pneumococcal vaccine in COPD is not strong, the argument for continued use is that the current vaccine provides coverage for 85% of pneumococcal strains causing invasive disease and the increasing rate of resistance of pneumococcus to selected antibiotics. Currently, administering the vaccine remains the standard of practice and is recommended by the Centers for Disease Control and Prevention and the American Lung Association. Repeated vaccination with the 23-valent product is not recommended for patients aged 2 to 64 years with chronic lung disease; however, revaccination is recommended for patients over 65 years of age if the first vaccination was more than 5 years earlier and the patient was younger than age 65. The GOLD guidelines recommend pneumococcal vaccine for all COPD patients 65 years and older and for patients less than 65 years only if the FEV_1 is less than 40% predicted.[52,53] In 2009, the CDC broadened their recommendations for the pneumococcal polysaccharide vaccine to include all persons ages 18 and over who smoke based on a higher risk of pneumococcal infection in these patients.

Long-Term Oxygen Therapy

❻ The use of supplemental oxygen therapy increases survival in COPD patients with chronic hypoxemia. Although long-term oxygen has been used for many years for patients with advanced COPD, it was not until 1980 that data became available documenting its benefits. At that time, the Nocturnal Oxygen Therapy Trial Group published its data comparing nocturnal oxygen therapy (NOT), 12 hours per day, with continuous oxygen therapy (COT), average of 20 hours per day.[54] Among patients who were followed for at least 12 months, the results revealed a mortality rate in the NOT group that was nearly double that of the COT group (51% vs 26%). Statistical estimates of the COT group suggest that COT may have added 3.25 years to a COPD patient's life. Additional data from the Nocturnal Oxygen Therapy Trial Group revealed that COT patients had fewer (but statistically insignificant) hospitalizations, improved quality of life and neuropsychological function, reduced hematocrit, and decreased pulmonary vascular resistance.[54]

The decline in mortality with oxygen therapy was further substantiated in 1981 in a study by the British Medical Research Council that compared 15 h/day of oxygen versus no supplemental oxygen in COPD patients.[55] Patients receiving oxygen therapy for at least part of the day had lower rates of mortality than those not receiving oxygen. Long-term oxygen therapy provides even more benefit in terms of survival after at least 5 years of use, and it improves the quality of life of these patients by increasing walking distance and neuropsychological condition and reducing time spent in the hospital.[56] Before patients are considered for long-term oxygen therapy, they should be stabilized in the outpatient setting, and pharmacotherapy should be optimized. Once this is accomplished, long-term oxygen therapy should be instituted if either of two conditions exists:

1. A resting PaO_2 of less than 55 mm Hg

2. Evidence of right-sided heart failure, polycythemia, or impaired neuropsychiatric function with a PaO_2 of less than 60 mm Hg

The most practical means of administering long-term oxygen is with the nasal cannula, at 1 to 2 L/min, which provides 24% to 28% oxygen. The goal is to raise the Pao_2 above 60 mm Hg. Patient education about flow rates and avoidance of flames (i.e., smoking) is of the utmost importance.

There are three different ways to deliver oxygen, including (1) in liquid reservoirs, (2) compressed into a cylinder, and (3) via an oxygen concentrator. Although conventional liquid oxygen and compressed oxygen are quite bulky, smaller, portable tanks are available to permit greater patient mobility. Oxygen concentrator devices separate nitrogen from room air and concentrate oxygen. These are the most convenient and the least expensive method of oxygen delivery. Oxygen-conservation devices are available that allow oxygen to flow only during inspiration, making the supply last longer. These may be particularly useful to prolong the oxygen supply for mobile patients using portable cylinders. However, the devices are bulky and subject to failure.

Adjunctive Therapies

In addition to supplemental oxygen, adjunctive therapies to consider as part of a pulmonary rehabilitation program are psychoeducational care and nutritional support. Psychoeducational care (such as relaxation) has been associated with improvement in the functioning and well-being of adults with COPD.[1,2] The role of nutritional support for patients with COPD is controversial. Several studies have shown an association among malnutrition, low BMI, and impaired pulmonary status among patients with COPD. However, a metaanalysis suggests that the effect of nutritional support on outcomes in COPD is small and not associated with improved anthropometric measures, lung function, or functional exercise capacity.[57]

■ PHARMACOLOGIC THERAPY

Results from numerous recent clinical trials have improved insight and understanding about the respective roles of various medications used in chronic COPD management; yet, some controversies still exist related to both effectiveness and safety. In contrast to the survival benefit conferred by supplemental oxygen therapy, there is no medication available for the treatment of COPD that has been shown to modify the progressive decline in lung function or prolong survival.[1] There is limited evidence that chronic treatment with long-acting inhaled β-agonists, inhaled corticosteroids, or the combination can reduce the rate of decline in spirometry in a subset of patients with more severe disease.[58] Currently, the primary goal of pharmacotherapy is to control patient symptoms and reduce complications, including the frequency and severity of exacerbations and improving the overall health status and exercise tolerance of the patient.

International guidelines recommend a stepwise approach to the use of pharmacotherapy based on disease severity[1,2], which is determined by the extent of airflow limitation and degree of symptoms. The impact of recurrent exacerbations on accelerating disease progression is increasingly recognized as an important factor to be considered. The primary goals of pharmacotherapy are to control symptoms (including dyspnea), reduce exacerbations, and improve exercise tolerance and health status. Currently, there is inadequate evidence to support the use of more aggressive pharmacotherapy early in the course of disease because of the lack of a disease modifying benefit. Because of the progressive nature of COPD, pharmacotherapy tends to be chronic and cumulative and step down approaches in stable patients are not successful. Patients exhibit variable responses to available therapies and the treatment approach should be individualized.

Pharmacotherapy of COPD typically involves the use of inhaled medications, requiring patient knowledge, understanding, and skills using the various inhalation devices. Several delivery devices are available (e.g., metered-dose inhalers, dry powder inhalers, nebulizers, and ancillary devices such as holding chambers), and the instructions about proper use vary. Comorbidities that are common for patients with COPD, including physical and mental conditions, can have a significant effect on the patient's ability to use the devices. Periodic and frequent reinforcement and observation by the clinician is required for the patient's benefit.

❼ Pharmacotherapy focuses on the use of bronchodilators to control symptoms. Bronchodilators relax bronchial smooth muscle, improve lung emptying, reduce thoracic hyperinflation at rest and during exercise, and improve exercise tolerance.[1] These effects can be seen in the absence of objective improvements on spirometry. There are several classes of bronchodilators to choose from, and no single class has been proven to provide superior benefit over other available agents. The initial and subsequent choice of medications should be based on the specific clinical situation and patient characteristics. Medications can be used as needed or on a scheduled basis depending on the clinical situation, and additional therapies should be added in a stepwise manner depending on the response and severity of disease. Considerations should be given to individual patient response, tolerability, adherence, and economic factors. A stepwise approach to the management of COPD has been proposed based on the stage of disease severity (Fig. 34–3).

According to the guidelines, patients with intermittent symptoms should be treated with short-acting bronchodilators. When symptoms become more persistent, long-acting bronchodilators should be initiated. For patients with an FEV_1 less than 50% and who experience frequent exacerbations, inhaled corticosteroids should be considered. Short-acting bronchodilators relieve symptoms and increase exercise tolerance. Long-acting bronchodilators relieve symptoms, reduce exacerbation frequency, and improve quality of life and health status. Patients have a variety of choices in using inhalational therapies, including metered dose inhalers (MDI), dry powder inhalers (DPI), or nebulizers. There is not a clear advantage of one delivery method over another, and it is recommended that patient-specific factors and preferences should be considered in selecting the device.[59]

Bronchodilators

Bronchodilator classes available for the treatment of COPD include β_2-agonists, anticholinergics, and methylxanthines. There is no clear benefit to one agent or class over others, although inhaled therapy generally is preferred. In general, it can be more difficult for patients with COPD to use inhalation devices effectively compared with other populations owing to advanced age and the presence of other comorbidities. Clinicians should advise, counsel, and observe patient technique with the devices frequently and consistently.

Bronchodilators generally work by reducing the tone of airway smooth muscle (relaxation), thus minimizing airflow limitation. For patients with COPD, the clinical benefits of bronchodilators include increased exercise capacity, decreased air trapping in the lungs, and relief of symptoms such as dyspnea. However, use of bronchodilators may not be associated with significant improvements in pulmonary function measurements such as FEV_1. In clinical studies, regular use of a long-acting inhaled bronchodilator (LABA or Anticholinergic) or ipratropium are associated with improved health status. Regular use of tiotropium also reduces exacerbation rates. In general, side effects of bronchodilator medications are related to their pharmacologic effects and are dose dependent. Because COPD patients are older and more likely to have comorbid

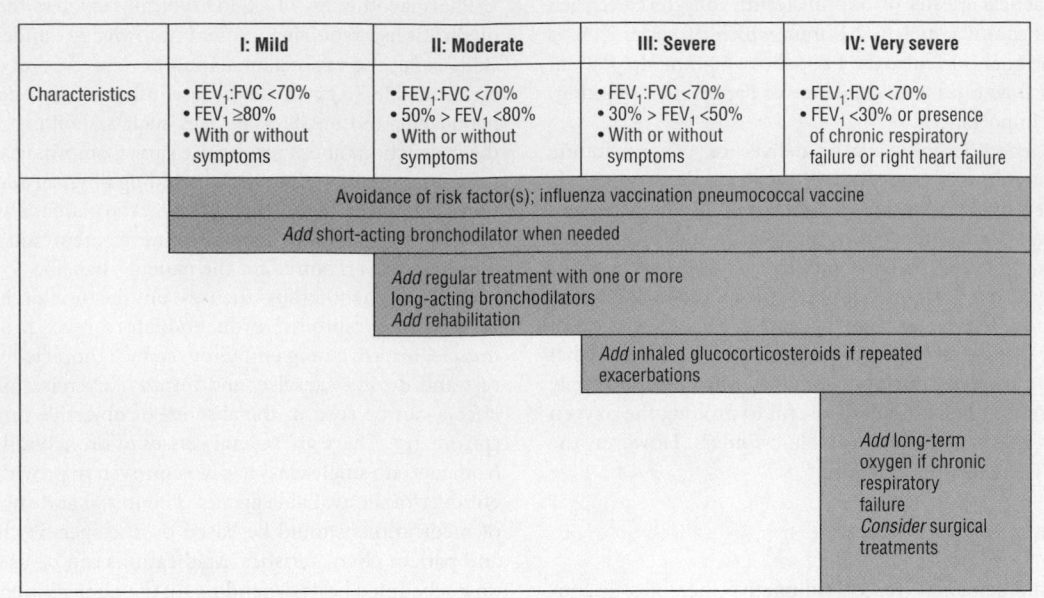

	I: Mild	II: Moderate	III: Severe	IV: Very severe
Characteristics	• FEV$_1$:FVC <70% • FEV$_1$ ≥80% • With or without symptoms	• FEV$_1$:FVC <70% • 50% > FEV$_1$ <80% • With or without symptoms	• FEV$_1$:FVC <70% • 30% > FEV$_1$ <50% • With or without symptoms	• FEV$_1$:FVC <70% • FEV$_1$ <30% or presence of chronic respiratory failure or right heart failure
	Avoidance of risk factor(s); influenza vaccination pneumococcal vaccine			
	Add short-acting bronchodilator when needed			
		Add regular treatment with one or more long-acting bronchodilators Add rehabilitation		
			Add inhaled glucocorticosteroids if repeated exacerbations	
				Add long-term oxygen if chronic respiratory failure Consider surgical treatments

FIGURE 34-3. Recommended therapy of stable COPD. (FEV$_1$, forced expiratory volume in the first second of expiration; FVC, forced vital capacity.) *(From reference 1.)*

conditions, the risk for side effects and drug interactions is higher compared with patients with asthma.

Short-Acting Bronchodilators The initial therapy for COPD patients who experience symptoms intermittently are short-acting bronchodilators. Among these agents, the choices are a short-acting beta$_2$ agonist or an anticholinergic. Either class of agents has a relatively rapid onset of action, relieves symptoms, and improves exercise tolerance and lung function. In general, both classes are equally effective.

Short-Acting Sympathomimetics (β_2-Agonists) A number of sympathomimetic agents are available in the United States. They vary in selectivity, route of administration, and duration of action. In COPD management, sympathomimetic agents with β_2-selectivity, or β_2-agonists, should be used as bronchodilators. β_2-Agonists cause bronchodilation by stimulating the enzyme adenyl cyclase to increase the formation of cyclic adenosine monophosphate (cAMP). cAMP is responsible for mediating relaxation of bronchial smooth muscle, leading to bronchodilation. In addition, they may improve mucociliary clearance. Although shorter-acting and less selective β-agonists are still used widely (e.g., metaproterenol, isoetharine, isoproterenol, and epinephrine), they should not be used owing to their shorter duration of action and increased cardiostimulatory effects. Short-acting, selective β_2-agonists such as albuterol, levalbuterol, and pirbuterol are preferred for therapy.

Sympathomimetics are available in inhaled, oral, and parenteral dosage forms. The preferred route of administration is by inhalation. The use of oral and parenteral β-agonists in COPD is discouraged because they are no more effective than a properly used metered-dose inhaler (MDI) or dry-powder inhaler (DPI), and the incidence of systemic adverse effects such as tachycardia and hand tremor is greater. Administration of β_2-agonists in the outpatient and emergency room settings via inhalers (MDIs or DPIs) is at least as effective as nebulization therapy and usually favored for reasons of cost and convenience.[59] Chapter 33 includes a complete description of the devices used for delivering aerosolized medication and a comparison β_2-agonist therapies.

Albuterol is the most frequently used β_2-agonist. It is available as an oral and inhaled preparation. Albuterol is a racemic mixture of (R)-albuterol, which is responsible for the bronchodilator effect, and (S)-albuterol, which has no therapeutic effect. (S)-Albuterol is considered by some clinicians to be inert, whereas others believe that it may be implicated in worsening airway inflammation and antagonizing the response to (R)-albuterol. Levalbuterol is a single-isomer formulation of (R)-albuterol. A retrospective evaluation of levalbuterol versus albuterol use for patients with asthma and COPD concluded that levalbuterol offered significant advantages over albuterol for hospitalized patients.[60] Other clinicians feel that there are no significant differences between the products and that the use of levalbuterol is not justified owing to its higher acquisition cost.[61] The effects of a single dose of levalbuterol have been compared with those of albuterol and ipratropium plus albuterol for patients with COPD. No significant differences in pulmonary function improvements or adverse effects were noted.[62]

In COPD patients, β_2-agonists exert a rapid onset of effect, although the response generally is less than that seen in asthma. Short-acting inhaled β_2-agonists cause only a small improvement in FEV$_1$ acutely but may improve respiratory symptoms and exercise tolerance despite the small improvement in spirometric measurements.[63] Patients with COPD can use quick-onset β_2-agonists as needed for relief of symptoms or on a scheduled basis to prevent or reduce symptoms. The duration of action of short-acting β_2-agonists is 4 to 6 hours.

Inhaled β_2-agonists are generally well tolerated. They can cause sinus tachycardia and rhythm disturbances in predisposed patients, but these are rarely reported. Skeletal muscle tremors can occur initially but subside as tolerance develops.

Short-Acting Anticholinergics When given by inhalation, anticholinergics such as ipratropium or atropine produce bronchodilation by competitively inhibiting cholinergic receptors in bronchial smooth muscle. This activity blocks acetylcholine, with the net effect being a reduction in cyclic guanosine monophosphate (cGMP), which normally acts to constrict bronchial smooth muscle. Muscarinic receptors on airway smooth muscle include M$_1$, M$_2$, and

M_3 subtypes. Activation of M_1 and M_3 receptors by acetylcholine results in bronchoconstriction; however, activation of M_2 receptors inhibits further acetylcholine release.

Ipratropium is the primary short-acting anticholinergic agent used for COPD in the United States. Atropine has a tertiary structure and is absorbed readily across the oral and respiratory mucosa, whereas ipratropium has a quaternary structure that is absorbed poorly. The lack of systemic absorption of ipratropium greatly diminishes the anticholinergic side effects such as blurred vision, urinary retention, nausea, and tachycardia associated with atropine. Ipratropium bromide is available as an MDI and a solution for inhalation. The MDI was recently reformulated with an HFA propellant and delivers 17 mcg per puff. Ipratropium is also available as an MDI in combination with albuterol and as a solution for nebulization at 200 mcg/mL. It provides a peak effect in 1.5 to 2 hours and has a duration of effect of 4 to 6 hours. Ipratropium has a slower onset of action and a more prolonged bronchodilator effect compared with standard β_2-agonists. Because of the slower onset of effect (15 to 20 minutes compared with 5 minutes for albuterol), it may be less suitable for as-needed use; however, it is often prescribed in that manner. The role of inhaled anticholinergics in COPD is well established.[64–66] However, results from the Lung Health Study showed that treatment with ipratropium did not affect the progressive decline in lung function.[40] Studies comparing ipratropium with inhaled β_2-agonists have generally reported similar improvements in pulmonary function. Others report a modest benefit with ipratropium, including a lower incidence of side effects such as tachycardia.[64,65]

Although the recommended dose of ipratropium is 2 puffs four times a day, there is evidence for a dose-response, so the dose can be titrated upward often to 24 puffs a day. Ipratropium has been shown to increase maximum exercise performance in stable COPD patients with doses of 8 to 12 puffs prior to exercise but not with doses of 4 puffs or less.[66,67] During sleep, ipratropium also has been shown to improve arterial oxygen saturation and sleep quality.[68] Ipratropium is well tolerated. The most frequent patient complaints are dry mouth, nausea, and an occasional metallic taste.

Clinicians differ about preference in choosing the initial short-acting bronchodilator therapy for the patient with COPD. Both a short-acting β_2-agonist and ipratropium represent reasonable choices for initial therapy.

❽ Long-Acting Bronchodilators For patients with moderate to severe COPD who experience symptoms on a regular and consistent basis, or in whom short-acting therapies do not provide adequate relief, long-acting bronchodilator therapies are the recommended treatment. Long-acting inhaled bronchodilator therapy can be administered as an inhaled β_2-agonist (LABA) or an anticholinergic. Long-acting, inhaled bronchodilator therapy is more convenient and effective, compared with short-acting agents, for patients with chronic symptoms. There are superior outcomes in lung function as measured by spirometry, symptoms including dyspnea, and, importantly, reductions in exacerbation frequency and improved quality of life.

Long-Acting Inhaled β_2-Agonists (LABAs) LABAs offer the convenience and benefit of a long duration of action for patients with persistent symptoms. Each of the currently available agents, salmeterol, formoterol, and arformoterol is dosed every 12 hours and provides sustained bronchodilation. Arformoterol and formoterol has an onset of action similar to albuterol (less than 5 minutes), whereas salmeterol has a slower onset (15 to 20 minutes); however, neither agent is recommended for acute relief of symptoms. There is no dose titration for any of these agents; the starting dose is the effective and recommended dose for all patients. The clinical benefits of long-acting inhaled β_2-agonists compared with short-acting therapies include similar or superior improvements in lung function and symptoms, as well as reduced exacerbation rates in some studies.[69–71] The use of the long-acting agents should be considered for patients with frequent and persistent symptoms. When patients require short-acting β_2-agonists on a scheduled basis, LABAs are more convenient based on dosing frequency but are also more expensive. Salmeterol and formoterol are available in dry powder inhalation devices, and formoterol and arformoterol as solutions for nebulization. An ultra-long-acting agent, indacaterol, which requires once daily dosing is in phase 3 and 4 clinical trials in 2009.

LABAs are also useful to reduce nocturnal symptoms and improve quality of life. When compared with short-acting bronchodilators or theophylline, both salmeterol and formoterol improve lung function, symptoms, exacerbation frequency, and quality of life.[72] These benefits are apparent even for patients with poorly reversible lung function and are related to improvements in inspiratory capacity.[73] Both salmeterol and formoterol have been compared with ipratropium. In separate studies, each agent improved FEV_1 compared with ipratropium and, in addition, the LABA was more effective for other selected outcomes (e.g., prolonged time to exacerbation for salmeterol while formoterol reduced symptoms and rescue inhaler use).[74,75]

Long-Acting Anticholinergics Tiotropium bromide, a long-acting quaternary anticholinergic agent, has been available in the United States since 2004. This agent blocks the effects of acetylcholine by binding to muscarinic receptors in airway smooth muscle and mucus glands, blocking the cholinergic effects of bronchoconstriction and mucus secretion. Tiotropium is more selective than ipratropium at blocking important muscarinic receptors. Tiotropium dissociates slowly from M_1 and M_3 receptors, allowing prolonged bronchodilation. The dissociation from M_2 receptors is much faster, allowing inhibition of acetylcholine release. Binding studies of tiotropium in the human lung show that it is approximately 10-fold more potent than ipratropium and protects against cholinergic bronchoconstriction for greater than 24 hours.[76]

When inhaled, tiotropium is minimally absorbed into the systemic circulation and results in bronchodilation within 30 minutes, with a peak effect in 3 hours. Bronchodilation persists for at least 24 hours, allowing for a once daily dosing. There is no titration of tiotropium dose; a regimen of 18 mcg inhaled once daily is recommended for all patients. In the United States, it is delivered via the HandiHaler, a single-load, dry-powder, breath-actuated device. Because it acts locally, tiotropium is well tolerated, with the most common complaint being a dry mouth. Other anticholinergic side effects that are reported include constipation, urinary retention, tachycardia, blurred vision, and precipitation of narrow-angle glaucoma symptoms.

The benefits of tiotropium have been evaluated in numerous trials of patients with COPD. Similar to long-acting β-agonists, tiotropium improves lung function and dyspnea, exacerbation frequency, and health-related quality of life.[77] In this study, tiotropium improved FEV_1 by an average of 12% to 22% compared with placebo. The tolerance that is demonstrated with chronic use of β-agonists does not occur with tiotropium therapy, as improvements in lung function are sustained with long-term therapy.[78]

There is a large body of evidence supporting the use of tiotropium as a long acting bronchodilator for COPD patients. Benefits have been demonstrated compared with placebo[79] and to ipratropium.[80] Tiotropium therapy is associated with a decreased risk of exacerbations compared with placebo or ipratropium, and equal or superior efficacy compared with LABAs in various studies.[81]

As a long-acting bronchodilator, tiotropium is an option to consider in addition to long-acting inhaled β_2-agonists for COPD management. Once-daily tiotropium has been compared with twice-daily salmeterol in two placebo-controlled trials of 6 months duration. Tiotropium reduced asthma exacerbations and hospital admissions and improved quality of life, whereas both active treatments improved lung function and reduced dyspnea.[79] In another 6-month randomized, controlled trial of patients with COPD, patients were randomized to receive either tiotropium once daily by DPI, salmeterol twice daily by MDI, or placebo.[82] Patients receiving tiotropium had greater improvements in trough FEV_1 and dyspnea scores than those receiving salmeterol. Patients also were more likely to have improvements in quality-of-life indicators with tiotropium than with salmeterol. However, no differences in frequency of exacerbations were noted among the three groups.

The most notable study involving the use of tiotropium in recent years for patients with COPD was the Understanding Potential Long-term Impacts on Function with Tiotropium(UPLIFT) trial.[83] This was a randomized, double-blind study of 4 years duration. A total of 5,993 subjects received either tiotropium 18 mcg daily inhaled via a HandiHaler device or a matching placebo. All other COPD therapies were allowed except for other anticholinergic therapies (e.g., ipratropium). The mean postbronchodilator FEV_1 among subjects was 1.32 L, and the primary outcome was the rate of decline in FEV_1 on spirometry. The results showed that tiotropium treatment resulted in prebronchodilator FEV_1 improvement of 87 to 103 ml, and postbronchodilator improvement of 47 to 65 mL, both of which were statistically significant. However, the rate of decline in the mean FEV_1 result was not statistically significant between the groups. Tiotropium-treated subjects benefited from treatment as reflected in improved quality-of-life scores, reduced exacerbation rates, fewer hospitalizations, and instances of respiratory failure. Tiotropium was associated with a lower overall risk of mortality, including deaths from respiratory and cardiac causes.

The safety of tiotropium documented in the UPLIFT trial is reassuring. Recently, retrospective analysis have reported an increased risk of cardiovascular events associated with ipratropium[84] and tiotropium use.[85] However, the UPLIFT study, which was a prospective trial over 4 years, did not report an increased cardiovascular risk associated with tiotropium use.[83]

Combination Anticholinergics and β-Agonists

Combination regimens of bronchodilators are used often in the treatment of COPD, especially as the disease progresses and symptoms worsen over time. Combining bronchodilators with different mechanisms of action allows the lowest possible effective doses to be used and reduces potential adverse effects from individual agents.[1] Combinations of both short- and long-acting β_2-agonists with ipratropium have been shown to provide added symptomatic relief and improvements in pulmonary function.[86-88] A combination of albuterol and ipratropium (Combivent) is available as an MDI in the United States for chronic maintenance therapy of COPD. This product offers the obvious convenience of two classes of bronchodilators in a single inhaler.

Although clinical practice guidelines recommend that combinations of long-acting bronchodilators are appropriate for patients who do not receive adequate benefit from a single agent, data to support the use of these combinations have been lacking. These approaches have been the focus of more recent research. Future combination inhalation products may contain long-acting β_2-agonists with tiotropium to reduce the need for frequent dosing. In a preliminary single-dose study, the combination of tiotropium and formoterol resulted in a faster and greater improvement in FEV_1 compared with either treatment alone.[89] In another trial, 95 subjects received either tiotropium 18 mcg or tiotropium plus formoterol 12 mcg either once or twice daily. All patients received each therapy for 2 weeks each in an open label, crossover design.

Both combination regimens improved lung function and reduced rescue therapy use compared with tiotropium alone.[90]

Methylxanthines

Methylxanthines, including theophylline and aminophylline, have been available for the treatment of COPD for at least five decades and at one time were considered first-line therapy. However, with the availability of long-acting inhaled β_2-agonists and inhaled anticholinergics, the role of methylxanthine therapy is significantly limited. Inhaled bronchodilator therapy is preferred for COPD. Because of the risk for drug interactions and the significant intrapatient and interpatient variability in dosage requirements, theophylline therapy generally is considered for patients who are intolerant or unable to use an inhaled bronchodilator. Theophylline is still an alternative to commonly used inhaled therapies partially due to the potential for multiple mechanisms (bronchodilation and antiinflammatory) and the possible benefit that systemic administration may exert on peripheral airways.[91]

The methylxanthines may produce bronchodilation through numerous mechanisms, including (1) inhibition of phosphodiesterase, thereby increasing cAMP levels, (2) inhibition of calcium ion influx into smooth muscle, (3) prostaglandin antagonism, (4) stimulation of endogenous catecholamines, (5) adenosine receptor antagonism, and (6) inhibition of release of mediators from mast cells and leukocytes.[92]

Chronic theophylline use for patients with COPD has been shown to exert improvements in lung function, including vital capacity (VC), FEV_1, minute ventilation, and gas exchange.[91] Subjectively, theophylline has been shown to reduce dyspnea, increase exercise tolerance, and improve respiratory drive in COPD patients.[91,92] Other nonpulmonary effects of theophylline that may contribute to improved overall functional capacity for patients with COPD include improved cardiac function and decreased pulmonary artery pressure.

Although theophylline is available in a variety of oral dosage forms, sustained-release preparations are most appropriate for the long-term management of COPD. These products have the advantages of improving patient compliance and achieving more consistent serum concentrations over rapid-release theophylline and aminophylline preparations. However, caution must be used in switching from one sustained-release preparation to another because there are considerable variations in sustained-release characteristics.[92] Aside from intravenous aminophylline, there is no need to use any of the various salts forms of theophylline.

Regular use of methylxanthines has not been shown to have either a beneficial or a detrimental effect on the progression of COPD. However, methylxanthines may be added to the treatment plan of patients who have not achieved an optimal clinical response to ipratropium and an inhaled β_2-agonist. Studies suggest that adding theophylline to a combination of albuterol and ipratropium provides added benefit for stable COPD patients, supporting the hypothesis that there is a synergistic bronchodilator effect.[93-95] The efficacy of combination therapy with salmeterol and theophylline for patients with COPD was reported to improve pulmonary function and reduce dyspnea better than either treatment alone.[96] Combination treatment also was associated with a reduced number of exacerbations only when compared with the theophylline group, suggesting that the salmeterol component was responsible for this beneficial effect.

As is the case with other bronchodilator therapy, parameters other than objective measurements, such as FEV_1, should be monitored to assess efficacy of theophylline in COPD. Subjective parameters, such as perceived improvements in symptoms of dyspnea and exercise tolerance, become increasingly important in assessing the acceptability of methylxanthines for COPD patients. Although objective improvement may be minimal, patients may experience an improvement in clinical symptoms, and thus benefit to the individual may be meaningful.

The role of theophylline in COPD is as maintenance therapy in the nonacutely ill patient. Therapy can be initiated at 200 mg twice daily and titrated upward every 3 to 5 days to the target dose. Most patients required daily doses of 400 to 900 mg. Dosage adjustments generally should be made based on serum concentration results. Traditionally, the therapeutic range of theophylline was identified as 10 to 20 mcg/mL; however, because of the frequency of dose-related side effects and the relatively minor benefit of higher concentrations, a more conservative therapeutic range of 8 to 15 mcg/mL often is targeted. This is especially preferable for the elderly. When concentrations are measured, trough measurements are most appropriate.

Once a dose is established, serum concentrations should be monitored once or twice a year unless the patient's disease worsens, medications that interfere with theophylline metabolism are added to therapy, or toxicity is suspected. The most common side effects of theophylline therapy are related to the gastrointestinal system, the cardiovascular system, and the central nervous system. Side effects are dose-related; however, there is overlap in side effects between the therapeutic and toxic ranges. Minor side effects include dyspepsia, nausea, vomiting, diarrhea, headache, dizziness, and tachycardia. More serious toxicities, especially at toxic concentrations, include arrhythmias and seizures.

Factors that decrease theophylline clearance and lead to reduced maintenance-dose requirements include advanced age, bacterial or viral pneumonia, left or right ventricular failure, liver dysfunction, hypoxemia from acute decompensation, and use of drugs such as cimetidine, macrolides, and fluoroquinolone antibiotics. Factors that may enhance theophylline clearance and result in the need for higher maintenance doses include tobacco and marijuana smoking, hyperthyroidism, and the use of such drugs as phenytoin, phenobarbital, and rifampin.

In summary, there are decades of experience with theophylline and other methylxanthine products in the management of patients with COPD. However, inhalation therapy is currently preferred based on superior efficacy and safety, as well as ease of use by the clinician. Theophylline is a challenging medication to dose, monitor, and manage due to the significant intrapatient and interpatient variability in pharmacokinetics and the potential for drug interactions and toxicities.

Corticosteroids

❾ Corticosteroid therapy has been studied and debated in COPD therapy for half a century; however, owing to the poor risk-to-benefit ratio, chronic systemic corticosteroid therapy should be avoided if possible.[1] Because of the potential role of inflammation in the pathogenesis of the disease, clinicians hoped that corticosteroids would be promising agents in COPD management. However, their use continues to be debated, especially in the management of stable COPD.

The antiinflammatory mechanisms whereby corticosteroids exert their beneficial effect in COPD include (1) reduction in capillary permeability to decrease mucus, (2) inhibition of release of proteolytic enzymes from leukocytes, and (3) inhibition of prostaglandins. Unfortunately, the clinical benefits of systemic corticosteroid therapy in the chronic management of COPD are often not evident, and the risk of toxicity is extensive and far-reaching. Currently, the appropriate situations to consider corticosteroids in COPD include (1) short-term systemic use for acute exacerbations and (2) inhalation therapy for chronic stable COPD.

The role of oral steroid use in chronic stable COPD patients was evaluated in a metaanalysis over a decade ago.[97] Investigators concluded that only a small fraction (10%) of COPD patients treated

with steroids showed clinically significant improvement in baseline FEV$_1$ (increase of 20%) compared with those treated with placebo. While a small number of COPD patients are considered responders to oral steroids, many of these patients actually may have an asthmatic, or reversible, component to their disease. The best predictors for response to oral steroids are the presence of eosinophils on sputum examination ($\geq$3%) and a significant response to sympathomimetics on pulmonary function tests.[98] Both the presence of eosinophils in sputum and the responsiveness to sympathomimetics suggest an asthmatic component to the disease process and thus may explain the clinical benefit seen with steroids.

Long-term adverse effects associated with systemic corticosteroid therapy include osteoporosis, muscular atrophy, thinning of the skin, development of cataracts, and adrenal suppression and insufficiency. The risks associated with long-term steroid therapy are much greater than the clinical benefits. If a decision to treat with long-term systemic corticosteroids is made, the lowest possible effective dose should be given once per day in the morning to minimize the risk of adrenal suppression. If therapy with oral agents is required, an alternate-day schedule should be used.

Previously, a common clinical practice was to administer a short course (2 weeks) of oral corticosteroids as a trial to predict which patients would benefit from chronic oral or inhaled corticosteroids. There is now sufficient evidence suggesting that this practice is not effective in predicting a long-term response to inhaled corticosteroids and should not be recommended.[99]

The use of chronic inhaled corticosteroid therapy has been of interest for the past decade. Their use has been common despite the lack of firm evidence about significant clinical benefit until recently. Inhaled corticosteroids have an improved risk-to-benefit ratio compared with systemic corticosteroid therapy. Using the model for asthma, it was hoped that the inhalation of potent corticosteroid would result in high local efficacy and limited systemic exposure and toxicity. In the latter part of the 1990s, several large international trials were initiated to evaluate the effect on inhaled corticosteroids in COPD. Unfortunately, the results of these major clinical trials failed to demonstrate any benefit from chronic treatment with inhaled corticosteroids in modifying long-term decline in lung function that is characteristic of COPD. Therefore, the role of inhaled corticosteroids in COPD continues to be debated in the literature, unlike in asthma, where their use is clearly advocated. Much of the debate centers on the appropriate outcome measures in this population of patients.

During the last decade, several studies of inhaled corticosteroids in COPD were designed to detect a benefit on slowing the progressive loss of lung function, but the results were disappointing.[101–106] None of the large national or international trials were able to demonstrate a benefit of high-dose inhaled corticosteroid therapy on this primary outcome. However, inhaled corticosteroids have been associated with other important benefits in some patients, including a decrease in exacerbation frequency and improvements in overall health status.[102,106,107] Clinicians continue to debate the most appropriate and relevant outcome measure to evaluate in COPD studies. Based on the results of clinical trials, consensus guidelines suggest that inhaled corticosteroid therapy should be considered for symptomatic patients with stage III or IV disease (FEV$_1$<50%) who experience repeated exacerbations.[1,2] These are the patients who demonstrated benefit in clinical trials and in whom a trial of inhaled corticosteroid therapy is warranted. There are also data from epidemiologic studies that suggest that chronic treatment with inhaled corticosteroids is associated with a lower risk of rehospitalization for a broader group of patients with COPD. Thus the debate about the appropriate role for this antiinflammatory therapy continues.

A metaanalysis evaluating randomized clinical trials involving inhaled corticosteroids for patients with COPD indicated that treatment was associated with a relative risk reduction in exacerbation frequency of 33%. The report indicated that 12 patients would require treatment for 20.8 months to prevent one exacerbation episode. The benefit was evident for patients with moderate to severe COPD.[108] This metaanalysis did not detect a mortality benefit.

Other investigators have reported a reduction in mortality for patients with COPD who were treated with inhaled corticosteroids. In an epidemiologic study of a Canadian database, patient mortality 3 months to 1 year following a hospitalization for a COPD exacerbation was evaluated for patients who received inhaled corticosteroids in the first 3 months compared with those who did not. For patients over 65 years of age, inhaled corticosteroid therapy reduced mortality by 25%. Much of the mortality reduction was reflected in deaths due to cardiovascular causes. Conversely, patients who received only bronchodilator therapy trended toward higher mortality rates, although not significant.[109] A pooled analysis of seven large trials also concluded that inhaled corticosteroids reduced all-cause mortality in COPD patients.[110]

Currently, the recommended role of inhaled corticosteroid therapy is for COPD patients with moderate to severe airflow obstruction (FEV_1 <50% predicted) and who experience frequent exacerbations despite bronchodilator therapy. Repeated exacerbations are described as 3 in 3 years. The initial hope that treatment with inhaled corticosteroids would prevent or slow the progressive decline in FEV_1 remains unproven; however, it is often argued that additional important outcomes for patients with COPD include relief of symptoms, fewer and less severe exacerbations, and improved quality of life.[111] Inhaled corticosteroids (ICs) do not prolong survival in COPD patients and there is good evidence to suggest that treatment with ICs increases the risk of pneumonia for patients with COPD.[112-114]

Although a dose-response relationship for ICs has not been demonstrated in COPD, the major clinical trials employed moderate to high doses for treatment. Side effects of ICs are relatively mild compared with the toxicity from systemic therapy. Hoarseness, sore throat, oral candidiasis, and skin bruising have been reported in the clinical trials. Severe side effects, such as adrenal suppression, osteoporosis, and cataract formation, have been reported less frequently than with systemic corticosteroids, but clinicians should monitor patients who are receiving high-dose chronic therapy.[115,116]

There is evidence supporting a dose relationship between inhaled corticosteroid use and the risk of fractures. In a cohort of over 1,600 subjects with a diagnosis of asthma or COPD (mean age 80 years), the risk of a fracture was 2.53 times higher (CI, 1.65-3.89) in those receiving a mean daily dose of inhaled corticosteroid of 601 mcg or greater.[117] However, the data are conflicting about this issue. A metaanalysis found no evidence supporting an increased risk of fractures or decreased bone mineral density with chronic inhaled corticosteroid use.[118] It appears prudent to suggest that, to minimize the risk of fracture, patients should be treated with the lowest effective dose of ICs.[119] It may also be helpful to recommend adequate intake of calcium and vitamin D and possibly periodic bone mineral density testing.

Combination Therapy: Bronchodilators and Inhaled Corticosteroids

Following the disappointing results of chronic inhaled corticosteroid studies and the progressive decline in lung function, investigators became interested in the combination of potent antiinflammatory therapies and long-acting bronchodilators. Subsequently, several studies have shown an additive benefit with long-acting bronchodilators.[120-123] In various studies, combination therapy with salmeterol plus fluticasone or formoterol plus budesonide was associated with greater improvements in clinical outcomes such as FEV_1,

health status, and frequency of exacerbations compared with ICs or long-acting bronchodilators alone. The availability of combination inhalers (e.g., salmeterol plus fluticasone and budesonide plus formoterol) makes administration of both ICs and long-acting bronchodilators more convenient for patients and decreases the total number of inhalations needed daily. An inhaled corticosteroid combined with a long acting β-agonist is superior to the individual components in reducing exacerbations, improving lung function and overall health status.[112] Therefore, there is growing evidence that inhaled corticosteroid and long-acting β-agonist combinations improve lung function, as well as reduce symptoms of dyspnea and exacerbation frequency.[122-124]

The combination of a long-acting β-agonist and inhaled corticosteroid has been compared with the long-acting β-agonist therapy alone. In a study involving nearly 1,000 patients with severe but stable COPD, subjects received either salmeterol 50 mcg/fluticasone 500 mcg twice daily or salmeterol 50 mcg twice daily for 44 weeks. Exacerbation frequency was significantly lower in the combination group (334 vs 464 episodes), which corresponded to a 35% reduction in the annualized rate. The time to the first exacerbation was also delayed with the combination therapy.[125] One finding of concern reported in this trial was the increased number of pneumonia cases for patients receiving combination therapy compared with salmeterol alone. There were 23 cases reported compared with 7 in the salmeterol group.[125] An increase in the risk for pneumonia was also reported in the Towards a Revolution in COPD Health (TORCH) study described below.[112]

The largest prospective study to date is referred to as the Towards a Revolution in COPD Health (TORCH) study.[112] This trial consisted of 6,112 patients who received one of four treatments for three years. Treatment groups were placebo, salmeterol 50 mcg twice daily, fluticasone 500 mcg twice daily, or the combination of salmeterol and fluticasone in a single inhaler. The primary outcome was death from any cause and secondary outcomes were exacerbation rates, lung function, and health status. None of the active treatments differed significantly from placebo, although the combination of salmeterol and fluticasone trended toward fewer deaths (P = .052). The combination also reduced exacerbation rates, and improved lung function and health status compared with the other treatments. Exacerbation rates were also significantly reduced with combination therapy compared with either single agent alone. Both treatment groups that included fluticasone had higher rates of pneumonia. Although this study did not reflect a mortality benefit, the authors indicated the risk of death was reduced by 17.5% with the combination and that the number needed to treat for 1 year to provide a benefit was 4.

For patients with an FEV_1 of less than 60% predicted, the individual agents and the combination decreased the rate of spirometry decline.[58]

In a head-to-head trial, a large study comparing a combination of salmeterol and fluticasone to tiotropium alone showed no difference in the exacerbation rates between the groups, although the combination therapy was associated with a higher study completion rate.[126]

Combinations of Long-Acting Bronchodilators Compared with Long-Acting Bronchodilators Plus Inhaled Corticosteroids

The combination of salmeterol and tiotropium has also been evaluated in a short-term crossover study involving only 22 subjects who received either salmeterol (50 mcg twice daily) plus fluticasone (500 mcg twice daily), fluticasone plus tiotropium (18 mcg once daily), or fluticasone, salmeterol, and tiotropium for 1 week. The triple combination provided a significant benefit of improved lung function compared with either of the dual treatments in subjects with moderate to severe COPD.[127] The benefit of triple therapy was evaluated in a 1 year randomized, double-blind, placebo control study involving 449 subjects with moderate to severe COPD. Treatment consisted of either tiotropium, tiotropium plus salmeterol, or tiotropium, salmeterol, and fluticasone.[128] There was no difference between treatments for the primary outcome of percentage of patients experiencing an exacerbation requiring systemic corticosteroids or antibiotics. The triple-drug regimen improved lung function, quality of life, and reduced hospitalization compared with tiotropium alone, while two-drug therapy did not offer any benefit in lung function improvement or hospitalization rates compared with the single agent. Another small study evaluated the addition of tiotropium for 1 month to a regimen of an inhaled corticosteroid and a long-acting β-agonist.[129] The addition of tiotropium improved lung function and quality-of-life scores, apparently by improving dynamics of lung capacity (inspiratory capacity). These effects were reversed when tiotropium therapy was discontinued. These data involving combinations of long acting bronchodilators are limited and preliminary. More research is required and should include other outcome parameters including relief of symptoms, exacerbation rates, and quality of life. Larger sample sizes and longer durations will provide insight into the value of combinations.

A retrospective cohort study of 42,090 patients in the Veterans Affairs healthcare system evaluated outcomes for patients with COPD who received tiotropium as part of a COPD regimen compared with a cohort of COPD patients who did not receive the medication. Patients who received tiotropium with ICs plus a long-acting β-agonist exhibited a 40% reduction in mortality compared with patients treated with ICs plus a long-acting β-agonist alone (95% CI of 0.45-0.79). Triple therapy patients also significantly reduced exacerbations and hospitalization rates. However, this same study demonstrated that tiotropium combined with two other medications (various) increased mortality and morbidity risks.[85]

α_1-Antitrypsin Replacement Therapy

For patients with inherited AAT deficiency-associated emphysema, treatment focuses on reduction of risk factors such as smoking, symptomatic treatment with bronchodilators, and augmentation therapy with replacement AAT. Based on knowledge about the relationship between serum concentrations of AAT and the risk of developing emphysema, the rationale for augmentation therapy is to maintain serum concentrations above the protective threshold throughout the dosing interval.[130] Indirect evidence of AAT activity in the interstitium of the lung has been demonstrated by measuring concentrations of the enzyme in epithelial lining fluid obtained during bronchoalveolar lavage. Augmentation therapy consists of weekly infusions of pooled human AAT to maintain AAT plasma levels over 10 micromolar. Much of the data supporting the use of AAT replacement is based on evidence of biochemical efficacy (e.g., administering the product and demonstrating protective serum concentrations of AAT).

Clinical evidence for slowing lung function decline or improving outcomes with augmentation therapy is sparse. Stated challenges to performing randomized clinical trials include the large sample size and long duration of follow-up required, and the expense of conducting such a trial. One observational study followed patients in the National Registry of Severe AAT Deficiency over a period of several years and documented clinical outcomes. In this study, patients who received weekly augmentation therapy with purified AAT had slower declines in FEV_1 and decreased mortality compared with patients who never received augmentation therapy.[131] However, this was an observational study of patients, not a randomized, placebo-controlled trial, and so direct cause-and-effect relationships cannot be concluded. One randomized,

placebo-controlled study of patients with severe AAT deficiency (ZZ phenotype) did show a significant reduction in lung tissue loss and destruction as measured by computed tomographic (CT) scan for patients receiving augmentation therapy.[132] Other measures of lung function and mortality were not recorded.

The recommended dosing regimen for replacement AAT is 60 mg/kg administered intravenously once a week at a rate of 0.08 mL/kg per minute, adjusted to patient tolerance. It has been estimated that this form of augmentation therapy will cost over $54,000 annually.[133] In the absence of alternative treatments, it is difficult to assess the cost-effectiveness using conventional criteria. There have been repeated problems with supply of this biologic replacement therapy (derived from pooled blood donors) related to production difficulty and contamination issues. Currently, there are three products available (Prolastin (Bayer), Aralast (Baxter), and Zemaira (ZLB Behring), which should minimize this problem in the future. Drug development research continues in the area of recombinant products and inhalational therapy.

The safety of AAT replacement therapy has been recently evaluated in two large observational studies. In the most recent study, 174 patients (n = 747) reported 720 adverse events, classified as severe in 8.8% of cases and moderate in 72.4% of cases.[134] Common complaints included headache, dizziness, nausea, dyspnea, and fever. The overall rate of adverse events was low (i.e., two events over 5 years).

TREATMENT

COPD Exacerbation

■ DESIRED OUTCOMES

🔟 The goals of therapy for patients experiencing exacerbations of COPD are (1) prevention of hospitalization or reduction in hospital stay, (2) prevention of acute respiratory failure and death, and (3) resolution of exacerbation symptoms and a return to baseline clinical status and quality of life.[135] Acute exacerbations can range from mild to severe. Factors that influence the severity, and subsequently the level of care required, include the severity of airflow limitation, presence of comorbidities and the history of previous exacerbations. Table 34–12 includes factors that warrant treatment in the hospital.

Various therapeutic options for exacerbation management are summarized in Table 34–13. Pharmacotherapy consists of intensification of bronchodilator therapy and a short course of systemic corticosteroids. Antimicrobial therapy is indicated in the presence of selected symptoms. Since the frequency and severity of exacerbations are closely related to each patient's overall health status, all patients should receive optimal chronic treatment, including smoking cessation, appropriate pharmacologic therapy, and preventative therapy such as vaccinations.

TABLE 34-12	Factors Favoring Hospitalization for Treatment of COPD Exacerbation

Presence of high risk comorbidity (e.g., pneumonia, arrhythmia, CHF, diabetes, renal or hepatic failure)
Suboptimal response to outpatient management
Marked worsening of dyspnea
Inability to eat or sleep due to symptoms
Worsening hypoxemia or hypercapnia
Mental status changes
Lack of home support for care
Uncertain diagnosis

Modified from ATS.

TABLE 34-13	Therapeutic Options for Acute Exacerbations of COPD
Therapy	**Comments**
Antibiotics	Recommended if two or more of the following are present: Increased dyspnea Increased sputum production Increased sputum purulence
Corticosteroids	Oral or intravenous therapy may be used. If intravenous is used, it should be changed to oral after improvement in pulmonary status. If continued longer than 14 days, then the dose should be tapered to avoid HPA Axis suppression.
Bronchodilators	MDIs and DPIs equal in efficacy to nebulization. β-Agonists also may increase mucociliary clearance. Long-acting β-agonists should not be used for quick relief of symptoms or on an as-needed basis.
Controlled oxygen therapy	Titrate oxygen to desired oxygen saturation (>90%). Monitor arterial blood gas for development of hypercapnia.
Noninvasive mechanical ventilation	Consider for patients with acute respiratory failure. Not appropriate for patients with altered mental status, severe acidosis, respiratory arrest, or cardiovascular instability.

■ NONPHARMACOLOGIC THERAPY

Controlled Oxygen Therapy

Oxygen therapy should be considered for any patient with hypoxemia during an exacerbation. Caution must be used, however, because many patients with COPD rely on mild hypoxemia to trigger their drive to breathe. In normal, healthy individuals, the drive to breathe is triggered by carbon dioxide accumulation. For patients with COPD who retain carbon dioxide as a result of their disease progression, hypoxemia rather than hypercapnia becomes the main trigger for their respiratory drive. Overly aggressive administration of oxygen to patients with chronic hypercapnia may result in respiratory depression and respiratory failure. Oxygen therapy should be used to achieve a Pao_2 of greater than 60 mm Hg or oxygen saturation of greater than 90%. However, an ABG should be obtained after oxygen initiation to monitor carbon dioxide retention owing to hypoventilation.

Noninvasive Mechanical Ventilation

Noninvasive positive-pressure ventilation (NPPV) provides ventilatory support with oxygen and pressurized airflow using a face or nasal mask with a tight seal but without endotracheal intubation. There have been numerous trials reporting the benefits of NPPV for patients with acute respiratory failure due to COPD exacerbations. In one metaanalysis of eight studies, NPPV was associated with lower mortality, lower intubation rates, shorter hospital stays, and greater improvements in serum pH in 1 hour compared with treatment with usual care alone.[136] The benefits seen with NPPV generally can be attributed to a reduction in the complications that often arise with invasive mechanical ventilation. Not all patients with COPD exacerbations are appropriate candidates for NPPV. Patients with altered mental status may not be able to protect their airway and thus may be at increased risk for aspiration. Patients with severe acidosis (pH <7.25), respiratory arrest, or cardiovascular instability should be not considered for NPPV. Patients failing a trial of NPPV or those considered poor candidates might be considered for intubation and mechanical ventilation.

■ PHARMACOLOGIC THERAPY

Bronchodilators

During exacerbations, intensification of bronchodilator regimens is used commonly. The doses and frequency of bronchodilators are increased to provide symptomatic relief. Short-acting β_2-agonists are preferred owing to rapid onset of action. Anticholinergic agents may be added if symptoms persist despite increased doses of β_2-agonists. In fact, combinations of these agents are employed often, although data are lacking about the benefit versus higher doses of one agent. Bronchodilators may be administered via MDIs or nebulization with equal efficacy. Nebulization may be considered for patients with severe dyspnea who are unable to hold their breath after actuation of an MDI. Clinical evidence supporting the use of theophylline during exacerbations is lacking, and thus theophylline generally should be avoided. However, addition of one of these agents may be considered for patients not responding to other therapies. The risk of adverse effects such as cardiac arrhythmias should be considered and serum levels monitored closely.

Corticosteroids

Until recently, the literature supporting the use of corticosteroids in acute exacerbations of COPD was sparse. However, since 1996, five studies have been performed that document the value of systemic corticosteroids in exacerbations of COPD.[137-141] The Systemic Corticosteroids in Chronic Obstructive Pulmonary Disease Exacerbations (SCCOPE) trial evaluated three groups of patients hospitalized for exacerbations of COPD.[137] The first group received an 8-week course of corticosteroids given as methylprednisolone 125 mg intravenously every 6 hours for 72 hours, followed by once-daily oral prednisone (60 mg on days 4 through 7, 40 mg on days 8 through 11, 20 mg on days 12 through 43, 10 mg on days 44 through 50, and 5 mg on days 51 through 57). The second group received a 2-week course given as methylprednisolone 125 mg intravenously every 6 hours for 72 hours, followed by oral prednisone (60 mg on days 5 through 7, 40 mg on days 8 through 11, and 20 mg on days 12 through 15) and placebo on days 16 through 57. The third group received placebo for all 57 days of study. Rates of treatment failure and hospital stay were significantly higher in the placebo group than in either treatment group at 30 and 90 days. Groups randomized to corticosteroid treatment also had a significantly shorter length of hospital stay compared with the placebo group. The 8-week regimen was not found to be superior to the 2-week regimen. Significant treatment benefits were no longer evident at 6 months.

Davies and colleagues[138] evaluated the oral use of corticosteroids in hospitalized patients with acute exacerbations of COPD. Patients received either 30 mg/day oral prednisolone or placebo for 14 days. Patients who were treated with corticosteroids had a significantly more rapid improvement in FEV_1 and a shorter hospital stay than did patients who received placebo. There was no significant difference between groups at 6-week follow-up.

In total, results from these trials suggest that patients with acute exacerbations of COPD should receive a short course of intravenous or oral corticosteroids. However, because of the large variability in dosage ranges, the optimal dose and duration of corticosteroid treatment are not known. It appears that short courses (9 to 14 days) are as effective as longer courses and have a lower risk of associated adverse effects owing to less time of exposure. Several trials used high initial doses of steroids before tapering to a lower maintenance dose. Adverse effects such as hyperglycemia, insomnia, and hallucinations may occur at higher doses. Depending on the clinical status of the patient, treatment may be initiated at a lower dose or tapered more quickly if these effects occur. It appears that a regimen of prednisone 40 mg orally daily (or equivalent) for 10 to 14 days can be effective for most patients.[142] If steroid treatment is continued for greater than 2 weeks, a tapering oral schedule should be employed to avoid hypothalamic-pituitary-adrenal (HPA) axis suppression.

Recent data suggest that ICs may be beneficial for treating COPD exacerbations, although this is not the standard of care. In one study, inhaled budesonide, alone or combined with formoterol, was as effective as oral corticosteroids in treating COPD exacerbations.[143]

Antimicrobial Therapy

⑪ It is thought that most acute exacerbations of COPD are caused by viral or bacterial infections. However, as many as 30% of exacerbations are caused by unknown factors.[1] A metaanalysis of nine studies evaluating the effectiveness of antibiotics in treating exacerbations of COPD determined that patients receiving antibiotics had a greater improvement in peak expiratory flow rate than those who did not.[144]

This metaanalysis concluded that antibiotics are of most benefit and should be initiated if at least two of the following three symptoms are present: increased dyspnea, increased sputum volume, and increased sputum purulence. The utility of sputum Gram stain and culture is questionable because some patients have chronic bacterial colonization of the bronchial tree between exacerbations.

The emergence of drug-resistant organisms has mandated that antibiotic regimens be chosen judiciously. Selection of empirical antimicrobial therapy should be based on the most likely organism(s) thought to be responsible for the infection based on the individual patient profile. The most common organisms for any acute exacerbation of COPD are *Hemophilus influenzae, Moraxella catarrhalis, Streptococcus pneumoniae,* and *Hemophilus parainfluenzae.* More virulent bacteria may be present for patients with more complicated acute exacerbations of COPD, including drug-resistant pneumococci, β-lactamase-producing *H. influenzae* and *M. catarrhalis,* and enteric gram-negative organisms, including *Pseudomonas aeruginosa.* Table 34–14 summarizes recommended antimicrobial therapy for exacerbations of COPD and the most common organisms based on patient presentation.[145]

Therapy with antibiotics generally should be continued for at least 7 to 10 days. Studies evaluating shorter treatment courses (usually 5 days) with the fluoroquinolones, second- and third-generation cephalosporins, and macrolide antimicrobials have demonstrated comparable efficacy with the longer treatment regimens.[146] If the patient deteriorates or does not improve as anticipated, hospitalization may be necessary, and more aggressive attempts should be made to identify potential pathogens responsible for the exacerbation.

COPD patients are at increased risk for pulmonary embolism during severe exacerbations requiring hospitalizations. An increased awareness of this risk and appropriate preventative measures are warranted.[147]

■ COMPLICATIONS

Cor Pulmonale

Cor pulmonale is right-sided heart failure secondary to pulmonary hypertension. Long-term oxygen therapy and diuretics have been the mainstays of therapy for cor pulmonale. Increasing the Pao$_2$ above 60 mm Hg with supplemental oxygen therapy decreases pulmonary hypertension and thus decreases the force against which the right ventricle has to work. While diuretics may help decrease fluid overload, caution should be used because patients with significant right-sided heart failure are highly dependent on preload for cardiac output. Therefore, the decision to use diuretics must be based on a risk-to-benefit ratio. Digitalis glycosides have no role in the treatment of cor pulmonale.

Other pharmacologic agents that have been investigated to treat cor pulmonale include hydralazine, calcium channel blockers, angiotensin-converting enzyme inhibitors, and angiotensin II antagonists. However, there is insufficient evidence to offer guidelines for the role of these agents in COPD patients with cor pulmonale.

Polycythemia

Polycythemia secondary to chronic hypoxemia in COPD patients can be improved by either oxygen therapy or periodic phlebotomy if oxygen therapy alone is not sufficient. COT was shown by the Nocturnal Oxygen Therapy Trial Group to reduce hematocrit values in treated patients.[31] Acute phlebotomy is indicated if the hematocrit is above 55% to 60% and the patient is experiencing central nervous system effects suggestive of sludging from high blood viscosity. Long-term oxygen then can be used to maintain a lower hematocrit.

TABLE 34-14 Recommended Antimicrobial Therapy in Acute Exacerbations of COPD

Patient Characteristics	Likely Pathogens	Recommended Therapy
Uncomplicated exacerbations 　<4 exacerbations per year 　No comorbid illness 　FEV$_1$ >50% of predicted	*S. pneumoniae* *H. influenzae* *M. catarrhalis* *H. parainfluenzae* Resistance uncommon	Macrolide (azithromycin, clarithromycin) Second- or third-generation cephalosporin Doxycycline Therapies not recommended[a]: TMP/SMX, amoxicillin, first-generation cephalosporins, and erythromycin
Complicated exacerbations: 　Age ≥ 65 and >4 exacerbations per year 　FEV$_1$ <50% but >35% of predicted	As above plus drug-resistant pneumococci, β-lactamase–producing *H. influenzae* and *M. catarrhalis*	Amoxicillin/clavulanate Fluoroquinolone with enhanced pneumococcal activity (levofloxacin, gemifloxacin, moxifloxacin)
Complicated exacerbations with risk of *P. aeruginosa* 　Chronic bronchial sepsis[b] 　Need for chronic corticosteroid therapy 　Resident of nursing home with <4 exacerbations per year 　FEV$_1$ <35% of predicted	Some enteric gram-negatives As above plus *P. aeruginosa*	Fluoroquinolone with enhanced pneumococcal and *P. aeruginosa* activity (levofloxacin) IV therapy if required: β-lactamase resistant penicillin with antipseudomonal activity 3rd- or 4th-generation cephalosporin with antipseudomonal activity

[a]TMP/SMX should not be used due to increasing pneumococcal resistance; amoxicillin and first-generation cephalosporins are not recommended due to β-lactamase susceptibility; and erythromycin is not recommended due to insufficient activity against *H. influenzae.*
[b]In sepsis, double antipseudomonal coverage should be considered (e.g., addition of aminoglycoside).
Modified and updated from reference 1.

■ OTHER PHARMACOLOGIC CONSIDERATIONS

A number of other treatments have been explored over the years. Among these therapies, either there is insufficient evidence to warrant recommending their use or they have been proven to not be beneficial in the management of COPD. A brief summary is provided because the clinician likely will encounter patients who are receiving or inquire about these treatments.

Suppressive Antimicrobial Agents

Because COPD patients often are colonized with bacteria and experience recurrent exacerbations of their condition, a common practice employed in the past has been the use of low-dose antimicrobial therapy as preventative or prophylaxis against these acute exacerbations. However, clinical studies over the past 40 years have failed to demonstrate any benefit from this practice.[1] The role of antimicrobial therapy is limited to acute exacerbations of COPD meeting specific criteria.

Expectorants and Mucolytics

Adequate water intake generally is acceptable to maintain hydration and assist in the removal of airway sections. Beyond this, the regular use of mucolytics or expectorants for COPD patients has no proven benefit.[148] This includes the use of saturated solutions of potassium iodide, ammonium chloride, acetylcysteine, and guaifenesin. In 2007, the FDA announced its intention to take action against several companies marketing unapproved timed-released formulations of guaifenesin. Two formulations are approved by the FDA (Humibid and Mucinex); however, data are lacking on their benefit.

Narcotics

Systemic (oral and parenteral) opioids, especially morphine, can relieve dyspnea for patients with end-stage COPD. Nebulized therapy is sometimes used in clinical practice although data about clinical benefit are lacking.[149] Opioids should be used carefully, if at all, to avoid adverse effects on ventilatory drive.

Respiratory Stimulants

There is no role for respiratory stimulants in the long-term management of COPD.[1] Agents that have shown some utility in the acute setting include almitrine and doxapram. However, almitrine is available only in Europe, and its usefulness is limited by neurotoxicity. Doxapram is available for intravenous use only and may be no better than intermittent NPPV.

Secondary pulmonary hypertension is a feature of severe COPD. This has prompted interest about the potential role of agents used to treat primary pulmonary hypertension. However, the use of an endothelin receptor antagonist (bosentan) failed to improve exercise tolerance and worsened hypoxemia in one trial.[150]

■ SURGICAL INTERVENTION

Various surgical options have been employed in the management of COPD. These include bullectomy, lung volume reduction surgery (LVRS), and lung transplantation. Bullectomy has been performed for many years and may be useful when large bullae (>1 cm) are noted on computerized axial tomography (CT or CAT) scan. The presence of bullae may contribute to complaints of dyspnea, and their removal can improve lung function and reduce symptoms, although there is no evidence of a mortality benefit. Because of the prevalence of COPD, it is the most frequent indication for lung transplantation. Intervention is considered when predicted survival

is less than 2 years, FEV_1 is <25% predicted, and hypoxemia, hypercapnia, and pulmonary hypertension exists despite medical management.[2] Experience to date shows 2-year survival of 655 to 90%, and 5-year survival of 415 to 53%.

Recent trials have evaluated the effect of bilateral lung volume reduction surgery (LVRS) for management of severe COPD. Short-term trials comparing the effects of pulmonary rehabilitation plus LVRS with pulmonary rehabilitation alone reported that the combination of treatments resulted in greater improvements in lung function, gas exchange, and quality of life at 3 months. Only recently have data evaluating the long-term effect of LVRS compared with pulmonary rehabilitation been published. The National Emphysema Treatment Trial (NETT), a prospective, randomized trial evaluating the long-term effects of LVRS plus pulmonary rehabilitation compared with pulmonary rehabilitation alone, followed 1,218 patients for 3 years.[151] The primary end points for the study were mortality and maximal exercise capacity 2 years after randomization. Secondary end points included pulmonary function, distance walked in 6 minutes, and quality-of-life measurements. At an interim analysis, patients with an FEV_1 of less than 20% of predicted or a carbon monoxide diffusing capacity of less than 20% of predicted were noted to be at high risk of death after surgery and subsequently were excluded from the study. Results of the study showed no mortality benefit with LVRS compared with pulmonary rehabilitation alone. Patients undergoing surgery had improved exercise capacity, lung function, and quality of life at 2 years, but these patients also had a higher risk of short-term morbidity and mortality associated with the surgery. A subgroup analysis of the study noted that patients with predominately upper-lobe emphysema and low exercise capacity undergoing surgery had lower mortality rates at 2 years compared with patients treated with medical therapy alone. Because of the costs and risks associated with LVRS, more studies are needed to better determine the ideal surgical candidates and identify subgroups of patients that would benefit most from surgery. The long-term benefits of LVRS are exhibited as improved Po_2 and decreased requirements for supplemental oxygen during treadmill walking as well as self-reported oxygen requirements for up to 24 months after the procedure.[152]

■ DIETARY SUPPLEMENTS

There has been increasing interest in the role of antioxidants, including vitamins E and C and β-carotene, in reducing the frequency of exacerbations. It is postulated that they may be beneficial in COPD as a result of an imbalance between oxidants and antioxidants that has been considered in the pathogenesis of smoking-induced lung disease. However, there is no good evidence that antioxidant therapies improve COPD symptoms or slow disease progression. Nutritional supplements, including creatine, have not proven beneficial to improve the benefit of pulmonary rehabilitation programs.[153]

■ INVESTIGATIONAL THERAPIES

Based on the knowledge about the importance of neutrophilic inflammation in COPD and potential therapeutic benefit of inhibition of neutrophil activity, a number of antiinflammatory compounds are being explored. Specifically, agents inhibiting leukotriene B_4, neutrophil elastase, and phosphodiesterases currently are being evaluated. To date, studies evaluating leukotriene-modifying therapies have been disappointing. Further studies are needed to evaluate the clinical benefit of such inhibitors for patients with COPD.

Phosphodiesterase 4 (PDE4) is the major phosphodiesterase found in airway smooth muscle cells and inflammatory cells and is responsible for degrading cAMP. Inhibition of PDE4 results in relaxation of airway smooth muscle cells and decreased activity of inflammatory cells and mediators such as TNF-α and IL-8. Two PDE4 inhibitors, cilomilast and roflumilast, have reached clinical trials. Cilomilast has been evaluated in several human trials and has been shown to improve expiratory airflow as measured by FEV_1 for patients with COPD when given at a dose of 15 mg twice daily for 6 weeks. To date, the results of clinical trials investigating these agents have been modest. Future studies of these agents should evaluate effects on other clinical outcomes such as health status, exacerbation frequency, and progression of disease.

Neutrophil elastase is implicated in the induction of bronchial disease, causing structural changes in lungs, impairment of muco-ciliary clearance, and impairment of host defenses. Protease inhibitors, namely, inhibitors of neutrophil elastase, are being investigated currently for the treatment of COPD.

Results have been disappointing in evaluating the benefit of infliximab, a tumor necrosis factor α-blocker, in treating COPD. A total of 234 patients with moderate to severe COPD received either infliximab 3 mg/kg or 5 mg/kg or placebo at baseline, 2, 6, 12, 18, and 24 weeks. Subjects completed a quality-of-life questionnaire [Chronic Respiratory Questionnaire (CRQ)] during treatment and out to 44 weeks. There were no differences on the CRQ or on any secondary end points including lung function, exercise capacity, or exacerbation rates. The discontinuation rate due to adverse events was high (20–27%) in the active treatment group.[154]

PHARMACOECONOMIC CONSIDERATIONS

The overall cost of therapy is an important consideration in contemporary medical practice. Meaningful cost analysis goes beyond the cost of the medication itself and incorporates the impact of a given therapeutic agent on overall healthcare cost. Because of the relative lack of benefit among objective outcome measures in COPD clinical trials, pharmacoeconomic studies can be useful in decision making about pharmacotherapy options. Pharmacoeconomic analyses in COPD, although limited, are available regarding antibiotic use in acute exacerbations and some therapies for management of chronic stable COPD.

The costs of managing an acute exacerbation of COPD in the ambulatory setting was evaluated in over 2,400 patients. Subjects were followed for 1 month following the diagnosis of the exacerbation. The overall relapse rate was 21%, with 31% and 16% of subjects requiring care in the emergency department and hospital, respectively. The overall costs for exacerbation treatment averaged $159, with 58% attributed to hospitalization.[155] These authors concluded that a significant cost savings would result from improving the successful ambulatory management of acute exacerbations.

Grossman and colleagues conducted a trial investigating the use of aggressive antimicrobial therapy (ciprofloxacin) compared with usual antibiotic therapy (defined as any nonquinolone) in the treatment of acute exacerbations of COPD.[156] Overall, the results indicated no preference for either treatment arm. However, for patients who were categorized as high risk (severe underlying lung disease, more than four exacerbations per year, duration of bronchitis greater than 10 years, elderly, significant comorbid illness), the use of aggressive antibiotic therapy was associated with improved clinical outcome, higher quality of life, and fewer costs. The results of this study are consistent with Table 34–14, which suggests that higher-risk patients are likely to have more resistant strains of organisms and thus require more aggressive antimicrobial treatment.

Few data are available about the cost-effectiveness of educational programs for patients with COPD. In an outpatient clinic, patients attending one 4-hour group session, followed by one to two individual sessions with a clinician, reported improved outcomes, and costs were reduced in an evaluation 12 months later.[157] Additional research is needed regarding the best model for education and also the specific self-management strategies to teach.

Friedman and colleagues conducted a post hoc pharmacoeconomic evaluation of two multicenter, randomized trials comparing the combination of ipratropium and albuterol with both drugs used as monotherapy.[158] Patients who received a combination of ipratropium and albuterol had lower rates of exacerbations, lower overall treatment costs, and improved cost-effectiveness compared with either drug used alone. With the introduction of new bronchodilator therapies and with no clearly consistent advantage of one class of agents over another, pharmacoeconomic analyses may be useful for clinicians in determining the most appropriate therapy for their patients.

CLINICAL CONTROVERSIES

In the United States, all products containing a LABA agent, either alone or in combination with ICs, include a black box warning about an increased risk of severe asthma attacks or death associated with their use. This caution applies to patients with asthma, and it is strongly recommended that LABAs use should always be in conjunction with another controller therapy (e.g., ICs) and that use should be limited in duration. This concern only applies to patients with asthma and is not relevant concerning the use of LABA therapy for COPD patients.

A combination product of a long-acting inhaled β-agonist (salmeterol) and an inhaled corticosteroid agent (fluticasone) is one of the most commonly prescribed medications for lung disease, including COPD. However, in expert guidelines, ICs are indicated only for patients with more severe disease who experience frequent exacerbations. Many patients now receiving therapy with the combination inhaler may be candidates for bronchodilator therapy alone, although the benefit of ICs continues to be a focus of clinical research, including the potential for a mortality benefit.

The role of systemic corticosteroids for acute exacerbations of COPD has been clarified in recent years. However, the appropriate dosage regimen is not well established. Regimens range from initial high doses (methylprednisolone 125 mg every 6 hours) to more conservative dosing (prednisone 40–60 mg/day). Consensus guidelines indicate that bronchodilator therapy is the focus of pharmacotherapy for COPD. However, there is no clear choice for the initial agent. For patients with daily but not persistent symptoms, either ipratropium or albuterol offers advantages as initial therapy. Both also have limitations if chosen as the initial therapy.

International guidelines recommend long-acting bronchodilator therapy for patients with moderate to very severe disease or when symptoms are not adequately managed with short-acting agents or as needed therapy. When response to a single long-acting bronchodilator is not optimal, guidelines recommend the use of combinations. However, data are lacking presently about the therapeutic benefit of combinations of long-acting bronchodilators, and this approach is associated with substantial costs.

EVALUATION OF THERAPEUTIC OUTCOMES

To evaluate therapeutic outcomes of COPD effectively, the practitioner must first delineate between chronic stable COPD and acute exacerbations. In chronic stable COPD, pulmonary function tests should be assessed periodically and with any therapy addition, change in dose, or deletion of therapy. Because objective improvements often are minimal, subjective assessments are important. Other outcome parameters are commonly evaluated, including dyspnea score, quality-of-life assessments, and exacerbation rates, including visits to the emergency department or hospitalization. In acute exacerbations of COPD, white blood cell count, vital signs, chest x-ray, and changes in frequency of dyspnea, sputum volume, and sputum purulence should be assessed at the onset and throughout treatment of an exacerbation. In more severe exacerbations, ABGs and oxygen saturation also should be monitored. As with any drug therapy, patient adherence to therapeutic regimens, side effects, potential drug interactions, and subjective measures of quality of life also must be evaluated.

END-OF-LIFE CARE

Based on the natural course of COPD, characterized by the progressive decline in lung function and development of complications, consideration should be given to end-of-life decisions and advanced directives.[159] Factors associated with expected mortality within 1 year have been identified. These include older age, diagnosis of depression, declining overall health status, hypercapnia, an FEV_1 of less than 30% predicted, ability to walk only a few steps without resting, more than one emergent hospitalization in the past year, and the presence of comorbidities, including congestive heart failure. An effective strategy to discuss end-of-life care involves the patient's participation in identifying advanced directives. Patients should be assured that symptoms, including pain, will be managed and their dignity will be preserved. Specific issues that should be addressed include location and provider for terminal care, desires to use or withhold mechanical ventilation, and involvement of other family members in decisions on behalf of the patient.

ABBREVIATIONS

AAT: α_1-antitrypsin

BMI: body mass index

COPD: chronic obstructive pulmonary disease

D_LCO: diffusion capacity for carbon monoxide

DPI: dry powder inhaler

FEV_1: forced expiratory volume in 1 second

FVC: forced vital capacity

GOLD: Global Initiative for Chronic Obstructive Lung Disease

Hg: mercury

LVRS: lung volume reduction surgery

MDI: metered-dose inhaler

NHLBI: National Heart, Lung, and Blood Institute

NPPV: noninvasive positive-pressure ventilation

Pao_2: pressure exerted by oxygen gas in arterial blood

$Paco_2$: pressure exerted by carbon dioxide gas in arterial blood

TORCH: toward a revolution in COPD health study

UPLIFT: understanding potential long-term impacts on function with tiotropium

WHO: World Health Organization

REFERENCES

1. Global Initiative for Chronic Obstructive Lung Disease. Global Strategy for the Diagnosis, Management, and Prevention of Chronic Obstructive Pulmonary Disease. NHLBI/WHO workshop report. Bethesda, MD: National Heart, Lung, and Blood Institute; April 2001. Updated November 2009, http://www.goldcopd.com/.
2. Celli BR, MacNee W, ATS/ERS Task Force. Standards for the diagnosis and treatment of patients with COPD: A summary of the ATS/ERS position paper. Eur Respir J 2004;23:932–946. Full report accessible at http://www.thoracic.org.
3. Rabe KF. Guidelines for chronic obstructive pulmonary disease treatment and issues of implementation. Proc Am Thorac Soc 2006;3:641–644.
4. Specialized Centers of Clinically Oriented Research (SCCOR). In: Chronic Obstructive Pulmonary Disease (COPD). RFA Number: REA-HL-05-008. Bethesda, MD; August 2004.
5. National Center for Health Statistics. National Health Interview Survey. Hyattsville, MD, U.S. Department of Health and Human Services, CDC, NCHS; 2001, www.cdc.gov/nchs/nhis.htm.
6. Mannino DM, Homa DM, Akinbami LJ, et al. Chronic obstructive pulmonary disease surveillance—United States, 1971–2000. Surveillance Summaries, August 2, 2002. MMWR 2002;51:1–16.
7. Wilt TJ, Niewoehner D, Kim C, et al. Use of spirometry for case finding, diagnosis, and management of chronic obstructive pulmonary disease (COPD). Evidence Report #121. Agency for Healthcare Research and Quality. AHRQ Publication 05-E017–1; August 2005.
8. Brown DW, Croft JB, Greenlund KJ, Giles WH. Deaths from Chronic Obstructive Pulmonary Disease—United States, 2000–2005. MMWR 2008;57:1229–1232.
9. Chronic Obstructive Pulmonary Disease: Data Fact Sheet. U.S. Department of Health and Human Services, National Institutes of Health. NHLBI, NIH Publication 03-5529. Bethesda, MD; March 2003.
10. Holguin F, Folch E, Redd SC, Mannino DM. Comorbidity and mortality in COPD-related Hospitalizations in the United States, 1979–2001. Chest; October 2005:2005–2011.
11. Chronic obstructive pulmonary disease (COPD) Fact sheet. American Lung Association. Feb 2010. Washington DC, available at www.lungusa.org/lung-disease/COPD/resources/fact-figures/COPD-Fact-Sheet.html. Accessed July 31, 2010.
12. National Institutes of Health. NHLBI Morbidity & Mortality: 2004 Chart Book on Cardiovascular, Lung, and Blood Diseases. U.S. Department of Health Services; May 2004, http://www.nhlbi.nih.gov/resources/docs/cht-book.htm.
13. Jansson SA, Andersson F, Borg S, Ericsson A, Jonsson E, Lundback B. Costs of COPD in Sweden according to disease severity. Chest 2002;122:1994–2002.
14. The Health Consequences of Smoking: A Report of the Surgeon General. Washington, DC; 2004.
15. Sandford AJ, Silverman EK. Chronic obstructive pulmonary disease. 1: Susceptibility factors for COPD the genotype-environment interaction. Thorax 2002;57:736–741.
16. Carrel RW, Lomas DA. Alpha-1 antitrypsin deficiency: A model for conformational diseases. N Engl J Med 2002;346: 45–53.
17. Hunninghake GM, Cho MH, Tesfaigzi Y, et al. MMP12, Lung Function, and COPD in High-Risk Populations. N Engl J Med 2009;361:2599–2608.
18. Barnes PJ. Chronic obstructive pulmonary disease. New Engl J Med 2000;343:269–280.
19. Stockley RA. Neutrophils and the pathogenesis of COPD. Chest 2002;121:151–155S.
20. Hogg JC. Pathophysiology of airflow limitation in chronic obstructive pulmonary disease. Lancet 2004;364:709–721.
21. Hill AT, Bayley D, Stockely RA. The interrelationship of sputum inflammatory markers in patients with chronic bronchitis. Am J Respir Crit Care Med 1999;160:893–898.

22. Ries AL. Impact of chronic obstructive pulmonary disease on quality of life: The role of dyspnea. Am J Med 2006;119:S12-S20.

23. MacNee W. Pathophysiology of cor pulmonale in chronic obstructive pulmonary disease. Part 2. Am J Respir Crit Care Med 1994;150:1158–1168.

24. Sin DD, Man SF. Why are patients with chronic obstructive pulmonary disease at increased risk of cardiovascular disease? The potential role of systemic inflammation in chronic obstructive pulmonary disease. Circulation 2003;107:1514–1519.

25. Casaburi R, ZuWallack R. Pulmonary Rehabilitation for Management of Chronic Obstructive Pulmonary Disease. N Engl J Med 2009;360:1329–1335.

26. Rodriguez-Roisin R. Toward a consensus definition for COPD exacerbations. Chest 2000;117(suppl 2):398S-401S.

27. Landbo C, Prescott E, Lange P, Vestbo J, Almdal TP. Prognostic value of nutritional status in chronic obstructive pulmonary disease. Am J Respir Crit Care Med 1999;160:1856–1861.

28. Ferris BG. Epidemiology standardization project (American Thoracic Society). Am Rev Respir Dis 1978;118:1–120.

29. Anzueto A. Clinical course of chronic obstructive pulmonary disease: Review of therapeutic interventions. Am J Med 2006;119:S46-S53.

30. Mannino DM, Doherty DE, Buist S. Global initiative on obstructive lung disease (GOLD) classification of lung disease and mortality: Findings from the atherosclerosis risk in communities (ARIC) study. Respir Med 2006;100:115–122.

31. Celli BR. The importance of spirometry in COPD and asthma. Chest 2000;117:15S-19S.

32. Andersson F, Borg S, Janson S-A, et al. The costs of exacerbations in chronic obstructive pulmonary disease (COPD). Respir Med 2002;96:700–708.

33. Anthonisen NR, Manfreda J, Warren CPW, et al. Antibiotic therapy in exacerbations of chronic obstructive pulmonary disease. Ann Intern Med 1987;106:196–204.

34. Groenewegen KH, Schols AMW, Wouters EFM. Mortality and mortality-related factors after hospitalization for acute exacerbation of COPD. Chest 2003;124:459–467.

35. Bach PB, Brown C, Gelfand SE, McCrory DC. Management of acute exacerbations of chronic obstructive pulmonary disease: A summary and appraisal of published evidence. Ann Intern Med 2001;134:600–620.

36. Almagro P, Calbo E, Ochoa de Echaguen A, et al. Mortality after hospitalization for COPD. Chest 2002;121:1441–1448.

37. Connors AF, Dawson NV, Thomas C, et al. Outcomes following acute exacerbation of severe chronic obstructive disease. Am J Respir Crit Care Med 1996;154:959–967.

38. Heffner JE, Fahy B, Hilling L, Barbieri C. Outcomes of advanced directive education of pulmonary rehabilitation patients. Am J Respir Crit Care Med 1997;155:1055–1059.

39. Parrott S, Godfrey C, Raw M, et al. Guidance for commissioners on the cost-effectiveness of smoking cessation interventions. Health International Authority. Thorax 1998;53(suppl 5):S1-S38.

40. Anthonisen NR, Connett JE, Kiley JP, et al. Effects of smoking intervention and the use of an inhaled anticholinergic bronchodilator on the rate of decline in FEV₁: The Lung Health Study. JAMA 1994;272:1497–1505.

41. Anthonisen NR, Skeans MA, Wise RA, Manfreda J, Kanner RE, Connett JE. The effects of a smoking cessation intervention on 14.5 year mortality: A randomized clinical trial. Ann Intern Med 2005;142:233–239.

42. Fiore MC, Jaén CR, Baker TB, et al. Treating Tobacco Use and Dependence: 2008 Update. Clinical Practice Guideline. Rockville, MD: U.S. Department of Health and Human Services. Public Health Service. May 2008, www.surgeongeneral.gov/tobacco.

43. Jorenby DE, Leischow SJ, Nides MA, et al. A controlled trial of sustained-release bupropion, a nicotine patch, or both for smoking cessation. New Engl J Med 1999;340:685–691.

44. Tonstad S, Tonnesen P, Hajek P, et al. Effect of maintenance therapy with varenicline on smoking cessation: a randomized controlled trial. JAMA 2006;296:64–71.

45. Celli BR, Halbert RJ, Nordyke RJ, Schan B. Airway obstruction in never smokers: Results from the Third National Health and Nutrition Examination Survey. Am J Med 2005;118:1364–1372.

46. Oroczo-Levi M, Garcia-Aymerich J, Villar J, Ramirez-Samiento A, Anto JM, Gea J. Wood smoke exposure and risk of chronic obstructive pulmonary disease. Eur Resp J 2006;27:542–546.

47. Casaburi R, ZuWallack R. Pulmonary rehabilitation for management of chronic obstructive pulmonary disease. N Engl J Med 2009;360:1329–1335.

48. American Thoracic Society. Pulmonary rehabilitation—1999: Official statement of the American Thoracic Society. Am J Respir Crit Care Med 1999;159:1666–1682.

49. Ringbaek TJ, Broendum L, Hemmingsen K, et al. Rehabilitation of patients with chronic obstructive pulmonary disease: Exercise twice a week is not sufficient! Respir Med 2000;94:150–154.

50. Nichol KL, Margolis KL, Wourenma J, Von Sternberg T. The efficacy and cost effectiveness of vaccination against influenza among elderly persons living in the community. New Engl J Med 1994;331:778–784.

51. Centers for Disease Control and Prevention. Prevention and control of influenza: Recommendations of the Advisory Committee on Immunization Practices (ACIP). MMWR 2006;55:1–42.

52. Jackson LA, Neuzil KM, Yu O, et al. Effectiveness of pneumococcal polysaccharide vaccine in older adults. N Engl J Med 2003;348:1747–1755.

53. Alfageme I, Vazquez R, Reyes N, et al. Clinical efficacy of anti-pneumococcal vaccination in patients with COPD. Thorax 2006;61:189–195.

54. Nocturnal Oxygen Therapy Trial Group. Continuous or nocturnal oxygen therapy in hypoxemic chronic obstructive lung disease. Ann Intern Med 1980;93:391–398.

55. Medical Research Council Working Party. Long-term domiciliary oxygen therapy in chronic hypoxic cor pulmonale complicating chronic bronchitis and emphysema. Lancet 1981;1:681–685.

56. O'Donohue WJ. Home oxygen therapy. Med Clin North Am 1996;80:611–622.

57. Ferreira IM, Brooks D, Lacasse Y, et al. Nutritional support for individuals with COPD: A meta-analysis. Chest 2000;117:672–678.

58. Celli BR, Thomas NE, Anderson JA, et al. Effect of pharmacotherapy on rate of decline of lung function in chronic obstructive pulmonary disease: Results from the TORCH study. Am J Respir Crit Care Med 2008; 178:332–338.

59. Dolovich MB, Ahrens RC, Hess DR, et al. Device selection and outcomes of aerosol therapy: Evidence-based guidelines. Chest 2005;127:335–371.

60. Truitt T, Witko J, Halpern M. Levalbuterol compared to racemic albuterol: efficacy and outcomes in patients hospitalized with COPD or asthma. Chest 2003;123:128–135.

61. Asmus MJ, Hendeles L. Levalbuterol nebulizer solution: Is it worth five times the cost of albuterol? Pharmacotherapy 2000;20:123–129.

62. Datta D, Vitale A, Lahiri B, ZuWallack R. An evaluation of nebulized levalbuterol in stable COPD. Chest 2003;124:844–849.

63. O'Donnel DE, Lam M, Webb KA. Measurement of symptoms, lung hyperinflation, and endurance during exercise in chronic obstructive pulmonary disease. Am J Respir Crit Care Med 1998;158:1557–1565.

64. Friedman M. A multicenter study of nebulized bronchodilator solutions in chronic obstructive pulmonary disease. Am J Med 1996;100(suppl 1A):30S-39S.

65. Wiggins J. The role of anticholinergics in "stable" chronic obstructive pulmonary disease: Unanswered questions. Respiration 1994;61:303–304.

66. Ikeda A, Nishimura K, Koyama H, et al. Dose-response study of ipratropium bromide aerosol on maximum exercise performance in stable patients with chronic obstructive pulmonary disease. Thorax 1996;51:48–53.

67. Tsukino M, Nishimura K, Ikeda A, et al. Effects of theophylline and ipratropium bromide on exercise performance in patients with stable chronic obstructive pulmonary disease. Thorax 1998;53:269–273.

68. Martin RJ, Bartelson BL, Smith P, et al. Effect of ipratropium bromide treatment on oxygen saturation and sleep quality in COPD. Chest 1999;115:1338–1345.

69. Mahler DA, Donohue JF, Barbee RA, et al. Efficacy of salmeterol xinafoate in the treatment of COPD. Chest 1999;115:957–965.

70. Rennard SI, Anderson W, ZuWallack R, et al. Use of a long-acting β_2-agonist, salmeterol xinafoate, in patients with chronic obstructive pulmonary disease. Am J Respir Crit Care Med 2001;163:1087–1092.

71. Van Noord JA, Smeets JJ, Raaijmakers JAM, et al. Salmeterol versus formoterol in patients with moderately severe asthma: Onset and duration of action. Eur Respir J 1996;9:1684–1688.

72. Dougherty JA, Didur BL, Aboussouan LS. Long-acting inhaled beta2 agonists for stable COPD. Ann Pharmacother 2003;37:1247–1255.

73. Bouros D, Kottakis J, LeGros V,Overend T, Della Cioppa G, Siafakas N. Effects of formoterol and salmeterol on resting inspiratory capacity in COPD patients with poor FEV₁ reversibility. Curr Med Res Opin 2004;20:581–586.

74. Rennard, SI, Anderson W, ZuWallack R, et al. Use of a long-acting inhaled beta2 adrenergic agoinist, salmeterol xinafoate, in patients with chronic obstructive pulmonary disease. Am J Respir Crit Care Med 2001;163:1087–1092.

75. Dahl R, Greefhorst LAPM, Nowak D, et al. Inhaled formoterol dry powder versus ipratropium bromide in chronic obstructive pulmonary disease. Am J Respir Crit Care Med 2001;164:778–784.

76. Barnes PJ. The pharmacological properties of tiotropium. Chest 2000;117:63S-66S.

77. Casaburi R, Mayler DA, Jones PW, et al. A long-term evaluation of once daily inhaled ipratropium in chronic obstructive pulmonary disease. Eur Respir J 2002;19:217–224.

78. Anzueto A, Tashkin D, Menjoge S, Kesten S. One year analysis of longitudinal changes in spirometry in patients with COPD receiving tiotropium. Pulm Pharmacol Ther 2005;18:75–81.

79. Brusasco V, Hodder R, Miravitlles M, Korducki L, Towse L, Kesten S. Health outcomes following treatment for six months with once daily tiotropium compared with twice daily salmeterol in patients with COPD. Thorax 2003;58:399–404.

80. Vincken W, Van Noord JA, Greefhorst APM, et al. Improved health outcomes in patients with COPD during one year treatment with tiotropium. Eur Respir J 2002;19:209–216.

81. Barr RG, Bourbeau J, Camargo CA Jr, Ram FSF. Tiotropium for stable chronic obstructive pulmonary disease: A meta-analysis. Thorax 2006;61:854–862.

82. Donohue JF, van Noord JA, Bateman ED, et al. A 6-month placebo-controlled study comparing lung function and health status changes in COPD patients treated with tiotropium or salmeterol. Chest 2002;122:47–55.

83. Tashkin DP, Celli B, Senn S, Burkhart D, Kesten S, Menjoge S, Decramer M. A 4 year trial of tiotropium in chronic obstructive pulmonary disease. N Engl J Med 2008;359:1543–1554.

84. Lee TA, Pickard S, Au DH, Bartle B, Weiss KB. Risk for death associated with medications for recently diagnosed chronic obstructive pulmonary disease. Ann Intern Med 2008;149:380–390.

85. Lee TA, Wilke C, Joo M, et al. Outcomes Associated with tiotropium use in patients with chronic obstructive pulmonary disease. Arch Intern Med 2009;169:1403–1410.

86. Van Noord JA, de Munck DRAJ, Bantje TA, et al. Long-term treatment of chronic obstructive pulmonary disease with salmeterol and the additive effect of ipratropium. Eur Respir J 2000;15:880–885.

87. Combivent Inhalation Aerosol Study Group. In chronic obstructive pulmonary disease, a combination of ipratropium and albuterol is more effective than either agent alone. Chest 1994;105:1411–1419.

88. D'Urzo AD, De Salvo MC, Ramirez-Rivera A, et al. In patients with COPD, treatment with a combination of formoterol and ipratropium is more effective than a combination of salbutamol and ipratropium. Chest 2001;119:1347–1356.

89. Cazzola M, Marco FD, Santus P, et al. The pharmacodynamic effects of single inhaled doses of formoterol, tiotropium, and their combination in patients with COPD. Pulm Pharmacol Ther 2004;17:35–39.

90. Van Noord JA, Aumann JL, Janssens E, et al. Effects of tiotropium with and without formoterol on airflow obstruction and resting hyperinfla-tion in patients with COPD. Chest 2006;129:509–517.

91. Barnes PJ. Theophylline in chronic obstructive pulmonary disease: new horizons. Proc Am Thorac Soc 2005;2:334–339.

92. Barnes PJ. Theophylline: new perspectives for an old drug. Am J Respir Crit Care Med 2003;167:813–818.

93. Man GC, Chapman KR, Ali SH, Darke AC. Sleep quality and nocturnal respiratory function with once-daily theophylline (Uniphyl) and inhaled salbutamol in patients with COPD. Chest 1996;110:648–653.

94. Nishimura K, Koyama H, Ikeda A, et al. The additive effect of theo-phylline on a high-dose combination of inhaled salbutamol and iprat-ropium bromide in stable COPD. Chest 1995;107:718–723.

95. Karpel JP, Kotch A, Zinny M, et al. A comparison of inhaled ipratro-pium, oral theophylline plus inhaled beta agonist, and the combination of all three in patients with COPD. Chest 1994;105:1089–1094.

96. ZuWallack RL, Mahler DA, Reilly D, et al. Salmeterol plus theo-phylline combination therapy in the treatment of COPD. Chest 2001;119:1661–1670.

97. Callahan CM, Dittus RS, Katz BP. Oral corticosteroid therapy for patients with stable chronic obstructive pulmonary disease: A meta-analysis. Ann Intern Med 1991;114:216–223.

98. Pizzichini E, Pizzichini MM, Gibson P, et al. Sputum eosinophilia predicts benefit from prednisone in smokers with chronic obstructive bronchitis. Am J Respir Crit Care Med 1998;158:1511–1517.

99. Senderovitz T, Vestbo J, Frandsen J, et al. Steroid reversibility test followed by inhaled budesonide or placebo in outpatients with stable chronic obstructive pulmonary disease. The Danish Society of Respiratory Medicine. Respir Med 1999;93:715–718.

100. Pauwels RA, Claes-Goran L, Latinen LA, et al. Long-term treatment with inhaled budesonide in persons with mild chronic obstruc-tive pulmonary disease who continue smoking. New Engl J Med 1999;340:1948–1953.

101. Vestbo J, Sorenson T, Lange P, et al. Long-term effect of inhaled budesonide in mild and moderate chronic obstructive pulmonary disease: A randomized, controlled trial. Lancet 1999;353:1819–1823.

102. Burge PS, Calverley PM, Jones PW, et al. Randomised, double-blind, placebo-controlled study of fluticasone propionate in patients with moderate to severe chronic obstructive pulmonary disease: The ISOLDE trial. Br Med J 2000;320:1297–1303.

103. Nishimura K, Koyama H, Ikeda A, et al. The effect of high-dose inhaled beclomethasone dipropionate in patients with stable COPD. Chest 1999;115:31–37.

104. Weir DC, Bale GA, Bright P, Sherwood Burge P. A double-blind pla-cebo-controlled study of the effect of inhaled beclomethasone dipro-pionate for 2 years in patients with nonasthmatic chronic obstructive pulmonary disease. Clin Exp Allergy 1999;29(suppl 2):125–128.

105. Paggiaro PL, Dahle R, Bakran I, et al. Multicentre, randomized, pla-cebo-controlled trial of inhaled fluticasone propionate in patients with chronic obstructive pulmonary disease. International COPD Study Group. Lancet 1998;351:773–780.

106. The Lung Health Study Research Group. Effect of inhaled triamci-nolone on the decline in pulmonary function in chronic obstructive pulmonary disease. New Engl J Med 2000;343:1902–1909.

107. Sutherland ER, Allmers H, Ayas NT, Venn AJ, Martin RJ. Inhaled corticosteroids reduce the progression of airflow limitation in chronic obstructive pulmonary disease: A meta-analysis. Thorax 2003;58:937–941.

108. Gartlehner G, Hansen RA, Carson SS, Lohr KN. Efficacy and safety of inhaled corticosteroids in patients with COPD: A systematic review and meta-analysis of health outcomes. Ann Fam Med 2006;4:253–262.

109. Macie C, Wooldrage K, Manfreda J, Anthonisen NR. Inhaled corticos-teroids and mortality in COPD. Chest 2006;130:640–646.

110. Sin DD, Wu L, Anderson JA, et al. Inhaled corticosteroids and mortality in chronic obstructive pulmonary disease. Thorax 2005;60:992–997.

111. Mapel DW, Hurley JS, Roblin D, et al. Survival of COPD patients using inhaled corticosteroids and long-acting beta agonists. Respir Med 2006;100:595–609.

112. Calverley PMA, Anderson JA, Celli B, et al. Salmeterol and fluticasone propionate and survival in chronic obstructive pulmonary disease. N Engl J Med 2007; 356:775–789.

113. Drummond MB, Dasenbrook EC, Pitz MW, Murphy DJ, Fan E. Inhaled corticosteroids in patients with stable chronic obstructive pulmonary disease: A systematic review and meta-analysis. JAMA 2008;300:2407–2416.

114. Singh S, Amin AV, Loke YK. Long-term use of inhaled corticosteroids and the risk of pneumonia in chronic obstructive pulmonary disease: A meta-analysis. Arch Intern Med 2009; 169:219–229.

115. Lipworth BJ. Systemic adverse effects of inhaled corticosteroid therapy: A systematic review and meta-analysis. Arch Intern Med 1999;159:941–955.

116. van Grunsven PM, van Schayck CP, Derenne JP, et al. Long-term effects of inhaled corticosteroids in chronic obstructive pulmonary disease: A meta-analysis. Thorax 1999;54:7–14.

117. Hubbard R, Tatterfield A, Smith C, et al. Use of inhaled corticosteroids and the risk of fracture. Chest 2006;130:1082–1088.

118. Jones A, Fay JK, Burr M, et al. Inhaled corticosteroid effects on bone metabolism in asthma and mild chronic obstructive pulmonary disease. Cochrane Database Syst Rev 2002;CD003537.

119. Decramer M, Ferguson G. Clinical Safety of long acting beta2 agonists and inhaled corticosteroid combination therapy in COPD. COPD 2006;3:163–171.

120. Calverly P, Pauwels R, Vestbo, J, et al. Combined salmeterol and fluticasone in the treatment of chronic obstructive pulmonary disease: A randomized, controlled trial. Lancet 2003;361:449–456.

121. Szafranski W, Cukier A, Ramirez A, et al. Efficacy and safety of budesonide/formoterol in the management of chronic obstructive pulmonary disease. Eur Respir J 2003;21:74–81.

122. Mahler DA, Wire P, Horstman D, et al. Effectiveness of fluticasone proprionate and salmeterol combination delivered via the Diskus device in the treatment of chronic obstructive pulmonary disease. Am J Respir Crit Care Med 2002;166:1084–1091.

123. Hanania NA, Darken P, Horstman D, et al. Efficacy and safety of fluticasone proprionate (250 mcg) and salmeterol (50 mcg) combined in the Diskus inhaler for the treatment of COPD. Chest 2003;124:834–843.

124. Calverley PM, Boonsawat W, Cseke Z, Zhong N, Peterson S., Olsson H. Maintenance therapy with budesonide and formoterol in chronic obstructive pulmonary disease. Eur Respir J 2003;22:912–919.

125. Kardos P, Wencker M, Glaab T, Vogelmeier C. Impact of salmeterol/fluticasone propionate versus salmeterol on exacerbations in severe chronic obstructive pulmonary disease. Am J Respir Crit Care Med 2007;175:144–149.

126. Wedzicha JA, Calverley PM, Seemungal TA, Hagan G, Ansari Z, Stockley RA, INSPIRE Investigators. The prevention of chronic obstructive pulmonary disease exacerbations by salmeterol/fluticasone propionate or tiotropium bromide. Am J Respir Crit Care Med 2008;177:19–26.

127. Baloria VA, Vialrino PC. Bronchodilator efficacy of combined salmeterol and tiotropium in patients with chronic obstructive pulmonary disease. Arch Bronchopneumol 2005;41:130–134.

128. Aaron SD, Vandemheen KL, Fergusson D, et al. Tiotropium in combination with placebo, salmeterol or fluticasone-salmeterol for treatment of chronic obstructive pulmonary disease. Ann Intern Med 2007;146:545–555.

129. Perng DW, Wu CC, Su KC, Lee YC, Perng RP, Tao CW. Additive benefits of tiotropium in COPD patients treated with long-acting beta2 agonists and corticosteroids. Respirology 2006;11:598–602.

130. Juvelekian GS, Stoller JK. Augmentation therapy for alpha1 antitrypsin deficiency. Drugs 2004;64: 1743–1756.

131. Alpha-1-Antitrypsin Deficiency Registry Study Group. Survival and FEV$_1$ decline in individuals with severe deficiency of alpha-1-antitrypsin. Am J Respir Crit Care Med 1998;158:49–59.

132. Dirksen A, Dijkman JH, Madsen F, et al. A randomized clinical trial of alpha-1-antitrypsin augmentation therapy. Am J Respir Crit Care Med 1999;160:1468–1472.

133. Gildea TR, Shermock KM, Singer ME, et al. Cost-effectiveness analysis of augmentation therapy for severe alpha1 antitrypsin deficiency. Am J Resp Crit Care Med 2003;167:1387–1392.

134. Stoller JK, Fallat R, Schluchter MD, et al. Augmentation therapy with alpha1 antitrypsin: patterns of use and adverse events. Chest 2003;123:1425–1434.

135. Quon BS, Gan WQ, Sin DD. Contemporary management of acute exacerbations of COPD: A systematic review and metaanalysis Chest 2008;133: 756–766.

136. Lightwoler JV, Wedzicha JA, Elliott MW, et al. Noninvasive positive pressure ventilation to treat respiratory failure resulting from exacerbations of chronic obstructive pulmonary disease: Cochrane systemic review and meta-analysis. Br Med J 2003;326: 185–189.

137. Niewoehner DE, Erbland ML, Deupree RH, et al. Effect of systemic glucocorticoids on exacerbations of chronic obstructive pulmonary disease. Department of Veterans Affairs Cooperative Study Group. New Engl J Med 1999;340:1941–1947.

138. Davies L, Angus RM, Calverley PMA. Oral corticosteroids in patients admitted to hospital with exacerbations of chronic obstructive pulmonary disease: A prospective, randomised, controlled trial. Lancet 1999;354:456–460.

139. Thompson WH, Nielson CP, Carvalho P, et al. Controlled trial of oral prednisone in outpatients with acute COPD exacerbation. Am J Respir Crit Care Med 1996;154:407–412.

140. Sayiner A, Aytemur ZA, Cirit M, et al. Systemic glucocorticoids in severe exacerbations of COPD. Chest 2001;119:726–730.

141. Aaron SD, Vandemheen KL, Hebert P, et al. Outpatient oral prednisone after emergency treatment of chronic obstructive pulmonary disease. New Engl J Med 2003;348:2618–2625.

142. Vondracek SF, Hemstreet BA. Is there an optimal corticosteroid regimen for the management of an acute exacerbation of chronic obstructive pulmonary disease? Pharmacotherapy 2006;26:522–532.

143. Stallberg B, Selroos O, Vogelmeier C, Andersson E, Ekstrom T, Larsson K. Budesonide/formoterol as effective as prednisolone plus formoterol in acute exacerbations of COPD: A double blind, randomized, non-inferiority, parallel group, multicenter study. Respir Res 2990;10:11.

144. Saint S, Bent S, Vittinghoff E, Grady D. Antibiotics in chronic obstructive pulmonary disease exacerbations: A meta-analysis. JAMA 1995;273:957–960.

145. Niederman MS. Antibiotic therapy for exacerbations of chronic bronchitis. Semin Respir Infect 2000;15:59–70.

146. Chodosh S, DeAbate C, Haverstock D, et al. Short-course moxifloxacin therapy for treatment of acute bacterial exacerbations of chronic bronchitis. Respir Med 2000;94:18–27.

147. Rizkallah J, Man SF, Sin DD. Prevalence of pulmonary embolism in acute exacerbations of COPD: A systematic review and metaanalysis. Chest 2009;135:786–793.

148. Poole PJ, Black PN. Mucolytic agents for chronic bronchitis or chronic obstructive pulmonary disease. Cochrane Database Syst Rev 2000;2, http://www updatusa.com.

149. Jenning AL, Davies AN, Higgins JP, Gibbs JS, Broadley KE. A systematic review of the use of opioids in the management of dyspnea. Thorax 2002;57:939–944.

150. Stolz D, Linka A, Di Valentino M, Meyer A, Brutsche M, Tamm M. A randomized, controlled trial of bosentan in severe COPD. Eur Respir J 2008;Sep;32:619–628.

151. National Emphysema Treatment Trial Research Group. New Engl J Med 2003;348:2059–2073.

152. Snyder ML, Goss CH, Neradilek B, et al. National Emphysema Treatment Trial Research Group. Changes in arterial oxygenation and self-reported oxygen use after lung volume reduction surgery. Am J Respir Crit Care Med 2008;178:339–345.

153. Deacon SJ, Vincent EE, Greenhaff PL, et al. Randomized controlled trial of dietary creatine as an adjunct therapy to physical training in chronic obstructive pulmonary disease. Am J Respir Crit Care Med 2008;178:233–239.

154. Rennard SI, Fogarty C, Kelsen S, et al. The safety and efficacy of infliximab in moderate to severe chronic obstructive pulmonary disease. AJRCCM 2007;175:926–934.

155. Miravitlles M, Murio C, Guerrero T, Gisbert R. Pharmacoeconomic evaluation of acute exacerbations of chronic bronchitis and COPD. Chest 2002;121:1449–1455.

156. Grossman RF, Mukerjee J, Vaughan D, et al. A one-year community-based health economic study of ciprofloxacin versus usual antibiotic treatment in acute exacerbations of chronic bronchitis. Chest 1998;113:131–141.

157. Gallefoss F. The effects of patient education in COPD in a 1-year follow-up randomized, controlled trial. Patient Educ Couns 2004;52:259–266.

158. Friedman M, Serby CW, Menjoge SS, et al. Pharmacoeconomic evaluation of a combination of ipratropium plus albuterol compared with ipratropium alone and albuterol alone in COPD. Chest 1999;115:635–641.

159. Hansen-Flashen J. Chronic obstructive pulmonary disease: The last year of life. Respir Care 2004; 49: 90–97.

REBECCA MOOTE, REBECCA L. ATTRIDGE, AND DEBORAH J. LEVINE

CHAPTER 35

Pulmonary Arterial Hypertension

KEY CONCEPTS

❶ Pulmonary arterial hypertension (PAH) may be defined as a mean pulmonary artery pressure (mPAP) ≥25 mm Hg at rest with a pulmonary wedge pressure (also known as pulmonary artery occlusion pressure) or left ventricular end diastolic pressure (LVEDP) ≤15 mm Hg measured by right cardiac catheterization.

❷ Regardless of the etiology, be it unknown or related to an associated medical condition, subgroups of PAH are based on similar clinical and pathological physiology.

❸ Diagnosis of PAH is growing due to increased awareness and knowledge of the disease state, leading to earlier and improved evaluation and identification.

❹ The underlying cause of PAH is a complicated amalgam of endothelial cell dysfunction, a procoagulant state, platelet activation, vasoconstriction, loss of relaxing factors, cellular proliferation, hypertrophy, fibrosis, and inflammation.

❺ Patients with PAH present with exertional dyspnea, fatigue, weakness, and exertion intolerance. As the disease progresses, symptoms of right heart dysfunction and failure, such as dyspnea at rest, lower extremity edema, chest pain, and syncope, are seen.

❻ The only way to make a definitive diagnosis of PAH is by right heart catheterization. The right heart catheterization provides important prognostic information and can be used to assess pulmonary vasoreactivity prior to initiating therapy.

❼ The goals of treatment are to alleviate symptoms, improve the quality of life, slow the progression of the disease, and improve survival.

❽ A general goal of PAH treatment is to correct the imbalance between vasoconstriction and vasodilation and prevent adverse thrombotic events to improve oxygenation and quality of life.

❾ Nonpharmacologic therapy is frequently used to address comorbid conditions that often accompany PAH.

❿ Conventional therapy of PAH includes oral anticoagulants, diuretics, oxygen, and digoxin.

⓫ Prostacyclin analogs such as epoprostenol, treprostinil, and iloprost induce potent vasodilation of pulmonary vascular beds.

⓬ Endothelin receptor antagonists, bosentan, ambrisentan, and sitaxsentan, improve exercise capacity, hemodynamics, and functional class in PAH.

⓭ Phosphodiesterase-5 inhibitors, including sildenafil and tadalafil, are potent and highly specific drugs that have been shown to reduce mPAP and improve functional class.

⓮ Only a very small number of patients with PAH demonstrate a favorable response to acute vasodilator testing. These are the only patients amenable to therapy with calcium channel blocker.

⓯ Combination therapy in PAH may address more than one mechanism causing this disease. Combination therapy in clinical trials has provided additional benefit but more studies are needed.

❶ Pulmonary arterial hypertension (PAH) may be defined as a mean pulmonary artery pressure (mPAP) ≥25 mm Hg at rest, with a pulmonary wedge pressure (also known as pulmonary artery occlusion pressure) or left ventricular end diastolic pressure (LVEDP) ≤15 mm Hg measured by cardiac catheterization.[1] PAH is a disorder that may occur either in the setting of underlying medical conditions or as an idiopathic disease that uniquely affects the pulmonary circulation. Historically, medical treatment of PAH has been problematic due to lack of effective therapy. Idiopathic PAH (IPAH), formerly known as primary pulmonary hypertension, has no known etiology or association with other diseases. Without medical therapy, it portends a poor prognosis (medial survival 2.8 years) after diagnosis.[2] Prior to the availability of disease-specific or targeted drug therapy for IPAH, survival rates for 1, 3, and 5 years were 68%, 48%, and 34%, respectively.[3] Others have found similar survival rates in registry studies.[4,5] Since 1995 when epoprostenol was approved by the FDA, a number of new therapeutic options have been developed. ❷ Regardless of the etiology, be it unknown or related to an associated medical condition, all subgroups of PAH are based on similar clinical and pathologic physiology. Several sets of guidelines exist to aid clinicians in diagnosis and management of PAH.[2,6–10]

EPIDEMIOLOGY

❸ In 2006, the prevalence of PAH was estimated to be 50,000 to 100,000 individuals in the United States.[7] Unfortunately, only 15,000 to 20,000 of the afflicted patients have an established diagnosis of

PAH and are currently receiving treatment. In a French registry study of more than 600 patients with PAH, Humbert et al. found that the most common cause of PAH was IPAH (approximately 40%), followed by PAH associated with connective tissue diseases (15.3%), congenital heart disease (11.3%), portal hypertension (10.4%), and familial PAH (FPAH) (3.9%).[5] Based on autopsy findings, PAH was found to occur in 0.13% of patients.[8]

ETIOLOGY

PAH most often originates with a predisposing state and one or more inciting stimuli that has been referred to as the "multiple hit hypothesis. Two or more hits may consist of a genetic disorder combined with one or more other genetic or environmental exposures or comorbidities.[11] Once a permissive and provocative environment exists, multiple mechanisms can be activated leading to vascular constriction, cellular proliferation, and a prothrombotic state resulting in PAH and its sequelae.[12] PAH can be associated with numerous conditions (Table 35–1) as well as being an idiopathic condition (IPAH). The World Health Organization

---

TABLE 35-1 World Health Organization Classification of Pulmonary Hypertension

1.0 Pulmonary arterial hypertension (PAH)
  1.1 Idiopathic (IPAH)
  1.2 Heritable
    1.2.1 BMPR2
    1.2.2 ALK-1, endoglin (with or without hereditary hemorrhagic telangiectasia)
    1.2.3 Unknown
  1.3 Drug and toxin induced
  1.4 Associated with (APAH):
    1.4.1 Connective tissue diseases
    1.4.2 HIV infection
    1.4.3 Portal hypertension
    1.4.4 Congenital heart diseases
    1.4.5 Schistosomiasis
    1.4.6 Chronic hemolytic anemia
  1.5 Persistent pulmonary hypertension of the newborn
  1.6 Pulmonary veno-occlusive disease (PVOD) and/or pulmonary capillary hemangiomatosis (PCH)
2.0 Pulmonary hypertension owing to left-heart disease
  2.1 Systolic dysfunction
  2.2 Diastolic dysfunction
  2.3 Valvular disease
3.0 Pulmonary hypertension owing to lung diseases and/or hypoxemia
  3.1 Chronic obstructive pulmonary disease
  3.2 Interstitial lung disease
  3.3 Other pulmonary diseases with mixed restrictive and obstructive pattern
  3.4 Sleep-disordered breathing
  3.5 Alveolar hypoventilation disorders
  3.6 Chronic exposure to high altitude
  3.7 Developmental abnormalities
4.0 Chronic thromboembolic pulmonary hypertension (CTEPH)
5.0 Pulmonary hypertension with unclear multifactorial mechanisms
  5.1 Hematologic disorders: myeloproliferative disorders, splenectomy
  5.2 Systemic disorders: sarcoidosis, pulmonary Langerhans cell histiocytosis: lymphangioleiomyomatosis, neurofibromatosis, vasculitis
  5.3 Metabolic disorders: glycogen storage disease, Gaucher disease, thyroid disorders
  5.4 Others: tumoral obstruction, fibrosing mediastinitis, chronic renal failure on dialysis

ALK-1, activin receptor-like kinase type-1; BMPR2, bone morphogenetic protein receptor 2; HIV, human immunodeficiency virus.

Reprinted from J Am Coll Cardiol, Vol. 54, Simonneau G, Robbins IM, Beghetti M, et al. Updated clinical classification of pulmonary hypertension, pages S43–S54, Copyright © 2009, with permission from Elsevier.

---

classification of PAH defines five groups: pulmonary arterial hypertension, pulmonary hypertension owing to left heart disease, pulmonary hypertension owing to lung diseases and/or hypoxia, chronic thromboembolic pulmonary hypertension (CTEPH), and pulmonary hypertension with unclear multifactorial mechanisms.[10] The incidence of IPAH is estimated to be five to six per 1 million in North America and Europe, with a marked female predominance (male-to-female ratio: 1:1.7) and a mean age at the time of recognition being approximately 37 years but with much variation.[12–15] PAH is a common complication of scleroderma, with 7% to 12% of patients developing PAH. Patients with scleroderma who develop PAH seem to have markedly worse outcomes in comparison with other PAH subgroups. PAH may also be a complication from other connective tissue disorders, including systemic lupus erythematosus, mixed connective tissue disease, and lung fibrosis. Patients with human immunodeficiency virus (HIV) infection can develop PAH with a prevalence of 0.46%. In patients with liver disease, portal hypertension may cause concurrent pulmonary hypertension in an estimated 2% to 6% of patients. Congenital heart diseases may also precipitate development of PAH.[10] Although uncommon in the United States, the most common forms of PAH worldwide are probably schistosomiasis and sickle cell disease followed by congenital heart disease and pulmonary hypertension of early childhood.[16] PAH can be a complication of sickle cell disease and is a major independent risk factor for death. Drugs and toxins that definitively precipitate PAH include anorexic drugs such as aminorex, fenfluramine, and dexfenfluramine.[16–18] Other drugs considered to be likely or possible causative agents for PAH include amphetamines, L-tryptophan, cocaine, and certain chemotherapeutic agents (mitomycin C, carmustine, etoposide, cyclophosphamide, bleomycin).[13,17] Rapeseed oil is also associated with PAH.[13]

Heritable PAH includes both IPAH with germline mutations and familial cases without an identified mutation. Germline mutations seen in PAH include bone morphogenetic protein receptor II (BMPR2) and activin receptor-like kinase type 1 (ALK-1). Mutations in the BMPR2 gene have been identified in approximately 70% of patients with familial PAH and in 11% to 40% of patients with IPAH.[10,19] Genetic testing for BMPR2 and ALK-1 may be offered and professional genetic counseling should be provided.[10]

PATHOPHYSIOLOGY

❹ The pathobiology of PAH involves several key biologic events, including endothelial cell dysfunction, a procoagulant state, platelet activation, constricting factors, loss of relaxing factors, cellular proliferation, hypertrophy, fibrosis, and inflammation—all combining to produce progressive and deleterious pulmonary vascular remodeling (Fig. 35–1).[20,21] Genetic substrates that are associated with PAH include BMPR2, ALK-1, nitric oxide synthase (ec-NOS), carbamylphosphate synthase gene, and 5-hydroxytryptamine (serotonin) transporter (5-HTT).[12,16,18] A mutation of BMPR2 receptor is an aberration of signal transduction in the pulmonary vascular smooth muscle cell that is postulated to alter apoptosis favoring cellular proliferation. ALK-1 is part of the transforming growth factor-β superfamily and is seen in hereditary hemorrhagic telangiectasia and PAH.[22] 5-HTT is associated with pulmonary artery smooth muscle cell proliferation and is present in IPAH in the homozygous form in 65% of patients.[23] Dysregulation of serotonin (5-HT) synthesis mediated via tryptophan hydroxylases (Tph1 and Tph2) is closely linked to the hypoxic PAH phenotype in mice, and both Tph1 and Tph2 may contribute to PAH development.[24] Known or suspected exposure to HIV infection should be explored.[19]

Molecular and cellular mechanisms are mediated by a variety of biologically active compounds, including prostacyclin (PGI$_2$), endothelin-1, nitric oxide, and serotonin. PGI$_2$ is a vasodilatory and

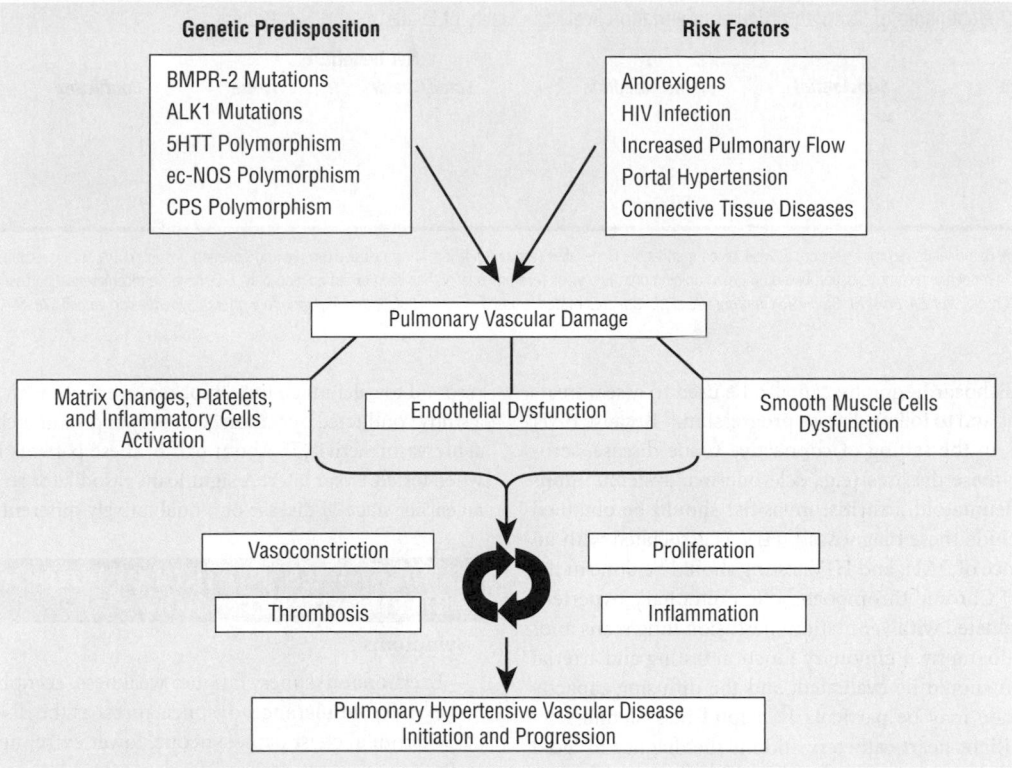

FIGURE 35-1. Pulmonary arterial hypertension; potential pathogenetic and pathobiologic mechanisms. (5-HTT, serotonin transporter gene; ALK-1, activin receptor-like kinase type 1 gene; BMPR-2, bone morphogenetic receptor 2 gene; CPS, carbamyl-phosphate synthase gene; ec-NOS, nitric oxide synthase gene; HIV, human immunodeficiency virus.) *(Reproduced with permission from Galie N, Torbicki A, Barst R. Guidelines on diagnosis and treatment of pulmonary arterial hypertension. Eur Heart J 2004;25:2243–2278.)*

antiproliferative substance that is produced by the endothelial cells, and the synthesis of PGI_2 and its circulating levels are reduced in PAH. Furthermore, thromboxane, a vasoconstrictor, is increased in PAH. Endothelin-1 is produced in the endothelium, and it possesses potent vasoconstrictor and mitogenic effects. Endothelin-1 levels are increased in PAH and clearance is reduced. Endothelin-1 acts via the endothelin receptors (ET_A and ET_B) to promote vascular smooth muscle proliferation and vasoconstriction.[1,20] Plasma levels of endothelin-1 correlate with severity of PAH and prognosis.[25] Nitric oxide (NO) is produced in the endothelium via NO synthase and leads to vasodilation and opening of cell membrane potassium channels to allow potassium ion efflux, membrane depolarization, and calcium channel inhibition. Voltage-dependent potassium channels (Kv 1.5) are inhibited by a number of stimuli that promote PAH, including hypoxia and fenfluramine, resulting in downregulated Kv 1.5 channels in patients with PAH. Entering calcium is a signal for release of sarcoplasmic calcium and activation of the contractile apparatus. NO promotes vasodilation through calcium channel inhibition. In PAH there is evidence of decreased NO synthase expression, leading to vasoconstriction and cell proliferation.[26] Alteration in NO is a therapeutic target, and treatment approaches include inhibition of phosphodiesterase-5 or calcium channel blockade. Elevated 5-HT has been observed and vasoconstriction mediated via the increased expression of the 5-HT_{1B} receptor is seen in PAH.[12]

Autoantibodies, proinflammatory cytokines, and inflammatory infiltrates may also participate in the pathogenesis of PAH. Coagulation is disordered in PAH as evidenced by increased levels of von Willebrand factor, plasma fibrinopeptide A, plasminogen activator inhibitor-1, serotonin, and thromboxane. Furthermore, tissue plasminogen activator, thrombomodulin, NO, and PGI_2 are decreased, leading to an imbalance favoring thrombosis. Endothelial dysfunction is the common denominator of mechanisms for PAH, and a variety of injuries, such as shear stress, inflammation, toxins, and hypoxia, are

thought to be involved. In IPAH endothelial dysfunction may occur as a result of proliferation of a monoclonal cell type leading to a plexiform lesion classically associated with this type of PAH. In addition, sleep-disordered breathing and obstructive sleep apnea are associated with cardiovascular morbidity. The reported range of prevalence of PAH in sleep-disordered breathing is 17% to 53%.[27]

5 The signs and symptoms of PAH are highly variable depending on the stage of the disease and comorbidities (Table 35–2). In patients with a clinical suspicion of PAH, Doppler echocardiography should be performed as a noninvasive screening test that can detect increased pulmonary pressures, although it may be imprecise in determining actual pressures compared with cardiac

TABLE 35-2 World Health Organization Functional Classification of Pulmonary Arterial Hypertension (PAH)

Class	Description
I	Patients with PAH in whom there is no limitation of usual physical activity; ordinary physical activity does not cause increased dyspnea, fatigue, chest pain, or presyncope.
II	Patients with PAH who have mild limitation of physical activity. There is no discomfort at rest, but normal physical activity causes increased dyspnea, fatigue, chest pain, or presyncope.
III	Patients with PAH who have marked limitation of physical activity. There is no discomfort at rest, but less than normal physical activity causes increased dyspnea, fatigue, chest pain, or presyncope.
IV	Patients with PAH who are unable to perform any physical activity at rest and who may have signs of right ventricular failure. Dyspnea and/or fatigue may be present at rest, and symptoms are increased by almost any physical activity.

Badesch DB, Abman SH, Simonneau G, Rubin LJ, McLaughlin W. Medical therapy for pulmonary arterial hypertension: Updated ACCP evidence-based clinical practice guidelines. Chest 2007; 131:1917–1928.

TABLE 35-3	Relationship of Strength of Recommendation Scale to Quality of Evidence and Net Benefit						
				Net Benefit			
Quality of Evidence	**Substantial**	**Intermediate**	**Small/Weak**	**None**	**Conflicting**	**Negative**	
Good	A	A	B	D	I	D	
Fair	A	B	C	D	I	D	
Low	B	C	C	I	I	D	
Expert opinion	E/A	E/B	E/C	I	I	E/D	

A, strong recommendation; B, moderate recommendation; C, weak recommendation; D, negative recommendation; I, inconclusive (no recommendation possible); E/A, strong recommendation based on expert opinion only; E/B, moderate recommendation based on expert opinion only; E/C, weak recommendation based on expert opinion only; E/D, negative recommendation based on expert opinion only.
Reprinted from J Am Coll Cardiol, Vol. 54, Barst RJ, Gibbs SR, Ghofrani HA, et al. Updated evidence-based treatment algorithm in pulmonary arterial hypertension, pages S78–S84, Copyright © 2009, with permission from Elsevier.

catheterization.[19] Echocardiography can also be used to assess treatment interventions and to follow disease progression.[17] Because PAH commonly occurs in the setting of connective tissue disease, serologic markers for these diseases (e.g., scleroderma, systemic lupus erythematosus, rheumatoid arthritis, myositis) should be obtained to confirm or exclude these diagnoses.[17] HIV is associated with an increased prevalence of PAH, and HIV testing should be done in the PAH workup.[1,17,19] Chronic thromboembolic pulmonary hypertension should be evaluated with ventilation–perfusion lung scans and/or pulmonary angiography. Pulmonary function testing and arterial blood oxygenation should be evaluated, and the diffusing capacity of carbon monoxide may be particularly helpful in systemic sclerosis and PAH.[17] Right-heart catheterization is the diagnostic "gold standard." It establishes the diagnosis of PAH, evaluates pulmonary vasoreactivity, and guides therapy.[17] In patients with PAH, serial determinations of functional class, exercise capacity (assessed by the 6-minute walk distance), and serial biomarkers provide benchmarks for disease severity, response to therapy, and progression.[19]

6 Right-heart catheterization provides important prognostic information and can be used to assess pulmonary vasoreactivity with the administration of fast-acting, short-duration vasodilators to determine the extent of vascular smooth muscle constriction and vasodilator response to calcium channel blockers (strength of recommendation: A for IPAH; E/C for associated pulmonary arterial hypertension [APAH]).[12] Table 35–3 lists the grading criteria for recommendations. Table 35–4 lists commonly used agents and their dosages. The consensus definition of a positive response is defined as reduction of mPAP by at least 10 mm Hg to a value of 40 mm Hg or less. Patients with this response are most likely to have a beneficial hemodynamic and clinical response to treatment with calcium channel blockers.[1,17] Those failing to achieve this response should not be treated with calcium channel blocker therapy. Those achieving this acute response may be treated with calcium channel blockers but need to be followed closely for safety and efficacy. Patients most likely to

respond to calcium channel blockers are those with IPAH.[17] Based on a study conducted by Sitbon et al. only approximately 13% will display acute vasoreactivity.[28] About half of these patients lose this response when tested 1 year later. A significant vasodilator response may reflect an earlier stage of disease or a qualitatively different disease process.[12]

CLINICAL PRESENTATION OF PULMONARY ARTERIAL HYPERTENSION

Symptoms

- Exertional dyspnea, fatigue, weakness, complaints of general exertion intolerance, dyspnea at rest as the disease progresses, exertional chest pain, syncope, lower extremity edema

- Symptoms of Related Conditions: Orthopnea, paroxysmal nocturnal dyspnea as a result of left-sided heart disease; Raynaud phenomenon, arthralgia, or swollen hands and other symptoms of connective tissue disease; a history of snoring as reported by the patient's partner may be a consequence of sleep-disordered breathing and can be associated with PAH.

Symptoms of Disease Progression

- Leg swelling, abdominal bloating and distension, anorexia, and more profound fatigue may develop as right ventricular dysfunction and tricuspid valve regurgitation evolve.

Signs

- Accentuated component of S_2 audible at the apex of the heart, early systolic ejection click, midsystolic ejection murmur, palpable left parasternal lift, right ventricular S_4 gallop, and a prominent "a" wave.

Signs of Advanced Disease

- Diastolic murmur of pulmonary regurgitation and holosystolic murmur of tricuspid regurgitation, hepatojugular reflux, a pulsatile liver, right ventricular S_3 gallop, marked distension of jugular veins, peripheral edema, low blood pressure, diminished pulse pressure, cool extremities suggesting markedly reduced cardiac output and peripheral vasoconstriction; cyanosis (suggests right-to-left shunting), digital clubbing, rales, dullness, decreased breath sounds, accessory muscle use, wheezing, prolonged exhalation; peripheral venous insufficiency (suggests venous thrombosis or pulmonary thrombotic disease).

Diagnostic Tests

- Electrocardiogram for chamber enlargement, chest radiography to detect enlarged pulmonary arteries, Doppler echocardiography to calculate right ventricular/right atrial pressure and pulmonary diastolic pressure, pulmonary function testing and arterial blood oxygenation; ventilation-perfusion scanning, computed tomography, or magnetic resonance imaging can be used to exclude other diagnoses; right-heart catheterization may be used to confirm the presence of PAH and to guide therapy.

- Tests for connective disease or other risk factors.

TABLE 35-4	Agent for Vasodilator Testing in Pulmonary Arterial Hypertension		
	Epoprostenol	**Adenosine**	**NO**
Route	IV	IV	Inhaled
Dose range	2–10 ng/kg/min	50–250 mcg/kg/min	10–80 ppm
Dosing increments	2 ng/kg/min every 15 minutes	50 mcg/kg/min every 2 minutes	10–80 ppm for 5 minutes
Common side effects	Headache, flushing, nausea	Chest tightness, dyspnea	None

NO, nitric oxide; IV, intravenous; ppm, parts per million.
Reprinted from J Am Coll Cardio, Vol. 53, McLaughlin VV, Archer SL, Badesch DB, et al. ACCF/AHA 2009 expert consensus document on pulmonary hypertension a report of the American College of Cardiology Foundation Task Force on Expert Consensus Documents and the American Heart Association developed in collaboration with the American College of Chest Physicians; American Thoracic Society, Inc.; and the Pulmonary Hypertension Association, pages 1573–1619, Copyright © 2009, with permission from Elsevier.

TREATMENT
Pulmonary Arterial Hypertension

■ DESIRED OUTCOMES

❼ The goals of treatment are alleviation of symptoms, improvement in the quality of life, prevention of disease progression, and improvement in survival.[13,29] While the first two outcomes are clearly obtainable based on data from randomized trials, controversy exists over improvement in survival with current treatment regimens. In a meta-analysis performed by Macchia et al. of 16 trials involving 1,962 patients, no change in total mortality was seen.[30] Up to 80% of the patients were in functional classes III/IV, with a median walking distance of 330 meters at baseline. Overall, experimental treatments were associated with a nonsignificant reduction in all-cause mortality, a minor but statistically significant improvement in exercise capacity, and an improved dyspnea status by at least one functional class. Changes in exercise capacity were not found to be predictive of a survival benefit.[30] Because most of the patients had advanced disease, the potential for a reduction in mortality may have been minimized, and less severely ill patients may have better outcomes.

However, a recent meta-analysis by Galie et al. of 21 trials including 3,140 patients found different results. In contrast to the previous meta-analysis, this study included six new randomized, controlled trials not previously evaluated and excluded one trial performed in lung fibrosis patients. Investigators found that active treatment of PAH resulted in a 43% reduction in mortality. Patients experienced an improvement in exercise capacity, determined by change in 6-minute walk distance. Approximately half of the patients were functional class III at baseline. With active treatment, functional class improved and number of hospitalizations was reduced. This meta-analysis offers support that treatment does improve survival; unfortunately, overall mortality remains high.[31] In addition, individual trials also show survival benefit, at least in the short term (i.e., 3 years).[32]

■ GENERAL APPROACH TO TREATMENT

Treatment of PAH may be categorized into nonpharmacologic, surgical, and pharmacologic interventions. ❽ The principal endothelial abnormalities that are current pharmacologic therapeutic targets include (a) supplementing endogenous vasodilators, (b) inhibiting endogenous vasoconstrictors, and (c) reducing endothelial platelet interaction and limiting thrombosis. Nonpharmacologic therapy can be quite broad and should be used when clinically appropriate. Surgical therapy is indicated in certain situations and includes atrial septostomy, pulmonary thromboendarterectomy for chronic thromboembolic pulmonary hypertension, and lung or heart–lung transplantation (for disease that is not responsive to medical therapy).[29]

■ NONPHARMACOLOGIC THERAPY

❾ Nonpharmacologic therapy is frequently used to address comorbid conditions that often accompany PAH. In patients with obstructive sleep apnea and PAH, positive airway pressure therapy should be provided.[6] Pulmonary thromboendarterectomy for PAH caused by chronic, recurrent thromboembolic disease improves hemodynamics, functional status, and survival. Pregnancy should be avoided; all females of child-bearing age should be counseled on the risks of pregnancy due to high mortality rates.[6] Immunization against influenza and pneumococcal disease should be provided according to standards for patients with serious cardiopulmonary disease.[13] Hypoxemia may aggravate vasoconstriction in patients with PAH, and it is advisable to avoid hypobaric hypoxia starting with altitudes between 1,500 and 2,000 meters. Commercial airplanes are pressurized to equivalent altitude between 1,600 and 2,500 meters and supplemental oxygen

in PAH patients should be considered.[18] Patients should adhere to a diet of 2,400 milligrams of sodium or less per day to avoid fluid retention (predisposing to right-heart failure).[13,19] Cardiopulmonary rehabilitation improves functional status and is safe and important for patients with PAH.[33] Patients with PAH are sensitive to anemia. Complete blood count should be monitored and anemia treated as appropriate.[18] Patients with long-standing hypoxia, such as those with right-to-left shunts, develop erythrocytosis. Phlebotomies may be indicated in symptomatic patients to prevent complications of hyperviscosity. PAH patients are affected by a variable degree of anxiety and/or depression that can have a profound impact on their quality of life. Support groups and psychological counseling can be helpful to improve understanding and acceptance of the disease.[18]

Patients with PAH are frequently anticoagulated with warfarin; therefore, patients should avoid drugs that interact with warfarin or those that potentially increase the risk of gastrointestinal hemorrhage (e.g., nonsteroidal anti-inflammatory drugs such as ibuprofen and aspirin), as anticoagulation in PAH is frequently considered. Nonsteroidal antiinflammatory drugs may also worsen renal function and are of particular concern in patients with low cardiac output or azotemia. Angiotensin-converting enzyme inhibitors, angiotensin receptor blockers, and β-blockers may cause hypotension and right-heart failure and should be used with caution in PAH.

■ PHARMACOLOGIC THERAPY

The number of potential therapies for PAH has expanded dramatically in the past decade. Multiple drugs have been developed specifically for treatment of PAH in addition to adjunctive therapy with anticoagulation and oxygen, as well as other therapies to treat comorbidities. Figure 35–2 illustrates the current recommended treatment algorithm based on the most recent guidelines.[6,29]

Conventional Pharmacologic Treatment

❿ Conventional therapy includes oral anticoagulants, diuretics, oxygen, and digoxin.[1,19] The rationale for oral anticoagulants in patients with PAH is based on the presence of traditional risk factors for venous thromboembolism, such as heart failure and sedentary lifestyle, as well as on the demonstration of thrombotic predisposition and thrombotic changes in the pulmonary microcirculation. The target international normalized ratio in most centers is 1.5 to 2.5.[1,17] In recent trials, 50% to 85% of patients have been anticoagulated; the highest prevalence has been in IPAH patients in New York Heart Association classes III and IV.[15] Anticoagulation is recommended for patients with IPAH (strength of recommendation: E/B).[13,19,29]

Diuretics are used in patients with decompensated right-heart failure and with associated findings of increased central venous pressure, abdominal organ congestion, peripheral edema, and ascites.[13] Appropriate diuretic therapy in right-heart failure allows clear symptomatic and clinical benefits in patients with PAH (strength of recommendation: E/A). Diuretics need to be used carefully as these patients should be maintained at as close to a euvolemic state as possible. There are no randomized trials of diuretic therapy in PAH. Approximately 50% to 70% of patients with PAH receive diuretic therapy.

Although oxygen saturation should be maintained at approximately 90%, there are no data currently available regarding the effects of long-term oxygen treatment in PAH (strength of recommendation: E/A). Oxygen treatment in patients with PAH associated with shunts (Eisenmenger syndrome) is controversial.[13]

Digoxin use in PAH is based on judgment rather than scientific evidence of efficacy. Digoxin can be used for PAH patients with right-heart failure as adjunctive therapy along with diuretics to control symptoms. Digoxin may be useful in PAH patients who develop atrial flutter to slow ventricular rate.[13,17] Current guidelines give digoxin a recommendation of E/C.[29] There are no long-term trials,

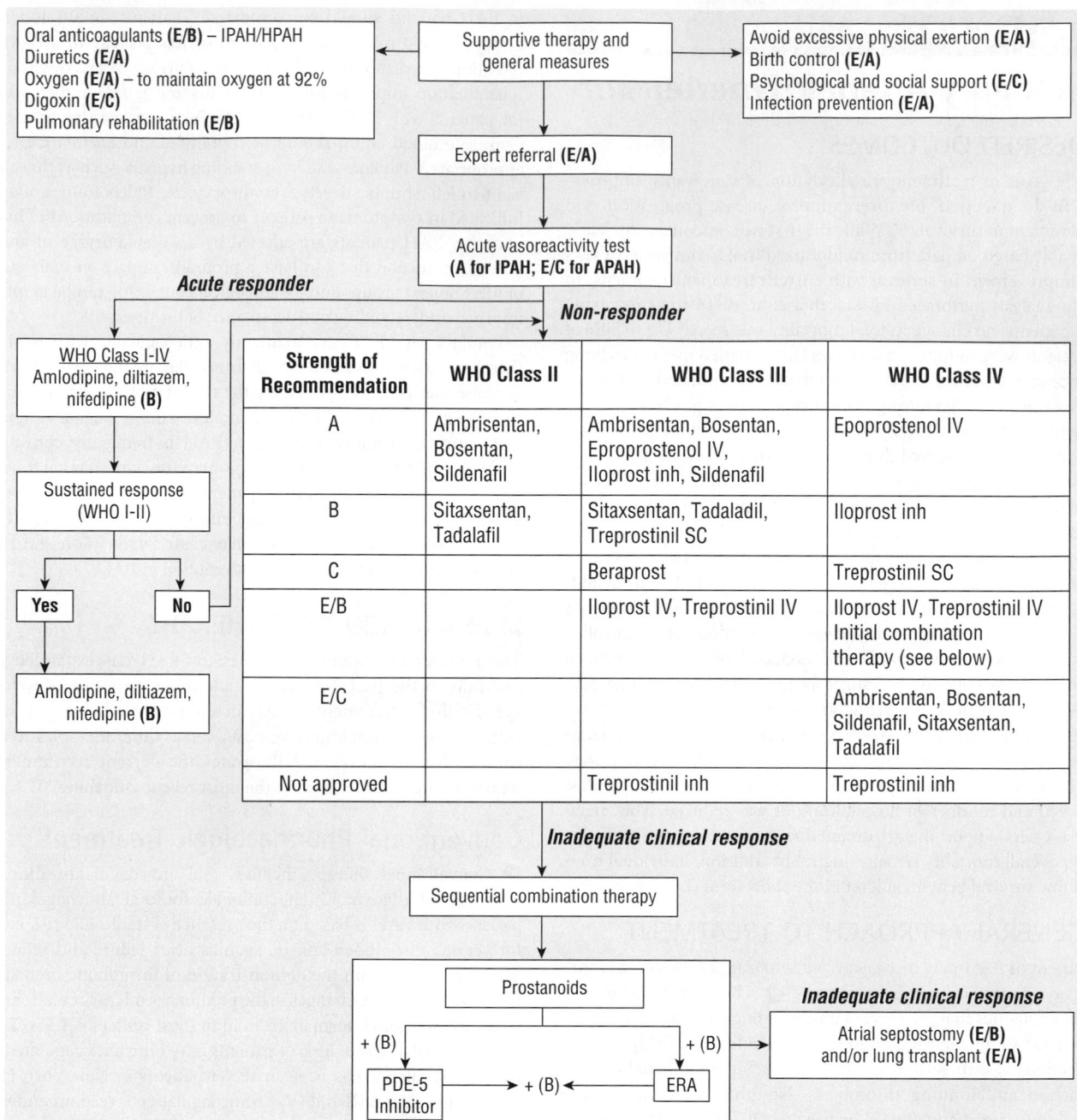

FIGURE 35-2. Treatment algorithm for pulmonary arterial hypertension (PAH). Designators (A), (B), (C), (D), (E/A), (E/B), and (E/C) are defined in Table 35–3. (CCB, calcium channel blocker; FC, functional class; IPAH, idiopathic pulmonary arterial hypertension; APAH, associated pulmonary arterial hypertension; HPAH, heritable pulmonary arterial hypertension.) *(Barst RJ, Gibbs SR, Ghofrani HA, et al. Updated evidence-based treatment algorithm in pulmonary arterial hypertension. JACC 2009;54(suppl S):S78–S84.)*

and benefit is uncertain. Optimal plasma concentrations for digoxin in PAH are unknown; however, in light of recent trials of digoxin in left systolic dysfunction, plasma concentrations should probably be in the range of 0.5 to 0.8 ng/mL. Patients on digoxin should receive periodic monitoring of potassium.

Specific Pharmacologic Therapy

In recent years, there has been a surge in availability of drug therapy for the treatment of PAH. Figure 35–3 illustrates the timeline of drug approval over the last few decades.

Synthetic Prostacyclin and Prostacyclin Analogs

⓫ Prostacyclin is produced predominantly by endothelial cells, and it induces potent vasodilation of all vascular beds. It is also a

potent inhibitor of platelet aggregation and possesses cytoprotective and antiproliferative activities. Prostacyclin synthase expression is reduced in pulmonary arteries, and urinary excretion of prostacyclin metabolites is reduced in PAH. Epoprostenol (Flolan) is a synthetic analog of prostacyclin and has a short half-life of 3 to 5 minutes; consequently, it must be given by continuous intravenous infusion. In controlled trials lasting up to 3 months, epoprostenol improved 6-minute walk distance, hemodynamics, and clinical events.[34-36] Long-term epoprostenol is initiated at a dose ranging from 2 to 4 ng/kg/min and increased at a rate limited by side effects (flushing, headache, diarrhea, jaw pain, backache, abdominal cramping, foot/leg pain, and, rarely, hypotension). Because the drug must be given by a pump to provide a continuous infusion, infection, catheter obstruction, and sepsis are potential complications. A Centers for Disease

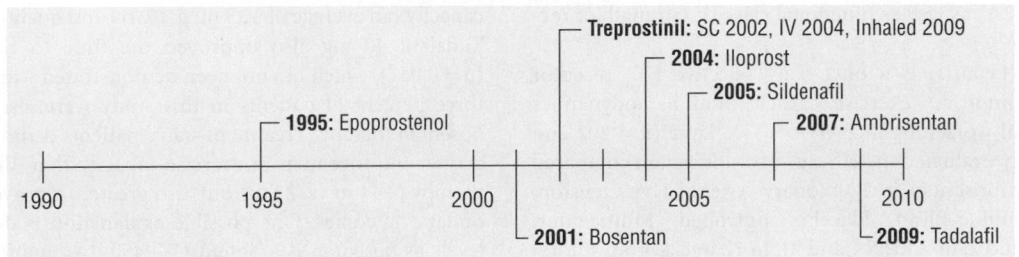

FIGURE 35-3. Timeline of pulmonary arterial hypertension (PAH) medication approvals. Epoprostenol: 1995; Treprostinil: SC 2002, IV 2004, Inhaled 2009, PO not approved; Iloprost: 2004; Bosentan: 2001; Ambrisentan: 2007; Sildenafil: 2005; Tadalafil: 2009.

Control and Prevention study found that bloodstream infections occurred with epoprostenol and treprostinil in the range of 0.3 to 2.1 per 1,000 medicine days (approximately one infection every 3 years) when these drugs are given by the intravenous route. The target dose for the first 2 to 4 weeks is around 10 to 15 ng/kg/min, and periodic dose increases are then required to maximize efficacy and to avoid tolerance. Optimal doses are variable but are in the range of 25 to 40 ng/kg/min.[13,18] Observational series have documented an improvement in survival in patients with IPAH compared with either historical control or predicted survival based on the National Institutes of Health Registry equation.[36,37] Based on current guidelines, epoprostenol is indicated for World Health Organization (WHO) functional class III and IV (strength of recommendation: A).[29]

Treprostinil (Remodulin) is a stable analog of prostacyclin given for subcutaneous (SC) or intravenous (IV) infusion approved for functional classes II, III, and IV.[13] The major advantages of treprostinil over epoprostenol include ease of use and increased safety due to a longer half-life, lowering the risk of rebound effects that may happen with drug interruption.[1] Treprostinil has been shown to improve 6-minute walk distance and hemodynamics with outcomes that are similar to epoprostenol.[38,39] In clinical trials, the greatest exercise improvement was observed in patients who were more compromised at baseline and in patients who could tolerate doses in the upper quartile (>13.8 ng/kg/min). The initial dose for treprostinil is 1.25 ng/kg/min by either the SC or the IV route. If not tolerated, the dose should be reduced to 0.625 ng/kg/min and retitration attempted at 4 weeks. If transitioning from epoprostenol to treprostinil, start with 10% of the epoprostenol dose. Dose may be increased by 1.25 ng/kg/min but no more than 2.5 ng/kg/min per week. Infusion site pain is the most common side effect of treprostinil, leading to discontinuation of the treatment in 8% of patients and limiting dose increase in other patients.[18] Other side effects are similar to epoprostenol. Based on international guidelines, treprostinil is recommended for functional class III (SC administration, strength of recommendation: B; IV administration, strength of recommendation: E/B), and functional class IV (SC administration, strength of recommendation: C; IV administration, strength of recommendation: E/B).[29]

Inhaled treprostinil (Tyvaso) was approved by the FDA in July 2009 to improve exercise capacity in functional class III patients. In a randomized, double-blind, 12-week trial, patients receiving inhaled treprostinil experienced a 20-meter improvement in 6-minute walk distance compared with those on placebo (p <0.0006). All patients included in the trial were concurrently receiving bosentan or sildenafil for at least 3 months.[40] An open-label extension of the trial found that inhaled treprostinil provided sustained benefit and was safe and efficacious over a 2-year period.[41] The approved dosing of inhaled treprostinil is 3 breaths (18 mcg each) four times daily during waking hours. The dose may be titrated based on patient tolerance at 1- to 2-week intervals to maximum dose of 9 breaths four times daily. While inhaled treprostinil avoids the infusion-related complications of the other prostacyclin analogs, use is cautioned in patients with

acute pulmonary infections or underlying lung disease. The most common adverse effects seen in clinical trials include throat irritation, cough, headache, nausea, dizziness, and flushing. Inhaled treprostinil may also cause systemic hypotension, and patients should be monitored carefully if they are concurrently on diuretics, antihypertensives, or other vasodilators. Further studies are being performed to evaluate the risk of oropharyngeal and pulmonary toxicities in patients on inhaled treprostinil. Current guidelines have not yet assigned a strength of recommendation for inhaled treprostinil use.[29] Iloprost (Ilomedin, Ventavis) is a prostacyclin analog that is given by inhalation using a dosing system provided by the manufacturer (ADD system) with the initial inhaled dose being 2.5 mcg 6 to 9 times/day up to every 2 hours during waking hours. The dose should be titrated and maintained at 5 mcg/dose if tolerated. In a 3-month, randomized, double-blind, placebo-controlled trial, iloprost via inhalation provided at least a 10% improvement in 6-minute walking distance and improvement in functional class.[42] Iloprost may also be used as add-on therapy to bosentan.[43] Adverse effects are similar to other prostacyclin analogs with the exception of infectious complications related to catheter use for drug delivery. Inhaled iloprost is indicated for functional class III (strength of recommendation: A) and functional class IV (strength of recommendation: B).[29]

Endothelin Receptor Antagonists ⓬ Endothelin-1 (ET-1), a peptide produced primarily by the vascular endothelial cells, is characterized as a powerful vasoconstrictor and mitogen for smooth muscle. Activation of the ET-1 system has been shown in both plasma and lung tissue of PAH patients. Bosentan (Tracleer) is an orally active dual ET_A and ET_B receptor antagonist that improves exercise capacity, functional class, hemodynamics, echocardiographic and Doppler variables, and time to clinical worsening.[44,45] In one of the larger studies with bosentan, patients were started on 62.5 mg twice daily for 4 weeks followed by 125 mg or 250 mg twice daily for a minimum of 12 weeks.[44] Both doses were better than placebo, and the higher dose provided greater improvement in 6-minute walking distance. Increases in hepatic aminotransferases occurred in 11% of patients and were dose dependent. The mechanism of increased liver enzymes is thought to be competition by bosentan and its metabolites with the biliary excretion of bile salts, resulting in retention of bile salts that can be cytotoxic to hepatocytes.[46] Bosentan should be started at 62.5 mg twice daily in adults and adolescents for 4 weeks. After 4 weeks of therapy, the dose should be increased to 125 mg twice daily. If liver function tests are confirmed to be in the range of three to five times the upper limit of normal, reduce the daily dose or interrupt treatment. If liver function tests return to pretreatment levels, bosentan may be continued or reintroduced if indicated. Liver function tests should be monitored at baseline and monthly thereafter, and monthly pregnancy testing is required in females (category X). Complete blood count should be monitored every 3 months as bosentan has been associated with anemia. Bosentan is indicated for WHO functional class II and III (strength of recommendation: A) as well as functional class IV (strength of recommendation: E/C).[29]

Ambrisentan (Letairis) is a once-daily selective ET_A receptor antagonist that improves exercise capacity and hemodynamics and delays clinical worsening in PAH.[47,48] Two large ($n = 202$ and 192) trials recently evaluated the efficacy of ambrisentan compared with placebo (Ambrisentan in Pulmonary Arterial Hypertension, Randomized, Double-Blind, Placebo-Controlled, Multicenter, Efficacy Study 1 and 2; or ARIES 1 and 2). In 12 weeks, both studies demonstrated a significant improvement in functional capacity at doses of 2.5 mg, 5 mg, and 10 mg daily (range of 31–59 m). However, greater response was seen with increased doses. All doses were well tolerated, with no patients on therapy experiencing an increase in liver function tests (LFTs) >3 times the upper limit of normal. Similar to bosentan, ambrisentan has liver toxicity and is category X for pregnancy. Liver toxicity is less with ambrisentan (0.8% in 12-week trials and 2.8% for up to 1 year), but monthly monitoring is still required.[13] Common side effects include peripheral edema, nasal congestion, flushing, and palpitations. Treatment should be initiated with 5 mg once daily and increased to 10 mg once daily if required. Ambrisentan is recommended for WHO functional class II and III (strength of recommendation: A) and may be used for WHO functional class IV (strength of recommendation: E/C).[29]

Sitaxsentan (Thelin) is a highly selective, orally active ET_A receptor antagonist shown to improve exercise capacity, hemodynamics, and clinical events in PAH at doses of 100 to 300 mg daily.[49-52] In clinical trials evaluating sitaxsentan 100 mg daily versus placebo, sitaxsentan therapy resulted in improvement in 6-minute walk distance and functional class.[53] Sitaxsentan may increase the international normalized ratio because of inhibition of cytochrome P450 2C9 if patients are also taking warfarin. Sitaxsentan may be associated with lower rates of hepatotoxicity than other endothelin antagonists.[52] Based on the 4th World Health Symposium, sitaxsentan is recommended for WHO functional class II and III (strength of recommendation: B) as well as class IV (strength of recommendation: E/C).[29] To date, sitaxsentan is not FDA approved in the United States.

Phosphodiesterase Inhibitors ⑬

Sildenafil (Revatio) is a potent and highly specific phosphodiesterase-5 inhibitor that is approved for erectile dysfunction but also has been shown to reduce mPAP and improve functional class. Sildenafil exerts its pharmacologic effect by increasing the intracellular concentration of cyclic guanosine monophosphate, leading to vasorelaxation and antiproliferative effects on vascular smooth muscle cells. In a recent trial, sildenafil induced a significant reduction in mPAP and vascular resistance, and functional capacity improved (an average of +37 m). Sildenafil improved endothelial dependent vasodilation, and reduced plasma concentrations of endothelin-1 (from 4.5 ± 0.6 to 3.1 ± 0.7 pg/mL; $p <0.0001$) and von Willebrand factor (from 183.1 ± 10.1 to 149.1 ± 17.6 mU/mL; $p <0.0001$).[54] In a year-long study, sildenafil in chronic thromboembolic pulmonary hypertension improved 6-minute walking distance and hemodynamics.[55] Other studies have found similar beneficial results.[56-58] The FDA-approved dose is 20 mg by mouth three times per day; however, much higher doses are routinely used clinically. Common adverse effects include headaches, flushing, epistaxis, dyspepsia, and diarrhea. Changes in vision have been reported, including blue-tinted vision and sudden loss of vision. In the event of sudden loss of vision, the drug should be stopped. Concurrent nitrate therapy may lead to excessive blood pressure reduction, and this combination should be avoided. Based on the current guidelines, sildenafil is recommended for functional class II and III patients with PAH (strength of recommendation: A) in addition to functional class IV patients (strength of recommendation: E/C).[29]

Another phosphodiesterase-5 inhibitor, tadalafil (Adcirca), was approved by the FDA in May 2009 for the treatment of PAH. In a 16-week study, tadalafil 40 mg daily significantly improved exercise capacity (an average of +33 m; $p <0.01$) and quality of life measures. Tadalafil 40 mg also improved the time to clinical worsening ($p = 0.041$), which has not been demonstrated with sildenafil. Fifty-three percent of patients in this study were also on background bosentan therapy. Treatment-naïve patients demonstrated not only greater improvement in exercise capacity than those on bosentan therapy (+44 m vs. 23 m) but also greater improvement on all secondary outcomes. One possible explanation is decreased tadalafil levels as bosentan is a potent CYP450 3A4 inducer. Higher doses of tadalafil may be required in patients on concurrent bosentan therapy.[59] The most commonly reported adverse events were headache, myalgia, and flushing. The recommended dose is 40 mg by mouth once a day.[59] Concurrent use with nitrate therapy should also be avoided with tadalafil. Current guidelines indicate tadalafil for functional class II and III (strength of recommendation: B) and functional class IV (strength of recommendation: E/C).[29]

Calcium Channel Blockers ⑭

A very small number of patients with IPAH demonstrating a favorable response to acute vasodilator testing will do well with calcium channel blockers (CCBs). As described previously, IPAH patients are most likely to respond to acute vasodilators and CCBs, but the number responding on long-term treatment is small (approximately 7%).[28] Large reductions in MPAP predict a better response to long-term CCBs. The preferred drugs are dihydropyridine CCBs as they lack the negative inotropic effects seen with verapamil. Diltiazem may be used in patients with tachycardia to slow heart rate through atrioventricular node blockade. If left ventricular systolic dysfunction is present, diltiazem and verapamil should not be used. Assessment of CCB therapy should occur soon after initiation, and if improvement in functional class to class I or II is not seen, additional or alternative PAH therapy should be instituted. CCBs should not be used empirically to treat PAH in the absence of demonstrated acute vasoreactivity.[29] In acute responders, calcium channel blockers may be used in WHO functional classes I through IV (strength of recommendation: B).[29] The doses of these drugs are relatively high—that is, up to 120 to 240 mg/day for nifedipine and 240 to 720 mg/day for diltiazem—however, initial doses should be much lower and titrated upward to response.[18]

Combination Therapy ⑮

Combination therapy is an attractive option to address the multiple pathophysiologic mechanisms in PAH, resulting in improvement in hemodynamics, symptoms, and exercise capacity. Combination therapy can be pursued by the simultaneous initiation of two (or more) treatments or by the addition of a second (or third) agent if previous treatment has been insufficient. Potential indications for combination therapy include signs of right-heart failure, 6-minute walk distance <380 m, and persistent functional class III or IV symptoms despite active treatment.[17] Hoeper found that following a goal-oriented treatment approach using combinations of bosentan, sildenafil, and inhaled iloprost significantly improved the combined end point of death, lung transplantation, and need for intravenous iloprost treatment.[60]

Bosentan, when combined with epoprostenol, improved hemodynamics, exercise capacity, and functional class, though this result was nonsignificant.[61] In patients with PAH who are deteriorating despite chronic treatment with prostanoids, the addition of bosentan or sildenafil results in improvement in pulmonary hemodynamics and exercise based on uncontrolled studies.[62,63] Addition of sildenafil to long-term epoprostenol therapy resulted in significant improvements in 6-minute walk distance, mPAP, cardiac output, and time to clinical worsening.[64] Two studies have evaluated the combination of inhaled iloprost with existing bosentan therapy, and one found a nonsignificant improvement in 6-minute walk distance. One study was terminated early due to a futility analysis of the predetermined sample size.[62] Addition of tadalafil to background bosentan therapy resulted in improvement in 6-minute walk distance.[59] Inhaled treprostinil in combination with bosentan or sildenafil also increased 6-minute walk distance.[40] An increase in adverse effects may be experienced with combination therapy.[64]

Sequential combination therapy is recommended for patients with inadequate clinical response to monotherapy; combinations of prostanoids, phosphodiesterase-5 inhibitors, and endothelin antagonists may be used (strength of recommendation: B).[29] Initial combination therapy may be necessary in WHO functional class IV patients (strength of recommendation: E/C).[29] More specific information concerning individual drugs used for PAH are shown in Table 35-5, and a summary of evidence for combination therapy is shown in Table 35-6.

TABLE 35-5 Drug Class Information

Drug	Mechanism of Action	Pharmacokinetics	Adverse Events	Drug–Drug Interactions	Dosing
Synthetic prostacyclin and prostacyclin analogs					
Epoprostenol (Flolan)	Potent vasodilator of all vascular beds	Metabolized to 2 major and 14 minor metabolites Half-life 3–5 minutes Stable for 8 hours at room temperature	Flushing, jaw pain, diarrhea, headache, backache, foot and leg pain, abdominal cramping, nausea, hypotension (rarely)	May increase risk of bleeding with anticoagulants Sympathomimetics antagonize vasodilatory effects Additive hypotensive effects with monoamine oxidase inhibitors	Starting dose 2–4 ng/kg/ min IV, titrate up to 20–40 ng/kg/min
IV/SC treprostinil (Remodulin)	Direct vasodilator of systemic and pulmonary vascular beds and inhibits platelet aggregation	Metabolized hepatically via CYP2C8 enzymes Half-life 4 hours	Cardiovascular dilation, diarrhea, nausea, headache, jaw pain, injection site pain, rash, and pruritus	May increase risk of bleeding with anticoagulants Sympathomimetics antagonize vasodilatory effects Additive hypotensive effects with monoamine oxidase inhibitors	Initially 1.25 ng/kg/min continuous SC or IV infusion Decrease to 0.625 ng/kg/min if not tolerated Increase by no more than 1.25 ng/kg/min weekly for the first 4 weeks of therapy and no more than 2.5 ng/kg/ min weekly for the duration of therapy
Inhaled treprostinil (Tyvaso)	Direct vasodilator of systemic and pulmonary vascular beds and inhibits platelet aggregation	Metabolized hepatically via CYP450 2C8 enzymes Half-life 4 hours	Throat irritation, cough, hemoptysis, pneumonia, syncope, flushing, nausea, headache	May increase risk of bleeding with anticoagulants Sympathomimetics antagonize vasodilatory effects Additive hypotensive effects with monoamine oxidase inhibitors	Initially 3 breaths (18 mcg) via oral inhalation four times daily during waking hours (approximately 4 hours apart) Reduce to 1–2 breaths if 3 breaths not tolerated; increase to 3 breaths when tolerance improves Goal maintenance dose is 9 breaths (54 mcg) per treatment four times daily; titrate by increasing 3 breaths at 1- to 2-week intervals as tolerated
Iloprost (Ventavis)	Dilates systemic and pulmonary arterial vascular beds, alters pulmonary vascular resistance and suppresses vascular muscle proliferation Potent endogenous inhibitor of platelet aggregation	Metabolized hepatically via beta oxidation of the carboxyl side chain Half-life 20–30 minutes	Flushing, hypotension, headache, nausea, trismus, cough, flulike syndrome, jaw pain	Increased hypotensive effects when used with vasodilators and antihypertensive medications Anticoagulants and antiplatelet medications may increase the risk of bleeding	Initially 2.5 mcg inhaled six to nine times daily (dosing at ≥2 hour intervals while awake) May titrate to 5 mcg per dose with a maximum daily dose of 45 mcg
Endothelin receptor antagonists					
Bosentan (Tracleer)	Competitive antagonist for type A and B endothelin receptors, which mediate vasoconstriction and vasodilation Lowers systemic vascular resistance, pulmonary vascular resistance, and mean pulmonary arterial pressure	Bioavailability 50% >98% protein bound Metabolized by CYP2C9 and 3A4; also inducer of CYP 2C9, 3A4, and 2C19 Half-life 5 hours	Headache, flushing, abnormal hepatic enzymes, edema, reduced hemoglobin concentrations Black box warning to monitor serum aminotransferases at baseline and monthly during therapy	Known substrates of CYP3A4 (e.g., cyclosporine A, glyburide, hormonal contraceptives) Known substrates of CYP2C9 (e.g., warfarin)	Initially 62.5 mg orally twice daily for 4 weeks Then increase to 125 mg orally twice daily Available through Tracleer Access Program

(continued)

TABLE 35-5	Drug Class Information (continued)				
Drug	**Mechanism of Action**	**Pharmacokinetics**	**Adverse Events**	**Drug–Drug Interactions**	**Dosing**
Ambrisentan (Letairis)	Selective antagonist for type A endothelin receptors, which mediates vasoconstriction and vasodilation Lowers systemic vascular resistance, pulmonary vascular resistance, and mean pulmonary arterial pressure	Bioavailability unknown 99% protein bound Metabolized by CYP3A4, 2C19, and uridine glucuronyltransferases, substrate of organic anion transport protein and P-glycoprotein Half-life-9 hours	Peripheral edema, flushing, palpitations, elevated hepatic enzymes, headache, nasal congestion	Cyclosporine will increase ambrisentan levels Known inhibitors of CYP3A4 (e.g., amiodarone, erythromycin) Known inhibitors of CYP2C19 (e.g., cimetidine, clopidogrel, efavirenz) Known inducers of CYP3A4 (e.g., carbamazepine, rifampin)	Initial dose 5 mg orally daily, titrated to maximum dose of 10 mg daily Available through Letairis Education and Access Program
Sitaxsentan (Thelin)	Selective antagonist for type A endothelin receptors, which mediates vasoconstriction and vasodilation Lowers systemic vascular resistance, pulmonary vascular resistance, and mean pulmonary arterial pressure	Bioavailability >90% >99% protein bound Moderate inhibitor of 2C9, 2C19, 3A4 Half-life 6.5 hours	Peripheral edema, nausea, decreased hemoglobin, fulminant hepatitis, increased aminotransferases, headache, dizziness, nasal congestion	Cyclosporine will increase sitaxsentan levels 2C9 inhibitor (will increase known 2C9 substrates, e.g., phenytoin, tolbutamide, warfarin) Increase risk of bleeding with warfarin	100–300 mg orally daily Not yet available in United States
Phosphodiesterase inhibitors					
Sildenafil (Revatio)	Increases the intracellular concentration of cyclic guanosine monophosphate (cGMP) resulting in vasorelaxation and antiproliferative effects on smooth muscle cells	Bioavailability 40% 96% protein bound Metabolized by CYP450 3A4 (major) and 2C9 (minor) Half-life 4 hours	Headache, flushing, dyspepsia, nasal congestion, dizziness, and rash	Known inhibitors of CYP3A4 and 2C9 (e.g., bosentan, cimetidine, fluvoxamine) Known inducers of CYP3A4 (e.g., rifampin, carbamazepine) Concurrent use with nitrates potentiates hypotensive effects	20 mg orally three times daily, taken at least 4–6 hours apart; 50 mg twice daily may be appropriate for more severe cases No greater efficacy with higher doses
Tadalafil (Adcirca)	Increases the intracellular concentration of cyclic guanosine monophosphate (cGMP) resulting in vasorelaxation and antiproliferative effects on smooth muscle cells	Bioavailability unavailable 94% protein bound Metabolized by CYP4503A4 (major) Half-life 15 hours	Headache, flushing, dyspepsia, myalgia, nausea, nasal congestion, nasopharyngitis, pain in extremity	Known inhibitors of CYP3A4 (e.g., bosentan, amiodarone) Known inducers of CYP3A4 (e.g., rifampin, carbamazepine) Concurrent use with nitrates potentiates hypotensive effects	40 mg orally once daily, with or without food Not recommended to divide the dose
Calcium channel blockers					
Nifedipine extended release (Procardia XL, Nifedical XL, Adalat CC)	Blocks the influx of extracellular calcium, causing vasodilation; more potent vasodilator than diltiazem	Bioavailability 90% Extensive first-pass effect reduces bioavailability to 86% Metabolized by CYP3A4 Half-life 2–5 hours	Peripheral edema, headache, dizziness, constipation, flushing	Known inhibitors of CYP3A4 (e.g., amiodarone, erythromycin) Known 3A4 inducers (e.g., rifampin, carbamazepine)	Start at reduced dose of 30 mg orally twice daily and titrate to 120–240 mg daily
Diltiazem (Cardia XT, Cardizem CD, LA, SR, Taztia XT)	Blocks the influx of extracellular calcium, causing vasodilation	Bioavailability 80% Extensive first pass effect reduces bioavailability to 40% to 60% Metabolized by CYP3A4 Half-life 4–6 hours	Gastrointestinal effects, negative inotropic effects, headache, flushing, peripheral edema	Known inducers of CYP3A4 (e.g., rifampin, carbamazepine) Known inhibitors of CYP3A4 (e.g., amiodarone, erythromycin)	Start at reduced dose of 60 mg orally three times daily and titrate to 240–720 mg daily
Amlodipine (Norvasc)	Blocks the influx of extracellular calcium, causing vasodilation; more potent vasodilator than diltiazem	Bioavailability 52% to 88% 93% protein bound Metabolized by CYP3A4 Half-life 35 hours	Palpitations, peripheral edema, fatigue, dizziness, headache, flushing	Known inducers of CYP3A4 (e.g., rifampin, carbamazepine) Known inhibitors of CYP3A4 (e.g., amiodarone, erythromycin)	Start at reduced dose of 2.5 mg orally daily, titrated to maximum dose of 40 mg daily

TABLE 35-6	Summary of Evidence on Combination Therapy	
Drug Combination	**Main Outcomes: Improvement in 6-Minute Walk Distance**	**Other Evaluations**
Bosentan ± inhaled iloprost		
STEP trial (*n* = 67)	26 m (*p* = 0.051)	Improvement in functional class, time to clinical worsening, and postinhalation hemodynamics (*p* <0.05)
COMBI trial (*n* = 40)	Terminated early due to futility analysis	
Epoprostenol ± oral therapy		
BREATHE-2 (*n* = 33) (Epoprostenol ± bosentan)	No difference	Trend toward improvement in hemodynamics, exercise capacity, and functional class at 16 weeks
PACES trial (*n* = 267) (Epoprostenol ± sildenafil)	28.8 m (*p* <0.001)	Improvement in mean pulmonary arterial pressure, cardiac output, time to clinical worsening, and health-related quality of life; no change in Borg dyspnea score
Oral therapy combination		
PHIRST trial (*n* = 405; *n* = 171 on background bosentan) (Tadalafil ± bosentan)	23 m	Improvement in time to clinical worsening, incidence of clinical worsening, and health-related quality of life
Oral Therapy ± Inhaled Treprostinil		
TRIUMPH I trial (*n* = 235)	20 m (*p* <0.0006)	No improvement in time to clinical worsening, change in functional class, or Borg dyspnea score

BREATHE-2, Bosentan Randomized Trial of Endothelin Antagonist Therapy; COMBI, Combination Therapy of Bosentan and Aerosolized Iloprost in Idiopathic Pulmonary Arterial Hypertension; PACES, The Efficacy and Safety of Sildenafil Citrate Used in Combination With Intravenous Epoprostenol in PAH; STEP, Iloprost Inhalation Solution Safety and Pilot Efficacy Trial in Combination with Bosentan for Evaluation in Pulmonary Arterial Hypertension; TRIUMPH I, Clinical Investigation Into Inhaled Treprostinil Sodium in Patients with Severe PAH

Data from Chin KM. Pulmonary arterial hypertension. J Am Coll Cardiol 2008;51:1527–1538 and Barst RJ, Gibbs JSR, Ghofrani HA, et al. Updated evidence-based treatment algorithm in pulmonary arterial hypertension. J Am Coll Cardiol 2009;54:S78–S84.

Investigational Therapy There are a few new agents within currently approved drug classes that are under investigation for use in PAH. Oral treprostinil is currently being evaluated in a series of studies known as the FREEDOM trials. FREEDOM-C (oral treprostinil in combination with an endothelin receptor antagonist and/or phosphodiesterase-5 inhibitor for the treatment of PAH) is a multicenter, randomized, double-blind trial evaluating oral treprostinil in patients already receiving an endothelin receptor antagonist and/or a phosphodiesterase-5 inhibitor. The trial found a nonsignificant improvement in 6-minute walk distance in patients on oral treprostinil for 16 weeks.[65] Macitentan, an ET_A/ET_B receptor antagonist, is under evaluation in a phase III trial (SERAPHIN).[20]

There are also novel pathways in the pathogenesis of PAH that may provide potential new targets for therapy. These include vasoactive intestinal polypeptide, Rho kinase inhibitors, serotonin receptor antagonists and transporter blockers, HMG-CoA reductase inhibitors, and platelet-derived growth factor.[17,20] Other strategies for PAH treatment include targeting angiogenesis, right ventricular remodeling, and endothelial progenitor cell therapy.[66]

■ EVALUATION OF THERAPEUTIC OUTCOMES

Response to treatment in PAH can be objectively measured by the 6-minute walk distance, echocardiography to assess pulmonary pressures, and right-heart catheterization as the gold standard to assess ventricular function and pulmonary pressures. The WHO functional classification system is clinically useful, but correlations to hemodynamics may be imprecise. Other outcomes that are useful in clinical trials include hospitalization for exacerbations of PAH and the development of complications and death.[67]

CLINICAL CONTROVERSY

The exact sequencing of drug therapy for PAH remains a matter of individual clinician preference given the paucity of randomized trial data to support selection of one drug over another in clinically worsening PAH. Of these sequencing dilemmas, the initiation of IV therapy is often the most controversial.

CONCLUSIONS

PAH is a challenging disease to manage; however, with the development of endothelin antagonists, phosphodiesterase inhibitors, and prostacyclin analogs, clinical improvement is possible in most patients, leading to a better quality of life and delay of disease progression. Patient education is important to improve acceptance of this disease and referral to specialty care centers that may provide the best outcomes.

ABBREVIATIONS

5-HTT: 5-hydroxytryptamine transporter

5-HT: serotonin

ALK-1: activin receptor-like kinase type 1

APAH: associated pulmonary arterial hypertension

BMPR2: bone morphogenetic protein receptor II

CCB: calcium channel blockers

CTEPH: chronic thromboembolic pulmonary hypertension

ec-NOS: nitric oxide synthase

FDA: Food and Drug Administration

FPAH: familial pulmonary arterial hypertension

HIV: human immunodeficiency virus

HPAH: heritable pulmonary arterial hypertension

IPAH: idiopathic pulmonary arterial hypertension

IV: intravenous

LVEDP: left ventricular end diastolic pressure

mPAP: mean pulmonary artery pressure

NO: nitric oxide

PAH: pulmonary arterial hypertension

PCH: pulmonary capillary hemangiomatosis

PVOD: pulmonary veno-occlusive disease

SC: subcutaneous

REFERENCES

1. Park MH. Advances in diagnosis and treatment in patients with pulmonary arterial hypertension. Catheter Cardiovasc Interv 2008;71:205–213.

2. Badesch DB, Abman SH, Ahearn GS, et al. Medical therapy for pulmonary arterial hypertension: ACCP evidence-based clinical practice guidelines. Chest 2004;126:35S–62S.

3. D'Alonzo GE. Survival in patients with primary pulmonary hypertension: Results from a national prospective registry. Ann Intern Med 1991;115:343–349.

4. Jing Z. Registry and survival study in Chinese patients with idiopathic and familial pulmonary arterial hypertension. Chest 2007;132:373–379.

5. Humbert M. Pulmonary arterial hypertension in France: Results from a national registry. Am J Respir Crit Care Med 2006;173:1023–1030.

6. Badesch DB, Abman SH, Simonneau G, Rubin LJ, McLaughlin VV. Medical therapy for pulmonary arterial hypertension: Updated ACCP evidence-based clinical practice guidelines. Chest 2007;131:1917–1928.

7. De Marco T. Pulmonary arterial hypertension and women. Cardiol Rev 2006;14:312–318.

8. Rubin LJ. Primary pulmonary hypertension. Chest 1993;104:236–250.

9. McLaughlin VV, Archer SL, Badesch DB, et al. ACCF/AHA 2009 expert consensus document on pulmonary hypertension: A report of the American College of Cardiology Foundation Task Force on Expert Consensus Documents and the American Heart Association: Developed in Collaboration with the American College of Chest Physicians, American Thoracic Society, Inc., and the Pulmonary Hypertension Association. Circulation 2009;119:2250–2294.

10. Simonneau G, Robbins IM, Beghetti M, et al. The 4th World Health Symposium. Updated clinical classification of pulmonary hypertension. J Am Coll Cardiol 2009;54:S43–S54.

11. Yuan JXJ. Pathogenesis of pulmonary arterial hypertension: The need for multiple hits. Circulation 2005;111:534–538.

12. McLaughlin VV, McGoon MD. Pulmonary arterial hypertension. Circulation 2006;114:1417–1431.

13. McLaughlin VV, Archer SL, Badesch DB, et al. ACCF/AHA 2009 expert consensus document on pulmonary hypertension a report of the American College of Cardiology Foundation Task Force on Expert Consensus Documents and the American Heart Association developed in collaboration with the American College of Chest Physicians; American Thoracic Society, Inc.; and the Pulmonary Hypertension Association. J Am Coll Cardiol 2009;53:1573–1619.

14. Haworth SG. Role of the endothelium in pulmonary arterial hypertension. Vascul Pharmacol 2006;45:317–325.

15. Rich S. Primary pulmonary hypertension: A national prospective study. Ann Intern Med 1987;107:216–223.

16. Humbert M. Update in pulmonary hypertension 2008. Am J Respir Crit Care Med 2009;179:650–656.

17. Chin KM. Pulmonary arterial hypertension. J Am Coll Cardiol 2008;51:1527–1538.

18. Galie N, Torbicki A, Barst R, et al. Guidelines on diagnosis and treatment of pulmonary arterial hypertension. The Task Force on Diagnosis and Treatment of Pulmonary Arterial Hypertension of the European Society of Cardiology. Eur Heart J 2004;25:2243–2278.

19. McGoon M, Gutterman D, Steen V, et al. Screening, early detection, and diagnosis of pulmonary arterial hypertension: ACCP evidence-based clinical practice guidelines. Chest 2004;126:14S–34S.

20. Olsson KM, Hoeper MM. Novel approaches to the pharmacotherapy of pulmonary arterial hypertension. Drug Discov Today 2009;14:284–290.

21. Murali S. Pulmonary arterial hypertension. Curr Opin Crit Care 2006;12:228–234.

22. Trembath RC. Clinical and molecular genetic features of pulmonary hypertension in patients with hereditary hemorrhagic telangiectasia. New Engl J Med 2001;345:325–334.

23. Eddahibi S. Serotonin transporter overexpression is responsible for pulmonary artery smooth muscle hyperplasia in primary pulmonary hypertension. J Clin Invest 2001;108:1141–1150.

24. Izikki M. Tryptophan hydroxylase 1 knockout and tryptophan hydroxylase 2 polymorphism: Effects on hypoxic pulmonary hypertension in mice. Am J Physiol Lung Cell Mol Physiol 2007;293:L1045–1052.

25. Rubens C. Big endothelin-1 and endothelin-1 plasma levels are correlated with the severity of primary pulmonary hypertension. Chest 2001;120:1562–1569.

26. Giaid A. Reduced expression of endothelial nitric oxide synthase in the lungs of patients with pulmonary hypertension. New Engl J Med 1995;333:214–221.

27. Atwood CW. Pulmonary artery hypertension and sleep-disordered breathing: ACCP evidence-based clinical practice guidelines. Chest 2004;126:72S–77S.

28. Sitbon O, Humbert M, Jais X, et al. Long-term response to calcium channel blockers in idiopathic pulmonary arterial hypertension. Circulation 2005;111:3105–3111.

29. Barst RJ, Gibbs JSR, Ghofrani HA, et al. Updated evidence-based treatment algorithm in pulmonary arterial hypertension. J Am Coll Cardiol 2009;54:S78–S84.

30. Macchia A, Marchioli R, Marfisi R, et al. A meta-analysis of trials of pulmonary hypertension: A clinical condition looking for drugs and research methodology. Am Heart J 2007;153:1037–1047.

31. Galie N, Manes A, Negro L, Palazzini M, Bacchi-Reggiani ML, Branzi A. A meta-analysis of randomized controlled trials in pulmonary arterial hypertension. Eur Heart J 2009;30:394–403.

32. McLaughlin VV, Presberg KW, Doyle RL, et al. Prognosis of pulmonary arterial hypertension: ACCP evidence-based clinical practice guidelines. Chest 2004;126:78S–92S.

33. Uchi M. Feasibility of cardiopulmonary rehabilitation in patients with idiopathic pulmonary arterial hypertension treated with intravenous prostacyclin infusion therapy. J Cardiol 2005;46:183–193.

34. Barst RJ. A comparison of continuous intravenous epoprostenol (prostacyclin) with conventional therapy for primary pulmonary hypertension. The Primary Pulmonary Hypertension Study Group. N Engl J Med 1996;334:296–302.

35. Rubin LJ, Mendoza J, Hood M, et al. Treatment of primary pulmonary hypertension with continuous intravenous prostacyclin (epoprostenol): results of a randomized trial. Ann Intern Med 1990;112:485–491.

36. Badesch DB, Tapson VF, McGoon MD, et al. Continuous intravenous epoprostenol for pulmonary hypertension due to the scleroderma spectrum of disease: a randomized, controlled trial. Ann Intern Med 2000;132:425–434.

37. Sitbon O. Long-term intravenous epoprostenol infusion in primary pulmonary hypertension: Prognostic factors and survival. J Am Coll Cardiol 2002;40:780–788.

38. Simonneau G. Continuous subcutaneous infusion of treprostinil, a prostacyclin analogue, in patients with pulmonary arterial hypertension: A double-blind, randomized, placebo-controlled trial. Am J Respir Crit Care Med 2002;165:800–804.

39. Gomberg-Maitland M, Tapson VF, Benza RL, et al. Transition from intravenous epoprostenol to intravenous treprostinil in pulmonary hypertension. Am J Respir Crit Care Med 2005;172:1586–1589.

40. McLaughlin VV, Rubin LJ, Benza RL, et al. TRIUMPH I: Efficacy and safety of inhaled treprostinil sodium in patients with pulmonary arterial hypertension (PAH) [abstract]. Am J Respir Crit Care Med 2008;177:A965.

41. Benza RL, Rubin LJ, McLaughlin VV, et al. TRIUMPH I: Long-term safety and efficacy of inhaled treprostinil sodium in patients with pulmonary arterial hypertension (PAH)—two year follow-up [abstract]. Am J Respir Crit Care Med 2009;179:A1041.

42. Olschewski H. Inhaled iloprost for severe pulmonary hypertension. N Engl J Med 2002;347:322–329.

43. McLaughlin VV, Ronald JO, Adaani F, Victor FT, Srinivas M, Richard NC. Randomized study of adding inhaled iloprost to existing bosentan in pulmonary arterial hypertension. Am J Respir Critical Care Med 2006;174:1257–1263.

44. Rubin LJ, Badesch DB, Barst RJ, et al. Bosentan therapy for pulmonary arterial hypertension. N Engl J Med 2002;346:896–903.

45. Channick RN, Simonneau G, Sitbon O, et al. Effects of the dual endothelin-receptor antagonist bosentan in patients with pulmonary hypertension: A randomised placebo-controlled study. Lancet 2001;358:1119–1123.

46. Fattinger K. The endothelin antagonist bosentan inhibits the canalicular bile salt export pump: A potential mechanism for hepatic adverse reactions. Clin Pharmacol Ther 2001;69:223–231.

47. Galie N. Ambrisentan therapy for pulmonary arterial hypertension. J Am Coll Cardiol 2005;46:529–535.

48. Barst RJ. A review of pulmonary arterial hypertension: Role of ambrisentan. Vasc Health Risk Manag 2007;3:11–22.

49. Barst RJ. Sitaxsentan therapy for pulmonary arterial hypertension. Am J Respir Crit Care Med 2004;169:441–447.

50. Barst RJ. Treatment of pulmonary arterial hypertension with the selective endothelin-A receptor antagonist sitaxsentan. J Am Coll Cardiol 2006;47:2049–2056.

51. Benza RL, Barst RJ, Galie N, et al. Sitaxsentan for the treatment of pulmonary arterial hypertension: A 1-year, prospective, open-label observation of outcome and survival. Chest 2008;134:775–782.

52. Waxman AB. A review of sitaxsentan sodium in patients with pulmonary arterial hypertension. Vasc Health Risk Manag 2007;3: 151–157.

53. Scott LJ. Sitaxentan: in pulmonary arterial hypertension. Drugs 2007;67:761–770; discussion 71–72.

54. Rossi R. Sildenafil improves endothelial function in patients with pulmonary hypertension. Pulm Pharmacol Ther 2008;21:172–177.

55. Reichenberger F. Long-term treatment with sildenafil in chronic thromboembolic pulmonary hypertension. Eur Respir J 2007;30: 922–927.

56. Lewis GD. Sildenafil improves exercise capacity and quality of life in patients with systolic heart failure and secondary pulmonary hypertension. Circulation 2007;116:1555–1562.

57. Galie N. Sildenafil citrate therapy for pulmonary arterial hypertension. N Engl J Med 2005;353:2148–2157.

58. Singh TP. A randomized, placebo-controlled, double-blind, crossover study to evaluate the efficacy of oral sildenafil therapy in severe pulmonary artery hypertension. Am Heart J 2006;151:851.e1–e5.

59. Galie N, Brundage BH, Ghofrani HA, et al. Tadalafil therapy for pulmonary arterial hypertension. Circulation 2009;119:2894–2903.

60. Hoeper MM. Goal-oriented treatment and combination therapy for pulmonary arterial hypertension. Eur Respir J 2005;26:858–863.

61. Humbert M, Barst RJ, Robbins IM, Channick RN, Galie N, Boonstra A. Combination of bosentan with epoprostenol in pulmonary arterial hypertension: BREATHE-2. Eur Respir J 2004;24:353–359.

62. Hoeper MM, Leuchte H, Halank M, et al. Combining inhaled iloprost with bosentan in patients with idiopathic pulmonary arterial hypertension. Eur Respir J 2006;28:691–694.

63. Ghofrani HA. Combination therapy with oral sildenafil and inhaled iloprost for severe pulmonary hypertension. Ann Intern Med 2002;136:515–522.

64. Simonneau Gr, Lewis JR, Nazzareno G, Robyn JB, Thomas RF, Adaani EF. Addition of sildenafil to long-term intravenous epoprostenol therapy in patients with pulmonary arterial hypertension: A randomized trial. Ann Intern Med 2008;149:521–530.

65. Tapson VF, Torres F, Kermeen F, et al. Results of the FREEDOM-C study: A pivotal study of oral treprostinil used adjunctively with an ERA and/or PDE-5 inhibitor for the treatment of PAH [abstract]. Am J Respir Crit Care Med 2009;179:A1040.

66. Ghofrani HA, Barst RJ, Benza RL, et al. Future perspectives for the treatment of pulmonary arterial hypertension. J Am Coll Cardiol 2009;54:S108–S117.

67. Badesch DB, Champion HC, Sanchez MAG, et al. Diagnosis and assessment of pulmonary arterial hypertension. J Am Coll Cardiol 2009;54:S55–S66.

36

Drug-Induced Pulmonary Diseases

HENGAMEH H. RAISSY, MICHELLE HARKINS, AND PATRICIA L. MARSHIK

KEY CONCEPTS

❶ Select populations may be more susceptible to toxicities associated with specific agents.

❷ Primary treatment is discontinuation of the offending agent and supportive care.

The manifestations of drug-induced pulmonary diseases span the entire spectrum of pathophysiologic conditions of the respiratory tract. As with most drug-induced diseases, the pathological changes are nonspecific. Therefore, the diagnosis is often difficult and, in most cases, is based on exclusion of all other possible causes. In addition, the true incidence of drug-induced pulmonary disease is difficult to assess as a result of the pathological nonspecificity and the interaction between the underlying disease state and the drugs.

Considering the physiologic and metabolic capacity of the lung, it is surprising that drug-induced pulmonary disease is not more common. The lung is the only organ of the body that receives the entire circulation. In addition, the lung contains a heterogeneous population of cells capable of various metabolic functions, including N-alkylation, N-dealkylation, N-oxidation, reduction of N-oxides, and C-hydroxylation.

Evaluation of epidemiologic studies on adverse drug reactions provides a perspective on the importance of drug-induced pulmonary disease. In a 2-year prospective survey of a community-based general practice, 41% of 817 patients experienced adverse drug reactions.[1] Four patients, or 0.5% of the total respondents, experienced adverse respiratory symptoms. Respiratory symptoms occurred in 1.2% of patients experiencing adverse drug reactions. In a recent retrospective analysis of clinical case series in France, 898 patients had reported drug allergy, with a bronchospasm incidence of 6.9%. When these patients were rechallenged with the suspected drug, only 241 (17.6%) tested positive. The incidence of bronchospasm in patients with positive provocation test was 7.9%.[2]

Adverse pulmonary reactions are uncommon in the general population but are among the most serious reactions, often requiring intervention. In a study of 270 adverse reactions leading to hospitalization from two populations, 3.0% were respiratory in nature.[3] Of the reactions considered to be life threatening, 12.3% were

Learning objectives, review questions, and other resources can be found at **www.pharmacotherapyonline.com**.

respiratory. An early report on death caused by drug reactions from the Boston Collaborative Drug Surveillance Program indicated that 7 of 27 drug-induced deaths were respiratory in nature.[4] This was confirmed in a follow-up study in which 6 of 24 drug-induced deaths were respiratory in nature.[5]

DRUG-INDUCED APNEA

Apnea may be induced by central nervous system depression or respiratory neuromuscular blockade (Table 36–1). Patients with chronic obstructive airway disease, alveolar hypoventilation, and chronic carbon dioxide retention have an exaggerated respiratory depressant response to narcotic analgesics and sedatives. In addition, the injudicious administration of oxygen in patients with carbon dioxide retention can worsen ventilation-perfusion mismatching, producing apnea.[6] Although the benzodiazepines are touted as causing less respiratory depression than barbiturates, they

TABLE 36-1	Drugs That Induce Apnea
	Relative Frequency of Reactions
Central nervous system depression	
Narcotic analgesics	F
Barbiturates	F
Benzodiazepines	F
Other sedatives and hypnotics	I
Tricyclic antidepressants	R
Phenothiazines	R
Ketamine	R
Promazine	R
Anesthetics	R
Antihistamines	R
Alcohol	I
Fenfluramine	R
L-Dopa	R
Oxygen	R
Respiratory muscle dysfunction	
Aminoglycoside antibiotics	I
Polymyxin antibiotics	I
Neuromuscular blockers	I
Quinine	R
Digitalis	R
Myopathy	
Corticosteroids	F
Diuretics	I
Aminocaproic acid	R
Clofibrate	R

F, frequent; I, infrequent; R, rare.

may produce a profound additive or synergistic effect when taken in combination with other respiratory depressants. Combining intravenous diazepam with phenobarbital to stop seizures in an emergency department frequently results in admissions to an intensive care unit for a short period of assisted mechanical ventilation, regardless of the drug administration rate. Too rapid intravenous administration of any of the benzodiazepines, even without coadministration of other respiratory depressants, will result in apnea. The risk appears to be the same for the various available agents (diazepam, lorazepam, and midazolam). Respiratory depression and arrests resulting in death and hypoxic encephalopathy have occurred following rapid intravenous administration of midazolam for conscious sedation prior to medical procedures. ❶ This has been reported more commonly in the elderly and the chronically debilitated or in combination with opioid analgesics. Concurrent use of inhibitors of cytochrome P450 3A4 with benzodiazepines is likely to lead to greater risk of respiratory depression.

❶ Prolonged apnea may follow administration of any of the neuromuscular blocking agents used for surgery, particularly in patients with hepatic or renal dysfunction. In addition, persistent neuromuscular blockade and muscle weakness have been reported in critically ill patients who are receiving neuromuscular blockers continuously for more than 2 days to facilitate mechanical ventilation.[7] This has resulted in delayed weaning from mechanical ventilation and prolonged intensive care unit stays. The prolonged neuromuscular blockade has been confined principally to pancuronium and vecuronium in patients with renal disease. Both agents have pharmacologic active metabolites that are excreted renally. The persistent muscular weakness is less well defined but appears to represent an acute myopathy.[7] High-dose corticosteroids appear to produce a synergistic effect, supported by animal studies showing that corticosteroids at dosages ≥2 mg/kg per day of prednisone produce atrophy in denervated muscle.[8] The fluorinated corticosteroids (e.g., triamcinolone) appear to be more myopathic.[9] Dose-dependent respiratory muscle weakness has been reported in chronic obstructive pulmonary disease (COPD) and asthma patients receiving repeated short courses of oral prednisone in the previous 6 months.[10]

Respiratory failure has been known to occur following local spinal anesthesia. Apnea from respiratory paralysis and rapid respiratory muscle fatigue has followed the administration of polymyxin and aminoglycoside antibiotics.[6] The mechanism appears to be related to the complexation of calcium and its depletion at the myoneural junction. Intravenous calcium chloride has been variably effective in reversing the paralysis.[6] The aminoglycosides competitively block neuromuscular junctions. This has resulted in life-threatening apnea when neomycin, gentamicin, streptomycin, or bacitracin has been ❶ administered into the peritoneal and pleural cavities.[6] The aminoglycosides will produce an additive blockade and ventilatory paralysis with curare or succinylcholine and in patients with myasthenia gravis or myasthenic syndromes.[6] Intravenous administration of aminoglycosides has resulted in respiratory failure in babies with infantile ❷ botulism. Treatment consists of ventilatory support and administration of an anticholinesterase agent (neostigmine or edrophonium).[6]

DRUG-INDUCED ASTHMA

Epidemiologic studies demonstrate an increase in the prevalence of asthma and COPD with increased use of acetaminophen. The use of aspirin or ibuprofen is not associated with asthma or COPD.[11] The association between use of acetaminophen in infancy and childhood and risk of childhood asthma was reported by the International Study of Asthma and Allergies in Childhood, including data from 31 countries.[12] Administration of acetaminophen in the first year of life was associated with a 46% increase in risk of asthma symptoms at the age of 6 to 7 years.[12] These findings should be interpreted with caution since confounding by indication may play a part in this association. The acetaminophen—asthma/COPD association may be explained by reduction of glutathione, an endogenous antioxidant enzyme in the airway epithelium resulting in oxidant damage in the lung.[11]

DRUG-INDUCED BRONCHOSPASM

Bronchoconstriction is the most common drug-induced respiratory problem. Bronchospasm can be induced by a wide variety of drugs through a number of disparate pathophysiologic mechanisms (Table 36–2). Regardless of the pathophysiologic mechanism, drug-induced bronchospasm is almost exclusively a problem of patients with preexisting bronchial hyperreactivity (e.g., asthma, COPD).[13] By definition, all patients with nonspecific bronchial hyperreactivity will experience bronchospasm if given sufficiently high doses of cholinergic or anticholinesterase agents. Severe asthmatics with a high degree of bronchial reactivity may wheeze following the inhalation of a number of particulate substances, such as the lactose in dry-powder inhalers and inhaled corticosteroids, presumably through direct stimulation of the central airway irritant receptors. Other pharmacologic mechanisms for inducing bronchospasm include β_2-receptor blockade and nonimmunologic histamine release from mast cells and basophils.[13] A large number of agents are capable of producing bronchospasm through immunoglobulin (Ig)E-mediated reactions.[13] These drugs can become a significant occupational hazard for pharmacists, nurses, and pharmaceutical industry workers.[13]

ASPIRIN-INDUCED BRONCHOSPASM

Aspirin sensitivity or intolerance occurs in 4% to 20% of all asthmatics.[14] The frequency of aspirin-induced bronchospasm increases with age. Patients older than age 40 years have a frequency approximately four times that of patients younger than 20 years.[14] The frequency increases to 14% to 23% in patients with nasal polyps.[14] Women predominate over men, and there is no evidence for a genetic or familial predisposition.[15,16] The classic description of the aspirin-intolerant asthmatic includes the triad of severe asthma, nasal polyps, and aspirin intolerance. The typical patient experiences intense vasomotor rhinitis, which may or may not be associated with aspirin exposure, beginning during the third or fourth decade of life.[17] Over a period of months, nasal polyps begin to appear, followed by severe asthma exacerbated by aspirin. Bronchospasm typically begins within minutes to hours following ingestion of aspirin and is associated with rhinorrhea, flushing of the head and neck, and conjunctivitis.[17] The reactions are severe and often life threatening.

All aspirin-sensitive asthmatics do not fit the classic "aspirin triad" picture, and not all patients with asthma and nasal polyps develop sensitivity to aspirin.[15,16] In most cases, aspirin-sensitive asthmatics are clinically indistinguishable from the general population of asthmatics except for their intolerance to aspirin and other nonsteroidal antiinflammatory drugs (NSAIDs). Aspirin-induced asthmatics are not at higher risk of having fatal asthma if aspirin and other NSAIDs are avoided.[18]

Diagnosis of aspirin-induced asthma requires a detailed medical history. The definitive diagnosis is made by aspirin provocation tests, which may be done via different routes.[15,16,19] An oral provocation test is used commonly where threshold doses of aspirin induce a positive

TABLE 36-2	Drugs That Induce Bronchospasm	
		Relative Frequency of Reactions
Anaphylaxis (IgE-mediated)		
Penicillins		F
Sulfonamides		F
Serum		F
Cephalosporins		F
Bromelin		R
Cimetidine		R
Papain		F
Pancreatic extract		I
Psyllium		I
Subtilase		I
Tetracyclines		I
Allergen extracts		I
ʟ-Asparaginase		F
Pyrazolone analgesics		I
Direct airway irritation		
Acetate		R
Bisulfite		F
Cromolyn		R
Smoke		F
N-acetylcysteine		F
Inhaled steroids		I
Precipitating IgG antibodies		
β-Methyldopa		R
Carbamazepine		R
Spiramycin		R
Cyclooxygenase inhibition		
Aspirin/nonsteroidal antiinflammatory drugs		F
Phenylbutazone		I
Acetaminophen		R
Anaphylactoid mast-cell degranulation		
Narcotic analgesics		I
Ethylenediamine		R
Iodinated-radiocontrast media		F
Platinum		R
Local anesthetics		I
Steroidal anesthetics		I
Iron–dextran complex		I
Pancuronium bromide		R
Benzalkonium chloride		I
Pharmacologic effects		
α-Adrenergic receptor blockers		I–F
Cholinergic stimulants		I
Anticholinesterases		R
β-Adrenergic agonists		R
Ethylenediamine tetraacetic acid		R
Unknown mechanisms		
Angiotensin-converting enzyme inhibitors		I
Anticholinergics		R
Hydrocortisone		R
Isoproterenol		R
Monosodium glutamate		I
Piperazine		R
Tartrazine		R
Sulfinpyrazone		R
Zinostatin		R
Losartan		R

F, frequent; I, infrequent; R, rare.

TABLE 36-3	Tolerance of Antiinflammatory and Analgesic Drugs in Aspirin-Induced Asthma	
Cross-Reactive Drugs		**Drugs with No Cross-Reactivity**
Diclofenac		Acetaminophen[a]
Diflunisal		Benzydamine
Fenoprofen		Chloroquine
Flufenamic acid		Choline salicylate
Flurbiprofen		Corticosteroids
Hydrocortisone hemisuccinate		Dextropropoxyphene
Ibuprofen		Phenacetin[a]
Indomethacin		Salicylamide
Ketoprofen		Sodium salicylate
Mefenamic acid		
Naproxen		
Noramidopyrine		
Oxyphenbutazone		
Phenylbutazone		
Piroxicam		
Sulindac		
Sulfinpyrazone		
Tartrazine		
Tolmetin		

[a]A very small percentage (5%) of aspirin-sensitive patients react to acetaminophen and phenacetin.

When lysine-aspirin bronchoprovocation was compared with oral aspirin provocation, both methods were equally sensitive.[21]

PATHOGENESIS

Aspirin-induced asthma is correctly classified as an idiosyncratic reaction in that the pathogenesis is still unknown. Patients with aspirin intolerance have increased plasma histamine concentrations after ingestion of aspirin and elevated peripheral eosinophil counts.[15,17] All attempts to define an immunologic mechanism have been unsuccessful. Chemically similar drugs such as salicylamide and choline salicylate do not cross-react, whereas a large number of chemically dissimilar NSAIDs do produce reactions.[15,17] Table 36–3 lists the analgesics that do and do not cross-react with aspirin.

The currently accepted hypothesis of aspirin-induced asthma is that aspirin intolerance is integrally related to inhibition of cyclooxygenase. This is supported by the following evidence: (a) All NSAIDs that inhibit cyclooxygenase produce reactions, (b) the degree of cross-reactivity is proportional to the potency of cyclooxygenase inhibition, and (c) each patient with aspirin sensitivity has a threshold dose for precipitating bronchospasm that is specific for the degree of cyclooxygenase inhibition produced, and once established, the dose of another cyclooxygenase inhibitor needed to induce bronchospasm can be estimated.[17]

The mechanism by which cyclooxygenase inhibition produces bronchospasm in susceptible individuals is unknown. Arachidonic acid metabolism through the 5-lipoxygenase pathway may lead to the excess production of leukotrienes C_4 and D_4.[16,18] Leukotrienes C_4, D_4, and E_4 produce bronchospasm and promote histamine release from mast cells.[17] The precise mechanism by which augmented leukotriene production occurs is unknown, and available hypotheses do not explain why only a small number of asthmatic patients react to aspirin and NSAIDs.

DESENSITIZATION

Patients with aspirin sensitivity can be desensitized. The ease of desensitization correlates with the sensitivity of the patient.[17] Highly sensitive patients who react initially to less than 100 mg aspirin require multiple rechallenges to produce desensitization.[15] Desensitization

reaction measured by a drop in forced expiratory volume in the first second of expiration (FEV_1) and/or the presence of symptoms.[19,20] A nasal provocation test is done by the application of one dose of lysine-aspirin, and aspirin sensitivity is manifested with clinical symptoms of watery discharge and a significant fall in inspiratory nasal flow.[19,20]

usually persists for 2 to 5 days following discontinuance, with full sensitivity reestablished within 7 days.[15] Cross-desensitization has been established between aspirin and all NSAIDs tested to date. Because patients may experience life-threatening reactions, desensitization should be attempted only in a controlled environment by personnel with expertise in handling these patients. In addition, there are reports of patients who have failed to maintain a desensitized state despite continued aspirin administration.[15,16] In one open follow-up trial in 172 aspirin-sensitive asthmatics who had undergone desensitization and continued daily aspirin treatment (1,300 mg/day) an improvement in nasal-sinus and asthma symptoms occurred after 6 months of treatment, which persisted up to 5 years.[22]

CROSS-SENSITIVITY WITH FOOD AND DRUG ADDITIVES

❶ Up to 80% of aspirin-sensitive asthmatics will have an adverse reaction to the yellow azo dye tartrazine (FD&C Yellow No. 5), which is used widely for coloring foods, drinks, drugs, and cosmetics.[14] However, the studies reporting high cross-reactivity were poorly controlled and often used only subjective criteria.[14,23] In double-blind, placebo-controlled trials using pulmonary function testing, sensitivity to tartrazine has proved to be a rare event.[23] Tartrazine sensitivity appears to occur only in aspirin-intolerant patients at a prevalence of 2%.[23] Although rare, owing to the severity of reaction and widespread use of tartrazine, the U.S. Food and Drug Administration (FDA) requires labeling for the products containing this dye.[24] The likely mechanism is dose-related histamine release, and the clinical presentation is the same as the reaction to aspirin in aspirin-sensitive patients.[24]

Reactions to other azo dyes, monosodium glutamate, parabens, and nonazo dyes have been reported much less frequently than reactions to tartrazine and have been equally difficult to confirm with controlled challenges.[23] Positive reactions to sodium benzoate, a food preservative, have been reported in as many as 23% of aspirin-sensitive individuals.[14] Acetaminophen is a weak inhibitor of cyclooxygenase. As such, approximately 5% of aspirin-sensitive asthmatics will experience reactions to acetaminophen.[14] Most aspirin-sensitive asthmatics can use acetaminophen as a safe alternative to aspirin. There is a growing body of evidence that selective cyclooxygenase-2 inhibitors may be used safely in aspirin-sensitive patients,[16,25-28] but long-term studies with these agents should be undertaken to confirm their safe use in aspirin-sensitive patients. At this point, the package inserts of these agents state that they are contraindicated for aspirin-sensitive asthmatics.[16,25-28] Sporadic cases of worsening bronchospasm and anaphylaxis have been reported in aspirin-sensitive asthmatics receiving intravenous hydrocortisone succinate, but such reactions have not been reported with use of other corticosteroids.[15] It is not known whether it is the hydrocortisone or the succinate that is the problem.

TREATMENT

Aspirin-Sensitive Asthma

❷ Therapy of aspirin-sensitive asthmatics takes one of two general approaches: desensitization or avoidance. Avoidance of triggering substances seldom alters the clinical course of patients' asthma. The therapy of asthma has been nonspecific; however, in theory, 5-lipoxygenase inhibitors such as zileuton or leukotriene antagonists should provide specific therapy. A few studies have investigated use of leukotriene modifiers to prevent aspirin-induced bronchospasm in aspirin-sensitive asthmatic patients.[29-33] Pretreatment with zileuton in eight aspirin-sensitive asthmatic patients protected them from

the same threshold-provoking doses of aspirin.[29] However, larger, escalating doses of aspirin above the threshold challenge doses were not examined in this study. Furthermore, when doses of aspirin were escalated above the threshold provocative doses, zileuton did not prevent formation of leukotrienes.[30] In a similar study, pretreatment with montelukast 10 mg/day did not protect patients when aspirin doses were increased above their threshold doses.[31] In another study, the mean provoking dose of aspirin did not differ in the asthmatics who were taking leukotriene modifiers and the control group (60.4 mg vs. 70.3 mg, respectively).[34] Although initial studies suggested that leukotriene modifiers blocked aspirin-induced reactions, it is now apparent that they merely shift the dose—response curve to the right, leaving the patient at risk at higher doses. Thus even patients who might benefit from leukotriene modifiers should avoid aspirin and all NSAIDs. A case of ibuprofen 400-mg—induced asthma was reported in an asthmatic patient on zafirlukast 20 mg twice daily.[35] Furthermore, most of the challenge studies are based on incremental doses of aspirin or NSAIDs, and exposure of patients to full clinical doses of aspirin or NSAIDs can overcome the antagonistic effect of leukotriene modifiers. The respiratory symptoms can be decreased but not prevented by pretreatment with antihistamines, cromolyn, and nedocromil.[15,36] The long-term asthma control of patients with aspirin sensitivity does not differ from that for other asthmatics. There is no evidence to support that aspirin-sensitive asthmatics respond better to leukotriene modifiers. In a double-blind, randomized, placebo-controlled study, aspirin-sensitive asthmatic patients on montelukast showed a 10% improvement in FEV_1 compared with the placebo group.[37] Similar results were reported when montelukast was compared with placebo in patients with intermittent or persistent asthma.[38]

β-BLOCKERS

❶ β-Adrenergic receptor blockers comprise the other large class of drugs that can be hazardous to a person with asthma. Even the more cardioselective agents such as acebutolol, atenolol, and metoprolol have been reported to cause asthma attacks.[13] Patients with asthma may take nonselective and β_1-selective blockers without incident for long periods; however, the occasional report of fatal asthma attacks resistant to therapy with β-agonists should provide ample warning of the dangers inherent in β-blocker therapy.[13]

If a patient with bronchial hyperreactivity requires β-blocker therapy, one of theselective β_1-blockers (e.g., acebutolol, atenolol, metoprolol, or pindolol) should be used at the lowest possible dose. In a meta-analysis of 29 clinical trials in patients with mild to moderate airway obstruction, cardioselective β-blockers did not produce any clinically significant respiratory effects in short term.[39] Celiprolol and betaxolol appear to possess greater cardioselectivity than currently marketed drugs.[40,41] Fatal status asthmaticus has occurred with the topical administration of the nonselective timolol maleate ophthalmic solution for the treatment of open-angle glaucoma.[42] Early investigations with ophthalmic betaxolol suggest that it is well tolerated even in timolol-sensitive asthmatics.[43,44]

SULFITES

Severe, life-threatening asthmatic reactions following consumption of restaurant meals and wine have occurred secondary to ingestion of the food preservative potassium metabisulfite.[23] Sulfites have been used for centuries as preservatives in wine and food. As antioxidants, they prevent fermentation of wine and discoloration of fruits and vegetables caused by contaminating bacteria.[45] Previously, sulfites had been given "generally recognized as safe" status by the FDA. Sensitive patients react to concentrations ranging from 5 to 100 mg, amounts that are consumed routinely by anyone eating in restaurants. Consumption of sulfites in U.S. diets is estimated to be 2 to 3 mg/day in the home with 5 to 10 mg per 30 mL of beer or wine consumed.[23] Anaphylactic or anaphylactoid reactions to sulfites in nonasthmatics are extremely rare. In the general asthmatic population, reactions to sulfites are ❶ uncommon. Approximately 5% of steroid-dependent asthmatics demonstrate sensitivity to sulfiting agents, but the prevalence is only around 1% in non—steroid-dependent asthmatic patients.[45]

MECHANISM

Three different mechanisms have been proposed to explain the reaction to sulfites in asthmatic patients.[45] The first is explained by the inhalation of sulfur dioxide, which produces bronchoconstriction in all asthmatics through direct stimulation of afferent parasympathetic irritant receptors. Furthermore, inhalation of atropine or the ingestion of doxepin protects sulfite-sensitive patients from reacting to the ingestion of sulfites. The second theory, IgE-mediated reaction, is supported by reported cases of sulfite-sensitive anaphylaxis reaction in patients with positive sulfite skin test. Finally, a reduced concentration of sulfite oxidase enzyme (the enzyme that catalyzes oxidation of sulfites to sulfates) compared with normal individuals has been demonstrated in a group of sulfite-sensitive asthmatics.

A number of pharmacologic agents contain sulfites as preservatives and antioxidants. The FDA now requires warning labels on drugs containing sulfites. Most manufacturers of drugs for the treatment of asthma have discontinued the use of sulfites. In addition, labeling is required on packaged foods that contain sulfites at 10 parts per million or more, and sulfiting agents are no longer allowed on fresh fruits and vegetables (excluding potatoes) intended for sale.

Pretreatment with cromolyn, anticholinergics, and cyanocobalamin have protected sulfite-sensitive patients.[45,46] Presumably, pharmacologic doses of vitamin B_{12} catalyze the nonenzymatic oxidation of sulfite to sulfate.

OTHER PRESERVATIVES

Both ethylenediamine tetraacetic acid (EDTA) and benzalkonium chloride, used as stabilizingand bacteriostatic agents, respectively, can produce bronchoconstriction.[47] In addition to producing bronchoconstriction, EDTA potentiates the bronchial responsiveness to histamine.[47] These effects presumably are mediated through calcium chelation by EDTA. Benzalkonium chloride is more potent than EDTA, and its mechanism appears to be a result of mast cell degranulation and stimulation of irritant C fibers in the airways.[47]

The bronchoconstriction from benzalkonium chloride can be blocked by cromolyn but not the anticholinergic ipratropium bromide.[48] Benzalkonium chloride is found in the commercial multiple-dose nebulizer preparations of ipratropium bromide and beclomethasone dipropionate marketed in the United Kingdom and Europe and is presumed to be in part responsible for paradoxical wheezing following administration of these agents.[47–49] Benzalkonium chloride is also found in albuterol nebulizer solutions marketed in the United States and has been implicated as a possible cause of paradoxical wheezing in infants receiving this preparation.[47] The effect of these agents on FEV_1 when used in the amount administered for treatment of acute asthma was evaluated in subjects with stable asthma.[50] Patients were assigned randomly to inhale up to four 600-mcg nebulized doses of EDTA and benzalkonium chloride and normal saline. The change in FEV_1 was not different between EDTA and the placebo group; however, benzalkonium chloride was associated with a statistically significant decrease in FEV_1 compared

with placebo. It is important to consider that these agents are always used in combination with bronchodilators and β_2-agonists, which are potent mast cell stabilizers, and the anecdotal reports have not yet been confirmed with controlled investigations.[47,48]

CONTRAST MEDIA

Iodinated radiocontrast materials are the most common cause of anaphylactoid reactions producing bronchospasm.[51] Chapter 95 discusses this topic.

NATURAL RUBBER LATEX ALLERGY

Allergy to natural rubber latex, first reported in 1989 in the United States, is a common cause of occupational allergy for healthcare workers.[52] Natural rubber is a processed plant product from the commercial rubber tree, *Hevea brasiliensis*.[53] Latex allergens are proteins found in both raw latex and the extracts used in finished rubber products. Latex gloves are the largest single source of exposure to the protein allergens.[53]

❶ The reported prevalence of latex allergy depends on the sample population. In the general population, latex allergy is less than 1%; however, the prevalence increases in healthcare workers to 5% to 15%.[53,54] Risk factors for latex allergy include frequent exposure to rubber gloves, history of atopic disease, and presence or history of hand dermatitis. Patients with spina bifida are at an increased risk of latex allergy, with an incidence of 24% to 60% as a result of early and repeated exposure to rubber devices during the surgical procedures.[53,54]

Clinical manifestations of latex allergy range from contact dermatitis and urticaria, rhinitis and asthma, and reported cases of anaphylaxis.[52,53] The early manifestation of rubber allergy is contact urticaria, which is an IgE-mediated reaction to rubber proteins following direct contact with the medical devices: mainly rubber gloves.[53] Contact dermatitis may occur within 1 to 2 days. Contact dermatitis is a cell-mediated delayed-type hypersensitivity reaction to the additive chemical component of rubber products.[53] Rhinitis and asthma may follow inhalation of allergens carried by cornstarch powder used to coat the latex gloves. Asthma caused by occupational exposure is seen mostly in atopic patients with histories of seasonal and perennial allergies and asthma.[53] Isolated cases of wheezing secondary to latex exposure in patients without a history of asthma have also been reported.[53]

The diagnosis of latex allergy is based on the presence of latex-specific IgE, as well as symptoms consistent with IgE-mediated ❷ reactions.[55] The mainstay of therapy for latex allergy is avoidance. The FDA requires appropriate labeling for all medical devices containing natural rubber latex to ensure avoidance and a latex-free environment. The role of pretreatment with antihistamines, corticosteroids, and allergen immunotherapy remains to be determined.[53,55] Specific immunotherapy for latex allergy (either subcutaneous or sublingual immunotherapy) has been evaluated. However, the frequency and severity of side effects remain high so immunotherapy for patients with moderate to severe asthma is contraindicated .[54,56]

ANGIOTENSIN-CONVERTING ENZYME INHIBITOR—INDUCED COUGH

❶ Cough has become a well-recognized side effect of angiotensin-converting enzyme (ACE) inhibitor therapy. According to spontaneous reporting by patients, cough occurs in 1% to 10% of patients receiving ACE inhibitors, with a preponderance of females. In a retrospective analysis, 14.6% of women had cough compared with 6.0% of the men on ACE inhibitors. It is suggested that women have a lower cough threshold, resulting in their reporting this adverse effect more commonly than men.[57] Studies specifically evaluating cough caused by ACE inhibitors report a prevalence of 19% to 25%.[58,59] Patients receiving ACE inhibitors had a 2.3 times greater likelihood of developing cough than a similar group of patients receiving diuretics.[58] Patients with hyperreactive airways do not appear to be at greater risk.[58] African Americans and Chinese have a higher incidence of cough.[57] When different disease states were compared, 26% of patients with heart failure had ACE inhibitor—induced cough compared with 14% of those with hypertension.[57] Cough can occur with all ACE inhibitors.[60]

The cough is typically dry and nonproductive, persistent, and not paroxysmal.[60] The severity of cough varies from a "tickle" to a debilitating cough with insomnia and vomiting. The cough can begin within 3 days or have a delayed onset of up to 12 months following initiation of ACE inhibitor therapy.[60] The cough remits within 1 to 4 days of discontinuing therapy but (rarely) can last up to 4 weeks and recur with rechallenge.[60] Patients should be given a 4-day withdrawal to determine if the cough is induced by ACE inhibitors. The chest radiograph is normal, as are pulmonary function tests (spirometry and diffusing capacity). Bronchial hyperreactivity, as measured by histamine and methacholine provocation, may be worsened in patients with underlying bronchial hyperreactivity such as asthma and chronic bronchitis. However, bronchial hyperreactivity is not induced in others.[60,61] The cough reflex to capsaicin is enhanced but not to nebulized distilled water or citric acid.[60]

The mechanism of ACE inhibitor—induced cough is still unknown. ACE is a nonspecific enzyme that also catalyzes the hydrolysis of bradykinin and substance P (see Chap. 19) that produce or facilitate inflammation and stimulate lung irritant receptors.[60] ACE inhibitors may also induce cyclooxygenase to cause the production of prostaglandins. NSAIDs, benzonatate, inhaled bupivacaine, theophylline, baclofen, thromboxane A_2 synthase inhibitor,[57,62] and cromolyn sodium all have been used to suppress or inhibit ACE inhibitor—induced cough.[60,63] The cough is generally unresponsive to cough suppressants or bronchodilator therapy. No long-term trials evaluating different treatment options for ACE inhibitor—induced cough exist. Cromolyn sodium may be considered first because it is the ❷ most studied agent and has minimal toxicity.[57] The preferred therapy is withdrawal of the ACE inhibitor and replacement with an alternative antihypertensive agent. Owing to their decrease in ACE inhibitor—induced side effects, angiotensin II receptor antagonists are often recommended in place of an ACE inhibitor; however, there are rare reports of this agent inducing bronchospasm.[64] The clinical trials suggest that angiotensin II receptor antagonists have the same incidence of cough as placebo. Furthermore, when angiotensin II receptor antagonists were compared with ACE inhibitors, cough occurred much less frequently. Reduction in the incidence of cough with angiotensin II receptor antagonists is likely caused by the lack of effect on clearance of bradykinin and substance P.[65] The use of alternative therapies to treat ACE inhibitor—induced cough is generally not recommended.[60]

PULMONARY EDEMA

Pulmonary edema may result from the failure of any of a number of homeostatic mechanisms. The most common cause of pulmonary edema is an increase in capillary hydrostatic pressure because of left ventricular failure. Excessive fluid administration in compensated

and decompensated heart failure patients is the most frequent cause of iatrogenic pulmonary edema. Besides hydrostatic forces, other homeostatic mechanisms that may be disrupted include the osmotic and oncotic pressures in the vasculature, the integrity of the alveolar epithelium, the interstitial pulmonary pressure, and the interstitial lymph flow.[6] The edema fluid in cardiogenic pulmonary edema contains a low amount of protein, whereas noncardiogenic pulmonary edema fluid has a high protein concentration.[6] This indicates that noncardiogenic pulmonary edema results primarily from disruption of the alveolar epithelium.

The clinical presentation of pulmonary edema includes persistent cough, tachypnea, dyspnea, tachycardia, rales on auscultation, hypoxemia from ventilation—perfusion imbalance and intrapulmonary shunting, widespread fluffy infiltrates on chest roentgenogram, and decreased lung compliance (stiff lungs). Noncardiogenic pulmonary edema may progress to hemorrhage; cellular debris collects in the alveoli, followed by hyperplasia and fibrosis with a residual restrictive mechanical defect.[6,66]

NARCOTIC-INDUCED PULMONARY EDEMA

The most common drug-induced noncardiogenic pulmonary edema is produced by the narcotic analgesics (Table 36–4).[6] Narcotic-induced pulmonary edema is associated most commonly with intravenous heroin use but also has occurred with morphine,

TABLE 36-4	Drugs That Induce Pulmonary Edema	
		Relative Frequency of Reactions
Cardiogenic pulmonary edema		
Excessive intravenous fluids		F
Blood and plasma transfusions		F
Corticosteroids		F
Phenylbutazone		R
Sodium diatrizoate		R
Hypertonic intrathecal saline		R
β_2-Adrenergic agonists		I
Noncardiogenic pulmonary edema		
Heroin		F
Methadone		I
Morphine		I
Oxygen		I
Propoxyphene		R
Ethchlorvynol		R
Chlordiazepoxide		R
Salicylate		R
Hydrochlorothiazide		R
Triamterene + hydrochlorothiazide		R
Leukoagglutinin reactions		R
Iron—dextran complex		R
Methotrexate		R
Cytosine arabinoside		R
Nitrofurantoin		R
Dextran 40		R
Fluorescein		R
Amitriptyline		R
Colchicine		R
Nitrogen mustard		R
Epinephrine		R
Metaraminol		R
Bleomycin		R
Iodide		R
Cyclophosphamide		R
VM-26		R

F, frequent; I, infrequent; R, rare.

methadone, meperidine, and propoxyphene use.[6,66,67] There have also been a few reported cases associated with the use of the opiate antagonist naloxone and nalmefene, a long-acting opioid antagonist.[66,68,69] The mechanism is unknown but may be related to hypoxemia similar to the neurogenic pulmonary edema associated with cerebral tumors or trauma or a direct toxic effect on the alveolar capillary membrane.[67] Initially thought to occur only with overdoses, most evidence now supports the theory that narcotic-induced pulmonary edema is an idiosyncratic reaction to moderate as well as high narcotic doses.[66,67]

Patients with pulmonary edema may be comatose with depressed respirations or dyspnea and tachypnea. They may or may not have other signs of narcotic overdose. Symptomatology varies from cough and mild crepitations on auscultation with characteristic radiologic findings to severe cyanosis and hypoxemia, even with supplemental oxygen. Symptoms may appear within minutes of intravenous administration but may take up to 2 hours to occur, particularly following oral methadone.[67] Hemodynamic studies in the first 24 hours have demonstrated normal pulmonary capillary wedge pressures in the presence of pulmonary edema.

Clinical symptoms generally improve within 24 to 48 hours, and radiologic clearing occurs in 2 to 5 days, but abnormalities in pulmonary function tests may persist for 10 to 12 weeks. Therapy consists of naloxone administration, supplemental oxygen, and ventilatory support if required. Mortality is less than 1%.[67]

Cough has been reported with intravenous administration of fentanyl.[70] A cohort of 1,311 adult patients undergoing elective surgery had 120 patients with vigorous cough within 20 seconds after administration of fentanyl.[70] The cough was associated with young age and absence of cigarette smoking.[70] Among anesthetic factors, it was associated with the absence of epidurally administered lidocaine and the absence of a priming dose of vecuronium.[70] A history of asthma or COPD had no predictive effect.[70] Further clinical trials are required to understand the mechanism of paradoxical cough with fentanyl and to identify the means to prevent it.

OTHER DRUGS THAT CAUSE PULMONARY EDEMA

A paradoxical pulmonary edema has been reported in a few patients following hydrochlorothiazide ingestion but not any other thiazide diuretic.[6] Acute pulmonary edema rarely has followed the injection of high concentrations of contrast medium into the pulmonary circulation during angiocardiography.[6] Rare occurrences of pulmonary edema have followed the intravenous administration of bleomycin, cyclophosphamide, and vinblastine.[6]

The selective β_2-adrenergic agonists terbutaline and ritodrine have been reported to induce pulmonary edema when used as tocolytics.[6] This disorder commonly occurs 48 to 72 hours after tocolytic therapy.[69] This has never occurred with their use in asthma patients, even in inadvertent overdosage. This reaction may result from excess fluid administration used to prevent the hypotension from β_2-mediated vasodilation or the particular hemodynamics of pregnancy. In a review of 330 patients who received tocolytic therapy and were monitored closely for their fluid status, no episode of pulmonary edema was reported.[69]

Interleukin-2, a cytokine used alone or in combination with cytotoxic drugs, has been reported to induce pulmonary edema. Although other cytokines have been associated with pulmonary edema, the problem is most significant with interleukin-2. A weight gain of 2 kg has been reported after treatment with interleukin-2.[69]

Pulmonary edema has occurred occasionally with salicylate overdoses. The serum salicylate concentrations are often greater than 45 mg/dL, and the patients have other signs of toxicity, although some cases have been associated with concentrations in the usual therapeutic range.[66,67]

PULMONARY EOSINOPHILIA

Pulmonary infiltrates with eosinophilia (Löffler syndrome) are associated with nitrofurantoin, *para*-aminosalicylic acid, methotrexate, sulfonamides, tetracycline, chlorpropamide, phenytoin, NSAIDs, and imipramine (Table 36–5).[6,71,72] The disorder is characterized by fever, nonproductive cough, dyspnea, cyanosis, bilateral pulmonary infiltrates, and eosinophilia in the blood.[6] Lung biopsy has revealed perivasculitis with infiltration of eosinophils, macrophages, and proteinaceous edema fluid in the alveoli. The symptoms and eosinophilia generally respond rapidly to withdrawal of the offending drug.

Sulfonamides were first reported as causative agents in users of sulfanilamide vaginal cream.[6] *para*-Aminosalicylic acid frequently produced the syndrome in tuberculosis patients being treated with this agent.[6] There are nine reported cases associated with sulfasalazine use in inflammatory bowel disease.[71] The drug associated most frequently with this syndrome is nitrofurantoin.[6,67] Nitrofurantoin-induced lung disorders appear to be more common in postmenopausal women.[67] Lung reactions made up 43% of 921 adverse reactions to nitrofurantoin reported to the Swedish Adverse Drug Reaction Committee between 1966 and 1976.[71] No apparent correlation exists between duration of drug exposure and severity or reversibility of the reaction.[71] Most cases occur within 1 month of therapy. Typical symptoms include fever, tachypnea, dyspnea, dry cough, and, less commonly, pleuritic chest pain. Radiographic findings include bilateral interstitial infiltrates, predominant in the bases and pleural effusions 25% of the time. Although there are anecdotal reports that steroids are beneficial, the usual rapid improvement following discontinuation of the drugs brings the usefulness of steroids into question. Complete recovery usually occurs within 15 days of withdrawal.

TABLE 36-5	Drugs That Induce Pulmonary Infiltrates with Eosinophilia (Löffler Syndrome)		
Drug	Relative Frequency of Reactions	Drug	Relative Frequency of Reactions
Nitrofurantoin	F	Tetracycline	R
para-Aminosalicylic acid	F	Procarbazine	R
Amiodarone	F	Cromolyn	R
Iodine	F	Niridazole	R
Captopril	F	Chlorpromazine	R
Bleomycin	F	Naproxen	R
L-tryptophan	F	Sulindac	R
Methotrexate	F	Ibuprofen	R
Phenytoin	F	Chlorpropamide	R
Gold salts	F	Mephenesin	R
Sulfonamides	I		
Penicillins	I		
Carbamazepine	I		
Granulocyte-macrophage colony stimulating factor	I		
Imipramine	I		
Minocycline	I		
Nilutamide	I		
Propylthiouracil	I		
Sulfazalazine	I		

F, frequent; I, infrequent; R, rare.

A few cases of pulmonary eosinophilia have been reported in asthmatics treated with cromolyn.[6,71] The significance of this is unknown in light of the occasional spontaneous occurrence of pulmonary eosinophilia in asthmatic patients. Cases of acute pneumonitis and eosinophilia have been reported to occur with phenytoin and carbamazepine therapy.[71] Patients have had other symptoms of hypersensitivity, including fever and rashes. The symptoms of dyspnea and cough subside following discontinuation of the drug.

OXYGEN TOXICITY

Because of the similarity to pulmonary fibrosis, oxygen-induced lung toxicity is reviewed briefly. More extensive reviews on this topic have been published.[73,74]

The earliest manifestation of oxygen toxicity is substernal pleuritic pain from tracheobronchitis.[74] The onset of toxicity follows an asymptomatic period and presents as cough, chest pain, and dyspnea. Early symptoms are usually masked in ventilator-dependent patients. The first noted physiologic change is a decrease in pulmonary compliance caused by reversible atelectasis. Then decreases in vital capacity occur, followed by progressive abnormalities in carbon monoxide diffusing capacity.[74] Decreased inspiratory flow rates, reflected in the need for high inspiratory pressures in ventilator-dependent patients, occur as the fractional concentration of inspired oxygen requirement increases. The lungs become progressively stiffer as the ability to oxygenate becomes more compromised.

The fraction of inspired oxygen and duration of exposure are both important determinants of the severity of lung damage. Normal human volunteers can tolerate 100% oxygen at sea level for 24 to 48 hours with minimal to no damage.[73] Oxygen concentrations of less than 50% are well tolerated even for extended periods. Inspired oxygen concentrations between 50% and 100% carry a substantial risk of lung damage, and the duration required is inversely proportional to the fraction of inspired oxygen.[73] Underlying disease states may alter this relationship. Lung damage may not be lasting and may improve months to years after the exposure.[75,76]

Oxygen-induced lung damage is generally separated into the acute exudative phase and the subacute or chronic proliferative phase. The acute phase consists of perivascular, peribronchiolar, interstitial, and alveolar edema with alveolar hemorrhage and necrosis of pulmonary endothelium and type I epithelial cells.[73] The proliferative phase consists of resorption of the exudates and hyperplasia of interstitial and type II alveolar lining cells. Collagen and elastin deposition in the interstitium of alveolar walls then leads to thickening of the gas-exchange area and the fibrosis.[73]

The biochemical mechanism of the tissue damage during hyperoxia is the increased production of highly reactive, partially reduced oxygen metabolites (Fig. 36-1).[74] These oxidants are normally produced in small quantities during cellular respiration and include the superoxide anion, hydrogen peroxide, the hydroxyl radical, singlet oxygen, and hypochlorous acid.[74] Oxygen free radicals are normally formed in phagocytic cells to kill invading microorganisms, but they are also toxic to normal cell components. The oxidants produce toxicity through destructive redox reactions with protein sulfhydryl groups, membrane lipids, and nucleic acids.[74]

The oxidants are products of normal cellular respiration that are normally counterbalanced by an antioxidant defense system that prevents tissue destruction. The antioxidants include superoxide dismutase, catalase, glutathione peroxidase, ceruloplasmin, and α-tocopherol (vitamin E). Antioxidants are ubiquitous in the body. Hyperoxia produces toxicity by overwhelming the antioxidant system. There is experimental evidence that a number of drugs and

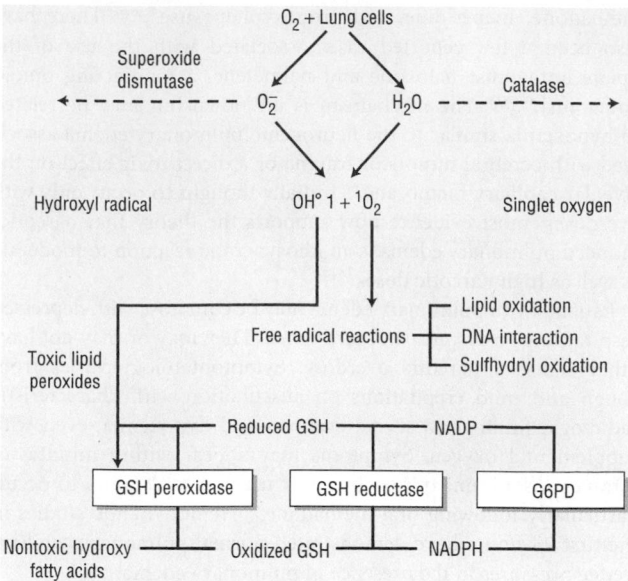

FIGURE 36-1. Schematic of the interaction of oxygen radicals and the antioxidant system. (GSH, glutathione; G6PD, glucose-6-phosphate dehydrogenase; NADP, nicotinamide-adenine dinucleotide phosphate; NADPH, reduced NADP.)

chemicals produce lung toxicity through increasing production of oxidants (e.g., bleomycin, cyclophosphamide, nitrofurantoin, and paraquat) and/or by inhibiting the antioxidant system (e.g., carmustine, cyclophosphamide, and nitrofurantoin).[77,78]

PULMONARY FIBROSIS

A large number of drugs are associated with chronic pulmonary fibrosis with or without a preceding acute pneumonitis (Table 36-6). The cancer chemotherapeutic agents make up the largest group and have been the subject of numerous reviews.[77,78]

TABLE 36-6	Drugs That Induce Pneumonitis and/or Fibrosis		
Drug	**Relative Frequency of Reactions**	**Drug**	**Relative Frequency of Reactions**
Oxygen	F	Chlorambucil	R
Radiation	F	Melphalan	R
Bleomycin	F	Lomustine and semustine	R
Busulfan	F	Zinostatin	R
Carmustine	F	Procarbazine	R
Hexamethonium	F	Teniposide	R
Paraquat	F	Sulfasalazine	R
Amiodarone	F	Phenytoin	R
Mecamylamine	I	Gold salts	R
Pentolinium	I	Pindolol	R
Cyclophosphamide	I	Imipramine	R
Practolol	I	Penicillamine	R
Methotrexate	I	Phenylbutazone	R
Mitomycin	I	Chlorphentermine	R
Nitrofurantoin	I	Fenfluramine	R
Methysergide	I	Leflunomide	R
Sirolimus	I	Mefloquine	R
Azathioprine, 6-mercaptopurine	R	Pergolide	R

F, frequent; I, infrequent; R, rare.

Although the mechanisms by which all the drugs produce pneumonitis and fibrosis are not known, the clinical syndrome, pulmonary function abnormalities, and histopathology present a relatively homogeneous pattern.[77] The histopathological picture closely resembles oxidant lung damage, and in some experimental cases, oxygen enhances the pulmonary injury.[67] Although the terms *pulmonary fibrosis* or *interstitial pneumonitis* have been used widely to describe pneumonia after bone marrow transplantation, in 1991, a National Institutes of Health workshop recommended that the term *idiopathic pneumonia syndrome* (IPS) should be used to avoid histopathological terms and to define the inherent heterogeneity of this disorder.[79] IPS accounts for more than 40% of deaths related to bone marrow transplantation.[79] Suggested causes of IPS include radiation or chemotherapy regimens prior to transplantation, graft-versus-host disease, unrecognized infections, and other inflammation-related lung injuries.[80,81] IPS is characterized by dyspnea, hypoxemia, nonproductive cough, diffuse alveolar damage, and interstitial pneumonitis in the absence of lower respiratory infection. IPS has been reported early and late, up to 24 months after bone marrow transplantation.[81]

The lung damage following ingestion of the contact herbicide paraquat classically resembles hyperoxic lung damage. Hyperoxia accelerates the lung damage induced by paraquat. Lung toxicity from paraquat occurs following oral administration in humans and aerosol administration and inhalation in experimental animals.[78] The pulmonary specificity of paraquat results in part from its active uptake into lung tissue. Paraquat readily accepts an electron from reduced nicotinamide-adenine dinucleotide phosphate and then is reoxidized rapidly, forming superoxide and other oxygen radicals.[78] The toxicity may be a result of nicotinamide-adenine dinucleotide phosphate depletion (see Fig. 36–1) and/or excess oxygen free radical generation with lipid peroxidation. Treatment with exogenous superoxide dismutase has had limited and conflicting results.[78]

A number of furans have been shown to produce oxidant injury to lungs.[78] Occasionally, patients with acute nitrofurantoin lung toxicity will progress to a chronic reaction leading to fibrosis, and rarely, a patient may develop chronic toxicity without an antecedent acute reaction. Like paraquat, nitrofurantoin undergoes cyclic reduction and reoxidation that may produce superoxide radicals or deplete nicotinamide-adenine dinucleotide phosphate. In addition, nitrofurantoin inhibits glutathione reductase, an enzyme involved in the glutathione antioxidant system (see Fig. 36–1). Table 36–7 lists possible nondrug causes of pulmonary fibrosis.

DRUGS ASSOCIATED WITH PULMONARY FIBROSIS

ANTINEOPLASTICS

A number of cancer chemotherapeutic agents produce pulmonary fibrosis. In an excellent review,[77] six predisposing factors for the development of cytotoxic drug—induced pulmonary disease were described: (a) cumulative dose, (b) increased age, (c) concurrent or previous radiotherapy, (d) oxygen therapy, (e) other cytotoxic drug therapy, and (f) preexisting pulmonary disease. Drugs that are directly toxic to the lung would be expected to show a dose—response relationship. Dose—response relationships have been established for bleomycin, busulfan, and carmustine (BCNU).[77] Bleomycin and busulfan exhibit threshold cumulative doses below which a very small percentage of patients exhibit toxicity, but carmustine shows a more linear relationship.[78] Older patients appear to be more susceptible, possibly as a result of a decrease in the antioxidant defense system.

TABLE 36-7 Possible Causes of Pulmonary Fibrosis

Idiopathic pulmonary fibrosis (fibrosing alveolitis)
Pneumoconiosis (asbestosis, silicosis, coal dust, talc berylliosis)
Hypersensitivity pneumonitis (molds, bacteria, animal proteins, toluene diisocyanate, epoxy resins)
Smoking
Sarcoidosis
Tuberculosis
Lipoid pneumonia
Systemic lupus erythematosus
Rheumatoid arthritis
Systemic sclerosis
Polymyositis/dermatomyositis
Sjögren syndrome
Polyarteritis nodosa
Wegener granuloma
Byssinosis (cotton workers)
Siderosis (arc welders' lung)
Radiation
Oxygen
Chemicals (thioureas, trialkylphosphorothioates, furans)
Drugs (see Tables 36–5, 36–6, and 36–8)

Excessive irradiation produces a pneumonitis and fibrosis thought to be caused by oxygen free radical formation.[77] Evidence for synergistic toxicity with radiation exists for bleomycin, busulfan, and mitomycin.[77] Hyperoxia has shown synergistic toxicity with bleomycin, cyclophosphamide, and mitomycin.[77] Carmustine, mitomycin, cyclophosphamide, bleomycin, and methotrexate all appear to show increased lung toxicity when they are part of multiple-drug regimens.

NITROSOUREAS

BCNU is associated with the highest incidence of pulmonary toxicity (20% to 30%).[77] The lung pathology generally resembles that produced by bleomycin and busulfan. Unique to BCNU is the finding of fibrosis in the absence of inflammatory infiltrates. BCNU preferentially inhibits glutathione reductase, the enzyme required to regenerate glutathione, thus reducing glutathione tissue stores.[77,78] The patients present with dyspnea, tachypnea, and nonproductive cough that may begin within a month of initiation of therapy but may not develop for as long as 3 years.[77] Most patients receiving BCNU develop fibrosis that may remain asymptomatic or become symptomatic any time up to 17 years after therapy.[82] The cumulative dose has ranged from 580 to 2,100 mg/m^2.[78] The disease is usually slowly progressive with a mortality rate from 15% to greater than 90% depending on the study and period of follow-up. In a retrospective study, the risk factors for development of IPS and prognostic factors for outcomes were evaluated in 94 patients with relapsed Hodgkin disease treated with BCNU containing high-dose chemotherapy and hematopoietic support. The risk factors for pulmonary fibrosis and mortality were female sex and dose of BCNU, with all deaths reported in those who received BCNU at doses of more than 475 mg/m^2.[83] Rapid progression and death within a few days occur in a small percentage of patients.[77] Corticosteroids do not appear to be effective in reducing damage.[77] Other nitrosoureas, lomustine, and semustine have also been reported to produce lung damage in patients receiving unusually high doses.[77]

BLEOMYCIN

Bleomycin is the best-studied cytotoxic pulmonary toxin. Because of its lack of bone marrow suppression, pulmonary toxicity is the dose-limiting toxicity of bleomycin therapy. The incidence of bleomycin lung toxicity is approximately 4%, which may be affected by the following risk factors: bleomycin cumulative dose, age, high concentration of inspired oxygen, radiation therapy, and multidrug regimens, particularly those with cyclophosphamide.[69] Age at the time of treatment with bleomycin may also be a risk factor; patients younger than 7 years of age at the time of receiving bleomycin therapy are more likely to develop pulmonary toxicity compared with older subjects.[69] The cumulative dose above which the incidence of toxicity significantly increases is 450 to 500 units.[77] However, rapidly fatal pulmonary toxicity has occurred with doses as low as 100 units.[77]

Experimentally, bleomycin generates superoxide anions, and the lung toxicity is increased by radiation and hyperoxia.[77] Pretreatment with superoxide dismutase and catalase reduces toxicity in experimental animals.[77] Bleomycin also oxidizes arachidonic acid, which may account for the marked inflammation. Bleomycin may also affect collagen deposition by its stimulation of fibroblast growth.[77] Combination of bleomycin with other cytotoxic agents, particularly regimens containing cyclophosphamide, may predispose patients to pulmonary damage.

There are two distinct clinical patterns of bleomycin pulmonary toxicity. Chronic progressive fibrosis is the most common; acute hypersensitivity reactions occur infrequently. Patients present with cough and dyspnea. The first physiologic abnormality seen is a decreased diffusing capacity of carbon monoxide.[77] Chest radiographs show a bibasilar reticular pattern, and gallium scans show marked uptake in the involved lung.[77] Chest radiographic changes lag behind pulmonary function abnormalities. Spirometry tests before each bleomycin dose are not predictive of toxicity. The single-breath diffusing capacity of carbon monoxide is the most sensitive indicator of bleomycin-induced lung disease. Although it is not absolutely predictive, a drop of 20% or greater in the diffusing capacity of carbon monoxide is an indication for using alternative therapies.[77] The prognosis of bleomycin lung toxicity has improved as a consequence of early detection, but the mortality rate is approximately 25%. Mild cases respond to discontinuation of bleomycin therapy.[69] Corticosteroid therapy appears to be helpful in patients with acute pneumonitis, although there have been no controlled trials. Patients with chronic fibrosis are less likely to respond. Although corticosteroids have been used for a number of drug-induced pulmonary problems, a study in mice showing a potential for worsening of lung damage when administered early during the repair stage should sound a word of caution against their indiscriminate use.[84]

MITOMYCIN

Mitomycin is an alkylating antibiotic that produces pulmonary fibrosis at a frequency of 3% to 12%.[77] The mechanism is unknown, but oxygen and radiation therapy appear to enhance the development of toxicity.[77] The clinical presentation and symptoms are the same as for bleomycin. The mortality rate is approximately 50%. Early withdrawal of the drug and administration of corticosteroids appear to improve the outcome significantly.

ALKYLATING AGENTS

A number of alkylating agents are associated with pulmonary fibrosis (see Table 36–5). The incidence of clinical toxicity is around 4%, although subclinical damage is apparent in up to 46% of patients at autopsy. The mechanism of toxicity is unknown; however, epithelial cell damage that triggers the arachidonic acid inflammatory cascade may be the initiating event.[77] The clinical presentation is insidious, with 4 years being the average durationof therapy before the onset of symptoms.[77] Patients present with low-grade fever, weight loss, weakness, dyspnea, cough, and rales.[77] Pulmonary function tests

initially show abnormal diffusion capacity followed by a restrictive pattern (low vital capacity). The histopathologic findings are nonspecific. The prognosis is one of slow progression with a mean survival of 5 months following diagnosis.[77] Although there is no direct dose-dependent correlation, patients receiving less than 500 mg of busulfan do not develop the syndrome without concomitant radiation or use of other pulmonary toxic chemotherapeutic agents.[77] There are anecdotal reports of beneficial responses to corticosteroids, but no controlled studies have been done.

Cyclophosphamide infrequently produces pulmonary toxicity. More than 20 well-documented cases have been reported to date. In animal models, cyclophosphamide produces reactive oxygen radicals. High oxygen concentrations produce synergistic toxicity with cyclophosphamide. The duration of therapy before the onset of symptoms is highly variable, and there may be a delay of several months between the onset of symptoms and discontinuation of the drug.[77] Cyclophosphamide may potentiate carmustine lung toxicity.[77] Clinical symptoms usually consist of dyspnea on exertion, cough, and fever. Inspiratory crackles and the bibasilar reticular pattern typical of cytotoxic drug-induced radiographic changes are present. Histopathological changes are also nonspecific. Approximately 60% of patients recover. Corticosteroid therapy has been reported to be beneficial; however, death despite corticosteroid administration has also been reported.

Chlorambucil, melphalan, and uracil mustard are also associated with pulmonary fibrosis. Of the alkylating agents, only nitrogen mustard and thiotepa have not been reported to cause fibrotic pulmonary toxicity.[77]

ANTIMETABOLITES

Methotrexate was first reported to induce pulmonary toxicity in 1969.[77] The pulmonary toxicity to methotrexate is unique in that discontinuation is not always necessary, and reinstitution of the drug may not produce recurrence of symptoms.[6] Methotrexate pulmonary toxicity most commonly appears to result from hypersensitivity,[71] and it can occur 3 or more years following methotrexate therapy.[85] Age, sex, underlying pulmonary disease, duration of therapy, or smoking is not associated with an increased risk of pneumonitis with methotrexate.[85] Serial pulmonary function tests did not help to identify pneumonitis in patients receiving methotrexate before the onset of clinical symptoms.[85] Reductions in diffusing capacity of carbon monoxide and lung volumes are the most common manifestations of methotrexate lung toxicity.[69] Pulmonary edema and eosinophilia are common, and fibrosis occurs in only 10% of the patients who develop acute pneumonitis.[77] Systemic symptoms of chills, fever, and malaise are common before the onset of dyspnea, cough, and acute pleuritic chest pain. Methotrexate is also associated with granuloma formation.[77]

The prognosis of methotrexate-induced pulmonary toxicity is good, with a 1% or less mortality rate.[71] Pulmonary toxicity has followed intrathecal as well as oral administration and has occurred after single doses as well as long-term daily and intermittent administration.[77] Pneumonitis has been reported to occur up to 4 weeks following discontinuation of therapy.[77] Numerous anecdotal reports have claimed dramatic benefit from corticosteroid therapy. It is unknown whether intermittent (weekly) dosing, as is done for rheumatoid arthritis, decreases the risk of methotrexate-induced pulmonary toxicity because pneumonitis has occurred with this form of dosing.

Rarely, azathioprine and its major metabolite 6-mercaptopurine have been reported to produce an acute restrictive lung disease. Procarbazine, a methylhydrazine associated more commonly with Löffler syndrome, rarely has been associated with pulmonary fibrosis.[71] The vinca alkaloids vinblastine and vindesine have been reported to produce severe respiratory toxicity in association with mitomycin. The incidence with the combination is 39% and may represent a true synergistic effect between these agents.[77]

NONCYTOTOXIC DRUGS

Pulmonary fibrosis associated with the ganglionic-blocking agent hexamethonium was first reported in 1954 (see Table 36-6).[6] Patients developed extreme dyspnea after several months on the drug. Pathological findings were consistent with bronchiectasis, bronchiolectasis, and fibrosis.[6] This phenomenon has occurred occasionally with use of the other ganglionic blockers (i.e., mecamylamine and pentolinium).[6]

In 1959, radiographic changes characteristic of diffuse pulmonary fibrosis were reported in 27 (87%) of 31 patients who had taken phenytoin for 2 years or more.[67] Since then, studies have been conflicting. If phenytoin does produce chronic fibrosis, it would appear to be a relatively rare event.

Gold salts (sodium aurothiomalate) used in the treatment of rheumatoid arthritis have produced pulmonary fibrosis with cough, dyspnea, and pleuritic pain 5 to 16 weeks following institution of therapy.[67] Pulmonary function tests show a restrictive defect, and patients generally have an eosinophilia. The reactions improve on discontinuation of the gold therapy and recur promptly on reexposure. The pulmonary deficit may not resolve completely.

AMIODARONE

Amiodarone, a benzofuran derivative, produces pulmonary fibrosis when used for supraventricular and ventricular arrhythmias (see Table 36-6).[86] The duration of amiodarone therapy before the onset of symptoms has ranged from 4 weeks to 6 years.[67,86,87] The estimated incidence is 1 in 1,000 to 2,000 treated patients per year. The clinical course is variable, ranging from acute onset of dyspnea with rapid progression into severe respiratory failure and death caused by slowly developing exertional dyspnea over a few months. Patients generally improve on discontinuation of the drug.[86,87] The majority of patients develop reactions while taking maintenance doses greater than 400 mg daily for more than 2 months or smaller doses for more than 2 years. The risk of amiodarone pulmonary toxicity is higher during the first 12 months of therapy even at a low dosage.[88] Other risk factors include cardiopulmonary surgery combined with the administration of high concentrations of oxygen.[88] Routine spirometry does not appear to be predictive of patients at risk.[89] Carbon monoxide diffusing capacity studies are sensitive indicators of amiodarone pulmonary toxicity but have only a 21% positive predictive value.[89] Clinical findings include exertional dyspnea, nonproductive cough, weight loss, and occasionally low-grade fever.[67,87,89] Radiographic changes are nondiagnostic and consist of diffuse bilateral interstitial changes consistent with a pneumonitis. Pulmonary function abnormalities include hypoxia, restrictive changes, and diffusion abnormalities.

The mechanism of amiodarone-induced pulmonary toxicity is multifactorial. Amiodarone and its metabolite can damage lung tissue directly by a cytotoxic process or indirectly by immunologic reactions.[88] Amiodarone is an amphiphilic molecule that contains both a highly apolar aromatic ring system and a polar side chain with a positively charged nitrogen atom.[86] Amphiphilic drugs characteristically produce a phospholipid storage disorder in the lungs of experimental animals and humans.[78] Chlorphentermine, an anorectic, is the prototype amphiphilic compound. The mechanism is currently believed to be the inhibition of lysosomal phospholipases.[78] The inflammation and fibrosis are thought to be a late finding resulting from nonspecific inflammation following the breakdown of phospholipid-laden macrophages.[86]

In a review of 39 cases, 9 patients died, and the remaining 30 patients had resolution of abnormalities after withdrawal of the drug.[86] Some patients have had resolution with lowering of the dosage, and therapy has been reinstituted at lower doses without problems in others. Of the patients who died, one half had received corticosteroids. There are reports of a protective effect with prophylactic corticosteroids and other reports of patients developing amiodarone lung toxicity while on corticosteroids.[86] At this time, any benefit of corticosteroids is unclear because most patients improve after stopping the drug.

MISCELLANEOUS PULMONARY TOXICITY

Drugs may produce serious pulmonary toxicity as part of a more generalized disorder. The pleural thickening, effusions, and fibrosis that occur as an extension of the retroperitoneal fibrotic reactions of methysergide and practolol or as part of a drug-induced lupus syndrome are the most common examples (Table 36-8).

Pleural and pulmonary fibrosis has been reported in one patient taking pindolol, a β-blocker structurally similar to practolol, an agent known to produce fibrosis.[67] Acute pleuritis with pleural effusions and fibrosis is a prominent manifestation of drug-induced lupus syndrome. Procainamide is associated with the largest number of pulmonary reactions, with 46% of patients with the lupus syndrome developing pulmonary complications.[6] Symptoms include pleuritic pain and fever with muscle and joint pain. Chest radiographs show bilateral pleural effusions and linear atelectasis. Patients have a positive antinuclear antibody test. Symptoms usually resolve within 6 weeks of drug withdrawal.[6]

Hydralazine is the next most common cause of lupus syndrome. Most patients who develop pleuropulmonary manifestations have antecedent symptoms of generalized lupus.[6] Other drugs that produce the lupus syndrome include isoniazid and phenytoin. Phenytoin can also produce hilar lymphadenopathy as part of a generalized pseudolymphoma or lymphadenopathy syndrome.[6]

TABLE 36-8	Drugs That May Induce Pleural Effusions and Fibrosis	
		Relative Frequency of Reactions
Idiopathic		
Methysergide		F
Practolol		F
Pindolol		R
Methotrexate		R
Nitrofurantoin		R
Drug-induced lupus syndrome		
Procainamide		F
Hydralazine		F
Isoniazid		R
Phenytoin		R
Mephenytoin		R
Griseofulvin		R
Trimethadione		R
Sulfonamides		R
Phenylbutazone		R
Streptomycin		R
Ethosuximide		R
Tetracycline		R
Pseudolymphoma syndrome		
Cyclosporine		R
Phenytoin		R

F, frequent; I, infrequent; R, rare.

MONITORING THERAPEUTIC OUTCOMES

Monitoring for drug-induced pulmonary diseases consists primarily of having a high index of suspicion that a particular syndrome may be drug induced. Most hypersensitivity or allergic reactions (bronchospasm) occur rapidly, within the first 2 weeks of therapy with the offending agent, and reverse rapidly with appropriate therapy (e.g., withdrawal of the offending agent and administration of corticosteroids and bronchodilators). Dyspnea associated with Löffler syndrome and acute pulmonary edema syndromes also improve rapidly in 1 to 2 days. However, some residual defect in diffusion capacity and the roentgenogram may persist for a few weeks. It is probably unnecessary to do follow-up spirometry or diffusion capacity determinations in these patients unless there is some concern that the syndrome will progress to pulmonary fibrosis (through the use of bleomycin or nitrofurantoin).

The routine monitoring of patients receiving known pulmonary toxins with dose-dependent toxicity such as amiodarone, bleomycin, or carmustine is still controversial. For chronic fibrosis, the diffusing capacity of carbon monoxide is the most sensitive test and may be useful in patients receiving bleomycin for detecting and preventing further deterioration of lung function with continued administration. Carmustine lung toxicity may be delayed up to 10 years following administration, and routine monitoring has not proved preventive. Monitoring patients receiving amiodarone in doses greater than 400 mg/day every 4 to 6 months may prove useful in detecting early disease that requires lowering the amiodarone or stopping the drug. Because there is no evidence of a cumulative dose effect once it has been established that the patient can tolerate the elevated dose, continued routine monitoring past the first year is unnecessary.

ABBREVIATIONS

ACE: angiotensin-converting enzyme

COPD: chronic obstructive pulmonary disease

EDTA: ethylenediamine tetraacetic acid

FDA: Food and Drug Administration

FEV_1: forced expiratory volume in the first second of expiration

IPS: idiopathic pneumonia syndrome

NSAIDs: nonsteroidal antiinflammatory drugs

REFERENCES

1. Martys CR. Adverse reactions to drugs in general practice. Br Med J 1979;2:1194–1197.
2. Messaad D, Sahla H, Benahmed S, Godard P, et al. Drug provocation tests in patients with a history suggesting an immediate drug hypersensitivity reaction. Ann Intern Med 2004;140:1001–1006.
3. Levy M, Kewitz H, Altwein W, et al. Hospital admissions due to adverse drug reactions: A comparative study from Jerusalem and Berlin. Eur J Clin Pharmacol 1980;17:25–31.
4. Shapiro S, Slone D, Lewis GP, et al. Fatal drug reactions among medical inpatients. JAMA 1971;216:467–472.
5. Porter J, Jick H. Drug-related deaths among medical inpatients. JAMA 1977;237:879–881.
6. Brewis RAL. Respiratory disorders. In: Davies DM, ed. Textbook of Adverse Drug Reactions, 2d ed. New York: Oxford University Press; 1981:154–178.
7. Hansen-Flaschen J, Cowen J, Raps EC. Neuromuscular blockade in the intensive care unit: More than we bargained for. Am Rev Respir Dis 1993;147:234–236.
8. Lieu F, Powers SK, Herb RA, et al. Exercise and glucocorticoid-induced diaphragmatic myopathy. J Appl Physiol 1993;75:763–771.
9. Dekhuijzen PNR, Gayan-Ramirez G, de Bock V, et al. Triamcinolone and prednisolone affect contractile properties and histopathology of rat diaphragm differently. J Clin Invest 1993;92:1534–1542.
10. Decramer M, Lacquet LM, Fagard R, et al. Corticosteroids contribute to muscle weakness in chronic airflow obstruction. Am J Respir Crit Care Med 1994;150:11–16.
11. McKeever TM, Lewis S, Smit HA, et al. The association of acetaminophen, aspirin, and ibuprofen with respiratory disease and lung function. Am J Respir Crit Care Med 2005;171;966–971.
12. Beasley R, Clayton T, Crane J, et al. Association between paracetamol use in infancy and childhood, and risk of asthma, rhinoconjunctivitis, and eczema in children aged 6–7 years: Analysis from Phase Three of the ISAAC programme. Lancet 2008;372:1039–1048.
13. Fisher HK. Drug-induced asthma syndromes. In: Weiss EB, Segal MS, Stein M, eds. Bronchial Asthma: Mechanisms and Therapeutics, 3d ed. Boston: Little, Brown; 1993:938–949.
14. Settipane GA. Aspirin and allergic diseases: A review. Am J Med 1983;74(suppl 6a):102–109.
15. Stevenson DD. Diagnosis, prevention, and treatment of adverse reactions to aspirin and nonsteroidal anti-inflammatory drugs. J Allergy Clin Immunol 1984;74:617–622.
16. Stevenson DD, Szczeklik A. Clinical and pathologic perspectives on aspirin sensitivity and asthma. J Allergy Clin Immunol. 2006;118:773–786.
17. Szczeklik A, Gryglewski RJ. Asthma and antiinflammatory drugs: Mechanisms and clinical patterns. Drugs 1983;25:533–543.
18. Matsuse H, Shimoda T, Matsua N, et al. Aspirin-induced asthma as a risk factor for asthma mortality. J Asthma 1997;34:314–317.
19. Szczezklik A, Nizankowaska E. Clinical features and diagnosis of aspirin induced asthma. Thorax 2000;55(suppl 2):S42–S44.
20. Dahlen B, Melillo G. Inhalation challenge in ASA-induced asthma. Respir Med 1998;92:378–384.
21. Dahlen B, Zetterstrom O. Comparison of bronchial and per oral provocation with aspirin in aspirin-sensitive asthmatics. Eur Respir J 1990;3:527–534.
22. Berges-Gimeno MP, Simon RA, Stevenson DD. Long term treatment with aspirin desensitization in asthmatic patients with aspirin-exacerbated respiratory disease. J Allergy Clin Immunol 2003;111:180–186.
23. Mathison DA, Stevenson DD, Simon RA. Precipitating factors in asthma: Aspirin, sulfites, and other drugs and chemicals. Chest 1985;87(suppl):50–54.
24. American Academy of Pediatrics, Committee on Drugs. "Inactive" ingredients in pharmaceutical products: Update. Pediatrics 1997;99:268–278.
25. Yoshida S, Ishizaki Y, Onuma K, et al. Selective cyclooxygenase 2 inhibitor in patients with aspirin-induced asthma. J Allergy Clin Immunol 2000;106:1201–1202.
26. Szczeklik A, Niankowska E, Bochenek G, et al. Safety of a specific COX-2 inhibitor in aspirin-induced asthma. Clin Exp Allergy 2001;31:219–225.
27. Dahlen B, Szczeklik A, Murray JJ. Celecoxib in patients with asthma and aspirin intolerance. N Engl J Med 2001;344:142.
28. Stevenson DD, Simon RA. Lack of cross-reactivity between rofecoxib and aspirin-sensitive patients with asthma. J Allergy Clin Immunol 2001;108:47–51.
29. Israel E, Fischer A, Rosenberg M, et al. The pivotal role of 5-lipoxygenase products in the reaction of aspirin-sensitive asthmatics to aspirin. Am Rev Respir Dis 1993;148:1447–1451.
30. Paul JD, Simon RA, Daffern PJ, et al. Lack of effect of the 5-lipoxygenase inhibitor zileuton in blocking oral aspirin challenges in aspirin-sensitive asthmatics. Ann Allergy Asthma Immunol 2000;85:40–45.
31. Stevenson DD, Simon RA, Mathison DA, Christiansen SC. Montelukast is only partially effective in inhibiting aspirin response in aspirin-sensitive asthmatics. Ann Allergy Asthma Immunol 2000;85:477–482.
32. Dahlén B, Nizankowska E, Szczeklik A, et al. Benefits from adding the 5-lipoxygenase inhibitor zileuton to conventional therapy in aspirin-intolerant asthmatics. Am J Respir Crit Care Med 1998; 157: 1187–1194.
33. Dahlén SE, Malmström K, Nizankowska E, et al. Improvement of aspirin-intolerant asthma by montelukast, a leukotriene antagonist:

A randomized, double-blind, placebo-controlled trial. Am J Respir Crit Care Med 2002;165:9–14.

34. Berges-Gimeno MP, Simon RA, Stevenson DD. The effect of leukotriene-modifier drugs on aspirin-induced asthma and rhinitis reactions. Clin Exp Allergy 2002;32:1491–1496.

35. Menendez R, Venzor J, Ortiz G. Failure of zafirlukast to prevent ibuprofen-induced anaphylaxis. Ann Allergy Asthma Immunol 1998;80:225–226.

36. Robuschi M, Gambaro G, Setini P, et al. Attenuation of aspirin-induced bronchoconstriction by sodium cromoglycate and nedocromil sodium. Am J Respir Crit Care Med 1997;155:1461–1464.

37. Dahlen S, Malmstrom K, Nizankowska E, et al. Improvement of aspirin-intolerant asthma by montelukast, a leukotriene antagonist: A randomized, double-blind, placebo-controlled trial. Am J Respir Crit Care Med 2002;165:9–14.

38. Reiss TF, Chervinsky P, Dockhorn RJ, et al. Montelukast, a once-daily leukotriene receptor antagonist, in the treatment of chronic asthma: A multicenter, randomized, double-blind trial. Arch Intern Med 1998;158:1213–1220.

39. Salpeter S, Ormiston T, Salpeter E. Cardioselective beta-blockers for reversible airway disease. Cochrane Database Syst Rev 2002;(4): CD002992.

40. Riddell JG, Shanks RG. Effects of betaxolol, propranolol, and atenolol on isoproterenol-induced β-adrenoceptor responses. Clin Pharmacol Ther 1985;38:554–559.

41. Hauck RW, Schulz CH, Emslander HP, Bohm M. Pharmacological actions of the selective and non-selective β-adrenoreceptor antagonists celiprolol, bisoprolol and propranolol on human bronchi. Br J Pharmacol 1994;113:1043–1049.

42. Fraunfeder FT, Barker AF. Respiratory effects of timolol. N Engl J Med 1984;311:1441.

43. Dunn TL, Gerber MJ, Shen AS, et al. The effect of topical ophthalmic instillation of timolol and betaxolol on lung function in asthmatic subjects. Am Rev Respir Dis 1986;133:264–268.

44. Anonymous. Systemic adverse reactions with betaxolol eye drops. Med J Aust 1995;162:84.

45. Simon RA. Update on sulfite sensitivity. Allergy 1998;53:78–79.

46. Anibarro B, Caballero T, Garcia-Ara C, et al. Asthma with sulfite intolerance in children: A blocking study with cyanocobalamin. J Allergy Clin Immunol 1992;90:103–109.

47. Beasley R, Rafferty P, Holgate ST. Adverse reactions to the nondrug constituents of nebulizer solutions. Br J Clin Pharmacol 1988;25: 283–287.

48. Zhang YG, Wright WJ, Tam WK, et al. Effect of inhaled preservatives on asthmatic subjects, II: Benzalkonium chloride. Am Rev Respir Dis 1990;141:1405–1408.

49. Beasley R, Fishwick, D, Miles JF, et al. Preservatives in nebulizer solutions: Risks without benefit. Pharmacotherapy 1998;18:130–139.

50. Asmus MJ, Barros MD, Liang J, et al. Pulmonary function response to EDTA, an additive in nebulized bronchodilators. J Allergy Clin Immunol 2001;107:68–72.

51. Greenberger PA. Contrast media reactions. J Allergy Clin Immunol 1984;74:600–605.

52. Tilles SA. Occupational latex allergy: Controversies in diagnosis and prognosis. Ann Allergy Asthma Immunol 1999;83:640–644.

53. Yunginger JW. Natural rubber latex allergy. In: Middleton E Jr, Reed CE, Ellis EF, et al., eds. Allergy Principles and Practice, 5th ed. St. Louis: CV Mosby; 1998;1073–1078.

54. Rolland JM, O'Hehir RE. Latex allergy: A model for therapy. Clin Exp Allergy 2008;38:898–912.

55. Poley GE, Slater JE. Latex allergy. J Allergy Clin Immunol 2000;105: 1054–1062.

56. Calamita Z, Saconato H, Pelá AB, Atallah AN. Efficacy of sublingual immunotherapy in asthma: Systematic review of randomized-clinical trials using the Cochrane Collaboration method. Allergy 2006;61:1162–1172.

57. Luque CA, Ortiz MV. Treatment of ACE inhibitor—induced cough. Pharmacotherapy 1999;19:804–810.

58. Sebastian JL, McKinney WP, Kaufman J, et al. Angiotensin-converting enzyme inhibitors and cough: Prevalence in an outpatient medical clinic population. Chest 1991;99:36–39.

59. Simon SR, Black HR, Moser M, Berland WE. Cough and ACE inhibitors. Arch Intern Med 1992;152:1698–1700.

60. Israili ZH, Hall WD. Cough and angioneurotic edema associated with angiotensin-converting enzyme inhibitor therapy: A review of the literature and pathophysiology. Ann Intern Med 1992;117:234–242.

61. Kaufman J, Casanova JE, Riendl P, et al. Bronchial hyperreactivity and cough due to angiotensin-converting enzyme inhibitors. Chest 1989;95:544–548.

62. Malini PL, Strocchi E, Zanardi M, et al. Thromboxane antagonism and cough induced by angiotensin-converting enzyme inhibitor. Lancet 1997;350:15–18.

63. Allen TL, Gora-Harper ML. Cromolyn sodium for ACE inhibitor-induced cough. Ann Pharmacother 1997;31:773–775.

64. Dicpinigaitis PV, Thomas SA, Sherman MB, et al. Losartan-induced bronchospasm. J Allergy Clin Immunol 1996;98:1128–1130.

65. Pylypchuk GB. ACE inhibitor- versus angiotensin II blocker—induced cough and angioedema. Ann Pharmacother 1998;32:1060–1066.

66. Lee-Chiong T Jr, Matthay RA. Drug-induced pulmonary edema and acute respiratory distress syndrome. Clin Chest Med 2004;25:95–104.

67. Cooper JAD, White DA, Matthay RA. Drug-induced pulmonary disease, II: Noncytotoxic drugs. Am Rev Respir Dis 1986;133:488–505.

68. Henderson CA, Reynolds JE. Acute pulmonary edema in a young male after intravenous nalmefene. Anesth Analg 1997;84:218–219.

69. Copper JA Jr. Drug-induced lung disease. Adv Intern Med 1997;42: 231–268.

70. Oshima T, Kasuya Y, Okumura Y, et al. Identification of independent risk factors for fentanyl-induced cough. Can J Anaesth 2006:53;753–758.

71. Obermiller T, Lakshminarayan S. Drug-induced hypersensitivity reactions in the lung. Immunol Allergy Clin North Am 1991;11:575–594.

72. Allen JN. Drug-induced eosinophilic lung disease. Clin Chest Med 2004;25:77–88.

73. Frank L, Massaro D. Oxygen toxicity. Am J Med 1980;69:117–126.

74. Jackson RM. Pulmonary oxygen toxicity. Chest 1985;88:900–905.

75. Elliott CG, Rasmusson BY, Crapo RO, et al. Prediction of pulmonary function abnormalities after adult respiratory distress syndrome (ARDS). Am Rev Respir Dis 1987;135:634–638.

76. Neff TA, Stocker R, Frey HR, et al. Long-term assessment of lung function in survivors of severe ARDS. Chest 2003;123:845–853.

77. Cooper JAD, White DA, Matthay RA. State of the art: Drug-induced pulmonary disease, I: Cytotoxic drugs. Am Rev Respir Dis 1986;133:321–340.

78. Kehrer JP, Kacew S. Systematically applied chemicals that damage lung tissue. Toxicology 1985;35:251–293.

79. Clark JG, Hansen JA, Hertz MI, et al. Idiopathic pneumonia syndrome after bone marrow transplantation. Am Rev Respir Dis 1993;147: 1601–1606.

80. Wiedemann HP. Toward an understanding of idiopathic pneumonia syndrome after bone marrow transplantation. Crit Care Med 1999;27:2040–2041.

81. Quabeck K. The lung as a critical organ in marrow transplantation. Bone Marrow Transplant 1994;14:S19–S28.

82. O'Driscoll BR, Hasleton PS, Taylor PM, et al. Active lung fibrosis up to 17 years after chemotherapy with carmustine (BCNU) in childhood. N Engl J Med 1990;323:378–382.

83. Rubio C, Hill ME, Milan S, et al. Idiopathic pneumonia syndrome after high-dose chemotherapy for relapsed Hodgkin's disease. Br J Cancer 1997;75:1044–1048.

84. Jantz MA, Sahn SA. Corticosteroids in acute respiratory failure. Am J Respir Crit Care Med 1999;160:1079–1100.

85. Lynch JP, McCune WJ. Immunosuppressive and cytotoxic pharmacotherapy for pulmonary disorders. Am J Crit Care 1997;155:395–420.

86. Rakita L, Sobol SM, Mostow N, et al. Amiodarone pulmonary toxicity. Am Heart J 1983;106:906–914.

87. Camus P, Martin WJ 2nd, Rosenow EC 3rd. Amiodarone pulmonary toxicity. Clin Chest Med 2004;25:65–75.

88. Jessurun GAJ, Boersma WG, Crijns HJGM. Amiodarone-induced pulmonary toxicity: Predisposing factors, clinical symptoms and treatment. Drug Saf 1998;18:339–344.

89. Gleadhill IC, Wise RA, Schonfeld SA, et al. Serial lung-function testing in patients treated with amiodarone: A prospective study. Am J Med 1989;86:4–10.

CHAPTER 37

Cystic Fibrosis

CHANIN C. WRIGHT AND YOLANDA Y. VERA

KEY CONCEPTS

❶ Good nutrition with appropriate pancreatic enzyme and vitamin supplementation are essential in the management of cystic fibrosis.

❷ Altered pharmacokinetics of cystic fibrosis patients can impact the dosing and clearance of pharmacologic therapy.

❸ Airway clearance and antiinflammatory therapies are key components to improve pulmonary health in cystic fibrosis patients.

❹ Antipseudomonal agents are the cornerstone of antibiotic therapy for chronic lung infections in the cystic fibrosis patient.

"Woe to that child which when kissed on the forehead tastes salty. He is bewitched and soon must die." This European adage accurately describes the fate of an individual diagnosed with cystic fibrosis during ancient times.[1]

Cystic fibrosis (CF) is a disease state resulting from a dysfunction in the cystic fibrosis transmembrane receptor (CFTR). It is the most common life-limiting disorder in the white population, with an incidence of 1 in 2,000 to 4,000 live births and a prevalence of 30,000 affected individuals in the United States.[2–7]

Currently with care, affected individuals have an expected life span of 36 years. Multiple organ systems are affected in CF individuals; especially, the lungs, the digestive system, and the reproductive organs. Mortality is most commonly due to chronic organ damage or resistant pulmonary infections.[8]

The pharmacist plays an essential role in the development and management of a pharmacotherapeutic care plan for the CF patient.

EPIDEMIOLOGY

CF is an autosomal recessive disease occurring in approximately 1 in 3,500 newborns. In the 1970s, patients only survived into their teen years. By 2006, progress in care had extended survival to 36 years. Institution of care at a young age impacts long-term survival; hence, timing of diagnosis and recognition of signs and symptoms is crucial.[2–7]

Learning objectives, review questions, and other resources can be found at **www.pharmacotherapyonline.com**.

Although CF occurs in all ethnicities, other ethnicities besides the white population display lower frequencies: 1 in 9,200 Hispanic Americans, 1 in 10,900 Native Americans, 1 in 15,000 African Americans, and 1 in 31,000 Asians. The carrier frequency is 1 in 28 for North American white populations, 1 in 29 Ashkenazi Jews, and 1 in 60 African Americans.[2]

ETIOLOGY

The cause of CF is due to a mutation of the CFTR gene. Extensive genetic studies have increased awareness regarding the large spectrum of mutations in the CF population. Over 15,000 mutations have been identified, however, typical panels screen for only 30 of them. The most common mutation identified in CF patients is ΔF508.[3]

Cystic fibrosis is an autosomal recessive disease, in which one mutation present on each allele of the CFTR gene results in presentation of the disease. The presentation of a mutation on only one allele of the CFTR gene will prevent the full expression of CF. Genetic studies have increased the understanding of genotype—phenotype relationships. Various mutations on the CFTR gene can result in various pathologies from primary lung disease to minor gastrointestinal (GI) involvement.[3]

PATHOPHYSIOLOGY

In order to treat CF successfully, a good understanding of the disease's underlying mechanism of action is crucial. It is well established that gene mutations cause an abnormality in the cystic fibrosis transmembrane conductance regulator. This initiates the sequence of events responsible for the manifestations of CF. Mucosal obstruction occurs in the distal airways of the lung and submucosal glands, which express the CFTR. The CFTR also performs numerous cellular functions, including the regulation of chloride transport across the cell membrane. Studies in genotype—phenotype relationships have shown that an abnormality on the CFTR contributes to the expression of other gene proteins involved with inflammatory responses, ion transport, and cell signaling. These various expressions result in differences in clinical severity among patients with the same mutations on the CFTR.[3,9–11]

Under normal conditions, the CFTR helps regulate ion transport and salt homeostasis in the sweat glands. Normally, the sodium ion is followed by the chloride ion and is reabsorbed from the lumen by the CFTR and apical sodium channels. As a result of the CFTR's malfunction in CF patients, chloride fails to be reabsorbed, which impacts the sodium ion reabsorption as well. This failed process produces sweat that contains high levels of salt. The end point of this process is a highly negatively charged lumen, which leads to an increased salt content in the sweat gland. This is also known as the transepithelial potential difference, which is 2 to 3 times as great in CF patients, as

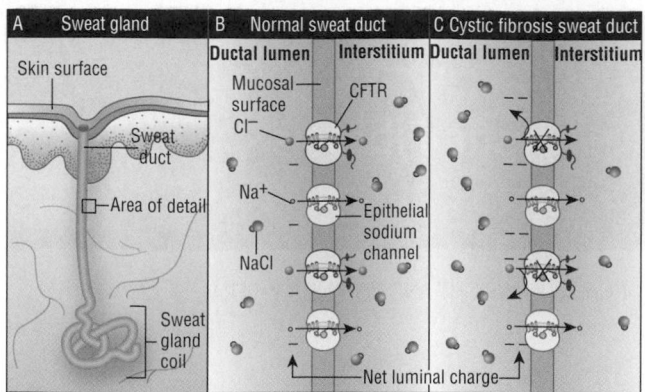

FIGURE 37-1. Mechanism of underlying elevated sodium chloride levels in the sweat of patients with cystic fibrosis. Sweat ducts (panel A) in patients with cystic fibrosis differ from those in people without the disease in the ability to reabsorb chloride before the emergence of sweat on the surface of the skin. A major pathway for Cl⁻ absorption is through CFTR, situated within luminal plasma membranes of cells lining the duct (i.e., on the apical, or mucosal, cell surface) (panel B). Diminished chloride reabsorption in the setting of continued sodium uptake leads to an elevated transepithelial potential difference across the wall of the sweat duct, and the lumen becomes more negatively charged because of a failure to reabsorb chloride (panel C). The result is that total sodium chloride flux is markedly decreased, leading to increased salt content. The thickness of the arrows corresponds to the degree of movement of ions.[10] *(Rowe SM, Miller S, Sorscher EJ. Cystic fibrosis. N Engl J Med 2005;352(19):1992–2001. Copyright © 2005 Massachusetts Medical Society. All rights reserved.)*

the potential difference in patients without the disease. These processes can lead to organ damage in the CF patient (Fig. 37–1).

There are several theories as to how mucosal obstruction occurs in the airways. One of these theories, known as the *low-volume model*, explains that the pulmonary surface epithelium behaves the opposite of a sweat gland in CF patients. There is an increased absorption of sodium, chloride, and fluid, which causes dehydration of the airway surfaces and defective mucociliary transport. An alternative theory known as the *high-salt model* indicates that the pulmonary surface epithelium behaves similarly to the sweat gland. A high salt content predisposes the CF patient to bacterial infections. Both theories agree that CF airways lack the ability to transport chloride through the CFTR.[9,12–13]

One of the common causes of morbidity and mortality in CF patients is mucosal obstruction of the exocrine glands. Mucosal obstruction causes the ducts to dilate, which results in the coating of lung surfaces by thick, viscous, neutrophil-dominated debris. These secretions initiate a cascade of events that lead to inflammation and formation of scar tissue in the lungs[14] (Fig. 37–2).

Other organ systems are impacted by the absence of CFTR activity as well. Ten percent of CF patients are born with meconium ileus, which is an intestinal obstruction that may be fatal if left untreated. Blockage of the pancreatic duct leads to complications such as chronic fibrosis and fatty replacement of the pancreatic gland. Bile duct obstruction causes cirrhosis of the liver, and CF male patients can experience infertility due to obstruction of the vas deferens in utero.[9]

CLINICAL PRESENTATION

In the classic presentation of CF, there are two mutations present (Table 37–1). The patients show signs and symptoms of chronic sinus and pulmonary infections, pancreatic insufficiency, and elevated sweat chloride levels. Patients with nonclassic CF have one mutation present, therefore retaining partial function of the CFTR and maintaining appropriate pancreatic function. (Fig. 37–3.)

SINUS AND PULMONARY PRESENTATION

CF patients will usually experience chronic infections and frequently develop polyps in the sinus cavity. Daily symptomatology includes shortness of breath and cough, with sputum production. A common finding in radiology chest films is a flat diaphragm with an increased chest diameter and air trapping. Pulmonary function tests will reflect a decrease in forced expiratory volume in 1 second (FEV_1). Older patients will experience digital clubbing, a deformity of the fingers and fingernails often associated with chronic hypoxia.

Bacterial growth in the lungs will often drive CF patients to a state of exacerbation, resulting in increased cough, a reduction in pulmonary function, and increased sputum production with a change in color.

GASTROINTESTINAL SYSTEM PRESENTATION

Newborns may present with meconium ileus, which is considered diagnostic of CF. Infants and small children will show an increase in frequency of small stools. Typically, steatorrhea, or greasy stools, is present and can lead to a failure to thrive, resulting in malnutrition. Older patients may experience constipation, abdominal cramping, and flatulence. This presentation is due to the obstruction of the pancreatic ducts and intestinal tract and their inability to digest essential nutrients. Patients with nonclassic CF will mostly maintain adequate pancreatic function and the ability to digest and absorb nutrients.

Pancreatic malfunction can also lead to an insulin deficiency, which is often a later finding detected by a loss in weight, an increase in blood glucose levels, and a failed oral glucose tolerance test (OGTT).

REPRODUCTIVE PRESENTATION

As patients reach adolescent and adult ages, tests may show azoospermia due to blockage of or the congenital bilateral absence of the vas deferens. Females may experience reduced fertility as cervical fluids have lower water content and decreased thinning during ovulation.[9,15–16]

DIAGNOSIS

CF newborn screening is required in all states as of 2010.[17] Depending on the state, this may include immunoreactive trypsin (IRT) screening and/or DNA analysis for genetic mutations. Abnormal values are followed up with sweat testing. The *quantitative pilocarpine iontophoresis sweat test* (QPIT) came about due to the risk of hyperpyrexia associated with older methods that utilized plastic body bags to make patients sweat. QPIT uses only a small area on the forearm, which is then stimulated to secrete sweat through the skin by iontophoresis of pilocarpine. Sweat from the stimulated area is then collected and analyzed for chloride content. Chloride concentrations are quantified as: normal: ≤39 mmol/L; intermediate: 40 to 59 mmol/L; abnormal: ≥60 mmol/L. Values ≥60 mmol/L are consistently diagnostic of CF. It is suggested that samples from two sites will increase the reliability of the diagnosis[3,7] (Fig. 37–4).

DESIRED OUTCOMES

Pharmacists play a vital role in assisting patients to reach the following goals, both long-term and short-term. Since CF affects multiple

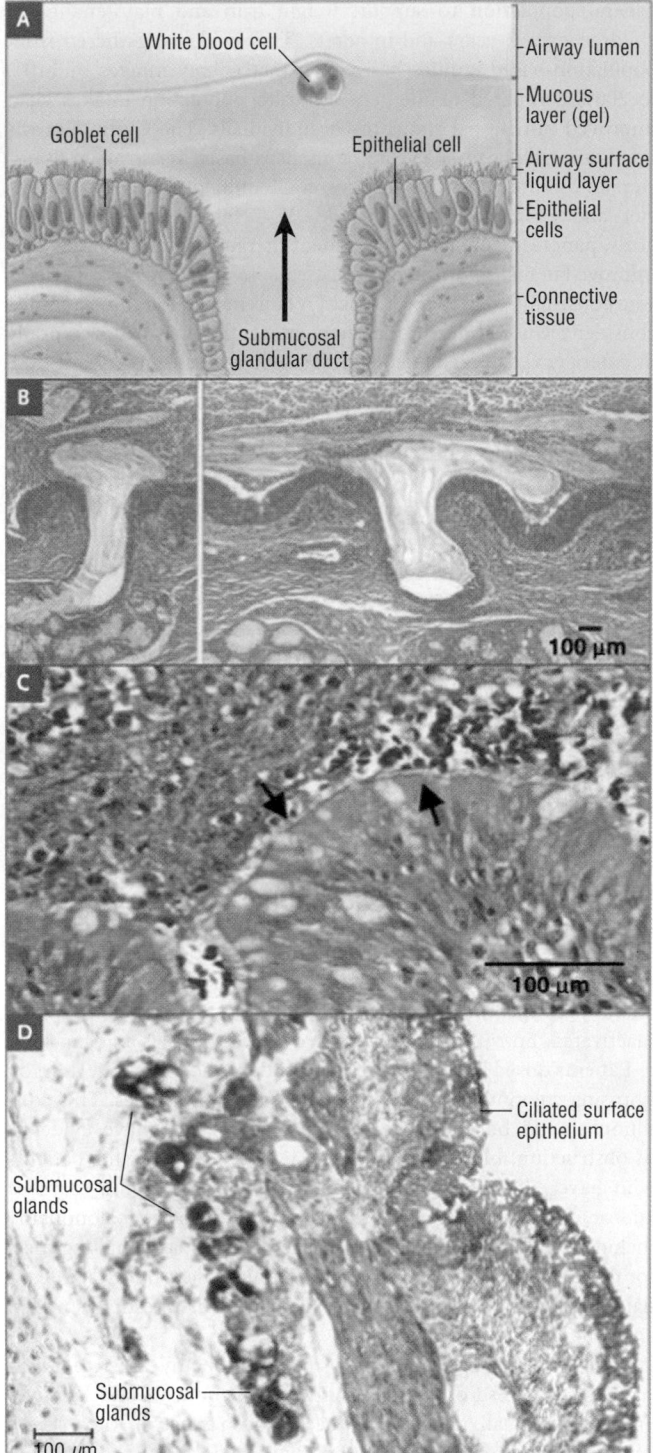

FIGURE 37-2. Extrusion of mucus secretion onto the epithelial surface of airways in cystic fibrosis. Panel A shows a schematic of the surface epithelium and supporting glandular structure of the human airway. In panel B, the submucosal glands of a patient with cystic fibrosis are filled with mucus, and mucopurulent debris overlies the airway surfaces, essentially burying the epithelium. Panel C is a higher-magnification view of a mucus plug tightly adhering to the airway surface, with arrows indicating the interface between infected and inflamed secretions and the underlying epithelium to which the secretions adhere. (Both panels B and C were stained with hematoxylin and eosin, with the colors modified to highlight structures.) Infected secretions obstruct airways and, over time, dramatically disrupt the normal architecture of the lung. In panel D, CFTR is expressed in surface epithelium and serous cells at the base of submucosal glands in a porcine lung sample, as shown by the dark staining, signifying binding by CFTR antibodies to epithelial structures (aminoethylcarbazole detection of horseradish peroxidase with hematoxylin counterstain).[10] (*Rowe SM, Miller S, Sorscher EJ. Cystic fibrosis. N Engl J Med 2005;352(19):1992–2001. Copyright © 2005 Massachusetts Medical Society. All rights reserved.*)

organ systems, there are several therapeutic goals that must be addressed for each system.[8]

SINOPULMONARY

- Prevent and treat sinusitis.
- Increase FEV_1 and promote optimal pulmonary function tests and prevent pulmonary exacerbations.
  - Promote effective airway clearance by providing counseling on use of appropriate medications and chest physiotherapy.
  - Prevent and treat colonization of the lungs with pathogens.
  - Prevent and treat acute exacerbations.

GASTROINTESTINAL

- Control pancreatic insufficiency by providing adequate enzyme supplementation.
- Optimize growth and nutritional status.
- Promote healthy bowel habits.
- Maintain normal vitamin levels.

REPRODUCTION

- Provide mutation analysis with appropriate genetic counseling at the time of diagnosis and periodically thereafter.

TABLE 37-1 Cystic Fibrosis Foundation Diagnosis Criteria and Clinical Presentation

A. Meets one or more of the following clinical features associated with the CF phenotype plus:
  a. Two CF mutations
  b. Two positive QPIT results
  c. An abnormal transepithelial potential difference value
B. The following are typical phenotypes associated with CF:
  a. Chronic sinopulmonary disease
    i. Persistent colonization/infection with pathogens typical of CF lung disease
    ii. Endobronchial disease manifested by
      1. Cough and sputum production
      2. Wheeze and air trapping
      3. Radiographic abnormalities
      4. Evidence of obstruction on pulmonary function test
      5. Digital clubbing
    iii. Chronic sinus disease
      1. Nasal polyps
      2. Radiographic changes
  b. Gastrointestinal/nutritional abnormalities
    i. Intestinal abnormalities
      1. Meconium ileus
      2. Exocrine pancreatic insufficiency
      3. Distal intestinal obstruction syndrome
      4. Rectal prolapse
      5. Recurrent pancreatitis
    ii. Chronic hepatobiliary disease manifested by clinical and/or laboratory evidence of
      1. Focal biliary cirrhosis
      2. Multilobar cirrohosis
    iii. Failure to thrive
    iv. Hypoproteinemia-edema
    v. Fat-soluble vitamin deficiencies
  c. Obstructive azoospermia in males
  d. Salt-loss syndromes
    i. Acute salt depletion
    ii. Chronic metabolic alkalosis
  e. CF in a first degree relative

PSYCHOSOCIAL

- Advocate activity in school and the workplace.
- Encourage compliance with pharmacologic and nonpharmacologic therapies in order to help prolong CF patient's lives.

NUTRITION

❶ In healthy individuals, the pancreas is vital to the absorption and digestion of essential nutrients for the body's growth and function. In pancreatic-insufficient CF individuals, the resulting inability to absorb these nutrients may lead to malnourishment. The focus of treatment lies in achieving and maintaining normal weight for adults and normal growth patterns for children. This is mostly achieved by managing GI and pulmonary symptoms, monitoring nutrient and energy intakes, and addressing psychosocial and financial issues. Numerous population-based studies have provided strong evidence to support optimization of nutritional status, due to its association with an improved pulmonary status. The Cystic Fibrosis Foundation, therefore, recommends that both children and adults maintain normal nutritional status in an effort to promote, healthy pulmonary function, including a better FEV_1 and an increase in survival.

To help meet this desired outcome, the Cystic Fibrosis Foundation recommends energy intakes greater than the standard for the general population to support weight gain and maintenance in children over 2 years and in adults. Trial evidence gathered from population-based studies has shown that energy intakes of 110% to 200% compared to the general health population intakes yield improved nutritional status in CF individuals. The Cystic Fibrosis Foundation has also established consensus-based assessment parameters to monitor nutritional status in CF individuals. These parameters and goals are listed under Table 37–2. In order to achieve these goals, pancreatic enzyme replacement therapy (PERT) is utilized to improve fat absorption due to pancreatic insufficiency. For patients who consistently fail to meet weight requirements, the clinician must consider the use of nutritional supplements that may be given orally or enterally via a percutaneous endoscopic gastrostomy tube (PEG).

PERT has been proven both safe and efficacious in improving nutritional status in CF patients and is recommended in addition to adequate dietary intake. Consensus-based guidelines have established a dose of 500 to 2,500 lipase units/kg of body weight per meal; or 10,000 units/kg/day; or 4,000 units/g of dietary fat per day. Generic enzyme supplements are not bioequivalent; therefore, the Cystic Fibrosis Foundation does not recommend their use.

Until recently, pancreatic enzymes were considered nutritional supplements and were not under the Food and Drug Administration (FDA) jurisdiction. New regulations required all pancreatic enzymes to obtain FDA approval by April 28th, 2010. To date, Creon®, and Zenpep®, and Pancreaze™ have been the only FDA approved preparations. Table 37–3 shows currently used enzyme preparations.[18–39]

Most preparations are capsules containing enteric-coated microspheres or enteric-coated tablets designed to withstand the acidic environment in the stomach allowing for absorption in the small intestine. Frequently CF patients require the addition of histamine receptor antagonists or proton pump inhibitors in order to create an alkaline environment in the intestine. Enteric-coated capsules should not be crushed but may be opened and mixed with nonalkaline food. However, if allowed to sit in food for a prolonged amount of time, the enteric coating will be lost and enzymes will be inactivated. Enzymes are administered prior to meals and snacks.[40]

Patients dosed beyond the recommended guidelines may develop fibrosing colonopathy, which leads to colonic strictures. This condition should be considered for individuals who have evidence of obstruction, bloody diarrhea, or ascites, as well as for patients who have a combination of abdominal pain, ongoing diarrhea and/or poor weight gain. Risk factors for fibrosing colonopathy include: age <12 years; enzyme dosage >6,000 lipase units/kg/meal for more than 6 months; history of meconium ileus or distal intestinal obstruction syndrome (DIOS); history of any intestinal surgery; and inflammatory bowel disease.

Patients who experience fibrosing colonopathy are treated by reducing the dose of enzyme supplements, or with oral laxatives and/or enemas, all of which have been proven effective. More severe cases may require surgical intervention.[41]

BONE HEALTH AND VITAMIN SUPPLEMENTATION

Increased longevity in CF patients has revealed bone disease as an emerging complication. Many studies have observed that 50% to 75% of CF adults have low bone density and increased rates of fractures. CF patients are especially at risk as a result of several contributing factors: malabsorption of vitamin D, poor nutritional status, physical inactivity, glucocorticoid therapy, delayed pubertal maturation, and early hypogonadism. Increased bone resorption and decreased bone formation are likely stimulated by elevated serum cytokine levels triggered by chronic pulmonary inflammation. Additionally, chronic infections lead to bone loss in patients

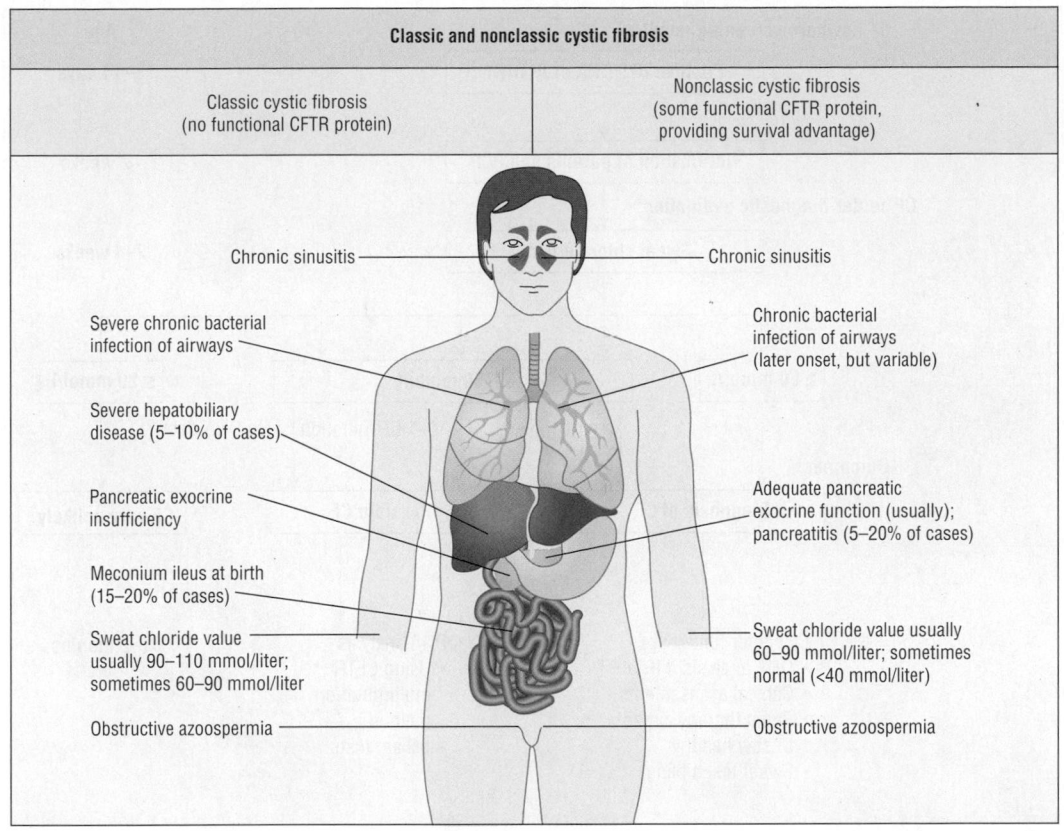

FIGURE 37-3. Classic and nonclassic cystic fibrosis. The findings in classic cystic fibrosis are shown on the left-hand side, and those of nonclassic cystic fibrosis on the right-hand side. Patients with nonclassic cystic fibrosis have better nutritional status and better overall survival. Although the lung disease is variable, patients with nonclassic cystic fibrosis usually have late-onset or more slowly progressive lung disease. Sweat-gland function, as evidenced by the sweat chloride test, is abnormal but not to the extent noted in classic cystic fibrosis. Pancreatitis may occur in patients with nonclassic disease. However, chronic sinusitis and obstructive azoospermia occur in both groups of patients. On the basis of these findings, one can infer that mutations in CTFR, perhaps coupled with other genetic or environmental factors, may confer a predisposition to sinusitis, pancreatitis, or congenital bilateral absence of the vas deferens (azoospermia) in the general population.[16] *(Knowles MR, Durie PR. What is cystic fibrosis? N Engl J Med 2002;347(6):439–442. Copyright © 2002 Massachusetts Medical Society. All rights reserved.)*

regardless of pancreatic sufficiency. Pancreatic insufficient CF patients have the inability to absorb fat-soluble vitamins A, D, E, and K. Decreased calcium absorption and intake can also compound this problem. As bone disease progresses, this can lead to exclusion from lung transplantation, which is often a life-saving operation for individuals with CF.

Appropriate bone density monitoring for CF patients requires a bone density scan in addition to obtaining levels of fat-soluble vitamins periodically. Special multivitamin formulations contain high amounts of fat-soluble vitamins designed to deliver the appropriate doses required. Even with these precautions, adequate vitamin D levels may be difficult to maintain due to altered absorption, reduced fat mass, and minimal exposure to sunlight. Medical management of CF patients can also contribute to bone disease by the administration of glucocorticoids, post-transplant immunosuppressant therapies, and antibiotic therapies that require protection from sunlight exposure.[42–50]

PULMONARY HEALTH AND TREATMENT

❸ One of the fundamentals of pulmonary care in CF patients is airway clearance. CF patients, in general, have impaired muco-ciliary clearance that results in thick sputum, predisposing them to chronic infections and inflammation. Effective airway clearance involves the use of a bronchodilator, a mucolytic medication, and chest percussion. It is recommended that airway clearance therapy (ACT) be initiated within the first few months of life Table 37–4).

Choosing a particular ACT routine for a patient is based on the patient's needs. There is no consensus on the optimal method of ACT. The regimen, including duration or number of treatments per day may be changed in response to acute illness or exacerbations.

Chest percussion was originally performed by hand, with a cupped hand pounding on the chest, which generates percussion or vibration. Currently, the most convenient method is the use of a percussion vest. Aerobic exercise is also effective and recommended for improved airway clearance.[51]

The recommended sequence of clearance therapy or "pulmonary toilet" regimen is as follows (note that these therapies are recommended for individuals ≥6 years of age and are administered concurrently with percussion therapy):

1. Bronchodilator: Albuterol is commonly used for this indication. It helps open up the airways and prevents bronchospasm.

2. Hypertonic saline (HyperSal™): It hydrates the airway mucus secretions and facilitates mucociliary function.

3. Dornase alfa (Pulmozyme®): Enzyme that cleaves extracellular DNA, which results in decreased viscosity of mucus.

4. Aerosolized antibiotics [tobramycin (TOBI®)]: If this therapy is indicated based on severity of lung disease and sputum cultures, it is administered after the CF patient completes percussion therapy.

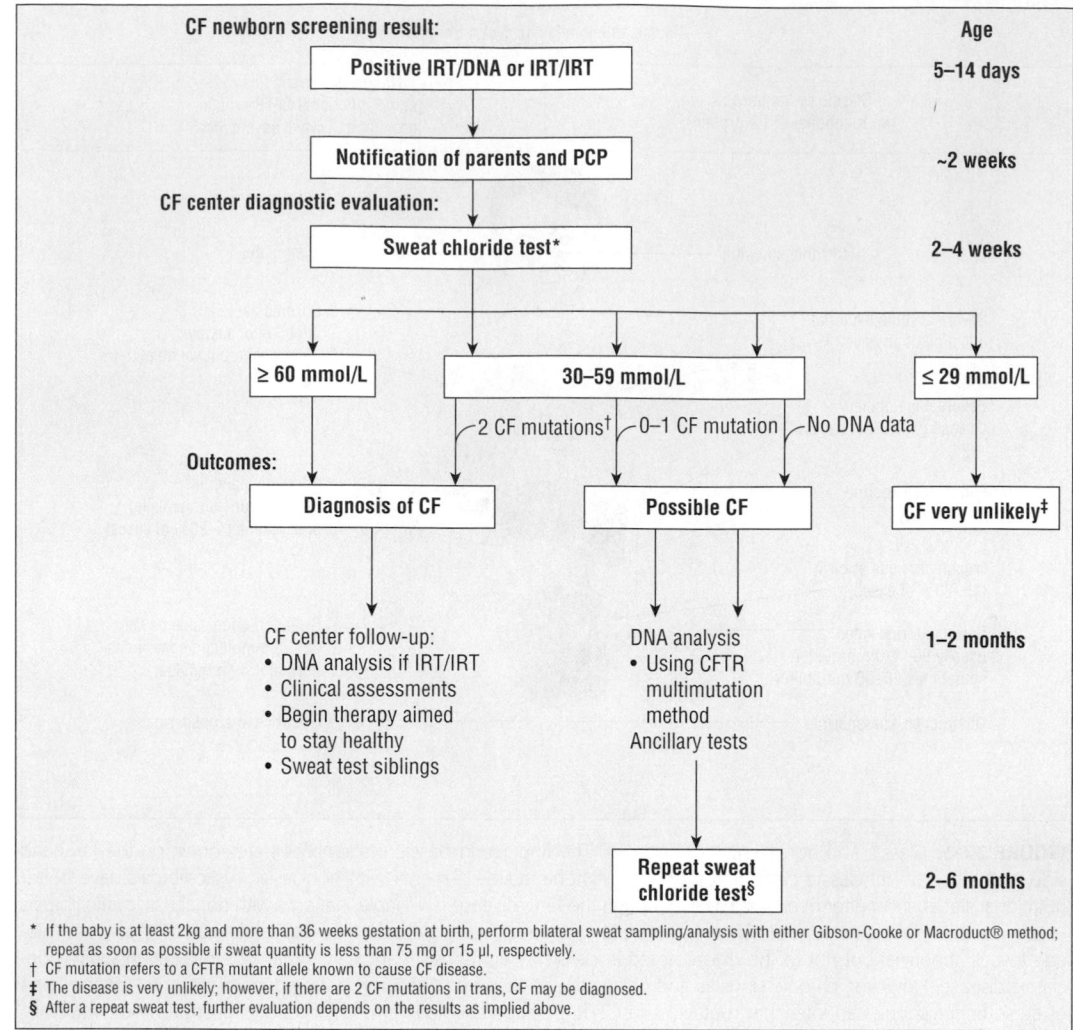

* If the baby is at least 2kg and more than 36 weeks gestation at birth, perform bilateral sweat sampling/analysis with either Gibson-Cooke or Macroduct® method; repeat as soon as possible if sweat quantity is less than 75 mg or 15 µl, respectively.
† CF mutation refers to a CFTR mutant allele known to cause CF disease.
‡ The disease is very unlikely; however, if there are 2 CF mutations in trans, CF may be diagnosed.
§ After a repeat sweat test, further evaluation depends on the results as implied above.

FIGURE 37-4. The CF diagnostic process for screened newborns.[3] (*Reprinted from J Pediatr, Vol. 153(2), Farrell PM, Rosenstein BJ, White TB, et al. Guidelines for the diagnosis of cystic fibrosis in newborns through older adults: Cystic Fibrosis Foundation Consensus Report, pages S4–14, Copyright © 2008, with permission from Elsevier.*)

Bronchodilator therapy is recommended for patients ≥6 years of age who demonstrate bronchiole hyperresponsiveness or a bronchodilator response. Chronic use of bronchodilator therapy is recommended to improve lung function by enhancing mucociliary action.[52–53]

| TABLE 37-2 | Cystic Fibrosis Foundation Nutritional Assessment Parameters and Recommendations |

- Age-appropriate BMI method should be utilized to assess weight and height.
- Better FEV_1 status at about 80% predicted or above was associated with BMI % at 50th percentile or higher.
- For children and adolescents aged 2 to 20 years, the CF Foundation recommends that weight-for-stature assessment use the BMI percentile method and that children and adolescents maintain a BMI at or above the 50th percentile.
- For children diagnosed before age 2 years, the CF Foundation recommends that children reach a weight-for-length status of 50th percentile by age 2 years.
- For adults aged 20 years and older, the CF Foundation recommends that weight-for-stature assessment use the BMI method and that women maintain a BMI ≥22, and men maintain a BMI ≥23.
- For adults aged 20 years and older, the CF Foundation recommends that unintentional weight loss be avoided. When encountered in patient care, unintentional weight loss should be evaluated in the context of the patient's usual weight and health status.

Inhaled hypertonic saline is a novel agent used for the treatment of CF. Hypertonic saline is recommended for patients ≥6 years of age. A study conducted in Australia showed that CF patients who surfed had better pulmonary outcomes than patients who did not surf.[54-55] Researchers believed that the inhalation of ocean water helped to improve FEV_1 in CF patients that surfed. In this study, 24 patients were randomly assigned to receive a daily treatment of 7% hypertonic saline with or without pretreatment of a control. Clearance and pulmonary function were measured during a 14-day period. Results showed significant improvement in FEV_1 and forced vital capacity (FVC), as well as improvement of respiratory symptoms in hypertonic saline patients. The study also demonstrated these patients were able to sustain mucus clearance for >8 hours. Other studies assessing the use of hypertonic saline have supported this study, showing an improvement in lung function and a 56% reduction in exacerbations.[52–56]

Dornase alfa (Pulmozyme®) is also recommended in all patients ≥6 years of age and is strongly recommended for patients with moderate to severe lung disease to improve lung function and reduce exacerbations. Three randomized controlled trials and a crossover trial involving 520 patients were conducted. Study results showed improvement in FEV_1 by 3.2% and a reduction in exacerbations.[52,57–58]

TABLE 37-3	Pancreatic Enzyme Supplements					
Trade Name	**Manufacturer**	**Lipase Units**	**Protease Units**	**Amylase Units**	**Dosage form**	**FDA Approval**
Creon® 6	Solvay Pharmaceuticals, Inc.	6,000	19,000	30,000	Delayed Release Capsule, enteric coated microspheres	Approved
Creon®12		12,000	38,000	60,000		Approved
Creon® 24		24,000	76,000	120,000		Approved
Pancreaze® MT-4	Johnson & Johnson	4,200	10,000	17,500	Capsule, enteric coated microtablets	Approved
Pancreaze® MT-10		10,500	25,000	43,750		Approved
Pancreaze® MT-16		16,800	40,000	70,000		Approved
Pancreaze® MT-20		21,000	37,000	61,000		Approved
Pancrecarb® MS-4	Digestive Care, Inc.	4,000	25,000	25,000	Delayed Release Capsule, enteric coated microspheres	Pending
Pancrecarb® MS-8		8,000	45,000	45,000		Pending
Pancrecarb® MS-16		16,000	52,000	52,000		Pending
Ultresa®	Axcan Scandipharm, Inc.	4,500	25,000	20,000	Capsule, enteric coated minitablets	Pending
Ultresa® MT-12		12,000	39,000	39,000		Pending
Ultresa® MT-18		18,000	58,500	58,500		Pending
Ultresa® MT-20		20,000	65,000	65,000		Pending
Viokase® 0.7g		16,800	70,000	70,000	Powder	Pending
Viokase® 8		8,000	30,000	30,000	Tablet	Pending
Viokase®16		16,000	60,000	60,000		Pending
Zenpep®	Eurand N.V.	5,000	17,000	27,000	Delayed release capsules, enteric coated beads	Approved
		10,000	34,000	55,000		Approved
		15,000	51,000	82,000		Approved
		20,000	68,000	109,000		Approved

ANTIINFLAMMATORY THERAPIES

Pulmonary inflammation begins early in life, as shown by the predominance of proinflammatory mediators that can be seen on bronchiolar lavage. A normal inflammatory response to bacteria becomes pathologic in CF patients who have both a prolonged and exaggerated reaction. Treatment of this inflammatory response is crucial to treating the CF patient.

Antiinflammatory therapies must address the neutrophil response and inhaled therapies will target the endobronchial location, which is the site of inflammation. Using medications that terminate the inflammatory process may be effective. Airway clearance and antibiotics will help control the inflammatory stimulation. Steroids and nonsteroidal antiinflammatory drugs (NSAIDs) are not widely used due to long-term safety concerns. High-dose ibuprofen (20 to 30 mg per kilogram of body weight twice daily) has proven efficacious in a study where patients showed less decline in pulmonary function when compared to patients given placebo. Patients on high-dose ibuprofen were able to maintain weight and had less hospital admissions. The benefits of this regimen exceed the risks of GI complications and nephrotoxicity. Despite these outcomes, less than 10% of CF patients in the United States are on this regimen. The low number of patients utilizing this proven therapy may be related to the requirement to obtain a specific therapeutic level of ibuprofen, which in turn requires frequent blood draws for pharmacokinetic monitoring.[52,59-62]

Studies with macrolides have shown an inhibition of the neutrophil migration and decrease in production of proinflammatory mediators. It is unclear at this point if the antiinflammatory

effects of macrolides are a combination of antimicrobial and/or immunomodulator mechanisms of action. A study conducted in Japan first demonstrated the benefit of macrolides against *P. aeruginosa*. Four randomized controlled trials have since demonstrated this effect with azithromycin (250 to 500 mg) given 3 times weekly, which has led to increased nutritional status and decreased pulmonary infections. Other treatments are under investigation, but larger studies are needed before they become recommended therapies.[52,59,63-64]

INFECTIOUS DISEASE

❹ Antibiotic therapy plays two integral roles in the treatment of CF patients: improving pulmonary function and preventing pulmonary failure. Oral, intravenous, and aerosolized antibiotic formulations are indicated and utilized for patients who experience acute pulmonary exacerbations, are chronically infected with *P. aeruginosa*, or require prevention of chronic *P. aeruginosa* infection. A major disadvantage of treatment in CF patients is that pathogens are not fully eradicated from the airways and will often develop resistance. Unfortunately, this limits antimicrobial selection and can contribute to deterioration of pulmonary function.

Early in life, patients will routinely be colonized with *S. aureus* and then later with *P. aeruginosa*.

Prophylaxis for *S. aureus* colonization is not recommended because in a 5- to 7-year study of cephalexin prophylaxis in young CF children, although the outcomes were favorable with respect to decreased *S. aureus* colonization, there was an increase in frequency of *P. aeruginosa* infections. Ultimately, this study showed no significant improvement in health outcomes.[65,66]

The finding of *P. aeruginosa* on sputum culture is a predictor of morbidity and mortality. There are relatively few antibiotics available for the treatment of *P. aeruginosa*. Antibiotics available include: extended-spectrum penicillins, select cephalosporins, select carbapenems, aztreonam, quinolones, colistimethate, and aminoglycosides. The only two mechanisms of action represented in this group are cell-wall destruction and inhibited cell-wall synthesis by ribosomal attachment. Standard practice is to combine

TABLE 37-4	Airway Clearance Therapies
Airway Clearance Medication	**Dose**
Albuterol	Two puffs prior to therapy 2–4 times a day
HyperSal™ (hypertonic saline)	4 mL delivered via nebulizer 2–4 times a day
Pulmozyme® (dornase alfa)	2.5 mg delivered via nebulizer 1–2 times a day

these two mechanisms for the best bactericidal results. It is not unusual for patients to have multiple organisms growing in their sputum. The clinician can review the quantitative sputum culture for both the organisms present and the amount or colony forming units grown. By targeting the organisms with the most numerous organisms present and reviewing the susceptibility panels, the clinician can choose the most appropriate regimen. After years of drug exposure, older CF patients will exhibit multidrug resistant *P. aeruginosa*. At this point, sputum cultures can be sent to specialized laboratories that will test combinations of antibiotics and report out any synergy results. Aerosolized antibiotics are directly deposited into the lung, providing concentrations that may overcome the standard measures of resistance.[67]

Other organisms that may be seen are *Alcaligenes, Stenotrophomonas, Mycobacteria, Aspergillus,* and *Burkholderia.* The importance of *Alcaligenes* as a pathogen is not well described. Originally only thought to have a prevalence of 2.7%, better lab testing and more studies have found infection rates closer to 8% in CF patients greater than 6 years old.[68-71] *Stenotrophomonas* is intrinsically multidrug resistant and pathogenic. A risk factor for acquiring this organism may be broad spectrum antibiotic use (carbapenems and cephalosporins).[72-73] Quite often this bacteria is misidentified and confirmatory testing may show *Burkholderia.* Prevalence in American CF patients is reported to be 8.4%; however, some centers report incidence to be as high as 25%.[74-76] Treatment choices are trimethoprim-sulfamethoxazole or doxycycline. *Mycobacteria* have been reported with more frequency in the last 10 years. Species include *M. tuberculosis,* nontuberculosis *M. chelonei, M. fortuitum,* and *M. avium-intracellulare* (MAI). The impact of *Mycobacteria* in the CF patient is unclear. Caseating granulomas have been found in some patients with clinical disease, while other patients with nontuberculosis mycobacterium have shown no adverse consequences.[77-80] *Aspergillus* species has a prevalence of 10% to 25% in American CF patients. During the TOBI trials, patients treated with aerosolized tobramycin appeared to be more at risk for colonization with *Aspergillus* than the placebo group. Although *Aspergillus* does not directly inhibit lung function, it may cause allergic bronchopulmonary aspergillosis, which is an immunologic mediated response to the presence of *Aspergillus* in the lungs.[81-82] *B. cepacia* is now known to be a bacterial species called *genomovars.* Currently, up to 9 species have been identified. This organism is commonly misidentified as *P. aeruginosa* or *Stenotrophomonas.*

The two typical antimicrobial choices to treat *B. cepacia* are ceftazidime and sulfamethoxazole-trimethoprim. It is important to recognize the transmission of *B. cepacia* from patient to patient has been shown and therefore proper infection control precautions should be taken. *B. cepacia* is usually transmitted via droplet route.[83-85]

Although CF patients are not more susceptible to respiratory viral infections, the outcome of such illnesses may be more severe. Decline in pulmonary function can be directly related to the number of annual viral infections. Newborns diagnosed with CF should receive respiratory syncytial virus (RSV) prevention with Synagis®, a monoclonal antibody, for the first 2 years of life. Synagis® is usually dosed at 15 mg/kg intramuscularly once a month during the RSV season. All CF patients who are 6 months of age or older should receive the annual influenza vaccine.[86-92]

Tobramycin (TOBI®) is recommended in all patients ≥6 years of age, and is strongly recommended for patients with moderate to severe lung disease and *Pseudomonas* present in sputum cultures. Aerosolized antibiotics deliver drugs locally to the lung while decreasing the risk of systemic side effects. In 1998, the FDA approved TOBI® for treating bacterial lung infections in patients with CF. Routine monitoring of serum aminoglycoside levels is unnecessary for patients with normal renal function using approved doses. It is recommended that CF patients use a preservative-free formulation of aerosolized antibiotics to prevent occurrence of bronchospasm.[93]

Gellar et al describe the pharmacokinetics of inhaled TOBI®, specifically looking at sputum concentrations in CF patients receiving three cycles of routine TOBI® (i.e., 28 days on, 28 days off), 300 mg twice a day. The study followed 258 patients for 24 weeks, and showed that approximately 95% of patients achieved sputum concentrations of >25 times the MIC of *Pseudomonas* isolates. This confirmed that inhaled TOBI® can be efficacious in helping prevent the progression of lung disease. At 25 times the MIC, tobramycin has a bactericidal effect.[94] (See Table 37–5.)

PHARMACOKINETICS

❷ CF patients are unique in respect to a larger volume of distribution and a faster rate of clearance. With a larger volume of distribution, patients may require larger antibiotic doses. Dosing intervals become shorter because drugs are eliminated faster. Critically ill patients may vary from their baseline function and require closer monitoring. However, as patients age, they tend to approach normal population parameters. Therapeutic drug monitoring and necessary dosage and regimen adjustments are critical to the successful treatment of CF patients.

Once daily dosing of aminoglycosides is preferred for ease of home care administration, and may actually work well in this setting. However, given the possibility of a shortened half-life, each patient's unique pharmacokinetic parameters must be calculated to determine if once daily dosing is appropriate.[95-97]

REPRODUCTION

Fertility discussions with older CF patients may arise during clinic visits, and these conversations should include genetic counseling and options for contraception. Drug-drug interactions between oral contraceptive pills (OCPs) and antibiotics should be monitored. Studies have shown that OCP use in CF patients is safe and effective in comparison with other contraception methods. Patches may not reliably adhere to the skin as a result of increased sweat on the surface of the skin.

The issues surrounding the use of contraception among CF men are similar to those among the normal population. CF men should not assume they are infertile and should adhere to using protective measures in order to prevent unwanted pregnancy and the spread of sexually transmitted diseases. Should a CF male with a nonfunctioning vas deferens desire to become a biological parent, microsurgical epididymal aspiration of spermatozoa with intracytoplasmic sperm injection into the oocyte can be performed.[16]

DIABETES

As CF patients live longer, glucose intolerance and CF-related diabetes (CFRD) are common complications. Even though it shares features of type 1 and type 2 diabetes, CFRD is unique because it is influenced by factors specific to CF, including: insulin deficiency, undernutrition, chronic and acute infection, elevated energy expenditure, glucagon deficiency, malabsorption, abnormal intestinal transit time, and liver dysfunction.[98] In comparison with the general CF population, patients with CFRD show a higher mortality rate. In a study of 448 patients, 60% of non-CFRD population and 25% of the CFRD population were alive at age 30. The average

TABLE 37-5 Anti-microbial agents utilized in CF

Antibiotic	Pediatric Dose (mg/kg/day)	Adult Dose	Frequency Range	Pathogens
Oral				
Ciprofloxacin	40	750 mg	Q 12 H	*Pseudomonas, Alcaligenes*
Sulfamethoxazole/Trimethoprim	15-20 mg of TMP	15-20 mg of TMP/kg/day	Q 6-8H	*Staphylococcus* (MRSA, MSSA),*Burkholderia Stenotrophomonas, Alcaligenes*
Doxycycline	2-4	Max 200 mg/day	Q12-24H	*Stenotrophomonas, Staphylococcus*
Intravenous				
Amikacin	22.5-30	15 mg/kg/day	Q8H	*Pseudomonas*
Aztreonam	200	2 grams	Q6-8H	*Pseudomonas*
Cefepime	150	2 grams	Q8H	*Pseudomonas*
Ceftazidime	150	2 grams	Q8H	*Pseudomonas, Burkholderia Alcaligenes*
Ciprofloxacin	30	400 mg	Q8H	*Pseudomonas, Alcaligenes*
Colistimethate	5-8	5-8 mg/kg/day	Q8H	*Pseudomonas*
Doxycycline	2-4	Max 200 mg/day	Q12-24H	*Stenotrophomonas, Staphylococcus*
Gentamicin	7.5-10	7.5-10 mg/kg/day	Q6-8H	*Pseudomonas*
Imipenem	60-100	2-4 grams	Q6H	*Pseudomonas, Burkholderia Alcaligenes*
Meropenem	30-50	1-2 grams	Q8H	*Pseudomonas, Burkholderia, Alcaligenes*
Piperacillin-Tazobactam	300-400 (piperacillin component)	4.5 grams	Q4-6H	*Pseudomonas, Alcaligenes, Staphylococcus* MSSA
Ticarcillin-Clavulanate	300-400 (ticarcillin component)	3.1 grams	Q4H	*Pseudomonas, Alcaligenes Staphylococcus* (MSSA)
Tobramycin	7.5-10	7.5-10 mg/kg/day	Q6-8H	*Pseudomonas*
Vancomycin	60	15 mg/kg	Q 6-12H	*Staphylococcus*(MRSA, MSSA)
Inhalation				
Tobramycin	60-600 mg/day	60-600 mg/day	Q12H	*Pseudomonas*
Colistimethate	75 mg/day	75 mg /day	Q12H	*Pseudomonas*
Aztreonam	225 mg/day	225 mg/day	Q8H	*Pseudomonas*

onset of CFRD is between 18 and 21 years, with a slight female predominance and is more commonly seen in CF gene mutation ΔF508.[98–102]

A desired goal in this population is to control hyperglycemia and hypoglycemia in order to reduce acute and chronic diabetes complications. Because insulin deficiency is the hallmark of CFRD, insulin is the recommended medical treatment. Insulin regimens are individualized based on the patient's lifestyle and circumstances. Exercise is encouraged because it can improve peripheral insulin sensitivity and have beneficial effects in overall health, pulmonary function, and well being.[99–102]

Oral antidiabetic agents have inconsistent results in literature, therefore, support for their use in therapy for CFRD patients is not recommended. Medications that help improve insulin sensitivity do not address the primary problem of insulin deficiency in CF. Metformin's mechanism of action is to improve hepatic and peripheral insulin sensitivity; however, it is contraindicated for patients with hypoxia due to the risk of fatal lactic acidosis. Additionally, metformin's multiple GI effects include anorexia, diarrhea, flatulence, and abdominal discomfort. Thiazolidinediones help to enhance peripheral insulin sensitivity, but there is serious potential for hepatic toxicity due to the underlying liver problems in CF patients. The use of acarbose is also discouraged due to its mechanism of action, which reduces postprandial glucose and insulin excursion by limiting intestinal absorption of glucose. This inhibits the energy absorption in malnourished individuals while causing diarrhea, anorexia, and abdominal discomfort. Sulfonylureas are being considered due to their ability to enhance insulin secretion by acting on a specific islet beta cell receptor, however, evidence has also shown that these agents bind and inhibit the CFTR. Use of sulfonylureas is not recommended at this time.[99,103]

SPECIAL POPULATIONS

PREGNANCY

As women with CF live longer, more choose to become pregnant. CF women considering pregnancy and their partners should both undergo genetic counseling. CF women who become pregnant are considered a high-risk pregnancy; therefore, several considerations should be addressed at the onset of and during pregnancy. At the beginning, both current medications and medications that might be used to treat exacerbations need to be considered. Several of these medications are classified as category C and may pose a potential harm to the fetus. These patients should also be screened and treated accordingly for CFRD.

Several complications that will arise during CF pregnancy include increases in minute ventilation, increased oxygen uptake, and increased blood volume and cardiac output. In a woman with severe lung disease, these changes can cause right-sided heart failure.

Other pharmacotherapy issues that are seen in this population are altered pharmacokinetics and increased maintenance of nutritional and pulmonary health.

The addition of the fetus impacts the CF woman's health by placing a strain on a precariously balanced state of being. The CF woman who chooses to breastfeed must take into account the additional nutritional requirement of approximately 500 kcal/day.[16]

PEDIATRICS

Education of the parents is emphasized in this population, concerning administration of pancreatic enzymes and infant formula. Parents are also counseled to encourage their child to adhere with pulmonary health and nutritional health practices. As the child grows into adolescence, compliance becomes an issue. Peer pressure and social restraints may interfere with CF compliance and may influence the patients to disregard their personal well being.

TRANSPLANT PATIENTS

Lung transplantation has become an option with a 5-year survival rate of approximately 50%. Criteria for selection of transplant candidates include not only an FEV_1 of <30%, but also gender, nutritional status, diabetic status, sputum microbiology, and number of pulmonary exacerbations. Factors affecting compliance to CF care and to immunosuppressant therapy may also be taken under consideration for candidacy.[16]

NEW THERAPIES

Currently being studied are attempts to restore normal airway hydration, either by inhaled osmotic agents that bring water to the airway surface or by inhaled agents that may inhibit ion transport. One such agent is mannitol, which works by creating an osmotic gradient; this is being studied as a dried powder inhaler. Amiloride inhibits ion transport, but its short half-life limits its usefulness. Compounds with similar structures are also being studied for potential use.

Due to antibiotic resistance, new therapies for CF often focus on new antibiotics. Tobramycin inhaled powder (TIP) and inhaled aztreonam (AZLI) are both currently in phase 3 trials. TIP's advantage is that it is administered faster than TOBI®. AZLI uses a new nebulizer to also reduce treatment time. A new inhaled antibiotic, Arikace, is now in phase 2 trials. This liposomal amikacin penetrates into CF mucus and delivers high concentrations of the drug to the site of infection.[108,109] Cayston® (aztreonam powder) has recently received approval from the European commission. It will use the Altera® nebulizer, which will decrease administration time from 30 minutes to 3 minutes. This would significantly improve compliance and have a positive impact on quality of life in CF patients.[110]

CLINICAL CONTROVERSIES

CF is a worldwide problem, with a variety of approaches toward treatment. Discussions regarding controversial methods are constantly being held while new therapies are tried. Due to the relatively small population of CF patients, any studies that are conducted are frequently small in number or do not accurately reflect this population. This makes it difficult to extrapolate and come to a consensus regarding therapy. Some of these controversies will be discussed.

Inhaled and/or oral N-acetylcysteine (NAC) is an antioxidant that may have some antiinflammatory effect. The CF Foundation does not recommend this therapy due to insufficient evidence; however, a few published studies have led some clinicians to utilize this therapy. To date, there is not enough information to identify an NAC dosing strategy that is tolerable.[52,59,104]

Bisphosphonate therapy is being added to bone health regimens in both adult and pediatric patients. Pediatric CF trials with these medications have not been conducted, although adult CF

trials indicated potential value. CF children will develop bone disease that forces clinicians to decide whether to utilize this controversial therapy. In adult CF patients, there have been a few studies assessing the use of injectable bisphosphonate. The use of intravenous pamidronate showed significant gains in bone mineral density (BMD), however there was a high incidence of adverse events, such as moderate-severe bone pain, fever, and phlebitis. Injectable formulations are useful to the CF population because they bypass the malabsorption issue. A once-a-week oral bisphosphonate trial is underway. There has been at least one promising adult study with oral alendronate; however, no study has been performed with risedronate.[42,49–50,105]

Colistimethate (Colistin®) is an antibiotic commonly used to treat pseudomonal infections. It is available in the injectable form that can be diluted and nebulized. Reports show a high incidence of bronchospasm and decline of FEV_1 in CF patients, especially in those with underlying reactive airway disease. Administration via inhalation can also be problematic due to low surface tension resulting in foaming of the solution. Thus, the recommended dose is questionable, due to variable drug delivery. However, for patients with multiple-drug-resistant pseudomonas, this may be the only alternative.[93,106–107]

SOCIAL

The social worker is an integral part of the CF team, due to the complex social issues that surround CF patients. Maintaining health insurance is a lifelong problem for CF patients. The inability to pay for CF meds may often influence compliance. Life insurance and homeowners insurance may never be obtainable. Maintaining employment is difficult because some employers may penalize for frequent hospitalizations. Thus, many CF patients have low paying jobs without insurance coverage.

Building relationships and confiding in others about personal health issues can be intimidating and difficult for CF patients. Children do not have opportunities to engage in friendships with other CF children. Due to infection control guidelines, group settings are limited. Support groups, although available, are restricted to online discussions. The decision to marry and have children is complicated by an awareness of a shortened life span.[16]

SUMMARY

Multidisciplinary care for CF patients should involve pulmonologists, gastroenterologists, pharmacists, social workers, respiratory therapists, and dieticians. Complexity of care requires good communication within the CF team. Although intravenous antibiotics have historically been a mainstay of therapy, recent focus has shifted to optimizing nutrition status and promoting effective pulmonary clearance. New treatment modalities such as inhaled antibiotics will necessitate greater involvement by pharmacists. As patients live longer, more issues that are social arise, and medical issues become more complex.

ABBREVIATIONS

ACT: airway clearance therapy

BMD: bone mineral density

BMI: body mass index

CF: cystic fibrosis

CFRD: cystic fibrosis-related diabetes

CFTR: cystic fibrosis transmembrane receptor

DIOS: distal intestinal obstruction syndrome

FDA: Food and Drug Administration

FEV$_1$: forced expiratory volume at 1 second

FVC: forced vital capacity

GI: gastrointestinal

IRT: immunoreactive trypsinogen

MIC: minimum inhibitory concentration

NAC: *N*-acetylcysteine

OGTT: oral glucose tolerance test

OCP: oral contraceptive pills

PEG: percutaneous endoscopic gastrostomy tube

PERT: pancreatic enzyme replacement therapy

QPIT: quantitative pilocarpine iontophoresis test

RSV: respiratory syncytial virus

REFERENCES

1. Quinton PM. Cystic fibrosis: Lessons from the sweat gland. Physiology 2007;22:212–225.
2. Moskowitz SM, Chmiel JF, Sternen DL, et al. Clinical practice and genetic counseling for cystic fibrosis and CFTR-related disorders. Genet Med 2008;10:851–866.
3. Farrell PM, Rosenstein BJ, White TB, et al. Guidelines for the diagnosis of cystic fibrosis in newborns through older adults: Cystic Fibrosis Foundation Consensus Report. J Pediatr 2008;153(2):S4–S14.
4. Sontag MK, Hammond KB, Zielenski J, et al. Two-tiered immunoreactive trypsinogen (IRT/IRT)-based newborn screening for cystic fibrosis in Colorado: Screening efficacy and diagnostic outcomes. J Pediatr 2005;147(suppl):S83–S88.
5. Parad RB, Corneau AM. Newborn screening for cystic fibrosis. Pediatr Ann 2003;32:528–535.
6. Corneau AM, Parad RB, Dorkin HL, et al. Population-based newborn screening for genetic disorders when multiple mutations DNA testing is incorporated: A cystic fibrosis newborn screening model demonstrating increased sensitivity but more carrier detections. Pediatrics 2004;113:1573–1581.
7. Cystic Fibrosis Foundation. Cystic fibrosis foundation patient registry, 2005 Annual Data Report to the Center Directors. Bethesda, MD: Cystic Fibrosis Foundation; 2006.
8. Cystic Fibrosis Foundation. Clinical Practice Guidelines for Cystic Fibrosis: Preventive and maintenance care for the patient with cystic fibrosis. May 2006; 1–24, *https://www.portcf.org/Resources/Consensus%20&%20Guidelines/Chapter%201.pdf*.
9. Rowe SM, Miller S, Sorscher EJ. Cystic fibrosis. N Engl J Med 2005;352(19):1992–2001.
10. Groman JD, Karczeski B, Sheridan M, et al. Phenotypic and genetic characterization of patients with features of "nonclassic" forms of cystic fibrosis. J Pediatr 2005;146:675–680.
11. Mickle JE, Cutting GR. Genotype-phenotype relationships in cystic fibrosis. Med Clin North Am 2000;84:597–607.
12. Mall M, Grubb BR, Harkema JR, et al. Increased airway epithelial Na+ absorption produces cystic fibrosis-like lung disease in mice. Nat Med 2004;10:487–493.
13. Smith JJ, Travis SM, Greenberg EP, et al. Cystic fibrosis airway epithelia fail to kill bacteria because of abnormal airway surface fluid. Cell 1996;85:229–236.
14. Engelhardt JF, Yankaskas JR, Ernst SA, et al. Submucosal glands are the predominant site of CFTR expression in the human bronchus. Nat Genet 1992;2:240–248.
15. Knowles MR, Durie PR. What is cystic fibrosis? N Engl J Med 2002;347:439–442.
16. Yankaskas JR, Marshall BC, Sufian B, et al. Cystic fibrosis adult care. Chest 2004;125:1S–S39.
17. Kerr M. Cystic fibrosis screening legislated for all newborns by 2010. Medscape Medical News 2009 Medscape, LLC. July 15, 2009, *http://www.medscape.com/viewarticle/705589_print*.
18. Stallings VA, Stark LJ, Robinson KA, et al. Evidence-based practice recommendations for nutrition-related management of children and adults with cystic fibrosis and pancreatic insufficiency: Results of a systematic review. J Am Diet Assoc 2008;108:832–839.
19. Steinkamp G, Demmelmair H, Ruhl-Bagheri I, et al. Energy supplements rich in linoleic acid improve body weight and essential fatty acid status of cystic fibrosis patients. J Pediatr Gastroenterol Nutr 2000;31:418–423.
20. Richardson I, Nyulasi I, Cameron K, et al. Nutritional status of an adult cystic fibrosis population. Nutrition 2000;16:255–259.
21. Stark LJ, Bowen AM, Tyc VL, et al. A behavioral approach to increasing calorie consumption in children with cystic fibrosis. J Pediatr Psychol 1990;15:309–326.
22. Stark LJ, Knapp LG, Bowen AM, et al. Increasing calorie consumption in children with cystic-fibrosis—Replication with 2-year follow-up. J Appl Beh Analysis 1993;26:435–450.
23. Lloyd-Still JD, Smith AE, Wessel HU. Fat intake is low in cystic fibrosis despite unrestricted dietary practices. JPEN J Parenter Enteral Nutr 1989;13:296–298.
24. Luder E, Kattan M, Thornton JC, et al. Efficacy of a nonrestricted fat diet in patients with cystic fibrosis. Am J Dis Child 1989;143:458–464.
25. Shepherd RW, Holt TL, Cleghorn G, et al. Short-term nutritional supplementation during management of pulmonary exacerbations in cystic fibrosis: A controlled study, including effects of protein turnover. Am J Clin Nutr 1988;48:235–239.
26. Hanning RM, Blimkie CJR, Baror O, et al. Relationships among nutritional status and skeletal and respiratory muscle function in cystic fibrosis: Does early dietary supplementation make a difference? Am J Clin Nutr 1993;57:580–587.
27. Bentur L, Kalnins D, Levison H, et al. Dietary intakes of young children with cystic fibrosis: Is there a difference? J Pediatr Gastroenterol Nutr 1996;22:254–258.
28. Vaisman N, Clarke R, Pencharz PB. Nutritional rehabilitation increases resting energy expenditure without affecting protein turnover in patients with cystic fibrosis. J Pediatr Gastroenterol Nutr 1991;13:383–390.
29. Van Biervliet S, De Waele K, Van Winekel M, et al. Percutaneous endoscopic gastrostomy in cystic fibrosis: Patient acceptance and effect of overnight tube feeding on nutritional status. Acta Gastroenterol Belg 2004;67:241–244.
30. Peterson ML, Jacobs DR Jr, Mills CE. Longitudinal changes in growth parameters are correlated with changes in pulmonary function in children with cystic fibrosis. Pediatrics 2003;112(3 Pt 1):588–592.
31. Konstan MW, Butler SM, Wohl ME, et al. Growth and nutritional indexes in early life predict pulmonary function in cystic fibrosis. J Pediatr 2003,142:624–630.
32. Thomson MA, Quirk P, Swanson CE, et al. Nutritional growth-retardation is associated with defective lung growth in cystic-fibrosis: A preventable determinant of progressive pulmonary dysfunction. Nutrition 1995;11:350–354.
33. Walker SA, Gozal D. Pulmonary function correlates in the prediction of long-term weight gain in cystic fibrosis patients with gastrostomy tube feedings. J Pediatr Gastroenterol Nutr 1998;27:53–56.
34. Navarro J, Rainisio M, Harms HK, et al. Factors associated with poor pulmonary function: Cross-sectional analysis of data from the ERCF. European Epidemiologic Registry of Cystic Fibrosis. Eur Respir J 2001;18:298–305.
35. Oliver MR, Heine RG, Ng CH, et al. Factors affecting clinical outcomes in gastrostomy-fed children with cystic fibrosis. Pediatr Pulmonol 2004;37:324–329.
36. Smith DL, Clarke JM, Stableforth DE. A nocturnal nasogastric feeding programme in cystic fibrosis adults. J Hum Nutr Diet 1994;7:257–262.

37. Williams SG, Ashworth F, McAlweenie A, et al. Percutaneous endoscopic gastrostomy feeding in patients with cystic fibrosis. Gut 1999;44:87–90.

38. Steinkamp G, von der Hardt H. Improvement of nutritional status and lung function after long-term nocturnal gastrostomy feedings in cystic fibrosis. J Pediatr 1994;124:244–249.

39. FDA approves pancreatic enzyme replacement product for marketing in United States: Creon designed to help those with cystic fibrosis, others with exocrine pancreatic insufficiency. U.S. Food and Drug Administration. U.S. Department of Health and Human Services 2009.

40. Cystic Fibrosis Foundation. Concepts in CF Care. Vol X, Section 1. Consensus Conferences. Bethesda, MD: Cystic Fibrosis Foundation; 2001.

41. Houwen RH, van der Doef HP, Sermer I, et al. Defining DIOS and constipation in cystic fibrosis with a multicentre study on the incidence, characteristics, and treatment of DIOS. J Pediatr Gastroenterol Nutr 2009;49:54–58.

42. Aris RM, Merkel PA, Bachrach LK, et al. Consensus statement: Guide to bone health and disease in cystic fibrosis. J Clin Endocrinol Metab 2005;90:1888–1896.

43. Elkin SL, Fairney A, Burnett S, et al. Vertebral deformities and low bone mineral density in adults with cystic fibrosis: A cross-sectional study. Osteoporos Int 2001;12:366–372.

44. Aris RM, Renner JB, Winders AD, et al. Increased rate of fractures and severe kyphosis: Sequelae of living to adulthood with cystic fibrosis. Ann Intern Med 1998;128:186–193.

45. Conway SP, Morton AM, Oldroyd B, et al. Osteoporosis and osteopenia in adults and adolescents with cystic fibrosis: Prevalence and associated factors. Thorax 2000;55:798–804.

46. Borowitz D, Baker RD, Stallings V. Consensus report on nutrition for pediatric patients with cystic fibrosis. J Pediatr Gastroenterol Nutr 2002;35:246–259.

47. Wilson DC, Rashid M, Durie PR, et al. Treatment of vitamin K deficiency in cystic fibrosis: Effectiveness of a daily fat-soluble vitamin combination. J Pediatr 2001;138:851–855.

48. Ontjes DA, Lark RK, Lester GE, et al. Vitamin D depletion and replacement in patients with cystic fibrosis. In: Norman A, Bouillon R, eds. Vitamin D endocrine system: Structural, biological, genetic and clinical aspects. Riverside, CA: Thomasset, University of California 2000;893–896.

49. Haworth CS, Selby PL, Adams JE, et al. Effect of intravenous pamidronate on bone mineral density in adults with cystic fibrosis. Thorax 2001;56:314–316.

50. Haworth CS, Selby PL, Webb AK, et al. Severe bone pain after intravenous pamidronate in adult patients with cystic fibrosis. Lancet 1998;86:1753–1754.

51. Flume PA, Robinson KA, O'Sullivan BP, et al. Cystic fibrosis pulmonary guidelines: Airway clearance therapies. Respir Care 2009;54:522–537.

52. Flume PA, O'Sullivan BP, Robinson KA, et al. Cystic fibrosis pulmonary guidelines: chronic medications for maintenance of lung health. Am J Respir Crit Care Med 2007;176:957–969.

53. Halfhide C, Evans HJ, Couriel J. Inhaled bronchodilators for cystic fibrosis. Cochrane Database Syst Rev 2008;4:CD003428.

54. Ratjen F. Restoring airway surface liquid in cystic fibrosis. N Engl J Med 2006;354:291–293.

55. Robinson M, Rose BR, et al. A controlled trial of long-term inhaled hypertonic saline in patients with cystic fibrosis. N Engl J Med 2006;354:229–240.

56. Ballmann M, von der Hart H. Hypertonic saline and recombinant human DNase: A randomised cross-over pilot study in patients with cystic fibrosis. J Cyst Fibros 2002;1:35–37.

57. Quan JM, Tiddens HA, Sy JP, et al. A two-year randomized, placebo-controlled trial of dornase alfa in young patients with cystic fibrosis with mild lung function abnormalities. J Pediatr 2001;139:813–820.

58. Nasr SZ, Kuhns LR, Brown RW, et al. Use of computerized tomography and chest x-rays in evaluating efficacy of aerosolized recombinant human DNase in cystic fibrosis patients younger than age 5 years: A preliminary study. Pediatr Pulmonol 2001;31:377–382.

59. Nichols DP, Konstan MW, Chmiel JF. Anti-inflammatory therapies for cystic fibrosis-related lung disease. Clin Rev Allerg Immunol 2008;35:135–153.

60. Lands LC, Milner R, Cantin AM, et al. High-dose ibuprofen in cystic fibrosis: Canadian safety and effectiveness trial. J Pediatr 2007;151:249–254.

61. Konstan MW, Schluchter MD, Xue W, et al. Clinical use of ibuprofen is associated with slower FEV_1 decline in children with cystic fibrosis. Am J Respir Crit Care Med 2007;176(11):1084–1089.

62. Konstan MW, Byard PJ, Hoppel CL, et al. Effect of high-dose ibuprofen in patients with cystic fibrosis. N Engl J Med 1995;332(13):848–854.

63. Saiman L, Marshall BC, Mayer-Hamblett N, et al. Azithromycin in patients with cystic fibrosis chronically infected with *Pseudomonas aeruginosa*: A randomized controlled trial. JAMA 2003;290(13):1749–1756.

64. Wolter J, Seeney S, Bell S, et al. Effect of long term treatment with azithromycin on disease parameters in cystic fibrosis: A randomised trial. Thorax 2002;57:212–216.

65. Saiman L, Siegel J. Infection control recommendations for patients with cystic fibrosis: Microbiology, important pathogens, and infection control practices to prevent patient-to-patient transmissions. Infect Control Hosp Epidemiol 2003;24:S6–S52.

66. Stutman HR, Lieberman JM, Nussbaum E, et al. Antibiotic prophylaxis in infants and young children with cystic fibrosis: A randomized controlled trial. J Pediatr 2002;140:299–305.

67. Saiman L, Mehar F, Niu WW, et al. Antibiotic susceptibility of multiply resistant *Pseudomonas aeruginosa* isolated from patients with cystic fibrosis, including candidates for transplantation. Clin Infect Dis 1996;23:532–537.

68. Cystic Fibrosis Foundation. Patient registry 1996. In: Annual Report. Bethesda, MD: Cystic Fibrosis Foundation; 1997.

69. Cystic Fibrosis Foundation. Patient registry 1997. In: Annual Report. Bethesda, MD: Cystic Fibrosis Foundation; 1998.

70. Burns JL, Emerson J, Stapp JR, et al. Microbiology of sputum from patients at cystic fibrosis centers in the United States. Clin Infect Dis 1998;27:158–163.

71. Saiman L, Chen Y, Tabibi S, et al. Identification and antimicrobial susceptibility of *Alcaligenes xylosoxidans* isolated from patients with cystic fibrosis. J Clin Microbiol 2001;39:3942–3945.

72. Sattler C, Mason EJ, Kaplan S. Nonrespiratory *Stenotrophomonas maltophilia* infection at a children's hospital. Clin Infect Dis 2000;31:1321–1330.

73. Elting LS, Khardori N, Bodey GP, et al. Nosocomial infection caused by *Xanthomonas maltophilia*: A case-control study of predisposing factors. Infect Control Hosp Epidemiol 1990;11:134–138.

74. Burde DR, Noble MA, Campbell ME, et al. *Xanthomonas maltophilia* misidentified as *Pseudomonas cepacia* in cultures of sputum from patients with cystic fibrosis: A diagnostic pitfall with major clinical implications. Clin Infect Dis 1995;20:445–448.

75. Demko CA, Stern RC, Doershuk CF. *Stenotrophomonas maltophilia* in cystic fibrosis: Incidence and prevalence. Pediatr Pulmonol 1998;25:304–308.

76. Denton M, Todd NJ, Kerr KG, et al. Molecular epidemiology of *Stenotrophomonas maltophilia* isolated from clinical specimens from patients with cystic fibrosis and associated environmental samples. J Clin Microbiol 1998;36:1953–1958.

77. Kilby JM, Gilligan PH, Yankaskas JR, et al. Nontuberculous mycobacteria in adult patients with cystic fibrosis. Chest 1992;102:70–75.

78. Torrens JK, Dawkins P, Conway SP, et al. Non-tuberculous mycobacteria in cystic fibrosis. Thorax 1998;53:182–185.

79. Tomashefski JF Jr, Stern RC, Demko CA, et al. Nontuberculous mycobacteria in cystic fibrosis. An autopsy study. Am J Respir Crit Care Med 1996;154:523–528.

80. Cullen AR, Cannon CL, Mark EJ, et al. *Mycobacterium abscessus* infection in cystic fibrosis. Colonization or infection? Am J Respir Crit Care Med 2003;167:828–834.

81. Equi A, Balfour-Lynn IM, Bush A, et al. Long term azithromycin in children with cystic fibrosis: A randomised, placebo-controlled cross-over trial. Lancet 2002;360(9338):978–980.

82. Bargon J, Dauletbaev N, Kohler B, et al. Prophylactic antibiotic therapy is associated with an increased prevalence of *Aspergillus*

colonization in adult cystic fibrosis patients. Respir Med 1999;93: 835–838.

83. Coenye T, Vandamme P, Govan JRW, et al. Taxonomy and identification of the *Burkholderia cepacia* complex. J Clin Microbiol 2001: 3427–3436.

84. Humphreys H, Peckham D, Patel P, et al. Airborne dissemination of *Burkholderia (Pseudomonas) cepacia* from adult patients with cystic fibrosis. Thorax 1994;49:11571159.

85. McMeamin JD, Zaccone TM, Coenye T, et al. Misidentification of *Burkholderia cepacia* in US cystic fibrosis treatment centers: An analysis of 1,051 recent sputum isolates. Chest 2000;117:1661–1665.

86. Ramsey BW, Gore EJ, Smith AL, et al. The effect of respiratory viral infections on patients with cystic fibrosis. Am J Dis Child 1989;143:662–668.

87. Hiatt PW, Grace SC, Kozinetz CA, et al. Effects of viral lower respiratory tract infection on lung function in infants with cystic fibrosis. Pediatr 1999;103:619–626.

88. Abman SH, Ogle JW, Harbeck RJ, et al. Early bacteriologic, immunologic, and clinical courses of young infants with cystic fibrosis identified by neonatal screening. J Pediatr 1991;119:211–217.

89. Synagis (Palivizumab) package insert. MedImmune Incorporated. July 2008.

90. Gruber WC, Campbell PW, Thompson JM, et al. Comparison of live attenuated and inactivated influenza vaccines in cystic fibrosis patients and their families: Results of a 3-year study. J Infect Dis 1994;169: 241–247.

91. Gross PA, Denning CR, Gaerlan PF, et al. Annual influenza vaccination: Immune response in patients over 10 years. Vaccine 1996;14: 1280–1284.

92. Fiore AE, Shay DK, Broder K, et al. Prevention and control of influenza. Recommendations of the Advisory Committee on Immunization Practices (ACIP). MMWR Recomm Rep 2008;57(RR07): 1–60.

93. Fiel SB. Aerosolized antibiotics in cystic fibrosis: Current and future trends. Expert Reviews of Respiratory Medicine. 2009 Medscape, LLC. 15 July 2009. *http://www.medscape.com/viewarticle/579507_print.*

94. Geller, David E, William H Pitlick, and Pasqua A Nardella. Pharmacokinetics and bioavailability of aerosolized tobramycin in cystic fibrosis. CHEST 122.1 (2002):219–226. Print.

95. Kuhn RJ, Kearns G. Cystic Fibrosis. Pediatric Pharmacotherapy Workbook. University of Kentucky Office of Continuing Pharmacy Education, 1998.

96. Yaffe S, Gerbracht LM, Mosovich LL, et al. Pharmacokinetics of methicillin in patients with cystic fibrosis. J Infect Dis 1977;135:828–831.

97. Powell SH, Thompson WL, Luthe MA, et al. Once-daily vs. continuous aminoglycoside dosing: Efficacy and toxicity in animal and clinical studies of gentamicin, netilmicin and tobramycin. J Infect Dis 1983;5:918–932.

98. Cystic Fibrosis Foundation. Diagnosis, screening, and management of cystic fibrosis related diabetes mellitus. Consensus Conferences. Vol IX Section II. Bethesda, MD: Cystic Fibrosis Foundation; 1999.

99. Rosenecker J, Eichler I, Kuhn L, et al. Genetic determination of diabetes mellitus in patients with cystic fibrosis. J Pediatr 1995;127:441–443.

100. Lanng S, Thorsteinsson B, Lund-Andersen C, et al. Diabetes mellitus in Danish CF patients: Prevalence and late diabetic complications. Acta Paediatr 1994;83:72–77.

101. Finkelstein SM, Wielinski CL, Elliott GR, et al. Diabetes mellitus associated with cystic fibrosis. J Pediatr 1988;112:373–377.

102. Geffner ME, Lippe BM, Maclaren NK, et al. Role of autoimmunity in insulinopenia and carbohydrate derangements with cystic fibrosis. J Pediatr 1988;112:419–421.

103. Sheppard DJ, Welsh MJ. Effect on ATP-sensitive K^+ channel regulators on cystic fibrosis transmembrane conductance regulator chloride currents. J Gen Physiol 1992;100:573–591.

104. Trouvanziam R, Conrad CK, Bottiglieri T, et al. High-dose oral *N*-acetylcysteine, a glutathione prodrug, modulates inflammation in cystic fibrosis. Proc Natl Acad Sci USA 103:4628–4633.

105. Aris RM, Lester GE, Camaniti M, et al. Alendronate for cystic fibrosis adults with low bone density: Results of a randomized, controlled trial. Am J Respir Crit Care Med 169:77–82.

106. Sexauer WP, Fiel SB. Aerosolized antibiotics in cystic fibrosis. Semin Respir Crit Care Med 2003;24:717–726.

107. Kuhn RJ. Pharmaceutical considerations in aerosol drug delivery. Pharmacotherapy 2002;22(3 Pt 2):S80–S85.

108. Rebelo K. ATS 2009: Inhalation powder tobramycin safe, effective to treat *Pseudomonas aeruginosa* in cystic fibrosis patients. Medscape Medical News. 2009 Medscape, LLC. 15 July 2009, *http://www.medscape.com/viewarticle/702973_print.*

109. Cystic Fibrosis Foundation. New antibiotics in the CF medicine chest. Bethesda, MD: Cystic Fibrosis Foundation; 2009. Aug 11, 2009 *http://www.cff.org.*

110. PARI's Altera Delivers Gilead's Cayston, approved by European Commission to treat cystic fibrosis. 2009 PARI Pharma. Sept 23, 2009, *http://www.paripharma.com.*

CHAPTER

38

Evaluation of the Gastrointestinal Tract

KEITH M. OLSEN AND GRANT F. HUTCHINS

KEY CONCEPTS

❶ The patient history is key to evaluating gastrointestinal (GI) tract disorders and should include the problem onset, the setting in which it developed, and its presentation. Patient warning signs and alarm symptoms should be identified quickly and referral for further evaluation should be obtained in a prompt manner.

❷ A complete physical examination should be performed, the severity and location of symptoms directing the focus of the examination.

❸ Contrast agents barium sulfate and gastrograffin allow evaluation of the hollow organs of the digestive tract for mucosally-based lesions as well as narrowing or strictures involving the GI tract.

❹ The upper GI series involves radiographic visualization of the esophagus, stomach, and small intestine; whereas the lower GI series involves visualization of the colon and rectum.

❺ Enteroclysis is used to evaluate the small bowel by introducing contrast agents by tube through the nose or mouth directly into the small intestine.

❻ Trans-abdominal ultrasound, computed tomography, and magnetic resonance imaging provide images of the gallbladder, liver, pancreas, and abdominal wall.

❼ Radionuclide imaging is sometimes useful to visualize and evaluate the liver, spleen, bile ducts, and gallbladder.

❽ The endoscope, an illuminated optical instrument, remains the cornerstone of gastrointestinal diagnosis and most importantly therapy. Common examples of endoscopic procedures include esophagastroduodenoscopy, colonoscopy, enteroscopy, endoscopic retrograde cholangiopancreatography, and endoscopic ultrasound.

Learning objectives, review questions, and other resources can be found at **www.pharmacotherapyonline.com**.

❾ Capsule endoscopy, a newer less invasive endoscopic technique, takes pictures of the GI tract in the assessment of the small bowel in particular.

❿ Ambulatory esophageal pH measurement is an important diagnostic test for gastroesophageal reflux disease and is often performed in conjunction with upper endoscopy. Most systems today are completely wireless and patient friendly.

⓫ Multichannel intraluminal impedance and pH monitoring combines acid exposure with impedance changes in resistant flow to aid the diagnosis of reflux in patients receiving a proton pump inhibitor and other antisecretory medications.

The gastrointestinal (GI) tract is composed of organs and tissues that have diverse forms and functions. It includes the esophagus, stomach, small intestine, large intestine, colon, rectum, biliary tract, gallbladder, liver, and pancreas. Despite the rapid proliferation of technology for the diagnosis of digestive diseases, the patient history and physical examination remain important for initial assessment, triage, and direction of further diagnostic interventions. When combined with a thorough patient history and physical examination, diagnostic procedures are essential in the evaluation of GI disorders. This chapter describes the most commonly used clinical tools to evaluate patients with GI tract–related diseases.

SYMPTOMS OF GASTROINTESTINAL DYSFUNCTION

A variety of symptoms can arise from GI tract dysfunction, including heartburn, dyspepsia, abdominal pain, nausea, vomiting, diarrhea, constipation, and gastrointestinal bleeding. Signs and symptoms of malabsorption, hepatitis, and GI infection are also commonly seen. All clinicians must recognize warning symptoms that include weight loss, intractable vomiting, anemia, dysphagia, and bleeding; and a patient presenting with any of these symptoms should be immediately referred for further diagnostic interventions. The following sections describe methods that are commonly used to assess patients with GI complaints. For specific details concerning each GI disease state, please consult that particular chapter in this book.

PATIENT HISTORY

1 A comprehensive patient history is the cornerstone in the evaluation of a patient with digestive complaints. A clear, detailed, chronologic account of the patient's problems should be gathered. This account should include the onset of the problem, the setting in which it developed, factors that alleviate and aggravate the problem, and its manifestations. The symptom onset often provides important information that helps to formulate a differential diagnosis. For example, biliary colic or pain, such as that encountered with symptomatic gallstone disease, typically evolves over minutes and is present for hours, but pain caused by pancreatitis evolves over hours and lasts for days. The setting is always relevant as it provides clues to the possible origin of the disorder. For example, in the patient with complaints of reflux or ulcer disease, when do the symptoms occur? Are they alleviated or worsened by food and does the pain diminish when administered acid-suppressive therapy? Is the patient immunosuppressed (opportunistic infection vs diseases such as diabetes mellitus)? Also aiding in the diagnosis is the identification of factors that alleviate or exacerbate the principal symptom. For instance, ingesting a meal often relieves the pain of duodenal ulcer, but worsens that of gastric ulcer. The healthcare professional should ask questions that address potential etiologic possibilities, including motility disorders, structural diseases, malignancies, infections, psychosocial factors, dietary factors, and travel-associated diseases.[1,2] Questions concerning past medical and family history detailing illnesses, surgical interventions, injuries, foreign travel, living conditions, and habits are valuable (Table 38-1). A good cardiopulmonary history is also extremely relevant and should be performed during the overall history. A thorough medication use history is vital as many agents cause GI injury (Table 38-2).

TABLE 38-1 General Questions in a Gastrointestinal History

1. Tell me about the problem that you are experiencing. When did it start? What were you doing when the symptoms began?
2. Where is your pain located? Please point to the area where you feel pain. How rapidly did the pain come on? Is your pain constant or intermittent? What factors exacerbate or alleviate your pain? Does the pain awaken you at night?
3. Have you had these symptoms in the past?
4. What medications are you taking to help alleviate the pain? How much do you take? Do these medications work?
5. What other medications are you currently taking? Why are you taking them?
6. Have you recently had a change in dietary intake? If so, please describe. Can you draw any correlation between the foods that you eat and your gastrointestinal (GI) complaint?
7. Have you recently had a change in bowel habits? Have you experienced any diarrhea or constipation lately? Do you experience painful bowel movements?
8. Have you experienced any nausea or vomiting lately? If so, please describe conditions centered around this event.
9. Have you experienced any recent change in weight? Was this intentional? How many pounds have you gained or lost and over what time period did this occur? How has your appetite been?
10. Have you passed any blood from your rectum or vomited blood? Have you noticed any dark, tarry stools?
11. Have you had any acid indigestion?
12. Do you have difficulty swallowing?
13. Has anyone in your family experienced similar GI complaints? If so, please describe. Does anyone in your family have a history of GI disorders, including cancer of the GI tract?
14. Describe your past medical history, including illnesses and surgeries.
15. Please describe any past injuries that you have experienced.
16. Have you recently traveled outside of the United States? If so, where? When? How long did you stay? What kind of living conditions did you experience? What foods and drinks did you ingest?

TABLE 38-2 Drugs That May Cause Gastrointestinal Injury[15-17]

Gastrointestinal mucosal injury
Aspirin
Bisphosphonates
Chemotherapeutic agents
Corticosteroids
Ethacrynic acid
Ethanol
Iron preparations
Nonsteroidal antiinflammatory agents
Pancreatic enzymes
Potassium chloride
Reserpine
Warfarin

Jaundice
Acetohexamide
Androgens
Chlorpropamide
Corticosteroids
Erythromycin
Estrogens
Ethanol
Gold salts
Nitrofurantoin
Phenothiazines
Warfarin

Liver damage
Acetaminophen
Allopurinol
Amiodarone
Aminosalicylic acid
Dapsone
Erythromycin
Ethanol
Glyburide
Isoniazid
Ketoconazole
Lovastatin
Methotrexate
Methyldopa
Monoamine oxidase inhibitors
Nevirapine
Niacin
Nifedipine
Nitrofurantoin
Phenazopyridine
Phenytoin
Propylthiouracil
Rifampin
Salicylates
Sulfonamides
Telithromycin
Tetracycline
Valproic acid
Verapamil
Warfarin
Zidovudine

Pancreatitis
Azathioprine
Corticosteroids
Didanosine
Estrogens
Ethacrynic acid
Ethanol
Furosemide
Metronidazole
Opiates
Pentamidine
Sulfonamides
Tetracycline
Thiazides

PHYSICAL EXAMINATION

❷ Many organ systems of the body interact and may provide important data needed for diagnosis, making it necessary to perform a thorough physical examination.[3] A comprehensive evaluation of the patient should be performed with notable attention to physical appearances and vital signs as they may suggest clues. A careful examination of the abdomen is an essential part of the gastrointestinal workup and classically includes inspection, auscultation, percussion, and palpation in this order. Inspection of the abdomen may reveal scars, hernias, bulges, or peristalsis. Auscultation is mainly focused on analysis of bowel sounds and identification of bruits and should be performed prior to percussion and/or palpation. Percussion of the abdomen allows for detection of tympany, measurement of visceral organ size, and detection of ascites. Palpation may allow the clinician to identify tenderness, rigidity, masses, and hernias. Moving from the abdominal exam, the digital rectal examination is used to detect rectal masses and tenderness, and to assess muscle tone. Stool on the examiner's glove obtained during rectal examination is often subjected to testing for detection of occult blood.[2,3] Patients presenting with upper gastrointestinal symptoms need more careful questioning to distinguish symptoms of reflux disease versus peptic ulcer disease. Additionally, once cardiovascular disease is eliminated, patients with chest pain may have a gastrointestinal source to their symptoms and further diagnostic workup may be needed.

LABORATORY AND MICROBIOLOGIC TESTS

Laboratory and microbiologic tests may be used to (a) assess organ function, (b) screen for certain GI disorders, and (c) evaluate the effectiveness of therapy. Laboratory testing should be viewed largely as supportive to an accurate history and physical examination. To achieve an accurate diagnosis and provide the best care, it is important to assess the patient's fluid and electrolyte status, nutritional status, and abdominal organ function. A complete blood cell count should be completed early in the evaluation to provide information concerning infection, malignancy, bone marrow suppression, anemia, and blood loss.[4] A serum chemistry panel provides clinicians with valuable information—involving several organ systems. For example, serum creatinine and blood urea nitrogen are often used as a measure of hydration status, as well as serving as indicators for renal function. Elevations in serum creatinine and blood urea nitrogen may be indicative of renal dysfunction or dehydration, and bleeding from the upper GI tract may lead to elevations in blood urea nitrogen. Albumin and prealbumin levels can be used to assess the patient's nutritional and hydration status and provide information concerning hepatic and renal function. Specifically, low albumin may be indicative of malnutrition, hepatic dysfunction, nephrotic syndromes, or protein-losing enteropathies. Serum measurements of sodium, chloride, and potassium are useful to determine electrolyte abnormalities associated with diarrheal illnesses.

More specific laboratory blood tests are often useful in classifying pancreaticobiliary disorders. Measurements of serum aspartate transaminase and alanine transaminase are elevated in most diseases of the liver, and serum alkaline phosphatase and bilirubin are often elevated in hepatobiliary disorders involving bile duct blockage. Prothrombin time and international normalized ratio are related to hepatocyte synthesis of vitamin K–dependent clotting factors and serve as indirect measurements of hepatic function. When evaluating patients with suspected pancreatitis, serum and urine measurements of amylase and lipase are important, because these will be elevated in many patients with acute pancreatitis (see Chapter 46).

Microbiologic and related studies are useful in evaluating patients with unexplained diarrhea, abdominal pain, and suspected GI infections. Stool may be examined to detect the presence of bacteria, parasites, or toxins. Pathogens most often responsible for infectious diarrhea and enteritis include bacteria such as *Shigella*, *Salmonella*, *Escherichia coli*, *Yersinia*, and *Clostridium difficile*. Viruses such as cytomegalovirus, especially in patients with acquired immune deficiency syndrome (AIDS), and parasites such as *Entamoeba histolytica* and *Giardia lamblia* are occasionally seen.[5] Patients presenting with watery diarrhea following antibiotic exposure within the previous 1 to 3 months should have their stool checked for *C difficile* toxins A and B. An additional organism *Helicobacter pylori* is a significant factor associated with peptic ulcer disease and MALT lymphomas; identification of this organism is critical in patients experiencing upper gastrointestinal symptoms and is often tested for during upper endoscopy (see Chapter 40).[5]

DIAGNOSIS

The patient's history, physical examination, and routine laboratory tests are valuable in establishing a diagnosis, but frequently more specific studies are required to confirm a clinical suspicion. The most appropriate diagnostic test depends on the anatomic region involved, the suspected abnormality, reliability of the test (e.g., sensitivity vs specificity), the patient's overall condition, and clinical manifestations of the patient. The next sections outline the most frequently used diagnostic studies and procedures and their roles in evaluating the GI tract.

RADIOLOGY

Radiologic procedures rely on the differential absorption of radiation of adjacent tissues to highlight anatomy and pathology. It is useful to divide radiologic testing into noncomputer- and computer-assisted procedures. Noncomputer-assisted radiologic procedures important in evaluating the GI tract include plain radiography, upper GI series with small bowel follow-through, lower GI series, and enteroclysis.[6,7]

Plain Radiography of the GI System

Radiographic evaluation of the GI tract often starts with plain films of the abdomen, which are noncontrast radiographs.[7] Specific abdominal structures that may be identified include the kidneys, ureters, and bladder. In addition, the esophagus, stomach, small and large intestine, and stones may be seen. Stones located within the gallbladder body and within the kidney are also sometimes seen on plain abdominal films. Plain films are often used to evaluate abdominal pain. Clinicians frequently employ plain radiographic fluoroscopy to guide and position other instruments that are used to evaluate and treat GI disorders; an example is the manipulation of dilation devices to treat esophageal strictures. Bowel obstruction and perforation are also sometimes seen using plain radiographic techniques, however the widespread availability of computed tomography (CT) scanning is gradually replacing these techniques.

Contrast Agents

❸ Barium sulfate and/or gastrograffin are the contrast agents of choice for studying the esophagus, stomach, and intestine.[7] Barium sulfate is a metallic material detected by radiography after swallowing the liquid agent; it is termed the *barium swallow*. Barium sulfate is not generally absorbed, and constipation is the most frequent adverse effect reported with its use. Barium sulfate and/or gastrograffin can reveal mucosal defects and lumen size, and is helpful in diagnosing hiatal hernias, strictures along the GI tract, polyps, tumors, and in some cases ulcers. Upper endoscopy is largely replacing the contrast studies in the diagnosis of upper

GI tract disorders, but in certain instances can be a valuable tool in establishing a diagnosis prior to endoscopic evaluation. The barium esophagram should not serve as a primary diagnostic tool for patients with heartburn.

Upper GI Series

❹ The upper GI series refers to the radiographic visualization of the esophagus, stomach, and small intestine. Patient preparation for an upper GI series usually consists of instructing patients to refrain from eating or drinking 8 to 12 hours prior to testing, which allows the upper GI tract to empty. A contrast agent such as barium sulfate or gastrograffin is administered to the patient at the beginning of the study. The observed swallowing of the contrast agent permits visualization and monitoring of esophageal structural and motor functions. As the contrast medium flows into the stomach and small intestine, several regional radiographic films are taken to inspect these areas. This tracking of contrast agents through the small intestine is referred to as the *small bowel follow-through*. The upper GI series with small bowel follow-through commonly uncovers gastric cancer, peptic ulcer disease, esophagitis, gastric outlet obstruction, and can be suggestive of Crohn's disease (Fig. 38–1). In general, the barium swallow is plagued by low sensitivity and specificity for many GI disorders and as mentioned is being replaced by upper endoscopic techniques.

Lower GI Series

The lower GI series is used to examine the colon and rectum and is particularly useful if a colonic obstruction is suspected. Patients complaining of lower abdominal pain, constipation, or diarrhea are often referred for a lower GI series, also called a barium enema. The

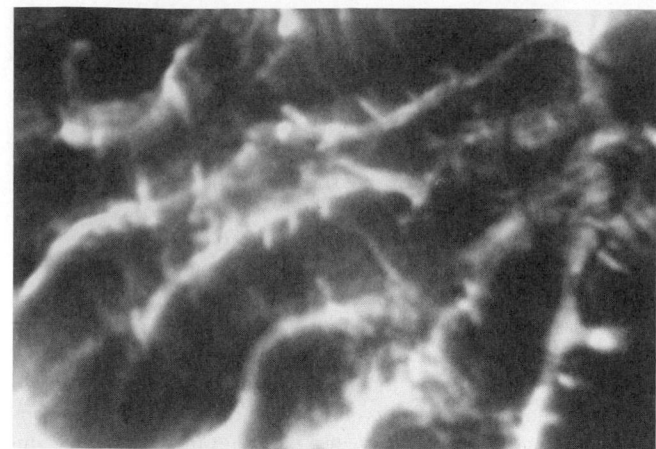

FIGURE 38-2. Normal small bowel enteroclysis. Contrast agents are instilled into the small bowel to highlight tumors, strictures, or other lesions. In this image, one can identify the normal circular folds.

colon is prepared for the procedure by instructing the patient to refrain from eating or drinking 8 to 12 hours before the procedure, and by administering bowel-cleansing agents such as bisacodyl, magnesium citrate, magnesium hydroxide, or polyethylene glycol electrolyte (PEG) solution. During a lower GI series, a barium sulfate enema is given to contrast the terminal large intestine and rectum. The lower GI series is sometimes useful to detect and evaluate enterocolitis, obstructions, volvulus, and mucosal and structural lesions.[7]

Small Bowel Enteroclysis

❺ Enteroclysis, or small bowel enema, refers to the technique of direct small bowel introduction of a contrast agent through a tube inserted through the patient's mouth or nose directly into the small intestine. Sequential radiographic films are taken of the small bowel as the contrast agent flows distally (Fig. 38–2). Because enteroclysis provides detailed imaging, it is an accurate method for evaluating the small bowel and for detecting small mucosal lesions that may be overlooked on the traditional small bowel follow-through.[9] Methylcellulose is used to enhance the detail of the small intestine in enteroclysis, thereby improving visualization. Patient preparation for this procedure involves instructing patients to refrain from eating or drinking 8 to 12 hours before testing and administering bowel-cleansing agents. The enteroclysis technique is a useful study for evaluation of the upper GI tract, but unfortunately it is not widely performed due to operator inexperience and is gradually being replaced by improved radiologic techniques such as CT or magnetic resonance imaging (MRI) enterography or more recently by small intestinal endoscopy known as single and double balloon enteroscopy.

IMAGING STUDIES

The second category of radiologic evaluation of the GI tract involves computer-assisted techniques, which allow a cross-sectional radiographic image of the body to be performed. Transabdominal ultrasonography, computed tomography, radionuclide scanning, and magnetic resonance imaging are frequently used imaging procedures for evaluating digestive disorders.[6,7]

Ultrasonography

❻ Ultrasonography provides images of deeper structures such as the gallbladder, liver, and kidneys and can also be very useful in helping to define vascular abnormalities in the intra-abdominal

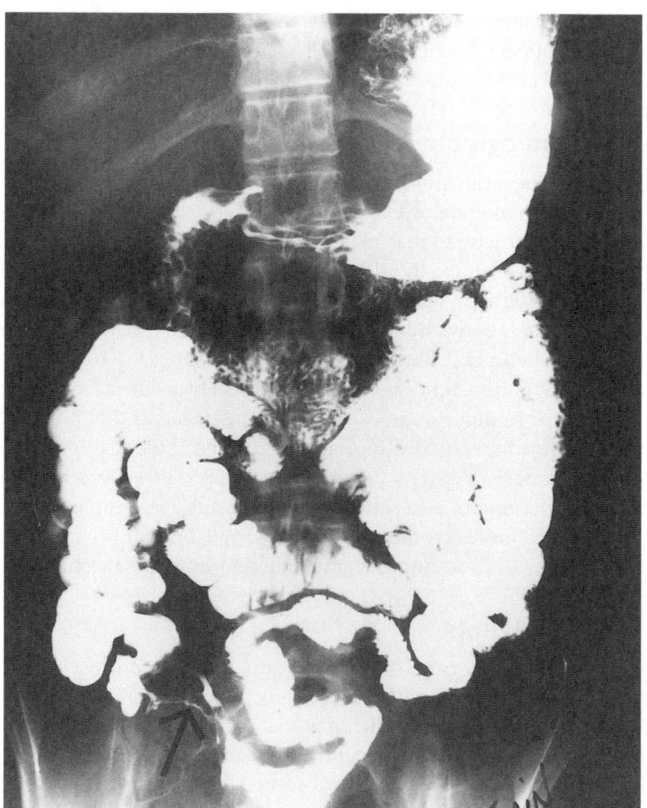

FIGURE 38-1. Upper GI series with small bowel follow-through demonstrating narrowed distal terminal ileum and separation of small bowel loops (*arrow*). These findings are consistent with Crohn's disease.

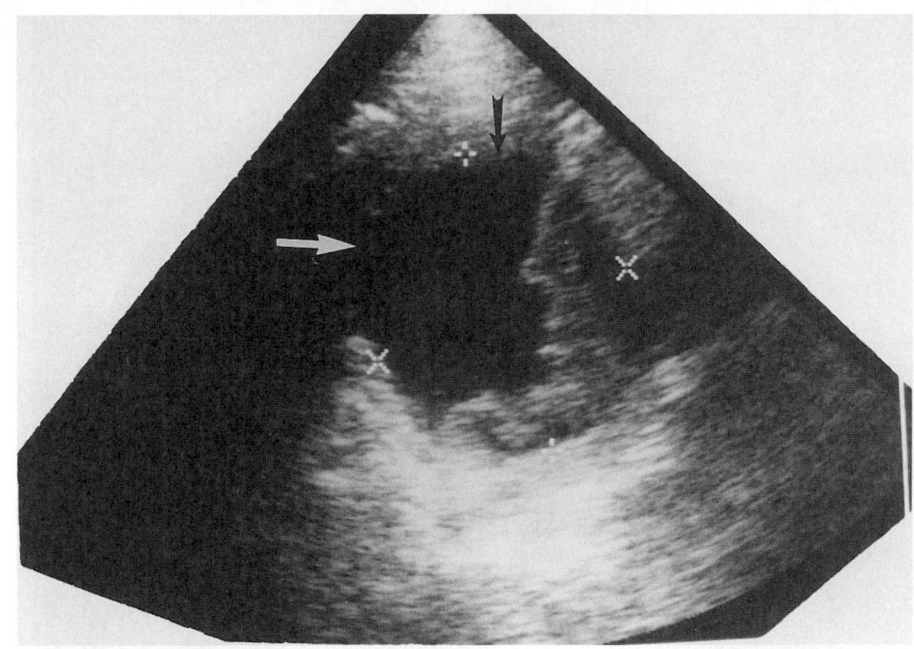

FIGURE 38-3. Abdominal ultrasonogram demonstrating a chronic pancreatic pseudocyst *(arrows)*.

cavity. Ultrasound involves the direction of a narrow beam of high-energy sound waves into the body and recording the reflections from the various organs and structures. Ultrasonography is noninvasive, relatively inexpensive, requires no ionizing radiation, and can be performed at bedside with a portable unit, and as such it is a well-accepted and useful technology. It accurately depicts gallstones presence within the gallbladder, helps define liver morphology, and is an excellent first test in the evaluation of the jaundiced patient to evaluate the absence or presence of biliary ductal dilation (Fig. 38–3). When combined with Doppler technologies, ultrasonography can image GI vascularity, in particular portal venous flow and in the early identification of aneurismal dilations of the abdominal aorta. Ultrasonography is limited by the presence of bowel gas and excessive amounts of body fat, particularly when evaluating deeper organs such as the pancreas.[6,7]

Computed Tomography

Computed tomography or computed axial tomography (CAT) scans provide detailed images of the GI system in which transverse planes of tissue are swept by a radiographic beam and a computer analysis of the variance in absorption produces a precise reconstructed image of that area.[6] Contrast agents may be added in a CT procedure to illuminate specific hollow structures and vascularity of the GI tract. The abdominal CT displays organs from the diaphragm down to the pelvic brim, and is especially valuable for detecting GI diseases of the liver, pancreas, spleen, and colon. Patient preparation for CT includes refraining from eating or drinking for a minimum of 4 hours before the test. The remarkable detail that CT offers in imaging organs and tissues adds to its popularity for evaluation of the GI system. CT scanning is rapidly replacing plane radiography of the abdomen due to its widespread availability, diminishing cost, and wealth of information gained. CT is useful in the identification of suspected intra-abdominal malignancy, pancreatitis, intra-abdominal abscesses, and cysts (Fig. 38–4).[6,7] Unlike ultrasonography, patient body size or the presence of gas does not limit the quality of imaging with CT. Contrast used during CT scanning is nephrotoxic and close attention to a patient's renal function is mandatory in these patients.

Radionuclide Imaging

7 Radionuclide imaging involves intravenous injections of a radiopharmaceutical imaging agent and the use of a computerized detection camera to gather images. A secretory agent is sometimes given in addition to the radiopharmaceutical agent to improve sensitivity. Although the choice of a radiopharmaceutical agent depends on the specific organ or function being studied, the most commonly used agent is technetium (^{99m}Tc) tagged to a carrier molecule. Radionuclide imaging is sometimes useful to visualize the liver and spleen (liver-spleen scan), bile ducts, gallbladder (HIDA [hepatoimin-odiacetic acid] scan), and gut (tagged red blood cell).[6,7] Cysts, abscesses, tumors, and obstructions are detected and displayed as areas of differential uptake of radioactivity.[6] Radionuclide bleeding scans may detect hemorrhages and may assist in localization to help with therapeutic intervention. Contrast media nephrotoxicity in patients with preexisting renal impairment remains a clinically significant problem. Pretest treatment in high-risk patients with pharmacologic agents has demonstrated mixed results.

Magnetic Resonance Imaging

Magnetic resonance imaging and magnetic resonance cholangiopancreatography (MRCP) places the patient in close proximity to a high-strength magnetic field through which pulses of radiofrequency radiation are projected, thereby exciting the nuclei of hydrogen, phosphorus, oxygen, and other elements. The radiofrequency signals are manipulated and recorded by a computer, and a two-dimensional image representing a section of the patient is produced.[6,7] MRI has greater sensitivity for identifying liver tumors than do ultrasonography, CT, and radionuclide imaging. Significant advances in MRI technology and imaging capabilities often make this a preferred diagnostic test, particularly in the evaluation of pancreaticobiliary disorders.[6,7]

Arteriography

Arteriography of the gut depicts the configuration of visceral blood vessels after intravenous administration of a contrast medium. Arteriography may be employed for vascular anomalies such as an aneurismal dilation and in the evaluation of obscure bleeding

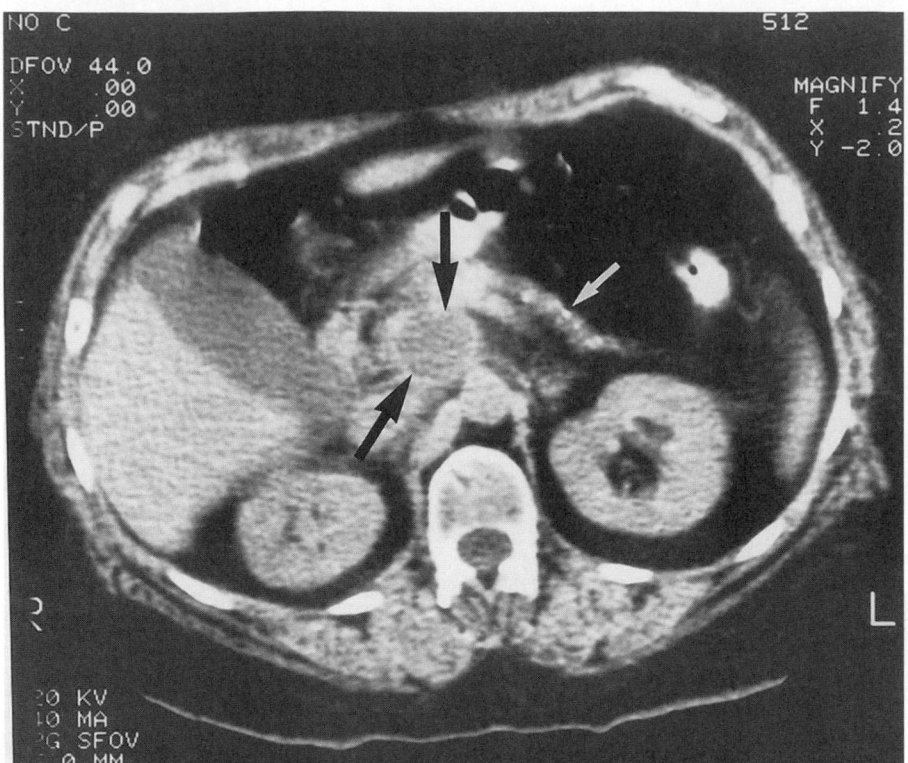

FIGURE 38-4. CT scan of the abdomen showing pancreatitis with calcification *(white arrow)* and pancreatic pseudocyst *(black arrows)*.

lesions. Therapeutic applications, including embolization of bleeding vessels, fistulas, and inoperable tumors.[6,7]

ENDOSCOPY

8 Refinement in optical engineering and fiber optics led to the development of the endoscope, which has revolutionized the management of GI disorders. Most endoscopic equipment today uses a computer chip device to provide high definition, detailed images of the particular lumen being examined. An endoscope is an illuminated white light and non-white light optical instrument designed to inspect the interior of the GI tract. Endoscopes enable the practitioner to inspect intraluminal mucosal lesions and to obtain biopsies and washings for cytology studies. Standard upper GI tract endoscopy (i.e., esophagogastroduodenoscopy [EGD]) is capable of inspecting the esophagus, stomach, and proximal small bowel. Lower GI tract endoscopic evaluation of the rectum and colon may be accomplished by colonoscopy or flexible-sigmoidoscopy. Standard upper and lower endoscopy can also be used to perform many therapeutic procedures and in addition many newer diagnostic and therapeutic endoscopic devices are now available.[8]

Preparation for endoscopic examinations includes instructing patients to refrain from eating or drinking for at least 8 to 12 hours prior to the endoscopic procedure. Bowel cleansing is necessary for colonoscopy and sigmoidoscopy using a variety of PEG-based solutions. Topical pharyngeal anesthetics, such as viscous lidocaine or benzocaine, usually improve patient acceptance of the upper endoscopic tube. Intravenous sedating agents, such as the benzodiazepines, lorazepam, midazolam, and, more recently, propofol, are among the most common agents used to induce differing levels of sedation, most commonly "conscious sedation" prior to the endoscopy. These sedating agents tend to improve patient acceptance and ease of the procedure. The agents should not be used without appropriate monitoring and the availability of flumazenil, a benzodiazepine antagonist. Serious adverse events

have occurred with these agents when used for conscious sedation. In addition, antimuscarinic agents such as atropine sulfate are occasionally used for their cardiovascular effects, such as increasing a patient's heart rate, or for their antispasmodic effects, such as reducing duodenal and colonic motility. Because of its effectiveness at reducing bowel motility, glucagon may be used. Endoscopy should be pursued with caution in patients with severe respiratory or cardiac failure, and endoscopy is contraindicated for patients with suspected perforated viscera. The most commonly used endoscopic studies are upper endoscopy (EGD), colonoscopy, flexible sigmoidoscopy, and endoscopic retrograde cholangiopancreatography (ERCP).[8] Newer endoscopic techniques include capsule endoscopy, endoscopic ultrasound (EUS), and single or double balloon enteroscopy. These techniques are outlined in detail below.

Esophagogastroduodenoscopy is used to examine the esophagus, stomach, and duodenum. Patient preparation for EGD includes fasting for at least 6 to 8 hours prior to the procedure and the administration of sedatives and topical anesthetics. Common indications include evaluation of suspected upper GI bleeding, obstructions, upper abdominal pain, and persistent vomiting. Evaluation of radiographic abnormalities is also a frequent procedural indication.[12] EGD can be used therapeutically in upper gastrointestinal bleeding for ligation procedures involving esophageal varices, sclerosing or vasoconstrictive agent administration at the site of the bleed in peptic ulcer induced bleeding, or via the use of a thermal device such as a gold probe or heater probe on a bleeding vessel. In addition to its therapeutic potential, EGD commonly uncovers peptic ulcer disease and is the method of choice to diagnose Barrett's esophagus, a premalignant condition of the esophagus and other esophageal ulcer erosive disorders (Fig. 38–5). Once viewed as the method of choice to diagnosis gastroesophageal reflux disease, upper endoscopy, although commonly used, is often times not performed before a trial of a proton pump inhibitor has been undertaken. The favorable side-effect profile of proton pump inhibitors in addition to their superior healing ability make these agents extremely power-

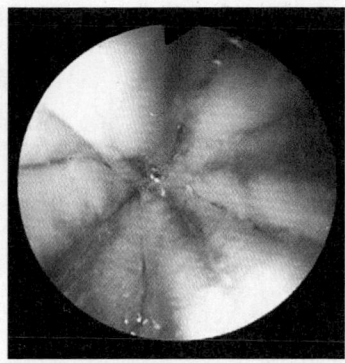

FIGURE 38-5. EGD demonstrating linear red streaks with a central white streak extended up the esophagus in peptic regurgitant esophagitis. *(From Kasper DL, Braunwald E, Hauser S, et al., eds. Harrison's Principles of Internal Medicine, 16th ed. New York: McGraw-Hill, 2005:1731, with permission.)*

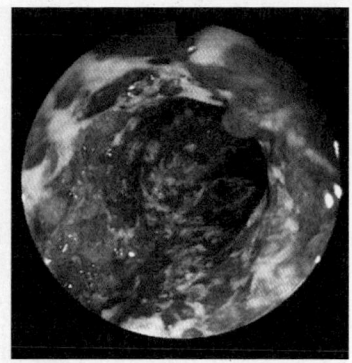

FIGURE 38-6. Sigmoidoscopic photograph demonstrating severe ulcerative colitis with diffuse ulceration, bleeding, and exudation. *(From Kasper DL, Braunwald E, Hauser S, et al., eds. Harrison's Principles of Internal Medicine, 16th ed. New York: McGraw-Hill, 2005:1732, with permission.)*

ful and widely prescribed by primary care physicians for heartburn and other symptoms attributed to gastroesophageal reflux disease. Primary care physicians usually refer patients for EGD only when they fail to respond to a course of proton pump inhibitor therapy, and by the time an endoscopy is performed the examination is likely to reveal normal-appearing mucosa. Even in patients undergoing upper endoscopy in the evaluation of reflux type symptomatology in the absence of proton pump inhibitor therapy, endoscopy will be normal in up to 50% of patients.[8]

Colonoscopy

Colonoscopy permits direct examination of the large intestine and rectum. To prepare for colonoscopy, the patient should fast for at least 8 to 12 hours prior to the examination, and bowel cleansing should be completed. Bowel preparations have traditionally involved a PEG-based or phosphate-based solution. However, because of concerns regarding phosphate-induced nephropathy, there has been a return to standard PEG-based solutions. A benzodiazepine and a short-acting narcotic agent are given to produce conscious sedation and in patients refractory or intolerant to conscious sedation agents, propofol is often administered to provide a deeper level of sedation. As with upper GI endoscopy, indications for lower GI endoscopy can be either diagnostic or therapeutic in nature. Common indications include evaluation and detection of abnormalities visualized by radiography, as well as diagnosis and therapy of GI hemorrhage, and importantly, screening patients for colorectal carcinoma. Additionally colonoscopy remains an invaluable procedure in the diagnosis, staging, and therapy of patients with inflammatory bowel disease (e.g., ulcerative colitis and Crohn's disease).[9]

Sigmoidoscopy

Flexible sigmoidoscopy is used to evaluate the sigmoid colon via the anorectum (Fig. 38-6). Flexible sigmoidoscopy has virtually replaced rigid sigmoidoscopy because of increased patient comfort and superior performance. The major indication for this examination is to evaluate symptoms related to the distal colon or rectum, such as hematochezia, painful defecation, and unexplained diarrhea. Flexible sigmoidoscopy is gradually being replaced by full colonoscopy in the evaluation and screening of patients for colorectal carcinoma. Patient preparation involves instructing patients to abstain from eating or drinking for at least 8 hours prior to the procedure and the administering of bowel-cleansing agents. Anoscopy is especially useful in evaluating the anus. The

major indications for anoscopic examination include symptoms related to the anus and rectum, such as bleeding, protruding anorectal lesions, pain with defecation in particular, and severe itching. Patients undergoing sigmoidoscopy or anoscopy generally do not require sedation.

Endoscopic Retrograde Cholangiopancreatography

Endoscopic retrograde cholangiopancreatography is an important procedure that is used to evaluate and treat diseases of the pancreaticobiliary tree. Common indications include common bile duct stone diagnosis and management, bile and pancreatic duct stricture management, and in the diagnosis and therapy of patients with biliary tract and/or pancreatic malignancies. Contrast injection following wire-guided bile or pancreatic duct cannulation reveals abnormalities such as obstruction due to malignancy or fluid collections, calculi, and strictures can be examined. ERCP also allows for the use of therapeutic techniques such as biliary or pancreatic sphincterotomy, removal of ductal stones from the common bile duct or main pancreatic duct, and in the stenting of biliary or pancreatic strictures. ERCP is also a useful method for tissue acquisition in the pancreaticobiliary tract using a variety of brush and biopsy devices. Recent advances in ERCP include the addition of direct bile duct or pancreatic duct visualization, a procedure which has greatly aided in the diagnosis and therapy of pancreaticobiliary disorders. Preparation for ERCP consists of conscious sedation and glucagon to relax gut motility and often requires the use of an anesthesiologist due to the complex and long procedural times associated with ERCP (Fig. 38-7).[7,9]

Endoscopic Ultrasound

Endoscopic ultrasound is a newer, exciting endoscopic technology which represents a marriage between upper endoscopy and standard ultrasound techniques. A high frequency ultrasound probe is attached to the working end of a diagnostic (radial array) or therapeutic (linear array) oblique viewing echoendoscope. Endoscopic ultrasound is commonly used to stage and diagnose upper GI tract malignancies such as those involving the esophagus, stomach, and pancreas. Upper GI tract locoregional tumor staging and tissue acquisition is highly sensitive and specific and provides a less invasive manner of tissue acquisition in many cases. Expanded uses of EUS include diagnosis and management of pancreatic fluid collections including pancreatic cystic neoplasms (non-pseudocystic), celiac plexus block vs neurolysis in pancreatic malignant and chronic pancreatitis patients, and in some centers in the direct instillation of antitumor agents into

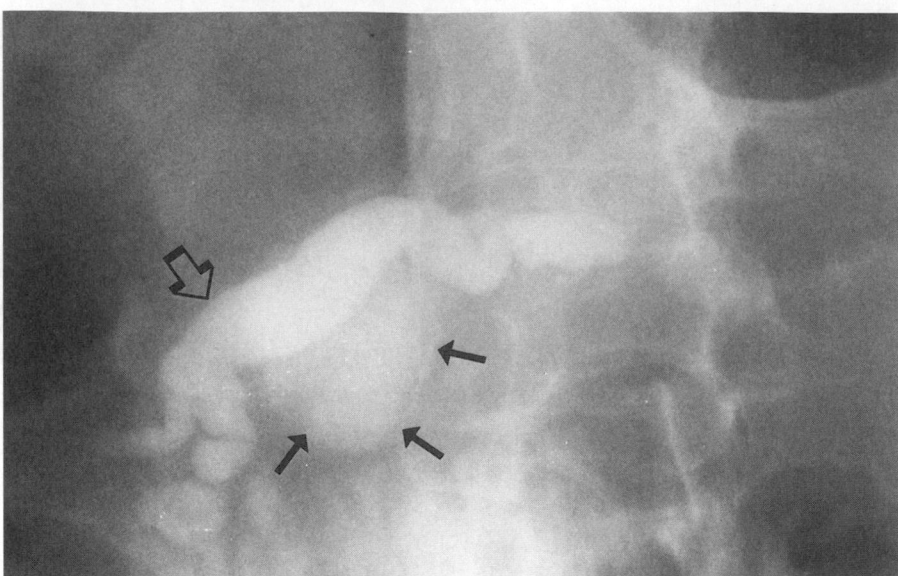

FIGURE 38-7. Endoscopic retrograde cholangiopancreatography (ERCP) demonstrating a dilated, irregular pancreatic duct with areas of stricturing *(large arrow)*. A pancreatic pseudocyst is visible immediately adjacent to the spine *(small arrows)*.

pancreatic malignancies. Lower GI tract EUS is also commonly performed most often in the diagnosis and locoregional staging of anorectal carcinoma and in evaluation of the anal sphincters. EUS is an invaluable tool in the management of GI tract disorders but does remain centered largely in academic, tertiary care referral institutions.

Enteroscopy

Enteroscopy, or direct visualization of the small intestine, has traditionally been limited to examination of the proximal most portions of the duodenum/jejunum because of excessive endoscope looping and discomfort to the patient during the examination. To overcome these difficulties two newer techniques, single and double balloon enteroscopy, have been developed. These particular enteroscopes involve sequential inflation and deflation of balloon attachment devices in order to sequentially "walk" the enteroscope down the small or large intestine. A combination of inflation, deflation, and endoscope reduction via torque and withdrawal allow for a pleating of the mucosal surface being examined. Complete traversal of the small intestine is routinely achieved via the oral route and significant traversal of the colon and distal small intestine is now possible from the rectal route. Common indications for these procedures include the evaluation of obscure GI bleeding, the diagnosis and evaluation of possible inflammatory bowel disease, and in the evaluation of radiologically discovered lesions such as mass or bowel wall thickening.

Capsule Endoscopy

❾ Capsule endoscopy allows the visualization of the esophagus, stomach, and small intestine. This device consists of a vitamin pill–sized video camera that is swallowed and acts as an endoscope (Fig. 38–8). As the video capsule travels naturally through the digestive tract, images are transmitted to a recording device placed on the patient's hip. Patients return the recording device to the practitioner so that the images can be downloaded to a computer and evaluated. Eventually, the camera is naturally excreted and not retrieved.[10] Capsule endoscopy represents a noninvasive means to evaluate the upper and lower GI tracts but unfortunately lacks therapeutic capability. Capsule endoscopy is often used in the evaluation of obscure GI bleeding and in the evaluation of suspected inflammatory bowel disease and is often times used in conjunction with single or double balloon enteroscopy.

MISCELLANEOUS TESTS

Esophageal Manometry

Esophageal manometry is used to evaluate diseases of the esophagus by assessing esophageal motor functions. Common indications for this procedure include dysphagia and obscure chest pain. A special catheter equipped with pressure transducers is placed into the esophagus to measure esophageal pressures and peristalsis. Provocative testing with pharmacologic agents such as edrophonium chloride, a cholinergic muscle stimulant, may be used to precipitate esophageal pain during this procedure. Typical indications for esophageal manometry include evaluating suspected esophageal dysmotility, nonobstructive dysphagia, obscure chest pain, intestinal pseudo-obstruction, achalasia, and aiding in the positioning instruments such as pH probes. Esophageal manometry almost always is performed following endoscopic evaluation of the upper GI tract and can be a valuable tool in diagnosing many nonspecific disorders of the upper GI tract.

Ambulatory Esophageal pH Monitoring

❿ Esophageal pH monitoring is considered by many clinicians as the gold standard in the evaluation of patients who complain

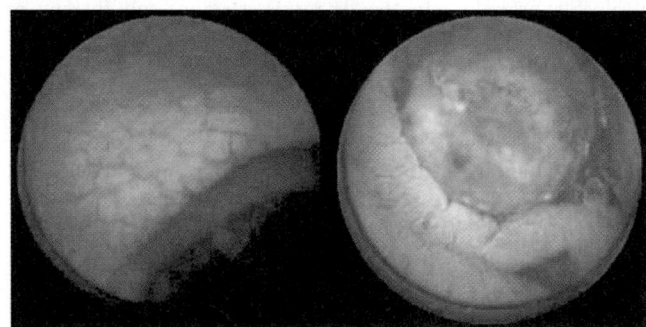

FIGURE 38-8. Capsule endoscopy images of a mildly scalloped jejuna fold (left) and an ileal tumor (right) in a patient with celiac sprue. *(From Kasper DL, Braunwald E, Hauser S, et al., eds. Harrison's Principles of Internal Medicine, 17th ed. New York: McGraw-Hill. http://www. acessmedicine.com. Images courtesy of Dr. Elizabeth Rajan; with permission.)*

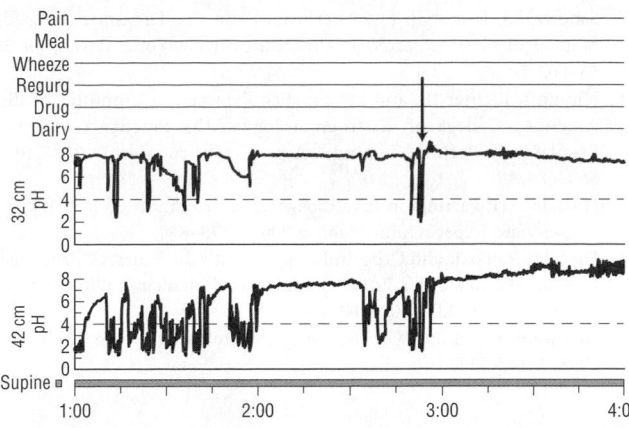

FIGURE 38-9. Ambulatory pH monitoring. The pH recordings from two esophageal probes are plotted over a 3-hour interval. Notice that the patient's symptom of regurgitation correlates with a low pH (<4) event (*arrow*).

of gastroesophageal reflux. Ambulatory 24-hour pH monitoring is an elegant way to link esophageal acid exposure, as detected by a probe in the esophagus, with patient symptoms. The pH probe is placed approximately 5 cm above the distal esophagus. Because intraesophageal pH is normally higher (pH 6) than that of the stomach (pH approximately 1–3), the pH probe will record a decrease in pH if gastroesophageal reflux occurs. The most accepted method to identify gastroesophageal reflux during monitoring is the sudden decrease in pH below 4.0. The ambulatory 24-hour pH study links the patient's symptom to an acid event (Fig. 38–9). Wireless pH monitoring systems have gradually replaced the older methods that required a wire probe placement. A capsule is attached to the distal esophagus by a delivery system. The capsule then transmits measured pH data to a receiver by radiotelemetry technique. Wireless systems offer the advantage of better patient acceptance and extended monitoring of up to 96 hours versus 24 hours of the wire method. There are limitations to ambulatory pH monitoring in patients receiving proton pump inhibitor therapy or in the detection of nonacidic or weakly acidic refluxate.[11]

⑪ Multichannel intraluminal impedance monitoring is an emerging technique to study acid and nonacid reflux. The method combines pH measurements with manometry that enables the measurement of and distinction between swallowing and reflux. In patients whose symptoms have not responded to empiric proton pump inhibitor therapy in GERD, the test can separate those in whom symptoms are associated with acid reflux from those in whom symptoms are associated with nonacid reflux. Outcomes studies are required to further evaluate the usefulness of this diagnostic method; however, accumulating data are extremely promising.[12,13]

The Bernstein test, an older procedure that is used to measure gastric fluid pH, has largely been replaced by ambulatory pH monitoring. The procedure requires inserting a nasogastric tube and administrating alternating dripped solutions of normal saline and 0.1 N hydrochloric acid (HCl) into the esophagus via the nasogastric tube. If patient symptoms are reproduced by the acid perfusion and not the saline, the study is considered abnormal and indicative of acid hypersensitivity.[14]

Laparoscopy

Laparoscopy uses a tube-like device with an elaborate optical system that permits distinct visualization of the peritoneal cavity. General anesthesia is often required and a surgical incision is made in the abdomen to allow the passage of the laparoscope. The exterior of the liver, gallbladder, spleen, peritoneum, diaphragm, and pelvic organs may be examined during the laparoscopic examination. Similar to the other endoscopic techniques mentioned, biopsies and therapeutic interventions may be performed during the laparoscopy. Laparoscopy, it is important to remember, is extremely invasive. Reasons for doing laparoscopy include evaluating patients with abdominal masses, chronic abdominal pain of unclear etiology, abnormalities indicated on liver-spleen scan, such as acute or chronic choleycystitis, and to aid in the diagnosis and management of intra-abdominal malignancy.

CONCLUSIONS

Evaluation of the GI tract begins with a careful history and comprehensive physical examination. It then proceeds in a deliberate and thoughtful manner to establish the correct diagnosis and appropriate management of a given GI tract problem. Laboratory and microbiologic testing in addition to appropriate radiologic evaluation are often the initial steps in the evaluation of a patient with a particular GI tract complaint. GI tract endoscopy using a wide range of endoscopic devices with both diagnostic and therapeutic potential has entered the GI tract mainstream in recent years. Despite the wide array of testing and procedures available clinicians need to continue to perform a thorough history and physical examination and should be keenly aware of warning signs and symptoms that require immediate referral for further diagnostic studies and possible therapeutic intervention.

ABBREVIATIONS

CAT: computed axial tomography

CT: computed tomography

EGD: esophagogastroduodenoscopy

ERCP: endoscopic retrograde colangiopancreatography

EUS: endoscopic ultrasound

MRCP: magnetic resonance cholangiopancreatography

MRI: magnetic resonance imaging

PEG: polyethylene glycol electrolyte solution

REFERENCES

1. Hasler WL, Owyang C. Approach to the patient with gastrointestinal disease. In: Fauci AS, Brunwald E, et al., eds. Harrison's Principles of Internal Medicine, 17th ed. New York: McGraw-Hill, 2008:1831–1836.
2. Proctor DD. Approach to the patient with gastrointestinal disease. In: Goldman L, Ausiello D, eds. Cecil's Textbook of Medicine, 23rd ed. Philadelphia, PA: WB Saunders, 2008:951–965.
3. Bates B. A Guide to Physical Examination, 10th ed. Bickely L, ed. Philadelphia, PA: Lippincott, 2008.
4. Farkas J, Farkas P, Hyde D. Liver and gastroenterology tests. In: Lee M, ed. Interpreting Laboratory Data. Bethesda, MD: American Society of Health-System Pharmacists, 2009:235–269.
5. Bouckengooghe AR, DuPont HL. Approach to the patient with diarrhea. In: Gorbach SL, Bartlett JG, Blacklow NR, eds. Infectious Diseases. Philadelphia, PA: Lippincott Williams & Wilkins, 2004:597–603.
6. Novelline RA. Squire's Fundamentals of Radiology. Cambridge, MA: Harvard University Press, 2004.
7. Pickhardt PJ. Diagnostic imaging procedures in gastroenterology. In: Goldman L, Ausiello D, eds. Cecil's Textbook of Medicine, 23rd ed. Philadelphia, PA: WB Saunders, 2008:965–969.

8. Tytgat GNJ. Upper gastrointestinal endoscopy. In: Yamada T, Alpers DH, Kaplowitz N, et al., eds. Gastroenterology. Philadelphia: Lippincott Williams & Wilkins, 2003:138:2825–2844.

9. Hay DW, Onion SK. Blackwell's Primary Care Essentials: Gastrointestinal and Liver Disease. Malden, MA: Blackwell Science, 2002:363.

10. Pasricha PJ. Gastrointestinal Endoscopy. In: Goldman L, Ausiello D, eds. Cecil's Textbook of Medicine, 23rd, ed. Philadelphia, PA: WB Saunders, 2008:970–976.

11. Lutsi B, Hirano I. Ambulatory pH monitoring: New advances and indications. Gastroenterol Hepatol 2006;2:825–842.

12. Tutuian R, Vela MF, Shay SS, Castell DO. Multichannel intraluminal impedance in esophageal function testing and gastroesophageal reflux monitoring. J Clin Gastroenterol 2003;37:206–215.

13. Sandler RS. Bernstein (acid perfusion) test. In: Drossman DA, ed. Manual of Gastroenterologic Procedures. New York: Raven, 1993: 56–60.

14. Hirano I, Richter JE, and the Practice Parameter Committee of the American College of Gastroenterology. ACG Practice Guideline: Esophageal Reflux Testing. Am J Gastroenterol 2007:102: 668–685.

15. Hussaini SH, Farrington EA. Idiosyncratic drug-induced liver injury: an overview. Expert Opin Drug Saf 2007;6:673–684.

16. Dienstag JL. Toxic and Drug-Induced Hepatitis. In: Fauci AS, Brunwald E, et al., eds. Harrison's Principles of Internal Medicine, 17th ed., New York: McGraw-Hill, 2008:1949–1955.

17. Nathwani RA, Kaplowitz N. Drug hepatotoxicity. Clin Liver Dis 2006;10:207–217.

CHAPTER 39

Gastroesophageal Reflux Disease

DIANNE B. WILLIAMS AND ROBERT R. SCHADE

KEY CONCEPTS

❶ Esophageal gastroesophageal reflux disease (GERD) syndromes can be described as symptom based or esophageal tissue injury based.

❷ Endoscopy is used to evaluate mucosal damage from GERD and to assess for the presence of Barrett esophagus or other complications; ambulatory pH monitoring (with or without impedance monitoring) is useful for confirming GERD for patients with persistent symptoms without evidence of mucosal damage or for patients with atypical symptoms; manometry is useful for patients who are candidates for antireflux surgery and for ensuring proper placement of pH probes.

❸ The goals of GERD treatment are to alleviate symptoms, decrease the frequency of recurrent disease, promote healing of mucosal injury, and prevent complications.

❹ GERD treatment is determined by disease severity and includes lifestyle changes and patient-directed therapy, pharmacologic treatment, and antireflux surgery.

❺ Patients with typical esophageal GERD syndromes should be treated with lifestyle modifications as appropriate and a trial of empiric acid-suppression therapy. Those who do not respond to empiric therapy or who present with alarm symptoms should undergo endoscopy.

❻ Surgical intervention is a viable alternative treatment for select patients when long-term pharmacologic management is undesirable.

❼ Acid suppression is the mainstay of GERD treatment. Proton pump inhibitors provide the greatest symptom relief and the highest healing rates, especially for patients with erosive disease or moderate to severe symptoms.

❽ Many patients with GERD will relapse if treatment medication is withdrawn; so long-term maintenance treatment may be required. A proton pump inhibitor is the drug of choice for maintenance of patients with moderate to severe GERD.

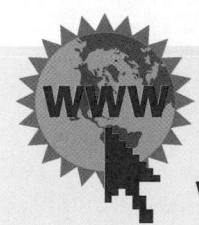

The complete chapter,
learning objectives, and other
resources can be found at
www.pharmacotherapyonline.com.

❾ Patient medication profiles should be reviewed for drugs that may aggravate GERD. Patients should be monitored for adverse drug reactions and potential drug–drug interactions.

Gastroesophageal reflux disease (GERD) is a common medical disorder. A consensus definition of GERD states it is "a condition that occurs when the refluxed stomach contents lead to troublesome symptoms and/or complications."[1] The key is that these troublesome symptoms adversely affect the well-being of the patient. Episodic heartburn that is not frequent enough or painful enough to be considered bothersome by the patient is not included in this definition of GERD.[1]

Esophageal GERD syndromes are classified as either symptom-based or tissue injury based depending on how the patient presents.[1] Symptom-based esophageal GERD syndromes may exist with or without esophageal injury and most commonly present as heartburn, regurgitation or dysphagia. Less commonly, odynophagia (painful swallowing) or hypersalivation may occur. Tissue injury–based syndromes may exist with or without symptoms. The spectrum of injury includes esophagitis (inflammation of the lining of the esophagus), Barrett esophagus (when tissue lining the esophagus is replaced by tissue similar to the lining of the intestine), strictures, and esophageal adenocarcinoma.[2] Esophagitis occurs when the esophagus is repeatedly exposed to refluxed gastric contents for prolonged periods of time. This can progress to erosion of the squamous epithelium of the esophagus (erosive esophagitis). Complications of long-term reflux may include the development of strictures, Barrett esophagus, or possibly adenocarcinoma of the esophagus.

Gastroesophageal reflux symptoms associated with disease processes in organs other than the esophagus are referred to as *extraesophageal reflux syndromes*. Patients with extraesophageal reflux syndromes may present with reflux chest pain syndrome, laryngitis, or asthma. An association between these syndromes and GERD should only be considered when they occur along with esophageal GERD syndrome because these extraesophageal symptoms are nonspecific and have many other causes.[1]

Inflammation of the esophagitis (reflux esophagitis) can sometimes progress to erosions of the squamous epithelium of the esophagus; this is known as *erosive esophagitis*. Many patients suffering from mild GERD do not go on to develop erosive esophagitis and are often managed with lifestyle changes, antacids, and nonprescription histamine-2 (H_2) receptor antagonists or nonprescription proton pump inhibitors. Those with more severe symptoms (with or without tissue injury) predictably follow a course of relapsing disease, requiring more intensive treatment with acid-suppression therapy followed by long-term maintenance therapy. Antireflux surgery offers an alternative for select patients in whom prolonged medical management is undesirable.

EPIDEMIOLOGY

Gastroesophageal reflux disease occurs in people of all ages but is most common in those older than age 40 years. Although mortality associated with GERD is rare, GERD symptoms may have a significant impact on quality of life. The true prevalence and incidence of GERD is difficult to assess because many patients do not seek medical treatment, symptoms do not always correlate well with the severity of the disease, and there is no standardized definition or universal gold standard method for diagnosing the disease. However, 10% to 20% of adults in Western countries suffer from GERD symptoms on a weekly basis.[3]

The prevalence of GERD varies depending on the geographic region but appears highest in Western countries.[3] Except during pregnancy, there does not appear to be a major difference in incidence between men and women. Although gender does not generally play a major role in the development of GERD, it is an important factor in the development of Barrett esophagus. Barrett esophagus is most prevalent in white adult males in Western countries and may increase the risk for adenocarcinoma of the esophagus especially in white males. Alarmingly, adenocarcinoma of the esophagus has increased two- to sixfold over the past 2 decades.[2] The relationship of adenocarcinoma to Barrett esophagus, or even just long-standing GERD, which may be an independent risk factor for esophageal adenocarcinoma, is not clear.

Other risk factors and comorbidities that may contribute to the development or worsening of GERD symptoms include family history, obesity, smoking, alcohol consumption, certain medications and foods, respiratory diseases, and reflux chest pain syndrome.

PATHOPHYSIOLOGY

The key factor in the development of GERD is the abnormal reflux of gastric contents from the stomach into the esophagus.[4] In some cases, gastroesophageal reflux is associated with defective lower esophageal sphincter (LES) pressure or function. Patients may have decreased gastroesophageal sphincter pressures related to (a) spontaneous transient LES relaxations, (b) transient increases in intraabdominal pressure, or (c) an atonic LES, all of which may lead to the development of gastroesophageal reflux. Problems with other normal mucosal defense mechanisms, such as abnormal esophageal anatomy, improper esophageal clearance of gastric fluids, reduced mucosal resistance to acid, delayed or ineffective gastric emptying, inadequate production of epidermal growth factor, and reduced salivary buffering of acid, may also contribute to the development of GERD. Substances that may promote esophageal damage upon reflux into the esophagus include gastric acid, pepsin, bile acids, and pancreatic enzymes. Thus the composition and volume of the refluxate, as well as duration of exposure, are important aggressive factors in determining the consequences of gastroesophageal reflux. Rational therapeutic regimens in the treatment of gastroesophageal reflux are designed to maximize normal mucosal defense mechanisms and attenuate the aggressive factors.

LOWER ESOPHAGEAL SPHINCTER PRESSURE

The lower esophageal sphincter is a manometrically defined zone at the distal esophagus with an elevated basal resting pressure. The sphincter is normally in a tonic, contracted state, preventing the reflux of gastric material from the stomach but relaxes on swallowing to permit the free passage of food into the stomach. Mechanisms by which defective LES pressure may cause

gastroesophageal reflux are threefold. First, and probably most importantly, reflux may occur following spontaneous transient LES relaxations that are not associated with swallowing. Although the exact mechanism is unknown, esophageal distension, vomiting, belching, and retching cause relaxation of the LES. While not thought to contribute significantly to erosive esophagitis, these transient relaxations, which are normal postprandially, may play an important role in symptom-based esophageal reflux syndromes. Transient decreases in sphincter pressure are responsible for more than half of the reflux episodes in patients with GERD. The propensity to develop gastroesophageal reflux secondary to transient decreases in LES pressure is probably dependent on numerous factors, including the degree of sphincter relaxation, efficacy of esophageal clearance, patient position (more common in recumbent position), gastric volume, and intragastric pressure. Second, reflux may occur following transient increases in intraabdominal pressure (stress reflux). An increase in intraabdominal pressure such as that occurring during straining, bending over, coughing, eating, or a Valsalva maneuver may overcome a weak LES, and thus may lead to reflux. Third, the LES may be atonic, thus permitting free reflux as seen in patients with scleroderma. Although transient relaxations are more likely to occur when there is normal LES pressure, the latter two mechanisms are more likely to occur when the LES pressure is decreased by such factors as fatty foods, gastric distension, smoking, or certain medications (Table 39–1).[5] Various foods aggravate esophageal reflux by decreasing LES pressure or by precipitating symptomatic reflux by direct mucosal irritation (e.g., spicy foods, orange juice, tomato juice, and coffee). Pregnancy is a condition in which reflux is common. There are many postulated reasons for the increased incidence of heartburn during pregnancy, including hormonal effects on esophageal muscle, LES tone, and physical factors (increased intraabdominal pressure) resulting from an enlarging uterus. A decrease in LES pressure resulting from any of the previously mentioned causes is not always associated with gastroesophageal reflux. Likewise, individuals who experience decreases in sphincter pressures and subsequently reflux, do not always develop GERD. The other natural defense mechanisms (anatomic factors, esophageal clearance,

TABLE 39-1	Foods and Medications That May Worsen GERD Symptoms

Decreased lower-esophageal sphincter pressure

Foods	Medications
Fatty meal	Anticholinergics
Carminatives (peppermint, spearmint)	Barbituates
Chocolate	Caffeine
Coffee, cola, tea	Dihydropyridine calcium channel
Garlic	blockers
Onions	Dopamine
Chili peppers	Estrogen
	Ethanol
	Nicotine
	Nitrates
	Progesterone
	Tetracycline
	Theophylline

Direct irritants to the esophageal mucosa

Foods	Medications
Spicy foods	Alendronate
Orange juice	Aspirin
Tomato juice	Nonsteroidal antiinflammatory
Coffee	drugs
	Iron
	Quinidine
	Potassium chloride

mucosal resistance, and other gastric factors) must be evoked to explain this phenomenon.

ANATOMIC FACTORS

Disruption of the normal anatomic barriers by a hiatal hernia (when a portion of the stomach protrudes through the diaphragm into the chest) was once thought to be a primary etiology of gastroesophageal reflux and esophagitis. Now it appears that a more important factor related to the presence or absence of symptoms in patients with hiatal hernia is the LES pressure. Patients with hypotensive LES pressures and large hiatal hernias are more likely to experience gastroesophageal reflux following abrupt increases in intraabdominal pressure compared with patients with a hypotensive LES and no hiatal hernia. Although anatomic factors are still considered significant by some, the diagnosis of hiatal hernia is currently considered a separate entity with which gastroesophageal reflux may simultaneously occur.

ESOPHAGEAL CLEARANCE

In many patients with GERD, the problem is not that they produce too much acid but that the acid produced spends too much time in contact with the esophageal mucosa. This is not surprising, because the symptoms and/or severity of damage produced by gastroesophageal reflux are partially dependent on the duration of contact between the gastric contents and the esophageal mucosa. This contact time is, in turn, dependent on the rate at which the esophagus clears the noxious material, as well as the frequency of reflux. The esophagus is cleared by primary peristalsis in response to swallowing, or by secondary peristalsis in response to esophageal distension and gravitational effects. Swallowing contributes to esophageal clearance by increasing salivary flow. Saliva contains bicarbonate that buffers the residual gastric material on the surface of the esophagus. The production of saliva decreases with increasing age, making it more difficult to maintain a neutral intraesophageal pH. Therefore, esophageal damage caused by reflux occurs more often in the elderly and similarly for patients with Sjögren syndrome or xerostomia. Swallowing is also decreased during sleep, making nocturnal GERD a problem in many patients.

MUCOSAL RESISTANCE

Within the esophageal mucosa and submucosa there are mucus-secreting glands that may contribute to the protection of the esophagus. Bicarbonate moving from the blood to the lumen can neutralize acidic refluxate in the esophagus. When the mucosa is repeatedly exposed to the refluxate in GERD, or if there is a defect in the normal mucosal defenses, hydrogen ions diffuse into the mucosa, leading to the cellular acidification and necrosis that ultimately cause esophagitis. In theory, mucosal resistance may be related not only to esophageal mucus but also to tight epithelial junctions, epithelial cell turnover, nitrogen balance, mucosal blood flow, tissue prostaglandins, and the acid–base status of the tissue. Saliva is also rich in epidermal growth factor, stimulating cell renewal.

GASTRIC EMPTYING

Delayed gastric emptying can contribute to gastroesophageal reflux. An increase in gastric volume may increase both the frequency of reflux and the amount of gastric fluid available to be refluxed. Gastric volume is related to the volume of material ingested, rate of gastric secretion, rate of gastric emptying, and amount and frequency of duodenal reflux into the stomach.

Factors that increase gastric volume and/or decrease gastric emptying, such as smoking and high-fat meals, are often associated with gastroesophageal reflux. This partially explains the prevalence of postprandial gastroesophageal reflux. Fatty foods may increase postprandial gastroesophageal reflux by increasing gastric volume, delaying the gastric emptying rate, and decreasing the LES pressure. Patients with gastroesophageal reflux, particularly infants, may have a defect in gastric antral motility. The delay in emptying may promote regurgitation of feedings, which might, in turn, contribute to two common complications of GERD in infants (e.g., failure to thrive and pulmonary aspiration).[6]

COMPOSITION OF REFLUXATE

The composition, pH, and volume of the refluxate are important aggressive factors in determining the consequences of gastroesophageal reflux. In animals, acid has two primary effects when it refluxes into the esophagus. First, if the pH of the refluxate is less than 2, esophagitis may develop secondary to protein denaturation. In addition, pepsinogen is activated to pepsin at this pH and may also cause esophagitis. Duodenogastric reflux esophagitis, or "alkaline esophagitis," refers to esophagitis induced by the reflux of bilious and pancreatic fluid. The term *alkaline esophagitis* may be a misnomer in that the refluxate may be either weakly alkaline or acidic in nature. An increase in gastric bile concentrations may be caused by duodenogastric reflux as a result of a generalized motility disorder, slower clearance of the refluxate, or after surgery.[7] Although bile acids have both a direct irritant effect on the esophageal mucosa and an indirect effect of increasing hydrogen ion permeability of the mucosa, symptoms are more often related to acid reflux than to bile reflux. Specifically, the percentage of time that the esophageal pH is <4 is greater for patients with severe disease as compared with those with mild disease. Esophageal pH monitoring in conjunction with 24-hour bile monitoring has shown a higher incidence of Barrett esophagus for patients who have both acid and alkaline reflux.[7] More study is needed to substantiate this finding. Nevertheless, the combination of acid, pepsin, and/or bile is a potent refluxate in producing esophageal damage.

COMPLICATIONS

Several complications may occur with gastroesophageal reflux, including esophagitis, esophageal strictures, Barrett esophagus, and esophageal adenocarcinoma. Strictures are common in the distal esophagus and are generally 1 to 2 cm in length. The use of nonsteroidal antiinflammatory drugs or aspirin is an additional risk factor that may contribute to the development or worsening of GERD complications.[3] Although GERD may lead to esophageal bleeding, the blood loss is usually chronic and low grade in nature, but anemia may occur. In some patients, the reparative process leads to the replacement of the squamous epithelial lining of the esophagus by specialized columnar-type epithelium (Barrett esophagus), which increases the incidence of esophageal strictures by as much as 30%. Additionally, the risk of esophageal adenocarcinoma may be higher for patients with Barrett esophagus as compared with the general population.[8]

The pathophysiology of gastroesophageal reflux is a complex cyclic process. It is difficult, if not impossible, to determine which occurs first: gastroesophageal reflux leading to defective peristalsis with delayed clearing or an incompetent LES pressure leading to gastroesophageal reflux. Understanding the factors associated with the development of GERD provides insight into the treatment modalities currently used to manage patients suffering from this disease.

CLINICAL PRESENTATION

❶ GERD syndromes can be described as symptom-based or esophageal tissue injury-based. Patients may also present with more complicated "alarm" symptoms which necessitates further diagnostic evaluation to differentiate other diseases as the cause. The spectrum of esophageal injury-based GERD syndromes includes esophagitis, strictures, Barrett esophagus and adenocarcinoma. The severity of the symptoms of gastroesophageal reflux does not always correlate with the degree of esophageal tissue injury, but it does correlate with the duration of reflux. Patients with symptom-based esophageal syndromes may have symptoms as severe as those with esophageal tissue injury. Patients may also present with extraesophageal syndromes that include atypical symptoms such as reflux chest pain syndrome, laryngitis, or asthma. It is important to distinguish GERD symptoms from those of other diseases, especially when chest pain or pulmonary symptoms are present. Interestingly, close to half of patients presenting with chest pain who have a normal electrocardiogram have GERD[9] and approximately half of patients with asthma have GERD.

The most useful tool in the diagnosis of gastroesophageal reflux is the clinical history, including presenting symptoms and associated risk factors. Patients presenting with typical symptoms of reflux do not usually require invasive esophageal evaluation. These patients generally benefit from an initial empiric trial of acid-suppression therapy. A clinical diagnosis of GERD can be assumed in patients who respond to appropriate therapy.[4] Further diagnostic evaluation is useful to prevent misdiagnosis, identify complications, and assess treatment failures.[2] Diagnostic tests should be performed in those patients who do not respond to therapy and for those who present with alarm symptoms (e.g., dysphagia, odynophagia, weight loss), which may be more indicative of more complicated disease.

❷ Useful tests in diagnosing GERD include endoscopy, ambulatory pH or impedance monitoring, and manometry. A camera-containing capsule swallowed by the patient offers the newest technology for visualizing the esophageal mucosa via endoscopy. The PillCam ESO is less invasive than traditional endoscopy and takes less than 15 minutes to perform in the clinician's office. Images of the esophagus are downloaded through sensors placed on the patient's chest that are connected to a data collector. The camera-containing capsule is later eliminated in the stool. Endoscopy is not useful as a screening tool for Barrett esophagus and esophageal adenocarcinoma for patients with long-standing GERD.[1] Unfortunately, the presence or absence of mucosal damage does not prove the patient's symptoms are reflux related; for that, ambulatory pH monitoring is useful. Ambulatory pH monitoring can be performed by passing a small pH probe transnasally and placing it approximately 5 cm above the LES.[10,11] Patients are asked to keep a diary of symptoms that later are correlated with the pH measurement corresponding to the time the symptom was reported.

Two recent developments related to ambulatory reflux monitoring include (1) the use of combined *impedance–pH monitoring* and (2) the use a wireless method of pH monitoring.[4] Whereas ambulatory pH monitoring only measures acid reflux, combined impedance–pH monitoring measures both acid and nonacid reflux. The wireless pH-monitoring involves attaching a radiotelemetry capsule to the esophageal mucosa. The advantages of this method are that a longer period of monitoring is possible (48 hours), it may demonstrate superior recording accuracy compared with some catheter designs, and it is more comfortable for the patient because a nasogastric tube is unnecessary.[1] Proton pump inhibitor therapy should be withheld for 7 days prior to performing ambulatory catheter pH, impendance–pH, or wireless pH monitoring when evaluating patients who have failed an initial empiric therapy and who have normal findings on endoscopy and manometry.[1]

CLINICAL CONTROVERSY

Professional organizations differ in their recommendation for or against endoscopy as a screening tool for patients with chronic symptoms of GERD for the purpose of detecting Barrett esophagus and thereby reducing the risk of esophageal adenocarcinoma.

CLINICAL PRESENTATION OF GERD

Symptom-based esophageal GERD syndromes (with or without esophageal tissue injury)

Typical symptoms (May be aggravated by activities that worsen gastroesophageal reflux such as recumbent position, bending over, or eating a meal high in fat.)

- Heartburn (hallmark symptom described as a substernal sensation of warmth or burning rising up from the abdomen that may radiate to the neck. May be waxing and waning in character.
- Water brash (hypersalivation)
- Belching
- Regurgitation

Alarm symptoms (These symptoms may be indicative of complications of GERD such as Barrett esophagus, esophageal strictures, or esophageal adenocarcinoma.)

- Dysphagia
- Odynophagia

Tissue injury–based esophageal GERD syndromes (with or without esophageal symptoms)

Symptoms (May present with alarm symptoms such as dysphagia, odynophagia or unexplained weight loss.)

- Esophagitis
- Strictures
- Barrett esophagus
- Esophageal adenocarcinoma

Extraesophageal GERD syndromes

Symptoms (These symptoms have an association with GERD, but causality should only be considered if a concomitant esophageal GERD syndrome is also present.)

- Chronic cough
- Laryngitis
- Asthma
- Dental enamel erosion

Diagnostic tests for GERD

Clinical history

- Generally sufficient to clinically diagnose GERD for patients with typical symptoms.

Endoscopy

- Preferred for assessing the mucosa for esophagitis, identifying Barrett esophagus and diagnosing complications.[6]
- Non-inflammatory GERD and major motor disorders may be missed by endoscopy.

- If no erosions, does not definitively show symptoms are GERD-related.

Ambulatory pH monitoring

- Identifies patients with excessive esophageal acid exposure and helps determine if symptoms are acid related.
- Useful for patients not responding to acid-suppression therapy.
- Documents the percentage of time the intraesophageal pH is <4 and determines the frequency and severity of reflux.
- Measures only acid reflux (not nonacid reflux).

Combined impedance–pH monitoring

- Measures both acid and nonacid reflux.

Manometry

- Ensure proper placement of esophageal pH probes (The recent advancement of the tubeless pH monitoring system using endoscopic landmarks for placement may negate the need for manometry for ensuring proper placement of esophageal pH probes.)
- Evaluate esophageal peristalsis and motility prior to antireflux surgery

Empiric trial of a proton pump inhibitor as a diagnostic test for GERD

- Less expensive and more convenient than ambulatory pH monitoring but lack standardized dosing regimen and duration of the diagnostic trial.

Barium radiography

- Not routinely used to diagnose GERD because lacks sensitivity and specificity; cannot identify Barrett esophagus.

Data from reference 2.

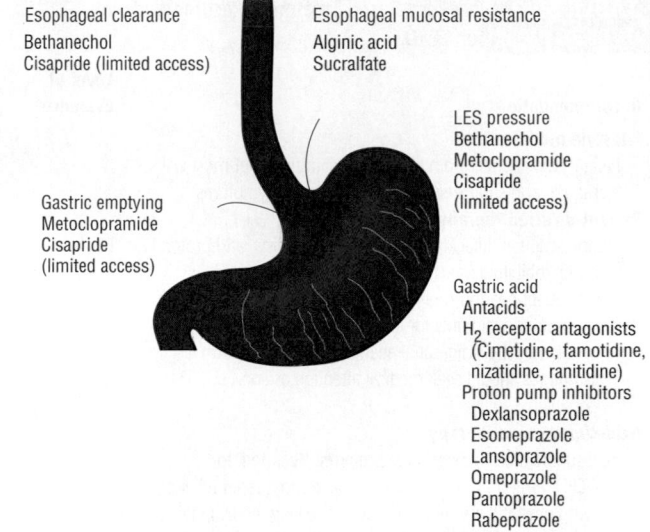

FIGURE 39-1. Therapeutic interventions in the management of gastroesophageal reflux disease. Pharmacologic interventions are targeted at improving defense mechanisms or decreasing aggressive factors (LES, lower esophageal sphincter).

TREATMENT

Therapeutic modalities used in the treatment of gastroesophageal reflux are targeted at reversing the various pathophysiologic abnormalities.

■ DESIRED OUTCOMES

❸ The goals of treatment are to (1) alleviate or eliminate the patient's symptoms, (2) decrease the frequency or recurrence and duration of gastroesophageal reflux, (3) promote healing of the injured mucosa, and (4) prevent the development of complications. Therapy is directed at augmenting defense mechanisms that prevent reflux and/or decrease the aggressive factors that worsen reflux or mucosal damage (Fig. 39–1). Therapy is directed at (1) decreasing the acidity of the refluxate, (2) decreasing the gastric volume available to be refluxed, (3) improving gastric emptying, (4) increasing LES pressure, (5) enhancing esophageal acid clearance, and (6) protecting the esophageal mucosa.

■ GENERAL APPROACH TO TREATMENT

❹ The treatment of GERD is categorized into one of the following modalities: (1) lifestyle modifications and patient-directed therapy with antacids, nonprescription H$_2$-receptor antagonists, and/or nonprescription proton pump inhibitors; (2) pharmacologic intervention with prescription-strength acid-suppression therapy; (3) and antireflux surgery (Table 39–2). The initial therapeutic modality used is in part dependent on the patient's condition (frequency of symptoms, degree of esophagitis, and presence of complications) (Table 39–3). Historically, a step-up approach was used, starting with noninvasive lifestyle modifications and patient-directed therapy and progressing to pharmacologic management or antireflux surgery. A step-down approach, starting with a proton pump inhibitor given once or twice daily instead of an H$_2$-receptor antagonist and then stepping down to the lowest dose of acid suppression (either an H$_2$-receptor antagonist or proton pump inhibitor) needed to control symptoms, is also effective. Neither the step-up nor the step-down approach has superior efficacy over the other. The clinician should determine the most appropriate approach for the individual patient. Every attempt should be made to aggressively control symptoms and to prevent relapses early in the course of the patient's disease in order to prevent the complications. For patients with moderate to severe GERD, especially those with erosive disease, starting with a proton pump inhibitor as initial therapy is advocated because of its superior efficacy over H$_2$-receptor antagonists.

While weight loss in obese patients and elevation of the head of the bed have proven beneficial for most GERD patients, recommending all lifestyle modifications to all patients is not recommended.[1] Instead, education on lifestyle modifications should be tailored to the individual needs of the patient. Table 39–4 lists many of the lifestyle modifications that can be recommended.[4]

❺ Patients who do not respond to lifestyle modifications and patient-directed therapy after 2 weeks should seek medical attention and are generally started on empiric therapy consisting of an acid-suppression agent. Acid-suppression therapy with proton pump inhibitors or H$_2$-receptor antagonists is the mainstay of GERD treatment. Patients presenting with moderate to severe symptoms (with or without esophageal erosions) should be started on a proton pump inhibitor as initial therapy because it provides the most rapid symptomatic relief and healing in the highest percentage of patients.[4] H$_2$-Receptor antagonists in divided doses are effective for patients with milder GERD symptoms. Standard H$_2$-receptor antagonist doses may be increased to 2 to 4 times the normal dose for patients who do not respond to standard doses. However, if this is necessary, it is more cost-effective and efficacious to switch to a proton pump inhibitor.

TABLE 39-2 Evidence-Based Treatment Recommendations for GERD

Recommendations	Level of Evidence[a]
Lifestyle modifications	
Patients may benefit from lifestyle modifications but most will require acid-suppression therapy to control symptoms.	IV
Patient-directed therapy	
Nonprescription antacids, H$_2$-receptor antagonists, and proton pump inhibitors may be used for patients with mild, infrequent heartburn or regurgitation. Patients experiencing continuous symptoms for longer than 2 weeks should be seen by their clinician. Patients experiencing alarm symptoms should seek medical attention as soon as possible.	IV
Acid-suppression therapy	
Acid-suppression therapy is the preferred treatment for GERD. Proton pump inhibitors provide more rapid relief of symptoms and are more effective at healing the esophageal mucosa compared to H$_2$-receptor antagonists in patients with moderate to severe GERD.	I
Promotility therapy	
Promotility therapy may be useful in some patients when combined with acid-suppression therapy. They are generally not recommended as monotherapy for patients with GERD.	II
Maintenance therapy	
Most patients with GERD will require continuous therapy to control symptoms and to prevent complications.	I
Surgery	
Antireflux surgery represents a viable maintenance option for patients with an established diagnosis of GERD.	II
Refractory GERD	
GERD that is refractory to adequate acid suppression is uncommon. In these cases, the diagnosis should be confirmed through further diagnostic tests.	IV

[a]Level of evidence: I, strong evidence from at least one published systematic review of multiple, well-designed, randomized, controlled trials; II, strong evidence from at least one published, properly designed, randomized, controlled trial of appropriate size and in an appropriate clinical setting. III, strong evidence from published, well-designed trials without randomization, single group, pre–post, cohort, time series, or matched case-controlled studies; IV, evidence from well-designed nonexperimental studies from more than one center or research group or opinion of respected authorities, based on clinical evidence, descriptive studies, or reports of expert consensus committees.

Data from reference 4.

Promotility agents are not as effective as acid-suppression agents. Combining promotility agents with acid-suppression drugs offers only modest improvements in symptoms over standard doses of H$_2$-receptor antagonists and should not be routinely recommended. In addition, the availability of a promotility agent that has an acceptable adverse effect profile is lacking. Mucosal protectants, such as sucralfate, have a very limited role in the treatment of GERD.

Maintenance therapy is generally necessary to control symptoms and to prevent complications. For patients with more severe symptoms (with or without esophageal erosions) or for patients with other complications, maintenance therapy with a proton pump inhibitor is most effective. Routine use of combination therapy has no role in maintenance therapy of GERD. GERD that is refractory to adequate acid suppression is uncommon. In these cases, the diagnosis should be confirmed through further diagnostic tests before long-term, high-dose therapy or antireflux surgery are considered.[4]

■ NONPHARMACOLOGIC THERAPY

Nonpharmacologic treatment of GERD includes lifestyle modifications and antireflux surgery, which may be viable maintenance modalities in select patients. Endoscopic therapies, such as endoscopic sewing devices and endoluminal application of radiofrequency heat energy, have fallen out of favor and not routinely recommended.

Lifestyle Modifications

The most common lifestyle modifications that a patient should be educated about include weight loss in obese patients and elevation of the head of the bed, especially for those patients who have symptoms while in a recumbent position. Other lifestyle modifications should be individualized based for the patient's specific situation. These include consumption of smaller meals and not eating 3 hours prior to sleeping, avoidance of foods or medications that exacerbate GERD; smoking cessation, avoidance of tight-fitting clothes, and avoidance of alcohol (Table 39–4).

Obesity increases the risk of GERD, most likely through increased intraabdominal pressure and possibly by disruption of the esophagogastric junction.[12] A high-fat meal will decrease LES pressure for 2 hours or more postprandially. In contrast, a high-protein, low-fat meal will elevate LES pressure. Consequently, weight loss and a low-fat diet may help to improve GERD symptoms. Elevating the head of the bed approximately 6 to 8 inches with a foam wedge under the mattress (not just elevating the head with pillows) decreases nocturnal esophageal acid contact time and should be recommended. Many foods may worsen the symptoms of GERD. Fats and chocolate can decrease LES pressure, whereas citrus juice, tomato juice, coffee, and pepper may irritate damaged endothelium.

It is important to evaluate patient profiles and to identify potential medications that may exacerbate GERD symptoms. Medications, such as anticholinergics, barbiturates, calcium channel blockers, and theophylline decrease LES pressure. Other medications, including aspirin, iron, nonsteroidal antiinflammatory drugs, quinidine, potassium chloride, and bisphosphonates can act as direct contact irritants to the esophageal mucosa. Patients taking bisphosphonates (e.g., alendronate) should be instructed to drink 6 to 8 oz of plain tap water and remain upright for at least 30 minutes following administration. Proper patient education can help prevent dysphagia or esophageal ulceration. Patients should be closely monitored for worsening symptoms when any of these medications are started. If symptoms worsen, alternative therapies may be warranted. The clinician must weigh the risks and benefits of continuing a drug known to worsen GERD and esophagitis.

Smoking can cause aerophagia, which leads to increased belching and regurgitation. However, data are lacking to show that symptoms improve for patients who quit smoking. Nevertheless, patients with GERD should be encouraged to quit smoking. Alcohol, although not thought to play a role in severe disease, decreases LES pressure and may exacerbate symptoms such as heartburn.

Many patients are noncompliant with lifestyle modifications, and even those who do comply generally continue to have symptoms that require acid-suppression therapy. Nonetheless, it is important to regularly stress the potential benefits of lifestyle modifications that would benefit each individual patient.

Interventional Approaches

Interventional approaches include antireflux surgery and endoscopic therapies.

Antireflux Surgery ❻ Surgical intervention is a viable maintenance alternative for select patients with well-documented GERD.[4] The goal of antireflux surgery is to re-establish the antireflux barrier, to position the lower esophageal sphincter within the abdomen where it is under positive (intraabdominal) pressure, and to close any associated hiatal defect. Antireflux surgery should be considered for patients (1) who fail to respond

TABLE 39-3 Therapeutic Approach to GERD in Adults

Patient Presentation	Recommended Treatment Regimen	Comments
Intermittent, mild heartburn	**Lifestyle modifications** **plus** **patient-directed therapy** Antacids • Maalox or Mylanta 30 mL as needed or after meals and at bedtime • Gaviscon 2 tabs after meals and at bedtime • Calcium carbonate 500 mg, 2–4 tablets as needed **and/or** Nonprescription H$_2$-receptor antagonists (taken up to twice daily) • Cimetidine 200 mg • Famotidine 10 mg • Nizatidine 75 mg • Ranitidine 75 mg **or** Nonprescription proton pump inhibitor (taken once daily) • Omeprazole 20 mg • Lansoprazole 15 mg	Lifestyle modifications should be individualized for each patient. Weight loss in obese patients and elevation of the head of the bed have been proven most beneficial. If symptoms are unrelieved with lifestyle modifications and nonprescription medications after 2 weeks, patient should seek medical attention.
Symptomatic relief of GERD	**Lifestyle modifications** **plus** **prescription-strength acid-suppression therapy** H$_2$-receptor antagonists (for 6–12 weeks) • Cimetidine 400 mg twice daily • Famotidine 20 mg twice daily • Nizatidine 150 mg twice daily • Ranitidine 150 mg twice daily **or** Proton pump inhibitors (for 4–8 weeks); all are given once daily • Dexlansoprazole 30 mg • Esomeprazole 20 mg • Lansoprazole 15 mg • Omeprazole 20 mg • Pantoprazole 40 mg • Rabeprazole 20 mg	For typical symptoms, treat empirically with prescription-strength acid-suppression therapy. If symptoms recur, consider maintenance therapy (MT). Note: Most patients will require standard doses for MT. Mild GERD can usually be treated effectively with H$_2$-receptor antagonists. Patients with moderate to severe symptoms should receive a proton pump inhibitor as initial therapy.
Healing of erosive esophagitis or treatment of patients presenting with moderate to severe symptoms or complications	**Lifestyle modifications** **Plus** Proton pump inhibitors for 4–16 weeks (up to twice daily) • Dexlansoprazole 60 mg daily • Esomeprazole 20–40 mg daily • Lansoprazole 30 mg daily • Omeprazole 20 mg daily • Rabeprazole 20 mg daily • Pantoprazole 40 mg daily **or** High-dose H$_2$-receptor antagonist (for 8–12 weeks) • Cimetidine 400 mg four times daily or 800 mg twice daily • Famotidine 40 mg twice daily • Nizatidine 150 mg four times daily • Ranitidine 150 mg four times daily	For atypical or alarm symptoms, obtain endoscopy (if possible) to evaluate mucosa. Give a trial of a proton pump inhibitor. If symptoms are relieved, consider MT. Proton pump inhibitors are the most effective maintenance therapy for patients with atypical symptoms, complications, and erosive disease. Patients not responding to pharmacologic therapy, including those with persistent atypical symptoms, should be evaluated via ambulatory reflux monitoring to confirm the diagnosis of GERD (if possible).
Interventional therapies	Antireflux surgery	

to pharmacologic treatment, (2) who opt for surgery despite successful treatment because of lifestyle considerations, including age, time, or expense of medications, (3) who have complications of GERD (e.g., Barrett esophagus, strictures), or (4) who have atypical symptoms and reflux documented with ambulatory pH monitoring. The antireflux surgical procedure chosen depends on the surgeon's expertise and preference, as well as on anatomic considerations. In general, 90% of patients have symptom resolution following successful Nissen fundoplication. The major complications with antireflux surgery include gas bloat syndrome (inability to belch or vomit), dysphagia, vagal denervation, splenic trauma, and, very rarely, death. In contrast, death has not occurred as a consequence of pharmacologic treatment with a proton pump inhibitor. Antireflux surgery is superior to medical management

with an H$_2$-receptor antagonist or a promotility agent. In a 7-year follow-up study of omeprazole compared with antireflux surgery for patients with esophagitis, symptoms (regurgitation and heartburn) were better controlled in the surgical group; however treatment failures were also higher in the surgical group. In addition, more patients in the surgical group complained of complications, such as inability to belch, flatulence, and dysphagia.[13] Long-term effectiveness of antireflux surgery is uncertain.

Endoscopic Therapies Endoscopic approaches for the management of GERD have included endoscopic sewing devices and endoluminal application of radiofrequency heat energy resulting in tissue injury or nerve ablation (the Stretta procedure).[14,15] Unfortunately, results from these endoscopic therapies have proven

TABLE 39-4 Nonpharmacologic Treatment of GERD with Lifestyle Modifications

Recommended lifestyle modifications for all GERD patients
- Elevate the head of the bed (increases esophageal clearance). Use 6- to 8-inch blocks under the head of the bed. Sleep on a foam wedge.
- Weight reduction (reduces symptoms) in obese patients

Recommended lifestyle modifications that should be individualized to specific patients
- Avoid foods that may decrease lower esophageal sphincter pressure (fats, chocolate, alcohol, peppermint, and spearmint)
- Include protein-rich meals in diet (augments lower esophageal sphincter pressure)
- Avoid foods that have a direct irritant effect on the esophageal mucosa. (spicy foods, orange juice, tomato juice, and coffee)
- Behaviors that may reduce esophageal acid exposure
  - Eat small meals and avoid eating immediately prior to sleeping (within 3 hours if possible; Decreases gastric volume)
  - Stop smoking (decreases spontaneous esophageal sphincter relaxation)
  - Avoid alcohol (increases amplitude of the lower esophageal sphincter, peristaltic waves, and frequency of contraction)
  - Avoid tight-fitting clothes
  - Take drugs that have a direct irritant effect on the esophageal mucosa with plenty of liquid if they cannot be avoided (bisphosphonates, tetracyclines, quinidine, and potassium chloride, iron salts, aspirin, nonsteroidal antiinflammatory drugs)

Data from reference 4.

disappointing and are not routinely recommended. Emergence of natural orifice transluminal surgery (NOTES) and surgical techniques may evolve.

PHARMACOLOGIC THERAPY

Pharmacologic treatment consists of (1) patient-directed therapy with nonprescription antacids, H_2-receptor antagonists, or proton pump inhibitors and (2) prescription-strength acid-suppression therapy or promotility medications.

Patient-Directed Therapy

Patient-directed therapy, where patients self-treat themselves with nonprescription medications, is appropriate for mild, intermittent symptoms. Patients with continuous symptoms lasting longer than 2 weeks should seek medical attention.

Antacids and Antacid–Alginic Acid Products

Patients should be educated that antacids are an appropriate component of treating milder GERD symptoms, even though documentation of their efficacy in placebo-controlled clinical trials is lacking.[4] Although the literature is somewhat controversial on the superiority of antacids to placebo, clinicians and patients clearly consider antacids to be effective for immediate symptomatic relief, and antacids are often used concurrently with other acid-suppression therapies. Maintaining the intragastric pH >4 decreases the activation of pepsinogen to pepsin, a proteolytic enzyme. Also, neutralization of gastric fluid leads to increased LES pressure. Patients who require frequent use of antacids for chronic symptoms should be treated with prescription-strength acid-suppression therapy because their illness is considered more significant.

An antacid product combined with alginic acid is not a potent neutralizing agent and does not enhance LES pressure; however, it does form a highly viscous solution that floats on the surface of the gastric contents. This viscous solution is thought to serve as a protective barrier for the esophagus against reflux of gastric contents. It also reduces the frequency of the reflux episodes. The combination product may be superior to antacids alone in relieving the symptoms of GERD.[4] Efficacy data indicating endoscopic healing are lacking.

Antacid or antacid combination products may cause gastrointestinal adverse effects (diarrhea or constipation, depending on the product), alterations in mineral metabolism, and acid–base disturbances. Aluminum-containing antacids may bind to phosphate in the gut and lead to bone demineralization. In addition, antacids interact with a variety of medications by altering gastric pH, increasing urinary pH, adsorbing medications to their surfaces, providing a physical barrier to absorption, or forming insoluble complexes with other medications. Antacids have clinically significant drug interactions with tetracycline, ferrous sulfate, isoniazid, quinidine, sulfonylureas, and quinolone antibiotics. Antacid–drug interactions are influenced by composition, dose, dosage schedule, and formulation of the antacid.

Dosage recommendations for antacids in the management of GERD are somewhat difficult to derive from the literature. Doses range from hourly to an as-needed basis (Table 39–3). In general, antacids have a short duration of action, which necessitates frequent administration throughout the day to provide continuous neutralization of acid. Taking antacids after meals can increase the duration of action from about 1 hour to 3 hours; however, nighttime acid suppression cannot be maintained with bedtime doses.

Nonprescription H_2-Receptor Antagonists and Proton Pump Inhibitors

Nonprescription H_2-receptor antagonists (cimetidine, famotidine, nizatidine, and ranitidine) are effective in diminishing gastric acid secretion when taken prior to meals and decrease GERD symptoms associated with exercise. Antacids may have a slightly faster onset of action, while the H_2-receptor antagonists have a much longer duration of action compared with antacids.

The proton-pump inhibitor omeprazole is available without a prescription. A dose of 20 mg/day is indicated for short-term treatment of heartburn. Lansoprazole 15 mg gives patients a second option in the proton pump inhibitor class that is now available without a prescription. Patients who do not respond to lifestyle modifications and patient-directed therapy after 2 weeks should be seen by their clinician.

Acid-Suppression Therapy

❼ Acid-suppression therapy with prescription-strength H_2-receptor antagonists and proton pump inhibitors are the mainstay of GERD treatment.

H_2-Receptor Antagonists (Cimetidine, Famotidine, Nizatidine, and Ranitidine) H_2-Receptor antagonists in divided doses are effective in treating patients with mild to moderate GERD.[4] The majority of the trials assessing the efficacy of standard doses of H_2-receptor antagonists indicate that symptomatic improvement is achieved in an average of 60% of patients after 12 weeks of therapy.[4] However, endoscopic healing rates tend to be lower, an average of 50% of patients at 12 weeks.[4]

The efficacy of H_2-receptor antagonists in the management of GERD is extremely variable and is frequently lower than desired. Response to the H_2-receptor antagonists is dependent on the (1) severity of disease, (2) dosage regimen used, and (3) duration of therapy. These factors are important to keep in mind when comparing clinical trials and/or assessing a patient's response to therapy. The severity of esophagitis at baseline has a profound impact on the patient's response to H_2-receptor antagonists. For symptomatic relief of mild GERD, low-dose, nonprescription H_2-receptor antagonists or standard doses given twice daily may be beneficial. Patients who do not respond to standard doses may be hypersecreters of gastric acid and will require higher doses. Although higher doses of H$_2$-receptor antagonists may provide higher symptomatic and endoscopic healing rates, limited information exists regarding the safety of these regimens, and they can be less effective and more costly than once daily proton pump inhibitors. Unlike duodenal ulcer disease, in which the duration of therapy is relatively short (e.g., 4 to 6 weeks), prolonged courses of H$_2$-receptor antagonists are frequently required in the treatment of GERD.

Because all of the H$_2$-receptor antagonists have similar efficacy, selection of the specific agent to use in the management of GERD should be based on factors such as differences in pharmacokinetics, safety profile, and cost. In general, the H$_2$-receptor antagonists are well tolerated. The most common adverse effects are headache, somnolence, fatigue, dizziness, and either constipation or diarrhea. Patients should be monitored for the presence of adverse effects as well as potential drug interactions, especially when on cimetidine. Cimetidine may inhibit the metabolism of theophylline, warfarin, phenytoin, nifedipine, and propranolol, among others. An alternate H$_2$-receptor antagonist should be selected if the patient is on any of these medications.

Proton Pump Inhibitors (Dexlansoprazole, Esomeprazole, Lansoprazole, Omeprazole, Pantoprazole, and Rabeprazole)

Proton pump inhibitors are superior to H$_2$-receptor antagonists in treating patients with moderate to severe GERD. This includes not only those patients with esophageal tissue injury (e.g., Barrett esophagus, strictures, or esophagitis), but also those patients with symptom-based GERD syndromes. A few trials have compared proton pump inhibitors with each other. In general, healing rates at 4 weeks and 8 weeks are similar; lansoprazole and rabeprazole, however, may relieve symptoms faster after the first dose when compared with omeprazole. Healing rates at 4 weeks and 8 weeks were similar. Symptomatic relief is seen in approximately 83% of patients with endoscopic evidence of injury after 8 weeks treated with a proton pump inhibitor, whereas the endoscopic healing rate at 8 weeks is 78%.[4] Proton pump inhibitors block gastric acid secretion by inhibiting gastric H$^+$/K$^+$-adenosine triphosphatase in gastric parietal cells.[16] This produces a profound, long-lasting antisecretory effect capable of maintaining the gastric pH >4, even during postprandial acid surges. A correlation appears to exist between the percentage of time the gastric pH remains >4 during the 24-hour period and healing erosive esophagitis.

The proton pump inhibitors are usually well-tolerated. Potential adverse effects include headache, dizziness, somnolence, diarrhea, constipation, nausea, and vitamin B$_{12}$ deficiency. The frequency of adverse events appears to be similar to that seen with the H$_2$-receptor antagonists. Of recent concern is the role proton pump inhibitors may play in the acquisition of *Clostridium difficile* infection during acid suppression. Acid suppression may result in loss of host defense against ingested spores and bacteria permitting a higher burden of exposure.[17,18] Patient selection is important to minimize this risk.

Drug interactions with the proton pump inhibitors vary slightly with each agent. All proton pump inhibitors can decrease the absorption of drugs such as ketoconazole or itraconazole, which require an acidic environment to be absorbed. All proton pump inhibitors are metabolized by the cytochrome P450 system to some extent, specifically by the CYP2C19 and CYP3A4 enzymes. While no interactions with lansoprazole, pantoprazole, or rabeprazole have been seen with CYP2C19 substrates such as diazepam, warfarin, and phenytoin, concerns have been raised regarding the concomitant use of proton pump inhibitors, especially omeprazole, with clopidogrel.[19,20] Clopidogrel, a prodrug, is converted to its active metabolite via the CYP2C19 and CYP3A4 enzyme.

Inhibition of CYP2C19 by proton pump inhibitors may decrease the effectiveness of clopidogrel causing cardiovascular adverse events. Further evaluation is needed to determine the extent of this drug interaction and the role polymorphic gene variation may play in patients on clopidogrel. In the mean time, careful review of the risk-to-benefit profile regarding the use of proton pump inhibitors for patients on clopidogrel should be considered. Using an alternative agent, such as an H$_2$-receptor antagonist may be prudent in this patient population.

CLINICAL CONTROVERSY

It is unclear which, if any, proton pump inhibitor is preferred for patients taking clopidogel due to potential drug interactions. Even pantoprazole, which does not affect CYP2C19, appears to have decrease the effectiveness of clopidogrel. Other mechanisms for this interaction have not been clearly established.

Esomeprazole does not appear to interact with warfarin or phenytoin, and an interaction with diazepam is generally not considered clinically relevant. Pantoprazole is also metabolized by a cytosolic sulfotransferase and is therefore less likely to have significant drug interactions compared with the other proton pump inhibitors. Although generally not a problem, omeprazole has the potential to inhibit the metabolism of warfarin, diazepam, and phenytoin, and lansoprazole may decrease theophylline concentrations. Patients taking warfarin should be monitored for potential bleeding. Drug interactions with omeprazole are of particular concern for patients who are considered "slow metabolizers" of omeprazole, which is more common in the Asian population but also found in approximately 3% of the caucasian population. Unfortunately, it is unclear which patients have the polymorphic gene variation that makes them slow metabolizers. Like omeprazole, the metabolism of esomeprazole may also be altered for patients with this polymorphic gene variation. Patients on potentially interacting drugs, such as warfarin, should be monitored closely for potential problems.

The proton pump inhibitors degrade in acidic environments and are therefore formulated in a delayed-release capsule or tablet formulation. Lansoprazole, esomeprazole, and omeprazole contain enteric-coated (pH-sensitive) granules in a capsule form. For patients who are unable to swallow the capsule or for pediatric patients, the contents of the delayed-release capsule can be mixed in applesauce or placed in orange juice. If a patient has a nasogastric tube, the contents of an omeprazole capsule can be mixed in 8.4% sodium bicarbonate solution. Esomeprazole granules can be dispersed in water. Lansoprazole comes in a packet for oral suspension and a delayed-release, orally disintegrating tablet. Although these dosage forms are beneficial for those who cannot swallow the capsule, such as elderly or pediatric patients, the packet for oral suspension should not be placed through a nasogastric tube. Patients taking pantoprazole or rabeprazole should be instructed not to crush, chew, or split the delayed-release tablets. Lansoprazole, esomeprazole, and pantoprazole are available in an intravenous formulation, which offers an alternative route of administration for patients who are unable to take an oral proton pump inhibitor. Importantly, the intravenous product is not more efficacious than oral proton pump inhibitors and is significantly more expensive. Careful patient selection is necessary to avoid the increased cost from the use of the intravenous product.

The newest dosage form of omeprazole is in a delayed-release tablet and a combination product with sodium bicarbonate in an immediate-release capsule and oral suspension (Zegerid). It is the first immediate-release proton pump inhibitor and should be taken on an empty stomach at least 1 hour before a meal. Zegerid offers an alternative to the delayed-release capsules or the intravenous formulation in adult patients with a nasogastric tube.

Dexlansoprazole is the newest proton pump inhibitor approved by the FDA. The capsule is a dual delayed-release formulation, with the first release occurring 1 to 2 hours after the dose and the second release occurring 4 to 5 hours after the dose. The clinical significance of this dual release is not known.

Patients should be instructed to take their proton pump inhibitor in the morning, 15 to 30 minutes before breakfast, to maximize efficacy, because these agents inhibit only actively secreting proton pumps. Dexlansoprazole can be taken without regards to meals. Patients with nocturnal symptoms may benefit from taking their proton pump inhibitor prior to the evening meal. If dosed twice daily, the second dose should be administered approximately 10 to 12 hours after the morning dose and prior to a meal or snack.

Promotility Agents

Promotility agents may be useful as an adjunct to acid-suppression therapy for patients with a known motility defect (e.g., LES incompetence, decreased esophageal clearance, delayed gastric emptying). Unfortunately, all available promotility agents are fraught with undesirable side effects and are not generally as effective as acid-suppression therapy. Extrapyramidal effects, sedation, and irritability are common with bethanechol and metoclopramide.

Cisapride Cisapride has comparable efficacy to H_2-receptor antagonists in treating patients with mild esophagitis. Unfortunately, cisapride is no longer available for routine use because of life-threatening cardiac arrhythmias when it is combined with certain medications and other disease states. It is currently available only through a limited access program from the manufacturer.

Metoclopramide Metoclopramide, a dopamine antagonist, increases LES pressure in a dose-related manner, and accelerates gastric emptying in gastroesophageal reflux patients. Unlike cisapride, however, metoclopramide does not improve esophageal clearance. Metoclopramide provides symptomatic improvement for some patients with gastroesophageal reflux disease; however, substantial data indicating that metoclopramide provides endoscopic healing are lacking. In addition, metoclopramide's side-effect profile and the incidence of tachyphylaxis with continued use limits its usefulness in treating many patients with GERD. The risk of adverse effects is much greater for elderly patients and for patients with renal dysfunction because the drug is primarily eliminated by the kidneys. Contraindications include Parkinson disease, mechanical obstruction, concomitant use of other dopamine antagonists or anticholinergic agents, and pheochromocytoma.

Bethanechol Bethanechol, a promotility drug, has limited value in the treatment of GERD because of unwanted side effects. Bethanechol is not routinely recommended for the treatment of GERD.

Other Promotility Drugs Under Investigation Other promotility drugs under investigation include domperidone, a dopamine antagonist, itopride, and baclofen. Because domperidone does not cross the blood–brain barrier, it does not cause the central nervous system effects seen with metoclopramide. However, it is not currently available in the United States. Baclofen, an aminobutyric acid (GABA) receptor type B agonist, may decrease esophageal acid exposure and the number of reflux episodes by decreasing the number of transient relaxations of the LES. However, this agent has many side effects, limiting its usefulness in GERD.

Mucosal Protectants

Sucralfate, a nonabsorbable aluminum salt of sucrose octasulfate, has very limited value in the treatment of GERD. Sucralfate is not routinely recommended for use in the treatment of GERD.

Combination Therapy

Combination therapy with an acid-suppression agent and a promotility agent or a mucosal protectant agent would seem logical given the multifactorial nature of the disease, particularly in light of the disappointing results seen with many monotherapy regimens. However, sufficient data to support combination therapy are limited, and this approach should not be routinely recommended unless a patient has GERD plus motor dysfunction occurring. The addition of an H_2-receptor antagonist at bedtime to proton pump inhibitor therapy for the treatment of nocturnal symptoms has been evaluated. The effectiveness of this strategy may decrease over time due to tachyphylaxis with H_2-receptor antagonists.[21]

Maintenance Therapy

❽ Although healing and/or symptomatic improvement may be achieved via many different therapeutic modalities, a large percentage of patients with gastroesophageal reflux will relapse following discontinuation of therapy, especially those with more severe disease. Patients who have symptomatic relapse following discontinuation of therapy or lowering of dose, including patients with complications such as Barrett esophagus, strictures, or esophagitis, should be considered for long-term maintenance therapy to prevent complications or worsening of esophageal function.[4] The goal of maintenance therapy is to improve quality of life by controlling the patient's symptoms and preventing complications. These goals cannot generally be achieved by decreasing the dose of the therapeutic modality used for initial healing or switching to a less potent acid-suppression agent. Most patients will require standard doses to prevent relapses. Patients should be counseled on the importance of complying with lifestyle changes and long-term maintenance therapy in order to prevent recurrence or worsening of disease.[4]

H_2-Receptor antagonists may be effective maintenance therapy for patients with mild disease.[4] The proton pump inhibitors are the drugs of choice for maintenance treatment of moderate to severe esophagitis or symptoms. Low doses of a proton pump inhibitor or alternate-day dosing may be effective in some patients with milder symptoms, thereby allowing titration in some cases. "On-demand" maintenance therapy, by which patients take their proton pump inhibitor only when they have symptoms, may be effective for patients with endoscopy-negative GERD.[4] Although not well studied, many patients with only mild to moderate symptoms may decide on their own to take their medication this way for the financial benefit. However, patients with more-persistent symptoms and/or complications should be maintained on standard doses of proton pump inhibitors.

Long-term chronic use of proton pump inhibitor doses higher than standard treatment doses is not indicated unless the patient has complicated symptoms, has erosive esophagitis per endoscopy, or has had further diagnostic evaluation to determine the level of acid exposure. Metoclopramide is not approved for maintenance therapy, and use is limited by adverse-effect profile. Antireflux surgery may also be considered a viable alternative to long-term drug therapy for maintenance of healing for patients who are candidates.

Maintenance Therapy with H$_2$–Receptor Antagonists The studies evaluating the efficacy of the H$_2$-receptor antagonists in maintaining GERD patients in remission have been disappointing. Currently, ranitidine 150 mg twice daily is the only H$_2$-receptor antagonist regimen that is FDA approved for maintenance of healing of erosive esophagitis.

Maintenance Therapy with Proton Pump Inhibitors Long-term use of the proton pump inhibitors are relatively safe, with no evidence of carcinoid tumors directly linked to their use. Prolonged hypergastrinemia leading to the development of colonic polyps, and potentially adenocarcinoma, was also a concern that has proven unfounded with long-term use.[22] However, the role of *Helicobacter pylori* status for patients with GERD has been questioned. As a consequence of the controversy surrounding *H. pylori* and GERD, specific guidelines on how to handle these patients are lacking. Most clinicians would probably opt to eradicate *H. pylori* infections once detected. Further studies are needed to determine the role of *H. pylori* for patients with GERD. Concern has been raised about the long-term use of proton pump inhibitors and the increased risk of bone fractures.[23] Data are conflicting, but the proposed mechanism is through inhibition by the H$^+$/K$^+$-ATPase pump indirectly inhibiting bone resorption. In addition, the increased pH may decrease calcium absorption, thereby putting patients at greater risk for fractures.[24,25]

SPECIAL POPULATIONS

There are several special populations that should be considered when discussing GERD, such as patients with atypical symptoms, pediatric patients, elderly patients, and patients with refractory symptoms.

PATIENTS WITH EXTRAESOPHAGEAL (ATYPICAL) GERD

Patients presenting with atypical symptoms may require higher doses and longer treatment courses as compared with patients with typical symptoms. Patients with suspected reflux chest pain syndrome may benefit from an empiric course of twice daily proton pump inhibitor therapy for 4 weeks once cardiac work up is known to be negative.[1] If symptoms continue, patients should be evaluated with manometry, ambulatory pH, or impedance-pH monitoring to rule out dysmotility or refractory symptoms.[1] Because there are many causes of asthma and laryngeal symptoms, a concomitant esophageal GERD syndrome must also be present to associate these symptoms with GERD. In practice, these patients may benefit from twice daily proton pump inhibitor for 3 to 4 months even though evidence supporting this regimen is not well established.[1] This recommendation is based more on pH monitoring data showing normalization of gastric pH with twice daily dosing.[1] For patients not responding to empiric therapy, pH monitoring may be beneficial in determining acid exposure as it relates to symptoms. The optimal dose of proton pump inhibition is not well-defined. Maintenance therapy is generally indicated for patients who respond to the therapeutic trial or have endoscopic evidence of reflux. Antireflux surgery may be an option in select patients. Without a concomitant esophageal GERD syndrome, acid-suppressing therapy is not well supported for patients with laryngitis or asthma symptoms.

PEDIATRIC PATIENTS WITH GERD

Many infants have physiologic reflux with little or no clinical consequence. Uncomplicated gastroesophageal reflux usually manifests as regurgitation or "spitting up" and resolves without incident by 12 to 14 months of life.[26] It usually responds to supportive therapy, including dietary adjustments, postural management, and reassurance for the parents. Thickened feedings may be useful in milder cases. While this does not decrease the time the pH is <4, it may decrease the incidence of regurgitation.[26] Chronic vomiting associated with gastroesophageal reflux must be distinguished from other causes, such as neurologic, metabolic, eating, and rumination disorders. Smaller, more frequent feedings may be beneficial. In formula-fed infants, an extensively hydrolyzed protein may help identify milk protein sensitivity as the cause of unexplained vomiting and crying.[26] Developmental immaturity of the LES is one suspected cause of gastroesophageal reflux in infants.[26] Like adults, transient LES relaxations seem to be the most common cause of gastroesophageal reflux in children. Other causes include impaired luminal clearance of gastric acid, neurologic impairment, and type of infant formula. Complications, although rare, include distal esophagitis, failure to thrive, esophageal peptic strictures, Barrett esophagus, and pulmonary disease.

The benefits of using a promotility medication, such as metoclopramide, erythromycin, domperidone, bethanachol, and baclofen, are outweighed by the potential adverse effects that may occur and, therefore, cannot be routinely recommended.[26] Ranitidine is commonly used at a dose of 2 mg/kg twice daily.[26] Tachyphylaxis may develop making the effectiveness of H$_2$-receptor antagonsists less than optimal. The use of proton pump inhibitor use in children is increasing, especially in those with esophagitis. Most patients will respond to once daily proton pump inhibiter dosing. Lansoprazole, esomeprazole and omeprazole are indicated for treating symptomatic and erosive GERD for pediatric patients older than age 1 year. Lanzoprazole 15 mg once daily is recommended for children who weigh 30 kg or less, and a dose of 30 mg once daily is recommended for those who weigh more than 30 kg. Esomeprazole may be dosed 10 to 20 mg daily for children 1 to 11 years old and 20 to 40 mg daily for children 12 to 17 years old. Omeprazole 5 mg daily may be used in children weighing between 5 to 10 kg, 10 mg for children weighing between 10 to 20 kg and 20 mg daily for children weighing >20 kg. Even though no major adverse events have been noted in children receiving proton pump inhibitors for up to 7 years, the relative safety of prolonged proton pump inhibitor use in children remains unknown.[27] Long-term use of a proton pump inhibitor without a clear diagnosis of GERD is not recommended.[26]

ELDERLY PATIENTS WITH GERD

Many elderly patients have decreased host defense mechanisms, such as saliva production. More aggressive therapy with a proton pump inhibitor may be warranted for patients older than 60 years of age with symptomatic GERD. Often these patients do not seek medical attention because they feel their symptoms are part of the normal aging process. They may also present with atypical symptoms such as chest pain, asthma, poor dentition, or jaw pain. Decreased GI motility is a common problem in elderly patients. Unfortunately, there are no good promotility agents available to these patients. Elderly patients are especially sensitive to the central nervous system effects of metoclopramide. They may also be sensitive to the central nervous system effects of H$_2$-receptor antagonists. Proton pump inhibitors appear to be the most useful treatment modality because they have superior efficacy and are dosed once daily, which is beneficial in all patients, but is especially beneficial in the elderly. Long-term risk of bone fractures may be of concern in this population. Patients at risk for bone fractures should be monitored appropriately.

PATIENTS WITH REFRACTORY GERD

GERD refractory to medical management is rare. Other causes for the patient's symptoms should be evaluated. The majority of patients with refractory symptoms experience nocturnal acid breakthrough. Other reasons for refractory symptoms may be related to timing of proton pump inhibitor and drug metabolism differences in certain patients. Because of this, switching to another proton pump inhibitor may be effective for refractory symptoms in some patients. Ambulatory pH monitoring is useful for patients who are not responding to therapy. Adding an H_2-receptor antagonist at bedtime for nocturnal symptoms has been suggested; however, the effect may be short-lived.[21] Antireflux surgery may also be considered in this patient population.

PHARMACOECONOMIC CONSIDERATIONS

In addition to the traditional clinical endpoints that demonstrate that a certain therapy is effective, the cost effectiveness of the therapy in relation to predicted outcomes and its effects on quality of life must be evaluated. For GERD, one must consider the primary goals of treatment: to relieve symptoms, to heal injury, to prevent recurrence, and to prevent complications. These factors must be evaluated separately, because different costs are associated with achieving each end point. For example, patients with complications associated with GERD, such as strictures, would be more likely to use medical resources as a consequence of revisits and diagnostic tests. Although effects on quality of life may be difficult to evaluate when your goal is preventing recurrence, untreated GERD has a more negative impact on psychological well-being than untreated hypertension, mild heart failure, angina pectoris, or menopause. Improving a patient's quality of life is a measure of treatment success and may help decide which therapy a patient receives.

The proton pump inhibitors are generally more expensive than the H_2-receptor antagonists or promotility agents. Omeprazole's generic availability and nonprescription availability of omeprazole and lansoprazole makes this less of an issue. However, the most expensive therapy is the one that is ineffective. If the H_2-receptor antagonist does not accomplish the treatment goals, then it costs more because the patient must be retreated.

Patient compliance is another factor that affects the outcome of drug therapy. Drug regimens that are easily managed improve compliance, and thus improve outcome for the patient. This especially can be a problem for patients who require high-dose therapy with H_2-receptor antagonists. Not only is the patient required to take the drug more often in higher doses, but there is also increased expense associated with such regimens. The patient may be unable to afford the drug. Choosing a drug that is least expensive and provides the greatest benefit related to dosing interval and number of tablets taken is the optimal regimen. Studies comparing various treatment strategies for GERD show that proton pump inhibitors are more cost-effective than H_2-receptor antagonists, especially for patients with moderate to severe disease.

Decision analysis has been used to evaluate the cost-effectiveness of lifestyle modifications and/or patient-directed therapy alone or combined with omeprazole 20 mg daily or ranitidine 150 mg twice daily for patients with persistent symptomatic GERD. A complex model that evaluated the influence of empiric versus definitive therapy, compliance, and efficacy of the three treatment regimens was employed. Although the retail cost of omeprazole was highest among the treatments evaluated, it was the most cost-effective strategy and was associated with the lowest overall cost. Studies also show that proton pump inhibitors improve quality-of-life measures in symptomatic patients with erosive esophagitis.[28] Additional studies are needed to evaluate the impact of various treatment regimens on quality-of-life issues and cost, and to compare long-term medical management with antireflux surgery and endoscopic therapies.

EVALUATION OF THERAPEUTIC OUTCOMES

❾ The long-term benefits of treatment are difficult to assess because of the limited information known about the epidemiology and natural history of GERD. Consequently, successful outcomes are generally measured in terms of three separate end points: (1) relieving symptoms, (2) healing the injured mucosa, and (3) preventing complications.

The short-term goal of therapy is to relieve symptoms such as heartburn and regurgitation to the point at which they do not impair the patient's quality of life. Patients should be educated regarding specific lifestyle modifications that are applicable to their individual situation including weight loss, raising the head of the bed, smoking cessation, eating smaller meals, and avoiding eating prior to bedtime. Patients should also be instructed to avoid or limit foods that aggravate GERD symptoms, such as fat and chocolate. In addition, the patient's drug profile should be reviewed to identify medications that may contribute to GERD symptoms. These agents should be avoided if possible. Table 39–5 has recommendations for providing pharmaceutical care to patients with GERD.

The clinician should take an active role in educating the patient about potential adverse effects and drug interactions that may occur with drug therapy. The frequency and severity of symptoms should be monitored and patients should be counseled on symptoms that suggest the presence of complications requiring immediate medical attention, such as dysphagia or odynophagia. Patients should also be monitored for the presence of atypical symptoms such as laryngitis asthma or chest pain. These symptoms require further diagnostic evaluation. Long-term maintenance treatment is indicated for patients who have strictures because the strictures commonly recur if reflux esophagitis is not treated.

The second goal is to heal the injured mucosa. Again, individualized lifestyle modifications and the importance of complying with the therapeutic regimen chosen to heal the mucosa should be stressed. Patients should be educated about the risk of relapse and the need for long-term maintenance therapy to prevent recurrence or complications.

TABLE 39-5	Recommendations for Providing Pharmaceutical Care to Patients with GERD

1. Assess the patient's symptoms to determine if patient-directed therapy is appropriate or whether patient should be evaluated by a clinician. Determine the type of symptoms, frequency, and exacerbating factors. Refer any patient with alarm or atypical symptoms to a clinician for further diagnostic workup.
2. Obtain a thorough history of prescription, nonprescription, and natural drug product use.
3. Counsel the patient on lifestyle modifications that will improve symptoms.
4. Recommend appropriate drug therapy based on patient presentation.
5. Develop a plan to assess effectiveness of acid-suppression therapy after an appropriate amount of time (8–16 weeks). Recommend alternative therapy if necessary.
6. Assess improvement in quality-of-life measures such as physical, psychologic, and social functioning and well-being.
7. Evaluate patient for the presence of adverse drug reactions, allergies, and drug interactions.
8. Stress the importance of compliance with the therapeutic regimen, including lifestyle modifications. Recommend a therapeutic regimen that is easy for the patient to accomplish.
9. Provide patient education with regard to disease state, lifestyle modifications, and drug therapy. Patients should be counseled on
   - What causes GERD and what things to avoid
   - When to take their medications
   - What potential adverse effects or drug interactions may occur
   - What alarm signs they should report to their clinician

The final, more long-term goal of therapy is to decrease the risk of complications (esophagitis, strictures, Barrett esophagus, and esophageal adenocarcinoma). A small subset of patients may continue to fail treatment despite therapy with high doses of H_2-receptor antagonists or a proton pump inhibitor. Patients should be monitored for the presence of continual pain, dysphagia, or odynophagia.

ABBREVIATIONS

GERD: gastroesophageal reflux disease

GI: gastrointestinal

H_2: histamine type-2

LES: lower esophageal sphincter

REFERENCES

1. The American Gastroenterological Association (AGA) Institute Medical Position Panel. American gastroenterological association medical position statement on the management of gastroesophageal reflux disease. Gastroenterology 2008;135:1383–1391.
2. Kahrilas PJ. Gastroesophageal reflux disease. N Engl J Med 2008;359:1700–1707.
3. Dent J, El-Serag HB, Wallander MA, Johansson S. Epidemiology of gastro-oesophageal reflux disease: a systematic review. Gut 2005;54:710–717.
4. DeVault KR, Castell DO. Updated guidelines for the diagnosis and treatment of gastroesophageal reflux disease. Am J Gastroenterol 2005;100:190–200.
5. DeVault KR. Review article: The role of acid suppression in patients with non-erosive reflux disease or functional heartburn. Aliment Pharmacol Ther 2006;23(suppl 1):33–39.
6. Rudolph CD, Mazur LJ, Liptak GS, et al. Guidelines for evaluation and treatment of gastroesophageal reflux in infants and children: Recommendations of the North American Society for Pediatric Gastroenterology and Nutrition. J Pediatr Gastroenterol Nutr 2001;32(suppl 2):1–31.
7. Hirano I. Review article: Modern technology in the diagnosis of gastrooesophageal reflux disease—Bilitec, intraluminal impedance and Bravo capsule pH monitoring. Aliment Pharmacol Ther 2006;23 (suppl 1):12–24.
8. Lagergren J, Bergstrom R, Lindgren A, Nyren O. Symptomatic gastroesophageal reflux as a risk factor for esophageal adenocarcinoma. N Engl J Med 1999;340:825–831.
9. Liu JJ, Carr-Lock DL, Osterman MT, et al. Endoscopic treatment for atypical manifestations of gastroesophageal reflux disease. Am J Gastroenterol 2006;101:440–445.
10. Pandolfino JE, Kahrilas PJ. Prolonged pH monitoring: Bravo capsule. Gastrointest Endosc Clin N Am 2005;15:307–318.
11. Pandolfino JE, Schreiner MA, Lee TJ, et al. Comparison of the Bravo wireless and Digitrapper catheter-based pH monitoring systems for measuring esophageal acid exposure. Am J Gastroenterol 2005;100:1466–1476.
12. Pandolfino JE, El-Serag HB, Zhang Q, et al. Obesity: A challenge to esophagogastric junction integrity. Gastroenterology 2006;130:639–649.
13. Lundell L, Miettinen P, Myrvold E, et al. Seven-year follow-up of a randomized clinical trial comparing proton-pump inhibition with surgical therapy for reflux oesophagitis. Br J Surg 2007;94:198–203.
14. Johnson DA. Endoscopic therapy for GERD—Baking, sewing, or stuffing: An evidence-based perspective. Rev Gastroenterol Disord 2003;3:142–149.
15. Pleskow D, Rothstein R, Lo S, et al. Endoscopic full-thickness plication for the treatment of GERD: 12-month follow-up for the North American open-label trial. Gastrointest Endosc 2005;61:643–649.
16. Horn J. The proton-pump inhibitors: Similarities and differences. Clin Ther 2000;22:266–280.
17. Aseeri M, Schroeder T, Kramer J, Zackula R. Gastric acid suppression by proton pump inhibitors as a risk factor for *Clostridium difficile*-associated diarrhea in hospitalized patients. Am J Gastroenterol 2008;013:2308–2313.
18. Dial S, Delaney JAC, Burkun AN, Suissa S. Use of gastric acid-suppressive agents and the risk of community-acquired *Clostridium difficile*-associated disease. JAMA 2005;294: 2989–2995.
19. Ho MP, Maddox TM, Wang L, et al. Risk of adverse outcomes associated with concomitant use of clopidogrel and proton pump inhibitors following acute coronary syndrome. JAMA 2009;301:937–944.
20. Stanek EJ, Aubert RE, Flockhart DA, et al. A national study of the effect of individual proton pump inhibitors on cardiovascular outcomes in patients treated with clopidogrel following coronary stenting: The clopidogrel Medco outcomes study, *http://scai.org/pdf/Stanek_Clopidogrel-PPI_SCAI_2009.pdf.*
21. Fackler WK, Ours TM, Vaezi MF, et al. Long-term effect of H2RA therapy on nocturnal gastric acid breakthrough. Gastroenterology 2002;122:625–632.
22. Garrett WR. Considerations for long-term use of proton-pump inhibitors. AJHP 1998;55:2268–2279.
23. Yu-Xiao Y, Lewis JD, Epstein S. Long-term proton pump inhibitor therapy and the risk of hip fracture. JAMA 2006;296:2947–2953.
24. Yu EW, Blackwell T, Ensrud KE, et al. Acid-suppressive medications and risk of bone loss and fracture in older adults. Calcif Tissue Int 2008;83:251–259.
25. Esomeprazole. Data on file. Wilmington, DE: AstraZeneca; 2008.
26. Vandenplas Y, Rudolph CD, Di Lorenzo C, et al. Pediatric gastroesophageal reflux clinical practice guidelines: Joint recommendations of the North American society for pediatric gastroenterology, hepatology, and nutrition (NASPGHAN) and the European society for pediatric gastroenterology, hepatology, and nutrition (ESPGHAN). J Pediatr Gastroenterol Nutr 2009;49:498–547.
27. Patel AS, Pohl JF, Easley DJ. Proton pump inhibitors in pediatrics. Pediatr Rev 2003;24:12–15.
28. Revicki D, Wood M, Maton PM, et al. The impact of gastroesophageal reflux disease on health-related quality of life. Am J Med 1998;104:252–258.

CHAPTER

40

Peptic Ulcer Disease

ROSEMARY R. BERARDI AND RANDOLPH V. FUGIT

KEY CONCEPTS

❶ Patients with peptic ulcer disease (PUD) should reduce psychological stress, cigarette smoking, and nonsteroidal antiinflammatory drug (NSAID) use and avoid foods and beverages that exacerbate ulcer symptoms.

❷ Eradication is recommended for all *Helicobacter pylori* (*H. pylori*)–positive patients with an active ulcer, a documented history of a prior ulcer, or a history of ulcer-related complications.

❸ The selection of an *H. pylori* eradication regimen should be based on efficacy, safety, antibiotic resistance, cost, and the likelihood of medication adherence. Treatment should be initiated with a proton pump inhibitor (PPI)–based three-drug regimen. If a second course of *H. pylori* therapy is required, the regimen should contain different antibiotics.

❹ PPI cotherapy reduces the risk of NSAID-related gastric and duodenal ulcers and is at least as effective as recommended dosages of misoprostol and superior to the histamine-2 receptor antagonists (H_2RA).

❺ Standard PPI dosages and a nonselective NSAID are as effective as a selective cyclooxygenase-2 (COX-2) inhibitor in reducing the risk of NSAID-induced ulcers and upper gastrointestinal (GI) complications.

❻ The eradication of *H. pylori* improves clinical outcomes and decreases the use of healthcare resources when compared with conventional antisecretory therapy. The cost effectiveness of misoprostol cotherapy is greatest for patients with the highest risk for GI complications. Cotherapy with PPIs and NSAIDs or selective COX-2 inhibitors is cost effective even in low-risk patients especially if the least costly PPI is used.

❼ Patients with PUD, especially those receiving *H. pylori* eradication or misoprostol cotherapy, require patient education regarding their disease and drug treatment to successfully achieve a positive therapeutic outcome.

❽ The recommended treatment for severe peptic ulcer bleeding after appropriate endoscopic treatment is the intravenous administration of a PPI loading dose followed by a 72-hour continuous infusion with a goal of maintaining an intragastric pH of 6 or greater.

❾ Critically ill patients at the highest risk of developing stress-related mucosal bleeding (SRMB) who require prophylactic drug therapy include those with respiratory failure on mechanical ventilation or those with coagulopathy.

❿ There are limited data to support the selection of a PPI over an intravenous H_2RA for SRMB prophylaxis. The decision should be based upon appropriate individual patient characteristics (e.g., nothing by mouth, presence of nasogastric tube, renal failure).

Learning objectives, review questions, and other resources can be found at **www.pharmacotherapyonline.com**.

PEPTIC ULCER DISEASE

Acid-related diseases (gastritis, erosions, and peptic ulcer) of the upper gastrointestinal (GI) tract require gastric acid for their formation.[1-3] Peptic ulcer disease (PUD) differs from gastritis and erosions in that ulcers typically extend deeper into the muscularis mucosa.[1] There are three common forms of peptic ulcers: *Helicobacter pylori* (*H. pylori*)-positive, nonsteroidal antiinflammatory drug (NSAID)-induced, and stress ulcers (Table 40–1). The term *stress-related mucosal damage* (SRMD) is preferred to stress ulcer or stress gastritis, because the mucosal lesions range from superficial gastritis and erosions to deep ulcers.

H. pylori–positive and NSAID-induced ulcers are chronic peptic ulcers that differ in etiology, clinical presentation, and tendency to recur (see Table 40–1). These ulcers develop most often in the stomach and duodenum of ambulatory patients (Fig. 40–1). Occasionally, ulcers develop in the esophagus, jejunum, ileum, or colon. The natural course of chronic PUD is characterized by frequent ulcer recurrence. The most important factors that influence ulcer recurrence are *H. pylori* infection and NSAID use. Other factors include cigarette smoking, alcohol use, ulcer-related complications, gastric acid hypersecretion, and patient noncompliance. The cause of ulcer recurrence is most likely multifactorial.

Peptic ulcers are also associated with Zollinger-Ellison syndrome (ZES), radiation, chemotherapy, vascular insufficiency, and other chronic diseases (Table 40–2).[1,3] Although a strong association exists between chronic pulmonary diseases, chronic renal failure, and cirrhosis, the pathophysiologic mechanisms of these associations remain unclear.[1] In contrast, SRMD occurs primarily in the stomach in critically ill patients (see Table 40–1).[1]

This chapter focuses on chronic PUD associated with *H. pylori* and NSAIDs. A brief discussion of ZES and upper GI bleeding related to PUD and SRMD is included.

TABLE 40-1	Comparison of Common Forms of Peptic Ulcer		
Characteristic	H. pylori Induced	NSAID Induced	SRMD
Condition	Chronic	Chronic	Acute
Site of damage	Duodenum > stomach	Stomach > duodenum	Stomach > duodenum
Intragastric pH	More dependent	Less dependent	Less dependent
Symptoms	Usually epigastric pain	Often asymptomatic	Asymptomatic
Ulcer depth	Superficial	Deep	Most superficial
GI bleeding	Less severe, single vessel	More severe, single vessel	More severe, superficial mucosal capillaries

H. pylori, Helicobacter pylori; NSAID, nonsteroidal antiinflammatory drug; SRMD, stress-related mucosal damage.

EPIDEMIOLOGY

The epidemiology of PUD is complicated and difficult to estimate given the variablity in the prevalence of H. pylori infection, NSAID use, and cigarette smoking as well as the various methods used to detect ulcers, e.g., endoscopy, radiology, symptoms, or complications.[1,4] The prevalence and incidence of PUD in the United States also reflects improvements in drug therapy, the dramatic shift to ambulatory management, and changes in the criteria and coding system for mortality and hospitalization data.[1] Recent trends suggest a shift from predominance in men to a similar occurrence in men and women with increasing rates of disease in older individuals and a decrease in the younger population.[1,4] Despite a modest decline in mortality, hospitalizations, and office visits, PUD remains one of the most common GI diseases, resulting in impaired quality of life, work loss, and high-cost medical care.

ETIOLOGY AND RISK FACTORS

Most peptic ulcers occur in the presence of acid and pepsin when H. pylori, NSAIDs, or other factors (see Table 40–2) disrupt the normal mucosal defense and healing mechanisms.[1] Hypersecretion of acid is the primary pathogenic mechanism in hypersecretory states such as ZES.[3] Benign gastric ulcers can occur anywhere in the stomach, although most are located on the lesser curvature, just distal to the junction of the antral and acid-secreting mucosa (see Fig. 40–1). Most duodenal ulcers occur in the first part of the duodenum (duodenal bulb).

HELICOBACTER PYLORI

H. pylori infection causes chronic gastritis in infected individuals and is causally linked to PUD, mucosa-associated lymphoid tissue (MALT) lymphoma, and gastric cancer (Fig. 40–2).[1,2,5–8] The majority of infected individuals remain asymptomatic, but 10% to 20% will develop PUD during their lifetime and about 1% will develop gastric cancer.[1,2,8] Host-specific cofactors and H. pylori strain variability play an important role in the pathogenesis of PUD and gastric cancer.[2,8] Although an association between H. pylori and PUD bleeding is less clear, there is evidence that eradication of H. pylori decreases recurrent bleeding.[5,9] No specific link has been established between H. pylori and dyspepsia, nonulcer dyspepsia (NUD), or gastroesophageal reflux disease (GERD).[5,9–11] However, some patients with dyspepsia and NUD may benefit from H. pylori eradication.[5,9] Although eradication of H. pylori may worsen GERD symptoms in some patients, eradication should not be withheld.[5,10] An association between H. pylori infection and iron deficiency anemia has been established, but cause and effect has not been proven, and whether H. pylori eradication is beneficial is uncertain.[5,11] There are insufficient data to support a link between H. pylori and extragastric manifestations including cardiovascular, hematologic, respiratory, hepatobiliary, and neurologic diseases.[5,11]

The prevalence of H. pylori varies by geographic location, socioeconomic conditions, ethnicity, and age. In developing countries, H. pylori prevalence is more common than in industrialized countries and correlates with lower socioeconomic levels.[2,5,6] The prevalence of H. pylori in the United States is 30% to 40% but is much higher in individuals over 60 years (50% to 60%) than in children under 12 years (10% to 15%) of age.[2,5] Although most individuals in the United States acquire H. pylori in childhood, the rate of acquisition in children is declining and most likely will continue to fall as a consequence of improved socioeconomic conditions.[2] Caucasians are infected with H pylori less frequently than African Americans and Hispanic persons, but this is thought to be related to lower socioecomonic status and living conditions. Infection rates do not differ with gender or smoking status.

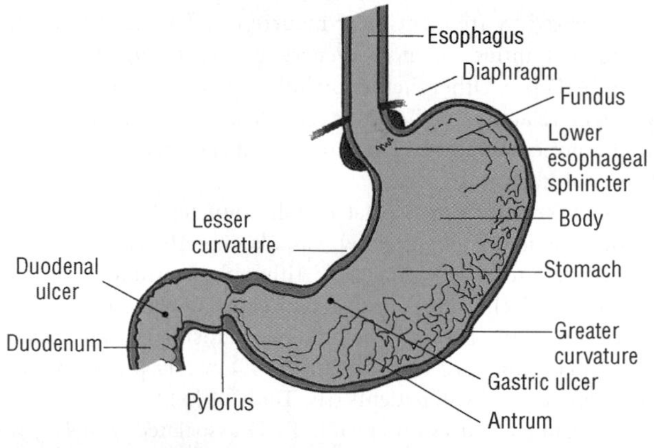

FIGURE 40-1. Anatomic structure of the stomach and duodenum and most common locations of gastric and duodenal ulcers.

TABLE 40-2	Potential Causes of Peptic Ulcer

Common causes
  Helicobacter pylori infection
  Nonsteroidal antiinflammatory drugs
  Critical illness (stress-related mucosal damage)
Uncommon causes of chronic peptic ulcer
  Idiopathic (non-*H. pylori*, non-NSAID peptic ulcer)
  Hypersecretion of gastric acid (e.g., Zollinger-Ellison syndrome)
  Viral infections (e.g., cytomegalovirus)
  Vascular insufficiency (e.g., crack cocaine associated)
  Radiation therapy
  Chemotherapy (e.g., hepatic artery infusions)
  Infiltrating disease (e.g., Crohn disease):
Diseases and medical conditions associated with chronic peptic ulcer
  Cirrhosis
  Chronic renal failure
  Chronic obstructive pulmonary disease
  Cardiovascular disease
  Organ transplantation

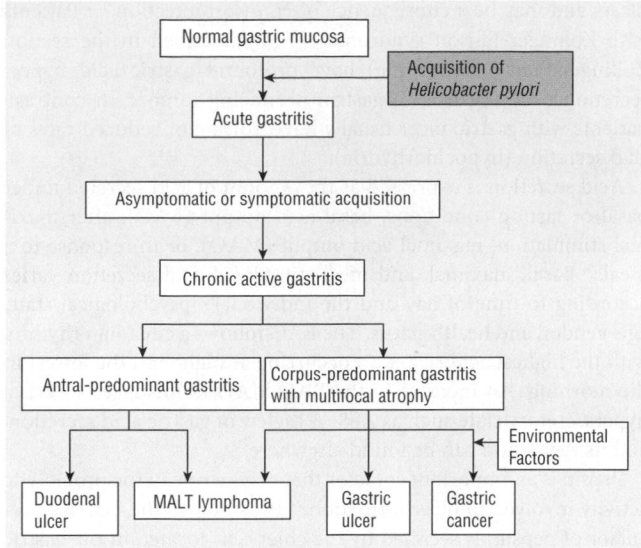

FIGURE 40-2. The natural history of *Helicobacter pylori* infection in the pathogenesis of gastric ulcer and duodenal ulcer, mucosa-associated lymphoid tissue (MALT) lymphoma, and gastric cancer.

TABLE 40-4	Risk Factors Associated with Nonsteroidal Antiinflammatory Drug (NSAID)–Induced Ulcers and Upper Gastrointestinal Complications[a]

Age >65
Previous peptic ulcer
Previous ulcer-related upper GI complication
High-dose NSAIDs
Multiple NSAID use
Selection of NSAID (e.g., COX-1 vs COX-2 inhibition)
NSAID-related dyspepsia
Aspirin (including cardioprotective dosages)
Concomitant use of NSAID plus low-dose aspirin
Concomitant use of oral bisphosphonates (e.g., alendronate)
Concomitant use of corticosteroids
Concomitant use of anticoagulant or coagulopathy
Concomitant use of antiplatelet drugs (e.g., clopidogrel)
Concomitant use of selective serotonin reuptake inhibitor
Chronic debilitating disorders (e.g., cardiovascular disease, rheumatoid arthritis)
Helicobacter pylori infection
Cigarette smoking
Alcohol consumption

[a]Combinations of risk factors are additive.
Data from references 1, 12 to 15, 20, and 29.

The most common route of *H. pylori* transmission is person to person either by gastro–oral (vomitus) or fecal–oral (diarrhea) contact which occurs primarily during childhood.[2] Members of the same household are likely to become infected when someone in the same household is infected.[2] *H. pylori* can also be transmitted by the use of inadequately sterilized endoscopes.

NONSTEROIDAL ANTIINFLAMMATORY DRUGS

NSAIDs (Table 40–3) are widely used in the United States, particularly in individuals over 60 years of age, to treat chronic pain and inflammation.[1] These agents include prescription and nonprescription medications and low-dose aspirin used for cardiovascular and cerebrovascular risk reduction.[1,12–14] There is overwhelming evidence linking chronic NSAID (including aspirin) use to a variety of upper GI tract injuries.[1,12–16] NSAIDs cause superficial (topical) mucosal damage consisting of petechiae (intramucosal hemorrhages) within minutes of ingestion, and progress to erosions with continued use.[1] These lesions typically heal within a few days and rarely cause ulcers or acute upper GI bleeding. Gastroduodenal ulcers develop in about 25% of chronic NSAID users with continued use.[12] Gastric ulcers are most common, occur primarily in the antrum, and are of greater concern because of their potential to cause ulcer-related upper GI complications (see Table 40–1). As many as 2% to 4% of patients with an NSAID ulcer will bleed or perforate.[12] Each year, NSAIDs account for at least 100,000 hospitalizations and between 7,000 and 10,000 deaths

TABLE 40-3	Selected Nonsteroidal Antiinflammatory Drugs (NSAIDs) and Cyclooxygenase-2 (COX-2) Inhibitors

Nonsalicylates[a]
  Nonselective (traditional) NSAIDs: indomethacin, piroxicam, ibuprofen, naproxen, sulindac, ketoprofen, ketorolac, flurbiprofen
  Partially selective NSAIDs: etodolac, nabumetone, meloxicam, diclofenac, celocoxib
  Selective COX-2 inhibitors: rofecoxib,[b] valdecoxib[b]
Salicylates
  Acetylated: aspirin
  Nonacetylated: salsalate, trisalicylate

[a]Based on COX-1/COX-2 selectivity ratio.
[b]Withdrawn from U.S. market.

in the United States.[12] NSAID-induced ulcers occur less frequently in the esophagus, small bowel, and colon.[16,17] How NSAIDs damage the lower GI tract is unclear, but the enteropathy is associated with lower GI bleeding.

Table 40–4 lists the risk factors associated with NSAID-induced ulcers and upper GI complications. Combinations of factors confer an additive risk.[12–16,18] Advanced age is an independent risk factor, and the incidence of NSAID-induced ulcers increases linearly with the age of the patient.[1] The high incidence of ulcer complications in older individuals may be explained by age-related changes in gastric mucosal defense. The relative risk of NSAID complications is increased for patients with a previous peptic ulcer and may be as high as 14-fold in those with a history of an ulcer-related complication.[1,16] The risk of adverse events is greatest during the first month after initiating continuous therapy and remains the same throughout treatment.[1]

NSAID ulcers and related complications are dose-dependent, but may occur with low doses of nonprescription NSAIDs and low cardioprotective dosages of aspirin (81 to 325 mg/day).[1,12–16] Factors such as NSAID potency, longer duration of effect, and a greater propensity to inhibit cyclooxygenase-1 (COX-1) versus COX-2 isoezymes are associated with increased risk (see Table 40–3).[1,16,18,19] NSAID-related dyspepsia, in itself, does not correlate directly with mucosal injury or clinical events. However, new-onset dyspepsia, changes in severity, or dyspepsia not relieved by antiulcer medications may suggest an ulcer or ulcer complication.[1] Nonacetylated salicylates (e.g., salsalate) may be associated with decreased GI toxicity.[1] Buffered or enteric-coated aspirin confers no added protection from upper GI events.[13]

NSAID ulcer and GI complication risk are increased with the use of multiple NSAIDs or the concomitant use of low-dose aspirin, oral bisphosphonates, corticosteroids, anticoagulants, antiplatelet drugs, and selective serotonin reuptake inhibitors.[1,12–16,20] The risk of an ulcer-related GI complication is greater when a NSAID or COX-2 inhibitor (see Table 40–3) is coadministered with low-dose aspirin than when either drug is taken alone.[1,13,16] The NSAID may also reduce the antiplatelet effects of aspirin, although NSAIDs vary in their effects on platelet function.[13–15] Corticosteroids, when used alone, do not potentiate the risk of ulcer or complications, but the relative risk is increased twofold in corticosteroid users who are also taking concurrent NSAIDs.[1,16] The relative risk of GI bleeding increases up to 20-fold when NSAIDs are taken concomitantly with anticoagulants (e.g., warfarin) and up to sixfold with the concurrent use of serotonin reuptake inhibitors.[16,17] When clopidogrel is taken in combination with aspirin, an NSAID, or an anticoagulant, the risk of GI bleeding is increased compared with when these agents are taken alone.[13,15,16] Even when prescribed as monotherapy, clopidogrel increases the risk of rebleeding for patients with history of a bleeding ulcer.[13,15,16]

H. pylori and NSAIDs act independently to increase ulcer risk and ulcer-related bleeding and appear to have additive effects.[5,16] Thus, the incidence of peptic ulcer is higher in *H. pylori*–positive NSAID users. Whether *H. pylori* infection is actually a risk factor for NSAID ulcers remains controversial.[1,5,16] However, eradication is reported to reduce the incidence of peptic ulcer if undertaken prior to starting the NSAID but does not reduce the risk for patients who were previously taking an NSAID.[1,5,16]

CIGARETTE SMOKING

Epidemiologic evidence links cigarette smoking to PUD, but it is uncertain whether smoking causes peptic ulcers.[1] Ulcer risk is proportional to the number of cigarettes smoked and is modest when fewer than 10 cigarettes are smoked per day. Cigarette smoking impairs ulcer healing, promotes ulcer recurrence, and increases ulcer risk.[1] The exact mechanism by which cigarette smoking contributes to PUD remains unclear. Possible mechanisms include inhibition of pancreatic bicarbonate secretion and increases in gastric acid secretion, but these effects are inconsistent. Whether nicotine or other components of smoke are responsible for these physiologic alterations is unknown.

PSYCHOLOGICAL STRESS

The importance of psychological factors in the pathogenesis of PUD remains controversial.[1] Clinical observation suggests that ulcer patients are adversely affected by stressful life events. However, results from controlled trials are conflicting and have failed to document a cause-and-effect relationship.[1] Emotional stress may induce behavioral risks such as smoking and the use of NSAIDs or alter the inflammatory response or resistance to *H. pylori* infection. The role of stress and how it affects PUD is complex and probably multifactorial.

DIETARY FACTORS

The role of diet and nutrition in PUD is uncertain.[1] Coffee, tea, cola beverages, beer, milk, and spices may cause dyspepsia but do not increase the risk for PUD. Beverage restrictions and bland diets do not alter the frequency of ulcer recurrence. Although caffeine is a gastric acid stimulant, constituents in decaffeinated coffee or tea, caffeine-free carbonated beverages, beer, and wine may also increase gastric acid secretion. In high concentrations, alcohol ingestion is associated with acute gastric mucosal damage and upper GI bleeding; however, there is insufficient evidence to confirm that alcohol causes ulcers.[1]

PATHOPHYSIOLOGY

A physiologic imbalance between aggressive (gastric acid and pepsin) and protective factors (mucosal defense and repair) remain important issues in the pathophysiology of gastric and duodenal ulcers.[1,21] Gastric acid is secreted by the parietal cells, which contain receptors for histamine, gastrin, and acetylcholine.[21] Acid (as well as *H. pylori* infection and NSAID use) is an independent factor that contributes to the disruption of mucosal integrity.[1] Increased acid secretion has been observed for patients with duodenal

ulcers and may be a consequence of *H. pylori* infection.[2,22] Patients with Zollinger-Ellison syndrome (ZES) (described in the section Zollinger-Ellison Syndrome) have profound gastric acid hypersecretion resulting from a gastrin-producing tumor.[3] In contrast, patients with gastric ulcer usually have normal or reduced rates of acid secretion (hypochlorhydria).

Acid secretion is expressed as the amount of acid secreted under basal or fasting conditions, basal acid output (BAO); after maximal stimulation, maximal acid output (MAO); or in response to a meal.[21] Basal, maximal, and meal-stimulated acid secretion varies according to time of day and the individual's psychological state, age, gender, and health status. The BAO follows a circadian rhythm, with the highest acid secretion occurring at night and the lowest in the morning. An increase in the BAO:MAO ratio suggests a basal hypersecretory state such as ZES. A review of gastric acid secretion, and its regulation can be found elsewhere.[21]

Pepsin is an important cofactor that plays a role in the proteolytic activity involved in ulcer formation.[21] Pepsinogen, the inactive precursor of pepsin, is secreted by the chief cells located in the gastric fundus (see Fig. 40–1). Pepsin is activated by acid pH (optimal pH of 1.8 to 3.5), inactivated reversibly at pH 4, and irreversibly destroyed at pH 7.

Mucosal defense and repair mechanisms (mucus and bicarbonate secretion, intrinsic epithelial cell defense, and mucosal blood flow) protect the gastroduodenal mucosa from noxious endogenous and exogenous substances.[1,21] The viscous nature and near-neutral pH of the mucus-bicarbonate barrier protect the stomach from the acidic contents in the gastric lumen. Mucosal repair after injury is related to epithelial cell restitution, growth, and regeneration. The maintenance of mucosal integrity and repair is mediated by the production of endogenous prostaglandins. The term *cytoprotection* is often used to describe this process, but *mucosal defense* and *mucosal protection* are more accurate terms, as prostaglandins prevent deep mucosal injury and not superficial damage to individual cells. Gastric hyperemia and increased prostaglandin synthesis characterize adaptive cytoprotection, the short-term adaptation of mucosal cells to mild topical irritants. This phenomenon enables the stomach to initially withstand the damaging effects of irritants. Alterations in mucosal defense that are induced by *H. pylori* or NSAIDs are the most important cofactors in the formation of peptic ulcers.

HELICOBACTER PYLORI

H. pylori is a spiral-shaped, pH-sensitive, gram-negative, microaerophilic bacterium that resides between the mucus layer and surface epithelial cells in the stomach, or any location where gastric-type epithelium is found.[2,22] The combination of its spiral shape and flagellum permits it to move from the lumen of the stomach, where the pH is low, to the mucus layer, where the local pH is neutral. *H. pylori* produces large amounts of urease, which hydrolyzes urea in the gastric juice and converts it to ammonia and carbon dioxide.[2] The local buffering effect of ammonia creates a neutral microenvironment within and surrounding the bacterium, which protects it from the lethal effect of gastric acid. *H. pylori* also produces acid-inhibitory proteins, which allows it to adapt to the low-pH environment of the stomach.[2]

H. pylori binds to specific regions within the stomach. It attaches to gastric-type epithelium by adherence pedestals, which prevent the organism from being shed during cell turnover and mucus secretion.[2] Colonization of the antrum and corpus (body) of the stomach is associated with gastric ulcer and cancer.[1,2,22] Antral organisms colonize gastric metaplastic tissue (gastric tissue that develops in the duodenum secondary to changes in gastric acid or bicarbonate secretion) leading to duodenal ulcer (see Fig. 40–2).[1,2] Although *H. pylori* causes chronic gastric mucosal inflammation in all infected individuals, only a minority actually develop an ulcer or gastric cancer.[1,2,8] The difference in the diverse clinical outcomes is related to variations in bacterial pathogenicity and host susceptability.[2,22]

Mucosal injury is produced by (1) elaborating bacterial enzymes (urease, lipases, and proteases), (2) adherence, and (3) *H. pylori* virulence factors.[2,22] Lipases and proteases degrade gastric mucus, ammonia produced by urease may be toxic to gastric epithelial cells, and bacterial adherence enhances the uptake of toxins into gastric epithelial cells. *H. pylori* induces gastric inflammation by altering the host inflammatory response and damaging epithelial cells directly by cell-mediated immune mechanisms or indirectly by activated neutrophils or macrophages attempting to phagocytose bacteria or bacterial products.[2,22] However, *H. pylori* strains are genetically diverse and account for differences in adaptation within the human host. Two of the most important are cytotoxin-associated gene protein (CagA) and vacuolating cytotoxin (VacA). About 60% of *H. pylori* strains in the United States possess CagA, but CagA-positive strains increase the risk for severe PUD, gastritis, and gastric cancer compared with CagA-negative strains.[2,22] The VacA gene codes for the Vac-A cytotoxin, a vacuolizating toxin. Although VacA is present in most all *H pylori* strains, strains vary in cytotoxicity and increased risk for peptic ulcer and gastric cancer.[2,22] Host polymorphisms are important markers of disease susceptibility and may identify high-risk patients.[2,22] Polymorphisms of interleukin (IL)-1β and its receptor antagonist, as well as tumor necrosis factor α (TNF-α) and IL-10, may be associated with increased gastric acid secretion and duodenal ulcer or acid suppression and gastric cancer.[2,22]

NONSTEROIDAL ANTIINFLAMMATORY DRUGS

NSAIDs, including aspirin (see Table 40–3), cause gastric mucosal damage by two important mechanisms: (1) direct or topical irritation of the gastric epithelium and (2) systemic inhibition of endogenous mucosal prostaglandin synthesis.[1,13] Although the initial injury is initiated topically by the acidic properties of many of the NSAIDs, systemic inhibition of the protective prostaglandins limits the ability of the mucosa to defend itself against injury and thus plays the predominant role in the development of gastric ulcer.[1,13]

Topical irritant properties are predominantly associated with acidic NSAIDs (e.g., aspirin) and their ability to decrease the hydrophobicity of the mucous gel layer in the gastric mucosa. Most nonaspirin NSAIDs have topical irritant effects, but aspirin is the most damaging. Although NSAID prodrugs, enteric-coated aspirin tablets, salicylate derivatives, and parenteral or rectal preparations are associated with less-acute topical gastric mucosal injury, they can cause ulcers and related GI complications as a result of their systemic inhibition of endogenous PGs.[1]

Cyclooxygenase (COX) is the rate-limiting enzyme in the conversion of arachidonic acid to prostaglandins and is inhibited by NSAIDs (Fig. 40–3). Two similar COX isoforms have been identified: cyclooxygenase-1 (COX-1) is found in most body tissue, including the stomach, kidney, intestine, and platelets; cyclooxygenase-2 (COX-2) is undetectable in most tissues under normal physiologic conditions, but its expression can be induced during acute inflammation and arthritis (Fig. 40–4).[1,13] COX-1 produces protective prostaglandins that regulate physiologic processes such as GI mucosal integrity, platelet homeostasis, and renal function. COX-2 is induced (unregulated) by inflammatory stimuli such as cytokines and produces prostaglandins involved with inflammation, fever, and pain. COX-2 is also constitutionally expressed in organs such as the brain, kidney, and reproductive tract. Adverse effects (e.g., GI or renal toxicity) of NSAIDs are primarily associated with the inhibition of COX-1, whereas antiinflammatory actions result primarily from NSAID inhibition of COX-2.[1,13]

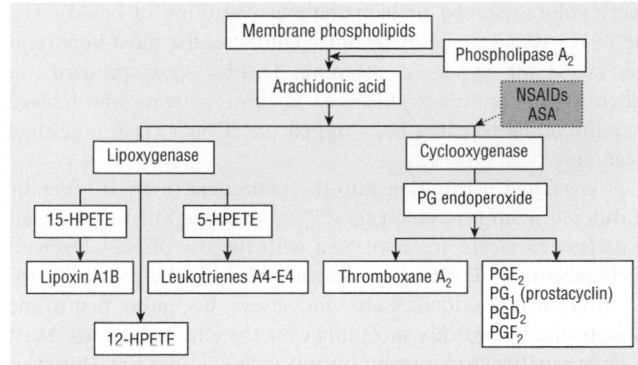

FIGURE 40-3. Metabolism of arachidonic acid after its release from membrane phospholipids. *Broken arrow* indicates inhibitory effects. (ASA, aspirin; HPETE, hydroperoxyeicosatetraenoic acid; NSAIDs, nonsteroidal antiinflammatory drugs; PG, prostaglandin.)

The COX-1-to-COX-2 inhibitory ratio determines the relative GI toxicity of a specific NSAID. Nonselective NSAIDs, including aspirin (see Table 40–3), inhibit both COX-1 and COX-2 to varying degrees and are associated with an increased propensity to cause gastric ulcers.[1,13] In contrast, the selective COX-2 inhibitors are associated with a reduction in ulcers and related GI complications, but the benefit of celecoxib, is less that that of rofecoxib and valdecoxib (see Table 40–3). The addition of aspirin to a selective COX-2 inhibitor reduces its ulcer-sparing benefit and increases ulcer risk.[1,13] Aspirin and nonaspirin NSAIDs irreversibly inhibit platelet COX-1, resulting in decreased platelet aggregation and prolonged bleeding times, thereby increasing the potential for upper and lower GI bleeding.[1,13,15] Coadministration of selected NSAIDs may reduce the antiplatelet effects of aspirin.[13–15] Clopidogrel and other medications that impair angiogenesis do not cause ulcers, per se, but may impair healing of gastric erosions leading to ulceration.[13,15]

COMPLICATIONS

Upper GI bleeding, perforation, and obstruction occur with *H. pylori*–associated and NSAID-induced ulcers and constitute the most serious, life-threatening complication of chronic PUD.[1,23] Bleeding is caused by the erosion of an ulcer into an artery. It may be occult (hidden) and insidious or may present as melena

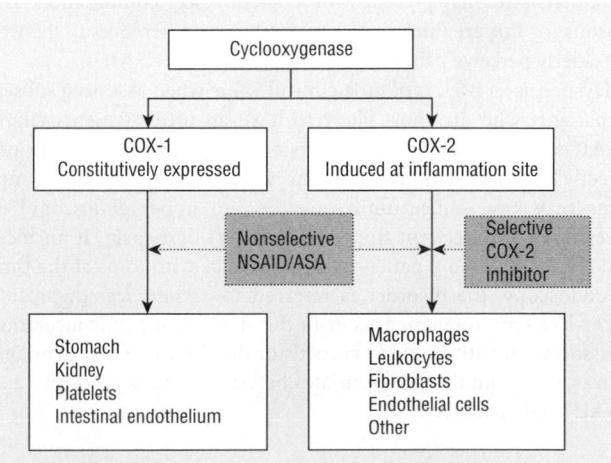

FIGURE 40-4. Tissue distribution and actions of cyclooxygenase (COX) isoenzymes. Nonselective nonsteroidal antiinflammatory drugs (NSAIDs) including aspirin (ASA) inhibit COX-1 and COX-2 to varying degrees; COX-2 inhibitors inhibit only COX-2. *Broken arrow* indicates inhibitory effects.

(black-colored stools) or hematemesis (vomiting of blood). The use of NSAIDs (especially in older adults) is the most important risk factor for upper GI bleeding. Deaths occur primarily in patients who continue to bleed or in those patients who rebleed after the initial bleeding has stopped (see Upper Gastrointestinal Bleeding).

Ulcer-related perforation into the peritoneal cavity is generally considered a surgical emergency.[1,23] About one third to one half of perforated ulcers are associated with the use of NSAIDs, with the highest mortality reported in the elderly.[23] The pain of perforation is usually sudden, sharp, and severe, beginning first in the epigastrium, but quickly spreading over the entire abdomen. Most patients experience ulcer symptoms prior to perforation. However, older patients who experience perforation in association with NSAID use may be asymptomatic. Penetration occurs when an ulcer burrows into an adjacent structure (pancreas, biliary tract, or liver) rather than opening freely into a cavity.

Gastric outlet obstruction is related to mechanical obstruction caused by scarring, muscular spasm or edema of the duodenal bulb usually resulting from chronic ulcercation.[1,23] Symptoms occur over several months and include early satiety, bloating, anorexia, nausea, vomiting, and weight loss. Perforation, penetration, and gastric outlet obstruction occur most often with long-standing PUD.

Treatment of PUD has improved so that even the most virulent ulcers can be managed with medication. Intractability to drug therapy is an infrequent manifestation of PUD and an infrequent indication for surgery.

SIGNS AND SYMPTOMS

The clinical presentation of PUD varies depending on the severity of epigastric pain and the presence of complications (Table 40–5).[1] Ulcer-related pain in duodenal ulcer often occurs 1 to 3 hours after meals and is usually relieved by food, but this is variable. In gastric ulcer, food may precipitate or accentuate ulcer pain. Antacids usually provide immediate pain relief in most ulcer patients. Pain usually diminishes or disappears during treatment; however, recurrence of epigastric pain after healing often suggests an unhealed or recurrent ulcer.

The presence or absence of epigastric pain does not define an ulcer.[1] Ulcer healing does not necessarily render the patient asymptomatic. Why symptoms remain is unclear, but it may relate to sensitization of afferent nerves in response to mucosal injury.[1] Conversely, the absence of pain does not preclude an ulcer diagnosis especially in the elderly who may present with a "silent" ulcer complication. The reasons for this are unclear, but may relate to differences in the way the elderly perceive pain or the analgesic effect of NSAIDs.

Dyspepsia in itself is of little clinical value when assessing subsets of patients who are most likely to have an ulcer. Patients taking NSAIDs often report dyspepsia, but dyspeptic symptoms do not directly correlate with an ulcer. Individuals with dyspeptic symptoms may have either uninvestigated (no upper endoscopy) or investigated (underwent upper endoscopy) dyspepsia. If an ulcer is not confirmed in a patient with ulcer-like symptoms at the time of endoscopy, the disorder is referred to as *nonulcer dyspepsia*.[9] Ulcer-like symptoms may occur in the absence of peptic ulceration in association with *H. pylori* gastritis or duodenitis. There is no one sign or symptom that differentiates between *H. pylori*–positive and NSAID-induced ulcer.

DIAGNOSIS

Routine laboratory tests are not helpful in establishing the diagnosis of PUD (see Table 40–5).[1]

TABLE 40-5	Clinical Presentation of Peptic Ulcer Disease

General
- Mild epigastric pain or acute life-threatening upper gastrointestinal complications

Symptoms
- Abdominal pain that is often epigastric and described as burning but may present as vague discomfort, abdominal fullness, or cramping
- A typical nocturnal pain that awakens the patient from sleep (especially between 12 AM and 3 AM)
- The severity of ulcer pain varies from patient to patient and may be seasonal, occurring more frequently in the spring or fall; episodes of discomfort usually occur in clusters, lasting up to a few weeks and followed by a pain-free period or remission lasting from weeks to years
- Changes in the character of the pain may suggest the presence of complications
- Heartburn, belching, and bloating often accompany the pain
- Nausea, vomiting, and anorexia are more common for patients with gastric ulcer than with duodenal ulcer but may also be signs of an ulcer-related complication

Signs
- Weight loss associated with nausea, vomiting, and anorexia
- Complications including ulcer bleeding, perforation, penetration, or obstruction

Laboratory tests
- Gastric acid secretory studies
- The hematocrit and hemoglobin are low with bleeding, and stool hemoccult tests are positive.
- Tests for *Helicobacter pylori* (see Table 40–6).

Diagnostic tests
- Fiberoptic upper endoscopy (esophagogastroduodenoscopy) detects more than 90% of peptic ulcers and permits direct inspection, biopsy, visualization of superficial erosions, and sites of active bleeding.
- Upper gastrointestinal radiography with barium has been replaced with upper endoscopy as the diagnostic procedure of choice for suspected peptic ulcer.

TESTS FOR *HELICOBACTER PYLORI*

The diagnosis of *H. pylori* infection can be made using endoscopic or nonendoscopic tests (Table 40–6).[2,5,24] The tests that require upper endoscopy are invasive, more expensive, and usually require a mucosal biopsy for histology, culture, or detection of urease activity. At least three tissue samples are taken from specific areas of the stomach, as patchy distribution of *H. pylori* infection can lead to false-negative results. Because certain medications may decrease the sensitivity of rapid urease test, antibiotics and bismuth salts should be withheld for 4 weeks and proton pump inhibitors (PPIs) for 1 to 2 weeks prior to endoscopic testing.[2,5] If the patient has been taking these medications, then a gastric biopsy for histology should be performed.[5]

Two types of nonendoscopic tests are available: tests that identify active infection and tests that detect antibodies (see Table 40–6). Antibody tests do not differentiate between active infection and previously eradicated *H. pylori*. The nonendoscopic tests include the urea breath test (UBT), serologic antibody detection tests, and the fecal antigen test. These tests are less invasive, more convenient, and less expensive than the endoscopic tests.[2,5,24]

The UBT is the most accurate noninvasive test and is based on *H. pylori* urease activity.[5] The ^{13}carbon (nonradioactive isotope) and ^{14}carbon (radioactive isotope) tests require that the patient ingest radiolabeled urea, which is then hydrolyzed by *H. pylori* (if present in the stomach) to ammonia and radiolabeled bicarbonate. The radiolabeled bicarbonate is absorbed in the blood and excreted in the breath. A mass spectrometer is used to detect ^{13}Carbon whereas ^{14}Carbon is measured using a scintillation counter. The fecal antigen test is less expensive and easier to perform than the UBT, and may

TABLE 40-6 Tests for Detection of Helicobacter pylori

Test	Description	Comments
Endoscopic tests		
Histology	Microbiologic examination using various stains	Gold standard; >95% sensitive and specific; permits classification of gastritis; results are not immediate; not recommended for initial diagnosis; tests for active *H. pylori* infection
Culture	Culture of biopsy	Enables sensitivity testing to determine appropriate treatment or antibiotic resistance; 100% specific; results are not immediate; not recommended for initial diagnosis; used after failure of second-line treatment; tests for active *H. pylori* infection
Biopsy (rapid) urease	*H. pylori* urease generates ammonia, which causes a color change	Test of choice at endoscopy; >90% sensitive and specific; easily performed; rapid results (usually within 24 hours); tests for active *H. pylori* infection
Polymerase chain reaction	*H. pylori* DNA detected gastric tissue	Test is highly specific and sensitive; high rate of false positives and false negatives; positive DNA does not directly equate top presence of the organism; considered a research technique
Nonendoscopic tests		
Antibody detection (laboratory based)	Detects antibodies to *H. pylori* in serum using laboratory-based enzyme-linked immunosorbent assay (ELISA) tests and latex agglutination techniques	Quantitative; less sensitive and specific than endoscopic tests; more accurate than in office; unable to determine if antibody is related to active or cured infection; antibody titers vary markedly among individuals and take 6 months to 1 year to return to the uninfected range; not affected by PPIs or bismuth; antibiotics given for unrelated indications may cure the infection, but antibody test will remain positive
Antibody detection (can be performed in office or near patient)	Detects IgG antibodies to *H. pylori* in whole blood or finger stick	Qualitative; quick (within 15 minutes); unable to determine if antibody is related to active or cured infection; most patients remain seropositive for at least 6 months to 1 year after *H. pylori* eradication; not affected by PPIs, bismuth, or antibiotics
Urea breath test	*H. pylori* urease breaks down ingested labeled C-urea, patient exhales labeled CO_2	Tests for active *H. pylori* infection; 95% sensitive and specific; results take about 2 days; antibiotics, bismuth, PPIs, and H_2RAs may cause false-negative results; withhold PPIs or H_2RAs (1–2 weeks) and bismuth or antibiotics (4 weeks) prior to testing; recommended test to confirm posttreatment eradication of *H. pylori*
Fecal antigen	Identifies *H. pylori* antigen in stool by enzyme immunoassay using polyclonal anti-*H. pylori* antibody	Tests for active *H. pylori* infection; sensitivity and specificity comparable to urea breath test when used for initial diagnosis; antibiotics, bismuth, and PPIs may cause false-negative results, but to a lesser extent than with the urea breath test; may be used posttreatment to confirm eradication, but patients may have a reluctance to obtain stool samples

H_2RA, H_2-receptor antagonist; PPI, proton pump inhibitor.
Data from references 2, 5, and 25.

be useful in children. Although comparable to the UBT in the initial detection of *H. pylori*, the fecal antigen test is less accurate when used to confirm *H. pylori* eradication posttreatment and is considered an alternative to the UBT.

Serologic tests are a cost-effective alternative for the initial diagnosis of *H. pylori* infection in the untreated patient.[2,5] Antibodies to *H. pylori* usually develop about 3 weeks after infection and remain present after successful eradication.[5] Therefore, serology should not be used to confirm *H. pylori* eradication.[2,5] Office-based tests are less expensive, widely available and provide rapid results, but the results are less accurate and more variable than the laboratory-based tests. Salivary and urine antibody tests are under investigation.[2]

Testing for *H. pylori* is only recommended if eradication is planned. Serologic antibody testing is a reasonable choice if endoscopy is not planned. The diagnostic accuracy of *H. pylori* tests for patients with an active bleeding ulcer has been questioned because of the potential for false-negative results. However, endoscopic biopsy-based tests such as the rapid urease test have a high degree of specificity in these patients (see Peptic Ulcer-Related Bleeding).[5]

Confirmation of eradication is indicated posttreatment of active ulcers, previous ulcers, MALT lymphoma, endoscopic resection of gastric cancer, and uninvestigated dyspepsia, but routine testing for all patients is neither cost-effective nor practical.[5] The decision to test posttreatment should be patient specific and take into consideration the patient's diagnosis, age, and ulcer history. The UBT is the preferred nonendoscopic test to confirm *H. pylori* eradication but must be delayed at least 4 weeks after the completion of treatment to avoid confusing bacterial suppression with eradication. The term *eradication* or *cure* is used when posttreatment tests conducted 4 weeks after the end of treatment do not detect the organism. Quantitative antibody tests are impractical for posttreatment as antibody titers remain elevated for long periods of time. A negative posttreatment antibody test, however, is considered reliable.

IMAGING AND ENDOSCOPY

The diagnosis of PUD depends on visualizing the ulcer crater either by upper GI radiography or upper endoscopy (see Table 40–5).[1] In the past, radiography was the initial diagnostic procedure of choice because of its lower cost, greater availability, and greater safety. Today, upper endoscopy has replaced radiography because it provides a more accurate diagnosis and permits direct visualization of the ulcer.

CLINICAL COURSE AND PROGNOSIS

The natural history of PUD is characterized by periods of exacerbations and remissions.[1] Ulcer pain is usually recognizable and episodic, but symptoms are variable, especially in older adults and for patients taking NSAIDs. Antiulcer medications, including the histamine-2 receptor antagonists (H_2RAs), PPIs, and sucralfate, relieve symptoms, accelerate ulcer healing, and reduce the risk of ulcer recurrence, but they do not cure the disease. Both duodenal and gastric ulcers recur unless the underlying cause (*H. pylori* or NSAID) is removed. Successful *H. pylori* eradication markedly decreases ulcer recurrence and complications. Prophylactic cotherapy or a COX-2 inhibitor decreases the risk of upper GI events for patients who are taking NSAIDs. GI bleeding, perforation, or obstruction remain troublesome complications of chronic PUD. Mortality for patients with gastric ulcer is slightly higher than in duodenal ulcer and the general population. The development of gastric cancer in *H. pylori*–infected individuals is a slow process that occurs over 20 to 40 years and is associated with a lifetime risk of less than 1%.[2,8]

TREATMENT

■ DESIRED OUTCOME

The treatment of chronic PUD varies depending on the etiology of the ulcer (*H. pylori* or NSAID), whether the ulcer is initial or recurrent, and whether complications have occurred (Fig. 40–5). Overall treatment is aimed at relieving ulcer pain, healing the ulcer, preventing ulcer recurrence, and reducing ulcer-related complications. The goal of therapy for *H. pylori*–positive patients with an active ulcer, a previously documented ulcer, or a history of an ulcer-related complication, is to eradicate *H. pylori*, heal the ulcer, and cure the disease. Successful eradication heals ulcers and reduces the risk of recurrence for most patients. The goal of therapy for a patient with a NSAID-induced ulcer is to heal the ulcer as rapidly as possible. Patients who are at high risk of developing NSAID ulcers should receive prophylactic cotherapy or be switched to a selective COX-2 inhibitor NSAID (if available) to reduce ulcer risk and related complications. When possible, the most cost-effective drug regimen should be used.

■ GENERAL APPROACH TO TREATMENT

The eradication of *H. pylori* infection with antimicrobials such as clarithromycin, metronidazole, amoxicillin, bismuth salts, and antisecretory drugs (PPIs or H$_2$RAs) relieve ulcer symptoms, heal the ulcer, and eradicate *H. pylori* infection. PPIs are preferred to H$_2$RAs or sucralfate for healing *H. pylori*–negative NSAID-induced ulcers because they accelerate ulcer healing and provide more effective relief of symptoms. Treatment with a PPI should be extended to 8 to 12 weeks if the NSAID must be continued. A PPI-based *H. pylori* eradication regimen is recommended when the patient with an active ulcer is taking an NSAID and is *H. pylori*–positive. Prophylactic cotherapy with either a PPI or misoprostol decreases ulcer risk and upper GI complications for patients taking nonselective NSAIDs. Selective COX-2 inhibitor NSAIDs (if available) may be used as an alternative to a nonselective NSAID, but their beneficial GI effect when taken with low-dose aspirin is negated and their association with adverse cardiovascular effects reduce their usefulness.

Dietary modifications are important for patients who are unable to tolerate certain foods and beverages. Lifestyle modifications such as

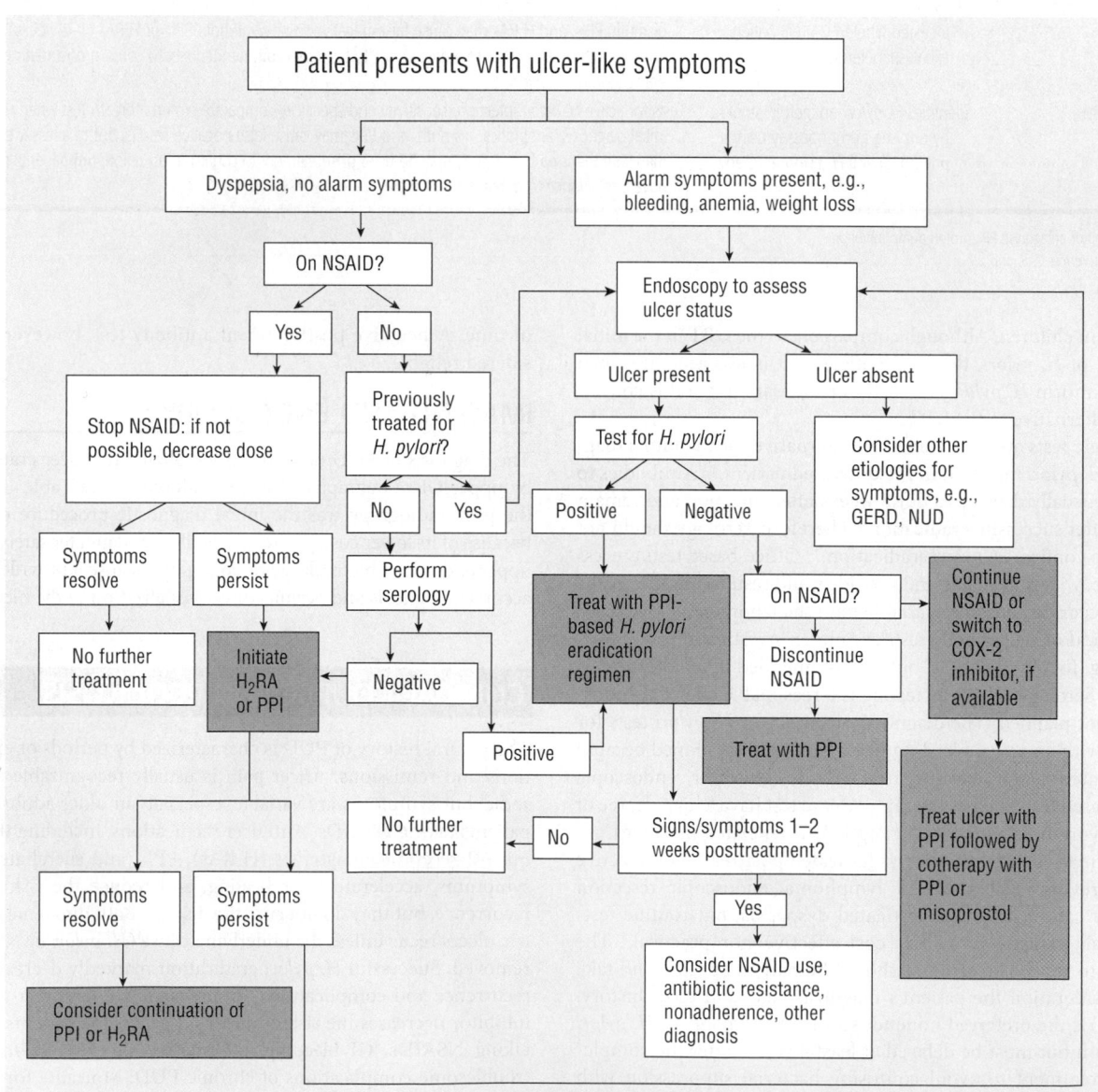

FIGURE 40-5. Algorithm. Guidelines for the evaluation and management of a patient who presents with dyspeptic or ulcer-like symptoms. (COX-2, cyclooxygenase-2; GERD, gastroesophageal reflux disease; *H. pylori, Helicobacter pylori*; H$_2$RA, H$_2$-receptor antagonist; PPI, proton pump inhibitor; NSAID, nonsteroidal antiinflammatory drug; NUD, nonulcer dyspepsia.)

reducing stress and stopping cigarette smoking is encouraged. Surgery may be necessary for patients with ulcer-related complications.

■ NONPHARMACOLOGIC THERAPY

❶ Patients with PUD should eliminate or reduce psychological stress, cigarette smoking, and the use of NSAIDs (including aspirin). Although there is no "antiulcer diet," the patient should avoid foods and beverages (e.g., spicy foods, caffeine, and alcohol) that cause dyspepsia or that exacerbate ulcer symptoms. If possible, alternative agents such as acetaminophen or nonacetylated salicylate (e.g., salsalate) should be used for relief of pain. Elective surgery for PUD is rarely performed today because of highly effective medical management. A subset of patients, however, may require emergency surgery for bleeding, perforation, or obstruction. In the past, surgical procedures were performed for medical treatment failures and included vagotomy with pyloroplasty or vagotomy with antrectomy.[23] Vagotomy (truncal, selective, or parietal cell) inhibits vagal stimulation of gastric acid. A truncal or selective vagotomy frequently results in postoperative gastric dysfunction and requires a pyloroplasty or antrectomy to facilitate gastric drainage. When an antrectomy is performed, the remaining stomach is anastomosed with the duodenum (Billroth I) or with the jejunum (Billroth II). A vagotomy is unnecessary when an antrectomy is performed for gastric ulcer. Postoperative consequences include postvagotomy diarrhea, dumping syndrome, anemia, and recurrent ulceration.

■ PHARMACOLOGIC THERAPY

Recommendations

❷ Table 40–7 presents guidelines for the eradication of infection in H. pylori–positive individuals. Table 40–8 lists regimens used to eradicate H. pylori infection.

❸ First-line therapy is usually initiated with a PPI-based three-drug regimen for 10 to 14 days. If a second course of treatment is required, the PPI-based three-drug regimen should contain different antibiotics or a four-drug regimen with a bismuth salt, metronidazole, tetracycline, and a PPI should be used.

TABLE 40-7	Guidelines for the Eradication of *Helicobacter pylori* Infection

Indications for treatment of *H. pylori* infection
- Established indications for the treatment of *H. pylori* include gastric or duodenal ulcer, mucosa-associated lymphoid tissue (MALT) lymphoma, after endoscopic resection of gastric cancer, and uninvestigated dyspepsia
- Controversial indications for the treatment of *H. pylori* infection include nonulcer dyspepsia, gastroesophageal reflux disease, individuals taking nonsteroidal antiinflammatory drugs (NSAIDs), individuals at high risk for gastric cancer, and unexplained iron deficiency anemia.

Initial treatment of *H. pylori* infection
- Use only those eradication regimens that are of proven effectiveness in the United States
- In the United States, first-line treatment should include a proton pump inhibitor (PPI), clarithromycin, and either amoxicillin or metronidazole (PPI-based triple therapy) for 10–14 days
- The PPI-based triple therapy amoxicillin-containing regimen is preferred initially because bacterial resistance to amoxicillin is almost absent, it has fewer adverse effects, and it leaves metronidazole as a backup agent for second-line therapy
- In penicillin allergic patients, metronidazole should be substituted for amoxicillin in the PPI- based triple therapy regimen and yields similar results when combined with clarithromycin
- An alternate initial strategy includes a PPI or H_2RA, bismuth salt, tetracycline, and metronidazole (bismuth-based quadruple therapy) for 10–14 days.
- Sequential therapy consisting of a PPI and amoxicillin for 5 days followed by a PPI, clarithromycin, and metronidazole for 5 days is an alternative to PPI-based triple therapy or PPI-based quadruple therapy, but requires further validation before it can be recommended as first-line therapy in the United States.

Eradication of *H. pylori* after initial treatment failure
- Avoid antibiotics that have been used in previous eradication regimens.
- Bismuth-based quadruple therapy with a bismuth salt, tetracycline, metronidazole, and a PPI or H_2RA for 10–14 days is an acceptable treatment regimen for persistent *H. pylori* infections.
- PPI-based triple therapy with levofloxacin and amoxicillin for 10 days may be more effective and better tolerated than PPI-based quadruple therapy with a bismuth salt, tetracycline, and metronidazole, but it requires further validation in the United States.

Data from references 5, 25 to 29.

TABLE 40-8	Drug Regimens Used to Eradicate *Helicobacter pylori*		
Drug #1	**Drug #2**	**Drug #3**	**Drug #4**
Proton pump inhibitor–based triple therapy[a]			
PPI once or twice daily[b]	Clarithromycin 500 mg twice daily	Amoxicillin 1 g twice daily *or* metronidazole 500 mg twice daily	
Bismuth-based quadruple therapy[a]			
PPI or H_2RA once or twice daily[b,c]	Bismuth subsalicylate[d] 525 mg 4 times daily	Metronidazole 250–500 mg 4 times daily	Tetracycline 500 mg 4 times daily
Sequential therapy[e]			
PPI once or twice daily on days 1–10[b]	Amoxicillin 1 g twice daily on days 1–5	Metronidazole 250–500 mg twice daily on days 6–10	Clarithromycin 250–500 mg twice daily on days 6–10
Second-line (salvage) therapy for persistent infections			
PPI or H_2RA once or twice daily[b,c]	Bismuth subsalicylate[d] 525 mg 4 times daily	Metronidazole 250–500 mg 4 times daily	Tetracycline 500 mg 4 times daily
PPI once or twice daily[b,f]	Amoxicillin 1 g twice daily	Levofloxacin 250 mg twice daily	

H_2RA, H_2-receptor antagonist; PPI, proton pump inhibitor.

[a]Although treatment is minimally effective if used for 7 days, 10–14 days is recommended. The antisecretory drug may be continued beyond antimicrobial treatment for patients with a history of a complicated ulcer, e.g., bleeding, or in heavy smokers.

[b]Standard PPI peptic ulcer healing dosages given once or twice daily (see Table 40–9).

[c]Standard H_2RA peptic ulcer healing dosages may be used in place of a PPI (see Table 40–9).

[d]Bismuth subcitrate potassium (biskalcitrate) 140 mg, as the bismuth salt, is contained in a prepackaged capsule (Pylera), along with metronidazole 125 mg and tetracycline 125 mg; three capsules are taken with each meal and at bedtime; a standard PPI dosage is added to the regimen and taken twice daily. All medications are taken for 10 days.

[e]Requires validation as first-line therapy in the United States.

[f]Requires validation as rescue therapy in the United States.

Data from references 5, 25 to 29.

TABLE 40-9 Oral Drug Regimens Used to Heal Peptic Ulcers and Maintain Ulcer Healing

Generic Name	Prescription Brand Name	Duodenal or Gastric Ulcer Healing (mg/dose)	Maintenance of Ulcer Healing (mg/dose)
Proton pump inhibitors			
Omeprazole	Prilosec, various	20–40 daily	20–40 daily
Omeprazole sodium bicarbonate	Zegerid	20–40 daily	20–40 daily
Lansoprazole	Prevacid, various	15–30 daily	15–30 daily
Rabeprazole	Aciphex	20 daily	20 daily
Pantoprazole	Pantoprazole, various	40 daily	40 daily
Esomeprazole	Nexium	20–40 daily	20–40 daily
Dexlansoprazole	Dexilant	30–60 daily	30 daily
H_2-receptor antagonists			
Cimetidine	Tagamet, various	300 four times daily 400 twice daily 800 at bedtime	400–800 at bedtime
Famotidine	Pepcid, various	20 twice daily 40 at bedtime	20–40 at bedtime
Nizatidine	Axid, various	150 twice daily 300 at bedtime	150–300 at bedtime
Ranitidine	Zantac, various	150 twice daily 300 at bedtime	150–300 at bedtime
Promote mucosal defense			
Sucralfate	Carafate, various	1 g 4 times daily 2 g twice daily	1–2 g twice daily 1 g 4 times daily

Patients with NSAID-induced ulcers should be tested to determine their *H. pylori* status. If *H. pylori*–positive, treatment should be initiated with a PPI-based three-drug regimen. If *H. pylori*–negative, the NSAID should be discontinued, and the patient treated with either a PPI, H_2RA, or sucralfate (see Table 40–9). If the NSAID is continued, treatment should be initiated with a PPI (if *H. pylori* negative) or with a PPI-based three-drug regimen (if *H. pylori* positive). Cotherapy with a PPI or misoprostol or switching to a selective COX-2 inhibitor (if available) is recommended for patients at risk of developing an ulcer-related complication (see Table 40–10).

Maintenance therapy with a PPI or H_2RA should be limited to high-risk patients with ulcer complications, patients who fail eradication, and those with *H. pylori*–negative ulcers. Treatment failure is associated with poor medication adherence, antimicrobial resistance, NSAID use, cigarette smoking, acid hypersecretion, or tolerance to the antisecretory effects of an H_2RA.

Treatment of *Helicobacter Pylori*–Positive Ulcers

This chapter focuses on the eradication of *H. pylori* in adults.[25–29] A discussion of the treatment of *H. pylori* infection in children is found elsewhere.[30,31]

The treatment of *H. pylori*–positive PUD should be effective, well tolerated, easy to adhere to, and cost-effective. Historically, none of these factors have been addressed in a systematic way making it difficult to identify the best evidence-based treatment regimens.[1] Successful eradication depends on the drug regimen, resistance to the antibiotics used, duration of therapy, medication adherence, and genetic polymorphism.[25–29] *H. pylori* regimens should have eradication (cure) rates of at least 80% based on intention-to-treat analysis or at least 90% based on per-protocol analysis, and they should minimize the potential for antimicrobial resistance.[1,25,29] Not one antibiotic, bismuth salt, or antiulcer drug achieves this goal, but clarithromycin is the single most effective antibiotic. Two-drug regimens that combine a PPI and either amoxicillin or clarithromycin have yielded marginal and variable eradication rates in the United States and are not recommended.[1,5] In addition, the use of only one antibiotic is associated with a higher rate of antimicrobial resistance.

Drug regimens (see Table 40–8) that combine an antisecretory drug with two antibiotics (triple therapy) or with two antibiotics and a bismuth salt (quadruple therapy) usually increase eradication rates to acceptable levels and reduce the risk of antimicrobial resistance.[5,25–29] When selecting an initial eradication regimen, an antibiotic combination should be used that permits second-line treatment (if necessary) with different antibiotics. The antibiotics that have been most extensively studied and found to be effective in various combinations include clarithromycin, amoxicillin, metronidazole, and tetracycline.[1] Because of insufficient data, ampicillin should not be substituted for amoxicillin, doxycycline should not be substituted for tetracycline,

TABLE 40-10 Guidelines for Reducing Gastrointestinal Risk for Patients Receiving Chronic NSAID Therapy

Gastrointestinal risk factors (see Table 40–4)

Cardiovascular Risk	No or Low GI Risk (No risk factors) Age < 65 years)	Moderate GI Risk (1–2 risk factors) Age ≥ 65 years High-dose NSAIDs Concomitant use of aspirin, corticosteroids, or anticoagulants	High GI Risk (>2 risk factors or prior ulcer or ulcer-related complication) Age ≥ 65 years Concomitant use of aspirin corticosteroids, or anticoagulants Dual antiplatelet therapy
No or low CV risk (patient does not require low-dose aspirin)	Nonselective NSAID or partially selective NSAID (see Table 40–3)	Nonselective NSAID or partially selective NSAID + PPI or misoprostol Selective COX-2 inhibitor NSAID (if available)	Avoid NSAID or selective COX-2 inhibitor, if possible; use alternative therapy Nonselective NSAID or partially selective NSAID + PPI or misoprostol Selective COX-2 inhibitor NSAID (if available) + PPI or misoprostol
High CV risk (patient requires low-dose aspirin, no NSAID)	No prophylaxis required	PPI or misoprostol	PPI or misoprostol
High CV risk (patient requires low-dose aspirin) and NSAID	Naproxen + PPI or misoprostol	Naproxen + PPI or misoprostol	Avoid NSAID or selective COX-2 inhibitor, if at all possible; use alternative therapy If antiinflammatory drug is needed and CV risk is >GI risk, use naproxen and aspirin + PPI or misoprostol If antiinflammatory drug and aspirin are needed and GI risk is >CV, use selective COX-2 inhibitor + PPI or misoprostol

COX-2, cycloxygenase-2 inhibitor; NSAID, nonsteroidal antiinflammatory drug; PPI, proton pump inhibitor; CV, cardiovascular; GI, gastrointestinal.
Data from references 12 to 15, 18, 19, and 59.

and azithromycin or erythromycin should not be substituted for clarithromycin. Antisecretory drugs enhance antibiotic activity and stability by increasing intragastric pH and by decreasing intragastric volume thereby enhancing the topical antibiotic concentration.[27]

Proton Pump Inhibitor–Based Three-Drug Regimens

PPI-based triple therapy (see Table 40–8) is the initial treatment of choice for eradicating *H. pylori* (see Table 40–7).[5,25–29] The regimens that combine either clarithromycin and amoxicillin or clarithromycin and metronidazole are more effective than the amoxicillin-metronidazole regimen. In most cases, increasing the antibiotic dosage does not improve eradication rates. The clarithromycin-amoxicillin regimen is preferred initially (see Table 40–7), but metronidazole should be substituted for amoxicillin for penicillin-allergic patients unless alcohol is consumed.[5,25–27] Unfortunately, eradication rates for PPI-based triple therapy have declined substantially in recent years in North America and Europe due primarily to an increase in clarithromycin-resistant *H. pylori* strains (see the section Factors that Contribute to Unsuccessful Eradication).[5,25–27] Other antibiotics and antibiotic combinations have been investigated, but these regimens should not be used as initial treatment in the United States until well-designed trials confirm their effectiveness.[5,27]

The recommended duration of therapy in the United States is 10 to 14 days, but the 14-day regimen is preferred in light of the decreasing eradication rate with the PPI-based triple therapy regimens containing clarithomycin.[5] Although a 7-day course has been approved by the FDA and is used in Europe, the longer treatment periods favor higher eradication rates and are less likely to be associated with antimicrobial resistance.[5,25–27]

CLINICAL CONTROVERSY

Some clinicians favor an initial 7-day *H. pylori* regimen even though clinical guidelines suggest a longer treatment course. These clinicians believe that the shorter treatment period enhances the compliance of a complicated drug regimen. Others adhere to clinical guidelines and recommend a 10- or 14-day treatment period that favors higher eradication rates in the compliant patient and is less likely to contribute to antimicrobial resistance.

The PPI is an integral part of the three-drug regimen and should be taken 30 to 60 minutes before a meal along with the two antibiotics (see Table 40–8).[5,32] Prolonged PPI treatment beyond 2 weeks after eradication is usually not necessary for ulcer healing. A single daily dose of a PPI may be less effective than a twice daily dose.[33] Substitution of one PPI for another is acceptable and does not enhance or diminish *H. pylori* eradication.[32,34] An H$_2$RA should not be substituted for a PPI, as H$_2$RA is associated with lower eradication rates.[35,36] Pretreatment with a PPI does not influence *H. pylori* eradication.[37]

Bismuth-Based Four-Drug Regimens

Bismuth-based quadruple therapy (see Table 40–8) is recommended as an alternative first-line eradication therapy (see Table 40–7) for those allergic to penicillin.[5,25–29] Although this regimen may be used initially, it is often reserved as a second-line therapy after treatment failure with the PPI-based clarithromycin-amoxicillin regimen (see the section Eradication of *H. Pylori* After Initial Treatment Failure). Eradication rates for bismuth-based quadruple therapy (bismuth salicylate, metronidazole, tetracycline, and either a PPI or H$_2$RA) are similar to those achieved with PPI-based triple therapy.[5,27,38]

Eradication rates are comparable when bismuth subcitrate potassium (biskalcitrate) is substituted for bismuth subsalicylate (see Table 40–8).[39] Substitution of amoxicillin for tetracycline lowers the eradication rate and is usually not recommended.[38] Substitution of clarithromycin 250 to 500 mg four times a day for tetracycline yields similar results but increases adverse effects. Bismuth salts have a topical antimicrobial effect.[1] The antisecretory drug hastens ulcer healing and relives pain in patients with an active ulcer. All medications except the PPI should be taken with meals and at bedtime.

The original bismuth-based regimens contained an H$_2$RA in place of a PPI, but a recent metaanalysis indicated that quadruple therapy with a PPI provides greater efficacy and permits a shorter treatment duration (7 days) when compared with the H$_2$RA-based regimens (10 to 14 days).[40] However. a 10- to 14-day duration is recommended in the United States as it generally provides higher eradication rates.[5] When treating an active ulcer, the antisecretory drug is usually continued for 2 (PPI) to 4 (H$_2$RA) weeks after stopping bismuth and antibiotics.

Bismuth-based quadruple therapy is the treatment of choice when medication costs are of overriding importance. However, major concerns include a 4-time-a-day dosing regimen (see Table 40–8), poor medication adherence, and frequent adverse effects. Although minor adverse effects are more common, the frequency of moderate or severe adverse effects is similar to those reported for the PPI-based triple therapy.[41]

Sequential Therapy Sequential therapy is a new form of eradication therapy whereby the antibiotics are administered in a sequence rather than all together.[5,26,29] The rationale for sequential therapy is to initially treat with antibiotics that rarely promote resistance (e.g., amoxicillin) to reduce the bacterial load and preexisting resistant organisms and then to follow with different antibiotics (e.g., clarithromycin and metronidazole) to kill the remaining organisms.[1] Treatment consists of a PPI and amoxicillin for 5 days followed by a PPI, clarithromycin, and metronidazole for an additional 5 days (see Table 40–8).[5,26,42] Although this regimen has achieved eradication rates that are superior to the PPI-based three-drug regimens containing clarithromycin,[42] the regimen requires a change in medication mid-treatment, which may contribute to nonadherence.[43] The advantages of sequential therapy need to be confirmed in the United States before it can be recommended as a first-line *H. pylori* eradication therapy (see Table 40–7).[5,26,27]

Eradication of *H. Pylori* After Initial Treatment Failure

H. pylori eradication is often more difficult after initial treatment fails and successful eradication after retreatment is extremely variable.[5,44] Treatment failures should be referred to a gastroenterologist for further diagnostic evaluation. Second-line (salvage) treatment should (a) use antibiotics that were not previously used during initial therapy; (b) use antibiotics that are not associated with resistance; (c) use a drug that has a topical effect such as bismuth; and (d) extend the duration of treatment to 14 days.[5,44,45] The most commonly used second-line therapy, after unsuccessful initial treatment with a PPI-amoxicillin-clarithromycin regimen, is a 14-day course of the PPI-based quadruple therapy (see Table 40–8).[5,26,27,45] A levofloxacin-containing regimen (see Table 40–8) may be an alternative second-line eradication regimen and may be better tolerated than PPI-based quadruple therapy (see Table 40–7).[46] Additionally, the levofloxacin regimen may serve as an alternative to PPI-clarithromycin-metronidazole usually recommended in penicillin allergic patients.[47] However, concerns about using fluoroquinolones for *H. pylori* eradication are related to the development of resistance and adverse effects such as tendonitis and hepatoxicity.[26] Other second-line regimens which include rifabutin and furazolidone are discussed elsewhere.[5,25–27]

Factors That Predict *H. Pylori* Eradication Outcomes

Factors that predict *H. pylori* eradication outcomes include antibiotic resistance, poor medication adherence, short duration of therapy, CagA status, high bacterial load, low intragastric pH, and genetic polymorphism.[5,45,48-50] Medication adherence decreases with multiple medications, increased frequency of administration, intolerable adverse effects, and costly drug regimens. One metaanalysis reported that CYP2C19 polymorphism may alter the effect of PPIs on gastric acid secretion thereby influencing eradication outcomes.[49] Tolerability varies with different regimens.[1,5] Common adverse effects include nausea, vomiting, abdominal pain, diarrhea and taste disturbances (metronidazole and clarithromycin). Adverse effects with metronidazole are dose-related (especially when >1 g/day) and include a disulfiram-like reaction with alcohol. Tetracycline may cause photosensitivity and should not be used in children because of possible tooth discoloration. Bismuth salts may cause darkening of the stool and tongue. Antibiotic-associated colitis occurs occasionally. Oral thrush and vaginal candidiasis may also occur.

An important predictor of *H. pylori* eradication is the presence or absence of resistant microorganisms.[5,50-52] United States data from 1993 to 1999 report resistance rates among *H. pylori* strains for metronidazole (37%), clarithromycin (10%), and amoxicillin (1.4%).[51] Data from 1998 to 2002 reveal rates of 25% for metronidazole, 13% for clarithromycin, and 0.9% for amoxicillin.[52] It is possible that the increased rate of clarithomycin resistance partially explains the decrease in efficacy of clarithomycin-containing regimens. The clinical importance of metronidazole resistance remains uncertain, as resistance can be overcome by using higher dosages and combining metronidazole with other antibiotics.[5] Resistance to tetracycline and amoxicillin is uncommon.[5] Resistance to bismuth has not been reported. The role of antibiotic sensitivity testing prior to initiating *H. pylori* treatment has not been established.

Probiotics

Probiotics (e.g., strains of *Lactobacillus* and *Bifidobacterium*) and foodstuffs (e.g., cranberry juice and some milk proteins) with bioactive components have been used proactively to control *H. pylori* colonization in at-risk individuals and, when taken as a supplement to eradication therapy, may have a role in improving *H. pylori* eradication and reducing the adverse effects of PPI-based triple therapy.[53-55] However, the administration of probiotics alone does not eradicate *H. pylori* infection. In the future, the regular intake of probiotics may constitute a low-cost alternative for individuals who are at-risk for *H. pylori* infection and, in combination with antibiotics, augment eradication rates. These preliminary data are encouraging and warrants more research in this area.

Treatment of NSAID-Induced Ulcers

Nonselective NSAIDs should be discontinued (when possible) upon confirmation of an active ulcer. If the NSAID is stopped, most uncomplicated ulcers heal with standard regimens of an H₂RA, PPI, or sucralfate (see Table 40–9).[1,13,29] However, the PPIs are usually preferred because they provide more rapid symptom relief and ulcer healing. If the NSAID is continued despite ulceration, consideration should be given to reducing the NSAID dose, switching to acetaminophen or a nonacetylated salicylate or to using a more selective COX-2 inhibitor (see Table 40–3). The PPIs are the drugs of choice when the NSAID is continued, as potent acid suppression is required to accelerate ulcer healing.[1,13,29] If the ulcer is *H. pylori*–positive, eradication should be initiated with a regimen that contains a PPI.[1,13,29]

Strategies to Reduce the Risk of NSAID Ulcer and GI Complications There are three therapeutic approaches to reducing the risk of NSAID ulcers and related upper GI complications (see Table 40–10). Medical cotherapy with either a PPI or misoprostol decreases ulcer risk and GI complications in high-risk patients.[12-14,16,19,29] The use of a selective COX-2 inhibitor instead of a nonselective NSAID also decreases risk of ulcers and upper GI events.[12-14,16,18,19,29] Unfortunately, these strategies do not completely eliminate ulcers and complications for patients at the "highest risk." When selecting a gastroprotective strategy, the GI benefits be must be balanced against the cardiovascular risks associated with selective COX-2 inhbitor NSAIDs, nonselective NSAIDs, and concomittant antiplatelet therapy.[12-16] Strategies aimed at reducing the topical irritant effects of nonselective NSAIDs, e.g., prodrugs, slow-release formulations, and enteric-coated products, do not prevent ulcers or GI complications.

Misoprostol Cotherapy Misoprostol, 200 mcg orally 4 times per day, reduces the risk of NSAID-induced gastric and duodenal ulcer, and related upper GI complications, but diarrhea and abdominal cramping limit its use.[12,16,56] Because a dosage of 200 mcg 3 times per day is comparable in efficacy to 800 mcg/day, the lower dosage should be considered for patients unable to tolerate the higher dose.[12,16] Reducing the misoprostol dosage to 400 mcg per day or less to minimize diarrhea compromises its gastroprotective effects. A fixed combination of misoprostol 200 mcg and diclofenac (50 mg or 75 mg) may enhance compliance, but the flexibility to individualize drug dosage is lost. A large clinical trial in rheumatoid arthritis patients provided the most compelling evidence that misoprostol reduces the risk of upper GI complications for high-risk patients.[57]

Proton Pump Inhibitor Cotherapy ❹ PPI cotherapy reduces NSAID-related gastric and duodenal ulcer risk and is better tolerated than misoprostol.[12-14,16,56] All PPIs are effective when used in standard dosages (see Table 40–9). Although head-to-head comparative trials are few, there are limited data to indicate that PPIs are superior to standard H₂RA dosages.[12,13,16] When lansoprazole (15 or 30 mg/day) was compared with misoprostol 800 mcg/day or placebo, both dosages of lansoprazole and misoprostol effectively reduced ulcer recurrence, although the PPI was better tolerated.[58] A greater proportion of those in the misoprostol group reported treatment-related adverse events and withdrew early from the study. Results from observational studies and metaanalyses indicate the PPIs reduce the risk of NSAID-related ulcer bleeding.[12,16,19,59]

H₂-Receptor Antagonist Cotherapy Standard H₂RA dosages (e.g., famotidine 40 mg/day) are effective in reducing NSAID-related duodenal ulcer but not gastric ulcer (the most frequent type of ulcer associated with NSAIDs).[12,13,16] Higher dosages (e.g., famotidine 40 mg twice daily, ranitidine 300 mg twice daily) may reduce the risk of gastric and duodenal ulcer, but studies comparing double dosages with PPIs or misoprostol are not available.[12,13] One study suggests that famotidine 20 mg twice daily may be an alternative to PPIs for patients taking low cardioprotective dosages of aspirin, but additional studies are required to confirm these findings.[60] The H₂RAs are not recommended as prophylactic cotherapy because it is likely that they are not as effective as the PPIs or misoprostol in preventing NSAID-induced gastric ulcer and related GI complications.[16] An H₂RA, however, may be used to relieve NSAID-related dyspepsia.

Cyclooxygenase-2 Inhibitors Two large outcome trials have compared celecoxib[61] and rofecoxib[62] to nonselective NSAIDs. Patients in the Celecoxib Long-term Arthritis Safety Study (CLASS) trial who were taking celecoxib and required cardioprotection (antiplatelet effects of aspirin) were permitted to take low-dose aspirin.[61] Although a 6-month analysis found a nonsignficant reduction in ulcer complications with celecoxib when compared with ibuprofen and diclofenac, results after 1 year found no difference between the groups. Today, celecoxib is not considered a selective COX-2 inhibitor (Table 40–3) by the FDA as it contains the same GI warnings as the nonselctive and patially selective NSAIDs.[63] A post hoc analysis confirmed that any gastroprotective benefits of celecoxib were negated in aspirin users. Similar effects have been observed with rofecoxib.

The Vioxx Gastrointestinal Outcomes Research (VIGOR) trial excluded aspirin users and found that ulcers and ulcer-related complications were significantly reduced with rofecoxib when compared with naproxen.[62] However, there was an increased number of nonfatal myocardial infarctions observed in the rofecoxib group compared with those taking naproxen. It was initially suggested that the lack of antiplatelet effects from rofecoxib, in contrast to the platelet inhibition associated with naproxen, was responsible for the increased thrombotic events observed in the rofecoxib group. Rofecoxib was later withdrawn from the market following an interim analysis of a study to prevent colorectal adenomas that revealed an increased risk of myocardial infarction and thrombotic stoke with rofecoxib when compared with placebo.[64] Subsequently, valdecoxib was withdrawn from the market amid concerns about cardiovascular risk.

Cardiovascular safety was also evaluated in the CLASS trial, but serious cardiovascular thromboembolic events were no different between celecoxib and the comparative nonselective NSAIDs. In contrast, the results of a metaanalysis of randomized trials of COX-2 inhbitor NSAIDs reported a dose-dependent increase in cardiovascular events with all COX-2 inhibitor NSAIDs, including celecoxib.[65] Increased cardiovascular risk appears to be dependent on a number of factors including increased COX-2 selectivity, higher dosages, and a longer duration of treatment.[12,18,19] Thus, the lowest effective celecoxib dose should be used for the shortest duration of time. Dyspepsia and abdominal pain, fluid retention, hypertension, and renal toxicity are associated with the COX-2 inhibitors and nonselective NSAIDs.[1]

COX-2 Inhibitor Versus NSAID plus PPI ⑤ There are limited data that suggest that for high-risk, H. pylori–negative patients, a COX-2 inhibitor NSAID may be as beneficial as a nonselective NSAID plus a PPI in reducing NSAID-related ulcer complications.[12,18,19] However, neither the COX-2 inhibitor NSAID nor the NSAID plus a PPI will eliminate upper GI events for these patients. Combining a COX-2 inhibitor NSAID with a PPI may be considered for very high-risk patients, but this regimen is likely to be of modest benefit.[12,18]

Gastrointestinal and Cardiovascular Safety Issues

There is no difference in cardiovascular risk between the selective COX-2 inhitor NSAIDs and the nonselective or partially selective NSAIDs, with the exception of naproxen[12,18,65] Thus, individual patient risk factors for NSAID-related GI bleeding and cardiovascular events must be weighed when determining treatment (see Table 40–10). Naproxen is preferred to nonnaproxen NSAIDs and COX-2 inhbitors because of its comparative cardiovascular safety and not because of its GI safety profile. There is insufficient evidence regarding the preferred NSAID for patients also taking low-dose aspirin.[14] Clopidogrel should not be substituted for low-dose aspirin in order to reduce recurrent GI bleeding as it is inferior to a PPI plus low-dose aspirin.[13] Despite limited evidence to suggest an interaction via the hepatic cytochrome P450 (CYP450) pathway, combining a PPI and clopidogrel with or without low-dose aspirin

results in less GI bleeding.[13] Ongoing studies for patients with cardiovascular disease should provide the necessary information to help resolve these issues. The lowest possible daily dose of a COX-2 inhibitor should be used as the cardiovascular risk may be dose dependent. However, no studies, to date, have evaluated the safety of low-dose COX-2 inhibitor NSAIDs for patients with or at risk for cardiovascular disease. In the future, there will be new formulations and classes of NSAIDs and COX-2 inhibitors with an improved GI and cardiovascular safety profile.[66] Until then patients who take NSAIDs or COX-2 inhibitors should be counseled about the signs and symptoms of upper GI bleeding and major cardiovascular events and what they should do if they occur.

Treatment of non-*H. Pylori*, non-NSAID Ulcers

Very few individuals have non-*H. pylori*, non-NSAID (idiopathic) ulcers.[29,67,68] Patients should be double-checked to verify that they are *H. pylori* negative and that they are not taking ulcerogenic medications. Possible explanations for *non-H.pylori*, non-NSAID ulcers include gastric hypersecretion, gastric outlet obstruction, genetic predisposition, concomitant diseases (see Table 40–2), and heavy tobacco use. Treatment should be initiated with conventional ulcer healing therapy (see Table 40–9). Although standard H_2RA or sucralfate dosage regimens heal the majority of gastric and duodenal ulcers in 6 to 8 weeks, PPIs provide comparable ulcer healing rates in 4 weeks.[32] A higher daily dose or a longer treatment duration is sometimes needed to heal larger gastric ulcers. Antacids are not used as single agents to heal ulcers because of the high volume and frequent doses required. When conventional antiulcer therapy is discontinued after ulcer healing, most patients develop a recurrent ulcer within 1 year.[32] Maintenance therapy may be required to prevent ulcer recurrence.

Long-Term Maintenance of Ulcer Healing

Continuous antiulcer therapy is aimed at the long-term maintenance of ulcer healing and the prevention of ulcer-related complications. Because *H. pylori* eradication dramatically decreases ulcer recurrence, continuous maintenance therapy is primarily used to treat high-risk patients who failed *H. pylori* eradication, have a history of ulcer-related complications, have frequent recurrences of *H. pylori*–negative ulcers, and are heavy smokers or NSAID users. For most patients, standard maintenance dosages (see Table 40–9) are effective.[32]

Treatment of Refractory Ulcers

Ulcers are considered refractory to therapy when symptoms, ulcers, or both persist beyond 8 to 12 weeks despite conventional treatment or when several courses of *H. pylori* eradication fail.[1,45] Poor patient compliance, antimicrobial resistance, cigarette smoking, NSAID use, gastric acid hypersecretion, or tolerance to the antisecretory effects of an H_2RA (see the section Antiulcer Agents) may contribute to refractory PUD. Patients with refractory ulcers should undergo upper endoscopy to confirm a nonhealing ulcer, exclude malignancy, and assess *H. pylori* status. *H. pylori*–positive patients should receive eradication therapy (see the secton Treatment of *Helicobacter pylori*–Associated Ulcers). In *H. pylori*–negative patients, higher PPI dosages (e.g., omeprazole 40 mg/day) heal the majority of ulcers. Continuous treatment with a PPI is often necessary to maintain healing, as refractory ulcers recur when therapy is discontinued or the dose is reduced. Switching from one PPI to another is not beneficial. Patients with refractory gastric ulcer may require surgery because of the possibility of malignancy.

Antiulcer Agents

Proton Pump Inhibitors The PPIs (omeprazole, esomeprazole, lansoprazole, dexlansoprazole, rabeprazole, and pantoprazole) dose-dependently inhibit basal and stimulated gastric acid secretion.[32] When PPI therapy is initiated, the degree of acid suppression increases over the first 3 to 4 days of therapy, as more proton pumps are inhibited.[32] Because PPIs inhibit only those proton pumps that are actively secreting acid, they are most effective when taken 30 to 60 minutes before meals.[32] The duration of acid suppression is a function of binding to the H^+/K^+-adenosine triphosphatase (ATPase) enzyme and is longer than their elimination half-lives.[32] Symptomatic acid rebound upon withdrawal of a PPI has been reported in healthy volunteers after 8 weeks of treatment.[1,69]

Various PPI dosage forms and formulations exist and (see Table 40-11) include the delayed-release enteric-coated dosage forms that have pH-sensitive granules contained in gelatin capsules (omeprazole, esomeprazole, prescription and nonprescription lansoprazole, and dexlansoprazole), rapidly disintegrating tablets (lansoprazole), and delayed release enteric-coated tablets (rabeprazole, pantoprazole, and nonprescription omeprazole).[32] The pH-sensitive enteric coating prevents degradation and premature protonation of the drug in stomach acid but dissolves at a higher pH in the duodenum where the drug is absorbed. Dexlansoprazole is formulated with a dual release mechanism that results in inhibition of proton pumps that become activated after initial release of the medication.[70,71] Omeprazole is also available as an immediate release formulation (oral suspension, oral capsule) containing sodium bicarbonate, which raises intragastric pH and protects omeprazole from acid degradation in the stomach thus permitting rapid absorption from the duodenum.[72] Intravenous products available in the United States include pantoprazole and esomeprazole.

Five of the PPIs provide similar rates of ulcer-healing (dexlansoprazole has not been labeled at this time for these indications), maintenance of ulcer healing, and symptom relief when used in recommended dosages (see Table 40-9). When higher dosages are indicated, the daily dose should be divided in order to obtain better 24-hour control of intragastric pH. A dosage reduction is unnecessary for patients with renal impairment or in older adults but should be considered in severe hepatic disease.[32] The short-term adverse effects of the PPIs are similar to those observed with the H_2RAs and include headache, nausea, and abdominal pain.[32] Because the immediate-release formulations contain sodium bicarbonate, they are contraindicated for patients with metabolic alkalosis and hypocalemia.[72] The sodium should also be taken into consideration for patients who are on sodium-restricted diets, e.g., congestive heart failure.

Drug Interactions All PPIs increase intragastric pH and may alter the bioavailability of orally administered drugs, such as ketoconazole (weak bases) and digoxin, or pH-dependent dosage forms.[32,73] This interaction is especially important with atazanavir, a protease inhibitor. Concomitant use with a PPI can significantly reduce the oral bioavailability of atazanavir and potentially lead to therapeutic failure and viral resistance in patients infected with HIV.[74] Omeprazole and esomeprazole selectively inhibit the hepatic CYP2C19 pathway and may decrease the elimination of phenytoin, warfarin, diazepam, and carbamazepine.[32] The PPIs may increase the metabolic clearance and decrease the GI absorption of levothyroxine resulting in increased thyroid-stimulating hormone levels and a corresponding increase in the levothyroxine dose.[75] A review of the FDA database for the years 1997 to 2001 reveals that drug interactions with PPIs are rare and usually do not constitute a major clinical risk.[76]

One of the most perplexing potential PPI drug interactions is with the antiplatelet drug clopidogrel. This interaction is especially important given recent consensus guidelines that recommend the use of a PPI for high-risk patients on antiplatelet therapies to prevent ulcers and related GI bleeding.[13] Clopidogrel, a prodrug, is converted to its active form through CYP2C19. PPIs may attenuate the antiplatelet effect of clopidogrel by inhibiting or competing for this metabolic pathway. FDA safety guidelines recommend that the coadministration of omeprazole, omeprazole/sodium bicarbonate, or esomeprazole with clopidogrel be avoided because they reduce the effectiveness of clopidogrel.[77-79] Details of new studies

---

TABLE 40-11 Proton Pump Inhibitor Formulations and Options for Administration

	Omeprazole	Esomeprazole	Lansoprazole	Pantoprazole	Rabeprazole	Dexlansoprazole
Commercially available oral formulations						
Capsule	X[a]	X	X			X[e]
Tablet	X[b]			X	X	
Oral disintegrating tablet			X			
Packet for oral suspension	X[c]	X[c]				
Extemporaneous oral preparations						
Pellets from capsule in water		X				
Pellets from capsule in applesauce	X		X			X
Pellets from capsule in juice	X	X[d]	X			
Extemporaneous preparation of delayed-release PPI in bicarbonate	X		X	X		
Parenteral formulations						
Intravenous	Not available in the United States	X		X		

X, product is available.

[a]Omeprazole is available as delayed-release enteric-coated pellets in a capsule or as immediate-release capsule that contains 20 or 40 mg of omeprazole with 1100 mg sodium bicarbonate (equivalent to 304 mg of sodium). Because 20 and 40 mg dosages contain the same amount of bicarbonate, two 20 mg capsules should not be substituted for the 40 mg immediate-release omeprazole-bicarbonate capsule.

[b]Omeprazole oral tablets are available as 20 mg delayed-release nonprescription tablets.

[c]Omeprazole oral suspension is available as 20 or 40 mg omeprazole with 1,680 mg sodium bicarbonate (equivalent to 460 mg of soidum). Because 20 and 40 mg dosages contain the same amount of bicarbonate, two 20 mg packets should not be substituted for the 40 mg immediate-release omeprazole-bicarbonate packet.

[d]No published information; based on omeprazole data.

[e]Dexlansoprazole is available as a dual delayed-release formulation in capsules for oral administration. The capsule contains dexlansoprazole in a mixture of two types of enteric-coated granules with different pH-dependent dissolution profiles.

Data from references 32, 70, and 72.

performed by the manufacturer and submitted to the FDA, as well as warnings regarding omeprazole, esomeprazole, and other interacting drugs (e.g., cimetidine) are contained in the clopidogrel package insert.[80] A reduced antiplatelet effect of clopidogrel may also result from genetic polymorphisms of the CYP2C19 pathway leading to decreased biotransformation of the drug to its active form.[81,82] Whether the use of other PPIs such as pantoprazole, lansoprazole, dexlansoprazole, and rebeprazole interact with clopidogrel remains uncertain as the capacity to inhibit CYP2C19 varies among these PPIs.[83,84] While some reports suggest a "class effect" among the different PPIs, other pharmacodynamic studies suggest an interaction with omeprazole and esomeprazole but not with pantoprazole.[83,84] Because of the uncertainty of the effect of the PPI-clopidogrel interaction on clinical outcomes and the extent to which other PPIs may interact with clopidogrel, caution is warranted. Until more compelling data becomes available, patients should have an acceptable indication for a PPI recognizing that risk versus benefit must be weighed on an individual basis. If a PPI is absolutely necessary, the use of omeprazole and esomeprazole should be avoided.

CLINICAL CONTROVERSY

Some clinicians believe that the antiplatelet effect of clopidogrel is attenuated by omeprazole and that there is an increased risk of adverse cardiac events when these medications are taken concomitantly. Strategies to avoid this interaction for patients at risk of NSAID-related GI events include switching omeprazole to another PPI or substituting an H_2RA for the PPI. Others believe that the use of a PPI (if indicated) and clopidogrel is not a safety concern and that it is not necessary to switch omeprazole to another PPI.

Potential Risks and Long-Term Safety Issues Numerous potential risks and safety issues (see Table 40–12) have been associated with the long-term use of PPIs as a consequence of prolonged hypergastrinemia and chronic hypochlorhydria.[32,85-88] In most cases, causality is difficult to ascertain because of the study design, confounding variables, and subject selection. All of the PPIs dose-dependently increase serum gastrin concentrations two- to fourfold as a function of their potent acid-inhibitory effect.[32,85] Fasting gastrin elevations are usually within the normal range and return to baseline within 1 month of discontinuing the drug. In humans, PPIs may lead to enterochromaffin-like (ECL) hyperplasia as a result of the hypergastrinemia, but there is no evidence that these changes result in dysplasia, carcinoid tumors, or gastric adenocarcinoma.[85,86] Although long-term PPI therapy in *H. pylori*–positive individuals is associated with progressive atrophic gastritis, there is insufficient data to link chronic PPI use with gastric cancer in *H. pylori*–positive patients.[85,86] Despite theoretical and in vitro data, there is no evidence to support an association between PPIs and colonic polyps or colorectal cancer.[85,86] Bacterial overgrowth occurs in the stomach as a consequence of hypochlorhydria and may lead to carcinogenic *N*-nitroso compounds in animals but is unlikely to result in significant gastric nitrosation in humans.[85,88]

Chronic PPI therapy may be associated with an increased risk of infection and nutritional deficiences.[85-87] Gastric acid (low stomach pH) plays an important role in the defense against bacterial colonization of the stomach and in nutrient absorption. Acid suppression has been implicated as a risk factor for community acquired pneumonia (CAP) and enteric infections (*Clostridium*

TABLE 40-12	Potential Risks and Safety Issues Associated with the Proton Pump Inhibitors

Gastric cancers or malignancy
    Carcinoid tumors
    Atrophic gastritis
    Adenocarcinoma
Bacterial overgrowth
    Increase in N-nitroso compounds from ingested nitrates (carcinogenic)
    Enteric infections (*Clostridium difficile, Salmonella typhimurium, and Campylobacter jejuni*)
    Community acquired pneumonia
Decreased nutrient absorption:
    Iron
    Calcium
    Cyanocobalamin (vitamin B12)
Osteoporosis and related fractures

Data from references 32, 85 to 88.

difficile, Salmonella, Campylobacter).[86] Three case-controlled studies demonstrate a higher adjusted relative risk of CAP for patients currently using PPIs compared with controls.[89-91] The results of these retrospectively designed studies, however, need to be interpreted cautiously because of the variability in the length of therapy for current PPI users and the inclusion of older (>60 years of age) patients with concomitant comorbidities. A systematic review of the literature has linked PPIs with various enteric infections, but the most convincing data was with *C. difficile*.[92] It is likely that sustained elevations in intragastric pH facilitate the survival of *C. difficile* spores. However, the magnitude of risk varies and causality is difficult to establish. The risk of various infections associated with PPI therapy can not be firmly established until the results of large prospective studies are made available.

The absorption of Vitamin B12, dietary iron, and calcium requires an acidic environment and may be adversely affected by PPI-induced prolonged hypochlorhydria.[86] Although a few studies have investigated the long-term use of PPIs on Vitamin B12 and iron absorption, the clinical importance of their effect on absorption has not been established, and monitoring of B12 and iron levels cannot be recommended.[86] However, adequate supplementation and monitoring should be considered in high risk populations (e.g., older patients, vegetarians, alcoholism) who may be already depleted.[85,86] High PPI dosage and long-term therapy have been associated with an increased risk of hip, wrist and spine fractures related to reduction in calcium absorption.[26,93] Although the results of the studies vary, the FDA has revised the warnings and precautions of prescription and nonprescription PPIs to reflect this potential risk.[93] Bone density tests for osteoporosis screening, calcium supplementation, or other precautions cannot be recommended solely based on chronic PPI therapy.[94] However, it is appropriate to screen and treat older patients for osteoporosis regardless of whether they are receiving long-term PPI therapy.

H_2-Receptor Antagonists Ulcer healing is comparable among H_2RAs (cimetidine, famotidine, nizatidine, and ranitidine) with equipotent multiple daily doses or a single full dose given after dinner or at bedtime (see Table 40-9), but tolerance to their antisecretory effect may occur.[95] Twice-daily administration suppresses daytime acid and benefits patients with daytime ulcer pain. Cigarette smokers may require higher doses or a longer duration of treatment. H_2RAs are eliminated renally and therefore a dosage reduction is recommended for patients with moderate to severe renal failure.[96] The short- and long-term safety of all four H_2RAs is similar.[1] Thrombocytopenia, the most common hematologic adverse effect, is reversible and occurs with all four H_2RAs. However, the propensity for H_2RAs to cause thrombocytopenia is likely overestimated.[97] Cimetidine inhibits several CYP450 isoenzymes, resulting in numerous drug interactions (e.g., theophylline, lidocaine, phenytoin, warfarin, and clopidogrel).[77,96] Ranitidine has less potential for hepatic CYP450 drug interactions, while famotidine and nizatidine do not interact with drugs metabolized by the hepatic CYP450 pathway.[96] The H_2RAs decrease acid secretion and may alter the bioavailability of orally administered drugs, similar to that seen with the PPIs.

Sucralfate Sucralfate heals peptic ulcers, but is not widely used today for this indication.[1] Deterrents to its use include the requirement for multiple doses per day, large tablet size, and the need to separate the drug from meals and potentially interacting medications. Drug interactions can be minimized by giving the interacting drug at least 2 hours before sucralfate. Alternative therapy is warranted for patients taking oral fluoroquinolones. Constipation may be troublesome especially in older individuals. Seizures may occur in dialysis patients taking aluminum-containing antacids. Hypophosphatemia may develop with long-term treatment. Gastric bezoar formation has also been reported.

Prostaglandins Misoprostol, a synthetic prostaglandin E_1 analog, moderately inhibits acid secretion and enhances mucosal defense.[1,98] Antisecretory effects are dose dependent over the range of 50 to 200 mcg; cytoprotective effects occur in humans at doses of greater than 200 mcg. Because protective effects occur at higher doses, it is difficult to establish the protective effect independent of the antisecretory action. Although not recommended in the United States, a dose of 200 mcg 4 times daily or 400 mcg twice daily heals duodenal ulcers and gastric ulcers comparable to standard H_2RA or sucralfate regimens. Diarrhea, the most troublesome adverse effect, is dose dependent and develops in 10% to 30% of patients.[1,98] Abdominal cramping, nausea, flatulence, and headache typically accompany the diarrhea. Taking the drug with or after meals and at bedtime may minimize the diarrhea. Misoprostol is contraindicated in pregnant women because it is uterotropic and produces uterine contractions that may endanger pregnancy.[98] If misoprostol is prescribed to women in their childbearing years, contraceptive measures must be confirmed and a negative serum pregnancy test should be documented within 2 weeks of initiating treatment. Patients should be counseled about the GI effects and the need to avoid magnesium antacids, as they may increase the propensity for GI adverse effects.

Bismuth Preparations Bismuth subsalicylate and bismuth subcitrate potassium (biskalcitrate) are the only available bismuth salts in the United States.[1,96] Possible ulcer-healing mechanisms include an antibacterial effect, a local gastroprotective effect, and stimulation of endogenous prostaglandins. Bismuth salts do not inhibit or neutralize acid. Bismuth subsalicylate is regarded as safe and has few adverse effects when taken in recommended dosages. Because renal insufficiency may decrease bismuth elimination, bismuth salts should be used with caution in older patients and in renal failure. Bismuth subsalicylate may cause salicylate sensitivity or bleeding disorders and should be used with caution for patients receiving concurrent salicylate therapy. Bismuth salts impart a black color to stool and possibly the tongue (liquid preparations).

Antacids Antacids neutralize gastric acid, inactivate pepsin, and bind bile salts.[96,98] Aluminum-containing antacids also suppress *H. pylori* and enhance mucosal defense. The GI adverse effects are most common and are dose dependent. Magnesium salts cause an osmotic diarrhea, whereas aluminum salts cause constipation. Diarrhea usually predominates with magnesium/aluminum

preparations. Aluminum-containing antacids (except aluminum phosphate) form insoluble salts with dietary phosphorus and interfere with phosphorus absorption. Hypophosphatemia occurs most often for patients with low dietary phosphate intake (e.g., malnutrition or alcoholism). Combined treatment with sucralfate may amplify the hypophosphatemia and aluminum toxicity.

Magnesium-containing antacids should not be used for patients with a creatinine clearance of less than 30 mL/min because magnesium excretion is impaired, which may lead to toxicity. Hypercalcemia may occur for patients with normal renal function taking more than 20 g/day of calcium carbonate and for patients with renal failure who are taking more than 4 g/day. The milk–alkali syndrome (hypercalcemia, alkalosis, renal stones, increased blood urea nitrogen, and increased serum creatinine concentration) occurs with high calcium intake for patients with systemic alkalosis produced by either ingestion of absorbable antacids (sodium bicarbonate) or prolonged vomiting. Antacids may alter the absorption and excretion of drugs when administered concomitantly.[96,98] Drug interactions may occur when antacids are administered with iron, warfarin, tetracycline, digoxin, quinidine, isoniazid, ketoconazole, or the fluoroquinolones. Most interactions can be avoided by separating the antacid from the oral drug by at least 2 hours.

Pharmacoeconomic Considerations

❻ The eradication of *H. pylori* improves clinical outcomes and decreases the use of healthcare resources when compared with conventional antisecretory therapy.[99] Thus the costs of continued treatment and recurrence far outweigh the cost of *H. pylori* drug regimens. The cost-effectiveness of misoprostol cotherapy is greatest for patients with the highest risk for NSAID-related GI complications.[100] The addition of a PPI to both nonselective and partially selective NSAIDs or selective COX-2 inhibitor NSAIDs (if available) is highly cost-effective even for patients with low GI risk especially when the least expensive PPI is used.[101]

EVALUATION OF THERAPEUTIC OUTCOMES

❼ Table 40–13 lists the recommendations for treating and monitoring patients with PUD. Relief of epigastric pain should be monitored throughout the course of treatment for patients with either *H. pylori*– or NSAID-related ulcers. Ulcer pain typically resolves in a few days when NSAIDs are discontinued and within 7 days upon initiation of antiulcer therapy. Most patients with uncomplicated PUD will be symptom free after treatment with any one of the recommended antiulcer regimens. The persistence, or recurrence, of symptoms within 14 days after the end of treatment suggests failure of ulcer healing or *H. pylori* eradication or an alternative diagnosis such as GERD. Most patients with uncomplicated *H. pylori*–positive ulcers do not require confirmation of ulcer healing or *H. pylori* eradication. However, eradication should be confirmed after treatment in individuals who are at risk for complications, for example, individuals who had a prior bleeding ulcer. The UBT is the preferred test to confirm *H. pylori* eradication when endoscopy is not indicated. Medication adherence should be assessed for patients who fail therapy. Because a large number of at-risk patients treated with NSAIDs do not receive adequate prophylaxis for GI complications, therapeutic outcomes can be improved by advocating preventive strategies. Patients on NSAIDs should be closely monitored for signs or symptoms of bleeding, obstruction, penetration, or perforation. A follow-up endoscopy is justified for patients with frequent symptomatic recurrence, refractory disease, complications, or suspected hypersecretory states.

TABLE 40-13	Recommendations for Treating and Monitoring Patients with *Helicobacter pylori*–Associated and Nonsteroidal Antiinflammatory Drug (NSAID)–Induced Ulcers

Helicobacter pylori-associated ulcer

1. Recommend drug treatment as presented in the chapter text. See Tables 40–7 and 40–8.
2. Assess patient allergies to determine if allergic to penicillin (or other antibiotics) so that drug regimens that contain penicillin (or other antibiotics) can be avoided. Avoid regimens that contain tetracycline in children.
3. Assess patient use of alcohol or alcohol-containing products with metronidazole and oral birth control medications with antibiotics and counsel appropriately.
4. Assess likelihood of nonadherence to the drug regimen as a cause of treatment failure.
5. Recommend a different antibiotic combination if *H. pylori* eradication fails and a second treatment is planned.
6. Inform the patient of change in stool color when bismuth salicylate is included in an *H. pylori* eradication regimen.
7. Assess and monitor patients for potential adverse effects, especially those associated with metronidazole, clarithromycin, and amoxicillin.
8. Assess and monitor patients for potential drug interactions, especially those receiving metronidazole, clarithromycin, or cimetidine.
9. Monitor patients for salicylate toxicity, especially patients receiving cotherapy with other salicylates and anticoagulants and patients with renal failure.
10. Monitor patients for persistent or recurrent symptoms within 14 days after completion of a course of *H. pylori* eradication therapy.
11. Provide patient education to patients who are receiving *H. pylori* eradication therapy and include why antibiotic and antiulcer combinations are used; when and how to take medications; adverse effects; alarm symptoms; the importance of adherence to the entire course of drug treatment; and contact their healthcare provider if alarm symptoms develop (e.g., blood in the stools, black tarry stools, vomiting, severe abdominal pain), or if symptoms persist or return after *H. pylori* eradication.

NSAID-induced ulcer

1. Recommend drug treatment as presented in the chapter text.
2. Assess risk factors for NSAID-induced ulcers and ulcer-related complications and recommend appropriate strategies for reducing ulcer risk (see Table 40–10).
3. Weigh patient risk factors for NSAID-related GI bleeding and cardiovascular events when selecting a strategy to reduce ulcer risk.
4. Recommend eradication treatment for *H. pylori*-positive patients taking NSAIDs.
5. Monitor patients for signs and symptoms of NSAID-related upper GI complications.
6. Assess and monitor patients for potential drug interactions and adverse effects (especially misoprostol).
7. Provide patient education to patients who are at risk of NSAID-induced ulcers or GI-related complications and include why cotherapy is used with nonselective NSAIDs; when and how to take medications; adverse effects; alarm symptoms; when to contact their healthcare provider; and the importance of adherence to drug treatment.

ZOLLINGER-ELLISON SYNDROME (ZES)

ZES is characterized by gastric acid hypersecretion and recurrent peptic ulcers that result from a gastrin-producing tumor (gastrinoma).[21,45] In the United States, ZES accounts for 0.1% to 1% of patients with duodenal ulcer; however, this may be an underestimation of the true incidence because of the heterogeneity of clinical manifestations.[21] Gastrinomas are classified as those associated with multiple endocrine neoplasia type 1 (MEN 1) or sporadic tumors, which have a greater tendency to behave as malignant tumors. In more than 80% of cases, gastrinomas are localized in an area referred to as the *triangle of gastrinomas*, which includes the convergence of the cystic duct and the common bile duct, the junction of the second and third portion of the duodenum, and the junction of the head and body of the pancreas.[21] More than 50% of the gastrinomas malignant, often with metastases to regional lymph nodes, liver, and bone.[21]

Zollinger-Ellison syndrome is suspected for patients with multiple ulcers and recurrent or refractory PUD, often accompanied by esophagitis or ulcer complications.[21,45] Ulcers occur most often in the duodenum but may involve the stomach or jejunum. Diarrhea occurs in about 50% of patients, and results from high concentrations of acid that overwhelm the duodenum's buffering capacity and damage to the mucosa.[21] Intraluminal acid also causes steatorrhea by inactivating pancreatic lipase and precipitating bile acids. Vitamin B12 malabsorption may result from reduced intrinsic factor activity. The diagnosis is established when the serum gastrin is higher than 1,000 pg/mL and the BAO ≥15 mEq/h for patients with an intact stomach (BAO ≥5 mEq/h for patients with previous gastric surgery) or when hypergastrinemia is associated with a gastric pH value of ≤2.[21] In situations in which the serum gastrin is between 100 and 1,000 pg/mL and gastric pH is ≤2, a secretin or calcium proactive test is used to aid the diagnosis.[21] Identification of the location of the tumor with imaging techniques is essential, as early surgical resection prior to liver metastases is often curative.[21] The widespread use of PPIs, although effective in reducing symptoms, may mask the clinical presentation and PPI-related hypergastrinemia may further complicate the diagnosis.[21]

Treatment is based on the presence or absence of peptic ulcers, esophagitis, diarrhea, and a gastrinoma, which may be malignant. The PPIs are the oral drugs of choice for managing gastric acid hypersecretion. Treatment should be instituted with omeprazole 60 mg/day (or an equivalent dose of the available PPIs) and should be adjusted based on individual patient response.[21] Dividing the daily dose and giving the PPI every 8 to 12 hours is most effective in controlling acid output and relieving symptoms. The goal of therapy for uncomplicated patients is to maintain BAO between 1 and 10 mEq/h, in the hour preceding the next dose of the PPI. In complicated cases, such as patients with MEN 1, GERD, or those who are undergoing partial gastrectomy, the BAO should be maintained below 5 mEq/h. A gradual reduction in PPI dose is recommended after the adequate control of gastric acid hypersecretion is achieved. Intravenous PPIs are used to suppress gastric acid secretion in patients who are unable to take oral PPIs. The somatostatin analogues, octreotide and lanreotide, directly inhibit the release of gastrin and gastric acid secretin and have been used with varying degrees of success.[21] However, these drugs are not considered first-line therapy as they are only available in the injectable form. Preliminary studies have found the long-acting depot formation of octreotide to be efficacious in the treatment of GI neuroendocrine tumors.[21] Patients with metastatic gastrinoma require tumor resection or treatment with chemotherapeutic agents.

UPPER GASTROINTESTINAL BLEEDING

There are about 160 cases of upper GI bleeding per 100,000 adults annually in the United States.[102] Despite a decreased incidence of PUD and improvements in the management of upper GI bleeding, the mortality rate associated with acute hemorrhage remains between 5% and 15%.[102-104] Upper GI bleeding is categorized as variceal or nonvariceal bleeding. Two common types of nonvariceal bleeding are bleeding from chronic peptic ulcers and bleeding from SRMD (stress gastritis, stress ulcer, or stress erosions), both of which are acid–peptic complications.[102-106] Upper GI bleeding associated with chronic PUD usually precedes hospital admission, whereas bleeding associated with SRMD develops in severely ill patients during hospitalization.[102,106]

The underlying pathophysiology of bleeding from a peptic ulcer or from SRMD is similar in that impaired mucosal defense in the presence of gastric acid and pepsin leads to mucosal damage. In chronic PUD, *H. pylori* infection and NSAID use are the most important etiologic factors, whereas the primary pathogenic factor of SRMD in critically ill patients is thought to be mucosal ischemia which is a result of reduced gastric blood flow (decreased oxygen and nutrient delivery) resulting from splanchnic hypoperfusion.[1,102,106-108] Defense mechanisms are normally in place to protect the gastric mucosa against the damaging effects of gastric acid, pepsin, and bile (see the section Pathophysiology of Chronic PUD). However, these defense mechanisms become diminished in the face of the overwhelming physiologic stress from critical illness and coupled with mucosal ischemia and subsequent reperfusion injury along with gastric acid result in the rapid development of mucosal lesions.[106-107] In contrast to chronic PUD, stress-related mucosal lesions are characteristically asymptomatic, numerous, located in the proximal stomach, and are unlikely to perforate.[107] Bleeding from SRMD occurs from superficial mucosal capillaries, whereas bleeding associated with chronic PUD usually results from a single vessel.[107]

The mortality rate associated with clinically important SRMB is approximately 50% and is related to the underlying severity of disease and comorbidities in this patient population.[105,107,109] In contrast, the mortality associated with chronic PUD-related bleeding is approximately 10% but can increase dramatically in select patient populations.[103,110,111] Although the initial management of acute upper GI bleeding focuses on aggressive resuscitative measures and ensuring hemodynamic stability, the medical management of PUD-related bleeding and SRMB is distinctly different.[102,103,106,107]

PEPTIC ULCER-RELATED BLEEDING

The most common presenting signs and symptoms of PUD-related bleeding are hematemesis (vomiting up blood) or melena (dark, tarry stools) or possibly both. When evaluating patients with PUD-related bleeding, the degree of risk for adverse outcomes must be rapidly assessed in order to determine if the patient's condition constitutes a medical emergency.[102,103] Two risk-stratification tools exist for early assessment and triage.[112,113] The Blatchford score is a newer risk-stratification scale and is used to evaluate the need for urgent endoscopic intervention for patients presenting with PUD-related bleeding.[112] The scale values range from 0 to 23, with higher scores indicating higher risk. The most well-known scale, however, is the Rockall Score.[113] This validated risk-assessment instrument is composed of two assessments: the clinical score, which is performed prior to endoscopy, and the endoscopic score. The use of these risk-stratification tools can reduce the requirement of endoscopic procedures and lead to early discharge for low-risk patients while ensuring rapid intervention for patients at higher risk.[102] These data will also allow the pharmacist to make appropriate pharmacotherapy decisions based on the patient's assessed level of risk. When considering the risk of death due to PUD-bleeding, the following patients generally have poorer prognoses and usually require more aggressive intervention including admission to an intensive care unit (ICU).[102,103,106,107]

- Older than 60 years of age
- Comorbid conditions (e.g., ischemic heart disease, congestive heart failure, renal failure, hepatic failure, metastatic cancer)
- High transfusion requirements
- Ongoing blood loss
- Presence of hypovolemic shock (i.e. tachycardia with a pulse of ≥100 beats per minute, hypotension with a systolic blood pressure of <100 mmHg with concomitant orthostatic changes, such as an increase in the heart rate of ≥20 beats per minute or decrease in systolic blood pressure of ≥20 mmHg upon standing from a sitting position)

- Prolonged prothrombin time [or increased international normalized ratio (INR)]
- Erratic mental status

Initial therapy for patients with defined hemostatic instability should focus on correcting fluid volume loss though appropriate volume resuscitative measures. This is usually accomplished with a continuous 0.9% sodium chloride infusion (or blood products if clinically indicated) through two large bore peripheral intravenous catheters (i.e., 16 to 18 gauge).[102,104] The use of nasogastric (NG) tubes remains controversial but may aid in early assessment and gastric lavage.[102]

Diagnostic endoscopy is usually performed as early as possible (preferably within 24 hours of presentation) to identify the source of the bleeding, assess the potential risk for rebleeding, and, if appropriate, employ therapeutic interventions to promote hemostasis.[102,104] Several endoscopic treatment approaches (e.g., thermocoagulation, laser therapy, injection sclerotherapy, hemoclipping, and ligation) can be used; however, to maximize the likelihood of positive outcomes, patients are usually treated with a combination of thermocoagulation and injection of lesions with epinephrine.[102-104] The appearance of the ulcer at the time of endoscopy is a prognostic indicator for the risk of rebleeding.[102,104,110] Clean-based and flat spot (pigmented) ulcers are most commonly seen and are associated with a low risk of rebleeding (5% and 10%, respectively).[104,110] In most cases, patients with clean base ulcers can be immediately discharged after endoscopy on antiulcer therapy (usually twice daily PPI), while patients with flat spot ulcers may be admitted to the general hospital ward for a brief observation period. Patients with an adherent clot overlying the ulcer base are at intermediate risk of rebleeding (22%), and controversy exists as to the appropriate management of these patients.[104,110] Adherent clots can be removed, and then the lesion be reclassified based on what is observed following clot removal.[104,110] Patients with a visible vessel or active bleeding are at the highest risk of rebleeding (43% and 55%, respectively) and should be managed within an ICU for at least 24 hours and then monitored on a general medical/surgical service for an additional 48 hours (total of 72 hours), as rebleeding significantly increases mortality.[102,103,110]

❽ Antisecretory therapy is often used as adjuvant therapy to endoscopic procedures to prevent PUD rebleeding in high-risk patients because acid impairs clot stability.[102] However, endoscopic hemostatis techniques remain the treatment of choice for patients with life-threatening bleeding, as this has been associated with better outcomes when compared with either placebo or pharmacotherapy alone.[102-104,109] H_2-Receptor antagonists are ineffective in preventing PUD rebleeding because they do not achieve an intragastric pH of 6 (which is needed to promote hemostatis and clot stability) and tolerance to their antisecretory effect develops rapidly (especially with high dose or intravenous therapy).[102-104,108,114,115] In contrast, PPIs reduce the incidence of rebleeding and need for surgery but have no significant impact on overall mortality.[102,103,114,115] Interestingly, subgroup analysis from two differing metaanalyses has suggested a mortality benefit with high-dose intravenous PPIs in a subpopulation of patients with the highest risk of rebleeding (i.e., nonbleeding visible vessel or active bleeding).[114,116]

The precise route (oral or intravenous) and the dose of PPI should be based on the clinical situation, risk of rebleeding, endoscopic identification of the lesion, and patient risk.[114,115] Because of the theoretical goal of maintaining intragastric pH values >6, and data from randomized, controlled trials, practice guidelines recommend that high-dose continuous infusion PPI (equivalent to omeprazole 80 mg given intravenously as a loading dose, followed by 8 mg/h continuous infusion for 72 hours) be used to reduce the risk of rebleeding in high-risk patients who have undergone endoscopy hemostasis.[102,103,114,115] Because intravenous omeprazole is not available in the United States and three small randomized, controlled trials have not demonstrated any evidence of improved outcomes between the available intravenous PPIs and omeprazole, most clinicians consider intravenous pantoprazole and esomeprazole to be equivalent to intravenous omeprazole on a milligram-per-milligram basis. Thus, intravenous pantoprazole and esomeprazole can be interchanged as there is currently no evidence to suggest that one PPI is superior to another.[115,117] The administration of high-dose continuous-infusion PPIs given prior to endoscopy hastens resolution of bleeding stigmata.[118] However, PPI therapy is not a replacement for interventional endoscopy for patients who are at high risk of rebleeding, as data demonstrate that the combination of a high-dose PPI continuous intravenous infusion with therapeutic endoscopy is superior to either strategy alone.[115,119] High-dose oral PPI therapy (omeprazole 80 mg/day for 5 days) is also effective; however, concerns exist as to whether critically ill patients will absorb the medication.[109,114] The risk of rebleeding is greatest within the first 72 hours (especially the first 24 hours), and it is during this time that antisecretory therapy to prevent rebleeding in high-risk patients should be employed.[102,103] Patients should be transitioned to an oral PPI upon completion of intravenous therapy. Somatostatin or octreotide have not demonstrated any significant benefit in treating nonvariceal bleeding and are not recommended at this time.[102,103]

Patients with upper GI bleeding should be tested for *H. pylori* at the time of endoscopy (see Tests for *Helicobacter Pylori*). However, the tests are associated with an increased rate of false-negatives when obtained during acute bleeding episodes.[120] If the initial results of the rapid urease test and/or histology are negative, a confirmatory test (^{14}C-urea breath test or serology) should be performed following the acute bleeding episode. There is no rationale for using intravenous therapy to eradicate *H. pylori*. Ulcer treatment, including *H. pylori* eradication, if appropriate, should be initiated after the acute bleeding episode has resolved (see Treatment of *Helicobacter Pylori*–Associated Ulcers and Treatment of NSAID-Induced Ulcers).

STRESS-RELATED MUCOSAL BLEEDING

Critically ill patients may develop SRMD leading to SRMB because of the homeostatic compromise that is associated with severe illness.[106,107] More than 75% (some studies suggesting up to 100%) of critically ill patients develop SRMD within the first 1 to 3 days of admission to an ICU, but the incidence of clinically important SRMB (defined as overt bleeding with concomitant hemodynamic instability and likely requirement for blood products) is 1% to 4%.[106,107,121] Clinically important bleeding increases the length of ICU stay by up to 11 days, results in excessive healthcare costs and is associated with increased mortality.[106,107,122] Thus, attempts to prevent SRMB are warranted in high-risk patients. Prophylactic therapy to prevent bleeding is most effective if initiated early in the patient's course.

❾ Patients who are at risk for SRMB include those with respiratory failure (need for mechanical ventilation for longer than 48 hours), coagulopathy (INR >1.5, platelet count <50,000 mm[3]), hypotension, sepsis, hepatic failure, acute renal failure, high-dose corticosteroid therapy (>250 mg/day hydrocortisone or equivalent), multiple trauma, severe burns (>35% of body surface area), head injury, traumatic spinal cord injury, major surgery, prolonged ICU admission (>7 days), or history of GI bleeding.[105–107,122] The relative importance of the various risk factors remains controversial, but most clinicians concur that patients with respiratory failure or coagulopathy should receive prophylaxis, as these two factors are independent risk factors for SRMB.[105,106] In the absence of these risk factors, some clinicians only administer prophylaxis to patients who

have two of the aforementioned risk factors.[105] Since not all patients in a hospital or ICU are at increased risk of SRMB, a cost-effective approach should be developed to target prophylactic therapy at high-risk patients.

CLINICAL CONTROVERSY

Some clinicians feel that stress-related mucosal bleeding prophylaxis is indicated for all critically ill patients given the associated mortality and increased length of stay for patients who develop this complication. Others adhere to clinical guidelines that suggest only high-risk patients such as those with respiratory failure requiring ventilation or patients with coagulopathy and perhaps those patients with two or more other risk factors will benefit from prophylaxis.

Prevention of SRMB includes resuscitative measures that restore mucosal blood and pharmacotherapy that either maintains an intragastric pH of >4 or provides gastric mucosal protection.[105–107] Although the benefits of enteral nutrition to patient outcome (e.g., improved nutritional status enhances mucosal integrity) are of overall clinical importance, its precise role as a sole modality to prevent SRMB remains controversial.[106–107] Therapeutic options for the prevention of SRMB include antacids (which are of historical interest, as they are no longer used because of cumbersome dosage schedules and side effects), antisecretory drugs (H2RAs and PPIs), and sucralfate (mucosal protectant).[105–107,109,122]

Antisecretory therapy is generally preferred for SRMB prophylaxis for several reasons. First, a large landmark study demonstrated that intravenous ranitidine was superior to oral sucralfate in preventing SRMB.[123] Second, ranitidine did not increase the risk for nosocomial pneumonia, as the incidence of pneumonia was not different between the two treatment groups.[123] Third, although sucralfate is an evidence based option, it is cumbersome, requiring multiple daily dosage administration (up to 4 times daily), which may occlude nasogastric tubes, cause constipation, interact with several medications, and/or increase the potential for aluminum toxicity in patients with renal dysfunction. Finally, sucralfate does not have any appreciable effect on reducing intragastric pH. Although data published in 2004 indicated that H2RAs were the most commonly prescribed antisecretory agents used to prevent SRMB,[124] it is now estimated that PPIs have become the mainstay of therapy.[106] Regardless, numerous studies and years of experience support the use of H2RAs, and they remain a recommended option for the prevention of SRMB.[105–107,124]

Parenteral H2RAs may be administered as either continuous infusions or intermittent bolus doses (see Table 40–14). Cimetidine, given as a continuous intravenous infusion, is the only FDA-labeled H2RA for the prevention of SRMB. Despite evidence suggesting that continuous infusions of the H2RAs are superior to intermittent dosing at maintaining an intragastric pH >4, there is no evidence to suggest better outcomes with respect to prevention of SRMB.[106] Thus, intermittent bolus doses of H2RAs are used more commonly than continuous infusions.[107,109] Drug interactions are more common with cimetidine, and for this reason the other H2RAs (famotidine, ranitidine) are used more frequently.[106] Adverse events associated with the use of H2RAs for the critically ill patient include thrombocytopenia, mental status changes (more common in older patients or individuals with renal or hepatic compromise), and tachyphylaxis (especially with parenteral or high dose therapy).[106] Given that the H2RAs are renally eliminates, dosage reductions are recommended for patients with renal dysfunction.

SECTION 4 · Gastrointestinal Disorders

TABLE 40-14	Pharmacotherapy Options for Prophylaxis of Stress-Related Mucosal Bleeding
Drug and Route	**Dosage**
Parenteral H₂RAs	
Cimetidine	300 mg IV loading dose followed by a 50 mg/h as a continuous infusion[a] or 300 mg IV every 6 to 8 hours
Ranitidine	6.25 mg/h as a continuous infusion or 50 mg IV every 6 to 8 hours
Famotidine	1.7 mg/h as a continuous infusion or 20 mg IV every 12 hours
Oral/NG PPIs	
Omeprazole	20–40 mg orally/NG[b] every 12 to 24 hours
Omeprazole/ bicarbonate powder for oral suspension	40 mg orally/NG to start, then followed by an additional 40 mg in 6 to 8 hours as a loading dose, and then 40mg every 24 hours
Lansoprazole	30 mg orally/NG[b,c] every 12 to 24 hours
Pantoprazole	40 mg orally/NG[b] every 12 to 24 hours
Parenteral PPIs	
Pantoprazole	40-80 mg IV every 12 to 24 hours
Esomprazole	40 mg IV every 12 to 24 hours

H₂RA, histamine-₂ receptor antagonist; PPI, proton pump inhibitor; IV, intravenous; NG, nasogastric tube.
[a]Product is FDA approved for the prevention of stress-related mucosal bleeding.
[b]Administered as an extemporaneously compounded suspension made with sodium bicarbonate.
[c]Administered as a rapidly disintegrating tablet given orally or by NG dissolved in 10 mL of water.

The PPIs are more potent than H₂RAs in inhibiting acid secretion and, unlike H₂RAs, tolerance does not develop.[106,107,109,122] Although there are limited data assessing the efficacy of PPIs for the prevention of SRMB, recent reports suggest that PPIs may be used as alternatives to H₂RAs or sucralfate.[122,125,126] Initial open-label studies of PPIs for SRMB prophylaxis were performed with omeprazole compounded suspensions given as 40 mg for two doses on the first day, followed by 20 mg/day thereafter in critically ill or trauma patients requiring mechanical ventilation and the presence of at least one additional risk factor.[127,128] The results of these studies demonstrated significant pH control above 4 and no GI bleeding in either trial. Because of the small number of subjects, no firm clinical outcomes can be derived from these studies. Since then, numerous extemporaneously compounded sodium bicarbonate suspensions of PPIs (see Table 40–11) have been used as cost-effective regimens for stress ulcer prophylaxis in patients with NG tubes.[106,109,122,129] In one study, immediate-release omeprazole–sodium bicarbonate suspension (40 mg × 2 doses, then 40 mg/day) was more effective than continuous infusion cimetidine in maintaining intragastric pH >4 in critically ill patients, but there was no difference in the incidence of clinically important SRMD between the two groups.[125] Based on meeting the prespecified criteria for noninferiority, immediate-release omeprazole gained FDA labeling for the prevention of SRMB.[125] In another trial of ICU patients requiring mechanical ventilation, patients were randomized to receive either lansoprazole 30 mg given as a rapidly disintegrating tablet mixed in 10 mL of water and administered via an NG tube or lansoprazole 30 mg given as an intravenous infusion (no longer available in the United Satates) once daily for 72 hours.[130] Enterally administered lansoprazole, despite having a lower bioavailability, resulted in superior intragastric pH control when compared with the intravenously administered lansoprazole.

One of the most compelling dose-finding pilot studies to evaluate the use of intravenous PPIs for SRMB prophylaxis was performed in over 200 ICU patients examining five different dosing strategies of pantoprazole (40 mg given every 8 hours, every 12 hours, and every 24 hours or 80 mg given every 12 hours or every 24 hours) versus cimetidine given as a 300 mg intravenous bolus followed by a 50 mg/h continuous infusion.[126] Each regimen was given for at least 48 hours and for up to 7 days. The time the intragastric pH was ≥4

increased from day 1 to day 2 in all the pantoprazole groups, whereas it actually decreased in the cimetidine group suggesting tachyphylaxis. No bleeding was identified in any of the treatment groups. The results suggest appropriate pH control can be obtained with doses of 80 mg given on day 1 and 40 mg given every 12 hours thereafter. The use of intravenous esomeprazole has also demonstrated efficacy in a small number of clinical studies.[106] Given the relatively limited data, the overall efficacy, optimal dosage, frequency, and route of administration for PPIs in the prevention of SRMB remains to be fully elucidated.[106,107] Based on the available evidence, several PPI dosing regimens for SRMB prophylaxis exist (see Table 40-14). Adverse events that have been described when the PPIs are used for this indication include an increased risk of enteric infections, including *C. difficile* associated diarrhea and noscomial pneumonia.[106]

❿ When deciding on the most appropriate pharmacotherapy plan for the prevention of SRMB for a specific patient, the clinical presentation of the patient and medication costs should be used as a guide. Patients who can take oral medication or have a working NG tube in place may be placed on an oral or compounded PPI suspension as a cost-effective measure. For most patients who are not able to utilize one of these routes, an intravenous H₂RA is appropriate. However, if the patient has renal dysfunction, develops thrombocytopenia, or mental status changes while on an H₂RA, then an intravenous PPI may be the most appropriate prophylaxis option. Consideration should be given to both the patient's clinical condition as well as the most cost effective option when developing protocols for preventing SRMB.

Improvement in the patient's overall medical condition (resolution of risk factors, discharge from the ICU, extubation, and oral intake) suggests that prophylactic therapy can be discontinued.[106] Too often the patient is continued on SRMB prophylaxis upon transition to the general medical/surgical unit and is often discharged on oral PPI therapy without an appropriate indication.[131] This results in unnecessary costs for the patient and the healthcare system.[131] Pharmacists should identify patients in which SRMB prophylaxis is no longer indicated.[106] If a patient develops clinically important bleeding, endoscopic evaluation of the GI tract is indicated along with aggressive antisecretory therapy (see the section Peptic Ulcer-Related Bleeding).

ABBREVIATIONS

BAO: basal acid output
COX-1: cyclooxygenase-1
COX-2: cyclooxygenase-2
CYP450: cytochrome P450
ECL: enterochromaffin-like
ELISA: enzyme-linked immunosorbent assay
GERD: gastroesophageal reflux disease
H. pylori: Helicobacter pylori
H₂RA: histamine-2 receptor antagonist
ICU: intensive care unit
MALT: mucosa-associated lymphoid tissue
MAO: maximal acid output
MEN: multiple endocrine neoplasia
NSAID: nonsteroidal antiinflammatory drug
NG: nasogastric
NUD: nonulcer dyspepsia
PG: prostaglandin
PPI: proton pump inhibitor

PUD: peptic ulcer disease

SRMB: stress-related mucosal bleeding

SRMD: stress-related mucosal damage

UBT: urea breath test

ZES: Zollinger-Ellison syndrome

REFERENCES

1. Soll AH, Graham DY. Peptic ulcer disease. In: Yamada T, Alpers DH, Kalloo KN, et al. eds. Textbook of Gastroenterology, 5th ed. Hoboken, NJ: Wiley-Blackwell; 2009:936–981.

2. Washington MK, Peek, RM. Gastritis and gastropathy. In: Yamada T, Alpers DH, Kalloo KN, et al. eds. Textbook of Gastroenterology, 5th ed. Hoboken, NJ: Wiley-Blackwell; 2009:1005–1025.

3. Del Valle J. Zollinger-Ellison syndrome. In: Yamada T, Alpers DH, Kalloo KN, et al. eds. Textbook of Gastroenterology, 5th ed. Hoboken, NJ: Wiley-Blackwell; 2009:982–1004.

4. Everhart JE, Ruhl CE. Burden of digestive diseases in the United States part I: Overall and upper gastrointestinal diseases. Gastroenterology 2009;136:376–386.

5. Chey WD, Wong BCY, and the Practice parameters committee of American College of Gastroenterology. Guideline on the management of Helicobacter pylori infection. Am J Gastroenterol 2007;102:1–18.

6. Azevedo NF, Huntington J, Goodman KJ. The epidemiology of Helicobacter pylori and public health implications. Helicobacter 2009;14(suppl 1):1–7.

7. Talley NJ, Fock KM, Moayyedi P. Gastric cancer concensus conference recommends Helicobacter pylori screening and treatment in asymptomatic persons from high-risk populations to prevent gastric cancer. Am J Gastroenterol 2008;103:510–514.

8. Leung WK, Ng EKW, Sung JJY. Tumors of the stomach. In: Yamada T, Alpers DH, Kalloo KN, et al. eds. Textbook of Gastroenterology, 5th ed. Hoboken, NJ: Wiley-Blackwell; 2009:1026–1053.

9. Talley NJ, Holtmann G. Approach to the patient with dyspepsia and related functional gastrointestinal complaints. In: Yamada T, Alpers DH, Kalloo KN, et al. eds. Principles of Clinical Gastroenterology, 1st ed. Hoboken, NJ: Wiley-Blackwell; 2008:38–61.

10. Furuta T, Delchier JC. Helicobacter pylori and non-malignant diseases. Helicobacter 2009;14 (suppl 1):29–35.

11. Pellicano R, Franceschi F, Saracco G, et al. Helicobacters and extragastric dseases Helicobacter 2009;14(suppl 1):58–68.

12. Lanza FL, Chan FKL, Quigley EMM, and the practice parameters committee of the American College of Gastroenterology. Guidelines for prevention of NSAID-related ulcer complications. Am J Gastroenterol 2009; 104:728–738.

13. Bhatt DL, Scheiman J, Abraham NS, et al. ACCF/ACG/AHA 2008 expert consensus document on reducing the gastrointetinal risks of antiplatelet therapy and NSAID use: A report of the American College of Cardiology Foundation Task Force on clinical expert consensus documents. Am J Gastroenterol 2008;103:2890–2907.

14. Chan FKL Abraham NS, Scheiman JM, Laine L. Management of patients on nonsteroidal anti-inflammatory drugs: A clinical practice recommendation from the First International Working Party on Gastrointestinal and Cardiovascular Effects of Nonsteroidal Anti-Inflammatory Drugs and Anti-platelet Agents. Am J Gastroenterol 2008;103:2908–2918.

15. Cryer B. Management of patients with high gastrointestinal risk on antiplatelet therapy. Gastroenterol Clin N Am 2009;38:289–303

16. Rostom A, Moayyedi P, Hunt R, and the Canadian Association of Gastroenterology Concensus Group. Canadian consensus guidelines on long-term nonsteroidal anti-inflammatory drug therapy and the need for gastroprotection: Benefits versus risks. Aliment Pharmacol Ther 2009;29:481–496.

17. Lanas A, Sopena F. Nonsteroidal anti-inflammatory drugs and lower gastrointestinal complication. Gastroenterol Clin N Am 2009;38: 333–352.

18. Chan FKL. The David Y. Graham Lecture: Use of nonsteroidal antiinflammatory drugs in a COX-2 restricted environment. Am J Gastroenterol 2008;103:221–227.

19. Scheiman JM. Balancing risks and benefits of cyclooxygenzse-2 selective nonsteroidal anti-inflammatory drugs. Gastroenterol Clin N Am 2009;38:305–314.

20. Loke YK, Trivedi AN, Singh S. Meta-analysis: Gastrointestinal bleeding due to interaction between selective serotonin uptake inhibitors and non-steroidal anti-inflammatory drugs. Aliment Pharmacol Ther 2008;27:31–40.

21. De Valle, Tedisco A. Gastric secretion. In: Yamada T, Alpers DH, Kalloo KN, et al. eds. Textbook of Gastroenterology, 5th ed. Hoboken, NJ: Wiley-Blackwell; 2009:284–329.

22. Costa AC, Figueiredo C, Touati E. Pathogenesis of Helicobacter pylori infection. Helicobacter 2009;14 (suppl 1):15–20.

23. Glasglow RE, Mulvihill SJ. Surgery for peptic ulcer disease and postgastrectomy syndromes. In: Yamada T, Alpers DH, Kalloo KN, et al. eds. Textbook of Gastroenterology, 5th ed. Hoboken, NJ: Wiley-Blackwell; 2009:1054–1070.

24. Monteiro L, Oleastro M, Lehours P, Megraud F. Diagnosis of Helicobacter pylori infection. Helicobacter 14 (suppl 1):8–14.

25. Malfertheiner P, Megraud F, O'Morain C, et al. Current concepts in the management of Helicobacter pylori infection—The Maastricht Maastrict III Consensus Report Gut 2007;56:772–781.

26. O'Connor A, Gisbert J, O'Morain C. Treatment of Helicobacter pylori infection. Helicobacter 2009;14(suppl 1):46–51.

27. Vakil N. H. pylori treatment: New wine in old bottles? Am J Gastroenterol 2009;104:26–30.

28. Rokkas P, Sechopoulos P, Robotis I, et al. Cumulative H. pylori eradication rates in clinical practice by adopting first and second-line regimens proposed by the Maastricht III Consensus and a third-line empirical regimen. Am J Gastroenterol 2009;104:21–25.

29. Malfertheiner P, Chan FKL, McColl KEL. Peptic ulcer disease. Lancet 2009;374:1449–1461.

30. Kindermann A, Lopes AI. Helicobacter pylori infection in pediatrics. Helicobacter 2009;14(suppl 1):52–57.

31. Francavilla R, Lionetti E, Cavallo L. Sequential treatment for Helicobacter pylori eradication in children. Gut 2008;57:1178.

32. Boparai V, Rajagopalan J, Triadafilopoulos G. Guide to the use of proton pump inhibitors in adult patients. Drugs 2008;68:925–947.

33. Vallve M, Vergara M, Gisbert JP, et al. Single vs. double dose of a proton pump inhibitor in triple therapy for Helicobacter pylori eradication: A meta-analysis. Aliment Pharmacol Ther 2002;16:1149–1156.

34. Vergara M, Vallve M, Gisbert JP, et al. Meta-analysis: Comparative efficacy of different proton-pump inhibitors in triple therapy for Helicobacter pylori eradication. Aliment Pharmacol Ther 2003;18:647–654.

35. Graham DY, Hammoud F, el-Zimaity HM, et al. Meta-analysis: Proton pump inhibitor or H_2-receptor antagonist for Helicobacter pylori eradication. Aliment Pharmacol Ther 2003;17:1229–1236.

36. Gisbert JP, Khorrami S, Calvet X, et al. Meta-analysis: Proton pump inhibitors vs. H_2-receptor antagonists—Their efficacy with antibiotics in Helicobacter pylori eradication. Aliment Pharmacol Ther 2003;18:757–766.

37. Janssen MJR, Laheij RJF, Boer WA, et al. Meta-analysis: The influence of pre-treatment with a proton pump inhibitor on Helicobacter pylori eradication. Aliment Pharmacol Ther 2005;21:341–345.

38. Gene E, Calvet X, Azagra R, et al. Triple vs quadruple therapy for treating Helicobacter pylori infection: A meta-analysis. Aliment Pharmacol Ther 2003;17:1137–1143.

39. Laine L, Hunt R, el-Zimaity H, et al. Bismuth-based quadruple therapy using a single capsule of bismuth biskalcitrate, metronidazole, and tetracycline given with omeprazole versus omeprazole, amoxicillin, and clarithromycin for eradication of Helicobacter pylori in duodenal ulcer patients: A prospective, randomized, multicenter, North American trial. Am J Gastroenterol 2003;98:562–567.

40. Fischbach LA, van Zanten S, Dickason J. Meta-analysis: The efficacy, adverse events, and adherence related to firstline anti-Helicobacter pylori quadruple therapies. Aliment Pharmacol Ther 2004;20: 1071–1082.

41. Laine L. Is it time for quadruple therapy to be first line? Can J Gastroenterol 2003;17(suppl B):33B–5B.

42. Jafri NS, Hornung CA, Howden CW. Meta-analysis: Sequential therapy appears superior to standard therapy for Helicobacter pylori infection in patients naive to treatment. Ann Intern Med 2008;148;1–9.

43. O'Morain CA, O'Connor JP. Is sequential therapy superior to standard triple therapy for the treatment of *Helicobacter pylori* infection? Nat Clin Pract Gastroenterol Hepatol 2009;6:8–9.

44. Megraud F, Lamouliatte H. Review article: The treatment of refractory *Helicobacter pylori* infection. Aliment Pharmacol Ther 2003;17:1333–1343.

45. Napolitano L. Refractory peptic ulcer disease. Gastroenterol Clin N Am 2009;38:267–288.

46. Saad RJ, Schoenfeld P, Kim HM, et al. Levofloxacin-based triple therapy versus bismuth-based quadruple therapy for persistent *Helicobacter pylori* infection: A meta-analysis. Am J Gastroenterol. 2006;101:488–496.

47. Gisbert JP, Perez-Aisa A, Castro-Fernandez M, et al. *Helicobacter pylori* first-line treatment and rescue option containing levofloxacin in patients allergic to penicillin. Dig Liver Dis 2010;42:287–290.

48. Suzuki T, Matsuo K, Sawaki A, et al. Systematic review and meta-analysis: Importance of CagA status for successful eradication of *Helicobacter pylori* infection. Aliment Pharmacol Ther 2006;24:273–280.

49. Padol S, Yuan Y, Thabane M, et al. The effect of CYP2C19 polymorphisms on *H pylori* eradication rate in dual and triple first-line PPI therapies: A meta-analysis. Am J Gastroenterol 2006;101:1467–1475.

50. Qasim A. O'Morain CA. Review article: Treatment of *Helicobacter pylori* infection and factors influencing eradication. Aliment Pharmacol Ther 2002;16(suppl 1):24–30.

51. Meyer JM, Silliman NP, Wang W, et al. Risk factors for *Helicobacter pylori* resistance in the United States: The surveillance of *H. pylori* antimicrobial resistance partnership (SHARP) study, 1993–1999. Ann Intern Med 2002;136:13–24.

52. Duck WM, Sobel J, Pruckler JM, et al. Antimicrobial resistance incidence and risk actors among *Helicobacter pylori*-infected persons in the United States. Emerg Infect Dis 2004;10:1088–1094.

53. Gotteland M, Brunser O, Cruchet S. Systematic review: Are probiotics useful in controlling gastric colonization by *Helicobacter pylori*. Aliment Pharmacol Ther 2006;23:1077–1086.

54. Kim MN, Kim N, Lee SH, et al. The effects of probiotics on PPI-triple therapy for *Helicobacter pylori* eradication. Helicobacter 2008;13:261–268.

55. Scaccianoce G, Zullo A, Hassan C, et al. Triple therapies plus different probiotics for *Helicobacter pylori* eradication. Eur Rev Med Pharmacol Sci 2008;12:251–256.

56. Targownik LE, Metge CJ, Leung S, et al. The relative efficacies of gastroprotective strategies in chronic users of nonsteroidal anti-inflammatory drugs. Gastroenterolgy 2008;134:937–944.

57. Silverstein FE, Graham DY, Senior JR, et al. Misoprostol reduces serious gastrointestinal complications in patients with rheumatoid arthritis receiving nonsteroidal anti-inflammatory drugs: A randomized, double-blind, placebo-controlled trial. Ann Intern Med 1995; 123:241–249.

58. Graham DY, Agrawal NM, Campbell DR, et al. Ulcer prevention in long-term users of nonsteroidal anti-inflammatory drugs: Results of a double-blind, randomized, multicenter, active- and placebo-controlled study of misoprostol vs lansoprazole. Arch Intern Med 2002;152:169–175.

59. Arora G, Singh G, Triadafilopoulos G. Proton pump inhibitors for gastroduodenal damagae related to nonsteroidal antiinflammatory drugs or aspirin: Twelve important questions for clinical practice. Clin Gastroenterol Hepatol 2009;7:725–736.

60. Taha AT, McCloskey C, Prasad R, Bezlyak V. Famotidine for the prevention of peptic ulcers and oesophagitis in patients taking low-dose aspirin (FAMOUS): A phase III, randomised, double-blind, placebo-controlled trial. Lancet 2009;374:119–125.

61. Silverstein F, Faich G, Goldstein JL, et al. Gastrointestinal toxicity with celecoxib vs nonsteroidal antiinflammatory drugs for osteoarthritis and rheumatoid arthritis. The CLASS study: A randomized controlled trial. JAMA 2000;284:1247–1255.

62. Bombardier C, Laine L, Reicin A, et al. Comparison of upper intestinal toxicity of rofecoxib and naproxen in patients with rheumatoid arthritis. VIGOR Study Group. N Engl J Med 2000;343:1520–1528.

63. US Food and Drug Administration: Drug Information. COX-2 Selective and Non-Selective Non-Steroidal Anti-Inflammatory Drugs (NSAIDs), *http://www.fda.gov/cder/drug/infopage/cox2/default.htm.*

64. Bresalier RS, Sandler RS, Quan H, et al. Cardiovascular events associated with rofecoxib in colorectal adenoma chemoprevention trial. N Engl J Med 2005:352:1092–1102.

65. Kearney PM, Baigent C, Godwin J, et al. Do selective cyclooxygenase-2 inhibitors and traditional non-steroidal antiinflammatory drugs increase the risk of atherothrombosis? Meta-analysis of randomized trials. BMJ 2006;322:1302–1308.

66. Fiorucci S. Prevention of nonsteroidal anti-inflammatory drug-induced ulcer: Looking forward to the future. Gastroenterol Clin N Am 2009;38:315–322.

67. McColl KEL. How I manage *H. pylori*-negative, NSAID/Aspirin-Negative Peptic Ulcers. Am J Gastroenterol 2009;104:190–193.

68. Gisbert JP, Calvert X. *Helicobacter pylori*-negative duodenal ulcer disease. Aliment Pharmacol Ther 2009;30;791–815.

69. Reimer C, Sondergaard G, Hilsted L, et al. Proton-Pump Inhibitor Therapy Induces Acid-Related Symptoms in Healthy Volunteers after Withdrawal of Therapy. Gastroenterology 2009;137:80–87.

70. Package insert. Kapidex (dexlansoprazole). Deerfield, IL. Takeda Pharmaceuticals America, Inc., *http://www.kapidex.com/PI.aspx.*

71. Metz DC, Valiky M, Dixit T, et al. Review article: Dual delayed release formulation of dexlansoprazole MR, a novel approach to overcome the limitations of conventional single release proton pump inhibitor therapy. Aliment Pharmacol Ther 2009;29:928–937.

72. Package insert. Zegerid (omeprazole/sodium bicarbonate). San Diego, CA. Santarus, Inc., *http://www.zegerid.com/assets/pdfs/prescribing_information.pdf.* Accessed Nov 3, 2009.

73. Lahner E, Annibale B, Fave GD. Systematic review: Impaired drug absorption related to the co-administration of antisecretory therapy. Aliment Pharmacol Ther 2009;29;219–229

74. Beique L, Giguere P, la Porte C, et al. Interactions between protease inhibitors and acid- reducing agents: A systematic review. HIV Medicine 2007;8:335–245.

75. Sachmechi I, Reich DM, Aninyei M, et al. Effect of proton pump inhibitors on serum thyroid-stimulating hormone level in euthyroid patients treated with levothyroxine for hypothyroidism. Endocr Pract 2007;13:345–349.

76. Labenz J, Petersen KU, Rosch W, Koelz HR. A summary of Food and Drug Administration-reported adverse events and drug interactions occurring during therapy with omeprazole, lansoprazole, and pantoprazole. Aliment Pharmacol Ther 2003;17:1015–1019.

77. U.S. Food and Drug Administration. Information for Healthcare Professionals: Update to the labeling of Clopidogrel Bisulfate (marketed as Plavix) to alert healthcare professionals about a drug interaction with omeprazole (marketed as Prilosec and Prilosec OTC), *http://www.fda.gov/Drugs/DrugSafety/PostmarketDrugSafetyInformationfor PatientsandProviders/DrugSafetyInformationforHeathcareProfessionals/ ucm190787.htm.*

78. U.S. Food and Drug Administration. Public Health Advisory: Updated Information about a drug interaction between Clopidogrel Bisulfate (marketed as Plavix) and omeprazole (marketed as Prilosec and Prilosec OTC), 2009, *http://www.fda.gov/Drugs/ DrugSafety/PublicHealthAdvisories/ucm190825.htm.* Accessed March 4, 2010

79. U.S. Food and Drug Administration. Information for healthcare professionals: update to the labelling of Clopidogrel Bisulfate (marketed as Plavix) to alert healthcare practitioners about a drug interaction with Omeprazole (marketed as Prilosec and Prilosec OTC). *http://www.fda.gov/Drugs/ DrugSafety/PostmarketDrugSafetyInformationforPatientsandProviders/ DrugSafetyInformationforHeathcareProfessionals/ucm19078.htm.* Accessed March 4, 2010

80. Plavix (clopidogrel bisulfate tablets). Bristol-Myers Squibb/ Sanofi Pharmaceuticals partnership, Bridgewater, NJ. Revised 2009, *http://products.sanofi-aventis.us/PLAVIX/plavix.pdf.* Accessed July 30, 2010

81. Mega JL, Close SL, Wiviott SD, et al. Cytochrome P-450 polymorphisms and response to clopidogrel. N Engl J Med. 2009;360:354–362.

82. Freedman JE, Hylek EM. Clopidogrel, genetics, and drug responsiveness. N Engl J Med 2009;360:411–413.

83. Last EJ, Sheehan AH. Review of recent evidence: Potential interaction between clopidogrel and proton pump inhibitors. Am J Health-Syst Pharm. 2009; 66:2117–2122.

84. Norgard NB, Mathews KD, Wall GC. Drug-drug interaction between clopidogrel and proton pump inhibitors. Ann Pharmacother 2009;43:1266–1274.

85. Laine L, Ahnen D, McClain C, et al. Review article: Potential gastrointestinal effects of long-term acid suppression with proton pump inhibitors. Aliment Pharmacol Ther 2000;14:651–668.

86. Ali T, Roberts DN, Tierney WM. Long-term safety concerns with proton pump inhibitors. Am J Med 2009;122:896–903.

87. Heidelbaugh JJ, Goldberg KL, Inadomi JM. Overutilization of proton pump inhibitors: A review of cost-effectiveness and risk. Am J Gastroenterol 2009;104:S27–S32.

88. Williams C, McColl KE. Review article: Proton pump inhibitors and bacterial overgrowth. Aliment Pharmacol Ther 2006;23:3–10.

89. Laheij RJF, Sturkenboom MCJM, Hassing R-J, et al. Risk of community-acquired pneumonia and use of gastric acid-suppressive drugs. JAMA 2004;292:1955–1960.

90. Gulmez SE, Holm A, Frederiksen H. et al. Use of proton pump inhibitors and the risk of community-acquired pneumonia: A population-based case-control study. Arch Intern Med 2007;167:950–955.

91. Sarkar M, Hennessy S, Yang YX. Proton-pump inhibitor use and the risk of community-acquired pneumonia. Ann Intern Med 2008;149:391–398.

92. Leonard J, Marshall JK, Moayyedi P. Systematic review of the risk of enteric infection in patients taking acid suppression. Am J Gastroenterol 2007;102:2047–2056.

93. US. Food and Drug administration, FDA safety communication: possible increase risk of fractures of the hip, wrist and spine with the use of proton pump inhibitors. *http://www.fda.gov/Drugs/DrugSafety/PostmarketDrugSafetyInformationforPatientsandProviders/ucm213206.htm.* Accessed May, 2010

94. Kahrilas PJ, Shaheen NJ, Vaezi MF. American Gastroenterological Association Medical Position Statement on Management of GERD. Gastroenterology 2008;135:1383–1391.

95. Furuta K, Adachi K, Komazawa Y, et al. Tolerance to H₂-receptor antagonist correlates well with the decline in efficacy against gastroesophageal reflux in patients with gastroesophageal reflux disease. J Gastroenterol Hepatol 2006;21:1581–1585.

96. Zweber A, Berardi RR. Heartburn and Dyspepsia. In: Handbook of Nonprescription Drugs, 16th ed. Washington, DC: American Pharmaceutical Association; 2009:231–246.

97. Wade EE, Rebuck JA, Healey MA, Rogers FB. H₂ antagonist-induced thrombocytopenia: Is this a real phenomenon? Intensive Care Med 2002;28:459–465.

98. Chong YS, Su LL, Arulkumaran S. Misoprostol: A quarter century of use, abuse and creative misuse. Obstet Gynecol Surg 2004;59:128–140.

98. Maton PN, Burton ME. Antacids revisited: A review of their clinical pharmacology and recommended therapeutic use. Drugs 1999;57:855–870.

99. Sonnenberg A, Schwartz JS, Cutler AF, et al. Cost savings in duodenal ulcer therapy through *Helicobacter pylori* eradication compared with conventional therapies: Results of a randomized, double-blind, multicenter trial. Arch Intern Med 1998;158:852–860.

100. Maetzel A, Ferraz MB, Bombardier C. The cost-effectiveness of misoprostol in preventing serious gastrointestinal events associated with the use of nonsteroidal anti-inflammatory drugs. Arthritis Rheum 1998;41:16–25.

101. Latimer N, Lord J, Grant RL, et al. Cost effectiveness of COX 2 selective inhibitors and traditional NSAIDs alone or in combination with a proton pump inhibitor for people with osteoarthritis. BMJ 2009;339:b2538.

102. Gralnek IM, Barkun AN, Bardou M. Management of acute bleeding from a peptic ulcer. N Engl J Med 2008;359:928–937.

103. Barkun AN, Bardou M, Marshall JK. Consensus recommendations for managing patients with nonvariceal upper gastrointestinal bleeding. Ann Intern Med 2003;139:843–857.

104. Bjorkman DJ. Endoscopic diagnosis and treatment of nonvariceal upper gastrointestinal hemorrhage. In: Yamada T, Alpers DH, Kalloo KN, et al. eds. Textbook of Gastroenterology, 5th ed. Hoboken, NJ: Wiley-Blackwell; 2009:3018–3031.

105. American Society of Health-System Pharmacists Therapeutic Guidelines on Stress Ulcer Prophylaxis. Am J Health Syst Pharm 1999;56:347–379.

106. Ali Tauseef, Harty RF. Stress-induced ulcer bleeding in critically ill patients. Gastroenterol Clin N Am 2009;38:245–265.

107. Stollman N, Metz DC. Pathophysiology and prophylaxis of stress ulcer in intensive care unit patients. J Crit Care 2005;20:35–45.

108. Laine L, Takeuchi K, Tarnawski A. Gastric mucosal defense and cytoprotection: Bench to bedside. Gastroenterology 2008;135:41–60.

109. Devlin JW, Welage LS, Olsen KM. Proton pump inhibitor formulary considerations in the acutely ill—Part 2: Clinical efficacy, safety, and economics. Ann Pharmacother 2005;39:1844–1851.

110. Elmunzer BJ, Inadomi JM, Elta GH. Risk stratification in upper gastrointestinal bleeding. J Clin Gastroenterol 2007;41:559–563.

111. Chiu PWY, Ng EKW. Predicting poor outcome from acute upper gastrointestinal hemorrhage. Gastroenterol Clin N Am 2009;38:215–230.

112. Blatchford O, Murray WR, Blatchford M. A risk score to predict need for treatment for upper-gastrointestinal haemorrhage. Lancet 2000;356:1318–1321.

113. Rockall TA, Logan RF, Devlin HB, et al. Risk assessment after acute upper gastrointestinal haemorrhage. Gut 1996;38:316–321.

114. Leontiadis GI, Sharma VK, Howden CW. Proton pump inhibitor therapy for peptic ulcer bleeding: Cochrane Collaboration meta-analysis of randomized controlled trials. Mayo Clin Proc 2007;82:286–296.

115. Leontiadis GI, Howden CW. The role of proton pump inhibitors in the management of upper gastrointestinal bleeding. Gastroenterol Clin N Am 2009;38:199–213.

116. Bardou M, Toubouti Y, Benhaberou-Brun D, et al. Meta-analysis: Proton-pump inhibitors in high-risk patients with acute peptic ulcer bleeding. Aliment Pharmacol Ther 2005;21:677–686.

117. Sung JYJ, Barkun A, Kuipers EJ, et al. Intravenous esomeprazole for prevention of recurrent peptic ulcer bleeding: A randomized trial. Ann Intern Med 2009;150:455–464.

118. Lau JY, Leung WK, Wu JCY, et al. Omeprazole before endoscopy in patients with gastrointestinal bleeding. N Engl J Med 2007;356:1631–1640.

119. Sung JJ, Chan FK, Lau JY. The effect of endoscopic therapy in patients receiving omeprazole for bleeding ulcers with nonbleeding visible vessels or adherent clots. Ann Intern Med 2003;139:237–243.

120. Gisbert JP, Abraiira V. Accuracy of *Helicobacter pylori* diagnostic tests in patients with bleeding peptic ulcer: A systematic review and meta-analysis. Am J Gastroenterol 2006;101:848–863.

121. Fennerty MB. Pathophysiology of the upper gastrointestinal tract in the critically ill patient: Rational for the therapeutic benefit of acid suppression. Crit Care Med 2002;30(suppl):S351–S355.

122. Jung R, MacLaren R. Proton-pump inhibitors for stress ulcer prophylaxis in critically ill patients. Ann Pharmacother 2002;36:1929–1937.

123. Cook D, Guyatt G, Marshall J, et al. A comparison of sucralfate and ranitidine for the prevention of upper gastrointestinal bleeding in patients requiring mechanical ventilation. N Engl J Med 1998;338:791–797.

124. Daley RJ, Rebuck JA, Welage LS, Rogers FB. Prevention of stress ulceration: Current trends in critical care. Crit Care Med 2004;32:2008–2013.

125. Conrad SA, Gabrielli A, Margolis B, et al. Randomized, double-blind comparison of immediate-release omeprazole oral suspension versus intravenous cimetidine for the prevention of upper gastrointestinal bleeding in critically ill patients. Crit Care Med 2005;33:760–765.

126. Somberg L, Morris J, Fantus R, et al. Intermittent intravenous pantoprazole and continuous cimetidine infusion: Effect on gastric pH control in critically ill patients at risk of developing stress-related mucosal disease. J Trauma 2008;64:1202–1210.

127. Phillips JO, Metzler MH, Palmirei MT, et al. A prospective study of simplified omeprazole suspension for the prophylaxis of stress-related mucosal damage. Crit Care Med 1996;24:1793–1800.

128. Lasky MR, Metzler MH, Phillips JO. A prospective study of omeprazole suspension to prevent clinically significant gastrointestinal bleeding from stress ulcers in mechanically ventilated trauma patients. J Trauma 1998;44:527–533.

129. Devlin JW, Welage LS, Olsen KM. Proton pump inhibitor formulary considerations in the acutely ill—Part 1: Pharmacology, pharmacodynamics and available formulations. Ann Pharmacother 2005;39:1667–1677.

130. Olsen KM, Devlin JW. Comparison of the enteral and intravenous lansoprazole phamacodynamic responses in critically ill patients. Aliment Pharmacol Ther 2008;28:326–333.

131. Heidelbaugh JJ, Goldberg KL, Inadomi JM. Overutilization of proton pump inhibitors: A review of cost-effectiveness and risk. Am J Gastroenterol 2009;104(suppl):S27–S32.

BRIAN A. HEMSTREET

CHAPTER 41

Inflammatory Bowel Disease

KEY CONCEPTS

❶ The exact cause of inflammatory bowel disease (IBD) is unknown, although there are components that appear to be infectious and other components that suggest immune dysregulation. Genetic variations explain some of the increased risk of disease occurrence.

❷ Ulcerative colitis (UC) is confined to the rectum and colon, causes continuous lesions, and affects primarily the mucosa and the submucosa. Crohn's disease (CD) can involve any part of the gastrointestinal (GI) tract, often causes discontinuous (skip) lesions, and is a transmural process that can result in fistulas, perforations, or strictures.

❸ Common GI complications of IBD include rectal fissures, fistulas (CD), perirectal abscess (UC), and colon cancer, while possible extraintestinal manifestations include hepatobiliary complications, arthritis, uveitis, skin lesions (including erythema nodosum and pyoderma gangrenosum), and aphthous ulcerations of the mouth.

❹ The severity of UC may be assessed by stool frequency, presence of blood in stool, fever, pulse, hemoglobin, erythrocyte sedimentation rate, C-reactive protein, abdominal tenderness, and radiologic or endoscopic findings. The severity of CD can be assessed using similar parameters, in addition to the CD activity index, which includes stool frequency, presence of blood in stool, endoscopic appearance, and physician's global assessment.

❺ The goals of IBD treatment are resolution of acute inflammation and complications, alleviation of systemic manifestations, maintenance of remission, and for some patients surgical palliation or cure.

❻ The first line of treatment for mild to moderate UC or Crohn's colitis consists of oral aminosalicylates, such as sulfasalazine or mesalamine; mesalamine or steroid enemas or suppositories may be used for distal disease. Certain delayed-release oral formulations of mesalamine may be used for Crohn's ileitis. Controlled-release budesonide may be used for CD confined to the ileum and/or ascending colon.

❼ Corticosteroids are often required for acute UC or CD. The duration of steroid use should be minimized and the dose tapered gradually over 3 to 4 weeks.

❽ Infliximab is a treatment option for patients with moderate to severe active UC and for those patients with UC who are dependent on corticosteroids. Azathioprine or mercaptopurine may be used for maintenance of remission as an alternative to infliximab for patients with UC who have failed aminosalicylates and for patients who are corticosteroid dependent.

❾ Intravenous continuous infusion of cyclosporine may be effective in treating severe colitis that is refractory to corticosteroids as an option to delay or prevent the need for surgery.

❿ Sulfasalazine and mesalamine derivatives can prevent recurrence of acute disease in many patients, while steroids are ineffective for this purpose.

⓫ Other drugs that are useful for treatment of CD include infliximab, adalimumab, and certolizumab (for moderate to severe or fistulizing disease); methotrexate, azathioprine, or mercaptopurine (for inadequate response or to reduce steroid dosage); metronidazole (for perineal disease); and cyclosporine (for refractory disease).

Learning objectives, review questions, and other resources can be found at **www.pharmacotherapyonline.com**.

There are two forms of idiopathic IBD: (1) UC, a mucosal inflammatory condition confined to the rectum and colon, and (2) CD, a transmural inflammation of the GI tract that can affect any part, from the mouth to the anus. The etiologies of both conditions are unknown, but they may have some common pathogenic mechanisms.

EPIDEMIOLOGY

Inflammatory bowel disease (IBD) is most prevalent in Western countries and in areas of northern latitude.[1] The reported rates of IBD are highest in Scandinavia, Great Britain, and North America.[2] Crohn's disease (CD) has an incidence of 3.6 to 8.8 per 100,000 persons in the United States and a prevalence of 20 to 40 per 100,000 people.[1-3] The incidence of CD varies considerably among studies, but has clearly increased dramatically over the last 3 or 4 decades.[3,4] Ulcerative colitis (UC) incidence ranges from 3 to 15 cases per 100,000 persons per year among the white population with a prevalence of 80 to 120 per 100,000.[4] The incidence of UC has remained relatively constant over many years.[2] Although most epidemiologic studies combine ulcerative proctitis with UC, 17% to 49% of cases are classified as proctitis.

Both sexes are affected equally with IBD, although some studies show slightly greater numbers of women with CD and males with UC.[2] UC and CD have bimodal distributions in age of initial

TABLE 41-1	Proposed Etiologies for Inflammatory Bowel Disease

Infectious agents
  Viruses (e.g., measles)
  L-Forms of bacteria
  Mycobacteria
  Chlamydia
Genetics
  Metabolic defects
  Connective tissue disorders
  Select genes and single nucleotide polymorphisms
Environmental Factors
  Diet
  Smoking (CD)
Immune defects
  Altered host susceptibility
  Immune-mediated mucosal damage
Psychological factors
  Stress
  Emotional or physical trauma
  Occupation

presentation. The peak incidence occurs in the second or third decades of life, with a second peak occurring between 60 and 80 years of age.[1,2] A high incidence of UC (4 to 5 times normal) occurs in Ashkenazi Jews, while blacks and Asians have a relatively low incidence of occurrence.[2,5,6]

ETIOLOGY

❶ Although the exact etiology of UC and CD is unknown, similar factors are believed responsible for both conditions (Table 41–1). The major theories of the cause of IBD involve a combination of infectious, genetic, and immunologic factors.[7] The inflammatory response with IBD may indicate abnormal regulation of the normal immune response or an autoimmune reaction to self-antigens. The microflora of the gastrointestinal tract may provide an environmental trigger to activate inflammation.[8] CD has been described as a disorder mediated by T lymphocytes that arise in genetically susceptible individuals as a result of a breakdown in the regulatory constraints on mucosal immune responses to enteric bacteria.[9]

INFECTIOUS FACTORS

Microorganisms are a likely factor in the initiation of inflammation in IBD.[8] However, no definitive infectious cause of IBD has been found, even though the presentation is similar to that caused by some invasive microbial pathogens. Patients with IBDs have increased numbers of surface-adherent and intracellular bacteria.[10] IBD may involve a loss of tolerance toward normal bacterial flora.[11] Other supporting evidence for an infectious etiology is that colitis does not appear to occur in genetically altered germ-free animals, intestinal lesions in IBD typically predominate in areas of highest bacterial exposure, and observed differences in the existing makeup of the resident luminal and muscosal bacterial flora in healthy subjects versus those with IBD.[8]

Suspect infectious agents include the measles virus, protozoans, mycobacteria such as *Mycobacterium paratuberculosis* or *avium*, and other bacteria such as *Listeria monocytogenes, Chlamydia trachomatis,* and *Escherichia coli.*[3,12] *Clostridium difficile* infection may lead to increases in frequency of relapses and enhanced severity of IBD.[3] Also, certain strains of bacteria produce toxins (necrotoxins, hemolysins, and enterotoxins) that cause mucosal damage. Bacteria elaborate peptides (e.g., formyl-methonyl-leucyl-phenylalanine) that have chemotactic properties and that cause an influx of inflammatory cells with subsequent release of inflammatory mediators and tissue destruction. Microbes may elaborate superantigens, which are capable of global T-lymphocyte stimulation and subsequent inflammatory response.[13] As many as 60% of patients with CD have circulating antibody to *Saccharomyces cerevisiae,* but this may not represent a disease mechanism.[9]

GENETIC FACTORS

Genetic factors predispose patients to IBDs, particularly CD. In studies of monozygotic twins, there has been a high concordance rate, with both individuals of the pair having an IBD (particularly CD).[9] Also, first-degree relatives of patients with IBD may have up to a 20-fold increase in the risk of disease.[10] Several genetic markers have been identified that occur more frequently for patients with IBD. The CARD15 gene on chromosome 16, formerly referred to as NOD2, is thought to account for 20% of the genetic predisposition to CD. Likewise, polymorphisms of the interleukin 23 receptor (IL23R) are strongly associated with CD and possibly UC.[15–17] Human leukocyte antigen (HLA) DR2 has been associated with UC in Japanese subjects, while HLA DR3 has been associated with UC in European subjects.[12,14] Additionally the multidrug resistance gene 1 (ABCB/MDR 1) on chromosome 7 has been identified as a potential susceptibility gene for UC.[15] As methods for identifying genetic variations have advanced, many other genes and single nucleotide polymorphisms have been associated with IBD, including DLG5, OCTN1, LC22A4, and CARD4, among others.[12,14,16,17] This represents an intense area of research focus as identifying means to alter or prevent the disease process.

IMMUNOLOGIC MECHANISMS

The immune system is known to play a critical role in the underlying pathogenesis of IBD. In CD the bowel wall is infiltrated with lymphocytes, plasma cells, mast cells, macrophages, and neutrophils. Similar infiltration has been observed in the mucosal layer of the colon in patients with UC. Inflammation in IBD is maintained by an influx of leukocytes from the vascular system into sites of active disease. This influx is promoted by expression of adhesion molecules (such as α_4 integrins) on the surface of endothelial cells in the microvasculature in the area of inflammation.[11,18] Many of the systemic manifestations of IBD have an immunologic etiology (e.g., arthritis or uveitis). Finally, IBD is typically responsive to immunosuppressive drugs (e.g., corticosteroids and azathioprine).

The immune theory of IBD assumes that IBD is caused by an inappropriate reaction of the immune system. Potential immunologic mechanisms include both autoimmune and nonautoimmune phenomena.[10,17] Autoimmunity may be directed against mucosal epithelial cells or against neutrophil cytoplasmic elements. Some patients with IBD have abnormal structural features of colonic epithelial cells even in the absence of active disease. Autoantibodies to these structures have been reported. Also, antineutrophil cytoplasmic antibodies are found in a high percentage of patients with UC (70%) and much less frequently with CD.[10] Presence of antineutrophil cytoplasmic antibodies in left-sided UC is associated with resistance to medical therapy.[19] Dysregulation of cytokines is a component of IBD. Specifically, Th_1 cytokine activity (which enhances cell-mediated immunity and suppresses humoral immunity) is excessive with CD, whereas Th_2 cytokine activity (which inhibits cell-mediated immunity and enhances humoral immunity) is excessive with UC.[17,20] The result is that patients have inappropriate T-cell responses to antigens from their own intestinal microflora.[17,20] The IL23 pathway has also been implicated in clonal expansion of Th_{17} cells, which produce various proinflammatory cytokines.[17] Expression of interferon-γ (a Th_1 derived cytokine) in intestinal mucosa of diseased patients is increased, while IL-4 (a Th2-derived cytokine) is reduced.[7,21]

Tumor necrosis factor-α (TNF-α) is a pivotal proinflammatory cytokine in both CD and UC. TNF-α can recruit inflammatory cells to inflamed tissues, activate coagulation, and promote the formation of granulomas. Production of TNF-α is increased in the mucosa and intestinal lumen of patients with CD.[7,10,21] Eicosanoids such as leukotriene B$_4$ are increased in rectal dialysates and tissues of IBD patients and are related to disease activity. Leukotriene B$_4$ enhances neutrophil adherence to vascular endothelium and acts as a neutrophil chemoattractant. These findings have led to the consideration of leukotriene inhibitor strategies for therapy.

PSYCHOLOGICAL FACTORS

Mental health changes appear to possibly correlate with remissions and exacerbations, especially of UC, but psychological factors overall are not thought to be an etiologic factor. There is a weak association between the number of stressful events experienced and the time to relapse of UC.[22,23]

DIET, SMOKING, AND NONSTEROIDAL ANTIINFLAMMATORY DRUG (NSAID) USE

Changes in diet by people in industrialized countries where CD is more common have not been consistently associated with the disease. Studies of increased intake of refined sugars or chemical food additives and reduced fiber intake have provided conflicting results regarding risk for CD. Smoking plays an important but contrasting role in UC and CD.

Smoking appears to be protective for UC.[10] The risk of developing UC in smokers is about 40% of that in nonsmokers.[2] Clinical relapses are associated with smoking cessation, and nicotine transdermal administration has been effective in improving symptoms for patients with UC.[24] In contrast, smoking is associated with a twofold increased frequency of CD.[2] Patients with CD who stop smoking have a more benign course than patients who continue smoking.[25] The mechanisms of these differing effects have not been identified.

Use of NSAIDs may trigger disease occurrence or lead to disease flares.[10,23,26] The effect of NSAIDs to inhibit prostaglandin production through cyclooxygenase inhibition may impair mucosal barrier protective mechanisms. The increased risk seems to be present for cyclooxygenase-2 inhibitors as well as cyclooxygenase-1 inhibitors; however, it is unclear whether cyclooxygenase-2 inhibitors may be somewhat safer in select patients with IBD.[27,28] The use of NSAIDs may be warranted in some patients with IBD, particularly those with concomitant arthritic symptoms, if the benefit is thought to outweigh the potential risk of disease flare.[23]

PATHOPHYSIOLOGY

UC and CD differ in two general respects: anatomic sites and depth of involvement within the bowel wall. There is, however, overlap between the two conditions, with a small fraction of patients showing features of both diseases. Confusion can occur, particularly when the inflammatory process is limited to the colon. Table 41-2 compares pathologic and clinical findings of the two diseases.

ULCERATIVE COLITIS

❷ UC is confined to the rectum and colon and affects the mucosa and the submucosa. In some instances, a short segment of terminal ileum may be inflamed; this is referred to as *backwash ileitis*. Unlike CD, the deeper longitudinal muscular layers, serosa, and regional

TABLE 41-2	Comparison of the Clinical and Pathologic Features of Crohn's Disease and Ulcerative Colitis	
Feature	**Crohn's Disease**	**Ulcerative Colitis**
Clinical		
Malaise, fever	Common	Uncommon
Rectal bleeding	Common	Common
Abdominal tenderness	Common	May be present
Abdominal mass	Common	Absent
Abdominal pain	Common	Unusual
Abdominal wall and internal fistulas	Common	Absent
Distribution	Discontinuous	Continuous
Aphthous or linear ulcers	Common	Rare
Pathologic		
Rectal involvement	Rare	Common
Ileal involvement	Very common	Rare
Strictures	Common	Rare
Fistulas	Common	Rare
Transmural involvement	Common	Rare
Crypt abscesses	Rare	Very common
Granulomas	Common	Rare
Linear clefts	Common	Rare
Cobblestone appearance	Common	Absent

lymph nodes are not usually involved.[1,10,11] Fistulas, perforation, or obstruction are uncommon because inflammation is usually confined to the mucosa and submucosa.

The primary lesion of UC occurs in the crypts of the mucosa (crypts of Lieberkuhn) in the form of a crypt abscess. Here, frank necrosis of the epithelium occurs; it is usually visible only with microscopy but may be seen grossly when coalescence of ulcers occurs. Extension and coalescence ulcers may surround areas of uninvolved mucosa. These islands of mucosa are called *pseudopolyps*. Other typical ulceration patterns include a "collar-button ulcer," which results from extensive submucosal undermining at the ulcer edge.[10,29,30] The extensive mucosal damage seen in UC can result in significant diarrhea and bleeding, although a small percentage of patients experience constipation.

❸ UC can be accompanied by complications that may be local (involving the colon or rectum) or systemic (not directly associated with the colon). With either type the complications may be mild, serious, or even life threatening. Local complications occur in the majority of UC patients. Other complications include hemorrhoids, anal fissures, or perirectal abscesses and are more likely to be present during active colitis. Enteroenteric fistulas are rare.

A major complication is toxic megacolon, which is a segmental or total colonic distension of greater than 6 cm with acute colitis and signs of systemic toxicity.[31] It is a severe condition that occurs in up to 7.9% of UC patients admitted to hospitals and results in death rates of up to 50%. With toxic megacolon, ulceration extends below the submucosa, sometimes even reaching the serosa. Vasculitis, swelling of the vascular endothelium, and thrombosis of small arteries occur; involvement of the muscularis propria causes loss of colonic tone, which leads to dilatation and potential perforation. The patient with toxic megacolon usually has a high fever, tachycardia, distended abdomen, and elevated white blood cell count, and a dilated colon is observed on x-ray.[7,31] Colonic perforation, however, may occur with or without toxic megacolon and is a greater risk with the first attack. Another infrequent major local complication is massive colonic hemorrhage. Colonic stricture, sometimes with clinical obstruction, may also complicate long-standing UC.

The risk of colonic carcinoma is much greater for patients with UC as compared with the general population and begins to increase

10 to 15 years after the diagnosis of UC. The absolute risk may be as high as 30% 35 years after diagnosis and as high as 49% for patients who have a long history of disease and who were less than 15 years of age at the time of diagnosis.

The inflammatory response seen in IBD has also been blamed for the systemic complications seen in both CD and UC. The systemic extraintestinal complications of UC are summarized in the next section.

Hepatobiliary Complications

Approximately 11% of patients with UC are reported to have hepatobiliary complications with overall frequencies ranging from 5% to 95% for patients with IBD.[32-35] Hepatic complications include fatty liver, pericholangitis, chronic active hepatitis, and cirrhosis. Biliary complications include primary sclerosing cholangitis, cholangiocarcinoma, and gallstones.

Fatty infiltration of the liver may be a result of malabsorption, protein-losing enteropathy, or concomitant steroid use. The most common hepatic complication is pericholangitis (acute inflammation surrounding the intrahepatic portal venules, bile ducts, and lymphatics), which occurs in up to one third of UC patients. This is associated with progressive fibrosis of intrahepatic and extrahepatic bile ducts in a small percentage of UC patients and is referred to as *primary sclerosing cholangitis*. Cirrhosis may be a sequela of cholangitis or of chronic active hepatitis. Often the severity of hepatic disease does not correlate with gastrointestinal disease activity.

Gallstones occur commonly for patients with CD (particularly with terminal ileal disease) and may be related to bile salt malabsorption. In addition, cholangiocarcinoma occurs 10 to 20 times more frequently in IBD patients as compared with the general population.[32]

Joint Complications

Arthritis commonly occurs in IBD patients and is typically asymmetric (unlike rheumatoid arthritis) and migratory, involving one or a few usually large joints.[32,34,35] The joints most often affected are the knees, hips, ankles, wrists, and elbows in decreasing frequency. Sacroiliitis also occurs commonly. Arthritis associated with UC is generally related to the severity of colonic disease, and resolution without recurrence is seen with proctocolectomy. In addition, arthritis in this setting is different from rheumatoid arthritis in that rheumatoid factors are generally not detected. It is nondeforming and nondestructive, even after multiple episodes.

Another potential joint complication is ankylosing spondylitis, which is often unresponsive to treatment. The incidence of ankylosing spondylitis in patients with UC is 30 times that of the general population and occurs most commonly for patients with the HLA-B27 phenotype.

Ocular Complications

Ocular complications including iritis, uveitis, episcleritis, and conjunctivitis occur in up to 10% of patients with IBD.[32,34,35] The most commonly reported symptoms with iritis and uveitis include blurred vision, eye pain, and photophobia. Episcleritis is associated with scleral injection, burning, and increased secretions. These complications may parallel the severity of intestinal disease, and recurrence after colectomy with UC is uncommon.

Dermatologic and Mucosal Complications

Skin and mucosal lesions associated with IBD include erythema nodosum, pyoderma gangrenosum, and aphthous ulceration. Five percent to 10% of IBD patients experience dermatologic or mucosal complications.[1,34,35]

Raised, red, tender nodules that vary in size from 1 cm to several centimeters are manifestations of erythema nodosum. They are typically found on the tibial surfaces of the legs and arms. These lesions are more commonly observed in CD patients and are noted to correlate with disease severity.

Pyoderma gangrenosum occurs more commonly for patients with UC (1% to 5% incidence) and is characterized by discrete skin ulcerations that have a necrotic center and a violaceous color of the surrounding skin.[34] They can be seen on any part of the body but are more commonly found on the lower extremities.

Oral lesions are found in 6% to 20% of patients with CD and 8% of patients with UC.[31] The most common lesion seen with CD is aphthous stomatitis. The severity of these lesions tends to parallel the disease course.

CROHN'S DISEASE

Crohn's disease is best characterized as a transmural inflammatory process. The terminal ileum is the most common site of the disorder, but it may occur in any part of the GI tract from mouth to anus. About two thirds of patients have some colonic involvement, and 15% to 25% of patients have only colonic disease.[10,13] Patients often have normal bowel separating segments of diseased bowel; that is, the disease is discontinuous.

Regardless of the site, bowel wall injury is extensive and the intestinal lumen is often narrowed. The mesentery first becomes thickened, edematous, and then fibrotic. Ulcers tend to be deep and elongated and extend along the longitudinal axis of the bowel, at least into the submucosa. The "cobblestone" appearance of the bowel wall results from deep mucosal ulceration intermingled with nodular submucosal thickening.

Complications of CD may involve the intestinal tract or organs unrelated to it. Small bowel stricture and subsequent obstruction is a complication that may require surgery. Fistula formation is common and occurs much more frequently than with UC.[12] Fistulas often occur in the areas of worst inflammation, where loops of bowel have become matted together by fibrous adhesions. Fistulas may connect a segment of the GI tract to skin (enterocutaneous fistula), two segments of the GI tract (enteroenteric fistula), or the intestinal tract with the bladder (enterovesicular fistula) or vagina. CD fistulae or abscesses associated with them frequently require surgical treatment.

Bleeding with CD is usually not as severe as with UC, although patients with CD may have hypochromic anemia. In addition, as with UC, the risk of carcinoma is increased but not as greatly as with UC.

Systemic complications of CD are common, and similar to those found with UC. Arthritis, iritis, skin lesions, and liver disease often accompany CD. Renal stones occur in up to 10% of patients with CD (less frequently with UC) and are caused by fat malabsorption, which allows for greater oxalate absorption and formation of calcium oxalate stones. Gallstones also occur with greater frequency in patients with ileitis, possibly because of bile acid malabsorption at the terminal ileum.

Nutritional deficiencies are common with CD.[36,37] Reported frequencies of various nutritional parameters are weight loss, 40% to 80%, up to 90% reported in children at the time of diagnosis; growth failure in children, 15% to 88%; iron deficiency anemia, 39%; vitamin B_{12} deficiency, 18.4%; folate deficiency, 19%; hypoalbuminemia, 17% to 76%; hypokalemia, 33%; and osteomalacia, 36%. There are usually decreased fat stores and lean tissue. Growth failure in children may also be associated with hypozincemia.

TABLE 41-3	Clinical Presentation of Ulcerative Colitis

Signs and symptoms
- Abdominal cramping
- Frequent bowel movements, often with blood in the stool
- Weight loss
- Fever and tachycardia in severe disease
- Blurred vision, eye pain, and photophobia with ocular involvement
- Arthritis
- Raised, red, tender nodules that vary in size from 1 cm to several centimeters

Physical examination
- Hemorrhoids, anal fissures, or perirectal abscesses may be present
- Iritis, uveitis, episcleritis, and conjunctivitis with ocular involvement
- Dermatologic findings with erythema nodosum, pyoderma gangrenosum, or aphthous ulceration

Laboratory tests
- Decreased hematocrit/hemoglobin
- Increased ESR or CRP
- Leukocytosis and hypoalbuminemia with severe disease
- (+) perinuclear antineutrophil cytoplasmic antibodies

CLINICAL PRESENTATION

The patterns of clinical presentation of IBD can vary widely. Patients may have a single acute episode that resolves and does not recur, but most patients experience acute exacerbations after periods of remission. With more severe disease, prolonged illness may occur.

ULCERATIVE COLITIS

Although a typical clinical picture of UC can be described, there is a wide range of presentation, from mild abdominal cramping with frequent small-volume bowel movements to profuse diarrhea (Table 41-3). Most patients with UC experience intermittent bouts of illness after varying intervals with no symptoms. Only a small percentage of patients has continuous unremitting symptoms or a single acute attack with no subsequent symptoms.

❹ Complex disease classifications are generally not used in clinical practice for UC. The arbitrarily determined distinctions of mild, moderate, and severe disease activity are generally used, and these are determined largely by clinical signs and symptoms.[38,39]

Mild: Fewer than 4 stools daily, with or without blood, with no systemic disturbance and a normal erythrocyte sedimentation rate (ESR).

Moderate: More than 4 stools per day but with minimal systemic disturbance.

Severe: More than 6 stools per day with blood, with evidence of systemic disturbance as shown by fever, tachycardia, anemia, or ESR of greater than 30 mm/h.

Fulminant: More than 10 bowel movements per day with continuous bleeding, toxicity, abdominal tenderness, requirement for transfusion, and colonic dilation.

It is also important to determine disease extent; that is, which part of the colon is involved—rectum, descending colon only, or the entire colon. Patients with "distal" disease have inflammation limited to areas distal to the splenic flexure (also referred to as *left-sided* disease), while those with "extensive disease" have inflammation extending proximal to the splenic flexure.[38,39] Likewise, inflammation confined to the rectal area is referred to as *proctitis*, while disease involving the rectum and sigmoid colon is referred to as *proctosigmoiditis*.[29] Inflammation of the majority of the colon is deemed *pancolitis*.

Two thirds of patients with UC have mild disease, which almost always starts in the rectum. Systemic signs and symptoms of the disease (e.g., arthritis, uveitis, or pyoderma gangrenosum) may be present in these patients and, in fact, may be the reason the patient seeks medical attention. Patients with mild disease are believed to be at lower risk of colon cancer. Moderate disease is observed in one fourth of patients.

With severe disease, the patient is usually found to be in acute distress, has profuse bloody diarrhea, and often has a high fever with leukocytosis and hypoalbuminemia. Often, the patient is dehydrated and therefore may be tachycardic and hypotensive. This presentation may have a sudden onset with rapid progression.

The diagnosis of UC is made on clinical suspicion and confirmed by biopsy, stool examinations, sigmoidoscopy or colonoscopy, or barium radiographic contrast studies. The presence of extracolonic manifestations such as arthritis, uveitis, and pyoderma gangrenosum may also aid in establishing the diagnosis.[38]

CROHN'S DISEASE

As with UC, the presentation of CD is highly variable. A single episode may not be followed by further episodes, or the patient may experience continuous, unremitting disease. The time between the onset of complaints and the initial diagnosis may be as long as 3 years. The patient typically presents with diarrhea and abdominal pain. Hematochezia occurs in about one half of the patients with colonic involvement and much less frequently when there is no colonic involvement. Commonly, a patient may first present with a perirectal or perianal lesion (Table 41-4). The diagnosis should also be suspected in children with growth retardation, especially with abdominal complaints.

Much like UC, guidelines classify the severity of active CD by the presence of several signs and symptoms.[40] Patients with mild to moderate CD are typically ambulatory and have no evidence of dehydration, systemic toxicity, loss of body weight, or abdominal tenderness, mass, or obstruction. Moderate to severe disease is considered for patients who fail to respond to treatment for mild to moderate disease or those with fever, weight loss, abdominal pain or tenderness, vomiting, intestinal obstruction, or significant anemia. Severe to fulminant CD is classified as the presence of persistent symptoms or evidence of systemic toxicity despite corticosteroid or biologic treatment or presence of cachexia, rebound tenderness, intestinal obstruction, or abscess. Disease activity may be assessed and correlated by evaluation serum C-reactive protein (CRP) concentrations.

The course of CD is characterized by periods of remission and exacerbation. Some patients may be free of symptoms for years, while others experience chronic problems in spite of medical therapy. As with UC, the diagnosis of CD involves a thorough evaluation using laboratory, endoscopic, and radiologic testing to detect the extent and characteristic features of the disease. Because of similarities that may exist between UC and CD confined to

TABLE 41-4	Clinical Presentation of Crohn's Disease

Signs and symptoms
- Malaise and fever
- Abdominal pain
- Frequent bowel movements
- Hemotachezia
- Fistula
- Weight loss and malnutrition
- Arthritis

Physical examination
- Abdominal mass and tenderness
- Perianal fissure or fistula

Laboratory tests
- Increased white blood cell count, ESR, and CRP
- (+) anti–Saccharomyces cerevisiae antibodies

the colon, a definitive diagnosis cannot be made in up to 15% of cases, even with pathologic specimens in hand. These patients may be referred to as *indeterminate colitis*. Small bowel involvement, strictures detected on radiographs, and presence of fistulas are characteristic of CD.

TREATMENT

Inflammatory Bowel Disease

■ DESIRED OUTCOME

⑤ To treat IBD properly, the clinician must have a clear concept of realistic therapeutic goals for each patient. These goals may relate to resolution of acute inflammatory processes, resolution of attendant complications (e.g., fistulas and abscesses), alleviation of systemic manifestations (e.g., arthritis), maintenance of remission from acute inflammation, or surgical palliation or cure. Treatment goals and the approach to the therapeutic regimen differ considerably between UC and CD.

When determining goals of therapy and selecting therapeutic regimens, it is important to understand the natural history of IBD.[40] Some cases of acute UC are self-limited. With mild to moderate acute colitis without systemic symptoms, 20% of patients may experience spontaneous improvement in their disease within a few weeks; however, a small percentage of patients may go on to experience more serious disease. With severe colitis, improvement without treatment cannot be expected. For instance, the response to medical management of toxic megacolon is variable and emergent colectomy may be required. When remission of UC is achieved, it is likely to last at least 1 year with medical therapy. In the absence of medical therapy, one half to two thirds of patients are likely to relapse within 9 months.[39] In some reports, remission rates with placebo have approached those found with active treatment.

Since CD is typified by a chronic relapsing course, approximately 20% of patients with CD will experience a relapse annually.[40] The chance of sustained remission is impacted by response to treatment. If patients remain in remission for 1 year, they have an 80% chance of remaining in remission the subsequent year, while 70% of patients will continue to have active disease in the year following a 12-month period in which they had active disease.[40] Thus inducing and maintaining remission for patients with IBD is an important aspect of treatment.

■ GENERAL APPROACH TO TREATMENT

⑥ Treatment of IBD centers on agents used to relieve the inflammatory process. Aminosalicylates, corticosteroids, antimicrobials, immunosuppressive agents, such as azathioprine, mercaptopurine, and methotrexate, and biologic agents are commonly used to treat active disease and for some agents to lengthen the time of disease remission. Information regarding the extent and distribution of the disease should be taken into account, as this will often dictate the route and formulation of drug therapy that will be most effective.

In addition to the use of drugs, surgical procedures are sometimes performed when active disease is inadequately controlled or when the required drug dosages pose an unacceptable risk of adverse effects. For most patients with IBD, nutritional considerations are also important because these patients are often malnourished. Finally, a variety of therapies may be used to address complications or symptoms of IBD. For example, antidiarrheals may be used in some patients with relatively well-controlled disease, although these are generally to be avoided in active moderate to severe UC because they may contribute to the development of toxic colonic

dilatation. Antimicrobial agents may be used in conjunction with drainage when abscesses are present or for patients with perianal disease. Iron supplementation may be required, particularly with UC, where blood loss from the colon can be significant.

■ NONPHARMACOLOGIC THERAPY

Nutritional Support

Proper nutritional support is an important aspect of the treatment of patients with IBD, not because specific types of diets are useful in alleviating the inflammatory conditions but because patients with moderate to severe disease are often malnourished, either because the inflammatory process results in significant malabsorption or maldigestion or because of the catabolic effects of the disease process. Elevated levels of interleukin-6 and TNF-α are known to increase protein turnover, resulting in protein loss and muscle wasting.[37] Malabsorption may occur in the patient with CD with inflammatory involvement of the small bowel, where many nutrients are absorbed, as well as in patients who have undergone multiple small bowel resections with subsequent reduction in absorptive surface ("short gut"). Maldigestion with accompanying diarrhea can occur if there is a bile salt deficiency in the gut.

Many specific diets have been tried to improve the condition of patients with IBD, but none has gained widespread acceptance. With each individual it may be helpful to eliminate specific foods that exacerbate symptoms. This elimination process must be conducted cautiously, as patients have been known to exclude a wide range of nutritious products without adequate justification. Some patients with IBD, although not the majority, have lactase deficiency; therefore, diarrhea may be associated with milk intake. For these patients, avoidance of milk or supplementation with lactase generally improves the patient's symptoms. Patients with small bowel strictures due to CD should avoid excessive high-residue foods, such as citrus fruits and nuts.[1]

The nutritional needs of the majority of patients can be adequately addressed with enteral supplementation.[36] In severe acute UC, enteral nutrition resulted in a significantly greater increase in serum albumin, fewer adverse effects related to the nutritional regimen, and fewer postoperative infections, as compared with isocaloric, isonitrogenous parenteral nutrition.[41] The regimens were similar with regard to remission rate and the need for colectomy. Consideration should be given to lipid administration for its caloric value, as well as in recognition of depleted peripheral fat stores in many IBD patients and the greater potential for fatty acid deficiency. The use of enteral nutrition for patients with CD is preferable, as favorable effects on modulation of proinflammatory cytokine production may lead to enhanced maintenance of nutritional stores and increased growth rates in children.[36,42,43] Likewise, use of enteral nutrition may facilitate induction of remission in up to 60% of patients with active CD and possibly reduce the use of corticosteroids.[36,42,44]

Parenteral nutrition may be used in the treatment of severe CD or UC. The use of parenteral nutrition allows complete bowel rest for patients with severe UC, which may alter the need for proctocolectomy. Parenteral nutrition has also been valuable in CD since remission may be achieved with parenteral nutrition in about 50% of patients.[45] In some patients, the disease may worsen when parenteral nutrition is stopped. Patients who have severe CD may require a course of parenteral nutrition to attain a reasonable nutritional status or in preparation for surgery, as poor perioperative nutritional status is associated with an increased incidence of postoperative complications.[37] Patients with enterocutaneous fistulas of various etiologies benefit from parenteral nutrition.[45] Parenteral nutrition may also be valuable in children or adolescents with growth retardation associated with CD, but surgery is often necessary with severe disease. Home parenteral nutrition may be required for patients requiring long-term therapy, particularly those with "short gut" as a consequence of surgical resection. Lastly, parenteral nutrition is more costly and is associated with more complications, such as serious infections, compared with enteral nutrition. Therefore, use should be limited to those patients for whom enteral nutrition is not preferred or feasible.

There is a growing interest in using probiotic approaches for IBD. Probiotics may lead to reestablishment of normal bacterial flora within the gut by oral administration of live bacteria such as nonpathogenic *Escherichia coli*, bifidobacteria, lactobacilli, or *Streptococcus thermophilus*. Probiotic formulations have been effective in maintaining remission in some trials for patients with UC; however differences in methodology, probiotics used, and underlying treatments for IBD make comparison of trials difficult.[46–48] A formulation of *Bifidiobacterium*, *Lactobacilli*, and *Streptococci* (VSL #3) is marketed specifically for use in UC as an adjunctive therapy and for patients who have a surgically constructed ileal pouch to prevent pouchitits.[47] Review of evidence for the probiotic use in the induction and maintenance of CD has led to recommendations not supporting widespread use, but rather further investigation.[48–52]

Surgery

Even with medical therapy 30% to 40% of patients with UC and 70% to 80% of patients with CD require surgical intervention at some point in their life.[53] Although surgery (proctocolectomy) is curative for UC, this is not the case for CD. Surgical procedures involve resection of segments of intestine that are affected, as well as correction of complications (e.g., fistulas) or drainage of abscesses.

For UC, colectomy may be necessary when the patient has disease uncontrolled by maximum medical therapy or when there are complications of the disease such as colonic perforation, toxic dilatation (megacolon), uncontrolled colonic hemorrhage, or colonic strictures. Colectomy may be indicated for patients with long-standing disease (greater than 8 to 10 years), as a prophylactic measure against the development of cancer, and for patients with premalignant changes (severe dysplasia) on surveillance mucosal biopsies. The most common surgical procedures include proctocolectomy (after which the patient is left with a permanent ileostomy) and abdominal colectomy, with removal of the mucosa of the rectum and anastomosis of an ileal pouch to the anus (ileal pouch-anal anastamosis).[53] The risk from surgery for these patients is relatively low if the operations are performed on a nonemergent basis.

The indications for surgery with CD are not as well established as for UC, and surgery is usually reserved for the complications of the disease. A recognized problem with intestinal resection for CD is the high rate of recurrence. Surgery may be appropriate in well-selected patients who have severe or incapacitating disease or obstruction in spite of aggressive medical management. The surgical procedures performed include resections of the major intestinal areas of involvement. For some patients with severe rectal or perianal disease, particularly abscesses, diversion of the fecal stream is performed with a colostomy. Other indications for surgery include strictures, colon cancer, an inflammatory mass, or intestinal perforations or fistulas.

■ PHARMACOLOGIC THERAPY

Drug therapy plays an integral part in the overall treatment of IBD. None of the drugs used for IBD are curative; at best, they serve to control the disease process. Therefore, a reasonable goal of drug therapy is resolution of disease symptoms such that the patient can carry on normal daily functions. The major types of drug therapy used in IBD include aminosalicylates, corticosteroids, immunosuppressive agents (azathioprine, mercaptopurine, cyclosporine, and methotrexate), antimicrobials (metronidazole and ciprofloxacin), and agents to inhibit TNF-α (anti-TNF-α antibodies) or leukocyte adhesion and migration (natalizumab).

Sulfasalazine, an agent that combines a sulfonamide (sulfapyridine) antibiotic and mesalamine (5-aminosalicylic acid) in the same molecule, has been used for many years to treat IBD but was originally intended to treat arthritis. Sulfasalazine is cleaved by gut bacteria in the colon to sulfapyridine (which is mostly absorbed and excreted in the urine) and mesalamine (which mostly remains in the colon and is excreted in stool).[44,54–56]

The active component of sulfasalazine is mesalamine, and the mechanism of action is not well understood.[44,54–56] Cyclooxygenase or lipoxygenase inhibition alone does not entirely account for the agent's effects. Aminosalicylates may block production of prostaglandins and leukotrienes, inhibit bacterial peptide-induced neutrophil chemotaxis and adenosine-induced secretion, scavenge reactive oxygen metabolites, and inhibit activation of the nuclear regulatory factor NF-κB.[10] Sulfasalazine is often used initially before oral mesalamine derivatives when expense is an issue; however, it is not tolerated as well as the mesalamine alternatives.

Because the mechanism of action of sulfasalazine is not related to the sulfapyridine component and since sulfapyridine is believed to be responsible for many of the adverse reactions to sulfasalazine, mesalamine alone can be used. Mesalamine can be used topically as an enema or suppository for the treatment of proctitis or given orally in slow-release formulations that deliver mesalamine to the small intestine and colon (Table 41–5 and Fig. 41–1). Slow-release

TABLE 41-5	Mesalamine Derivatives for Treatment of Inflammatory Bowel Disease			
Product	**Trade Name(s)**	**Formulation**	**Dose per Day**	**Site of Action**
Sulfasalazine	Azulfidine, Azulfidine Entabs, Sulfazine, Sulfazine EC	Immediate release or enteric coated tablets	4–6 g	Colon
Mesalamine	Rowasa	Enema	1–4 g	Rectum, distal colon
	Asacol, Asacol HD	Mesalamine tablet coated with Eudragit-S (delayed-release acrylic resin)	2.4–4.8 g	Distal ileum and colon
	Pentasa	Mesalamine capsules encapsulated in ethylcellulose microgranules	2–4 g	Small bowel and colon
	Lialda	Mesalamine tablet formulated with MMX delayed-release technology (pH-dependent outer coat with polymeric matrix core); allows for once daily dosing	1.2–4.8 g	Colon
	Apriso	Mesalamine capsule formulated with enteric-coated granules in a delayed-release polymer matrix; allows for once daily dosing	1.5 g	Colon
	Canasa	Mesalamine suppository	500–1000 mg	Rectum
Olsalazine	Dipentum	Dimer of 5-aminosalicylic acid oral capsule	1.5–3 g	Colon
Balsalazide	Colazal	Capsule	6.75 g	Colon

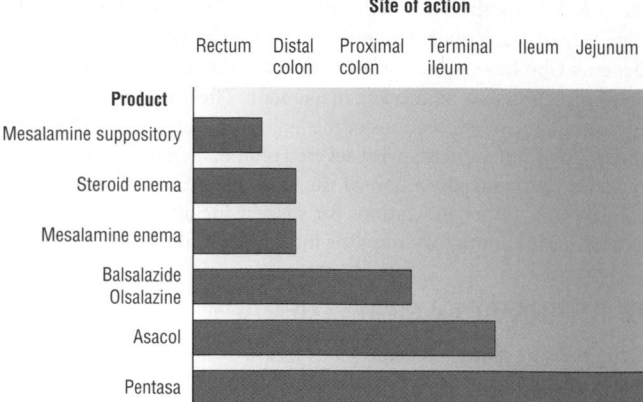

FIGURE 41-1. Site of activity of various agents used to treat inflammatory bowel disease.

oral formulations of mesalamine, such as Pentasa, release mesalamine from the duodenum to the ileum, with up to 59% of the drug passing into the colon.[54] A tablet formulation of mesalamine (Lialda), uses a pH-dependent coating in combination with a polymeric matrix core, and releases drug evenly throughout the colon, also allowing for once daily dosing.[55,56] A once daily capsule formulation of mesalmine (Apriso) utilizes enteric-coated mesalamine granules in a polymer matrix for delayed and extended delivery of mesalamine to the colon.[56] The use of the once daily oral mesalamine preparations may help to enhance adherence thus improving long-term outcomes. Olsalazine is a dimer of two 5-aminosalicylate molecules linked by an azo bond. Mesalamine is released in the colon after colonic bacteria cleave olsalazine. Balsalazide is a mesalamine prodrug that couples mesalamine with the inert carrier molecule 4-aminobenzoyl-B-alanine and is enzymatically cleaved in the colon to release mesalamine. The recommended daily doses of the oral mesalamine derivatives are intended to approximate the molar equivalent of mesalamine present in 4 g of sulfasalazine. Because the oral mesalamine formulations are coated tablets or granules, they should not be crushed or chewed. Unlike sulfasalazine, all of these agents are safe to use for patients with sulfonamide allergies.

Corticosteroids and adrenocorticotropic hormone have been widely used for the treatment of UC and CD, given parenterally, orally, or rectally.[57] Corticosteroids modulate the immune system and inhibit production of cytokines and mediators. It is not clear whether the most important steroid effects are systemic or local (mucosal). Budesonide is a corticosteroid that is administered orally in a controlled-release formulation designed to release in the terminal ileum. The drug undergoes extensive first-pass

metabolism; so systemic exposure is thought to be minimized.[58] Immunosuppressive agents such as azathioprine, mercaptopurine, methotrexate, or cyclosporine are also used for the treatment of IBD (Table 41–6).

Azathioprine and mercaptopurine are effective for long-term treatment of both CD and UC.[39,40,44,59] These agents are generally reserved for patients who are refractory to or dependent upon corticosteroids. They are usually used in conjunction with mesalamine derivatives and/or steroids and must be used for extended periods of time, ranging from a few weeks up to 12 months, before benefits may be observed.[59] Early use of azathioprine in combination with infliximab for patients with CD who are naive to treatment with immunosuppressive agents or corticosteroids improves outcomes versus use of these agents individually.[60]

Azathioprine and mercaptopurine may be associated with serious adverse effects such as lymphomas, pancreatitis, or nephrotoxicity.[59] Predisposition to development of these adverse effects may be related to polymorphisms in the enzyme thiopurine methyl transferase (TPMT), which is partially responsible for activation and metabolism of these drugs.[61] The Food and Drug Administration recommends that patients be tested for TPMT genotype and phenotype or activity prior to initiating therapy to identify patients that may have reduced TPMT activity and thus be at risk for toxicity. Adjusting azathioprine and mercaptopurine doses by measuring concentrations of metabolites, particularly 6-thioguanine (6-TGN), may be useful, with higher levels associated with greater remission rates.[61]

Cyclosporine has also been of short-term benefit in treatment of acute, severe UC when used in a continuous intravenous infusion. Lower dose continuous infusions (2 mg/kg vs 4 mg/kg daily), or oral daily doses of 5 to 6 mg/kg in conjunction with steroids may be an effective option for those with fulminant disease.[62] The agent poses a risk of nephrotoxicity and neurotoxicity. Some studies evaluating tacrolimus for the treatment of IBD suggest a potential role for use for patients with fistulizing CD, for patients unresponsive to steroids or infliximab, or in management of some extraintestinal manifestations.[63] Methotrexate 25 mg given intramuscularly or subcutaneously once weekly is useful for treatment and maintenance of CD and may result in steroid sparing effects, while data supporting use in UC are lacking.[40,64,65]

Antimicrobial agents, particularly metronidazole, are frequently used in attempts to control CD but are not typically useful in UC.[40,52,66] Metronidazole is of value for some patients with active CD, particularly involving the perineal area or when fistulas or abscesses are present.[52,66] Likewise, there may be a role for use of metronidazole in combination with azathioprine to reduce postsurgical recurrence of CD.[52] The mechanism of metronidazole's

TABLE 41-6	Immunomodulator, Immunosuppressive, and Biologic Agents for the Treatment of Inflammatory Bowel Disease		
Product	**Trade Name(s)**	**Indication(s)**[a]	**Dose**
Azathioprine	Imuran, Azasan	CD, UC	1.5–2.5 mg/kg per day orally
Mercaptopurine	Purinethol	CD, UC	1.5–2.5 mg/kg per day orally
Methotrexate	Rheumatrex, Trexall	CD	15–25 mg weekly (IM[a]/SC[a]/orally)
Cyclosporine	Sandimmune	CD, UC	4 mg/kg per day IV[a] continuous infusion
Infliximab	Remicade	CD, UC	Induction: 5 mg/kg IV at 0, 2, and 6 weeks; 10 mg/kg per dose IV for non-responders
			Maintenance: 5 mg/kg IV every 8 weeks
Adalimumab	Humira	CD	Induction: 160 mg SC day 1 (given as four 40 mg injections in 1 day or as two 40 mg injections per day for 2 consecutive days), then 80 mg SC 2 weeks later (day 15)
			Maintenance: 40 mg SC every other week, starting on day 29 of therapy
Certolizumab	Cimzia	CD	Induction: 400mg SC initially, then 400 mg SC at 2 and 4 weeks
			Maintenance: 400 mg SC every 4 weeks if initial response
Natalizumab	Tysabri	CD	Induction/maintenance: 300 mg IV every 4 weeks

[a]CD = Crohn's disease, UC = ulcerative colitis, IV = intravenous, SC = subcutaneous, IM = intramuscular

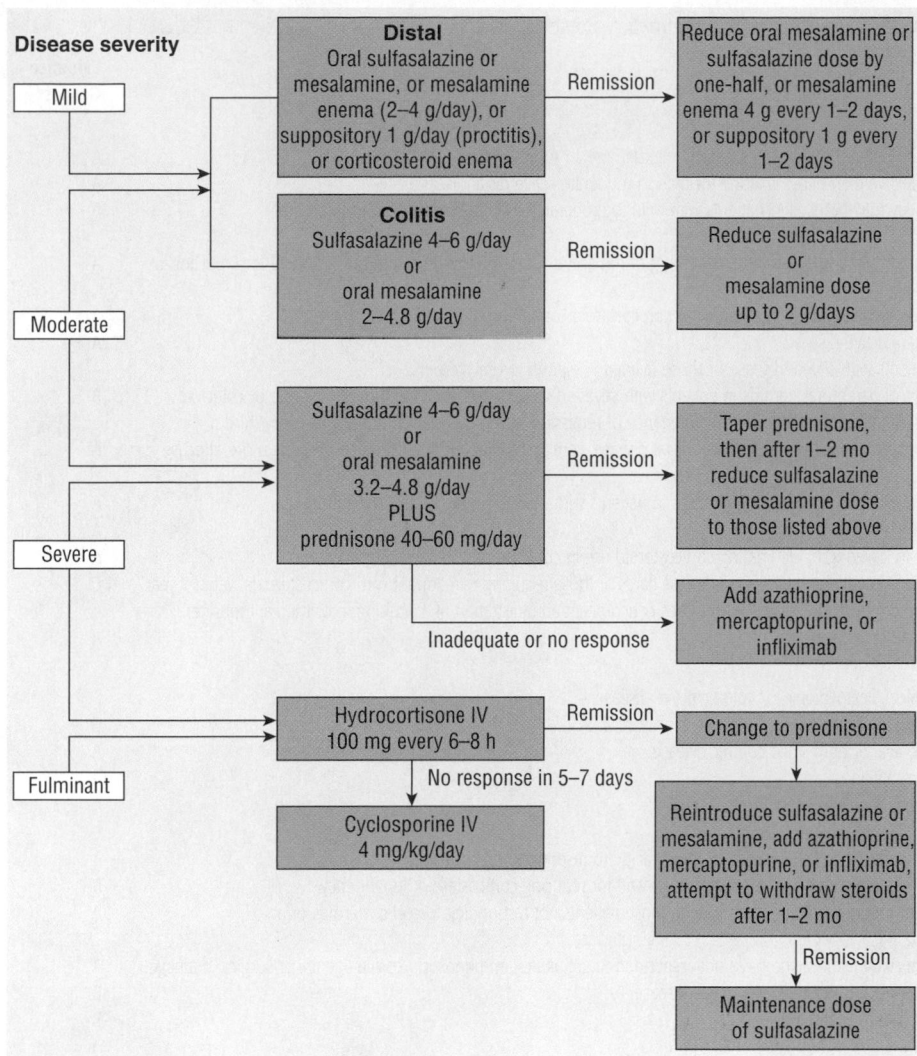

FIGURE 41-2. Treatment approaches for ulcerative colitis.

effect on CD has not been determined but is theorized to relate to interruption of a bacterial role in the inflammatory process. Ciprofloxacin has also been used for treatment of IBD, with some studies demonstrating efficacy for CD when used in combination with metronidazole.[40] Rifaximin, a nonabsorbable antibiotic, has also shown some efficacy in treatment of both UC and CD.[40,52,66]

Three biologic agents are now available for treatment of IBD that target TNF-α.[67] Infliximab is an IgG$_1$ chimeric monoclonal antibody that is administered intravenously and binds TNF-α and inhibits its inflammatory effect in the gut. The agent is useful for moderate to severe active CD and UC disease, as well steroid-dependent or fistulizing disease, as both an induction and maintenance therapy. Adalimumab is also an IgG1 antibody to TNF-α; however, this agent, unlike infliximab, is fully humanized and contains no murine sequences. Theoretically, the lack of a murine component in adalimumab reduces antibody development seen with use of infliximab. This agent can be administered subcutaneously. Adalimumab is a treatment option for patients with moderate to severe active CD previously treated with infliximab who have lost response. Certolizumab pegol is a humanized pegylated Fab fragment directed against TNF-α that is administered subcutaneously and demonstrates similar efficacy to adalimumab and infliximab.[67]

Lastly, natalizumab is a novel biologic agent that inhibits leukocyte adhesion and migration by targeting α_4 integrin.[18,67] This agent can be used in the treatment of CD for patients who are unresponsive to other therapies, including corticosteroids and TNF-α inhibitors.

Ulcerative Colitis

Mild to Moderate Disease Most patients with active UC that have mild to moderate disease can be managed on an outpatient basis with oral or topical (rectal) therapies (Fig. 41–2, Table 41–7). The first line of drug therapy for patients with extensive disease is oral sulfasalazine or an oral mesalamine derivative.[39] Topical mesalamine in an enema or suppository formulation is more effective than oral mesalamine or topical steroids for distal disease.[29,39] The combination of oral and topical mesalamine is more effective than either alone for active distal disease.[29,39,68,69] When given orally, usually 4 to 6 g/day, and possibly up to 8 g/day, of sulfasalazine is required to attain control of active inflammation. There does not appear to be an increased rate of response with increased dosage over 6 g/day, although side effects increase. Even with the use of adequate doses, patient improvement usually takes 4 weeks and sometimes longer.[39] The dosage of sulfasalazine that can be given is usually limited by the patient's tolerance of the agent; most adverse effects of sulfasalazine are dose related (GI disturbances, headache, and arthralgia).[38] Sulfasalazine therapy should be instituted at 500 mg/day and increased every few days up to 4 g/day or the maximum tolerated. It should not be used for patients with allergy to sulfonamide-containing drugs.

TABLE 41-7 Levels of Evidence for Therapeutic Interventions in Inflammatory Bowel Disease

Interventions	Evidence Grades[a]
Ulcerative colitis	
Mild to moderate active distal disease may be treated with oral aminosalicylates, topical mesalamine, or topical steroids.	A
Combined oral and topical aminosalicylates are more effective than either is alone for mild to moderate active distal disease.	A
Oral prednisone in doses of 40–60 mg/day or 1 mg/kg/day may be used in patients with mild to moderate distal disease unresponsive to oral or topical aminosalicylates.	B
Sulfasalazine in doses of 4–6 g/day or an alternate aminosalicylate in doses of up to 4.8 g/g of the active 5-aminosalicylate moiety are effective for induction of mild to moderate extensive colitis.	A
Infliximab is effective for moderate to severe disease in those patients not responding to corticosteroids or an immunosuppressive agent.	A
Systemic corticosteroids are effective in moderate to severe active disease.	A
Hospitalization for parenteral steroids is indicated for patients with severe disease or those failing to respond to oral steroids.	A
Failure to demonstrate improvement following 7–10 days of parenteral steroids in patients with severe disease is an indication for cyclosporine or colectomy; mesalamine suppositories (proctitis) and enemas (distal colitis) are effective in maintenance of remission with doses as infrequently as every third night.	B
Sulfasalazine, mesalamine, or balsalazide are effective in maintenance of remission of distal disease; combining oral and topical mesalamine is more effective than is either alone.	A
Sulfasalazine, olsalazine, mesalamine, and balsalazide are effective in preventing relapses in patients with mild to moderate extensive disease.	A
Corticosteroids are not effective as maintenance treatment.	A
Azathioprine, mercaptopurine, or infliximab are effective in lowering or eliminating corticosteroid use in corticosteroid-dependent patients.	A
Azathioprine, mercaptopurine, or infliximab may be effective in patients with severe disease flares or those requiring retreatment with corticosteroids within 1 year.	C
Oral cyclosporine is effective for patients with corticosteroid refractory disease but requires concomitant administration of azathioprine or mercaptopurine.	C
Infliximab therapy is effective for maintenance if there is an initial response.	A
Crohn's disease	
Oral aminosalicylates are effective for mild to moderate ileal, ilealocolonic, or colonic active disease.	D
Metronidazole may be effective in patients not responding to sulfasalazine.	D
Ileal release budesonide is effective for mild to moderate ileal or right-sided colonic disease.	A
Topical hydrocortisone is effective for distal colonic inflammation.	A
Systemic corticosteroids are effective in moderate to severe active disease.	A
Systemic corticosteroids are not effective for patients with perianal fistulas.	C
Hospitalization for parenteral steroids is indicated for patients with severe disease or those failing to respond to oral steroids.	A
Parenteral methotrexate is effective for induction of remission in patients with active disease and for reducing corticosteroid dependency.	B
Infliximab, adalimumab, and certolizumab are effective for moderate to severe disease in those patients not responding to corticosteroids or an immunosuppressive agent.	A
Infliximab and adalimumab are effective for those patients with fistulas who have not responded to antibiotics, immunosuppressive agents, or surgical drainage.	A
High-dose oral cyclosporine (7.6 mg/kg) has short-term efficacy in patients with active disease.	B
Intravenous cyclosporine is effective for the treatment of fistulizing disease.	B
Corticosteroids are not effective as maintenance treatment.	A
Budesonide is effective as short-term maintenance therapy (3 months) but not long term.	A
Azathioprine, mercaptopurine, or infliximab are effective in lowering or eliminating corticosteroid use in corticosteroid-dependent patients.	A
Azathioprine, mercaptopurine, or infliximab may be effective in patients with severe disease flares or those requiring retreatment with corticosteroids within 1 year.	A
Azathioprine or mercaptopurine is effective for maintenance of remission regardless of disease distribution.	A
Azathioprine or mercaptopurine may be effective for treating perianal or enteric fistulae.	C
Methotrexate maintenance therapy (15–25 mg IM weekly) is effective for patients whose active disease has responded to IM methotrexate.	A
Methotrexate 25 mg IM for up to 16 weeks followed by 15 mg IM weekly is effective for patients with chronic active disease.	A
Infliximab, adalimumab, and certolizumab therapy is effective for maintenance if there is an initial response.	A

[a]A, Homogenous evidence from multiple well-designed, randomized (therapeutic) or cohort (descriptive) controlled trials, each involving a number of participants to be of sufficient statistical power; B, evidence from at least 1 large well-designed clinical trial with or without randomization from cohort or case control analytic studies or well-designed metaanalysis; C, evidence based on clinical experience, descriptive studies, or reports of expert committees; D, not rated.
From references 29, 36, 40, and 76.

Oral mesalamine derivatives (such as those listed in Table 41–5) are reasonable alternatives to sulfasalazine for treatment of mild to moderate UC. Oral mesalamine products are used for patients with extensive disease, while topical agents, such as enemas and suppositories, are used for distal disease. Mesalamine is more effective than placebo but no more effective than sulfasalazine for extensive disease.[70,71] Mesalamine preparations are typically better tolerated, and the majority of patients intolerant to sulfasalazine or topical steroids should tolerate one of the other oral mesalamine derivatives.[38,39] Dose-related effects do exist, and when used orally for active extensive disease, the equivalent of 4.8 g of the active 5-aminosalicylic acid moiety should be administered when possible.[39,70,71] Studies comparing daily doses of 2.4 g versus 4.8 g of mesalamine (Asacol formulation) for patients with moderate active UC demonstrated greater efficacy at 6 weeks of therapy (58% vs 72%, *P* <0.05).[68,72,73] While the dosage range for Pentasa is 2 to 4 g/day, 4 g/day appears to be more effective.[70] Olsalazine is effective for treatment of mild to moderate UC, however, 15% to 25% of patients taking olsalazine experience severe diarrhea, often necessitating discontinuation of the drug. This results from a direct osmotic effect of the drug to induce small bowel fluid secretion. For this reason it is not the drug of first choice.[39] Balsalazide is effective for treatment of mild to moderate UC.[74,75] The new once daily formulations of mesalamine offer similar efficacy in mild to moderate UC with the benefit of once daily dosing and potentially lower pill burden.[55,56] When used topically, mesalamine suppositories will only reach to approximately 10 to 20 cm with the lower GI tract and therefore should be reserved for patients with proctitis. Enema formulations will reach to the splenic flexure and therefore can be used for distal disease.[29,39]

Moderate to Severe Disease ❼ Systemic corticosteroids have a place in the treatment of moderate to severe active UC regardless of disease location or of those patients who are unresponsive to maximal doses of oral and/or topical mesalamine derivatives.[39,76] Oral steroids (usually up to 1 mg/kg per day of prednisone equivalent or 40 to 60 mg daily) may be used for patients who do not have an adequate response to sulfasalazine or mesalamine.[39] The response to steroids may be evident sooner than sulfasalazine or the aminosalicylates. Oral steroids should not be used as initial therapy for mild to moderate UC, mainly because of the known risks of steroid use. If steroids are used to attain remission, tapered drug withdrawal should be accomplished to minimize long-term steroid exposure.

Topically administered steroids given as suppositories, enemas, or foams can be used as initial therapy for patients with ulcerative proctitis or distal colitis. Topical agents are also beneficial for treatment of tenesmus. With these agents, local actions are believed to be responsible for drug effects. Topical steroids are effective in the treatment of active, distal UC. However, rectal mesalamine is more effective than rectal steroids for inducing remission.[29,39,68,69,76]

Infliximab is another viable option for patients with moderate to severe active UC who are unresponsive to steroids or other immunosuppressive agents.[67,68,76,77] For outpatients with moderately active UC, infliximab demonstrated response rates of up to 69% at 8 weeks following initial doses of 5 mg/kg.[78] Studies in hospitalized patients have shown mixed results, with some demonstrating reduced rates of colectomy for patients receiving infliximab.[67,77,79,80]

Nicotine has been proposed as a treatment for UC (but not as a treatment for CD) based on the observation of the onset of a flare of UC after smoking cessation in some individuals. While less effective than aminosalicylates, transdermal nicotine in daily doses of 15 to 25 mg may improve symptoms for patients with mild to moderate active UC, particularly for patients who are ex-smokers, and can be considered as an adjunctive therapy in both distal and extensive disease.[24,29,39,81]

Severe or Fulminant Disease Patients with uncontrolled severe colitis or who have incapacitating symptoms require hospitalization for effective management. Under these conditions, patients generally receive nothing by mouth to put the bowel at rest. Most medication is given by the parenteral route. Sulfasalazine or mesalamine derivatives are not beneficial for treatment of severe colitis because of rapid elimination of these agents from the colon with diarrhea, thereby not allowing sufficient time for gut bacteria to cleave the molecules. It is difficult to evaluate drugs in this setting, because patients with severe disease almost always receive additional medications including steroids.

Steroids have been valuable in the treatment of severe disease because the use of these agents may allow some patients to avoid colectomy. Intravenous hydrocortisone 300 to 400 mg daily in three divided doses or methylprednisolone 48 to 60 mg once daily are considered first-line agents.[39,76] Methylprednisolone is typically preferred due to its lesser mineralocorticoid effects. A trial of steroids is warranted in most patients before proceeding to colectomy, unless the condition is grave or rapidly deteriorating. The length of the medical trial before consideration of surgery is open to debate. Steroids increase surgical risk, particularly infectious risk, if an operation is required later. After a colectomy is performed, steroids should no longer be required for the disease; however, they must be withdrawn gradually (usually over 3 to 4 weeks) to avoid hypoadrenal crisis due to adrenal suppression.

❽ Patients who are unresponsive to parenteral corticosteroids after 7 to 10 days should receive cyclosporine by intravenous infusion. Seventy percent to 80% of hospitalized patients who are unresponsive to corticosteroids will respond to cyclosporine.[62]

Continuous intravenous infusion of cyclosporine (4 mg/kg per day) is typically effective in steroid-resistant acute severe UC and may reduce the need for emergent colectomy.[62,82] Intravenous cyclosporine has also been recommended as an alternative to steroids for patients with severe attacks of UC (fulminant colitis).[83] Patients who are controlled on intravenous cyclosporine can then be switched to an oral cyclosporine taper regimen with subsequent transition to azathioprine or mercaptopurine.[76] As mentioned earlier, infliximab is also an alternative to cyclosporine and may also deter the need for colectomy for patients with severe disease not responsive to steroids.[67,76–79]

Maintenance of Remission

❾ After remission from active disease is achieved, the goal of therapy is to then maintain remission. The major agents used for maintenance of remission are sulfasalazine and the mesalamine derivatives.[70,84] The value of sulfasalazine in preventing recurrences has been documented in several placebo-controlled trials.[84] Sulfasalazine, most commonly dosed at 2 g/day, was superior to mesalamine when using the main end point of failure to maintain endoscopic or clinical remission [OR 1.29 (95% CI, 1.05-1.57)].[84] Sulfasalazine also appears to be more effective in maintaining remission compared with the newer agents, such as olsalazine.

For patients with distal disease or proctitis, mesalamine enemas or suppositories are considered first-line agents.[29,39,69] The frequency of administration of topical agents may possibly be lessened to every third night over time. Oral agents, including sulfasalazine, mesalamine, and balsalazide, are also effective options if patients do not wish to use topical preparations.[29,39,69] The combination of topical and oral mesalamine is superior to either regimen alone for maintenance therapy.

CLINICAL CONTROVERSY

A major question about the use of aminosalicylates for maintenance of remission of UC is whether they reduce the patient's risk of developing colorectal cancer. It has been suggested that mesalamine, in doses >1.2 g/day, is protective against the development of colorectal cancer; however, this is not entirely supported by controlled trials. Given the often slow development of colorectal cancer and the relapsing nature of UC, these significantly limit the ability to conduct long-term surveillance studies for patients in remission.

Steroids do not have a role in the maintenance of remission with UC because they are ineffective.[39] Steroids should be gradually withdrawn after remission is induced (over 3 to 4 weeks). If they are continued, the patient will be at risk for steroid-induced adverse effects without likelihood of benefits. For patients who require chronic steroid use (steroid dependency), there is a strong justification for alternative therapies or colectomy. Azathioprine is effective in preventing relapse of UC for periods exceeding 4 years.[59,72,76,85] However, 3 to 6 months may be required before beneficial effects are noted. For patients who initially respond to infliximab, continued dosing of 5 mg/kg as maintenance therapy every 8 weeks is another alternative for corticosteroid-dependent patients or those failing immunosuppressive therapy.[67,76,77]

▪ CROHN'S DISEASE

Management of CD often proves more difficult than management of UC, partly because of the greater complexity of presentation with

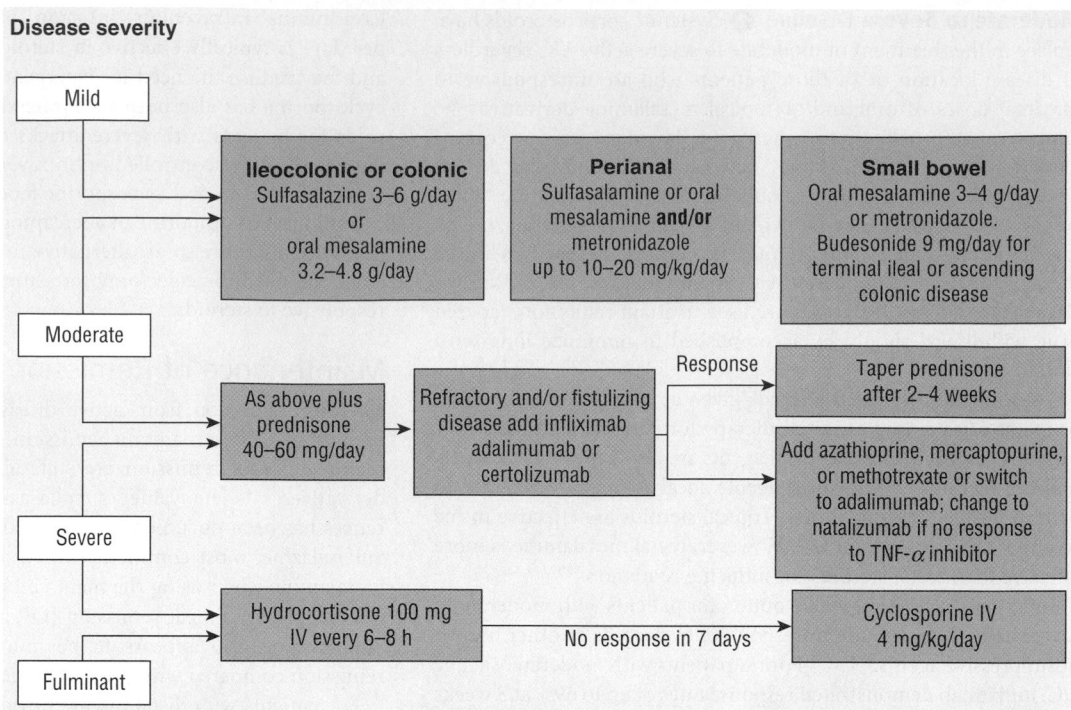

FIGURE 41-3. Treatment approaches for Crohn's disease.

CD[86] (Fig. 41–3, Table 41–6). The disease may involve any segment of the GI tract, from mouth to anus, and may involve other visceral structures and soft tissues through fistulization. There is a greater reliance on drug therapy with CD because resection of all involved intestine may not be possible. Unfortunately, recurrence of CD is common following surgery with reported rates of up to 64% recurrence following surgical resection of affected areas of bowel.[53]

Mild to Moderate Active Crohn's Disease

The goal of treatment for active CD is to achieve remission; however, in many patients, reduction of symptoms so the patient may carry out normal activities or reduction of the steroid dose required for control is a significant accomplishment. In the majority of patients, mild to moderate active CD is treated with sulfasalazine or mesalamine derivatives, while steroids, azathioprine, mercaptopurine, methotrexate, biologic agents, or metronidazole are frequently for moderate to severe disease.

Sulfasalazine, when administered in daily doses of 3 to 6 g, is slightly superior to placebo for patients with mild to moderate CD and is more effective when CD involves the colon.[40,87] Mesalamine formulations such as Pentasa or Asacol have the ability to release mesalamine in the small bowel thus targeting ileal disease, yet have demonstrated variable results for patients with active CD.[86,87] Only a few small trials utilizing Asacol at 3.8 g/day or Pentasa at 4g/day have demonstrated superiority to placebo for treatment of active CD.[86,87] Despite variable effectiveness, the mesalamine derivatives may be better tolerated than sulfasalazine, particularly at higher doses. Thus, a trial of sulfasalazine or an oral mesalamine derivative is reasonable as initial therapy for patients with mild to moderate active CD with ileal, ileocolonic, or colonic involvement.[39]

Systemic corticosteroids are frequently used for the treatment of active CD, particularly with more moderate to severe presentations; however, controlled release budesonide (Entocort) is a viable first-line option for patients with mild to moderate ileal or right-sided (ascending colonic) disease.[40,58,76,87,88] This agent is superior to placebo and has demonstrated superiority to mesalamine and reported rates of remission rates of up 69% at 8 weeks in some trials.[40,87,88]

For this reason, recent guidelines advocate use of budesonide 9 mg/day as a first-line option for patients with CD confined to the ileum and/or right colon.[40]

Metronidazole (given orally up to 20 mg/kg per day in divided doses) has demonstrated variable efficacy but may possibly be useful in some patients with CD, particularly for patients with colonic or ileocolonic involvement or for those patients with perineal disease.[66,86,87,89] For most patients with colonic or perineal disease, metronidazole would be added to a mesalamine product or steroids as adjunctive therapy, where satisfactory control of CD is not gained with first-line agents, or in attempts to reduce steroid dosage.[52,66] Ciprofloxacin 1 g/day has gained attention as an alternative to metronidazole and has demonstrated some efficacy in small trials only.[52,66,77,86,87] The combination of ciprofloxacin with metronidazole appears to be efficacious in some patients with perianal disease.[66,87,89] Antibiotics demonstrate minimal efficacy in mild to moderate active CD and thus are not recommended for routine use.[40,87]

Moderate to Severe Active Crohn's Disease

Oral systemic steroids, such as prednisone 60 mg/day, are generally considered first-line therapies for moderate to severe active CD and are effective in inducing remission for up to 70% of patients. Oral systemic steroids should be reserved for patients with moderate to severe disease who have failed aminosalicylates or budesonide.[40,76,86] Hospitalized patients with severe or fulminant disease or those who are unable to tolerate oral therapy are candidates for administration of parenteral steroids.[40,76] Systemic steroids do not appear to be effective for treatment of perianal fistulas.[76,89]

❿ The immunomodulators (azathioprine and mercaptopurine) are effective in maintaining steroid-induced remission and are generally limited to use for patients not achieving adequate response to standard medical therapy or to reduce steroid doses when high steroid doses are required.[59,76,86,90] Azathioprine and mercaptopurine have both demonstrated long-term benefits for patients with CD.[59,85] The usual doses of azathioprine is 2 to 3 mg/kg per day, and for mercaptopurine to 1.5 mg/kg per day.[76] Starting doses are typically 50 mg/day and increased at 2-week intervals; however, complete blood counts with differential should be monitored every 2 weeks while doses are being titrated.[76] The onset of therapeutic effects are delayed with both azathioprine and mercaptopruine, and a minimum of 3 to 4 months is often required to see clinical benefits.[76,86]

As mentioned previously, clinical response to mercaptopurine may be related to whole-blood concentrations of the metabolite 6-TGN, while toxicity is correlated with concentrations of another metabolite, 6-methylmercaptopurine.[14,59,61,91] Determination of TPMT activity is recommended to determine which patients require lower doses of these agents.[15,59,76] Alternatively, a newer strategy for evaluating a patient's risk for toxicity is to perform a TPMT genotype or phenotype.[59,76,91] This is recommended prior to therapy with subsequent dose adjustments based on the patient's genotypic profile.[76]

CLINICAL CONTROVERSY

While thiopurines, such as azathioprine and mercaptopurine, are effective for maintenance of remission of CD, it is debated how long treatment should be continued once remission is achieved. Evidence has demonstrated efficacy of these agents in maintaining remission for greater than 4 years; however, some authors argue that long-term exposure to these potentially toxic agents outweighs the benefit.

⓫ Although mostly used in the setting of maintenance therapy, methotrexate is another option for use as induction therapy for patients with moderate to severe CD.[86] Use of a weekly intramuscular or subcutaneous injection of 25 mg has demonstrated efficacy for induction of remission in CD and has also demonstrated corticosteroid-sparing effects.[40,76,86,92] While there are risks of bone marrow suppression, hepatotoxicity, and pulmonary toxicity, use of low-dose methotrexate appears relatively safe when continued as maintenance therapy if proper monitoring is implemented.

Infliximab is a well-established treatment option for moderate to severe active CD for patients failing immunosuppressive therapy, in those who are corticosteroid dependent, and for treatment of fistulizing disease.[60,67,76,93] In large trials, a 5 mg/kg single intravenous infusion of infliximab resulted in clinical improvement in 58% of patients at 2 weeks and 65% of patients at 8 weeks.[67,93] Continued dosing of 5 mg/kg at 2 and 6 weeks following the initial dose leads to higher response rates and is recommended as the regimen of choice for induction therapy in active disease.[76] Response rates of up to 62% in the reduction of number of draining fistulas have been reported following induction therapy and continued maintenance dosing with infliximab.[67,93,94] Patients who receive infliximab often develop antibodies to infliximab (ATI), which can result in increases in the occurrence of serious infusion reactions and loss of response to the drug. Up to 10% of patients per year require discontinuation of infliximab due to adverse effects and loss of efficacy related to development of ATIs.[67] Strategies to reduce ATI formation include administration of a second dose within 8 weeks of the first dose, concurrent administration of steroids (hydrocortisone 200 mg intravenously on the day of the infusion or oral prednisone the day prior), and use of concomitant immunosuppressive agents.[67,76,93] Induction of tolerance utilizing a dose escalation technique was also effective in administering infliximab to patients with previous severe infusion reactions.[95] As mentioned previously, use of infliximab in combination with azathioprine may lead to better outcomes in steroid or immunosuppressive naive patients.[60]

Adalimumab is another viable option for moderate to severe CD. Trials evaluating treatment with adalimumab for patients with moderately to severely active CD who have lost response to infliximab have demonstrated up to a 54% complete response in some instances.[67,96–98] Certolizumab has also demonstrated efficacy in moderate to severe CD with patients who have a baseline CRP of greater than 10 mg/dL exhibiting the best response rates, reported as 37% at 6 weeks versus 26% for placebo.[67,99] Natalizumab is reserved for patients who do not respond to steroids or the TNF-α inhibitors. Patients who initially responded to natalizumab treatment had rates of sustained response reported as 61% versus 28% for placebo at week 36.[100]

Cyclosporine is typically not recommended for treatment of CD except for acute management of patients with severe fistulizing disease.[76,94,101] Up to 83% of patients with refractory fistulas responded to intravenous cyclosporine (4 mg/kg per day) within a mean of 7.9 days.[86] The dose of cyclosporine is important in determining efficacy. An oral dose of 5 mg/kg per day is ineffective, whereas 7.6 mg/kg per day has demonstrated effectiveness in some trials.[76,101] However, toxic effects limit the routine use of this higher dosage. At present, the therapeutic blood or plasma concentration range for cyclosporine has not been established for CD, but whole-blood trough concentrations of 300 to 500 ng/mL for intravenous therapy or 200 to 400 ng/mL for oral therapy have been established.[76,86] When using cyclosporine clinicians should recognize the accompanying long-term risk of renal toxicity and infection, as well as the potential for drug interactions.

Maintenance of Remission

Prevention of recurrence of disease is typically more difficult with CD than with UC. There is minimal evidence to support that sulfasalazine and oral mesalamine derivatives are effective therapies for maintenance of CD following medically-induced remission.[86,87,102,103] Despite these findings, an attempt to maintain remission with sulfasalazine and oral mesalamine following a medically-induced remission is reasonable given the favorable side-effect profile and cost of these drugs compared with the immunosuppressive and biologic agents.[86] Mesalamine does appear to have some efficacy in preventing post surgical relapse following resection, with absolute risk reductions of 10% to 15% for relapse reported in some studies.[103,104]

Systemic steroids have no place in the prevention of recurrence of CD. These agents do not appear to alter the long-term course of the disease and predispose patients to serious adverse effects with long-term use.[40,76,105] Budesonide at maintenance doses of 6 mg/day has demonstrated efficacy in maintaining remission at 3 months; however, use longer than this is generally not recommended, as a loss of efficacy is seen after this time frame.[76,106] Despite this recommendation, use of budesonide as maintenance therapy for up to 1 year results in low rates of clinically important adverse effects.[107]

Azathioprine, mercaptopurine, and methotrexate are useful for some patients with CD to maintain remission. Azathioprine and mercaptopurine are effective in maintaining remission in CD for up to 4 years, particularly in steroid-induced remission, and therefore these drugs are generally considered first-line agents.[40] Patients who may benefit from these agents include those with quiescent disease who are steroid dependent or refractory, in postsurgical patients to prevent recurrence, those with frequent flares requiring steroids, and those patients with perianal or enteric fistulas.[59,76,86] For patients who initially respond to methotrexate, continued dosing at 15 mg intramuscularly once weekly is also effective in maintaining remission.[76,86] This agent has steroid sparing effects and thus represents an alternative therapy to azathioprine and mercaptopurine.

Infliximab infusion given at a dose of 5 mg/kg every 8 weeks is more effective than placebo in maintaining remission for patients who initially respond to infliximab for active CD.[67,68,76,78,93] An increase in the dose to 10 mg/kg is possible if loss of efficacy over time is evident. Additionally, infliximab is the effective maintenance therapy for fistulizing disease; however, given the high cost of this agent, some have questioned whether this approach is the most cost effective.[94] Adalimumab is also a treatment option for maintenance therapy of CD. Following induction therapy, doses of 40 mg subcutaneously every other week have resulted in clinical remission rates of 36% to 46% after 56 weeks of therapy.[108,109] Certolizumab is also effective for maintenance of CD, with remission rates for patients who initially responded reported as 49% at 26 weeks versus 29% with placebo[67,110] For patients treated with natalizumab who initially respond, maintenance therapy led to response rates of 44% compared with 26% for placebo ($P = 0.001$).[100]

CLINICAL CONTROVERSY

Use of immunomodulator agents, such as azathioprine and mercaptopurine, is becoming more common earlier in the course of IBD and for patients who may not fully respond to aminosalicylates. For patients that are receiving aminosalicylates who are started on immunomodulator agents it is unclear as to whether the aminosalicylate should be continued once the immunomodulator becomes effective. Continued use of aminosalicylates may aid in prevention of colorectal cancer; however, the effects of continued use on disease control drug toxicity and adherence to therapy are not known.[111]

SELECTED COMPLICATIONS

TOXIC MEGACOLON

The treatment required for toxic megacolon includes general supportive measures to maintain vital functions, consideration for early surgical intervention, and use of drugs (steroids, cyclosporine, and antimicrobials).[31,39] Aggressive fluid and electrolyte management is required for dehydration. Fluids and electrolytes may be lost through vomiting, diarrhea, and nasogastric intubation, as well as through fluid accumulation in the bowel. If the patient has lost significant amounts of blood, transfusion may be necessary. Opiates and medications with anticholinergic properties should be discontinued because these agents enhance colonic dilatation, thereby increasing the risk of bowel perforation. Broad spectrum antimicrobials that include coverage for gram-negative bacilli and intestinal anaerobes should be used as preemptive therapy in the event that perforation occurs.[31] Fortunately, perforation occurs in only 2% to 3% of cases.[39] If the patient is not on steroids, then high doses intravenous therapy should be administered to reduce acute inflammation. Emergent surgical intervention, mainly an abdominal colectomy with formation of an ileostomy, is an important consideration for patients with toxic megacolon and prevents death in some patients.[31,39,53]

SYSTEMIC MANIFESTATIONS

The common systemic manifestations of IBD include arthritis, anemia, and skin manifestations such as erythema nodosum and pyoderma gangrenosum, uveitis, and liver disease. These problems may be related to the inflammatory process. For some of these manifestations specific therapies can be instituted, whereas for others the treatment that is used for the GI inflammatory process also addresses the systemic manifestations.

Anemia occurs when there is significant blood loss from the GI tract. If the patient can consume oral medication, ferrous sulfate

should be administered. If the patient is unable to take oral medication and the patient's hematocrit is sufficiently low, blood transfusions or intravenous iron infusions may be required.[34,35] Anemia may also be related to malabsorption of vitamin B12 or folic acid, particularly for patients who have had ileal resection, so these may also be required. Patients with IBD are also at high risk for bone loss, osteoporosis, and fractures.[35,112] Screening for osteoporosis via DXA is recommended for patients using steroids for >3 months, in postmenopausal females, males over age 50, and those who have sustained a low-stress fracture.[35,112] If the patient is deemed high risk for osteoporosis, vitamin D and calcium should be instituted. If osteoporosis is present, then calcium, vitamin D, and a bisphosphonate are recommended.[35,112] Corticosteroid use should be limited, and weight-bearing exercise initiated.

There are no consistently recommended therapies for apthous ulcers, liver disease, episcleritis, or uveitis associated with IBD. These manifestations are worse during exacerbations of the intestinal disease, and measures improving intestinal disease will improve these systemic manifestations. Unfortunately, this association has not been demonstrated consistently. For arthritis associated with IBD, aspirin or another NSAID may be beneficial, as might be steroids. However NSAID use may exacerbate the underlying IBD. Liver transplantation is being used more frequently for definitive treatment of primary sclerosing cholangitis. Infliximab and the other TNF-α inhibitors may alleviate some arthritic and skin manifestations of IBD such as ankylosing spondylitis, erythema nodosum, and pyoderma gangrenosum.[35,113]

SPECIAL CONSIDERATIONS

PREGNANCY

Either the occurrence or consideration of pregnancy may cause significant concerns for the patient with IBD. Patients with IBD have similar infertility rates as the general female population, thus the rate of normal childbirth is similar to that for healthy populations.[114-116] Some studies have noted a greater risk of spontaneous abortions for patients with IBD. Furthermore, there is a greater incidence of low-birth-weight infants for mothers with chronic idiopathic UC.[114] Pregnancy has minimal effects on the course of IBD.[114-116] Likewise, IBD appears to have little effect on the course of pregnancy, particularly if the IBD is quiescent at the time of conception.[114-116] Patients who are pregnant experience IBD recurrence rates similar to those of nonpregnant females. In addition, there is no justification for therapeutic abortion with IBD because termination of the pregnancy has not been observed to improve the disease.

Steroids and sulfasalazine may be administered during pregnancy with the same guidelines that would be applied to the non-pregnant patient.[114-116] Steroids given systemically do not appear to be detrimental to the fetus. Sulfasalazine is generally well tolerated; however, it does interfere with folate absorption, so supplementation with folic acid 1 mg twice daily should be used during the pregnancy.[114] Interestingly, sulfasalazine causes decreased sperm counts and reduced fertility in males.[114] This effect is reversible on discontinuation of the drug, and it is not reported with mesalamine. Immunosuppressive drugs (azathioprine and mercaptopurine) may be associated with fetal deformities in humans and are classified as pregnancy category D; however, they have been used commonly in IBD without detriment for most patients.[114-116] Infliximab, adalimumab, and certolizumab are classified as pregnancy category B drugs and appear to be relatively safe for use in pregnant patients.[114-116] Natalizumab is a pregnancy category C drug, and thus may be used if benefit is thought to outweigh risk. Metronidazole may be used for short courses for treatment of trichomoniasis, but prolonged use should be avoided due to potential mutagenic effects.[114] Methotrexate should not be used during pregnancy, as it is a known abortifacient (category X).[76,114-116]

Although prednisone and prednisolone can be detected in breast milk, breast-feeding is believed to be safe for the infant when low doses of prednisone are used.[115] Sulfasalazine does not pose a risk of kernicterus, as levels of sulfapyridine in breast milk are low or undetectable. Metronidazole should not be given to nursing mothers because it is excreted into breast milk.[115,116]

ADVERSE DRUG EFFECTS

Drug intolerance often limits the usefulness of agents used to treat IBD. Many patients receiving sulfasalazine, mesalamine, corticosteroids, metronidazole, azathioprine, mercaptopurine, methotrexate, or biologic agents may experience undesired effects. In some cases, these adverse effects can be significant and require discontinuation of the therapy. Knowledge of the common or important adverse reactions will assist in avoiding or minimizing their effects.

Sulfasalazine is often associated with adverse drug effects, and these effects may be classified as either dose related or idiosyncratic.[117,118] The sulfapyridine portion of the sulfasalazine molecule is believed to be responsible for much of the sulfasalazine toxicity.[117] Dose-related side effects usually include GI disturbances such as nausea, vomiting, diarrhea, or anorexia but may also include headache and arthralgia. These adverse reactions tend to occur more commonly on initiation of therapy and decrease in frequency as therapy is continued. Approaches to the management of these adverse effects include discontinuing the agent for a short period and then reinstituting therapy at a reduced dosage with subsequent slower dose escalation, administration with food, or substituting another enteric-coated 5-ASA product.[117,118] Folic acid absorption is impaired by sulfasalazine, which may lead to anemia. Patients receiving sulfasalazine should receive oral folic acid supplementation.

Adverse effects that are idiosyncratic are not dose related and most commonly include rash, fever, or hepatotoxicity, as well as relatively uncommon but serious reactions such as bone marrow suppression, thrombocytopenia, pancreatitis, pneumonitis, interstitial nephritis, and hepatitis. For most patients with idiosyncratic reactions, sulfasalazine must be discontinued. In some patients who have experienced allergic reactions to sulfasalazine, a desensitization procedure can be instituted. By gradually increasing sulfasalazine dosage over weeks to months, patient tolerance has been improved.[118]

Oral mesalamine derivatives may impose a lower frequency of adverse effects as compared with sulfasalazine. Up to 80% to 90% of patients who are intolerant to sulfasalazine will tolerate oral mesalamine derivatives.[117] However, olsalazine may cause watery diarrhea in up to 25% of patients, often requiring drug discontinuation.[117]

Adverse reactions to corticosteroids are well recognized and may occur when corticosteroids are used for any indication. However, there is a greater potential for adverse effects when corticosteroids are used for the treatment of IBD because high doses must often be used for extended periods. The well-appreciated adverse effects of corticosteroids include hyperglycemia, hypertension, osteoporosis, acne, fluid retention, electrolyte disturbances, myopathies, muscle wasting, increased appetite, psychosis, and reduced resistance to infection. In addition, corticosteroid use may cause adrenocortical suppression. To minimize corticosteroid effects, clinicians have used alternate-day steroid therapy; however, some patients do not do well clinically on the days when no steroid is given. For most patients a single daily corticosteroid dose suffices,

and divided daily doses are unnecessary. Another problem with corticosteroids is adrenal insufficiency after abrupt steroid withdrawal. This necessitates gradual tapering of steroid therapy for patients using these agents daily for more than 2 to 3 weeks.[117] Due to its lower bioavailability and lower potential for adverse effects, budesonide may be used as alternate steroid therapy in CD involving the ileum or right colon or may be substituted for prednisone in CD patients who are steroid dependent or require long-term therapy.[36,40,106]

Immunomodulators, such as azathioprine and mercaptopurine, have a significant potential for adverse reactions and have resulted in withdrawal rates in clinical trials of up to 20%.[59] Adverse events to thiopurines are typically divided into two groups, type A and type B.[59] Type A are dose related and include malaise, nausea, infectious complications, hepatitis, and myelosuppression. As mentioned earlier, the myelosuppression from azathioprine and mercaptopurine is related to a deficiency of TPMT with subsequent accumulation of toxic metabolites. Type B reactions are considered idiosyncratic and include fever, rash, arthralgia, and pancreatitis (3% to 15% of patients).[59,117] 6-Mercaptopurine causes adverse reactions similar to azathioprine; however, there are fewer reports of lymphomas with this agent. Some data suggest that mercaptopurine may be used successfully for patients who are intolerant to azathioprine.[119]

Most patients receiving metronidazole for CD tolerate the agent fairly well; however, mild adverse effects occur frequently. They commonly include nauseas, metallic taste, urticaria, and glossitis.[66,117] More serious effects that occur with long-term use include development of paresthesias and reversible peripheral neuropathy.[66,117] Other effects include a disulfiram-like reaction if alcohol is ingested in conjunction.

The TNF-α inhibitors may be associated with development of serious adverse effects and carry similar adverse profiles for the available agents. Infliximab use has been associated with infusion reactions. Premedication with acetaminophen, diphenhydramine, and possibly corticosteroids may reduce the incidence and severity of these reactions.[40,120,121] Due to administration via the subcutaneous route, adalimumab and certolizumab may be more associated with injection site reactions versus infusion-related reactions. Serum sickness has occurred for patients who received infliximab doses separated by a long period of time.[67,76,121] Autoimmune phenomena, such as lupus and hemolytic anemia, may also occur during infliximab therapy, as well as an increase in the incidence of adverse neurologic events such as optic neuritis and demyelinating syndrome.[120] Risk of hepatosplenic T-cell lymphoma may be increased with use of infliximab, particularly if used in combination with immunomodulators such as azathioprine. Young male patients appear to be at higher risk for development of lymphoma.[40,120,121] Infliximab may also cause worsening of heart failure and thus is contraindicated for patients with New York Heart Association Class III or IV heart failure.

All TNF-α inhibitors predispose patients to development of serious infections. Patients with clinically significant active infections should not receive TNF-α inhibitors. Sepsis and tuberculosis may occur because of the inhibition of TNF-protective mechanisms. Patients should receive a tuberculin skin test [purified protein derivative (PPD)] ORA QuantiFERON® test and a chest x-ray prior to initiating therapy to rule out undiagnosed tuberculosis.[67,121] Reactivation of hepatitis B may occur; thus, patients should also be screened for hepatitis B virus infection prior to initiating therapy.[121] Patients should also be screened for hepatitis C infection, although it does not appear that use of TNF-α inhibitors alter the disease course.[121] Lastly, use of natalizumab is associated with development of progressive multifocal leukoencephalopathy and is only available via the manufacturer's TOUCH prescribing program.[67] Patients receiving natalizumab should be monitored for development of adverse neurologic events and undergo MRI of the brain should development of progressive multifocal leukoencephalopathy be suspected.

EVALUATION OF THERAPEUTIC OUTCOMES

The success of therapeutic regimens to treat IBD can be measured by patient-reported complaints, signs, and symptoms; by direct clinician examination (including endoscopy); by history and physical examination; by selected laboratory tests; and by quality-of-life measures. Evaluation of IBD severity is difficult because much of the assessment is subjective.[122] To create more objective measures, disease rating scales or indices have been created. The CD Activity Index (CDAI) is a commonly used scale, particularly for evaluation of patients during clinical trials.[123] The scale incorporates eight elements: (1) number of stools in the past 7 days, (2) sum of abdominal pain ratings from the past 7 days, (3) rating of general well-being in the past 7 days, (4) use of antidiarrheals, (5) body weight, (6) hematocrit, (7) finding of abdominal mass, and (8) a sum of extraintestinal symptoms present in the past week. Elements of this index provide a guide for those measures that may be useful in assessing the effectiveness of treatment regimens. A subsequent scale was developed specifically for Perianal CD, known as the *Perianal CD Activity Index* (PDAI).[122] The PDAI includes five items: presence of discharge, pain, restriction of sexual activity, type of perianal disease, and degree of induration.

Standardized assessment tools have also been constructed for UC.[124,125] Elements in these scales include (1) stool frequency, (2) presence of blood in the stool, (3) mucosal appearance (from endoscopy), and (4) physician's global assessment based on physical examination, endoscopy, and laboratory data.

Additional studies that are often useful include direct endoscopic examination of affected areas and/or radiocontrast studies. For patients with acute disease, assessment of fluid and electrolyte status is important, because these may be lost during diarrheal episodes. Other laboratory tests, such as serum albumin, transferrin, or other markers of visceral protein status as well as markers of inflammation (ESR or CRP), may be used.

Assessment of the IBD patient must include consideration of adverse drug effects. Because many of the agents used have a relatively high probability of causing adverse effects, particularly corticosteroids and other immunosuppressive agents, patient assessment should include collection of history and physical and laboratory data that are necessary to prevent or recognize adverse drug effects.

Finally, a patient quality-of-life assessment should be performed regularly.[122] Agents that appear clinically equivalent may differ substantially in resulting quality of life. Inquiry should be made regarding general well-being, emotional function, and social function. Social function may include assessment of the ability to perform routine daily functions and to maintain occupational activities, sexual function, and recreation. The most common tool used to assess quality of life is the Inflammatory Bowel Disease Questionnaire (IBDQ), a 32-item questionnaire that covers four disease dimensions: bowel function, emotional status, systemic symptoms, and social function.[122,125] The IBDQ has shown good correlation with the CDAI.[122] A shortened version has also been developed for use in the community practice setting.[125] A lesser used tool is the Rating Form of Inflammatory Bowel Disease Patient Concerns.[122]

Quality-of-life studies have been conducted with infliximab. To balance the exceptionally high cost of this therapy, CD patients who receive infliximab have improved quality of life, have fewer emergency room visits, have a reduced requirement for surgery, and are more likely to be employed.[126,127]

ABBREVIATIONS

6-MP: 6-mercaptopurine

6-TGN: 6-thioguanine

ATI: antibodies to infliximab

CD: Crohn's disease

CRP: C-reactive protein

ESR: erythrocyte sedimentation rate

HLA: human leukocyte antigen

IBD: inflammatory bowel disease

NSAID: nonsteroidal antiinflammatory drug

TPMT: thiopurine S-methyltransferase

TNF-α: tumor necrosis factor-alpha

UC: ulcerative colitis

REFERENCES

1. Langmead L, Rampton D. A GP guide to inflammatory bowel disease. Practitioner 2001;245:224–229.
2. Sandler RS, Eisen GM. Epidemiology of inflammatory bowel disease. In: Kirsner JB, ed. Inflammatory Bowel Diseases. Philadelphia, PA: WB Saunders; 2000:89–112.
3. Shanahan F, Bernstein CN. The evolving epidemiology of inflammatory bowel disease. Current Opinion. Gastroenterol 2009,25:301–305.
4. Feldman M: Sleisenger and Fordtran's Gastrointestinal and Liver Disease, 7th ed. New York, NY: Elsevier; 2002.
5. Cross RK, Jung C, Wasan S, et al Racial differences in disease phenotypes in patients with Crohn's Disease. Inflamm Bowel Dis 2006;12:192–198.
6. Straus WL, Eisen Gm, Sandler RS, et al. Crohn's Disease: Does race matter? Am J Gastroenterol 2000;95:479–483.
7. Viscido A, Aratari A, Maccioni F, et al. Inflammatory bowel diseases: clinical update of practical guidelines. Nucl Med Comm 2005;26:649–655.
8. Seksik P, Sokol H, Lepage P, et al. Review article: the role of bacteria in onset and perpetuation of inflammatory bowel disease. Aliment Pharmacol Ther 2006;24 (suppl 3):11–18.
9. Shanahan F. Crohn's disease. Lancet 2003;359:62–69.
10. Podolsky DK. Inflammatory bowel disease. N Engl J Med 2002;347:417–429.
11. Farrell RJ, Peppercorn MA. Ulcerative colitis. Lancet 2002;359:331–340.
12. Lakatos PL, Fischer S, Lakatos L, et al. Current concept on the pathogenesis of inflammatory bowel disease-crosstalk between genetic and microbial factors: Pathogenic bacteria and altered bacterial sensing or changes in mucosal integrity take "toll". World J Gastroenterol 2006;12:1829–1841.
13. Shanahan F. Pathogenesis of ulcerative colitis. Lancet 1993;342:407–411.
14. Vermeire S. Review article: Genetic susceptibility and application of genetic testing in clinical management of inflammatory bowel disease. Aliment Pharmacol Ther 2006;24(suppl 3):2–10.
15. Herrlinger KR, Jewell DP. Review article: interactions between genotype and response to therapy in inflammatory bowel diseases. Aliment Pharmacol Ther 2006;24:1403–1412.
16. Edouard LE, Libioulle C, Renaers C, Belaiche J, Georges M. Genetics of UC: The come-back of interleukin 10. Gut 2009;58:1173–1175.
17. Abraham C, Cho JH. IL-23 and Autoimmunity: New insights into the pathogenesis of inflammatory bowel disease. Annu. Rev. Med. 2009;60:97–110.
18. Lanzaratto F, Carpani M, Chaudhary R, Ghosh S. Novel treatment options for inflammatory bowel disease: Targeting a4 integrin. Drugs 2006;66:1179–1189.
19. Sandborn WJ, Landers CJ, Tremaine WJ, Targan BR. Association of antineutrophil cytoplasmic antibodies with resistance to treatment of

left-sided ulcerative colitis: Results of a pilot study. Mayo Clin Proc 1996;71:431–436.

20. Blumberg RS, Strober W. Prospects for research in inflammatory bowel disease. JAMA 2001;285:643–647.

21. MacDonald TT, DiSabatino A, Gordon JN. Immunopathogenesis of Crohn's Disease. J Parent Ent Nutr 2005;29:S118–S125.

22. Bitton A, Sewitch MJ, Peppercorn MA, et al. Psychosocial determinants of relapse in UC: A longitudinal study. Am J Gastroenterol 2003;98:2112–2115.

23. Singh S, Graff LA, Bernstein CN. Do NSAIDs, Antibiotics, Infections, or Stress Trigger Flares in IBD? Am J Gastroenterol 2009;104:1298–1313.

24. McGrath J, McDonald JWD, MacDonald JK. Transdermal nicotine for induction of remission in ulcerative colitis. Cochrane Database of Systematic Reviews 2004, Issue 4. Art. No. : CD004722. DOI: 10. 1002/14651858. CD004722. pub2.

25. Cosnes J, Beaugerie L, Carbonnel F, Gendre JP. Smoking cessation and the course of Crohn's disease: An intervention study. Gastroenterology 2001;120:1093–1099.

26. Cipolla G, Crema F, Sacco S, et al. Nonsteroidal anti-inflammatory drugs and inflammatory bowel disease: Current perspectives. Pharmacol Res 2002;46:1–6.

27. Mahadevan U, Loftus EV, Tremaine WJ, Sandborn WJ. Safety of selective cyclooxygenase inhibitors in inflammatory bowel disease. Am J Gastroenterol 2002;97:910–914.

28. Bonner, GF. Using COX-2 inhibitors in IBD: Anti-inflammatories inflame a controversy (Editorial). Am J Gastroenterol 2002;97:783–785.

29. Regueiro M, Loftus, EV, Steinhart H, Cohen RD. Clinical guidelines for the medical management of left-sided ulcerative colitis and ulcerative proctitis: Summary statement. Inflamm Bowel Dis 2006;12:972–978.

30. Geboes K. Review article: What are the important endoscopic lesions for detection of dysplasia in inflammatory bowel disease? Aliment Pharmacol Ther 2006;24(suppl 3):50–55.

31. Gan SI, Beck PL. A new look at toxic megacolon: An update and review of incidence, etiology, pathogenesis, and management. Am J Gastroenterol 2003;98:2363–2371.

32. Monsen V, Sorstad J, Hellers G, et al. Extracolonic diagnosis in ulcerative colitis: An epidemiologic study. Am J Gastroenterol 1990;85:711–716.

33. Harmatz A. Hepatobiliary manifestations of inflammatory bowel disease. Med Clin North Am 1994;78:1387–1398.

34. Rankin GB. Extraintestinal and systemic manifestations of inflammatory bowel disease. Med Clin North Am 1990;74:39–50.

35. Kethu SR. Extraintestinal manifestations of inflammatory bowel diseases. J Clin Gastroenterol 2006;40:467–475.

36. Hartman C, Eliakim R, Shamir R. Nutritional status and nutritional therapy in inflammatory bowel diseases. World J Gastroenterol 2009;15:2570–2578.

37. Filippi J, Al-Jaouni R, Wiroth JB, et al. Nutritional deficiencies in patients with Crohn's Disease in remission. Inflamm Bowel Dis 2006;12:185–191.

38. Collins P, Rhodes J. Ulcerative colitis: diagnosis and management. BMJ 2006;333:340–343.

39. Kornbluth A, Sachar DB. Ulcerative practice guidelines in adults (Update): American College of Gastroenterology, Practice Parameters Committee. Am J Gastroenterol 2004;99:1371–1385.

40. Lichtenstein GR, Hanauer SB, Sandborn WJ, The Practice Parameters Committee of the American College of Gastroenterology. Management of Crohn's Disease in Adults. Am J Gastroenterol 2009;104:465–483.

41. Gonzalez-Huix F, Fernandez-Banares F, Esteve-Comas M, et al. Enteral versus parenteral nutrition as adjunct therapy in acute ulcerative colitis. Am J Gastroenterol 1993;88:227–232.

42. Griffiths AM. Enteral nutrition in the management of Crohn's Disease. J Parent Ent Nutr 2005;29:S108–S117.

43. Sanderson IR, Croft NM. The anti-inflammatory effects of enteral nutrition. J Parent Ent Nutr 2005;29:S134–S140.

44. Buning C, Lochs H. Conventional therapy for Crohn's Disease. World J Gastroenterol 2006;12:4794–4806.

45. Lewis JD, Fisher RL. Nutritional support in inflammatory bowel disease. Med Clin North Am 1994;78:1443–1456.

46. Gassull MA. Review article: The intestinal lumen as a therapeutic target in inflammatory bowel disease. Aliment Pharmacol Ther 2006;24(suppl 3):90–95.

47. Sullivan A, Nord CE. Probiotics and gastrointestinal diseases. J Intern Med 2005;257:78–92.

48. Zigra PI, Maipa VE, Alamanos YP. Probiotics and remission of ulcerative colitis: A systematic review. Neth J Med 2007;65:411–418.

49. Butterworth AD, Thomas AG, Akobeng AK. Probiotics for induction of remission in Crohn's disease. Cochrane Database of Systematic Reviews 2008, Issue 3. Art. No. : CD006634. DOI: 10. 1002/14651858. CD006634. pub2.

50. Rolfe VE, Fortun PJ, Hawkey CJ, Bath-Hextall FJ. Probiotics for maintenance of remission in Crohn's disease. Cochrane Database of Systematic Reviews 2006, Issue 4. Art. No. : CD004826. DOI: 10. 1002/14651858. CD004826. pub2.

51. Rahimi R, Nikfar S, Rahimi F, et al. A meta-analysis on the efficacy of probiotics for maintenance of remission and prevention of clinical and endoscopic relapse in Crohn's disease. Dig Dis Sci 2008;53:2524–2531.

52. Prantera C, Scribano ML. Antibiotics and probiotics in inflammatory bowel disease: Why, when, and how. Current Opin Gastroenterol 2009;25:329–333

53. Hancock L, Windsor AC, Mortensen. Inflammatory bowel disease: the view of the surgeon. Colorectal Dis 2006;8(suppl 1):10–14.

54. Sandborn WJ, Hanauer SB. Systematic review: The pharmacokinetic profiles of oral mesalazine formulations and mesalazine pro-drugs used in the management of ulcerative colitis. Aliment Pharmacol Ther 2003;17:29–42.

55. Tindall WN. New approaches to adherence issues when dosing oral aminosalicylates in ulcerative colitis. Am J Health-Syst Pharm. 2009;66:451–457.

56. Lakatos PL. Use of new once-daily 5-aminosalicylic acid preparations in the treatment of ulcerative colitis: Is there anything new under the sun? World J Gastroenterol 2009;15:1799–1804.

57. Friend Dr. Review article: Issues in oral administration of locally acting glucocorticoids for the treatment of inflammatory bowel disease. Aliment Pharmacol Ther 1998;12:591–603.

58. Hofer KN. Oral budesonide in the management of Crohn's Disease. Ann Pharmacother 2003;37;1457–1464.

59. Derijks LJJ, Gilissen LPL, Hooymans PM, Hommes DW. Review article: thiopurines in inflammatory bowel disease. Aliment Pharmcol Ther 2006;24:715–729.

60. GA, Vermeire S, Rutgeerts P. Immunosuppression in inflammatory bowel disease: Traditional, biological or both? Current Opinion in Gastroenterology 2009;25:323–328.

61. Osterman MT, Kundu R, Lichtenstein GR, et al. Association of 6-thioguanine nucleotide levels and inflammatory bowel disease activity: A meta-analysis. Gastroenterology. 2006;130:1047–1053.

62. Durai D. Hawthorne AB. Review article: how and when to use ciclosporin in ulcerative colitis. Aliment Pharmacol Ther 2005;22:907–916.

63. Gonzalez-Lama Y, Gisbert JP, Mate J. The role of tacrolimus in inflammatory bowel disease: A systematic review. Dig Dis Sci 2006;51:1833–1840.

64. Schroder O, Stein J. Low dose methotrexate in inflammatory bowel disease: Current status and future directions. Am J Gastroenterol 2003;98:530–537.

65. Vandell AG, DiPiro JT. Low-dose methotrexate for treatment and maintenance of remission in patients with inflammatory bowel disease. Pharmacotherapy 2002;22:613–620.

66. Guslandi M. Antibiotics for inflammatory bowel disease: Do they work? Eur J Gastroenterol Hepatol 2005;17:145–147.

67. Rutgeerts P, Vvermeire Ss, Van Assche G. Biological Therapies for Inflammatory Bowel Diseases. Gastroenterol 2009;136:1182–1197.

68. Sandborn WJ. What's new: innovative concepts in inflammatory bowel disease. Colorectal Dis 2006;8(suppl 1):3–9.

69. Gionchetto P, Rizzello F, Morselli C, et al. Review article: Aminosalicylates for distal colitis. Aliment Pharmacol Ther 2006;24(suppl 3):41–44.

70. Hanauer SB. Review article: high dose aminosalicylates to induce and maintain remission in ulcerative colitis. Aliment Pharmacol Ther 2006;24(suppl 3):37–40.

71. Sutherland L,MacDonald JK. Oral 5-aminosalicylic acid for induction of remission in ulcerative colitis. Cochrane Database of Systematic Reviews 2006, Issue 2. Art. No. : CD000543. DOI: 10. 1002/14651858. CD000543. pub2.

72. Hanauer SB, Sandborn WJ, Kornbluth A, et al. Delayed-release oral mesalamine 4. 8g/day (800mg tablet) versus 2. 4g/day (400mg tablet) for treatment of moderately active ulcerative colitis: Combined analysis of two randomized, double blind, controlled trials. Gastroenterology 2005;128:A75–A75.

73. Hanauer SB, Sandborn WJ, Kornbluth A et al. Delayed-release oral mesalamine 4. 8g/day (800mg tablet) for treatment of moderately active ulcerative colitis. The ASCEND II Trial. Am J Gastroenterol 2005;100:2478–2485.

74. Rahimi R Nikfar S Rezaie A, Abdollahi M. Comparison of Mesalazine and Balsalazide in Induction and Maintenance of Remission in Patients with Ulcerative Colitis: A Meta-Analysis. Dig Dis Sci 2009;54: 712–721.

75. Pruitt R, Hanson J, Safdi M, et al. Balsalazide is superior to mesalamine in the time to improvement of signs and symptoms of acute mild-to-moderate ulcerative colitis. Am J Gastroenterol 2002;97:3078–3086.

76. American Gastroenterological Association Institute technical review on corticosteroids, immunomodulators, and infliximab in inflammatory bowel disease. Gastroenterology 2006;130;940–987.

77. Lawson MM, Thomas AG, Akobeng AK. Tumor necrosis factor alpha blocking agents for induction of remission in ulcerative colitis. Cochrane Database of Systematic Reviews 2006, Issue 3. Art. No. : CD005112. DOI: 10. 1002/14651858. CD005112. pub2.

78. Rutgeerts P, Sandborn WJ, Feagan BG, et al. Infliximab for induction and maintenance therapy for ulcerative colitis. N Engl J Med 2005;353;2462–2476.

79. Janerot G, Hertervig E, Friis-Liby I, et al. Infliximab as rescue therapy in severe to moderately severe ulcerative colitis: A randomized, placebo controlled study. Gastroenterology 2005;1805–1811.

80. Regueiro M, Curtis J, Plevy S. Infliximab for hospitalized patients with severe ulcerative colitis. J Clin Gastroenterol 2006;40:476–481.

81. McGilligan VE, Wallace JM, Heavey PM, Ridley DL, Rowland IR. Hypothesis about mechanisms through which nicotine might exert its effect on the interdependence of inflammation and gut barrier function in ulcerative colitis. Inflamm Bowel Dis. 2007;13:108–115.

82. Shibolet O, Regushevskaya E, Brezis M, Soares-Weiser K. Cyclosporine A for induction of remission in severe ulcerative colitis. Cochrane Database of Systematic Reviews 2005, Issue 1. Art. No. : CD004277. DOI: 10. 1002/14651858. CD004277. pub2.

83. D'Haens G, Lemmens L, Geboes K, et al. Intravenous cyclosporine versus corticosteroids as single therapy for severe attacks of ulcerative colitis. Gastroenterology 2001;120:1323–1329.

84. Sutherland L, MacDonald JK. Oral 5-aminosalicylic acid for maintenance of remission in ulcerative colitis. Cochrane Database of Systematic Reviews 2006, Issue 2. Art. No. : CD000544. DOI: 10. 1002/14651858. CD000544. pub2.

85. Holtmann MH, Krummenauer F, Claas C, et al. Long-term effectiveness of azathioprine in IBD beyond 4 years: A European multicenter study in 1,176 patients. Dig Dis Sci 2006;51:1516–1524.

86. Gionchetti P. Conventional therapy for Crohn's Disease. World J Gastroenterol 2006;12:4794–4806.

87. Sandborn WJ, Feagan BG, Lichtenstein GR. Medical management of mild to moderate Crohn's disease: Evidence-based treatment algorithms for induction and maintenance of remission. Aliment Pharmacol Ther 207;26:987–1003.

88. Otley A, Steinhart AH. Budesonide for induction of remission in Crohn's disease. Cochrane Database of Systematic Reviews 2005, Issue 4. Art. No. : CD000296. DOI: 10. 1002/14651858. CD000296. pub2.

89. AGA Technical review on perianal Crohn's Disease. Gastroenterology 2003;125:1508–1530.

90. Sandborn W, Sutherland L, Pearson D, May G, Modigliani R, Prantera C. Azathioprine or 6-mercaptopurine for induction of remission in Crohn's disease. Cochrane Database of Systematic Reviews 2000, Issue 3. Art. No. : CD000545. DOI: 10. 1002/14651858. CD000545.

91. Dubinsky MC, Lamothe S, Yang HY, et al. Pharmacogenomics and metabolite measurement for 6-mercaptopurine therapy in inflammatory bowel disease. Gastroenterology 2000;18:705–713.

92. Alfadhli AAF, McDonald JWD, Feagan BG. Methotrexate for induction of remission in refractory Crohn's disease. Cochrane Database of Systematic Reviews 2004, Issue 4. Art. No. : CD003459. DOI: 10. 1002/14651858. CD003459. pub2.

93. Kamm Ma. Review article: biological drugs in Crohn's Disease. Aliment Pharmacol Ther 2006;24(suppl 3):80–89.

94. Bressler B, Sands BE. Review article: medical therapy for fistulizing Crohn's Disease. Aliment Pharmacol Ther 2006;24:1283–1293.

95. Duburque C, Lelong J, Iacob R, et al. Successful induction of tolerance to infliximab in patients with Crohn's Disease and prior severe infusion reactions. Aliment Pharmacol Ther 2006;24:851–858.

96. Konstantinos AP, Shaye OA, Vasiliaukas EA, Ippoliti A, Dubinsky, et al. Safety and efficacy of adalimumab (D2E7) in Crohn's Disease patients with an attenuated response to infliximab. Am J Gastrenterol 2005;100:75–79.

97. Sandborn WJ, Rutgeerts P, Enns R, et al. Adalimumab induction therapy for Crohn's Disease previously treated with infliximab. Ann Intern Med 2007;146:829–838.

98. Hanauer SB, Sandborn WJ, Rutgeerts P, et al. Human Anti-Tumor necrosis factor monocolonal antibody (adalimumab) in Crohn's Disease: The CLASSIC-I Trial. Gastroenterology 2006;130:323–333.

99. Sandborn WJ, Feagan BG, Stoinov S, et al. Certolizumab pegol for the treatment of Crohn's disease. N Engl J Med 2007;357:228–238.

100. Sandborn WJ, Colombel JF, Enns R, et al. Natalizumab induction and maintenance therapy for Crohn's disease. N Engl J Med 2005;353:1912–1925.

101. McDonald JWD, Feagan BG, Jewell D, Brynskov J, Stange EF, MacDonald JK. Cyclosporine for induction of remission in Crohn's disease. Cochrane Database of Systematic Reviews 2005, Issue 2. Art. No. : CD000297. DOI: 10. 1002/14651858. CD000297. pub2.

102. Akobeng AK, Gardener E. Oral 5-aminosalicylic acid for maintenance of medically-induced remission in Crohn's Disease. Cochrane Database of Systematic Reviews 2005, Issue 1. Art. No. : CD003715. DOI: 10. 1002/14651858. CD003715. pub2.

103. Feagan BG. Maintenance therapy for inflammatory bowel disease. Am J Gastroenterol 2003;98:S6–S17.

104. Lemann M. Review article: can post-operative recurrence in Crohn's Disease be prevented? Aliment Pharm Ther 2006;24 (suppl 3):22–28.

105. Steinhart AH, Ewe K, Griffiths AM, Modigliani R, Thomsen OO. Corticosteroids for maintenance of remission in Crohn's disease. Cochrane Database of Systematic Reviews 2003, Issue 4. Art. No. : CD000301. DOI: 10. 1002/14651858. CD000301.

106. Benchimol EI, SeowCH, Otley AR, Steinhart AH. Budesonide for maintenance of remission in Crohn's disease. Cochrane Database of Systematic Reviews 2009, Issue 1. Art. No. : CD002913. DOI: 10. 1002/14651858. CD002913. pub2.

107. Lichtenstein GR, Bengtsson B, Hapten-White L, Rutgeerts P. Oral budesonide for maintenance of remission of Crohn's disease: a pooled safety analysis. Aliment Pharmacol Ther 2009;643–653.

108. Hanauer SB, Sandborn WJ, Rutgeerts P, Fedorak RN, Lukas, et al. Adalimumab for maintenance treatment of Crohn's Disease: Results of the ClASSIC-II Trial. Gut 2007;56:1232–1239.

109. Colombel J, Sandborn WJ, Rutgeerts P, et al. Adalimumab for maintenance of clinical response and remission in patients with Crohn's Disease: The CHARM Trial. Gasteroenterology 2007;132:52–65.

110. Schreiber S, Khaliq-Kareemi M, Lawrance IC, et al. Maintenance therapy with certolizumab pegol for Crohn's disease. N Engl J Med 2007;357:239–250.

111. Andrews JM, Travis SPL, Gibson PR, Gasche C. Systematic review: Does concurrent therapy with 5-ASA and immunomodulators in inflammatory bowel disease improve outcomes? Aliment Pharmacol Ther 2009;29:459–469.

112. American Gastroenterological Association medical position statement: Guidelines on osteoporosis in gastrointestinal diseases. Gastroenterol 2003;124:791–794.

113. Padovan M, Castellino G, Govoni M, Trotta F. The treatment of the rheumatological manifestations of the inflammatory bowel diseases. Rheumatol Int 2006;26:953–958.

114. Steinlauf AF, Present DH. Medical management of the pregnant patient with inflammatory bowel disease. Gastroenterol Clin N Am 2004;33:361–385.

115. Ferrero S, Ragni N. Inflammatory bowel disease: Management issues during pregnancy. Arch Gynecol Obstet 2004;270:79–85.

116. Dubinsky M, Abraham B, Mahadevan U. Management of the pregnant IBD patient. Inflamm Bowel Dis 2008;14:1736–1750.

117. Navarro F, Hanauer SB. Treatment of inflammatory bowel disease: Safety and tolerability issues. Am J Gastroenterol 2003;98(suppl): S18–S23.

118. Kung SJ, Choudhary C, McGeady SJ, Cohn JR. Lack of cross-reactivity between 5-aminosalicylic acid-based drugs: A case report and review of the literature. Ann All Asthma Immunol 2006;97: 284–287.

119. Hindorf W, Johansson M, Eriksson A, Kvifors E, Almer SHC. Mercaptopurine treatment should be considered in azathioprine intolerant patients with inflammatory bowel disease. Aliment Pharmacol Ther 2008;29:654–661.

120. Pascal Juillerat P, Pittet V, Felley C, et al. Drug Safety in Crohn's Disease. Digestion 2007;76:161–168. K.

121. Papa A, Mocci G, Bonizzi M, Felice C, Andrisani G, De Vitis I. Use of Infliximab in Particular Clinical Settings: Management Based on Current Evidence. Am J Gastroenterol 2009;104:1575–1586.

122. Sostegni R, Daperno M, Scaglione N. Review article: Crohn's Disease: Monitoring disease activity. Aliment Pharmacol Ther 2006;17(suppl 2):11–17.

123. Best WR, Becktel JM, Singleton JW, et al. Development of a Crohn's disease activity index. Gastroenterology 1976;70:439–444.

124. Sanborn WJ, Tremaine WJ, Schroeder KW, et al. Cyclosporine enemas for treatment-resistant, mildly to moderately active, left-sided ulcerative colitis. Am J Gastroenterol 1993;88:640–645.

125. Irvine EJ, Zhou Q, Thompson AK. The short inflammatory bowel disease questionnaire: A quality of life instrument for community physicians managing inflammatory bowel disease. CERPT investigators. Canadian Crohn's relapse prevention trial. Am J Gastroenterol 1996;91:1571–1578.

126. Lichtenstein GR, Yan S, Balla M, Hanauer S. Remission in patients with Crohn's disease is associated with improvement in employment and quality of life and a decrease in hospitalizations and surgeries. Am J Gastroenterol 2004;99:91–96.

127. Rubenstein JH, Chong RY, Cohen RD. Infliximab decreases resource use among patients with Crohn's disease. J Clin Gastroenterol 2002;35:151–156.

42

Nausea and Vomiting

CECILY V. DIPIRO AND ROBERT J. IGNOFFO

KEY CONCEPTS

❶ Nausea and/or vomiting is often a part of the symptom complex for a variety of gastrointestinal, cardiovascular, infectious, neurologic, metabolic, or psychogenic processes.

❷ Nausea or vomiting is caused by a variety of medications or other noxious agents.

❸ The overall goal of treatment should be to prevent or eliminate nausea and vomiting regardless of etiology.

❹ Treatment options for nausea and vomiting include drug and nondrug modalities such as relaxation, biofeedback, and self-hypnosis.

❺ The primary goal with chemotherapy-induced nausea and vomiting (CINV) is to prevent nausea and/or vomiting. Optimal control of acute nausea and vomiting positively impacts the incidence and control of delayed and anticipatory nausea and vomiting.

❻ The emetic risk of the chemotherapeutic regimen is the primary factor to consider when selecting prophylactic antiemetics for CINV.

❼ Patients at high risk of vomiting should receive prophylactic antiemetics for postoperative nausea and vomiting.

❽ Patients receiving single-exposure, high-dose radiation therapy to the upper abdomen or receiving total or hemibody irradiation, should receive prophylactic antiemetics for radiation-induced nausea and vomiting.

Nausea and vomiting are common complaints in individuals of all ages. (Disorders are discussed in Etiology section.) However, because of the variable etiologies of these problems, management can be quite simple or detailed and complex, essentially innocuous or associated with therapy-induced adverse reactions. This chapter provides an overview of nausea and vomiting, two multifaceted problems.

Nausea is usually defined as the inclination to vomit or as a feeling in the throat or epigastric region alerting an individual that vomiting is imminent. Vomiting is defined as the ejection or expulsion of gastric contents through the mouth and is often a forceful

event. Either condition may occur transiently with no other associated signs or symptoms; however, these conditions also may be only part of a more complex clinical presentation.

ETIOLOGY

❶ Nausea and vomiting may be associated with a variety of conditions, including gastrointestinal (GI), cardiovascular, infectious, neurologic, or metabolic disease processes. Nausea and vomiting may be a feature of such conditions as pregnancy, or may follow operative procedures or administration of certain medications, such as those used in cancer chemotherapy. Psychogenic etiologies of these symptoms may be present, especially in young women with an underlying emotional disturbance. Anticipatory etiologies may be involved, such as in patients who have previously received cytotoxic chemotherapy. Table 42–1 lists specific etiologies associated with nausea and vomiting.[1]

The etiology of nausea and vomiting may vary with the age of the patient. For example, vomiting in the newborn during the first day of life suggests upper digestive tract obstruction or an increase in intracranial pressure. Other illnesses associated with vomiting in children include pyloric stenosis, duodenal ulcer, stress ulcer, adrenal insufficiency, septicemia, and diseases of the pancreas, liver, or biliary tree. ❷ Drug-induced nausea and vomiting are of particular concern, especially with the increasing number of patients receiving cytotoxic treatment. A four-level classification system defines the risk for emesis with specific cytotoxic agents (Table 42–2).[2] Although some agents may have greater emetic risk than others, combinations of agents, high doses, clinical settings, psychological conditions, prior treatment experiences, and unusual stimulus of sight, smell, or taste may alter a patient's response to drug treatment. In this setting, nausea and vomiting may be unavoidable and some patients experience these problems so intensely that chemotherapy is postponed or discontinued.

Cancer patients undergoing chemotherapy may experience breakthrough nausea and/or vomiting despite receiving prophylactic antiemetics. Historically, breakthrough emesis occurs in 10% to 40% treated with modern-day antiemetics. Anticipatory nausea or vomiting (ANV) is believed to be a learned, conditioned, or psychological response to a poor outcome from a previous event. It may be triggered by tastes, odors, sights, thoughts, or anxiety associated with chemotherapy.[3] In the setting of optimal antiemetic prophylaxis, chemotherapy-induced ANV can occur in up to 10% and 20% of patients receiving chemotherapy but rarely occurs unless the patient has previously experienced post-treatment nausea or vomiting.[4,5] In addition to the emetic risk of various cytotoxic regimens, other common etiologies have been proposed for the development of nausea and vomiting in cancer patients (Table 42–3).[6,7]

TABLE 42-1	Specific Etiologies of Nausea and Vomiting

Gastrointestinal mechanisms
  Mechanical obstruction
    Gastric outlet obstruction
    Small bowel obstruction
  Functional gastrointestinal disorders
    Gastroparesis
    Nonulcer dyspepsia
    Chronic intestinal pseudoobstruction
    Irritable bowel syndrome
  Organic gastrointestinal disorders
    Peptic ulcer disease
    Pancreatitis
    Pyelonephritis
    Cholecystitis
    Cholangitis
    Hepatitis
  Acute gastroenteritis
    Viral
    Bacterial

Cardiovascular diseases
  Acute myocardial infarction
  Congestive heart failure
  Radiofrequency ablation

Neurologic processes
  Increased intracranial pressure
  Migraine headache
  Vestibular disorders

Metabolic disorders
  Diabetes mellitus (diabetic ketoacidosis)
  Addison disease
  Renal disease (uremia)

Psychiatric causes
  Psychogenic vomiting
  Anxiety disorders
  Anorexia nervosa

Therapy-induced causes
  Cytotoxic chemotherapy
  Radiation therapy
  Theophylline preparations
  Anticonvulsant preparations
  Digitalis preparations
  Opiates
  Antibiotics
  Volatile general anesthetics

Drug withdrawal
  Opiates
  Benzodiazepines

Miscellaneous causes
  Pregnancy
  Noxious odors
  Operative procedures

Reprinted and adapted from Hasler WL, Chey WD. Gastroenterology, 2003, Vol. 25, 1860–1867.

TABLE 42-2	Emetic Risk of Intravenous Cytotoxic Agents

Emetic Risk (If No Prophylactic Medication is Administered)	Cytotoxic Agent (in Alphabetical Order)
High (>90%)	Carmustine
	Cisplatin
	Cyclophosphamide ≥1,500 mg/m²
	Dacarbazine
	Dactinomycin
	Mechlorethamine
	Streptozotocin
Moderate (30%–90%)	Carboplatin
	Cytarabine >1 g/m²
	Cyclophosphamide <1,500 mg/m²
	Daunorubicin
	Doxorubicin
	Epirubicin
	Idarubicin
	Ifosfamide
	Irinotecan
	Oxaliplatin
	Procarbazine
Low (10%–30%)	Bortezomib
	Capecitabine
	Cetuximab
	Cytarabine ≤1 g/m²
	Docetaxel
	Erlotinib
	Etoposide
	Fluorouracil
	Gemcitabine
	Lapatinib
	Methotrexate
	Mitomycin
	Mitoxantrone
	Paclitaxel
	Pemetrexed
	Sorafenib
	Sunitinib
	Temozolamide
	Topotecan
	Trastuzumab
Minimal (<10%)	Bevacizumab
	Bleomycin
	Busulfan
	2-Chlorodeoxyadenosine
	Fludarabine
	Rituximab
	Vinblastine
	Vincristine
	Vinorelbine

Data from Prevention of chemotherapy and radiotherapy-induced emesis. Results of the 2004 Perugia International Antiemetic Consensus Conference. Ann Oncol 2006;17:20–28, by permission of Oxford University.

PATHOPHYSIOLOGY

The three consecutive phases of emesis include nausea, retching, and vomiting. Nausea, the imminent need to vomit, is associated with gastric stasis and may be considered a separate and singular symptom. Retching is the labored movement of abdominal and thoracic muscles before vomiting. The final phase of emesis is vomiting, the forceful expulsion of gastric contents caused by GI retroperistalsis. The act of vomiting requires the coordinated contractions of the abdominal muscles, pylorus, and antrum, a raised gastric cardia, diminished lower esophageal sphincter pressure, and esophageal dilatation.[8] Vomiting should not be confused with regurgitation, an act in which the gastric or esophageal contents rise to the pharynx because of pressure differences caused by, for example, an incompetent lower esophageal sphincter. Accompanying autonomic symptoms of pallor, tachycardia, and diaphoresis account for many of the distressing feelings associated with emesis.

Vomiting is triggered by afferent impulses to the vomiting center, a nucleus of cells in the medulla. Impulses are received from sensory centers, which include the chemoreceptor trigger zone (CTZ), cerebral cortex, and visceral afferents from the pharynx and GI tract. These afferent impulses are integrated by the vomiting center, resulting in efferent impulses to the salivation center, respiratory center, and the pharyngeal, GI, and abdominal muscles, leading to vomiting.

TABLE 42-3	Nonchemotherapy Etiologies of Nausea and Vomiting in Cancer Patients

Fluid and electrolyte abnormalities
   Hypercalcemia
   Volume depletion
   Water intoxication
   Adrenocortical insufficiency
Drug induced
   Opiates
   Antibiotics
   Antifungals
Gastrointestinal obstruction
Increased intracranial pressure
Peritonitis
Metastases
   Brain
   Meninges
   Hepatic
Uremia
Infections (septicemia, local)
Radiation therapy

Data from Stephenson and Davies,[6] and American Society of Health-System.[7]

TABLE 42-4	Presentation of Nausea and Vomiting

General
   Depending on severity of symptoms, patients may present in mild to severe distress
Symptoms
   Simple: Self-limiting, resolves spontaneously and requires only symptomatic therapy
   Complex: Not relieved after administration of antiemetics; progressive deterioration of patient secondary to fluid–electrolyte imbalances; usually associated with noxious agents or psychogenic events
Signs
   Simple: Patient complaint of queasiness or discomfort
   Complex: Weight loss; fever; abdominal pain
Laboratory tests
   Simple: None
   Complex: Serum electrolyte concentrations; upper/lower GI evaluation
Other information
   Fluid input and output
   Medication history
   Recent history of behavioral or visual changes, headache, pain, or stress
   Family history positive for psychogenic vomiting

The CTZ, located in the area postrema of the fourth ventricle of the brain, is a major chemosensory organ for emesis and is usually associated with chemically induced vomiting. Because of its location, bloodborne and cerebrospinal fluid toxins have easy access to the CTZ. Therefore, cytotoxic agents primarily stimulate this area rather than the cerebral cortex and visceral afferents. Similarly, pregnancy-associated vomiting probably occurs through stimulation of the CTZ.

Numerous neurotransmitter receptors are located in the vomiting center, CTZ, and GI tract, including cholinergic, histaminic, dopaminergic, opiate, serotonergic, neurokinin, and benzodiazepine receptors. Chemotherapeutic agents, their metabolites, or other emetic compounds theoretically trigger the process of emesis through stimulation of one or more of these receptors. Effective antiemetics are able to antagonize or block the emetogenic receptors.

CLINICAL PRESENTATION

Because it is impossible to discuss all clinical settings in which the presence of nausea and vomiting might be a pertinent finding, these processes are presented in Table 42–4 as they might occur together, and also as *simple* or *complex* in presentation.

TREATMENT

■ DESIRED OUTCOME

❸ The overall goal of antiemetic therapy is to prevent or eliminate nausea and vomiting. This should be accomplished without adverse effects or with clinically acceptable adverse effects. Although this goal may be accomplished easily in patients with simple nausea and vomiting, patients with more complex problems require greater assistance. In addition to these clinical goals, appropriate cost issues should be considered, particularly in the management of chemotherapy-induced and postoperative nausea and vomiting.

■ GENERAL APPROACH TO TREATMENT

❹ Treatment options for nausea and vomiting include drug and nondrug modalities. The treatment of nausea and vomiting

is quite varied depending on the associated medical situation. Even though a number of potentially effective measures are available, most patients receive a medication at some point in their care. For simple nausea and vomiting, patients may choose to do nothing or to select from a variety of nonprescription drugs. As symptoms become worse or are associated with more serious medical problems, patients are more likely to benefit from prescription antiemetic drugs. When prescribed according to reliable clinical information, these agents often provide acceptable relief; however, some patients will never be totally free of symptoms. This lack of relief is most disabling when it is associated with an unresolved medical problem or when the necessary therapy for this condition is the cause of the nausea or vomiting, as in the case of patients who are receiving chemotherapy of moderate or high emetic risk.

■ NONPHARMACOLOGIC MANAGEMENT

Nonpharmacologic management of nausea and vomiting involves the use of a variety of dietary, physical, or psychological strategies that are consistent with the etiology of nausea and vomiting. For patients with simple complaints, perhaps resulting from excessive or disagreeable food or beverage consumption, avoidance or moderation in dietary intake may be preferable. Patients suffering symptoms of systemic illness may improve dramatically as their underlying condition resolves. Finally, patients in whom these symptoms result from labyrinthine changes produced by motion may benefit quickly by assuming a stable physical position.

Nonpharmacologic interventions are classified as behavioral interventions and include relaxation, biofeedback, self-hypnosis, cognitive distraction, guided imagery, acupuncture, and systematic desensitization.[9,10] The reader is referred to references 11 to 13 for a more complete discussion on nonpharmacological strategies.

■ PHARMACOLOGIC THERAPY

❹ Although many approaches to the treatment of nausea and vomiting have been suggested, antiemetic drugs (nonprescription and prescription) are most often recommended. These agents represent a variety of pharmacologic and chemical classes, as well as dosage regimens and routes of administration. With so many treatment possibilities available, factors that enable the clinician to

TABLE 42-5 Common Antiemetic Preparations and Adult Dosage Regimens

Drug	Adult Dosage Regimen	Dosage Form/Route	Availability
Antacids			
Antacids (various)	15–30 mL every 2–4 h prn	Liquid/oral	OTC
Antihistaminic–anticholinergic agents			
Cyclizine (Marezine)	50 mg before departure; may repeat in 4–6 h prn	Tab	OTC
Dimenhydrinate (Dramamine)	50–100 mg every 4–6 h prn	Tab, chew tab, cap	OTC
Diphenhydramine (Benadryl)	25–50 mg every 4–6 h prn	Tab, cap, liquid	Rx/OTC
	10–50 mg every 2–4 h prn	IM, IV	
Hydroxyzine (Vistaril, Atarax)	25–100 mg every 4–6 h prn	IM (unlabeled use)	Rx
Meclizine (Bonine, Antivert)	12.5–25 mg 1 h before travel; repeat every 12–24 h prn	Tab, chew tab	Rx/OTC
Scopolamine (Transderm Scop)	1.5 mg every 72 h	Transdermal patch	Rx
Trimethobenzamide (Tigan)	300 mg 3–4 times daily	Cap	Rx
	200 mg 3–4 times daily	IM	
Benzodiazepines			
Alprazolam (Xanax)	0.5–2 mg three times daily prior to chemotherapy	Tab	Rx (C-IV)
Lorazepam (Ativan)	0.5–2 mg on night before and morning of chemotherapy	Tab	Rx (C-IV)
Butyrophenones			
Haloperidol (Haldol)	1–5 mg every 12 h prn	Tab, liquid, IM, IV	Rx
Droperidol (Inapsine)[a]	2.5 mg; additional 1.25 mg may be given	IM, IV	Rx
Cannabinoids			
Dronabinol (Marinol)	5–15 mg/m^2 every 2–4 h prn	Cap	Rx (C-III)
Nabilone (Cesamet)	1–2 mg twice daily	Cap	Rx (C-II)
Histamine (H$_2$) antagonists			
Cimetidine (Tagamet HB)	200 mg twice daily prn	Tab	OTC
Famotidine (Pepcid AC)	10 mg twice daily prn	Tab	OTC
Nizatidine (Axid AR)	75 mg twice daily prn	Tab	OTC
Ranitidine (Zantac 75)	75 mg twice daily prn	Tab	OTC
5-hydroxytryptamine-3 receptor antagonists (see Tables 42–6 for CINV dosing and 42–8 for PONV dosing)			
Miscellaneous agents			
Metoclopramide (Reglan), for delayed CINV	20–40 mg 3–4 daily	Tab	Rx
Olanzapine (Zyprexa)	2.5–5 mg twice daily	Tab	Rx
Phenothiazines			
Chlorpromazine (Thorazine)	10–25 mg every 4–6 h prn	Tab, liquid	Rx
	25–50 mg every 4–6 h prn	IM, IV	
Prochlorperazine (Compazine)	5–10 mg 3–4 daily prn	Tab, liquid	Rx
	5–10 mg every 3–4 h prn	IM	
	2.5–10 mg every 3–4 h prn	IV	Rx
	25 mg twice daily prn	Supp	Rx
Promethazine (Phenergan)	12.5–25 mg every 4–6 h prn	Tab, liquid, IM, IV, supp	Rx

C-II, C-III, C-IV, controlled substance schedule 2, 3, and 4, respectively; cap, capsule; chew tab, chewable tablet; CINV, chemotherapy-induced nausea and vomiting; liquid, oral syrup, concentrate, or suspension; OTC, nonprescription; PONV, postoperative nausea and vomiting; Rx, prescription; supp, rectal suppository; tab, tablet.
[a]See text for current warnings.

discriminate among various choices include (a) the suspected etiology of the symptoms; (b) the frequency, duration, and severity of the episodes; (c) the ability of the patient to use oral, rectal, injectable, or transdermal medications; and (d) the success of previous antiemetic medications. Please see Table 42–5 for dosing information of commonly available antiemetic preparations.

The treatment of simple nausea and vomiting usually requires minimal therapy. For these symptoms, patients may choose from a lengthy list of nonprescription products. Both nonprescription and prescription drugs useful in the treatment of simple nausea and vomiting are usually effective in small, infrequently administered doses. Side effects and toxic effects in these settings are also usually minimal. Although suitable for occasional simple nausea and vomiting, nonprescription agents are often abandoned by the patient as symptoms continue or become progressively worse. As the patient's condition warrants, prescription medications may be chosen, either as single-agent therapy or in combination.

The management of complex nausea and vomiting, for example, in patients who are receiving cytotoxic chemotherapy, may require combination therapy. In combination regimens, the goal is to achieve symptomatic control through administration of agents with different pharmacologic mechanisms of action.

Antacids

Patients who are experiencing simple nausea and vomiting may use various antacids. In this setting, single or combination nonprescription antacid products, especially those containing magnesium hydroxide, aluminum hydroxide, and/or calcium carbonate, may provide sufficient relief, primarily through gastric acid neutralization.

Common antacid regimens for the relief of acute or intermittent nausea and vomiting include one or more 15 to 30 mL doses of single- or multiple-agent products. Potential adverse effects from antacids are usually related to the presence of magnesium, aluminum, or calcium salts. Specifically, osmotic diarrhea from magnesium and constipation from aluminum or calcium salts may be of concern to patients, particularly those self-medicating with high or frequently administered antacid doses. Generally, however, when used occasionally for acute episodic relief of nausea and vomiting, antacids do not produce serious toxicities.

Antihistamine–Anticholinergic Drugs

Antiemetic drugs from the antihistaminic–anticholinergic category appear to interrupt various visceral afferent pathways that stimulate nausea and vomiting and may be appropriate in the treatment of simple nausea and vomiting. Adverse reactions associated with the use of the antihistaminic–anticholinergic agents primarily include drowsiness, confusion, blurred vision, dry mouth, and urinary retention, and possibly tachycardia, particularly in elderly patients. Also, as doses are increased or are more frequently administered, patients with narrow-angle glaucoma, prostatic hyperplasia, or asthma are at greater risk of complications from the anticholinergic effects of these drugs.

Benzodiazepines

Since nausea and vomiting are often associated with chemotherapy, radiotherapy, and surgery, anticipatory anxiety may occur prior to these therapies and may exacerbate symptoms. Benzodiazepines may be useful in this setting.

Benzodiazepines are relatively weak antiemetics and are primarily used to prevent anxiety or ANV in patients receiving highly emetogenic chemotherapy. They are also useful against akathisia associated with metoclopramide therapy. Both alprazolam and lorazepam are used as adjuncts to other antiemetics in patients treated with cisplatin-containing regimens. Lorazepam significantly reduced the incidence of ANV in cisplatin-treated patients. Lorazepam caused both mild sedation and amnesia.[14] Alprazolam is usually given orally and has an onset of about 60 minutes, while lorazepam is given orally or sublingually, which has a more rapid onset.

Buterophenones

Two buterophenone compounds that have antiemetic activity are haloperidol and its congener droperidol; both block dopaminergic stimulation of the CTZ. Although each agent is effective in relieving nausea and vomiting, haloperidol is not considered first-line therapy for uncomplicated nausea and vomiting but has been used in palliative care situations.[15] The current labeling of droperidol recommends that all patients should undergo a 12-lead electrocardiogram prior to administration, followed by cardiac monitoring for 2 to 3 hours after administration because of the possibility of the development of potentially fatal QT prolongation and/or torsade de pointes.[16] The clinical use of droperidol has effectively ceased outside of clinical trials in anesthesia.

Cannabinoids

Cannabinoids have complex effects on the central nervous system (CNS) and their effects at receptors in neural tissues may explain efficacy in chemotherapy-induced nausea and vomiting (CINV). Oral dronabinol and nabilone are one of several therapeutic options when CINV is refractory to other antiemetics; they are not indicated as first-line agents.

Chemotherapy use with over 1,300 patients in 30 randomized, controlled trials from 1975 to 1996 was analyzed to quantify the antiemetic efficacy and adverse effects of several cannabinoids.[17] Oral nabilone, oral dronabinol, and intramuscular levonantradol were compared with conventional antiemetics (prochlorperazine, metoclopramide, chlorpromazine, thiethylperazine, haloperidol, domperidone, and alizapride) or placebo. Across all trials, cannabinoids were slightly more effective than active comparators and placebo when the chemotherapy regimen was of moderate emetogenic potential, and patients preferred them. No dose–response relationships were evident to the authors. Side effects included euphoria, drowsiness, sedation, somnolence, dysphoria, depression, hallucinations, and paranoia.

Corticosteroids

Corticosteroids have demonstrated antiemetic efficacy since the initial recognition that patients who received prednisone as part of their Hodgkin disease protocol appeared to develop less nausea and vomiting than did those patients who were treated with protocols that excluded this agent. Methylprednisolone has also been used as a component of an antiemetic regimen, but the majority of trials have included dexamethasone. The site and mechanism of action of corticosteroids for CINV is unknown.

Dexamethasone is the most commonly used corticosteroid in the management of chemotherapy-induced and postoperative nausea and vomiting (PONV), either as a single agent or in combination with 5-hydroxytryptamine-3 receptor antagonists (5-HT$_3$-RA). For CINV, dexamethasone is effective in the prevention of both cisplatin-induced acute emesis and when used alone or in combination for the prevention of delayed nausea and vomiting associated with CINV.[18-21] Corticosteroids affect almost every organ system. Insomnia, gastrointestinal symptoms, agitation, and appetite stimulation are some of the more common side effects reported in this patient population. For patients with simple nausea and vomiting, steroids are not indicated and may be associated with unacceptable risks.

H$_2$-Receptor Antagonists

Histamine$_2$-receptor antagonists work by decreasing gastric acid production and are used to manage simple nausea and vomiting associated with heartburn or gastroesophageal reflux. Except for potential drug interactions with cimetidine, these agents cause few side effects when used for episodic relief.

5-Hydroxytryptamine-3 Receptor Antagonists

5-HT$_3$-RAs block presynaptic serotonin receptors on sensory vagal fibers in the gut wall, effectively blocking the acute phase of CINV. These agents do not completely block the acute phase of CINV and are less efficacious in preventing the delayed phase, but they are the standard of care in the management of CINV, PONV, and radiation-induced nausea and vomiting (RINV). Issues involved in the use of dolasetron, granisetron, ondansetron, and palonosetron are reviewed in detail in the sections that follow. The most common side effects associated with these agents are constipation, headache, and asthenia.

Metoclopramide

Metoclopramide, a procainamide congener, provides significant antiemetic effects by blocking the dopaminergic receptors centrally in the CTZ. Metoclopramide increases lower esophageal sphincter tone, aids gastric emptying, and accelerates transit through the small bowel, possibly through the release of acetylcholine. Metoclopramide is used for its antiemetic properties in patients with diabetic gastroparesis and with dexamethasone for prophylaxis of delayed CINV. Its use as prophylaxis for acute chemotherapy-induced nausea and vomiting was supplanted by the introduction of the 5-HT$_3$-RAs in the early 1990s. These agents have greater efficacy and decreased toxicity compared with metoclopramide in patients who are receiving cisplatin-based regimens.[22,23]

Olanzapine

Olanzapine is an antipsychotic that blocks several neurotransmitters including dopamine at D$_2$ and 5-HT$_3$-RA. Use of olanzapine, in combination with palonosetron and dexamethasone, effectively prevented acute CINV, while continued monotherapy with olanzapine prevented most cases of delayed nausea and vomiting in patients receiving moderately and highly emetogenic chemotherapy in a single-arm, phase 2 clinical trial in 40 patients.[24] The National Comprehensive Cancer Network (NCCN) antiemesis practice guideline includes olanzapine as one of many options in patients who experience breakthrough nausea and/or vomiting following prophylaxis for CINV.[25] Sedation is the most common side effect with olanzapine.

Phenothiazines

Phenothiazines have been the most widely prescribed antiemetic agents and appear to block dopamine receptors, most likely in the CTZ. Phenothiazines are marketed in an array of dosage forms, none of which appears to be more efficacious than another. These agents may be most practical for long-term treatment and are inexpensive in comparison with newer drugs. Rectal administration is a reasonable alternative in patients in whom oral or parenteral administration is not feasible.

Phenothiazines are most useful in adult patients with simple nausea and vomiting. Intravenous prochlorperazine provided quicker and more complete relief with less drowsiness than intravenous promethazine in adult patients treated in an emergency department for nausea and vomiting associated with uncomplicated gastritis or gastroenteritis.[26] There are numerous potential side effects with these medications, including extrapyramidal reactions, hypersensitivity reactions with possible liver dysfunction, bone marrow aplasia, and excessive sedation.

Substance P/Neurokinin 1 Receptor Antagonists

Substance P is a peptide neurotransmitter in the neurokinin (NK) family whose preferred receptor is the NK_1 receptor.[27] The acute phase of CINV is believed to be mediated by both serotonin and substance P, whereas substance P is believed to be the primary mediator of the delayed phase. Aprepitant is the first substance P/NK_1 receptor antagonist in clinical use; others are in development. The efficacy of aprepitant was demonstrated in patients receiving high-dose cisplatin-based chemotherapy[20,21] and in patients receiving doxorubicin and cyclophosphamide,[28] a regimen of moderate to high emetic risk. The three-drug regimen of aprepitant, dexamethasone, and ondansetron provided improved protection from vomiting for the 5 days after chemotherapy administration as compared with the combination of dexamethasone and ondansetron.

Aprepitant has the potential for numerous drug interactions because it is a substrate, moderate inhibitor, and an inducer of cytochrome isoenzyme CYP3A4 and an inducer of CYP2C9. Aprepitant can increase serum concentrations of many drugs metabolized by CYP3A4, including docetaxel, paclitaxel, etoposide, irinotecan, ifosfamide, imatinib, vinorelbine, vincristine, and vinblastine. In clinical studies, aprepitant was concomitantly administered with etoposide, vinorelbine, or paclitaxel, with no adjustment in the doses of these agents to account for potential drug interactions. The efficacy of oral contraceptives may be reduced when given with aprepitant. Concomitant administration with warfarin may result in a clinically significant decrease in the international normalized ratio.[29] The dose of oral dexamethasone should be reduced 50% when coadministered with aprepitant, because of the 2.2-fold increase in observed area under the plasma-concentration-versus time curve.[30] Aprepitant is not approved for use in children.

Fosaprepitant, an injectable form of aprepitant, has been approved by the FDA as an intravenous substitute for oral aprepitant on day 1 of the standard 3-day CINV prevention regimen, with oral aprepitant administered on days 2 and 3.[31]

■ CHEMOTHERAPY-INDUCED NAUSEA AND VOMITING

There are five categories of CINV: acute, delayed, anticipatory, breakthrough, and refractory. ❺ Nausea and vomiting that occurs within 24 hours of chemotherapy administration is defined as acute, whereas when it starts more than 24 hours after chemotherapy administration, it is defined as delayed. The primary goal with CINV is to *prevent* nausea and/or vomiting. Optimal control of acute nausea and vomiting impacts positively on the incidence and control of delayed and anticipatory nausea and vomiting.[32]

Emesis occurring during previous chemotherapy predisposes for the risk of developing ANV.[4] Breakthrough nausea and vomiting is defined as emesis occurring despite prophylactic administration of antiemetics, requiring use of rescue antiemetics. Poor response to multiple antiemetic regimens is defined as refractory nausea and vomiting.

Clinical practice guidelines for the use of antiemetics in CINV have been published.[2,25,33] Despite the demonstrated improvement in outcomes with the use of these practice guidelines, they are underutilized by a high percentage of practitioners.[34] Furthermore, product availability and recommended doses are often institution-specific and may vary considerably from the doses listed in Table 42–6.

Factors to consider when selecting an antiemetic for CINV include the following:

- The emetic risk of the chemotherapy agent or regimen (see Table 42–2)
- Patient-specific factors
- Patterns of emesis after administration of specific chemotherapy agents or regimens

Prophylaxis of Acute CINV

❻ The emetic risk of the chemotherapeutic agent (see Table 42–2) is the primary factor to consider when deciding whether to administer prophylactic agents and which antiemetic(s) to select. Table 42–6 summarizes recommendations from version 4 of the 2009 NCCN antiemetic guidelines.[25] Antiemetic guidelines published by other groups are in overall agreement with the NCCN guidelines.

Patients receiving chemotherapy that is classified as being of high emetic risk should receive a combination of three antiemetic drugs on the day of chemotherapy administration (day 1) including a 5-HT_3-RA (e.g., dolasetron, granisetron, ondansetron, or palonosetron) + dexamethasone + an NK_1 receptor antagonist (e.g., aprepitant). Patients receiving regimens that are classified as moderate emetic risk should receive a two-drug combination antiemetic regimen containing a 5-HT_3-RA + dexamethasone on day 1. The exception to this is patients who are receiving an anthracycline plus cyclophosphamide and select patients receiving other chemotherapies of moderate emetic risk, for example, carboplatin, cisplatin, doxorubicin, epirubicin, ifosfamide, irinotecan or methotrexate; these patients should receive the triple-drug combination described for regimens of high emetic risk.

For chemotherapy regimens that are low emetic risk, dexamethasone or any of the following: prochlorperazine, metoclopramide, and/or diphenhydramine, and/or lorazepam alone is recommended for prophylaxis.[25] When equivalent doses are used for the prevention of acute emesis, all 5-HT_3-RAs are considered to be of

TABLE 42-6	Dosage Recommendations for CINV for Adult Patients	
Emetic Risk	Prophylaxis of Acute Phase of CINV (One Dose Administered Prior to Chemotherapy)	Prophylaxis of Delayed Phase of CINV
High (including the AC regimen[a])	5-HT$_3$ receptor antagonists (5-HT$_3$-RA): Dolasetron 100 mg orally or 100 mg IV or 1.8 mg/kg IV Granisetron 2 mg orally or 1 mg IV or 0.01 mg/kg IV or 34.3 mg transdermal patch Ondansetron 16–24 mg orally or 8–12 mg IV (maximum 32 mg) Palonosetron 0.25 mg IV	
	and Dexamethasone 12 mg orally or IV	Dexamethasone 8–12 mg orally days 2–4
	and Aprepitant 125 mg orally or Fosaprepitant 115 mg IV	Aprepitant 80 mg orally days 2 and 3 after chemotherapy
Moderate	5-HT$_3$-RA: Dolasetron 100 mg orally or 100 mg IV or 1.8 mg/kg IV	5-HT$_3$-RA : Dolasetron 100 mg orally daily[b]
	Granisetron 2 mg orally or 1 mg IV or 0.01 mg/kg IV or 34.3 mg transdermal patch	Granisetron 1–2 mg orally daily[b]
	Ondansetron 16–24 mg orally or 8–12 mg IV (max. 32 mg) Palonosetron 0.25 mg IV Palonosetron 0.5 mg orally	Ondansetron 8 mg orally daily or twice daily[b]
	and Dexamethasone 8–12 mg orally or IV	Dexamethasone 8–12 mg orally daily[b]
	and in select patients[c] Aprepitant 125 mg orally or Fosaprepitant 115 mg IV	Aprepitant 80 mg orally days 2 and 3 if used on day 1
Low	Dexamethasone 8–12 mg orally or IV	None
Minimal	None	None

[a]See reference 33.
[b]For 2–3 days following chemotherapy.
[c]Patients receiving other chemotherapies of moderate emetic risk, for example, carboplatin, cisplatin, doxorubicin, epirubicin, ifosfamide, irinotecan, or methotrexate.
Doses included in the above table reflect the recommendations from published guidelines (references 2, 25, 33). These doses may differ from manufacturer labeling; they reflect the consensus of the guideline participants.
CINV, chemotherapy-induced nausea and vomiting.

equivalent efficacy and safety. When available in both oral and intravenous dosage forms, oral agents are equally effective as intravenous products. The decision as to which 5-HT$_3$-RA to use should be based on patient-specific factors and cost.

Prophylaxis of Delayed CINV

Management of delayed CINV has historically challenged practitioners. The best strategy for preventing delayed CINV (nausea and/or vomiting occurring 24 or more hours after chemotherapy) is to control acute CINV and provide adequate prophylaxis for delayed CINV.[35] Aprepitant, dexamethasone, and metoclopramide are effective in preventing delayed CINV, whereas 5-HT$_3$-RAs are

inconsistent.[27] However, palonosetron controlled delayed emesis more effectively than granisetron, suggesting that another 5-HT$_3$-RA should not be prescribed as a rescue medication when palonosetron is given prophylactically for acute CINV.[36]

Patients receiving cisplatin and other agents are at highest risk for experiencing delayed CINV. The addition of aprepitant in the recommended three-drug combination on the day of cisplatin administration and additional doses of aprepitant and dexamethasone on days two and three after cisplatin administration improved the control of delayed vomiting as compared with patients who received dexamethasone alone postchemotherapy (51% vs 72%).[20,21] Use of aprepitant also decreased delayed CINV in patients receiving an anthracycline plus cyclophosphamide, as compared with twice-daily ondansetron (49% vs 55%).[28] Current practice guidelines recommend administration of aprepitant and dexamethasone on days 2 and 3 and dexamethasone with or without lorazepam on day 4.[2,25]

The incidence of delayed CINV following chemotherapy with agents of moderate emetic risk is less well defined. The current NCCN recommendation is to give aprepitant or any of the following: dexamethasone, a 5-HT$_3$-RA, and/or lorazepam and/or a histamine-2 blocker or a proton pump inhibitor on days 2 and 3.[25] The American Society of Clinical Oncology (ASCO) and Multinational Association of Supportive Care in Cancer (MASCC) practice guidelines do not include aprepitant on days 2 and 3.

A second-generation 5-HT$_3$-RA, palonosetron, has a prolonged serum half-life and higher receptor binding affinity that may offer another option for prophylaxis of delayed CINV. Palonosetron given once every 7 days protected more patients from delayed emesis than either ondansetron or dolasetron in adult patients receiving chemotherapy of moderate emetic risk.[37-39] Subsequently, a large randomized, blinded study in patients receiving chemotherapy of high emetic risk showed that palonesetron plus dexamethasone was not inferior to granisetron plus dexamethasone for controlling acute CINV but was superior for delayed CINV.[36] Palonosetron may also be better than ondansetron in patients receiving multi-day chemotherapy, but a larger randomized, prospective trial is needed to substantiate the finding of a recent study.[40]

Treatment of Anticipatory Nausea and Vomiting

ANV is more difficult to control than acute or delayed CINV. A key principle in the treatment of ANV is that effective management of delayed CINV or ANV requires adequate control of acute CINV.[41] In addition, ANV may be prevented with behavioral therapy or pharmacotherapy.[42] The benzodiazepines, lorazepam and alprazolam, are effective in preventing ANV and improve outcomes in both acute and delayed emesis.

Treatment of Breakthrough CINV

Breakthrough nausea and/or vomiting occurs in 10% to 40% of patients receiving chemotherapy despite the use of multi-agent prophylaxis.[32] All patients receiving chemotherapy should be prescribed antiemetics for rescue of breakthrough nausea and vomiting. Rescue medications used in adult patients include prochlorperazine, promethazine, lorazepam, metoclopramide, haloperidol, benzodiazepines such as lorazepam, 5-HT$_3$-RAs, dexamethasone, and cannabinoids such as dronabinol or olanzapine.[25,43]

Around-the-clock dosing of rescue antiemetics should be considered rather than as-needed administration. The choice of agent should be based on patient-specific factors, including potential adverse drug reactions and cost. Chlorpromazine, lorazepam, and dexamethasone are recommended for pediatric patients.[44]

Treatment of Refractory Nausea and Vomiting

The general approach to the management of refractory CINV is to upgrade the antiemetic strategy to the next level of prophylaxis or to add breakthrough antiemetics to the regimen.[45] Some patients will experience nausea and vomiting despite optimal acute and delayed prophylaxis and failure of rescue antiemetics. Addition of another agent from a different pharmacologic class is recommended and routes other than the oral route may be required. Agents such as corticosteroids, haloperidol, olanzapine, and nabilone in alternating schedules or by alternating routes are recommended.[25]

Prophylaxis of Anticipatory Nausea and Vomiting

As stated earlier, ANV rarely occurs unless the patient has previously experienced post-treatment nausea or vomiting. ANV may also be prevented with prophylactic pharmacotherapy using benzodiazepines the night before and morning of chemotherapy. A large observational study done after the introduction of 5-HT$_3$-RAs in patients receiving granisetron as antiemetic therapy evaluated ANV as an outcome.[7] An incidence of anticipatory nausea was observed in 10% and anticipatory vomiting in 2% of patients, which is substantially lower than reported prior to the application of effective antiemetic regimens.[46]

CLINICAL CONTROVERSY

The prevention of CINV in patients receiving multi-day chemotherapy is complicated by the overlap of acute and delayed emesis after the first day of chemotherapy. There are few studies and a lower complete control rate using standard antiemetic prophylaxis for patients receiving multi-day chemotherapy regimens.[47] While acute emesis can be controlled adequately, delayed emesis occurs in 50% or more of patients. Agents such as palonosetron, aprepitant, dexamethasone, and olanzapine are effective for both acute and delayed emesis and may have the greatest potential for success in multiday chemotherapy regimens. While the latest NCCN guidelines provide suggestions in this setting, further research is necessary before definitive recommendations can be made.

■ POSTOPERATIVE NAUSEA AND VOMITING

Postoperative nausea and vomiting (PONV) in adults complicates surgical procedures for approximately 25% to 30% of patients undergoing anesthesia.[48] PONV usually occurs within 24 hours after anesthesia, with the highest incidence during the first 2 hours. Most patients undergoing an operative procedure do not require preoperative prophylactic antiemetic therapy and universal PONV prophylaxis is not cost-effective. Table 42–7 summarizes the risk factors for PONV. The use of a risk assessment tool can improve emetic outcomes in patients undergoing surgery by identifying the patients most likely to benefit from prophylaxis.[49]

Adherence to consensus guidelines for prophylaxis and treatment of PONV decreases emetic episodes.[50,51] In addition to using prophylactic antiemetics in high-risk patients, other strategies include using regional rather than systemic anesthesia, propofol, and hydration, as well as avoiding nitrous oxide, volatile anesthetics, and opioids. Total intravenous anesthesia reduced the risk of PONV similar to the prophylactic administration of a single antiemetic.[52]

TABLE 42-7	Risk Factors for Postoperative Nausea and Vomiting (PONV)

Factors unrelated to anesthesia
History of motion sickness
Metabolic factors:
    Uremia
    Diabetes mellitus
    Electrolyte disturbances

Patient-related factors
Age
Female gender (2 to 3 times greater incidence of PONV versus males)
Nonsmoker
History of PONV or motion sickness (3-fold increase in incidence of PONV)
Hydration status

Factors related to anesthesia
Use of volatile anesthetics
Nitrous oxide
Use of opioids (intraoperative or postoperative)

Factors related to surgery
Operative site (higher incidence of PONV after eye, oral, plastic, ear, nose and throat, head and neck, gynecological, obstetric, laparoscopic, and abdominal procedures)
Duration of surgery

Adapted from Kovac[48] and Gan et al.[50]

Prophylaxis of PONV

The most important independent predictors for PONV are female, nonsmoking, a history of PONV or motion sickness, and use of postoperative opioids. A simplified risk model allows clinicians to estimate the risk for PONV among patient groups.[49] Patients with 0 or 1 of these 4 risk factors present are at lowest risk (10–20%) and those with 3 or 4 risk factors are at highest risk for PONV (60–80%). Moderate risk is defined by this model as the presence of 2 risk factors. ❼ Although the optimal management of PONV is not known, patients at highest risk of vomiting should receive prophylactic antiemetics. Patients at low risk for PONV are unlikely to benefit from prophylaxis and may potentially experience adverse reactions from the medications.

Patients at moderate risk for PONV should receive one or two prophylactic antiemetics, and those at high risk should receive two prophylactic antiemetic agents from different classes.[50,52] Optimal dosing of agents used in combination has not been determined. When the different combinations were compared, no differences were found between 5-HT$_3$-RA plus droperidol; 5-HT$_3$-RA plus dexamethasone; and droperidol plus dexamethasone.[53]

Cyclizine, dexamethasone, dolasetron, droperidol, granisetron, metoclopramide, ondansetron, tropisetron, scopolamine, and palonosetron are as effective as placebo for the prophylaxis of PONV.[54–56] Table 42–8 summarizes the doses for prophylactic antiemetics from the consensus guidelines.[50]

Dexamethasone is an effective, inexpensive prophylactic agent when administered either alone or in combination with other antiemetic drugs before the induction of anesthesia.[52,54,57] Although droperidol is one of the most effective agents for PONV prophylaxis, concerns about the development of torsade de pointes severely limit its use.[58] With equivalent efficacy and safety profiles, acquisition cost was the primary factor that differentiated the 5-HT$_3$-RAs from each other.[50] 5-HT$_3$-RAs appear to be most effective when given at the end of surgery.

The NK$_1$ antagonist aprepitant was approved for the prevention of PONV at a dose of 40 mg given orally within 3 hours prior to induction of anesthesia.[29] Aprepitant is equivalent to ondansetron 4 mg IV in the incidence of nausea and reducing the need for rescue in the 24 hours after surgery, but was significantly better than ondansetron for preventing vomiting in the 24 and 48 hours after surgery.[59]

TABLE 42-8 Recommended Prophylactic Doses of Selected Antiemetics for Postoperative Nausea and Vomiting in Adults and Postoperative Vomiting in Children

Drug	Adult Dose	Pediatric Dose (IV)	Timing of Dose[a]
Aprepitant[b]	40 mg orally	Not labeled for use in pediatrics	Within 3 h prior to induction
Dexamethasone	4–5 mg IV	150 mcg/kg up to 5 mg	At induction
Dimenhydrinate	1 mg/kg IV	0.5 mg/kg up to 25 mg	Not specified
Dolasetron	12.5 mg IV	350 mcg/kg up to 12.5 mg	At end of surgery
Droperidol[d]	0.625–1.25 mg IV	10–15 mcg/kg up to 1.25 mg	At end of surgery
Granisetron	0.35–1.5 mg IV	40 mcg/kg up to 0.6 mg	At end of surgery
Haloperidol	0.5–2 mg (IM or IV)	c	Not specified
Ondansetron	4 mg IV	50–100 mcg/kg up to 4 mg	At end of surgery
Palonosetron[b]	0.075 mg IV	Not labeled for patients < 18 y	At induction
Prochlorperazine	5–10 mg IM or IV	c	At end of surgery
Promethazine[d]	6.25–25 mg IV	c	At induction
Scopolamine	Transdermal patch	c	Prior evening or 4 h before surgery
Tropisetron	2 mg IV	0.1 mg/kg up to 2 mg	At end of surgery

[a]Based on recommendations from consensus guidelines; may differ from manufacturer's recommendations.
[b]Labeled for use in PONV but not included in consensus guidelines.
[c]Pediatric dosing not included in consensus guidelines.
[d]See Food and Drug Administration (FDA) "black box" warning.
From Gan et al.[50]

Treatment of PONV

Patients who experience PONV after receiving prophylactic treatment with a 5-HT$_3$-RA plus dexamethasone should receive rescue therapy from a different drug class such as a phenothiazine, metoclopramide, or droperidol.[50] Repeating the agent given for PONV prophylaxis within 6 hours of surgery is of no additional benefit.[60] Furthermore, a repeated dose of a 5-HT$_3$-RA is not effective in treatment of PONV.[61,62] An emetic episode occurring more than 6 hours postoperatively can be treated with any of the drugs used for prophylaxis except dexamethasone and transdermal scopolamine.[50]

If no prophylaxis was given, the recommended treatment is low-dose 5-HT$_3$-RA as follows: dolasetron 12.5 mg, granisetron 0.1 mg, ondansetron 1 mg, and tropisetron 0.5 mg. Alternative treatments for established PONV include dexamethasone 2 to 4 mg IV, droperidol 0.625 mg IV, or promethazine 6.25 to 12.5 mg IV.[63]

■ RADIATION-INDUCED NAUSEA AND VOMITING (RINV)

Nausea and vomiting associated with radiation therapy is not well understood. It is neither as predictable nor as severe as CINV, and many patients receiving radiation therapy will not experience nausea or vomiting. Risk factors associated with the development of RINV include the site of radiation, the dose, dose rate, and area of the body to be irradiated.

❽ Patients receiving single-exposure, high-dose radiation therapy to the upper abdomen, or total or hemibody irradiation, should receive prophylactic antiemetics for RINV.

Prophylaxis of RINV

Four radiotherapy-induced emesis risk groups have been defined by the Antiemetic Subcommittee of the MASCC and the ASCO antiemetic practice guidelines.[2,33] Both groups recommend preventive therapy with a 5-HT$_3$-RA and dexamethasone in patients who are receiving total body irradiation (high emetic risk). The efficacy of oral granisetron 2 mg and ondansetron 8 mg was demonstrated in 34 patients who underwent hyperfractionated total body irradiation.[64] Patients undergoing radiation therapy procedures with moderate to low emetic risk should receive a 5-HT$_3$-RA prior to each fraction.

■ DISORDERS OF BALANCE

Disorders of balance include vertigo, dizziness, and motion sickness. The etiology of these complaints may include diseases that are infectious, postinfectious, demyelinative, vascular, neoplastic, degenerative, traumatic, toxic, psychogenic, or idiopathic. Symptoms of imbalance perceived by the patient present a particular clinical challenge. Whether associated with a minor or complex disorder, motion sickness may be associated with nausea and vomiting.

Beneficial therapy for patients in this setting can most reliably be found among the antihistaminic–anticholinergic agents. However, the precise mechanisms of action of these agents are currently unknown. Neither the antihistaminic nor the anticholinergic potency appears to correlate well with the ability of these agents to prevent or treat the nausea and vomiting associated with motion sickness. When used for their depressant effects on labyrinth excitability, these agents produce variable efficacy and safety profiles. Oral regimens of antihistaminic–anticholinergic agents given one to several times each day may be effective, especially when the first dose is administered prior to motion.

Scopolamine is commonly used to prevent nausea or vomiting caused by motion. The usefulness of scopolamine in preventing motion sickness was enhanced with the development of the transdermal system (patch) that increased patient satisfaction and decreased untoward side effects. A review of 12 randomized, controlled studies showed that scopolamine provided better protection from motion-induced sickness than did placebo, but was not superior to antihistamines and combinations of scopolamine and ephedrine.[65]

■ ANTIEMETIC USE DURING PREGNANCY

As many as 75% of pregnant women experience nausea and vomiting to some degree during the first trimester of pregnancy. The severity of the symptoms varies considerably, from mild nausea to incapacitating nausea and vomiting. Severity may be decreased by taking a multiple vitamin at the time of conception. The etiology of nausea and vomiting of pregnancy (NVP) is not well understood. For the majority of women, these symptoms are self-limited, although approximately 1% to 3% develop hyperemesis gravidarum, a serious condition marked by severe physical symptoms and/or medical complications requiring hospitalization. In its most severe state, hyperemesis gravidarum may result in volume contraction, starvation, and electrolyte abnormalities.

Initial management of NVP often involves dietary changes and/or lifestyle modifications. Nonpharmacologic interventions for NVP include ginger[66] and acupressure, although efficacy trials for acupressure are lacking. Persistent nausea and/or vomiting leads to the consideration of drug therapy at a time when teratogenic potential of each agent must be considered.

Treatment recommendations for the management of NVP are available from the American College of Obstetricians and Gynecologists (ACOG).[67] A comprehensive review of treatment options for NVP was published.[68] Pyridoxine (10–25 mg 1–4 times daily), with or without doxylamine (12.5–20 mg 1–4 times daily), is recommended as first-line therapy. In cases of refractory NVP, addition of a histamine$_1$-receptor antagonist such as dimenhydrinate (50–100 mg orally or rectally every 4–6 hours as needed), diphenhydramine (25–50 mg orally or 10–50 mg IV every 4–6 hours as needed), or meclizine (25 mg orally every 4–6 hours as needed) is recommended. Dopamine antagonists can also be added if symptoms continue (metoclopramide 5–10 mg IV every 8 hours as needed; promethazine 12.5–25 mg IV every 4 hours as needed; prochlorperazine 5–10 mg orally every 6 hours as needed).

Patients with persistent NVP or who show signs of dehydration should receive intravenous fluid replacement with thiamine. Ondansetron 2 to 8 mg orally/IV every 8 hours as needed may alleviate NVP, but intravenous ondansetron was no more effective than promethazine for treatment of severe NVP.[69] Corticosteroids should be reserved for patients with refractory NVP or hyperemesis gravidarum; methylprednisolone 16 mg orally/IV every 8 hours for 3 days followed by a 2-week taper is recommended. This regimen may be repeated if necessary, but treatment should not exceed a total of 6 weeks.

ANTIEMETIC USE IN CHILDREN

CINV

Practice guidelines recommend that a corticosteroid (such as dexamethasone) plus a 5-HT$_3$-RA be administered to children receiving chemotherapy of high or moderate emetic risk.[33] Although studies show there is a wide variation in metabolism and clearance of 5-HT$_3$-RAs, higher weight-based doses have not been adequately studied in pediatric patients.[70]

Consensus guidelines suggest that there are no differences between 5-HT$_3$-RAs in safety or efficacy. However, a randomized, comparative study demonstrated that one dose of palonosetron 0.25 mg IV provided better complete control than ondansetron (8 mg/m^2 IV) in children treated with moderate to highly emetogenic chemotherapy.[71] This study needs to be confirmed in a larger randomized trial.

Gastroenteritis

For nausea and vomiting associated with pediatric gastroenteritis, emphasis should be placed on oral rehydration therapy (ORT); several products are commercially available. However, a recent meta-analyses has shown that pharmacotherapy may be a useful adjunct to ORT.[72] One double-blind study suggested that a single dose of ondansetron may facilitate ORT and reduced the need for IV fluids in children with gastroenteritis who were unable to tolerate oral intake.[73,74] While promethazine given in suppository form was the most often prescribed antiemetic for pediatric gastroenteritis, the Food and Drug Administration added a black box warning due to serious adverse events reports in children and adolescents, including death.[75,76]

PHARMACOECONOMIC CONSIDERATIONS

Cost of antiemetic drugs for the treatment of nausea and vomiting is only one variable to consider in a pharmacoeconomic outcome assessment. Other variables include the cost of managing complications and the impact on loss of work, functionality, and productivity as well as delays of potentially curable therapies. Inadequately controlled emesis can lead to unexpected hospitalizations for potentially serious complications including electrolyte deficiencies, dehydration, esophageal tears, and wound dehiscence.

It is economically and clinically important to develop antiemetic protocols based on appropriate decision analysis to optimize clinical outcomes. The clinical practice guidelines that have been previously described are valuable tools when developing institution-specific antiemetic protocols. The need to control antiemetic costs for health systems is universal and formulary management strategies have been described.[77]

CINV

A large study based on claims data was used to determined the costs associated with CINV over one cycle of chemotherapy.[78] Direct medical cost in the uncontrolled CINV group was estimated to be $1,300 (in 2006 U.S. dollars), or 30% higher than in the controlled CINV group. A sensitivity analysis demonstrated that a new antiemetic agent that could decrease the uncontrolled CINV rate from 50% to 10% would be cost-effective as long as the new drug cost is $500 or less.

PONV

As was presented earlier, the risk of developing PONV increases as the number of risk factors increase. Any occurrence of PONV would likely delay patient discharge from the post-anesthesia unit with a potential increase in the cost of patient care. Prophylactic antiemetic therapy was cost effective with a number needed to treat (NNT) of 3 to 4 (an NNT <5 is considered cost-effective).[79] In low-risk patients, the NNT was about 20 and not cost-effective.

EVALUATION OF EMETIC OUTCOMES

In assessing emetic outcomes, standardized monitoring criteria should include the subjective assessment of the patient's severity of nausea, as well as objective parameters, such as changes in patient weight, the number of vomiting episodes each day, the volume of vomitus lost, and evaluation of fluid, acid–base balance, and electrolyte status, with particular attention to serum sodium, potassium, and chloride concentrations. In addition, evaluation of renal function may become important, particularly in patients with volume contraction and progressive electrolyte disturbances. Specific parameters include daily urine volume, urine specific gravity, and urine electrolyte concentrations. Physical assessment of patients should include evaluation of mucous membranes and skin turgor, because dryness of these tissues may be indicative of significant volume loss.

For patients on chemotherapy, evaluation of emetic outcomes should occur after the administration of each chemotherapy cycle. Adherence to outpatient antiemetic regimens occurs in about 65% of patients. Delayed nausea and vomiting occurs in 15% to 40% of patients, depending on the emetic risk of the chemotherapy and the antiemetic regimen used for prophylaxis. Patients receiving high risk regimens are most likely to report symptoms of nausea and vomiting on day 3 after chemotherapy.[80] Symptom management assessments should be performed on the third or fourth day after chemotherapy. Documentation of a nausea and/or vomiting event will assist the clinician in modifying the antiemetic regimen for the next cycle of chemotherapy.

In the postsurgical anesthesia setting, assessment of nausea and vomiting is important for detecting dehydration, decreased blood pressure, or cardiac arrhythmias. Other complications of PONV include suture line tension, wound dehiscence, and increased bleeding under surgical flaps.[81]

ABBREVIATIONS

ACOG: American College of Obstetricians and Gynecologists

ANV: Anticipatory nausea and vomiting

ASCO: American Society of Clinical Oncology

CINV: chemotherapy-induced nausea and vomiting

CTZ: chemoreceptor trigger zone

MASCC: Multinational Association of Supportive Care in Cancer

NCCN: National Comprehensive Cancer Network

NK_1: neurokinin 1

NNT: number needed to treat

NVP: nausea and vomiting of pregnancy

ORT: oral rehydration therapy

PONV: postoperative nausea and vomiting

RINV: radiation-induced nausea and vomiting

$5\text{-}HT_3RA$: 5-hydroxytryptamine-3 receptor antagonist

REFERENCES

1. Hasler WL, Chey WD. Nausea and vomiting. Gastroenterology 2003;125:1860–1867.
2. Prevention of chemotherapy and radiotherapy-induced emesis. Results of the 2004 Perugia International Antiemetic Consensus Conference. Ann Oncol 2006;17:20–28.
3. Schwartzberg, L. Chemotherapy-induced nausea and vomiting: State of the art in 2006. J Support Oncol 2006;4:3–8.
4. Aapro MS, Molassiotis A, Olver I. Anticipatory nausea and vomiting. Support Care Cancer 2005;13:117–121.
5. Aapro MS, Kirchner V, Terrey JP. The incidence of anticipatory nausea and vomiting after repeat cycle chemotherapy: the effect of granisetron. Br J Cancer 1994;69:957–960.
6. Stephenson J, Davies A. An assessment of etiology-based guidelines for the management of nausea and vomiting in patients with advanced cancer. Support Care Cancer 2006;14:348–353.
7. American Society of Health-System (ASHP) therapeutic guidelines on the pharmacologic management of nausea and vomiting in adult and pediatric patients receiving chemotherapy or radiation therapy or undergoing surgery. Am J Health-Syst Pharm 1999;56:729–764.
8. Lee M. Nausea and vomiting. In: Feldman M, ed. Sleisenger and Fordtran's Gastrointestinal and Liver Disease: Pathophysiology/Diagnosis/Management. St. Louis, MO: Elsevier, 2006:119–130.
9. Mundy EA, DuHamel KN, Montgomery GH. The efficacy of behavioral interventions for cancer treatment-related side effects. Semin Clin Neuropsychiatr 2003;8:253–275.
10. Matteson S, Roscoe J, Hickok J, Morrow GR. The role of behavioral conditioning in the development of nausea. Am J Obstet Gynecol 2002;186:S239–S243.
11. Morrow GR, Carroll J, Ryan EP, et al. Behavioral interventions in treating anticipatory nausea and vomiting. J Natl Compr Canc Netw 2007;5:44–50.
12. Lee J, Dodd M, Dibble S, Abrams D. Review of acupressure studies for chemotherapy-induced nausea and vomiting Control. J Pain Symp Manage 2008;36:529–544.
13. Lotfi-Jam K, Carey M, Jefford M, et al. Nonpharmacologic strategies for managing common chemotherapy adverse effects: A systematic review. J Clin Oncol 2008;26:5618–5629.
14. Antonarakis ES, Hain RD. Nausea and vomiting associated with cancer chemotherapy: Drug management in theory and in practice. Arch Dis Child 2004;89:877–880.
15. Critchley P, Plach N, Grantham M, et al. Efficacy of haloperidol in the treatment of nausea and vomiting in the palliative patient: A systematic review. J Pain Symptom Manage 2001;22:631–634.
16. Inapsine (droperidol). www.fda.gov/medwatch/SAFETY/2001/inapsine.htm.
17. Tramer MR, Carroll D, Campbell FA, et al. Cannabinoids for control of chemotherapy induced nausea and vomiting: Quantitative systematic review. BMJ 2001;323:1–8.
18. Italian Group for Antiemetic Research. Double-blind, dose-finding study of four intravenous doses of dexamethasone in the prevention of cisplatin-induced acute emesis. J Clin Oncol 1998;16:2937–2942.
19. Ioannidis JT, Hesketh PJ, Lau J. Contribution of dexamethasone to control of chemotherapy-induced nausea and vomiting: A meta-analysis of randomized evidence. J Clin Oncol 2000;18:3409–3422.
20. Poli-Bigelli S, Rodrigues-Pereira J, Carides AD, et al. Addition of the neurokinin 1 receptor antagonist aprepitant to standard antiemetic therapy improves control of chemotherapy-induced nausea and vomiting. Results from a randomized, double-blind, placebo-controlled trial in Latin America. Cancer 2003;97:3090–3098.
21. Hesketh PJ, Grunbert SM, Gralla RJ, et al. The oral neurokinin-1 antagonist aprepitant for the prevention of chemotherapy-induced nausea and vomiting: A multinational, randomized, double-blind, placebo controlled trial in patients receiving high-dose cisplatin—The Aprepitant Protocol 052 Study Group. J Clin Oncol 2003;21:4112–4119.
22. De Mulder PH, Seynaeve C, Vermorken JB, et al. Ondansetron compared with high-dose metoclopramide in prophylaxis of acute and delayed cisplatin-induced nausea and vomiting: A multicenter, randomized, double-blind, crossover study. Ann Intern Med 1990;113:834–840.
23. Heron JF, Goedhals L, Jordaan JP, et al. Oral granisetron alone and in combination with dexamethasone: A double-blind randomized comparison against high-dose metoclopramide plus dexamethasone in prevention of cisplatin-induced emesis. Ann Oncol 1994;5:579–584.
24. Navari RM, Einhorn LH, Loehrer PJ Sr, et al. A phase II trial of olanzapine, dexamethasone, and palonosetron for the prevention of chemotherapy-induced nausea and vomiting: a Hoosier oncology group study. Support Care Cancer 2007;15:1285–1291.
25. National Comprehensive Cancer Network. Clinical Practice Guidelines in Oncology. Antiemesis. Version 2; 2010. http://www.nccn.org/professionals/physician_gls/PDF/antiemesis.pdf.
26. Ernst A, Weiss SJ, Park S, et al. Prochlorperazine versus promethazine for uncomplicated nausea and vomiting in the emergency department: A randomized, double-blind clinical trial. Ann Emerg Med 2000;36:89–94.
27. Stahl SM. The ups and downs of novel antiemetic drugs, Part 1: Substance P, 5-HT, and the neuropharmacology of vomiting. J Clin Psychol 2003;64:498–499.
28. Warr, DG, Hesketh PJ, Gralla RJ, et al. Efficacy and tolerability of aprepitant for the prevention of chemotherapy-induced nausea and vomiting in patients with breast cancer after moderately emetogenic chemotherapy. J Clin Oncol 2005;23:2822–2830.
29. Emend [package insert]. Whitehouse Station, NJ: Merck & Co, July 2009.
30. McCrea JB, Majumdar AK, Goldberg MR, et al. Effects of the neurokinin-1 receptor antagonist aprepitant on the pharmacokinetics of dexamethasone and methylprednisolone. Clin Pharmacol Ther 2003;74:17–24.
31. Van Belle S, Cocquyt V. Fosaprepitant dimeglumine (MK-0517 or L-785,298), an intravenous neurokinin-1 antagonist for the prevention of chemotherapy induced nausea and vomiting. Expert Opin Pharmacother 2008;9:3261–3270.
32. Kris MG, Hesketh PJ, Herrstedt J, et al. Consensus proposals for the prevention of acute and delayed vomiting and nausea following high-emetic-risk chemotherapy. Support Care Cancer 2005;13:85–96.
33. Kris MG, Hesketh PJ, Somerfield MR, et al. American Society of Clinical Oncology guideline for antiemetics in oncology: Update 2006. J Clin Oncol 2006;24:2932–2947.

34. Grunberg, SM, Deuson, RR, Mavros, P, et al. Incidence of chemotherapy-induced nausea and emesis after modern antiemetics. Cancer 2004;100:2261–2268.

35. Ihbe-Heffinger A, Ehlken B, Bernard R, et al. The impact of delayed chemotherapy-induced nausea and vomiting on patients, health resource utilization and costs in German cancer centers. Ann of Oncol 2004;15:526–536.

36. Saito M, Aogi K, Sekine I, et al. Palonosetron plus dexamethasone versus granisetron plus dexamethasone for prevention of nausea and vomiting during chemotherapy: a double-blind, double-dummy, randomised, comparative phase III trial. Lancet Oncol 2009;10: 115–124.

37. Aloxi [package insert]. Bloomington, MI: MGI PHARMA Inc., April 2008.

38. Eisenberg P, Figueroa-Vadillo J, Zamora R, et al. Improved prevention of moderately emetogenic chemotherapy-induced nausea and vomiting with palonosetron, a pharmacologically novel 5-HT3 receptor antagonist : Results of a phase III, single-dose trial versus dolasetron. Cancer 2003;98:2473–2482.

39. Gralla R, Lichinitser M, Van Der Vegt S, et al. Palonosetron improves prevention of chemotherapy-induced nausea and vomiting following moderately emetogenic chemotherapy: Results of a double-blind randomized phase III trial comparing single doses of palonosetron with ondansetron. Ann Oncol 2003;14:1570–1577.

40. Musso M, Scalone R, Bonanno V, et al. Palonosetron (Aloxi) and dexamethasone for the prevention of acute and delayed nausea and vomiting in patients receiving multiple-day chemotherapy. Support Care Cancer 2009;17:205–209.

41. Schnell FM. Chemotherapy-induced nausea and vomiting: The importance of good antiemetic control. Oncologist 2003;8:187–198.

42. Malik IA, Khan WA, Qazilbash M, et al. Chemotherapy-induced Nausea and Vomiting: Challenges and Opportunities for Improved Outcomes. Am J Clin Oncol 1995;18:170–175.

43. Hawkins R, Grunberg S. Chemotherapy-induced Nausea and Vomiting: Challenges and Opportunities for Improved Outcomes. Clin J Oncol Nurs 2009;13:54–64.

44. Dupuis LL, Nathan PC. Options for the prevention and management of acute chemotherapy-induced nausea and vomiting in children. Paediatr Drugs 2003;5:597–613.

45. Lohr L. Chemotherapy-induced nausea and vomiting. Cancer J 2008;14:85–93.

46. Wilcox PM, Fetting JH, Nettesheim KM, Abeloff MD. Anticipatory vomiting in women receiving cyclophosphamide, methotrexate, and 5-FU (CMF) adjuvant chemotherapy for breast carcinoma. Cancer Treat Rep 1982;66:1601–1604.

47. Navari RM. Prevention of emesis from multiday and high dose chemotherapy regimens. J Natl Compr Canc Netw 2007;5:51–59.

48. Kovac AL. Prevention and treatment of postoperative nausea and vomiting. Drugs 2000;59:213–243.

49. Kapoor R, Hola, ET Adamson RT, Mathis AS. Comparison of two instruments for assessing risk of postoperative nausea and vomiting. Am J Health-Syst Pharm. 2008;65:448–453.

50. Gan TJ, Meyer TA, Apfel CC, et al. Society for ambulatory anesthesia guidelines for the management of postoperative nausea and vomiting. Anesth Analg 2007;105:1615–1628.

51. White PF, O'Hara JF, Roberson CR, Wender RH, MD, Candiotti KA, and The POST-OP Study Group. The impact of current antiemetic practices on patient outcomes: A prospective study on high-risk patients. Anesth Analg 2008;107:452–458.

52. Apfel CA, Korttila K, Abdalla M, et al. A factorial trial of six interventions for the prevention of postoperative nausea and vomiting. N Engl J Med 2004;350:2441–2451.

53. Habib AS, El-Moalem HE, Gan TJ. The efficacy of the 5-HT3 receptor antagonists combined with droperidol for PONV prophylaxis is similar to their combination with dexamethasone. A meta-analysis of randomized controlled trials. Can J Anaesth 2004;51:311–319.

54. Carlisle JB, Stevenson CA. Drugs for preventing postoperative nausea and vomiting. Cochrane Database Syst Rev 2006;3:CD004125.

55. Kranke P, Morin AM, Roewer N, Wulf H, Eberhart LH. Palonosetron 04–07 Study Group. A randomized, double-blind study to evaluate the efficacy and safety of three different doses of palonosetron versus placebo in preventing postoperative nausea and vomiting over a 72-hour period. Anesth Analg 2008;107:439–444.

56. Candiotti KA, Kovac AL, Melson TI, et al: The Palonosetron 04-06 Study Group. A randomized, double-blind study to evaluate the efficacy and safety of three different doses of palonosetron versus placebo for preventing postoperative and post-discharge nausea and vomiting. Anesth Analg 2008;107:445–451.

57. Wang JJ, Ho ST, Tzeng JI, Tang CS. The effect of timing of dexamethasone administration on its efficacy as a prophylactic antiemetic for postoperative nausea and vomiting. Anesth Analg 2000;91: 136–139.

58. Hill RP, Lubarsky DA, Phillips-Bute B, et al. Cost-effectiveness of prophylactic antiemetic therapy with ondansetron, droperidol or placebo. Anesthesiology 2000;92:958–967.

59. Gan TJ, Apfel C, Kovac A, et al. A randomized, double-blind comparison of the NK$_1$ antagonist, aprepitant versus ondansetron for the prevention of postoperative nausea and vomiting. Anesth Analg 2007;104:1082–1089.

60. Kovac AL, O'Connor TA, Pearman MH, et al. Efficacy of repeat intravenous dosing of ondansetron in controlling postoperative nausea and vomiting: A randomized, double-blind, placebo-controlled multicenter trial. J Clin Anesth 1999;11:453–459.

61. Kreisler NS, Spiekermann BF, Ascari CM, et al. Small-dose droperidol effectively reduces nausea in a general surgical adult patient population. Anesth Analg 2000;91:1256–1261.

62. Candiotti KA, Nhuch F, Kamat A, et al. Granisetron versus ondansetron treatment for breakthrough postoperative nausea and vomiting after prophylactic ondansetron failure: a pilot study. Anesth Analg 2007;104:1370–1373.

63. Habib AS, Gan TJ. The effectiveness of rescue antiemetics after failure of prophylaxis with ondansetron or droperidol: a preliminary report. J Clin Anesth 2005;17:62–65.

64. Spitzer TR, Friedman CJ, Bushnell W, et al. Double-blind, randomized, parallel-group study on the efficacy and safety of oral granisetron and oral ondansetron in the prophylaxis of nausea and vomiting in patients receiving hyperfractionated total body irradiation. Bone Marrow Transplant 2000;26:203–210.

65. Spinks AB, Wasiak J, Villaneuva EV, Bernath V. Scopolamine for preventing and treating motion sickness. Cochrane Database Syst Rev 2004;3:CD002851.

66. Portnoi G, Chng LA, Karimi-Tabesh L, et al. Prospective comparative study of the safety and effectiveness of ginger for the treatment of nausea and vomiting in pregnancy. Am J Obstet Gynecol 2003;189: 1374–1377.

67. Nausea and vomiting of pregnancy. ACOG Practice Bulletin No. 52. American College of Obstetricians and Gynecologists. Obstet Gynecol 2004;103:803–815.

68. Badell ML, Ramin SM, Smith JA. Treatment options for nausea and vomiting during pregnancy. Pharmacotherapy 2006;26:1273–1287.

69. Sullivan CA, Johnson CA, Roach H,, et al. A pilot study of intravenous ondansetron for hyperemesis gravidarum. Am J Obstet Gynecol 1996;174:1565–1568.

70. Wade I, Takeda T, Sato M, et al. Pharmacokinetics of granisetron in adults and children with malignant diseases. Biol Pharm Bull 2001;24:432–435.

71. Sepulveda-Vildosola AC, Betanzos-Cabrera Y, Lastiri GG, et al. Palonosetron hydrochloride is an effective and safe option to prevent chemotherapy-induced nausea and vomiting in children. Arch Med Res 2008;39:601–606.

72. DeCamp LR, Byerley JS, Doshi N, Steiner MJ. Use of antiemetic agents in acute gastroenteritis: a systematic review and meta-analysis. Arch Pediatr Adolesc Med 2008;162:858–865.

73. Freedman SB, Adler M, Seshadri R, Powell EC. Oral ondansetron for gastroenteritis in a pediatric emergency department. N Engl J Med 2006;354:1698–1705.

74. Roslund G, Hepps TS, McQuillen KK. The role of oral ondansetron in children with vomiting as a result of acute gastritis/gastroenteritis who have failed oral rehydration therapy: a randomized controlled trial. Ann Emerg Med 2008;52:22–29.

75. Kwon KT, Rudkin SE, Langdorf MI. Antiemetic use in pediatric gastroenteritis: A national survey of emergency physicians,

pediatricians, and pediatric emergency physicians. Clin Pediatr 2002;41: 641–652.

76. Starke PR, Weaver J, Chowdhury BA. Boxed warning added to promethazine labeling for pediatric use. N Engl J Med 2005;352:2653.

77. Lucarelli CD. Formulary management strategies for type 3 serotonin receptor antagonists. Am J Health Syst Pharm 2003;60:S4-S11.

78. Shih YT, Xu Y, Elting LS. Costs of uncontrolled chemotherapy-induced nausea and vomiting among working-age cancer patients receiving highly or moderately emetogenic chemotherapy. Cancer 2007;110:678–685.

79. Kranke P, Schuster F, Eberhart LH. Recent advances, trends and economic consideration in the risk assessment, prevention and treatment of postoperative nausea and vomiting. Expert Opin Pharmacother 2007;8:3217–3235.

80. Shih V, Wan HS, Chan A. Clinical predictors of chemotherapy-induced nausea and vomiting in breast cancer patients receiving adjuvant doxorubicin and cyclophosphamide. Ann Pharmacother 2009;43:444–452.

81. Gundzik K. Nausea and vomiting in the ambulatory surgical setting. Orthop Nurs 2008;27,182–188.

CHAPTER

43

Diarrhea, Constipation, and Irritable Bowel Syndrome

PATRICIA H. POWELL AND VIRGINIA H. FLEMING

KEY CONCEPTS

❶ Diarrhea is caused by many viral and bacterial organisms. It is most often a minor discomfort, not life threatening, and usually self-limited.

❷ The four pathophysiologic mechanisms of diarrhea have been linked to the four broad diarrheal groups, which are secretory, osmotic, exudative, and altered intestinal transit. The three mechanisms by which absorption occurs from the intestines are active transport, diffusion, and solvent drag.

❸ Management of diarrhea focuses on preventing excessive water and electrolyte losses, dietary care, relieving symptoms, treating curable causes, and treating secondary disorders.

❹ Bismuth subsalicylate is marketed for indigestion, relieving abdominal cramps, and controlling diarrhea, including traveler's diarrhea, but may cause interactions with several components if given in excess.

❺ Underlying causes of constipation should be identified when possible and corrective measures taken (e.g., alteration of diet or treatment of diseases such as hypothyroidism).

❻ The foundation of treatment of constipation is dietary fiber or bulk-forming laxatives that provide 10–15 g/day of raw fiber.

❼ Irritable bowel syndrome (IBS) is one of the most common gastrointestinal disorders characterized by lower abdominal pain, disturbed defecation, and bloating. Many nongastrointestinal manifestations also exist with IBS. Visceral hypersensitivity is a major culprit in the pathophysiology of the disease.

❽ Dietary-predominant IBS should be managed by dietary modification and drugs such as loperamide when diet changes alone are insufficient to promote control of symptoms.

❾ Several drug classes are useful in the treatment of the pain associated with IBS including tricyclic compounds and the gut-selective calcium channel blockers.

Learning objectives, review questions, and other resources can be found at **www.pharmacotherapyonline.com**.

DIARRHEA

Diarrhea is a troublesome discomfort that affects most individuals in the United States at some point in their lives and can be thought of as both a symptom and a sign. Usually diarrheal episodes begin abruptly and subside within 1 or 2 days without treatment. This chapter focuses primarily on noninfectious diarrhea, with only minor reference to infectious diarrhea (see Chap. 122 for a discussion of gastrointestinal infections). Diarrhea is often a symptom of a systemic disease, and not all possible causes of diarrhea are discussed in this chapter. Acute diarrhea is commonly defined as <14 days' duration, persistent diarrhea as more than 14 days' duration, and chronic diarrhea as more than 30 days' duration.

To understand diarrhea, one must have a reasonable definition of the condition; unfortunately, the literature is extremely variable on this. Simply put, diarrhea is an increased frequency and decreased consistency of fecal discharge as compared to an individual's normal bowel pattern. Frequency and consistency are variable within and between individuals. For example, some individuals defecate as often as three times per day, whereas others defecate only two or three times per week. A Western diet usually produces a daily stool weighing between 100 and 300 g, depending on the amount of nonabsorbable materials (mainly carbohydrates) consumed. Patients with serious diarrhea may have a daily stool weight in excess of 300 g; however, a subset of patients experience frequent small, watery passages. Additionally, vegetable fiber-rich diets, such as those consumed in some Eastern cultures (e.g., those in Africa), produce stools weighing more than 300 g/day.

Diarrhea may be associated with a specific disease of the intestines or secondary to a disease outside the intestines. For instance, bacillary dysentery directly affects the gut, whereas diabetes mellitus causes neuropathic diarrheal episodes. Furthermore, diarrhea can be considered as acute or chronic disease. Infectious diarrhea is often acute; diabetic diarrhea is chronic. Congenital disorders in gastrointestinal ion-transport mechanisms are another cause of chronic diarrhea.[1] Whether acute or chronic, diarrhea has the same pathophysiologic causes that help in identification of specific treatments.

EPIDEMIOLOGY

The epidemiology of diarrhea varies in developed versus developing countries.[2] In the United States, diarrheal illnesses are usually not reported to the Centers for Disease Control and Prevention (CDC) unless associated with an outbreak or an unusual organism or condition. For example, the acquired immunodeficiency syndrome (AIDS) has been identified with protracted diarrheal illness. Diarrhea is a major problem in daycare centers and nursing homes, probably because early childhood and senescence plus environmental conditions are risk factors. Although an exact epidemiologic profile in the United States is not available through the CDC or published literature, chronic diarrhea affects approximately 5% of the adult population and ranges from 3% to 20% in children worldwide.[3-5] In developing countries, diarrhea is a leading cause of illness and death in children, creating a tremendous economic strain on healthcare costs.

❶ Most cases of acute diarrhea are caused by infections with viruses, bacteria, or protozoa and are generally self-limited.[6] Although viruses are more commonly associated with acute gastroenteritis, bacteria are responsible for more cases of acute diarrhea.

Evaluation of a noninfectious cause is considered if diarrhea persists and no infectious organism can be identified, or if the patient falls into a high-risk category for metabolic complications with persistent diarrhea. Common causative bacterial organisms include *Shigella, Salmonella, Campylobacter, Staphylococcus,* and *Escherichia coli*. Foodborne bacterial infection is a major concern, as several major food poisoning episodes have occurred that were traced to poor sanitary conditions in meat-processing plants. Acute viral infections are attributed mostly to the Norwalk and rotavirus groups.

PHYSIOLOGY

In the fasting state, 9 L of fluid enters the proximal small intestine each day. Of this fluid, 2 L are ingested through diet, while the remainder consists of internal secretions. Because of meal content, duodenal chyme is usually hypertonic. When chyme reaches the ileum, the osmolality adjusts to that of plasma, with most dietary fat, carbohydrate, and protein being absorbed. The volume of ileal chyme decreases to about 1 L/day upon entering the colon, which is further reduced by colonic absorption to 100 mL daily. If the small intestine water absorption capacity is exceeded, chyme overloads the colon, resulting in diarrhea. In humans, the colon absorptive capacity is about 5 L daily. Colonic fluid transport is critical to water and electrolyte balance.

Absorption from the intestines back into the blood occurs by three mechanisms: active transport, diffusion, and solvent drag. Active transport and diffusion are the mechanisms of sodium transport. Because of the high luminal sodium concentration (142 mEq/L), sodium diffuses from the sodium-rich gut into epithelial cells, where it is actively pumped into the blood and exchanged with chloride to maintain an isoelectric condition across the epithelial membrane.

Hydrogen ions are transported by an indirect mechanism in the upper small intestine. As sodium is absorbed, hydrogen ions are secreted into the gut. Hydrogen ions then combine with bicarbonate ions to form carbonic acid, which then dissociates into carbon dioxide and water. Carbon dioxide readily diffuses into the blood for expiration through the lung. The water remains in the chyme.

Paracellular pathways are major routes of ion movement. As ions, monosaccharides, and amino acids are actively transported, an osmotic pressure is created, drawing water and electrolytes across the intestinal wall. This pathway accounts for significant amounts of ion transport, especially sodium. Sodium plays an important role in stimulating glucose absorption. Glucose and amino acids are actively transported into the blood via a sodium-dependent cotransport mechanism. Cotransport absorption mechanisms of glucose-sodium and amino acid-sodium are extremely important for treating diarrhea.

Gut motility influences absorption and secretion. The amount of time in which luminal content is in contact with the epithelium is under neural and hormonal control. Neurohormonal substances, such as angiotensin, vasopressin, glucocorticoid, aldosterone, and neurotransmitters also regulate ion transport.

PATHOPHYSIOLOGY

❷ Four general pathophysiologic mechanisms disrupt water and electrolyte balance, leading to diarrhea, and are the basis of diagnosis and therapy. These are (a) a change in active ion transport by either decreased sodium absorption or increased chloride secretion; (b) change in intestinal motility; (c) increase in luminal osmolarity; and (d) increase in tissue hydrostatic pressure. These mechanisms have been related to four broad clinical diarrheal groups: secretory, osmotic, exudative, and altered intestinal transit.

Secretory diarrhea occurs when a stimulating substance either increases secretion or decreases absorption of large amounts of water and electrolytes. Substances that cause excess secretion include vasoactive intestinal peptide (VIP) from a pancreatic tumor, unabsorbed dietary fat in steatorrhea, laxatives, hormones (such as secretion), bacterial toxins, and excessive bile salts. Many of these agents stimulate intracellular cyclic adenosine monophosphate and inhibit Na$^+$/K$^+$-adenosine triphosphatase (ATPase), leading to increased secretion. Also, many of these mediators inhibit ion absorption simultaneously. Secretory diarrhea is recognized by large stool volumes (>1 L/day) with normal ionic contents and osmolality approximately equal to plasma. Fasting does not alter the stool volume in these patients.

Poorly absorbed substances retain intestinal fluids, resulting in osmotic diarrhea. This process occurs with malabsorption syndromes, lactose intolerance, administration of divalent ions (e.g., magnesium-containing antacids), or consumption of poorly soluble carbohydrate (e.g., lactulose). As a poorly soluble solute is transported, the gut adjusts the osmolality to that of plasma; in so doing, water and electrolytes flux into the lumen. Clinically, osmotic diarrhea is distinguishable from other types, as it ceases if the patient resorts to a fasting state.

Inflammatory diseases of the gastrointestinal tract discharge mucus, serum proteins, and blood into the gut. Sometimes bowel movements consist only of mucus, exudate, and blood. Exudative diarrhea affects other absorptive, secretory, or motility functions to account for the large stool volume associated with this disorder.

Altered intestinal motility produces diarrhea by three mechanisms: reduction of contact time in the small intestine, premature emptying of the colon, and bacterial overgrowth. Chyme must be exposed to intestinal epithelium for a sufficient time period to enable normal absorption and secretion processes to occur. If this contact time decreases, diarrhea results. Intestinal resection or bypass surgery and drugs (such as metoclopramide) cause this type of diarrhea. On the other hand, an increased time of exposure allows fecal bacteria overgrowth. A characteristic small intestine diarrheal pattern is rapid, small, coupling bursts of waves. These waves are inefficient, do not allow absorption, and rapidly dump chyme into the colon. Once in the colon, chyme exceeds the colonic capability to absorb water.

Etiologic Examination of the Stool

Stool characteristics are important in assessing the etiology of diarrhea. A description of the frequency, volume, consistency, and color provides diagnostic clues. For instance, diarrhea starting in the small intestine produces a copious, watery or fatty (greasy), and foul-smelling stool; contains undigested food particles; and is usually free from gross blood. Colonic diarrhea appears as small, pasty, and sometimes bloody or mucoid movements. Rectal tenesmus with flatus accompanies large intestinal diarrhea.

CLINICAL PRESENTATION

Table 43–1 outlines the clinical presentation of diarrhea and Table 43–2 shows common drug-induced causes of diarrhea.

TABLE 43-1	Clinical Presentation of Diarrhea

General
- Usually, acute diarrheal episodes subside within 72 hours of onset, whereas chronic diarrhea involves frequent attacks over extended time periods.

Signs and symptoms
- Abrupt onset of nausea, vomiting, abdominal pain, headache, fever, chills, and malaise.
- Bowel movements are frequent and never bloody, and diarrhea lasts 12 to 60 hours.
- Intermittent periumbilical or lower right quadrant pain with cramps and audible bowel sounds is characteristic of small intestinal disease.
- When pain is present in large-intestinal diarrhea, it is a gripping, aching sensation with tenesmus (straining, ineffective, and painful stooling). Pain localizes to the hypogastric region, right or left lower quadrant, or sacral region.
- In chronic diarrhea, a history of previous bouts, weight loss, anorexia, and chronic weakness are important findings.

Physical examination
- Typically demonstrates hyperperistalsis with borborygmi and generalized or local tenderness.

Laboratory tests
- Stool analysis studies include examination for microorganisms, blood, mucus, fat, osmolality, pH, electrolyte and mineral concentration, and cultures.
- Stool test kits are useful for detecting gastrointestinal viruses, particularly rotavirus.
- Antibody serologic testing shows rising titers over a 3- to 6-day period, but this test is not practical and is nonspecific.
- Occasionally, total daily stool volume is also determined.
- Direct endoscopic visualization and biopsy of the colon may be undertaken to assess for the presence of conditions such as colitis or cancer.
- Radiographic studies are helpful in neoplastic and inflammatory conditions.

TABLE 43-2	Drugs Causing Diarrhea

Laxatives
Antacids containing magnesium
Antineoplastics
Auranofin (gold salt)
Antibiotics
  Clindamycin
  Tetracyclines
  Sulfonamides
  Any broad-spectrum antibiotic
Antihypertensives
  Reserpine
  Guanethidine
  Methyldopa
  Guanabenz
  Guanadrel
  Angiotensin-converting enzyme inhibitors
Cholinergics
  Bethanechol
  Neostigmine
Cardiac agents
  Quinidine
  Digitalis
  Digoxin
Nonsteroidal antiinflammatory drugs
Misoprostol
Colchicine
Proton pump inhibitors
H_2-receptor blockers

A medication history is extremely important in identifying drug-induced diarrhea. Many agents, including antibiotics and other drugs, cause diarrhea or, less commonly, pseudomembranous colitis. Self-inflicted laxative abuse for weight loss is popular.

Most acute diarrhea is self-limiting, subsiding within 72 hours. However, infants, young children, the elderly, and debilitated persons are at risk for morbid and mortal events in prolonged or voluminous diarrhea. These groups are at risk for water, electrolyte, and acid-base disturbances, and potentially cardiovascular collapse and death. The prognosis for chronic diarrhea depends on the cause; for example, diarrhea secondary to diabetes mellitus waxes and wanes throughout life.

TREATMENT

Diarrhea

■ PREVENTION

Acute viral diarrheal illness often occurs in daycare centers and nursing homes. Because person-to-person contact is the mechanism by which viral disease spreads, isolation techniques must be initiated. For bacterial, parasitic, and protozoal infections, strict food handling, sanitation, water, and other environmental hygiene practices can prevent transmission. If diarrhea is secondary to another illness, controlling the primary condition is necessary. Antibiotics and bismuth subsalicylate are advocated to prevent traveler's diarrhea, in conjunction with treatment of drinking water and caution with consumption of fresh vegetables.[7]

■ DESIRED OUTCOME

❸ If prevention is unsuccessful and diarrhea occurs, therapeutic goals are to (a) manage the diet; (b) prevent excessive water, electrolyte, and acid-base disturbances; (c) provide symptomatic relief; (d) treat curable causes; and (e) manage secondary disorders causing diarrhea (Figs. 43–1 and 43–2).

Clinicians must clearly understand that diarrhea, like a cough, may be a body defense mechanism for ridding itself of harmful substances or pathogens. The correct therapeutic response is not necessarily to stop diarrhea at all costs.

■ NONPHARMACOLOGIC MANAGEMENT

Dietary management is a first priority in the treatment of diarrhea. Most clinicians recommend discontinuing consumption of solid foods and dairy products for 24 hours. However, fasting is of questionable value, as this treatment modality has not been extensively studied. In osmotic diarrhea, these maneuvers control the problem. If the mechanism is secretory, diarrhea persists. For patients who are experiencing nausea and/or vomiting, a mild, digestible, low-residue diet should be administered for 24 hours. If vomiting is present and uncontrollable with antiemetics (see Chap. 42), nothing is taken by mouth. As bowel movements decrease, a bland diet is begun.

Feeding should continue in children with acute bacterial diarrhea. Fed children have less morbidity and mortality, whether or not they receive oral rehydration fluids. Studies are not available in the elderly or in other high-risk groups to determine the value of continued feeding in bacterial diarrhea.

Water and Electrolytes

Rehydration and maintenance of water and electrolytes are primary treatment goals until the diarrheal episode ends. If the patient is volume depleted, rehydration should be directed at replacing water

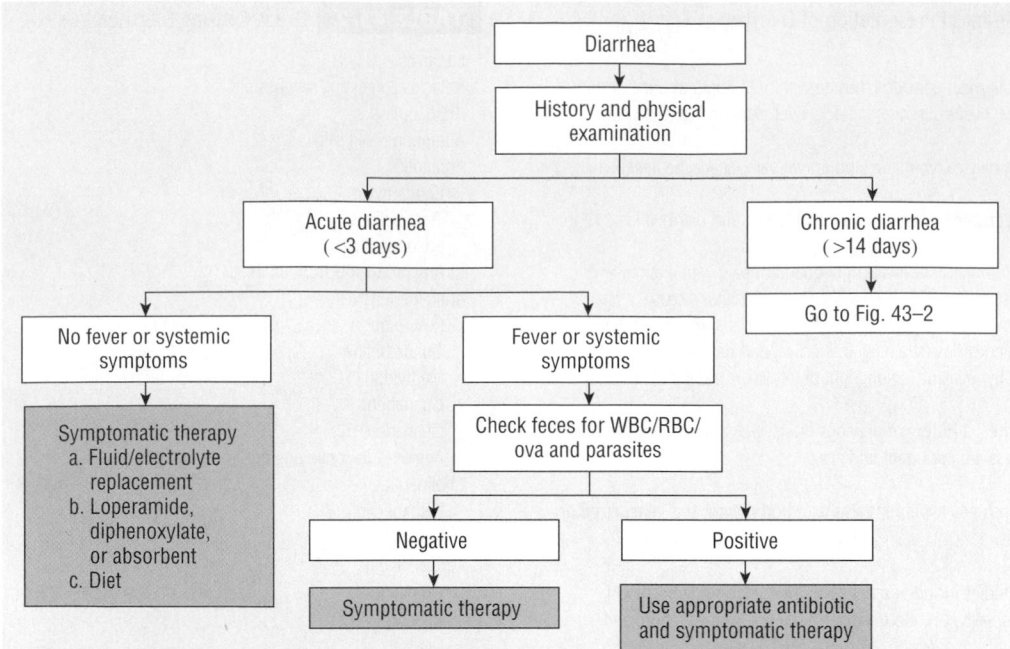

FIGURE 43-1. Recommendations for treating acute diarrhea. Follow these steps: (a) Perform a complete history and physical examination. (b) Is the diarrhea acute or chronic? If chronic diarrhea, go to Figure 43–2. (c) If acute diarrhea, check for fever and/or systemic signs and symptoms (i.e., toxic patient). If systemic illness (fever, anorexia, or volume depletion), check for an infectious source. If positive for infectious diarrhea, use appropriate antibiotic/ anthelmintic drug and symptomatic therapy. If negative for infectious cause, use only symptomatic treatment. (d) If no systemic findings, then use symptomatic therapy based on severity of volume depletion, oral or parenteral fluid/electrolytes, antidiarrheal agents (see Table 43–4), and diet. (RBC, red blood cells; WBC, white blood cells.)

and electrolytes to normal body composition. Then water and electrolyte composition are maintained by replacing losses. Many patients will not develop volume depletion and therefore will only require maintenance fluid and electrolyte therapy. Parenteral and enteral routes may be used for supplying water and electrolytes. If vomiting and dehydration are not severe, enteral feeding is the less costly and preferred method. In the United States, many commercial oral rehydration preparations are available (Table 43–3).

Because of concerns about hypernatremia, physicians continue to hospitalize patients and use intravenous fluids to correct fluid and electrolyte deficits in severe dehydration. Oral solutions are strongly recommended.[8–10] In developing countries, the World Health Organization Oral Rehydration Solution (WHO-ORS) saves the lives of millions of children annually.

During diarrhea, the small intestine retains its ability to actively transport monosaccharides such as glucose. Glucose actively carries sodium with water and other electrolytes. The WHO now recommends an ORS with a lower osmolarity, sodium content, and glucose load (see Table 43–3).[11] A separate oral supplement of zinc 20 mg daily for 14 days in addition to ORS significantly reduces the severity and duration of acute diarrhea in developing countries.[8,12] ORS is a lifesaving treatment for millions afflicted in developing countries. Acceptance in developed countries is less enthusiastic; however, the advantage of this product in reducing hospitalizations may prove its use as a cost-effective alternative, saving millions of dollars in healthcare expenditures.

■ PHARMACOLOGIC THERAPY

Various drugs have been used to treat diarrheal attacks (Table 43–4), including antimotility agents, adsorbents, antisecretory compounds, antibiotics, enzymes, and intestinal microflora. Usually these drugs are not curative but palliative.

Opiates and Their Derivatives

Opiates and opioid derivatives (a) delay the transit of intraluminal contents or (b) increase gut capacity, prolonging contact and absorption. Enkephalins, which are endogenous opioid substances, regulate fluid movement across the mucosa by stimulating absorptive processes. Limitations to the use of opiates include an addiction potential (a real concern with long-term use) and worsening of diarrhea in selected infectious diarrhea.

Most opiates act through peripheral and central mechanisms with the exception of loperamide, which acts only peripherally. Loperamide is antisecretory; it inhibits the calcium-binding protein calmodulin, controlling chloride secretion. Loperamide, available as 2 mg capsules or 1 mg/5 mL solution (both are nonprescription products), is suggested for managing acute and chronic diarrhea. The usual adult dose is initially 4 mg orally, followed by 2 mg after each loose stool, up to 16 mg/day. Used correctly, this agent has rare side effects, such as dizziness and constipation. If the diarrhea is concurrent with a high fever or bloody stool, the patient should be referred to a physician. Also, diarrhea lasting 48 hours beyond initiating loperamide warrants medical attention. Loperamide can also be used in traveler's diarrhea. It is comparable to bismuth subsalicylate for treatment of this disorder.[7]

Diphenoxylate is available as a 2.5 mg tablet and as a 2.5 mg/5 mL solution. A small amount of atropine (0.025 mg) is included in the product to discourage abuse. In adults, when taken as 2.5 to 5 mg three or four times daily, not to exceed a 20 mg total daily dose, diphenoxylate is rarely toxic. Some patients may complain of atropinism (blurred vision, dry mouth, and urinary hesitancy). Like loperamide, it should not be used in patients who are at risk of bacterial enteritis with *E. coli, Shigella,* or *Salmonella.*

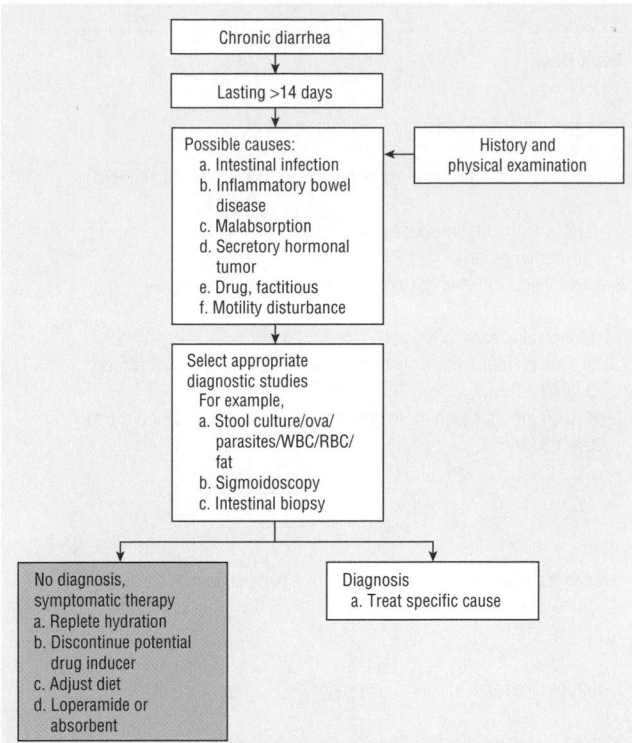

FIGURE 43-2. Recommendations for treating chronic diarrhea. Follow these steps: (a) Perform a careful history and physical examination. (b) The possible causes of chronic diarrhea are many. These can be classified into intestinal infections (bacterial or protozoal), inflammatory disease (Crohn disease or ulcerative colitis), malabsorption (lactose intolerance), secretory hormonal tumor (intestinal carcinoid tumor or vasoactive intestinal peptide-secreting tumor [VIPoma]), drug (antacid), factitious (laxative abuse), or motility disturbance (diabetes mellitus, irritable bowel syndrome, or hyperthyroidism). (c) If the diagnosis is uncertain, selected appropriate diagnostic studies should be ordered. (d) Once diagnosed, treatment is planned for the underlying cause with symptomatic antidiarrheal therapy. (e) If no specific cause can be identified, symptomatic therapy is prescribed. (RBC, red blood cells; WBC, white blood cells.)

Difenoxin, a diphenoxylate derivative also chemically related to meperidine, is also combined with atropine and has the same uses, precautions, and side effects. Marketed as a 1 mg tablet, the adult dosage is 2 mg initially, followed by 1 mg after each loose stool, not to exceed 8 mg/day.

Paregoric, camphorated tincture of opium, is marketed as a 2 mg/5 mL solution and is indicated for managing both acute and chronic diarrhea. It is not widely prescribed today because of its abuse potential.

CLINICAL CONTROVERSY

Long-term use of oral opiates is not routinely recommended for several pharmacologic reasons. Some opioids such as morphine and codeine have the tendency to cause constipation by slowing down the peristaltic action of the bowels, which can also result in a functional ileus. This effect can be minimized by administering laxatives and/or stool softeners in patients who require long-term opiate therapy. Prokinetic agents may also be helpful in treating opiate-related constipation.

Adsorbents

Adsorbents are used for symptomatic relief. These products, many not requiring a prescription, are nontoxic, but their effectiveness remains unproven. Adsorbents are nonspecific in their action; they adsorb nutrients, toxins, drugs, and digestive juices. Polycarbophil absorbs 60 times its weight in water and can be used to treat both diarrhea and constipation. It is a nonprescription product and is sold as a 500 mg chewable tablet. This hydrophilic, nonabsorbable product is safe and may be taken four times daily, up to 6 g/day in adults. See Table 43–4 for selected antidiarrheal preparations.

Antisecretory Agents

Bismuth subsalicylate appears to have antisecretory, antiinflammatory, and antibacterial effects. As a nonprescription product, it is marketed for indigestion, relieving abdominal cramps, and controlling diarrhea, including traveler's diarrhea. Bismuth subsalicylate dosage strengths are a 262 mg chewable tablet, 262 mg/5 mL liquid, and 524 mg/15 mL liquid. The usual adult dose is 2 tablets or 30 mL every 30 minutes to 1 hour up to 8 doses per day.

❹ Bismuth subsalicylate contains multiple components that might be toxic if given excessively to prevent or treat diarrhea. For instance, an active ingredient is salicylate, which may interact with anticoagulants or may produce salicylism (tinnitus, nausea, and vomiting). Bismuth reduces tetracycline absorption and may interfere with select gastrointestinal radiographic studies. Patients may complain of a darkening of the tongue and stools with repeat

TABLE 43-3	Oral Rehydration Solutions				
	WHO-ORS[a]	Pedialyte[b] (Ross)	Rehydralyte[b] (Ross)	Enfalyte (Mead Johnson)	Resol[b] (Wyeth)
Osmolality (mOsm/L)	245	249	304	200	269
Carbohydrates[b] (g/L)	13.5	25	25	30[c]	20
Calories (cal/L)	65	100	100	126	80
Electrolytes (mEq/L)					
Sodium	75	45	75	50	50
Potassium	20	20	20	25	20
Chloride	65	35	65	45	50
Citrate	–	30	30	34	34
Bicarbonate	30	–	–	–	–
Calcium	–	–	–	–	4
Magnesium	–	–	–	–	4
Sulfate	–	–	–	–	–
Phosphate	–	–	–	–	5

[a]World Health Organization reduced osmolarity Oral Rehydration Solution.
[b]Carbohydrate is glucose.
[c]Rice syrup solids are carbohydrate source.

TABLE 43-4 Selected Antidiarrheal Preparations

	Dose Form	Adult Dose
Antimotility		
Diphenoxylate	2.5 mg/tablet	5 mg four times daily; do not exceed 20 mg/day
	2.5 mg/5 mL	
Loperamide	2 mg/capsule	Initially 4 mg, then 2 mg after each loose stool; do not exceed 16 mg/day
	2 mg/capsule	
Paregoric	2 mg/5 mL (morphine)	5–10 mL one to four times daily
Opium tincture	10 mg/mL (morphine)	0.6 mL four times daily
Difenoxin	1 mg/tablet	2 tablets, then 1 tablet after each loose stool; up to 8 tablets/day
Adsorbents		
Kaolin-pectin mixture	5.7 g kaolin + 130.2 mg pectin/30 mL	30–120 mL after each loose stool
Polycarbophil	500 mg/tablet	Chew 2 tablets four times daily or after each loose stool; do not exceed 12 tablets/day
Attapulgite	750 mg/15 mL	1200–1500 mg after each loose bowel movement or every 2 hours; up to 9000 mg/day
	300 mg/7.5 mL	
	750 mg/tablet	
	600 mg/tablet	
	300 mg/tablet	
Antisecretory		
Bismuth subsalicylate	1050 mg/30 mL	Two tablets or 30 mL every 30 min to 1 h as needed up to 8 doses/day
	262 mg/15 mL	
	524 mg/15 mL	
	262 mg/tablet	
Enzymes (lactase)	1,250 neutral lactase units/4 drops	3–4 drops taken with milk or dairy product
	3,300 FCC lactase units per tablet	
Bacterial replacement (*Lactobacillus acidophilus, Lactobacillus bulgaricus*)		2 tablets or 1 granule packet three to four times daily; give with milk, juice, or water
Octreotide	0.05 mg/mL	Initial: 50 mcg subcutaneously
	0.1 mg/mL	One to two times per day and titrate dose based on indication up to 600 mcg/day in two to four divided doses
	0.5 mg/mL	

administration. Salicylate can induce gout attacks in susceptible individuals.

Bismuth subsalicylate suspension has been evaluated in the treatment of secretory diarrhea of infectious etiology as well. In a dose of 30 mL every 30 minutes for eight doses, unformed stools decrease in the first 24 hours. Bismuth subsalicylate may also be effective in preventing traveler's diarrhea.

Octreotide, a synthetic octapeptide analog of endogenous somatostatin, is effective for the symptomatic treatment of carcinoid tumors and other peptide-secreting tumors, dumping syndrome, and chemotherapy-induced diarrhea.[13] It has had limited success in patients with AIDS-associated diarrhea and short-bowel syndrome, does not appear to have an advantage over various opiate derivatives in the treatment of chronic idiopathic diarrhea, and has the disadvantage of being administered by injection.[14] Metastatic intestinal carcinoid tumors secrete excessive amounts of vasoactive substances, including histamine, bradykinin, serotonin, and prostaglandins. Primary carcinoid tumors occur throughout the gastrointestinal tract, with most in the ileum. Predominant signs and symptoms experienced by patients with these tumors are attributable to excessive concentrations of 5-hydroxytryptophan and serotonin. The totality of their clinical effects is termed the carcinoid syndrome. Some patients have a violent, watery diarrhea with abdominal cramping. Initially, diarrhea might be managed with various agents such as codeine, diphenoxylate, cyproheptadine, methysergide, phenoxybenzamine, or methyldopa. But octreotide is now considered first-line therapy for carcinoid syndrome.

Octreotide blocks the release of serotonin and many other active peptides and has been effective in controlling diarrhea and flushing. It is reported to have direct inhibitory effects on intestinal secretion and stimulatory effects on intestinal absorption. Non—gastrin-secreting adenomas of the pancreas are tumors associated with profuse watery diarrhea. This condition has been referred to as Verner-Morrison syndrome, WDHA (watery diarrhea, hypokalemia, and achlorhydria) syndrome, pancreatic cholera, watery diarrhea syndrome, and vasoactive intestinal peptide-secreting tumor (VIPoma). Excessive secretion of VIP from a retroperitoneal or pancreatic tumor produces most of the clinical features. Surgical tumor dissection is the treatment of choice. In nonsurgical candidates, the profuse watery diarrhea and other symptoms commonly encountered are managed with octreotide.

The dose of octreotide varies with the indication, disease severity, and patient response.[13] For managing diarrhea and flushing associated with carcinoid tumors in adults, the initial dosage range is 100 to 600 mcg/day in two to four divided doses subcutaneously for 2 weeks. For controlling secretory diarrhea of VIPomas, the dosage range is 200 to 300 mcg/day in two to four divided doses for 2 weeks. Some patients may require higher doses for symptomatic control. Patients responding to these initial doses may be switched to Sandostatin LAR Depot, a long-acting octreotide formulation. This product consists of microspheres containing the drug. Initial doses consist of 20 mg given intramuscularly intragluteally at 4-week intervals for 2 months. It is recommended that during the first 2 weeks of therapy the short-acting formulation also be administered subcutaneously. At the end of 2 months, patients with good symptom control may have the dose reduced to 10 mg every 4 weeks, while those without sufficient symptom control may have the dose increased to 30 mg every 4 weeks. For patients experiencing recurrence of symptoms on the 10 mg dose, dosage adjustment to 20 mg should be made. It is not uncommon for patients with carcinoid tumors or VIPomas to experience periodic exacerbation of symptoms. Subcutaneous octreotide for several days should be reinstituted in these individuals. In so-called carcinoid crisis, octreotide is given as an intravenous infusion at 50 mcg/h for 8 to 24 hours.

Because octreotide inhibits many other gastrointestinal hormones, it has a variety of intestinal side effects. With prolonged use, gallbladder and biliary tract complications such as cholelithiasis have been reported. Approximately 5% to 10% of patients complain of nausea, diarrhea, and abdominal pain. Local injection pain occurs with about an 8% incidence. With high doses, octreotide may reduce dietary fat absorption, leading to steatorrhea.

Two other somatostatin analogs, lanreotide and vapreotide, have been studied.[14,15] Lanreotide is approved for use in the United States for acromegaly. The starting dose is 90 mg subcutaneously every 4 weeks for 3 months, then the dose is adjusted based upon growth hormone and insulin-like growth factor levels.[16] Vapreotide is an orphan drug that is indicated for pancreatic and gastrointestinal fistulas as well as esophageal variceal bleeding.

Miscellaneous Products

Probiotics are microorganisms that have been used for many years to replace colonic microflora. This supposedly restores normal intestinal function and suppresses the growth of pathogenic microorganisms. *Saccharomyces boulrdii, Lactobacillus GG,* and *Lactobacillus acidophilus* have been shown to decrease the duration of infectious and antibiotic-induced diarrhea in adults and children.[17] A combination probiotic product, VSL#3 (which contains multiple strains of lactobacilli and bifidobacteria) may have benefit in preventing radiation-induced diarrhea when given three times a day.[18] The dosage of probiotic preparations varies depending on the brand used. Intestinal flatus is the primary patient complaint experienced with this modality.

Anticholinergic drugs such as atropine block vagal tone and prolong gut transit time. Drugs with anticholinergic properties are present in many nonprescription products. Their value in controlling diarrhea is questionable and limited because of side effects. Angle-closure glaucoma, selected heart diseases, and obstructive uropathies are relative contraindications to the use of anticholinergic agents.

Lactase enzyme products are helpful for patients who are experiencing diarrhea secondary to lactose intolerance. Lactase is required for carbohydrate digestion. When a patient lacks this enzyme, eating dairy products causes an osmotic diarrhea. Several products are available for use each time a dairy product, especially milk or ice cream, is consumed.

Investigational Drugs

Several new classes of compounds are undergoing clinical trials for efficacy in acute diarrhea.[19] Enkephalins are endogenous opiate compounds in the gut that have antisecretory and proabsorptive activity in the small intestine. They promote sodium and chloride reabsorption via stimulation of a nonadrenergic, noncholinergic neurotransmitter. Enkephalinase inhibitors are compounds that slow down the enzymatic (i.e., enkephalinase) breakdown of endogenous enkephalins found in the small intestines. They exert an antisecretory effect without affecting GI motility or CNS-related effects/side effects. One specific compound, originally called acetorphan but now referred to as racecadotril, has been extensively tested in humans and found to be equal to other opiate antidiarrheals such as loperamide, while causing less GI motility side effects such as abdominal bloating, pain, and constipation.[20–22] Racecadotril is currently licensed only in France and a few developing countries with a high incidence of childhood diarrhea.

Vaccines are a new therapeutic frontier in controlling infectious diarrheas, especially in developing countries.[23–24] An oral vaccine for cholera is licensed and available in other countries (Dukoral from SBL Vaccines) and appears to provide somewhat better immunity and has fewer adverse effects than the previously available parenteral vaccine. However, the CDC does not recommend cholera vaccines for most travelers, nor is the vaccine available in the United States.

Oral *Shigella* vaccine, although effective under field conditions, requires 5 weekly oral doses and repeat booster doses, thereby limiting its practicality for use in developing nations. With about 1,500 serotypes for *Salmonella*, a vaccine is not currently available for humans. There are two newer typhoid vaccine formulations, one a parenteral inactivated whole-cell vaccine and the other an oral live-attenuated (Ty21a) vaccine that is administered in four doses on days 1, 3, 5, and 7, to be completed at least 1 week before exposure. Two rotavirus vaccines have been shown to prevent gastroenteritis due to rotavirus infection in infants and children.[25] The pentavalent human-bovine reassortant vaccine (RotaTeq from Merck) is administered as a three-oral-dose sequence, and the monovalent human vaccine (Rotarix from GlaxoSmithKline) is administered as a two-oral-dose sequence. A rotavirus vaccine program has been formed to reduce child morbidity and mortality from diarrheal disease by accelerating the availability of rotavirus vaccines appropriate for use in developing countries.

■ EVALUATION OF THERAPEUTIC OUTCOMES

General Outcomes Measures

Therapeutic outcomes are directed toward key symptoms, signs, and laboratory studies. Constitutional symptoms usually improve within 24 to 72 hours. Monitoring for changes in the frequency and character of bowel movements on a daily basis in conjunction with vital signs and improvement in appetite are of utmost importance. Also, the clinician needs to monitor body weight, serum osmolality, serum electrolytes, complete blood cell counts, urinalysis, and culture results (if appropriate).

Acute Diarrhea

Most patients with acute diarrhea experience mild to moderate distress. In the absence of moderate to severe dehydration, high fever, and blood or mucus in the stool, this illness is usually self-limiting within 3 to 7 days. Mild to moderate acute diarrhea is usually managed on an outpatient basis with oral rehydration, symptomatic treatment, and diet. Elderly persons with chronic illness as well as infants may require hospitalization for parenteral rehydration and close monitoring.

Severe Diarrhea

In the urgent/emergent situation, restoration of the patient's volume status is the most important outcome. Toxic patients (fever dehydration, hematochezia, or hypotension) require hospitalization, intravenous fluids and electrolyte administration, and empiric antibiotic therapy while awaiting culture and sensitivity results. With timely management, these patients usually recover within a few days.

CONSTIPATION

Constipation is a commonly encountered medical condition in the United States for which many patients initiate self-treatment. Constipation also accounts for many emergency room, primary care, gasteroenterologist, and pediatrician visits each year in the United States.[26] Though often considered more of a minor uncomfortable or unpleasant problem, constipation can have serious consequences and be costly to the healthcare system. One of the major underlying problems contributing to constipation in the Western world is lack of adequate dietary fiber. An additional contributing factor is public misconception about normal bowel function. Many people believe that daily bowel movements are required for normal health or that accumulation of toxic substances will occur with infrequent defecation. Inappropriate laxative use by the general public may result from these misconceptions.

Constipation does not have a single, generally agreed upon definition. A general definition from the American Gastroenterology Association (AGA) defines functional constipation as a bowel disorder characterized by difficult, infrequent, or seemingly incomplete defecation that does not meet criteria for irritable bowel syndrome (IBS).[27] The lay public and healthcare professionals often define/describe constipation in a number of both quantitative and qualitative ways. Physicians often use stool frequency to define constipation (most commonly fewer than three bowel movements per week); however, the "normal" frequency of bowel movement is not well established (and can vary from person to person). Patients more often describe constipation in terms of symptoms or a combination of quantitative and qualitative descriptors that are difficult to quanitfy: bowel movement frequency, stool size or consistency (hard or lumpy stools), straining upon defecation, inability to defecate at will, and symptoms such as sensation of incomplete evacuation.

Examples of definitions of constipation that have been used in clinical studies include the following: (a) fewer than three stools per week for women and five stools per week for men despite a high-residue diet, or a period of more than 3 days without a bowel movement; (b) straining (incomplete evacuation, hard/lumpy stools, etc.) at stool greater than 25% of the time and/or two or fewer stools per week; or (c) straining at defecation and less than one stool daily with minimal effort. A symptom-based system for classifying functional constipation (and other functional gastrointestinal disorders) called the Rome criteria is often used to define constipation in clinical trials today. The Rome criteria encompass both quantitative (frequency) and qualitative (stool consistency, etc.) symptoms associated with constipation. The most current revision of the criteria, Rome III, was released in 2006 and is outlined in Table 43–5.

EPIDEMIOLOGY

A systematic review of the epidemiology of constipation in North America reported a prevalence range for constipation of 1.9% to 27%, with most reported estimates ranging from 12% to 19%.[28] Prevalence estimates by gender were female-to-male ratio of 2.2:1.[28] Similarly, in a multinational survey of 13,879 adult participants from seven countries, the rate of self-reported constipation was 12.3% overall (range 5% to 18%). Constipation was more common in women (2.4-fold more likely) and the elderly.[29] Other factors associated with constipation in some reports include inactivity, lower socioeconomic class, lower income, non-Caucasian race, symptoms of depression, and history of physical or sexual abuse.[28,30]

Although bowel movement frequency does not decrease as a consequence of aging, there is an age-related increase in laxative use and self-reported constipation rates.[28,31] Factors associated with the increased prevalence of constipation in the elderly include a higher number of daily medications, increased incidence of chronic comorbidities, changes in mobility status, changes in diet/lifestyle, and institutuionalization.

PATHOPHYSIOLOGY

Constipation may be primary or secondary. Primary constipation occurs without an identifiable underlying cause, whereas secondary constipation may be the result of constipating drugs, lifestyle factors, or medical disorders (Table 43–6). Three primary constipation subtypes exist–normal transit, slow transit, and disordered defecation (also referred to by various other names such as pelvic floor dysfunction, anorectal dyssynergia, outlet constipation, dyscoordinated pelvic muscle activity).[30] Normal transit constipation is the most common and often referred to as "functional constipation." These patients have normal GI motility and stool frequency but may experience difficulty evacuating, passage of hard stools, or bloating and abdominal discomfort. Slow transit constipation represents an abnormality of GI transit time that leads to infrequent defecation. Dysfunction of the pelvic floor muscles and/or

TABLE 43-6	Possible Causes of Constipation
Conditions	**Possible Causes**
GI disorders	Irritable bowel syndrome
	Diverticulitis
	Upper GI tract diseases
	Anal and rectal diseases
	Hemorrhoids
	Anal fissures
	Ulcerative proctitis
	Tumors
	Hernia
	Volvulus of the bowel
	Syphilis
	Tuberculosis
	Helminthic infections
	Lymphogranuloma venereum
	Hirschsprung's disease
Metabolic and endocrine disorders	Diabetes mellitus with neuropathy
	Hypothyroidism
	Panhypopituitarism
	Pheochromocytoma
	Hypercalcemia
	Enteric glucagon excess
Cardiac disorders	Heart failure
Pregnancy	Depressed gut motility
	Increased fluid absorption from colon
	Use of iron salts
Lifestyle factors	Dietary changes
	Inadequate fluid intake
	Low dietary fiber
	Decreased physical activity
Neurogenic causes	CNS diseases
	Trauma to the brain (particularly the medulla)
	Spinal cord injury
	CNS tumors
	Cerebrovascular accidents
	Parkinson disease
Psychogenic causes	Ignoring or postponing urge to defecate
	Psychiatric diseases
Drug induced	See Table 43–7

TABLE 43-5	Diagnostic Criteria for Functional Constipation[27,a]

1. Must include two or more of the following:
   a. Straining during at least 25% of defecations
   b. Lumpy or hard stools in at least 25% of defecations
   c. Sensation of incomplete evacuation for at least 25% of defecations
   d. Sensation of anorectal obstruction/blockage for at least 25% of defecations
   e. Manual maneuvers to facilitate at least 25% of defecations (e.g., digital evacuation, support of the pelvic floor)
   f. Fewer than three defecations per week
2. Loose stools are rarely present without the use of laxatives
3. There is insufficient evidence for IBS

[a]Criteria fulfilled for the last 3 months with symptoms onset at least 6 months prior to diagnosis

anal sphincter are the most frequently encountered reasons for disordered defecation. In patients with defecatory disorders, these muslces/sphinter (which normally relax during defecation) contract and impede evacuation of stool. It is common for the subtypes to overlap in a single patient.

❺ Approaches to the treatment of constipation should begin with attempts to determine its cause. Disorders of the GI tract (IBS or diverticulitis), metabolic disorders (diabetes), or endocrine disorders (hypothyroidism) or other secondary causes may be involved. Constipation commonly results from a diet low in fiber or from use of constipating drugs such as opiates. Finally, constipation may sometimes be psychogenic in origin. Each of these causes is discussed in the following sections.

Constipation is a frequently reported problem in the elderly, probably the result of improper diets (low in fiber and liquids), increasing number of daily medications, diminished abdominal wall muscular strength, and possibly diminished physical activity. However, as previously stated, the frequency of bowel movements is not decreased with normal aging.

Drug-Induced Constipation

Use of drugs that inhibit the neurologic or muscular function of the GI tract, particularly the colon, may result in constipation. The majority of cases of drug-induced constipation are caused by opiates, various agents with anticholinergic properties, and antacids containing aluminum or calcium. With most of the agents listed in Table 43–7, the inhibitory effects on bowel function are dose dependent, with larger doses clearly causing constipation more frequently.

Opiates have effects on all segments of the bowel, but effects are most pronounced on the colon. The major mechanism by which opiates produce constipation has been proposed to be prolongation of intestinal transit time by causing spastic, nonpropulsive contractions. An additional contributory mechanism may be an increase in electrolyte absorption.

All opiate derivatives are associated with constipation, but the degree of intestinal inhibitory effects seems to differ between agents. Orally administered opiates appear to have greater inhibitory effects than parenterally administered products. Orally administered enkephalins (endogenous opiate-like polypeptides) have antimotility properties. In some reports, transdermal fentanyl has been associated with less constipation than oral sustained-release morphine.[32]

TABLE 43–7 Drugs Causing Constipation

Analgesics
  Inhibitors of prostaglandin synthesis
  Opiates
Anticholinergics
  Antihistamines
  Antiparkinsonian agents (e.g., benztropine or trihexyphenidyl)
  Phenothiazines
  Tricyclic antidepressants
Antacids containing calcium carbonate or aluminum hydroxide
Barium sulfate
Calcium channel blockers
Clonidine
Diuretics (non-potassium-sparing)
Ganglionic blockers
Iron preparations
Muscle blockers (D-tubocurarine, succinylcholine)
Nonsteroidal antiinflammatory agents
Polystyrene sodium sulfonate

TABLE 43–8 Clinical Evaluation of Constipation

History and physical examination

- Clarify what the patient means by constipation, identifying specific signs and symptoms (i.e., infrequent bowel movements, stools that are hard, small, or dry; difficulty or pain of defecation, feeling of abdominal discomfort or bloating, incomplete evacuation, etc.)
- Ask specifically about presence of Alarm signs and symptoms
- Evaluate general health, psychological status, medications, diet, comorbidities, onset of symptoms, and what treatments have been tried
- Identify underlying secondary causes or conditions (Table 43–6)
- Perform rectal exam for presence of anatomical abnormalities (such as fistulas, fissures, hemorrhoids, rectal prolapse) or abnormalities of perianal descent. Digital examination of rectum to check for fecal impaction, anal stricture, or rectal mass.

Laboratory tests

- No routine recommendations for lab testing—as indicated by clinical discretion
- In patients with signs and symptoms suggestive of organic disorder, specific testing may be performed (i.e., thyroid-function tests, electrolytes, glucose, complete blood count) based on clinical presentation
- In patients with alarm signs and symptoms or when structural disease is a possibility, select appropriate diagnostic studies:
  1. Protoscopy
  2. Sigmoidoscopy
  3. Colonoscopy
  4. Barium enema

CLINICAL PRESENTATION

See Table 43–8.

TREATMENT

Constipation

■ GENERAL APPROACH TO TREATMENT

Evaulation of constipation should attempt to clarify the patient's specific symptoms (i.e., exactly what the patient means by constipation). The patient should be asked about the frequency of bowel movements and the chronicity of constipation. Constipation occurring recently in an adult may indicate significant colon pathology such as malignancy. Constipation present since early infancy may be indicative of neurologic disorders. The patient should also be carefully questioned about usual diet and laxative regimens. Does the patient have a diet consistently deficient in high-fiber items and containing mainly highly refined foods? What laxatives or cathartics has the patient used to attempt relief of constipation? The patient should be questioned about other concurrent medications, with interest focused on agents that might cause constipation. Each patient should be questioned specifically to identify any "alarm symptoms" that would warrant further diagnostic workup[33] (Table 43–9). Evaulation should also include assessment of general health status, signs of underlying medical illness (i.e., hypothyroidism), and psychological status (e.g., depression or other psychological illness).

For most patients who complain of constipation, a thorough physical examination is not required after it is established that constipation (a) is not a chronic problem, (b) is not accompanied by signs of significant GI disease (i.e., alarm symptoms such as rectal bleeding or anemia), and (c) does not cause severe discomfort. In these circumstances, the patient may be referred directly to the first-line therapies for constipation described in the next section (mainly

TABLE 43-9	Alarm Signs and Symptoms in Patients with Constipation

1. Hematochezia
2. Melena
3. Family history of colon cancer
4. Family history of inflammatory bowel disease
5. Anemia
6. Weight loss
7. Anorexia
8. Nausea and vomiting
9. Severe, persistent constipation that is refractory to treatment
10. New onset or worsening of constipation in elderly patients without evidence of a possible primary cause

bulk-forming laxatives and dietary fiber with occasional use of saline or stimulant laxatives). Patients with alarm symptoms, with a family history of colon cancer, or those >50 years old with new symptoms may need further diagnostic evaluation. Table 43–10 presents a general treatment algorithm for the management of constipation.

⑥ The proper management of constipation requires a number of different modalities; however, the basis for therapy should be dietary modification in most cases. The major dietary change should be an increase in the amount of fiber consumed daily. In addition to dietary management, patients should be encouraged to alter other aspects of their lifestyle if necessary. Important considerations are to encourage patients to exercise (achieved even by brisk walking after dinner) and to adjust bowel habits so that a regular and adequate time is made to respond to the urge to defecate. Another general measure is to increase fluid intake. This is generally recommended and believed beneficial, although there is little objective evidence to support this measure.

TABLE 43-10	Constipation Treatment Algorithm

History
- Stool frequency
- Stool consistency
- Difficulty of defecation

Possible causes
- Diet deficient in high-fiber items and consisting mainly of highly refined foods
- GI disorders
- Metabolic and endocrine disorders
- Pregnancy
- Neurogenic
- Psychogenic
- Drug induced
- Laxative abusers

Symptoms seen with chronic constipation
- Fluid and electrolyte imbalances (hypokalemia)
- Protein-losing gastroenteropathy with hypoalbuminemia
- Syndromes resembling colitis

Select appropriate diagnostic studies
- Proctoscopy
- Sigmoidoscopy
- Colonoscopy
- Barium enema

Diagnosis
1. Treat specific cause
2. No diagnosis, symptomatic therapy
   A. Bulk-forming agents
   B. Dietary modification
   C. Alter lifestyle (exercise)
   D. Increase fluid intake
   F. Discontinue potential drug inducer

If an underlying disease is recognized as the cause of constipation, attempts should be made to correct it. GI malignancies may be removed via surgical resection. Endocrine and metabolic derangements should be corrected by the appropriate methods. For example, when hypothyroidism is the cause of constipation, cautious institution of thyroid-replacement therapy is the most important treatment measure.

As discussed earlier, many drug substances may cause constipation. If a patient is consuming medications well known to cause constipation, consideration should be given to alternative agents. For some medications (e.g., antacids), nonconstipating alternatives exist. If no reasonable alternatives exist to the medication thought to be responsible for constipation, consideration should be given to lowering the dose. If a patient must remain on constipating medications, then more attention must be given to general measures for prevention of constipation, as discussed in the next section.

■ NONPHARMACOLOGIC THERAPY

Dietary Modification and Bulk-Forming Agents

The most important aspect of therapy for constipation for the majority of patients is dietary modification to increase the amount of fiber consumed. Fiber, the portion of vegetable matter not digested in the human GI tract, increases stool bulk, retention of stool water, and rate of transit of stool through the intestine. The result of fiber therapy is an increased frequency of defecation. Also, fiber decreases intraluminal pressures in the colon and rectum, which is thought to be beneficial for diverticular disease and for IBS. The specific physiologic effects of fiber are not well understood. Patients should be advised to gradually increase daily fiber intake to 20 to 25 grams, either through dietary changes or fiber supplement products.[30] Fruits, vegetables, and cereals typically have the highest fiber content. Bran, a by-product of milling of wheat, is often added to foods to increase fiber content and contains a high amount of soluble fiber, which may be extremely constipating in larger doses. Raw bran is generally 40% fiber. Medicinal products, often called "bulk-forming agents," such as psyllium hydrophilic colloids, methylcellulose, or polycarbophil, have properties similar to those of dietary fiber and may be taken as tablets, powders, or granules.

A trial of dietary modification with high-fiber content should be continued for at least 1 month before effects on bowel function are determined. Most patients begin to notice effects on bowel function 3 to 5 days after beginning a high-fiber diet, but some patients may require a considerably longer period of time. Patients should be cautioned that abdominal distension and flatus may be particularly troublesome in the first few weeks of fiber therapy, particularly with high bran consumption. Gradually increasing dietary fiber over a few weeks to the goal of 20 to 25 grams may help reduce some of the adverse abdominal effects. In most cases these problems resolve with continued use.

Bulk-forming laxatives have few adverse effects. The only major caution in the use of bulk-forming laxatives is that obstruction of the esophagus, stomach, small intestine, and colon has been reported when the agents have been consumed without sufficient fluid and in patients with intestinal stenosis.

Surgery

In a small percentage of patients who present with complaints of constipation, surgical procedures are necessary because of the presence of colonic malignancies or GI obstruction from a number of other causes. In each case, the involved segment of intestine may be resected or revised. Surgery may be required in some endocrine disorders that cause constipation, such as pheochromocytoma, which requires removal of a tumor.

Biofeedback

Patients with constipation due to pelvic floor dysfunction/disordered defecation may have a less favorable response to fiber therapy than other constipation subtypes.[34] Many adult patients with functional defecatory disorders appear to benefit from pelvic floor retraining with biofeedback therapy. Success rates of 65–80% have been reported in controlled and uncontrolled studies.[35] The value of biofeedback in children with chronic constipation has not been well demonstrated.[36]

■ PHARMACOLOGIC THERAPY

Drug Regimens of Choice

For most patients, treatment and prevention of constipation should consist of bulk-forming agents in addition to dietary modifications that increase dietary fiber.[30,37] A variety of products are available that provide adequate bulk. Whichever agent is chosen, it should be used daily and continued indefinitely in most patients, particularly those with chronic constipation.

For most persons with acute constipation, infrequent use (less than every few weeks) of laxative products is acceptable. Acute constipation may be relieved by the use of a tap-water enema or a glycerin suppository; if neither is effective, the use of oral sorbitol, low doses of bisacodyl or senna, low-dose polyethylene glycol (PEG) (Miralax), or saline laxatives (e.g., milk of magnesia) may provide relief. If laxative treatment is required for longer than 1 week, the person should be advised to consult a physician to determine if there is an underlying cause of constipation that requires treatment with other modalities.

For bedridden or geriatric patients, or others with chronic constipation, bulk-forming laxatives remain the first line of treatment, but the use of more potent laxatives may be required relatively frequently. When other than bulk-forming laxatives are used, they should be administered in the lowest effective dose and as infrequently as possible to maintain regular bowel function (more than three stools per week). Agents that may be used in these situations include "osmotic" laxatives such as sorbitol, lactulose, low-dose PEG, or perhaps milk of magnesia (magnesium hydroxide). "Stimulant" laxatives such as senna and bisacodyl may also be used but because these agents can have a less desirable side effect profile, they may be reserved for patients who fail to respond to osmotic laxatives and increased daily fiber.[30,38] Mineral oil should be avoided, particularly in bedridden patients, because of the risk of aspiration and lipoid pneumonia. Some patients with chronic constipation may present with fecal impactions. Before vigorous oral laxatives can be used, the impaction needs to be removed using mechanical methods, including tap-water or saline enemas and digital extraction.

In the hospitalized patient without GI disease, constipation may be related to the use of general anesthesia and/or opiate substances. Most orally or rectally administered laxatives may be used in these situations. For prompt initiation of bowel evacuation, either a tap-water enema, glycerin suppository, or oral milk of magnesia is recommended. Several new agents that are peripheral opioid-receptor antagonists may be used in specific patient populations (postsurgical, hospitalized, and/or palliative care patients receiving chronic opioid therapy).

With infants and children, constipation may occur commonly. In patients with persistent problems, the underlying etiology may be neurologic, metabolic, or secondary to anatomic abnormalities. Management of constipation in this age group should consist

TABLE 43-11	Dosage Recommendations for Laxatives and Cathartics
Agent	**Recommended Dose**
Agents that cause softening of feces in 1–3 days	
Bulk-forming agents/osmotic laxatives	
Methylcellulose	4–6 g/day
Polycarbophil	4–6 g/day
Psyllium	Varies with product
Polyethylene glycol 3350	
Emollients	
Docusate sodium	50–360 mg/day
Docusate calcium	50–360 mg/day
Docusate potassium	100–300 mg/day
Lactulose	15–30 mL orally
Sorbitol	30–50 g/day orally
Mineral oil	15–30 mL orally
Agents that result in soft or semifluid stool in 6–12 h	
Bisacodyl (oral)	5–15 mg orally
Senna	Dose varies with formulation
Magnesium sulfate (low dose)	<10 g orally
Agents that cause watery evacuation in 1–6 h	
Magnesium citrate	18 g 300 mL water
Magnesium hydroxide	2.4–4.8 g orally
Magnesium sulfate (high dose)	10–30 g orally
Sodium phosphates	Varies with salt used
Bisacodyl	10 mg rectally
Polyethylene glycol–electrolyte preparations	4 L

of dietary modification with an emphasis on high-fiber foods or treatment of underlying cause. For acute constipation in most age groups, a tap-water enema or glycerin suppository may be helpful. Occasional use of osmotic or stimulant laxatives in low doses is justified as well.

Drug Classes

The traditional classification system for laxatives and cathartics by suspected mode of action may not be very useful, as the mode of action is not clearly understood for many agents. In general, most of these products induce bowel evacuation by one or more of the mechanisms associated with the etiology of diarrhea, including active electrolyte secretion, decreased water and electrolyte absorption, increased intraluminal osmolarity, and increased hydrostatic pressure in the gut. Laxatives convert the intestine from primarily an organ that absorbs water and electrolytes to an organ that secretes these substances. Identification of laxative agents by traditional classification system however, is important as this nomenclature is often used by other healthcare practitioners and in the medical literature (Table 43–11).

The three general classes of laxatives are discussed in this section: (a) those causing softening of feces in 1 to 3 days (bulk-forming laxatives, docusates, the poorly absorbable sugars (lactulose and sorbitol), and low-dose PEG; (b) those that result in soft or semifluid stool in 6 to 12 hours (diphenylmethane derivatives and anthraquinone derivatives; "stimulant-type" laxatives); and (c) those causing water evacuation in 1 to 6 hours (saline cathartics, castor oil, and high-dose polyethylene glycol-electrolyte lavage solution).

Emollient Laxatives

Emollient laxatives are surfactant agents, docusate in its various salts, which work by facilitating mixing of aqueous and fatty materials within the intestinal tract. They may increase water and electrolyte secretion in the small and large bowel. Increased stool moisture content should lead to a softer, easier-to-pass stool. These products are generally given orally, although docusate potassium has also been used rectally. With these products, softening of stools occurs within 1 to 3 days of therapy.

Emollient laxatives are ineffective in treating constipation but are used mainly to prevent this condition. They may be helpful in situations in which straining at stool should be avoided, such as after recovery from myocardial infarction, with acute perianal disease, or after rectal surgery. It is unlikely that these agents would be effective in preventing constipation if major causative factors (e.g., heavy opiate use, uncorrected pathology, or inadequate dietary fiber) are not concurrently addressed.

Although docusates are generally safe, a few adverse effects have been noted. They may increase the intestinal absorption of agents administered concurrently and alter toxic potential. Reports of increased fecal soiling associated with docusate use in elderly patients may limit their use in this population.[38]

Mineral Oil

Mineral oil is the only lubricant laxative in routine use. This agent, obtained from petroleum refining, acts by coating stool and allowing for easier passage. It inhibits colonic absorption of water, thereby increasing stool weight and decreasing stool transit time. Mineral oil may be given orally or rectally in a dose of 15 to 45 mL. Generally, the effect on bowel function is noted after 2 or 3 days of use.

Mineral oil is helpful in situations similar to those suggested for docusates: to maintain a soft stool and to avoid straining for relatively short periods of time (a few days to 2 weeks); however, it possesses a much greater potential for adverse effects, and its routine use should be discouraged. Mineral oil may be absorbed systemically and can cause a foreign-body reaction in lymphoid tissue. Also, in debilitated or recumbent patients, mineral oil may be aspirated, causing lipoid pneumonia.[30,38] Mineral oil may decrease the absorption of fat-soluble vitamins (A, D, E, and K) with chronic use by causing retention in the GI tract. Finally, even when given orally, mineral oil may leak from the anal sphincter, causing pruritus and soiling of clothing.

Lactulose and Sorbitol

Lactulose is a nonabsorbable disaccharide that is used orally or rectally. It is metabolized by colonic bacteria to low-molecular-weight acids, resulting in an osmotic effect whereby fluid is retained in the colon. The fluid retained in the colon lowers the pH and increases colonic peristalsis. Lactulose increases stool frequency and consistency in patients with chronic constipation (vs. placebo) and may be more effective than fiber alone. Head-to-head studies suggest that lactulose is slightly less effective than low-dose PEG or some combination laxative agents (such as those containing fiber plus senna–not currently available in the United States). Lactulose is generally not recommended as a first-line agent for the treatment of constipation because it is costly, requires a prescription, and is associated with adverse effects such as flatulence, nausea, and abdominal discomfort or bloating–though it can be useful in some patients. It may be justified as an alternative for acute constipation or in patients with an inadequate response to increased dietary fiber and bulking agents. In some patients with more complex disease or nonmodifiable risk factors for constipation (such as beridden, elderly patients with chronic or debilitating illnesses and constipating medications), lactulose may be required on a more regular basis. In addition to the adverse abdominal effects associated with lactulose, diarrhea and electrolyte imbalances can occasionally occur.[38] Sorbitol, a monosaccharide, also exerts its effect by osmotic action and has been recommended as a cost-effective alternative to lactulose. It is as effective as lactulose but may cause less nausea and is much less expensive.[37,38]

Diphenylmethane and Anthraquinone Derivatives

Bisacodyl, the only remaining diphenylmethane derivative with the withdrawal of phenolphthalein, exerts its therapeutic effect by stimulating the mucosal nerve plexus of the colon and may also affect intestinal fluid secretion by altering fluid and electrolyte transport. Bisacodyl exhibits significant interpatient variability in effective dose, with doses that cause no effect in one patient or resulting in excessive cramping and fluid evacuation in others. Bisacodyl is generally reserved for intermittent use (every few weeks) to treat constipation or as a bowel preparation before diagnostic procedures in which cleansing of the colon is necessary. It may be administered orally or as a suppository, both recommended once daily. Bisacodyl may sometimes cause severe abdominal cramping as well as significant fluid and electrolyte imbalances with chronic use.

Senna or sennosoids are the only remaining anthraquinone derivatives after removal of cascara sagrada and casanthrone (cascara extracts). Laxative effects are limited to the colon, and stimulation of the Auerbach plexus may be involved. As with bisacodyl, senna is only generally recommended for intermittent use. Senna-containing products are given orally.

In the past, clinicians have hesitated to use stimulant-type laxatives on a regular basis due to claims that the colon was harmed by chronic use. Stimulant laxatives were thought to cause cathartic colon, damage the enteric nervous system, and lead to a physical dependence on laxatives for defecation. There is little evidence that stimulant laxatives given in appropriate doses (not more than once daily) cause intestinal/enteric damage or physical dependency (the role of psychological dependency is a separate issue discussed in the laxative abuse section).[30] Excessive use or abuse of stimulant laxatives, however, is a concern with these agents and can result in large-volume watery diarrhea, fluid loss, and electrolyte disturbances. Melanosis coli, a change in colon pigmentation with chronic anthraquinone therapy once thought to be linked to colon cancer, is now known to be a benign and reversible condition. Though safety may be of less concern than previously thought, because of their risk of adverse effects (abdominal cramping and fluid/electrolyte imbalance), stimulants are typically reserved for intermittent use or in patients who fail to respond adequately to bulking and osmotic laxatives. However, some patients with severe chronic constipation and nonmodifiable risk factors may use these agents on a more regular basis.

Saline Cathartics

Saline cathartics are composed of relatively poorly absorbed ions such as magnesium, sulfate, phosphate, and citrate, which produce their effects primarily by osmotic action causing retention of fluid in the GI tract. Magnesium also stimulates the secretion of cholecystokinin, a hormone that causes stimulation of bowel motility and fluid secretion. These agents may be given orally or rectally. A bowel movement may result within a few hours after oral doses and in 1 hour or less after rectal administration.

These agents should be used primarily for acute evacuation of the bowel, which may be necessary before diagnostic examinations, after poisonings, and in conjunction with some anthelmintics to eliminate parasites. Such agents as milk of magnesia (an 8% suspension of magnesium hydroxide) may be used occasionally (every few weeks) to treat constipation in otherwise healthy adults. Saline cathartics should not be used on a routine basis. The enema formulations of these agents may be useful in fecal impactions.

As with most laxatives, these agents may cause fluid and electrolyte depletion. Also, magnesium or sodium accumulation may occur when magnesium-containing cathartics are used in patients with renal dysfunction or when sodium phosphate is used in patients with congestive heart failure. These risks increase with long-term use.

Castor Oil

Castor oil is metabolized in the GI tract to an active compound, ricinoleic acid, which stimulates secretory processes, decreases glucose absorption, and promotes intestinal motility, primarily in the small intestine. Castor oil usually results in a bowel movement within 1 to 3 hours of administration. Because the agent has such a strong purgative action, it should not be used for the routine treatment of constipation.

Glycerin

Glycerin is usually administered as a 3 g suppository and exerts its effect by osmotic action in the rectum. As with most agents given as suppositories, the onset of action is usually less than 30 minutes. Glycerin is considered a safe laxative, although it may occasionally cause rectal irritation. Its use is acceptable on an intermittent basis for constipation, particularly in children.

Polyethylene Glycol-Electrolyte Lavage Solution

Whole-bowel irrigation with polyethylene glycol-electrolyte lavage solution (PEG-ELS) has become popular for colon cleansing before diagnostic procedures or colorectal operations. Various preparations are available (of varying molecular weights) with and without electrolytes.

Four liters of this solution is administered over 3 hours to obtain complete evacuation of the GI tract. The lavage solution is not recommended for routine treatment of constipation, and its use should be avoided in patients with intestinal obstruction.

Low doses of PEG, however, are FDA-approved for treatment of constipation. For this indication, PEG is administered in smaller volumes (10–30 g or 17–34 g per 120–240 mL) usually once (or twice) daily. With lesser volumes and slower ingestion, PEG has a much lower incidence of the adverse abdominal effects or electrolyte disturbances associated with whole-bowel lavage. PEG may also have fewer side effects than other "osmotic" agents because it is not absorbed systemically or metabolized by colonic bacteria.[39] PEG has been safely tolerated even when used for longer durations of therapy (up to 6 months). PEG was first approved as a prescription laxative for occasional constipation in 1999. In 2006, PEG 3350 gained FDA approval for nonprescription treatment of occasional constipation under the brand name Miralax.

Lubiprostone

Lubiprostone is the first new drug in a class called "chloride channel activators," which are designed to act locally in the gut to open chloride channels on the GI luminal epithelium, which, in turn, stimulates chloride-rich fluid secretion into the intestinal lumen. Increased intraluminal fluid secretion helps to soften stool and accelerate GI transit time.[40] Lubiprostone (Amitiza) was first approved in 2006 for "chronic idiopathic constipation in adults" at a recommended dose of one 24 mg capsule twice daily with food. In 2008, Lubiprostone also received FDA approval for treatment of patients with constipation-predominant irritable bowel sydnrome (IBS-C). Clinical trials have shown a significant increase in spontaneous bowel movements in patients treated with lubiprostone versus placebo as well as improvement in straining, stool consistency, and overall constipation severity.[41] For most patients, bowel movements occur within 24 to 48 hours of lubiprostone administration. Common adverse effects include headache (13%), diarrhea, and nausea.[40] Because of its high cost (especially relative to other available laxative agents) and lack of comparative data with other laxative therapies, lubiprostone will likely be reserved for patients with chronic constipation that fail conventional first-line agents.

Prucalopride

Prucalopride is a selective 5 hydroxytriptamine-4 (5HT-4) receptor agonist being developed for treatment of chronic constipation and IBS-C. Prucalopride demonstrates proenterokinetic effects (increased colonic motility and transit), specifically in the GI tract. Prucalopride, however, is more selective than the previously available serotonergic agonist cisapride and tegaserod with higher affinity for the 5HT-4 receptor. Receptor selectivity is thought to improve the safety profile of prucalopride over cisapride and tegaserod, which were removed from the market due to concerns for adverse cardiovascular events. In clinical trials, prucalopride significantly increased the number of complete, spontaneous bowel movements in adults with chronic constipation.[42] Constipation symptoms and quality of life were also improved with prucalopride. This agent has been safely tolerated in clinical trials with no adverse cardiovascular effects versus placebo (though data are limited). Prucalopride has not yet been approved by the FDA.

Opioid-Receptor Antagonists

Alvimopan (Entereg) is an oral gastrointestinal-specific mu-receptor antagonist approved for short-term use in hospitalized patients to accelerate recovery of bowel function after large or small bowel resection. Causes of postoperative ileus are multifactorial, with the effects of opioids considered to be a significant contributing factor. Alvimopam antagonizes the GI (peripheral) effects of opioids without affecting analgesia because it does not cross the blood-brain barrier. Alvimopan is only available through a special use program (ENTEREG access support and education; EASE), which requires hospitals to register and meet all requirements before the drug can be administered. Additionally, alvimopan is contraindicated in patients receiving therapeutic doses of opioids for more than seven consecutive days prior to surgery (as they may be more sensitive to the drug's effects). Dosing for alvimopan is as follows: 12 mg capsule adminstered 30 min to 5 hours before surgery and then 12 mg twice daily for up to 7 days or until discharge (maximum of 15 doses).

Methylnaltrexone (Relistor) is mu receptor-antagonist approved for opioid-induced constipation in patients with advanced disease receiving palliative care or when response to laxative therapy has been insufficient. This agent does not cross the blood-brain barrier or antagonize analgesia; it acts on peripheral mu receptors to antagonize unwanted opioid side effects such as constipation. It is administered at a weight-based dose as a subcutaneous injection, usually every other day (no more than once daily), and is contraindicated in patients with known or suspected gastrointestinal obstruction.

Naltrexone and naloxone are opioid antagonists but are not used in constipation because they do cross the blood-brain barrier and reverse CNS effects of opioids (respiratory depression and analgesia).

Other Agents

Tap-water enemas may be used to treat simple constipation. The administration of 200 mL of tap water by enema to an adult often results in a bowel movement within 30 minutes. Soap-suds enemas are no longer recommended as their use may result in proctitis or colitis.

Prevention

For certain groups of patients, such as those recovering from myocardial infarction or rectal surgery, straining at defecation is to be avoided. The basis of preventive therapy in these patients should be bulk-forming laxatives. Additionally, the use of docusate is popular, although its effectiveness is debated. In pregnant patients, constipation may result because of alterations in anatomy or iron supplementation. As described earlier, bulk-forming laxatives and docusates should be the first line of prevention.

LAXATIVE ABUSE SYNDROME

Misconceptions about normal bowel patterns and the effect of laxatives have contributed to a syndrome of laxative abuse that is relatively common in the United States. The availability of laxatives over the counter and as chocolates or gums conveys to the public that the use of these agents is without adverse consequences. Abuse of laxatives has occurred traditionally in persons trying to maintain daily bowel function, but has extended to others who use laxatives for the purpose of controlling weight. In either case, the consistent abuse of strong laxatives and cathartics may lead to serious illness.

Laxative abuse for the purpose of maintaining daily bowel function begins with misconceptions about the frequency, quantity, or consistency of stools. With the use of strong purgatives, the colon may be so thoroughly cleansed that a bowel movement may not occur normally until a few days later. This delay reinforces the need for more purgatives, and the cycle of laxative dependence is begun. Eventually the patient may require daily laxatives to maintain bowel function. A variation of laxative abuse is seen in persons who use them as a means of weight loss.

The laxative abuser may present with contradictory findings of diarrhea and weight loss. In addition, long-term abusers of laxatives tend to have vomiting, abdominal pain, lassitude, weakness, thirst, edema, and bone pain (caused by osteomalacia). With prolonged use of laxatives a number of serious illnesses may arise, including fluid and electrolyte imbalances (e.g., acid-base imbalances and hypokalemia), protein-losing gastroenteropathy with hypoalbuminemia, and syndromes resembling colitis.

The determination of laxative abuse syndrome can be difficult because many laxative abusers vigorously deny laxative use. Middle-aged women tend to be the most common laxative abusers. The chronic laxative abuse problem should be addressed by a combination of measures, including psychiatric evaluation, dietary modification with reliance on bulk-forming laxatives, and specific guidelines to the patient for the withdrawal of stimulant laxatives.

EVALUATION OF THERAPEUTIC OUTCOMES

The ultimate goal of treatment for constipation is alteration of lifestyle (particularly diet) and modifiable secondary causes (drugs, etc.) to prevent further episodes of constipation. Short-term goals include alleviation of acute constipation with relief from symptoms. For patients with chronic constipation, the goals are more long term and include use of proper diet and decreased reliance on laxatives in addition to relief of symptoms for the patient so that quality of life is not diminished. Effective treatment of constipation requires the patient to become more knowledgeable about the causes of constipation, proper diet, and appropriate use of laxatives.

IRRITABLE BOWEL SYNDROME

IBS is a gastrointestinal syndrome characterized by chronic abdominal pain and altered bowel habits in the absence of any organic cause. It is the most commonly diagnosed gastrointestinal condition.

EPIDEMIOLOGY

The prevalence of IBS is approximately 10% to 15% based on North American and European population-based studies; however, there is a wide variation in prevalence by individual country.[43-46] IBS affects men and women, young patients, and the elderly with an overall 2:1 female predominance in North America.[45] However, younger patients and women are more likely to be diagnosed with IBS. Although only 15% of those affected actually seek medical attention, IBS is the cause of between 25% and 50% of all referrals to gastroenterologists.[43]

PATHOPHYSIOLOGY

Although the exact pathophysiologic abnormalities with IBS are still being actively investigated, IBS likely results from altered somatovisceral and motor dysfunction of the intestine from a variety of causes. Abnormal central nervous system processing of afferent signals may lead to visceral hypersensitivity, with the specific nerve pathway affected determining the exact symptomatology expressed. This visceral hypersensitivity is a neuroenteric phenomenon that is independent of motility and psychological disturbances.[47] Factors known to contribute to these alterations include genetics, motility factors, inflammation, colonic infections, mechanical irritation to local nerves, stress, and other psychological factors.

Serotonin-Type Receptors

The enteric nervous system contains a significant percentage of the body's 5-hydroxytryptamine (serotonin, 5-HT).[48] Two types of serotonin exist within the gut: serotonin type 3 (HT_3) and serotonin type 4 (HT_4), which are responsible for secretion, sensitization, and motility.[49] There is an increase in the postprandial levels of 5-HT in those who suffer from diarrhea-predominant IBS when compared with nonsufferers.[48] Therefore, stimulation and antagonism of these serotonin receptors have become a focused area for research on new drug therapies for both diarrhea- and constipation-predominant disease.

CLINICAL PRESENTATION

❼ IBS presents as either diarrhea-predominant or constipation-predominant disease and can be defined as lower abdominal pain, disturbed defecation (constipation, diarrhea, or an alternating pattern of both), and bloating in the absence of structural or biochemical factors that might explain these symptoms (Table 43–12).

TABLE 43-12 Clinical Presentation of Irritable Bowel Syndrome

Signs and symptoms
- Lower abdominal pain
- Abdominal bloating and distension
- Diarrhea symptoms, >3 stools/day
- Extreme urgency
- Passage of mucus
- Constipation symptoms, <3 stools/wk, straining, incomplete evacuation
- Psychological symptoms such as depression and anxiety

Nongastrointestinal symptoms
- Urinary symptoms
- Fatigue
- Dyspareunia

Other concurrent conditions
- Fibromyalgia
- Functional dyspepsia
- Chronic fatigue syndrome

Reduced health-related quality of life

| TABLE 43-13 | Symptom-Based Criteria for Irritable Bowel Syndrome |

The manning criteria[50]

Chronic or recurrent abdominal pain for at least 6 months and two or more of the following:
1. Abdominal pain relieved with defecation
2. Abdominal pain associated with more frequent stools
3. Abdominal pain associated with looser stools
4. Abdominal distension
5. Feeling of incomplete evacuation after defecation
6. Mucus in stools

Rome III diagnostic criteria for irritable bowel syndrome[27]

Recurrent abdominal pain or discomfort at least 3 days per month in the last 3 months associated with two or more of the following:
1. Relieved with defecation
2. Onsest associated with a change in frequency of stool
3. Onset associated with a change in form (appearance) of stool

Because IBS can consist of a variable number of signs and symptoms, two diagnostic criteria "check lists" are commonly used to aid in the workup of a patient suspected of having IBS. The Manning criteria were first proposed in 1978, whereas the Rome criteria were initially proposed in 1999 and revised as recently as 2006 by an international working group in an effort to help standardize the diagnostic criteria used in clinical research protocols. Table 43–13 shows the symptom criteria for both of the Manning[50] and Rome III[27] symptom-based criteria.

Additional diagnostic steps that can be taken include sigmoidoscopy or colonoscopy; examination of the stool for occult blood and ova and parasites; complete blood cell count; erythrocyte sedimentation rate; and serum electrolytes. In some cases, radiographic imaging studies, such as computed tomography scans or barium swallows or enemas, may also be necessary if the findings of the foregoing assessment are not typical for IBS.[43]

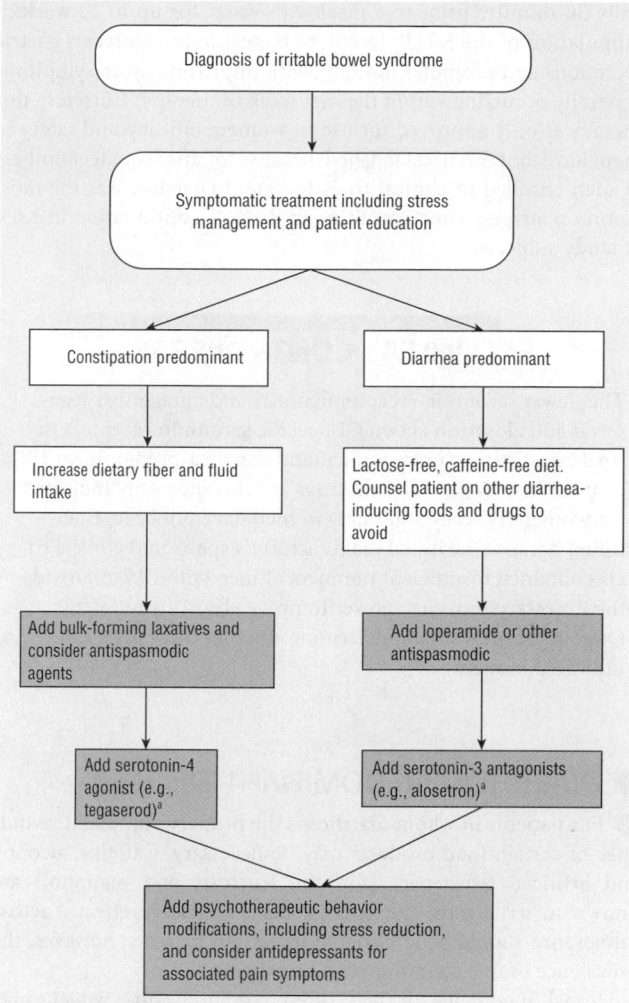

FIGURE 43-3. A general stepwise approach to the management of both constipation- and diarrhea-predominant irritable bowel syndrome. [a]Consider manufacturer sponsored patient access program.

TREATMENT

Irritable Bowel Syndrome

■ GENERAL APPROACH TO TREATMENT

The treatment approach to IBS is based upon the predominant symptoms and their severity (Fig. 43–3). Milder, less frequent episodes can be managed with dietary restrictions and a higher-fiber diet, with addition of bulk-forming laxatives, if necessary. More persistent disease may require as-needed uses of various antispasmodic or antidiarrheal agents such as loperamide. Lastly, the most-severe forms of this disease may call for pharmacologic agents directed specifically at the underlying neurohormonal imbalance, such as the 5-HT$_4$ agonists (e.g., tegaserod), or the 5-HT$_3$ receptor antagonists (e.g., alosetron).

Alosetron, a 5-HT$_3$ receptor antagonist, was withdrawn from the U.S. market in 2000 as a result of serious adverse effects, including severe constipation and ischemic colitis that did not appear in the initial clinical trials. It was reintroduced in 2002 and is now limited to an FDA-approved restricted-use program in lower initial doses, and requires extensive postmarketing surveillance. Results of these trials are necessary to definitively determine alosetron's true safety profile, especially with regard to its association with or causation of fatal ischemic colitis.

■ CONSTIPATION-PREDOMINANT DISEASE

In the constipation-predominant patient, dietary fiber may be beneficial. Patients should be instructed to begin with 1 tablespoonful of fiber with one meal daily and gradually increase the dose to include fiber with two and three meals a day until the desired outcome is achieved. End points that the patient should aim for include bulkier and more easily passed stools. For patients unable to tolerate dietary bran, bulking agents such as psyllium may be substituted.[51] Laxative use is not encouraged in these patients, and it should only be used in the smallest dose for the least amount of time in cases of severe constipation.

The 5-HT$_4$ partial agonist tegaseride was the first therapy approved by the FDA specifically for short-term, intermittent treatment of IBS-C.[52] Tegaseride was suspended from marketing in early 2007 at the request of the FDA due to an analysis of clinical trial data showing a small, yet significant, increase in ischemia events (MI, cerebrovascular accident (CVA), and unstable angina) in patients with preexisting cardiovascular disease and/or cardiovascular risk factors. In July 2007, the drug's manufacturer, Novartis, began a tegaseride (Zelnorm) restricted-access program for patients in the United States. Tegaseride is a serotonin derivative that activates 5-HT$_4$ receptors on the neurons in the gastrointestinal tract, increasing GI motility and decreasing visceral sensations. It is approved as 2 mg or 6 mg doses given twice daily 30 minutes prior to a meal with water for up to 12 weeks.[53] Stimulation of the 5-HT$_4$ receptors by tegaseride increases gastric secretions and promotes motility, with improvement in symptoms generally occurring within the first week of therapy. Currently this therapy is only approved for use in women; efficacy and safety in men have not been established because of inadequate numbers of men enrolled in clinical trials to date.[54] Diarrhea was the most common adverse effect, resulting in drug discontinuation in 1.6% of study subjects.

CLINICAL CONTROVERSY

The newer serotonin receptor agonists and antagonists tegaserod and alosetron act on GI-specific serotonin receptors to treat constipation-predominant and diarrhea-predominant IBS, respectively. However, both drugs are currently only indicated for women. Efficacy and safety in men have not been established because the initial manufacturer's sponsored clinical trials contained insufficient numbers of men with IBS to provide the necessary statistical power to prove efficacy and safety. Ongoing studies should determine whether these drugs are indicated in men.

■ DIARRHEA-PREDOMINANT DISEASE

❽ For patients in whom diarrhea is the primary complaint, avoidance of certain food products may be necessary. Caffeine, alcohol, and artificial sweeteners (sorbitol, fructose, and mannitol) are known to irritate the gut and produce a laxative effect. Lactose intolerance should be considered in certain patients; however, the prevalence of this condition may be exaggerated.

Herbal medicines or teas often contain senna, which may produce diarrhea. In patients with disease persistence following dietary modification, loperamide may be used for episodic management of urgent diarrhea, or in situations in which the patient wishes to avoid the possibility of an acute onset of symptoms.[53] Loperamide decreases intestinal transit, enhances water and electrolyte absorption, and strengthens rectal sphincter tone. Some patients may require continuous therapy, and careful dosage titration can usually be undertaken to prevent the development of constipation.

Diarrhea-predominant IBS caused by excessive stimulation of the 5-HT$_3$ receptor can be relieved by the drug alosetron. Alosetron was the first effective treatment for diarrhea-predominant IBS.[55] However, in November 2000 it was voluntarily withdrawn from the market because of severe GI adverse effects, including 113 reported cases of serious constipation and 8 cases of possible ischemic colitis and death. This decision was met with a great public outcry, as many who had suffered for years had experienced relief for the first time. Because this drug was highly effective in many patients, the FDA approved restricted use of alosetron in June 2002. Alosetron is now available via an FDA-approved restricted-use program in conjunction with GlaxoSmithKline as detailed at *http://www.lotronex.com*. It is now indicated, in lower initial doses of 0.5 mg twice daily, for women with diarrhea-predominant symptoms of longer than 6 months' duration that are not relieved by conventional therapy. Healthcare providers must use extreme caution in therapy with this drug and must follow strict FDA-mandated guidelines.

Probiotics (see earlier Diarrhea) such as *Lactobacillus* and *Bifidobacterium* reduced IBS symptoms in several investigative trials.[17] Another 5-HT$_3$ antagonist, cilansetron, has demonstrated efficacy similar to that of alosetron in phase II trials and enrolled enough male patients to show benefit in males as well.[55]

Use of Antidepressants in Irritable Bowel Syndrome

Tricyclic antidepressants have shown some benefit in treatment of diarrhea-predominant IBS associated with moderate to severe abdominal pain, by modulating perception of visceral pain, altering GI transit time, and treating underlying comorbidities.[56,57] Selective serotonin reuptake inhibitors are less-well studied, with only one report with paroxetine showing some improvement in stool passage and "well-being" but no decrease in abdominal pain.[58-60]

Figure 43–3 shows a general stepwise approach to the management of both constipation and diarrhea-predominant IBS.

■ PAIN IN IRRITABLE BOWEL SYNDROME

❾ Some patients with IBS suffer significant pain associated with their disease. Data supporting the use of antispasmodic agents in these patients are conflicting.[43] A trial of low-dose antidepressant therapy is indicated, especially if pain is associated with eating. Both tricyclic antidepressants and serotonin reuptake inhibitors produce analgesia and may relieve depressive symptoms if present. Preprandial doses of drugs containing anticholinergic properties may suppress pain (and/or diarrhea) associated with an overactive postprandial gastrocolonic response. Tricyclic antidepressants should be avoided in patients with pain and constipation. In addition, psychotherapy, including cognitive behavioral therapy, relaxation therapy, and hypnotherapy, has been shown to decrease IBS symptoms.[61]

■ EVALUATION OF THERAPEUTIC OUTCOMES

IBS is usually classified as constipation-predominant, diarrhea-predominant, or IBS with abdominal pain and bloating. Therapeutic goals in IBS should focus on the patient's primary complaint. Dietary and drug therapy goals should focus on end-organ treatment to relieve abdominal pain (antispasmodic drugs) or disturbed bowel habits (antidiarrheals and bulk-forming agents). Additionally, severe symptoms from central nervous system dysregulation should be treated with antidepressants, psychotherapy, relaxation/stress management, cognitive behavior treatment, and/or hypnosis aimed at specific affective disorders.[43] Lastly, the serotonin receptor agonists and antagonists can be used in carefully selected patients whose symptoms are not adequately controlled with other agents. The American Gastroenterology Association recommends that patients with severe IBS consider psychological treatments such as psychotherapy, relaxation/stress management, and/or cognitive behavior treatment.

ABBREVIATIONS

AGA: American Gastroenterology Association

AIDS: acquired immunodeficiency syndrome

CDC: Centers for Disease Control and Prevention

CVA: Cerebrovascular Accident

5-HT: serotonin

IBS: irritable bowel syndrome

IBS-C: constipation-predominant irritable bowel syndrome

ORS: oral rehydration solution

PEG-ELS: polyethylene glycol-electrolyte lavage solution

PHM: peptide histidine methionine

VIP: vasoactive intestinal peptide

REFERENCES

1. Binder HJ. Causes of chronic diarrhea. N Engl J Med 2006;355(3): 236–239.

2. Cheng AC, McDonald JR, Thielman NM. Infectious diarrhea in developed and developing countries. J Clin Gastroenterol 2005;39(9): 757–773.

3. Sandler RS, Stewart WF, Liberman JN, Ricci JA, Zorich NL. Abdominal pain, bloating, and diarrhea in the United States: Prevalence and impact. Dig Dis Sci 2000;45(6):1166–1171.

4. Scallan E, Majowicz S, Hall G, et al. Prevalence of diarrhoea in the community in Australia, Canada, Ireland, and the United States. Int J Epidemiol 2005;34:454–460.

5. Jones T, McMillian M, Scallan E, et al. A population-based estimate of the substantial burden of diarrhoeal disease in the United States; Food Net, 1996–2003. Epidemiol Infect 2007;135:293–301.

6. Musher DM, Musher BL. Contagious acute gastrointestinal infections. N Engl J Med 2004;351(23):2417–2427.

7. DuPont HL, Ericsson CD, Farthing MJG, et al. Expert review of the evidence base for self-therapy of travelers' diarrhea. J Travel Med 2009;16(3):161–171.

8. Bhatnagar S, Bhandari N, Mouli U, Bhan M. Consensus Statement of IAP National Task Force: Status Report on Management of Acute Diarrhea. Indian Pediatrics 2004;41:335–348.

9. Atia AN, Buchman AL. Oral rehydration solutions in non-cholera diarrhea: A review. Am J Gastroenterol 2009;104(10):2596–2604.

10. Fine KD, Schiller LR. AGA technical review on the evaluation and management of chronic diarrhea. Gastroenterology 1999;116(6): 1464–1486.

11. World Health Organization. WHO/UNICEF Joint Statement: Clinical Management of Acute Diarrhea (WHO/FCH/CAH/04.7); Geneva, Switzerland: World Health Organization; 2004.

12. Bhandari N, Mazumder S, Taneja S, et al. Effectiveness of zinc supplementation plus oral rehydration salts compared with oral rehydration salts alone as a treatment for acute diarrhea in a primary care setting: A cluster randomized trial. Pediatrics 2008 2008;121(5):e1279–1285.

13. Harris AG, Odorisio TM, Woltering EA, et al. Consensus statement—octreotide dose titration in secretory diarrhea—Diarrhea Management Consensus Development Panel. Dig Dis Sci 1995;40(7):1464–1473.

14. Schiller LR. Review article: Anti-diarrheal pharmacology and therapeutics. Aliment Pharmacol Ther 1995;9(2):87–106.

15. Ruszniewski P, Ducreux M, Chayvialle JA, et al. Treatment of the carcinoid syndrome with the longacting somatostatin analogue lanreotide: A prospective study in 39 patients. Gut 1996;39(2): 279–283.

16. Lombardi G, Minuto F, Tamburrano G, et al. Efficacy of the new long-acting formulation of lanreotide (lanreotide Autogel) in somastatin analogue-naive patients with acromegaly. J Endocrinol Invest 2009;32(3):202–209.

17. Floch MH, Walker WA, Guandalini S, et al. Recommendations for probiotic use—2008. J Clin Gastroenterol 2008;42:S104–S108

18. Delia P, Sansotta G, Donato V, et al. Use of probiotics for prevention of radiation-induced diarrhea. World J Gastroenterol 2007;13(6): 912–915.

19. Farthing MJ. Antisecretory drugs for diarrheal disease. Dig Dis 2006;24(1–2):47–58.

20. Gallelli L, Colosimo M, Tolotta G, et al. Prospective randomized double-blind trial of racecadotril compared with loperamide in elderly people with gastroenteritis living in nursing homes. Eur J Clin Pharmacol 2010;66(2):137–144.

21. Wang H, Shieh M, Liao K. A blind, randomized comparison of racecadotril and loperamide for stopping acute diarrhea in adults. World J Gastroenterol 2005;11(10):1540–1543.

22. Prado D. A multinational comparison of racecadotril and loperamide in the treatment of acute watery diarrhoea in adults. Scand J Gastroenterol 2002;37(6):656–661.

23. Thompson RF, Bass DM, Hoffman SL. Travel vaccines. Infect Dis Clin North Am 1999;13(1):149–167.

24. Tacket CO, Kotloff KL, Losonsky G, et al. Volunteer studies investigating the safety and efficacy of live oral El Tor Vibrio cholerae 01 vaccine strain CVD 111. Am J Trop Med Hyg 1997;56(5):533–537.

25. CDC. Prevention of rotavirus gastroenteritis among infants and children Recommendations of the Advisory Committee on Immunization Practices (ACIP). MMWR 2009;58(No. RR-2):1–26.

26. Shah N, Chitkara D, Locke G, Meek P, Talley N. Ambulatory Care for Constipation in the United States, 1993–2004. Am J Gastroenterol 2008;103:1746–1753.

27. Longstreth G, Thompson W, Chey W, Houghton L, Mearin F, Spiller R. Functional bowel disorders. Gastroenterology. 2006;130(5): 1480–1491.

28. Higgins P, Johanson J. Epidemiology of constipation in North America: A systematic review. Am J Gastroenterol 2004;99(4):750–759.

29. Wald A, Scarpignato C, Mueller-Lissner S, et al. A multinational survey of prevalence and patterns of laxative use among adults with self-defined constipation. Aliment Pharmacol Ther 2008;28(7):917.

30. Lembo A, Camilleri M. Chronic constipation. N Engl J Med 2003;349(14):1360–1368.

31. Harari D, Gurwitz JH, Avorn J, Bohn R, Minaker KL. Bowel habit in relation to age and gender: Findings from the National Health Interview Survey and Clinical Implications. Arch Intern Med 1996;156(3): 315–320.

32. Allan L, Richarz U, Simpson K, Slappendel R. Transdermal fentanyl versus sustained release oral morphine in strong-opioid naive patients with chronic low back pain. Spine 2005;30(22):2484–2490.

33. Brandt L, Prather C, Quigley E, Schiller L, Schoenfeld P, Talley N. Systematic review on the management of chronic constipation in North America. Am J Gastroenterol 2005:S5–S21.

34. Voderholzer W, Schatke W, Muhldorfer B, Klauser A, Birkner B, Muller-Lissner S. Clinical response to dietary fiber treatment of chronic constipation. Am J Gastroenterol 1997;92(1):95–98.

35. Bharucha A, Wald A, Enck P, Rao S. Functional anorectal disorders. Gastroenterology 2006;130(5):1510–1518.

36. Bassotti G, Chistolini F, Sietchiping-Nzepa F, De Roberto G, Morelli A, Chiarioni G. Biofeedback for pelvic floor dysfunction in constipation. BMJ 2004;328(7436):393.

37. Foxx-Orenstein A, McNally M, Odunsi S. Update on constipation: One treatment does not fit all. Clev Clin J Med 2008;75(11):813–824.

38. Gallagher PF, O'Mahony D, Quigley EM. Management of chronic constipation in the elderly. Drugs & Aging 2008;25(10):807–821.

39. DiPalma J, vB Cleveland M, McGowan J, Herrera J. A randomized, multicenter, placebo-controlled trial of polyethylene glycol laxative for chronic treatment of chronic constipation. Am J Gastroenterol 2007;102:1436–1441.

40. Lacy B, Chey W. Lubiprostone: chronic constipation and irritable bowel syndrome with constipation. Expert Opin Pharmacother 2009;10(1):143–152.

41. Cash B, Lacy B. Systematic review: FDA-approved prescription medications for adults with constipation. Gastroenterol Hepatol 2006;2(10):736–749.

42. Camilleri M, Kerstens R, Rykx A, Vandeplassche L. A placebo-controlled trial of prucalopride for severe chronic constipation. N Engl J Med 2008;358(22):2344–2354.

43. Brandt L, Chey W, Foxx-Orenstein A, et al. An evidence-based position statement on the management of irritable bowel syndrome. Am J Gastroenterol 2009;104(S1):S1–S35.

44. Hungin A, Chang L, Locke G, Dennis E, Barghout V. Irritable bowel syndrome in the United States: Prevalence, symptom patterns and impact. Aliment Pharmacol Ther 2005;21(11):1365–1375.

45. Brandt L, Bjorkman D, Fennerty M, et al. Systematic review on the management of irritable bowel syndrome in North America. Am J Gastroenterol 2002;97(s11):S7–S26.

46. Hungin A, Whorwell P, Tack J, Mearin F. The prevalence, patterns and impact of irritable bowel syndrom: An international survey of 40,000 subjects. Aliment Pharmacol Ther 2003;17(5):643–650.

47. Gerson CD, Gerson M-J, Awad RA, et al. Irritable bowel syndrome: An international study of symptoms in eight countries. Eur J Gastroenterol Hepatol 2008;20(7):659–667.

48. Bearcroft CP, Perrett D, Farthing MJG. Postprandial plasma 5-hydroxytryptamine in diarrhoea predominant irritable bowel syndrome: A pilot study. Gut 1998;42(1):42–46.

49. Chey WD. Tegaserod and other serotonergic agents: What is the evidence? Rev Gastroenterol Disord 2003;3(suppl 2):S35–40.

50. Manning A, Thompson W, Heaton K, Morris A. Towards positive diagnosis of the irritable bowel. Br Med J 1978;2(6138):653–654.

51. Thompson WG. Irritable bowel syndrome: A management strategy. Best Pract Res Clin Gastroenterol 1999;13(3):453–460.

52. Camilleri M. Review article: Tegaserod. Aliment Pharmacol Ther 2001;15(3):277–289.

53. Tougas G, Snape WJ, Otten MH, et al. Long-term safety of tegaserod in patients with constipation-predominant irritable bowel syndrome. Aliment Pharmacol Ther 2002;16(10):1701–1708.

54. Muller-Lissner SA, Fumagalli I, Bardhan KD, et al. Tegaserod, a 5-HT4 receptor partial agonist, relieves symptoms in irritable bowel syndrome patients with abdominal pain, bloating and constipation. *Aliment Pharmacol Ther* 2001;15(10):1655–1666.

55. Ford AC, Brandt LJ, Young C, Chey WD, Foxx-Orenstein AE, Moayyedi P. Efficacy of 5-HT3 antagonists and 5-HT4 agonists in irritable bowel syndrome: systematic review and meta-analysis. Am J Gastroenterol 2009;104(7):1831–1843.

56. Rahimi R, Nikfar S, Rezaie A, Abdollahi M. Efficacy of tricyclic antidepressants in irritable bowel syndrome: A meta-analysis. W J Gastroenterol 2009;15(13):1548–1553.

57. Abdul-Baki S, El Hajj I, ElZahabi L, et al. A randomized controlled trial of imipramine in patients with irritable bowel syndrome. W J Gastroenterol 2009;15(29):3636–3642.

58. Tabas G, Beaves M, Wang J, Friday P, Mardini H, Arnold G. Paroxetine to treat irritable bowel syndrome not responding to high-fiber diet: A double-blind, placebo-controlled trial. Am J Gastroenterol 2004;99(5):914–920.

59. Han C, Masand PS, Krulewicz S, et al. Childhood abuse and treatment response in patients with irritable bowel syndrome: A post-hoc analysis of a 12-week, randomized, double-blind, placebo-controlled trial of paroxetine controlled release. J Clin Pharm Ther 2009;34(1):79–88.

60. Masand PS, Pae C-U, Krulewicz S, et al. A double-blind, randomized, placebo-controlled trial of paroxetine controlled-release in irritable bowel syndrome. Psychosomatics 2009;50(1):78–86.

61. Heymann-Monnikes I, Arnold R, Florin I, Herda C, Melfsen S, Monnikes H. The combination of medical treatment plus multicomponent behavioral therapy is superior to medical treatment alone in the therapy of irritable bowel syndrome. Am J Gastroenterol 2000;95(4):981–994.

CHAPTER

44

Portal Hypertension and Cirrhosis

JULIE M. SEASE

KEY CONCEPTS

❶ Cirrhosis is a severe, chronic, irreversible disease associated with significant morbidity and mortality. However, the progression of cirrhosis secondary to alcohol abuse can be interrupted by abstinence. It is therefore imperative for the clinician to educate and support abstinence from alcohol as part of the overall treatment strategy of the underlying liver disease.

❷ Patients with cirrhosis should receive endoscopic screening for varices, and certain patients with varices should receive primary prophylaxis with nonselective β-adrenergic blockade therapy to prevent variceal hemorrhage.

❸ When nonselective β-adrenergic blocker therapy is used to prevent rebleeding, β-blocker therapy can be titrated to achieve a goal heart rate of 55 to 60 beats per minute or the maximal tolerated dose.

❹ Octreotide is the preferred vasoactive agent for the medical management of variceal bleeding. Endoscopy employing endoscopic band ligation is the primary therapeutic tool for the management of acute variceal bleeding.

❺ The combination of spironolactone and furosemide is the recommended initial diuretic therapy for patients with ascites.

❻ All patients who have survived an episode of spontaneous bacterial peritonitis should receive long-term antibiotic prophylaxis.

❼ The mainstay of therapy of hepatic encephalopathy involves therapy to lower blood ammonia concentrations and includes diet therapy, lactulose, and antibiotics alone or in combination with lactulose.

Chronic liver injury causes damage to normal liver tissue resulting in the development of regenerative nodules surrounded by fibrous bands.[1] Fibrosis, defined as the encapsulation or replacement of injured tissue by collagenous scar, results from an abnormal perpetuation of the normal wound healing process. If fibrotic liver disease advances, collagen bands progress to bridging fibrosis and eventually frank hepatic cirrhosis.[2] The word *cirrhosis* is derived from the Greek *kirrhos*, meaning orange-yellow, and refers to the color of the cirrhotic liver as seen upon autopsy or during surgery.[3] Cirrhosis is

an advanced stage of liver fibrosis.[1] The advanced fibrosis of cirrhosis leads to shunting of the portal and arterial blood supply directly into hepatic outflow through the central veins, and exchange between hepatic sinusoids and hepatocytes is compromised. Clinical consequences of cirrhosis include impaired hepatocyte function, the increased intrahepatic resistance of portal hypertension, and hepatocellular carcinoma. Circulatory irregularities such as splanchnic vasodilation, vasoconstriction and hypoperfusion of the kidneys, water and salt retention, and increased cardiac output also occur.

❶ While cirrhosis has many causes (Table 44–1), in the Western world, excessive alcohol intake and hepatitis C are the most common causes.[1,3,4] This chapter elucidates the pathophysiology of cirrhosis and the resultant effects on human anatomy and physiology. Treatment strategies for managing the most commonly encountered clinical complications of cirrhosis are discussed.

EPIDEMIOLOGY

The exact prevalence of cirrhosis is unknown, but a reasonable estimate is that 1% of populations have histologically diagnosable cirrhosis.[1] Cirrhosis was responsible for over 28,000 deaths in America in 2007, and chronic liver disease continues to be ranked twelfth among the leading causes of death in the United States.[5] Acute variceal bleeding and spontaneous bacterial peritonitis are among the immediately life-threatening complications of cirrhosis. Associated conditions causing significant morbidity include ascites and hepatic encephalopathy. Approximately 50% of patients with cirrhosis develop ascites during 10 years of observation and, within 2 years, nearly half of patients who develop ascites will die.[6]

TABLE 44–1	Etiology of Cirrhosis

Chronic alcohol consumption
Chronic viral hepatitis (types B, C, and D)
Metabolic liver disease
   Hemochromatosis
   Wilson's disease
   Alpha 1-antitrypsin deficiency
   Nonalcoholic steatohepatitis ("fatty liver")
   Cystic fibrosis
Immunologic disease
   Autoimmune hepatitis
   Primary biliary cirrhosis
   Primary sclerosing cholangitis (90% associated with ulcerative colitis)
Vascular disease
   Budd-Chiari
   Cardiac failure
Drugs
   Isoniazid, methyldopa, amiodarone, methotrexate, tamoxifen, retinol (vitamin A), propylthiouracil, didanosine

Data from references 1, 2, and 3.

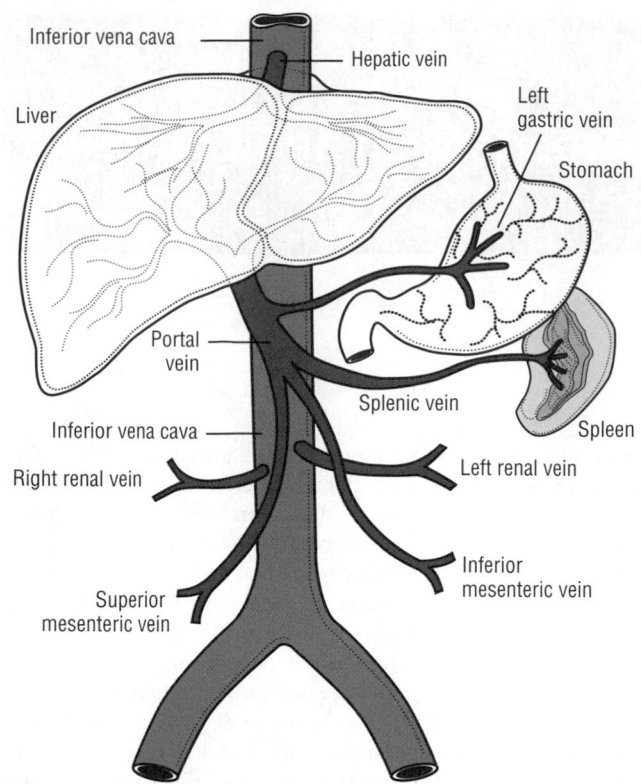

FIGURE 44-1. The portal venous system.

PATHOPHYSIOLOGY OF CIRRHOSIS

Any discussion of cirrhosis must be based on a firm understanding of hepatic anatomy and vascular supply. Conceptually, the liver can be thought of as an elaborate blood filtration system receiving blood from the hepatic artery and the portal vein (Fig. 44–1), with portal blood originating from the mesenteric, gastric, splenic, and pancreatic veins.[7] Blood enters the liver via the portal triad, which contains branches of the portal vein and hepatic artery, bile ducts, and lymphatic and nerve tissue. It then drains through the sinusoidal spaces (also known as the space of Disse) of the hepatic lobule (Fig. 44–2), which are lined by the workhorses of the liver, the hepatocytes. Individual hepatocytes are arranged in plates that are one cell thick. The six or more surfaces of each individual hepatocyte make contact with adjacent hepatocytes, border the bile canaliculi, or are exposed to the sinusoidal space. Filtered blood travels into the terminal hepatic venules, also called central veins, and then empties into larger hepatic veins and eventually into the inferior vena cava. Functional gradients of hepatocytes based on oxygen saturation have been reported. Hepatocytes closest to the portal triad, which contains the hepatic artery, have twice the oxygen saturation of those hepatocytes nearer to the terminal hepatic venule. Those hepatocytes closest to the portal triad also have higher levels of peroxisomes, glucose-6-phosphatase activity, urea cycle activity, bile acid uptake, glutathione content, and glycogen synthesis.

Normally, hepatic stellate cells function to store vitamin A and help to maintain the normal matrix in the sinusoidal space.[8] During chronic liver disease, however, hepatic stellate cells undergo an "activation" process, which is the central event in the development of hepatic fibrosis. Activation causes stellate cells to lose vitamin A, become highly proliferative, and synthesize fibrotic scar tissue, which accumulates in the sinusoidal space. This leads to loss of hepatocyte microvilli, loss of sinusoidal endothelial fenestrae,

deterioration of hepatocyte function, and, if fibrosis progresses, eventual cirrhosis.

Cirrhosis causes changes to the splanchnic vascular bed as well as the systemic circulation.[9] Splanchnic vasodilation, decreased responsiveness to vasoconstrictors, and the formation of new blood vessels contribute to an increased splanchnic blood flow, formation of gastroesophageal varices, and variceal bleeding. All of these components are part of the portal hypertensive syndrome. Portal hypertension is characterized by hypervolemia, increased cardiac index, hypotension, and decreased systemic vascular resistance. This is a so-called hyperkinetic syndrome, which leads to a marked activation of neurohumoral vasoactive factors, a response that occurs in an effort to maintain the arterial blood pressure within normal limits. Activation of neurohumoral vasoactive factors is a main component in the pathophysiology of the ascites and renal dysfunction that often accompany chronic liver disease. Portal-systemic shunting may also occur and is involved in hepatic encephalopathy and other complications.

In summary, cirrhosis results from fibrotic changes within the hepatic sinusoids and results in changes in the levels of vasodilatory and vasoconstrictor mediators and an increase in blood flow to the splanchnic vasculature.

ANATOMIC AND PHYSIOLOGIC EFFECTS OF CIRRHOSIS

Cirrhosis and the pathophysiologic abnormalities that cause it result in the commonly encountered problems of ascites, portal hypertension, esophageal varices, hepatic encephalopathy, and coagulation disorders. Other less commonly seen problems in patients with cirrhosis include hepatorenal syndrome, hepatopulmonary syndrome, and endocrine dysfunction. These are discussed in the section dealing with the management of cirrhotic complications.

ASCITES

Ascites is the accumulation of an excessive amount of fluid within the peritoneal cavity.[10] It is the most commonly occurring major complication of cirrhosis.[6] Approximately half of all cirrhotic patients develop ascites within 10 years of diagnosis. Several hypotheses have been offered to explain the mechanism for the development of ascites in decompensated cirrhosis.[10] Most acceptable theories state that ascites formation begins as a result of the development of sinusoidal hypertension and portal hypertension. Portal hypertension activates vasodilatory mechanisms that are mediated mostly by nitric oxide overproduction. This leads to splanchnic and peripheral arteriolar vasodilation and, in advanced disease, a drop in arterial pressure. Baroreceptor-mediated activation of the renin-angiotensin-aldosterone system, activation of the sympathetic nervous system, and release of antidiuretic hormone occur in response to the resulting arterial hypotension in an effort to restore normal blood pressure (Fig. 44–3). These changes cause renal sodium and water retention. Additionally, ongoing splanchnic vasodilation increases splanchnic lymph production beyond the capacity of the lymph transportation system. Leakage of lymphatic fluid into the peritoneal cavity occurs. Persistent renal sodium and water retention, increased splanchnic vascular permeability, and lymph leakage into the peritoneal cavity combine to create the sustained ascites formation of end-stage liver disease.

PORTAL HYPERTENSION AND VARICES

Sinusoidal portal hypertension is most often caused by alcohol-induced cirrhosis.[11] It is associated with acute variceal bleeding, a medical emergency that carries a mortality rate of 20% at 6 weeks and is among the most severe complications of cirrhosis.[12] Portal

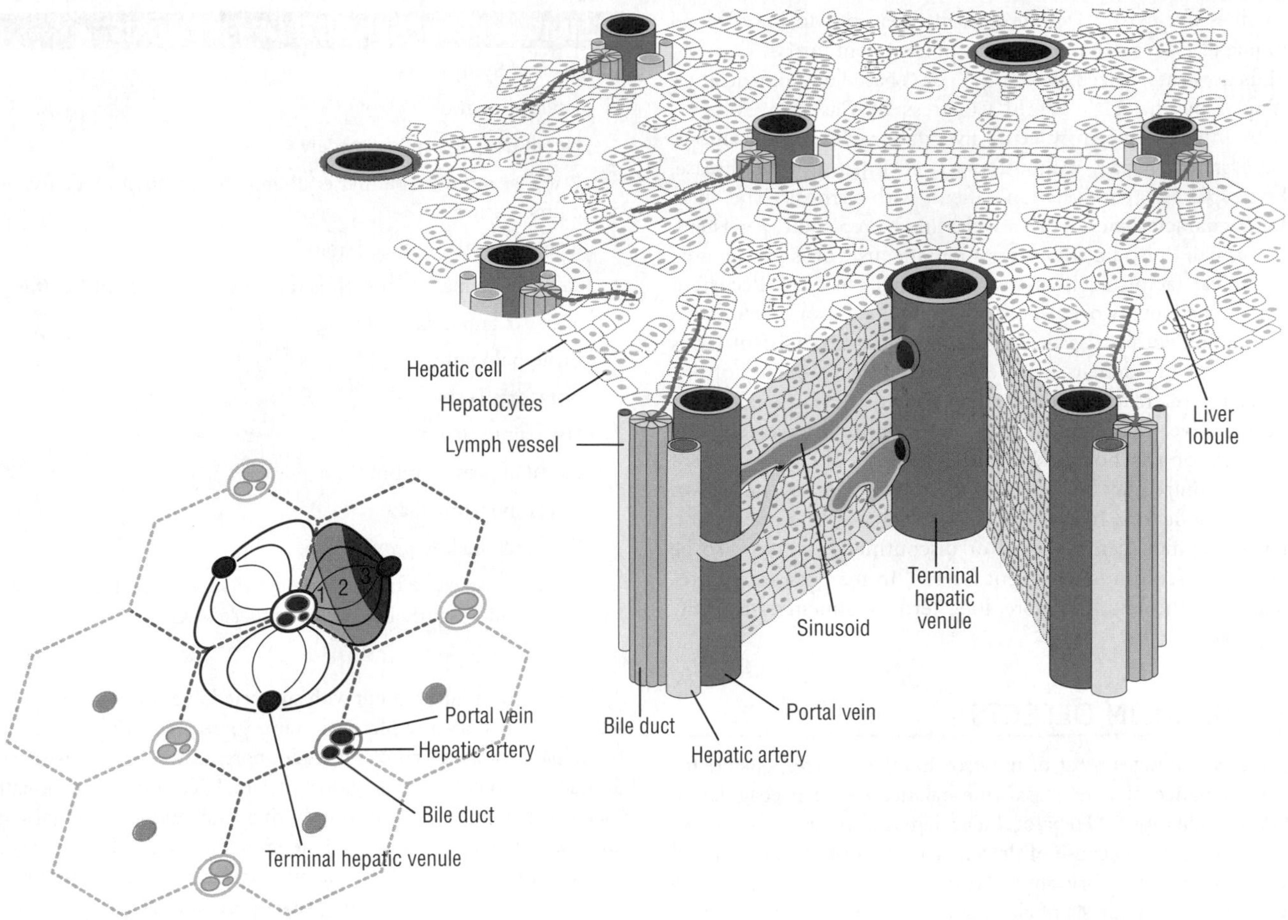

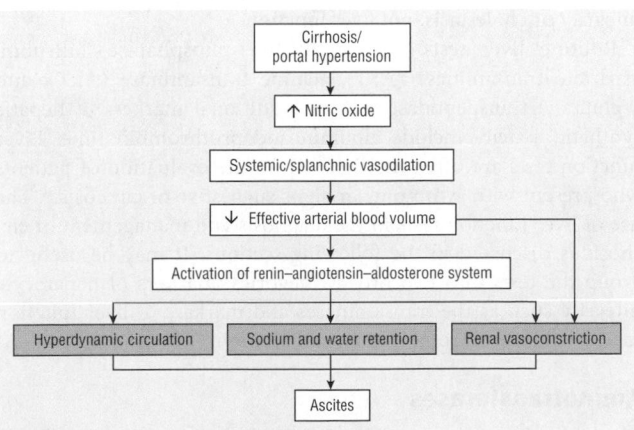

Hepatic cell
Hepatocytes
Lymph vessel

Portal vein
Hepatic artery

Bile duct

Terminal hepatic venule

Liver lobule

Terminal hepatic venule

Sinusoid

Bile duct

Portal vein

Hepatic artery

FIGURE 44-2. The hepatic lobule.

hypertension is defined by the presence of a gradient of greater than 5 mmHg between the portal and central venous pressures (see Fig. 44–1).[11] The gradient is called the hepatic venous pressure gradient (HVPG). Esophageal and gastric varices arise after the pressure gradient of 8 to 10 mm Hg is reached, and bleeding can occur from these varices once the gradient rises above 12 mmHg. Varices occur because of the body's need to find collateral outlets to relieve the increased pressure of portal hypertension. Other outlets, besides esophageal and gastric varices, include retroperitoneal vessels, the hemorrhoidal venous plexus, a recanalized umbilical vein, and intrahepatic shunts. Five percent of patients with cirrhosis are expected to develop varices within 1 year, and 28% will develop

them within 3 years. Acute variceal bleeding occurs in 25% to 40% of cirrhosis patients and is the cause of death for one third of these patients.

Progression to bleeding can be predicted by Child-Pugh score, red wale markings on the varices, and an alcoholic etiology of liver disease. Twelve percent of patients with small varices at initial endoscopy will experience variceal bleeding within 2 years. Twenty to 29% of patients with variceal bleeding will die within 30 days. Rebleeding is common following initial hemorrhage, especially within the first 72 hours. More than 50% of recurrent bleeding episodes occur within the first 10 days of the initial bleed, and risk returns to baseline after 6 weeks. Primary prevention of bleeding is a major goal in the therapy of portal hypertension, and strategies include both pharmacologic and surgical approaches.

HEPATIC ENCEPHALOPATHY

The term *hepatic encephalopathy* (HE) describes a wide range of neuropsychiatric symptoms that are associated with liver failure.[13] Symptoms of HE are thought to result from an accumulation of gut-derived nitrogenous substances in the systemic circulation as a consequence of decreased hepatic functioning and shunting through portosystemic collaterals bypassing the liver.[14] Once these substances enter the central nervous system, they cause alterations of neurotransmission that affect consciousness and behavior. Ammonia is the most commonly cited culprit in the pathogenesis of HE, but glutamate, benzodiazepine receptor agonists, and manganese are also potential causes.[13,14] Arterial ammonia levels are increased commonly in both acute and chronic liver disease, but an established correlation between blood ammonia levels and mental

Cirrhosis/
portal hypertension

↑ Nitric oxide

Systemic/splanchnic vasodilation

↓ Effective arterial blood volume

Activation of renin–angiotensin–aldosterone system

Hyperdynamic circulation

Sodium and water retention

Renal vasoconstriction

Ascites

FIGURE 44-3. Pathogenesis of ascites.

status does not exist.[14] Despite this, interventions to lower blood ammonia levels remain the mainstay of treatment for HE.

HE is now categorized as type A, B, or C based on nomenclature developed by the 11th World Congress of Gastroenterology.[13] Type A is HE induced by acute liver failure, Type B is due to portal-systemic bypass without associated intrinsic liver disease, and type C is HE that occurs in patients with cirrhosis. The duration and characteristics of HE are classified as episodic, persistent, and minimal. Episodic HE occurs spontaneously or is precipitated by a clinical factor, such as gastrointestinal bleeding. Recurrent HE is defined by two episodes of spontaneous or precipitated HE occurring within 1 year, and the hallmark of persistent HE is chronic cognitive deficits that decrease a patient's quality of life. Minimal HE refers to cirrhotic patients who do not suffer clinically overt cognitive dysfunction but who are found to have cognitive impairment on psychological studies. The onset of HE in a patient with liver failure may be related to the presence of several known precipitating factors. In cases of HE associated with a precipitant, if that precipitant can be cured or discontinued, it may also be possible to discontinue treatment for HE. In many cases, no precipitant is found and, therefore, long-term treatment of HE may be required.

COAGULATION DEFECTS

The liver synthesizes most of the proteins that are responsible for the maintenance of hemostasis (the balance between coagulation and anticoagulation).[15] Hepatocellular damage can lead to a disruption in hemostasis because of defects it may cause in the function of coagulation and fibrinolytic factors. These defects include a reduction in the synthesis of clotting factors, excessive fibrinolysis, disseminated intravascular coagulation, thrombocytopenia, and platelet dysfunction. Most coagulation factors are created in the liver, and the levels of these factors can be significantly reduced in chronic liver disease associated with extensive hepatocellular damage. Factor VII is the first factor to decrease as liver function declines due to its short half-life. A reduction in clotting factor VII is common in end-stage liver disease, affecting 60% of patients. Low factor VII activity is prognostic for reduced survival, and the prothrombin time is a standard component of the Child-Pugh scoring system. Accelerated intravascular coagulation and fibrinolysis can be detected in some patients with cirrhosis. The coexistence of sepsis, shock, surgery, trauma, or ascites may cause a progression from accelerated intravascular coagulation to disseminated intravascular coagulation. In patients with cirrhosis, disseminated intravascular coagulation involves increased release of procoagulants, impaired removal of activated coagulation factors and endotoxins produced by gut bacteria, and reduced synthesis of coagulation inhibitors. Both platelet number and function may also be affected in cirrhosis. Platelet numbers are reduced by multiple mechanisms, including splenomegaly due to portal hypertension and sequestration of platelets in the spleen, reduced hepatic production of thrombopoietin, bone marrow suppression, and increased platelet destruction. Mild to moderate thrombocytopenia occurs in 15% to 70% of patients with cirrhosis. The net effect of the coagulation disorders that occur in cirrhosis is the development of bleeding.

CLINICAL PRESENTATION

Cirrhotic patients may present in a variety of ways, from asymptomatic with abnormal radiographic or laboratory studies to decompensated with ascites, spontaneous bacterial peritonitis, hepatic encephalopathy, or variceal bleeding.[16]

CLINICAL PRESENTATION OF CIRRHOSIS

Signs and Symptoms

- Asymptomatic
- Hepatomegaly, splenomegaly
- Pruritis, jaundice, palmar erythema, spider angiomata, hyperpigmentation
- Gynecomastia, reduced libido
- Ascites, edema, pleural effusion, and respiratory difficulties
- Malaise, anorexia, and weight loss
- Encephalopathy

Laboratory Tests

- Hypoalbuminemia
- Elevated prothrombin time
- Thrombocytopenia
- Elevated alkaline phosphatase
- Elevated aspartate transaminase (AST), alanine transaminase (ALT), and γ-glutamyl transpeptidase (GGT)

The approach to a patient with suspected liver disease begins with a thorough history and physical exam. Some presenting characteristics of patients with cirrhosis include anorexia, weight loss, weakness, fatigue, jaundice, pruritus, gastrointestinal bleeding, coagulopathy, increasing abdominal girth with shifting flank dullness, mental status changes, and vascular spiders. Osteoporosis, as a result of vitamin D malabsorption and resultant calcium deficiency, can also occur.

A thorough history including risk factors that predispose patients to cirrhosis should be taken.[16] Quantity and duration of alcohol intake should be determined. Risk factors for hepatitis B and C transmission should be inquired about. These include birthplace in endemic areas, sexual history, intranasal or intravenous drug use, body piercing or tattooing, and accidental contamination of body tissues or blood. Information concerning any history of transfusions, as well as any personal history of autoimmune or hepatic diseases, should be gathered. A family history should also be taken, looking especially for any family member with a prior history of autoimmune or hepatic diseases.

LABORATORY ABNORMALITIES

There are no laboratory or radiographic tests of hepatic function that can accurately diagnose cirrhosis.[16] Despite this, liver function tests, a complete blood count with platelets, and a prothrombin time test should be performed if liver disease is suspected. Tests that measure the level of serum liver enzymes are usually referred to as liver function tests.[17] However; these tests actually reflect hepatocyte integrity or cholestasis, not liver function.

Routine liver tests include alkaline phosphatase, bilirubin, aspartate transaminase (AST), alanine transaminase (ALT), and γ-glutamyl transpeptidase (GGT). Additional markers of hepatic synthetic activity include albumin and prothrombin time. Liver function tests are often the first step in the evaluation of patients who present with symptoms or signs suggestive of cirrhosis.[16] The use of liver function tests in the diagnosis and management of cirrhosis is discussed in the following sections. It may be useful to group the tests into two broad categories: markers of hepatocyte integrity such as the transaminases and markers of liver function mass such as prothrombin time and albumin.[17]

Aminotransferases

The aminotransferases, AST and ALT, are enzymes that are highly concentrated in the liver. Liver injury, whether acute or chronic, results, at some point in the course of the disease, in increases in the serum concentrations of the aminotransferase enzymes. The degree of elevation, rate of rise, and nature of the course of alteration in aminotransferase serum levels are helpful in suggesting possible etiologies. Liver function tests will typically be elevated to the highest levels in acute viral, ischemic, or toxic liver injury. Chronic hepatitis and cirrhosis patients may present with elevated aminotransferase levels, but they may also present with aminotransferase levels within the normal reference range. The degree of aminotransferase level elevation is dependent upon the course of the hepatic injury being experienced by the patients and also depends on when the enzyme levels are tested. In a landmark study by Cohen and Kaplan, alcoholic liver disease resulted in AST elevations of only six to seven times the upper limit of normal in 98% of patients.[18] The ratio of AST to ALT also provides information in patients with suspected alcoholic liver disease. Seventy percent of patients with alcoholic liver disease in the study by Cohen and Kaplan had ratios greater than two, whereas 92% of patients had ratios greater than one.

Alkaline Phosphatase and Gamma-Glutamyl Transpeptidase

Elevated serum levels of alkaline phosphatase and GGT occur in cases of liver injury with a cholestatic pattern and therefore accompany conditions such as primary biliary cirrhosis, primary sclerosing cholangitis, drug-induced cholestasis, bile duct obstruction, autoimmune cholestatic liver disease, and metastatic cancer of the liver.[17] Neither alkaline phosphatase nor GGT is found solely in the liver, and elevations in either of these biomarkers can occur in a variety of disease states affecting other bodily tissues. However, the combination of an elevation in alkaline phosphatase level with a concomitant elevation in GGT level increases clinical suspicion of hepatic etiology.

Child-Pugh Classification and Model for End-Stage Liver Disease Score

The Child-Pugh classification system has gained widespread acceptance as a means of quantifying the myriad effects of the cirrhotic process on the laboratory and clinical manifestations of this disease.[19] Recommended drug dosing adjustments for patients in liver failure, when available, are normally based upon the Child-Pugh score. The newer Model for End-stage Liver Disease (MELD) scoring system is now the accepted classification scheme used by the United Network for Organ Sharing (UNOS) in the allocation livers for transplantation.[20] The Child-Pugh classification system employs a combination of physical and laboratory findings (Table 44–2), whereas the MELD score calculation takes into account a patient's serum creatinine, bilirubin, international normalized ratio (INR), and etiology of liver disease omitting the more subjective reports of ascites and encephalopathy used

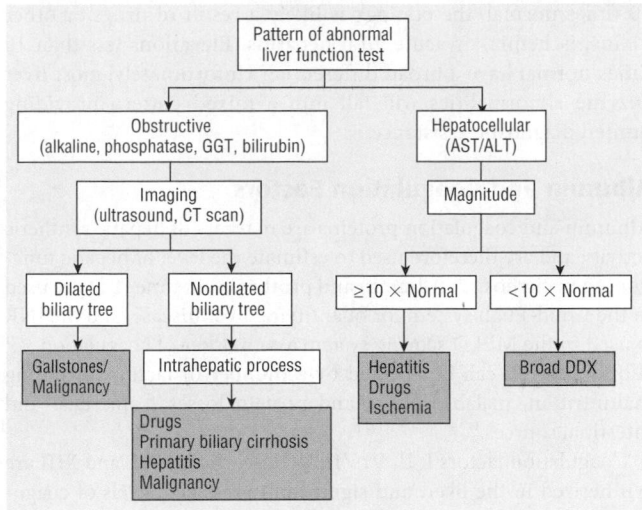

FIGURE 44-4. Interpretation of liver function tests. DDX; differential diagnosis.

in the Child-Pugh system. The MELD scoring calculation is as follows:[21]

$$MELD\ score = 0.957 \times Log_e(creatinine\ mg/dL) + 0.378$$
$$\times\ Log_e(bilirubin\ mg/dL)$$
$$+ 1.120 \times Log_e(INR) + 0.643*$$

These classification systems are important because they are used to assess and define the severity of the cirrhosis, and as a predictor for patient survival, surgical outcome, and risk of variceal bleeding.

Bilirubin

Bilirubin is the product of the breakdown of hemoglobin molecules in the reticuloendothelial system.[17] Elevations in serum conjugated bilirubin indicate that the liver has lost at least half of its excretory capacity and are usually a sign of liver disease. When found in conjunction with markedly elevated AST and ALT, conjugated hyperbilirubinemia indicates the possible presence of acute viral hepatitis, autoimmune hepatitis, toxic liver injury, or ischemic liver injury. Elevated conjugated bilirubin levels with concomitant increases in alkaline phosphatase and normal aminotransferase levels are a sign of cholestatic disease and possible cholestatic drug reactions. Causes of elevations in unconjugated bilirubin include hemolysis, Gilbert syndrome, hematoma reabsorption, and ineffective erythropoiesis. Causes of conjugated hyperbilirubinemia include bile duct obstruction, hepatitis, cirrhosis, primary sclerosing cholangitis, primary biliary cirrhosis, total parenteral nutrition, drug toxins, and vanishing bile duct syndrome. When cirrhosis has been established, the degree of bilirubin elevation has prognostic significance and is used as a component of the Child-Pugh and MELD scoring systems for quantifying the degree of cirrhosis.[19,21]

Figure 44–4 describes a general algorithm for the interpretation of liver function tests. The algorithm first separates the tests into two categories based on the underlying pathology (pattern of elevations): obstructive (alkaline phosphatase, GGT, and bilirubin) versus hepatocellular (AST and ALT). If a hepatocellular pattern predominates, the magnitude of elevation provides diagnostic assistance. If the degree of elevation is greater than

TABLE 44-2	Criteria and Scoring for the Child-Pugh Grading of Chronic Liver Disease		
Score	**1**	**2**	**3**
Total bilirubin (mg/dL)	1–2	2–3	>3
Albumin (g/dL)	>3.5	2.8–3.5	<2.8
Ascites	None	Mild	Moderate
Encephalopathy (grade)	None	1 and 2	3 and 4
Prothrombin time (seconds prolonged)	1–4	4–6	>6

Grade A, <7 points; grade B, 7–9 points; grade C, 10–15 points.
Data from reference 19.

---

*Multiply the score by 10 and round to the nearest whole number. (Laboratory values less than 1 are rounded up to 1 for the purposes of the MELD calculation.)

10 times normal, the etiology is likely a result of drugs or other toxins, ischemia, or acute viral hepatitis. Elevations less than 10 times normal have a broad differential. Unfortunately, most liver enzyme abnormalities will fall into a mixed pattern providing limited diagnostic assistance.

Albumin and Coagulation Factors

Albumin and coagulation proteins are markers of hepatic synthetic activity and are therefore used to estimate the level of hepatic functioning in cirrhosis.[17] Albumin and prothrombin time (PT) are used in the Child-Pugh system for quantifying liver disease, and the INR is used in the MELD scoring system as a marker of coagulation.[19,21] Albumin levels can be affected by a number of factors, including malnutrition, malabsorption, and protein losses from renal and intestinal sources.[17]

Coagulation factors I, II, V, VII, VIII, IX, X, XI, XII, and XIII are synthesized in the liver, and significantly reduced levels of coagulation factors II, V, VII, and XIII have been observed in patients with chronic liver disease and systemic bleeding unrelated to portal hypertension.[15] PT prolongation has also been observed in patients with chronic liver disease also have PT prolongation. The PT has been used in cases of acetaminophen-induced hepatic failure, viral hepatitis, and drug reactions as a prognostic laboratory value.[22] A PT over 100 seconds correlates with poor prognosis in acetaminophen-induced hepatic failure, and over 50 seconds indicates a poor prognosis in cases of viral hepatitis and drug reactions.

Thrombocytopenia

Thrombocytopenia (generally defined as a platelet count less than 150,000) is a common feature of chronic liver disease found in 15% to 70% of cirrhotic patients depending on the stage of liver disease and definition of thrombocytopenia.[15] The etiology of thrombocytopenia in liver disease is multifactorial, involving primarily splenomegaly due to portal hypertension with pooling of platelets in the spleen. A decrease in thrombopoietin due to decreased hepatic synthesis occurs as well as an immune-mediated destruction of platelets. Additionally, bone marrow suppression related to the hepatitis C virus or interferon antiviral treatment may exist and lead to thrombocytopenia associated with the cirrhotic process.

ENDOSCOPIC AND RADIOGRAPHIC ABNORMALITIES

While no radiographic test is considered a diagnostic standard for cirrhosis, radiographic studies may be used to detect ascites, hepatosplenomegaly, hepatic or portal vein thromboses, and hepatocellular carcinoma.[16] Ultrasonography, because it does not require radiation exposure or intravenous contrast and is relatively low cost, should be the first radiographic study in the evaluation of a patient with suspected cirrhosis. Hepatic nodularity, irregularity, increased echogenicity, and atrophy are all ultrasonographic findings indicative of cirrhosis. Ascites may also be detected on ultrasound. Computed tomography and magnetic resonance imaging can demonstrate liver nodularity as well as atrophic and hypertrophic changes. Ascites and varices may also be detected on computed tomography or magnetic resonance imaging scans. Portal vein patency can be assessed by computer tomography imaging.

LIVER BIOPSY

Liver biopsy should be considered after a thorough noninvasive workup has failed to confirm a diagnosis in suspected cirrhosis. Liver biopsy has a sensitivity and specificity of 80% to 100% for

an accurate diagnosis of cirrhosis and its etiology. The success of biopsy as a diagnostic tool is dependent upon the number of histologic samples retrieved as well as the sampling method used.

TREATMENT

Cirrhosis

■ GENERAL APPROACHES TO TREATMENT

General approaches to therapy in cirrhosis should include the following:

1. Identify and eliminate, where possible, the causes of cirrhosis (e.g., alcohol abuse).

2. Assess the risk for variceal bleeding and begin pharmacologic prophylaxis when indicated. Prophylactic endoscopic therapy can be used for patients with high-risk medium and large varices as well as in patients with contraindications or intolerance to nonselective β-adrenergic blockers. Endoscopic therapy is also appropriate for patients suffering acute bleeding episodes. Variceal obliteration with endoscopic techniques in conjunction with pharmacological intervention is the recommended treatment of choice in patients with acute bleeding.

3. Evaluate the patient for clinical signs of ascites and manage with pharmacologic therapy (e.g., diuretics) and paracentesis. Careful monitoring for spontaneous bacterial peritonitis (SBP) should be used in patients with ascites who undergo acute deterioration.

4. Hepatic encephalopathy is a common complication of cirrhosis and requires clinical vigilance and treatment with dietary restriction, elimination of central nervous system depressants, and therapy to lower ammonia levels.

5. Frequent monitoring for signs of hepatorenal syndrome, pulmonary insufficiency, and endocrine dysfunction is necessary.

■ DESIRED OUTCOMES

The desired therapeutic outcomes can be viewed in two categories: *resolution of acute complications* such as tamponade of bleeding and resolution of hemodynamic instability for an episode of acute variceal hemorrhage and *prevention of complications* through lowering of portal pressure with medical therapy using β-adrenergic blocker therapy or supporting abstinence from alcohol. Treatment end points and desired therapeutic outcomes are presented for each of the recommended therapies discussed.

■ MANAGEMENT OF PORTAL HYPERTENSION AND VARICEAL BLEEDING

The management of varices involves three strategies: (a) primary prophylaxis (prevention of the first bleeding episode); (b) treatment of acute variceal hemorrhage; and (c) secondary prophylaxis (prevention of rebleeding in patients who have previously bled).[12]

Primary Prophylaxis

β-Adrenergic Blockade The mainstay of primary prophylaxis is the use of nonselective β-adrenergic blocking agents such as propranolol or nadolol.[11] These agents reduce portal pressure by reducing portal venous inflow via two mechanisms: a decrease in cardiac output through β_1-adrenergic blockade and a decrease in splanchnic blood flow through β_2-adrenergic blockade.[23]

Meta-analysis of 12 trials of the nonselective β-adrenergic blockers propranolol or nadolol demonstrated the effectiveness of these agents in the prevention of bleeding, especially in patients with medium- or large-sized varices, over a median follow-up of 2 years with a trend toward a reduction in mortality.[24] This analysis indicated that one bleeding episode is avoided for every 10 patients treated with a nonselective β-adrenergic blocker. Mortality was lowered in cirrhotic patients with esophageal varices who have never bled when those patients are treated with a β-adrenergic blocker.[25] In this analysis, it was found that one life was saved for every 17 patients treated with a β-adrenergic blocker. Nadolol reduces the rate of growth of small esophageal varices in patients with cirrhosis.[26] However, β-adrenergic blocker therapy does not prevent the formation of first varices.[23] Screening esophagogastroduodenoscopy (EGD) is recommended for the diagnosis of esophageal and gastric varices when the diagnosis of cirrhosis is made, repeated every 2 to 3 years in patients who have no varices upon initial surveillance, or repeated annually in the event of decompensation.[27,28] Once started, β-adrenergic blocker therapy should be continued for life unless it is not tolerated.[29]

Treatment Recommendations: Variceal Bleeding—Primary Prophylaxis

❷ All patients with cirrhosis should be screened for varices upon diagnosis.[28] For patients with small varices (less than 5 mm) who have not bled and who have no criteria for increased risk of bleeding (increased risk includes those with Child-Pugh score of B or C or the presence of red wale marks on varices), β-adrenergic blocker therapy may be instituted, although long-term benefit has not been established. Patients with small varices plus risk factors for variceal hemorrhage should receive prophylaxis therapy with a nonselective β-adrenergic blocker (such as propranolol). All patients found to have medium to large varices (varices greater than 5 mm) that have not bled but have high risk for hemorrhage should receive prophylaxis therapy with a nonselective β-adrenergic blocker or endoscopic variceal ligation (EVL). Patients with medium and large varices who have not bled and who are at lower risk for hemorrhage should receive prophylaxis with nonselective β-adrenergic blocker therapy instead of EVL; although, EVL may be used in patients who are intolerant or nonadherent or who have contraindications to β-blocker therapy. Initiate therapy with oral propranolol 20 mg twice daily or nadolol 40 mg once daily and titrate to maximal tolerated dose. In most studies, the dose of nonselective β-adrenergic blocker was titrated to decrease the heart rate by 25% of baseline. Heart rate does not correlate with reduction in HVPG, and direct HVPG measurement is not widely available; therefore, titration of β-blocker therapy to the maximal tolerated dose is now recommended.[28,30]

Patients with contraindications to therapy with nonselective β-adrenergic blockers (i.e., those with asthma, insulin-dependent diabetes with episodes of hypoglycemia, and peripheral vascular disease) or intolerance to β-adrenergic blockers should be considered for alternative prophylactic therapy with EVL.[28] EVL has been compared to nonselective β-adrenergic blocker therapy in patients with large varices and found to be associated with a significantly lower incidence of first variceal bleed.[31,32] EVL is equivalent to nadolol and propranolol for prevention of first variceal bleed.[33–35] Current guidelines place EVL as a possible first option for primary prophylaxis in patients with high-risk medium to large varices.[28] EVL is the recommended secondary option for patients with lower-risk medium to large varices who are intolerant to, are nonadherent to, or have contraindications to nonselective β-adrenergic blocker therapy. Nitrates are no longer recommended as alternative therapy for primary prophylaxis

against variceal bleeding in patients with intolerance to nonselective β-adrenergic blockers.[28] In fact, isosorbide mononitrate was found in one study to result in a greater 1- and 2-year probability of first variceal bleed with no difference in survival as compared to placebo.[36] At this time, there is also insufficient evidence to support the use of other therapies and procedures (such as combination nonselective β-adrenergic blocker therapy with isosorbide mononitrate, combination nonselective β-adrenergic blocker therapy with spironolactone, combination nonselective β-adrenergic blocker therapy with EVL, shunt surgery, and endoscopic sclerotherapy) for primary prevention of variceal hemorrhage.[28] Nonselective β-adrenergic blocker therapy remains the mainstay of therapy in portal hypertension patients with known varices to avoid first variceal bleeding.

■ ACUTE VARICEAL HEMORRHAGE

Variceal hemorrhage is a medical emergency that carries a mortality rate of 15% to 20%, requires admission to an intensive care unit, and is one of the most feared complications of cirrhosis.[28,37] It is important to note that variceal bleeding secondary to portal hypertension can occur in patients without signs of liver disease; for example, in patients with chronic portal vein thrombosis.[38] Treatment of acute variceal bleeding includes general stabilizing and assessment measures as well as specific measures to control the acute hemorrhage and prevent early recurrence.[28,37]

Management of Acute Variceal Hemorrhage

Initial treatment goals include (a) adequate blood volume resuscitation, (b) protection of airway from aspiration of blood, (c) correction of significant coagulopathy and/or thrombocytopenia with fresh frozen plasma and platelets, (d) prophylaxis against SBP and other infections, (e) control of bleeding, (f) prevention of rebleeding, and (g) preservation of liver function.[28] Prompt stabilization of blood volume with a goal of maintaining hemodynamic stability and a hemoglobin of 8 g/dL should be undertaken. Volume should be expanded to maintain a systolic blood pressure of 90 to 100 mm Hg and a heart rate of less than 100 beats per minute, but vigorous resuscitation with saline solution should generally be avoided because this may lead to recurrent variceal hemorrhage or accumulation of ascites and/or fluid at other anatomical sites.[28,37] Use of recombinant factor VIIa therapy is not recommended in cirrhotic patients with GI hemorrhage at this time. Airway management is critical in patients with variceal hemorrhage, especially those with concomitant hepatic encephalopathy or severe bleeding.[28] Elective or more emergent intubation may be required prior to diagnostic endoscopy. Combination pharmacological therapy plus endoscopic therapy with preferably EVL, or sclerotherapy if EVL is not technically feasible, is considered the most rational approach to the treatment of acute variceal bleeding.[12,28]

Vasoactive drug therapy (usually octreotide) is routinely used early to stop or slow bleeding for patient management as soon as a diagnosis of variceal bleeding is suspected, and potentially even before EGD. Antibiotic therapy to prevent SBP and other infections, as well as to prevent rebleeding and decrease mortality, should be implemented. Figure 44–5 presents an algorithm for the management of variceal hemorrhage.

Drug Therapy

Drugs employed to manage acute variceal bleeding in the United States include (a) the somatostatin analogue octreotide and (b) vasopressin. These agents work as splanchnic vasoconstrictors, thus decreasing portal blood flow and pressure. Agents available

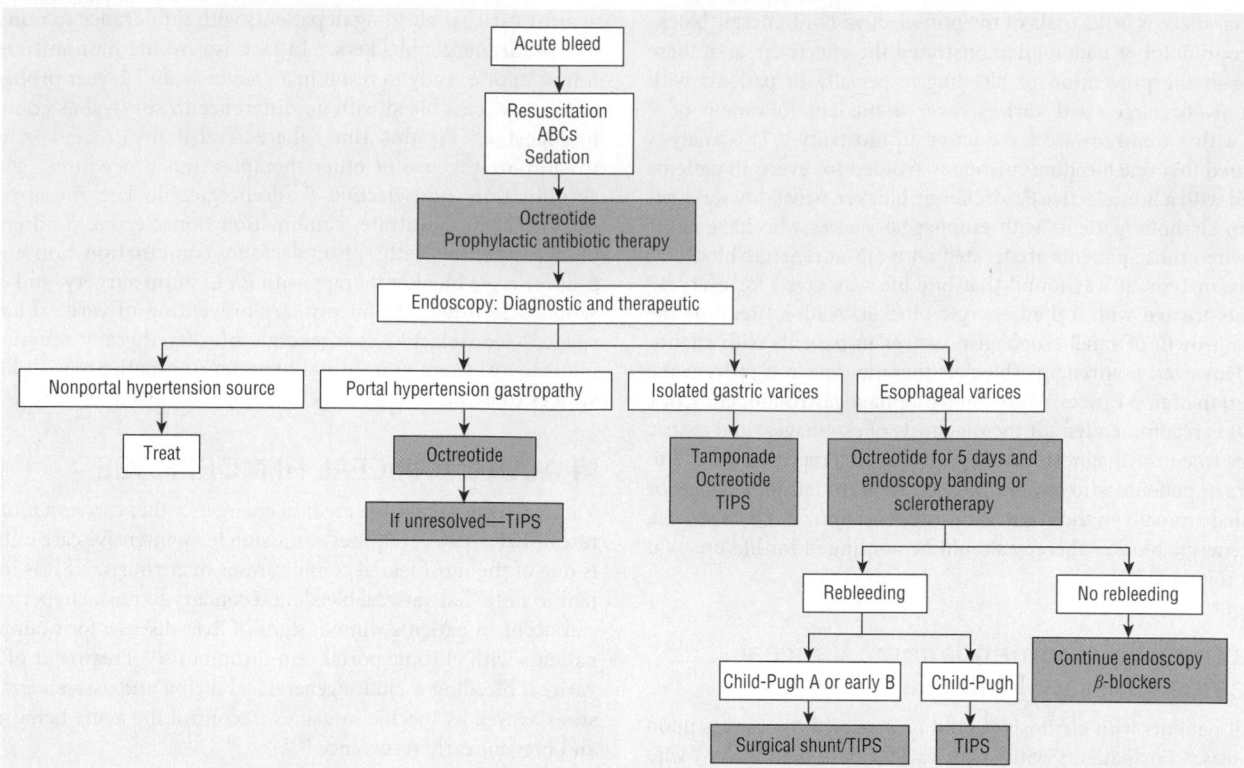

FIGURE 44-5. Management of acute variceal hemorrhage.

in other countries also include terlipressin, which is an analogue of vasopressin, and another somatostatin analogue, vapreotide.

Somatostatin and Octreotide Somatostatin is a naturally occurring tetradecapeptide hormone, and octreotide is a synthetic octapeptide that shares a four–amino acid segment with somatostatin and has similar pharmacologic activity with greater potency and longer duration of action as compared with somatostatin.[39] Somatostatin and octreotide cause a reduction in portal pressure and port-collateral blood flow through inducing splanchnic vasoconstriction without causing the systemic effects associated with vasopressin.[28,39] The splanchnic vasoconstriction found with somatostatin and octreotide therapy is due to inhibition of the release of vasodilatory peptides like glucagon; however, octreotide has a local vasoconstrictive effect confined to the splanchnic vasculature.[28] Somatostatin and somatostatin analogues are associated with fewer side effects as compared with vasopressin.[24] Octreotide is available as both subcutaneous and intravenous injection, though the most recent recommended dosing of octreotide for variceal bleeding consists of an initial intravenous bolus of 50 mcg followed by a continuous intravenous infusion of 50 mcg per hour.[28,37] Because octreotide is safe for continuation for multiple days and because around half of early recurrent bleeding occurs within in the first 3 to 5 days, guidelines suggest continuation of octreotide for 5 days after acute variceal bleeding.[28,37,40] Studies have been conducted comparing octreotide with placebo, with balloon tamponade, with vasopressin, and with glypressin for the treatment of acute variceal bleeding with somewhat mixed results.[41–46] While studies comparing octreotide with placebo or with balloon tamponade did not find octreotide to be superior for controlling bleeding, octreotide was significantly better for survival as compared with balloon tamponade.[41,42] No significant differences in bleeding control or mortality were found in studies comparing octreotide with vasopressin or terlipressin.[43–46] A meta-analysis of studies

of somatostatin analogues in general also failed to showed a beneficial effect.[47] A meta-analysis comparing either endoscopic therapy (with sclerotherapy or EVL) alone or endoscopic therapy plus octreotide, somatostatin, or vapreotide showed improved initial control of bleeding and 5-day hemostasis with combination therapy without any differences in mortality or severe adverse events.[48] Octreotide used alone may be less effective for controlling bleeding due to tachyphylaxis and a more transient effect relative to terlipressin.[49,50]

Vasopressin (also known as antidiuretic hormone) is a potent, nonselective vasoconstrictor that reduces portal pressure by causing splanchnic vasoconstriction, which reduces splanchnic blood flow.[39] Unfortunately, the vasoconstrictive effects of vasopressin are nonselective—the vasoconstriction is not restricted to the splanchnic vascular bed. Potent systemic vasoconstriction induces peripheral resistance, which reduces cardiac output, heart rate, and coronary blood flow. These effects on cardiac hemodynamics can lead to myocardial ischemia or infarction, arrhythmias, mesenteric ischemia, ischemia of the limbs, and cerebrovascular accidents. A meta-analysis of four randomized, controlled clinical trials of vasopressin for variceal hemorrhage demonstrated that vasopressin was significantly more effective than no treatment at controlling bleeding; however, mortality was not affected.[24] Adverse effects were reported in one to two thirds of patients, and vasopressin was discontinued in about 25% of patients secondary to adverse effects. A meta-analysis comparing vasopressin and somatostatin in the management of acute esophageal variceal hemorrhage found somatostatin more efficacious for controlling acute hemorrhage from esophageal varices with significantly less adverse effects.[51] Only four patients must be treated with somatostatin over vasopressin for one to derive additional benefit in terms of initial control of bleeding, and only nine patients need to be treated with somatostatin instead of vasopressin in order for one to experience benefit in terms of avoidance of rebleeding. Though somatostatin is not available in the United States today, its analogue octreotide is commonly used instead of vasopressin for acute variceal hemorrhage.

A recommended dosing strategy for vasopressin is a continuous intravenous infusion of 0.2 to 0.4 units per minute, which can be increased to a maximal dose of 0.8 units per minute.[28] Vasopressin should only be used at the highest effective dose continuously for a maximum of 24 hours and should always be administered with intravenous nitroglycerin at a starting dose of 40 mcg per minute (which can be increased to a maximum of 400 mcg per minute and adjusted to maintain systolic blood pressure over 90 mm Hg) in order to minimize the risk of serious adverse events. With the recent addition of safer and equally effective treatment alternatives, vasopressin, alone or combined with nitroglycerin, can no longer be recommended as first-line therapy for the management of variceal hemorrhage.[28] Terlipressin, a synthetic analogue of vasopressin, has fewer side effects and a longer duration of action than vasopressin. It reduces mortality in acute variceal hemorrhage but is not currently available in the United States.[24]

Cirrhotic patients with active bleeding are at high risk of severe bacterial infections such as SBP.[28] Short-term prophylactic antibiotic therapy to reduce the risk of infection during episodes of bleeding not only reduces the likelihood of development of SBP and other infections, it also reduces the incidence of rebleeding and increases short-term survival.[52-54] Prophylactic antibiotic therapy should be prescribed for all patients with cirrhosis and acute variceal bleeding.[28] A short course (7 days maximum) of oral norfloxacin 400 mg twice daily or intravenous ciprofloxacin when the oral route is not available is recommended. Alternatively, in patients with severe cirrhosis in areas with high quinolone resistance, intravenous ceftriaxone 1 g per day may be preferable.

Endoscopic Interventions: Sclerotherapy and Band Ligation

The Baveno IV Consensus Report recommended that endoscopy be performed as soon as possible following admission in cases of suspected variceal hemorrhage, especially in cases of significant bleeding and in patients with suspected cirrhosis.[12] Endoscopy is used to diagnose variceal bleeding, and endoscopic techniques, such as EVL and sclerotherapy, can be used in an attempt to stop variceal bleeding. EVL consists of placement of rubber bands around the varix through a clear plastic channel attached to the end of the endoscope. After the rubber bands are in place, the varix will slough off after 48 to 72 hours. Typically, the EVL procedure is repeated every 1 to 2 weeks until variceal obliteration is attained. Surveillance endoscopy is then performed 1 to 3 months after obliteration and then repeated every 6 to 12 months indefinitely.[28,37] Endoscopic sclerotherapy involves injection of 1 to 4 mL of a sclerosing agent into the lumen of the varices to tamponade blood flow. EVL is more effective than sclerotherapy with greater control of hemorrhage, less risk for rebleeding, and lower likelihood of adverse events.[32,55] No difference in mortality has been found between these two endoscopic procedures; however. HVPG is increased following both EVL and sclerotherapy, though HVPG decreases to baseline within 2 days following EVL and remains elevated for longer following sclerotherapy.[56] Consensus recommendation calls for EVL (in conjunction with pharmacological therapy) as the recommended form of endoscopic therapy for acute variceal bleeding, though endoscopic sclerotherapy may be employed if ligation is technically difficult.[12]

Endoscopic injection of the tissue adhesive N-butyl-cyanoacrylate to control acute gastric variceal bleeding as well as EVL was associated with a lower rate of rebleeding as compared with EVL in one

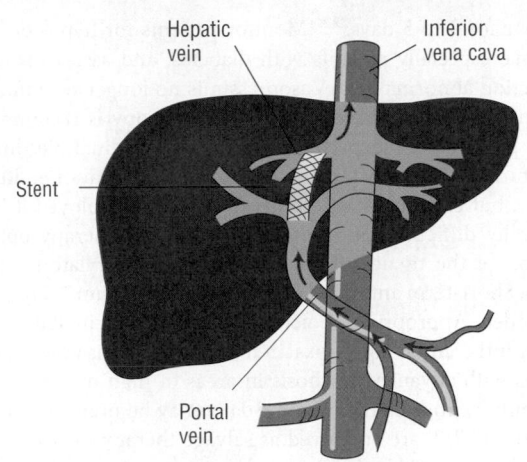

FIGURE 44-6. Transjugular intrahepatic portosystemic shunt (TIPS).

trial.[57] Endoscopic therapy with 2-octyl cyanoacrylate is effective for initial control of bleeding from fundal varices as well as prevention of rebleeding.[58] Therefore, endoscopic therapy with these agents is recommended for patients with acute bleeding from gastric varices.[12,28]

Interventional and Surgical Treatment Approaches

Standard therapy fails to control initial bleeding or early rebleeding in 10% to 20% of patients with acute variceal hemorrhage.[37] In these cases, a salvage procedure, such as balloon tamponade or transjugular intrahepatic portosystemic shunt (TIPS), is necessary. Balloon tamponade is effective in controlling variceal bleeding temporarily; however, rebleeding is common after balloon deflation, and complications result in mortality rates of up to 20% with balloon tamponade.[37] Sengstaken-Blakemore tubes are recommended for used in esophageal variceal bleeding. Linton tubes are preferred for bleeding from fundal gastric varices. Balloon tamponade should be reserved as a temporizing measure until a more definitive treatment, such as TIPS, can be performed.

In patients with acute variceal bleeding refractory to pharmacologic or endoscopic therapy, a decrease in portal pressure through use of the TIPS procedure is effective in controlling bleeding and preventing rebleeding.[59] The TIPS procedure involves the placement of one or more stents between the hepatic vein and the portal vein (Fig. 44-6). TIPS (preferably with polytetrafluoroethylene-covered stents) is recommended for patients who fail to achieve hemostasis after a second attempt at endoscopic therapy.[12] TIPS provides an effective decompressive shunt without laparotomy and can be employed regardless of Child-Pugh score, unlike shunt surgery, which is restricted to Child-Pugh class A patients.[28] TIPS decreased the incidence of variceal rebleeding and decreased the incidence of deaths due to rebleeding.[60] There was a significantly increased rate of posttreatment encephalopathy found in TIPS-treated patients.

Treatment Recommendations: Variceal Hemorrhage

Patients require cautious resuscitation with colloids and blood products to correct intravascular losses and to reverse existing coagulopathies.[12,28,37] ❹ Drug therapy with octreotide should be initiated early to control bleeding and facilitate diagnostic and therapeutic endoscopy. Therapy is initiated with an intravenous bolus of 50 mcg and is followed by a continuous infusion of 50 mcg per hour for 3 to 5 days.[28,37] Monitor patients for hypo- or hyper-glycemia, especially patients with diabetes, and assess for cardiac conduction abnormalities. Vasopressin is no longer recommended for control of variceal bleeding.[12,28,37] Endoscopy is recommended in any patient with suspected upper gastrointestinal bleeding due to ruptured varices. EVL is the recommended form of endoscopic therapy, but endoscopic sclerotherapy may be employed if EVL is technically difficult. An additional endoscopic therapy option is injection of the tissue adhesive N-butyl-cyanoacrylate for gastric varices. Short-term antibiotic prophylaxis (maximum 7 days) is recommended. Appropriate choices include norfloxacin 400 mg twice daily or intravenous ciprofloxacin if the oral route is unavailable. In patients with advanced cirrhosis in areas of high quinolone resistance, intravenous ceftriaxone 1 g daily may be preferred. Surgical shunts and TIPS are employed as salvage therapy in patients who have failed repeated endoscopy and vasoactive drug therapy.

Secondary Prophylaxis: Prevention of Rebleeding Because rebleeding after initial control of variceal hemorrhage occurs in a median of 60% of patients within 1 to 2 years without treatment and because rebleeding carries a mortality rate of 33%, it is inappropriate to simply observe patients for evidence of further bleeding.[24,61] Only patients who underwent shunt surgery or TIPS to control their initial acute bleeding require no further intervention as secondary prophylaxis.[28,37] Patients who underwent one of these procedures to treat their initial bleed should be referred for transplantation if they are a candidate.[28] Candidates include those with a Child-Pugh score greater than or equal to 7 or MELD score greater than or equal to 15. Combination therapy with β-adrenergic blockers and chronic EVL to eradicate varices is the best treatment option for secondary prophylaxis of variceal bleeding.[12,28,37] Secondary prophylaxis should be started as soon as possible following the acute bleed once the patient has had no bleeding for at least 24 hours and before the patient is discharged from the hospital. Alternatives for the secondary prevention of rebleeding include surgical or interventional shunting, but pharmacologic plus endoscopic interventions should be used as first-line therapy to prevent rebleeding.

Drug Therapy The combination of EVL and a nonselective β-adrenergic blocking agent provides the most rational approach for secondary prophylaxis because nonselective β-adrenergic blocking agents can protect against variceal rebleeding before variceal obliteration can be accomplished through EVL, and β-adrenergic blocking agents will also delay variceal recurrence.[28,37] EVL plus nonselective β-adrenergic blocker has been compared with EVL alone for the prevention of rebleeding.[62,63] Rebleeding rates were significantly lower in patients treated with combination therapy (23% and 14%) versus EVL alone (47% and 38%). A meta-analysis comparing combination endoscopic therapy (with either sclerotherapy or EVL) and nonselective β-adrenergic blocker versus either therapy alone found that combination therapy reduces overall and variceal rebleeding better than either therapy alone.[64] The combination of EVL and nonselective β-adrenergic blocker should be employed in any patient who experiences first or recurrent variceal bleeding while on either EVL or nonselective β-adrenergic blocker alone.[28,37]

The lowest rate of variceal rebleeding occurs in patients when pharmacologic therapy leads to a reduction in HVPG of greater than 20% of baseline or to a measurement less than 12 mm Hg.[61,65] Ideally, portal pressure monitoring would help to assess the response to nonselective β-adrenergic blocker therapy and identify responders from nonresponders earlier in the treatment course. In order to utilize the HVPG measurement for clinical decision making, the technique used to make this measurement would first have to be standardized, including the best time to perform the repeat HVPG measurement.[28,37]

The combination of nonselective β-adrenergic blocker and isosorbide mononitrate could be more effective than nonselective β-adrenergic blocker therapy alone for lowering HVPG. Only one trial has evaluated nonselective β-adrenergic blocker plus isosorbide mononitrate verus nonselecive β-adrenergic blocker alone.[66] Rebleeding rates were lower with combination therapy, but no statistically significant difference in rebleeding rates were attained. A randomized, controlled trial comparing variceal rebleeding in patients treated with combination therapy plus EVL versus patients treated with combination therapy alone found rebleeding rates that were significantly lower with combination therapy plus EVL versus combination therapy alone.[67] However, patients treated with combination therapy plus EVL had similar rebleeding rates compared with those treated with nonselective β-adrenergic blocker plus EVL. Patients treated with combination therapy are more likely to discontinue therapy than patients treated with nonselective β-adrenergic blocker therapy alone.[66] Whether nitrate therapy should be added to nonselective β-adrenergic blocker therapy in patients with prior history of variceal bleeding remains controversial, especially in patients who are able to undergo EVL. The unresolved questions surrounding HVPG measurement further compound this quandary.

Treatment Recommendations: Secondary Prophylaxis The combination of EVL plus pharmacologic therapy to prevent rebleeding is currently considered the most rational therapeutic approach.[28,37] Pharmacologic therapy should be initiated with a nonselective β-blocker such as propranolol 20 mg twice daily or nadolol at a dose of 20 mg once daily.[37] ❸ β-Blocker therapy can be titrated to achieve a goal heart rate of 55 to 60 beats per minute or the maximal tolerated dose. Monitor patients for evidence of heart failure, bronchospasm, and glucose intolerance, particularly hypoglycemia in patients with insulin-dependent diabetes. EVL should be conducted every 1 to 2 weeks until variceal obliteration, and then the patient should be followed by surveillance endoscopy in 1 to 3 months and then every 6 to 12 months. Combination therapy with nonselective β-blocker plus isosorbide mononitrate can be considered in patients who are unable to undergo EVL. Patients who cannot tolerate or who fail pharmacologic and endoscopic interventions can be considered for TIPS or surgical shunting to prevent bleeding. A summary of evidence-based treatment recommendations regarding portal hypertension and variceal bleeding is found in Table 44–3.

Ascites and Spontaneous Bacterial Peritonitis

Patients with cirrhosis experience overt fluid retention and ascites as liver disease progresses.[10] The classic physical exam findings of ascites are a bulging abdomen with shifting flank dullness.[6] The development of ascites in patients with cirrhosis is an indication of advanced liver disease and is a poor prognostic sign.[6,10] The principle therapeutic goals for patients with ascites are to control the ascites; to prevent or relieve ascites-related symptoms such as dyspnea, abdominal pain, and abdominal distention; and to prevent life-threatening complications such as SBP and the hepatorenal syndrome.[10] Treatment of ascites is expected to have little effect on survival, however.[37] Workup includes a history and physical exam, abdominal paracentesis and/or ultrasound,

TABLE 44-3	Evidence-Based Table of Selected Treatment Recommendations: Variceal Bleeding in Portal Hypertension	
Recommendation		**Grade**
Prevention of variceal bleeding		
Nonselective β-blocker therapy should be initiated in:		
Patients with small varices and criteria for increased risk of hemorrhage		IIaC
Patients with medium/large varices without high risk of hemorrhage		IA
Endoscopic variceal ligation (EVL) should be offered to patients who have contraindications or intolerance to nonselective β-blockers		IA
EVL may be recommended for prevention in patients with medium/large varices at high risk of hemorrhage instead of nonselective β-blocker therapy		IA
Treatment of variceal bleeding		
Short-term antibiotic prophylaxis should be instituted upon admission		IA
Vasoactive drugs should be started as soon as possible, prior to endoscopy, and maintained for 3–5 days		IA
Endoscopy should be performed within 12 hours to diagnose variceal bleeding and to treat bleeding with either sclerotherapy or EVL		IA
Secondary prophylaxis of variceal bleeding		
Nonselective β-blocker therapy plus EVL is the best therapeutic option for prevention of recurrent variceal bleeding		IA

Recommendation grading:

Class I—Conditions for which there is evidence and/or general agreement

Class II—Conditions for which there is conflicting evidence and/or a divergence of opinion

Class IIa—Weight of evidence/opinion is in favor of efficacy

Class IIb—Efficacy less well established

Class III—Conditions for which there is evidence and/or general agreement that treatment is not effective and/or potentially harmful

Level A—Data from multiple randomized trials or meta-analyses

Level B—Data derived from single randomized trial or nonrandomized studies

Level C—Only consensus opinion, case studies, or standard of care

Data from reference 28.

and ascitic fluid analysis.[6] The treatment of ascites is based on oral diuretics and is carried out in a slow, stepwise fashion.[37] Treatment of ascites should be initiated only in stable patients (e.g.; those without ongoing variceal hemorrhage, bacterial infection, or renal dysfunction).

SBP is an infection of ascitic fluid that occurs in the absence of any evidence of an intra-abdominal, surgically treatable source of infection.[6] SBP is a common complication that develops in 10% to 20% of patients hospitalized with severe liver disease, cirrhosis, and ascites.[37] The key mechanism behind the development of SBP is thought to be bacterial translocation.[68] Decreased motility of the gastrointestinal tract with disturbances of the gut flora, changes in the structure of the gastrointestinal tract, and reduced local and humoral immunity combine to lead to the free flow of microorganisms and endotoxins to the mesenteric lymph nodes. Most episodes of SBP are caused by *Escherichia coli*, *Klebsiella pneumonia*, and pneumococci.[6] Symptoms and signs of SBP include fever, abdominal pain, abdominal tenderness, rebound, encephalopathy, renal failure, acidosis, peripheral leukocytosis, and altered mental status.[6,68] Paralytic ileus, hypotension, and hypothermia are poor prognostic indicators.[68] Thirteen percent of patients with SBP present with no symptoms. For this reason, a diagnostic paracentesis with analysis of ascitic fluid should be performed in all patients admitted with ascites.[6] Spontaneous bacterial peritonitis is diagnosed when there is possible ascitic fluid bacterial culture and ascitic fluid cell counts show an absolute polymorphonuclear (PMN) leukocyte count of greater than or equal to 250 cells/mm³.

Management of Ascites and Spontaneous Bacterial Peritonitis

The following treatment guidelines for the management of adult patients with ascites and spontaneous bacterial peritonitis were updated and approved by the Practice Guidelines Committee of the American Association for the Study of Liver Diseases (AASLD).

Ascites In adult patients with new-onset ascites as determined by physical exam or radiographic studies, abdominal paracentesis should be performed, and ascitic fluid analysis should include a cell count with differential, ascitic fluid total protein, and a serum-ascites albumin gradient (SAAG). If infection is suspected, ascitic fluid cultures should be obtained at the time of the paracentesis. The SAAG can accurately determine whether ascites is a result of portal hypertension or another process.[69] If the SAAG is greater than 1.1 g/dL, the patient almost certainly has portal hypertension and will usually be responsive to salt restriction and diuretics. If the SAAG is less than 1.1 g/dL, the patient likely does not have portal hypertension and, except in cases of nephrotic syndrome, is less likely to respond to salt restriction and diuretics. The treatment of ascites secondary to portal hypertension is relatively straightforward and includes abstinence from alcohol, sodium restriction, and diuretics.[6]

❶ Abstinence from alcohol is an essential element of the overall treatment strategy. Abstinence from alcohol can result in improvement of the reversible component of alcoholic liver disease, resolution of ascites, or improved responsiveness of ascites to medical therapy. Patients with cirrhosis not caused by alcohol have less reversible liver disease, and, by the time ascites is present, these patients may be best managed with liver transplantation rather than protracted medical therapy.

Beyond avoidance of alcohol, the primary treatment of ascites due to portal hypertension and cirrhosis is salt restriction and oral diuretic therapy. Fluid loss and weight change depend directly on sodium balance in these patients. Evaluation of urinary sodium excretion, preferably utilizing a 24-hour urine collection, may be helpful when rapidity of weight loss is less than desired.[69,70] Severe hyponatremia, defined as serum sodium less than a threshold of 120 to 125 mEq/L, does warrant fluid restriction.[6] However, rapid correction of asymptomatic hyponatremia is not recommended as patients with cirrhosis are usually asymptomatic until their serum sodium concentrations are less than 110 mEq/L or unless the decline in serum sodium is rapid.

Diuretic Therapy ❺ The AASLD practice guidelines recommend that diuretic therapy be initiated with the combination of spironolactone and furosemide. At one time, spironolactone was commonly recommended for initial therapy as a single agent. However, due to the likelihood for development of drug-induced hyperkalemia with spironolactone when used as monotherapy, the drug is now recommended only for use as a lone diuretic agent in patients with minimal fluid overload. If tense ascites is present, paracentesis should be performed prior to institution of diuretic therapy and salt restriction. For patients who respond to diuretic therapy, this approach is preferred over the use of serial paracenteses. In patients with refractory ascites, serial paracenteses may be employed. Albumin infusion postparacentesis is controversial, but reasonable for extraction volumes exceeding 5 liters. Laboratory tests for renal function and electrolytes need to be monitored during therapy. Referral for liver transplantation should be made in patients with refractory ascites. TIPS is a therapeutic modality for the treatment of refractory ascites that may be considered in appropriately selected patients. Peritoneovenous shunting may be considered in treatment refractory patients who are not candidates for paracenteses, transplant, or TIPS.

Spontaneous Bacterial Peritonitis

Relatively broad-spectrum antibiotic therapy that adequately covers the three most commonly encountered pathogens (*Escherichia coli*, *Klebsiella pneumoniae*, and pneumococci) is warranted in patients with documented or suspected SBP.[6,37,68] Empirical therapy should not be delayed while awaiting culture results. In some patients, signs and symptoms of infection are present such as fever, abdominal pain, and unexplained encephalopathy at the bacterascites stage (i.e., signs and symptoms are present before the PMN count in the ascitic fluid is elevated).[6] In these patients, signs and symptoms of infection justify empiric antibiotic therapy until culture results are known, regardless of the PMN count in the ascitic fluid.

Cefotaxime 2 g every 8 hours, or a similar third-generation cephalosporin, is considered the drug of choice for SBP.[6] Cefotaxime is more effective than the combination of ampicillin and tobramycin.[71] A 5-day course of antibiotic therapy was as efficacious as 10 days of therapy in a randomized trial involving 100 patients with SBP.[72] Ofloxacin 400 mg every 12 hours administered orally for an average of 8 days is equivalent to intravenous cefotaxime for treatment of SBP in patients without vomiting, shock, significant hepatic encephalopathy, or serum creatinine over 3 mg/dL.[73] Intravenous ciprofloxacin offers another potential treatment alternative.[74] Patients with SBP who previously received quinolone therapy as prophylaxis should be treated with an alternative agent since patients who have received quinolone therapy may become infected with quinolone-resistant flora.[6]

Secondary bacterial peritonitis, ascitic fluid infection caused by a surgically treatable intraabdominal source, can masquerade as SBP. Free perforation should be considered when multiple or atypical organisms are cultured, a very high ascitic fluid PMN count is seen, or when at least two of the following are seen on ascitic fluid analysis: total protein greater than 1 g/dL, lactate dehydrogenase greater than the upper limit of normal for serum, and glucose less than 50 mg/dL.[75] A 48-hour follow-up PMN count that rises above pretreatment levels despite antibiotic treatment is indicative of secondary nonperforation peritonitis.[76] Patients with free perforation or nonperforation secondary peritonitis should receive a third-generation cephalosporin plus anaerobic coverage in addition to undergoing laparotomy.[75]

Treatment Recommendations: Ascites and Spontaneous Bacterial Peritonitis

Adult patients admitted to the hospital with new-onset ascites should have an abdominal paracentesis performed to establish the SAAG, the ascitic fluid cell count and differential, and the ascitic fluid total protein. If ascitic fluid infection is suspected, ascitic fluid should be cultured at the bedside. ❶ Patients who drink alcohol should be strongly discouraged from further alcohol use. ❺ Sodium restriction to 2,000 mg/day, together with spironolactone and furosemide, is the main stay of therapy. Diuretic therapy should be initiated with single morning doses of spironolactone 100 mg and furosemide 40 mg administered orally. Titrate diuretic therapy every 3 to 5 days using the 100 mg:40 mg ratio to attain adequate natriuresis and weight loss (reasonable daily weight loss goal is 0.5 kg).[77] Maximum daily doses are 400 mg spironolactone and 160 mg furosemide.[69,70] This combination ratio is used because it usually maintains normokalemia.[6] Fluid restriction, unless the serum sodium is less than 120 to 125 mEq/L, and bed rest are not recommended. Monitor urinary sodium excretion using a 24-hour urine collection and monitor serum potassium and renal function frequently. Avoid rapid correction of asymptomatic hyponatremia in patients with cirrhosis. If tense ascites is present, paracentesis should be performed prior to institution of diuretic therapy and salt restriction. For patients who respond to diuretic therapy, this approach is preferred over the use of serial paracenteses. Discontinue diuretic therapy in patients who experience uncontrolled or recurrent encephalopathy, severe hyponatremia (serum sodium less than 120 mEq/L) despite fluid restriction, or renal insufficiency (serum creatinine greater than 2 mg/dL). Serial paracenteses may be considered for patients with refractory ascites and albumin infusion of 6 to 8g/L of fluid removed can be considered postparacentesis when paracentesis volumes exceed 5 L.

Patients with ascitic fluid PMN counts greater than or equal to 250 cells/mm³ should receive empiric antibiotic therapy with intravenous cefotaxime 2 g every 8 hours or a similar third-generation cephalosporin. Oral ofloxacin 400 mg twice daily may be an alternative option in patients without prior exposure to quinolones, vomiting, shock, severe encephalopathy, or serum creatinine over 3 mg/dL. Patients with ascitic fluid PMN counts less than 250 cells/mm³ but with signs and symptoms of infection (symptoms such as abdominal pain, abdominal tenderness, and fever) should also receive empiric antibiotic treatment. Patients with ascitic fluid PMN counts greater than or equal to 250 cells/mm³ and suspicion of SBP should also receive 1.5 g of albumin per kilogram body weight within 6 hours of detection and 1 g per kilogram body weight on day 3 if they also have a serum creatinine over 1 mg/dL, blood urea nitrogen over 30 mg/dL, or total bilirubin over 4 mg/dL.

❻ All patients who have survived an episode of SBP should receive long-term antibiotic prophylaxis with daily norfloxacin 400 mg or double strength trimethoprim-sulfamethoxazole. Long-term prophylaxis should also be considered for the prevention of SBP in patients with low-protein ascites (less than 1.5 g/dL) who also have one of the following: serum creatinine greater than or equal to 1.2 mg/dL, blood urea nitrogen greater than or equal to 25 mg/dL, serum sodium less than or equal to 130 mEq/L, or Child-Pugh score of greater than or equal to 9 with bilirubin greater than or equal to 3 mg/dL. Short-term prophylaxis (7 days) is indicated in patients with cirrhosis and gastrointestinal hemorrhage. A summary of evidence-based treatment recommendations regarding ascites and SBP is found in Table 44–4.

◼ HEPATIC ENCEPHALOPATHY

The clinical manifestations of HE vary widely.[78] Patients with minimal HE do not suffer from clinically overt cognitive dysfunction; nevertheless, it adversely affects their ability to function socially and perform in the workplace, and it may also affect their ability to drive safely.[13] Episodic HE refers to precipitated, spontaneous, or recurrent acute episodes of HE. *Recurrent HE* refers to two spontaneous or precipitated episodes of HE that occur within 1 year. Persistent HE refers to mild, severe, or treatment-dependent symptoms that are chronic in nature and negatively impact a patient's quality of life.

The prevalence of HE among cirrhotics is variable but may be found in up to 70% of patients. To determine the severity of HE, a grading system that relates neurologic and neuromuscular signs can be used (Table 44–5). Presently, the primary substances thought to be involved in the development of HE are ammonia, glutamate, manganese, and the γ-aminobutyric acid (GABA)-benzodiazepine receptor agonists.[13,78]

Management of Hepatic Encephalopathy

Episodic HE may develop in a clinically stable cirrhotic patient as the result of a precipitating event.[13] Table 44–6 lists the most commonly encountered precipitating factors and suggests general treatment alternatives. Table 44–7 describes the treatment goals for patients with HE and contrasts the differences between episodic

TABLE 44-4 Evidence-Based Table of Selected Treatment Recommendations: Ascites and Spontaneous Bacterial Peritonitis

Recommendation	Grade
Ascites	
Paracentesis should be performed in patients with apparent new-onset ascites	IC
Sodium restriction of 2,000 mg/day should be instituted as well as oral diuretic therapy with spironolactone and furosemide	IIaA
Diuretic-sensitive patients should be treated with sodium restriction and diuretics rather than serial paracentesis	IIaC
Refractory ascites	
Serial therapeutic paracenteses may be performed	IC
Postparacentesis albumin infusion of 6 to 8 g/L of fluid removed can be considered if more than 5 L are removed during paracentesis	IIaC
Treatment of SBP	
If ascitic fluid PMN counts are greater than 250 cells/mm³, empiric antibiotic therapy should be instituted (cefotaxime 2 g every 8 hours)	IA
If ascitic fluid PMN counts are less than 250 cells/mm³, but signs or symptoms of infection exist, empiric antibiotic therapy should be initiated while awaiting culture results	IB
Ofloxacin 400 mg twice daily may be substituted for cefotaxime in patients without vomiting, shock, grade II or higher encephalopathy, or serum creatinine greater than 3 mg/dL and if there is no prior exposure to quinolones	IIaB
If ascitic fluid polymorphonuclear leukocyte counts are greater than 250 cells/mm³, clinical suspicion of SBP is present, and the patient has a serum creatinine greater than 1 mg/dL, blood urea nitrogen greater than 30 mg/dL, or total bilirubin over 4 mg/dL, 1.5 g/kg albumin should be infused within 6 hours of detection and 1 g/kg albumin infusion should also be given on day 3	IIaB
Prophylaxis against SBP	
Short-term antibiotic prophylaxis should be used for 7 days to prevent SBP in cirrhosis patients with gastrointestinal hemorrhage	IA
Patients who survive an episode of SBP should receive long-term prophylaxis with either daily norfloxacin or trimethoprim-sulfamethoxazole	IA
Patients with low protein ascites (less than 1.5 g/dL) plus at least one of the following: serum creatinine greater than or equal to 1.2 mg/dL, blood urea nitrogen greater than or equal to 25 mg/dL, serum sodium less than or equal to 130 mEq/L, or Child-Pugh score of greater than or equal to 9 with bilirubin greater than or equal to 3 mg/dL may also justifiably receive long-term norfloxacin or sulfamethoxazole/trimethoprim as prophylaxis	IB

Recommendation grading:

Class I—Conditions for which there is evidence and/or general agreement

Class II—Conditions for which there is conflicting evidence and/or a divergence of opinion

Class IIa—Weight of evidence/opinion is in favor of efficacy

Class IIb—Efficacy less well established

Class III—Conditions for which there is evidence and/or general agreement that treatment is not effective and/or potentially harmful

Level A—Data from multiple randomized trials or meta-analyses

Level B—Data derived from single randomized trial or nonrandomized studies

Level C—Only consensus opinion, case studies, or standard of care

Data from reference 6.

and persistent HE. The general approach to the management of HE is to first identify and treat any precipitating factors, and, when associated with a precipitant, the clinical features of HE may resolve after the precipitating factor is treated or removed.[13,14] The development of overt HE in cirrhosis is associated with increased mortality.[79]

Treatment approaches for episodic and persistent HE include (a) reducing ammonia blood concentrations by dietary restrictions and drug therapy aimed at inhibiting ammonia production or enhancing its removal and (b) inhibition of the γ-aminobutyric acid (GABA)-benzodiazepine receptors. Additionally, treatment for persistent HE should include avoidance and prevention of precipitating factors in an effort to avoid acute decompensation.[14]

Hyperammonemia

❼ Treatment interventions to reduce ammonia blood concentrations are recommended in patients with HE.[14] Decreasing ammonia blood concentrations by reducing the nitrogenous load from the gut remains a mainstay of therapy for patients with HE. Treatment options most commonly used to decrease ammonia load from the gut include nutritional management, nonabsorbable disaccharides, and antibiotics.

Guidelines for nutritional support of patients with liver disease have been published by the European Society for Parenteral and Enteral Nutrition.[80] Protein withdrawal is a cornerstone of treatment for patients during acute episodes of HE.[14] However, prolonged restriction can lead to malnutrition and poorer prognosis among HE patients. Therefore, once successful reversal of HE symptoms is achieved, protein is added back to the diet in combination with other therapies until a target of 1 to 1.5 g/kg per day is reached. Vegetable-source and dairy-source protein may be preferable to meat-source protein because the latter contains a higher calorie to nitrogen ratio. Also, the higher fiber content of vegetable protein lowers colonic pH, increasing catharsis. Most patients will tolerate at least 1 g/kg/day of standard proteins without becoming encephalopathic.[81] Branched-chain amino acid (BCAA) formulations may provide a better-tolerated source of protein in those patients with protein intolerance.[14] Bowel cleansing using cathartics or lactulose enemas (see following discussion) results in rapid removal of ammonia substrate from the colon and may be combined with dietary intervention to help the patient eliminate ammonia and tolerate dietary protein.

The use of lactulose, a nonabsorbable disaccharide, is standard therapy for both acute and chronic HE. Lactulose, when administered orally through ingestion or a nasogastric tube, passes through the gastrointestinal tract and reaches the colon unchanged. It can also be administered by retention enema. Lactulose is metabolized by gut flora into acetic acid and lactic acid, which lower colonic pH and create a cathartic effect.

Lactulose administration lowers ammonia levels in the blood in several ways: (a) through creation of a laxative effect that reduces

TABLE 44-5 Grading System for Hepatic Encephalopathy

Grade	Level of Consciousness	Personality/Intellect	Neurologic Abnormalities
0	Normal	Normal	None
1	Inverted sleep patterns/restless	Mild confusion, euphoria or depression, decreased attention, irritable, slowing of ability to perform mental tasks	Slight tremor, apraxia, incoordination
2	Lethargic, drowsy, intermittent disorientation (usually for time)	Obvious personality changes, inappropriate behavior, gross deficits in ability to perform mental tasks	Asterixis, abnormal reflexes
3	Somnolent but arousable, markedly confused, disorientation to time and/or place, amnesia	Unable to perform mental tasks, occasional fits of rage, speech present but incomprehensible	Abnormal reflexes
4	Coma/unarousable	None	Decerebrate, Babinski sign present

Data from reference 13.

TABLE 44-6 Portosystemic Encephalopathy: Precipitating Factors and Therapy

Factor	Therapy Alternatives
Gastrointestinal bleeding	
Variceal	Band ligation/sclerotherapy
	Octreotide
Nonvariceal	Endoscopic therapy
	Proton pump inhibitors
Infection/sepsis	Antibiotics
	Paracentesis
Electrolyte abnormalities	Discontinue diuretics
	Fluid and electrolyte replacement
Sedative ingestion	Discontinue sedatives/tranquilizers
	Consider reversal (flumazenil/naloxone)
Dietary excesses	Limit daily protein
	Lactulose
Constipation	Cathartics
	Bowel cleansing/enema
Renal insufficiency	Discontinue diuretics
	Discontinue NSAIDs, nephrotoxic antibiotics
	Fluid resuscitation

Data from reference 13, 14, and 78.

the time period available for ammonia absorption, (b) through leaching of ammonia from the circulation into the colon and increasing bacterial uptake of ammonia by colonic bacteria, and (c) through reducing ammonia production by the small intestine by interfering directly with the uptake of glutamine by the intestinal wall and its subsequent metabolism to ammonia.[82] Upon evaluation of the numerous clinical trials studying the effectiveness of lactulose in the treatment of HE, one may determine that the standards of evidence-based medicine have not been met.[14,83,84] In fact, lactulose plus neomycin was not better than placebo for the management of acute HE.[85] Despite this and because reevaluation of lactulose for the management of HE (especially acute HE) would require a new clinical trial, bowel cleansing through lactulose administration remains a cornerstone in HE therapy.[14] Inhibiting the activity of urease-producing bacteria by using neomycin or metronidazole can decrease production of ammonia.[86,87] Neomycin at doses of 3 to 6 g daily can be given for 1 to 2 weeks during an acute episode of HE.[14] For persistent HE, a dose of 1 to 2 g daily could be used with periodic renal and annual auditory monitoring. Despite poor absorption, chronic use of neomycin can lead to irreversible ototoxicity, nephrotoxicity, and the possibility of staphylococcal superinfection. As such, neomycin should not be considered first-line therapy for HE. In patients with an inadequate response to lactulose alone, combination therapy with neomycin may be tried. Metronidazole initiated at 250 mg twice daily may also produce a favorable clinical response in HE. However, neurotoxicity caused by impaired hepatic clearance of the drug may be problematic.

TABLE 44-7 Treatment Goals: Episodic and Persistent Hepatic Encephalopathy

Episodic HE	Persistent HE
Control precipitating factor	Reverse encephalopathy
Reverse encephalopathy	Avoid recurrence
Hospital/inpatient therapy	Home/outpatient therapy
Maintain fluid and hemodynamic support	Manage persistent neuropsychiatric abnormalities
	Manage chronic liver disease
Expect normal mentation after recovery	High prevalence of abnormal mentation after recovery

Ammonia generated by *Helicobacter pylori* in the stomach may be associated with precipitating or worsening HE in patients with cirrhosis.[88] However, a prospective clinical trial showed no significant improvement in mental status or serum ammonia levels in patients with HE who underwent *H. pylori* eradication.[89] Therefore, routine eradication of *H. pylori* is not recommended.[14]

Rifaximin is a synthetic antibiotic structurally similar to rifamycin with a systemic absorption of only 0.4%.[82] Rifaximin lowers blood ammonia levels and improves neuropsychiatric symptoms in HE. Rifaximin 1,200 mg/day has been compared with lactitol 60 g/day in patients with grade I to III HE for 5 to 10 days.[90] Comparable percentages of patients showed clinical improvement at the end of the treatment period; however, improvements in blood ammonia concentrations and in the HE index were significantly greater among rifaximin-treated patients. There was also a higher number of patients who showed complete resolution of their neuropsychiatric symptoms with rifaximin treatment versus the nonabsorbable disaccharide lactitol. Rifaximin has also been compared with neomycin in patients with grade I to III HE.[91] In this randomized, double-blind comparison, patients were treated for 21 days with either rifaximin 1,200 mg daily or neomycin 3 g/day. While significant improvements were seen in both groups, improvements in psychometric performance and blood ammonia concentrations were significantly greater in patients treated with rifaximin. Also, while no adverse events were reported in the rifaximin-treatment group, nearly a fourth of neomycin-treated patients experienced increases in blood urea nitrogen and serum creatinine levels, and nearly a third reported nausea, abdominal pain, and vomiting.

CLINICAL CONTROVERSY

Rifaximin has been shown to be effective in the treatment of HE and has a favorable side effect profile as compared with other antibiotics in use for HE today.[91] It has been found to be more effective in some HE-related measurement parameters as compared with lactitol.[90] Though studies to date have enrolled relatively small numbers of patients and even though it does not carry the indication for HE in the United States, rifaximin is largely considered second-line therapy for patients with HE who fail therapy or have inadequate results with lactulose. Whether or not rifaximin should be considered as first-line therapy over lactulose or whether rifaximin should be considered first-line therapy in addition to lactulose remains controversial. Rifaximin costs approximately 12 times more than lactulose.[82] However, if rifaximin is more effective than lactulose and prevents other costs, such as hospitalizations, treatment with rifaximin or rifaximin plus lactulose may actually be more cost effective than therapy with lactulose alone. A large multicenter trial comparing rifaximin plus lactulose with placebo plus lactulose in patients with recurrent episodic HE is under way and should provide some further information about rifaximin and its place in the therapy of HE in the future.

Ammonia removal can be enhanced by stimulating its detoxification. This is done by supporting alternative metabolic pathways, which can reduce blood ammonia concentrations. L-Ornithine L-aspartate stimulates residual hepatic urea cycle activity and promotes peripheral glutamine synthesis.[92] Intravenous L-Ornithine L-aspartate is effective in cirrhotic patients with grade 1 and grade 2 HE to reduce blood ammonia and improve clinical symptoms of

HE with clinical response rates similar to those of lactulose.[93] Oral L-Ornithine L-aspartate is effective at reducing blood ammonia and improving clinical symptoms in patients with grade 2 HE.[94]

Zinc is a cofactor of urea cycle enzymes and can be deficient in cirrhotic patients, especially in cases of malnourishment.[14] Zinc replacement has mixed results for decreasing ammonia levels and improving symptoms of HE.[95,96] In a controlled trial in cirrhotic patients with mild HE, the administration of zinc sulfate 600 mg/day for 3 months resulted in increased urea formation and lower ammonia levels along with improvement in psychological test scores.[96] Other therapies studied in HE to lower the ammonia load from the gut include sodium benzoate and probiotics like *Lactobacillus acidophilus* and *Enterococcus faecium* SF 68.[14]

Drugs Affecting Neurotransmission

The GABA-receptor complex is the primary inhibitory neural network within the central nervous system. An enhanced GABA-ergic tone and an increased amount of endogenous benzodiazepines may contribute to HE.[97] Based on evidence of an increase in benzodiazepine receptor ligands in patients with hepatic encephalopathy, flumazenil has been evaluated for the treatment of HE.[98] Among five prospective, placebo-controlled trials, three reported benefit with flumazenil, whereas two found no difference when compared to placebo. With dosages of 0.2 to 15 mg IV, response rates were variable, ranging from 17% to 78%. Improvements, however, were often transient. Flumazenil 1 mg intravenous bolus may be considered for short-term therapy in refractory patients with suspected benzodiazepine intake, but cannot be recommended for routine clinical use.[14]

Alterations of dopaminergic neurotransmission have also been thought to play a role in the symptoms of HE, particularly the extrapyramidal signs.[14] Improvements of extrapyramidal symptoms have been reported with bromocriptine therapy.[99] Bromocriptine 30 mg twice daily is indicated for chronic HE treatment in patients who are unresponsive to other therapies.[14] Prolactin levels may become elevated during bromocriptine treatment, and ototoxicity is possible.[14,82] Bromocriptine should be avoided in patients with ascites.[82]

Treatment Recommendations: Hepatic Encephalopathy

Treatment recommendations depend on the type of HE being managed: episodic HE, persistent HE, or minimal HE.[37] The general approach to the management of HE is first to identify patients with acute episodic HE and then to provide aggressive management of any precipitating events (see Table 44–7).[14] When the precipitating event has been discovered and appropriate therapy initiated, then steps to rapidly reverse the encephalopathy should be implemented.

❼ The mainstay of therapy of HE involves measures to lower blood ammonia concentrations and includes diet therapy, lactulose, and antibiotics alone or in combination with lactulose. Other commonly used adjunctive therapies include zinc replacement in patients with zinc deficiency, flumazenil, and possibly bromocriptine.

In patients with episodic HE, protein is withheld or limited while maintaining the total caloric intake until the clinical situation improves. Then dietary protein is titrated back up based on tolerance, increasing gradually to a total of 1 to 1.5 g/kg per day. Consider the substitution of meat-source protein with vegetable or dairy protein. Zinc sulfate supplementation at a dose of 220 mg twice daily is recommended for long-term management in patients with cirrhosis who are zinc deficient.

In episodic HE, lactulose is initiated at a dose of 45 mL orally every hour (or by retention enema: 300 mL lactulose syrup in 1 L water held for 60 minutes) until catharsis begins. The dose is then decreased to 15 to 45 mL orally every 8 to 12 hours and titrated to

produce two to three soft stools per day. The enema is retained for 1 hour with the patient in the Trendelenburg position. For chronic encephalopathy, dosing is the same except that the initial hourly administration is not required. Patients are maintained on this regimen to prevent recurrence of episodic HE. Monitor electrolytes periodically, follow patients for changes in mental status, and titrate to the number of stools as already described.

Antibiotic therapy with either metronidazole (initiated at 250 mg twice daily but titrated up to four times daily in the literature) or neomycin (dose at 3 to 6 g/day for 1 to 2 weeks for episodic HE and 1 to 2 g/day for persistent HE) are reserved for patients who have not responded to diet and lactulose therapy and when the combination may provide additive effects and improved clinical response. Because rifaximin 400 mg three times daily provides similar effectiveness and has less risk of side effects as compared with other antibiotic options, rifaximin is often used today as second-line therapy for patients who have inadequate response to lactulose or are unable to tolerate or adhere to therapy with lactuose.[37]

■ SYSTEMIC COMPLICATIONS

In addition to the more common complications of chronic liver disease discussed earlier, other complications can occur, including hepatorenal syndrome, hepatopulmonary syndrome, coagulation disorders, and endocrine dysfunction.

Hepatorenal syndrome, which is a functional renal failure in the setting of cirrhosis, occurs in the absence of structural kidney damage.[100] It develops in patients with cirrhosis as a result of intense renal vasoconstriction, which results from extreme systemic vasodilatation. The resultant reduction in blood supply to the kidneys causes avid sodium retention and oliguria. As liver disease progresses, systemic vasodilatation worsens and, subsequently, increased renal vasoconstriction occurs and renal blood flow is further decreased. As this occurs, the heart's response becomes insufficient to maintain perfusion pressure, which the kidneys rely heavily upon at this point to maintain adequate blood flow. Hepatorenal syndrome is common and develops in approximately 20% of hospitalized patients with cirrhosis.

Management of hepatorenal syndrome begins with a first step of discontinuing diuretics and any other medication that could potentially decrease effective blood volume and to expand the intravascular volume with intravenous albumin at a dose of 1 g/kg up to a maximum of 100 g.[37] Precipitating factors such as infection, fluid loss, and blood loss should be investigated and treated if found. Liver transplantation is the only definitive therapy for hepatorenal syndrome and the only therapy that will prolong survival. Therapies used to bridge patients until transplantation include arteriolar vasoconstrictor based treatments with terlipressin or midodrine plus octreotide used in addition to intravenous albumin infusion as already discussed.

Hepatopulmonary syndrome affects somewhere between 5% and 32% of patients with cirrhosis.[101] This abnormality is characterized by a defect in arterial oxygenation, which is caused by the pulmonary vascular dilatation that occurs in the presence of liver disease. Less commonly, pleural and pulmonary arteriovenous shunting can occur as well as portopulmonary venous anastomoses. These patients present with dyspnea on exertion, at rest, or both. Cirrhotic patients with these findings should be evaluated for hepatopulmonary syndrome, which is diagnosed based upon the presence of arterial hypoxemia. Arterial hypoxemia is defined based on measurements of the partial pressure of oxygen that are performed with patients sitting and at rest. Testing for an increased alveolar–arterial oxygen gradient is also particularly important as this gradient can rise abnormally before the patient's partial pressure of oxygen measurement becomes abnormally low. Long-term management requires supportive therapy with supplemental oxygen. The prognosis for these patients is poor. Ultimately, liver transplantation offers the best chance for long-term recovery.

Coagulation disorders occur in patients with chronic liver disease because the liver plays a central role in the maintenance of hemostasis since it is the site for synthesis of a majority of the proteins involved in the regulation of coagulation and fibrinolysis.[15] These disorders increase the risk of bleeding and tend to become more profound as the liver failure becomes more severe. Correction of the coagulopathy is essential for patients actively bleeding. The pathophysiology of the coagulopathy is complex and involves impaired synthesis of clotting factors, excessive fibrinolysis, disseminated intravascular coagulation, thrombocytopenia, and platelet dysfunction. Acute therapy involves platelet transfusions for thrombocytopenia and fresh frozen plasma for prolongation of the PT because of clotting factor deficiencies.[37]

The presence of cirrhosis can produce abnormal circulating levels of various hormones.[102] Hypogonadism, diabetes mellitus, osteoporosis, and thyroid disorders are among the endocrine disorders that may develop related to advanced liver disease. Erectile dysfunction related to hypogonadism can be treated with the administration of testosterone and the removal of causative factors such as alcohol.

■ LIVER TRANSPLANTATION

The complications seen in patients with chronic liver disease are essentially functional as a secondary effect of the circulatory and metabolic changes that accompany liver failure. Consequently, liver transplantation is the only treatment that can offer a cure for complications of end-stage cirrhosis.

PHARMACOKINETIC AND PHARMACODYNAMIC CHANGES IN LIVER FAILURE

Cirrhosis modulates the behavior of drugs in the body by inducing kinetic alterations in drug absorption, distribution, and clearance.[103] Additionally, patients with cirrhosis may exhibit pharmacodynamic changes with increased sensitivity to the effects of certain drugs, namely opiates, benzodiazepines, and nonsteroidal antiinflammatory drugs (NSAIDs). These pharmacodynamic changes are separate and distinct from the enhancement of drug effects seen in cirrhosis patients as a result of pharmacokinetic changes. Hepatic drug clearance is primarily dependent upon protein binding, hepatic blood flow, and metabolic enzyme activity. The pathophysiologic changes that occur in patients with cirrhosis, including reduced liver blood flow, intra- and extrahepatic portal-systemic shunting, diminished metabolic and synthetic function, and capillarization of the sinusoids, can have a significant impact on each of these factors. The consequence of these changes is a reduction in intrinsic metabolic activity, a reduction in the delivery of blood to the liver that decreases clearance and prolongs half-life, and a reduction in the degree of protein binding that increases the fraction of unbound drug in the serum. Finally, patients with cirrhosis frequently accumulate large amounts of interstitial fluid resulting in substantial changes in the volume of distribution, which also prolongs drug half-life. These changes occur most commonly in combination in patients with cirrhosis and are dynamic throughout the disease course. The effect that these changes will have depends on the drug and the type of biotransformation that the drug undergoes.

Drugs with a high extraction ratio (high-extraction drugs) are dependent on blood flow for metabolism, and the rate of metabolism will be sensitive to changes in blood flow. Drugs with a low extraction ratio (low-extraction drugs) are dependent on intrinsic metabolic activity for metabolism, and the rate of metabolism

will reflect changes in intrinsic clearance and protein binding. Furthermore, hepatic biotransformation involves two types of metabolic processes: phase I reactions and phase II reactions. Phase I reactions involve the cytochrome P450 system and include hydrolysis, oxidation, dealkylation, and reduction reactions. Phase II reactions involve conjugation of the drug with an endogenous molecule such as sulfate or an amino acid, rendering it more water soluble and enhancing its elimination. Drugs metabolized by phase I reactions, especially oxidation, tend to be significantly impaired in patients with cirrhosis, whereas drugs eliminated by conjugation are relatively unaffected.

The variability and complexity of the interaction between the extent and severity of liver disease and individual characteristics of the drug make it difficult to predict the degree of pharmacokinetic perturbation in an individual patient. Unfortunately, there are no sensitive and specific clinical or biochemical markers that allow us to quantify the extent of liver insufficiency or the degree of metabolic activity. In addition, renal insufficiency and alterations that commonly accompany cirrhosis further complicate empiric dosing recommendations in these patients. Dosing recommendations are most commonly nonspecific, with recommendations labeled for patients with mild to moderate liver impairment. Dosing information for patients with more severe liver impairment is not available. As a result, when patients with cirrhosis require therapy with drugs that undergo hepatic metabolism (e.g., benzodiazepines), monitoring response to therapy and anticipating drug accumulation and enhanced effects is essential. In the case of benzodiazepines, selection of an agent such as lorazepam, an intermediate-acting agent that is metabolized via conjugation and has no active metabolites, is easier to monitor than a drug such as diazepam, a long-acting benzodiazepine that is oxidized in the liver and has an active metabolite with a long half-life of its own.

PHARMACOECONOMIC CONSIDERATIONS

Two studies, both related to the prevention of variceal bleeding and published recently, are mentioned here.[104,105] A recent analysis provides evidence that HVPG monitoring is not cost-effective for use in patients with varices and no history of variceal bleeding as compared to treatment with standard β-blocker therapy without invasive monitoring.[104] A cost-utility evaluation of secondary prophylaxis therapies concluded that patients are best served by treatment with either endoscopic band ligation or endoscopic band ligation plus medical management as compared with TIPS placement.[105] Because treatment approaches for patients with cirrhosis can range from supportive medical therapy to repeated endoscopic procedures with serious complications to liver transplantation, the need for application of economic analysis is obvious. Of critical importance is the question of when, in the course of chronic liver disease, the various treatment interventions are employed and whether liver transplantation should be attempted earlier, thereby avoiding most of the complications associated with chronic liver disease.

EVALUATION OF THERAPEUTIC OUTCOMES

Table 44–8 summarizes the management approach for patients with cirrhosis, including monitoring parameters and therapeutic outcomes. Cirrhosis is generally a chronic progressive disease that requires aggressive medical management to prevent or delay common complications. Table 44–8 also lists monitoring criteria that need to be carefully followed in order to achieve the maximum benefit from the medical therapies employed and prevent adverse effects. A therapeutic plan including therapeutic end points for each medical and diet therapy needs to be developed and discussed with the patient.

TABLE 44-8 Management Approach and Outcome Assessments

Complication	Treatment Approach	Monitoring Parameter	Outcome Assessment
Ascites	Diet, diuretics, paracentesis, TIPS	Daily assessment of weight	Prevent or eliminate ascites and its secondary complications
Spontaneous bacterial peritonitis	Antibiotic therapy, prophylaxis if undergoing paracentesis	Evidence of clinical deterioration (e.g., abdominal pain, fever, anorexia, malaise, fatigue)	Prevent/treat infection to decrease mortality
Variceal bleeding	Pharmacologic prophylaxis	Child-Pugh score, endoscopy, CBC	Appropriate reduction in heart rate and portal pressure
	Endoscopy, vasoactive drug therapy (octreotide), ligation or sclerotherapy, volume resuscitation, pharmacologic prophylaxis	CBC, evidence of overt bleeding	Acute: control acute bleedChronic: variceal obliteration, reduce portal pressures
Coagulation disorders	Blood products (PPF, platelets), vitamin K	CBC, prothrombin time, platelet count	Normalize PT time, maintain/improve hemostasis
Hepatic encephalopathy	Ammonia reduction (lactulose, antibiotics), elimination of drugs causing CNS depression, limit excess protein in diet	Grade of encephalopathy, EEG, psychological testing, mental status changes, concurrent drug therapy	Maintain functional capacity, prevent hospitalization for encephalopathy, decrease ammonia levels, provide adequate nutrition
Hepatorenal syndrome	Eliminate concurrent nephrotoxins (NSAIDs), decrease or discontinue diuretics, volume resuscitation, liver transplantation	Serum and urine electrolytes, concurrent drug therapy	Prevent progressive renal injury by preventing dehydration and avoiding other nephrotoxins Liver transplantation for refractory hepatorenal syndrome
Hepatopulmonary syndrome	Paracentesis to relieve ascites, O_2 therapy	Dyspnea, presence of ascites	Acute: relief of dyspnea and hypoxiaChronic: manage ascites as above

CBC, complete blood cell count; CNS, central nervous system; EEG, electroencephalogram; PT, prothrombin time; NSAID, nonsteroidal antiinflammatory drug; PPF, plasma protein fraction; TIPS, transjugular intrahepatic portosystemic shunt.

ABBREVIATIONS

AAA: aromatic amino acid

AASLD: American Association for the Study of Liver Diseases

ALT: alanine transaminase

AST: aspartate transaminase

BCAA: branched-chain amino acid

EGD: esophagogastroduodenoscopy

EVL: endoscopic variceal ligation

GABA: γ-aminobutyric acid

GGT: γ-glutamyl transpeptidase

HE: hepatic encephalopathy

HVPG: hepatic venous pressure gradient

MELD: Model for End-stage Liver Disease

NSAIDs: non-steroidal anti-inflammatory drugs

PMN: polymorphonuclear

PT: prothrombin time

SAAG: serum-ascites albumin gradient

SBP: spontaneous bacterial peritonitis

TIPS: transjugular intrahepatic portosystemic shunt

UNOS: United Network for Organ Sharing

REFERENCES

1. Schuppan D, Afdhal NH. Liver cirrhosis. Lancet 2008;371(9615): 838–851.
2. Bataller R, Brenner DA. Liver fibrosis. Journal Clin Invest 2005;115(2):209–218.
3. Guha IN, Iredale JP. Clinical and diagnostic aspects of cirrhosis. In: Rodés J, Benhamou J, Blei A, eds. Textbook of Hepatology: From Basic Science to Clinical Practice. 3rd ed. Malden, MA: Blackwell Publishing; 2007.
4. Abboud G, Kaplowitz N. Drug-induced liver injury. Drug Safety 2007;30(4):277–294.
5. Xu J, Kochanek KD, Tejada-Vera B. Deaths: Preliminary data for 2007. National Vital Statistics Reports 2009;58(1):1–51.
6. Runyon BA. Management of adult patients with ascites due to cirrhosis: An update. Hepatology 2009;49(6):2087–2107.
7. Malarkey DE, Johnson K, Ryan L, et al. New insights into functional aspects of liver morphology. Toxicologic Pathology 2005;33: 27–34.
8. Friedman SL. Hepatic fibrosis—role of hepatic stellate cell activation. Medscape General Medicine 2002;4(3), http://www.medscape.com/viewarticle/436461_print.
9. Bosch J, Berzigotti A, Garcia-Pagan JC, et al. The management of portal hypertension: Rational basis, available treatments and future options. Journal of Hepatology 2008;48:S68–S92.
10. Kashani A, Landaverde C, Medici V, et al. Fluid retention in cirrhosis:pathophysiology and management. Q J Med 2008;101:71–85.
11. Wright AS, Rikkers LF. Current management of portal hypertension. J Gastrointest Surg 2005;9:992–1005.
12. de Franchis R. Evolving consensus in portal hypertension: Report of the Baveno IV consensus workshop on methodology of diagnosis and therapy in portal hypertension. J Hepatol 2005;43:167–176.
13. Stewart CA, Cerhan J. Hepatic encephalopathy: A dynamic or static condition. Metabolic Brain Disease 2005;20(3):193–204.
14. Blei AT, Cordoba J, and The Practice Parameters Committee of the American College of Gastroenterology. Hepatic encephalopathy. Am J Gastroenterol 2001;96:1968–1976.
15. Peck-Radosavljevic M. Review article: Coagulation disorders in chronic liver disease. Aliment Pharmacol Ther 2007;26(suppl 1):21–28.
16. Heidelbaugh JJ, Bruderly M. Cirrhosis and chronic liver failure, I: Diagnosis and evaluation. Am F Physician 2006;74:756–762, 781.
17. Giannini EG, Testa R, and Savarino V. Liver enzyme alteration: A guide for clinicians. Can Med Assoc J 2005;172(3):367–379.
18. Cohen JA, Kaplan MM. The SGOT/SGPT ratio—an indicator of alcoholic disease. Dig Dis Sci 1979;24:835–838.
19. Pugh RNH, Murray-Lyon IM, Dawson JL, et al. Transection of the oesophagus for bleeding oesophagus varices. Br J Surg 1973;60: 646–649.
20. About the MELD/PELD calculator, http://www.unos.org/resources/MeldPeldCalculator.asp?index=97.
21. MELD/PELD calculator documentation, http://www.unos.org/SharedContentDocuments/MELD_PELD_Calculator_Documentation.pdf.
22. O'Grady JG, Alexander GJM, Hayllar KM, et al. Early indicators of prognosis in fulminant hepatic failure. Gastroenterology 1989;97(2):439–445.

23. Groszmann RJ, Guadalupe G, Bosch J, et al. Beta-blockers to prevent gastroesophageal varices in patients with cirrhosis. N Engl J Med 2005;353:2254–2261.

24. D'Amico G, Pagliaro L, Bosch J. Pharmacological treatment of portal hypertension: An evidence-based approach. Semin Liver Dis 1999;19:475–505.

25. Chen W, Nikolova D, Frederiksen SL, et al. Beta-blockers reduce mortality in cirrhotic patients with oesophageal varices who have never bled (Cochrane review). J Hepatol 2004;40(suppl 1):67 (abstract).

26. Merkel C, Marin R, Angeli P, et al. A placebo-controlled clinical trial of nadolol in the prophylaxis of growth of small esophageal varices in cirrhosis. Gastroenterology 2004;127:476–484.

27. de Franchis R. Updated consensus in portal hypertension: Report of the Baveno III consensus workshop on definitions, methodology and therapeutic strategies in portal hypertension. J Hepatol 2000;33:846–852.

28. Garcia-Tsao G, Sanyal AJ, Grace ND, et al. Prevention and management of gastroesophageal varices and variceal hemorrhage in cirrhosis. Hepatology 2007;46(3):922–938.

29. Abraczinkas DR, Ookubo R, Grace ND, et al. Propranolol for the prevention of first variceal hemorrhage: A lifetime commitment? Hepatology 2001;34:1096–1102.

30. Garcia-Tsao G, Grace N, Groszmann RJ, et al. Short term effects of propranolol on portal venous pressure. Hepatology 1986;6:101–106.

31. Khuroo MS, Khuroo NS, Farahat KL, et al. Meta-analysis: endoscopic variceal ligation for primary prophylaxis of oesophageal variceal bleeding. Aliment Pharmacol Ther 2005;21:347–361.

32. Garcia-Pagan JC, Bosch J. Endoscopic band ligation in the treatment of portal hypertension. Nat Clin Pract Gastroenterol Hepatol 2005;2:526–535.

33. Lo GH, Chen WC, Chen MH, et al. Endoscopic ligation vs. nadolol in the prevention of first variceal bleeding in patients with cirrhosis. Gastrointest Endosc 2004;59:333–338.

34. Schepke M, Kleber G, Nurnberg D, et al. Ligation versus propranolol for the primary prophylaxis of variceal bleeding in cirrhosis. Hepatology 2004;40:65–72.

35. Lay CS, Tsai YT, Lee FY, et al. Endoscopic variceal ligation versus propranolol for the primary prophylaxis of first variceal bleeding in patients with cirrhosis. J Gastroenterol Hepatol 2006;21:413–419.

36. Garcia-Pagan JC, Villanueva C, Vila MC, et al. Isosorbide mononitrate in the prevention of first variceal bleed in patients who cannot receive beta-blockers. Gastroenterology 2001;121:908–914.

37. Garcia-Tsao G, Lim J, and Members of the Veterans Affairs Hepatitis C Resource Center Program. Management and treatment of patients with cirrhosis and portal hypertension: Recommendations from the Department of Veterans Affairs hepatitis C resource center program and the national hepatitis C program. Am J Gastroenterol 2009;104:1802–1829.

38. Chawla Y, Duseja A, Dhiman RK. Review article: Modern management of portal vein thrombosis. Aliment Pharmacol Ther 2009 August 12 [Epub ahead of print].

39. de Franchis, R. Somatostatin, somatostatin analogues and other vasoactive drugs in the treatment of bleeding oesophageal varices. Digestive and Liver Disease 2005;36(suppl 1):S93–S100.

40. D'Amico G, de Franchis R. Upper digestive bleeding in cirrhosis: Post-therapeutic outcome and prognostic indicators. Hepatology 2003;38:599–612.

41. Burroughs AK and the International Octreotide Varices Study Group. Double blind RCT of 5 days octreotide versus placebo, associated with sclerotherapy for trial/failures. AASLD Abstracts. Hepatology 1996;24:352A.

42. McKee R. A study of octreotide in oesophageal varices. Digestion 1990;45:60–65.

43. Hwang SJ, Lin HC, Change CF, et al. A randomized controlled trial comparing octreotide and vasopressin in the control of acute esophageal variceal bleeding. J Hepatol 1992;16:320–325.

44. Huang CC, Sheen IS, Chu CM, et al. A prospective randomized controlled trial of sandostatin and vasopressin in the management of acute bleeding esophageal varices. Chang Gung Med J 1992;15:78–83.

45. Silvain C, Carpentier S, Sautereau D, et al. Terlipressin plus transdermal nitroglycerin vs. octreotide in the control of acute bleeding from esophageal varices: A multicenter randomized trial. Hepatology 1993;18:61–65.

46. Pedretti G, Elia G, Calzetti C, et al. Octreotide versus terlipressin in the acute variceal hemorrhage in cirrhosis: Emergency control and prevention of early rebleeding. Clin Invest 1994;72:653–659.

47. Gotzsche PC, Hrobjartsson A. Somatostatin analogues for acute bleeding oesophageal varices. Cochrane Database Syst Rev 2005, CD000193.

48. Bañares R, Albillos A, Rincon D, et al. Endoscopic treatment versus endoscopic plus pharmacologic treatment for acute variceal bleeding: A meta-analysis. Hepatology 2002;305:609–615.

49. Escorsell A, Bandi JC, Andreu V, et al. Desensitization to the effects of intravenous octreotide in cirrhotic patients with portal hypertension. Gastroenterology 2001;120:161–169.

50. Baik SK, Jeong PH, Ji SW, et al. Acute hemodynamic effects of octreotide and terlipressin in patients with cirrhosis: A randomized comparison. Am J Gastroenterol 2005;100:631–635.

51. Imperiale TF, Teran JC, McCullough AJ. A meta-analysis of somatostatin versus vasopressin in the management of acute esophageal variceal hemorrhage. Gastroenterology 1995;109(4):1289–1294.

52. Bernard B, Grange JD, Khac EN, et al. Antibiotic prophylaxis for the prevention of bacterial infections in cirrhotic patients with gastrointestinal bleeding: A meta-analysis. Hepatology 1999;29:1655–1661.

53. Soares-Weiser K, Brezis M, Tur-Kaspa R, et al. Antibiotic prophylaxis for cirrhotic patients with gastrointestinal bleeding (Cochrane Review). The Cochrane Library 2002, Issue 2:CD002907.

54. Hou MC, Lin HC, Liu TT, et al. Antibiotic prophylaxis after endoscopic therapy prevents rebleeding in acute variceal hemorrhage: A randomized trial. Hepatology 2004;39:746–753.

55. Villanueva C, Piqueras M, Aracil C, et al. A randomized controlled trial comparing ligation and sclerotherapy as emergency endoscopic treatment added to somatostatin in acute variceal bleeding. J Hepatol 2006;45:560–567.

56. Avgerinos A, Armonis A, Stefanidis G, et al. Sustained rise of portal pressure after sclerotherapy, but not band ligation, in acute variceal bleeding in cirrhosis. Hepatology 2004;39:1623–1630.

57. Tan PC, Hou MC, Lin HC, et al. A randomized trial of endoscopic treatment of acute gastric variceal hemorrhage: N-butyl-2-cyanoacrylate injection versus band ligation. Hepatology 2006;43:690–697.

58. Rengstorff DS, Binmoeller KF. A pilot study of 2-octyl cyanoacrylate injection for treatment of gastric fundal varices in humans. Gastrointest Endosc 2004;59:553–558.

59. Wong F. The use of TIPS in chronic liver disease. Ann Hepatol 2006;5(1):5–15.

60. Zheng M, Chen Y, Bai J, et al. Transjugular intrahepatic portosystemic shunt versus endoscopic therapy in the secondary prophylaxis of variceal rebleeding in cirrhotic patients meta-analysis update. J Clin Gastroenterol 2008;42(5):507–516.

61. Bosch J, Garcia-Paga JC. Prevention of variceal rebleeding. Lancet 2003;361:952–954.

62. Lo GH, Lai KH, Cheng JS, et al. Endoscopic variceal ligation plus nadolol and sucralfate compared with ligation alone for the prevention of variceal rebleeding: A prospective, randomized trial. Hepatology 2000;32:461–465.

63. De la Pena J, Bullet E, Sanchez-Hernandez E, et al. Variceal ligation plus nadolol compared with ligation for prophylaxis of variceal rebleeding: A multicenter trial. Hepatology 2005;41:572–578.

64. Gonzalez R, Zamora J, Gomez-Camarero J, et al. Meta-analysis: Combination endoscopic and drug therapy to prevent variceal rebleeding in cirrhosis. Ann Intern Med 2008;149:109–122.

65. D'Amico G, Garcia-Pagan JC, Luca A, et al. HVPG reduction and prevention of variceal bleeding in cirrhosis: A systematic review. Gastroenterology 2006;131:1611–1624.

66. Gournay J, Masliah C, Martin T, et al. Isosorbide mononitrate and propranolol compared with propranolol alone for the prevention of variceal rebleeding. Hepatology 2000;31:1239–1245.

67. Garcia Pagan JC, Villanueva C, Albillos A, et al. Nadolol plus isosorbide mononitrate alone or associated with band ligation in the prevention of variceal rebleeding: A multicenter randomized controlled trial. Gut 2009;58(8):1144–1150.

68. Koulaouzidis A, Bhat S, Saeed AA. Spontaneous bacterial peritonitis. World J Gastroenterol 2009;15(9):1042–1049.

69. Runyon BA. Ascites and spontaneous bacterial peritonitis. In: Feldman M, Friedman LS, Brandt LJ, eds. Sleisenger and Fortran's Gastrointestinal and Liver Disease. 8th ed. Philadelphia, PA: Saunders; 2006:1935–1964.

70. Runyon BA. Care of patients with ascites. N Engl J Med 1994;330: 337–342.

71. Felisart J, Rimola A, Arroyo V, et al. Randomized comparative study of efficacy and nephtrotoxicity of ampicillin plus tobramycin versus cefotaxime in cirrhotics with severe infections. Hepatology 1985;5:457–462.

72. Runyon BA, McHutchison JG, Antilon MR, et al. Short-course vs long-course antibiotic treatment of spontaneous bacterial peritonitis: A randomized controlled trial of 100 patients. Gastroenterology 1991;100:1737–1742.

73. Navasa M, Follo A, Llovet JM, et al. Randomized, comparative study of oral ofloxacin versus intravenous cefotaxime in spontaneous bacterial peritonitis. Gastroenterology 1996;111:1011–1017.

74. Angeli P, Guarda S, Fasolato S, et al. Switch therapy with ciprofloxacin vs intravenous ceftazidime in the treatment of spontaneous bacterial peritonitis in patients with cirrhosis: Similar efficacy at lower cost. Aliment Pharmacol Ther 2006;23:75–84.

75. Akriviadis EA, Runyon BA. The value of an algorithm in differentiating spontaneous from secondary bacterial peritonitis. Gastroenterology 1990;98:127–133.

76. Pache I, Bilodeau M. Severe haemorrhage following abdominal paracentesis for ascites in patients with liver failure. Aliment Pharmacol Ther 2005;21:525–529.

77. Pockros PJ, Reynolds TB. Rapid diuresis in patients with ascites from chronic liver disease: The importance of peripheral edema. Gastroenterology 1986;90:1827–1833.

78. Mas A. Hepatic encephalopathy: From pathophysiology to treatment. Digestion 2006;73(suppl 1):86–93.

79. Bustamante J, Rimola A, Ventura PJ, et al. Prognostic significance of hepatic encephalopathy in patients with cirrhosis. J Hepatol 1999;30:890–895.

80. Plauth M, Cabré E, Kondrup J, et al. ESPEN guidelines on parenteral nutrition: Hepatology. Clin Nutr 2009;28(4):436–444.

81. Charlton M. Branched-chain amino acid enriched supplements as therapy for liver disease. J Nutr 2006;136:295S–298S.

82. Morgan MY, Blei A, Grüngreiff K, et al. The treatment of hepatic encephalopathy. Metab Brain Dis 2007;22:389–405.

83. Cordoba J, Blei AT. Treatment of hpatic encephalopathy. Am J Gastroenterol 1997;92:1429–1439.

84. Riordan SM, Williams R. Treatment of hepatic encephalopathy. N Engl J Med 1997;337:473–479.

85. Blanc P, Daures JP, Liautard J, et al. Lactulose–neomycin combination versus placebo in the treatment of acute hepatic encephalopathy: Results of a randomized controlled trial. Gastroenterol Clin Biol 1994;18:1063–1068.

86. Hawkins RA, Jessy J, Mans AM, et al. Neomycin reduces the intestinal production of ammonia from glutamine. Adv Exp Med Biol 1994;368:125–134.

87. Morgan MH, Read AE, Speller DC. Treatment of hepatic encephalopathy with metronidazole. Gut 1982;23:1–7.

88. Gubbins GP, Moritz TE, Marsano LS, et al. Helicobacter pylori is a risk factor for hepatic encephalopathy in acute alcoholic hepatitis: The ammonia hypothesis revisited. The Veterans Administration cooperative study group no. 275. Am J Gastroenterol 1993;88:1906–1910.

89. Vasconez C, Elizalde JI, Llach J, et al. Helicobacter pylori, hyperammonemia and subclinical portosystemic encephalopathy: Effects of eradication. J Hepatol 1999;30:260–264.

90. Mas A, Rodes J, Sunyer L, et al. Comparison of rifaximin and lactitol in the treatment of acute hepatic encephalopathy: Results of a randomized, double-blind, double-dummy, controlled clinical trial. J Hepatol 2003;38:51–58.

91. Pedretti G, Calzetti C, Missale G, et al. Rifaximin versus neomycin on hyperammoniemia in chronic portal systemic encephalopathy in cirrhotics: A double-blind, randomized trial. Ital J Gastroenterol 1991;23:175–178.

92. Butterworth RF. Pathophysiology of hepatic encephalopathy: A new look at ammonia. Metab Brain Dis 2002;17:221–227.

93. Kircheis G, Nilium R, Held C, et al. Therapeutic efficacy of L-Ornithine-L-aspartate infusions in patients with cirrhosis and hepatic encephalopathy: Results of a placebo-controlled, double-blind study. Hepatology 1997;25:1351–1360.

94. Stauch S, Kircheis G, Adler G, et al. Oral L-ornithine-L-aspartate therapy of chronic hepaticencephalopathy: Results of a placebo-controlled double-blind study. J Hepatol 1998;28:856–864.

95. Riggio O, Ariosto F, Merli M, et al. Short-term oral zinc supplementation does not improve chronic hepatic encephalopathy: Results of a double-blind crossover trial. Dig Dis Sci 1991;36:1204–1208.

96. Marchesini G, Favvri A, Bianchi G, et al. Zinc supplementation and amino acid–nitrogen metabolism in patients with advanced cirrhosis. Hepatology 1996;23:1084–1092.

97. Basile AS, Hughes RD, Harrison PM, et al. Elevated brain concentrations of 1,4-benzodiazepines in fulminant hepatic failure. N Engl J Med 1991;325:473–478.

98. Als-Nielson B, Kjaergard LL, Glaudd C. Benzodiazepine receptor antagonists for acute and chronic hepatic encephalopathy. Cochrane Database Syst Rev 2001;4:CD002798.

99. Uribe M, Farca A, Marquez MA, et al. Treatment of chronic portal systemic encephalopathy with bromocriptine: A double-blind controlled trial. Gastroenterology 1979;76:1347–1351.

100. Garcia-Tsao G, Parikh CR, Viola A. Acute kidney injury in cirrhosis. Hepatology 2008;48:2064–2077.

101. Rodriquez-Roisin R, Krowka MJ. Hepatopulmonary syndrome—a liver-induced lung vascular disorder. New Engl J Med 2008;358:2378–2387.

102. Minemura M, Tajri K, Shimizu Y. Systemic abnormalities in liver disease. World J Gastroenterol 2009;15(24):2960–2974.

103. Verbeeck RK. Pharmacokinetics and dosage adjustment in patients with hepatic dysfunction. Eur J Clin Pharmacol 2008;64:1147–1161.

104. Hicken BL, Sharara AI, Abrams GA, et al. Hepatic venous pressure gradient measurements to assess response to primary prophylaxis in patients with cirrhosis: a decision analytical study. Aliment Pharmacol Ther 2003;17:145–153.

105. Rubenstein JH, Eisen GM, Inadomi JM. A cost-utility analysis of secondary prophylaxis for variceal hemorrhage. Am J Gastroenterol 2004;99:1274–1288.

WILLIAM R. KIRCHAIN AND RONDALL E. ALLEN

CHAPTER

45

Drug-Induced Liver Disease

KEY CONCEPTS

❶ The liver itself through its normally functioning enzymes and processes often causes a drug to become toxic through a process known as bioactivation.

❷ Drug-induced liver disease occurs as several different clinical presentations: idiosyncratic reactions, allergic hepatitis, toxic hepatitis, chronic active toxic hepatitis, toxic cirrhosis, and liver vascular disorders.

❸ The mechanisms of drug-induced liver disease are diverse, representing many phases of biotransformation, and are susceptible to genetic polymorphism.

❹ A fulminant or severe drug-induced reaction within the liver usually involves the immune system and is marked by large scale cell necrosis.

❺ The assessment of a possible liver injury caused by drugs should include what is known in the literature, the timing involved, the clinical course, and, always, an exploration for preexisting conditions that may have encouraged the lesion's development.

❻ Liver enzyme assays can help to determine if a particular type of liver damage is present.

❼ Monitoring for drug-induced liver disease must be tailored to the drug and the patient's potential risk factors.

Learning objectives, review questions, and other resources can be found at **www.pharmacotherapyonline.com**.

The number of drugs associated with adverse reactions involving the liver is extensive.[1] One of the more common reasons for the withdrawal of a drug from the marketplace is an elevation of serum concentrations of liver enzymes.[2] Its impact on the pharmaceutical industry has led regulatory agencies to withdraw drugs from the market, restrict the use of certain medications, and issue black box warnings.[3]

Alcohol-induced liver disease is the most common type of drug-induced liver disease. All other drugs together account for less than 10% of patients hospitalized for elevated liver enzymes.[4] Drug-induced liver disease accounts for as much as 20% of acute liver failure in pediatric populations and at least that many of adults with acute liver failure.[5] In approximately 75% of these cases liver transplantation is ultimately required for patient survival.[2] Of patients who required liver transplantation according to the United Network for Organ Sharing, acetaminophen, isoniazid, antiepileptics, and antibiotics collectively account for just over 60% of cases.[6] In a prospective analysis of 1,200 patients admitted to a hospital in South Carolina for liver dysfunction, isoniazid accounted for 21 of 132 cases with various antibiotics and sulfa drugs accounting for another 30 cases.[7] Overall, the reported incidence of drug-induced liver disease is around 1 in 10,000 to 1 in 100,000 patients.[1]

The liver's function affects almost every other organ system in the body, but there are no specific diagnostic tests for drug-induced liver disease or a means to single out an implicated drug. Therefore it is important to know the patterns of drug-related pathology in order to assess adverse reactions when they occur. ❶ The liver's normal metabolic outcome is to decrease the reactivity of a drug or toxin, in effect deactivating it. In many of the patterns of damage that this chapter will review, the first step is a net increase in reactivity that results from the normal processes of metabolism in the liver. This now bioactivated compound if left unconjugated or otherwise unbound is free to react in uncontrolled ways within the cell.

PATTERNS OF DRUG-INDUCED LIVER DISEASE

HEPATOCELLULAR INJURY

Hepatocellular injury is characterized by significant elevations in the serum aminotransferases which usually precede elevations in total bilirubin levels and alkaline phosphatase levels.[8] Most injuries occur within 1 year of initiating the offending agent. Hepatocellular injury can lead to fulminant hepatitis with a corresponding 20% survival rate with supportive care.[9] For those patients who present with the combination of hepatocellular injury and jaundice, there is a 10% mortality rate.[10] Acarbose, allopurinol, fluoxetine, and losartan are capable of causing hepatocellular injury.[8]

❷ Hepatocellular injuries can be further subdivided by specific histologic patterns and clinical presentations. Centrolobular necrosis, steatohepatitis (steatonecrosis), phospholipidosis, and generalized hepatocellular necrosis are each identifiable by particular biopsy results and subtle differences in clinical presentation.

CENTROLOBULAR NECROSIS

❷ Centrolobular necrosis is often a dose-related, predictable reaction; however, it also can be associated with idiosyncratic reactions. Also called direct or metabolite-related hepatotoxicity, centrolobular necrosis is usually the result of the production of a toxic metabolite (Fig. 45–1). The damage spreads outward from the middle of a lobe of the liver.

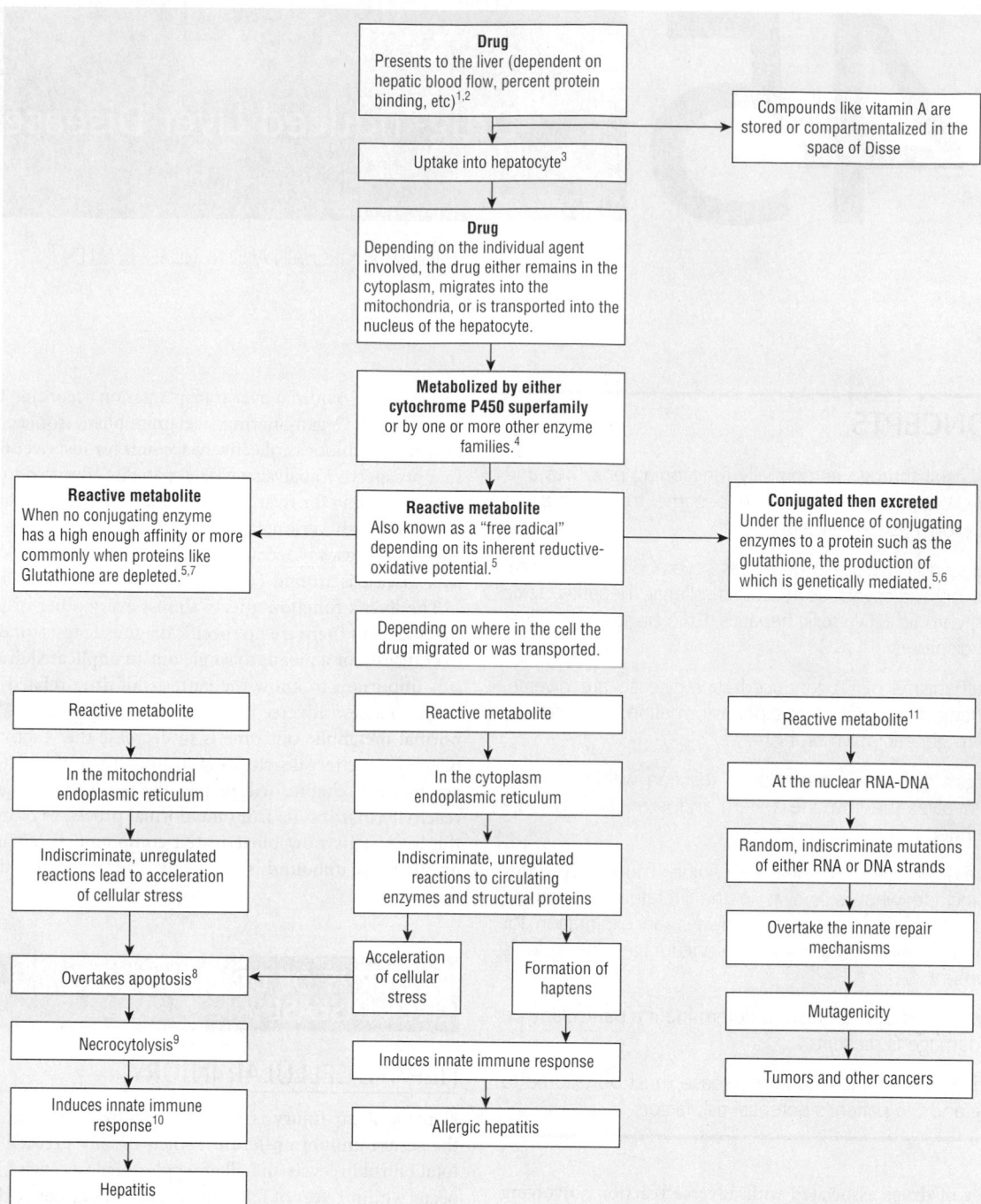

FIGURE 45-1. A general diagram of biotransformation. (1) Hepatic blood flow, which changes proportionately with changes in cardiac output, delivers the drug to the liver. (2) Protein binding is most affected by nutritional status and competing drugs. (3) The drug is actively transported into the hepatocyte by the organic anion transport pump, a transmembrane protein. (4) The metabolite (drug) interacts with one of a number of enzymes, the most common being CYP2C9, 2C19, 2D6, and 3A4. This family of enzymes is regulated by the complementary DNA xenobiotic receptor. The xenobiotic receptor is in turn upregulated by other drugs, changes in cholesterol catabolism, and bile acids. The immediate result of the action of these phase I enzymes is the production of a reactive metabolite. (5) The unstable metabolite then reacts with glucuronidase, various transferases, or hydroxylases to form a conjugated metabolite. The efficacy of these enzymes is affected by the patient's nutritional state and genetic polymorphism, leading to variations in individual risk for toxicity. (6) The conjugated metabolite is removed from the hepatocyte by the canalicular membrane export pump, one of a large family of membrane proteins (other members of this family pump conjugated metabolites back into the blood for excretion by the kidney). These proteins are subject to genetic polymorphism as well, again leading to some patients having an increased risk for toxicity. (7) If unable to form a conjugate, the unstable metabolite can participate in oxidative reactions that damage lipids, proteins, or even DNA. (8) The normal process of cellular aging, death, and reabsorption by surrounding cells. (9) Widespread, rapid cellular death with the creation of multiple antigens. (10) Activation Kupffer cells, killer cells, B-cells, and other T-cells with the associated production of inflammatory cytokines the relative numbers of which and the innate activity of each mediated by genetic polymorphism. (11) Drugs or active metabolites that are transported or diffuse into the mitochondria or the nucleus can damage DNA, leading to mutagenicity and ultimately hepatic cancers.

Patients suffering from centrolobular necrosis tend to present in one of two ways, depending on the extent of necrosis. Mild drug reactions, involving only small amounts of parenchymal liver tissue, may be detected as asymptomatic elevations in the serum aminotransferases. If the reaction is diagnosed at this stage, most of these patients will recover with minimal cirrhosis and thus minimal chronic liver impairment. More severe forms of centrolobular necrosis are accompanied by nausea, vomiting, upper abdominal pain, and jaundice.[11,12]

These reactions are predictable, often dose-related effects in the liver caused by specific agents. When taken in overdose, acetaminophen becomes bioactivated to a toxic intermediate known as N-acetyl-p-benzoquinone imine (NAPQI). NAPQI is very reactive, with a high affinity for sulfhydryl groups. The protein glutathione provides a ready source of available sulfhydryl groups within the hepatocyte. When the liver's glutathione stores are depleted and there are no longer sulfhydryl groups available to detoxify this metabolite, it begins to react directly with the hepatocyte (see Fig. 45–1). In addition, the depletion of glutathione changes the mitochondrial oxidized to reduced glutathione ratio resulting in catastrophic shifts in mitochondrial function, accelerating cell necrocytolysis.[13] Replenishing the liver's sulfhydryl capacity through the administration of N-acetylcysteine early after ingestion of the overdose halts this process.[13] During the first hours after ingestion, some patients report mild symptoms of nausea and vomiting, but no elevations of the commonly measured liver enzymes are seen. Serum elevations in the liver enzymes begin 40 to 50 hours after ingestion.[14]

Reye syndrome is an aggressive form of toxic hepatitis often associated with aspirin use in children. Valproate toxicity can also present in this pattern. Early in the process of Reye syndrome, mitochondrial dysfunction leads to the depletion of acyl-coenzyme A and carnitine. Fatty acids accumulate and gluconeogenesis is impaired, resulting in hypoglycemia. A concurrent disruption of the urea cycle occurs, leading to a decrease in the removal of ammonia and a slowing of protein use. A threefold rise in the blood ammonia level and an increase in the prothrombin time are common findings. In advanced stages of Reye's syndrome, many patients develop intracranial hypertension that can be life-threatening and refractory to therapy.[15,16]

NONALCOHOLIC STEATOHEPATITIS

Nonalcoholic steatohepatitis (NASH), also known as steatohepatitis and steatonecrosis, results from the accumulation of fatty acids in the hepatocyte. In the pre-acute stages this is known as nonalcoholic fatty liver disease (NAFLD). Drugs or their metabolites that cause NAFLD do so by affecting fatty-acid esterification and oxidation rates within the mitochondria of the hepatocyte (see Fig. 45–1). Hepatic vesicles become engorged with fatty acids, eventually disrupting hepatocyte homeostasis. In patients with diabetes, various dyslipidemias and even hypertension, the de novo production of free fatty acids from excess circulating carbohydrates, accelerates this process of accumulation. The liver biopsy is marked by a massive infiltration by polymorpho-nuclear leukocytes, degeneration of the hepatocytes, and the presence of Mallory bodies.[4]

Alcohol is the drug that most commonly produces steatonecrotic changes in the liver. When alcohol is converted into acetaldehyde, the synthesis of fatty acids is increased.[17,18] The hepatocyte can become completely engorged with microvesicular fat, resulting in alcoholic fatty liver. Metabolically this type of de novo free fatty acid synthesis depletes NADPH in favor of NADP+ and reduces the hepatocytes' ability to respond to stress, bypassing normal apoptosis and increasing the rate of necrocytolysis. In NAFLD, the same end point is often achieved through oxidation of lipid peroxidases.[19] If the offending agent is withdrawn before significant numbers of hepatocytes become necrotic, the process is completely reversible

without long-term sequelae. If not, then ever increasing rates of necrocytolysis will induce an innate immune response and result in hepatitis.

Tetracycline produces NAFLD and NASH.[20] The lesions are characterized by large vesicles of fat found diffused throughout the liver. The development of this reaction is related to the high concentrations achieved when tetracycline is given intravenously and in doses greater than 1.5 g/day. The mortality of tetracycline steatohepatitis is high (70%–80%), and those who do survive often develop cirrhosis. Sodium valproate also can produce steatonecrosis through the process of bioactivation. ❶ Cytochrome P450 converts valproate to delta-4-valproic acid, a potent inducer of microvesicular fat accumulation.[21]

Patients experiencing steatohepatitis may present with abdominal fullness or pain as their only complaint. Patients with more severe steatonecrosis will present with all the symptoms characteristic of alcoholic hepatitis such as nausea, vomiting, steatorrhea, abdominal pain, pruritus, and fatigue.

PHOSPHOLIPIDOSIS

Phospholipidosis is the accumulation of phospholipids instead of fatty acids. The phospholipids usually engorge the lysosomal bodies of the hepatocyte.[22] Amiodarone is associated with this reaction. Patients treated with amiodarone who develop overt hepatic disease tend to have received higher doses of the drug. These patients also have higher amiodarone-to-N-desethyl-amiodarone ratios, indicating a greater accumulation of the parent compound. Amiodarone and its major metabolite N-desethyl-amiodarone remain in the liver of all patients for several months after therapy is stopped. Usually the phospholipidosis develops in patients treated for more than 1 year. The patient can present with either elevated aminotransferases or hepatomegaly; jaundice is rare.[4,23]

GENERALIZED HEPATOCELLULAR NECROSIS

Generalized hepatocellular necrosis mimics the changes associated with the more common viral hepatitis. The onset of symptoms is usually delayed as much as a week or more after exposure to toxin. Bioactivation is often important for toxic hepatitis to develop. Many drugs that are associated with toxic hepatitis produce metabolites that are not inherently toxic to the liver. Instead, they bind with proteins to create haptens, which serve as neoantigens and induce the innate immune response (see Fig. 45–1).[24]

❶ The rate of bioactivation can vary between males and females and between individuals of the same sex.[25,26] The superfamily of cytochrome P450 (CYP450) enzymes metabolize lipophilic substrates that are actively pumped into the hepatocyte by an organic anion (or cation) transporting protein. The CYP450 subspecies 2C, 2D, 3A, and 4A are regulated by the highly inducible xenobiotic receptor on complementary DNA. The receptor is found in the liver, and to a lesser extent in the cells lining the intestinal tract, and is responsible for cholesterol catabolism and bile acid homeostasis. ❸ The activity of this receptor is subject to genetic polymorphism. This results in a wide variation in the sensitivity of the population to hepatic damage.[27]

The long-term administration of isoniazid can lead to hepatic dysfunction in 10% to 20% of those receiving the drug. Yet severe toxic hepatitis develops in only 1% or less of this population.[28] ❸ The N-acetyltransferase 2 (NAT2) genotype appears to play a role in determining a patient's relative risk. In one study, patients with the slow-type NAT2 genotype had a 28-fold greater risk of developing serum aminotransferase elevations than did patients with the fast-type NAT2 genotype.[29] Isoniazid is metabolized by several pathways, acetylation being the major pathway. It is acetylated to acetylisoniazid, which, in turn, is hydrolyzed to acetylhydrazine.[30] The acetylhydrazine, and to a lesser extent the acetylisoniazid, are directly toxic to the cellular proteins in the hepatocyte, but rapid acetylators detoxify acetylhydrazine very rapidly, converting it to diacetylhydrazine (a nontoxic metabolite). Therefore, it is the rate and efficiency of this reaction sequence that ultimately determines if hepatocellular damage will ensue.

Isoniazid simultaneously is an example of the potential predictability of drug-induced liver disease based on single nucleotide polymorphism and a lesson in the limitations of our current understanding. ❸ There are definite links to NAT2 genotype and toxicity.[31] The risk for this reaction is also influenced heavily by the age of the patient, with older patients having a much higher risk than younger patients. In fact, age may be more important than genotype.[28,29,31] In one prospective series focused on drug-induced liver disease, cases involving isoniazid had a median onset at 6 months of therapy with around 30% of isoniazid-induced liver disease clustered between 6 to 8 months.[7]

Ketoconazole produces generalized hepatocellular necrosis or milder forms of hepatic dysfunction in 1% to 2% of patients treated for fungal infections. The onset is usually early in therapy. In immunocompromised patients in whom ketoconazole is used, special care should be taken to watch for changes in liver function.[32]

TOXIC CIRRHOSIS

The scarring effect of hepatitis in the liver leads to the development of cirrhosis. Some drugs tend to cause such a mild case of hepatitis that it may not be detected. Mild hepatitis can be easily mistaken for a more routine generalized viral infection. If the offending drug or agent is not discontinued, this damage will continue to progress. The patient eventually presents not with hepatitis, but with cirrhosis.

Methotrexate causes periportal fibrosis in most patients who experience hepatotoxicity. ❶ The lesion results from the action of a bioactivated metabolite produced by CYP450.[33] This process occurs most commonly in patients treated for psoriasis and arthritis. The extent of damage can be reduced or controlled by increasing the dosage interval to once weekly or by routine use of folic acid supplements.[33] Vitamin A is normally stored in liver cells, and causes significant hypertrophy and fibrosis when taken for long periods in high doses. Hepatomegaly is a common finding, along with ascites and portal hypertension. In patients with vitamin A toxicity, gingivitis and dry skin are also very common. This is accelerated by ethanol, which competes with retinol for aldehyde dehydrogenase.[17]

CHOLESTATIC INJURY

❷ A second pattern of hepatic damage is an injury that primarily involves the bile canalicular system and is known as cholestatic injury. Cholestatic disease is more often seen in patients over the age of 60 and is slightly more common in males.[34] In cholestatic disease, disturbance of the subcellular actin filaments around the canaliculi prevents the movement of bile through the canalicular system.[35] The inability of the liver to remove bile causes intrahepatic accumulation of toxic bile acids and excretion products.[36] Although rare, some patients develop progressive destruction of the cholangiocytes leading to the vanishing bile duct syndrome.

Drug-induced cholestasis can occur as an acute disorder (e.g., cholestasis with or without hepatitis and cholestasis with bile duct injury) or as a chronic disorder (e.g., vanishing bile duct syndrome, sclerosing cholangitis, and cholelithiasis).[37] However, the most common form of drug-induced cholestasis is cholestasis with hepatitis. Most patients with this acute disorder present with nausea, malaise, jaundice, and pruritus.[8] Elevations in serum alkaline phosphatase levels are more prominent and usually precede the elevations of

other liver enzymes in serum.[5] A liver biopsy is not usually required, but is sometimes pursued when other causes of cholestatic disease are suspected.[38] Although the antipsychotic drug chlorpromazine appears to be the prototype drug for this disorder, other medications are associated with other forms of cholestatic injury, such as erythromycin estolate, amoxicillin-clavulanic acid, and carbamazepine.[9]

Cholestatic injury, also known as cholestatic jaundice or cholestasis, can be classified by the area of the bile canalicular or ductal system that is impaired. Canalicular cholestasis is often associated with long-term, high-dose estrogen therapy. These patients are often asymptomatic and present with mild to moderate elevations of serum bilirubin.[39] An intravenous form of vitamin E, α-tocopherol acetate, causes cholestatic jaundice, primarily involving the canalicular duct in premature infants. The incidence of this reaction in those receiving this formulation was high (>10%) and the mortality even higher (>50%).[40]

The administration of total parenteral nutrition for periods greater than 1 week induces cholestatic changes and nonspecific enzyme elevations in some patients. Patients with low serum albumin concentrations may be at greater risk than patients with normal serum albumin concentrations.[4] This reaction also has been reported to occur rarely with sulfonamides, sulfonylureas, erythromycin estolate and ethylsuccinate, captopril, lisinopril, and other phenothiazines.[41]

MIXED HEPATOCELLULAR AND CHOLESTATIC INJURY

❶ The final pattern of hepatic damage is a combining of the previous two patterns. This presentation can be the result of three different processes. In some patients, an injury may begin as hepatocellular (or cholestatic) and simply spread so rapidly that by the time the patient presents for diagnosis and treatment, all areas of the liver are affected. In other patients, the underlying mechanism of damage is such that cells are injured regardless of their anatomical location or primary metabolic role.

LIVER VASCULAR DISORDERS

Focal lesions in hepatic venules, sinusoids, and portal veins occur with various drugs. The most commonly associated drugs are the cytotoxic agents used to treat cancer, the pyrrolizidine alkaloids, and the sex hormones. A centralized necrosis often follows and can result in cirrhosis. Azathioprine and herbal teas that contain comfrey (a source of pyrrolizidine alkaloids) are associated with the development of venoocclusive disease. The exact incidence is rare and may be dose related.[4] Peliosis hepatitis is a rare type of hepatic vascular lesion that can be seen as both an acute and a chronic disease. The liver develops large, blood-filled lacunae (space or cavity) within the parenchyma. Rupture of the lacunae can lead to severe peritoneal hemorrhage. Peliosis hepatitis is associated with exposure of the liver to androgens, estrogens, tamoxifen, azathioprine, and danazol. Androgens with a methyl alkylation at the 17-carbon position of the testosterone structure are the most frequently reported agents that cause peliosis hepatitis, usually after at least 6 months of therapy.[42]

MECHANISMS OF DRUG-INDUCED LIVER DISEASE

STIMULATION OF AUTOIMMUNITY

❹ Autoimmune injuries involve antibody mediated cytotoxicity or direct cellular toxicity.[38,43] This type of injury occurs when enzyme drug adducts migrate to the cell surface and form neoantigens. The liver plays host to all of the cells that make up the innate immune response system in the body along with Kupffer cells which are a type of macrophage. These cells sit in anticipation around the hepatocytes, in the space of Disse and elsewhere waiting for antigens (or neoantigens) to present themselves. The neoantigens serve as targets for cytolytic attack by killer T-cells, and others.[7] Halothane, sulfamethoxazole, carbamazepine, and nevirapine are associated with autoimmune injuries.[35] Stimulation of autoimmunity is often associated with fulminant presentations.

Dantrolene, isoniazid, phenytoin, nitrofurantoin, and trazodone are associated with a type of autoimmune-mediated disease in the liver called *chronic active hepatitis*.[11] Patients experience periods of symptomatic hepatitis followed by periods of convalescence, only to repeat the experience months later. It is a progressive disease with a high mortality rate and is more common in females than males. Antinuclear antibodies appear in most patients. These drugs appear to form antiorganelle antibodies.[23] The exact identification of a causative agent is sometimes difficult as diagnosis requires multiple episodes occurring long after exposure to the offending drug.

IDIOSYNCRATIC REACTIONS

Idiosyncratic drug-related hepatotoxicity is rare and usually occurs in a small proportion of individuals. These adverse reactions are often categorized into allergic and nonallergic reactions. ❹ The allergic reactions are characterized by fever, rash, and eosinophilia. They are usually dose-related and have a short latency period (<1 month). Upon reexposure to the offending agent, the patient will experience rapid recurrence of hepatotoxicity. Studies show that minocycline, nitrofurantoin, and phenytoin can cause allergic reactions.[3]

Unlike the allergic reactions, the nonallergic idiosyncratic reactions are devoid of the hypersensitivity features and usually have a long latency period (several months). These patients often have normal liver function tests for 6 months or longer and then suddenly develop hepatotoxicity. Dependent on the medication, the incident can be independent of dose or dose related. Amiodarone, isoniazid, and ketoconazole are associated with nonallergic drug-related hepatotoxicity.[3]

DISRUPTION OF CALCIUM HOMEOSTASIS AND CELL MEMBRANE INJURY

Drug-induced damage to the cellular proteins that are involved with calcium homeostasis can lead to an influx of intracellular calcium that causes a decline in adenosine triphosphate levels and disruption of the actin fibril assembly. The resulting impact on the cell is blebbing of the cell membrane, rupture, and cell lysis.[36] Lovastatin, venlafaxine, and phalloidin, which is the active component of mushrooms, impair calcium homeostasis.[36,43]

METABOLIC ACTIVATION OF THE CYTOCHROME P450 ENZYMES

Most hepatocellular injuries involve the production of high-energy reactive metabolites by the CYP450 system. These reactive metabolites are capable of forming covalent bonds with cellular proteins (enzymes) and nucleic acids that lead to adduct formation. In the case of acute toxicity, the enzyme-drug adduct can cause cell injury or cell lysis. Adducts that form with DNA can cause long-term consequences such as neoplasia. Acetaminophen, furosemide, and diclofenac are examples of this mechanism of liver injury.[44] Individual genetic differences can play a role in the significance of this process. Patients with a single nucleotide polymorphism (SNP) that codes for slow-reacting variants of CYP450 will react differently from those with a SNP that codes for very fast-reacting variants.

STIMULATION OF APOPTOSIS

Apoptosis represents a distinct pattern of cell lysis that is characterized by cell shrinkage and fragmentation of nuclear chromatin. Apoptotic pathways are triggered by interactions between death ligands (tumor necrosis factor and Fas ligand) and death receptors (tumor necrosis factor receptor 1 and Fas). These interactions activate caspases which cleave cellular proteins and eventually lead to cell death.[45] Cumulative doses of acetaminophen cause apoptosis.[43]

MITOCHONDRIAL INJURY

Drugs that impair mitochondrial structure, function, or DNA synthesis can disrupt β-oxidation of lipids and oxidative energy production within the hepatocyte.[35] In acute disease, prolonged interruption of β-oxidation leads to microvesicular steatosis, whereas, in chronic disease, macrovesicular disease is present.[9] Severe damage to the mitochondria eventually leads to hepatic failure and death. Aspirin, valproic acid, and tetracycline cause mitochondrial injury by inhibiting β-oxidation and amiodarone via disruption of oxidative phosphorylation.[36]

LIVER NEOPLASTIC DISEASE

A large body of the current literature on adverse reactions and the liver addresses the development of neoplasms following drug therapy. Both carcinoma- and sarcoma-like lesions have been identified. Fortunately, hepatic tumors associated with drug therapy are usually benign and remit when drug therapy is discontinued. Except in rare instances, these lesions are associated with long-term exposure to the offending agent.[46] Androgens, estrogens, and other hormonal-related agents are the most frequently associated causes of neoplastic disease. The model for drug-induced hepatic cancer is polyvinyl chloride exposure. Used in the production of many types of plastic products, polyvinyl chloride induces angiosarcoma in exposed workers after as few as 3 years of exposure.[47]

ASSESSMENT

The best and most important technique for assessing and monitoring drug-induced liver disease is the patient's history. ❺ Questions addressing the patient's drug use along with a thorough review of systems are essential. The use of a protocol, such as that proposed by Danan and Benichou, can significantly improve the accuracy of the assessment (Table 45–1).[48] Drugs for recreational purposes must not be overlooked. Cocaine has been directly linked to liver disease.[49] Ecstasy, the street name of methylenedioxymethamphetamine, has induced fulminant hepatitis, which has led to death in some cases.[50] The more pervasive impact of street drugs on the incidence of hepatic disease is the concomitant injection or ingestion of adulterants. Many of these adulterants are either directly toxic or serve to enhance the toxicity of the drug.

It is also important to determine nondrug hepatic disease risk from occupational or environmental exposure. Arsenic, for example, is known to induce both acute and chronic hepatic reactions.[50] Even if exposure to an environmental toxin does not produce a hepatic reaction, it may predispose a patient to a hepatic reaction when a drug is added. Table 45–2 lists some of the more common hepatic toxins found in occupational or environmental exposures that can add to the risk for developing a hepatic lesion.[51] Immune-mediated chronic liver diseases can often be tracked to geographic clusters that correspond to known toxic waste sites around the world.[51]

TABLE 45-1 An Approach to Evaluating a Suspected Hepatotoxic Reaction Using a Clinical Diagnostic Scale

Patient Presents with Elevated Liver Enzymes	Score	Component Subscore
Literature		
Literature supports this drug (drug combination) and pattern of liver enzyme elevation	+2	
No literature supports this, but the drug has been on the market less than 5 years	+0	–
No literature supports this and the drug has been on the market for 5 years or more	–3	
Alternative causes		
Alternative causes (e.g., viral, alcohol) are completely ruled out	+3	
Alternative causes are partially ruled out	+0	–
Alternative causes cannot be ruled out and are possible or even probable	–1	
Presentation		
The presentation includes 4 or more extrahepatic (fever, malaise, etc.) symptoms	+3	
The presentation includes 2–3 extrahepatic symptoms	+2	–
The presentation includes only 1 identifiable extrahepatic symptom	+1	
The presentation is essentially a laboratory abnormality, with no extrahepatic symptoms	+0	
Temporality		
Initiation of drug therapy to onset is 4–56 days	+3	
Initiation of drug therapy to onset is <4 or >56 days	+1	
Discontinuance of therapy to onset is 0–7 days	+3	–
Discontinuance of therapy to onset is 8–15 days	+0	
Discontinuance of therapy to onset is >15 days	–1	
Rechallenge		
Rechallenge was positive	+3	–
Rechallenge was negative or not attempted	+0	
Total Score		–

The likelihood that this presentation is an adverse reaction in the liver increases linearly with an increasing score. The maximum score is 14, and scores below 7 are associated with an ever decreasing likelihood that the drug or drug combination in question caused the problem. This approach is not designed for the assessment of hepatic cancers or cirrhotic conditions.

Reprinted from J Clin Epidemiol, Vol 46, Danan G, Benichou C. Causality assessment of adverse reactions to drugs–I. A novel method based on the conclusions of international consensus meetings: Application to drug-induced liver injuries: pages 1323–1330, Copyright 1993, with permission from Elsevier.

A person's use of alternative medicine must be solicited. In the prospective series of cases noted earlier, from an area of the country where traditional medicine usage is commonplace, herbal remedies and other traditional medicines accounted for 14 of 132 cases of

TABLE 45-2 Environmental Hepatotoxins and Associated Occupations at Risk for Exposure

Hepatotoxin	Associated Occupations at Risk for Exposure
Arsenic	Chemical plant, agricultural workers
Carbon tetrachloride	Chemical plant workers, laboratory technicians
Copper	Plumbers, sculpture artists, foundry workers
Dimethylformamide	Chemical plant workers, laboratory technicians
2,4-Dichlorophenoxyacetic acid	Horticulturists
Fluorine	Chemical plant workers, laboratory technicians
Toluene	Chemical plant, agricultural workers, laboratory tech
Trichloroethylene	Printers, dye workers, cleaners, laboratory technicians
Vinyl chloride	Plastics plant workers; also found as a river pollutant

drug-induced liver disease.[7] Comfrey tea is a common cause of hepatocellular damage. As in the case of the Chinese remedy *jin bu huan*, or as in the case of the more elegantly presented chaparral capsules containing grease wood leaves, the end of therapy with these types of agents is occasionally severe disability or death from fulminant hepatic failure.[52] Pennyroyal oil, margosa oil, and clove oil cause a dose-related hepatotoxicity.[52]

The nutritional status of a patient can be as important to the development of a drug-induced liver disease as the hepatotoxin itself.[50] Patients who are malnourished because of illness or long-term alcohol abuse make up the most troublesome group.[53] Low serum levels of vitamins E and C, along with lutein and the α- and β-carotenes are associated with asymptomatic elevations in transaminases. Conversely, high serum iron, transferrin, and selenium levels are also associated with asymptomatic elevations of transaminases.[54]

All potential drug reactions should be judged as to the timing of the reaction versus drug administration, pharmacokinetic considerations, the information in the literature records about previous reactions, the inclusion of alternative nondrug causes, and close clinical observation when the drug in question is stopped. It is also important to keep in mind that most elevations in liver enzymes will not be associated with a drug. In a study of all patients admitted to a hospital in the United Kingdom with elevated liver aminotransferases, only 9% of cases involved a drug other than alcohol as the possible cause.[3] In all cases, titers of serum antibodies to hepatitis A, B, and C should be drawn. Even in cases in which the drug is absolutely targeted as the cause, viral hepatitis may be a complication.

Often there is no good clinical test available to determine the exact type of hepatic lesion, short of liver biopsy. ❻ There are certain patterns of enzyme elevation that have been identified and can be helpful (Table 45–3).[55,56] The specificity of any serum enzyme depends on the distribution of that enzyme in the body. Alkaline phosphatase is found in the bile duct epithelium, bone, and intestinal and kidney cells. 5'-Nucleotidase is more specific for hepatic disease than alkaline phosphatase, because most of the body's store of 5'-nucleotidase is in the liver. Glutamate dehydrogenase is a good indicator of centrolobular necrosis because it is found primarily in centrolobular mitochondria. Most hepatic cells have extremely high concentrations of transaminases. Aspartate aminotransferase (AST) and alanine aminotransferase (ALT) are commonly measured in serum. Because of their high concentrations and easy liberation from the hepatocyte cytoplasm, AST and ALT are sensitive indicators of necrotic lesions within the liver. After an acute hepatic lesion is established, it may take weeks for these concentrations to return to normal.[56]

Serum bilirubin concentration is a sensitive indicator of most hepatic lesions and has significant prognostic value. High peak bilirubin concentrations are associated with poor survival. Other important findings that indicate poor survival are a peak prothrombin time greater than 40 seconds, elevated serum creatinine, and low arterial pH. The presence of encephalopathy or prolonged jaundice are not good signs for the survival of the patient and are strong indicators for transplantation.[57]

Bilirubin concentrations and serum enzyme elevations give a static picture of the liver's condition and are not good indicators of hepatic function. Clinically available tests to predict hepatic function include measurement of serum proteins (albumin or transferrin). As a hepatic function decreases, serum protein concentrations in the body decrease at a rate determined by each protein's own elimination rate. Overhydration and starvation can also decrease serum protein concentrations. Changes in the prothrombin time often occur earlier than the changes in albumin or transferrin. The response of the prothrombin time to the administration of 10 mg of parenteral vitamin K is often used to differentiate between hepatic and extrahepatic disease.

TABLE 45-3 Relative Patterns of Hepatic Enzyme Elevation versus Type of Hepatic Lesion

Enzyme	Abbreviations	Necrotic	Cholestatic	Chronic
Alkaline phosphatase	Alk Phos, AP	↑	↑↑↑	↑
5′-Nucleotidase	5-NC, 5NC	↑	↑↑↑	↑
γ-Glutamyltransferase	GGT, GGTP	↑	↑↑↑	↑↑
Aspartate aminotransferase	AST, SGOT	↑↑↑	↑	↑↑
Alanine aminotransferase	ALT, SGPT	↑↑↑	↑	↑↑
Lactate dehydrogenase	LDH	↑↑↑	↑	↑

↑, <100% of normal; ↑↑, >100% of normal, ↑↑↑, >200% of normal.

MEASUREMENT OF LIVER FUNCTION

A good compound for a liver function test would theoretically be (a) nontoxic and lacking any pharmacologic effect; (b) either rapidly and completely absorbed orally or easily administered via a peripheral vein; (c) eliminated only by the liver; and (d) easily measured (drug and its metabolite) in blood, saliva, or urine.[58]

Several tests are used in research settings and in liver transplant patients to indicate liver function. Tests such as sulfobromophthalein, indocyanine green, or sorbitol measure qualities of hepatic clearance. There are also a few drugs that have been used to test liver function. The advantage of sorbitol over indocyanine green is a much lower incidence of allergic reactions. It is partially cleared by the kidney, and urine levels must also be determined during the test.[58] A good estimate of hepatic clearance can be obtained by serial blood levels of a variety of hepatically eliminated drugs if an assay is locally available. Ultrasound and computed tomographic imaging can be used on a periodic basis to monitor for the development of fibrosis or vascular lesions in the liver and for hepatocellular carcinomas.[60]

If a liver biopsy has been performed, the injury should be classified by the histologic findings. ❻ In cases in which there is no biopsy, the pattern of liver enzyme elevation can estimate the type of injury. Hepatocellular injuries are marked by elevations in transaminase that are at least two times normal. If the alkaline phosphatase is also elevated, a hepatocellular lesion is still suspected when the elevation of ALT is notably higher than the elevation of alkaline phosphatase. If the magnitude of elevation is nearly equal between ALT and alkaline phosphatase, the lesion is likely cholestatic.

A liver injury is acute if it lasts less than 3 months; it is considered chronic after 3 months of consistent symptoms or enzyme elevation. A liver injury is severe if the patient has marked jaundice, if the prothrombin time does not improve by more than 50% after the administration of vitamin K, or if encephalopathy is detectable. If an acute liver injury progresses from normal to severe in a matter of a few days or weeks, it is considered fulminant.[61,62]

MONITORING

The serum transaminases AST and ALT are the most commonly used transaminases in the clinical setting. There are often no set rules available for a particular drug. ❼ The general guidelines found in Table 45–4 can help in determining a monitoring schedule for drugs where no prior recommendations are published. Concentrations of these enzymes should be obtained approximately every 4 weeks, depending on the reported characteristics of the reaction in question. Methotrexate should be monitored every 4 weeks, because toxicity usually develops over a period of several weeks to months.[60] In addition, some recommend that sulfobromophthalein or indocyanine green excretion studies be performed on a regular basis and that patients treated for very long periods of time should have a liver biopsy performed every 12 months.[63]

ABBREVIATIONS

ALT: alanine aminotransferase

AST: aspartate aminotransferase

CYP450: cytochrome P450 liver enzyme system

NAFLD: nonalcoholic fatty liver disease

TABLE 45-4 An Approach to Determining a Drug-Monitoring Plan to Detect Hepatotoxicity in Patients Initiated on Hepatotoxic Drugs

Draw a baseline set of blood samples for liver enzymes, bilirubin, and albumin before beginning the drug

↓

Is the patient pregnant?
Is the patient older than age 60 years?
Is the patient exposed to an environmental hepatotoxin at work or at home?
Is the patient drinking more than one alcoholic beverage per day or bingeing?
Is the patient using any injected recreational drug?
Is the patient using herbal remedies or tisanes that are associated with hepatic damage?
Is the patient's diet deficient in magnesium, vitamin E, vitamin C, or α- or β-carotenes?
Is the patient's diet excessive in vitamin A, iron, or selenium?
Does the patient have hypertriglyceridemia or type 2 diabetes mellitus?
Does the patient have juvenile arthritis or systemic lupus erythematosus?
Does the patient have chronic or chronic remitting viral hepatitis (hepatitis B or C)?

↓

Yes to one to two risk factors	No
↓	↓
Redraw liver enzymes every 180 days depending on the drug, for the first year	Redraw liver enzymes if other signs or symptoms manifest

Does the patient have more than two risk factors?
Is the drug identified as one that may cause a predictable hepatotoxic reaction?[a]

Yes	No	No
↓	↓	↓
Redraw liver enzymes every 60–90 days depending on the drug, for the first year	Redraw liver enzymes every 180 days as directed above for the first year	Redraw liver enzymes if other signs or symptoms manifest

If no toxicity is manifested during the first year of therapy, then redraw liver enzymes every 6–12 months; assess liver for cirrhosis every 1–2 years by ultrasound and every 4–6 years by CT or MRI scan; biopsy as directed by other findings

[a]A drug can become a predictable risk if it is administered concurrently with another drug or food that is known to induce or inhibit its metabolism.

NAPQI: *N*-acetyl-*p*-benzoquinone imine

NASH: nonalcoholic steatohepatitis

NAT2: *N*-acetyltransferase 2 genotype

SNP: single nucleotide polymorphism

REFERENCES

1. Biour M, Jaillon PJ. [Drug-induced hepatic diseases]. Pathol Biol (Paris) 1999;47:928–937.

2. Lee W. Drug-induced hepatotoxicity. N Engl J Med 2003;349:474–485.

3. Kaplowitz N. Idiosyncratic drug hepatotoxicity. Nat Rev Drug Discov 2005;4:489–499.

4. Lewis J. Drug-induced liver disease. Med Clin North Am 2000;84: 1275–1311.

5. Murray KF. Drug-related hepatotoxicity and acute liver failure. J Pediatr Gastroenterol Nutr 2008;47:395–405.

6. Mindikoglu AL. Magder LS, Regev A. Oucome of liver transplantation for drug-induced acute liver failure in the United States: Analysis of the united network for organ sharing database. Liver Transpl 2009;15:675–676, 719–729.

7. Reuben A, Koch DG, Lee WM. Acute liver failure (ALF) secondary to drug induced liver injury (DILI): Causes & consequences. Hepatology 2009;50:347A.

8. Navarro V, Senior J. Drug-related hepatotoxicity. N Engl J Med 2006;354:731–739.

9. Rmachandran R, Kakar S. Histological patterns in drug-induced liver disease. J Clin Pathol 2009;62:481–492.

10. Bjornsson E. Drug-induced liver injury: Hy's rule revisited. Clin Pharmacol Ther 2006;79:521–528.

11. Fernandes NF, Martin RR, Schenker S. Trazodone-induced hepatotoxicity: A case report with comments on drug-induced hepatotoxicity. Am J Gastroenterol 2000;95:532–535.

12. Fontana RJ, McCashland TM, Benner KG, et al. Acute liver failure associated with prolonged use of bromfenac leading to liver transplantation. The Acute Liver Failure Study Group. Liver Transpl Surg 1999;5:480–484.

13. Riemer J, Bulleid N, Herrmann JM. Dissulfide formation in the ER and mitchondria: Two solutions to a common process. Science 2009;324:1284–1287.

14. Tan H, Chang CY, Martin P. Acetaminophen hepatotoxicity: Current management. Mt Sinai J Med 2009;76:75–83.

15. Belay ED, Bresee JS, Holman RC, et al. Reye's syndrome in the United States from 1981 through 1997 [see comments]. N Engl J Med 1999;340:1377–1382.

16. Monto AS. The disappearance of Reye's syndrome—A public health triumph [editorial; comment] [see comments]. N Engl J Med 1999;340:1423–1424.

17. Leo MA, Lieber CSJ. Alcohol, vitamin A, and beta-carotene: Adverse interactions, including hepatotoxicity and carcinogenicity. Am J Clin Nutr 1999;69:1071–1085.

18. Agarwal DP, Goedde HW. Human aldehyde dehydrogenases: Their role in alcoholism. Alcohol 1989;6:517–523.

19. Bohan A, Boyer J. Mechanisms of hepatic transport of drugs: Implications for cholestatic drug reactions. Semin Liver Dis 2002;22:123–136.

20. Lee WM. Acute hepatic failure. N Engl J Med 1993;329:1862–1872.

21. Konig SA, Schenk M, Sick C, et al. Fatal liver failure associated with valproate therapy in a patient with Friedreich's disease: Review of valproate hepatotoxicity in adults. Epilepsia 1999;40:1036–1040.

22. Lullman H, Lullman R, Wasserman O. Drug-induced phospholipidosis, II. Tissue distribution of the amphiphilic drug chlorphentermine. CRC Crit Drug Rev Toxicol 1975;4:185–218.

23. Chang CC, Petrelli M, Tomashefski JF Jr, McCullough AJJ. Severe intrahepatic cholestasis caused by amiodarone toxicity after withdrawal of the drug: A case report and review of the literature. Arch Pathol Lab Med 1999;123:251–256.

24. Beane PH, Bourdi M. Autoantibodies against cytochrome P450 in drug-induced autoimmune hepatitis. Ann NY Acad Sci 1993;685: 641–645.

25. Evans WE, Relling MV. Pharmacogenomics: Translating functional genomics into rational therapeutics. Science 1999;286:487–491.

26. Hunt CM, Westerkam WR, Stave GM. Effect of age and gender on the activity of human hepatic CYP3A. Biochem Pharmacol 1992;44: 275–283.

27. Liddle C, Goodwin B. Regulation of hepatic drug metabolism: Role of nuclear receptors PXR and CAR. Semin Liver Dis 2002;22:115–122.

28. Tsagaropoou-Stinga H, Mataki-Emmanouilidon R, Karida-Kavalioti S, et al. Hepatotoxic reactions in children with severe tuberculosis treated with isoniazid-rifampin. Pediatr Infect Dis 1985;4:270–273.

29. Ohno M, Yamaguchi I, Yamamoto I, et al. Slow *N*-acetyltransferase 2 genotype affects the incidence of isoniazid and rifampicin-induced hepatotoxicity. Int J Tuberc Lung Dis 2000;4:256–261.

30. Kergueris MF, Bourin M, Larousse C. Pharmacokinetics of isoniazid: Influence of age. Eur J Clin Pharm 1986;30:335–340.

31. Vuilleumier N, Rossier MF, Chiappe A, et al. CYP2E1 genotype and isoniazid-induced hepatotoxicity in patients treated for latent tuberculosis. Eur J Clin Pharmacol 2006;62:423–429.

32. Van Puijenbroek EP, Metselaar HJ, Berghuis PH, et al. [Acute hepatocytic necrosis during ketoconazole therapy for treatment of onychomycosis. National Foundation for Registry and Evaluation of Adverse Effects.] Ned Tijdschr Geneeskd 1998;142:2416–2418.

33. Gunawan B, Kaplowitz N. Mechanisms of drug-induced liver disease. Clin Liver Dis 2007;11:459–475.

34. Lucena MI, Adrarde RJ, Kaplowitz N, Garcia-Cortes M, Fernandez MC, et al. Phenotypic characterization of idiosyncratic drug-inudced liver injury: The influence of age and sex. Hepatology 2009;49: 2001–2009.

35. Leonard PA, Clegg DO, Carson CC, et al. Low dose pulse methotrexate in rheumatoid arthritis: An 8-year experience with hepatotoxicity. Clin Rheumatol 1987;6:575–582.

36. Cullen P. Mechanistic classification of liver injury. Toxicol Pathol 2005;33:6–8.

37. Jaeschke H, Gores G, Cederbaum A, et al. Mechanisms of hepatotoxicity. Toxicol Sci 2002;65:166–176.

38. Clinical Practice Guidelines Panel. Beuers U, Boberg KM, Chapman RW, Chazouilleres O, Invernizzi P, et al. EASL Clinical Practice Guidelines: Management of cholestatic liver diseases. J Hepatology 2009;51:237–267.

39. Foitl DR, Hyman G, Leftowitch JH. Jaundice and intrahepatic cholestasis following high-dose megestrol acetate for breast cancer. Cancer 1989;63:438–439.

40. Lorch V, Murphy D, Hoersten L, et al. Unusual syndrome among premature infants: Associated with a new intravenous vitamin E product. Pediatrics 1985;75:598–601.

41. Olsson R, Wiholm BE, Sand C, et al. Liver damage from flucloxacillin, cloxacillin and dicloxacillin. J Hepatol 1992;15:154–161.

42. Soe KL, Soe M, Gluud CN. [Liver pathology associated with anabolic androgenic steroids]. Ugeskr Laeger 1994;156:2585–2588.

43. Chang C, Schiano T. Review Article: Drug Hepatoxicity. Aliment Pharmacol Ther 2007;25:1135–1151.

44. Tarantino G, DiMinno M, Capone D. Drug-induced liver injury: Is it somehow forseeable? World J Gastroenterol 2009;15(23): 2817–2833.

45. Malhi H, Gores G, Lemasters J. Apoptosis and necrosis in the liver: A tale of two deaths? Hepatology 2006;43:S31-S44.

46. Lee FI, Smith PM, Bennett B, Williams DMJ. Occupationally related angiosarcoma of the liver in the United Kingdom 1972–1994. Gut 1996;39:312–318.

47. Anonymous. Epidemiologic notes and reports: Angiosarcoma of the liver among polyvinyl chloride workers—Kentucky. MMWR Morb Mortal Wkly Rep 1997;46:99–101.

48. Danan G, Benichou C. Causality assessment of adverse reactions to drugs—I. A novel method based on the conclusions of international consensus meetings: Application to drug-induced liver injuries. J Clin Epidemiol 1993;46:1323–1330.

49. Van Thiel DH, Perper JA. Hepatotoxicity associated with cocaine abuse. Recent Dev Alcohol 1992;10:335–341.

50. Jones AL, Simpson KJJ. Review article: Mechanisms and management of hepatotoxicity in ecstasy (MDMA) and amphetamine intoxications. Aliment Pharmacol Ther 1999;13:129–133.

51. Stanca CM, Babar J, Singal V. Pathogenic role of environmental toxins in immune-mediated liver diseases. J Immunotoxicol 2008;5:59–68.

52. Steadman C. Herbal hepatotoxicity. Semin Liver Dis 2002;22: 195–206.

53. Seef LB, Cuccherin BA, Zimmerman HJ, et al. Acetaminophen hepatotoxicity in alcoholics: A therapeutic misadventure. Ann Intern Med 1986;104:399–404.

54. Ruhl CE, Everhart JE. Relation of elevated serum alanine aminotransferase activity with iron and antioxidant levels in the United States. Gastroenterology 2003;124:1821–1829.

55. Whitehead MW, Haukes ND, Hainesworth I, Kingham JGC. A prospective study of causes of notably raised aspartate aminotransferase of liver origin. Gut 1999;45:129–133.

56. Choppa S, Griffin PH. Laboratory tests and diagnostic procedures in evaluation of liver disease. Am J Med 1985;79:221–230.

57. O'Grady JG, Alexander GJM, Hayllar KM, Williams R. Early indicators of prognosis in fulminant hepatic failure. Gastroenterology 1989;97:439–445.

58. Barstow L, Smith RE. Liver function assessment by drug metabolism. Pharmacotherapy 1990;10:280–288.

59. Zech J, Lange H, Bosch J, et al. Steady-state extrarenal sorbitol clearance as a measure of hepatic plasma flow. Gastroenterology 1988;95:749–759.

60. Mathieu D, Kobeiter H, Maison P, et al. Oral contraceptive use and focal nodular hyperplasia of the liver. Gastroenterology 2000;118:560–564.

61. Anonymous. Standardization of definitions and criteria of causality assessment of adverse drug reactions, drug-induced liver disorders: Report of an international consensus meeting. Int J Clin Pharmacol Ther Toxicol 1990;28:317–322.

62. Newman M, Auerbach R, Feiner H, et al. The role of liver biopsies in psoriatic patients receiving long-term methotrexate treatment: Improvement in liver abnormalities after cessation of treatment. Arch Dermatol 1989;125:1218–1224.

63. O'Connor GT, Olmstead EM, Sug K, et al. Detection of hepatotoxicity associated with methotrexate therapy for psoriasis. Arch Dermatol 1989;125:1209–1217.

SCOTT BOLESTA AND PATRICIA A. MONTGOMERY

CHAPTER 46

Pancreatitis

KEY CONCEPTS

ACUTE PANCREATITIS

❶ Patients with severe acute pancreatitis require early and aggressive intravenous fluid resuscitation and should be managed similarly to patients with sepsis.

❷ Factors that can contribute to acute pancreatitis should be corrected, including discontinuation of medications that could be potential causes.

❸ Parenteral opioid analgesics are used to control abdominal pain associated with acute pancreatitis.

❹ Meperidine is not recommended as a first-line agent for the treatment of pain from acute pancreatitis due to the risk of adverse effects and the resultant dosing limitations.

❺ The only definitive indication for antibiotic use in acute pancreatitis is to treat known or suspected infection.

CHRONIC PANCREATITIS

❻ Chronic pain, malabsorption with resultant steatorrhea, and diabetes mellitus are the hallmark complications and symptoms of chronic pancreatitis.

❼ Pain from chronic pancreatitis can initially be treated with nonopioid analgesics, but opioids will eventually be required as the disease progresses.

❽ Pancreatic enzyme supplementation and reduction in dietary fat intake are the primary treatments for malabsorption due to chronic pancreatitis.

❾ Enteric-coated pancreatic enzyme supplements are the preferred dosage form in the treatment of malabsorption and steatorrhea due to chronic pancreatitis.

❿ The addition of an antisecretory agent to pancreatic enzyme supplementation may increase the effectiveness of enzyme therapy for malabsorption and steatorrhea due to chronic pancreatitis.

Learning objectives, review questions, and other resources can be found at **www.pharmacotherapyonline.com**.

Pancreatitis is inflammation of the pancreas with variable involvement of regional tissues or remote organ systems.[1] Acute pancreatitis is characterized by severe pain in the upper abdomen and elevations of pancreatic enzymes in the blood.[1–3] In the majority of patients, acute pancreatitis is a mild, self-limiting disease that resolves spontaneously without complications. Approximately 20% of adults have a severe course, and 10% to 30% of those with severe acute pancreatitis die.[1] Although exocrine and endocrine pancreatic function may remain impaired for variable periods after an attack, acute pancreatitis seldom progresses to chronic pancreatitis.[1,2]

Chronic pancreatitis is characterized by long-standing inflammation that eventually leads to a loss of pancreatic exocrine and endocrine function.[4–6] It is a progressive disease that often goes unnoticed for many years. Usually patients first present with complaints of chronic abdominal pain. Later in the disease process malabsorption with resultant steatorrhea occurs. This leads to malnutrition and weight loss. Finally, patients develop diabetes mellitus due to a loss of pancreatic endocrine function.[4,5]

EPIDEMIOLOGY

The prevalence of pancreatitis varies widely with geographic, etiologic (e.g., alcohol consumption), environmental, and genetic factors. The reported prevalence of acute pancreatitis among men and women in the United States is less than 1%.[7] Approximately six per 100,000 population will develop chronic pancreatitis with a peak incidence between ages 35 and 54 and about 85% of cases occurring in men.[6] However, this incidence may be underestimated due to diagnostic difficulties and various classification systems. Also, the prevalence of chronic pancreatitis varies widely based on geographic location.[4,6] Hospitalizations for acute pancreatitis have increased in the United States, most likely related to an increase in gallstones in association with obesity.[8] The incidence of gallstone-related acute pancreatitis has increased among white women older than age 60 years.[9] Hospitalization for chronic pancreatitis has also doubled in the past decade, with black patients being almost two to three times as likely to be hospitalized for chronic pancreatitis than for alcoholic cirrhosis.[6]

PANCREATIC EXOCRINE PHYSIOLOGY

The pancreas possesses both endocrine and exocrine functions. The islets of Langerhans, which contain the cells of the endocrine pancreas, secrete insulin, glucagon, somatostatin, and other polypeptide hormones. The exocrine pancreas is composed of acini and ductules that secrete about 2.5 L/day of isotonic fluid that contains water, electrolytes, and pancreatic enzymes necessary for digestion. Bicarbonate and other electrolytes are secreted primarily by

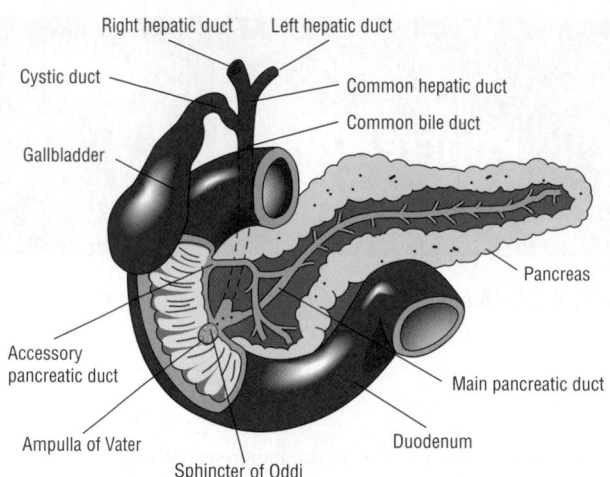

FIGURE 46-1. Anatomic structure of the pancreas and biliary tract.

the centroacinar (ductular) cells in order to neutralize gastric acid. Pancreatic juice is delivered to the duodenum via the pancreatic ducts (Fig. 46–1) where the alkaline secretion neutralizes gastric acid and provides an appropriate pH for maintaining the activity of pancreatic enzymes.[10]

The major pancreatic exocrine enzyme groups are as follows:

- Amylolytic: amylase
- Lipolytic: lipase, procolipase, prophospholipase A_2, and carboxylesterase
- Proteolytic: trypsinogen, chymotrypsinogen, procarboxypeptidase, and proelastase
- Nucleolytic: ribonuclease, deoxyribonuclease
- Other: trypsin inhibitor

Amylase is responsible for digestion of starches and glycogen through hydrolysis. The lipolytic enzymes break down triglycerides, cholesterol, and other fats in the digestive tract. Specifically, lipase hydrolyzes triglycerides into fatty acids and monoglycerides. Colipase and bile acids facilitate this process by allowing lipase to act on the hydrophobic surface of fat droplets in the mainly hydrophilic environment. Phospholipase A_2 and carboxylesterase continue to break down fatty acids, cholesterol, monoglycerides, and other products of fat digestion. Proteolytic enzymes digest proteins into oligopeptides and free amino acids, while nucleases break down nucleic acids.[10,11]

The production of proteolytic enzymes in the pancreas occurs in a manner that prevents self-digestion of the pancreas. These enzymes are synthesized within the acinar cells and secreted into the duodenum as zymogens (inactive enzymes). Enterokinase secreted by the duodenal mucosa converts trypsinogen to trypsin, which then activates all other proteolytic zymogens along with procolipase and prophospholipase A_2. Thus two important mechanisms protect the pancreas from the potential degradative action of its own digestive enzymes. First, the synthesis of proteolytic enzymes as zymogens requires extrapancreatic activation by trypsin. Second, pancreatic juice contains a low concentration of trypsin inhibitor, which inactivates any autocatalytically formed trypsin within the pancreas. Proteolytic activity of trypsin in the intestinal lumen is not inhibited because the concentration of trypsin inhibitor is minimal. Lipase, amylase, ribonuclease, and deoxyribonuclease are secreted by the acinar cells in their active form.[10]

The regulation of exocrine pancreatic secretion is a complex interplay of neurohormonal feedback with three distinct phases. The first phase is the cephalic phase where the sight, smell, and taste of food produce pancreatic enzyme secretion through stimu-

lus of the vagus nerve. Vasoactive intestinal peptide (VIP) and gastrin-releasing peptide (GRP) released from efferent vagus nerve terminals bind to receptors on the acinar cells stimulating enzyme release.[10] Water and bicarbonate are also released from ductal cells due to VIP stimulation. The gastric phase occurs due to gastric distension from food entering the stomach. This results primarily in secretion of digestive enzymes from the pancreas. Once chyme enters the duodenum the intestinal phase begins. The chyme causes secretin to be released from the duodenal mucosa when its pH is less than 4.5. Secretin results in water and bicarbonate secretion from the pancreas, which is necessary since lipolytic enzymes are inactivated at a pH below 5.[11] Digestive enzymes are released from the pancreas due to the presence of fatty acids, peptides, amino acids, and glucose in the duodenum.[10]

The feedback mechanism for continued release of pancreatic enzymes involves the hormone cholecystokinin (CCK). When products of fat, protein, and starch digestion enter the upper small intestine they stimulate release of CCK from I cells into the blood. Elevated levels of CCK in the serum activate a vagovagal reflex causing further release of VIP and GRP, leading to enhanced pancreatic enzyme secretion. Inhibition of this feedback loop is thought to be due to trypsin. After digestion is complete unoccupied trypsin is thought to inhibit the release of CCK.[10] A more in-depth discussion of pancreatic physiology can be found elsewhere.[10]

ACUTE PANCREATITIS

Acute pancreatitis varies from mild to severe disease. The morphological appearance of the pancreas and surrounding tissue ranges from interstitial edema and inflammatory cells (interstitial pancreatitis) to pancreatic and extrapancreatic necrosis (necrotizing pancreatitis). Necrotizing pancreatitis has a higher risk of infection, organ failure, and mortality.[2] The rupture of blood vessels within or around the pancreas can also lead to a collection of blood in the retroperitoneal space.

ETIOLOGY

Table 46–1 lists the etiologic risk factors associated with acute pancreatitis. Obstruction caused by gallstones is the most common

TABLE 46-1	Etiologic Risk Factors Associated with Acute Pancreatitis
Structural	Gallstone disease, sphincter of Oddi dysfunction, pancreas divisum, pancreatic tumors
Toxins	Alcohol (ethanol) consumption, scorpion bite, organophosphate insecticides
Infectious	Bacterial, viral (including AIDS), parasitic
Metabolic	Hypertriglyceridemia, chronic hypercalcemia
Genetic	Cystic fibrosis, α_1-antitrypsin deficiency, hereditary (trypsinogen gene mutations)
Medications	See Table 46–2 for specific drugs
Iatrogenic	Abdominal surgery, ERCP
Kidney disease	Chronic kidney disease, dialysis-related
Trauma	Blunt abdominal trauma
Vascular	Vasculitis, atherosclerosis, cholesterol emboli, coronary artery bypass surgery
Other etiologies	Congenital, Crohn disease, autoimmune, tropical, solid organ transplantation (e.g., liver, kidney, heart), refeeding syndrome
Idiopathic	Undetermined cause

AIDS, acquired immune deficiency syndrome; ERCP, endoscopic retrograde cholangiopancreatography.
Data from references 1, 2, 8, 13, 15.

TABLE 46-2　Medications Associated with Acute Pancreatitis

Class I (Definite Association)	Class II (Probable Association)	Class III (Possible Association)	
5-Aminosalicylic acid	Acetaminophen	Aldesleukin	Indomethacin
Asparaginase	Carbamazepine	Amiodarone	Infliximab
Azathioprine	Cisplatin	Calcium	Ketoprofen
Corticosteroids	Erythromycin	Celecoxib	Ketorolac
Cytarabine	Hydrochlorothiazide	Clozapine	Lipid emulsion
Didanosine	Interferon alpha-2b	Cholestyramine	Lisinopril
Enalapril	Lamivudine	Cimetidine	Mefenamic acid
Estrogens	Octreotide	Ciprofloxacin	Metformin
Furosemide	Sitagliptin	Clarithromycin	Methyldopa
Mercaptopurine		Clonidine	Metolazone
Opiates		Cyclosporine	Metronidazole
Pentamidine		Danazol	Nitrofurantoin
Pentavalent antimonials		Diazoxide	Omeprazole
Sulfasalazine		Etanercept	Ondansetron
Sulfamethoxazole and trimethoprim		Ethacrynic acid	Oxyphenbutazone
Sulindac		Exenatide	Paclitaxel
Tetracycline		Famciclovir	Pravastatin
Valproic acid/salts		Glyburide	Propofol
		Gold therapy	Propoxyphene
		Granisetron	Rifampin
		Ibuprofen	Sertraline
		Indinavir	Zalcitabine

Data from references 27, 125–127.

cause of acute pancreatitis and alcohol abuse the second; together they account for 70% to 80% of all cases of acute pancreatitis.[6] There has been an increase in identification of genetic and autoimmune causes of acute pancreatitis.[12] Most of the remaining cases are idiopathic.[9,13] Acute pancreatitis occurs in 1.8% to 7.2% of all patients who have undergone endoscopic retrograde cholangiopancreatography (ERCP), and in 30% to 40% of high-risk patients.[8,13,14] End-stage kidney disease increases the risk of acute pancreatitis, with patients who are receiving chronic peritoneal dialysis being at higher risk than those receiving hemodialysis.[15] Cigarette smoking appears to increase the risk of pancreatitis, especially in alcohol-related disease.[16] Pregnancy is not considered a cause of acute pancreatitis; however, pregnant women develop pancreatitis as a result of a coincident process, most commonly cholelithiasis. In pediatric patients, the common etiologies are systemic illness, biliary disease, trauma, and medications.[17]

Medications

Drug-induced acute pancreatitis should be suspected when other causes have been excluded and there is a temporal relationship with the initiation of a medication that has been implicated as a cause. The percentage of acute pancreatitis cases caused by medications is 0.1 to 2%.[18] Most information on drug-induced acute pancreatitis is obtained from case reports.[19–24] Proton pump inhibitors and histamine$_2$-receptor antagonists may be initiated in response to early symptoms of unrecognized pancreatitis and may confound the association between the drug and the disease. However, a retrospective cohort study does not support an association between acute pancreatitis and proton pump inhibitors or histamine$_2$-receptor antagonists.[19] Medications such as propofol and tamoxifen are associated with pancreatitis from hyperlipidemia.[22,24] There is a higher incidence of drug-induced acute pancreatitis in U.S. patients with human immunodeficiency virus (HIV) treated with antiretroviral therapy.[25] However, there was no increase in acute pancreatitis associated with antiretroviral use in a well-controlled trial including data from 33,742 person-years.[26] Medications used in the treatment of inflammatory bowel disease and type 2 diabetes mellitus have also been associated with a higher incidence of drug-induced acute

pancreatitis.[18,27] Metformin is associated with acute pancreatitis at toxic serum concentrations.[23] The onset after initiation of these medications ranges from a few months to several years, with a median of 5 weeks; onset after rechallenge can occur within hours. The onset may differ according to the mechanism. Clinicians should be especially suspicious of drug-induced acute pancreatitis in high-risk patients, such as those receiving multiple medications or immunomodulating drugs, and in geriatric, HIV-positive, and cancer patients.[27]

Numerous drugs are believed to cause acute pancreatitis, but ethical and practical considerations prevent rechallenge with suspected agents.[28] Table 46–2 lists specific agents associated with acute pancreatitis based on known association. Class I (definite association) implies a temporal relationship of drug administration to abdominal pain and hyperamylasemia in at least 20 reported cases with at least one positive response to rechallenge with the offending agent. Class II medications are implicated in more than ten, but less than 20, reported cases of acute pancreatitis and suggest a probable association. Class III includes medications with a possible association, defined as fewer than 10 published cases or unpublished reports in pharmaceutical or U.S. Food and Drug Administration files. Table 46–2 includes only selected class III medications. A comprehensive list of class III drugs can be found elsewhere.[29]

Mechanisms of drug-induced pancreatitis are not clearly defined but may fall into several general categories, including direct toxic effects of the drug or its metabolites, hypersensitivity, drug-induced hypertriglyceridemia, and alterations of cellular function in the pancreas and pancreatic duct.[18] Once the process is initiated, disease severity is determined by the propagation of proinflammatory mediators. Although acute pancreatitis is an infrequent complication of drug therapy it is prudent to withdraw medication when an association is suspected.

PATHOPHYSIOLOGY

The pathophysiology of acute pancreatitis is based on events that initiate injury and secondary events that establish and perpetuate the injury (Fig. 46–2). Alcohol abuse and gallstones cause different

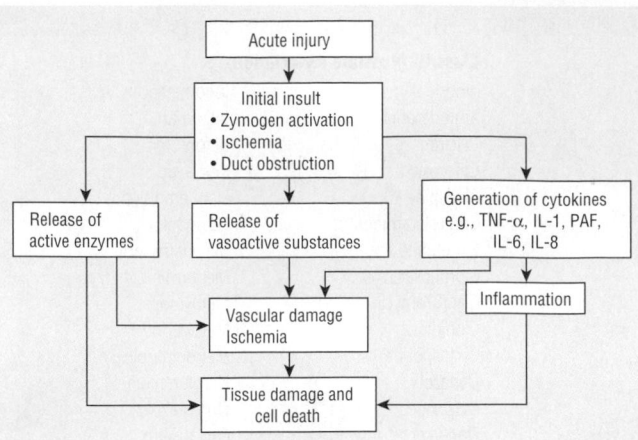

FIGURE 46-2. Pathophysiology of acute pancreatitis: initiating and secondary events. (IL-1β, interleukin-1β; IL-6, interleukin-6; IL-8, interleukin-8; PAF, platelet-activating factor; TNF-α, tumor necrosis factor-α.)

initial insults to the pancreas. However, acute pancreatitis of any etiology involves the premature activation of trypsinogen to trypsin within the pancreas, leading to activation of other digestive enzymes and autodigestion of the gland.[1,2] The lysosomal proteinase, cathepsin B, and intracellular calcium may be involved in the activation of trypsinogen as well as decreased activity of trypsin inhibitor.[30] Genetic abnormalities in pathways that protect the pancreas from autodigestion also play a pathophysiologic role in the development of some forms of acute pancreatitis, and may be the differentiating factor in the minority of alcoholics that develop disease.[1,31]

In addition to increased production, activated enzymes are retained in the acinar cells in higher concentrations than normal.[32] Activated pancreatic enzymes released into the pancreas and surrounding tissues produce damage and necrosis to the pancreatic tissue, the surrounding fat, the vascular endothelium, and adjacent structures. Lipase damages the fat cells, producing noxious substances that cause further pancreatic and peripancreatic injury. The release of cytokines by acinar cells directly causes their injury and enhances the inflammatory response.[30] Injured acinar cells liberate chemoattractants that recruit neutrophils, macrophages, and other cells to the area of inflammation. These immune responses cause a systemic inflammatory response syndrome (SIRS). Vascular damage and ischemia cause the release of kinins, which make capillary walls permeable and promote tissue edema. The release of damaging oxygen-free radicals appears to correlate with the severity of pancreatic injury.[2] Finally, pancreatic infection may result from increased intestinal permeability and translocation of colonic bacteria.[31,33]

COMPLICATIONS

Early complications are a result of fluid losses and SIRS. Hypotension results from hypovolemia, hypoalbuminemia, the release of kinins, and sepsis. Even patients with mild disease have significant fluid losses. Renal complications are usually caused by hypovolemia. Pulmonary complications develop when fluid accumulates within the pleural space compressing the lungs, and with development of the acute respiratory distress syndrome (ARDS), which limits gas exchange. The differential diagnosis for hypoxemia should include ARDS in patients with acute pancreatitis who do not have a history of pulmonary disease.[3] Pleural effusions occur in 4% to 17% of patients, more frequently on the left.[2] Gastrointestinal bleeding occurs secondary to numerous causes, including rupture of a pseudocyst (collection of pancreatic secre-

tions and tissue debris enclosed by a wall of fibrous or granulation tissue). Severe acute pancreatitis is also associated with confusion and coma.

Local complications including acute fluid collection, pancreatic necrosis, infection, abscess (collection of pus in or adjacent to the pancreas), and pseudocyst develop approximately 3 to 4 weeks after the initial attack. Pancreatic infections occur in 15% to 30% of those with pancreatic necrosis and are usually secondary infections of necrotic tissue.[8] Pancreatic ascites occur when pancreatic secretions spread throughout the peritoneal cavity. Systemic complications include cardiovascular, renal, pulmonary, metabolic, hemorrhagic, and central nervous system abnormalities.[2] Long-term complications include glucose intolerance and recurrence of acute pancreatitis.[34]

CLINICAL PRESENTATION

Signs and Symptoms

The clinical presentation of acute pancreatitis varies depending on the severity of the inflammatory process and whether damage is confined to the pancreas or involves local and systemic complications (Table 46–3).[2,8,9]

Diagnosis

Most guidelines agree that the diagnosis should be made within 48 hours based on characteristic abdominal pain and amylase, lipase, or both being elevated to at least three times the upper limit of normal. Lipase is more sensitive and specific than amylase and is preferred. Contrast-enhanced computed tomography (CECT) of the abdomen may be used to confirm the diagnosis, including in patients with amylase or lipase levels that are not three times the upper limit of normal. Some guidelines consider ultrasonography to be an acceptable alternative to CECT.[2,35] However, it is best used to ascertain the presence of gallstones. The diagnosis of acute pancreatitis should also be considered when evaluating patients with SIRS (see Table 46–3).[1,2,35–37] For further information on laboratory tests and abdominal imaging refer to Table 46–3.

Prediction of Disease Severity Prediction of severity of acute pancreatitis is useful for decisions involving the need for aggressive treatment, including admission to intensive care units. The risk for severe acute pancreatitis should be assessed upon admission and on an ongoing basis.[2,3] Several recognized scoring systems have been developed to assess the likelihood of severe disease (Table 46–4). However, development and validation of such systems remains an ongoing area of research. The Ranson criteria scoring system was developed for pancreatitis and assesses 11 variables that must be monitored at the time of admission and during the initial 48 hours of hospitalization.[2,9] Severe acute pancreatitis is characterized by three or more criteria. Patients with fewer than three Ranson criteria have a mortality rate of less than 1%, whereas those with six or more have a 100% mortality rate.[2] The Ranson criteria are complete only after 48 hours. The Atlanta scoring system was developed based on consensus opinions; it consolidates clinical indicators, organ failure, and local complications to provide an ongoing assessment of disease severity.[8,9] The Acute Physiology and Chronic Health Evaluation II (APACHE II) system uses 12 indicators of physiologic and biochemical function, age, and previous health status to predict mortality in critically ill patients, but it is not specific to pancreatitis. The APACHE II score is calculated within the first 24 hours and is considered among the best predictors of severity on admission. A score greater than or equal to 8 points is considered the threshold for severe acute pancreatitis.[2,8,9] A modification, called the APACHE-O, improves predictive value in acute pancreatitis by adding points for a body mass index of 26 kg/m^2 or more.[38]

TABLE 46-3 Presentation and Diagnosis of Acute Pancreatitis

General
- The patient may have acute mild symptoms or present with a severe acute attack with life-threatening complications.

Symptoms
- The patient may present initially with moderate abdominal discomfort to excruciating pain, nausea, shock, and respiratory distress.
- Abdominal pain occurs in 95% of patients. The pain is usually epigastric and radiates to either of the upper quadrants or the back in two thirds of patients. In gallstone pancreatitis, the pain is typically sudden and quite severe, and the intensity is often described as "knife-like" or "boring." The pain usually reaches its maximum intensity within 30 minutes and may persist for hours or days. Repositioning the patient relieves very little of the pain. In alcohol abuse and other cases, the onset of pain may be less abrupt and poorly localized. Pain may not be the dominant symptom if it is masked by multiorgan failure.
- Nausea and vomiting occur in 85% of patients and usually follow the onset of abdominal pain. Vomiting does not provide relief of the abdominal pain.

Signs
- Marked epigastric or diffuse tenderness on palpation with rebound tenderness and guarding in severe cases. The abdomen is often distended and tympanic, with bowel sounds decreased or absent in severe disease.
- Vital signs may be normal, but hypotension, tachycardia, and low-grade fever are sometimes observed, especially with widespread pancreatic inflammation and necrosis.
- Dyspnea and tachypnea are often signs of acute respiratory complications. Jaundice and altered mental status may be present and have multiple causes. Other signs of alcoholic liver disease may be present in patients with alcoholic pancreatitis.

Laboratory tests
- Leukocytosis is frequently present; hyperglycemia or hypoalbuminemia may be present. Liver transaminases, alkaline phosphatase, and bilirubin are usually elevated in gallstone pancreatitis and in patients with intrinsic liver disease. Elevated serum triglycerides may also be a possible etiology.
- The hematocrit may be normal, but hemoconcentration results from multiple factors (e.g., vomiting). In patients with third-space fluid loss, hemoconcentration is present and a reasonably accurate marker of severe disease. A hemoglobin concentration of >47% predicts severe acute pancreatitis and one of <44% predicts mild disease. Further, failure to reverse hemoconcentration has been associated with pancreatic necrosis.
- The total serum calcium is usually normal initially, but hypocalcemia disproportionate to the hypoalbuminemia may develop. Marked hypocalcemia is an indication of severe necrosis and a poor prognostic sign.
- The serum amylase concentration usually rises within 4 to 8 hours of the initial attack, peaks at 24 hours, and returns to normal over the next 8 to 14 days. Serum amylase concentrations greater than three times the upper limit of normal are highly suggestive of acute pancreatitis. Persistent elevations suggest extensive pancreatic necrosis and related complications. Normal concentrations may be observed if testing is delayed (i.e., amylase may have returned to normal) or in patients with hyperlipidemic pancreatitis (i.e., marked triglyceride elevations may interfere with amylase assay). In addition, many nonpancreatic diseases may be associated with hyperamylasemia, including salivary, kidney, hepatobiliary, metabolic, female reproductive tract, and neoplastic diseases.[2,8]
- Serum lipase is specific to the pancreas, and concentrations are elevated and parallel the elevations in serum amylase. Levels remain elevated with pancreatic inflammation and return to normal when the inflammatory process resolves. Because of its longer half-life, elevations of serum lipase can be detected after the serum amylase has returned to normal.
- C-reactive protein (CRP) is a widely available test and levels greater than 150 mg/L at 48–72 hours predict severe acute pancreatitis with accuracy similar to that of APACHE II. Newer markers (e.g., urinary trypsinogen activation peptide) provide both diagnostic and prognostic information but are not routinely used in practice.
- Thrombocytopenia and an increase in the international normalized ratio are seen in some patients with severe acute pancreatitis and associated liver disease.

Abdominal imaging
- CECT is used to identify the cause of pancreatitis and confirm the diagnosis. It is less accurate for evaluating the gallbladder and biliary ducts. The test distinguishes interstitial from necrotizing pancreatitis but does not distinguish between fat necrosis and acute fluid collection. Tests that are performed in the first few days may miss necrosis. A CECT performed too early may result in unnecessary exposure to risk and increased cost. Formal scoring systems may be used to evaluate the findings.
- Magnetic resonance imaging is used to grade the severity of acute pancreatitis, to identify biliary duct problems that are not seen on CT, or if there are contraindications to CECT. Patients over the age of 40 with pancreatitis of an unknown etiology should be evaluated for pancreatic malignancy with CT or endoscopic ultrasonography.
- Ultrasonography of the abdomen is useful to determine pancreatic enlargement and peripancreatic fluid collections. It is also sensitive for detecting dilated biliary ducts and stones in the gallbladder.

APACHE, acute physiologic and chronic health evaluation; CECT, contrast-enhanced computed tomography; CT, computed tomography.
Data from references 8, 38, 45, 128.

Some studies have found obesity to be an independent risk factor for complications of acute pancreatitis.[38] Mortality from acute pancreatitis is strongly correlated with additional organ failure, especially persistent multisystem organ failure. Research continues for a sensitive scoring system that can be used early in the course of acute pancreatitis.[39]

CLINICAL COURSE AND PROGNOSIS

The clinical course of acute pancreatitis varies from a mild transitory disorder to a severe necrotizing disease. Mild acute pancreatitis is self-limiting and subsides spontaneously within 3 to 5 days. Mortality increases with unfavorable early prognostic signs, local complications, and organ failure. Pancreatic necrosis carries a 10% mortality, but this increases to 30% to 40% with infected necrosis.[2] Mortality is influenced by etiology, as idiopathic and postoperative acute pancreatitis have higher rates than gallstone- or alcoholically-induced disease. First and second occurrences also carry a higher mortality than subsequent episodes. Death during the first few days results from SIRS and multiorgan failure. When death occurs after this period, it is usually a result of infected necrosis, pancreatic abscess, and sepsis.[2]

TREATMENT

Acute Pancreatitis

■ DESIRED OUTCOME

Treatment of acute pancreatitis is aimed at relieving abdominal pain and nausea, replacing fluids, correcting electrolyte, glucose, and lipid abnormalities, minimizing systemic complications, and preventing pancreatic necrosis and infection. Management varies depending on the severity of the attack (Fig. 46–3). Patients with mild acute pancreatitis respond very well to the initiation of supportive care and the reduction of pancreatic secretions. Patients with severe acute pancreatitis should be treated aggressively and monitored closely.

TABLE 46-4 Prognostic Indicators for Severe Acute Pancreatitis

Prognostic Factor	Criterion
Ranson criteria	
On admission	
Age (y)	>55
WBC (cells/mm³)	>16,000
Glucose (mg/dL)	>200
LDH (IU/L)	>350
AST (units/L)	>250
Within 48 hours	
Decrease in hematocrit (% points)	>10
Increase in BUN (mg/dL)	>5
Calcium (mg/dL)	<8
PaO₂ (mm Hg)	<60
Base deficit (mmol/L)	>4
Estimated fluid deficit (L)	>6
Atlanta criteria	
Unfavorable prognostic signs	
Ranson criteria	≥3
APACHE II score	≥8
Organ failure (shock)	
SBP (mm Hg)	<90
Pulmonary insufficiency (PaO₂ mm Hg)	<60
Kidney failure after hydration [serum creatinine (mg/dL)]	>2
Gastrointestinal tract bleeding (mL in 24 h)	>500
Systemic complications	
Disseminated intravascular coagulation	
Platelets (mm³)	≤100,000
Fibrinogen (g/L)	<1
Fibrin-split products (m/mL)	>80
Metabolic disturbance	
Calcium (mg/dL)	≤7.5
Local complications	
Pseudocyst	Present
Necrosis	Present
Abscess	Present

WBC, white blood cells; LDH, lactate dehydrogenase; AST, aspartate aminotransferase; BUN, blood urea nitrogen; PaO₂, partial pressure of arterial oxygen; APACHE, Acute Physiology and Chronic Health Evaluation; SBP, systolic blood pressure.

Data from Topazian and Gorelick[36] and Whitcomb.[9]

GENERAL APPROACH TO TREATMENT

All patients with acute pancreatitis should receive supportive care, including intravenous fluid resuscitation, adequate nutrition, and effective relief of pain and nausea. The use of nasogastric aspiration offers no clear advantage in patients with mild acute pancreatitis, but it is beneficial in patients with profound pain, severe disease, paralytic ileus, and intractable vomiting.[2] Patients predicted to follow a severe course will require treatment of cardiovascular, respiratory, renal, and metabolic complications.[1] Aggressive fluid resuscitation is essential to correct intravascular volume depletion. However, specific recommendations cannot be made from the current literature, and this is a subject of ongoing research.[40] The prognosis of the patient often depends on the rapidity and adequacy of volume restoration, as large quantities of fluid are sequestered within the peritoneal and retroperitoneal spaces ❶. Vasodilatation from the inflammatory response, vomiting, and nasogastric suction contributes to hypovolemia and fluid and electrolyte abnormalities. Intravenous colloids may be required to maintain intravascular volume and blood pressure because fluid losses are high in protein. Patients with pancreatitis and SIRS should be treated according to SIRS guidelines. Intravenous potassium, calcium, and magnesium are used to correct electrolyte deficiency states. Insulin is used to treat hyperglycemia. Local complications resolve as the inflammatory process subsides. However,

patients with necrotizing pancreatitis may require antibiotics and surgical intervention.[2] Medications listed in Table 46–2 should be discontinued if possible ❷.

NONPHARMACOLOGIC THERAPY

Nonpharmacologic therapy includes ERCP for removal of any underlying biliary tract stones, surgery, and nutritional support. Surgery is indicated in patients with pancreatic pseudocyst or abscess or to drain the pancreatic bed if hemorrhagic or necrotic material is present. The need for admission to an intensive care unit should also be addressed.

Nutrition and Probiotics

Nutritional support plays an important role in the management of patients with mild or severe disease as acute pancreatitis creates a catabolic state that promotes nutritional depletion. This can impair recovery, increase the risk of complications, and prolong hospitalization.[41,42] Patients with mild acute pancreatitis can begin oral feeding when bowel sounds have returned and pain has resolved.[8] In severe or complicated disease, nutritional deficits develop rapidly and are complicated by tissue necrosis, organ failure, and surgery. Nutritional support should begin when it is anticipated that oral nutrition will be withheld for more than 1 week.[43,44] In the past, there was concern that enteral feeding stimulated pancreatic enzyme secretion and exacerbated the underlying disease. However, numerous studies have shown that enteral feeding in severe acute pancreatitis is as safe and effective as parenteral nutrition, attenuates the acute inflammatory response, and improves disease severity.[41,43,44] The mechanisms for this include protection of the gut barrier and prevention of colonization with pathogenic bacteria, both of which may prevent translocation of bacteria and infection.[45] Therefore, the enteral route is preferred over the parenteral in patients with severe acute pancreatitis, provided that it can be tolerated. More specifically, the nasojejunal route may be preferred,[2] but the nasogastric route also appears to be safe and effective.[37,42,46] If enteral feeding is not possible or if the patient is unable to obtain sufficient nutrients, parenteral nutrition should be implemented before protein and calorie depletion become advanced. Intravenous lipids should not be withheld unless the serum triglyceride concentration is greater than 500 mg/dL.[2] Preliminary data suggest that the early nasojejunal administration of probiotics, such as lactobacillus, with enteral nutrition may reduce bacterial translocation and possibly decrease pancreatic necrosis and abscess.[47,48]

PHARMACOLOGIC THERAPY

Recommendations

Besides fluid resuscitation and nutritional support patients with acute pancreatitis require treatment for pain and nausea. Pain and nausea can be treated with intravenous analgesics and antiemetics. Antisecretory agents may be used to prevent stress-related mucosal bleeding. Octreotide may be tried in severe acute pancreatitis, but its efficacy remains uncertain (see Fig. 46–3). The use of prophylactic antibiotics is controversial and most guidelines do not support this practice.[2,37]

Relief of Abdominal Pain

Parenteral opioid analgesics are used to control abdominal pain associated with acute pancreatitis ❸. The most important factors to consider in selecting an analgesic are efficacy and safety. Although the administration of some opioids is associated with mild and transient increases in serum amylase and lipase, these effects

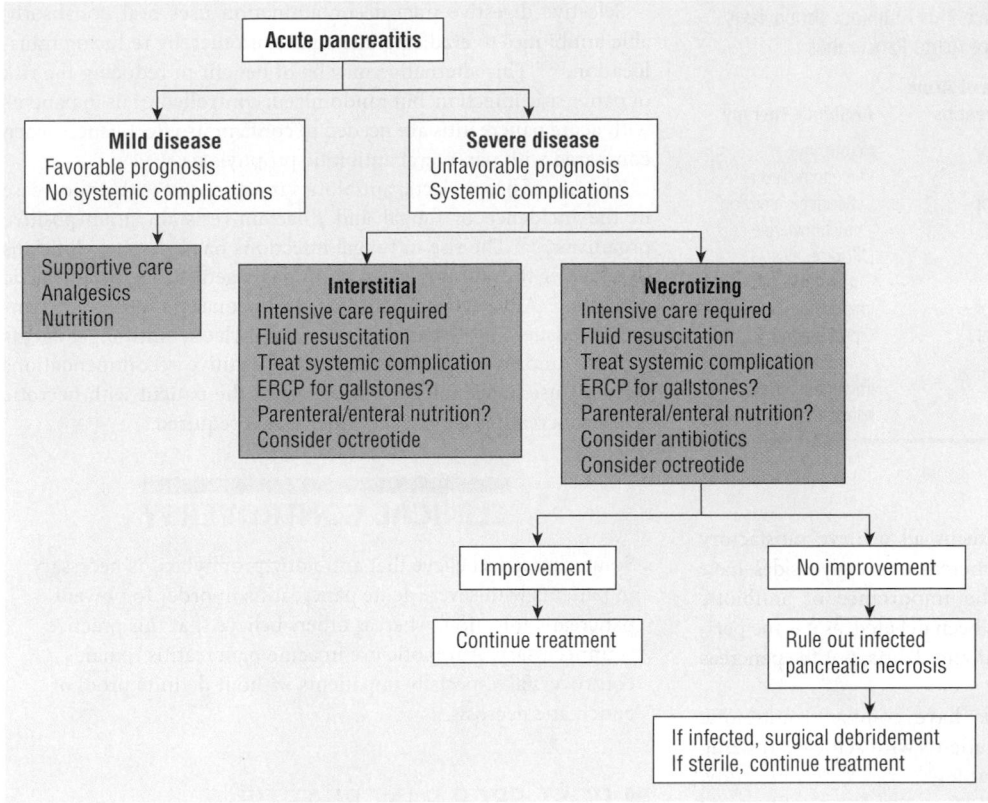

FIGURE 46-3. Algorithm of guidelines for evaluation and treatment of acute pancreatitis. (ERCP, endoscopic retrograde cholangiopancreatography.)

are not deleterious to the patient. Traditionally, treatment was initiated with parenteral meperidine (50 to 100 mg every 3 to 4 hours) because it did not significantly alter the function of the sphincter of Oddi (see Fig. 46–1), thereby worsening the disease course.[49,50] However, meperidine is not recommended as a first-line agent because of the risk of adverse effects and dosing limitations ❹. As a result many hospitals have either restricted or eliminated the use of meperidine. Active metabolites of meperidine accumulate with kidney dysfunction and may cause seizures or psychosis. The maximum recommended parenteral dose of meperidine is 600 mg/day in divided doses in patients with normal kidney function, but it should not be used in patients with kidney dysfunction.

Parenteral morphine is often recommended for pain control because it provides a longer duration of pain relief than meperidine with less risk of seizures. However, its use in acute pancreatitis is sometimes avoided because it is thought to cause spasm of the sphincter of Oddi, increases in serum amylase, and, rarely, pancreatitis.[2] Although morphine increases biliary pressure, there is no evidence to indicate that it is contraindicated for use in acute pancreatitis as no studies have compared clinical outcomes of acute pancreatitis using various analgesics.[50] Hydromorphone may be used because it also has a longer half-life than meperidine. Patient-controlled analgesia should be considered in patients who require frequent opioid dosing (e.g., every 2 to 3 hours). Dosing of pain medications should be monitored carefully and adjusted daily. There is no evidence that antisecretory agents, such as histamine$_2$-receptor antagonists or proton pump inhibitors, prevent an exacerbation of abdominal pain.[51]

Limitation of Systemic Complications and Prevention of Pancreatic Necrosis

A number of agents have been investigated to limit disease progression by either directly or indirectly reducing pancreatic secretion, inhibiting the action of circulating inflammatory mediators, or increasing pancreatic microcirculation.[52–54] The use of parenteral

histamine$_2$-receptor antagonists or proton pump inhibitors does not improve the overall outcome of patients with acute pancreatitis.[8] Similarly, corticosteroids are not useful in limiting systemic complications and altering the course of the disease.[52] Clinical studies with protease inhibitors such as aprotinin and gabexate have failed to show a mortality reduction in acute pancreatitis, and their use is not supported by guidelines.[2,8,35,37,52,53] Neither agent is currently available in the United States. Conflicting or inconclusive data exist regarding the efficacy of atropine, lexipafant, low-molecular-weight dextran, antioxidants such as N-acetylcysteine, indomethacin, interleukin-10, and infliximab.[52,54]

Somatostatin and its synthetic analog octreotide are potent inhibitors of pancreatic enzyme secretion and have been used to interrupt the inflammatory process. Several studies and a meta-analysis that evaluated the efficacy of somatostatin and octreotide suggest a slight trend toward benefit in patients with severe pancreatitis.[2,55] Limitations of these studies include small numbers of patients, no placebo, and inclusion of patients with mild disease.[53] There are insufficient data to support the routine use of somatostatin or octreotide in the treatment of acute pancreatitis, and guidelines do not recommend their use.[37]

Prevention of Infection

Prophylactic antibiotics do not offer any benefit in cases of mild acute pancreatitis or when there is no necrosis. Use of antibiotics in patients with severe acute pancreatic necrosis, but without infection, is not currently supported by randomized, controlled trials ❺. This is true with or without the presence of pancreatic necrosis.

Antibiotic prophylaxis in early clinical trials showed no benefit, but these studies were limited due to inclusion of patients with a wide range of disease severity and insufficient enrollment of patients with severe necrotizing pancreatitis.[1,52] In addition, they used ampicillin, which does not penetrate well into pancreatic tissue.[52] Imipenem-cilastatin, metronidazole, cefotaxime, piperacillin,

TABLE 46-5	Clinical Trials of Intravenous Antibiotic Prophylaxis in Patients with Severe Acute Pancreatitis		
Primary Author	**Patients (n)**	**Cause of Acute Pancreatitis**	**Antibiotic Therapy**
Sainio et al.[58]	30	Alcohol	Cefuroxime
Pederzoli et al.[57]	74	Biliary	Imipenem-cilastin
Delcenserie et al.[59]	23	Alcohol	Ceftazidime, amikacin, metronidazole
Schwarz et al.[60]	26	Biliary	Ofloxacin plus metronidazole
Nordback et al.[61]	58	Alcohol	Imipenem-cilastin
Isenmann et al.[62]	114	Alcohol	Ciprofloxacin plus metronidazole
Rokke et al.[64]	73	Any	Imipenem-cilastin
Dellinger et al.[63]	100	Any	Meropenem

mezlocillin, ofloxacin, and ciprofloxacin all achieve satisfactory bactericidal tissue concentrations, whereas aminoglycosides have poor penetration.[52,53,56] However, the importance of antibiotic penetration into pancreatic tissue has been debated, as it is the peripancreatic retroperitoneal necrotic fat and debris, not the pancreas itself, that becomes infected.

Several randomized clinical trials have compared antibiotic prophylaxis with no prophylaxis in patients with acute necrotizing pancreatitis with varying results (Table 46–5).[57-64] In one study, prophylaxis with cefuroxime lowered mortality, length of hospital stay, and the overall infection rate.[58] However, the decrease in total infections was attributed to fewer urinary tract infections in the antibiotic group. In contrast, other antibiotic regimens decreased the incidence of infections but had no effect on mortality.[57,59,60,63,64] The carbapenem agent imipenem-cilastatin has been used in two trials. A single-blind trial with 58 patients found a reduction in the need for surgery but no effect on mortality or sepsis.[61] An unblinded trial with 73 patients found a lower rate of infections but no difference in the need for surgery or mortality.[64] In contrast, a double-blind trial with 100 patients found no benefit from early antibiotic therapy using another carbapenem agent, meropenem.[63] Studies that included severe acute pancreatitis without computed tomography (CT) demonstration of necrosis failed to show a beneficial effect on mortality.[59,62] The two largest trials, which were also double-blind, did not demonstrate any benefit with prophylaxis.[62,63] Two meta-analyses and a Cochrane review concluded that prophylaxis with broad-spectrum antibiotics decreases sepsis and mortality in patients with severe acute pancreatitis and necrosis.[65-67] However, these were conducted prior to publication of two trials demonstrating no benefit.[63,64] A meta-analysis that included these two trials found prophylactic antibiotics do not reduce infected necrosis or mortality.[68] In addition, overuse of antibiotics increases microbial resistance. Currently, use of antibiotics in necrotizing pancreatitis is not recommended in the absence of infection.

Because the source of bacterial contamination in acute pancreatitis is most likely the colon, the choice of antibiotic should be broad spectrum, covering the range of enteric aerobic gram-negative bacilli and anaerobic microorganisms. Treatment should be initiated within the first 48 hours and continued for 2 to 3 weeks. Imipenem-cilastatin (500 mg every 8 hours) has been widely used because of its good penetration into the pancreas and one positive prophylaxis study.[64] However, it has been replaced on many hospital formularies by one of the newer carbapenems. Fluoroquinolones, such as ciprofloxacin or levofloxacin, combined with metronidazole should be considered for penicillin-allergic patients.[1,52]

Selective digestive tract decontamination uses oral nonabsorbable antibiotics to eradicate intestinal flora thereby reducing translocation.[56,69] This alternative may be of benefit in reducing the risk of pancreatic infection, but randomized, controlled trials in patients with acute pancreatitis are needed to confirm its effectiveness when compared with parenteral antibiotic prophylaxis.[1,2,52,56]

The use of prophylactic antibiotics is associated with an increase in the incidence of fungal and β-lactam-resistant gram-positive organisms.[70,71] The rise in fungal infections has led some clinicians to consider the addition of an antifungal agent to the prophylactic regimen.[72] Although agents such as fluconazole penetrate pancreatic tissue,[73] the effectiveness of prophylactic antifungal agents remains unproven, and there are no definitive recommendations for their use. Once infection develops in the patient with necrotic acute pancreatitis, surgical debridement is required.

CLINICAL CONTROVERSY

Some clinicians believe that antibiotic prophylaxis is necessary in patients with severe acute pancreatitis in order to prevent pancreatic infection, whereas others believe that this practice is unnecessary. Antibiotic use in acute pancreatitis remains controversial, especially in patients without definite proof of pancreatic necrosis.

■ POST-ERCP PANCREATITIS

The clinical characteristics of post-ERCP pancreatitis are similar to those of acute pancreatitis from other causes. In most cases the disease course is mild and resolves in several days. Pretreatment with octreotide, corticosteroids, calcium channel blockers, allopurinol, natural β-carotene, and aprotinin has been disappointing.[1,74,75] However, some benefit has been demonstrated with somatostatin, diclofenac suppositories, and gabexate.[1,76,77] To date, there have not been any studies to evaluate the cost-effectiveness of prophylactic therapy.[14,78,79]

CHRONIC PANCREATITIS

Chronic pancreatitis results from long-standing pancreatic inflammation resulting in irreversible destruction of pancreatic tissue with fibrin deposition, leading to a loss of exocrine and endocrine function.[4-6] It has four different stages, beginning with a preclinical inflammatory stage in which patients remain asymptomatic or have indistinguishable symptoms.[6] In the second stage patients present with acute attacks that often resemble those of acute pancreatitis. The third stage consists of episodes of intermittent or constant abdominal pain. Finally, in the burnout stage patients present with diminished or absent pain but develop malabsorption syndrome due to loss of pancreatic exocrine function and diabetes mellitus from loss of endocrine function.

ETIOLOGY

Chronic alcohol consumption, especially heavy drinking, remains the leading cause of chronic pancreatitis in Western society, accounting for approximately 70% to 80% of cases.[6,80] Generally, consumption of 100 to 150 g/day of alcohol over 10 to 15 years posses a significant risk of chronic pancreatitis.[81] Twenty percent of the remaining cases can be classified as idiopathic, while 10% are due to rare causes, such as autoimmune, hereditary, and tropical pancreatitis.[6,81] Various genetic alterations have also been associated with the occurrence of chronic pancreatitis, including mutations of the

TABLE 46-6	M-ANNHEIM Classification of Risk Factors for Chronic Pancreatitis
Pancreatitis with Multiple risk factors	
Alcohol	Excessive consumption (>80 g/day)
	Increased consumption (20–80 g/day)
	Moderate consumption (<20 g/day)
Nicotine	Quantitated in pack-years for current smokers
Nutritional factors	High fat and protein diet
	Hyperlipidemia (esp. hypertriglyceridemia)
Hereditary factors	Hereditary pancreatitis
	Familial pancreatitis
	Early- and late-onset idiopathic pancreatitis
	Tropical pancreatitis
	Possible gene mutations (e.g., *PRSS1*, *SPINK1*, and *CFTR*)
Efferent duct factors	Pancreas divisum
	Annular pancreas/congenital abnormalities
	Pancreatic duct obstruction
	Posttraumatic pancreatic duct scars
	Sphincter of Oddi dysfunction
Immunologic factors	Autoimmune pancreatitis
Miscellaneous and rare factors	Hypercalcemia and hyperparathyroidism
	Chronic kidney disease
	Medications
	Toxins

PRSS1, cationic trypsinogen; *SPINK1*, serine protease inhibitor Kazal type 1; *CFTR*, cystic fibrosis transmembrane conductance regulator.
Adapted with kind permission of Springer Science and Business Media from Schneider A, Lohr JM, Singer MV, Table 46–2, copyright 2007.[89]

cationic trypsinogen (*PRSS1*), serine protease inhibitor Kazal type 1 (*SPINK1*), and the cystic fibrosis transmembrane conductance regulator (*CFTR*) genes.[81-84] There is also a demonstrated risk of chronic pancreatitis with cigarette smoking that appears to be dose dependent and may contribute to mortality from chronic pancreatitis.[80,85-88] A proposed classification system called the M-ANNHEIM classification takes into account the various risk factors for chronic pancreatitis (Table 46–6).[89]

PATHOPHYSIOLOGY

Although the exact mechanism for the pathogenesis of chronic pancreatitis is unknown several theories have been proposed. The oxidative stress theory proposes that the pancreas is exposed to by-products of mixed-function oxidases that lead to an inflammatory reaction.[81,90] Increased activity of hepatic and pancreatic oxidases may be due to increased exposure to substrates (e.g., fat), inducers (e.g., alcohol), or other substances. A comparison of serum oxidative markers in chronic pancreatitis patients versus healthy volunteers supports this theory.[91] A toxic-metabolic theory focuses on alcohol as a primary causative agent where by-products of its metabolism in the pancreas lead to lipid accumulation in acinar cells and eventual fatty degeneration of the pancreas.[90] Ductal obstruction theories state that alcohol leads to obstruction of pancreatic ductals secondary to increased protein deposition and stone formation. This leads to scarring of ductal epithelial cells, which potentiates further obstruction and eventually results in acinar atrophy and fibrin deposition. The final major theory suggests that periductular necrosis from repeated episodes of acute pancreatitis eventually leads to ductal obstruction and stone formation with subsequent acinar atrophy and fibrosis.

Regardless of the pathophysiologic mechanism several pieces of evidence now point to activation of pancreatic stellate cells as the cause of fibrin deposition in chronic pancreatitis. Various toxins, oxidative stress, and inflammatory mediators have been shown to activate pancreatic stellate cells.[90,92] Cellular signaling pathways involved in this activation are modulated by hydroxymethylglutaryl-coenzyme A reductases and peroxisome proliferator-activated receptor-gamma nuclear receptors.[93] As an example, exposure of the pancreas to alcohol and its metabolites leads to the production of various mediators and proinflammatory cytokines, especially tumor necrosis factor alpha and interleukins 1 and 6.[92,93] These then activate pancreatic stellate cells, which initiate fibrinogenesis. Other mediators generated by the stellate cells themselves perpetuate continued stellate cell activation.

The pathogenesis of pain in chronic pancreatitis has long been thought to be the result of increased pancreatic parenchymal pressure from obstruction, inflammation, and necrosis.[94,95] A neurogenic mechanism may also be responsible. Continued activation of trypsin not only damages afferent neurons but also has effects on sensory pain receptors within the pancreas.[94] Changes also occur within the central nervous system that further contribute to the neurogenic mechanism of pain.[94,96,97] Therefore, compression of pancreatic nerve fibers after a meal along with continuous firing of peripheral and central neurons may explain the burning and shooting pain of chronic pancreatitis.[96]

CLINICAL PRESENTATION

Chronic pain, malabsorption with resultant steatorrhea, and diabetes mellitus are the hallmark complications and symptoms of chronic pancreatitis **6**. Although abdominal pain is the most common symptom at any stage, patients may present with various signs and symptoms depending on the stage of the disease. A more comprehensive list of the common signs and symptoms is presented in Table 46–7.

Diagnosis

The diagnosis of chronic pancreatitis is based primarily on presenting signs and symptoms in combination with either imaging or pancreatic function studies (see Table 46–7). Although histology would be the best diagnostic test it is difficult and risky to perform and is generally not recommended.[82] Therefore, testing usually begins with noninvasive and inexpensive studies such as serum trypsinogen, fecal elastase, mixed triglyceride breath test, and abdominal ultrasonography.[4,98,99] However, these tests are usually useful only in advanced disease.[4] Magnetic resonance cholangiopancreatography or CT may be used next. The most sensitive studies are the secretin and CCK stimulation tests for exocrine pancreatic insufficiency.[5,81,82] Performing these studies is uncomfortable for patients and they are not widely available, so they are usually reserved to rule out chronic pancreatitis if imaging studies are nondiagnostic.[4,5] The gold standard invasive study is ERCP.[5,81] However, due to the risks associated with this procedure endoscopic ultrasonography (EUS) has become an accepted alternative for the diagnosis of chronic pancreatitis.[5,81,82,100]

Clinical Course and Prognosis

The clinical course of chronic pancreatitis depends upon the etiology. The median age at onset is as early as 10 years for hereditary chronic pancreatitis, whereas alcoholic and late-onset idiopathic chronic pancreatitis have median onsets of 36 and 62 years, respectively.[101] Exocrine insufficiency, which occurs when lipase secretion is less than 10% of normal,[4,81] develops about 5 years after diagnosis in alcoholic chronic pancreatitis and 22 years in hereditary chronic pancreatitis. Diabetes mellitus was shown to occur about 8 years after diagnosis of alcoholic chronic pancreatitis and up to 27 years after diagnosis of early-onset idiopathic chronic

TABLE 46-7	Signs, Symptoms, and Diagnosis of Chronic Pancreatitis

Signs
- Malnutrition (especially in chronic alcoholism)
- Abdominal mass (may indicate a pancreatic pseudocyst)
- Jaundice may be seen
- Splenomegaly (rare)

Symptoms
- Abdominal pain
  - Commonly in epigastric area
  - May radiate to the back
  - Described as deep and penetrating
  - May be relieved by bending/leaning forward or bringing knees to the chest
  - Often occurs with meals and at night
  - May be associated with nausea and vomiting
- Steatorrhea
  - Patients describe bulky or foul-smelling stools often with obvious oil droplets
  - Usually have an average of three to four stools per day
  - May be associated with deficiencies in fat-soluble vitamins
  - Watery diarrhea, excess gas, and abdominal cramps are uncommon
- Pancreatic diabetes mellitus
- Diarrhea (associated with steatorrhea)
- Weight loss
  - May be due to severe malabsorption or acute/chronic pain
  - Substantial loss may be due to associated or unrelated malignancy
- Dyspepsia

Laboratory studies
- CBC to rule out infection (i.e., infected pseudocyst)
- Serum amylase and lipase
  - Low specificity for chronic pancreatitis
  - May be elevated in acute exacerbations
  - Usually are normal or only slightly elevated
- Total bilirubin, alkaline phosphatase, and hepatic transaminases may be elevated with ductal obstruction
- Fasting serum glucose
- Pancreatic function tests
  - Serum trypsinogen (<20 ng/mL is abnormal)
  - Fecal elastase (<200 mcg/g of stool is abnormal)
  - Fecal fat estimation (>7 g/day is abnormal; need to collect 72 hours of stool)
  - Secretin stimulation (evaluates duodenal bicarbonate secretion)
  - ^{13}C-mixed triglyceride breath test
- Serum albumin (may be low with malnutrition)
- Serum calcium (may be low with malnutrition)

Imaging studies
- Noninvasive
  - Abdominal ultrasound
  - Computed tomography (CT)
  - Magnetic resonance cholangiopancreatography (MRCP)
- Invasive
  - Endoscopic ultrasonography (EUS)
  - Endoscopic retrograde cholangiopancreatography (ERCP)

CBC, complete blood count.
Data from references 4, 5, 129.

pancreatitis. Resolution of pain from pancreatic burnout tended to coincide with exocrine insufficiency.

The life expectancy of patients with chronic pancreatitis is shorter than that of the general population. The 10-year survival is 70%, while the 20-year rate was 45%.[6] However, death in patients with chronic pancreatitis most commonly results from cardiovascular disease, infection, or malignancy rather than from the disease itself.[6,101] One of the most significant complications of long-standing disease is pancreatic cancer. Patients with alcoholic chronic pancreatitis are 15 times as likely as the general population to develop pancreatic cancer, while 40% of those with hereditary chronic pancreatitis may be diagnosed.[6,81]

TREATMENT

Chronic Pancreatitis

■ DESIRED OUTCOME

The major goals in the treatment of uncomplicated chronic pancreatitis are relief of abdominal pain, treatment of the associated complications of malabsorption and diabetes mellitus, and improvement in quality of life. Secondary goals include treating associated disorders such as depression and malnutrition.

■ GENERAL APPROACH TO TREATMENT

Treatment of chronic pancreatitis and its complications involves various nonpharmacologic and pharmacologic interventions. Lifestyle modifications should include abstinence from alcohol and smoking cessation.[5,81] Also, patients with steatorrhea may need to eat smaller, more frequent meals and reduce dietary fat intake.[4,5] The majority of patients require analgesics and pancreatic enzyme supplementation.[5,81,82] Pain can initially be controlled with medications but may require more aggressive medical and surgical therapies as the disease progresses. Patients with malabsorption require pancreatic enzymes to reduce steatorrhea and maintain adequate nutrient absorption.[5,81] An antisecretory agent may be added to the regimen when enzymes alone provide an inadequate reduction in steatorrhea.[4,5,81]

■ NONPHARMACOLOGIC THERAPY

In addition to medical management the treatment of chronic pancreatitis includes both lifestyle and dietary modifications. Patients should be counseled to abstain from alcohol use, and smoking cessation should be advocated. It is unclear if cessation of alcohol use reduces pain in patients with alcoholic chronic pancreatitis, but its use hastens disease progression.[4] Patients with steatorrhea should be counseled to eat small and frequent meals.[102] A reduction in dietary fat is not needed empirically, but a decrease to 0.5 g/kg/day is recommended for those whose symptoms are uncontrolled with enzyme supplementation. Patients who do not consume adequate calories from their normal diet may be given whole protein or peptide-based oral nutritional supplements. Supplementation with medium-chain triglycerides, which do not require lipolysis, should be considered for patients with steatorrhea who are unable to gain weight. Complete enteral nutrition is recommended for patients who cannot consume adequate calories, have continued weight loss, experience complications, or require surgery. A jejunal feeding tube is the recommended route for administration of enteral nutrition in chronic pancreatitis patients; it increases patient weight and decreases abdominal pain and opioid use.[103]

Invasive procedures and surgery are primarily used to treat uncontrolled pain and the associated complications of chronic pancreatitis. Stents placed via ERCP may be used to treat pancreatic duct strictures in order to relieve parenchymal pressure and reduce pain.[95,100,104] Extracorporeal shock wave lithotripsy can be used to break up pancreatic stones with ultrasonic vibration prior to removal by ERCP.[95,100,104,105] However, combining these procedures to treat pain provides no additional benefit and increases cost.[106] Blockade of pain signals through the celiac plexus may be achieved utilizing EUS.[82,95,100,104] Some complications of chronic pancreatitis that can be treated endoscopically include common bile duct strictures, duodenal obstructions, and pancreatic pseudocysts.[100,104] Various surgical techniques, including total pancreatectomy, may also be used to relieve pain associated with chronic pancreatitis.[5,95,107] Surgery is more effective at relieving pain compared with endoscopic procedures, but these trials have a number of limitations.[108,109]

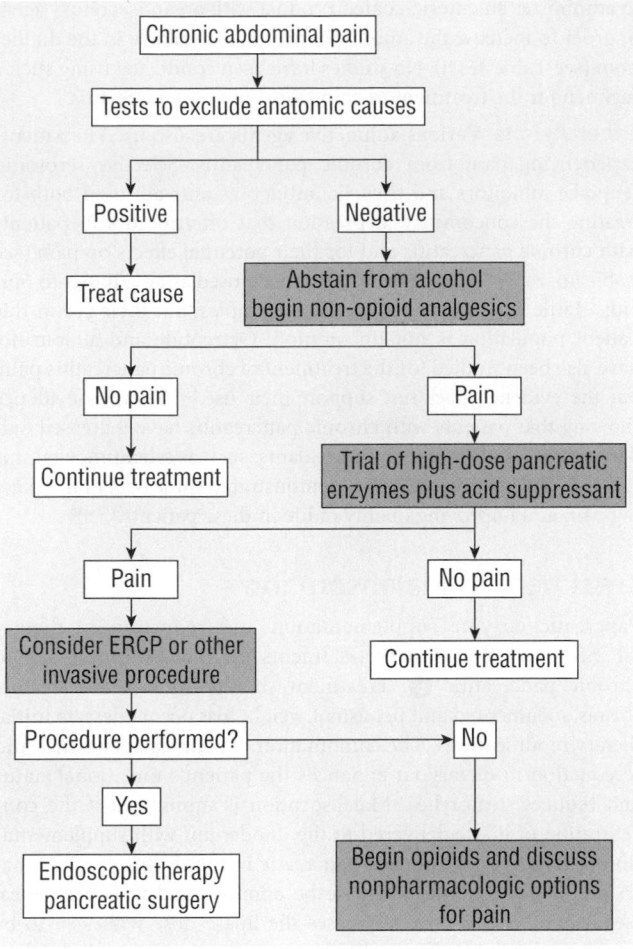

FIGURE 46-4. Algorithm for the treatment of abdominal pain in chronic pancreatitis. (ERCP, endoscopic retrograde cholangiopancreatography.)

Finally, total pancreatectomy with transplantation of pancreatic islet cells to reduce the need for exogenous insulin is a possible option for the treatment of pain due to chronic pancreatitis.[82,110]

■ PHARMACOLOGIC THERAPY

General Recommendations

Pharmacologic therapy of chronic pancreatitis is aimed at controlling pain, treating malabsorption and associated steatorrhea, and controlling diabetes mellitus. Once other causes have been excluded nonopioid analgesics should be tried initially for pain management (Fig. 46–4).[4,5] Patients unresponsive to nonopioid analgesics may be given a trial of pancreatic enzyme supplements prior to addition of opioids.[4,82,95] If these measures fail, an oral opioid should be added to the drug regimen. Opioids administered by nonoral routes should be reserved for patients who cannot take oral medications or whose pain is unresponsive to oral opioids. Additional agents may be considered for added pain control and disorders associated with chronic pancreatitis.

Most patients with malabsorption will require a modification in diet along with pancreatic enzyme supplementation in order to achieve adequate nutritional status and reduction in steatorrhea (Fig. 46–5). An antisecretory agent should be added to the regimen when there is an inadequate response to enzyme therapy alone.[4] If these measures are ineffective, documentation of the diagnosis and exclusion of other diseases should be undertaken. Exogenous insulin is the primary pharmacologic agent used in the treatment of diabetes mellitus associated with chronic pancreatitis.[4] However,

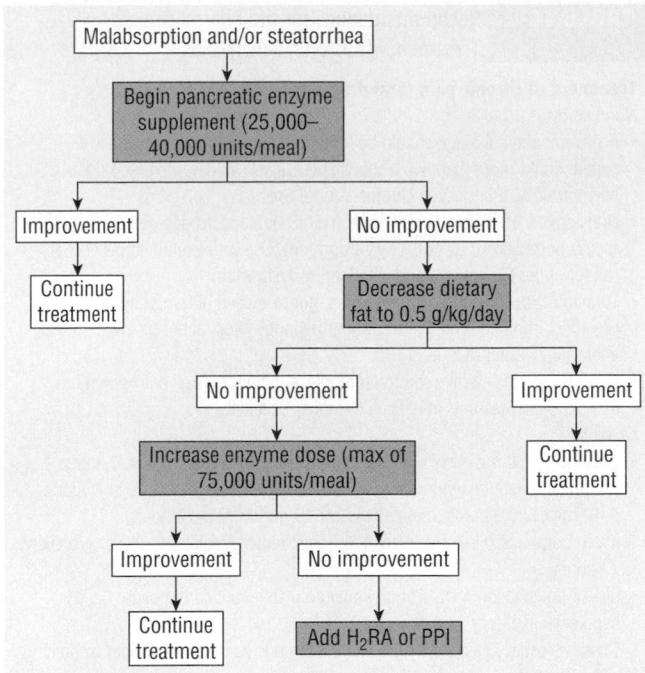

FIGURE 46-5. Algorithm for the treatment of malabsorption and steatorrhea in chronic pancreatitis. (H$_2$RA, hitamine$_2$-receptor antagonist; PPI, proton pump inhibitor.)

some patients may have favorable results with the use of oral agents for control of blood glucose.

Relief of Chronic Abdominal Pain

Analgesics Pain from chronic pancreatitis can initially be treated with nonopioid analgesics, but opioids will eventually be required as the disease progresses ❼. Therapy should begin with acetaminophen or nonsteroidal antiinflammatory drugs (NSAIDs) (Table 46–8).[4,5] Regimens should be individualized and should begin with the lowest effective dose. The dosage regimen should be maximized before adding or substituting agents. Analgesics should be scheduled around the clock rather than as needed in order to maximize efficacy. Also, scheduling analgesics prior to meals should help decrease postprandial pain. When nonopioid analgesics fail to control pain low-potency opioids (e.g., hydrocodone) should be added to the regimen (see Table 46–8). Tramadol has also been used successfully to treat pain in patients with chronic pancreatitis, but at a higher dose than that approved in the United States.[4] Severe pain unresponsive to these therapies necessitates the use of opiate analgesics. Although opioids carry about a 10% to 30% risk of addiction in this population their use should not be withheld.[4] Unless contraindicated, oral opioids should be used before parenteral, transdermal, or other dosage forms. Although oxycodone was found to relieve pain better than morphine in a study of simulated chronic pancreatitis pain, adequate trials comparing agents have not been conducted.[111] Therefore, the choice of agent should be based on cost, compliance, and avoidance of adverse drug events (e.g., allergic reactions).

CLINICAL CONTROVERSY

Since the evidence supporting the use of pancreatic enzyme supplements for treating pain associated with chronic pancreatitis is not overwhelming, clinicians debate over their use for this purpose. Often the decision to use enzyme supplements for the treatment of pain comes from clinical experience and the knowledge that their use carries minimal risk of adverse effects.

TABLE 46-8 Recommendations for the Pharmacologic Treatment of Chronic Pancreatitis

Treatment of chronic pain (oral drug regimens)

Nonopioids
- Acetaminophen: Dosage should be limited to 500 mg four times a day if patient drinks more than two alcoholic beverages per day; increased risk of hepatotoxicity, especially in chronic alcohol use
- Nonsteroidal antiinflammatory drugs (NSAIDs): Standard dosage regimens of aspirin or traditional NSAIDs (e.g., ibuprofen). Use with caution in patients at risk for upper GI bleeding and with kidney dysfunction
- Tramadol: 50–100 mg every 4–6 hours, not to exceed 400 mg/day; has opioid-like effect; contraindicated in alcohol or hypnotic intoxication; be aware of drug interactions; expensive
- Consider use of selective serotonin reuptake inhibitors (e.g., paroxetine) or tricyclic antidepressants in difficult-to-manage patients

Opioids
- Codeine 30–60 mg every 6 hours; hydrocodone 5–10 mg every 4–6 hours; morphine sulfate (extended-release) 30–60 mg every 8–12 hours; oxycodone 5–10 mg every 6 hours; methadone 2.5–10 mg every 8–12 hours; hydromorphone 0.5–1 mg every 4–6 hours; fentanyl patch 25–100 mcg/h every 72 hours
- Risk of potentiation with alcohol; impaired respiration; constipation; hypotension; allergy
- Dosing is usually based on providing continuous pain relief; consider combining with acetaminophen or NSAIDs; opioid dependence is common; abuse is a concern in alcoholics; tolerance may develop

Pancreatic enzymes
- Four to eight tablets of a preferred product (see Table 46-9) with each meal plus either a histamine$_2$-receptor antagonist or proton pump inhibitor; no clinical trials support such a regimen for pain management

Treatment of malabsorption and steatorrhea
- Start with 25,000–40,000 USP units of lipase with each meal of a preferred product (see Table 46-9); administer dose during or just after meals
- Increase dose to a maximum of 75,000 USP units per meal
- Products containing enteric-coated microspheres or minimicrospheres may be more effective than other dose forms

Acid suppression agents
- May improve efficacy of enzyme therapy for malabsorption and steatorrhea
- May allow a lower dose of enzyme supplements to be used

USP, United States Pharmacopeia
From references 4, 5, 11, 95, 117, 118, 120, 121.

Pancreatic Enzymes Although pancreatic enzymes are primarily used to treat malabsorption associated with chronic pancreatitis they are also used to treat pain from the disease. Relief of pain using pancreatic enzymes is thought to be due to their ability to break down CCK.[4,11,82,95] Normally, the release of CCK, which causes an increase in pancreatic secretion, is inhibited by trypsin. However, there is a decrease in the production of trypsin in patients with chronic pancreatitis. This leads to a loss of negative feedback on the release of CCK and thus an increase in pain due to unabated pancreatic secretion. The proteases in pancreatic enzyme supplements are thought to act as substitutes for endogenous trypsin, leading to a decrease in CCK release.

Despite this intuitive mechanism there were mixed results from trials investigating pancreatic enzyme supplements for the treatment of pain from chronic pancreatitis. This may be due to the differences between the various enzyme formulations used in the trials as well as the small number of subjects enrolled.[4,11,82,95] A meta-analysis that pooled the results of all six prospective trials found no benefit with the use of enzyme supplements for pain relief.[112] However, the two trials that used non-enteric-coated enzyme formulations demonstrated a benefit in the treatment of pain.[4,11,82,95] Enteric-coated formulations may not release enough proteases in the duodenum to inhibit CCK release. However, non-enteric-coated products are no longer available in the United States. Therefore, it may be reasonable

to administer an enteric-coated product with an antisecretory agent in order to increase the amount of proteases available in the duodenum (see Table 46–8). No studies have been conducted using such a regimen for the treatment of pain from chronic pancreatitis.

Other Agents Various adjunctive agents are also used in patients experiencing pain from chronic pancreatitis. Selective serotonin reuptake inhibitors and tricyclic antidepressants are used both for treating the concomitant depression that often occurs in patients with chronic pancreatitis and for their potential effects on pain (see Table 46–8).[4,95] Gabapentin has also been used as an adjunct to opioids.[4] Little evidence supports these therapies, but their use in this patient population is not uncommon. Octreotide and allopurinol have also been studied for the treatment of chronic pancreatitis pain, but the evidence does not support their use.[4,95] There is evidence showing that patients with chronic pancreatitis have increased oxidative stress, and the use of antioxidants, such as selenium, vitamins C and E, and beta-carotene, has demonstrated some benefit in relieving pain and improving quality of life in these patients.[113–116]

Treatment of Malabsorption

Pancreatic enzyme supplementation and reduction in dietary fat intake are the primary treatments for malabsorption due to chronic pancreatitis ❽. Treatment should begin when steatorrhea is documented and persistent weight loss occurs despite initial dietary modifications. The combination of pancreatic enzymes and a reduction in dietary fat enhances the patient's nutritional status and reduces steatorrhea. Malabsorption is minimized if the concentration of lipase delivered to the duodenum with supplementation is about 10% of normal pancreatic output.[4] This requires that 25,000 to 40,000 units of lipase be administered with each meal (see Table 46–8).[11] In many cases the lipase dose will need to be increased due to insufficient lipolytic activity, but doses greater than 75,000 units per meal are not recommended.

There is little evidence regarding the optimal dosage form and administration of pancreatic enzyme supplements. Most studies have compared them to placebo rather than to other enzyme products and have used quantitation of fat absorption or elimination rather than weight gain as a primary measure of efficacy.[117] Although they improve fat absorption, they may not completely eliminate steatorrhea.[117,118] However, they improve the quality of life of patients with chronic pancreatitis.[119] Since most exogenous lipase is rapidly and irreversibly destroyed at low intragastric pH, enteric-coated products are preferred for the treatment of malabsorption and steatorrhea ❾. The enteric coating dissolves at a pH greater than 5.5, which allows a sufficient quantity of enzymes to remain intact until dissolution of the coating in the duodenum.[11] However, enzymes must also be emptied from the stomach into the duodenum at the same rate and time as ingested food. The size of the enteric-coated enzyme preparation influences the rate of enzyme delivery to the duodenum.[4,11] Likewise, the administration time relevant to a meal influences the timing of enzyme delivery. Products that contain enzymes in small enteric-coated microspheres or minimicrospheres are often the best products because they are thought to mix effectively with chyme, thus leaving the stomach at a similar rate.[11] Also, the optimal administration time of enzymes containing minimicrospheres appears to be either with a meal or just after.[4,120]

Despite enzyme therapy patients may continue to have steatorrhea and fail to gain sufficient weight. Compliance should be assessed in these patients as the number of capsules required with each meal can lead to noncompliance. Alternative products with higher lipase content can be tried in order to reduce the number of capsules needed. If this fails the dose of lipase should be increased. Finally, addition of an antisecretory agent may be tried to increase the availability of active enzymes in the duodenum.[121]

TABLE 46-9 Commercially Available Pancreatic Enzyme (Pancrelipase) Preparations

Product	Enzyme Content per Unit Dose (USP Units)		
	Lipase	Amylase	Protease
Enteric-coated microspheres			
Ultrase	4,500	20,000	25,000
Enteric-coated microspheres with bicarbonate buffer			
Pancrecarb MS-4	4,000	25,000	25,000
Pancrecarb MS-8	8,000	40,000	45,000
Pancrecarb MS-16	16,000	52,000	52,000
Enteric-coated minimicrospheres			
Creon 6,000 lipase units[a]	6,000	30,000	19,000
Creon 12,000 lipase units[a]	12,000	60,000	38,000
Creon 24,000 lipase units[a]	24,000	120,000	76,000
Enteric-coated minitablets			
Ultrase MT 12	12,000	39,000	39,000
Ultrase MT 18	18,000	58,500	58,500
Ultrase MT 20	20,000	65,000	65,000

USP, United States Pharmacopeia.
[a]FDA-approved product.

Pancreatic Enzyme Supplements Until recently none of the commercially available pancreatic enzyme supplements were approved by the FDA because they predated enactment of the Food, Drug, and Cosmetic Act of 1938. Since the FDA announced in 2004 that all products would have to seek approval only one has been approved and three others have submitted new drug applications.[122] Dosage forms of products currently available in the United States include enteric-coated microspheres, bicarbonate-buffered microspheres, enteric-coated minimicrospheres, and enteric-coated minitablets encased in a cellulose or gelatin capsule (Table 46–9). Enzymes are easily administered to patients able to swallow the capsules or their contents. However, administration to patients with enteral feeding tubes presents a challenge. Products containing microspheres may be administered through feeding tubes in an applesauce or apple juice mixture.[11] Clinicians must be aware, however, that available products are not equivalent and should consider this before substituting products in patients who require administration through a nonoral route.

Adverse reactions from pancreatic enzyme supplements are generally benign. High doses can lead to nausea, diarrhea, and intestinal upset.[11] One of the more serious adverse effects of these products is fibrosing colonopathy. It occurs when the enzymes cause deposition of fibrin in the colon, leading to colonic stricture. This reaction is uncommon and has been reported mostly in children with cystic fibrosis who received high doses of enzymes for prolonged periods.[11] Certain enteric coatings may specifically invoke this reaction. Another concern with pancreatic enzymes is the risk of possible viral infection due to contamination of these porcine-derived products.[122] Finally, pancreatic enzymes have been associated with deficiencies in fat-soluble vitamins, and appropriate monitoring and supplementation, especially of vitamin D, should be instituted.[4,81]

Adjuncts to Enzyme Therapy The addition of a histamine$_2$-recpetor antagonist or proton pump inhibitor to pancreatic enzyme supplementation may increase the effectiveness of enzyme therapy for malabsorption and steatorrhea ❿. The beneficial effects of these agents result from an increase in gastric and duodenal pH.[11,81] This is thought to result in an increase in the amount of active enzymes available in the duodenum. Traditionally, their use has been advocated with non-enteric-coated enzyme products.[4,11] However, their use in combination with enteric-coated preparations results in similar efficacy between standard and low-dose enzyme regimens.[121]

■ PHARMACOECONOMIC CONSIDERATIONS

The pharmacoeconomic issues associated with the medical treatment of acute pancreatitis and chronic pancreatitis have not been extensively examined. Aggressive medical and surgical care decreases mortality in acute pancreatitis, but the overall cost-effectiveness of a specific treatment is unknown. The relief of abdominal pain in acute pancreatitis and chronic pancreatitis, as well as pancreatic enzyme supplementation in patients with chronic pancreatitis, improves quality of life and nutritional status.[119,123]

With so few FDA-approved pancreatic enzyme supplements currently available pricing should remain fairly competitive. However, if cost is based on the total number of capsules per day, rather than the cost of a single capsule, high-potency preparations may help minimize cost. The addition of a histamine$_2$-receptor antagonist or proton pump inhibitor may actually be cost-effective for patients with chronic pancreatitis who are inadequately controlled on maximal enzyme therapy. They reduce the amount of enzymes needed and they may improve efficacy.[121]

EVALUATION OF THERAPEUTIC OUTCOMES

ACUTE PANCREATITIS

Hydration status, serum electrolytes, pain control, and nutritional status should be assessed periodically in patients with mild acute pancreatitis, depending on the degree of abdominal pain and fluid loss. Patients with severe acute pancreatitis should receive intensive care and close monitoring of vital signs, fluid and electrolyte status, white blood cell count, blood glucose, lactate dehydrogenase, aspartate aminotransferase, serum albumin, hematocrit, blood urea nitrogen, serum creatinine, and international normalized ratio. Continuous hemodynamic and arterial blood gas monitoring is essential. Serum lipase, amylase, and bilirubin require less frequent monitoring. The patient should also be monitored for signs of infection, relief of abdominal pain, and adequate nutritional status. Severity of disease and patient response should be assessed using an evidence-based method, for example APACHE II.

CHRONIC PANCREATITIS

The severity and frequency of abdominal pain should be assessed periodically in patients with chronic pancreatitis using a standardized scale to determine the efficacy of pain therapy. Patients receiving opioids should be prescribed scheduled bowel regimens and be monitored for constipation. Patients receiving pancreatic enzymes for malabsorption should have their weight and stool frequency and consistency monitored periodically. More objective assessments of fecal fat content, such as the ^{13}C-mixed triglyceride breath test, can be utilized but are usually unnecessary and impractical in general clinical practice.[4,98,124] Blood glucose must be closely monitored in patients with diabetes mellitus, and those with long-standing disease should receive appropriate monitoring for nephropathy, retinopathy, and neuropathy.[4]

ACKNOWLEDGMENT

The authors wish to acknowledge the contributions of Rosemary R. Berardi, Pharm.D., FCCP, FASHP, to previous editions of this chapter.

ABBREVIATIONS

ARDS: acute respiratory distress syndrome

CT: computed tomography

CCK: cholecystokinin

CECT: contrast-enhanced computed tomography

CFTR: cystic fibrosis transmembrane conductance regulator gene

ERCP: endoscopic retrograde cholangiopancreatography

EUS: endoscopic ultrasonography

GRP: gastrin-releasing peptide

HIV: human immunodeficiency virus

NSAID: nonsteroidal antiinflammatory drug

PRSS1: cationic trypsinogen gene

SIRS: systemic inflammatory response syndrome

SPINK1: serine protease inhibitor Kazal type 1 gene

VIP: vasoactive intestinal peptide

REFERENCES

1. Mitchell RM, Byrne MF, Baillie J. Pancreatitis. Lancet 2003;361(9367): 1447–1455.
2. Forsmark CE, Baillie J. AGA Institute technical review on acute pancreatitis. Gastroenterology 2007;132(5):2022–2044.
3. Cappell MS. Acute pancreatitis: etiology, clinical presentation, diagnosis, and therapy. Med Clin North Am 2008;92(4):889–923, ix–x.
4. Forsmark CE. Chronic Pancreatitis. In: Feldman M, Friedman LS, Brandt LJ, eds. Gastrointestinal and Liver Disease: Pathophysiology, Diagnosis, Management. 8th ed. Philadelphia: Saunders; 2006: 1271–1308.
5. Nair RJ, Lawler L, Miller MR. Chronic pancreatitis. Am Fam Physician 2007;76(11):1679–1688.
6. Spanier BW, Dijkgraaf MG, Bruno MJ. Epidemiology, aetiology and outcome of acute and chronic pancreatitis: An update. Best Pract Res Clin Gastroenterol 2008;22(1):45–63.
7. Etemad B, Whitcomb DC. Chronic pancreatitis: Diagnosis, classification, and new genetic developments. Gastroenterology 2001;120(3):682–707.
8. Lowenfels AB, Maisonneuve P, Sullivan T. The changing character of acute pancreatitis: Epidemiology, etiology, and prognosis. Curr Gastroenterol Rep 2009;11(2):97–103.
9. Whitcomb DC. Clinical practice: Acute pancreatitis. N Engl J Med 2006;354(20):2142–2150.
10. Pandol SJ. Pancreatic Secretion. In: Feldman M, Friedman LS, Brandt LJ, es. Gastrointestinal and Liver Disease: Pathophysiology, Diagnosis, Management. 8th ed. Philadelphia: Saunders; 2006:1189–1201.
11. Ferrone M, Raimondo M, Scolapio JS. Pancreatic enzyme pharmacotherapy. Pharmacotherapy 2007;27(6):910–920.
12. Finkelberg DL, Sahani D, Deshpande V, Brugge WR. Autoimmune pancreatitis. N Engl J Med 2006; 355(25):2670–2676.
13. Lee JK, Enns R. Review of idiopathic pancreatitis. World J Gastroenterol 2007;13(47):6296–6313.
14. Cooper ST, Slivka A. Incidence, risk factors, and prevention of post-ERCP pancreatitis. Gastroenterol Clin North Am 2007;36(2):259–276, vii–viii.
15. Quraishi ER, Goel S, Gupta M, Catanzaro A, Zasuwa G, Divine G. Acute pancreatitis in patients on chronic peritoneal dialysis: An increased risk? Am J Gastroenterol 2005;100(10):2288–2293.
16. Morton C, Klatsky AL, Udaltsova N. Smoking, coffee, and pancreatitis. Am J Gastroenterol 2004;99(4):731–738.
17. Lowe ME, Greer JB. Pancreatitis in children and adolescents. Curr Gastroenterol Rep 2008;10(2):128–135.
18. Balani AR, Grendell JH. Drug-induced pancreatitis: Incidence, management and prevention. Drug Saf 2008;31(10):823–837.
19. Eland IA, Alvarez CH, Stricker BH, Rodriguez LA. The risk of acute pancreatitis associated with acid-suppressing drugs. Br J Clin Pharmacol 2000;49(5):473–478.
20. Blomgren KB, Sundstrom A, Steineck G, Genell S, Sjostedt S, Wiholm BE. A Swedish case-control network for studies of drug-induced morbidity—acute pancreatitis. Eur J Clin Pharmacol 2002;58(4):275–283.
21. Blomgren KB, Sundstrom A, Steineck G, Wiholm BE. Obesity and treatment of diabetes with glyburide may both be risk factors for acute pancreatitis. Diabetes Care 2002;25(2):298–302.
22. Lin HH, Hsu CH, Chao YC. Tamoxifen-induced severe acute pancreatitis: A case report. Dig Dis Sci 2004;49(6):997–999.
23. Mallick S. Metformin induced acute pancreatitis precipitated by renal failure. Postgrad Med J 2004;80(942):239–240.
24. Devlin JW, Lau AK, Tanios MA. Propofol-associated hypertriglyceridemia and pancreatitis in the intensive care unit: An analysis of frequency and risk factors. Pharmacotherapy 2005;25(10):1348–1352.
25. Fessel J, Hurley LB. Incidence of pancreatitis in HIV-infected patients: Comment on findings in EuroSIDA cohort. AIDS 2008;22(1): 145–147.
26. Smith CJ, Olsen CH, Mocroft A, et al. The role of antiretroviral therapy in the incidence of pancreatitis in HIV-positive individuals in the EuroSIDA study. AIDS 2008;22(1):47–56.
27. Dhir R, Brown DK, Olden KW. Drug-induced pancreatitis: A practical review. Drugs Today (Barc) 2007;43(7):499–507.
28. Eland IA, van Puijenbroek EP, Sturkenboom MJ, Wilson JH, Stricker BH. Drug-associated acute pancreatitis: Twenty-one years of spontaneous reporting in the Netherlands. Am J Gastroenterol 1999;94(9):2417–2422.
29. Trivedi CD, Pitchumoni CS. Drug-induced pancreatitis: An update. J Clin Gastroenterol 2005;39(8):709–716.
30. Criddle DN, McLaughlin E, Murphy JA, Petersen OH, Sutton R. The pancreas misled: Signals to pancreatitis. Pancreatology 2007;7(5–6): 436–446.
31. Vonlaufen A, Wilson JS, Apte MV. Molecular mechanisms of pancreatitis: Current opinion. J Gastroenterol Hepatol 2008;23(9):1339–1348.
32. Gorelick F. Pancreatic protease-activated receptors: Friend and foe. Gut 2007;56(7):901–902.
33. Weiss FU, Halangk W, Lerch MM. New advances in pancreatic cell physiology and pathophysiology. Best Pract Res Clin Gastroenterol 2008;22(1):3–15.
34. Sand J, Nordback I. Acute pancreatitis: Risk of recurrence and late consequences of the disease. Nat Rev Gastroenterol Hepatol 2009;6(8):470–477.
35. Pezzilli R, Uomo G, Zerbi A, et al. Diagnosis and treatment of acute pancreatitis: The position statement of the Italian Association for the study of the pancreas. Dig Liver Dis 2008;40(10):803–808.
36. Topazian M, Gorelick F. Acute pancreatitis. In: Yamada T, Alpers D, Kaplowitz N, Laine L, Owyang C, Powell D, eds. Textbook of Gastroenterology. 4th ed. Philadelphia: Lippincott Williams & Wilkins; 2003:2026–2060.
37. UK Working Party on Acute Pancreatitis. UK guidelines for the management of acute pancreatitis. Gut 2005;54(suppl 3):iii, 1–9.
38. Mofidi R, Patil PV, Suttie SA, Parks RW. Risk assessment in acute pancreatitis. Br J Surg 2009;96(2):137–150.
39. Harrison DA, D'Amico G, Singer M. The Pancreatitis Outcome Prediction (POP) Score: A new prognostic index for patients with severe acute pancreatitis. Crit Care Med 2007;35(7):1703–1708.
40. Gardner TB, Vege SS, Pearson RK, Chari ST. Fluid resuscitation in acute pancreatitis. Clin Gastroenterol Hepatol 2008;6(10):1070–1076.
41. McClave SA, Chang WK, Dhaliwal R, Heyland DK. Nutrition support in acute pancreatitis: A systematic review of the literature. J Parenter Enteral Nutr 2006;30(2):143–156.
42. Meier RF, Beglinger C. Nutrition in pancreatic diseases. Best Pract Res Clin Gastroenterol 2006;20(3):507–529.
43. Al-Omran M, Groof A, Wilke D. Enteral versus parenteral nutrition for acute pancreatitis. Cochrane Database Syst Rev 2003;(1):CD002837.
44. Marik PE, Zaloga GP. Meta-analysis of parenteral nutrition versus enteral nutrition in patients with acute pancreatitis. BMJ 2004;328(7453):1407.
45. Banks PA, Freeman ML. Practice Guidelines in Acute Pancreatitis. Am J Gastroenterol 2006;101(10):2379–2400.

46. Petrov MS, van Santvoort HC, Besselink MG, van der Heijden GJ, Windsor JA, Gooszen HG. Enteral nutrition and the risk of mortality and infectious complications in patients with severe acute pancreatitis: A meta-analysis of randomized trials. Arch Surg 2008;143(11): 1111–1117.

47. Olah A, Belagyi T, Issekutz A, Gamal ME, Bengmark S. Randomized clinical trial of specific lactobacillus and fibre supplement to early enteral nutrition in patients with acute pancreatitis. Br J Surg 2002;89(9):1103–1107.

48. Penner R, Fedorak RN, Madsen KL. Probiotics and nutraceuticals: Non-medicinal treatments of gastrointestinal diseases. Curr Opin Pharmacol 2005;5(6):596–603.

49. Isenhower HL, Mueller BA. Selection of narcotic analgesics for pain associated with pancreatitis. Am J Health Syst Pharm 1998;55(5):480–486.

50. Thompson DR. Narcotic analgesic effects on the sphincter of Oddi: A review of the data and therapeutic implications in treating pancreatitis. Am J Gastroenterol 2001;96(4):1266–1272.

51. Banks PA. Practice guidelines in acute pancreatitis. Am J Gastroenterol 1997;92(3):377–386.

52. Norton ID, Clain JE. Optimising outcomes in acute pancreatitis. Drugs 2001;61(11):1581–1591.

53. Yousaf M, McCallion K, Diamond T. Management of severe acute pancreatitis. Br J Surg 2003;90(4):407–420.

54. Fantini L, Tomassetti P, Pezzilli R. Management of acute pancreatitis: Current knowledge and future perspectives. World J Emerg Surg 2006;1:16.

55. Andriulli A, Leandro G, Clemente R, et al. Meta-analysis of somatostatin, octreotide and gabexate mesilate in the therapy of acute pancreatitis. Aliment Pharmacol Ther 1998;12(3):237–245.

56. Lankisch PG, Lerch MM. The role of antibiotic prophylaxis in the treatment of acute pancreatitis. J Clin Gastroenterol 2006;40(2): 149–155.

57. Pederzoli P, Bassi C, Vesentini S, Campedelli A. A randomized multicenter clinical trial of antibiotic prophylaxis of septic complications in acute necrotizing pancreatitis with imipenem. Surg Gynecol Obstet 1993;176(5):480–483.

58. Sainio V, Kemppainen E, Puolakkainen P, et al. Early antibiotic treatment in acute necrotising pancreatitis. Lancet 1995;346(8976):663–667.

59. Delcenserie R, Yzet T, Ducroix JP. Prophylactic antibiotics in treatment of severe acute alcoholic pancreatitis. Pancreas 1996;13(2):198–201.

60. Schwarz M, Isenmann R, Meyer H, Beger HG. Antibiotic use in necrotizing pancreatitis: Results of a controlled study. Dtsch Med Wochenschr 1997;122(12):356–361.

61. Nordback I, Sand J, Saaristo R, Paajanen H. Early treatment with antibiotics reduces the need for surgery in acute necrotizing pancreatitis—a single-center randomized study. J Gastrointest Surg 2001;5(2):113–118.

62. Isenmann R, Runzi M, Kron M, et al. Prophylactic antibiotic treatment in patients with predicted severe acute pancreatitis: A placebo-controlled, double-blind trial. Gastroenterology 2004;126(4):997–1004.

63. Dellinger EP, Tellado JM, Soto NE, et al. Early antibiotic treatment for severe acute necrotizing pancreatitis: A randomized, double-blind, placebo-controlled study. Ann Surg 2007;245(5):674–683.

64. Rokke O, Harbitz TB, Liljedal J, et al. Early treatment of severe pancreatitis with imipenem: A prospective randomized clinical trial. Scand J Gastroenterol 2007;42(6):771–776.

65. Golub R, Siddiqi F, Pohl D. Role of antibiotics in acute pancreatitis: A meta-analysis. J Gastrointest Surg 1998;2(6):496–503.

66. Sharma VK, Howden CW. Prophylactic antibiotic administration reduces sepsis and mortality in acute necrotizing pancreatitis: A meta-analysis. Pancreas 2001;22(1):28–31.

67. Villatoro E, Bassi C, Larvin M. Antibiotic therapy for prophylaxis against infection of pancreatic necrosis in acute pancreatitis. Cochrane Database Syst Rev 2006;(4):CD002941.

68. Bai Y, Gao J, Zou DW, Li ZS. Prophylactic antibiotics cannot reduce infected pancreatic necrosis and mortality in acute necrotizing pancreatitis: Evidence from a meta-analysis of randomized controlled trials. Am J Gastroenterol 2008;103(1):104–110.

69. Luiten EJ, Bruining HA. Antimicrobial prophylaxis in acute pancreatitis: Selective decontamination versus antibiotics. Baillieres Best Pract Res Clin Gastroenterol 1999;13(2):317–330.

70. Gloor B, Muller CA, Worni M, et al. Pancreatic infection in severe pancreatitis: The role of fungus and multiresistant organisms. Arch Surg 2001;136(5):592–596.

71. Howard TJ, Temple MB. Prophylactic antibiotics alter the bacteriology of infected necrosis in severe acute pancreatitis. J Am Coll Surg 2002;195(6):759–767.

72. De Waele JJ, Vogelaers D, Blot S, Colardyn F. Fungal infections in patients with severe acute pancreatitis and the use of prophylactic therapy. Clin Infect Dis 2003;37(2):208–213.

73. Shrikhande S, Friess H, Issenegger C, et al. Fluconazole penetration into the pancreas. Antimicrob Agents Chemother 2000;44(9):2569–2571.

74. Poon RT, Fan ST. Antisecretory agents for prevention of post-ERCP pancreatitis: Rationale for use and clinical results. J Pancreas 2003;4(1):33–40.

75. Lavy A, Karban A, Suissa A, Yassin K, Hermesh I, Ben-Amotz A. Natural beta-carotene for the prevention of post-ERCP pancreatitis. Pancreas 2004;29(2):e45–e50.

76. Murray B, Carter R, Imrie C, Evans S, O'Suilleabhain C. Diclofenac reduces the incidence of acute pancreatitis after endoscopic retrograde cholangiopancreatography. Gastroenterology 2003;124(7):1786–1791.

77. Hoogerwerf WA. Pharmacological management of pancreatitis. Curr Opin Pharmacol 2005;5(6):578–582.

78. Bai Y, Gao J, Zou DW, Li ZS. Prophylactic octreotide administration does not prevent post-endoscopic retrograde cholangiopancreatography pancreatitis: A meta-analysis of randomized controlled trials. Pancreas 2008;37(3):241–246.

79. Zheng M, Chen Y, Bai J, Xin Y, Pan X, Zhao L. Meta-analysis of prophylactic allopurinol use in post-endoscopic retrograde cholangiopancreatography pancreatitis. Pancreas 2008;37(3):247–253.

80. Yadav D, Hawes RH, Brand RE, et al. Alcohol consumption, cigarette smoking, and the risk of recurrent acute and chronic pancreatitis. Arch Intern Med 2009;169(11):1035–1045.

81. Tattersall SJ, Apte MV, Wilson JS. A fire inside: Current concepts in chronic pancreatitis. Intern Med J 2008;38(7):592–598.

82. Draganov P, Toskes PP. Chronic pancreatitis: Controversies in etiology, diagnosis and treatment. Rev Esp Enferm Dig 2004;96(9): 649–654.

83. Keiles S, Kammesheidt A. Identification of CFTR, PRSS1, and SPINK1 mutations in 381 patients with pancreatitis. Pancreas 2006;33(3): 221–227.

84. Weiss FU, Simon P, Bogdanova N, et al. Complete cystic fibrosis transmembrane conductance regulator gene sequencing in patients with idiopathic chronic pancreatitis and controls. Gut 2005;54(10): 1456–1460.

85. Maisonneuve P, Lowenfels AB, Mullhaupt B, et al. Cigarette smoking accelerates progression of alcoholic chronic pancreatitis. Gut 2005;54(4):510–514.

86. Maisonneuve P, Frulloni L, Mullhaupt B, et al. Impact of smoking on patients with idiopathic chronic pancreatitis. Pancreas 2006;33(2): 163–168.

87. Seicean A, Tantau M, Grigorescu M, Mocan T, Seicean R, Pop T. Mortality risk factors in chronic pancreatitis. J Gastrointestin Liver Dis 2006;15(1):21–26.

88. Tolstrup JS, Kristiansen L, Becker U, Gronbaek M. Smoking and risk of acute and chronic pancreatitis among women and men: A population-based cohort study. Arch Intern Med 2009;169(6):603–609.

89. Schneider A, Lohr JM, Singer MV. The M-ANNHEIM classification of chronic pancreatitis: Introduction of a unifying classification system based on a review of previous classifications of the disease. J Gastroenterol 2007;42(2):101–119.

90. Stevens T, Conwell DL, Zuccaro G. Pathogenesis of chronic pancreatitis: An evidence-based review of past theories and recent developments. Am J Gastroenterol 2004;99(11):2256–2270.

91. Verlaan M, Roelofs HM, van-Schaik A, et al. Assessment of oxidative stress in chronic pancreatitis patients. World J Gastroenterol 2006;12(35):5705–5710.

92. Talukdar R, Tandon RK. Pancreatic stellate cells: New target in the treatment of chronic pancreatitis. J Gastroenterol Hepatol 2008;23(1):34–41.

93. Talukdar R, Saikia N, Singal DK, Tandon R. Chronic pancreatitis: Evolving paradigms. Pancreatology 2006;6(5):440–449.

94. Anaparthy R, Pasricha PJ. Pain and chronic pancreatitis: Is it the plumbing or the wiring? Curr Gastroenterol Rep 2008;10(2):101–106.

95. Gachago C, Draganov PV. Pain management in chronic pancreatitis. World J Gastroenterol 2008;14(20):3137–3148.

96. Drewes AM, Krarup AL, Detlefsen S, Malmstrom ML, Dimcevski G, Funch-Jensen P. Pain in chronic pancreatitis: The role of neuropathic pain mechanisms. Gut 2008;57(11):1616–1627.

97. Drewes AM, Gratkowski M, Sami SA, Dimcevski G, Funch-Jensen P, rendt-Nielsen L. Is the pain in chronic pancreatitis of neuropathic origin? Support from EEG studies during experimental pain. World J Gastroenterol 2008;14(25):4020–4027.

98. Sun DY, Jiang YB, Rong L, Jin SJ, Xie WZ. Clinical application of 13C-Hiolein breath test in assessing pancreatic exocrine insufficiency. Hepatobiliary Pancreat Dis Int 2003;2(3):449–452.

99. Conwell DL, Banks PA. Chronic pancreatitis. Curr Opin Gastroenterol 2008;24(5):586–590.

100. Adler DG, Lichtenstein D, Baron TH, et al. The role of endoscopy in patients with chronic pancreatitis. Gastrointest Endosc 2006;63(7):933–937.

101. Mullhaupt B, Truninger K, Ammann R. Impact of etiology on the painful early stage of chronic pancreatitis: A long-term prospective study. Z Gastroenterol 2005;43(12):1293–1301.

102. Meier R, Ockenga J, Pertkiewicz M, et al. ESPEN Guidelines on Enteral Nutrition: Pancreas. Clin Nutr 2006;25(2):275–284.

103. Stanga Z, Giger U, Marx A, DeLegge MH. Effect of jejunal long-term feeding in chronic pancreatitis. J Parenter Enteral Nutr 2005;29(1):12–20.

104. Kowalczyk LM, Draganov PV. Endoscopic therapy for chronic pancreatitis: Technical success, clinical outcomes, and complications. Curr Gastroenterol Rep 2009;11(2):111–118.

105. Guda NM, Partington S, Freeman ML. Extracorporeal shock wave lithotripsy in the management of chronic calcific pancreatitis: A meta-analysis. Journal of the Pancreas 2005;6(1):6–12.

106. Dumonceau JM, Costamagna G, Tringali A, et al. Treatment for painful calcified chronic pancreatitis: Extracorporeal shock wave lithotripsy versus endoscopic treatment: A randomised controlled trial. Gut 2007;56(4):545–552.

107. Deviere J, Bell RH, Jr., Beger HG, Traverso LW. Treatment of chronic pancreatitis with endotherapy or surgery: critical review of randomized control trials. J Gastrointest Surg 2008;12(4):640–644.

108. Dite P, Ruzicka M, Zboril V, Novotny I. A prospective, randomized trial comparing endoscopic and surgical therapy for chronic pancreatitis. Endoscopy 2003;35(7):553–558.

109. Cahen DL, Gouma DJ, Nio Y, et al. Endoscopic versus surgical drainage of the pancreatic duct in chronic pancreatitis. N Engl J Med 2007;356(7):676–684.

110. Garcea G, Weaver J, Phillips J, et al. Total pancreatectomy with and without islet cell transplantation for chronic pancreatitis: A series of 85 consecutive patients. Pancreas 2009;38(1):1–7.

111. Staahl C, Dimcevski G, Andersen SD, et al. Differential effect of opioids in patients with chronic pancreatitis: An experimental pain study. Scand J Gastroenterol 2007;42(3):383–390.

112. Brown A, Hughes M, Tenner S, Banks PA. Does pancreatic enzyme supplementation reduce pain in patients with chronic pancreatitis: A meta-analysis. Am J Gastroenterol 1997;92(11):2032–2035.

113. Cullen JJ, Mitros FA, Oberley LW. Expression of antioxidant enzymes in diseases of the human pancreas: Another link between chronic pancreatitis and pancreatic cancer. Pancreas 2003;26(1):23–27.

114. Bhardwaj P, Thareja S, Prakash S, Saraya A. Micronutrient antioxidant intake in patients with chronic pancreatitis. Trop Gastroenterol 2004;25(2):69–72.

115. Kirk GR, White JS, McKie L, et al. Combined antioxidant therapy reduces pain and improves quality of life in chronic pancreatitis. J Gastrointest Surg 2006;10(4):499–503.

116. Bhardwaj P, Garg PK, Maulik SK, Saraya A, Tandon RK, Acharya SK. A randomized controlled trial of antioxidant supplementation for pain relief in patients with chronic pancreatitis. Gastroenterology 2009;136(1):149–159.

117. Waljee AK, Dimagno MJ, Wu BU, Schoenfeld PS, Conwell DL. Systematic review: Pancreatic enzyme treatment of malabsorption associated with chronic pancreatitis. Aliment Pharmacol Ther 2009;29(3):235–246.

118. Safdi M, Bekal PK, Martin S, Saeed ZA, Burton F, Toskes PP. The effects of oral pancreatic enzymes (Creon 10 capsule) on steatorrhea: A multicenter, placebo-controlled, parallel group trial in subjects with chronic pancreatitis. Pancreas 2006;33(2):156–162.

119. Czako L, Takacs T, Hegyi P, et al. Quality of life assessment after pancreatic enzyme replacement therapy in chronic pancreatitis. Can J Gastroenterol 2003;17(10):597–603.

120. Dominguez-Munoz JE, Iglesias-Garcia J, Iglesias-Rey M, Figueiras A, Vilarino-Insua M. Effect of the administration schedule on the therapeutic efficacy of oral pancreatic enzyme supplements in patients with exocrine pancreatic insufficiency: A randomized, three-way crossover study. Aliment Pharmacol Ther 2005;21(8):993–1000.

121. Vecht J, Symersky T, Lamers CB, Masclee AA. Efficacy of lower than standard doses of pancreatic enzyme supplementation therapy during acid inhibition in patients with pancreatic exocrine insufficiency. J Clin Gastroenterol 2006;40(8):721–725.

122. Traynor K. First FDA-approved pancrelipase product may mark new era for providers, patients. Am J Health Syst Pharm 2009;66(12):1066, 1068.

123. Wehler M, Nichterlein R, Fischer B, et al. Factors associated with health-related quality of life in chronic pancreatitis. Am J Gastroenterol 2004;99(1):138–146.

124. Dominguez-Munoz JE, Iglesias-Garcia J, Vilarino-Insua M, Iglesias-Rey M. 13C-mixed triglyceride breath test to assess oral enzyme substitution therapy in patients with chronic pancreatitis. Clin Gastroenterol Hepatol 2007;5(4):484–488.

125. Bain SC, Stephens JW. Exenatide and pancreatitis: An update. Expert Opin Drug Saf 2008;7(6):643–644.

126. Ahmad SR, Swann J. Exenatide and rare adverse events. N Engl J Med 2008;358(18):1970–1971.

127. U.S. Food and Drug Administration. Information for healthcare professionals—acute pancreatitis and sitagliptin (marketed as Januvia and Janumet). 2009, *http://www.fda.gov/Drugs/DrugSafety/PostmarketDrugSafetyInformationforPatientsandProviders/DrugSafetyInformationforHeathcareProfessionals/ucm183764.htm*.

128. Balthazar EJ. Staging of acute pancreatitis. Radiol Clin North Am 2002;40(6):1199–1209.

129. Chen WX, Zhang WF, Li B, et al. Clinical manifestations of patients with chronic pancreatitis. Hepatobiliary Pancreat Dis Int 2006;5(1):133–137.

47

Viral Hepatitis

PAULINA DEMING

KEY CONCEPTS

❶ Hepatitis A is transmitted via the fecal–oral route. Transmission is most likely to occur through travel to countries with high rates of hepatitis A, poor sanitation and hygiene, and over-crowded areas.

❷ Hepatitis A causes an acute, self-limiting illness and does not lead to chronic infection. There are three stages of infection: incubation, acute hepatitis, and convalescence. Rarely, the infection progresses to liver failure.

❸ Treatment of hepatitis A consists of supportive care. There is no role for antiviral agents in treatment.

❹ Hepatitis B causes both acute and chronic infection. Infants and children are at high risk for chronic infection.

❺ Several therapies are available for hepatitis B, including lami-vudine, interferon α2b, pegylated interferon α2a, entecavir, adefovir, telbivudine, and tenofovir. Patient status, extent of disease, viral load, and viral resistance are all considered when deciding on treatment.

❻ Chronic hepatitis B patients may require long-term therapy. Long-term therapy poses a challenge because of the potential for developing resistance. Resistance to lamivudine and telbivudine is most common, although resistance mutations to adefovir and entecavir have also been seen. Optimal treatment of resistant strains is unknown.

❼ Prevention of hepatitis B infections focuses on immunization of all children and at-risk adults.

❽ Hepatitis C is an insidious, blood-borne infection. Injection drug use is the major mode of transmission in the United States.

❾ Combination pegylated interferon and ribavirin therapy is the treatment of choice for hepatitis C. Treatment duration for hepatitis C infections is 48 weeks for viral genotype 1, and 24 weeks for genotypes 2 and 3. However, therapy may be optimized based on infecting genotype and virologic response. Viral genotype 1 is most difficult to treat.

❿ Side effects of hepatitis C therapy pose a significant obstacle to completion of therapy and chance for cure. Adjunct pharmacologic therapy and dose reductions may be necessary to prevent premature cessation of treatment.

Learning objectives, review questions, and other resources can be found at **www.pharmacotherapyonline.com**.

The major hepatotrophic viruses responsible for viral hepatitis are hepatitis A, hepatitis B, hepatitis C, delta hepatitis, and hepatitis E. All share clinical, biochemical, immunoserologic, and histologic findings. Both hepatitides A and E are spread through fecal–oral contamination; whereas hepatitides B, C, and delta are transmitted parenterally. Infection with delta hepatitis requires coinfection with hepatitis B. Although the rates of acute infection have declined, viral hepatitis remains a major cause of morbidity and mortality with a significant impact on healthcare costs in the United States. Significant therapeutic advances have occurred with hepatitis B with the approval of new agents and updated guidelines for care. For hepatitis C, the challenge remains of increasing successful outcomes while minimizing side effects of therapy. This chapter focuses on hepatitides A, B, and C.

HEPATITIS A

Hepatitis A virus (HAV), or infectious hepatitis, is often a self-limiting and acute viral infection of the liver posing a health risk worldwide. The infection is rarely fatal. According to the Centers for Disease Control and Prevention (CDC), the 2,979 reported cases of acute clinical hepatitis A infection in the United States in 2007 were the lowest in recorded history.[1] Although vaccine preventable, HAV continues to be one of the most commonly reported infections.

EPIDEMIOLOGY

Various patient groups are at increased risk for infection with HAV. Children pose a particular problem with the spread of the disease because they often remain clinically asymptomatic and are infectious for longer periods of time than adults. Traditionally, the most likely patient group affected is household or close personal contacts of an infected person. ❶ Infection primarily occurs through the fecal–oral route, by person-to-person, or by ingestion of contaminated food or water. Incidentally, HAV's prevalence is linked to regions with low socioeconomic status and specifically to those with poor sanitary conditions and overcrowding. Rarely, the virus can be spread through blood or blood products. Despite being detectable in saliva, there are no data to suggest transmission through this mode of contact.[2] International travel and immigration also mitigate potential exposure to the virus.

International travel, in particular travel to HAV endemic areas, continues to be a major risk factor for HAV infection. Although rates have declined as a result of successful vaccination programs to a record low of 1.0 cases per 100,000 people in 2007, the proportion of HAV rates among international travelers continues to rise. Other identified risk factors include sexual and household contact with a HAV infected person, men who have sex with men (MSM), and injection drug users (IDUs).[1] Additional patient groups that are at risk include patients with chronic liver disease and persons working with nonhuman primates. For half of all identified HAV cases in 2007, no risk factor was identified.[1] In pregnant women, acute HAV infection may be associated with maternal complications and preterm labor.[3] Food-borne outbreaks also occur; a 2003 outbreak in Pennsylvania was associated with more than 500 persons infected and 3 deaths, and was linked to green onions imported from Mexico.[4]

HAV infections acquired through international travel create significant HAV-associated costs in terms of loss of work time and healthcare costs. Despite low endemic rates and successful vaccinations of at-risk populations in the United States, unvaccinated children acquiring HAV infections abroad can serve as reservoirs of the virus upon return to the United States, even while remaining clinically asymptomatic themselves. Nearly 40% of children younger than age 15 years with HAV had international travel as a risk factor in 2004.[1] According to the CDC, the majority of travel-related cases correspond to travel to Central and South America and Mexico.[1] Most Americans traveling to Mexico do not consider that country to be a risk in part because of Mexico's proximity to the United States. Moreover, most tourists falsely believe that higher-end resorts imply safety and that short visits to foreign countries are not associated with a risk for infection. In fact, frequent, short visits will have a cumulative risk for infection that should not be ignored.[6]

ETIOLOGY

Hepatitis A is a RNA virus belonging to the genus *Hepatovirus* of the *Picornaviridae* family. Humans are the only known reservoir for the virus and transmission occurs primarily through the fecal–oral route.[7] The virus is stable in the environment for at least a month and requires heating foods to a minimum of 85°C (185°F) for 1 minute or disinfecting with a 1:100 dilution of sodium hypochlorite (bleach) in tap water for inactivation.[2,8]

Multiple genotypes of the virus exist and although the clinical implications of infection by particular type are unknown, types I and III are the most commonly identified in human outbreaks.[7]

PATHOPHYSIOLOGY

HAV infection is usually acute, self-limiting, and confers lifelong immunity. HAV's life cycle in the human host classically begins with ingestion of the virus. Absorption in the stomach or small intestine allows entry into the circulation and uptake by the liver. Replication of the virus occurs within hepatocytes and gastrointestinal epithelial cells. New virus particles are released into the blood and secreted into bile by the liver. The virus is then either reabsorbed to continue its cycle or excreted in the stool. The enterohepatic cycle will continue until interrupted by antibody neutralization.[7] The exact mechanism of replication and secretion is unknown; however, the initial viral expansion does not seem to be associated with hepatic injury as peak viral fecal excretion precedes clinical signs and symptoms of infection.[2]

On biopsy, acute hepatitis is marked by hepatocellular degeneration, inflammatory infiltrate, and hepatocyte regeneration. Hepatocellular degeneration occurs as a result of immune-mediated injury and not as a direct cytopathic effect of the virus.[9] Clinical symptoms of HAV typically identify the onset of the immune response. Cytolytic T cells mediate hepatocyte lysis to eradicate the virus and mark the cellular immune response with rising hepatic enzyme levels.[7]

TABLE 47-1	Clinical Presentation of Acute Hepatitis A

Signs and symptoms
- The preicteric phase brings nonspecific influenza-like symptoms consisting of anorexia, nausea, fatigue, and malaise
- Abrupt onset of anorexia, nausea, vomiting, malaise, fever, headache, and right upper quadrant abdominal pain with acute illness
- Icteric hepatitis is generally accompanied by dark urine, acholic (light-colored) stools, and worsening of systemic symptoms
- Pruritus is often a major complaint of icteric patients

Physical examination
- Icteric sclera, skin, and secretions
- Mild weight loss of 2–5 kg
- Hepatomegaly

Laboratory tests
- Positive-serum immunoglobulin M anti-hepatitis A virus
- Mild elevations of serum bilirubin, γ-globulin, and hepatic transaminase (alanine transaminase and aspartate transaminase) values to about twice normal in acute anicteric disease
- Elevations of alkaline phosphatase, γ-glutamyl transferase, and total bilirubin in patients with cholestatic illness

CLINICAL PRESENTATION

❷ The incubation period of HAV is approximately 28 days, with a range of 15 to 50 days. Viremia occurs within 1 to 2 weeks of exposure as patients begin to shed the virus.[2] Table 47–1 summarizes the clinical features of acute hepatitis A. Peak fecal shedding of the virus precedes the onset of clinical symptoms and elevated liver enzymes. Acute hepatitis follows, beginning with the preicteric or prodromal period. The phase is marked by an abrupt onset of nonspecific symptoms, some very mild.[2] Other, more unusual symptoms include chills, myalgia, arthralgia, cough, constipation, diarrhea, pruritus, and urticaria. The phase generally lasts 2 months. There are no specific symptoms unique to HAV. Liver enzyme levels rise within the first weeks of infection, peaking approximately in the fourth week and normalizing by the eighth week. Conjugated bilirubinemia, or dark urine, precedes the onset of the icteric period. The concentration of virus declines at this point and patients are generally considered noninfectious approximately 1 week after the onset of jaundice.[10] Gastrointestinal (GI) symptoms may persist or subside during this time and some patients may have hepatomegaly. Duration of the icteric period varies and corresponds to disease duration. It averages between 7 and 30 days.[7]

Symptoms and severity of HAV vary according to age. Children younger than 6 years of age typically are asymptomatic. Symptoms, if they do occur, do not include jaundice. In older children and adults, the majority of patients present with symptoms that last less than 2 months and 70% of adults experience jaundice. Peak viral shedding precedes the onset of GI symptoms in adults. In young children, shedding can occur for months following diagnosis.[2] Because children are often asymptomatic and will shed the virus for long periods of time they can serve as a reservoir for the spread of HAV.

HAV RNA is detectable in the serum for an average of 17 days before peak alanine aminotransferase (ALT) levels and can persist for an average of 79 days after the onset of symptoms. In some patients, serum HAV is detectable for more than a year.[11] Immunoglobulin (Ig) M antibody to HAV (anti-HAV) is required for a diagnosis of acute infection. Serum HAV becomes detectable 5 to 10 days before the onset of symptoms and can persist for months. IgG anti-HAV replaces IgM and indicates host immunity following the acute phase of the infection. Serologic tests exist but should be interpreted with caution.[8] FDA-approved assays for serologic testing detect IgM and total anti-HAV (IgG and IgM). Patients who have detectable total anti-HAV and a negative IgM have resolved their infection. Although patients who are successfully immunized will have IgG, assays are not sensitive enough to detect anti-HAV in most patients. Similarly, patients who receive intramuscular (IM) Ig will also have anti-HAV but concentrations are below the level of detection of most assays.[2,8] Concentrations of antibody often fall to 10 to 100 times lower than what would be expected after a natural course of infection. Although a positive anti-HAV result confirms protection, undetectable concentration of anti-HAV may not necessarily imply that protective levels were not achieved.[8]

HAV does not lead to chronic infections. Some patients may experience symptoms for up to 9 months. Rarely, patients experience complications from HAV, including relapsing hepatitis, cholestatic hepatitis, and fulminant hepatitis. Fatalities from HAV are generally rare though more likely in patients older than age 50 years and in persons with preexisting liver disease.[8] Fulminant hepatitis occurs mostly in young children and adults with chronic liver disease. Although occurring in 0.01% of clinical infections, fulminant hepatitis has a high fatality rate and therapy consists of supportive care.[9]

Diagnosis

A diagnosis of HAV is based on clinical criteria of an acute onset of fatigue, abdominal pain, loss of appetite, intermittent nausea and vomiting, jaundice or elevated serum aminotransferase levels, and serologic testing for IgM anti-HAV. Serologic testing is necessary to differentiate the diagnosis from other types of hepatitis.

TREATMENT

Hepatitis A Virus

■ DESIRED OUTCOME

❸ The majority of people infected with HAV can be expected to fully recover without clinical sequelae.[7] Nearly all individuals will have clinical resolution within 6 months of the infection, and a majority will have done so by 2 months. Rarely, symptoms persist for longer or patients relapse. The ultimate goal of therapy is complete clinical resolution. Other goals include reducing complications from the infection, normalization of liver function, and reducing infectivity and transmission.

■ GENERAL APPROACH TO TREATMENT

No specific treatment options exist for HAV infections. Instead, patients should receive general supportive care. In patients who develop liver failure, transplant is the only option. Although hepatocellular damage occurs through immune-mediated responses, steroid use is not recommended.[12] Prevention and prophylaxis are key to managing the virus. The importance of good hand hygiene cannot be overemphasized in preventing disease transmission. Immunoglobulin is used for pre- and postexposure prophylaxis, and offers passive immunity. Active immunity is achieved through vaccination. Vaccines were approved for use in 1995 and implemented in the routine vaccination of children, as well as at-risk adults, to reduce the overall incidence of HAV.[8]

Prevaccination serologic testing to determine susceptibility is generally not recommended. In some cases, testing may be cost effective if the cost of the test is less than that of the vaccine and if the person is from a moderate to high endemic area and likely to have prior immunity. Prevaccination serologic testing of children is not recommended. Similarly, because of high vaccine response, postvaccine serologic testing is not recommended.[8]

TABLE 47-2	Recommendations for Hepatitis A Virus (HAV) Vaccination

All children at 1 year of age

Children and adolescents age 2–18 y who live in states or communities where routine hepatitis A vaccination has been implemented because of high disease incidence

Persons traveling to or working in countries that have high or intermediate endemicity of infection[a]

Men who have sex with men

Illegal drug users

Persons with occupational risk for infection (e.g., persons who work with HAV-infected primates or with HAV in a research laboratory)

Persons who have clotting factor disorders

Persons with chronic liver disease

[a] Travelers to Canada, Western Europe, Japan, Australia, or New Zealand are at no greater risk for infection than they are in the United States. All other travelers should be assessed for HAV risk.
From Centers for Disease Control and Prevention.[8,13]

PREVENTION OF HEPATITIS A

HAV is easily preventable with vaccination. Because children often serve as reservoirs of the disease, vaccine programs have targeted children as the most effective means to control HAV. Two vaccines for HAV are available and are incorporated into the routine childhood vaccination schedule. In October 2005, the FDA reduced the minimum age for the vaccines to 12 months of age. In response, the Advisory Committee on Immunization Practices recommended expanding vaccine coverage to all children, including catch-up programs for children living in areas without existing vaccination programs. The new recommendations were enacted in the attempt to further reduce HAV incidence rates and possibly to eradicate the virus.[13] In 2007, the U.S. Department of Health and Human Services issued a health advisory after receiving reports of HAV from international adoptees. Guidelines for international adoptees and their adoptive parents are available from the CDC. Adult vaccination recommendations also exist (Table 47–2).

Routine prevention of HAV transmission includes regular hand washing with soap and water after using the bathroom, changing a diaper, and before food preparation. For travelers to countries with high endemic rates of HAV, even short-term stays in urban and upscale resorts are not risk free.[8] In particular, contaminated water and ice, fresh produce, and any uncooked foods pose a risk.[7]

Vaccines to Prevent Hepatitis A

Two inactivated virus vaccines are currently licensed in the United States: Havrix and Vaqta. Both vaccines are inactivated virus and are available for pediatric and adult use. The differences in the two vaccines are in the use of a preservative and in expression of antigen content. Vaqta is formulated without a preservative and uses units of HAV antigen to express potency. Havrix uses 2-phenoxyphenol as a preservative and antigen content is expressed as enzyme-linked immunosorbent assay units. Pediatric dosing is indicated for children 12 months of age through 18 years of age, and adult dosing is for patients ages 19 years and older (Table 47–3).[8] Although high seroconversion rates of ≥94% are achieved with the first dose, both vaccines recommend a booster shot to achieve the highest possible antibody titers. In situations of postexposure prophylaxis, previously only immunoglobulin was indicated but recent guidelines changes allow the use of vaccines for this indication. The change to the use of the vaccine is advantageous as vaccination confers the benefit of long-term immunity against HAV.[13] Both vaccines may be given concomitantly with immunoglobulin and the two brands are interchangeable for booster shots.[8]

TABLE 47-3	Recommended Dosing of Havrix and Vaqta				
Vaccine	Age (y)	Dose	No. of Doses	Schedule (mo)
Havrix	1–18	720 ELISA units	2	0, 6–12
	≥19	1,440 ELISA units	2	0, 6–12
Vaqta	1–18	25 units	2	0, 6–18
	≥19	50 units	2	0, 6–18

ELISA, enzyme-linked immunoabsorbent assay.
From Centers for Disease Control and Prevention.[13]

Vaccine efficacy may be reduced in certain patient populations. In HIV (human immunodeficiency virus)-infected patients, greater immunogenic response may correlate with higher baseline CD4 cell counts. Response to the HAV vaccine as determined by detection of anti-HAV after vaccination found that among HIV patients, females and patients with CD4 counts >200 cells/mm^3 at vaccination had a higher response rate.[16]

The most common side effects of the vaccines include soreness and warmth at the injection site, headache, malaise, and pain. Reported serious adverse events include anaphylaxis, Guillain-Barré syndrome, brachial plexus neuropathy, transverse myelitis, multiple sclerosis, encephalopathy, and erythema multiforme. However, causality of these reported events has not been established. Furthermore, incidence of serious adverse events in the vaccinated population did not differ from the incidence in nonvaccinated populations. It is important to note that more than 65 million doses of the vaccine have been administered and despite routine monitoring for adverse events, there are no data to suggest a greater incidence of serious adverse events among vaccinated people compared with nonvaccinated. The vaccine is considered safe.[8]

Twinrix is a bivalent vaccine for hepatitides A and B that was approved by the FDA in 2001. The vaccine is approved for people ages 18 and older and is given at 0, 1, and 6 months. Although seroconversion exceeds 90% for HAV after the first dose, the full three-dose series is required for maximal hepatitis B virus (HBV) seroconversion. An accelerated dosing schedule is available but requires a total of four doses for optimal response. The combined vaccine offers the advantage of immunization against both types of hepatitis in a single vaccine.

Immunoglobulin

Ig is used when pre- or postexposure prophylaxis against HAV infection is needed in persons for whom vaccination is not an option. Immunoglobulin is preferred for children <12 months of age and for postexposure prophylaxis in patients aged >40 years, patients with chronic liver disease, and persons allergic to any part of the vaccine. A sterile preparation of concentrated antibodies against HAV, Ig provides protection by passive transfer of antibody. Ig is most effective if given in the incubation period of the infection. Receipt of Ig within the first 2 weeks of infection will reduce infectivity and moderate the infection in 85% of patients. Patients who receive at least 1 dose of the HAV vaccine at least 1 month earlier do not need pre- or postexposure prophylaxis with Ig.[8] Ig is available both as an intravenous (IV) and IM injection but for HAV exposure, only the IM is used. If given to infants or pregnant women, the thimerosal-free formulation should be used.

International travelers are the major patient population receiving preexposure prophylaxis with Ig. HAV vaccination or prophylaxis with Ig is recommended for travelers to countries with high endemic rates of HAV. Serious adverse events are rare. Anaphylaxis has been reported in patients with Ig A deficiency. Patients who had an anaphylaxis reaction to Ig should not receive it. There is no contraindication for use in pregnancy or lactation.

Dosing of Ig is the same for adults and children. For postexposure prophylaxis and for short-term preexposure coverage of <3 months, a single dose of 0.02 mL/kg is given intramuscularly. For long-term preexposure prophylaxis of ≤5 months, a single dose of 0.06 mL/kg is used. Either the deltoid or gluteal muscle may be used. In children younger than 24 months of age, Ig can be given in the anterolateral thigh muscle.[8]

For people who were recently exposed to HAV and who had not been previously vaccinated, Ig is indicated in the following situations: (a) when in close personal contact with an HAV-infected person; (b) all staff and attendees of daycare centers when HAV is documented; (c) if they were involved in a common source exposure; for example, in a food-borne outbreak with an HAV-infected food handler, other food handlers at the location should receive Ig; if the case person handled food and had poor hygiene or diarrhea, patrons of the location should also receive Ig if they can be identified and located within the 2 weeks of the exposure; (d) classroom contacts of an index case patient; and (e) schools, hospitals, and work settings where close personal contact occurred with the case patient.[8]

Ig can be given concomitantly with the HAV vaccine. Although the antibody titer will be lower than if the vaccine were administered alone, the response is still protective. However, Ig can interfere with the response of other vaccines and should be delayed. The measles, mumps, and rubella (MMR) vaccine should be delayed for a minimum of 3 months after receipt of Ig. The varicella vaccine must be delayed for 5 months. Conversely, Ig should not be given to patients who received the MMR within 2 weeks or the varicella vaccine within 3 weeks. In situations where the benefits of Ig outweigh the benefits of the other vaccines, revaccination can be performed after Ig administration. For the MMR, revaccination should be at least 3 months later, and for the varicella vaccine, at least 5 months later.[8] In general, Ig does not interfere with inactivated vaccines and may be administered safely with other vaccines traditionally given to travelers to some developing countries, such as the oral poliovirus or yellow fever vaccine.[8]

PHARMACOECONOMIC CONSIDERATIONS

Although the costs of an HAV outbreak are significant, routine vaccination of all individuals is not cost-effective. Rather, by targeting at-risk populations, the majority of cases can be prevented. Children play a pivotal role in disease persistence. The use of the HAV vaccine is cost-effective in children and offers the most benefit to the personal contacts of children, reflecting the role of children as a reservoir for the disease.[16] The use of the combined HAV-HBV vaccine is effective in reducing costs associated with HAV among persons who are at increased risk for infection. Among 100,000 healthcare workers in high endemic states, the vaccine was anticipated to reduce the number of related work loss days from 34,463 to 4,667 days, an estimated savings of $6.1 million.[16] Nearly $2 million in savings could be seen in costs associated with HAV treatment. In a sexually transmitted diseases clinic serving 1 million patients, the combined vaccine was expected to prevent 2,263 occult infections and cost $13,397 per quality-adjusted life-year (QALY).[17] Both studies predicted between $2 million and $2.5 million in savings associated with HAV treatment, realized mostly in reduced hospitalizations. The risk of HAV from food transmission in the United States is low and can be avoided in many cases by adherence to basic hygiene practices.

HEPATITIS B

Although a vaccine was made available in 1981, HBV has acutely infected more than 2 billion people globally, leading to chronic infection in more than 350 million people.[18] Chronic infection with HBV is a major public health issue as it serves as a reservoir for continued HBV transmission and poses a significant risk of death resulting from liver disease. More than 1 million people per year die as a result of liver cirrhosis and hepatocellular carcinoma(HCC).

EPIDEMIOLOGY

According to the CDC, only 12% of the global population lives in an area of low prevalence for hepatitis B, defined as an area where <2% of the population is HBsAg (hepatitis B surface antigen)-positive.[18] Prevalence can vary regionally; however, areas commonly associated with high infectivity rates include sub-Saharan Africa, most of Asia, as well as the Amazon and southern parts of Eastern and Central Europe.[18] Areas of high prevalence, approximately 45% of the global population, are of special concern because most infections are of infants and children and >90% of cases lead to a chronic carrier state. Although less than 1% of people have chronic infection in both Western Europe and North America,[18] in the United States HBV is the second most common type of acute viral hepatitis and the third most reported preventable disease, second only to HAV.[19] Rates of infection in the South are highest, however overall rates of infection in the United States continue to decline. There are approximately 1.25 million chronically infected HBV people in the United States. In 2007, an estimated 43,000 people developed new infections. Annually, 3,000 to 5,000 people die from chronic liver disease attributable to HBV.[1]

HBV is transmitted sexually, parenterally, and perinatally. In areas of high HBV prevalence, perinatal transmission from mother to infant is most common, whereas in areas of intermediate prevalence, horizontal transmission from child to child is most common. Sexual contact, both homosexual and heterosexual, and injection drug use are the predominant forms of transmission in low-endemic countries such as the United States.[20] Concentration of HBV is high in blood, serum, and wound exudates of infected persons. The virus is detectable in moderate quantities in semen, vaginal fluid, and saliva, and is present in low concentrations in urine, feces, sweat, tears, and breast milk.[19,21] Transmission can occur through contact with infected body fluids in the absence of blood, as the virus may be stable in the environment for a number of days.[21,22] In the United States in 2007, no risk factor could be identified for the majority of acute infections with HBV. Among patients with identifiable risk factors, the most common risk was sexual contact, specifically multiple sexual partners, MSM, and sexual contact with a known HBV-positive person. Sexual contact was a consistent risk among all patients but especially among those aged 45 years or younger. Other known risk factors include IDU and household contact of HBV-positive person. A previously identified risk includes international travel, and was the largest overall risk factor in 2004 among children younger than 15 years of age.[5] No cases were documented for patients receiving transfusions or on hemodialysis.[18] Among racial and ethnic groups, HBV is highest among non-Hispanic blacks. Hispanics and non-Hispanic whites have similarly low rates, while Asians/Pacific Islanders have the lowest HBV rates.[5]

The mode of transmission has clinical implications because chronic infections are associated with infection acquired in younger patients, especially those infected perinatally and in early childhood.[21]

ETIOLOGY

The HBV is a DNA virus of the family *Hepadnaviridae*. It is a partially double-stranded, circular DNA with 3,200 base pairs that typically infects liver cells, although it has been found in kidney, pancreas, and mononuclear cells.[23,24] Seven HBV genotypes exist

TABLE 47-4	Worldwide Distribution of Hepatitis B Virus Genotypes
Genotype	**Geographic Distribution**
A	Northern/Central Europe, North America, sub-Saharan Africa
B, C	Southeast Asia, Japan
D	Mediterranean region, Middle East, India
F	Central and South America, North American Indians, Polynesia
G	France, North America
H	Central America

Data from Ganne-Carrie N, Williams V, Kaddouri H, et al. Significance of hepatitis B virus genotypes A to F in a cohort of patients with chronic hepatitis B in the Seine Saint Denis district of Paris (France). J Med Virol 2006;78:335–340.

(A to H) with distinct geographic distribution (Table 47–4). It is possible that genotype prevalence may be dependent on mode of transmission as types B and C are found in areas where vertical transmission is the primary mode of infection.[25] Correlations between clinical outcomes and HBV genotypes have been suggested, with genotype C associated with more severe liver injury, including liver cirrhosis and progression to HCC.[25] Noted limitations of studies are frequently small sample sizes and a predominance of research from Asia, primarily comparing genotypes B and C.[25] Nonetheless, a study of a diverse patient immigrant population infected with genotypes A, B, C, D, and E, confirmed that more severe liver fibrosis was significantly higher in HBV genotypes A, C, and D-infected patients. Genotype B may be more benign because it is associated with faster seroconversion, although clinical studies suggest genotype A may have equivalent, if not higher rates of seroconversion.[26,27] Resistance mutations may contribute to genotype virulence and hence impact severity of liver disease in infection.[28]

PATHOPHYSIOLOGY

Upon infection, replication of the virus begins by attachment of the virion to the hepatocyte cell surface receptors. The particles are transported to the nucleus where the DNA is converted into closed, circular DNA that serves as a template for pregenomic RNA. Viral RNA is then transcribed and transported back to the cytoplasm where it can alternatively serve as a reservoir for future viral templates or bud into the intracellular membrane with the viral envelope proteins and infect other cells.[23,27] The viral genome has four reading frames coding for various proteins and enzymes required for viral replication and spread. Several of these proteins are used diagnostically (Table 47–5). The HBsAg is the most abundant of the three surface antigens and is detectable at the onset of clinical symptoms. Its persistence past 6 months after initial detection corresponds to chronic infection and poses an increased risk for cirrhosis, hepatic decompensation, and HCC. Development of antibody to HBsAg (anti-HBsAg) confers immunity to the virus and clearance of HBsAg is associated with favorable outcomes.[24,29] The precore polypeptide encodes for the secretory protein hepatitis B e antigen (HBeAg) and the hepatitis B core antigen (HBcAg) proteins. Although HBeAg's role in infection is nebulous, it is present in an acute infection and is replaced by antibodies (anti-HBeAg) once an infection is resolved. HBeAg was assumed to be a marker of viral replication and infectivity; however, it is now known that some viral mutants exist that are unable to have or have downregulated expression of HBeAg, although their ability to replicate is not affected.[27] HBeAg-negative mutants pose a particular clinical challenge because they are refractory to treatment. The HBcAg is a nucleocapsid protein that, when expressed on hepatocytes, promotes immune-mediated cell death. High levels of antibodies (IgM anti-HBcAg) are detectable during acute infections. The detection of IgM anti-HBcAg is also a reliable assay for diagnosing fulminant acute hepatitis where HBsAg and

TABLE 47-5 Interpretation of Serologic Tests in Hepatitis B Virus

Tests	Result	Interpretation
HBsAg	(−)	
Anti-HBc	(−)	Susceptible
Anti-HBs	(−)	
HBsAg	(−)	
Anti-HBc	(+)	Immune because of natural infection
Anti-HBs	(+)	
HBsAg	(−)	Immune because of vaccination (valid only if test performed 1–2 mo after third vaccine dose)
Anti-HBc	(−)	
Anti-HBs	(+)	
HBsAg	(+)	
Anti-HBc	(+)	Acute infection
IgM anti-HBc	(+)	
HBsAg	(+)	
Anti-HBc	(+)	Chronic infection
IgM anti-HBc	(−)	
Anti-HBs	(−)	
HBsAg	(−)	Four interpretations possible:
Anti-HBc	(+)	1. Recovery from acute infection
Anti-HBs	(−)	2. Distant immunity and test not sensitive enough to detect low level of HBs in serum
		3. Susceptible with false-positive anti-HBc
		4. May have undetectable level of HBsAg in serum and be chronically infected

HBc, hepatitis B core; HBs, hepatitis B surface; HBsA, hepatitis B surface associated; HBsAg, hepatitis B surface antigen; IgM, immunoglobulin M.
From Centers for Disease Control and Prevention: Hepatitis B Serology. http://www.cdc.gov/ncidod/ diseases/hepatitis/b/Bserology.htm.

TABLE 47-6 Factors Associated with Hepatitis B Virus (HBV) Cirrhosis and Disease Progression

Persistence of HBV serum DNA
Infection with genotype C
Co-infection with HCV, delta hepatitis, or HIV
Age at diagnosis
Severity of liver disease at diagnosis
Male sex
Frequency of severe hepatic flares
Alcohol use
Laboratory/physical findings of abnormal liver function

HCV, hepatitis C virus; HIV, human immunodeficiency virus
Data from Fattovich,[26] Lok and McMahon,[27] and Wright.[34]

HBV DNA are often undetectable.[23,30] Patients who respond to vaccine will have anti-HBsAg only.[8]

HBV itself does not seem to be pathogenic to cells; rather, it is thought that the immune response to the virus is cytotoxic to hepatocytes. Antigen nonspecific inflammatory responses triggered by T cells may be responsible for most hepatic injury, with progression to cirrhosis and HCC.[21,23] The immune response includes major histocompatibility complex (MHC) class I CD8 cytotoxic T cells and MHC class II CD4 T-helper cells. In both an acute and chronic infection, the antibody response is strong. In an acute infection, however, the cytotoxic T-cell response is critical to viral clearance. If the response is weak, chronic infection is likely.[23] Moreover, liver injury is likely caused by secondary, nonspecific inflammation activated by the initial cytotoxic lymphocyte response and as an attempt by the immune system to clear the virus by destroying HBV antigen presenting hepatocytes. Destruction of hepatocytes results in release of circulating, and hence increased, ALT levels.

Cirrhosis

Cirrhosis results as the liver attempts to regenerate while in an environment of persistent inflammation. Like in other viral hepatitis-induced cirrhoses, continued alcohol consumption exacerbates hepatocellular damage. Most patients with compensated cirrhosis are either asymptomatic or have mild symptoms of epigastric pain and dyspepsia.[26] During cirrhosis, the liver enters a cycle of ongoing liver damage, fibrosis, and attempts at regeneration. The classical appearance of a small and knobby liver reflects the irreversible effect of nodules of regenerating cells integrated with infiltrates of inflammatory induced fibrous tissue. Both viral and clinical factors affect the outcome of cirrhosis (Table 47–6). The development of cirrhosis is mostly insidious and patients can remain stable for years before disease progression. An estimated 20% of all chronic hepatitis B patients develop complications of hepatic insufficiency and portal hypertension as their compensated cirrhosis progresses

to decompensated cirrhosis within a 5-year period.[27] Typically, the initial clinical findings of decompensated cirrhosis are ascites, jaundice, variceal bleed, encephalopathy, or a combination of symptoms.[26] Damage is irreversible. Treatment is supportive care and patients are candidates for liver transplantation.

Hepatocellular Carcinoma

HBV is a known risk factor for the development of HCC and in areas of high HBV endemicity, a major complication of the infection.[21,23] The development of HCC can be insidious, occurring in the absence of cirrhosis or in the presence of clinically silent, compensated cirrhosis. Many patients with HCC have no signs of decompensated cirrhosis.[26] The virus itself is not likely the causative agent of the cancer. In most cases, HCC develops after years of inflammatory processes provoked by ongoing HBV infection. Compared to hepatitis C virus (HCV), however, HBV does seem to provoke a more direct carcinogenic effect as evidenced by its presence in less-severe liver disease, and among patients with advanced HCC, HBV infection is associated with a worse survival rate.[31] Several factors influence the development of HCC, as well as predict survival (see Table 47–6). HCC is more prevalent in males; in older patients; in patients coinfected with HCV or delta hepatitis; and in patients with serologic markings of past or present HBV infection, preexisting cirrhosis, or continued alcohol ingestion. Risks for death and decompensation increase with underlying liver disease. Other host-specific or environmental factors may impact the course of liver disease. In Asian patients, HCC tumors are commonly seen in otherwise healthy patients, whereas HCC is typically seen in white patients with chronic liver disease.[32] Persistently elevated HBV DNA levels (≥10,000 copies/mL) predict HCC development, even after adjusting for sex, age, cigarette smoking, alcohol consumption, HBeAg status, ALT level, and liver cirrhosis.[33] HBeAg status is not a risk factor. In otherwise healthy patients without coinfection or who do not have HCC or decompensation at the time of seroclearance, HBsAg seroclearance does predict a favorable long-term outcome.[29] Additional predictors of survival include younger age and maintenance of liver function as evidenced by laboratory findings.[26]

CLINICAL PRESENTATION

❹ The clinical symptoms and course of an HBV infection are indistinguishable from other types of viral hepatitis. Three phases of an HBV infection exist. During the initial or acute phase of a HBV infection in adults and older children, the HBV enters a 4- to 10-week incubation period, during which antibodies toward the HBV core are produced and the virus replicates profusely. Active viral replication results in high serum HBV DNA levels and HBeAg secretion.[23] ALT levels may rise slightly, but most patients will remain asymptomatic. Symptoms, if they do occur, include fever, anorexia, nausea, vomiting, jaundice, dark urine, clay-colored or pale stools, and abdominal pain. Most neonates and children are anicteric and have no clinical symptoms, whereas up to half of adult patients are icteric.[26] HBsAg does not become detectable until after significant viremia. The initial phase is considered immunotolerant because no hepatic injury is sustained, as evidenced by generally normal ALT levels. Patients are highly infectious during this time.[25] In perinatally acquired infections, and in young children, the phase can last for decades–until adulthood.[24] Infected children pose a particular risk because they are often asymptomatic, undiagnosed, and highly infectious.

The immunoactive phase marks a decrease in HBV DNA levels with ongoing secretion of HBeAg. Patients are symptomatic with intermittent flares of hepatitis and marked increases in ALT levels. More frequent flares are associated with disease progression.[34] The phase can last a few weeks in acute disease, and for years in patients with chronic disease. As the host immune system attempts to gain control of the infection by stopping active viral replication, serum HBV DNA levels drop to undetectable, ALT levels normalize, and liver necroinflammation resolves.[26]

If the infection is self-limiting, HBV DNA quickly subsides, HBeAg disappears within weeks, and HBsAg usually resolves within 4 months. The final phase is seroconversion and is defined by the replacement of HBeAg with anti-HBeAg. Factors favoring seroconversion include female sex, older age, biochemical activity, and genotype. Flares of hepatitis with ALT levels >5 times the upper limits of normal, compared to <5 times the upper limits of normal, correspond to increased immune system activity and precede seroconversion. Some studies suggest that the A and B genotypes are associated with earlier seroconversion than genotypes C and D but the data are inconclusive and no recommendations exist for genotype testing in clinical practice.[25,27]

Chronic HBV

❹ Patients who continue to have detectable HBsAg and HBeAg and a high serum titer of HBV DNA for more than 6 months have chronic HBV.[26] Table 47–7 lists the clinical features of chronic hepatitis B. The most predictive factor for developing a chronic infection is age. Perinatal infections almost always result in chronic

infections because of immune tolerance to the virus.[35] Risks of chronicity decline to a rate of 30% in infants and to less than 5% of acute adult infections.[24]

Chronic infections can be controlled in many cases, but cure is not possible because the HBV template is integrated into the host genome. In patients with recurring cycles of viral expression and host immune response, progressive liver damage ensues.[35] Patients can be divided into two types of chronic hepatitis B: those who are HBeAg-positive and those who are HBeAg-negative. The ability to express HBeAg by the virus differentiates the two types of chronic infection. Patients are considered to be in the "immune tolerant" phase when HBeAg is positive, high serum HBV DNA levels are detected, and ALT levels are normal. Typically these patients were infected early in life and develop elevated ALT levels later in life. Spontaneous HBeAg clearance is possible and is associated with older age, higher ALT, and infection with HBV genotype B.[27]

Patients who are HBeAg-negative can be further subdivided into the active or inactive carrier. HBeAg-negative chronic HBV patients who are active carriers have high serum HBV DNA, elevated ALT levels, and liver necroinflammation.[26] The clinical course tends to be worse with a very low rate of spontaneous remission. Patients may have long periods of disease remission but recurring flares of hepatitis with increased frequency and severity can progress to cirrhosis and HCC. HBeAg-negative chronic HBV patients who are inactive carriers have detectable HBsAg and anti-HBeAg, normal ALT, and either low or undetectable levels of HBV DNA. This patient population usually experiences a more benign course of disease, with the possibility of long-term remission, even seroconversion, although reactivation is possible with the progression to cirrhosis and HCC. Rarely, patients will resolve their infection. Patients with undetectable HBsAg but with anti-HBsAg and anti-HBcAg represent a small portion of patients who are not likely to experience reinfection or reactivation unless immunosuppressed.[26] Up to 20% of patients in the inactive carrier state may revert to detectable HBeAg, emphasizing the need for life-long follow-up to confirm quiescence.[27]

HBV MUTATIONS

❻ Among the DNA viruses, HBV is notable for its significantly higher mutation rate.[27] Long-term therapy is problematic because of the high likelihood of developing viral resistance. One of the most common mutations consists of a nucleotide substitution either preventing or causing downregulation of the production of HBeAg. The mutation results in a chronic infection that may have a poorer long-term prognosis. Typically, the mutation emerges during the infection and represents a later stage in the course of chronic HBV infection with more advanced liver disease. Variants in the precore or core promoter region are thought to be responsible for the mutation.[27]

The selective pressures of the L-nucleoside analog antivirals, including lamivudine, cause the YMDD mutation. The mutation is associated with the active site of the DNA polymerase and causes an altered active site. The incidence of lamivudine resistance increases with each subsequent year of therapy and may be associated with a more severe disease progression.[27] An added risk of developing resistance is the retention of the mutation within the virus even four years after lamivudine therapy.[36] Cross-resistance of lamivudine-resistant YMDD mutants to telbivudine has been demonstrated and patients treated with lamivudine and telbivudine showed resistance mutations to both drugs. Telbivudine-specific resistance can also occur at rates lower than that seen in lamivudine.[37] Other mutations include resistance to adefovir and entecavir. Resistance to adefovir is associated with substitutions of aspargine by threonine (rtN236T) and substitution of alanine by valine or threonine (rtA181V/T), as well as other

---

TABLE 47-7	Clinical Presentation of Chronic Hepatitis B[a]

Signs and symptoms
- Easy fatigability, anxiety, anorexia, and malaise
- Ascites, jaundice, variceal bleeding, and hepatic encephalopathy can manifest with liver decompensation
- Hepatic encephalopathy is associated with hyperexcitability, impaired mentation, confusion, obtundation, and eventually coma
- Vomiting and seizures

Physical examination
- Icteric sclera, skin, and secretions
- Decreased bowel sounds, increased abdominal girth, and detectable fluid wave
- Asterixis
- Spider angiomata

Laboratory tests
- Presence of hepatitis B surface antigen >6 mo
- Intermittent elevations of hepatic transaminase (alanine transaminase and aspartate transaminase) and hepatitis B virus DNA >20,000 IU/mL (10^5 copies/mL)
- Liver biopsies for pathologic classification as chronic persistent hepatitis, chronic active hepatitis, or cirrhosis

[a]Chronic hepatitis B can be present even without all the signs, symptoms, and physical examination findings listed being apparent.

possible mutations to the HBV polymerase gene. The addition of lamivudine in adefovir resistance may overcome resistance, although the optimal management of either adefovir- or entecavir-resistant strains is not clear.[27,38]

PREVENTION OF HEPATITIS B

Despite the introduction of the HBV vaccine in 1981 and recommendations on vaccination in 1982, rates of HBV did not decline in the early 1980s. Initial declines in incidence were likely attributable to behavioral changes among high-risk groups as a result of the acquired immune deficiency syndrome (AIDS) epidemic. A 94% decline in rates between 1990 and 2004 was seen in children and adolescents, which began with the initiation of screening of pregnant women and subsequent immunizations of infants and recommendations set forth in the 1990s to immunize adolescents. Regulations enacted by Occupational Safety and Health Administration (OSHA) further reduced overall U.S. rates by 75%.[19,22]

❼ Prophylaxis against HBV can be achieved by vaccination or by passive immunity in postexposure cases with hepatitis B immunoglobulin. Vaccination is the most effective strategy to prevent infection and a comprehensive vaccination strategy has been implemented in the United States (Table 47–8). Vaccines use HBsAg for the antigen via recombinant DNA technology using yeast to prompt active immunity. More than 60 million adolescents and more than 40 million infants and children have received a HBV vaccine in the United States since 1982. The vaccine is considered safe. Since 2000, vaccines licensed in the United States either contain none or trace amounts of thimerosal as a preservative. Available vaccines include two single-antigen products and three combination products. The two single-antigen products are Recombivax HB and Engerix-B. Twinrix is a combination vaccine for HAV and HBV in adults. Comvax and Pediarix are used for children and are used for HBV along with other scheduled vaccines.

Passive immunity in the form of anti-HBsAg offers temporary protection against HBV and is used in conjunction with the hepatitis B vaccine for postexposure prophylaxis.[22]

TABLE 47-8 Recommendations for Hepatitis B Virus (HBV) Vaccination

Infants
Adolescents including all previously unvaccinated children <19 y
All unvaccinated adults at risk for infection
All unvaccinated adults seeking vaccination (specific risk factor not required)
Men and women with a history of other sexually transmitted diseases and persons with a history of multiple sex partners (>1 partner/6 mo)
Men who have sex with men
Current or recent injection drug users
Household contacts and sex partners of persons with chronic hepatitis B infection and healthcare and public safety workers with exposure to blood in the workplace
Clients and staff of institutions for the developmentally disabled
International travelers to regions with high or intermediate levels (HBsAg prevalence ≥2%) of endemic HBV infection
Recipients of clotting-factor concentrates
Sexually transmitted disease clinic patients
HIV patient/HIV-testing patients
Drug-abuse treatment and prevention clinic patients
Correctional facilities inmates
Chronic dialysis/ESRD patients including predialysis, peritoneal dialysis, and home dialysis patients
Persons with chronic liver disease

ESRD, end-stage renal disease; HIV, human immunodeficiency virus.
From Centers for Disease Control.[22]

TREATMENT
Hepatitis B Virus

■ DESIRED OUTCOME

HBV infections are not curable; rather, the goals of therapy are to increase the chances for seroclearance, prevent disease progression to cirrhosis and HCC, and to minimize further injury in patients with ongoing liver damage.

■ GENERAL APPROACH TO TREATMENT

❺ Response to therapy is monitored by biochemical (normalization of ALT levels), histologic examination of liver cells from biopsy (a minimum 2-point decrease in histology activity compared with baseline biopsy), and virologic response (undetectable serum HBV DNA levels and loss of HBeAg in HBeAg-positive patients).[27] Maintenance of viral suppression is defined as durability of response. In HBeAg-positive patients, successful therapy includes loss of HBeAg status and seroconversion to anti-HBeAg. Other serologic markers are typically not evaluated in clinical trials. Recommendations for treatment consider the patient's age, serum HBV DNA and ALT levels, as well as histologic evidence and clinical progression of disease (Figs. 47–1 and 47–2). Not all chronic HBV patients are candidates for treatment. Some patients may be best managed with periodic monitoring for disease progression because the chances for therapeutic response are unlikely and do not outweigh the risks and costs associated with treatment. Various guidelines have been published and updates made as more drugs are indicated for use in HBV.[27,30,39]

■ NONPHARMACOLOGIC THERAPY

All chronic HBV patients should be counseled on preventing disease transmission. Sexual and household contacts should be vaccinated. To minimize further liver damage, all chronic HBV patients should avoid alcohol and be immunized against HBV. No level of alcohol use has been established as safe.[27] Moreover, patients are encouraged to consult their medical provider before using any new medications, including herbals and nonprescription drugs.[22]

Herbal medicines are an intriguing option to many patients. Four common preparations include *Phyllanthus*, milk thistle, glycyrrhizin (licorice root extract), and a mixture of herbs known as Liv 52. Although some of the products may have some benefits, the methodologic qualities of the trials evaluating the herbs are poor. Randomized, placebo-controlled studies and long-term followup data are lacking. Meta-analysis of existing studies demonstrated that milk thistle and Liv 52 do not affect the course of liver disease. Herbal treatment is not recommended for patients with chronic hepatitis B.[40]

■ PHARMACOLOGIC THERAPY

❺ Because hepatic damage is sustained by ongoing viral replication, drug therapy aims to suppress viral replication by either immune mediating or antiviral agents. In the United States, interferon (IFN)-α2b, lamivudine, telbivudine, adefovir, entecavir, pegylated (peg) IFN-α2a, and tenofovir are all approved as first-line therapy options for chronic HBV.[27]

Interferon

Interferon-α2b therapy was the first approved therapy for treatment of HBV and improves long-term outcomes and survival.[21] Acting as a host cytokine, it has antiviral, antiproliferative, and

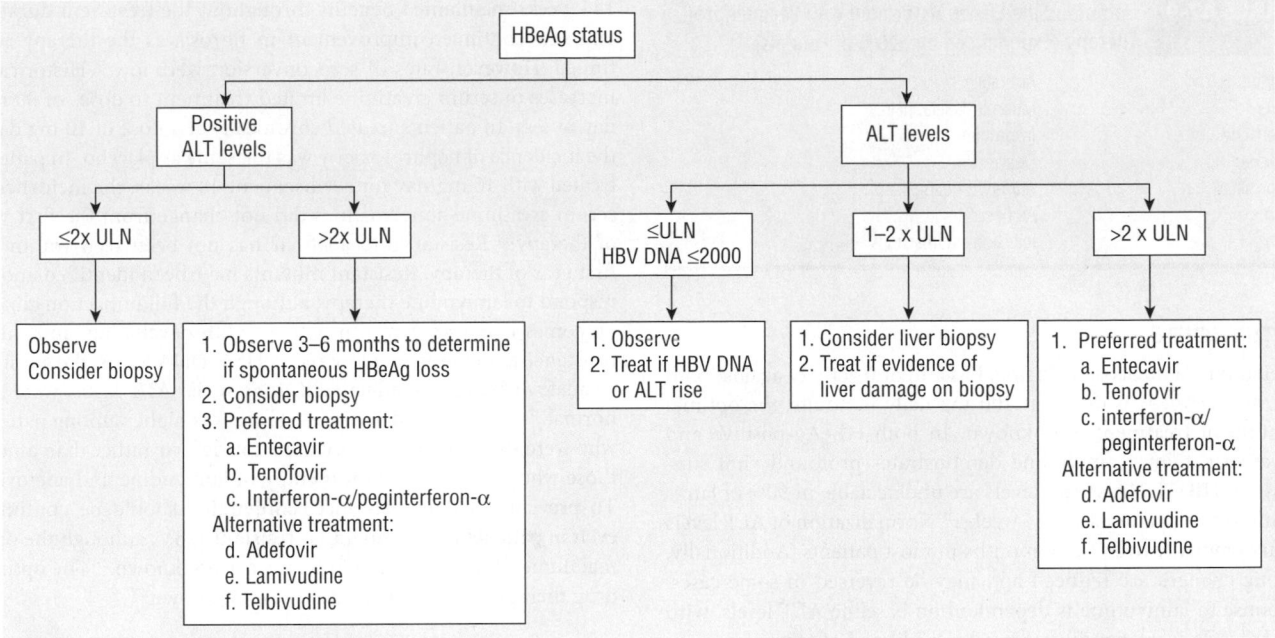

FIGURE 47-1. Suggested treatment algorithm for chronic hepatitis B virus infection based on the recommendations of the American Association for the Study of Liver Diseases. (ALT, alanine transaminases; HBeAg, hepatitis B e antigen; PegIFN, pegylated interferon.) *(Adapted from reference 27.)*

immunomodulatory effects in chronic HBV.[41] Several factors correlate with improved response to interferon therapy, including increased ALT and HBV DNA levels, high histologic activity score

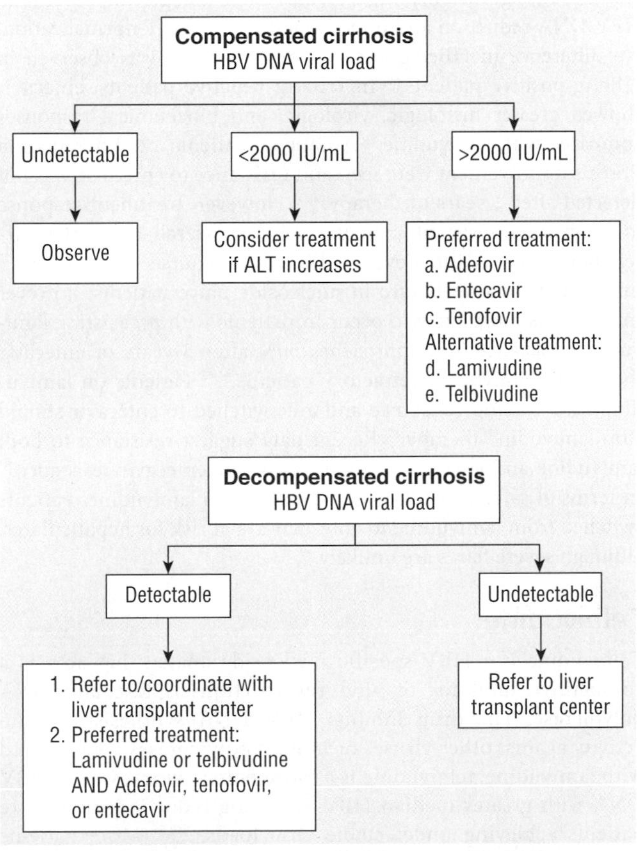

Compensated cirrhosis
HBV DNA viral load

Undetectable → Observe

<2000 IU/mL → Consider treatment if ALT increases

>2000 IU/mL → Preferred treatment:
a. Adefovir
b. Entecavir
c. Tenofovir
Alternative treatment:
d. Lamivudine
e. Telbivudine

Decompensated cirrhosis
HBV DNA viral load

Detectable → 1. Refer to/coordinate with liver transplant center
2. Preferred treatment: Lamivudine or telbivudine AND Adefovir, tenofovir, or entecavir

Undetectable → Refer to liver transplant center

FIGURE 47-2. Suggested treatment algorithm based on the recommendations of the American Association for the Study of Liver Diseases for chronic hepatitis B virus-infected patients with cirrhosis. *(Adapted from reference 27.)*

at biopsy, and being non-Asian. Asian patients tend to have more normal ALT levels in chronic infection, confounding the actual impact of ethnicity on infection.[41]

Patients who respond to interferon therapy tend to have a more durable response than that seen with lamivudine, likely as a consequence of interferon's stimulation of the immune response for seroconversion. Seroconversion rates range from 30% to 40% and are often permanent, although relapse is more likely in HBeAg-negative patients.[35,42] The duration of therapy is finite, although the optimal duration of treatment is unclear. Treatment for a minimum of 12 months is associated with greater sustained virologic response rates than treatment for 4 to 6 months. Seroconversion can occur during or after therapy is complete. An extended treatment duration of 24 months may benefit the difficult-to-treat HBeAg-negative patient.[35] Additional benefits of interferon-based therapy in responsive patients is a reduction in cirrhosis, HCC, and death.[27] Conventional interferon therapy is plagued with numerous problems, including the inconvenience of thrice-weekly injections; however, standard interferon therapy has virtually been replaced by the use of pegylated interferon (peg interferon) because of the benefits in ease of administration, decreased side effect profile, and improvements in efficacy. Compared with conventional interferon, peginterferon has a longer half-life enabling once-weekly injections. For HBV treatment, the approved peg-interferon formulation is pegIFN-α2a. Studies comparing pegIFN-α2a monotherapy with peginterferon-α2a–lamivudine combination therapies suggest that combination therapy caused greater HBV DNA suppression than peginterferon-α2a monotherapy; peginterferon-α2a monotherapy better achieved HBeAg seroconversion than lamivudine monotherapy with no difference in combination therapy; and combination therapy resulted in less lamivudine resistance than lamivudine monotherapy. Interferon-based therapies are still limited by multiple adverse effects (Table 47–9). The high risk of infection precludes use of interferon in decompensated cirrhotic patients.[27] In patients with compensated cirrhosis, interferon appears to be safe and effective, although it can provoke hepatic flares and precipitate hepatic decompensation.[27,35] The optimal role of interferon-based therapies in HBV treatment is not defined.

TABLE 47-9	Common Side Effects Associated with Peginterferon Therapy (Experienced by >20% of Patients)
Fatigue	Arthralgia
Fever	Musculoskeletal pain
Headache	Insomnia
Nausea	Depression
Anorexia	Anxiety/emotional lability
Rigors	Alopecia
Myalgia	Injection site reactions

Lamivudine

Lamivudine, a nucleoside analog, has antiviral activity against both HIV and HBV. It is dosed at 100 mg daily in adults; the optimal duration of treatment is unknown. In both HBeAg-positive and -negative patients, lamivudine demonstrates profound viral suppression. HBV DNA serum levels are undetectable in 90% of lamivudine-treated patients after 4 weeks.[35] Normalization of ALT levels occurs gradually over 3 to 6 months in most patients. Additionally, fibrotic changes are reduced and may be reversed in some cases. Response to lamivudine is dependent on baseline ALT levels, with higher levels corresponding to greater likelihood of seroconversion. Seroconversion rates increase with duration of therapy and are at 50% by the fifth year of therapy.[27] The advantages of lamivudine-based therapy include its safety profile and patient tolerability and the convenience of an oral tablet. Moreover, lamivudine can safely be used in immunosuppressed and cirrhotic patients.[42] Patients who can maintain long-term viral suppression have reduced and possibly reversed cirrhotic changes. However, lamivudine therapy is not without problems. There is no clear duration of treatment and HBeAg-negative patients have a less than 20% viral suppression rate after 12 months of therapy. Serum HBV DNA levels return to baseline upon cessation of therapy.[43] Seroconversion rates are less than 20% after 1 year of therapy and will relapse in up to 58% of patients. Relapse rates are highest among Asian patients.[42] Resistance is inevitable and can undermine the value of treatment. The emergence of YMDD mutants increases with each subsequent year of therapy, with rates approaching 70% after 4 years of therapy, and is associated with returns of serum HBV DNA and elevated ALT levels.[21,23] Relapse is associated with reversion of histological benefits.[27] Although seroconversion can occur even after the appearance of resistant mutants,[23] the prognosis is poor for most patients who develop resistance.[35] In HBeAg-negative chronic hepatitis B, where therapy is long term and the exact duration of therapy unknown, resistance is an especially daunting problem.[27]

Patients on lamivudine therapy require monitoring for breakthrough infection. If patients have confirmed lamivudine-resistant mutations, therapy should be changed to include agents with activity against lamivudine-resistant HBV.[27]

Adefovir

Adefovir dipivoxil is an acyclic nucleotide analog of adenosine monophosphate. The drug acts by inhibiting HBV DNA polymerase. It is dosed at 10 mg daily for 1 year in adults, although the optimal duration of therapy is unknown.[27] A 48-week course of treatment is effective in improving histologic findings, reducing serum HBV DNA and ALT levels, and increasing HBeAg seroconversion in both HBeAg-negative and -positive patients.[44,45] The durability of the response is likely related to a long duration of treatment following seroconversion.[46] Further suppression of HBV DNA and ALT levels occurred in long-term therapy over 4 to 5 years with improved histologic findings.[38] In HBeAg-negative patients treated for 48 weeks, the benefits of therapy were lost within 4 weeks of stopping adefovir. In contrast, patients treated for

144 weeks maintained benefits throughout the treatment duration and saw continued improvement in fibrosis as the therapy continued. However, rates of seroconversion were low.[38] Historically, increases in serum creatinine limited treatment to doses of 30 mg/day or less. In patients treated chronically at a dose of 10 mg daily, the incidence of nephrotoxicity was the same as placebo. In patients treated with 10 mg/day for a subsequent 48 weeks, the incidence of serum creatinine abnormalities did not change from the first year of therapy.[38] Resistance to adefovir has not been seen within the first year of therapy. Resistant mutants have been identified and do respond to lamivudine therapy, although the full impact on clinical outcomes is not known.[27] In patients with developing lamivudine resistance as demonstrated by rising HBV DNA levels, the addition of adefovir was more effective if done while ALT levels were still normal.[47] The risk of adefovir resistance was higher among patients who were switched from lamivudine to adefovir rather than among those who had combination therapy of lamivudine and adefovir.[48] To prevent adefovir resistance, lamivudine should be continued even in patients with lamivudine-resistant HBV, although the optimal duration for combination therapy is not known.[27] The optimal drug therapy in adefovir resistance is not known.[27]

Entecavir

Entecavir is a guanosine nucleoside analog that acts by inhibiting HBV polymerase. An oral agent, it is more potent than lamivudine and adefovir in suppressing serum HBV DNA levels and is effective in lamivudine-resistant HBV.[27,49] Rates of HBeAg seroconversion are higher in patients with elevated baseline ALT.[27] The drug is dosed at 0.5 mg daily for adults with treatment-naive or non-lamivudine-resistant infections and at 1 mg daily in lamivudine-refractory patients. In a 48-week trial comparing it to lamivudine, entecavir resulted in significantly higher rates of histologic improvement, HBV DNA reduction and undetectability, and ALT normalization. No difference in HBeAg loss or seroconversion was observed in HBeAg-positive patients.[50] In HBeAg-negative patients, entecavir showed greater histologic, virologic, and biochemical responses compared with lamivudine.[51] Among all patients, no differences in fibrosis improvement were seen and resistance to entecavir was not detected after 2 years of therapy.[50,51] However, treatment response in lamivudine-resistant patients is lower overall and entecavir-resistant mutants can develop during the course of treatment.[27] Entecavir resistance is rare in nucleoside naïve patients; however resistance is most likely to occur in patients with preexisting lamivudine resistance and approaches 50% after 5 years of entecavir therapy in lamivudine refractory patients.[47,52] Patients on lamivudine who develop resistance and are switched to entecavir should stop lamivudine therapy.[27] Recent data suggest resistance to both lamivudine and adefovir is a risk factor for entecavir resistance.[53] In terms of safety, entecavir is comparable to lamivudine. Patients switched from lamivudine to entecavir are at risk for hepatic flares, although severe flares are unlikely.[49]

Telbivudine

Telbivudine is a HBV-specific nucleoside analog that acts as a competitive inhibitor of viral reverse transcriptase and DNA polymerase. The drug inhibits HBV DNA synthesis with no activity against other viruses or human polymerases.[37] Compared with lamivudine, telbivudine is a more potent suppressor of HBV DNA with greater median HBV DNA log reductions and more patients achieving undetectable viral loads.[37,49,54] More patients also experienced a normalization of ALT levels. Although more telbivudine-treated patients experienced seroconversion, the difference was not significant even at 2 years of therapy. Treatment failure, including an inability to suppress HBV DNA levels below

5 log, occurred statistically more often in lamivudine treated patients than in telbivudine treated ones.[54] Compared with adefovir, telbivudine significantly reduced HBV DNA levels, although no difference was seen for HBeAg loss or ALT normalization.[52] Resistance may limit telbivudine's efficacy, although long-term data are needed.[49] Telbivudine selects for the YMDD mutations. During a 2-year evaluation, resistance increased substantially from year 1 at 5% to 25.1% in year 2 in HBeAg-positive patients and from 2.3% to 10.8% in HBeAg-negative patients.[54,55] In comparison, lamivudine resistance increased from 11% to 39.5% among HBeAg-positive patients and from 10.7% to 25.9% in HBeAg-negative patients.[54,55] Varying degrees of hepatic impairment do not alter the kinetics of the drug, nor does the coadministration of lamivudine or adefovir.[56,57] Combination therapy of telbivudine and lamivudine did demonstrate greater seroconversion rates but the difference was not statistically different from monotherapy.[58] Telbivudine monotherapy is comparable with lamivudine in safety with few case reports of myopathy and elevations of creatinine kinase.[54,55]

Tenofovir

Tenofovir is a nucleotide analog first approved for use in HIV and approved for HBV in 2008. It is available either as a single agent oral tablet or as a combination therapy with emtricitabine. Tenofovir is similar to adefovir but without the nephrotoxicity seen with adefovir, permitting adult dosing to be 300 mg versus 10 mg of adefovir. The higher dosing strategy likely confers several advantages to tenofovir in comparison with adefovir. Among HBeAg-positive patients, more patients treated with tenofovir had undetectable HBV DNA, ALT normalization, and loss of HBsAg than the adefovir-treated group. Rates of histologic response and seroconversion were similar. Among HBeAg-negative patients, more patients treated with tenofovir had undetectable HBV DNA, but there was no difference in ALT normalization, histologic response, and no patients lost HBsAg.[59] In lamivudine-resistant chronic hepatitis B, tenofovir showed an earlier and greater suppression of HBV DNA than adefovir. There are limited data on tenofovir resistance. Tenofovir can overcome adefovir treatment failure but adefovir mutants persist, suggesting cross-resistance.[60] The long-term impact of tenofovir resistance or optimal management to prevent resistance is unknown at this time. Toxicity is minimal compared with adefovir. [42]

■ ALTERNATIVE DRUG TREATMENTS

Emtricitabine is a cytosine analog approved for use in HIV and with activity against HBV. It is currently not approved for HBV but has been used in combination with tenofovir. In a comparative study with placebo, emtricitabine showed a significant decrease in viral load to undetectable in 54% of patients, normalization of ALT levels in 65% of patients, and improvement in necroinflammatory score. However, seroconversion to anti-HBeAg and HBeAg loss did not differ between placebo and emtricitabine. Emtricitabine safety was comparable to placebo. At the end of the 48-week treatment, 20 emtricitabine-treated patients had YMDD or YMDD-related resistance mutations.[61] Emtricitabine is similar to lamivudine and thus likely to induce similar mutations.[27]

Combination therapy has been proposed to increase drug effectiveness and to counter the issues of resistance. Potential disadvantages for combination therapy include costs, toxicity, and drug interactions. Currently no data exist that combination therapy improves effectiveness. Data for preventing resistance is mixed as complete suppression of resistance has not been achieved with combination therapy. Combination therapy with interferon and lamivudine creates less resistance than lamivudine monotherapy,

but the combination did not change the post-therapy viral response in comparison to interferon monotherapy.[27] YMDD mutants remain susceptible to adefovir.[47] Adding adefovir to patients on lamivudine when HBV DNA levels began to increase better maintained normal ALT levels and suppressed HBV DNA than waiting to add adefovir until after ALT levels increased.[46] Adding adefovir to lamivudine when lamivudine resistance develops in HBeAg-negative patients was associated with improved ALT normalization and a lower likelihood for virological breakthrough or development of adefovir resistance. Both groups had similar rates of virologic response.[48] In a comparison study of lamivudine monotherapy versus lamivudine-adefovir combination therapy in treatment-naïve patients, similar rates of seroconversion, HBV DNA suppression, and rates of ALT normalization were observed. There was a lower rate of YMDD mutation resistance in the combination therapy group at 15% versus 43% in the lamivudine monotherapy group.[62] A comparison study of telbivudine, lamivudine, or a combination of telbivudine and lamivudine did not find any benefit to combination therapy as compared with telbivudine monotherapy. Resistance was not reported.[63] The American Association for the Study of Liver Disease recommends combination therapy with lamivudine or telbivudine plus adefovir, tenofovir, or entecavir for decompensated cirrhotic patients with chronic HBV regardless of HBV DNA levels or HBeAg status.[27] Moreover, current guidelines suggest combination therapy with two or more agents in patients who develop antiviral resistant HBV.[27]

■ SPECIAL POPULATIONS

The decision to treat cirrhotic patients depends on disease progression. Patients with decompensated cirrhosis require referral for liver transplant. Most recently updated guidelines suggest lamivudine, telbivudine, adefovir, tenofovir, and entecavir are possible agents for use in cirrhotic patients (see Fig. 47–2).[27]

In patients co-infected with HCV, the clinical practice is to treat the more dominant form of the hepatitis virus. There are no current recommendations on management of HBV/HCV co-infection. Previously published recommendations suggested treating HCV according to published guidelines and to consider the addition of entecavir or adefovir if HBV DNA levels remained stable or rose.[27]

Patients co-infected with hepatitis D, which requires infection with hepatitis B, may be treated with high-dose interferon alfa or peginterferon.[27] There is an overall paucity of data on HBV-HDV co-infection treatment. Lamivudine has not been shown to be effective, neither has ribavirin, a drug used in combination therapy with interferon for HCV treatment.[64,65]

In HIV coinfected patients, therapy should be tailored specifically to the patient. If the patient is being treated for HIV, certain regimens may be optimized to include drugs with efficacy against HBV, including tenofovir, emtricitabine, or lamivudine. If patients are on a stable regimen that does not include HBV-active drugs or are not considered for highly active anti-retroviral therapy (HAART), peginterferon-α or adefovir may be used.[27] Because of neutropenia associated with peginterferon-α, patients considered for interferon therapy should have CD4 counts >500 cells/uL. In patients being considered for HAART, combination therapy is recommended for HBV with either tenofovir and lamivudine or tenofovir and emtricitabine. Patients with confirmed lamivudine resistance should have tenofovir added to their regimens.[27]

Although the majority of chronic HBV patients are adults, children may be treated. Lamivudine is indicated for children age 2 years and older and interferon is approved for use in children age 1 year and older. Entecavir is approved for adolescents age 16 years and older, whereas pegylated interferon and adefovir do not have indications for pediatric dosing.

PHARMACOECONOMIC CONSIDERATIONS

Cost considerations in HBV include the cost-effectiveness of the HBV vaccine and available antiviral treatments. The use of a combined HAV/HBV vaccine is cost-effective.[17] Routine use of the HBV vaccine in HIV counseling and testing sites, including sexually transmitted disease clinics, showed it to be an effective and cost-effective measure in preventing HBV among high-risk groups. The model, which considered four different strategies in vaccination, including no vaccination, found that routine vaccination would cost $4,400 per QALY and per life-year saved. When costs of HBV treatment and transplants were included, the cost decreased to $2,200 per QALY, further supporting routine vaccination as a cost-effective measure.[58]

The cost-effectiveness of therapy for chronic HBV patients must address the approval of new agents for treatment. For noncirrhotic chronic HBV patients with elevated ALT levels, the most cost-effective therapy consisted of initiating treatment with lamivudine and switching to adefovir with the development of lamivudine resistance. The salvage strategy cost $8,447 per QALY. Pegylated interferon was not compared.[66] In chronic HBV patients with cirrhosis, entecavir was the most effective, yet more expensive option. Entecavir cost $25,626 per QALY as compared with adefovir's $19,731 per QALY. Salvage therapy was not found to be cost-effective in this patient population.[67] Pegylated interferon was not compared for initial treatment because of its relative novelty in HBV treatment; because interferon is not considered a treatment option for cirrhosis, it was not included in the analysis of cirrhotic patients.

CLINICAL CONTROVERSY

Although previously published guidelines do not support the use of IFN in cirrhosis because of the potential for an IFN-induced hepatic flare progressing to decompensation, some experts suggest peg-IFN-α2a may be an option for some patients with compensated cirrhosis. Moreover, some experts argue that lamivudine, although indicated for use in cirrhosis, may cause clinical decompensation because of the drug's high risk for resistance and, hence, viral rebound triggering decompensation.

HEPATITIS C

HCV is approximately 5 times as common as HIV and is responsible for an estimated 10,000 chronic liver disease-associated deaths per year.[1] More than 190,000 deaths from HCV-related disease are expected between 2010 and 2019, with projected costs exceeding $10 billion.[68] Most acute infections are asymptomatic and the course of the infection is insidious. As a result, many patients are not diagnosed until significant disease progression.

EPIDEMIOLOGY

❽ HCV is the most common blood-borne pathogen. In the United States, approximately 3.2 million people are chronically infected with HCV.[1] An estimated 17,000 new HCV infections occurred in 2007; however, because of the clinically silent nature of acute infections and the 20- to 30-year disease progression to cirrhosis, it is the 200,000 patients infected per year in the late 1980s who contribute to today's HCV burden.[68] Considering that HCV infection is prevalent in high-risk populations such as prisoners, IDUs, and the homeless, and that this population is generally excluded from most surveys, the actual number of chronically infected people is significantly higher. Nearly 75% of infected people may not be identified.[68] The single largest risk factor for infection is injection drug use. Some experts also consider other illicit drug use, for example intranasal cocaine, as a risk factor because of the possible contamination of drug paraphernalia not limited to syringes and needles.[4] Historically, blood transfusion posed a major risk for infection. Patients who received blood transfusions or transplants before 1992, clotting factors before 1987, or were ever on chronic hemodialysis represent a majority of chronic HCV infections.[1] Improved screening of blood in 1992 decreased the risk of transfusion-related HCV.[70] Currently hemodialysis and transfusions both represent less than 1% of risk factors in known HCV exposures.[4] Healthcare associated transmission is rare; however, a much publicized outbreak linked to an endoscopy center in Nevada in 2007 prompted an examination of HCV outbreaks associated with healthcare. Since 1998, over 58,000 patients have been screened for possible exposure to HCV in non-hospital healthcare venues, including the Nevada incident. The identified risk in Nevada was unsafe injection practices.[1] Although sexual transmission is an often-identified risk factor, the actual risk is very low and may be confounded by other behaviors. Studies of monogamous couples in long-term relationships do not support the use of barrier methods for preventing transmission. Testing of sexual partners in a monogamous relationship is mainly recommended for ease of mind.[70] Although sexual contact is considered an inefficient means of HCV transmission, multiple sexual partners and co-infection with sexually transmitted diseases, including HIV, increase the risk for HCV sexual transmission.[71]

Screening

Although acute HCV infections are often not recognized and many progress to chronic infections, routine screening for infection is not recommended. Various guidelines and position papers for the screening and treatment of chronic HCV infection exist. Screening is warranted in patients who are at high risk for infection (Table 47-10). Although the risk of HCV in monogamous relationships is very low and barrier methods are not recommended, sexual partners are recommended to be tested for the sake of reassurance.[70] The risk of infection from other needle-borne exposures, such as acupuncture, tattooing, and body piercing, is unclear and at this time not an indication for routine screening for HCV.[70]

ETIOLOGY

HCV is a single-stranded RNA virus of the family *Flaviviridae* notable for lacking a proofreading polymerase and enabling frequent viral mutations.[68,72] The virus replicates within hepatocytes and like hepatitis B, is not directly cytopathic. HCV replicates copiously

TABLE 47-10	Recommendations for Hepatitis C Virus (HCV) Screening

Current or past use of injection drug use
Co-infection with HIV
Received blood transfusions or organ transplantations before 1992
Received clotting factors before 1987
Patients who have ever been on hemodialysis
Patients with unexplained elevated ALT levels or evidence of liver disease
Healthcare and public safety workers after a needlestick or mucosal exposure to HCV-positive blood
Children born to HCV-positive mothers
Sexual partners of HCV-positive patients

ALT, alanine transaminase; HIV, human immunodeficiency virus.
Data from Hoofnagle.[72]

TABLE 47-11 Worldwide Hepatitis C Virus Genotype Distribution

Genotype	Region
1	Worldwide, especially United States, Northern Europe
2	Worldwide, especially Northern Europe, Japan
3	India
4	Middle East, Africa
5	South Africa
6	Hong Kong, Southeast Asia

From Hoofnagle.[72]

with an estimated serum half-life of 2 to 3 hours. The result is a proliferate, persistently mutating virus posing an immense challenge for immune-mediated control.[72]

HCV is differentiated into six major genotypes, numbered 1 to 6, and varying in nucleotide sequence by 30% to 50%. Genotypes are further classified into subtypes (a, b, c, etc.), which differ by 10% to 30% in nucleotide sequence. The most widely distributed genotypes are 1 and 2, with genotype 1 the most common (Table 47–11). In the United States, the majority of infections are caused by genotypes 1a and 1b, followed by genotypes 2 and 3. Although infection caused by any of the genotypes can lead to cirrhosis, end-stage liver disease (ESLD), or HCC, the significance of the infecting genotype is related to therapeutic response. Genotypes 2 and 3 are at least twice as likely to respond to therapy as genotype 1. Genotypes 4, 5, and 6 are not well understood but are expected to respond with rates similar to genotype 1.[72]

PATHOPHYSIOLOGY

In the vast majority of cases, an acute HCV infection leads to chronic infection. The immune response in an acute HCV infection is mostly insufficient to eradicate the virus. During the early phases of infection, natural killer cells are activated as HCV RNA levels rapidly rise. A combined effort of HCV specific CD4 and CD8 T lymphocytes and interferon co-expression decrease viral replication. The eradication of HCV by cytotoxic T lymphocytes may occur either as a result of induced apoptosis by infected hepatocytes or by the release of interferon to stifle viral replication. The extent of hepatocyte apoptosis may correlate with the course of the disease. Liver damage and HCC are associated with high levels of hepatocyte apoptosis. Low levels of apoptosis are associated with viral persistence. Moreover, CD4 T-helper cells are unlikely to mediate liver injury, but rather may promote an environment conducive for other immune responses damaging to the liver. Bystander killing may also play a role in hepatic damage. Although HCV infects less than 10% of hepatocytes, up to 20% of cells are activated for apoptosis.[64]

HCV poses a daunting challenge for immune control because of its rapid viral diversification. HCV genomic mutations are detectable within 1 year of infection. Resolved cases of HCV are defined by a vigorous T-cell response with highly active CD8 and persistent CD4 cell response. It is hypothesized that the CD8 activity mediates protective immunity but requires the aid of CD4 cells to maintain the response during viral mutations.[64]

CLINICAL PRESENTATION

In an acute HCV infection, most patients are asymptomatic and undiagnosed. HCV RNA is detectable within 1 to 2 weeks of exposure and levels rise quickly during the initial weeks. The HCV RNA levels plateau at 10^5 to 10^7 international units/mL and precede a peak in ALT levels and the onset of symptoms. Rising ALT levels indicate hepatic injury and cell necrosis. It is not unusual for levels to exceed values 10 times the upper limits of normal.[72] Although HCV RNA serum levels can show interpatient variability, the levels tend to be stable for the individual patient.[65] Typically, symptoms occur 7 weeks after the infection, with a range of 3 to 12 weeks. Approximately one third of adults will experience some mild and nonspecific symptoms, including fatigue, anorexia, weakness, jaundice, abdominal pain, or dark urine.[68,72] Acute infections rarely progress to fulminant hepatitis, although the course can be severe and prolonged. If the infection is self-limiting, symptoms last several weeks as ALT and HCV RNA levels subside. Almost all patients, including immunosuppressed patients, will develop antibodies to HCV. Typically, antibodies are not detectable until either at the time of or shortly after the development of symptoms and are not used diagnostically in an acute infection because a third of infected patients may test negative at the onset of symptoms despite infection.[72]

Up to 85% of acutely infected patients will go on to develop a chronic HCV infection, defined as persistently detectable HCV RNA for 6 months or more. HCV RNA levels and ALT levels can fluctuate and even have periods of undetectable HCV RNA and normal ALTs. Most patients will have few, if any symptoms. The most common symptom is persistent fatigue. Additional symptoms include right upper quadrant pain, nausea, or poor appetite. On physical examination, hepatomegaly is usually present. With advanced disease, stigmata of liver disease is evident, such as spider nevi, splenomegaly, palmar erythema, testicular atrophy, and caput medusae. However, almost all patients with chronic HCV will have some degree of necroinflammatory disease on liver biopsy. The extent of structural damage varies considerably.[72] Chronic inflammation of the liver from chronic HCV infection may result in fibrosis. Fibrosis is defined by altered hepatic perfusion creating a distorted structure and affecting normal function.[75] The speed of fibrosis progression can vary and is not necessarily predicative of cirrhosis development. An estimated 20% of chronic HCV patients will develop cirrhosis and half of those patients will progress to either decompensated cirrhosis or HCC. Historically, one third of untreated patients may expect to develop cirrhosis within 20 years, while another third of patients may delay the onset of cirrhosis for 50 years or never develop it.

It is currently not possible to definitively identify patients at risk for disease progression.[75] Several factors may correlate with a decreased risk for chronicity. Being younger than 40 years old, female, non-black, not immunosuppressed, and with a symptomatic acute HCV infection decreases the risk of developing a chronic infection. Being older than age 20 years at infection triples the risk for chronic HCV. Blacks, especially black men, are more likely to develop chronic infection and have lower treatment responses.[76] Becoming symptomatic and having jaundice is associated with a lower likelihood of chronic infection, perhaps correlating to a stronger immune response to the acute infection. Finally, immunosuppressed patients, such as those with HIV, are more prone to chronic infection although they are not inherently unable to clear the infection.[72] Recently a variation on a gene encoding for endogenous interferon has been described which is associated with a difference in response to treatment and may explain differences in response between patients of African American and European ancestry.[77] Similarly, disease progression is associated with increased age, male sex, continued alcohol intake, obesity, and HIV coinfection. Diabetes, as well as steatosis, may also potentiate fibrosis progression. Viral load and genotypes other than genotype 3 are not factors. Genotype 3 may be associated with fibrosis progression.[75] The development of HCV cirrhosis poses a 30% risk over 10 years for the development of ESLD, as well as a 1% to 2% risk per year of developing HCC.[70] Progression to cirrhosis is the primary concern in patients infected with HCV for 2 decades or longer. Unfortunately, because acute infections are typically not recognized, the diagnosis of HCV is often not made until disease progression.

HCV is also rarely associated with extrahepatic manifestations. The most common is cryoglobulinemia, a local deposition of immune complexes that cause vasculitis. Typical manifestations involve the skin and internal organ damage, predominantly affecting the kidneys. Symptoms of cryoglobulinemia include fatigue, skin rash, purpura, arthralgias, renal disease, and neuropathy.[72] Other, more rare symptoms include B-cell non-Hodgkin lymphoma, Sjögren syndrome, glomerulonephritis, arthritis, corneal ulcers, thyroid disease, neuropathies, and porphyria cutanea tarda.[78]

For many patients, a diagnosis of hepatitis C is incidental. Some patients are diagnosed after finding persistently abnormal transaminases. Unfortunately, those patients who present with symptoms typically have advanced disease. A diagnosis of chronic HCV is confirmed with a reactive enzyme immunoassay for anti-HCV. Testing for anti-HCV is not routinely recommended because of the low prevalence of HCV in the general population and the nonspecificity of the test. Although many professional associations advocate testing for both symptomatic and asymptomatic persons with risk factors for HCV, the U.S. Preventative Task Force does not recommend routine screening of high-risk individuals.[79]

TREATMENT

Hepatitis C Virus

■ DESIRED OUTCOME

The primary goal of therapy is to eradicate HCV infection. Resolving the infection prevents the development of chronic HCV infection sequelae including death. Even patients who are unable to achieve cure may see histological improvements with therapy.[69]

■ GENERAL APPROACH TO TREATMENT

Treatment for HCV is necessary because nearly 85% of acutely infected patients develop chronic infections and are at risk of developing cirrhosis, ESLD, and HCC. Moreover, HCV infection is the most common indication for liver transplant. Treatment is indicated for patients previously untreated who have chronic HCV, circulating HCV RNA, increased ALT levels, evidence on biopsy of moderate to severe hepatic grade and stage, and compensated liver disease.[69] According to the American Association for the Study of Liver Diseases, among chronic HCV patients, symptomatic cryoglobulinemia is an indication for HCV antiviral therapy irrespective of the stage of liver disease.[70] Therapy is not without risk, and in some cases may not be recommended, such as in patients with decompensated liver disease, a history of severe uncontrolled psychiatric disorder, and in patients with severe hematologic cytopenias.[69] Table 47–12 lists the contraindications to therapy.

Before therapy is initiated, quantitative HCV testing, genotyping, and a liver biopsy are performed. Quantitative amplification

TABLE 47-12	Contraindications to Hepatitis C Virus Combination Therapy

Autoimmune hepatitis
Decompensated liver disease
Pregnant or unwilling to comply with contraception
Patients with untreated thyroid disease
Patients with serum creatinine >1.5 mg/dL or on hemodialysis
Patients with major, uncontrolled depression
Patients with severe concurrent medical disease
Patients with solid organ transplant including renal, heart, or lung

assays for HCV RNA are performed in patients who are candidates for therapy to obtain baseline information on the viral load. A baseline HCV RNA level serves as a prognostic indicator for response and is used to monitor virologic response once therapy is initiated. Genotyping is also necessary for treatment candidates because response to therapy and duration of therapy vary depending on the infecting genotype. Liver biopsy is used to determine histologic grade and stage and to guide therapy.[70] Because most chronic HCV patients are not diagnosed for years, a biopsy can provide clinical information on the extent of hepatic damage incurred since infection and offer baseline data to assess disease progression.[69] In some patients, liver biopsy may support a decision to delay treatment.

Overall, the greatest predictor of treatment response is infection with nongenotype 1. Adherence to therapy is a crucial component in response, especially among genotype 1-infected patients. Patients who take at least 80% of their medications for at least 80% of the treatment time are more likely to successfully respond to therapy.[80] Treatment response is monitored according to the following terminology:

Rapid virological response (RVR): a patient with undetectable viral load at week 4 of treatment

Early virological response (EVR): patient who experiences at least a 2-log reduction in viral load by the 12th week of treatment (partial EVR) or a patient with undetectable viral load by the 12th week of treatment (complete EVR)

End-of-treatment response (ETR): patient with no detectable viral load at the end of treatment

Sustained virological response (SVR): patient with no detectable viral load at the conclusion of therapy and 24 weeks later

Relapser: patient who responds to therapy but whose viral load becomes detectable at the conclusion of therapy

Nonresponder: patient with a detectable viral load after 24 weeks of therapy

Null responder: patient with a viral load that never decreased by >2 logs after 24 weeks of therapy

Partial responder: patient with at least a 2-log reduction in viral load but detectable viral levels after 24 weeks of therapy

Patients who achieve a RVR are highly likely to achieve cure; however, patients who do not achieve RVR should not be assumed to be nonresponsive. A negative RVR does not imply inability to achieve SVR, rather it indicates patients will require a full course of therapy and potentially an extended duration of therapy. Patients who experience a complete EVR are more likely to also have an SVR. Less than 3% of patients who fail to have an EVR can be expected to achieve an SVR.[69,70] Achieving a complete EVR is a better marker of SVR than achieving a partial EVR. If the goal of therapy is viral eradication and an EVR is not achieved, therapy may be discontinued at 12 weeks. In some patients, however, histologic benefits can occur without an EVR and histologic improvements alone may warrant continuation of therapy.[69]

■ NONPHARMACOLOGIC THERAPY

All chronic HCV patients should be vaccinated against hepatitides A and B. Lifestyle changes are an important factor in reducing health consequences in hepatitis C. Continued alcohol use is a known risk factor for disease progression and severity. There is no established lower limit of alcohol consumption at which disease progression is not seen. Obesity is also a factor and patients should be encouraged to eat a balanced diet and exercise regularly to maintain a normal weight. Progression of fibrotic changes is

TABLE 47-13	Recommended Hepatitis C Virus Treatment Dosing			
Genotype	Peg-IFN Dose		Ribavirin Dose	Duration[a]
1, 4	Peginterferon-α2a 180 mcg/wk	≤75 kg[b]	1,000 mg	48 weeks
	or	>75 kg	1,200 mg	
	Peginterferon-α2b 1.5 mcg/wk	≤65 kg	800 mg	48 weeks
		>65–85 kg	1000 mg	
		>85–105 kg	1200 mg	
		>105 kg	1,400 mg	
2, 3	Peginterferon-α2a 180 mcg/wk		800 mg	24 weeks
	or			
	Peginterferon-α2b 1.5 mcg/wk		800 mg	24 weeks

[a] Actual treatment duration may be different depending on virological response.
[b] Patient weight.

associated with obesity. Moreover, obesity and decreased insulin resistance contribute to decreased response to interferon. Smoking may also contribute to disease progression. Patients should be encouraged to maintain good overall health, stop smoking, and avoid alcohol and illicit drugs.[70,81] The use of herbal therapy is ineffective.[40] Patients should consult with their physician prior to initiating any herbal therapies and minimize prescriptive drug use if possible.[70]

■ PHARMACOLOGIC THERAPY

❾ The current standard of care for chronic HCV patients is a combination therapy of a once-weekly injection of peginterferon and a daily oral dose of ribavirin. Overall response rates are greatest with combination therapy at an SVR rate of 54% to 56%.[69] Therapy is optimized based on genotype, patient weight, and response to therapy. Table 46–13 lists current therapeutic regimens. For genotype 1, evaluation for RVR at 4 weeks is recommended as an indicator of the probability of achieving an SVR. Patients who do not achieve a RVR should be evaluated for virologic response at 12 weeks (EVR). Because therapy is not without a significant side-effect profile and because failure to achieve a complete EVR is so strongly correlated with treatment failure, some clinicians will terminate therapy early in genotype 1 patients (Fig. 47–3). Patients who achieve complete viral suppression between weeks 12 and 24 may be treated for as long as 72 weeks.[70] Conversely, because genotypes 2 and 3 respond so well to therapy, there are data to support early treatment termination in patients who show an EVR at 4 weeks (Fig. 47–3).[82] Current guidelines suggest patients with genotypes 2 and 3 be treated for the full 24 weeks of therapy.[70]

Interferon

Historically, treatment of HCV involved the use of interferon-α. Although interferon monotherapy resulted in an SVR in less than 10% of patients, the response was durable. The addition of a pegylated moiety to interferon improved the pharmacokinetic profile of the drug to reduce injection frequency from 3 times to once a week, and doubled SVR rates. Even among cirrhotic patients, peginterferon was safe and effective.[69] Two peginterferons are available, peginterferon-α2a (Pegasys) and peginterferon-α2b (PEG-Intron). Table 47–14 lists the differences between the two drugs. It is unclear which therapy is superior. Achievement of SVR may be more likely in patients with an early and intense viral suppression. The current guidelines do not address which formulation of interferon should be preferentially used in HCV treatment.

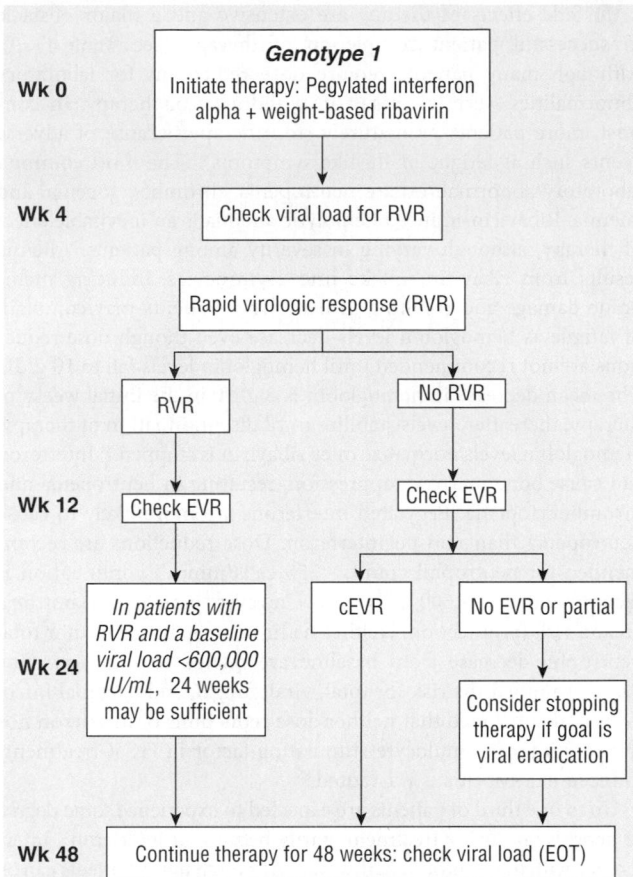

FIGURE 47-3. Suggested response-optimized chronic hepatitis C virus infection treatment regimens based on the recommendations of the American Association for the Study of Liver Diseases.[70] EOT, end of treatment. (Adapted from reference 70.)

Ribavirin

Ribavirin, a synthetic guanosine analog, is ineffective as a monotherapy for HCV and its exact mechanism of action is unknown. When added to interferon, ribavirin significantly increases SVR rates, especially among genotypes 2 and 3. Ribavirin is dosed based on weight for optimal response in genotype 1 and 4 infections. Although monotherapy with peginterferon is an option for patients with contraindications to ribavirin, ribavirin is ineffective as monotherapy and should not be used alone. However, SVR rates are highest among patients treated with a combination of peginterferon and ribavirin at >40% for genotype 1 patients and at approximately 80% for genotypes 2 and 3.[69]

TABLE 47-14	Pegylated Interferon Comparison	
	Pegasys	**PEG-Intron**
Interferon	Alfa-2a	Alfa-2b
Indications	HBV, HCV	HCV
PEG moiety (weight)	Branched (40 kDa)	Linear (12 kDa)
Distribution	8–12 L; highest concentration in liver, spleen, kidneys	Body-weight dependent: 1 L/kg; distributes throughout body
Metabolism	Liver	Liver
Excretion	Renal	Renal
Dosing	Fixed: 180 mcg/wk subcutaneously	Weight dependent: 1.5 mcg/kg/wk subcutaneously

HBV, hepatitis B virus; HCV, hepatitis C virus.

➓ Side effects of therapy are extensive and a major obstacle to successful patient completion of therapy (see Table 47–9). Although many patients require dose reductions for laboratory abnormalities, very few result in withdrawal of therapy. In contrast, more patients prematurely stop therapy because of adverse events such as fatigue or flu-like symptoms.[84] The most common laboratory abnormalities are neutropenia, thrombocytopenia, and anemia. Ribavirin-induced hemolytic anemia is an inevitable effect of therapy, although varying in severity among patients. Anemia results from ribavirin uptake into erythrocytes, inducing membrane damage and resulting in hemolysis. Patients may complain of fatigue as hemoglobin levels decrease even though dose reductions are not recommended until hemoglobin levels fall to 10 g/dL. The mean decrease in hemoglobin is 3 g/dL in the initial weeks of therapy; thereafter, levels stabilize until discontinuation of therapy. Hemoglobin levels normalize once ribavirin is stopped.[84] Interferon can cause bone marrow suppression, resulting in neutropenia and thrombocytopenia. Pegylated interferons are more likely to cause neutropenia than non-peginterferon. Dose reductions are recommended for neutrophil counts <750 cells/mm; discontinuation is recommended at <500 cells/mm. However, patients are not at a greater risk for infection. Neither nadir neutrophil counts nor total neutrophil decrease from baseline are related to infection. One study examined the risk for total, viral, fungal, and bacterial infections and concluded that neither dose reductions of interferon nor the addition of granulocyte-stimulating factor in HCV-treatment-induced neutropenia is warranted.[85]

Up to one third of patients are expected to experience some degree of depression during treatment, partly because of interferon's interference with the serotonin pathways.[70] Although many patients can be managed with selective serotonin reuptake inhibitors, various degrees of counseling and psychiatric consultations may be necessary. Severe depression and suicidal behaviors are rare but not undocumented. More common side effects include flu-like symptoms, which can be managed by acetaminophen or nonsteroidal inflammatory drugs.[69]

Alternative Treatments

Currently, investigated drug treatments for chronic HCV include taribavirin, various formulations of interferon, protease inhibitors, and polymerase inhibitors. Taribavirin is a ribavirin prodrug designed to concentrate within the liver with the goal of minimizing ribavirin-induced anemia. Longer acting versions of interferon, such as albuferon, are also being investigated. Telaprevir, previously referred to as VX-950, is a reversible, selective, and specific HCV RNA protease inhibitor. It is an oral drug and current data suggest optimal dosing to be three times per day. Although telaprevir demonstrated great viral load reduction even among previous interferon nonresponders, when taken alone it demonstrated viral breakthrough within 2 weeks of initiation.[86] Bocepravir is also a serine protease inhibitor currently being investigated in nonresponders. Early studies demonstrated profound viral suppression; however, the role of these agents will likely be as adjuncts to current therapy. Several other protease inhibitors are in various stages of development. A number of polymerase inhibitors are also in various stages of investigation. Studies in treatment-naïve and treatment-refractory patients are ongoing.[87]

Special Populations

Clinical trials are conducted with a patient population that generally does not reflect the patient spectrum encountered in clinical practice. There are no contraindications to the treatment of injection drug users, prisoners, persons with substance abuse issues, or persons with psychiatric disorders. However, barriers exist that can prevent access to care. A multidisciplinary approach to HCV treatment that includes mental health and substance abuse professionals should be considered in providing care to special populations.[88]

Published recommendations for treatment in various populations are as follows.[70]

Patients with Normal ALTs The decision to treat patients with normal ALTs is somewhat controversial and made on an individual patient basis. Clinicians should consider the risks and benefits of therapy, including histologic data, genotype, likelihood for response, and other factors, such as patient willingness to undergo therapy. Successful treatment significantly improves patient quality of life and reduces fatigue.[88] Moreover, the definition of normal can vary by reporting laboratory.

Patients with Decompensated Cirrhosis Patients with evidence of decompensation are candidates for liver transplantation. Therapy is generally not recommended unless administered by experienced clinicians. Serious adverse events including neutropenia and anemia are more likely in cirrhotics and may be managed through the use of growth factors.

Relapsed Patients The decision to retreat should consider the previous therapeutic regimen. Patients with prior treatment with interferon monotherapy or interferon and ribavirin should be considered for retreatment with peginterferon and ribavirin. The likelihood for SVR is lower, but may be as high as 50%. Retreatment with peginterferon and ribavirin after a previously failed course of peginterferon and ribavirin is not recommended.

Nonresponders Retreatment with peginterferon and ribavirin can increase SVR rates in patients previously treated with interferon monotherapy or interferon and ribavirin. Previous adherence, treatment tolerance, severity of underlying liver disease, as well as factors affecting treatment response, such as genotype, should be considered before deciding to retreat.

Accidental Needle-Stick Exposures Prophylactic treatment immediately following an accidental needle-stick exposure is not recommended for multiple reasons. Risk of transmission is considered low and among those infected, a percentage will successfully seroconvert and not require treatment. Because an initial delay in therapy does not increase the risk for developing a chronic infection, most experts wait 8 to 12 weeks before initiating treatment to allow for spontaneous remission. No formal guidelines exist as the optimal duration of treatment is unknown. Treatment is suggested for 12 to 24 weeks.

Injection Drug Users Injection drug use is a major factor in the cycle of HCV transmission. There are no recommendations against treatment for active IDUs although ongoing drug abuse can create many complications and expert opinion dictates that the decision to treat be made on a case-by-case basis. Treatment is recommended for recovering drug users, including those in drug treatment programs assuming patients are willing to comply with close monitoring and contraception requirements. Reinfection rates are low among injection drug users who achieve SVR.[89] It is recommended that patients continue ongoing drug abuse and psychiatric counseling while on HCV therapy.

Alcoholism Because continued alcohol use affects disease progression and severity and thus response to therapy, the cessation of alcohol use during therapy is recommended. Moreover, a period of abstinence before initiation of therapy is also recommended.

End-Stage Renal Disease The role of chronic HCV treatment is not defined for patients with end-stage renal disease. Hemodialysis is a risk factor for acquiring HCV infection yet a contraindication for ribavirin use. Patients with mild renal insufficiency (GFR ≥60 mL/min) may be treated with combination peginterferon and ribavirin. Monotherapy with interferon is an option in patients with renal insufficiency or with end-stage renal disease as ribavirin is contraindicated in these patients due to risks of ribavirin accumulation and severe hemolytic anemia. Peginterferon can pose toxicity problems and requires careful monitoring.

HIV Co-Infection A large portion of HIV-infected patients who acquired the virus via injection drug use will be coinfected with HCV. Treatment poses additional problems because of hepatotoxicity issues associated with highly active antiretroviral treatment, hepatic complications from HIV-associated diseases, as well as flares in hepatitis as CD4 counts recover. Current guidelines recommend a 48-week course of therapy regardless of genotype. The prognosis for an SVR is worse than in patients infected with HCV only. In general, treatment is recommended and both HIV and HCV therapies can be coadministered with the exception of didanosine and zidovudine. The combination of ribavirin and didanosine can result in fatal lactic acidosis. Ribavirin causes hemolytic anemia and when combined with zidovudine can result in severe anemia.[91]

Children Currently therapy is indicated for children age 2 years and older and consists of peginterferon-α2b dosed at 60 mcg/m^2 weekly in combination with ribavirin 15 mg/kg daily for 48 weeks. Ribavirin is available in a liquid formulation. Pediatric patients tend to better tolerate therapy than adults. Pediatric patients should be evaluated as candidates for therapy similarly to the criteria for adults (Table 47–12).

African Americans Response rates of African Americans to HCV therapy is lower than rates observed with Caucasians and non-Hispanic whites, and genetic mutations of HCV may partially explain the discrepancies. African Americans have higher rates of chronic HCV than non-Hispanic whites and Hispanics and have greater rates of baseline neutropenia. African Americans with HCV should be evaluated for treatment and treated according to current guidelines. Baseline neutropenia (ANC <1500 mm^3) should not exclude patients from treatment.

PREVENTION

No vaccine is available for HCV. It is unlikely that a vaccine will be developed in the near future because of the mutagenesis of the virus. Patients infected with HCV should be counseled on not being blood, organ, or semen donors. Although the likelihood of household transmission is small, patients should minimize risks by avoiding possible blood or mucus exposure, such as not sharing razors or toothbrushes and covering open wounds. Patients who continue to use illegal drugs should avoid sharing all drug paraphernalia, as risk of transmission is not limited to needles and syringes.

PHARMACOECONOMIC CONSIDERATIONS

The progression of HCV-induced liver disease is highly variable and identifying which patients will progress remains a clinical challenge. Because not all patients will develop clinical sequelae, therapy may not be necessary in all patients. Given the relative unreliability of treatment to achieve an SVR, the costs associated with therapy, and the side-effect profile of the drugs, the cost-effectiveness of therapy may be questioned. Several studies have assessed the economic values of treating chronically infected HCV patients.

Issues of cost-effectiveness must weigh the public health impact of HCV against the costs of therapy. Despite the decreased incidence of acute HCV infections, epidemiologic data suggest the greatest disease burden will occur in 2015, reflecting the slow progression of disease in patients infected in the late 1970s and early 1980s. At the same time, HCV-related mortality is expected to triple.[92] A projected 720,000 patient-years will be lost as a result

of decompensated cirrhosis and HCC. Predicted costs exceed $21 billion from the development of clinical sequelae. In patients who are younger than age 65 years, the costs associated with premature death are even higher—an expected $54 billion.[68] Although not all patients will develop HCV-related liver disease, it is not currently possible to identify which patients will have disease progression. Moreover, HCV-infected patients are prone to high levels of fatigue and neuropsychiatric and cognitive impairment, further contributing to decreased patient quality of life.[92]

Treatment with peginterferon therapy compared with traditional interferon is a cost-effective approach among noncirrhotic patients who are infected with any of the genotypes, especially in patients who are infected with nongenotype 1.[93] A review of studies published on the cost-effectiveness of therapies for HCV found that HCV therapy is cost-effective most of the time. Reduced cost-effectiveness was seen in patients treated with normal transaminases and healthy biopsies. However, most clinicians would opt not to treat such patients. Moreover, evaluating virologic response by week 12 and terminating therapy if no response is evident substantially lowers treatment costs by more than $15,000. Overall, various studies found that HCV treatment falls within the accepted cost-effectiveness margin, defined as less than $50,000 per QALY. The studies concluded that antiviral therapy costs offset costs associated with disease sequelae.[91]

CLINICAL CONTROVERSIES

In patients with advanced disease, a biopsy may be risky and offer no additional clinical information of whether to treat or not. Some clinicians believe that if therapy is to be initiated regardless, the liver biopsy offers no additional information. In patients with genotype 2 or 3, because response to therapy is so high and most clinicians treat despite biopsy results, there may not be a reason for biopsy.

Histologic improvement is not limited to patients who experience an SVR. Some clinicians believe interferon-based antiviral therapies, regardless of response, can decrease the incidence of HCC development.

Although ribavirin dosing is different for the treatment of genotype 1 depending on the formulation of pegylated interferon, most clinicians will dose ribavirin according to patient weight, irrespective of the formulation.

New data from clinical practice studies in Europe suggest peginterferon-α2a may achieve greater rates of SVR in genotype 1 patients. Data are in abstract form and contradict a recently published trial.

ABBREVIATIONS

AASLD: American Association for the Study of Liver Diseases

ALT: alanine aminotransferase

ANC: absolute neutrophil count

Anti-HAV: antibody to hepatitis A virus

CDC: Centers for Disease Control and Prevention

ESLD: end-stage liver disease

ETR: end-of-treatment response

EVR: early virological response

FDA: Food and Drug Administration

GI: gastrointestinal

HAART: highly active anti-retroviral therapy

HAV: hepatitis A virus

HBcAg: hepatitis B core antigen

HBeAg: hepatitis B e antigen

HBsAg: hepatitis B surface antigen

HBV: hepatitis B virus

HCC: hepatocellular carcinoma

HCV: hepatitis C virus

HIV: human immunodeficiency virus

IDU: injection drug user

IFN: interferon

Ig: immunoglobulin

MHC: Major histocompatibility complex

MMR: measles, mumps, rubella

MSM: men who have sex with men

peg: pegylated [polyethylene glycol]

QALY: quality-adjusted life-year(s)

RVR: rapid virological response

SVR: sustained virological response

ULN: upper limit of normal

REFERENCES

1. Centers for Disease Control and Prevention. Surveillance for acute viral hepatitis-United States, 2007. MMWR Morb Mortal Wkly Rep 2009;58(SS03):1–27.
2. Nainan OV, Xia G, Vaughan G, Margolis HA. Diagnosis of hepatitis A virus infection: A molecular approach. Clin Microbiol Rev 2006;19: 63–79.
3. Elinav E, Ben-Dov IZ, Shapira Y, et al. Acute hepatitis A infection in pregnancy is associated with high rates of gestational complications and preterm labor. Gastroenterol 2006;130:1129–1134.
4. Centers for Disease Control and Prevention. Hepatitis A outbreak associated with green onions at a restaurant—Monaca, Pennsylvania, 2003. MMWR Morb Mortal Wkly Rep 2003;2002;52(47):1155–1157.
5. Centers for Disease Control and Prevention. Hepatitis Surveillance Report No. 61. Atlanta, GA: U.S. Department of Health and Human Services, Centers for Disease Control and Prevention, 2006.
6. Steffen R. Changing travel-related global epidemiology of hepatitis A. Am J Med 2005;118(Suppl 10A):46s–49s.
7. Cuthbert JA. Hepatitis A. Old and new. Clin Microbiol Rev 2001; 14:38–58.
8. Centers for Disease Control and Prevention. Prevention of hepatitis A through active or passive immunizations: Recommendations of the Advisory Committee on Immunization Practices (ACIP). MMWR Morb Mortal Wkly Rep 1999;48(RR-12):1–37.
9. World Health Organization position paper: Hepatitis A vaccines. Wkly Epidemiol Rec 2000;5:37–44.
10. Leach CT. Hepatitis A in the United States. Pediatr Infect Dis J 2004;23:551–552.
11. Bower WA, Nainan OV, Han X, Margolis HS. Duration of viremia in hepatitis A virus infection. J Infect Dis 2000;182:12–17.
12. Rawls RA, Vega KJ. Viral hepatitis in minority America. J Clin Gastroenterol 2005;39:144–151.
13. Centers for Disease Control and Prevention. Update: Prevention of hepatitis A after exposure to hepatitis A virus and in international travelers. Updated recommendations of the Advisory Committee on Immunization Practices (ACIP). MMWR Morb Mortal Wkly Rep 2007;56(41):1080–1084.
14. Centers for Disease Control and Prevention. Health advisory—hepatitis A infections linked to children adopted from Ethiopia and their family contacts. HealthAlert Network, July 18, 2007. http://www2a.cdc.gov/HAN/ArchiveSys/ViewMsgV.asp?AlertNum=00263.
15. Weissman S, Feucht C, Moore BA. Response to hepatitis A vaccine in HIV-positive patients. J Viral Hepat 2006;13:81–86.
16. Jacobs RJ, Gibson GA, Meyerhoff AS. Cost-effectiveness of hepatitis A/B vaccine versus hepatitis B vaccine for healthcare and public safety workers in the western United States. Infect Control Hosp Epidemiol 2004;25:563–569.
17. Jacobs RD, Meyerhoff AS. Cost-effectiveness of hepatitis A/B vaccine versus hepatitis B vaccine in public sexually transmitted disease clinics. Sex Transm Dis 2003;30:859–865.
18. World Health Organization. Hepatitis B. Fact Sheet No. 204, 2000. http//www.who.int/mediacentre/factsheets/fs204/en.
19. Centers for Disease Control and Prevention. Hepatitis B Slide Kit. Division of Viral Hepatitis, 2003. http//www.cdc.gov/ncidod/ diseases/ hepatitis/slides/index.htm.
20. Lok ASF. Chronic hepatitis B. N Engl J Med 2002;346:1682–1683.
21. Lavanchy D. Hepatitis B virus epidemiology, disease burden, treatment, and current and emerging prevention and control measures. J Viral Hepat 2004;11:97–107.
22. Centers for Disease Control. A comprehensive immunization strategy to eliminate transmission of hepatitis B virus infection in the United States: Recommendations of the Advisory Committee on Immunization Practices (ACIP). Part 1: Immunization of infants, children, and adolescents. MMWR Morb Mortal Wkly Rep 2005;54 (RR-16):1–31.
23. Ganem D, Prince AM. Hepatitis B virus infection—Natural history and clinical consequences. N Engl J Med 2004;350:1118–1129.
24. Lee WM. Hepatitis B virus infection. N Engl J Med 1997;337: 1733–1745.
25. Kao JH. Hepatitis B viral genotypes: Clinical relevance and molecular characteristics. J Gastroenterol Hepatol 2002;17:643–650.
26. Fattovich G. Natural history of hepatitis B. J Hepatol 2003;39:s50–s58
27. Lok ASF, McMahon BJ. AASLD practice guidelines: Chronic hepatitis B. Hepatology 2001;34:1225–1241.
28. Ganne-Carrie N, Williams V, Kaddouri H, et al. Significance of hepatitis B virus genotypes A to E in a cohort of patients with chronic hepatitis B in the Seine Saint Denis district of Paris (France). J Med Virol 2006;78:335–340.
29. Arase Y, Ikeda K, Suzuki F, et al. Long-term outcome after hepatitis B surface antigen seroclearance in patients with chronic hepatitis B. Am J Med 2006;119:71.e9–71e.16.
30. Raimondo G, Pollicino T, Squadrito G. Clinical virology of hepatitis B virus infection. J Hepatol 2003;39(Suppl 1):s26–s30.
31. Cantarini MC, Trevisani F, Morselli-Labate AM, et al. Effect of the etiology of viral cirrhosis on the survival of patients with hepatocellular carcinoma. Am J Gastroenterol 2006;101:91–98.
32. Bruxi J, Llovet JM. Hepatitis B virus and hepatocellular carcinoma. J Hepatol 2003;39(Suppl 1):s59–s63.
33. Chen CJ, Yang HI, Su J, et al. Risk of hepatocellular carcinoma across a biological gradient of serum hepatitis B virus DNA level. JAMA 2006;295:65–73.
34. Wright TL. Introduction to chronic hepatitis B infection. Am J Gastroenterol 2006;101(Suppl 1):s1–s6.
35. Farrell GC, Teoh NC. Management of chronic hepatitis B virus infection: A new era of disease control. Intern Med J 2006;36:100–113.
36. Yim HJ, Hussain M, Liu Y, et al. Evolution of multi-drug resistant hepatitis B virus during sequential therapy. Hepatology 2006;44:703–712.
37. Kim JW, Park SH, Louie SG. Telbivudine: A novel nucleoside analog for chronic hepatitis B. Ann Pharmacother 2006;40:472–478.
38. Hadziyannis SJ, Tassopoulos NC, Heathcote EJ, et al. Long-term therapy with adefovir dipivoxil for HBeAg-negative chronic hepatitis B. N Engl J Med 2005;352:2673–2681.
39. Lok ASF, McMahon BJ. Chronic hepatitis B. Update of recommendations. Hepatology 2004;39:1–5.
40. Dhiman RK, Chawla YK. Herbal medicines for liver diseases. Dig Dis Sci 2005;50:1807–1812.
41. Asmuth DM, Nguyen HH, Melcher GP, et al. Treatments for hepatitis B. Clin Infect Dis 2004;39:1353–1362.
42. Craxi A, Antonucci G, Camma C. Treatment options in HBV. J Hepatol 2006;44(Suppl 1):s77–s83.
43. Jacobson IM. Therapeutic options for chronic hepatitis B: considerations and controversies. Am J Gastroenterol 2006;101(Suppl 1):s13–s18.

44. Marcellin P, Chang TT, Lim SG, et al. Adefovir dipivoxil for the treatment of hepatitis B e antigen-positive chronic hepatitis B. N Engl J Med 2003;348:808–816.

45. Hadziyannis SJ, Tassopoulos NC, Heathcote EJ, et al. Adefovir dipivoxil for the treatment of hepatitis B e antigen-negative chronic hepatitis B. N Engl J Med 2003;348:800–807.

46. Wu IC, Shiffman ML, Tong MJ, et al. Sustained hepatitis B e antigen seroconversion in patients with chronic hepatitis B after adefovir dipivoxil treatment: analysis of precore and basal core promoter mutants. Clin Infect Dis 2008;47(10):1305–1311.

47. Lampertico P, Vigano M, Manenti E, et al. Adefovir rapidly suppresses hepatitis B in HBeAg-negative patients developing genotypic resistance to lamivudine. Hepatology 2005;42:1414–1419.

48. Vassiliadis TG, Giouleme O, Koumerkeridis G, et al. Adefovir plus lamivudine are more effective than adefovir alone in lamivudine-resistant HBeAg- chronic hepatitis B patients: a 4-year study. J Gastroenterol Hepatol 2010;25:54-60.

49. Dienstag JL. Looking to the future: New agents for chronic hepatitis B. Am J Gastroenterol 2006;101(Suppl 1):s19–s25.

50. Chang TT, Gish RG, de Man R, et al. A comparison trial of entecavir and lamivudine for HBeAg-positive chronic hepatitis B. N Engl J Med 2006;354:1001–1010.

51. Lai CL, Shouval D, Lok AS, et al. Entecavir versus lamivudine for patients with HBeAg-negative chronic hepatitis B. N Engl J Med 2006;354:1011–1020.

52. Jones R, Nelson M. Novel anti-hepatitis B agents: A focus on telbivudine. Int J Clin Pract 2006;60:1295–1299.

53. Shim JH, Suh DJ, Kim KM, et al. Efficacy of entecavir in patients with chronic hepatitis B resistant to both lamivudine and adefovir or to lamivudine alone. Hepatololgy 2009;50:1064–1071.

54. Liaw YF, Gane E, Leung N, et al. 2-year GLOBE trial results: telbivudine is superior to lamivudine in patients with chronic hepatitis B. Gastroenterology 2009;136:486–495.

55. Lai CL, Gane E, Liaw YF, et al. Telbivudine versus lamivudine in patients with chronic hepatitis B. N Engl J Med 2007;357:2576–2588.

56. Zhou XJ, Marbury TC, Alcorn HW, et al. Pharmacokinetics of telbivudine in subjects with various degrees of hepatic impairment. Antimicrob Agents Chemother 2006;50:1721–1726.

57. Zhou XJ, Fielman BA, Lloyd DM, Chao GC, Brown NA. Pharmacokinetics of telbivudine in healthy subjects and absence of drug interaction with lamivudine or adefovir dipivoxil. Antimicrob Agents Chemother 2006;50:2309–2315.

58. Kim SY, Billah K, Lieu TA, et al. Cost effectiveness of hepatitis B vaccination at HIV counseling and testing sites. Am J Prev Med 2006;30:498–506.

59. Marcellin P, Heathcote EJ, Buti M, et al. Tenofovir disoproxil fumarate versus adefovir dipivoxil for chronic hepatitis B. N Engl J Med 2008;359:2442–2455.

60. Tan J, Degertekin B, Wong SN, et al. Tenofovir monotherapy is effective in hepatitis B patients with antiviral treatment failure to adefovir in the absence of adefovir-resistant mutants. J Hepatology 2008;48:391–398.

61. Lim SG, Ng TM, Kung N, et al. A double-blind placebo-controlled study of emtricitabine in chronic hepatitis B. Arch Intern Med 2006;166:49–56.

62. Sung JJY, Lai JY, Zeuzem S. Lamivudine compared with lamivudine and adefovir dipivoxil for the treatment of HBeAg-positive chronic hepatitis B. J Hepatol 2008;48:728–735.

63. Lai CL, Leung N, Teo EK, et al. A 1-year trial of telbivudine, lamivudine, and the combination in patients with hepatitis B e antigen-positive chronic hepatitis B. Gastroenterology 2005;129:528–536.

64. Niro G, Ciancio A, Gaeta GB, et al. Pegylated interferon alpha-2b as monotherapy or in combination with ribavirin in chronic hepatitis delta. Hepatology 2006;44:713–720.

65. Yurdaydin C, Bozkaya H, Onder FO, et al. Treatment of chronic delta hepatitis with lamivudine vs lamivudine + interferon vs interferon. J Viral Hepat 2008;15:314–321.

66. Kanwal F, Gralnek IM, Martin P, et al. Treatment alternatives for chronic hepatitis B virus infection: A cost-effectiveness analysis. Ann Intern Med 2005;142:821–831.

67. Kanwal F, Farid M, Martin P, et al. Treatment alternatives for hepatitis B cirrhosis: A cost-effectiveness analysis. Am J Gastroenterol 2006;101:2076- 2089.

68. McHutchison JG, Bacon BR. Chronic hepatitis C: An age wave of disease burden. Am J Manag Care 2005;11(Suppl 10):s286–s295.

69. Dienstag JL, McHutchison JG. American Gastroenterological Association technical review of the management of hepatitis C. Gastroenterology 2006;130:231–264.

70. Ghany, MG, Strader DB, Thomas DL, et al. American Association for the Study of Liver Diseases Practice Guidelines: Diagnosis, management, and treatment of hepatitis C. Hepatology 2009;49:1335–1174.

71. Terrault NA. Sexual activity as a risk factor for hepatitis C. Hepatology 2002;36(5 Suppl 1):s99–s105.

72. Hoofnagle JH. Course and outcome of hepatitis C. Hepatology 2002;36(5 Suppl 1):s21–s29.

73. Kanto T, Hayashi N. Immunopathogenesis of hepatitis C virus infection: Multifaceted strategies subverting innate and adaptive immunity. Intern Med 2006;45:183–191.

74. National Institutes of Health Consensus Development Conference Statement: Management of hepatitis C. 2002–June 10–12. Hepatology 2002;36(Suppl 1):s3–s20.

75. Massard J, Ratziu V, Thabut D, et al. Natural history and predictors of disease severity in chronic hepatitis C. J Hepatol 2006;44:s19–s24.

76. Muir AJ, Bornstein JD, Killenberg PG, Peginterferon alfa-2b and ribavirin for the treatment of chronic hepatitis C in blacks and non-Hispanic whites. N Engl J Med 2004;350:2265–2271.

77. Ge D, Fellay J, Thompson AJ, et al. Genetic variation in IL28B predicts hepatitis C treatment-induced viral clearance. Nature 2009;461:399–401.

78. Mayo, MJ. Extrahepatic manifestations of hepatitis C infection. Am J Med Sci 2002;325:135–148.

79. U.S. Preventive Services Task Force. Screening for hepatitis C virus infection in adults: Recommendation statement. Ann Intern Med 2004;140:462–464.

80. McHutchison JG, Manns M, Patel K, et al. Adherence to combination therapy enhances sustained response in genotype-1 infected patients with chronic hepatitis C. Gastroenterology 2002;123:1061–1069.

81. Seeff LB. Natural history of chronic hepatitis C. Hepatology 2002;36(Suppl 1):s35–s46.

82. Mangia A, Santoro R, Minerva N, et al. Peginterferon alfa-2b and ribavirin for 12 vs. 24 weeks in HCV genotype 2 or 3. N Engl J Med 2005;352:2609–2617.

84. Fried MW. Side effects of therapy of hepatitis C and their management. Hepatology 2002;36(Suppl 1):s237–s244.

85. Cooper CL, Al-Bedwawi S, Lee C, Garber G. Rate of infectious complications during interferon-based therapy for hepatitis C is not related to neutropenia. Clin Infect Dis 20063;42:1674–1678.

86. Reesink HW, Zeuzem S, Weegink CJ, et al. Rapid decline of viral RNA in hepatitis C patients treated with VX-950: A phase 1b, placebo-controlled, randomized study. Gastroenterology 2006;131:997–1002.

87. Qureshi SA, Qureshi H, Hameed A. Hepatitis C therapy—the future looks bright. Eur J Clin Microbiol Infect Dis 2009;28:1409-1413.

88. Geppert CMA, Arora S, Ethical issues in the treatment of hepatitis C. Clin Gastroenterol Hepatol 2005;3:937–944.

89. Arora S, O'Brien C, Zeuzem S, et al. Treatment of chronic hepatitis C patients with persistently normal alanine aminotransferase levels with the combination of peginterferon alpha-2a (40 kDa) plus ribavirin: Impact on health-related quality of life. J Gastroenterol Hepatol 2006;21:406–412.

90. Grebely J, Conway B, Raffa JD, et al. Hepatitis C virus reinfection in injection drug users. Hepatology 2006;44:1139–1145.

91. Swan T. Care and Treatment for Hepatitis C and HIV Coinfection. U.S. Department of Health and Human Services Health Resources and Services Administration HIV/AIDS Bureau, April 2006. *http://hab.hrsa.gov/tools/coninfection/indexhtml.*

92. Wong JB. Hepatitis C: Cost of illness and considerations for the economic evaluation of antiviral therapies. Pharmacoeconomics 2006;24:661–672.

93. Sullivan SD, Craxi A, Alberti A, et al. Cost-effectiveness of peginterferon alpha-2a plus ribavirin versus interferon alpha-2b plus ribavirin as initial therapy for treatment-naïve chronic hepatitis C. Pharmacoeconomics 2004;22:257–265.

48

Drug Therapy Individualization in Patients with Hepatic Disease and Genetic Alterations in Drug Metabolizing Activity

Y. W. FRANCIS LAM

KEY CONCEPTS

❶ Hepatic elimination of drugs is primarily dependent on three variables: activity of metabolizing enzymes, plasma protein binding, and liver blood flow, each of which could be altered significantly in patients with liver diseases.

❷ Hepatic extraction ratio represents a conceptual measure of the efficiency of extraction of drug from the blood by the liver, and is not a measure of the metabolic capacity of the liver per se.

❸ Increased systemic bioavailability is primarily a concern for orally administered drugs that have a high hepatic extraction ratio.

❹ Both phase I and II enzymes have been associated with altered drug exposure.

❺ Evaluation of patient's liver function for assessment of need of dosage adjustment is difficult, with most clinicians opting for use of the Child-Pugh classification.

❻ Genetic polymorphisms affecting the drug metabolizing enzymes represent an additional patient-specific factor to consider in optimization of drug therapy.

❼ There are few examples of how metabolic genotypes or phenotypes can determine dosage of individual drugs.

❽ There have been increased attempts to incorporate pharmacogenetics in clinical studies during drug development and in regulatory review.

Although there are different patient-related variables that can change the pharmacokinetics of drugs and potentially require dosage regimen modification, the most common dosing changes likely occur with alterations in elimination capacity of the two primary eliminating organs, the liver and the kidneys. This chapter will focus on the changes in drug pharmacokinetics and pharmacodynamics resulting from altered hepatic drug metabolism in patients with hepatic dysfunction, and the implications for dosing. In addition, genetic changes in metabolic capacity of the patient also affect drug elimination from the liver, and examples of how pharmacogenetics have impacted dose modification and labeling is discussed in this chapter.

> Learning objectives, review questions, and other resources can be found at **www.pharmacotherapyonline.com**.

DRUG ELIMINATION BY THE LIVER

❶ Drugs are primarily eliminated from the body by metabolism and excretion. The liver plays a pivotal role in the metabolism of drugs and formation of metabolites prior to their excretion by the kidneys. The overall capacity of the liver to carry out its metabolic role is primarily dependent on three factors: activity of the metabolizing enzymes within the smooth endoplasmic reticulum and the cytosol of the hepatocyte; the degree of drug protein binding in the blood, which affects the amount of unbound drugs available for uptake into the hepatocyte; and liver blood flow, which delivers drugs to the hepatocyte via the portal vein for orally administered drugs and via the systemic circulation for drugs administered by other routes. Thus, patient-specific factors that affect enzymatic activity, protein binding, or liver blood flow would potentially result in significant alterations in drug disposition and therapeutic response. An understanding of the pharmacokinetic basis of hepatic drug elimination/metabolism is a foundational premise from which one can conceptualize and quantify altered drug disposition in patients with liver dysfunction.

PHARMACOKINETIC BASIS OF HEPATIC DRUG CLEARANCE

Only unbound drugs can be transported from the vasculature to the hepatocyte, where biotransformation, which is dependent on the activity of the relevant metabolic enzymes occurs. Therefore, blood flow to the liver, the degree of plasma protein binding, and the intrinsic metabolic activity, all affect the efficiency of the liver to metabolize a specific drug. The intrinsic metabolic activity, defined as the ability of the hepatocyte to eliminate a given drug in the absence of drug supply limitations such as plasma protein binding and blood flow, reflects the inherent activity of the relevant drug metabolizing enzymes and is quantified as intrinsic clearance (Cl_{int}). The hepatic clearance (Cl_H) is related to the three physiological determinants by the following mathematical relationship:

$$Cl_H = \frac{Q_H \times fu_B \times Cl_{int}}{Q_H + fu_B \times Cl_{int}}$$

where Q_H is hepatic blood flow and fu_B is unbound drug fraction in the blood.

Based on this mathematical relationship, when enzyme activity (Cl_{int}) and fu_B are very low relative to hepatic blood flow, they will become the primary determinants and rate limiting process for hepatic clearance, as $Cl_H \sim fu_B \times Cl_{int}$. On the other hand, when enzyme activity and fu_B are very high in relation to blood flow, Cl_H would approximate hepatic blood flow and be the rate limiting process for hepatic clearance. A more detailed discussion of the complex mathematical relationship between hepatic clearance and the three

TABLE 48-1 Examples of High-Extraction Drugs with Corresponding Reported Percentage Increase in Bioavailability in the Presence of Cirrhosis, and Low-extraction Drugs

High-Extraction Ratio (≥ 0.7) Flow Dependent		Low-Extraction Ratio (≤0.3) Flow Independent
	Reported increases in bioavailability in presence of cirrhosis	
Labetalol	91%	Diazepam
Midazolam	100%	Erythromycin
Morphine	115%	Phenytoin
Nifedipine	78%	Theophylline
Propranolol	67%	Valproic acid
Verapamil	60%	Warfarin

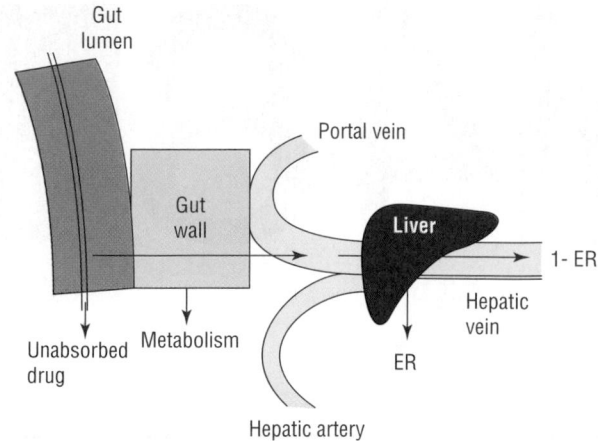

FIGURE 48-1. Schematic representation of the liver integrating the concept of hepatic extraction and first pass effect.

physiological determinants, as well as the different pharmacokinetic models used to explain the physiological approaches to hepatic drug clearance, are provided in the review by Wilkinson.[1]

❷ The hepatic clearance for any drug can also be conceptualized as the product of blood flow across the liver and the hepatic extraction ratio (ER_H) for that drug. The ER_H is a semi-quantitative measure of the efficiency of extraction of drug from the blood by the liver that has a numerical value that ranges from zero to 1. High-extraction ratio drugs which have an ER_H ≥0.7 are readily cleared from the blood and more sensitive to changes in, and rate-limited by, hepatic blood flow. Examples of high-extraction ratio drugs with this flow-dependent elimination characteristic are metoprolol, nitroglycerin, and verapamil. Low-extraction ratio drugs—those with an ER_H ≤0.3 are more sensitive to changes in the degree of plasma protein binding and/or intrinsic metabolic activity, and rate-limited by these two factors rather than by hepatic blood flow. They are thus also considered to demonstrate flow-independent elimination. Warfarin, diazepam, and valproic acid are representative examples of low-extraction ratio drugs (Table 48–1).

Although it seems confusing that extensively metabolized drugs such as warfarin, phenytoin, and theophylline are classified as "low-extraction" drugs, it is important to remember that the ER_H does not measure metabolic capacity per se, rather it is a conceptual semi-quantitative measure to help define the ease of extraction of a drug by the liver as the drug is delivered to the hepatocyte. Based on the degree of plasma protein binding, drugs with low-extraction ratio are sometimes further subgrouped as binding sensitive (e.g., phenytoin) and binding insensitive (e.g., theophylline). As such, the mathematical relationship discussed in the preceding paragraph would dictate that hepatic clearance of a highly protein-bound, low-extraction ratio drug would depend on both intrinsic clearance and the degree of plasma protein binding; in contrast, the intrinsic clearance of a drug that is minimally bound to plasma proteins is the primary factor affecting its hepatic clearance.

ALTERED HEPATIC DRUG CLEARANCE IN LIVER DISEASES

Based on the overview of the pharmacokinetic basis of hepatic drug clearance, changes in drug metabolism can result from alterations in hepatic blood flow, plasma protein binding, or intrinsic metabolic activity. While many different pathophysiological liver diseases can result in reduced functional capacity, most acute entities such as hepatitis, liver cancer, and hepatosplenic schistosomiasis are usually not associated with significant or prolonged alterations in drug metabolism. Jorga et al.[2] showed that in patients with moderate

chronic hepatitis, there was no difference in the unbound clearance of tolcapone compared with that in healthy volunteers. In contrast, patients with nonalcoholic cirrhosis showed a significant decrease in unbound clearance of tolcapone. In fact, most clinical studies that have investigated the effect of liver diseases on drug disposition have primarily been conducted in patients with cirrhosis.[3]

CHANGES IN HEPATIC BLOOD FLOW

❸ The liver is primarily perfused by blood from the hepatic artery, which carries oxygenated blood from the aorta, and the portal vein, which carries nutrient-rich blood from the gastrointestinal tract. The terminal branches of the hepatic artery and the portal vein merge into the hepatic sinusoids and serve as the vascular capillaries of the hepatocyte. The hepatic vein is the conduit by which blood from the liver enters into the inferior vena cava and then the systemic circulation. The portal vein provides about 75% of the liver's total blood supply of about 1.5 L/min in healthy adults. Therefore, the liver is the first site of metabolism for orally administered drugs even before they reach the systemic circulation (Fig. 48–1). This "first pass effect" primarily affects high extraction ratio drugs and the extent of drug elimination can be significant, resulting in low systemic bioavailability (Table 48–1). Simply put, under the assumptions of complete drug dissolution, absence of drug degradation in the gastrointestinal tract, and absence of gut wall metabolism, a drug with ER_H of 70%, will have a bioavailability of 30%. Although the extent of drug metabolism can be circumvented by oral administration of a higher dose compared with that for intravenous administration, the oral bioavailability of some drugs could be very low and variable, necessitating administration by alternative routes such as the sublingual route for nitroglycerin.

In patients with cirrhosis, due to any of the multiplicity of causes (see Chapter 43), blood flow across the liver is usually decreased.[4,5] In addition, cirrhosis also causes alteration of vasculature within the liver, resulting in intra- and extra-hepatic portasystemic shunting. Shunt formation has been shown to allow up to 80% of blood supply to bypass the hepatocytes,[5] and thus does not come in contact with the metabolizing enzymes located therein. Furthermore, the permanent loss of hepatocyte function in patients with cirrhosis also results in reduced metabolic capacity. These two pathological processes together decrease hepatic clearance significantly for orally administered high extraction ratio drugs, and the reduced first pass effect results in a dramatic increase in systemic bioavailability (Table 48–1).[3] Pentikainen et al.[6] reported that in patients without cirrhosis, the oral bioavailability of midazolam is 38%. In patients with cirrhosis, the bioavailability is 76%, representing a two-fold increase. This can have a significant impact on the likelihood of the patient experiencing an adverse drug reaction and warrant dosage adjustment for patients with liver diseases which will be discussed later in this chapter. In contrast, low-extraction ratio drugs tend to have minimal first pass effects and therefore exhibit high bioavailability after oral administration. As long as additional biological processes, such as gastrointestinal absorption, are not altered then bioavailability will be minimally affected.

CHANGES IN METABOLIC CAPACITY

In addition to altering the liver vasculature, cirrhosis also has been associated with irreversible hepatic damage and cell death. Although extensive hepatic damage is associated with reduced drug metabolism as evidenced by a decrease in Cl_{int} the extent of impairment is variable not only among patients, but also among different metabolic enzymes.

❹ In general, phase I oxidative metabolism mediated by the cytochrome P450 (CYP) enzyme system is more sensitive to the effect of cirrhosis than phase II conjugation reactions, especially glucuronidation.[7] For example, among the benzodiazepines, the clearance of diazepam and midazolam, but not of oxazepam and temazepam, are reduced in patients with cirrhosis.[3] This differential effect between phase I oxidation and phase II conjugation reactions may be related to greater sensitivity of the CYP enzyme system to hypoxia as the result of impaired uptake of oxygen caused by sinusoidal capillarization.[8] Indeed hypoxia has been shown to have an important role in suppressing CYP-mediated drug metabolism in both animal[9] and human[10] studies. Frommes et al.[11] have shown that oxygen administration via a face mask in cirrhotic patients resulted in normalization of clearance of the phase I substrate theophylline but not of acetaminophen, a phase II substrate. Other factors that may contribute to the variable sparing effect include activation of latent UDP-glucuronosyltransferase (UGT), increased extrahepatic glucuronidation, differences between specific glucuronidation pathways, and similar to the CYP enzyme system, a differential effect on individual UGT isoforms.[7] Despite the general belief of "sparing" of phase II conjugation reactions in patients with cirrhosis, it is important to note that more recent studies have shown conjugation reactions can be reduced in patients with liver dysfunction, especially those with severe liver cirrhosis (Table 48–2).[2,12–14] The conflicting result between the study of Sonne et al.[13] and Shull et al.[15] could be related to the difference in severity of liver diseases in the two study populations.

Given the presence of multiple isoforms of human cytochrome P450 enzymes, different studies have investigated whether there are selective differences in expression and activity of individual isoenzymes. George et al.[16,17] found that the total CYP amount in the livers obtained from 50 patients with different degrees of end-stage liver disease, Child-Pugh class A to C, was reduced when compared with healthy individuals. Based on the Child-Pugh classification, four of the 50 patients had class A, 17 had class B, and 29 had class C cirrhosis. In addition, 18 patients also had cholestasis.

Selective and variable alterations in amount, catalytic activities, and mRNA level among CYP1A2, CYP2C8/10, CYP2E1, and

CYP3A were reported in these 50 patients, and the presence or absence of cholestasis also had an effect on the observed changes. CYP1A2 amount and catalytic activity were significantly reduced with a corresponding decrease in mRNA level in patients with both cholestatic and noncholestatic cirrhosis. CYP3A4 amount, catalytic activity, and mRNA were significantly reduced only in patients without cholestasis. The amount and catalytic activity of CYP2E1 were decreased only in cirrhotic patients with cholestasis, whereas the CYP2E1 mRNA level was lower in both types of cirrhosis. In contrast, CYP2C8/10 amount and catalytic activity were not reduced in either type of cirrhosis. Although the corresponding levels of mRNA were shown to be decreased in both cirrhosis types, the use of a nonspecific polyclonal antibody to identify CYP2C8/10 might have recognized other 2C isoenzymes and produced erroneous results. In summary, while it is clear that based on in vitro studies at the protein level,[16,17] the extent of hepatic dysfunction-induced impairment in drug metabolism is dependent on both severity and type of disease, as well as the specific isoenzyme affected, the exact mechanism for this differential effect remains to be elucidated. In addition, the ability to extrapolate these results to the patient care setting and possible dosage recommendation would likely require incorporation of the effect of additional patient-specific variables such as concurrent medications and disease states.

CHANGES IN EXTENT OF PLASMA PROTEIN BINDING

An additional complicating factor occurs for low-extraction, protein-binding sensitive drugs. In patients with cirrhosis, production of drug-binding proteins such as albumin and alpha-1-acid glycoprotein are decreased, resulting in an increase in the unbound concentration of acidic and basic drugs, respectively. The magnitude and duration of the elevated unbound concentration is difficult to predict.

BILIARY EXCRETION AND HEPATIC TRANSPORT OF DRUGS

The biliary tract is important not only for bile secretion, but also for excretion of drugs and metabolites mediated by the APT-binding cassette superfamily of hepatic transporters. Drugs and metabolites that are excreted into the bile reach the small intestine via the biliary tract. Within the small intestine, these metabolites, especially the glucuronides, can be converted back to the parent compound, resulting in reabsorption of both parent and metabolites and thus complete the enterohepatic circulation. Therefore, interruption of this enterohepatic circulation could reduce systemic drug exposure. There is little information on the contribution of biliary excretion to the overall drug elimination and the effect of liver diseases on biliary excretion of drugs is poorly quantitated.

The role of hepatic transport proteins in mediating drug uptake into the hepatocytes and biliary excretion of drugs has been recognized in recent years. Among these hepatic transporters, the organic

TABLE 48-2	Example of Drugs with Documented Changes in Phase 2 Metabolic Capacity in Patients with Liver Diseases			
Drug	**Types or Severity of Liver Disease**	**Changes in Pharmacokinetic Parameters**	**Recommended Dosing Modification**	**References**
Diflunisal	Histologically proven cirrhosis	36% reduction in clearance of unbound diflunisal		12
		38% reduction in formation of phenolic and acyl glucuronides		
Oxazepam	Biopsy proven cirrhosis	54% reduction in oral clearance		13
Tolcapone	Child-Pugh class B	44% reduction in unbound clearance	50% dose reduction	2
Zidovudine	Child-Pugh class B or C	73% reduction in oral clearance	50% dose reduction	14

anion transporting polypeptide (OATP) and the P-glycoprotein multidrug transporter, or MDR1, have been the most studied. OATP is an uptake transporter which is responsible for the hepatic uptake of organic anions primarily, whereas P-glycoprotein is an efflux transporter that is responsible for the biliary excretion of cationic drugs. Although different human diseases are known to be associated with loss of transporter function,[18] currently there is little specific information regarding how liver disease affects the function of these proteins and therefore hepatic transport in humans. Nevertheless, reduced expression of transporters including OATP2 and MRP2 have been observed in patients with cholestatic liver diseases,[19,20] which could impair excretory liver function. On the other hand, intermittent hypoxia could up-regulate hepatocellular P-glycoprotein expression.[21]

ADDITIONAL EFFECTS OF LIVER DISEASES ON DRUG DISPOSITION AND EFFECTS

EFFECT ON DRUG ABSORPTION

Delayed gastric emptying possibly related to altered action of gastrointestinal hormones, has been shown to occur in patients with cirrhosis.[22] While this will delay the rate of absorption, the extent of drug absorption is generally not reduced. Although the liver has no functional role in affecting the absorption of drug from the gastrointestinal tract per se, its unique anatomical positioning within the circulating system makes it a primary site of loss for orally administered drug prior to its entry into the systemic circulation. As previously discussed, drugs with a high extraction ratio tend to undergo significant "pre-systemic metabolism" or "first pass effect," resulting in low systemic bioavailability. In patients who have cirrhosis with associated portasystemic shunting and/or reduction in metabolic capacity, oral administration of these drugs could result in a significant increase in their systemic bioavailability and hence pharmacodynamic effect. In contrast, drugs with low extraction ratios have been noted to be negligibly affected.

EFFECT ON DRUG EXCRETION

Reduced glomerular filtration rate and renal plasma flow have been observed in patients with liver cirrhosis[23] and patients with liver transplant,[24] potentially accounting for reported decreased renal elimination of commonly used drugs[3] In addition, in individual patients, advanced liver disease can be complicated by the presence of hepatorenal syndrome. In these patients, dosage reduction would need to be considered even for drugs that are primarily excreted unchanged by the kidney. For example, the elimination of the antiepileptic agent levetiracetam is primarily dependent on the kidney, yet a 50% dosage reduction was recommended for patients with severe cirrhosis.[25] It is difficult to assess renal function in patients with liver cirrhosis.[23,24] Most serum creatinine-based equations tend to overestimate the true glomerular filtration rate. This has led some investigators to suggest the use of inulin or iothalamate to measure GFR in patients with advanced liver diseases.[23]

EFFECT ON DRUG PHARMACODYNAMICS

Changes in therapeutic response to a drug can occur in patients with liver disease even in the absence of any changes in pharmacokinetics. Increased drug sensitivity can occur as a result of altered affinity of the drug to its target, altered binding to the target, alteration in the target itself, altered permeability of the blood brain barrier, or increases in GABA-ergic activity or GABA receptors. Altered pharmacodynamic responses have been reported in the literature with analgesics, benzodiazepines, loop diuretics, and beta-blockers.[26]

Bakti et al.[27] reported that with similar unbound triazolam concentration at 2.25 hours after drug administration, cirrhotic patients have an average of 30% greater impairment in psychometric performance tests, including digit symbol substitution test, flicker sensitivity, and pursuit rotor, when compared with healthy control subjects. Test performance was similar in both groups prior to administration of triazolam. The study results suggest that the increased sensitivity is not due to altered pharmacokinetics and might explain why clinically some cirrhotic patients develop encephalopathy and other CNS effects even when administered standard doses of benzodiazepines, cimetidine,[28] and quinolones.[29]

On the other hand, resistance to the pharmacodynamic effects of loop diuretics in patients with cirrhosis has been reported for bumetamide, furosemide, torasemide, and triamterene.[26] For these drugs, the sigmoidal curve that describes the relationship between drug concentration and pharmacological response is shifted to the right, indicating a reduced response compared with healthy individuals. Down-regulation of β_2-adrenoreceptors in patients with cirrhosis[30] has been suggested as a possible mechanism of lower therapeutic response observed with metipranolol[31] in patients with cirrhosis.

LIVER FUNCTION ASSESSMENT

In contrast to renal impairment, accurate quantification of liver function in patients with hepatic impairment is difficult to perform, especially for the purpose of drug dosage adjustment. The severity of liver function impairment is usually assessed clinically with the Pugh modification of the Child-Turcotte classification.[32] Based on the clinical evidence of ascites and encephalopathy and laboratory parameters that measure the liver's synthetic and excretory functions, patients are assigned different scores in accordance to the level of impairment in these parameters (Table 48–3). The classification is easy to use and useful for following the clinical course of an individual patient or comparing groups of patients among studies. It is noteworthy that the Child-Pugh classification does not include assessment of renal function, an important prognostic factor in liver disease. The Model for End-stage Liver Disease (MELD) is a more recently developed, and potentially more objective scoring system for liver disease severity and includes variables such as serum bilirubin, creatinine, and the international normalized ratio (INR) of prothrombin time.[33] However, alterations in the synthesis of albumin

TABLE 48-3	Severity of Liver Disease Based on the Child-Pugh Classification		
Clinical or Laboratory Parameters	1 Point	2 Points	3 Points
Ascites	Absent	Mild	Moderate
Encephalopathy (grade)	Absent	Grade 1 or 2	Grade 3 or 4
Serum albumin	>3.5 g/dL (>35 g/L)	2.8–3.5 g/dL (28–35 g/L)	<2.8 g/dL (<28 g/L)
Serum bilirubin	1–2 mg/dL (17.1–34.2 mmol/L)	2–3 mg/dL (34.2–51.3 mmol/L)	>3 mg/dL (>51.3 mmol/L)
Prothrombin time (sec > control)	1–4	4–10	>10

A value of 5 suggests absence of liver impairment, whereas 15 would indicate severe liver failure. Child-Pugh class A = 5 to 6 points, class B = 7 to 9 points, and class C = 10 to 15 points. The original Child-Turcotte classification consisted of grades A, B, and C, with grade C being the most severe liver disease. Similar to the Pugh modification, the Child-Turcotte classification includes albumin, bilirubin, and ascites, plus assessment of nutrition and neurological disorder.

or clotting factors and the corresponding changes in their respective laboratory parameters as well as the presence of patient-specific variables such as nutritional status and vitamin K intake complicate the utility of these parameters in the MELD functional assessment tool. In addition, in contrast to renal impairment, none of the clinically used liver function tests, including those used in the Child-Pugh classification and MELD,[33] correlate well with drug pharmacokinetic parameters. This not only is a result of their inability to quantify the primary physiological determinants of hepatic clearance, including intrinsic clearance and hepatic blood flow, but also a reflection of the complex and multiple physiological processes not being accurately accounted for by any individual laboratory test.

The inability of endogenous markers to provide a quantitative measurement of the liver capacity to metabolize drugs has led to the administration of exogenous model substrates and calculation of their clearances or the extent or rate of formation of their respective metabolite as quantitative liver function measurements.[34] Based on the physiological determinants of hepatic clearance discussed previously, these exogenously administered model substrates can be generally categorized into flow dependent, e.g., indocyanine green, lidocaine, and sorbitol; and flow independent, e.g., aminopyrine, antipyrine, caffeine, and erythromycin.[25] However, none of these markers have been shown to be better than the Child-Pugh classification for assessing liver function in patients. The time required for performing these tests, as well as the invasiveness of some of the procedures associated with specific tests, also limit their clinical utility. Indeed, to date, they have not gained widespread acceptance for predicting drug kinetics and aiding dosage adjustment in patients with liver dysfunction.

Furthermore, studies showed that administration of a flow-dependent and flow-independent model substrate in the same subjects did not result in an independent measure of the physiological determinants of hepatic clearance. Rather, a correlation between the two test measures was unexpectedly obtained.[35,36] Since cirrhosis causes both irreversible hepatic cell damage and altered vasculature via portasystemic shunting, the pharmacokinetic profile of a drug can be affected by changes in hepatic blood flow and drug metabolizing enzyme activity. However, it is not known to what extent reduced hepatocyte function would impact elimination of flow-dependent drugs. Nevertheless, the "intact hepatocyte hypothesis," which suggests the presence of intra-hepatic shunts in chronic liver disease, has been proposed as a possible explanation for the reduced extraction of flow-dependent drugs. This may account for the observed positive correlation between the clearances of both flow-dependent and flow-independent drugs.[35,36] In addition, given the complexity of the CYP enzyme system, simultaneous administration of several model substrates which have specificity for different metabolic enzymes has been advocated and can be accomplished by the administration of various combinations of drugs.[37–39] This so-called "cocktail approach" has been primarily used in the research environment to characterize changes in metabolic capacities in patients with liver dysfunction.

DRUG DOSING IN PATIENTS WITH LIVER IMPAIRMENT

Similar to dosing considerations in patients with kidney dysfunction, drug dosage regimen adjustment in patients with liver diseases can in general be accomplished by either dose reduction, extending the dosing interval, or a combination of both strategies. However, the lack of a clinical laboratory test that correlates well with the metabolic capacity of the liver has hampered the development of dosing guidelines or algorithms. The U.S. Food and Drug Administration (FDA), through official guidance, has suggested the need of dosage adjustment for drugs that exhibit a greater than two-fold increase in AUC in patients with hepatic impairment,[40] although no specific recommendation (e.g., percentage dose reduction or extent of liver impairment) has been provided.

Nevertheless, based on an understanding of the pharmacokinetic basis of hepatic drug metabolism, knowledge of the likely etiology of liver dysfunction (reduced liver blood flow, porta-systemic shunting, or hepatic failure), and characteristics of the drug in question (flow dependent or flow independent, extent of plasma protein binding), a conceptual framework for rational dosing can be made. For orally administered drugs with a high ER_H the initial and maintenance doses in patients with cirrhosis need to be reduced because of the likely significant decrease in first pass effect caused by porta-systemic shunting and decreased hepatic blood flow. The challenge in adopting this conceptual framework to clinical practice is our inability to predict the magnitude of dose reduction needed. Given the data of Pentikainen[6] and the ranges of reported percentage increase in bioavailability for some commonly used drugs (Table 48–1), one prudent approach is to assume 100% bioavailability unless there is specific bioavailability data or dosage adjustment recommendations. If this is the case one can estimate the reduced maintenance dose proportionally by using the following mathematical expression: $D_H/D_N = F/100$, where F is the known bioavailability of the drug in patients without liver disease available from the literature or the manufacturer, and D_H and D_N are the doses used in patients with liver dysfunction and normal liver function, respectively. If drugs with a high ER_H were administered intravenously, then only the maintenance dose would need to be reduced as a result of reduced hepatic blood flow. For drugs with a low ER_H, changes in bioavailability is minimal after oral administration and the initial dose for both oral and intravenous routes could be the same as patients with normal liver function. On the other hand, the maintenance dose for both administration routes would need to be reduced in patients with cirrhosis based on the estimated reduction in metabolic capacity.

For example, the oral dose of theophylline can be reduced by up to 50%, because the clearance is 0.042 L/kg/h in patients with cirrhosis as compared with 0.062 L/kg/h in patients with normal liver function.[41] Similarly, the dosage of tolcapone also is recommended to be reduced by 50% because of the difference in unbound clearance in patients with Child-Pugh class B cirrhosis relative to normal volunteers.[2] Obviously, this dose modification strategy serves only as a starting point. The therapeutic index of the drug in question and good clinical judgment with an awareness of other factors that can further change the metabolic capacity (for example, in the case of theophylline, viral illness, smoking, drug—drug interaction, congestive heart failure) would greatly enhance the ability of a clinician to optimize drug therapy in patients with liver dysfunction.

5 Since there is no equivalent of serum creatinine or creatinine clearance for assisting dosage adjustment in patients with liver dysfunction, the Child-Pugh classification, despite its limitation, is still used primarily by clinicians to assess the extent of liver dysfunction and dose adjustment if needed.[42] Since a total Child-Pugh score of 5 and 15 represent, respectively, normal liver function and severe hepatic impairment, it is reasonable to reduce the maintenance dose by 25% for a drug that is primarily dependent on the liver for elimination (≥65% to 70%) in a patient with a score of 8 to 9. A dose reduction of at least 50% would be prudent for a patient with a score of ≥10. Likewise, Child-Pugh B and C classifications[32,43] could result in similar 50% and 75% reductions, respectively, of the daily maintenance dose. For both classification systems, depending on the severity of the liver dysfunction and clinical judgment, extension of the dosing interval should also be considered. Again, based on the assumption of 100% bioavailability, the extended dosing interval can be estimated proportionally by the following mathematical expression: $T_N/T_H = F/100$, where F is the known bioavailability of the drug in patients without liver disease available from the literature or the manufacturer, and T_H and T_N are the dosing intervals used in patients with hepatic dysfunction and normal liver function, respectively.

Since the FDA official guidance recommends the use of the Child-Pugh classification to categorize the extent of hepatic impairment in patients,[40] this classification has been employed during drug development as the foundation for the development of dosage recommendations for patients with liver diseases. For example, two- to four-fold increases, respectively, in the AUC of atomoxetine in patients with Child-Pugh B and C classifications, have led to the labeling recommendations of 50% and 75% reduction of the normal dose used in patients with normal liver function.[32,44] A summary of dosage recommendations for 23 recently approved drugs has been published; however, the utility of these data to guide drug therapy decisions in clinical practice is unknown.[45]

PHARMACOGENETIC ALTERATION IN DRUG METABOLIZING ENZYME ACTIVITIES

⑥ While many factors, including age, gender, smoking, and diet, can influence drug disposition and therapeutic response in individual patients, recent research emphasis has focused on the effect of pharmacogenetics on drug pharmacokinetics and pharmacodynamics. For a more in-depth discussion of the concept of pharmacogenetics and how drug disposition and response are related to specific genotypes and/or phenotypes, please refer to Chapter 9. In that chapter, there is also a tabulation of the most commonly utilized diagnostic substrates for those drug-metabolizing enzymes which exhibit genetic variability. The focus of the subsequent sections of this chapter is to provide information on how pharmacogenetic testing has been reported in the literature and its impact on drug therapy individualization or labeling changes for those drugs that are metabolized by polymorphic enzymes.

Pharmacogenetic testing to identify the presence of altered metabolic activity can be achieved by phenotyping and/or genotyping. In general, a genotype is a trait marker of an individual's metabolic activity for a specific polymorphic enzyme and is independent of time and external factors such as concurrent medications, smoking status, or diet. Phenotyping, on the other hand, represents the metabolic activity at a specific time, which could be susceptible to changes associated with concurrent drug therapy. For most patients receiving concurrent therapy, the phenotype might be the more useful and relevant assessment of metabolic capacity and, hence, the foundational information to guide dosing considerations. For example, in the presence of a potent CYP2D6 inhibitor, the CYP2D6 metabolic capacity of a genotypic extensive metabolizer (EM) could be significantly decreased to a level similar to that of a poor metabolizer (PM).[46] In such a scenario, the metabolic capacity would be more accurately reflected by the phenotype, and the dose of the given CYP2D6 substrate drug in a genotypic EM might need to be reduced.

DOSING IN PATIENTS WITH GENETICALLY ALTERED METABOLIC CAPACITIES

ALTERATION IN PHASE ONE ENZYMES

CYP2C9

Metabolism of the pharmacologically active S-warfarin is almost exclusively mediated by the polymorphic CYP2C9, with the *3 allele having a greater influence on its disposition than the *2 allele. A meta-analysis of 39 studies involving 7,907 genotyped patients reported that racemic warfarin doses in patients carrying either of these two allelic variants were 20% to 78% lower compared to those

with the wild-type *1 allele.[47] Aithal et al.[48] and Margaglione et al.[49] reported higher incidence of bleeding complications in patients with the *2 or the *3 allele compared with patients with the *1 allele. While these studies[47–50] demonstrate a role for the CYP2C9 polymorphism in determining warfarin dose requirement and minimizing toxicity, polymorphisms in other target genes could also be relevant. Examples of additional polymorphisms include those affecting the activities of vitamin K 2,3-epoxide reductase complex, subunit 1 (VKORC1), γ-glutamyl carboxylase, epoxide hydrolase, calumenin, and protein C, as well as the uptake of vitamin K.[51] Incorporation of the relevant covariates of warfarin dosing in dosing algorithm could further optimize warfarin dosing in clinical practice.[52] Of these, the VKORC1 polymorphism is mostly defined, with the G/G genotype as the homozygous wild-type requiring higher warfarin doses than G/A and A/A genotypes. Current data suggest that both VKORC1 and CYP2C9 are major determinants of warfarin dose, whereas the other genes contribute up to 10% of variation.[51] In August 2007, the FDA revised the warfarin product label to include pharmacogenetic information, and subsequently approved different genetic tests for warfarin dosing.

A recent study using a pharmacogenetic algorithm that incorporated clinical and genetic data to estimate initial dose of warfarin showed better correlation between predicted dose and actual dose requirement, in particular for patients requiring low (≤21 mg/wk) and high (≥49 mg/wk) doses, than a clinical algorithm or a fixed-dose approach.[53] Two recent studies utilized modeling techniques to simulate the potential clinical and economic outcomes of pharmacogenomic-guided dosing in hypothetical patient cohorts treated with warfarin for the first time, and concluded that the relatively high cost ($326 to $570 for CYP2C9 and VKORC1 bundled testing) of genotype-guided dosing is associated with modest improvements with respect to quality-adjusted life-years, survival rates, and total adverse event rates. Nevertheless, the investigators also suggested that cost-effectiveness of pharmacogenomic-guided warfarin dosing could be improved in several ways. This includes decreasing genotyping cost by 50%, achieving greater effectiveness in INR-control in clinical outcomes (quality-adjusted life-years, survival rates, and total adverse event rates) with genotype-guided dosing, and applying the genotype-guided dosing algorithm in patients with out-of-range INRs and/or at high risk for hemorrhage.[54,55]

CLINICAL CONTROVERSY

Although scientific evidence suggests the value of clinical testing for CYP2C9 and VKORC1 when prescribing warfarin, many clinicians argue against routine use of the genotyping tests until there is evidence of improvement in long-term outcome.[56,57]

CYP2C19

Despite the fact that CYP2C19 mediates the metabolism of several drugs, including proton pump inhibitors (PPIs), diazepam, and voriconazole, its clinical utility has not been examined as extensively as that of the CYP2D6 polymorphism. The polymorphic CYP2C19 is the primary isoenzyme responsible for the metabolism for PPIs. Although there are up to 10-fold differences in systemic exposure between carriers of the CYP2C19*1 allele versus *2 and *3 alleles, patients possessing one or two of these variant alleles did not experience higher incidence of concentration-related toxicity. This is likely a reflection of the wide margin of safety for these drugs. Rather, the clinical relevance of the CYP2C19 polymorphism is related to the efficacy of PPIs in eradicating H pylori. Compared with CYP2C19 PMs, higher PPI doses are required in CYP2C19 EMs to achieve similar drug exposure, intragastric pH, and efficacy.[58] Similar to CYP2D6*2, a recently identified CYP2C19*17 allele is associated with a very rapid metabolism phenotype and carriers of this allelic variant would likely require higher doses of PPIs for acid suppression.[59,60] Although one study showed no association between *CYP2C19*17* genotype and eradication of *H pylori* for pantoprazole,[61] another study predicted that omeprazole AUC would be lower by about 40% in homozygous carriers of *CYP2C19*17*.[62] Given the higher affinity of omeprazole to CYP2C19 compared with pantoprazole,[63] further studies using omeprazole are required to clarify the clinical relevance of *CYP2C19*17* genotype in determining the success rate of treatment of acid-related disorders.

Furata et al.[64] reported the results of pharmcogenomic-based tailored lansoprazole regimens designed to achieve sufficient acid inhibition for eradication of *H pylori*. Based on 24-hour intragastric pH monitoring in healthy volunteers, lansoprazole dosage regimens that achieved intragastric pH ≥5.0 were documented to be 30 mg 3 times daily for homozygous carriers of the **1* allele, 15 mg 3 times daily for heterozygous carriers of the **1* allele, and 15 mg twice daily for homozygous carriers of the **2* or **3* alleles. For achieving intragastric pH ≥5.8, the corresponding dosage regimens in the three *CYP2C19* genotypes groups were 30 mg 4 times daily, 15 mg 4 times daily, and 15 mg twice daily, respectively. Three hundred *H pylori*-positive patients were then randomly assigned to receive either the standard regimen consisting of lansoprazole 30 mg, clarithromycin 400 mg, and amoxicillin 750 mg, all given twice daily; or the pharmacogenomics-based regimen consisting of lansoprazole dosed according to patient's *CYP2C19* genotype and antibiotic regimen according to genetic testing of bacterial susceptibility to clarithromycin. The eradication rate for the pharmacogenomics-based regimen was 96% (144 of 150 patients), significantly higher than the 70% (105 of 150 patients) achieved with the standard regimen (P < 0.001). Including the cost of the genotyping test, the per-patient cost for successful eradication of *H pylori* for the genotype-based regimen ($669) was similar to that of the standard regimen ($657), lending support not only to the clinical usefulness, but also the cost-effectiveness of pharmacogenomic-based therapeutic approach as well.

CYP2C19 polymorphism has also been associated with dosing of the antiplatelet drug clopidogrel, which requires biotransformation to its active metabolite. In 162 healthy subjects, those with at least one reduced-function *CYP2C19* allele had 32.4% lower AUC of the active metabolite, reduced inhibition of platelet aggregation, and decreased pharmacological response (P < 0.001). In addition, in 1,477 patients with acute coronary syndromes, higher incidences of cardiovascular events following myocardial infarction were noted in patients with reduced *CYP2C19* function when compared with noncarriers of the reduced-function alleles.[65] This and six other studies were cited in the revised clopidrogel FDA-approved product label (updated May 5, 2009) which noted a 30% to 50% reduction in AUC of the active metabolite in *CYP2C19* intermediate and poor metabolizers after a loading dose of 300 or 600 mg and a maintenance dose of 75 mg daily.[65]

CYP2D6

The report of a female patient found to be resistant to normal doses of nortriptyline[66] represented one of the earliest indications of how altered metabolic capacity can impact drug dosing and response. The clinical observation and subsequent metabolic phenotyping and genotyping identified three extra copies of the *CYP2D6* gene in the patient,[67] thereby accounting for her extremely high dose requirement of 500 mg/day. This patient and others with similar high *CYP2D6* activity were subsequently categorized as ultrarapid metabolizers (UM).

This clinical observation led to a dramatic increase in the identification, cloning, and investigation of the functional significance of numerous additional *CYP2D6* alleles. To date, it is probably safe to label *CYP2D6* as the most studied but yet most variable gene.

TABLE 48-4	Dosage Adjustment (Percentage of Normal Dose) of Selected Antidepressants and Antipsychotics Based on CYP2D6 Genotypes			
Drugs	**EM**	**IM**	**PM**	**UM**
Desipramine	130	80	30	260
Imipramine	130	80	30	
Venlafaxine	130	80	30	
Olanzapine	140	60	40	
Maprotiline	130	80	40	
Trimipramine	130	80	40	
Amitriptyline	120	90	50	
Nortriptyline	120	90	50	230
Risperidone	110	100	50	
Clomipramine	120	90	60	
Fluvoxamine	120	90	60	
S-Flupenthixol	120	90	70	
Fluoxetine	110	90	70	
Mianserine	110	90	70	300
Paroxetine	110	90	70	
Zuclopenthixol	110	90	70	
Haloperidol	110	100	80	

Table adapted from Kirchheiner et al.[70]

The presence of multiple alleles with significant interindividual (20%–96%) and intraindividual (12%–140%) variabilities in enzyme activity[68,69] may be partially responsible for the time gap between the nortriptyline case report and subsequent attempts to utilize metabolic genotype or phenotype to generate antidepressant dose recommendations.[70] The investigators compared the pharmacokinetic profiles of 32 CYP2D6- and CYP2C19-dependent antidepressants in subjects with an array of *CYP2D6* and *CYP2C19* genotypes. The analysis took into consideration the contribution of the polymorphic isoenzymes to the overall elimination of each antidepressant, and provided dose recommendation for 14 of the 32 antidepressants in EMs, intermediate metabolizers (IMs), and PMs of *CYP2D6* (Table 48–4) or *CYP2C19*. In general, PMs need about 50% of normal dose of tricyclic antidepressants, whereas the dose reduction was smaller for the selective serotonin reuptake inhibitors (SSRIs).

Using the approach proposed by Kirchheiner et al.,[70] nortriptyline maintenance dose requirements for attainment of comparable systemic exposure were estimated to be 50% in PMs and up to 230% of the average dose in UMs. Though there are multiple literature reports of increased incidence of antidepressant adverse effects in PMs of *CYP2D6*, there were no other documented reports of therapeutic failure for CYP-dependent antidepressants in UMs. Kirchheiner et al.[70] acknowledged the lack of data preclude any dose recommendation in UMs for most antidepressants, with the exception of nortriptyline, desipramine, and mianserin. They further noted that only five of 54 reviewed studies included evaluation of efficacy in relation to genotypes, and only the study of Mihara et al.[71] showed a significant relationship (P = 0.023). More recently, Brockmoller et al.[72] reported that the clearance of S-mirtazapine in UMs was 12.6-fold higher than in PMs, and suggested that poor response might occur in UMs as a result. Although this data suggests the need for a higher dosage for UMs, no specific recommendations were made.

The formation of the active metabolite O-desmethyltramadol from tramadol is dependent on CYP2D6, and similar to codeine, analgesic relief from tramadol has been reported to be lower in PMs.[73] Although tramadol also possess other opioid and non-opioid-dependent mechanisms for its analgesic effect, Stamer et al.[74] have shown in a prospective study of 300 patients recovering from abdominal surgery, a significant difference in the percentage of nonresponders (based on need for rescue pain medication and patient's satisfaction upon interview) between *CYP2D6* PMs (46.7%) and EMs (21.6%)

($P = 0.005$). They also reported a difference in the postoperative analgesic dose requirement of tramadol between the two groups: 144.7 ± 22.6 mg in PMs and 108.2 ± 56.9 mg in EMs ($P < 0.001$). In the recovery room 43.3% of genotypic PMs compared with 21.6% of genotypic EMs required rescue medication. The authors concluded that PMs required higher analgesic consumption to achieve pain relief. Even though there are likely other significant pharmacogenetic variables affecting opioid analgesic response, the difference in dosing requirement shown in this study suggests that 30% dose increases might be necessary in patients who are *CYP2D6*-poor metabolizers. Similar to the PMs, the presence of *CYP2D6*10* allele in intermediate metabolizers has also been associated with reduced tramadol efficacy.[75]

The anticancer drug tamoxifen is metabolized by *CYP2D6* to its active metabolite endoxifen. Recently, a robust correlation between the *CYP2D6* genotype and endoxifen concentration was noted; PMs had a reduced relapse-free time and disease-free survival rate.[76,77] Although many studies had tested for an association between the *CYP2D6* genotype and clinical response to tamoxifen, most of the trials involved a relatively small number of patients. Currently, the FDA has not revised the product label of tamoxifen.

CLINICAL CONTROVERSY

Currently there is no consensus about the use of *CYP2D6* genotyping testing in patients prescribed tamoxifen. Some clinicians advocated its use, especially in postmenopausal women who are *CYP2D6* PM, where aromatase inhibitors would be a valid alternative therapeutic choice. Opponents of the practice argue that routine use of the genotype test should await more reliable evidence from well-designed studies. On the other hand, the clinical implication of *CYP2D6* metabolic status is more relevant for prescribing concurrent therapy that might interact with tamoxifen via *CYP2D6* inhibition. When prescribing antidepressants in breast cancer patients for management of depression and/or vasomotor symptoms, choice of antidepressants should take into consideration their inhibitory effect on CYP2D6.[46,78]

CYP3A

Despite the existence of significant interindividual variability in activity, evaluations of the role of *CYP3A* genes (*CYP3A4*, *CYP3A5*, and *CYP3A7*) in mediating disposition and response have not been conclusive. The most convincing evidence showing a genetic influence on tacrolimus pharmacokinetics has been demonstrated in patients with the *3 allele of *CYP3A5*3*. Homozygous carriers of the *3 allele had a higher plasma tacrolimus concentration compared to patients with the *CYP3A5*1* allele, although considerable overlap was noted.[79,80] MacPhee et al.[81] showed that homozygous and heterozygous carriers of the *CYP3A5*1* allele required a longer time to achieve therapeutic concentrations and suggested these individuals be prescribed an initial tacrolimus dose that is twice normal. Given that it is common clinical practice to measure tacrolimus concentrations, this genotype-based dose modification recommendation could be readily tested. Based on current pharmacogenetic information, dosing information cannot be predicted nor are dosage modifications recommended for cyclosporine or sirolimus.[82]

ALTERATION IN PHASE 2 ENZYMES

Thiopurine Methyltransferase

6-Mercaptopurine and azathioprine are used in the management of childhood acute lymphoblastic leukemia and autoimmune and inflammatory diseases such as rheumatoid arthritis. S-methylation of these drugs is mediated by the polymorphic thiopurine S-methyltransferase (TPMT). PMs and IMs with two and one deficient *TPMT* allele, respectively, are prone to significant hematopoietic adverse effects when given standard doses. Currently, it is well established that PMs and IMs would need a maximum of 10% to 15% and 50%, respectively, of the normal dose of thiopurines.[83] The identification of a patient's *TPMT* genotype prior to therapy initiation has been adopted as a standard procedure in some hospitals in the United States.[84] In a recent study, Fargher et al.[85] reported that 67% of National Health Service clinicians in England routinely utilize *TPMT* phenotyping compared with approximately 5% who use genotyping to guide prescribing and monitoring of azathioprine. Investigators reported that screening for *TPMT* gene mutations for all patients prior to starting azathioprine is cost-neutral if only homozygous carriers of the mutation suffer from myelosuppression. Screening would become cost beneficial if heterozygous carriers of the mutations also experienced myelosuppression.[86] Additional documentation of cost-effectiveness of the strategy,[86,87] expanded education of clinicians, and further availability of commercial tests for determination of *TPMT* genotype and phenotype may make it easier to justify and implement genotype-based thiopurine dosing into clinical practice.

Uridine Diphosphate Glucuronosyltransferase

The uridine diphosphate glucuronosyltransferase 1A1 (UGT1A1) is involved in the glucuronidation of several anticancer drugs including irinotecan. Irinotecan is a prodrug and the pharmacologically active moiety, SN-38, is inactivated by UGT1A1. Thus, PMs of UGT1A1 have a higher incidence of dose-limiting toxicities.[88] A prospective clinical pharmacogenetic study has shown a correlation between the development of grade 4 neutropenia and patients who are homozygous carriers of the *UGT1A1*28* allele.[89] In fact, the product label for irinotecan has been updated to reflect the need of reducing initial dose by at least one level (e.g., from 250 mg/m^2 to 125 mg/m^2) in homozygous carriers of the *UGT1A1*28* allele (Table 48–4).

N-Acetyltransferase

The bimodal distribution of isoniazid's acetylation capacity, which was demonstrated several decades ago, explained the higher incidence of peripheral neuropathy and hepatotoxicity seen in slow acetylators (SAs) compared with rapid acetylators (RAs).[90] Years later, genotyping studies confirmed an inverse relationship between the numbers of active *NAT2* allele and the risk of hepatotoxicity: 28-fold and 4-fold increases in relative risk were noted for patients with no active and one active *NAT2* allele, respectively, when compared to patients with two active *NAT2* alleles.[91,92] Currently two large phase III studies of isoniazid in European and Asian countries are enrolling patients to determine the utility of *NAT* genotype-based dosing (2.5 mg/kg twice weekly for SAs and 7.5 mg/kg twice weekly for RAs) in reducing toxicity in SAs and early treatment failure in RAs. The trials are expected to be completed in late 2011 to early 2012. (See Isoniazid Dose Adjustment According to NAT2 Genotype, *http://www.clinicaltrials.gov*.)

POTENTIALS, CHALLENGES, AND LIMITATIONS OF PHARMACOGENETIC SCREENING AS A PHARMACOTHERAPY DOSING TOOL

❽ The above cited examples suggest that there is great potential value associated with the use of pharmacogenetic screening of patients to optimize therapy. The value of early detection of patients with deficient metabolic genotype and/or phenotype is clearly demonstrated with the thiopurines and irinotecan, whereas clinical experience with nortriptyline[66,67] and ondansetron[93] showed that optimal therapeutic response can be achieved earlier in UMs. Given the data on poorer clinical outcome in *CYP2D6* PMs receiving tamoxifen,[76,77] it will likely be of significant value to implement this pharmacogenetic knowledge into clinical practice. Although there is no documented report of an association between metabolic polymorphisms and SSRI efficacy, PMs were shown to have significant side effects with venlafaxine[94] and paroxetine.[95] Given the high incidence of nonadherence to antidepressants,[96,97] one can also make a case that genotype-based dose reduction in PMs might improve therapeutic outcome, lower the incidence of side effects, and improve adherence to the medication regimen.

❼ Despite the expanding body of beneficial evidence, the pace of incorporation of pharmacogenetic-guided individualized therapy into clinical practice has been slow.[98] Currently, pharmacogenetic screening for deficiency in TPMT is one of the few examples of how pharmacogenetics can enhance the individualization of thiopurine drug therapy.[85] The updated product labels of irinotecan and clopidogrel lack specific and quantitative information regarding dose reduction for homozygous or heterozygous carriers of the respective reduced-function alleles and to date genotype-based dosing information is not available for most other drugs. Given the extensive literature on genotype-related differences in drug pharmacokinetics, the incorporation of dosing information into clinical practice has been slow. For example, clearance of tolbutamide in homozygous carriers of *CYP2C9*3* was 84% lower than that in subjects with the *CYP2C9*1/*1* genotype, whereas heterozygous carriers of the *2* allele have about 50% lower clearance.[99] Based on these results, dose reductions of about 90% and 50% would seem to be an appropriate recommendation in these patients for controlled clinical trials to evaluate whether the goal of genotype-based therapy could be achieved in clinical practice. However, to date, such a prospective trial has not been carried out. Since efficacy of the oral sulphonylureas can be evaluated easily in clinical practice, implementation of these dose recommendations in clinics or physician's office in lieu of expensive and time consuming clinical trials might be the first step to take in achieving pharmacogenetic-based dosing and therapy individualization.

Yet it is clear that not all drugs are candidates for genotype-guided dose recommendation. The drug in question not only has to be primarily metabolized by a polymorphic enzyme, it also needs to have a narrow therapeutic index. Based on the knowledge of their pharmacology, the SSRIs would not be good candidates, and it is not surprising that the Evaluation of Genomic Applications in Practice and Prevention Working Group does not recommend the application of pharmacogenomics for these agents.[100] In the study of Brockmoller et al.,[101] although there was a trend towards lower

haloperidol efficacy in UMs and higher efficacy in the PMs, there was significant overlap in the haloperidol daily doses among the four metabolic groups, with 14 ± 10 mg in UMs versus 13 ± 9 mg in the PMs. This could be due to the complex metabolic disposition of haloperidol that includes CYP2D6- and CYP3A4-mediated oxidation, glucuronidation, and interconversion with reduced haloperidol. The clinical utility of *CYP2D6* genotyping is further minimized by significant interethnic variabilities in metabolic disposition,[102] and possibly the difficulty of relating rating scale-based changes in psychotic symptoms to specific metabolic genotypes. In addition, as demonstrated with risperidone, the presence of an active metabolite would also make it difficult to demonstrate the clinical relevance of genotype-based dose recommendation for the parent compound.

❽ Nevertheless, it is encouraging to find that pharmaceutical companies have chosen to include pharmacogenetic screening to identify special populations for evaluation of pharmacokinetics, pharmacodynamics, and clinical outcomes during the drug development process.[103] As an example, *CYP2D6* genotype was one of the patient-related variables included in the evaluation of differences in systemic exposure of atomoxetine and an 8- to 10-fold increase in AUC and higher incidence of adverse effects was noted in the PM population.[104] Although no specific dose recommendation arose from the results, the information was incorporated into the drug labeling.[44]

As additional data regarding the clinical relevance of pharmacogenetic screening for dosing and therapy individualization become available, the information can be incorporated not only for drugs in development but also for drugs that have been approved. It is noteworthy that over the years, the FDA has updated the product labels of more than 200 drugs to include pharmacogenetic information. This information is in general divided into three categories: pharmacogenetic test either (1) required or (2) recommended for therapeutic decision making, and (3) the availability of pharmacogenetic test is for information purposes only. Specifically, the labeling of 5-mercaptopurine, azathioprine, irinotecan, and clopidogrel were revised to reflect the risk of toxicity and/or the lack of efficacy, as well as the need of dosage adjustment in PMs and IMs. The FDA has also approved the AmpliChip CYP genotyping test (Roche Diagnostics) for screening of common *CYP2C19* and *CYP2D6* alleles, and the UGT1A1 Molecular Assay (Third Wave Technologies) for genotyping *UGT1A1* alleles.[105,106] However, due to lack of study data using patients' individualized genotypes, the revised label information does not specifically address the precise dose reduction for patients receiving any of these drugs (Table 48–5).

TABLE 48-5	Examples of Label Changes Incorporating Pharmacokinetic Data or Therapeutic Response in Patients with Liver Diseases or Genetic Alteration in Metabolic Capacity	
Drug	**Relevant Pharmacokinetic Data or Therapeutic Response as a Result of Patient-Specific Alteration in Disposition**	**Label Information Incorporating Study Data**
Atomoxetine[104]	4-fold and 2-fold increases in AUC in patients with Child-Pugh C and B classification, respectively	Reduce normal dose by 75% and 50%, respectively, in the two groups of patients.
	5 to 10-fold increases in c_{max} and AUC in CYP2D6 PMs	Blood levels in PMs are similar to those attained by taking strong inhibitors of CYP2D6. The higher blood levels in PMs lead to a higher rate of some adverse effects.
6-Mercaptopurine[83]	6-MP is inactivated via TPMT to the inactive metabolite methyl-6-MP. TPMT activity is controlled by a genetic polymorphism, with a defined correlation between deficiency in TPMT activity and myelotoxicity	Patients with intermediate TPMT activity may be at increased risk of myelotoxicity if receiving conventional doses of 6-MP. Patients with low or absent TPMT activity are at an increased risk of developing severe, life-threatening myelotoxicity if receiving conventional doses of 6-MP. TPMT genotyping or phenotyping (red blood cell TPMT activity) can help identify patients who are at an increased risk for developing 6-MP toxicity. The optimal starting dose for homozygous deficient patients has not been established.
Irinotecan[89]	Irinotecan is converted to the active metabolite SN-38, which is subsequently inactivated by UGT1A1. Irinotecan toxicity is related to SN-38 exposure	Individuals homozygous for the *UGT1A1*28* allele are at increased risk for Neutropenia after irinotecan administration. A reduction in the starting dose by at least 1 level of irinotecan should be considered for patients known to be homozygous for the *UGT1A1*28* allele. The appropriate dose reduction in this patient population is not known.

CONCLUSION

Pharmacogenetics has the potential to improve drug therapy in patients. However, variations in multiple genes that affect both the pharmacokinetics and pharmacodynamics of the candidate drugs present significant challenges in identifying specific gene-variant combinations that can help clinicians achieve optimal therapeutic outcomes for their patients. In addition, few studies address the cost-effectiveness of genomic-guided dosing. Additional clinical trials, similar to the study of Furuta et al.[64] and the ongoing *NAT2* genotype-guided treatment evaluation need to be done before pharmacogenetics-guided dosing can be routinely recommended in clinical practice.

ABBREVIATIONS

AUC: area under the curve

Cl_H: hepatic clearance

Cl_{int}: intrinsic clearance

CYP: cytochrome P450

EM: extensive metabolizer

ER_H: hepatic extraction ratio

fu_B: unbound drug fraction in the blood

IM: intermediate metabolizer

NAT: *N*-acetyltransferase

PM: poor metabolizer

Q_H: hepatic blood flow

TPMT: thiopurine *S*-methyltransferase

UGT: uridine diphosphate glucuronosyltransferase

UM: ultrarapid metabolizer

REFERENCES

1. Wilkinson GR. Clearance approaches in pharmacology. Pharmacol Rev 1987;39(1):1–47.
2. Jorga KM, Kroodsma JM, Fotteler B, et al. Effect of liver impairment on the pharmacokinetics of tolcapone and its metabolites. Clin Pharmacol Ther 1998;63(6):646–654.
3. Verbeeck RK. Pharmacokinetics and dosage adjustment in patients with hepatic dysfunction. Eur J Clin Pharmacol 2008;64(12):1147–1161.
4. Miyajima H, Nomura M, Muguruma N, et al. Relationship among gastric motility, autonomic activity, and portal hemodynamics in patients with liver cirrhosis. J Gastroenterol Hepatol 2001;16(6):647–659.
5. Groszmann R, Kotelanski B, Cohn JN, Khatri IM. Quantitation of portasystemic shunting from the splenic and mesenteric beds in alcoholic liver disease. Am J Med 1972;53(6):715–722.
6. Pentikainen PJ, Valisalmi L, Himberg JJ, Crevoisier C. Pharmacokinetics of midazolam following intravenous and oral administration in patients with chronic liver disease and in healthy subjects. J Clin Pharmacol 1989;29(3):272–277.
7. Elbekai RH, Korashy HM, El-Kadi AO. The effect of liver cirrhosis on the regulation and expression of drug metabolizing enzymes. Curr Drug Metab 2004;5(2):157–167.
8. Morgan DJ, McLean AJ. Therapeutic implications of impaired hepatic oxygen diffusion in chronic liver disease. Hepatology 1991;14(6):1280–1282.
9. Fradette C, Batonga J, Teng S, Piquette-Miller M, du Souich P. Animal models of acute moderate hypoxia are associated with a down-regulation of CYP1A1, 1A2, 2B4, 2C5, and 2C16 and up-regulation of CYP3A6 and P-glycoprotein in liver. Drug Metab Dispos 2007;35(5):765–771.
10. Richer M, Lam YW. Hypoxia, arterial pH and theophylline disposition. Clin Pharmacokinet 1993;25(4):283–299.
11. Froomes PR, Morgan DJ, Smallwood RA, Angus PW. Comparative effects of oxygen supplementation on theophylline and acetaminophen clearance in human cirrhosis. Gastroenterology 1999;116(4):915–920.
12. Macdonald JI, Wallace SM, Mahachai V, Verbeeck RK. Both phenolic and acyl glucuronidation pathways of diflunisal are impaired in liver cirrhosis. Eur J Clin Pharmacol 1992;42(5):471–474.
13. Sonne J, Andreasen PB, Loft S, Dossing M, Andreasen F. Glucuronidation of oxazepam is not spared in patients with hepatic encephalopathy. Hepatology 1990;11(6):951–956.
14. Taburet AM, Naveau S, Zorza G, et al. Pharmacokinetics of zidovudine in patients with liver cirrhosis. Clin Pharmacol Ther 1990;47(6):731–739.
15. Shull HJ, Wilkinson GR, Johnson R, Schenker S. Normal disposition of oxazepam in acute viral hepatitis and cirrhosis. Ann Intern Med 1976;84(4):420–425.
16. George J, Murray M, Byth K, Farrell GC. Differential alterations of cytochrome P450 proteins in livers from patients with severe chronic liver disease. Hepatology 1995;21(1):120–128.
17. George J, Liddle C, Murray M, Byth K, Farrell GC. Pre-translational regulation of cytochrome P450 genes is responsible for disease-specific changes of individual P450 enzymes among patients with cirrhosis. Biochem Pharmacol 1995;49(7):873–881.
18. Ho RH, Kim RB. Transporters and drug therapy: implications for drug disposition and disease. Clin Pharmacol Ther 2005;78(3):260–277.
19. Kullak-Ublick GA, Baretton GB, Oswald M, Renner EL, Paumgartner G, Beuers U. Expression of the hepatocyte canalicular multidrug resistance protein (MRP2) in primary biliary cirrhosis. Hepatol Res 2002;23(1):78–82.
20. Zollner G, Fickert P, Silbert D, et al. Adaptive changes in hepatobiliary transporter expression in primary biliary cirrhosis. J Hepatol 2003;38(6):717–727.
21. Dopp JM, Moran JJ, Abel NJ, et al. Influence of intermittent hypoxia on myocardial and hepatic P-glycoprotein expression in a rodent model. Pharmacotherapy 2009;29(4):365–372.
22. Ishizu H, Shiomi S, Kawamura E, et al. Gastric emptying in patients with chronic liver diseases. Ann Nucl Med 2002;16(3):177–182.
23. Proulx NL, Akbari A, Garg AX, Rostom A, Jaffey J, Clark HD. Measured creatinine clearance from timed urine collections substantially overestimates glomerular filtration rate in patients with liver cirrhosis: a systematic review and individual patient meta-analysis. Nephrol Dial Transplant 2005;20(8):1617–1622.
24. Tangri N, Alam A, Edwardes MD, Davidson A, Deschenes M, Cantarovich M. Evaluating cimetidine for GFR estimation in liver transplant recipients. Nephrol Dial Transplant 2010;25(4):1285–1289.
25. Brockmoller J, Thomsen T, Wittstock M, Coupez R, Lochs H, Roots I. Pharmacokinetics of levetiracetam in patients with moderate to severe liver cirrhosis (Child-Pugh classes A, B, and C): characterization by dynamic liver function tests. Clin Pharmacol Ther 2005;77(6):529–541.
26. Verbeeck RK, Horsmans Y. Effect of hepatic insufficiency on pharmacokinetics and drug dosing. Pharm World Sci 1998;20(5):183–192.
27. Bakti G, Fisch HU, Karlaganis G, Minder C, Bircher J. Mechanism of the excessive sedative response of cirrhotics to benzodiazepines: model experiments with triazolam. Hepatology 1987;7(4):629–638.
28. Kimelblatt BJ, Cerra FB, Calleri G, Berg MJ, McMillen MA, Schentag JJ. Dose and serum concentration relationships in cimetidine-associated mental confusion. Gastroenterology 1980;78(4):791–795.
29. Chapuis L, Cadranel JF, Nordmann P, et al. Grand mal seizures as a complication of treatment with pefloxacin in patients with cirrhosis. A report of three cases. J Hepatol 1993;19(3):383–384.
30. Gerbes AL, Remien J, Jungst D, Sauerbruch T, Paumgartner G. Evidence for down-regulation of beta-2-adrenoceptors in cirrhotic patients with severe ascites. Lancet 1986;1(8495):1409–1411.
31. Janku I, Perlik F, Tkaczykova M, Brodanova M. Disposition kinetics and concentration-effect relationship of metipranolol in patients with cirrhosis and healthy subjects. Eur J Clin Pharmacol 1992;42(3):337–340.
32. Pugh RN, Murray-Lyon IM, Dawson JL, Pietroni MC, Williams R. Transection of the oesophagus for bleeding oesophageal varices. Br J Surg 1973;60(8):646–649.

33. Cholongitas E, Marelli L, Shusang V, et al. A systematic review of the performance of the model for end-stage liver disease (MELD) in the setting of liver transplantation. Liver Transpl 2006;12(7):1049–1061.

34. Burra P, Masier A. Dynamic tests to study liver function. Eur Rev Med Pharmacol Sci 2004;8(1):19–21.

35. Colli A, Buccino G, Cocciolo M, Parravicini R, Scaltrini G. Disposition of a flow-limited drug (lidocaine) and a metabolic capacity-limited drug (theophylline) in liver cirrhosis. Clin Pharmacol Ther 1988;44(6):642–649.

36. Forrest JA, Finlayson ND, Adjepon-Yamoah KK, Prescott LF. Antipyrine, paracetamol, and lignocaine elimination in chronic liver disease. Br Med J 1977;1(6073):1384–1387.

37. Frye RF, Matzke GR, Adedoyin A, Porter JA, Branch RA. Validation of the five-drug "Pittsburgh cocktail" approach for assessment of selective regulation of drug-metabolizing enzymes. Clin Pharmacol Ther 1997;62(4):365–376.

38. Chainuvati S, Nafziger AN, Leeder JS, et al. Combined phenotypic assessment of cytochrome p450 1A2, 2C9, 2C19, 2D6, and 3A, N-acetyltransferase-2, and xanthine oxidase activities with the "Cooperstown 5+1 cocktail". Clin Pharmacol Ther 2003;74(5):437–447.

39. Jerdi MC, Daali Y, Oestreicher MK, Cherkaoui S, Dayer P. A simplified analytical method for a phenotyping cocktail of major CYP450 biotransformation routes. J Pharm Biomed Anal 2004;35(5):1203–1212.

40. Food and Drug Administration. Guidance for industry: pharmacokinetics in patients with impaired hepatic function: study design, data analysis, and impact on dosing and labeling. www.fda.gov/downloads/Drugs/GuidanceComplianceRegulatoryInformation/Guidances/UCM072123.pdf

41. Piafsky KM, Sitar DS, Rangno RE, Ogilvie RI. Theophylline disposition in patients with hepatic cirrhosis. N Engl J Med 1977;296(26):1495–1497.

42. Lucena MI, Andrade RJ, Tognoni G, Hidalgo R, Sanchez de la Cuesta F. Drug use for non-hepatic associated conditions in patients with liver cirrhosis. Eur J Clin Pharmacol 2003;59(1):71–76.

43. Child C, Turcotte J. Surgery and portal hypertension. In: Child C, ed. The Liver and Portal Hypertension. Philadelphia, PA: WB Saunders, 1964:1–85.

44. Food and Drug Administration. Atomoxetine clinical pharmacology review. 2002.

45. Spray JW, Willett K, Chase D, Sindelar R, Connelly S. Dosage adjustment for hepatic dysfunction based on Child-Pugh scores. Am J Health Syst Pharm 2007;64(7):690, 692–693.

46. Alfaro CL, Lam YW, Simpson J, Ereshefsky L. CYP2D6 status of extensive metabolizers after multiple-dose fluoxetine, fluvoxamine, paroxetine, or sertraline. J Clin Psychopharmacol 1999;19(2):155–163.

47. Lindh JD, Holm L, Andersson ML, Rane A. Influence of CYP2C9 genotype on warfarin dose requirements—a systematic review and meta-analysis. Eur J Clin Pharmacol 2009;65(4):365–375.

48. Aithal GP, Day CP, Kesteven PJ, Daly AK. Association of polymorphisms in the cytochrome P450 CYP2C9 with warfarin dose requirement and risk of bleeding complications. Lancet 1999;353(9154):717–719.

49. Margaglione M, Colaizzo D, D'Andrea G, et al. Genetic modulation of oral anticoagulation with warfarin. Thromb Haemost 2000;84(5):775–778.

50. Higashi MK, Veenstra DL, Kondo LM, et al. Association between CYP2C9 genetic variants and anticoagulation-related outcomes during warfarin therapy. JAMA 2002;287(13):1690–1698.

51. Wadelius M, Chen LY, Eriksson N, et al. Association of warfarin dose with genes involved in its action and metabolism. Hum Genet 2007;121(1):23–34.

52. Gage BF, Eby C, Milligan PE, Banet GA, Duncan JR, McLeod HL. Use of pharmacogenetics and clinical factors to predict the maintenance dose of warfarin. Thromb Haemost 2004;91(1):87–94.

53. Klein TE, Altman RB, Eriksson N, et al. Estimation of the warfarin dose with clinical and pharmacogenetic data. N Engl J Med 2009;360(8):753–764.

54. Eckman MH, Rosand J, Greenberg SM, Gage BF. Cost-effectiveness of using pharmacogenetic information in warfarin dosing for patients with nonvalvular atrial fibrillation. Ann Intern Med 2009;150(2):73–83.

55. You JH, Tsui KK, Wong RS, Cheng G. Potential clinical and economic outcomes of CYP2C9 and VKORC1 genotype-guided dosing in patients starting warfarin therapy. Clin Pharmacol Ther 2009;86(5):540–547.

56. Anderson DC, Jr. Pharmacogenomics and warfarin. Am J Health Syst Pharm 2009;66(2):121.

57. Bussey HI, Wittkowsky AK, Hylek EM, Walker MB. Genetic testing for warfarin dosing? Not yet ready for prime time. Pharmacotherapy 2008;28(2):141–143.

58. Furuta T, Sugimoto M, Shirai N, Ishizaki T. CYP2C19 pharmacogenomics associated with therapy of Helicobacter pylori infection and gastro-esophageal reflux diseases with a proton pump inhibitor. Pharmacogenomics 2007;8(9):1199–1210.

59. Baldwin RM, Ohlsson S, Pedersen RS, et al. Increased omeprazole metabolism in carriers of the CYP2C19*17 allele; a pharmacokinetic study in healthy volunteers. Br J Clin Pharmacol 2008;65(5):767–774.

60. Hunfeld NG, Mathot RA, Touw DJ, et al. Effect of CYP2C19*2 and *17 mutations on pharmacodynamics and kinetics of proton pump inhibitors in Caucasians. Br J Clin Pharmacol 2008;65(5):752–760.

61. Kurzawski M, Gawronska-Szklarz B, Wrzesniewska J, Siuda A, Starzynska T, Drozdzik M. Effect of CYP2C19*17 gene variant on Helicobacter pylori eradication in peptic ulcer patients. Eur J Clin Pharmacol 2006;62(10):877–880.

62. Sim SC, Risinger C, Dahl ML, et al. A common novel CYP2C19 gene variant causes ultrarapid drug metabolism relevant for the drug response to proton pump inhibitors and antidepressants. Clin Pharmacol Ther 2006;79(1):103–113.

63. Li XQ, Andersson TB, Ahlstrom M, Weidolf L. Comparison of inhibitory effects of the proton pump-inhibiting drugs omeprazole, esomeprazole, lansoprazole, pantoprazole, and rabeprazole on human cytochrome P450 activities. Drug Metab Dispos 2004;32(8):821–827.

64. Furuta T, Shirai N, Kodaira M, et al. Pharmacogenomics-based tailored versus standard therapeutic regimen for eradication of H. pylori. Clin Pharmacol Ther 2007;81(4):521–528.

65. Mega JL, Close SL, Wiviott SD, et al. Cytochrome p-450 polymorphisms and response to clopidogrel. N Engl J Med 2009;360(4):354–362.

66. Bertilsson L, Aberg-Wistedt A, Gustafsson LL, Nordin C. Extremely rapid hydroxylation of debrisoquine: a case report with implication for treatment with nortriptyline and other tricyclic antidepressants. Ther Drug Monit 1985;7(4):478–480.

67. Bertilsson L, Dahl ML, Sjoqvist F, et al. Molecular basis for rational megaprescribing in ultrarapid hydroxylators of debrisoquine. Lancet 1993;341(8836):63.

68. Kashuba AD, Nafziger AN, Kearns GL, et al. Quantification of intraindividual variability and the influence of menstrual cycle phase on CYP2D6 activity as measured by dextromethorphan phenotyping. Pharmacogenetics 1998;8(5):403–410.

69. Labbe L, Sirois C, Pilote S, et al. Effect of gender, sex hormones, time variables and physiological urinary pH on apparent CYP2D6 activity as assessed by metabolic ratios of marker substrates. Pharmacogenetics 2000;10(5):425–438.

70. Kirchheiner J, Brosen K, Dahl ML, et al. CYP2D6 and CYP2C19 genotype-based dose recommendations for antidepressants: a first step towards subpopulation-specific dosages. Acta Psychiatr Scand 2001;104(3):173–192.

71. Mihara K, Otani K, Tybring G, Dahl ML, Bertilsson L, Kaneko S. The CYP2D6 genotype and plasma concentrations of mianserin enantiomers in relation to therapeutic response to mianserin in depressed Japanese patients. J Clin Psychopharmacol 1997;17(6):467–471.

72. Brockmoller J, Meineke I, Kirchheiner J. Pharmacokinetics of mirtazapine: enantioselective effects of the CYP2D6 ultra rapid metabolizer genotype and correlation with adverse effects. Clin Pharmacol Ther 2007;81(5):699–707.

73. Poulsen L, Arendt-Nielsen L, Brosen K, Sindrup SH. The hypoalgesic effect of tramadol in relation to CYP2D6. Clin Pharmacol Ther 1996;60(6):636–644.

74. Stamer UM, Lehnen K, Hothker F, et al. Impact of CYP2D6 genotype on postoperative tramadol analgesia. Pain 2003;105(1-2):231–238.

75. Wang G, Zhang H, He F, Fang X. Effect of the CYP2D6*10 C188T polymorphism on postoperative tramadol analgesia in a Chinese population. Eur J Clin Pharmacol 2006;62(11):927–931.

76. Kiyotani K, Mushiroda T, Imamura CK, et al. Significant effect of polymorphisms in CYP2D6 and ABCC2 on clinical outcomes of adjuvant tamoxifen therapy for breast cancer patients. J Clin Oncol 2010;28(8):1287–1293.

77. Goetz MP, Rae JM, Suman VJ, et al. Pharmacogenetics of tamoxifen biotransformation is associated with clinical outcomes of efficacy and hot flashes. J Clin Oncol 2005;23(36):9312–9318.

78. Kelly CM, Juurlink DN, Gomes T, et al. Selective serotonin reuptake inhibitors and breast cancer mortality in women receiving tamoxifen: a population based cohort study. BMJ 2010;340:c693. doi: 10.1136/bmj.c693.

79. Haufroid V, Mourad M, Van Kerckhove V, et al. The effect of CYP3A5 and MDR1 (ABCB1) polymorphisms on cyclosporine and tacrolimus dose requirements and trough blood levels in stable renal transplant patients. Pharmacogenetics 2004;14(3):147–154.

80. Zheng H, Zeevi A, Schuetz E, et al. Tacrolimus dosing in adult lung transplant patients is related to cytochrome P4503A5 gene polymorphism. J Clin Pharmacol 2004;44(2):135–140.

81. MacPhee IA, Fredericks S, Tai T, et al. The influence of pharmacogenetics on the time to achieve target tacrolimus concentrations after kidney transplantation. Am J Transplant 2004;4(6):914–919.

82. Wang Y, Wang C, Li J, et al. Effect of genetic polymorphisms of CYP3A5 and MDR1 on cyclosporine concentration during the early stage after renal transplantation in Chinese patients co-treated with diltiazem. Eur J Clin Pharmacol 2009;65(3):239–247.

83. Teml A, Schaeffeler E, Herrlinger KR, Klotz U, Schwab M. Thiopurine treatment in inflammatory bowel disease: clinical pharmacology and implication of pharmacogenetically guided dosing. Clin Pharmacokinet 2007;46(3):187–208.

84. Relling MV, Pui CH, Cheng C, Evans WE. Thiopurine methyltransferase in acute lymphoblastic leukemia. Blood 2006;107(2):843–844.

85. Fargher EA, Tricker K, Newman W, et al. Current use of pharmacogenetic testing: a national survey of thiopurine methyltransferase testing prior to azathioprine prescription. J Clin Pharm Ther 2007;32(2):187–195.

86. Tavadia SM, Mydlarski PR, Reis MD, et al. Screening for azathioprine toxicity: a pharmacoeconomic analysis based on a target case. J Am Acad Dermatol 2000;42(4):628–632.

87. Oh KT, Anis AH, Bae SC. Pharmacoeconomic analysis of thiopurine methyltransferase polymorphism screening by polymerase chain reaction for treatment with azathioprine in Korea. Rheumatology (Oxf) 2004;43(2):156–163.

88. Rouits E, Boisdron-Celle M, Dumont A, Guerin O, Morel A, Gamelin E. Relevance of different UGT1A1 polymorphisms in irinotecan-induced toxicity: a molecular and clinical study of 75 patients. Clin Cancer Res 2004;10(15):5151–5159.

89. Innocenti F, Undevia SD, Iyer L, et al. Genetic variants in the UDP-glucuronosyltransferase 1A1 gene predict the risk of severe neutropenia of irinotecan. J Clin Oncol 2004;22(8):1382–1388.

90. Evans DA. Genetic variations in the acetylation of isoniazid and other drugs. Ann N Y Acad Sci 1968;151(2):723–733.

91. Ohno M, Yamaguchi I, Yamamoto I, et al. Slow N-acetyltransferase 2 genotype affects the incidence of isoniazid and rifampicin-induced hepatotoxicity. Int J Tuberc Lung Dis 2000;4(3):256–261.

92. Huang YS, Chern HD, Su WJ, et al. Polymorphism of the N-acetyltransferase 2 gene as a susceptibility risk factor for antituberculosis drug-induced hepatitis. Hepatology 2002;35(4):883–889.

93. Candiotti KA, Birnbach DJ, Lubarsky DA, et al. The impact of pharmacogenomics on postoperative nausea and vomiting: do CYP2D6 allele copy number and polymorphisms affect the success or failure of ondansetron prophylaxis? Anesthesiology 2005;102(3):543–549.

94. Lessard E, Yessine MA, Hamelin BA, O'Hara G, LeBlanc J, Turgeon J. Influence of CYP2D6 activity on the disposition and cardiovascular toxicity of the antidepressant agent venlafaxine in humans. Pharmacogenetics 1999;9(4):435–443.

95. Murphy GM, Jr., Kremer C, Rodrigues HE, Schatzberg AF. Pharmacogenetics of antidepressant medication intolerance. Am J Psychiatry 2003;160(10):1830–1835.

96. Kaplan EM. Antidepressant noncompliance as a factor in the discontinuation syndrome. J Clin Psychiatry 1997;58(Suppl 7):31–35; discussion 36.

97. Thompson C, Peveler RC, Stephenson D, McKendrick J. Compliance with antidepressant medication in the treatment of major depressive disorder in primary care: a randomized comparison of fluoxetine and a tricyclic antidepressant. Am J Psychiatry 2000;157(3):338–343.

98. Zineh I, Pebanco GD, Aquilante CL, et al. Discordance between availability of pharmacogenetics studies and pharmacogenetics-based prescribing information for the top 200 drugs. Ann Pharmacother 2006;40(4):639–644.

99. Kirchheiner J, Bauer S, Meineke I, et al. Impact of CYP2C9 and CYP2C19 polymorphisms on tolbutamide kinetics and the insulin and glucose response in healthy volunteers. Pharmacogenetics 2002;12(2):101–109.

100. Recommendations from the EGAPP Working Group: testing for cytochrome P450 polymorphisms in adults with nonpsychotic depression treated with selective serotonin reuptake inhibitors. Genet Med 2007;9(12):819–825.

101. Brockmoller J, Kirchheiner J, Schmider J, et al. The impact of the CYP2D6 polymorphism on haloperidol pharmacokinetics and on the outcome of haloperidol treatment. Clin Pharmacol Ther 2002;72(4):438–452.

102. Lam YW, Jann MW, Chang WH, et al. Intra- and interethnic variability in reduced haloperidol to haloperidol ratios. J Clin Pharmacol 1995;35(2):128–136.

103. Chou M, Huang S, Sahajwalla C, Lesko L. An informal survey of pharmacogenetics/pharmacogenomics (PGTX) in a sample of INDs and NDAs [abstract]. Clin Pharmacol Ther 2003;73:P33.

104. Sauer JM, Ponsler GD, Mattiuz EL, et al. Disposition and metabolic fate of atomoxetine hydrochloride: the role of CYP2D6 in human disposition and metabolism. Drug Metab Dispos 2003;31(1):98–107.

105. Food and Drug Administration. Medical devices, clinical chemistry and clinical toxicology devices: Drug metabolizing enzyme genotyping system. Final rule. Federal Register 2005;70:865–867.

106. Hasegawa Y, Sarashina T, Ando M, et al. Rapid detection of UGT1A1 gene polymorphisms by newly developed invader assay. Clin Chem 2004;50(8):1479–1480.

ROBERT A. MANGIONE AND PRITI N. PATEL

CHAPTER 49

Celiac Disease

KEY CONCEPTS

❶ Celiac disease is a chronic, inflammatory autoimmune disorder caused by intolerance to gluten found in wheat, barley, rye, and other foods when a genetically predisposed person is exposed to the environmental trigger, gluten.

❷ Celiac disease is common in Europe and North America, affecting between 1 in 100 to 1 in 120 adults, and 1 in 80 to 1 in 300 children.

❸ The integrity of the tissue junctions of the intestinal epithelium is compromised in patients with celiac disease; this enables gluten to reach the lamina propria. The presence of gluten in the lamina propria and an inherited combination of genes contribute to the heightened immune sensitivity to gluten that is found in patients with celiac disease.

❹ The classic presenting symptom in adults is diarrhea, which may be accompanied by abdominal pain or discomfort; however, it is noteworthy that during the last decade it has been reported that diarrhea has been the main presenting symptom of celiac disease in less than 50% of cases.

❺ Dermatitis herpetiformis is a skin manifestation of celiac disease. All patients with celiac disease will not develop dermatitis herpetiformis; however, all patients with dermatitis herpetiformis are considered to have celiac disease.

❻ The frequency of diagnosis of patients with celiac disease has increased; however, the majority of patients with this condition remain undiagnosed.

❼ A confirmed diagnosis of celiac disease requires both positive findings on duodenal biopsy and a positive response to a gluten-free diet. The most common serologic markers that are used for screening patients are serum immunoglobulin (IgA) endomysial antibodies and IgA serum anti-tissue transglutaminase antibodies.

❽ Strict, lifelong adherence to a gluten-free diet is the only treatment for celiac disease.

❾ Clinicians must evaluate the patient with celiac disease for nutritional deficiencies (including folic acid, vitamin B12, fat-soluble vitamins, iron, and calcium) due to malabsorption. Iron-deficiency anemia may be the only presenting sign of disease in patients without diarrhea.

---

❶ Celiac disease is a chronic, inflammatory autoimmune disorder caused by an intolerance to ingested gluten, a storage protein found in wheat, barley, and rye. Genetic, environmental, and immune factors all play a role in the development of celiac disease. The mainstay of treatment of the disease is strict adherence to a gluten-free diet.

A disease resembling celiac disease was first described by a Greek physician in the second century AD.[1] In the mid-1900s, the connection between the ingestion of cereals and celiac disease was made. For many years, celiac disease was considered a disease of childhood with primarily gastrointestinal symptoms. It is now recognized as a disease of all ages with varied presentation.

Also known as celiac sprue, nontropical sprue, and gluten-sensitive enteropathy, the disease is characterized by both gastrointestinal and extraintestinal symptoms. Chronic inflammation caused by exposure to gluten leads to gastrointestinal discomfort, nutrient malabsorption, and systemic complications. Gastrointestinal symptoms, including diarrhea, cramping, bloating, and flatulence, are the "classic" symptoms; however, a patient with celiac disease may initially present with a variety of extraintestinal symptoms. Patients with silent celiac disease have no or minimal symptoms but manifest mucosal damage on biopsy and have positive serologic testing. Patients with celiac disease classified as latent are asymptomatic patients who may show positive serology, have the human leukocyte antigen (HLA)-DQ2 and/or DQ8 haplotype, but have normal mucosa on biopsy.[2]

Adherence to a gluten-free diet is essential because it improves symptoms and prevents long-term complications of celiac disease, which include T-cell lymphomas, small bowel adenocarcinoma, and esophageal and oropharyngeal carcinomas.[3]

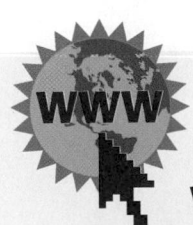

The complete chapter, learning objectives, and other resources can be found at **www.pharmacotherapyonline.com**.

CHAPTER

50

Clinical Assessment of Kidney Function

THOMAS C. DOWLING

KEY CONCEPTS

❶ The stage of chronic kidney disease (CKD) should be determined for all individuals based on the level of kidney function, independent of etiology, according to the National Kidney Foundation (NKF) Kidney Disease/Dialysis Outcome Quality Initiative CKD classification system.

❷ Persistent proteinuria indicates the presence of CKD.

❸ Quantitation of urine protein excretion, such as the measurement of a spot urine albumin-to-creatinine ratio, is recommended for determining the severity of CKD and monitoring the rate of disease progression.

❹ The glomerular filtration rate (GFR) is the single best indicator of kidney function.

❺ Measurement of the GFR is most accurate when performed following the exogenous administration of inulin, iothalamate, or radioisotopes such as technetium 99m diethylenetriamine pentaacetic acid (^{99m}Tc-DTPA).

❻ Equations to estimate creatinine clearance or GFR are commonly used in ambulatory and inpatient settings and incorporate patient laboratory and demographic variables, such as serum creatinine, cystatin C, age, gender, weight, and ethnicity.

❼ Longitudinal assessment of GFR and proteinuria is important for monitoring the efficacy of therapeutic interventions, such as angiotensin-converting enzyme inhibitors and angiotensin receptor blockers, which are used to slow or halt the progression of kidney disease.

❽ The measurement of S_{cr} alone, evaluation of a plot of the reciprocal of S_{cr} versus time, and serum cystatin C concentration should be used with caution to estimate the rate of

decline in renal function in patients with CKD, as these indices do not consider patient age, lean body mass, gender, diet, concomitant diseases and drug therapy, circadian rhythm, stability of kidney function, or tubular secretion of creatinine.

❾ Other assessments of the kidney, such as radiography, computed tomography, magnetic resonance imaging, sonography, and biopsy, are mainly used for determining the diagnosis of a given condition, as they provide evidence of the functional and structural changes associated with kidney disease.

Chronic kidney disease (CKD) is an increasingly alarming worldwide health concern, with nearly 2 million people in the United States alone estimated to require hemodialysis or kidney transplantation by 2030. In response to this widespread problem, the National Kidney Foundation (NKF) has developed a standardized approach for the identification and classification of individuals with CKD and their subsequent stratification into risk categories for end-stage renal disease (ESRD) (see Chapter 52).[1,2] These efforts have heightened the awareness of the need for early identification of patients with CKD and the importance of monitoring kidney function in the clinical setting.

Assessment of renal function using both qualitative and quantitative methods is an important part of the evaluation of patients and an essential characterization of individuals who participate in clinical research investigations. Estimation of creatinine clearance (CL_{cr}) has been considered the clinical standard for assessment of renal function for more than 40 years; however, new methods to estimate the glomerular filtration rate (GFR) are now used in many clinical settings to identify patients with CKD. Other tests, such as urinalysis, radiographic procedures, and biopsy, are also useful for determining the pathology and etiology of kidney disease. Urinalysis, for example, may give clues to the primary location (e.g., glomerular or tubular) of the renal disease. Follow-up studies, such as imaging procedures and kidney biopsy, may then further differentiate the specific cause, thereby guiding the selection of the optimal therapeutic intervention.

❶ Quantitative indices of GFR or CL_{cr} are considered the most useful diagnostic tools for the identification of the presence of CKD. These measures can also be used to quantify changes in function that may occur as a result of disease progression, therapeutic

Learning objectives, review questions, and other resources can be found at **www.pharmacotherapyonline.com**.

intervention, or a toxic insult.[3] The measurement or estimation of creatinine clearance, however, remains the most commonly used index for individualizing medication dosage regimens in patients with acute and chronic kidney disease. Furthermore, CL_{cr} has been the chief index used to stratify patients in pharmacokinetic studies that serve as the basis for the design of renal dosing algorithms in Food and Drug Administration (FDA) approved package inserts and tertiary drug information sources.[4] The composite term *renal function* includes the processes of filtration, secretion, and reabsorption, as well as endocrine and metabolic functions. Alterations of all five renal functions, whether declining or improving, are associated primarily with GFR. This chapter critically evaluates the various methods that can be used for the quantitative assessment of kidney function in individuals with normal renal function, as well as in those with CKD and acute renal failure (Table 50–1). Where appropriate, discussion regarding the qualitative assessment of renal function is also presented, including specialized tests such as kidney biopsy.

EXCRETORY FUNCTION

The most important contribution of the kidney to overall maintenance of body homeostasis is the urinary excretion of water, electrolytes, endogenous substances such as urea, and environmental toxins. Through the combined processes of glomerular filtration, tubular secretion, and reabsorption, the nephron, as the functional unit of the kidney, regulates the output of water, electrolytes, and solutes from the body and is the key organ responsible for maintenance of homeostasis despite fluctuations in dietary ingestion.

TABLE 50-1	Markers of Renal Function
Renal plasma/blood flow	*p*-aminohippurate (PAH)
	^{131}I-orthoiodohippurate (^{131}I-OIH)
	^{99m}Tc-mercaptoacetyltriglycine (^{99m}Tc-MAG3)
Glomerular filtration rate	Inulin, sinistrin
	Iothalamate
	Iohexol
	^{99m}Tc-diethylenetriaminepentaacetic acid (^{99m}Tc-DTPA)
	^{125}I-iothalamate
	Creatinine
	Cystatin C
Tubular function	*p*-aminohippurate (PAH)
	N^1-methylnicotinamide (NMN)
	Tetraethylammonium (TEA)
	β_2-microglobulin
	Retinol-binding protein (RBP)
	Protein HC (α_1-microglobulin)
	N-acetylglucosaminidase (NAG)
	Alanine aminopeptidase (AAP)
	Adenosine-binding protein (ABP)

FILTRATION

Glomerular filtration is a passive process by which water and small molecular weight ions (<5–10 kDa) and molecules diffuse across the glomerular capillary membrane into the Bowman capsule and then enter the proximal tubule (Fig. 50–1). Because most proteins are too large (>60 kDa) to be substantially filtered, or their filtration is impeded by the electronegative charge on the epithelial surface of the glomerulus, compounds presented to the glomerulus in the protein-bound state are not filtered and thus remain in the peritubular circulation.

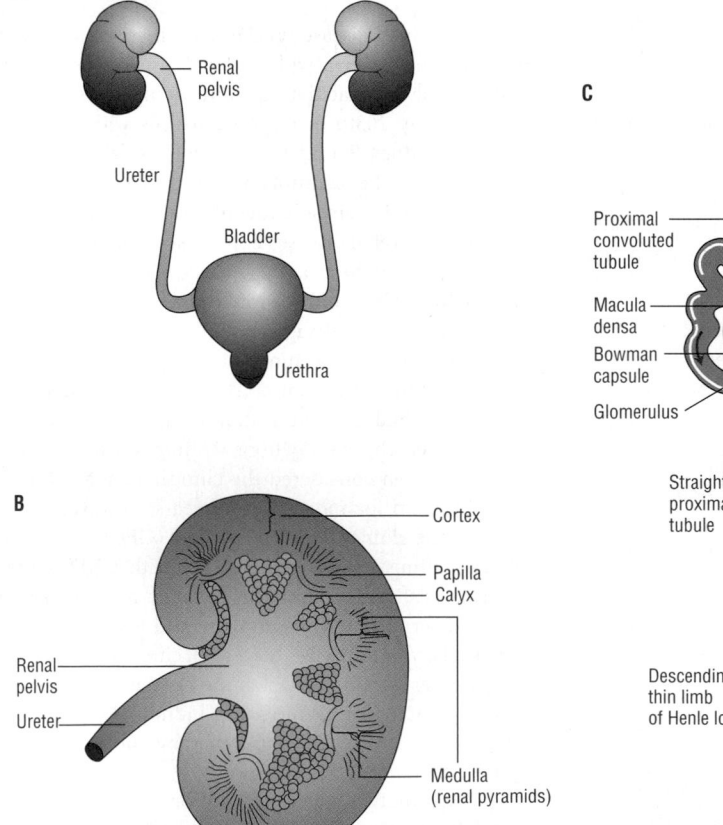

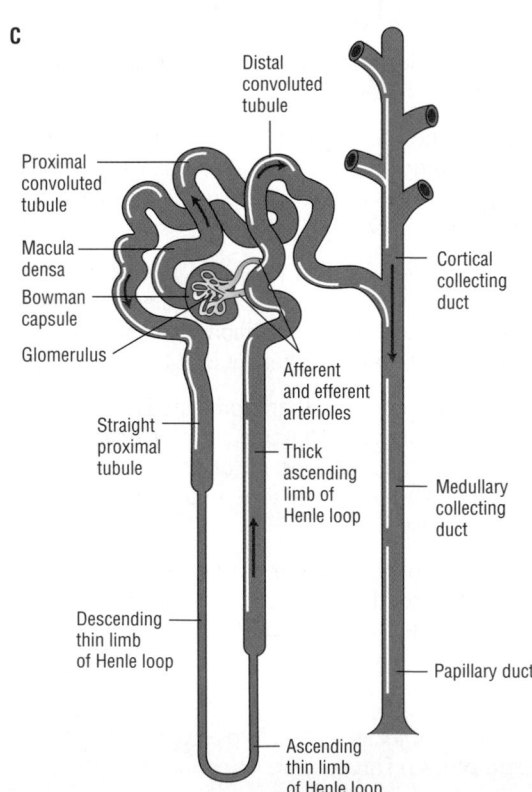

FIGURE 50-1. Structures of the *(A)* urinary system, *(B)* kidney, and *(C)* nephron, the functional unit of the kidney.

SECRETION

Secretion is an active process that mainly takes place in the proximal tubule and facilitates the elimination of compounds from the renal circulation into the tubular lumen. Several highly efficient anionic and cationic transport systems for a wide range of endogenous and exogenous substances have been identified, and the renal clearance of these actively secreted entities can greatly exceed GFR; for example, their clearance may be in the range of 600 to 1,000 mL/min (10–16.7 mL/s). Probenecid, p-aminohippurate (PAH), and penicillin are examples of anionic substances; creatinine, cimetidine, and procainamide are well-characterized cations.[5] These transport systems are not mutually exclusive, as probenecid has been observed to compete with the tubular secretion of cimetidine.[6] Other transport pathways, such as P-glycoprotein and multidrug resistance protein, are also present in several tissues, including the kidney, liver, jejunum, colon, and brain. These efflux proteins are now recognized as important contributors to the renal elimination of many drugs.[7] For example, P-glycoprotein, which is located on the apical membrane of the proximal tubule, plays an important role in the renal elimination of a wide range of drugs, such as cimetidine, digoxin, and procainamide. Blockade of P-glycoprotein could result in decreased renal elimination of such compounds, leading to an increased drug exposure. Verapamil and cyclosporine are the two most widely studied agents that reduce the activity of this tubular transport mechanism.[8] The net process of tubular secretion for drugs is therefore likely a result of multiple secretory pathways acting simultaneously.

REABSORPTION

Reabsorption of water and solutes occurs throughout the nephron, whereas the reabsorption of most medications occurs predominantly along the distal tubule and collecting duct. Urine flow rate and physiochemical characteristics of the molecule influence these processes: highly ionized compounds are not reabsorbed unless pH changes within the urine increase the fraction unionized, so that reabsorption may be facilitated.

INTACT NEPHRON HYPOTHESIS

The intact nephron hypothesis described by Bricker,[9] which was published more than 40 years ago, proposes that kidney function of patients with renal disease is the net result of a reduced number of appropriately functioning nephrons. As the number of nephrons is reduced from the initial complement of 2 million, those that are unaffected compensate; that is, they hyperfunction. The cornerstone of this hypothesis is that glomerulotubular balance is maintained, such that those nephrons capable of functioning will continue to perform in an appropriate fashion. Extensive studies have shown that single-nephron GFR increases in the unaffected nephrons; thus, the whole-kidney GFR, which represents the sum of the single-nephron GFRs of the remaining functional nephrons, may remain close to normal until there is extensive injury. Based on this, we would presume that a measure of one component of nephron function could be used as an estimate of all renal functions. This, indeed, has been and remains our clinical approach.

FILTRATION CAPACITY

GFR is dependent on numerous factors, one of which is protein load. Bosch[10] suggested that an appropriate comprehensive evaluation of renal function should include the measurement of "filtration capacity" of the kidney. This is similar in context to a cardiac stress test. The patient may have no hypoxic symptoms, for example, angina while resting, but it may become quite evident when the patient begins to exercise. Subjects with normal renal function administered an oral or IV protein load prior to measurement of GFR have been noted to increase their GFR by as much as 50%. As renal function declines, the kidneys usually compensate by increasing the single-nephron GFR. The renal reserve, the maximal degree by which GFR can be increased, will be reduced in those individuals whose kidneys are already functioning at higher than normal levels because of preexisting renal injury. Thus, this may be a complementary, insightful index of renal function reserve for many individuals with as yet unidentified CKD.

Not only is quantification of renal function an important component of a diagnostic evaluation, but it also serves as an important parameter for monitoring therapy directed at the etiology of the diminished function itself, thereby allowing for objective measurement of the success or failure of treatment. Measurement of renal function also serves as a useful indicator of the ability of the kidneys to eliminate drugs from the body. Furthermore, alterations of drug distribution and metabolism have been associated with the degree of renal function. A discussion of pharmacokinetic changes in renal disease is extensively reviewed in Chapter 57. Although several indices have been used for the quantification of filtration capacity or GFR in the research setting, estimations of creatinine clearance and GFR are the primary approaches used in the clinical arena.

ENDOCRINE FUNCTION

The kidney synthesizes and secretes many hormones involved in maintaining fluid and electrolyte homeostasis. Secretion of renin by the cells of the juxtaglomerular apparatus and production and metabolism of prostaglandins and kinins are among the kidney's endocrine functions. In addition, in response to decreased oxygen tension in the blood, which is sensed by the kidney, erythropoietin is produced and secreted by peritubular fibroblasts. Because these functions are related to renal mass, decreased endocrine activity is associated with the loss of viable kidney cells. In the presence of stages 3 to 5 CKD and moderate to severe acute renal injuries, secretion of erythropoietin is impaired, leading to reduced red blood cell formation; normocytic anemia, and symptoms of reduced oxygen delivery to tissues, such as fatigue, dyspnea, and angina (see Chapters 52 and 53). Renal anemia is clearly associated with many comorbidities, such as left ventricular hypertrophy, which is present in over 40% of patients with CKD.[11] Indeed, anemia-induced renal hypoxia results indirectly in erythropoietin gene activation, tubular necrosis, and apoptosis, thereby contributing to further renal cell injury.[12] This cyclic relationship between kidney disease, suppression of erythropoietin secretion, and cardiovascular disease is also referred to as the cardiorenal anemia syndrome.

METABOLIC FUNCTION

The kidneys perform a variety of metabolic functions, including the activation of vitamin D_3, gluconeogenesis, and metabolism of endogenous compounds such as insulin, steroids, and xenobiotics. Impaired renal function results in decreased formation of activated vitamin D_3 and decreased insulin metabolism. It is common for patients with diabetes and chronic renal failure to have reduced requirements for exogenous insulin,[13] and supplemental therapy with activated vitamin D_3 (calcitriol) or other vitamin D analogues (paricalcitol and doxercalciferol) is often necessary to avert the bone loss and pain associated with renal osteodystrophy.[14] Cytochrome

TABLE 50-2 Presentation of Chronic Kidney Disease (CKD)

	Early CKD (Stages 1–2)	Late CKD (Stages 3–4)
General	Patient may not appear in distress	Patient may have edema
Symptoms	Not likely present	Patient may have fatigue, malaise, pruritus, and/or nausea
Signs	Not likely present	May present with fluid retention, anemia, dyspnea, or reduced urine output
Laboratory tests	Microalbuminuria Mildly elevated serum creatine and blood urea nitrogen	Persistent proteinuria Reduced glomerular filtration rate or creatine clearance rate Abnormal urinalysis
Other diagnostic tests		Renal ultrasound shows reduced kidney mass

P450 (CYP), *N*-acetyltransferase, glutathione transferase, renal peptidases, and other enzymes responsible for the degradation and activation of selected endogenous and exogenous substances have been identified in the kidney. The CYP enzymes in the kidneys are as active as that in the liver, when corrected for organ mass. In vitro studies have demonstrated impaired function of CYP3A4 and CYP2C9, whereas CYP1A2, CYP2C19, and CYP2D6 are not affected. These data are supported by recent clinical trials in patients with ESRD receiving hemodialysis, where hepatic CYP3A activity was reported to be reduced by 28% from values observed in age-matched controls; partial correction was noted following the hemodialysis procedure.[15,16] See Chapter 57 for a more detailed discussion.

QUALITATIVE AND SEMIQUANTITATIVE INDICES OF KIDNEY FUNCTION

Patients who develop CKD remain relatively asymptomatic until impairment has progressed to the point that systemic manifestations and/or secondary complications become evident (Table 50–2). As renal function declines, patients may develop de novo or experience an exacerbation of hypertension, edema, electrolyte abnormalities, anemia, or other complications (see Chapters 52 and 53). The National Kidney Foundation (NKF) currently recommends that all patients with CKD, and those at increased risk for CKD, undergo at least yearly a comprehensive laboratory assessment composed of (a) serum creatinine to estimate GFR; (b) albumin-to-creatinine ratio in a spot urine specimen; (c) examination of urine sediment for red blood cell and white blood cell counts; (d) renal ultrasonography; (e) serum electrolytes, including sodium, potassium, chloride, and bicarbonate; (f) urine pH; and (g) urine-specific gravity.[17] The roles of each of these indices in the identification and monitoring of CKD are discussed in detail below.

LABORATORY PROCEDURES TO DETECT THE PRESENCE OF KIDNEY DISEASE

Urinalysis is an important tool for detecting and differentiating various aspects of kidney disease, which often goes unnoticed as the result of its asymptomatic presentation. It can be used to detect and monitor the progression of diseases such as diabetes mellitus, glomerulonephritis, and chronic urinary tract infections.[17-19] A typical urinalysis provides information about physical and chemical composition, most of which can be completed quickly and inexpensively by visual observation (volume and color) and dipstick testing. Microscopic urinalysis requires use of a light microscope to determine cellular content, as described below.

Chemical Analysis of Urine

pH The normal urine pH typically ranges from 4.5 to 7.8; an elevation above this may suggest the presence of urea-splitting bacteria. In patients with renal tubular acidosis, urine pH is usually >5.5 because of impaired hydrogen ion secretion in the distal tubule or collecting duct.

Glucose Glucose is usually not present in the urine because the kidney normally completely reabsorbs all the glucose filtered at the glomerulus. When a patient's blood glucose concentration exceeds the maximum threshold for glucose reabsorption in the kidney (~180 mg/dL [~10 mmol/L]), glucosuria will be present. Routine assessment of glucosuria has been replaced by newer methods of direct blood glucose measurements. Urine glucose testing is now used mainly as a screening tool for the detection of diabetes.

Ketones Acetoacetate and acetone normally are not found in the urine; they are, however, excreted in patients with diabetic ketoacidosis. They are also present under conditions of fasting or starvation. Typically, values of acetone excretion are reported as small (<20 mg/dL [<3.4 mmol/L]), moderate (30–40 mg/dL [5.2–6.9 mmol/L]), and large (>80 mg/dL [>13.8 mmol/L]).

Nitrite Nitrite usually is not present in urine. The presence of nitrite is most commonly the result of conversion from urinary nitrate by bacteria in the urine. The presence of nitrite thus suggests that the patient has a urinary tract infection, commonly caused by gram-negative rods such as *Escherichia coli*. Although false-positive results are very rare, false-negative results are more common and may be caused by a lack of dietary nitrate, reduced urine nitrate concentration as a consequence of diuresis, or infections caused by bacteria, such as enterococci and *Acinetobacter,* which do not reduce nitrate, and pseudomonads, which convert nitrate to nitrogen gas.

Leukocyte Esterase Leukocyte esterase is released from lysed granulocytes in the urine; its presence is suggestive of urinary tract infection. False-positive tests can result from delayed processing of the urine sample, contamination of the sample with vaginal secretions (e.g., blood or heavy mucus discharge), or by *Trichomonas* infection (e.g., trichomoniasis). False-negative tests can be produced by the presence of high levels of protein or ascorbic acid.

Heme The heme test indicates the presence of hemoglobin or myoglobin in the urine. A positive test without the presence of red blood cells suggests either red cell hemolysis or rhabdomyolysis.

Protein or Albumin Persistent proteinuria or albuminuria, that is, observation of its presence on at least three occasions over a period of 3 to 6 months, is now considered the principal marker of kidney damage.[16,17]

❷ Evaluation of urinary protein or albumin is now a standard tool used to characterize the severity of CKD and to monitor the rate of disease progression or regression. Under normal conditions, plasma proteins remain in the glomerular capillaries as blood perfuses the kidney and thus do not cross the glomerular basement membrane or enter the urinary space. Some of these proteins, such as albumin and globulins, are not filtered by the glomerulus as a result of charge and size selectivity (>40 kDa). Smaller proteins (<20 kDa) pass across the glomerular basement membrane but are readily reabsorbed in the proximal tubule. Most healthy individuals excrete between 30 and 150 mg/day of total protein consisting of approximately 30 mg of albumin. The remainder of the protein in the urine is secreted by the tubules (Tamm-Horsfall, immunoglobulin A, and urokinase) or comprised of smaller proteins, such as β_2-microglobulin, apoproteins, enzymes, and peptide hormones. Increased excretion of these low molecular weight proteins in the urine is considered a sensitive marker of tubulointerstitial disease.

Historically, the sulfosalicylic acid test was used as a crude measure of proteinuria. This test is performed by adding sulfosalicylic acid to urine and then visually comparing this admixture with a tube of untreated urine; the presence of turbidity indicates the qualitative presence of proteinuria. Dipstick tests are now the most common means to determine in a semiquantitative fashion a patient's daily urine protein or albumin excretion. False-positive results can occur in the presence of alkaline urine (pH >7.5), when the dipstick is immersed too long, in those with highly concentrated urine, in the presence of drugs such as penicillin, sulfonamides, and tolbutamide, as well as blood, pus, semen, and vaginal secretions. False-negative results occur with dilute urine (specific gravity <1.015) and when proteinuria is caused by nonalbumin or low molecular weight proteins such as heavy or light chains or Bence Jones proteins. The results of these dipstick tests are graded as negative (<10 mg/dL [<100 mg/L]), trace (10–20 mg/dL [100–200 mg/L]), 1+ (30 mg/dL [300 mg/L]), 2+ (100 mg/dL [1,000 mg/L]), 3+ (300 mg/dL [3,000 mg/L]), or 4+ (>1,000 mg/dL [>10,000 mg/L]). Portable desktop analyzers such as the Chemstrip 101 Urine Analyzer (Roche Diagnostics) and Clinitek 50 Urine Chemistry Analyzer (Bayer Corporation) can also be used as an alternative to visual urinalysis test strip evaluation.

❸ Because most dipstick methods are not specific for albumin, test strips that are specific for low levels of albuminuria (30–300 mg/day) should be employed. Microalbuminuria test strips, such as the Chemstrip Micral-Test II (Roche Diagnostics), when dipped into a urine sample assume a color ranging from white (0 mg/L) to red (100 mg/L), depending on the amount of albumin present in the sample. In patients with a positive protein or albumin dipstick test, a 24-hour urine collection with measurement of albumin excretion can be used to further define the degree of albuminuria. However, this method requires a high degree of patient compliance and is being replaced by a similarly accurate but less cumbersome technique: calculation of the ratio of protein or albumin (in milligrams) to creatinine (in grams [or millimoles]) obtained from an untimed (spot) urine specimen. The normal ratio is <30 mg albumin or <200 mg protein per gram of creatinine (<3.4 mg albumin or <22.6 mg protein per millimole of creatinine) in the urine, with values between 30 and 300 mg of albumin per gram of creatinine (3.4–22.6 mg of albumin per millimole of creatinine) considered to be in the microalbuminuria range.[17] Positive test results should be repeated, particularly in patients without an underlying cause for renal disease, such as diabetes or hypertension. Monitoring of the degree of glomerular injury in patients with CKD should use the albumin-to-creatinine ratio, whereas for patients with clinical proteinuria, that is, excretion of >500 mg per day or an albumin-to-creatinine ratio >500 mg/g (>56.6 mg/mmol), the protein-to-creatinine ratio can be used.

CLINICAL CONTROVERSY

In the past, measurement of the urinary protein excretion rate was accomplished using a 24-hour urine collection in patients who were at risk for CKD. However, many now advocate the use of an untimed "spot" urine sample with either an albumin-specific dipstick or measurement of the albumin-to-creatinine ratio.

Specific Gravity Specific gravity is a measure of urine weight relative to water (1.00) that is performed using a refractometer. Thus, specific gravity is dependent on water intake and urine-concentrating ability. Normal values range from 1.003 to 1.030. Osmolality, which is a measure of the number of solute particles in the urine, is a more accurate measure of the kidney's ability to make a concentrated urine. Generally, the two values correlate; however, when large quantities of heavier molecules, such as glucose, are in the urine, the specific gravity may be elevated relative to the osmolality. These tests are used in the assessment of urine-concentrating ability and are most informative when interpreted along with the hydration status of the patient and plasma osmolality.

Microscopic Analysis of Urine Formed elements that may be detected in the urine include erythrocytes and leukocytes, casts, and crystals. An important consideration in the assessment of hematuria is whether the cells are of renal origin. More than two cells per high-power field is abnormal, and the presence of dysmorphic cells suggests renal parenchymal origin because of damage as they pass through the glomerulus or during exposure to the varying osmotic environments of the tubular lumen. White blood cells may be present in the urine in association with infection or inflammatory conditions, such as interstitial nephritis. More than one cell per high-power field is usually considered abnormal. Contamination of the sample should also be considered when there are many cells; such contamination may be the result of menses or of inadequate sample collection. Casts are cylindrical forms composed of protein, with or without cells that take the shape of the collecting tubules, where they are formed. Casts without cells are labeled *hyaline casts* and consist of the Tamm-Horsfall mucoprotein, secreted by the renal tubules. They are nonspecific and may appear in concentrated urine. In the presence of red or white blood cells, casts may be formed that include the cells, indicating that the cells were of renal origin. Solubility of the Tamm-Horsfall protein is increased as urine pH rises; therefore, sample collection for casts should occur with the first morning void when the urine is most acidic. Otherwise, casts may dissolve and elude detection.

A variety of crystals may be present in the urine, including uric acid, calcium oxalate, calcium phosphate, calcium magnesium ammonium pyrophosphate, and cystine. Many of these have a unique crystalline form, which permits them to be identified with microscopy.

Serum or Blood Urea Nitrogen

Amino acids metabolized to ammonia are subsequently converted in the liver to urea, the production of which is dependent on protein availability (diet) and hepatic function. Urea undergoes glomerular filtration followed by reabsorption of up to 50% of the filtered load in the proximal tubule. The reabsorption rate of urea is mainly dependent on the reabsorption of water. The excretion of urea may therefore be decreased under conditions that necessitate water conservation, such as dehydration, although the GFR may be normal or only slightly reduced. This condition is evident when a patient exhibits prerenal azotemia, or an increase of the blood urea nitrogen to a greater extent than the serum creatinine. The normal blood urea nitrogen (BUN)-to-creatinine ratio is 10 to 15:1 using conventional units (1:25 to 1:16 using SI units), and an elevated ratio (decreased ratio using SI units) is suggestive of a decreased effective circulating volume, which stimulates increased water and hence urea reabsorption. Creatinine is not reabsorbed to any significant extent by the kidneys. Despite these limitations, BUN is usually used in combination with the serum creatinine concentration as a simple screening test for the detection of renal dysfunction.

Serum Creatinine

Creatinine is the primary standard endogenous biomarker used for the detection of kidney disease. The third National Health and Nutrition Examination Survey (NHANES III) revealed a mean serum creatinine of 0.96 mg/dL (85 μmol/L) in women and 1.16 mg/dL (103 μmol/L) in men in the United States.[20] Values were lower among Mexican Americans and higher among non-Hispanic blacks. For all groups, the serum creatinine increased with age. The report also noted that among community-dwelling adults, 10.9 million have a serum creatinine greater than 1.5 mg/dL (133 μmol/L), 3 million have a serum creatinine greater than 1.7 mg/dL (150 μmol/L), and 0.8 million have a serum creatinine greater than 2 mg/dL (177 μmol/L). Although the serum creatinine concentration alone is not an optimal measure of kidney function, it is often used as a marker for referral to a nephrologist. There is presently no accepted single standard for an "abnormal" serum creatinine level, as it is dependent on gender, race, age, and lean body mass.

The concentration of creatinine in serum is a function of creatinine production and renal excretion. Creatinine is a product of creatine metabolism from muscle; therefore, its production is directly dependent on muscle mass. At steady state, the "normal" serum creatinine concentration range is 0.5 to 1.5 mg/dL (44–133 μmol/L) for men and women. Creatinine is eliminated primarily by glomerular filtration, and as GFR declines, the serum creatinine concentration rises (Fig. 50–2).

Several methods are used to determine serum creatinine concentration, most of which use the nonspecific Jaffe reaction, a colorimetric method based on the reaction of creatinine with alkaline picrate. This nonspecific method also reacts with noncreatinine chromogens in the serum, which may result in a falsely increased serum creatinine concentration.[18] Noncreatinine chromogens are not present in the urine in sufficient quantities to interfere with the urinary creatinine measurement, because the concentration of creatinine in urine is several-fold greater than the serum concentration. The impact of this interference is seen with the creatinine clearance (CL_{cr}) calculation:

$$CL_{cr} = (U_{cr} \times V)/(S_{cr} \times t)$$

where U_{cr} = urine creatinine concentration, V = urine volume, S_{cr} = serum creatinine concentration, and t = duration of the urine collection.

This "normal" interference results in an increase in the serum creatinine concentration of ~10%; therefore, the measured creatinine

TABLE 50-3	Factors that may alter Creatinine Clearance Determinations
Analytical	**Physiologic**
Acetoacetate	Age, weight, gender
Ascorbic acid	Diet
Cephalosporins (cephalothin, cefazolin, cephalexin, cefoxitin, cefaclor, cephradine)	Diurnal variation
Clavulonic acid	Cimetidine
Dobutamine	Trimethoprim
Dopamine	Probenecid
5-flucytosine	Exercise
Fructose	
Glucose	
Protein	
Pyruvate	
Uric acid	

clearance would underestimate the true GFR by 10%. In subjects with normal renal function, this tends to counterbalance the effect of the contribution of tubular secretion of creatinine, which increases urine creatinine by nearly 10%. Thus, CL_{cr} has been proposed to serve as a good measure of GFR in subjects with normal renal function. However, this false increase in serum creatinine becomes less noticeable as the true creatinine concentration rises, due to the increasing contribution of tubular secretion to the renal clearance of creatinine.[21] This becomes significant when kidney function is reduced to less than 50% of normal.

Diabetic ketoacidosis may produce increased concentrations of acetoacetate, which serves as a chromophore in the Jaffe reaction, thereby increasing the serum creatinine concentration. Other substances that react with this procedure in the serum are glucose, protein, pyruvate, fructose, uric acid, and ascorbic acid (Table 50–3). In addition, some antibiotics are associated with a false increase in serum creatinine concentration, including cephalothin, cefazolin, cephalexin, cefoxitin, cefaclor, cephradine, and clavulanic acid.[22,23] Other agents, such as the fluoroquinolones (ciprofloxacin, fleroxacin, lomefloxacin, ofloxacin, levofloxacin, sparfloxacin, and temafloxacin), do not produce a false elevation in serum creatinine.[24] The degree of interference is dependent on the serum concentration of the antibiotic, so blood samples for creatinine should be obtained when the antibiotic concentration is lowest (at the end of a dosing interval). These interferences are not observed when the serum creatinine is measured using an enzymatic technique. The antifungal agent 5-flucytosine causes an increase in serum creatinine when measured using the Ektachem (Eastman Kodak) enzymatic system, but it does not interact with the Jaffé method.[25] Daly et al.[26] reported a false-negative effect of dobutamine and dopamine on the serum creatinine value when measured using the Ektachem system. The interference is concentration dependent and results in a 10% to 100% decrease in serum creatinine concentration. The authors hypothesized that both drugs compete with the chromogenic dye for oxidation by hydrogen peroxide in a concentration-dependent manner. The problem is most evident when blood samples are contaminated with residual IV solution containing the interfering drug. These differences emphasize the need to standardize a method within the clinic setting and require the clinician to be aware of the methods employed in the laboratory for the determination of creatinine concentrations.

Other compounds are known to interfere with serum creatinine concentration by inhibiting the active tubular secretion of creatinine. Among these are cimetidine and trimethoprim, which compete for creatinine secretion at the cationic transport system in a dose-dependent fashion. Cimetidine, given as a single 400 mg

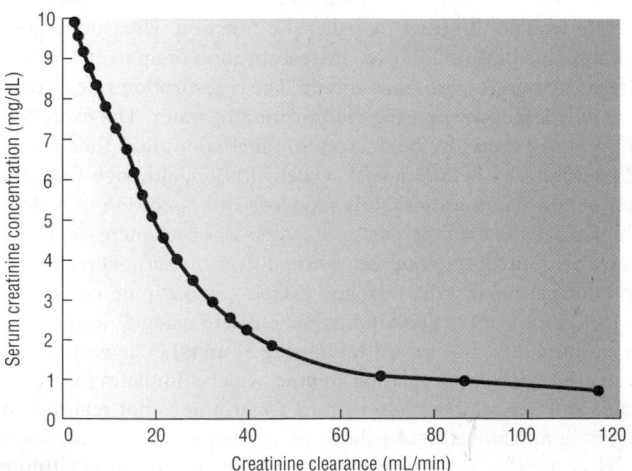

FIGURE 50-2. Relationship between serum creatinine and creatinine clearance.

dose, can result in a reduction of the CL_{cr}-to-inulin clearance ratio from 1.30 to 1.03, without a change in inulin clearance. Ranitidine, an H_2-receptor antagonist similar to cimetidine, however, does not have a similar effect on creatinine secretion following single doses of 300 to 1,200 mg.[27]

Serum creatinine concentration is dependent on the "input" function, or formation rate, and "output" function, or elimination rate. Its formation rate depends on the zero-order production from creatine metabolism, as well as input from other sources, such as dietary intake. Creatine metabolism is directly proportional to muscle mass; therefore, individuals with more muscle mass have a higher serum creatinine concentration at any given degree of kidney function than those with less muscle mass. Strenuous exercise is associated with an increase of ~10% in the level of serum creatinine. In contrast, cachectic patients, as the result of minimal muscle mass, will have very low serum creatinine concentrations, as do those with spinal cord injuries.[28] Elderly patients and those with poor nutrition may also have low serum creatinine concentrations (<1.0 mg/dL [88 μmol/L]) secondary to decreased muscle mass. Dietary intake of creatine also influences serum creatinine concentration. During the cooking of meat, some creatine is converted to creatinine, which is rapidly absorbed following ingestion.

Serum creatinine concentrations may rise as much as 50% within 2 hours of a meat meal and remain elevated for as long as 8 to 24 hours.[29] Ingestion of creatine as an ergogenic dietary supplement is currently popular. There are conflicting reports as to the effect of creatine ingestion on serum creatinine concentration. Poortsmans and Francaux[30] evaluated a short-term regimen of 20 g creatine per day for 5 days in healthy subjects and reported no significant change in serum creatinine concentration, creatinine excretion rate, or creatinine clearance. Robinson et al.,[31] however, reported a 25% to 40% increase in serum creatinine concentration after ingestion of 20 g creatine per day for either 5 days or 8 weeks. The renal excretion rate of creatinine was not measured. The issue of whether creatine ingestion adversely affects kidney function was studied by Edmunds et al.[32] They noted that creatine supplementation led to an increase in renal disease progression in a rat model for renal cystic disease, suggesting that creatine supplementation may be a risk factor in patients with preexisting renal disease. These conditions present a problem only when a single serum creatinine concentration is used to represent the entire 24-hour collection period, which is usually the case. An alternative is to obtain multiple samples and calculate the area under the serum concentration time curve and divide this by the collection time interval to obtain the average plasma creatinine concentration. This is rarely done in clinical practice, but it points out the need to question patients regarding dietary intake for the 24 hours preceding the measurement of CL_{cr}.

Diurnal variation in serum creatinine concentration may also affect the accuracy of the CL_{cr} determination. Although the fluctuation is minimal, the observed peak plasma creatinine concentration generally occurs at approximately 7:00 PM, whereas the nadir is in the morning. To minimize this effect, the CL_{cr} is usually performed over a 24-hour period with the plasma creatinine obtained in the morning, as long as the patient has stable kidney function. Collection of urine remains a limiting factor in the 24-hour CL_{cr} because of incomplete collections and interconversion between creatinine and creatine that can occur if the urine is not maintained at a pH <6.

Serum and Urinary Cystatin C

Cystatin C is a 132 amino acid (13.3 kDa) cysteine protease inhibitor produced by all nucleated cells of the body that is considered a biomarker of renal function. It is freely filtered at the glomerulus and undergoes both reabsorption and catabolism in the proximal tubule. The renal handling of this biomarker is distinctly different from creatinine and exogenous GFR markers, such as inulin, iohexol, and iothalamate. Originally introduced in Europe, it was recommended as a marker of kidney function because of findings that serum concentrations significantly correlated with GFR as well as serum creatinine. It was hypothesized that because cystatin C production was not limited to muscle mass, it would provide a more reliable estimate of renal function than creatinine. However, it has now been shown that serum cystatin C concentrations can be altered by many factors other than kidney function, such as age, nutritional status, gender, weight, height, cigarette smoking, serum C-reactive protein levels, steroid therapy, and rheumatoid arthritis.[33–35] Recent studies have reported that it may be a more sensitive index of kidney disease or acute injury compared with serum creatinine. Comparison of ^{125}I-iothalamate with serum creatinine and cystatin C showed that the serum creatinine began to increase when the GFR was <75 mL/min/1.73 m² (0.72 mL/s/m²), whereas cystatin C concentrations began to rise when the GFR dropped below 88 mL/min/1.73 m² (0.85 mL/s/m²).[33] The recent development of an automated immunoassay technique has resulted in the development of suggested reference ranges of 0.70 to 1.38 mg/L in children older than 1 year of age and 0.55 to 1.37 mg/L in adults. However, Keevil et al.[36] reported that serum cystatin C had greater intraindividual variability than serum creatinine in healthy individuals, which may limit its use in longitudinal evaluations of renal function.

The utility of cystatin C as a quantitative measure of GFR is still largely unkown. In a 4-year longitudinal study in 30 Pima Indians without CKD, the reciprocal cystatin C index (100/cystatin C) was shown to be a better predictor of declining GFR than was reciprocal serum creatinine, estimated GFR, or CL_{cr}.[37] However in patients being treated for malignant disease, Page et al.[38] reported increased cystatin C concentrations that were independent of CL_{cr}. Cystatin C concentrations were also noted to be independent of GFR and weakly associated with measured creatinine clearance, in pediatric and adult renal transplant recipients, possibly due to the formation of cystatin–immunoglobulin complexes or reduced tubular catabolism.[39,40] Two additional studies have shown a strong association between serum cystatin C and cardiovascular disease in elderly and non-CKD patients, suggesting that it may provide useful prognostic information in some populations.[41,42]

In addition to longitudinal monitoring of serum cystatin C values, at least five equations have been proposed to determine estimated GFR (eGFR) using serum cystatin C (CysC) and demographic variables including lean body mass (LM), age, gender, race, and serum creatinine (S_{cr}):[43–46]

$$\text{eGFR (mL/min)} = 77.24 \times (\text{CysC in mg/L})^{-1.2623}$$

$$\text{Log}_{10}\text{eGFR (mL/min)} = 2.222 + \left(-0.802 \times \sqrt{\text{CysC in } \frac{mg}{L}}\right) + (0.009876 \times \text{LM})$$

$$\text{eGFR (mL/min/1.73 m}^2) = 127.7 \times (\text{CysC in mg/L})^{-1.17} \times (\text{age in years})^{-0.13} \times 0.91 \text{ [if female]} \times 1.06 \text{ [if black]}$$

$$\text{eGFR (mL/min/1.73 m}^2) = 76.7 \times (\text{CysC in mg/L})^{-1.19}$$

$$\text{eGFR (mL/min/1.73 m}^2) = 177.6 \times (S_{cr} \text{ in mg/dL})^{-0.65} \times (\text{CysC in mg/L})^{-0.57} \times (\text{age in years})^{-0.20} \times 0.82 \text{ [if female]} \times 1.11 \text{ [if black]}$$

Conversion from eGFR conventional units of mL/min/1.73 m² to eGFR SI units of mL/s/m² requires multiplication by 0.00963; conversion from eGFR conventional units of mL/min to eGFR SI units of mL/s requires multiplication by 0.0167. Serum creatinine in μmol/L can be converted to mg/dL by multiplication using 0.0113 as the conversion factor.

Recent studies by MacDonald et al.[43] and Vupputuri et al.[46] reported that body weight is a significant covariate in GFR determination using cystatin C. Using GFR measured as plasma inulin clearance, lean body mass accounted for at least 16.3% of the variance in GFR values obtained using cystatin C ($P < 0.001$). When using a cystatin C-based estimate of GFR, which incorporates the CysC, age, race, and gender, a higher prevalence of CKD was reported in obese patients when compared with the MDRD4 equation.[46] Thus, a rigorous evaluation of the impact of body composition and obesity on GFR estimates using cystatin C is needed.

Alternative Methodologies

Urinary biomarkers such as KIM-1, NGAL, and cystatin C have shown promise in detecting early kidney injury.[47] Because it is normally reabsorbed and catabolized in the renal proximal tubule, it is hypothesized that tubular damage would lead to increased urinary excretion of cystatin C. Koyner et al.[48] showed that postoperative cardiac surgery patients with early elevated urinary cystatin C concentrations (corrected for urinary creatinine) had the highest prevalence of developing acute kidney injury (AKI). Here, plasma creatinine concentrations did not peak until 48 hours after admission to the intensive care unit, suggesting that urinary biomarkers such as cystatin C may be beneficial in early diagnosis of AKI. Use of cystatin C as a quantitative measure of GFR requires further study and may yield useful information for comprehensive evaluations of health and cardiovascular status, including detection of acute and chronic changes in kidney function.

Beta-trace protein (BTP) has recently been proposed as a new alternate endogenous marker of GFR.[49-51] Similar to cystatin C, it is a low molecular weight glycoprotein (168 amino acids) that is filtered through the glomerular basement membrane and reabsorbed in the renal proximal tubule. Elevated concentrations of BTP in serum have been reported in patients with CKD,[52] kidney transplant recipients,[53] and children.[54] Equations to estimate GFR that incorporate BTP concentrations in adults and pediatric populations are currently being evaluated.[55]

MEASUREMENT OF KIDNEY FUNCTION

The gold standard quantitative index of kidney function is a measured GFR. A variety of methods may be used to measure and estimate kidney function in the acute care and ambulatory settings. Estimation of GFR is important for early recognition and monitoring of patients with CKD. Estimation of CL_{cr} is important as a guide for drug dose adjustment in the presence of renal impairment.

It is important to recognize conditions that may alter renal function independent of underlying renal pathology. For example, protein intake, such as oral protein loading or an infusion of amino acid solution, may increase GFR.[10] As a result, inter- and intrasubject variability must be considered when it is used as a longitudinal marker of renal function. Dietary protein intake has been demonstrated to correlate with GFR in healthy subjects. Brändle et al.[56] evaluated renal function in four groups of healthy volunteers, each ingesting a diet controlled for protein over a 4-month period. The GFR was nonlinearly related to urine nitrogen excretion, with an observed maximum of 181.7 mL/min (3.03 mL/s) at a urinary nitrogen excretion rate of 20 g/day (1.43 mol/d), or 125 g/day protein intake. Subjects who are vegetarian have a lower GFR than individuals who consume a similar caloric but normal protein content diet because of their reduced dietary protein intake. When challenged with a protein load, the vegetarian subjects are able to increase their GFR to the "normal" range.[10] Findings from the Nurses' Health Study[57] indicate that longitudinal changes in GFR are independent of the source of protein (nondairy animal, dairy, or vegetable) in women with normal renal function. However, women with mild renal insufficiency (GFR 71 ± 7 mL/min [1.18 ± 0.12 mL/s]) who consumed the highest amount of protein (93 g/day) had a threefold greater risk of a ≥ 5 mL/min (≥ 0.08 mL/s) decline in GFR compared with the lowest protein group (60 g/day); rates of decline were highest in those consuming nondairy animal protein. The increased GFR following a protein load is the result of renal vasodilation accompanied by an increased renal plasma flow. The exact mechanism of the renal response to protein is unknown but may be related to extrarenal factors such as glucagon, prostaglandins, and angiotensin II, or to intrarenal mechanisms, such as tubular transport and tubuloglomerular feedback.[58,59] Despite the evidence of a "renal reserve," standardized evaluation techniques have not been developed. Therefore, assessment of the standard GFR measurement technique must consider the dietary protein status of the patient at the time of the study.

CLINICAL CONTROVERSY

The estimation of creatinine clearance in elderly patients with low serum creatinine values is controversial. Some clinicians advocate correction of serum creatinine to 1 mg/dL to account for reduced muscle mass. The impact of this correction factor on GFR estimates using MDRD4 or other equations has yet to be evaluated in this population.

MEASUREMENT OF THE GLOMERULAR FILTRATION RATE

❹ A measured GFR remains the single best index of functioning renal mass. As renal mass declines in the presence of age-related loss of nephrons or coexisting disease states such as hypertension and diabetes, there is a progressive decline in GFR. The rate of decline in GFR can be used to predict the time to onset of stage 5 CKD, as well as the risk of complications of CKD. Accurate measurement of GFR in clinical practice is a critical variable for the individualization of the dosage regimens of renally excreted medications so as to maximize their therapeutic efficacy and avoid potential toxicity.

The GFR is expressed as the volume of plasma filtered across the glomerulus per unit time, based on total renal blood flow and capillary hemodynamics. The normal values for GFR are 127 ± 20 mL/min/1.73 m² (1.22 ± 0.19 mL/s/m²) and 118 ± 20 mL/min/1.73 m² (1.14 ± 0.19 mL/s/m²) in healthy men and women, respectively. For example, if the normal renal blood flow was ~1 L/min/1.73 m² (0.01 mL/s/m²), plasma volume was 60% of blood volume, and filtration fraction across the glomerulus was 20%, then the normal GFR would be ~120 mL/min/1.73 m² (1.16 mL/s/m²).

Because GFR cannot be measured directly in humans, clearance methods that use substances that are freely filtered without additional clearance because of tubular secretion or reduction as the result of reabsorption are required. Additionally, the substance should not be susceptible to metabolism within renal tissues and should not alter renal function. Given these conditions, the GFR is equivalent to the renal clearance of the solute marker:

$$\text{GFR} = \text{renal CL} = (A_e)/\text{AUC}_{0-t}$$

where renal CL is renal clearance of the marker, A_e is the amount of marker excreted in the urine in a specified period of time, t, and AUC_{0-t} is the area under the plasma concentration-versus-time curve of the marker.

TABLE 50-4 Sensitivity and Clinical Utility of Renal Function Tests

	Accuracy	Clinical Utility	Cost
Inulin clearance	++++	+	$$$$
Radiolabeled markers	+++	+	$$$
Nonisotopic contrast agents	+++	++	$$$
Creatinine clearance	++	+++	$$
Serum creatinine	+	++++	$

+ = least acceptable, ++ = adequate, +++ = better, ++++ = best.

Under steady-state conditions, for example, during a continuous infusion of the marker, the expression simplifies to

$$GFR = renal\ CL = (A_e)/(C_{ss} \times t)$$

where C_{ss} is the steady-state plasma concentration of the marker achieved during continuous infusion. The continuous infusion method can also be employed without urine collection, where plasma clearance is calculated as $CL = $ infusion rate$/C_{ss}$. Requirements of this method include steady-state plasma concentrations and accurate measurement of infusate concentrations. Plasma clearance can also be determined following a single-dose IV injection with multiple samplings of blood to estimate area under the curve ($AUC_{0-\infty}$). Here, clearance is calculated as $CL = $ dose$/AUC$. These plasma clearance methods commonly yield clearance values 10% to 15% higher than urine collection methods.[60,61]

❺ Several markers have been used for the measurement of GFR, including both exogenous and endogenous compounds. Those administered as exogenous agents, such as inulin, iothalamate, iohexol, and radioisotopes, require specialized administration techniques and detection methods for the quantification of function, but they generally provide a more accurate measure of GFR. Methods that employ endogenous compounds, such as creatinine, require less technical expertise but produce results with greater variability. The marker of choice depends on the purpose and cost of the test (e.g., ^{125}I-iothalamate costs $2,000 per vial [Glofil-125, QOL Medical]); research protocols will generally use a more accurate test than one used in the clinical setting (Table 50–4).

Inulin Clearance

Inulin is a large fructose polysaccharide (5,200 Da) obtained from the Jerusalem artichoke, dahlia, and chicory plants. It is not bound to plasma proteins, is freely filtered at the glomerulus, is not secreted or reabsorbed, and is not metabolized by the kidney. The volume of distribution of inulin approximates extracellular volume, or 20% of ideal body weight. Because it is eliminated by glomerular filtration, its elimination half-life is dependent on renal function and is ~1.3 hours in subjects with normal renal function. Measurement of plasma and urine inulin concentrations can be performed using high-performance liquid chromatography.[62] Sinistrin, another polyfructosan, has similar characteristics to inulin; it is filtered at the glomerulus and not secreted or reabsorbed to any significant extent. It is a naturally occurring substance derived from the root of the North African vegetable red squill, *Urginea maritime,* which has a much higher degree of water solubility than inulin. Assay methods for sinistrin have been described using enzymatic procedures, as well as high-performance liquid chromatography with electrochemical detection.[63]

Iothalamate Clearance

Alternatives have been sought for inulin as a marker for GFR because of the problems of availability, high cost, sample preparation, and assay variability. Iothalamate is an iodine-containing radiocontrast agent that is available in both radiolabeled (^{125}I) and nonradiolabeled

forms. This agent is handled in a manner similar to that of inulin; it is freely filtered at the glomerulus and does not undergo substantial tubular secretion or reabsorption. The nonradiolabeled form is most widely used to measure GFR in ambulatory and research settings and can safely be administered by IV bolus, continuous infusion, or subcutaneous injection.[64] Plasma and urine iothalamate concentrations can be measured using high-performance liquid chromatography.[65] A reported slight positive bias of ~10 mL/min (0.17 mL/s) suggests that there is some degree of nonrenal clearance of this agent. However, plasma iothalamate clearance methods that do not require urine collections have been shown to be highly correlated with iothalamate renal clearance, making them particularly well suited for longitudinal evaluations of renal function.[66]

Iohexol

Iohexol, a nonionic, low osmolar, iodinated contrast agent, has also been used for the determination of GFR. It is eliminated almost entirely by glomerular filtration, and plasma and renal clearance values are similar to observations with other marker agents: strong correlations of 0.90 or greater and significant relationships such as $CL_{iohexol} = 0.90\ CL_{iothalamate} + 6.8$ mL/min have been reported.[67-69] These data support iohexol as a suitable alternative marker for the measurement of GFR. One key advantage of this agent is that a single plasma sample can be used to quantify iohexol clearance, provided sufficient time has elapsed since injection. For patients with a reduced GFR, more time must be allotted—more than 24 hours if the estimated GFR is less than 20 mL/min (0.33 mL/s).[67]

Radiolabeled Markers

The GFR has also been quantified using radiolabeled markers, such as ^{125}I-iothalamate (614 Da, radioactive half-life of 60 days), ^{99m}Tc-diethylenetriamine pentaacetic acid (^{99m}Tc-DPTA; 393 Da, radioactive half-life of 6.03 hours), and ^{51}Cr-ethylenediaminetetraacetic acid (^{51}Cr-EDTA; 292 Da, radioactive half-life of 27 days).[70] These relatively small molecules are minimally bound to plasma proteins and do not undergo tubular secretion or reabsorption to any significant degree. ^{125}I-iothalamate and ^{99m}Tc-DPTA are used in the United States, whereas ^{51}Cr-EDTA is used extensively in Europe. The use of radiolabeled markers allows one to determine the individual contribution of each kidney to total renal function.[71] Various protocols exist for the administration of these markers and subsequent determination of GFR using either plasma or renal clearance calculation methods. The nonrenal clearance of these agents appears to be low (3–8 mL/min [0.05–0.13 mL/s]), suggesting that plasma clearance is an acceptable technique except in patients with severe renal insufficiency (GFR <30 mL/min [<0.50 mL/s]). Indeed, highly significant correlations between renal clearance among radiolabeled markers has been demonstrated.[72] Although total radioactive exposure to patients is usually minimal, use of one of these agents does require compliance with radiation safety committees and appropriate biohazard waste disposal.

Estimation of GFR

A series of equations for estimating GFR have been proposed over the past 10 years (Table 50–5). The most commonly used equations are those proposed by Levey and colleagues,[73-77] which have gained widespread support for the estimation of GFR as a tool for the identification and risk categorization of CKD in many patient populations. The initial equations were derived from multiple regression analysis of data obtained from the 1,628 patients enrolled in the Modification of Diet in Renal Disease Study (MDRD), where GFR was measured by renal clearance of ^{125}I-iothalamate. The first regression model yielded

TABLE 50-5	Equations for the Estimation of Creatinine Clearance and GFR in Adults with Stable Renal Function
Cockroft and Gault[89]	Men: $CL_{cr} = (140 - age) \, ABW/(S_{cr} \times 72)$ Women: $CL_{cr} \times 0.85$
Jelliffe[95]	Men: $CL_{cr} = (100/S_{cr}) - 12$ Women: $CL_{cr} = (80/S_{cr}) - 7$
Jelliffe[95]	Men: $CL_{cr} = 98 - [0.8 \, (age - 20)]/S_{cr}$ Women: $CL_{cr} \times 0.9$
Mawer et al.[94]	Men: IBW $[29.3 - (0.203 \times age)] \, [1 - (0.03 \times S_{cr})]/(14.4 \times S_{cr})$ Women: IBW $[25.3 - (0.175 \times age)] \, [1 - (0.03 \times S_{cr})]/$ $(14.4 \times S_{cr})$
Hull et al.[96]	Men: $CL_{cr} = [(145 - age)/S_{cr}] - 3$ Women: $Cl_{cr} \times 0.85$
Levey et al. (MDRD6)[73]	GFR $= 170 \times (S_{cr})^{-0.999} \times [age]^{-0.176} \times [0.762$ if patient is female$] \times [1.180$ if patient is black$] \times [SUN]^{-0.170} \times [Alb]^{0.318}$
Levey et al. (MDRD4)[74]	GFR $= 186 \times (S_{cr})^{-1.154} \times [age]^{-0.203} \times [0.742$ if patient is female$] \times [1.210$ if patient is black$]$
Levey et al. (MDRD4-IDMS)[74]	GFR $= 175 \times (S_{cr})^{-1.154} \times [age]^{-0.203} \times [0.742$ if patient is female$] \times [1.210$ if patient is black$]$
Levey et al. (CKD-EPI)[81]	GFR $= 141 \times \min (S_{cr}/\kappa, 1)^{\alpha} \times \max (S_{cr}/\kappa, 1)^{-1.209} \times 0.993^{Age} \times 1.018$ [if female] $\times 1.159$ [if black]
Rule et al. (MCQ)[82]	GFR $= \exp [1.911 + \dfrac{5.249}{S_{cr}} - \dfrac{2.114}{S_{cr}^2} - 0.00686$ $\times$ Age $- 0.205$ (if female)]

κ is 0.7 for women and 0.9 for men, α is −0.329 for women and −0.411 for men; min indicates the minimum of S_{cr}/κ or 1, and max indicates the maximum of S_{cr}/κ or 1. (If S_{cr} <0.8 mg/dL, use 0.8 for S_{cr}.)
ABW = actual body weight, Alb = serum albumin concentration (g/dL), CL_{cr} = creatinine clearance in mL/min, GFR = glomerular filtration rate, IBW = ideal body weight (kg), S_{cr} = serum or plasma creatinine (mg/dL), SUN = serum urea nitrogen concentration (mg/dL).

a six-variable Modification of Diet in Renal Disease Study (MDRD6) equation.[74,75] This new equation had a higher correlation coefficient ($r^2 = 0.902$) and thus provided a more precise estimate of GFR than measured CL_{cr} ($r^2 = 0.866$) or CL_{cr} estimated by the Cockcroft-Gault equation ($r^2 = 0.842$) in the MDRD population. A newer modified, four-variable version of the original MDRD equation (MDRD4), based on plasma creatinine, age, gender, and race, was shown to provide a similar estimate of GFR results compared with the six-variable equation predecessor[74] and has been subsequently updated based on the calibrated serum creatinine (IDMS) assay.[75] The MDRD4 equation is now recommended by the NKF and the National Kidney Disease Education Program (NKDEP) for calculating the estimated GFR (eGFR) in patients with a history of CKD risk factors and a GFR <60 mL/min/1.73 m² (<0.58 mL/s/m²). The performance of the MDRD equations has been assessed in a variety of patient populations with GFR <60 mL/min/1.73m² (<0.58 mL/s/m²), including those with diabetic nephropathy and renal transplant patients. However, the MDRD equations have been shown to be less accurate in healthy subjects, diabetic patients with normal GFR (88–182 mL/min/1.73 m² [0.85–1.75 mL/s/m²]), and healthy potential kidney donors.[76] In a small study of elderly subjects (age >68 years) with mild/moderate CKD (GFR 53 ± 18 mL/min/1.73 m² [0.51 ± 0.17 mL/s/m²]), the MDRD6 equation was slightly positively biased compared with the Cockcroft-Gault equation (8% vs. 10%), but precision was similar between methods relative to measured GFR.[77] Beddhu et al.[78] reported that the MDRD6 equation, like the Cockcroft-Gault equation, is dependent on creatinine production and is susceptible to bias in malnourished patients with ESRD. In patients with GFR values >60 mL/min/1.73 m² (>0.58 mL/s/m²), the values provided by the MDRD4 equation have been shown to be highly variable and less accurate then other traditional estimation methods, perhaps

in part because the original study population consisted only of patients with low GFR values (<60 mL/min/1.73m² [<0.58 mL/s/m²]). The study also included few Asians, elderly patients, those with diabetes, or ill, hospitalized patients;[79] thus, the MDRD4 should be used with caution in children, the elderly, and those with extremes in muscle mass (cachectic and obese) until further performance data are available.

CLINICAL CONTROVERSY

Some practitioners are advocating the use of the MDRD4 equation in patients without CKD, although it appears to have a weaker correlation with GFR than the Cockcroft-Gault equation. Recent evidence suggests that the MDRD4 equation should be reserved for patients with a GFR <60 mL/min. The use of newer equations, such as the CKD-EPI, may have improved accuracy in patients with GFR >60 mL/min; however, further studies are required.

A single GFR equation may not be best suited for all populations, and choice of equation has been shown to affect CKD prevalence estimates.[80] This has led to a revitalized interest in the areas of nephrology, epidemiology, and development of new GFR equations over the past 5 years. The newest equations to be proposed for the estimation of GFR have been derived from wider CKD populations than the MDRD study and include the CKD-EPI[81] and Mayo Clinic Quadratic (MCQ) equations.[82] The CKD-EPI equation was developed from pooled study data involving 5,500 patients, with mean GFR values of 68 ± 40 mL/min/1.73 m² (0.65 ± 0.39 mL/s/m²) (range 2–190 mL/min/1.73m² [0.02–1.83 mL/s/m²]). It has been reported that the CKD-EPI equation is less biased (2.5 vs. 5.5 mL/min/1.73 m² [0.024 vs. 0.053 mL/s/m²]) but similarly imprecise compared with MDRD4. Rule et al.[82] developed the MCQ equation to estimate GFR from a population of CKD ($n = 320$) and healthy individuals ($n = 580$), using $1/S_{cr}$, $1/S_{cr}^2$, age, and gender as the covariates. Using the NHANES database, Snyder et al.[80] reported that MCQ GFR values resulted in 28% fewer patients being categorized as CKD stage 3 or 4 when compared with MDRD4. Thus, further evaluation of these newer GFR equations, including those incorporating "correction factors" for Japanese[83] and Chinese[84] populations, is needed. A variety of online resources that provide GFR calculators are available, such as the NKDEP website,[85] which provides GFR using the MDRD4 and MDRD4-IDMS equations. It should be noted that one must verify that a given equation is appropriate for the institutional creatinine reporting method.

The approach to standardize serum creatinine assays, and thereby improve the accuracy of eGFR results, has been implemented in most hospital clinical laboratories.[75] This IDMS assay calibration, called isotope dilution-mass spectrometry, is designed to reduce the interlaboratory variability in serum creatinine values. In settings using IDMS calibration, the revised MDRD-IDMS equation should be used based on the estimated 5% to 20% reduction in creatinine values. Recent recommendations from the NKDEP include reporting serum creatinine values in mg/dL to two decimal places (e.g., 0.93 mg/dL) and values in μmol/L to the nearest whole number (e.g., 84 μmol/L). This practice will likely reduce rounding errors that in the past contributed to bias between creatinine-based GFR or CL_{cr} estimates, but it does not improve GFR estimation in those without CKD. The impact of this new creatinine reporting approach on the accuracy of automated GFR results, calculated by a specified method, remains to be determined.

Measured Creatinine Clearance

Although the measured (24-hour) CL_{cr} has served as the basis of developing CL_{cr} estimation equations in the past, it has limited clinical utility for estimation of GFR. Short-duration witnessed CL_{cr} correlates with iothalamate clearance performed using the single-injection technique. In a multicenter study[86] of 136 patients with type I diabetic nephropathy, the correlations of simultaneous CL_{cr}, Cockcroft-Gault CL_{cr}, and 24-hour CL_{cr} (compared with $CL_{iothalamate}$) were 0.81, 0.67, and 0.49, respectively, indicating increased variability with the 24-hour clearance determination. In a selected group of 110 patients, measurement of a 4-hour CL_{cr} during water diuresis provided the best estimate of the GFR as determined by the $CL_{iothalamate}$. Furthermore, the ratio of CL_{cr} to $CL_{iothalamate}$ did not appear to increase as the GFR decreased. These data suggest that a short collection period with a water diuresis may be the best method for estimation of GFR by creatinine clearance.

A limitation of using creatinine as a filtration marker is that it undergoes varying degrees of tubular secretion. Tubular secretion augments the filtered creatinine by ~10% in subjects with normal kidney function. If the nonspecific Jaffe reaction is used, which overestimates the serum creatinine concentration by ~10% because of the noncreatinine chromogens, then the creatinine clearance is a very good measure of GFR in patients with normal kidney function. Tubular secretion, however, increases to as much as 100% in patients with renal insufficiency.[21] As renal impairment develops, the remaining nephrons hypertrophy, and the degree of tubular secretion decreases less than the decrease in filtration. The result is an overestimation of creatinine clearance as a function of GFR assessed by inulin or iothalamate clearance. For example, Bauer et al.[21] reported that the CL_{cr}-to-CL_{inulin} ratio in subjects with mild impairment was 1.20; for moderate impairment, it was 1.87; and for severe impairment, it was 2.32. Thus, creatinine clearance is a poor indicator of GFR in patients with moderate to severe renal insufficiency.

Because cimetidine blocks the tubular secretion of creatinine, the potential role of several oral cimetidine regimens to improve the accuracy and precision of creatinine clearance as an indicator of GFR has been evaluated. The CL_{cr}-to-CL_{DPTA} ratio declined from 1.33 with placebo to 1.07 when 400 mg of cimetidine was administered four times daily for 2 days prior to and during the clearance determination.[87] Similar results were observed when a single 800 mg dose of cimetidine was given 1 hour prior to the simultaneous determination of CL_{cr} and $CL_{iothalamate}$; the ratio of CL_{cr} to $CL_{iothalamate}$ was reduced from a mean of 1.53 to 1.12.[88] Thus, a single oral dose of cimetidine 800 mg should provide adequate blockade of creatinine secretion to improve the accuracy of a creatinine clearance measurement as an eGFR in patients with stages 3 to 5 CKD.

Estimation of Creatinine Clearance

❼ Many equations describing the mathematical relationships between various patient factors and CL_{cr} have been reported over the past 3 decades. Most equations incorporate factors such as age, gender, weight, and serum creatinine concentration, without the need for urine collection. The most widely used of these estimators is the Cockcroft-Gault equation,[89] which identified age and body mass as factors that significantly contribute to the estimate of CL_{cr}. This relationship was based on observations from 249 male patients with stable kidney function in whom the creatinine production rates were estimated. Estimated creatinine clearance, using the Cockcroft-Gault equation, remains the most common approach for stratifying patients in pharmacokinetic studies in clinical development and is reported most often in FDA-approved package inserts for new drug entities.[4]

The issue of which if any modified weight index should be used in the Cockcroft-Gault equation remains controversial, and approaches vary widely among clinical practitioners. For obese individuals, defined as those weighing >30% their ideal body weight (IBW), it is generally recommended that IBW be used in place of actual body weight (ABW)[90] in the Cockcroft-Gault equation, where

$$IBW (kg, men) = 50 + 2.3 (height\ in\ inches > 60)$$

$$IBW (kg, women) = 45 + 2.3 (height\ in\ inches > 60)$$

An alternative approach for estimating CL_{cr} (mL/min) in obese patients is the Salazar-Corcoran equation, which has been shown to be unbiased and superior to the Cockcroft-Gault equation in this population.[90,91] In the morbidly obese population, such as those with body mass index (BMI) ≥ 40 kg/m[2], use of lean body weight was recently reported to improve the accuracy of the Cockcroft-Gault equation in predicting 24-hour CL_{cr}.[92] Regardless of the approach used to estimate renal function in obese patients, it is imperative that drug therapy outcomes be monitored closely in this special population.

Luke et al.[93] evaluated the ability of the Cockcroft-Gault method and four other methods to predict CL_{cr}, with inulin clearance being considered the standard measure of GFR. The simultaneously determined inulin and creatinine clearances correlated best, $r^2 = 0.85$, and the CL_{cr} overestimated CL_{inulin} by ~15% due to tubular secretion of creatinine. For the five calculated clearances, Cockcroft-Gault and Mawer et al.[94] correlated the best with inulin clearance. The Cockcroft-Gault method showed a linear relationship with CL_{inulin} equal to 1.121 of CL_{cr} plus 20.6 mL/min (0.34 mL/s) ($r^2 = 0.66$), whereas for Mawer et al., the relationship was CL_{inulin} equal to 1.051 of CL_{cr} plus 18.3 mL/min (0.31 mL/s) ($r^2 = 0.66$). Other methods, such as Jelliffe[95] and Hull et al.,[96] consistently underestimated the CL_{cr}. As kidney function declined, there was an increase in the fraction of creatinine eliminated by secretion as measured by the CL_{cr}-to-CL_{inulin} ratio, consistent with earlier reports. Gault et al.[97] also evaluated the performance of the Cockcroft-Gault estimator of renal function compared with inulin and ^{99m}Tc-DPTA. Except for conditions of unstable kidney function, it performed like the 24-hour creatinine clearance method (Table 50–5).

Patients undergoing screening for participation in the African American Study of Kidney Disease (AASK) were evaluated for kidney function based on an estimated CL_{cr} compared with the simultaneous ^{125}I-iothalamate and measured 24-hour CL_{cr}.[98] The simultaneous CL_{cr} provided the best estimate of GFR. Cockcroft-Gault was the preferred method for estimation of GFR, based on performance and ease of use. This method was noted to underestimate the GFR by 9%, perhaps because of the increased excretion rate of creatinine by black patients.[98,99]

Administration of cimetidine has also resulted in improved performance of the Cockcroft-Gault equation to predict GFR. Ixkes et al.[100] gave patients three 800 mg doses of cimetidine in 24 hours and measured creatinine plasma levels from 3 to 7 hours following the final dose. During this 4-hour period, the $CL_{iothalamate}$ was determined as the measure of GFR. The Cockcroft-Gault calculations were performed with the plasma creatinine measurement 3 hours after the last dose of cimetidine. The ratio of the Cockcroft-Gault estimated CL_{cr}-to-$CL_{iothalamate}$ ratio decreased from 1.28 ± 0.21 to 0.98 ± 0.11 in the presence of cimetidine. This cimetidine dosing schedule also improved the accuracy of Cockcroft-Gault estimates relative to GFR in renal transplant patients with GFR values ranging from 20 to 80 mL/min/1.73 m^2 (0.19–0.77 mL/s/m^2).[101,102]

Liver Disease

The prediction of CL_{cr} or GFR is particularly problematic in patients with preexisting liver disease and renal impairment. Lower than expected serum creatinine values may result from reduced muscle mass, protein-poor diet, diminished hepatic synthesis of creatine (a precursor of creatinine), and fluid administration and can lead to significant overestimation of creatinine clearance. Orlando et al.[103] evaluated 10 healthy subjects, 10 patients with mild liver disease, and 10 with severe liver disease and observed a measured CL_{cr}-to-CL_{inulin} ratio of 1.05, 1.03, and 1.04 for each group, respectively. When the CL_{cr} of patients with severe liver disease was estimated using the Cockcroft-Gault equation, the resultant ratio (CL_{cr} Cockcroft-Gault to CL_{inulin}) was 1.23. Lam et al.[104] likewise noted an overprediction by Cockcroft-Gault of the measured CL_{cr} in patients with severe disease, by 40% to 100%.

Studies of renal function in patients with severe hepatic disease confirm the earlier observations of Hull et al.[95] and Caregaro et al.,[105] who reported that measured CL_{cr} overestimated GFR by 50% in hepatic patients with a GFR of 56 ± 19 mL/min/1.73 m^2 (0.54 ± 0.18 mL/s/m^2) because of increased tubular secretion of creatinine. The effect of cimetidine administration on measured CL_{cr} was recently evaluated in a small study by Sansoe et al.[106] In 12 patients with compensated cirrhosis, serum creatinine values increased from 0.68 ± 0.11 to 0.94 ± 0.14 mg/dL (69 ± 10 μmol/L to 83 ± 12 μmol/L) during coadministration of cimetidine (1,000 mg given as 400 mg × 1, then 200 mg every 3 hours) during a 9-hour clearance period. The CL_{cr} was reduced from 138 ± 20 to 89 ± 13 mL/min (2.30 ± 0.33 to 1.49 ± 0.22 mL/s), with no change in measured GFR.

CLINICAL CONTROVERSY

In patients with liver disease, falsely low serum creatinine values frequently occur as a result of malnourishment, muscle wasting, and enhanced tubular secretion of creatinine. Preliminary data suggest that the use of cimetidine may improve the accuracy of measured creatinine clearance compared with measured GFR in patients with cirrhosis. However, the effect of this approach on methods to estimate CL_{cr} or GFR is unknown.

DeSanto et al.[107] studied 19 patients with mild liver disease whose inulin and creatinine clearances were 90 ± 4.4 and 122 ± 7 mL/min/1.73 m^2 (0.87 ± 0.042 and 1.17 ± 0.067 mL/s/m^2), respectively. The degree of overestimation of GFR by creatinine clearance was inversely correlated with GFR ($r = 0.452$, $P < 0.04$). In cirrhotic patients being evaluated for liver transplant (GFR 58 ± 5.1 mL/min/1.73 m^2 [0.56 ± 0.049 mL/s/m^2]), the MDRD4, MDRD6, and Cockcroft-Gault equations significantly overestimated GFR by 30% to 50% and were imprecise estimates of GFR before and after liver transplantation.[108,109] Thus, measurement of renal function in patients with hepatic disease should be performed using a method specific for glomerular filtration, and estimation equations for GFR or creatinine clearance should be avoided.

Other Special Populations

Davis and Chandler[110] confirmed the accuracy of the Cockcroft-Gault equation to predict CL_{cr} in trauma patients with stable kidney function, and Thakur et al.[28] demonstrated its successful use in 42 paraplegic subjects. Renal transplant recipients are frequently monitored for renal function, as numerous complications may occur during the life of the allograft. Goerdt et al.[111] assessed the bias and precision with which several nomographic methods predicted GFR (iohexol clearance) in 127 patients with stable kidney function. The Cockcroft-Gault method performed poorly, overestimating iohexol clearance. This is expected, as iohexol clearance provides a true measure of GFR, whereas the Cockcroft-Gault CL_{cr} estimate is falsely high because of the tubular secretion of creatinine. Huang et al.[112] reported the inability of several CL_{cr} equations to predict renal function in hospitalized patients with advanced human immunodeficiency virus (HIV) disease. All of the prediction methods overestimated the measured 24-hour CL_{cr}. The reasons for the poor predictability of these methods are unclear, although 24-hour collection methods result in increased variability, often because of inadequate collection of urine.

Renal function assessment during pregnancy is usually performed using a 24-hour creatinine clearance determination. Quadri et al.[113] evaluated the Cockcroft-Gault method during each trimester in 34 pregnant women and compared these estimates with the measured 24-hour CL_{cr}. Prepregnancy weights were used throughout the study for the Cockcroft-Gault method, and results correlated well with the measured clearances ($r^2 = 0.76$). The maximal CL_{cr} occurred during the second trimester for both methods.

Unstable Renal Function

Patients with unstable kidney function present a unique situation because serum creatinine values are changing, and steady state cannot be assumed when estimating CL_{cr}. It can take several days for serum creatinine values to reach steady state in early acute renal failure, but this time can be reduced when renal function is improving. In patients with previously normal renal function, a change in the serum creatinine concentration >50% over a period of 1 day is suggestive of unstable renal function. In patients with preexisting CKD (GFR <60 mL/min/1.73 m^2 [<0.58 mL/s/m^2]), an increase in serum creatinine by 30% or more than 1 mg/dL [88 μmol/L] over a 24- to 48-hour period indicates the presence of acute renal failure. Methods to measure GFR in this population, such as ^{125}I-iothalamate clearance, are cumbersome and costly, especially in the acute care setting. Table 50–6 lists several equations for estimating renal function under these conditions.[114–116] Although these equations are commonly used to estimate CL_{cr} in patients with acute renal failure, a rigorous evaluation of the accuracy and precision of each of these proposed methods is lacking. Also lacking is a method to estimate GFR, an equivalent to the MDRD equation for patients with CKD, for patients with acute renal failure.

TABLE 50-6 Equations for the Estimation of Creatine Clearance in Adults with Unstable Renal Function

		Equations	
Reference	Units	Men	Women
Jelliffe[114]	mL/min	$E^{ss} = wt[29.3 - 0.203(age)]$	$E^{ss} = wt[25.1 - 0.175(age)]$
		$E^{ss}_{corr} = E^{ss}[1.035 - 0.0337(S_{cr})]$	$E^{ss}_{corr} = E^{ss}[1.035 - 0.0337(S_{cr})]$
		$E = E^{ss}_{corr} - \dfrac{[4wt(S_{cr2} - S_{cr1})]}{\Delta t \; day}$	$E = E^{ss}_{corr} - \dfrac{[4wt(S_{cr2} - S_{cr1})]}{\Delta t \; day}$
		$CL_{cr} = \dfrac{E}{14.4(S_{cr})}$	$CL_{cr} = \dfrac{E}{14.4(S_{cr})}$
Chiou et al.[115]	mL/min	$V_d = 0.6 \; L(wt^a)$	$V_d = 0.6 \; L(wt^a)$
		$CL_{cr} = \dfrac{2[28 - 0.2(age)]}{14.4(S_{cr1} + S_{cr2})}$	$CL_{cr} = \dfrac{2wt^a[22.4 - 0.16(age)]}{14.4(S_{cr1} + S_{cr2})}$
		$+ \dfrac{2[V_d(S_{cr1} - S_{cr2})]}{(S_{cr1} + S_{cr2})\Delta t \; min} - [CrCl^{NR} \times wt^a]$	$+ \dfrac{2[V_d(S_{cr1} - S_{cr2})]}{(S_{cr1} + S_{cr2})\Delta t \; min} - [CrCl^{NR} \times wt^a]$
Brater[116]	mL/min per 70 kg	$CL_{cr} = \dfrac{[293 - (age) \times [1.035 - 0.01685(S_{cr1} + S_{cr2})]]}{(S_{cr1} + S_{cr2})}$	$CL_{cr} =$ Male value $\times 0.86$
		$+ \dfrac{49(S_{cr1} - S_{cr2})}{(S_{cr1} + S_{cr2})\Delta t \; day}$	

CL_{cr} = creatinine clearance, $CrCl^{NR}$ = nonrenal clearance of creatinine (0.048 mL/min per kg), E = creatinine excretion, E^{ss} = steady-state creatinine excretion, E^{ss}_{corr} = corrected steady-state creatinine excretion, Δt day, = time in days between S_{cr1} and S_{cr2}, Δt min = time in minutes between S_{cr1} and S_{cr2}, S_{cr1} = first serum creatinine value, S_{cr2} = second serum creatinine value, S_{cr} = average of S_{cr1} and S_{cr2}, V_d = volume distribution of creatinine.

The equation proposed by Jelliffe is a revised dynamic model of creatinine kinetics based on theoretical estimates of creatinine production and adjusted for age and changes in serum creatinine; however, its ability to predict changes in drug clearance (and dose adjustments) has not been evaluated.[114] In the acute setting, factors previously discussed that may alter the serum creatinine concentration must be evaluated to avoid misinterpretation. The inappropriate use of the Cockcroft-Gault equation in those with acute renal failure can significantly overestimate the value of CL_{cr} when compared with equations that are designed to account for changes in serum creatinine in patients with unstable renal function.[117] It is thus, ultimately, most important to recognize that renal function in patients with acute renal failure is generally markedly lower than one would estimate using steady-state methods, and dose adjustments should be made if necessary to avoid drug toxicity (see Chapter 51 and Tables 50–7 and 50–8).

CLINICAL CONTROVERSY

Serum creatinine values can fluctuate widely in patients with unstable renal function. Although some practitioners advocate the Cockcroft-Gault equation using the highest of the two serum creatinine values, others recommend calculation of CL_{cr} using either the Brater[116] or Jelliffe equation.[114]

Kidney Function in Children

Kidney function in the neonate is difficult to assess because of difficulty in urine and blood collection, the frequent presence of a non–steady-state serum creatinine, and the apparent disparity between the development of glomerular and tubular function. Preterm infants demonstrate significantly reduced GFR prior to 34 weeks, which rapidly increases and becomes similar to term infants within the first week of life.[118] Evaluation of GFR in preterm infants on day 3 of life, using an inulin infusion, failed to identify a relationship between patient weight and GFR.

Gestational age, which ranged from 23.4 to 36.9 weeks (mean 30.2 weeks), however, correlated with both GFR and the reciprocal of serum creatinine. The inulin clearance increased from 0.67 to 0.85 mL/min (0.011–0.014 mL/s) in those with gestational age younger than 28 weeks versus those of 32 to 37 weeks of age, whereas S_{cr} decreased from 1.05 to 0.73 mg/dL (93–65 μmol/L), respectively. Creatinine was measured using a specific enzymatic method to avoid interference from bilirubin or drugs.[119] Creatinine clearance has also been evaluated in infants younger than 1 week of age, and values of 17.8 mL/min/1.73 m² (0.171 mL/s/m²) on day 1 increased to 36.4 mL/min/1.73 m² (0.351 mL/s/m²) by day 6.[120] In light of these rapid changes in GFR, estimation of GFR is not recommended for infants younger than 1 week of age. Kidney function expressed as GFR standardized to body surface area

TABLE 50-7 Scenario A (Worsening Renal Function)

J.R. is a 50-year-old man (weight 70 kg, body surface area 1.73 m²) admitted to the intensive care unit following an automobile accident. His renal function was normal prior to admission; however, his serum creatinine has increased from 0.6 mg/dL to 3.0 mg/dL over the past 24 hours.

Equation	Cl_{cr}	Assumptions
Jelliffe[114]	24.4 mL/min	E^{ss} = 1341.2 mg/day
		E^{ss}_{corr} = 1306 mg/day
		S_{cr} = 1.8 mg/dL
		S_{cr1} = 0.6 mg/dL
		S_{cr2} = 3.0 mg/dL
		Δt = 1 day
		Wt = 70 kg
Brater[116]	19.1 mL/min	S_{cr1} = 0.6 mg/dL
		S_{cr2} = 3.0 mg/dL
		Δt = 1 day
Cockcroft-Gault[89]	29.2 mL/min	S_{cr2} = 3.0 mg/dL
		Wt = 70 kg

Cl_{cr} = creatinine clearance rate, Δt = time between S_{cr1} and S_{cr2}, E^{ss} = steady-state creatinine excretion, E^{ss}_{corr} = steady-state creatinine excretion corrected, S_{cr} = average serum creatinine, S_{cr1} = first serum creatinine value, S_{cr2} = second serum creatinine value, Wt = weight.

TABLE 50-8 Scenario B (Improving Renal Function)

J.R. has been in the intensive care unit for 1 week, and his status is improving. His serum creatinine has decreased from 3.0 mg/dL to 1.0 mg/dL over the past 24 hours.

Approach	Cl_{cr} mL/min	Assumptions
Jelliffe[114]	64.5 mL/min	E^{ss} = 1341.2 mg/day
		E^{ss}_{corr} = 1297.7 mg/day
		S_{cr} = 2.0 mg/dL
		S_{cr1} = 3.0 mg/dL
		S^{cr2} = 1.0 mh/dL
		Δt = 1 day
		Wt = 70 kg
Brater[116]	78.7 mL/min	S_{cr1} = 3.0 mg/dL
		S_{cr2} = 1.0 mg/dL
		Δt = 1 day
Cockcroft-Gault[89]	87.5 mL/min	S_{cr} = 1.0 mg/dL
		Wt = 70 kg

Cl_{cr} = creatinine clearance rate, Δt = time between S_{cr1} and S_{cr2}, E^{ss} = steady-state creatinine excretion, E^{ss}_{corr} = steady-state creatinine excretion corrected, S_{cr} = serum creatinine, S_{cr1} = first serum creatinine value, S_{cr2} = second serum creatinine value, Wt = weight.

increases with age and stabilizes at ~1 year. In older children, GFR is best assessed using standard measurement techniques for GFR. Subcutaneous administration of ^{125}I-iothalamate has been effectively used to measure GFR in children ranging in age from 1 to 20 years.[121]

Estimation of CL_{cr} as described by Schwartz et al.[122] is dependent on the child's age and length:

$$GFR = [length\ (cm) \times k]/(S_{cr}\ in\ mg/dL)$$

where k is defined by age group: infant (1–52 weeks) = 0.45, child (1–13 years) = 0.55, adolescent male = 0.7, and adolescent female = 0.55.

Subsequent studies verified these relationships in children with normal renal function or mild renal impairment. However, variability increases at clearance values <50 mL/min (<0.84 mL/s). Al-Harbi and Lireman[123] reported a good correlation of the predicted CL_{cr} with measured 4-hour CL_{cr} and ^{99m}Tc-DPTA ($r = 0.75$) in 48 pediatric renal allograft recipients 3 to 19 years of age. However, predictive performance measures of bias and precision were not reported. Fong et al.[124] evaluated the method in critically ill children (mean age 5.6 years; range 0.1–20.8 years) and concluded that the method significantly overestimated the measured CL_{cr} (bias = 45%). Pierrat et al.[125] compared the MDRD, Schwartz, and Cockcroft-Gault equations in children 3 to 19 years of age. In children younger than 12 years, the Schwartz and MDRD equations were significantly more biased than Cockcroft-Gault, and Cockcroft-Gault provided the best prediction of GFR in children older than 12 years. Because the MDRD equation was developed in the adult population, the results of these investigations suggest that further studies will be needed to clarify the value of any of these predictive methods in children. More recently, an equation for GFR based on BTP was shown to yield similar values of GFR compared with the Schwartz equation in 387 pediatric patients (age 10.7 ± 7.1 years) who underwent a ^{99m}TC-DTPA GFR scan.[55] Dose adjustments and other therapeutic decisions based on kidney function warrant appropriate measures of renal status to avoid incorrect decisions.

Kidney Function in the Elderly

Cross-sectional studies demonstrate decreased GFR as a function of age when GFR is measured as inulin, iothalamate, or creatinine clearance.[126,127] The Baltimore Longitudinal Study on Aging,[127] an evaluation of 254 normal healthy subjects, revealed

that creatinine clearance decreases at the rate of approximately 0.75 mL/min/1.73 m²/y (0.0072 mL/s/m²/y) beginning in the fourth decade of life. These subjects were evaluated prospectively for up to 23 years. Interestingly, approximately one-third of the subjects showed no change in renal function from their baseline value, and a small number showed an increased clearance. These changes may be a result of normal physiologic changes or of subclinical insults to the kidneys initiating the events leading to chronic progressive loss of renal function. Fliser et al.[128] studied renal functional reserve in healthy young (age 23–32 years) and elderly (age 61–82 years) volunteers using an amino acid infusion technique. Inulin clearance was used as the measure of GFR, which increased 16% in young and 17% in elderly subjects following the infusion. Renal functional reserve thus appears to be maintained in healthy elderly individuals.

Interpretation of the serum creatinine concentration alone is difficult in the elderly patient primarily because of the decreased muscle mass and resultant lower production rate of creatinine. Thus, the level of serum creatinine often remains within the normal range despite a reduction in the number of functional nephrons. As renal function declines, the kidneys excrete a larger fraction of creatinine. This perpetuates the "normal" serum creatinine. Recent recommendations, such as the adoption of standardized creatinine assays by clinical laboratories and reporting of serum creatinine values to two decimal places, will likely improve the accuracy of renal function estimation in the elderly population.[75]

The Cockcroft-Gault formula[89] can be used to estimate the CL_{cr} of elderly patients. Smythe et al.[129] estimated CL_{cr} in 23 patients older than 60 years using seven different methods and compared the results with a measured 24-hour CL_{cr} determination. Estimations were performed with the actual serum creatinine concentration and also with the serum creatinine rounded up to 1 mg/dL (88 μmol/L) if the actual value was <1 mg/dL (<88 μmol/L). Rounding the serum creatinine to 1 mg/dL (88 μmol/L) resulted in a significantly lower estimate of measured creatinine clearance (−28.8 mL/min [−0.481 mL/s]) compared with the unadjusted serum creatinine (+2.3 mL/min [+0.038 mL/s]). When capping serum creatinine values at 0.68 mg/dL (60 μmol/L), estimation of GFR using the MDRD equation overestimated creatinine clearance by up to 50 mL/min (0.84 mL/min).[130] Until further data are available, fixing or rounding serum creatinine concentration to an arbitrary value in elderly patients is not recommended.

An alternative to the estimation of GFR or a 24-hour clearance determination is a 4-hour clearance performed during water diuresis. This approach correlated with the inulin clearance as well as with an inpatient 24-hour CL_{cr}.[86] However, one must be aware of the potential risk of hyponatremia in the geriatric patient who is unable to tolerate an oral water load, as well as the need for complete bladder emptying to ensure accurate results. O'Connell et al.[131] assessed the accuracy of 2- and 8-hour urine collections compared with 24-hour creatinine clearance determinations in 45 hospitalized patients older than 65 years with indwelling urethral catheters. Single, timed urine collections for CL_{cr} showed minimal bias with the 8-hour collection compared with the 24-hour value, whereas the 2-hour determination was both biased and imprecise.

APPLICATION OF RENAL FUNCTION ESTIMATION EQUATIONS FOR DRUG DOSING

As stated previously, creatinine clearance estimated using the Cockcroft-Gault equation remains the most common approach for stratifying patients in pharmacokinetic studies in clinical development and is reported most often in FDA-approved package inserts for new drug entities.[4] A recent survey of pharmacy practitioners indicated that over 95% of individuals use the Cockcroft-Gault equation, or a variation using ideal or lean body weight in obese patients, when applied to renal drug dosing. Use of other equations to estimate CL_{cr} may result in drug-dosing errors. For example, Wright et al.[132] showed that use of the Jelliffe equation in place of the Cockcroft-Gault to calculate the carboplatin dose resulted in obese patients having a 62% lower frequency of dose reductions and toxicity, yet a higher rate of cancer progression, when compared with nonobese patients. Thus, underestimation of GFR resulted in a lower carboplatin dose when compared with the Cockcroft-Gault method. Other modifications to the Cockcroft-Gault equation, including adjustments (or rounding) in serum creatinine to account for "low" serum creatinine values in the elderly, may also result in drug-dosing errors. In patients older than 60 years with serum creatinine < 1 mg/dL (<88 μmol/L), rounding the serum creatinine value up to 1 mg/dL (88 μmol/L) resulted in dose estimates for gentamicin that were significantly lower (−90 ± 67 mg/day) than doses calculated based on the actual serum creatinine value.[129] In a study by Roberts et al.[130] of elderly subjects (age 65 ± 13 years), rounding serum creatinine values up to a minimum of 0.68 mg/dL (60 μmol/L) resulted in CLcr estimates that were highly correlated with gentamicin clearance. Although the impact of this rounding approach on errors in drug dosing was not reported, the evidence to date indicates that rounding of serum creatinine values to an arbitrary value should be avoided because of the potential for underdosing drugs, especially in the elderly.

The automated reporting of eGFR in the clinical setting has led some practitioners to consider substituting eGFR in place of CL_{cr} for renal dose adjustments. Concerns with this approach include the uncertainty of applying eGFR values to CL_{cr}-based algorithms in package inserts and potential dosing errors and toxicity, especially for drugs with narrow therapeutic indices.[133-135] Recent studies in over 1,200 patients with renal disease have shown that overestimation of renal function using the MDRD equation results in 30% to 60% higher doses for digoxin, amantadine, and various antimicrobials compared with doses calculated using CL_{cr} estimates.[136-139] A recent study by Stevens et al.[140] reported that use of a back-corrected value of eGFR, based on a calculated body surface area (BSA), yields dose calculations that are similar to those calculated using a measured (iothalamate) GFR. Use of this back-correction approach has not been validated, and calculating BSA in clinical settings is inconvenient and unlikely to occur. Without back-correction of the eGFR value, the significantly higher estimate of renal function may result in dosing errors; this approach is therefore not warranted until studies are conducted to assess the relationship between eGFR estimations and a drug's pharmacokinetic parameters and/or pharmacodynamic end points. A more detailed discussion of application of renal function estimates and renal dosing approaches is provided in Chapter 56.

ASSESSMENT OF PROGRESSION

Chronic kidney disease (see Chapter 52) will eventually lead to end-stage renal disease (see Chapter 53), necessitating dialysis (see Chapter 54) or transplantation for survival (see Chapter 98). The rate of progression can be slowed and in some cases halted through dietary modification, strict blood pressure control, initiation of angiotensin-converting enzyme inhibitor or angiotensin receptor blocker therapy to reduce urinary protein excretion, and improved glucose control in patients with diabetes mellitus (see Chapter 52). The efficacy of these interventions is optimally assessed with the sequential measurement of an accurate and sensitive index of GFR, such as iohexol, iothalamate, or radioisotope clearance.[141]

❽ Alternatively, newer methods to estimate GFR, such as cystatin C and the MDRD4 equation, and traditional methods, such

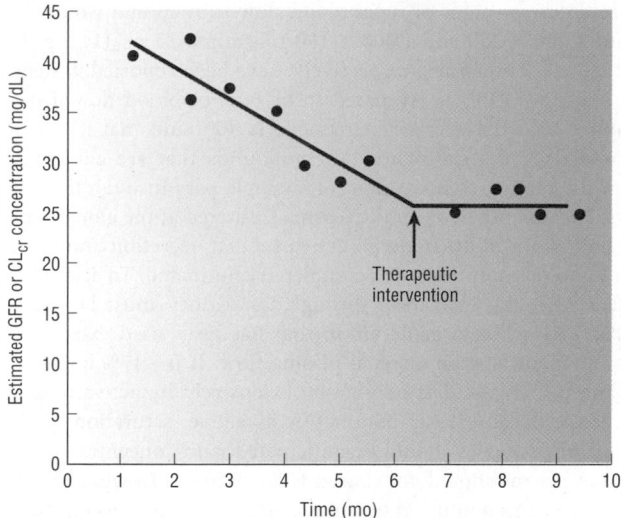

FIGURE 50-3. Illustration of the estimated glomerular filtration rate (eGFR) or creatinine clearance (CL_{cr}) decline over time and change in renal function in a hypothetical patient with progressive renal impairment. The *arrow* indicates a change in the rate of progression, which may be related to a therapeutic intervention.

as the linear decline in the reciprocal of the serum creatinine concentration as a function of time, are simple clinical tools that can be used to evaluate the rate of progression of renal disease and to predict the time when dialysis will be needed.[2,20]

Figure 50–3 depicts the change in estimated GFR or CL_{cr} over time in a typical patient with progressive CKD. Clinicians can use the eGFR or CL_{cr} plotted as a function of time as a prognostic tool, to predict when dialysis may be needed (CL_{cr} <20 mL/min [<0.33 mL/s]) or as a marker for evaluating the success of therapeutic interventions to alter the rate of decline in renal function. Several factors, such as changes in dietary intake of creatinine and decreased muscle mass, which are associated with a reduction in the production of creatinine, may alter the utility of the relationship. Microalbuminuria has been identified as an early marker of renal disease in patients with diabetic nephropathy[142] and numerous other conditions, such as hypertension and obesity.[143,144] Albuminuria is a more sensitive marker than total protein for monitoring CKD progression, as well as a modifiable risk factor for renal disease progression and cardiovascular disease.[41] Thus, patients with microalbuminuria (30–300 mg/day) on at least two or three occasions or overt albuminuria (>300 mg/day) should begin to receive pharmacotherapy. For children, microalbuminuria is considered present if albumin excretion exceeds 0.36 mg/kg/day, and overt albuminuria has been defined as an excretion rate that exceeds 4 mg/kg/day. The urinary albumin-to-creatinine ratio is also an accurate predictor of 24-hour proteinuria, a marker of renal disease. Guidelines for monitoring indicate that a urine albumin-to-creatinine ratio of >30 mg/g (>3.4 mg/mmol) places the patient at increased risk of developing diabetic nephropathy and is an indication for the initiation of pharmacotherapeutic intervention.[19] Microalbuminuria has also been suggested as a risk factor for renal dysfunction among patients with essential hypertension.[145]

MEASUREMENT OF RENAL PLASMA AND BLOOD FLOW

Measurement of renal plasma and blood flow is rarely if ever determined in the clinical setting; rather, it is reserved for research settings to evaluate hemodynamic changes related to disease or drug therapy. The kidneys receive ~20% of cardiac output, and representative values of renal blood flow in men and women of about 1,200 ± 250 and 1,000 ± 180 mL/min/1.73 m² (11.6 ± 2.4 and 9.6 ± 1.7 mL/s/m²), respectively, have been reported.[146] Renal plasma flow (RPF) is estimated to be 60% of blood flow if it is assumed that the average hematocrit is 40% and that it can be measured by the use of model compounds that are eliminated from the plasma compartment on a single pass through the kidneys. Because only 20% of the plasma is filtered at the glomerulus, the compound must undergo active tubular secretion and minimal to no reabsorption to be completely eliminated. To accurately reflect RPF, the extraction through the kidney must be nearly 100%. PAH is an organic anion that has been used extensively for the quantification of renal plasma flow. It is ~17% bound to plasma proteins and is eliminated extensively by active tubular secretion. Because PAH elimination is active, saturation of the transport processes should be anticipated, and concentrations of PAH in plasma should not exceed 10 to 20 mg/L. Dowling et al.[147] used a sequential infusion technique and observed concentration-dependent renal clearance of PAH at concentrations >100 mg/dL (1,000 g/L). Furthermore, PAH is also metabolized, possibly within the kidney, to N-acetyl-PAH, and it is important for the analytical method to differentiate the parent compound and metabolite.[65] Prescott et al.[148] noted that the renal clearance of PAH decreases at low plasma concentrations, whereas the clearance of the acetyl metabolite increases. Further studies are necessary to evaluate the mechanisms and significance of these findings. The extraction ratio (ER) for PAH is 70% to 90% at plasma concentrations of 10 to 20 mg/L; hence, the term *effective renal plasma flow* (ERPF) has been used when the clearance of PAH is not corrected for the extraction ratio or if it is assumed to be 1.[5] Normal values are about 650 ± 160 mL/min (10.9 ± 2.7 mL/s) for men and 600 ± 150 mL/min (10.0 ± 2.5 mL/s) for women.[146] Children will reach normalized adult values by 3 years of age, and ERPF will begin to decline as a function of age after 30 years, reaching about one-half of its peak value by 90 years of age. The method for calculation of ERPF is based on the relationship among organ clearance, ER, and flow:

$$ERPF = renal\ PAH\ CL = RPF \times ER$$

Effective renal blood flow (ERBF) can be estimated from ERPF by assuming the extraction ratio is 1 and correcting for the red blood cell volume of the blood (hematocrit [HCT]):

$$ERBF = ERPF/(1 - HCT)$$

ERPF can also be measured using the radioisotope ^{131}I-orthoiodohippurate (^{131}I-OIH) or ^{99m}Tc-mercaptoacetyltriglycine (^{99m}Tc-MAG3).[149] One important advantage of this method is its ability to measure ERPF in total or for each kidney independently, as well as its ability to produce renal images. Russell and Dubovsky,[150] using a single-injection technique, compared clearance methods with and without urine collection and showed similar results with each method.

QUANTITATIVE ASSESSMENT OF TUBULAR FUNCTION

Although GFR is the best overall indicator of renal function, it may not provide an accurate measure of tubular function, either secretory capacity or cellular function, suitable for use in the research environment.[151] Tubular secretory function can be assessed by measuring PAH transport as the prototype marker of the organic anion secretory system. N^1-methylnicotinamide (NMN) and tetraethylammonium are prototype compounds secreted by the cationic transport system and may be used as markers of cationic secretory capacity. Edwards et al.[152] demonstrated delayed recovery of

NMN clearance among patients with psoriasis treated with low-dose cyclosporine, as compared with the recovery of GFR and renal blood flow. Earlier studies with NMN suggested its use to assess the effects of selected renal diseases on drug handling by the kidneys.[153] Dowling et al.[147] explored the usefulness of famotidine as a marker for cationic transport but was unable to demonstrate saturation, perhaps due to the contribution from other parallel secretory pathways, such as P-glycoprotein and multidrug resistance protein 2 (MRP2).

Furthermore, Karyekar et al.[154] demonstrated that itraconazole, a P-glycoprotein inhibitor, significantly reduced the renal tubular secretion of cimetidine in healthy individuals, suggesting that cimetidine may be used as an in vivo probe of renal P-glycoprotein function. It should also be recognized that these transport systems are not necessarily mutually exclusive. Indeed, probenecid, which is secreted by the anionic pathway, inhibits the secretion of cationic compounds. Quantitative measures of tubular transport capacity are currently limited primarily to the research setting.

Other measures of tubular function are less specific and are regarded primarily as indices of damage within the nephron. Low molecular weight proteins located in the proximal tubule, such as β_2-microglobulin, can be used as urinary biomarkers to detect early tubular toxicity for drugs such as carboplatin, ifosfamide, and etoposide.[155] The rise in β_2-microglobulin is related to an early functional defect in the proximal tubular cell. This is followed by a rise in the excretion of enzymes released as a result of structural damage of the cells and, finally, by the formation and excretion of cellular casts. Other low molecular weight proteins used as markers of tubular function are retinol-binding protein (21 kDa), protein HC (also known as α_1-microglobulin, 27 kDa), KIM-1, NGAL, interleukin-18, and fatty-acid binding proteins (FABPs).[47,156,157] These proteins are normally freely filtered at the glomerulus and then completely reabsorbed by the proximal tubule. Increases in their excretion are thus suggestive of tubular dysfunction but are not diagnostic, as an increased production rate or GFR less than 30 mL/min may lead to increased excretion. In each case, the maximal reabsorptive capacity may be exceeded, leading to net excretion of the protein.

Numerous urinary enzymes such as N-acetylglucosaminidase, alanine aminopeptidase, alkaline phosphatase, γ-glutamyltransferase, pyruvate kinase, glutathione transferase, lysozyme, and pancreatic ribonuclease have been used as diagnostic markers for renal disease. Jung et al.[158] compared the ability of five enzymes (N-acetylglucosaminidase, alanine aminopeptidase, alkaline phosphatase, γ-glutamyltransferase, and lysozyme) to detect early rejection episodes in kidney transplant patients. Only N-acetylglucosaminidase and alanine aminopeptidase were early predictors of rejection. N-acetylglucosaminidase is an enzyme contained within the lysosome of the tubular cell and is released when the lysosome is damaged, whereas alanine aminopeptidase is an enzyme of the brush border. Both markers were increased approximately 2 days earlier than serum creatinine in patients with transplant rejection.

QUALITATIVE DIAGNOSTIC PROCEDURES

Radiologic Studies

❾ The etiology of kidney disease can be evaluated using several qualitative diagnostic techniques, including radiography, ultrasonography, magnetic resonance imaging (MRI), and biopsy. The standard radiograph of the kidneys, ureters, and bladder provides a gross estimate of kidney size and identifies the presence of calcifications.[70] Although an easy test to perform, the value of the information is minimal, and more detailed evaluations are often necessary. The intravenous urogram (formerly known as intravenous pyelogram) involves the administration of a contrast agent to facilitate visualization of the urinary collecting system. It is primarily used in the assessment of structural changes that may be associated with hematuria, pyuria, or flank pain, resulting from recurrent urinary tract infections, obstruction, or stone formation. For patients with low GFRs, retrograde administration of dye into the ureters may be performed to facilitate visualization of the collecting system. Contrast agents are also employed during renal angiography for the assessment of renovascular disease. As a test for the diagnosis of renovascular hypertension, the captopril (angiotensin-converting enzyme inhibitor) test is a useful adjunct. Under conditions of unilateral renal artery stenosis, the affected kidney produces large quantities of angiotensin II, which constricts the efferent arteriole to maintain GFR. The administration of an angiotensin-converting enzyme inhibitor results in reduced uptake of the contrast agent because the efferent arteriole is dilated, thereby decreasing the perfusion pressure of the affected kidney. For patients with bilateral disease, a decrease in uptake is observed in both kidneys.[159] Computed tomography (CT) is a cross-sectional anatomical imaging procedure based on x-ray data. The procedure is frequently performed with contrast to enhance imaging. Spiral, or helical, CT, a more recent technique, provides for three-dimensional reconstruction of tissues. CT is performed as a test for the evaluation of obstructive uropathy, malignancy, and infections of the kidney.

Renal Ultrasonography

Ultrasonography uses sound waves to generate a two-dimensional image. The echogenicity of the kidney is compared with that of an adjacent organ—liver on the right and spleen on the left—with an increased echogenicity indicating an abnormal finding. Ultrasonography can distinguish the renal pyramids, medulla, and cortex, as well as abnormalities in structure, such as those that occur with obstruction. Renal ultrasonography is also used as a guide for site localization during percutaneous kidney biopsy.

Magnetic Resonance Imaging

MRI is based on aligning hydrogen nuclei in the body with the use of a powerful magnet and applying radiofrequency pulses. The signals emitted by the hydrogen nuclei during realignment on repeated pulses allows for generation of the tissue image. Realignment times can also be altered with the use of contrast agents (gadolinium and gadopentetate), leading to increased signal intensity and improved imaging. MRI is useful for the assessment of obstruction, malignancy, and renovascular lesions. The relative advantages and limitations of these procedures are discussed in more detail in recent reviews.[70,160]

Biopsy

Renal biopsy is used in several conditions to facilitate diagnosis when clinical, laboratory, and imaging findings prove inconclusive. Proteinuria and hematuria are both associated with renal parenchymal disease. When less invasive studies are unsuccessful in differentiating the cause, and the possible causes have different therapeutic approaches, biopsy may be indicated. The functional status of the kidney is not assessed with biopsy, and the severity of disease and progression are best measured using the quantitative tests discussed above. Contraindications to renal biopsy include a solitary kidney, severe hypertension, bleeding disorder, severe anemia, cystic kidney, and hydronephrosis. Complications resulting from biopsy primarily include hematuria, which may last for several days, and perirenal hematoma.[19]

CONCLUSION

The prevalence of kidney disease has increased dramatically over the past 2 decades, indicating a need for early identification, risk classification, and monitoring of renal function in patients with CKD. Comprehensive approaches to evaluating renal function in the clinical setting include the Cockcroft-Gault equation for estimating creatinine clearance and drug dosing, estimation of GFR in patients with CKD, and measurement of urinary protein excretion or albumin-to-creatinine ratio as a marker of the integrity of the glomerular basement membrane. The optimal care of patients identified as having CKD involves treatment modalities aimed at slowing or halting the progression of disease, as described in Chapter 51. Accurate measurement of GFR using exogenous administration of inulin, iothalamate, or radioisotope techniques such as ^{99m}Tc-DPTA is typically reserved for research settings to assess drug therapy outcomes and the progression of disease. Use of qualitative assessments of renal function, such as radiography, CT, MRI, sonography, and biopsy, can help to determine the underlying cause of kidney disease.

ABBREVIATIONS

AUC: Area under the plasma concentration versus time curve

CKD: Chronic kidney disease

CKD-EPI: Chronic kidney disease epidemiology collaboration

CL: Clearance

CL_{cr}: Creatinine clearance

C_{ss}: Concentration of a substance in plasma under steady-state conditions

CT: Computed tomography

eGFR: Estimated glomerular filtration rate

ER: Extraction ratio

ERBF: Effective renal blood flow

ERPF: Effective renal plasma flow

GFR: Glomerular filtration rate

HCT: Hematocrit

IBW: Ideal body weight

MDRD: Modification of Diet in Renal Disease study

NKF: National Kidney Foundation

PAH: Para-aminohippuric acid

S_{cr}: Serum creatinine

U_{cr}: urine creatinine concentration

REFERENCES

1. Levey AS, Eckardt KU, Tsukamoto Y, et al. Definition and classification of chronic kidney disease: A position statement from Kidney Disease: Improving Global Outcomes (KDIGO). Kidney Int 2005;67(6):2089–2100.

2. Stevens LA, Coresh J, Greene T, Levey AS. Assessing kidney function—Measured and estimated glomerular filtration rate. N Engl J Med 2006;354(23):2473–2483.

3. Campens D, Buntinx F. Selecting the best renal function tests. Int J Technol Assess Health Care 1997;13:343–356.

4. Dowling TC, Matzke GR, Murphy JE, Burckart GJ. Evaluation of renal drug dosing approaches: Label information and clinical pharmacist approaches. Pharmacotherapy 2010;30(8):776–786.

5. Sica DA, Schoolwerth AC. Renal handling of organic anions and cations: Excretion of uric acid. In: Brenner BM, ed. Brenner and Rector's The Kidney. 6th ed. Philadelphia, PA: WB Saunders; 2000:680–700.

6. Hsyu PH, Gisclon LG, Hui AC, Giacomini KM. Interactions of organic anions with the organic cation transporter in renal BBMV. Am J Physiol 1988;254:F56–F61.

7. Bendayan R. Renal drug transport: A review. Pharmacotherapy 1996;16:971–985.

8. Sikic BI. Pharmacologic approaches to reversing multidrug resistance. Semin Hematol 1997;34:40–47.

9. Bricker NS. On the meaning of the intact nephron hypothesis. Am J Med 1969;46:1–11.

10. Bosch JP. Renal reserve: A functional view of glomerular filtration rate. Semin Nephrol 1995;15:381–385.

11. Levin A, Singer J, Thompson CR, Ross H, Lewis M. Prevalent left ventricular hypertrophy in the predialysis population: Identifying opportunities for intervention. Am J Kidney Dis 1996;27:347–354.

12. Lacombe C, Mayeux P. The molecular biology of erythropoietin. Nephrol Dial Transplant 19 99;1994;14(Suppl 2):22–28.

13. Alvestrand A. Carbohydrate and insulin metabolism in renal failure. Kidney Int Suppl 1997;62:S48–S52.

14. Martin KJ, Olgaard K, Coburn JW, et al. Diagnosis, assessment, and treatment of bone turnover abnormalities in renal osteodystrophy. Am J Kidney Dis 2004;43(3):558–565.

15. Dowling TC, Briglia AE, Fink JC, et al. Characterization of hepatic cytochrome P4503A (CYP3A) activity in ESRD patients. Clin Pharmacol Ther 2003;73(5):427–434.

16. Nolin TD, Appiah K, Kendrick SA, Le P, McMonagle E, Himmelfarb J. Hemodialysis acutely improves hepatic CYP3A4, metabolic activity. J Am Soc Nephrol 2006;17(9):2363–2367.

17. Keane WF, Eknoyan G. Proteinuria, albuminuria, risk, assessment, detection, elimination (PARADE): A position paper of the National Kidney Foundation. Am J Kidney Dis 1999;33:1004–1010.

18. Kasiske BL, Keane WF. Laboratory assessment of renal disease: Clearance, urinalysis, and renal biopsy. In: Brenner BM, ed. Brenner and Rector's The Kidney. 6th ed. Philadelphia, PA: WB Saunders; 2000:1129–1170.

19. Rose BD, Renneke HG. Renal Pathophysiology—The Essentials. Baltimore, MD: Williams & Wilkins 1994.

20. Jones CA, McQuillan GM, Kusek JW, et al. Serum creatinine levels in the US population: Third National Health and Nutrition Examination Survey. Am J Kidney Dis 1998;32:992–999.

21. Bauer JH, Brooks CS, Burch RN. Clinical appraisal of creatinine clearance as a measurement of glomerular filtration rate. Am J Kidney Dis 1982;2:337–346.

22. Green AJE, Halloran SP, Mould GP, et al. Interference by newer cephalosporins in current methods for measuring creatinine. Clin Chem 1990;36:2139–2140.

23. Hanser AM, Parent X. Interference of clavulanic acid in the assay of creatinine using the Jaffe method on the Dade/RXL analyzer. Ann Biol Clin 2000;58(6):735–737.

24. Massoomi F, Matthews HG III, Destache CJ. Effect of seven fluoroquinolones on the determination of serum creatinine by the picric acid and enzymatic methods. Ann Pharmacother 1993;27:586–588.

25. Young DS, ed. Effects of Drugs on Clinical Laboratory Tests. 4th ed. Washington, DC: AACC Press; 1995:3.190–3.211.

26. Daly TM, Kempe KC, Scott MG, et al. "Bouncing" creatinine levels [Letter]. N Engl J Med 1996;334:1749–1750.

27. Van den Berg, Koopman MG, Arisz L. Ranitidine has no influence on tubular creatinine secretion. Nephron 1996;74:705–708.

28. Thakur V, Reisin E, Solomonow M, et al. Accuracy of formula-derived creatinine clearance in paraplegic subjects. Clin Nephrol 1997;47:237–242.

29. Mayersohn M, Conrad KA, Achari R. The influence of a cooked meat meal on creatinine plasma concentration and creatinine clearance. Br J Clin Pharmacol 1983;15:227–230.

30. Poortsmans JR, Francaux M. Long-term oral creatine supplementation does not impair renal function in healthy athletes. Med Sci Sports Exerc 1999;31:1108–1110.

31. Robinson TM, Sewell DA, Casey A, et al. Dietary creatine supplementation does not affect some haematological indices, or indices of muscle damage and renal function. Br J Sports Med 2000;34:284–288.

32. Edmunds JW, Jayapalan S, DiMarco NM, et al. Creatine supplementation increases renal disease progression in Han:SPRD-cy Rats. Am J Kidney Dis 2001;37:73–78.

33. Coll E, Botey A, Alvarez L, et al. Serum cystatin C as a new marker for noninvasive estimation of glomerular filtration rate and as a marker for early renal impairment. Am J Kidney Dis 2000;36:29–34.

34. Knight EL, Verhave JC, Spiegelman D, et al. Factors influencing serum cystatin C levels other than renal function and the impact on renal function measurement. Kidney Int 2004;65:1416–1421.

35. Levin A. Cystatin C, serum creatinine, and estimates of kidney function: Searching for better measures of kidney function and cardiovascular risk. Ann Intern Med 2005;142:586–588.

36. Keevil BG, Kilpatrick ES, Nichols SP, Maylor PW. Biological variation of cystatin C: Implications for the assessment of glomerular filtration rate. Clin Chem 1998;44(7):1535–1539.

37. Perkins BA, Nelson RG, Ostrander BE, et al. Detection of renal function decline in patients with diabetes and normal or elevated GFR by serial measurements of serum cystatin C concentration: Results of a 4-year follow-up study. J Am Soc Nephrol 2005;16:1404–1412.

38. Page MK, Bükki B, Luppa P, Neumeier D. Clinical value of cystatin C determination. Clin Chim Acta 2000;297:67–72.

39. Bokenkamp A, Domanetzki M, Zinck R, et al. Cystatin C serum concentrations underestimate glomerular filtration rate in renal transplant recipients. Clin Chem 1999;45:1866–1868.

40. Akbas SH, Yavuz A, Tuncer M, et al. Serum cystatin C as an index of renal function in kidney transplant patients. Transplant Proc 2004;36(1):99–101.

41. Brosius FC, Hostetter TH, Kelepouris E, et al. Detection of chronic kidney disease in patients with or at increased risk of cardiovascular disease: A science advisory from the American Heart Association Kidney and Cardiovascular Disease Council; the Councils on High Blood Pressure Research, Cardiovascular Disease in the Young, and Epidemiology and Prevention; and the Quality of Care and Outcomes Research Interdisciplinary Working Group: Developed in collaboration with the National Kidney Foundation. Circulation 2006;114(10):1083–1087.

42. Shlipak MG, Katz R, Sarnak MJ, et al. Cystatin C and prognosis for cardiovascular and kidney outcomes in elderly persons without chronic kidney disease. Ann Intern Med 2006;145(4):237–246.

43. MacDonald J, Marcora S, Jibani M, et al. GFR estimation using cystatin C is not independent of body composition. Am J Kidney Dis 2006;48:412–419.

44. Larsson A, Malm J, Grubb A, Hansson LO. Calculation of glomerular filtration rate expressed in mL/min from plasma cystatin C values in mg/L. Scand J Clin Lab Invest 2004;64:25–30.

45. Stevens LA, Coresh J, Schmid CH, et al. Estimating GFR using serum cystatin C alone and in combination with serum creatinine: A pooled analysis of 3,418 individuals with CKD. Am J Kidney Dis 2008;51:395–406.

46. Vupputuri S, Fox CS, Coresh J, et al. Differential estimation of CKD using creatinine- versus cystatin C-based estimating equations by category of body mass index. Am J Kidney Dis 2009;53:993–1001.

47. Coca SG, Parikh CR. Urinary biomarkers for acute kidney injury: Perspectives on translation. Clin J Am Soc Nephrol 2008;3:481–490.

48. Koyner JL, Bennett MR, Worcester EM, et al. Urinary cystatin C as an early biomarker of acute kidney injury following adult cardiothoracic surgery. Kidney Int 2008;74:1059–1069.

49. Vaidya VS, Waikar SS, Ferguson MA, et al. Urinary biomarkers for sensitive and specific detection of acute kidney injury in humans. Clin Transl Sci 2008;1:200–208.

50. Huber AR, Risch L. Recent developments in the evaluation of glomerular filtration rate: is there a place for beta-trace? Clin Chem 2005;51:1329–1330.

51. White CA, Akbari A, Doucette S, et al. Estimating GFR using serum beta trace protein: accuracy and validation in kidney transplant and pediatric populations. Kidney Int 2009;76:784–791.

52. White CA, Akbari A, Doucette S et al. A novel equation to estimate glomerular filtration rate using beta-trace protein. Clin Chem 2007;53:1965–1968.

53. Poge U, Gerhardt T, Stoffel-Wagner B, et al. Beta-trace protein-based equations for calculation of GFR in renal transplant recipients. Am J Transplant 2008;8:608–615.

54. Kobata M, Shimizu A, Rinno H, et al. Beta-trace protein, a new marker of GFR, may predict the early prognostic stages of patients with type 2 diabetic nephropathy. J Clin Lab Anal 2004;18:237–239.

55. Benlamri A, Nadarajah R, Yasin A, Lepage N, Sharma AP, Filler G. Development of a beta-trace protein based formula for estimation of glomerular filtration rate. Pediatr Nephrol 2010;25(3):485–490.

56. Brändle E, Sieberth HG, Hautman RE. Effect of chronic dietary protein intake on the renal function in healthy subjects. Eur J Clin Nutr 1996;50:734–740.

57. Knight EL, Stampfer MJ, Hankinson SE, Spiegelman D, Curhan GC. The impact of protein intake on renal function decline in women with normal renal function or mild renal insufficiency. Ann Intern Med 2003;138(6):460–467.

58. Brenner BM, Lawler EV, Mackenzie HS. The hyperfiltration theory: A paradigm shift in nephrology. Kidney Int 1996;49:1774–1777.

59. Woods LL. Intrarenal mechanisms of renal reserve. Semin Nephrol 1995;15:386–395.

60. Dowling TC, Frye RF, Fraley DS, Matzke GR. Comparison of iothalamate clearance methods for measuring GFR. Pharmacotherapy 1999;19(8):943–950.

61. Florijn KW, Barendregt JNM, Lentjes EGWM, et al. Glomerular filtration rate measurement by "single-shot" injection of inulin. Kidney Int 1994;46:252–259.

62. Dall'Amico R, Montini G, Pisanello L, et al. Determination of inulin in plasma and urine by reverse-phase high-performance liquid chromatography. J Chromatogr B Biomed Appl 1995;672:155–159.

63. Soper CPR, Bending MR, Barron JL. An automated enzymatic inulin assay, capable of full sinistrin hydrolysis. Eur J Clin Chem Clin Biochem 1995;33:497–501.

64. Agarwal R. Ambulatory GFR measurement with cold iothalamate in adults with chronic kidney disease. Am J Kidney Dis 2003;41(4):752–759.

65. Dowling TC, Frye RF, Zemaitis MA. Simultaneous determination of p-aminohippuric acid, acetyl-p-aminohippuric acid and iothalamate in human plasma and urine by high-performance liquid chromatography. J Chromatogr B Biomed Sci Appl 1998;716(1–2):305–313.

66. Agarwal R, Bills JE, Yigazu PM, et al. Assessment of iothalamate plasma clearance: duration of study affects quality of GFR. Clin J Am Soc Nephrol 2009;4:77–85.

67. Frennby B, Sterner G, Almán T, et al. The use of iohexol clearance to determine GFR in patients with severe chronic renal failure—A comparison between different clearance techniques. Clin Nephrol 1995;43:35–46.

68. Rocco MV, Buckalew VM Jr, Moore LC, Shihabi ZK. Measurement of glomerular filtration rate using nonradioactive iohexol: Comparison of two one-compartment models. Am J Nephrol 1996;16:138–143.

69. Lundqvist S, Hietala SO, Groth S, Sjödin JG. Evaluation of single sample clearance calculations in 902 patients. A comparison of multiple and single sample techniques. Acta Radiol 1997;38(1):68–72.

70. Hricak H, Meux M, Reddy GP. Radiologic assessment of the kidney. In: Brenner BM, ed. Brenner and Rector's The Kidney. 6th ed. Philadelphia, PA: WB Saunders; 2000:1171–1200.

71. Frennby B, Almén T, Lilja B, et al. Determination of the relative glomerular filtration rate of each kidney in man. Acta Radiol 1995;36:410–417.

72. Morton K, Pisani DE, Whiting JH Jr, et al. Determination of glomerular filtration rate using technitium-99m-DTPA with differing degrees of renal function. J Nucl Med Technol 1997;25:110–114.

73. Levey AS, Bosch JP, Lewis JB, et al. A more accurate method to estimate glomerular filtration rate from serum creatinine: A new prediction equation. Ann Intern Med 1999;130:461–470.

74. Levey AS, Greene T, Kusek J, Beck G. A simplified equation to predict glomerular filtration rate from serum creatinine. J Am Soc Nephrol 2000;11:155A.

75. Myers GL, Miller WG, Coresh J, et al. Recommendations for improving serum creatinine measurement: A report from the Laboratory Working Group of the National Kidney Disease Education Program. Clin Chem 2006;52:5–18.

76. Rule AD, Gussak HM, Pond GR, et al. Measured and estimated GFR in healthy potential kidney donors. Am J Kidney Dis 2004;43(1):112–119.

77. Lamb EJ, Webb MC, Simpson DE, Coakley AJ, Newman DJ, O'Riordan SE. Estimation of glomerular filtration rate in older patients with chronic renal insufficiency: Is the modification of diet in renal disease formula an improvement? J Am Geriatr Soc 2003;51(7):1012–1017.

78. Beddhu S, Samore MH, Roberts MS, et al. Creatinine production, nutrition, and glomerular filtration rate estimation. J Am Soc Nephrol 2003;14(4):1000–1005.

79. Poggio ED, Nef PC, Wang X, et al. Performance of the Cockcroft-Gault and modification of diet in renal disease equations in estimating GFR in ill hospitalized patients. Am J Kidney Dis 2005;46(2):242–252.

80. Snyder JJ, Foley RN, Collins AJ. Prevalence of CKD in the United States: A sensitivity analysis using the National Health and Nutrition Examination Survey (NHANES) 1999–2004. Am J Kidney Dis 2009;53(2):218–228.

81. Levey AS, Stevens LA, Schmid CH, et al. A new equation to estimate glomerular filtration rate. Ann Intern Med. 2009;150:604–612.

82. Rule AD, Larson TS, Bergstralh EJ, et al. Using serum creatinine to estimate glomerular filtration rate: Accuracy in good health and in chronic kidney disease. Ann Intern Med 2004;141:929–937.

83. Matsuo S, Imai E, Horio M, et al. Revised equations for estimated GFR from serum creatinine in Japan. Am J Kidney Dis 2009;53(6):982–992.

84. Li H, Zhang X, Xu G, et al. Determination of reference intervals for creatinine and evaluation of creatinine-based estimating equation for Chinese patients with chronic kidney disease. Clin Chim Acta 2009;403(1–2):87–91.

85. National Kidney Disease Education Program. 2009. *http://www.nkdep.nih.gov/professionals/gfr_calculators/index.htm.*

86. Lemann J, Bidani AK, Bain RP, et al. Use of the serum creatinine to estimate glomerular filtration rate in health and early diabetic nephropathy. Am J Kidney Dis 1990;16:236–243.

87. Roubenoff R, Drew H, Moyer M, et al. Oral cimetidine improves the accuracy and precision of creatinine clearance in lupus nephritis. Ann Intern Med 1990;113:501–506.

88. Zaltzman JS, Whiteside C, Cattran D, et al. Accurate measurement of impaired glomerular filtration using single-dose oral cimetidine. Am J Kidney Dis 1996;27:504–511.

89. Cockroft DW, Gault MH. Prediction of creatinine clearance from serum creatinine. Nephron 1976;16:31–41.

90. Spinler SA, Nawarskas JJ, Boyce EG, et al. Predictive performance of ten equations for estimating creatinine clearance in cardiac patients. Iohexol Cooperative Study Group. Ann Pharmacother 1998;32(12):1275–1283.

91. Salazar DE, Corcoran GB. Predicting creatinine clearance and renal drug clearance in obese patients from estimated fat-free body mass. Am J Med 1988;84(6):1053–1060.

92. Demirovic JA, Pai AB, Pai MP. Estimation of creatinine clearance in morbidly obese patients. Am J Health Syst Pharm 2009;66(7):642–648.

93. Luke DR, Halstenson CE, Opsahl JA, et al. Validity of creatinine clearance estimates in the assessment of renal function. Clin Pharmacol Ther 1990;48:503–508.

94. Mawer CE, Knowles BR, Lucas SB, et al. Computer-assisted prescribing of kanamycin for patients with renal insufficiency. Lancet 1972;1:12–15.

95. Jelliffe RW. Creatinine clearance: Bedside estimate. Ann Intern Med 1973;79:604–605.

96. Hull JH, Hak LJ, Koch GC, et al. Influence of range of renal function and liver disease on predictability of creatinine clearance. Clin Pharmacol Ther 1981;29:516–521.

97. Gault MH, Longerich LL, Harnett JD, et al. Predicting glomerular function from adjusted serum creatinine. Nephron 1992;62:249–256.

98. Coresh J, Toto RD, Kirk KA, et al. Creatinine clearance as a measure of GFR in screens for the African-American study of kidney disease. Am J Kidney Dis 1998;32:32–42.

99. Goldwasser P, Aboul-Magd A, Maru M. Race and creatinine excretion in chronic renal insufficiency. Am J Kidney Dis 1997;30:16–22.

100. Ikkes MCJ, Koopman MG, van Acker BAC, et al. Cimetidine improves GFR-estimation by the Cockcroft-Gault formula. Clin Nephrol 1997;47:229–236.

101. Schiff J, Paraskevas S, Keith D, et al. Prediction of the glomerular filtration rate using equations in kidney-pancreas transplant patients receiving cimetidine. Transplantation 2006;81(3):469–472.

102. Kemperman FA, Surachno J, Krediet RT, Arisz L. Cimetidine improves prediction of the glomerular filtration rate by the Cockcroft-Gault formula in renal transplant recipients. Transplantation 2002;73(5): 770–774.

103. Orlando R, Floreani M, Padrini R, Palatini P. Evaluation of measured and calculated creatinine clearances as glomerular filtration markers in different stages of liver cirrhosis. Clin Nephrol 1999;51:341–347.

104. Lam NP, Sperelakis R, Kuk J, et al. Rapid estimation of creatinine clearances in patients with liver dysfunction. Dig Dis Sci 1999;44:1222–1227.

105. Caregaro L, Menon F, Angeli P, et al. Limitations of serum creatinine level and creatinine clearance as filtration markers in cirrhosis. Arch Intern Med 1994;154:201–205.

106. Sansoe G, Ferrari A, Castellana CN, Bonardi L, Villa E, Manenti F. Cimetidine administration and tubular creatinine secretion in patients with compensated cirrhosis. Clin Sci 2002;102(1):91–98.

107. DeSanto NG, Anastasio P, Loguercio C, et al. Creatinine clearance: An inadequate marker of renal filtration in patients with early posthepatitic cirrhosis (Child A) without fluid retention and muscle wasting. Nephron 1995;70:421–424.

108. Skluzacek PA, Szewc RG, Nolan CR, et al. Prediction of GFR in liver transplant candidates. Am J Kidney Dis 2003;42(6):1169–1176.

109. Gonwa TA, Jennings L, Mai ML, et al. Estimation of glomerular filtration rates before and after orthotopic liver transplantation: Evaluation of current equations. Liver Transpl 2004;10(2):301–309.

110. Davis GA, Chandler MHH. Comparison of creatinine clearance estimation methods in patients with trauma. Am J Health Syst Pharm 1996;53:1028–1032.

111. Goerdt PJ, Heim-Duthoy KL, Macres M, Swan SK. Predictive performance of renal function equations in renal allografts. Br J Clin Pharmacol 1997;44:261–265.

112. Huang E, Hewitt R, Shelton M, Morse GD. Comparison of measured and estimated creatinine clearance in patients with advanced HIV disease. Pharmacotherapy 1996;16:222–229.

113. Quadri KH, Bernardini J, Greenberg A, et al. Assessment of renal function during pregnancy using a random urine protein to creatinine ratio and Cockcroft-Gault formula. Am J Kidney Dis 1994(3);24: 416–420.

114. Jelliffe RW. Estimation of creatinine clearance in patients with unstable renal function, without a urine specimen. Am J Nephrol 2002;22(4):320–324.

115. Chiou WL, Hsu FH. A new simple rapid method to monitor renal function based on pharmacokinetic considerations of endogenous creatinine. Res Commun Chem Pathol Pharmacol 1975;10: 315–330.

116. Brater DC. Drug Use in Renal Disease. Balgowlah, Australia: ADIS Health Science Press; 1983:22–56.

117. Bouchard J, Macedo E, Soroko S, et al. Comparison of methods for estimating glomerular filtration rate in critically ill patients with acute kidney injury. Nephrol Dial Transplant 2010;25(1):102–107.

118. Arant BS Jr. Developmental patterns of renal functional maturation compared in the human neonate. J Pediatr 1978;92:705–712.

119. van den Anker, de Groot R, Broerse HM, et al. Assessment of glomerular filtration rate in preterm infants by serum creatinine: Comparison with inulin clearance. Pediatrics 1995;96:1156–1158.

120. Sertel H, Scopes J. Rates of creatinine clearance in babies less than one week of age. Arch Dis Child 1973;48:717–720.

121. Bajaj G, Alexander SR, Browne R, et al. ^{125}Iodine-iothalamate clearance in children: A simple method to measure glomerular filtration. Pediatr Nephrol 1996;10:25–28.

122. Schwartz GJ, Brion LP, Spitzer A. The use of plasma creatinine concentration for estimating glomerular filtration rate in infants, children, and adolescents. Pediatr Clin North Am 1987;34:571–590.

123. Al-Harbi N, Lireman D. Comparison of three different methods of estimating the glomerular filtration rate in children after renal transplantation. Am J Nephrol 1997;17:68–71.

124. Fong J, Johnston S, Valentino T, Notterman D. Length/serum creatinine ratio does not predict measured creatinine clearance in critically ill children. Clin Pharmacol Ther 1995;58:192–197.

125. Pierrat A, Gravier E, Saunders C, et al. Predicting GFR in children and adults: A comparison of the Cockcroft-Gault, Schwartz, and modification of diet in renal disease formulas. Kidney Int 2003;64(4):1425–1436.

126. Lindeman RD, Tobin J, Shrock NW. Longitudinal studies on the rate of decline in renal function with age. J Am Geriatr Soc 1985;33:278–281.

127. Lindeman RD. Assessment of renal function in the old: Special considerations. Clin Lab Med 1993;13:269–277.

128. Fliser D, Ritz E, Franek E. Renal reserve in the elderly. Semin Nephrol 1995;15:463–467.

129. Smythe M, Hoffman J, Kizy K, et al. Estimating creatinine clearance in elderly patients with low serum creatinine concentrations. Am J Hosp Pharm 1994;51:198–204.

130. Roberts GW, Ibsen PM, Schiøler CT. Modified diet in renal disease method overestimates renal function in selected elderly patients. Age Ageing 2009;38(6):698–703.

131. O'Connell MB, Wong MO, Bannick-Mohrland SD, et al. Accuracy of 2- and 8-hour urine collections for measuring creatinine clearance in the hospitalized elderly. Pharmacotherapy 1993;13:135–142.

132. Wright JD, Tian C, Mutch DG, et al. Carboplatin dosing in obese women with ovarian cancer: a Gynecologic Oncology Group study. Gynecol Oncol 2008;109(3):353–358.

133. Spruill WJ, Wade WE, Cobb HH. Estimating glomerular filtration rate with a modification of diet in renal disease equation: implications for pharmacy. Am J Health-Syst Pharm 2007;64:652–660.

134. Wolowich WR, Raymo L, Rodriguez JC. Problems with the use of the Modified Diet in Renal Disease formula to estimate renal function. Pharmacotherapy 2005;25:1283–1285.

135. Bauer L. Creatinine clearance versus glomerular filtration rate for the use of renal drug dosing in patients with kidney dysfunction. Pharmacotherapy 2005;25:1286–1287.

136. Wargo KA, Eiland EH, Hamm W, et al. Comparison of the modification of diet in renal disease and Cockcroft-Gault equations for antimicrobial dosage adjustments. Ann Pharmacother 2006;40 (7–8):1248–1253.

137. Gill J, Malyuk R, Djurdjev O, Levin A. Use of GFR equations to adjust drug doses in an elderly multi-ethnic group—A cautionary tale. Nephrol Dial Transplant 2007;22(10):2894–2899.

138. Golik MV, Lawrence KR. Comparison of dosing recommendations for antimicrobial drugs based on two methods for assessing kidney function: Cockcroft-Gault and modification of diet in renal disease. Pharmacotherapy 2008;28(9):1125–1132.

139. Hermsen ED, Maiefski M, Florescu MC, Qiu, Rupp ME. Comparison of the Modification of Diet in Renal Disease and Cockcroft-Gault equations for dosing antimicrobials. Pharmacotherapy 2009;29:649–655.

140. Stevens LA, Nolin TD, Richardson MM. Comparison of drug dosing recommendations based on measured GFR and kidney function estimating equations. Am J Kidney Dis 2009;54(1):33–42.

141. Agodoa L, Eknoyan G, Ingelfinger J, et al. Assessment of structure and function in progressive renal disease. Kidney Int Suppl 1997;63:S144–S150.

142. Rossing P, Astrup AS, Smidt UM, et al. Monitoring kidney function in diabetic nephropathy. Diabetologia 1994;37:708–712.

143. Valensi P, Assayag M, Busby M, et al. Microalbuminuria in obese patients with or without hypertension. Int J Obes Relat Metab Disord 1996;20:574–579.

144. Berrut G, Bouhanick B, Fabbri P, et al. Microalbuminuria as a predictor of a drop in glomerular filtration rate in subjects with non-insulin-dependent diabetes mellitus and hypertension. Clin Nephrol 1997;48:92–97.

145. Mimran A, Ribstein J, DuCailar G. Is microalbuminuria a marker of early intrarenal vascular dysfunction in essential hypertension? Hypertension 1994;23:1018–1021.

146. Dworkin LD, Sun AM, Brenner BM. The renal circulations. In: Brenner BM, ed. Brenner and Rector's The Kidney. 6th ed. Philadelphia, PA: WB Saunders; 2000:277–318.

147. Dowling TC, Frye RF, Fraley DS, Matzke GR. Characterization of tubular functional capacity in humans using para-aminohippurate and famotidine. Kidney Int 2001;59:295–303.

148. Prescott LF, Freestone S, McAuslane JAN. The concentration-dependent disposition of intravenous p-aminohippurate in subjects with normal and impaired renal function. Br J Clin Pharmacol 1993;35:20–29.

149. Taylor A, Manatunga A, Morton K, et al. Multicenter trial validation of a camera-based method to measure Tc-99m mercaptoacetyltriglycine, or Tc-99m MAG$_3$, clearance. Radiology 1997;204:47–54.

150. Russell CD, Dubovsky EV. Comparison of single-injection multi-sample renal clearance methods with and without urine collection. J Nucl Med 1995;36:603–606.

151. Nassseri K, Daley-Yates PT. A comparison of N-1-methylnicotinamide clearance with 5 other markers of renal function in models of acute and chronic renal failure. Toxicol Lett 1990;53:243–245.

152. Edwards BD, Maiza A, Daley-Yates PT, et al. Altered clearance of N-1-methylnicotinamide associated with the use of low doses of cyclosporine. Am J Kidney Dis 1994;23:23–30.

153. Maiza A, Daley-Yates PT. Estimation of the renal clearance of drugs using endogenous N-1-methylnicotinamide. Toxicol Lett 1990;53: 231–235.

154. Karyekar CS, Eddington ND, Briglia AE, Gubbins PO, Dowling TC. Renal interaction between itraconazole and cimetidine. J Clin Pharmacol 2004;44:919–927.

155. Daw NC, Gregornik D, Rodman J, et al. Renal function after ifosfamide, carboplatin and etoposide (ICE) chemotherapy, nephrectomy and radiotherapy in children with Wilms tumor. Eur J Cancer 2009;45(1):99–106.

156. Jung K, Diego J, Strobelt V, et al. Diagnostic significance of some urinary enzymes for detecting acute rejection crises in renal transplant recipients: Alanine aminopeptidase, alkaline phosphatase, γ-glutamyl transferase, N-acetyl-β-glucosaminidase, and lysozyme. Clin Chem 1986;32:1807–1811.

157. Rosner MH. Urinary biomarkers for the detection of renal injury. Adv Clin Chem 2009;49:73–97.

158. Jung K. Urinary enzymes and low-molecular-weight proteins as markers of tubular dysfunction. Kidney Int Suppl 1994;47:S29–S33.

159. Taylor A, Nally JV. Clinical applications of renal scintigraphy. AJR Am J Roentgenol 1995;164:31–41.

160. Higgins TJ, Mindell HJ, Fairbank JT. Kidney imaging techniques. In: Greenberg A, ed. Primer on Kidney Diseases. 4th ed. Philadelphia, PA: Elsevier Saunders; 2005:47–55.

CHAPTER 51

Acute Kidney Injury

WILLIAM DAGER AND JENANA HALILOVIC

KEY CONCEPTS

❶ Risk, Injury, Failure, Loss of Kidney Function, and End-Stage Renal Disease (RIFLE) and Acute Kidney Injury Network (AKIN) criteria are two classification systems used to stage the severity of AKI. Both RIFLE and AKIN classes are based on separate criteria for serum creatinine (S_{cr}) and urine output.

❷ Acute kidney injury (AKI) is a common complication in the hospitalized patient and is associated with a high mortality rate.

❸ AKI is predominantly categorized based on the anatomical area of injury or malfunction: (a) prerenal—decreased renal blood flow, (b) intrinsic—a structure within the kidney is damaged, and (c) postrenal—an obstruction is present within the urine collection system.

❹ Conventional formulas used to calculate the glomerular filtration rate (GFR) and creatinine clearance should not be used to estimate renal function in patients with AKI. Instead, a change in S_{cr} from baseline and urine output information are more useful in determining the trend and severity of AKI. Currently, several novel biomarkers are being explored to aid in early detection and outcome prediction of AKI.

❺ Prevention is key; there are very few therapeutic options for the management of established AKI.

❻ Supportive management remains the primary approach to prevent or reduce the complications associated with severe AKI. Supportive therapies include renal replacement therapies (RRTs), nutritional support, avoidance of nephrotoxins, and blood pressure and fluid management.

❼ For those patients with prolonged or severe AKI, RRTs are the cornerstone of support and facilitate an aggressive approach to fluid, electrolyte, and waste management.

❽ Diuretic resistance is a common phenomenon in the patient with severe AKI and can be addressed with aggressive sodium restriction, combination diuretic therapy, or a continuous infusion of a loop diuretic.

❾ Drug-dosing regimens for AKI patients receiving intermittent hemodialysis (IHD) are predominantly extrapolated from data derived from patients with chronic kidney disease (CKD); however, important pharmacokinetic differences exist in patients with severe AKI that should be considered.

❿ Drug-dosing guidelines for AKI patients receiving continuous renal replacement therapies (CRRTs) are poorly characterized, and individualized doses may need to be determined by estimating the clearance of medications associated with a high risk of toxicity by the patient and the CRRT procedure.

The development of acute kidney injury (AKI) leading to acute renal failure (ARF) presents a difficult challenge to the clinician because there are many possible causes, and the onset may be asymptomatic. A thorough patient workup is often necessary and includes past medical and surgical history, medication use, physical examination, and multiple laboratory tests. The consequences of AKI can be serious, especially in hospitalized patients, among whom complications and mortality are particularly high. Supportive therapy is the focus of management for those with established AKI, as there is no therapy that directly reverses the injury associated with its numerous causes. Management goals include maintenance of blood pressure, fluid, and electrolyte homeostasis, all of which may be dramatically altered. Additional therapies designed to eliminate or minimize the insult that precipitated AKI include discontinuation of the offending drug (i.e., the nephrotoxin), aggressive hydration, maintenance of renal perfusion, and specific maneuvers to limit or reverse the kidney injury. Because of the poor clinical outcomes and lack of specific therapies, the importance of preventing AKI cannot be overemphasized. Individuals at highest risk, such as those with pre-existing organ failure, including chronic kidney disease (CKD), and the elderly with chronic medical conditions, need to be identified and their exposure to harmful diagnostic or therapeutic procedures or medications minimized.

Renal replacement therapies (RRTs), such as hemodialysis and peritoneal dialysis, have been available for decades but have not resulted in dramatic improvements in the outcomes of patients with AKI. However, newer RRT modalities, including an array of continuous renal replacement therapies (CRRTs), appear to offer some benefits, although available resources may limit their use, and drug dosing is challenging due to a paucity of data. Despite the supportive care that CRRTs offer, the development of AKI is frequently a catastrophic event. In this chapter, the epidemiology and multiple etiologies of AKI, as well as the clinical features associated with the most common types of AKI, are presented. Methods to recognize and identify the extent of functional loss are also discussed. Finally, preventive strategies and management approaches for those with established AKI are reviewed.

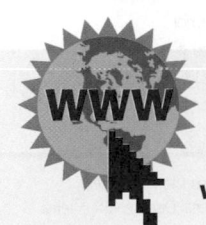

DEFINITION OF ACUTE KIDNEY INJURY

Before the first consensus definition of acute kidney injury was published in 2004, there was no agreement on the diagnostic criteria of this complex disorder. Acute renal failure (ARF) was the term commonly used to describe an abrupt decrease in the glomerular filtration rate (GFR) or the more clinically available index of renal function, creatinine clearance (CL_{cr}). The major challenge of using the term ARF was the lack of a universally accepted clinically relevant definition. In fact, more than 30 definitions for ARF have been reported in the medical literature, making comparisons and understanding of epidemiology, treatment, and patient outcome between studies difficult.[1] In 2004, the Acute Dialysis Quality Initiative (ADQI) group published a new consensus-derived definition and classification system for ARF called the Risk, Injury, Failure, Loss of Kidney Function, and End-Stage Kidney Disease (RIFLE) classification. The Risk, Injury, and Failure classes describe the three grades of renal dysfunction based on increasing severity. The patient is assigned a class based on the more severe change in the separate criteria of serum creatinine (S_{cr}) or urine output. Because the S_{cr} criteria are based on its change from baseline, the patient's renal function prior to the development of renal failure needs to be known. If the baseline measure of S_{cr}, CL_{cr}, or GFR is not available, and the patient has no history of renal dysfunction, one can estimate the baseline S_{cr} value by using the Modification of Diet in Renal Disease (MDRD) equation with an assumed normal GFR of 75 mL/min/1.73 m². The last two components of the RIFLE classification are Loss of Kidney Function, defined as the need for RRT for more than 4 weeks, and End-Stage Kidney Disease (ESKD), defined as the need for RRT for more than 3 months.[2]

In 2007, the Acute Kidney Injury Network (AKIN) slightly modified the RIFLE criteria (see Table 51-1 for an overview of both classification systems). The term acute renal failure was replaced by acute kidney injury to emphasize that the disorder exists along a wide continuum, ranging from mild renal dysfunction to the need for RRT. RIFLE-Risk, RIFLE-Injury, and RIFLE-Failure were replaced by AKIN stages 1, 2, and 3, respectively; Loss and End-Stage Kidney Disease were removed from the staging system but retained as outcomes. Also, a time frame of 48 hours was added as a diagnostic criterion to ensure that the process was indeed acute in nature. In an effort to increase the sensitivity of the RIFLE criteria, the change in S_{cr} was lowered from 0.5 mg/dL (44 μmol/L) to 0.3 mg/dL (27 μmol/L) for RIFLE-Risk class. Finally, AKIN criteria place all patients receiving RRT automatically into AKIN stage 3.[3]

❶ So far, the RIFLE classification has gained more recognition than the AKIN staging system, mostly because of the greater number of validation studies published. In addition, the few studies that have compared the RIFLE scoring system with the newly proposed AKIN criteria in critically ill patients have noted no difference in sensitivity or ability to predict outcome.[4,5]

Since the consensus guidelines on AKI were published, multiple studies have validated the ability of the RIFLE criteria to predict certain patient outcomes, particularly hospital mortality.[6,7] When compared with patients without AKI, mortality increases proportionally with the severity of renal dysfunction.[8] This increased risk of death may even persist in patients who recover their renal function after an AKI episode.[9] In addition, AKI is associated with increased length of hospital stay, ventilator days, need for RRT, and development of CKD and ESKD.[10]

Even though the RIFLE and AKIN staging systems have led to a standardized and widely accepted classification of AKI, their dependence on S_{cr} and urine output as the main diagnostic criteria is associated with some inherent weaknesses. An increase in S_{cr} is usually evident about 1 or 2 days after development of AKI. This lag time in S_{cr} rise may significantly delay diagnosis of AKI and adversely affect patient outcomes. Urine output reduction emerges earlier in AKI but is a very nonspecific marker because it may not always be present. In fact, patients with AKI can either be anuric (urine output <50 mL/day), oliguric (urine output <500 mL/day), or nonoliguric (urine output >500 mL/day). Urine output will also vary with volume status, diuretic administration, and presence of obstruction.[11]

EPIDEMIOLOGY

The epidemiology of AKI has been poorly characterized in part due to the lack of a standardized definition, differences in the population under study, and geographical location. AKI is considered to be an uncommon condition in the community-dwelling, generally healthy population, with an annual incidence depending on the definition that ranges from 0.01% to 0.06% (Table 51-2).[12] On the other hand, AKI is significantly more common in hospitalized individuals, with a reported incidence of 7% to 18%. Intensive care unit (ICU) patients have the highest risk of developing AKI, with 36% to 67% of critically ill patients being affected.[6,7]

❷ Increased mortality and morbidity are two well-recognized complications of AKI. Any degree of renal dysfunction is associated with an increased risk of death, particularly if the patient does not recover his or her baseline renal function at the time of hospital discharge.[13] The odds of death increase further with the severity of the RIFLE category.[14] For survivors of AKI, the development of

TABLE 51-1	RIFLE and AKIN Classification Schemes for Acute Kidney Injury[a]	
RIFLE category	**S_{cr} or GFR criteria**	**Urine output criteria**
Risk	S_{cr} increase to 1.5-fold or GFR decrease >25% from baseline	<0.5 mL/kg/h for ≥6 h
Injury	S_{cr} increase to 2-fold or GFR decrease >50% from baseline	<0.5 mL/kg/h for ≥12 h
Failure	S_{cr} increase to 3-fold or GFR decrease >75% from baseline, or S_{cr} ≥4 mg/dL (≥354 μmol/L) with an acute increase of at least 0.5 mg/dL (44 μmol/L)	Anuria for ≥12 h
Loss	Persistent acute renal failure = complete loss of function (RRT) for >4 weeks	
ESKD	RRT >3 months	
AKIN criteria	**S_{cr} criteria**	**Urine output criteria**
Stage 1	S_{cr} increase ≥0.3 mg/dL (≥27 μmol/L) or 1.5- to 2-fold from baseline	<0.5 mL/kg/h for ≥6 h
Stage 2	S_{cr} increase >2- to 3-fold from baseline	<0.5 mL/kg/h for ≥12 h
Stage 3	S_{cr} increase >3-fold from baseline or S_{cr} ≥4 mg/dL (≥354 μmol/L), with an acute increase of at least 0.5 mg/dL (44 μmol/L) or need for RRT	<0.3 mL/kg/h for ≥24 h or anuria for ≥12 h

[a]AKIN criteria require a time constraint of 48 hours for diagnosis. GFR decreases are specified only by RIFLE. In both cases, the criterion that leads to the worst possible diagnosis should be used.
AKIN = Acute Kidney Injury Network, ESKD = end-stage kidney disease, GFR = glomerular filtration rate, RIFLE = Risk, Injury, Failure, Loss of Kidney Function, and End-Stage Renal Disease, RRT = renal replacement therapy, S_{cr}, serum creatinine.

TABLE 51-2	Incidence and Outcomes of Acute Kidney Injury		
	Community-Acquired AKI	**Hospital-Acquired AKI**	**ICU-Acquired AKI**
Incidence	Low (<1%)	Moderate (7–20%)	High (35–70%)
Cause	Single	Single or multiple	Multifactorial
Overall mortality rate (%)	~15%	15–40%	30–90%
Common risk factors	Poor fluid intake, dehydration, drugs (ACEIs, ARBs, diuretics, NSAIDs, chemotherapy), infection, trauma, rhabdomyolysis	Volume depletion, hypotension, low cardiac output, nephrotoxic drugs, radiocontrast dyes	Sepsis/septic shock, major surgery, multiorgan failure, hypotension, low cardiac output, nephrotoxic drugs

ACEIs, angiotensin-converting enzyme inhibitors; AKI, ACE = angiotensin-converting enzyme, AKI = acute kidney injury, ARBs = angiotensin receptor blockers, ICU = intensive care unit; NSAIDs = nonsteroidal antiinflammatory drugs.

some degree of CKD and need for RRT are other important considerations.[15] Long-term follow-up studies indicate that patients continue to recover renal function up to 6 months after hospital discharge. Even though the majority of patients will recover normal kidney function, ~25% will have CKD, and 12.5% will remain dialysis-dependent.[16]

ETIOLOGY

❸ The etiology of AKI can be divided into broad categories based on the anatomic location of the injury associated with the precipitating factor(s). The management of patients presenting with this disorder is largely predicated on identification of the specific etiology responsible for the patient's current AKI (Fig. 51–1). Traditionally, the causes of AKI have been categorized as (a) prerenal, which results from decreased renal perfusion in the setting of undamaged parenchymal tissue, (b) intrinsic, the result of structural damage to the kidney, most commonly the tubule from a ischemic or toxic insult, and (c) postrenal, caused by obstruction of urine flow downstream from the kidney (Fig. 51–2).

Community-acquired AKI most commonly occurs secondary to renal hypoperfusion from volume depletion (dehydration, vomiting, and diarrhea), heart failure, or the ingestion of medications such as angiotensin-converting enzyme (ACE) inhibitors and angiotensin receptor blockers (ARBs). Other less common causes include infection (e.g., human immunodeficiency virus [HIV] nephropathy), trauma, rhabdomyolysis, and vascular events.[12,17] The most common cause of hospital- and intensive care unit (ICU)–acquired AKI is intrinsic, occurring as the result of ischemic or toxic acute tubular necrosis (ATN). The presence of underlying CKD increases the risk of AKI threefold. Other risk factors for developing AKI are advanced age (>65 years), multisystem organ failure, sepsis, preexisting chronic diseases, drugs, infection, surgery, malignancy, and bone marrow or solid organ transplantation.[12,18] It has been suggested that certain genetic polymorphisms responsible for vascular and inflammatory processes may contribute to the large variability in patient susceptibility to AKI.[19] However, evidence has been relatively inconclusive, and more research with higher quality studies will be necessary to confirm current findings.

PATHOPHYSIOLOGY

PSEUDORENAL KIDNEY INJURY

Pseudorenal AKI is characterized by a rise in either the blood urea nitrogen (BUN) or the S_{cr}, which misleadingly may suggest the presence of renal dysfunction, when in fact GFR is not diminished. This could be the result of cross-reactivity with the assay used to measure the BUN or S_{cr} or selective inhibition of the secretion of

creatinine into the proximal tubular lumen by certain medications (see Chapter 50). The initiation or discontinuation of such agents should be considered in the assessment for acute changes in renal function and should be looked for as part of the workup in any patient who is suspected of having AKI.

PRERENAL ACUTE KIDNEY INJURY

Prerenal AKI or prerenal azotemia results from hypoperfusion of the renal parenchyma, with or without systemic arterial hypotension. Renal hypoperfusion with systemic arterial hypotension may be caused by a decline in either the intravascular volume or the effective circulating blood volume. Intravascular volume depletion may result from several conditions, including hemorrhage, excessive gastrointestinal (GI) losses (severe vomiting or diarrhea), dehydration, extensive burns, and diuretic therapy. Effective circulating blood volume may be reduced in conditions associated with a decreased cardiac output and systemic vasodilation (e.g., sepsis). Renal hypoperfusion without systemic hypotension is most commonly associated with bilateral renal artery occlusion or unilateral occlusion in a patient with a single functioning kidney.

Patients with a mild reduction in effective circulating blood volume or volume depletion are generally able to maintain a normal GFR by activating several compensatory mechanisms. Those initial physiologic responses by the body stimulate the sympathetic nervous and the renin–angiotensin–aldosterone system and release antidiuretic hormone if hypotension is present. These responses work together to directly maintain blood pressure via vasoconstriction and stimulation of thirst, which in conscious patients results in increased fluid intake, as well as sodium and water retention. Additionally, GFR may be maintained by afferent arteriole dilation (mediated by intrarenal production of vasodilatory prostaglandins, kallikrein, kinins, and nitric oxide) and efferent arteriole constriction (mainly mediated by angiotensin II). In concert, these homeostatic mechanisms are often able to maintain arterial pressure and renal perfusion, potentially averting the progression to AKI.[20] If, however, the decreased renal perfusion is severe or prolonged, these compensatory mechanisms may be overwhelmed, and prerenal AKI will then be clinically evident.

Patients at risk for prerenal AKI are particularly susceptible to changes in the afferent and efferent arteriolar tone, as they may not be able to compensate as readily. Certain drug classes can interfere with these renal adaptive responses that are normally responsible for maintaining adequate renal perfusion. The resulting reduction in the glomerular hydrostatic pressure precipitates an abrupt decline in GFR and is sometimes referred to as functional AKI. A common cause of this syndrome is a decrease in efferent arteriolar resistance as the result of initiation of an ACE inhibitor or ARB (see Chapter 55) For example, individuals with heart failure are often given an ACE inhibitor or ARB to help improve left ventricular function, but if the dose is titrated too rapidly, they may experience

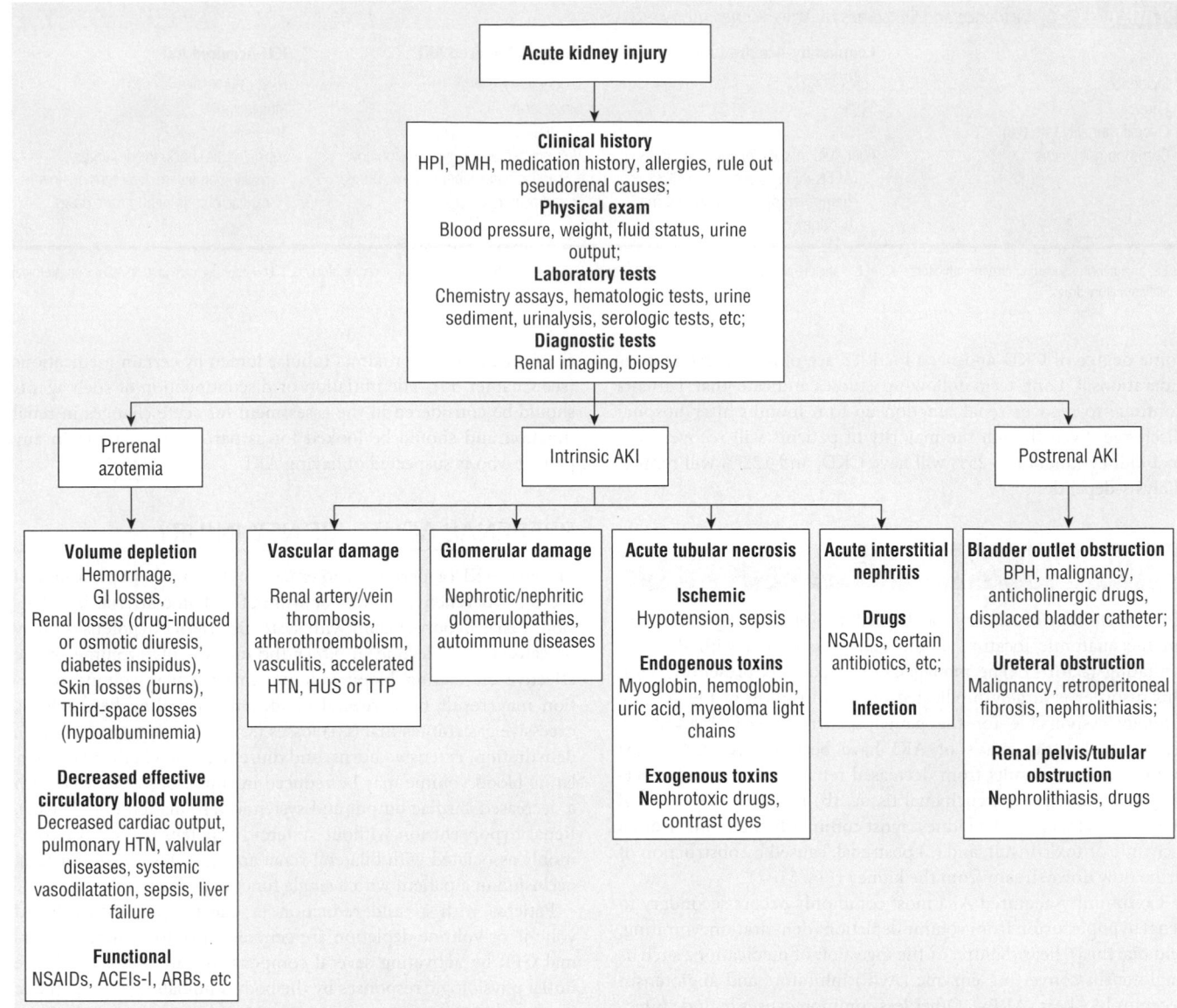

FIGURE 51-1. Classification of acute kidney injury (AKI) based on etiology. (ACEIs, angiotensin-converting enzyme inhibitors; ARBs, angiotensin receptor blockers; BPH, benign prostatic hyperplasia; GI, gastrointestinal; HTN, hypertension; HUS, hemolytic uremic syndrome; NSAIDs, nonsteroidal antiinflammatory drugs; TTP, thrombotic thrombocytopenic purpura.

a decline in their GFR. If the increase in the S_{cr} is less than 30% from baseline, the medication can be continued. Another classic example is initiation of ACE inhibitors or ARBs in patients with renovascular disease. It is estimated that ACE inhibitor–induced renal failure occurs in 6% to 23% of patients with bilateral renal artery stenosis and in ~38% of patients with unilateralstenosis who have a single kidney.[21] As a result, administration of ACE inhibitor or ARB therapy in the presence of those conditions is contraindicated. Nonsteroidal antiinflammatory drugs (NSAIDs) may also initiate AKI in susceptible individuals. NSAIDs inhibit renal prostaglandin production and afferent arteriolar vasodilation, which some patients rely on to maintain renal perfusion and GFR. Patients at risk for NSAID-induced AKI include those with CKD, volume depletion, and decreased effective circulating blood volume.[22]

If the causes of renal hypoperfusion are promptly corrected, prerenal AKI can be reversed and renal function returned to the patient's normal baseline in a matter of days. Prolonged prerenal azotemia, in contrast, can cause direct (and potentially irreversible) injury to the renal parenchyma and lead to development of ischemic ATN[23] (see the review of intrinsic AKI below).

INTRINSIC ACUTE KIDNEY INJURY

Intrinsic AKI results from direct damage to the kidney and is categorized on the basis of the injured structures within the kidney: the renal vasculature, glomeruli, tubules, and interstitium. Many diverse mechanisms associated with the development of intrinsic AKI are categorized in Figure 51–1.

Renal Vasculature Damage

Occlusion of the larger renal vessels resulting in AKI is not common but can occur if large atheroemboli or thromboemboli occlude the bilateral renal arteries or one vessel of the patient with a single kidney. Atheroemboli most commonly develop during vascular procedures that cause atheroma dislodgement, such as angioplasty and aortic manipulations. Thromboemboli may arise from dislodgement of a mural thrombus in the left ventricle of a patient with severe heart failure or from the atria of a patient with atrial fibrillation. Renal artery thrombosis may occur in a similar fashion to coronary thrombosis, in which a thrombus forms in conjunction with an atherosclerotic plaque.

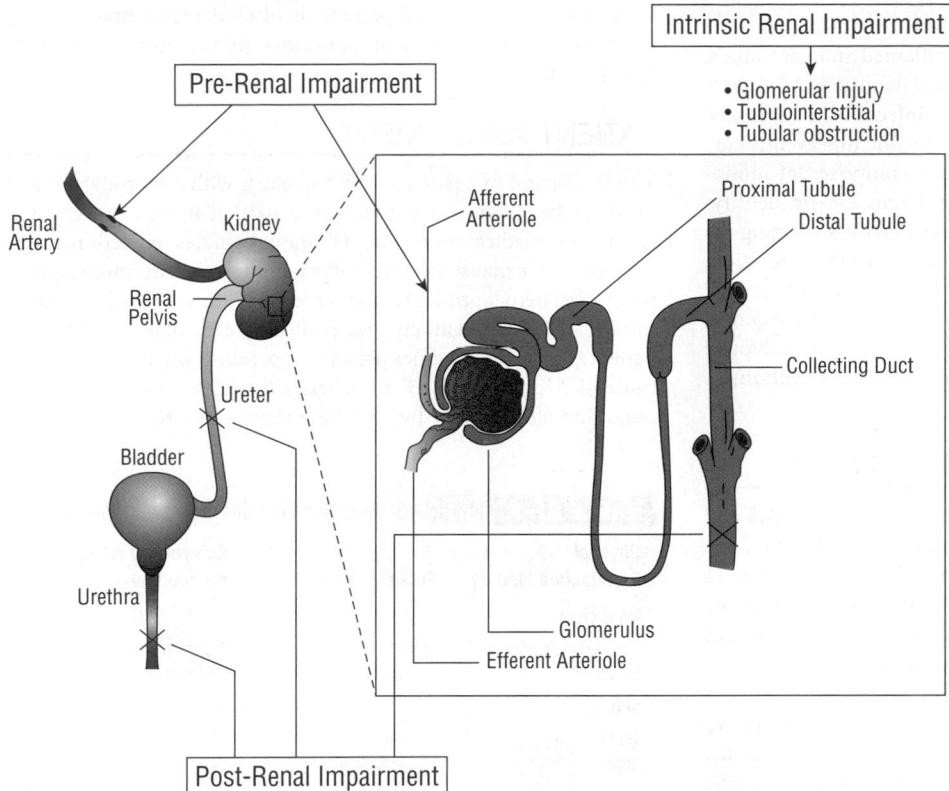

FIGURE 51-2. Physiologic classification of AKI. Blood flows through the afferent arteriole, to the glomerulus, and exits through the efferent arteriole. The formation of glomerular ultrafiltrate is dependent on the surface area of the capillaries within the glomerular region, their permeability, and the net hydrostatic pressure across the capillary wall. A decrease in blood flow and renal perfusion can lead to a prerenal reduction in renal function. Under conditions in which renal blood flow is diminished, the kidney maintains glomerular ultrafiltration by vasodilating the afferent and vasoconstricting the efferent arterioles. Medications that may interfere with these processes may result in an abrupt decline in glomerular filtration. Damage to the glomerular or tubular regions leads to intrinsic AKI. Obstruction of urine flow once in the collecting tubule, ureter, bladder, or urethra is termed postrenal impairment.

Although smaller vessels can also be obstructed by atheroemboli or thromboemboli, the damage is limited to the vessels involved, and the development of significant AKI is unlikely. However, these small vessels are susceptible to inflammatory processes that lead to microvascular damage and vessel dysfunction when the renal capillaries are affected. Neutrophils invade the vessel wall, causing damage that can include thrombus formation, tissue infarction, and collagen deposition within the vessel structure. Diffuse renal vasculitis can be mild or severe, with severe forms promoting concomitant ischemic ATN. The S_{cr} is usually elevated when the lesions are diffuse; thus, the area of damage is large. Accelerated hypertension that is not treated may also compromise renal microvascular blood flow, causing diffuse renal capillary damage.

Glomerular Damage

Only 5% of the cases of intrinsic AKI are of glomerular origin. The glomerulus is one of two capillary beds in the kidney. It serves to filter fluid and solute into the tubules while retaining proteins and other large blood components in the intravascular space. Because the glomerulus is a capillary system, similar damage observed in the renal vasculature by the same mechanisms can occur in addition to severe inflammatory processes specific to the glomerulus. The pathophysiology and specific therapeutic approaches to glomerulonephritis are described in detail in Chapter 56.

Tubular Damage

Approximately 85% of all cases of intrinsic AKI are caused by ATN, of which 50% are a result of renal ischemia, often arising from an extended prerenal state. The remaining 35% are the result of exposure to direct tubule toxins, which can be endogenous (myoglobin, hemoglobin, or uric acid) or exogenous (contrast agents, aminoglycoside antibiotics, etc.). The tubules located within the medulla of the kidney are particularly at risk from ischemic injury, as this portion of the kidney is metabolically active and thus has high oxygen requirements, yet even in the best of situations, receives relatively low oxygen delivery (as compared with the cortex). Thus, ischemic conditions caused by severe hypotension or exposure to vasoconstrictive drugs preferentially affect the tubules more than any other portion of the kidney.

The clinical evolution of ATN is characterized by three distinct phases: initiation, maintenance, and recovery. The hallmarks of the initiation phase are ischemic injury and GFR reduction, both of which occur as a result of the interplay of several different pathophysiologic processes. Ischemic injury causes tubular epithelial cell necrosis or apoptosis and is followed by an extension phase with continued hypoxia and an inflammatory response involving the nearby interstitium. The loss of epithelial cells between the filtrate and the interstitium leaves the basement membrane denuded and unable to appropriately regulate fluid and electrolyte transfer across the tubular lumen. As a result, the glomerular filtrate starts leaking back into the interstitium and is reabsorbed into the systemic circulation. Additionally, urine flow is obstructed by accumulation of sloughed epithelial cells, cellular debris, and formation of casts. The onset of ATN can occur over hours to days, depending on the factors responsible for the damage to the tubular epithelial cells. Regardless of the etiology; tubular injury, back leakage, and obstruction lead to a loss in the ability to concentrate urine, decreased urine output, and, ultimately, reduction in the GFR. Continued kidney hypoxia or toxin exposure after the original insult kills more cells and propagates the inflammatory response; it also can extend the injury and delay the recovery process. With prolonged ischemia, the tubular epithelial cells in the corticomedullary junction are damaged and die.[23] When the toxin or ischemia is removed, a maintenance phase ensues and may last anywhere from a few weeks to several months. The maintenance phase is eventually followed by a recovery phase, during which new tubule cells are regenerated. The recovery phase is associated with a notable diuresis, which requires prompt attention to maintain fluid balance, or a secondary prerenal injury may occur. However, if the ischemia or injury is extremely severe or prolonged, cortical necrosis may occur, limiting tubule cell regrowth in the affected areas.[21]

Interstitial Damage

If the renal interstitium becomes severely inflamed and edematous, it can lead to development of acute interstitial nephritis (AIN). AIN may be caused by drugs (see Chapter 55), infections, and, rarely, autoimmune idiopathic diseases. Whatever the inciting event, acute interstitial injury is characterized by lesions comprised of monocytes, eosinophils, macrophages, B cells, or T cells, clearly identifying an immunologic response as the injurious process affecting the interstitium. If AIN is caused by a drug hypersensitivity reaction, most patients will regain normal renal function within several weeks if the offending drug is promptly discontinued. If symptoms of AIN remain unrecognized, and the exposure to the causative agent continues, persistent renal dysfunction associated with interstitial fibrosis and tubular atrophy may develop.[24]

POSTRENAL ACUTE KIDNEY INJURY

Postrenal AKI accounts for less than 5% of all cases of AKI and may develop as the result of obstruction at any level within the urinary collection system from the renal tubule to the urethra (see Fig. 51–1).[23] However, if the obstructing process is above the bladder, it must involve both kidneys (one kidney in a patient with a single functioning kidney) to cause significant AKI, as one functioning kidney can generally maintain a near normal GFR. Bladder outlet obstruction, the most common cause of obstructive uropathy, is often the result of a prostatic process (hypertrophy, cancer, or infection), producing a physical impingement on the urethra and thereby preventing the passage of urine. It may also be the result of an improperly placed urinary catheter. Neurogenic bladder or anticholinergic medications may prevent bladder emptying and cause AKI. The blockage may occur at the ureter level, secondary to nephrolithiasis, blood clots, sloughed renal papillae, or physical compression by an abdominal process, such as retroperitoneal fibrosis, cancer, or an abscess. Crystal deposition within the tubules from oxalate and some medications severe enough to cause AKI is uncommon, but it is possible in patients with severe volume contraction and in those receiving large doses of a drug with relatively low urine solubility (see Chapter 55). In these cases, patients have insufficient urine volume to prevent crystal precipitation in the urine.[25] Extremely elevated uric acid concentrations from chemotherapy-induced tumor lysis syndrome can cause obstruction and direct tubular injury as well. Wherever the location of the obstruction, urine will accumulate in the renal structures above the obstruction and cause increased pressure upstream. The ureters, renal pelvis, and calyces all expand, and the net result is a decline in GFR. If renal vasoconstriction ensues, a further decrement in GFR will be observed.

CLINICAL PRESENTATION

The initiating sign or symptom prompting the clinical suspicion of AKI is highly variable and largely dependent on the underlying etiology. It may be a change in urinary habits (e.g., decreased urine output or urine discoloration), sudden weight gain, or severe abdominal or flank pain. Early recognition and cause identification are critical, as they directly affect the outcome of AKI. One of the first steps in the diagnostic process is to determine if the renal complication is acute, chronic, or the result of an acute change in a patient with known CKD (also called acute-on-chronic renal failure). Patients should also be promptly evaluated for any changes in their fluid and electrolyte status. Patients presenting with AKI in the outpatient environment may have very nonspecific or seemingly unrelated symptoms so that the time of onset of the injury can be difficult to determine. On the other hand, AKI in hospitalized patients is often detected much earlier in its course due to frequent laboratory studies and daily patient assessment.

PATIENT ASSESSMENT

The assessment of a patient with AKI starts with a thorough review of his or her medical records, with a particular focus on chronic conditions, medication history, laboratory studies, procedures, and surgeries. An exhaustive review of prescription and nonprescription medicines, herbal products, and recreational drugs may help determine if AKI was potentially precipitated by drug ingestion. Overall, patient presentation varies widely, depending on the underlying cause of AKI. Table 51–3 summarizes the most common physical exam findings associated with different types of AKI.

TABLE 51–3	Physical Examination Findings in Acute Kidney Injury	
Physical Examination Finding	**Possible Diagnosis**	**Category of Acute Kidney Injury**
Vital signs		
Orthostatic hypotension	Volume depletion	Prerenal
Febrile	Sepsis	Intrinsic: tubule necrosis
Skin		
Tenting	Volume depletion	Prerenal
Rash	Hypersensitivity reaction	Intrinsic: interstitial nephritis
Petechiae	Thrombotic: thrombocytopenic purpura	Intrinsic: vasculitis
	Hemolytic uremic syndrome	
	Sepsis	Intrinsic: tubule necrosis
Splinter hemorrhages	Endocarditis	Intrinsic: glomerulonephritis
Janeway lesions		
Osler nodes		
Edema	Total-body volume overload	Intrinsic or prerenal because of heart failure
		Other types of prerenal unlikely
HEENT		
Hollenhorst plaque	Cholesterol emboli	Intrinsic: vascular
Roth spots	Endocarditis	Intrinsic: glomerulonephritis
	Heart failure	
Elevated jugular venous pressure	Pulmonary hypertension	Prerenal
Heart		
S$_3$ heart sound	Heart failure	Prerenal
New or increased murmur	Endocarditis	Intrinsic: glomerulonephritis
Lung		
Rales	Heart failure	Prerenal
Abdomen		
Renal artery bruit	Renal artery stenosis	Prerenal
Ascites	Liver failure or right-heart failure	Prerenal Hepatorenal syndrome
Bladder distension	Bladder outlet obstruction	Postrenal
Genitourinary		
Prostatic enlargement	Prostatic hypertrophy or cancer	Postrenal
Gynecologic		
Abnormal bimanual examination	Possible bilateral ureteral obstruction or cervical cancer	Postrenal

HEENT = head, eyes, ears, nose, and throat.

During the initial patient evaluation, presumptive signs and symptoms of AKI need to be differentiated from a potential new diagnosis of CKD. A past medical history for renal disease–related chronic conditions (e.g., poorly controlled hypertension and diabetes mellitus), previous laboratory data documenting the presence of proteinuria or an elevated S_{cr}, and the finding of bilateral small kidneys on renal ultrasonography suggest the presence of CKD rather than AKI. However, it is important to note that patients with CKD may develop episodes of AKI as well. In that case, an abrupt rise in the patient's baseline S_{cr} is one of the most useful indicators of the presence of an acute insult to the kidneys.

An acute change in urinary habits is another common and noticeable symptom associated with AKI. The presence of cola-colored urine is indicative of blood in the urine, a finding commonly associated with acute glomerulonephritis. In hospitalized patients, changes in urine output may be helpful in characterizing the cause of the patient's AKI. Acute anuria is typically caused by either complete urinary obstruction or a catastrophic event (e.g., shock or acute cortical necrosis). Oliguria, which often develops over several days, suggests prerenal azotemia, whereas nonoliguric renal failure usually results from acute intrinsic renal failure or incomplete urinary obstruction.

Depending on the underlying cause of AKI, patients may present with a variety of symptoms affecting virtually any organ system of the body. Constitutional symptoms such as nausea, vomiting, fatigue, and malaise are common but nonspecific. The onset of flank pain is suggestive of a urinary stone; however, if bilateral, it may suggest swelling of the kidneys secondary to acute glomerulonephritis or acute interstitial nephritis. Complaints of severe headaches may suggest the presence of severe hypertension and vascular damage. The presence of fever, rash, and arthralgias may be indicative of drug-induced acute interstitial nephritis or lupus nephritis. A recent increase in the patient's weight or complaints of tight-fitting rings secondary to salt and water retention indicate prerenal causes and may be helpful in defining the time of onset of kidney injury.

A thorough physical examination is an important step in evaluating individuals with AKI, as clues regarding the etiology can be evident from the patient's head (eye exam) to toe (evidence of dependent edema) assessment. Observations will either support or refute the cause as prerenal, intrinsic, or postrenal. Evaluation of the volume and hemodynamic status is critical as well, as it will guide patient management. For example, patients with prerenal AKI can present with either volume depletion or fluid overload. Volume depletion may be evidenced by the presence of postural hypotension, decreased jugular venous pressure (JVP), and dry mucous membranes. Fluid overload, on the other hand, is often reflected by elevated JVP, pitting edema, ascites, and pulmonary crackles.

LABORATORY TESTS AND INTERPRETATION

CONVENTIONAL MARKERS OF KIDNEY FUNCTION

❹ The commonly available laboratory tests used to evaluate the patient with renal insufficiency are described in Chapter 50, and those of particular value in the assessment of renal function in patients with AKI are highlighted in Table 51–4. Over the past 3 decades, S_{cr} has been the most widely used laboratory test for estimating creatinine clearance (by the Cockroft-Gault equation), which, in turn, was used as a surrogate marker for GFR. Only in the last 10 years has the multiple versions of the Modification of Diet in Renal Disease (MDRD) equation been used as an alternative method for determining GFR in patients with CKD.[26] Numerous other equations and markers have been proposed to estimate GFR

TABLE 51-4	Diagnostic Parameters for Differentiating Causes of Acute Kidney Injury[a]		
Laboratory Test	**Prerenal Azotemia**	**Acute Intrinsic Kidney Injury**[b]	**Postrenal Obstruction**
Urine sediment	Hyaline casts, may be normal	Graunular casts, cellular debris	Cellular debris
Urinary RBC	None	2–4+	Variable
Urinary WBC	None	2–4+	1+
Urine Na (mEq/L or mmol/L)	<20	>40	>40
FE_{Na} (% [fraction])	<1 [<0.01]	>2 [>0.02]	Variable
Urine/serum osmolality	>1.5	<1.3	<1.5
Urine$_{cr}$/S$_{cr}$	>40:1	<20:1	<20:1
BUN/S$_{cr}$ (SI units)	>20 (<1:12.4)	~15 (~1:16)	~15 (~1:16)
Urine-specific gravity	>1.018	<1.012	Variable

[a]Common laboratory tests are used to classify the cause of acute kidney injury (AKI). Functional AKI, which is not included in this table, would have laboratory values similar to those seen in prerenal azotemia. However, the urine osmolality-to-plasma osmolality ratios may not exceed 1.5, depending on the circulating levels of antidiuretic hormone.
[b]The laboratory results listed under Acute Intrinsic Kidney Injury are those seen in acute tubular necrosis, the most common cause of such injury.
BUN = blood urea nitrogen, FE_{Na} = fractional excretion of sodium, RBC = red blood cell, S_{cr} = serum creatinine, WBC = white blood cell.

accurately.[27] However, the Cockroft-Gault and MDRD 4-variable equations have so far remained the most widely used for estimating renal function in clinical practice.

There are several limitations associated with its use. S_{cr} varies widely with a patient's age, gender, muscle mass, diet, and hydration status. For example, patients with reduced creatinine production, such as those with low muscle mass, may have very low S_{cr} values (<0.6 mg/dL [<53 μmol/L]); thus, the presence of a gradual S_{cr} rise to normal values (0.8–1.2 mg/dL [71–106 μmol/L]) may actually indicate reduced GFR. When coupled with a decline in urine output, this might suggest the presence of AKI. However, in the presence of improved nutrition and a large muscle mass, an S_{cr} of 1.2 mg/dL (106 μmol/L) may be a true representation of a person's current renal status. Instead of using fixed numbers to determine renal function, changes in the value from a patient's baseline need to be reviewed. S_{cr} is normally inversely proportional to GFR. However, rapid changes in GFR (as they occur in AKI) disrupt this equilibrium and make S_{cr} a very insensitive marker. In fact, changes in S_{cr} will lag behind the GFR's decline due to slow accumulation, increased tubular secretion, and increased extrarenal clearance.[28] This can lead to a significant overestimation of the patient's GFR in the early stages of AKI and consequently a potential delay in the diagnosis of the disorder.

An example of this phenomenon is illustrated by an acute renal artery thrombus that results in abrupt cessation of GFR in one kidney as a consequence of the complete obstruction of blood flow to that kidney (Fig. 51–3). Although 5 minutes following the event GFR is decreased 50% (assuming the other kidney is functioning and unaffected), the S_{cr} remains unchanged. Assuming a standard daily creatinine production of ~20 mg/kg of lean body weight, one can expect ~1.4 g of creatinine production in a 24-hour period in a 70 kg individual. In pharmacokinetic terms, daily creatinine production is analogous to a continuous infusion, and GFR determines the elimination rate of creatinine. In a patient with normal renal function (GFR of 120 mL/min [2.00 mL/s]), the half-life of creatinine is 3.5 hours, with 95% of steady state achieved in ~14 hours. If GFR declines to 50%, 25%, or 10% of normal, the half-life of creatinine increases, resulting in prolongation of the time to reach 95% of steady state, specifically taking 1, 2, and 4 days, respectively.[29]

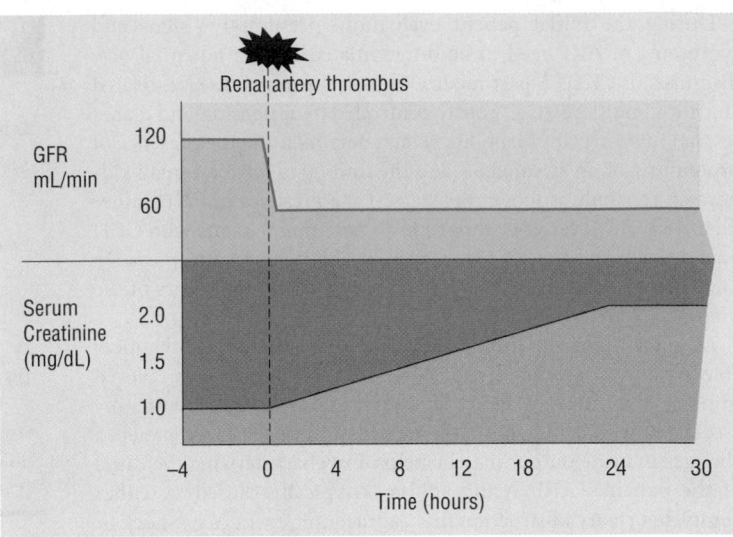

FIGURE 51-3. Glomerular filtration rate (GFR; mL/min) and serum creatinine (S_cr; g/dL) versus time following acute renal injury. Prior to time 0, a GFR of 120 mL/min and an S_cr of 1 g/dL exist. At time 0, an abrupt renal artery thrombus forms, depriving one kidney of renal blood flow. Composite GFR immediately declines by 50% to ~60 mL/min. However, S_cr does not increase immediately, as it is dependent on creatinine production and attainment of steady-state serum concentrations. For comparison of values to SI units, multiply serum creatinine in mg/dL by 88.4 to give units of μmol/L; multiply GFR in mL/min by 0.0167 to give units of mL/s.

Because of the challenges associated with the accuracy of S_{cr} in AKI, several GFR calculation methods, such as the Cockcroft-Gault, MDRD, and Chronic Kidney Disease Epidemiology Collaboration (CKD-EPI) equations, should not be used in AKI patients with unstable renal function. These equations will typically overestimate GFR when the AKI is worsening and underestimate it when the AKI is resolving. Instead, it may be useful to evaluate changes in S_{cr} values from the patient's baseline and also consider the S_{cr} sequence values to determine if renal function is potentially improving (values declining) or worsening (values rising). The most recent S_{cr} value reflects the time-averaged kidney function over the preceding time period. Several mathematical approaches to estimate GFR in patients with unstable S_{cr} that incorporate the principles of creatinine accumulation and elimination have been proposed and are discussed in detail in Chapter 50.[30,31] These methods have not been extensively validated in the setting of acute alterations in renal function, and their value for adjusting medication dosing is questionable. Additionally, these equations are complex and are not commonly used in the clinical setting.

Two other widely available markers of renal function are BUN and urine output. BUN is widely used to assess hemodialysis adequacy in chronic hemodialysis patients. However, its use in AKI is very limited because urea's production and renal clearance are heavily influenced by extrarenal factors such as critical illness, volume status, protein intake, and medications. Urine output measured over a specified period of time (e.g., 4–24 hours) allows for short-term assessment of kidney function, but its utility is limited to cases in which it is significantly decreased. The presence of anuria suggests complete kidney failure, whereas oliguria indicates some level of kidney damage. Urine output needs to be interpreted with caution, as it is dependent on several factors, such as hydration status and medications. As mentioned earlier in the chapter, a patient may have AKI and still maintain a normal urine output; this condition is referred to as nonoliguric AKI.

Another approach to measuring renal function when S_{cr} values alone are not reflective of function is to directly measure creatinine clearance over a short period of time, for example, 4 to 12 hours.[32] Although potentially precise and fairly simple to do, accuracy is questionable because the urine output is generally low, and if the collection is incomplete, the lost urine can have a dramatic impact on the clearance determination.

Currently, in addition to BUN and S_{cr}, selected blood tests, urinary chemistry, and urinary sediment are routinely used to differentiate the cause of AKI and guide patient management. For example, a complete blood cell count with differential can help rule out infectious causes of AKI. Serum electrolyte values are likely to be abnormal because of the acute decline of the kidney's ability to regulate electrolyte excretion, and particular attention should be paid to serum potassium and phosphorus values, which can be markedly elevated and cause life-threatening complications.

In individuals with normal renal function, the ratio between BUN and S_{cr} is usually less than 15:1 using conventional units (1:16 using SI units). In the presence of prerenal AKI, reabsorption of BUN exceeds that of creatinine; thus, one often sees a ratio greater than 20:1 (1:12.4). Given the limited usefulness of solely using S_{cr} or BUN concentrations to differentiate the etiology of AKI, urinary electrolytes and osmolality should be determined, and both a microscopic and chemical analysis of the urine should be performed (Table 51–5). The finding of a high urinary specific gravity, in the absence of glucosuria or mannitol administration, suggests an intact urinary concentrating mechanism and that the cause of the patient's AKI is likely prerenal azotemia. The presence of urinary protein is often difficult to interpret, especially in the setting of acute or chronic renal failure. A patient with CKD may have a baseline proteinuria, thus clouding the clinical presentation, unless this is known at the time of AKI assessment. Classically, proteinuria is a hallmark of glomerular damage. However, tubular damage can also result in proteinuria, as the tubules are responsible for reabsorbing small proteins that are normally filtered by all glomeruli. The presence of blood also results in a positive urine protein test, so this confounder must always be assessed when a positive urine protein is obtained. Hematuria suggests acute intrinsic AKI secondary to glomerular injury, infection, or a kidney stone. On microscopic examination, the key findings are cells, casts, and crystals, and the presence of one or more of these suggest specific etiologies of the AKI (Table 51–5). The presence of crystals may suggest nephrolithiasis and a postrenal obstruction. If red blood cells or red blood cell casts are present, one should consider the presence of a physical injury to the glomerulus, renal parenchyma, or vascular beds. The finding of white blood cells or white blood cell casts suggests interstitial inflammation (i.e., interstitial nephritis), which can be secondary to an allergic, granulomatous, or infectious process.

Simultaneous measurement of urine and serum electrolytes is also helpful in the setting of AKI (see Table 51–4). From these values, a

TABLE 51-5 Urinary Findings as a Guide to the Etiology of Acute Kidney Injury

Type of Urinary Evaluation	Presence of	Suggestive of
Urinalysis	Leukocyte esterases	Pyelonephritis
	Nitrites	Pyelonephritis
	Protein	
	Mild (<0.5 g/day)	Tubular damage
	Moderate (0.5–3 g/day)	Glomerulonephritis, pyelonephritis, tubular damage
	Large (>3 g/day)	Glomerulonephritis, nephrotic syndrome
	Hemoglobin	Glomerulonephritis, pyelonephritis, renal infarction, renal tumors, kidney stones
	Myoglobin	Rhabdomyolysis-associated tubular necrosis
	Urobilinogen	Hemolysis-associated tubular necrosis
Urine sediment	Microorganisms	Pyelonephritis
Cells	Red blood cells	Glomerulonephritis, pyelonephritis, renal infarction, papillary necrosis, renal tumors, kidney stones
	White blood cells	Pyelonephritis, interstitial nephritis
	Eosinophils	Drug-induced interstitial nephritis, renal transplant rejection
	Epithelial cells	Tubular necrosis
Casts	Granular casts	Tubular necrosis
	Hyaline casts	Prerenal azotemia
	White blood cell casts	Pyelonephritis, interstitial nephritis
	Red blood cell casts	Glomerulonephritis, renal infarct, lupus nephritis, vasculitis
Crystals	Urate	Postrenal obstruction
	Calcium phosphate	Postrenal obstruction

fractional excretion of sodium can be calculated. The equation for the calculation of the fractional excretion of sodium (FE_{Na}) is

$$FE_{Na} = (\text{excreted Na/filtered Na}) \times 100$$
$$= (U_{vol} \times U_{Na})/(GFR \times S_{Na}) \times 100$$

where

$$GFR = (U_{vol} \times U_{cr})/(S_{cr} \times t)$$

Thus,

$$FE_{Na} = (U_{Na} \times S_{cr} \times 100)/(U_{cr} \times S_{Na})$$

where U_{vol} is urine volume; U_{cr} is urine creatinine concentration; U_{Na} is urine sodium; S_{cr} is serum creatinine concentration; S_{Na} is serum sodium concentration, which usually does not vary much; GFR is the glomerular filtration rate; and t is the time period over which the urine is collected.

The fractional excretion of sodium is one of the better diagnostic parameters to differentiate the cause of AKI. A low urinary sodium concentration (<20 mEq/L [<20 mmol/L]) and low fractional excretion of sodium (<1%) in a patient with oliguria suggest that there is stimulation of the sodium-retentive mechanisms in the kidney and that tubular function is intact. These findings are most characteristic of prerenal azotemia. Unfortunately, diuretic use in the preceding days limits the usefulness of the fractional excretion of sodium calculation by increasing natriuresis, even in hypovolemic patients. The fractional excretion of urea (FE_{Urea}), which can be calculated like FE_{Na}, is sometimes used as an alternative means to assess tubular function.

The inability to concentrate urine results in a high fractional excretion of sodium (>2%), suggesting tubular damage is the primary cause of the intrinsic AKI. Diagnosing the type of AKI using fractional excretion of sodium is not absolute, as there are some intrinsic causes that can be associated with a low fractional excretion of sodium (e.g., contrast nephropathy, myoglobinuria, and interstitial nephritis). Highly concentrated urine (>500 mOsm/kg [>500 mmol/kg]) suggests stimulation of antidiuretic hormone and intact tubular function. These findings are consistent with prerenal azotemia.

NOVEL BIOMARKERS OF KIDNEY FUNCTION

A number of new serum and urinary biomarkers are currently under investigation for early detection and prediction of prognosis of AKI. They represent a heterogeneous group in their ability to detect, classify, and predict the clinical course of AKI. However, they all allow for a significantly earlier diagnosis of AKI compared with conventional methods, in most cases, 48 hours before a rise in S_{cr} is observed. Currently, these tests are not routinely available in most clinical practice sites. Table 51–6 summarizes the characteristics of the six most promising biomarkers that are currently under investigation.

One such marker, serum cystatin C (see Chapter 50), is an endogenous cysteine proteinase that is released into the plasma by all nucleated cells in the body at a relatively constant rate and is then freely filtered by the glomerulus.[26] It does not undergo any significant secretion or reabsorption, but is instead completely metabolized by the proximal renal tubules.[33] Thus, a reduction in GFR will result in a rise in plasma and urine concentrations of cystatin C. Cystatin C levels may be altered by certain disease states (e.g., thyroid dysfunction and systemic inflammation) and possibly patient demographics (age, weight, gender, etc.).[34-36]

Another relatively novel biomarker is neutrophil gelatinase–associated lipocalin (NGAL), a transporter protein found on cell surfaces of neutrophils and various epithelial cells. So far, NGAL has been associated with several physiologic functions, such as iron metabolism, immunity, and kidney development.[37] The 2-hour urine NGAL levels correlate well with the severity and duration of AKI and may predict length of stay, need for RRT, and death in patients undergoing cardiopulmonary bypass.[38] Although NGAL appears to be a very sensitive, specific, and early biomarker of AKI, its levels may be influenced by the presence of CKD, infection, and inflammation.[39,40] Interleukin (IL)-18, a proinflammatory cytokine, is found in elevated urinary concentrations following AKI. In fact, it seems to be specific for ischemic ATN and can distinguish it from CKD, prerenal azotemia, nephrotic syndrome, and urinary tract infections.[41] Certain systemic inflammatory and immune-mediated diseases are associated with increased plasma IL-18 levels; however, their impact on urinary IL-18 is still unknown.[40] Kidney injury molecule 1 (KIM-1) is a biomarker upregulated in the proximal tubules and released into the urine in response to ischemic and nephrotoxic ATN. One advantage of KIM-1 is that it is not expressed in healthy kidney tissue or detected in plasma. Its production may be induced by exposure to nephrotoxins and the presence of CKD.[42,43] Another novel biomarker of AKI is the liver-type fatty acid binding protein (L-FABP), which is found in proximal tubular cells and is involved in fatty acid metabolism in the kidney. Elevated urinary L-FABP levels can be found in CKD as well as in response to oxidative stress and tubulointerstitial damage.[44,45] So far, human studies have been limited but have yielded promising results.[46,47] Recently, beta trace protein (BTP), also referred to as lipocalin-type prostaglandin D synthase, has been introduced as a potential marker of GFR. BTP is a glycoprotein expressed in several tissues, most notably in cerebrospinal fluid. It catalyzes conversion of

TABLE 51-6 Summary of Selected Novel Biomarkers for Early Detection of Acute Kidney Injury

Biomarker	Sample Source	Detection Time After Surgery or Constrast Dye Administration (Hours)	Detection Time before a Change in S_{cr} Is Observed (Hours)	Advantages	Disadvantages
Cystatin C	Plasma and urine	12–14 (plasma) 6 (urine)	24–48 (plasma)	Good marker for early diagnosis of AKI / Superior to S_{cr} for GFR estimation / Commercial assay available / Most validated (besides S_{cr})	Does not differentiate between different types of AKI / Plasma levels may be influenced by thyroid dysfunction, inflammation, corticosteroids, age, gender, height, weight
NGAL	Plasma and urine	2–4 (plasma and urine)	24–72 (plasma and urine)	Good marker for early diagnosis of AKI / Commercial assay available	Does not differentiate between different types of AKI / Plasma levels may be influenced by CKD, inflammation, malignancy, infection
IL-18	Urine	4–12	24–48	Good marker of ischemic ATN / Predictor of AKI-associated mortality	Impact of elevated serum IL-18 levels on urine levels unknown / Needs further validation
KIM-1	Urine	12–24	N/A	Good marker of intrinsic AKI / Predictor of AKI-associated mortality	Levels may be influenced by CKD and nephrotoxins / No studies in ICU/septic patients
L-FABP	Urine	4–6	N/A	Good marker of tubulointerstitial injury	Levels may be influenced by CKD / No studies in ICU/septic patients
BTP	Plasma and urine	N/A	N/A	Potentially useful marker of GFR and renal injury	Limited human studies

AKI = acute kidney injury, ATN = acute tubular necrosis, BTP = beta trace protein, CKD = chronic kidney disease, GFR = glomerular filtration rate, ICU = intensive care unit, IL-18 = interleukin-18, KIM-1 = kidney injury molecule 1, L-FABP = liver-type fatty acid binding protein, N/A = not available, NGAL = neutrophil gelatinase–associated lipocalin, S_{cr} = serum creatinine.

prostaglandin H_2 to prostaglandin D_2 and is freely filtered at the glomerulus.[48] So far, serum BTP as a marker of GFR has been studied in renal transplant recipients with good success.[49] In addition, urinary BTP may be useful in predicting renal injury in diabetic patients.[50]

DIAGNOSTIC PROCEDURES

When the source of renal injury is unclear after a history, physical examination, and assessment of laboratory values, then imaging techniques such as abdominal radiography, including the kidneys, ureters, and bladder (KUB), computed tomography (CT), and ultrasonography may be helpful. These may reveal small, shrunken kidneys indicative of CKD, and postrenal obstruction can often be identified with a renal ultrasonogram and/or CT scan. Renal ultrasonography is useful in detecting obstruction or hydronephrosis. Nephrolithiases as small as 5 nm or a narrowing of the ureteral tract can be detected by ultrasonography or more sensitive tests, such as KUB and CT. No contrast dye is required, and it is noninvasive, simple, portable, and rapid to accomplish. In selected conditions under the guidance of a nephrologist, more invasive procedures, such as cystoscopy and biopsy, may be considered to detect the presence of malignancy, prostate hypertrophy, uterine fibroids, nephrolithiases, or ureterolithiases.

If insertion of a urinary catheter into the patient's bladder after the patient has voided or attempted to void does not yield a large volume of urine (>500 mL), then one can usually exclude postrenal obstruction distal to the bladder as the cause of AKI. Cystoscopy with retrograde pyelography may be helpful if the possibility of obstruction exists, and the insertion of a catheter did not result in a significant volume of urine.

In cases in which the cause of ARF is not evident, renal biopsies are useful in determining the cause in the majority of patients. Because of the associated risk of bleeding, a renal biopsy is rarely undertaken and should only be performed in those circumstances when a definitive diagnosis is needed to guide therapy, such as the precise etiology of glomerulonephritis (see Chapter 50).

PREVENTION OF AKI

■ DESIRED OUTCOME

❺ Given the dismal outcome of established AKI, it is critical to identify patients at risk and implement prevention strategies when possible. Once AKI occurs, treatment is largely supportive and mainly consists of removing the cause of kidney injury, minimizing subsequent complications, and allowing kidney function to recover. Consequently, the goals of AKI prevention and treatment are to (a) prevent AKI and its complications, (b) avoid or minimize further renal insults that would worsen the existing injury or delay recovery, and (c) provide supportive measures until kidney function returns.

■ GENERAL APPROACH TO PREVENTION

The preventive strategy will depend on the type of renal insult. Clearly, complete avoidance of all potential causes of injury is the most effective preventive method; however, it may not always be possible to implement. Sometimes, the risk of renal injury is predictable, such as decreased perfusion secondary to coronary bypass surgery or secondary to the administration of a radiocontrast dye prior to a diagnostic procedure. In these situations, the potential insult to the kidneys cannot be avoided but may be preventable with aggressive hydration and removal of any additional insults. In the outpatient setting, all healthcare professionals should educate the patient on preventive measures for AKI. Patients should receive counseling regarding their optimal daily fluid intake (~2 L/day) to avoid dehydration, especially if they are

TABLE 51-7	Prevention of Acute Kidney Injury

Therapies of definite/possible benefit
Normal saline infusion
Sodium bicarbonate infusion
Ascorbic acid
N-acetylcysteine

Therapies where more data are needed
Anaritide (low-dose)

Not recommended therapies
Dopamine (low-dose)
Loop diuretics
Renal replacement therapy
Epoietin alfa

to receive a potentially nephrotoxic medication. In the inpatient setting, hydration, maintenance of a target mean arterial pressure in the critically ill, and avoidance of nephrotoxic medications are commonly implemented strategies for the prevention of AKI.

Generally, prevention strategies are categorized into nonpharmacologic and pharmacologic therapies. It is important to recognize that the strength of supporting evidence varies between the different preventive measures described in the following sections. (See Table 51-7 for a list of proposed therapies and recommendations based on current evidence.)

■ NONPHARMACOLOGIC THERAPIES

Hydration

Hydration is one of the primary interventions that has consistently shown benefit and is routinely used in the prevention of AKI. Fluids have largely been studied in association with contrast-induced nephropathy (CIN), a common cause of ATN in the inpatient setting (see Chapter 55 for a detailed discussion of CIN). Typically, an increase in the S_{cr} is noted within 24 hours for CIN, peaking after 5 days. CIN is associated with increased mortality especially in individuals with CKD, diabetes, volume depletion, concurrent nephrotoxic drug therapy, or hemodynamic instability.[51] Hydration is thought to counterbalance some of the deleterious effects of radiocontrast dyes by diluting the contrast media, preventing renal vasoconstriction that contributes to hypoxia and ischemia, and minimizing tubular obstruction.[52] Current evidence supports use of isotonic saline over hypotonic saline and use of parenteral over the oral route of administration in high-risk individuals.[53,54] Sodium bicarbonate infusion has recently been evaluated for the prevention of CIN. The hypothesized mechanism for protection is that sodium bicarbonate may reduce the formation of oxygen free radicals by alkalinizing renal tubular fluid. So far, studies have produced mixed results.[55–57] Several meta-analyses have reported reduced incidences of CIN with sodium bicarbonate over isotonic saline; however, they also acknowledged that significant heterogeneity existed between studies, such as differences in the definition of CIN, cumulative dosages of sodium bicarbonate used, and study populations.[58,59] Either sodium bicarbonate or isotonic saline may be used in high-risk individuals receiving radiocontrast media. A common sodium bicarbonate regimen is 154 mEq/L (154 mmol/L) infused at 3 mL/kg/h for 1 hour before the procedure and at 1 mL/kg/h for 6 hours after the procedure.[56] The rate and duration of normal saline infusion vary, but one commonly cited regimen is 1 mL/kg/h for 12 hours before and 12 hours after the procedure.[53] The rate of administration may be adjusted depending on the patient's cardiopulmonary and volume status.

Extracorporeal Blood Purification

Another potential approach for the prevention of CIN is extracorporeal blood purification, that is, prophylactic administration of RRT to patients who are at high risk of AKI. Radiocontrast media are eliminated by the kidneys, but their clearance is delayed in patients with renal dysfunction, thereby increasing their risk for nephrotoxicity. RRT use is based on its ability to enhance radiocontrast dye clearance and thus potentially prevent nephrotoxicity. So far, studies have yielded conflicting results, some showing potential benefit, others indicating harm.[60,61] A recent meta-analysis showed no benefit of extracorporeal blood purification in decreasing the incidence of CIN.[62] In fact, there was a trend toward increased risk of harm when the analysis was limited to studies of hemodialysis. However, the meta-analysis also found that dialysis was initiated at least 1 hour after administration of the contrast media in the majority of the studies. The timing of dialysis is an important consideration, as tubular damage may start to occur after only 15 minutes of exposure to radiocontrast media.[62] Other, more practical issues associated with using prophylactic RRT are cost and the labor-intensive and invasive nature of the procedure itself.

Overall, evidence to date does not demonstrate any consistent significant benefit with the routine use of extracorporeal blood purification to prevent CIN over standard medical therapy.

■ PHARMACOLOGIC THERAPIES

Loop Diuretics

There is significant controversy surrounding the use of loop diuretics in the prevention of AKI. Early experimental studies proposed that loop diuretics had the following theoretical advantages: decreased risk of tubular obstruction secondary to an increased urine flow and flushing out of debris; increased urine output that may be beneficial in itself, as nonoliguric AKI is associated with better outcomes than oliguric AKI; decreased risk of ischemic injury as the result of inhibition of the sodium/potassium chloride cotransporter and thus a reduction in oxygen demand; and enhanced renal blood flow due to increased availability of renal prostaglandins.[63] However, clinical studies have been less favorable. Even though the majority of studies demonstrate that loop diuretics increase urine output, they lack beneficial effects on patient outcomes, such as mortality, need for RRT, and renal recovery.[63–65] There is even some evidence of potential harm associated with their use, in particular, ototoxicity and possibly mortality in certain clinical settings.[66] The proposed explanations for such lack of benefit are twofold. Loop diuretics may not be reaching the proximal tubule as their site of action due to tubular obstruction from debris, increased extrarenal clearance secondary to hypoalbuminemia, and increased urinary protein binding due to albuminuria. Also, loop diuretics may actually decrease renal blood flow by reducing effective circulating arterial volume, which, in turn, may stimulate the adrenergic and the renin-angiotensin systems.[63]

CLINICAL CONTROVERSY

Loop diuretics are widely used for the management of volume overload in critically ill patients, including those with concomitant AKI. Although volume overload is certainly an appropriate indication for loop diuretics, current evidence does not support their use for prevention of AKI or treatment of oliguria.

Dopamine Agonists

Dopamine is a nonselective dopamine receptor agonist that, in high doses, also stimulates the adrenergic receptors. Low doses of intravenous (IV) dopamine (≤ 2 mcg/kg/min) increase renal blood flow, induce natriuresis and diuresis, and might be expected to increase GFR. Theoretically, this could be considered beneficial, as an increase in renal perfusion and oxygenation might limit ischemic cell injury, inhibition of sodium transport might reduce oxygen demand, and an enhanced GFR might flush nephrotoxins and casts from the tubules. Despite these theoretical suggestions, controlled studies have found that low-dose dopamine did not prevent AKI, need for dialysis, or mortality compared with placebo.[67,68] Thus, current evidence does not support the use of low-dose dopamine for prevention of AKI.

CLINICAL CONTROVERSY

Despite most studies not showing improved patient outcomes with its use, low-dose dopamine continues to be commonly used. The risks associated with dopamine (extravasation and the potential for significant dosing errors) suggest that its use should be avoided whenever possible.

Fenoldopam mesylate is a selective dopamine A-1 receptor agonist that increases renal blood flow, natriuresis, and diueresis. Although fenoldopam seems ineffective in preventing CIN, it may have some benefit in preventing AKI in critically ill patients or those undergoing surgery.[69,70]

Antioxidants

Ascorbic Acid Ascorbic acid has mainly been studied in the prevention of CIN, as its antioxidant properties are thought to alleviate oxidative stress caused by CIN-associated ischemia reperfusion injury.[71] Studies have not consistently demonstrated benefit when ascorbic acid was given to patients with CKD for the prevention of CIN.[72,73] However, its excellent safety profile and low cost make it an attractive option for high-risk individuals. The recommended dose of ascorbic acid is 3 g orally before the procedure, then 2 g orally twice daily for two doses after the procedure.

N-Acetylcysteine N-acetylcysteine (NAC) is another antioxidant that has been widely studied in the prevention of CIN in patients with renal insufficiency. However, a therapeutic benefit has not been consistently demonstrated, and large heterogeneity in results across different studies makes it difficult to determine whether NAC is truly effective or not.[72,74] Similar to ascorbic acid, NAC's low cost, safety profile, tolerability, and possible benefit make it a reasonable option for patients at risk for CIN. The recommended dosing regimen for prevention of CIN is 600 to 1,200 mg orally every 12 hours for four doses, with the first two doses administered prior to contrast exposure. NAC has also been evaluated for the prevention of AKI in postoperative patients, but studies have failed to demonstrate any benefit.[75,76] Thus, use of NAC should be reserved for prevention of CIN only and not for other types of AKI.

Glycemic Control

Glycemic control in critically ill patients is of utmost importance, as both hyper- and hypoglycemia are associated with increased mortality.[77] Hyperglycemia is common during critical illness, and one of its key features in that setting is insulin resistance. The causes of insulin resistance are multifactorial but include impaired glucose

homeostasis due to loss of the kidney's metabolic function, as well as decreased hepatic and peripheral glucose uptake secondary to uremia. Hyperglycemia has also been associated with increased risk of renal injury, but the exact mechanisms by which glucose may contribute to renal toxicity are not fully elucidated.[78] Experimental studies indicate increased sensitivity to renal ischemia reperfusion injury, glucose overload in the kidney causing tissue damage, and increased inflammation.[79] Patients may also be at higher risk for hypoglycemia, as the kidneys are the primary metabolic site of insulin.

The target blood glucose concentrations in critically ill patients are controversial. A prospective, randomized controlled study by van den Berghe et al.[80] demonstrated a 41% reduction in the development of AKI and reduced mortality in the intensive insulin therapy group (80–110 mg/dL [4.4–6.1 mmol/L]) compared with the standard control (<200 mg/dL [<11.1 mmol/L]) group of surgical intensive care (ICU) patients. Several other studies, particularly those in nonsurgical ICU patients, failed to reproduce these results.[81,82] A recent large multicenter randomized study conducted in medical and surgical ICU patients revealed that intensive glucose control was associated with significantly greater 90-day mortality rates and higher risk of hypoglycemia compared with conventional insulin therapy (144–180 mg/dL [8–10 mmol/L]). Although the study did not report the incidence of ICU-acquired AKI, no significant difference in the need for RRT between the two groups was noted.[83] Thus, current evidence suggests that moderate control of blood glucose to levels of 144 to 180 mg/dL (8.0–10.0 mmol/L) may be more appropriate in the critical care setting. Specifically for patients with AKI, it should be recognized that they are at increased risk for hypoglycemia as well as insulin resistance due to altered renal function, so that more frequent glucose monitoring may be required.

■ OTHER APPROACHES TO PREVENTION

Several other therapies have been investigated for the prevention of AKI. Most of them have shown promising results in experimental studies but the experience in using them in humans is still either inconclusive or limited. One such example is theophylline, which may attenuate adenosine-mediated renal vasoconstriction and GFR reduction in patients with CIN. A systematic review of nine randomized trials indicated a trend toward reduced incidence of CIN with theophylline use. These findings require cautious interpretation as definitions of CIN as well as hydration and theophylline protocols varied markedly.[84] Thus, evidence is currently inconclusive and more research is needed to assess the role of theophylline as a modality for CIN prevention.

Erythropoietin alfa (EPO) is another agent under study for the prevention of AKI. EPO is a primary regulator of red blood cell production and is widely used to treat anemia in patients with CKD and cancer. Experimental models have demonstrated the tissue-protective role of EPO against ischemic renal injury.[85] One small prospective randomized trial has reported that a single dose of EPO (300 units/kg) significantly decreased the risk of postoperative AKI from 29% to 8% after coronary artery bypass surgery.[86] However, a recent double-blind placebo-controlled trial found no difference in the outcome of AKI among 529 enrolled ICU patients.[87] Larger clinical trials would be necessary to demonstrate its safety and efficacy before EPO can be recommended for the prevention of AKI.

Natriuretic peptides, specifically atrial natriuretic peptide (ANP) and B-type natriuretic peptide (BNP), are also being explored for the prevention of AKI in certain clinical settings. Both ANP and BNP mediate vasodilation and natriuresis, as well as increase renal perfusion and GFR. Clinical studies with anaritide (human recombinant ANP) and nesiritide have been relatively inconclusive, but there seems to be growing evidence that lower doses (50 ng/kg/min of anaritide and 0.005 µg/kg/min of nesiritide) and longer infusion times may reduce the risk of postoperative AKI.[88,89] The proposed explanation for these differences in response is that lower doses of anaritide and nesiritide are associated with lower risks of hypotension, which, if present, may adversely affect renal perfusion and counterbalance any protective effects these drugs may have. Large multicenter, randomized studies are warranted to further clarify the role of natriuretic peptides in the prevention of AKI.

TREATMENT OF AKI

■ DESIRED OUTCOMES

Short-term goals include minimizing the degree of insult to the kidney, reducing extrarenal complications, and expediting the patient's recovery of renal function. The ultimate goal is to have the patient's renal function restored to his or her pre-AKI baseline.

■ GENERAL APPROACH TO TREATMENT

Prerenal sources of AKI should be managed with hemodynamic support and volume replacement. If the cause is immune related, as may be the case with interstitial nephritis or glomerulonephritis, appropriate immunosuppressive therapy must be promptly initiated. Postrenal therapy focuses on removing the cause of the obstruction. It is important to approach the treatment of established AKI with an understanding of the patient's comorbidities and baseline renal function. Loss of kidney function combined with other clinical conditions, such as cardiac and liver failure, are associated with higher mortality than that associated with the development of AKI alone.[90] At times, the most efficacious remedy for AKI is management of the comorbid precipitating event. Appreciation of the baseline renal function is also important at the outset of AKI management, because the presence of CKD indicates the highest degree of renal function that can be attained after AKI resolution. Finally, the presence of CKD indicates that the kidneys have less reserve; thus, there is a greater likelihood that the individual may not fully recover from the current insult.

❻ Supportive care is the mainstay of AKI management regardless of etiology. RRT may be necessary to maintain fluid and electrolyte balance while removing accumulating waste products. The slow process of renal recovery cannot begin until there are no further insults to the kidney. In the case of ATN, the recovery process typically occurs within 10 to 14 days after resolution of the last insult. The recovery period will be prolonged if the kidney is exposed to repeated insults.

■ NONPHARMACOLOGIC

Initial modalities to reverse or minimize prerenal AKI include eliminating medications associated with diminished renal blood flow, improving cardiac output, and removing a prerenal obstruction. If dehydration is evident, then appropriate fluid replacement therapy, as described later in this chapter, should be initiated. Moderately volume-depleted patients can be given oral rehydration fluids; however, if IV fluid is required, isotonic normal saline is the replacement fluid of choice, and large volumes may be necessary to provide adequate fluid resuscitation. Typically, IV fluid challenges are initiated with 250 to 500 mL of normal saline over 15 to 30 minutes with an assessment after each challenge of the patient's volume status. Unless profound dehydration is present, as may be seen in diabetic ketoacidosis and hyperosmolar hyperglycemic states, 1 to 2 L is usually adequate. Patients with diabetic ketoacidosis or a hyperosmolar hyperglycemic state often have a 10% to 15% total-body water deficit, and more aggressive fluid replacement is

necessary. The patient should be monitored for pulmonary edema, peripheral edema, adequate blood pressure (diastolic blood pressure >60 mm Hg), normoglycemia, and electrolyte balance. Urine output may not be promptly observed, as the kidney continues to retain sodium and water until rehydration is achieved. Up to 10 L may be required in the septic patient during the first 24 hours, because of the profound increase in vascular capacitance and fluid leakage into the extravascular, interstitial space.[91]

Patients with AKI on top of preexisting CKD should not be expected to produce urine beyond their preexisting baseline. In patients with anuria or oliguria, slower rehydration, such as 250 mL boluses or 100 mL/h infusions of normal saline, should be considered to reduce the risk for pulmonary edema, especially if heart failure or pulmonary insufficiency exists. Other replacement fluids may be considered if the dehydration is accompanied by a severe electrolyte imbalance amenable to large and relatively rapid infusions. For example, dehydration resulting from severe diarrhea is often accompanied by metabolic acidosis caused by bicarbonate losses. A reasonable IV rehydration fluid in this situation is 5% dextrose with 0.45% sodium chloride (NaCl) plus 50 mEq (50 mmol) of sodium bicarbonate per liter, administered as boluses as described above, followed by a brisk continuous infusion (200 mL/h) until rehydration is complete, acidosis corrected, and diarrhea resolved. This fluid will remain mostly in the intravascular space, providing the necessary perfusion pressure to the kidneys, as well as a substantial amount of bicarbonate to correct the acidosis.

If the prerenal AKI is a result of blood loss or is complicated by symptomatic anemia, red blood cell transfusion to a hematocrit no higher than 30% is the treatment of choice.[92] Although albumin is sometimes used as a resuscitative agent, its use should be limited to individuals with severe hypoalbuminemia (e.g., liver disease and nephritic syndrome) who are resistant to crystalloid therapy. These patients have severe hypoalbuminemia-associated third spacing that complicates fluid management, and albumin may be useful in this setting.

The most common interventions that must be made when treating patients with intrinsic or postobstructive AKI involve fluid and electrolyte management. Most patients with these types of AKI, as well as those with a prerenal cause who are excessively fluid resuscitated, ultimately become fluid overloaded. This means drug infusions and nutrition solutions must be maximally concentrated. So-called keep vein open or maintenance IV infusions should be minimized unless the patient is euvolemic or is receiving RRT to maintain fluid balance. Supportive care goals for the hospitalized patient with any type of AKI include maintenance of adequate cardiac output and blood pressure to allow adequate tissue perfusion. However, a fine balance must be maintained in anuric and oliguric patients unless the patient is hypovolemic or is able to achieve fluid balance via RRT. If fluid intake is not minimized, edema may rapidly develop, especially in hypoalbuminemic patients. In contrast, a continuous IV infusion of vasopressors, such as dopamine, at doses of ≥2 mcg/kg/min, or norepinephrine when used to maintain adequate tissue perfusion, may also induce kidney hypoxia as the result of a reduction in renal blood flow. Consequently, hemodynamic monitoring may be necessary for critically ill patients (see Chapter 30).

Because there is no current definitive therapy for AKI, supportive management remains the primary approach to prevent or reduce associated complications or death. In the presence of severe AKI, RRTs are commonly prescribed to manage uremia, metabolic acidosis, hyperkalemia, and complications of excess fluid retention, such as pulmonary edema and accumulation of renally cleared medications. Although precise indications for starting RRT are unclear, some general guidelines for therapy have been proposed (Table 51–8).

TABLE 51-8	The AEIOUs That Describe the Indications for Renal Replacement Therapy	
Indication for Renal Replacement Therapy	**Clinical Setting**	
A Acid–base abnormalities	Metabolic acidosis resulting from the accumulation of organic and inorganic acids	
E Electrolyte imbalance	Hyperkalemia, hypermagnesemia	
I Intoxications	Salicylates, lithium, methanol, ethylene glycol, theophylline, phenobarbital	
O fluid overload	Postoperative fluid gain	
U Uremia	High catabolism of acute renal failure	

Renal Replacement Therapies

❼ RRTs can be administered either intermittently or continuously. The optimal mode for hemodialysis is unclear and varies depending on the clinical presentation of the patient.[93] Some recent data suggest that more aggressive approaches using RRTs in a more liberal fashion or use of a bioartificial membrane consisting of renal proximal tubule cells may improve survival in critically ill patients with AKI.[93,94] The choice of continuous versus intermittent RRTs is a matter of considerable debate and is usually determined by physician preference and the resources available at the hospital.

Intermittent Hemodialysis

Intermittent hemodialysis (IHD) is the most frequently used RRT and has several advantages. IHD machines are readily available in most acute care facilities, and healthcare workers are commonly familiar with their use. Hemodialysis treatments usually last 3 to 4 hours, with blood flow rates to the dialyzer typically ranging from 200 to 400 mL/min. Advantages of IHD include rapid removal of volume and solute and rapid correction of most of the electrolyte abnormalities associated with AKI. IHD can be scheduled at times that maximize staffing availability and treatments per day per machine, while minimizing inconvenience to the patient. The primary disadvantage is hypotension, typically caused by rapid removal of intravascular volume over a short period of time. Venous access for dialysis can be difficult in hypotensive patients and can limit the effectiveness of IHD, leading to ineffective solute clearance, lack of acidosis correction, continued volume overload, and delayed recovery because of further renal ischemia insults. If hemodialysis is carefully monitored and hypotension avoided, better patient outcomes can be achieved.[95] Patients with stage 5 CKD generally achieve adequate solute and volume control with dialysis done three times weekly, but hypercatabolic, fluid-overloaded patients with AKI may require daily hemodialysis treatments.[96] The use of daily versus three times weekly IHD in the setting of AKI has been associated with a reduction in dialysis-related hypotension and a shorter period of time to full recovery of kidney function.[97] Chapter 54 provides a detailed explanation of the principles and processes of hemodialysis.

Continuous Renal Replacement Therapies

In contrast to IHD, CRRTs that were developed over the past 15 years have proven to be a viable management approach for hemodynamically unstable patients with AKI.[98] Several CRRT variants have been developed, including continuous venovenous hemofiltration (CVVH), continuous venovenous hemodialysis (CVVHD), and continuous venovenous hemodiafiltration (CVVHDF). They differ in the degree of solute and fluid clearance that can be clinically achieved as a result of the use of diffusion, convection, or a combination of both. Although solute removal is slower, a greater amount can be removed over a 24-hour period compared with IHD, which is associated with improved outcomes in critically ill patients with AKI.[99]

In CVVH, solute and fluid clearance is primarily a result of convection, in which passive diffusion of fluids containing solutes is removed, while volume absent of the solutes is replaced (Fig. 51–4). CVVHD provides extensive solute removal primarily by diffusion, in which solute molecules at a higher concentration (plasma) pass through the dialysis membrane to a lower concentration (dialysate), and some fluid is removed as a function of the ultrafiltration coefficient of the dialyzer. Because the dialysate flows in a countercurrent direction to the plasma flow on the other side of the membrane, the concentration gradient is maximized. CVVHD is associated with a lower incidence of clotting than CVVH because of reduced hemoconcentration, as there is less fluid removal during the process. CVVHDF combines both convection or hemofiltration and hemodialysis, achieving even higher solute and fluid removal rates (Fig. 51–4). The ultrafiltration rate is an important determinant of the effectiveness of all three forms of CRRT; achievement of a removal rate of 35 mL/kg/h is associated with improved survival.[99] However, in direct comparisons of ultrafiltration rates of 25 to 40 mL/kg/h or higher, no difference in mortality has been observed, and there was a tendency toward prolonged need for renal replacement in those who received the higher ultrafiltration rate.[100,101]

Because of the reduced blood flow rates relative to IHD, thrombosis is a significant concern with CRRT; thus, some form of anticoagulation during RRT is generally necessary for almost all patients. Typical anticoagulation is achieved by the administration of unfractionated heparin, or in some cases, a low molecular weight heparin, direct thrombin inhibitor, or citrate solution.[102] Replacement fluids can be infused either just before or after the dialyzer/hemofilter. Infusing fluids after the hemofilter can result in hemoconcentration within the filter, a factor associated with an increased risk of thrombosis of the dialyzer. Replacing fluids before the filter reduces thrombosis risk, but it also reduces solute clearance.

Disadvantages of CRRT are that not all hospitals have the special equipment necessary to provide these treatments, they require intensive nursing care around the clock, and they are more expensive than IHD because of the need to individualize the IV replacement and dialysate fluids. There is also very little known about drug-dosing requirements for those who are receiving these therapies.[103] CRRT use is most commonly considered for those patients with higher acuity because of their intolerance of IHD-associated hypotension. In one meta-analysis, no difference in clinical outcomes between the two approaches was seen until there was an adjustment for severity of illness. CRRT was then found to be associated with a lower mortality rate.[104] Because patients treated with continuous therapies are almost always more critically ill than those treated by IHD, comparisons of outcome must control for illness severity.

CRRT and hybrid extended-duration intermittent hemodialysis are now being commonly used for critically ill patients with AKI. With CRRT, more solute and water removal can be achieved than with the hemodialysis treatments given three times per week for patients with ESKD. This has influenced how dialysis is prescribed in the intensive care unit for hypercatabolic patients with AKI. Daily IHD is associated with improved survival and faster resolution of AKI compared with dialysis given every other day.[90] Daily delivery of IHD presents challenges to clinicians prescribing drug and nutrition therapy, as most of these dosing guidelines are based on dialysis given three times per week in CKD patients. Thus, application of these guidelines in patients with AKI may yield suboptimal outcomes.

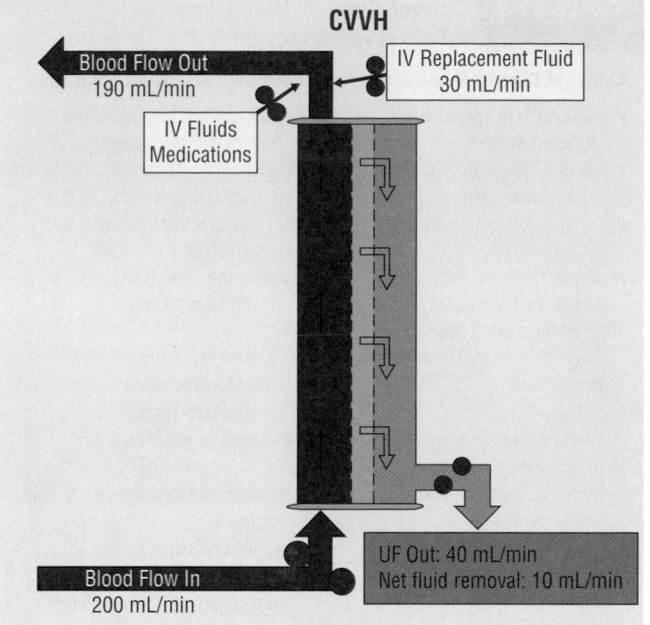

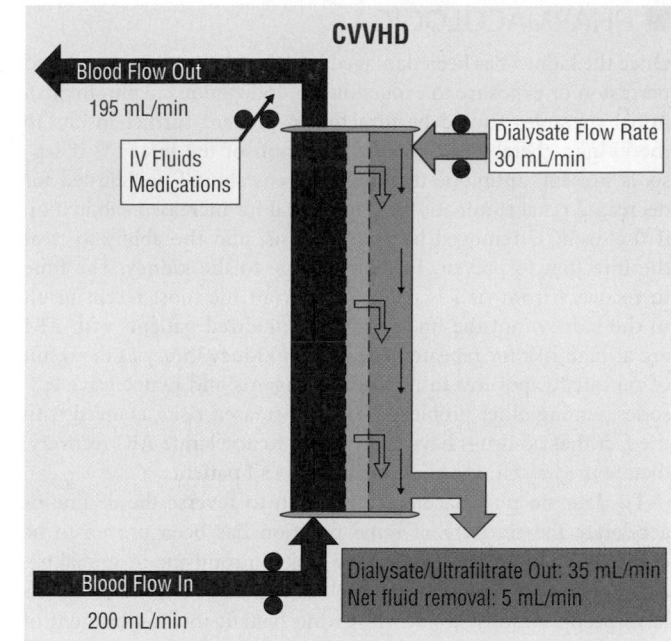

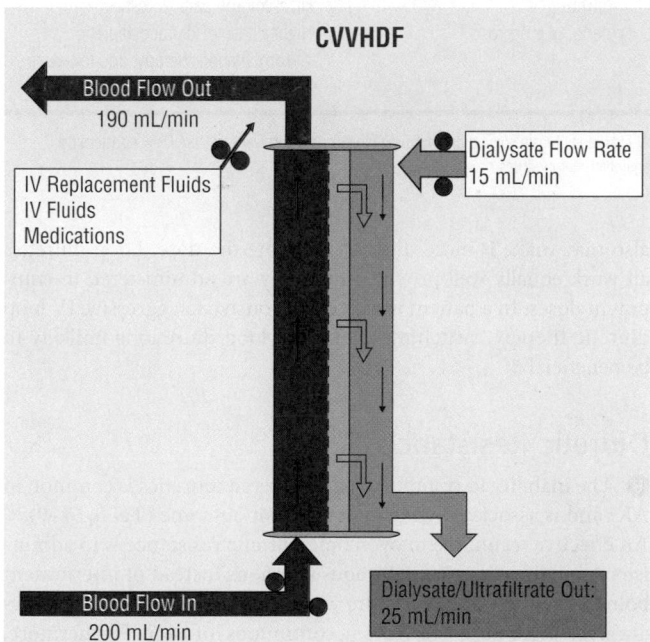

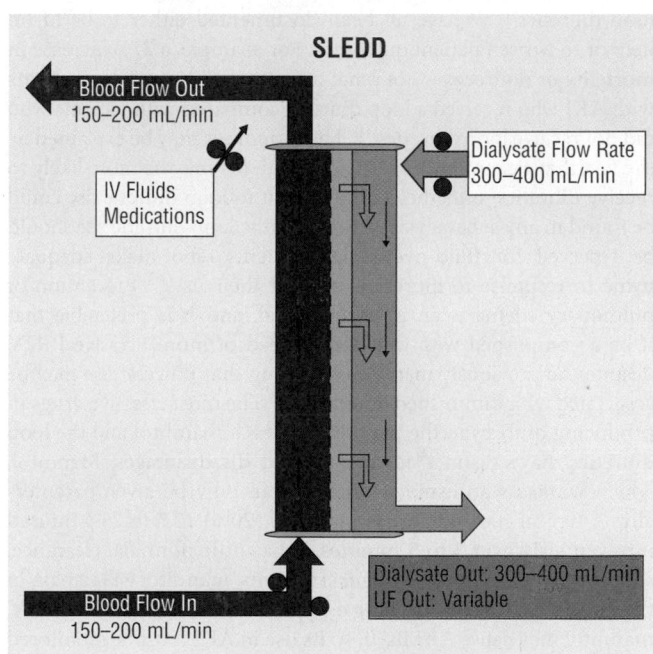

FIGURE 51-4. Several renal replacement therapies are commonly used in patients with AKI, including one of the three primary continuous renal replacement therapy (CRRT) variants: (a) continuous venovenous hemofiltration (CVVH), (b) continuous venovenous hemodialysis (CVVHD), (c) continuous venovenous hemodiafiltration (CVVHDF), and the hybrid intermittent hemodialysis therapy (d) slow extended daily dialysis (SLEDD). The blood circuit in each diagram is represented in red, the hemofilter/dialyzer membrane is yellow, and the ultrafiltration/dialysate compartment is brown. Excess body water and accumulated endogenous waste products are removed solely by convection when CVVH is employed. With CVVHD, waste products are predominantly removed as the result of passive diffusion from the blood, where they are in high concentration to the dialysate. The degree of fluid removal that is accomplished by convection is usually minimal. CVVHDF uses convection to a degree similar to that employed during CVVH as well as diffusion, and thus is often associated with the highest clearance of drugs and waste products. Finally, SLEDD employs lower blood and dialysate flow rates than intermittent hemodialysis (IHD), but because of its extended duration, it is a gentler means of achieving adequate waste product and fluid removal.

Hybrid IHD therapies have a variety of names, with the two most common being sustained low-efficiency dialysis[105] and slow, extended, daily dialysis (see Fig. 51–4).[106] These therapies use lower blood (150–200 mL/min) and dialysate (300–400 mL/min) flow rates with extended treatment periods of 6 to 12 hours. Unlike CRRT, these therapies do not require any new equipment. Anticoagulation is still required, but the amount necessary compared with CRRT is lower.[106] Although the use of hybrid hemodialysis therapies is increasing, our knowledge of the impact of these therapies on drug removal remains limited.[107,108]

CLINICAL CONTROVERSY

Some clinicians believe that CRRTs are preferable to IHD because they provide more consistent fluid and waste product removal. Others suggest that IHD is preferable because the nursing and medical staff is more familiar with its use, and round-the-clock nursing is not needed. New hybrid approaches with slower removal over a prolonged time period may potentially appeal to both groups.

■ PHARMACOLOGIC

Once the kidney has been damaged by an acute insult (e.g., reduced perfusion or exposure to exogenous or endogenous nephrotoxins), initial therapies should be directed to prevent further insults to the kidney, thereby minimizing extension of the injury.[109] If sepsis is present, antibiotic therapy regimens should be adjusted for decreased renal elimination, the potential for increased elimination if the agent is removed by hemodialysis, and the ability to treat the infection to prevent further damage to the kidney. The time to recovery from AKI is determined from the most recent insult to the kidney, not the first insult. Hospitalized patients with AKI are at high risk for repeated episodes of kidney injury as the result of repeated exposures to nephrotoxic agents and hypotensive episodes, among other problems. These increased risks, coupled with the fact that no drugs have been found to accelerate AKI recovery, dictate the way clinicians approach the AKI patient.

To date, no pharmacologic approach to reverse the decline or accelerate the recovery of renal function has been proven to be clinically useful. Many agents have looked promising in animal trials, only to be found ineffective in human trials. Numerous agents have been investigated and shown no benefit in the treatment of established AKI.[110] In recent years thyroxine,[111] dopamine,[67,112] and loop diuretics[113-115] have all been documented either to be of no help or to worsen patient outcomes. For example, a 77% increase in mortality or nonrecovery of renal function was reported in patients with AKI who received a loop diuretic compared with patients who did not receive loop diuretics.[115] These findings may be explained by the fact that sicker, fluid-overloaded patients may be more likely to receive diuretics; nonetheless, no benefit to loop diuretic use could be found in any subanalysis. Consequently, loop diuretic use should be reserved for fluid-overloaded patients who make adequate urine in response to diuretics to merit their use.[113] Prevention of pulmonary edema is an important goal, and it is preferable that it be accomplished with diuretics instead of more invasive RRTs, despite the previously mentioned finding that diuretic use may be associated with diminished outcomes.[115] The most effective drugs in producing diuresis in the patient with AKI, mannitol and the loop diuretics, have distinct advantages and disadvantages. Mannitol, which works as an osmotic diuretic, can only be given parenterally. A typical starting dose is mannitol (20%) 12.5 to 25 g infused intravenously over 3 to 5 minutes. It has little nonrenal clearance, so when given to anuric or oliguric patients, mannitol will remain in the patient, potentially causing a hyperosmolar state. Additionally, mannitol may cause AKI itself, so its use in AKI must be monitored carefully by measuring urine output and serum electrolytes and osmolality.[116] Adequately designed comparative trials of mannitol to normal saline currently do not exist. Because of these limitations of mannitol, some clinicians recommend that it be reserved for the management of cerebral edema.[117]

Furosemide and bumetanide are the most frequently used loop diuretics in patients with AKI. Ethacrynic acid is typically reserved for patients who are allergic to sulfa compounds. Furosemide is the most commonly used loop diuretic because of its lower cost, availability in oral and parenteral forms, and reasonable safety and efficacy profiles. A disadvantage with furosemide is its variable oral bioavailability in many patients and potential for ototoxicity with high serum concentrations that may be attained with rapid, high-dose bolus infusions. Consequently, initial furosemide doses, which should not exceed 40 to 80 mg, are usually administered intravenously to assess whether the patient will respond. Torsemide and bumetanide have better oral bioavailability than furosemide and are more potent; 4:1 and 40:1 respectively compared to furosemide. Torsemide has a longer duration of activity than the other loop diuretics, which allows for less-frequent administration but which

TABLE 51-9	Common Causes of Diuretic Resistance in Patients with Severe AKI
Causes of Diuretic Resistance	**Potential Therapeutic Solutions**
Excessive sodium intake (sources may be dietary, IV fluids, and drugs)	Remove sodium from nutritional sources and medications
Inadequate diuretic dose or inappropriate regimen	Increase dose, use continuous infusion or combination therapy
Reduced oral bioavailability (usually furosemide)	Use parenteral therapy; switch to oral torsemide or bumetanide
Nephrotic syndrome (loop diuretic protein binding in tubule lumen)	Increase dose, switch diuretics, use combination therapy
Reduced renal blood flow	
Drugs (NSAIDs, ACEIs, vasodilators)	Discontinue these drugs if possible
Hypotension	Intravascular volume expansion and/or vasopressors
Intravascular depletion	Intravascular volume expansion
Increased sodium resorption	
Nephron adaptation to chronic diuretic therapy	Combination diuretic therapy, sodium restriction
NSAID use	Discontinue NSAID
Heart failure	Treat heart failure, increase diuretic dose, switch to better-absorbed loop diuretic
Cirrhosis	High-volume paracentesis
Acute tubular necrosis	Higher dose of diuretic, diuretic combination therapy; add low-dose dopamine

ACEIs = angiotensin-converting enzyme inhibitors, IV = intravenous, NSAIDs = nonsteroidal antiinflammatory drugs.

also may make it more difficult to titrate the dose. Loop diuretics all work equally well provided that they are administered in equipotent doses. In a patient who is unresponsive to aggressive IV loop diuretic therapy, switching to another loop diuretic is unlikely to be beneficial.

Diuretic Resistance

8 The inability to respond to administered diuretics is common in AKI and is associated with a poor patient outcome (Table 51-9).[115] An effective technique to overcome diuretic resistance is to administer loop diuretics via continuous infusions instead of intermittent boluses. Less natriuresis occurs when equal doses of loop diuretics are given as a bolus instead of as a continuous infusion. Furthermore, adverse reactions from loop diuretics (myalgia and hearing loss) occur less frequently in patients receiving continuous infusion compared with those receiving intermittent boluses, ostensibly because higher serum concentrations are avoided. However, these adverse effects still may occur with continuous infusion of loop diuretics and should be monitored.[118] The finding that the continuous infusions of loop diuretics have efficacy that is at least as good as intermittent bolus dosing, with fewer adverse effects, appears to be consistent for all agents, including furosemide,[119] bumetanide,[120] and torsemide.[121] When a continuous loop diuretic infusion is used, an initial loading dose is given (equivalent to furosemide 40–80 mg) prior to the initiation of a continuous infusion at 10 to 20 mg/h of furosemide or its equivalent. Patients with low creatinine clearances may have much lower rates of diuretic secretion into the tubular fluid; consequently, higher doses are generally used in patients with renal insufficiency.[117] Diuretic resistance may occur simply because excessive sodium intake overrides the ability of the diuretics to eliminate sodium. However, other reasons for diuretic resistance often exist in this population. Patients with ATN have a reduced number of functioning nephrons on which the diuretic may exert its action. Other clinical states, such as glomerulonephritis, are associated with heavy proteinuria. Intraluminal loop diuretics cannot exert their effect in the loop of Henle because they are extensively bound to proteins present in the urine. Still other patients may have greatly reduced bioavailability of oral furosemide because of intestinal edema, often associated with high preload states, which further reduces oral furosemide absorption. Table 51–9 includes possible therapeutic options to counteract each form of diuretic resistance. Combination therapy of loop diuretics plus a diuretic from a different pharmacologic class may be an alternative approach in the setting of AKI.[122] Loop diuretics increase the delivery of NaCl to the distal convoluted tubule and collecting duct. With time, these areas of the nephron compensate for the activity of the loop diuretic and increase sodium and chloride resorption. Diuretics that work at the distal convoluted tubule (chlorothiazide and metolazone) or the collecting duct (amiloride, triamterene, and spironolactone) may have a synergistic effect when administered with loop diuretics by blocking the compensatory increase in sodium and chloride resorption. The combination of loop diuretics and usual doses of thiazide diuretics may be effective in renal disease despite the accumulation of endogenous organic acids in renal disease that blocks the transport of loop diuretics into the lumen. If oral thiazides cannot be given to the patient, chlorothiazide 500 mg, a more expensive option, can be administered parenterally.

Several drug combinations with loop diuretics have been investigated, including the addition of one or more of the following: theophylline, acetazolamide, spironolactone, thiazides, or metolazone.[116] Of these combinations, oral metolazone is used most frequently with furosemide. Metolazone, unlike other thiazides, produces effective diuresis at a GFR <20 mL/min (0.33 mL/s). This combination of metolazone and a loop diuretic has been used successfully in the management of fluid overload in patients with heart failure, cirrhosis, and nephrotic syndrome. Despite a lack of supporting evidence, oral metolazone at a dose of 5 mg is commonly administered 30 minutes prior to an IV loop diuretic to allow time for absorption. Additionally, this combination has been found to be efficacious in pediatric patients in addition to adults.[123] The combination of mannitol plus IV loop diuretics is used by some practitioners,[124] but no convincing evidence of the superiority of this combination regimen to conventional dosing of either diuretic alone exists.

■ ELECTROLYTE MANAGEMENT

Hypernatremia and fluid retention are frequent complications of AKI; thus, sodium restriction is a necessary intervention. In general, patients should receive no more than 3 g of sodium per day from all sources, including IV fluids, drugs, and enteral intake. Clinicians should be vigilant about sources of sodium. Excessive sodium intake is a common reason diuretic therapy fails. Commonly administered IV antibiotics, as well as other medications, may contain significant amounts of sodium; for example, 1 L of 0.9% NaCl yields 154 mEq (154 mmol; 3.5 g) of sodium. At usual doses, IV metronidazole provides 1.3 g of sodium per day, ampicillin up to 800 mg, piperacillin ~700 mg, and fluconazole 500 mg. The cumulative effect of a few sodium-containing medications and fluids can be significant.

In continuous and intermittent RRTs, there usually is less concern about hyponatremia developing because these therapies often incorporate isonatremic (135–140 mEq/L [135–140 mmol/L] of sodium) solutions as the dialysate or ultrafiltrate replacement solutions. Serum sodium concentrations should be monitored daily. Hyperkalemia, hyperphosphatemia, and, to a lesser extent, hypermagnesemia are electrolyte disorders that are frequently seen in patients with AKI. Higher ultrafiltration rates can potentially increase the risk for hyperphosphatemia. The shift in electrolytes is generally not a serious concern in those who are receiving RRT, but electrolytes should be monitored closely in all patients with AKI.

The most common electrolyte disorder encountered in AKI patients is hyperkalemia, as >90% of potassium is renally eliminated. Life-threatening cardiac arrhythmias may occur with serum potassium concentrations >6 mEq/L (6 mmol/L), so potassium restriction is essential. All patients with AKI should have serum potassium monitored at least daily, and twice daily for those who are seriously ill. This frequency is a consequence of the seriousness of the potential arrhythmias, the dynamic nature of potassium serum concentrations in the acutely ill patient, the potential for metabolic acidosis leading to increased extracellular potassium concentrations, and potassium's ubiquitous presence in foods and some medications. Commonly encountered medications that contain substantial amounts of potassium include oral phosphorous replacement powders (e.g., Neutra-Phos and Neutra-Phos-K) and alkalinizers (Polycitra) (see Chapter 59). Many foods are high in potassium, including potatoes, beans, and various fruits. Some medications may promote potassium retention by the kidneys and should also be avoided or closely monitored (see Chapter 55 and 60). Typically, no potassium should be added to parenteral solutions unless hypokalemia is documented. Patients receiving enteral nutrition should be limited to a 3 g potassium diet. Patients receiving RRT should also have their serum potassium concentration measured at least daily. Some centers add no potassium to their CRRT solutions, and hypokalemia can result unless one is prospectively monitoring for its development. Chapter 60 discusses the treatment of hyperkalemia in detail.

Other electrolytes that require monitoring are phosphorus and magnesium. Both are eliminated by the kidneys and are not removed efficiently by dialysis. In the early stages of AKI, hyperphosphatemia may be more common than hypophosphatemia. Patients who have significant tissue destruction (e.g., trauma, rhabdomyolysis, and tumor lysis syndrome) may have significant phosphorus released from the destroyed tissue. Treatment of the hyperphosphatemic state can include CRRT. Calcium-containing antacids should be avoided to prevent precipitation of calcium phosphate in the soft tissues. Typically, the dietary intake of phosphorus and magnesium is restricted, but in patients receiving prolonged renal replacement, deficiency states can occur, particularly in pediatric patients because of their reduced body stores. In contrast to the patient with CKD, calcium balance is usually not an important issue for the patient with AKI because of the limited duration of the illness. One exception to this is seen in patients who are receiving CRRT with citrate as the anticoagulant. Citrate binds to serum calcium, and without an adequate concentration of calcium, blood cannot form a clot. Citrate is thus typically infused before the dialyzer/hemofilter to maintain the dialyzer circuit calcium levels between 0.70 and 1 mEq/L (0.35–0.50 mmol/L). Calcium chloride (10 g of CaCl diluted in 500 mL normal saline) or gluconate (20 g of calcium gluconate to 500 mL normal saline) is then administered prior to returning the blood to the patient to maintain systemic ionized calcium levels between 2.22 and 2.62 mEq/L (1.11–1.31 mmol/L).[125] The citrate that reaches the systemic circulation is subsequently metabolized by the liver. Severe hypocalcemia can result in arrhythmias, even death, so frequent monitoring of unbound serum calcium concentrations is essential.

■ NUTRITIONAL INTERVENTIONS

Nutritional management of critically ill patients with AKI can be extremely complex, as it needs to account for metabolic derangements resulting from both renal dysfunction and underlying disease processes, as well as the effects of RRT on nutrient balance. Stress, inflammation, and injury lead to hypermetabolic and hypercatabolic states and may alter the nutritional requirements. In addition, severe malnutrition found in up to 42% of patients with AKI is a risk factor for increased hospital mortality and length of stay.[126] Thus, patient outcomes can be significantly improved if the nutritional status is optimized (see Chapter 153).

Loss of the normal physiologic and metabolic functions of the kidney and the hypercatabolic response to stress and injury will have a significant impact on the metabolism of nutrients. Derangements in glucose, lipid, and protein metabolism result in hyperglycemia and insulin resistance, hypertriglyceridemia, and protein catabolism and negative nitrogen balance (see Chapter 153 for a detailed discussion). The latter, in particular, is problematic to manage, as increased amino acid turnover and skeletal muscle breakdown lead to muscle wasting and malnutrition and do not respond well to increasing exogenous protein supplementation. CRRT is often employed in this patient population to help manage complications such as fluid overload, electrolyte abnormalities, and azotemia. However, CRRT may also remove small water-soluble molecules such as amino acids and certain micronutrients. As a result, patients receiving CRRT will typically have higher protein requirements (1.5–2.5 g/kg/day) and may require additional micronutrient supplementation to account for these losses. The degree of amino acids lost through CRRT depends on the type and modality of CRRT used, duration of dialysis, dialysate flow rate, effluent rate, and type of hemodiafilter membrane.[127]

Another nutritional consideration for patients receiving CRRT is the heat loss as a consequence of the cooling of the patient's blood as it traverses the extracorporeal circuit.[128] Even though the blood cooling effect by CRRT is widely recognized in clinical practice, its prevention and effect on energy and nutritional requirements have not been well studied. Limited research on CRRT-induced hypothermia is difficult to compare because of inconsistencies in the definition of hypothermia, as well as differences in types, modalities, and circuit configurations used. It has been proposed that the heat loss can be attenuated by warming the IV ultrafiltrate replacement solution, but other investigators found no benefit in using fluid warmers to prevent CRRT-induced hypothermia.[129] The blood-cooling effect is reported to occur more frequently with venovenous modalities, higher dialysate, and lower blood flow rates. Also, certain patient characteristics, such as female gender, low normal baseline temperature, and low body weight, have been identified as risk factors for hypothermia.[128,129] In summary, CRRT should be recognized as a potential source of heat loss. However, no recommendations are currently available for prevention or define the nutritional supplementation that may be necessary as the result of CRRT-induced blood cooling.

■ DRUG-DOSING CONSIDERATIONS

❾ Optimization of drug therapy for patients with AKI is often quite challenging. The multiple variables influencing responses to the drug regimen include the patient's residual drug clearance, the accumulation of fluids, which can markedly alter a drug's volume of distribution, and delivery of CRRT or IHD, which can increase drug clearance and affect the patient's fluid status to further complicate the clinician's projection of the optimal dosage regime. For renally eliminated drugs (>30% excreted unchanged in the urine), particularly for agents with a narrow therapeutic range, serum drug concentration measurements and assessment of pharmacodynamic responses are likely to be necessary. If hepatic function is intact, choosing an agent eliminated primarily by the liver may be preferred. However, any renally eliminated active metabolites may accumulate to a point where they can elicit an undesired

pharmacologic effect. Renal failure can also independently impair nonrenal drug elimination that includes metabolism.[130] Clinical experiences and pharmacokinetic studies in patients with established AKI are fairly limited. The use of dosing guidelines based on data derived from patients with stable CKD, however, may not reflect the clearance and volume of distribution in critically ill AKI patients (see Chapter 57).[103,131]

CLINICAL CONTROVERSY

In the volume-depleted patient requiring a renally eliminated medication, dosing regimens based on the initial S_{cr} prior to fluid therapy have the potential to underestimate renal function and drug elimination, resulting in subtherapeutic serum concentrations. Although not accepted as a standard practice, an initial 24-hour dosing regimen with a bolus might be optimal for many patients.

Edema, which is common in AKI, can significantly increase the volume of distribution of many drugs, particularly water-soluble ones with relatively small volumes of distribution. Increased fluid distribution into the tissues (i.e., sepsis and anasarca in heart failure) can also contribute to a larger volume of distribution for many drugs and thereby reduce the proportion of drug in the plasma that is available to be removed by CRRT or IHD. Because AKI frequently occurs in critically ill patients, multisystem organ failure is often an accompanying problem. Reductions in cardiac output or liver function in addition to volume overload can significantly alter the pharmacokinetic profile of many drugs, such as vancomycin, aminoglycosides, and low molecular weight heparins.[132,133]

In almost all cases where rapid onset of activity is desired, a loading dose may be necessary to promptly achieve desired serum concentrations because the expanded volume of distribution and the prolonged elimination half-life result in an extended time (3.5 times the half-life) until steady-state concentrations are achieved. Maintenance dosing regimens should be reassessed frequently and be based on the patient's current renal function. A dose that provides the desired serum concentration on one day may be inappropriate only a few days later if the patient's fluid status, RRT prescription or renal function has changed dramatically.

CLINICAL CONTROVERSY

Some clinicians use a standard ESKD dosage regimen despite the fact that renal function can fluctuate, such that the patient's renal function may be in one dosing range one day and in another the next. Others believe, however, that the patient's clinical need for the drug and any change in the volume of distribution or the RRT therapy should be considered if one has any chance of achieving the target serum concentrations.

Drug therapy individualization for the AKI patient who is receiving any form of renal replacement therapy is complicated by the fact that patients with AKI may have a higher residual nonrenal clearance than patients with CKD who have a similar CL_{cr}.[103] This has been reported with some drugs, such as ceftriaxone, imipenem, and vancomycin.[134–138] Alterations in the activity of some, but not all, cytochrome P450 enzymes have been demonstrated in patients with CKD.[130] The nonrenal clearance of imipenem in patients with AKI (91 mL/min [1.52 mL/s]) is between the values observed in stage 5 CKD patients (50 mL/min [0.84 mL/s]) and those with normal renal function (120 mL/min [2 mL/s]).[138] This may be the result of less accumulation of uremic waste products that may alter hepatic function. A nonrenal clearance value in a patient with AKI that is higher than anticipated based on data from individuals with CKD would result in lower than expected, possibly subtherapeutic, serum concentrations. For example, to maintain comparable serum concentrations, the imipenem dose requirement in patients with AKI would be 2,000 mg daily as compared with the recommended dosage for patients with ESKD of 1,000 mg daily.[138] As AKI persists, the nonrenal clearance values appear to approach those observed in patients with CKD.[136,138,139] Finally, the clearance of aminoglycosides has been reported to be higher and the elimination half-life shorter in those with severe AKI compared with ESKD patients requiring hemodialysis.[131] Another challenge is that much of the dosing-related data was acquired in patients with CKD, with initial pharmacokinetic assessments done after single-dose administration. The determination of pharmacokinetic parameters using a single-dose model may result in more rapid initial drug removal estimates secondary to distribution from the plasma to the tissue as well. Thus, application of dosing regimens derived from studies in patients with CKD and ESKD may result in underdosing of these agents and thereby contribute to less than optimal clinical outcomes.

IHD Compared with CRRT

In addition to patient-specific differences, there are marked differences between IHD and the three primary types of CRRT—CVVH, CVVHD, and CVVHDF—with regard to drug removal.[140-142]

CRRT During CVVH, drug removal primarily occurs via convection/ultrafiltration (the passive transport of drug molecules at the concentration at which they exist in plasma water into the ultrafiltrate). Convective removal is most efficient for smaller agents, typically less than 15,000 Da (15 kDa) in size, and those that are primarily unbound in the plasma. The clearance of a drug by either of these methods is thus a function of the membrane permeability for the drug, which is called the sieving coefficient (SC) and the rate of ultrafiltrate formation (UFR). Alteration in the pore size of the filter and surface charge relative to the molecule being removed may vary between different dialyzers. If diffusion of the drug is not dependent on the filter pore size, then the SC can be calculated as follows:

$$SC = (2 \times C_{UF})/[(C_a) + (C_v)]$$

where C_a and C_v are the concentrations of the drug in the plasma going into and returning from the dialyzer/hemofilter, respectively, and C_{UF} is the concentration in the ultrafiltrate. The SC is often approximated by the fraction unbound (f_u) because this information may be more readily available. Thus, the clearance by CVVH can be calculated as

$$Cl_{CVVH} = UFR \times SC$$

or approximated as

$$Cl_{CVVH} = UFR \times f_u$$

In CVVHDF, clearance is a combination of both diffusion and convection. The Cl_{CVVHDF} can be mathematically approximated, providing the blood flow rate is greater than 100 mL/min and the dialysate flow rate (DFR) is between 8 and 33 mL/min, as

$$Cl_{CVVHDF} = (UFR \times f_u) + Cl_{diffusion}$$

where $Cl_{diffusion}$ is the clearance via diffusion from plasma water to the dialysate. In the clinical setting, it is not possible to separate these two components (UFR and DFR) of Cl_{CVVHDF}. In essence the Cl_{CVVHDF} is calculated as the product of the combined ultrafiltrate and dialysate volume (V_{df}) and the concentration of the drug in this fluid (C_{df}) divided by the plasma concentration (C_p^{mid}) at the midpoint of the V_{df} collection period.

❿ Individualization of therapy for a patient receiving CRRT is dependent on the patient's residual renal function and the clearance of the drug by the mode of CRRT the patient is receiving. There are differences in the rate of drug removal, not only between the three primary modes of CRRT, but also within each mode.[135,140-143] This is a result of differences in the filter membrane composition, variable degrees of drug binding to the membrane, and permeability characteristics of the membrane.[143-147] The primary factors that influence drug clearance during CRRT are thus the ultrafiltration rate, blood flow rate, and dialysate flow rate. For example, clearance in CVVH is directly proportional to the ultrafiltration rate, whereas clearance during CVVHDF, which depends on both the ultrafiltration rate and the dialysate flow rate, increases as either flow rate increases. An increase in the ultrafiltration flow rate (5–45 mL/min) and dialysate flow rate (8.3–33.3 mL/min), however, can have dramatic effects on the clearance of agents such as ceftazidime during CVVH and CVVHD, respectively (Fig. 51–5).[147] Another factor that changes drug dosing is the type of RRT used in the patient. CRRT can rapidly remove excess fluid from edematous patients, thereby changing the volume of distribution (V_D) of drugs with limited distribution (low V_D suggesting a greater proportion in the plasma or extracellular fluid) fairly rapidly. Drug clearances attained by IHD, CRRTs, and hybrid RRTs all differ from each other and must be added to any endogenous drug clearance that the patient generates.[135] An algorithmic approach for drug dosage adjustment in patients undergoing CRRT has been proposed.[141] In CRRT, the clearance of a given agent may be ascertained from published reports.[141,148,149] Table 51–10 summarizes the sieving coefficients of frequently used drugs. These data can be used to design initial dosage regimens for patients receiving CVVH.[140,143]

For example, IM is a 48-year-old, 60 kg man with an S_{cr} that has increased from 2.3 mg/dL to 7.2 mg/dL (203–636 µmol/L) over 3 days. The residual Cl_{cr} value in this patient, calculated using the Jeliffe equation (see Chapter 49), is 4.8 mL/min (0.080 mL/s). The consulting nephrologist recommends that CVVHDF be initiated

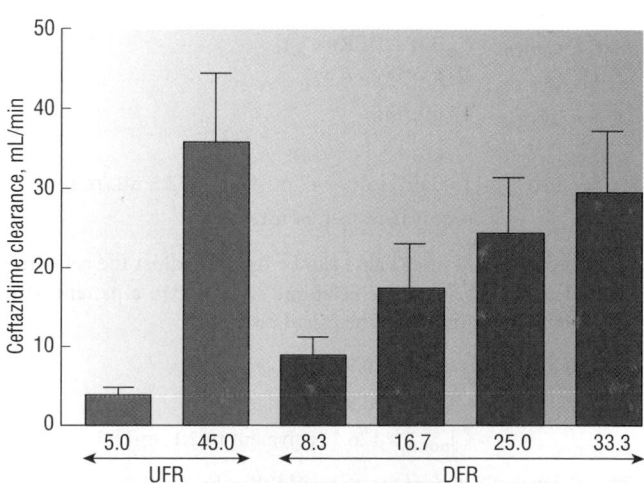

FIGURE 51-5. The effect of increasing ultrafiltration rate (UFR in milliliters per minute) and dialysate flow rate (DFR in milliliters per minute) on the clearance of ceftazidime. *(Adapted from reference 147.)*

TABLE 51-10 Predicted and Measured Sieving Coefficients of Selected Drugs[103,140-143,148,149]

Drug	Predicted	Measured
Amikacin	0.95	0.88
Amphotericin	0.01	0.32–0.4
Ampicillin	0.80	0.6–0.69
Cefepime	0.97	0.47–0.97
Cefoperazone	0.10	0.27–0.69
Cefotaxime	0.62	0.55–1.1
Cefoxitin	0.30	0.32
Ceftazidime	0.90	0.38–0.78
Ceftriaxone	0.10	0.71–0.82
Clindamycin	0.25	0.49–0.98
Digoxin	0.75	0.96
Erythromycin	0.25	0.37
5-fluorocytosine	0.96	0.98
Gentamicin	0.95	0.81–0.75
Imipenem	0.80	0.78
Metronidazole	0.80	0.80
Mezlocillin	0.68	0.68
N-acetylprocainamide	0.80	0.92
Nafcillin	0.20	0.47
Netilmicin	–	0.85
Oxacillin	0.05	0.02
Phenobarbital	0.60	0.86
Phenytoin	0.10	0.45
Procainamide	0.80	0.86
Theophylline	0.47	0.85
Tobramycin	0.95	0.78–0.86
Vancomycin	0.90	0.5–0.8

using a Fresenius F-80 filter at blood, ultrafiltrate, and dialysate flow rates of 150, 15, and 33.3 mL/min, respectively. The patient is to receive cefepime while on CVVHDF. The patient's residual cefepime clearance (Cl_{RES}) can be estimated using the following regression equation relating Cl_{cr} and cefepime clearance:

$$Cl_{RES} \text{ (mL/min)} = [0.96 \times (Cl_{cr})] + 10.9$$
$$Cl_{RES} = [0.96 \times (4.8)] + 10.9$$
$$= 15.5 \text{ mL/min (equivalent to 0.26 mL/s)}$$

The total clearance while on CVVHDF would be the sum of the patient's residual clearance and the cefepime clearance associated with CVVHDF (which can be approximated as described above) as follows:

$$Cl_{CVVHDF} = [(UFR + DFR) \times f_u)]$$
$$Cl_{CVVHDF} = [(15 + 33) \times 0.97]$$
$$Cl_{CVVHDF} = 47 \text{ mL/min}$$
$$Cl_T = CL_{RES} + CL_{CVVHDF}$$
$$Cl_T = 15.5 \text{ mL/min} + 47 \text{ mL/min} = 62.5 \text{ mL/min}$$
$$\text{(equivalent to 1.04 mL/s)}$$

This patient's clearance value can be used to adjust the cefepime dose as described below. The cefepime clearance in a patient with normal renal function would be calculated as:

$$Cl_{norm} \text{(mL/min)} = [0.96 \times (Cl_{cr})] + 10.9$$
$$Cl_{norm} = [0.96 \times 120] + 10.9$$
$$Cl_{norm} = 126.1 \text{ (eqivalent to 2.11 mL/s)}$$

The dosage adjustment factor would then be

$$Q = Cl_T/Cl_{norm}$$
$$Q = 62.5 \div 126 = 0.49$$

For this patient's situation, the normal regimen of cefepime would be 2,000 mg (D_n) every 12 hours (τ_n). If one wanted to maintain D_n and extend the dosing interval (τ_n), then τ_f would be calculated as:

$$\tau_f = \tau_n/Q$$
$$\tau_f = 12 \text{ hours}/0.49$$
$$\tau_f \approx 24 \text{ hours}$$

This approach suggests the patient should receive cefepime 2,000 mg every 24 hours. If the additional clearance associated with CVVHDF (40.2 mL/min [0.67 mL/s]) was not considered, the calculated dosing interval would have been considerably longer. Several variables can affect the outcome of these calculations, including the multiple variables within the dialysis therapy—for example, UFR, blood flow rate, and DFR—and interpatient variability in nonrenal and renal drug clearance, to name just two.

Intermittent Hemodialysis Limitations of IHD-based dosing charts include variability in the patient's individual pharmacokinetic parameters, differences in the dialysis prescription, such as dialyzer blood flow or duration, and the use of new IHD dialyzers. The approach to hemodialysis may also change on a daily basis, especially in unstable individuals with ARF. This could include, for example, the dialyzer/filter used, the duration, the degree of hemofiltration compared with convection, and the blood flow rate. Individualization of a dosing regimen may require daily assessment of the clinical status of the patient and any planned or recently administered hemodialysis.

Overall, there are numerous potential pharmacokinetic and pharmacodynamic alterations to be aware of in the patient with AKI. Unfortunately, there is a dearth of data to quantify these changes, and even less evidence to prove that if one incorporates these considerations into patient care, the associated outcomes will be improved.

EVALUATION OF THERAPEUTIC OUTCOMES

Vigilant monitoring of patients with AKI is essential, particularly in those who are critically ill (Table 51–11). Once the laboratory-based tests (e.g., urinalysis and fractional excretion of sodium

TABLE 51-11 Key Monitoring Parameters for Patients with Established Acute Kidney Injury

Parameter	Frequency
Fluid ins/outs	Every shift
Patient weight	Daily
Hemodynamics (blood pressure, heart rate, mean arterial pressure, etc.)	Every shift
Blood chemistries	
Sodium, potassium, chloride, bicarbonate, calcium, phosphate, magnesium	Daily
Blood urea nitrogen/serum creatinine	Daily
Drugs and their dosing regimens	Daily
Nutritional regimen	Daily
Blood glucose	Daily (minimum)
Serum concentration data for drugs	After regimen changes and after renal replacement therapy has been instituted
Times of administered doses	Daily
Doses relative to administration of renal replacement therapy	Daily
Urinalysis	
Calculate measured creatinine clearance	Every time measured urine collection performed
Calculate fractional excretion of sodium	Every time measured urine collection performed
Plans for renal replacement	Daily

calculations) have been conducted to diagnose the cause of AKI, they usually do not have to be repeated. In established AKI, daily measurements of urine output, fluid intake, and weight should be performed. Vital signs should be monitored at least daily, more often if patient acuity of illness is high. Daily blood tests for electrolytes, BUN, and a complete blood cell count should be considered routine for hospitalized patients.

Therapeutic drug monitoring should be performed for drugs that have a narrow therapeutic window that can be measured by the hospital laboratory. If results from these serum drug concentrations cannot be obtained in a timely fashion (<24 hours), then their value is limited. When considering approaches to measuring serum concentrations, consensus is limited. Measuring a serum drug concentration prior to hemodialysis has the advantage of allowing time for the result to be reported and redosing done shortly after dialysis with minimal delay. This is especially important if the desired pharmacologic effects are lost during or after hemodialysis is complete because the serum concentrations have become subtherapeutic. Knowledge based on previous observations of how a particular agent is removed for a given dialysis approach and any prehemodialysis serum concentration of the agent can assist in estimating the amount removed and predicting any necessary post-dialysis dose. Serum concentrations drawn after hemodialysis may reflect plasma concentrations that are transiently depressed until the drug can reequilibrate from the tissues (plasma rebound effect). The advantage with an after-dialysis level is the greater accuracy in determining how much drug was cleared during hemodialysis, but this may delay reestablishing target effects. Greater therapeutic drug monitoring may be necessary in patients with AKI than what is done routinely for other patients because of the potential changes in dynamic status (changing volume status, changing renal function, and RRTs) of patients with AKI.

PHARMACOECONOMIC CONSIDERATIONS

AKI is a large financial burden on the healthcare system. Much of this cost is incurred because of extended ICU stays which are inherently expensive. Healthcare costs may also vary by the modality of dialysis a patient is receiving. A post-hoc analysis of a multicenter, multinational study conducted in 2000-01 estimated that the total cost difference between continuous and intermittent RRT in critically ill patients ranges from $3630/day more with continuous RRT to $379/day more with intermittent RRT.[155] In addition, it is estimated that an S_{cr} increase ≥ 0.5mg/dL (≥ 44 μmol/L) is associated with a 6.5-fold increase in odds for mortality, 3.5-day increase in length of stay, and $7,500 (1998 dollars) in excess hospital costs, and average hospital costs in patients requiring RRT are around $50,000.[150,151] Higher costs have been associated with the severity of AKI using the RIFLE criteria.[152] Most patients who survive AKI regain life-sustaining renal function, but the 5% who do not regain renal function[23] continue to incur the economic and personal costs of dialysis or kidney transplantation. The financial burden is estimated to be over $50,000 per year greater than the non-dialysis-dependent patient whose kidneys recovered from AKI. Nonetheless, patients who required RRT for their AKI generally have a good quality of life after recovery.[151]

Medical intervention costs can be normalized to assess total costs using quality-adjusted life-years (QALYs) gained by the intervention. The use of a QALY approach to treatment of critically ill patients with AKI indicates that treating these patients is very expensive relative to other common medical interventions.[153] For example, in 2001, the treatment of critically ill AKI patient cost per QALY was $168,711, compared with treatment of acute myocardial infarction cost per QALY of $45,000, and the routine treatment of hypertension cost per QALY of $31,321.[154] A typical cost per QALY of <$100,000 is considered cost-effective. Another study found that daily hemodialysis was cost effective when compared to alternate-day hemodialysis with about $5000 per QALY gained.[156] Overall, more research needs to be done to improve the AKI survival rate to reduce this cost per QALY. Furthermore, it underscores the need to prevent the occurrence of AKI in the first place.

CONCLUSION

The unique characteristics of AKI compared with CKD can lead to notable differences in how renal function is measured and how treatment regimens are developed. Most management approaches currently involve prevention and support of the patient once AKI is established, so as to minimize the potential for additional harm to either the patient or the kidney. Monitoring approaches and pharmacologic regimens should consider frequent changes in the clinical presentations, with most decisions considered short term. Understanding the constantly changing status inherent to AKI and how to adjust management regimens is a key component to optimizing therapy.

ACKNOWLEDGMENT

We gratefully acknowledge Ann Spencer, PharmD, and Bruce Mueller, PharmD, for their contributions to the prior editions of this chapter.

ABBREVIATIONS

ACE: Angiotensin-converting enzyme

AIN: Acute interstitial nephritis

AKI: Acute kidney injury

AKIN: Acute Kidney Injury Network

ANP: Atrial natriuretic peptide

ARB: Angiotensin receptor blocker

ARF: Acute renal failure

ATN: Acute tubular necrosis

BTP: Beta trace protein

BUN: Blood urea nitrogen

CIN: Contrast-induced nephropathy

CKD: Chronic kidney disease

CL_{cr}: Creatinine clearance

CRRT: Continuous renal replacement therapy

CT: Computed tomography

CVVH: Continuous venovenous hemofiltration

CVVHD: Continuous venovenous hemodialysis

CVVHDF: Continuous venovenous hemodiafiltration

EPO: Erythropoietin alpha

ESKD: End-stage kidney disease

FE_{Na}: Fractional excretion of sodium

GFR: Glomerular filtration rate

ICU: Intensive care unit

IHD: Intermittent hemodialysis

IL-18: Interleukin-18

KIM-1: Kidney injury molecule 1

KUB: Kidney ureter bladder

L-FABP: Liver-type fatty acid binding protein

NAC: *N*-acetylcysteine

NGAL: Neutrophil gelatinase-associated lipocalin

NSAID: Nonsteroidal antiinflammatory drug

QALY: Quality-adjusted life-year

RIFLE: Risk, Injury, Failure, Loss of Kidney Function, and End-Stage Kidney Disease

RRT: Renal replacement therapy

S_{cr}: Serum creatinine

REFERENCES

1. Kellum JA, Levin N, Bouman C, Lameire N. Developing a consensus classification system for acute renal failure. Curr Opin Crit Care 2002;8(6):509–514.

2. Bellomo R, Ronco C, Kellum JA, Mehta RL, Palevsky P. Acute renal failure—Definition, outcome measures, animal models, fluid therapy and information technology needs: The Second International Consensus Conference of the Acute Dialysis Quality Initiative (ADQI) Group. Crit Care 2004;8(4):R204–R212.

3. Mehta RL, Kellum JA, Shah SV, et al. Acute Kidney Injury Network: Report of an initiative to improve outcomes in acute kidney injury. Crit Care 2007;11(2):R31.

4. Chang CH, Lin CY, Tian YC, et al. Acute kidney injury classification: Comparison of AKIN and RIFLE criteria. Shock 2009.

5. Bagshaw SM, George C, Bellomo R. A comparison of the RIFLE and AKIN criteria for acute kidney injury in critically ill patients. Nephrol Dial Transplant 2008;23(5):1569–1574.

6. Bagshaw SM, George C, Dinu I, Bellomo R. A multi-centre evaluation of the RIFLE criteria for early acute kidney injury in critically ill patients. Nephrol Dial Transplant 2008;23(4):1203–1210.

7. Hoste EA, Clermont G, Kersten A, et al. RIFLE criteria for acute kidney injury are associated with hospital mortality in critically ill patients: A cohort analysis. Crit Care 2006;10(3):R73.

8. Ricci Z, Cruz D, Ronco C. The RIFLE criteria and mortality in acute kidney injury: A systematic review. Kidney Int 2008;73(5):538–546.

9. Bihorac A, Yavas S, Subbiah S, et al. Long-term risk of mortality and acute kidney injury during hospitalization after major surgery. Ann Surg 2009;249(5):851–858.

10. Bagshaw SM, George C, Bellomo R. Early acute kidney injury and sepsis: a multicentre evaluation. Crit Care 2008;12(2):R47.

11. Ricci Z, Ronco C. Year in review 2007: Critical care—Nephrology. Crit Care 2008;12(5):230.

12. Lameire N, Van Biesen W, Vanholder R. The changing epidemiology of acute renal failure. Nat Clin Pract Nephrol 2006;2(7):364–377.

13. Liano F, Felipe C, Tenorio MT, et al. Long-term outcome of acute tubular necrosis: A contribution to its natural history. Kidney Int 2007;71(7):679–686.

14. Uchino S, Bellomo R, Goldsmith D, Bates S, Ronco C. An assessment of the RIFLE criteria for acute renal failure in hospitalized patients. Crit Care Med 2006;34(7):1913–1917.

15. Coca SG, Yusuf B, Shlipak MG, Garg AX, Parikh CR. Long-term risk of mortality and other adverse outcomes after acute kidney injury: A systematic review and meta-analysis. Am J Kidney Dis 2009;53(6):961–973.

16. Goldberg R, Dennen P. Long-term outcomes of acute kidney injury. Adv Chronic Kidney Dis 2008;15(3):297–307.

17. Kaufman J, Dhakal M, Patel B, Hamburger R. Community-acquired acute renal failure. Am J Kidney Dis 1991;17(2):191–198.

18. Pisoni R, Wille KM, Tolwani AJ. The epidemiology of severe acute kidney injury: From BEST to PICARD, in acute kidney injury—New concepts. Nephron Clin Pract 2008;109(4):C188–C191.

19. Lu JC, Coca SG, Patel UD, Cantley L, Parikh CR. Searching for genes that matter in acute kidney injury: A systematic review. Clin J Am Soc Nephrol 2009;4(6):1020–1031.

20. Badr KF, Ichikawa I. Prerenal failure: A deleterious shift from renal compensation to decompensation. N Engl J Med 1988;319(10):623–629.

21. Lameire N. The pathophysiology of acute renal failure. Crit Care Clin 2005;21(2):197–210.

22. Gambaro G, Perazella MA. Adverse renal effects of anti-inflammatory agents: Evaluation of selective and nonselective cyclooxygenase inhibitors. J Intern Med 2003;253(6):643–652.

23. Clarkson MRF, Eustace JA, Rabb H. Acute kidney injury. In: Brenner BM, ed. Brenner and Rector's The Kidney. Vol 1. 8th ed. Philadelphia, PA: WB Saunders; 2007:943–975.

24. Remuzzi GP, N;De Broe, M.E. Tubulointerstitial diseases. In: Brenner BM, ed. Brenner and Rector's The Kidney. Vol 1. 8th ed. Philadelphia, PA: WB Saunders; 2007:1174–1202.

25. Perazella MA. Drug-induced nephropathy: An update. Expert Opin Drug Saf 2005;4(4):689–706.

26. Levey AS, Bosch JP, Lewis JB, Greene T, Rogers N, Roth D. A more accurate method to estimate glomerular filtration rate from serum creatinine: A new prediction equation. Modification of Diet in Renal Disease Study Group. Ann Intern Med 1999;130(6):461–470.

27. Soares AA, Eyff TF, Campani RB, Ritter L, Camargo JL, Silveiro SP. Glomerular filtration rate measurement and prediction equations. Clin Chem Lab Med 2009;47(9):1023–1032.

28. Bagshaw SM, Bellomo R. Early diagnosis of acute kidney injury. Curr Opin Crit Care 2007;13(6):638–644.

29. Trombetta DPF, E.F. The Kidneys. In: Lee M, ed. Basic Skills in Interpreting Laboratory Data. 4th ed. Bethesda, MD: American Society of Health-System Pharmacists; 2009:161–178.

30. Jelliffe RW, Jelliffe SM. Estimation of creatinine clearance from changing serum-creatinine levels. Lancet. 1971;2(7726):710.

31. Chiou WL, Hsu FH. Pharmacokinetics of creatinine in man and its implications in the monitoring of renal function and in dosage regimen modifications in patients with renal insufficiency. J Clin Pharmacol 1975;15(5–6):427–434.

32. Baumann TJ, Staddon JE, Horst HM, Bivins BA. Minimum urine collection periods for accurate determination of creatinine clearance in critically ill patients. Clin Pharm 1987;6(5):393–398.

33. Herget-Rosenthal S, Poppen D, Husing J, et al. Prognostic value of tubular proteinuria and enzymuria in nonoliguric acute tubular necrosis. Clin Chem 2004;50(3):552–558.

34. Knight EL, Verhave JC, Spiegelman D, et al. Factors influencing serum cystatin C levels other than renal function and the impact on renal function measurement. Kidney Int 2004;65(4):1416–1421.

35. Manetti L, Pardini E, Genovesi M, et al. Thyroid function differently affects serum cystatin C and creatinine concentrations. J Endocrinol Invest 2005;28(4):346–349.

36. Rule AD, Bergstralh EJ, Slezak JM, Bergert J, Larson TS. Glomerular filtration rate estimated by cystatin C among different clinical presentations. Kidney Int 2006;69(2):399–405.

37. Soni SS, Cruz D, Bobek I, et al. NGAL: A biomarker of acute kidney injury and other systemic conditions. Int Urol Nephrol 2009.

38. Bennett M, Dent CL, Ma Q, et al. Urine NGAL predicts severity of acute kidney injury after cardiac surgery: A prospective study. Clin J Am Soc Nephrol 2008;3(3):665–673.

39. Mitsnefes MM, Kathman TS, Mishra J, et al. Serum neutrophil gelatinase-associated lipocalin as a marker of renal function in children with chronic kidney disease. Pediatr Nephrol 2007;22(1):101–108.

40. Devarajan P. Emerging urinary biomarkers in the diagnosis of acute kidney injury. Expert Opin Med Diagn 2008;2(4):387–398.

41. Parikh CR, Jani A, Melnikov VY, Faubel S, Edelstein CL. Urinary interleukin-18 is a marker of human acute tubular necrosis. Am J Kidney Dis 2004;43(3):405–414.

42. van Timmeren MM, van den Heuvel MC, Bailly V, Bakker SJ, van Goor H, Stegeman CA. Tubular kidney injury molecule-1 (KIM-1) in human renal disease. J Pathol 2007;212(2):209–217.

43. Zhou Y, Vaidya VS, Brown RP, et al. Comparison of kidney injury molecule-1 and other nephrotoxicity biomarkers in urine and kidney following acute exposure to gentamicin, mercury, and chromium. Toxicol Sci 2008;101(1):159–170.

44. Kamijo A, Sugaya T, Hikawa A, et al. Clinical evaluation of urinary excretion of liver-type fatty acid-binding protein as a marker for the monitoring of chronic kidney disease: A multicenter trial. J Lab Clin Med 2005;145(3):125–133.

45. Yokoyama T, Kamijo-Ikemori A, Sugaya T, Hoshino S, Yasuda T, Kimura K. Urinary excretion of liver type fatty acid binding protein accurately reflects the degree of tubulointerstitial damage. Am J Pathol 2009;174(6):2096–2106.

46. Kato K, Sato N, Yamamoto T, Iwasaki YK, Tanaka K, Mizuno K. Valuable markers for contrast-induced nephropathy in patients undergoing cardiac catheterization. Circ J 2008;72(9):1499–1505.

47. Portilla D, Dent C, Sugaya T, et al. Liver fatty acid-binding protein as a biomarker of acute kidney injury after cardiac surgery. Kidney Int 2008;73(4):465–472.

48. Kobata M, Shimizu A, Rinno H, et al. Beta-trace protein, a new marker of GFR, may predict the early prognostic stages of patients with type 2 diabetic nephropathy. J Clin Lab Anal 2004;18(4):237–239.

49. White CA, Akbari A, Doucette S, et al. Estimating GFR using serum beta trace protein: accuracy and validation in kidney transplant and pediatric populations. Kidney Int 2009;76(7):784–791.

50. Uehara Y, Makino H, Seiki K, Urade Y. Urinary excretions of lipocalin-type prostaglandin D synthase predict renal injury in type-2 diabetes: A cross-sectional and prospective multicentre study. Nephrol Dial Transplant 2009;24(2):475–482.

51. McCullough PA. Contrast-induced acute kidney injury. J Am Coll Cardiol 2008;51(15):1419–1428.

52. Weisbord SD, Palevsky PM. Prevention of contrast-induced nephropathy with volume expansion. Clin J Am Soc Nephrol 2008;3(1):273–280.

53. Mueller C, Buerkle G, Buettner HJ, et al. Prevention of contrast media-associated nephropathy: Randomized comparison of 2 hydration regimens in 1620 patients undergoing coronary angioplasty. Arch Intern Med 2002;162(3):329–336.

54. Trivedi HS, Moore H, Nasr S, et al. A randomized prospective trial to assess the role of saline hydration on the development of contrast nephrotoxicity. Nephron Clin Pract 2003;93(1):C29–C34.

55. From AM, Bartholmai BJ, Williams AW, Cha SS, Pflueger A, McDonald FS. Sodium bicarbonate is associated with an increased incidence of contrast nephropathy: A retrospective cohort study of 7977 patients at mayo clinic. Clin J Am Soc Nephrol 2008;3(1):10–18.

56. Merten GJ, Burgess WP, Gray LV, et al. Prevention of contrast-induced nephropathy with sodium bicarbonate: A randomized controlled trial. JAMA 2004;291(19):2328–2334.

57. Vasheghani-Farahani A, Sadigh G, Kassaian SE et al. Sodium bicarbone in preventing contrast nephropathy in patients at risk for volume overload: a randomized controlled trial. J Nephrol 2010 Mar-Apr;23(2):216–223.

58. Kanbay M, Covic A, Coca SG, Turgut F, Akcay A, Parikh CR. Sodium bicarbonate for the prevention of contrast-induced nephropathy: A meta-analysis of 17 randomized trials. Int Urol Nephrol 2009;41(3):617–627.

59. Navaneethan SD, Singh S, Appasamy S, Wing RE, Sehgal AR. Sodium bicarbonate therapy for prevention of contrast-induced nephropathy: A systematic review and meta-analysis. Am J Kidney Dis 2009;53(4):617–627.

60. Reinecke H, Fobker M, Wellmann J, et al. A randomized controlled trial comparing hydration therapy to additional hemodialysis or N-acetylcysteine for the prevention of contrast medium-induced nephropathy: The Dialysis-versus-Diuresis (DVD) Trial. Clin Res Cardiol 2007;96(3):130–139.

61. Marenzi G, Marana I, Lauri G, et al. The prevention of radiocontrast-agent-induced nephropathy by hemofiltration. N Engl J Med 2003;349(14):1333–1340.

62. Cruz DN, Perazella MA, Bellomo R, et al. Extracorporeal blood purification therapies for prevention of radiocontrast-induced nephropathy: A systematic review. Am J Kidney Dis 2006;48(3):361–371.

63. Karajala V, Mansour W, Kellum JA. Diuretics in acute kidney injury. Minerva Anestesiol 2009;75(5):251–257.

64. Ho KM, Sheridan DJ. Meta-analysis of frusemide to prevent or treat acute renal failure. BMJ 2006;333(7565):420.

65. Cantarovich F, Rangoonwala B, Lorenz H, Verho M, Esnault VL. High-dose furosemide for established ARF: A prospective, random-ized, double-blind, placebo-controlled, multicenter trial. Am J Kidney Dis 2004;44(3):402–409.

66. Venkataraman R. Can we prevent acute kidney injury? Crit Care Med 2008;36(4 Suppl):S166–S171.

67. Bellomo R, Chapman M, Finfer S, Hickling K, Myburgh J. Low-dose dopamine in patients with early renal dysfunction: A placebo-controlled randomised trial. Australian and New Zealand Intensive Care Society (ANZICS) Clinical Trials Group. Lancet 2000;356(9248):2139–2143.

68. Friedrich JO, Adhikari N, Herridge MS, Beyene J. Meta-analysis: Low-dose dopamine increases urine output but does not prevent renal dysfunction or death. Ann Intern Med 2005;142(7):510–524.

69. Landoni G, Biondi-Zoccai GG, Tumlin JA, et al. Beneficial impact of fenoldopam in critically ill patients with or at risk for acute renal failure: A meta-analysis of randomized clinical trials. Am J Kidney Dis 2007;49(1):56–68.

70. Briguori C, Colombo A, Airoldi F, et al. N-acetylcysteine versus fenoldopam mesylate to prevent contrast agent-associated nephrotoxicity. J Am Coll Cardiol 2004;44(4):762–765.

71. Cetin M, Devrim E, Serin Kilicoglu S, et al. Ionic high-osmolar contrast medium causes oxidant stress in kidney tissue: Partial protective role of ascorbic acid. Ren Fail 2008;30(5):567–572.

72. Briguori C, Airoldi F, D'Andrea D, et al. Renal Insufficiency Following Contrast Media Administration Trial (REMEDIAL): A randomized comparison of 3 preventive strategies. Circulation 13 2007;115(10):1211–1217.

73. Boscheri A, Weinbrenner C, Botzek B, Reynen K, Kuhlisch E, Strasser RH. Failure of ascorbic acid to prevent contrast-media induced nephropathy in patients with renal dysfunction. Clin Nephrol 2007;68(5):279–286.

74. Amini M, Salarifar M, Amirbaigloo A, Masoudkabir F, Esfahani F. N-acetylcysteine does not prevent contrast-induced nephropathy after cardiac catheterization in patients with diabetes mellitus and chronic kidney disease: A randomized clinical trial. Trials 2009;10:45.

75. Sisillo E, Ceriani R, Bortone F, et al. N-acetylcysteine for prevention of acute renal failure in patients with chronic renal insufficiency undergoing cardiac surgery: A prospective, randomized, clinical trial. Crit Care Med 2008;36(1):81–86.

76. Ho KM, Morgan DJ. Meta-analysis of N-acetylcysteine to prevent acute renal failure after major surgery. Am J Kidney Dis 2009;53(1):33–40.

77. Mehta RL, Pascual MT, Soroko S, et al. Spectrum of acute renal failure in the intensive care unit: The PICARD experience. Kidney Int 2004;66(4):1613–1621.

78. Mehta RL. Glycemic control and critical illness: Is the kidney involved? J Am Soc Nephrol 2007;18(10):2623–2627.

79. Vanhorebeek I, Gunst J, Ellger B, et al. Hyperglycemic kidney damage in an animal model of prolonged critical illness. Kidney Int 2009.

80. van den Berghe G, Wouters P, Weekers F, et al. Intensive insulin therapy in the critically ill patients. N Engl J Med 2001;345(19):1359–1367.

81. Arabi YM, Dabbagh OC, Tamim HM, et al. Intensive versus conventional insulin therapy: A randomized controlled trial in medical and surgical critically ill patients. Crit Care Med 2008;36(12):3190–3197.

82. Van den Berghe G, Wilmer A, Hermans G, et al. Intensive insulin therapy in the medical ICU. N Engl J Med 2006;354(5):449–461.

83. Finfer S, Chittock DR, Su SY, et al. Intensive versus conventional glucose control in critically ill patients. N Engl J Med 2009;360(13):1283–1297.

84. Bagshaw SM, Ghali WA. Theophylline for prevention of contrast-induced nephropathy: A systematic review and meta-analysis. Arch Intern Med 2005;165(10):1087–1093.

85. Johnson DW, Pat B, Vesey DA, Guan Z, Endre Z, Gobe GC. Delayed administration of darbepoetin or erythropoietin protects against ischemic acute renal injury and failure. Kidney Int 2006;69(10):1806–1813.

86. Song YR, Lee T, You SJ, et al. Prevention of acute kidney injury by erythropoietin in patients undergoing coronary artery bypass grafting: A pilot study. Am J Nephrol 2009;30(3):253–260.

87. Endre ZH, Walker RJ, Pickering JW et al. Early intervention with erythropoietin does not affect the outcome of acute kidney injury. Kidney Int 2010 Jun;77(11):1020–1030.

88. Sackner-Bernstein JD, Kowalski M, Fox M, Aaronson K. Short-term risk of death after treatment with nesiritide for decompensated heart failure: A pooled analysis of randomized controlled trials. JAMA 2005;293(15):1900–1905.

89. Morikawa S, Sone T, Tsuboi H, et al. Renal protective effects and the prevention of contrast-induced nephropathy by atrial natriuretic peptide. J Am Coll Cardiol 2009;53(12):1040–1046.

90. McAlister FA, Ezekowitz J, Tonelli M, Armstrong PW. Renal insufficiency and heart failure: Prognostic and therapeutic implications from a prospective cohort study. Circulation 2004;109(8):1004–1009.

91. Ognibene FP. Hemodynamic support during sepsis. Clin Chest Med 1996;17(2):279–287.

92. Hebert PC, Wells G, Blajchman MA, et al. A multicenter, randomized, controlled clinical trial of transfusion requirements in critical care. Transfusion Requirements in Critical Care Investigators, Canadian Critical Care Trials Group. N Engl J Med 1999;340(6):409–417.

93. Bell M. Acute kidney injury: New concepts, renal recovery. Nephron Clin Pract 2008;109(4):C224–C228.

94. Ding F, Humes HD. The bioartificial kidney and bioengineered membranes in acute kidney injury. Nephron Exp Nephrol 2008;109(4): E118–E122.

95. Schortgen F, Soubrier N, Delclaux C, et al. Hemodynamic tolerance of intermittent hemodialysis in critically ill patients: Usefulness of practice guidelines. Am J Respir Crit Care Med 2000;162(1):197–202.

96. Clark WR, Mueller BA, Kraus MA, Macias WL. Extracorporeal therapy requirements for patients with acute renal failure. J Am Soc Nephrol 1997;8(5):804–812.

97. Schiffl H, Lang SM, Fischer R. Daily hemodialysis and the outcome of acute renal failure. N Engl J Med 2002;346(5):305–310.

98. Ronco C, Bellomo R, Kellum JA. Continuous renal replacement therapy: Opinions and evidence. Adv Ren Replace Ther 2002;9(4):229–244.

99. Ronco C, Bellomo R, Homel P, et al. Effects of different doses in continuous veno-venous haemofiltration on outcomes of acute renal failure: A prospective randomised trial. Lancet 2000;356(9223):26–30.

100. Bellomo R, Cass A, Cole L, et al. Intensity of continuous renal-replacement therapy in critically ill patients. N Engl J Med 2009;361(17): 1627–1638.

101. Casey ET, Gupta BP, Erwin PJ, Montori VM, Murad MH. The dose of continuous renal replacement therapy for actute renal failure: a systematic review and meta-analysis. Ren Fail 2010 Jun;32(5):555–561.

102. Oudemans-van Straaten HM, Wester JP, de Pont AC, Schetz MR. Anticoagulation strategies in continuous renal replacement therapy: Can the choice be evidence based? Intensive Care Med 2006;32(2): 188–202.

103. Heintz BH, Matzke GR, Dager WE. Antimicrobial dosing concepts and recommendations for critically ill adult patients receiving continuous renal replacement therapy or intermittent hemodialysis. Pharmacotherapy 2009;29(5):562–577.

104. Kellum JA, Angus DC, Johnson JP, et al. Continuous versus intermittent renal replacement therapy: A meta-analysis. Intensive Care Med 2002;28(1):29–37.

105. Marshall MR, Golper TA, Shaver MJ, Alam MG, Chatoth DK. Urea kinetics during sustained low-efficiency dialysis in critically ill patients requiring renal replacement therapy. Am J Kidney Dis 2002;39(3):556–570.

106. Kumar VA, Craig M, Depner TA, Yeun JY. Extended daily dialysis: A new approach to renal replacement for acute renal failure in the intensive care unit. Am J Kidney Dis 2000;36(2):294–300.

107. Dager WE. Filtering out important considerations for developing drug-dosing regimens in extended daily dialysis. Crit Care Med 2006;34(1):240–241.

108. Manley HJ, Bailie GR, McClaran ML, Bender WL. Gentamicin pharmacokinetics during slow daily home hemodialysis. Kidney Int 2003;63(3):1072–1078.

109. Sutton TA, Fisher CJ, Molitoris BA. Microvascular endothelial injury and dysfunction during ischemic acute renal failure. Kidney Int 2002;62(5):1539–1549.

110. Pruchnicki MC, Dasta JF. Acute renal failure in hospitalized patients: Part 2. Ann Pharmacother 2002;36(9):1430–1442.

111. Acker CG, Singh AR, Flick RP, Bernardini J, Greenberg A, Johnson JP. A trial of thyroxine in acute renal failure. Kidney Int 2000;57(1):293–298.

112. Schrier RW, Wang W. Acute renal failure and sepsis. N Engl J Med 2004;351(2):159–169.

113. Bagshaw SM, Delaney A, Haase M, Ghali WA, Bellomo R. Loop diuretics in the management of acute renal failure: A systematic review and meta-analysis. Crit Care Resusc 2007;9(1):60–68.

114. Davis A, Gooch I. Best evidence topic report: The use of loop diuretics in acute renal failure in critically ill patients to reduce mortality, maintain renal function, or avoid the requirements for renal support. Emerg Med J 2006;23(7):569–570.

115. Stevens MA, McCullough PA, Tobin KJ, et al. A prospective randomized trial of prevention measures in patients at high risk for contrast nephropathy: Results of the P.R.I.N.C.E. study. Prevention of radiocontrast induced nephropathy clinical evaluation. J Am Coll Cardiol 1999;33(2):403–411.

116. Better OS, Rubinstein I, Winaver JM, Knochel JP. Mannitol therapy revisited (1940–1997). Kidney Int 1997;52(4):886–894.

117. Brater DC. Diuretic therapy. N Engl J Med 1998;339(6):387–395.

118. Howard PA, Dunn MI. Severe musculoskeletal symptoms during continuous infusion of bumetanide. Chest 1997;111(2):359–364.

119. Schuller D, Lynch JP, Fine D. Protocol-guided diuretic management: comparison of furosemide by continuous infusion and intermittent bolus. Crit Care Med 1997;25(12):1969–1975.

120. Rudy DW, Voelker JR, Greene PK, Esparza FA, Brater DC. Loop diuretics for chronic renal insufficiency: A continuous infusion is more efficacious than bolus therapy. Ann Intern Med 1991;115(5):360–366.

121. Kramer WG, Smith WB, Ferguson J, et al. Pharmacodynamics of torsemide administered as an intravenous injection and as a continuous infusion to patients with congestive heart failure. J Clin Pharmacol 1996;36(3):265–270.

122. Ellison DH. Diuretic resistance: Physiology and therapeutics. Semin Nephrol 1999;19(6):581–597.

123. Segar JL, Chemtob S, Bell EF. Changes in body water compartments with diuretic therapy in infants with chronic lung disease. Early Hum Dev 1997;48(1–2):99–107.

124. Sirivella S, Gielchinsky I, Parsonnet V. Mannitol, furosemide, and dopamine infusion in postoperative renal failure complicating cardiac surgery. Ann Thorac Surg 2000;69(2):501–506.

125. Amanzadeh J, Reilly RF, Jr. Anticoagulation and continuous renal replacement therapy. Semin Dial 2006;19(4):311–316.

126. Cano N, Fiaccadori E, Tesinsky P, et al. ESPEN guidelines on enteral nutrition: Adult renal failure. Clin Nutr 2006;25(2):295–310.

127. Btaiche IF, Mohammad RA, Alaniz C, Mueller BA. Amino acid requirements in critically ill patients with acute kidney injury treated with continuous renal replacement therapy. Pharmacotherapy 2008;28(5):600–613.

128. Yagi N, Leblanc M, Sakai K, Wright EJ, Paganini EP. Cooling effect of continuous renal replacement therapy in critically ill patients. Am J Kidney Dis 1998;32(6):1023–1030.

129. Rickard CM, Couchman BA, Hughes M, McGrail MR. Preventing hypothermia during continuous veno-venous haemodiafiltration: A randomized controlled trial. J Adv Nurs 2004;47(4):393–400.

130. Vilay AM, Churchwell MD, Mueller BA. Clinical review: Drug metabolism and nonrenal clearance in acute kidney injury. Crit Care 2008;12(6):235.

131. Dager WE, King JH. Aminoglycosides in intermittent hemodialysis: pharmacokinetics with individual dosing. Ann Pharmacother 2006;40(1):9–14.

132. Haas CE, Nelsen JL, Raghavendran K, et al. Pharmacokinetics and pharmacodynamics of enoxaparin in multiple trauma patients. J Trauma 2005;59(6):1336–1343, discussion 1343–1334.

133. Kane-Gill SL, Feng Y, Bobek MB, Bies RR, Pruchnicki MC, Dasta JF. Administration of enoxaparin by continuous infusion in a naturalistic setting: Analysis of renal function and safety. J Clin Pharm Ther 2005;30(3):207–213.

134. Tegeder I, Bremer F, Oelkers R, et al. Pharmacokinetics of imipenem-cilastatin in critically ill patients undergoing continuous venovenous hemofiltration. Antimicrob Agents Chemother 1997;41(12): 2640–2645.

135. Mueller BA, Pasko DA, Sowinski KM. Higher renal replacement therapy dose delivery influences on drug therapy. Artif Organs 2003;27(9):808–814.

136. Macias WL, Mueller BA, Scarim SK. Vancomycin pharmacokinetics in acute renal failure: preservation of nonrenal clearance. Clin Pharmacol Ther 1991;50(6):688–694.

137. Heinemeyer G, Link J, Weber W, Meschede V, Roots I. Clearance of ceftriaxone in critical care patients with acute renal failure. Intensive Care Med 1990;16(7):448–453.

138. Mueller BA, Scarim SK, Macias WL. Comparison of imipenem pharmacokinetics in patients with acute or chronic renal failure treated with continuous hemofiltration. Am J Kidney Dis 1993;21(2):172–179.

139. Macias WL, Mueller BA, Scarim SK, Robinson M, Rudy DW. Continuous venovenous hemofiltration: An alternative to continuous arteriovenous hemofiltration and hemodiafiltration in acute renal failure. Am J Kidney Dis 1991;18(4):451–458.

140. Bugge JF. Pharmacokinetics and drug dosing adjustments during continuous venovenous hemofiltration or hemodiafiltration in critically ill patients. Acta Anaesthesiol Scand 2001;45(8):929–934.

141. Joy MS, Matzke GR, Armstrong DK, Marx MA, Zarowitz BJ. A primer on continuous renal replacement therapy for critically ill patients. Ann Pharmacother 1998;32(3):362–375.

142. Veltri MA, Neu AM, Fivush BA, Parekh RS, Furth SL. Drug dosing during intermittent hemodialysis and continuous renal replacement therapy : Special considerations in pediatric patients. Paediatr Drugs 2004;6(1):45–65.

143. Bohler J, Donauer J, Keller F. Pharmacokinetic principles during continuous renal replacement therapy: Drugs and dosage. Kidney Int Suppl 1999(72):S24–S28.

144. Joy MS, Matzke GR, Frye RF, Palevsky PM. Determinants of vancomycin clearance by continuous venovenous hemofiltration and continuous venovenous hemodialysis. Am J Kidney Dis 1998;31(6):1019–1027.

145. Kronfol NO, Lau AH, Barakat MM. Aminoglycoside binding to polyacrylonitrile hemofilter membranes during continuous hemofiltration. ASAIO Trans 1987;33(3):300–303.

146. Lau AH, Kronfol NO. Determinants of drug removal by continuous hemofiltration. Int J Artif Organs. 1994;17(7):373–378.

147. Matzke GR, Frye RF, Joy MS, Palevsky PM. Determinants of ceftazidime clearance by continuous venovenous hemofiltration and continuous venovenous hemodialysis. Antimicrob Agents Chemother 2000;44(6):1639–1644.

148. Bressolle F, Kinowski JM, de la Coussaye JE, Wynn N, Eledjam JJ, Galtier M. Clinical pharmacokinetics during continuous haemofiltration. Clin Pharmacokinet 1994;26(6):457–471.

149. Reetze-Bonorden P, Bohler J, Keller E. Drug dosage in patients during continuous renal replacement therapy. Pharmacokinetic and therapeutic considerations. Clin Pharmacokinet 1993;24(5):362–379.

150. Chertow GM, Burdick E, Honour M, Bonventre JV, Bates DW. Acute kidney injury, mortality, length of stay, and costs in hospitalized patients. J Am Soc Nephrol 2005;16(11):3365–3370.

151. Korkeila M, Ruokonen E, Takala J. Costs of care, long-term prognosis and quality of life in patients requiring renal replacement therapy during intensive care. Intensive Care Med 2000;26(12):1824–1831.

152. Dasta JF, Kane-Gill SL, Durtschi AJ, Pathak DS, Kellum JA. Costs and outcomes of acute kidney injury (AKI) following cardiac surgery. Nephrol Dial Transplant 2008;23(6):1970–1974.

153. Hamel MB, Phillips RS, Davis RB, et al. Outcomes and cost-effectiveness of initiating dialysis and continuing aggressive care in seriously ill hospitalized adults. SUPPORT Investigators: Study to Understand Prognoses and Preferences for Outcomes and Risks of Treatments. Ann Intern Med 1997;127(3):195–202.

154. Pruchnicki MC, Dasta JF. Acute renal failure in hospitalized patients: Part 1. Ann Pharmacother 2002;36(7–8):1261–1267.

155 Srisavat N, Lawsin L, Uchino S, Bellomo R, Kellum JA. Cost of acute renal replacement therapy in the intensive care unit: results from The Beginning and Ending Supportive Therapy for the Kidney (BEST Kidney) Study. Crit Care 2010;14(2):R46.

156 Desai AA, Baras JB, Berk BB, et al. Management of acute kidney injury in the intensive care unit. Arch Intern Med 2008;168(16):1761–1767.

CHAPTER

52

Chronic Kidney Disease: Progression-Modifying Therapies

VIMAL K. DEREBAIL, ABHIJIT V. KSHIRSAGAR, AND MELANIE S. JOY

KEY CONCEPTS

❶ The prevalence of chronic kidney disease (CKD) is estimated at nearly 25 million people in the United States.

❷ Because the development of CKD is a complex phenomenon, the Kidney Disease Outcomes Quality Initiative (K/DOQI) has recommended categorizing risk factors associated with CKD as susceptibility, initiation, and progression factors.

❸ Reduction of kidney mass, development of glomerular hypertension, and intratubular proteinuria are key mechanisms responsible for the progression of CKD.

❹ CKD is classified into five stages based on the presence of kidney structural damage (e.g., proteinuria) and/or kidney function (glomerular filtration rate). Stage 1 is indicative of mild structural changes with "normal" kidney function, while stage 5 is analogous to end-stage renal disease when patients are approaching the need for dialysis or kidney transplantation.

❺ Serum creatinine concentration is not a reliable marker of kidney function among the elderly, the malnourished, and children. Therefore, it is important to estimate the glomerular filtration rate rather than just measuring the serum creatinine, especially in these three populations.

❻ Stage 5 CKD manifests as asterixis, pruritus, dysgeusia, nausea, vomiting, anorexia, weight loss, and susceptibility to bleeding. These signs and symptoms of uremia drive the decision to implement kidney replacement therapy.

❼ The progression of CKD can be slowed by optimizing blood pressure control and among diabetics blood glucose control.

❽ Diabetic patients with or without hypertension who demonstrate persistent microalbuminuria despite intensive insulin therapy should have their angiotensin-converting enzyme inhibitor (ACEI) or angiotensin receptor blocker (ARB) dose titrated to achieve maximal suppression of urinary albumin excretion to halt or slow CKD progression.

❾ ACEIs and ARBs are key pharmacologic treatments of chronic kidney disease because of their hemodynamic and blood pressure reduction effects, which help to limit kidney disease progression.

❿ Dietary protein restriction, lipid-lowering interventions, cessation of smoking, and symptom control of anemia have been suggested to slow the rate of progression of CKD; however, the utility of these interventions remains unclear.

Under normal conditions each of the 2 million nephrons of the kidneys work in an organized fashion to filter, reabsorb, and excrete various solutes and water. The kidney is the primary regulator of sodium and water balance, as well as of acid-base homeostasis. The kidney also produces hormones necessary for red blood cell synthesis and calcium homeostasis. Dysregulation of kidney function is classified as acute kidney disease and chronic kidney disease. Acute kidney failure refers to the rapid loss of kidney function over days to weeks. Chronic kidney disease (CKD), also called *chronic renal insufficiency* or *progressive kidney disease* by some, is defined as a progressive loss of function occurring over several months to years and is characterized by the gradual replacement of normal kidney architecture with parenchymal fibrosis.

The working group of the National Kidney Foundation's (NKF) Kidney Dialysis Outcomes and Quality Initiative (K/DOQI) has developed a CKD classification system based on the presence of structural kidney damage and/or functional changes in glomerular filtration rate (GFR) present for a period of 3 months or more.[1] CKD is categorized by the level of kidney function (as defined by GFR) into stages 1 through 5, with each increasing number indicating a more advanced stage of the disease (Table 52–1).[1] The use of GFR versus serum creatinine concentration (henceforth, serum creatinine) to define the stages of CKD was chosen because the serum creatinine alone is an inaccurate index of kidney function and there is marked variability in GFR among subjects with similar serum creatinine values (see Chap. 50). Although the stages are defined functionally by the GFR, the classification system also accounts for

TABLE 52-1	Definition and Prevalence of the Stages of Chronic Kidney Disease[2,3]	
Stage	**Glomerular Filtration Rate[a]**	**Prevalence[c]**
1	≥90[b]	3,600,000[d]
2	60–89	6,500,000[d]
3	30–59	15,500,000
4	15–29	700,000
5	<15 (includes only patients on dialysis)[e]	519,100[e]

[a]Glomerular filtration rate in milliliters per minute per 1.73 m² (mL/min/m²) body surface area. To convert to mL/s/m² multiply values by 0.00963.

[b]Chronic kidney disease can be present with a normal or near normal GFR if other markers of kidney disease are present, such as proteinuria, hematuria, biopsy results showing kidney damage, or anatomic abnormalities (e.g., cysts).

[c]Applied to 2000 U.S. Census.

[d]Based on persistent elevated albumin-to-creatinine ratio and eGFR.

[e]ESRD prevalent patients from USRDS data through 2007 (USRDS 2009 Annual Data Report).

structural evidence of kidney damage. Normal kidney function in adults is approximately 120 mL/min/1.73 m² (1.16 mL/s/m²) based on measured GFR. Even though a GFR of >90 mL/ min/1.73 m² (>0.87 mL/s/m²) is considered normal kidney function, a patient can be diagnosed with stage 1 CKD if the patient has proteinuria, hematuria, or evidence via a kidney biopsy of structural damage. Stage 5 CKD was previously referred to as end-stage renal disease (ESRD) or end-stage kidney disease. As a note to the clinician, a Medicare ICD-9 code exists for stage 6 CKD and is primarily for the purposes of billing for services. This designation represents patients with ESRD [eGFR<15mL/min/1.73m² (<0.14 mL/s/m²)] receiving renal replacement therapy. In this chapter, stage 5 CKD will refer to patients with eGFR<15mL/min/1.73m² (<0.14 mL/s/m²) or patients receiving replacement therapy in order to maintain consistency with the CKD literature.

EPIDEMIOLOGY OF CKD

❶ The epidemiology of stage 5 CKD, or ESRD, has been well documented through the efforts of the USRDS, a national data system that collects, analyzes, and distributes information about U.S. patients on hemodialysis and peritoneal dialysis, as well as kidney transplant recipients.[2] Beginning in 2008, the USRDS Report has also included data regarding the earlier stages of CKD, drawing from both National Health and Nutrition Examination Survey (NHANES) data and claims data. In NHANES III and subsequent populations, the prevalence of CKD at any stage using present definitions is estimated between 13% and 16%, representing over 25 million individuals.[2,3] Stage 3 CKD [eGFR <60mL/min/1.73 m²] has risen from 5.7% in NHANES III (1988–1994) to 8.1% in the more recent NHANES population (2003–2006).[4] Claims data for 2006 suggest that CKD prevalence among those 65 years or older is 6.4% using traditional claims codes and 4.2% using the more recent coding system.[4] Although less than that in NHANES, the data represent a significant increase in CKD prevalence likely due in part to increases in awareness and reporting. The CKD prevalence is similar to that of other chronic conditions such as hypertension, diabetes mellitus, and cardiovascular disease.

In the United States alone, there are several major epidemiologic studies in progress to better describe the natural history of CKD, its progression, and concurrent morbidities. One study targets individuals with polycystic kidney disease,[5] while another study targets African Americans with hypertensive nephrosclerosis.[6] The Chronic Renal Insufficiency Cohort (CRIC) study, funded by the National Institutes of Health[7] and the Fresenius and Amgen, Inc. cosponsored study (Stride Registry)[8] are investigating progressive CKD and its relationship with comorbid cardiovascular disease. The NKF has recognized the importance of early detection and initiated the Kidney Early Evaluation Program (KEEP)[9] to provide free screening and education for people at high risk of developing kidney disease. Baseline characteristics have largely confirmed the previously reported demographic and clinical factors associated with CKD.[10,11] Perhaps some of the most alarming data from KEEP was the low awareness of the disease. Less than 10% of patients were aware of this diagnosis, and even among those with later stages of CKD (stages 3 to 5) only 11% of patients were aware of the diagnosis.[11]

USRDS estimates of new cases of stage 5 CKD necessitating renal replacement therapy increased by 5% to 10% per year during the two decades spanning 1980 to 2000.[2] However, since 2002, the rate of increase had declined to less than 1% to 2% per year.[2] A potential factor attributed to this decline has been the implementation of angiotensin-converting enzyme inhibitor (ACEI) and angiotensin receptor blocker (ARB) therapy as a standard of care for those with early stage CKD.[12] At present, the four most

TABLE 52-2	Risk Factors Associated with Chronic Kidney Disease
Risk Factor	
Susceptibility	
Advanced age	
Reduced kidney mass and low birth weight	
Racial/ethnic minority	
Family history	
Low income or education	
Systemic inflammation	
Dyslipidemia	
Initiation	
Diabetes mellitus	
Hypertension	
Glomerulonephritis	
Progression	
Hyperglycemia (among diabetic patients)	
Hypertension	
Proteinuria	
Obesity	
Smoking	

common causes of incident stage 5 CKD in the United States are diabetes mellitus (158 cases per million), hypertension (101 cases per million), glomerulonephritis (25 cases per million), and polycystic kidney disease (9 cases per million).[2]

❷ It is often assumed that all patients with stage 1 or 2 CKD progress continuously toward stage 5. Thus, information on risk factors obtained from USRDS data is assumed to be generalizable to all stages of CKD. Early data from the KEEP and CRIC studies offer some support for this assumption.[10,11] However, further complicating these issues is the fact that the development and progression of the early stages of CKD is a complex phenomenon.[13] The risk factors associated with CKD are numerous and varied and many of these are not those one would traditionally consider as having a direct influence on the causal pathway. The working group of K/DOQI has recommended categorizing CKD risk factors as susceptibility factors, initiation factors, or progression factors to help clinicians stratify the overall risks of individual patients (Table 52–2).[14]

In this chapter the initiation and progression factors associated with the development of CKD are reviewed. Because diabetes mellitus and hypertension are the two most prevalent etiologies for CKD, the course and treatments that have been proven to slow the progressive kidney function decline are critically evaluated. This chapter focuses on the early CKD stages, that is, stages 1, 2, and 3, which are the critical battleground if one hopes to minimize the number of patients who ultimately require renal replacement therapy. CKD is a continuous and progressive disease state that often results in the appearance of several concomitant complications that commence at various stages in the progression of the disease. The pathophysiology, consequences, and complications of CKD that tend to become evident in those with stage 4 or 5 CKD are discussed in Chap. 53 along with treatment options and monitoring parameters.

ETIOLOGY

SUSCEPTIBILITY FACTORS

CKD susceptibility factors include advanced age,[15] low income or education,[16,17] and racial/ethnic minority status,[18] as well as reduced kidney mass,[19] low birth weight,[19,20] and family history of CKD.[21] These factors have not been proven to directly cause kidney damage. Novel proposed susceptibility factors are systemic inflammation[22,23] and dyslipidemia.[24,25] Although, most of these susceptibility factors are not amenable to pharmacologic or lifestyle interventions, they are useful for identifying populations that are at high risk of CKD.

INITIATION FACTORS

❸ Initiation factors are conditions that directly result in kidney damage and are modifiable by pharmacologic therapy. Diabetes mellitus, hypertension, autoimmune diseases, polycystic kidney disease, systemic infections, urinary tract infections, urinary stones, lower urinary tract obstruction, and nephrotoxicity are all considered initiation factors. Because diabetes mellitus, hypertension, and glomerular diseases are, respectively, the three most common causes of CKD in the United States, the following discussion focuses on these conditions.

Diabetes Mellitus

Approximately 20% to 40% of those with diabetes mellitus will develop diabetic CKD.[26] Given the greater prevalence of type 2 diabetes mellitus, the majority of patients who develop diabetes-associated CKD are those with type 2 disease. Although not all individuals with diabetic nephropathy progress to stage 5 CKD, the lifetime risk is considerable. A prospective study of over 300,000 individuals screened from the Multiple Risk Factor Intervention Trial estimated that approximately 3% of individuals with diabetes mellitus will develop stage 5 CKD.[27] Diabetics have a 12-fold greater relative risk of developing stage 5 CKD than those without diabetes. Diabetics also have an increased risk of developing CKD as the result of a "nondiabetic" cause, suggesting an underlying genetic susceptibility to kidney diseases.[28]

Hypertension

Hypertension also increases the risk of CKD, although the exact role as a cause or consequence is often debated as the kidney has a role in the development and modulation of high blood pressure. Hypertension generally develops concomitantly with progressive kidney disease. In the NHANES III survey, a serum creatinine of 1.6 mg/dL (141 μmol/L) or higher for men and 1.4 mg/dL (124 μmol/L) or higher for women was more common in persons with hypertension (9.1%) than in persons without hypertension (1.1%).[29] Recent data suggest that among patients with an estimated GFR of 20 to 70 mL/min/1.73 m², over 85% have concomitant hypertension.[30]

Prospective studies have shown that elevated blood pressure increases the risk for the development of CKD among subjects without initial kidney disease. In a study of 316,675 adult managed-care patients with normal baseline kidney function, the likelihood of incident ESRD (stage 5 CKD) was increased in those with elevated baseline blood pressure. The likelihood of CKD development was twofold higher for those with relatively minor elevations in blood pressure, 120 to 129 mm Hg systolic over 80 to 84 mm Hg diastolic as compared with those with blood pressure lower than 120/80 mm Hg. For those with blood pressure greater than 210/120 mm Hg, the likelihood of CKD was fourfold higher.[31]

Data from the Multiple Risk Factor Intervention Trial, a primary prevention trial in coronary heart disease, demonstrated that the overall lifetime risk of developing stage 5 CKD for individuals with hypertension was 5.6%.[32] The risk varied dramatically by level of blood pressure, from 0.33% in those with stage 1 hypertension (systolic blood pressure 140 to 150 mm Hg and/or diastolic blood pressure 90 to 100 mm Hg) to 4.5% for systolic blood pressure levels greater than 180 mm Hg or diastolic blood pressure levels greater than 110 mm Hg over a follow-up period of approximately 16 years.[32]

Glomerulonephritis

Glomerular diseases are also considered initiation factors of CKD. The epidemiology and pathophysiology of glomerular diseases are variable, and thus all diseases should not be lumped into one disease category. Some conditions, such as Goodpasture's disease or Wegener's granulomatosus, may progress rapidly to stage 5 CKD and thus may best be categorized as causes of acute renal failure. Other conditions such as immunoglobulin A (IgA) nephropathy, membranous nephropathy, focal segmental glomerulosclerosis, and lupus nephritis are more indolent and are considered causes of CKD (see Chap. 56). The chronic glomerular diseases progress at variable rates, with loss of GFR ranging from 0.9 to 9.8 mL/min per year.[33–35]

PROGRESSION FACTORS

❹ Progression risk factors are those associated with further declines in renal function. Persistence of the underlying initiation factors (e.g., hypertension, diabetes mellitus, glomerulonephritis, and polycystic kidney disease) themselves may serve as the most important predictors of progressive CKD. Other factors associated with progression include those that may be consequent to the underlying renal disease (hypertension, proteinuria, hyperlipidemia) or independent of the underlying renal disease (smoking, obesity).

Hypertension

The early treatment of hypertension and the achievement of aggressive target values has been demonstrated to slow the rate of progression of CKD.[36] Bakris et al. demonstrated a direct correlation between the level of achieved blood pressure and preservation of kidney function in diabetic patients.[37] Their analysis included 10 studies measuring a change in GFR for diabetic patients treated with various antihypertensive agents. An inverse linear relationship was observed between average attained blood pressure at study completion and average GFR; lower final mean arterial blood pressure resulted in a lower average decline in GFR. Specifically, a systolic blood pressure of 180 mm Hg was associated with a 14 mL/min per year decline in GFR as compared with only a 2 mL/min per year decline in GFR among those with a systolic blood pressure of 135 mm Hg.[37]

An extended follow-up analysis of the MDRD original cohort showed that patients assigned to lower blood pressure target (mean arterial pressure <92 mm Hg) were 32% less likely to develop stage 5 CKD than those in the usual target blood pressure (mean arterial pressure <107 mm Hg).[38] Therefore, low blood pressure slowed the progression of nondiabetic kidney disease even for patients with an existing moderately to severely decreased GFR.

Diabetes Mellitus

Hyperglycemia is an initiation and progression risk factor for CKD. Diabetic nephropathy represents the most common cause for ESRD.[2] In the NHANES population 1999 to 2006, the diagnosis of diabetes is associated with a 2.51 (2.07–3.02, P<0.001) odds ratio for CKD, representing the greatest risk factor after older age.[2] The likelihood of developing overt nephropathy varies between type 1 and type 2 diabetes mellitus. Without treatment, nearly 80% of patients with type 1 diabetes and microalbuminuria will develop overt nephropathy and nearly 50% of those with type 1 diabetes, nephropathy and hypertension will develop ESRD within 10 years.[26,39] In contrast, only 20% to 40% of those with type 2 diabetes for over 15 years will demonstrate progressive disease.[26] A recent evaluation of participants in the Diabetes Control and Complications Trial (DCCT) and the Epidemiology of Diabetes Interventions and Complications (EDIC) study suggests the historical estimates of diabetic nephropathy may be inflated, since 17% to 25% of their type 1 diabetic participants developed diabetic nephropathy after 30 years.[40] It is not clear whether the lower incidence represents an improvement in overall care or simply is a by-product of enrollment in these studies. Progression of diabetic nephropathy likely has multiple determinants including both hypertensive and glycemic control and therefore occurs at a variable rate. As will be discussed, control of both blood pressure and hyperglycemia may attenuate progression of diabetic CKD.

Proteinuria

The importance of proteinuria in the progression of both diabetic and nondiabetic kidney disease has been well documented.[41] In diabetic kidney disease (types 1 and 2), an albumin excretion rate higher than 30 mg per 24 hours (microalbuminuria) strongly predicted the development of overt nephropathy (proteinuria) and subsequent loss of kidney function.[42] In nondiabetic kidney disease, the Modification of Diet in Renal Disease (MDRD) Study-a randomized clinical trial examining oral protein restriction and blood pressure control on progression of preexisting CKD, demonstrated that a patient's baseline level of proteinuria strongly predicted future loss of GFR.[43] Furthermore, individuals with the highest levels of baseline proteinuria benefited most from pharmacologic reduction of blood pressure. Another study of more than 1,800 individuals with varying stages of CKD demonstrated a strong, graded risk of CKD based on the level of proteinuria; a fivefold increased risk of progression was observed for each 1.0 g/day increase in proteinuria.[44]

The joint role of blood pressure and proteinuria in the progression of CKD was investigated by Jafar et al. using data from 11 randomized, controlled trials that compared the efficacy of antihypertensive regimens for patients with predominantly nondiabetic kidney disease.[45] Patients with higher systolic blood pressures and urine protein excretion greater than 1.0 g/day had greater risk for progression of CKD. ($P<0.006$).[45]

Smoking

Although the adverse effects of smoking on cardiovascular disease are well documented, only recently have the consequences of smoking on the progression of CKD been recognized. Smoking is associated with an acute reduction in GFR and increased heart rate and blood pressure, likely secondary to nicotine exposure.[46] Nicotine has also been associated with an increase in urinary albumin excretion.[46] Significant data exist to suggest that smoking may promote initiation and progression of CKD in subjects with type 1 and type 2 diabetes.[46,47] The "cigarette pack years" was an independent predictive factor for CKD progression among diabetic subjects.[48] In addition, smoking has also been associated with the diagnosis of CKD in those with hypertension, especially among black subjects.[49] Some studies have demonstrated an association between smoking and albuminuria[50] and the development of stage 5 CKD.[51] Baseline data from the aforementioned CRIC study also demonstrate a modest association between smoking and CKD.[10] Smoking has also been identified as a risk factor for progression in patients with IgA nephropathy, polycystic kidney disease, and systemic lupus erythematosus.[46,52]

Hyperlipidemia

Dyslipidemia may be associated with kidney disease. CKD with or without nephrotic syndrome is frequently accompanied by abnormalities in lipoprotein metabolism. The prevalence of hyperlipidemia appears to increase as kidney function declines, and hyperlipidemia is a characteristic of the nephrotic syndrome.[53] Elevated plasma total and low-density lipoprotein cholesterol occurs in 85% to 90% of patients with decreased kidney function and proteinuria greater than 3 g/day. Approximately 50% of these patients have low levels [<35 mg/dL (<0.91 mmol/L)] of high-density lipoprotein cholesterol, and 60% have triglyceride concentrations greater than 200 mg/dL (2.26 mmol/L).[53] Three epidemiologic studies[24,25,54] demonstrated that dyslipidemia predicts incident CKD among individuals considered at low risk for CKD.[55]

Obesity

Several studies have evaluated the association between obesity and development of CKD.[56,57] Iseki et al. examined the relationship between body mass index (BMI) and the development of ESRD from a large population of Japanese subjects participating in a community-based screening.[57] BMI was associated with an increased risk of the development of ESRD in men but not in women. Population data from Kaiser Permanente revealed an increased risk of ESRD in overweight and obese subjects.[56] The risk of ESRD was directly related to the magnitude of obesity and remained even after adjustment for diabetes and hypertension.[56] Another study showed that a BMI ≥25 kg/m^2 at age 20 years is associated with a threefold increase in risk of CKD compared with a BMI lower than 25 kg/m^2. Obesity (BMI ≥30 kg/m^2) among men and morbid obesity (BMI ≥35 kg/m^2) among women were associated with three- to fourfold increases in risk.[58]

More recent studies have provided some conflicting data. The Framingham Offspring Study demonstrated an increased risk for CKD among the obese (BMI ≥30 kg/m^2) but not among the overweight (BMI ≥25 kg/m^2 to <30 kg/m^2).[59] However, this association was not apparent after adjustment for traditional cardiovascular risk factors of diabetes, hypertension, and dyslipidemia. A study of Korean men without diabetes or hypertension demonstrated a fourfold increase in the risk for CKD among those gaining >0.75kg/year, even with normal weight at baseline.[60] Other studies have demonstrated elevated inflammatory markers associated with CKD in those with higher BMI.[61,62] Finally a meta-analysis of 16 cohort studies of body weight and kidney disease demonstrated a higher risk among the overweight and obese, particularly in women.[63] These conflicting data highlight a need for further study to this potential relationship between body weight and kidney disease risk.

OTHER FACTORS

Other potential risk factors associated with CKD include hyperuricemia,[64,65] periodontal disease,[23,66,67] lead exposure,[68] and illicit drug use.[69] Genetic studies have suggested apolipoprotein E variants are associated with progression of CKD in both whites and blacks,[70] and they have identified the nonmuscle myosin heavy-chain type II isoform A (MYH9) gene in association with nondiabetic kidney disease in African Americans.[71,72] The exact role and importance of these factors in initiating or sustaining renal damages are not yet clear and require additional study.

PATHOPHYSIOLOGY

As evidenced by the variety of initiation and progression factors, kidney damage can result from heterogeneous causes. Diabetic nephropathy is characterized by glomerular mesangial expansion; in hypertensive nephrosclerosis, the kidney's arterioles have arteriolar hyalinosis; and renal cysts develop in polycystic kidney disease. Therefore, the initial structural damage may depend on the primary disease affecting the kidney. However, the majority of progressive nephropathies share a final common pathway to irreversible renal parenchymal damage and ESRD (Fig. 52–1).[73] The key elements of this pathway are (1) loss of nephron mass, (2) glomerular capillary hypertension, and (3) proteinuria.

The exposure to any of the initiation risk factors can result in loss of nephron mass. The remaining nephrons hypertrophy to compensate for the loss of renal function and nephron mass.[73] Initially, this compensatory hypertrophy may be adaptive. Over time, the hypertrophy can lead to the development of intraglomerular hypertension, possibly mediated by angiotensin II.[74]

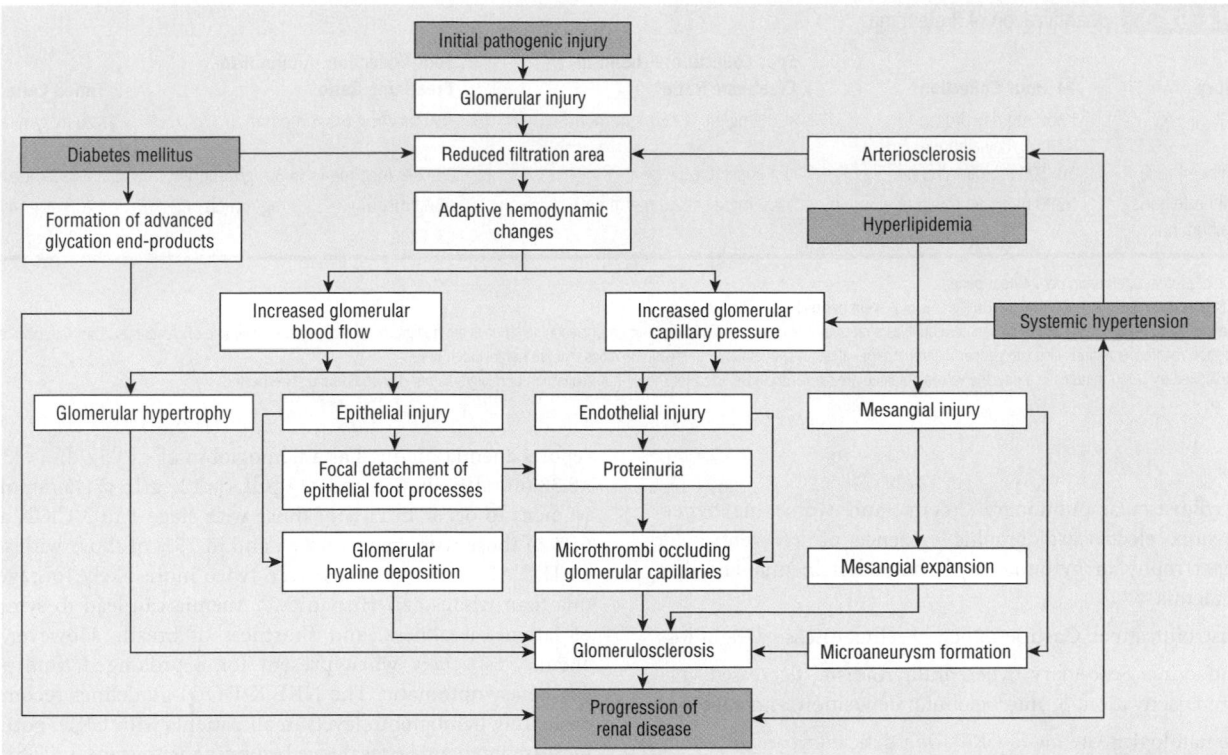

FIGURE 52-1. Proposed mechanisms for progression of renal disease.

Angiotensin II is a potent vasoconstrictor of both afferent and efferent arterioles, but it preferentially affects the efferent arterioles, leading to increased pressure within the glomerular capillaries and consequent increased filtration fraction. The development of intraglomerular hypertension usually correlates with the development of systemic arterial hypertension. High intraglomerular capillary pressure impairs the size-selective function of the glomerular permeability barrier, resulting in increased urinary excretion of albumin and frank proteinuria.[74] Angiotensin II may also mediate renal disease progression through nonhemodynamic effects.[75]

Proteinuria alone may promote progressive loss of nephrons as a result of direct cellular damage[73,75] Filtered proteins such as albumin, transferrin, complement factors, immunoglobulins, cytokines, and angiotensin II are toxic to kidney tubular cells. Numerous studies have demonstrated that the presence of these proteins in the renal tubule activates tubular cells, which leads to the upregulated production of inflammatory and vasoactive cytokines, such as endothelin, monocyte chemoattractant protein (MCP-1), and CCL5 [regulated upon activation, normal T-cell expressed and secreted (RANTES)].[76] Proteinuria is also associated with the activation of complement components on the apical membrane of proximal tubules. Accumulating evidence now suggests that intratubular complement activation may be the key mechanism of damage in the progressive proteinuric nephropathies.[76] These events ultimately lead to scarring of the interstitium, progressive loss of structural nephron units, and reduction in GFR.

CLINICAL PRESENTATION

❺ CKD is often asymptomatic, and should be suspected in individuals with conditions such as diabetes, hypertension, genitourinary abnormalities, and autoimmune diseases. In addition, individuals of older age and those with a family history of kidney disease should be considered for CKD screening. Recommended screening studies include serum creatinine and

GFR measurement, urinalysis, and/or imaging studies of the kidneys. A novel tool known as SCreening for Occult REnal Disease (SCORED) may also help to identify those with CKD in a cost-effective and noninvasive manner.[77] This self-administered survey predicts that nearly 20% of individuals with all risk factors of diabetes mellitus, advanced age, hypertension, and cardiovascular disease will have an eGFR<60mL/min/1.73m².[78] Abnormal elevations of serum creatinine, reflecting decreases in GFR, or presence of urinary or imaging study abnormalities are indications for a full evaluation of CKD.[1] Furthermore, the rate of GFR loss can vary in CKD because of differences in the underlying disease process and extent of kidney damage, treatment responsiveness, and compliance with therapies.

CLINICAL PRESENTATION OF CKD STAGES 1 TO 4

General

- CKD development and progression may be insidious in onset, often without noticeable symptoms. The diagnosis of CKD requires measurement of serum creatinine, estimation of GFR, and assessment of the urine (urinalysis) for protein and/or albumin excretion.

- CKD stages 3, 4, and 5 require further workup to identify the presence of CKD complications of anemia, cardiovascular disease, metabolic bone disease, malnutrition, and disorders of fluids and electrolytes.

Symptoms

- Symptoms are generally absent in CKD stages 1 and 2 and may be minimal during stages 3 and 4. General symptoms associated with stages 1 to 4 include edema, cold intolerance, shortness of breath, palpitations, cramping and muscle pain, depression, anxiety, fatigue, and sexual dysfunction. The classic symptoms associated with stage 5 CKD are discussed in chapters 53 and 54.

TABLE 52-3	Quantification of Proteinuria				
Category	**24-Hour Collection**[a]	**Spot Collection: Protein-to-Creatinine Ratio**[b]	**Spot Collection: Albumin-to-Creatinine Ratio**[c]		**Timed Collection**[d]
Normal	<300 mg/day protein <30 mg/day albumin	<200 mg/g (<22.6 mg/mmol)	<30 mcg/mg (<3.4 mg/mmol)		<20 mcg/min
Microalbuminuria	30–300 mg/day albumin	Not applicable	30–299 mcg/mg (<33.8 mg/mmol)		20–199 mcg/min
Clinical proteinuria or albuminuria	≥300 mg/day protein or albumin	>200 mg/g (>22.6 mg/mmol)	≥300 mcg/mg (<33.9 mg/mmol)		≥200 mcg/min

[a]Milligrams of protein or albumin per 24-hour period.
[b]Milligrams of protein per gram of creatinine (milligrams of protein per millimole of creatinine).
[c]Micrograms of albumin per milligram of creatinine (equal, as a ratio, to milligrams of albumin per gram of creatinine; SI units are milligrams of albumin per millimole of creatinine). The National Kidney Foundation recommendations also cite gender differences for values of spot albumin-to-creatinine ratios that are not included here.
[d]When multiplied by 1,440 minutes in a day, the values obtained are similar to those listed for the 24-hour collection of milligrams per day of albumin, as expected.

Signs

- Cardiovascular-pulmonary: Edema and worsening hypertension, electrocardiographic evidence of left ventricular hypertrophy, arrhythmias, hyperhomocysteinemia, and dyslipidemia
- Gastrointestinal: Gastroesophageal reflux disease, weight loss
- Endocrine: Secondary hyperparathyroidism, decreased vitamin D activation, β_2-microglobulin deposition, and gout
- Hematologic: Anemia of CKD, iron deficiency, and bleeding
- Fluid/electrolytes: Hyper- or hyponatremia, hyperkalemia, and metabolic acidosis

The NKF K/DOQI defines kidney damage in reference to the presence of clinical proteinuria, in addition to the GFR. Clinicians should be aware of the methods available to detect and interpret proteinuria and albuminuria (Table 52–3). In addition, Chap. 50 provides a detailed discussion of the relative merits of the various methods currently available for the detection of urinary protein.

❻ Patients with stage 1 or 2 CKD disease usually do not have any symptoms or metabolic derangements such as acidosis, anemia, and bone disease. In addition, the most common measure of impairment of kidney function, serum creatinine, may be only slightly elevated in these early CKD stages. Consequently, estimation of the GFR and assessment for urinary protein is imperative for recognition of early stages of CKD. Because the early stages of CKD are often undetected, the diagnosis requires a high level of suspicion for patients with chronic conditions such as hypertension and diabetes. Signs and symptoms associated with CKD become more prevalent in stages 3 to 5. Anemia, abnormalities of calcium and phosphorus metabolism (secondary hyperparathyroidism), malnutrition, and fluid and electrolyte abnormalities become more common as kidney function deteriorates (see Chap. 53).

ANEMIA

Because the kidneys secrete 90% of the endogenous hormone erythropoietin, a hormone necessary for erythropoiesis, declining kidney function can lead to erythropoietin deficiency and anemia. The prevalence of anemia at specific stages of CKD is difficult to ascertain because of limited available data and use of various definitions.[1] Estimates of anemia [hemoglobin of less than 12 g/dL (120g/L; 7.45 mmol/L)] prevalence for patients with a GFR greater than 80 mL/min per 1.73 m² (0.77 mL/s/m²) range from 1 to 30%.[79] The true prevalence rate estimation is unclear as other factors, such as ethnicity, age, and gender, can also contribute to anemia. Data from the KEEP study targeting a higher risk population,

reports anemia [defined as a hemoglobin of <13.5g/dL (<135 g/L; <8.38 mmol/L) in men and <12g/dL ([<120 g/L; <7.45 mmol/L) in women] to occur in 20% of those with stage 1 to 3 CKD, almost 65% of those with stage 4 CKD, and in 75% of those with stage 5 CKD.[80] African Americans were twice more likely to have anemia than whites and Hispanics.[80] Anemia can lead to symptoms of fatigue, weakness, and shortness of breath. However, mild anemia, especially when present for a prolonged time period, can be asymptomatic. The NKF K/DOQI guidelines recommend evaluating hemoglobin levels in all patients with CKD, noting the increase in anemia prevalence beginning with stage 3.[81] The treatment of anemia can improve or resolve symptoms and may help to stabilize kidney function.[82] Chapter 53 discusses the management of anemia in CKD.

CARDIOVASCULAR DISEASE

CKD is associated with a high rate of cardiovascular morbidity and mortality.[83] An epidemiologic study of more than 300,000 individuals demonstrated a strong relationship between GFR and cardiovascular disease: The lower the level of GFR, the higher the incidence of cardiovascular events.[84] In fact, individuals with stages 2 to 4 CKD were more likely to die from cardiovascular disease complications than to survive to the initiation of renal replacement therapy.[85] A recent evaluation of a large database of over 400,000 individuals demonstrated a nearly twofold risk of cardiovascular death among those with CKD.[86] Data from NHANES and KEEP also demonstrate a greater risk of myocardial infarction, stroke, and death among those with CKD.[87] Interestingly, two other recent studies have demonstrated elevated cardiovascular risk among those with a CKD diagnosis based separately on reduced GFR or albuminuria.[88,89] In both studies, those with diminished GFR were considered as a different population than those with only albuminuria, suggesting that reduced GFR and albuminuria may provide separate cardiovascular risk information.[88,89] Consequently, monitoring for the presence or development of cardiovascular disease for patients with CKD is an important aspect of their care. Appropriate traditional and nontraditional cardiovascular risk factor assessments are necessary in the evaluation of the patient with CKD. Guidelines for the evaluation, monitoring, and treatment of cardiovascular diseases for patients with CKD have been published.[83]

DISORDERS OF CALCIUM AND PHOSPHORUS HOMEOSTASIS

Abnormalities in calcium and phosphorus metabolism typically occur in stages 3 to 5 CKD. Secondary hyperparathyroidism, however, can develop earlier despite normal serum calcium and phosphorus levels, at a GFR of 80 mL/min per 1.73 m² or below.[90] Thus, to detect secondary hyperparathyroidism and limit the bone complications, it is recommended that parathyroid hormone concentration, vitamin D levels, and calcium and phosphorus be monitored beginning in stage 3 CKD.[91] Additional systemic benefits of correcting abnormalities in calcium, phosphorus, and parathyroid hormone may include cardiovascular risk reduction. A recent controlled study of 24 CKD patients reported reductions in urinary protein excretion and high-sensitivity C-reactive protein with paricalcitol treatment.[92] Additionally, an uncontrolled study of 10 IgA nephropathy patients reported a 25% reduction in urinary protein after initiation of twice weekly calcitriol therapy to existing angiotensin converting enzymes inhibitors.[93] These studies show preliminary data suggesting the need for more extensive evaluations regarding any protective role of vitamin D on kidney function decline. Chapter 53 discusses the management of bone disease caused by CKD.

MALNUTRITION

Anorexia and malnutrition are complications of CKD. Although there are limited data defining exactly at which stage malnutrition develops, the NKF K/DOQI guidelines recommend evaluating for signs of malnutrition when the GFR is lower than 60 mL/min per 1.73 m² (stages 3, 4, and 5).[94] An investigation for malnutrition should include a dietary assessment for protein and calorie intake, serum albumin, and/or assessment of protein appearance in the urine (as a marker of protein intake). Chapter 149 discusses the interpretation of these tests, and Chap. 153 discusses nutritional recommendations for patients with CKD.

TREATMENT

Chronic Kidney Disease

■ GOAL OF THERAPY

The goal of therapy is to delay the progression of CKD, thereby minimizing the development or severity of associated complications including cardiovascular disease and ultimately limiting the progression to ESRD. Both nonpharmacologic and pharmacologic interventions are available to slow the rate of CKD progression and may also decrease the incidence and prevalence of ESRD.

❼ In addition to pharmacologic therapy, the patient with CKD usually will benefit from modest dietary protein. The main purpose of pharmacologic therapy is to control the underlying conditions (such as diabetes mellitus and hypertension) that have incited kidney damage to prevent further loss of kidney function. Patients generally require a multimodality treatment approach irrespective of the cause of their kidney disease. Therapy with ACEIs and/or ARBs is a nearly universal key therapeutic component.

Nonpharmacologic Therapy

Dietary Protein Restriction Experimental studies of kidney disease in animals suggest that dietary protein restriction may delay the rate of progression of kidney function decline.[95] This hypothesis was tested in humans in the MDRD study, a randomized, controlled trial that evaluated the benefits of dietary protein restriction and blood pressure reduction on the rate of CKD progression.[43,96] Most enrolled subjects had nondiabetic kidney disease, and 24% of them had a diagnosis of polycystic kidney disease. Subjects with moderate CKD (GFR of 25 to 55 mL/min per 1.73 m²) were randomized by dietary protein intake groups (1.3 g/kg per day or 0.58 g/kg per day), in addition to blood pressure grouping, for a total of four groups. Subjects with advanced

CKD [GFR 13 to 24 mL/min per 1.73 m²] were randomized to a low-protein diet (0.58 g/kg/day) or a very-low-protein diet (0.28 g/kg/day) with a ketoamine acid supplement, in addition to blood pressure, also for a total of four groups. After a mean followup of 2.2 years, protein restriction failed to show a statistical benefit in slowing the progression of CKD in any of the study groups. However, a secondary analysis of the MDRD study was conducted and revealed that in those patients with a GFR of less than 25 mL/min per 1.73 m² a protein intake of 0.6 g/kg per day was significantly associated with a decreased rate of progressive renal disease.[96] In addition, this analysis showed that the rate of progression to ESRD was significantly reduced by 41% for each 0.2 g/kg per day reduction in dietary protein intake. The discrepancy in results between the primary and secondary analyses can be explained by the different statistical methods used in each of the two analyses, in that the later analysis evaluated participants who were actually compliant with their dietary prescription. The most recent follow-up of the advanced CKD group found no difference in progression to kidney failure but perhaps suggested an increased risk of death in the very-low-protein group. However, data on protein intake at the time of follow-up was not available.[97]

Because of concerns regarding the inadequate statistical power of individual studies, recent meta-analyses have been performed to determine the effect of protein restriction on the progression of CKD.[98–100] The studies have had varying conclusions, although the reduction in loss of GFR was relatively nominal. The most recent randomized trial in diabetic nephropathy[101] was not able to demonstrate renoprotection of a low-protein diet but, most importantly, noted the difficulty that patients had adhering to the requirements of a low-protein diet.

Thus, the available data suggest only a relatively small benefit from dietary protein restriction in CKD patients. Because low-protein diets may lead to malnutrition for patients with advanced CKD and those with nephrotic-range proteinuria, the NKF K/DOQI has advocated a dietary protein intake of 0.6 g/kg per day for patients with a GFR <25 mL/min per 1.73 m².[94] Titration of protein intake up to 0.75 g/kg per day is suggested for patients who cannot achieve or maintain adequate nutritional status with the lower protein (0.6 g/kg per day) diet.[94]

Smoking Cessation

Although the effectiveness of smoking cessation on limiting progressive CKD has not been prospectively evaluated, one study suggested that smoking cessation resulted in a protective effect against proteinuria and reduced GFR.[102] This later study showed that although current smokers had a significantly higher albumin excretion (and reduced GFR) versus nonsmokers, those patients who quit smoking had a statistical association with only microalbuminuria.[102] Based on the evolving data concerning the detrimental effects of smoking on the kidney and the well-documented associations with cardiovascular disease, the clinician should educate patients regarding this risk and institute appropriate therapeutic options, both nonpharmacologic and pharmacologic, for smoking cessation. These options are discussed in further detail in Chap. 75.

Pharmacologic Therapy

Guidelines for CKD treatment usually recognize the differences in pathogenesis and course of diabetic and nondiabetic CKD. Consequently, pharmacologic interventions are discussed separately for these conditions within this chapter. The major focus of this chapter is on the impact of ACEI and ARB therapies on progressive CKD. Pharmacologic therapies specific for glomerulonephritis are discussed in Chap. 56, while therapies for the treatment of complications of kidney disease are covered in Chap. 53.

Diabetic Chronic Kidney Disease

■ INTENSIVE INSULIN THERAPY

Several large prospective studies performed in the 1990s showed the benefits of blood glucose control in both the development and progression of microvascular complications. The largest of these studies, the DCCT enrolled 1,441 patients with type 1 diabetes mellitus who were randomized to conventional blood glucose control or to intensive glucose control.[103] Conventional control consisted of up to two insulin injections per day guided by blood glucose levels. Intensive control consisted of three or more times daily injections or external insulin pump to a goal hemoglobin A_{1c} ≤6.0% (≤0.06). The main outcome measure of efficacy was retinopathy, a marker of microvascular disease often associated with diabetic nephropathy among individuals with type 1 diabetes mellitus. Roughly half of the patients had mild retinopathy. Intensive insulin control reduced the risk of new occurrences of retinopathy by 76% among those without baseline retinopathy and reduced the risk of progressive retinopathy by 54% among those with baseline retinopathy. Intensive therapy was also associated with a 39% reduction in the development of "microalbuminuria" (urinary albumin excretion ≥40 mg/day) and a 54% reduction in the development of "frank albuminuria" (urinary albumin excretion ≥300 mg/day) compared with conventional therapy. The beneficial effect of intensive therapy on the development of proteinuria persisted even 7 to 8 years after completion of the randomized phase of the DCCT.[104] Individuals initially randomized to the intensive therapy had a 59% reduction in the development of new microalbuminuria, and 84% reduction in the development of albuminuria compared with the conventional group. In the intensive therapy group, follow-up after 30 years of diabetes demonstrated a lower cumulative incidence of diabetic nephropathy (9% vs 25%).[40] However, at least one episode of hypoglycemia occurred in 65% of intensive insulin therapy patients as compared with 35% in the standard treatment group.[104]

The Intensive Glucose Control Study of the United Kingdom Prospective Diabetes Study (UKPDS) also evaluated prevention of microvascular complications among individuals with type 2 diabetes mellitus.[105] Individuals newly diagnosed with type 2 diabetes mellitus were randomized to intensive therapy [goal fasting plasma glucose of <108 mg/dL (<6 mmol/L)] or conventional therapy [goal fasting plasma glucose of <270 mg/dL (<15 mmol/L)] after 3 months of dietary counseling. Individuals in either group could use oral sulfonylureas or insulin. After 10 years of followup, the intensive group had an 11% reduction in median hemoglobin A_{1c} and a 12% reduction in any diabetes-related end point compared with the conventional group. Most of the observed benefit was in a reduction in microvascular end points, primarily proliferative retinopathy.[105]

The DCCT, the UKPDS, and their long-term follow-up provide support for reducing microvascular complications, including nephropathy, with intensive therapy for patients with type 1 and type 2 diabetes mellitus. Intensive therapy can include insulin or oral drugs but employs testing of blood sugar at least three times daily. Furthermore, goals of therapy included an A_{1c} of <7% (<0.07) and preprandial plasma and peak postprandial blood glucose of 92 to 130 mg/dL (5.1 to 7.2 mmol/L) and <180 mg/dL (10.0 mmol/L), respectively.[106] However, recent data suggest that more aggressive glycemic goals [Hgb A_{1c} of <6.0% (<0.06)] may be associated with increased mortality.[107] Clinician's are encouraged to review Chap. 83 for a thorough review of dosing, monitoring, and goals of therapies to treat diabetes mellitus.

■ OPTIMAL HYPERTENSION CONTROL

The Seventh Joint National Committee on Prevention, Detection, Evaluation, and Treatment of High Blood Pressure recommends a goal blood pressure of less than 130/80 mm Hg for patients with CKD.[108] Elevated blood pressure is often more difficult to control for patients with CKD than for those with normal kidney function. Therefore, to achieve adequate blood pressure goals, three or more different blood pressure medications are usually required.[109] Figure 52–2 depicts the proposed algorithm for the management of hypertension for people with CKD and diabetes. The selection of individual classes of drugs for limiting progression of CKD is presented in the following sections.

Reduction of blood pressure in type 1 and type 2 diabetic patients has been associated with lower rates of CKD progression.[37,110–120] The UKPDS,[118] a randomized trial of captopril or atenolol among 1,148 hypertensive type 2 diabetic patients, evaluated the effect of blood pressure reduction to a level of less than 150/85 mm Hg versus less than 180/105 mm Hg on macrovascular and microvascular outcomes. Reductions of 24% in diabetes-related end points, 32% in deaths related to diabetes, 44% in strokes, and 37% in microvascular end points were observed after a median follow-up of 8.4 years.[118] The benefit of blood pressure control has been confirmed in subsequent studies of type 2 diabetic subjects with microalbuminuria.[114,119,121–125] These seminal studies used either ACEI (Table 52–4) or ARB (Table 52–5) classes of drugs, which likely have nonhemodynamic beneficial effects on CKD progression, as discussed below, as well as blood-pressure-lowering effects. In type 1 diabetes with nephropathy, a rigorous blood pressure goal (MAP of ≤92 mm Hg) leads to decreased proteinuria.[126]

Patients diagnosed with both hypertension and diabetes mellitus have been estimated to have up to a sixfold higher risk of developing ESRD than do those patients with diabetes mellitus alone.[109] Adequate blood pressure control can reduce the rate of decline in GFR and the degree of albuminuria for hypertensive type 1 and type 2 diabetic patients.[109] Although all interventions that reduce blood pressure have historically shown reductions in urinary albumin and protein excretion, the ACEIs were the first agents shown to reduce glomerular capillary pressure and volume, which have resulted in preservation of renal function in animal models and human studies.[127,128] Table 52–6 summarizes the documented effects of the other various available antihypertensive agents on renal blood flow and GFR.[129,130]

Antihypertensive Drug Choice ❽ Several studies have confirmed the beneficial effects of ACEIs on renal function for patients with and without diabetes and both ACEIs and ARBs remain the mainstay of therapy. Table 52–4 shows the results of the key studies that evaluated more than 100 diabetic subjects followed over 2 to 6 years.[110–112,114–116,131] These studies show that the benefit of ACEI use in CKD is seen in both type 1 and 2 diabetic subjects, across different degrees of kidney damage (normoalbuminuria, microalbuminuria, frank proteinuria, and reduction in GFR), and are drug-class specific. These findings consistently support the role of ACEI therapy in the management of CKD. It is customary to begin at low doses and increase the dose at 4-week intervals to control the level of proteinuria. The dose is usually increased until proteinuria is reduced by 30% to 50% or the development of side effects such as elevations in serum creatinine or potassium occurs.

A meta-analysis that pooled several of the small and large randomized, controlled studies showed beneficial effects of ACEI therapy on diabetic nephropathy.[132] Progression to proteinuria was reduced by 65% for patients with diabetes mellitus and microalbuminuria, and progression of nephropathy (doubling of serum creatinine) was reduced by 40% for patients with overt proteinuria (comprised of 30% diabetics and 70% nondiabetics) (Fig. 52–3).[132] However, a meta-analysis of 127 studies with more than 30,000 subjects suggests

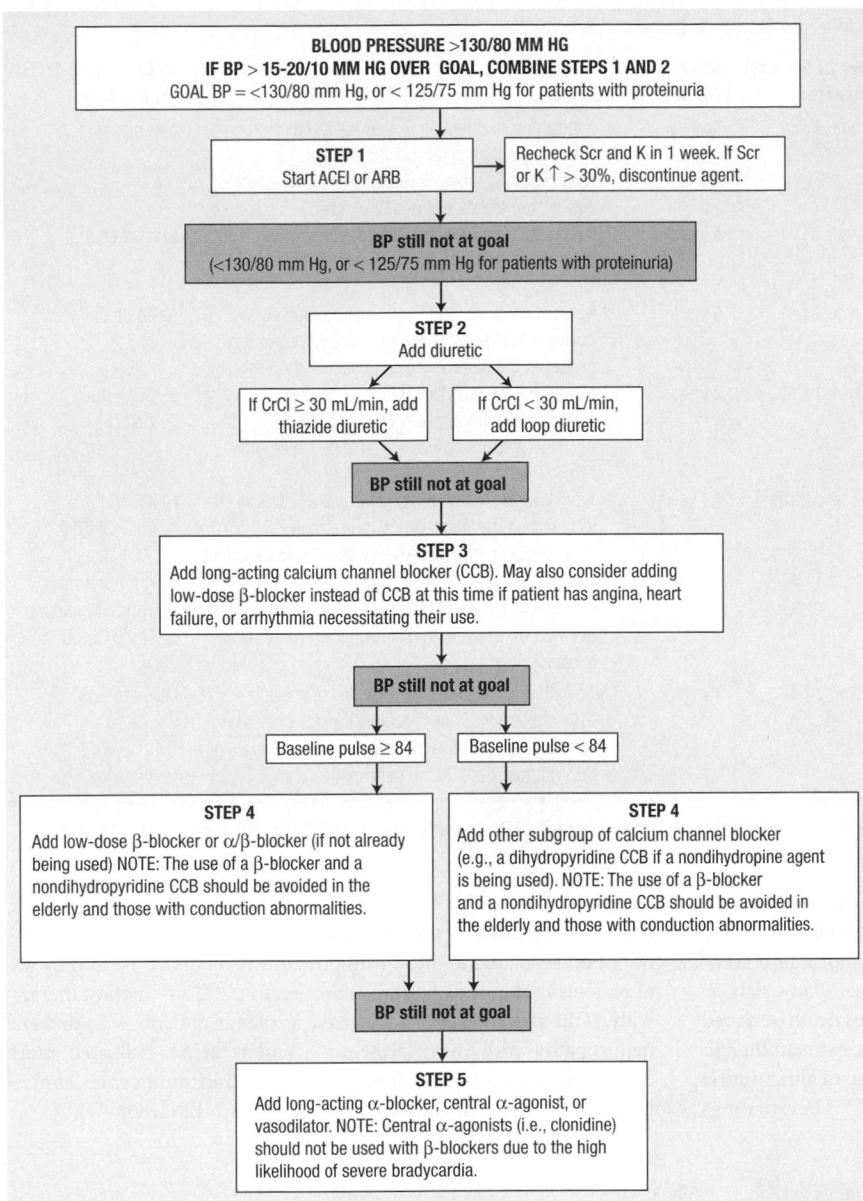

BLOOD PRESSURE >130/80 MM HG
IF BP > 15-20/10 MM HG OVER GOAL, COMBINE STEPS 1 AND 2
GOAL BP = <130/80 mm Hg, or < 125/75 mm Hg for patients with proteinuria

STEP 1
Start ACEI or ARB

Recheck Scr and K in 1 week. If Scr or K ↑ > 30%, discontinue agent.

BP still not at goal
(<130/80 mm Hg, or < 125/75 mm Hg for patients with proteinuria)

STEP 2
Add diuretic

If CrCl ≥ 30 mL/min, add thiazide diuretic

If CrCl < 30 mL/min, add loop diuretic

BP still not at goal

STEP 3
Add long-acting calcium channel blocker (CCB). May also consider adding low-dose β-blocker instead of CCB at this time if patient has angina, heart failure, or arrhythmia necessitating their use.

BP still not at goal

Baseline pulse ≥ 84

Baseline pulse < 84

STEP 4
Add low-dose β-blocker or α/β-blocker (if not already being used) NOTE: The use of a β-blocker and a nondihydropyridine CCB should be avoided in the elderly and those with conduction abnormalities.

STEP 4
Add other subgroup of calcium channel blocker (e.g., a dihydropyridine CCB if a nondihydropine agent is being used). NOTE: The use of a β-blocker and a nondihydropyridine CCB should be avoided in the elderly and those with conduction abnormalities.

BP still not at goal

STEP 5
Add long-acting α-blocker, central α-agonist, or vasodilator. NOTE: Central α-agonists (i.e., clonidine) should not be used with β-blockers due to the high likelihood of severe bradycardia.

FIGURE 52-2. Hypertension management algorithm for patients with CKD. Dosage adjustments should be made every 2 to 4 weeks as needed. The dose of one agent should be maximized before another is added. (ACEI, angiotensin-converting enzyme inhibitor; ARB, angiotensin receptor blocker; BP, blood pressure; CAD, coronary artery disease; CCB, calcium channel blocker; CHF, congestive heart failure; MI, myocardial infarction; UP:Cr, urinary protein-to-creatinine ratio.) *(Lewis EJ, Hunsicker LG, Bain RP, Rohde RD. The effect of angiotensin-converting-enzyme inhibition on diabetic nephropathy. The Collaborative Study Group. N Engl J Med. 1993 Nov 11;329(20):1456–1462. Copyright © 1993 Massachusetts Medical Society. All rights reserved.)*

that the benefit of ACEIs and ARBs over other pharmacologic agents is related to blood pressure attained during the study rather than to special properties of the ACEI or ARB (e.g., antiproteinuric effects).[133]

The ARBs have also been shown to slow the progression of diabetic kidney disease.[122-125] Table 52-5 summarizes data from several key studies (with at least 100 patients) evaluating ARB efficacy in type 2 diabetes. All patients in these trials had at least a level of proteinuria consistent with microalbuminuria and all were hypertensive. With the exception of one, the studies were of a sufficiently long duration to determine the beneficial effects of ARBs on nephropathy. Of note, the beneficial effect of delaying the onset of diabetic nephropathy was significant in type 2 diabetic patients who received irbesartan 300 mg daily for up to 2 years.[123] A similar trend (although not statistically significant) was observed in those subjects who received a lower dose of irbesartan (150 mg daily). Currently, the data show efficacy of both ACEIs and ARBs in type 2 diabetes, whereas only ACEIs have been adequately evaluated for patients with type 1 diabetes. Although no data exist comparing ACEIs and ARBs in head-to-head trials in type 2 diabetes, in practice these agents are used somewhat interchangeably. ACEIs are typically started as first line with a change to an ARB if not tolerated.

The lack of response among some patients to ACEI or ARB therapy with regards to blood pressure or proteinuria may be due to aldosterone escape in renin-angiotensin-aldosterone system blockade. Type 2 diabetic subjects with nephropathy who had increased aldosterone plasma levels during a mean 35-month treatment with losartan had a faster decline in the rate of GFR compared with those without aldosterone escape.[134] With the thought that further aldosterone blockade may improve outcomes, combination therapy with both ACEIs and ARBs has been investigated in both studies and subsequent metaanalyses.[135-138] In summary, these studies demonstrate a greater reduction in proteinuria with the combination of these agents, with some studies demonstrating a trend to higher serum potassium and serum creatinine concentrations. Unfortunately, none of these are of sufficient duration to determine if the reduction in proteinuria translates to preservation of renal function. It was recently suggested that polymorphisms in the cytochrome P450 (*CYP2C9*) drug metabolizing gene may result in less favorable therapeutic response to the ARB losartan.[139] The Arg144Cys and Ile359Leu polymorphisms are reported to reduce CYP2C9 activity,[140,141] and this may result in formation of metabolites with less pharmacological activity than E-3174.

A recent study has raised concerns with the use of combination ACEI/ARB. The Ongoing Telmisartan Alone and in Combination

TABLE 52-4 Key Angiotensin-Converting Enzyme Inhibitor Studies in Diabetic Patients

Drug, Dose, and Study Design	Baseline Renal Characteristics	Number of Subjects and Disease	Study Duration	Outcome	Reference and Study Name
Captopril 25 mg three times a day; randomized, placebo-controlled trial	UPE ≥500 mg/day, S_{cr}≤2.5 mg/dL (≤221 µmol/L)	409 type 1 DM	3 years	Risk reduction of doubling S_{cr} was 48% with captopril treatment; subanalysis showed a larger risk reduction with more elevated S_{cr} (76% when the S_{cr} was greater than 2 mg/dL [177 µmol/L])	Lewis et al.[110]
Enalapril once daily; randomized, placebo-controlled trial	Normotensive, UAE 20–200 mcg/min	103 type 2 DM	5 years	Risk reduction of 66.7% for progression to clinical albuminuria with enalapril	Ahmad et al.[111]
Enalapril 10 mg once daily; randomized, placebo-controlled trial	Normotensive, UAE ≤30 mg/day	156 type 2 DM	6 years	Risk reduction of 12.5% for microalbuminuria with enalapril treatment; GFR reductions were two times greater in the placebo-treated patients at 6 years	Ravid et al.[112]
Lisinopril 10 mg once daily with titration to BP; placebo-controlled trial	Normotensive patients with either normoalbuminuria or microalbuminuria	530 type 1 DM	2 years	18.8% lower UPE with lisinopril treatment; greater treatment effect in those with baseline microalbuminuria (34.2 mcg /min vs 1 mcg /min)	EUCLID Study Group[113]
Ramipril 10 mg once daily; randomized, placebo-controlled trial	Normoalbuminuria or microalbuminuria	3,577 type 2 DM	4.5 years	Ramipril lowered risk of overt nephropathy with and without baseline microalbuminuria (relative risk of 0.8); lower UP:Cr at 1 and 4.5 years with ramipril treatment	HOPE and MICROHOPE[114]
Captopril 50 mg twice a day; randomized, placebo-controlled trial	Normotensive patients with microalbuminuria	143 type 1 DM	2 years	Risk reduction of 67.8% for clinical proteinuria with captopril treatment; GFR reductions of 7.9 mL /min per 1.73 m² per year in placebo group while stable in captopril group	North American Microalbuminuria Study Group[115]
Enalapril 5 mg once daily, titrated to BP; placebo-controlled trial	Hypertensive, GFR of 30–100 mL/min per 1.73 m² (0.29–0.96 mL/s/m²)	121 type 2 DM	3 years	Clinical albuminuria progression in 7% of enalapril versus 21% of placebo group; enalapril therapy preserved GFR, whereas placebo treatment resulted in a loss of 0.33 mL/min per 1.73 m² per month	Lebovitz et al.[116]

BP, blood pressure; DM, diabetes mellitus; GFR, glomerular filtration rate; S_{cr}, serum creatinine; UAE, urinary albumin excretion; UP:Cr, urinary protein-to-creatinine ratio; UPE, urinary protein excretion.

with Ramipril Global Endpoint Trial (ONTARGET) randomized 25,620 patients with established atherosclerotic vascular disease or diabetes with end-organ damage to telmisartan, ramipril, or a combination of the two drugs.[142] The composite outcome of any dialysis, renal transplantation, doubling of serum creatinine, or death occurred more frequently for patients receiving combination treatment than in either of the two other groups, despite a lower degree of albuminuria and less progression to micro- or macroalbuminuria.[142] These findings have led some to advise against the combination of these two agents, however, criticisms of the study have argued that these findings cannot be extrapolated to those with proteinuric renal disease as only 4% of patients in the study had overt proteinuria.[143] Combination therapy with ACEI and ARB likely does have a role for patients with diabetic nephropathy with overt proteinuria and is being evaluated more closely in an ongoing randomized double-blind multicenter clinical trial of Veterans Administration patients (VA NEPHRON D).[144]

TABLE 52-5 Key Angiotensin Receptor Blocker Studies in Diabetic Patients

Drug, Dose, and Study Design	Baseline Characteristics	Number of Subjects and Disease	Duration	Outcomes	Reference and Study Name
Irbesartan 300 mg once daily; amlodipine 10 mg once daily, randomized, placebo-controlled trial	Hypertensive, UPE ≥900 mg/day	1,715 type 2 DM	2.6 years	Irbesartan therapy resulted in a 20% (for placebo) and 23% (for amlodipine) risk reduction in primary composite end point of doubling of S_{cr}, development of ESRD, or death	Lewis et al.[122]
Irbesartan 150 mg once daily; irbesartan 300 mg once daily; randomized, placebo-controlled trial	Hypertensive, AER of 20–200 mcg/min	590 type 2 DM	2 years	Irbesartan 150 mg resulted in a 24% reduction in UAE; irbesartan 300 mg resulted in a 38% reduction in UAE; placebo resulted in a 2% decrease; hazard ratio for diabetic nephropathy was 0.56 and 0.32 in the 150 mg and 300 mg irbesartan groups, respectively	Parving et al.[123]
Losartan 50–100 mg once daily; randomized placebo-controlled trial	Hypertensive, UA:U$_{cr}$ of at least 300 mg/g (33.9 mg/mmol) and S_{cr} 1.3–3 mg/dL (115–265 µmol/L)	1,513 type 2 DM	3.4 years	Losartan therapy resulted in a 16% risk reduction of primary composite end point of doubling of S_{cr}, ESRD, or death; level of proteinuria declined by 35% with losartan therapy	Brenner et al.[124]
Irbesartan 150 mg twice a day; randomized, placebo-controlled trial, crossover study	Hypertensive and normotensive, microalbuminuria	128 type 2 DM	120 days	Irbesartan had a beneficial effect on reducing AER in both hypertensive and normotensive patients with type 2 diabetes	Sasso et al.[125]

AER, albumin excretion rate; DM, diabetes mellitus; ESRD, end-stage renal disease; S_{cr}, serum creatinine; UA:U$_{cr}$, urinary albumin-to-urinary creatinine ratio; UAE, urinary albumin excretion; UPE, urinary protein excretion.

TABLE 52-6	Effects of Antihypertensive Agents on Renal Blood Flow (RBF) and Glomerular Filtration Rate (GFR)	
Antihypertensive Agents	**Mechanism of Action**	**Effects on Renal Hemodynamics**
Diuretics	Sodium and volume depletion	↓ GFR and RBF
	↑ Vasodilatory prostaglandin levels (IV loop diuretics)	↑ RBF
	Renal vasoconstriction (IV thiazide diuretics)	↓ GFR and RBF
β-Adrenergic blockers	↓ Cardiac output	↓ GFR and RBF
	↑ Renal vascular resistance (nonselective agents)	↓ GFR and RBF
	↑ Renal vascular resistance (β_1-selective agents)	No change in GFR and RBF
Centrally acting antiadrenergic drugs	↓ Renal vascular resistance (methyldopa)	No change in GFR and RBF
	↓ Renal perfusion pressure (clonidine, α_2-adrenergic agonist)	↓ GFR and RBF
Peripherally acting antiadrenergic drugs	Direct vasodilation (postsynaptic α_1-adrenoreceptor blocking agents)	No change in GFR and RBF
Direct vasodilator agents	↓ Renal vascular resistance (hydralazine, minoxidil)	↑ RBF and no effect on GFR
	Arterial vasodilation plus dilatation of venous capacitance vessels (nitroprusside)	↓ GFR and RBF (acute effect)
Calcium channel blockers		
Nondihydropyridine	↓ Renal vascular resistance by vasodilation of efferent arterioles (hypertensive patients)	↑ RBF and no change in GFR
Dihydropyridine (L-type)	↓ Renal vascular resistance by vasodilation of afferent arterioles (amlodipine, felodipine)	↑ RBF and ↑ GFR
Dihydropyridine (T-type)	↓ Renal vascular resistance by vasodilation of efferent arterioles (manidipine, efonidipine)	↑ RBF and no change in GFR
Renin-angiotensin-aldosterone system inhibitors (RAAS inhibitors)		
Angiotensin-converting enzyme inhibitors, angiotensin receptor blockers, direct renin inhibitors.	↓ Renal vascular resistance by vasodilation of efferent arterioles	↑ RBF and no change in GFR[a]

↓, decrease; ↑, increase
[a]In some instances, may see a decrease in GFR with use of ACEIs and ARBs.

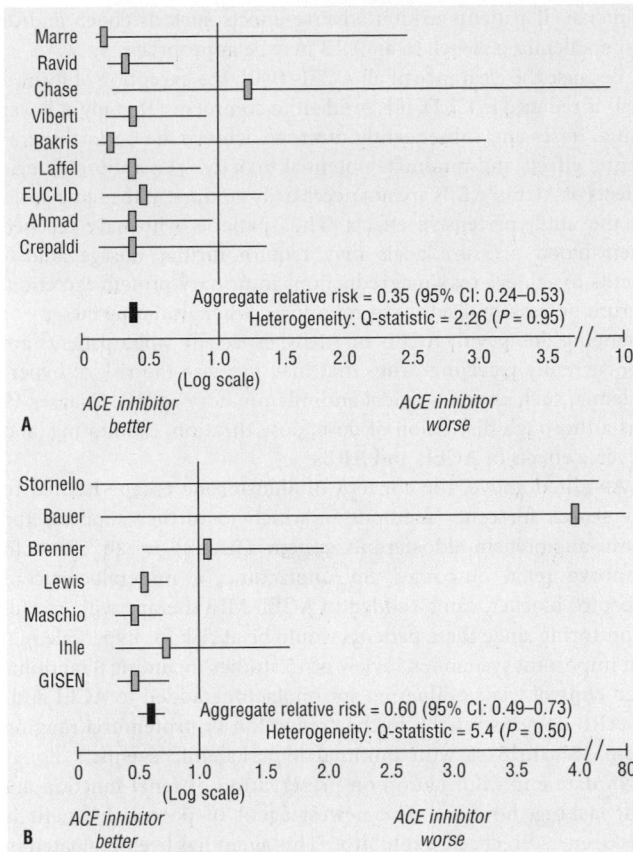

FIGURE 52-3. Therapeutic strategies to prevent progression of renal disease in diabetic individuals. (Blood glucose of 70 to 120 mg/dL corresponds to 3.9 to 6.7 mmol/L.) (A) Relative risk for developing *microalbuminuria* with 95% confidence intervals (CIs) in each study, and the aggregate *relative risk* with 95% CIs for all studies (N = 642 with diabetes). (B) Relative risk for doubling serum creatinine concentration or development of ESRD with 95% CIs in each study, and aggregate relative risk with 95% CIs for all studies (N = 1,277; 479 with diabetes). (ACE, angiotensin-converting *enzyme*.) *(Reprinted from Am J Kideny Dis, Vol. 35(4), Kshirsagar AV, Joy MS, Hogan SL, Falk RJ, Colindres RE. Effect of ACE inhibitors in diabetic and nondiabetic chronic renal disease: a systematic overview of randomized placebo-controlled trials, pages 695–707, Copyright © 2000, with permission from Elsevier.)*

Studies suggest that no individual ACEI drug is truly superior to any other ACEI,[132] and the same holds true for ARBs.[145,146] For patients with hypertension, the primary goal is to optimally treat the blood pressure to target, and the secondary goal is to control proteinuria. For normotensive patients with microalbuminuria, one should titrate the ACEI/ARB to reduce the degree of microalbuminuria. However, patients with hypertension and proteinuria may still exhibit side effects associated with blood pressure lowering, and dosages should be titrated to the maximum reduction of proteinuria without reducing blood pressure to a level associated with adverse events including renal function compromise. Patients should be initiated on the lowest possible dose of ACEI/ARB and titrated to blood pressure control and proteinuria reduction. A specific recommendation regarding the dose to initiate therapy with a specific ACEI/ARB has not been established; consequently, the lowest recommended dose for the management of hypertension may be appropriate until such information is available. In addition, one needs to consider the presence of other concomitant diseases and past history of treatment, as well as any side effects demonstrated with particular agents. Generally, ACEIs are more cost-effective than ARBs because of the availability of generic formulations, and individual patient insurance coverage should be reviewed by the

CLINICAL CONTROVERSY

ACEI and ARBs have been advocated for treatment of hypertension in CKD for the reduction of proteinuria. Early studies suggested that a combination of ACEI and ARB may have additional benefit; however, recent data suggest that the combination may be associated with a higher incidence of adverse outcomes including frequent hyperkalemia and need for acute dialysis. However, many would still advocate for combined ACEI and ARB therapy for patients with overt proteinuria.

clinician. If patients exhibit adverse effects such as cough and/or hyperkalemia, a switch to an ARB may be appropriate.

Because the clearance of all ACEIs (with the exception of fosinopril) is reduced in CKD, it is prudent to commence therapy at lower initial doses and subsequently titrate to achieve the optimal therapeutic effects and minimize potential toxicity. The antiproteinuric effects of ACEIs/ARBs are not necessarily attained at the same doses as the antihypertensive effects. Thus patients who have reached their blood pressure goals may require further dosage adjustments to achieve maximal reductions in urinary protein excretion. Serum potassium needs to be monitored when initiating therapy or changing doses with ACEIs or ARBs, especially when patients are concurrently receiving drugs that may increase the risk of hyperkalemia, such as nonsteroidal antiinflammatory agents. Chapter 19 has a thorough discussion of dose, dose titration, monitoring, and adverse effects of ACEIs and ARBs.

As noted above, the concept of aldosterone escape has led to the search for other methods in which to further suppress the renin-angiotensin-aldosterone system (RAAS) in an effort to improve renal outcomes. Spironolactone, a mineralocorticoid receptor blocker, can be added to ACEI/ARB therapy with careful monitoring since these patients would be at risk for hyperkalemia. An important systematic review of 15 studies including 8 randomized control trials evaluating spironolactone added to ACEI and/or ARB demonstrated a further reduction in proteinuria ranging from 15% to 54% with minimal hyperkalemic events.[147] Long-term data and information on preservation of renal function are still lacking, however. The newest agent of potential benefit is aliskiren, a direct renin inhibitor. This agent has been evaluated in three trials, two in combination with an ARB and one in combination with a diuretic.[148-150] Proteinuria was reduced in all of these studies although data regarding long-term benefit are lacking. The exact role of both these agents-whether to be used alone, with an ACEI or ARB, or added to ACEI/ARB combination-is still to be determined.

Some calcium channel blockers (CCBs) decrease glomerular injury without negatively changing renal hemodynamics.[128] The postulated mechanisms for this decrease in renal injury include suppression of glomerular hypertrophy, inhibition of platelet aggregation, and decrease in salt accumulation.[128] Although the data regarding dihydropyridine CCBs do not suggest any beneficial effects beyond those attributable to reducing blood pressure, there is some suggestion that the nondihydropyridine agents (diltiazem and verapamil) may have beneficial effects on proteinuria, although not as profoundly as ACEIs.[151] These agents are used occasionally in combination with ACEIs or ARBs, although data are limited to support this. In general, nondihydropyridine CCBs are used as second-line antiproteinuric drugs when ACEIs or ARBs are not tolerated. Efonidipine and manidipine, novel dihydropyridine CCBs that affect T-type calcium channels rather than L-type calcium channels, reduce intraglomerular pressure and may have antiproteinuric effects as well.[130,151] However, these drugs are not presently available in the United States, and how to best utilize these agents is not yet known.

Nondiabetic Chronic Kidney Disease

■ ANTIHYPERTENSIVE AGENTS

❾ Reduction of blood pressure is key to decreasing cardiovascular and renal sequelae. However, all antihypertensive agents are not equal in their ability to preserve kidney function despite similar efficacy in terms of blood pressure reduction. Among the different antihypertensives available, ACEIs and ARBs are currently also considered the first choice for patients with nondiabetic CKD because they reduce intraglomerular pressure. Several short- and long-term clinical trials have assessed the effect of ACEIs on renal function for patients without diabetes; Table 52–7 summarizes these trials.[131,152-155] These studies vary in length from 12 weeks to 7 years, and

TABLE 52-7	Key Studies with Angiotensin-Converting Enzyme Inhibitors in Patients Without Diabetes				
Drug, Dose, and Study Design	**Baseline Characteristics**	**Number of Subjects and Disease**	**Duration**	**Outcomes**	**Reference and Study Name**
Benazepril 10 mg once daily; randomized, placebo-controlled trial	Mild [GFR 46–60 mL/min (0.77–1.00 mL/s) Moderate [GFR 30–45 mL/min (0.50–0.75 mL/s)] renal insufficiency	583 Patients with various renal disorders including diabetes mellitus	3 years	Benazepril afforded a 53% risk reduction in primary end point of doubling of S_{cr} or requirement for dialysis; 71% and 46% risk reductions in the mild and moderate renal insufficiency groups, respectively	Maschio et al.[152]
Ramipril 2.5 mg once daily and titrated to BP; randomized, placebo-controlled trial	GFR 20–70 mL/min per 1.73 m² [0.19–0.67 mL/s/m²] UPE ≥1 g/day	352 Proteinuric patients	5 years	Rate of loss of GFR was 0.89 mL/min per month in placebo group versus 0.39 mL/min per month in ramipril group; twice the numbers of patients receiving placebo versus ramipril reached primary composite end point of doubling of S_{cr} or ESRD	The GISEN Group[131]
Enalapril 20 mg once daily versus losartan 50 mg once daily; randomized trial	Proteinuria	93 Hypertensives	12 weeks	UP:Cr was reduced by 43% in losartan group versus 23% in enalapril group ($P = 0.05$)	Nielsen et al.[153]
Enalapril 5–40 mg daily versus other antihypertensive agents; randomized, controlled trial	UPE ≥0.5 g/day S_{cr} ≤1.5 mg/dL (≤132 μmol/L)	44 IgAN patients	7 years	Renal survival was significantly better in the enalapril group (100%) versus the other antihypertensive group (70%) after 4 years, and 92% versus 55% respectively, after 7 years; proteinuria significantly decreased in the enalapril group, whereas it tended to increase in the control group	Praga et al.[154]
Ramipril 1.25–5 mg daily versus conventional therapy; randomized controlled trial	Proteinuria 1–3 g/day	186 Chronic nephropathies	31 months	Progression to use ESRD was half as common in the ramipril group; patients with GFR ≤45 mL/min per 1.73 m² (0.43 mL/s/m²) and proteinuria ≥1.5 g/24 hours had the greatest benefit from ramipril therapy	Ruggeneti et al.[155]

ESRD, end-stage renal disease; GFR, glomerular filtration rate; IgAN, immunoglobulin A nephropathy; S_{cr}, serum creatinine; UP:Cr, urinary protein-to-creatinine ratio; UPE, urinary protein excretion.

several enrolled a small number of subjects. Most patients had nephropathy associated with proteinuria and advanced CKD. Significant reductions in the risk of doubling serum creatinine, requirement for dialysis, and/or proteinuria were demonstrated for patients receiving the ACEIs. These studies and the summary results of a meta-analysis revealed that ACEIs conferred a 40% reduction in the risk of developing ESRD or doubling of serum creatinine for patients with overt proteinuria (>300 mg protein per 24 hours) and renal disease of various etiologies (see Fig. 52–3).[132] However, a meta-analysis failed to show a significant benefit of ACEI and/or ARBs over other antihypertensive agents in CKD progression.[133] A post hoc analysis of the African American Study of Kidney Disease and Hypertension (AASK), which evaluated two different blood pressure targets and three different treatment regimens in subjects with a GFR between 20 and 65 mL/min per 1.73 m² showed that the change in the level of proteinuria over 6 months of treatment predicted the progression of hypertensive CKD.[156] In addition, a post hoc analysis of the Antihypertensive and Lipid-Lowering Treatment to Prevent Heart Attack Trial (ALLHAT), where hypertensive subjects were randomized to chlorthalidone, amlodipine, or lisinopril for a mean of 4.9 years, revealed similar incident rates of ESRD in the three treatment groups irrespective of the cause of renal disease.[157] Therefore, although the drug class versus absolute blood pressure reduction is an evolving area of investigation, current treatment guidelines recommend use of ACEI or ARBs in subjects with CKD.

The ARBs, although evaluated to a lesser extent than ACEIs, appear to have similar efficacy in terms of kidney protection for patients with several forms of glomerulonephritis (Table 52–8).[158,159] Proteinuria reduction on the order of 25% to 47% was shown with ARB therapy. However, these studies employed small numbers of patients with short follow-up time frames as compared with studies in diabetic patients. Despite these limitations, most clinicians use either ACEI or ARB therapy as the standard of care for patients with nondiabetic CKD and proteinuria. The combination use of ARBs with ACEIs, similar to data in diabetic kidney disease, results in a greater decrease in proteinuria than that seen with either agent alone.[160] The Combination Treatment of Angiotensin-II Receptor Blocker and Angiotensin-Converting Enzyme Inhibitor in Non-diabetic Renal Disease (COOPERATE) study prospectively evaluated the use of losartan 100 mg daily alone, trandolapril 3 mg daily alone, or the combination of the two in 336 patients with nondiabetic kidney diseases. The primary end point, time to doubling of serum creatinine or ESRD, was observed in 11% of combination therapy patients and in 23% of each of the single-agent treatment groups.[161] However, this study has drawn several criticisms.[162,163] In light of the ONTARGET study findings above,[142] combination therapy may be dangerous and perhaps is best used in the setting of overt proteinuria and with close supervision. The selection of ACEIs versus ARBs in the control of proteinuria in nondiabetic kidney disease is essentially predicated on cost of therapy, patient tolerance, and clinician preference. As with diabetic kidney disease, modulation of RAAS with mineralocorticoid blockers, such as spironolactone,[147] and perhaps the direct renin inhibitor, aliskiren, may have a role in kidney disease with overt proteinuria.

The CCBs are also effective treatments for hypertension for patients with nondiabetic CKD. However, as was mentioned previously, only the nondihydropyridine CCBs have been studied and shown to reduce the rate of decline of kidney function. There are currently no data to suggest that higher doses of nondihydropyridine CCBs are needed to elicit a reduction in proteinuria as compared with a reduction in blood pressure. The role of dihydropyridine T-type CCBs remains uncertain.

Although diuretics are commonly used to treat fluid overload and hypertension for patients with CKD, there are minimal data to suggest any renal protection in terms of proteinuria regression or a reduction in the rate of progression. A single randomized, controlled trial has demonstrated an additive benefit of hydrochlorothiazide, a thiazide diuretic, to an ACEI regimen in reducing proteinuria in nondiabetic proteinuric kidney disease.[164] Chapter 58 addresses the use of diuretics for managing volume overload. Other available antihypertensive agents are used to control blood pressure in patients with kidney disease. Additional central and peripherally acting antihypertensive agents can be used for patients with CKD. One must consider the need for dosage reductions caused by decreases in GFR for drugs that are excreted by the kidneys and/or supplemental doses as a consequence of dialysis removal of hydrophilic β-blockers such as nadolol, acebutolol, and atenolol.

Regardless of the treatment regimen, hypertension should be treated to the currently accepted targets for patients with CKD. If proteinuria is present, the use of ACEIs, ARBs, and possibly nondihydropyridine CCBs may be superior to conventional agents in decreasing proteinuria and glomerular hypertension.

As precipitous reductions in blood pressure may be deleterious to kidney function for patients with underlying CKD, blood pressure targets in these patients should be achieved over several weeks to allow the kidney to adapt to reduced perfusion pressures.[108] Typically there is an acute but sustained reduction in GFR of approximately 25% to 30% within 3 to 7 days after initiation of ACEI therapy as a result of a reduction in intraglomerular pressure.[165] If a sustained increase in the serum creatinine by more than 30% after ACEI therapy initiation is observed, reduction of the dose or even discontinuation of ACEI therapy should be strongly considered (see Chap. 55). It is necessary to realize that although ACEI therapy may be effective in reducing the rate of nephropathy progression, one needs to consider their propensity for hyperkalemia and potential for acute GFR reduction especially for patients who already have compromised GFR.

TABLE 52-8	Key Studies with Angiotensin Receptor Blockers in Patients Without Diabetes				
Drug, Dose, and Study Design	**Baseline Characteristics**	**Number of Subjects and Disease**	**Duration**	**Outcomes**	**Reference**
Losartan 50 mg once daily versus control	Normotensive, proteinuria	23 FSGS patients	1 year	Proteinuria decreased 47% in the losartan group at 1 year, while there was a significant increase in proteinuria in the control group; total serum protein and albumin concentrations also increased in the losartan group; cholesterol levels of the losartan group were significantly reduced	Usta et al.[158]
Losartan 25 mg once daily versus enalapril 10 mg once daily; randomized, controlled trial	GFR 36–93 mL/min	34 Primary glomerulonephritis	3 months	Proteinuria reduced 25% versus 45% in losartan and enalapril groups, respectively; significant decline in GFR in enalapril group and no change in losartan group	Tylicki et al.[159]

FSGS, focal segmental glomerulosclerosis; GFR, glomerular filtration rate; UPE, urinary protein excretion.

CLINICAL CONTROVERSY

Some clinicians fail to prescribe ACEI or ARB medications when the GFR is less than 20 to 30 mL/min per 1.73 m² because they fear the patient may develop a further elevation in serum creatinine, whereas other clinicians prescribe these medications and evaluate serum creatinine closely after therapy initiation and dosage increases.

Other Interventions to Limit Disease Progression

❿ Other interventions such as lipid-lowering regimens and anemia management have been suggested to slow the progression of CKD.

Hyperlipidemia Treatment Although several drugs are available for lipid lowering, the β-hydroxy-β-methylglutaryl coenzyme A (HMG-CoA) reductase inhibitors, or statins, and gemfibrozil have been most often used in dyslipidemic patients with CKD with and without proteinuria.[166] The primary goal of treatment is to decrease the risk for progressive atherosclerotic cardiovascular disease. Additionally, a prior meta-analysis of 13 studies of lipid-lowering agents also showed a reduction in the rate of CKD progression by 0.156 mL/min per month.[167] Mechanisms for this effect are unknown, but statins may reduce proteinuria, inflammation and fibrosis.[168] In animal models of hyperlipidemia and kidney disease, lipid-lowering agents can decrease the extent of glomerular injury.[169] Recent clinical data have provided less certainty. A post hoc analysis of the ALLHAT[170] demonstrated no difference in ESRD rates among those treated with pravastatin versus those treated with usual care. A Cochrane systematic review demonstrated a decline in proteinuria and all-cause cardiovascular mortality but no attenuation of the decline of renal function.[168] However, this would not preclude appropriate treatment of hyperlipidemia. Additional therapies that show favorable benefits on lipids are cholestyramine, carnitine, fish oil, low-molecular-weight heparins, and exercise.[171,172] The National Cholesterol Education Program III and NKF K/DOQI guidelines should be consulted for a thorough review of lipid reduction and cardiovascular disease for patients with CKD.[83,173] Therefore, treatment of lipid abnormalities for patients with CKD may have a beneficial effect on slowing the rate of progression of the kidney disease.

Anemia Treatment Prolonged anemia is associated with left ventricular hypertrophy and heart failure. It has been suggested that anemia may increase the rate of CKD progression.[174] Researchers have coined the phrase "cardiorenal anemia syndrome" to describe the interrelationship between anemia, heart failure, and CKD.[174] Tissue hypoxia associated with anemia could be a stimulus for continued renal injury in those with stages 3 to 5 CKD. Although, at present, no definitive studies have been performed, some have hypothesized that the treatment of heart failure and anemia may reduce the progression of both heart failure and CKD.[175] Chapter 53 discusses anemia as a complication of CKD.

PHARMACOECONOMIC CONSIDERATIONS

The financial and societal costs of the care of individuals with CKD are disproportionately high. Excluding those with ESRD, patients with CKD comprise less than 10% of the Medicare population, yet account for nearly 28% of Medicare expenditures or over $57 billion.[2] These statistics suggest that the spectra of CKD is responsible for nearly one third of total Medicare expenditures.

There have been several evaluations of the potential pharmacoeconomic impact of screening for microalbuminuria in various populations. Generally speaking, the cost-effectiveness of screening is most apparent when targeted to high-risk populations including those with hypertension or diabetes or those over the age of 60.[176-178] When applied to diabetes, screening actually appears to have associated cost savings.[177,178] When compared with other conventional measures, such as screening for cervical cancer, screening for proteinuria in appropriate populations is similar or more favorable.[178] Intensive management of diabetes and hypertension beyond screening also appear to cost-effective.[177] As a caveat, these analyses employ simulated models whose results remain to be prospectively confirmed.

With regard to choice of pharmacologic agent, the majority of focus has been on agents employed in RAAS blockade. Both ARBs and ACEIs have been evaluated in the setting of diabetic kidney disease and appear to be favorable from the standpoint of cost and quality-adjusted life years gained.[176,177] ACEIs have demonstrated similar cost benefit in nondiabetic kidney disease.[179] One study provides data to suggest that even the more novel and expensive direct renin inhibitor, aliskiren, may have an beneficial cost profile in hypertensive diabetics with proteinuria.[180] In summary, screening and optimal therapy with intensive glycemic control and RAAS blockade may limit progression to ESRD and death with reasonable costs to society.

CONCLUSIONS

DIABETICS

Based on the available clinical and experimental data, pharmacologic interventions can help to limit the progression of CKD in diabetic patients. Figure 52–4 summarizes these interventions. All patients with type 1 diabetes for a duration of more than 5 years and all type 2 diabetics should be screened yearly for microalbuminuria (urinary albumin excretion or urinary albumin-to-creatinine ratio).[106] Blood glucose should be maintained within or close to the normal range by frequent insulin doses or by using a continuous subcutaneous insulin infusion while minimizing the risk of hypoglycemia by frequent blood glucose monitoring.[106] ACEI therapy should be initiated in normotensive and hypertensive type 1 or type 2 diabetic patients with persistent microalbuminuria (30 to 300 mg/day) or overt albuminuria (greater than 300 mg/day). ACEIs should be titrated every 1 to 3 months to achieve a maximal reduction in urinary albumin excretion. Within 1 week of initiating or increasing the dose of an ACEI, serum creatinine and potassium should be evaluated to detect abrupt reductions in GFR or development of hyperkalemia. ARBs should be considered as another first-line therapy for type 2 diabetic patients for the reduction of persistent proteinuria or albuminuria. A nondihydropyridine CCB may be an effective secondary alternative agent for patients who are unable to tolerate either an ACEI or an ARB. A combination of an ACEI with an ARB may result in a greater reduction in proteinuria or albuminuria than either agent alone and thus may be a therapeutic alternative for patients who are not maximally responding to single-agent therapy. Addition of an aldosterone receptor blocker may be considered in subjects with documented aldosterone escape. Direct renin inhibition represents a novel approach whose role is still to be determined.

NONDIABETIC PATIENTS

Figure 52–5 summarizes therapeutic interventions for nondiabetic patients with CKD. Nutritional management should be monitored frequently, regardless of the amount of protein intake prescribed,

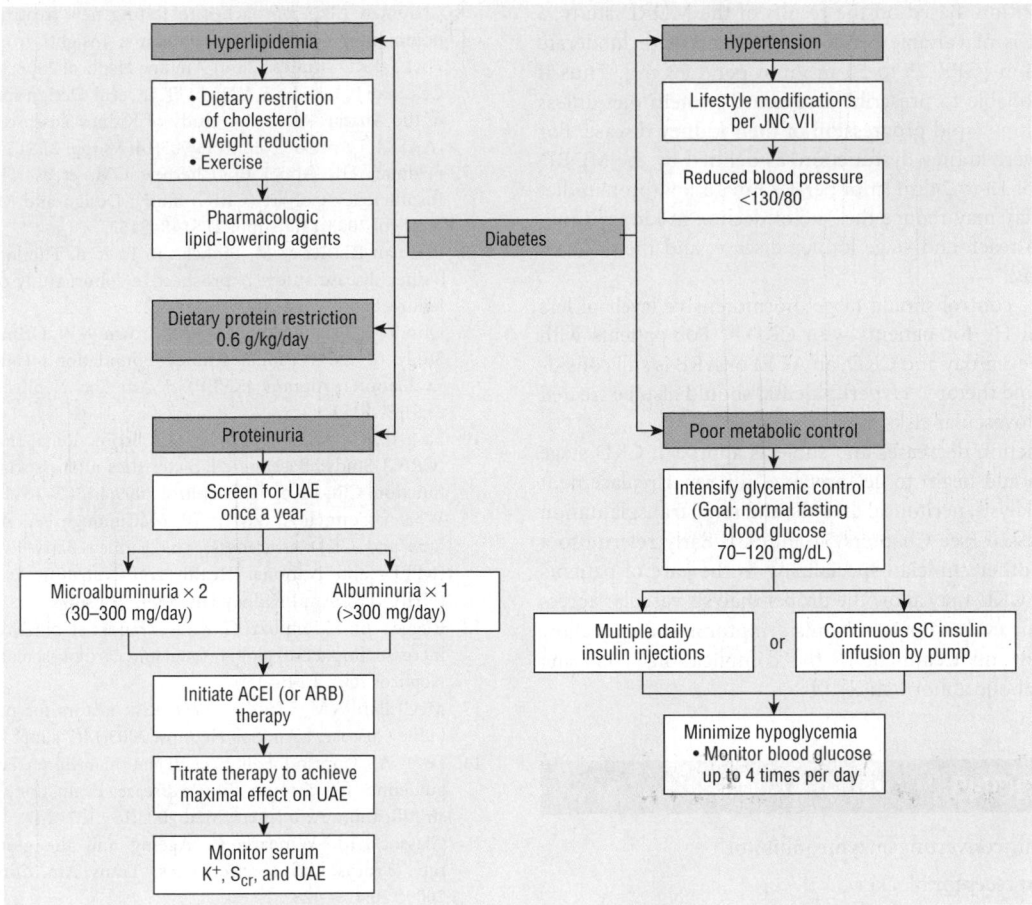

FIGURE 52-4. Therapeutic strategies to prevent progression of renal disease in diabetic individuals. (ACEI, angiotensin-converting enzyme inhibitor; ARB, angiotensin receptor blocker; UAE, urinary albumin excretion; SC, subcutaneous).

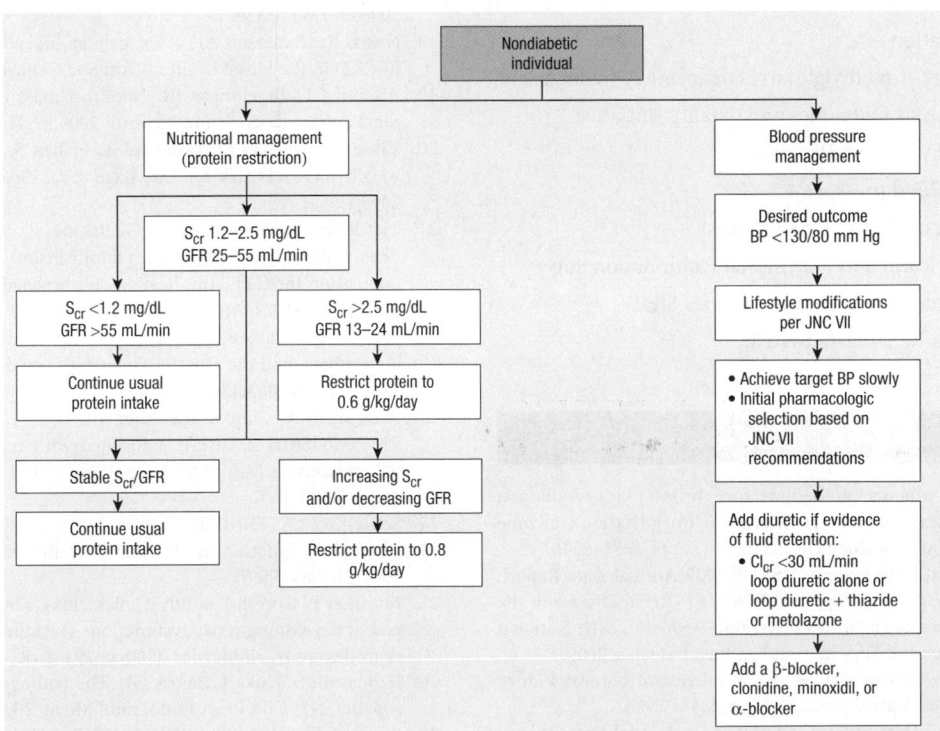

FIGURE 52-5. Therapeutic strategies to prevent progression of renal disease in nondiabetic individuals. (*ACEI*, angiotensin-converting *enzyme* inhibitor; ARB, angiotensin receptor blocker; BP, blood pressure; *GFR, glomerular filtration rate*; CL_{cr}, *creatinine clearance*; MAP, *mean arterial pressure*; S_{cr}, serum creatinine.

to avoid malnutrition. Based on the results of the MDRD study, a low-protein diet is of variable benefit for patients with moderate kidney dysfunction [GFR 25 to 55 mL/min per 1.73 m²]. Thus it is probably reasonable to prescribe a standard-protein diet unless the patient develops rapid progression of their kidney disease. For patients with severe kidney dysfunction, as defined by the MDRD study as a GFR of 13 to 24 mL/min per 1.73 m², a low-protein diet of 0.6 g/kg per day may reduce the rate of decline in kidney function, the time to reach end-stage kidney disease, and the onset of uremic symptoms.[96]

Blood pressure control should target normotensive levels of less than 130/80 mm Hg for patients with CKD.[108] For patients with proteinuria above 3 g/day and CKD, an ACEI or ARB is still considered to be first-line therapy. Hyperlipidemia should also be treated to decrease cardiovascular risks.

As kidney function decreases and subjects approach CKD stage 4, the patient should begin to get prepared for renal replacement therapy. Hemodialysis, peritoneal dialysis, and renal transplantation need to be discussed (see Chapters 54 and 98). Early referral to a nephrologist or other clinician specializing in the care of patients with progressive CKD may allow the proper dialysis vascular access placement and the evaluation for uremia symptoms and may allow for identification and treatment of the complications including anemia and metabolic abnormalities.[181]

ABBREVIATIONS

ACEI: angiotensin-converting enzyme inhibitor

ARB: angiotensin receptor blocker

CCB: calcium channel blocker

CKD: chronic kidney disease

CRIC: Chronic Renal Insufficiency Cohort

DCCT: Diabetes Control and Complications Trial

ESRD: end-stage renal disease

GFR: glomerular filtration rate

HMG-CoA: β-hydroxy-β-methylglutaryl coenzyme A (reductase)

K/DOQI: Kidney Dialysis Outcomes and Quality Initiative

KEEP: Kidney Early Evaluation Program

MAP: mean arterial blood pressure

MDRD: Modification of Diet in Renal Disease

NHANES: National Health and Nutritional Examination Survey

UKPDS: United Kingdom Prospective Diabetes Study

USRDS: United States Renal Data System

REFERENCES

1. K/DOQI clinical practice guidelines for chronic kidney disease: Evaluation, classification, and stratification. Kidney Disease Outcome Quality Initiative. Am J Kidney Dis 2002;39(2 suppl 2):S1–S246.

2. United States Renal Data System. USRDS 2009 Annual Data Report: Atlas of Chronic Kidney Disease and End-Stage Renal Disease in the United States. National Institutes of Health. Bethesda, MD: National Institute of Diabetes and Digestive and Kidney Diseases; 2009.

3. Coresh J, Selvin E, Stevens LA, et al. Prevalence of chronic kidney disease in the United States. Jama 2007;298:2038–2047.

4. United States Renal Data System. USRDS 2008 Annual Data Report: Atlas of Chronic Kidney Disease and End-Stage Renal Disease in the United States. National Institutes of Health, Bethesda, MD: National Institute of Diabetes and Digestive and Kidney Diseases; 2008.

5. Chapman AB. Approaches to testing new treatments in autosomal dominant polycystic kidney disease: Insights from the CRISP and HALT-PKD studies. Clin J Am Soc Nephrol 2008;3:1197–1204.

6. Gassman JJ, Greene T, Wright JT, Jr., et al. Design and statistical aspects of the African American Study of Kidney Disease and Hypertension (AASK). J Am Soc Nephrol 2003;14(7 suppl 2):S154–S165.

7. Feldman HI, Appel LJ, Chertow GM, et al. The Chronic Renal Insufficiency Cohort (CRIC) Study: Design and Methods. J Am Soc Nephrol 2003;14(7 suppl 2):S148–S153.

8. Perlman RL, Kiser M, Finkelstein F, et al. The longitudinal chronic kidney disease study: A prospective cohort study of predialysis renal failure. Semin Dial 2003;16:418–423.

9. Ohmit SE, Flack JM, Peters RM, Brown WW, Grimm R. Longitudinal Study of the National Kidney Foundation's (NKF) Kidney Early Evaluation Program (KEEP). J Am Soc Nephrol 2003;14(7 suppl 2):S117–S121.

10. Lash JP, Go AS, Appel LJ, et al. Chronic Renal Insufficiency Cohort (CRIC) Study: Baseline characteristics and associations with kidney function. Clin J Am Soc Nephrol 2009;4:1302–1311.

11. Whaley-Connell A, Sowers JR, McCullough PA, et al. Diabetes mellitus and CKD awareness: The Kidney Early Evaluation Program (KEEP) and National Health and Nutrition Examination Survey (NHANES). Am J Kidney Dis 2009;53(4 suppl 4):S11–S21.

12. Ruggenenti P, Remuzzi G. Kidney failure stabilizes after a two-decade increase: Impact on global (renal and cardiovascular) health. J Am Soc Nephrol 2007;2:146–150.

13. McClellan WM, Flanders WD. Risk factors for progressive chronic kidney disease. J Am Soc Nephrol 2003;14(7 suppl 2):S65–S70.

14. Levey AS, Coresh J, Balk E, et al. National Kidney Foundation practice guidelines for chronic kidney disease: Evaluation, classification, and stratification. Ann Intern Med 2003;139:137–147.

15. Glassock RJ, Winearls C. Ageing and the glomerular filtration rate: Truths and consequences. Trans Am Clin Climatol Assoc 2009;120:419–428.

16. Shoham DA, Vupputuri S, Diez Roux AV, et al. Kidney disease in life-course socioeconomic context: The Atherosclerosis Risk in Communities (ARIC) Study. Am J Kidney Dis 2007;49:217–226.

17. Shoham DA, Vupputuri S, Kaufman JS, et al. Kidney disease and the cumulative burden of life course socioeconomic conditions: The Atherosclerosis Risk in Communities (ARIC) study. Soc Sci Med 2008;67:1311–1320.

18. Norris K, Nissenson AR. Race, gender, and socioeconomic disparities in CKD in the United States. J Am Soc Nephrol 2008;19:1261–1270.

19. Abitbol CL, Ingelfinger JR. Nephron mass and cardiovascular and renal disease risks. Semin Nephrol 2009;29:445–454.

20. Vikse BE, Irgens LM, Leivestad T, Hallan S, Iversen BM. Low birth weight increases risk for end-stage renal disease. J Am Soc Nephrol 2008;19:151–157.

21. McClellan WM, Satko SG, Gladstone E, Krisher JO, Narva AS, Freedman BI. Individuals with a family history of ESRD are a high-risk population for CKD: Implications for targeted surveillance and intervention activities. Am J Kidney Dis 2009;53(3 suppl 3):S100–S106.

22. Erlinger TP, Tarver-Carr ME, Powe NR, et al. Leukocytosis, hypoalbuminemia, and the risk for chronic kidney disease in US adults. Am J Kidney Dis 2003;42:256–263.

23. Kshirsagar AV, Moss KL, Elter JR, Beck JD, Offenbacher S, Falk RJ. Periodontal disease is associated with renal insufficiency in the Atherosclerosis Risk In Communities (ARIC) study. Am J Kidney Dis 2005;45:650–657.

24. Schaeffner ES, Kurth T, Curhan GC, et al. Cholesterol and the risk of renal dysfunction in apparently healthy men. J Am Soc Nephrol 2003;14:2084–2091.

25. Muntner P, Coresh J, Smith JC, Eckfeldt J, Klag MJ. Plasma lipids and risk of developing renal dysfunction: The atherosclerosis risk in communities study. Kidney Int 2000;58:293–301.

26. Dronavalli S, Duka I, Bakris GL. The pathogenesis of diabetic nephropathy. Nat Clin Pract Endocrinol Metab 2008;4:444–452.

27. Brancati FL, Whelton PK, Randall BL, Neaton JD, Stamler J, Klag MJ. Risk of end-stage renal disease in diabetes mellitus: A prospective cohort study of men screened for MRFIT. Multiple Risk Factor Intervention Trial. Jama. 1997;278:2069–2074.

28. Freedman BI. End-stage renal failure in African Americans: Insights in kidney disease susceptibility. Nephrol Dial Transplant 2002;17:198–200.

29. Coresh J, Wei GL, McQuillan G, et al. Prevalence of high blood pressure and elevated serum creatinine level in the United States: Findings from the third National Health and Nutrition Examination Survey (1988–1994). Arch Intern Med 2001;161:1207–1216.

30. Muntner P, Anderson A, Charleston J, et al. Hypertension Awareness, Treatment, and Control in Adults With CKD: Results from the Chronic Renal Insufficiency Cohort (CRIC) Study. Am J Kidney Dis 2009.

31. Hsu CY, McCulloch CE, Darbinian J, Go AS, Iribarren C. Elevated blood pressure and risk of end-stage renal disease in subjects without baseline kidney disease. Arch Intern Med 2005;165:923–928.

32. Klag MJ, Whelton PK, Randall BL, et al. Blood pressure and end-stage renal disease in men. N Engl J Med. 1996;334:13–18.

33. Cattran DC, Reich HN, Beanlands HJ, Miller JA, Scholey JW, Troyanov S. The impact of sex in primary glomerulonephritis. Nephrol Dial Transplant 2008;23:2247–2253.

34. Hladunewich MA, Troyanov S, Calafati J, Cattran DC. The natural history of the non-nephrotic membranous nephropathy patient. Clin J Am Soc Nephrol 2009;4:1417–1422.

35. Mackinnon B, Fraser EP, Cattran DC, Fox JG, Geddes CC. Validation of the Toronto formula to predict progression in IgA nephropathy. Nephron Clin Pract 2008;109:c148–c153.

36. Ravera M, Re M, Deferrari L, Vettoretti S, Deferrari G. Importance of blood pressure control in chronic kidney disease. J Am Soc Nephrol 2006;17(4 suppl 2):S98–S103.

37. Bakris GL. A practical approach to achieving recommended blood pressure goals in diabetic patients. Arch Intern Med 2001;161:2661–2667.

38. Sarnak MJ, Greene T, Wang X, et al. The effect of a lower target blood pressure on the progression of kidney disease: Long-term follow-up of the modification of diet in renal disease study. Ann Intern Med 2005;142:3423–3451.

39. Raile K, Galler A, Hofer S, et al. Diabetic nephropathy in 27,805 children, adolescents, and adults with type 1 diabetes: Effect of diabetes duration, A1C, hypertension, dyslipidemia, diabetes onset, and sex. Diabetes Care 2007;30:2523–2528.

40. Nathan DM, Zinman B, Cleary PA, et al. Modern-day clinical course of type 1 diabetes mellitus after 30 years' duration: The diabetes control and complications trial/epidemiology of diabetes interventions and complications and Pittsburgh epidemiology of diabetes complications experience (1983–2005). Arch Intern Med 2009;169:1307–1316.

41. Bakris GL. Slowing nephropathy progression: Focus on proteinuria reduction. Clin J Am Soc Nephrol 2008;3 suppl 1:S3–S10.

42. Keane WF. Proteinuria: Its clinical importance and role in progressive renal disease. Am J Kidney Dis 2000;35(4 suppl 1):S97–105.

43. Klahr S, Levey AS, Beck GJ, et al. The effects of dietary protein restriction and blood-pressure control on the progression of chronic renal disease. Modification of Diet in Renal Disease Study Group. N Engl J Med. 1994;330:877–884.

44. Jafar TH, Stark PC, Schmid CH, et al. Proteinuria as a modifiable risk factor for the progression of non-diabetic renal disease. Kidney Int 2001;60:1131–1140.

45. Jafar TH, Stark PC, Schmid CH, Landa M, Maschio G, de Jong PE, de Zeeuw D, Shahinfar S, Toto R, Levey AS. Progression of chronic kidney disease: The role of blood pressure control, proteinuria, and angiotensin-converting enzyme inhibition: A patient-level meta-analysis. Ann Intern Med 2003;139:244–252.

46. Orth SR. Effects of smoking on systemic and intrarenal hemodynamics: Influence on renal function. J Am Soc Nephrol 2004;15 (suppl 1):S58–S63.

47. Ejerblad E, Fored CM, Lindblad P, et al. Association between smoking and chronic renal failure in a nationwide population-based case-control study. J Am Soc Nephrol 2004;15:2178–2185.

48. Sawicki PT, Didjurgeit U, Muhlhauser I, Bender R, Heinemann I, Berger M. Smoking is associated with progression of diabetic nephropathy. Diabetes Care. 1994;17:126–131.

49. Bakris G, Rahman M, Lea J, Ward H, Massry S, Wang S, AASK Study Group. Associations between cardiovascular risk factors and glomerular filtration rate at baseline in the African American Study of Kidney Disease (AASK) trial. J Am Soc Nephrol. 1998;10:A0717.

50. Hogan SL, Vupputuri S, Guo X, et al. Association of cigarette smoking with albuminuria in the United States: The third National Health and Nutrition Examination Survey. Ren Fail 2007;29:133–142.

51. Haroun MK, Jaar BG, Hoffman SC, Comstock GW, Klag MJ, Coresh J. Risk factors for chronic kidney disease: A prospective study of 23,534 men and women in Washington county, Maryland. J Am Soc Nephrol 2003;14:2934–2941.

52. Ward MM, Studenski S. Clinical prognostic factors in lupus nephritis. The importance of hypertension and smoking. Arch Intern Med. 1992;152:2082–2088.

53. Kasiske BL. Hyperlipidemia in patients with chronic renal disease. Am J Kidney Dis. 1998;32(5 suppl 3):S142–S156.

54. Fox CS, Larson MG, Leip EP, Culleton B, Wilson PW, Levy D. Predictors of new-onset kidney disease in a community-based population. Jama 2004;291:844–850.

55. Cases A, Coll E. Dyslipidemia and the progression of renal disease in chronic renal failure patients. Kidney Int Suppl 2005:S87–S93.

56. Hsu CY, McCulloch CE, Iribarren C, Darbinian J, Go AS. Body mass index and risk for end-stage renal disease. Ann Intern Med 2006;144:21–28.

57. Iseki K, Ikemiya Y, Kinjo K, Inoue T, Iseki C, Takishita S. Body mass index and the risk of development of end-stage renal disease in a screened cohort. Kidney Int 2004;65:1870–1876.

58. Ejerblad E, Fored CM, Lindblad P, Fryzek J, McLaughlin JK, Nyren O. Obesity and risk for chronic renal failure. J Am Soc Nephrol 2006;17:1695–1702.

59. Foster MC, Hwang SJ, Larson MG, et al. Overweight, obesity, and the development of stage 3 CKD: The Framingham Heart Study. Am J Kidney Dis 2008;52:39–48.

60. Ryu S, Chang Y, Woo HY, Kim SG, et al. Changes in body weight predict CKD in healthy men. J Am Soc Nephrol 2008;19:1798–1805.

61. Wolkow PP, Niewczas MA, Perkins B, et al. Association of urinary inflammatory markers and renal decline in microalbuminuric type 1 diabetics. J Am Soc Nephrol 2008;19:789–797.

62. Ramos LF, Shintani A, Ikizler TA, Himmelfarb J. Oxidative stress and inflammation are associated with adiposity in moderate to severe CKD. J Am Soc Nephrol 2008;19:593–599.

63. Wang Y, Chen X, Song Y, Caballero B, Cheskin LJ. Association between obesity and kidney disease: A systematic review and meta-analysis. Kidney Int 2008;73:19–33.

64. Obermayr RP, Temml C, Gutjahr G, Knechtelsdorfer M, Oberbauer R, Klauser-Braun R. Elevated uric acid increases the risk for kidney disease. J Am Soc Nephrol 2008;19:2407–2413.

65. Weiner DE, Tighiouart H, Elsayed EF, Griffith JL, Salem DN, Levey AS. Uric acid and incident kidney disease in the community. J Am Soc Nephrol 2008;19:1204–1211.

66. Fisher MA, Taylor GW, Shelton BJ, et al. Periodontal disease and other nontraditional risk factors for CKD. Am J Kidney Dis 2008;51:45–52.

67. Shultis WA, Weil EJ, Looker HC, et al. Effect of periodontitis on overt nephropathy and end-stage renal disease in type 2 diabetes. Diabetes Care 2007;30:306–311.

68. Lin JL, Lin-Tan DT, Hsu KH, Yu CC. Environmental lead exposure and progression of chronic renal diseases in patients without diabetes. N Engl J Med 2003;348:277–286.

69. Vupputuri S, Batuman V, Muntner P, et al. The risk for mild kidney function decline associated with illicit drug use among hypertensive men. Am J Kidney Dis 2004;43:629–635.

70. Hsu CC, Kao WH, Coresh J, et al. Apolipoprotein E and progression of chronic kidney disease. Jama 2005;293:2892–2899.

71. Kopp JB, Smith MW, Nelson GW, et al. MYH9 is a major-effect risk gene for focal segmental glomerulosclerosis. Nat Genet 2008;40:1175–1184.

72. Kao WH, Klag MJ, Meoni LA, et al. MYH9 is associated with non-diabetic end-stage renal disease in African Americans. Nat Genet 2008;40:1185–1192.

73. Remuzzi G, Benigni A, Remuzzi A. Mechanisms of progression and regression of renal lesions of chronic nephropathies and diabetes. J Clin Invest 2006;116:288–2896.

74. Campbell RC, Ruggenenti P, Remuzzi G. Halting the progression of chronic nephropathy. J Am Soc Nephrol 2002;13(suppl 3):S190–S195.

75. Aros C, Remuzzi G. The renin-angiotensin system in progression, remission and regression of chronic nephropathies. J Hypertens suppl 2002;20:S45–S53.

76. Abbate M, Zoja C, Remuzzi G. How does proteinuria cause progressive renal damage? J Am Soc Nephrol 2006;17:2974–2984.

77. Bang H, Vupputuri S, Shoham DA, et al. SCreening for Occult REnal Disease (SCORED): A simple prediction model for chronic kidney disease. Arch Intern Med 2007;167:374–381.

78. Kshirsagar AV, Bang H, Bomback AS, et al. A simple algorithm to predict incident kidney disease. Arch Intern Med 2008;168:2466–2473.

79. Hsu CY, McCulloch CE, Curhan GC. Epidemiology of anemia associated with chronic renal insufficiency among adults in the United States: Results from the Third National Health and Nutrition Examination Survey. J Am Soc Nephrol 2002;13:504–510.

80. McFarlane SI, Chen SC, Whaley-Connell AT, et al. Prevalence and associations of anemia of CKD: Kidney Early Evaluation Program (KEEP) and National Health and Nutrition Examination Survey (NHANES) 1999–2004. Am J Kidney Dis 2008;51(4 suppl 2):S46–S55.

81. KDOQI Clinical Practice Guidelines and Clinical Practice Recommendations for Anemia in Chronic Kidney Disease. Am J Kidney Dis 2006;47(5 suppl 3):S11–S145.

82. Jungers P, Choukroun G, Oualim Z, Robino C, Nguyen AT, Man NK. Beneficial influence of recombinant human erythropoietin therapy on the rate of progression of chronic renal failure in predialysis patients. Nephrol Dial Transplant 2001;16:307–312.

83. K/DOQI clinical practice guidelines for cardiovascular disease in dialysis patients. Am J Kidney Dis 2005;45(4 suppl 3):S1–S153.

84. Go AS, Chertow GM, Fan D, McCulloch CE, Hsu CY. Chronic kidney disease and the risks of death, cardiovascular events, and hospitalization. N Engl J Med 2004;351:1296–1305.

85. Keith DS, Nichols GA, Gullion CM, Brown JB, Smith DH. Longitudinal follow-up and outcomes among a population with chronic kidney disease in a large managed care organization. Arch Intern Med 2004;164:659–663.

86. Wen CP, Cheng TY, Tsai MK, et al. All-cause mortality attributable to chronic kidney disease: A prospective cohort study based on 462 293 adults in Taiwan. Lancet 2008;371(9631):2173–2182.

87. McCullough PA, Li S, Jurkovitz CT, et al. CKD and cardiovascular disease in screened high-risk volunteer and general populations: The Kidney Early Evaluation Program (KEEP) and National Health and Nutrition Examination Survey (NHANES) 1999–2004. Am J Kidney Dis 2008;51(4 suppl 2):S38–S45.

88. Hallan S, Astor B, Romundstad S, Aasarod K, Kvenild K, Coresh J. Association of kidney function and albuminuria with cardiovascular mortality in older vs younger individuals: The HUNT II Study. Arch Intern Med 2007;167:2490–2496.

89. Cirillo M, Lanti MP, Menotti A, et al. Definition of kidney dysfunction as a cardiovascular risk factor: Use of urinary albumin excretion and estimated glomerular filtration rate. Arch Intern Med 2008;168:617–624.

90. Martinez I, Saracho R, Montenegro J, Llach F. The importance of dietary calcium and phosphorous in the secondary hyperparathyroidism of patients with early renal failure. Am J Kidney Dis. 1997;29:496–502.

91. Foundation NK. K/DOQI clinical practice guidelines for bone metabolism and disease in chronic kidney disease. Am J Kidney Dis 2003;42(4 suppl 3):S1–S201.

92. Alborzi P, Patel NA, Peterson C, et al. Paricalcitol reduces albuminuria and inflammation in chronic kidney disease: A randomized double-blind pilot trial. Hypertension 2008;52:249–255.

93. Szeto CC, Chow KM, Kwan BC, Chung KY, Leung CB, Li PK. Oral calcitriol for the treatment of persistent proteinuria in immunoglobulin A nephropathy: An uncontrolled trial. Am J Kidney Dis 2008;51:724–731.

94. Kopple JD. National kidney foundation K/DOQI clinical practice guidelines for nutrition in chronic renal failure. Am J Kidney Dis 2001;37(1 suppl 2):S66–S70.

95. Brenner BM. Hemodynamically mediated glomerular injury and the progressive nature of kidney disease. Kidney Int. 1983;23:647–655.

96. Levey AS, Adler S, Caggiula AW, et al. Effects of dietary protein restriction on the progression of advanced renal disease in the Modification of Diet in Renal Disease Study. Am J Kidney Dis. 1996;27:652–663.

97. Menon V, Kopple JD, Wang X, Beck GJ, et al. Effect of a very low-protein diet on outcomes: Long-term follow-up of the Modification of Diet in Renal Disease (MDRD) Study. Am J Kidney Dis 2009;53:208–217.

98. Fouque D, Laville M. Low protein diets for chronic kidney disease in non diabetic adults. Cochrane Database Syst Rev 2009:CD001892.

99. Pan Y, Guo LL, Jin HM. Low-protein diet for diabetic nephropathy: A meta-analysis of randomized controlled trials. Am J Clin Nutr 2008;88:660–666.

100. Robertson L, Waugh N, Robertson A. Protein restriction for diabetic renal disease. Cochrane Database Syst Rev 2007:CD002181.

101. Koya D, Haneda M, Inomata S, et al. Long-term effect of modification of dietary protein intake on the progression of diabetic nephropathy: A randomised controlled trial. Diabetologia 2009;52:2037–2045.

102. Pinto-Sietsma SJ, Mulder J, et al. Smoking is related to albuminuria and abnormal renal function in nondiabetic persons. Ann Intern Med 2000;133:585–91.

103. The effect of intensive treatment of diabetes on the development and progression of long-term complications in insulin-dependent diabetes mellitus. The Diabetes Control and Complications Trial Research Group. N Engl J Med. 1993;329:977–986.

104. Sustained effect of intensive treatment of type 1 diabetes mellitus on development and progression of diabetic nephropathy: The Epidemiology of Diabetes Interventions and Complications (EDIC) study. Jama 2003;290:2159–2167.

105. Intensive blood-glucose control with sulphonylureas or insulin compared with conventional treatment and risk of complications in patients with type 2 diabetes (UKPDS 33). UK Prospective Diabetes Study (UKPDS) Group. Lancet. 1998;352(9131):837–853.

106. American Diabetes Association Standards of medical care in diabetes-2007. Diabetes Care 2007;30(suppl 1):S4–S41.

107. Gerstein HC, Miller ME, Byington RP, et al. Effects of intensive glucose lowering in type 2 diabetes. N Engl J Med 2008;358:2545–2559.

108. Chobanian AV, Bakris GL, Black HR, et al. Seventh report of the Joint National Committee on Prevention, Detection, Evaluation, and Treatment of High Blood Pressure. Hypertension 2003;42:1206–1252.

109. Bakris GL, Williams M, Dworkin L, et al. Preserving renal function in adults with hypertension and diabetes: A consensus approach. National Kidney Foundation Hypertension and Diabetes Executive Committees Working Group. Am J Kidney Dis 2000;36:646–661.

110. Lewis EJ, Hunsicker LG, Bain RP, Rohde RD. The effect of angiotensin-converting-enzyme inhibition on diabetic nephropathy. The Collaborative Study Group. N Engl J Med. 1993;329:1456–1462.

111. Ahmad J, Siddiqui MA, Ahmad H. Effective postponement of diabetic nephropathy with enalapril in normotensive type 2 diabetic patients with microalbuminuria. Diabetes Care. 1997;20:1576–1581.

112. Ravid M, Brosh D, Levi Z, Bar-Dayan Y, Ravid D, Rachmani R. Use of enalapril to attenuate decline in renal function in normotensive, normoalbuminuric patients with type 2 diabetes mellitus. A randomized, controlled trial. Ann Intern Med. 1998;128:982–988.

113. Randomised placebo-controlled trial of lisinopril in normotensive patients with insulin-dependent diabetes and normoalbuminuria or microalbuminuria. The EUCLID Study Group. Lancet. 1997;349(9068):1787–1792.

114. Effects of ramipril on cardiovascular and microvascular outcomes in people with diabetes mellitus: Results of the HOPE study and MICRO-HOPE substudy. Heart Outcomes Prevention Evaluation Study Investigators. Lancet 2000;355(9200):253–259.

115. Laffel LM, McGill JB, Gans DJ. The beneficial effect of angiotensin-converting enzyme inhibition with captopril on diabetic nephropathy in normotensive IDDM patients with microalbuminuria. North American Microalbuminuria Study Group. Am J Med. 1995;99:497–504.

116. Lebovitz HE, Wiegmann TB, Cnaan A, et al. Renal protective effects of enalapril in hypertensive NIDDM: Role of baseline albuminuria. Kidney Int suppl. 1994;45:S150–S155.

117. Tight blood pressure control and risk of macrovascular and microvascular complications in type 2 diabetes: UKPDS 38. UK Prospective Diabetes Study Group. Bmj. 1998;317(7160):703–713.

118. Efficacy of atenolol and captopril in reducing risk of macrovascular and microvascular complications in type 2 diabetes: UKPDS 39. UK Prospective Diabetes Study Group. Bmj. 1998;317(7160):713–720.

119. Savage S, Johnson Nagel N, Estacio RO, et al. The ABCD (Appropriate Blood Pressure Control in Diabetes) trial. Rationale and design of a

trial of hypertension control (moderate or intensive) in type II diabetes. Online J Curr Clin Trials. 1993 Nov 24;Doc No 104:[6250 words; 128 paragraphs].

120. Bakris GL, Weir MR, Shanifar S, et al. Effects of blood pressure level on progression of diabetic nephropathy: Results from the RENAAL study. Arch Intern Med 2003;163:1555–1565.

121. Viberti G, Wheeldon NM. Microalbuminuria reduction with valsartan in patients with type 2 diabetes mellitus: A blood pressure-independent effect. Circulation 2002;106:672–678.

122. Lewis EJ, Hunsicker LG, Clarke WR, et al. Renoprotective effect of the angiotensin-receptor antagonist irbesartan in patients with nephropathy due to type 2 diabetes. N Engl J Med 2001;345:851–860.

123. Parving HH, Lehnert H, Brochner-Mortensen J, Gomis R, Andersen S, Arner P. The effect of irbesartan on the development of diabetic nephropathy in patients with type 2 diabetes. N Engl J Med 2001;345: 870–878.

124. Brenner BM, Cooper ME, de Zeeuw D, et al. Effects of losartan on renal and cardiovascular outcomes in patients with type 2 diabetes and nephropathy. N Engl J Med 2001;345:861–869.

125. Sasso FC, Carbonara O, Persico M, et al. Irbesartan reduces the albumin excretion rate in microalbuminuric type 2 diabetic patients independently of hypertension: A randomized double-blind placebo-controlled crossover study. Diabetes Care 2002;25:1909–1913.

126. Lewis JB, Berl T, Bain RP, Rohde RD, Lewis EJ. Effect of intensive blood pressure control on the course of type 1 diabetic nephropathy. Collaborative Study Group. Am J Kidney Dis. 1999;34:809–817.

127. Parving HH. Impact of blood pressure and antihypertensive treatment on incipient and overt nephropathy, retinopathy, and endothelial permeability in diabetes mellitus. Diabetes Care. 1991;14:260–269.

128. Dworkin LD, Benstein JA, Parker M, Tolbert E, Feiner HD. Calcium antagonists and converting enzyme inhibitors reduce renal injury by different mechanisms. Kidney Int. 1993;43:808–814.

129. Schlueter WA, Batlle DC. Renal effects of antihypertensive drugs. Drugs. 1989;37:900–925.

130. Wenzel RR. Renal protection in hypertensive patients: Selection of antihypertensive therapy. Drugs 2005;65(suppl 2):29–39.

131. Randomised placebo-controlled trial of effect of ramipril on decline in glomerular filtration rate and risk of terminal renal failure in proteinuric, non-diabetic nephropathy. The GISEN Group (Gruppo Italiano di Studi Epidemiologici in Nefrologia). Lancet. 1997;349(9069):1857–1863.

132. Kshirsagar AV, Joy MS, Hogan SL, Falk RJ, Colindres RE. Effect of ACE inhibitors in diabetic and nondiabetic chronic renal disease: A systematic overview of randomized placebo-controlled trials. Am J Kidney Dis 2000;35:695–707.

133. Casas JP, Chua W, Loukogeorgakis S, et al. Effect of inhibitors of the renin-angiotensin system and other antihypertensive drugs on renal outcomes: Systematic review and meta-analysis. Lancet 2005;366(9502):2026–2033.

134. Schjoedt KJ, Andersen S, Rossing P, Tarnow L, Parving HH. Aldosterone escape during blockade of the renin-angiotensin-aldosterone system in diabetic nephropathy is associated with enhanced decline in glomerular filtration rate. Diabetologia 2004;47:1936–1939.

135. Mogensen CE, Neldam S, Tikkanen I, et al. Randomised controlled trial of dual blockade of renin-angiotensin system in patients with hypertension, microalbuminuria, and non-insulin dependent diabetes: The candesartan and lisinopril microalbuminuria (CALM) study. Bmj 2000;321(7274):1440–1444.

136. Jennings DL, Kalus JS, Coleman CI, Manierski C, Yee J. Combination therapy with an ACE inhibitor and an angiotensin receptor blocker for diabetic nephropathy: A meta-analysis. Diabet Med 2007;24:486–493.

137. MacKinnon M, Shurraw S, Akbari A, Knoll GA, Jaffey J, Clark HD. Combination therapy with an angiotensin receptor blocker and an ACE inhibitor in proteinuric renal disease: A systematic review of the efficacy and safety data. Am J Kidney Dis 2006;48:8–20.

138. Kunz R, Friedrich C, Wolbers M, Mann JF. Meta-analysis: Effect of monotherapy and combination therapy with inhibitors of the renin angiotensin system on proteinuria in renal disease. Ann Intern Med 2008;148:30–48.

139. Joy MS, Dornbrook-Lavender K, Blaisdell J, et al. CYP2C9 genotype and pharmacodynamic responses to losartan in patients with primary and secondary kidney diseases. Eur J Clin Pharmacol 2009;65:947–953.

140. Yasar U, Forslund-Bergengren C, Tybring G, et al. Pharmacokinetics of losartan and its metabolite E-3174 in relation to the CYP2C9 genotype. Clin Pharmacol Ther 2002;71:89–98.

141. Yasar U, Tybring G, Hidestrand M, et al. Role of CYP2C9 polymorphism in losartan oxidation. Drug Metab Dispos 2001;29:1051–1056.

142. Mann JF, Schmieder RE, McQueen M, et al. Renal outcomes with telmisartan, ramipril, or both, in people at high vascular risk (the ONTARGET study): A multicentre, randomised, double-blind, controlled trial. Lancet 2008;372(9638):547–553.

143. Ruggenenti P, Remuzzi G. Proteinuria: Is the ONTARGET renal substudy actually off target? Nat Rev Nephrol 2009;5:436–437.

144. Fried LF, Duckworth W, Zhang JH, et al. Design of combination angiotensin receptor blocker and angiotensin-converting enzyme inhibitor for treatment of diabetic nephropathy (VA NEPHRON-D). Clin J Am Soc Nephrol 2009;4:361–368.

145. Bakris G, Burgess E, Weir M, Davidai G, Koval S. Telmisartan is more effective than losartan in reducing proteinuria in patients with diabetic nephropathy. Kidney Int 2008;74:364–369.

146. Galle J, Schwedhelm E, Pinnetti S, Boger RH, Wanner C. Antiproteinuric effects of angiotensin receptor blockers: Telmisartan versus valsartan in hypertensive patients with type 2 diabetes mellitus and overt nephropathy. Nephrol Dial Transplant 2008;23:3174–3183.

147. Bomback AS, Kshirsagar AV, Amamoo MA, Klemmer PJ. Change in proteinuria after adding aldosterone blockers to ACE inhibitors or angiotensin receptor blockers in CKD: A systematic review. Am J Kidney Dis 2008;51:199–211.

148. Persson F, Rossing P, Schjoedt KJ, Juhl T, et al. Time course of the antiproteinuric and antihypertensive effects of direct renin inhibition in type 2 diabetes. Kidney Int 2008;73:1419–1425.

149. Parving HH, Persson F, Lewis JB, Lewis EJ, Hollenberg NK. Aliskiren combined with losartan in type 2 diabetes and nephropathy. N Engl J Med 2008;358:2433–2446.

150. Persson F, Rossing P, Reinhard H, et al. Renal effects of aliskiren compared to and in combination with irbesartan in patients with type 2 diabetes, hypertension and albuminuria. Diabetes Care 2009 Jul 8.

151. Hart P, Bakris GL. Calcium antagonists: Do they equally protect against kidney injury? Kidney Int 2008;73:795–796.

152. Maschio G, Alberti D, Janin G, et al. Effect of the angiotensin-converting-enzyme inhibitor benazepril on the progression of chronic renal insufficiency. The Angiotensin-Converting-Enzyme Inhibition in Progressive Renal Insufficiency Study Group. N Engl J Med. 1996;334:939–945.

153. Nielsen S, Dollerup J, Nielsen B, Jensen HA, Mogensen CE. Losartan reduces albuminuria in patients with essential hypertension. An enalapril controlled 3 months study. Nephrol Dial Transplant. 1997;12 suppl 2:19–23.

154. Praga M, Gutierrez E, Gonzalez E, Morales E, Hernandez E. Treatment of IgA nephropathy with ACE inhibitors: A randomized and controlled trial. J Am Soc Nephrol 2003;14:1578–1583.

155. Ruggenenti P, Perna A, Gherardi G, et al. Renoprotective properties of ACE-inhibition in non-diabetic nephropathies with non-nephrotic proteinuria. Lancet. 1999;354(9176):359–364.

156. Lea J, Greene T, Hebert L, et al. The relationship between magnitude of proteinuria reduction and risk of end-stage renal disease: Results of the African American study of kidney disease and hypertension. Arch Intern Med 2005;165:947–953.

157. Rahman M, Pressel S, Davis BR, et al. Renal outcomes in high-risk hypertensive patients treated with an angiotensin-converting enzyme inhibitor or a calcium channel blocker vs. a diuretic: A report from the Antihypertensive and Lipid-Lowering Treatment to Prevent Heart Attack Trial (ALLHAT). Arch Intern Med 2005;165:936–946.

158. Usta M, Ersoy A, Dilek K, et al. Efficacy of losartan in patients with primary focal segmental glomerulosclerosis resistant to immunosuppressive treatment. J Intern Med 2003;253:329–334.

159. Tylicki L, Rutkowski P, Renke M, Rutkowski B. Renoprotective effect of small doses of losartan and enalapril in patients with primary glomerulonephritis. Short-term observation. Am J Nephrol 2002;22: 356–362.

160. Wolf G, Ritz E. Combination therapy with ACE inhibitors and angiotensin II receptor blockers to halt progression of chronic renal disease: Pathophysiology and indications. Kidney Int 2005;67:799–812.

161. Nakao N, Yoshimura A, Morita H, Takada M, Kayano T, Ideura T. Combination treatment of angiotensin-II receptor blocker and angiotensin-converting-enzyme inhibitor in non-diabetic renal disease (COOPERATE): A randomised controlled trial. Lancet 2003;361(9352): 117–124.

162. Kunz R, Wolbers M, Glass T, Mann JF. The COOPERATE trial: A letter of concern. Lancet 2008;371(9624):1575–1576.

163. Bidani A. Controversy about COOPERATE ABPM trial data. Am J Nephrol 2006;26:629 (author reply -32).

164. Vogt L, Waanders F, Boomsma F, de Zeeuw D, Navis G. Effects of dietary sodium and hydrochlorothiazide on the antiproteinuric efficacy of losartan. J Am Soc Nephrol 2008;19:999–1007.

165. Apperloo AJ, de Zeeuw D, de Jong PE. A short-term antihypertensive treatment-induced fall in glomerular filtration rate predicts long-term stability of renal function. Kidney Int. 1997;51:793–797.

166. Piecha G, Adamczak M, Ritz E. Dyslipidemia in chronic kidney disease: Pathogenesis and intervention. Pol Arch Med Wewn 2009;119:487–492.

167. Fried LF, Orchard TJ, Kasiske BL. Effect of lipid reduction on the progression of renal disease: A meta-analysis. Kidney Int 2001;59:260–269.

168. Navaneethan SD, Pansini F, Perkovic V, et al. HMG CoA reductase inhibitors (statins) for people with chronic kidney disease not requiring dialysis. Cochrane Database Syst Rev 2009:CD007784.

169. Keane WF. The role of lipids in renal disease: Future challenges. Kidney Int Suppl 2000;75:S27–S31.

170. Rahman M, Baimbridge C, Davis BR, et al. Progression of kidney disease in moderately hypercholesterolemic, hypertensive patients randomized to pravastatin versus usual care: A report from the Antihypertensive and Lipid-Lowering Treatment to Prevent Heart Attack Trial (ALLHAT). Am J Kidney Dis 2008;52:412–424.

171. Kshirsagar AV, Shoham DA, Bang H, Hogan SL, Simpson RJ, Jr., Colindres RE. The effect of cholesterol reduction with cholestyramine on renal function. Am J Kidney Dis 2005;46:812–819.

172. Massy ZA, Ma JZ, Louis TA, Kasiske BL. Lipid-lowering therapy in patients with renal disease. Kidney Int. 1995;48:188–198.

173. Executive Summary of The Third Report of The National Cholesterol Education Program (NCEP) Expert Panel on Detection, Evaluation, And Treatment of High Blood Cholesterol In Adults (Adult Treatment Panel III). Jama 2001;285:2486–2497.

174. Silverberg D, Wexler D, Blum M, Wollman Y, Iaina A. The cardio-renal anaemia syndrome: Does it exist? Nephrol Dial Transplant 2003;18(suppl 8):viii, 7–12.

175. Silverberg DS, Wexler D, Iaina A, Schwartz D. The correction of anemia in patients with the combination of chronic kidney disease and congestive heart failure may prevent progression of both conditions. Clin Exp Nephrol 2009;13:101–106.

176. Palmer AJ, Valentine WJ, Chen R, et al. A health economic analysis of screening and optimal treatment of nephropathy in patients with type 2 diabetes and hypertension in the USA. Nephrol Dial Transplant 2008;23:1216–1223.

177. Howard K, White S, Salkeld G, et al. Cost-Effectiveness of Screening and Optimal Management for Diabetes, Hypertension, and Chronic Kidney Disease: A Modeled Analysis. Value Health 2009 Oct 29.

178. Powe NR, Boulware LE. Population-based screening for CKD. Am J Kidney Dis 2009;53(3 suppl 3):S64–S70.

179. Vegter S, Perna A, Hiddema W, et al. Cost-effectiveness of ACE inhibitor therapy to prevent dialysis in nondiabetic nephropathy: Influence of the ACE insertion/deletion polymorphism. Pharmacogenet Genomics 2009;19:695–703.

180. Delea TE, Sofrygin O, Palmer JL, et al. Cost-effectiveness of aliskiren in type 2 diabetes, hypertension, and albuminuria. J Am Soc Nephrol 2009;20:2205–2213.

181. Eknoyan G, Levin N. NKF-K/DOQI Clinical Practice Guidelines: Update 2000. Foreword. Am J Kidney Dis 2001;37(1 suppl 1): S5–S6.

JOANNA Q. HUDSON

KEY CONCEPTS

❶ The number of patients with chronic kidney disease (CKD) is increasing, and it is expected that the number of patients with end-stage renal disease (ESRD) will exceed 780,000 by the year 2020.

❷ Common complications of stages 4 and 5 CKD include anemia, CKD–mineral and bone disorder (MBD) and renal osteodystrophy, fluid and electrolyte abnormalities, metabolic acidosis, and malnutrition.

❸ Anemia of CKD, which is primarily caused by a deficiency in the production of endogenous erythropoietin by the kidney, is a common complication observed in patients with stages 4 and 5 CKD.

❹ CKD-MBD and renal osteodystrophy are common in patients with CKD and contribute to extravascular calcifications and an increased risk of cardiovascular mortality.

❺ Cardiovascular complications are prevalent in the CKD population and are the leading cause of mortality in patients with ESRD. Thus at the initiation of dialysis, all ESRD patients should be assessed for cardiovascular disease, which includes assessment for coronary artery disease, cardiomyopathy, valvular heart disease, cerebrovascular disease, and peripheral vascular disease in addition to screening for both traditional and nontraditional cardiovascular risk factors.

❻ The management of CKD and the associated secondary complications should be initiated prior to development of ESRD.

❼ Guidelines by the National Kidney Foundation Kidney Disease/Dialysis Outcomes Quality Initiative (NKF-K/DOQI) and Kidney Disease: Improving Global Outcomes (KDIGO) provide information to assist health care providers in clinical decisions and the design of appropriate therapy to manage complications.

❽ Patient education plays a critical role in the appropriate management of patients with stage 4 or 5 CKD and related complications. A multidisciplinary team structure is a rational approach to provide this education and effectively design and implement the extensive nonpharmacologic and pharmacologic interventions required.

❾ Management of anemia includes administration of erythropoietic-stimulating agents (ESAs) (epoetin alfa and darbepoetin alfa) and regular iron supplementation (oral or intravenous administration) to achieve a target hemoglobin of 11 to 12 g/dL (110–120 g/L; 6.83–7.45 mmol/L). There is now evidence indicating a higher risk of cardiovascular events when hemoglobin is targeted to greater than 12 g/dL (120 g/L; 7.45 mmol/L).

❿ Management of CKD-MBD includes dietary phosphorus restriction, prudent use of phosphate-binding agents, vitamin D, and calcimimetic therapy.

The clinical syndrome that develops insidiously as kidney function declines to stages 4 and 5 chronic kidney disease (CKD), begins with nonspecific symptoms such as nausea and vomiting, which become progressively worse as the glomerular filtration rate (GFR) drops below 15 mL/min/1.73 m^2 (0.14 mL/s/m^2). At this level of GFR renal replacement therapy, either dialysis (see Chap. 54) or transplantation (see Chap. 98), is indicated. The patient with stage 5 CKD requiring chronic dialysis or renal transplantation is said to have end-stage renal disease (ESRD). In this chapter, ESRD refers specifically to patients who are receiving chronic dialysis.

The staging system for CKD was primarily designed to help clinicians identify individuals in need of appropriate interventions to delay progression of CKD, as discussed in Chapter 52.[1] Often complications of CKD are unrecognized or are inappropriately managed, and for many patients this contributes to significant morbidity, premature mortality, or a poor prognosis by the time they reach ESRD.[2] The most frequent complications of CKD include fluid and electrolyte abnormalities, anemia, CKD-related mineral and bone disorder (CKD-MBD) and renal osteodystrophy, hypertension, hyperlipidemia, and metabolic acidosis. Miscellaneous complications resulting from the effects of CKD on other organ systems also occur. Table 53–1 lists other complications of CKD that are not specifically covered in this chapter. Cardiovascular disease is also common in patients with CKD and requires early and aggressive intervention.[3] This chapter discusses the epidemiology of CKD and the pathophysiology and pharmacotherapeutic management of the complications and comorbidities that occur frequently in adult patients with stage 4 and 5 CKD.

Learning objectives, review questions,
and other resources can be found at
www.pharmacotherapyonline.com.

EPIDEMIOLOGY

❶ Approximately 26 million people in the United States are estimated to have CKD, a number that has increased in the last 2 decades as the prevalence of diabetes and hypertension has

TABLE 53-1 Other Complications of Chronic Kidney Disease

Organ System or Complication	Effects
Amyloidosis	Accumulation of β_2-microglobulin
	Manifests as carpal tunnel syndrome
Uremic bleeding	Potentially a result of platelet abnormalities
Endocrine	Thyroid function–symptoms of hypothyroidism
	Hypothermia
	Glycemic control–↑ in hypoglycemic episodes as kidney disease progresses (result of ↓ degradation of insulin by the kidney)
Gastrointestinal	Nausea, vomiting, diarrhea, anorexia, GI bleeding
Immune system	Impaired cell-mediated immunity
	Lymphopenia
Neurologic	Peripheral neuropathies
	Restless leg syndrome
	Uremic encephalopathy

increased.[4] The 2009 report of the United States Renal Data System (USRDS), indicates that in 2007, the latest year for which data are available, a total of 111,000 new cases of ESRD were reported (incidence) and the number of individuals with ESRD (prevalence) as of the end of 2007 was 527,283, including 368,544 patients on dialysis and 158,739 with a functioning kidney after transplantation.[2] Incidence rates of ESRD are higher in African Americans (3.7 times greater) and Native Americans (1.8 times greater) compared with whites, a trend that has persisted over the last decade. The incidence in Hispanics is 1.5 times greater than that observed in non-Hispanics.[2] The incident rate has also increased dramatically in patients 65 years of age and older over the last decade and the prevalence has increased 24% since 2000. Although the overall number of patients with ESRD is substantial now, it is projected that by the year 2020 the number will exceed 780,000 patients, with the majority of cases attributable to diabetes. Total Medicare costs for ESRD in 2007 were approximately $24 billion, a 6.1% increase from the previous year, which accounted for 5.8% of the total Medicare budget in 2007.[2]

The mortality rate in the ESRD population increases substantially with age and is much greater than age-matched individuals in the general population for every age group. In fact, ESRD patients have a mortality rate 7 to 8.5 times higher than age-matched individuals without kidney disease.[2] Associated predictors of mortality and hospitalization in hemodialysis patients include decreased serum albumin, elevated phosphorus, low hemoglobin level, catheter use for dialysis access, and the presence of comorbidities, such as diabetes and cardiovascular disease.[2,5] The association of mortality with these factors highlights the need to address complications as soon as they are detected, ideally prior to development of ESRD.

CKD was identified as one of the public health priorities for the nation in the Healthy People 2010 and the Healthy People 2020 disease prevention and health promotion objectives.[6,7] The proposed goals of this 2020 initiative as it relates to CKD are as follows: (a) reduce the rate of new cases of ESRD, (b) reduce deaths in persons with ESRD, (c) increase the proportion of CKD patients receiving care from a nephrologist at least 12 months before the start of renal replacement therapy, (d) reduce kidney failure due to diabetes, (e) increase the proportion of persons with diabetes and CKD who receive recommended medical evaluation and who receive medical treatment with angiotensin-converting enzyme inhibitors or angiotensin II receptor blockers, (f) improve cardiovascular care in persons with CKD, (g) reduce the percentage of the U.S. population with CKD, (h) reduce the death rate among people with CKD, and (i) increase the percentage of persons with CKD who know they have impaired renal function.[6,7]

ETIOLOGY

Many clinical conditions and diseases lead to progressive kidney damage and ESRD (see Chaps. 52 and 56). Diabetes mellitus continues to be the leading cause of CKD and ultimately of ESRD in the United States, accounting for 54% of new ESRD cases in 2007.[2] Hypertension, as the second leading cause of ESRD in the United States, accounts for approximately 33% of new cases of ESRD.[2] Glomerulonephritis, which includes a wide variety of lesions caused by immunologic, vascular, and other idiopathic diseases (see Chap. 56) is the third leading cause of ESRD in the United States. Other diseases and conditions causing CKD are cystic kidney disease, Wegener granulomatosis, vascular diseases, and acquired immunodeficiency syndrome (AIDS) nephropathy.

PATHOPHYSIOLOGY

Progression of CKD to ESRD occurs over years to decades in the majority of cases, with the precise mechanism of kidney damage dependent on the etiology of the disease (see Chaps. 52 and 56). The consequences and complications of marked reductions in kidney function are fairly uniform irrespective of the underlying etiology. The mechanisms of progression of CKD and measures to delay progression are essential elements for primary care clinicians to consider as they design intervention strategies for their patients. Those clinicians who care for patients with ESRD or stages 4 and 5 CKD must also have a clear understanding of the pathogenesis, clinical presentation, and management strategies for secondary complications and comorbidities to improve quality of care and outcomes.

No single toxin is responsible for all of the signs and symptoms of uremia observed in patients with stage 4 or 5 CKD. Accumulation of one or several of these known and potential toxins may be the result of increased secretion, as with the biologically active substances such as parathyroid hormone (PTH) and atrial natriuretic peptide; decreased clearance because of reduced metabolism within the kidney for compounds such as PTH, gastrin, growth hormone, glucagon, somatostatin, prolactin, calcitonin, and insulin; and/or decreased renal clearance of metabolic by-products of protein metabolism. The buildup of these uremic toxins ultimately results in altered organ and immune function and leads to a myriad of secondary complications.

❷ Altered fluid and electrolyte homeostasis, metabolic acidosis, anemia of CKD, CKD-MBD and renal osteodystrophy, and cardiovascular disease are among the common complications associated with a substantial decline in GFR. The pathophysiology of these complications is described here.

FLUID AND ELECTROLYTE ABNORMALITIES

Sodium and Water

In persons with normal kidney function, sodium balance is maintained at a sodium intake of 120 to 150 mEq/day (120–150 mmol/day). The fractional excretion of sodium (FE_{Na}) ranges from approximately 1% to 3% (see Chap. 58 for more information). Water balance is also maintained with a normal range of urinary osmolality of 50 to 1,200 mOsm/kg (50–1,200 mmol/kg); average range 500–800 mOsm/kg [500–800 mmol/kg]. In most individuals with CKD and stable kidney function, total body sodium and water increase modestly, but may not be clinically obvious. Free water clearance is generally maintained until the more advanced stages of CKD when patients have a reduced ability to concentrate or dilute their urine. In patients with severe CKD (stages 4 and 5), serum sodium concentration is generally maintained as the result of an increase in FE_{Na} by as much as 30%, but results in a volume-expanded state.[8] Significant sodium retention is more common when the GFR is less than 10 mL/min./1.73 m² (0.10 mL/s/m²). Volume overload with pulmonary edema can result, but the most common manifestation of increased intravascular volume is hypertension, which may further contribute to progressive kidney damage.

Individuals with CKD may also have impaired ability to conserve sodium and water. As a result they are prone to develop prerenal acute kidney injury when conditions of volume depletion occur (e.g., vomiting, blood loss, diarrhea, etc.). Thus FE_{Na} and urine osmolality may be less useful in patients with advanced CKD who develop acute on chronic CKD to differentiate prerenal from an intrinsic acute kidney injury.

Potassium Homeostasis

Serum potassium is freely filtered at the glomerulus, reabsorbed in the proximal tubule and loop of Henle, and actively secreted into the urine at the cortical collecting duct. The kidneys normally excrete 90% to 95% of the daily potassium dietary load. The fractional excretion of potassium (FE_K) is approximately 25% (0.25) (see Chap. 60). Normally only 5% to 10% of ingested potassium is excreted through the gut. Potassium homeostasis is also maintained by shifting extracellular potassium intracellularly immediately following ingestion of a potassium load. In patients with CKD, potassium balance is maintained by an increase in distal tubular potassium secretion in which aldosterone plays an important role; FE_K can increase to as high as five times normal.[8] Thus the serum potassium concentration is usually maintained in the normal range until the GFR is less than 20 mL/min/1.73 m² (0.19 mL/s/m²), at which point mild hyperkalemia is likely to develop. Mild elevations are observed in stage 3 CKD, but more significant (and life-threatening) elevations are likely to be observed in those with stage 4 and 5 CKD. A significant increase in potassium secretion by the colon also contributes to the maintenance of potassium balance, but this adaptation cannot compensate fully for the decrease in renal potassium excretion that occurs with advanced kidney disease.

METABOLIC ACIDOSIS

Individuals with normal kidney function generate enough hydrogen ion to reclaim all filtered bicarbonate and to secrete approximately 1 mEq/kg per day (1 mmol/kg per day) of hydrogen ions, which are generated from the metabolism of dietary proteins (see Chap. 61). As a result, a constant body fluid pH is maintained through the buffering of hydrogen ion by proteins, hemoglobin, phosphate, and bicarbonate. Renal ammoniagenesis and phosphate excretion buffer the urine and facilitate acid excretion. In advanced CKD, all filtered bicarbonate is reclaimed, but the ability of the kidneys to synthesize ammonia is impaired. This decrease in urinary buffer results in decreased net acid excretion and continuous positive hydrogen ion balance; consequently, metabolic acidosis develops. Clinically significant metabolic acidosis is commonly seen when the GFR drops below 30 mL/min/1.73 m² (0.29 mL/s/m²) (stage 4 CKD) and the plasma bicarbonate concentration tends to stabilize at 15 to 20 mEq/L (15 to 20 mmol/L). Treatment is required to maintain the bicarbonate at the recommended target of 22 mEq/L (22 mmol/L) in this population.[9]

ANEMIA OF CHRONIC KIDNEY DISEASE

❸ The primary cause of anemia in CKD patients is a decrease in production of erythropoietin by the proximal tubular cells of the kidney, where approximately 90% of production occurs. Plasma concentrations of erythropoietin increase exponentially in response to decreased oxygenation in individuals with normal kidney function as hemoglobin and hematocrit decline. In contrast, there is no correlation between the degree of anemia and erythropoietin concentrations in anemic ESRD patients. The result is a normochromic (normal colored red cell), normocytic (normal size red cell) anemia.[10] There is a strong correlation between the prevalence of anemia and the stage of CKD, with prevalence estimates of approximately 50% in stage 4 CKD and 75% for stage 5 CKD patients at the start of dialysis.[10]

Iron demands increase when red blood cell production is stimulated by an erythropoietin stimulating agent (ESA) such as epoetin alfa; therefore, iron deficiency is common in individuals with CKD and is the leading cause of resistance to ESAs. Iron supplementation is often necessary to correct and prevent iron deficiency. Hepcidin is a hormone produced by the liver that is responsible for regulation of iron. This hormone directly inhibits the protein ferroportin that transports iron out of storage cells. When iron stores are high, hepcidin production is increased to block the transfer of iron from enterocytes to the plasma. Conversely hepcidin production is decreased when iron stores are low. Hepcidin production is also induced by inflammation or infection. As a result the increase in hepcidin in inflammatory conditions may lead to a sequestering of iron and ineffective red blood cell production (e.g., iron-restricted erythropoiesis). The fact that hepcidin plays such a role in iron regulation has prompted the development of hepcidin antagonists to potentially alter iron transport.[11]

Additional factors contributing to the development of anemia of CKD are the decreased red cell life span (from the normal of 120 days to approximately 60 days in individuals with stage 5 CKD), vitamin B_{12} and folate deficiencies, and blood loss from regular laboratory testing and hemodialysis for patients requiring this modality of renal replacement therapy. A schematic of the process of red blood cell production is shown in Figure 53–1 that includes factors that impair this process in individuals with CKD.[12]

Anemia in the CKD population has been associated with decreased quality of life, increased hospitalizations, and cardiovascular disease.[13,14] ESAs have been shown to reduce these morbidities; however, there is now increasing evidence that treatment of anemia to hemoglobin targets above 12 g/dL (120 g/L; 7.45 mmol/L) may lead to increased risk of cardiovascular events and death.[15,16] Thus treatment approaches have shifted to less aggressive use of ESAs and more conservative goals for Hb in the CKD population.[17]

CKD-MINERAL AND BONE DISORDER (CKD-MBD) AND RENAL OSTEODYSTROPHY

❹ Disorders of mineral and bone metabolism are common in the CKD population and include abnormalities in parathyroid hormone (PTH), calcium, phosphorus, the calcium-phosphorus product, vitamin D and bone turnover, as well as soft tissue calcifications. Historically these abnormalities have been described as classic characteristics of secondary hyperparathyroidism and renal osteodystrophy (ROD). Recently the term *CKD-mineral and bone disorder (CKD-MBD)* has been advocated to encompass the abnormalities in mineral and bone metabolism as well as associated calcifications.[18]

The pathophysiology of CKD-MBD is complex (Fig. 53–2). Calcium and phosphorus homeostasis is mediated through the effects of four hormones on bone, the GI tract, kidney, and parathyroid gland. These hormones include PTH, the precursor

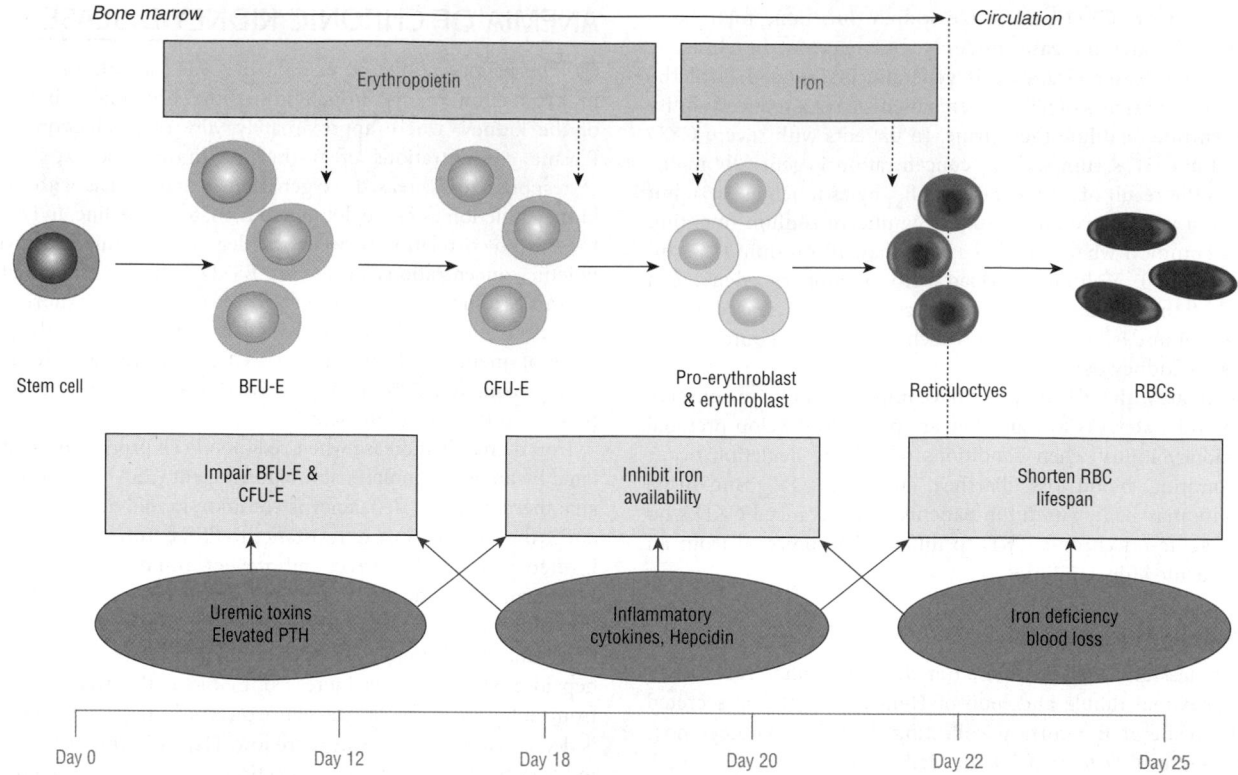

FIGURE 53-1. The process of red blood cell production (erythropoiesis) in the bone marrow requires erythropoietin and iron. This process is impaired due to factors that occur in advanced CKD such as accumulation of uremic toxins and inflammation (shown in the rectangles and ovals). (BFU-E, burst-forming unit erythroid; CFU-E, colony-forming unit erythroid; RBC, red blood cells.) (*Reprinted from Adv Chronic Kidney Dis, Vol. 16:2, Kalantar-Zadeh, et al., Intravenous Iron Versus Erythropoiesis-Stimulating Agents: Friend or Foe in Treating Chronic Kidney Disease Anemia?, 143, Copyright © 2009, with permission from Elsevier.*)

form of vitamin D known as 25-hydroxyvitamin D (25-OHD), active vitamin D or 1,25-dihydroxyvitamin D (calcitriol), and fibroblast growth factor-23 (FGF-23). As kidney function declines there is a decrease in phosphorus elimination, which results in hyperphosphatemia and a reciprocal decrease in serum calcium concentration. Hypocalcemia is the primary stimulus for secretion

of PTH by the parathyroid glands. PTH secretion is suppressed by the interaction of ionized calcium with the calcium-sensing receptor on the chief cells of the parathyroid gland. Hyperphosphatemia also increases PTH synthesis and release through its direct effects on the parathyroid gland and production of prepro-PTH messenger RNA.[19] In an attempt to normalize ionized calcium, PTH decreases

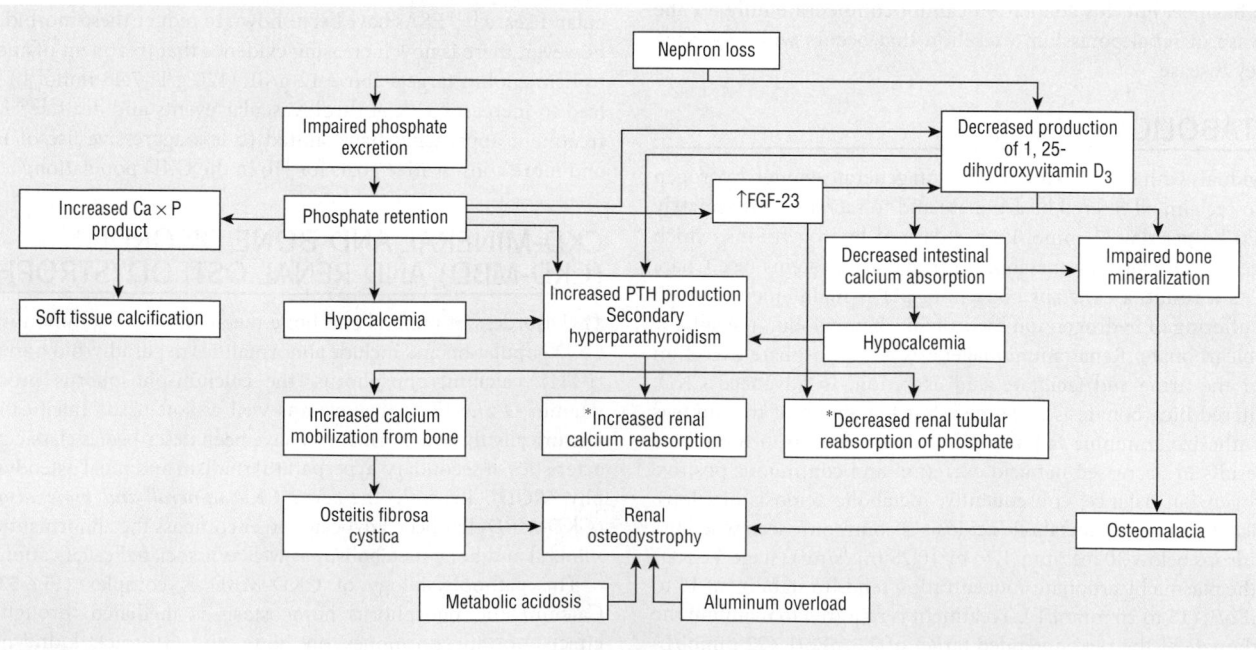

FIGURE 53-2. Pathogenesis of CKD-MBD and renal osteodystrophy. (*These adaptations are lost as kidney disease progresses.)

phosphorus reabsorption and increases calcium reabsorption by the proximal tubules of the kidney (at least until the GFR falls to less than approximately 30 mL/min) and also increases calcium mobilization from bone. FGF-23 production in bone also increases and promotes phosphate excretion by the kidney. The result is a resetting of the calcium and phosphorus homeostasis set point, at least in the early stages of CKD; however, this occurs at the expense of an elevated PTH ("the trade-off hypothesis"). With advanced kidney disease the kidney fails to respond to PTH or to FGF-23. The increase in PTH is most notable when GFR is less than 60 mL/min/1.73 m^2 (0.58 mL/s/m^2) (stage 3 CKD) and worsens as kidney function further declines.[20] Elevated PTH levels have been reported in approximately 21% of patients with an estimated GFR between 60 and 69 mL/min/1.73 m^2 (0.58 and 0.66 mL/s/m^2) and in 56% of patients with stage 3, 4, or 5 CKD.[20]

The most active form of vitamin D (1,25-dihydroxyvitamin D$_3$ or calcitriol) promotes increased intestinal absorption of calcium, which helps to normalize ionized calcium. Calcitriol also works directly on the parathyroid gland to suppress PTH production. The enzyme 1 α-hydroxylase is responsible for the final hydroxylation and conversion of the vitamin D precursor, 25-hydroxyvitamin D, to the active form in the kidney. As kidney disease progresses the process is impaired and the resultant vitamin D deficiency leads to reduced intestinal calcium absorption and worsening hyperparathyroidism. Increases in FGF-23, which facilitate excretion of phosphorus, may also promote calcitriol deficiency.[21] Calcitriol deficiency is observed at all levels of GFR but is more prevalent in individuals with stage 3 CKD.[20] Many individuals with CKD are also deficient in 25-OH vitamin D. This may be the result of decreased dermal synthesis of vitamin D, decreased exposure to sunlight, and reduced dietary intake of vitamin D.[22] In patients with stage 3 or 4 CKD, 25-OH deficiency (levels of <30 ng/mL [<75 nmol/L]) are associated with increased PTH. Evaluation of 25-OH levels and supplementation with a vitamin D precursor (e.g., ergocalciferol or cholecalciferol) in patients with observed deficiencies are recommended for stages 3 and 4 CKD (opinion-based recommendation).[22]

The abnormalities of CKD-MBD lead to bone abnormalities and other associated consequences. The continuous high rate of production of PTH by the parathyroid glands promotes parathyroid hyperplasia. Nodular tissue demonstrates more rapid growth potential and appears to be associated with fewer vitamin D and calcium-sensing receptors, resulting in resistance to the effects of calcium and vitamin D therapy and subsequent development of ROD.[19] Bone abnormalities are found almost universally in ESRD patients and in the majority of those with stages 3–5 CKD.[18] The skeletal complications associated with the bone abnormalities include osteitis fibrosa cystica (high bone turnover disease), osteomalacia (low bone turnover disease), and adynamic bone disease. Osteitis fibrosa cystica is most common and is characterized by areas of peritrabecular fibrosis. Bone marrow fibrosis and decreased erythropoiesis are also consequences of severe osteitis fibrosa cystica. Osteomalacia was historically noted in hemodialysis patients with aluminum toxicity, a finding less common today due to the decreased use of aluminum-containing phosphate binders and changes in the processing of dialysate solutions to decrease aluminum absorption. Adynamic lesions are characterized by low amounts of fibrosis or osteoid tissue and low bone formation rates. The incidence of adynamic lesions has increased over the last 10 years and may be present in as many as 50% of dialysis patients.[23] Multiple risk factors for the development of this bone disease have been identified: high concentrations of dialysate calcium along with high doses of calcium-containing phosphate binders, aggressive management with vitamin D therapy, diabetes, aluminum toxicity, and advanced age.[23] Symptoms of ROD are often not evident until after significant skeletal damage has developed; consequently,

prevention is the key to minimize the consequences of long-term complications. When symptoms such as bone pain and skeletal fractures occur, the disease is not easily amenable to treatment.

Of concern with CKD-MBD is the increased mortality associated with this complication. Secondary hyperparathyroidism (sHPT) as evidenced by PTH levels >495 pg/mL (>495 ng/L) in CKD patients is associated with increased morbidity and mortality and sudden death in hemodialysis patients.[24] Elevations of serum phosphorus, even within the upper limits of the normal range, have been associated with increased risk of cardiovascular events and/or mortality (all-cause or cardiovascular mortality) in patients with stages 3–5 CKD.[18,25] An elevated calcium times phosphorus product (Ca × P) is also associated with poor outcomes, including vascular calcification, cardiovascular disease, calciphylaxis, and death.[26] In two large, national, cross-sectional samples of hemodialysis patients who had received dialysis for at least 1 year, elevated serum phosphorus levels and Ca × P were associated with increased risk of death.[26,27] Patients with a Ca × P above 72 mg^2/dL^2 (5.8 mmol^2/L^2) were found to have a 34% higher risk of death compared with patients with a Ca × P in the desired range of 43 to 52 mg^2/dL^2 (3.5 to 4.2 mmol^2/L^2).[26] Calcium scores, as measured by electron-beam computed tomography, were significantly higher in hemodialysis patients than in patients without kidney disease who had proven coronary artery disease. Intake of calcium from calcium-based binders also appears to be a significant contributor to coronary artery calcification, even in young dialysis patients.[28] The incidence of calciphylaxis in patients with ESRD has increased over the last decade and has also been linked to elevated Ca × P product, although a direct cause and effect relationship has not been established.[29] These data underscore the need to consider all the consequences of elevated PTH, calcium, and phosphorus, not just their effects on bone.

CARDIOVASCULAR DISEASE

❺ Patients with CKD are at increased risk of cardiovascular disease, independent of the etiology of their kidney disease. Mortality secondary to cardiovascular disease is 10 to 30 times greater in dialysis patients than in the general population.[30] Higher mortality has also been observed in individuals with stages 3–5 CKD. In a study with data from over 1,120,295 individuals from a Kaiser Permanente Renal Registry higher mortality and risk of cardiovascular events were reported for individuals with stage 3–5 CKD compared to those with an estimated GFR above 60 mL/min/1.73 m^2 (0.58 mL/s/m^2) (reference group).[31] The rate of death from any cause was 17% greater for individuals with stage 3 CKD and 600% greater in those with stage 5 CKD not requiring dialysis. The rate of cardiovascular events was also greater compared with the reference group, with an increase of 43% observed for those with stage 3 CKD and 343% for individuals with stage 5 CKD. A cardiovascular event was defined as hospitalization for coronary heart disease, heart failure, ischemic stroke, and peripheral arterial disease.

Although a clearly unique pathogenesis of cardiovascular disease specific to CKD has not been identified, it is known that manifestations of kidney disease are contributory.[30] Like diabetes CKD is considered a "coronary heart disease equivalent."[32] In addition to traditional cardiac risk factors such as hypertension and hyperlipidemia, diabetes, tobacco use, and physical inactivity, patients with kidney disease have other unique risk factors. Among these are hyperhomocysteinemia, elevated levels of C-reactive protein, increased oxidant stress, and hemodynamic overload.[3] Complications of CKD such as anemia and metabolic disorders (i.e., CKD-MBD) are also contributory. In particular, arterial vascular disease (e.g., atherosclerosis) and cardiomyopathy are the primary types of cardiovascular disorders present in the CKD population.[3,30] These disorders lead to development of ischemic heart disease and its manifestations including myocardial infarction. As a predominant comorbidity, cardiovascular disorders and their sequelae are the leading cause of death in the ESRD population.[2,3]

Hypertension

The pathogenesis of hypertension in CKD is multifactorial, but for many, fluid retention is a major contributor. In addition to the other pathophysiologic mechanisms responsible for the development of hypertension, patients with ESRD may also have increased sympathetic activity, decreased activity of vasodilators such as nitric oxide, elevated levels of endothelin-1, chronic use of an ESA, hyperparathyroidism, and structural changes in the arteries (e.g., metastatic calcification) as contributing factors.[3] Patients with ESRD also display an abnormal diurnal blood pressure rhythm as evidenced by the fact that their blood pressure does not decrease during the nighttime hours.[3] It is unclear what causes this disturbance in the diurnal rhythm, but this "nondipping" phenomenon indicates sustained elevations in blood pressure are present over a prolonged period of time when compared with the general population.

Based on data from the 2009 USRDS, nine in ten Medicare CKD patients age 65 and older have a diagnosis of hypertension, an increase from 72% in 1995.[2] Hypertension induced by volume expansion and increased systemic vascular resistance increases myocardial work and contributes to development of left ventricular hypertrophy (LVH). A "U-shaped" relationship between blood pressure and mortality has been observed, such that higher mortality is associated with the highest and lowest levels of blood pressure.[3]

Hyperlipidemia

CKD with or without nephrotic syndrome is frequently accompanied by abnormalities in lipoprotein metabolism. It is well established that dyslipidemias cause atherosclerotic cardiovascular disease, and there are many compelling reasons to aggressively treat these disorders. A clear association between hypercholesterolemia, hypertriglyceridemia, or other lipoprotein changes in patients with CKD and cardiovascular disease has not been demonstrated in large prospective studies because individuals with kidney disease are usually excluded from these trials. It is likely that the same lipoprotein abnormalities that confer increased risk of cardiovascular disease in the general population would also be harmful to patients with kidney disease. This is supported by information from the Atherosclerosis Risk in Communities (ARIC) study.[33] In this study, the association between the severity of dyslipidemia and risk of future cardiovascular events evaluated over a 10.5-year follow-up period was similar to that in patients who had normal kidney function.[33]

A low or declining serum cholesterol in patients with ESRD is also associated with higher mortality, a paradoxical effect.[3] These findings beg the question of whether aggressive lipid lowering is warranted in this population. Further analysis, however, shows that low cholesterol levels were observed in conjunction with inflammation and malnutrition, factors that increase mortality. In the absence of these confounding factors, it is the higher cholesterol levels, not the lower levels, that were associated with increased mortality.

The lipid panel generally observed in patients with CKD without nephrotic syndrome is a normal total and low-density lipoprotein (LDL) cholesterol, low high-density lipoprotein (HDL), and high triglycerides (plasma concentrations >200 mg/dL [>2.26 mmol/L]).[34] Although the concentrations of LDL are not uniformly increased in patients with kidney disease, these patients appear to produce small, dense LDL particles that are more susceptible to oxidation and more atherogenic than larger LDL subfractions. Other lipoprotein abnormalities include changes in apoprotein content of lipoprotein molecules and increased very-low-density and intermediate-density

lipoproteins. For patients with CKD and a urinary protein excretion greater than 3 g/day (as in nephrotic syndrome), the major lipid abnormalities are elevation of plasma total and LDL cholesterol, with or without low HDL cholesterol (<35 mg/dL [<0.91 mmol/L]) and elevated triglycerides. Treatment of proteinuria resolves the hyperlipidemia in most patients with nephrotic syndrome.

CLINICAL PRESENTATION

Damage to the kidney has detrimental consequences for many other organ systems, particularly once patients develop ESRD. The subjective and objective findings of CKD that may be present in an individual are dependent on the severity of disease (i.e., stage of CKD). At the time of referral to a nephrologist patients may present with some, but rarely all, of the signs and symptoms associated with uremia and secondary complications of CKD, unless they are in stage 4 or 5 CKD. It is apparent that management of CKD requires treatment of multiple secondary complications. Unfortunately many CKD patients are not diagnosed with the disease until they reach stage 5 CKD and are at or near the point of requiring renal replacement therapy. This problem has prompted automated reporting of the estimated glomerular filtration rate (eGFR) by clinical labs as determined by the MDRD equation for the purpose of identifying individuals with CKD earlier (see Chaps. 50 and 52). Clinicians must understand how to interpret the eGFR appropriately to stage individuals with kidney disease and determine the best options to delay progression and manage the associated complications.

CLINICAL PRESENTATION OF STAGE 4 OR 5 CHRONIC KIDNEY DISEASE

Symptoms

- Uremic symptoms (fatigue, weakness, shortness of breath, mental confusion, nausea and vomiting, bleeding, and loss of appetite), as well as itching, cold intolerance, weight gain, and peripheral neuropathies are common in patients with stage 5 disease.

Signs

- Edema, changes in urine output (volume and consistency), "foaming" of urine (indicative of proteinuria), and abdominal distension.

Laboratory Tests[a]

- *Decreased*: creatinine clearance, bicarbonate (metabolic acidosis), hemoglobin/hematocrit (anemia), iron stores (iron deficiency), vitamin D levels, albumin (malnutrition), glucose (may result from decreased degradation of insulin with impaired kidney function or poor oral intake), calcium (in early stages of CKD), HDL.

- *Increased*: serum creatinine, blood urea nitrogen, potassium, phosphorus, PTH, blood pressure (hypertension is a common cause and result of CKD), glucose (uncontrolled diabetes is a cause of CKD), low-density lipoprotein and triglycerides, calcium (in ESRD)

- *Other*: May be hemoccult-positive if GI bleeding occurs secondary to uremia.

Other Diagnostic Tests

- Left ventricular hypertrophy may be observed, as well as increased homocysteine levels and increased C-reactive protein.

TABLE 53-2	Target Hb and Iron Indices for Anemia Management in Chronic Kidney Disease[53]	
Parameter	ND-CKD and PD-CKD	HD-CKD
Hb	11–12 g/dL (110–120 g/L; 6.83–7.45 mmol/L)	11–12 g/dL (110–120 g/L; 6.83–7.45 mmol/L
TSat	>20% (>0.20)	>20% (>0.20)
CHr	–	>29 pg/cell
Serum ferritin[a]	>100 ng/mL (>100 µg/L)	>200 ng/mL (>200 µg/L)

ND-CKD, nondialysis CKD patients; PD-CKD, peritoneal dialysis patients; HD-CKD, hemodialysis patients;

CHr, content of hemoglobin in reticulocytes; CKD, chronic kidney disease; Hb, hemoglobin; TSat, transferrin saturation.

[a]Serum ferritin is an acute phase reactant—use clinical judgment when above 500 ng/mL (500 µg/L).

ANEMIA OF CHRONIC KIDNEY DISEASE

Since many individuals with anemia of CKD are asymptomatic upon presentation, laboratory evaluation is commonly the initial approach to diagnosing anemia of CKD. According to the KDOQI guidelines for anemia management in CKD the hemoglobin (Hb) should be measured in all individuals with CKD regardless of stage.[35] The diagnosis of anemia is made and further workup of anemia is required when the Hb is less than 13.5 g/dL (135 g/L; 8.38 mmol/L) for adult males and less than 12 g/dL (120 g/L; 7.45 mmol/L) for adult females. Iron deficiency is the primary cause of resistance to treatment of anemia with ESAs; therefore, assessment of the iron status is required. The iron indices transferrin saturation (TSat) and serum ferritin provide information on iron immediately available for use in the bone marrow for red blood cell production (TSat) and storage iron (serum ferritin). The TSat is calculated as ([serum iron/TIBC] × 100), where TIBC is the total iron-binding capacity. If the TSat and serum ferritin values are below the desired threshold (Table 53–2), iron supplementation is warranted.

Additional workup includes evaluation for the presence of other potential causes of anemia such as blood loss, deficiencies in vitamin B_{12} or folate, or other disease states that contribute to anemia, including human immunodeficiency virus infection and malignancies. Red blood cell indices (mean corpuscular hemoglobin, mean corpuscular volume, mean corpuscular hemoglobin concentration), white blood cell count, differential and platelet count, and absolute reticulocyte count should also be assessed. A stool guaiac test should be performed to rule out GI bleeding.

Iron supplementation is required by most CKD patients receiving an ESA because of the increased iron demand that results from stimulation of red blood cell production. As CKD worsens, a progressive decline in Hb despite ESA therapy may be observed. Consequently, regular evaluation of Hb and iron status is warranted to ensure the desired outcomes are met and to make necessary dose adjustments in ESAs and iron therapy. Iron supplementation may also be required in individuals with anemia who have *iron restricted erythropoiesis*. In this condition the individual

with anemia may have a TSat below goal (less than 20% [0.20]); however, the serum ferritin may be at goal (e.g., above 100–200 ng/mL [100–200 µg/L]) or even elevated. It has been shown that anemic hemodialysis patients with a TSat less than 25% (0.25) and serum ferritin between 200 and 1200 ng/mL (200–1200 µg/L) had an improved response to ESAs when they also received a 1 g course of IV iron.[36]

Signs and symptoms of anemia of CKD include, but are not limited to, fatigue, shortness of breath, cold intolerance, chest pain, tingling in the extremities, tachycardia, headaches, and general malaise. The effects of anemia and decreased oxygen delivery on other comorbid conditions, including LVH, have been considered given the burden of cardiovascular complications in this population. Despite associations of worsening anemia with development of LVH, there are no prospective studies demonstrating that early and aggressive treatment improves cardiovascular end points or LVH in the CKD population. Improvements in quality of life have been observed with increased Hb, but such improvements must be weighed against reported risks of more aggressive anemia management to achieve higher Hb levels in the CKD population.[37]

CKD-MINERAL AND BONE DISORDER (CKD-MBD) AND RENAL OSTEODYSTROPHY

The K/DOQI clinical practice guidelines for bone metabolism and disease have been available since 2003 and provide recommendations for the workup and treatment of CKD-MBD.[22] In 2009 the KDIGO clinical practice guidelines for CKD-MDB were published.[18] Recommendations from both the K/DOQI and KDIGO are presented here. It should be noted that many of the recommendations are based on opinion or limited evidence given the lack of randomized, controlled studies to evaluate outcomes of treating the biochemical abnormalities to specific targets.

The biochemical abnormalities of CKD-MBD should be evaluated in patients with stage 3 CKD and include an evaluation of serum phosphorus, calcium, Ca × P product, and PTH. The recommended frequencies of monitoring calcium, phosphorus, and PTH by CKD stage based on the K/DOQI and KDIGO guidelines are shown in Table 53–3.[18,22] The KDIGO guidelines also recommend monitoring bone-specific alkaline phosphatase annually in stage 4 and 5 CKD patients. The frequency of monitoring these parameters may increase once a diagnosis of CKD-MDB is made and further information is needed to assess the patient's response to treatment and to guide decisions about changes in therapy.

Clinicians involved in the care of patients with CKD should know which PTH assays are available in their facilities. PTH is secreted from the parathyroid gland as intact PTH, an 84-amino-acid peptide chain (1–84 PTH) that is biologically active, and as smaller carboxy-terminal PTH fragments.[38] Circulating levels of these fragments (e.g., 7–84 PTH) may increase substantially in patients with CKD and actively antagonize the effects to 1–84 PTH. The available immunoradiometric assays, known as second-generation assays,

TABLE 53-3	Recommended Frequency of Monitoring Calcium, Phosphorus, PTH , and 25 OHD by Stage of CKD (K/DOQI and KDIGO Guidelines)[18,22]					
	Calcium and Phosphorus			PTH		25-Hydroxyvitamin D
CKD Stage	K/DOQI	KDIGO	K/DOQI	KDIGO	K/DOQI	KDIGO
3	Annually	Every 6–12 months	Annually	Baseline, then based on CKD progression	If PTH above target	Baseline level; correct deficiencies as in general population
4	Every 3 months	Every 3–6 months	Every 3 months	Every 6–12 months	Not measured	
5	Monthly	Every 1–3 months	Every 3 months	Every 3–6 months		

KDIGO, Kidney Disease: Improving Global Outcomes; K/DOQI, Kidney Disease Outcomes Quality Initiative; PTH, parathyroid hormone.

TABLE 53-4	Guidelines for Calcium, Phosphorus, Calcium Phosphorus Product, and Intact Parathyroid Hormone[a,18,22]		
	Chronic Kidney Disease		
Parameter	**Stage 3**	**Stage 4**	**Stage 5**
Corrected calcium	"Normal"	"Normal"	8.4–9.5 mg/dL[b] (2.10–2.38 mmol/L)
Phosphorus	2.7–4.6 mg/dL (0.87–1.49 mmol/L)	2.7–4.6 mg/dL (0.87–1.49 mmol/L)	3.5–5.5 mg/dL (1.13–1.78 mmol/L)
Ca × P	<55 mg²/dL² [4.4 mmol²/L²]	<55 mg²/dL² (4.4 mmol²/L²)	<55 mg²/dL² (4.4 mmol²/L²)
Intact parathyroid hormone	35–70 pg/mL (35–70 ng/L)	70–110 pg/mL (70–110 ng/L)	150–300 pg/mL (150–300 ng/L)

[a]Differences with Kidney Disease: Improving Global Outcomes (KDIGO) described in text (see CKD-MBD Desired Outcome section).
[b]Recommend normal range for laboratory used, but keeping target at lower end of range.

measure not only the intact PTH molecule but also fragments, which may lead to overestimation of biologically active PTH. A correction factor for these fragments cannot be established since commercially available assays measure different types and amounts of these fragments and give inconsistent results. For this reason KDIGO did not specify a particular PTH target, but rather advocated looking at trends in serum PTH to make treatment decisions. For the dialysis population KDIGO recommends a general PTH range of two to nine times the upper limit of the normal range for the assay.[18] This differs from the K/DOQI guidelines which recommend specific ranges for each stage of CKD (Table 53-4). The risks associated with sustained elevations in PTH that would be permitted by following the KDIGO guidelines have raised concern and, at present, the K/DOQI recommendations continue to serve as the basis for treating CKD-MBD.

In addition to monitoring for biochemical abnormalities that define CKD-MBD and are associated with negative outcomes, evaluation of bone architecture is also necessary in some cases. Individuals with stages 3–5 CKD and metabolic abnormalities of CKD-MBD (e.g., abnormal phosphorus, calcium, PTH, and vitamin D) with bone involvement are said to have renal osteodystrophy. The gold standard test for diagnosing renal osteodystrophy is bone biopsy for histologic analysis; however, this is an invasive test that is not easily performed. Both K/DOQI and KDIGO guidelines recommend bone biopsy only in patients in whom the etiology of symptoms is not clear or in individuals with more unique biochemical abnormalities.[18,22] This includes patients experiencing unexplained fractures, persistent hypercalcemia, and possible aluminum toxicity.[22] If aluminum concentrations are elevated (60 to 200 μg/L [2.2 to 7.4 μmol/L]) a deferoxamine test should be done. KDIGO also suggests a bone biopsy be considered in CKD patients prior to beginning treatment with bisphosphonates since adynamic bone disease is a contraindication to the use of these agents. Bone biopsy findings are described on the basis of turnover rate, mineralization, and volume. High bone turnover disease, or *osteitis fibrosa*, is a common pattern observed with renal osteodystrophy, although individuals may also have low bone turnover disease. Bone mineral density testing is not generally recommended in patients with advanced CKD since this test has not been shown to predict fracture risk and does not indicate the type of renal osteodystrophy.[18]

Abnormalities in mineral metabolism are highly associated with vascular and soft-tissue calcifications, known risk factors for mortality; therefore, diagnostic testing for calcifications should be considered in the evaluation for CKD-MBD. Electron-beam computed tomography (EBCT) is a noninvasive and sensitive method available for detecting cardiovascular calcifications and has been used clinically and in studies in the CKD population. Other methods advocated include lateral abdominal radiographs to detect vascular calcification and echocardiogram to detect valvular calcification. KDIGO suggests these tests are reasonable alternatives to EBCT based on the sensitivity to detect calcifications and lower cost.[18]

METABOLIC ACIDOSIS

Metabolic acidosis generally does not occur until stage 4 CKD. The complete evaluation of acid–base status requires measurement of serum electrolytes and arterial blood gases when acidosis is suspected. A complete medical history and review of medications is necessary to determine whether there are other potential causes of acid–base disturbances (e.g., diabetic ketoacidosis, ingestion of toxins, or GI disorders). The anion gap, indicating the differences in unmeasured cations and anions, should also be calculated (see Chap. 61). An elevated anion gap (>17 mEq/L [>17 mmol/L]) is often present in patients with stage 4 or 5 CKD because of the accumulation of organic anions, phosphates, and sulfates. Treatment of metabolic acidosis in patients with CKD generally includes administration of bicarbonate to correct acidemia with the time course for correction depending on the severity of the acidosis. Asymptomatic patients with mild acidosis (bicarbonate of 12 to 20 mEq/L [12 to 20 mmol/L; pH of 7.2 to 7.4) generally do not require emergent therapy, and gradual correction with oral bicarbonate administration over days to weeks is appropriate.

CARDIOVASCULAR DISEASE

Individuals with CKD are at increased risk for CVD; thus screening for the presence of cardiovascular risk factors is a high priority in this population. Individuals with stage 4 CKD should be assessed for cardiovascular risk factors and considered in the highest risk group for cardiovascular events. The risk of developing congestive heart failure increases in both young and elderly CKD patients.[2] Modifiable cardiovascular risk factors in patients with CKD are hypertension, diabetes mellitus, hyperlipidemia, and smoking.[33] The K/DOQI guidelines for stage 5 dialysis patients recommend that all patients starting dialysis be assessed for cardiovascular disease (including coronary artery disease, cardiomyopathy, valvular heart disease, cerebrovascular disease, and peripheral vascular disease) and be screened for traditional (e.g., hypertension and hyperlipidemia) and nontraditional cardiovascular risk factors.[3]

Hypertension

As in the general population patients with CKD may not have symptoms of elevated blood pressure; therefore, blood pressure monitoring is essential. Edema and other indications of volume expansion may be observed in individuals with hypertension as a result of volume overload. Patients with stages 4 and 5 CKD should have their blood pressure evaluated at every clinic visit and at home, if feasible. Patients with ESRD should have their blood pressure monitored at every scheduled clinic visit (or hemodialysis session), and they should also be encouraged to learn how to monitor their blood pressure while at home. Patients who have required extensive surgeries in both arms to establish vascular accesses should have blood pressure measured in the thighs or legs. Blood pressure should be measured with an appropriate-size cuff prior to insertion of the needles for hemodialysis.

Blood pressure monitoring performed in the clinical setting has been shown to both overestimate and underestimate true blood pressure in CKD patients.[39,40] Ambulatory blood pressure monitoring (ABPM) is recommended in individuals with CKD to better determine variations in blood pressure throughout the day and to detect the "nondipping phenomenon" (loss of the protective decline in blood pressure that occurs during sleep) that is more common in the CKD population. ABPM has also been shown to better correlate with end organ damage (e.g., proteinuria) than blood pressure readings measured in the clinical setting. ABPM is also recommended for dialysis patients since both pre- and postdialysis blood pressures are poor indicators of interdialytic blood pressure.[39]

Hyperlipidemia

A complete fasting lipid profile including total cholesterol, LDL, HDL, and triglycerides should be done in all CKD patients. Lipoprotein levels may be influenced by several factors, including GFR and proteinuria. It is recommended that CKD patients have their lipid profile assessed more frequently than the general population to identify abnormalities and treat them early. In patients on hemodialysis the lipid profile should be done prior to dialysis or on nondialysis days.[41] Patients should also be evaluated for other conditions that are known to cause dyslipidemias (e.g., liver disease).

TREATMENT

Chronic Kidney Disease

Once a patient is diagnosed with CKD, implementation of therapy to address the primary cause (e.g., diabetes, hypertension, or glomerulonephritis) and to delay progression is a priority. The key concepts involved in the management of disease progression are discussed in detail in Chapter 52. When patients reach stage 4 CKD, progression to ESRD is almost inevitable, although the process may be delayed if appropriate therapy is initiated. It is during stage 4 CKD that planning for renal replacement therapy (hemodialysis or peritoneal dialysis) should begin, including patient education about dialysis modalities and options for transplantation (see Chap. 54 and 98).

6 Individuals with CKD should be evaluated for secondary complications (e.g., anemia and CKD-MBD) and comorbid conditions and receive treatment for these complications prior to development of ESRD. Historically, the common complications of anemia and CKD-MBD have not been diagnosed or appropriately managed in the earlier stages of CKD.[2] Late referral to a nephrologist may in part account for this poor management; however, even in ideal clinical environments such as nephrology clinics, these secondary complications may be overlooked. There are opportunities for other health care professionals to make recommendations for appropriate workup and management of CKD and its associated complications.

■ DESIRED OUTCOME

The overall goal of therapy in individuals with stage 2, 3, and the early phase of stage 4 CKD is to delay or prevent progression of the disease and the associated comorbidities. Patients who reach CKD stage 4 almost inevitably experience progression to ESRD and thus at some time in the near future will require dialysis or transplantation to sustain life. The primary goal is to sustain a good quality of life and prevent adverse outcomes by aggressively managing complications of advanced CKD.

■ GENERAL APPROACH TO PATIENT CARE

7 Management of the existent complications and consequences of CKD should be based on the most current consensus guidelines and the best clinical practices such as those developed by the NKF-K/DOQI, KDIGO, Cochrane Renal group, and other relevant professional associations. The K/DOQI guidelines and recommendations were developed based on evidence, when available, or the opinion of an expert group of individuals when sufficient evidence was lacking. Recommendations based primarily on opinion have been subject to some criticism. With this in mind, the K/DOQI guidelines should not replace clinical judgment, but should provide a basis upon which treatment decisions can be made in the context of both evidence and opinion. The secondary complications that are addressed in the currently available clinical practice guidelines include anemia of CKD, bone metabolism and disease, cardiovascular disease in dialysis patients, dyslipidemias, hypertension, and nutrition.

8 Appropriate management of secondary complications of CKD ideally involves a multidisciplinary approach to address the nonpharmacologic and pharmacologic interventions, dietary education, and social/financial concerns. The typical team includes physicians (nephrologists), nurses, dietitians, and social workers in outpatient dialysis facilities. In some outpatient dialysis centers pharmacists are also active members of the care team, although this is more common in dialysis units associated with healthcare institutions.

Reducing the incidence and risk of drug-related problems (DRPs) is one of the primary goals in caring for the CKD patient. ESRD patients are prescribed an average of 8 to 10 medications, which increases the potential of DRPs.[42] This risk is further compounded by the fact that many patients see practitioners outside of the dialysis unit and receive prescriptions from these providers in addition to the medications they require during dialysis. Medication reconciliation is essential to reduce the risk of DRPs and requires that pharmacists and other practitioners consult with the dialysis facilities to get a complete medication history. Pharmacists in the community must be prepared to provide medication therapy management (MTM) for individuals with CKD since this population receives medications and care in the community settings. Frequent medication reviews are paramount to reduce DRPs and patient exposure of these patients to nephrotoxic agents (see Chap. 54). Drug-dosing guidelines based on the degree of kidney function should be followed, and a complete medication history of prescription and nonprescription medications, as well as herbals and nutritional supplements, should be obtained and routinely updated. Chronic use of nonsteroidal antiinflammatory drugs and cyclooxygenase-2 inhibitors should be avoided when possible. Patients should be instructed on all brand and generic names of these classes of medications to reduce the risk of exposure. Appropriate measures should also be taken for hospitalized patients to decrease the risk of nephrotoxicity from radiocontrast agents (for procedures requiring such dyes), and antibiotics such as aminoglycosides, as well as from nonsteroidal antiinflammatory drugs and angiotensin-converting enzyme inhibitors (ACEIs) (see Chaps. 51 and 55).

Continued patient education, initiated prior to development of ESRD, is essential to help patients become active participants in their own care and to become knowledgeable about medications which they often require on a chronic basis. Pharmacists involved with the dialysis population have identified many specific drug-related problems (e.g., inappropriate dose or indication for a medication, adverse drug reactions) that commonly occur in the ESRD population and have demonstrated that clinical pharmacy services reduce such problems and improve patient quality of life.[42]

■ FLUID AND ELECTROLYTE ABNORMALITIES

Maintenance of fluid volume, osmolarity, electrolyte balance, and acid–base status are all regulated in large part by the kidney and their homeostasis is altered in patients with impaired kidney function. A comprehensive discussion of fluid and electrolyte disorders and treatment options is presented in Chapters 58–60. The unique aspects of treatment of sodium, water, and potassium disorders in stage 4 CKD and dialysis patients are highlighted here.

Desired Outcomes

Sodium and Water Homeostasis The goal in the individual with CKD is to maintain sodium and water balance as indicated by serum sodium concentrations in the normal range (i.e., 135 to 145 mEq/L [135 to 145 mmol/L]) and a euvolemic state. By achieving these goals, the risk of developing or worsening hypertension secondary to volume overload is reduced. Achievement of these goals is also warranted to prevent complications in individuals with congestive heart failure or other conditions that may be affected by volume status.

Potassium Homeostasis The focus is on prevention of hyperkalemia and its acute adverse consequences, particularly cardiac effects, while maintaining potassium concentrations of approximately 4 to 5.5 mEq/L (4 to 5.5 mmol/L). This is often achieved through dietary restriction of potassium, minimizing exposure to medications that may increase serum potassium, and use of sodium–potassium exchange resins when indicated. If hyperkalemia develops, management options are based on the rapidity and degree to which potassium is elevated (see Chap. 60).

Nonpharmacologic Therapy

Sodium and Water Homeostasis The ability of the kidney to adjust to abrupt changes in sodium intake is greatly diminished in patients with severe CKD. Sodium restriction beyond a no-added-salt diet should generally not be recommended. The kidney maintains the ability to lower urinary sodium content to essentially zero, but this can only be accomplished by very gradual sodium restriction over a period of several days. Hospitalized patients with CKD should not routinely be sodium restricted because they have adapted to their outpatient intake. Negative sodium balance and its resultant volume contraction can cause decreased kidney perfusion and an acute decline in GFR.

Fluid restriction is generally unnecessary for CKD patients not requiring dialysis provided sodium intake is controlled. An intact thirst mechanism maintains total-body water and effective plasma osmolality near normal. Large amounts of free water administered orally or as IV fluid may induce hyponatremia and volume overload. Sodium retention and volume expansion also contribute to hypertension in many patients with severe CKD, and diuretic therapy may be necessary to control edema or blood pressure. Saline-containing IV solutions should also be used cautiously in patients with CKD because the kidney's ability to excrete a salt load is impaired and the kidneys are prone to volume overload. Sodium restriction (e.g., less than 2 g per day) is warranted in the ESRD population to help control volume status.

Potassium Homeostasis Hyperkalemia is more common in patients with stage 5 CKD and in those who require dialysis. The majority of patients can be managed with a dietary potassium restriction of 50 to 80 mEq/day (50 to 80 mmol/day) and a reduction in dialysate potassium concentrations (see Chap. 54). Hyperkalemia is less common in the peritoneal dialysis population because of the more extensive removal of potassium by the peritoneal dialysis procedure and therefore, these patients are often allowed more liberal dietary potassium intake.

Pharmacologic Therapy

Sodium and Water Homeostasis Diuretic therapy is often necessary to prevent edema and the associated symptoms from volume overload. Loop diuretics increase urine volume and renal sodium excretion even in individuals with stage 4 CKD. Diuretic resistance can occur and requires use of higher doses of loop diuretics. In these situations a combination of a loop diuretic with the thiazide diuretic, metolazone, can substantially increase excretion of sodium and water (see Chap. 58). When a patient develops ESRD diuretics become ineffective as residual kidney function is lost and dialysis becomes necessary to control volume status.

Potassium Homeostasis The definitive treatment of severe hyperkalemia for a dialysis-dependent ESRD patient is hemodialysis. In reality, there is often a delay between diagnosis of hyperkalemia and institution of dialysis, which necessitates the use of other temporizing measures, such as IV calcium gluconate, insulin and glucose, nebulized β_2-adrenergic agonists (albuterol), and sodium polystyrene sulfonate (see Chap. 60). Unfortunately, shifting potassium into the intracellular fluid compartment with insulin and glucose or with albuterol makes removal of potassium via dialysis more difficult. Multiple dialysis sessions may be necessary following potassium redistribution to the extracellular space. Sodium polystyrene sulfonate, a potassium–sodium exchange resin, can be given orally in doses of 30 to 60 g to increase potassium excretion via the ileum and colon. Sodium bicarbonate therapy is no longer advocated in the treatment of ESRD hyperkalemia unless severe metabolic acidosis is also present because the potassium-lowering effect is unreliable. Loop diuretics, a standard pharmacologic treatment option for hyperkalemia, are ineffective in patients with ESRD.

Each patient's medications should routinely be reviewed to identify those that increase serum potassium. This includes potassium-sparing diuretics, β-blockers, which interfere with the extra-renal translocation of potassium into cells, and ACEIs, which may cause hyperkalemia by reducing aldosterone production. Polycitra, used for the treatment of metabolic acidosis, contains potassium citrate and should not be prescribed for patients with severe CKD. The contribution of dialysis modalities to potassium homeostasis in patients with ESRD must also be considered (see Chap. 54). Constipation in patients with CKD can interfere with colonic potassium excretion; therefore a good bowel regimen is also important.

Evaluation of Therapeutic Outcomes

Monitoring of volume status and serum electrolyte levels should be done at each clinic visit in patients with stages 4 and 5 CKD. This should include an evaluation of signs and symptoms of extracellular fluid volume expansion (e.g., pitting edema, rales, ascites, shortness of breath, and increased weight) and consequences of volume overload (e.g., hypertension, pulmonary edema) and hyperkalemia (e.g., arrhythmias). Blood pressure monitoring in the clinic setting and at home, if feasible, is recommended to detect onset or worsening of hypertension and to monitor the efficacy of the antihypertensive regimens. As kidney disease progresses dietary intervention and diuretic therapy will likely become necessary.

Serum electrolytes are generally measured monthly in the dialysis population. Additional monitoring in the hemodialysis population includes assessment of the predialysis weight compared to a patient's dry weight (the target weight following hemodialysis at which the patient is hemodynamically stable). The greater the difference in weight, the more volume an individual has accumulated since the last hemodialysis session. While the hemodialysis prescription can be altered acutely to remove more volume by increasing ultrafiltration (see Chap. 54), a patient consistently gaining excessive weight between dialysis sessions will require counseling on restriction of sodium and water.

■ ANEMIA OF CHRONIC KIDNEY DISEASE

Desired Outcome

The desired outcomes of anemia management are to increase oxygen-carrying capacity, decrease signs and symptoms of anemia, improve the patient's quality of life, and decrease the need for blood transfusions. Achievement of these goals requires a combination of an ESA and iron supplementation to promote and maintain erythropoiesis. Hemoglobin (Hb) is the preferred monitoring parameter for red blood cell production because, unlike Hct, its concentration is not affected by blood storage conditions and instrumentation used for analysis. Table 53–2 lists the target Hb and iron indices for those stage 5 CKD patients who are dialysis dependent as well as those not yet receiving dialysis.

Target Hemoglobin The recommended target Hb in all stage 5 CKD patients receiving ESAs is 11 to 12 g/dL (110–120 g/L; 6.83–7.45 mmol/L).[17] This target range is clearly below the "normal Hb" range and has been a topic of much debate for several years. Observational studies and USRDS data have shown decreased hospitalizations, lower mortality, and improved quality of life with Hb levels above 11 g/dL (110 g/L; 6.83 mmol/L).[43–45] "Normalization" of Hb to levels above 12 g/dL (120 g/L; 7.45 mmol/L) with ESA therapy, however, has resulted in increased risk of mortality and cardiovascular events compared with patients maintained in the 11 to 12 g/dL (110–120 g/L; 6.83–7.45 mmol/L) range. These conclusions were based on results reported in 2006 from clinical trials (CHOIR and CREATE trials) that included individuals with early stage CKD and from previous data reported in the hemodialysis population (Normal Hematocrit Cardiac Trial, NHCT).[15,16,46] A summary of these key trials is shown in Table 53–5. An increased risk of all-cause mortality with ESA treatment was also reported in a meta-analysis of nine randomized, controlled trials that included over 5,100 CKD patients treated to Hb targets in the range of 12 to

---

TABLE 53-5 Trials Evaluating ESAs and Target Hb/Hct

Study	Study Population and End Points	ESA	Target Hb or Hct	Results	Comments
Normal Hematocrit Cardiac Trial (NHCT)[16,131]	1,265 ESRD patients with CHF or ischemic heart disease on hemodialysis *Primary end points:* Length of time to death or first MI	Epoetin alfa	Low Hct 32% (0.32) ($n = 631$) "Normal" Hct 42% (0.42) ($n = 634$)	Study was stopped before completion when the group randomized to a higher Hct target showed a trend toward higher mortality and nonfatal MI [relative risk (RR) 1.28, 95% CI 0.92–1.78]	Higher Hct target in the hemodialysis population with cardiovascular disease was not supported.
Correction of Hb and Outcomes in Renal Insufficiency (CHOIR)[15]	1432 Stage 3-4 CKD patients *Primary end points:* Composite of death, MI, hospitalization for congestive heart failure, and stroke	Epoetin alfa	Low Hb 11.3 g/dL (113 g/L; 7.01 mmol/L) ($n = 717$) High Hb 13.5 g/dL (135 g/L; 8.38 mmol/L) ($n = 715$)	Study stopped before completion because of a higher risk of the composite of death, stroke, MI, and hospitalization for CHF in the group randomized to higher Hb target [hazard ratio 1.34; 95% CI 1.03–1.74]	Mean Hb for high Hb group was 12.6 g/dL (126 g/L; 7.82 mmol/L); mean Hb for low Hb group was 11.3 g/dL (113 g/L; 7.01 mmol/L). Those who reached the target Hb in the higher Hb group received larger doses of epoetin alfa (10,694 Units) compared to those who achieved the target Hb in the lower Hb group (6,057 Units).
Cardiovascular Risk Reduction by Early Anemia Treatment with Epoetin Beta (CREATE)[46]	603 CKD patients (primarily Stage 4) *Primary end point:* Composite cardiovascular events	Epoetin beta	Partial anemia correction group: Hb 10.5–11.5 g/dL (105–115 g/L; 6.52–7.14 mmol/L) ($n = 302$) Complete anemia correction group: Hb 13.0–15.0 g/dL (130–150 g/L; 8.07–9.31 mmol/L) ($n = 301$)	No significant difference in the risk of a first cardiovascular event between the complete correction and partial correction groups (hazard ratio: 0.78; 95% CI: 0.53 to 1.14; $P = 0.20$)	More frequent dialysis initiation (42 vs 37%, $P = 0.03$) and hypertension (30 vs 20%, $P = 0.005$) in the group randomized to a higher Hb target
Trial to Reduce Cardiovascular Events with Aranesp Therapy (TREAT)[52]	4,038 stage 3–4 CKD pts with type 2 DM *Primary end points:* Composite outcomes of death or a cardiovascular event and of death or ESRD	Darbepoetin alfa or placebo	13 g/dL (130 g/L; 8.07 mmol/L) for darbepoetin group ($n = 2,012$) Placebo group received darbepoetin as rescue therapy if Hb <9 g/dL (<90 g/L; 5.59 mmol/L) ($n = 2,026$)	No evidence of benefit with darbepoetin alfa and a trend toward harm: Death or a cardiovascular event (hazard ratio for darbepoetin vs. placebo, 1.05; 95% CI, 0.94 to 1.17; $P = 0.41$). Death or ESRD (hazard ratio, 1.06; 95% CI, 0.95 to 1.19; $P = 0.29$). Fatal or nonfatal stroke (hazard ratio, 1.92; 95% CI, 1.38–2.68; $P < 0.001$).	Median Hb achieved was 12.5 g/dL (125 g/L; 7.76 mmol/L) in darbepoetin group and 10.6 g/dL (106 g/L; 6.58 mmol/L) in placebo group. Patients with a history of cancer in the higher Hb group also had a higher risk of death.

CHF, congestive heart failure; DM, diabetes mellitus; ESA, erythropoietic-stimulating agent; ESRD, end-stage renal disease.

16 g/dL (120–160 g/L; 7.45–9.93 mmol/L).[47] There was also a higher risk of dialysis access thrombosis and uncontrolled blood pressure in the higher Hb group. Following the release of CHOIR and CREATE the Centers for Medicare and Medicaid Services (CMS), which pays dialysis facilities for a significant portion of services, changed the reimbursement structure for ESAs to reduce payment by 50% if the Hb remained above 13 g/dL (130 g/L; 8.07 mmol/L) for 3 months or greater to promote more conservative and less costly use of ESAs.

The association of poor outcomes with dose of ESA used in the aforementioned studies has also raised concern. Subsequent analysis of the CHOIR study showed that high-dose ESA use was associated with greater risk of death.[48] Those individuals able to achieve the target Hb in the CHOIR study did not have worse outcomes. Further analysis of the NHCT data also showed a reduction in mortality by 60% for those individuals who responded to epoetin therapy compared with nonresponders.[49] Higher mortality with higher ESA dose has also been reported in other observational studies.[50] Such findings have led to discussion of whether hyporesponsiveness to ESAs due to other conditions such as inflammation may explain the higher event rates in this group of individuals. The overall negative cardiovascular outcomes observed with higher Hb targets in the randomized trials has prompted much discussion about the potential causes, including not only ESA dose and Hb target but also the rate of rise in Hb and the variability in Hb over time (e.g., degree of fluctuation in Hb).[51]

Additional discussion on this topic has also been stimulated by the initial results from the Trial to Reduce Cardiovascular Events with Aranesp Therapy (TREAT), a trial initiated prior to the release of data from the CHOIR and CREATE studies (Table 53–5).[52] Despite the association between anemia and reduction in hospitalization and cardiovascular events that prompted many to expect positive outcomes from this study, individuals treated to the higher Hb target did not have a reduction in the defined primary end points compared with the lower Hb group. In addition, there was also an almost twofold increase in the risk of stroke (5% in the treatment group vs 2.6 % in the placebo group). Those patients with a history of cancer in the higher Hb group also had a higher risk of death, a finding that requires additional investigation. These findings further support the recommendation of adhering to the recommendations in the labeling of not exceeding a Hb of 12 g/dL (120 g/L; 7.45 mmol/L).

CLINICAL CONTROVERSY

The higher risk of mortality and cardiovascular events in CKD patients treated to achieve a higher Hb with an ESA has led to an update in targets for Hb. There is a discrepancy, however, in the FDA target Hb (10–12 g/dL [100–120 g/L; 6.21–7.45 mmol/L]) stated in the labeling for ESAs and the K/DOQI target Hb (11–12 g/dL [110–120 g/L; 6.83–7.45 mmol/L]), not to exceed 13 g/dL (130 g/L; 8.07 mmol/L). There are also practitioners who advocate that for patients without specific cardiovascular risk factors (e.g., atherosclerosis) a Hb of 12–13 g/dL (120–130 g/L; 7.45–8.07 mmol/L) achieved with low-dose ESA is reasonable. Healthcare providers must weigh the risks and benefits of ESA use in individual patients and consider the reimbursement structure for ESAs and iron in the practice environment when making decisions about anemia management.

Iron Status Iron indices that should be monitored include the TSat, an indicator of iron immediately available for delivery to the bone marrow, and serum ferritin, an indirect measure of storage iron. The content of hemoglobin in reticulocytes (CHr) is also recommended as a parameter to assess iron status in hemodialysis patients, although it is not as commonly used in clinical practice as the TSat (see Table 53–2). Transferrin is the carrier protein for iron and, as a protein, may be affected by nutritional status. Serum ferritin is an acute-phase reactant, meaning it may be elevated under certain inflammatory conditions and give a false indication of storage iron. The higher recommended level for serum ferritin in hemodialysis patients is based on the information showing lower ESA doses and improved response to iron at this level of ferritin.[53] Previous versions of the K/DOQI anemia guidelines recommended an upper level for TSat of 50% (0.50) and serum ferritin of 800 ng/mL (800 μg/L) to reduce the risk of iron overload. No upper level for these iron indices has been established in the current recommendations; however, the guidelines state that there is insufficient evidence to recommend routine administration of IV iron if the patient's serum ferritin level is greater than 500 ng/mL (500 μg/L).[53] There is now evidence, however, to support administration of IV iron in anemic hemodialysis patients (Hb less than 11 g/dL [110 g/L; 6.83 mmol/L]) with a low TSat (less than 25% [0.25]) and elevated ferritin (500–1200 ng/mL[500–1200 μg/L]).[36] Since ferritin is an acute-phase reactant the decision of whether to give IV iron in conditions of elevated ferritin must be based on objective parameters such as TSat and Hb in addition to the clinical condition of the patient (e.g., infection, inflammation).

Nonpharmacologic Therapy

Nonpharmacologic therapy for anemia of CKD includes maintaining adequate dietary intake of iron as well folate and B_{12}. Patients on hemodialysis or peritoneal dialysis should be routinely supplemented with water-soluble vitamins (including B_{12} and folate) as these vitamins are often depleted with dialysis therapy. A relatively small amount of dietary iron, approximately 1 to 2 mg (or approximately 10%), is absorbed each day, primarily in the duodenum. Although there is some debate as to whether GI absorption of iron is significantly altered in patients with severe CKD, it is clear that oral intake from dietary sources alone is insufficient to meet the increased iron requirements from initiation of ESA therapy.[53]

Pharmacologic Therapy

❾ Pharmacologic therapy for anemia of CKD is based upon a foundation of ESA therapy to correct erythropoietin deficiency and iron supplementation to correct and prevent iron deficiency caused by ongoing blood loss and increased iron demands associated with the initiation of erythropoietic therapy (Figs. 53–3 and 53–4). Iron therapy is first-line therapy for anemia of CKD if iron deficiency is diagnosed, and for some patients the target Hb may be achieved without concomitant ESA therapy. For most individuals with advanced CKD, however, combined therapy with iron and an ESA is often required to effectively stimulate erythropoiesis.

Iron Supplementation Options for iron supplementation include oral and IV therapy (Tables 53–6 and 53–7). Oral iron preparations differ in their content of elemental iron: ferrous salts (ferrous sulfate, ferrous fumarate, and ferrous gluconate), polysaccharide iron complex, and a heme iron polypeptide formulation. Five IV iron products are currently available in the United States (see Table 53–7): two composed of iron dextran (INFeD, molecular weight [MW] 96 kDa; and Dexferrum, MW 265 kDa), sodium ferric gluconate (Ferrlecit, MW 350 kDa), iron sucrose (Venofer, MW 43 kDa), and ferumoxytol (Feraheme, MW 750 kDa).[54–56]

Pharmacology and Mechanism of Action. Iron supplements provide the elemental iron required for production of hemoglobin and its subsequent incorporation in red blood cells,

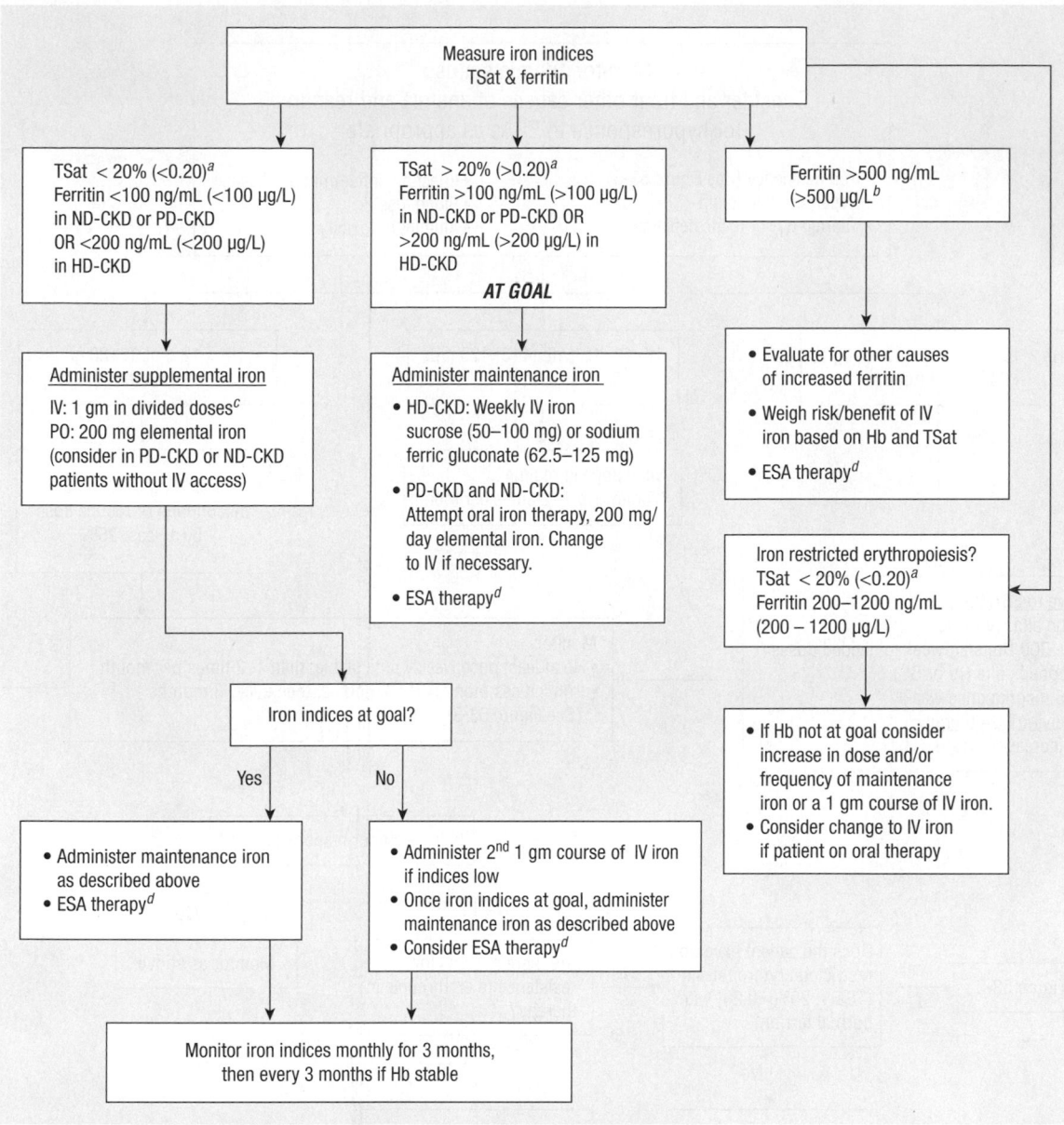

ND-CKD = nondialysis CKD patients; PD-CKD = peritoneal dialysis patients; HD-CKD = hemodialysis patients

[a] Or CHr < 29 pg/cell in hemodialysis patients

[b] Clinical judgement should be used to determine if iron supplementation should be continued when ferritin > 500 ng/mL (>500 µg/L)

[c] Sodium ferric gluconate, iron sucrose, and iron dextran may be administered in divided doses over 8–10 HD sessions for HD-CKD patients.
Administer in divided doses over a prolonged administration time (e.g. up to 400 mg iron sucrose over 2.5 hrs) for PD-CKD and ND-CKD patients.
Ferumoxytol may be administered as two 510-mg doses. Test dose required for iron dextran.

[d] See Figure 53-4.

FIGURE 53-3. Algorithm for iron therapy in the management of the anemia of CKD. (ESA, erythropoietic-stimulating agent; Hb, hemoglobin; TSat, transferrin saturation; ND-CKD, nondialysis CKD patients; PD-CKD, peritoneal dialysis patients; HD-CKD, hemodialysis patients.)

the net result of which is an increase in the transportation of oxygen to tissues.

Bioavailability. Approximately 10% of orally administered iron is absorbed in the duodenum and upper jejunum. Absorption of iron is decreased by food and achlorhydria. The heme form of oral iron binds to a different receptor in the GI tract than nonheme iron, is absorbed to a greater extent, and may be better tolerated.[57] Some oral iron formulations also include ascorbic acid to enhance iron absorption.

Intravenous iron preparations are colloids that consist of an iron-containing core that is surrounded by a carbohydrate shell to stabilize the iron complex. Available agents differ in the size of the core and the composition of the surrounding carbohydrate. These differences affect the rate of dissociation of iron from the complex to phagocytes within the reticuloendothelial system where iron is either stored or released to the extracellular carrier protein transferrin, which transports iron to the bone marrow for red blood cell production. The half-lives of the available IV iron formulations differ: ferric gluconate (1 hour), iron sucrose (6 hours), ferumoxytol (15 hours), and iron dextran (40 to 60 hours).[54,56,58]

Efficacy, Dosage, and Administration. Although supplementation using oral preparations may seem more practical than IV administration, oral iron therapy is limited by poor absorption and nonadherence with therapy primarily due to adverse effects and,

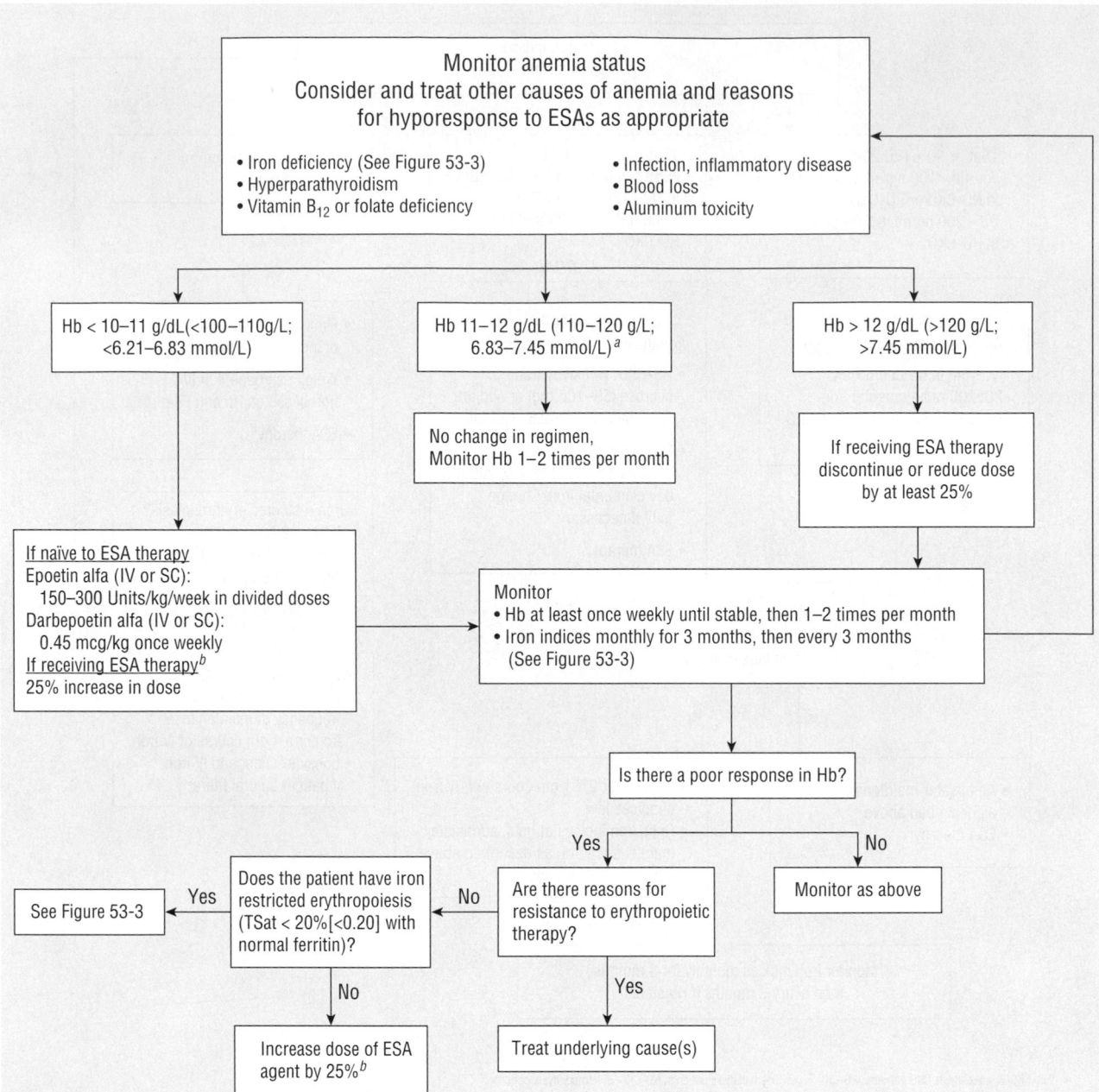

FIGURE 53-4. Algorithm for erythropoietic stimulating agent therapy in the management of the anemia of CKD. (ESA, erythropoietic-stimulating agent; Hb, hemoglobin; SC, subcutaneous; TSat, transferrin saturation.)

[a]Note that the goal Hb is 10–12 g/dL (100–120 g/L; 6.21–7.45 mmol/L) based on FDA labeling for ESAs

[b]Do not adjust ESA dose more frequently than every 4 weeks as a general rule

thus, it is a challenge to achieve goal iron indices. If oral therapy is initiated, the recommended dose is 200 mg of elemental iron per day (see Table 53–6). Either oral or IV administration of iron is recommended in early-stage CKD and the peritoneal dialysis population. Oral iron supplementation is more convenient for these patients, who do not have regular IV access; however, at some point they are likely to require IV iron supplementation to meet iron needs and correct absolute iron deficiency, especially if receiving an ESA.

In patients with ESRD, GI absorption of iron is often inadequate to meet the increase in iron demand from ESA therapy and chronic blood loss in the hemodialysis population. K/DOQI guidelines recommend IV iron as the preferred route of administration in the hemodialysis population.[53] Parenteral iron improves the responsiveness to ESA therapy and reduces the dose required to

achieve and maintain the target Hb in hemodialysis patients. For the hemodialysis population typical repletion dosing regimens are 100 mg as iron sucrose or iron dextran over 10 dialysis sessions, or 125 mg of sodium ferric gluconate over 8 dialysis sessions (see Table 53–7). Ferumoxytol is administered as 510 mg at a rate not to exceed 30 mg per second (1 mL per second) with a second dose given within 3 to 8 days.[56] Administration of 1 g of IV iron is recommended to initially replete hemodialysis patients with an absolute iron deficiency; however, without ongoing iron supplementation, many patients quickly become iron deficient. To prevent iron deficiency maintenance doses of IV iron are administered in hemodialysis patients (e.g., iron sucrose or iron dextran 25 to 100 mg/wk; sodium ferric gluconate 62.5 to 125 mg/wk) based on evidence of improved Hb and lower ESA doses with these regimens.[53,59]

TABLE 53-6 Oral Iron Preparations

Iron Product	Common Agents and Available Units	Amount of Elemental Iron Per Unit	Number of Units Per Day[a]
Ferrous sulfate	Fer-In-Sol (75 mg/0.6 mL)	75 mg	2–3
	Feosol (200 mg)	65 mg	3–4
	Ferrous sulfate, various preparations (325 mg)	65 mg	3–4
	Slow FE (160 mg)	50 mg	4
Ferrous fumarate	Ferrous fumarate, various preparations (300 mg)	99 mg	2
	Femiron (63 mg)	20 mg	10
	Nephro-Fer (350 mg)	115 mg	2
	Vitron-C (65–125 mg)	65 mg	3
Ferrous gluconate	Ferrous gluconate, various (325 mg)	36 mg	5
	Fergon (240 mg)	27 mg	6
Polysaccharide iron	Niferex (50 mg)	50 mg	4
	Hytinic (150 mg)	150 mg	1–2
Heme iron polypeptide	Proferrin-ES (12 mg)	12 mg	17

[a]Number of units per day depends on the amount of elemental iron per unit; 200 mg elemental iron per day is recommended.

Iron administration in patients with what is known as *iron restricted erythropoiesis* (also referred to as *functional iron deficiency*) is more questionable. Under these conditions a trial of IV iron therapy may be warranted if the Hb is less than the target of 11 g/dL (110 g/L; 6.83 mmol/L). A recent study conducted in ESA-treated anemic hemodialysis patients with a low TSat (<25% [<0.25]) and an elevated serum ferritin (>500 ng/mL [>500 μg/L]) showed a significantly greater Hb response rate in patients who received a 1 g course of IV iron as sodium ferric gluconate in conjunction with a 25% increase in ESA dose than in those who only received an increase in the ESA dose.[36]

Adverse Effects. Adverse effects of oral iron are primarily GI in nature and include constipation, nausea, and abdominal cramping. These adverse effects are more likely as the dose is escalated and may be present in more than 50% of patients receiving 200 mg of elemental iron per day. These unfavorable effects often discourage patients from taking these medications on a chronic basis. Some of these GI side effects can be minimized if oral iron products are taken with food; however, food decreases absorption of oral iron. Patients should initially be instructed to take oral iron on an empty stomach; however, if side effects lead to intolerance and nonadherence these agents can be administered with food, or an alternative agent may be prescribed.

Adverse effects of IV iron include allergic reactions, hypotension, dizziness, dyspnea, headaches, lower back pain, arthralgia, syncope, and arthritis. Some of these reactions, in particular hypotension, can be minimized by decreasing the dose or rate of infusion of iron. The most concerning potential consequence of IV iron administration is anaphylaxis. Anaphylactoid reactions to iron dextran have been reported in up to 1.8% of patients, with serious reactions including respiratory complications and cardiovascular collapse occurring in approximately 0.6%.[60] Such reactions are believed to be partly a response to antibody formation to the dextran component. Adverse reactions have been reported two to eight times more frequently in those receiving Dexferrum compared with INFeD.[61] Based on the labeling for all iron dextran products clinicians should (a) administer a test dose of 25 mg prior to the first therapeutic dose; if there are no signs or symptoms of an anaphylactic-type reaction then administer the full therapeutic dose; (b) observe for signs or symptoms of anaphylactic-type reactions during and after every administration; and (c) note that patients with a history of drug

TABLE 53-7 Intravenous Iron Preparations

Iron Compounds	FDA-Approved Indications	FDA-Approved Dosing	Warnings	Dose Ranges[a]
Iron Dextran (INFeD, Watson Pharma Inc., Morrisontown, NJ, and DexFerrum, American Regent, Inc., Shirley, NY)[b]	Patients with iron deficiency in whom oral iron is unsatisfactory	IV push: 100 mg over 2 min (25-mg test dose required)	Black box (risk of anaphylactic reactions)	25–1,000 mg
Sodium ferric gluconate (Ferrlecit, Sanofi-Aventis, Dagenham, Essex, England)[c]	Adult and pediatric HD patients age 6 years and older receiving ESA therapy	IV push (adult): 125 mg over 10 min IV infusion (adult): 125 mg in 100 mL of 0.9% NaCl over 60 min IV infusion (pediatric): 1.5 mg/kg in 25 mL of 0.9% NaCl over 60 min; maximum dose 125 mg	General	62.5–1,000 mg
Iron sucrose (Venofer, American Regent, Inc., Shirley, NY)[d]	HD patients with CKD receiving ESA therapy	IV push: 100 mg over 2–5 min IV infusion: 100 mg in maximum of 100 mL of 0.9% NaCl over 15 min	General	25–1,000 mg
	Nondialysis-CKD patients receiving or not receiving ESA therapy	IV push: 200 mg over 2–5 min on 5 different occasions within 14-day period		
	PD patients receiving ESA therapy	IV infusion: 2 infusions, 14 days apart, of 300 mg in a maximum of 250 mL of 0.9% NaCl over 1.5 h, followed by 1 infusion, 14 days later, of 400 mg in a maximum of 250 mL of 0.9% NaCl over 2.5 h		
Ferumoxytol (Feraheme, AMAG Pharmaceuticals, Lexington, MA)[e]	Adult patients with iron-deficiency anemia associated with chronic kidney disease	IV: 510 mg (17 mL) as a single dose, followed by a second 510 mg dose 3–8 days after the initial dose (rate of 1 mL or 30 mg/second)	General	510 mg

CKD, chronic kidney disease; ESA, erythropoietin-stimulating agent; HD, hemodialysis; PD, peritoneal dialysis.
[a]Small dosing ranges (e.g., 25–150 mg per week) generally used for maintenance regimens. Larger doses (e.g., 1 g) should be administered in divided doses.
[b]Supplied in 2-mL single-dose vials containing 50 mg of elemental iron per mL.
[c]Available in colorless glass ampules containing 62.5 mg elemental iron (12.5 mg/mL).
[d]Supplied in 5-mL single-dose vials containing 100 mg elemental iron (20 mg/mL).
[e]Supplied as a 17-mL single-use vial containing 510 mg elemental iron (30 mg/mL).

allergies may be at increased risk of anaphylactic-type reactions.[62,63] The potential for increased risk of reactions with concomitant use of angiotensin-converting enzyme inhibitors and iron dextran is also highlighted in the labeling for iron dextran, and a statement is included to clarify that there are differences in the chemical characteristics and clinical effects of available iron dextran products (e.g., Dexferrum and INFeD) since these agents are often erroneously considered interchangeable.[63]

The risk of adverse events with iron dextrans was particularly influential in product selection prior to the availability of sodium ferric gluconate, iron sucrose, and ferumoxytol. These IV iron formulations have a better safety record than either of the iron dextran products, based on their history of use in Europe over the last 4 decades (sodium ferric gluconate and iron sucrose) and data in the United States since these products were approved.[61,64] These newer agents do not require administration of a test dose prior to administration of the full dose. As a precaution with all IV preparations, patients should be observed during and immediately following administration for any adverse reactions.

Administration of IV iron also introduces a risk of iron overload. Deposition of excess iron may affect several organ systems, leading to hepatic, pancreatic, and cardiac dysfunction. Bone marrow biopsy provides the most definitive diagnosis of iron overload, but because it is an extremely invasive procedure, it is not widely employed in most clinical settings. Maintaining serum ferritin and TSat values that demonstrate efficacy in preventing iron deficiency yet are safe is the most reasonable approach to minimize the risk of iron toxicity. The challenge is in defining these upper limits, particularly for serum ferritin, which may be elevated in inflammatory conditions and not reflective of true iron stores in such situations. If symptomatic overload does occur, deferoxamine (Desferal) or phlebotomy may be necessary.

Dosage Considerations.

The safety and efficacy of high-dose IV iron regimens have been evaluated to determine the most cost-effective and efficacious dosing strategies. Iron dextran has been safely administered to dialysis patients in total-dose infusions ranging from 400 mg to 2 g.[65] Similar high-dose regimens of 500 mg have also been safely administered to patients with stage 3 or 4 CKD.[66] Sodium ferric gluconate has been safely administered at doses of 250 mg infused over 1 hour (4.2 mg/min).[67] In this same evaluation, 19 doses greater than 250 mg were administered; 1 dose of 312.5 mg, 14 doses of 375 mg, and 4 doses of 500 mg, with infusion rates varying from 1.22 mg/min to 25 mg/min. No serious adverse events were reported, although nonserious events, such as pruritus, did occur in 4 of the 144 patients who received the 250 mg dose. If doses higher than those currently approved are used in practice, they should be administered over a prolonged time period (e.g., at least 2–3 hours). Iron sucrose at doses of up to 500 mg administered over 3 hours on consecutive days has been successful in maintaining iron stores without causing serious adverse events.[68] When administered over a shorter time period this same dose was associated with dizziness, hypotension, and nausea.[69] In this same evaluation the administration of lower doses of 200 to 300 mg given over 2 hours resulted in fewer adverse events. Higher-dose regimens for iron sucrose have been approved in patients with early-stage CKD and peritoneal dialysis patients (see Table 53–7), populations in whom administration of higher doses are more convenient as these patients are seen less frequently by healthcare providers than the hemodialysis population.[58] Ferumoxytol was approved in 2009 for use in the adult CKD population, including dialysis and nondialysis patients. The approved dose is 510 mg administered at a rate of up to 30 mg per second, a higher dose and administration rate compared with other available IV iron formulations.[70,71]

Although there are conflicting reports, most clinicians believe that exposure to iron may contribute to the risk of bacterial infection because iron is used by microorganisms for metabolic functions. The association of IV iron with oxidative stress, acceleration of atherosclerosis, and other cardiovascular conditions has also been suggested.[72,73] These potential long-term risks of IV iron therapy are not clearly defined, and there are no data confirming unequivocally that aggressive use of IV iron in CKD patients treated with ESA therapy increases patient morbidity or mortality.

As a superparamagnetic oxide, ferumoxytol may affect the diagnostic ability of magnetic resonance imaging studies; therefore, these imaging studies should be done prior to administration of ferumoxytol when possible. These effects may persist for up to 3 months following administration of ferumoxytol. Ferumoxytol will not interfere with x-ray, computed tomography, positron emission tomography, single photon emission computed tomography, ultrasonography, or nuclear medicine imaging.[56]

Erythropoietic-Stimulating Agent Therapy

Pharmacology and Mechanism of Action.

Erythropoietic-stimulating agents (ESAs) are glycoproteins manufactured by recombinant DNA technology that have the same biologic activity as endogenous erythropoietin. Available ESAs in the United States include epoetin alfa (distributed as Epogen by Amgen, Inc., Thousand Oaks, CA; and Procrit by Ortho Biotech, Johnson & Johnson, Raritan, NJ) and darbepoetin alfa (Aranesp by Amgen, Inc., Thousand Oaks, CA). Epoetin beta is available from several sources outside the United States (e.g., NeoRecormon, F. Hoffmann–La Roche).

Since 1989, epoetin alfa has been the mainstay of therapy for anemia of CKD. Darbepoetin alfa was approved for treatment of anemia of CKD in September 2001. Darbepoetin alfa differs from epoetin alfa by the addition of two N-linked carbohydrate side chains, which increases the molecular weight (~37 kDa for darbepoetin compared with 30.4 kDa for epoetin alfa). The increase in sialic acid content decreases the affinity of darbepoetin for the erythropoietin receptor, but extends the half-life compared with epoetin alfa.[74]

Pharmacokinetics and Pharmacodynamics.

Epoetin alfa may be administered by either the IV or the subcutaneous (SC) route. Although bioavailability with SC administration is approximately 30% to 36% that of IV, the prolonged absorption phase leads to an extended half-life of 24 hours with SC administration compared to 8.5 hours with IV administration.[75,76] The prolonged half-life with SC administration leads to a more sustained physiologic stimulation of erythroid precursors. Trials have shown that the same target Hb can be achieved and maintained at SC epoetin doses 15 to 30% lower than IV doses.[53,77] Darbepoetin alfa has a longer half-life than does epoetin alfa (25.3 hours and 48.8 hours after IV and SC administration, respectively).[78] More recent information based on studies with prolonged sampling times compared with the original pharmacokinetic studies have reported an even longer half-life of darbepoetin of 70 to 105 hours with SC administration.[75] The prolonged half-life of darbepoetin offers the advantage of less-frequent dosing, starting at once a week or once every other week when given IV or SC. This is of particular benefit in stage 4 and 5 CKD patients who are not yet receiving dialysis and those receiving peritoneal dialysis. Prolonged dosing intervals, as infrequent as once every 4 weeks, have also been effective in maintaining target Hb in many CKD patients, including nondialysis CKD and ESRD patients.[79,80]

The pharmacodynamics of epoetin and darbepoetin are important to consider when evaluating response to therapy. With initiation of ESA therapy or a change in dose, the Hb may begin to rise as the result of demargination of reticulocytes; however, it takes approximately 10 days before erythrocyte progenitor cells mature and are released into the circulation. The Hb continues to increase until the life span of the cells stimulated by epoetin or darbepoetin is reached (mean 2 months; range 1 to 4 months in patients with ESRD). At this point a new steady state is achieved (i.e., the rate at which red blood cells are being produced equals the rate at which they are leaving the circulation). For this reason it is important to evaluate the Hb response over several weeks as opposed to making changes in the dosing regimen prematurely.

Efficacy. Patients will generally respond to ESA therapy in a dose-related fashion unless there are confounding factors present that may cause resistance to therapy or failure to respond as defined by the K/DOQI guidelines.[53] The most common causes of resistance are iron deficiency, acute illness, catheter insertion, hypoalbuminemia, elevated C-reactive protein, chronic bleeding, aluminum toxicity, malnutrition, hyperparathyroidism, cancer and chemotherapy, AIDS, inflammation, and infection. Erythropoietic therapy may be continued in the infected or postoperative patient, even though increased doses are often required to maintain or slow the rate of decline in Hb. Deficiencies in folate and vitamin B_{12} should also be considered as potential causes of resistance to ESA therapy, as both are essential for optimal erythropoiesis.

Medicare has developed new clinical performance measures (CPMs) for ESRD providers that emphasize both an upper and a lower limit of Hb. Of note the limits advocated in the new CPMs are based on FDA labeling (Hb 10–12 g/dL[100–120 g/L; 6.21–7.45 mmol/L]) as opposed to the K/DOQI guidelines (Hb 11–12 g/dL [110–120 g/L; 6.83–7.45 mmol/L]).[81]

Adverse Effects. Hypertension is the most common adverse event reported with epoetin alfa and darbepoetin alfa and may be associated with the rate of rise in Hb.[53] Protocols established in some clinical settings, primarily in outpatient dialysis clinics, sometimes recommend withholding ESA therapy if blood pressure is above a defined threshold. K/DOQI guidelines for anemia do not recommend withholding ESA therapy for elevated blood pressure, but instead advocate more judicious use of antihypertensive agents and dialysis to control blood pressure; however, according to FDA-approved product labeling ESAs should not be used in those with uncontrolled blood pressure.[74,76,82] Seizures have occurred in patients treated with epoetin, particularly within the first 90 days of starting therapy. Vascular access thrombosis may also be more frequent during ESA therapy.[76,83] The potential for these adverse effects calls for close monitoring of the rate of rise in Hb, changes in blood pressure, and monitoring neurologic symptoms following initiation of therapy or a change in ESA dose.

Data demonstrating a higher risk of adverse outcomes in CKD patients treated more aggressively to Hb targets above 12 g/dL (120 g/L; 7.45 mmol/L) with ESAs prompted the FDA to issue a warning in March 2007 about safety concerns of higher Hb targets. Manufacturers revised the ESA product labeling to include updated warnings, a new boxed warning, and modifications to the dosing instructions. The new boxed warning advises healthcare providers to monitor Hb and to adjust the ESA dose to maintain the lowest hemoglobin level needed to avoid blood transfusions. Of note the Hb target in the product labeling for ESAs is 10 to 12 g/dL (100–120 g/L; 6.21–7.45 mmol/L),[74,76,82] An FDA-approved medication guide describing the risks of ESA use must also be given to patients receiving ESA therapy.

Neutralizing antibodies to ESAs have been identified in a relatively small number of patients treated with ESAs; approximately 200 cases were reported between 1998 and 2004.[84] These patients develop antibody-mediated pure red cell aplasia (PRCA), which results in an absolute resistance to ESA therapy and reliance on blood transfusions as the primary therapeutic option. Cases were mostly reported between 1998 and 2002 and occurred in parallel with the increase

in SC administration, primarily with one epoetin alfa product manufactured outside the United States, Eprex (Johnson & Johnson, Manati, Puerto Rico). Differences in this formulation that were noted at the time of the increase in PRCA cases were the substitution of human albumin with polysorbate 80 and use of uncoated rubber stoppers in the single-dose syringes, factors that in combination may have increased the immunogenicity of SC-administered epoetin alfa. Changes in packaging of these syringes led to a decrease in PRCA case reports. Although the case reports of antibody-associated PRCA are relatively few in number, further evaluation for PRCA should be considered for patients receiving ESA therapy who develop a rapid decrease in Hb level (rate of 0.5–1.0 g/dL/wk [5–10 g/L/wk; 0.31–0.62 mmol/L/wk]), become transfusion dependent, and have an absolute reticulocyte count of less than 10,000/μL (10 × 10⁹/L) with a normal platelet and white blood cell count. Discontinuation of ESA therapy is recommended in antibody-mediated PRCA because antibodies are cross-reactive and continued exposure may lead to anaphylactic reactions. Immunosuppressive therapy has been effective in up to 50% of patients with PRCA.[84] A peptide-based erythropoietin-receptor agonist, hematide, an investigational agent that has a different amino acid sequence than native or recombinant erythropoietin, has been shown to stimulate erythropoiesis in patients with PRCA or hyporesponsiveness due to antierythropoietin antibodies and may provide another option in the future for individuals with PRCA.[85]

Drug–Drug Interactions. No significant drug interactions have been reported with the available ESAs.

Dosing and Administration. Recommended starting doses of epoetin alfa are 50 to 100 Units/kg IV or SC three times per week for hemodialysis patients.[76] Less frequent dosing is preferred for stage 4 CKD patients and peritoneal dialysis patients since these patients are seen in the outpatient clinic setting on a relatively infrequent basis.[86,87] Improved erythropoiesis and reduced transfusion requirements were observed in patients with anemia (Hb <10 g/dL [<100 g/L; <6.21 mmol/L]) who received once-weekly SC doses of 10,000 Units of epoetin alfa.[86] Monthly dosing intervals for epoetin alfa SC have also been effective in maintaining target Hb values in this population.[87]

The starting dose of darbepoetin alfa in patients not previously receiving ESA therapy is 0.45 mcg/kg IV or SC administered once weekly. A conversion table for patients who are to be switched from epoetin alfa (Units per week) to darbepoetin alfa (micrograms per week) is available in the package insert for darbepoetin.[74] The usual dosing frequency of darbepoetin is weekly for patients previously receiving epoetin two to three times per week and every other week for patients receiving epoetin once weekly. Extended dosing intervals of darbepoetin as infrequent as every 4 weeks have been successful in maintaining Hb levels.[75]

The IV route of administration is preferred for most hemodialysis patients.[53] Subcutaneous administration of ESAs is preferable for peritoneal dialysis patients and the nondialysis CKD population because these patients do not usually have regular IV access. Dose adjustments should be made based on Hb response with consideration of the recent data on risks associated with higher Hb levels and rate of rise in Hb. A general recommendation is to reduce the ESA dose by 25% if the Hb is approaching 12 g/dL (120 g/L; 7.45 mmol/L) or if the Hb increases by more than 1 g/dL (10 g/L; 0.62 mmol/L) in any 2-week period. A 25% increase in dose may be considered if the Hb is below target range and has not increased by 1 g/dL (10 g/L; 0.62 mmol/L) after 4 weeks of ESA treatment and if no causes of resistance to the ESA have been identified.[74,82] Figures 53–3 and 53–4 provide an algorithmic approach to management of anemia using ESAs and iron therapy in patients with ESRD.

Transfusions and Adjunct Therapies Red blood cell transfusions are currently a third-line treatment option for anemia of

CKD. Red blood cell transfusions carry many risks and therefore should only be used in select situations, such as acute management of symptomatic anemia, following significant acute blood loss, and prior to surgical procedures that carry a high risk of blood loss, with the goal of preventing inadequate tissue oxygenation or cardiac failure. l-Carnitine supplementation and vitamin C were previously suggested as adjunctive treatments of anemia associated with kidney disease but are not recommended in the K/DOQI guidelines because of the lack of evidence supporting improved anemia management with these therapies.[88]

Pharmacoeconomic Considerations

Pharmacoeconomic considerations in the management of anemia of CKD relate primarily to the costs associated with ESAs and IV iron to sustain erythropoiesis. In the outpatient dialysis environment there is a fee-for-service reimbursement system that was implemented by the federal government through the Medicare system. As a general practice, dialysis facilities are reimbursed for ESAs and IV iron at a rate based on the success of maintaining Hb within specific targets, which have changed as guidelines and clinical performance measures for anemia management have been updated. This fee-for-service reimbursement system led to an increase in average ESA doses; the Medicare cost of ESAs was $1.8 billion in 2007.[2] USRDS data indicate that these costs have stabilized. This is due, in part, to changes in the composite rate administered to dialysis facilities, limits on reimbursement for ESAs if Hb levels exceed upper limits, and the recent warnings about ESA safety, which have led to a decrease in ESA use and target Hb levels.

The results of CHOIR, CREATE, and the NHCT prompted CMS to develop a plan for bundling ESAs along with other separately billable drugs into a single payment system to provide an incentive for dialysis facilities to use ESAs more sparingly and reduce costs. This "bundling" of payments for dialysis services is designed to reduce financial incentives for utilization of ESAs and other previously separately billable drugs. Included in the bundled payment are services provided for the dialysis procedure itself that were included in the previous composite rate, separately billable injectable drugs administered during the dialysis procedure (such as ESAs, vitamin D analogs, iron, antibiotics) and their oral equivalents, and separately billable laboratory tests related to the treatment of ESRD. The proposed payment plan for this bundling system was released in the fall of 2009 and is currently in draft form. Once finalized this bundling system is planned for implementation in January 2011.

Evaluation of Therapeutic Outcomes

Iron status should be assessed every month during initial ESA treatment, and every 3 months for those receiving a stable ESA regimen or for those hemodialysis patients not treated with an ESA.[53] For all ESAs, the initial dose and subsequent adjustments should be determined by the patient's Hb level relative to the target Hb level, and the most recent observed rate of increase in Hb. Hemoglobin should be monitored at least monthly in patients receiving ESA therapy, although more frequent monitoring (e.g., every 1–2 weeks) is warranted after initiation of an ESA or following a dose change until the Hb is stable. The response to ESA therapy should be evaluated at least over 2 to 4 weeks before a change in the dose of epoetin alfa or darbepoetin alfa is made. New FDA and CMS recommendations now advise healthcare providers to withhold ESA therapy if the Hb is >12 g/dL (>120 g/L; >7.45 mmol/L); some clinicians, however, may institute a dosage reduction of ≥25% to prevent drastic shifts in Hb levels. An algorithm for anemia management is depicted in Figures 53–3 and 53–4.

■ CKD-MINERAL AND BONE DISORDER (CKD-MBD) AND RENAL OSTEODYSTROPHY

Desired Outcome

The overall goal for management of CKD-MBD is to "normalize" the biochemical parameters and prevent the detrimental consequences, including renal osteodystrophy, cardiovascular and extravascular calcifications, and the associated morbidity and mortality. Unfortunately prospective trials to evaluate the effect of controlling CKD-MBD on these outcomes are limited. At present the K/DOQI (U.S. guidelines) and KDIGO (international guidelines) can be used to guide clinical decision making; however, there are notable differences in these guidelines.[18,22]

CLINICAL CONTROVERSY

K/DOQI clinical practice guidelines for bone metabolism and disease in CKD have been available in the United States since 2003. Targets for calcium, phosphorus, calcium-phosphorus product, and PTH are defined based on opinion and evidence, when available, and have led to development of standardized protocols. In 2009 KDIGO international guidelines for CKD-MBD were published. Given the lack of randomized, controlled trials to support specific target levels for calcium, phosphorus, and PTH the recommendations for target levels and treatment approaches are much more general. Healthcare providers are left to use clinical judgment and new information as it becomes available to sort out the discrepancies in these guidelines where they exist.

The K/DOQI recommended targets for calcium, phosphorus, Ca × P product, and PTH based on the stage of CKD are shown in Table 53–4.[22] The calcium should be corrected for albumin level. The recommended corrected serum calcium for patients with stage 3 or 4 CKD is within the normal range, whereas the proposed range for patients with stage 5 CKD is slightly lower than the normal range. This lower range for calcium in stage 5 CKD patients is based on observations of an increased risk of soft tissue and vascular calcifications in this population, particularly in those individuals with an elevated Ca × P product. Serum phosphorus concentrations should be within the normal range, with higher concentrations acceptable in stage 5 CKD, in part, because of the challenges of lowering phosphorus. The proposed Ca × P product of 55 mg^2/dL^2 (4.4 mmolL^2/L^2) is much lower than the previous recommendation of 65 to 70 mg^2/dL^2 (5.2 to 5.7 mmolL^2/L^2). The PTH values recommended for patients with stage 4 or 5 CKD are above the normal range to prevent oversuppression of PTH and reduce the risk of adynamic bone disease. Serum aluminum levels should also be maintained below 20 μg/L (0.74 μmol/L) to minimize the risk of developing aluminum toxicity, a contributing factor to bone disease.[22]

Based on a lack of randomized, controlled trials showing improved outcomes with control of calcium, phosphorus, and PTH within narrowly defined ranges, KDIGO does not define specific targets for these parameters. KDIGO recommends maintaining serum phosphorus within the normal range for stage 3 to 5 CKD patients and lowering phosphorus toward the normal range for dialysis patients. They propose that calcium should be maintained within the normal range for all CKD patients. KDIGO also supports evaluation of trends in calcium and phosphorus values individually as opposed to attempting to achieve a target Ca × P product.[18] Overall, these recommendations for calcium and phosphorus do not differ drastically from K/DOQI. Clinicians do need to consider risk of calcifications in the stage 5 CKD population and whether a lower target calcium is warranted in individual patients. No specific PTH target range is advocated by KDIGO, but rather the recommendation is to evaluate trends and consider intervention in individuals with values above the upper range for the assay method used. In the dialysis population a broad range for PTH of two to nine times the upper normal limit of the assay is suggested.

❿ Management of PTH, phosphorus, and calcium balance is important in preventing CKD-MBD, ROD, and cardiovascular and extravascular calcifications. Patients with ESRD usually require a combination of dietary intervention, phosphate-binding medications, vitamin D, and calcimimetic therapy to achieve these goals.

Nonpharmacologic Therapy

Dietary Phosphorus Restriction Dietary phosphorus restriction should be a first-line intervention for management of hyperphosphatemia in patients with CKD and should be initiated for most patients with stage 3, 4, or 5 CKD. The K/DOQI guidelines recommend phosphorus restriction to 800 to 1,000 mg/day when the upper levels of serum phosphorus are reached (see Table 53–4).[22] This recommendation also applies to patients with PTH levels above the recommended range given the evidence that lowering phosphorus ingestion directly decreases PTH synthesis and secretion.[89] The challenge with dietary restriction of phosphorus is providing enough protein to prevent malnutrition, a common problem in the ESRD population because foods high in phosphorus are generally high in protein. Examples of foods or beverages that contain high amounts of phosphorus include meats, dairy products, dried beans, nuts, colas, peanut butter, and beer. Nutritional goals must be evaluated on an individual basis, preferably by a dietitian specializing in the care of CKD patients. Dialysis patients require a higher protein intake (1.2–1.3 g/kg per day), making restriction of phosphorus even more challenging. Removal of phosphorus does occur with peritoneal dialysis and hemodialysis (approximately 2–3 g/wk, dependent on the dialysis prescription); however, intermittent dialysis alone does not usually control hyperphosphatemia.

One of the most common obstacles to the success of dietary phosphorus restriction is patient noncompliance because of the poor palatability and inconvenience. Regular counseling by a dietitian is necessary to design a realistic diet that works with the patient's lifestyle.

Dialysis Hemodialysis and peritoneal dialysis lower serum phosphorus and calcium, the extent to which is dependent on the concentration of both entities in the dialysate and the duration of dialysis. K/DOQI recommends the dialysate calcium concentration in hemodialysis or peritoneal dialysis should be 2.5 mEq/L (1.25 mmol/L).[22] KDIGO suggests a dialysate calcium concentration of 2.5 to 3.0 mEq/L (1.25–1.50 mmol/L).[18] Dialysis alone cannot control these parameters, and dietary and pharmacologic interventions are also required in the majority of dialysis-dependent ESRD patients.

Parathyroidectomy Parathyroidectomy is a therapeutic option for patients with severe CKD-MBD who do not respond to pharmacologic therapy. The K/DOQI guidelines recommend surgery for those patients with persistently elevated PTH (PTH >800 pg/mL [>800 ng/L]) associated with hypercalcemia and/or hyperphosphatemia that are refractory to medical therapy.[22] Surgical approaches include either subtotal parathyroidectomy or total parathyroidectomy with autotransplantation of parathyroid tissue to an accessible site, such as the forearm. Postoperative hypocalcemia, hypophosphatemia, and hypomagnesemia may occur because of a marked increase in bone production in relation to bone

absorption ("hungry bone syndrome"). Following surgery frequent monitoring of calcium and phosphorus is necessary as described in Chapter 59. Treatment with supplemental calcium and vitamin D may be required for weeks or months.

Pharmacologic Therapy
Phosphate-Binding Agents

Pharmacology and Mechanism of Action. Drugs that bind dietary phosphorous in the GI tract form insoluble phosphate compounds that are excreted in feces, thus reducing phosphorus absorption and serum phosphorus concentrations. A variety of phosphate-binding agents are available, including elemental calcium-, lanthanum-, aluminum-, and magnesium-containing compounds, and the nonelemental agent sevelamer carbonate (Table 53–8). Patients must be instructed to take these agents with meals to maximize the binding of phosphorus in the GI tract.

Efficacy. Oral calcium compounds are well established as first-line agents for control of both serum phosphorus and calcium concentrations, at least in the early stages of CKD when hypocalcemia is more common. Calcium carbonate and calcium acetate are the primary preparations used; calcium citrate is also available but is not recommended since the citrate component increases aluminum absorption. The chloride salt is also not recommended because it is very astringent and unpalatable, and absorbed chloride may contribute to systemic acidosis. Calcium carbonate is marketed in a variety of dosage forms (see Table 53–8) and is relatively inexpensive. Unfortunately, many calcium carbonate products are considered food supplements and thus are not required by law to meet United States Pharmacopeia (USP) disintegration and dissolution requirements. In general, nationally advertised brands meet USP quality standards for disintegration and dissolution, but it is difficult to determine whether private label or house brands conform to these standards. Variability in gastric pH may also affect disintegration or dissolution, and thus phosphate-binding efficacy. Calcium carbonate is more soluble in an acidic medium and therefore should be administered prior to meals when stomach acidity is highest. In addition, acid-suppressing agents such as ranitidine and proton pump inhibitors may reduce the phosphate-binding activity of calcium carbonate by increasing gastric pH. Calcium acetate binds approximately twice as much phosphorus as calcium carbonate at comparable doses of elemental calcium.[22] Increased binding potency limits GI calcium absorption; however, calcium acetate is more soluble, and therefore better absorbed than calcium carbonate in an alkaline pH, which may explain the similar incidence of hypercalcemia with these agents. For patients with hypocalcemia, calcium carbonate or calcium acetate may also be given as a calcium supplement taken between meals to promote calcium absorption.

Although calcium-containing phosphate-binding agents continue to be used as first-line therapy, their chronic use may increase the risk for vascular and tissue calcification.[28] The K/DOQI guidelines recommend that the total dose of elemental calcium provided by calcium-containing binders not exceed 1,500 mg per day and the total daily intake of elemental calcium from all sources not exceed 2,000 mg.[22] Calcium-containing binders are not recommended for dialysis patients who have persistent elevations in serum calcium >10.2 mg/dL (>2.55 mmol/L) or PTH values <150 pg/mL (150 ng/L).[22] KDIGO guidelines suggest restricting the dose of calcium-containing binders in stage 3 to 5 CKD patients if hypercalcemia is present or if arterial calcification or adynamic bone disease (low bone turnover disease) is evident.[18] Since both of these recommendations regarding calcium intake are based primarily on opinion, clinicians in essence have to rely on their past experiences and clinical judgment as they individualize therapy for their patients.

TABLE 53-8 Phosphate-Binding Agents Used for the Treatment of Hyperphosphatemia in CKD Patients

Compound	Trade Name	Compound Content (mg)	Dose Titration[a]	Starting Doses	Comments
Calcium carbonate[b] (40% elemental calcium)	Tums Oscal-500 Caltrate 600	500, 750, 1,000, 1,250 1,250 1,500	Increase or decrease by 500 mg per meal (200 mg elemental calcium)	0.5–1 g (elemental calcium) three times a day with meals	First-line agent; dissolution characteristics and phosphate binding may vary from product to product; Approximately 39 mg phosphorus bound per 1 g calcium carbonate
Calcium acetate (25% elemental calcium)	PhosLo	667	Increase or decrease by 667 mg per meal (168 mg elemental calcium)	0.5–1 g (elemental calcium) three times a day with meals	First-line agent; comparable efficacy to calcium carbonate with half the dose of elemental calcium; Approximately 45 mg phosphorus bound per 1 g calcium acetate; By prescription only
Sevelamer carbonate *Available as tablet and powder for oral suspension	Renvela	800	Increase or decrease by 800 mg per meal	800–1,600 mg three times a day with meals	First-line agent; lowers low-density lipoprotein cholesterol; More expensive than calcium products; consider in patients at risk for extraskeletal calcification; Associated with a lower risk of acidosis and GI adverse events than Renagel.
Sevelamer Hydrochloride	Renagel	400, 800	Increase or decrease by 1 tablet per meal	Same as Renvela	Same as Renvela, plus acidosis
Lanthanum carbonate	Fosrenol	500, 750, 1,000	Increase or decrease by 750 mg per day	750–1,500 mg daily in divided doses with meals	First-line agent; Available as chewable tablets
Aluminum hydroxide[b]	Alterna GEL	600 mg/5 mL	–	300–600 mg three times a day with meals	Not a first line agent; do not use concurrently with citrate-containing products; Reserve for short-term use (4 weeks) in patients with hyperphosphatemia not responding to other binders

[a]Based on phosphorus levels, titrate every 2 to 3 weeks until phosphorus goal reached.
[b]Multiple preparations available that are not listed.

Sevelamer is a nonabsorbable, nonelemental hydrogel phosphate-binding agent. The hydrochloride salt of sevelamer was approved by the FDA in 2000; however, its use was associated with the development of acidosis in some CKD patients. The manufacturer therefore developed the carbonate formulation that provides an added buffering capacity and does not contribute to acidosis.[90] This formulation is available as a tablet and powder for oral suspension and will eventually replace sevelamer hydrochloride. Sevelamer effectively lowers phosphorus and has also been shown to significantly lower LDL and increase HDL cholesterol.[90,91] Whether sevelamer lowers the risk of calcification compared with calcium-containing binders is an issue of some debate. There are studies to support use of sevelamer over calcium-containing binders to decrease progression of arterial calcification in both dialysis and nondialysis CKD patients.[92] These findings have been refuted by other studies showing that sevelamer is associated with similar rates of vascular calcification compared with calcium acetate.[93] K/DOQI guidelines suggest using a noncalcium-containing binder in dialysis patients with severe vascular or soft tissue calcifications, although these are opinion-based recommendations.[22] KDIGO states that binder choice be made considering the stage of CKD, other factors of CKD-MBD such as risk of calcifications, and other therapies.[18]

Lanthanum carbonate is a phosphate binder approved for patients with ESRD. Short-term (6–28 weeks) and long-term (2–3 years) therapy with lanthanum has demonstrated efficacy in controlling phosphorus and maintaining PTH in the target range with less risk of hypercalcemia than calcium-containing binders.[94,95] Initial daily doses are in the range of 750 to 1,500 mg (administered in divided doses with meals) with doses of 1,500 to 3,000 mg often being required to maintain target phosphorus in ESRD patients. The poor GI absorption, which limits systemic effects, and high binding capacity with phosphorus makes this an attractive phosphate-binding agent, particularly when options other than calcium-containing binders are needed. Lanthanum is available as a chewable tablet, which may be appealing for some patients. Lanthanum carbonate (2,250 to 3,000 mg/day) was as effective in lowering serum phosphorus as sevelamer hydrochloride (4,800 to 6,400 mg/day) in hemodialysis patients.[96] The effect of lanthanum on progression of calcification has not been evaluated in clinical trials.

Aluminum salts were widely used in the 1980s as phosphate-binding agents because of their high binding potency. They should no longer be used as first line agents but rather reserved for acute treatment of severe hyperphosphatemia or used at low doses in combination with either calcium-containing binding agents or sevelamer in cases of hyperphosphatemia that is not responding to therapy with a single agent. According to K/DOQI guidelines, the duration of aluminum therapy should be limited to four weeks if these agents are used at all.[22]

Magnesium-containing antacids are also effective phosphate binders and may decrease the amount of calcium-containing binders necessary for control of phosphorus; however, their use is limited by the frequent occurrence of GI side effects (i.e., diarrhea) and the potential for magnesium accumulation.

Adverse Effects. Adverse effects of all phosphate binders are generally limited to GI side effects, including constipation, diarrhea, nausea, vomiting, and abdominal pain. The risk of hypercalcemia may necessitate restriction of calcium-containing binders use and/or a reduction in dietary intake. Aluminum binders have been associated with CNS toxicity and the worsening of anemia, whereas magnesium binder use may lead to hypermagnesemia and hyperkalemia.

Drug–Drug and Drug–Food Interactions. Calcium-containing phosphate-binding agents interfere with the absorption of several oral medications that are commonly prescribed for CKD patients, including iron, zinc, and quinolone antibiotics. No drug interaction studies have been performed with sevelamer carbonate; however, studies with sevelamer hydrochloride have shown no drug interactions with digoxin, warfarin, metoprolol, enalapril, or iron. Coadministration with ciprofloxacin did, however, result in a 50% decrease in bioavailability of the antibiotic. This information is reported in the labeling for the newer formulation sevelamer carbonate.[97] Potential interactions between sevelamer and cyclosporine (decreased bioavailability of cyclosporine) and altered phosphorus binding in the presence of agents that increase gastric pH (e.g., omeprazole) have been reported.[98,99] Drug interaction studies with lanthanum, although limited, have shown that coadministration with warfarin, digoxin, and metoprolol did not affect the bioavailability of those agents.[100] In general, it is rational to separate the administration time of oral medications for which a reduction in bioavailability has a clinically significant effect (e.g., quinolones) from phosphate binders by at least 1 hour before or 3 hours after administration of the phosphate binder. This is a key patient-counseling recommendation as patients are often switched from one phosphate binder to another, and it is easier for them to remember this general concept regarding phosphate binders and other medications. Many phosphate binders are marketed as antacids or calcium supplements, and often CKD patients do not know why they have been prescribed these agents. Regular patient counseling is essential to improve adherence and minimize the potential for drug interactions.

Dosing and Administration. Initial dosing regimens for phosphate-binding agents and suggested dose titration schemes are shown in Table 53–8. Doses should be titrated to achieve the recommended serum phosphorus concentrations based on the patient's stage of CKD. The daily dose of elemental calcium should be limited in individuals with elevated calcium levels.

Vitamin D Therapy Vitamin D compounds include ergocalciferol (vitamin D_2) and cholecalciferol (vitamin D_3) that must be converted to the active form in the kidney. Calcitriol (1,25-dihydroxyvitamin D_3) is the most active form of vitamin D and is available as an oral formulation (Rocaltrol) as well as an IV formulation (Calcijex). The currently available vitamin D analogs include paricalcitol (19-nor-1,25-dihydroxyvitamin D_2; Zemplar) and doxercalciferol (1α-hydroxyvitamin D_2; Hectorol). Calcitriol or one of the vitamin D analogs is required for patients with severe kidney disease because these agents do not require conversion by the kidney to the biologically active form.

Pharmacology and Mechanism of Action. Active vitamin D suppresses PTH secretion by stimulating absorption of serum calcium by intestinal cells and through direct activity on the parathyroid gland to decrease PTH synthesis. As a result, the serum calcium concentration is raised and the parathyroid glands decrease the rate of secretion and formation of PTH. The set point for calcium (i.e., the calcium concentration at which PTH secretion is decreased by 50%), which is generally raised in CKD-MBD, is lowered when active vitamin D therapy is initiated. This indicates that a lower ionized calcium concentration is effective at suppressing secretion of PTH. All of these actions are mediated by the interaction of vitamin D with vitamin D receptors, which are located in many organs, including the parathyroid gland, GI tract, and kidney. Calcitriol also upregulates vitamin D receptors, which ultimately may reduce parathyroid hyperplasia. Unfortunately, the enhanced GI absorption of calcium and phosphorus with calcitriol therapy frequently leads to hypercalcemia and hyperphosphatemia. There is also evidence that hyperphosphatemia results in resistance to the PTH-suppressing effects of vitamin D and directly stimulates PTH release. These actions contribute to the increase in the

Ca × P product, which is associated with soft-tissue and vascular calcifications.[22,25] Consequently, reasonable control of calcium and phosphorus must be achieved before initiation and during continued vitamin D therapy. This does not mean that vitamin D therapy should be withheld or discontinued in patients with a Ca × P product greater than 55 mg^2/dL^2 (4.4 $mmoL^2/L^2$). Rather interventions with agents with a lower risk of hypercalemia and hyperphosphatemia, and more prudent use of phosphate binders to lower calcium and phosphorus, may be necessary in such patients.

The unique interactions of vitamin D with the vitamin D receptors have been a focus of research and have led to the development of vitamin D analogs, which vary in their affinity for these receptors and result in less hypercalcemia while retaining the positive physiologic actions on bone and parathyroid tissue. Paricalcitol and doxercalciferol are D_2 compounds that effectively lower PTH.[101] Paricalcitol differs from calcitriol by the absence of the exocyclic carbon 19 and the fact that it is a vitamin D_2 derivative. Doxercalciferol is a prohormone that needs to be hydroxylated in the liver to 1,25-dihydroxyvitamin D_2. These agents are available in an IV formulation for use in patients with stage 5 CKD and in oral forms that are approved for use in those with stage 3 to 5 CKD.

Pharmacokinetics. Calcitriol can be administered orally as well as by IV injection. Oral absorption occurs rapidly; therefore oral and IV therapies are both reasonable options for treatment of CKD-MBD. When paricalcitol is administered IV, its half-life is similar to that of calcitriol (up to 30 hours). The half-life of paricalcitol after oral administration is 17 to 20 hours in patients with stage 3 and 4 CKD.[102] Doxercalciferol has a slightly prolonged half-life of 45 hours.[103]

Efficacy. Administration of calcitriol by either the oral or the IV route may be based on conventional dosing (usually 0.25–0.5 mcg/day) or pulse dosing (0.5–2 mcg two to three times per week). Logistically, IV dosing is more practical in hemodialysis patients, whereas oral therapy is more practical for nondialysis CKD and peritoneal dialysis patients. Conventional daily oral doses of calcitriol may be more frequently associated with hypercalcemia and hyperphosphatemia, because vitamin D receptors are located in intestinal mucosa where direct stimulation can occur.

Although hypercalcemia is less likely with the newer analogs (paricalcitol and doxercalciferol), elevated calcium concentrations have been observed with these agents in patients with ESRD. However, some of these cases were associated with excessive dosing of these agents and oversuppression of PTH, a condition more likely to promote hypercalcemia. When administered at doses 10 times that of calcitriol and at a dose equivalent to doxercalciferol, paricalcitol has been less frequently associated with hypercalcemia in animal studies and in human trials.[104,105] Intestinal calcium absorption was 14% lower in paricalcitol-treated hemodialysis patients compared with those treated with calcitriol.[106] Doxercalciferol and paricalcitol have also been evaluated in patients with stages 3 and 4 CKD. They are effective in reducing PTH to target levels; however, differences in the magnitude of elevations of calcium and phosphorus have not been directly compared in this population.[107,108]

Although comparisons between vitamin D analogs are relatively limited the incidence of hyperphosphatemia with paricalcitol was lower than with doxercalciferol when administered at high doses to hemodialysis patients.[105] A more rapid suppression of PTH was also observed in paricalcitol-treated patients compared to those who received calcitriol. The more clinically significant finding from this study was the decrease in incidence of hypercalcemia and elevated Ca × P in the paricalcitol-treated patients.[109] Nontraditional effects of vitamin D, including a potential survival benefit, have also been reported.[101] An improvement in 3-year survival in a large dialysis population receiving paricalcitol was observed compared with a

TABLE 53-9 Available Vitamin D Agents

Generic Name	Trade Name	Form of Vitamin D	Dosage Range	Dosage Forms	Frequency of Administration
Vitamin D precursor					
Ergocalciferol[a]	Vitamin D$_2$	D$_2$	400–50,000 IU	PO	Daily (doses of 400–2000 IU)
Cholecalciferol[a]	Vitamin D$_3$	D$_3$			Weekly or monthly for higher doses (50,000 IU)
Active vitamin D					
Calcitriol	Calcijex		0.5–5 mcg	IV	Three times per week
	Rocaltrol		0.25–5 mcg	PO	Daily, every other day, or three times per week
Vitamin D analogs					
Paricalcitol	Zemplar		1–4 mcg	PO	Daily or three times per week
			2.5–15 mcg	IV	Three times per week
Doxercalciferol	Hectorol		5–20 mcg	PO	Daily or three times per week
			2–8 mcg	IV	Three times per week

[a]Multiple preparations are available that are not listed.

historic cohort that received calcitriol.[110] This survival advantage was also observed for hemodialysis patients who received vitamin D (either calcitriol or paricalcitol) compared with no vitamin D and was independent of calcium, phosphorus, and PTH.[111] The relationship between all available vitamin D agents (calcitriol, doxercalciferol, and paricalcitol) and mortality was further evaluated in a retrospective analysis of more than 7,700 hemodialysis patients.[112] After a median follow-up of 37 weeks, all-cause mortality and atherosclerotic cardiovascular mortality were similar for doxercalciferol- and paricalcitol-treated patients and similar to the calcitriol-treated patients when adjusted for laboratory values (e.g., calcium, PTH, albumin, phosphorus) and standardized mortality for the dialysis clinics included in this study. Vitamin D therapy, regardless of agent, was associated with lower mortality. It must be noted that these are observational studies and that prospective, randomized, controlled trials are required to better understand survival benefits associated with vitamin D therapy. Antiproteinuric effects of paricalcitol have also been reported in patients with stages 3 and 4 CKD.[113] These findings are of interest when considering other potential effects of vitamin D beyond suppression of PTH.

Adverse Effects. Although all agents are effective in suppressing PTH levels, they differ in the degree to which they cause other metabolic abnormalities. Adverse effects of note with vitamin D therapy in patients treated for CKD-MBD include hypercalcemia and hyperphosphatemia. Differences in calcitriol and vitamin D analogs have been demonstrated in animal studies and in clinical trials evaluating their effect on reduction of PTH while minimizing the risk of these adverse consequences.[105,106]

Drug–Drug and Drug–Food Interactions. Cholestyramine may reduce the absorption of orally administered calcitriol and doxercalciferol. In vitro data suggest that paricalcitol is metabolized by the hepatic enzyme CYP3A4 and has the potential to interact with other agents that are metabolized by this enzyme. When ketoconazole, a CYP3A4 inhibitor, was given concomitantly, paricalcitol serum concentrations doubled.[114] Caution is also advised when CYP3A4 inhibitors are given to those receiving doxercalciferol. No other significant interactions have been reported.

Dosing and Administration. Recommendations for vitamin D therapy differ based on the stage of CKD. Because deficiency in the vitamin D precursor, 25-hydroxyvitamin D, is common in patients with CKD, K/DOQI guidelines recommend measuring 25-hydroxyvitamin D levels in patients with stage 3 or 4 CKD who have PTH values above the upper recommended ranges (see Table 53–4). If the 25-hydroxyvitamin D level is less than 30 ng/mL (75 nmol/L), a vitamin D precursor (e.g., ergocalciferol or cholecalciferol) is recommended. The dose and duration of treatment are dependent on the severity of the deficiency. To prevent vitamin D

insufficiency, doses of 600 to 800 units per day of ergocalciferol are recommended. Calcitriol, doxercalciferol, or paricalcitol should be administered orally when PTH remains elevated despite the achievement of adequate 25-hydroxyvitamin D levels.

Initial oral doses of vitamin D recommended in patients with stage 3 or 4 CKD are 0.25 mcg calcitriol, 1 mcg doxercalciferol, or 1 mcg paricalcitol administered daily.[115] For paricalcitol the recommended daily dose is 2 mcg if the PTH is greater than 500 pg/mL (500 ng/L). If these agents are administered intermittently (generally three times per week), the recommended initial oral dose is twice the daily dose. Higher starting doses may be required based on the severity of CKD-MBD. Prior to starting therapy the serum calcium and phosphorus should be within the normal range to minimize the risk of hypercalcemia and an elevated Ca × P. In patients with ESRD there is a clearly defined role for treatment with active vitamin D or a vitamin D analog because the conversion of precursors to active vitamin D is impaired. The active vitamin D agents available in the United States vary markedly with regard to the oral and IV dosage regimens that are recommended for CKD patients (Table 53–9). Serum calcium and Ca × P should be monitored regularly while the patient is receiving therapy. Dose adjustments should be made every 2 to 4 weeks based on PTH concentrations.[22] For patients who need to be converted from calcitriol to paricalcitol, a dosing conversion ratio of 1:4 of IV calcitriol to paricalcitol has been proposed; however, some clinicians suggest a ratio of 1:3 to avoid oversuppression of PTH.

Calcimimetics

Pharmacology and Mechanism of Action. Cinacalcet hydrochloride (Sensipar) is a calcimimetic agent approved for treatment of secondary hyperparathyroidism in ESRD patients and for treatment of hypercalcemia in patients with parathyroid carcinoma. Cinacalcet is the first agent in this class to receive FDA approval. This compound acts on the calcium-sensing receptor on the surface of the chief cells of the parathyroid gland to mimic the effect of extracellular ionized calcium and increase the sensitivity of the calcium-sensing receptor to calcium, subsequently reducing PTH secretion. Cinacalcet does not increase intestinal calcium and phosphorus absorption. In fact, the reduction in PTH with cinacalcet is associated with a decrease in serum calcium.[116]

Pharmacokinetics. The maximum plasma concentration of cinacalcet is achieved in approximately 2 to 6 hours following oral administration. The half-life is approximately 30 to 40 hours. Cinacalcet has a large volume of distribution (approximately 1,000 L), and is 93% to 97% bound to plasma proteins, both characteristics indicating that removal by dialysis is negligible. Cinacalcet is metabolized by the liver, specifically by the cytochrome P450 isoenzymes CYP3A4, CYP2D6, and CYP1A2.[117]

Efficacy. In placebo-controlled clinical trials conducted in dialysis patients (predominantly those receiving hemodialysis) cinacalcet significantly decreased PTH and the Ca × P product within the 6-month study period, regardless of the severity of secondary hyperparathyroidism.[116] The starting dose of 30 mg per day was titrated every 3 or 4 weeks to a maximum dose of 180 mg per day to achieve the target PTH of ≤250 pg/mL (≤250 ng/L) and avoid hypocalcemia. Approximately 66% and 93% of patients in the clinical trials were receiving concurrent vitamin D and phosphate binders, respectively. If a patient experienced symptoms of hypocalcemia or had a serum calcium <8.4 mg/dL (<2.10 mmol/L), calcium supplements and/or calcium-based phosphate binders could be increased. If ineffective, the vitamin D dose could be increased. The median dose required to achieve the desired PTH by the end of the study period was 90 mg. This agent is not approved for use in patients with early stage CKD (stages 3–5 CKD not requiring dialysis) due to the risk of hypocalcemia. Because cinacalcet was approved after the K/DOQI guidelines on bone disease became available, the challenge to clinicians is in deciding how to most effectively use cinacalcet in conjunction with other therapies to manage CKD-MBD. KDIGO guidelines endorse the use of cinacalcet alone or in conjunction with vitamin D therapy to lower PTH in the dialysis population.[18] There are no studies evaluating the effect of cinacalcet on vascular calcification in humans.

Adverse Effects. The most frequently reported adverse events with cinacalcet were nausea and vomiting. Although nausea and vomiting occurred more frequently with cinacalcet, these events were generally transient, mild to moderate in nature, and infrequently led to withdrawal from clinical trials.[117]

Because cinacalcet lowers serum calcium and may cause hypocalcemia, this agent should not be started if the serum calcium is less than the lower limit of normal, approximately 8.4 mg/dL (2.10 mmol/L). Serum calcium should be measured within 1 week after initiation or following a dose adjustment of cinacalcet. Once the maintenance dose is established, serum calcium should be measured approximately monthly. Potential manifestations of hypocalcemia include paresthesia, myalgia, cramping, tetany, and convulsions.

Drug–Drug and Drug–Food Interactions. Because cinacalcet is metabolized by multiple hepatic enzymes there is potential for drug interactions. Cinacalcet is also a potent inhibitor of the enzyme CYP2D6. As a result, dose adjustments of concomitant medications that are predominantly metabolized by this enzyme and have a narrow therapeutic index, such as flecainide, thioridazine, vinblastine, and most tricyclic antidepressants (e.g., amitriptyline) may be required.[117]

Several agents commonly used in the CKD population have been evaluated for interactions with cinacalcet. Coadministration of calcium carbonate or sevelamer did not affect the pharmacokinetics of cinacalcet. Pantoprazole did not alter the pharmacokinetics of cinacalcet. This is an important finding because pantoprazole alters gastric pH, and the solubility of cinacalcet decreases as the gastric pH rises over 5.5. Coadministration of cinacalcet with warfarin also did not affect the pharmacokinetics of warfarin. Coadministration of cinacalcet and ketoconazole, a strong inhibitor of cytochrome P450 (CYP) 3A4, resulted in an increase in the area under the curve and maximum concentration of 2.3 and 2.2 times, respectively. Concurrent administration of cinacalcet with amitriptyline increased amitriptyline exposure and nortriptyline (active metabolite) exposure by approximately 20% in CYP2D6-extensive metabolizers.[117]

Food has been shown to increase absorption of cinacalcet by up to 81% compared with fasting; therefore this medication should be taken with meals to achieve the maximal effect.

Dosing and Administration. The recommended starting oral dose of cinacalcet is 30 mg once daily. The dose should be titrated every two to four weeks to a maximum dose of 180 mg once daily to achieve the desired PTH levels and to maintain near-normal serum calcium concentrations. Patients with hepatic disease may require lower doses, as studies have shown a decrease in metabolism of cinacalcet in this patient population. Cinacalcet is available as a film-coated tablet containing 30, 60, or 90 mg.

Pharmacoeconomic Considerations

Pharmacoeconomic considerations in the management of CKD-MBD and ROD include medication costs, the cost associated with laboratory monitoring, bone biopsies when indicated, and the medical expenditures associated with the management of calcifications and bone fractures. If the associated complications such as vascular and soft-tissue calcifications that may increase morbidity and hospitalizations can be significantly reduced, the additional medication costs may be of minimal consequence.

The pattern of vitamin D product use in U.S. dialysis units has been strongly influenced by Medicare reimbursement. Currently, IV vitamin D products are separately reimbursable expenses for dialysis programs. In fact, dialysis programs often generate significant profit from the IV administration of these agents. In contrast, oral administration of vitamin D is more convenient for patients with stage 3 or 4 CKD and the peritoneal dialysis population; however, these agents are not separately reimbursable. The fact that these agents must be purchased by the patient makes noncompliance with therapy an issue. The payment system for the hemodialysis population is all subject to change as the new "bundling" of payments for dialysis services, designed to reduce financial incentives for utilization of "unnecessary" dialysis services, is implemented in outpatient dialysis facilities (see Pharmacoeconomic Considerations for the anemia management section). In the bundling system currently proposed, the financial reimbursement a dialysis unit receives per dialysis session ($14 per dialysis treatment) would now also include costs of oral drugs such as phosphate binders and cinacalcet. There are concerns in the nephrology community about the effect the new system would have on treatment for CKD-MBD. Dialysis providers may advocate changing patients from more expensive, noncalcemic phosphate binders (e.g., sevelamer carbonate, and lanthanum carbonate) to less expensive calcium-containing binders. Calcitriol, which is more likely to cause hypercalcemia and hyperphosphatemia, may be used more in the ESRD population since both the IV and oral form are less expensive than paricalcitol and doxercalciferol. It is also anticipated that the use of cinacalcet may be reduced because of the cost of this oral calcimimetic. These changes in prescribing to reduce cost burden on dialysis facilities could potentially increase the incidence of hypercalcemia, calcifications, and morbidity in the ESRD population.

■ CHRONIC METABOLIC ACIDOSIS

Desired Outcome

The goals of therapy for patients with CKD are to normalize the pH of the blood (pH of approximately 7.35–7.45) and maintain the serum bicarbonate within the normal range (22–26 mEq/L [22–26 mmol/L]). In patients on hemodialysis, the goal of therapy is to maintain a predialysis or stabilized bicarbonate concentration at or above 22 mEq/L (22 mmol/L).[9] Metabolic acidosis appears to stimulate protein catabolism, which can contribute to a negative nitrogen balance and lower albumin concentrations. Lower serum bicarbonate levels in peritoneal dialysis patients have also been associated with a higher hospitalization rate and longer hospital stays.[9] Severe acidemia (blood pH <7.1–7.2) suppresses myocardial contractility, predisposes patients to cardiac arrhythmias, and may lead to a decrease in total peripheral vascular resistance and blood pressure, reduced hepatic blood flow, and impaired oxygen delivery.[118] The prevention and treatment of severe metabolic acidosis in patients with kidney disease are also important to prevent the development of CKD-MBD since chronic metabolic acidosis has been shown to alter bone metabolism and decrease the effectiveness of vitamin D therapy.[22]

Nonpharmacologic Therapy

Therapy for metabolic acidosis requires pharmacologic intervention to correct the acidemia. Treatment of other underlying disorders that may be contributory is also warranted.

Pharmacologic Therapy

In patients with stage 4 or 5 CKD, the use of alkalinizing salts, such as sodium bicarbonate or citrate/citric acid preparations, is useful to replenish depleted body bicarbonate stores. Sodium bicarbonate tablets are manufactured in 325- and 650-mg strengths (a 650-mg tablet contains 7.6 mEq [7.6 mmol] sodium and 7.6 mEq [7.6 mmol] bicarbonate). Shohl solution and Bicitra contain 1 mEq/mL (1 mmol/mL) of sodium and the equivalent of 1 mEq/mL (1 mmol/mL) of bicarbonate as sodium citrate/citric acid. Citrate is metabolized in the liver to bicarbonate, and citric acid is metabolized to CO_2 and water. Polycitra, which contains potassium citrate (1 mEq/mL [1 mmol/mL] of sodium, 1 mEq/mL [1 mmol/mL] of potassium, and 2 mEq/mL [2 mmol/mL] of bicarbonate) should not be used in patients with severe CKD because of the risk of hyperkalemia.

The replacement dose of alkali (base) needed to restore the serum bicarbonate concentration to normal (24 mEq/L [24 mmol/L]) can be approximated by multiplying the volume of distribution of bicarbonate (0.5 L/kg) by the patient's body weight (in kilograms) and the patient's base deficit (difference between the patient's serum bicarbonate value and the normal value of 24 mEq/L [24 mmol/L]). The calculated amount of bicarbonate replacement therapy (in milliequivalents [or in mmols]) should be administered over several days to prevent volume overload from excessive sodium intake. After the serum bicarbonate has normalized, a maintenance regimen of bicarbonate to neutralize daily acid production may be all that is necessary (12 to 20 mEq/day [12 to 20 mmol/day] in divided doses). Doses are subsequently titrated to maintain normal plasma bicarbonate concentrations. Patients with renal tubular acidosis may require higher doses of alkalinizing agents (see Chap. 61). Fluid balance should be monitored carefully because of the sodium content of these agents. Citrate-containing solutions should not be used in combination with aluminum-containing compounds because they can enhance aluminum absorption and increase the risk of aluminum intoxication. Excessive doses of alkalinizing agents may cause metabolic alkalosis, as well as lethargy or cardiac depression secondary to a decrease in ionized serum calcium concentration. Gastrointestinal distress characterized by gastric distension and flatulence is relatively common with high doses of oral sodium bicarbonate. Patients with severe acidemia (serum bicarbonate <8 mEq/L [<8 mmol/L]; pH <7.2) will likely require IV therapy (see Chap. 61).

Metabolic acidosis in both adult and pediatric patients undergoing dialysis is usually managed by tailoring the patient's dialysis prescription. Increasing the concentration of bicarbonate (or acetate) in the dialysate to values above the serum bicarbonate concentration causes diffusion of the bicarbonate across the dialyzer and is an effective chronic treatment for metabolic acidosis in the dialysis population (see Chap. 54). Administration of oral bicarbonate salts may also be necessary for some dialysis patients.

Evaluation of Therapeutic Outcomes

Regular monitoring of serum electrolytes and arterial blood gases is necessary to determine the effectiveness of therapy. A gradual correction of serum bicarbonate is appropriate to avoid overcorrection

and subsequent complications such as alkalosis and other electrolyte abnormalities (see Chap. 61). Laboratory measurement of serum bicarbonate is associated with several technical problems. Blood collection techniques, transportation, and assay methodology can affect the measured concentrations. Blood samples should not have contact with air, process delays should be avoided, and consistent analytical methods should be used with serial measurements to improve accuracy.[9]

■ CARDIOVASCULAR DISEASE

Specific recommendations regarding the management of cardiovascular disease in the ESRD population are included in K/DOQI guidelines. This includes recommendations for management of coronary artery disease, acute coronary syndromes, valvular heart disease, cardiomyopathy, dysrhythmias, cerebrovascular disease, and peripheral vascular disease. Differences in management of these disorders in dialysis patients compared with the general population are emphasized. Guidelines for management of cardiovascular risk factors are also included. Two of the most common medication amenable risk factors for cardiovascular disease in the CKD population—hypertension and hyperlipidemia—are discussed here.

Desired Outcome

Hypertension The goal blood pressure for cardiovascular risk reduction in patients with early-stage CKD is less than 130/80 mm Hg.[118] The target blood pressure in patients with ESRD is not well defined; however, the K/DOQI guidelines propose a predialysis blood pressure of less than 140/90 mm Hg and a postdialysis blood pressure of less than 130/80 mm Hg, although this recommendation is not based on data from prospective, controlled studies.[3] The targets may need to be individualized for patients who experience intradialytic hypotension (hypotension during the hemodialysis process). These goals can rarely be achieved using lifestyle modifications alone and aggressive antihypertensive therapy is often required.

Hyperlipidemia Based on strong evidence of risk reduction and the benefits of lipid-lowering therapy in the general population, the consensus is that CKD patients are among the highest-risk group for cardiovascular conditions (i.e., equivalent to that of patients with known coronary heart disease) and should be treated aggressively for dyslipidemia to an LDL cholesterol goal below 100 mg/dL (2.59 mmol/L).[41,119] The decision to lower LDL cholesterol to less than 70 mg/dL (1.81 mmol/L) based on more recent data in high-risk populations is a therapeutic option, although this approach is not supported by strong evidence from clinical trials in CKD. Table 53–10 lists the goals and suggested course of therapy based on the K/DOQI guidelines for patients with stage 5 CKD based on their lipid abnormality.

Nonpharmacologic Therapy

Hypertension Fluid intake should be restricted in patients with volume overload, particularly in patients on hemodialysis who are at risk for substantial fluid accumulation between dialysis sessions. Regular dietary counseling is critical to the success of nonpharmacologic interventions, given the large number of lifestyle changes typically required by CKD patients. Other lifestyle modifications, including regular exercise, weight loss, and smoking cessation, are also recommended but difficult to implement.

A primary nonpharmacologic intervention for management of hypertension in patients with ESRD is sodium restriction to approximately 2 g/day. In hemodialysis patients, achievement of an individual's "dry weight" is necessary to control blood pressure and may be done through dietary intervention, increased

TABLE 53-10 Management of Dyslipidemia in Patients with Chronic Kidney Disease[41]

Dyslipidemia	Goal	Initial Therapy	Modification in Therapy[a]	Alternative[a]
TG ≥500 mg/dL (≥5.56 mmol/L)	TG <500 mg/dL (<5.56 mmol/L)	TLC	TLC + fibrate or niacin	Fibrate or niacin
LDL 100–129 mg/dL (2.56–3.34 mmol/L)	LDL <100 mg/dL (<2.56 mmol/L)	TLC	TLC + low-dose statin	Bile acid sequestrant or niacin
LDL ≥130 mg/dL (≥3.36 mmol/L)	LDL <100 mg/dL (<2.56 mmol/L)	TLC + low-dose statin	TLC + maximum-dose statin	Bile acid sequestrant or niacin
TG ≥200 mg/dL (≥2.26 mmol/L) and non-HDL ≥130 mg/dL (≥3.36 mmol/L)	Non-HDL <130 mg/dL (<3.36 mmol/L)	TLC + low-dose statin	TLC + maximum-dose statin	Fibrate or niacin

HDL, high-density lipoprotein; LDL, low-density lipoprotein; Non-HDL, total cholesterol minus HDL cholesterol; TG, triglycerides; TLC, therapeutic lifestyle changes.
[a]Dosing of selected agents by class: fibrate (gemfibrozil 600 mg twice a day); niacin (1.5–3 g/day of immediate-release product); statin (simvastatin 10–40 mg/day if glomerular filtration rate [GFR] <30 mL/min [<0.50 mL/s], 20–80 mg/day if GFR >30 mL/min [>0.50 mL/s]); bile acid sequestrant (cholestyramine 4–16 g/day). See Chapter 28 for more complete dosing information.

ultrafiltration, and longer dialysis sessions (see Chap. 54). Aggressive ultrafiltration in hemodialysis patients has shown beneficial effects of lowering blood pressure and decreasing left ventricular mass index. Prolonged hemodialysis also better maintains normal blood pressure, improves survival, and reduces the need for antihypertensive medications; however, the majority of hemodialysis programs in the United States use shorter dialysis sessions (3- to 4-hour sessions three times per week).[3]

Hyperlipidemia In patients with elevated triglyceride levels (≥500 mg/dL [≥5.65 mmol/L]) and/or LDL between 100 and 129 mg/dL (2.56–3.34 mmol/L), lifestyle changes without pharmacologic therapy are recommended as initial therapy (see Chap. 28). Unfortunately, most patients with CKD have already been advised to adhere to difficult dietary regimens, which may include protein, phosphorus, sodium, potassium, and fluid restrictions. Thus, although diet therapy is a reasonable first-step approach, it may not be successful in many patients with CKD because of noncompliance. A dietitian who is well versed in the management of kidney disease should be consulted.

Pharmacologic Therapy

Hypertension Most patients with hypertension and advanced CKD (GFR <30 mL/min/1.73 m² [<0.29 mL/s/m²]) require three or more antihypertensive agents to achieve target blood pressure.[118] Blood pressure reductions can be achieved with agents in all antihypertensive classes, although there is a preference for agents that inhibit the renin–angiotensin system, and choice should be guided by the individual patient's concomitant disease states.

Diuretic therapy is beneficial for management of blood pressure in patients with early CKD; however, thiazide diuretics are not generally effective in patients with a GFR of <30 mL/min (<0.50 mL/s). Loop diuretics can be used throughout all stages of CKD; however, patients with ESRD who have minimal to no residual kidney function will often not respond to these agents.

ACEIs or angiotensin receptor blockers are the preferred agents for patients with progressive CKD and proteinuria. They are also preferred in certain patients with ESRD because of their potential benefits including regression of LVH, reduction in sympathetic nerve activity and pulse-wave velocity, improvement in endothelial function, and reduced oxidative stress.[3] Lower initial doses of these agents may be necessary because the elimination half-lives of the parent compound (captopril and lisinopril) or active metabolite (enalapril, benazepril, and ramipril) are prolonged in ESRD patients. Available angiotensin receptor blockers do not require dosage adjustment for decreased kidney function, and they are not effectively removed by hemodialysis.

Calcium channel blockers that selectively lower systemic vascular resistance also appear to be effective in the treatment of hypertension in patients with ESRD and are associated with decreased total and cardiovascular mortality.[3] β-Blockers may be particularly useful in hypertensive CKD patients given the beneficial effects after myocardial infarction. Agents such as esmolol, timolol,

pindolol, metoprolol, and labetalol, which are metabolized and not significantly removed by dialysis, may be easier to dose titrate than agents that are both dialyzable and extensively eliminated unchanged by the kidney (e.g., acebutolol, atenolol, bisoprolol, and nadolol). Agents requiring less-frequent dosing may be used to improve patient compliance.

Use of other antihypertensive agents in the patient with CKD should be based on recommendations in the general population (see Chap. 19). In the ESRD population, agents that act on the sympathetic nervous system, such as prazosin, terazosin, doxazosin, clonidine, guanabenz, and guanfacine, may be required in patients who are unresponsive to ACEIs, calcium channel blockers, or β-blocker therapy, and used in conjunction with adequate dialysis. Central α₂-agonists such as clonidine appear to be the safest of these agents; however, adverse effects, such as dry mouth, may lead to extra fluid consumption in some patients. Postsynaptic α-blockers (e.g., prazosin) are associated with postural hypotension following hemodialysis. Guanethidine and methyldopa should be avoided because of potential complications, including severe postural hypotension, severe dialysis-related hypotension, and impotence. The addition of vasodilators such as minoxidil may prove useful in patients resistant to combinations of the previously mentioned agents.

Based on claims data from the USRDS approximately 75% of stage 3 to 5 CKD patients with hypertension (excluding the ESRD population) received an ACEI or angiotensin receptor blocker within a year after diagnosis of CKD. The data also indicated that β-blockers and nondihydropyridine calcium channel blockers were used in approximately 50% and 40% of CKD patients, respectively. Loop diuretic use was reported in approximately 40% of stage 3 to 5 CKD patients and thiazide-like diuretics were prescribed for approximately 35%.[2]

Hyperlipidemia Management of dyslipidemia in patients with CKD is based on the report from the National Cholesterol Education Program and the K/DOQI guidelines for dyslipidemia in patients with CKD.[41,119] If lifestyle changes are not effective in achieving goal triglyceride and LDL levels after a few months, drug therapy is warranted (see Table 53–10 and Chap. 28). Drug therapy is also recommended for those with more extreme elevations in LDL (≥130 mg/dL [≥3.36 mmol/L]).

Drug classes that may prove useful in treatment of lipid disorders include 3-hydroxy-3-methylglutaryl coenzyme A (HMG-CoA) reductase inhibitors (statins), bile acid sequestrants, nicotinic acid, and fibric acids (gemfibrozil and clofibrate). Statins are the most effective drugs for lowering LDL and total cholesterol in patients with kidney disease (with or without nephrotic syndrome) and generally should be regarded as the drugs of first choice, keeping in mind the controversies in the ESRD population (see below). Drug therapy for hypertriglyceridemia includes a fibrate or nicotinic acid; in general, fibrates are better tolerated. Patients receiving sevelamer as a phosphate binder may also benefit from its cholesterol-lowering effects.

Several potential drug interactions and/or adverse effects have been observed in those CKD patients receiving antilipemic therapy. The nonselective binding activity of bile acid sequestrants may reduce absorption of corticosteroids, digoxin, thiazide diuretics, warfarin, and other commonly used medications. Myositis and myalgia, along with increased serum creatine phosphokinase (CPK), may occur in ESRD patients who use clofibrate. Determining the optimal dose of clofibrate in this patient population is difficult as plasma protein-binding changes markedly affect free concentrations of the active metabolite clofibric acid, which has a prolonged half-life in patients with stage 5 CKD. Gemfibrozil may be a safer alternative, as the half-life is not altered with kidney dysfunction. Lower doses of 300 mg twice a day with close monitoring of CPK are recommended by some clinicians, based on an association of standard dose therapy with increases in CPK concentrations in dialysis patients.

Although statins are remarkably free of adverse effects in otherwise healthy subjects, one should be cognizant of the potential myotoxic effects of these drugs, especially when administered with interacting agents, such as azole antibiotics, cyclosporine, gemfibrozil, and niacin, and in the presence of hepatic disease.[119] There is increased risk of rhabdomyolysis with combined fibrate and statin therapy in patients with CKD, and diligent monitoring by prescribers and patients is necessary. Dose reductions are warranted for lovastatin and rosuvastatin in stage 4 CKD and with simvastatin in ESRD patients because of their reduced renal elimination.[120]

Statins in Early-Stage CKD. Statins are effective agents in patients with early-stage CKD, although there is little documented clinical trial data.[3] Atorvastatin therapy targeted to achieve an LDL of 80 mg/dL (2.07 mmol/L) or a maximum dose of 80 mg per day decreased cardiovascular risk in individuals with coronary heart disease and stage 3 CKD.[121] This effect was similar to that achieved in individuals without CKD. These results are similar to those from the Treating to New Targets trial, which evaluated atorvastatin (80 mg vs 10 mg per day) on cardiovascular events in patients with ($n = 3,107$) and without ($n = 6,549$) CKD.[122] Atorvastatin 80 mg reduced the relative risk of major cardiovascular events by 32% in patients with CKD over the median follow-up period of 5 years. Thus statin therapy clearly can reduce cardiovascular risk for patients with stage 3 CKD. Evidence of these benefits for those with stage 4 CKD, however, is lacking.

Statins in the ESRD Population. Data on statin use in the ESRD population are not consistently favorable as they are in early CKD. Although observational studies in hemodialysis patients receiving statins indicated a significant benefit: 31% relative risk reduction in overall mortality and a 23% reduction in cardiac causes of death,[123] the findings from prospective studies have not been encouraging.[124,125] Results from a 4-year study evaluating the effect of atorvastatin therapy on cardiac mortality in more than 1,200 hemodialysis patients with type 2 diabetes showed no significant benefit in the composite end point compared with the placebo group.[124] In fact, there was a significantly greater relative risk of fatal stroke in the atorvastatin-treated patients. These findings do not support initiation of statin therapy in ESRD patients, especially those with type 2 diabetes. The AURORA trial assessed the impact of rosuvastatin 10 mg daily or placebo on the primary end points of death from cardiovascular causes, nonfatal MI, or nonfatal stroke. Despite a 43% reduction in cholesterol in the rosuvastatin group there was no difference in the primary end points.[125] It is evident from these trials that information from the general population regarding statin therapy cannot be directly extrapolated to the ESRD population. Results from an ongoing trial known as the Study of Heart and Renal Protection (SHARP) trial will provide additional information on the use of the combination of simvasta-

tin and ezetimibe both in those with early-stage CKD as well as in hemodialysis patients.[126]

CLINICAL CONTROVERSY

While observational studies have reported decreased mortality associated with statin use in the dialysis population, this has not been demonstrated in prospective trials (4D and AURORA trials). Critics of these prospective trials argue that these trials included patients with preexisting cardiovascular disease (e.g., history of MI) and speculate whether a study designed for primary prevention of cardiovascular events would have yielded positive results. There is also the argument that LDL cholesterol levels in the populations studied were relatively low and the effect of statins in individuals with higher LDL cholesterol levels (above 150 mg/dL [3.88 mmol/L]) was not adequately studied. For these reasons some practitioners support use of statins for primary prevention of cardiovascular events in the dialysis population and for individuals with LDL cholesterol levels well above 150 mg/dL (3.88 mmol/L).

Pharmacoeconomic Considerations

Hypertension Compliance and economic factors must be considered in the selection of antihypertensive therapy for CKD patients. Patients with ESRD are prescribed a median of eight medications.[32] Choosing agents that can be administered once or twice daily may improve patient compliance. In addition, there are now many options within some antihypertensive classes such as calcium channel blockers, ACEIs, angiotensin receptor blockers, and β-blockers, which allow for less-frequent dosing. In most cases, no clear therapeutic advantage has been demonstrated with any particular agent within a class. Therefore, selecting the least costly agent that can be administered once or twice daily is reasonable.

A meta-analysis of studies done in the hemodialysis population evaluating the effect of blood pressure lowering on cardiovascular outcomes showed that blood pressure lowering was associated with a decreased risk of cardiovascular events and all-cause and cardiovascular mortality.[127] As more information becomes available from studies evaluating the effects of long-term therapy of hypertension on cardiovascular events in patients with CKD, cost benefits from potentially decreasing the occurrence of such events and their comorbidities may be quantified.

Hyperlipidemia Statin therapy for treatment of dyslipidemias has been shown to be cost-effective in patients at high risk for coronary heart disease. Although this has not specifically been evaluated in patients with CKD, this population is considered in the highest-risk group for coronary heart disease and cardiovascular events. It may be reasonable, at least in theory, to extrapolate this information on the cost benefits of therapy to the CKD population, although findings from the trials in the ESRD population contradict this rationale.

Evaluation of Therapeutic Outcomes

Hypertension Blood pressure monitoring to determine the effectiveness of therapy should be done at each clinic visit, particularly following initiation of therapy (nonpharmacologic or pharmacologic), and at home when feasible. Patients on hemodialysis should have blood pressure measured before, during, and after dialysis to determine the effect of changes in their volume status on blood pressure. Some hemodialysis patients experience a paradoxical rise in blood pressure during dialysis. In these cases, the effect of dialysis on removal of antihypertensive agents and the dosing times relative to the dialysis procedure need to be evaluated. Similarly, patients may need to adjust the time of administration of antihypertensive therapy relative to the dialysis session if intradialytic hypotension occurs. Such decisions should be based on the pharmacokinetic profile of the antihypertensive agent in patients with ESRD. Chapter 19 discusses more specifics of monitoring blood pressure and associated complications.

Hyperlipidemia Patients should have their lipid profile reassessed 2 to 3 months following a change in treatment and at least annually thereafter.[41] Periodic evaluations of cardiovascular performance, as described in Chapters 17 and 28, are also warranted.

◼ OTHER COMPLICATIONS

Nutritional Status

Protein-energy malnutrition is very common among patients with advanced CKD (stages 4 and 5).[9] Causes of malnutrition in these patients include inadequate food intake secondary to anorexia, altered taste sensation, and the unpalatability of prescribed diets. Other factors in the ESRD population, such as the effect of the dialysis procedure on removal of nutrients, hypercatabolism induced by other inflammatory conditions, and blood loss are also contributory. Protein restriction as an intervention to potentially delay progression of kidney disease in patients with stage 3 or 4 CKD may also lead to protein malnutrition by the time a patient reaches ESRD; therefore the risks versus the benefits of this intervention must be considered on an individual basis (see Chap. 52) as hypoalbuminemia and malnutrition have a strong association with mortality in chronic dialysis patients.

Patients with ESRD have increased nutritional needs relative to the general population, based on the effect of the disease state and the dialysis procedure on nutritional status. The recommended dietary protein intake in chronic hemodialysis patients is 1.2 g/kg body weight per day.[9] The recommended intake for chronic peritoneal dialysis patients is at least 1.2 to 1.3 g/kg body weight per day, based on the increased protein loss that occurs with this dialysis modality. Protein requirements are higher in patients who are acutely ill (see Chap. 149). The recommended total daily energy intake in both hemodialysis and peritoneal dialysis patients is 35 kcal/kg (147 kJ/kg) body weight per day. For peritoneal dialysis patients, this includes intake from both diet and the glucose absorbed from peritoneal dialysate. For patients older than 60 years of age this criterion differs, because increasing age is generally associated with reduced physical activity and lean body mass. Daily energy intake for these patients is 30 to 35 kcal/kg (126–147 kJ/kg) body weight per day. Nutritional support should be considered for those patients who cannot achieve these goals with oral intake alone. Another option for nutritional supplementation in patients on hemodialysis includes interdialytic parenteral nutrition (see Chap. 151).

Vitamin requirements for ESRD patients receiving dialysis differ from those of a healthy person because of dietary modifications, kidney dysfunction, and dialysis therapy. The plasma concentrations of vitamins A and E are elevated in ESRD, whereas those of the water-soluble vitamins (B_1, B_2, B_6, B_{12}, niacin, pantothenic acid, folic acid, biotin, and vitamin C) tend to be low in large part because many are dialyzable. The goal for vitamin supplementation should be to prevent subclinical and frank deficiency and to avoid pathology from overdosage. Special vitamin supplements have been formulated for the dialysis population, which primarily include B vitamins with C and folic acid.

Supplementation with l-carnitine has been advocated for its potential benefits in patients with ESRD, including management of hypertriglyceridemia, hypercholesterolemia, and anemia.[128]

Although some of these benefits have been demonstrated, the evidence does not strongly support routine supplementation. Cost and the addition of yet another medication to the already complex regimen prescribed for many of these patients also mitigate against the routine use of this agent.

Uremic Bleeding

Bleeding complications in patients with CKD are usually mild but can result in major hemorrhagic events. The primary mechanisms underlying the hemostatic problem are platelet biochemical abnormalities and alterations in platelet–vessel wall interactions. Decreased platelet aggregation and adhesiveness have been shown in a number of studies in ESRD patients.[129] Additionally, there is a decreased plasma concentration and defective binding of the large multimer of von Willebrand factor which results in abnormal platelet–blood vessel wall interactions. Patients on hemodialysis are at even greater risk of bleeding, not only because of the hemodialysis process itself but from administration of other medications. Heparin is frequently administered during dialysis procedures to prevent clotting during dialysis. Patients who are at high risk for bleeding may require alternative anticoagulation procedures rather than traditional hemodialysis with systemic heparinization. In addition, dialysis patients often receive systemic anticoagulation (warfarin) or antiplatelet therapy (aspirin or clopidogrel) for prevention of access clotting or other cardiovascular disorders. This complication is discussed in additional detail in Chapter 54.

CONCLUSIONS

The number of patients with and at risk for CKD is increasing, with a substantial rise in the population with stage 5 CKD expected in the next decade. Although efforts to delay progression of CKD are paramount, measures to diagnose and manage the associated secondary complications and comorbid conditions early in the course of the disease are also essential. Common complications of stages 4 and 5 CKD include anemia, CKD-MBD and renal osteodystrophy, fluid and electrolyte abnormalities, metabolic acidosis, and malnutrition. Cardiovascular complications are also prevalent in the population with CKD, and are the leading cause of mortality in patients with stage 5 disease. Patient education plays a critical role in the appropriate management of CKD and related complications.

A multidisciplinary team structure is a rational approach to providing this education and effectively designing and implementing the required extensive nonpharmacologic and pharmacologic interventions. Pharmacists are among the healthcare providers who contribute substantially to this team as shown by their activities in identifying and resolving drug-related problems, improving patient adherence with drug therapy, and providing more cost-effective medication use in dialysis facilities.[42,130] There are many opportunities for pharmacists to become involved in both the outpatient dialysis or ambulatory care settings as well as the inpatient environment to improve the management of patients with CKD and the associated complications.

ABBREVIATIONS

ACEI: Angiotensin-converting enzyme inhibitor

ABPM: Ambulatory blood pressure monitoring

AIDS: Acquired immunodeficiency syndrome

ARIC: Atherosclerosis Risk in Communities study

Ca × P: Calcium phosphorus product; serum calcium multiplied by serum phosphorus

CPK: Creatine phosphokinase

CPMs: Clinical performance measures

CMS: Centers for Medicare and Medicaid Services

CKD: Chronic kidney disease

DRPs: Drug-related problems

eGFR: Estimated glomerular filtration rate

EBCT: Electron-beam computed tomography

ESA: Erythropoietic-stimulating agent

ESRD: End-stage renal disease

FE_K: Fractional excretion of potassium

FE_{Na}: Fractional excretion of sodium

GFR: Glomerular filtration rate

Hb: Hemoglobin

HCT: Hematocrit

HDL: High-density lipoprotein

HMG-CoA: 3-hydroxy-3-methylglutaryl coenzyme A (reductase)

KDIGO: Kidney Disease: Improving Global Outcomes

K/DOQI: Kidney Disease Outcomes Quality Initiative

LDL: Low-density lipoprotein

LVH: Left ventricular hypertrophy

MBD: Mineral and bone disorder

MTM: Medication therapy management

PRCA: Pure red cell aplasia

PTH: Parathyroid hormone

ROD: Renal osteodystrophy

SHARP: Study of Heart and Renal Protection

sHPT: Secondary hyperparathyroidism

TREAT: Trial to Reduce Cardiovascular Events with Aranesp Therapy

TSat: Transferrin saturation

USRDS: United States Renal Data System

REFERENCES

1. K/DOQI clinical practice guidelines for chronic kidney disease: Evaluation, classification, and stratification. Am J Kidney Dis 2002;39(2 suppl 1):S1–266.
2. U.S. Renal Data System, USRDS 2009 Annual Data Report: Atlas of End-Stage Renal Disease in the United States. Bethesda, MD: National Institutes of Health, National Institute of Diabetes and Digestive and Kidney Diseases; 2009.
3. K/DOQI Clinical Practice Guidelines for Cardiovascular Disease in Dialysis Patients. Am J Kidney Dis 2005;45(3 Pt 2):16–153.
4. Coresh J, Selvin E, Stevens LA, et al. Prevalence of chronic kidney disease in the United States. JAMA 2007;298(17):2038–2047.
5. Lacson E Jr, Wang W, Hakim RM, et al. Associates of mortality and hospitalization in hemodialysis: Potentially actionable laboratory *variables and vascular access.* Am J Kidney Dis 2009;53(1):79–90.
6. U.S. Department of Health and Human Services. Healthy People 2010. 2nd ed. With Understanding and Improving Health and Objectives for Improving Health—Focus Area 4: Chronic Kidney Disease. 2 vols. Washington, DC: U.S. Government Printing Office; 2000.
7. U.S. Department of Health and Human Services. Proposed Healthy People 2020 Objectives, *www.healthypeople.gov/HP2020/Objectives/TopicAreas.aspx.*
8. Brenner RM, Brenner BM. Adaptation to renal injury. In: Kasper DL, Braunwald E, Fauci AS, et al, eds. Harrison's Principles of Internal Medicine. New York: McGraw-Hill;2005:1639–1644.
9. Clinical practice guidelines for nutrition in chronic renal failure. K/DOQI, National *Kidney Foundation.* Am J Kidney Dis 2000;35(6 suppl 2):S1–140.
10. Thomas R, Kanso A, and Sedor JR. Chronic kidney disease and its complications. Prim Care 2008;35(2):329–344, vii.
11. Ganz T. Hepcidin and its role in regulating systemic iron metabolism. Hematology Am Soc Hematol Educ Program 2006:507:29–35.
12. Kalantar-Zadeh K, Streja E, Miller JE, Nissenson AR. Intravenous iron versus erythropoiesis-stimulating agents: Friends or foes in treating chronic kidney disease anemia? Adv Chronic Kidney Dis 2009;16(2):143–151.
13. Li S, Foley RN, Collins AJ. Anemia, hospitalization, and mortality in patients receiving peritoneal dialysis in the United States. Kidney Int 2004;65(5):1864–1869.
14. Levin A, Hemmelgarn B, Culleton B, et al. Guidelines for the management of chronic kidney disease. CMAJ 2008;179(11):1154–1162.
15. Singh, AK, Szczech L, Tang KL, et al. Correction of anemia with epoetin alfa in chronic kidney disease. N Engl J Med 2006;355(20):2085–2098.
16. Besarab A, Bolton WK, Browne JK, et al. The effects of normal as compared with low hematocrit values in patients with cardiac disease who are receiving hemodialysis and epoetin. N Engl J Med 1998;339(9):584–590.
17. KDOQI Clinical Practice Guideline and Clinical Practice Recommendations for anemia in chronic kidney disease: 2007 update of hemoglobin target. Am J Kidney Dis 2007;50(3):471–530.
18. KDIGO clinical practice guideline for the diagnosis, evaluation, prevention, and treatment of chronic kidney disease-mineral and bone disorder (CKD-MBD). Kidney Int Suppl 2009;(113):S1–130.
19. Fukagawa M, Nakanishi S, Kazama JJ. Basic and clinical aspects of parathyroid hyperplasia in chronic kidney disease. Kidney Int Suppl 2006;(102):S3–7.
20. Levin A, Bakris GL, Molitch M, et al. Prevalence of abnormal serum vitamin D, PTH, calcium, and phosphorus in patients with chronic kidney disease: Results of the study to evaluate early kidney disease. Kidney Int 2007;71(1):31–38.
21. Gutierrez O, Isakova T, Rhee E, et al. Fibroblast growth factor-23 mitigates hyperphosphatemia but accentuates calcitriol deficiency in chronic kidney disease. J Am Soc Nephrol 2005;16(7):2205–2215.
22. Eknoyan G, Levin A, Levin NW. Bone metabolism and disease in chronic kidney disease. Am J Kidney Dis 2003;42(4 suppl 3):1–201.
23. Coen G. Adynamic bone disease: An update and overview. J Nephrol 2005;18(2):117–122.
24. Ganesh SK, Stack AG, Levin NW, et al. Association of elevated serum PO(4), Ca × PO(4) product, and parathyroid hormone with cardiac mortality risk in chronic hemodialysis patients. J Am Soc Nephrol 2001;12(10):2131–2138.
25. Kestenbaum B, Belozeroff V. Mineral metabolism disturbances in patients with chronic kidney disease. Eur J Clin Invest 2007;37(8):607–622.
26. Block GA, Hulbert-Shearon TE, Levin NW, Port FK. Association of serum phosphorus and calcium × phosphate product with mortality risk in chronic hemodialysis patients: A national study. Am J Kidney Dis 1998;31(4):607–617.
27. Block GA, Port FK. Re-evaluation of risks associated with hyperphosphatemia and hyperparathyroidism in dialysis patients: Recommendations for a change in management. Am J Kidney Dis 2000;35(6):1226–1237.
28. Goodman WG, Goldin J, Kuizon BD, et al. Coronary-artery calcification in young adults with end-stage renal disease who are undergoing dialysis. N Engl J Med 2000;342(20):1478–1483.
29. Rogers NM, Coates PT. Calcific uraemic arteriolopathy: An update. Curr Opin Nephrol Hypertens 2008;17(6):629–634.
30. Sarnak MJ, Levey AS, Schoolwerth AC, et al. Kidney disease as a risk factor for development of cardiovascular disease: a statement from the American Heart Association Councils on Kidney in Cardiovascular Disease, High Blood Pressure Research, Clinical Cardiology, and Epidemiology and Prevention. Hypertension 2003;42(5):1050–1065.
31. Go AS, Chertow GM, Fan D, et al. Chronic kidney disease and the risks of death, cardiovascular events, and hospitalization. N Engl J Med 2004;351(13):1296–1305.

815

32. U.S. Renal Data System, USRDS 2008 Annual Data Report: Atlas of End-Stage Renal Disease in the United States. Bethesda, MD: National Institutes of Health, National Institute of Diabetes and Digestive and Kidney Diseases; 2008.

33. Muntner P, He J, Astor BC, et al. Traditional and nontraditional risk factors predict coronary heart disease in chronic kidney disease: Results from the atherosclerosis risk in communities study. J Am Soc Nephrol 2005;16(2):529–538.

34. Ritz E, Wanner C. Lipid changes and statins in chronic renal insufficiency. J Am Soc Nephrol 2006;17(12 suppl 3):S226–230.

35. KDOQI Clinical Practice Guidelines and Clinical Practice Recommendations for Anemia in Chronic Kidney Disease. Am J Kidney Dis 2006;47(5 suppl 3):S11–145.

36. Coyne DW, Kapoian T, Suki W, et al. Ferric gluconate is highly efficacious in anemic hemodialysis patients with high serum ferritin and low transferrin saturation: Results of the Dialysis Patients' Response to IV Iron with Elevated Ferritin (DRIVE) Study. J Am Soc Nephrol 2007;18(3):975–984.

37. Fishbane S. Erythropoiesis-stimulating agent treatment with full anemia correction: A new perspective. Kidney Int 2009;75(4):358–365.

38. Herberth J, Fahrleitner-Pammer A, Obermayer-Pietsch B, et al. Changes in total parathyroid hormone (PTH), PTH-(1–84) and large C-PTH fragments in different stages of chronic kidney disease. Clin Nephrol 2006;65(5):328–334.

39. Agarwal R. Home and ambulatory blood pressure monitoring in chronic kidney disease. Curr Opin Nephrol Hypertens 2009;18(6):507–512.

40. Thompson AM, Pickering TG. The role of ambulatory blood pressure monitoring in chronic and end-stage renal disease. Kidney Int 2006;70(6):1000–1007.

41. K/DOQI Clinical Practice Guidelines for managing dyslipidemias in patients with chronic kidney disease. Am J Kidney Dis 2003;41(4 suppl 3):S1–S91.

42. Pai AB, Boyd A, Depczynski J, et al. Reduced drug use and hospitalization rates in patients undergoing hemodialysis who received pharmaceutical care: A 2-year, randomized, controlled study. Pharmacotherapy 2009;29(12):1433–1440.

43. U.S. Renal Data System, USRDS 2007 Annual Data Report: Atlas of End-Stage Renal Disease in the United States. Bethesda, MD: National Institutes of Health, National Institute of Diabetes and Digestive and Kidney Diseases; 2007.

44. Collins AJ. Influence of target hemoglobin in dialysis patients on morbidity and mortality. Kidney Int Suppl 2002;(80):44–48.

45. Finkelstein FO, Story K, Firanek C, et al. Health-related quality of life and hemoglobin levels in chronic kidney disease patients. Clin J Am Soc Nephrol 2009;4(1):33–38.

46. Drueke TB, Locatelli F, Clyne N, et al. Normalization of hemoglobin level in patients with chronic kidney disease and anemia. N Engl J Med 2006;355(20):2071–2084.

47. Phrommintikul A, Haas SJ, Elsik M, Krum H. Mortality and target haemoglobin concentrations in anaemic patients with chronic kidney disease treated with erythropoietin: A meta-analysis. Lancet 2007;369(9559):381–388.

48. Szczech LA, Barnhart HX, Inrig JK, et al. Secondary analysis of the CHOIR trial epoetin-alpha dose and achieved hemoglobin outcomes. Kidney Int 2008;74(6):791–798.

49. Kilpatrick RD, Critchlow CW, Fishbane S, et al. Greater epoetin alfa responsiveness is associated with improved survival in hemodialysis patients. Clin J Am Soc Nephrol 2008;3(4):1077–1083.

50. Zhang Y, Thamer M, Stefanik K, et al. Epoetin requirements predict mortality in hemodialysis patients. Am J Kidney Dis 2004;44(5):866–876.

51. Unger EF, Thompson AM, Blank MJ, Temple R. Erythropoiesis-stimulating agents—Time for a reevaluation. N Engl J Med 2010;362(3):189–192.

52. Pfeffer MA, Burdmann EA, Chen CY, et al. A trial of darbepoetin alfa in type 2 diabetes and chronic kidney disease. N Engl J Med 2009; 361(21):2019–2032.

53. Clinical practice guidelines and clinical practice recommendations for anemia in chronic kidney disease in adults. Am J Kidney Dis 2006;47(5 suppl 3):S16–85.

54. Danielson BG. Structure, chemistry, and pharmacokinetics of intravenous iron agents. J Am Soc Nephrol 2004;15(suppl 2):S93–98.

55. Ferrlecit. Package Insert. Corona, CA: Watson Pharma; 2006.

56. Feraheme. Package Insert. Lexington, MA: AMAG Pharmaceuticals; 2009.

57. Nissenson AR, Berns JS, Sakiewicz P, et al. Clinical evaluation of heme iron polypeptide: Sustaining a response to rHuEPO in hemodialysis patients. Am J Kidney Dis 2003;42(2):325–330.

58. Venofer. Package Insert. Shirley, NY: American Regent Laboratories; 2008.

59. Schiesser D, Binet I, Tsinalis D, et al. Weekly low-dose treatment with intravenous iron sucrose maintains iron status and decreases epoetin requirement in iron-replete haemodialysis patients. Nephrol Dial Transplant 2006;21(10):2841–2845.

60. Fishbane S. Safety in iron management. Am J Kidney Dis 2003;41(5 suppl):18–26.

61. Chertow GM, Mason PD, Vaage-Nilsen O, Ahlmen J. Update on adverse drug events associated with parenteral iron. Nephrol Dial Transplant 2006;21(2):378–382.

62. Dexferrum. Package Insert. Shirley, NY: American Regent Laboratories; 2008.

63. In FeD. Package Insert. Florham Park, NJ: Watson Pharma; 2009.

64. Singh A, Patel T, Hertel J, et al. Safety of ferumoxytol in patients with anemia and CKD. Am J Kidney Dis 2008;52(5):907–915.

65. Auerbach M, Winchester J, Wahab A, et al. A randomized trial of three iron dextran infusion methods for anemia in EPO-treated dialysis patients. Am J Kidney Dis 1998;31(1):81–86.

66. Dahdah K, Patrie JT, Bolton WK. Intravenous iron dextran treatment in predialysis patients with chronic renal failure. Am J Kidney Dis 2000;36(4):775–782.

67. Folkert VW, Michael B, Agarwal R, et al. Chronic use of sodium ferric gluconate complex in hemodialysis patients: Safety of higher-dose (> or = 250 mg) administration. Am J Kidney Dis 2003;41(3): 651–657.

68. Blaustein DA, Schwenk MH, Chattopadhyay J, et al. The safety and efficacy of an accelerated iron sucrose dosing regimen in patients with chronic kidney disease. Kidney Int Suppl 2003;(87): S72–77.

69. Chandler G, Harchowal J, Macdougall IC. Intravenous iron sucrose: Establishing a safe dose. Am J Kidney Dis 2001;38(5):988–991.

70. Provenzano R, Schiller B, Rao M, et al. Ferumoxytol as an intravenous iron replacement therapy in hemodialysis patients. Clin J Am Soc Nephrol 2009;4(2):386–393.

71. Spinowitz BS, Kausz AT, Baptista J, et al. Ferumoxytol for treating iron deficiency anemia in CKD. J Am Soc Nephrol 2008;19(8): 1599–1605.

72. Hayat A. Safety issues with intravenous iron products in the management of anemia in chronic kidney disease. Clin Med Res 2008;6(3–4):93–102.

73. Aronoff GR. Safety of intravenous iron in clinical practice: implications for anemia management protocols. J Am Soc Nephrol 2004;15(suppl 2):S99–106.

74. Aranesp. Package Insert. Thousand Oaks, CA: Amgen; 2008.

75. Macdougall IC, Padhi D, Jang G. Pharmacology of darbepoetin alfa. Nephrol Dial Transplant 2007;22(suppl 4):iv2–iv9.

76. Epogen. Package Insert. Thousand Oaks, CA: Amgen; 2008.

77. Besarab A. Optimizing anaemia management with subcutaneous administration of epoetin. Nephrol Dial Transplant 2005;20(suppl 6):vi10–5.

78. Macdougall IC, Gray SJ, Elston O, et al. Pharmacokinetics of novel erythropoiesis stimulating protein compared with epoetin alfa in dialysis patients. J Am Soc Nephrol 1999;10(11): 2392–2395.

79. Theodoridis M, Passadakis P, Kriki P, et al. Efficient monthly subcutaneous administration of darbepoetin in stable CAPD patients. Perit Dial Int 2005;25(6):564–569.

80. Agarwal AK, Silver MR, Reed JE, et al. An open-label study of darbepoetin alfa administered once monthly for the maintenance of haemoglobin concentrations in patients with chronic kidney disease not receiving dialysis. J Intern Med 2006;260(6):577–585.

81. Wish JB. Past, present, and future of chronic kidney disease anemia management in the United States. Adv Chronic Kidney Dis 2009;16(2):101–108.

82. Procrit. Package Insert. Raritan, NJ: Ortho Biotech; 2008.

83. Lee YK, Koo JR, Kim JK, et al. Effect of route of EPO administration on hemodialysis arteriovenous vascular access failure: A randomized controlled trial. Am J Kidney Dis 2009;53(5):815–822.

84. Pollock C, Johnson DW, Horl WH, et al. Pure red cell aplasia induced by erythropoiesis-stimulating agents. Clin J Am Soc Nephrol 2008;3(1):193–199.

85. Macdougall IC, Rossert J, Casadevall N, et al. A peptide-based erythropoietin-receptor agonist for pure red-cell aplasia. N Engl J Med 2009;361(19):1848–1855.

86. Provenzano R, Garcia-Mayol L, Suchinda P, et al. Once-weekly epoetin alfa for treating the anemia of chronic kidney disease. Clin Nephrol 2004;61(6):392–405.

87. Spinowitz B, Germain M, Benz R, et al. A randomized study of extended dosing regimens for initiation of epoetin alfa treatment for anemia of chronic kidney disease. Clin J Am Soc Nephrol 2008;3(4):1015–1021.

88. NKF-K/DOQI Clinical Practice Guidelines for Anemia of Chronic Kidney Disease: update 2000. Am J Kidney Dis 2001;37(1 suppl 1):S182–238.

89. Moe SM, Drueke TB. Management of secondary hyperparathyroidism: the importance and the challenge of controlling parathyroid hormone levels without elevating calcium, phosphorus, and calcium-phosphorus product. Am J Nephrol 2003;23(6):369–379.

90. Pai AB, Shepler BM. Comparison of sevelamer hydrochloride and sevelamer carbonate: risk of metabolic acidosis and clinical implications. Pharmacotherapy 2009;29(5):554–561.

91. Delmez J, Block G, Robertson J, et al. A randomized, double-blind, crossover design study of sevelamer hydrochloride and sevelamer carbonate in patients on hemodialysis. Clin Nephrol 2007;68(6):386–391.

92. Block GA, Spiegel DM, Ehrlich J, et al. Effects of sevelamer and calcium on coronary artery calcification in patients new to hemodialysis. Kidney Int 2005;68(4):1815–1824.

93. Qunibi W, Moustafa M, Muenz LR, et al. A 1-year randomized trial of calcium acetate versus sevelamer on progression of coronary artery calcification in hemodialysis patients with comparable lipid control: The Calcium Acetate Renagel Evaluation-2 (CARE-2) study. Am J Kidney Dis 2008;51(6):952–965.

94. Hutchison AJ, Maes B, Vanwalleghem J, et al. Long-term efficacy and tolerability of lanthanum carbonate: Results from a 3-year study. Nephron Clin Pract 2006;102(2):c61–71.

95. Joy MS, Kshirsagar A, Candiani C, et al. Lanthanum carbonate. Ann Pharmacother 2006;40(2):234–240.

96. Sprague SM, Ross EA, Nath SD, et al. Lanthanum carbonate vs. sevelamer hydrochloride for the reduction of serum phosphorus in hemodialysis patients: A crossover study. Clin Nephrol 2009; 72(4):252–258.

97. Renvela. Package Insert. Cambridge, MA: Genzyme Corporation; 2009.

98. Guillen-Anaya MA, Jadoul M. Drug interaction between sevelamer and cyclosporin. Nephrol Dial Transplant 2004;19(2):515.

99. Capitanini A, Lupi A, Osteri F, et al. Gastric pH, sevelamer hydrochloride and omeprazole. Clin Nephrol 2005;64(4):320–322.

100. Fosrenol. Package Insert. Wayne, PA: Shire U.S. Inc.; 2008.

101. Andress D. Nonclassical aspects of differential vitamin D receptor activation: Implications for survival in patients with chronic kidney disease. Drugs 2007;67(14):1999–2012.

102. Zemplar Capsules Package Insert. Abbott Park, IL: Abbott Laboratories Inc.; 2009.

103. Bailie GR, Johnson CA. Comparative review of the pharmacokinetics of vitamin D analogues. Semin Dial 2002;15(5):352–357.

104. Brown AJ, Finch J, Slatopolsky E. Differential effects of 19-nor-1,25-dihydroxyvitamin D(2) and 1,25-dihydroxyvitamin D(3) on intestinal calcium and phosphate transport. J Lab Clin Med 2002;139(5):279–284.

105. Joist HE, Ahya SN, Giles K, et al. Differential effects of very high doses of doxercalciferol and paricalcitol on serum phosphorus in hemodialysis patients. Clin Nephrol 2006;65(5):335–341.

106. Lund RJ, Andress DL, Amdahl M, et al. Differential effects of paricalcitol and calcitriol on intestinal calcium absorption in hemodialysis patients. Am J Nephrol 2009;31(2):165–170.

107. Coburn JW, Maung HM, Elangovan L, et al. Doxercalciferol safely suppresses PTH levels in patients with secondary hyperparathyroidism associated with chronic kidney disease stages 3 and 4. Am J Kidney Dis 2004;43(5):877–890.

108. Coyne D, Acharya M, Qiu P, et al. Paricalcitol capsule for the treatment of secondary hyperparathyroidism in stages 3 and 4 CKD. Am J Kidney Dis 2006;47(2):263–276.

109. Sprague SM, Llach F, Amdahl M, et al. Paricalcitol versus calcitriol in the treatment of secondary hyperparathyroidism. Kidney Int 2003;63(4):1483–1490.

110. Teng M, Wolf M, Lowrie E, et al. Survival of patients undergoing hemodialysis with paricalcitol or calcitriol therapy. N Engl J Med 2003;349(5):446–456.

111. Teng M, Wolf M, Ofsthun MN, et al. Activated injectable vitamin D and hemodialysis survival: A historical cohort study. J Am Soc Nephrol 2005;16(4):1115–1125.

112. Tentori F, Hunt WC, Stidley CA, et al. Mortality risk among hemodialysis patients receiving different vitamin D analogs. Kidney Int 2006;70(10):1858–1865.

113. Agarwal R, Acharya M, Tian J, et al. Antiproteinuric effect of oral paricalcitol in chronic kidney disease. Kidney Int 2005;68(6):2823–2828.

114. Zemplar Injection Package Insert. Abbott Park, IL: Abbott Laboratories Inc.; 2009.

115. Hudson JQ. Secondary hyperparathyroidism in chronic kidney disease: Focus on clinical consequences and vitamin D therapies. Ann Pharmacother 2006;40(9):1584–1593.

116. Quarles LD. Cinacalcet HCl: A novel treatment for secondary hyperparathyroidism in stage 5 chronic kidney disease. Kidney Int Suppl 2005;(96):S24–28.

117. Sensipar (cinacalcet HCl) Tablets Package Insert. Thousand Oaks, CA: Amgen Inc.; 2009.

118. Abosaif NY, Arije A, Atray NK, et al. K/DOQI clinical practice guidelines on hypertension and antihypertensive agents in chronic kidney disease. Am J Kidney Dis 2004;43(5 suppl 1):S1–290.

119. Executive Summary of The Third Report of The National Cholesterol Education Program (NCEP) Expert Panel on Detection, Evaluation, and Treatment of High Blood Cholesterol in Adults (Adult Treatment Panel III). JAMA 2001;285(19):2486–2497.

120. Harper CR, Jacobson TA. Managing dyslipidemia in chronic kidney disease. J Am Coll Cardiol 2008;51(25):2375–2384.

121. Koren MJ, Davidson MH, Wilson DJ, et al. Focused atorvastatin therapy in managed-care patients with coronary heart disease and CKD. Am J Kidney Dis 2009;53(5):741–750.

122. Shepherd J, Kastelein JJ, Bittner V, et al. Intensive lipid lowering with atorvastatin in patients with coronary heart disease and chronic kidney disease: The TNT (Treating to New Targets) study. J Am Coll Cardiol 2008;51(15):1448–1454.

123. Andreucci VE, Fissell RB, Bragg-Gresham JL, et al. Dialysis Outcomes and Practice Patterns Study (DOPPS) data on medications in hemodialysis patients. Am J Kidney Dis 2004;44(5 suppl 2):61–67.

124. Wanner C, Krane V, Marz W, et al. Atorvastatin in patients with type 2 diabetes mellitus undergoing hemodialysis. N Engl J Med 2005;353(3):238–248.

125. Fellstrom BC, Jardine AG, Schmieder RE, et al. Rosuvastatin and cardiovascular events in patients undergoing hemodialysis. N Engl J Med 2009;360(14):1395–1407.

126. Baigent C, Landry M. Study of Heart and Renal Protection (SHARP). Kidney Int Suppl 2003;(84):S207–210.

127. Heerspink HJ, Ninomiya T, Zoungas S, et al. Effect of lowering blood pressure on cardiovascular events and mortality in patients on dialysis: A systematic review and meta-analysis of randomised controlled trials. Lancet 2009;373(9668):1009–1015.

128. Matera M, Bellinghieri G, Costantino G, et al. History of L-carnitine: implications for renal disease. J Ren Nutr 2003;13(1):2–14.

129. Kaw D, Malhotra D. Platelet dysfunction and end-stage renal disease. Semin Dial 2006;19(4):317–322.

130. Joy MS, DeHart RM, Gilmartin C, et al. Clinical pharmacists as multidisciplinary health care providers in the management of CKD: A joint opinion by the Nephrology and Ambulatory Care Practice and Research Networks of the American College of Clinical Pharmacy. Am J Kidney Dis 2005;45(6):1105–1118.

131. Besarab A, Goodkin DA, Nissenson AR. The normal hematocrit study—Follow-up. N Engl J Med 2008;358(4):433–434.

CHAPTER 54

Hemodialysis and Peritoneal Dialysis

KEVIN M. SOWINSKI AND MARIANN D. CHURCHWELL

KEY CONCEPTS

❶ The hemodialysis procedure involves the perfusion of blood and dialysate on opposite sides of a semipermeable membrane. Substances are removed from the blood by diffusion and convection. Excess plasma water is removed via ultrafiltration.

❷ The native arteriovenous fistula is the preferred access for hemodialysis because of fewer complications and a longer survival rate. Venous catheters are plagued by complications such as infection and thrombosis and often deliver relatively poor blood flow rates.

❸ Adequacy of hemodialysis can be assessed by the Kt/V and urea reduction ratio (URR). The National Kidney Foundation's Kidney Disease Outcomes Quality Initiative has set the minimum goal Kt/V at greater than 1.2 per treatment and the URR at greater than 65%. In practice, most patients on hemodialysis exceed this goal.

❹ During hemodialysis, patients commonly experience hypotension and cramps. Other more serious complications include infection and thrombosis of the vascular access.

❺ The peritoneal dialysis procedure involves the instillation of dialysate into the peritoneal cavity via a permanent peritoneal catheter. The peritoneal membrane lines the highly vascularized abdominal viscera and acts as the semipermeable membrane across which diffusion and ultrafiltration occur. Substances are removed from the blood across the peritoneum via diffusion and ultrafiltration. Excess plasma water is removed via ultrafiltration created by osmotic pressure generated by various dextrose or icodextrin concentrations.

❻ Patients on peritoneal dialysis are required to instill and drain, manually or via automated systems, several liters of fresh dialysate each day. The more exchanges a patient completes each day, the greater the solute removal.

❼ Patients on peritoneal dialysis are required to instill and drain, manually or via automated systems, several liters of fresh dialysate each day. The more exchanges a patient completes each day, the greater the solute removal.

❽ Nasal carriage of *Staphylococcus* aureus is associated with an increased risk of catheter-related infections and peritonitis. Prophylaxis with intranasal mupirocin (twice a day for 5 days every month) or mupirocin (daily) at the exit site can effectively reduce S. aureus infections.

The three primary treatment options for patients with end-stage renal disease (ESRD) are hemodialysis (HD), peritoneal dialysis (PD), and kidney transplantation. The United States Renal Data System (USRDS) is the national system that "collects, analyzes, and distributes" data relating to patients with ESRD or stage 5 chronic kidney disease (CKD) in the U.S.[1] According to the 2009 USRDS, at the end of 2007, there were more than 527,000 patients in the United States with ESRD. Of these, 341,264 and 26,340 patients were being treated with HD and PD, respectively, and 151,502 had a functioning kidney transplant. In 2007, nearly 111,000 new patients started therapy for ESRD (dialysis or transplantation) and over 88,000 patients died. The vast majority of new dialysis patients are treated with HD. The number of patients treated with PD has decreased by over 7% since 2000.[1] Although the number of patients who have received a kidney transplant has risen steadily, transplantation has not kept pace with the growing prevalence of ESRD in the United States.

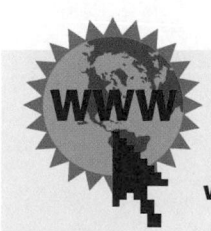

The complete chapter, learning objectives, and other resources can be found at **www.pharmacotherapyonline.com**.

THOMAS D. NOLIN AND JONATHAN HIMMELFARB

CHAPTER 55

Drug-Induced Kidney Disease

KEY CONCEPTS

❶ The initial diagnosis of drug-induced kidney disease typically involves detection of elevated serum creatinine and blood urea nitrogen, for which there is a temporal relationship between the toxicity and use of a potentially nephrotoxic drug.

❷ Drug-induced kidney disease is best prevented by avoiding the use of potentially nephrotoxic agents for patients at increased risk for toxicity. However, when exposure to these drugs cannot be avoided, recognition of risk factors and specific techniques, such as hydration, may be used to reduce potential nephrotoxicity.

❸ Acute tubular necrosis is the most common presentation of drug-induced kidney disease in hospitalized patients. The primary agents implicated are aminoglycosides, radiocontrast media, cisplatin, amphotericin B, and osmotically active agents.

❹ Angiotensin-converting enzyme inhibitors and nonsteroidal antiinflammatory drugs are associated with hemodynamically-mediated kidney injury, the pathogenesis of which is a decrease in glomerular capillary hydrostatic pressure.

❺ Acute allergic interstitial nephritis is observed in up to 27% of kidney biopsies performed for hospitalized patients with unexplained acute kidney injury. Clinical manifestations of allergic interstitial nephritis typically present approximately 14 days after initiation of therapy and include fever, maculopapular rash, eosinophilia, arthralgia, often with pyuria, hematuria, proteinuria, and oliguria.

Numerous diagnostic and therapeutic agents have been associated with the development of drug-induced kidney disease (DIKD) or nephrotoxicity. It is a relatively common complication with variable presentations depending on the drug and clinical setting, inpatient or outpatient. Manifestations of DIKD include acid–base abnormalities, electrolyte imbalances, urine sediment abnormalities, proteinuria, pyuria, and/or hematuria.[1] However, the most common manifestation of DIKD is a decline in the glomerular filtration rate (GFR), which results in a rise in serum creatinine (S_{cr}) and blood urea nitrogen (BUN) and several other indicators of acute

Learning objectives, review questions, and other resources can be found at **www.pharmacotherapyonline.com**.

and chronic kidney injury (see Chaps. 50 and 51). Initial diagnosis of DIKD is often delayed as it typically is based on the detection of elevated S_{cr} and BUN, for which there is a temporal relationship between the kidney injury and exposure to the potentially nephrotoxic drug. This is consistent with classic qualitative definitions of acute renal failure, which have relied on either an abrupt increase in S_{cr} or an abrupt decline in urine output (see Chaps. 50 and 51).[2] The clinical use of numerous definitions of acute renal failure and nephrotoxicity based on quantitative changes in the S_{cr} concentration and other clinical end points made it extraordinarily difficult to ascertain their true incidence.[3] Relatively new diagnostic criteria based on a combination of physiologic measurements (e.g., S_{cr} and urine output) have been recently introduced and are now being incorporated into clinical practice and research.[4–6] This has resulted in replacement of the term *acute renal failure* with *acute kidney injury* (AKI) and will likely lead to epidemiologic data about DIKD that are more accurate in the future.

Nephrotoxicity is often reversible if one discontinues the use of the offending agent, but in some cases there may still be an AKI and progression to stage 5 chronic kidney disease (CKD) which is also termed *end-stage renal disease* (ESRD). Currently, many different mechanisms are responsible for the pathogenesis of DIKD, and the introduction of new drugs with novel mechanisms of action provides the potential for the identification of new presentations of AKI and CKD. This chapter reviews the epidemiology, pathophysiology, risk factors, and basic principles of prevention of DIKD. Detailed discussions of these issues plus management strategies are presented for the most commonly used agents that have been associated with a moderate to high likelihood of DIKD.

EPIDEMIOLOGY

The incidence and characteristics of outpatient or community-acquired DIKD are not well understood since mild toxicity is often unrecognized in this setting. However, the acquisition of data regarding the pharmacoepidemiology of these effects has become more important as care increasingly shifts to the outpatient setting. The incidence of community-based AKI that required dialysis was recently reported to be 29.5 per 100,000 person years and 522.4 per 100,000 person years for patients not requiring dialysis.[7] Although the incidence of drug-induced AKI was not specifically reported, earlier studies have implicated community-acquired DIKD in up to 20% of hospital admissions due to AKI.[8] Conversely, AKI has been reported in up to 7% of hospitalized patients,[9] and as many as 20% to 30% of critically ill patients may experience AKI during their hospitalization.[10,11] Drug-induced causes have been implicated in up to 60% of all cases of in-hospital AKI and as such are a recognized source of significant morbidity and mortality.[12] Although the incidence of in-hospital antibiotic-induced AKI alone has been reported to be as high as 36%,[1] it appears to be declining, while cases of in-hospital AKI due to nonselective nonsteroidal antiinflammatory drugs (NSAIDs), angiotensin-converting enzyme inhibitors (ACEIs), chemotherapeutic agents, and antiviral drugs are increasing.[2]

CLINICAL PRESENTATION OF DRUG-INDUCED KIDNEY DISEASE

General

- The most common manifestation is a decline in GFR leading to a rise in S_{cr} and BUN.
- Alterations in renal tubular function without loss of glomerular filtration may be evident.

Symptoms

- Patients may complain of malaise, anorexia, vomiting, shortness of breath, or edema, particularly in the outpatient setting.

Signs

- Decreased urine output may be an early sign of toxicity, particularly with radiographic contrast media, NSAIDs, and ACEIs, with progression to volume overload and hypertension.
- Proximal tubular injury: Metabolic acidosis with bicarbonaturia; glycosuria in the absence of hyperglycemia; and reductions in serum phosphate, uric acid, potassium, and magnesium due to increased urinary losses.
- Distal tubular injury: Polyuria from failure to maximally concentrate urine, metabolic acidosis from impaired urinary acidification, and hyperkalemia from impaired potassium excretion.

Laboratory Tests

- An abrupt (within 48 hours) reduction in kidney function defined as an absolute increase in S_{cr} of ≥0.3 mg/dL (27 µmol/L), a percentage increase in S_{cr} of ≥50% (1.5-fold from baseline), or a reduction in urine output (documented oliguria of less than 0.5 ml/kg per hour for more than 6 hours)],[13] when correlated temporally with the initiation of drug therapy may indicate drug-induced AKI.

Other Diagnostic Tests

- Urinary excretion of N-acetyl-β-D-glucosaminidase, γ-glutamyl transpeptidase, glutathione S-transferase, and interleukin (IL)-18 are markers of proximal tubular injury and have been used for the early detection of AKI in critically ill patients.
- Kidney injury molecule-1 (KIM-1) is expressed in the proximal tubule and is upregulated for patients with ischemic acute tubular necrosis, appearing in the urine within 12 hours after the ischemic insult.
- Neutrophil gelatinase-associated lipocalin (NGAL) protein may be detected in the urine within 3 hours of ischemic injury.

❶ Because the most common manifestation of DIKD is a decline in GFR leading to a rise in S_{cr} and BUN, the onset of toxicity in hospitalized, acutely ill patients is most often recognized by routine laboratory monitoring. Decreased urine output may also be an early sign of toxicity, particularly with radiographic contrast media, NSAIDs, and ACEIs. In the outpatient setting, nephrotoxicity is often recognized by the development of symptoms such as malaise, anorexia, vomiting, volume overload (shortness of breath or edema),

and hypertension. S_{cr} or BUN concentrations and urine collection for creatinine clearance may subsequently be measured to quantify the degree of decline in GFR. Marked intrasubject between-day variability of S_{cr} values have been noted (±20% for values within the normal range; see Chap. 50). Furthermore, they may be altered as the result of dietary changes and initiation of drug therapy, which may interfere with the assay procedure. Thus changes in S_{cr} or urine output consistent with the diagnostic criteria for AKI (see Chap. 51),[13] when correlated temporally with the initiation of drug therapy, are a common threshold for the identification of DIKD.

Nephrotoxicity may also be evidenced by primary alterations in renal tubular function without a corresponding loss of glomerular filtration (Table 55–1). In this setting, urinary enzymes and low-molecular-weight proteins may be used as earlier and more specific biomarkers of nephrotoxicity compared with S_{cr} and BUN, which are relatively insensitive markers of kidney injury.[14] S_{cr} and BUN are used as surrogates of kidney function, not injury per se, and typically significant kidney injury must have occured days before a rise in either is evident. Urinary excretion of kidney injury molecule-1 (KIM-1), N-acetyl-β-glucosaminidase, γ-glutamyl transpeptidase, glutathione S-transferase, neutrophil gelatinase-associated lipocalin (NGAL), and interleukin-18 are markers of proximal tubular injury and have been used for the early detection of acute kidney damage

TABLE 55–1	Drug-Induced Renal Structural–Functional Alterations and Examples
Tubular epithelial cell damage	
Acute tubular necrosis	• Pentamidine
• Aminoglycoside antibiotics	• Foscarnet
• Radiographic contrast media	• Zoledronate
• Cisplatin, carboplatin	Osmotic nephrosis
• Amphotericin B	• Mannitol
• Cyclosporine, tacrolimus	• Dextran
• Adefovir, cidofovir, tenofovir	• Intravenous immunoglobulin
Hemodynamically-mediated kidney injury	
• Angiotensin-converting enzyme inhibitors	• Nonsteroidal anti-inflammatory drugs
	• Cyclosporine, tacrolimus
• Angiotensin II receptor blockers	• OKT3
Obstructive nephropathy	
Intratubular obstruction	Nephrolithiasis
• Acyclovir	• Sulfonamides
• Sulfonamides	• Triamterene
• Indinavir	• Indinavir
• Foscarnet	Nephrocalcinosis
• Methotrexate	• Oral sodium phosphate solution
Glomerular disease	
• Gold	• Nonsteroidal antiinflammatory drugs, cyclooxygenase-2 inhibitors
• Lithium	
	• Pamidronate
Tubulointerstitial disease	
Acute allergic interstitial nephritis	Chronic interstitial nephritis
• Penicillins	• Cyclosporine
• Ciprofloxacin	• Lithium
• Nonsteroidal anti-inflammatory drugs, cyclooxygenase-2 inhibitors	• Aristolochic acid
	Papillary necrosis
• Proton pump inhibitors	• NSAIDs, combined phenacetin, aspirin, and caffeine analgesics
• Loop diuretics	
Renal vasculitis, thrombosis, and cholesterol emboli	
Vasculitis and thrombosis	• Methamphetamines
• Hydralazine	• Cyclosporine, tacrolimus
• Propylthiouracil	• Adalimumab
• Allopurinol	• Bevacizumab
• Penicillamine	Cholesterol emboli
• Gemcitabine	• Warfarin
• Mitomycin C	• Thrombolytic agents

in several patient populations.[14-16] For example, the transmembrane protein KIM-1 is upregulated for patients with ischemic acute tubular necrosis, appearing in the urine within 12 hours after the ischemic insult.[16] Urinary N-acetylglucosamine (NAG) concentrations are a highly sensitive indicator of AKI and have been shown to detect AKI in critically ill patients up to 4 days prior to a rise in S_{cr} was observed.[16] Similarly, urinary NGAL is an early marker of AKI, preceding a rise in S_{cr} by up to 3 days. In the future, urinary biomarkers such as KIM-1, NAG, and NGAL may facilitate the earlier detection of kidney injury and diagnosis of nephrotoxicity and minimize the long-term consequences of this common drug-induced disorder.[14,16]

PRINCIPLES FOR PREVENTION OF DRUG-INDUCED NEPHROPATHY

❷ The primary principle for prevention of DIKD is to avoid the use of nephrotoxic agents for patients at increased risk for toxicity. Therefore, an awareness of potentially nephrotoxic drugs and knowledge of risk factors that increase renal vulnerability is essential.[17] Exposure to these drugs often cannot be avoided, so several interventions have been proposed to reduce the potential for the development of nephrotoxicity, for example, adjustment of medication dosage regimens based on accurate estimates of renal function, and careful and adequate hydration to establish high urine flow rates.[12,18] Other preventative strategies are still theoretical and/or investigational and relate directly to the specific nephrotoxic mechanisms of a given drug. For example, cidofovir and adefovir are antiretroviral drugs that are actively transported by human organic anion transporter 1 (OAT1).[1,19] Competitive inhibition of OAT1-mediated transport with probenecid minimizes intracellular accumulation of cidofovir and adefovir in renal proximal tubule cells and reduces the likelihood of nephrotoxicity.[1,20]

Table 55-1 lists the several specific drug-induced renal structural–functional alterations that are responsible for the vast majority of cases of DIKD. This chapter discusses the pathophysiologic mechanisms responsible for the development of DIKD with these agents in detail, along with clinical presentation, prevention strategies, therapeutic management approaches, and relevant monitoring plans.

TUBULAR EPITHELIAL CELL DAMAGE

❸ Drugs that lead to renal tubular epithelial cell damage typically do so via direct cellular toxicity or ischemia. Damage is most often localized in the proximal and distal tubular epithelia and is termed *acute tubular necrosis* (ATN) when cellular degeneration and sloughing from proximal and distal tubular basement membranes are observed.[21,22] This classically manifests as cellular debris-filled, muddy-brown, granular casts in the urinary sediment.[22,23] Specific indicators of proximal tubular injury include metabolic acidosis with bicarbonaturia; glycosuria in the absence of hyperglycemia; and reductions in serum phosphate, uric acid, potassium, and magnesium as a result of increased urinary losses. Indicators of distal tubular injury include polyuria from failure to maximally concentrate urine (i.e., nephrogenic diabetes insipidus), metabolic acidosis from impaired urinary acidification, and hyperkalemia from impaired potassium excretion.[1] ATN is the most common presentation of DIKD in the inpatient setting. The primary agents associated with this type of injury are aminoglycosides, radiocontrast media, cisplatin, amphotericin B, foscarnet, and osmotically active agents such as immunoglobulins, dextrans, and mannitol.[1,11,24,25]

ACUTE TUBULAR NECROSIS

Aminoglycoside Nephrotoxicity

Incidence Aminoglycoside antibiotic-associated nephrotoxicity has been reported to occur in between 10% and 25% of patients receiving a therapeutic course.[11,26,27] Critically ill patients appear to have a higher risk for nephrotoxicity with reported rates as high as 58%.[26] The large variance is in part a result of the use of different definitions of toxicity, variability between agents in the class, and the risk factors present in the study population.

Clinical Presentation Clinical evidence of aminoglycoside-associated nephrotoxicity is typically seen within 5 to 10 days after initiation of therapy and manifests as a gradual progressive rise in S_{cr} and BUN and decrease in creatinine clearance.[11] Patients usually present with nonoliguria, i.e., they maintain urine volumes greater than 500 mL/day and sometimes have microscopic hematuria and proteinuria.[11,25] Although renal magnesium wasting can occur (i.e., daily excretion of more than 10 to 30 mg), the risk of symptomatic hypomagnesemia is generally low. Full recovery of renal function is common if aminoglycoside therapy is discontinued immediately upon discovering signs of toxicity.[11] However, severe AKI may develop occasionally, and for these individuals renal replacement therapy may be required (see Chap. 51). The diagnosis of aminoglycoside-associated nephrotoxicity is often difficult, particularly in critically ill patients with multiple comorbidities and is confounded by other factors that are independently associated with the development of AKI.[26] For instance, concurrent dehydration, sepsis, hypotension, ischemia, and use of other nephrotoxic drugs frequently contribute to AKI in patients who are receiving aminoglycosides.[22]

Pathogenesis Aminoglycoside-associated ATN is primarily due to accumulation of high drug concentrations within proximal tubular epithelial cells, and subsequent generation of reactive oxygen species that produce mitochondrial injury, which leads to cellular apoptosis and necrosis.[17,25] This results in cell sloughing from proximal tubular basement membranes into the tubular lumen, which can result in tubular obstruction and back leakage of the glomerular filtrate across the damaged tubular epithelium. Toxicity is related to cationic charge of the drugs in this class, which facilitates their binding to negatively charged renal tubular epithelial membrane phospholipids in the proximal tubules, followed by intracellular transport and concentration in lysosomes. The number of cationic groups on the drug molecule appear to correlate with the degree of nephrotoxicity, which is consistent with the observation of higher rates of toxicity with neomycin versus gentamicin, followed by tobramycin, then amikacin.[1,11,17]

Risk Factors Multiple risk factors for aminoglycoside-associated nephrotoxicity have been identified: the aggressiveness of aminoglycoside dosing, synergistic toxicity as the result of combination drug therapy and preexisting clinical conditions of the patient (Table 55-2).[11,17,26]

Prevention Aminoglycoside-associated ATN may be prevented by careful and cautious selection of patients and the use of alternative antibiotics whenever possible and as soon as microbial sensitivities are known. Commonly used alternatives include fluoroquinolones (e.g., ciprofloxacin or levofloxacin) and third- or fourth-generation cephalosporins (e.g., ceftazidime or cefepime). When aminoglycosides are necessary, gentamicin, tobramycin, and amikacin are most commonly used, but therapy should be selected to optimize antimicrobial efficacy.[28] Furthermore, it is imperative to avoid volume depletion, limit the total aminoglycoside dose administered, and avoid concomitant therapy with other nephrotoxic drugs. Future therapeutic alternatives may include new aminoglycoside congeners that retain the desired bactericidal activity and yet are devoid

TABLE 55-2 Potential Risk Factors for Aminoglycoside Nephrotoxicity

A. Related to aminoglycoside dosing:
    Large total cumulative dose
    Prolonged therapy
    Trough concentration exceeding 2 mg/L[a]
    Recent previous aminoglycoside therapy
B. Related to synergistic nephrotoxicity. Aminoglycosides in combination with
    Cyclosporine
    Amphotericin B
    Vancomycin
    Diuretics
    Iodinated radiographic contrast agents
    Cisplatin
    NSAIDs
C. Related to predisposing conditions in the patient:
    Preexisting kidney disease
    Diabetes
    Increased age
    Poor nutrition
    Shock
    Gram-negative bacteremia
    Liver disease
    Hypoalbuminemia
    Obstructive jaundice
    Dehydration
    Hypotension
    Potassium or magnesium deficiencies

[a]The equivalent concentration in SI molar units are 4.3 μmol/L for tobramycin, 4.2 μmol/L for gentamicin, and 1.4 μmol/L for vancomycin.

of nephrotoxicity,[29] and may also include concurrent use of antioxidant compounds such as vitamin E and *N*-acetylcysteine.[30]

Prospective, individualized pharmacokinetic monitoring has been used for more than three decades, and its use has been associated with a decrease in the incidence of aminoglycoside-associated nephrotoxicity.[31] These studies, however, were often small and statistically underpowered. High-dose intermittent dosing of aminoglycosides, termed *once daily dosing*, used in combination with other antibiotics, has been intensively investigated as a practical cost-effective method to maintain antimicrobial efficacy while reducing AKI.[32] The reduction in incidence may be the result of limited proximal tubular aminoglycoside uptake during the transient, high-peak serum concentrations, and because of the presence of low aminoglycoside concentrations for a greater proportion of the dosing interval which facilitates excretion of the aminoglycoside.[28] Although greater clinical efficacy and reduced nephrotoxicity may be realized with once daily compared with standard dosing, seriously ill, immunocompromised, and elderly patients, as well as those with preexisting kidney disease, are not ideal candidates for this approach.[32]

Management Aminoglycoside use should be discontinued or the dosage regimen revised if AKI is evident [i.e., there is an S_{cr} increase of 0.5 mg/dL (44 μmol/L) or more that is not attributable to another cause]. Other nephrotoxic drugs should be discontinued if possible, and the patient should be maintained adequately hydrated and hemodynamically stable.[10] Short-term renal replacement therapy may be necessary, but ESRD has rarely been reported to be solely the result of aminoglycoside toxicity.

Radiographic Contrast Media Nephrotoxicity

Incidence The incidence of radiographic contrast media-induced nephrotoxicity (CIN) has declined over the last decade from approximately 15% to 7% of all patients receiving iodinated contrast; yet it remains the third leading cause of hospital-acquired AKI,

accounting for up to 11% of cases.[33,34] The incidence varies depending on the population studied and presence of risk factors; rising from <2% for patients with normal renal function up to 50% for patients with a high risk, such as those with CKD or diabetes mellitus.[35,36] As the number of risk factors associated with CIN increases, there is a proportional increase in the incidence of nephrotoxicity and in short- and long-term mortality rates.[34,37] A 5.5-fold increased risk of death has been reported for patients who develop CIN compared with those who do not, with the highest mortality rates observed for patients who develop AKI and require renal replacement therapy.[34,37] In-hospital and 2-year mortality rates of 36% and 81%, respectively, have been reported for patients who develop CIN and require dialysis; an in-hospital mortality rate of only 7% was observed in those with nephrotoxicity not requiring dialysis.[34]

Clinical Presentation CIN is usually transient in nature, presenting most commonly as nonoliguria with kidney injury apparent within the first 24 to 48 hours after the administration of contrast. The S_{cr} concentration usually peaks between 3 and 5 days after exposure, with recovery after 7 to 10 days.[33,35,38] However, irreversible oliguric (urine volume <500 mL/day) AKI requiring dialysis has been reported in high-risk patients.[37] Urinalysis typically reveals tubular enzymuria with hyaline and granular casts but may also be completely void of casts. The urine sodium concentration and fractional excretion of sodium are frequently low, with the latter typically <1% (<0.01).[1]

Pathogenesis The primary mechanisms by which contrast media induces nephrotoxicity are renal ischemia and direct cellular toxicity.[34,35] Renal ischemia likely results from systemic hypotension and simultaneous acute vasoconstriction caused by disruption of normal prostaglandin synthesis and the release of adenosine, endothelin, and other renal vasoconstrictors. Subsequently, a 50% sustained reduction in renal blood flow that lasts for several hours immediately following contrast administration may be evident.[34] This reduced renal blood flow leads to increased concentrations of contrast in the renal tubules and exacerbates the direct cytotoxicity and ATN. The extent of cellular toxicity is directly related to the duration of tubular cell exposure to contrast. Thus, preservation of high urinary flow rates with adequate hydration before, during, and after contrast administration is vital to keep renal blood flow as high as reasonably possible to minimize tubular cell exposure to the contrast agent.[34,35] In humans, plasma osmolality is normally between 275 and 290 mOsm/kg (275 and 290 mmol/kg). Since low- and high-osmolar contrast agents are hyperosmolar to plasma [i.e., 600 to 800 mOsm/kg (600 to 800 mmol/kg) and ~2,000 mOsm/kg (~2,000 mmol/kg)] respectively, their use may result in osmotic diuresis, dehydration, renal ischemia, and increased blood viscosity caused by red blood cell aggregation. Oxidative stress has also been implicated in the development of ATN after contrast administration,[39] which may explain the possible benefit of the antioxidant *N*-acetylcysteine.[40–42]

Risk Factors Decreased renal blood flow exacerbates the ischemic and direct cytotoxic effects of contrast media on the renal tubules. Therefore, preexisting kidney disease, particularly in those with estimated GFR <60 mL/min/1.73 m² (<0.58 mL/s/m²), is the most important risk factor present in up to 60% of patients who develop CIN.[34,35] Other patients' specific risk factors include conditions associated with decreased renal blood flow (i.e., congestive heart failure, dehydration/volume depletion, and hypotension), and patients with atherosclerosis and reduced effective circulating arterial blood volume appear to also have an elevated risk.[38,43] Diabetes is also a significant risk factor, likely due to coexisting kidney disease (diabetic nephropathy). The presence of multiple myeloma has traditionally been considered a relative contraindication for contrast use, but the risk appears to be associated with concomitant dehydration, kidney disease, or hypercalcemia rather than the diagnosis itself.[35] Larger volumes or doses of contrast and use of low- and high-osmolar contrast agents are also independent predictors of CIN. Intraarterial administration of contrast confers greater risk than intravenous administration.[34] Lastly, concurrent use of nephrotoxins and drugs that alter renal hemodynamics such as NSAIDs and ACEIs also increases risk.[38] Risk factors are additive, and there is a proportional increase in the incidence of CIN and associated mortality as the number of risk factors increases.[34,37]

Prevention CIN can be anticipated in the majority of patients who are at risk; so the use of preventative procedures is justified for virtually all patients. Table 55–3 lists the recommended interventions for prevention of contrast nephrotoxicity. All patients scheduled to receive contrast media should be assessed for risk factors, and the risk-to-benefit ratio should be considered.[33–35,38,41,43,44] High-risk patients can be identified by evaluating medical history and indication for the contrast study, along with their most recent S_{cr} concentrations. Nephrotoxicity is best prevented in high-risk patients by using alternative imaging procedures (e.g., ultrasound, noncontrast magnetic resonance imaging, and nuclear medicine scans).[41] However, if contrast media must be used, the smallest adequate volume should be administered. If the ratio of the volume of contrast to be infused relative to the patient's creatinine clearance is ≥3.7 (≥222 if creatinine clearance is expressed in units of milliliters per second), the likelihood of nephrotoxicity is markedly increased.[45] Therefore, in general, the volume of contrast (in milliliters per second) administered should not be greater than twice the baseline estimated creatinine clearance.[34]

Low-osmolar (600 to 800 mOsm/kg; 600 to 800 mmol/kg) nonionic (iohexol and iopamidol) and ionic (ioxaglate) contrast agents may be used to prevent or minimize the incidence of nephrotoxicity. Standard hyperosmolar contrast media (e.g., low- and high-osmolar agent) are not reabsorbed in the kidney and cause osmotic diuresis, which contributes to the renal toxicity observed with these agents. Low-osmolar contrast agents have less than half the osmolality of high-osmolar (~2,000 mOsm/kg; ~2,000 mmol/kg) agents and are associated with less toxicity, especially when used for patients with preexisting kidney disease.[46] However, use of low-osmolar agents does not preclude the development of nephrotoxicity. Even low-osmolar agents are hyperosmolar to plasma, which is likely the reason they are associated with greater nephrotoxicity than the iso-osmolar nonionic contrast agent iodixanol.[47] Iodixanol has been shown to have the lowest risk for CIN for patients with CKD and diabetes.[34,46]

CLINICAL CONTROVERSY

Some clinicians believe that low- or iso-osmolar contrast media should be used for virtually all patients at risk for toxicity. Others believe that the cost-to-benefit ratio of using low-osmolar contrast agents to prevent nephrotoxicity is questionable except for patients at high risk.

Volume expansion and correction of dehydration prior to contrast administration is a mainstay of preventive therapy.[41,48] Parenteral hydration with isotonic saline before and after contrast administration reduces the incidence of toxicity, particularly in high-risk patients, and is currently the most widely accepted preventative intervention.[35,48] Volume expansion may exert its beneficial effects through dilution of contrast media, prevention of renal vasoconstriction leading to ischemia, preservation of high urine flow rates, decreased tubular cell exposure to contrast, and avoidance of tubular obstruction.[48] Hydration with isotonic sodium bicarbonate has been shown to provide more protection than saline, perhaps by reducing the formation of pH-dependent oxygen free radicals,[49,50] but recent studies reported contradictory findings.[41,51] Larger, adequately powered studies are needed to confirm these findings and to demonstrate conclusively that bicarbonate based hydration is superior to saline.[48] The use of oral hydration regimens has also been proposed but also requires further study to clarify its role and is not currently recommended in lieu of parenteral hydration.[41,48]

N-acetylcysteine is a thiol-containing antioxidant that may effectively reduce the risk of developing CIN for patients with preexisting kidney disease. Despite the publication of more than 30 clinical trials and 10 metaanalyses, a therapeutic benefit of NAC has not been consistently demonstrated, and its therapeutic role remains controversial.[41,42] Nevertheless, its use should be considered, along with hydration, for all patients who are at high risk of toxicity.[35,40,42,44,50,52] The recommended *N*-acetylcysteine dosing regimen for prevention of CIN is to give four doses of 600 mg to 1,200 mg orally every 12 hours, with the first dose administered prior to contrast exposure (see Table 55–3).[34,42,50,52] Finally, other nephrotoxic drugs should be discontinued if possible, and subsequent contrast studies appropriately timed to minimize cumulative toxicity.

TABLE 55–3	Recommended Interventions for Prevention of Contrast Nephrotoxicity[33,34,42,48,50,52]	
Intervention	**Recommendation**	**Recommendation Grade**[a]
Contrast	• Minimize contrast volume/dose	A-1
	• Use noniodinated contrast studies	A-2
	• Use low- or iso-osmolar contrast agents	A-2
Medications	• Avoid concurrent use of potentially nephrotoxic drugs, e.g., NSAIDs, aminoglycosides	A-2
Isotonic sodium chloride (0.9%)	• Initiate infusion 3–12 hours prior to contrast exposure and continue 6–24 hours postexposure	A-1
	• Infuse at 1–1.5 mL/kg/h adjusting postexposure as needed to maintain urine flow rate of ≥150 mL/h	
	• Alternatively, in urgent cases, initiate infusion at 3 mL/kg/h, beginning 1 hour prior to contrast exposure, then continue at 1 mL/kg/h for 6 hours postexposure	
Isotonic sodium bicarbonate [154 mEq/L (154 mmol/L)]	• Initiate and maintain infusion as per isotonic sodium chloride above	B-2
	• Alternatively, initiate infusion at 3 mL/kg/h, beginning 1 hour prior to contrast exposure, then continue at 1 mL/kg/h for 6 hours postexposure	
N-acetylcysteine	• Administer 600–1,200 mg by mouth (PO) every 12 hours, 4 doses beginning prior to contrast exposure (i.e., 1 dose prior to exposure and 3 doses postexposure)	B-1

[a]Strength of recommendations: A, B, and C are good, moderate, and poor evidence to support recommendation, respectively. Quality of evidence: 1, evidence from more than 1 properly randomized, controlled trial; 2, evidence from more than 1 well-designed clinical trial with randomization, from cohort or case-controlled analytic studies or multiple time series, or dramatic results from uncontrolled experiments; 3 evidence from opinions of respected authorities, based on clinical experience, descriptive studies, or reports of expert communities.

CLINICAL CONTROVERSY

Some clinicians believe that insufficient evidence exists to justify use of *N*-acetylcysteine for the prevention of contrast-induced nephrotoxicity, while others feel that its safety profile, ease of use, low cost, and potential for benefit are adequate justification for use for all patients.

Continuous venovenous hemofiltration (CVVH) may also be an effective means of preventing CIN.[53,54] However, because of the logistical issues (e.g., technical difficulty) and high cost of CVVH, currently this approach is not widely used and should be considered only for the highest risk patients in whom contrast exposure is unavoidable. Use of mannitol and furosemide for prevention may be harmful, and recent evidence indicates that fenoldopam, dopamine, and calcium channel blockers are ineffective in the prevention of CIN in CKD patients.[33,34] Consequently, these approaches are generally not recommended for the prevention of CIN.

Management Currently there is no specific therapy available for managing established CIN. Care is supportive as described in Chap. 51. Renal function (e.g., S_{cr}, urine output), electrolytes (e.g., sodium, potassium), and volume status should be closely monitored, and renal replacement therapy should be used as needed for patients when indicated (see Chap. 51).

Cisplatin Nephrotoxicity

Incidence Cisplatin is one of the most important and widely used antineoplastic drugs for the treatment of solid tumors, often demonstrating exceptional efficacy (i.e., cure rates over 90% in testicular cancers).[55,56] Unfortunately, the primary dose-limiting toxicity of platin-containing compounds is nephrotoxicity. The incidence of cisplatin nephrotoxicity was extremely high early in its development, with more than 70% of patients developing AKI in the 1980s.[55] Current estimates are much lower, primarily the result of limiting the total drug dose, reducing the rate of administration, and aggressively hydrating patients, yet it still occurs in 20% to 30% of patients and remains a significant cause of morbidity.[56,57] Carboplatin, a second-generation platinum analog, is associated with a lower incidence of nephrotoxicity than cisplatin and thus is the preferred agent in high-risk patients.[58]

Clinical Presentation Cisplatin administration results in impaired tubular reabsorption and decreased urinary concentration ability, leading to increased excretion of salt and water (i.e., polyuria) within 24 hours of treatment. Polyuria persists, and a decrease in GFR evidenced by a rise in S_{cr} concentration may be seen within 72 to 96 hours after cisplatin administration.[55,57] Serum creatinine peaks approximately 10 to 14 days after initiation of therapy, with recovery by 21 days. As many as 25% of patients may have reversible elevations in S_{cr} and BUN for 2 weeks after cisplatin treatment. However, kidney damage is dose related and cumulative with subsequent cycles of therapy, so the S_{cr} concentration may continue to rise, and irreversible kidney injury may result.[57] Hypomagnesemia is a hallmark finding of cisplatin nephrotoxicity, due to impaired magnesium reabsorption and thus increased urinary losses.[55] Hypomagnesemia is often accompanied by hypocalcemia and hypokalemia and may be severe, leading to seizures, neuromuscular irritability, or personality changes. Urinalysis typically reveals leukocytes, renal tubular epithelial cells, and granular casts.[57]

Pathogenesis The pathogenesis of cisplatin nephrotoxicity is multifactorial in nature and likely begins with cellular uptake and accumulation of the drug in proximal tubular epithelial cells to concentrations that may reach five times the serum concentration.[56,57]

Tubular cell exposure to cisplatin then activates a series of cell signaling pathways, including the mitogen-activated protein kinase (MAPK) pathway, p53, caspase, and the generation of reactive oxygen species, that collectively promote tubular cell injury and death via necrosis and/or apoptosis. Simultaneous production of proinflammatory cytokines such as tumor necrosis factor-α (TNF-α) within tubular cells activates an inflammatory response which may worsen the renal insult.[56] Although tubular damage is evident in both the proximal and distal segments, the majority occurs in the proximal tubules and is followed by a progressive loss of glomerular filtration capacity and impaired distal tubular function. Renal biopsies generally reveal necrosis of proximal and distal tubules and collecting ducts, with no obvious morphological changes to the glomeruli.[57]

Risk Factors Risk factors include increased age, dehydration, renal irradiation, concurrent use of nephrotoxic drugs, large cumulative doses, and alcohol abuse.[55,57]

Prevention The best renoprotective strategy during cisplatin treatment incorporates a combination of interventions, including prospective dose reduction and decreased frequency of administration, which usually requires using the platin compounds in combination with other chemotherapeutic agents, avoiding concurrent use of other nephrotoxic drugs, and ensuring patients are euvolemic or somewhat hypervolemic prior to initiating treatment.[55,56] Vigorous hydration with isotonic saline should be used for all patients with a goal of maintaining at least 100 to 150 mL/h of urine output during and after cisplatin treatment. Hydration should be initiated 12 to 24 hours prior to and continued for 2 to 3 days after cisplatin administration at rates of 100 to 250 mL/h, as tolerated, to maintain a urine flow of 3 to 4 L/day.[55] Concurrent use of diuretics such as furosemide and mannitol to maintain urine flow has not been consistently demonstrated to be renoprotective; thus, their use is no longer recommended.[55]

Amifostine, an organic thiophosphate that is converted to an active metabolite, chelates cisplatin in normal cells and reduces the nephrotoxicity, neurotoxicity, ototoxicity, and myelosuppression associated with cisplatin and carboplatin therapy. It is also thought to serve as a thiol donor, thereby reducing intracellular reactive oxygen species and corresponding oxidative stress that plays a critical role in the development of cellular injury.[30,56] Pretreatment with amifostine should be considered for patients who are at high risk for kidney injury, particularly patients who are elderly, volume depleted, have CKD, or are receiving other nephrotoxic drugs concurrently. The current recommended dose of amifostine is 910 mg/m^2 administered intravenously over 15 minutes, beginning 30 minutes prior to cisplatin administration.[59] Common toxicities include acute hypotension, nausea, and fatigue.

Promising investigational techniques include the use of hypertonic saline (e.g., administration of each dose in 250 mL of 3% saline) to reduce tubular cisplatin uptake, *N*-acetylcysteine to reduce oxidative damage by acting as a sulfhydryl donor, and disulfiram metabolite diethyldithiocarbamate to reduce cytochrome P450 2E1-mediated generation of hydroxyl radicals.[55,56,60] Recently, the protective effect of melatonin and the ability of cisplatin-incorporated polymeric micelles to maintain antitumor activity while reducing nephrotoxicity were demonstrated. Finally, reduced renal exposure can be achieved with the use of localized intraperitoneal administration in conjunction with systemic administration of sodium thiosulfate for those with peritoneal tumors.[55]

Management AKI caused by cisplatin therapy is usually partially reversible with time and supportive care, including dialysis. Renal function indices should be closely followed, with S_{cr} and BUN concentrations checked daily. Serum magnesium, potassium, and calcium concentrations should be monitored daily and corrected as needed.[57] Hypocalcemia and hypokalemia may be difficult to reverse until hypomagnesemia is corrected. Progressive kidney disease caused by cumulative nephrotoxicity may be irreversible and in some cases may lead to ESRD and require chronic dialysis support.

Amphotericin B Nephrotoxicity

Incidence Variable rates of amphotericin B nephrotoxicity have been reported that correspond in large part to the cumulative dose administered. Nephrotoxicity may be seen in nearly 30% of patients receiving median cumulative doses as low as 240 mg[61] and reaches an incidence of >80% when cumulative doses approach 5 g.[61,62] Although numerous studies demonstrate lower rates of nephrotoxicity with liposomal formulations compared with conventional amphotericin B, it is difficult to compare rates of toxicity between products and studies because of the variability in the study populations, doses administered, and inconsistent definitions of nephrotoxicity and methods of assessment.[63]

Clinical Presentation Dose-dependent nephrotoxicity is often evident after administration of cumulative doses of 2 to 3 g as nonoliguria, renal tubular potassium, sodium, and magnesium wasting, impaired urinary concentrating ability, and distal renal tubular acidosis.[1,11] Although the cumulative dose is a significant risk factor, the time to onset of kidney injury varies considerably, ranging from a few days to weeks.[61] Tubular dysfunction usually manifests 1 to 2 weeks after treatment is begun, and potassium and magnesium replacement may be necessary. This is typically followed by a decrease in GFR and a rise in S_{cr} and BUN concentrations.[64] Consequently, renal function indices should be closely followed, with S_{cr} and BUN concentrations checked daily, and serum magnesium, potassium, and calcium concentrations monitored every other day and corrected as needed.

Pathogenesis Amphotericin B nephrotoxicity occurs predominantly via two mechanisms. The first is direct tubular epithelial cell toxicity resulting from interaction of amphotericin B with ergosterol in the cell membrane, leading to increased tubular cell membrane permeability, lipid peroxidation, and eventual necrosis of proximal tubular cells.[61] Tubular injury appears to be exacerbated by ischemic injury, which is a result of a reduction in renal blood flow and GFR due to afferent arteriolar vasoconstriction.[11,61]

Risk Factors Risk factors that impact the likelihood of developing amphotericin B nephrotoxicity include preexisting kidney disease, large individual and cumulative doses, short infusion times, volume depletion, hypokalemia, increased age, and concomitant administration of diuretics and other nephrotoxins (cyclosporine in particular).[11,61,64]

Prevention Permanent decrements in GFR are best prevented by incorporating a low threshold [i.e., if S_{cr} reaches 2 mg/dL (177 μmol/L) on 2 consecutive days] for stopping amphotericin B or switching to a liposomal formulation.[65] Several liposomal amphotericin B formulations are now available and should be used in most high-risk patients as they have been reported to reduce nephrotoxicity by enhancing drug delivery to sites of infection and reducing interaction with tubular epithelial cell membranes.[61] Nephrotoxicity can also be minimized by limiting the cumulative dose, increasing the infusion time, ensuring the patient is well hydrated, and avoiding concomitant administration of other nephrotoxins.[11] Administration of 1 L intravenous 0.9% sodium chloride daily during the course of therapy appears to reduce toxicity and a single infusion of saline 10 to 15 mL/kg prior to administration of each dose of amphotericin B are generally recommended.[61] A number of other antifungal agents such as itraconazole, voriconazole, and caspofungin are viable alternatives and are now routinely used in lieu of amphotericin B for patients at high risk of developing nephrotoxicity.[11,65]

Management Amphotericin B nephrotoxicity is best treated by discontinuation of therapy and substitution of alternative antifungal therapy, if possible. Renal tubular dysfunction and glomerular filtration will improve gradually to some degree in most patients, but damage may be irreversible. Renal function indices should be closely followed, with S_{cr} and BUN concentrations checked daily, and serum magnesium, potassium, and calcium concentrations should be monitored daily and corrected as needed.[11]

OSMOTIC NEPHROSIS

The term *sucrose nephrosis* was first used in 1940 to describe renal lesions observed at autopsy in patients who died of severe AKI following parenteral administration of hyperosmolar sucrose.[67] The lesions were characterized by severe swelling and vacuolization of the proximal tubular epithelial cells. Subsequently, the term *osmotic nephrosis* was used to describe the lesion in light of the suspected mechanism, an osmotic gradient between the tubular lumen and epithelial cells.[67] It is now known that several drugs, including mannitol, low-molecular-weight dextran, hydroxyethyl starch, and radiographic contrast media, or drug vehicles, such as sucrose, maltose, and propylene glycol, are associated with osmotic nephrosis, which may rarely lead to ATN and AKI.[24,67–69] Since osmotic nephrosis does not necessarily negatively affect proximal tubular function, its presence may often go undetected in patients without overt signs of ATN. This likely contributes to the extremely low incidence of osmotic nephrosis reported for causative agents.[67] Intravenous immunoglobulin solutions containing hyperosmolar sucrose may cause osmotic nephrosis and AKI in 1% to 10% of cases, which is usually reversible shortly after discontinuing therapy.[67,70] Recently, maltose-based intravenous immunoglobulin solutions have also been implicated in the development of osmotic nephrosis.[68,71] Although intravenous immunoglobulin-induced nephropathy is the modern prototype for osmotic nephrosis, it is understood that the vehicle (i.e., sucrose or maltose) is the culprit and not the immunoglobulins themselves.

The clinical presentation of osmotic nephrosis is often subtle. While tubular proteinura or vacuolated tubular cells may be observed on urinalysis for patients with AKI, the definitive diagnosis of osmotic nephrosis is only made via a kidney biopsy.[67] Intravenous immunoglobulin-induced AKI typically presents as oliguria after 3 to 4 days of treatment and may persist for up to 2 weeks.[24] Kidney injury occurs via uptake of the offending agent through pinocytosis into proximal tubular epithelial cells, subsequent formation of vacuoles, and accumulation of lysosomes, which collectively results in an oncotic gradient and thus cellular swelling, tubular luminal occlusion, and compromised cellular integrity.[24,67] Renal replacement therapy may be necessary for up to 40% of patients developing osmotic nephrosis-associated AKI.[67] However, it is usually reversible, with 80% of patients recovering normal renal function following withdrawal of the offending drug.[24]

Risk factors for osmotic nephrosis include excessive doses of offending agents, preexisting kidney disease, ischemia, older age (>65 years), and concomitant use of other nephrotoxins, particularly cyclosporine.[24,67] Nephrotoxicity may be prevented by limiting the dose, reducing the rate of infusion, and avoiding dehydration and concomitant nephrotoxins.

HEMODYNAMICALLY MEDIATED KIDNEY INJURY

④ Hemodynamically mediated kidney injury generally refers to any cause of AKI resulting from an acute decrease in intraglomerular pressure, including "prerenal" states leading to reduced effective renal blood flow (e.g., hypovolemia, congestive heart failure) and medications that affect the renin–angiotensin system.[11,12,23] The kidneys receive approximately 25% of resting cardiac output, which renders them particularly susceptible to alterations in renal blood flow and enhances their exposure to circulating drugs.[17] Within each nephron, blood flow and pressure are regulated by glomerular afferent and efferent arterioles to maintain intraglomerular capillary hydrostatic pressure, glomerular filtration, and urine output. Afferent and efferent arteriolar vasoconstrictions are primarily mediated by angiotensin II, whereas afferent vasodilation is primarily mediated by prostaglandins (Fig. 55–1).[72] This specialized blood flow is precisely regulated by interrelations between arachidonic acid metabolites, natriuretic factors, nitric oxide, the sympathetic nervous system, the renin–angiotensin system, and the macula densa response to distal tubular solute delivery.[72,73] Drug-induced causes of hemodynamic kidney injury typically stem from constriction of glomerular afferent arterioles and/or dilation of glomerular efferent arterioles. ACEIs, angiotensin II receptor blockers, and NSAIDs are the agents that have been most commonly implicated.

ANGIOTENSIN-CONVERTING ENZYME INHIBITORS AND ANGIOTENSIN II RECEPTOR BLOCKERS

Incidence

The incidence of ACEI- or angiotensin II receptor blocker (ARB)-mediated kidney injury has not been established. Patients with renal artery stenosis, volume depletion, and congestive heart failure and those with preexisting kidney disease, including diabetic nephropathy, are most likely to experience a significant decline in renal function when therapy with one of these agents is initiated.[74] For example, between 20% to 25% of hospitalized patients with congestive heart failure develop AKI after treatment with ACEIs is initiated.[75,76] The incidence of ACEI induced AKI may be as high as 23% for patients with bilateral renal artery stenosis and up to 38% for patients with unilateral renal artery stenosis.[10]

Clinical Presentation

Therapy with ACEIs and ARBs will acutely reduce GFR; so a moderate rise in S_{cr} after initiation of therapy should be anticipated.[74] Importantly, a distinction must be made between a potentially detrimental reduction in GFR and a normal, predictable rise in S_{cr}. An increase in S_{cr} of up to 30% is commonly observed within 3 to 5 days of initiating therapy and is an indication that the drug has begun to exert its desired pharmacologic effect.[11,74] The increase in S_{cr} typically stabilizes within 1 to 2 weeks and is usually reversible upon stopping the drug. Furthermore, an association exists between acute increases in S_{cr} of ≤30% from baseline that stabilize within the first 2 months of initiating therapy and preservation of renal function. The S_{cr} threshold for discontinuation of ACEI or ARB therapy is unclear.[74] However, an increase in S_{cr} of more than 30% above baseline in the course of 1 to 2 weeks may necessitate discontinuation of the offending drug.

Pathogenesis

The pathogenesis of ACEI- or ARB-mediated kidney injury is the result of disruption of normal autoregulation of intraglomerular capillary hydrostatic pressure.[11] Normally, the kidney attempts to maintain GFR by dilating the afferent arteriole and constricting the efferent arteriole in response to a decrease in renal blood flow. During states of reduced blood flow, the juxtaglomerular apparatus increases renin secretion. Plasma renin converts angiotensinogen to angiotensin I, and ultimately angiotensin II by angiotensin-converting enzyme. Angiotensin II constricts the afferent and efferent arterioles, but has a greater effect on the efferent arterioles, resulting in a net increase in intraglomerular pressure.[74] Additionally, renal prostaglandins, prostaglandin E_2 in particular, are released and induce a net dilation of the afferent arteriole, thereby improving blood flow into the glomerulus. Together these processes maintain GFR and urine output (Fig. 55–2).[23,72,73]

ACEI- or ARB-mediated kidney injury is the result of a decrease in glomerular capillary hydrostatic pressure sufficient to reduce

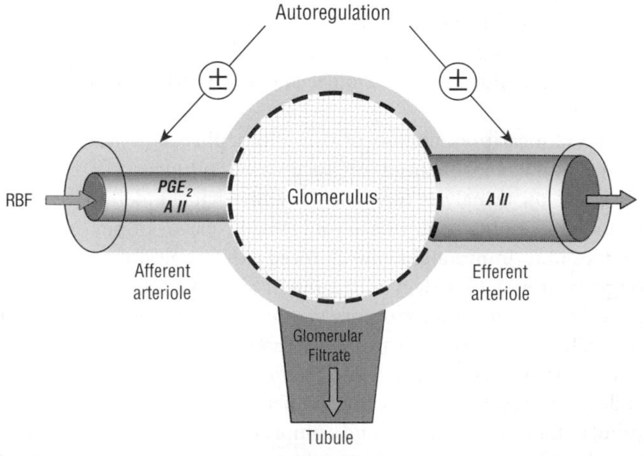

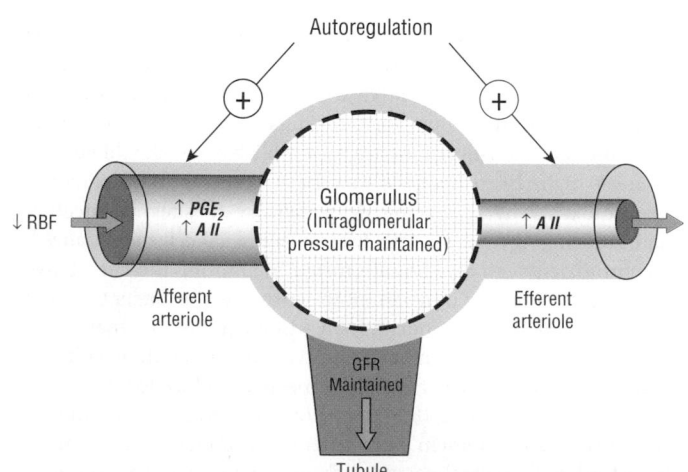

FIGURE 55-1. Normal glomerular autoregulation serves to maintain intraglomerular capillary hydrostatic pressure, glomerular filtration rate (GFR), and, ultimately, urine output. (A II, angiotensin II; PGE_2, prostaglandin E_2; RBF, renal blood flow.)

FIGURE 55-2. Glomerular autoregulation during "prerenal" states (i.e., reduced blood flow). (A II, angiotensin II; GFR, glomerular filtration rate; PGE_2, prostaglandin E_2; RBF, renal blood flow.)

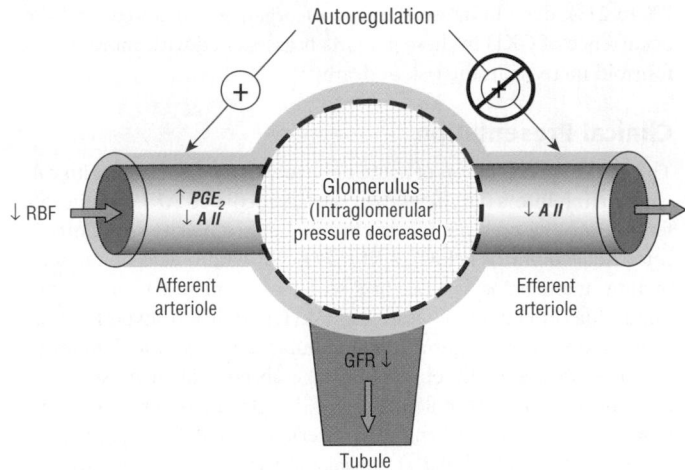

FIGURE 55-3. Pathogenesis of angiotensin-converting enzyme inhibitor (ACEI) nephropathy. (A II, angiotensin II; GFR, glomerular filtration rate; PGE$_2$, prostaglandin E$_2$; RBF, renal blood flow.)

glomerular ultrafiltration.[24] When ACEI therapy (e.g., enalapril or ramipril) is initiated, the synthesis of angiotensin II is decreased, thereby preferentially dilating the efferent arteriole. This reduces outflow resistance from the glomerulus and decreases hydrostatic pressure in the glomerular capillaries, which alters Starling forces across the glomerular capillaries to decrease intraglomerular pressure and GFR and then often leads to nephrotoxicity, particularly in the setting of reduced renal blood flow or effective arterial blood volume (Fig. 55–3), that is, prerenal settings in which glomerular afferent arteriolar blood flow is reduced and the efferent arteriole is vasoconstricted to maintain sufficient glomerular capillary hydrostatic pressure for ultrafiltration.[12,24]

Risk Factors

Patients at greatest risk are those dependent on angiotensin II and renal efferent arteriolar constriction to maintain blood pressure and GFR.[24,74] These include patients with bilateral renal artery stenosis or stenosis in a single kidney (i.e., renal transplant); patients with decreased effective arterial blood volume (i.e., prerenal states), especially those with congestive heart failure, volume depletion from excess diuresis or gastrointestinal fluid loss, hepatic cirrhosis with ascites, and nephrotic syndrome; patients with preexisting kidney disease; and patients receiving concurrent nephrotoxic drugs, particularly other drugs that affect intraglomerular autoregulation.[12,74]

Prevention

Hemodynamically mediated AKI caused by ACEIs or ARBs is frequently preventable by recognizing the presence of preexisting kidney disease or decreased effective renal blood flow as a result of volume depletion, heart failure, or liver disease. A common strategy for at-risk patients is to initiate therapy with very low doses of a short-acting ACEI (e.g., captopril 6.25 mg to 12.5 mg), then gradually titrate the dose upward and convert to a longer-acting agent after patient tolerance has been demonstrated. Outpatients may be started on low doses of long-acting ACEIs (e.g., enalapril 2.5 mg) with gradual dose titration every 2 to 4 weeks until the maximum dose or desired response is achieved. Renal function indices and serum potassium concentrations must be monitored carefully, daily for hospitalized patients and every 2 to 3 days for outpatients. Monitoring may need to be more frequent during outpatient initiation of ACEI or ARB therapy for patients with preexisting kidney disease, congestive heart failure, or suspected renovascular disease.

Use of concurrent hypotensive agents and other drugs that affect renal hemodynamics (e.g., NSAIDs, diuretics) should be discouraged and dehydration avoided.

Management

Acute decreases in renal function and the development of hyperkalemia usually resolve over several days after ACEI or ARB therapy is discontinued. Occasionally patients will require management of severe hyperkalemia, as described in detail in chapter 60.

ACEI or ARB therapy may frequently be reinitiated, particularly for patients with congestive heart failure, after intravascular volume depletion has been corrected or diuretic doses reduced. Slight reductions in renal function [maintenance of a S$_{cr}$ concentration of 2 to 3 mg/dL (177 to 265 μmol/L)] may be an acceptable trade-off for hemodynamic improvement in certain patients with severe congestive heart failure or renovascular disease not amenable to revascularization.[77]

NONSTEROIDAL ANTIINFLAMMATORY DRUGS AND SELECTIVE CYCLOOXYGENASE-2 INHIBITORS

Incidence

The overall safety of NSAIDs is evidenced by the nonprescription availability in the United States of several drugs in the class (e.g., ibuprofen, naproxen, ketoprofen). Although potential adverse renal effects from nonprescription NSAIDs had been a concern, conventional nonselective NSAIDs and selective cyclooxygenase-2 (COX-2) inhibitors are unlikely to acutely affect kidney function in the absence of renal ischemia or excess renal vasoconstrictor activity.[11,78,79] Nevertheless, given their general safety and widespread availability, NSAIDs are among the most commonly used drugs. More than 30 million people take NSAIDs daily worldwide.[78] Although the incidence of NSAID-induced AKI is unclear, historical reports suggest that 500,000 to 2.5 million people develop some degree of NSAID nephrotoxicity in the United States annually.[80]

Clinical Presentation

NSAID- and COX-2-induced AKI can occur within days of initiating therapy, particularly with a short-acting agent such as ibuprofen, or within days of some other precipitating event (e.g., intravascular volume depletion). Patients typically present with complaints of diminished urine output, weight gain, and/or edema. Urine sodium concentrations [<20 mEq/L (<20 mmol/L)] and fractional excretion of sodium [<1% (0.01)] are usually low, and BUN, S$_{cr}$, potassium, and blood pressure are typically elevated.[22,81] The urine sediment is usually bland and unchanged from baseline but may show occasional granular casts.

Pathogenesis

The pathogenesis of NSAID- and COX-2-induced AKI lies in the disruption of normal intraglomerular autoregulation.[11,79,81] Specifically, NSAIDs inhibit cyclooxygenase (COX)-catalyzed synthesis of vasodilatory prostaglandins, including prostaglandins I$_2$ (prostacyclin) and E$_2$, from arachidonic acid.[79] These prostaglandins are synthesized in the renal cortex and medulla by vascular endothelial and glomerular mesangial cells, and their effects are primarily local and result in net afferent arteriolar vasodilation.[79,81] Vasodilatory prostaglandins have limited activity in states of normal renal blood flow, but in states of decreased renal blood flow their synthesis is increased and they serve a vital autoregulatory role in the protection against renal ischemia and hypoxia by antagonizing renal arteriolar vasoconstriction due to angiotensin

II, norepinephrine, endothelin, and vasopressin.[24,79] Thus, administration of NSAIDs in the setting of reduced renal blood flow will blunt the usual compensatory increase in prostaglandin activity, altering the normal autoregulatory balance in favor of renal vasoconstrictors, thereby promoting renal ischemia and a reduction in glomerular filtration.[81]

Risk Factors

Risk factors for NSAID- and COX-2-induced AKI include age >60 years, preexisting kidney disease, hepatic disease with ascites, congestive heart failure, intravascular volume depletion/dehydration, concurrent diuretic therapy, or systemic lupus erythematosus.[11,24,81] The elderly are at higher risk because of multiple comorbidities, multiple-drug therapies, and reduced renal hemodynamics. Combined use of NSAIDs or COX-2 inhibitors and concurrent nephrotoxic drugs, particularly other drugs that affect intraglomerular autoregulation should be avoided in high-risk patients.[11]

Prevention

NSAID- and COX-2 inhibitor-induced AKI can be prevented by recognizing high-risk patients, avoiding potent compounds such as indomethacin and using analgesics with less prostaglandin inhibition, such as acetaminophen, nonacetylated salicylates, aspirin, and possibly nabumetone.[11,81] Nonnarcotic analgesics (e.g., tramadol) may also be useful but do not provide antiinflammatory activity. When NSAID therapy is essential for high-risk patients, the minimal effective dose should be used for the shortest duration possible, and NSAIDs with short half-lives should be considered (e.g., sulindac) along with optimal management of predisposing medical problems and frequent renal function monitoring.[11] Moreover, use of concurrent hypotensive agents and other drugs that affect renal hemodynamics (e.g., ACEIs, ARBs, diuretics) should be discouraged in high-risk patients and dehydration avoided.

Traditional, nonselective NSAIDs inhibit COX-1 and COX-2, whereas the selective drugs meloxicam, celecoxib, and valdecoxib preferentially inhibit COX-2. COX-2 inhibitors were anticipated to be beneficial in high-risk patients. However, recent data indicate that they affect renal function similarly to nonselective NSAIDs, and thus caution is warranted with their use, particularly in high-risk patients.[11,81]

Management

NSAID-induced AKI is treated by discontinuation of therapy and supportive care. Kidney injury is rarely severe, and recovery is usually rapid. Occasionally, the hemodynamic insult is sufficiently severe to cause ATN, which can prolong injury.[24]

CYCLOSPORINE AND TACROLIMUS

The calcineurin inhibitors cyclosporine and tacrolimus have dramatically enhanced the success of solid-organ transplantation. As many as 94% of kidney transplant patients are prescribed a calcineurin inhibitor-based immunosuppressive regimen.[82] Nephrotoxicity, however, remains a major dose-limiting adverse effect of both drugs. Although delayed chronic interstitial nephritis has also been reported, acute hemodynamically mediated kidney injury is an important mechanism of calcineurin inhibitor-induced nephrotoxicity.

Incidence

Historically, reversible AKI occurred frequently in transplant recipients during the first 6 months of cyclosporine therapy. The 5-year risk of CKD after transplantation of a nonrenal organ ranges from 7% to 21%, depending on the type of organ transplanted, and the occurrence of CKD in these patients is associated with more than a fourfold increase in the risk of death.[83]

Clinical Presentation

The clinical presentation of acute nephrotoxicity associated with calcineurin inhibitors (i.e., hemodynamically mediated AKI) is quite different from the presentation of chronic nephrotoxicity (see Chronic Interstitial Nephritis below). AKI may occur within days of initiating therapy, manifesting as a rise in S_{cr} concentration and a corresponding decline in creatinine clearance.[11,84] Hypertension, hyperkalemia, sodium retention, oliguria, renal tubular acidosis, and hypomagnesemia are frequently observed in the absence of urine sediment abnormalities or morphologic lesions.[11,82] On the other hand, renal biopsy may reveal thickening of arterioles, mild focal glomerular sclerosis, proximal tubular epithelial cell vacuolization and atrophy, and interstitial fibrosis. Biopsy is most useful to distinguish acute calcineurin inhibitor nephrotoxicity from acute cellular rejection of the transplanted kidney, the latter being evidenced by interstitial infiltrates composed of activated lymphocytes (see Chap. 98).[84]

Pathogenesis

The acute hemodynamic changes associated with calcineurin inhibitor nephrotoxicity result from an increase in potent vasoconstrictors including thromboxane A_2 and endothelin, activation of the renin–angiotensin and sympathetic nervous systems, as well as a reduction in the vasodilators nitric oxide, prostacyclin, and prostaglandin E_2.[82,84] The net effect is an imbalance in afferent and efferent tone, resulting in predominantly afferent vasoconstriction with reduced renal plasma flow and GFR.[11] The mechanism of acute nephrotoxicity is generally thought to be dose related, since renal function improves rapidly following dose reduction.[11]

Risk Factors

Risk factors include age over 65, higher dose, concomitant therapy with nephrotoxic drugs (particularly NSAIDs), and interacting drugs that inhibit calcineurin inhibitor metabolism and transport and thus increase systemic exposure, older kidney allograft age, salt depletion, diuretic use, and polymorphic expression of P-glycoprotein.[82] The incidence of AKI with potential progression to chronic nephropathy has decreased since the introduction of lower-dose-therapy regimens. Unfortunately, there has been no apparent reduction in the incidence of the slow, dose-dependent decline in glomerular filtration.[84]

Prevention

Because acute hemodynamically mediated kidney injury secondary to cyclosporine and tacrolimus appears to be concentration related, pharmacokinetic and pharmacodynamic monitoring is an important means of preventing toxicity.[82] However, the persistent presence of therapeutic or low cyclosporine concentrations does not totally preclude the development of nephrotoxicity. Calcium channel blockers may antagonize the vasoconstrictor effect of cyclosporine by dilating glomerular afferent arterioles and preventing acute decreases in renal blood flow and glomerular filtration.[82] Lastly, decreased doses of cyclosporine or tacrolimus, primarily when used in combination with other nonnephrotoxic immunosuppressants, may minimize the risk of toxicity, but this may increase the risk of chronic rejection.[84]

Management

AKI usually improves with dose reduction and treatment of contributing illness or the discontinuation of interacting drugs.

CKD is usually irreversible, but progressive toxicity may be limited by discontinuation of cyclosporine (or tacrolimus) therapy or dose reduction, with the continuation of other immunosuppressants.[82,84] S_{cr} and BUN should be closely monitored (daily if possible), as should cyclosporine or tacrolimus concentrations, to ensure that serum concentrations are within the narrow therapeutic range.

CRYSTAL NEPHROPATHY

Crystal nephropathy is caused by precipitation of drug crystals in distal tubular lumens, which commonly leads to intratubular obstruction, interstitial nephritis, and occasionally superimposed ATN. Nephrolithiasis is a type of crystal nephropathy that results from abnormal crystal precipitation in the renal collecting system, potentially causing urinary tract obstruction with kidney injury. Numerous medications have been associated with development of crystal nephropathy (Table 55–4).

INTRATUBULAR OBSTRUCTION

Drugs may induce crystal nephropathy with subsequent intratubular obstruction and AKI by direct (precipitation of the drug itself) and indirect means (i.e., promoting release and precipitation of tissue-degradation products). Antineoplastic drugs may cause acute renal tubular obstruction indirectly by inducing tumor lysis syndrome, hyperuricemia, and intratubular precipitation of uric acid crystals.[85] Acute oliguric or anuric kidney injury develops rapidly.

TABLE 55-4	Drugs Associated with Allergic Interstitial Nephritis	
Antimicrobials		
Acyclovir	Indinavir	
Aminoglycosides	Rifampin	
Amphotericin B	Sulfonamides	
β-Lactams	Tetracyclines	
Erythromycin	Trimethoprim-sulfamethoxazole	
Ethambutol	Vancomycin	
Diuretics		
Acetazolamide	Loop diuretics	
Amiloride	Triamterene	
Chlorthalidone	Thiazide diuretics	
Neuropsychiatric		
Carbamazepine	Phenytoin	
Lithium	Valproic acid	
Phenobarbital		
Nonsteroidal antiinflammatory drugs		
Aspirin	Ketoprofen	
Indomethacin	Phenylbutazone	
Naproxen	Diclofenac	
Ibuprofen	Zomepirac	
Diflunisal	Cyclooxygenase-2 inhibitors	
Piroxicam		
Miscellaneous		
Acetaminophen	Lansoprazole	
Allopurinol	Methyldopa	
Interferon-alfa	Omeprazole	
Aspirin	P-aminosalicylic acid	
Azathioprine	Phenylpropanolamine	
Captopril	Propylthiouracil	
Cimetidine	Radiographic contrast media	
Clofibrate	Ranitidine	
Cyclosporine	Sulfinpyrazone	
Glyburide	Warfarin sodium	
Gold		

The diagnosis is supported by a urine uric acid-to-creatinine ratio greater than 1. Uric acid precipitation can be prevented by vigorous pretreatment hydration with normal saline, beginning at least 48 hours prior to chemotherapy, to maintain urine output 100 mL/h in adults, administration of allopurinol 100 mg/m^2 thrice daily (maximum of 800 mg/day) started 2 to 3 days prior to chemotherapy, and urinary alkalinization to pH 7.0.[86]

Drug-induced rhabdomyolysis is another form of indirect toxicity, which can lead to intratubular precipitation of myoglobin and, if severe, AKI.[87] The most common cause of drug-induced rhabdomyolysis is direct myotoxicity from 3-hydroxy-3-methylglutaryl-coenzyme A (HMG-CoA) reductase inhibitors or statins, including lovastatin and simvastatin. The risk of rhabdomyolysis is increased when these drugs are administered concurrently with gemfibrozil, niacin, or inhibitors of the CYP3A4 metabolic pathway (e.g., erythromycin and itraconazole).[88]

Intratubular precipitation of drugs or their metabolites can also directly cause AKI. Precipitation of drug crystals is due primarily to supersaturation of a low urine volume with the offending drug or relative insolubility of the drug in either alkaline or acidic urine.[89] Volume depletion is an important risk factor for the development of AKI. Urine pH decreases to approximately 4.5 during maximal stimulation of renal tubular hydrogen ion secretion. Certain solutes can precipitate and obstruct the tubular lumen at this acid pH, particularly when urine is concentrated, such as for patients with volume depletion. For example, several antiviral drugs have been associated with intratubular precipitation and AKI.[19,89,90] Acyclovir is relatively insoluble at physiologic urine pH and is associated with intratubular precipitation in dehydrated oliguric patients.[19,89] Foscarnet complexation with ionized calcium may result in precipitation of calcium-foscarnet salt crystals in renal glomeruli, causing primarily a crystalline glomerulonephritis. The salt crystals may then secondarily precipitate in the renal tubules causing tubular necrosis. The protease inhibitor indinavir has been associated with crystalluria, crystal nephropathy, dysuria, urinary frequency, back and flank pain, or nephrolithiasis in approximately 8% of treated patients.[89,90] Intratubular indinavir crystal precipitation can be prevented in nearly 75% of treated patients if one assures that the patient consumes at least 2 to 3 L of fluid per day.[89] Sulfadiazine, when used at high doses, and methotrexate may also precipitate in acidic urine and can cause oligoanuric kidney injury.[89] Massive administration of ascorbic acid can also result in obstruction of renal tubules with calcium oxalate crystals. Oxalate, a poorly soluble ascorbic acid metabolite, can also precipitate and worsen renal function when ascorbic acid is administered to patients with AKI, congenital nephrotic syndrome, and renal transplant patients.[89,91,92] Triamterene and the quinolone antibiotic ciprofloxacin may also precipitate in renal tubules and cause kidney injury.[89]

Kidney injury caused by intratubular precipitation of most tissue-degradation products or drugs and their metabolites can be largely prevented and possibly treated by administering the drug after vigorously prehydrating the patient, maintaining a high urine volume, and urinary alkalinization.[89]

NEPHROCALCINOSIS

Nephrocalcinosis is a clinical–pathologic condition characterized by extensive tubulointerstitial precipitation and deposition of calcium phosphate crystals leading to marked tubular calcification.[93–95] It is most commonly seen in clinical conditions associated with hypercalcemia and hypercalciuria, such as hyperparathyroidism, malignancy, and less frequently increased intake of calcium or vitamin D. However, nephrocalcinosis can also result from hyperphosphatemia and hyperphosphaturia in the absence of hypercalcemia, as is known to occur for patients who have received oral sodium phosphate solution (OSPS) as a bowel preparation.[94,96]

Acute Phosphate Nephropathy

The term *acute phosphate nephropathy* was coined specifically to describe OSPS-induced nephrocalcinosis, as its pathogenesis is the result of increased phosphate intake rather than hypercalcemia.[95] During the last decade, several cases of nephrocalcinosis have been reported after use of OSPS for bowel preparation prior to gastrointestinal procedures,[93,95,97-99] and strong associations have recently been demonstrated between exposure to OSPS and a decline in kidney function, particularly in the elderly and those with preexisting kidney disease.[100-102] The incidence of acute phosphate nephropathy is between 1 in 1,000 and 1 in 5,000 exposures, translating to roughly 1,400 to 7,000 new cases annually.[96] Patients usually present with AKI several days to months after exposure to OSPS. Patients in one cohort of 21 cases of acute phosphate nephropathy presented with AKI and a mean S_{cr} of 3.9 mg/dL (345 μmol/L) at a median of 1 month after colonoscopy.[95] Low-grade proteinuria (<1.0 g/day), normocalcemia, and bland urinary sediment are usually observed. Extensive deposition of calcium phosphate in the distal tubules and collecting ducts without glomerular or vascular injury is the hallmark of acute phosphate nephropathy.[93,95] Risk factors include advanced age, preexisting kidney disease, female sex, hypertension, diabetes, bowel conditions associated with prolonged intestinal transit, high sodium phosphate dosage, volume depletion, and medications that affect renal perfusion or function (e.g., diuretics, lithium, NSAIDs, ACEIs, or ARBs).[94]

NEPHROLITHIASIS

Nephrolithiasis (formation of renal calculi or kidney stones) does not present as classic nephrotoxicity since GFR is usually not decreased. Drug-induced nephrolithiasis can be the result of abnormal crystal precipitation in the renal collecting system, potentially causing pain, hematuria, infection, or, occasionally, urinary tract obstruction with kidney injury. The overall prevalence of drug-induced nephrolithiasis is estimated to be 1%.[103]

Kidney stone formation, possibly also accompanied by intratubular precipitation of crystalline material, has been a rare complication of drug therapy. Until the acquired immune deficiency syndrome (AIDS) era, triamterene had been the drug most frequently associated with kidney stone formation, with a prevalence of 0.4%.[103] Sulfadiazine is a poorly soluble sulfonamide that has caused symptomatic acetylsulfadiazine crystalluria with stone formation and flank or back pain, hematuria, or kidney injury in up to 29% of patients treated with the drug.[89] A high urine volume and urinary alkalinization to pH >7.15 may be protective. Numerous other drugs have been implicated in the development of nephrolithiasis, including the antiviral drugs nelfinavir and foscarnet, the antibacterial agents ciprofloxacin, amoxicillin, and nitrofurantoin, and various products containing ephedrine, norephedrine, and pseudoephedrine.[103] Most recently, a catastrophic outbreak of nephrolithiasis occurred in China stemming from consumption of melamine-contaminated dairy products. Most of those affected were children younger than 3 years of age. The now classic presentation consisted of dysuria, hematuria, occasional proteinuria, and stone passage: AKI occurred in 2.5% of the cases.[104]

GLOMERULAR DISEASE

Proteinuria, particularly nephrotic range proteinuria (defined as urine protein excretion greater than 3.5 g/day per 1.73 m²) with or without a decline in the GFR is a hallmark sign of glomerular injury (see Chap. 56).[105] Several different glomerular lesions may occur, including minimal change disease, focal segmental glomerulosclerosis, and membranous nephropathy, mostly by immune mechanisms rather than direct cellular toxicity. Although drug-induced glomerular disease is uncommon, a variety of agents have been implicated.[106]

Minimal Change Glomerular Disease

Drug-induced minimal change glomerular disease is frequently accompanied by interstitial nephritis and is most common during NSAID therapy.[105] Lithium, quinolone antibiotics, and interferon-α have also been implicated.[24,25,106] Patients present abruptly with nephrotic range proteinuria, hypoalbuminemia, and hyperlipidemia and rarely with hematuria and hypertension.[25,105] The pathogenesis is unknown, but nephrotic range proteinuria as a consequence of NSAID therapy is frequently associated with a T-lymphocytic interstitial infiltrate, suggesting disordered cell-mediated immunity. Proteinuria usually resolves rapidly after discontinuation of the offending drug, and a 3- to 4-week course of corticosteroids may help resolve the lesion. More than 90% of adults achieve complete remission over the course of several months.[105]

Focal Segmental Glomerulosclerosis

Focal segmental glomerulosclerosis (FSGS) is characterized by patchy areas (i.e., only some glomeruli are partially affected by the disease) of glomerular sclerosis with interstitial inflammation and fibrosis (see Chap. 56). FSGS is becoming the most common cause of nephrotic syndrome in African Americans and whites in the United States.[105] It represents a pattern of glomerular injury, not a disease per se, and is the final common pathway by which normal glomerular components are replaced by fibrous scar tissue. FSGS has been described in the setting of chronic heroin abuse (known as *heroin nephropathy*).[107] The pathogenesis is unknown but may include direct toxicity by heroin or adulterants and injury from bacterial or viral infections accompanying intravenous drug use. The bisphosphonates pamidronate and zoledronate, commonly used to treat osteoporosis, malignancy-associated hypercalcemia, and Paget disease, are associated with the development of a particularly aggressive variant of FSGS called *collapsing glomerulopathy*.[108] It presents with massive proteinuria (>8 g/day), and it is typically characterized by rising S_{cr} at diagnosis and rapid progression to ESRD.[105,109] Patients receiving intravenous formulations, high doses, or prolonged therapy are at highest risk.[108]

Membranous Nephropathy

Membranous nephropathy is characterized by subepithelial immune complex formation along glomerular capillary loops and, although rarely seen, has classically been associated with gold therapy, penicillamine, captopril, and NSAID use.[25,106] Patients present with nephrotic range proteinuria and microscopic hematuria, with hypertension and elevated S_{cr} apparent for patients with more advanced disease.[105] The pathogenesis may involve damage to proximal tubule epithelium with antigen release, antibody formation, and glomerular immune complex deposition. Proteinuria usually resolves slowly after discontinuing the offending drug. Patients who remain nephrotic after 6 months should be treated with a 6 to 12 month course of immunosuppressive therapy, which typically consists of prednisone and cyclophosphamide.[105]

TUBULOINTERSTITIAL NEPHRITIS

Tubulointerstitial nephritis refers to diseases in which the predominant changes occur in the renal interstitium rather than the tubules. The presentation may be acute and reversible with interstitial edema, rapid loss of renal function, and systemic symptoms or chronic and irreversible, associated with interstitial fibrosis and minimal to no systemic symptoms.[21,25]

ACUTE ALLERGIC INTERSTITIAL NEPHRITIS

Incidence

⑤ The incidence of drug-induced acute allergic interstitial nephritis (AIN) is unclear and likely varies with clinical setting. For example, the incidence has been estimated to be 0.7 cases per 100,000 young outpatient men but from 10% to 27% of kidney biopsies performed in hospitalized patients with unexplained AKI demonstrate AIN.[110-112] Multiple drugs have been implicated in the development of AIN (Table 55–4).[21,24,25] It usually manifests 2 weeks after exposure to a drug but may occur sooner if the patient was previously sensitized.[113]

Clinical Presentation Although methicillin-induced AIN is the prototype for AIN, it is now recognized that AIN is associated with all β-lactam antibiotics (including cephalosporins) and numerous other antimicrobials. Clinical signs present approximately 14 days after initiation of therapy and include (with their approximate incidence) fever (27% to 80%), maculopapular rash (15% to 25%), eosinophilia (23% to 80%), arthralgia (45%), and oliguria (50%).[110,112,113] Systemic hypersensitivity findings of the classic triad of fever, rash, and arthralgia, often along with eosinophilia and eosinophiluria, strongly suggest the diagnosis of AIN. However, this constellation of findings is not consistently reliable as one or more are frequently absent; so caution is warranted in basing diagnosis on hypersensitivity findings alone.[110,112] Eosinophiluria, an important marker of drug-induced AIN, is frequently absent, possibly because of fragility of eosinophils in urine and inadequate laboratory methodology. Anemia, leukocytosis, and elevated immunoglobulin E levels may occur. Tubular dysfunction may be manifested by acidosis, hyperkalemia, salt wasting, and concentrating defects.[21,113] The clinical presentation of AIN caused by proton pump inhibitors, which has recently been observed, is similar to that of β-lactams.[114-116]

NSAID-induced AIN has a different clinical presentation than that seen with most other drugs.[24] Patients are typically over 50 years of age (reflecting NSAID use for degenerative joint disease), the onset is delayed a mean of 6 months from initiation of therapy compared with 2 weeks with β-lactams, and there is a much lower incidence of fever, rash, and eosinophilia, which collectively may be observed in <10% of patients.[24,110,112] Concomitant nephrotic syndrome (proteinuria >3.5 g/day) occurs in more than 70% of patients. Prompt diagnosis of AIN is important as discontinuation of the offending drug may prevent irreversible renal damage.[21] Renal biopsy is the most definitive method for diagnosis.

Pathogenesis The pathogenesis of the majority of cases of AIN is considered to be an allergic hypersensitivity response. This is supported by the fact that AIN is characterized as a diffuse or focal interstitial infiltrate of lymphocytes, eosinophils, and occasional polymorphonuclear neutrophils.[21,113] Granulomas and tubular epithelial cell necrosis are relatively common with drug-induced AIN. Occasionally a humoral antibody-mediated mechanism is implicated by the presence of circulating antibody to a drug hapten–tubular basement membrane complex, low serum complement levels, and deposition of immunoglobulin G and complement in the tubular basement membrane.[21] More commonly, a cell-mediated immune mechanism is suggested by the absence of these findings and the presence of a predominantly T-lymphocyte.[113]

Risk Factors No specific risk factors have been identified because these are idiosyncratic hypersensitivity reactions. Individuals with other drug allergies may have increased risk and warrant close monitoring.

Prevention No specific preventive measures are known because of the idiosyncratic nature of these reactions. Patients must be monitored carefully to recognize the signs and symptoms, because promptly discontinuing the offending drug often leads to full recovery.[21]

Management Corticosteroid therapy is beneficial and should be initiated immediately or soon after diagnosis of AIN along with discontinuance of the offending drug to avoid the risk of incomplete recovery of renal function. While various regimens have been used, high-dose oral prednisone 1 mg/kg/day for 8 to 14 weeks with a stepwise taper has been used successfully.[111,115] Typical renal function indices (e.g., S_{cr}, BUN) and signs and symptoms of AIN should be monitored closely for improvement.

CHRONIC INTERSTITIAL NEPHRITIS

Lithium, analgesics, calcineurin inhibitors, aristolochic acid, and only a few other drugs have been reported to cause chronic interstitial nephritis, which is usually a progressive and irreversible lesion.[1,21]

Lithium

Incidence The prevalence of non-dialysis-dependent CKD stemming from chronic lithium nephrotoxicity in the general population of patients treated with lithium was recently estimated to be 1.2%.[117] The prevalence of lithium-induced ESRD among all ESRD patients is between 0.2% and 0.8%.[117,118] Several renal tubular lesions are associated with lithium therapy: an impaired ability to concentrate urine (nephrogenic diabetes insipidus) is seen in up to 87% of patients with biopsy proven nephrotoxicity,[113] and incomplete distal renal tubular acidosis is observed in up to 50% of these patients.[119]

Clinical Presentation Lithium-induced nephrotoxicity is typically asymptomatic and develops insidiously during years of therapy. Blood pressure is normal and urinary sediment is bland, making detection difficult until the disease progresses significantly.[120] It is usually recognized by rising BUN or S_{cr} concentrations or the onset of hypertension. Polydipsia (excessive thirst) and polyuria (excessive urination) are observed in 40% and 20%, respectively, of patients with nephrogenic diabetes insipidus (see Chap. 58).[119] Although interstitial fibrosis may be observed as early as 5 years after beginning therapy, lithium-induced CKD usually occurs after 10 to 20 years of lithium treatment.[120]

Pathogenesis The precise mechanism of chronic lithium-induced nephrotoxicity is not well characterized. Impaired ability to concentrate urine is a result of a decrease in collecting duct response to antidiuretic hormone, which may be related to downregulation of aquaporin 2 water channel expression during lithium therapy.[120] Chronic tubulointerstitial nephritis attributed to lithium is evidenced most commonly by biopsy findings of interstitial fibrosis, tubular atrophy, and glomerular sclerosis.[21,118] The pathogenesis may involve cumulative direct lithium toxicity since duration of therapy correlates with the decline in the GFR.

Risk Factors It is now established that long-term lithium therapy is associated with nephrotoxicity in the absence of episodes of acute intoxication, and that the duration of therapy is the major determinant of chronic nephrotoxicity.[118,120] Increased age may also be a risk factor, but daily dose is not.[120]

Prevention Prevention of acute and chronic toxicity includes maintaining lithium concentrations as low as therapeutically possible, avoiding dehydration, and monitoring renal function. It is unknown whether progression to CKD can be prevented by stopping lithium use when mild kidney injury is first recognized. This poses a dilemma as lithium is highly effective for affective disorders and the risks and potential benefits of discontinuing such a beneficial drug need to be carefully considered.[120] However, if lithium therapy is continued, renal function must be monitored and therapy discontinued if it continues to decline. Amiloride has been used for prevention and treatment of lithium-induced nephrogenic diabetes insipidus, since it blocks epithelial sodium transport of lithium into the cortical collecting duct in the distal nephron.[120,121]

Management Symptomatic polyuria and polydipsia can be reversed by discontinuation of lithium therapy or ameliorated with amiloride 5 to 10 mg daily during continued lithium therapy (see Chap. 58).[119,121] If polyuria does not resolve within 7 to 10 days of therapy, then the amiloride dose should be increased to 20 mg daily. Progressive chronic interstitial nephritis is treated by discontinuation of lithium therapy, adequate hydration, and avoidance of other nephrotoxic agents. Lithium serum concentrations, as well as renal function indices, including urine output, BUN, and S_{cr}, should be monitored closely for resolution of signs and symptoms of toxicity.[120]

Cyclosporine and Tacrolimus

Delayed chronic tubulointerstitial nephritis, considered the Achilles' heel of calcineurin inhibitor based immunosuppressive regimens, has been reported after several months of therapy and can result in irreversible kidney disease.[82] Toxicity is progressive and usually manifests as a slowly rising S_{cr} concentration and decreased creatinine clearance that may not reflect the severity of histopathologic changes. All three compartments of the kidney can be affected, evidenced by typical biopsy findings that include arteriolar hyalinosis, glomerular sclerosis, and a striped pattern of tubulointerstitial fibrosis.[82,84,119] The pathogenesis appears to involve sustained renal arteriolar endothelial cell injury and increased extracellular matrix synthesis, which ultimately result in chronic ischemia of the tubulointerstitial compartment because of increased release of endothelin-1, decreased production of nitric acid, and upregulation of transforming growth factor-β.[82] Unlike acute nephrotoxicity, chronic toxicity is not dose dependent.

Aristolochic Acid

Incidence In the early 1990s, a cluster of young women with rapidly progressive kidney disease leading to ESRD were reported in Brussels, Belgium. The patients had strikingly similar pathologic findings of interstitial fibrosis with tubular atrophy on renal biopsy. Further investigation revealed that all the women were patients of the same weight-loss clinic and had received a weight-loss treatment containing Chinese herbs.[122] Subsequent analysis of the herb-based treatment demonstrated significant amounts of *Aristolochia fangchi* (Guang fang ji), known to contain aristolochic acid, the major alkaloid of the botanical species *Aristolochia*.[122] Although the true incidence is unknown, approximately 3% to 5% of patients who received the weight-loss regimen developed disease, and numerous additional cases of aristolochic acid nephropathy have been reported worldwide.[122]

Clinical Presentation Patients with aristolochic acid nephropathy typically present with mild to moderate hypertension, mild proteinuria, glucosuria, and moderately elevated S_{cr} concentrations.[122] Anemia and shrunken kidneys are also common on initial presentation. The overwhelming majority of cases reported to date have been in women. The main pathologic lesions observed in the kidneys are interstitial fibrosis with atrophy and destruction of proximal tubules throughout the renal cortex; in general, the glomeruli are not affected. Perhaps the most remarkable feature of

aristolochic acid nephropathy is the rate at which it progresses. In most individuals, ESRD requiring dialysis or transplantation develops within 6 to 24 months of exposure. An alarming high prevalence (approximately 40% to 45%) of urothelial transitional cell carcinoma has been observed in Belgian patients who underwent renal transplantation.[122]

Pathogenesis Although the precise mechanism of aristolochic acid nephropathy and urothelial carcinoma has yet to be characterized. The major components of aristolochic acid are metabolized to mutagenic compounds called *aristolactam I* and *aristolactam II*, respectively, which have been demonstrated to form aristolochic acid–DNA adducts in humans. Recent data indicate that these adducts cause direct DNA damage and may lead to proximal tubular atrophy and apoptosis.[122]

Prevention The primary means of preventing aristolochic acid nephropathy appears to be the limitation of exposure to compounds containing aristolochic acids. Several countries, including the United Kingdom, Canada, Australia, and Germany, have banned the use of *Aristolochia*-containing herbs.[122]

PAPILLARY NECROSIS

Papillary necrosis is a form of chronic tubulointerstitial nephritis characterized by necrosis of the renal papillae, the regions of the kidney where the collecting ducts enter the renal pelvis, which leads to progressive kidney disease.[21,123] Papillary necrosis is associated with diabetes, sickle cell disease, obstruction and infection of the urinary tract, and most commonly analgesic use.[21,124]

Analgesic Nephropathy

Incidence Prototypical analgesic nephropathy is characterized by chronic tubulointerstitial nephritis with papillary necrosis.[21] Chronic excessive consumption of combination analgesics, particularly those containing phenacetin, was believed to be the major cause and led to the removal of phenacetin and phenacetin mixtures from most world markets. However, contemporary analgesics, particularly aspirin, acetaminophen, and NSAIDs, alone or in combination, are also associated with the development of analgesic nephropathy, but there is insufficient causative evidence to definitively link these nonphenacetin-containing analgesics with nephropathy.[123] The incidence of analgesic nephropathy has declined significantly since removal of phenacetin from many countries, with the prevalence estimated to now be <5% in the United States adult ESRD population.[124]

Clinical Presentation Analgesic nephropathy is a progressive disease that evolves slowly over several years.[124] It is difficult to recognize in the early stages of the disease because patients are often asymptomatic,[125] and it may be underdiagnosed as a cause of ESRD. It is seen more commonly in women than men.[21] Early manifestations are generally nonspecific and may include headache and upper gastrointestinal symptoms; later manifestations include impaired urinary concentrating ability, dysuria, sterile pyuria, microscopic hematuria, mild proteinuria (<1.5 g/day), and lower back pain. As disease progresses, hypertension, atherosclerotic cardiovascular disease, renal calculi, and bladder stones are common, and pyelonephritis is a classic finding in advanced analgesic nephropathy.[123,125] The most sensitive and specific diagnostic criteria include (1) a history of chronic daily habitual analgesic ingestion (daily use for at least 3 to 5 years); (2) intravenous pyelography, renal ultrasound, or renal computed tomography imaging, which reveals decreased renal mass and bumpy renal contours; (3) elevated S_{cr}, i.e., up to 4 mg/dL (354 μmol/L); and (4) papillary calcifications.[123,124]

Pathogenesis Analgesic nephropathy originates in the papillary tip as a result of accumulated toxins, drugs and metabolites, decreased blood flow, and impaired cellular energy production. The metabolism of phenacetin to acetaminophen, which is then oxidized to toxic free radicals that are concentrated in the papilla, appears to be the initiating factor that causes toxicity by mechanisms analogous to acetaminophen hepatotoxicity via glutathione depletion.[21,119] Cortical interstitial nephritis develops secondary to papillary necrosis. Salicylates potentiate these effects by also depleting renal glutathione, and inhibiting prostaglandin-mediated vasodilation, thus further predisposing the renal medulla to ischemic injury.[21,119]

Risk Factors The epidemiology of analgesic use and analgesic nephropathy continues to evolve. The classic concept persists that risk for ESRD increases with cumulative consumption of combination analgesics, phenacetin, or acetaminophen and aspirin or NSAIDs. Caffeine contained in combination analgesics may increase risk, but the role is not clear.[123,124] Chronic use of therapeutic doses of NSAIDs alone, but not aspirin or salicylates alone, can cause analgesic nephropathy. High-dose acetaminophen use alone is associated with an increased risk for ESRD. However, these associations remain inconclusive as a consequence of study design flaws, as acetaminophen has been the preferentially prescribed analgesic for patients with chronic kidney disease.[123,124]

Prevention Prevention has depended primarily on public health efforts to restrict the sale of phenacetin and combination analgesics. This has effectively reduced analgesic nephropathy in Australia and Europe.[123] However, risk continues with ongoing availability of nonprescription combination analgesics containing aspirin, acetaminophen, and caffeine in the United States and throughout the world.

Individuals requiring chronic analgesic therapy may reduce risk by limiting the total dose, avoiding combined use of two or more analgesics, and maintaining good hydration to prevent renal ischemia and decrease the papillary concentration of toxic substances. Acetaminophen remains the preferred nonopiate analgesic for patients with preexisting kidney disease.

Management Treatment of established nephrotoxicity requires cessation of analgesic consumption.[119] This can prevent progression and may improve renal function. Renal function indices, including urine output, BUN, and S_{cr}, should be monitored every several months. Patients should also be monitored for the development of transitional cell carcinoma of the renal pelvis, calyces, ureters, and bladder, which may present years after analgesic nephropathy is diagnosed.[21]

RENAL VASCULITIS, THROMBOSIS, AND CHOLESTEROL EMBOLI

RENAL VASCULITIS

Drug-induced renal vascular disease commonly presents as vasculitis, thrombotic microangiopathy, or cholesterol emboli. Vasculitis implies inflammation of the vessel wall, capillaries, or glomeruli and is typically classified according to vessel size (i.e., small, medium, or large vessel vasculitis).[25] Small vessel vasculitides usually affect multiple organ systems, including the kidneys and lungs, and are associated with nonspecific inflammatory symptoms such as fever, malaise, myalgias, arthralgias, and weight loss.[105] Numerous drugs are associated with the development of renal vasculitis, including hydralazine, propylthiouracil, allopurinol, phenytoin, sulfasalazine, penicillamine, and minocycline (Table 55–1).[25,126] Most drug-induced cases of vasculitis, including hydralazine, propylthiouracil, allopurinol, and penicillamine, have been implicated in the

development of antineutrophil cytoplasmic antibody (ANCA)-positive vasculitis.[25,127] Recently, the antitumor necrosis factor-α drug adalimumab was associated with the development of ANCA-associated renal vasculitis.[126,128] Patients present with hematuria, proteinuria, oliguria, and red cell casts, frequently along with fever, malaise, myalgias, and arthralgias.[25,105] Treatment typically consists of withdrawing the offending drug and administration of corticosteroids or other immunosuppressive therapy, and usually leads to resolution of symptoms within weeks to months.[126]

Thrombotic Microangiopathy

Thrombotic microangiopathy is characterized clinically by microangiopathic hemolytic anemia, fragmented red cells, and thrombocytopenia and pathologically by vascular endothelial proliferation, endothelial cell swelling, and intraluminal platelet thrombi in the small vessels, particularly affecting the renal and cerebral capillaries and arterioles.[24,25,129] The absence of inflammation in vessel walls distinguishes thrombotic microangiopathy from vasculitis. Numerous medications, including oral contraceptive agents, cyclosporine, tacrolimus, muromonab-CD3, many cancer chemotherapeutic agents including mitomycin C, cisplatin, and gemcitabine, interferon-α, ticlopidine, clopidogrel, and quinine are associated with the development of thrombotic microangiopathy.[24,25,129] Recently, bevacizumab, a humanized monoclonal antibody against vascular endothelial growth factor, was reported to cause thrombotic microangiopathy,[130] and other drugs in the class have also been implicated in vascular adverse reactions.[131] Patients may present with fever, neurological dysfunction, elevated S_{cr} and BUN, and hypertension, along with microangiopathic hemolytic anemia and thrombocytopenia.[25] Kidney injury can be severe and irreversible, although corticosteroids, antiplatelet agents, plasma exchange, plasmapheresis, and high-dose intravenous immunoglobulin G have each induced clinical improvement.

Cholesterol Emboli

Anticoagulants (particularly warfarin) and thrombolytics (e.g., urokinase, streptokinase, tissue-plasminogen activator) are associated with cholesterol embolization of the kidney.[1,132] These drugs act to remove or prevent thrombus formation over ulcerative plaques or may induce hemorrhage within clots, thereby causing showers of cholesterol crystals that lodge in small diameter arteries of the kidney (renal arterioles and glomerular capillaries). Cholesterol crystal emboli induce an endothelial inflammatory response, which leads to complete obstruction, ischemia, and necrosis of affected vessels within weeks to months after initiation of therapy.[1,132] Purple discoloration of the toes and mottled skin over the legs are important clinical clues. Treatment is supportive in nature, since kidney injury is generally irreversible.

COSTS OF DRUG-INDUCED KIDNEY DISEASE

The costs of DIKD are not well defined, but recent data indicate that the pharmacoeconomic implications are enormous. An increase in S_{cr} of ≥0.5 mg/dL (44 μmol/L) is independently associated with a 6.5-fold increase in the odds of death, a 3.5-day increase in length of hospital stay, and nearly \$7,500 in excess hospital costs even after adjusting for age, sex, and measures of comorbidity.[9] A recent report indicates that amphotericin B-induced AKI leads to a mean increased length of hospital stay of 8.2 days and adjusted additional costs of \$29,823 per patient.[133] Lastly, the mean additional in-hospital cost for each episode of contrast-induced AKI has been estimated to be \$10,345 per case. The major driver of the increased costs associated with contrast-induced AKI was the cost of the longer initial hospital stay.[34] The increased availability of automated clinical decision support systems and computer-guided medication dosing for hospital inpatients may improve the safety of potentially harmful drugs and minimize the occurrence of nephrotoxicity in this setting, thereby potentially lowering the corresponding economic consequences.[133]

ABBREVIATIONS

ACEI: angiotensin-converting enzyme inhibitor

AIDS: acquired immune deficiency syndrome

AIN: allergic interstitial nephritis

AKI: acute kidney injury

ARB: angiotensin II receptor blocker

BUN: blood urea nitrogen

CIN: contrast media-induced nephrotoxicity

CKD: chronic kidney disease

COX: cyclooxygenase

CYP: cytochrome P450

ESRD: end-stage renal disease

FSGS: focal segmental glomerulosclerosis

GFR: glomerular filtration rate

HIV: human immunodeficiency virus

KIM-1: kidney injury molecule-1

NGAL: neutrophil gelatinase-associated lipocalin

NSAID: nonsteroidal antiinflammatory drug

OSPS: oral sodium phosphate solution

S_{cr}: serum creatinine

REFERENCES

1. Choudhury D, Ahmed Z. Drug-associated renal dysfunction and injury. Nat Clin Pract Nephrol 2006;2:80–91.
2. Himmelfarb J, Ikizler TA. Acute kidney injury: Changing lexicography, definitions, and epidemiology. Kidney Int 2007;71:971–976.
3. Zappitelli M, Parikh CR, Akcan-Arikan A, et al. Ascertainment and epidemiology of acute kidney injury varies with definition interpretation. Clin J Am Soc Nephrol 2008;3:948–954.
4. Warnock DG. Towards a definition and classification of acute kidney injury. J Am Soc Nephrol 2005;16:3149–3150.
5. Hoste EA, Kellum JA. Acute kidney injury: Epidemiology and diagnostic criteria. Curr Opin Crit Care 2006;12:531–537.
6. Ricci Z, Cruz D, Ronco C. The RIFLE criteria and mortality in acute kidney injury: A systematic review. Kidney Int 2008;73:538–546.
7. Hsu CY, McCulloch CE, Fan D, et al. Community-based incidence of acute renal failure. Kidney Int 2007;72:208–212.
8. Elasy TA, Anderson RJ. Changing demography of acute renal failure. Semin Dial 1996;9:438–443.
9. Chertow GM, Burdick E, Honour M, et al. Acute kidney injury, mortality, length of stay, and costs in hospitalized patients. J Am Soc Nephrol 2005;16:3365–3370.
10. Lameire N, Van Biesen W, Vanholder R. Acute renal failure. Lancet 2005;365:417–430.
11. Pannu N, Nadim MK. An overview of drug-induced acute kidney injury. Crit Care Med 2008;36:S216–S223.
12. Schetz M, Dasta J, Goldstein S, Golper T. Drug-induced acute kidney injury. Curr Opin Crit Care 2005;11:555–565.
13. Mehta RL, Kellum JA, Shah SV, et al. Acute kidney injury network: Report of an initiative to improve outcomes in acute kidney injury. Crit Care 2007;11:R31.
14. Goodsaid FM, Blank M, Dieterle F, et al. Novel biomarkers of acute kidney toxicity. Clin Pharmacol Ther 2009;86:490–496.
15. Coca SG, Parikh CR. Urinary biomarkers for acute kidney injury: Perspectives on translation. Clin J Am Soc Nephrol 2008;3:481–490.
16. Vaidya VS, Ferguson MA, Bonventre JV. Biomarkers of acute kidney injury. Annu Rev Pharmacol Toxicol 2008;48:463–493.
17. Perazella MA. Renal vulnerability to drug toxicity. Clin J Am Soc Nephrol 2009;4:1275–1283.
18. Naughton CA. Drug-induced nephrotoxicity. Am Fam Physician 2008;78:743–750.
19. Izzedine H, Launay-Vacher V, Deray G. Antiviral drug-induced nephrotoxicity. Am J Kidney Dis 2005;45:804–817.
20. Doan ML, Mallory GB, Kaplan SL, et al. Treatment of adenovirus pneumonia with cidofovir in pediatric lung transplant recipients. J Heart Lung Transplant 2007;26:883–889.
21. Silva FG. Chemical-induced nephropathy: A review of the renal tubulointerstitial lesions in humans. Toxicol Pathol 2004;32(suppl 2):71–84.
22. Khalil P, Murty P, Palevsky PM. The patient with acute kidney injury. Prim Care 2008;35:239–264, vi.
23. Abuelo JG. Normotensive ischemic acute renal failure. N Engl J Med 2007;357:797–805.
24. Perazella MA. Drug-induced nephropathy: An update. Expert Opin Drug Saf 2005;4:689–706.
25. John R, Herzenberg AM. Renal toxicity of therapeutic drugs. J Clin Pathol 2009;62:505–515.
26. Oliveira JF, Silva CA, Barbieri CD, et al. Prevalence and risk factors for aminoglycoside nephrotoxicity in intensive care units. Antimicrob Agents Chemother 2009;53:2887–2891.
27. Martinez-Salgado C, Lopez-Hernandez FJ, Lopez-Novoa JM. Glomerular nephrotoxicity of aminoglycosides. Toxicol Appl Pharmacol 2007;223:86–98.
28. Drusano GL, Ambrose PG, Bhavnani SM, et al. Back to the future: Using aminoglycosides again and how to dose them optimally. Clin Infect Dis 2007;45:753–760.
29. Sandoval RM, Reilly JP, Running W, et al. A non-nephrotoxic gentamicin congener that retains antimicrobial efficacy. J Am Soc Nephrol 2006;17:2697–2705.
30. Koyner JL, Sher Ali R, Murray PT. Antioxidants. Do they have a place in the prevention or therapy of acute kidney injury? Nephron Exp Nephrol 2008;109:e109–e117.
31. Greenwood BC, Szumita PM, Lowry CM. Pharmacist-driven aminoglycoside quality improvement program. J Chemother 2009;21:42–45.
32. Olsen KM, Rudis MI, Rebuck JA, et al. Effect of once-daily dosing vs. multiple daily dosing of tobramycin on enzyme markers of nephrotoxicity. Crit Care Med 2004;32:1678–1682.
33. Barrett BJ, Parfrey PS. Clinical practice. Preventing nephropathy induced by contrast medium. N Engl J Med 2006;354:379–386.
34. McCullough PA. Contrast-induced acute kidney injury. J Am Coll Cardiol 2008;51:1419–1428.
35. Rudnick MR, Kesselheim A, Goldfarb S. Contrast-induced nephropathy: How it develops, how to prevent it. Cleve Clin J Med 2006;73:75–77.
36. Brar SS, Shen AY, Jorgensen MB, et al. Sodium bicarbonate vs sodium chloride for the prevention of contrast medium-induced nephropathy in patients undergoing coronary angiography: A randomized trial. JAMA 2008;300:1038–1046.
37. Rudnick M, Feldman H. Contrast-induced nephropathy: What are the true clinical consequences? Clin J Am Soc Nephrol 2008;3:263–272.
38. Maeder M, Klein M, Fehr T, Rickli H. Contrast nephropathy: Review focusing on prevention. J Am Coll Cardiol 2004;44:1763–1771.
39. Pflueger A, Abramowitz D, Calvin AD. Role of oxidative stress in contrast-induced acute kidney injury in diabetes mellitus. Med Sci Monit 2009;15:RA125–RA136.
40. Marenzi G, Assanelli E, Marana I, et al. N-acetylcysteine and contrast-induced nephropathy in primary angioplasty. N Engl J Med 2006;354:2773–2782.
41. Ellis JH, Cohan RH. Prevention of contrast-induced nephropathy: An overview. Radiol Clin North Am 2009;47:801–811, v.
42. Fishbane S. N-acetylcysteine in the prevention of contrast-induced nephropathy. Clin J Am Soc Nephrol 2008;3:281–287.

43. Solomon R. Contrast-induced acute kidney injury (CIAKI). Radiol Clin North Am 2009;47:783–788.

44. Kelly AM, Dwamena B, Cronin P, et al. Meta-analysis: Effectiveness of drugs for preventing contrast-induced nephropathy. Ann Intern Med 2008;148:284–294.

45. Laskey WK, Jenkins C, Selzer F, et al. Volume-to-creatinine clearance ratio: A pharmacokinetically based risk factor for prediction of early creatinine increase after percutaneous coronary intervention. J Am Coll Cardiol 2007;50:584–590.

46. Heinrich MC, Haberle L, Muller V, et al. Nephrotoxicity of iso-osmolar iodixanol compared with nonionic low-osmolar contrast media: Meta-analysis of randomized controlled trials. Radiology 2009;250:68–86.

47. Jo SH, Youn TJ, Koo BK, et al. Renal toxicity evaluation and comparison between visipaque (iodixanol) and hexabrix (ioxaglate) in patients with renal insufficiency undergoing coronary angiography: The RECOVER study: A randomized controlled trial. J Am Coll Cardiol 2006;48:924–930.

48. Weisbord SD, Palevsky PM. Prevention of contrast-induced nephropathy with volume expansion. Clin J Am Soc Nephrol 2008;3:273–280.

49. Merten GJ, Burgess WP, Gray LV, et al. Prevention of contrast-induced nephropathy with sodium bicarbonate: A randomized controlled trial. JAMA 2004;291:2328–2334.

50. Briguori C, Airoldi F, D'Andrea D, et al. Renal Insufficiency Following Contrast Media Administration Trial (REMEDIAL): A randomized comparison of 3 preventive strategies. Circulation 2007;115:1211–1217.

51. From AM, Bartholmai BJ, Williams AW, et al. Sodium bicarbonate is associated with an increased incidence of contrast nephropathy: A retrospective cohort study of 7977 patients at mayo clinic. Clin J Am Soc Nephrol 2008;3:10–18.

52. Schweiger MJ, Chambers CE, Davidson CJ, et al. Prevention of contrast induced nephropathy: Recommendations for the high risk patient undergoing cardiovascular procedures. Catheter Cardiovasc Interv 2006;69:135–140.

53. Marenzi G, Marana I, Lauri G, et al. The prevention of radiocontrast-agent-induced nephropathy by hemofiltration. N Engl J Med 2003;349:1333–1340.

54. Marenzi G, Lauri G, Campodonico J, et al. Comparison of two hemofiltration protocols for prevention of contrast-induced nephropathy in high-risk patients. Am J Med 2006;119:155–162.

55. Launay-Vacher V, Rey JB, Isnard-Bagnis C, et al. Prevention of cisplatin nephrotoxicity: State of the art and recommendations from the European Society of Clinical Pharmacy Special Interest Group on Cancer Care. Cancer Chemother Pharmacol 2008;61:903–909.

56. Pabla N, Dong Z. Cisplatin nephrotoxicity: Mechanisms and renoprotective strategies. Kidney Int 2008;73:994–1007.

57. Yao X, Panichpisal K, Kurtzman N, Nugent K. Cisplatin nephrotoxicity: A review. Am J Med Sci 2007;334:115–124.

58. Hartmann JT, Lipp HP. Toxicity of platinum compounds. Expert Opin Pharmacother 2003;4:889–901.

59. Hensley ML, Hagerty KL, Kewalramani T, et al. American Society of Clinical Oncology 2008 clinical practice guideline update: Use of chemotherapy and radiation therapy protectants. J Clin Oncol 2009;27:127–145.

60. Al Ghamdi SS, Chatterjee PK, Raftery MJ, et al. Role of cytochrome P4502E1 activation in proximal tubular cell injury induced by hydrogen peroxide. Ren Fail 2004;26:103–110.

61. Goldman RD, Koren G. Amphotericin B nephrotoxicity in children. J Pediatr Hematol Oncol 2004;26:421–426.

62. Bates DW, Su L, Yu DT, et al. Mortality and costs of acute renal failure associated with amphotericin B therapy. Clin Infect Dis 2001;32:686–693.

63. Ullmann AJ. Nephrotoxicity in the setting of invasive fungal diseases. Mycoses 2008;51(suppl 1):25–30.

64. Saliba F. Antifungals and renal safety—getting the balance right. Int J Antimicrob Agents 2006;27(suppl 1):21–24.

65. Slavin MA, Szer J, Grigg AP, et al. Guidelines for the use of antifungal agents in the treatment of invasive Candida and mould infections. Intern Med J 2004;34:192–200.

66. Kleinberg M. What is the current and future status of conventional amphotericin B? Int J Antimicrob Agents 2006;27(suppl 1):12–16.

67. Dickenmann M, Oettl T, Mihatsch MJ. Osmotic nephrosis: Acute kidney injury with accumulation of proximal tubular lysosomes due to administration of exogenous solutes. Am J Kidney Dis 2008;51:491–503.

68. Chacko B, John GT, Balakrishnan N, et al. Osmotic nephropathy resulting from maltose-based intravenous immunoglobulin therapy. Ren Fail 2006;28:193–195.

69. Welles CC, Tambra S, Lafayette RA. Hemoglobinuria and acute kidney injury requiring hemodialysis following intravenous immunoglobulin infusion. Am J Kidney Dis 2010;55:148–151.

70. Szeto CC, Chow KM. Nephrotoxicity related to new therapeutic compounds. Ren Fail 2005;27:329–333.

71. Huter L, Simon TP, Weinmann L, et al. Hydroxyethylstarch impairs renal function and induces interstitial proliferation, macrophage infiltration and tubular damage in an isolated renal perfusion model. Crit Care 2009;13:R23.

72. Kobori H, Nangaku M, Navar LG, Nishiyama A. The intrarenal renin-angiotensin system: From physiology to the pathobiology of hypertension and kidney disease. Pharmacol Rev 2007;59:251–287.

73. Cupples WA, Braam B. Assessment of renal autoregulation. Am J Physiol Renal Physiol 2007;292:F1105–F1123.

74. Ryan MJ, Tuttle KR. Elevations in serum creatinine with RAAS blockade: Why isn't it a sign of kidney injury? Curr Opin Nephrol Hypertens 2008;17:443–449.

75. Chittineni H, Miyawaki N, Gulipelli S, Fishbane S. Risk for acute renal failure in patients hospitalized for decompensated congestive heart failure. Am J Nephrol 2007;27:55–62.

76. Cruz CS, Cruz LS, Silva GR, Marcilio de Souza CA. Incidence and predictors of development of acute renal failure related to treatment of congestive heart failure with ACE inhibitors. Nephron Clin Pract 2007;105:c77–c83.

77. Epstein BJ. Elevations in serum creatinine concentration: Concerning or reassuring? Pharmacotherapy 2004;24:697–702.

78. Cheng HF, Harris RC. Renal effects of non-steroidal anti-inflammatory drugs and selective cyclooxygenase-2 inhibitors. Curr Pharm Des 2005;11:1795–1804.

79. House AA, Silva Oliveira S, Ronco C. Anti-inflammatory drugs and the kidney. Int J Artif Organs 2007;30:1042–1046.

80. Whelton A. Nephrotoxicity of nonsteroidal anti-inflammatory drugs: Physiologic foundations and clinical implications. Am J Med 1999;106:13S–24S.

81. Barkin RL, Buvanendran A. Focus on the COX-1 and COX-2 agents: Renal events of nonsteroidal and anti-inflammatory drugs-NSAIDs. Am J Ther 2004;11:124–129.

82. Naesens M, Kuypers DR, Sarwal M. Calcineurin inhibitor nephrotoxicity. Clin J Am Soc Nephrol 2009;4:481–508.

83. Ojo AO, Held PJ, Port FK, et al. Chronic renal failure after transplantation of a nonrenal organ. N Engl J Med 2003;349:931–940.

84. Liptak P, Ivanyi B. Primer: Histopathology of calcineurin-inhibitor toxicity in renal allografts. Nat Clin Pract Nephrol 2006;2:398–404.

85. Lameire N, Van Biesen W, Vanholder R. Acute renal problems in the critically ill cancer patient. Curr Opin Crit Care 2008;14:635–646.

86. Tosi P, Barosi G, Lazzaro C, et al. Consensus conference on the management of tumor lysis syndrome. Haematologica 2008;93:1877–1885.

87. Bagley WH, Yang H, Shah KH. Rhabdomyolysis. Intern Emerg Med 2007;2:210–218.

88. Molden E, Skovlund E, Braathen P. Risk management of simvastatin or atorvastatin interactions with CYP3A4 inhibitors. Drug Saf 2008;31:587–596.

89. Yarlagadda SG, Perazella MA. Drug-induced crystal nephropathy: An update. Expert Opin Drug Saf 2008;7:147–158.

90. Izzedine H, Harris M, Perazella MA. The nephrotoxic effects of HAART. Nat Rev Nephrol 2009;5:563–573.

91. Parasuraman R, Venkat KK. Crystal-induced kidney disease in 2 kidney transplant recipients. Am J Kidney Dis 2010;55:192–197.

92. Gabardi S, Munz K, Ulbricht C. A review of dietary supplement-induced renal dysfunction. Clin J Am Soc Nephrol 2007;2:757–765.

93. Gonlusen G, Akgun H, Ertan A, et al. Renal failure and nephrocalcinosis associated with oral sodium phosphate bowel cleansing: Clinical patterns and renal biopsy findings. Arch Pathol Lab Med 2006;130:101–106.

94. Heher EC, Thier SO, Rennke H, Humphreys BD. Adverse renal and metabolic effects associated with oral sodium phosphate bowel preparation. Clin J Am Soc Nephrol 2008;3:1494–1503.

95. Markowitz GS, Stokes MB, Radhakrishnan J, D'Agati VD. Acute phosphate nephropathy following oral sodium phosphate bowel purgative: An underrecognized cause of chronic renal failure. J Am Soc Nephrol 2005;16:3389–3396.

96. Markowitz GS, Radhakrishnan J, D'Agati VD. Towards the incidence of acute phosphate nephropathy. J Am Soc Nephrol 2007;18: 3020–3022.

97. Desmeules S, Bergeron MJ, Isenring P. Acute phosphate nephropathy and renal failure. N Engl J Med 2003;349:1006–1007.

98. Markowitz GS, Whelan J, D'Agati VD. Renal failure following bowel cleansing with a sodium phosphate purgative. Nephrol Dial Transplant 2005;20:850–851.

99. Beloosesky Y, Grinblat J, Weiss A, et al. Electrolyte disorders following oral sodium phosphate administration for bowel cleansing in elderly patients. Arch Intern Med 2003;163:803–808.

100. Russmann S, Lamerato L, Motsko SP, et al. Risk of further decline in renal function after the use of oral sodium phosphate or polyethylene glycol in patients with a preexisting glomerular filtration rate below 60 ml/min. Am J Gastroenterol 2008;103:2707–2716.

101. Hurst FP, Bohen EM, Osgard EM, et al. Association of oral sodium phosphate purgative use with acute kidney injury. J Am Soc Nephrol 2007;18:3192–3198.

102. Khurana A, McLean L, Atkinson S, Foulks CJ. The effect of oral sodium phosphate drug products on renal function in adults undergoing bowel endoscopy. Arch Intern Med 2008;168:593–597.

103. Daudon M, Jungers P. Drug-induced renal calculi: Epidemiology, prevention and management. Drugs 2004;64:245–275.

104. Hau AK, Kwan TH, Li PK. Melamine toxicity and the kidney. J Am Soc Nephrol 2009;20:245–250.

105. Beck LH, Jr., Salant DJ. Glomerular and tubulointerstitial diseases. Prim Care 2008;35:265–296, vi.

106. Izzedine H, Launay-Vacher V, Bourry E, et al. Drug-induced glomerulopathies. ExpertOpinDrug Saf 2006;5:95–106.

107. Jaffe JA, Kimmel PL. Chronic nephropathies of cocaine and heroin abuse: A critical review. Clin J Am Soc Nephrol 2006;1:655–667.

108. Perazella MA, Markowitz GS. Bisphosphonate nephrotoxicity. Kidney Int 2008;74:1385–1393.

109. Albaqumi M, Soos TJ, Barisoni L, Nelson PJ. Collapsing glomerulopathy. J Am Soc Nephrol 2006;17:2854–2863.

110. Baker RJ, Pusey CD. The changing profile of acute tubulointerstitial nephritis. Nephrol Dial Transplant 2004;19:8–11.

111. Gonzalez E, Gutierrez E, Galeano C, et al. Early steroid treatment improves the recovery of renal function in patients with drug-induced acute interstitial nephritis. Kidney Int 2008;73:940–946.

112. Clarkson MR, Giblin L, O'Connell FP, et al. Acute interstitial nephritis: Clinical features and response to corticosteroid therapy. Nephrol Dial Transplant 2004;19:2778–2783.

113. Markowitz GS, Perazella MA. Drug-induced renal failure: A focus on tubulointerstitial disease. Clin Chim Acta 2005;351:31–47.

114. Harmark L, van der Wiel HE, de Groot MC, van Grootheest AC. Proton pump inhibitor-induced acute interstitial nephritis. Br J Clin Pharmacol 2007;64:819–823.

115. Ricketson J, Kimel G, Spence J, Weir R. Acute allergic interstitial nephritis after use of pantoprazole. CMAJ 2009;180:535–538.

116. Brewster UC, Perazella MA. Acute kidney injury following proton pump inhibitor therapy. Kidney Int 2007;71:589–593.

117. Bendz H, Schon S, Attman PO, Aurell M. Renal failure occurs in chronic lithium treatment but is uncommon. Kidney Int 2010;77: 219–224.

118. Presne C, Fakhouri F, Noel LH, et al. Lithium-induced nephropathy: Rate of progression and prognostic factors. Kidney Int 2003;64: 585–592.

119. Braden GL, O'Shea MH, Mulhern JG. Tubulointerstitial diseases. Am J Kidney Dis 2005;46:560–572.

120. Grunfeld JP, Rossier BC. Lithium nephrotoxicity revisited. Nat Rev Nephrol 2009;5:270–276.

121. Bedford JJ, Weggery S, Ellis G, et al. Lithium-induced nephrogenic diabetes insipidus: Renal effects of amiloride. Clin J Am Soc Nephrol 2008;3:1324–1331.

122. Debelle FD, Vanherweghem JL, Nortier JL. Aristolochic acid nephropathy: A worldwide problem. Kidney Int 2008;74:158–169.

123. Vadivel N, Trikudanathan S, Singh AK. Analgesic nephropathy. Kidney Int 2007;72:517–520.

124. De Broe ME, Elseviers MM. Over-the-counter analgesic use. J Am Soc Nephrol 2009;20:2098–2103.

125. Brix AE. Renal papillary necrosis. Toxicol Pathol 2002;30:672–674.

126. Wiik A. Drug-induced vasculitis. Curr Opin Rheumatol 2008;20: 35–39.

127. Aloush V, Litinsky I, Caspi D, Elkayam O. Propylthiouracil-induced autoimmune syndromes: Two distinct clinical presentations with different course and management. Semin Arthritis Rheum 2006;36:4–9.

128. Simms R, Kipgen D, Dahill S, et al. ANCA-associated renal vasculitis following anti-tumor necrosis factor alpha therapy. Am J Kidney Dis 2008;51:e11–e14.

129. Dlott JS, Danielson CF, Blue-Hnidy DE, McCarthy LJ. Drug-induced thrombotic thrombocytopenic purpura/hemolytic uremic syndrome: A concise review. Ther Apher Dial 2004;8:102–111.

130. Eremina V, Jefferson JA, Kowalewska J, et al. VEGF inhibition and renal thrombotic microangiopathy. N Engl J Med 2008;358: 1129–1136.

131. Gurevich F, Perazella MA. Renal effects of anti-angiogenesis therapy: Update for the internist. Am J Med 2009;122:322–328.

132. Meyrier A. Cholesterol crystal embolism: Diagnosis and treatment. Kidney Int 2006;69:1308–1312.

133. Hug BL, Witkowski DJ, Sox CM, et al. Occurrence of adverse, often preventable, events in community hospitals involving nephrotoxic drugs or those excreted by the kidney. Kidney Int 2009;76:1192–1198.

ALAN H. LAU

CHAPTER 56

Glomerulonephritis

KEY CONCEPTS

❶ Glomerulonephritis is a collection of glomerular diseases mediated by different immunologic pathogenic mechanisms, resulting in varied clinical presentation and therapeutic outcomes.

❷ The signs and symptoms associated with glomerulonephritis can be nephritic in nature, characterized by inflammatory injury, or nephrotic in nature, characterized by proteinuria.

❸ In the absence of specific and effective therapy for many types of glomerulonephritis, supportive treatments for edema, hypertension, hyperlipidemia, and intravascular thrombosis play important roles in reducing the complications associated with the disease.

❹ To maximize therapeutic benefits and minimize drug-induced complications, patients have to be monitored closely to assess their therapeutic responses as well as the development of any treatment-induced toxicities.

❺ Among all the types of glomerulonephritis, minimal-change nephropathy is most responsive to treatment. Steroids can induce good responses in most patients during initial treatment as well as relapse.

❻ Because of the lack of consistently effective treatment for primary focal segmental glomerular sclerosis, angiotensin-converting enzyme inhibitors or angiotensin receptor blockers are commonly used for patients with mild disease to control symptoms. Steroids and immunosuppressive agents are reserved for patients with severe disease.

❼ The optimal treatment for lupus nephritis depends on the underlying lesion and disease activity, as well as the severity and duration of the clinical presentation.

❽ The treatment of poststreptococcal glomerulonephritis is mainly supportive and symptomatic. Antibiotic therapy does not prevent subsequent diseases but may reduce the severity.

Learning objectives, review questions, and other resources can be found at **www.pharmacotherapyonline.com**.

The precise pathogenetic mechanisms of many glomerular diseases remain unknown, and the available therapeutic regimens are still far from optimal. This chapter provides an overview of the primary causes of glomerulonephritis with a focus on their etiology, the pathophysiologic mechanisms responsible for glomerular injury, and the clinical presentation of the eight predominant types of glomerulonephritis. Treatment options and monitoring approaches for each of these types of glomerulonephritis are also discussed. Diabetes mellitus is an important secondary cause of glomerular injury, and a thorough discussion of the pathophysiology and management of this condition can be found in Chap. 83.

NORMAL GLOMERULAR ANATOMY AND FUNCTION

The glomerulus, which is enclosed within the Bowman capsule, consists of two important components: the filtration barrier and the mesangium (Fig. 56–1). The capillary wall, which serves as a filtration barrier, consists of three well-defined layers: fenestrated endothelium, glomerular basement membrane (GBM), and epithelial cell layer. The epithelial cells, also known as podocytes, have specialized foot processes embedded in the outer layer of the GBM. It is across this barrier that fluid flows and ultimately becomes the ultrafiltrate. Under normal conditions, the GBM functions as a compact hydrated gel of matrix proteins with a pore-like structure. The mesangium, which consists of mesangial cells embedded in an extracellular matrix, provides support for the glomerular capillaries and also modulates blood flow through the capillaries.

The unique capillary bed of the glomerulus allows small nonprotein plasma constituents up to the size of inulin, which has a molecular weight of 5.2 kDa, to pass freely while excluding macromolecules equal to or larger than albumin, which has a molecular weight of 69 kDa. The ease of passage of solutes through the glomerular membrane is impacted by both the size and charge of the solute. Fixed,

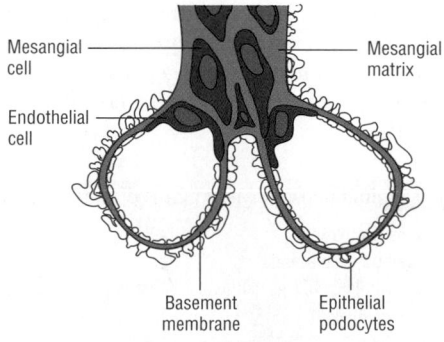

FIGURE 56-1. Microanatomy of the glomerulus.

negatively charged sites are found within the glomeruli in all three layers of the capillary wall: the endothelium, the epithelium, and the GBM. The movement of negatively charged molecules is thus restricted more than that of neutral or positively charged molecules. Different glomerular diseases affect this size- and charge-selective barrier to different extents; consequently, glomerulopathies present with varied clinical features and solute-excretion patterns.

Some of the glomerular cells, such as the epithelial cells, have phagocytic function that can remove macromolecules trapped within the filtration barrier. They are also capable of synthesizing the GBM. In contrast, the mesangial cells regulate glomerular hemodynamics in response to angiotensin II and by producing prostaglandins. These cells also synthesize and respond to various cytokines and thus play a key role in immune-mediated glomerular diseases. Resident phagocytes in the mesangium are responsible for moving macromolecules trapped in the basement membrane into the urinary space. They are also involved in the development of both immune and nonimmune glomerular injury.

EPIDEMIOLOGY AND ETIOLOGY

In the United States in 2007, glomerulonephritis was the third most common cause of end-stage renal disease (ESRD), accounting for approximately 15% of all the living ESRD patients. About 7,500 patients (6.8% of all patients) develop stage 5 chronic kidney disease, which is also called end-stage renal disease (ESRD), because of glomerulonephritis each year.[1]

Humoral and cellular immunologic mechanisms participate in the pathogenesis of most glomerulonephritis. Abnormalities in coagulation and metabolism, as well as hereditary and vascular diseases, also contribute to glomerular damage. The histopathologic manifestations vary substantially among the different types of glomerulonephritis. An overview of the primary pathogenetic mechanisms is presented in this section, and specific abnormalities for each of the primary types of glomerulonephritis are presented in subsequent sections.

PATHOPHYSIOLOGY

❶ The glomerular lesion may be diffuse (involving all glomeruli), focal (involving some but not all glomeruli), or segmental, also known as local (involving part of the individual glomerulus). The pathologic manifestations may also be described as proliferative (overgrowth of epithelium, endothelium, or mesangium), membranous (thickening of GBM), and/or sclerotic.

The glomerular capillary wall is particularly susceptible to immune-mediated injury. Antigen and antibody tend to localize in the glomerulus, probably because of its high blood flow and capillary hydrostatic pressure. Parenchymal damage can be induced as a result of humoral- and cell-mediated immune reactions (Table 56-1). Antibodies and sensitized T lymphocytes are the primary mediators of glomerular injury.[2,3]

Production of antibodies to endogenous or exogenous antigens that are recognized as foreign by the host is the first step in humoral immunologic damage to the glomerulus. Endogenous antigens may be intrinsic glomerular antigens, such as Heymann antigen on the epithelial cell or Goodpasture antigen on the GBM, or previously sequestered antigens, such as DNA or thyroglobulin. Exogenous antigens are most often viral, bacterial, parasitic, or fungal in origin. Antineutrophil cytoplasmic autoantibodies (ANCAs) (i.e., autoantibodies that react to the cytoplasmic components of neutrophils and monocytes) are found in patients with idiopathic crescentic glomerulonephritis and also in the accompanying vasculitis.

Complexes of antigens and antibodies may be formed in the circulation and then passively entrapped in the glomerular capillary or mesangium. Alternately, experimental antibodies may combine with endogenous glomerular antigens or exogenous antigens entrapped in the glomerulus to form complexes locally, or in situ.[3] The type and extent of glomerular damage are dependent on the location of the immune complex formation and the rate at which it is removed. Impaired removal facilitates the growth of the complex and thus increases the likelihood of glomerular damage.

Subsequent to antigen–antibody formation, a series of biologic events is triggered that ultimately leads to glomerular injury. Noninflammatory lesions can result from the binding of noncomplement-fixing antibody to the glomerular epithelial cell (mechanism 1) or from the activation of the complement system to form the C5b-9 membrane attack complex (mechanism 2).[3] Both mechanisms can damage the glomerular epithelial cell and result in capillary wall injury and proteinuria. Inflammatory lesions are induced by glomerular infiltration of circulating inflammatory cells such as neutrophils, monocytes/macrophages, and platelets (mechanism 3) or by proliferation of resident glomerular mesangial cells (mechanism 4), resulting in GBM damage.[3] The migration of neutrophils and monocytes to the glomerular tufts is promoted by chemoattractants such as complement fragments (C3a and C5a), platelet-activating factor, interleukin-8, and monocyte chemotactic protein-1.[4] Various cytokines, chemokines, and growth factors are then released to participate in the inflammatory process.[2]

T cells sensitized to glomerular antigen, macrophages, and resident mesangial cells are important participants in cell-mediated injury. Sensitized T cells can cause glomerular hypercellularity in the absence of antibody deposition.[2-4] Cytotoxic T cells may bind with the target cells and destroy them. Alternatively, a delayed-type hypersensitivity reaction may be initiated by activated T cells through the release of lymphokines to attract, activate, and transform monocytes into macrophages.[3] These humoral and cellular mediators, in conjunction with a host of toxic molecular entities including reactive oxygen species, proteinases, eicosanoids, and procoagulants, which are secreted by neutrophils, macrophages, platelets, and resident glomerular cells can alter the permeability, blood flow, and function of the glomeruli. Vascular constriction and occlusion follow and result in the eventual destruction of the glomeruli.

Acute forms of glomerular injury frequently lead to chronic and persistent renal dysfunction, even though the original immune factors that induced the initial glomerular injury have resolved. Experimental and clinical investigations suggest that a variety of factors may participate in the progression of renal injury. These factors include systemic and glomerular hypertension, high dietary protein intake, proteinuria, glomerular hypertrophy, hyperlipidemia, activation of the coagulation system, abnormalities of calcium and phosphorus balance, and tubulointerstitial injury. The degree of proteinuria not only is an index of the severity of glomerular disease but also has been associated with an increased the rate of progression of renal injury. Heavy

---

TABLE 56-1 Immunologic Mechanisms of Glomerular Injury

Circulating immune complexes
In situ antigen–antibody interaction
    Intrinsic glomerular antigen; e.g., glomerular basement membrane antigens
    Exogenous planted antigens
Cell-mediated mechanism

TABLE 56-2 Tendencies of Glomerular Diseases to Manifest Nephrotic and Nephritic Features

	Nephrotic Features	Nephritic Features
Minimal-change nephropathy	++++	–
Membranous nephropathy	++++	+
Diabetic glomerulosclerosis	++++	+
Amyloidosis	++++	+
Focal segmental glomerulosclerosis	+++	++
Mesangioproliferative glomerulonephritis	++	++
Membranoproliferative glomerulonephritis	++	+++
Proliferative glomerulonephritis	++	+++
Acute poststreptococcal glomerulonephritis	+	++++
Crescentic glomerulonephritis[a]	+	++++

[a]Can be immune complex-mediated, antiglomerular basement membrane antibody-mediated, or associated with antineutrophil cytoplasmic autoantibodies.

proteinuria is an indicator of poor prognosis in various glomerular diseases.

Proteinuria is also accompanied by an increased flux of macromolecules across the mesangium. The mesangial overload may then lead to structural damage. The passage of serum components, such as complement, across the GBM may have a pathophysiologic effect on the glomerular epithelial cells and alter the integrity of the glomerular filtration barrier. The damaging effects of macromolecules other than albumin, such as immunoglobulins, lipoproteins, transferrin, and complement, remain to be characterized.

CLINICAL PRESENTATION

❷ Although patients with glomerular disease may present with an array of signs and symptoms, they are often categorized into one of two broad classifications: nephritic syndrome or nephrotic syndrome (Table 56–2). The unique clinical presentation characteristics of the predominant glomerulopathies are described in the individual disease sections, presented later in the chapter.

Nephritic syndrome reflects glomerular inflammation and frequently results in hematuria. White cells and cellular and granular casts are commonly found in the urine. In contrast, nephrotic syndrome reflects noninflammatory injury to the glomerular structures and results in few cells or cellular casts in the urine. Initially, there may be limited or no reduction in renal excretory function.

Hematuria occurs when red blood cells leak through the openings of the GBM. The presence of red cell casts is highly indicative of glomerulonephritis or vasculitis. The presence of dysmorphic red blood cells in the urine is suggestive of glomerular disease. The red blood cells are damaged as they pass through the openings in the GBM or the cells may sustain osmotic injury as they travel through the different osmotic environments within the lumen of the kidney tubules.

The presence of proteinuria indicates a defect of the size- and/or charge-selective barriers within the GBM. Normal urinary protein excretion is between 40 and 80 mg/day, with a maximum of 150 mg. Fewer than 20 mg of the excreted proteins are albumin. Most of the albumin that enters the glomerular filtrate is either reabsorbed or catabolized by the tubular epithelium. The dipsticks that are commonly used to identify proteinuria detect only albumin; they become positive when protein excretion is more than 300 to 500 mg/day. They are therefore unable to detect the early stages of renal injury secondary to diabetes mellitus or hypertension, which often result in microalbuminuria with urinary albumin excretion ranges between 30 and 300 mg/day. Chemstrip Micral-Test II (Roche

Diagnostics, Indianapolis, IN), a simple immunoassay on a dipstick, permits specific and semiquantitative determination of urinary albumin concentrations at five levels: 0, 10, 20, 50, and 100 mg/L. Another qualitative test, Micro-Bumintest (Bayer Diabetes Care, Mishawaka, IN), registers a positive reading when the urine albumin concentration is greater than 40 mg/L.

Hypertension is common for patients with glomerular diseases, as a result of renal salt retention causing plasma volume expansion. In contrast, increased activity of vasoconstrictors such as angiotensin II is often the cause for patients with chronic glomerular diseases. Scarring of the glomerulus resulting in regional ischemia is thought to be responsible for the hypertension. Activation of the sympathetic nervous system and the release of vasoconstrictor substances may also contribute.

NEPHRITIC SYNDROME

Glomerular bleeding resulting in hematuria is typical in nephritic syndrome. Dysmorphic red cells, especially acanthocytes, are a sensitive and specific marker of glomerular bleeding. The presence of pus and cellular and granular casts in the urine is common. The extent of proteinuria is variable. Patients with severe nephritic glomerular injury have renal function impairment because of the reduced glomerular surface area available for filtration, as a result of constriction of the capillary lumen by proliferating mesangial cells or inflammatory cells.

CLINICAL PRESENTATIONS OF NEPHRITIC AND NEPHROTIC SYNDROMES

General

☐ The patients are generally not in acute distress

Symptoms

☐ The patients may not experience any major symptoms

Nephritic Signs	**Nephrotic Signs**
☐ Hematuria	☐ Edema
☐ Hypertension and edema as renal function declines	☐ Weight gain
	☐ Fatigue
Laboratory Tests	
☐ Proteinuria up to 3 g/day	☐ Proteinuria, >3.5 g/day/1.73 m²
☐ Pus, cellular and granular casts in urine is common	☐ Hyperlipidemia
☐ Hypoproteinemia	☐ Lipiduria
☐ Hypercoagulable state for some patients	

NEPHROTIC SYNDROME

Nephrotic syndrome is characterized by proteinuria greater than 3.5 g/day per 1.73 m², hypoproteinemia, edema, and hyperlipidemia. A hypercoagulable state may also be present in some patients. The syndrome may be the result of primary diseases of the glomerulus, or be associated with systemic diseases such as diabetes mellitus, lupus, amyloidosis, and preeclampsia. Hypoproteinemia, especially hypoalbuminemia, results from increased urinary loss of albumin and an increased rate of catabolism of filtered albumin by proximal tubular cells. The compensatory increase in hepatic synthesis of albumin is insufficient to replenish the protein loss, probably because of malnutrition.

Edema formation in patients with nephrotic syndrome was traditionally thought to be driven by the reduced plasma oncotic pressure secondary to hypoalbuminemia. If the oncotic pressure is low, the movement of fluid from the vascular space to the interstitial compartment results in a reduction of the plasma volume, which can trigger compensatory renal sodium and water retention through the activation of the renin–angiotensin–aldosterone axis, vasopressin, and the sympathetic nervous system (the "underfill" mechanism). However, experimental data reveal that the plasma volume is actually normal or elevated. Hypoalbuminemia may not cause edema until the serum albumin concentration is less than 2 g/dL (20 g/L). In addition, the transcapillary oncotic pressure gradient is not as high as previously thought because increased lymphatic flow reduces the interstitial oncotic pressure by removing protein and fluid from the interstitium, thereby reducing the transcapillary oncotic pressure gradient.[5] Instead, fluid retention is likely mediated by a primary increase in sodium reabsorption at the distal nephron, which is probably caused by tubular resistance to the action of atrial natriuretic peptide (the "overflow" mechanism).[6] It is likely that both mechanisms may contribute to nephrotic edema in different patients.[6]

Albuminuria greater than 3 g daily is associated with a significant increase in serum cholesterol concentrations for patients with primary glomerular disease.[7] Hyperlipidemia in nephrotic syndrome is characterized by elevated serum total cholesterol and triglyceride concentrations, with increased very-low-density lipoprotein (VLDL) and low-density lipoprotein (LDL) cholesterol concentrations. Lipoprotein (a) levels may also be increased. The reduced plasma oncotic pressure as a result of hypoalbuminemia may stimulate hepatic synthesis of lipids and lipoproteins. The increased VLDL production and increased liver cholesterol synthesis, along with a decrease in LDL receptor activity, can then lead to an increase in LDL cholesterol concentrations. In addition, reduced serum albumin or the loss of a liporegulatory substance may result in reduced VLDL clearance.[8] Nephrotic patients with hyperlipidemia, especially those with concomitant hypertension, are presumed to have an increased risk for atherosclerotic vascular disease. Hyperlipidemia also promotes the progression of glomerular injury, as evidenced by glomerulosclerosis, mesangial expansion, and hyalinosis.[8,9]

Many patients with nephrotic syndrome have a hypercoagulable state caused by defects of several control proteins in the coagulation cascade. The concentration of the coagulation inhibitor antithrombin III is reduced because of increased loss in the urine. A reduced amount of the coagulation inhibitors proteins C and S, along with increased concentrations of factors V and VIII, increased fibrinogen concentrations and abnormal platelet function, may also contribute to the hypercoagulable state. The net result of these alterations in coagulation is an increased risk for arterial and venous thrombosis, especially in the deep veins and renal veins. As many as 25% of patients with membranous nephropathy may have renal vein thrombosis.

DIAGNOSIS

Patients with suspected glomerular disease should have an extensive medical history obtained to identify potential systemic causes (Table 56–3). Medication, environmental, and occupational histories may also help identify possible exposure to potentially nephrotoxic agents. A carefully conducted physical examination and laboratory evaluation may reveal the presence of systemic diseases that may contribute to the development of glomerular disease (Fig. 56–2). In addition, the patient's age, gender, and ethnic background may be helpful in pinpointing the specific type of glomerular disease. Many of the conditions are more prevalent

TABLE 56-3	Evaluation of Patients Suspected of Having Glomerular Disease

Medical history
To identify symptoms of medical conditions that may cause glomerular disease
- Diabetes mellitus
- Amyloidosis
- Systemic lupus erythematosus
- Other familial conditions associated with renal disease
To identify symptoms suggestive of nephrotic syndrome
- Reduced appetite
- Fatigue
- Weight gain
- Edema

Medication, environmental, and occupational histories
To identify possible exposure to potentially nephrotoxic drugs, toxins, or chemicals

Physical examination
To identify signs and symptoms associated with systemic diseases
- Hypertension
- Rash
- Arthritis
- Retinopathy
- Neuropathy
- Lymphadenopathy
- Hepatomegaly
- Malignancy

Laboratory evaluation
Urinalysis
- To determine nephrotic nature of glomerular disease
  - Proteinuria, >3.5 g/day/1.73 m²
  - Lipiduria
- To determine nephritic nature of glomerular disease
  - Hematuria
  - Pyuria
  - Cellular, granular casts
Glomerular filtration rate
- To determine extent of glomerular damage
Other tests
- To identify type and etiology of glomerular disease
  - Serum complement concentration
  - Antinuclear and anti-DNA antibodies
  - Antistreptolysin antibodies
  - Circulating antiglomerular basement membrane antibodies
  - Cryoglobulins

Percutaneous renal biopsy
- To provide definitive diagnosis of glomerular disease

in certain age groups, although they may occur at any age. For example, proliferative glomerulonephritis is more common in those younger than 40 years of age, whereas the incidence of membranous glomerulonephritis is dramatically higher in those older than 50 years of age.

Laboratory evaluation such as urinalysis can help differentiate the nephrotic or nephritic nature of the disease. The glomerular filtration rate (GFR) may be used to determine the extent of glomerular damage. In the early stages of the disease, the GFR may remain normal. Initial injury to the glomerulus primarily lowers the permeability coefficient (K_f) of the GBM by reducing the surface area available for filtration and/or the unit permeability of the membrane. The reduced permeability is compensated by an elevation in the glomerular capillary hydrostatic pressure through afferent arteriolar dilation and efferent arteriolar constriction. Extensive glomerular damage may therefore be present before a substantial reduction of total GFR is evident.

Although the cause of glomerular disease may be established from clinical and laboratory evaluation, sometimes percutaneous renal biopsy may be needed to provide a definitive diagnosis.

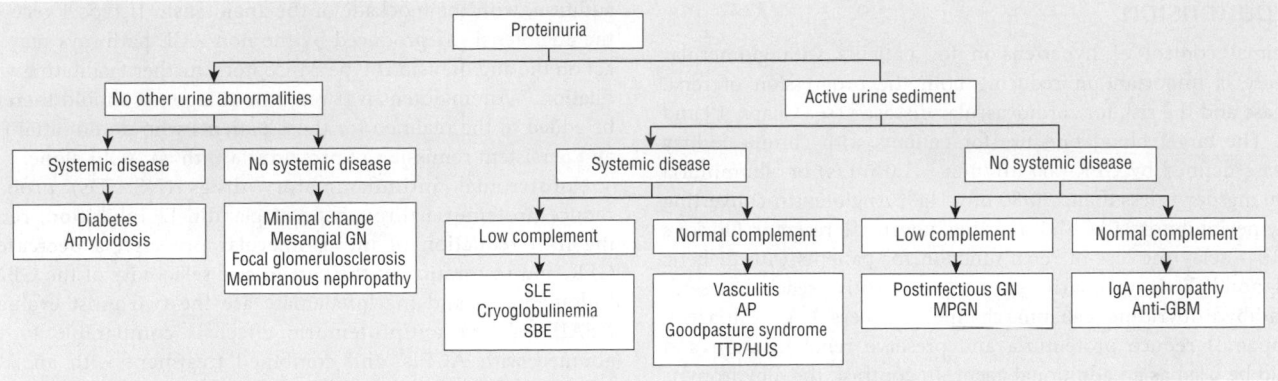

FIGURE 56-2. Clinical presentations of glomerulonephritis. (AP, anaphylactoid purpura; GBM, glomerular basement membrane; GN, glomerulonephritis; HUS, hemolytic uremic syndrome; IgA, immunoglobulin A; MPGN, membranoproliferative glomerulonephritis; SBE, subacute bacterial endocarditis; SLE, systemic lupus erythematosus; TTP, thrombotic thrombocytopenic purpura.)

TREATMENT

Glomerulonephritis

◼ GENERAL APPROACH TO TREATMENT

The management of patients with glomerulonephritis involves specific pharmacologic therapy for the glomerular disease and supportive measures to prevent and/or treat the pathophysiologic sequelae, namely, hypertension, edema, and progression of renal disease. For patients with nephrotic syndrome, supportive therapy should also address the management of extrarenal complications of heavy proteinuria, namely, hypoalbuminemia, hyperlipidemia, and thromboembolism. Because patients with significant proteinuria tend to have more rapid decline of renal function, reduction of proteinuria thus becomes critical in delaying the rate of progression toward ESRD.

Immunosuppressive agents, alone or in combination, are commonly used to alter the immune processes that are responsible for the glomerulonephritides. Corticosteroids, in addition to their immunosuppressive effect, also possess antiinflammatory activities. They reduce the production and/or release of many substances that mediate the inflammatory process, such as prostaglandins, leukotrienes, platelet-activating factors, tumor necrosis factors, and interleukin-1 (IL-1). Movement of leukocytes and macrophages to the site of inflammation is also inhibited. The immunosuppressive effects of corticosteroids are mediated through the inhibition of the release of IL-1 and tumor necrosis factor by activated macrophages, and interleukin-2 (IL-2) by activated T cells. In addition, the actions of migration-inhibiting factor and γ-interferon are inhibited. Processing of antigens is thus affected by the presence of corticosteroids. Cytotoxic agents, such as cyclophosphamide, chlorambucil, or azathioprine, are commonly used to treat glomerular diseases. Cyclosporine can reduce lymphokine production by activated T lymphocytes, and it may decrease proteinuria by improving the permselectivity of the GBM. Mycophenolate mofetil is useful in different glomerulonephritides because of its effects on T- and B-cell lymphocytes.

Because many immune factors are implicated in the pathogenesis of glomerulonephritis, plasmapheresis may be used to remove these mediators. During the procedure, whole blood is removed from the body and centrifugation is used to separate the cellular elements from the plasma. The cells are then infused back to the patient after resuspension in saline or plasma substitute. The plasma proteins, presumably including the pathogenic immune factors, are thereby removed from the patient.

Recently, many novel targets were identified and new agents are being evaluated for their usefulness to control the disease, preserve renal function, and improve patient outcome. To stay abreast of the expanding availability of treatment options, one can routinely consult one of the clinical trial registries, such as *www.clinicaltrials.gov*.[10]

◼ SUPPORTIVE THERAPY

❸ For patients with nephrotic syndrome, dietary measures involve restriction of sodium intake to 50 to 100 mEq/day (50 to 100 mmol/day),[11] protein intake of 0.8 to 1 g/day,[11,12] and a low-lipid diet of less than 200 mg cholesterol. Total fat should account for less than 30% of daily total calories.[11] Sodium restriction is important not only in the control of edema, but also in the control of hypertension and proteinuria. Similarly, protein restriction not only helps to reduce proteinuria but also has a potential role in retarding the progression of renal disease. Patients should also stop smoking because a dose-dependent increase in risk for developing ESRD was observed in men with primary inflammatory (immunoglobulin A glomerulonephritis) or noninflammatory (polycystic kidney disease) renal diseases.[13]

Edema

Management of nephrotic edema involves salt restriction, bedrest, and use of support stockings and diuretics. However, severe salt restriction is difficult to achieve and prolonged bedrest could predispose nephrotic patients to thromboembolism. Hence the use of a loop diuretic such as furosemide is frequently required. Although the delivery of diuretic to the kidney tubules is normal, the presence of large amounts of protein in the urine promotes drug binding, and thereby reduces the availability of the diuretic to the luminal receptor sites. In addition, reduced sodium delivery to the distal tubule secondary to decreased glomerular perfusion may also alter diuretic effectiveness. Large doses of the loop diuretic, such as 160 to 480 mg of furosemide, may be needed for patients with moderate edema (see Chap. 58). In some instances, a thiazide diuretic or metolazone may be added to enhance natriuresis.[11,14] Alternatively, continuous intravenous infusion of a loop diuretic, such as furosemide 160 to 480 mg/day, may be employed.[15] For patients with morbid edema, albumin infusion may be used to expand plasma volume and to increase diuretic delivery to the renal tubules, thus enhancing diuretic effect. However, it may precipitate congestive heart failure and may also reduce therapeutic response to steroid in minimal-change nephropathy. For patients with significant edema, the goal of treatment should be a daily loss of 1 to 2 lb (0.45 to 0.9 kg) of fluid until the patient's desired weight has been obtained.

Hypertension

Optimal control of hypertension for patients with glomerular disease is important in reducing both the progression of renal disease and the risk for cardiovascular disease[12] (see Chaps. 19 and 52). The target blood pressure for patients with chronic kidney disease defined by GFR <60 mL/min (<1.0 mL/s) or albuminuria >300 mg/day is less than 130/80 mm Hg.[16] Angiotensin-converting enzyme inhibitors (ACEIs) and angiotensin II receptor blockers (ARBs) delay the loss of renal function for patients with diabetic and nondiabetic (primarily glomerulonephritis) renal diseases.[17] Nondihydropyridine calcium channel blockers (e.g., diltiazem, verapamil) reduce proteinuria and preserve renal function and could be used as an additional agent. In contrast, the dihydropyridine calcium channel blockers (e.g., nifedipine, amlodipine, or nisoldipine) are effective in lowering blood pressure, but without the benefit of proteinuria reduction.[18]

Proteinuria

Dietary protein restriction reduces proteinuria and may retard renal function deterioration. Secondary analysis of the Modification of Diet in Renal Disease Study for patients with moderate renal insufficiency [GFR of 25 to 55 mL/min/1.73 m² (0.24 to 0.53 mL/s/m²)] revealed that reduced protein intake (0.66 g/kg/day) delayed the rate of GFR deterioration for patients with severe renal insufficiency [GFR of 13 to 24 mL/min/1.73 m² (0.13 to 0.23 mL/s/m²)].[19] Consequently, modest protein restriction of 0.8 g/kg/day is reasonable for patients with moderate renal insufficiency. Decreasing dietary protein also reduces the intake of phosphorus and potassium. In many instances, the potential benefits of protein restriction have to be balanced against the need for protein intake to overcome nutritional deficiencies. For nondialyzed patients who have GFRs of less than 25 mL/min/1.73 m² (0.24 mL/s/m²), dietary protein intake should be reduced to 0.6 g/kg/day.[12]

It is now recognized that proteinuria is an independent risk factor for renal function decline and cardiovascular disease.[20] Reducing proteinuria can retard renal function loss and delay the progression to ESRD.[21] The antiproteinuric effect of ACEIs is associated with a fall in filtration fraction, suggesting a reduction in intraglomerular pressure. Recent studies show that ACEIs and ARBs may also have direct effects on podocytes, resulting in reduction of proteinuria and glomerular scarring. [22] In addition, angiotensin-converting enzyme (ACE) inhibition may also reduce the effect of angiotensin II on renal cell proliferation, thereby reducing sclerosis. These beneficial effects on proteinuria are beyond what can be attributed by the drug's antihypertensive effects (see Chap. 52).[23,24]

CLINICAL CONTROVERSY

Are there differences in the proteinuria reduction and renal protective effects of ACEIs and ARBs? Would combined use of the agents be justified?

The combined use of an ACEI and an ARB reduces the rate of renal function decline more than either treatment alone.[17] A meta-analysis of 21 randomized, controlled studies revealed that combination therapy enhanced the reduction of proteinuria in both diabetic and nondiabetic patients.[25] Combination therapy maximizes blockade of the renin–angiotensin system by counteracting the effects of angiotensin II produced by non-ACE pathways. In addition, with the blockade of the angiotensin II type 1 receptor, the angiotensin II produced by the non-ACE pathways may still act on the angiotensin II type 2 receptors, further facilitating vasodilation.[26] An angiotensin II receptor antagonist should therefore be added to the regimen for those patients who do not attain full and persistent remission of proteinuria with an ACEI alone.

Nonsteroidal antiinflammatory drugs (NSAIDs) probably reduce proteinuria through prostaglandin E_2 inhibition, resulting in a reduction of intraglomerular pressure, a decrease in GFR, and restoration of the barrier size selectivity of the GBM.[11] Indomethacin and meclofenamate are the two most evaluated NSAIDs. Their antiproteinuric effect is comparable to that attained with ACEIs, and combined treatment with an ACEI results in additional proteinuria reduction.[27] However, adherence to a low-sodium diet or concurrent use of a diuretic is needed to maximize the antiproteinuric effect. Because of their potential for nephrotoxicity, especially for patients with poor renal function, long-term use of an NSAID for renoprotection is not preferred.[23]

Hyperlipidemia

An abnormal lipoprotein profile increases the risk of atherosclerosis and coronary heart disease for patients with nephrotic syndrome. It is therefore important to treat patients with persistent nephrotic syndrome and sustained dyslipidemia, especially those with high VLDL and LDL cholesterol levels in the presence of a normal or low high-density lipoprotein cholesterol level (see Chaps. 28 and 53). Therapy is especially needed for those with concurrent atherosclerotic cardiovascular disease, or with additional risk factors for atherosclerosis, such as smoking and hypertension.[8]

A low-fat diet is usually not sufficient to correct hyperlipoproteinemia.[11] β-Hydroxy-β-methylglutaryl-coenzyme A (HMG-CoA) reductase inhibitors, also known as "statins" such as lovastatin, pravastatin, simvastatin, and fluvastatin, are considered the treatment of choice.[11] They reduce total plasma cholesterol concentration, LDL cholesterol, and total plasma triglyceride concentrations.[8] Aside from the lipid-lowering effects, statins may confer renoprotection through different mechanisms, including reduction of cell proliferation and mesangial matrix accumulation and antiinflammatory and immunomodulatory effects.[28] Recent clinical studies show that they can reduce proteinuria and delay renal function loss.[29,30] The combined use of an ACEI with a statin may offer additional benefits in controlling nephrotic hyperlipidemia.[19]

Anticoagulation

Renal vein thrombosis, pulmonary emboli, or other thromboembolic events, are serious and common complications of nephrotic syndrome, and are frequently seen in those with membranous nephropathy. Although patients who have documented thromboembolic episodes should be anticoagulated with warfarin until remission of nephrotic syndrome, the use of prophylactic anticoagulation is controversial. A decision analysis study suggested that prophylactic anticoagulation is beneficial for patients with membranous nephropathy.[31] Prophylactic anticoagulation is not recommended for all patients, rather a "selective" approach or individualized assessment should be conducted to identify those at high risk [i.e., those with severe nephrotic syndrome and a serum albumin concentration <2.0 to 2.5 g/dL (<20 to 25 g/L)].[31] Also at risk are those who require prolonged bedrest, those receiving high-dose intravenous steroid therapy, and individuals who are dehydrated as well as post surgical patients.[11]

■ DISEASE PROGRESSION AND TREATMENT CONSIDERATIONS

The course and prognosis of the different glomerular diseases are extremely variable and depend on the underlying etiology. In glomerular diseases with a secondary cause, such as poststreptococcal glomerulonephritis, after the initiating factor is removed, the prognosis of the renal disease is often good. In contrast, the rates of renal function deterioration among the primary glomerulonephritides vary according to the form of glomerulonephritis. The majority of patients with minimal-change disease, IgA nephropathy, and membranous nephropathy have a fairly good prognosis. However, those with focal segmental glomerulosclerosis who are resistant to therapy, as well as those with rapidly progressive glomerulonephritis who are untreated, are likely to experience rapid loss of renal function. In some instances, half of the renal function may be lost within a 3-month period. Certain glomerulonephritides, such as minimal-change nephropathy, are very responsive to treatment. In contrast, for some other types of glomerulonephritis, such as membranous proliferative glomerulonephritis, consistently effective therapy has yet to be found.

Because of the variable courses exhibited by the different glomerulonephritides, specific treatment approaches have been developed for each disease. The natural history of the glomerulonephritis has to be well delineated before a promising regimen can be evaluated, from both therapeutic and economic perspectives. Otherwise, patients will be exposed to unnecessary treatment-related toxicities if they have a type of glomerulonephritis that is likely to undergo spontaneous remission. The potential therapeutic benefits of treatment regimens should always be weighed against the risks to which the patients are being exposed. It is therefore imperative to identify patients who are most likely to benefit from treatment, especially those who have other risk factors that may contribute to the deterioration of their renal function. In those instances in which satisfactory regimens are not available to treat the primary disease, appropriate supportive measures should be employed. Optimization of systemic and glomerular pressure, reducing proteinuria, and possibly controlling hyperlipidemia may all improve the long-term outcome as well as the quality of life of these patients.

Evaluation of Therapeutic Outcomes

4 Patients should be monitored closely for therapeutic response as well as the development of treatment-related toxicities. Although the rate of renal function deterioration is an important indicator of the long-term success of treatment, resolution of nephrotic and nephritic signs and symptoms associated with the glomerulopathies is an important short-term therapeutic target.

Serum creatinine concentration as well as creatinine clearance should be evaluated prior to and during treatment; 24-hour urine outflow should be collected to determine the extent of proteinuria. Alternatively, the daily urine protein excretion may be estimated from the urinary total protein-to-creatinine concentration ratio. After establishing the correlation between the 24-hour urinary protein excretion and the protein-to-creatinine ratio, single, random urine specimens may be used in place of a 24-hour urine collection. Blood pressure should be monitored periodically to assess the need for and the adequacy of antihypertensive therapy. The pressures should also be evaluated in conjunction with clinical signs and symptoms of edema and fluid overload to gauge the need for volume control as well as diuretic use. For patients with nephrotic syndrome, serum lipid concentrations should be monitored. If the patient has hematuria, urinalysis and a complete blood count should be obtained. The clinician should also be aware of the patient's appetite and energy level, because these are indicators of the patient's overall state of well-being. At times, renal biopsy is needed to assess response to treatment and disease progression, to determine future treatment strategy, and to confirm the initial diagnosis.

Patients receiving cytotoxic drug treatment should be evaluated for drug-related toxicities every week during the initial treatment period. After 1 month of treatment, the frequency of monitoring may be reduced. When the patient is on long-term steroid treatment, monthly visits are often required for assessment of both efficacy and toxicities. If a favorable response is obtained after a course of treatment, the patient may be evaluated every 3 to 4 months. The patient's renal function, proteinuria, urinalysis, blood pressure, lipid profile, and the overall state of health should be assessed during these regular follow-up visits.

INDIVIDUAL GLOMERULOPATHIES

MINIMAL-CHANGE NEPHROPATHY

Epidemiology and Etiology

Minimal-change nephropathy (also termed nil disease or minimal-change disease) is commonly found in children, accounting for about 85% to 90% of all cases of nephrotic syndrome in children between 1 and 4 years of age. The percentage drops gradually to less than 50% after age 10 years and accounts for less than 20% of all cases of idiopathic nephrotic syndrome in adults. Secondary causes of minimal-change nephropathy include NSAIDs, lupus, and various T-cell–related disorders, such as Hodgkin disease and leukemias.

Pathophysiology

Minimal-change disease is characterized by the absence of definitive pathologic changes observed under light and immunofluorescence microscopy. The characteristic lesion in patients with minimal-change disease, as visualized under electron microscopy, is the spreading and fusion of the foot processes of epithelial cells over an unchanged GBM. Lipoid nephrosis is another term that has been used to describe this type of glomerular disease because lipids, as well as renal tubular cells, are found in the urine. The pathogenesis of minimal-change disease is unknown. Altered cell-mediated immunologic response, specifically T-cell dysfunction or changes in the T-cell subpopulations, may be responsible. The activated lymphocytes are thought to secrete lymphokines that reduce the production of anions in the GBM. The permeability of the GBM to plasma albumin is increased through a reduction of electrostatic repulsion. The loss of anionic charges also results in fusion of the epithelial cell foot processes. Other vascular permeability factors, such as hemopexin, IL-4, and vascular endothelial growth factor, also have been suggested to be responsible.

Clinical Presentation

Most patients present initially with edema, frequently acute in onset, following a nonspecific upper respiratory tract infection, allergic reaction, or vaccinations, which might have activated the T lymphocytes. Nephrotic syndrome with massive proteinuria (substantially more than 40 mg/m^2 per hour for children and greater than 3-3.5 g/day for adults), edema, hypoalbuminemia, and hyperlipidemia is common. The patient's weight may increase dramatically because of sodium and fluid retention. Nephritic features, such as gross hematuria, are uncommon. Hypertension and decreased renal function are uncommon in children but are more common in older adults.[32] For some patients, volume depletion may result in mild to moderate azotemia.

TREATMENT

Minimal-Change Nephropathy

■ PHARMACOLOGIC THERAPY

Steroids

Initial Therapy ❺ Minimal-change disease is most responsive to initial treatment with corticosteroids. In children, steroid therapy is expected to reduce proteinuria in approximately 90% of the patients, with >95% 10-year renal survival.[33] Because of the excellent response to initial therapy with steroids and the prevalence of this glomerular disease in children, reduction of proteinuria secondary to steroid treatment is considered diagnostic for minimal-change disease without the need for biopsy. Prednisone is commonly administered at 60 mg/m² per day initially for 4 to 6 weeks. The dose is then reduced to 40 mg/m² per day every other day for another 4 to 6 weeks, with or without tapering afterward (Fig. 56–3).[34] Proteinuria will disappear in 50% of patients after 1 week and in 90% of patients after 4 weeks of treatment. Different versions of the steroid regimen are available as there is no consensus on the optimal dose and duration. Studies are being conducted to identify the best strategy to induce remission, reduce disease recurrence, and minimize adverse effects of the therapy. Commonly, the initial episode is treated with an extended course (months) of therapy, followed by shorter treatment (weeks) for relapses.[35]

For adults, prednisone 1 mg/kg per day is given initially for 4 weeks with a reduction to 0.75 mg/kg every other day for the next 4 weeks. Proteinuria will disappear in 50% to 60% of patients after 8 weeks of treatment, and complete remission will be attained in 80% of patients after 28 weeks of therapy.[32]

Relapse As many as 85% of the patients who respond to initial steroid therapy (steroid sensitive) will experience a relapse of proteinuria, mostly within 6 to 12 months after disease onset. The risk of relapse is affected by the duration of initial steroid therapy.[11,34] Children who were asymptomatic with proteinuria diagnosed during routine urine screening tend to have less-frequent relapses and a more favorable clinical course. In those who relapse, 50% to 65% may have steroid-responsive relapse episodes over the subsequent 3- to 5-year period. The dose and duration of steroid treatment for the relapse do not influence the subsequent rate of relapse.[11,34] Commonly, 60 mg/m² per day of prednisone is given until the urine is free of protein for 3 days, to be followed by 4 weeks of alternate-day prednisone at 40 mg/m² per dose.[34]

Frequent Relapse Approximately 10% to 20% of children will experience three or four relapses that are responsive to steroid. Half of them will then relapse frequently and become steroid dependent, requiring continuous low-dose alternate-day prednisone to maintain an extended relapse-free period.[34] A small number of patients eventually develop resistance to steroids, and a biopsy done at that time often reveals another pathology such as focal segmental glomerulosclerosis. It is controversial whether minimal-change disease progresses into focal segmental glomerulosclerosis or whether the glomerulosclerosis that was present at the time of initial diagnosis was inadvertently diagnosed as minimal-change nephropathy because of tissue-sampling error during the renal biopsy.

Cytotoxic Agents

Cytotoxic agents are often considered for patients who are steroid resistant, as well as for those who require large doses of steroids to sustain remission (steroid dependent). These agents are also beneficial for pediatric patients who experience growth inhibition secondary to chronic use of steroid.[11] Cytotoxic agents are effective in inducing remission and the duration of remission tends to be longer than that induced by steroid. In those patients who relapse after cytotoxic therapy, they may respond to steroid better than before.

Cyclophosphamide at 2 mg/kg per day for 10 to 12 weeks given alone or with prednisone (50 to 75 mg/m²) is very effective in inducing remission and restoring steroid responsiveness for patients who

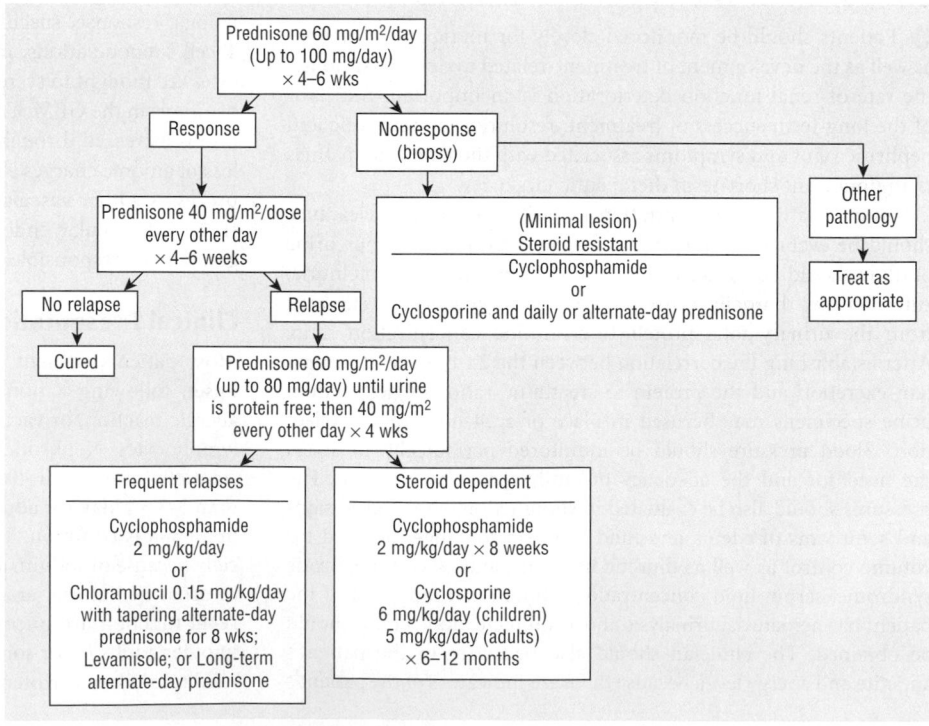

FIGURE 56-3. Treatment algorithm for minimal-change nephropathy. (*Reprinted by permission from Macmillan Publishers Ltd: Bargman JM. Management of minimal lesion glomerulonephritis: Evidence-based recommendations. Kidney Int Suppl 1999;55:S3–S16.*)

were previously steroid dependent and then became steroid resistant. Alternatively, chlorambucil at 0.1 to 0.2 mg/kg per day may be used. This agent, however, is associated with more adverse effects than cyclophosphamide. Azathioprine has also been used; however, treatment for 6 to 12 months is often needed before any favorable response is apparent.

The immunosuppressive effect of cytotoxic agents, with or without the concurrent use of steroids, can result in serious infections, which are the primary cause of death for patients with minimal-change nephropathy. Other toxicities associated with cyclophosphamide include gonadal fibrosis, which results in sterility, hemorrhagic cystitis, alopecia, and a potential to develop malignancy in those on long-term treatment.

Cyclosporine

Cyclosporine decreases lymphokine production by activated T lymphocytes and thereby reduces proteinuria by reversing the lymphokine-induced alterations in the anionic charge and permeability of the GBM to albumin. For patients with steroid-sensitive or steroid-dependent disease, cyclosporine induces remission in 80% to 85% of patients. However, the disease-free period is not often sustained, and relapse, which is usually not as responsive to cyclosporine retreatment, may occur as soon as the drug is tapered or discontinued. The steroid-sparing effect of cyclosporine is also useful for steroid-dependent patients, especially those who have experienced significant adverse effects.

The usual starting dose of cyclosporine for remission induction is 5 mg/kg per day for adults and 100 to 150 mg/m² per day for children. Similar dosages are used to maintain remission long term. The optimal cyclosporine blood concentrations, as well as the need to monitor them, are controversial. No correlation has been found between the severity of the cyclosporine-induced tubulointerstitial lesions and the mean dose or trough drug concentration. However, monitoring of the area under the serum concentration–time curve has been suggested and target exposures have been proposed.[36] Testing the in vitro sensitivity of peripheral blood lymphocytes to cyclosporine in the presence of a T-cell mitogen may offer a novel method to predict response and individualize therapy.[37]

Adverse events such as rise in serum creatinine, hypertrichosis, and gingival hyperplasia are quite common. Long-term therapy may result in persistent hypertension and progressive renal failure. Cyclosporine should not therefore be given for more than 4 months in the absence of any beneficial effect. Consequently, it is indicated for patients (1) who relapse frequently or are steroid dependent, after failing to respond to a course of cyclophosphamide; (2) for whom cyclophosphamide is contraindicated or when gonadal toxicity is a concern; (3) who are steroid dependent when a "steroid holiday" is needed for catch-up growth and puberty; or (4) who have steroid-resistant disease.[34]

Levamisole

Levamisole, an immunostimulant, can promote the maturation of young T cells and restore the function of T cells and phagocytes when the immune system is depressed. It may also inhibit the production of an immunosuppressive lymphokine. Levamisole was found to have a steroid-sparing effect and was capable of maintaining remission in children who had frequent relapse steroid-dependent nephrotic syndrome.[38] In addition, it is as effective as cyclophosphamide in reducing relapse rate and steroid dosages.[39] The most serious adverse effect of levamisole is neutropenia, which is generally reversible. At present the drug is no longer available in the United States; however, it is still used elsewhere in the world for select steroid-dependent patients.

Mycophenolate Mofetil

Mycophenolate mofetil is an immunosuppressant that can suppress T- and B-cell lymphocyte proliferation, B-lymphocyte antibody production, and expression of adhesion molecules. It is reported to have steroid-sparing effects and to be useful in steroid-dependent patients, as well as in those who fail cytotoxic thereapy.[40,41]

Therapeutic Outcomes

The long-term prognosis of most patients with minimal-change disease is good. The majority of pediatric patients will not experience any relapse of the disease 10 years after the initial onset, and most will be free of the proteinuria after puberty. In adults, an 85% to 90% survival rate is seen 10 years after disease onset. Although this condition may spontaneously remit in up to 70% of untreated adults, life-threatening complications may be associated with untreated nephrotic syndrome. Significant deterioration in renal function is uncommon in both adult and pediatric patients and is observed only in those who are steroid resistant or steroid dependent. Because of the overall favorable outcome of the disease and the relatively uncommon progression into chronic renal failure, aggressive use of cytotoxic agents is not indicated even for most patients with frequent relapses. Toxicities associated with aggressive therapy do not justify the need to induce remission in those patients who fail to respond to steroids and the nonaggressive use of cytotoxic agents. Symptomatic therapy with diuretics to control edema, in conjunction with a low-salt diet and albumin infusion as needed for acute development of anasarca, is often a more rewarding therapeutic approach. NSAIDs and ACEIs may also be used to reduce the proteinuria.

FOCAL SEGMENTAL GLOMERULOSCLEROSIS

Etiology and Epidemiology

Focal segmental glomerulosclerosis (FSGS) is a clinicopathologic condition that can be idiopathic (primary) or secondary to a variety of causes. FSGS accounts for less than 15% of the cases of idiopathic nephrotic syndrome in children and approximately 15% to 20% in adults; however, it may account for 36% to 80% of the cases in African Americans.[42] The incidence of FSGS has been rapidly increasing, so that it now is the most common glomerular disease that ultimately leads to ESRD. Conditions such as sickle cell disease, cyanotic congenital heart disease, and morbid obesity can induce hemodynamic stress on an initially normal nephron population and result in FSGS. Severe glomerular injury can also be seen in patients with nephropathy associated with heroin abuse, human immunodeficiency virus (HIV) infection, and genetic mutations involving the podocin and WT1 genes.[42] A recent case series identified the association of FSGS and proteinuria in bodybuilders after long-term anabolic steroid abuse.[43] The primary and secondary sclerotic lesions may be morphologically similar, but they represent diseases with different courses and responses to therapy.

Pathophysiology

Sclerotic lesions are characteristically found in some of the glomeruli (focal) and usually involve only a portion of the glomeruli (segmental).[44] Similar to minimal-change disease, fusion of foot processes is commonly seen in those glomeruli that are not sclerotic. It is thought that both minimal-change disease and FSGS share similar pathogenetic mechanisms, with FSGS resulting in severe injury to the glomerular epithelial cells. During the early stage of FSGS, only a small number of glomeruli may have the segmental sclerotic lesion, and the disease may be confined to the juxtamedullary region. If an inadequate number of glomeruli are sampled during renal biopsy, the diagnosis of FSGS may be missed, or the patient may be thought to have minimal-change disease. Resistance to steroid therapy may thus be one of the first clues that the patient, indeed, has FSGS rather than minimal-change disease. Alternatively, a patient may have the steroid-sensitive minimal-change disease initially, which subsequently progresses to steroid-resistant FSGS.

Clinical Presentation

Almost all the patients present with proteinuria, and many of them have all the features of nephrotic syndrome. The proteinuria is non-selective, containing albumin and other higher-molecular-weight proteins, and is usually less severe when compared to patients who have minimal-change disease. Hypertension, microscopic hematuria, and renal dysfunction may be seen in up to half of the patients. Reduced renal function becomes more prevalent as the disease progresses.

The presenting clinical features in nephrotic adults with minimal-change nephropathy can be indistinguishable from that of FSGS, and renal biopsy is therefore critical in the diagnosis of adults with nephrotic syndrome. African Americans have a fourfold higher risk of developing FSGS than white or Asian patients. They tend to develop the disease earlier and present with nephrotic range proteinuria more often. They are less responsive to steroids and are more likely to experience a rapid decline in renal function, resulting in ESRD.

TREATMENT

Focal Segmental Glomerulosclerosis

■ PHARMACOLOGIC THERAPY

Steroids

❻ The treatment of FSGS is controversial because of the lack of data from randomized, prospective, controlled trials. A course of prednisone (1 to 2 mg/kg per day) with tapering after 3 to 4 months of treatment is first used for nephrotic patients.[42,44] Urinary protein excretion and serum albumin concentration should be monitored to assess efficacy. The median time to induce complete remission is 3 to 4 months, although 5 to 9 months may be needed in some patients.[42] In general, 30% to 40% of all patients can be expected to attain complete remission; for those who are not responding, treatment should be continued for 6 months before they are considered steroid resistant.[45]

If the patient develops a relapse after an adequate response to the initial treatment, a second course of steroids is generally sufficient.[42] However, if relapse occurs frequently, cytotoxic agents or cyclosporine would be indicated.

For patients who are not nephrotic, their relatively favorable prognosis does not support using steroids or other immunosuppressive agents. However, close follow-up and good blood pressure control with ACEIs are necessary to minimize disease progression.[44]

Most of the studies conducted thus far include mostly white patients. In a recent retrospective review of 72 patients that included 65 African-American patients, steroid use was not associated with renal survival or the induction of proteinuria remission.[46] The initial creatinine level, blood pressure, and severity of renal lesion are significant factors for renal survival. About one third of the patients

who received steroids developed complications such as diabetes and significant weight gain.

Cytotoxic Agents

When used with steroids during initial therapy, cytotoxic agents were not found to offer any additional beneficial effect.[42] For those patients who are not responding to steroids during initial therapy, cytotoxic agents such as cyclophosphamide (2 mg/kg/day) and chlorambucil (0.1 to 0.2 mg/kg/day) have been used with pulse methylprednisolone to induce remission. Response rates as high as 66% have been reported in uncontrolled trials, although such favorable responses have not been universally observed.[42]

Calcineurin and Rapamycin Inhibitors

In steroid-resistant patients, cyclosporine therapy has produced a complete or partial remission in 70% of patients, with a relapse rate of 47%.[47] Encouraging results have also been reported with the concurrent use of cyclosporine and steroid.[42] Adverse effects of cyclosporine commonly include gingival hyperplasia, hypertrichosis, hypertension, and renal insufficiency. In an attempt to minimize the long-term side effects, a regimen that included periodic cyclosporine dose reduction when given with steroid, cyclophosphamide, and mycophenolate mofetil was developed, and favorable effects were observed.[48] Tacrolimus has also been used to induce remission and reduce proteinuria for patients with refractory disease.[49] The effect of sirolimus on proteinuria has been found to be conflicting, however, it may cause a rapid decline in GFR, and hence, its use for FSGS in not recommended.[50]

Mycophenolate Mofetil

Mycophenolate mofetil has been reported to have favorable effects for patients who were steroid resistant, many of whom had failed to respond to other cytotoxic agents and cyclosporine.[51] Forty-four percent of the patients had reduced proteinuria and the improvement was sustained in 50% for up to 1 year. Deterioration of renal function was not observed. Other investigators have reported similar experiences. Further studies are needed to define the role of this agent among the various treatment options.

Symptomatic Therapy

Because of the lack of a consistently effective regimen for primary FSGS, many patients with mild disease are treated conservatively. ACEIs and ARBs are effective in reducing proteinuria and in stabilizing renal function in many patients with primary or secondary FSGS.[42] For patients who have nephrotic range proteinuria, an elevated serum creatinine concentration and interstitial scarring on biopsy, corticosteroids with or without immunosuppressive agents are often used.

THERAPEUTIC OUTCOMES

ESRD develops within 10 years in 10% or less of the 30% to 50% of adults and children who had attained complete remission.[47] For those patients who are resistant to therapy, the rate of renal function deterioration to ESRD may be rapid, within 1 year, or slow, over as long as 10 to 20 years; approximately 50% develop ESRD within 10 years. Those patients with severe proteinuria (>10 to 15 g/day), high serum creatinine concentration at diagnosis, initial steroid resistance, or interstitial fibrosis on renal biopsy are likely to have a more rapid decline in renal function.[44] African-American patients may also have a higher risk. Kidney transplantation is often indicated for those patients who develop ESRD; however, FSGS has recurred in 20% to 50% of the renal allografts soon after transplantation. Children and those with severe disease or rapid progression to ESRD prior to transplantation are more likely to experience a recurrence. The proteinuria may reappear within hours after transplantation, and graft failure may occur in one third to one half of the patients. The median time to recurrence was reported to be 14 days in one study. Although cyclosporine is ineffective in preventing the recurrence of nephrotic syndrome after transplantation, a high dose of the agent (up to 35 mg/kg per day) induces a remission of the recurrent disease. ACEIs and plasmapheresis are also used to prolong graft survival. The effectiveness of these therapies and the rapid recurrence of the disease in the transplanted kidney substantiate the possibility that a circulating humoral mediator is responsible for the nephropathy.

MEMBRANOUS NEPHROPATHY

Etiology and Epidemiology

Membranous nephropathy is the most common disorder responsible for idiopathic nephrotic syndrome in adults, accounting for about 20% to 25% of cases. It is also a frequent cause of renal failure secondary to glomerulonephritis. The hallmark histologic features of membranous nephropathy are glomerular capillary wall thickening with subepithelial deposits under light and electron microscopy. Most cases are idiopathic, but approximately 25% of adults and 80% of children have secondary causes.[52,53] In the United States, the most common etiologies are autoimmune diseases (e.g., lupus), infection (e.g., hepatitis B and C), syphilis, neoplasm (e.g., carcinoma of the lung, breast, gastrointestinal tract, or kidney), and medications (e.g., gold, penicillamine, or captopril). Malaria and schistosomiasis are common causes in other parts of the world. De novo membranous nephropathy can also occur in the allografts of renal transplant patients. Because the responses to therapy as well as the prognosis for idiopathic and secondary membranous nephropathy are different, it is important to identify any potential underlying causes for the nephropathy prior to treatment. Although this glomerular disease can occur at any age, the peak incidence is between ages 30 and 50 years and is especially likely in patients older than age 50 years who present with nephrotic syndrome.[52]

Pathophysiology

Examination of kidney tissue under light microscopy reveals normal mesangium and normocellularity. The glomerular capillary wall may be thickened in well-developed lesions. In the advanced stage, the capillary wall is markedly thickened, and intramembranous deposits are found. Progressive changes in capillary lumen patency parallel those in the GBM, resulting in glomerulosclerosis with capillary collapse and tubular atrophy in end-stage membranous nephropathy. Immunofluorescence microscopy shows strong capillary wall staining of IgG and C3 on the epithelial side of the basement membrane. Antibody-mediated immune injury appears to be the main pathogenetic mechanism. The immune complex can be formed in situ or deposited from circulating immune complexes.

Clinical Presentation

Most patients with membranous nephropathy present with heavy proteinuria (exceeding 3.5 g/day). Those patients excreting large amounts of IgG and α_1-microglobulin, indicating more significant tubulointerstitial damage, have a lower remission rate and are more likely to progress toward renal failure.[52]

The signs and symptoms are usually insidious in onset and may consist of anorexia, malaise, edema, anasarca, or ascites, and pericardial and pleural effusions may also be present. As a result of a hypercoagulable state, pulmonary embolism may develop but rarely results in death. The incidence of renal vein thrombosis varies from 5% to 62%,[53] and membranous nephropathy should be suspected when there is a sudden onset of hematuria, loin pain, pulmonary embolus, fluctuating or worsening proteinuria or GFR, renal tubular acidosis, or an increase in leg edema. Hypertension is found in approximately 30% of patients and is more common with renal insufficiency or in advanced disease.

In addition to heavy proteinuria, urinalysis often reveals lipiduria and oval fat bodies. Microhematuria is seen in fewer than 25% of patients, and gross hematuria and red cell casts are rare. In idiopathic membranous nephropathy, the serum complement concentrations are normal. Low levels of complement should alert one to search for secondary causes, such as lupus, hepatitis B infection, or an alternative diagnosis. Similarly, antinuclear antibodies, anti-DNA antibodies, rheumatoid factor, hepatitis B serologies, and serum cryoglobulins are generally negative in idiopathic membranous nephropathy. Occult malignancy has been found in as many as 10% of elderly patients with membranous nephropathy.

The natural course of idiopathic membranous nephropathy is variable. Up to 30% of the patients experience spontaneous remission, commonly within 2 years of disease onset. Half of the remaining patients have persistent proteinuria with long-term preservation of renal function, while the other half has gradual loss of renal function.[52] Heavy proteinuria (>10 g/day), male gender, elevated serum creatinine concentration at the time of presentation; poorly controlled hypertension, advanced age at onset of disease, non-Asian race, certain human leukocyte antigen phenotypes, and tubulointerstitial fibrosis on initial renal biopsy are associated with progressive renal disease.[52,53] A predictive algorithm, incorporating the level of proteinuria, initial creatinine clearance, as well as the slope of renal function decline over 6 months, has been developed to determine the risk for disease progression.[52]

In general, patients with idiopathic membranous nephropathy have a relatively benign course with mean 10-year survival of approximately 70%. Those who present with persistent nonnephrotic proteinuria seldom develop renal insufficiency and have a normal life expectancy. Fewer than 10% of patients develop a remitting and relapsing course.[53] The prognosis for secondary membranous nephropathy depends on the underlying cause. Remission occurs when the infection resolves or when the causative medication is withdrawn.

TREATMENT

Membranous Nephropathy

The treatment of idiopathic membranous nephropathy is controversial and ranges from supportive therapy to immunosuppression. Conservative management of patients with mild disease includes edema control with salt restriction and diuretics[5] and reduction of proteinuria with protein restriction and ACEIs (Fig. 56–4).[53] Management of hypertension and hyperlipidemia is required for most patients, whereas prophylactic anticoagulation, despite having benefits shown to outweigh the risks, is usually given only for patients with renal vein thrombosis or documented pulmonary embolus.[31,53]

■ PHARMACOLOGIC THERAPY

Steroids

Remission of proteinuria, whether spontaneously or treatment related, may confer a good prognosis. Corticosteroids alone were

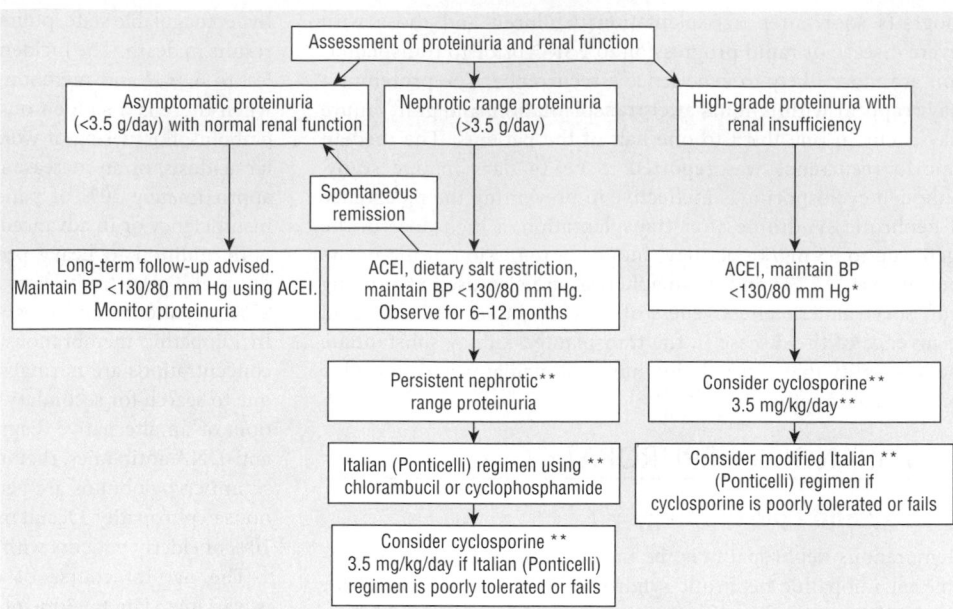

FIGURE 56-4. Treatment algorithm for idiopathic membranous neph-ropathy. Patients may change from one category to another during the course of follow-up. (*, supported by evidence from controlled trials; **, introduction of risk reduction strategies for both secondary effects of disease and adverse effects of immuno-therapy; ACEI, angiotensin-converting enzyme inhibitor; BP, blood pressure.) (*This article was published in Semin Nephrol, 20, Geddes CC, Cattran DC, The treatment of idiopathic mem-branous nephropathy, 299–308, Copyright © Elsevier 2000.*)

ineffective in improving proteinuria remission rate in all controlled trials and in preventing progression in all but one study.[51] The result of a metaanalysis also confirmed the lack of efficacy of steroids when used alone.

Cytotoxic Agents

Cytotoxic agents, when used in conjunction with corticosteroids, are effective in increasing the remission rate of proteinuria and preserving renal function. Ponticelli and colleagues devised such a regimen by combining intravenous methylprednisolone (1 g) for 3 days followed by oral methylprednisolone (0.4 mg/kg) for the subsequent 27 days of months 1, 3, and 5. Oral chlorambucil (0.2 mg/kg) is to be given daily in months 2, 4, and 6.[54] The 10-year renal survival was increased to 92% when compared with 60% in the con-trol group. They later substituted cyclophosphamide (2.5 mg/kg per day) for chlorambucil, which resulted in similar rates of proteinuria remission and relapse, but with fewer serious side effects in those who received cyclophosphamide.[55]

Results from a recent metaanalysis of randomized, controlled trials affirmed that cytotoxic agents, but not steroids, are effective in reducing nephrotic-range proteinuria, with cyclophosphamide having fewer adverse effects than chlorambucil.[56]

Cyclosporine

A controlled trial found that cyclosporine, given at a dose of 3 to 4 mg/kg/day for 6 months, was effective for patients with medium risk for disease progression.[52] For patients with severe nephrotic syndrome and deteriorating renal function who do not respond to cytotoxic therapy, cyclosporine may offer some benefits; however, the risk for cyclosporine nephrotoxicity is of concern, especially during long-term therapy. A 12-month course of cyclosporine (mean dose: 3.8 mg/kg/day) was found to reduce proteinuria as well as the rate of renal deterioration.[57] In a recent study of 41 patients who received cyclosporine, many with concurrent steroid and ACEI therapy, the median treatment time to complete remission was 225 days among the 34% of patients who attained complete remission.[58] During such long-term treat-ment, hypertension may be exacerbated and the serum creatinine concentration may be increased because of nephrotoxicity. When

the renal function declines, the dose of cyclosporine should be reduced.

Alternative Therapeutic Options

Because spontaneous remission is common and only approxi-mately 25% of patients with new-onset idiopathic membranous nephropathy ultimately develop ESRD in 20 to 30 years, it is pru-dent not to aggressively treat all patients at the onset of the disease. Patients who have a low risk for renal disease progression can be managed with observation and symptomatic therapy. Normalizing the blood pressure and reducing proteinuria with ACEIs and/or ARBs are important as both hypertension and proteinuria are inde-pendent risk factors for the progression of renal failure.[52] Patients with low risk for renal disease progression include children 2 to 16 years of age, adult males with proteinuria less than 2 g/day, or adult females with proteinuria less than 5 g/day and normal renal func-tion. In contrast, patients who have a high risk of developing renal failure, including those with proteinuria greater than 10 g/day with or without impaired renal function, and patients with symptomatic nephrotic syndrome with a plasma albumin of less than 2 g/dL (20 g/L) should be aggressively treated to induce remission. An alkylat-ing agent such as cyclophosphamide or chlorambucil, combined with steroids, should be given to induce remission. Recently, ritux-imab was shown to be effective in treating small number of patients, while eculizumab was not effective.[59-61] Mycophenolate mofetil was not more effective or better tolerated than cyclophosphamide.[62] Tetracosactide, a synthetic analog of adrenocorticotropic hormone, has also been shown in small studies to offer results superior to the cytotoxic–steroid combination regimen.[63]

The cytotoxic–steroid combination regimen may be effective in inducing remission in the 30% to 40% of the medium-risk patients who relapse within 2 years after treatment discontinuation. Alternately, cyclosporine may be used with similar effectiveness.[52] The cyclophosphamide–steroid combination should also be used for relapse in high-risk patients.

For patients with a transplanted kidney, both de novo and recur-rent membranous nephropathy may occur. Patients with primary membranous nephropathy are more at risk. Recurrence is typically associated with nephrotic syndrome and a high risk of allograft failure from disease and/or rejection.

MEMBRANOPROLIFERATIVE GLOMERULONEPHRITIS

Etiology, Epidemiology, and Pathophysiology

Membranoproliferative glomerulonephritis (MPGN) is one of the least-common renal morphologic entities that occur in older children and adults. For some unclear reason, the incidence of MPGN has been decreasing over the past few decades in the United States and Europe. However, in Africa and Asia, idiopathic MPGN is still common, perhaps secondary to exposure to unrecognized infectious and parasitic agents.

The several types of MPGN are classified according to the pathologic features. Type I MPGN, also known as mesangiocapillary glomerulonephritis, is characterized by diffuse thickening of glomerular capillary walls and mesangial hypercellularity. Immune complexes are presumed to have a major role in the pathogenesis of type I MPGN, which is the most common type of primary, idiopathic MPGN.

Type II MPGN is also known as dense-deposit disease (DDD) because of the presence of dense deposits of C3 within the GBM, which gives rise to a ribbon-like appearance. Other variants of the disease include type III MPGN, which is seen rarely and consists of subendothelial and subepithelial deposits with lamination and disruption of the lamina densa of the GBM.

Type I MPGN is a slowly progressive disease that accounts for 80% of all MPGN, but only 5% to 15% of all cases of nephrotic syndrome seen in pediatric and adult patients. It occurs most frequently for patients between 5 and 30 years of age, and because remissions are rare, many patients eventually develop ESRD. The renal survival is 60% to 65% at 10 years, and the presence of nephrotic syndrome, interstitial disease, and hypertension are poor prognostic indicators.[64] Type II MPGN is a more aggressive disease that constitutes approximately 15% of all patients with MPGN. Only 20% of patients remain stable for more than a few years, and the median time before the development of ESRD is 7 years.

Clinical Presentation

Nephrotic syndrome is the most common presenting condition although some patients may also have a nephritic component (hematuria), hypertension, and renal insufficiency. Hypocomplementemia is commonly seen.

TREATMENT

Membranoproliferative Glomerulonephritis

■ STEROIDS

The efficacy of corticosteroids, cyclophosphamide, antiplatelet drugs, and anticoagulants has been evaluated for the treatment of MPGN. In children, prednisone 40 mg/m² given on alternate days is effective, when compared with placebo, in reducing the decline in GFR.[65] This observation was confirmed by other uncontrolled studies.[64] Consequently, prednisone should be given for 6 to 12 months to children with MPGN, proteinuria (more than 3 g/day), and/or impaired renal function.[64] Other studies suggest that this regimen may also be beneficial in children with mild proteinuria.

Although the effect of steroids has not been proven in adults, antiplatelet drugs, such as dipyridamole and aspirin, as well as warfarin, were found in randomized controlled trials to reduce proteinuria but had no effect on GFR.[64] Subcutaneous heparin has also been used in a small number of patients with favorable results.[66] Adult patients with idiopathic MPGN, heavy proteinuria, and/or impaired renal function should be given dipyridamole or aspirin. Unfortunately, no controlled study comparing the effect of steroids with antiplatelet agents is yet available.

■ CYTOTOXIC AGENTS

Cyclophosphamide and azathioprine were found to have no beneficial effect. Cyclosporine was evaluated in a limited number of patients with MPGN with some beneficial effect; however, the trials were not controlled or randomized. In addition, the risks for developing adverse effects were high. Figure 56–5 presents an algorithm for treatment and follow-up of MPGN.

■ ANTIPLATELET AGENTS

Although several studies have shown dipyridamole and aspirin to reduce proteinuria, reduction of GFR decline was not generally observed.[64] Consequently, antiplatelet therapy should be considered

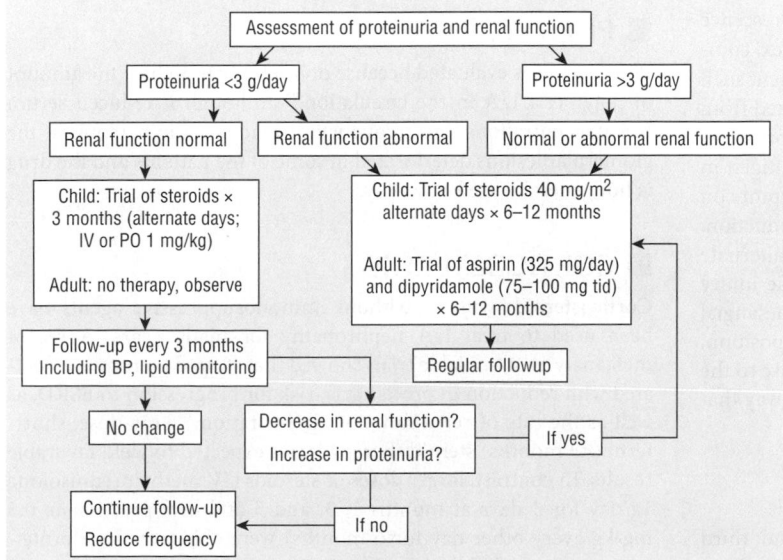

FIGURE 56-5. Treatment algorithm for membranoproliferative glomerulonephritis. (BP, blood pressure.) (*Reprinted by permission from Macmillan Publishers Ltd: Levin A. Management of membranoproliferative glomerulonephritis: Evidence-based recommendations. Kidney Int Suppl 1999;55:S41–S46.*)

as a viable option only for those patients with significant proteinuria. There should be periodic follow up of patients to assess proteinuria and renal function.

Since steroids are not known to be effective for type II disease other yet-to-be-proven strategies such as rituximab, eculizumab, sulodexide, and plasma infusion or exchange may be considered.[67] It is difficult to conduct large-scale controlled trials for MPGN because of the low incidence of the disease. Based on the available studies, many of the drugs evaluated do not have any consistent, beneficial effect on renal function and proteinuria. Renal transplantation is an alternative; however, the recurrence rate is close to 100% for type II MPGN and is approximately 20% to 30% for type I MPGN. Half of the allografts ultimately fail.

IMMUNOGLOBULIN A NEPHROPATHY

Etiology and Epidemiology

IgA nephropathy, also known as *Berger disease*, was first described in France in 1968. It now is the most common primary glomerulonephritis in the world and accounts for 10% of patients with ESRD in many countries. The prevalence among patients with glomerulonephritis or patients who had kidney biopsy varies from as high as 50% in Japan and East Asia to 10% to 30% in Europe. In the United States, the overall prevalence is approximately 10% to 15% but is as high as 35% among Native Americans living in New Mexico.[68] These differences in prevalence may reflect variations in genetic predisposition, as well as the criteria used for urinary screening and kidney biopsy.

IgA nephropathy is more frequently seen in younger adults and is two to six times more common in males than in females. It is uncommon in blacks, both in the United States and in Africa.[68] IgA nephropathy was once thought to be a benign disease presenting with asymptomatic hematuria; however, its ability to present with any clinical syndrome associated with glomerular disease is now recognized. Some patients will develop ESRD over variable periods of time.

Pathophysiology

Primary IgA nephropathy is an immune-complex–mediated disease in which IgA deposits and other pathologic lesions are found in kidney tissues. In contrast, Henoch-Schönlein purpura, a systemic disease that is believed to be closely linked to IgA nephropathy, shares similar immunohistologic findings in the kidneys. Both typically have vasculitis affecting the joints, skin, and gastrointestinal tract, which may result from the same pathologic process of IgA nephropathy. The diagnosis of IgA nephropathy is established by the presence of mesangial IgA deposits upon immunofluorescence examination of the kidney biopsy. The IgA immune complex, composed of IgA antibody bound with an environmental antigen, such as a virus, bacteria, or food substances, is presumed deposited from the systemic circulation. Alternately, the complex may be formed in situ, with the IgA antibody bound with an endogenous antigen in the mesangium. In the mesangium, IgA can bind with receptors on the mesangial cells to induce proliferation and cytokine production. In addition, IgA can activate complement through the alternate pathway to induce glomerular damage.[69] The extent of the injury depends on the characteristics of the IgA that favor mesangial deposition, the susceptibility of the mesangium toward deposition, the ability of the patient to mount an inflammatory response to the deposits, and the response of the kidney to the injury in a way that favors progressive renal damage.[70]

Clinical Presentation

IgA nephropathy commonly presents in the second and third decades of life, but it can occur at any age. Many patients have microscopic hematuria and proteinuria for years, persistently or intermittently, during the early stages of the disease. About half of the patients present with gross hematuria concurrent with an infection, commonly in the upper respiratory tract.[68] The hematuria may occur 1 to 2 days after the onset of infection symptoms, which is different from the 10- to 14-day delay seen after the pharyngitis in poststreptococcal glomerulonephritis. Proteinuria is common, and nephrotic range often indicates advanced disease. Hypertension and edema are infrequent but are common in poststreptococcal glomerulonephritis.

Renal dysfunction is uncommon at the initial presentation; however, approximately 10% to 20% of the patients develop ESRD within 10 years, and 30% develop it after 20 years.[71] Hypertension, severe proteinuria, renal function impairment, old age, and the severity of histologic lesions are all predictive factors for poor long-term outcome.[69-71]

TREATMENT

Immunoglobulin A Nephropathy

Spontaneous remission is seen in only 10% to 25% of children and 5% to 7.5% of adults. Unfortunately, no therapy is known to be consistently effective for the treatment of IgA nephropathy. Because of the slow progression of the disease to ESRD, it is very difficult to conduct trials to evaluate the long-term effectiveness of specific treatments. The lack of understanding of the pathogenetic mechanisms and the unavailability of appropriate animal models severely limit the development of rational treatment regimens.

■ NONPHARMACOLOGIC THERAPY: LOW-GLUTEN DIET AND TONSILLECTOMY

Restriction of dietary gluten is effective for patients with celiac disease but not for patients with no identifiable nephritogenic antigens.[72] Removal of the tonsils, which produce IgA_1 and may contribute to IgA nephropathy, may reduce proteinuria and hematuria. This is especially helpful for patients who developed recurrent macroscopic hematuria as provoked by bacterial tonsillitis. There are limited studies to show the long-term renoprotective effects of tonsillectomy; however, larger studies with longer follow-up are needed to affirm such beneficial effect.[70]

■ PHENYTOIN

Phenytoin was evaluated because of its ability to reduce the amount of polymeric IgA in the circulation.[72] Although it reduced serum IgA concentrations and frequency of macroscopic hematuria, the glomerular lesions deteriorated in some of the patients and the drug is not generally used nowadays.

■ CORTICOSTEROIDS

Corticosteroids with or without immunosuppressive agents have been used to treat IgA nephropathy for many years. A recent metaanalysis of available trials showed that steroid therapy is associated with reduction in proteinuria, risk for progression to ESRD, as well as the rate of renal function deterioration.[73] Low-dose, short-term (<3 months) steroid therapy is not expected to yield favorable results. In contrast, larger doses of steroids (IV methylprednisolone 1g/day for 3 days at months 1, 3, and 5 and oral prednisone 0.5 mg/kg every other day for 6 months) were able to reduce proteinuria and renal function deterioration.[74] However, the dose of the steroids and the risk for toxicity might be considered high by many.[70] Patients with nephrotic range proteinuria and impaired renal function are likely candidates for steroid therapy; however, the responses to such treatment are not favorable.

CYTOTOXIC AGENTS

Several studies have evaluated the efficacy of azathioprine and cyclophosphamide. In some of the studies, cyclophosphamide was used in conjunction with dipyridamole, heparin and warfarin. It is difficult to assess which of these agents contributed to the limited favorable effects observed. In addition, in many of these studies, blood pressure control and ACE inhibition were not always optimal. At present, there is no clear evidence to support the use of these cytotoxic agents for IgA nephropathy, except perhaps for those patients with advanced rapidly progressive disease.[70]

CLINICAL CONTROVERSY

Is fish oil effective for IgA nephropathy?

FISH OIL

The third approach is to reduce glomerular inflammation and glomerulosclerosis induced by IgA deposits. Antiinflammatory agents, antiplatelet drugs, and anticoagulants have been tried without success to decrease the production or action of mediators responsible for IgA immune-complex–induced glomerular damage.

However, the *n*-3 fatty acids in fish oil reduce the production or action of prostaglandins and leukotrienes, thus limiting the renal damage caused by inflammation, platelet aggregation, and vasoconstriction.[24] In a controlled trial on patients with heavy proteinuria and mildly impaired renal function, daily use of fish oil delayed the progression of renal failure with modest reduction in proteinuria.[75] A metaanalysis of five controlled studies indicated that a minor, but not statistically significant, beneficial effect on renal function may be observed.[76] Results from several recent studies failed to confirm the beneficial effects reported earlier, and further studies are needed to confirm the role as well as the optimal dose. In many of the studies, 4 to 12 g/day were given for 2 or more years. Some of the fish oil preparations are rich in cholesterol; thus, it is appropriate to monitor the LDL cholesterol levels for patients receiving therapy.

ANGIOTENSIN-CONVERTING ENZYME INHIBITION

Because hypertension is a negative prognostic indicator of IgA nephropathy and many of these patients already have left ventricular diastolic malfunction despite being normotensive, early antihypertensive intervention with ACEIs or ARBs is important.[68,69] If a single agent is insufficient to reduce proteinuria and maintain blood pressure at 125/75 mm Hg, combined use of ACEI and ARB should be instituted.[70]

ALTERNATIVE THERAPEUTIC APPROACHES

Patients with IgA nephropathy have abnormal production of IgA and several different immunoglobulins. Immunoglobulins, administered intravenously initially and then intramuscularly, may have beneficial effects through immunomodulation, increased catabolism of autoantibodies, and blockade of receptors.[77] The

doses in this experimental trial, which has not been independently replicated, were very high: 1 g/kg/day for 2 days IV for the first three months, then 0.35 mL/kg IM every 15 days for the next six months. Plasmapheresis with albumin replacement was performed before the 2- to 12-hour IV infusions to avoid serum sickness. Reduction in proteinuria, hematuria, GFR decline, and histologic activity index were observed for 11 patients with a progressive course of the disease. Renal survival was prolonged for eight of these patients who were followed for 3 to 10 years.[78] Larger, randomized, controlled trials are needed before one can recommend this regimen with confidence.

Urokinase, danazol, dapsone, sodium cromoglycate, and plasma exchange have also been evaluated, but none is consistently effective nor shown to affect renal function.[71,77] Cyclosporine treatment was found in a limited number of studies to reduce proteinuria; however, renal function decreased during treatment. Consequently, its use is limited by the potential for nephrotoxicity.[24,77]

The HMG-CoA reductase inhibitor fluvastatin was reported to reduce urinary protein excretion in moderately proteinuric (0.6 to 1.6 g/day) patients who had IgA nephropathy with normal renal function.[79] Creatinine clearance remained stable during the 6-month study. Although evaluation for a longer term in a larger patient population is needed to confirm this beneficial effect, statin use is an obvious choice for hyperlipidemic patients with IgA.

Antiplatelet agents are commonly used in Japan and rarely outside of Asia for IgA nephropathy.[80] A recent metaanalysis of seven trials (four in Japan and three in Hong Kong) revealed that these agents reduced proteinuria and stabilized renal function.[81] Mycophenolate mofetil and several new strategies are being evaluated as experimental treatments for IgA nephropathy on the premise that they may reduce IgA synthesis and mesangial uptake and/or suppress the effects of proinflammatory or profibrogenic mediators.[81]

Normotensive patients with normal renal function, isolated microhematuria, and proteinuria less than 1 g/day should be observed closely without specific treatment.[69] Patients with minimal proteinuria of 0.5 to 1 g/day receive fish oil and an ACEI or ARB (Fig. 56–6) to attain BP of <103/80 mmHg and urinary protein excretion of <500 mg/day.[24] Combined ACEI and ARB seems to be more effective than monotherapy. Because corticosteroids reduce proteinuria, a course of alternate-day prednisone (1 mg/kg/day) with subsequent tapering is indicated for patients with proteinuria greater than 3 g/day who have good renal function [>70 mL/min (>1.17 mL/s)].[71] A more aggressive IV or oral steroid regimen may be considered, even though its efficacy has not been definitively established. For patients with a slow progressive decline in creatinine clearance [<70 mL/min (<1.17 mL/s)], fish oil should be given. Azathioprine, cyclophosphamide, mycophenolate mofetil, or dipyridamole/warfarin therapy may also be used, although

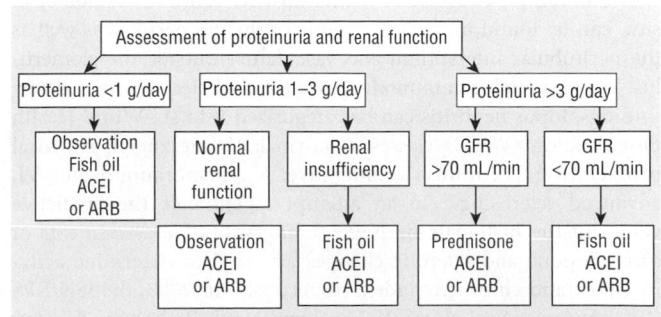

FIGURE 56-6. Treatment algorithm for biopsy-proven IgA nephropathy. (ACE, angiotensin-converting enzyme; ARB, angiotensin receptor blocker; GFR, glomerular filtration rate.) *(Modified from reference 71.)*

the efficacy of these agents has not been firmly established. If the patient experiences rapid GFR decline of more than 2 mL/min (0.033 mL/s) per month, immunoglobulin therapy may be considered despite the fact that only limited data are available. Other therapies that may be considered for these patients include pulse steroids, a cyclophosphamide–steroid combination, mycophenolate mofetil, and plasmapheresis.[24,69,71,82]

■ THERAPEUTIC OUTCOMES

Urinary protein excretion and the mean arterial blood pressure at follow-up correlate well with the progression of disease. The risk of developing ESRD is proportional to the amount of proteinuria, under the influence of ACEI and ARB therapy, after 1 year of follow-up.[83] For those patients who develop end-stage renal failure, transplantation is appropriate, especially for young adults. Recurrence of IgA mesangial deposits in the renal allograft may occur in up to 50% of patients in 5 years and be universally present at 10 years or more posttransplant, but the recurrence of clinical disease is only approximately 10% to 15%.[68,69] There is also no correlation between the aggressiveness of the primary disease and the rate of recurrence.[68] Use of ACEI may improve graft survival[84] while immunosuppression with corticosteroids, azathioprine, and/or cyclosporine is not expected to prevent the recurrent nephropathy.

LUPUS NEPHRITIS

Etiology and Epidemiology

Glomerulonephritis is one of the most serious complications of systemic lupus erythematosus (SLE) and accounts for much of the morbidity and mortality of patients afflicted with the disease. SLE predominantly affects young women between 15 and 40 years of age, with an incidence of 1 in 2,000 women in the United States. African Americans are more susceptible; they develop the disease at a younger age, have nephritis earlier in the course, and are more likely to progress to end-stage kidney disease.

The renal manifestations of lupus nephritis are variable and encompass a wide spectrum of histopathologic lesions.[85] The underlying histopathology is associated with different prognoses and responses to therapy, which can not be predicted solely based on clinical manifestations. Thus, a renal biopsy is required to assess the severity of the disease and to predict the short-term and long-term outcomes associated with therapy. Drugs, such as hydralazine and procainamide, are known to precipitate a lupus syndrome; however, they are unlikely to cause disease that affects the kidney.

Pathophysiology

Immune complex deposits, whether formed in the circulation or in situ, can be found in various regions of the glomerulus, as well as the peritubular interstitium and vasculature outside the glomerulus. Based on light, immunofluorescence, and electron microscopy findings, lupus nephritis can be categorized into six World Health Organization (WHO) classes: I, normal; II, mesangial; III, focal proliferative; IV, diffuse proliferative; V, membranous; and VI, advanced sclerosing.[86] In an attempt to enhance the predictive values of the histologic findings, semiquantitative assessments of active lesions and sclerotic changes are used to determine activity index and chronicity index, respectively. In 2003, the ISN/RPS (International Society of Nephrology/Renal Pathology Society) classification was developed to reduce interobserver reproducibility and provide a practical and standardized approach to biopsy interpretation so that outcome data can be compared worldwide.[87]

The hallmark feature in the pathogenesis of SLE is B-cell hyperactivity and the dysregulated production of autoantibodies against multiple antigens in the body, including DNA and various ribonucleoproteins.[85,88] The size and location of the immune complexes in the glomerulus correlate with the nature and severity of renal injury. Deposition of small numbers of stable immune complexes of intermediate size in the mesangium tends to produce less severe inflammation in the glomerulus. The sequestration of the immune complexes in the mesangium prevents them from activating inflammatory mediators. Hence, the lesion is noninflammatory in nature. In contrast, large numbers of intermediate-sized or large immune complexes result in infiltration of inflammatory cells and release of necrotizing enzymes.

Clinical Presentation

Females have a higher risk for developing lupus, especially in the adult years. Nephritis is commonly seen within the first 4 years of diagnosis of SLE but may also be the first manifestation of the disease. The clinical presentation ranges from minimal hematuria and proteinuria to severe, rapidly progressive diffuse glomerulonephritis. Proteinuria is very common, and nephrotic syndrome is seen in most patients with membranous lesions. Microscopic hematuria is almost always present, whereas macroscopic hematuria, which commonly indicates severe renal involvement, is rare.[86] Active urinary sediments (red cell casts, dysmorphic red cells, and hematuria) are suggestive of the diffuse proliferative lesion.[85] Hypertension is present in 25% to 45% of patients and is associated with a worse prognosis. Recent studies affirm the poor prognosis and higher risk for renal involvement among African-American and Texan-Hispanic patients, compared with white and Puerto Rican–Hispanic patients, due to the greater severity of disease at baseline, presence of certain autoantibodies, and socioeconomic considerations.[89] Other conditions found to be associated with poor prognosis include elevated serum creatinine concentration, heavy proteinuria, anemia [hematocrit <26% (<0.26)], and disease onset during childhood or in those >60 years of age. Most patients have hypocomplementemia and increased antibody titers for anti-double-stranded DNA, particularly those with focal or diffuse proliferative lesions. Serum creatinine concentration at the time of diagnosis is most predictive of short-term outcome.

■ TREATMENT

Lupus Nephritis

❼ The choice of therapy depends on the underlying lesion and the activity, as well as the chronicity indices. Acute life-threatening disease involving multiple organs requires induction treatment that can suppress the disease promptly. In contrast, long-term management of chronic indolent disease requires therapy with more acceptable side-effect profiles. Corticosteroids are the cornerstone of therapy. However, for severe lupus nephritis, primarily the diffuse proliferative type, alkylating agents may be needed to reduce or prevent the progression to ESRD. Newer alternatives with fewer side effects are now available.

Optimal blood pressure control is important. ACE inhibitor or ARB has been shown to reduce proteinuria. Patients with normal renal function and less than 2 g of proteinuria usually do not require therapy, except for the management of extrarenal lupus manifestations. The prognosis of these patients is generally good, and renal biopsy can be delayed. However, close follow-up of renal function and urinalysis is required.

■ ACUTE INDUCTION TREATMENT

Steroids and Cytotoxic Agents

Patients with more than 2 g of proteinuria, deteriorating renal function, and/or active urinary sediments require a renal biopsy to define the underlying lesion and determine the activity and chronicity of disease. Patients with proliferative lesions, class IV and class III with subendothelial deposits and signs of severe disease activity, should be treated with pulse intravenous methylprednisolone followed by low-dose oral steroids. Cyclophosphamide is used concurrently because it is a powerful B-cell inhibitor and can suppress the resynthesis of autoantibodies to normal levels.[86] Combined use of intravenous cyclophosphamide and methylprednisolone is more effective than either agent alone in inducing remission.[88,90] Cyclophosphamide is given orally in some of the regimens.[91] Azathioprine has also been used in conjunction with cyclophosphamide. The risk for adverse events, such as infection, gonadal damage, amenorrhea, and cervical dysplasia, and malignancy is increased with the cytotoxic regimens.[88] Studies show that cyclophosphamide toxicities may be related to the cumulative doses rather than the route of administration.[91] Because oral doses of cyclophosphamide tend to accrue easily, it is prudent to use it only for those who are high risk and had failed other therapies.

Mycophenolate Mofetil

> ### CLINICAL CONTROVERSY
>
> Should mycophenolate mofetil be used in place of cyclophosphamide for lupus nephritis?

Several trials have found that mycophenolate mofetil with concurrent steroid therapy is an effective agent for induction therapy.[92] It was as effective as cyclophosphamide in inducing remission but with fewer side effects. A recent meta-analysis of the literature corroborates to the fact that it is an excellent agent for the induction of remission and that continued use may reduce risk for death or development of ESRD.[89] However, many of these trials were conducted in Asia, and the results may not be reproducible in American patients. Two recent trials that included African Americans, who are known to have a poorer prognosis, also show that mycophenolate mofetil was more efficacious than intravenous cyclophosphamide and resulted in fewer adverse effects.[88,93] Based on these data, mycophenolate mofetil seems to be a viable alternative to intravenous cyclophosphamide, especially for patients with mild to moderate focal or diffuse lupus nephritis or membranous lupus nephritis (WHO class III, IV, or V) and preserved renal function. However, the duration of follow-up in these trials was not as long as the trials that were conducted to establish the efficacy of cyclophosphamide-based regimens. The ability of mycophenolate mofetil to sustain the remission long term is still unclear (Fig. 56–7).

■ CHRONIC MAINTENANCE TREATMENT

Steroids and Cytotoxic Agents

Oral steroid is most frequently used for maintenance treatment (prednisolone 5 to 15 mg/day or equivalent).[86] Alternate-day regimens, although not evaluated, are often used in children to minimize growth retardation. Monthly pulse IV steroids in conjunction with cyclophosphamide resulted in more sustained remission, fewer relapses, and no significant increase in side effects.[94] Meta-analysis shows this combination to be more beneficial than steroid

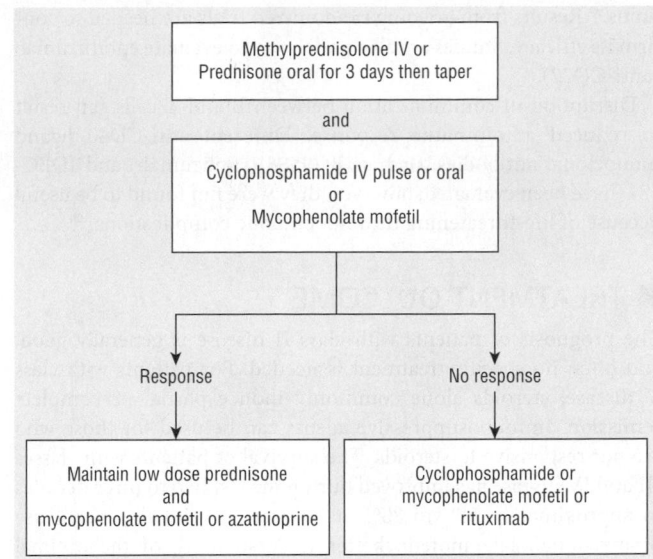

FIGURE 56-7. Treatment algorithm for proliferative lupus nephritis.

or cyclophosphamide alone. Cyclophosphamide, because of its bladder and gonadal toxicity, has been given as monthly and then bimonthly intravenous injection, instead of daily administration, for 2 or more years. However, toxicity is still a concern. A study conducted in Europe showed that after initial lower pulse doses of IV cyclophosphamide, oral azathioprine was able to attain remission rates similar to those of higher initial pulse doses of cyclophosphamide with quarterly follow-up doses.[95] Recently, daily doses of mycophenolate mofetil or azathioprine for 2 years have been shown to be more effective than intravenous pulses of cyclophosphamide in reducing relapse while being less toxic.[96]

Cyclosporine

Cyclosporine may reduce proteinuria and lupus activity, stabilize renal function, and improve kidney morphology. It has been shown to have comparable efficacy and safety with azathioprine in preventing relapse for patients with diffuse proliferative lupus nephritis.[97]

■ ALTERNATIVE THERAPEUTIC AGENTS

Many new agents have been developed to target the various pathways, costimulatory molecules, and immune mediators responsible for the pathologic autoantibody production.

LJP-394 (Riquent, abetimus sodium), composed of four double-stranded oligodeoxynucleotides, render specific B lymphocytes unresponsive to immunogen by cross-linking with the surface immunoglobulin receptors, thereby reducing anti-DNA antibody production. It may reduce renal and systemic SLE flares in a subgroup of patients whose anti-DNA antibodies are bound avidly to the compound.[98] However, a subsequent study did not reveal such a beneficial effect when compared with placebo.[88]

Rituximab is a monoclonal antibody directed against CD20, which is a membrane-associated glycoprotein on B lymphocytes. It causes B-lymphocyte depletion without affecting plasma cells, which do not have CD20. For patients, the B-cell depletion correlates with clinical response. The drug has been reported to have 75% response rate in refractory lupus or lupus nephritis. However, these studies are uncontrolled, and different regimens were used in heterogeneous groups of patients.[60,88] In the first randomized trial rituximab failed to show a superior response for patients receiving glucocorticoids and other background immunosuppressant therapy for remission induction in moderately to severely active nonrenal lupus.[99] Results from ongoing randomized trials are needed to confirm its efficacy. Studies are also under way to evaluate epratuzumab (anti-CD22).

Disruption of communication between B and T cells can result in reduced autoimmune response. Different anti-CD40 ligand monoclonal antibodies, such as BG9588 (ruplizumab) and IDEC-131, have been evaluated; however, they were not found to be useful because of life-threatening thromboembolic complications.[100]

■ TREATMENT OUTCOME

The prognosis of patients with class II disease is generally good, and often no specific treatment is needed. For patients with class V disease, steroids alone commonly induce partial or complete remission. Immunosuppressive agents can be used for those who are not responsive to steroids. The survival of patients with classes III and IV disease has improved during the last two to three decades to approximately 74% to 80% at 10 years.[85] With the recent use of mycophenolate mofetil, better understanding of the optimal cytotoxic regimens, the use of lower steroid dosages, and better management of complications such as hypertension, infections, hyperlipidemia, and other metabolic complications of the disease, the long-term outcome has became more favorable. Lupus patients with end-stage kidney disease on dialysis fare as well as those with non-lupus–related renal disease. In those patients who received a renal transplant, the allograft outcome of patients with lupus nephritis is favorable and comparable to those without lupus. Recurrence of lupus in the renal allograft can occur but is usually of minor clinical importance.

RAPIDLY PROGRESSIVE GLOMERULONEPHRITIS

Etiology and Epidemiology

Rapidly progressive glomerulonephritis (RPGN) describes a clinicopathologic syndrome of rapid loss of renal function—usually a greater than 50% decrement of the GFR within 3 months. The predominant histologic finding of RPGN is extensive crescent formation, usually in more than 50% of the glomeruli. Hence, it is also known as *crescentic glomerulonephritis*. RPGN accounts for 2% to 7% of all renal biopsy findings and is responsible for up to 5% of patients with end-stage kidney disease. The age ranges of susceptible patients vary with the type of RPGN. For example, types I and II RPGN are more common in younger patients, whereas type III is seen more frequently in older individuals.

RPGN is not a single disease entity. A variety of glomerulonephritides with or without systemic diseases may present as RPGN, including anti-GBM glomerulonephritis, Goodpasture syndrome, lupus nephritis, poststreptococcal glomerulonephritis, membranoproliferative glomerulonephritis, IgA nephropathy, polyarteritis nodosa, Wegener granulomatosis, and idiopathic crescentic glomerulonephritis.

Primary RPGN is categorized according to the immunofluorescence microscopic findings, indicating different immunopathogenesis, therapeutic approaches, and clinical outcome. Type I is characterized by the linear localization of immunoglobulins, mainly IgG, along the GBM, signifying anti-GBM antibody-induced injury. Type II is defined by the coarse granular deposition of immunoglobulins and complement within the capillary walls and mesangium, indicating immune-complex–mediated injury. Type III is characterized by scanty or complete lack of immune complex deposits; consequently, it is also known as *pauci-immune RPGN*. Circulating ANCAs are often detected in type III RPGN.

Pathophysiology

Different etiologic factors are implicated as the cause of RPGN: toxins, drugs, viral and bacterial infections, neoplasms, autoimmune mechanisms, and various immunogenetic factors.[101] Regardless of the etiology and type of RPGN, damage in the glomerular capillary wall by both humoral and cellular pathways of inflammation is common. Activation of the terminal C5b-9 (membrane-attacking complex) of the complement system produces severe capillary wall injury. Proteinases and reactive oxygen species released by neutrophils and macrophages may result in severe glomerular injury. Platelets and the coagulation system are activated and result in capillary thrombosis. The ruptured capillaries release fibrinogen and procoagulants that may come into contact with thrombogenic tissue debris and lead to fibrinoid changes. In anti-GBM glomerulonephritis, the direct attack of the anti-GBM antibody on the GBM is responsible for the capillary wall injury.[101] For patients with ANCA-associated disease, the interaction of ANCAs with neutrophils and monocytes, which have been primed by concurrent infections or inflammatory processes, can lead to activation of these leukocytes and release of toxic oxygen species and lytic enzymes, resulting in vascular injury.

The disruption of the capillary wall allows movement of macrophages and other plasma constituents into Bowman space and stimulates the formation of crescents, which are composed mainly of parietal epithelial cells, as well as macrophages and fibroblasts. Crescent formation indicates the severity of the glomerular capillary disease but not its pathogenesis.

Clinical Presentation

Among the crescentic glomerulonephritides, the pauci-immune RPGN (type III) is the most frequent, accounting for more than 50% of cases, whereas the anti-GBM antibody-mediated RPGN (type I) is the least frequent, occurring in roughly 10% to 20% of patients. Of patients with type I RPGN, 60% to 70% may have concurrent pulmonary hemorrhage and Goodpasture syndrome, which is caused by antibodies directed against the pulmonary alveolar basement membrane. Most patients with immune-complex–mediated RPGN (type II) have collagen vascular disease, systemic infections, or a severe form of primary glomerular disease. Approximately 70% of patients with type III RPGN also present with evidence of systemic vasculitis, such as Wegener granulomatosis and polyarteritis nodosa. Some patients have only renal manifestations and are said to have idiopathic crescentic glomerulonephritis or renal vasculitis.

The clinical presentation is dominated by progressive renal insufficiency with complaints of tea-colored urine, malaise, anorexia, low-grade fever, and migratory polyarthropathy. Type I RPGN is more common in younger patients, whereas patients with ANCA-mediated disease tend to be older.[102] Urinalysis commonly shows nephritic sediments with hematuria, erythrocyte casts, and proteinuria. However, overt nephrotic syndrome is rare.

Serologic analysis is very useful in distinguishing the different types of RPGN. The detection of serum anti-GBM antibodies with the appropriate clinical presentation confirms the diagnosis of anti-GBM glomerulonephritis. More than 80% of patients with pauci-immune or idiopathic crescentic glomerulonephritis have circulating ANCAs. ANCAs are autoantibodies specific for the cytoplasmic constituents of neutrophil granules and monocyte lysosomes. Patients with ANCA-associated disease limited to renal involvement often have P-ANCA (perinuclear staining), whereas patients with Wegener granulomatosis tend to have C-ANCA (cytoplasmic staining). Both the anti-GBM antibody and the ANCAs are absent in patients with type II RPGN. Measurements of circulating immune complexes are not useful for making a specific diagnosis, but detection of specific serum antibodies known to mediate immune complex–associated nephritis is helpful, using anti-DNA antibody as a marker for lupus nephritis and elevated antistreptolysin O titers for poststreptococcal glomerulonephritis.

TREATMENT

Rapidly Progressive Glomerulonephritis

Early aggressive therapy has improved the renal prognosis of patients with crescentic glomerulonephritis. The rapid deterioration of renal function and the paucity of a large number of patients make randomized controlled studies very difficult to conduct. Based on the available data, immunosuppressive therapy alone appears to be ineffective for type I RPGN, while types II and III RPGN respond well to high-dose steroid therapy.[101,103] Regardless of the type of RPGN, poor response to therapy and an ominous renal survival are expected if the patient presents with oliguria, has a serum creatinine concentration greater than 6 or 7 mg/dL (530 or 619 μmol/L), is dialysis dependent, or has a renal biopsy showing advanced chronic parenchymal disease.[104] Because of the differences in response, the therapeutic approaches for each type of RPGN are presented separately below.

◼ ANTIGLOMERULAR BASEMENT MEMBRANE GLOMERULONEPHRITIS (TYPE I)

Steroids and cyclophosphamide, in conjunction with plasma exchange, have been used effectively to control the disease. Plasma exchanges remove the pathogenic anti-GBM antibodies in circulation and are conducted for 2 weeks or until the antibodies disappear. Steroids (prednisolone 1 mg/kg/day, tapered over 6 months) and cyclophosphamide (2 to 3 mg/kg/day for 3 months) are then given to prevent new antibody production.[102,103] Patients with mild disease generally respond well to plasma exchange alone or immunosuppression (steroid and/or cytotoxic agents). For patients with severe disease (poor renal function and extensive crescent formation), most are expected to respond to the combination of plasma exchange and steroid/cytotoxic drug therapy. Pulse intravenous administration of corticosteroids (methylprednisolone 30 mg/kg/day for 3 days) has been used successfully to alleviate pulmonary hemorrhage, but the results are not as convincing for glomerulonephritis.[101,103] Because of the rapid decline in renal function, diagnosis should be established early so that therapy can proceed without delay. When the serum creatinine concentration is 6 mg/dL (530 μmol/L) or above or the patient is oliguric or requires dialysis, the response to therapy is usually poor, and the patient should be treated conservatively.[102,103] Poor response should also be expected when crescents are found in more than 85% of the glomeruli.

◼ IMMUNE-COMPLEX–MEDIATED GLOMERULONEPHRITIS (TYPE II)

Patients with postinfectious RPGN generally have a favorable prognosis even without treatment. Complete spontaneous recovery occurs in 50% of cases, whereas chronic renal failure develops in 32%.[101] Pulse doses of methylprednisolone (30 mg/kg/day, every other day × 3), followed by oral prednisone (1 mg/kd/day, tapered over several months) and then tapering, are beneficial in type II RPGN, with a response rate of 85% for patients with acute disease and 70% in those with more chronic disease.[101,103] Plasmapheresis does not appear to provide any additional benefit.[103]

◼ ANTINEUTROPHIL CYTOPLASMIC AUTOANTIBODY-ASSOCIATED GLOMERULONEPHRITIS (TYPE III)

Combined use of high-dose corticosteroids and cyclophosphamide induces remission in more than 90% of patients.[104] Cyclophosphamide, if given intravenously, is associated with fewer infectious complications while being as effective as the oral route in inducing remission; however, the risk of relapse may be higher.[105] Because approximately 30% of the patients may relapse, cyclophosphamide also has been used for maintenance therapy. Mycophenolate mofetil and methotrexate are now being used, and they have been shown in limited studies to be effective.[103,105] Plasmapheresis is not expected to have any additional benefits for patients with mild to moderate disease who are receiving immunosuppressive therapy. However, as an adjunct to immunosuppressive therapy, it may be beneficial for patients with severe disease presenting with acute renal failure, especially those with pulmonary hemorrhage.[105]

◼ RENAL TRANSPLANTATION

Anti-GBM nephritis may recur in up to 55% of patients who received a renal transplant. However, only 25% of these patients showed clinical disease activity, with rare allograft failure. Because the frequency of recurrence and its severity are related to the presence of circulating anti-GBM antibody, it is recommended that transplantation should not be performed until the anti-GBM antibody is undetectable for at least 6 to 12 months. The recurrence rate of ANCA-associated nephritis is 17%, with the average time to relapse from transplantation of 31 months.[106]

POSTSTREPTOCOCCAL GLOMERULONEPHRITIS

Etiology and Epidemiology

Poststreptococcal glomerulonephritis (PSGN) and glomerulonephritis caused by other infectious agents, such as bacteria, viruses, and parasites, were once common. Improved sanitation, personal hygiene, medical care, and public health measures helped to decrease the incidence of group A streptococcal infection both in the United States and in other developed countries, resulting in a decline of PSGN. In contrast, glomerulonephritis secondary to other infectious agents, such as hepatitis C and HIV, is seen with increasing frequency.

PSGN is now the most common form of glomerulonephritis in children but is less common than the other types of glomerulonephritis in adults. PSGN is seen mostly in children aged between 5 and 15 years and is uncommon in children younger than 2 years of age and in adults older than 50 years of age. It normally follows pharyngeal or skin infection caused by the nephritogenic strains of group A streptococci; however, other strains of streptococci, such as groups C and G, have also been reported to cause PSGN. Streptococcal pharyngitis is more common in winter and early spring, whereas skin infection is frequently found in the summer. The risk for developing acute glomerulonephritis secondary to the nephritogenic strains of bacteria is approximately 10% to 15% for infected patients. However, three to four times more patients may experience a subclinical form of the disease.

Pathophysiology

Streptococcal antigens may induce changes in the glomerular components rendering them immunogenic or autologous IgG may be altered to become antigenic. Alternately, the streptococcal antigens may induce antibodies that react with glomerular antigens. In situ immune complexes are then formed and result in a complement-mediated inflammatory response. The kinin and coagulation cascades are activated, and chemotactic factors are released to recruit neutrophils and monocytes, resulting in acute glomerular lesions.

Examination of the acute PSGN kidneys reveals hypercellular glomeruli with proliferation of mesangial and endothelial cells. Infiltration of neutrophils, monocytes, and eosinophils is apparent within the capillary lumen and also in the mesangial areas. Crescent formation may be seen for patients with severe disease, and if found in more than 30% of the glomeruli, RPGN may be present concurrently.[107] The prognosis is generally poor for these patients, and complete recovery is unlikely. Immunofluorescence examination reveals diffuse granular deposits of IgG and C3 along the GBM and also in the mesangium.

Clinical Presentation

The nephritis is preceded by a latent period following a streptococcal infection. The latent period is commonly 7 to 14 days for pharyngitis and 14 to 28 days for skin infection. An acute nephritic syndrome then develops, commonly with hematuria and edema. Gross hematuria is seen in 70% of patients, and microscopic hematuria can be found in all patients. Hypertension is usually mild to moderate and results from sodium and water retention. Many patients have signs and symptoms associated with volume overload, which include dyspnea, orthopnea, and cough. Urinalysis of patients with PSGN reveals hematuria, dysmorphic red blood cells, and red cell casts. Proteinuria is common but often not in the nephrotic range. Renal function is frequently mildly impaired.

Throat or skin culture may be positive for group A streptococci, despite the latent period following the initial infection. However, antibiotic therapy may render the culture result negative. Serologic measurements of antibodies to different streptococcal antigens can confirm recent exposure to the infection. Titers that can be measured include antistreptolysin O (ASO), antistreptokinase, antihyaluronidase (AHase), antideoxyribonuclease B (ADNase B), and antinicotyladenine dinucleotidase (NADase).[108] For most patients with streptococcal pharyngitis, the ASO titers begin to rise about 10 to 14 days later, peak at 3 to 4 weeks, and persist for several months before decreasing. The rise in ASO titers can be reduced by antibiotic treatment and may not be seen for patients with streptococcal skin infection in whom the streptolysin may be bound to skin lipids. ADNase B and AHase titers should be used instead because they are specific and are positive in the majority of patients. The streptozyme test is a combined assay for ASO, ADNase B, NADase, and AHase. Antibodies to other antigens such as zymogen, streptococcal cationic proteinase exotoxin B (SPEB), and plasmin receptor (Plr) were evaluated recently.[109]

Serum complement levels are often decreased for patients with PSGN. If the C3 level is depressed for more than 6 to 8 weeks, MPGN, lupus nephritis, or glomerulonephritis related to endocarditis or occult visceral abscess should be suspected. Renal biopsy is not normally indicated unless the patient has prolonged hematuria, proteinuria, or depressed C3 level. Renal biopsy is needed to detect other types of glomerulonephritis such as lupus, RPGN, or MPGN.

TREATMENT

Poststreptococcal Glomerulonephritis

❽ The treatment of PSGN is mainly supportive and symptomatic. Early antibiotic therapy does not prevent subsequent PSGN, but it may reduce the severity of the disease. It can, however, prevent the spread of the streptococcal infection to other family members. Antibiotic prophylaxis is not recommended because infected patients will develop long-lasting, often lifelong immunity against the strain of streptococci. Exposure to another nephritogenic strain of streptococci is possible, but unlikely.

Supportive measures should be used to control fluid volume and blood pressure. Because the hypertension is of the low-renin type, ACEIs and β-blockers are not expected to be useful. If the patient has crescentic disease, use of pulse steroids and/or immunosuppressive agents can be considered; however, the efficacy and safety of these agents have not been established for this condition.

The acute manifestations of PSGN are normally self-limited, and for more than 95% of patients renal function has returned to baseline within 3 to 6 weeks. Diuresis usually begins 7 to 10 days after onset of the acute episode, whereas hypertension and azotemia resolve in 1 to 2 weeks. Gross hematuria lasts for 1 to 2 weeks, and proteinuria usually resolves within 6 months in more than 90% of children. However, microscopic hematuria may persist for up to 2 years. In general, children have more rapid recovery than adults. Prognosis is often better when PSGN occurs during an epidemic than in cases found sporadically. Most of the children will recover fully and be free from chronic complications of PSGN if they have no preexisting renal disorder, heavy proteinuria, or crescentic glomerular lesions or did not require hospitalization during the acute episode. In contrast, adult patients have a less favorable long-term outcome. As many as 50% of the patients may develop persistent proteinuria, hypertension, and renal insufficiency, with some resulting in end-stage renal failure.

PHARMACOECONOMIC CONSIDERATIONS

Prospective, randomized, controlled comparative trials need to be conducted in a sizable patient population before the efficacy and economic implications of a new regimen can be established. This type of large-scale study is potentially feasible for the more common forms of glomerulonephritis, such as minimal-change disease, IgA nephropathy, and membranous nephropathy. In contrast, prospective controlled trials are difficult to conduct for the relatively uncommon glomerulonephritides such as membranous proliferative glomerulonephritis. After defining the natural history and the optimal drug regimen for each glomerulonephritis, in conjunction with the incidence of drug-induced complications, the economic implications of the individual treatment approach can be assessed. However, the optimal approaches for treating most types of glomerulonephritis have not been identified, and the economic implications of the individual treatment regimens thus remain to be established.

CONCLUSIONS

A better understanding of the pathogenetic mechanisms leading to glomerular injury has improved the treatment of glomerulonephritis. However, the glomerulopathies are a heterogeneous group of immune disorders with different clinical courses, prognoses, and responses to current immunologic and non-immunologic therapies. The clinician should understand the natural history and prognosis of each subgroup of glomerulonephritis, the efficacy of different immunomodulation regimens in inducing disease remission and preserving renal function, and the characteristics of at-risk patients who warrant aggressive therapy. Judicious use of immunosuppressive agents with careful monitoring of their adverse effects cannot be overemphasized.

In addition, treatment of the disease complications and control of factors that lead to progression of renal disease are important in reducing the morbidity and mortality of patients with glomerulonephritis.

ABBREVIATIONS

ACE: angiotensin-converting enzyme

ADNase B: antideoxyribonuclease B

AHase: antihyaluronidase

ANCA: antineutrophil cytoplasmic autoantibody

ARB: angiotensin II receptor blocker

ASO: antistreptolysin O

ESRD: end-stage renal disease

GBM: glomerular basement membrane

GFR: glomerular filtration rate

FSGS: focal segmental glomerulosclerosis

HIV: human immunodeficiency virus

HMG-CoA: hydroxymethylglutaryl coenzyme A (reductase)

IL: interleukin

LDL: low-density lipoprotein (cholesterol)

MPGN: membranoproliferative glomerulonephritis

NADase: antinicotyladenine dinucleotidase

PSGN: poststreptococcal glomerulonephritis

RPGN: rapidly progressive glomerulonephritis

SLE: systemic lupus erythematosus

VLDL: very-low-density lipoprotein (cholesterol)

WHO: World Health Organization

REFERENCES

1. U.S. Renal Data System 2009 Annual Data Report. Minneapolis, MN: USRDS Coordinating Center; 2009, *http://www.usrds.org*.

2. Schena FP, Gesualdo L, Grandaliano G, Montinaro V. Progression of renal damage in human glomerulonephritides: Is there sleight of hand in winning the game? Kidney Int 1997;52:1439–1457.

3. Couser WG. Mediation of immune glomerular injury. J Am Soc Nephrol 1990;1:13–29.

4. Remuzzi G, Zoja C, Perico N. Proinflammatory mediators of glomerular injury and mechanisms of activation of autoreactive T cells. Kidney Int Suppl 1994;44:S8–S16.

5. Humphreys MH. Mechanisms and management of nephrotic edema. Kidney Int 1994;45:266–281.

6. Schrier RW, Fassett RG. A critique of the overfill hypothesis of sodium and water retention in the nephrotic syndrome. Kidney Int 1998;53:1111–1117.

7. Warwick GL, Fox JG, Boulton-Jones JM. The relationship between urinary albumin excretion rate and serum cholesterol in primary glomerular disease. Clin Nephrol 1994;41:135–137.

8. Wheeler DC, Bernard DB. Lipid abnormalities in the nephrotic syndrome: Causes, consequences, and treatment. Am J Kidney Dis 1994;23:331–346.

9. Kaysen GA, De Sain-van der Verlden M. New insights into lipid metabolism in the nephrotic syndrome. Kidney Int Suppl 1999;71:S18–S21.

10. Nachman PH, Martin J. Developments in the immunotherapy of glomerular disease. J Pharm Prac 2002;15:472–489.

11. Ponticelli C, Passerini P. Treatment of the nephrotic syndrome associated with primary glomerulonephritis. Kidney Int 1994;46:595–604.

12. Klahr S, Levey A, Beck G, et al. The effects of dietary protein restriction and blood pressure control on the progression of chronic renal disease. N Engl J Med 1994;330:877–884.

13. Orth SR, Stockmann A, Conradt C, et al. Smoking as a risk factor for end-stage renal failure in men with primary renal disease. Kidney Int 1998;54:926–931.

14. Fliser D, Schroter M, Neubeck M. Coadministration of thiazides increases the efficacy of loop diuretics even in patients with advanced renal failure. Kidney Int 1994;46:482–488.

15. Rudy DW, Voelker JR, Greene PK, et al. Loop diuretics for chronic renal insufficiency: A continuous infusion is more efficacious than bolus therapy. Ann Intern Med 1991;115:360–366.

16. Chobanian AV, Bakris GL, Black HR, et al. The seventh report of the joint national committee on prevention, detection, evaluation and treatment of high blood pressure: The JNC 7 report. JAMA 2003;289:2560–2572.

17. Ruggenenti P, Remuzzi G. Is therapy with combined ACE inhibitor and angiotensin receptor antagonist the new gold standard of treatment for nondiabetic, chronic proteinuric nephropathies? NephSAP 2003;2:235–237.

18. Gashti CN, Bakris GL. The role of calcium antagonists in chronic kidney disease. Curr Opin Nephrol Hypertens 2004;18:155–161.

19. Levey AS, Adler S, Caggiula AW, et al. Effects of dietary protein restriction on the progression of advanced renal disease in the Modification of Diet in Renal Disease Study. Am J Kidney Dis 1996;27:652–663.

20. Toto R. Proteinuria reduction: Mandatory consideration or option when selecting an antihypertensive agent? Curr Hypertens Rep 2005;7:374–378.

21. The GISEN group (Gruppo Italiano di Studi Epidemiologici in Nefrologia). Randomized placebo-controlled trial effect of ramipril on decline in glomerular filtration rate and risk of terminal renal failure in proteinuric, non-diabetic nephropathy. Lancet 1997;349:1857–1863.

22. Jefferson JA, Shank SJ. Glomerular disease: The podocyte is ready for prime time and may already be center stage. NephSAP 2006;331–338.

23. Vogt L, Navis G, de Zeeuw D. Renoprotection: A matter of blood pressure reduction or agent-characteristics? J Am Soc Nephrol 2002;13(suppl 3):S202–S207.

24. Alexopoulos E. Treatment of primary IgA nephropathy. Kidney Int 2004;65:341–355.

25. MacKinnon M, Shurraw S, Akbari A, Knoll GA, Jaffey J, Clark HD. Combination therapy with an angiotensin receptor blocker and an ACE inhibitor in proteinuric renal disease: A systematic review of the efficacy and safety data. Am J Kidney Dis 2006;48:8–20.

26. Taal MV, Brenner BM. Combination ACEI and ARB therapy: Additional benefit in renoprotection? Curr Opin Nephrol Hypertens 2002;11:377–381.

27. Perico N, Remuzzi A, Sangalli F, et al. The antiproteinuric antagonism in human IgA nephropathy is potentiated by indomethacin. J Am Soc Nephrol 1998;9:2308–2317.

28. Oda H, Keane WF. Recent advances in statins and the kidney. Kidney Int Suppl 1999;71:S2–S5.

29. Tonelli M, Moyé L, Sacks FM. Effect of pravastatin on loss of renal function in people with moderate chronic renal insufficiency and cardiovascular disease. J Am Soc Nephrol 2003;14:1605–1613.

30. Agarwal R. Effects of statins on renal function. Am J Cardiol 2006;97:748–755.

31. Glassock RJ. Prophylactic anticoagulation in nephrotic syndrome: A clinical conundrum. J Am Soc Nephrol 2007;18:2221–2225.

32. Nolasco F, Cameron JS, Heywood EF, et al. Adult-onset minimal-change nephrotic syndrome: A long-term follow-up. Kidney Int 1986;29:1215–1223.

33. Jennette JC, Mandal AK. The nephrotic syndrome. In: Mandal AK, Jennette JC, eds. Diagnosis and Management of Renal Disease and Hyper-tension, 2nd ed. Durham, NC: Carolina Academic Press; 1994:235–272.

34. Bargman JM. Management of minimal lesion glomerulonephritis: Evidence-based recommendations. Kidney Int Suppl 1999;70:S3–S16.

35. Tune BM, Mendoza SA. Treatment of the idiopathic nephrotic syndrome: Regimens and outcomes in children and adults. J Am Soc Nephrol 1997;8:824–832.

36. Rinaldi S, Sesto A, Barsotti P, Faraggiana T, Sera F, Rizzoni G. Cyclosporine therapy monitored with abbreviated area under curve in nephrotic syndrome. Pediatr Nephrol 2005;20:25–29.

37. Yoshida M, Yoshikawa N, Akashi M, et al. Lymphocyte drug sensitivity is useful for prediction of the antiproteinuric effect and relapse rate in cyclosporine treatment for frequent-relapse minimal change nephrotic syndrome. Kidney Blood Press Res 2005;28:226–229.

38. Fu LS, Shien CY, Chi CS. Levamisole in steroid-sensitive nephrotic syndrome children with frequent relapses and/or steroid dependency: Comparison of daily and every-other-day usage. Nephron Clin Pract 2004;97:c137–c141.

39. Alsaran K, Grisaru S, Stephens D, et al. Levamisole vs. cyclophosphamide for frequently-relapsing steroid-dependent nephrotic syndrome. Clin Nephrol 2001;56:289–294.

40. Novak I, Frank R, Vento S, et al. Efficacy of mycophenolate mofetil in pediatric patients with steroid-dependent nephrotic syndrome. Pediatr Nephrol 2005;20:1265–1268.

41. Day CJ, Cockwell P, Lipkin GW, et al. Mycophenolate mofetil in the treatment of resistant idiopathic nephrotic syndrome. Nephrol Dial Transplant 2002;17:2011–2013.

42. Korbet SM. Treatment of primary focal segmental glomerulosclerosis. Kidney Int 2002;62:2301–2310.

43. Leal C. Herlitz, Glen S. et al. Development of focal segmental glomerulosclerosis after anabolic steroid abuse. J Am Soc Nephrol 2010;21:163–172

44. Korbet SM. Primary focal segmental glomerulosclerosis. J Am Soc Nephrol 1998;9:1333–1340.

45. Burgess E. Management of focal segmental glomerulosclerosis: Evidence-based recommendations. Kidney Int Suppl 1999;70:S26–S32.

46. Crook ED, Habeeb D, Gowdy O, et al. Effects of steroids in focal segmental glomerulosclerosis in a predominantly African-American population. Am J Med Sci 2005;330:19–24.

47. Frassinetti Castelo Branco Camurça Fernandes P, Bezerra Da Silva G Jr, De Sousa Barros FA, et al. Treatment of steroid-resistant nephrotic syndrome with cyclosporine: Study of 17 cases and a literature review. J Nephrol 2005;18:711–720.

48. El-Reshaid K, El-Reshaid W, Madda J. Combination of immunosuppressive agents in treatment of steroid-resistant minimal change disease and primary focal segmental glomerulosclerosis. Ren Fail 2005;27:523–530.

49. Westhoff TH, Schmidt S, Zidek W, Beige J, van der GM. Tacrolimus in steroid-resistant and steroid-dependent nephrotic syndrome. Clin Nephrol 2006;65:393–400.

50. Cho ME, Hurley JK, Kopp JB Sirolimus therapy of focal segmental glomerulosclerosis is associated with nephrotoxicity. Am J Kidney Dis 2007;49:310–317.

51. Cattran DC, Wang GG, Appel GB, et al. Mycophenolate mofetil in the treatment of focal segmental glomerulosclerosis. Clin Nephrol 2004;62:405–411.

52. Cattran D. Management of membranous nephropathy: When and what for treatment J Am Soc Nephrol 2005;16:1188–1194.

53. Geddes CC, Cattran DC. The treatment of idiopathic membranous nephropathy. Semin Nephrol 2000;20:299–308.

54. Ponticelli C, Zucchelli P, Passerini P, et al. A 10-year follow-up of a randomized study with methylprednisolone and chlorambucil in membranous nephropathy. Kidney Int 1995;48:1600–1604.

55. Ponticelli C, Altieri P, Scolari F, et al. A randomized study comparing methylprednisolone plus chlorambucil versus methylprednisolone plus cyclophosphamide in idiopathic membranous nephropathy. J Am Soc Nephrol 1998;9:444–450.

56. Perna A, Schieppati A, Zamora J, et al. Immunosuppressive treatment for idiopathic membranous nephropathy: A systematic review. Am J Kidney Dis 2004;44:385–401.

57. Cattran DC, Greenwood C, Ritchie S, et al. A controlled trial of cyclosporine in patients with progressive membranous nephropathy. Kidney Int 1995;47:1130–1135.

58. Fritsche L, Budde K, Farber L, et al. Treatment of membranous glomerulopathy with cyclosporin A: How much patience is required? Nephrol Dial Transplant 1999;14:1036–1038.

59. Ruggenenti P, Chiurchiu C, Abbate M, et al. Rituximab for idiopathic membranous nephropathy: Who can benefit? Clin J Am Soc Nephrol 2006;1:738–748.

60. Jayne D. Role of Rituximab therapy in glomerulonephritis. J Am Soc Nephrol 2010;21:14–17.

61. Appel G, Nachman P, Hogan S, et al. Eculizumab (C5 complement inhibitor) in the treatment of idiopathic membranous nephropathy [abstract]. J Am Soc Nephrol 2002;13:668A.

62. Branten AJ, du Buf-Vereijken PW, Vervloet M, Wetzels JF. Mycophenolate mofetil in idiopathic membranous nephropathy: A clinical trial with comparison to a historic control group treated with cyclophosphamide. Am J Kidney Dis 2007;50:248–256.

63. Ponticelli C, Passerini P, Salvadori M, et al. A randomized pilot trial comparing methylprednisolone plus a cytotoxic agent versus synthetic adrenocorticotropic hormone in idiopathic membranous nephropathy. Am J Kidney Dis 2006;47:233–240.

64. Levin A. Management of membranoproliferative glomerulonephritis: Evidence-based recommendations. Kidney Int Suppl 1999;70:S41–S46.

65. Tarshish P, Bernstein J, Tobin JN, et al. Treatment of mesangiocapillary glomerulonephritis with alternate-day prednisone—A report of the International Study of Kidney Disease in Children. Pediatr Nephrol 1992;6:123–130.

66. Appel GB, Cook HT, Hageman G, et al. Membranoproliferative glomerulonephritis type II (dense deposit disease): An update. J Am Soc Nephrol 2005;16:1392–1404.

67. Smith RJ, Alexander J, Barlow PN, et al. New approaches to the treatment of dense deposit disease. J Am Soc Nephrol 2007;18:2447–2456.

68. Donadio JV, Grande JP. Immunoglobulin A nephropathy. N Engl J Med 2002;347:738–748.

69. Floege J, Feehally J. IgA nephropathy: Recent developments. J Am Soc Nephrol 2000;11:2395–2403.

70. Barratt J, Feehally J. IgA nephropathy. J Am Soc Nephrol 2005;16:2088–1097.

71. Nolin L, Courteau M. Management of IgA nephropathy: Evidence-based recommendations. Kidney Int Suppl 1999;70:S56–S62.

72. Glassock RJ. The treatment of IgA nephropathy at the end of the millennium. J Nephrol 1999;12:288–296.

73. Samuels JA, Strippoli GF, Craig JC, et al. Immunosuppressive treatments for immunoglobulin A nephropathy: A meta-analysis of randomized controlled trials. Nephrology (Carlton) 2004;9:177–185.

74. Pozzi C, Andrulli S, Del Vecchio L, et al. Corticosteroids effectiveness in IgA nephropathy: Long-term results of a randomized, controlled trial. J Am Soc Nephrol 2004;15:157–163.

75. Donadio JV, Jr., Grande JP, Bergstralh EJ, et al. The long-term outcome of patients with IgA nephropathy treated with fish oil in a controlled trial. Mayo Nephrology Collaborative Group. J Am Soc Nephrol 1999;10:1772–1777.

76. Dillon JJ. Fish oil therapy for IgA nephropathy: Efficacy and interstudy variability. J Am Soc Nephrol 1997;8:1739–1744.

77. Glassock GJ. The treatment of IgA nephropathy: Status at the end of the millennium. J Nephrol 1999;12:288–296.

78. Rasche FM, Keller E, Lepper PM, et al. High-dose intravenous immunoglobulin pulse therapy in patients with progressive immunoglobulin A nephropathy: A long-term follow-up. Clin Exp Immunol 2006;146:47–53.

79. Buemi M, Allegra A, Corica F, et al. Effect of fluvastatin on proteinuria in patients with immunoglobulin A nephropathy. Clin Pharmacol Ther 2000;67:427–431.

80. Taji Y, Kuwahara T, Shikata S, et al. Meta-analysis of antiplatelet therapy for IgA nephropathy. Clin Exp Nephrol 2006;10:268–273.

81. Lai KN. Future directions in the treatment of IgA nephropathy. Nephron 2002;92:263–270.

82. Sanz-Guajardo D. Plasmapheresis in the treatment of glomerulonephritis: Indications and complications. Am J Kidney Dis 2000;36:liv–lvi.

83. Donadio JV, Bergstralh EJ, Grande JP, et al. Proteinuria patterns and their association with subsequent end-stage renal disease in IgA nephropathy. Nephrol Dial Transplant 2002;17:1197–1203.

84. Courtney AE, McNamee PT, Nelson WE, Maxwell AP. Does angiotensin blockade influence graft outcome in renal transplant recipients with IgA nephropathy? Nephrol Dial Transplant 2006;21:3550–3554.

85. Contreras G, Roth D, Pardo V, et al. Lupus nephritis: A clinical review for practicing nephrologists. Clin Nephrol 2002;57:95–107.

86. Cameron JS. Lupus nephritis. J Am Soc Nephrol 1999;10:413–424.

87. Weening JJ, D'Agati VD, Schwartz MM, et al. The classification of glomerulonephritis in systemic lupus erythematosus revisited. Kidney Int 2004;65:521–530.

88. Waldman M, Appel GB. Update on the treatment of lupus nephritis. Kidney Int 2006;70:1403–1412.

89. Alarcon GS, McGwin G Jr, Petri M, et al. Time to renal disease and end-stage renal disease in PROFILE: A multiethnic lupus cohort. PLoS Med 2006;3:e396.

90. Gourley MF, Austin HA, Scott D, et al. Methylprednisolone and cyclophosphamide, alone or in combination, in patients with lupus nephritis. A randomized, controlled trial. Ann Intern Med 1996;125:549–557.

91. Lai KN, Tang SCW, Mok CC. Treatment for lupus nephritis: A revisit. Nephrology (Carlton) 2005;10:180–188.

92. Walsh M, James M, Jayne D, Tonelli M, Manns BJ, Hemmelgarn BR. Mycophenolate mofetil for induction therapy of lupus nephritis: A systematic review and meta-analysis. Clin J Am Soc Nephrol 2007;2:968–975

93. Ginzler EM, Dooley MA, Aranow C, et al. Mycophenolate mofetil or intravenous cyclophosphamide for lupus nephritis. N Engl J Med 2005;353:2219–2228.

94. Illei GG, Austin HA, Crane M, et al. Combination therapy with pulse cyclophosphamide plus pulse methylprednisolone improves long-term renal outcome without adding toxicity in patients with lupus nephritis. Ann Intern Med 2001;135:248–257.

95. Houssiau FA, Vasconcelos C, D'Cruz D, et al. Immunosuppressive therapy in lupus nephritis: The Euro-Lupus Nephritis Trial, a randomized trial of low-dose versus high-dose intravenous cyclophosphamide. Arthritis Rheum 2002;46:2121–2131.

96. Contreras G, Pardo V, Leclercq B, et al. Sequential therapies for proliferative lupus nephritis. N Engl J Med 2004;350:971–980.

97. Moroni G, Doria A, Mosca M, et al. A randomized pilot trial comparing cyclosporine and azathioprine for maintenance therapy in diffuse lupus nephritis over four years. Clin J Am Soc Nephrol 2006;1:925–932.

98. Alarcon-Segovia D, Tumlin JA, Furie RA, et al. LJP 394 for the prevention of renal flare in patients with systemic lupus erythematosus: Results from a randomized, double-blind, placebo-controlled study. Arthritis Rheum 2003;48:442–454.

99. Merrill JT, Neuwelt CM, Wallace DJ, et al. Efficacy and safety of rituximab in moderately-to-severely active systemic lupus erythematosus: The randomized, double-blind, phase ii/iii systemic lupus erythematosus evaluation of rituximab trial. Arthritis Rheum. 2010;62:222–233.

100. Boumpas DT, Furie R, Manzi S, et al. A short course of BG9588 (anti-CD40 ligand antibody) improves serologic activity and decreases hematuria in patients with proliferative lupus glomerulonephritis. Arthritis Rheum 2003;48:719–727.

101. Couser WG. Rapidly progressive glomerulonephritis: Classification, pathogenetic mechanisms, and therapy. Am J Kidney Dis 1988;11:449–464.

102. Little MA, Pusey CD. Rapidly progressive glomerulonephritis: Current and evolving treatment strategies. J Nephrol 2004;17:10–19.

103. Bolton WK. Treatment of glomerular disease: ANCA-negative RPGN. Semin Nephrol 2000;20:244–255.

104. Jennette JC. Rapidly progressive crescentic glomerulonephritis. Kidney Int 2003;63:1164–1177.

105. de Groot K, Adu D, Savage CO. The value of pulse cyclophosphamide in ANCA-associated vasculitis: Meta-analysis and critical review. Nephrol Dial Transplant 2001;16:2018–2027.

106. Nachman PH, Segelmark M, Westman K, et al. Recurrent ANCA-associated small-vessel vasculitis after transplantation: A pooled analysis. Kidney Int 1999;56:1544–1550.

107. Couser WG, Johnson RJ. Postinfective glomerulonephritis. In: Neilson EG, Couser WG, eds. Immunologic Renal Diseases, 2nd ed. Philadelphia, PA: Lippincott-Raven; 2001:899–929.

108. Rodriguez-Iturbe B, Parra G. Glomerulonephritis associated with infection: Poststreptococcal glomerulonephritis. In: Massry SG, Glassock RJ, eds. Massry & Glassock's Textbook of Nephrology, 4th ed. Philadelphia, PA: Lippincott Williams & Wilkins, 2001:667–671.

109. Rodriguez-Iturbe B. Nephritis-associated streptococcal antigens: Where are we now? J Am Soc Nephrol 2004;15:1961–1962.

57

Drug Therapy Individualization for Patients with Chronic Kidney Disease

GARY R. MATZKE

KEY CONCEPTS

❶ Chronic kidney disease has been demonstrated to result in minimal alterations in the absorption or bioavailability of only a few drugs.

❷ The volume of distribution of many drugs is increased in the presence of acute and chronic kidney disease (CKD) as a consequence of volume expansion and reduced protein binding.

❸ In addition to the expected decrement in renal clearance, nonrenal clearance (i.e., gastrointestinal and hepatic drug metabolism) of several drugs is also reduced in patients with CKD.

❹ Individualization of a drug dosage regimen for a patient with reduced kidney function is based on the pharmacodynamic/pharmacokinetic characteristics of the drug and the patient's degree of residual renal function.

❺ The drug dosing guidelines for patients with CKD in many drug information resources are highly variable and thus many are not optimal for clinical use.

❻ The effect of hemodialysis or peritoneal dialysis on drug elimination is dependent on the characteristics of the drug and the dialysis prescription.

❼ The application of hemodialysis clearance data to guide drug dosage regimen design for hemodialysis patients is limited and prospective monitoring of serum concentrations is often warranted.

Patients with chronic kidney disease (CKD) are commonly encountered in clinical practice. Indeed, it is estimated that nearly 15 million adults in the United States have serum creatinine values of 1.5 mg/dL (133 mmol/L) or greater.[1] In older adults, age-related declines in renal function combine with an increased use of medications to make this patient group particularly susceptible to adverse effects secondary to the lack of appropriate pharmacotherapy individualization.[2,3] The presence of a marked reduction in kidney function, whether it is an acute kidney injury (AKI) or CKD in any patient, necessitates that the clinician individualize drug therapy to maximize therapeutic outcomes.

Learning objectives, review questions, and other resources can be found at **www.pharmacotherapyonline.com**.

CKD is often accompanied by the development of anemia, hyperparathyroidism, hyperlipidemia, hypertension, and changes in gastrointestinal tract integrity (see Chapters 52 and 53). Thus CKD patients are often prescribed an extensive array of medications. There are now many reports that document changes in the disposition of some drugs in patients with CKD as the result of changes in bioavailability,[4,5] distribution volume,[6,7] and metabolic activity.[8–11] Thus drug therapy individualization is warranted for most patients with CKD. If a drug is predominantly renally eliminated unchanged, a dosage regimen adjustment may be calculated on the basis of the ratio of the patient's residual renal function relative to an age and gender normal value for estimated creatinine clearance or glomerular filtration rate.[12] However, for medications that are extensively metabolized or for which dramatic changes in protein binding and/or distribution volume have been noted, a more complex adjustment strategy may need to be employed.[7,13] Furthermore, because of the physiologic and biochemical changes associated with progressive CKD, patients may respond to a given dose or serum concentration of a drug differently than patients with normal renal function.[4]

Clinicians thus design individualized therapeutic regimens to optimize therapeutic outcomes and minimize adverse events, if they use basic pharmacokinetic principles combined with the drug's disposition properties and the patient's clinical characteristics. In this chapter, the influence of CKD on drug absorption, distribution, metabolism, and elimination is characterized. The array of drug information resources for the adjustment of the dosage regimens for patients with CKD is critiqued. A practical framework for drug dosage individualization for patients with CKD based on continuous versus categorical classifications is presented and the influences of peritoneal dialysis and hemodialysis on drug disposition are discussed. Finally, drug administration strategies for those receiving hemodialysis are presented. Drug dosage regimen adjustment strategies for patients with AKI, including those who are receiving continuous renal replacement therapy are presented in Chapter 51.

EFFECT ON DRUG ABSORPTION

❶ There is little quantitative information regarding the influence of CKD on drug absorption and bioavailability. Changes in gastrointestinal transit time and gastric pH, edema of the gastrointestinal tract, vomiting and diarrhea (frequent complications of severe renal insufficiency), and antacid administration have all been proposed as a rationale for alterations in the bioavailability of drugs in CKD patients. Evaluations of bioavailability are generally conducted in those with severe stable renal insufficiency, that is, stage 5 CKD, which is also called end-stage renal disease (ESRD). The assessment of bioavailability in this patient population is, however, complicated, because most of these patients are prescribed multiple medications (often in excess of 10 to 12 different agents), many of which cannot be discontinued during the course of a bioavailability study.

Many of the drug absorption so-called "bioavailability" studies in ESRD patients were not designed to provide an assessment of the drug's absolute bioavailability (i.e., they did not include a comparison of oral to intravenous administration of the drug). Rather, the principal outcomes were the documentation of alterations in the peak concentration (C_{max}), time at which the peak concentration was attained (t_{max}), or in the fractional amount of drug recovered in the urine in a finite time period. Unfortunately, this limited information has been extrapolated by some into a general conclusion that drug absorption is slowed and/or that the extent of absorption is reduced as the result of the development of CKD.[5]

In fact, the absolute bioavailability of only a few drugs is affected by ESRD and many of these are rarely used.[4,7] An increase in bioavailability as the result of a decrease in metabolism during the drug's first pass through the gastrointestinal tract and liver has been noted for some β-blockers (e.g., bufuralol, oxprenolol, propranolol, and tolamolol), dextropropoxyphene, and dihydrocodeine.[4,7] Although the bioavailability of these compounds is increased, clinical consequences (development of excessive or unexpected adverse effects) have only been demonstrated with dextropropoxyphene and dihydrocodeine.

EFFECT ON DRUG DISTRIBUTION

The volume of distribution of many drugs is increased in patients with moderate to severe CKD as well as those with preexisting CKD who develop AKI (Table 57–1).[7,14,15] This increase in distribution volume may be the result of decreased protein binding, increased tissue binding, or pathophysiologic alterations in body composition (e.g., fluid overload).

Generally, the plasma protein binding of acidic drugs (e.g., warfarin and phenytoin) is decreased in those with ESRD,[3,6,16] whereas the binding of basic drugs (e.g., quinidine and lidocaine) is usually

TABLE 57-2 Unbound Fraction of Selected Drugs in Patients with Normal Renal Function and End-Stage Renal Disease

Acidic Drugs	Normal	ESRD	Change from Normal (%)
Abecarnil	4	15	275
Azlocillin	63	75	20
Cefazolin	16	29	81
Cefoxitin	27	59	119
Ceftriaxone	10	20	100
Clofibrate	3	9	200
Dicloxacillin	3	9	200
Diflunisal	12	44	267
Doxycycline	12	28	133
Furosemide	4	6	50
Methotrexate	57	64	12
Metolazone	5	10	100
Moxalactam	48	64	33
Pentobarbital	34	41	21
Phenytoin	10	22	115
Salicylate	8	20	150
Sulfamethoxazole	34	58	71
Valproic acid	8	23	188
Warfarin	1	2	100

Basic Drugs	Normal	ESRD	Change from Normal (%)
Decreased			
Clonidine	56	48	−14
Disopyramide	32	28	−13
Propafenone	3	2	−29
Increased			
Amphotericin B	3.5	4.1	17
Chloramphenicol	45	64	42
Diazepam	2	8	300
Fluoxetine	5.5	6.5	18
Ketoconazole	1	1.5	50
Rosiglitazone	0.16	0.22	38
Triamterene	19	43	126

TABLE 57-1 Volume of Distribution of Selected Drugs in Patients with End-Stage Renal Disease

Drug	Normal (L/kg)	ESRD (L/kg)	Change from Normal (%)
Increased			
Amikacin	0.20	0.29	45
Azlocillin	0.21	0.28	33
Cefazolin	0.13	0.17	31
Cefoxitin	0.16	0.26	63
Cefuroxime	0.20	0.26	30
Clofibrate	0.14	0.24	71
Dicloxacillin	0.08	0.18	125
Erythromycin	0.57	1.09	91
Furosemide	0.11	0.18	64
Gentamicin	0.20	0.32	60
Isoniazid	0.6	0.8	33
Minoxidil	2.6	4.9	88
Nalmefene	7.9	14.7	86
Phenytoin	0.64	1.4	119
Trimethoprim	1.36	1.83	35
Vancomycin	0.64	0.85	33
Decreased			
Chloramphenicol	0.87	0.60	−31
Digoxin	7.3	4.0	−45
Ethambutol	3.7	1.6	−57

normal or only slightly decreased or increased (Table 57–2).[3,6] The decrease in binding of acidic drugs has been attributed to qualitative changes in the binding sites, accumulation of endogenous inhibitors of binding, and/or decreased concentrations of albumin. The first two of these mechanisms appear to account for most of the observed changes in binding. In addition, the high concentrations of metabolites of some compounds that accumulate in patients with ESRD may compete for protein binding sites with the parent compound.

❷ The unbound fraction of many acidic drugs increases in CKD patients as the result of a decrease in protein binding. A new equilibrium is ultimately established as a result of increased drug elimination/distribution, such that the unbound concentrations remain comparable to those observed in patients with normal renal function despite the fact that total concentrations are reduced. Thus, the net effect is an alteration in the relationship between total drug concentration and pharmacodynamic effect; it is commonly seen with the anticonvulsant phenytoin. The protein binding of this acidic drug, which binds to albumin, is significantly reduced and this change alters the relationship between total phenytoin concentration and desired effect as well as toxicity.[17] The resulting increase in unbound fraction, from values of 10% in those with normal renal function to ~20% or more in those with stage 5 CKD, results in increased hepatic clearance and decreased total concentrations. Thus, in patients with CKD, the therapeutic range based on total phenytoin concentration is shifted downward from normal values of 10 to 20 mg/L (10–20 mcg/mL; 40–79 mmol/L) to values as low as 4 to 8 mg/L (4–8 mcg/mL; 16–32 mmol/L). Since the unbound concentration therapeutic range is the same for all patients, 1 to 2 mg/L (1–2 mcg/mL; 4–8 mmol/L), such a measurement provides the best target for individualizing phenytoin therapy in patients with CKD.

When unbound concentration measurements are not clinically available, one can approximate the equivalent "total" phenytoin concentration in an ESRD patient relative to an individual with normal renal function.[17] Although these approaches have not been rigorously evaluated, they may be useful in some clinical settings to predict dosage requirements.

The principal binding protein for several basic drugs is α_1-acid glycoprotein, an acute-phase reactant protein whose plasma concentrations are increased in CKD patients.[3,7] As a result of this increase, the unbound fraction of some basic drugs may be significantly decreased in ESRD patients.

Altered tissue binding may also affect the apparent volume of distribution of a drug. For example, the distribution volume of digoxin has been reported to be reduced by 30% to 50% from normal values in patients with stage 5 CKD, as well as in hemodialysis patients.[18] This reduction in the distribution volume may be secondary to a decrease in tissue binding as a result of competitive inhibition by endogenous or exogenous substances. Acidosis or the presence of digoxin-like immunoreactive substances that bind to and inhibit membrane adenosine triphosphatase may also contribute to this phenomenon.[19] In this situation, the absolute amount of digoxin bound to the receptor is reduced and the resultant serum digoxin concentration is higher than anticipated. Multiple methods have been proposed to estimate the degree of reduction in digoxin's distribution volume.[18]

Thus, in patients with renal insufficiency, particularly in those with stage 5 CKD, a "normal" total drug concentration may be associated with either an adverse reaction secondary to elevated unbound drug concentrations, or a subtherapeutic response because of an altered plasma-to-tissue drug concentration ratio. The monitoring of unbound drug concentrations in CKD patients is thus warranted for those drugs that have a narrow therapeutic range, are highly protein bound (free fraction of <20%), and for which marked variability in the free fraction has been reported (e.g., phenytoin and disopyramide).

Finally, the method used to calculate the volume of distribution may be influenced by renal insufficiency. The three most commonly used volume of distribution terms are: volume of the central compartment (V_c), volume of the terminal phase (V_β and V_{area}), and volume of distribution at steady state (V_{ss}). The V_c for many drugs approximates extracellular fluid volume and thus may be increased or decreased by acute changes. Oliguric acute renal failure is often accompanied by fluid overload and a resultant increased V_c for many drugs. The V_{area} or V_β represents the proportionality constant between plasma concentrations in the terminal elimination phase and the amount of drug remaining in the body. V_β is affected by both distribution characteristics, as well as by the terminal elimination rate constant. V_β and V_{ss} will often be similar in magnitude, with V_β being slightly larger. Because V_{ss} has the advantage of being independent of drug elimination, it is the most appropriate volume term to use when one desires to compare drug distribution volumes between patients with renal insufficiency and those with normal renal function.[21]

EFFECT ON METABOLISM

❸ A decrease in the renal clearance of drugs in patients with CKD is well appreciated. However, there is now good preclinical and emerging clinical evidence that CKD may lead to alterations in nonrenal clearance of many medications as the result of alterations

TABLE 57-3	Nonrenal Clearance of Many Drugs is Reduced in Patients with End-Stage Renal Disease	
Acyclovir	Guanadrel	Repaglinide
Aztreonam	Imipenem	Rosuvastatin
Bufuralol	Isoniazid	Roxithromycin
Bupropion	Ketoprofen	Simvastatin
Captopril	Ketorolac	Telithromycin
Carvedilol	Lomefloxacin	Valsartan
Cefipime	Losartan	Vancomycin
Cefmetazole	Lovastatin	Verapamil
Cefonicid	Metoclopramide	Zidovudine
Cefotaxime	Minoxidil	
Ceftriaxone	Morphine	
Ceftizoxime	Nicardipine	
Cervistatin	Nimodipine	
Cilastatin	Nitrendipine	
Cimetidine	Nortriptyline	
Ciprofloxacin	Procainamide	
Didanosine	Quinapril	
Didanosine	Quinapril	
Encainide	Reboxetine	
Erythromycin	Raloxifene	

in the activities of uptake and efflux transporters as well as cytochrome P450 (CYP) enzymes in the liver and other organs[8–11,22,23] (Table 57–3). However, the effect(s) of renal insufficiency on nonrenal drug clearance also appears to depend on whether the reduction in renal function is acute or chronic in nature. The degree of reduction in those with AKI does not appear to be as great as that observed in ESRD patients.[14]

Although the early studies should be interpreted with caution because concurrent drug intake, age, smoking status, and alcohol intake were often not well controlled, those published in the last few years provide strong evidence of a significant independent effect of CKD on drug metabolism, predominantly for those drugs which are metabolized by CYP3A4[9] (Table 57–4). CYP3A activity as measured by the erythromycin breath test (EBT) is 28% lower in ESRD patients as compared with healthy controls.[24] Although baseline CYP3A activity was lower in these patients, the increase in CYP3A activity observed following enzyme induction with rifampin was similar.[24] Nolin and colleagues have recently shown that EBT results are reduced more in those ESRD patients with higher blood urea nitrogen concentrations and that hemodialysis is associated with an acute improvement in the patient's metabolic activity.[9] These data indicate that CKD has a detrimental effect on this important pathway of hepatic drug metabolism in humans.

Prediction of the effect of renal insufficiency on the metabolism of a particular drug is however difficult and there is currently no quantitative strategy to predict changes for one drug based on data from another in the same class. However, some qualitative insight can be gained if one knows what enzyme is involved in the metabolism of the drug of interest and how the enzyme(s) or transporter(s) is affected by the presence of CKD.

Investigations of the effect of chronic renal failure on hepatic enzyme activity in animals have demonstrated reductions in some, but not all, pathways of drug metabolism.[9,22,23] The mechanism(s) by which CKD affects hepatic drug metabolism is not clearly known, but may relate to accumulation of endogenous inhibitors (e.g., uremic toxins) or to the fact that CKD patients exist in a chronic inflammatory state and have increased levels of oxidative stress,[25] and other factors known to downregulate CYP enzymes.[26] In rat models of chronic renal failure, protein expression of several CYP enzymes, including CYP3A1 and CYP3A2 (corresponding to human CYP3A4), is reduced in the liver by as much as 75%. The mechanism of this decrease in protein content and messenger ribonucleic acid

TABLE 57-4 Drugs which are Predominantly Metabolized for which a Decrease in Nonrenal Clearance has been Observed in CKD Patients

Drug	Renal Function	CL$_{total}$[a]	CL$_{renal}$[a]	CL$_{nonrenal}$[a]	Metabolic Pathway(s)
Cibenzyline	Normal	707 mL/min	344	363	CYP2D6, CYP3A4
	ESRD	224	0	224	
Cyclophosphamide	Normal	79 mL/min	15	64	CYP2B6, CYP2C9, CYP3A4,
	CKD	47	2.4	44.6	
Felbamate	Normal	0.5 mL/min/kg	0.15	0.35	CYP2E1, CYP3A4
	CKD	0.25	0.02	0.23	
Reboxetine	Normal	37 mL/min	3	34	CYP3A4
	CKD	12	1	11	
Roxithromycin	Normal	48.8 mL/min	5.5	43.3	CYP3A4
	CKD	25.4	0.4	25.0	
Telithromycin	Normal	79.2 L/h	9.3	69.9	CYP3A4
	CKD	50.0	2.6	47.4	

[a]Clearance in mL/min can be converted to mL/s through multiplication by 0.0167.

expression suggests transcriptionally mediated downregulation or post-translational inhibition of the metabolic pathway.[9,22]

Thus, current data suggest a differential effect on the individual CYP enzymes with the activity of some enzymes (e.g., CYP3A4 and CYP2C9) being reduced, while others (e.g., CYP2E1) are not affected.[9,10] This differential effect on individual enzymes may help to explain some of the conflicting reports of whether drug metabolism is altered in the presence of CKD.

EFFECT OF RENAL INSUFFICIENCY ON METABOLITE ELIMINATION

Patients with severe renal insufficiency who are receiving chronic treatment with some agents may experience accumulation of metabolite(s) as well as parent compound. Metabolites of several drugs have been reported to have significant pharmacologic and/or toxicologic activity. However, the pharmacokinetics and pharmacodynamics of metabolites are not often fully elucidated. In a sense, the patient with severe CKD is being exposed to a new pharmacologic entity since the sum of the serum concentrations of the metabolite and the parent compound are markedly different than those reported in patients with normal renal function.

The metabolite may have pharmacologic activity similar to that of the parent drug and thus contribute significantly to clinical response; that is true, for example, of oxypurinol. Alternatively, the metabolite may have qualitatively dissimilar pharmacologic action; for example, normeperidine has central nervous system (CNS) stimulatory activity that reportedly produces seizures, whereas meperidine has CNS depressant actions.[27] Because of the multiplicity of potential interactions of compounds that are primarily metabolized, the practical consequences of metabolite accumulation are difficult to predict and are most often identified in those patients at risk by trial and error.

EFFECT OF CKD ON RENAL DRUG EXCRETION

Renal clearance (CL$_R$) of a drug is the composite of GFR, tubular secretion, and reabsorption [(CL$_R$ = (GFR × f_u) + (CL$_{secretion}$ − CL$_{reabsorption}$)], where f_u is the fraction of the drug unbound to plasma proteins. Drug elimination by filtration occurs by diffusion; while tubular secretion and reabsorption are bidirectional processes that involve carrier-mediated renal transport systems.[28] Renal transport systems have been broadly classified on the basis of substrate selectivity into the anionic and cationic renal transport systems, which are responsible for the transport of a number of organic acidic and

basic drugs, respectively (see Chapter 50). Renal organic anion transport is mediated by transporters, transporting polypeptides, and multidrug resistance-associated protein transporters.[29] Several drugs, including β-lactam antibiotics, diuretics, and nonsteroidal antiinflammatory drugs, are actively secreted by one or more of these transporter families which also have an essential role in the elimination of glucuronide metabolites. Organic cation transport systems mediate the reabsorption and excretion of endogenous cationic compounds and drugs (e.g., cimetidine, famotidine, and quinidine). The P-glycoprotein transport system in the kidney is also involved in the secretion of cationic and hydrophobic drugs (e.g., digoxin and vinca alkaloids).[29] Other important renal transport systems include the peptide transporters, which are involved in the uptake of peptide-like drugs including β-lactam antibiotics and angiotensin-converting enzyme inhibitors, while nucleoside transporter proteins are involved in uptake of nucleosides and nucleoside analogs (e.g., zidovudine and dideoxyinosine).

Alterations in filtration, secretion, or reabsorption, secondary to CKD may have a dramatic effect on drug disposition: for drugs that are primarily filtered, a reduction in glomerular filtration rate will result in a proportional decrease in renal drug clearance. However, for drugs that are extensively renally secreted (CL$_R$ >300 mL/min [>5.00 mL/s]), the loss of filtration clearance (up to 120 mL/min [2.00 mL/s]) will have less of an impact. In the absence of data delineating the contribution of tubular function to renal clearance, the clinical measurement or estimation of creatinine clearance remains the guiding factor for drug dosage regimen design.[7,12] The importance of an alteration in renal function on drug elimination depends on two factors: the fraction of drug normally eliminated by the kidney unchanged and the degree of renal insufficiency. Quantitation of the patient's renal function can be accomplished by measurement of CL$_{cr}$ or GFR or estimation of CL$_{cr}$ or GFR based on the stable serum creatinine concentration (see Chapter 50). Because of the time delay involved and problems in obtaining complete urine collections, measured CL$_{cr}$ or GFR values are infrequently used for initial drug dosage regimen design. Therefore the calculation of initial drug dosage regimens relies on the estimation of CL$_{cr}$ or GFR in adults and children from such routinely available clinical data as age, gender, height, weight, and serum creatinine. Although several methods have been proposed to estimate GFR from routinely available clinical data (see Chapter 50) the usefulness of an estimated GFR (eGFR) to guide drug dosing has only recently been extensively evaluated.[30–33] The results of these investigations have yielded controversial findings and future prospective studies of the relationship between estimated CL$_{cr}$ and GFR and the total body clearance of medications will likely be needed to resolve this issue. At the present time the use of CL$_{cr}$ is preferred but the use of eGFR is likely better than not

TABLE 57-5	Stepwise Approach to Adjust Drug Dosage Regimens for Patients with Renal Insufficiency
Step 1	Obtain history and relevant demographic/clinical information	Record demographic information, obtain past medical history including history of renal disease, and record current laboratory information (e.g., serum creatinine)
Step 2	Estimate creatinine clearance	Use Cockcroft-Gault equation to estimate creatinine clearance, or calculate creatinine clearance from timed urine collection
Step 3	Review current medications	Identify drugs for which individualization of the treatment regimen will be necessary
Step 4	Calculate individualized treatment regimen	Determine treatment goals (see text); calculate dosage regimen based on pharmacokinetic characteristics of the drug and the patient's renal function
Step 5	Monitor	Monitor parameters of drug response and toxicity; monitor drug levels if available/applicable
Step 6	Revise regimen	Adjust regimen based on drug response or change in patient status (including renal function) as warranted

considering the potential influence of CKD on drug dosage regimen design. These relationships are most accurate for individuals of average muscle mass for their age, weight, and height. The CL_{cr} and eGFR of emaciated and obese adult patients is difficult to predict, and incorrect estimates have been obtained with most methods.

Several methods are also available for estimating creatinine clearance in adults with acute renal failure using age, height, weight, serum creatinine, and time data (see Chapter 50). These methods have not been independently validated and their usefulness for approximating renal function in complex patient situations is not currently recommended.

DRUG DOSAGE REGIMEN DESIGN FOR PATIENTS WITH CHRONIC KIDNEY DISEASE

❹ An approach for designing a dosage regimen for a patient with CKD is depicted in Table 57–5. The design of the optimal dosage regimen is dependent on the availability of an accurate characterization of the relationship between the pharmacokinetic parameters of the drug and renal function and an accurate assessment of the patient's renal function (CL_{cr}). Prior to 1998 there was no consensus regarding the explicit criteria for characterization of the relationship between the pharmacokinetics and pharmacodynamics of a drug and renal function. The U.S. Food and Drug Administration (FDA) industry guidance issued in May 1998[34] and the European Medicines Agency guidance of 2004[35] provided a framework to help companies decide when they should conduct such a "characterization" study and proposed explicit recommendations for study design, data analysis, and assessment of the impact of the study results on drug dosing. Thus the quality of data available to clinicians has improved dramatically in the last 10 years. A new draft FDA guidance was proposed in 2010 and characterization of the influence of CKD on the pharmacokinetics and pharmacodynamics of a broader range of medications, including many that are predominantly metabolized, is now recommended.[36] The availability of this critical information for many new medications will increase the proportion of patients for whom drug dosage individualization will then be practical.

Most dosage-adjustment guidelines have proposed the use of a fixed dose or interval for patients with broad ranges of renal function that are different from those that are the foundation of the CKD staging scheme (see Chapter 52).[3,13,15,29,37–39] Indeed,

normal renal function has often been ascribed to anyone who has a CL_{cr} >80–90 mL/min (>1.34–1.50 mL/s), even though the population normal CL_{cr} values range from 115 to 125 mL/min/1.73 m² (>1.11–1.20 mL/s/m²). Mild renal insufficiency encompasses the range of 60 to 89 mL/min (1.00–1.49 mL/s), moderate renal insufficiency the CL_{cr} range of 30 to 59 mL/min (0.50–0.99 mL/s), while severe renal insufficiency and ESRD often are defined as a CL_{cr} of 15 to 29 mL/min (0.25–0.49 mL/s) and <15 mL/min (<0.25 mL/s), respectively. Each of these categories encompasses a broad range in renal function, and thus the calculated drug regimen may not be optimal for all patients whose renal function lies within the given category of renal function.

❺ Secondary references, such as the American Hospital Formulary Service Drug Information Service,[37] the British National Formulary,[38] and Drug Prescribing in Renal Failure,[39] are generally touted as excellent sources of information about a drug's pharmacokinetic characteristics in subjects with normal and impaired renal function. A recent analysis of several of these sources suggests a need for a consistent quantitative approach to drug dosage regimen individualization for those with CKD.[40] The authors concluded that the remarkable variation in recommendations along with the paucity of details of the methods used to generate the dosing advice made these sources of drug information less than optimal for clinical use. None of these sources consistently provide the explicit relationships of the kinetic parameters of interest (total body clearance, elimination rate constant, and distribution volume) with a continuous index of renal function, such as CL_{cr}. To find this information, one may need to identify the original research study that assessed the drug's disposition or a comprehensive review article on the class of drugs of interest. This is a time consuming process that may be difficult to carry out for each drug and patient combination in real time. Ideally, one should be able to identify a relationship between total body clearance (CL) or elimination rate constant (k) with an eGFR or CL_{cr}, such as those depicted in Table 57–6. This information, along with the patient's estimated CL_{cr} or GFR is the foundation upon which one can formulate a therapeutic regimen to attain the desired therapeutic outcome.

If specific literature recommendations and/or the relationship of kinetic parameters to eGFR or CL_{cr} are not available, then one can estimate the CL or k of the patient with the method of Rowland and Tozer,[12] provided the fraction of the drug that is eliminated renally unchanged (f_e) in subjects with normal renal function is known.[14]

| TABLE 57-6 | Relationship Between Creatinine Clearance and Total-Body Clearance and Terminal Elimination Rate Constant of Selected Drugs |

Drug	Elimination Rate Constant	Total Body Clearance[a]
Acyclovir		CL = 3.37 (CL_{cr}) + 0.41
Amikacin	$k = (0.0024 \times CL_{cr}) + 0.01$	CL = 0.6 (CL_{cr}) + 9.6
Aztreonam		CL = 0.8 (CL_{cr}) + 26.6
Cefazolin	$k = (0.0028 \times CL_{cr}) + 0.022$	CL = 0.34 (CL_{cr}) + 6.6
Ceftazidime	$k = (0.004 \times CL_{cr}) + 0.004$	CL = 1.15 (CL_{cr}) + 10.6
Ciprofloxacin		CL = 2.83 (CL_{cr}) + 363
Digoxin		CL = 0.88 (CL_{cr}) + 23
Gentamicin	$k = (0.0029 \times CL_{cr}) + 0.015$	CL = 0.983 (CL_{cr})
Imipenem		CL = 1.42 (CL_{cr}) + 54
Lithium		CL = 0.20 (CL_{cr})
Ofloxacin		CL = 1.04 (CL_{cr}) + 38.7
Piperacillin	$k = (0.0049 \times CL_{cr}) + 0.21$	CL = 1.36 (CL_{cr}) + 1.50
Tobramycin	$k = (0.0029 \times CL_{cr}) + 0.01$	CL = 0.801 (CL_{cr})
Vancomycin	$k = (0.00083 \times CL_{cr}) + 0.0044$	CL = 0.69 (CL_{cr}) + 3.7

CL, total-body clearance; CL_{cr}, creatinine clearance.
[a]Clearance in mL/min can be converted to mL/s through multiplication by 0.0167.

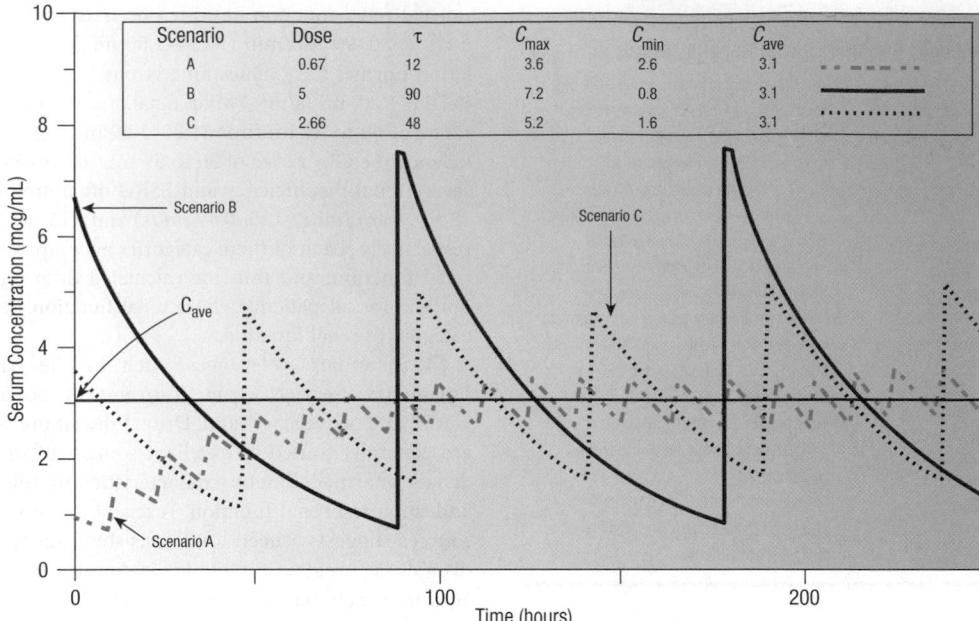

FIGURE 57-1. Although the average steady-state concentrations (C_{ave}) are identical regardless of which dosage-adjustment strategy one decides to implement, the concentration–time profile will be markedly different if one changes the dose and maintains the dosing interval (τ) constant *(Scenario A)*, versus changing the dosing interval and maintaining the dose constant *(Scenario B)* or changing both *(Scenario C)*.

This approach assumes that the change in CL and k are proportional to CL_{cr}, that renal disease does not alter the drug's metabolism, that the metabolites, if formed, are inactive and nontoxic, that the drug obeys first-order (linear) kinetic principles, and that it is adequately described by a one-compartment model. If these assumptions are true, then the kinetic parameter/dosage-adjustment factor (Q) can be calculated as:

$$Q = 1 - [f_e(1 - KF)]$$

where KF is the ratio of the patient's CL_{cr} to the assumed normal value of 120 mL/min (equivalent to 2.00 mL/s). Thus for a drug that is 85% eliminated renally unchanged in a patient who has a CL_{cr} of 10 mL/min (0.17 mL/s), the Q factor would be:

$$Q = 1 - [0.85(1 - (10/120))]$$
$$= 1 - [0.85(0.92)]$$
$$= 1 - 0.78$$
$$= 0.22$$

The best method for dosage regimen adjustment must then be selected. Specifically, one must determine whether the desired goal is the maintenance of a similar peak, trough, or average steady-state drug concentration. If there is a significant relationship between peak concentration and clinical response[41] (e.g., aminoglycosides) or toxicity[42] (e.g., quinidine, phenobarbital, and phenytoin), then attainment of the specific target values is critical. If, however, no specific target values for peak or trough concentrations have been reported (e.g., antihypertensive agents and benzodiazepines), then a regimen goal of attaining the same average steady-state concentration may be appropriate.

Although several methods have been proposed to attain the desired average steady-state concentration profile, the principal choices are to decrease the dose or prolong the dosing interval. If the size of the dose is reduced while the dosing interval remains unchanged, the desired average steady-state concentration will be similar; however, the peak will be lower and the trough higher

(Fig. 57–1). Alternatively, if the dosing interval is increased and the dose size remains unchanged, the peak and trough concentrations in the patient with reduced renal function will be similar to those in the patient with normal renal function. This dosage adjustment method is often recommended because it is likely to yield cost savings as a result of a reduction in nursing and pharmacy time, as well as a reduction in the supplies associated with frequent drug administration. Finally, the dose and dosing interval may both need to be changed to allow the administration of a clinically feasible dose (500 mg vs a calculated value of 487 mg) or a practical dosing interval, for example, 12 hours instead of 17 hours.

If the relationship between the pharmacokinetic parameters of the drug and renal function are known, the first step in the process is to estimate the drug disposition parameters in the patient with renal insufficiency. The dosage-adjustment factor (Q) can then be calculated as the ratio of the estimated elimination rate constant or total body clearance of the patient relative to subjects with normal renal function (CL_{cr} = 120 mL/min [2.00 mL/s]). This parameter may be used to determine the dose or dosing interval alterations necessary for the patient.

For example, the following relationship between total-body clearance (CL) and creatinine clearance (expressed in conventional units of mL/min) has been reported for ganciclovir:[43]

$$CL(mL/min/1.8\ m^2) = 1.25(CL_{cr}) + 8.57$$

Thus, CL for a subject with normal renal function (CL_{norm}) would be calculated as:

$$CL_{norm} = [1.25(120)] + 8.57$$
$$CL_{norm} = 158.6\ mL/min\ per\ 1.8\ m^2$$

Clearance (CL_{fail}) for a patient with a creatinine clearance of 10 mL/min would be:

$$CL_{fail} = [1.25(10)] + 8.57$$
$$CL_{fail} = 21.1\ mL/min\ per\ 1.8\ m^2$$

Ganciclovir is commonly used in solid-organ transplantation patients as prophylaxis against or treatment for cytomegalovirus infection.[44] The inhibitory concentration (IC_{50}) of ganciclovir against 50% of clinical isolates of cytomegalovirus ranges from approximately 0.1 - 2.8 mg/L (0.4 to 11 mmol/L).[43] Consequently, trough concentrations should be maintained within this range, but caution is warranted as neutropenia has been associated with the attainment of ganciclovir trough concentrations exceeding 2.6 mcg/mL (2.6 mg/L; 10 mmol/L).[45] If a patient with ESRD received the ganciclovir dose intended for a patient with normal renal function, the predicted trough concentrations would approach 5.2 mcg/mL (5.2 mg/L; 20 mmol/L). Consequently, a dosage modification would be necessary to avoid potential toxicity. The dosing regimen can be modified using the ratio of the predicted clearance values. The quotient or Q for this patient can be calculated as:

$$Q = CL_{fail}/CL_{norm}$$
$$Q = 21.1/158.6$$
$$Q = 0.133$$

where CL_{norm} is the clearance in a patient with normal renal function and CL_{fail} is the clearance of the patient with impaired renal function.

The maintenance dose (D_f) for the patient or the adjusted dosing interval (τ_f) may then be calculated from the following relationships, where D_n is the normal dose and τ_n is the normal dosing interval:

$$D_f = D_n \times Q$$
$$\tau_f = \tau_n/Q$$

For this patient situation, the normal dose and dosing interval of ganciclovir would be 5 mg/kg and 12 hours, respectively. If we wanted to maintain the dosing interval at 12 hours, then D_f would be calculated as:

$$D_f = (5 \text{ mg/kg}) \times (0.133) = 0.67 \text{ mg/kg}$$

This regimen would result in decreased peak and trough concentrations compared to a patient with this degree of renal insufficiency who received a normal dosage regimen (Fig. 57–1, Scenario A). However, the peak concentrations would be lower and the trough concentrations higher than those observed when a patient with normal renal function received a standard regimen.

If one maintains D_n and extends the dosing interval, τ_f would be calculated as:

$$\tau_f = \tau_n/Q = 12/0.133 = 90 \text{ hours}$$

This regimen would yield similar peak and trough concentrations in the renally impaired patient as in the patient with normal renal function, but there is a risk of missed doses with such an unorthodox interval (Fig. 57–1, Scenario B). In addition, the prolonged period below the steady-state drug concentration (C_{ss}) average concentration may be less than optimal.

Finally, a practical dosing interval (τ_p) may be selected and then a dose based on that interval can be calculated. If a dosage interval τ_f of 24 hours were selected, because in many institutions there is an increased risk of missed doses with longer dosing intervals, then the D_f would be calculated as follows:

$$D_f = [D_n \times Q \times \tau_f]/\tau_p$$
$$= [(5 \text{ mg/kg}) \times (0.133) \times (24)]/12$$
$$= 1.33 \text{ mg/kg}$$

This method would be most appropriate, as prolonged subtherapeutic concentrations are avoided and troughs are reduced (Fig. 57–1, Scenario C). The selection of which dosage-adjustment method to use to calculate an optimal regimen depends on the drug characteristics and the patient care situation. This dosage-adjustment method assumes that the protein binding and volume of distribution of the drug are not significantly altered by renal insufficiency. Thus, this approach cannot be used with accuracy for those drugs with demonstrated differences in these pharmacokinetic parameters.

If the volume of distribution (V_D) of a drug is significantly altered in CKD patients or in whom one desires to attain a specific maximum or minimum concentration, the estimation of a dosage regimen becomes more complex. If the relationship between V_D and CL_{cr} has been characterized, then V_D may be estimated. If one assumes that a one-compartment linear model can describe the drug, the predicted V_D may then be used with the predicted elimination rate constant (k) of the drug to yield an adjusted-dosing interval and intravenous or oral dose. For orally administered drugs, the τ_f can be calculated and the dose can then be approximated as:

$$\tau_f = [(-1/k_f)(\ln[C_{min}/C_{max}])] + t_{peak}$$
$$\text{Dose}_{po} = [FC_p^t V_D(k_a - k)]/[k_a(e^{-kt}/1 - e^{-k\tau})(e^{-kat}/1 - e^{-ka\tau})]$$

where, F equals bioavailability, C_p^t equals the desired plasma concentration at time t, and k_a is the absorption rate constant. This approach allows for the individualization of an oral dosage regimen for attainment of specific peak and trough serum concentrations. If the drug is absorbed extremely rapidly, one can approximate the τ_f and the dose using equations originally proposed for IV dosing as:

$$\tau_f = (-1/k_f)(\ln[C_{min}/C_{max}])$$
$$\text{Dose}_{po} = V_D \times (C_{max} - C_{min})$$

Digoxin is a frequently used oral medication for which the V_D is decreased in CKD patients and for which one usually desires to closely control the plasma concentration time profile. The V_D and CL_{fail} of digoxin can be estimated for a 70-kg (154 lb) patient with a CL_{cr} of 12 mL/min per 1.73 m² (0.11 mL/s/m²) as summarized by Job[18]:

$$V_D = 226 + [(298(CL_{cr}))/(29.1 + CL_{cr})]$$
$$= 226 + [(298(12))/(29.1 + 12)]$$
$$= 226 + 87.0$$
$$= 313 \text{ L}$$
$$CL_{fail} = (0.88 \times CL_{cr}) + 23 \text{ mL/min}$$
$$= 10.6 + 23$$
$$= 33.6 \text{ mL/min}$$
$$k_f = CL_{fail}/V_D$$
$$= (33.6 \text{ mL/min} \times 1440 \text{ min/d})/313 \text{ L}$$
$$= (48.3 \text{ L/d})/313 \text{ L}$$
$$= 0.154 \text{ day}^{-1}$$

The t_{peak} is generally at 2 hours, and the k_a from the literature is about 0.76 hour^{-1} or 18 day^{-1}.[15] Thus, one now has all the information needed to calculate the τ_f and dose for this patient assuming the desired C_{min} and C_{max} are 0.8 and 1.4, respectively:

$$\tau_f = [(-1/k_f)(\ln[C_{min}/C_{max}])] + t_{peak}$$
$$= [(-1/0.154)(\ln[0.8/1.4])] + 2 \text{ hours}$$
$$= [(-6.49)(-0.56)] + 2 \text{ hours}$$
$$= 3.6 \text{ days} + 2 \text{ hours}$$
$$\cong 4 \text{ days}$$
$$\text{Dose}_{po} = [(1)(1.4)(313)(18 - 0.154)]/[18(e^{-0.154(0.083)}/1 -$$
$$e^{-0.154(4)}) - (e^{-18(0.083)}/1 - e^{-18(4)})]$$
$$= 0.226 \text{ mg or}$$
$$\cong \text{one 0.25 mg oral capsule every 4 days}$$

Alternatively, the predicted volume of distribution and elimination rate constant or the total-body clearance may be used to calculate a dose regimen that will maintain the desired average C_{ss} of the drug:

$$\text{Dose(mg/h)} = C_{ss}[(k_f \times V_D) \text{ or } (CL_f)]$$

Depending on how much variance above and below the average steady state one desires, the dosing interval may range from hourly to as infrequently as every 48 hours or longer. For example, if the calculated dose were 10 mg/h, the desired average steady-state concentration would be maintained with a dosing interval of 60 mg every 6 hours or 480 mg every 48 hours.

PATIENTS RECEIVING CONTINUOUS RENAL REPLACEMENT THERAPY

Continuous renal replacement therapies are used for the management of fluid overload and the removal of uremic toxins in patients with acute renal failure and other conditions.[46] The several forms of continuous renal replacement therapy in clinical use today are extensively described in Chapter 51 and several dosage regimen individualization approaches are presented and critiqued. Which of these therapies will be optimal for a given patient is dependent on several factors, including bleeding risk, degree of hypercatabolism, acid–base balance, and experience of the healthcare provider team.

PATIENTS RECEIVING CHRONIC PERITONEAL DIALYSIS

Peritoneal dialysis, like other dialysis modalities, has the potential to affect drug disposition; however, drug therapy individualization is often less complicated in these patients as a result of the limited drug clearances achieved with the variants of this procedure (see Chapter 54). In general, hemodialysis is more effective in removing drugs than peritoneal dialysis such that if a drug is not removed by hemodialysis, it is unlikely to be significantly removed by peritoneal dialysis.

Many of the factors that are important in determining drug dialyzability for other treatment modalities pertain to peritoneal dialysis as well.[48,49] Peritoneal dialysis involves the instillation of 1 to 3 L of dialysis solution into the peritoneal cavity. Waste products and other substances, including drugs, move from the blood and surrounding tissues into the dialysis solution by means of diffusion and ultrafiltration. Factors that influence drug dialyzability by peritoneal dialysis include drug-specific characteristics such as molecular weight, solubility, degree of ionization, protein binding, and volume of distribution. The intrinsic properties of the peritoneal membrane that affect drug removal include blood flow and peritoneal membrane surface area, which is approximately equal to the body surface area. There is an inverse relationship between peritoneal drug clearance and molecular weight, protein binding, and volume of distribution. Also, drug compounds that are ionized at physiologic pH will diffuse across the membrane more slowly than unionized compounds. Detailed reviews of the disposition of several drugs in chronic peritoneal dialysis patients are reported elsewhere.[47,48] Anti-infective agents are the most commonly studied drugs because of their primary role in the treatment of peritonitis[48,50] (see Chapter 54). Most other drugs can generally be dosed based on the residual renal function of the patient because the additional clearance by peritoneal dialysis is so small.

PATIENTS RECEIVING CHRONIC HEMODIALYSIS

Although many new hemodialyzers have been introduced in the past 20 years and more than 100 different ones were available in the

United States in 2010, the effect of hemodialysis on drug disposition is rarely reevaluated after it is initially reported. Thus, most of the literature, especially for older medications, probably represents an underestimation of the impact of hemodialysis on its disposition.[51]

❻ The impact of hemodialysis on a patient's drug therapy is dependent on several factors, including the characteristics of the drug, the dialysis conditions, and the clinical situation for which dialysis is performed. Drug-related factors that affect dialyzability include the molecular weight or size, degree of protein binding, and distribution volume.[7] The vast majority of dialysis filters in use in the United States up until the mid-1990s were composed of cellulose, cellulose acetate, or regenerated cellulose (cuprophane) (see Chapter 54), and they were generally impermeable to drugs with a molecular weight greater than 1,000 Da. Drugs that are small but highly protein bound also are not well dialyzed because both of the principal binding proteins, α_1-acid glycoprotein and albumin, have a very high molecular weight. Finally, those drugs that are widely distributed, V_D greater than 2 L/kg, are poorly removed by hemodialysis.

The hemodialysis procedure, be it acute for the management of AKI, intermittent 3 times a week or daily for an extended period or some combination thereof for the management of ESRD as well as the prescription for the patient can also dramatically affect the dialysis clearance of a medication.[52] The primary factors that vary between patients are the composition of the dialysis filter, the filter surface area, the blood and dialysate flow rates, and whether or not the dialysis unit reuses the dialysis filter. Dialysis membranes in the 21st century are predominantly composed of semisynthetic or synthetic materials (e.g., polysulfone, polymethylmethacrylate, or polyacrylonitrile). High-flux dialysis membranes have the largest pore sizes and more closely mimic the filtration characteristics of the human kidney. This allows the passage of most solutes, including drugs, that have a molecular weight of 20,000 Da or less.[53] Thus, high-molecular-weight drugs such as vancomycin are extensively cleared by this mode of dialysis. An increase in removal has also been reported with several other drugs that have lower molecular weights (Table 57–7).[51] The impact of hemodialysis on drug therapy should thus not be viewed as a generic procedure such that a certain percentage of a drug is removed with each dialysis session; neither should a "yes" answer regarding the dialyzability of drugs be considered sufficient information to make therapeutic decisions, since this provides no quantification of the impact of hemodialysis. Characteristics of the dialysis procedure that was utilized in the drug study, such as membrane composition and surface area and blood and dialysis flow rates, are thus critical data that should be

TABLE 57-7	Drug Disposition during Dialysis Depends on Dialyzer Characteristics[51]			
	Hemodialysis Clearance (mL/min)[a]		**Half-Life during Dialysis (h)**	
Drug	**Conventional**	**High Flux**	**Conventional**	**High Flux**
Cefazolin	15.1	30–38	NR	NR
Ceftazidime	60	155[b]	3.3	1.2[b]
Cefuroxime	NR	103[c]	3.8	1.6[c]
Foscarnet	183	253[c]	NR	NR
Gentamicin	58.2	116[c]	3.0	4.3[c]
Netilmicin	46	87–109	5.0–5.2	2.9–3.4
Ranitidine	43.1	67.2[c]	5.1	2.9[c]
Vancomycin	9–21	40–150[c]	35–38	4.5–11.8[c]
		72–116[d]		NR

NR, not reported.
[a]Clearance in mL/min can be converted to mL/s through multiplication by 0.0167.
[b]Polyamide filter.
[c]Polysulfone filter.
[d]Polymethylmethacrylate.

known before one uses the hemodialysis clearance data to prospectively design a drug dosing regimen for a hemodialysis patient.

The quantitative impact of hemodialysis on drug disposition can be calculated in several ways.[7] The most commonly utilized means for assessing the effect of hemodialysis is to calculate the dialyzer clearance (CL_D) of the drug. The CL_D can be calculated by several approaches. The CL^b_D from blood can be calculated as $CL^b_D = Q_b [(A_b - V_b)/A_b]$, where Q_b is blood flow through the dialyzer, A_b is the concentration of drug in blood going into the dialyzer, and V_b is the blood concentration of drug leaving the dialyzer. This equation is valid only if the drug concentrations are measured in whole blood and if the drug rapidly and completely distributes into red blood cells. Because drug concentrations are generally determined in plasma, the previous equation is usually modified to $CL^p_D = Q_p [(A_p - V_p)/A_p]$ where p represents plasma and Q_p is plasma flow, which equals $Q_b (1 - \text{hematocrit})$. This clearance calculation most accurately reflects dialysis drug clearance as most drugs do not significantly penetrate red blood cells or bind to formed blood elements. However, one must keep in mind that venous plasma concentrations may be artificially high and CL^p_D will be low if plasma water is removed from the blood at a faster rate than drug. This tends to occur when extensive ultrafiltration is performed simultaneously with diffusion during dialysis.

The recovery clearance approach remains the benchmark for the determination of dialyzer clearance and it can be calculated as:[7]

$$CL^r_D = R/AUC_{0-t}$$

where R is the total amount of drug recovered unchanged in the dialysate and AUC_{0-t} is the area under the predialyzer plasma concentration–time curve during the period of time that the dialysate was collected. To determine the AUC_{0-t}, at least two and preferably three to four plasma concentrations should be obtained during dialysis.

The hemodialysis clearance values reported in the literature may vary significantly depending on which of these methods were used to calculate CL_D. The principal reason for this is that for most medications we do not know the degree and rapidity with which the drug crosses the red blood cell membrane. Because the CL^r_D method incorporates no assumption of the degree of red blood cell permeability, it can be reliably used as the benchmark value. The primary limitation of this calculation is that the concentrations of the drug in the dialysate may be below the sensitivity limits of the assay.

The following principles may be used to generate a drug dosage regimen recommendation for hemodialysis patients by using a value of CL_D that is reported in the literature.[7,51] Because clearance terms are additive, the total clearance during dialysis can be calculated as the sum of the patient's residual renal and nonrenal clearance during the interdialytic period (CL_{RES}) and dialyzer clearance (CL_D):

$$CL_T = CL_{RES} + CL_D$$

The half-life during the period between dialysis treatments and during dialysis can then be calculated from the following relationships using an estimate of the drug's distribution volume (V_D), which can be obtained from the literature:[14]

$$t_{1/2,\text{offHD}} = 0.693[V_D/CL_{RES}]$$
$$t_{1/2,\text{onHD}} = 0.693[V_D/(CL_{RES} + CL_D)]$$

Once the key pharmacokinetic parameters have been estimated/calculated, they may be used to simulate the plasma concentration–time profile of the drug for the individual patient and then one can ascertain how much drug to administer and when. This approach to drug therapy individualization can be accomplished in a stepwise fashion assuming first-order elimination of the drug and a one-compartment model.

For example, a 34-year-old male with ESRD was admitted to a hospital from the outpatient hemodialysis unit, where he experienced shaking and chills and had a temperature of 40°C (104°F). He weighed 70 kg (154 lb) and was 69 inches (175 cm) tall, had a residual CL_{cr} of 3 mL/min (0.05 mL/s), and received high-flux dialysis for 3 hours 3 times a week on an F80 polysulfone dialyzer. He received 140 mg of gentamicin at the end of his most recent hemodialysis treatment, which ended less than an hour prior to admission to the hospital.

The first step is to estimate this patient's pharmacokinetic parameters of gentamicin on the basis of published population data.[14] The volume of distribution in this patient is 23.1 L (0.33 L/kg × 70 kg),[54] and his residual total body clearance (CL_{RES}) estimated from the relationship between CL and creatinine clearance [$CL_{RES} = CL_{cr} \times 0.98$] is 3 mL/min (0.05 mL/s) or 0.176 L/h. The elimination rate constant can be approximated as:

$$k = CL_{RES} \div V_D$$
$$= 0.176 \text{ L/h} \div 23.1 \text{ L}$$
$$= 0.0076 \text{ hr}^{-1}$$

The hemodialysis clearance of gentamicin is dependent on the dialyzer and a value of 116 mL/min is a reasonable estimate for this dialyzer.[51]

One now can predict what the plasma concentrations of gentamicin will be over the next 24 to 48 hours, assuming the infusion time for the drug (t') was 30 minutes. The concentration at the end of the 30-minute infusion (C_{max}) would be:

$$C_{max} = \frac{(\text{Dose}/t')(1 - e^{-kt'})}{CL_{RES}}$$
$$C_{max} = \frac{(280 \text{ mg/h})(1 - e^{-(0.0076)0.5})}{0.176 \text{ L/h}}$$
$$C_{max} = (1{,}944 \text{ mg/L})(0.003) = 6.0 \text{ mg/L}$$

The plasma concentration prior to the next dialysis session (C_{bD}), which is 44 hours away, and the concentration four hours later after dialysis (C_{aD}) can be calculated as:

$$C_{bD} = C_{max} \times e^{-(CL_{RES}/V_D) \times t}$$
$$= 6.0 \times e^{-0.0076 \times 44}$$
$$= 4.3 \text{ mg/L}$$
$$C_{aD} = C_{bD} \times e^{-((CL_{RES} + CL_D)/V_D) \times t}$$
$$= 4.3 \times e^{-((0.176 + 6.96)/23.1) \times 4}$$
$$= 4.3 \times e^{-0.309 \times 4}$$
$$= 1.25 \text{ mg/L}$$

On the basis of these data, a second dose will likely be required at the end of the next dialysis session as one generally desires to have gentamicin concentrations fall below 2 mg/L (2 mcg/mL; 4.2 mmol/L) before administering another dose.

During this interdialytic interval, several blood samples were collected to characterize this patient's residual gentamicin clearance, distribution volume, and the clearance of gentamicin during dialysis. Blood samples were therefore collected at the following times after the first dose:

DAY 1: 7 PM (2 hours after dose)	6.5 mg/L or mcg/mL (13.6 mmol/L)
DAY 2: 8 AM (39 hours after dose; just before dialysis)	4.1 mg/L or mcg/mL (8.6 mmol/L)
DAY 3: 12 noon (immediately after dialysis)	2.0 mg/L or mcg/mL (4.2 mmol/L)

The C_{max} can be calculated by back-extrapolation to the end of the infusion as described in Chapter 8. The elimination rate during the interdialytic period (k_{ID}) and during dialysis (k_{DD}), and the V_D can be calculated as:

$$k_{ID} = (\ln C_1/C_2)/\Delta t$$

$$k_{ID} = (\ln 6.5/4.1)/37 = 0.0125/h$$

$$V_D = \frac{Dose/t'}{k_{ID}} \quad \frac{1 - e^{-k_{ID}t'}}{(C_{max} - C_{min}e^{-k_{ID}t'})}$$

$$V_D = \frac{140/0.5}{0.0125} \quad \frac{1 - e^{-(0.0125)0.5}}{(6.7 - 0.0e^{-(0.0125)0.5})}$$

$$V_D = \frac{134.4}{6.7} = 20 \text{ L}$$

$$k_{DD} = (\ln C_2/C_3)/\Delta t$$

$$k_{DD} = (\ln 4.1/2.0)/4 = 0.179/h$$

where Δt is the time in hours between the two measured concentrations and C_{min} the gentamicin concentration in plasma prior to the administration of the first dose is zero.

The patient's residual clearance (CL_{RES}) of gentamicin can then be calculated as:

$$CL_{RES} = V_D \times k_{ID}$$

$$CL_{RES} = 20.0 \text{ L} \times 0.0125 = 0.25 \text{ L/h or } 4.2 \text{ mL/min}$$

The dialyzer clearance (CL_D) can be calculated as follows because one knows the total clearance during dialysis (CL_T) and CL_{RES}:

$$CL_D = CL_T - CL_{RES}$$

$$CL_D = (k_{DD} \times V_D) - 4.2 \text{ mL/min}$$

$$CL_D = (0.179/h \times 20.0 \text{ L}) - 4.2 \text{ mL/min}$$

$$CL_D = (3.6 \text{ L/h or } 59.6 \text{ mL/min}) - 4.2 \text{ mL/min}$$

$$CL_D = 55.4 \text{ mL/min}$$

The ultimate reason for measuring the plasma concentrations of aminoglycosides and several other agents is to individualize the patient's dosage regimen to achieve a bacteriologic cure while preserving residual renal function. Thus there remains one important step in our evaluation: the calculation of the dose this patient should receive next. The two factors that enter into this decision are the desired peak and trough concentrations and the degree of rebound in drug concentrations, after the end of dialysis. Because gentamicin concentrations have been noted to increase by approximately 25% within 1.5 to 2 hours after the end of hemodialysis, the trough concentration of this patient can be considered to be 2.5 mg/L (2.0 mg/L × 1.25). Although this value is higher than one might like to maintain in an individual with normal renal function, a prolonged period of almost 24 hours would be required just to have the concentration drop below 2.0 mg/L (2.0 mcg/mL; 4.2 mmol/L). Assuming the desired peak concentration was 7.0 mg/L (7.0 mcg/mL; 14.6 mmol/L), the postdialysis dose this patient would need can then be calculated using the simplified approach below, because the elimination half-life is extremely prolonged relative to the infusion time, and thus minimal drug is eliminated during the infusion period:

$$Dose = V_D \times (C_{max} - C_{min})$$

$$= 20.0 \text{ L} \times (7.0 - 2.5) = 90 \text{ mg}$$

❼ It is common practice in most hemodialysis units to administer drugs after the patient has received dialysis on the premise that it is desirable to minimize the loss of drug that would result from the additional clearance during hemodialysis. Certainly, administration of antihypertensive agents and vasoactive drugs should be avoided in the hours prior to a hemodialysis session to minimize the likelihood of hypotension. However, emerging pharmacokinetic and pharmacodynamic considerations suggest that this may not be the optimal approach for several other agents, such as aminoglycosides[55-57] and vancomycin.[58-60] Two evaluations of predialysis and one of intradialytic dosing of aminoglycosides indicate that similar peak concentrations, a prime indicator of efficacy, can be obtained in these scenarios relative to those observed with postdialysis dosing.[55-56] The area under the concentration-time curve during the dosing interval and the subsequent predialysis concentrations were noted to be significantly reduced and thus the risk of ototoxicity and further renal injury may be minimized. The best dosing schedule, a dose roughly twice that traditionally employed for postdialysis administration, in the 26 patients evaluated by Teigen et al., resulted in the achievement of the desired peak and area under the concentration–time curve in approximately 90% of patients.[56] The administration of traditional doses of tobramycin (1.5 mg/kg) or vancomycin (1,000 mg) during dialysis has been associated with markedly lower areas under the concentration–time curve than those observed when the same dose was administered postdialysis; consequently, higher dosage regimens are usually necessary to compensate for the additional loss of drug during the dialysis procedure. It is highly recommended that aminoglycoside and vancomycin concentrations in hemodialysis patients be measured after the first dose and dialysis session and so that the dosage regimen can be individualized accordingly using Bayesian methodology whenever possible.

CONCLUSIONS

Subtherapeutic or supratherapeutic responses to drugs in patients with renal insufficiency are often misinterpreted and not recognized as such. The adverse outcomes associated with inappropriate drug dosing have not been quantified but do warrant future investigations. Sound pharmacokinetic principles, used in concert with reliable population pharmacokinetic estimates, should ultimately yield the optimal approach to drug dosage regimen design for patients with renal insufficiency. Individualization of therapy should be undertaken whenever clinical therapeutic monitoring tools are available. The key action step is to use the knowledge we have to improve patient outcomes. The recent study of van Dijk et al. is an unfortunate reminder of how far we still have to go.[61] They observed that although dosage adjustments based on renal function were warranted in 24% of the prescriptions of the patients with CL_{cr} less than 51 mL/min (0.85 mL/s), such adjustments were only performed in 59% of cases.

ABBREVIATIONS

A_b: concentration of drug in blood going into the dialyzer (arterial side)

A_p: concentration of drug in plasma going into the dialyzer (arterial side)

AUC_{0-t}: the area under the predialyzer plasma concentration–time curve during hemodialysis

C_a: concentration of the drug in the plasma going into a filter

C_{aD}: plasma concentration after dialysis

C_{ave}: average plasma concentration

C_{bD}: plasma concentration prior to the next dialysis session

C_{df}: concentration of drug in the dialysis fluid

C_{ss}: average steady-state plasma concentration

CL: total-body clearance

CL^b_D: dialyzer clearance from blood

CL_{cr}: creatinine clearance

CL_D: dialyzer clearance

CL_{fail}: clearance of a drug in patients with impaired renal function

CL_{norm}: clearance of a drug in patients with normal renal function

CL^p_D: dialyzer clearance from plasma

CL_{PT}: estimated total body clearance for a given patient

CL_R: net renal excretion

$CL_{reabsorption}$: tubular reabsorption

CL_{RES}: residual drug clearance in a dialysis patient

$CL_{secretion}$: tubular secretion

C_{max}: peak drug concentration

CNS: central nervous system

C^t_p: desired plasma concentration at time t

CYP: cytochrome P450 enzymes

D_f: maintenance dose for a patient with renal insufficiency

D_n: dose for a patient with normal renal function

ESRD: end-stage renal disease

f_e: fraction of drug eliminated unchanged in the urine

f_u: fraction of drug unbound to plasma proteins

GFR: glomerular filtration rate

IC_{50}: inhibitory concentration of 50%

k_a: absorption rate constant

k: elimination rate constant

k_{DD}: elimination rate constant during dialysis

k_f: ratio of the patient's creatinine clearance to the assumed normal value of 120 mL/min

k_{ID}: elimination rate constant between dialysis sessions (interdialytic)

Q: kinetic parameter/dosage-adjustment factor

Q_b: blood flow through the dialyzer

Q_p: plasma flow through the dialyzer = Q_b (1-hct)

R: the total amount of drug recovered unchanged in the dialysate

τ_f: dosing interval in a patient with renal failure

τ_p: practical dosing interval for a patient with renal failure

τ_n: dosing interval in a patient with normal renal function

t_{max}: time-to-peak drug concentration

$t_{1/2}$: half-life

$t_{1/2,onHD}$: half-life during dialysis

$t_{1/2,offHD}$: half-life off dialysis

V_{area}: volume of distribution area

V_β: volume of distribution

V_c: volume of the central compartment

V_D: volume of distribution

V_{ss}: volume of distribution at steady state

REFERENCES

1. Jones CA, McQuillan GM, Kusek JW, et al. Serum creatinine levels in the U.S. population: Third National Health and Nutrition Examination Survey. Am J Kidney Dis 1998;32:992–999.

2. Mangoni AA, Jackson SH. Age-related changes in pharmacokinetics and pharmacodynamics: Basic principles and practical applications. Br J Clin Pharmacol 2004;57:6–14.

3. Olyaei, AJ, WM Bennett. Drug dosing in the elderly patients with chronic kidney disease. Clin Geriatr Med 2009;25:459–527.

4. Matzke GR, Frye RF. Drug administration in patients with renal insufficiency: Minimising renal and extrarenal toxicity. Drug Saf 1997;16:205–231.

5. Cusack BJ. Pharmacokinetics in older persons. Am J Geriatr Pharmacother 2004;2(4):274–302.

6. Grandison MK, Boudinot FD. Age-related changes in protein binding of drugs: Implications for therapy. Clin Pharmacokinet 2000;38:271–290.

7. Matzke GR, Comstock TJ. Influence of renal disease and dialysis on pharmacokinetics. In: Evans WE, Schentag JJ, Burton ME, eds. Applied Pharmacokinetics: Principles of Therapeutic Drug Monitoring, 4th ed. Baltimore, MD: Lippincott Williams & Wilkins, 2005:187–212.

8. Nolin TD, Frye RF, Matzke GR. Hepatic drug metabolism and transport in patients with kidney disease. Am J Kidney Dis 2003;42:906–925.

9. Nolin, DT. Altered Nonrenal Drug Clearance in ESRD. Curr Opin Nephrol Hypertens 2008;17:255–559.

10. Dreisbach, AW. The influence of chronic renal failure on drug metabolism and transport. Clin Pharmaco Ther 2009;86:553–556.

11. Nolin DT, Frye RF, Le Phuong, et el. ESRD impairs nonrenal clearance of fexofenadine but not midazolam. J Am Soc Nephrol 2009;20:2269–2276.

12. Rowland M, Tozer TN. Clinical Pharmacokinetics: Concepts and Applications, 3rd ed. Philadelphia, PA: Lea & Febiger, 1995:156–183.

13. Matzke GR, Dowling TD. Dosing concepts in renal dysfunction. In: Murphy JE, ed. Clinical Pharmacokinetics Pocket Reference, 4th ed. Bethesda, MD: American Society of Health-System Pharmacists, 2008:427–443.

14. Matzke GR, Clermont G. Clinical pharmacology and therapeutics. In: Murray PT, Brady HR, Hall JB, eds. Intensive Care in Nephrology. Boca Raton, FL: Taylor & Francis, 2006:245–265.

15. Thummel KE, Shen DD, Isoherranen N, Smith HE. Design and optimization of dosage regimens: Pharmacokinetic data. In: Hardman JG, Limbird LE, Goodman GA, eds. Goodman & Gilman's The Pharmacological Basis of Therapeutics, 11th ed. New York: McGraw-Hill, 2006:1787–1888.

16. Meijers BKI, Bammens B, Verbeke K, Evenepoel P. A review of albumin binding in CKD. Am J Kidney Dis 2008;51:839–850.

17. Winter ME. Phenytoin and Fosphenytoin. In: Murphy JE, ed. Clinical Pharmacokinetics Pocket Reference, 4th ed. Bethesda, MD: American Society of Health-System Pharmacists, 2008:247–259.

18. Job ML. Digoxin. In: Murphy JE, ed. Clinical Pharmacokinetics Pocket Reference, 4th ed. Bethesda, MD: American Society of Health-System Pharmacists, 2008:139–147.

19. Malini PL, Strocchi E, Feliciangeli G, et al. Digitalis receptors and digoxin sensitivity in renal failure. Clin Exp Pharmacol Physiol 1985;12:115–120.

20. Lam YW, Banerji S, Hatfield C, Talbert RL. Principles of drug administration in renal insufficiency. Clin Pharmacokinet 1997;32:30–57.

21. Koup J. Disease states and drug pharmacokinetics. J Clin Pharmacol 1989;29:674–679.

22. Leblond F, Guevin C, Demers C, et al. Downregulation of hepatic cytochrome P450 in chronic renal failure. J Am Soc Nephrol 2001;12:326–332.

23. Leblond FA, Giroux L, Villeneuve JP, Pichette V. Decreased in vivo metabolism of drugs in chronic renal failure. Drug Metab Dispos 2000;28:1317–1320.

24. Dowling TC, Briglia AE, Fink JC, et al. Characterization of hepatic cytochrome P4503A activity in patients with end-stage renal disease. Clin Pharmacol Ther 2003;73:427–434.

25. Himmelfarb J, Stenvinkel P, Ikizler TA, Hakim RM. The elephant in uremia: Oxidant stress as a unifying concept of cardiovascular disease in uremia. Kidney Int 2002;62:1524–1538.

26. Morgan ET, Li-Masters T, Cheng PY. Mechanisms of cytochrome P450 regulation by inflammatory mediators. Toxicology 2002;181–182:207–210.

27. Murphy EJ. Acute pain management for the patient with concurrent renal or hepatic disease. Anaesth Intensive Care 2005;33(3):311–322.

28. Lee W, Kim RB. Transporters and renal drug elimination. Annu Rev Pharmacol Toxicol 2004;44:137–166.

29. Verbeeck, RK, FT Musuamba. Pharmacokinetics and dosage adjustment in patients with renal dysfunction. Eur J Clin Pharmacol 2009;65:757–773.

30. Wargo KA, Eiland EH, Hamm W, English TM, Phillippe HM. Comparison of the modification of diet in renal disease and Cockroft-Gault equations for antimicrobial dosage adjustments. Ann Pharmacotherapy 2006;40:1248–1253.

31. Spruill WJ, Wade WE, Cobb HH. Estimating glomerular filtration rate with a modification of diet in renal disease equation: implications for pharmacy. Am J Health Syst Pharm 2007;64:652–660.

32. Hermsen ED, Malefski M, Florescu MC, Qui, Rupp ME. Comparison of the modification of diet in renal disease and Cockroft-Gault equations for dosing antimicrobials. Pharmacother 2009;29:649–655.

33. Stevens LA Stevens LA, Nolin TD, Richardson MM. Comparison of drug, closing recommendations based on measured GFR and kidney function estimating equations. Am J Kidney Dis 2009l;54: 33–42.

34. Anonymous. Characterization of the relationship between the pharmacokinetics and pharmacodynamics of a drug and renal function. U.S. Department of Health and Human Services, FDA Guidance, May 1998. http://www.fda.gov/cber/guidelines.htm.

35. Anonymous. Note for guidance on the evaluation of the pharmacokinetics of medicinal products in patients with impaired renal function. European Medicines Agency, 2004. http://www.emea.eu.int.

36. Anonymous. Pharmacokinetics in patients with impaired renal function – study design, data analysis, and impact on dosing and labeling. U.S. Department of Health and Human Services, Draft FDA Guidance, March 2010. http://www.fda.gov/cber/guidelines.htm.

37. McEvoy GK, Litvak K, Welsh OH, et al. American Hospital Formulary Service, Drug Information. Bethesda, MD: American Society of Hospital Pharmacists, 2001.

38. Joint formulary committee. British National Formulary, 48th ed. London: British Medical Association and Royal Pharmaceutical Society of Great Britain, 2004. http://www.bnf.org/bnf/.

39. Aronoff GR, Bennett WM, Berns JS, et al. Drug Prescribing in Renal Failure: Dosing Guidelines for Adults and Children, 5th ed. Philadelphia, PA: American College of Physicians-American Society of Internal Medicine, 2007.

40. Vidal L, Shavit M, Fraser A, Paul M, Leibovici L. Systematic comparison of four sources of drug information regarding adjustment of dose for renal function. BMJ 2005;331:263–266.

41. Craig WA. Pharmacokinetic/pharmacodynamic parameters: Rationale for antibacterial dosing of mice and men. Clin Infect Dis 1998; 26:1–12.

42. Murphy JE. Clinical Pharmacokinetics Pocket Reference, 4th ed. Bethesda, MD: American Society of Health-System Pharmacists, 2008.

43. Scott JC, Partovi N, Ensom MH. Ganciclovir in solid organ transplant recipients: Is there a role for clinical pharmacokinetic monitoring? Ther Drug Monit 2004;26:68–77.

44. Pescovitz MD, Pruett TL, Gonwa T, et al. Oral ganciclovir dosing in transplant recipients and dialysis patients based on renal function. Transplantation 1998;66:1104–1107.

45. Balfour HH. Management of cytomegalovirus disease with antiviral drugs. Rev Infect Dis 1990;12:S849-S860.

46. Heintz BH, Matzke GR, Dager WE. Antimicrobial dosing concepts and recommendations for critically ill adult patients receiving continuous renal replacement therapy or intermittent hemodialysis. Pharmacother 2009;29:562–577.

47. Taylor CA, Abdel-Rahman E, Zimmerman SW, Johnson CA. Clinical pharmacokinetics during continuous ambulatory peritoneal dialysis. Clin Pharmacokinet 1996;31:293–308.

48. Manley HJ, Bailie GR. Treatment of peritonitis in APD: pharmacokinetic principles. Semin Dial 2002;15:418–421.

49. Veltri MA, Neu AM, Fivush BA, et al. Drug dosing during intermittent hemodialysis and continuous renal replacement therapy: special considerations in pediatric patients. Paediatr Drugs 2004;6:45–65.

50. Li PKT, Szeto CC, Piraino B, et al. Peritoneal dialysis-related infections recommendations: 2010 update. Perit Dial Int 2010;30:393–423.

51. Matzke GR. Status of hemodialysis of drugs in 2002. J Pharm Pract 2002;15:405–418.

52. Secker BS, Mueller BA, Sowinski KM. Drug dosing considerations in alternative hemodialysis. Adv Chronic Kidney Dis 2007;14:e17–e26.

53. Cheung AK. Hemodialysis and hemofiltration. In: Greenberg A, Cheung AK, Coffman TM, Falk RJ, Jennette JC, eds. Primer on Kidney Disease, 5th ed. Philadelphia, PA: WB Saunders, 2008.

54. Dager WE, King, JH. Aminoglycosides in intermittent hemodialysis: pharmacokinetics with individual dosing. Ann Pharmacother 2006;40:9–14.

55. Matsuo H, Hayashi J, Ono K, et al. Administration of aminoglycosides to hemodialysis patients immediately before dialysis: A new dosing modality. Antimicrob Agents Chemother 1997;41:2597–2601.

56. Teigen MMB, Duffull S, Dang L, Johnson DW. Dosing of gentamicin in patients with end-stage renal disease receiving hemodialysis. J Clin Pharmacol 2006;46:1259–1267.

57. Mohamed OHK, Wahba IM, Watnick S, et al. Administration of tobramycin in the beginning of the hemodialysis session: A novel intradialytic dosing regimen. Clin J Am Soc Nephrol 2007;2:694–699.

58. Scott Mk, Macias WL, Kraus MA, et al. Effects of dialysis membrane on intradialytic vancomycin administration. Pharmacotherapy 1997;17(2):256–262.

59. Ariano RE, Fine A, Sitar DS, Rexrode S, Zelenitsky SA. Adequacy of a vancomycin dosing regimen in patients receiving high-flux hemodialysis. Am J Kidney Dis 2005;46;681–687.

60. Crawford BS, Largen RF, Walton T, Doran JJ. Once-weekly vancomycin for patients receiving high-flux hemodialysis. Am J Health-Syst Phar 2008;65:1248–1253.

61. van Dijk EA, Drabbe NRG, Kruijtbosch M, De Smet PAGM. Drug dosage adjustments according to renal function at hospital discharge. Ann Pharmacother 2006;40:1254–1260.

58

Disorders of Sodium and Water Homeostasis

JAMES D. COYLE AND GARY R. MATZKE

KEY CONCEPTS

❶ Hypovolemic hypotonic hyponatremia is relatively common in patients taking thiazide diuretics. Thiazide-induced hyponatremia is usually mild and relatively asymptomatic. Hyponatremia rarely if ever occurs with loop diuretics.

❷ The syndrome of inappropriate secretion of antidiuretic hormone causes euvolemic hypotonic hyponatremia. Common causes of this syndrome include lung cancer, central nervous system disorders, pulmonary disorders, and a variety of drugs.

❸ Symptoms of hyponatremia are usually neurologic in nature and symptom severity depends both on the magnitude of the decrease in serum sodium concentration and the rate at which it developed. Treatment of hyponatremia is associated with a risk of osmotic demyelination syndrome, a severe neurologic complication that can develop if the rate of serum sodium correction exceeds 8 to 12 mEq/L (8–12 mmol/L) within 24 hours.

❹ Asymptomatic or mildly symptomatic hyponatremic patients should generally be managed conservatively with treatment directed at the underlying cause. A 0.9% sodium chloride infusion can be cautiously used to correct the serum sodium in patients with hypovolemic hypotonic hyponatremia and moderate to severe symptoms. A 3% sodium chloride infusion can be cautiously used in patients with euvolemic or hypervolemic hypotonic hyponatremia and moderate to severe symptoms.

❺ Hypernatremia most commonly occurs when increased water or hypotonic fluid losses are not offset by increased water intake or administration. For example, patients with diabetes insipidus excrete large volumes of dilute urine, but usually develop hypernatremia only if their water intake does not increase to offset the increased water losses.

❻ Symptoms of hypernatremia are usually neurologic in nature, and range in severity from weakness, lethargy, restlessness, irritability, and confusion to twitching, seizures, coma, and death. The severity of symptoms depends on both the magnitude of the increase in serum sodium and the rate at which it developed.

❼ The treatment goals in patients with hypernatremia include cautious correction of the serum sodium concentration and, when appropriate, restoration of a normal extracellular fluid volume. Too rapid correction of the serum sodium can result in cerebral edema, seizures, neurologic damage, and possibly death. To minimize the risk of these complications, the serum sodium concentration should be corrected at a maximum rate of 0.5 to 1 mEq/L (0.5–1 mmol/L) per hour, depending on the rate of hypernatremia development, and be limited to no more than 10 mEq/L (10 mmol/L) per day.

❽ Patients with central diabetes insipidus should be treated with intranasal desmopressin acetate, with goals of decreasing urine volume to less than 2 L per day while maintaining the serum sodium concentration between 137 and 142 mEq/L (137 and 142 mmol/L). Patients with nephrogenic diabetes insipidus should be treated by correcting the underlying cause when possible, and sodium chloride restriction in conjunction with a thiazide diuretic to decrease the extracellular fluid volume by approximately 1 to 1.5 L.

❾ Edema can develop as a primary defect in renal sodium handling or as a response to a decreased effective circulating volume. It is usually first detected in the feet or pretibial areas of ambulatory patients. Pulmonary edema, evidenced by auscultatory crackles, can be life-threatening.

❿ Diuretics are the primary pharmacologic means for achieving the desired therapeutic outcomes of minimization of edema and improving organ function. Diuretic resistance can be overcome by using an increased dose or by using a combination of a loop diuretic and a thiazide or thiazide-like diuretic.

The human body tightly regulates blood volume and plasma osmolality as both are essential for normal cellular function. Blood volume is important because it is a determinant of effective tissue perfusion which is required to deliver oxygen and nutrients to and remove metabolic waste products from tissues. Plasma osmolality is an important determinant of intracellular volume. Maintenance of normal intracellular volume is particularly critical in the brain, where alterations can result in significant neural dysfunction and potentially death.

The homeostatic mechanisms for regulating blood volume and plasma osmolality involve control of sodium and water balance.[1] Interestingly, the homeostatic mechanisms for controlling blood volume are focused on controlling sodium balance. In contrast, the homeostatic mechanisms for controlling plasma osmolality, which is largely determined by serum sodium concentration, are focused on controlling water balance. Thus, sodium and water balance are closely related and are frequently considered together. Disorders of sodium and water homeostasis are common and potentially serious.

It is important for clinicians to understand these disorders because they can both be caused by and treated with medications. This chapter reviews the etiology, classification, clinical presentation, and therapy for disorders of sodium and water homeostasis.

SODIUM AND WATER HOMEOSTASIS

Hypo- and hypernatremia are syndromes of altered plasma tonicity and cell volume that reflect a change in the ratio of total exchangeable body sodium to total body water. Many factors affect tonicity and water balance and a sound understanding of the pathogenesis and evaluation approaches are of utmost importance if one is to successfully prevent and manage these syndromes.

Sixty percent of total body water is located intracellularly, whereas 40% is contained in the extracellular space.[1] Sodium and its accompanying anions, chloride and bicarbonate, comprise more than 90% of the total osmolality of the extracellular fluid (ECF), whereas intracellular osmolality is primarily dependent on the concentration of potassium and its accompanying anions (mostly organic and inorganic phosphates). The differential concentrations of sodium and potassium in the intra- and extracellular fluid are maintained by the sodium-potassium-adenosine triphosphatase (Na^+-K^+-ATPase) pump.[1,2] Most cell membranes are freely permeable to water, and thus the osmolality of intra- and extracellular body fluids is the same.

Solutes that cannot freely cross cell membranes, such as sodium, are referred to as effective osmoles. The concentration of effective osmoles in the ECF determines the tonicity of the ECF, which directly affects the distribution of water between the extra- and intracellular compartments.[1] Addition of an isotonic solution to the ECF will result in no change in intracellular volume because there will be no change in the effective osmolality of the ECF. Addition of a hypertonic solution to the ECF, however, will result in a decrease in cell volume, whereas addition of a hypotonic solution to the ECF will result in an increase in cell volume. Table 58–1 summarizes the composition of commonly used intravenous solutions and their respective distribution into extracellular and intracellular compartments following infusion.

The serum sodium concentration is tightly regulated, and usually varies by no more than 2% to 3%. Regulation of serum sodium concentration occurs indirectly via mechanisms that control its determinants, plasma osmolality, and blood volume.[1] The kidney regulates water excretion through a feedback mechanism with the hypothalamus, such that the serum osmolality remains relatively constant (275–290 mOsm/kg [275–290 mmol/kg]) despite day-to-day variations in water intake. Plasma osmolality is largely determined by the concentrations of sodium and the accompanying anions chloride and bicarbonate, and can be estimated as:

$$Sosm = (2 \times S_{Na}) + (B_{glucose}/18) + (BUN/2.8)$$

where Sosm = serum osmolality in milliosmoles per kilogram; S_{Na} = serum sodium concentration in mEq/L; $B_{glucose}$ = glucose

concentration in mg/dL; and BUN = blood urea nitrogen concentration in mg/dL.[1,3]

Alternatively, when using SI units the equation becomes:

$$Sosm = (2 \times S_{Na}) + (B_{glucose}) + (BUN)$$

where Sosm = serum osmolality in millimoles per kilogram; S_{Na} = serum sodium concentration in mmol/L; $B_{glucose}$ = glucose concentration in mmol/L; and BUN = blood urea nitrogen concentration in mmol/L.[1,3]

Arginine vasopressin (AVP), commonly known as antidiuretic hormone (ADH), is released from the posterior pituitary when the plasma osmolality increases by 1% to 2% or more.[1] AVP binds to the vasopressin 2 (V2) receptors on the basolateral surface of renal tubular epithelial cells, resulting in the insertion of water channels (aquaporin 2) into the apical tubular lumen surface of the cell.[4] Water can then pass through the cell into the peritubular capillary space where it is then reabsorbed into the systemic circulation. An increase in serum osmolality sensed in the hypothalamus results not only in AVP release, but also in stimulation of thirst. The combination of an increase in water intake and a decrease in water excretion results in a decrease in the serum osmolality and inhibition of AVP secretion once the plasma osmolality is restored to normal.

Nonosmotic release of AVP occurs when a decrease in a person's effective circulating blood volume results in a decrease in systemic blood pressure.[1] The effective circulating volume is that part of the ECF that is located in the arterial system and is responsible for organ perfusion.[1] A decrease in the effective circulating volume (more accurately, the pressure associated with that volume) activates arterial baroreceptors in the carotid sinus and glomerular afferent arterioles, resulting in stimulation of the renin-angiotensin system and increased synthesis of angiotensin II. Angiotensin II stimulates both nonosmotic release of AVP and thirst. This volume stimulus overrides osmotic inhibition of AVP release, and conservation of water fosters restoration of effective circulating volume and blood pressure at the expense of hypo-osmolality.

Proper assessment of a patient with an abnormal serum sodium concentration requires knowledge of the fact that changes in the serum sodium concentration do not necessarily correlate with changes in ECF volume or sodium content as the sodium concentration is determined by the ratio of the ECF sodium content and ECF volume.[1] Although hyponatremia and hypernatremia can be associated with conditions of high, low, or normal ECF sodium and volume, both conditions are most commonly the result of abnormalities of water metabolism.[1]

HYPONATREMIA

EPIDEMIOLOGY AND ETIOLOGY

Hyponatremia (serum sodium <135 mEq/L [<135 mmol/L]) is the most common electrolyte abnormality encountered in clinical

---

TABLE 58-1 Composition of Intravenous Replacement Solutions

Solution	Dextrose	[Na⁺] (mEq/L or mmol/L)	[Cl⁻] (mEq/L or mmol/L)	Tonicity	Distribution		
					% ECF	% ICF	Free Water/L
D_5W	5 g/dL (50 g/L)	0	0	Hypotonic	40	60	1,000 mL
0.45% sodium chloride	0	77	77	Hypotonic	73	37	500 mL
0.9% sodium chloride	0	154	154	Isotonic	100	0	0 mL
3% sodium chloride^a	0	513	513	Hypertonic	100	0	−2,331 mL

Cl⁻, chloride; D_5W, 5% dextrose in water; ECF, extracellular fluid; ICF, intracellular fluid; Na⁺, sodium.
^{a}This solution will result in osmotic removal of water from the intracellular space.

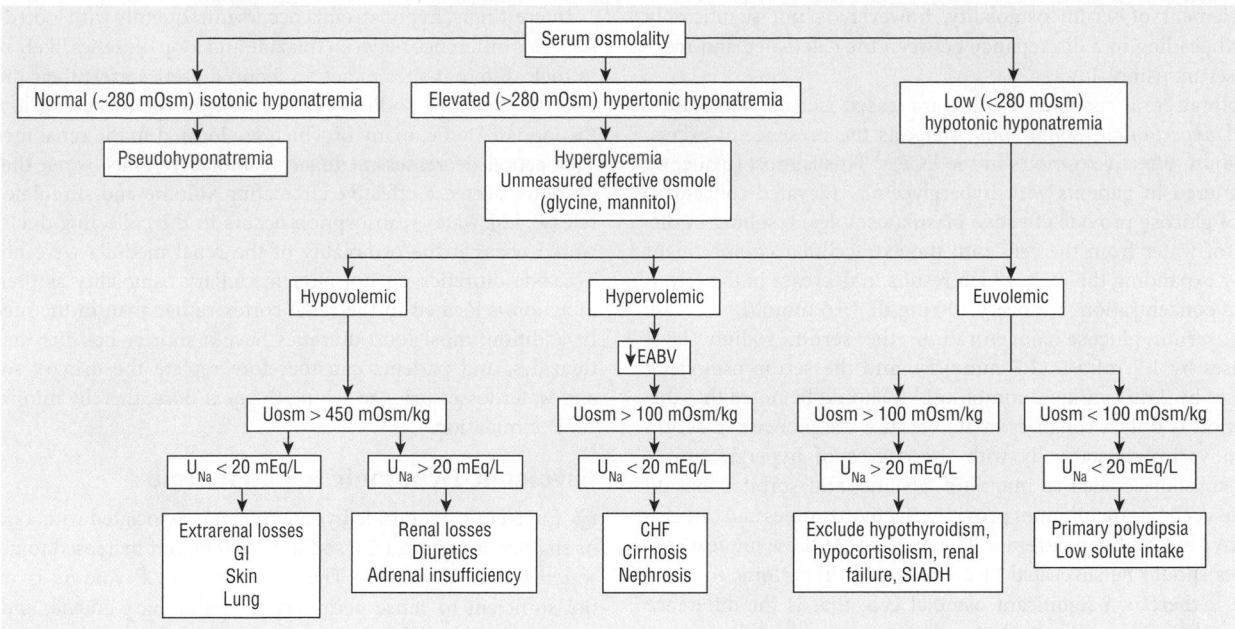

FIGURE 58-1. Diagnostic algorithm for the evaluation of hyponatremia. (CHF, congestive heart failure; SIADH, syndrome of inappropriate secretion of antidiuretic hormone; U_{Na}, urine sodium concentration [values in mEq/L are numerically equivalent to mmol/L]; Uosm, urine osmolality [values in mOsm/kg are numerically equivalent to mmol/kg].)

practice.[5,6] Although its prevalence is not well established and varies with the patient population studied, it has been estimated to be as high as 28% in patients admitted to an acute care hospital. Mild hyponatremia (serum sodium <136 mEq/L [<136 mmol/L]) was observed in 42.6%, while 6.2% of patients had values <126 mEq/L (<126 mmol/L), and only 1.2% had values <116 mEq/L (<116 mmol/L). The incidence has been reported to be as high as 21% in patients seen in ambulatory hospital clinics, and 7% in community clinics.[7] Drug-induced hyponatremia, especially that associated with diuretics and psychotropic medications, is more commonly seen in women than men. Increasing age (>30 years) is also clearly a risk factor for hyponatremia, independent of gender.[7]

Hyponatremia incidence in the nursing home setting is 2-fold higher than that observed in similar aged-community dwelling individuals.[5] Over 75% of these episodes were precipitated by increased fluid intake of hypotonic oral or intravenous fluids. Similarly, the ingestion of excessive quantities of fluids has been identified as a key risk factor in marathon runners who develop hyponatremia. Although women had a 3-fold higher rate of hyponatremia, smaller body size and longer racing time, not gender, appear to be the principle factors which account for the increased incidence.[8]

Recognition of the high prevalence of hyponatremia is important because this condition is associated with significant morbidity and mortality.[9,10,11] Transient or permanent brain dysfunction can result from either the acute effects of hypo-osmolality or from too rapid correction of hypo-osmolality in patients with symptomatic hyponatremia. Hyponatremia is predominantly the result of an excess of extracellular water relative to sodium because of impaired water excretion. The kidney normally has the capacity to excrete large volumes of dilute urine after ingestion of a water load. Nonosmotic release of AVP, however, can lead to retention of water and to a drop in serum sodium concentration, despite a fall in both serum and intracellular osmolality. The causes of nonosmotic release of AVP include hypovolemia, decreased effective circulating volume as seen in patients with chronic heart failure (CHF), nephrosis, and cirrhosis. The syndrome of inappropriate antidiuretic hormone secretion (SIADH) is also a common cause of hyponatremia which is associated with oncologic disease, especially small cell lung cancer.[10] The

pathophysiology, clinical features, and management of hyponatremia are detailed below.

PATHOPHYSIOLOGY

Hyponatremia can be associated with normal, increased, or decreased plasma osmolality, depending on its cause (Fig. 58-1).[1,3] Hyponatremia in patients with normal serum osmolality can be caused by hyperlipidemia or hyperproteinemia. Historically, this form of hyponatremia, termed *pseudohyponatremia*, was an artifact of the method of serum sodium concentration measurement. This laboratory artifact is uncommon today and has been overcome with the use of ion-specific electrodes to measure the serum sodium concentration. If the sodium concentration in a laboratory is still measured by flame photometry, the volume of serum will be overestimated because the elevated lipids or proteins account for a greater proportion of the total volume of the sample (Fig. 58-2). Because the sodium is distributed in only the water component of serum, the measured serum sodium concentration is falsely decreased. The

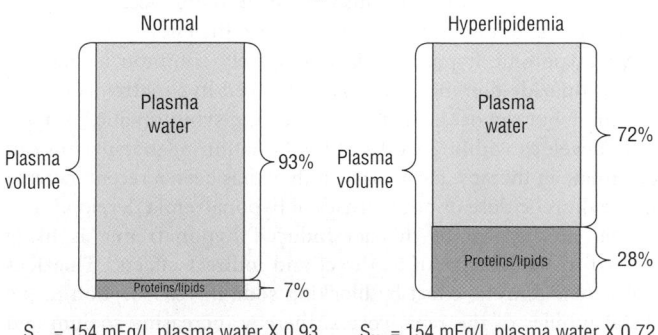

FIGURE 58-2. Elevated lipids or proteins result in a larger discrepancy between the volume of the sample and plasma water, leading to a falsely low measurement of the serum sodium concentration when using the method of flame photometry. (S_{Na}, serum sodium concentration [values in mEq/L are numerically equivalent to mmol/L].)

measurement of serum osmolality, however, is not significantly affected, leading to a discrepancy between the calculated and measured serum osmolality.

Hyponatremia associated with increased serum osmolality, termed *hypertonic hyponatremia*, suggests the presence of excess, nonsodium-effective osmoles in the ECF.[1,3] This is most frequently encountered in patients with hyperglycemia. Elevated concentrations of glucose provide effective plasma osmoles, resulting in diffusion of water from the cells into the extracellular compartment thereby expanding the ECF, which results in decrease in the serum sodium concentration. For every 100 mg/dL (5.6 mmol/L) increase in the serum glucose concentration, the serum sodium level decreases by 1.7 mEq/L (1.7 mmol/L), and the serum osmolality increases by 2 mOsm/kg (2 mmol/kg).[3] It should be noted that this correction is only a rough estimate because the increase in serum sodium varies substantially with the degree of hyperglycemia.[12] Other substances such as mannitol, glycine, and sorbitol that do not cross cellular membranes provide effective osmoles and can also cause hypertonic hyponatremia. The presence of these unmeasured osmoles should be suspected in patients with hypertonic hyponatremia if there is a significant osmolal gap, that is the difference between the measured and calculated plasma osmolality.[1]

Hyponatremia associated with decreased plasma osmolality, termed *hypotonic hyponatremia*, is the most common form of hyponatremia and has many potential causes (see Fig. 58–1).[1,3] An important step in the diagnostic evaluation of patients with hypotonic hyponatremia is clinical assessment of the patient's extracellular fluid volume.[3] Categorization of these patients into one of three groups (decreased, increased, or clinically normal ECF volume) is very helpful in identifying the pathophysiologic mechanisms responsible for the hyponatremia and an appropriate treatment regimen.

Hypovolemic Hypotonic Hyponatremia

Most patients with ECF volume contraction lose fluids that are hypotonic relative to plasma and thus can be transiently hypernatremic. This includes patients with fluid losses caused by diarrhea, excessive sweating, and diuretics. This transient hypernatremic hyperosmolality results in osmotic release of AVP and stimulation of thirst. If sodium and water losses continue, more AVP is released as a result of hypovolemia. Patients who then drink water or who are given hypotonic fluids intravenously retain water and develop hyponatremia. These patients typically have a urine osmolality greater than 450 mOsm/kg (greater than 450 mmol/kg), reflecting the presence of AVP and formation of a concentrated urine.[13] The urine sodium concentration is <20 mEq/L (<20 mmol/L) when sodium losses are extrarenal, as in patients with diarrhea, and >20 mEq/L (>20 mmol/L) in patients with renal sodium losses, as occurs in the setting of diuretic use or adrenal insufficiency.[13]

❶ Hypotonic hyponatremia is relatively common in patients taking thiazide diuretics.[14] Thiazide-induced hyponatremia is usually mild, but can occasionally be severe and symptomatic.[15] It typically develops within 2 weeks of the initiation of therapy, but can occur late in therapy, particularly if there has been a recent increase in the diuretic dose or other causes of hyponatremia develop.[1,15]

The mechanism of thiazide-induced hyponatremia is likely related to the balance of its direct and indirect effects.[1] Thiazides exert their diuretic effect by blocking sodium reabsorption in the distal tubules of the renal cortex, thereby increasing sodium and water removal from the body. The resulting decrease in effective circulating volume stimulates AVP release. Increased AVP release results in increased reabsorption of free water in the collecting duct, as well as increased water intake because of stimulation of thirst. Hyponatremia develops when the net result of these effects is the loss of more sodium than water.

Interestingly, hyponatremia occurs infrequently with loop diuretics.[1] This difference between thiazide and loop diuretics likely relates to their different sites of action. Loop diuretics exert their diuretic effect by blocking sodium reabsorption in the ascending limbs of the loop of Henle, many of which are located in the renal medulla. This action decreases medullary osmolality. Thus, when the loop diuretics decrease effective circulating volume and stimulate AVP release, less water reabsorption occurs in the collecting ducts than would occur if the osmolality of the renal medulla were normal. Thiazide diuretics do not alter medullary osmolality as their site of action is located in the renal cortex rather than in the medulla. In addition, most loop diuretics have a shorter half-life than the thiazides, and patients can therefore replete the urinary sodium and water losses prior to taking the next dose, thereby minimizing AVP stimulation.

Euvolemic Hypotonic Hyponatremia

❷ Euvolemic hypotonic hyponatremia is associated with a normal or slightly decreased ECF sodium content and increased total body water and ECF volume. The increase in ECF volume is usually not sufficient to cause peripheral or pulmonary edema, and thus patients appear clinically euvolemic. Euvolemic hyponatremia is most commonly the result of SIADH release. In this syndrome, water intake exceeds the capacity of the kidneys to excrete water, either because of an increased release of AVP via nonosmotic and/or nonphysiologic processes or enhanced renal sensitivity to AVP.[16] The urine osmolality in patients with SIADH is generally greater than 100 mOsm/kg (greater than 100 mmol/kg), and the urine sodium concentration is usually greater than 20 mEq/L (greater than 20 mmol/L) as a result of the ECF volume expansion.

The most common causes of SIADH include tumors such as small cell lung cancer, central nervous system disorders (e.g., head trauma, stroke, meningitis, and pituitary surgery), as well as pulmonary disease.[3] Patients with renal insufficiency, adrenal insufficiency, and hypothyroidism can also present with euvolemic hyponatremia, and the evaluation of patients with suspected SIADH should always include consideration of these disorders. A wide variety of drugs can also cause SIADH by enhancing AVP release, the renal effect of AVP or by unknown mechanisms.[3,10,11,17,18] (Table 58–1) The differential diagnosis of euvolemic hypotonic hyponatremia also includes primary or psychogenic polydipsia. Patients with this disorder drink more water (usually >20 L/day) than the kidneys can excrete as solute-free water. Unlike SIADH, however, AVP is suppressed, resulting in a urine osmolality that is less than 100 mOsm/kg (less than 100 mmol/kg). The urine sodium is typically low (<15 mEq/L [<15 mmol/L]) as a result of urinary dilution.[19] Hyponatremia can develop with more modest water intake in patients who are ingesting a very low-solute diet, such as a low-sodium vegetarian diet.

Hypervolemic Hypotonic Hyponatremia

Hyponatremia associated with an increase in ECF volume occurs in conditions in which renal sodium and water excretion are impaired. Patients with cirrhosis, congestive heart failure, and nephrotic syndrome have an expanded ECF volume and edema, but a decreased effective circulating volume. This decreased volume results in renal sodium retention, and eventually ECF volume expansion and edema. At the same time, there is nonosmotic release of AVP and retention of water in excess of sodium, which perpetuats the hyponatremia.

CLINICAL PRESENTATION

❸ Patients with chronic, mild hyponatremia (serum sodium concentration greater than 125–130 mEq/L [greater than

125–130 mmol/L]) are usually asymptomatic, with hyponatremia being discovered incidentally when serum electrolytes are measured for other purposes.[1,3,20] However, recent data from a small number of carefully evaluated patients suggest that it might be more accurate to say that symptoms of mild hyponatremia are frequently unnoticed by both physician and patient.[21] These data suggest that chronic, mild hyponatremia is associated with impairment of attention, posture, and gait, all of which contribute to a substantially increased risk of falls. Even those who seem to be "asymptomatic" when formally tested can be shown to have impaired attention and gait to a degree that is compatible with a blood alcohol level of 0.06% (13 mmol/L).[22,23]

Patients with moderate (serum sodium concentration of 115–125 mEq/L [115–125 mmol/L]) to severe (serum sodium concentration less than 110–115 mEq/L [110–115 mmol/L]) or rapidly developing hypotonic hyponatremia often present with a range of neurologic symptoms resulting from hypoosmolality-induced volume expansion of brain cells.[1,3,20] Classic symptoms include nausea and malaise, headache, lethargy, restlessness, and disorientation, and in some seizures, coma, permanent brain damage, respiratory arrest, brainstem herniation, and death.

The presence of these symptoms and their severity depend on both the magnitude of the hyponatremia and the rate at which the hyponatremia developed.[1,3,20] The magnitude of the hyponatremia is important because serum osmolality decreases in direct proportion to the serum sodium concentration, and water movement into brain cells increases as serum osmolality decreases. The rate of osmolality change is an important factor because brain cells are able to adjust their intracellular osmolality to minimize cellular volume changes in response to volume changes, but time is required for this adaptation to occur.[1,24] When a decline in plasma osmolality causes movement of water into brain cells, sodium, potassium, and *organic osmolytes* move out of the cells to decrease intracellular osmolality and minimize intracellular water movement. Organic osmolytes, such as myoinositol, are osmotically active substances that contribute substantially to controlling intracellular osmolality without directly altering cellular function.[24] The various components of this adaptive mechanism occur over different time frames, with sodium and potassium efflux occurring over minutes to several hours and organic osmolyte efflux occurring over hours to days.[24] Maximal compensation for a decrease in plasma osmolality typically requires up to 48 hours. Thus, acute changes in plasma osmolality are not compensated for instantaneously and are more likely to be associated with symptoms. Patients with concurrent respiratory failure and hypoxemia are at greater risk for adverse neurologic outcomes because hypoxemia diminishes the capacity of the brain to actively transport solute out of cells, leading to a higher incidence of cerebral edema.[25] Children and women have been noted to have poor clinical outcomes relative to adults and males. For example, women have a 25-fold higher risk of death or permanent neurological damage than men.[26]

In addition to neurologic symptoms, patients with hypovolemic hyponatremia can present with signs and symptoms of hypovolemia, including dry mucous membranes, decreased skin turgor, tachycardia, decreased jugular venous pressure, and orthostatic hypotension. These findings are helpful in identifying the type of hyponatremia.

The brain's adaptation to changes in plasma osmolality is also associated with symptoms that can develop if hyponatremia is corrected too rapidly (i.e., >12 mEq/L [>12 mmol/L] per day). These patients might experience an acute decrease in brain cell volume, which contributes to the pathogenesis of *osmotic demyelination syndrome*.[27,28] Patients with this complication might develop para- or quadriparesis, pseudo-bulbar palsy, and locked-in syndrome

5 to 7 days after treatment because of demyelination lesions in the pons.[28,29] Patients who have a significant degree of cerebral adaptation to hypotonic hyponatremia are at higher risk of experiencing this syndrome.[28] This is presumably because these patients have lower intracellular osmolalities at the initiation of therapy, which results in greater decreases in intracellular volume when the plasma osmolality is raised rapidly. Brain adaptation to increases in plasma osmolality requires time, just as was true for its initial adaptation to a decrease in serum sodium concentration.

CLINICAL PRESENTATION OF HYPONATREMIA

General

- Hyponatremia is asymptomatic in most patients. Symptoms directly attributable to hyponatremia include neurologic dysfunction associated with cerebral edema.

Symptoms

- The presence and severity of symptoms are related both to the magnitude and rapidity of onset of the hyponatremia. Nausea and malaise are the earliest findings, followed by headache, lethargy, restlessness, and disorientation, and eventually seizures, coma, permanent brain damage, respiratory arrest, brainstem herniation, and death if hyponatremia is severe or develops rapidly. Other symptoms that can be seen with hyponatremia are those attributable to its underlying cause, such as volume depletion in patients with hypovolemic hypotonic hypo-osmolality or volume excess in patients with hypervolemic hypotonic hyponatremia.

Signs

- General: Dry mucous membranes, decreased skin turgor, tachycardia, decreased jugular venous pressure, and postural hypotension can be present in hypovolemic patients.

- Pulmonary: Noncardiogenic pulmonary edema has been described.

- Neurologic: Depressed reflexes. Rapid correction of hyponatremia can result in an acute decrease in brain cell volume resulting in demyelinating brain injury.

Laboratory Tests

- Serum sodium values <135 mEq/L (<135 mmol/L) are present. Plasma osmolality and urine sodium concentration can be helpful in diagnosing the cause. Tests including but not limited to serum glucose and lipids and tests to assess kidney and thyroid function should be conducted to identify or rule out potential causes.

TREATMENT

Hyponatremia

■ DESIRED OUTCOME

❹ The goal of treating patients with hypovolemic hypotonic hyponatremia is to resolve the underlying cause of the sodium and ECF volume deficits, and safely correct the hyponatremia. The treatment goals for hypervolemic and euvolemic hypotonic patients depend on the underlying cause of the hyponatremia and the severity of the patient's symptoms. Patients with an acute onset of hyponatremia or severe symptoms require more aggressive therapy to correct the hypotonicity. The initial goal for these patients is to increase plasma tonicity enough to control the severe symptoms; this typically requires a relatively small increase in serum sodium concentration of approximatley 5%.[3] Once control of the severe symptoms is achieved, full correction of the serum sodium concentration should be achieved at a controlled rate. Asymptomatic patients and patients with mild to moderate symptoms do not require rapid correction of the serum sodium and the treatment is dictated by the underlying etiology. In all cases the goal is to avoid an increase in the serum sodium concentration more than 12 mEq/L (more than 12 mmol/L) in 24 hours.[1,3,30] Some recommend that the maximal rate of correction not exceed 8 mEq/L (8 mmol/L) in 24 hours.[20]

■ GENERAL APPROACH TO TREATMENT

The following principles serve as general guidelines for the treatment of patients with hyponatremia:[1,3,13,20,30] (1) It is important for both the short- and long-term management of the patient to treat the underlying cause of hyponatremia. (2) Appropriate treatment of patients with hypotonic hyponatremia requires balancing the risks of the hyponatremia versus the risk of osmotic demyelination syndrome. In general, patients who acutely developed moderate to severe hyponatremia and/or patients who have severe symptoms are at greatest risk and potentially benefit most from more rapid correction of their hyponatremia. (3) Active correction of hypovolemic hypotonic hyponatremia is usually best accomplished with 0.9% sodium chloride solution as these patients have both sodium and water deficits. (4) Active correction of euvolemic and hypervolemic hypotonic hyponatremia in patients who do not require rapid correction is usually best accomplished by water restriction. Demeclocycline, vasopressin V2-receptor antagonists (vaptans), or sodium chloride plus a loop diuretic, can be used if the initial response to water restriction is not adequate. In patients with severe symptoms, 3% sodium chloride solution (possibly combined with furosemide) should initially be used to more rapidly correct the hyponatremia. Furosemide can be administered concurrently to enhance the serum sodium correction by increasing the excretion of water. (5) Long-term management is required for patients in whom the underlying cause of hyponatremia cannot be corrected. This can include water restriction, increasing sodium intake, and/or the use of an AVP antagonist. Application of these principles to the treatment of patients with various forms of hypotonic hyponatremia is discussed in the following sections.

ACUTE OR SEVERELY SYMPTOMATIC HYPOTONIC HYPONATREMIA

A patient who has or is at high risk of experiencing severe symptoms caused by hyponatremia should receive either 3% or 0.9% sodium chloride solution until severe symptoms resolve.[1,3,13,20,30] Resolution of severe symptoms frequently requires only a small, 5% increase in serum sodium, although some suggest that the initial target should be to increase serum sodium to approximately 120 mEq/L (120 mmol/L).[3,31] The relative concentrations of urine sodium and potassium (osmotically effective urine cations) must be compared with those of the infusate in planning a treatment regimen for patients with hypotonic hyponatremia. For the serum sodium to increase after infusion of a solution of sodium chloride, the concentration of sodium in the infusate must exceed the sum of the sodium and potassium concentration in the urine to effect net-free water excretion.

Patients with SIADH often have urinary concentrations of osmotically effective urine cations that exceed the sodium concentration of 0.9% sodium chloride (154 mEq/L [154 mmol/L]), and thus these patients should be preferentially treated with 3% sodium chloride (513 mEq/L [513 mmol/L]). In this case use of isotonic sodium chloride carries the potential hazard of actually worsening hypona-

tremia.[1,31] The relatively high concentration of urinary sodium in patients with SIADH stems from the fact that the ECF is expanded, thus minimizing reabsorption of sodium along the nephron. When the urine osmolality exceeds 300 mOsm/kg (300 mmol/kg), it is generally advisable to add an intravenous loop diuretic, not only to increase the excretion of solute-free water, but also to prevent volume overload, which can result from infusion of hypertonic sodium chloride. Intravenous furosemide, initially at a dose of 40 mg every 6 hours, is generally sufficient to prevent volume overload and to decrease the concentration of osmotically active urine cations to less than 150 mEq/L (less than 150 mmol/L).

Patients with hypovolemic hypotonic hyponatremia, conversely, can be treated with 0.9% sodium chloride solution. In contrast to patients with SIADH, patients with this condition avidly reabsorb sodium throughout the nephron when the effective circulating blood volume is decreased. Thus the urine osmolality is primarily comprised of urea, and the concentration of urine sodium is often less than 20 mEq/L (less than 20 mmol/L), which is substantially less than the sodium concentration in 0.9% sodium chloride solution. Use of 3% sodium chloride solution will also effectively correct hyponatremia in these patients, but its use should be reserved for situations requiring very rapid correction.

Hypervolemic hypotonic hyponatremic patients are particularly problematic to manage acutely because the sodium and volume required to minimize the risk of cerebral edema or seizures can worsen their already compensated hepatic, cardiac, or renal function. It is generally agreed that these patients should be treated with hypertonic sodium chloride and prompt initiation of fluid restriction. Loop diuretic therapy will also likely be required to facilitate urinary excretion of free water.

■ DETERMINATION OF SODIUM CHLORIDE INFUSION REGIMEN

Several methods for determining the correct sodium chloride solution infusion regimen for a hyponatremic patient have been proposed.[1,3,32–36] It is important to recognize that usual approaches provide only a rough estimate of the correct infusion regimen as their use involves known but yet incorrect assumptions. More accurate equations have recently been derived, but the benefits of this more complex approach relative to the approach outlined below remain to be determined.[33,34]

One commonly used approach for estimation of the change in plasma sodium resulting from the infusion of 1 L of 3% or 0.9% sodium chloride solution is:[3,32]

Change in S_{Na} with 1 L of infusate

$$= [IV_{Na} - S^1_{Na}] \div (BW + IV_{vol})$$

where S^1_{Na} = initial patient serum sodium concentration; IV_{Na} = sodium concentration of infusate (154 mEq/L [154 mmol/L] for 0.9% sodium chloride or 513 mEq/L [513 mmol/L] for 3% sodium chloride); IV_{vol} = 1 L of infusate; and BW = total body water (in liters), which can be estimated as a fraction of body weight (kilograms) as follows[37]:

0.6 × body weight for children and men <70 years old
0.5 × body weight for men ≥70 years old and females <70 years old
0.45 × body weight for women ≥70 years old

The appropriate infusion volume for a given patient can then be estimated based on the proportion of the estimated change that would result from a 1-L infusion that is actually desired in that patient. Finally, an appropriate infusion rate can be calculated for this infusion volume to control the rate of increase in the serum sodium concentration.

For example, consider the case of a 170 centimeter (5 feet 7 inch), 60 kilogram (132 pound), 66-year-old woman who presents with nausea, vertigo, and disorientation that have developed over the past several days. She was started on carbamazepine 10 days ago for the treatment of trigeminal neuralgia. Her serum sodium is currently 108 mEq/L (108 mmol/L). Assuming this woman has carbamazepine-induced SIADH, an initial approach to treatment might include discontinuing her carbamazepine and partially correcting her hyponatremia by raising her serum sodium to approximately 120 mEq/L (120 mmol/L) over the first 24 hours of hospitalization. This should be an adequate response to alleviate her current symptoms, decrease the risk of more severe symptoms, and minimize the risk of osmotic demyelination syndrome. Assuming that use of 3% sodium chloride solution is appropriate, the infusion regimen required to increase her serum sodium to 120 mEq/L (120 mmol/L) over the next 24 hours can be calculated as follows:

Change in S^1_{Na} with 1 L of infusate =

$$(513 \text{ mEq/L} - 108 \text{ mEq/L}) \div [(0.5 \text{ L/kg} \times 60 \text{ kg}) + 1.0 \text{ L}]$$
$$= 13.1 \text{ mEq/L or } 1.31 \text{ mEq/100 mL}$$

In SI units:

$$(513 \text{ mmol/L} - 108 \text{ mmol/L}) \div [(0.5 \text{ L/kg} \times 60 \text{ kg}) + 1.0 \text{ L}]$$
$$= 13.1 \text{ mmol/L or } 1.31 \text{ mmol/100 mL}$$

Because infusion of 1 L of 3% sodium chloride solution would produce a 13.1 mEq/L (13.1 mmol/L) rise in the serum sodium, and we desire only a 12 mEq/L (12 mmol/L) increase, the appropriate infusion volume is 916 mL [(12 mEq/L ÷ 13.1 mEq/L) × 1,000 mL] or in SI units [(12 mmol/L ÷ 13.1 mmol/L) × 1,000 mL]. The approach to this calculation would be similar if 0.9% sodium chloride solution were used, except that the expected increase in serum sodium concentration would be only 1.5 mEq/L (1.5 mmol/L) per liter infused, and an infusion volume of approximately 8 L would be required to achieve the targeted serum sodium concentration.

In the presence of symptoms, the serum sodium should be increased by approximately 1.5 mEq/L (1.5 mmol/L) per hour over the first 2 to 4 hours (for a total of 3 to 6 mEq/L [3 to 6 mmol/L]) or until the symptoms have resolved. Thus, an initial infusion rate of 114 mL/h [1.5 mEq/L per hour ÷ 1.31 mEq/L per 100 mL] or [1.5 mmol/L per hour ÷ 1.31 mmol/L per 100 mL] for SI units for the first 2 to 4 hours, followed by an infusion rate of approximately 23 to 31 mL/h for the next 20 to 22 hours, respectively, would be a reasonable initial treatment plan.

CLINICAL CONTROVERSY

Clinicians often disagree whether or not to administer 3% sodium chloride to patients with symptomatic hypotonicity. Advantages of 3% sodium chloride include more rapid correction of serum sodium concentration and smaller infusion volumes. The disadvantage of 3% sodium chloride is a higher risk of exceeding maximum recommended rates of correction and causing osmotic demyelination syndrome. The clinician must carefully consider the cause of the patient's hyponatremia as well as the relative risk of slower correction of the hyponatremia versus the development of osmotic demyelination syndrome.

■ EVALUATION OF THERAPEUTIC OUTCOMES

Patients with severely symptomatic hypotonic hyponatremia should be admitted to the intensive care unit or to a highly monitored setting for close monitoring of neurologic and volume status. Serial physical examinations of the heart, lungs, and neurologic status should be performed several times over the initial 12 hours of hospitalization. The serum sodium concentration should be measured every 2 to 4 hours, and the urine osmolality, sodium, and potassium should be measured every 4 to 6 hours over the first day of therapy. The rate of administration of the infusate should then be adjusted to avoid exceeding a rise in the serum sodium greater than 12 mEq/L (greater than 12 mmol/L) per day.

NONEMERGENT HYPOVOLEMIC HYPOTONIC HYPONATREMIA

Most patients with hypovolemic hypotonic hyponatremia do not require rapid correction of their hyponatremia because they are either asymptomatic or have only mild-to-moderate symptoms. Many of these patients are at higher risk of developing osmotic demyelination syndrome if serum sodium correction occurs too rapidly because they have chronic hyponatremia that has been maximally compensated for by the brain's osmotic adaptation. The combination of the adaptive decrease in intracellular osmolality and rapid increase in serum osmolality results in excessive movement of water out of the brain cells, intracellular volume depletion, and thereby an increased risk of osmotic demyelination syndrome. Treatment of these patients should include correction of the underlying condition, if possible. When direct treatment of the hyponatremia is justified, a 0.9% solution of sodium chloride should be used.[1] This solution effectively replaces both the sodium and water deficits that characterize these patients and presents a lower risk of an excessive rate of correction than 3% sodium chloride solution.

A patient's ECF volume deficit (ECFVd) can be estimated based on sex, change in body weight, and age. For example, consider the case of a 56-year-old woman who was started on hydrochlorothiazide 10 days ago for the treatment of hypertension. She is 173 cm (5 ft 8 in) tall and weighed 62 kg (137 lb) at that time. Today she presents with complaints of mild nausea and "feeling dizzy" when she stands up. Her weight is now 55.5 kg (122 lb). Physical examination reveals dry mucous membranes and orthostatic hypotension. Her serum sodium is 125 mEq/L (125 mmol/L). The patient's ECFVd could be estimated as follows:[38]

$$\text{ECFVd} = \text{ECFV}_{norm} - \text{ECFV}_{current}$$
$$\text{ECFVd} = [\text{TBW}_{norm} \times 0.5 \text{ L/kg} \times 0.33] - [\text{TBW}_{current} \times 0.5 \text{ L/kg} \times 0.33]$$
$$\text{ECFVd} = [62 \text{ kg} \times 0.5 \text{ L/kg} \times 0.33] - [55.3 \text{ kg} \times 0.5 \text{ L/kg} \times 0.33]$$
$$\text{ECFVd} = 1.1 \text{ L}$$

If the patient's previous weight were not known, it could be roughly estimated based on clinical signs and symptoms. The presence of hyponatremia suggests an ECFVd of 5% or more, whereas the presence of orthostatic hypotension suggests an ECFVd of at least 10% to 15%. A 0.9% solution of sodium chloride is considered to be isotonic and thus is optimal to correct the volume deficit because it will remain in the ECF space (see Table 58–1).

The expected increase in the serum sodium concentration following infusion of 1 L of 0.9% sodium chloride (154 mEq/L [154 mmol/L]) can be estimated as:

Change in S_{Na} with 1 L of infusate = $[IV_{Na} - S^1_{Na}] \div (BW + IV_{vol})$
$$= [154 \text{ mEq/L} - 125 \text{ mEq/L}] \div [(0.5 \text{ L/kg} \times 55.3 \text{ kg}) + 1.0 \text{ L}]$$
$$= 1.0 \text{ mEq/L}$$

In SI units:

$$= [154 \text{ mmol/L} - 125 \text{ mmol/L}] \div [(0.5 \text{ L/kg} \times 55.3 \text{ kg}) + 1.0 \text{ L}]$$
$$= 1.0 \text{ mmol/L}$$

The patient's sodium serum concentration can thus be predicted to be 126 mEq/L (125 mEq/L + 1.0 mEq/L) or 126 mmol/L (125 mmol/L + 1.0 mmol/L) following the infusion.

Because the overriding initial treatment goal is to restore effective circulating volume, it might be necessary to infuse 0.9% sodium chloride at 200 to 400 mL/h until symptoms of hypovolemia moderate. The infusion rate can then be decreased to 100 to 150 mL/h so that the serum sodium level increases by no more than 12 mEq/L (12 mmol/L) over the initial 24 hours. Infusion of 0.9% sodium chloride at rates greater than 250 mL/h should be used cautiously in patients with a history of left ventricular dysfunction or renal insufficiency. It is important to recognize that the rate of increase in the serum sodium concentration can substantially increase once hypovolemia has been corrected if infusion rates are not decreased.[1] Once the ECF volume is restored, AVP secretion will cease, and a rapid water diuresis can ensue, which can potentially result in an increase in the serum sodium at a rate greater than 12 mEq/L (greater than 12 mmol/L) per day. Ideally, the potential for this increase in correction rate is recognized prospectively and infusion rates are appropriately adjusted. Estimation of the patient's ECFVd at the initiation of therapy can help in this regard. If the serum sodium is observed to be increasing at a rate greater than 12 mEq/L (greater than 12 mmol/L) per day, the infusate should be changed to 0.45% sodium chloride, and the infusion rate set to one that approximates urine output (approximately 1.5–2 mL/kg per hour is a reasonable initial rate), to slow the rate of increase in the serum sodium concentration.[3]

■ EVALUATION OF THERAPEUTIC OUTCOMES

Patients presenting with evidence of volume depletion should be reexamined frequently during the initial few hours of therapy. The serum sodium concentration should be measured every 2 to 4 hours to allow timely adjustment of the rate and composition of intravenous fluids to avoid an increase in the serum sodium greater than 12 mEq/L (greater than 12 mmol/L) per day. Intravenous 0.9% sodium chloride should be administered judiciously in patients with a history of congestive heart failure or renal insufficiency, with frequent assessments of the cardiopulmonary examination so the infusion rate can be appropriately decreased at the earliest sign of pulmonary congestion.

NONEMERGENT EUVOLEMIC HYPOTONIC HYPONATREMIA

The fact that an individual's neurolgical performance is restored to normal with correction of their hyponatremia provides a rationale for therapeutic management of all patients to maintain their serum sodium above 135 mEq/L (135 mmol/L).[5] Long-term management is thus required for patients in whom the underlying cause of hyponatremia is not readily correctable. The treatment of SIADH always involves water restriction and correction of the underlying cause, if possible. Drugs that could be contributing should be identified and discontinued. The goal is to induce negative water balance by restricting water intake to less than 1,000 to 1,200 mL/day, such that water losses from insensible sources (skin and lung) and from obligate urine and fecal losses exceed intake. Daily insensible water losses via skin and lungs are approximately 900 mL/day, whereas approximately 200 mL and a minimum of 500 mL/day is lost in stool and in urine output, respectively. Because approximately 850 mL of water per day is ingested in food, and an additional 350 mL are generated from oxidative processes, the water intake reduction should result in a negative water balance of several hundred milliliters per day.[1] Other goals include maintenance of the serum sodium level above 125 mEq/L (125 mmol/L) to prevent symptoms of hypotonicity, and avoidance of iatrogenic hypo- or hypervolemia.

Patients with chronic SIADH who are unable to restrict water sufficiently to maintain the serum sodium greater than 120 to 125 mEq/L (greater than 120–125 mmol/L) can be treated by increasing solute intake with sodium chloride and/or loop diuretics.[3] Sodium chloride or urea tablets increase the obligatory daily solute excretion, which augments the capacity for renal water excretion. The goal is to increase the daily solute intake and excretion to approximately 900 mOsm (900 mmol) per day. Because an average diet contains approximately 600 mOsm (600 mmol), 9 grams of sodium chloride would be required to increase the osmolar excretion to 900 mOsm/day (900 mmol/day) (each 1-g sodium chloride tablet contains 17 mmol of sodium and 17 mmol of chloride). Because extracellular volume expansion is an expected adverse effect, a loop diuretic should be administered concurrently to avoid pulmonary congestion and peripheral edema. Loop diuretics also enhance water excretion by limiting the formation of the medullary concentration gradient.[39]

Demeclocycline is another treatment option for patients who are not adequately controlled by fluid restriction alone. Demeclocycline inhibits tubular AVP activity, resulting in increased water excretion.[1,40] The usual dose of demeclocycline is 300 mg 2 to 4 times daily. Because of its delayed onset of action (3–6 days), this agent has no role in the acute management of severe hyponatremia, and dosage changes should be made no more frequently than every 3 to 4 days during its use.[1,40] Demeclocycline should not be used in patients with liver disease or compromised fluid intake, who are at high risk for demeclocycline-induced renal tubular toxicity and acute renal failure, or in children because it can interfere with bone development.[1,41]

The historic therapeutic options of water restriction, diuretic therapy, and increased sodium intake have recently been augmented with the introduction of AVP antagonists or "vaptans" (Table 58–2). These agents can be used to treat SIADH, as well as other causes of euvolemic and hypervolemic hypotonic hyponatremia.[42–45]

Blockade of AVP binding can occur at one or more of its three distinct AVP receptors: V1, which are predominantly found in the liver, central nervous system, and cardiomyocytes; V2, located in the distal nephron; and V3, which are localized in the anterior pituitary and pancreas. Selective antagonism of the V2 receptor prevents aquaporin-2 water channel transport to the apical surface, thereby decreasing AVP-dependent water reabsorption in the collecting duct. This results in an increase in urine output and free-water excretion along with a decrease in urine osmolality and an increase in serum sodium. These positive outcomes are achieved without significantly increasing the excretion of electrolytes and thus these agents have been called "aquaretics."[43] Conivaptan, a mixed vasopressin V1- and V2-receptor antagonist, was approved by the FDA in 2006 for treatment of acute euvolemic hyponatremia in hospitalized patients. Because it is available only for intravenous administration and is not approved for use in patients with heart failure, its utility for the treatment of chronic hyponatremia is very limited. Several selective V2 antagonists have been investigated recently and show promise for the treatment of several chronic hyponatremic syndromes.[42–48]

Tolvaptan (Samsca; Otsuka America Pharmaceutical Company, Ltd.) is an orally active selective AVP V2-receptor blocker that received FDA marketing approval in May 2009 for the treatment of clinically significant (serum sodium <125 mEq/L [<125 mmol/L]) euvolemic or hypervolemic hyponatremia or less marked symptomatic hyponatremia that has been nonresponsive to other therapeutic interventions in patients with heart failure, cirrhosis, and SIADH.[49] It appears to be safe and effective at promoting aquaresis and raising

TABLE 58-2 Vasopressin Receptor Antagonists in Development

Drug	Company	Approval Status	Mode of Action Adminstration Route	Indication
Conivaptan (Vaprisol)	Astellas	Approved in U.S.	V1- & V2-receptor antagonist Nonselective IV limited to 4 days of use	Euvolemic hyponatremia
Tolvaptan (Samsca)	Otsuka	Approved in U.S.	V2-receptor antagonist Selective Oral	Euvolemic and hypervolemic hyponatremia
Stavaptan (SR-121463)	Sanofi-Synthelabo	Phase III	V2-receptor antagonist Selective Oral	Euvolemic and hypervolemic hyponatremia
Lixivaptan (VPA-985)	Cardiokine	Phase III	V2-receptor antagonist Selective Oral	Euvolemic and hypervolemic hyponatremia
Mozavaptan (Physuline)	Otsuka	Approved in Japan	V2-receptor antagonist Selective Oral	Euvolemic hyponatremia SIADH

serum sodium levels in both short- and intermediate-term studies (SALT-1 and SALT-2) when given alone.[48] When used alone it is superior to furosemide or fluid restriction and when given in combination synergistic effects have been noted.[50]

Tolvaptan is primarily metabolized by the CYP3A4 and less than 1% is renally eliminated unchanged; thus physicians should avoid its use in those receiving potent inhibitors of CYP3A4 such as ketaconazole, clarithromycin, itraconazole, ritonivir, etc. Concomitant therapy with P-gp inhibitors and grapefruit juice has also been noted to result in increased serum concentrations. In contrast, the optimal benefits of tolvaptan therapy may not be realized, and its dosage may need to be increased for those patients who are receiving CYP3A4 inducers such as phenytoin and St. John's Wort, etc.[49] Dose linearity has been observed within the therapeutic range and minimal accumulation, as was expected, based on its terminal half-life of 5 to 9 hours after seven plus days of therapy.[51]

Tolvaptan's recommended starting dosage is 15 mg orally once daily. If, after 24 hours, a greater increase in serum sodium concentration is needed, the dosage may be increased to 30 mg once daily and after another 24 hours, to a maximum of 60 mg once daily. Tolvaptan therapy is contraindicated in those needing rapid correction of their serum sodium concentration, those unable to sense or respond appropriately to thirst, patients with hypovolemic hyponatremia, patients taking strong CYP3A4 inhibitors, and patients who are not excreting urine.[49] Among clinical trial participants who had a serum sodium concentration of less than 125 mEq/L (less than 125 mmol/L) at the start of tolvaptan therapy, the most common adverse events were thirst, dry mouth, weakness, constipation, hyperglycemia, and urinary frequency. Although these adverse events have rarely necessitated discontinuation of therapy, FDA-approved labeling has a boxed warning stating that tolvaptan therapy should begin or resume only in a hospital where clinicians can closely monitor the patient's serum sodium concentration. The labeling also states that healthcare providers must review the product's medication guide with every patient receiving tolvaptan therapy.

The vaptans have dramatic effects on water excretion and tolvaptan represents the greatest breakthrough in the therapy of hyponatremia and disorders of fluid homeostasis since the introduction of loop diuretics. The role of vaptans in the clinical management of patients with SIADH, heart failure, and cirrhosis will likely expand as further experience is gained.

It is important to recognize that vasopressin receptor antagonists are contraindicated in hypovolemic patients as their use would worsen the hypovolemia.

■ EVALUATION OF THERAPEUTIC OUTCOMES

The serum sodium level should be measured every 24 to 48 hours after the water restriction is initiated until it stabilizes at a concentration of greater than 125 mEq/L (greater than 125 mmol/L). A continued decline in the serum sodium level would indicate either nonadherence to the prescribed restriction or the need for a more stringent restriction. Once the serum sodium level has stabilized above 125 mEq/L (125 mmol/L), patients should then be seen every 2 to 4 weeks to assess neurologic status and to obtain serum and urine for sodium, potassium, and osmolality. Again, attention should be given to volume status (i.e., blood pressure, mucous membranes, skin turgor, and heart and lung examination), particularly in patients who are being treated with sodium chloride tablets and loop diuretics.

NONEMERGENT HYPERVOLEMIC HYPOTONIC HYPONATREMIA

The initial treatment goals for patients with asymptomatic or minimally symptomatic hypotonic hyponatremia and an expanded ECF volume include achieving a negative water balance while minimizing rapid changes in cell volume until the serum sodium is greater than 125 mEq/L (greater than 125 mmol/L). This entails correction of the underlying cause when possible, as well as restriction of water intake to a volume less than 1,000 to 1,200 mL/day. Dietary intake of sodium should be restricted to 1,000 to 2,000 mg/day, depending on the degree of ECF volume expansion and edema.

Patients with hypervolemic hypotonic hyponatremia caused by congestive heart failure should be treated with measures that can potentially improve cardiac contractility and improve the effective circulating volume, thereby limiting the nonosmotic release of AVP. Therapeutic options include digitalis or afterload reduction with angiotensin-converting enzyme inhibitors (ACEIs) or angiotensin II receptor blockers (ARBs). Of these, only ACEIs have been shown in clinical trials to be of benefit in partially correcting hyponatremia in patients with congestive heart failure.[52] No specific ACE inhibitor offers any particular advantage for this indication, and the dose should be titrated to keep the systolic blood pressure in the 110 to 130 mm Hg range. Dose-limiting adverse effects include hyperkalemia (serum potassium >5.5 mEq/L [>5.5 mmol/L]), as well as a decline in renal function. The benefits and risks of continuing ACE inhibition must be weighed carefully in each case, but a decrease in glomerular filtration rate (GFR) of less than 30% that stabilizes within 2 months of therapy initiation generally does not require dosage reduction or discontinuation of the ACE inhibitor.[53]

CLINICAL CONTROVERSY

Some clinicians regard any increase in serum creatinine in patients on ACEIs as a reason to decrease dosage or discontinue the medication. ACEIs selectively dilate the afferent arteriole, causing a decrease in intraglomerular pressure and reduced GFR. Although this might be viewed negatively, many experts suggest that the decrease in pressure is likely renoprotective, and that one does not need to reduce the dosage or discontinue therapy unless the resulting decrease in GFR is greater than 30% and does not stabilize within 2 months.

Other potentially treatable causes of asymptomatic hyponatremia associated with an expanded ECF volume include nephrotic syndrome and cirrhosis. ACEIs can be used to decrease proteinuria in patients with nephrotic syndrome, leading to partial correction of hypoalbuminemia and to a decrease in nonosmotic AVP release. Patients with advanced cirrhosis can benefit from placement of a transjugular intrahepatic portosystemic shunt, which can increase the effective circulating volume and thus reduce the nonosmotic release of AVP. This procedure can potentially exacerbate or precipitate hepatic encephalopathy, and should be avoided in patients with a history of encephalopathy.

Vasopressin receptor antagonists have also been proposed for the treatment of hypervolemic hypotonic hyponatremia in patients with congestive heart failure and cirrhosis.[42–45,54,55] The effectiveness of tolvaptan in the short-term management of heart failure patients with hypervolemic hyponatremia has been evidenced by decreased body weight, increased urine output, decreased pulmonary capillary wedge pressure, and decreases in urine osmolality.[56–61] Longstanding beneficial effects, reduction in hospitalization or death, or progression of heart failure have not been observed in several pivotal trials.[58,60,62] Prolonged use of tolvaptan leads to increased endogenous levels of AVP and some have theorized that this overstimulation of V(1A)-receptors could lead to increased afterload and progression of HF.[63] However, after 52 weeks of tolvaptan therapy (30 mg daily) no worsening of left ventricular dilatation was observed by Udelson and colleagues.[62]

■ EVALUATION OF THERAPEUTIC OUTCOMES

Patients should initially be evaluated on a daily basis for lung congestion, ascites, peripheral edema, and signs or symptoms of hyponatremia. The serum sodium concentration should be measured daily until it stabilizes above 125 mEq/L (125 mmol/L) following initiation of water restriction. Patients should then be assessed 1 week following discharge, and then every 2 to 4 weeks to assess compliance with the water restriction and other treatment measures, volume status, and hyponatremia-related symptoms.

HYPERNATREMIA

EPIDEMIOLOGY AND ETIOLOGY

❺ Hypernatremia (serum sodium >145 mEq/L [>145 mmol/L]) is always associated with hypertonicity and results from a deficit of water relative to ECF sodium content.[1] Hyperosmolar states are

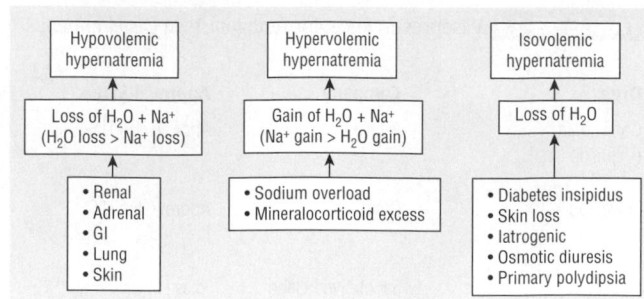

FIGURE 58-3. Common etiologies of hypernatremia. (H_2O, water; Na^+, sodium.)

a potent stimulus for thirst, and therefore hypernatremia is most commonly observed in patients with an impaired thirst response or in those without access to water. Infants and comatose patients, as well as elderly or disabled patients with an impaired sensorium or functional status are therefore at highest risk for this disorder.[64] The incidence of hypernatremia in general medical-surgical hospital patients and intensive care unit patients has been estimated to be at least 1% and 7.9%, respectively.[65,66] Outcome generally depends on the rapidity with which the hypernatremia developed. Mortality from acute hypernatremia in children, which develops in less than 72 hours, ranges from 10% to 70%. In contrast, chronic hypernatremia in children, defined as that which develops over 3 or more days, has a mortality rate of 10%.[67] An acute increase in serum sodium in adults to greater than 160 mEq/L (greater than 160 mmol/L) is associated with a 75% mortality rate.[35] Adults in whom the hypernatremia developed at a slower rate have a lower but still high mortality rate of approximately 60%. Hypernatremia in adults is often associated with a serious underlying illness, which likely contributes to the high mortality rate.

PATHOPHYSIOLOGY

Hypernatremia can result from either loss of water or hypotonic fluids, or less commonly from administration of hypertonic fluids or ingestion of sodium. Patients develop hypovolemic, hypervolemic, or isovolemic hypernatremia depending on the relative magnitude of sodium and water loss or gain caused by the underlying condition (Fig. 58–3).

Water loss commonly occurs as a result of insensible losses (evaporative losses of water through the skin and lungs) in patients deprived of water. Hospitalized patients who are febrile or receiving mechanical ventilation are often treated with intravenous fluids containing insufficient free water to replace insensible losses. Hypernatremia can be observed in patients with hypotonic gastrointestinal losses (diarrhea or vomiting) or in patients who have been exposed to high temperatures who suffer large water losses from both sweat and insensible losses.

Diabetes insipidus (DI) is a condition characterized by decreased AVP secretion or decreased renal response to AVP.[1,68,69] Patients excrete large volumes (3 to 20 L/day) of dilute urine, resulting in large urinary losses of water. DI is classified as either central (decreased AVP secretion) or nephrogenic (decreased renal response to AVP). Table 58–3 summarizes the causes of DI. Patients with central DI often present with sudden onset of polyuria, whereas patients with nephrogenic DI develop polyuria more gradually.

Administration of hypertonic sodium chloride can result in hypernatremia and an expanded ECF volume. This is typically iatrogenic, and can follow administration of sodium bicarbonate, use of hypertonic sodium chloride enemas, or intrauterine injection of hypertonic sodium chloride. Rarely, patients with hyperaldosteronism spontaneously present with an expanded ECF and mild hypernatremia.[64]

TABLE 58-3	Causes of Diabetes Insipidus
Central DI	**Nephrogenic DI**
Idiopathic	Lithium toxicity
Familial	Hypercalcemia
Neurosurgery	Hypokalemia
Head trauma	Cidofovir
CNS malignancy	Foscarnet
Hypoxic encephalopathy	Inherited aquaporin-2 defect
Sheehan syndrome	Inherited vasopressin V2-receptor defect
	Demeclocycline

CNS, central nervous system; DI, diabetes insipidus.

CLINICAL PRESENTATION

❻ The symptoms of hypernatremia are primarily caused by a decrease in neuronal cell volume and can include weakness, lethargy, restlessness, irritability, and confusion.[1,64] Symptoms of more severe or rapidly developing hypernatremia include twitching, seizures, coma, and death. Hypernatremia results in movement of water from the intracellular space to the extracellular fluid. As discussed above, neurons can adapt to ECF tonicity changes by adjusting intracellular osmolality, including decreasing or increasing the concentration of organic osmolytes. In the case of hypernatremia, ECF hypertonicity results in generation of intracellular organic osmolytes within 24 hours of onset. This increase in intracellular fluid tonicity then draws water into the neurons, thus limiting the decrease in cell volume. Patients with chronic hypernatremia are therefore less likely to present with symptoms caused by this cerebral adaptation than patients with acute hypernatremia.

CLINICAL PRESENTATION OF HYPERNATREMIA

General

☐ The rise in the plasma sodium concentration and osmolality causes acute water movement from the intracellular to the extracellular fluid. In the brain this decrease in volume can cause rupture of the cerebral veins, leading to focal intracerebral and subarachnoid hemorrhages and possible irreversible neurologic damage.

Symptoms

☐ The clinical manifestations of this disorder begin with lethargy, weakness, confusion, restlessness, and irritability, and can progress to twitching, seizures, coma, and death. Severe symptoms usually require an acute elevation in the plasma sodium concentration to above 160 mEq/L (160 mmol/L). Values >180 mEq/L (>180 mmol/L) are associated with a high mortality rate.

Signs

☐ Signs of hypernatremia can include postural hypotension, tachycardia, dry oral mucosa, diminished skin turgor, and reduced or increased output of dilute or concentrated urine, depending on cause.

☐ Signs associated with chronic hypernatremia are often difficult to detect because most affected adults have underlying neurologic disease.

Laboratory Tests

☐ Serum sodium levels are generally >145 mEq/L (>145 mmol/L). Measurement of urine volume and osmolality may be helpful in diagnosing the cause.

Hypernatremia is often associated with serious underlying illness, and signs and symptoms related to that illness can also be present. Patients with a history of severe diarrhea or vomiting can present with ECF volume depletion. Elderly patients deprived of water after sustaining a stroke or hip fracture often present with mental status changes and signs of ECF volume depletion. Clinically detectable extracellular fluid volume depletion, however, might not be evident until the serum sodium concentration exceeds 160 mEq/L (160 mmol/L), because these patients primarily have water loss, two thirds of which is derived from the intracellular space. The urine is concentrated, osmolality often exceeds 450 mOsm/kg (450 mmol/kg), as a result of both osmotic and nonosmotic release of AVP. The first step in evaluating patients with hypernatremia is the clinical assessment of the ECF volume, urine volume, and urine osmolality (Fig. 58–4).

Patients with a contracted ECF volume and a low urine output include those who have sustained insensible water losses that exceed intake, as well as those with extrarenal losses of hypotonic fluids. On physical examination, one should search for postural hypotension, diminished skin turgor, and delayed capillary refill. The daily urine output is typically less than 1 L.

A recent multicenter, case-control study examined the clinical presentation of hypernatremia in 150 elderly patients in geriatric care facilities.[70] Low blood pressure, tachycardia, dry oral mucosa, decreased skin turgor, and recent changes in consciousness were all more common in hypernatremic patients than in controls. Perhaps not surprisingly in this mixed patient population, the presence of signs of dehydration was variable, with orthostatic hypotension and decreased subclavicular and forearm skin turgor present in at least 60% of patients. Abnormal subclavicular and thigh skin turgor, dry oral mucosa, and recent change in consciousness were significantly and independently associated with hypernatremia.

Osmotic Diuresis

Patients undergoing an osmotic diuresis generally have urine volumes greater than 3 L/day. Excessive urinary excretion of glucose, sodium, urea, or an exogenously administered solute such as mannitol are identified either by history or by direct measurement of serum and urinary concentrations of the suspected solute. Patients with postobstructive diuresis, such as those with bladder outlet obstruction caused by prostatic hypertrophy, are usually volume expanded as a result of retained excess solute because of a decline in the GFR.[1] The osmotic diuresis that follows alleviation of the obstruction is appropriate in that it promotes excretion of the excess retained solute. Patients with severe hyperglycemia, conversely, present with signs of volume depletion, and the diuresis is therefore inappropriate, further exacerbating the degree of ECF volume contraction.

Diabetes Insipidus

Patients with DI tend to maintain a normal ECF volume as long as they are conscious and have free access to water. Patients typically have only a slight elevation in the serum sodium concentration (usually in the 141–145 mEq/L [141–145 mmol/L] range), and a daily urine volume greater than 3 L.[71] A water deprivation test is sometimes recommended to aid in the differential diagnosis between central and nephrogenic DI.[30] This consists of depriving patients of water for 8 to 12 hours. Urine osmolality, urine volume, and body weight are then measured before and after subcutaneous administration of 5 mcg of desmopressin acetate. Patients with central DI will show a prompt increase in urine osmolality to approximately 600 mOsm/kg (600 mmol/kg) and a decrease in urine volume after desmopressin administration. Those with nephrogenic DI will be unable to increase the urine osmolality above 300 mOsm/kg (300 mmol/kg).[1] The direct measurement of

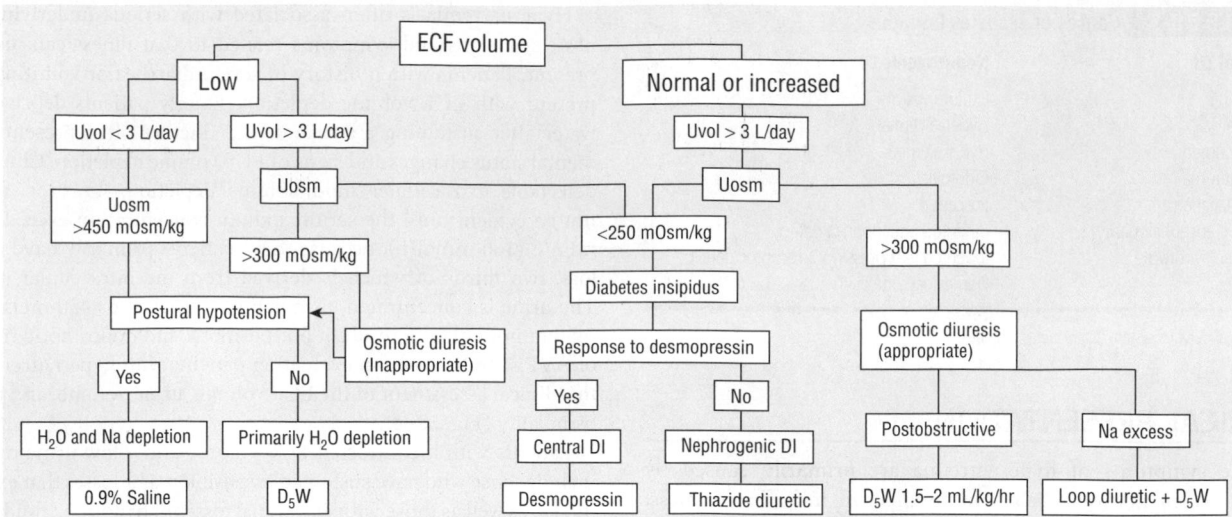

FIGURE 58-4. Diagnostic and treatment algorithm for hypernatremia. (D₅W, 5% dextrose in water; ECF, extracellular fluid; H₂O, water; Na, sodium; Uosm, urine osmolality [values in mOsm/kg are numerically equivalent to mmol/kg]; Uvol, daily urine volume.) See text for guidelines regarding calculations of infusion rates for intravenous solutions.

vasopressin levels after infusion of 5% sodium chloride at a rate of 0.05 mL/kg/min for no more than 2 hours improves the accuracy of diagnosis, but carries a high risk of ECF volume overload.[72]

The value of performing a water deprivation test in patients with polyuria and hypernatremia, such as patients with DI, has recently been questioned.[73] Because hypernatremia provides a maximal stimulus for AVP secretion, discriminating between nephrogenic and central DI can be based on plasma vasopressin concentration and urinary response to desmopressin without the need for water deprivation. The water deprivation test is thus likely to only be of diagnostic value in patients with polyuria and a normal serum sodium concentration.

Sodium Overload

Patients who have ingested large amounts of sodium (>4 tablespoons [1,400 mEq or 1,400 mmol Na⁺] of sodium chloride) or who have received greater than 5 L of hypertonic fluids are volume expanded, although this may not always be clinically evident as edema. This results in an osmotic diuresis, polyuria, and a urine osmolality greater than 300 mOsm/kg (greater than 300 mmol/kg). The excess sodium will be excreted in the urine in patients with normal renal function.

TREATMENT

Hypernatremia

■ DESIRED OUTCOME

❼ The desired goals for patients with hypernatremia include correction of the serum sodium concentration at a rate that restores and maintains cell volume as close to normal as possible, as well as normalizing the ECF volume in states of ECF volume depletion or expansion. Adequate treatment should result in the resolution of symptoms associated with hypovolemia. Careful titration of fluids and medications should minimize the adverse effects from too rapid correction. Rapid correction can result in movement of excessive water into the brain cells, resulting in cerebral edema, seizures, neurologic damage, and potentially death.[1] Modulation of dietary sodium intake and sodium replacement can be necessary to prevent recurrence of hypernatremia.

■ PHARMACOLOGIC THERAPY

Hypovolemic Hypernatremia

Hypovolemic hypernatremia should initially be treated with 0.9% sodium chloride until hemodynamic stability is restored. An initial infusion rate of 200 to 300 mL/h will likely be appropriate for many patients. Once intravascular volume is restored, 0.45% sodium chloride or 5% dextrose in water can then be infused to correct the water deficit,[38] the volume of which can be estimated as:

$$\text{Water deficit} = \text{Present TBW} \times [(S^1_{Na}/140) - 1]$$

where TBW = total body water; S^1_{Na} = initial patient serum sodium concentration (in mEq/L [or mmol/L]); and 140 = normal or goal S_{Na} (in mEq/L [or mmol/L]).

The rate of correction depends on the rapidity with which the hypernatremia developed. Hypernatremia that has developed over a few hours can be initially corrected at a rate of approximately 1 mEq/L (1 mmol/L) per hour, whereas a rate of 0.5 mEq/L (0.5 mmol/L) per hour should be used when it has developed more slowly.[20,64] The rate of correction should generally be limited to no more than 10 mEq/L (10 mmol/L) per day.[30,64]

Treatment of hyperglycemia-induced osmotic diuresis consists of correcting the hyperglycemia with insulin, as well as administering 0.9% sodium chloride until signs of ECF volume depletion resolve. Once hemodynamic stability is restored, the water deficit should be corrected in a manner analogous to that described for patients with hypovolemic hypernatremia above. The corrected serum sodium level should be calculated by adding 1.7 mEq/L (1.7 mmol/L) for every 100 mg/dL (5.6 mmol/L) increase in the serum glucose concentration before estimating the water deficit.[3]

Hypernatremia in patients undergoing a postobstructive diuresis should be treated with infusion of hypotonic fluids such as 0.45% sodium chloride at maintenance rates of approximately 1.5 mL/kg per hour. It is important to avoid the temptation to administer fluids to replace urine output on a 1:1 volume basis, because this tends to perpetuate the diuresis.

The serum sodium concentration and fluid status should be monitored every 2 to 3 hours over the first 24 hours of admission in patients with symptomatic hypernatremia to permit appropriate adjustment in the rate of infusion of hypotonic fluids. After

TABLE 58-4	Drugs Used to Manage Central and Nephrogenic Diabetes Insipidus	
Drug	**Indication**	**Dose**
Desmopressin acetate	Central and nephrogenic	5–20 mcg intranasally every 12–24 h
Chlorpropamide	Central	125–250 mg orally daily
Carbamazepine	Central	100–300 mg orally bid
Clofibrate	Central	500 mg orally qid
Hydrochlorothiazide	Central and nephrogenic	25 mg orally q 12–24 h
Amiloride	Lithium-related nephrogenic	5–10 mg orally daily
Indomethacin	Central and nephrogenic	50 mg orally q 8–12 h

symptoms resolve and the serum sodium is less than 148 mEq/L (less than 148 mmol/L), serum sodium determinations every 6 to 12 hours and fluid status assessment every 8 to 24 hours are generally sufficient to follow the course of therapy.

Central Diabetes Insipidus

8 Patients with central DI should generally receive AVP replacement therapy with desmopressin, an AVP analog.[1,20] Because of variable absorption of oral desmopressin, DI is best treated with the intranasal formulation 1-desamino-8-D-arginine vasopressin (DDAVP); however, oral tablets are available and can be useful in some patients. The beginning intranasal dose should be 10 mcg once daily. Ultimately, the dose may need to be titrated up to 10 mcg twice daily for most adults. Each insufflation of intranasal DDAVP delivers 10 mcg of desmopressin acetate at a concentration of 100 mcg/mL. Several medications with antidiuretic properties have been used successfully in the management of central and nephrogenic DI (Table 58–4). They can be used as an alternative to DDAVP or adjunctively.

The desmopressin dose should be adjusted to achieve adequate urinary concentration during sleep to prevent nocturia, to result in a daily urine volume of approximately 1.5 to 2 L, and to maintain the serum sodium concentration in the 137 to 142 mEq/L (137–142 mmol/L) range. The serum sodium concentration should be measured every 3 to 4 days during the initial dose titration period, and then every 2 to 4 months. Administration of desmopressin results in nonsuppressible AVP activity and presents a risk of water intoxication caused by excess water retention.[1] Patients using desmopressin should therefore be monitored for signs and symptoms of hyponatremia and hypervolemia. It has been suggested that patients using desmopressin who experience water intoxication can minimize the risk of a second episode by delaying a dose of desmopressin each week until polyuria and thirst develop, thus demonstrating the need for additional desmopressin doses.[20]

Nephrogenic Diabetes Insipidus

Hypercalcemia and hypokalemia should be corrected, and medications that contribute to the pathogenesis should be discontinued. One key goal in treating nephrogenic DI is to induce a mild ECFVd (1–1.5 L) with a thiazide diuretic and dietary sodium restriction (85 mEq [85 mmol] Na+ or 2,000 mg sodium chloride per day), which often can decrease urine volume by as much as 50% (see Table 58–4). This will increase proximal water reabsorption, decrease the volume of filtrate delivered to the distal nephron, and decrease urine volume. NSAIDs such as indomethacin at a dose of 50 mg 3 times a day can potentiate the activity of AVP and can be used as adjunctive therapy.[1,74] Patients with lithium-induced nephrogenic DI can derive particular benefit from amiloride at a dose of 5 to 10 mg daily; amiloride directly inhibits uptake of lithium from the tubular lumen into principal cells in the cortical collecting duct.[1,75]

■ EVALUATION OF TREATMENT OUTCOMES

Physical examination with attention to volume status and measurement of serum and urine sodium concentration and osmolality should be assessed every 2 to 3 months during chronic therapy. A 24-hour urine collection to measure urine volume and sodium excretion will help guide therapy with diuretics and determine adherence to sodium restriction.

Sodium Overload

Treatment of sodium overload consists of administration of loop diuretics to facilitate excretion of the excess sodium, as well as intravenous D_5W. The latter should be infused at a rate that will decrease the serum sodium at approximately 0.5 mEq/L (0.5 mmol/L) per hour, or 1 mEq/L (1 mmol/L) per hour in cases in which the hypernatremia developed rapidly over several hours.[64] The volume of infusate may be estimated as described previously. Furosemide should be administered at a dose of 20 to 40 mg intravenously every 6 hours.

The serum sodium should initially be measured every 2 to 4 hours, and the diuretic continued until signs of ECF volume overload (pulmonary congestion and edema) resolve. The serum sodium concentration can be determined every 6 to 12 hours once the serum sodium level is less than 148 mEq/L (less than 148 mmol/L) and symptoms of hypertonicity resolve.

EDEMA

The body closely monitors blood volume to help ensure adequate tissue perfusion. A decline in the effective circulating volume (actually the blood pressure resulting from that volume) results in decreased sodium and water excretion by the kidney.[1] Under these conditions, the kidneys retain all the water and sodium ingested until the effective circulating volume is restored to normal. An increase in dietary sodium is accompanied by an increase in water intake caused by the initial increase in serum osmolality and stimulation of thirst. The resultant increase in ECF volume augments renal perfusion, effecting a transient increase in GFR which leads to enhanced sodium filtration and excretion.[76] These homeostatic mechanisms are crucial in maintaining sodium balance, as retention of just a few milliequivalents (mmoles) of sodium per day can eventually lead to an expanded ECF volume and edema formation.

PATHOPHYSIOLOGY

9 Edema may be defined as a clinically detectable increase in interstitial fluid volume. Clinical detectability in adults generally requires an interstitial volume increase of at least 2.5 to 3 L.[1] Edema develops when excess sodium is retained either as a primary defect in renal sodium excretion, or as a response to a decrease in the effective circulating volume despite a normal or expanded ECF volume. An increase in the capillary hydrostatic pressure because of an expansion of the ECF volume, or an increase in central venous pressure may lead to edema formation. Edema may also occur when there is an alteration in Starling forces within the capillary.[77] The Starling equation denotes the relationship between factors affecting the movement of fluid between the capillary and interstitium and is discussed in detail in Chapter 30.

Edema may develop rapidly in those with an acute decompensation in myocardial contractility which leads to an elevation in pulmonary venous pressure that is transmitted back to the pulmonary capillaries and ultimatley results in acute pulmonary edema. Edema may also develop insidiously as in the case of renal sodium and water retention due to diminished effective circulating volume which leads to a rise in the ECF volume and edema formation in both peripheral and pulmonary interstitial tissues.

Edema formation in patients with nephrotic syndrome is primarily related to renal sodium and water retention. A decrease in capillary oncotic pressure does not appear to play a major role until the serum albumin concentration less than 2 g/dL (less than 20 g/L). This is explained by the fact that both capillary and interstitial oncotic pressure decrease proportionately above a serum albumin concentration of 2 g/dL (20 g/L), and thus the transcapillary oncotic gradient is not significantly altered.[78]

Patients with cirrhosis initially develop ascites as a result of an increase in the pressure in the portal circulation proximal to the diseased liver. Sequestration of fluid in the abdominal cavity (ascites) and peripheral vasodilation as a consequence of increased levels of circulating cytokines, result in a decrease in the effective circulating volume, activation of the sympathetic nervous system, and secondary hyperaldosteronism. Therefore, renal sodium retention leads to worsened ascites and edema.

CLINICAL PRESENTATION

Edema is usually first detected in the feet or pretibial area of ambulatory patients and in the presacral area of bed-bound individuals. Edema is described as "pitting" when a depression created by exerting pressure for several seconds over a bony prominence such as the tibia does not rapidly refill. The severity of the edema should be rated on a semi-quantitative scale of 1+ to 4+ depending on the depth of the pit (1+ = 2 mm, 2+ = 4 mm, 3+ = 6 mm, and 4+ = 8 mm).

The extent of the edema should also be quantified according to the area of involvement. Pretibial edema, for example, should be quantified according to how far it extends up the lower leg (e.g., one-third up the lower leg). Pulmonary edema, an increase in lung interstitial and alveolar water, is often evidenced by crackles (also called rales) upon auscultation. It should be quantified according to how far the crackles extend from the dependent portion of the lung(s). So, for example, edema limited to the ankles and feet would indicate less severe edema than edema that extends halfway up the lower legs, and crackles limited to the base of both lungs in an upright person would indicate less severe pulmonary edema than crackles throughout both lung fields.

TREATMENT

Edema

■ GENERAL APPROACH TO TREATMENT

❿ The goals of therapy are to minimize tissue edema and thus improve organ function, as well as to relieve symptoms of edema such as dyspnea in patients with CHF or abdominal distention in patients with ascites. It is important to emphasize that the presence of edema does not always dictate the need for instituting pharmacologic (diuretic) therapy. Only pulmonary edema requires immediate pharmacologic treatment because it is life-threatening. Other forms of edema may be treated gradually, with a comprehensive approach that includes not only diuretics, but also sodium restriction and treatment of the underlying disease state. Sodium intake should generally be restricted to 1,000 to 2,000 mg/day. A slow, more judicious approach in non-life-threatening situations will help to minimize complications of diuretic therapy and excessive fluid removal. These may include impaired vital organ perfusion, azotemia, and impaired cardiac output due to a fall in the left ventricular end-diastolic filling pressure.

■ PHARMACOLOGIC THERAPY

Diuretics are the primary pharmacologic therapy for the management of edema. Patients with expanded ECF volume and edema often require therapy with diuretics when treatment of the underlying disease and daily sodium restriction are insufficient to relieve the edema. Diuretics can be categorized according to the site in the nephron where sodium reabsorption is inhibited. Loop diuretics inhibit the sodium-potassium-chloride (Na^+-K^+-$2Cl^-$) carrier in the loop of Henle. Thiazide diuretics inhibit the Na^+-Cl^- carrier in the distal tubule. Finally, potassium-sparing diuretics inhibit the sodium channel in the cortical collecting duct either directly (triamterene and amiloride), or by interfering with aldosterone activity (spironolactone and eplerenone). The efficacy of a diuretic depends on the presence of several factors, including the amount of filtered solute normally reabsorbed at the site of action, the amount of solute reabsorbed distal to the site of action, and adequate delivery of drug to the site of action in the nephron.

Loop diuretics are the most potent diuretics, as evidenced by the fact that they increase peak fractional excretion of sodium (FeNa) to 20% to 25% (0.20–0.25). Thiazide- and potassium-sparing diuretics are less potent and increase peak FeNa to 3% to 5% (0.03–0.05) and 1% to 2% (0.01–0.02), respectively.[1] Although

TABLE 58-5	Maximal Effective Dose and Dosing Interval for Edema Management with Loop Diuretics						
Diuretic	Dosing Interval	Normal	Cirrhosis	CHF	Nephrotic Syndrome	GFR (10–50 mL/min)	GFR (<10 mL/min)
Furosemide							
IV	6–8 h	10–40 mg	40 mg	40–80 mg	120 mg	80 mg	200 mg
Oral	6–8 h	20–80 mg	80 mg	80–160 mg	240 mg	160 mg	320–400 mg
Bumetanide							
IV/Oral	6–8 h	1 mg	1 mg	2–3 mg	3 mg	2–3 mg	8–10 mg
Torsemide							
IV/Oral	24 h	15–20 mg	10–20 mg	20–50 mg	50 mg	20–50 mg	50–100 mg

CHF, congestive heart failure; GFR, glomerular filtration rate.

a large portion of the filtered sodium is reabsorbed in the proximal nephron, the efficacy of proximal-acting diuretics such as acetazolamide is limited by reabsorption of the excess fluid and sodium in the loop of Henle.

The effectiveness of thiazide and loop diuretics is dependent on the concentration of the drug in the tubular lumen. These diuretics are delivered to the tubular lumen of the kidney by active transport by the proximal tubular cells. Osmotic diuretics, conversely, are freely filtered into the tubular lumen in the proximal tubule, whereas spironolactone gains access to mineralocorticoid receptors in the cortical collecting duct through diffusion from the systemic circulation.

A threshold concentration of loop or thiazide diuretic must be delivered to the active site (e.g., loop of Henle or distal tubule) to achieve a natriuresis.[1,79] Once this concentration is achieved, further increases in diuretic dose will not elicit an increase in diuretic response. Thus a ceiling dose of these diuretics is recognized. Administration of 40 mg of intravenous furosemide to a normal subject will result in excretion of 200 to 250 mEq (200–250 mmol) of sodium in 3 to 4 L of urine over a 3- to 4-hour period.[79] Table 58–5 summarizes the maximal effective doses and dosing intervals for loop diuretics in patients with cirrhosis, CHF, nephrotic syndrome, as well as those with reduced renal function.

Patients with renal insufficiency often require larger doses of diuretics to achieve adequate concentrations of the drug at the active site. The natriuretic response is decreased in patients with renal insufficiency because the filtered load of sodium falls proportionately as GFR declines. This can be partially overcome by dosing diuretics more frequently, as well as by using continuous infusions in critically ill hospitalized patients.[1,80,81] The latter will maintain more consistent levels of the diuretic above the threshold concentration. Patients who are diuretic resistant should be treated with both a loop and a thiazide-type diuretic. Patients with CHF and a normal GFR may have impaired oral absorption of furosemide. An adequate diuresis is most readily sustained by increasing the frequency of diuretic administration (Fig. 58–5).

Diuretic resistance can be caused by increased uptake of sodium in the distal tubule, impaired delivery of diuretics to the site of action, or decreased intrinsic diuretic activity. Animal studies have demonstrated binding of furosemide to albumin in the tubular lumen, which decreases the availability of the drug to the active site.[82] Human studies, however, have demonstrated that when albumin binding is inhibited by concurrent administration of sulfasoxazole, diuretic resistance persists, suggesting a decrease in intrinsic tubular sensitivity to loop diuretics.[83] This impaired natriuretic response can be overcome by using higher diuretic doses to increase the delivery of free drug to the secretory site in the nephron.[80,81] Combinations of loop diuretics with distally acting diuretics are generally necessary to promote a natriuresis that exceeds tubular sodium reabsorption for those with nephrotic syndrome (Fig. 58–6).

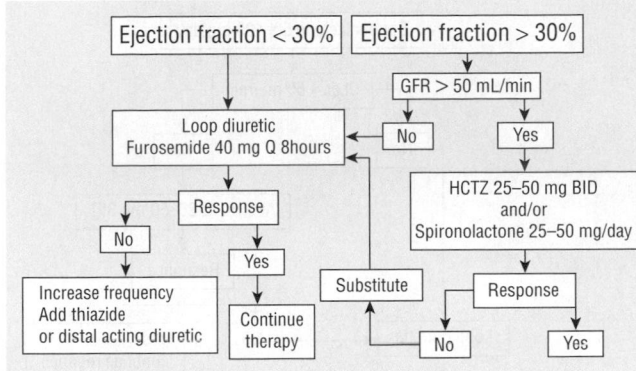

FIGURE 58-5. Therapeutic algorithm for diuretic use in patients with congestive heart failure. (GFR, glomerular filtration rate [50 mL/min is equivalent to 0.84 mL/s]; HCTZ, hydrochlorothiazide.)

CLINICAL CONTROVERSY

Some clinicians advocate using combinations of diuretics in cases of diuretic resistance associated with nephrotic syndrome, while others prefer to use larger-than-average doses of single agents to overcome enhanced protein binding in the tubular lumen associated with proteinuria.

Secondary hyperaldosteronism plays a major role in the pathogenesis of edema in patients with cirrhosis. Therefore, these patients should initially be treated with spironolactone in the absence of impaired GFR and hyperkalemia. Thiazides can then be added for patients with a creatinine clearance >50 mL/min (>0.84 mL/s). For those patients who remain diuretic resistant, a loop diuretic can replace the thiazide. Patients with impaired GFR (creatinine clearance of <40 mL/min [<0.67 mL/s]) can require a loop diuretic, with addition of a thiazide in those who do not achieve adequate diuresis.[81] Care should be taken to avoid hypokalemia, which can precipitate hepatic encephalopathy by increasing ammoniagenesis (Fig. 58–7).[84]

Complications of loop and thiazide diuretic therapy include hypokalemia, excess depletion of ECF volume, hyponatremia, hypomagnesemia, metabolic alkalosis, and hyperuricemia. Thiazides can also cause hypercalcemia, particularly in patients with mild subclinical hyperparathyroidism. Chronic therapy with potassium-sparing diuretics, including triamterene, amiloride, and spironolactone, can cause a mild metabolic acidosis and can precipitate hyperkalemia. Patients with moderate to severe kidney dysfunction or those receiving NSAIDs, ACEIs, or ARBs are

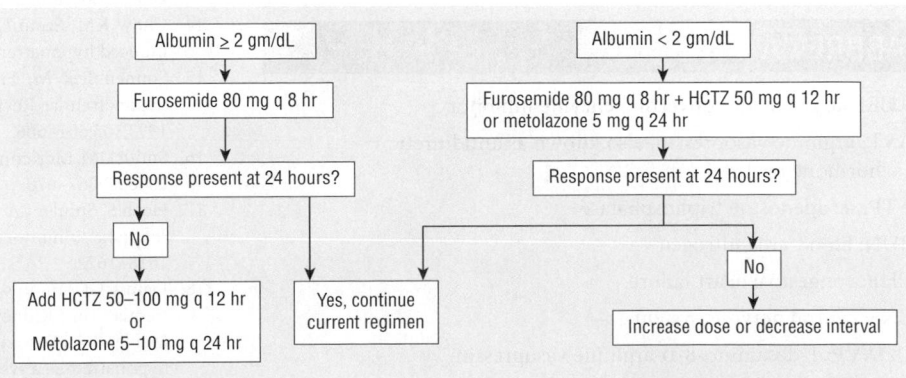

FIGURE 58-6. Therapeutic algorithm for diuretic therapy in patients with nephrotic syndrome. Albumin concentration of 2 gm/dL is equivalent to 20 g/L. (HCTZ, hydrochlorothiazide.)

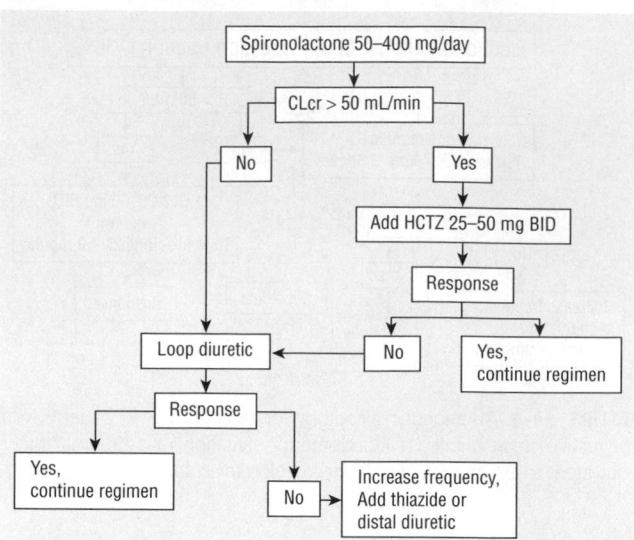

FIGURE 58-7. Therapeutic algorithm for diuretic use in patients with cirrhosis. (CL_{cr}, creatinine clearance [50 mL/min is equivalent to 0.84 mL/s]; HCTZ, hydrochlorothiazide.)

at highest risk for this complication. In addition, spironolactone can cause reversible gynecomastia in patients receiving therapy for more than several weeks. This side effect, however, has not been associated with eplerenone, a newly available aldosterone antagonist.[85]

EVALUATION OF THERAPEUTIC OUTCOMES

Patients should be monitored by careful history and intermittent physical examinations to detect signs and symptoms of edema as well as adverse effects of treatment. Physical examination should include measurement of blood pressure and pulse in either supine or seated positions and after standing for 2 to 3 minutes. ECF volume can be estimated based on the height of the jugular venous pressure, extent of edema, auscultation of the heart and lungs, and skin mobility. Followup monitoring (10–14 days after initiation of therapy) should include determinations of serum sodium, potassium, chloride, bicarbonate, magnesium, calcium, BUN, serum creatinine, and uric acid. A new steady state will have developed over that time period and further fluctuations in ECF volume and electrolyte balance should not occur in the absence of a change in clinical status, diuretic dose, or dietary intake. Repeated blood tests are not necessary at every visit unless there is a change in the patient's clinical status.

ABBREVIATIONS

ACEI: angiotensin-converting enzyme inhibitor

AVP: arginine vasopressin, also known as antidiuretic hormone or ADH

ATPase: adenosine triphosphatase

BUN: blood urea nitrogen

CHF: congestive heart failure

CNS: central nervous system

DDAVP: 1-desamino-8-D-arginine vasopressin

D_5W: 5% dextrose in water

DI: diabetes insipidus

ECF: extracellular fluid

ECFVd: extracellular fluid volume deficit

$ECFV_{current}$: current extracellular fluid volume

$ECFV_{norm}$: normal extracellular fluid volume

FeNa: fractional excretion of sodium

GFR: glomerular filtration rate

IV_{Na}: sodium concentration of infusate

IV_{vol}: volume of infusate

NSAID: nonsteroidal antiinflammatory drug

S^1_{Na}: initial patient serum sodium concentration

SIADH: syndrome of inappropriate secretion of antidiuretic hormone

TBW: total-body water

$TBW_{current}$: current total-body water

TBW_{norm}: normal total-body water

REFERENCES

1. Rose DR, Post TW. Clinical Physiology of Acid-Base and Electrolyte Disorders, 5th ed. New York: McGraw-Hill, 2001.
2. Andreoli TE. Water: Normal balance, hyponatremia, and hypernatremia. Ren Fail 2000;2:711–735.
3. Androgué HJ, Madias NE. Hyponatremia. N Engl J Med 2000;342:1581–1589.
4. Deen PM, Verdijk MA, Knoers NV, et al. Requirement of human renal water channel aquaphorin-2 for vasopressin-dependent concentration of urine. Science 1994;264:92–95.
5. Upadhyay A, Jaber BL, Madias NE. Incidence and prevalence of hyponatremia. Am J Med 2006;119(7A):S30-S35.
6. Upadhyay A, Jaber BL, Madias NE. Epidemiology of hyponatremia. Semin Nephrol 2009;29(3):227–238.
7. Hawkins RC. Age and gender as risk factors for hyponatremia and hypernatremia. Clin Chim Acta 2003;337:169–172.
8. Almond CSD, Shin AY, Fortescue EB, et al. Hyponatremia among runners in the Boston Marathon. N Engl J Med 2005;352:1550–1556.
9. Asadollahi K, Beeching N, Gill G. Hyponatremia as a risk factor for hospital mortality. Q J Med 2006;99:877–880.
10. Kacprowicz RF, Lloyd JD. Electrolyte complications of malignancy. Emerg Med Clin N Am 2009;27:257–269.
11. Nzerue CM, Baffoe-Bonnie H, You W, et al. Predictors of outcome in hospitalized patients with severe hyponatremia. J Natl Med Assoc 2003;95:335–343.
12. Kurtz I, Nguyen MK. Evolving concepts in the quantitative analysis of the determinants of the plasma water sodium concentration and the patho-physiology and treatment of dysnatremias. Kidney Int 2005;68:1982–1993.
13. Reynolds RM, Seckl JR. Hyponatremia for the clinical endocrinologist. Clin Endocrinol 2005;63:366–374.
14. Chow KM, Szeto CC, Wong, TY-H, et al. Risk factors for thiazide-induced hyponatremia. Q J Med 2003;96:911–917.
15. Sonnenblick M, Friedlander Y, Rosin AJ. Diuretic-induced severe hyponatremia: Review and analysis of 129 reported patients. Chest 1993;103:601–606.
16. Smith DM, McKenna K, Thompson CJ. Hyponatremia. Clin Endocrinol 2000;52:667–678.
17. Jacob S, Spinler SA. Hyponatremia associated with selective serotonin reuptake inhibitors in older adults. Ann Pharmacother 2006;40:1618–1622.
18. Liamis G, Milionis H, Elisaf M. A review of drug-induced hyponatremia. Am J Kidney Dis 2008;52:144–153.
19. Meulendijks D, Mannesse CK, Jansen PA, et al. Antipsychotic-induced hyponatremia: a systematic review of the published evidence. Drug Saf 2010;33:101–114.

20. Reynolds RM, Padfield PL, Seckl JR. Disorders of sodium balance. BMJ 2006;332:702–705.

21. Decaux G. Is asymptomatic hyponatremia really asymptomatic? Am J Med 2006;119(7A):S79-S82.

22. Kinsella S, Moran S, Sullivan MO, et al. Hyponatremia independent of osteoporosis is associated with fracture occurrence. Clin J Am Soc Nephrol 2010;5:275–280.

23. Ayus JC, Morits ML. Bone disease as a new complication of hyponatremia: moving beyond brain injury. Clin J Am Soc Nephrol 2010;5:167–168.

24. Sterns RH, Silver SM. Brain volume regulation in response to hypoosmolality and its correction. Am J Med 2006;119(7A):S12-S16.

25. Ayus JC, Arrief AI. Chronic hyponatremic encephalopathy in postmenopausal women—Association of therapies with morbidity and mortality. JAMA 1999;281:2299–2304.

26. Castilla-Guerra L, Fernandez-Moreno MC, Lopez-Chozas JM, et al. Electrolyte disturbances and seizures. Epilepsia 2006;47:1990–1998.

27. Sterns RH. Severe symptomatic hyponatremia: Treatment and outcome: A study of 64 cases. Ann Intern Med 1987;107:656–664.

28. Murase TM, Sugimura Y, Takefuji S, et al. Mechanisms and therapy of osmotic demyelination. Am J Med 2006;119(7A):S69-S73.

29. Sterns RH, Riggs JE, Schochet SS Jr. Osmotic demyelination syndrome following correction of hyponatremia. N Engl J Med 1986;314:1535–1542.

30. Ellison DH. Core curriculum in nephrology: Disorders of sodium and water. Am J Kidney Dis 2005;46:356–361.

31. Decaux G, Soupart A. Treatment of symptomatic hyponatremia. Am J Med Sci 2003;326:25–30.

32. Androgue HJ, Madias NE. Aiding fluid prescription for dysnatremias. Intensive Care Med 1997;23:309–316.

33. Nguyen MK, Kurtz I. A new quantitative approach to the treatment of the dysnatremias. Clin Exp Nephrol 2003;7:125–137.

34. Kurtz I, Nguyen MK. Evolving concepts in the quantitative analysis of the determinants of the plasma water sodium concentration and the pathophysiology and treatment of the dysnatremias. Kidney Int 2005;68:1982–1993.

35. Kraft MD, Btaiche IF, Sacks GS, Kudsk KA. Treatment of electrolyte disorders in adult patients in the intensive care unit. Am J Health Syst Pharm 2005;62:1663–1682.

36. Liamis G, Kalogirou M, Saugos V, Moses E. Therapeutic approach in patients with dysnatremias. Nephrol Dial Transplant 2006;21:1564–1569.

37. Fanestil DD, Moore FD. Compartmentation of body water. In: Narins RG, ed. Maxwell and Kleeman's Fluid and Electrolyte Metabolism, 5th ed. New York: McGraw-Hill, 1994:1–20.

38. Mange K, Matsuura D, Cizman B, et al. Language guiding therapy: The case of dehydration versus volume depletion. Ann Intern Med 1997;127:848–853.

39. Decaux G, Waterlot Y, Genette F, Mockel J. Treatment of the syndrome of inappropriate secretion of antidiuretic hormone with furosemide. N Engl J Med 1981;304:329–330.

40. Verbalis JG. Hyponatremia and hyposmolar disorders. In: Greenberg A, ed. Primer on Kidney Diseases, 5th ed. Philadelphia, PA: WB Saunders, 2009:52–60.

41. Curtis NJ, van Heyningen C, Turner JJ. Irreversible nephrotoxicity from demeclocycline in the treatment of hyponatremia. Age Ageing 2002;31:151–152.

42. Greenberg A, Verbalis JG. Vasopressin receptor antagonists. Kidney Int 2006;69:2124–2130.

43. Palmer BF, Sterns RH. Syllabus: fluid, electrolyte and acid-base disorders. Nephrol Self Assess Program 2009;8(2):121–142.

44. Palm CP, Pistrosch F, Herbrig K, Gross P. Vasopressin antagonists as aquaretic agents for the treatment of hyponatremia. Am J Med 2006;119(7A):S87-S92.

45. Schrier RW, Gross P, Gheorghiade M, et al. Tolvaptan, a selective oral vasopressin V_2-receptor antagonist, for hyponatremia. N Engl J Med 2006;355:2099–2112.

46. Goldsmith SR. Treatment options for hyponatremia in heart failure. Heart Fail Rev 2009;14:65–73.

47. Oghlakian G, Klapholz M. Vaospressin and vasopressin receptor antagonists in heart failure. Cardiol Rev 2009;17:10–15.

48. Costello-Boerriger LC, Boerriger G, Burnett JC. Pharmacology of vasopressin antagonists. Heart Fail Rev 2009;14:75–82.

49. Samsca [package insert]. Rockville, MD: Otsuka America Pharmaceutical, Inc.; July 2009.

50. Shoaf SE, Graumer SL, Briemont P, et al. Pharmacokinetic and pharmacodynamic interaction between tolvaptan, an ono-peptide AV antagonist and furosemide or hydrochlorthiazide. J Cardiovasc Pharmacol 2007;50:213–222.

51. Hauptman PJ, Zimmer C, Udelson J, et al. Comparison of two doses and dosing regimens of tolvaptan in congestive heart failure. J Cardiolvasc Pharmacol 2005;46:609–614.

52. Elisaf M, Theodorou J, Pappas C, Siamopoulos K. Successful treatment of hyponatremia with angiotensin-converting enzyme inhibitors in patients with congestive heart failure. Cardiology 1995;86:477–480.

53. Bakris GL, Weir MR. Angiotensin-converting enzyme inhibitor-associated elevation of creatinine: Is this a cause for concern? Arch Intern Med 2000;160:685–693.

54. Gerbes AL, Gulberg V, Gines P, et al. Therapy of hyponatremia in cirrhosis with a vasopressin receptor antagonist: A randomized double-blind multicenter trial. Gastroenterology 2003;124:933–939.

55. Berl T, Quittnet-Pelletier F, Verbalis JG, et al. Oral tolvaptan is safe and effective in chronic hyponatremia. J Am Soc Nephrol 2010;21:705–712.

56. Dixon MB, Lien YH. Tolvaptan and its potential in the treatment of hyponatremia. Therapeut Clin Risk Management 2008;4:1149–1155.

57. Gheorghaide M, Niazi I, Quyang J, et al. Vasopressin V2-receptor blockage with tolvaptan in patients with chronic heart failure: results from a double-blind randomized trial. Circulation 2003;107:2690–2696.

58. Gheorghaide M, Gattis WA, O'Connor CM, et al. Effects of tolvaptan, a vasopressin antagonist, in patients hospitalized with worsening heart failure: a randomized controlled trial. JAMA 2004;291:1963–1971.

59. Gheorghiade M, Konstam MA, Burnett JC Jr, et al. Short-term clinical effects of tolvaptan, an oral vasopressin antagonist, in patients hospitalized for heart failure: the EVEREST Clinical Status Trials. JAMA 2007;297:1332–1343.

60. Konstam MA, Gheorghiade M, Burnett JC Jr, et al. Effects of oral tolvaptan in patients hospitalized for worsening heart failure: the EVEREST Outcome Trial. JAMA 2007;297:1319–1331.

61. Udelson JE, Orlandi C, Quyang J, et al. Acute hemodynamic effects of tolvaptan, a vasopressin V2 receptor blocker, in patients with symptomatic heart failure and systolic dysfunction: the ECLIPSE international, multi-center, randomized, placebo-controlled trial. Heart Failure Society of America; September 19, 2007; Washington, DC.

62. Udelson JE, McGrew FA, Flores E, et al. Multicenter, randomized, double-blind, placebo-controlled study on the effect of oral tolvaptan on left ventricular dilation and function in patients with heart failure and systolic dysfunction. J Am Coll Cardiol 2005;49:2151–2159.

63. Costello-Boerriger LC, Smith WB, Boerriger G, et al. Vasopressin-2-receptor antagonism augments water excretion without changes in renal hemodynamics or sodium and potassium excretion in human heartfailure. Am J Physiol Renal Physiol 2005;290:F273- F278.

64. Dennen P, Linas S. Hypernatremia. In: Greenberg A, ed. Primer on Kidney Diseases, 5th ed. Philadelphia, PA: WB Saunders, 2009:60–69.

65. Palevsky PM, Bhagrath R, Greenberg A. Hypernatremia in hospitalized patients. Ann Intern Med 1996;124:197–203.

66. Aiyagari V, Deibert E, Diringer MN. Hypernatremia in the neurologic intensive care: How high is too high? J Crit Care 2006;21:163–172.

67. Moritz ML, Ayus JC. The changing pattern of hypernatremia in hospitalized children. Pediatrics 1999;104:435–439.

68. Sands JM, Bichet DG. Nephrogenic diabetes insipidus. Ann Intern Med 2006;144:186–194.

69. Garofeanu CG, Weir M, Rosas-Arellano P, et al. Causes of reversible nephrogenic diabetes insipidus: A systematic review. Am J Kidney Dis 2005;45:626–637.

70. Chassagne P, Druesne L, Capet C, Menard JF, Bercoff E. Clinical presentation of hypernatremia in elderly patients: A case control study. J Am Geriatr Soc 2006;54:1225–1230.

71. Andreoli TE. The polyuric syndromes. Nephrol Dial Transplant 2001;16(Suppl 6):10–12.

72. Zerbe RL, Robertson GL. A comparison of plasma vasopressin measurements with a standard indirect test in the differential diagnosis of polyuria. N Engl J Med 1981;304:1539–1546.

73. Moritz ML. A water deprivation test is not indicated in the evaluation of hypernatremia [letter]. Am J Kidney Dis 2005;46:1150–1151.

74. Monnens L, Jonkman A, Thomas C. Response to indomethacin and hydrochlorothiazide in nephrogenic diabetes insipidus. Clin Sci 1984;66:709–715.

75. Battle DC, Von Riotte AB, Gaviria M, Grupp M. Amelioration of polyuria by amiloride in patients receiving long-term lithium therapy. N Engl J Med 1985;312:408–414.

76. Bonventre JV, Leaf A. Sodium homeostasis: Steady states without a setpoint. Kidney Int 1982;21:880–883.

77. Taylor AE. Capillary fluid filtration: Starling forces and lymph flow. Circ Res 1981;49:557–575.

78. Schrier RW. Pathogenesis of sodium and water retention in high-output and low-output cardiac failure, nephrotic syndrome, cirrhosis, and pregnancy. N Engl J Med 1988;319:1127–1134.

79. Sarafidis PA, Georgianos PI, Lasaridis AN. Diuretics in clinical practice. Part I: mechanism of action, pharmacological effects and clinical indications of diuretic compounds. Expert Opin Drug Saf 2010;9: 243–257.

80. Rudy DW, Voelker JR, Greene PK, et al. Loop diuretics for chronic renal insufficiency: A continuous infusion is more efficacious than bolus therapy. Ann Intern Med 1991;115:360–366.

81. Ellison DH. Edema and the clinical use of diuretics. In: Greenberg A, ed. Primer on Kidney Diseases, 5th ed. Philadelphia, PA: WB Saunders, 2009:135–147.

82. Kirchner KA, Voelker JR, Brater DC. Intratubular albumin blunts the response to furosemide—A mechanism for diuretic resistance in the nephrotic syndrome. J Pharmacol Exp Ther 1990;252: 1097–1101.

83. Agarwal R, Gorski JC, Sundblad K, Brater DC. Urinary protein binding does not affect response to furosemide in patients with nephrotic syndrome. J Am Soc Nephrol 2000;11:1100–1105.

84. Weiner ID, Wingo CS. Hypokalemia—Consequences, causes, and correction. J Am Soc Nephrol 1997;8:1179–1188.

85. Liew D, Martin J, Krum H. Eplerenone. Pharmacia. Curr Opin Investig Drugs 2003;4:316–322.

CHAPTER 59

Disorders of Calcium and Phosphorus Homeostasis

AMY BARTON PAI

KEY CONCEPTS

❶ Severe acute hypercalcemia can result in cardiac arrhythmias, whereas chronic hypercalcemia can lead to calcium deposition in soft tissues including blood vessels and the kidney.

❷ The correction of hypercalcemia can include multiple pharmacotherapeutic modalities such as hydration, diuretics, bisphosphonates, and steroids, depending on the etiology and acuity of the hypercalcemia.

❸ Hypocalcemia is typically associated with an insidious onset; however, some drugs such as cinacalcet are associated with rapid decreases in serum calcium.

❹ Acute treatment of hypocalcemia requires calcium supplementation whereas chronic management may require other therapies such as vitamin D to maintain serum calcium values.

❺ Hyperphosphatemia occurs most frequently in patients with chronic kidney disease.

❻ Treatment of nonemergent hyperphosphatemia includes the use of phosphate binders to decrease absorption of phosphorus from the gastrointestinal tract.

❼ Hypophosphatemia is a relatively common complication among critically ill patients.

❽ Treatment of acute hypophosphatemia usually requires intravenous supplementation of phosphorous salts.

Disorders of calcium and phosphorus are common complications of multiple acute and chronic diseases. These disorders are frequently seen in the acute care setting; however, they are also often present in ambulatory patients, usually in a less severe state. The consequences of electrolyte disorders can range from asymptomatic to life-threatening, requiring hospitalization and emergent treatment. The maintenance of fluid and electrolyte homeostasis requires adequate functioning and modulation by multiple hormones on tissues of multiple organ systems.

There are many common drug therapies that can disturb the normal homeostatic mechanisms that maintain calcium and phosphorous balance. In addition, with some drug therapies, toxicity is

Learning objectives, review questions, and other resources can be found at **www.pharmacotherapyonline.com**.

enhanced when underlying electrolyte disorders are present. Drug-induced disorders typically respond well to discontinuation of the offending agent(s); however, additional therapies are sometimes required to correct the disorder. This chapter reviews the etiology, classification, clinical presentation, and therapy for the most common disorders of calcium and phosphorus homeostasis.

DISORDERS OF CALCIUM HOMEOSTASIS

The maintenance of physiologic calcium concentrations in the intracellular and extracellular spaces is vital for the preservation and function of cell membranes; propagation of neuromuscular activity; regulation of endocrine and exocrine secretory functions; blood coagulation cascade; platelet adhesion process; bone metabolism; muscle cell excitation/contraction coupling; and mediation of the electrophysiologic slow-channel response in cardiac and smooth-muscle tissue.

The disorders of calcium homeostasis are related to the calcium content of the extracellular fluid, which is tightly regulated and comprises less than 0.5% of the total body stores of calcium. Skeletal bone contains more than 99% of total body stores of calcium.[1] Extracellular fluid (ECF) calcium is moderately bound to plasma proteins (46%), primarily albumin.[2] Ionized or free calcium is the physiologically active form and is the fraction that is homeostatically regulated.[3] Extracellular calcium, however, is most commonly measured as the total serum calcium level, which includes both bound and unbound calcium.[2] The normal total calcium serum concentration range is 8.5 to 10.5 mg/dL (2.13–2.63 mmol/L).[3]

Proper assessment of total serum calcium concentrations includes measurement of the patient's serum albumin concentration. Hypoalbuminemia, which can be associated with many chronic disease states, is probably the most common cause of "laboratory hypocalcemia." Patients remain asymptomatic because the unbound or ionized fraction of serum calcium remains normal (normal range, 4.4–5.4 mg/dL [1.10–1.35 mmol/L]). A corrected total serum calcium (S_{ca}) concentration can be calculated based on the measured total serum calcium and the difference between a patient's measured albumin concentration and the normative value of 4 g/dL (40 g/L) by the following equations:

$$\text{Corrected } S_{ca} \text{ (mg/dL)} = \text{measured } S_{ca} \text{ (mg/dL)} + [0.8 \times (4.0 \text{ g/dL} - \text{measured albumin (g/dL)})]$$

Or

$$\text{Corrected } S_{ca} \text{ (mmol/L)} = \text{measured } S_{ca} \text{ (mmol/L)} + [0.02 \times (40 \text{ g/L} - \text{measured albumin (g/L)})]$$

The concentration of ionized calcium is closely regulated by the interactions of parathyroid hormone (PTH), phosphorus,

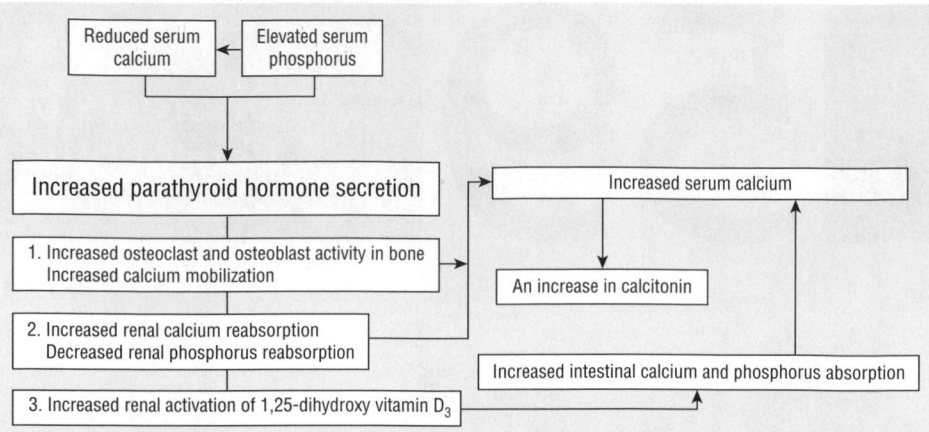

FIGURE 59-1. Homeostatic mechanisms to maintain serum calcium concentrations.

vitamin D, and calcitonin (Fig. 59–1). PTH increases serum calcium concentrations by stimulating calcium release from bone, increasing renal tubular reabsorption, and enhancing absorption in the gastrointestinal tract secondary to increased renal production of 1,25-dihydroxy vitamin D_3. Vitamin D directly increases serum calcium, as well as phosphorus concentrations, by increasing gastrointestinal absorption. Indirectly, it can also lead to calcium release from bone and reduced renal excretion. Calcitonin inhibits osteoclastic bone resorption. Its plasma concentrations are increased when ionized calcium concentrations are high as the body attempts to return the calcium level to the normal range. Disruption of these homeostatic mechanisms results in the clinical manifestations of hypercalcemia or hypocalcemia.

Alteration of the concentration of albumin or its binding of calcium can be expected to change the unbound fraction of total serum calcium. The most significant cause of changes in calcium binding to albumin is a change in extracellular fluid pH. In the presence of acute metabolic alkalosis the fraction of calcium bound to albumin is increased, thus reducing the plasma concentration of ionized calcium. This can result in symptomatic hypocalcemia; that is, paresthesia, muscle cramping and spasms, memory loss, and seizures.[1] Conversely, metabolic acidosis decreases calcium binding to albumin and results in increased ionized calcium. Hypoalbuminemic states are probably the most common cause of "laboratory hypocalcemia." When the albumin level is decreased, the ionized calcium concentration can be normal although total serum calcium concentration is low. Each 1 g/dL (10 g/L) drop in the serum albumin concentration below 4 g/dL (40 g/L) will result in a decrease of total serum calcium concentration by 0.8 mg/dL (0.20 mmol/L).[1,2] This approach of calculating an albumin-adjusted calcium concentration has been found to overestimate the degree of hypercalcemia and usually fails to identify hypocalcemia in critically ill patients, therefore ionized calcium values should be used to assess calcium status in these patients.[4,5]

HYPERCALCEMIA

There are multiple and diverse causes of hypercalcemia (total serum calcium >10.5 mg/dL [2.62 mmol/L]) (Table 59–1). The most common causes of hypercalcemia are cancer and primary hyperparathyroidism. The reported incidence of primary hyperparathyroidism in the United States ranges from 10 to 30 cases per 100,000 people.[6] Hypercalcemia of cancer occurs in approximately 20% to 40% of cancer patients at some time during the course of their disease.[7] Cancer-associated hypercalcemia

is predominantly encountered in hospitalized patients, whereas primary hyperparathyroidism accounts for the vast majority of cases in the outpatient setting.[8,9]

PATHOPHYSIOLOGY

Hypercalcemia is the result of one or a combination of three primary mechanisms: increased bone resorption, increased gastrointestinal absorption, or increased tubular reabsorption by the kidneys (see Fig. 59–1).

Many tumors secrete PTH–related protein (PTHrP), which binds to the PTH receptors in bone and renal tissues, leading to increased bone resorption and renal tubular reabsorption.[10] Tumors can also secrete substances such as vitamin D, transforming growth factor, interleukins, prostaglandins, interferon, tumor necrosis factor, and granulocyte-macrophage colony–stimulating factor, which are associated with the development of hypercalcemia.[7] Hypercalcemia of malignancy is a common complication of squamous cell carcinomas of the lung, head, and neck, hematologic malignancies such as multiple myeloma and

TABLE 59-1	Etiologies of Hypercalcemia
Neoplasms	**Medications**
Bone metastasis	Thiazides
Breast	Lithium
Multiple myeloma	Vitamin D
Lymphoma	Vitamin A
Leukemia	Calcium
Humoral induced	Aluminum/magnesium antacids
Ovary	Theophylline
Kidney	Tamoxifen
Pheochromocytoma	Ganciclovir
Multiple endocrine neoplasia	**Granulomatous disease**
Lung	Sarcoidosis
Head and neck	Tuberculosis
Esophagus	Cryptococcus
Cervix	Berylliosis
Lymphoproliferative disease	Histoplasmosis
Hyperparathyroidism	Coccidioidomycosis
Primary	Leprosy
Tertiary	**Endocrine disease**
Miscellaneous	Adrenal insufficiency
Immobilization	Hyperthyroidism
Paget's disease	Acromegaly
Familial hypocalciuric hypercalcemia	
Adolescence	
Rhabdomyolysis	

T-cell lymphomas, and carcinomas of ovary, kidney, bladder, and breast. The most frequent types of malignancy associated with hypercalcemia are carcinomas of the lung and breast.[9] Breast and squamous cell lung carcinomas secrete PTHrP which binds to the type I PTH receptor (PTHR1) and enhances bone resorption. In contrast, up to 40% of patients with multiple myeloma develop hypercalcemia principally as the result of osteoclast-mediated bone destruction.[9]

Primary hyperparathyroidism is the most common cause of chronic hypercalcemia in the general population. Benign parathyroid adenomas account for 80% to 85% of these cases of hyperparathyroidism, parathyroid hyperplasia accounts for 15%, and parathyroid carcinoma is the cause in less than 1% of cases.[8]

Other causes of chronic hypercalcemia include medications, endocrine and granulomatous disorders, physical immobilization, high bone-turnover states (adolescence and Paget disease), and rhabdomyolysis. Increased gastrointestinal absorption can be the result of excessive ingestion of vitamin D analogs, calcium supplements, and lithium. Lithium and vitamin A therapy can increase bone resorption, whereas increased renal tubular reabsorption of calcium can occur with thiazide and lithium therapy. The exact mechanism of lithium-induced hypercalcemia is not known but may include competitive inhibition of calcium influx into cells, increasing the threshold sensitivity of the calcium-sensing receptor and subsequent inhibition of PTH gene transcription.[9] Addison's disease, acromegaly, and thyrotoxicosis are endocrine disorders that can lead to hypercalcemia because of increased renal tubular reabsorption and increased bone resorption. Finally, the granulomatous disorders (sarcoidosis, tuberculosis, histoplasmosis, and leprosy) are associated with hypercalcemia caused by an increase in gastrointestinal and renal tubular absorption secondary to granuloma production of 1,25-dihydroxy vitamin D_2.[12] Milk-alkali syndrome is the term applied to those situations where an individual develops hypercalcemia following the ingestion of calcium and absorbable alkali (e.g., calcium carbonate) and is an important cause of hypercalcemia in patients who are not on dialysis.[13,14]

CLINICAL PRESENTATION

Patients with mild to moderate hypercalcemia, that is, total serum calcium concentrations above the upper threshold of normal but less than 13 mg/dL (<3.25 mmol/L) or ionized calcium concentrations less than 6.0 mg/dL (<1.50 mmol/L), can often be asymptomatic. This is typically the case for the vast majority of patients who have drug-induced hypercalcemia or primary hyperparathyroidism.[8,15,16] In fact, one study noted normocalcemia in approximately 20% of patients with a diagnosis of primary hyperparathyroidism, suggesting target tissue resistance to PTH.[16]

❶ The presenting signs and symptoms of severe hypercalcemia that occur if the total serum calcium concentration is >13 mg/dL (>3.25 mmol/L) may differ depending on the acuity of onset.[2] Hypercalcemia of malignancy usually develops quickly and is accompanied by a classic symptom complex of anorexia, nausea and vomiting, constipation, polyuria, polydipsia, and nocturia.[15] Polyuria and nocturia secondary to a urinary-concentrating defect constitute some of the most frequent renal effects of hypercalcemia.[15] Hypercalcemic crisis is characterized by an acute elevation of total serum calcium to a value >15 mg/dL (>3.75 mmol/L), acute renal insufficiency, and obtundation (inability to arouse).[15] If untreated, hypercalcemic crisis can progress to oliguric renal failure, coma, and life-threatening ventricular arrhythmias.[15] The primary complications associated with chronic hypercalcemia (hyperparathyroidism) include metastatic calcification, hypercalciuria, and chronic renal insufficiency secondary to interstitial nephrocalcinosis.[15]

CLINICAL PRESENTATION OF HYPERCALCEMIA

General

- The signs and symptoms of hypercalcemia depend on severity and on the rapidity of onset.

Symptoms

- Symptoms include fatigue, weakness, anorexia, depression, anxiety, cognitive dysfunction, vague abdominal pain, and constipation. Renal symptoms can include polyuria, polydipsia, and nocturia. Rarely, severe hypercalcemia leads to acute pancreatitis

Signs

- Renal: The most important renal manifestations which are generally the result of chronic hypercalcemia are nephrolithiasis; renal tubular dysfunction, particularly decreased concentrating ability; and acute and chronic renal insufficiency.

- Cardiovascular: Long-standing hypercalcemia can lead to the deposition of calcium in heart valves, coronary arteries, and myocardial fibers. Hypercalcemia also directly shortens the myocardial action potential, which is reflected in a shortened QT interval and coving of the ST-T wave. Spontaneous ventricular tachyarrhythmias and elevations in blood pressure have also been reported.

- Musculoskeletal: A number of rheumatologic complaints have been described in hyperparathyroidism, including gout, pseudo-gout, and chondrocalcinosis. The relative roles of hypercalcemia and PTH excess in these problems are not known.

Laboratory Tests

- Serum calcium concentrations of >10.5 mg/dL (>2.63 mmol/L) are considered to represent hypercalcemia. Patients with values up to 13 mg/dL (3.25 mmol/L) are generally considered to have mild or moderate hypercalcemia, whereas those with values greater than this indicate the presence of severe hypercalcemia.

Calcium and/or calcium-phosphorus complex deposition in blood vessels and multiple organs is a complication of chronic hypercalcemia and/or concomitant hyperphosphatemia and hyperparathyroidism. Calcium deposits in atherosclerotic lesions contribute to cardiac disease.[17] Intracardiac and arterial calcifications have been found in patients with Paget disease who have normal renal function. It is hypothesized that similar calcification processes occur in both bone and vascular tissue, leading to cardiovascular diseases including heart failure, systolic hypertension, and ischemic heart disease.[18]

The electrocardiographic changes associated with hypercalcemia include shortening of the QT interval and coving of the ST-T wave.[15] Very high serum calcium concentrations can cause T-wave widening, indicating a repolarization defect that may be associated with spontaneous ventricular tachyarrhythmias.[15] Hypertension and arrhythmias have occurred in the setting of hypercalcemia. The effects of digoxin on cardiac conduction including lowering of the excitation threshold, shortening of the effective refractory period and increased atrioventricular refractoriness, can be potentiated by hypercalcemia.[19]

Nephrolithiasis (kidney stones) and nephrocalcinosis (calcium deposits in the kidney) are the primary renal complications arising from long-standing hypercalcemia, as the result of primary hyperparathyroidism. Stone formation is dependent on a favorable milieu within the kidney or urinary tract such as, oversaturation of the urine and/or reduced concentrations of endogenous inhibitors of crystal formation (e.g., citrate or pyrophosphate). It is estimated that hyperparathyroidism accounts for 2% to 8% of all patients with calcium stones.[20,21] Of note, in those patients with low glomerular filtration rates (GFRs), the 24-hour urinary calcium will actually diminish secondary to decreased production of 1,25-dihydroxy vitamin D_2. However, the fractional excretion of calcium might increase.[21] Sarcoidosis is the other hypercalcemic condition frequently associated with calcium stones.[20] Other causes of nephrolithiasis with calcium-containing stones include hypocitraturia, renal tubular acidosis, hyperoxaluria, and hyperuricosuria.[22,23] Stone formers who have primary hyper-parathyroidism are more likely to be female, older than 50 years of age, and have a family history of multiple endocrine disorders.[20] High dietary sodium intake can also raise urinary calcium concentrations, perhaps due to a reduction in calcium reabsorption in the kidney, thus predisposing patients to calcium stones. Although chronic renal failure can be the ultimate result of persistent stones, it is the primary cause of renal disease in <2% of the end-stage renal disease population.

TREATMENT

Hypercalcemia

■ DESIRED OUTCOME

The indications for the treatment of acute hypercalcemia are dependent on the severity of hypercalcemia, acuity of its development, and presence or absence of symptoms requiring emergent treatment (e.g., necrotizing pancreatitis). The therapeutic intervention plan should be crafted to reverse signs and symptoms, restore normocalcemia, and correct or manage the underlying cause of hypercalcemia.

Chronic hypercalcemia is usually caused by an underlying medical condition or prescribed pharmacotherapies that can be resolved by successful treatment of the condition or withdrawal of the offending agent. Acute hypercalcemic episodes induced by malignancies may be mitigated by chemotherapy and/or radiation treatment. Effective surgical or drug treatment of primary hyperparathyroidism should reduce serum calcium concentrations as well as reduce the development of long-term complications such as vascular complications, chronic kidney disease (CKD), and kidney stones.

■ NONPHARMACOLOGIC THERAPY

Hypercalcemic crisis and acute symptomatic severe hypercalcemia should be considered medical emergencies and treated immediately (Fig. 59–2).

These patients may require immediate-acting interventions to promptly reduce the serum calcium concentration if they are experiencing ECG changes, neurologic manifestations, or pancreatitis. Pharmacologic therapy consisting of volume expansion and enhancement of urinary calcium excretion with loop diuretics is usually the initial management strategy. Hemodialysis against a zero- or low-calcium dialysate solution should be considered for patients with severely impaired renal function (CKD stage 4 or 5) who cannot tolerate large fluid loads and in whom diuretics have limited efficacy.[22]

Effective treatment of moderate to severe hypercalcemia in the absence of life-threatening symptoms begins with attention to the underlying disorder and correction of associated fluid and electrolyte abnormalities. Patients with primary hyperparathyroidism may require surgery, particularly if they have systemic manifestations. Patients with malignancy often require surgical or chemotherapeutic reduction of tumor load to control the exogenous supply of cytokines and hormones (e.g. PTHrP) that cause hypercalcemia. In contrast, patients with drug-induced hypercalcemia generally respond to discontinuation of the offending agent.

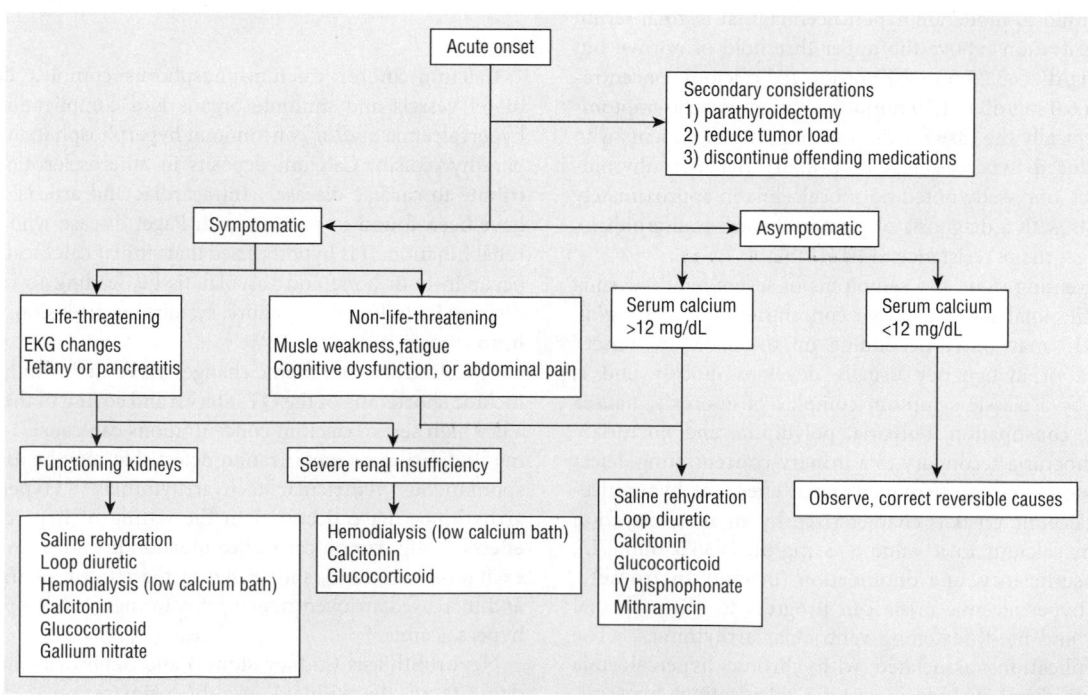

FIGURE 59-2. Pharmacotherapeutic options for the acutely hypercalcemic patient. Serum calcium of 12 mg/dL is equivalent to 3.00 mmol/L.

Drug	Starting Dosage	Time Frame to Initial Response	Contraindications	Adverse Effects
0.9% saline ± electrolytes	200–300 mL/hour	24–48 hours	Renal insufficiency; congestive heart failure	Electrolyte abnormalities; fluid overload
Loop diuretics	40–80 mg IV q 1–4 hours	N/A	Allergy to sulfas (use ethacrynic acid)	Electrolyte abnormalities
Calcitonin	4 units/kg q 12 hours SC/IM 10–12 units/hours IV	1–2 hours	Allergy to calcitonin	Facial flushing, nausea/vomiting, allergic reaction
Pamidronate	30–90 mg IV over 2–24 hours	2 days	Renal insufficiency	Fever
Etidronate	7.5 mg/kg/day IV over 2 hours	2 days	Renal insufficiency	Fever
Zoledronate	4–8 mg IV over 15 min	1–2 days	Renal insufficiency	Fever, fatigue, skeletal pain
Ibandronate	2–6 mg IV bolus	2 days	Renal insufficiency	Fever, musculoskeletal pain
Gallium nitrate	200 mg/m²/day	?	Severe renal insufficiency	Nephrotoxicity; hypophosphatemia; nausea/vomiting/diarrhea; metallic taste
Mithramycin	25 mcg/kg IV over 4–6 hours	12 hours	Decreased liver function; renal insufficiency; thrombocytopenia	Nausea/vomiting; stomatitis; thrombocytopenia; nephrotoxicity; hepatotoxicity
Glucocorticoids	40–60 mg oral prednisone equivalents daily	3–5 days	Serious infections; hypersensitivity	Diabetes; osteoporosis; infection

SC, subcutaneous.

■ PHARMACOLOGIC THERAPY

CLINICAL CONTROVERSY

Although dialysis is the most effective method for rapidly reducing highly elevated serum calcium in patients with CKD, many clinicians choose normal saline and/or a loop diuretic approach as the initial therapy.

❷ For those patients with normal to moderately impaired renal function (CKD stages 3 and 4), the cornerstone of initial treatment of severe hypercalcemia or hypercalcemic crisis is volume expansion with normal saline to increase natriuresis and ultimately urinary calcium excretion (see Table 59–2). Patients with symptomatic hypercalcemia are often extracellular volume depleted secondary to vomiting and polyuria; thus rehydration with saline-containing fluids is necessary to interrupt the stimulus for sodium and calcium reabsorption in the renal tubule.[24] Rehydration can be accomplished by the infusion of normal saline at rates of 200 to 300 mL/h, until the patient is fluid resuscitated and serum calcium approaches the upper limit of the normal range. The precise rate depends on concomitant conditions (primarily cardiovascular and renal) and magnitude of hypercalcemia. The saline infusion rate can be decreased to a rate that approximates the patient's intake of oral or intravenous fluids. (See Chapter 58 for a thorough discussion of the concepts and calculations of water deficit.) Adequacy of hydration is assessed by measuring fluid intake and output or by central venous pressure monitoring.[9] Loop diuretics such as furosemide (40–80 mg IV every 1–4 hours) or ethacrynic acid (for patients with sulfa allergies) can also be instituted to increase urinary calcium excretion and to minimize the development of volume overload from the administration of saline[9] (Fig. 59–2 and Table 59–2). Loop diuretics such as furosemide block calcium (and sodium) reabsorption in the thick ascending limb of the loop of Henle and augment the calciuric effect of saline alone. The importance of rehydration prior to loop diuretic use is critical because if dehydration persists or becomes worse the serum calcium can actually increase because of enhanced proximal tubule calcium reabsorption.[2] Potassium chloride, 10 to 20 mEq/L (10–20 mmol/L), should be added to the saline solution after rehydration is accomplished to maintain

normokalemia in the presence of diuretic therapy. Serum magnesium levels should also be monitored, and magnesium replacement instituted if magnesium levels fall below 1.8 mg/dL (0.74 mmol/L). Rehydration with saline and administration of furosemide can result in a decrease of 2 to 3 mg/dL (0.50–0.75 mmol/L) in total serum calcium within 24 to 48 hours.[9]

In those patients in whom saline hydration therapy is contraindicated (e.g., those with severe chronic heart failure [CHF] or moderate to severe renal dysfunction), short-term therapy with calcitonin is a viable alternative agent to initiate reduction of serum calcium levels within 24 to 48 hours. Calcitonin has a rapid onset of action (within 1–2 hours); however, the degree and extent of serum calcium level reduction are often unpredictable.[2] Calcitonin decreases serum calcium concentrations, primarily by inhibiting bone resorption. It can also reduce renal tubular reabsorption of calcium, thus promoting calciuresis.[25] Recently, the calcitonin receptor has been shown to play an important role in calcium homeostasis, particularly in states of calcium stress (e.g., vitamin D toxicity).[25] Calcitonin from salmon sources is most commonly administered subcutaneously or intramuscularly (for larger volumes) in a starting dose of 4 units/kg every 12 hours. The side effects from intravenously administered calcitonin (facial flushing, nausea, and vomiting) limit patient acceptability. Allergic reactions, although rare, do occur; therefore a test dose (intradermal injection of 0.1 mL of a 10-units/mL solution) is recommended prior to starting therapy. If marked erythema and/or wheal formation does not occur within 15 minutes after administration, therapy can begin. Salmon calcitonin therapy is associated with tachyphylaxis caused by antibody formation to foreign proteins or molecules resembling the calcitonin polypeptide.[25] Tachyphylaxis has been primarily documented in patients receiving therapy for more than 4 months and thus might not be clinically significant in the acute care setting. The addition of corticosteroid therapy or conversion to human calcitonin increases effectiveness.[2]

Finally, intravenous phosphate was used historically to rapidly reduce ionized calcium concentrations through the formation of insoluble calcium-phosphate salts. However, intravenous phosphate is extremely hazardous because extraskeletal (e.g., intraluminal and intrarenal) precipitation of calcium-phosphate can result in metastatic calcification, hypotension, acute renal failure, or death and thus it currently does not have a role in the management of acute hypercalcemia.[2]

Bisphosphonates block bone resorption very efficiently, render the hydroxyapatite crystal of bone mineral resistant to hydrolysis by phosphatases, and also inhibit osteoclast precursors from attaching to the mineralized matrix, thus blocking their transformation into mature functioning osteoclasts.[15,26] The antiresorptive properties of this class of agents can provide long-term control of serum calcium and are the first-line therapy for cancer-associated hypercalcemia.

Pamidronate is very effective in controlling hypercalcemia associated with malignancy and slightly more effective than etidronate.[7] The usual dose of pamidronate is 30 to 90 mg as an IV infusion given over 2 to 24 hours. Pamidronate also has the advantage of single-day therapy.[9] Etidronate, when administered in doses of 7.5 mg/kg per day by slow intravenous infusion over at least 2 hours for 3 days, is effective in the therapy of hypercalcemia of malignancy.[9] Zoledronate and ibandronate are the newest high-potency bisphosphonates with demonstrated effectiveness in the treatment of hypercalcemia of malignancy. Complete response has been reported in 88.4% to 86.7% of zoledronate-versus 69.7% of pamidronate-treated patients.[27,28] Zoledronate intravenous doses of 4 to 8 mg given over 5 minutes have resulted in normalization of serum calcium concentrations.[28] Intravenous infusions of 0.02 or 0.04 mg/kg diluted in 5% dextrose (given over 20–50 minutes) have also been effective.[29] A similar hypocalcemic response has been noted with ibandronate in comparison with pamidronate (76.5% vs 75.8%); however, the time period to a relapse of hypercalcemia was longer with ibandronate (14 days vs 4 days), suggesting a therapeutic advantage for ibandronate.[30] In contrast to other bisphosphonates, ibandronate can be administered by bolus injection. Single doses of 4 to 6 mg when administered every 3 to 4 weeks have been effective in managing hypercalcemia of malignancy.[31] The onset of serum calcium concentration decline is slower with bisphosphonate therapy (concentrations begin to decline in 2 days and reach a nadir in 7 days); thus calcitonin therapy can be necessary if rapid serum level reduction is required.[9,31] Duration of normocalcemia varies, but usually does not exceed 2 to 3 weeks. It appears to be dependant on the severity and treatment response of the underlying malignancy.[2] The duration of response has been suggested to be longer with zoledronate (4–5 weeks), although the data is sparse.[29] Fever is a common side effect of intravenous bisphosphonate therapy. Although oral bisphosphonates are useful for the treatment of bone turnover in Paget disease, there are insufficient data to suggest their use for the initial treatment of hypercalcemia. The use of oral bisphosphonates for maintenance therapy in patients predisposed to hypercalcemia (malignancy) has been successful in some cases.[32] The safety of continuous bisphosphonate therapy in patients with moderate to severe renal insufficiency is currently unknown. Renal function monitoring (serum creatinine) is advised with the use of bisphosphonates, as cases of acute tubular necrosis have been reported.[33,34] Although there are no published guidelines for frequency of serum creatinine monitoring, it is advisable to evaluate serum creatinine within a week after the infusion and just prior to the next scheduled dose.

CLINICAL CONTROVERSY

Bisphosphonates are renally eliminated and prescribing information advises that they be used with caution in patients with a GFR less than 30 mL/min (<0.5 mL/s); however, many clinicians use these agents for first-line treatment of cancer-related hypercalcemia.

Gallium nitrate is indicated for the treatment of symptomatic hypercalcemia of malignancy not responsive to hydration therapy.[35] However, because of its adverse side-effect profile, it is generally reserved for those who fail to respond to less toxic agents. Gallium nitrate inhibits bone resorption, and may be superior to calcitonin in inducing normocalcemia. It can provide a longer duration of normocalcemia as compared with etidronate. The initial dose is usually a continuous IV infusion of 200 mg/m^2 per day for 5 consecutive days. Gallium nitrate can be more effective in achieving normocalcemia in patients with epidermoid (squamous) cancers.[36] Because gallium nitrate is nephrotoxic, the initial dose should be conservative and the patient's renal function closely monitored if it is coadministered with other nephrotoxic drugs, including some chemotherapeutic agents, nonsteroidal anti-inflammatory drugs (NSAIDs), and antibiotics (e.g., gentamicin). Other common adverse effects include hypophosphatemia, nausea, vomiting, diarrhea, hypocalcemia, and metallic taste.

Mithramycin (plicamycin) is a potent cytotoxic antibiotic that inhibits osteoclast-mediated bone resorption and thereby reduces hypercalcemia. Mithramycin can be administered at a dose of 25 mcg/kg via intravenous infusion over 4 to 6 hours in saline or 5% dextrose solutions. This therapy can be repeated daily for 3 to 4 days or on alternating days for 3 to 8 doses.[9,37] Serum calcium levels begin to fall within 12 hours of a mithramycin dose, with the peak effect generally occurring over 48 to 96 hours.[2,9] Single doses are usually well tolerated.[37] Common dose-related adverse effects of mithramycin include nausea, vomiting, stomatitis, thrombocytopenia, inhibition of platelet function, and renal and hepatotoxicity can be avoided by limiting the number of doses administered to less than four.[2] Mithramycin is usually limited to short-term therapy (typically one to two doses) in patients who have not responded to alternative therapies. Complete blood count, liver function, and renal function should be monitored within 1 to 2 days after administration. Mithramycin should be avoided in patients with thrombocytopenia and liver and renal insufficiency (creatinine clearance <30 mL/min [<0.5 mL/s]).[9]

Denosumab is a monoclonal antibody that inhibits the receptor activator of nuclear factor kappa-light-chain-enhancer of activated B cells (NF-κB) ligand (RANKL), a principal mediator of osteoclast survival. Denosumab is in phase III clinical trials for the treatment of osteoporosis. Recently, denosumab has been investigated in patients with malignancies and bone metastases (without hypocalcemia) who were either bisphosphonate naïve or who had previous exposure to bisphosphonates. Patients were randomized to receive an IV bisphosphonate every 4 weeks (91% received zoledronic acid) or a fixed dose of denosumab every 4 weeks (30, 120, 180 mg) or every 12 weeks (60, 180 mg) to investigate the effect on the primary outcome measure of urinary-N-telopeptide, a marker for bone turnover. Patients who were bisphosphonate naïve had similar decline in markers of bone turnover. In patients with previous exposure to bisphosphonates, treatment with denosumab produced significantly greater reductions in bone turnover compared with an IV bisphosphonate. These preliminary results indicate that denosumab reduces bone turn over and may be efficacious in preventing or treating hypercalcemia of malignancy.[38]

Prednisone or an equivalent agent in the corticosteroid class is usually effective in the treatment of hypercalcemia resulting from multiple myeloma, leukemia, lymphoma, sarcoidosis, and hypervitaminoses A and D.[2,26,37] These agents are effective because they reduce gastrointestinal calcium absorption and decrease renal tubular calcium reabsorption.[37] Corticosteroids may also prevent tachyphylaxis to salmon calcitonin.[25] Daily doses of 40 to 60 mg of prednisone or the equivalent are effective at reducing serum calcium within 3 to 5 days followed by a reduction in urinary calcium excretion within 7 to 10 days. The disadvantages of corticosteroid therapy are its relatively slow onset of action and the

TABLE 59-3	Treatment of Nephrolithiasis Associated with Chronic Hypercalcemia and Hypercalciuria	
Intervention	Indications	Comments
Extracorporeal shock wave lithotripsy		
Uses sound waves to break up stones which then can pass spontaneously	Obstruction of the urinary tract especially with stones >5 mm	Consider adjunctive use of potassium citrate to inhibit aggregation of residual fragments
Prevention of Stone Formation		
Alkalinizing agents	Treatment for nonemergent active stones Can also be used for prevention	Potassium citrate preferred over sodium citrate as it decreases urinary calcium, inhibits calcium oxalate precipitation, and increases urinary citrate more
Potassium citrate PO 20 mEq twice daily Sodium citrate PO 20–30 mEq twice daily		
Decrease urinary calcium excretion		
Thiazide diuretics Hydrochlorothiazide PO 50 mg every day Indapamide PO 25 mg every day Chlorthalidone PO 25 mg every day	Prevention	Drug of choice in patients with low bone density
Binding intestinal calcium		
Cellulose sodium phosphate (Calcibind) Calcium binding ion-exchange resin that decreases gastrointestinal absorption of calcium: PO 5 g twice daily with oxalate restriction	Prevention for those with absorptive hypercalciuria	Alternative to thiazides if intolerant or ineffective, monitor bone density
Inhibition of crystal formation		
Phyllanthus nituri plant extract Inhibits calcium oxalate stone formation by incorporating glycosaminoglycans into the calculi: PO 2 g daily	Prevention, after shock wave lithotripsy	Commercial preparations with *P nituri* as the sole ingredient can be difficult to obtain
Low calcium diet		
Less than 400 mg per day	Prevention	Monitor bone density prior to and periodically during treatment, limit oxalate restriction, can increase hyperoxaluria, data suggest high calcium intake may actually be more beneficial

potential for diabetes mellitus, osteoporosis, and increased susceptibility to infection.[39]

Asymptomatic patients with mild hypercalcemia may be carefully observed, especially if treatment for the underlying condition (malignancy) is initiated. The calcimimetic agent cinacalcet HCl was recently approved for its calcium-lowering effect in the management of parathyroid carcinoma.[40,41] It binds to the calcium-sensing receptor, and increases the sensitivity for receptor activation by extracellular calcium. This results in reduced PTH and serum calcium concentrations.[40,41] Cinacalcet HCl administered at a starting dose of 30 mg orally twice daily has been used for the treatment of hypercalcemia secondary to parathyroid carcinoma. The dosage is titrated every 2 to 4 weeks in 30-mg increments until the desired serum calcium level is achieved. The maximum approved dosage is 90 mg 3 to 4 times daily. Patients should have serum calcium measured within 1 week after starting or increasing the dose of this agent.[42,43]

Subcutaneous administration of salmon calcitonin, 50 to 100 international units daily or 3 times weekly, has been used to manage mild hypercalcemia in patients with Paget disease.[44] The intranasal formulation of calcitonin has been used in doses of 200 to 400 international units daily; unfortunately, this has resulted in only mild decreases in serum calcium. The lack of significant efficacy of the synthetic intranasal formulation is the result of the lower potency and shorter duration of action as compared to salmon calcitonin. Patients who develop nephrolithiasis from hypercalciuria are most often treated with sodium citrate to prevent stone formation, thiazide diuretics to decrease urinary calcium excretion, or shock wave lithotripsy (Table 59–3).

HYPOCALCEMIA

❸ Hypocalcemia occurs infrequently in the outpatient setting and is most common in elderly, malnourished patients and those who have received sodium phosphate as a bowel preparation agent. The incidence of hypocalcemia in intensive care unit patients ranges from 70% to 90% based on total serum calcium values less than 8.5 mg/dL (<2.13 mmol/L) to 15% to 50% based on the observation of ionized calcium concentrations less than 4.4 mg/dL (<1.10 mmol/L).[3] Emergent treatment of hypocalcemia is rarely warranted unless life-threatening symptoms are present (e.g., frank tetany or seizures).

PATHOPHYSIOLOGY

Hypocalcemia is the result of alterations in the effect of PTH and vitamin D on the bone, gut, and kidney (see Fig. 59–1). The primary causes of hypocalcemia are postoperative hypoparathyroidism and vitamin D deficiency. Other causes include magnesium deficiency, thyroid surgery, medications, hypoalbuminemia, blood transfusions, peripheral blood progenitor cell harvesting, tumor lysis syndrome, and mutations in the calcium-sensing receptor.[45–50] PTH concentrations are elevated in conditions of hypocalcemia, with the exception of hypoparathyroidism and hypomagnesemia.[51]

Vitamin D Deficiency

Vitamin D and its metabolites play an important role in the maintenance of extracellular calcium concentrations and in normal skeletal structure and mineralization. Vitamin D is necessary for the optimal absorption of calcium and phosphorus. On a worldwide basis, the most common cause of chronic hypocalcemia is nutritional vitamin D deficiency. In malnourished populations, manifestations include rickets and osteomalacia. Nutritional vitamin D deficiency is uncommon in Western societies because of the fortification of milk with ergocalciferol. The most common cause of vitamin D deficiency in Western societies is gastrointestinal disease.[15] Gastric surgery, chronic pancreatitis, small-bowel disease, intestinal resection, and bypass surgery are associated with decreased concentrations of vitamin D and its metabolites.[15] Vitamin D replacement therapy might need to be administered by the intravenous route if poor oral bioavailability is noted. Decreased production of 1,25-dihydroxyvitamin D_3 can occur as a result of a hereditary defect resulting in vitamin D–dependent rickets. Recently, polymorphisms of the vitamin D receptor have been identified, and these genetic variations can contribute to increased risk of rickets associated with vitamin D and calcium deficient diets, especially in certain African and East Asian populations.[53] It also can occur secondary to chronic kidney disease if there is insufficient production of the 1-α-hydroxylase enzyme for the production of the most active metabolite, 1,25-dihydroxy vitamin D_3.[54] Treatment of hypocalcemia associated with CKD is reviewed in Chapter 53.

Hypomagnesemia

Hypomagnesemia of any cause can be associated with severe symptomatic hypocalcemia that is unresponsive to calcium replacement therapy (see Chapter 60). Reduced serum magnesium concentrations can impair PTH secretion and induce resistance of target organs to the actions of PTH.[15] Normalization of serum calcium concentrations in these patients is thus dependent on appropriate replacement of magnesium.

Tissue Consumption of Calcium

Decreased total serum calcium concentrations are seen in up to 10% of patients with acute pancreatitis, principally due to low serum albumin concentrations. These patients typically have more severe attacks, a poorer prognosis, and increased mortality rates.[55] The mechanisms responsible for the development of true hypocalcemia in pancreatitis have not been completely elucidated but may include binding of calcium to liberated fatty acids or possibly transcellular shifts induced by gram-negative endotoxin translocated from the gastrointestinal tract.[55] The etiology of sepsis-associated hypocalcemia may be the result of inflammatory mediators affecting calcium homeostasis.[56] Finally, rhabdomyolysis and tumor lysis syndrome can result in acute elevations of serum phosphorus that can bind ionized calcium.

Hungry Bone Sydrome

An acute, symptomatic rapid fall in total serum calcium concentration (to values <7 mg/dL [<1.75 mmol/L]) is common in patients who have recently had a parathyroidectomy or thyroidectomy. Hypocalcemia in these postsurgical patients is generally transient in nature.[52] The "hungry bone syndrome" is a condition of profound hypocalcemia whereby the bone avidly incorporates calcium and phosphorus from the blood in an attempt to recalcify bone. Serum calcium concentrations should be monitored every 6 hours during the 24 to 48 hours following such surgeries, and pharmacologic doses of calcium can be necessary to prevent or minimize the drop in serum calcium. Additionally, mild to moderate hypocalcemia can be a long-term consequence of parathyroidectomy in hemodialysis patients.[52]

Drug-Induced Hypocalcemia

Drug-induced hypocalcemia has been reported in patients receiving furosemide, calcitonin, bisphosphonates, gallium nitrate, mithramycin, cinacalcet, fluoride, ketoconazole, and pentamidine.[43,57] Oral phosphorus therapy, commonly used to treat patients with malabsorption syndromes caused by gastrointestinal diseases, can also result in hypocalcemia. The anticonvulsants phenobarbital and phenytoin cause hypocalcemia by increasing catabolism of vitamin D and thereby impairing calcium release from bone and reducing intestinal calcium absorption.[45] Drugs that cause hypomagnesemia (aminoglycosides, amphotericin B, cyclosporine, diuretics, foscarnet, and cisplatin) are also associated with an increased risk of hypocalcemia. Chelating agents in blood (citrate) and in radiographic contrast media (ethylenediamine tetraacetate) can also cause transient hypocalcemia.[45,46,58] Concentrated citrate is increasingly being used in hemodialysis catheter locks and to anticoagulate the dialysis circuit during continuous renal replacement therapy. Symptomatic hypocalcemia (ionized calcium <2.4 mg/dL [<0.60 mmol/L]) has been reported in patients exposed to citrate solutions, which appears to be related to the concentration of the citrate solution.[59] Injection of citrate solutions greater than the volume of the dead space of the catheter lumen or accidental injection of citrate catheter lock solutions that are not intended for systemic administration have been associated with serious cardiovascular problems such as hypotension or cardiac arrest.[60]

Hypoparathyroidism

Hypoparathyroidism can be caused by autoimmune disease, congenital defects, or iatrogenically by inadvertent removal during thyroidectomy or from damage with radiation therapy. Chronic hypothyroidism produces an insidious development of hypocalcemia and thus most patients remain asympotomatic. The chronic hypocalcemia may ultimately present as visual impairment secondary to cataracts.[61]

CLINICAL PRESENTATION

The clinical manifestations of hypocalcemia are quite variable. The more acute the drop in ionized calcium concentration, the more likely the patient will develop symptoms.[51] Increases in plasma pH enhances the binding of calcium to albumin thus alkalosis can result in rapid decreases in ionized calcium. Concomitant hypomagnesemia, hypokalemia, hyponatremia, and additive side effects from prescribed medications also increase the likelihood of symptomatic presentation.

Hypocalcemia can manifest as neuromuscular, CNS, dermatologic, and cardiac sequelae.[15] Acute hypocalcemia is more likely to manifest as neuromuscular (paresthesia, muscle cramps, tetany, and laryngeal spasm) and cardiovascular symptoms, whereas chronic hypocalcemia often presents as CNS (e.g., depression, anxiety, memory loss, confusion, hallucinations, and tonic-clonic seizures) and dermatologic symptoms (hair loss, grooved and brittle nails, and eczema).[45] The hallmark sign of acute hypocalcemia is tetany caused by enhanced peripheral neuromuscular irritability.[15] Tetany manifests as paresthesia around the mouth and in the extremities, muscle spasms and cramps, carpopedal (hands and feet) spasms, and rarely as laryngospasm and bronchospasm.[15] Chvostek's and/or Trousseau's signs can be elicited during physical examination.[45] Chvostek's sign is elicited by tapping the facial nerve anterior to the ear and eliciting twitching of facial muscles. Trousseau's sign is elicited by inflating a blood pressure cuff above systolic blood pressure for 3 minutes and observing whether a carpal spasm is induced.

The cardiovascular manifestations of hypocalcemia result in electrocardiographic changes characterized by a prolonged QT interval and symptoms of decreased myocardial contractility often associated with congestive heart failure.[45] Both acute and chronic hypocalcemia can result in a reversible syndrome characterized by acute myocardial failure or refractory congestive heart failure. Other cardiovascular manifestations include arrhythmias, bradycardia, and hypotension that are unresponsive to fluid and pressor administration.[45]

CLINICAL PRESENTATION OF HYPOCALCEMIA

General

☐ Hypocalcemia is caused in part by disorders of vitamin D or PTH. Acute causes of hypocalcemia result in rapid decreases in serum ionized calcium and can be associated with sepsis, alkalosis, or drugs. Parathyroidectomy or thyroidectomy are also associated with a rapid reduction in serum calcium. Vitamin D deficiency associated with malnutrition should not be overlooked as an etiology of chronic hypocalcemia.

Symptoms

☐ The symptoms of hypocalcemia, usually associated with an acute decrease in serum calcium, include tetany, paresthesia, muscle cramps, and laryngeal spasms. Chronic hypocalcemia is usually associated with the symptoms of depression, anxiety, memory loss, and confusion.

Signs

☐ Neurologic: The hallmark of acute hypocalcemia is tetany, which is characterized by neuromuscular irritability including seizure potential. Extrapyramidal disorders, mainly parkinsonism but also dystonia, hemiballismus, choreoathetosis, and oculogyric crises occur in 5% to 10% of patients with idiopathic hypoparathyroidism. Chvostek's and/or Trousseau's signs can be elicited during physical examination.

☐ Dermatologic: The skin can be dry, puffy, and coarse. Other dermatologic manifestations can include hyperpigmentation, dermatitis, eczema, and psoriasis. Hair and skin signs including coarse, brittle, and sparse hair with patchy alopecia and brittle nails can also appear.

☐ Ophthalmologic: Cataract development has been reported to occur with hypocalcemia.

☐ Dental manifestations: These are usually associated with the presence of chronic hypocalcemia in early development. Signs include dental hypoplasia, failure of tooth eruption, defective enamel and root formation, and abraded carious teeth.

☐ Cardiovascular: Hypotension, decreased myocardial performance, and congestive heart failure have been reported. A prolonged QT interval, arrhythmias, and bradycardia can also occur but are more common with acute or very severe hypocalcemia.

☐ Gastrointestinal: Steatorrhea can be associated with chronic hypocalcemia.

☐ Musculoskeletal: Although patients with chronic hypocalcemic disorders have skeletal abnormalities, such findings do not appear to be direct consequences of hypocalcemia. Some patients with hypocalcemia have myopathy.

☐ Endocrine: Hypocalcemia alone can impair insulin release. In addition, idiopathic hypoparathyroidism can be associated with polyglandular autoimmune syndromes.

Laboratory Tests

☐ Serum calcium levels of less than 8.5 mg/dL (<2.13 mmol/L) are considered to represent hypocalcemia if ionized calcium values are also less than 4.4 mg/dL (<1.1 mmol/L).

TREATMENT

Hypocalcemia

■ DESIRED OUTCOME

❹ The goals of therapy for patients with normal renal function are the resolution of signs and symptoms of hypocalcemia, restoration of normocalcemia, management of associated electrolyte abnormalities, and treatment of the underlying cause of hypocalcemia. The goals for patients with chronic kidney disease are different and are discussed in detail in Chapter 53. Asymptomatic hypocalcemia associated with hypoalbuminemia requires no treatment because ionized (physiologically active) plasma calcium concentrations are normal. Treatment of hypocalcemia is dependent on identification of the pathogenesis of the underlying disorder, acuteness of onset, and presence and severity of symptoms. Acute symptomatic hypocalcemia requires parenteral administration of soluble calcium salts (Fig 59–3).

■ PHARMACOLOGIC THERAPY

The initial therapeutic intervention for patients with acute symptomatic hypocalcemia is to administer 100 to 300 mg of elemental calcium intravenously over 5 to 10 minutes.[62] This can be accomplished by the administration of 1 g of calcium chloride (27% elemental calcium) or 2 to 3 g of calcium gluconate (9% elemental calcium). Calcium gluconate is generally preferred over calcium chloride for peripheral venous administration because calcium gluconate is less irritating to veins. The use of calcium gluconate provides a less predictable and slightly smaller increase in plasma ionic calcium compared with calcium chloride. Calcium should not be infused at a rate greater than 60 mg of elemental calcium per minute because severe cardiac dysfunction, including ventricular fibrillation, can result.[62] Intravenous calcium administration should be used with caution in patients receiving digitalis glycosides because of the possibility of bradycardia or atrioventricular (A-V) block.[3] The bolus dose of calcium is only effective for 1 to 2 hours and should be followed by a continuous infusion of elemental calcium at a rate of 0.5 to 2 mg/kg per hour.[3] The calcium concentrations should be monitored every 4 to 6 hours during the intravenous infusions. The ionized calcium concentration usually normalizes within 4 hours, and the maintenance infusion rate of elemental calcium can then be decreased to 0.3 to 0.5 mg/kg per hour to maintain the desired calcium concentration.[1] Calcium should not be added to bicarbonate- or phosphate-containing solutions because of the possibility of precipitation.

Once acute hypocalcemia is corrected by parenteral administration, further treatment modalities should be individualized according to the cause of hypocalcemia. If hypomagnesemia is present, magnesium supplementation is indicated (see Chapter 60). Hypocalcemia secondary to hungry bone syndrome following parathyroidectomy has been attenuated by pretreatment with bisphosphonates.[63] Asymptomatic and chronic hypocalcemia associated with hypoparathyroidism and vitamin D–deficient states can be managed by oral calcium and vitamin D supplementation (see Chapter 53). Therapy is begun with 1 to 3 g/day of elemental calcium.[1] Average maintenance doses range

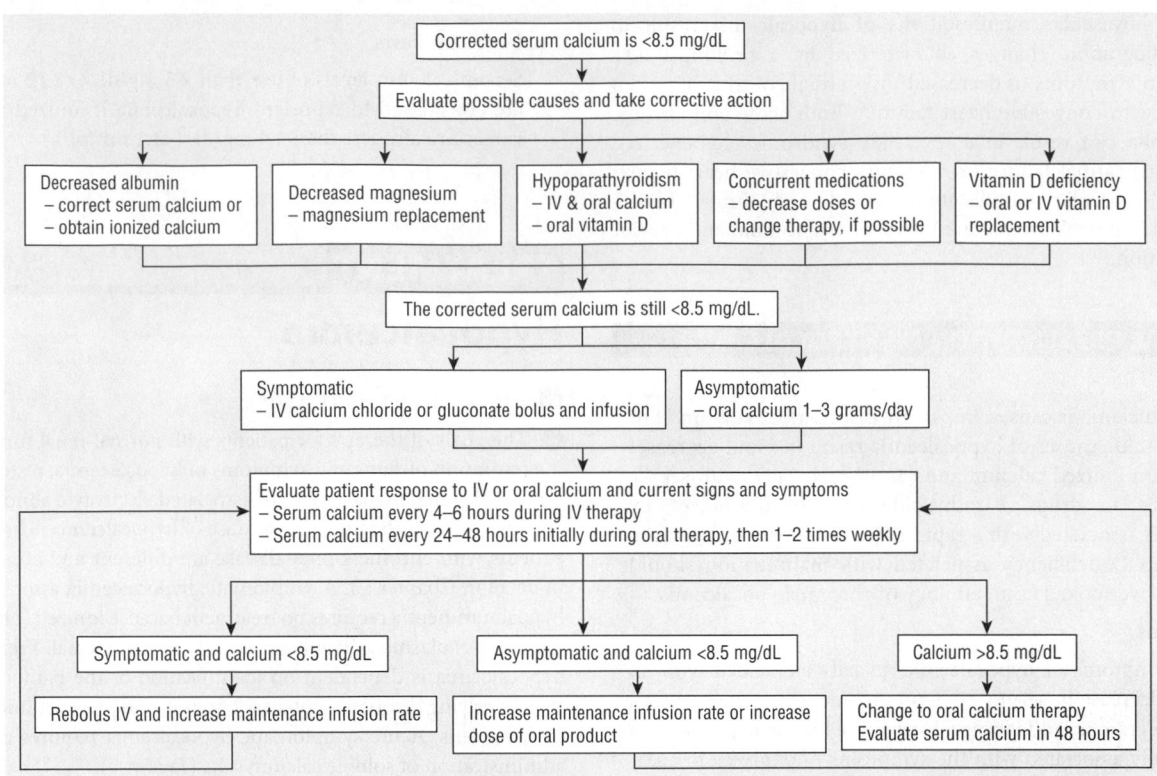

FIGURE 59-3. Hypocalcemia diagnostic and treatment algorithm. Serum calcium of 8.5 mg/dL is equivalent to 2.13 mmol/L.

from 2 to 8 g of elemental calcium per day in divided doses. If serum calcium does not normalize, a vitamin D preparation may need to be added.

Treatment of hypocalcemia associated with vitamin D–deficient states should be individualized. In patients with malabsorption, vitamin D requirements vary markedly, and large doses can be required. In contrast, vitamin D deficiency associated with anticonvulsant medication can be corrected with smaller doses of vitamin D. Oral doses of 1,25-dihydroxy vitamin D_3 usually range from 0.5 to 3 mcg daily. The usual initial oral dose of ergocalciferol is 50,000 international units daily.[62] Vitamin D doses are usually adjusted approximately every 4 weeks. Vitamin D deficiency is highly prevalent especially in areas of low sun exposure and limited dietary sources of vitamin D.[64] New data suggest that current dietary recommendations are not sufficient to maintain 25-hydroxy vitamin D_3 concentrations at or above 32 mcg/L (90 mmol/L).[64] The treatment of vitamin D deficiency associated with CKD generally requires the administration of 1,25-dihydroxy vitamin D_3 or another synthetic vitamin D_2 analog such as paricalcitol or doxercalciferol. Patients who have reduced 25-hydroxylase activity (e.g., hepatic disease) can also require treatment with calcitriol (1,25-dihydroxy vitamin D_3). The newer vitamin D_2 analogs (paricalcitol and doxercalciferol) were developed to preferentially suppress PTH secretion with less effect on serum calcium concentration and thus their efficacy for the management of hypocalcemia may be minimal. In selected cases, increasing calcium ingestion can be required if vitamin D replacement alone is ineffective in returning calcium concentrations to normal.

Adverse effects of oral calcium and vitamin D supplementation include hypercalcemia and hypercalciuria, especially in the hypoparathyroid patient, in whom the renal calcium-sparing effect of PTH is absent. Hypercalciuria can increase the risk of calcium stone formation and nephrolithiasis in susceptible patients. One maneuver to help prevent calcium stones is to maintain the urine calcium excretion below 300 mg per day. Intermittently monitoring

24-hour urine collections for total calcium excretion can help to minimize the occurrence of hypercalciuria. The addition of thiazide diuretics for patients at risk for stone formation can result in an increase in tubular calcium reabsorption and reduction of vitamin D requirements.[62]

DISORDERS OF PHOSPHORUS HOMEOSTASIS

Inorganic phosphorus in the form of phosphate is an essential element in phospholipid cell membranes, nucleic acids, and phosphoproteins, which are required for mitochondrial function.[65] Phosphorus regulates the intermediary metabolism of carbohydrates, fats, and proteins. Phosphorus also regulates enzymatic reactions including glycolysis, ammoniagenesis, and the 1-hydroxylation of 25-hydroxy vitamin D_3.[65] In addition, phosphorus is required for the generation of 2,3-diphosphoglycerate (2,3-DPG) in red blood cells, which is required for normal oxygen-hemoglobin dissociation and delivery of oxygen to the tissues.[66] Phosphorus is the source of the high-energy bonds of adenosine triphosphate (ATP), thus fueling a wide variety of physiologic processes, including muscle contractility, electrolyte transport, neurologic function, and other important biochemical reactions.[65] Considering its diverse biologic importance, it is not difficult to appreciate the clinical implications of disorders of phosphorus homeostasis.

Phosphate, the major intracellular anion, is present in living organisms mainly as organic phosphate esters such as 2,3-DPG, adenosine, guanosine triphosphate, and fructose 1,6-diphosphate.[65] Only a small fraction of intracellular phosphorus exists as inorganic phosphate; however, this fraction is critical because it is the source from which ATP is resynthesized.[65] The majority of inorganic phosphate is located in the extracellular space where it is the prime determinant of intracellular phosphate; thus, small increments in the organic phosphate levels can profoundly alter both the extracellular and intracellular phosphate levels. Metabolic disturbances (acidosis, alkalosis, and ketoacidosis), hydrogen ion shifts, and hormones (PTH, calcitonin, cortisol, and vitamin D) all can cause transcellular shifts in phosphorus concentrations. Because of these phenomena, the serum phosphorus level does not accurately reflect total body stores.[66]

The typical Western diet provides a daily intake of 800 to 1,600 mg of phosphorus. Approximately 60% to 80% of this is absorbed in the gastrointestinal tract by passive and active transport (vitamin D mediated). PTH, 1,25-dihydroxy vitamin D_3, and low-phosphate diets mediate increased absorption. Decreased absorption occurs under conditions of increased dietary intake of phosphorus and magnesium, glucocorticoid therapy, and hypothyroidism. The normal serum phosphorus concentration in adults is 2.5 to 4.5 mg/dL (0.81–1.45 mmol/L) and for children younger than 12 years old it is 4 to 5.6 mg/dL (1.29–1.81 mmol/L). Influx via the gastrointestinal tract and bone and tubular reabsorption by the kidney are the most important regulators of steady-state serum phosphorus concentrations. Renal excretion of phosphorus is a two-step process: glomerular filtration and proximal tubular reabsorption by passive transport coupled to sodium. Under normal conditions, 85% to 90% of filtered phosphate is reabsorbed, the majority in the early proximal tubule. Renal tubular reabsorption of phosphate is inhibited by PTH and 1,25-dihydroxy vitamin D_3.[65] There are increasing data in the literature that indicate fibroblast growth factor 23 (FGF23) is a key regulator of phosphate homeostasis.[68,69] FGF23 acts principally to decrease tubular reabsorption of phosphate and inhibit 1α-hydroxylase, thereby reducing the concentration of active vitamin D. FGF23-mediated receptor activation requires klotho, a transmembrane protein. The tissue specificity for FGF23 effects appears to be defined by klotho-FGF23 coexpression. Conversely, phosphate reabsorption in the renal tubule is increased by growth hormone, insulin and insulin-like growth factor 1.[65] Internal phosphorus balance (transcellular phosphate distribution) is also of importance in the maintenance of normal serum phosphate. The serum phosphate level can vary by as much as 2 mg/dL (0.65 mmol/L) throughout the day, primarily as the result of changes in carbohydrate intake, insulin secretion, and diurnal variation.[65]

HYPERPHOSPHATEMIA

Hyperphosphatemia typically results from either renal failure or endogenous intracellular phosphate release. Hyperphosphatemia occurs frequently in patients with acute renal failure and is a nearly universal finding in those with advanced stages of CKD (e.g., stages 4 and 5). Tumor lysis syndrome is a complication of chemotherapy associated with massive lysis of cells and release of intracellular contents. The incidence of tumor lysis syndrome has been reported to be as high as 40% in patients treated for non-Hodgkin lymphoma.[65] Other causes of hyperphosphatemia include hemolysis and rhabdomyolysis.

Pathophysiology

❺ The most common cause of hyperphosphatemia is a failure of renal tubular reabsorption to maintain serum phosphate when GFR is markedly inpaired (e.g., GFR <25 mL/min [<0.42 mL/s]).[65] Retention of phosphate decreases vitamin D synthesis and induces hypocalcemia, which leads to an increase in PTH, a finding that can be seen in those with stage 2 to 3 CKD. This physiologic response inhibits further tubular reabsorption of phosphorus as the kidney attempts to correct hyperphosphatemia and normalize serum calcium concentrations. Patients with excessive exogenous phosphate administration or who experience massive tissue breakdown or cell lysis in the setting of acute renal failure can rapidly develop moderate to severe hyper-phosphatemia (serum phosphate

>6.5 mg/dL [>2.10 mmol/L]).[65] Severe hyperphosphatemia (serum phosphate >7.0 mg/dL [>2.26 mmol/L]) is commonly encountered in patients with CKD, especially those with GFRs less than 15 mL/min per 1.73 m² (0.14 mL/min/m²) (see Chapter 53).

Hyperphosphatemia caused by an increase in renal tubular reabsorption associated with hypoparathyroidism and associated decreases in PTH is usually less severe than that observed in patients with severe renal failure or excessive exogenous or endogenous introduction of phosphate into the ECF. Acromegaly (mediated by growth hormone) and thyrotoxicosis (mediated by catecholamines) can also cause hyperphosphatemia by increasing tubular phosphate reabsorption.

Exogenous Phosphate Loads

Iatrogenic causes of hyperphosphatemia have been widely reported, and clinicians should be aware of the phosphorus content of intravenous, oral, and rectally administered products. Large doses of phosphate administered intravenously to treat hypercalcemia can ultimately result in severe life-threatening hyperphosphatemia. Although less-well recognized, oral and rectal administration of phosphate-containing solutions such as sodium phosphate (Fleet Phospho-Soda) can also result in severe and life-threatening hyperphosphatemia, especially in patients with moderate and severe renal insufficiency.[67,70] The risk of mortality is dependent on the amount of phosphorus absorbed from the administered product, however, fatalities have occurred at lower phosphate concentrations.[67] Acute phosphate nephropathy and renal failure have also been reported with the use of oral sodium phosphate bowel preparations. Recently the FDA issued a safety warning regarding the use of these products in patients at risk (the elderly, those with CKD) or on medications known to effect renal hemodynamics (e.g., diuretics, NSAIDs or renin-angiotensin-aldosterone system inhibitors).[71] Intravenous or oral vitamin D therapy can increase absorption of phosphorus in the gastrointestinal tract by up to 50%. High-dose etidronate (10–20 mg/kg/d) therapy has been associated with increased serum phosphate concentrations apparently mediated by drug-related increase in tubular phosphate reabsorption.[72] Acute phosphorus poisoning as a result of ingestion of laundry detergents is a rare and often unrecognized cause of elevated phosphate concentrations.

Rapid Tissue Catabolism

Any disorder that results in necrosis of skeletal muscle (i.e., rhabdomyolysis) can generate the release of large amounts of intracellular phosphate into the systemic circulation. This condition is frequently associated with acute kidney injury (see Chapter 51) and thus severe hyperphosphatemia can develop because of increased endogenous phosphate release coupled with the impaired proximal tubule reabsorption such that phosphaturic hormones (e.g., PTH, FGF23) become ineffective. Bowel infarction, malignant hyperthermia, and severe hemolysis are also conditions that can increase endogenous release of phosphate.

Moderate hyperphosphatemia is also commonly observed in patients undergoing treatment for acute leukemia and lymphomas.[73] Chemotherapeutic treatment of acute lymphoblastic leukemia can result in the release of large amounts of phosphate into the systemic circulation secondary to lysis of lymphoblasts. Initiation of chemotherapy for Burkitt lymphoma results in tumor lysis syndrome, a rapid lysis of malignant cells that results in hyperphosphatemia, hyperuricemia, hyperkalemia, and hypocalcemia.[73]

Acid–Base Disorders

Lactic acidosis and diabetic ketoacidosis can trigger the transcellular shift of endogenous intracellular phosphate into the extracellular space and thereby dramatically increases serum phosphorous concentrations. In one study, hyperphosphatemia was present in more than 90% of patients with diabetic ketoacidosis prior to the initiation of treatment.[74] After the institution of treatment, serum phosphate levels should be checked hourly as they can decrease rapidly, and patients can ultimately develop hypophosphatemia.

Clinical Presentation

The severe acute onset of hyperphosphatemia can result in calcium and phosphate complexation and lead to the precipitation of calcium phosphate into soft tissues, intrarenal calcification, nephrolithiasis, or obstructive uropathy. Other symptoms associated with moderate to severe hyperphosphatemia include nausea, vomiting, diarrhea, lethargy, and seizures. The major effects of long-term hyperphosphatemia are related to the development of hypocalcemia (caused by phosphate inhibition of renal 1-α-hydroxylase) and its related consequences, as well as vascular and organ damage resulting from the deposition of calcium-phosphate crystals. Extravascular calcification can result in band keratopathy, "red eye," pruritus, and periarticular calcification, especially in CKD patients. In addition, soft-tissue calcifications in the conjunctiva, skin, heart, cornea, lung, gastric mucosa, and kidney have been observed, primarily in CKD patients with chronic disordered mineral metabolism.[64] Hyperphosphatemia associated with CKD can result in renal osteodystrophy because of overproduction of PTH. This condition is discussed in detail in Chapter 53.

CLINICAL PRESENTATION OF HYPERPHOSPHATEMIA

General

- As the serum phosphate concentration is primarily determined by the ability of the kidneys to reabsorb phosphate, hyperphosphatemia is uncommon in patients with normal kidney function.

Symptoms

- Acute symptoms include GI disturbances, lethargy, obstruction of the urinary tract, and rarely seizures. Symptoms associated with chronic hyperphosphatemia are associated with deposition of calcium-phosphate crystals and include "red eye" and pruritus.

Signs

- The elevated calcium-phosphate product results in precipitation in arteries, joints, soft tissues, and the viscera. This can result in tissue necrosis, termed *calciphylaxis*.

Laboratory Tests

- Serum phosphate levels >4.5 mg/dL (>1.45 mmol/L) represent hyperphosphatemia.

TREATMENT

Hyperphosphatemia

■ DESIRED OUTCOME

Management of patients with acutely elevated serum phosphate should be directed at avoiding gastrointestinal and neurologic symptoms and preventing deposition in the urinary tract to avoid the development of acute renal failure. The treatment of hyperphosphatemia is focused on returning serum phosphate concentrations to the normal or near normal (for those with CKD) range, with the hope that one can minimize the long-term cardiovascular consequences of

calcium-phosphate crystal deposition in the vasculature. Calcium-phosphate crystals are likely to form in vivo when the product of the serum calcium and phosphate concentrations exceeds 50 to 60 mg²/dL² (4.0–4.8 mmol²/L²). The National Kidney Foundation's Dialysis Outcomes Quality Initiative guidelines for bone metabolism and disease defines the goal calcium-phosphorus product as less than 55 mg²/dL² (4.4 mmol²/L²).[68] Furthermore, serum phosphate concentrations greater than 6.5 mg/dL (2.10 mmol/L) have been independently associated with increased morbidity and mortality.[75] Serum phosphate concentrations should be maintained in the 2.7 to 4.6 mg/dL (0.87–1.49 mmol/L) range for those with stages 3 and 4 CKD, whereas for patients in stage 5 CKD the goal is to maintain values between 3.5 and 5.5 mg/dL (1.13–1.78 mmol/L).[76]

■ PHARMACOLOGIC THERAPY

Severe symptomatic hyperphosphatemia manifesting as hypocalcemia and tetany should be treated by the intravenous administration of calcium salts. Although this can seem counterintuitive in a patient with a phosphate of 16 mg/dL (5.17 mmol/L) and a calcium of 7 mg/dL (1.75 mmol/L) (the calcium-phosphorus product is 112 mg²/dL² [9.0 mmol²/L²]), correction of severe hypocalcemia is of primary importance because of the critical nature of this disorder. If calcium concentrations are not critically low, the initial management strategy should include limitation of all exogenous sources of phosphate and efforts to block further absorption should be initiated. Dialysis can be initiated if the patient remains symptomatic despite these interventions.

❻ In general, the most effective way to treat nonemergent hyperphosphatemia is to decrease phosphate absorption from the GI tract by the use of phosphate-binding agents.[65] Antacids containing divalent and trivalent cations (calcium, lanthanum, magnesium, and aluminum), or sevelamer are the agents most frequently used in the prevention and treatment of hyperphosphatemia (see Table 53–8).[77,78] Long-term treatment with aluminum hydroxide and aluminum carbonate should be discouraged because the use of these agents has been associated with anemia, CNS disorders, and bone disease.[79] Short-term therapy with these agents is effective and safe. Aluminum and calcium are available in oral suspension formulations, which can aid administration in acutely ill patients with G-tubes. The most frequent adverse effect from phosphate-binding agents (especially calcium) is constipation (see Table 53–8). Calcium salts are the preferred phosphate-binding agents except when there is concomitant hypercalcemia. Therapy with the polymer agent (sevelamer) or lanthanum carbonate might avoid the detrimental effects associated with aluminum, magnesium, or calcium therapy.

CLINICAL CONTROVERSY

Emerging data suggest that noncalcium, nonaluminum phosphate binders can slow progression of cardiac calcification in chronic hemodialysis patients; however, there are no data to suggest that there are any benefits to using sevelamer for the management of those who develop acute hyperphosphatemia. Thus, a more cost-effective approach to phosphate binding in acute situations would be use of calcium- or aluminum-based binders.

HYPOPHOSPHATEMIA

Mild to moderate hypophosphatemia is typically found in patients with serum phosphate concentrations of 1 to 2 mg/dL (0.32–0.65 mmol/L), whereas severe hypophosphatemia that is frequenly symptomatic is correlated with a phosphorus concentration of less than 1 mg/dL (0.32 mmol/L).[66] Hypophosphatemia has been observed in approximately 1% to 3% of the laboratory screening panels of patients who have been admitted to a hospital.[66] The incidence in hospitalized critically ill patients is 18% to 28%.[81] Unlike its severe form, mild or moderate hypophosphatemia seldom causes recognizable signs and symptoms.[73]

PATHOPHYSIOLOGY

❼ Hypophosphatemia can be the result of decreased gastrointestinal absorption, reduced tubular reabsorption, or extracellular to intracellular redistribution.[65] Although mild to moderate hypophosphatemia is common and can occur in inpatients and outpatients, severe hypophosphatemia is predominantly encountered in the acute care setting and can be associated with life-threatening symptoms, including seizures, coma, and rhabdomyolysis (Table 59–4).

Phosphate-binding substances such as sucralfate, calcium carbonate, sevelamer, lanthanum carbonate, and aluminum- or magnesium-containing antacids have the potential to bind large amounts of phosphorus in the gut, thereby preventing absorption. If phosphate-binding agents are ingested on a chronic basis in conjunction with a dietary phosphorus deficiency, hypophosphatemia can result.[73] Patients who are receiving long-term phosphate-binding agents, those with peptic ulcer disease or CKD, and those who may be predisposed to moderate hypophosphatemia (alcoholics) are at highest risk for the development of severe hypophosphatemia. Hyperparathyroidism can cause hypophosphatemia as a result of decreased gastrointestinal absorption of dietary phosphorus.

Reduced tubular reabsorption of phosphate can occur in hyperparathyroid (primary and secondary) patients with normal renal function and those with vitamin D deficiency or elevated FGF23 concentrations. Elevated PTH levels lead to an increase in serum calcium concentrations and decreased serum phosphate concentrations. Serum phosphorus is decreased as the result of a reduction in renal tubular reabsorption.[82] Recovery from extensive third degree burns is associated with development of an anabolic state as stress levels decrease and nutritional therapies take effect as well as a marked diuretic phase associated with an impressive renal loss of phosphate.[82] Because phosphate is rapidly incorporated into the new cells, this can contribute to the severity of the hypophosphatemia. Drugs that cause increased renal elimination of phosphate include diuretics (acetazolamide and osmotic diuretics), glucocorticoids, and sodium bicarbonate.

Rapid refeeding of malnourished patients with high-carbohydrate, high-calorie diets with inadequate amounts of supplemental phosphate can result in severe symptomatic hypophosphatemia. This phenomenon is especially prevalent in patients with other underlying risk factors for the development of hypophosphatemia, such as alcoholism.[82] The etiology of severe hypophosphatemia associated with hyperalimentation and nutritional recovery can be separated into two phases: acute, rapid hypophosphatemia secondary to intracellular shifts of phosphate resulting from glucose-induced insulin secretion; and the gradual decrease in serum phosphate concentration over 5 to 10 days secondary to tissue repair in the presence of phosphate deprivation.[83] The development of severe hypophosphatemia secondary to hyperalimentation can be prevented by the administration of 12 to 15 mmol of phosphate per liter of hyperalimentation solution or 15 mmol per 1,000 calories (4.2 kJ) of dextrose.[83] Transcellular shifts in phosphate also occur after parathyroidectomy, causing severe hypocalcemia and hypophosphatemia because of hungry bone syndrome (deposition of phosphate and calcium in the bone).

Severe and prolonged respiratory alkalosis (a result of hyperventilation, pain, anxiety, and sepsis) can cause hypophosphatemia.[66] Respiratory alkalosis is thought to contribute significantly to the hypophosphatemia observed during alcohol withdrawal.[66] Although patients with diabetic ketoacidosis may present with hyperphosphatemia, the institution of therapy to correct it can cause serum phosphate concentrations to decrease rapidly as phosphate shifts back into the intracellular compartment. In addition, the acidosis associated with the diabetic ketoacidotic state can cause a decomposition of organic compounds inside the cell and a release of inorganic phosphate into the plasma and subsequently into the urine.[65] The combination of intracellular phosphate breakdown and the shift of phosphate into cells on initiation of treatment can lead to severe hypophosphatemia. Drugs associated with transcellular shifts in phosphate include dextrose solutions, glucagon, insulin, catecholamines, calcitonin, erythropoietic agents, and anabolic steroids.

Chronic ethanol abusers are prone to a variety of serum electrolyte disorders including hypocalcemia, hypomagnesemia, hypokalemia, and hypophosphatemia. The etiology of hypophosphatemia in the alcoholic patient is multifactorial. Malnutrition, poor dietary

---

TABLE 59-4	Conditions Associated with the Development of Hypophosphatemia

Decreased gastrointestinal absorption
Phosphate-binding drugs
  Sucralfate
  Calcium carbonate
  Aluminum/magnesium antacids
  Sevelamer
  Lanthanum carbonate
Decreased dietary phosphorus intake
Glucocorticoids
Vitamin D deficiency/resistance
Hypoparathyroidism
Chronic diarrhea
Steatorrhea

Reduced tubular reabsorption
Hyperparathyroidism (primary and secondary)
Elevated FGF23
Recovery from burns
Rickets
Malignant neoplasms
Fanconi syndrome
Acute volume expansion
Metabolic acidosis
Renal transplantation
Vitamin D deficiency and/or resistance
Diuretics
  Acetazolamide
  Osmotic agents
Glucocorticoids
Sodium bicarbonate

Internal redistribution
Refeeding syndrome
Parenteral nutrition
Parathyroidectomy (hungry bone syndrome)
Alcoholism
Respiratory alkalosis
Diabetic ketoacidosis (correction)
Dextrose solutions
Insulin
Catecholamines
Anabolic steroids
Glucagon
Calcitonin
Erythropoietin

intake, diarrhea, vomiting, and the use of phosphate-binding antacids can all contribute to the hypophosphatemia of alcoholism.[65] In addition, serum phosphate concentrations may decrease after hospitalization in the alcoholic patient with the institution of dextrose-containing intravenous fluids as a result of an intracellular shift of phosphate.[65,83] Hyperventilation associated with the alcohol withdrawal syndrome can also contribute to the development of hypophosphatemia.[73,83] Alcoholic patients are particularly susceptible to the complications of hypophosphatemia such as rhabdomyolysis, which is often seen during withdrawal or refeeding.[73,83] Thus, serum phosphate concentrations should be routinely monitored in alcoholic patients.

CLINICAL PRESENTATION

The clinical manifestations of severe hypophosphatemia are diverse and many organ systems can be affected. It is likely that two primary biochemical abnormalities are responsible for most of the clinical manifestations of severe hypophosphatemia.[65] First, intracellular energy stores may be decreased secondary to depletion of intracellular ATP. This can result in disruptions in cellular function. Second, reduced red blood cell 2,3-DPG concentrations are associated with a shift to the left of the oxyhemoglobin saturation curve. This shift is associated with a decrease in the release of oxygen to peripheral tissues (increased oxygen affinity for hemoglobin) and may result in tissue hypoxia.[65] These metabolic disorders can be seen in a wide variety of organ systems.

Neurologic (CNS) manifestations of severe hypophosphatemia result in a metabolic encephalopathy syndrome. This progressive syndrome of irritability, apprehension, weakness, numbness, paresthesia, dysarthria, confusion, obtundation, seizures, and coma has been described in patients with severe hypophosphatemia.[73,82] Neuropsychiatric disturbances include apathy, delirium, hallucinations, and paranoia. Peripheral neuropathy and symptoms resembling Guillain-Barré syndrome have also been reported.[73]

Severe hypophosphatemia can result in significant dysfunction of skeletal muscle ranging from myalgia, bone pain, and weakness, with chronic hypophosphatemia, to potentially fatal rhabdomyolysis with severe acute hypophosphatemia.[82] Laboratory evaluations can help to distinguish between chronic and acute on chronic hypophosphatemia. Elevated alkaline phosphatase, normal creatine phosphokinase, and normal to low phosphate and calcium are present in cases of chronic hypophosphatemia. In contrast, hyperkalemia, hyperuricemia, elevated blood urea nitrogen and creatinine, hypercalcemia, and myoglobinuria are often present in cases in which rhabdomyolysis complicates the acute or chronic hypophosphatemia.[82] Hypophosphatemia can result in acute respiratory failure secondary to respiratory muscle weakness and diaphragmatic contractile dysfunction. Thus frequent assessment of serum phosphate concentration is indicated in patients at risk for respiratory failure. Likewise, adequate treatment of hypophosphatemia in respiratory failure can aid in successful weaning from the ventilator.[66] Dysphagia and ileus have also been attributed to hypophosphatemia.[66]

Myocardial dysfunction has been reported to be impaired in the setting of hypophosphatemia and has resulted in congestive cardiomyopathy. This has been reported in alcoholics, and postoperative and intensive care patients. A depletion in cardiac ATP stores has been hypothesized as the cause of this syndrome.[82] Arrhythmias have also been reported in patients with hypophosphatemia. Because hypophosphatemia is a potentially reversible cause of heart failure, it should be considered in patients who experience an acute deterioration in ventricular function.

Hematologic manifestations of hypophosphatemia include decreased levels of 2,3-DPG, decreased red blood cell ATP, and membrane rigidity.[65] When red blood cell ATP decreases to below 15% of normal, cells become spherocytic and rigid, and are trapped and destroyed in the spleen.[65] Therefore, hemolysis can be a manifestation of severe hypophosphatemia. Reduction in ATP content of white blood cells can result in mobility, chemotaxis, phagocytosis, and bactericidal dysfunction.[73] These changes can contribute to an increased risk of infection in hypophosphatemic patients. Animal studies also demonstrate platelet abnormalities in the setting of hypophosphatemia.[74] The implications of hypophosphatemia for human platelet function, however, have not been determined.

Finally, prolonged hypophosphatemia may result in osteopenia and osteomalacia because of enhanced osteoclastic resorption of bone and limited crystallization constituents (phosphate), respectively. Glucose intolerance from hypophosphatemia caused by tissue insensitivity to insulin has also been described.

CLINICAL PRESENTATION OF HYPOPHOSPHATEMIA

General

☐ The manifestations of hypophosphatemia depend on the chronicity and severity of the phosphate depletion. The major conditions associated with symptomatic hypophosphatemia are chronic alcoholism, intravenous hyperalimentation without adequate phosphate supplementation, and the chronic ingestion of antacids. Severe hypophosphatemia can also be seen during treatment of diabetic ketoacidosis and with prolonged hyperventilation.

Symptoms

☐ Except for the effects on mineral metabolism, the symptoms of hypophosphatemia are caused by two consequences (reduction of red cell 2,3-DPG and reduction of intracellular ATP levels), and can impact virtually all organ systems. The symptoms are predominantly neurological and can include irritability, apprehension, weakness, numbness, paresthesia, and confusion. Severe acute development of hypophosphatemia can result in seizures or coma.

Signs

☐ The initial response of bone to hypophosphatemia contributes to hypercalcemia and hypercalciuria. Prolonged hypophosphatemia can also result in rickets and osteomalacia.

☐ Neurologic: Severe hypophosphatemia can lead to a metabolic encephalopathy.

☐ Cardiopulmonary: Impaired myocardial contractility, respiratory failure secondary to ATP depletion, congestive heart failure, new onset or worsening of an existing condition.

☐ Musculoskeletal: Proximal myopathy, dysphagia, and ileus have been reported. Acute hypophosphatemia superimposed on preexisting severe phosphate depletion can lead to rhabdomyolysis.

☐ Hematologic: Alterations in the hematopoietic system can also occur, resulting in hemolysis, reduction in phagocytotic and granulocyte chemotactic ability, as well as defective clot retraction and thrombocytopenia.

Laboratory Tests

☐ Serum phosphate levels <2.4 mg/dL (<0.78 mmol/L) are indicative of hypophosphatemia; however, symptomatic hypophosphatemia typically is not evident until serum phosphate <1 mg/dL (<0.32 mmol/L).

TABLE 59-5 Phosphorus Replacement Therapy

Product (Salt)	Phosphate Content	Initial Dosing Based on Serum K
Oral therapy (potassium phosphate + sodium phosphate)		
Neutra-Phos (7 mEq/packet each of Na and K)	250 mg (8 mmol)/packet	1 packet 3 times daily[a]
Neutra-Phos-K (14.25 mEq/packet of K)	250 mg (8 mmol)/packet	Serum K >5.5 mEq/L (>5.5 mmol/L); not recommended
K-Phos Neutral (13 mEq/tablet Na and 1.1 mEq/tablet K)	250 mg (8 mmol)/tablet	Serum K >5.5 mEq/L (>5.5 mmol/L) 1 tablet 3 times daily
Uro-KP-Neutral (10.9 mEq/tablet Na and 1.27 mEq/tablet K)	250 mg (8 mmol)/tablet	Serum K >5.5 mEq/L (>5.5 mmol/L) 1 tablet 3 times daily
Fleets Phospho-soda (Sodium phosphate solution)	4 mmol/mL	Serum K >5.5 mEq/L (>5.5 mmol/L) 2 mL 3 times daily
Intravenous therapy		
Sodium PO$_4$ (4.0 mEq/mL Na)	3 mmol/mL	Serum K >3.5 mEq/L (>3.5 mmol/L) 15–30 mmol IVPB
Potassium PO$_4$ (4.4 mEq/mL K)	3 mmol/mL	Serum K <3.5 mEq/L (<3.5 mmol/L) 15–30 mmol IVPB

IVPB, intravenous piggyback; K, potassium; Na, sodium; PO$_4$, phosphate.
[a]Monitor serum K closely + intravenous piggy back.

TREATMENT

Hypophosphatemia

■ DESIRED OUTCOME

The goals of therapy are the reversal of signs and symptoms of hypophosphatemia, normalization of serum phosphate concentrations, and management of underlying conditions. Awareness of the clinical situations in which hypophosphatemia is anticipated (alcoholism, diabetic ketoacidosis, and parenteral nutrition) is of vital importance in preventing iatrogenic hypophosphatemia. The routine addition of phosphate in concentrations of 12 to 15 mmol/L to intravenous hyperalimentation solutions is of utmost importance for the prevention of severe hypophosphatemia in hospitalized patients.

■ PHARMACOLOGIC THERAPY

8 Severe (<1 mg/dL [<0.32 mmol/L]) or symptomatic hypophosphatemia should be treated with parenteral phosphate replacement. Oral phosphate supplementation is usually reserved for patients who are asymptomatic or who exhibit mild to moderate hypophosphatemia. Estimation of total body phosphate deficit is difficult because phosphate is an intracellular electrolyte. Dosage and infusion recommendations, as well as response to parenteral phosphate replacement, are highly variable.[81] The infusion of 15 mmol of phosphate in 250 mL 5% dextrose or 0.9% sodium chloride over 3 hours is a safe and effective treatment for severe hypophosphatemia.[81] Mean increases in serum phosphate of 0.5 to 0.8 mg/dL (0.16–0.26 mmol/L) have been reported. Doses of 15 to 30 mmol of phosphate can be given over 1 to 3 hours in patients without hypercalcemia (serum calcium >10.5 mg/dL [>2.63 mmol/L]).[84] Other authors recommend a wider dosage range of 0.08 to 0.64 mmol/kg body weight (5–45 mmol in a 70-kg [154 lb] patient) given over 4 to 12 hours.[85] Intravenous phosphate therapy produces the desired increase in serum phosphate at 24 hours in 20% to 80% of patients. Response is dependent on the degree of phosphate depletion and replacement dose administered.[65] Furthermore, the initial success is often followed in 48 to 72 hours by recurrent hypophosphatemia, necessitating close monitoring of serum phosphate and repeated administration of phosphate products as warranted.

Parenteral phosphate supplementation is associated with risks of hyperphosphatemia, metastatic soft tissue deposition of calcium-phosphate product, hypomagnesemia, hypocalcemia, and hyperkalemia or hypernatremia (caused by intravenous phosphate salt) (Table 59-5). Inappropriate administration of large doses of parenteral phosphate over relatively short time periods has resulted in symptomatic hypocalcemia and soft-tissue calcification.[65] The rate of infusion and choice of initial dosage should therefore be based on severity of hypophosphatemia, presence of symptoms, and coexistent medical conditions. Patients should be closely monitored with frequent (every 6 hours) serum phosphate determinations for 48 to 72 hours after starting intravenous therapy. It can be necessary to continue administration of intravenous phosphate for several days in some patients, although other patients may be able to tolerate an oral maintenance regimen. Monitoring should also include assessment of serum potassium, calcium, and magnesium concentrations. Hypomagnesemia secondary to intracellular shifts occurs frequently (27%–80%) in severely hypophosphatemic patients.[81] Therapy with parenteral phosphate should be undertaken with great caution and at reduced dosage for patients with hypercalcemia or renal dysfunction.[73,83]

Mild to moderate or asymptomatic hypophosphatemia can be treated by the administration of oral phosphate salts in doses of 1.5 to 2 g (50–60 mmol) daily in divided doses (see Table 59-5). Phosphate concentrations should be monitored daily, with the goal of correcting the reduced phosphate concentration in approximately 7 to 10 days. The primary dose-limiting adverse effect associated with oral phosphate replacement is the development of osmotic diarrhea. Patients with mild to moderate hypophosphatemia and moderate to severe renal insufficiency should receive reduced daily oral doses (i.e., 1 g or approximately 30 mmol of phosphate) with careful monitoring of serum phosphate concentration because they are predisposed to phosphate retention. In addition to phosphate supplementation for hypophosphatemia, dipyridamole can decrease renal phosphate leaking and increase serum phosphate. Doses of 75 mg 4 times daily have resulted in increases in serum 1,25-dihydroxy vitamin D$_3$ and decreases in serum calcium and urolithiasis events.[86]

CONCLUSIONS

Clinicians play an integral part in the management of fluid and electrolyte abnormalities. Initial treatment strategy should be based on acuity of onset and severity of symptoms. Because the etiologies of calcium and phosphate disorders are diverse, it is important to integrate the known or anticipated pathophysiologic disease course into the treatment strategy. The patient's medication history should be comprehensively assessed to determine whether the electrolyte abnormality may be drug induced. After resolution or treatment of the calcium or phosphate disorder, the medication regimen should be evaluated periodically. This proactive interventional approach will facilitate the management of mild disorders in the community and can reduce the need for hospitalization.

ABBREVIATIONS

ATP: adenosine triphosphate

CHF: congestive heart failure

CKD: chronic kidney disease

CNS: central nervous system

FGF23: fibroblast growth factor 23

2,3-DPG: 2,3-diphosphoglycerate

NSAID: nonsteroidal anti-inflammatory drug

PTH: parathyroid hormone

PTHrP: PTH-related protein

S_{ca}: serum calcium

REFERENCES

1. Copper MS, Gittoes NJL. Diagnosis and management of hypocalcemia. BMJ 2008;336:1298–1302.
2. Nussbaum SR. Pathophysiology and management of severe hypercalcemia. Endocrinol Metab Clin North Am 1993;22:343–362.
3. Dickerson RN, Treatment of moderate to severe acute hypocalcemia in critically ill trauma patients. J Parenter Enteral Nutr 2007;21:228–233.
4. Slomp J, van der Voort PH, Gerritsen RT, et al. Albumin-adjusted calcium is not suitable for diagnosis of hyper- and hypocalcemia in the critically ill. Crit Care Med 2003;31:1389–1393.
5. Byrnes MC, Huynh K, Helmer SD, et al. A comparison of corrected serum calcium levels to ionized calcium levels among critically ill surgical patients. Am J Surg 2005;189:310–314.
6. Levine MA. Primary hyperparathyroidism: 7,000 years of progress. Cleve Clin J Med 2005;72:1084–1097.
7. Lumachi F, Brunello A, Roma A, et al. Medical treatment of malignancy-associated hypercalcemia. Curr Med Chem 2008;15:415–421.
8. Rifai MA, Moles JK, Harrington DP. Lithium-induced hypercalcemia and parathyroid dysfunction. Psychosomatics 2001;42:359–361.
9. Fraser WD. Hyperparathyroidism. Lancet 2009;374:145–158.
10. McMahan J. A case of resistant hypercalcemia of malignancy with a proposed treatment algorithm. Ann Pharmacother 2009;43:1532–1538.
11. Strewler GJ. The physiology of parathyroid hormone-related protein. N Engl J Med 2000;342:177–185.
12. Pecherstorfer M, Brenner K, Zojer N. Current management strategies for hypercalcemia. Treat Endocrinol 2003;2:273–292.
13. Picolis MK, Lavis VR, Orlander PR. Milk-alkali is a major cause of hypercalcemia. Clin Endocrinol (Oxf) 2005;63:566–576.
14. Beall DP, Henslee HB, Webb HR, et al. Milk-alkali syndrome: A historical review and description of the modern version of the syndrome. Am J Med Sci 2006;331:233–242.
15. Moe SM. Disorders involving calcium, phosphorus and magnesium. Prim Care 2008;35:215–237, v–vi.
16. Maruani G, Hertig A, Paillard M, Houillier P. Normocalcemic primary hyperparathyroidism: Evidence for a generalized target-tissue resistance to parathyroid hormone. J Clin Endocrinol Metab 2003;88:4641–4648.
17. Abedin M, Tintut Y, Demer LL. Vascular calcification: Mechanisms and clinical ramifications. Arterioscler Thromb Vasc Biol 2004;24:1161–1170.
18. Bevilacqua M, Dominguez LJ, Rosini S, Barbagallo M. Bisphosphonates and atherosclerosis: Why? Lupus 2005;14:773–779.
19. Vella A, Gerber TC, Hayes DL, et al. Digoxin, hypercalcemia and cardiac conduction. Postgrad Med 1999;75:554–556.
20. Rodman JS, Mahler RJ. Kidney stones as a manifestation of hypercalcemic disorders. Hyperparathyroidism and sarcoidosis. Urol Clin North Am 2000;27:275–285.
21. Yamashita H, Noguchi S, Uchino S, et al. Influence of renal function on clinico-pathological features of primary hyperparathyroidism. Eur J Endocrinol 2003;148:597–602.
22. Ralston SH, Coleman R, Fraser WD, et al. Medical management of hypercalcemia. Calcif Tissue Int 2004;74:1–11.
23. Lumachi F, Brunello A, Roma A, Basso U. Cancer-induced hypercalcemia. Anticancer Res 2009;29:1551–1555.
24. Davey RA, Turner AG, McManus JF, et al. Calcitonin plays a physiological role to protect against hypercalcemia in mice. J Bone Miner Res 2008;23:1182–1193.
25. Grauer A, Ziegler R, Raue F. Clinical significance of antibodies against calcitonin. Exp Clin Endocrinol Diabetes 1995;103:345–351.
26. Stewart AF. Hypercalcemia associated with cancer. N Engl J Med 2005;352:373–379.
27. Wellington K, Goa KL. Zoledronic acid: A review of its use in the management of bone metastases and hypercalcemia of malignancy. Drugs 2003;63:417–437.
28. Major P, Lortholary A, Hon J, et al. Zoledronic acid is superior to pamidronate in the treatment of hypercalcemia of malignancy: A pooled analysis of two randomized, controlled clinical trials. J Clin Oncol 2001;19:558–567.
29. Body JJ, Lortholary A, Romieu G, et al. A dose-finding study of zoledronate in hypercalcemic cancer patients. J Bone Miner Res 1999;14:1557–1561.
30. Pecherstorfer M, Steinhauer EU, Rizzoli R, et al. Efficacy and safety of ibandronate in the treatment of hypercalcemia of malignancy: A randomized multicenter comparison to pamidronate. Support Care Cancer 2003;11:539–547.
31. Guay DR. Ibandronate, an experimental intravenous bisphosphonate for osteoporosis, bone metastases and hypercalcemia of malignancy. Pharmacotherapy 2006;26:655–673.
32. Costa L, Lipton A, Coleman RE. Role of bisphosphonates for the management of skeletal complications and bone pain from skeletal metastases. Support Cancer Ther 2006;3:143–153.
33. Banerjee D, Asif A, Striker L, et al. Short-term, high-dose pamidronate-induced acute tubular necrosis: The postulated mechanisms of bisphosphonate nephrotoxicity. Am J Kidney Dis 2003;41:E18.
34. Markowitz GS, Fine PL, Stack JI, et al. Toxic acute tubular necrosis following treatment with zoledronate (Zometa). Kidney Int 2003;64:281–289.
35. Leyland-Jones B. Treatment of cancer-related hypercalcemia: The role of gallium nitrate. Semin Oncol 2003;30(2 Suppl 5):13–19.
36. Cvitkovic F, Armand JP, Tubiana-Hulin M, et al. Randomized, double-blind, phase II trial of gallium nitrate compared with pamidronate for acute control of cancer-related hypercalcemia. Cancer J 2006;12:47–52.
37. Edelson GW, Kleerekoper M. Hypercalcemic crisis. Med Clin North Am 1995;79:79–92.
38. Body JJ, Lipton A, Gralow J, et al. Effects of denosumab in patients with bone metastases, with and without previous bisphosphonate exposure. J Bone Miner Res 2010;25:440–446.
39. Silverman SL, Lane NE. Glucocorticoid-induced osteoporosis. Curr Osteoporos Rep 2009;7:23–26.
40. Silverberg SJ, Rubin MR, Faiman et al. Cinacalcet hydrochloride reduces the serum calcium concentration in inoperable parathyroid carcinoma. J Clin Endocrinol Metab 2007;92:3803–3808.
41. Franceschini N, Joy MS, Kshirsagar A. Cincacet HCl: A calcimimetic agent for the management of primary and secondary hyperparathyroidism. Expert Opin Investig Drugs 2003;12:1413–1421.
42. Sensipar (cinacalcet HCl) [package insert]. Thousand Oaks, CA: Amgen, Inc; 2004.
43. Cinacalcet: New drug. Secondary hyperparathyroidism: Where are the clinical data? Prescrire Int 2006;15:90–93.
44. Inzerillo AM, Zaidi M, Huang CL. Calcitonin: physiological actions and clinical applications. J Pediatr Endocrinol Metab 2004;17:931–940.
45. Guise TA, Mundy GR. Evaluation of hypocalcemia in children and adults. J Clin Endocrinol Metab 1995;80:1473–1478.
46. Jawan B, de Villa V, Luk HN, et al. Ionized calcium changes during living-donor liver transplantation in patients with and without administration of blood-bank products. Transpl Int 2003;16:510–514.
47. Kishimoto M, Ohto H, Shikama Y, et al. Treatment for the decline of ionized calcium levels during peripheral blood progenitor cell harvesting. Transfusion 2002;42:1340–1347.
48. Yarpuzlu AA. A review of clinical and laboratory findings and treatment of tumor lysis syndrome. Clin Chim Acta 2003;333:13–18.

49. Alvarez-Hernandez D, Santamaria I, Rodriguez-Garcia M, et al. A novel mutation in the calcium-sensing receptor responsible for autosomal dominant hypocalcemia in a family with two uncommon parathyroid hormone polymorphisms. J Mol Endocrinol 2003;31:255–262.

50. Hu J, Mora S, Colussi G, et al. Autosomal dominant hypocalcemia caused by a novel mutation in the loop 2 region of the human calcium receptor extracellular domain. J Bone Miner Res 2002;17:1461–1469.

51. Peacock M. Calcium metabolism in health and disease. Clin J Am Soc Nephrol 2010;5:S23-S30.

52. Fischer PR, Thacher TD, Pettifor JM, et al. Vitamin D polymorphisms and nutritional rickets in Nigerian children. J Bone Miner Res 2000;15:2206–2210.

53. Fouser L. Disorders of calcium, phosphorus and magnesium. Pediatr Ann 1995;24:38,41–46.

54. Ariyan CE, Sosa JA. Assessment and management of patients with abnormal calcium. Crit Care Med 2004;32:S146-S154.

55. Ammori BJ, Barclay GR, Larvin M. Hypocalcemia in patients with acute pancreatitis: a putative role for systemic endotoxin exposure. Pancreas 2003;26:213–217.

56. Lind L, Carlstedt F, Rastad J, et al. Hypocalcemia and parathyroid hormone secretion in critically ill patients. Crit Care Med 2000;28:93–99.

57. Maalouf NM, Heller HJ, Odvina CV, et al. Bisphosphonate-induced hypocalcemia: Report of 3 cases and review of the literature. Endocr Pract 2006;12:48–53.

58. Choyke PL, Knopp MV. Pseudohypocalcemia with MR imaging contrast agents: A cautionary tale. Radiology 2003;227:639–646.

59. Uhl L, Maillet S, King S, Kruskall MS. Unexpected citrate toxicity and severe hypocalcemia during apheresis. Transfusion 1997;37:1063–1065.

60. Polaschegg HD, Sodemann K. Risks related to catheter locking solutions containing concentrated citrate. Nephrol Dial Transplant 2003;18:2688–2689.

61. Marx SJ. Hyperparathyroid and hypoparathyroid disorders. N Engl J Med 2000;343:1863–1875.

62. Dickerson RN. Treatment of hypocalcemia in critical illness–part 2. Nutrition 2007;23:436–437.

63. Lee I, Sheu WH, Tu ST, et al. Bisphosphonate pretreatment attenuates hungry bone syndrome postoperatively in subjects with primary hyperparathyroidism. J Bone Miner Metab 2006;24:255–258.

64. Hollis BW. Circulating 25-hydroxy vitamin D levels indicative of vitamin D sufficiency: Implications for establishing a new effective dietary intake recommendation for vitamin D. J Nutr 2005;135:317–322.

65. DeMeglio LA, White KE, Econs MJ. Disorders of phosphate metabolism. Endocrinol Metab Clin North Am 2000;29:591–609.

66. Uribarri J. Phosphorus homeostasis in normal health and in chronic kidney disease patients with special emphasis on dietary phosphorus. Semin Dial 2007;20:295–301.

67. Fine A, Patterson J. Severe hyperphosphatemia following phosphate administration for bowel preparation in patients with renal failure: Two cases and a review of the literature. Am J Kidney Dis 1997;29:103–105.

68. Liu S, Quarles LD. How fibroblast growth factor 23 works. J Am Soc Nephrol 2007;18:1637–1647.

69. Prie D, Torres PU, Friedlander G. Latest findings in phosphate homeostasis. Kidney Int 2009;75:882–889.

70. Aydogan T, Kanbay M, Uz B, et al. Fatal hyperphosphatemia secondary to a phosphosoda bowel preparation in a geriatric patient with normal renal function. J Clin Gastroenterol 2006;40:177.

71. U.S. Food and Drug Administration. Oral Sodium Phosphate (OSP) Products for Bowel Cleansing. FDA Alert, 2006. http://www.fda.gov/cder/drug/infopage/osp_solution/default.htm.

72. Didronel (etidronate sodium) [package insert]. Cincinnati, OH: Procter & Gamble Pharmaceuticals, Inc.; October 2007.

73. Amanzadeh J, Reilly RF. Hypophosphatemia: An evidence-based approach to its clinical consequences and management. Nat Clin Pract Nephrol 2006;2:136–148.

74. Kelsler R, McDonald RD, Cadnapaphornchai P. Dynamic changes in serum phosphorus levels in diabetic ketoacidosis. Am J Med 1985;79:571–576.

75. Eknoyan G, Levin A, Levin NW. K/DOQI clinical practice guidelines for bone metabolism and disease in chronic kidney disease. Am J Kidney Dis 2003;42(Suppl 3):S1–S201.

76. Block GA, Klassen PS, Lazarus JM, et al. Mineral metabolism, mortality and morbidity in maintenance hemodialysis. 2004;15:2208–2218.

77. Joy MS, Finn WF. Randomized, double-blind, placebo-controlled, dose-titration, Phase III study assessing the efficacy and tolerability of lanthanum carbonate: A new phosphate binder for the treatment of hyperphosphatemia. Am J Kidney Dis 2003;42:96–107.

78. D'Haese PC, Spasovski GB, Sikole A, et al. A multicenter study on the effects of lanthanum carbonate (Fosrenol) and calcium carbonate on renal bone disease in dialysis patients. Kidney Int 2003;85:S73-S78.

79. Coladonato JA. Control of hyperphosphatemia among patients with ESRD. J Am Soc Nephrol 2005;16:S107-S114.

80. Chertow GM, Burke SK, Raggi P. Sevelamer attenuates the progression of coronary and aortic calcification in hemodialysis patients. Kidney Int 2002;62:245–252.

81. Perreault MM, Ostrop NJ, Tierney MG. Efficacy and safety of intravenous phosphate replacement in critically ill patients. Ann Pharmacother 1997;31:683–688.

82. Subramanian R, Khardori R. Severe hypophosphatemia. Pathophysiologic implications, clinical presentation, and treatment. Medicine (Baltimore) 2000;79:1–78.

83. Amanzadeh J, Reilly RF. Hypophosphatemia: an evidence-based approach to its clinical consequences and management. Nat Clin Pract Nephrol 2006;2:136–148.

84. Charron T, Bernard F, Skrobik Y, et al. Intravenous phosphate in the intensive care unit: More aggressive repletion regimens for moderate and severe hypophosphatemia. Intensive Care Med 2003;29:1273–1278.

85. Clark CL, Sacks GS, Dickerson RN, et al. Treatment of hypophosphatemia in patients receiving specialized nutrition support using a graduated dosing scheme: Results from a prospective clinical trial. Crit Care Med 1995;23:1504–1511.

86. Prie D, Blanchet FB, Essig M, et al. Dipyridamole decreases renal phosphate leak and augments serum phosphorus in patients with low renal phosphate threshold. J Am Soc Nephrol 1998;9:1264–1269.

DONALD F. BROPHY AND JANE FRUMIN

CHAPTER 60

Disorders of Potassium and Magnesium Homeostasis

KEY CONCEPTS

❶ Potassium is the primary intracellular ion in the human body.

❷ The normal serum potassium concentration range is 3.5 to 5 mEq/L (3.5–5 mmol/L).

❸ Potassium regulates many biochemical processes in the body and is a key ion for electrical action potentials across cellular membranes.

❹ In patients with concomitant hypokalemia and hypomagnesemia, it is imperative to correct the hypomagnesemia before the hypokalemia.

❺ Potassium chloride is the preferred potassium supplement for the most common causes of hypokalemia.

❻ Hyperkalemia is a common occurrence in patients with acute or chronic kidney disease.

❼ Magnesium is an important cofactor for many cellular functions.

❽ The normal serum magnesium concentration range is 1.4 to 1.8 mEq/L (0.70–0.90 mmol/L).

❾ Hypomagnesemia is commonly caused by excessive gastrointestinal or renal magnesium wasting.

❿ Hypermagnesemia is commonly observed in patients with acute or chronic kidney disease.

Potassium and magnesium are electrolytes that are responsible for numerous metabolic activities. Disorders of these electrolytes are frequently seen in both the acute care and community ambulatory care settings. Therefore, clinicians need a firm understanding of the etiology, pathophysiology, symptoms, pharmacotherapy, and monitoring of these disorders. This chapter describes the homeostatic mechanisms that are responsible for the maintenance of normal potassium and magnesium serum concentrations. The clinical disorders responsible for the development of hyperkalemia, hypermagnesemia, hypokalemia, and hypomagnesemia are also reviewed.

Learning objectives, review questions, and other resources can be found at **www.pharmacotherapyonline.com**.

POTASSIUM

❶ Potassium is the most abundant cation in the body, with estimated total-body stores of 3,000 to 4,000 mEq (3,000–4,000 mmol).[1] Ninety-eight percent of this amount is contained within the intracellular compartment, and the remaining 2% is distributed within the extracellular compartment. The sodium potassium adenosine triphosphatase (Na^+-K^+-ATPase) pump located in the cell membrane is responsible for the compartmentalization of potassium. This pump is an active transport system that maintains increased intracellular stores of potassium by transporting sodium out of the cell and potassium into the cell at a ratio of 3:2. Consequently, the pump maintains a higher concentration of potassium inside the cell.

❷ The normal serum concentration range for potassium is 3.5 to 5.0 mEq/L (3.5–5.0 mmol/L), whereas the intracellular potassium concentration is usually approximately 150 mEq/L (150 mmol/L).[2] Approximately 75% of the intracellular potassium is located in skeletal muscle; the remaining 25% is located in the liver and red blood cells. Extracellular potassium is distributed throughout the serum and interstitial space. Potassium is dynamic in that it is constantly moving between the intracellular and extracellular compartments according to the body's needs. Thus the serum potassium concentration alone does not accurately reflect the total-body potassium content.

❸ Potassium has many physiologic functions within cells, including protein and glycogen synthesis and cellular metabolism and growth. It is also a determinant of the electrical action potential across the cell membrane.[1] The ratio of the intracellular to extracellular potassium concentration is the major determinant of the resting membrane potential across the cell membrane. Thus the resting membrane potential is greatly affected by variations in extracellular potassium concentration. Serum potassium concentrations outside the normal range can have disastrous effects on neuromuscular activity, in particular cardiac conduction. Hypo- and hyperkalemia are both associated with potentially fatal cardiac arrhythmias, along with other neuromuscular disturbances. Finally, potassium is integral to maintaining healthy blood pressure balance; indeed, both the National High Blood Pressure Education Program and the Institute of Medicine recommend potassium supplementation as strategies for preventing and treating hypertension.[3–5]

CONTROL OF POTASSIUM HOMEOSTASIS

Potassium homeostasis, the maintenance of serum potassium within the normal range, is affected by dietary intake, gastrointestinal and urinary excretion, hormones, acid–base balance, body fluid tonicity and a highly integrated feedback mechanism.[6,7]

The recommended daily allowance for dietary potassium intake is approximately 50 mEq/day. Potassium is found in abundance in fruits, vegetables, and meats. The typical American ingests approximately 50 to 150 mEq (50–150 mmol) of potassium daily. Nearly all of this is absorbed, with only 10 to 20 mEq/day (10–20 mmol/day) eliminated in feces. The amount eliminated in the feces increases, however, in patients with diarrhea and in those with chronic kidney disease (CKD).[7]

The kidney is the primary route of potassium elimination. Potassium is freely filtered but almost all of it is reabsorbed passively in the proximal tubule and the thick ascending limb of the loop of Henle.[8] Therefore urinary potassium excretion is primarily determined by potassium secretion from the luminal cells of the distal tubule and collecting duct. Although the amount of potassium filtered by the glomerulus approaches 700 mEq (700 mmol) per day, only approximately 10% to 20% is actually excreted in the urine.[8] However, this amount can vary based on dietary intake, serum potassium concentration, and aldosterone activity. For example, more potassium is renally excreted in conditions that result in high aldosterone activity (e.g., dehydration) when the body is attempting to conserve sodium or when there is an increase in dietary potassium intake.

Hormones such as insulin, catecholamines, and aldosterone dramatically affect potassium homeostasis. Insulin is the most important hormonal mediator of potassium balance because it stimulates the cellular Na^+-K^+-ATPase pump to increase transport of potassium into liver, muscle, and adipose tissue.[6] There is a complex negative feedback loop in which insulin secretion tightly regulates serum potassium concentrations: an increase of only a few tenths of a milliequivalent of potassium stimulates pancreatic insulin secretion in an attempt to prevent hyperkalemia from developing.[1] If hyperkalemia does occur, glucagon is released from the liver to protect against insulin-induced hypoglycemia. Conversely, hypokalemia inhibits insulin secretion, a finding that explains why some patients receiving diuretics develop hyperglycemia.

An elevation in circulating catecholamines such as epinephrine usually results in the intracellular movement of potassium by two mechanisms.[8] They stimulate the β-receptor, which directly activates the Na^+-K^+-ATPase pump. Second, they stimulate glycogenolysis, which raises blood glucose concentrations, thereby increasing insulin secretion. This dual mechanism is often used therapeutically in patients with hyperkalemia to normalize serum potassium concentrations.

Aldosterone, a mineralocorticoid that is secreted from the adrenal glands in response to high serum potassium concentrations, promotes urinary potassium excretion. Aldosterone works in the distal tubule and collecting duct to promote the reabsorption of sodium and water in exchange for potassium. Aldosterone may also have extrarenal activity by stimulating cellular Na^+-K^+-ATPase pump activity.[8]

Changes in acid–base status significantly affect the serum potassium concentration. For example, the infusion of metabolic inorganic acids, such as hydrochloric acid, results in an increase in serum potassium. The body compensates for excessive hydrogen ions by moving them from the serum into the cell in exchange for intracellular potassium, to maintain electroneutrality. The process by which this occurs is complex, and a cellular H^+-K^+-ATPase pump has been identified. The efflux of potassium into the serum can result in hyperkalemia. A commonly quoted approximation of the pH effect is that for every 0.1 unit decrease in pH, there is a corresponding increase in serum potassium of 0.6 to 0.8 mEq/L (0.6–0.8 mmol/L) (with a wide range of 0.2–1.7).[5] This is often referred to as *false hyperkalemia* because there is not a true excess of total-body potassium. Metabolic acidosis associated with lactic acidosis and ketoacidosis, does not result in hyperkalemia, because both cations and anions enter the cell, thus maintaining electroneutrality.[1] Respiratory acidosis also does not significantly affect the serum potassium concentration.

Conversely, metabolic alkalosis has been associated with hypokalemia. As a result of a net loss of hydrogen ion from the serum, intracellular hydrogen ions enter the serum to increase the acidity of the blood. To maintain electroneutrality extracellular potassium ions are shifted intracellularly. This creates a relative deficiency of potassium in the serum. Serum potassium decreases approximately 0.6 mEq/L (0.6 mmol/L) for each 0.1 unit increase in blood pH. This is frequently termed *false hypokalemia* because there is not a true deficiency in total-body potassium.

Finally, hyperosmolality can result in enhanced movement of potassium from the cell into the extracellular fluid. This occurs most likely because of the associated cell shrinkage and water loss, which increases the intracellular-to-extracellular potassium gradient.[3] This is seen most commonly in conditions such as diabetic ketoacidosis. Conversely, hypo osmolality does not seem to affect potassium distribution.

HYPOKALEMIA

Epidemiology

Hypokalemia (defined as a serum potassium concentration <3.5 mEq/L [<3.5 mmol/L]) is a commonly encountered electrolyte abnormality in clinical practice. Hypokalemia can be categorized as mild (serum potassium 3.1–3.5 mEq/L [3.1–3.5 mmol/L]), moderate (serum potassium 2.5–3.0 mEq/L [2.5–3.0 mmol/L]), or severe (<2.5 mEq/L [<2.5 mmol/L]).[9] When hypokalemia is detected, a diagnostic workup that evaluates the patient's comorbid disease states and concomitant medications should be initiated. Hypokalemia is virtually nonexistent in healthy adults. This is due in part to the relatively high potassium content in the typical Western diet as well as the body's effective potassium-sparing mechanisms, which tightly regulate the serum potassium concentration. However it has been estimated that as many as 50% of patients who receive thiazide or loop diuretics have serum potassium concentrations less than 3.5 mEq/L (3.5 mmol/L).[10]

Etiology and Pathophysiology

Hypokalemia results when there is a total-body potassium deficit, or when serum potassium is shifted into the intracellular compartment. Total-body deficits occur in the setting of poor dietary intake of potassium, or when there are excessive renal and gastrointestinal losses of potassium.

Maintaining a consistent dietary intake of potassium is important because the body has no effective method for storing potassium. At steady state, potassium excretion matches potassium intake; approximately 90% of ingested potassium is renally excreted, whereas 10% is excreted in feces.[8] This underscores the importance of eating a well-balanced diet. Elderly patients with chronic diseases and those undergoing surgery are at increased risk for developing hypokalemia because of insufficient intake or losses resulting from surgery.

Many drugs can cause hypokalemia by a variety of mechanisms including intracellular potassium shifting and increased renal or stool losses (Table 60–1). The most common cause of drug-induced hypokalemia is loop and thiazide diuretic administration as these agents inhibit renal sodium reabsorption, which results in increased sodium delivery to the distal tubule. Consequently, hypokalemia develops because the distal tubule selectively reabsorbs sodium, and excretes potassium down its concentration gradient. Second, because diuretics result in volume contraction, aldosterone is secreted which further promotes the renal excretion of potassium. If concomitant potassium supplements are not provided to patients receiving loop and thiazide diuretics, mild to moderate hypokalemia is inevitable.

The second most common etiology of hypokalemia is excessive loss of potassium-rich GI fluid as a result of diarrhea and/or

TABLE 60-1	Mechanism of Drug-Induced Hypokalemia	
Transcellular Shift	**Enhanced Renal Excretion**	**Enhanced Fecal Elimination**
β_2-Receptor agonists	**Diuretics**	**Laxatives**
Epinephrine	Acetazolamide	Sodium polystyrene sulfonate
Albuterol	Thiazides	Phenolphthalein
Terbutaline	Indapamide	Sorbitol
Pirbuterol	Metolazone	
Salmeterol	Furosemide	
Isoproterenol	Torsemide	
Ephedrine	Bumetanide	
Pseudoephedrine	Ethacrynic acid	
Tocolytic agents	**High-dose penicillins**	
Ritodrine	Nafcillin	
Nylidrin	Ampicillin	
Theophylline	Penicillin	
Caffeine	**Mineralocorticoids**	
Insulin overdose	**Miscellaneous**	
	Aminoglycosides	
	Amphotericin B	
	Cisplatin	

vomiting. The typical potassium loss in feces is approximately 10 mEq (10 mmol) per day.[7] In diarrheal states, this amount increases proportionally with the volume of stool output. Vomiting also accounts for substantial potassium losses, which have been estimated to be as high as 30 to 50 mEq (30–50 mmol) per liter of vomitus.[10] Metabolic alkalosis can also occur in cases of severe diarrhea and vomiting as a result of loss of these bicarbonate-rich fluids. This causes an intracellular shifting of potassium, which lowers the serum concentration of potassium even further. Prolonged diarrhea and vomiting can significantly affect children and elderly patients because their kidneys are unable to effectively maintain adequate fluid status.

❹ Hypomagnesemia, which is present in more than 50% of cases of clinically significant hypokalemia, contributes to the development of hypokalemia because it reduces the intracellular potassium concentration and promotes renal potassium wasting.[11] While the precise mechanism of the accelerated renal loss is unknown, many believe that the intracellular potassium concentration may decrease because hypomagnesemia impairs the function of the Na^+-K^+-ATPase pump thereby promoting K+ wasting. Alternatively, the combination of increased sodium delivery to the distal tubule, elevated aldosterone concentrations, and hypomagnesemia may cause the renal outer medullary potassium channels to excrete potassium.[11] What is clear is that hypokalemia and hypomagnesemia often coexist as a result of drugs (diuretic administration) or disease states (diarrhea). When concomitant hypokalemia and hypomagnesemia occur, the magnesium deficiency should be corrected first, otherwise full repletion of the potassium deficit is difficult.

CLINICAL PRESENTATION OF HYPOKALEMIA

General

- The signs and symptoms of hypokalemia are usually nonspecific and highly variable between patients.

Symptoms

- Symptoms are highly dependent on the degree of hypokalemia and its rapidity of onset.
- Mild hypokalemia is often asymptomatic.
- Moderate hypokalemia is associated with cramping, weakness, malaise, and myalgias.

Signs

- Cardiovascular: In severe hypokalemia, electrocardiogram (ECG) changes often include ST-segment depression or flattening, T-wave inversion, and U-wave elevation. Clinical arrhythmias include heart block, atrial flutter, paroxysmal atrial tachycardia, ventricular fibrillation, and digitalis-induced arrhythmias.
- Musculoskeletal: Cramping and impaired muscle contraction.

Laboratory Tests

- Serum potassium concentration <3.5 mEq/L (<3.5 mmol/L) is diagnostic. Hypomagnesemia (serum magnesium concentration <1.7 mg/dL [<0.70 mmol/L]) can also be present.

TREATMENT

Hypokalemia

■ DESIRED OUTCOME

The goals of hypokalemia management are to prevent its development, treat serious life-threatening complications, normalize the serum potassium concentration, identify and correct the underlying cause of hypokalemia, and finally prevent overcorrection of the serum potassium concentration.

■ GENERAL APPROACH TO THERAPY

The general approach to therapy depends on the degree and rapidity with which hypokalemia developed and the presence of symptoms. Serum potassium concentrations between 3.5 and 4 mEq/L (3.5 and 4 mmol/L) are a sign of early potassium depletion. No pharmacologic therapy is recommended at this point; however, these patients should be encouraged to increase their dietary intake of potassium-rich foods. When the serum potassium concentration is between 3.0 and 3.5 mEq/L (3.0 and 3.5 mmol/L), it is debatable whether pharmacologic therapy should be initiated. Oral potassium supplementation should be initiated in patients with underlying cardiac conditions that predispose them to cardiac arrhythmias.[12] This includes patients receiving concomitant digoxin therapy. Patients with serum potassium concentrations below 3.0 mEq/L (3.0 mmol/L) should always be treated to achieve values between 4.0 and 4.5 mEq/L (4.0 and 4.5 mmol/L). In asymptomatic patients, oral therapy is the preferred route of administration. Intravenous (IV) potassium can be necessary in symptomatic patients with severe depletion, or in patients who are intolerant to oral supplementation. In patients with concomitant moderate to severe hypomagnesemia, the magnesium deficit should be corrected before potassium supplementation, to prevent refractory hypokalemia.[8,13]

■ NONPHARMACOLOGIC THERAPY

Various nonpharmacologic therapies have been used to prevent and treat hypokalemia. The best and most abundant source of potassium supplementation comes from dietary sources, in particular, fresh fruits and vegetables, fruit juices, and meats.[13] Table 60–2 lists foods that are excellent sources of potassium. Salt substitutes that contain potassium chloride are another effective, inexpensive source of potassium. Increased dietary intake of foods with high potassium content however is not recommended long term for many patients because it can add unwanted calories to the patient's diet. Moreover, dietary potassium is almost entirely coupled with

TABLE 60-2 Foods That Are High in Potassium

High content (>250 mg/100 g)	Highest content (>1,000 mg/100 g)
Vegetables	Dried figs
Spinach	Molasses
Tomatoes	**Very high content (>500 mg/100 g)**
Broccoli	Dried fruits (dates, prunes)
Squash	Nuts
Beets	Avocados
Cauliflower	Bran cereals
Carrots	Lima beans
Potatoes	
Fruits	
Bananas	
Cantaloupe	
Kiwi	
Oranges	
Mangos	
Meats	
Ground beef	
Steak	
Pork	
Lamb	
Veal	

phosphate, rather than chloride, so it is not as effective in correcting potassium loss associated with hypochloremic conditions such as vomiting, nasogastric suctioning, and diuretic therapy.[13]

■ PHARMACOLOGIC THERAPY

Formal guidelines for potassium supplementation were last published by the National Council on Potassium in Clinical Practice in 2000 (Table 60–3).[13] These guidelines provide a comprehensive framework for potassium administration as a prophylactic and therapeutic replacement in many distinct patient populations. When deciding how to design the optimal regimen one must consider: (1) the patient's normal baseline potassium concentration; (2) underlying medical conditions that can affect potassium balance; (3) concomitant medications that can affect potassium balance; (4) the patient's dietary and salt intake; and (5) the patient's ability to comply with the therapeutic regimen.[13]

A general rule for potassium replacement is that for every 1 mEq/L (1 mmol/L) decrease of potassium below 3.5 mEq/L (3.5 mmol/L), there is a corresponding total-body potassium deficit of 100 to 400 mEq (100–400 mmol). Because of the wide variance in projected deficits, each patient's therapy must be individualized and adjustments made on the basis of the patient's signs, symptoms, and frequent measurements of serum potassium. In patients receiving chronic loop or thiazide diuretic therapy, 40 to 100 mEq (40–100 mmol) of oral potassium supplementation can correct mild to moderate potassium deficits. Doses up to 120 mEq (120 mmol) can be required in more severe deficiencies. When providing oral potassium supplementation, the total daily dose should be divided into three to four doses to minimize the development of GI side effects. Patients receiving diuretics can become chronically hypokalemic and can benefit from combination potassium-sparing diuretic therapy.

CLINICAL CONTROVERSY

The replacement of potassium intravenously can be accomplished by IV piggyback or Buretrol administration. A pharmacist usually prepares the potassium IV piggyback, double checks the concentration and fluid, and then dispenses the final product to the medical unit. However, with Buretrol administration, essentially any clinician (e.g., nurse or physician) can prepare the solution on the medical unit and infuse the potassium solution into the patient. The Joint Commission and the United States Pharmacopeia 797 Standards now advocate that all parenteral products be compounded in a sterile, laminar flow environment, and be double-checked by a pharmacist to assure patient safety. Many hospitals to date have not adapted these recommendations, which were developed to improve patient safety.

❺ Whenever possible, potassium supplementation should be administered by mouth. Three salts are available for oral potassium supplementation: chloride, phosphate, and bicarbonate. Potassium phosphate should be used when patients are both hypokalemic and hypophosphatemic; potassium bicarbonate is most commonly used when potassium depletion occurs in the setting of metabolic acidosis. Potassium chloride, however, is the primary salt form used because it is the most effective treatment for the most common causes of potassium depletion (i.e., diuretic-induced and diarrhea-induced) as these conditions are associated with potassium and chloride losses.

TABLE 60-3 General Consensus Guidelines for Potassium Replacement

Guideline	Comment
Potassium replacement therapy should accompany dietary consumption of potassium-rich foods.	Potassium-rich foods often cannot completely replace potassium associated with chloride losses (vomiting, diuretics, or nasogastric suction) because it is almost entirely coupled to phosphate. Furthermore, increasing dietary intake of these foods can lead to unwanted weight gain.
Potassium replacement is recommended for sodium sensitive and hypertensive patients.	A high-sodium diet often results in excessive urinary potassium excretion.
Potassium replacement is recommended in patients who are subject to vomiting, diarrhea, or diuretic/laxative abuse.	These conditions promote excessive renal and GI potassium loss.
Potassium supplementation is best administered orally in divided doses over several days to achieve full repletion.	
Laboratory measurement of serum potassium is convenient but not always accurate.	Clinicians should be aware of the factors that result in transcellular potassium shifts. Monitoring 24-hour urinary potassium excretion can be necessary in high-risk patients.
Patient adherence to potassium replacement can be increased with compliance-enhancing regimens.	Microencapsulated products have no bitter smell or aftertaste and have much better GI tolerance. Regimens should be made as simple as possible to follow.
A potassium dosage of 20 mEq/day (20 mmol/day) is usually sufficient to prevent hypokalemia from occurring. Doses of 40–100 mEq (40–100 mmol) are usually sufficient to treat hypokalemia.	

TABLE 60-4 Differentiation of Available Potassium Supplements

Supplement	Comment
Controlled-release microencapsulated tablet	Disintegrates better in GI tract; fewer GI erosions as compared to wax-matrix tablets
Encapsulated controlled-release microencapsulated particles	Fewer erosions as compared to wax-matrix tablets
Potassium chloride elixir	Inexpensive, poor taste, poor compliance, immediate effect
Potassium chloride effervescent tablets for solution	More expensive than elixir, convenient
Wax-matrix extended-release tablets	Easier to swallow; more GI erosions as compared to other therapies

Potassium chloride can be administered in either tablet or liquid formulations (Table 60-4). The liquid forms are generally less expensive; however, patient compliance can be low because of their strong, unpleasant taste. Two sustained-release solid dosage forms are currently available in the United States: a wax-matrix formulation, and a microencapsulated formulation. The microencapsulated tablet is generally preferred because it disintegrates better in the stomach and is associated with less GI irritation.[13] Intravenous potassium use should be limited to: (1) severe cases of hypokalemia (serum concentration <2.5 mEq/L [<2.5 mmol/L]); (2) patients exhibiting signs and symptoms of hypokalemia such as ECG changes or muscle spasms; or (3) patients unable to tolerate oral therapy. Intravenous supplementation is more dangerous than oral therapy because it is more likely to result in hyperkalemia, phlebitis, and pain at the site of infusion.

The vehicle in which IV potassium is administered is important. Whenever possible, potassium should be prepared in saline-containing solutions (e.g., 0.9% or 0.45% sodium chloride [NaCl]). Dextrose-containing solutions stimulate insulin secretion, which can cause intracellular shifting of potassium, worsening the patient's hypokalemia, and should be avoided whenever possible.[14] Generally, 10 to 20 mEq (10–20 mmol) of potassium is diluted in 100 mL 0.9% NaCl for IV administration. These concentrations are safe when administered through a peripheral vein over one hour. When infusion rates exceed 10 mEq/h (10 mmol/h), ECG monitoring should be performed to detect cardiac changes. The serum potassium concentration should be evaluated following the infusion of each 30 to 40 mEq (30–40 mmol) to direct further potassium replacement requirements. Multiple doses of potassium can be repeated as needed until the serum potassium concentration normalizes. To allow adequate time for the potassium to equilibrate between the intra- and extracellular spaces, the clinician should wait at least 30 minutes from the end of each infusion before obtaining a serum concentration. Care should be taken to avoid sampling from the same line in which the potassium was infused, as this can result in a spuriously high potassium concentration.

In cases of severe potassium depletion, patients can require as much as 300 to 400 mEq/day (300–400 mmol/day). In this instance, it is common practice to dilute 40 to 60 mEq (40–60 mmol) in 1,000 mL 0.45% NaCl and infuse at a rate not exceeding 40 mEq/h (40 mmol/h). This should be performed in an intensive care unit under continuous ECG monitoring. Because of the high potassium concentration, and the risk for burning pain and peripheral venous sclerosis, the infusion should be through a central venous catheter into a large vein (e.g., superior vena cava) but care must be taken not to place the tip of the catheter into the right atrium.[15] Directly delivering high potassium concentrations into the heart can result in cardiac arrhythmias. Given the volume required to infuse this dose of

potassium, this infusion strategy might be impractical in certain clinical situations (e.g., patients requiring fluid restriction). A reasonable alternative is to split the potassium dose between the oral and IV routes. For example, if a symptomatic patient requires 120 mEq (120 mmol) of potassium, the clinician can give 60 mEq (60 mmol) as the immediate-release potassium liquid, and the other 60 mEq (60 mmol) can be given through the IV route (20 mEq/100 mL/h [20 mmol/100mL/h] in three doses). When giving large potassium doses, serum monitoring should be performed following the administration of half the dose to guide the clinician as to the need for additional potassium. This can also help avoid the development of hyperkalemia.

In the rare circumstances when cardiac arrest from hypokalemia is imminent, IV bolus dosing of potassium 10 mEq (10 mmol) over 5 minutes can be initiated and repeated once, if necessary.[15]

■ ALTERNATIVE THERAPIES

Potassium-sparing diuretics are an alternative to chronic exogenous potassium supplementation, especially when patients are concomitantly receiving drugs that are known to deplete potassium (e.g., diuretics or amphotericin B). Spironolactone inhibits the effect of aldosterone in the distal convoluted tubule, thereby decreasing potassium elimination in the urine. Spironolactone is especially effective as a potassium-sparing agent in patients with primary or secondary hyperaldosteronism. Amiloride and triamterene act by an aldosterone-independent mechanism; however, the precise mechanism of their potassium sparing is unknown.

Spironolactone is available as 25-mg, 50-mg, and 100-mg tablets. The usual starting dose is 25 to 50 mg daily, and can be titrated to a maximum dose of 400 mg/day. The potassium-retaining effects generally take approximately 48 hours to occur. Important side effects include hyperkalemia, gynecomastia, breast tenderness, and impotence in men.

Triamterene is available as 50-mg and 100-mg capsules. The usual starting dose is 50 mg twice daily, which can be titrated to 100 mg twice daily. Triamterene 50 mg is available as a combination product with hydrochlorothiazide 25 mg and is commonly used for the treatment of hypertension. Common side effects include hyperkalemia, sodium depletion, and metabolic acidosis.

Amiloride is available as a 5-mg tablet. The usual starting dose is 5 mg daily; however, 10 mg can be given in those with severe hypokalemia. This is also available as a combination product with hydrochlorothiazide 50 mg. The most common side effects are hyperkalemia and metabolic acidosis.

Generally, concomitant use of potassium supplementation with potassium-sparing diuretics is not necessary. There is a significant risk of hyperkalemia during combination therapy, especially in patients with underlying renal insufficiency or diabetes mellitus.

While there have been no pharmacoeconomic evaluations of the different pharmacotherapeutic alternatives to manage hypokalemia, the most convenient source of chronic potassium supplementation is appropriate dietary intake of potassium-rich foods.

■ EVALUATION OF THERAPEUTIC OUTCOMES

Serum potassium concentrations should be monitored regularly while the patient is receiving potassium supplementation. For patients receiving prophylactic potassium supplementation during diuretic therapy, the serum potassium and magnesium concentrations, as well as renal function should be monitored every 1 to 2 months in stable patients. In hospitalized patients receiving oral therapy for mild hypokalemia, the potassium concentration should be monitored every 2 to 3 days. Generally, the potassium concentration begins to increase within 72 hours. If it does not increase by at least 1 mEq/L (1 mmol/L) within 96 hours, the clinician should suspect concomitant magnesium depletion. Patients receiving IV potassium supplementation require close ECG monitoring if the infusion rate is >20 mEq/h (>20 mmol/h). Doses greater than this should be administered only in the presence of continuous ECG monitoring. Additionally, the patient should have potassium concentrations obtained halfway through, and 30 minutes following completion of the total potassium dose to guide further potassium dosing. Finally, the patient should be assessed for adverse effects such as pain at the infusion site or phlebitis.

HYPERKALEMIA

Hyperkalemia, defined as a serum potassium concentration greater than 5.0 mEq/L (>5.0 mmol/L), can be further classified according to its severity: mild hyperkalemia (5.1–5.9 mEq/L [5.1–5.9 mmol/L]), moderate hyperkalemia (6.0–7.0 mEq/L [6.0–7.0 mmol/L]), and severe hyperkalemia (>7 mEq/L [>7 mmol/L]).[18]

Epidemiology

6 Hyperkalemia is much less common than hypokalemia. In fact, if all patients with acute and chronic kidney disease were excluded, the true prevalence of hyperkalemia would be insignificant. The incidence of hyperkalemia in hospitalized patients is highly variable, and reports have ranged from 1.4% to 10%.[13] Most cases of hyperkalemia are the result of overcorrection of hypokalemia with IV potassium supplements. Severe hyperkalemia occurs more commonly in elderly patients with renal insufficiency who receive chronic oral potassium supplementation.[17,18]

Etiology and Pathophysiology

Hyperkalemia develops when potassium intake exceeds excretion (true hyperkalemia) (i.e., elevated total-body stores), or when the transcellular distribution of potassium is disturbed (i.e., normal total-body stores). The four primary causes of hyperkalemia— (1) increased potassium intake, (2) decreased potassium excretion, (3) tubular unresponsiveness to aldosterone, and (4) redistribution of potassium into the extracellular space—are discussed below.

Hyperkalemia Associated with Increased Potassium Intake

Hyperkalemia in this setting is almost always associated with renal insufficiency. Patients with stage 4 or 5 CKD and dialysis patients who are noncompliant with dietary potassium restrictions often present with life-threatening hyperkalemia. Many of these patients do not realize that fresh fruits and vegetables contain large amounts of potassium. Anecdotally, in many dialysis centers the incidence of hyperkalemia peaks during the summer months, when fresh garden produce is available. Another common dietary source associated with the development of hyperkalemia is potassium chloride salt substitutes. Many dialysis patients are instructed to use salt substitutes to avoid excessive sodium intake in an attempt to control volume overload. These patients unwittingly become hyperkalemic because these products contain approximately 10 to 15 mEq (10–15 mmol) potassium per gram, or 200 mEq (200 mmol) per tablespoon. Finally, many over-the-counter herbal and alternative medicine products may contain significant concentrations of potassium.[19–20]

It is essential for patients with CKD to receive education regarding dietary sources of potassium as well as information on the potassium content of herbal products because the ingestion of these can lead to hyperkalemia.

Hyperkalemia Associated with Decreased Renal Potassium Excretion
The kidneys excrete 80% of the daily potassium intake. Therefore, when the kidney is unable to excrete potassium appropriately, as in acute kidney injury (AKI) and stage 4 to 5 CKD, potassium is retained and often results in hyperkalemia. Finally, many drugs can inhibit the kidney's ability to excrete potassium by inhibiting aldosterone and thus contribute to an increase in serum potassium concentrations.

Severe hyperkalemia is more common in AKI than in CKD because patients are often hypercatabolic and can have underlying disorders, such as rhabdomyolysis or tumor lysis syndrome, which result in release of potassium from injured or lysed cells.[21] Severe hyperkalemia is rare in stable CKD patients, perhaps because of enhanced GI and renal potassium excretion.[22] Data suggest that hyperkalemia directly stimulates renal K^+ excretion through an effect that is independent of, and additive to, that of aldosterone.[22] Although the overall incidence of hyperkalemia is higher in patients with CKD when compared to patients without CKD, due to these adaptive mechanisms and their decreased susceptibility to cardiac effects of chronic hyperkalemia, it has been associated with a lower mortality rate.[18] Renal excretion of potassium is also inhibited by various endocrinologic disorders, including adrenal insufficiency, Addison's disease, and selective hypoaldosteronism. All of these disorders involve a decreased production of aldosterone, which results in the retention of potassium.

Several drugs have profound effects on the kidney's ability to regulate potassium.[23] Four drug classes in particular have specific effects on the kidney: angiotensin-converting enzyme inhibitors (ACEIs), angiotensin-II receptor blockers (ARBs), potassium-sparing diuretics, and prostaglandin inhibitors such as nonsteroidal anti-inflammatory drugs (NSAIDs). Although hyperkalemia with these drugs is typically dose dependent, the rates of hyperkalemia have been reported to range from 5% to 10% in most clinical trials. Other commonly used drugs that can cause hyperkalemia are digoxin, cyclosporine, tacrolimus, trimethoprim-sulfamethoxazole, heparin, and pentamidine.[23]

Tubular Unresponsiveness to Aldosterone
Certain medical conditions, such as sickle cell anemia, systemic lupus erythematosus, and amyloidosis, can produce a defect in tubular potassium secretion, possibly as the result of an alteration in the aldosterone-binding site. The exact mechanism of the tubular unresponsiveness is unknown.

Redistribution of Potassium into the Extracellular Space
The efflux of potassium from within the cell into the extracellular fluid, which is associated with no change in total-body potassium stores, is to be expected in the presence of metabolic acidosis, diabetes mellitus, chronic renal failure, or lactic acidosis. β-Blockers can also result in a transcellular potassium shift.[23]

The serum potassium concentration can also be falsely elevated in some conditions, and not reflect the actual in vivo potassium concentration. This is termed *pseudohyperkalemia*. Pseudohyperkalemia occurs most commonly in the setting of extravascular hemolysis of red blood cells. When a blood specimen is not processed promptly and cellular destruction occurs, intracellular potassium is released into the serum. Pseudohyperkalemia can also occur in conditions of thrombocytosis or leukocytosis. If severe hyperkalemia is found in a patient who is asymptomatic with an otherwise normal laboratory report, the hyperkalemia is most likely pseudohyperkalemia, and a repeat blood sample should be evaluated. Truly elevated potassium concentrations are normally associated with other laboratory abnormalities, such as low carbon dioxide (acidosis) or elevated blood urea nitrogen and creatinine concentrations (indicating renal insufficiency).

CLINICAL PRESENTATION OF HYPERKALEMIA

General

- Related to the effects of excessive potassium on neuromuscular, cardiac, and smooth muscle cell function.

Symptoms

- Frequently asymptomatic.
- The patient might complain of heart palpitations or skipped heartbeats.

Signs

- ECG changes (see Fig. 60–1 for description).

Laboratory Tests

- Serum potassium concentration >5.5 mEq/L (>5.5 mmol/L).

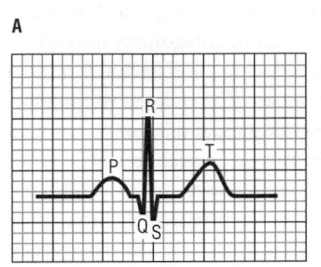
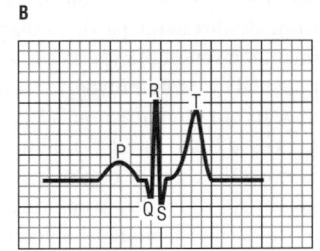
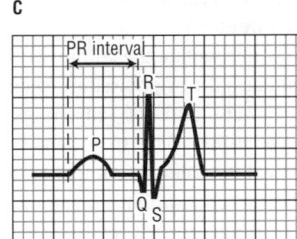
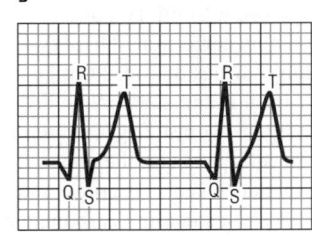
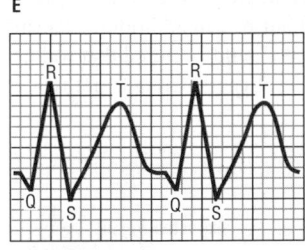
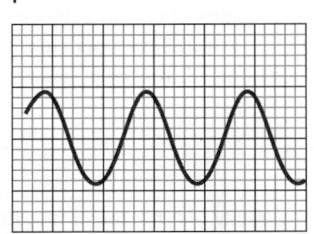

FIGURE 60-1. The earliest electrocardiographic manifestation of hyperkalemia is an increase in the rate of ventricular repolarization, which results in a peaking of the T wave at serum potassium concentrations of ~5.5 to 6 mEq/L (~5.5–6 mmol/L) *(B)*, relative to the normal ECG presentation *(A)*. Further increases in the serum potassium concentration above 6 mEq/L (6 mmol/L) result in conduction delays through the His-Purkinje system, the atrial myocardium, and the ventricular myocardium. The ECG manifestations of these conduction delays and the sequence in which they occur are a widening of the PR interval *(C)*, delay through the His-Purkinje system, a loss of the P wave *(D)*, delay through the atrial myocardium, a widening of the QRS complex *(E)*, and delay through the ventricular myocardium. Finally, there is a merging of the QRS complex with the T wave *(F)*, which results in a sine-wave appearance.

TREATMENT

Hyperkalemia

■ DESIRED OUTCOME

The goals of therapy for the treatment of hyperkalemia are to antagonize adverse cardiac effects, reverse signs and symptoms that are present, and return the serum and total-body stores of potassium to normal. The design of the treatment approach is determined by the severity of hyperkalemia, the rapidity of its development, and the patient's clinical condition. Although ECG changes are directly proportional to the plasma potassium concentration and its rate of increase, they may not be present in all patients. In contrast, ventricular fibrillation may be the first cardiac manifestation of hyperkalemia in some patients.[24] Asymptomatic patients with mild hyperkalemia usually require no specific therapy other than dietary education to control intake, and monitoring of serum potassium daily if an inpatient or weekly if an outpatient to assure resolution. Severe hyperkalemia (>7 mEq/L [>7 mmol/L]) or moderate hyperkalemia (6.0–6.9 mEq/L [6.0–6.9 mmol/L]), when associated with clinical symptoms or ECG changes, requires immediate treatment. Initial treatment of severe and moderate symptomatic hyperkalemia is focused on antagonism of the cardiac membrane actions of hyperkalemia (e.g., with calcium). Secondarily, one should attempt to decrease extracellular potassium concentration by promoting its intracellular movement (e.g., with glucose, insulin, β_2-receptor agonists, or sodium bicarbonate) or enhance its removal from the body by hemodialysis, the oral administration of cation-exchange resins, and/or the use of loop diuretics. In any case, the underlying cause of hyperkalemia should be identified and reversed, and exogenous potassium must be withheld.

■ GENERAL APPROACH TO TREATMENT

A general treatment approach for patients with hyperkalemia is outlined in Figure 60–2. In patients who have acute ECG changes, IV calcium should be administered to prevent or treat any cardiac manifestations of hyperkalemia. At the same time, the serum potassium concentration should be rapidly decreased to <5.0 mEq/L (<5.0 mmol/L) within minutes by administering drugs that cause an intracellular shift, followed by those that increase the elimination of potassium from the body.[24] If the patient is asymptomatic, rapid correction may not be necessary, and will likely depend on the clinical context associated with the rise in serum potassium concentration. If one anticipates the need to reduce total-body potassium stores, an ion exchange resin (e.g., sodium polystyrene sulfonate [SPS]) that results in removal of potassium from the body over several hours to days should be initiated shortly after the emergent care has been instituted.

■ NONPHARMACOLOGIC THERAPY

A recent study suggested that hemodialysis patients who ingested foods supplemented with glycyrrhetinic acid, the active ingredient in licorice, were better able to maintain plasma potassium concentrations within the normal range compared to hemodialysis patients given placebo.[25,26] Glycyrrhetinic acid inhibits the enzyme 11β-hydroxy-steroid dehydrogenase II, thereby increasing cortisol availability in the colon. The net result is enhanced potassium elimination in the feces. Other nonpharmacologic therapies, specifically available for dialysis-dependent patients with end-stage renal disease (ESRD), are the institution of intermittent dialysis or hemofiltration therapy.

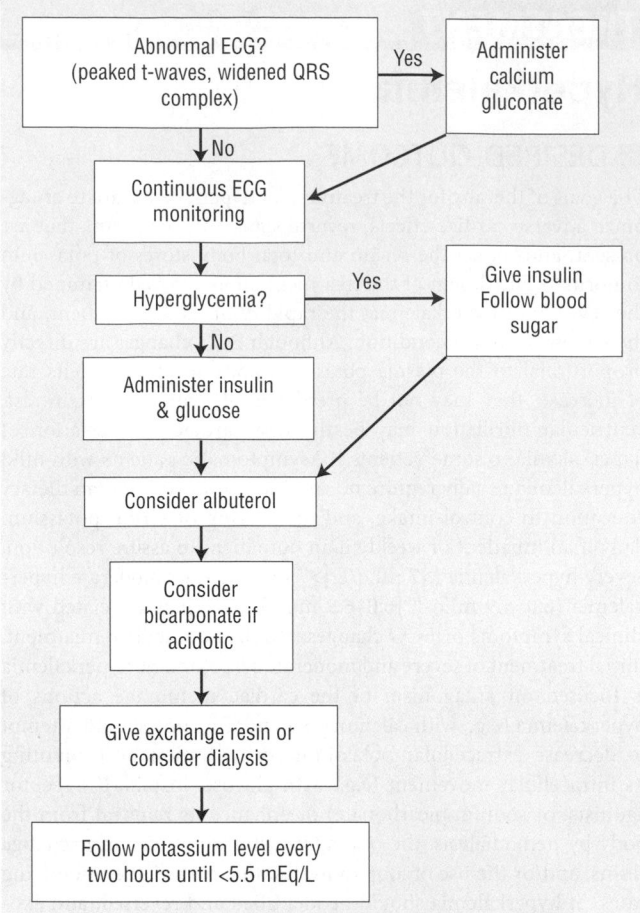

FIGURE 60-2. Treatment approach for hyperkalemia. (Serum potassium of 5.5 mEq/L is equivalent to 5.5 mmol/L.)

■ PHARMACOLOGIC THERAPY

Various drug therapies have been used to lower the serum potassium concentration. The optimal regimen for a given patient is dependent on the rapidity and degree of lowering that is necessary. Table 60–5 provides an overview of the available therapies, and their respective onset and duration of action one can expect.

While specific treatment recommendations vary, it is generally accepted that asymptomatic patients with potassium concentrations <6.0 mEq/L (<6.0 mmol/L) can be treated conservatively. In patients with normal renal function, or those with stage 3 or 4 CKD, this typically involves the administration of furosemide to promote

urinary potassium excretion. When given IV at a dosage of 40 to 80 mg, urine flow usually increases within minutes and persists for approximately 4 to 6 hours. Close monitoring of the patient's volume status and other electrolyte concentrations is required while the patient is receiving furosemide or other loop diuretic therapy. Alternatively, SPS (Kayexalate) a cation-exchange resin can be administered orally or rectally by enema. SPS is available in powder form or prepackaged as a 33% sorbitol suspension. The oral route is more effective than the enema and is better tolerated by the patient. As the resin passes through the intestines, each gram of SPS exchanges 1 mEq (1 mmol) of sodium for 1 mEq (1 mmol) of potassium ions, which are in a relatively higher concentration in the large intestine. The onset of action of SPS is within 1 hour, and it can be repeated every 4 hours as needed. The sorbitol component of the suspension promotes the excretion of the cationically modified potassium exchange resin by inducing diarrhea. The usual oral SPS dose is 15 to 60 g in the 33% sorbitol suspension. A retention enema prepared by mixing 60 to 100 g SPS in 100 to 200 mL of a 30% sorbitol or 10% dextrose suspension warmed to body temperature will usually remove 0.5 mEq of potassium per gram of SPS.[27] The enema may be retained in the rectum for several hours as tolerated by the patient.

In symptomatic patients, or in those with severe hyperkalemia, emergency care is indicated. Initial therapy in this setting is the administration of IV calcium chloride or gluconate 1 g to protect the heart from life-threatening arrhythmias.[24] Calcium antagonizes the cardiac membrane effect of hyperkalemia by reducing the electrical threshold potential for cardiac myocytes and reverses ECG changes within minutes. Its duration of action is 30 to 60 minutes, and it can be repeated as needed based on ECG findings. Intravenous calcium can be given as either the chloride or gluconate salt; each is available as a 10% solution by weight. Calcium chloride provides approximately three times more calcium than equal volumes of the gluconate salt; however, it can cause tissue necrosis if extravasation occurs. For this reason, calcium gluconate is more commonly administered, with the standard dose being 10-mL IV bolus over 5 to 10 minutes.

Rapid correction of hyperkalemia may necessitate the administration of drugs that result in an intracellular shift of potassium, such as insulin and dextrose, sodium bicarbonate, and a β_2-adrenergic receptor agonist (e.g., albuterol or terbuatline). The treatment of choice depends on the underlying medical disorders accompanying hyperkalemia. For example, in patients with concomitant metabolic acidosis, a sodium bicarbonate bolus or infusion of 50 to 100 mEq (50–100 mmol) is the preferred therapy (see Chapter 61 for additional information). Sodium bicarbonate helps to correct the metabolic acidosis by raising the extracellular pH, in addition to causing a rapid intracellular potassium shift. It should be noted that sodium bicarbonate is much less effective when hyperkalemia is not related

TABLE 60-5	Therapeutic Alternatives for the Management of Hyperkalemia					
Medication	**Dose**	**Route of Administration**	**Onset/Duration of Action**	**Acuity**	**Mechanism of Action**	**Expected Result**
Calcium	1 g	IV over 5–10 min	1–2 min/10–30 min	Acute	Raises cardiac threshold potential	Reverses electrocardiographic effects
Furosemide	20–40 mg	IV	5–15 min/4–6 h	Acute	Inhibits renal Na⁺ reabsorption	Increased urinary K⁺ loss
Regular insulin	5–10 units	IV or SC	30 min/2–6 h	Acute	Stimulates intracellular K⁺ uptake	Intracellular K⁺ redistribution
Dextrose 10%	1,000 mL (100 g)	IV over 1–2 h	30 min/2–6 h	Acute	Stimulates insulin release	Intracellular K⁺ redistribution
Dextrose 50%	50 mL (25 g)	IV over 5 min	30 min/2–6 h	Acute	Stimulates insulin release	Intracellular K⁺ redistribution
Sodium bicarbonate	50–100 mEq (50–100 mmol)	IV over 2–5 min	30 min/2–6 h	Acute	Raises serum pH	Intracellular K⁺ redistribution
Albuterol	10–20 mg	Nebulized over 10 min	30 min/1–2 h	Acute	Stimulates intracellular K⁺ uptake	Intracellular K⁺ redistribution
Hemodialysis	4 h	N/A	Immediate/variable	Acute	Removal from serum	Increased K⁺ elimination
Sodium polystyrene sulfonate	15–60 g	Oral or rectal	1 h/variable	Nonacute	Resin exchanges Na⁺ for K⁺	Increased K⁺ elimination

K⁺, potassium ion; Na⁺, sodium ion; SC, subcutaneous.

to metabolic acidosis.[21] Sodium bicarbonate is also less effective in patients with ESRD, in whom a decrease in serum potassium may not be seen for as long as 4 hours.[27] Sodium bicarbonate can also lead to sodium and volume overload in patients with stage 4 or 5 CKD. Administration of a fast-acting (e.g., Insulin Lispro) or regular insulin (5–10 units IV and dextrose (10% or 50%) is an effective method of reducing potassium. Insulin increases the activity of the Na^+-K^+-ATPase pump, thereby intracellularly shifting potassium. Glucose should be given with insulin unless the serum glucose is >250 mg/dL (>13.9 mmol/L) because hypoglycemia can develop as a result of the effects of the insulin therapy. An IV bolus of 10 units of regular insulin and 25 g of dextrose usually lowers the serum potassium concentration by 0.6 mEq/L (0.6 mmol/L) in dialysis-dependent patients.[24] β_2-Adrenergic agonists have a dual mechanism for lowering serum potassium. First, they stimulate the Na^+-K^+-ATPase pump to promote intracellular potassium uptake. Second, they stimulate pancreatic β-receptors to increase insulin secretion. Albuterol can be administered via IV (0.5 mg given over 15 minutes) or via nebulizer (10–20 mg nebulized over 10 minutes); however, it should be noted that injectable albuterol is not available in the United States. In ESRD patients, decreases in plasma potassium concentration of 0.6 mEq/L (0.6 mmol/L) and 1.0 mEq/L (1.0 mmol/L) can be anticipated after inhalation of 10 mg and 20 mg of albuterol, respectively. Of note, the doses of inhaled albuterol used for hyperkalemia are at least 4 times higher than those typically used for bronchospasm.[24] There are important limitations with albuterol therapy, most notably variable bioavailability via the inhaled route (leading to potential over- or under-dosing and unpredictability of response) and second, cardiac side effects such as tachycardia which are undesirable in patients who already have an abnormal ECG. Furthermore, as many as 40% of patients may be resistant to the hypokalemic effects of albuterol and patients already receiving a nonselective β_2-receptor antagonist may not respond. Therefore, albuterol should not be used alone for the urgent treatment of hyperkalemia in CKD patients.[24] The use of subcutaneous terbutaline in a small group of dialysis patients with hyperkalemia has also been shown to be effective.[28]

A Cochrane Review evaluated the emergency treatment of hyperkalemia.[29] Many of the reviewed studies were small, and not all intervention groups had sufficient data for meta-analysis to be performed. However, given these limitations, inhaled and nebulized β-agonists, and IV insulin-and-glucose were all deemed effective. The combination of nebulized β-agonists with IV insulin and glucose appeared to be more effective than either agent alone. The meta-analysis results were equivocal for IV bicarbonate, and notably, SPS was not effective by 4 hours.

A major problem with drawing conclusions from this meta-analysis is the heterogeneity of the study population. Most of the data were from nonrandomized, noncontrolled observational studies and case reports. Doses of the drugs were not standardized and follow-up was often lacking. Therefore, the clinician should exercise caution when extrapolating these findings to his or her clinical practice. This underscores the need for clinicians to be able to interpret the limitations of the published literature. Nonetheless, the Cochrane database review corroborates the approach detailed in Figure 60–2.

CLINICAL CONTROVERSY

SPS suspension pre-mixed in 33% sorbitol is commonly stocked in hospital pharmacies for the management of hyperkalemia, however, its clinical effectiveness is now being reconsidered.[29] More important, emerging data suggest its use may be associated with GI necrosis.[30-31] Clinicians should reserve SPS use until other alternative treatments have failed.

■ EVALUATION OF THERAPEUTIC OUTCOMES

The evaluation of therapeutic outcomes differs based on the severity of hyperkalemia. For example, mild or moderate asymptomatic hyperkalemia is observed much more frequently compared with symptomatic, severe hyperkalemia. Many drugs such as ACEIs, ARBs, and spironolactone result in asymptomatic hyperkalemia. In patients with normal renal function, once these drugs are initiated and the dose titrated, clinicians should check the potassium concentration at least monthly. For those patients with renal dysfunction, monitoring should be more frequent, such as biweekly until the dose is stabilized. In the case where the patient has been on a stable dose for a long period of time and hyperkalemia develops, the clinician should attempt to downward titrate the dose or switch to another medication without hyperkalemia as a side effect (e.g., calcium channel blocker).

In patients who have acute symptomatic hyperkalemia (e.g., ECG changes), frequent potassium concentration and ECG monitoring is warranted. The patient should receive continuous ECG telemetry monitoring until the serum potassium concentration decreases below 5.0 mEq/L (5.0 mmol/L), and the ECG abnormalities resolve. Similarly, while the patient is receiving emergent therapy, serial serum potassium concentrations should be obtained hourly until the potassium concentration decreases below 5.0 mEq/L (5.0 mmol/L). For patients who receive insulin and dextrose therapy for hyperkalemia, blood glucose monitoring should be performed hourly, or more frequently if patients demonstrate signs and symptoms of hypoglycemia. For patients who receive large doses of sodium bicarbonate therapy for hyperkalemia, an arterial blood gas or serum chemistry profile should be obtained to assess their acid–base status. Furthermore, the patient should be evaluated for signs of fluid overload secondary to the high sodium load. Patients receiving albuterol or terbutaline therapy should be questioned regularly regarding the development of palpitations and tachycardia. The patient's medication records should be reviewed to assure the patient is not receiving drug therapy that increases the serum potassium concentration. Furthermore, the patient should be questioned regarding the occurrence of diarrheal stool output.

DISORDERS OF MAGNESIUM HOMEOSTASIS

❼ Magnesium plays a central role in cellular function and is an important cofactor in more than 300 biochemical reactions in the body, especially those systems that are dependent on adenosine triphosphate. Mitochondrial function, protein synthesis, cell membrane function, parathyroid hormone (PTH) secretion, and glucose metabolism are just a few important functions affected by magnesium.[32] It is the fourth most abundant extracellular cation and second most abundant intracellular cation, after potassium. Disorders of magnesium homeostasis are commonly encountered in clinical situations and most frequently are manifested as alterations in cardiovascular and neuromuscular function. Life-threatening conditions such as paralysis and cardiac arrhythmias can occur, making the proper recognition and treatment of these problems of paramount importance. Altered magnesium balance also plays a key role in chronic disease states such as diabetes mellitus, chronic kidney disease, osteoporosis, development of kidney stones, as well as heart and vascular disease.[33]

❽ Magnesium is principally distributed in bone (67%) and muscle (20%). Because of its predominantly intracellular distribution, measurement of magnesium in the extracellular compartment may not accurately reflect the total-body magnesium content. The majority of magnesium in the extracellular fluid is in the ionized form as only 20% is bound to serum proteins. The normal range for serum magnesium is 1.4 to 1.8 mEq/L, which is equivalent to 1.7 to 2.3 mg/dL or 0.70 to 0.95 mmol/L.[33,34]

The recommended daily dietary magnesium intake for adults is approximately 420 mg/day and 320 mg/day for men and women, respectively.[33] The maintenance of magnesium homeostasis depends on the balance between intake and output. Thirty percent to 40% of ingested magnesium is absorbed in the small bowel. The absorption of magnesium decreases as the dietary intake increases. Reductions in absorption have also been noted in the elderly and those with CKD. A small amount is present in intestinal secretions and reabsorbed in the sigmoid colon. The kidneys play a major role in maintaining magnesium balance. Approximately 95% of the filtered magnesium is reabsorbed, thus in most patients less than 5% is excreted in the urine.[34] Renal magnesium handling is unique in that approximately 20% of the filtered magnesium is reabsorbed in the proximal tubule; the majority of reabsorption occurs in the thick ascending limb of the loop of Henle. This explains why loop diuretics often cause profound urinary magnesium wasting. Unlike most other important electrolytes, there is no hormonal regulation of the distribution of magnesium between bone and circulating or intracellular magnesium pools. Because of this, both hypomagnesemia and hypermagnesemia commonly occur.

HYPOMAGNESEMIA

Epidemiology

Hypomagnesemia is a common problem in both ambulatory and hospitalized patients. Although the exact prevalence is difficult to estimate, it has been reported that up to 65% of intensive care unit patients are magnesium deficient.[35] Although serum magnesium concentrations are not a reliable index of total-body magnesium content, they remain the primary diagnostic tool to evaluate body stores.

Etiology and Pathophysiology

❾ Hypomagnesemia is usually associated with disorders of the intestinal tract or kidney.[34] Drugs or conditions that interfere with intestinal absorption or increase renal excretion of magnesium can result in hypomagnesemia (Table 60–6). Decreased intestinal absorption as a result of small bowel disease is the most common cause of hypomagnesemia worldwide. These disorders include regional enteritis; radiation enteritis; ulcerative colitis; acute and chronic diarrhea; pancreatic insufficiency and other malabsorptive syndromes; small-bowel bypass surgery; and chronic laxative abuse. Hypomagnesemia is commonly associated with alcoholism. The etiology is often multifactorial, including reduced intake, pancreatic insufficiency, chronic vomiting and diarrhea, and urinary magnesium wasting. In addition, patients who are hospitalized for acute alcohol withdrawal often receive IV glucose and can experience even greater reductions in their serum magnesium concentration.

Primary renal magnesium wasting can be caused by a defect in renal tubular magnesium reabsorption, or inhibition of sodium reabsorption in those segments in which magnesium transport follows passively. The former condition is associated with hypercalciuria, nephrolithiasis, and progressive renal disease. The latter is associated with Gitelman's and Bartter's syndromes.[34] Much more common than these is renal magnesium wasting secondary to thiazide and loop diuretics.[33] Other commonly used drugs that can cause renal magnesium wasting include aminoglycosides, amphotericin B, cyclosporine, digoxin, tacrolimus, cisplatin, pentamidine, and foscarnet.

TABLE 60–6	Causes of Hypomagnesemia

Gastrointestinal
Reduced intake
  Protein-calorie malnutrition
  Prolonged parenteral fluid administration without magnesium
  Alcoholism
Reduced absorption
  Primary hypomagnesemia
  Malabsorption syndromes (e.g., tropical sprue, celiac disease, radiation enteritis, or intestinal lymphectasia)
  Short-bowel syndrome (e.g., small-bowel resection or ileal bypass)
  Pancreatic insufficiency
Increased loss
  Excessive vomiting
  Prolonged nasogastric suction
  Excessive laxative use
  Intestinal and biliary fistulas
  Prolonged diarrhea (ulcerative colitis, Crohn disease, or cancer of the colon)

Renal
Primary tubular disorders
  Primary renal magnesium wasting
  Bartter's syndrome
  Renal tubular acidosis
  Diuretic phase of acute tubular necrosis
  Postobstructive diuresis
  Postrenal transplant diuresis
Glomerulonephritis
Pyelonephritis
Drug-induced renal losses
  Aminoglycosides
  Amphotericin B
  Cyclosporine
  Tacrolimus
  Diuretics
  Digitalis
  Cisplatin
  Pentamidine
  Forscarnet
Hormone-induced renal losses
  Primary hyperparathyroidism
  Hyperthyroidism
  Aldosteronism
  "Hungry bone syndrome" after parathyroidectomy

Internal redistribution
Diabetic ketoacidosis
Glucose, amino acid, or insulin administration
Massive blood transfusion (citrate)
Pancreatitis with lipidemia (magnesium soap)

Other
Excessive sweating and lactation
Hypercalcemia and hypercalciuria
Phosphate depletion
Chronic alcoholism
Extracellular fluid volume expansion

CLINICAL PRESENTATION OF HYPOMAGNESEMIA

General
- The dominant organ systems affected by hypomagnesemia are the neuromuscular and cardiovascular systems.

Symptoms
- Neuromuscular symptoms such as tetany, twitching, and generalized convulsions are common.
- Cardiac symptoms include heart palpitations.

Signs

- Neuromuscular: Presence of Chvostek's sign, Trousseau's sign, tremor, and tetany.
- Cardiovascular: Cardiac arrhythmias (ventricular fibrillation, torsade de pointes, or digoxin-induced arrhythmias), sudden cardiac death, and hypertension can be present. ECG abnormalities include widened QRS complex and peaked T waves with mild hypomagnesemia; and prolonged PR interval, progressive widening of QRS complex, and flattened T waves with moderate to severe hypomagnesemia.

Laboratory Tests

- Serum magnesium concentration less than 1.4 mEq/L (0.70 mmol/L). Serum potassium and calcium concentrations can also be low.

TREATMENT

Hypomagnesemia

■ DESIRED OUTCOME

The treatment goals in the management of hypomagnesemia are (1) resolution of the corresponding signs and symptoms, (2) restoration of normal magnesium concentrations, (3) correction of concomitant electrolyte abnormalities, and (4) identification and correction of the underlying cause of magnesium depletion.

■ GENERAL APPROACH TO TREATMENT

Nearly all of the data regarding magnesium replacement therapy have been derived from reports in acutely ill, hospitalized patients. Magnesium supplementation can be given by the oral, IM, or IV route. Table 60–7 outlines one approach to the hypomagnesemic

TABLE 60-7	Guidelines for Treatment of Magnesium Deficiency in Adults

1. Serum magnesium <1 mEq/L (<1.2 mg/dL [<0.5 mmol/L]) with life-threatening symptoms (seizure or arrhythmia)

Day 1

2 g magnesium sulfate (1 g magnesium sulfate = 8.1 mEq Mg²⁺) mixed with 6 mL 0.9% NaCl in 10-mL syringe and administer IV push over 1 min

Follow with 1.0 mEq Mg²⁺/kg lean body weight IV infusion over 24 h

Days 2–5

0.5 mEq [0.25 mmol] Mg²⁺/kg lean body weight per day divided in maintenance IV fluids

2. Serum magnesium <1 mEq/L (<1.2 mg/dL [<0.5 mmol/L]) without life-threatening symptoms

Day 1

Total of 1 mEq (0.5 mmol) Mg²⁺/kg lean body weight per day as continuous IV infusion, or divided and given IM q 4 h for five doses

Days 2–5

0.5 mEq (0.25 mmol) Mg²⁺/kg lean body weight IV infusion per day as continuous IV infusion or divided and given IM every 6–8 h

3. Serum magnesium >1 mEq/L (>1.2 mg/dL [>0.5 mmol/L]) and <1.5 mEq/L (<1.8 mg/dL [<0.75 mmol/L]) without symptoms

As in no. 2 above, or

Milk of magnesia 5 mL 4 times daily as tolerated, or

Magnesium-containing antacid 15 mL 3 times daily as tolerated, or

Magnesium oxide tablets 400 mg 4 times daily; increase to two tablets 4 times daily as tolerated

Mg²⁺, magnesium ion; NaCl, sodium chloride.

TABLE 60-8	Common Magnesium Products and Their Elemental Magnesium Content
Product	**Elemental Magnesium Content**
Magnesium oxide	242 mg in a 400-mg tablet
Magnesium hydroxide	167 mg in a 400-mg tablet or 5-mL oral suspension
Magnesium citrate	48 mg in the 290 mg/5 mL oral solution
Magnesium gluconate	27 mg in a 500-mg tablet
Magnesium lactate	84 mg in a 84 mg-tablet

patient. The severity of the magnesium depletion and the presence of severe signs and symptoms should dictate the route of administration. Because IM administration is painful, it should be reserved for those patients with severe hypomagnesemia and limited venous access. IV bolus administration is associated with flushing, sweating, and a sensation of warmth; thus bolus administration should be avoided if possible. Additionally, because calcium forms a complex with the sulfate moiety, which is then excreted, large amounts of IV magnesium sulfate should be administered with caution to hypocalcemic patients, as it can further exacerbate calcium deficiency.[33] There have been no clinical trials assessing the optimal regimen for magnesium replacement, however, it is widely accepted that 8 to 12 g of magnesium sulfate be administered in the first 24 hours followed by 4 to 6 g per day for 3 to 5 days to adequately replete body stores.[35] Even if severe magnesium depletion is present, approximately 50% of the administered dose is excreted in the urine. Consequently, magnesium replacement should be performed over 3 to 5 days, and continued supplementation should be provided for patients unable to eat and for those patients with continued magnesium wasting. Table 60–8 lists the commonly prescribed magnesium oral supplements and their respective elemental magnesium content.

■ PHARMACOLOGIC THERAPY

It is currently controversial whether all asymptomatic patients require magnesium supplementation.[34] However, should treatment be warranted, those patients with serum magnesium concentrations greater than 1 mEq/L (1.2 mg/dL [0.5 mmol/L]), can be treated with oral supplements, such as magnesium-containing antacids or laxatives, or magnesium oxide tablets or capsules. The typical dose of magnesium oxide is 400 (242 mg elemental magnesium) to 800 mg (484 mg elemental magnesium) given 3 or 4 times daily until repleted. However, as expected, diarrhea is the most common dose-limiting side effect of oral therapy, which can greatly reduce patient compliance. Moreover, many oral products contain very little magnesium, which necessitates frequent dosing (Table 60–8).

In cases of severe magnesium depletion (serum concentrations <1 mEq/L [<0.5 mmol/L]), or if signs and symptoms are present regardless of the serum concentration, IV magnesium should be administered. A 50% solution of magnesium sulfate is available for injection in 2-mL or 10-mL ampules (4 mEq/mL [2 mmol/mL]). The 50% solution should be diluted to 20% before injection to prevent venous sclerosis and pain. Therapy should be continued until the signs and symptoms have completely resolved. In patients with renal insufficiency, the dose should be reduced by 50%.

■ EVALUATION OF THERAPEUTIC END POINTS

In patients with acute, asymptomatic mild to moderate hypomagnesemia receiving therapy, serum magnesium concentrations should be obtained at least daily during their hospitalization.

Patients receiving oral magnesium therapy should be questioned regarding GI tolerance and the occurrence of diarrhea. Patients being treated for symptomatic severe hypomagnesemia should have their serum magnesium concentration monitored hourly until the serum concentration reaches 1.5 mEq/L (0.75 mmol/L) and the symptoms resolve. At that point, the serum magnesium concentration can be monitored every 6 to 12 hours for the next 24 hours while receiving magnesium supplementation. Once the magnesium concentration is stable in the normal range, a concentration can be obtained daily. It should be reiterated that it typically takes 3 to 5 days to fully replete total-body magnesium stores. Patients receiving oral magnesium-containing antacids or supplements should be asked regularly about the occurrence of diarrhea.

HYPERMAGNESEMIA

Epidemiology

🔟 Hypermagnesemia (serum magnesium >2 mEq/L [>1.0 mmol/L]) is a rare occurrence that is generally seen in patients with stage 4 or 5 CKD when magnesium intake exceeds the excretory capacity of the kidneys. Elderly patients are prone to hypermagnesemia because of their reduced glomerular filtration rate (GFR) and because of their tendency to consume magnesium-containing antacids and vitamins.

Etiology and Pathophysiology

Because absolute magnesium excretion decreases as GFR declines, serum magnesium concentrations tend to increase in patients with moderate to severe CKD. Indeed, magnesium concentrations steadily increase as the GFR decreases below 30 mL/min/1.73m² (0.29 mL/s/m²). As long as the patient maintains a normal diet, the serum magnesium concentration typically stabilizes at approximately 2.5 mEq/L (1.25 mmol/L). If patients with stage 4 or 5 CKD are taking concomitant magnesium-containing antacids, the serum concentration can approach 6 mEq/L (3 mmol/L), a value associated with signs and symptoms of toxicity. Critically ill patients with multiorgan system failure receiving enteral or parenteral nutrition are also prone to develop hypermagnesemia. Finally, the parenteral treatment of eclampsia with magnesium sulfate can lead to hypermagnesemia. Table 60–9 lists other causes of hypermagnesemia.

Clinical Presentation

The signs and symptoms of hypermagnesemia reflect magnesium's action on the neuromuscular and cardiovascular systems.[35,36] The main symptoms include lethargy, confusion, arrhythmias, and

TABLE 60-9	Causes of Hypermagnesemia

Decreased renal excretion
Acute renal failure
Chronic kidney disease with exogenous intake

Excessive intake
Treatment of toxemia of pregnancy
Ureteral irrigants (hemiacidrin)
Cathartics

Other
Lithium therapy
Hypothyroidism
Milk-alkali syndrome
Addison disease
Viral hepatitis
Acute diabetic ketoacidosis

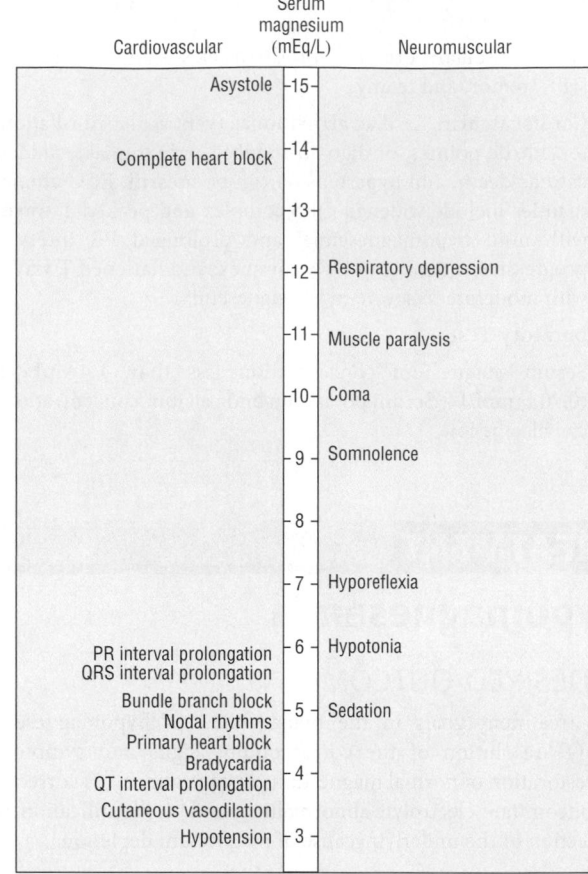

FIGURE 60-3. Clinical findings associated with hypermagnesemia. (Serum magnesium levels in mmol/L can be determined by multiplying the serum magnesium value expressed in mEq/L by 0.5.)

muscle weakness. Symptoms are rare when the serum concentration is <4 mEq/L (<2 mmol/L) (Fig. 60–3).

TREATMENT

Hypermagnesemia

■ DESIRED OUTCOME

The goals of therapy are to (1) reverse the neuromuscular and cardiovascular manifestations of hypermagnesemia, (2) decrease the magnesium concentration toward normal values, and (3) identify and treat the underlying cause of hypermagnesemia.

■ PHARMACOLOGIC THERAPY

There are three primary means of treating hypermagnesemia: (1) reduce magnesium intake, (2) enhance elimination of magnesium, and (3) antagonize the physiologic effects of magnesium. The optimal treatment regimen for the management of hypermagnesemia depends on the severity of the patient's signs and symptoms and the degree of serum concentration elevation. Intravenous elemental calcium doses of 100 to 200 mg directly antagonize the neuromuscular and cardiovascular effects of hypermagnesemia. Oral calcium is not effective because of its relatively poor bioavailability and slow onset of action. The clinical effect of calcium is immediate, but the effect is transient; hence, repeated IV doses of 100 to 200 mg of elemental calcium (e.g., 2 g of calcium gluconate) might need to be administered hourly until the signs or symptoms abate and the magnesium concentration

TABLE 60-10	Magnesium Content of Selected Foods
Food	**Elemental Magnesium Content (mg)**
Halibut, cooked, 3 oz	90
Almonds, dry roasted, 1 oz	80
Cashews, dry roasted, 1 oz	75
Spinach, one-half cup	75
Shredded wheat cereal, two biscuits	55
Instant oatmeal, 1 cup	55
Baked potato with skin (medium)	50
Peanuts, dry roasted, 1 oz	50
Yogurt, plain, skim milk, 8 oz	45
Brown rice, long-grained, one-half cup	40
Banana (medium)	30

is normalized. Supportive care with cardiac pacing, vasopressors, and mechanical ventilation can be necessary in life-threatening situations. In patients with normal renal function, or those with stage 1, 2, or 3 CKD, forced diuresis with saline and loop diuretics can promote magnesium elimination. An initial IV bolus of furosemide 40 mg or a similar equivalent can be used. Subsequent dosing can be determined based on the patient's clinical response. Patients with CKD can require long-term loop diuretic therapy to maintain adequate fluid and electrolyte balance. In dialysis patients, their hemodialysis prescription should be changed to employ magnesium-free dialysate.

■ EVALUATION OF THERAPEUTIC END POINTS

Patients who are receiving IV calcium salts for the treatment of severe, symptomatic hypermagnesemia should have their serum magnesium concentration evaluated hourly until symptoms abate and the magnesium concentration decreases below 4 mg/dL (1.64 mmol/L). Furthermore, the patient should be continuously monitored to detect ECG changes. In CKD patients who can produce urine, forced diuresis with saline and furosemide should reduce the serum magnesium concentration within 6 to 12 hours. Close monitoring of the urine output and physical examination for signs of volume overload are important. Emergency hemodialysis will usually correct the hypermagnesemia within 4 hours and is a reasonable option for those who are currently receiving hemodialysis. To prevent further episodes of hypermagnesemia, the patient should receive dietary education regarding foods and beverages that contain large quantities of magnesium (Table 60-10).

In conclusion, disorders of potassium and magnesium are frequently encountered in both the acute care and community ambulatory care settings. If severe, these disorders can have catastrophic results. Clinicians should be able to identify patients at risk for these common electrolyte disorders and quickly design appropriate pharmacotherapy and monitoring regimens to optimize patient outcomes.

ABBREVIATIONS

ACEI: angiotensin-converting enzyme inhibitor

AKI: acute kidney injury

ARB: angiotensin-II receptor blocker

CKD: chronic kidney disease

ECG: electrocardiogram

ESRD: end-stage renal disease

GI: gastrointestinal

IV: intravenous

NSAID: nonsteroidal anti-inflammatory drug

PTH: parathyroid hormone

SPS: sodium polystyrene sulfonate

REFERENCES

1. Peterson LN, Levi M. Disorders of potassium metabolism. In: Schrier RW, ed. Renal and Electrolyte Disorders, 6th ed. Philadelphia, PA: Lippincott Williams & Wilkins, 2003:171–215.
2. Schaefer TJ, Wolford RW. Disorders of potassium. Emerg Med Clin North Am 2005;23:723–747.
3. Whelton PK, He J, Appel LJ, et al. Primary prevention of hypertension: clinical and public health advisory from the National High Blood Pressure Education Program. JAMA 2002;288:1882–1888.
4. Panel on Dietary Reference Intakes for Electrolytes and Water. Dietary Reference Intakes for Water, Potassium, Sodium, Chloride, and Sulfate. Food and Nutrition Board, Institute of Medicine; Washington, DC: National Academies Press, 2005.
5. Adrogue HJ, Madias NE. Sodium and potassium in the pathogenesis of hypertension. N Engl J Med 2007;356:1966–1978.
6. Greenlee M, Wingo CS, McDonough AA, Youn JH, Kone BC. Narrative review: evolving concepts in potassium homeostasis and hypokalemia. Ann Intern Med 2009;150:619–625.
7. Palmer BF, Sterns RH. Fluid, electrolyte and acid–base disturbances: hypokalemia. In: Palmer BF, Sterns RH, eds. NephSAP® Nephrology Self-Assessment Program. Washington, DC: American Society of Nephrology, 2009:70–88.
8. Malnic G, Muto S, Giebisch G. Regulation of potassium excretion. In: Alpern RJ, Hebert SC, eds. Seldin and Giebisch's The Kidney, 4th ed. Amsterdam: Elsevier, 2008:1301–1347.
9. Gennari FJ. Disorders of potassium homeostasis: Hypokalemia and hyperkalemia. Crit Care Clin 2002;18:273–288.
10. Gennari FJ. Hypokalemia. N Engl J Med 1998;339:451–458.
11. Huang CL, Kuo E. Mechanism of hypokalemia in magnesium deficiency. J Am Soc Nephrol 2007;18:2649–2652.
12. Sica DA, Struthers AD, Cushman WC, et al. Importance of potassium in cardiovascular disease. J Clin Hypertens 2002;4:198–206.
13. Cohn JN, Kowey PR, Whelton PK, Prisant LM. New guidelines for potassium replacement in clinical practice: A contemporary review by the National Council on Potassium in Clinical Practice. Arch Intern Med 2000;160:2429–2436.
14. Agarwal A, Wingo CS. Treatment of hypokalemia [letter]. N Engl J Med 1999;340:154–155.
15. 2005 American Heart Association Guidelines for Cardiopulmonary Resuscitation and Emergency Cardiovascular Care. Part 10.1. Life threatening emergencies. Circulation 2005;112:IV-121–IV-125.
16. Rastegar A, Soleimani M. Hypokalemia and hyperkalemia. Postgrad Med J 2001;77:759–764.
17. Luckey AE, Parsa CJ. Fluid and electrolytes in the aged. Arch Surg 2003;138:1055–1060.
18. Einhorn LA, Zhan M, Hsu VD, et al. The frequency of hyperkalemia and its significance in chronic kidney disease. Arch Int Med 2009;169:1156–1162.
19. Burrowes JD, Van Houten G. Use of alternative medicine by patients with stage 5 chronic kidney disease. Adv Chronic Kidney Dis 2005;12:312–325.
20. Mueller BA, Scott MK, Sowinski KM, Prag KA. Noni juice (Morinda citrifolia): Hidden potential for hyperkalemia? Am J Kidney Dis 2000;35:310–312.
21. Chmielewski CM. Hyperkalemic emergencies: Mechanisms, manifestations and management. Crit Care Nurs Clin North Am 1998;10:449–458.
22. Gennari FJ, Segal AS. Hyperkalemia: An adaptive response in chronic renal insufficiency. Kidney Int 2002;62:1–9.
23. Perazella MA. Drug-induced hyperkalemia: Old culprits and new offenders. Am J Med 2000;109:307–314.
24. Weisberg LS. Management of severe hyperkalemia. Crit Care Med 2008;36:3246–3251.

25. Farese S, Jruse A, Pasch A, et al. Glycyrrhetinic acid food supplementation lowers serum potassium concentration in chronic hemodialysis patients. Kidney Int 2009;76;877–884.

26. Ferrari P. Licorice: a sweet alterantive to prevent hyperkalemia in dialysis patients? Kidney Int 2009;76;811–812.

27. Ahmed J, Weisberg LS. Hyperkalemia in dialysis patients. Semin Dial 2001;15:348–356.

28. Sowinski KM, Cronin D, Mueller BA, Kraus MA. Subcutaneous terbuatline use in CKD to reduce potassium concentrations. Am J Kidney Dis 2005;45:1040–1045.

29. Mahoney BA, Smith WAD, Lo DS, et al. Emergency interventions for hyperkalemia. Cochrane Database Syst Rev 2005;18:CD003235.

30. McGowan CE, Saha S, Chu G, et al. Intestinal necrosis due to sodium polystyrene sulfonate (Kayexalate) in sorbital. South Med J 2009;102:493–497.

31. Sterns RH, Rojas M, Bernstein P, Chennupati S. Ion-exchange resin for the treatment of hyperkalemia: Are they safe and effective? J Am Soc Nephrol 2010;21:733–735.

32. Drueke TB, Lacour B. Disorders of calcium, phosphorus and magnesium metabolis, In: Feehally J, Floege J, Johnson RJ, eds. Comprehensive Clinical Nephrology, 3rd ed. Philadelphia, PA: Mosby Elsevier, 2007:123–140.

33. Musso CG. Magnesium metabolism in health and disease. Int Urol Nephrol 2009;41:357–362.

34. Martin KJ, Gonzalez EA, Slatopolsky E. Clinical consequences and management of hypomagnesemia. J Am Soc Nephrol 2009;20:2291–2295.

35. Topf JM, Murray PT. Hypomagnesemia and hypermagnesemia. Rev Endocr MetabDisord 2003;4:195–206.

36. Moe SM. Disorders involving calcium, phosphorus and magnesium. Primary Care 2008;35:215–237.

61

Acid–Base Disorders

JOHN W. DEVLIN AND GARY R. MATZKE

KEY CONCEPTS

❶ The kidney plays a central role in the regulation of acid–base homeostasis through the excretion or reabsorption of filtered bicarbonate (HCO_3^-), the excretion of metabolic fixed acids, and generation of new HCO_3^-.

❷ Metabolic acidosis and metabolic alkalosis are generated by a primary change in the serum bicarbonate concentration. In metabolic acidosis, bicarbonate is lost or a nonvolatile acid is gained, whereas metabolic alkalosis is characterized by a gain in bicarbonate or a loss of nonvolatile acid.

❸ Arterial blood gases, along with serum electrolytes, physical findings, medical and medication history, and the clinical condition of the patient, are the primary tools to determine the cause of an acid–base disorder and to design and monitor a course of therapy.

❹ Renal tubular acidosis refers to a group of disorders characterized by impaired tubular renal acid handling despite normal or near-normal glomerular filtration rates. These patients often present with hyperchloremic metabolic acidosis.

❺ Respiratory compensation for a primary metabolic acidosis begins rapidly (within 15–30 minutes) but does not reach a steady state for 12 to 24 hours after the onset of metabolic acidosis.

❻ Primary therapy of most acid–base disorders must include treatment or elimination of the underlying cause, not just correction of the pH and electrolyte disturbances.

❼ Potassium supplementation is always necessary for patients with chronic metabolic acidosis, as the bicarbonaturia resulting from alkali therapy increases renal potassium wasting.

❽ Effective treatment of the underlying cause of some organic acidoses (e.g., ketoacidosis) can result in the regeneration of bicarbonate within hours, thus mitigating the need for alkali therapy.

❾ Loss of gastric acid from vomiting or nasogastric suctioning is often responsible for the development of a metabolic alkalosis, characterized by hypochloremia and hyperbicarbonatemia.

❿ Aggressive diuretic therapy can produce a metabolic alkalosis, and the accompanying hypokalemia can be serious.

⓫ The patient's response to volume replacement can be predicted by the urine chloride concentration and permits the differential diagnosis of metabolic alkalosis.

⓬ Management of sodium chloride-resistant metabolic alkaloses usually consists of treatment of the underlying cause of mineralocorticoid excess. In patients in whom the mineralocorticoid excess cannot be corrected, chronic pharmacologic therapy can be required.

⓭ In most cases of acute metabolic acidosis, such as following cardiopulmonary arrest, sodium bicarbonate therapy is not indicated and can be detrimental. Blood gas analysis should guide therapy.

Acid–base disorders are common and often serious disturbances that can result in significant morbidity and mortality. This chapter reviews the mechanisms responsible for the maintenance of acid–base balance and the laboratory analyses that aid clinicians in their assessment of acid–base disorders. The pathophysiology of the four primary acid–base disturbances is presented, the therapeutic options are critiqued, and guidelines for the achievement of the desired therapeutic outcomes are presented. Because many drugs affect acid–base homeostasis and many acid–base abnormalities are potentially preventable, clinicians must anticipate drug-related problems to avoid or minimize the clinical consequences of acid base disorders, and when necessary, design appropriate treatment regimens.

ACID–BASE CHEMISTRY

An acid (in this equation, hydrochloric acid) is a substance that can *donate* protons (hydrogen ion [H^+]):

$$\text{(acid) HCl} \rightarrow H^+ + \text{chloride ion (Cl}^-)$$

A base (in this equation, ammonia [NH_3]) is a substance that can *accept* protons (hydrogen ion [H^+]):

$$\text{Ammonia (NH}_3) + H^+ \rightarrow NH_4^+ \text{ (base)}$$

The acid–base pairs commonly encountered in clinical practice are listed in Table 61–1.

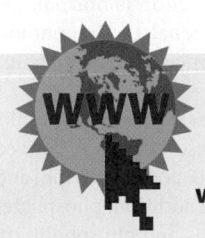

The complete chapter, learning objectives, and other resources can be found at **www.pharmacotherapyonline.com**.

TABLE 61-1	Acid–Base Pairs
Carbonic acid/bicarbonate	H_2CO_3/HCO_3^-
Monobasic/dibasic phosphate	H_2PO_4/HPO_4^-
Ammonium/ammonia	NH_4^+/NH_3
Lactic acid/lactate	$H_6C_5O_2/H_5C_5O_2^-$

The acidity of body fluids is quantified in terms of the hydrogen ion concentration. By convention, the degree of acidity is expressed as pH, or the negative logarithm (base 10) of the hydrogen ion concentration. Thus hydrogen ion concentration and pH are inversely related. Normally, the pH of blood is maintained at 7.40 ($[H^+]$ of 4×10^{-8} M) with a range of 7.35 to 7.45. A pH of less than 6.7 ($[H^+]$ of 2×10^{-7} M), representing a five-fold increase in hydrogen ion concentration, or greater than 7.7 ($[H^+]$ of 2×10^{-8} M), representing a 50% decrease in hydrogen ion concentration, are considered incompatible with life.

The hydrogen ion concentration in blood may not be indicative of that in other body compartments. For example, the pH within cells, within the cerebrospinal fluid, or on the surface of bone can all be altered without causing an alteration in blood pH.[1] Recognizing this caveat, the acid–base status of the body is usually analyzed based on measurement of blood pH. Alterations in blood pH serve as the basis for the diagnosis of acid–base disorders.

Because the dissociation of acid–base pairs is an equilibrium reaction, the relationship between hydrogen ion concentration or pH and the relative concentrations of the acid and base can be described mathematically in terms of the dissociation constant for the acid–base buffer pair. When expressed as a logarithmic relationship, where pK is the negative logarithm of the dissociation constant K, this is known as the Henderson-Hasselbalch equation:

$$pH = pK + \log([base]/[acid])$$

BUFFERS

The ability of a weak acid and its corresponding anion (base) to resist change in the pH of a solution on the addition of a strong acid or base is referred to as *buffering*. An acid–base pair is most efficient in functioning as a buffer at a pH close to its pK. The principal extracellular buffer is the carbonic acid/bicarbonate (H_2CO_3/HCO_3^-) system. Other physiologic buffers include plasma proteins, hemoglobin, and phosphates. Because the isohydric principle requires that all buffer systems remain in chemical equilibrium, the complex buffering of biologic fluids can be analyzed based on a single buffer pair.

The carbonic acid/bicarbonate buffer system plays a unique role in acid–base homeostasis. In addition to being the most abundant extracellular buffer, the components of this buffer pair are under dynamic regulation by the body. In the presence of carbonic anhydrase, carbonic acid, $[H_2CO_3]$ is in equilibrium with carbon dioxide (CO_2) gas. Changes in ventilation that alter the partial pressure of CO_2 (PCO_2) in the blood regulates the carbonic acid level in the blood. The bicarbonate concentration is independently regulated by the kidney. Because the pK for the carbonic acid/bicarbonate system is 6.1, the relationship between pH, carbonic acid, and bicarbonate concentrations can be described by the Henderson-Hasselbalch equation. The concentration of carbonic acid is directly proportional to the amount of CO_2 dissolved in blood, which is equal to the product of PCO_2 and its solubility in physiologic fluids, ($PCO_2 \times 0.03$ for PCO_2 expressed in mm Hg [or $PCO_2 \times 0.226$ for PCO_2 expressed in kPa). This term

can therefore be substituted into the equation below in place of $[H_2CO_3]$.

$$pH = 6.1 + ([HCO_3^-]/[H_2CO_3])$$
$$pH = 6.1 + \log([HCO_3^-]/(PCO_2 \times 0.03)) \text{ for } PCO_2 \text{ in mm Hg}$$

or

$$pH = 6.1 + \log([HCO_3^-]/(PCO_2 \times 0.226)) \text{ for } PCO_2 \text{ in kPa}$$

Thus, hydrogen ion concentration and pH are determined not by the absolute amounts of bicarbonate and PCO_2, but by their ratio.[1] Under normal physiologic conditions, the kidneys maintain the serum bicarbonate at approximately 24 mEq/L (24 mmol/L), whereas the lungs maintain the PCO_2 at approximately 40 mm Hg (5.3 kPa). The normal physiologic pH is thus 7.4:

$$pH = 6.1 + \log[24/(0.03 \times 40)] \text{ (or } pH = 6.1 + \log[24/(0.226 \times 5.3)])$$
$$pH = 6.1 + 1.3 = 7.4$$

If, in response to an acid load, the serum bicarbonate concentration were to decrease to 12 mEq/L (12 mmol/L), the predicted pH would be:

$$[HCO_3^-] = 12 \text{ mEq/L (12 mmol/L)}$$
$$PCO_2 = 40 \text{ mm Hg(5.3 kPa)}$$
$$pH = 6.1 + \log[12/(0.03 \times 40)] \text{ or}$$
$$pH = 6.1 + \log[12/(0.226 \times 5.3)]$$
$$pH = 6.1 + 1.0 = 7.1$$

However, the normal respiratory response to an acid load is hyper-ventilation. As a result, if the PCO_2 decreased to approximately 26 mm Hg, the change in pH would be less:

$$[HCO_3^-] = 12 \text{ mEq/L (12 mmol/L)}$$
$$PCO_2 = 26 \text{ mm Hg(3.5 kPa)}$$
$$pH = 6.1 + \log[12/(0.03 \times 26)]$$
$$(\text{or } pH = 6.1 + \log[12/(0.226 \times 3.5)])$$
$$pH = 6.1 + 1.19 = 7.29$$

Thus, the physiologic regulation of both PCO_2 and $[HCO_3^-]$ permit the carbonic acid/bicarbonate system to provide more effective buffering of the extracellular fluids than could be achieved on the basis of chemical buffering alone.

REGULATION OF ACID–BASE HOMEOSTASIS

Cellular metabolism results in the production of large quantities of hydrogen that need to be excreted to maintain acid–base balance. In addition, small amounts of acid and alkali are also presented to the body through the diet. The bulk of acid production is in the form of CO_2, with the average adult producing approximately 15,000 mmol of CO_2 each day from the catabolism of carbohydrate, protein, and fat.[2] When respiratory function is normal, the amount of CO_2 produced metabolically is equal to the amount lost by respiration, and the blood CO_2 concentration remains constant.

Digestion of dietary substances and tissue metabolism also results in the production of nonvolatile acids. These acids are derived primarily from the sulfur-containing amino acids cysteine and methionine, as well as from ingested sulfur. In addition, phosphates are generated from the metabolism of proteins and phospholipids.

Neutral substances such as glucose can also be incompletely metabolized to intermediates, such as lactic and pyruvic acid, and fatty acids can be incompletely metabolized to acetoacetic acid and β-hydroxybutyric acid. These dietary and metabolic fixed acids are excreted, primarily by the kidney, to maintain acid–base homeostasis. On average, daily fixed acid excretion is approximately 0.8 mEq/kg per day (0.8 mmol/kg per day).[3]

Three mechanisms, each of which vary in their onset, collectively maintain acid–base balance: extracellular buffering, ventilatory regulation of carbon dioxide elimination, and renal regulation of hydrogen ion and bicarbonate excretion. Extracellular buffering occurs rapidly and is the body's first defense against a sudden increase in hydrogen ion concentration. Hyperventilation will then result in a decrease in P_{CO_2}, returning blood pH toward normal. Finally, the kidney will excrete the excess hydrogen ion, with the resultant return of acid–base balance to normal over a period of day(s).

EXTRACELLULAR BUFFERING

The body's buffering system can be divided into three components: bicarbonate/carbonic acid, proteins, and phosphates. The bicarbonate buffer is the most important of the body's buffers, because (1) there is more bicarbonate present in the extracellular fluid (ECF) than any other buffer component; (2) the supply of carbon dioxide is unlimited; and (3) the acidity of ECF can be regulated by controlling either the bicarbonate concentration or the P_{CO_2}.

Carbonic acid represents the respiratory component of the buffer pair because its concentration is directly proportional to the P_{CO_2}, which is determined by ventilation. Bicarbonate represents the metabolic component because the kidney may alter its concentration by reabsorption, generating new bicarbonate, or altering elimination.[4] The bicarbonate buffer system easily adapts to changes in acid–base status by alterations in ventilatory elimination of acid (P_{CO_2}) and/or renal elimination of base (HCO_3^-).

The phosphate buffer system consists of serum inorganic phosphate (3.5 to 5 mg/dL [1.13–1.62 mmol/L]), intracellular organic phosphate, and calcium phosphate in bone. Extracellular phosphate is present only in low concentrations, so its usefulness as a buffer is limited; however, as an intracellular buffer, phosphate is more useful. Calcium phosphate in bone is relatively inaccessible as a buffer, but prolonged metabolic acidosis will result in the release of phosphate from bone.

Intracellular and extracellular proteins also act as buffering systems. The charged side chains of amino acids provide the buffering action. Because the concentration of protein is much greater intracellularly than extracellularly, protein is much more important as an intracellular buffer.

RESPIRATORY REGULATION

The second mechanism for maintenance of acid–base homeostasis is control of ventilation. Both the rate and depth of ventilation can be varied to allow for excretion of CO_2 generated by diet and tissue metabolism. Medullary chemoreceptors in the brainstem sense changes in P_{CO_2} and in pH and modulate the control of breathing. Increasing minute ventilation (the total amount of air exhaled over a 1-minute period), by increasing respiratory rate and/or tidal volume (the amount of air exhaled in one breath), will increase CO_2 excretion and decrease the blood P_{CO_2}. Conversely, decreasing minute ventilation decreases CO_2 excretion and increases blood P_{CO_2}. This system rapidly adjusts within minutes to changes in acid–base balance.[2]

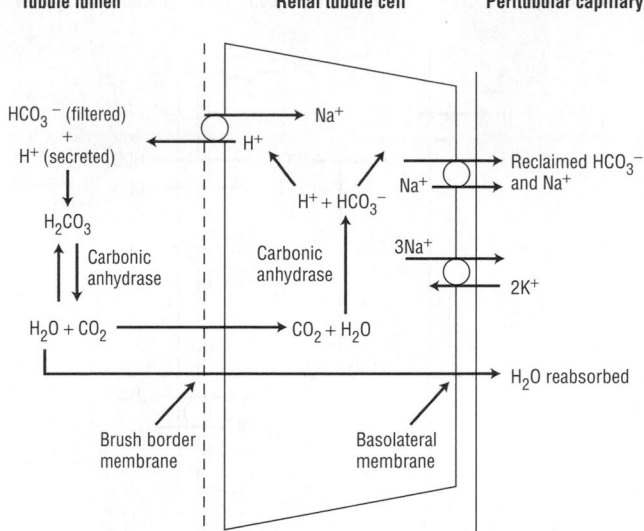

FIGURE 61-1. Proximal tubular bicarbonate reabsorption. In the tubular lumen, filtered bicarbonate (HCO_3^-) combines with hydrogen ion (H^+) secreted by an apical sodium ion (Na^+)-H^+ exchanger to form carbonic acid (H_2CO_3). The carbonic acid is rapidly broken down to carbon dioxide (CO_2) and water by carbonic anhydrase located on the luminal surface of the brush border membrane. The CO_2 then diffuses into the proximal tubular cell, where it reforms carbonic acid in the presence of intracellular carbonic anhydrase. The carbonic acid dissociates the former hydrogen ion that can again be secreted into the tubular lumen, and bicarbonate that exits the cell across the basolateral membrane and enters the peritubular capillary.

RENAL REGULATION

❶ Because bicarbonate is a small ion, it is freely filtered at the glomerulus. The bicarbonate load delivered to the nephron is approximately 4,500 mEq/day (4,500 mmol/day). To maintain acid–base balance, this entire filtered load must be reabsorbed. Bicarbonate reabsorption occurs primarily in the proximal tubule (Fig. 61–1). In the tubular lumen, filtered bicarbonate combines with hydrogen ion secreted by the apical sodium ion (Na^+)-H^+-exchanger to form carbonic acid. The carbonic acid is rapidly broken down to CO_2 and water by carbonic anhydrase located on the luminal surface of the brush border membrane. The CO_2 then diffuses into the proximal tubular cell, where it reforms carbonic acid in the presence of intracellular carbonic anhydrase. The carbonic acid dissociates to form hydrogen ion, that can again be secreted into the tubular lumen, and bicarbonate that exits the cell across the basolateral membrane and enters the peritubular capillary.

Excretion of metabolic fixed acids and generation of new HCO_3^- is achieved through renal ammoniagenesis and distal tubular hydrogen ion secretion. Ammoniagenesis plays a critical role in acid–base homeostasis, with ammonium (NH_4^+) excretion comprising approximately 50% of renal net acid excretion. Ammonium is generated from the deamination of glutamine in the proximal tubule. For each ammonium ion excreted in the urine, one bicarbonate ion is regenerated and returned to the circulation.[5]

Distal tubular hydrogen ion secretion accounts for the remaining 50% of net acid excretion (Fig. 61–2). In the distal tubular cell, CO_2 combines with water in the presence of intracellular carbonic anhydrase to form carbonic acid, which dissociates to H^+ and HCO_3^-. The H^+ is actively transported into the tubular lumen by a H^+-adenosine triphosphatase (ATPase). The

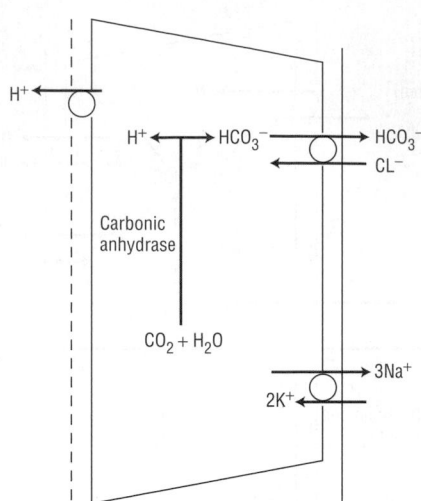

FIGURE 61-2. Collecting duct acid excretion. Hydrogen ion (H⁺) and bicarbonate (HCO₃⁻) are generated intracellularly from carbon dioxide (CO₂) and water, in the presence of intracellular carbonic anhydrase. The hydrogen ion is actively secreted into the tubular lumen by H⁺-adenosine triphosphatase (ATPase) located in the apical (luminal) membrane. Bicarbonate exits the cell across the basolateral membrane and enters the peritubular capillary. (Cl⁻, chloride ion; Na⁺, sodium ion.)

bicarbonate exits the cell across the basolateral membrane and enters the circulation.[5]

ACID–BASE DISTURBANCES

❷ Alterations in blood pH are designated by the suffix "-emia"; *acidemia* is an arterial blood pH <7.35 and *alkalemia* is an arterial blood pH >7.45. The pathophysiologic processes that result in alterations in blood pH are designated by the suffix "-osis." These disturbances are classified as either metabolic or respiratory in origin. In metabolic acid–base disorders, the primary disturbance is in the plasma bicarbonate concentration. Metabolic acidosis is characterized by a decrease in the plasma bicarbonate concentration whereas in metabolic alkalosis the plasma bicarbonate concentration is increased. Respiratory acid–base disorders are caused by alterations in alveolar ventilation that produce corresponding changes in the partial pressure of carbon dioxide from arterial blood (Paco₂). In respiratory acidosis, the Paco₂ is elevated; in respiratory alkalosis, it is decreased. Each disturbance has a compensatory (secondary) response that attempts to correct the HCO₃⁻: Paco₂ ratio toward normal and mitigate the change in pH (Table 61–2). Although the time course of the respiratory compensatory responses to metabolic disturbances is rapid, the metabolic compensation for respiratory

TABLE 61-2	Interpretation of Simple Acid–Base Disorders		
Acid–Base Disorder	**pH**	**Primary Disturbances**	**Compensation**
Acidosis			
Respiratory	Decrease	Increase Paco₂	Increase HCO₃⁻
Metabolic	Decrease	Decrease HCO₃⁻	Decrease Paco₂
Alkalosis			
Respiratory	Increase	Decrease Paco₂	Decrease HCO₃⁻
Metabolic	Increase	Increase HCO₃⁻	Increase Paco₂

HCO₃⁻, bicarbonate; Paco₂, partial pressure of carbon dioxide from arterial blood.

TABLE 61-3	Normal Blood Gas Values	
	Arterial Blood	**Mixed Venous Blood**
pH	7.40 (7.35–7.45)	7.38 (7.33–7.43)
Po₂	80–100 mm Hg (10.6–13.3 kPa)	35–40 mm Hg (4.7–5.3 kPa)
Sao₂	95%	70%–75%
Pco₂	35–45 mm Hg (4.7–6.0 kPa)	45–51 mm Hg (4.7–6.8 kPa)
HCO₃⁻	22–26 mEq/L (22–26 mmol/L)	24–28 mEq/L (24–28 mmol/L)

HCO₃⁻, bicarbonate; Pco₂, partial pressure of carbon dioxide; Po₂, partial pressure of oxygen; Sao₂, saturation of arterial oxygen.

disturbances is slow. As a result, respiratory disturbances are characterized as acute (minutes to hours in duration), indicating that there has not been sufficient time for metabolic compensation, or chronic (days), indicating sufficient time for metabolic compensation has elapsed.

CLINICAL ASSESSMENT OF ACID–BASE STATUS

❸ Blood gases are measured to determine the patient's oxygenation and acid–base status. Under normal circumstances, there is no clinically significant difference in pH between arterial and mixed venous blood. Arterial samples are designated with the letter "a" (e.g., partial pressure of oxygen from arterial blood [Pao₂] and Paco₂), whereas mixed venous samples are labeled with the letter "v" or not labeled (e.g., partial pressure of oxygen from venous blood [Pvo₂] and partial pressure of carbon dioxide from venous blood [Pvco₂]). The normal values for arterial and venous blood gases are shown in Table 61–3. Arterial blood reflects how well the blood is being oxygenated by the lungs (an accurate measurement of Pao₂), whereas venous blood reflects how much oxygen tissues are using. Arterial blood rather than venous blood should be used whenever possible because venous blood obtained from an extremity can provide misleading information. If metabolism in the extremity is altered by hypoperfusion, exercise, infection, or some other cause, the difference in the amount of dissolved oxygen between arterial and venous blood can be dramatic. The venous pH and Pco₂ during cardiopulmonary resuscitation, might be significantly lower and higher, respectively, than the arterial pH and arterial Pco₂. This indicates a severe tissue acidosis from CO₂ accumulation caused by hypoperfusion.

ANALYSIS OF ARTERIAL BLOOD GAS DATA

Arterial blood gases provide an assessment of the patient's acid–base status.[6] Low pH values (<7.35) indicate an acidemia, whereas high pH values (>7.45) indicate an alkalemia (Fig. 61–3). In a metabolic acidosis, the pH is decreased in association with a decreased serum bicarbonate concentration and a compensatory decrease in Paco₂. In a respiratory acidosis, the pH is decreased; the Paco₂, however, is elevated. The serum bicarbonate concentration is variable, depending on whether it is an acute disturbance (minimal increase in serum bicarbonate) or a chronic respiratory acidosis (substantial increase in serum bicarbonate). In a metabolic alkalosis, the pH is elevated in association with an increased bicarbonate concentration and a compensatory increase in Paco₂. In respiratory alkalosis, the pH is also elevated; the Paco₂, however, is decreased. As with respiratory acidosis, the metabolic compensation is variable, with a minimal decrease in serum bicarbonate in acute respiratory alkalosis and a larger decrease in [HCO₃⁻] in chronic respiratory alkalosis. Although

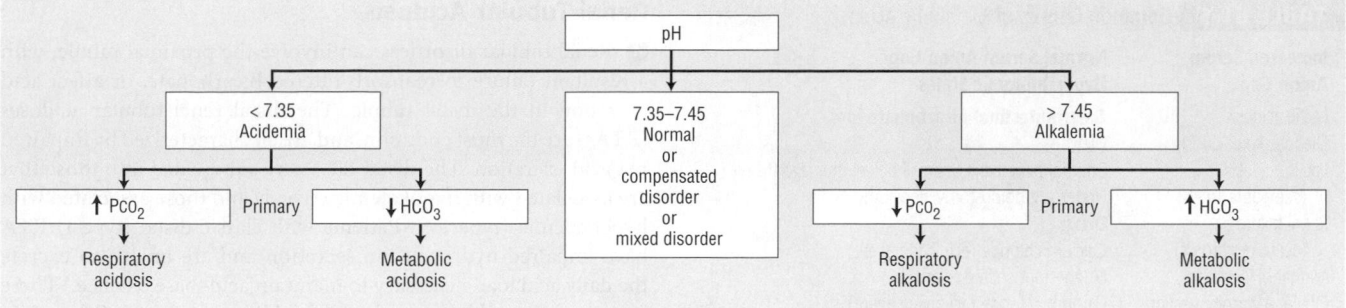

FIGURE 61-3. Analysis of arterial blood gases. (HCO_3^-, bicarbonate; P_{CO_2}, partial pressure of carbon dioxide.)

each measurement has a normal range (see Table 61–3), it is often easiest to consider the midpoint of each range as the normal value. This would correlate to a pH of 7.4, $Paco_2$ of 40 mm Hg (5.3 kPa) and HCO_3^- of 24 mEq/L (24 mmol/L). Steps in acid–base interpretation are described in Table 61–4.

When arterial blood gases differ significantly from those expected on the basis of the patient's clinical condition and previous laboratory determinations, additional venous blood samples should be drawn to assess plasma electrolyte concentrations. The bicarbonate calculated from the patient's $Paco_2$ and pH of the blood gas should be compared with the measured total CO_2 content (the amount of CO_2 gas extractable from plasma, consisting of HCO_3^-, H_2CO_3, and Pco_2). Ordinarily, the blood gas bicarbonate value is approximately 1 to 2 mEq/L (1–2 mmol/L) less than total CO_2 content.[3] If these values do not correspond, the results should be interpreted with caution because the difference can reflect an error in the blood collection or storage of the sample, or in the calibration of the blood gas analyzer.

METABOLIC ACID–BASE DISORDERS

METABOLIC ACIDOSIS

Pathophysiology

Metabolic acidosis is characterized by a decrease in pH as the result of a primary decrease in serum bicarbonate concentration. This can result from the buffering (consumption of HCO_3^-) of an exogenous acid, an organic acid accumulating because of a metabolic disturbance (e.g., lactic acid or ketoacids), or the progressive accumulation of endogenous acids secondary to impaired renal function (e.g., phosphates and sulfates).[7] The serum HCO_3^- can also be decreased as the result of a loss of bicarbonate-rich body fluids (e.g., diarrhea, biliary drainage, or pancreatic fistula) or occur secondary to the rapid administration of non-alkali–containing intravenous fluids (dilutional acidosis).[8]

TABLE 61-4	Steps in Acid–Base Diagnosis

1. Obtain arterial blood gases (ABGs) and electrolytes simultaneously.
2. Compare $[HCO_3^-]$ on ABG and electrolytes to verify accuracy.
3. Calculate anion gap (AG).
4. Is acidemia (pH <7.35) or alkalemia (pH >7.45) present?
5. Is the primary abnormality respiratory (alteration in $Paco_2$) or metabolic (alteration in HCO_3^-)?
6. Estimate compensatory response (Table 60–7).
7. Compare change in $[Cl^-]$ with change in $[Na^+]$.

$[Cl^-]$, chloride ion; $[HCO_3^-]$, bicarbonate; $[Na^+]$, sodium ion; $Paco_2$, partial pressure of carbon dioxide from arterial blood.

The serum anion gap (SAG), as defined below, can be used to infer whether an organic or mineral acidosis is present.

$$SAG = [Na^+] - [Cl^-] - [HCO_3^-]$$

To maintain electroneutrality, the total concentration of cations in the serum must equal the total concentration of anions.

$$[Na^+] + [UCs] = ([Cl^-] + [HCO_3^-]) + [UAs]$$

The cation concentration is equal to the sodium concentration plus that of "unmeasured" cations (UCs), predominantly magnesium, calcium, and potassium. The anion concentration is equal to the concentrations of chloride, bicarbonate, and "unmeasured" anions (UAs), including proteins, sulfates, phosphates, and organic anions. Therefore, as the result of the combination of the two equations above, the SAG can be expressed as:

$$SAG = [UAs] - [UCs]$$

The normal SAG is approximately 9 mEq/L (9 mmol/L), with a range of 3 to 11 mEq/L (3–11 mmol/L). This value is lower than the value of 12 mEq/L (12 mmol/L) cited in the literature in the past because of changes in the instrumentation for measurement of serum electrolytes.[7] Increases in the anion gap to values in excess of 17 to 20 mEq/L (17–20 mmol/L) are indicative of the accumulation of unmeasured anions in ECF.

These unmeasured anions are generated as the result of the consumption of HCO_3^- by endogenous organic acids such as lactic acid, acetoacetic acid, or β-hydroxybutyric acid or from the ingestion of toxins such as methanol or ethylene glycol. The degree of elevation in the SAG is dependent on the clearance of the anion, as well as the multiple factors that influence HCO_3^- concentrations. Thus the SAG is a relative rather than an absolute indication of the cause of metabolic acidosis. The SAG can also be elevated in the metabolic acidosis because of renal failure, as the result of the accumulation of various organic anions, phosphates, and sulfates.

In hyperchloremic metabolic acidosis, bicarbonate losses from the ECF are replaced by chloride, and the SAG remains normal. This decrease in bicarbonate may be due to gastrointestinal tract losses, dilution of bicarbonate in the ECF as the result of the addition of sodium chloride solutions or chloride-containing acids. Common causes of metabolic acidosis with an increased or a normal SAG are listed in Table 61–5.

Hyperchloremic Metabolic Acidosis

Hyperchloremic metabolic acidosis can result from increased gastrointestinal bicarbonate loss, renal bicarbonate wasting, impaired renal acid excretion, or exogenous acid gain. Gastrointestinal

TABLE 61-5	Common Causes of Metabolic Acidosis
Increased Serum Anion Gap	**Normal Serum Anion Gap/ Hyperchloremic States**
Lactic acidosis	**Gastrointestinal bicarbonate loss**
Diabetic ketoacidosis	Diarrhea
Lactic acidosis	External pancreatic or small bowel drainage (fistula)
(see Table 61–6)	Ureterosigmoidostomy, ileostomy
Renal failure	**Drugs**
(acute or chronic)	Calcium chloride (acidifying agent)
Methanol ingestion	Magnesium sulfate (diarrhea)
Ethylene glycol ingestion	Calcium chloride (acidifying agent)
Salicylate overdosage	**Renal tubular acidosis**
Starvation	Hypokalemia
	Proximal renal tubular acidosis (type II)
	Distal renal tubular acidosis (type I)
	Carbonic anhydrase inhibitors
	(e.g., acetazolamide)
	Hypokalemia
	Generalized distal nephron dysfunction (type IV)
	Mineralocorticoid deficiency or resistance
	Tubulointerstitial disease
	Drug-induced hyperkalemia
	Potassium-sparing diuretics (amiloride, spironolactone, triamterene)
	Trimethoprim
	Pentamidine
	Heparin
	Angiotensin-converting enzyme inhibitors and receptor blockers
	Nonsteroidal anti-inflammatory drugs
	Cyclosporin A
	Other
	Acid ingestion (ammonium chloride, hydrochloric acid, hyperalimentation)
	Expansion acidosis (rapid saline administration)

disorders such as diarrhea, biliary or pancreatic drainage through either a surgical drain or fistula can result in the loss of large volumes of bicarbonate-containing fluids. Severe diarrhea, the most common cause of hypochloremic metabolic acidosis, can lead to a daily loss of 5 to 10 L of fluid containing 100 to 140 mEq/L (100–140 mmol/L) of sodium, 20 to 40 mEq/L (20–40 mmol/L) of potassium, 80 to 100 mEq/L (80–100 mmol/L) of chloride, and 30 to 50 mEq/L (30–50 mmol/L) of bicarbonate.[4] Patients who have undergone ureteral diversion into the sigmoid colon or isolated ileal loop can also develop a hyperchloremic metabolic acidosis. This is the result of a net loss of bicarbonate given that chloride is reabsorbed and bicarbonate is secreted by gastrointestinal epithelial cells in the presence of the urine that is retained in the colon or bowel loop.

Hyperchloremic metabolic acidosis caused by renal bicarbonate wasting is the defining disturbance in proximal renal tubular acidosis and is a complication of therapy with carbonic anhydrase inhibitors. During the treatment of diabetic ketoacidosis, renal loss of β-hydroxybutyrate and acetoacetate, which would otherwise be metabolized to yield bicarbonate, can contribute to the development of hyperchloremic metabolic acidosis. Impaired renal acid excretion that occurs as a result of distal tubular dysfunction in patients with distal renal tubular acidoses can also occur in patients with moderate to severe renal insufficiency from other causes. The metabolic acidosis of renal insufficiency is initially hyperchloremic but can progress to an anion-gap acidosis as the renal insufficiency worsens and sulfates, phosphates, and other anions accumulate. Hyperchloremic metabolic acidosis can also result from the exogenous administration of acid (hydrochloric acid, ammonium chloride) or the unbuffered administration of acid salts from the amino acids in total parenteral nutrition fluids.

Renal Tubular Acidosis

❹ Renal tubular disorders can involve the proximal tubule, with a resultant failure to reabsorb filtered bicarbonate, or affect acid excretion in the distal tubule. The distal renal tubular acidoses (RTAs) are the most common, and are all characterized by impaired net acid excretion. The distal RTAs are subdivided into those that are associated with hypokalemia (type I) and those associated with hyperkalemia (type IV). Patients with classic distal (type I) RTA have impaired hydrogen ion secretion and are unable to excrete the daily acid load necessary to maintain acid–base balance.[4] These patients are unable to maximally acidify their urine (i.e., attain urine pH <5.5), even in the face of an acid challenge. Type I RTA may be the result of a primary tubular defect or develop secondary to a wide variety of disorders including hypercalcemia, multiple myeloma, systemic lupus erythematosus, Sjögren syndrome, sickle-cell disease, and renal transplant rejection, or following the administration of amphotericin B or ingestion of toluene. The primary form of this disorder usually occurs in children and can result in severe acidosis, slowed growth, nephrocalcinosis, and kidney stones.[7,9] In adults, clinical complications include osteomalacia, nephrocalcinosis, and recurrent kidney stones. The hypokalemia associated with classic distal (type I) RTA results from secondary hypoaldosteronism associated with volume depletion. The renal potassium wasting decreases considerably if bicarbonate therapy is administered.

The hyperkalemic distal (type IV) RTAs are a heterogeneous group of disorders characterized by hypoaldosteronism or generalized distal tubule defects. The most common form of type IV RTA is hyporeninemic hypoaldosteronism. This syndrome is most commonly associated with mild renal insufficiency caused by diabetic nephropathy, but can also be seen in a variety of other disorders, including chronic interstitial nephritis, sickle-cell disease, human immunodeficiency virus (HIV) nephropathy, and obstructive uropathy. The clinical presentation of this syndrome is often exacerbated by pharmacologic therapy with agents that can interfere with the renin-angiotensin-aldosterone axis, such as β-adrenergic blockers, angiotensin-converting enzyme inhibitors, angiotensin receptor blockers, and nonsteroidal antiinflammatory drugs. Heparin can induce the syndrome by inhibiting adrenal aldosterone biosynthesis. Patients with this form of RTA are able to maximally acidify their urine (urine pH <5.5).[9] The primary defect in acid excretion is impaired ammoniagenesis caused by mild renal insufficiency. Hyperaldosteronism predisposes to the development of hyperkalemia, which results in further impairment of ammoniagenesis. Treatment to control the hyperkalemia is usually sufficient to reverse the metabolic acidosis, and mineralocorticoid replacement is frequently unnecessary.

Hyperkalemic distal (type IV) RTA resulting from generalized distal tubule defects is less common than hyporeninemic hypoaldosteronism but is more common than classic distal (type I) RTA. Patients with this defect have impaired tubular potassium secretion in addition to impaired urinary acidification (urine pH >5.5, despite acidemia or acid loading). Urinary obstruction is the most frequent cause of this disorder, which can also be associated with sickle-cell nephropathy, systemic lupus erythematosus, HIV nephropathy, analgesic abuse nephropathy, amyloidosis, renal transplant rejection, and chronic cyclosporine nephrotoxicity.

Proximal (type II) RTA is characterized by defects in proximal tubular reabsorption of bicarbonate. Normally, more than 85% of filtered bicarbonate is reabsorbed in the proximal tubule. Defects in proximal tubular bicarbonate reabsorption result in increased delivery of bicarbonate to the distal nephron, which has a limited capacity for bicarbonate reabsorption. As a result, at a normal serum bicarbonate concentration, the filtered bicarbonate load is incompletely reabsorbed, and is lost in the urine. As the serum bicarbonate concentration decreases, the filtered load of bicarbonate is proportionately decreased. A new equilibrium is established in which the kidney is able to reabsorb the filtered bicarbonate load, albeit at a reduced serum bicarbonate concentration. Thus patients with proximal RTA present with a chronic, nonprogressive hyperchloremic metabolic acidosis. These patients are able to acidify their urine in response to an acid load, but develop bicarbonaturia at a reduced serum bicarbonate concentration following bicarbonate loading. The impaired bicarbonate reabsorption results in salt wasting and secondary hyperaldosteronism. Hypokalemia, which can be severe, usually develops as a result of the hyperaldosteronism and bicarbonaturia.[4,7] Unlike patients with classic distal (type I) RTA, the hyperkalemia if present in proximal RTA is exacerbated by alkali replacement. Proximal RTA can develop as an isolated defect, or it can be associated with generalized proximal tubular dysfunction (Fanconi syndrome), with impaired proximal tubular glucose, phosphate, and amino acid reabsorption. Proximal RTA usually presents as an acquired disorder, secondary to a variety of diseases (amyloidosis, multiple myeloma, or nephrotic syndrome) or exposure to toxins (lead, cadmium, mercury, or outdated tetracyclines). Pharmacologic therapy with carbonic anhydrase inhibitors produces an iatrogenic form of proximal RTA.

Elevated Anion Gap Metabolic Acidosis

Metabolic acidosis with an increased SAG commonly results from increased endogenous organic acid production. In lactic acidosis, lactic acid accumulates as a by-product of anaerobic metabolism. Accumulation of the ketoacids β-hydroxybutyric acid and acetoacetic acid defines the ketoacidosis of uncontrolled diabetes mellitus, alcohol intoxication, and starvation (see Table 61–5). In advanced renal failure, accumulation of phosphate, sulfate, and organic anions is responsible for the increased SAG, which is usually less than 24 mEq/L (24 mmol/L).[10] The severe metabolic acidosis seen in myoglobinuric acute renal failure caused by rhabdomyolysis may be caused by the metabolism of large amounts of sulfur-containing amino acids released from myoglobin.

The presence of mild elevations in the SAG cannot be automatically attributed to the presence of a high SAG metabolic acidosis. Elevations in the SAG are commonly seen in hospitalized patients, especially those who are critically ill.[10] A variety of factors can contribute to this nonspecific elevation in the SAG, including the presence of alkalemia, which increases the anionic charge of albumin and other plasma proteins. The usefulness of the SAG as a marker of acid–base status is dependent on proper interpretation of a patient's clinical status.[5,11] Despite these limitations, when the SAG exceeds 20 to 25 mEq/L (20–25 mmol/L) a significant organic acidosis is likely to be present.

High anion gap metabolic acidosis can develop in many clinical settings, including uncontrolled diabetes mellitus (see Chapter 83), alcohol intoxication (see Chapters 44 and 75), and starvation (see Chapter 72). Toxic ingestions of methanol and ethylene glycol, are also associated with high anion gap metabolic acidosis and can be differentiated from other causes of SAG because of the presence of an elevated osmolar gap. The mechanisms responsible for the development of acidosis in these settings are diverse.[12] (See type I diabetes + ketoacidosis case in Casebook.)

Lactic Acidosis Lactic acidosis is one of the most common causes of high SAG metabolic acidosis and can impact approximately 1% of hospitalized patients. Lactic acid is the end product of anaerobic metabolism of glucose (glycolysis).[13] In normal individuals, lactic acid derived from pyruvate enters the circulation in small amounts and is promptly removed by the liver. In the liver, and to a lesser

TABLE 61-6 Causes of Lactic Acidosis

Primary decrease in tissue oxygenation
Shock
Severe anemia
Congestive heart failure
Asphyxia
Carbon monoxide poisoning

Deranged oxidative metabolism
Medications
Catecholamines
Linezolid
Metformin
Nalidixic acid
Nucleoside-analog reverse transcriptase inhibitors (didanosine, stavudine, zidovudine)
Overdose (iron, isoniazid, salicylates, theophylline)
Propofol infusion syndrome
Propylene glycol toxicity (IV lorazepam)
Sodium nitroprusside (secondary to cyanide toxicity)
Streptozocin
Diabetes mellitus
Malignancy
Seizures
Methanol, ethanol, or ethylene glycol
Disorders associated with inborn errors of metabolism

extent in the kidney, lactic acid is reoxidized to pyruvic acid, which is then metabolized to CO_2 and H_2O. The normal plasma lactate concentration in healthy subjects is approximately 1 mEq/L (1 mmol/L).[3,12,13] The diagnosis of lactic acidosis should be considered in all patients with metabolic acidosis associated with an increased SAG. Lactic acidosis is considered to be present when lactate concentrations exceed 4 to 5 mEq/L (4–5 mmol/L) in an acidemic patient.

Classically, lactic acidosis has been differentiated into disorders associated with tissue hypoxia (type A lactic acidosis) and disorders associated with deranged oxidative metabolism (type B lactic acidosis), although the distinction between them is blurred (Table 61–6). The etiologies of lactic acidosis can also be categorized on the basis of changes in lactate production and/or utilization.[12,13] Metabolic disturbances can result in increased tissue pyruvate production or impaired utilization, with proportional increases in lactate concentrations. Increased lactate production is more commonly associated with alterations in tissue redox state, resulting in preferential conversion of pyruvate to lactate. During anaerobic metabolism, reduced nicotinamide adenine dinucleotide accumulates, driving the conversion of pyruvate to lactate and increasing the lactate:pyruvate ratio. States of enhanced metabolic activity (e.g., grand mal seizures, strenuous exercise, or hyperthermia), decreased tissue oxygen delivery (e.g., severe anemia, hypoxia, circulatory shock, or carbon monoxide poisoning) or impaired oxygen utilization (e.g., cyanide toxicity) all are associated with lactic acidosis. Impaired hepatic clearance of lactate, as seen in hypoperfusion states, liver failure, and alcohol intoxication, can also result in lactic acidosis.

Cardiovascular and septic shock, with resultant tissue hypoperfusion, are the most common causes of lactic acidosis. Poor tissue perfusion and hypoxia influence enzymatic pyruvate and lactate metabolism to stimulate anaerobic glycolysis and to decrease lactate utilization. This leads to hyperlactatemia and lactic acidosis. The mortality rate of this type of lactic acidosis can be as high as 80% and correlates with the degree of hyperlactatemia.

Lactic acidosis associated with liver disease, toxins, and congenital enzyme deficiency can be caused by deranged oxidative metabolism or impaired lactate clearance.[4,13] The exact role of diabetes mellitus in the induction of lactic acidosis is not clear. It may involve a decrease in pyruvate dehydrogenase activity, the enzyme responsible for pyruvate metabolism. Lactic acidosis in neoplastic disease is uncommon and reported mostly in patients with myeloproliferative disorders. Leukocytes and neoplastic cells in general have high rates of glycolysis. In the case of a large tumor or tightly packed bone marrow, oxygenation can be decreased, favoring the accumulation of lactate. Lactic acidosis has been reported in patients with massive liver tumors, and it has been postulated that the liver uptake of lactate is decreased in these patients. Lactic acidosis associated with seizures is usually transient and occurs because of excessive muscle activity.[13]

A number of medications can cause lactic acidosis.[13-23] Two of the most common medications associated with the development of lactic acidosis are nucleoside-analog reverse transcriptase inhibitors (NRTIs) (3.9 cases per 1,000 person-years) and metformin (0.03 cases per 1,000 person-years).[15-18] The proposed mechanism of NRTI-induced lactic acidosis is the inhibition of the enzyme DNA polymerase gamma that is responsible for mitochondrial DNA synthesis.[15] Disruption of this enzyme can inhibit the transport of lactate into the mitochondria, leading to an accumulation in the cytoplasm. Stavudine is the NRTI most frequently associated with lactic acidosis; however, the combination of stavudine and didanosine confers the highest risk.

The primary suspected mechanism for metformin-induced lactic acidosis is inhibition of liver gluconeogenesis as the result of its inhibitory effects on pyruvate carboxylase which is necessary for the conversion of pyruvate to glucose.[16,17] Other possible pathways for metformin-associated lactic acidosis include a decrease in both hepatic intracellular pH and cardiac output and an increase in lactate production in the gut and increased renal loss of bicarbonate.[14] Risk factors for metformin-induced lactic acidosis include renal insufficiency, liver disease, dehydration, advanced age, alcohol consumption, and supratherapeutic dosing. Metformin should be discontinued during periods of tissue hypoxia (e.g., myocardial infarction, sepsis), for 3 days after contrast media has been administered or 2 days before general anesthesia administration. In the latter two cases, metformin should only be reinstituted when the patient's renal function is stable.

Propylene glycol is commonly used as a solubilizing agent in intravenous drug preparations (e.g., lorazepam, pentobarbital) and is predominantly metabolized to lactic acid via the hepatic enzyme alcohol dehydrogenase. The administration of large doses of propylene glycol, particularly to patients with renal or liver insufficiency, can lead to a lactic acidosis with an osmolar gap and thus serial measurement of the osmolar gap can be used to detect propylene glycol accumulation.[18,19]

Reports of the association between propofol and lactic acidosis were initially described in children.[20] This association is now recognized in adults and has come to be known as the propofol-related infusion syndrome. In addition to lactic acidosis, cardiac failure, rhabdomyolysis, and renal failure have been observed primarily because of uncoupling of oxidative phosphorylation and impaired oxidation of free fatty acids. This syndrome is most frequently seen in patients receiving propofol at high doses (>5 mg/kg/h) for more than 2 days.

CLINICAL CONTROVERSY

The incidence of the propofol infusion syndrome among critically ill patients administered propofol is unknown and the role that worsening critical illness plays in patients with suspected propofol infusion remains unclear.

CLINICAL PRESENTATION

Chronic metabolic acidosis is usually not associated with severe acidemia and is relatively asymptomatic. The major manifestations are in the bones, where chronic acidemia causes bone demineralization with the development of rickets in children and osteomalacia and osteopenia in adults. In infants and children, chronic metabolic acidosis is associated with growth failure and short stature and can be associated with nonspecific symptoms including anorexia, nausea, weight loss, and muscle weakness.

Severe metabolic acidosis is usually associated with acute processes. The manifestations of severe acidemia (pH <7.20) involve the cardiovascular, respiratory, and central nervous systems. Hyperventilation is often the first sign of metabolic acidosis. At a pH of 7.2, pulmonary ventilation increases approximately fourfold, and an eightfold increase has been noted at a pH of 7.[24,25] Respiratory compensation can occur as Kussmaul respirations—the deep, rapid respirations seen commonly in patients with diabetic ketoacidosis. In extremely severe acidosis (pH <6.8), CNS function is disrupted to such a degree that the respiratory center is depressed.

CNS depression correlates more closely with spinal fluid pH than with blood pH. For this reason, neurologic symptoms tend to occur more frequently and to a greater degree in patients with respiratory acidosis because the CO_2 accumulated in the respiratory form readily crosses the blood-brain barrier to cause acidosis in the CNS.[1] Because of the slow penetration of administered bicarbonate into the CNS, the CNS pH fails to normalize as rapidly as blood pH. Therefore patients continue to hyperventilate because of sustained CNS acidity, and severe respiratory alkalosis can occur. Sustained lowering of the $Paco_2$ within 12 to 36 hours is to be anticipated during the correction of any metabolic acidosis.[1]

Systemic acidosis can cause peripheral arteriolar dilatation, characterized by flushing, a rapid heart rate, and wide pulse pressure. Initially, cardiac output can be increased, but as acidosis becomes more severe, myocardial contractility becomes impaired, and cardiac output decreases. The effects of vagal stimulation are also enhanced at pH levels lower than 7.1, probably as a consequence of inhibition of acetylcholinesterase. This increases the danger of vagally mediated bradycardia and heart block during acidosis.

Gastrointestinal symptoms of metabolic acidosis include loss of appetite, nausea, and vomiting. Severe acidosis (pH <7.1) interferes with carbohydrate metabolism and insulin utilization, and results in hyperglycemia. Metabolic acidosis alters potassium homeostasis and contributes to the development of hyperkalemia. The magnitude of the effect on serum potassium depends on the type of acidosis: Acidosis caused by mineral acids (e.g., hydrochloric acid) are associated with a greater change in potassium levels than acidosis caused by organic acids (e.g., lactic acidosis), in which the increase in potassium attributable to the acidosis per se is minimal.

CLINICAL PRESENTATION OF METABOLIC ACIDOSIS

General

- The patient is usually relatively asymptomatic if the acidosis is acute and mild. In those with severe acidemia (pH <7.15–7.20) the cardiovascular, respiratory, and central nervous systems can be affected.

Symptoms

- The patient may complain of loss of appetite, nausea, and vomiting.

Signs

- Cardiac: Flushing, a rapid heart rate, wide pulse pressure, and an increase in cardiac output can be seen initially. This can be followed by a reduction in cardiac output, blood pressure, and liver and kidney blood flow.

■ Cerebral: Obtundation or coma.

■ Metabolic: Insulin resistance; increased protein degradation; increased metabolic demands.

■ Gastrointestinal: Nausea, vomiting, loss of appetite.

■ Respiratory: Dyspnea, hyperventilation with deep, rapid respirations is seen in those with severe acidosis.

■ Chronic acidemia causes bone demineralization with the development of rickets in children and osteomalacia and osteopenia in adults.

Laboratory Tests

Serum CO_2 is low. Hyperglycemia and hyperkalemia are common. Patients with a pH <7.2 are deemed to have a severe acidosis.

COMPENSATION

❺ The patient's primary means to compensate for metabolic acidosis is to increase carbon dioxide excretion by increasing respiratory rate. This results in a decrease in $Paco_2$. This ventilatory compensation results from stimulation of the respiratory center by changes in cerebral bicarbonate concentration and pH.[1] For every 1-mEq/L (1 mmol/L) decrease in bicarbonate concentration below the average of 24, the $Paco_2$ decreases by approximately 1 to 1.5 mm Hg (0.13–0.20 kPa) from the normal value of 40 (5.3 kPa) (Table 61–7).

TABLE 61-7	Guidelines for Initial Interpretation of Acid–Base Disorders
Acidosis	
Metabolic	$Paco_2$ in mm Hg should decrease by 1.3 times the fall in plasma $[HCO_3^-]$ (in mEq/L)
	$Paco_2$ in kPa should decrease by 0.17 times the fall in plasma $[HCO_3^-]$ (in mmol/L)
Acute respiratory	The plasma $[HCO_3^-]$ should increase by 0.1 times the increase in $Paco_2$ ± 3 in mm Hg
	The plasma $[HCO_3^-]$ should increase by 0.75 times the increase in $Paco_2$ ± 0.4 in kPa
Chronic respiratory	The plasma $[HCO_3^-]$ should increase by 0.35 times the increase in $Paco_2$ ± 4 in mm Hg
	The plasma $[HCO_3^-]$ should increase by 2.6 times the increase in $Paco_2$ ± 0.5 in kPa
Alkalosis	
Metabolic	$Paco_2$ in mm Hg should increase by 0.4–0.6 times the rise in plasma $[HCO_3^-]$ (in mEq/L)
	$Paco_2$ in kPa should increase by 0.05–0.08 times the rise in plasma $[HCO_3^-]$ (mmol/L)
Acute respiratory	The plasma $[HCO_3^-]$ should decrease by 0.2 times the decrease in $Paco_2$ in mm Hg but usually not to <18 mEq/L
	The plasma $[HCO_3^-]$ should decrease by 1.5 times the decrease in $Paco_2$ in kPa but usually not to <18 mmol/L
Chronic respiratory	The plasma $[HCO_3^-]$ should fall by 0.35 times the decrease in $Paco_2$ in mm Hg but usually not to <14 mEq/L
	The plasma $[HCO_3^-]$ should fall by 2.6 times the decrease in $Paco_2$ in kPa but usually not to <14 mmol/L

HCO_3^-, bicarbonate; $Paco_2$, partial pressure of carbon dioxide from arterial blood.
Adapted from Kamel S, Razeen-Davids M, Lin, SH et al. Interpretation of electrolytes and acid-base parameters in blood and urine. In: Bremmer BM, ed. Bremmer and Rector's The Kidney, 8th ed. New York: Saunders, 2007:898–923. Copyright © Elsevier 2007.

The anticipated $Paco_2$ associated with a given bicarbonate concentration for patients with uncomplicated metabolic acidosis can be calculated as[25]:

$$Paco_2 = (1.5 \times [HCO_3^-]) + 8] \pm 2 \text{ for } Paco_2 \text{ in mm Hg}$$
$$(Paco_2 = (0.2 \times [HCO_3^-]) + 1.1] \pm 0.3 \text{ for } Paco_2 \text{ in kPa})$$

For example, 95% of patients with a plasma bicarbonate of 16 mEq/L (16 mmol/L) should have an arterial Pco_2 of 30 to 34 mm Hg (4.0–4.6 kPa). An observed arterial Pco_2 within this range is consistent with physiologic respiratory compensation for a metabolic acidosis and suggests that there is no respiratory disturbance. In contrast, if the Pco_2 is less than 30 mm Hg (4.0 kPa), a superimposed respiratory alkalosis can be present, whereas if the Pco_2 is greater than 34 mm Hg (4.6 kPa), a superimposed respiratory acidosis is likely present.

TREATMENT

Metabolic Acidosis

■ CHRONIC METABOLIC ACIDOSIS

❻ Asymptomatic patients with mild to moderate degrees of acidemia (plasma bicarbonate of 12 to 20 mEq/L ([12–20 mmol/L]; pH 7.2–7.4) do not require emergent therapy. They can usually be managed with gradual correction of the acidemia, over a period of days to weeks, using oral sodium bicarbonate or other alkali preparations (Table 61–8). In all forms of chronic metabolic acidosis, primary therapy should be directed at treating the underlying disease state. Gastrointestinal pathology should be treated to reduce ongoing bicarbonate losses, and factors that exacerbate RTA should be treated. If acidemia persists, alkali therapy should be instituted with the goal of normalization of blood pH. The loading dose (LD) of alkali to initially correct the acidemia can be calculated as follows where V_D is the volume of distribution of bicarbonate[26]:

$$LD(\text{mEq or mmol/L}) = (V_D HCO_3^- \times \text{body weight [BW]})$$
$$\times (\text{desired } [HCO_3^-] - \text{current } [HCO_3^-])$$

For a 60-kg patient with a serum bicarbonate of 15 mEq/L (24–15 mmol/L), the loading dose is calculated thus:

$$LD(\text{mEq}) = (0.5 \text{ L/kg} \times 60 \text{ kg}) \times (24 \text{ mEq/L} - 15 \text{ mEq/L})$$
$$= 30 \text{ L} \times 9 \text{ mEq/L}$$
$$= 270 \text{ mEq/L}(270 \text{ mmol/L})$$

The calculated loading dose of alkali should be administered over several days to avoid volume overload from the accompanying sodium load. For this scenario, a regimen of 60 to 70 mEq (60–70 mmol) three times a day for 3 to 5 days should result in an increase in HCO_3^- levels toward normal. In addition to the calculated loading dose, supplemental alkali must also be provided to replace ongoing losses, which can be approximated to be 2 mEq/kg (2 mmol/kg) per day or 40 mEq (40 mmol) 3 times a day. In patients with associated volume depletion, bicarbonate replacement can be provided simultaneous with volume resuscitation by substituting bicarbonate for chloride in intravenous crystalloid solutions.

In patients with chronic metabolic acidosis because of gastrointestinal bicarbonate losses, maintenance therapy should provide sufficient alkali to replace ongoing bicarbonate losses. The magnitude of this replacement is variable and can be substantial (>10 mEq/kg [>10 mmol/kg] per day). In addition, associated losses of other electrolytes, such as potassium and magnesium, may need to be replaced (see Chapter 60).

TABLE 61-8 Therapeutic Alternatives for Oral Alkali Replacement

Generic Name	Trade Name(s)	Milliequivalents of Alkali	Dosage Form(s)	Comment
Shohl's solution Sodium citrate/citric acid	Bicitra (Willen)	1 mEq Na/mL; equivalent to 1 mEq bicarbonate	Solution (500 mg Na citrate, 334 mg citric acid/5 mL)	Citrate preparations increase absorption of aluminum
Sodium bicarbonate	Various (e.g., Sodamint)	3.9 mEq bicarbonate/tablet (325 mg)	325 mg tablet	Bicarbonate preparations can cause bloating because of CO_2 production
		7.8 mEq bicarbonate/tablet (650 mg)	650 mg tablet	
	Baking soda (various)	60 mEq bicarbonate/tsp (5 g/tsp)	Powder	
Potassium citrate	Urocit-K (Mission)	5 mEq citrate/tablet	5 mEq tablet	See above
Potassium bicarbonate/ potassium citrate	K-Lyte (Bristol)	25 mEq bicarbonate/tablet	25 mEq tablet (effervescent)	
	K-Lyte DS (Bristol)	50 mEq bicarbonate/tablet (double strength)	50 mEq tablet (effervescent)	See above
Potassium citrate/ citric acid	Polycitra-K (Willen)	2 mEq K/mL; equivalent to 2 mEq bicarbonate	Solution (1,100 mg K citrate, 334 mg citric acid/5 mL)	See above
		30 mEq bicarbonate/ unit dose packet	Crystals for reconstitution (3,300 mg K citrate, 1,002 mg citric acid/unit dose packet)	
Sodium citrate/ potassium citrate/ citric acid	Polycitra (Willen) Polycitra-LC (Willen)	1 mEq K, 1 mEq Na/mL; equivalent to 2 mEq bicarbonate	Syrup (Polycitra) solution (Polycitra-LC) (Both contain 550 mg K citrate, 500 mg Na citrate, 334 mg citric acid/5 mL)	See above

Proximal (type II) RTA is a bicarbonate-wasting disorder that requires the administration of large maintenance doses of alkali (10–15 mEq/kg [10–15 mmol/kg] per day). As alkali replacement raises the serum bicarbonate concentration toward normal, the proximal tubule's capacity to reabsorb bicarbonate is overwhelmed, and renal bicarbonate wasting increases. In children, aggressive therapy of proximal RTA is necessary to avoid growth retardation and osteopenia. Because this is generally a mild, nonprogressive acidosis in adults, the benefit of alkali therapy is frequently outweighed by the risks of increased potassium wasting. In patients with classic distal (type I) RTA, maintenance therapy usually requires only enough alkali to buffer the amount of acid generated from dietary intake and metabolism. This usually approximates 1 to 3 mEq/kg per day (1–3 mmol/kg).

❼ After initial potassium deficits are replaced, ongoing potassium supplementation may not be required, as renal potassium losses decrease following initiation of appropriate alkali therapy. The use of potassium alkali salts can, however, be desirable in patients with associated nephrolithiasis, because sodium salts can increase urinary calcium excretion.

The metabolic acidosis associated with hyperkalemic distal (type IV) RTA with hyporeninemic-hypoaldosteronemia that is often seen in patients with diabetes mellitus can be corrected by the treatment of hyperkalemia alone (see Chapter 60). The use of supplemental alkali (1–2 mEq/kg [1–2 mmol/kg] per day) to increase sodium intake and stimulate distal tubular potassium secretion can be beneficial. A minority of patients require the administration of pharmacologic amounts of fludrocortisone.[4] Type IV RTA resulting from a generalized distal tubular disorder often responds to low doses of alkali (1.5–2.0 mEq/kg [1.5–2.0 mmol/kg] per day).[27] Corrections of the acidosis along with modest dietary potassium restriction (to 1 mEq/kg [1 mmol/kg] per day) will often result in the maintenance of serum potassium levels of 5 mEq/L (5 mmol/L) or less.

ACUTE SEVERE METABOLIC ACIDOSIS

❽ The management of patients with life-threatening acute metabolic acidosis (plasma bicarbonate of 8 mEq/L [8 mmol/L] and pH <7.20) is dependent on the underlying cause and the patient's cardiovascular status. In some cases patients will require emergent hemodialysis therapy (see Chapter 51). Patients with hyperchloremic acidosis (e.g., diarrhea-induced) are unable to regenerate bicarbonate, and the generation of new bicarbonate by the kidneys can require several

days before one can observe a meaningful change in their status.[11] Thus intravenous alkali therapy is often required for these patients.

Although conventional wisdom recommends the use of alkali replacement in patients with severe acidemia because of the deleterious effects of acidemia on circulatory function,[6,10–12] studies have not demonstrated that its administration improves patient outcomes.[28–31] Alkali therapies may either improve or worsen clinically relevant endpoints such as [H^+], $Paco_2$, lactate concentrations, and cardiac output. The specific patient populations most likely to benefit or be harmed from alkalinizing therapy are presented in Table 61–9.

There are several therapeutic alternatives available for the acute correction of severe metabolic acidosis. Sodium acetate, sodium citrate, and sodium lactate are unreliable sources of alkali because their alkalinizing effect is dependent on their oxidative conversion to bicarbonate. This process is often impaired in critically ill patients, especially those with liver disease or circulatory failure. Although sodium bicarbonate is the most widely used intravenous alkalotic agent,[11] several studies suggest that it is frequently ineffective and can actually be deleterious, especially in patients with lactic acidosis.[28–31] Two of the three remaining alternatives (Carbicarb and dichloroacetate) are investigational and not available in most clinical settings. Tromethamine, or THAM, is a carbon dioxide-consuming, commercially available solution that buffers respiratory as well as metabolic acids.

SODIUM BICARBONATE

While sodium bicarbonate administration provides fluid and electrolyte replacement and increases arterial pH, neither animal nor

TABLE 61-9 Patients Likely to Benefit or Be Harmed from Alkalinizing Therapy

Potential for Benefit	Potential for Harm
Distal (type 1) renal tubular acidosis	Hypernatremia
Severe hypchloremic metabolic acidosis secondary to diarrhea or surgical diversion	Hypernatremia
	Acute renal failure
	Congestive heart failure
Specific poisonings and intoxications (e.g., salicylate overdose with metabolic acidosis)	Pulmonary disease resulting in decreased ventilation
	Acute lung injury where lung-protective ventilation strategy is used
	Diabetic ketoacidosis

clinical studies demonstrate an improvement in cardiac function, organ perfusion, or intracellular pH.[28-31] In addition, sodium bicarbonate administration can actually have paradoxical adverse effects on intracellular pH. When bicarbonate is given by IV infusion, the carbon dioxide generated diffuses more readily than bicarbonate across cell membranes and into cerebrospinal fluid. Therefore, the intracellular pH can actually be decreased by administration of bicarbonate.[4]

CLINICAL CONTROVERSY

Although it has been recommended that sodium bicarbonate be administered to raise the arterial pH to approximately 7.20, there are no controlled clinical trials demonstrating that sodium bicarbonate administration is significantly better than general supportive care in reducing morbidity and mortality in these patients.[4,11,20-23]

Excessive sodium bicarbonate administration can result in (1) a shift of the oxyhemoglobin saturation curve to the left thereby impairing oxygen release from hemoglobin to tissues; (2) sodium and water overload, with subsequent pulmonary congestion and hypernatremia; (3) paradoxical tissue acidosis as a result of the production of CO_2 that freely diffuses into myocardial and cerebral cells[32]; and (4) decreased ionized calcium with a resultant decrease in myocardial contractility. If there is an endogenous source of bicarbonate, such as can occur in the case of ketoacidosis or lactic acidosis, a bicarbonate "overshoot" can develop because the ketoacids (acetoacetic acid and β-hydroxybutyric acid) or lactic acid are converted in the liver to bicarbonate once the underlying cause of acidosis is corrected.[10,11,33] Alkalosis can also result if too much sodium bicarbonate is administered too quickly.

If intravenous sodium bicarbonate is used, one must be mindful that the goals are to increase, not normalize, pH (to approximately 7.20) and plasma bicarbonate (to 8–10 mEq/L [8–10 mmol/L]). There is no calculative method that will assure attainment of these goals with a given dose of sodium bicarbonate because of the multiplicity of competing processes that can affect acid–base status (e.g., vomiting, potential increases in endogenous acid production, and renal failure) and the marked variability in the volume of distribution of bicarbonate (50% of body weight in patients with mild acidosis to approximately 100% in those with severe acidosis).[10,32-33] Adrogue and Madias[12] recommended that the dose of sodium bicarbonate be calculated using a distribution volume of 50% of body weight for all patients to avoid overtreatment. The total dose calculated as described previously in the RTA section should be administered as an infusion over one-half to several hours. Follow-up monitoring of arterial blood gases, beginning no sooner than 30 minutes after the end of the infusion, should be used to guide further therapeutic decisions.

Bicarbonate therapy is generally not necessary for patients with cardiac arrest, even if the initial arrest was unmonitored. The American Heart Association's Advanced Cardiac Life Support (ACLS) provider manual states that sodium bicarbonate is not useful or effective during resuscitation in hypoxic patients with lactic acidosis. Additionally, sodium bicarbonate is considered to be not useful or effective in those who are undergoing prolonged resuscitation with effective ventilation.[34] Furthermore, if sodium bicarbonate is used, it should be used only after defibrillation, cardiac compression, support of ventilation including intubation, and drug therapies such as epinephrine and antiarrhythmic agents have been employed.[35] The intial dose of sodium bicarbonate in this situation is 1 mEq/kg [1 mmol/kg]) administered by rapid, direct intravenous injection.[36] Subsequent doses of sodium bicarbonate should be based on measurements of arterial blood pH and $Paco_2$ given the propensity for it to cause alkalemia.[37]

TROMETHAMINE

THAM, available as a 0.3 N solution, is a highly alkaline, sodium-free organic amine that acts as a proton acceptor to prevent or correct acidosis.[39] THAM combines with hydrogen ions from carbonic acid to form bicarbonate and a cationic buffer. THAM also acts as an osmotic diuretic to increase urine flow, urine pH, and the excretion of fixed acids, CO_2, and electrolytes. At pH 7.4, 30% of THAM is not ionized and therefore can penetrate into cells and neutralize acidic anions of the intracellular fluid. Intracellular pH increases have been noted within 1 hour after the infusion of THAM. There is, however, no clinical or physiologic evidence that this action is beneficial, or that THAM is more efficacious than sodium bicarbonate.[28,39]

When THAM is used, it must be administered slowly, with careful monitoring to avoid alkalosis. The usual empiric dosage range for tromethamine is 1 to 5 mmol/kg administered intravenously over 1 hour, but doses up to 1.25 mmol/kg can be given over 5 to 15 minutes in acute situations. The dose of THAM can be individualized using the following equation[39]:

$$\text{Dose of THAM (in mL)} = 1.1 \times BW \text{(in kilograms)} \times \text{base deficit}$$

where base deficit = normal $[HCO_3^-]$ minus current $[HCO_3^-]$.

The need for additional THAM is determined by serial measurements of the serum bicarbonate concentration and calculation of the base deficit. Large doses can cause respiratory depression as a result of an increase in blood pH and a decrease in $Paco_2$ concentration.[38] THAM solution is highly alkaline and can cause severe inflammation, vascular spasm, or tissue damage (necrosis, sloughing, pain, chemical phlebitis, or thrombosis) if infiltration occurs. Hyperkalemia, hypoglycemia, hypocalcemia, and impaired coagulation have also been reported.[28,39] This agent should only be used with extreme caution in patients with severe liver or kidney failure.

CARBICARB

Carbicarb is an equimolar mixture of sodium carbonate (Na_2CO_3) and sodium bicarbonate ($NaHCO_3$).[39,40] Given that the carbonate ion is a stronger base than bicarbonate, Carbicarb preferentially buffers hydrogen ions resulting in the formation of bicarbonate rather than CO_2. Thus Carbicarb limits, but does not eliminate, the generation of CO_2. Unlike bicarbonate, which can produce a paradoxical intracellular acidosis and thereby impair cardiac function, Carbicarb appears to correct intracellular acidosis if present.[41,42] Despite these effects, there are no consistent data on the effects of carbicarb on hemodynamic endpoints and this agent is not available for use in humans.[28]

DICHLOROACETATE

Dichloroacetate (DCA), another investigational agent, facilitates aerobic lactate metabolism by stimulating the activity of lactate dehydrogenase, thus reversing hyperlactatemia and elevating blood pH.[43,44] DCA, when compared to conventional management in controlled studies, however, has not been shown to improve hemodynamic parameters or clinical outcomes.[43,45,46] DCA can cause mild drowsiness and peripheral neuropathy that can be ameliorated or prevented with thiamine supplementation.[44] The future role of DCA in the management of metabolic acidosis, particularly lactic acidosis, remains to be clarified.[28]

METABOLIC ALKALOSIS

Pathophysiology

Metabolic alkalosis is a simple acid–base disorder that presents as alkalemia (increased arterial pH) with an increase in plasma bicarbonate. It is an extremely common entity in hospitalized patients with acid–base disturbances. Under normal circumstances, the kidney is readily able to excrete an alkali load. Thus evaluation of patients with metabolic alkalosis must consider two separate issues: (1) the initial process that generates the metabolic alkalosis; and (2) alterations in renal function that maintain the alkalemic state.[47]

❾ The generation of metabolic alkalosis can also result from excessive losses of hydrogen ion from the kidneys or stomach or from a gain secondary to the ingestion or administration of bicarbonate-rich fluids. Gastric juice, rich in chloride and hydrogen ion, is secreted at a rate of less than 50 mL/h in the basal state, but can increase up to five-fold with stimulation.[8] In the gastric parietal cells, hydrogen ion and bicarbonate are generated from CO_2 and water.[47] The hydrogen ion is secreted into gastric fluid, and the bicarbonate is retained in the ECF. Normally, an amount of bicarbonate equal to the bicarbonate generated in the stomach is eliminated in the alkaline pancreatic and small-bowel secretions, maintaining hydrogen ion balance. With vomiting and nasogastric suctioning, hydrogen ion is lost externally and metabolic alkalosis results. Diarrhea, as seen with secretory villous adenomas and other secretory diarrheas, often results in excessive gastrointestinal losses of chloride-rich, bicarbonate-poor fluid and thus leads to the generation of metabolic alkalosis.

❿ Diuretic agents acting on the thick ascending limb of the loop of Henle (e.g., furosemide, bumetanide, and torsemide) and distal convoluted tubule (e.g., thiazides), have most commonly been associated with the generation of metabolic alkalosis.[48] These agents promote the excretion of sodium and potassium almost exclusively in association with chloride, without a proportionate increase in bicarbonate excretion. Collecting duct hydrogen ion secretion is stimulated directly by the increased luminal flow rate and sodium delivery, and indirectly by intravascular volume contraction, which results in secondary hyperaldosteronism. Renal ammoniagenesis can also be stimulated by concomitant hypokalemia, further augmenting net acid excretion.

Increased renal acid excretion can also be the result of excess mineralocorticoid activity. Elevated mineralocorticoid levels directly stimulate collecting duct hydrogen ion secretion and indirectly increase ammoniagenesis by causing hypokalemia.[47] Increased mineralocorticoid activity can result from Cushing syndrome, primary hyperaldosteronism, or hyperaldosteronism secondary to increased renin activity (e.g., malignant hypertension). In Bartter and Gitelman syndromes, defects in sodium transport in the loop of Henle (Bartter) or distal convoluted tubule (Gitelman) lead to hypokalemia, secondary hyperaldosteronism, and metabolic alkalosis.[47] In Liddle's syndrome, enhanced sodium reabsorption by the cortical collecting duct epithelial sodium channel results in a syndrome of pseudo-hyperaldosteronism.[47] Administration of high doses of penicillins (e.g., ticarcillin) can produce metabolic alkalosis because they act as nonreabsorbable anions. High concentrations of poorly reabsorbable anions in the distal renal tubule increase luminal flow rate and luminal electronegativity, which enhances the secretion of potassium and hydrogen ion and results in hypokalemia and metabolic alkalosis.

Metabolic alkalosis can also be generated by the gain of exogenous alkali. This can be seen as a result of bicarbonate administration or from the infusion of organic anions that are metabolized to bicarbonate, such as acetate, lactate, and citrate. The milk-alkali syndrome was historically a common cause of metabolic alkalosis in patients with peptic ulcer disease secondary to the ingestion of large quantities of milk products and antacids. With the advent of alternative therapies for dyspeptic syndromes that are far more effective than milk, this syndrome is now rarely seen.

TABLE 61-10	Causes of Metabolic Alkalosis Differentiated on the Basis of Their Responsiveness to Sodium Chloride

Sodium chloride–responsive (urinary chloride concentration <10 mEq/L [<10 mmol/L])
Gastrointestinal disorders
   Vomiting
   Gastric drainage
   Villous adenoma of the colon
   Chloride diarrhea
Diuretic therapy
Correction of chronic hypercapnia
Cystic fibrosis
Excessive bicarbonate therapy of an organic acidosis
Mild/moderate potassium deficiency

Sodium chloride–resistant (urinary chloride concentration >20 mEq/L [>20 mmol/L])
Excess mineralocorticoid activity
   Hyperaldosteronism
   Cushing syndrome
   Bartter syndrome
   Gitelman syndrome
Excessive black licorice intake
Profound potassium depletion
Magnesium deficiency
Liddle syndrome
Estrogen therapy

Unclassified
Alkali administration
Milk-alkali syndrome
Massive blood or plasma protein fraction transfusion
Nonparathyroid hypercalcemia
Carbohydrate refeeding after starvation
Large doses of penicillin

Metabolic alkalosis is predominantly maintained because of an abnormality in renal function. Normally, the kidneys are capable of excreting all of the excess bicarbonate presented to them, even during periods of increased bicarbonate loads.[4] As the serum bicarbonate concentration increases, the filtered bicarbonate load exceeds the maximal rate for bicarbonate reabsorption, and the excess bicarbonate is excreted in the urine. Under normal circumstances, the excess bicarbonate is rapidly excreted, and metabolic alkalosis does not occur or is corrected in a matter of hours.[47]

⓫ Several mechanisms can impair renal bicarbonate excretion and contribute to the maintenance phase of metabolic alkalosis.[47] In general, these mechanisms can be divided into volume-mediated processes (sodium chloride–responsive) and volume-independent processes (sodium chloride–resistant) that are predominantly associated with excess mineralocorticoid activity and hypokalemia (Table 61–10). Intravascular volume depletion maintains metabolic alkalosis through a number of mechanisms. Decreases in the glomerular filtration rate reduce the filtered load of bicarbonate at any given serum concentration, thereby decreasing the kidney's ability to excrete a bicarbonate load. Although this can play a role in patients with chronic kidney disease, it is also an important factor in patients in whom intravascular volume contraction accompanies metabolic alkalosis. Decreased effective arterial blood volume also enhances proximal and distal tubular sodium reabsorption. Sodium reabsorption must be coupled with reabsorption of an anion, such as chloride or bicarbonate, or exchange with a cation, such as potassium or hydrogen, to maintain charge neutrality. In the proximal tubule, increased sodium reabsorption stimulates bicarbonate reabsorption. In the distal nephron, enhanced sodium reabsorption, particularly in the setting of hypokalemia, stimulates hydrogen ion secretion.

Mineralocorticoid excess also plays a significant role in the maintenance of metabolic alkalosis. In patients with volume-responsive metabolic alkalosis, intravascular volume depletion stimulates aldosterone secretion. As discussed earlier, excess mineralocorticoid activity can also underlie the generation of metabolic alkalosis. In either situation, the increased mineralocorticoid effect stimulates collecting duct hydrogen ion secretion. Metabolic alkalosis can also be maintained by persistent hypokalemia, enhancing proximal tubular bicarbonate reabsorption, stimulating ammoniagenesis, and increasing distal tubular hydrogen ion secretion.[47]

Clinical Presentation

There are no unique signs or symptoms associated with mild to moderate metabolic alkalosis, but patients may complain of symptoms related to the underlying cause of the disorder (e.g., muscle weakness with hypokalemia or postural dizziness with volume depletion). They may have a history of vomiting, gastric drainage, or diuretic use, all of which contribute to the development of metabolic alkalosis. Severe alkalemia (blood pH >7.60) has been associated with cardiac arrhythmias, particularly in patients with heart disease, hyperventilation, and hypoxemia.[49] Neuromuscular irritability can be present, with signs of tetany or hyperactive reflexes, possibly caused by the decreased ionized calcium concentration that occurs secondary to the increase in pH. This decrease in ionized calcium may be caused by a conformational change in the albumin molecules to which the calcium is bound, resulting in increased binding, or by decreased competition from hydrogen ions for binding sites on the albumin molecule. Mental confusion, muscle cramping, and paresthesia can also occur. Lastly, patients will be more difficult to liberate from mechanical ventilation. (Please see metabolic alkalosis case 59 from Casebook.)

Compensation

The respiratory response to metabolic alkalosis is hypoventilation, which results in an increased $PaCO_2$. Respiratory compensation is initiated within hours when the central and peripheral chemoreceptors sense an increase in pH. The $PaCO_2$ increases 6 to 7 mm Hg (0.8–0.9 kPa) for each 10-mEq/L (10 mmol/L) increase in bicarbonate, up to a $PaCO_2$ of approximately 50 to 60 mm Hg (6.7–8.0 kPa) (see Table 61–7) before hypoxia sensors react to prevent further hypoventilation. If the $PaCO_2$ is normal or less than normal, one should consider the presence of a superimposed respiratory alkalosis, which can be secondary to fever, gram-negative sepsis, or pain.

TREATMENT

Metabolic Alkalosis

Because the body tolerates alkalemia far less well than acidemia, treatment of metabolic alkalosis is nearly always required and should be aimed at correcting the factor(s) responsible for the maintenance of the alkalosis.[23,49] For example, vomiting should be treated with antiemetics, gastric losses of hydrogen ion during nasogastric suction can be modulated by giving histamine blockers such as ranitidine or proton pump inhibitors such as omeprazole, and reducing or discontinuing diuretic therapy.[47,50] Metabolic alkalosis will persist until the renal mechanism responsible for maintaining the disorder is corrected, despite the fact that the original cause of the elevated plasma bicarbonate may have resolved. For example, hypovolemia should be treated with sodium chloride (i.e., diuretic abuse or nasogastric suction) to allow excretion of bicarbonate by the kidney. However, patients with severely compromised cardiovascular function may not be able to tolerate this therapeutic approach. In situations such as this and/or the presence of life-threatening alkalosis, some have advocated reduction in pH by control of ventilation.[4] Although controlled hypoventilation, sometimes using inspired CO_2 with supplemental oxygen to prevent hypoxia can be life-saving,[4] this approach is not universally accepted.[33] Therapy for metabolic alkalosis can be conceptualized on the basis of the sodium chloride responsiveness of the disorders as shown in Figure 61–4.

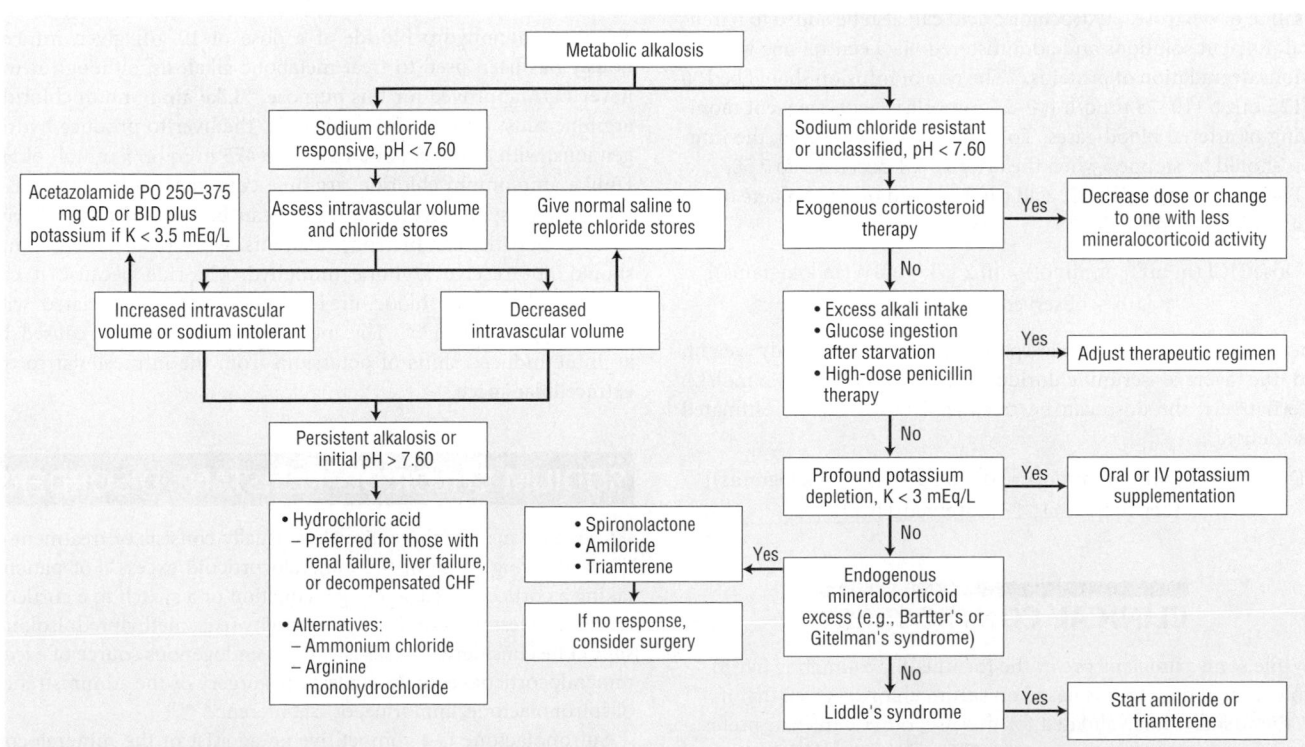

FIGURE 61-4. Treatment algorithm for patients with primary metabolic alkalosis. (BID, twice daily; CHF, chronic heart failure; K, potassium [serum potassium in mEq/L is numerically equivalent to mmol/L]; PO, orally; QD, every day.)

SODIUM CHLORIDE–RESPONSIVE DISORDERS

Sodium chloride–responsive disorders usually result from volume depletion and chloride loss, which can accompany severe vomiting, prolonged nasogastric suction, and diuretic therapy. Initially therapy is directed at expanding intravascular volume and replenishing chloride stores. Sodium and potassium chloride–containing solutions should be administered to patients who can tolerate the volume load.[47,49] Patients with metabolic alkalosis who are volume overloaded or intolerant to volume administration because of congestive heart failure can benefit from the carbonic anhydrase inhibitor acetazolamide. This agent inhibits the action of carbonic anhydrase, thereby inhibiting renal bicarbonate reabsorption. Unfortunately, it also increases the renal losses of potassium and phosphate. Administration of acetazolamide (250–375 mg once or twice daily) can promote a sufficient bicarbonate diuresis and return the pH toward normal.[57] However, because the clinical effectiveness of the drug declines as the HCO_3^- concentration decreases, only rarely will this approach fully correct the alkalosis.[47]

Acidifying agents including hydrochloric acid, ammonium chloride, and arginine monohydrochloride can be used to treat severe (pH >7.6) symptomatic metabolic alkalosis.[52] In general, this management is reserved for patients who are unresponsive to conventional fluid and electrolyte management or who are unable to tolerate the requisite volume load because of decompensated congestive heart failure or advanced renal failure.[47] Alternatively, hemodialysis using a low-bicarbonate dialysate can be used for the rapid correction of metabolic alkalosis.

HYDROCHLORIC ACID

Hydrochloric acid is usually infused intravenously via a large central vein as a 0.1 to 0.25 N HCl solution in either 5% dextrose or normal saline, although sterile water has also been used. Extemporaneously prepared solutions can be made by adding 100 to 250 mEq (100–250 mmol) of HCl through a 0.22-mm filter into a glass container of saline or dextrose. Hydrochloric acid can also be added to parenteral nutrient solutions and administered via a central line without serious degradation of proteins.[53] The rate of infusion should be 100 to 125 mL/h (10–25 mEq/h [10–25 mmol/h]), with frequent monitoring of arterial blood gases. To prevent overcorrection, the infusion should be stopped when the arterial pH decreases to 7.50.[47]

The dose of hydrochloric acid can be based on an estimate of the total body chloride deficit[36]:

$$\text{Dose HCl (in mEq or mmol)} = [0.2 \text{ L/kg} \times \text{BW(in kilograms)}] \times [103 - \text{observed serum chloride}]$$

where the estimated chloride space is 0.2 times the body weight, and the average serum chloride is 103 mEq/L (103 mmol/L). Alternatively, the dose can be calculated based on the estimated base deficit[49]:

$$\text{Dose HCl (in mEq or mmol)} = [0.5 \text{ L/kg} \times \text{BW (in kilograms)}] \times (\text{desired}[HCO_3^-] - \text{observed}[HCO_3^-])$$

CLINICAL CONTROVERSY

While some clinicians prefer the formula for estimating hydrochloric acid dose that is based on serum chloride given that it is the first formula validated for this use; other clinicians prefer the formula that uses the serum HCO_3^- given that HCO_3^- is a goal of therapy when initiating hydrochloric acid therapy.

The dose of hydrochloric acid is usually infused intravenously over 12 to 24 hours.[54] A severe transient respiratory acidosis can occur if the hydrochloric acid is infused too quickly because of a slower reduction of the elevated bicarbonate concentration in the cerebrospinal fluid than in the extracellular fluid. Improvement is usually seen within 24 hours of initiating therapy. Arterial blood gases and serum electrolytes should be drawn every 4 to 8 hours to evaluate and adjust therapy.

AMMONIUM CHLORIDE

Ammonium chloride has a limited role in the treatment of metabolic alkalosis. The liver converts ammonium chloride (NH_4Cl) to urea and free hydrochloric acid[36]:

$$2NH_4Cl + 2HCO_3^- \rightarrow CO(NH_2)_2 + CO_2 + 3H_2O + 2Cl^-$$

The dose of ammonium chloride can be calculated on the basis of the chloride deficit using the same method as for HCl and assuming that 20 g ammonium chloride will provide 374 mEq (374 mmol) of H^+. However, only one half of the calculated dose of ammonium chloride should be administered so as to avoid ammonia toxicity. Ammonium chloride is available as a 26.75% solution containing 100 mEq (100 mmol) of H^+ in 20 mL, which should be further diluted prior to administration. A dilute solution can be prepared by adding 20 mL of ammonium chloride to 500 mL of normal saline and infusing the solution at a rate of no more than 1 mEq/min (1 mmol/min). Improvement in metabolic status is usually seen within 24 hours. CNS toxicity, marked by confusion, irritability, seizures, and coma, has been associated with more rapid rates of administration. Ammonium chloride must be administered cautiously to patients with renal or hepatic impairment. In patients with hepatic dysfunction, impaired conversion of ammonia to urea can result in increased ammonia levels and worsened encephalopathy. In patients with renal failure, the increased urea synthesis can exacerbate uremic symptoms.[36]

ARGININE MONOHYDROCHLORIDE

Arginine monohydrochloride at a dose of 10 g/h given intravenously has been used to treat metabolic alkalosis, although it was never FDA approved for this purpose.[36] Like ammonium chloride, arginine must undergo metabolism by the liver to produce hydrogen ions, with a conversion of 100 g to 475 mEq (475 mmol) of H^+. Unlike ammonium chloride, arginine combines with ammonia in the body to synthesize urea; thus it can be used in patients with relative hepatic insufficiency. Patients with renal insufficiency should not receive arginine monohydrochloride because it can significantly elevate blood urea nitrogen and is associated with severe hyperkalemia.[36,47] The increase in potassium is caused by arginine-induced shifts of potassium from the intracellular to the extracellular space.

SODIUM CHLORIDE–RESISTANT DISORDERS

⑫ Management of these disorders usually consists of treatment of the underlying cause of the mineralocorticoid excess. For patients taking a corticosteroid, a dosage reduction or a switch to a corticosteroid with less mineralocorticoid activity (e.g., methylprednisolone) should be considered. Patients with an endogenous source of excess mineralocorticoid activity can require surgery or the administration of spironolactone, amiloride, or triamterene.[47,49,55]

Spironolactone is a competitive antagonist of the mineralocorticoid receptor. Amiloride and triamterene are potassium-sparing diuretics that inhibit the epithelial sodium channel in the distal convoluted tubule and collecting duct. All three agents inhibit aldosterone-stimulated sodium reabsorption in the collecting duct. In addition, spironolactone directly inhibits aldosterone stimulation of the hydrogen ion secretory pump. Thus, most patients with mineralocorticoid excess, including Bartter and Gitelman syndromes, respond to therapy with these agents.[47,55–57] Liddle syndrome, which is a form of pseudohypoaldosteronism caused by overactivity of the epithelial sodium channel, is not responsive to spironolactone but can be treated with either amiloride or triamterene. Although experience is limited, some patients with Bartter and Gitelman syndromes may respond to nonsteroidal anti-inflammatory agents or angiotensin-converting enzyme inhibitors.[55–57] Finally, aggressive potassium repletion can correct the alkalosis in those who have not responded to the approaches outlined above.

RESPIRATORY ACID–BASE DISORDERS

As with the metabolic acid–base disturbances, there are two cardinal respiratory acid–base disturbances: respiratory acidosis and respiratory alkalosis. These disorders are generated by a primary alteration in carbon dioxide excretion, which changes the concentration of carbon dioxide, and therefore the carbonic acid concentration in body fluids. A primary reduction in $Paco_2$ causes an increase in pH (respiratory alkalosis), and a primary increase in $Paco_2$ causes a decrease in pH (respiratory acidosis). Unlike the metabolic disturbances, for which respiratory compensation is rapid, metabolic compensation for the respiratory disturbances is slow. Hence, these disturbances can be further divided into acute disorders, with a duration of minutes to hours, and where metabolic compensation has yet to occur, and chronic disorders that have been present long enough for metabolic compensation to be complete.

RESPIRATORY ALKALOSIS

Respiratory alkalosis is characterized by a primary decrease in $Paco_2$ that leads to an elevation in pH. The $Paco_2$ decreases when the excretion of CO_2 by the lungs exceeds the metabolic production of CO_2. It is the most frequently encountered acid–base disorder, occurring physiologically in normal pregnancy and in persons living at high altitudes.[59] Respiratory alkalosis also occurs frequently among hospitalized patients (Table 61–11).

TABLE 61-11 Causes of Respiratory Alkalosis
Central stimulation of respiration
Anxiety
Pain
Fever
Brain tumors, vascular accidents
Head trauma
Pregnancy
Progesterone
Catecholamines, theophylline, nicotine
Salicylates
Hypoxemia or tissue hypoxemia
High altitude
Decreased $Paco_2$
Pneumonia
Pulmonary edema
Severe anemia
Peripheral stimulation of respiration
Pulmonary emboli
Asthma

$Paco_2$, partial pressure of carbon dioxide from arterial blood.

Pathophysiology

A decrease in $Paco_2$ occurs when ventilatory excretion exceeds metabolic production. Because endogenous production of CO_2 is relatively constant, negative CO_2 balance is primarily caused by an increase in ventilatory excretion of CO_2 (hyperventilation). The metabolic production of CO_2, however, can be increased during periods of stress or with excess carbohydrate administration (e.g., parenteral nutrition). Hyperventilation can develop from an increase in neurochemical stimulation via either central or peripheral mechanisms, or be the result of voluntary or mechanical (iatrogenic) hyperventilation.

A decrease in $Paco_2$ can occur in patients with cardiogenic, hypovolemic, or septic shock because oxygen delivery to the carotid and aortic chemoreceptors is reduced. This relative deficit in Pao_2 stimulates an increase in ventilation. The hyperventilation in sepsis is also mediated via a central mechanism. Hyperventilation-induced respiratory alkalosis with an elevation in cardiac index and hypotension without peripheral vasoconstriction can therefore be an early sign of sepsis.

Clinical Presentation

Although most patients are asymptomatic, respiratory alkalosis can cause adverse neuromuscular, cardiovascular, and gastrointestinal effects.[59] During periods of decreased $Paco_2$, there is a decrease in cerebral blood flow, which can be responsible for symptoms of light-headedness, confusion, decreased intellectual functioning, syncope, and seizures. Nausea and vomiting can occur, probably as a result of cerebral hypoxia. In severe respiratory alkalosis, cardiac arrhythmias can occur because of sensitization of the myocardium to the arrhythmogenic effects of circulating catecholamines.[2] Acute respiratory alkalosis has no effect on blood pressure or cardiac output in awake individuals. Anesthetized patients, however, can experience a decrease in both cardiac output and blood pressure, possibly owing to the lack of a tachycardic response.[59]

The concentration of serum electrolytes can also be altered secondary to the development of respiratory alkalosis. The serum chloride concentration is usually slightly increased, and serum potassium concentration can be slightly decreased. Clinically significant hypokalemia can be a consequence of extreme respiratory alkalosis, although the effect is usually very small or negligible.[2,59] Serum phosphorus concentration can decrease by as much as 1.5 to 2.0 mg/dL (0.48–0.65 mmol/L) because of the shift of inorganic phosphate into cells. Reductions in the blood ionized calcium concentration can be partially responsible for symptoms such as muscle cramps and tetany. Approximately 50% of calcium is bound to albumin, and an increase in pH results in an increase in binding.[54]

CLINICAL PRESENTATION OF RESPIRATORY ALKALOSIS
General
The patient is usually asymptomatic if the condition is chronic and mild.
Symptoms
The patient may complain of light-headedness, confusion, muscle cramps and tetany, and decreased intellectual functioning.
Nausea and vomiting can occur, probably as a result of cerebral hypoxia.
Signs
In severe respiratory alkalosis pH >7.60
Syncope and seizures
Cardiac arrhythmias
Hyperventilation

Laboratory Tests

▫ Serum chloride concentration is usually slightly increased. Serum ionized calcium, potassium, and phosphorus concentration can be decreased.

Compensation

The initial response of the body to acute respiratory alkalosis is chemical buffering: hydrogen ions are released from the body's buffers—intracellular proteins, phosphates, and hemoglobin—and titrate down the serum bicarbonate concentration. This process occurs within minutes. Acutely, the bicarbonate concentration can be decreased by a maximum of 3 mEq/L (3 mmol/L) for each 10-mm Hg (1.3 kPa) decrease in $Paco_2$[24] (see Table 61–7). When only physicochemical buffering has occurred, the disturbance is referred to as acute respiratory alkalosis.

Metabolic compensation occurs when respiratory alkalosis persists for more than 6 to 12 hours. In response to the alkalemia, proximal tubular bicarbonate reabsorption is inhibited, and the serum bicarbonate concentration decreases. Renal compensation is usually complete within 1 to 2 days. The renal bicarbonaturia, as well as decreased NH_4^+ and titratable acid excretion, are direct effects of the reduced $Paco_2$ and pH on renal reabsorption of chloride and bicarbonate.[2] The acuity of the respiratory alkalosis can be assessed on the basis of the degree of renal compensation (see Table 61–7). In fully compensated respiratory alkalosis, the bicarbonate concentration decreases by 4 mEq/L (4 mmol/L) below 24 for each 10-mm Hg (1.3 kPa) drop in $Paco_2$. For example, a sustained decrease in $Paco_2$ of 20 mm Hg (2.7 kPa) will lower serum bicarbonate from 24 to 14 mEq/L (24–14 mmol/L) with a resultant pH of 7.46. Bicarbonate concentrations differing from those anticipated using the preceding guidelines suggest a mixed acid–base disorder.

TREATMENT

Respiratory Alkalosis

Because most patients with respiratory alkalosis, especially chronic cases, have few or no symptoms and pH alterations are usually mild (pH not exceeding 7.50), treatment is often not required.[49] The first consideration in the treatment of acute respiratory alkalosis with pH >7.50 is the identification and correction of the underlying cause. Relief of pain, correction of hypovolemia with intravenous fluids, treatment of fever or infection, treatment of salicylate overdose, and other direct measures can prove effective. A rebreathing device, such as a paper bag, can be useful in controlling hyperventilation in patients with the anxiety/hyperventilation syndrome.[54] Oxygen therapy should be initiated in patients with severe hypoxemia. Patients with life-threatening alkalosis (pH >7.60), particularly if it is a mixed respiratory and metabolic condition and they have complications such as arrhythmia or seizures can require mechanical ventilation with sedation and/or paralysis to control hyperventilation.

Respiratory alkalosis in patients receiving mechanical ventilation is usually iatrogenic. It can often be corrected by decreasing either the set respiratory rate or tidal volume, although other measures can also be employed. The use of a capnograph and spirometer in the breathing circuit enables a more precise adjustment of the ventilator settings. Another method of treating respiratory alkalosis is to increase the amount of dead space in the ventilator circuit by placing a known length of tubing between the artificial airway and the "Y" piece of the ventilator. This results in "rebreathing" of expired gas, and therefore an increase

TABLE 61-12 Causes of Acute Respiratory Acidosis

Central
Drugs (anesthetics, opioids, sedatives)
Stroke
Head injury
Infection
Status epilepticus
Perfusion abnormalities
Massive pulmonary embolism
Cardiac arrest
Airway and pulmonary abnormalities
Airway obstruction: foreign body, laryngeal edema
Aspiration of vomitus
Asthma
Chronic pulmonary obstructive disease
Severe pulmonary edema
Severe pneumonia
Adult respiratory distress syndrome
Smoke inhalation
Pneumothorax
Neuromuscular abnormalities
Brainstem or cervical cord injury
Guillain-Barré syndrome
Myasthenia gravis
Mechanical ventilator
Ventilator malfunction
Inadequate frequency or tidal volume settings
Large dead space
Total parenteral nutrition (increased CO_2 production)

in the inspired carbon dioxide concentration, which should increase the carbon dioxide tension of the patient, correcting the respiratory alkalosis. In patients breathing more rapidly than the ventilator settings, sedation with or without paralysis can be employed.

RESPIRATORY ACIDOSIS

Pathophysiology

Respiratory acidosis occurs when the lungs fail to excrete carbon dioxide resulting in a lower pH. This can be the result of conditions that centrally inhibit the respiratory center, diseases that interfere with pulmonary perfusion or neuromuscular function, and intrinsic airway or parenchymal pulmonary disease (Table 61–12). Acute respiratory acidosis with hypoxemia, hypercarbia, and acidosis is life-threatening. Those disorders that produce an increase in $Paco_2$ and hypoxemia to a degree compatible with life (e.g., chronic obstructive pulmonary disease), with or without oxygen therapy, can result in chronic respiratory acidosis (Table 61–13). These patients can function normally without noticeable neurologic

TABLE 61-13 Causes of Chronic Respiratory Acidosis

Neuromuscular abnormalities
Brainstem infarct
Obesity-hypoventilation (Pickwickian) syndrome
Tumors
Poliomyelitis
Multiple sclerosis
Diaphragmatic paralysis
Perfusion abnormalities
Chronic obstructive pulmonary disease
Kyphoscoliosis
Interstitial pulmonary disease
Overzealous parenteral feeding

defects with $Paco_2$ concentrations in the range of 90 to 100 mm Hg (12–13.3 kPa) (normal, 40 mm Hg [5.3 kPa]), provided adequate oxygenation is maintained.[59]

Clinical Presentation

Respiratory acidosis can produce neurologic symptoms, including altered mental status, abnormal behavior, seizures, stupor, and coma. Hypercapnia can mimic stroke or CNS tumors by producing headache, papilledema, focal paresis, and abnormal reflexes. These CNS symptoms are attributable to the vasodilator effects of CO_2 in the brain that result in an increase in cerebral blood flow.[2] The CNS response to hypercapnia is extremely variable between patients and is most influenced by the acuity of presentation. Given that chronic hypercapnia blunts the usual respiratory stimulus of an elevated $Paco_2$, hypoxemia rather than hypercapnia provides the primary ventilatory stimulus in patients with severe chronic respiratory acidosis.[59]

The degree to which cardiac contractility and heart rate are altered depends on the severity of the acidosis and the rapidity with which it develops. Modest acute hypercapnia ($Paco_2$ of 50–55 mm Hg [6.7–7.3 kPa]) stimulates a stress-like response, with elevated catecholamines and corticosteroid hormone levels, and can result in increased cardiac output and pulmonary artery pressure.[59] As the severity increases, cardiac output declines and vascular resistance decreases leading to refractory hypotension in some patients.[2]

In respiratory acidosis, the serum potassium concentration increases modestly secondary to cellular shifts. The increases are less than those seen with inorganic metabolic acidosis and are difficult to predict for individual patients (see Chapter 60).

CLINICAL PRESENTATION OF RESPIRATORY ACIDOSIS

General

The patient is usually symptomatic.

Symptoms

The patient may complain of confusion or difficulty thinking and headache.

Signs

In severe respiratory acidosis:

Cardiac: Increased cardiac output if moderate that decreases if severe. Refractory hypotension can be present in some patients.

CNS: Abnormal behavior, seizures, stupor, and coma. Papilledema, focal paresis, and abnormal reflexes can also be present.

Laboratory Tests

Serum potassium concentration can be modestly increased. Hypercapnia can be moderate ($Paco_2$ of 50–55 mm Hg [6.7–7.3 kPa]) to severe ($Paco_2$ of >80 mm Hg [>10.6 kPa]). Hypoxia (Pao_2 is <70 mm Hg [<9.3 kPa]) is often present.

Compensation

The body responds to acute respiratory acidosis with chemical buffering. The increase in $Paco_2$ results in increased carbonic acid levels. The carbonic acid dissociates, releasing hydrogen ions, which are buffered by nonbicarbonate buffers (i.e., proteins, phosphate, and hemoglobin) and bicarbonate. Thus, on the basis of physicochemical factors, increases in $Paco_2$ raise the serum bicarbonate concentration. In general, in acute respiratory acidosis,

the bicarbonate concentration increases by 1 mEq/L (1 mmol/L) above 24 for each 10-mm Hg (1.3 kPa) increase in $Paco_2$ above 40 (5.3 kPa) (see Table 61–7).

Metabolic compensation occurs when respiratory acidosis is prolonged beyond 12 to 24 hours. In response to hypercapnia and acidemia, proximal tubular bicarbonate reabsorption, ammoniagenesis, and distal tubular hydrogen secretion are enhanced, resulting in an increase in the serum bicarbonate concentration that raises the pH toward normal. Renal compensation for chronic hypercapnia generally results in the plasma bicarbonate concentration increasing by 4 mEq/L (4 mmol/L) above 24 for each 10-mm Hg (1.3 kPa) increase in $Paco_2$ above 40 (5.3 kPa) (see Table 61–7). The new steady state in acid–base values is generally achieved within 5 days of the onset of hypercapnia in dogs; the time interval necessary for compensation in humans has not been established.

TREATMENT

Respiratory Acidosis

The treatment of respiratory acidosis is dependent on the chronicity of the patient's condition. Respiratory decompensation in patients with chronic elevations in $Paco_2$ are frequently seen in those with acute infections and those recently started on narcotic analgesics or oxygen therapy.[49] Aggressive treatment of these conditions can offer considerable benefit and should be initiated. Furthermore, tranquilizers and sedatives should be avoided and supplemental oxygen, if used, should be minimized.

ACUTE RESPIRATORY ACIDOSIS

⓭ When carbon dioxide excretion is severely impaired ($Paco_2$ >80 mm Hg [>10.6 kPa]) and/or life-threatening, hypoxia is present (Pao_2 <40 mm Hg [<5.3 kPa]); the immediate therapeutic goal is to provide adequate oxygenation. Under these circumstances, hypoxia, not acidemia, is the principal threat to life. A patent airway needs to be established, which can necessitate intubation. Excessive secretions must be cleared from the airway and oxygen administered to restore adequate oxygenation. Mechanical ventilation is usually required.

The underlying cause of the acidosis should be treated aggressively (e.g., bronchodilators for treatment of severe bronchospasm; narcotic or benzodiazepine antagonists to reverse the deleterious effects of these agents on the respiratory center). Bicarbonate administration is rarely necessary in the treatment of respiratory acidosis. Furthermore, rapid correction of acidosis with bicarbonate can eliminate the patient's respiratory drive or precipitate metabolic alkalosis. Cautious use of alkali (bicarbonate or THAM) can restore the responsiveness of bronchial muscles to β-adrenergic agonists and thus can be beneficial for those patients with severe bronchospasm.[49] Arterial blood gases should be monitored closely to ensure that the respiratory acidosis is resolving without creating a metabolic alkalosis as the result of compensatory elevation in HCO_3^- and decrease in $Paco_2$. Arterial blood gases should be obtained every 2 to 4 hours during the acute phase and less frequently (every 12–24 hours) as the acidosis improves.

ACUTE RESPIRATORY ACIDOSIS IN A COMPENSATED CHRONIC RESPIRATORY ACIDOTIC PATIENT

Patients with a history of chronic respiratory acidosis (e.g., those with chronic obstructive pulmonary disease) can experience an acute worsening of their respiratory acidosis. This can result in severe life-threatening hypoxemia. As with acute respiratory acidosis, the goals of therapy are maintenance of a patent airway and adequate oxygenation. Individuals with chronic respiratory acidosis are routinely able to tolerate a low Pao_2 and an elevated $Paco_2$ because of compensation (increased number of red blood cells, hemoglobin content, and 2,3-diphosphoglycerate). The drive to breathe in these patients is dependent on hypoxemia rather than hypercarbia. Administration of oxygen to a patient with chronic respiratory acidosis can eliminate this drive to breathe and result in the syndrome of carbon dioxide narcosis. In this case, if the Pao_2 is 50 mm Hg (6.7 kPa), no oxygen treatment is necessary. If the Pao_2 is <50 mm Hg (<6.7 kPa), oxygen therapy should be initiated carefully using a controlled flow of oxygen.[2]

Arterial blood gases should be checked periodically to ensure adequate oxygenation. If the $Paco_2$ increases during oxygen therapy, it can be a sign of impending carbon dioxide narcosis and oxygen therapy may need to be discontinued. The underlying cause of the acute exacerbation should be aggressively managed. Pulmonary infections should be treated with the appropriate antibiotics and bronchodilators administered as necessary. Excess secretions should be cleared from the airway to allow proper gas exchange. This can involve increasing oral fluid intake to decrease the viscosity of secretions, deep breathing, and postural drainage, suction, or bronchoscopy.

MIXED ACID–BASE DISORDERS

DIAGNOSIS

The diagnosis of a mixed disorder depends on an understanding of the appropriate quantitative response of the compensatory mechanisms for each of the simple acid–base disturbances. To diagnose mixed disorders, one must know how each of the four simple disorders alters pH, $Paco_2$, and $[HCO_3^-]$ (see Table 61–7). If a given set of blood gases does not decrease within the range of expected responses for a simple acid–base disturbance, a mixed disorder should be suspected. In addition to laboratory information, a thorough history and physical examination of the patient will often lead to the diagnosis, even before the laboratory data are available. Examples of common mixed disturbances follow.

Mixed Respiratory Acidosis and Metabolic Acidosis

In mixed respiratory and metabolic acidosis, there is a failure of compensation. The respiratory disorder prevents the compensatory decrease in $Paco_2$ expected in the defense against metabolic acidosis. The metabolic disorder prevents the buffering and renal mechanisms from raising the bicarbonate concentration as expected in the defense against respiratory acidosis. In the absence of these compensatory mechanisms the pH decreases markedly.

Mixed respiratory and metabolic acidosis may develop in patients with cardiorespiratory arrest, in those with chronic lung disease who are in shock, and in metabolic acidosis patients who develop respiratory failure. When treating this mixed disorder, clinicians need to respond to both the respiratory and metabolic acidosis. Improved oxygen delivery must be initiated to improve hypercarbia and hypoxia. Mechanical ventilation may be needed to reduce $Paco_2$. During the initial stage of therapy, appropriate amounts of alkali should be given to reverse the metabolic acidosis (see Treatment, Metabolic Acidosis above).

Mixed Respiratory Alkalosis and Metabolic Alkalosis

The combination of respiratory and metabolic alkalosis is the most common mixed acid–base disorder. This mixed disorder occurs frequently in critically ill surgical patients with respiratory alkalosis caused by mechanical ventilation, hypoxia, sepsis, hypotension, neurologic damage, pain, or drugs, and with metabolic alkalosis caused by vomiting or nasogastric suctioning and massive blood transfusions. It can also occur in patients with hepatic cirrhosis who hyperventilate, receive diuretics, or vomit, as well as in patients with chronic respiratory acidosis and an elevated plasma bicarbonate concentration who are placed on mechanical ventilation and undergo a rapid decrease in $Paco_2$.

The renal excretion of bicarbonate that usually occurs as compensation for the respiratory alkalosis is prevented by the complicating metabolic alkalosis. Likewise, the retention of $Paco_2$ expected to compensate for metabolic alkalosis is prevented by the primary respiratory alkalosis. The failure of compensation that occurs with mixed respiratory and metabolic alkalosis can result in a severe alkalemia.

Administration of sodium chloride and potassium chloride solutions will help correct the metabolic component of this disorder and adjustment of the ventilator and/or treatment of an underlying disorder that is causing hyperventilation can correct or ameliorate the respiratory component of this mixed disorder.

Mixed Metabolic Acidosis and Respiratory Alkalosis

This mixed disorder is often seen in patients with advanced liver disease, salicylate intoxication, and pulmonary-renal syndromes. The respiratory alkalosis will decrease the $Paco_2$ beyond the appropriate range for the respiratory compensation usually seen with metabolic acidosis. The plasma bicarbonate concentration also decreases below the level expected in compensation for a simple respiratory alkalosis. In a sense, the defense of pH for either disorder alone is enhanced; thus the pH can be normal or close to normal, with a low $Paco_2$ and a low $[HCO_3^-]$. Treatment of this disorder should be directed at the underlying cause. Because of the enhanced compensation, the pH is usually closer to normal than in either of the two simple disorders.

Mixed Metabolic Alkalosis and Respiratory Acidosis

This mixed disorder often occurs in patients with chronic obstructive pulmonary disease and chronic respiratory acidosis who are treated with salt restriction, diuretics, and possibly glucocorticoids. When diuretics are initiated, the plasma bicarbonate may increase because of increased renal bicarbonate generation and reabsorption, providing mechanisms for both generating and maintaining metabolic alkalosis. The elevated pH diminishes respiratory drive and may therefore worsen the respiratory acidosis.

Although the pH may not deviate significantly from normal, treatment may need to be initiated to maintain Pao_2 and $Paco_2$ at acceptable levels. Because it is often difficult to correctly identify this mixed disorder, it is helpful to observe the patient's response to discontinuation of diuretics and administration of sodium and potassium chloride.[2] If the patient has a simple metabolic alkalosis, the $Paco_2$ will normalize, but it will only minimally affect the $Paco_2$ if it is a mixed disorder. Treatment should be aimed at decreasing the plasma bicarbonate with sodium and potassium chloride therapy, thereby allowing the renal excretion of retained bicarbonate from the diuretic-induced metabolic alkalosis. This therapy should be used cautiously to avoid exacerbating any underlying congestive heart failure.

EVALUATION OF THERAPEUTIC OUTCOMES

Because acid–base disorders are such a common and widespread problem, pharmacists can play a key role in identifying, preventing, and properly treating acid–base abnormalities. Acid–base disorders do not occur only in the intensive care unit setting. Patients in ambulatory and extended care settings have many chronic conditions and drug therapies that commonly affect acid–base balance. Thus pharmacists in all practice settings should use their knowledge to identify patients at high risk for developing drug-related problems which affect acid–base balance and to undertake appropriate prevention and treatment measures to improve the quality of life of the patients they care for.

ABBREVIATIONS

BW: body weight

CNS: central nervous system

DCA: dichloroacetate

ECF: extracellular fluid

H^+: hydrogen ion

HCO_3^-: bicarbonate

H_2CO_3: carbonic acid

HIV: human immunodeficiency virus

NH_4^+: ammonium

$Paco_2$: partial pressure of carbon dioxide from arterial blood

Pao_2: partial pressure of oxygen from arterial blood

pH: the negative logarithm (base 10) of the hydrogen ion concentration

pK: the negative logarithm of the dissociation constant

$Pvco_2$: partial pressure of carbon dioxide from venous blood

Pvo_2: partial pressure of oxygen from venous blood

RTA: renal tubular acidosis

SAG: serum anion gap

THAM: tromethamine (*Tris*[hydroxymethyl]-aminomethane)

UCs: unmeasured cations

UAs: unmeasured anions

REFERENCES

1. Stewart PA. Goals, definitions and basic principles. In: Kellum JA, Ebers Paul WG, ed. Stewart's Textbook of Acid-Base, 2nd ed. Amsterdam: Elsevier, 2007:36–62.

2. Constable P. Clinical acid-base chemistry. In: Ronco C, ed. Critical Care Nephrology, 2nd ed. Philadelphia, PA: Elsevier, 2009:581–614.

3. Dubose TD. Disorders of acid-base balance. In: Bremmer BM, ed. Bremmer and Rector's The Kidney, 8th ed. New York: Saunders, 2007:612–672.

4. Kamel S, Razeen-Davids M, Lin, SH et al. Interpretation of electrolytes and acid-base parameters in blood and urine. In: Bremmer BM, ed. Bremmer and Rector's The Kidney, 8th ed. New York: Saunders, 2007:898–923.

5. Morgan TJ. Unmeasured ions and the strong ion gap. In: Kellum JA, Ebers PWG, eds. Stewart's Textbook of Acid-Base, 2nd ed. Amsterdam: Elsevier, 2007:324–335.

6. Boniatti MM, Cardozo PR, Castilho RK et al. Acid-base disorders evaluation in critically ill patients: we can improve our diagnostic ability. Intensive Care Med 2009;35(8):1377–1382.

7. Adrogue HJ. Metabolic acidosis: pathophysiology, diagnosis and management. J Nephrol 2006;19(Suppl 9):S62–S69.

8. Gennari FJ, Weise WJ. Acid-base disturbances in gastrointestinal disease. Clin J Am Soc Nephrol 2008;3(6):1861–1868.

9. Ring T. Renal tubular acidosis. In: Kellum JA, Ebers PWG, eds. Stewart's Textbook of Acid-Base, 2nd ed. Amsterdam: Elsevier, 2007:408–423.

10. Schoolwerth AC, Kaneko TM, Sedlacek M et al. Acid-base disturbances in the intensive care unit: metabolic acidosis. Semin Dial 2006;19(6):492–495.

11. Morris CG, Low J. Metabolic acidosis in the critically ill: part 1. Classification and pathophysiology. Anaesthesia 2008;63(3):294–301.

12. Adrogue HJ, Madias NE. Management of life-threatening acid–base disorders I. N Engl J Med 1998;338:26–34.

13. Mizock BA. Lactic acidosis. In: Kellum JA, Ebers PWG, eds. Stewart's Textbook of Acid-Base, 2nd ed. Amsterdam: Elsevier, 2007: 376–392.

14. Topcu I, Yentur EA, Kefi A, et al. Seizures, metabolic acidosis and coma resulting from acute isoniazid intoxification. Anaesth Intensive Care 2005;33(4):518–520.

15. Lactic Acidosis International Study Group. Risk factors for lactic acidosis and severe hyperlactimia in HIV-1-infected adults exposed to antiretroviral therapy. AIDS 2007 30;21(18):2455–2464.

16. Almirall J, Briculle M, Gonzalez-Clemente JM. Metformin-associated lactic acidosis in type 2 diabetes mellitus: incidence and presentation in common clinical practice. Nephrol Dial Transplant 2008;23(7): 2436–2438.

17. Bodner M, Meier C, Krahenbuhl S, et al. Metformin, sulfonylureas, or other antidiabetes drugs and the risk of lactic acidosis or hypoglycemia: A nested case-control analysis. Diabetes Care 2008;31(11): 2086–2091.

18. Yahwak JA, Riker RR, Fraser GL, et al. Determination of a lorazepam dose threshold for using the osmol gap to monitor for propylene glycol toxicity. Pharmacotherapy 2008;28(8):984–991.

19. Bledsoe KA, Kramer AH. Propylene glycol toxicity complicating use of barbiturate coma. Neurocrit Care 2008;9(1):122–124.

20. Corbett SM, Montoya IS, Moore FA. Propofol-related infusion syndrome in intensive care patients. Pharmacotherapy 2008;28(2):250–258.

21. Zietse R, Zoutendijk R, Hoorn EJ. Fluid, electrolyte and acid-base disorders associated with antibiotic therapy. Nat Rev Nephrol 2009;5(4):193–202.

22. Kato K, Sugiura S, Yano K, et al. The latent risk of acidosis in commercially available total parenteral nutrition (TPN) products: a randomized clinical trial in postoperative patients. J Clin Biochem Nutr 2009;45(1):68–73.

23. Shiber JR. Severe non-anion gap metabolic acidosis induced by topiramate: A case-report. J Emerg Med 2010;38(4):494–496.

24. Adrogues HJ. Mixed acid-base disturbances. J Nephrol 2006;19 (Suppl 9):S97–S103.

25. Albert MS, Dell RB, Winters RW. Quantitative displacement of acid–base equilibrium in metabolic acidosis. Ann Intern Med 1964;66: 312–322.

26. Kraut JA. The role of metabolic acidosis in the pathogenesis of renal osteodystrophy. Adv Ren Replace Ther 1995;2:40–51.

27. Chadra V, Alon US. Hereditary renal tubular disorders. Semin Nephrol 2009;29(4):399–411.

28. Thomas KW, Schmidt GA. Alkanizing therapy in the management of acid-base disorder. In: Ronco C, ed. Critical Care Nephrology, 2nd ed. Philadelphia, PA: Elsevier, 2009:685–713.

29. Cooper DJ, Walley KR, Wiggs BR, Russell JA. Bicarbonate does not improve hemodynamics in critically ill patients who have lactic acidosis: A prospective controlled clinical study. Ann Intern Med 1990;112:492–498.

30. Kaplan LJ, Frangos S. Clinical review: Acid–base abnormalities in the intensive care unit-part II. Crit Care 2005;9:198–203.

31. Forsythe SM, Schmidt GA. Sodium bicarbonate for the treatment of lactic acidosis. Chest 2000;117:260–267.

32. Adrogue HJ, Rashad MN, Gorin AB, et al. Assessing acid–base status in circulatory failure: Differences between arterial and central venous blood. N Engl J Med 1989;320:1312–1316.

33. Kellum JA. Disorders of acid-base balance. Crit Care Med 2007;35(11):2630–2636.

34. Emergency Cardiac Care Committee and Subcommittees, American Heart Association. Guidelines for cardiopulmonary resuscitation and emergency cardiovascular care. Circulation 2005;112:IV-1–IV-211.

35. Spohr F, Wenzel V, Bottinger BW. Thrombolyis and other drugs during cardiopulmonary resuscitation. Curr Opin Crit Care 2008;14(3): 292–298.

36. McEvoy GK, Litvak K, Welsh OH, et al. American Hospital Formulary Service, Drug Information. Bethesda, MD: American Society of Health-System Pharmacists, 2011.

37. Geraci MJ, Klipa D, Heckman MG et al. Prevalence of sodium bicarbonate-induced alkalemia in cardiopulmonary arrest patients. Ann Pharmacother 2009;43:1245–1250.

38. Hoste EA, Colpaert K, Vanholder RC et al. Sodium bicarbonate versus THAM in ICU patients with mild metabolic acidosis. J Nephrol 2005;18(3):303–307.

39. Leung JM, Landow L, Franks M, et al. Safety and efficacy of intravenous Carbicarb in patients undergoing surgery: Comparison with sodium bicarbonate in the treatment of mild metabolic acidosis. Crit Care Med 1994;22:1540–1549.

40. Shapiro JI. Functional and metabolic responses of the isolated heart during acidosis: Effects of sodium bicarbonate and Carbicarb. Am J Physiol 1990;258:H1835–H1839.

41. Shapiro JI. Pathogenesis of cardiac dysfunction during metabolic acidosis: Therapeutic implications. Kidney Int 1997;51:47–51.

42. Bersin RM, Arieff AI. Improved hemodynamic function during hypoxia with Carbicarb, a new agent for the management of acidosis. Circulation 1988;77:227–233.

43. Stacpoole PW, Wright EC, Baumgartner TG, et al. A controlled clinical trial of dichloroacetate for treatment of lactic acidosis. N Engl J Med 1992;327:1564–1569.

44. Stacpoole PW, Nagaraja NV, Hutson AD. Efficacy of dichloroacetate as a lactate-lowering drug. J Clin Pharmacol 2003;43:683–691.

45. Shangraw RE, Lohan-Mannion D, Hayes A, et al. Dichloroacetate stabilizes the intraoperative acid-base balance during liver transplantation. Liver Transpl 2008;14(7):989–998.

46. Vary TC, Siegel JH, Zechnich A, et al. Pharmacologic reversal of abnormal glucose regulation, BCAA utilization, and muscle catabolism in sepsis by dichloroacetate. J Trauma 1988;28:1301–1311.

47. Khanna A, Kurtzman NA. Metabolic alkalosis. J Nephrol 2006;19 (Suppl 9):S86–S96.

48. Mikhalidis G, Mikhailidis DP, Elisaf M. Acid-base and electrolyte abnormalities observed in patients receiving cardiovascular drugs. J Cardiovasc Pharmacol Ther 2003;8:267–279.

49. Adrogue HJ, Madias NE. Management of life-threatening acid–base disorders II. N Engl J Med 1998;338:107–111.

50. Barton CH, Vaziri ND, Ness RL, et al. Cimetidine in the management of metabolic alkalosis induced by nasogastric drainage. Arch Surg 1979;1:70–74.

51. Mazur JE, Devlin JW, Peters MJ, et al. Single versus multiple doses of acetazolamide for metabolic alkalosis in critically ill medical patients: a randomized, double-blind trial. Crit Care Med 1999;27(7):1257–1261.

52. Rowlands BJ, Tindall SF, Elliot DJ. The use of dilute hydrochloric acid and cimetidine to reverse severe metabolic alkalosis. Postgrad Med J 1978;54:118–123.

53. Mirtallo JM, Rogers KR, Johnson JA, et al. Stability of amino acids and the availability of acid in total parenteral nutrition solutions containing hydrochloric acid. Am J Hosp Pharm 1981;38:1729–1731.

54. Foster GT, Vaziri ND, Sassoon CS. Respiratory alkalosis. Respir Care 2001;46:384–391.

55. Roser M, Eibl N, Eisenhaber B, et al. Gitelman síndrome. Hypertension 2009;53(6):893–897.

56. Hene RJ, Koomans HA, Dorhout Mees EJ, et al. Correction of hypokalemia in Bartter's syndrome by enalapril. Am J Kidney Dis 1987;9:200–205.

57. Vinci JM, Gill JR Jr, Bowden RE, et al. The kallikrein-kinin system in Bartter's syndrome and its response to prostaglandin synthetase inhibition. J Clin Invest 1987;61:1671–1682.

58. Goldfarb S, Sharma K. Acid-base balance. In: Fishman AP, et al, ed. Fishman's Pulmonary Diseases and Disorders, 4th ed. New York: McGraw-Hill, 2008:717–742.

CHAPTER

62

Evaluation of Neurologic Illness

SUSAN C. FAGAN AND FENWICK T. NICHOLS

KEY CONCEPTS

❶ The clinical neurologic history and examination are the cornerstones of neurologic diagnosis and management.

❷ Through the patient's history one can determine the main symptoms, the mode of onset (gradual or sudden), progression over time (maximal at onset or steadily gaining intensity), and associated illnesses/risk factors.

❸ The neurologic examination is directed at localization of the disease process so that evaluation and management may be planned appropriately.

❹ The neurologic examination of a specific patient may be adapted to the patient's specific deficit. For example, a patient with double vision may warrant an extensive cranial nerve examination but a less extensive assessment of finger strength.

To contribute most effectively to the care of patients with neurologic illness, one must understand the tools used in the diagnosis and management of these patients. In addition, clinicians must be able to gather their own data through a targeted neurologic examination and history taking to ensure optimal pharmacotherapy in neurologic patients. Despite technologic advances that have led to the development of sensitive diagnostic tests in neuroscience, the clinical neurologic history and examination are still the cornerstones of the neurologic diagnosis and management.[1]

SIGNS AND SYMPTOMS

❶ As in all of medicine, obtaining an accurate and complete history is of utmost importance in the evaluation of neurologic diseases. In many instances, the diagnosis can be made on the basis

Learning objectives, review questions, and other resources can be found at **www.pharmacotherapyonline.com**.

of the history, and the neurologic examination can be tailored to optimally evaluate the patient and confirm the diagnosis. The clinician depends on the patient or family for the details of the illness. Care must be taken to avoid "leading" the patient. Obtaining an accurate history may be difficult because a number of neurologic diseases may affect patients' speech and memory. ❷ Through the patient's history one can determine the main symptoms, the mode of onset (gradual or sudden), progression over time (maximal at onset or steadily gaining intensity), and associated illnesses/risk factors (recent head injury from a motor vehicle accident). The physical examination is important because it can reveal evidence of systemic disease that may have affected the nervous system secondarily (e.g., a seizure in a patient with elevated temperature and stiff neck may suggest meningitis). The neurologic examination is only one component of a complete general physical examination.

THE NEUROLOGIC EXAMINATION

❸ An assessment of patient effort is necessary to interpret the results of the neurologic examination. It can identify any abnormalities, particularly asymmetry of function, and help to localize the lesion within the nervous system (central versus peripheral and specific location within the central nervous system [CNS] or the peripheral nervous system). The neurologic examination consists of six main components: higher cortical function (mental status), cranial nerves, motor function, reflexes, sensory function, and gait. Table 62–1 describes the common approaches to assessing each of the six domains and includes examples of the diseases in which abnormal findings are common.

❹ A targeted neurologic examination can be performed when a specific deficit is suspected. Table 62–2 describes the cranial nerve examination in more detail. The reader is encouraged to consult other references to better understand the intricacies of the neurologic examination. The clinician must synthesize the results of the history and physical examination to arrive at an anatomic localization of the lesion and create a differential diagnosis.

PROCEDURES USED IN THE DIAGNOSIS

In addition to the neurologic examination, certain imaging techniques and procedures may be essential in the diagnosis of neurologic disorders. Lumbar puncture is used to obtain cerebrospinal

TABLE 62-1 The Neurologic Examination

Domain	Tests Performed	Diseases
Mental status	While obtaining the history: general mental and emotional status, speech, memory, alertness, abstract reasoning, ability to follow commands (motor integration), ability to communicate	Dementias, stroke, metabolic encephalopathies
Cranial nerves	Visual acuity, visual fields, eye movements, jaw strength, corneal reflex, facial symmetry, auditory acuity, gag reflex, shoulder and neck strength	Myasthenia gravis, Parkinson's disease, stroke, amyotrophic lateral sclerosis (ALS)
Motor function	Motor strength with and without resistance, coordination (rapid alternating movements, finger-to-nose), tremors, atrophy, fasciculations	Stroke, myasthenia gravis, Parkinson's disease, ALS
Reflexes	Biceps, triceps, tendon reflexes, plantar response (Babinski sign is an upgoing toe and is abnormal), superficial cutaneous reflexes (abdominal)	Stroke, spinal cord lesions, endocrine diseases (e.g., diabetes, hypothyroidism), peripheral neuropathy
Sensory function	Asymmetry to pinprick, vibration, temperature	Stroke, peripheral neuropathy, migraine aura, diabetes, spinal cord lesions
Gait	Walking, standing (Romberg test = eyes closed, which will accentuate disequilibrium)	Stroke, Parkinson's disease, spinal cord lesions

TABLE 62-2 Cranial Nerve Function and Examples of Testing

I. Olfactory nerve. Smell: identify odors (coffee, cinnamon, lemon; test each nostril separately).
II. Optic nerve. Visual acuity: eye chart. Visual fields: peripheral vision and blind spot; funduscopic exam; pupil size and reaction; color vision (rarely done)
III. Oculomotor (cranial nerves III, IV, and VI have similar functions and are tested as a unit). Eye movements: patient is asked to watch a light as it moved up, down, and on both sides, while eye movements are observed.
IV. Trochlear. See III.
V. Trigeminal nerve. Motor: tests power of jaw opening and sideways deviation against the resistance of a hand placed against the jaw. Sensory: test corneal reflex by touching cornea (also nasal mucosa) with a wisp of cotton.
VI. Abducens. See III.
VII. Facial nerve. Observe asymmetry of face at rest or on speaking, baring teeth, raising eyebrows, or wrinkling forehead. Reflex eye closure to a threatening movement. Glabellar tap: repetitive tapping over bridge of nose–initial blinking should cease after the first few taps.
VIII. Auditory nerve. Vestibular division: observe for nystagmus, positional testing. Auditory division: test acuity with light sound; watch, whisper, rubbing of fingers close to ear.
IX. Glossopharyngeal nerve. Test for gag reflex by touching back of throat with tongue depressor; test swallowing and coughing and note any drooling or pooling of saliva. Test symmetry of palate movement on vocalizing "ah."
X. Vagus nerve. Test gag reflex as in IX.
XI. Spinal accessory nerve. Trapezius and sternomastoid muscles: test power of shrugging shoulders and turning the head to one side against resistance.
XII. Hypoglossal nerve. Motor function of tongue. Look for wasting and abnormal movements.

fluid (CSF). It is used most often as an evaluation of CNS infections such as meningitis and encephalitis, but it is also useful in subarachnoid hemorrhage, multiple sclerosis, and dementia. Opening pressure, cell count and differential, glucose concentration, total protein concentration, and culture and sensitivity are obtained routinely. A space-occupying lesion in the brain with mass effect is a relative contraindication to lumbar puncture because herniation could result. Prior to performing a lumbar puncture, the patient should be checked for papilledema, which may indicate increased intracranial pressure. The opening CSF pressure usually is less than 180 mm H_2O. Normal CSF is clear and colorless and should not contain any red blood cells or polymorphonuclear cells. The presence of up to five mononuclear cells is considered normal. Total protein in the CSF usually is 45 mg/dL or less. Protein may increase with infection, breakdown of the blood–brain barrier (e.g., tumors, stroke, and trauma), and diabetes.

Electroencephalography (EEG) records the electrical activity of the brain. The record is interpreted by observing the basic rhythms and waveforms, the symmetry of the recording, and abnormal electrical discharges. It also may be used to assess the response to photic stimulation or hyperventilation. It is used primarily in the diagnosis of seizures and may be helpful in the evaluation of patients with altered mental status. EEG also may be used to measure evoked potentials. The evoked potentials are the EEG response to repetitive stimuli (visual, auditory, or tactile) and provide information about the presence of abnormalities and disturbances (but not the cause) in the specific pathways tested.

Electromyography (EMG) and nerve conduction velocities (NCVs) are used to assess the function of the peripheral nerves, neuromuscular junction, and muscles. NCVs are measured by stimulating the nerve and recording the speed of conduction of the impulse. NCVs can be used to detect the presence of localized peripheral nerve injuries (e.g., carpal tunnel) or diffuse symmetric neuropathies (which may be inherited or acquired). EMG assesses muscle dysfunction as a result of primary muscle disease or secondary to nerve injury. This test is used to diagnose peripheral neuropathies (inherited and acquired), Guillain-Barré syndrome, myasthenia gravis, amyotrophic lateral sclerosis, radiculopathies, and muscle diseases.

The cerebral circulatory system can be imaged or evaluated in a number of different ways depending on the type and location of the abnormality suspected. Imaging techniques can be used to identify local arterial stenosis, aneurysms, or arteriovenous malformations. Atherosclerosis of the extracranial arteries, a frequent cause of stroke, can be evaluated using ultrasound (referred to as duplex sonography, carotid Doppler, or color-flow Doppler), magnetic resonance angiography (MRA), spiral computed tomographic angiography (CTA), or intraarterial angiography. The intracranial arterial circulation can be evaluated using transcranial Doppler, MRA, CTA, or intraarterial angiography. Each technique has its own advantages and disadvantages. Intraarterial angiography provides the best imaging of the smaller arteries of the cerebral circulation but is more invasive than the other measures.

Computed tomography (CT) uses x-rays to produce images of "slices" of the brain that are 1 to 10 mm in thickness. CT revolutionized the practice of neurology by allowing direct imaging of the brain anatomy. CT is currently available in most communities and is used to evaluate patients with intracranial disease. CT scans are used to identify tumors, hemorrhages, infarctions, hydrocephalus, and atrophy. Intravenous contrast agents (a contrast-enhanced scan) can be administered to enhance the image of blood vessels and areas of blood–brain barrier damage that may be caused by abscesses, other inflammatory conditions, tumors, or stroke.

Magnetic resonance imaging (MRI) uses the magnetic properties of the hydrogen atom nucleus and proton to produce computer-processed scans that provide improved anatomic detail when compared with CT scans. MRI offers the advantages of better differentiating between white and gray matter and delineating lesions close to bone (brainstem and cerebellum) and has no radiation risk;

however, it is not as readily available as CT and is more expensive. MRI has a proven advantage over CT in evaluating lesions in the posterior fossa and in detecting lesions in the white matter, such as plaques in multiple sclerosis. MRI is also useful in the diagnosis of tumors and very early ischemic stroke (diffusion-weighted imaging). Imaging of the spinal canal and its contents can be accomplished either by MRI myelography or CT myelography.

Other imaging techniques such as positron emission tomography (PET) and single-photon emission computed tomography (SPECT) are considered tests of brain function. These tests are being studied extensively in epilepsy as well as in cerebrovascular disorders, cerebral tumors, movement disorders, and dementia. PET scans use a positron-emitting isotope to display chemical activity and the rates of biologic processes within the brain. This method can assess regional metabolic changes in the brain. The expense, technical complexity (a cyclotron is needed), and limited availability of this technique limit its clinical usefulness.

SPECT scans measure radiotracer uptake by tissues and provide cross-sectional images of the brain. This technique has been used extensively to assess cerebral blood flow. Although the resolution of SPECT is not as good as PET, the availability has led to wide clinical use in disorders such as stroke, dementia, and epilepsy.

CONCLUSION

Assessment of the patient with neurologic disease is challenging. The patient by virtue of the neurologic deficit, may or may not be able to provide reliable information regarding medication history or extent of illness. The clinician must develop alternate strategies to obtain a complete data set and develop a pharmacotherapy plan. Ability to interpret and synthesize the results of the neurologic examination and other diagnostic tests will help a great deal in this quest.

ABBREVIATIONS

CNS: central nervous system

CSF: cerebrospinal fluid

CT: computed tomography

CTA: computed tomography angiography

EEG: electroencephalogram

EMG: electromyography

MRA: magnetic resonance angiography

MRI: magnetic resonance imaging

NCVs: nerve conduction velocities

PET: positron-emission tomography

SPECT: single-photon emission computed tomography

REFERENCE

1. Campbell WW. DeJong's The Neurologic Examination, 6th ed. Philadelphia, PA: Lippincott Williams & Wilkins, 2005.

CHAPTER

63

Alzheimer's Disease

PATRICIA W. SLATTUM, RUSSELL H. SWERDLOW, AND ANGELA MASSEY HILL

KEY CONCEPTS

❶ Alzheimer's disease (AD) is the most common form of dementing illness, and the prevalence of AD increases with each decade of life.

❷ The etiology of AD is unknown, and current pharmacotherapy neither cures nor arrests the pathophysiology.

❸ Neuritic plaques and neurofibrillary tangles are the pathologic hallmarks of AD; however, the definitive cause of this disease is yet to be determined.

❹ AD affects multiple areas of cognition and is characterized by a gradual onset with a slow, progressive decline.

❺ A thorough physical examination (including neurologic examination), as well as laboratory and imaging studies, is required to rule out other disorders and diagnose AD before considering drug therapy.

❻ Pharmacotherapy for AD focuses on impacting three domains: cognition, behavioral and psychiatric symptoms, and functional ability.

❼ Nondrug therapy and social support for the patient and family are the primary treatment interventions for AD.

❽ Cholinesterase inhibitors and memantine are used to treat cognitive symptoms of AD; other medications have been suggested to be beneficial because of their potential preventive or cognitive effects.

❾ Appropriate management of vascular disease risk factors may reduce the risk for developing AD and may prevent the worsening of dementia in patients with AD.

❿ A thorough behavioral assessment and plan with careful examination of environmental factors should be conducted before initiating drug therapy for behavioral symptoms.

⓫ Pharmacotherapy may reduce the total cost of treating AD by delaying cognitive decline and time to nursing home placement.

"I now begin the journey that will lead me into the sunset of my life."
Ronald Reagan

Learning objectives, review questions, and other resources can be found at **www.pharmacotherapyonline.com**.

Alzheimer's disease (AD), first characterized by Alois Alzheimer in 1907, is a gradually progressive dementia affecting cognition, behavior, and functional status. The exact pathophysiologic mechanisms underlying AD are not entirely known, and no cure exists.[1] Although drugs may reduce AD symptoms for a time, the disease is eventually fatal.

AD profoundly affects the family as well as the patient. The need for supervision and assistance increases until the late stages of the disease, when AD patients become totally dependent on a family member, spouse, or other caregiver for all of their basic needs. These are the all-too-common experiences of the millions of people in the United States who care for someone with AD.

EPIDEMIOLOGY

❶ AD is the most common cause of dementia, accounting for 50% to 60% of cases of late-life cognitive dysfunction. Its prevalence among dementia patients increases to 80% if AD lesions in conjunction with other pathologic brain lesions are considered.[2] Table 63–1 lists the most common types of dementia among older adults. Dementia in an individual can result from multiple etiologies. This chapter focuses exclusively on dementia of the Alzheimer's type. However, the reader is encouraged to use the nonpharmacologic approaches and management of behavioral problems outlined in this chapter as a general treatment approach for other types of dementia that may share similar features with AD.

Approximately 5.3 million Americans have AD.[3,4] By the year 2050, 1 in 5 people will be older than age 65 years, and the number of AD patients is projected to be 13.2 million (Fig. 63–1). Most cases present in persons older than age 65 years, but approximately 5% of cases occur in persons younger than age 65 years. Onset can be as early as age 40 years, resulting in the arbitrary age classifications of early onset (age 40–64 years) and late onset (age 65 years and older).[4,5]

Increasing age is the greatest risk factor for AD.[4] The prevalence of AD increases exponentially with age, affecting approximately 7% of individuals age 65 to 74 years, 53% of those age 75 to 84 years, and 40% of persons age 85 years and older.[3] Genetic inheritance is also a significant risk factor, although other factors may contribute. Factors determining age of onset and rate of progression remain largely undefined.

TABLE 63-1	Common Types of Dementia in Late Life

Alzheimer's disease
Vascular dementia
Lewy body dementia
Frontotemporal dementia, including Pick's disease
Reversible causes of dementia (e.g., normal-pressure hydrocephalus, thyroid dysfunction, vitamin B_{12} deficiency, depression)

Data from Reisberg,[90] Rubin,[47] and Chapman et al.[91]

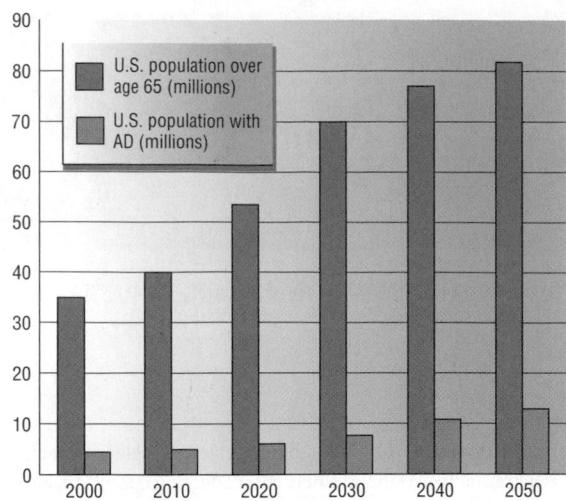

FIGURE 63-1. Our aging population. The percentage of U.S. population older than age 65 years and the percentage with AD projected from years 2000 to 2050. (*Estimates based on data from references 88 and 89.*)

Survival following AD diagnosis is typically 4 to 6 years.[4] AD is the fifth leading cause of death for those age 65 years and older in the United States.[4] AD may not cause death directly. The most common cause of death in patients with AD is pneumonia, possibly resulting from eating problems in the terminal stage of the disease.[6,7]

ETIOLOGY AND GENETICS

❷ The exact etiology of AD is unknown; however, several genetic and environmental factors have been explored as potential causes of AD. Dominantly inherited forms of AD account for less than 1% of cases.[4,8] More than half of early-onset, dominantly inherited cases of AD can be attributed to alterations on chromosomes 1, 14, or 21. The majority and most aggressive early-onset cases are attributed to mutations of a gene located on chromosome 14, which produces a protein called presenilin 1.[5] A structurally similar protein, presenilin 2, is produced by a gene on chromosome 1. Both presenilin 1 and presenilin 2 encode for membrane proteins that may be involved in amyloid precursor protein (APP) processing. Scientists have identified more than 160 mutations in presenilin genes, and these mutations appear to result in reduced activity of γ-secretase, an enzyme important in β-amyloid peptide (βAP) formation.[5] APP is encoded on chromosome 21. Only a small number of early-onset familial AD cases have been associated with mutations in the *APP* gene, resulting in overproduction of βAP or an increase in the proportion of βAP ending at residue 42.[5]

Genetic susceptibility to sporadic, late-onset AD is thought to be primarily linked to the apolipoprotein E (*APOE*) genotype.[5,8,9] Thus far, the contribution of other candidate genes appears to be minor, although AD may be a heterogeneous disease resulting from complex interactions among multiple susceptibility genes and environmental factors. The gene responsible for the production of *APOE* is located on chromosome 19. There are three major subtypes or alleles of *APOE* (e.g., *2, *3, and *4). Humans inherit one copy of the *APOE* gene from each parent. Inheritance of the *APOE*4* allele is believed to account for much of the genetic risk in sporadic AD. The mechanism through which *APOE*4* confers an increased risk is unknown, although *APOE*4* is associated with other factors that may contribute to AD pathology, such as abnormalities in mitochondria, cytoskeletal dysfunction, and low glucose usage.[5] The risk for AD is 2- to 3-fold higher in individuals with one *APOE*4* allele and 12-fold higher in individuals with

two *APOE*4* alleles compared to those with no *APOE*4* alleles.[9] Moreover, onset of symptoms occurs at a relatively younger age as compared with patients having zero or only one copy of *APOE*4* in their genotype.[9] The strength of association is not the same across all races however.[1] Although inheritance of the *APOE*4* allele increases the risk of AD, it is not diagnostic or even essential for disease presence.

Genetic factors have been linked to both early- and late-onset AD. Alterations to chromosomes 1, 14, and 21 are associated with early-onset AD, whereas the presence of *APOE*4* alleles increases risk of developing late-onset AD. Genetic explanatory factors continue to be investigated.[5,8] However, genetic causes of AD have been directly associated with only a small percentage of Alzheimer's patients, and the exact cause of AD remains unknown.

ENVIRONMENTAL AND OTHER FACTORS

A number of environmental factors are associated with an increased risk of AD, including age, decreased reserve capacity of the brain (reduced brain size, low educational level, and reduced mental and physical activity in late life), head injury, Down syndrome, depression, herpes simplex, and risk factors for vascular disease (hypercholesterolemia, hypertension, atherosclerosis, coronary heart disease, elevated homocysteine, obesity, and diabetes).[1,4] Whether these vascular risk factors are true causal risk factors for AD contributing to AD pathology, or whether they result in cerebrovascular pathology that, in turn, contributes to the symptoms of AD, remains to be established.

The incidence of AD rises with increasing age, so that among centenarians the histopathologic and clinical changes needed to justify a diagnosis of AD probably coexist in more than 90% of these individuals.[10–12] One oft-quoted study concluded that almost half those older than age 85 years have AD.[13] AD may develop in individuals over the course of decades,[14,15] suggesting that AD is a disease most people are in the process of developing throughout adulthood. The debate about whether tangle-and-plaque dementia is a distinct disease or part of aging remains unresolved. An in-depth discussion of the aging—AD controversy is not possible in this chapter; it is reviewed elsewhere.[16,17]

PATHOPHYSIOLOGY

❸ The signature lesions in AD are neuritic plaques and neurofibrillary tangles (NFTs) located in the cortical areas and medial temporal lobe structures of the brain.[1] Along with these lesions, degeneration of neurons and synapses, as well as cortical atrophy occurs. Plaques and NFTs may also be present in other diseases, even in normal aging, but at least in younger demographics there tends to be a higher burden of plaques and NFTs in AD-affected subjects than there is in age-matched controls. Several mechanisms have been proposed to explain changes in the brain that result in the symptoms of AD, including misfolding of proteins (βAP aggregation and deposition leading to the formation of plaques and hyperphosphorylation of tau protein leading to NFT development); synaptic failure and depletion of neurotrophin and neurotransmitters; and mitochondrial dysfunction (oxidative stress, impaired insulin signaling in the brain, vascular injury, inflammatory processes, loss of calcium regulation, and defects in cholesterol metabolism).[2]

AMYLOID CASCADE HYPOTHESIS

Neuritic plaques (also termed amyloid or senile plaques) are extracellular lesions found in the brain and cerebral vasculature. Plaques from AD brains largely consist of a protein called β-amyloid protein (Aβ). Aβ peptides consisting of 36 to 43 amino acids are produced via processing of a larger protein, APP. Aβ_{42} is less common than other Aβ peptides, but is prone to aggregation and plaque formation.[2] The amyloid cascade hypothesis states that there is an imbalance between the production and clearance of Aβ peptides resulting in aggregation that causes accumulation of Aβ and ultimately leading to AD.[2] Studies on the genetic forms of AD, including early-onset AD and Down syndrome led to the formulation of the amyloid cascade hypothesis. The amyloid cascade hypothesis has substantially evolved since it was initially proposed. While Aβ sequestered in plaques was at first believed to represent the critical toxic species, more recent versions of the hypothesis assume Aβ that is not sequestered in plaques actually drives the disease.[2] Even so, the amyloid cascade hypothesis seems most applicable in cases of early-onset, autosomal dominant AD. However, such cases comprise less than 1% of AD, and it is not clear whether it is reasonable to etiologically extrapolate to the late-onset form (which afflicts the vast majority of those affected). Whether individuals with late-onset AD also carry genetic variations that promote a primary Aβ amyloidosis remains to be shown. If this turns out not to be the case, the possibility that amyloidosis in late-onset AD is secondary to a more upstream event will require consideration. Before this conceptual conundrum is laid to rest, however, the amyloid cascade hypothesis will likely undergo a therapy-based practical test. If treatments that efficiently reduce βAP production or remove brain βAP fail to arrest disease progression, it would argue amyloidosis is not the primary pathology in most of those with AD.

NEUROFIBRILLARY TANGLES

As Aβ was being identified in plaques, other researchers showed that NFTs are commonly found in the cells of the hippocampus and cerebral cortex in persons with AD and are composed of abnormally hyperphosphorylated tau protein. Tau protein provides structural support to microtubules, the cell's transportation and skeletal support system.[2] When tau filaments undergo abnormal phosphorylation at a specific site, they cannot bind effectively to microtubules, and the microtubules collapse. Without an intact system of microtubules, the cell cannot function properly and eventually dies. The density of the NFTs correlates well with the severity of the dementia, because they are a hallmark of neuronal death.[2] NFTs are found in other dementing illnesses besides AD, and may represent a common method by which various inciting factors culminate in cell death.[2]

INFLAMMATORY MEDIATORS

Inflammatory or immunologic paradigms are often viewed as a corollary of the amyloid cascade hypothesis. Certainly, brain amyloid deposition associates with local inflammatory and immunologic alterations. This line of observation led some to propose that inflammation is relevant to AD neurodegeneration.[2] The inflammatory/immunologic hypotheses argue that although Aβ may have direct neurotoxicity, at least some of its toxicity might actually be an indirect consequence of an Aβ protofibril-induced microglia activation and astrocyte recruitment. This inflammatory response may represent an attempt to clear amyloid deposition. However, it is also associated with release of cytokines, nitric oxide, and other radical species, and complement factors that can both injure neurons and promote ongoing inflammation.[2] Indeed, levels of multiple cytokines and chemokines are elevated in AD brains, and certain proinflammatory gene polymorphisms are reported to be associated with AD.[2]

Consistent with these molecular observations are epidemiologic data suggesting that exposure to nonsteroidal antiinflammatory drugs (NSAIDs) may reduce AD risk.[18,19] However, multiple prospective short duration trials of NSAIDs in AD prevention and of NSAIDs as AD treatment have been therapeutically disappointing.[2] Interestingly, the conceptual impetus for trying NSAIDs in AD has radically shifted in recent years. Rather than postulate that clinical benefits (if any are shown to exist) might derive from an antiinflammatory effect, current thinking is that any observed benefits would reflect the ability of some NSAIDs to alter APP processing away from its 42-amino-acid degradation product (Aβ_{42}).

THE CHOLINERGIC HYPOTHESIS

Multiple neuronal pathways are destroyed in AD. Neuronal damage can be seen in conjunction with plaque structures.[2] Widespread cell dysfunction or degeneration results in a variety of neurotransmitter deficits, with cholinergic abnormalities being the most prominent.[2] Loss of cholinergic activity correlates with AD severity. In late AD, the number of cholinergic neurons is reduced, and there is loss of nicotinic receptors in the hippocampus and cortex. Presynaptic nicotinic receptors control the release of acetylcholine, as well as other neurotransmitters important for memory and mood, including glutamate, serotonin, and norepinephrine.[2]

The discovery of vast cholinergic cell loss led to the development of a cholinergic hypothesis linked to the pathophysiology of AD. The cholinergic hypothesis targeted cholinergic cell loss as the source of memory and cognitive impairment in AD. Consequently, it was presumed that increasing cholinergic function would improve symptoms of memory loss. This approach is flawed for two reasons. First, cholinergic cell loss appears to be a secondary consequence of Alzheimer's pathology, not the disease-producing event; second, cholinergic neurons are only one of many neuronal pathways destroyed in AD. It is increasingly clear that simple addition of acetylcholine cannot compensate for the loss of neurons, receptors, and other neurotransmitters lost during the course of the illness. Thus the goal is to minimize or improve symptoms through augmentation of neurotransmission at remaining synapses.

OTHER NEUROTRANSMITTER ABNORMALITIES

Although the cholinergic system has received particular attention in AD pharmaceutical research, deficits also exist in other neuronal pathways. For example, serotonergic neurons of the raphe nuclei and noradrenergic cells of the locus ceruleus are lost, while monoamine oxidase type B activity is increased. Monoamine oxidase type B is found predominantly in the brain and in platelets, and is responsible for metabolizing dopamine. In addition, abnormalities appear in glutamate pathways of the cortex and limbic structures, where a loss of neurons leads to a focus on excitotoxicity models as possible contributing factors to AD pathology.

Glutamate is the major excitatory neurotransmitter in the cortex and hippocampus. Many neuronal pathways essential to learning and memory use glutamate as a neurotransmitter, including the pyramidal neurons (a layer of neurons with long axons carrying information out of the cortex), hippocampus, and entorhinal cortex. Glutamate and other excitatory amino acid neurotransmitters have been implicated as potential neurotoxins in AD.[20] In experimental models if glutamate is allowed to remain in the synapse for extended periods of time, it can destroy nerve cells. Toxic effects are thought to be mediated through increased intracellular calcium and accumulation of intracellular free radicals.[20] Dysregulated glutamate activity is thought to be one of the primary mediators of neuronal injury after stroke or acute brain injury. Although intimately involved in cell injury, the role of excitatory amino acids in AD is as yet unclear; however, blockade of N-methyl-D-aspartate (NMDA) receptors decreases activity of glutamate in the synapse and may hypothetically lessen the degree of cellular injury in AD.

BRAIN VASCULAR DISEASE AND HIGH CHOLESTEROL

There is growing evidence of a causal association between cardiovascular disease and its risk factors and the incidence of AD. Cardiovascular risk factors that are also risk factors for dementia include hypertension, elevated low-density lipoprotein cholesterol, low high-density lipoprotein cholesterol, and, particularly, diabetes.[21] Brain vascular disease may augment the cognitive impairment observed for a given amount of AD pathology in the brain. Dysfunctional blood vessels may impair nutrient delivery to neurons and reduce clearance of Aβ from the brain.[2] In addition, vascular disease may accelerate amyloid deposition and increase amyloid toxicity to neurons.[44] Controlling high blood pressure is associated with reduced rate of progression of dementia.[45] Diabetes may increase the risk of dementia through factors related to "metabolic syndrome" (dyslipidemia and hypertension), effects of potentially toxic glucose metabolites on the brain and vasculature, and through insulin itself.[21] Disturbances in insulin-signaling pathways, both in the periphery and the brain, have been linked to AD. Insulin may also regulate the metabolism of Aβ and tau protein.[2]

Research has found multiple links between cholesterol and the occurrence of AD. Apolipoprotein E is a lipoprotein that is synthesized in the liver, central nervous system, and cerebrospinal fluid. It is responsible for transporting cholesterol in the blood through the brain. It is carried by low-density lipoprotein into neurons and binds to NFTs. Apo E4 is associated with increasing deposition of Aβ and is thought to act as an accelerating modulator in the course of vascular dementia. The elevated cholesterol levels in brain neurons may alter membrane functioning and result in the cascade leading to plaque formation and AD.

OTHER MECHANISMS

Other hypotheses proposed to explain AD pathogenesis include oxidative stress, mitochondrial dysfunction, and postmenopausal loss of estrogen in women. Each of these mechanisms may contribute to AD pathogenesis, but the extent of the contribution is uncertain. There is a growing body of evidence of a role for oxidative stress and the accumulation of free radicals in the brain of AD patients.[2] Some epidemiologic studies suggest vitamin E, and possibly the combination of vitamin E and vitamin C, may reduce AD risk while others do not.[2] Mitochondrial dysfunction may result in disruption of energy metabolism in the neuron.[2] Estrogen is thought to be involved in promoting neuronal growth, and in preventing oxidative damage, which would benefit cells exposed to Aβ.[22] Estrogen receptors are present in the brain, and are distributed in a pattern consistent with areas destroyed in AD.[22] Estrogen may be important in maintaining normal cholinergic neurotransmission.[22] Estrogen may also increase NMDA receptor numbers in brain areas involved in recording new memories and prevent cell damage by acting as an antioxidant.[22] Additional mechanisms postulated for estrogen's involvement in maintaining memory function are related to the fact that it increases cerebral blood flow and glucose use, reduces plasma levels of Apo E, and blunts stress-related glucocorticoid release. Postmenopausal loss of estrogen may, therefore, impact maintenance of memory functions.

A single common mechanism for producing AD does not exist. Regardless of the source, however, the features remain the same: degeneration of neurons in higher brain areas; accumulation of NFTs and neuritic plaques; profound destruction of cholinergic pathways; and an insidious dementia, slowly progressive until death.

TABLE 63-2	Stages of Alzheimer's Disease
Mild (MMSE score 26–18)	Patient has difficulty remembering recent events. Ability to manage finances, prepare food, and carry out other household activities declines. May get lost while driving. Begins to withdraw from difficult tasks and to give up hobbies. May deny memory problems.
Moderate (MMSE score 17–10)	Patient requires assistance with activities of daily living. Frequently disoriented with regard to time (date, year, season). Recall for recent events is severely impaired. May forget some details of past life and names of family and friends. Functioning may fluctuate from day to day. Patient generally denies problems. May become suspicious or tearful. Loses ability to drive safely. Agitation, paranoia, and delusions are common.
Severe (MMSE score 9–0)	Patient loses ability to speak, walk, and feed self. Incontinent of urine and feces. Requires care 24 hours a day, 7 days a week.

MMSE, Mini-Mental Status Examination.
Data from Burns and Iliffe,[1] Alzheimer's Association,[4] Rubin.[47]

CLINICAL PRESENTATION OF ALZHEIMER'S DISEASE

❹ The onset of AD is almost imperceptible, without abrupt changes in cognition or function. Deficits occur progressively over time, affecting multiple areas of cognition.[1,4] For treatment and assessment purposes, it is helpful to divide Alzheimer's symptoms into two basic categories: cognitive symptoms and noncognitive (behavioral) symptoms. Cognitive symptoms are present throughout the illness, whereas behavioral symptoms are less predictable. Table 63–2 summarizes the stages of AD.

CLINICAL PRESENTATION OF ALZHEIMER'S DISEASE

General

☐ The patient may have vague memory complaints initially, or the patient's significant other may report that the patient is "forgetful." Cognitive decline is gradual over the course of illness. Behavioral disturbances may be present in moderate stages. Loss of daily function is common in advanced stages.

Symptoms

Cognitive

☐ Memory loss (poor recall and losing items)

☐ Aphasia (circumlocution and anomia)

☐ Apraxia

☐ Agnosia

☐ Disorientation (impaired perception of time and unable to recognize familiar people)

☐ Impaired executive function

Noncognitive

☐ Depression, psychotic symptoms (hallucinations and delusions)

☐ Behavioral disturbances (physical and verbal aggression, motor hyperactivity, uncooperativeness, wandering, repetitive mannerisms and activities, and combativeness)

Functional

☐ Inability to care for self (dressing, bathing, toileting, and eating)

Laboratory Tests

☐ Rule out vitamin B$_{12}$ and folate deficiency

☐ Rule out hypothyroidism with thyroid function tests

☐ Blood cell counts, serum electrolytes, liver function tests

Other Diagnostic Tests

☐ CT or MRI scans may aid diagnosis

DIAGNOSIS

A family member often first brings memory complaints to the attention of a primary care clinician. Up to 50% of patients who meet criteria for dementia are not given a diagnosis in the primary care setting, leading some to believe that an appropriate screening tool may be helpful in aiding diagnosis and leading to earlier treatment.[23,24] Despite the phenomenon of underdiagnosis, the United States Preventative Services Task Force concluded that there are insufficient data to recommend for or against cognitive screening for AD, because it could not be determined if the benefits outweigh the risks.[23]

Until recently the only way to confirm a clinical diagnosis of AD was through direct examination of brain tissue at autopsy or biopsy, although the recent development of in vivo plaque detection methods may change this. Several criteria have been developed for the detection and diagnosis of dementia, including the *Diagnostic and Statistical Manual of Mental Disorders*, Fourth Edition, Text Revision (DSM-IV-TR) criteria,[25] the Agency for Healthcare Research and Quality (AHRQ) Guidelines,[26] the American Academy of Neurology Guidelines,[27] the National Institute of Neurological Disorders and Stroke (NINDS) criteria,[28] and the National Institute of Neurological Communicative Disorders and Stroke (NINCDS) and the Alzheimer's Disease and Related Disorders Association (ADRDA) Criteria.[29]

AD is still primarily a clinical diagnosis.[4] The patient's examination should suggest that cognitive decline from a previously higher baseline has occurred. The history should corroborate this, and further indicate cognitive decline has reached the point where changes in social or occupational functioning are present. It is possible to administer a sophisticated exam that defines cognitive domain strengths and weaknesses, and enables a neuroanatomic localization of the observed deficits. Ideally, evidence of defective retention memory (amnesia) will implicate bimesiotemporal dysfunction. Evidence of parietal cortical dysfunction (visuospatial dysfunction), dorsolateral prefrontal dysfunction (executive dysfunction), or lateral temporal dysfunction (language dysfunction) should also be present. When approached in this way, the exam can indicate a pattern of cognitive decline that is consistent with what would be expected in AD, and assist with rendering a diagnosis that is as much a diagnosis of inclusion as it is of exclusion.

Objectively defining social or occupational dysfunction can prove tricky in the older patient who may be retired, and who may also lead a socially restricted lifestyle for reasons of frailty. For such patients, the minimal requirement is to establish a change in activities of daily living. Early on, this usually involves a change in instrumental activities of daily living (handling finances, organizing medications) rather than basic activities of daily living (hygiene, dressing). Some AD subspecialists use a detailed, standardized, semistructured interview of a nonpatient informant as the most critical piece of the diagnostic evaluation.[30]

Almost any medication can contribute to cognitive impairment in vulnerable individuals, but certain classes of medication are more commonly implicated. Benzodiazepines and other sedative hypnotics, anticholinergics, opioid analgesics, antipsychotics, and anticonvulsants have been associated with cognitive impairment.[31,32] NSAIDs, histamine H$_2$-receptor antagonists, digoxin, amiodarone, antihypertensives, and corticosteroids have been implicated in cases of delirium.[31] Because medications are a reversible cause of cognitive symptoms, medication review and management are essential.

❺ For patients who meet criteria for the dementia syndrome (whether the underlying cause is ultimately felt to be AD or not), current recommendations from the American Academy of Neurology include a neuroimaging study (computed tomography or magnetic resonance imaging), as well as a serologic evaluation that includes blood cell counts, serum electrolytes, liver function tests, a test of thyroid function, and a vitamin B$_{12}$ level.[27] Earlier guidelines included a serologic test for syphilis, but this requirement has since been downgraded to optional. When circumstances suggest AD is not the leading entity on the differential diagnosis, other neurologic tests such as spinal fluid analysis or electroencephalogram can occasionally be justified. Neuropsychological testing is also optional, but can prove quite useful for the diagnosis of AD by helping to establish a neuroanatomical localization for the patient's cognitive deficits.

Efforts to define the role of other AD diagnostic tests are ongoing. Positron emission tomography scanning may reveal a pattern of hypometabolism typical of AD (bitemporoparietal hypometabolism), but by itself the diagnostic accuracy of positron emission tomography scanning still lags behind that of the clinical examination and history.[33] *APOE* genotyping by itself is also insufficient to make or break a diagnosis of AD, but demonstrating an *APOE*4* allele in a suspected patient increases the specificity of the diagnosis and can help predict which patients with mild cognitive impairment are most likely to progress to a full-blown diagnosis of AD over the next several years.[34] Unless the patient developed dementia prior to age 60 years and also had a parent that developed AD before age 60 years, presenilin 1, presenilin 2, or *APP* genotyping is usually not indicated.

MILD COGNITIVE IMPAIRMENT

It has long been recognized that aging individuals experience changes in cognitive function. Mild cognitive impairment (MCI) constitutes a syndromic designation that categorizes patients with cognitive complaints insufficient to warrant a diagnosis of dementia. Persons diagnosed with MCI carry a 10% to 15% chance per year of progressing to an AD diagnosis.[35] A logical extension of this is that what clinicians are actually seeing in most people with MCI is the initial manifestation of a progressive degenerative dementia that will eventually meet AD diagnostic criteria.[1,35] However, it is important to note that not everyone meeting MCI criteria does or will have AD. As the MCI designation is increasingly applied, MCI criteria continue to evolve.[35]

TREATMENT

Alzheimer's Disease

■ DESIRED OUTCOMES

❻ The primary goal of treatment in AD is to symptomatically treat cognitive difficulties and preserve patient function as long as possible. Secondary goals include treating the psychiatric and behavioral sequelae that occur as a result of the disease. Current AD treatments have not been shown to prolong life, cure AD, or halt or reverse the pathophysiologic processes of the disorder.[36]

GENERAL TREATMENT APPROACH

Clinical trials have consistently demonstrated modest benefits of early and continuous treatment with cholinesterase inhibitors.[36] Memantine added in moderate to severe disease may also provide benefit. Following this approach allows for maximum gain and maintenance of cognition and activities of daily living. A symptomatic approach is used to treat behavioral symptoms as they arise.

Provision of education to the patient and family at the time of diagnosis, including discussion of the course of illness, realistic expectations of treatment, and the importance of legal and financial planning, are essential to appropriate treatment. Good communication skills are important to maintain a therapeutic environment and minimize stress throughout the course of illness.

NONPHARMACOLOGIC THERAPY

❼ AD has a profound effect on both the patient and family, so appropriate treatment, both nonpharmacologic and pharmacologic, is needed. Nonmedication interventions are the current primary interventions for management of AD, and medications should be used in the context of multimodal interventions. Behavioral and psychiatric symptoms are among the most challenging and distressing symptoms of the disease and may be the determining factor in a family's decision to seek institutional care. Symptoms such as sleep disturbances, wandering, urinary incontinence, agitation, and aggression in patients with dementia are best managed using behavioral interventions rather than medications whenever possible.[37,38]

Upon initial diagnosis, the patient and caregiver should be educated on the course of illness, prognosis, available treatments, legal decisions, and quality-of-life issues. Education, including short- and long-term programs, improves caregiver knowledge and confidence, and in some cases, delays time to nursing home placement.[39] Table 63–3 lists basic principles of care for the AD patient. Communication between the patient and family members is essential in order to minimize stress on everyone.

The general approach to developing nonmedication strategies for behavioral symptoms is to identify the symptom, identify causative factors, and adapt the caregiving environment to remedy the situation.[4] Environmental triggers may include noise, glare, an insecure space, and too much background distraction, including television. Personal discomfort may also trigger behaviors, so it is important to monitor for pain, hunger, thirst, constipation, full bladder, fatigue, infections and skin irritation, comfortable temperature, fears, and frustrations.[4] Medical comorbidity is a major source of functional and cognitive impairment in patients with AD, so general health maintenance is warranted.[44] Interventions should redirect the patient's attention rather than be confrontational and should specifically address known triggers. Creating

TABLE 63-3	Basic Principles of Care for the Alzheimer's Patient

- Consider vision, hearing, or other sensory impairments.
- Find optimal level of autonomy and adjust expectations for patient performance over time.
- Avoid confrontation. Remain calm, firm, and supportive if the patient becomes upset.
- Maintain a consistent, structured environment with stimulation level appropriate to the individual patient.
- Provide frequent reminders, explanations, and orientation cues. Employ guiding, demonstration, and reinforcement.
- Reduce choices, keep requests and demands of the patient simple, and avoid complex tasks that lead to frustration.
- Bring sudden declines in function and the emergence of new symptoms to professional attention.

Data from Alzheimer's Association,[4] Rubin,[47] and Lyketsos et al.[57]

TABLE 63-4	Resources for Caregivers of Persons with Alzheimer's Disease

The following organizations provide educational literature and information on diagnosis, treatment, social support, and ongoing research in Alzheimer's disease:

U.S. Administration on Aging, National Family Caregiver Support Program
http://www.aoa.gov
National Institute on Aging Alzheimer's Disease Education & Referral Center (ADEAR)
http://www.nia.nih.gov/alzheimers
The Alzheimer's Association
http://www.alz.org
The Alzheimer's Research Forum
http://www.alzforum.org
AARP
http://www.aarp.org
National Family Caregivers Association
http://www.thefamilycaregiver.org
ElderCare Online
http://www.ec-online.net

a calm environment and removing stressors and triggers is key. Caregivers should be referred to support services, such as the Alzheimer's Association, for assistance in developing nonpharmacologic strategies for managing difficult behaviors.

The caregiver must be prepared to face the changes in life that will occur, and acceptance of this does not come easily. Denial on the part of the patient and rationalization on the part of the family are common. The clinician should encourage the family to address legal and financial matters and designate a durable power of attorney for execution of financial and medical decisions once the patient is incompetent. The caregiver will need to address issues such as respite services to provide time for rest, relaxation, and conduct of personal business. Caregiver stress impacts the health and quality of life of the caregiver as well as the patient. Eventually, the caregiver will need to face critical questions with respect to institutionalization. This is probably the most difficult decision for the caregiver. Clinician support and referral to social services is vitally important in assisting the caregiver at that moment. The family should also be referred to local resources, such as the Alzheimer's Association, that can provide detailed information regarding support services. Table 63–4 lists some referral sources for caregivers.

Education, communication, and planning are the key nonpharmacologic components of caring for an AD patient. Preparation in the early stages of illness will lessen some of the caregiver stress as the illness progresses.

PHARMACOLOGIC THERAPY

Pharmacotherapy for Cognitive Symptoms

❽ Table 63–5 presents a treatment algorithm for managing cognitive symptoms in AD. Cholinesterase inhibitors and NMDA-receptor

TABLE 63-5	Treatment Options for Cognitive Symptoms in Alzheimer's Disease

- In mild to moderate disease, consider therapy with a cholinesterase inhibitor:
  - Donepezil or
  - Rivastigmine or
  - Galantamine
- Titrate to recommended maintenance dose as tolerated.
- In moderate to severe disease, consider adding antiglutamatergic therapy:
  - Memantine
- Titrate to recommended maintenance dose as tolerated.
- Alternatively, consider memantine or cholinesterase inhibitor therapy alone.
- Behavioral symptoms may require additional pharmacologic approaches.

Data from Burns and Iliffe,[1] Lleó et al,[44] and Lyketsos et al.[57]

antagonists are indicated for treatment of AD. The latest treatment guideline recommends the use of cholinesterase inhibitors for AD, with no preference for a specific agent.[40–42] Donepezil, rivastigmine, and galantamine are indicated in mild to moderate AD, while donepezil is also indicated in severe disease. Memantine is indicated for moderate to severe AD; current evidence does not support its use in earlier stages of the disease.[43] Additional benefit may be achieved when memantine is added to cholinesterase inhibitor therapy in moderate to severe AD.[44,70] There is no evidence supporting combination therapy of more than one cholinesterase inhibitor.

Disagreement exists about how to determine effectiveness of treatments for AD. Selection of qualitative versus quantitative assessment may bias a clinician's impression of response. Subtle changes are often detected only by psychometric testing rather than with routine questioning. Because no standard has been suggested to define the effectiveness of these medications, great variation exists between clinicians and the duration of treatment ranges from months to years. Realistic expectations for treatment success may include short-term improvement of symptoms and less decline in behavioral, functional, and cognitive abilities over the longer term.[36]

Unfortunately, clinical trials have failed to provide answers to key questions in treating AD patients. Information from clinical trials is insufficient to know if a cholinesterase inhibitor dose—response relationship exists, or if additional cognitive improvement may be gained by increasing to the maximum tolerated dose, rather than continuing with the usual recommended daily dosage. Guidance in extrapolating data related to changes in cognition is needed so that a reasonable duration of clinical treatment with cholinesterase inhibitors and NMDA-antagonists can be determined.

In natural disease progression studies, scores on the Alzheimer's Disease Assessment Scale—Cognition (ADAS-cog) have been shown to worsen (increase) by an average of 4 points over 6 months and 7 points over 1 year. Based on these findings, the general consensus is that a 4-point change in the ADAS-cog represents a clinically significant change. Therefore, if a pharmacotherapeutic agent decreases the ADAS-cog by 4 points, one could think of this as having reversed progression of disease symptoms by 6 months. The usefulness of the ADAS-cog in clinical practice is limited because of the time required for administration; it is much more practical to assess changes in disease severity using the Mini-Mental Status Examination (MMSE).

An untreated patient has an average decline of 2 to 4 points in MMSE score per year. Consequently, successful treatment would reflect a decline of less than 2 points a year. It is reasonable to change to a different cholinesterase inhibitor if the decline in MMSE score is greater than 2 to 4 points after 1 year with the initial agent.

❽ Cholinesterase Inhibitors In the early 1980s, researchers began to examine means to enhance cholinergic activity in patients with AD by inhibiting the hydrolysis of acetylcholine through reversible inhibition of cholinesterase. Tacrine was the first such drug to be examined in a systematic fashion. However, tacrine is fraught with significant side effects, including hepatotoxicity, that severely limit its usefulness. For all practical purposes the use of tacrine has been replaced by the use of safer, more tolerable cholinesterase inhibitors. The newer cholinesterase inhibitors donepezil, rivastigmine, and galantamine show similar efficacy and adverse event profiles to one another and are generally well tolerated. The most frequent adverse events associated with these agents are mild to moderate gastrointestinal symptoms (nausea, vomiting, and diarrhea).[44] Other cholinergic side effects are generally dose related and include urinary incontinence, dizziness, headache, syncope, bradycardia, muscle weakness, salivation, and sweating. Gradual dose titration over several months can improve tolerability.[42] Abrupt discontinuation can lead to worsening cognition and behavior in some patients.[45,46] Concurrent use of anticholinergic medications with cholinesterase inhibitors should be avoided.

Table 63–6 summarizes the clinical pharmacology of the cholinesterase inhibitors. The mechanism of action differs slightly between drugs in this class.[47] Donepezil specifically and reversibly inhibits acetylcholinesterase. Rivastigmine inhibits both butyrylcholinesterase and acetylcholinesterase. Galantamine is a selective, competitive, reversible acetylcholinesterase inhibitor and also enhances the action of acetylcholine on nicotinic receptors. The clinical relevance of these differences is unknown. Choice of cholinesterase inhibitor therapy for an individual patient is based on ease of use, patient preference, cost, and safety issues such as potential for drug interactions.[40,41] In 2008, galantamine became available in generic form, which has reduced the cost of galantamine therapy. A generic form of donepezil has also been approved by the U.S. Food and Drug Administration (FDA) in December 2009, and (as of this writing) may become available as early as 2010.

TABLE 63-6	Clinical Pharmacology of Cognitive Enhancing Medications			
	Donepezil	**Rivastigmine**	**Galantamine**	**Memantine**
Brand Name	Aricept	Exelon	Razadyne	Namenda
Dosage Forms	Tablet Orally disintegrating tablet	Capsule Oral solution Patch	Tablet Oral solution Extended-release (ER) capsule	Tablet Oral solution (Extended-release formulation in development)
Starting Dose	5 mg daily in the evening	1.5 mg twice a day 4.6 mg/day (patch)	4 mg twice a day 8 mg daily for (ER)	5 mg once daily
Maintenance Dose	5–10 mg daily 23 mg daily in moderate to severe AD	3–6 mg twice a day 9.5 mg/day (patch)	8–12 mg twice a day (16–24 mg daily for ER)	10 mg twice a day
Meals	Can be taken with or without food	Take with meals	Take with meals	Can be taken with or without food
Mechanism of Action	Reversible inhibition of acetylcholinesterase	Reversible inhibition of acetylcholinesterase and butyrylcholinesterase	Reversible inhibition of acetylcholinesterase and modulation of nicotinic receptors	Antagonism of N-methyl-D-aspartate (NMDA) receptors
Half-Life	70 hours	1.5 hours	7 hours	60–80 hours
Protein Binding	96%	40%	18%	45%
Metabolism	Substrate (minor) of CYP2D6 and 3A34; glucuronidation	Cholinesterase-mediated hydrolysis	Substrate (minor) of CYP2D6 and 3A34; glucuronidation	Glucuronidation
Renal Elimination	Yes	Major pathway	Yes	Yes

Data from references 48 and 92–95.

❽ Antiglutamatergic Therapy Memantine is the only NMDA-antagonist currently available. At concentrations achieved at least under in vitro conditions, memantine blocks glutamatergic neurotransmission by antagonizing NMDA receptors. Glutamate is an excitatory neurotransmitter in the brain implicated in long-term potentiation, a neuronal mechanism important for learning and memory.[44] Under experimental conditions, blocking NMDA receptors can mitigate excitotoxic neurotoxicity and provide neuroprotection. There is currently no evidence to indicate memantine confers neuroprotection in AD.[43,44]

Memantine has been studied in patients with moderate and severe AD as monotherapy and in combination with donepezil with modest favorable results on cognition and function.[43] It is currently indicated for use in AD patients with moderate to severe illness. Studies of memantine alone and in combination with cholinesterase inhibitors in mild AD performed to date have provided insufficient evidence to support an indication for mild AD.[4]

Memantine has 100% bioavailability regardless of administration with or without food. Protein binding is low. Memantine is not metabolized by the liver and does not inhibit cytochrome P450. Memantine is primarily excreted unchanged in the urine. The half-life ranges from 60 to 80 hours.[44]

Overall, memantine has been well tolerated in clinical trials. The most common adverse events associated with memantine include constipation, confusion, dizziness, headache, hallucinations, coughing, and hypertension.[48]

Memantine is likely to be used as monotherapy and also in combination with cholinesterase inhibitors in patients with moderate to severe AD. Memantine should be initiated at 5 mg once a day and increased weekly by 5 mg a day to the effective dose of 10 mg twice daily.[48] It may be given with or without food. Dosing of 10 mg daily is recommended in patients with severe renal impairment (creatinine clearance of 5–29 mL/min [0.08 to 0.49 ml/s]).[48]

Role of Combination Therapy Combination therapy with memantine added to cholinesterase inhibitor therapy is generally prescribed for patients with moderate to severe AD. The rationale for this add-on therapy is that the drug classes have different mechanisms of action. The clinical effectiveness of using combination therapy with a cholinesterase inhibitor plus memantine was compared to using a cholinesterase inhibitor alone and no treatment.[49] This study showed significant decreases in the rate of progression of dementia across the treatment groups, such that patients who received combination therapy showed the least decline in cognitive function, followed by the group that only received cholinesterase inhibitors. The group that received combination also had the lowest rate of decline in functional status. Another combination trial assessed the efficacy and safety of memantine versus placebo in patients with moderate to severe AD already receiving stable treatment with donepezil.[50] Patients randomized to combination therapy with memantine and donepezil showed significant improvements in cognition and function in this 6-month study. However, in patients with mild to moderate AD, there were no benefits seen when memantine therapy was added to a cholinesterase inhibitor.

Available data suggest treatment strategies currently under investigation will at best slow rather than arrest cognitive decline.[52] It therefore seems reasonable to predict that for the foreseeable future combination therapy will become increasingly common in AD, especially as drugs or treatments with unique mechanisms of action become available, and drugs with neuroprotective modes of action are concomitantly used with symptomatic drugs.

Effect of Current Treatments on Neurodegenerative Processes AD is a progressive disorder. Affected individuals typically experience some degree of cognitive decline and histologic change years (if not decades) before a diagnosis is made. Therefore, the ideal treatment will be one that not only reverses symptoms by enhancing cognitive function (a symptomatic treatment), but also arrests the neurodegeneration-relevant molecular processes that underlie cognitive decline (a disease-modifying treatment).

Clinical trials for AD prompt consideration of whether positive outcomes suggest either a symptomatic or disease-modifying effect. Any rapid performance improvement on cognitive ability, activities of daily living, or behavioral end points is indicative of a symptomatic effect. All cholinesterase inhibitor agents and memantine demonstrate this pattern. On the other hand, arrest of decline or a sustained reduction in the slope of decline would argue the presence of a disease-modifying effect. It has not been possible to unequivocally demonstrate this in trials of the currently approved treatments. Definitive trials evaluating whether cholinesterase inhibitors or memantine have disease-modifying effects are difficult to perform, because doing so requires continuing a placebo arm over an extended period, well beyond demonstration of symptomatic benefit. Also, subject attrition over an extended study would complicate both intent-to-treat and observed cases analyses.

With the currently approved AD drug treatments, placebo-controlled pivotal trials were followed by open-label extension studies. Published studies have lasted as long as 5 years, and as part of these studies, decline in the treatment group was compared with "projected" placebo groups based on the placebo groups followed during the 6-month randomized phase of the efficacy study, as well as natural history cohorts from the pre-cholinesterase inhibitor therapy era. Although analyses of this sort conclude that, for up to at least 5 years, persons receiving treatment exceed their projected nontreatment cognitive performance, no convincing evidence of a disease-modifying effect emerges.[53-56]

Management of Brain Vascular Health

9 Guidelines for the principles of care of patients with AD support the management of vascular brain disease and its associated risk factors as part of the treatment of AD.[57] There is a growing body of evidence that brain vascular disease plays an important role in the progression of dementia. For a given level of Alzheimer's pathology, vascular disease in the brain may add to the degree of cognitive impairment.[57] Management of brain vascular disease includes monitoring blood pressure, glucose, cholesterol, and homocysteine and initiation of appropriate interventions.[57] Guidelines recommend initiation of low-dose aspirin therapy in patients with AD with significant brain vascular disease.[57] Elevated homocysteine levels correlate with decreased performance on cognitive tests, but there remains insufficient evidence of a benefit of B vitamin supplementation (B_6, B_{12}, and folic acid) on cognitive function in patients with AD.[58] Reducing the risk for developing brain vascular disease may also be an important strategy in reducing the risk for developing AD. The Alzheimer's Association's Maintain Your Brain campaign is designed to increase awareness of the importance of brain health as a part of healthy aging and recommends staying physically, mentally, and socially active; adopting a low-fat, low-cholesterol diet rich in dark vegetables and fruit; and managing body weight, blood pressure, cholesterol, and blood sugar to reduce the risk of heart disease, stroke, and diabetes.[4] Appropriate management of vascular disease risk factors may reduce the risk for developing AD.[59]

Other Potential Treatment Approaches

Estrogen Estrogen replacement has been studied extensively for the treatment and prevention for AD. Most, but not all, retrospective epidemiologic studies show a lower incidence of AD in women who took estrogen replacement therapy postmenopausally.

Prospective clinical trials have not supported the use of estrogen as a treatment for cognitive decline and longer trials tend to suggest harm. Overall, the evidence does not support the use of estrogen to treat or prevent dementia.[41,60]

Antiinflammatory Agents Retrospective epidemiologic studies suggest a protective effect against AD in patients who have taken NSAIDs. The benefits of antiinflammatory agents have been less compelling in prospective clinical studies. NSAIDs have had no cognitive benefit in AD patients or else benefits so minimal the risk of harm exceeds the potential benefit.[61-63] Tolerability is problematic.[61-64] Additionally, prednisone treatment was associated with worsening behavioral symptoms.[64] Because there is a lack of compelling data and also a significant incidence of adverse effects, particularly gastritis and the possibility of gastrointestinal bleeds, NSAIDs and prednisone are not recommended for general use in the treatment or prevention of AD at the present time.

Lipid-Lowering Agents A potential AD protective effect has been postulated for lipid-lowering agents, particularly the 3-hydroxy-3-methylglutaryl-coenzyme A-reductase inhibitors. Longitudinal epidemiologic studies suggest an association between elevated midlife total cholesterol levels and AD.[21] Increased risk of dementia does not appear to be associated with hypercholesterolemia in late life however.[21] Other studies note that the incidence of AD is lower in patients who have taken either a statin or another lipid-lowering agent, but not in patients who were taking other cardiovascular medications.[21] It is important to note that not all epidemiologic studies suggest an association between cholesterol and AD.[21]

Randomized controlled trials of statin therapy given in late life to patients at risk for vascular disease indicate that statins do not prevent AD.[65] Several randomized controlled trials of statins for the treatment of mild to moderate AD have been completed or are ongoing. Thus far, these trials have not demonstrated a significant

benefit of statin therapy, but results of ongoing trials should help to clarify the role of statins in the treatment of AD.[66] Interestingly, cognitive impairment has been recognized as a rare adverse event associated with statin therapy. The extent of cognitive impairment may depend on the lipid solubility of the drug, regulating the amount of drug that is able to cross the blood—brain barrier. As simvastatin and lovastatin have the highest lipophilicity, they may be the most likely candidates to cause memory impairment.[67] More research is needed to understand the complex relationship between cholesterol, statin therapy, and cognitive functioning. For now these agents should be reserved for patients who have other indications for their use.[57]

Dietary Supplements

Vitamin E Based on pathophysiologic theories involving oxidative stress and the accumulation of free radicals in AD, significant interest has evolved regarding the use of antioxidants in the treatment of AD. For a period starting in the late 1990s, vitamin E was frequently recommended as adjunctive treatment for AD patients. This was based on data from the only published clinical trial to date, which evaluated the time to critical end points (i.e., death, institutionalization, loss of ability to perform activities of daily living, or severe dementia) in patients treated with vitamin E, selegiline, the combination, or placebo.[68] Although vitamin E and selegiline were superior to placebo, this study has been criticized because of differences in baseline cognitive severity, calling the validity of the results into question. Because of vitamin E's perceived safety (at that time) and low cost, doses of up to 2,000 IU per day were commonly recommended.

Evidence related to vitamin E's role in prevention of AD is mixed. Epidemiologic studies in individuals without AD have yielded conflicting results, with some studies showing delay in the onset of AD in individuals taking vitamin E supplements, but others failing to find this association.[44] Some studies have also found that dietary intake of vitamin E is associated with reduced risk, while others have not.[44] A study in patients with mild cognitive impairment failed to show that vitamin E had a significant effect on slowing the progression to AD.[68]

Vitamin E treatment may also be associated with risks. Side effects observed with vitamin E administration include impaired hemostasis, fatigue, nausea, diarrhea, abdominal pain, and falls.[68] A meta-analysis found that high-dose vitamin E increases mortality in supplemented subjects.[69] In light of these findings, vitamin E supplementation is not recommended for the treatment of AD.[41]

Nutraceuticals, Supplements, and Medical Foods *Ginkgo biloba* for the prevention and treatment of AD has been extensively studied. Rationales for studying Ginkgo for AD have included its potential to increase blood flow, decrease blood viscosity, antagonize platelet-activating factor receptors, increase anoxia tolerance, inhibit monoamine oxidase, and serve as an antioxidant. Active ingredients in *G biloba* include flavonoids, the Ginkgoflavone glycosides, and bioflavonoids. Most studies reporting benefit in patients with AD have studied a standardized extract, EGb 761, in doses of 120 mg per day for at least 4 to 6 weeks. Those advocating the use of Ginkgo for AD suggest doses of 120 to 240 mg of the standard leaf extract twice per day be used, and note 12 weeks of consistent dosing may be needed to observe an effect.[70] However, a large trial of *G biloba* in which the 120 mg twice a day dose was studied did not reduce either the overall incidence rate of dementia or AD incidence in elderly individuals with normal cognition or MCI.[71] Side effects reported from EGb 761 studies were typically mild but did include nausea, vomiting, diarrhea, headaches, dizziness, palpitations, restlessness, and weakness. Because EGb also has a potent antiplatelet effect, it should be avoided by individuals taking anticoagulant or antiplatelet therapies, and should be used cautiously in patients taking NSAIDs.[70,72] Further, the content of retail herbal products is poorly standardized, and significant variation in purported active ingredient content can exist from lot to lot and between manufacturers. Current practice guidelines do not recommend Ginkgo for the prevention or treatment of AD.[57]

Huperzine A is an alkaloid isolated from the Chinese club moss, *Huperzia serrata*. It reversibly inhibits acetylcholinesterase and is administered orally in doses of 50 to 200 mcg 2 to 4 times daily. Nondefinitive clinical studies suggest huperzine A may have efficacy in the symptomatic treatment of AD, but more studies are needed to determine its place in therapy. In a medium-sized, randomized, double-blind, placebo-controlled multicenter study in patients with mild to moderate AD performed in China, treatment with huperzine A at doses of 400 mcg/day for 12 weeks resulted in improvement in cognition by an average of 4.6 points assessed by ADAS-cog ($P = 0.000$), 2.7 points on the MMSE, and 1.5 points on the Alzheimer's Disease Assessment Scale—noncognition ($P = 0.008$).[73] Replication of these study results are still pending. The current consensus is that huperzine A has not been adequately studied for use in AD, its consistency in retail products remains a concern, and potential side effects could be substantial, especially in those taking cholinesterase inhibitors.[70,74] Huperzine A is not currently recommended for AD treatment.

Arguments that omega-3 fatty acids found in fish oil, such as docosahexaenoic acid, could benefit AD subjects have existed for some years. A large prospective, placebo-controlled trial of docosahexaenoic acid in AD subjects was recently reported. For the most part, results were disappointing, and although it could not be ruled out that population subsets did benefit, the primary study end points were negative.[75] At the time of this chapters' preparation, testing of other dietary supplements, such as curcumin, is ongoing.[70]

Currently, the only dietary agent approved by the FDA for the treatment of AD is AC1202, which is sold under the commercial name Axona. AC1202 is a modification of medium-chain triglyceride formulations used decades ago for the treatment of pediatric epilepsy; such formulations contain mixtures of C5–C12 fatty acids. AC1202 consists primarily of the C8 fatty acid, caprylic acid. AC1202 is converted by the liver to a ketone body, betahydroxybutyrate, which is secreted into the blood stream. Betahydroxybutyrate crosses the blood—brain barrier and can be used as an oxidative phosphorylation substrate by neuron mitochondria. Due to its ability to support brain bioenergetics, which is impaired in AD, betahydroxybutyrate was first proposed as a potential AD treatment in 1989.[76] Support for AC1202 efficacy in the treatment of AD comes mostly from a phase IIb trial in which subjects randomized to 40 mg per day of AC1202 for 45 days performed relatively better on the cognitive portion of ADAS-cog than did subjects randomized to a placebo.[77] A subanalysis of these data revealed this benefit was entirely driven by subjects who did not have an *APOE*4* allele. For *APOE*4* carriers, ADAS-cog performance between subjects receiving AC1202 and placebo were comparable at all time points studied. Gastrointestinal-related side effects were common but in general side effects were felt to be mild. Based on these data and on the established safety track record of medium-chain triglyceride oil, in 2009 the FDA gave permission for AC1202 to be marketed as a medical food for the treatment of AD. Medical foods constitute a unique category that consists of ingestible entities specifically intended for the treatment of diseases that have "specific nutritional requirements" and in which the medical food may manipulate disease-relevant pathophysiology. Although medical foods regulatory approval standards are not nearly as rigorous as those required for approvals of new medications, medical foods are not available over-the-counter and are obtained only by prescription.

CLINICAL CONTROVERSY

The compound tramiprosate (homotaurine), or Alzhemed, showed promise as a treatment of Alzheimer's disease in early development. In animal studies, homotaurine demonstrated the ability to interfere with the actions of Aβ early in the amyloid cascade, subsequently preventing amyloid plaque formation and subsequent degeneration of neuronal cells. Phase III trials were disappointing, and the FDA refused to approve marketing of homotaurine as a prescription drug. Homotaurine is naturally occurring in seaweed, and its manufacturer decided to remarket the product as the dietary supplement, Vivimind for age-associated memory impairment. Controversy exists between those who advocate for availability of dietary supplements to consumers and those who advocate for evidence-based medicine. The major concern is the marketing of potentially ineffective products to those suffering from memory loss or dementia.[96]

Drugs and Treatment Strategies in Development

Current drug development strategies fall broadly into one of two categories. The first category includes treatments specifically designed to reduce levels of brain Aβ or manipulate its configuration. The second category includes all other strategies.

To reduce brain amyloid levels, approaches to both reducing Aβ production and enhancing its removal have been and still are undergoing evaluation. Aβ is produced through enzymatic processing of APP by two enzyme complexes, the β- and γ-secretases. β-Secretase inhibitors have entered phase II human trials. Agents that specifically inhibit γ-secretase could prove problematic from a side-effect perspective, as γ-secretase is also critical for processing Notch3, a protein of developmental importance and perhaps brain maintenance. Certain NSAIDs (ibuprofen and flurbiprofen) influence the γ-secretase but do not inhibit it outright. In general, these NSAIDs alter where γ-secretase cuts the APP protein. An enantiomer of flurbiprofen, tarenflurbil, recently completed a large phase III efficacy trial in which no evidence of efficacy was seen.[52]

Immunotherapy approaches have been studied as a way to enhance Aβ removal. The most extensive investigation involved AN1792, a Aβ-based vaccine. A phase II trial in humans was prematurely halted after a substantial percentage of those mounting a robust immune response to the vaccine experienced encephalitis, a potentially life-threatening brain inflammation. The most comprehensive, long-term clinicopathologic study of subjects receiving AN1792 later concluded vaccinated subjects show a predictable rate of cognitive decline and that despite reducing brain plaque burdens, AN1792 vaccination is unlikely to meaningfully benefit those with the common form of late-onset, sporadic AD.[78]

Most proponents of the amyloid cascade hypothesis currently claim the species of Aβ that is most likely to prove relevant to AD neurodegeneration are Aβ oligomers. Aβ oligomers are formed through limited aggregation of Aβ monomers. Aβ oligomers are too small to form fibrils and may retain aqueous solubility. A drug called tramiprosate was previously created to prevent Aβ oligomer formation and tested clinically in a large phase III trial. No evidence of efficacy was seen.[52]

Despite these failures, the next generation of amyloid clearance therapies are currently under development. This generation includes modifications of the active immunization approach that, hopefully, will not trigger encephalitis. Passive immunization approaches via antibody infusions are also under investigation. At the time of this writing, results of a phase III trial of bapineuzumab, an Aβ antibody, are expected in 2010. The usefulness of treating

AD subjects with intravenous immunoglobulin preparations, which naturally contain antibodies to $A\beta$, is under evaluation.[52]

The second category of AD treatment development includes efforts not specifically intended to reduce brain $A\beta$ levels. Neuroscientists are unraveling intracellular pathways involved in cell information processing, and drugs that can modulate these pathways are under development. Drugs that retard neurofibrillary tangle formation in mice expressing mutant human *tau* transgenes, such as valproic acid, were recently tested in humans, although no evidence of efficacy was seen. Other "anti-tangle" drugs are in various stages of development.[52] The thiazolidinedione drugs rosiglitazone and pioglitazone, which reduce insulin resistance and which may also have antiinflammatory effects, were recently tested in humans with AD, although the most definitive of these trials showed no evidence of efficacy. Despite this, efforts at treating AD through modification of insulin signaling pathways are ongoing.[52]

A phase II trial of latrepirdine (dimebon) recently generated much attention.[79] Suggestions of efficacy in phase II trials in no way ensures efficacy will be seen in phase III trials. This caveat seems especially pertinent in AD drug development, as phase II trials of flurbiprofen, tramiprosate, and rosiglitazone all reported some evidence of efficacy that did not bear out in phase III studies. However, in the initial 6-month placebo-controlled trial, which was conducted in Russia, AD subjects randomized to dimebon performed better on cognitive and overall performance measures than those randomized to placebo. Subjects subsequently enrolled in a 6-month open-label continuation study continued to perform above their pre-study baseline. This was the first study in which AD subjects have been reported to perform above their pre-treatment baseline over the course of a full year. At concentrations achieved in human subjects dimebon does not appear to act as a cholinesterase inhibitor or NMDA-receptor antagonist. It does not appear to reduce $A\beta$ production and indeed in animal models appears to increase $A\beta$ production. There are data that suggest nanomolar concentrations of dimebon affect mitochondrial function. Unfortunately, results from a phase III Dimebon study reported in Spring 2010 failed to show efficacy in the treatment of AD.

Obviously, successful development of new AD treatments depends on elucidating AD's true underlying pathophysiology. If AD is a primary amyloidosis, as is postulated by the amyloid cascade hypothesis, then reducing $A\beta$ would seem a rational way to proceed with drug development. If AD is not a primary amyloidosis, then the impact antiamyloid therapies have on the disease will be limited at best. Finally, at genetic and epidemiologic levels, it is now possible to define several different Alzheimer's "diseases." It is not unreasonable to consider whether treatments useful in one type of AD may not benefit patients with another type.

■ PHARMACOTHERAPY OF NONCOGNITIVE SYMPTOMS

The majority of patients with AD manifest noncognitive symptoms at some point in the illness.[37] These symptoms can be roughly divided into three categories: psychotic symptoms, inappropriate or disruptive behavior, and depression. Effective management of these problems is important because behavioral symptoms are distressing to both the patient and the caregiver, necessitate increased caregiver supervision and patience, and are a leading reason for nursing home placement. In fact, presence of neuropsychiatric symptoms increases caregiver burden more than loss of cognition or self-care.

❿ Strategies for treatment of psychotic or behavioral symptoms should include environmental interventions first, then pharmacologic interventions if warranted. The need for medications may exist when neuropsychiatric symptoms are of sufficient

severity to cause significant distress to the patient or caregiver, interfere with function or cause disability, impede delivery of necessary care, or pose a danger to self or others.[41,57] The balance between risks of the medication and expected benefits must be acceptable to the patient or surrogate decision maker. Medications should be used cautiously, with adequate monitoring for efficacy and adverse events.

Despite the high prevalence of noncognitive symptoms in AD, little research has been conducted in these patients. Data from clinical trials of antidepressants, cholinesterase inhibitors, and antipsychotics are now emerging, but clearly more research is needed. Because of limited clinical data, treatment is primarily empiric, with side-effect profiles used as a guide in selecting the appropriate treatment. Psychotropic medications with anticholinergic effects should be avoided because they may actually worsen cognition and interfere with cholinesterase inhibitor therapy. Other side effects in the elderly include sedation, medication-induced postural instability, and extrapyramidal side effects, which can decrease the clinical usefulness of traditional psychotropic agents.

General guidelines governing therapy can be summarized as follows: use reduced doses, monitor closely, titrate dosage slowly, and document carefully. Caregivers often have erroneous expectations regarding the effects of psychotropic medications, and the anticipated benefits and risks of therapy should be clearly explained. Disruptive behaviors and delusions wax and wane with disease progression. Attempts to slowly taper and discontinue antipsychotic medication should be undertaken regularly in minimally symptomatic patients, because some patients improve on medication withdrawal.[57] Table 63–7 outlines suggested doses of medications.

Cholinesterase Inhibitors and Memantine

Clinical trials with cholinesterase inhibitors have consistently reported modest benefit in managing neuropsychiatric symptoms, although these are generally not the primary outcomes studied in the trials.[80-82] Any benefits in symptoms such as agitation may accrue gradually over time, since cholinesterase inhibitors may not significantly reduce agitation when administered to patients experiencing acute agitation.[83] Memantine shows modest behavioral benefits as well, either alone or in combination with cholinesterase

TABLE 63-7	Medications Used for Noncognitive Symptoms of Dementia			
Drugs	**Starting Dose (mg)**	**Maintenance Dose in Dementia (mg/d)**	**Target Symptoms**	
Antipsychotics			Psychosis: hallucinations, delusions, suspiciousness	
Haloperidol	0.25	1–3		
Olanzapine	2.5	5–10	Disruptive behaviors: agitation, aggression	
Quetiapine	25	100–300		
Risperidone	0.25	0.75–2		
Ziprasidone	20	40–160		
Antidepressants			Depression: poor appetite, insomnia, hopelessness, anhedonia, withdrawal, suicidal thoughts, agitation, anxiety	
Citalopram	10	10–20		
Escitalopram	5	20–40		
Fluoxetine	5	10–40		
Paroxetine	10	10–40		
Sertraline	25	75–100		
Venlafaxine	25	75–225		
Trazodone	25	75–150		
Anticonvulsants			Agitation or aggression	
Carbamazepine	100	200–600		
Valproic Acid	125	500–1,000		

Data from Lleó et al,[44] Benoit et al,[37] and Grossberg and Desai.[97]

inhibitors, and may also spare the use of antipsychotics to treat agitation.[80,81] These treatments can provide modest short-term improvement and possibly slow the development and progression of behavioral symptoms. Cholinesterase inhibitors also have a small beneficial effect on caregiver burden and active time use among caregivers of persons with AD.[84] These benefits should be considered along with cognitive benefits in treatment decisions. Long-term effects on behavior have not been demonstrated to date, and further research is needed.

Antipsychotics

Antipsychotics are widely used in the management of neuropsychiatric symptoms in AD. There is modestly convincing evidence that most of the atypical antipsychotics provide some benefit for particular neuropsychiatric symptoms, but these data have been insufficient to gain FDA approval as an indication for the management of behavioral symptoms in AD. Based on a recent meta-analysis, only 17% to 18% of dementia patients show a treatment response to atypical antipsychotics.[85] In a double-blind, placebo-controlled trial of 421 outpatients with AD and psychosis, aggression, or agitation randomized to receive olanzapine, quetiapine, risperidone, or placebo for up to 36 weeks, there were no significant differences among the treatments in time to discontinuation of treatment or improvement in the Clinical Global Impression of Change scale. The investigators concluded that adverse effects offset advantages in the efficacy of atypical antipsychotic drugs for treatment of psychosis, aggression, or agitation in patients with AD.[85] Adverse events are common with atypical and typical antipsychotics in patients with AD. These adverse events associated with atypical antipsychotics include somnolence, extrapyramidal symptoms, abnormal gait, worsening cognition, cerebrovascular events, and increased risk of death.[86] Typical antipsychotics may also be associated with a small increased risk of death, as well as more severe extrapyramidal effects and hypotension. Chapter 76 has a more detailed discussion of antipsychotic adverse events. Overall, there is a modest expectation of treatment benefit and potential for significant harm associated with antipsychotic use in patients with AD. Individual risk and benefit must be considered when initiating therapy. Diligent monitoring during treatment is essential along with frequent reassessment of continued need.

CLINICAL CONTROVERSY

Antipsychotic medications have been widely used to treat disruptive behaviors and psychosis in AD patients, although the evidence supporting their modest benefit for some symptoms is limited.[86] Use of antipsychotics to treat severe neuropsychiatric symptoms in AD remains controversial. Recent studies indicate that atypical and typical antipsychotics have been associated with infrequent but serious adverse events, including a small increased risk of death.[81,85] These findings resulted in a FDA-mandated "black box warning" concerning the use of atypical antipsychotics in the treatment of AD. Careful consideration of risk versus benefit in individual patients is warranted.

Antidepressants

Depressive symptoms are common in patients with AD, occurring in as many as 50% of patients.[44] Apathy may be even more frequent, but these symptoms may be difficult to distinguish in patients with dementia. Many trials have studied the efficacy of antidepressants in treating depression in patients with AD, but the results are conflicting. Small sample size, short duration of treatment, and differing

measures of therapy outcomes limit comparison across studies and may account in part for conflicting study results.[44] Improvement in patients receiving placebo is also common. In practice, treatment with selective serotonin reuptake inhibitors (SSRIs) is initiated most commonly in patients with AD, based on side-effect profile and evidence of efficacy.[41] Among the SSRIs, the best evidence exists for sertraline and citalopram.[81] Buproprion, venlafaxine, and mirtazapine may be alternatives.[41] Serotonergic function may also play a role in some of the other behavioral symptoms of AD, and some studies support the use of SSRIs in the management of these behaviors, even in the absence of depression.[81] Tricyclic antidepressants have efficacy similar to the SSRIs, but should generally be avoided because of their anticholinergic activity.[41] There is little evidence for the use of trazodone to manage behavioral or depressive symptoms, but it is commonly recommended to treat insomnia in patients with AD.[41]

Chapter 77 has a more complete discussion of treatment of depression.

Miscellaneous Therapies

Because antipsychotic and antidepressant therapy has shown only modest efficacy and poses a risk of undesirable side effects, medications traditionally used to treat disruptive behaviors and aggression in other psychiatric and neurologic disorders have been suggested as potential alternatives. These alternatives include benzodiazepines, buspirone, and antiepileptics.[81]

Benzodiazepines have been used to treat anxiety, agitation, and aggression, but the benefit is generally modest.[41] Because benzodiazepines impair cognition, worsen breathing disorders, and may increase the risk of falls in AD patients, their routine use is not advised, except on an "as needed basis" for infrequent episodes of agitation.[41] "Mood stabilizer" anticonvulsants such as carbamazepine, valproic acid, or gabapentin may be appropriate alternatives, but evidence is conflicting.[81] Clearly, more rigorous placebo-controlled studies are needed to determine the relative efficacy and place in therapy for these medication alternatives.

Noncognitive symptoms are often the most difficult aspect of AD for the caregiver. When nonpharmacologic approaches fail, selected antipsychotics and antidepressants have been useful for effective management of behavioral, psychotic, and depressive symptoms, thereby easing caregiver burden and allowing the patient to spend additional time at home. Alternative treatments are available in case initial choices are not successful. Adverse events remain an important concern in this population.

PHARMACOECONOMIC CONSIDERATIONS

The economic and social costs of AD are staggering. It is the third most expensive illness in the United States after heart disease and cancer, and the majority of medical and caregiving expenses are left to the patients' families and to government programs (state and federal). The total national cost of AD is estimated at approximately $148 billion annually.[4] In 2005, annual Medicare costs were estimated at $91 billion and Medicaid costs for institutionalized AD patients were estimated at $21 billion.[4] With life expectancy and the number of AD cases increasing, the cost of AD is projected to quadruple over the next 50 years.[4] The potential financial burden of this disease on the healthcare system could reach crisis proportions in the near future unless more effective avenues are developed to provide care for these individuals, to prevent the disease from occurring, or to slow its progression.

Seventy-five percent of care for AD patients is provided by family and friends.[4] Higher levels of home care have been associated with poorer health and higher rates of emotional stress in caregivers, increasing the likelihood of placing patients in institutionalized care, which is considered the greatest financial cost in treating patients with AD.[4] On average, the cost of yearly nursing home care is $70,000 to $77,000 per year depending on the area of the country where care is provided.[4] Clearly, the greatest economic burden for the home-living AD patient is the time spent in caring for the patient, whereas in the nursing home the burden is the cost for others to provide care.

Economic data on the cost benefit of medications in AD are growing. Few studies provide prospective cost data from randomized controlled trials, and the data that does exist is for relatively short durations of therapy. Two clinical trials suggest that there is no benefit or disadvantage of donepezil compared to placebo in the cost of healthcare resource use.[42] There are no similar data for galantamine or rivastigmine. One cost analysis trial of memantine found that there was a trade-off between lower costs borne by the caregiver during treatment and higher drug costs borne by the patient.[43] Cost-effectiveness would be established if medications were shown to reduce the cost of care, particularly institutional care, but current randomized controlled trials have not been of sufficient duration to establish this.[42] Most estimates of cost related to AD therapy are based on pharmacoeconomic models involving extrapolation of results from short-term trials, epidemiologic data, and data on resource use in various healthcare delivery models.[87] Each analysis employs different assumptions and incorporates different aspects of cost, making comparisons across analyses difficult. Until long-term data are available, the true cost benefit of various treatment approaches remains unknown.

⓫ Data from current pharmacoeconomic studies in AD suggest that medication therapy may reduce costs of treating this illness; however, the true cost-effectiveness of these therapies has yet to be established. If AD treatments delay cognitive decline and time to nursing home placement, then they not only have potential economic benefit, but significant effects on the quality of life of patients and caregivers. Future studies, including prospective pharmacoeconomic trials of longer duration and more detailed cost-evaluation modeling, are needed to determine the role and benefits of pharmacotherapy on AD.

EVALUATION OF THERAPEUTIC OUTCOMES

An evaluation of therapeutic outcomes in the patient with AD begins with a thorough assessment at baseline and a clear definition of therapeutic goals. Cognitive status, physical status, functional performance, mood, and behavior all need to be evaluated before initiation of drug therapy. The clinician should interview both the patient and the caregiver to assess response to drug therapy. In evaluating response to cognitive agents, the clinician should ask questions about the patient's ability to perform daily functional tasks and about mood and behavior, as well as questions about memory and orientation. Objective assessments such as MMSE for cognition assessment and the Functional Activities Questionnaire for assessment of activities of daily living, can be used to quantify changes in symptoms and function.

Because target symptoms of psychiatric disorders may respond differently in dementia patients, a detailed list of symptoms to be treated should be documented in the pharmacotherapy plan to aid in monitoring. These could include, for example, "striking at spouse because patient believes spouse is an impostor," "verbal threats and refusal to allow clothes to be changed," and so on, as opposed to documenting vague symptoms such as "aggression" or "delusions." To make an accurate assessment of depression, multiple symptoms (e.g., sleep, appetite, and activity and interest levels) need to be assessed in addition to the patient's stated mood.

The patient should be observed carefully for potential side effects of drug therapy. The specific side effects to be monitored and the method and frequency of monitoring should be documented. Periodic assessments for drug effectiveness, side effects, compliance, need for dosage adjustment, and change in treatment should occur at least monthly. However, patients need to be treated for an adequate duration to see a therapeutic effect from a given intervention. Because the effects of cognition-enhancing medications are not great, a treatment period of several months to a year may be necessary before it can be determined whether therapy is beneficial. Cognitive effects of the drug are often noticed only as a plateauing during treatment or as deterioration following drug discontinuation. In general, cognitive agents should be continued if the patient is demonstrating no change in clinical status. However, if there is doubt, the medication can be slowly tapered and discontinued, and the patient monitored off the drug for 4 to 6 weeks to determine the need for continued therapy.

ABBREVIATIONS

Aβ: beta-amyloid peptide

AD: Alzheimer's disease

ADAS-cog: Alzheimer's Disease Assessment Scale—Cognition

Apo E: apolipoprotein E

APP: amyloid precursor protein

DSM-IV-TR: *Diagnostic and Statistical Manual of Mental Disorders*, Fourth Edition, Text Revision

MMSE: Mini-Mental Status Examination

NFT: neurofibrillary tangle

NMDA: *N*-methyl-D-aspartate

NSAID: nonsteroidal antiinflammatory drug

SSRI: selective serotonin reuptake inhibitor

REFERENCES

1. Burns A, Iliffe S. Alzheimer's disease. BMJ 2009;339:b158.
2. Querfurth HW, LaFerla FM. Alzheimer's disease. N Engl J Med 2010;362:329–344.
3. Hebert LE, Scherr PA, Bienias JL, et al. Alzheimer's disease in the U.S. population: Prevalence estimates using the 2000 census. Arch Neurol 2003;60:1119–1122.
4. Alzheimer's Association. *http://www.alz.org/*.
5. Williamson J, Goldman J, Marder KS. Genetic aspects of Alzheimer's disease. Neurologist 2009;15:80–86.
6. Brunnström HR, Englund EM. Cause of death in patients with dementia disorders. Eur J Neurol 2009;16:488–492.
7. Mitchell SL, Teno JM, Kiely DK, et al. The clinical course of advanced dementia. N Engl J Med 2009;361:1529–1538.
8. Bertram L, Tanzi RE. Genome-wide association studies in Alzheimer's disease. Hum Mol Genet 2009;18:R137–R145.
9. Kim J, Basak J, Holtzman DM. The role of apolipoprotein E in Alzheimer's disease. Neuron 2009;63:287–303.
10. Jicha GA, Parisi JE, Dickson DW, et al. Alzheimer's and Lewy body pathology in centenarian case series. Neurology 2005;6(Suppl 1):A275.
11. Thomassen R, van Schaick HW, Blansjaar BA. Prevalence of dementia over age 100. Neurology 1998;50:283–286.
12. Blansjaar BA, Thomassen R, Van Schaick HW. Prevalence of dementia in centenarians. Int J Geriatr Psychiatry 2000;15:219–225.
13. Evans DA, Funkenstein HH, Albert MS, et al. Prevalence of Alzheimer's disease in a community population of older persons. Higher than previously reported. JAMA 1989;262:2551–2556.

14. Snowdon DA, Kemper SJ, Mortimer JA, et al. Linguistic ability in early life and cognitive function and Alzheimer's disease in late life. Findings from the Nun Study. JAMA 1996;275:528–532.

15. Smyth KA, Fritsch T, Cook TB, et al. Worker functions and traits associated with occupations and the development of AD. Neurology 2004;63:498–503.

16. Swerdlow RH. Is aging part of Alzheimer's disease, or is Alzheimer's disease part of aging? Neurobiol Aging 2007;28:1465–1480.

17. Kern A, Behl C. The unsolved relationship of brain aging and late-onset Alzheimer disease. Biochim Biophys Acta 2009;1790:1124–1132.

18. McGreer PL, McGreer EG. NSAIDs and Alzheimer disease: epidemiological, animal model and clinical studies. Neurobiol Aging 2007;28:639–647.

19. Vlad SC, Miller DR, Kowall NW, et al. Protective effects of NSAIDs on the development of Alzheimer disease. Neurology 2008;70:1672–1677.

20. Parsons CG, Stöffler A, Danysz W. Memantine: a NMDA receptor antagonist that improves memory by restoration of homeostasis in the glutamatergic system—to little activation is bad, too much is even worse. Neuropharmacology 2007;53:699–723.

21. Dickstein DL, Walsh J, Brautigam H, et al. Role of vascular risk factors and vascular dysfunction in Alzheimer's disease. Mt Sinai J Med 2010;77:82–102.

22. Simpkins JW, Singh M. More than a decade of estrogen neuroprotection. Alzheimer Dement 2008;4:S131–S136.

23. Boustani M, Peterson B, Hanson L, et al. Screening for dementia in primary care: A summary of the evidence for the U.S. Preventive Services Task Force. Ann Intern Med 2003;138:927–937.

24. Milne A, Cluverwell A, Guss R, et al. Screening for dementia in primary care: a review of the use, efficacy and quality of measures. Int Psychogeriatr 2008;20:911–926.

25. American Psychiatric Association. Diagnostic and Statistical Manual of Mental Disorders, Fourth Edition, Text Revision. Washington, DC: American Psychiatric Association, 2000.

26. Costa PT Jr, Williams TF, Somerfield M, et al. Early Identification of Alzheimer's Disease and Related Dementias. Clinical Practice Guidelines, Quick Reference Guide for Clinicians, No. 19. Rockville, MD: U.S. Department of Health and Human Services, Public Health Service, Agency for Health Care Policy and Research, 1996.

27. Knopman DS, DeKosky ST, Cummings JL, et al. Practice parameter: Diagnosis of dementia (an evidence-based review): Report of the Quality Standards Subcommittee of the American Academy of Neurology. Neurology 2001;56:1143–1153.

28. Roman GC, Tatemichi TK, Erkinjuntti T, et al. Vascular dementia: Diagnostic criteria for research studies. Report of the NINDS-AIREN international workshop. Neurology 1993;43:250–260.

29. McKhann G, Drachman D, Folstein M, et al. Mental and clinical diagnosis of Alzheimer's disease: Report of the NINCDS-ADRDA Work Group under the auspices of the Department of Health and Human Services Task Force on Alzheimer's disease. Neurology 1984;34:939–944.

30. Fillenbaum GG, Peterson B, Morris JC. Estimating the validity of the Clinical Dementia Rating Scale: The CERAD experience. Consortium to Establish a Registry for Alzheimer's Disease. Aging 1996;8:379–385.

31. Moore AR, O'Keeffe ST. Drug-induced cognitive impairment in the elderly. Drugs Aging 1999;15:15–28.

32. Boustani M, Campbell N, Munger S. Impact of anticholinergics on the aging brain: a review and practical application. Aging Health 2008;4:311–320.

33. Coleman RE. Positron emission tomography diagnosis of Alzheimer's disease. Neuroimaging Clin N Am 2005;15:837–846.

34. Schipper HM. Apolipoprotein E: Implications for AD neurobiology, epidemiology and risk assessment. Neurobiol Aging 2009; doi:10.1016j.neurobiolaging.2009.04.021.

35. Peterwen RC, Roberts RO, Knopman DS, et al. Mild cognitive impairment: Ten years later. Arch Neurol 2009;66:1447–1455.

36. Geldmacher DS, Frolich L, Doody RS, et al. Realistic expectations for treatment success in Alzheimer's disease. J Nutr Health Aging 2006;10:417–429.

37. Benoit M, Arbus C, Blanchard F, et al. Professional consensus on the treatment of agitation, aggressive behaviour, oppositional behaviour and psychotic disturbances in dementia. J Nutr Health Aging 2006;10:410–415.

38. Ayalon L, Gum AM, Feliciano L, Arean PA. Effectiveness of nonpharmacological interventions for the management of neuropsychiatric symptoms in patients with dementia: A systematic review. Arch Intern Med 2006;166:2182–2188.

39. Doody RS, Stevens JC, Beck C, et al. Practice parameter: Management of dementia (an evidence-based review). Neurology 2001;56:1154–1166.

40. Qaseem A, Snow V, Cross JT Jr, et al. Current pharmacologic treatment of dementia: A clinical practice guideline from the American College of Physicians and the American Academy of Family Physicians. Ann Intern Med 2008;148:370–378.

41. APA Work Group on Alzheimer's Disease and other Dementias; Rabins PV, Blacker D, Rovner BW, et al. American Psychiatric Association practice guideline for the treatment of patients with Alzheimer's disease and other dementias, second edition. Am J Psychiatry 2007;164:5–56.

42. Birks J. Cholinesterase inhibitors for Alzheimer's disease. Cochrane Database Syst Rev 2006;1:CD005593.

43. McShane R, Areosa Sastre A, Minakaran N. Memantine for dementia. Cochrane Database Syst Rev 2006;2:CD003154.

44. Lleó A, Greenberg SM, Growdon JH. Current pharmacotherapy for Alzheimer's disease. Annu Rev Med 2006;57:513–533.

45. Singh S, Dudley C. Discontinuation syndrome following donepezil cessation. Int J Geriatr Psychiatry 2003;18:282–284.

46. Lee J, Monette J, Sourial N, et al. The use of a cholinesterase inhibitor review committee in long-term care. J Am Med Dir Assoc 2007;8:243–247.

47. Rubin CD. The primary care of Alzheimer's disease. Am J Med Sci 2006;332:314–333.

48. Namenda (memantine hydrochloride) [package insert]. St. Louis, MO: Forest Laboratories; 2007.

49. Atri A, Shaughnessy LW, Locascio JJ, Growdon JH. Long-term course and effectiveness of combination therapy in Alzheimer disease. Alzheimer Dis Assoc Disord 2008;22:209–221.

50. Tariot PN, Farlow MR, Grossberg GT, et al. Memantine treatment in patients with moderate to severe Alzheimer's disease already receiving donepezil: A randomized controlled trial. JAMA 2004;291:317–324.

51. Porsteinsson AP, Grossberg GT, Mintzer J, Olin JT. Memantine treatment in patients with mild to moderate Alzheimer's disease already receiving a cholinesterase inhibitor: A randomized, double-blind, placebo-controlled trial. Curr Alzheimer Res 2008;5:83–89.

52. Rafii MS, Aisen PS. Recent developments in Alzheimer's disease therapeutics. BMC Med 2009;7:7.

53. Rogers SL, Doody RS, Pratt RD, Ieni JR. Long-term efficacy and safety of donepezil in the treatment of Alzheimer's disease: Final analysis of a US multicentre open-label study. Eur Neuropsychopharmacol 2000;10(3):195–203.

54. Raskind MA, Peskind ER, Truyen L, et al. The cognitive benefits of galantamine are sustained for at least 36 months: A long-term extension trial. Arch Neurol 2004;61:252–256.

55. Farlow MR, Lilly ML; ENA713 B352 Study Group. Rivastigmine: An open-label, observational study of safety and effectiveness in treating patients with Alzheimer's disease for up to 5 years. BMC Geriatr 2005;5:3.

56. Reisberg B, Doody R, Stoffler A, et al. A 24-week open-label extension study of memantine in moderate to severe Alzheimer's disease. Arch Neurol 2006;63:49–54.

57. Lyketsos CG, Colenda CC, Beck C, et al. Position statement of the American Association for Geriatric Psychiatry regarding principles of care for patients with dementia resulting from Alzheimer's disease. Am J Geriatr Psychiatry 2006;14:561–573.

58. Balk EM, Raman G, Tatsioni A, et al. Vitamin B_6, B_{12}, and folic acid supplementation and cognitive function: A systematic review of randomized trials. Arch Intern Med 2007;167:21–30.

59. Middleton LE, Yaffe K. Promising strategies for the prevention of dementia. Arch Neurol 2009;66:1210–1215.

60. Barrett-Conner, E, Laughlin GA. Endogenous and exogenous estrogen, cognitive function and dementia in postmenopausal women: Evidence from epidemiologic studies and clinical trials. Semin Reprod Med 2009;27:275–282.

61. Bennett DA, Whitmer RA. NSAID exposure and risk of Alzheimer disease: Is timing everything? Neurology 2009;72(22):1884–1885.

62. in t'Veld BA, Ruitenberg A, Hofman A, et al. Nonsteroidal antiin-flammatory drugs and the risk of Alzheimer's disease. N Engl J Med 2001;345(21):1515–1521.

63. Arvanitakis Z, Grodstein F, Bienias JL, et al. Relation of NSAIDs to incident AD, change in cognitive function, and AD pathology. Neurology 2008;70(23):2219–2225.

64. Aisen PS, Davis KL, Berg JD, et al. A randomized controlled trial of prednisone in Alzheimer's disease. Neurology 2000;54:588–593.

65. McGuinness B, Bullock CD, Passmore P. Statins for the prevention of dementia [review]. Cochrane Database Syst Rev 2009;2:CD003160.

66. Kandiah N, Feldman HH. Therapeutic potential of statins in Alzheimer's disease. J Neurol Sci 2009;283:230–234.

67. Wagstaff L, Mitton M, Mclendon B, et al. Statin-associated memory loss: Analysis of 60 case reports and review of the literature. Pharmacotherapy 2003;23(7):871–880.

68. Isaac MGEKN, Quinn R, Tabet N. Vitamin E for Alzheimer's disease and mild cognitive impairment. Cochrane Database Syst Rev 2008;3:CD002854.

69. Miller ER 3rd, Pastor-Barriuso R, Riemersma RA, et al. Meta-analysis: high-dosage vitamin E supplementation may increase all-cause mortality. Ann Intern Med 2005;142:37–46.

70. Kelley BJ, Knopman DS. Alternative medicine and Alzheimer disease. Neurologist 2008;14:299–306.

71. DeKosky ST, Williamson JD, Fitzpatrick AL, et al. *Gingko biloba* for prevention of dementia. A randomized controlled trial. JAMA 2008;300:2253–2262.

72. Marcolina S. The use of ginkgo biloba for Alzheimer's dementia. Alternative Medicine Alert 2006;9(6):61–72.

73. Zhang Z, Wang X, Chen Q, et al. Clinical efficacy and safety of huperzine Alpha in treatment of mild to moderate Alzheimer disease, a placebo-controlled, double-blind, randomized trial. Zhonghua Yi Xue Za Zhi 2002;82:941–944.

74. Li J. Wu HM, Zhou GJ, et al. Huperzine A for Alzheimer's disease. Cochrane Database Syst Rev 2008;2:CD005592.

75. Quinn JF, Raman R, Thomas RG, et al. A clinical trial of docosahexaenoic acid (DHA) for the treatment of Alzheimer's disease [abstract]. Alzheimer Dement 2009;5:P84.

76. Swerdlow R, Marcus DL, Landman J, et al. Brain glucose and ketone body metabolism in patients with Alzheimer's disease. Clin Res 1989;37:461A.

77. Henderson ST, Vogel JL, Barr LJ, et al. Study of the ketogenic agent AC-1202 in mild to moderate Alzheimer's disease: a randomized, double-blind, placebo-controlled, multicenter trial [abstract]. Nutr Metab 2009;6:31.

78. Holmes C, Boche D, Wilkinson D, et al. Long-term effects of Abeta42 immunisation in Alzheimer's disease: follow-up of a randomized, placebo-controlled phase I trial. Lancet 2008;372:216–223.

79. Doody RS, Gavrilova SI, Sano M, et al. Effect of dimebon on cognition, activities of daily living, behavior, and global function in patients with mild-to-moderate Alzheimer's disease: a randomized, double-blind, placebo-controlled study. Lancet 2008;372:207–215.

80. Cummings JL, Mackell J, Kaufer D. Behavioral effects of current Alzheimer's disease treatments: a descriptive review. Alzheimer Dement 2008;4:49–60.

81. Passmore MJ, Gardner DM, Polak Y, et al. Alternatives to atypical antipsychotics for the management of dementia-related agitation. Drugs Aging 2008;25:381–398.

82. Rodda J, Morgan S, Walker Z. Are cholinesterase inhibitors effective in the management of the behavioral and psychological symptoms of dementia in Alzheimer's disease? A systematic review of randomized, placebo-controlled trials of donepezil, rivastigmine and galantamine. Int Psychogeriatr 2009;21:813–824.

83. Howard RJ, Juszczak E, Ballard CG, et al. Donepezil for the treatment of agitation in Alzheimer's disease. N Engl J Med 2007;357:1382–1392.

84. Lingler JH, Martire LM, Schulz R. Caregiver-specific outcomes in antidementia clinical drug trials: A systematic review and meta-analysis. J Am Geriatr Soc 2005;53:983–990.

85. Schneider LS, Tariot PN, Dagerman KS, et al. Effectiveness of atypical antipsychotic drugs in patients with Alzheimer's disease. N Engl J Med 2006;355:1525–1538.

86. Schneider LS, Dagerman K, Insel PS. Efficacy and adverse effects of atypical antipsychotics for dementia: Meta-analysis of randomized, placebo-controlled trials. Am J Geriatr Psychiatry 2006;14:191–210.

87. Cohen JT, Neumann PJ. Decision analytic models for Alzheimer's disease: State of the art and future directions. Alzheimer Dement 2008;4:212–222.

88. Blennow K, deLeon MJ, Zetterberg H. Alzheimer's disease. Lancet 2006;368:387–403.

89. U.S. Census Bureau, Population Division. U.S. Interim Projections by Age, Sex, Race, and Hispanic Origin: 2000–2050; Table 2a, Projected Population of United States, by Age and Sex: 2000–2050. *http://www.census.gov/population/www/projections/usinterimproj/*.

90. Reisberg B. Diagnostic criteria in dementia: a comparison of current criteria, research challenges, and implications for DSM-V. J Geriatr Psychiatry Neurol 2006;19:137–146.

91. Chapman DP, Williams SM, Strine TW, et al. Dementia and its implications for public health. Prev Chronic Dis [serial online] 2006. *http://www.cdc.gov/pcd/issues/2006/apr/05_0167.htm*.

92. Aricept (donepezil hydrochloride) [package insert]. Teaneck, NJ: Eisai Co., Ltd.; 2006.

93. Exelon (rivastigmine tartrate) [package insert]. East Hanover, NJ: Novartis Pharmaceuticals; 2006.

94. Razadyne (galantamine hydrobromide) [package insert]. Titusville, NJ: Ortho-McNeil-Janssen Pharmaceuticals; 2008.

95. Exelon (rivastigmine) Patch [package insert]. East Hanover, NJ: Novartis Pharmaceutical; 2009.

96. Swanoski MT. Homotaurine: A failed drug for Alzheimer's disease and now a nutraceutical for memory protection. Am J Health Syst Pharm 2009;66:1950–1953.

97. Grossberg GT, Desai AK. Management of Alzheimer's disease. J Gerontol A Biol Sci Med Sci 2003;58A:331–353.

64

Multiple Sclerosis

JACQUELYN L. BAINBRIDGE AND JOHN R. CORBOY

KEY CONCEPTS

❶ The etiology of multiple sclerosis (MS) is unknown, and currently there is no cure.

❷ Multiple sclerosis is characterized by central nervous system demyelination and axonal damage, and appears to be autoimmune in nature.

❸ Multiple sclerosis is classified by the nature of progression over time into several categories which have different clinical presentations and responses to therapy.

❹ Diagnosis of MS requires evidence of dissemination of lesions over time and in multiple parts of the central nervous system and/or optic nerve, and is made primarily on the basis of clinical symptoms and examination. Diagnostic criteria also allow for the use of magnetic resonance imaging, spinal fluid evaluation, and evoked potentials to aid in the diagnosis.

❺ Acute exacerbations or relapses of MS can be disabling. When this is the case, acute exacerbations and relapses are treated with high-dose glucocorticoids, such as methylprednisolone, intravenously, with onset of clinical response typically within 3 to 5 days.

❻ Treatment of relapsing-remitting MS with the disease-modifying therapies (DMTs) interferon β (Avonex, Betaseron, Rebif, Extavia), glatiramer acetate (Copaxone), natalizumab (Tysabri), mitoxantrone (Novantrone), and fingolimod (Gilenya) can reduce annual relapse rate, lessen severity of relapses, slow progression of changes on magnetic resonance imaging scans, slow progression of disability, and slow cognitive decline. In addition, they have been shown to reduce the likelihood of developing a second attack after a first clinically isolated syndrome consistent with MS.

❼ In most cases, treatment with DMTs should begin promptly after the diagnosis of relapsing-remitting MS, or after a clinically isolated syndrome if the brain magnetic resonance imaging is suggestive of high risk of further attacks. Natalizumab, and other choices that have been associated with problematic adverse events, should be reserved for those patients who have failed one or more standard therapies and those with poor prognostic signs.

❽ The definition of treatment inadequacy for relapsing-remitting MS remains unclear, and therapy changes after "treatment failure" should be individualized.

❾ Although studies do not support the general use of any of the FDA-approved DMTs in patients with progressive forms of the illness, information derived from multiple studies suggests younger patients with progressive illness and those with either superimposed acute relapses or enhancing lesions on magnetic resonance imaging scans may benefit from some of the presently used DMTs.

❿ Patients suffering with MS frequently have symptoms such as spasticity, bladder dysfunction, fatigue, neuropathic pain, cognitive dysfunction, and depression that can require treatment. Patients must be counseled that therapies such as interferon β and glatiramer acetate will not relieve these symptoms. Depression is common in MS and can pose the risk of suicide.

Multiple sclerosis (MS) is an inflammatory disease of the central nervous system (CNS) that affects approximately 1 in 200 women and somewhat fewer men in the United States.[1] The term multiple sclerosis refers to two characteristics of the disease: the numerous affected areas of the brain and spinal cord producing multiple neurologic symptoms that accrue over time, and the characteristic plaques or sclerosed areas that are the hallmark of the disease.

❶ Although MS was first described almost 140 years ago, the cause remains a mystery, and a cure is still unavailable. Nevertheless, many advances have been made in treating and managing the complications of the disease and improving the quality of life of individuals affected by MS.

EPIDEMIOLOGY

Epidemiologic aspects of MS have been reviewed in a variety of publications.[1-5] MS usually is diagnosed in patients between the ages of 15 and 45 years, and the peak incidence occurs in the fourth decade of life. There are approximately 10,000 new cases diagnosed per year in the United States. Women are afflicted more than men by a ratio of approximately 2:1. Men usually develop the first signs of MS at a later age than women and are also more likely to develop the progressive form of the disease. The most important factors in the determination of risk for developing the disease are geography, age, environmental influences, and genetics. In general, disease prevalence is higher the greater the distance from the equator. Within the United States, the prevalence of MS is higher in states above the 37th parallel. Multiple sclerosis occurs more frequently in whites of Scandinavian ancestry than in other ethnic groups. Epidemiologic and experimental data have suggested an inverse relationship between MS risk and 25-hydroxyvitamin D levels.[1,6]

ETIOLOGY

It is thought that genetically susceptible individuals ≤15 years of age who have lived in a high-risk area for at least 2 years and were exposed to a crucial environmental agent are at risk for developing MS. Interestingly, an individual who migrates from a low- to a high-risk area prior to the age of 15 years acquires the same chance of developing MS as those who live in a high-risk area all their lives.[2] If the move is made from a high- to a low-risk area, the individual retains the high risk if the move is made after the age of 15 years but acquires the lower risk if the move is made prior to this age.[2] Smoking cigarettes has been associated with both an increased risk of developing MS and with more severe progression of disability.[5,7]

Viral or bacterial infections may be an important environmental cause of MS. Although no clear association has been identified, infections might cause either a direct attack on myelin and the oligodendrocyte, or stimulation of an autoimmune response leading to demyelination. Evidence to support a viral etiology includes increased immunoglobulin G (IgG) synthesis in the CNS, increased antibody titers to certain viruses, and epidemiologic studies that indicate a childhood exposure factor, suggesting that "viral" infections may precipitate exacerbations. In addition, viruses have been shown to cause diseases with prolonged incubation periods, myelin destruction, and a relapsing-remitting course in both humans and experimental animal models.[1,8]

Although numerous viruses have been proposed as associated with MS, the greatest evidence is for Epstein-Barr virus (EBV). Antibody titers to Epstein-Barr nuclear antigen (EBNA) complex are higher in MS patients vs controls, especially if blood is collected ≥5 years before onset. These titers increase over time in MS patients vs controls (controls are unchanged), and a 4-fold increase in EBNA titers over time results in a 3-fold increased risk of developing MS (almost 18-fold increase in those with first samples before age 20).[9] Interestingly, one paper notes individuals positive for *HLA DRB1*1501* have a 24-fold increased risk of developing MS when they also have antibodies to certain epitopes within EBNA-1 compared with others.[10] This is consistent with a genetic-environmental interaction. In addition, anti-EBNA titers have been associated with relapsing-remitting MS (RRMS), conversion of clinically isolated syndrome (CIS) to RRMS, and with magnetic resonance imaging (MRI) measures such as gadolinium-enhancing lesions, change in T2 lesion volume ($r = 0.27$; $P = 0.044$), and Expanded Disability Status Scale (EDSS) score ($r = 0.3$; $P = 0.035$). Zivadinov et al. also found anti-EBNA and anti-vascular cell adhesion (VCA) titers associated with gray matter atrophy in MS.[11] While Serafini et al. have claimed to identify evidence of abortive infection in a significant number of MS patients,[12] others have not been able to replicate these findings.[13] The majority of the data would lead to a conclusion that exposure to EBV is somehow associated with developing MS, but does not support the concept of an active or aborting EBV infection directly causing MS.

The familial recurrence rate of MS is approximately 5%, with siblings being the most commonly reported relationship,[4] and a concordance rate among monozygotic twins of approximately 25%.[14] This is consistent with the idea that an environmental agent is important in the etiology of MS, but also suggests a role for one or more genes. Genes that lie within the major histocompatibility complex (MHC), which is located on the sixth chromosome in humans, have been linked to MS.[1,4] Recent data show a significant association of risk with mutations in the IL-2α and IL-7α receptor genes.[15,17] African Americans are significantly less likely to

be diagnosed with MS compared with whites, though there is emerging evidence that they are more likely to have a severe disease course[18] and respond less well to interferon therapy.[19] A locus on chromosome 1 may be associated with increased susceptibility in African Americans.[20]

PATHOPHYSIOLOGY

❷ The basic physiologic derangement in MS is the stripping of the myelin sheath surrounding CNS axons. This activity is associated with an inflammatory, perivenular infiltrate consisting of T and B lymphocytes, macrophages, antibodies, and complement.[8] Demyelination renders axons susceptible to damage, which becomes irreversible when they are severed. Irreversible axonal damage correlates with disability and can be visualized as hypointense lesions, or "black holes," on T_1-weighted MRI.[21,22]

It is now well accepted that MS lesions are heterogeneous, which may be in part due to differences in the stage of evolution of the lesions over time, differences in underlying immunopathogenesis, or a combination of the two. Briefly stated, acute lesions show demyelination and axonal destruction with lymphocytic activity consistent with an inflammatory state. In contrast, more chronic lesions display less inflammatory lymphocytes with active remyelination.[8] Although traditional descriptions have focused on the white matter as the sole location of MS lesions, more recent studies have clearly identified cortical and subcortical gray matter lesions both pathologically[23] and radiographically.[24] In addition, a subset of patients with progressive MS are noted to have abnormalities consistent with B-cell follicles in the meninges.[25]

Just as the full dimensions of the neuropathology are uncertain, so is the pathogenesis of the MS lesion. There is substantial evidence, however, to suggest it is an autoimmune process directed against myelin and oligodendrocytes, the cells that make myelin in the CNS[8] (Fig. 64–1). A new concept of T-cell entry into the CNS suggests that the initial lymphocyte invasion in MS may proceed through the ventricles, towards the choroid plexus along a CCL 20 gradient that attracts activated Th17 cells.[26] The actual mediator of myelin and axonal destruction has not been established, but may reflect a combination of macrophages, antibodies, destructive cytokines, and reactive oxygen intermediates. The exact trigger for the activation of the T cells in the periphery remains unclear, but the T cells in MS patients recognize myelin basic protein (MBP), proteolipid protein, myelin oligodendrocyte glycoprotein, and myelin-associated glycoprotein. T-helper subtypes can be either pathogenic or protective in MS. Furthermore, theory holds that certain T-cell subsets are not terminally differentiated, but instead engender a level of plasticity that allows for their conversion from pathogenic to protective and vice versa under certain conditions (Fig. 64–2).[27] In patients with stable or mild disease, increased numbers of cells are found that express messenger RNA (mRNA) for transforming growth factor-β (TGF-β) and interleukin-10 (IL-10) compared with patients with severe disease. Conversely, a reduction in the number of T-regulatory (Treg) cells, which exhibit suppressor activity, is associated with active MS and can be found in patients with progressive disease. It should be noted, however, that Treg ratios do not always correlate with disease activity. Of note, there is experimental evidence that associates high 25-hydroxyvitamin D levels with improved Treg function, favoring the Th2 phenotype in the Th1/Th2 balance.[28] Finally, the significance of one of the immunological hallmarks of MS, the intrathecal synthesis of multiple clones of immunoglobulins, remains unclear. The antigen(s) against which these immunoglobulins are directed remain unknown, but do not appear to include common CNS myelin antigens.[29] The complex interplay of a variety of cells, antibodies, and cytokines remains to be elucidated.

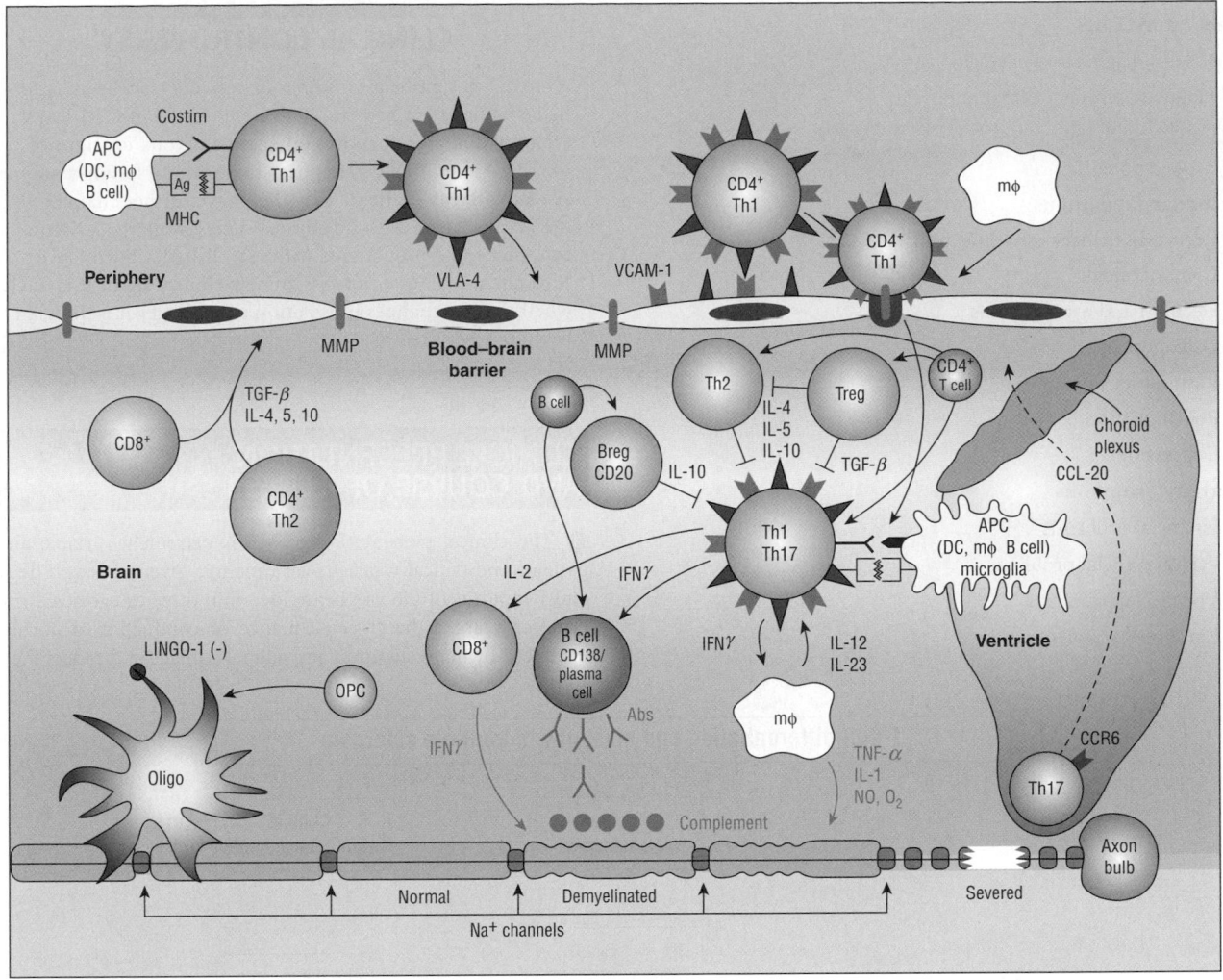

FIGURE 64-1. Autoimmune theory of the pathogenesis of multiple sclerosis (MS). In MS, the immunogenic cells tend to be more myelin-reactive, and these T-cells produce cytokines mimicking a Th1-mediated pro-inflammatory reaction. T-helper cells (CD4+) appear to be key initiators of myelin destruction in MS. These autoreactive CD4+ cells, especially of the T-helper cell type 1 (Th1) subtype, are activated in the periphery, perhaps following a viral infection, and express adhesion molecules on their surfaces that allow them to attach and roll along the endothelial cells that constitute the blood–brain barrier. In order for this reaction to occur, costimulation and MHC along with an antigen on an APC (macrophage, dendrite cell, B cell) must be present. The activated T cells also produce MMP that help to create openings in the blood–brain barrier, allowing entry of the activated T cells past the blood–brain barrier and into the CNS. Once inside the CNS, the T cells produce pro-inflammatory cytokines, especially interleukins (ILs) 1, 2, 12, 17, and 23, tumor necrosis factor-α (TNF-α), and interferon-γ (INF-γ), which further create openings in the blood–brain barrier, allowing entry of B cells, complement, macrophages, and antibodies. The T cells also interact within the CNS with the resident microglia, astrocytes, and macrophages, further enhancing production of proinflammatory cytokines and other potential mediators of CNS damage, including reactive oxygen intermediates and nitric oxide. The role of modulating, or downregulating, cytokines such as IL-4, IL-5, IL-10, and transforming growth factor-β (TGF-β) also has been described. These cytokines are the products of CD4+, CD8+, and Th1 cells.[8] New pathogenic mechanisms involve, but are not limited to, receptor-ligand mediated T-cell entry via choroid plexus (CCR6-CCL20 axis),[26] coupling of key receptor-ligands for inhibition of myelination/demyelination (LINGO-1/NOGO66/p75 or TROY complex, Jagged-Notch signaling). (Ag, antigens; APC, antigen presenting cell; DC, dendrite cell; IgG, immunoglobulin G; Mϕ, macrophage; NA+, sodium ion; MMP, matrix metalloproteinases; MHC, major histocompatibility complex; OPC, oligodendrocyte precursor cell; VLA, very late antigen; VCAM, vascular cell adhesion molecule.)

CLINICAL PRESENTATION OF MULTIPLE SCLEROSIS

General

 Most patients with multiple sclerosis present with nonspecific complaints. Many have problems with their vision or paresthesias.

Primary Symptoms/Signs

 Visual complaints/optic neuritis

 Gait problems and falls

 Paresthesias

 Pain

 Spasticity

 Weakness

 Ataxia

 Speech difficulty

 Psychological changes

 Cognitive changes

 Fatigue

 Bowel/bladder dysfunction

 Sexual dysfunction

 Tremor

Laboratory Tests

☐ MS is a diagnosis of exclusion

☐ Magnetic resonance imaging

☐ Cerebrospinal fluid studies

☐ Evoked potentials

Secondary Symptoms

☐ Recurrent urinary tract infections

☐ Urinary calculi

☐ Decubiti and osteomyelitis

☐ Osteoporosis

☐ Respiratory infections

☐ Poor nutrition

☐ Depression

Tertiary Symptoms

☐ Financial problems

☐ Personal/social problems

☐ Vocational problems

☐ Emotional problems

CLINICAL CONTROVERSY

A small but significant number of patients have been identified who have not had clear MS symptoms, but MRI scans, typically done for purposes other than to look for signs of MS, have identified what appear to be typical lesions consistent with MS. Patients may then have further changes on MRI scans, again with no clinical signs. Similarly, a significant percentage of patients with established MS will have MRI changes unassociated with new clinical signs. It is unclear whether MRI changes in isolation should trigger a clinician to begin or alter therapy.

CLINICAL PRESENTATION AND COURSE OF ILLNESS

❸ The clinical presentation of MS is extremely variable among patients and typically varies over time in a given patient. The signs and symptoms of MS can be divided into three categories. Primary symptoms are a direct consequence of conduction disturbances produced by demyelination and axonal damage and reflect the area

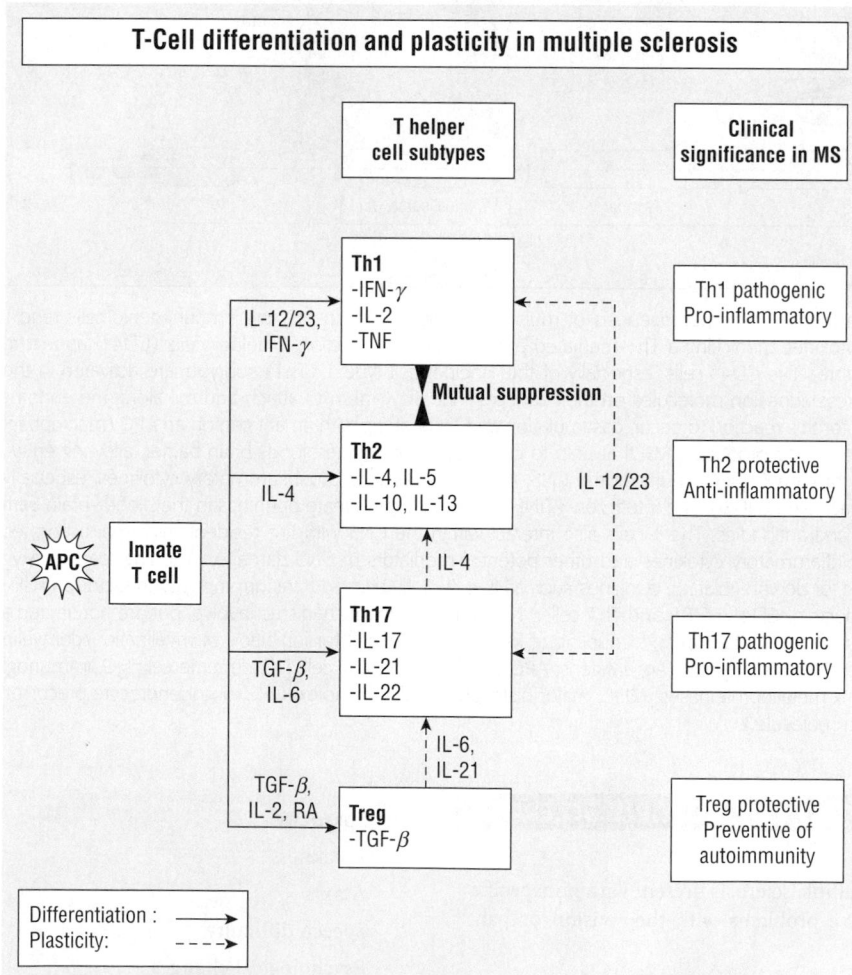

FIGURE 64-2. Upon interaction with an antigen-laden APC and specific cytokines, the innate T-cells undergo differentiation into a few lineages (subtypes). Four subtypes significant for MS pathophysiology are illustrated here (Th1, Th2, Th17, Treg). Th1 and Th17 are pro-inflammatory, Th2 is antiinflammatory, and Treg is regulatory. Th1 and Th2 are mutually suppressive and are relatively stable differentiated subtypes. In contrast, Th17 and Treg subtypes are recently found to exhibit "plasticity." In other words, they can undergo phenotypic conversion to another T-cell subtype (Th1 or Th2) in the presence of specific cytokine conditions. This plasticity of Th17 and Treg is the immunologic basis for development of therapeutic agents to favor the production of suitable Th subtypes for combating microbial invasion and also concurrently achieving neurocellular recovery after an infection.[27] (APC, antigen presenting cell.)

of the brain or spinal cord that is damaged. Secondary symptoms are complications resulting from primary symptoms. For example, urinary retention, a primary symptom, can lead to frequent urinary tract infections, a secondary symptom. Tertiary symptoms relate to the effect of the disease on the patient's everyday life.[30]

The clinical course of MS is classified into four categories.[31] At the onset of symptoms, about 85% of patients have attacks—new symptoms lasting at least 24 hours and separated from other new symptoms by at least 30 days—followed by remissions (complete or incomplete). Attacks frequently are referred to as relapses or exacerbations, and the first attack is called a clinically isolated syndrome. This course is called relapsing-remitting MS. During the RRMS phase, there is a correlation between new brain MRI lesions and clinical attacks, but typically there are many more new MRI lesions than new clinical symptoms. In RRMS patients, attack frequency tends to decrease over time and becomes independent of the development of progressive disabilities.[32] Neurologic recovery following an acute exacerbation is often quite good early in the disease course, but following repeated relapses, recovery tends to be less complete. In addition, there is a new concept of a radiologically isolated syndrome (RIS), referring to individuals who have clinical scenarios not typical of MS, yet obtain MRI scans for other reasons (e.g., headache) and have radiological signs suggestive of MS. Some percentage of these patients convert to typical MS over time,[33] although when to start treatment remains unclear.

Up to 10% to 20% of RRMS patients have a benign course, characterized by few relapses, often sensory, with minimal disability accruing over time. Most RRMS patients eventually enter a progressive phase in which attacks and remissions generally are difficult to identify. This is referred to as secondary-progressive MS (SPMS). Disability tends to accumulate more significantly during this phase of the illness. New brain MRI lesions, especially those seen only after the injection of contrast material, are less common, and brain atrophy and T1 holes increase.[34]

Approximately 15% of patients never have acute attacks and remissions but have progressive disease from the outset, known as primary-progressive MS (PPMS). These patients will have symptoms, especially spastic paraparesis, that may worsen rapidly or relatively slowly over time, and they accrue progressively more disability. Patients with PPMS are diagnosed at a later age, and the number of males is roughly equal to that of females. In general, PPMS patients tend to have a worse prognosis than those who present initially with RRMS, although more recent data suggest progression is variable.[35] Many clinical trials have suggested that a significant portion of patients with PPMS do not receive benefit from studied therapies. However, a recent article using rituximab suggests a subgroup of PPMS patients who are less than 51 years of age and have at least one gadolinium-enhancing lesion may benefit from this therapy.[36] Finally, a small percentage of patients may have a mixture of both progression and relapses, referred to as progressive-relapsing MS (PRMS). These are generally treated as relapsing patients.

Progression of the illness throughout the lifetime of the individual can be measured in many ways. The most widely used clinical rating scale in MS is the EDSS, which uses a numerical value ranging from 0 (no disability) to 10 (death from MS) to evaluate several neurologic functions.[37] The limitations of this scale are the relative insensitivity to clinical changes not involving impairment of gait and ambulation, such as changes in cognition, fatigue, and affect. Other tools, such as the Multiple Sclerosis Functional Composite (MSFC), are being evaluated for possible increased sensitivity and utility in describing changes in MS-related disability over time.[38] Increasingly, MRI is being used as an index of both disease activity and progression.[8] Specifically, the appearance of new lesions or changes in lesion number, size, and volume are being used as

TABLE 64-1	Prognostic Indicators in Multiple Sclerosis	
Indicator	**Favorable Prognosis**	**Unfavorable Prognosis**
Age at onset	<40 years	>40 years
Gender	Female	Male
Initial symptoms	Optic neuritis or sensory symptoms	Motor or cerebellar symptoms
Attack frequency in early disease	Low	High
Course of disease	Relapsing/remitting	Progressive

Data from Swanson,[42] McDonald et al.,[43] and Polman et al.[44]

outcome measures in research studies. Optical coherence tomography measures the retinal neural fiber layer thickness, and may also be a measurable sign of pathological progression over time.[39]

The unpredictable nature of MS makes it impossible to anticipate when an exacerbation will occur. However, certain factors may aggravate symptoms or lead to an acute attack (new episode of demyelination), including infections, heat (including fever), sleep deprivation, stress, malnutrition, anemia, concurrent organ dysfunction, exertion, and childbirth. Interestingly, many patients experience a significant reduction in acute relapses during the third trimester of pregnancy, followed by a relative increase postpartum.[40]

Multiple sclerosis usually does not directly diminish life expectancy. The development of secondary complications such as pneumonia or septicemia (secondary to aspiration of mouth contents with swallowing difficulties, decubitus ulcers, or urinary tract infections) or rapid progression of primary lesions affecting respiratory function can lead to a shorter than expected life span. Most of this decrease in life span is seen in patients with rapidly progressive disease. Suicide rates as high as 7 times that expected in the general population have been reported.[41] Clinical and demographic factors used to predict prognosis of MS are listed in Table 64–1.[5,42] Several MRI features also have been shown to correlate with progression of disease (see below).[44–46]

DIAGNOSIS

❹ Multiple sclerosis is a diagnosis of exclusion; symptoms frequently can be attributed to other neurologic diseases, just as many syndromes can mimic MS. Some patients may have typical symptoms consistent with classic CIS, whereas many others may have symptoms that are more vague. The diagnosis remains primarily a clinical one that requires the demonstration of "lesions separated in space and time," referring to the occurrence of at least two episodes of neurologic disturbance reflecting distinct sites of damage in the CNS that cannot be explained by another mechanism.[43] An international panel of MS experts was convened in 2000 to reevaluate current diagnostic criteria and to incorporate new data. The result of this panel's work is the McDonald criteria,[43] which allow brain MRI lesions, cerebrospinal fluid (CSF) abnormalities, and visual-evoked potential (VEP) studies to substitute for clinical lesions in defining "separated in space and time." A recent reevaluation of the McDonald criteria has simplified the use of these laboratory studies.[44] In the new scheme, diagnostic categories are MS, possible MS (for those individuals at high risk of developing MS), and not MS. The new criteria allow for earlier diagnosis.[47] Newer, simpler MRI criteria defining dissemination in time and space may be somewhat more sensitive and equally specific.[48,49] A consensus panel of the American Association of Neurology endorses the utility of MRI for diagnostic purpose,[47] and the U.S. Food and Drug Administration (FDA) has approved several of the immunotherapies to be used after a single attack of demyelination in the context of an appropriately abnormal brain MRI.

LABORATORY STUDIES

To date, there are no tests specific for MS. Evidence provided by MRI of the brain and spine, CSF evaluation, and evoked potentials, used in conjunction with the physical examination and history, aids in establishing the diagnosis of MS.

Imaging Studies

MRI produces images of the brain and spine that reflect damage in the CNS that is characteristic of MS plaques in multiple forms, for instance, in the periventricular white matter areas of the brain, as well as more generalized abnormalities such as brain atrophy. MRI is the preferred technique and is much more sensitive than computed tomography. It is useful for establishing diagnosis and prognosis. Patients with a single, typical attack of demyelination (possible MS or CIS, e.g., optic neuritis) and three or more T_2-weighted lesions on the brain MRI have an almost 90% likelihood of developing a second attack (clinically definite MS) over 15 years.[45] Optic neuritis is a common first symptom of MS and is indicative of a lesion or lesions localizing on the optic nerve. In contrast, similar individuals with normal brain MRIs have only a 19% likelihood of developing MS over 15 years.[45] Total volume of T_2-weighted lesions (called T_2 burden of disease) at the onset of CIS also appears to correlate with the development of disability.[45] Lesions that enhance after injection of the contrast material gadolinium indicate new lesions and disruption of the blood—brain barrier and are associated with early conversion to MS in CIS/possible MS patients,[45] but do not correlate well over time with progression of disability. Brain atrophy, even early in the course of the illness, probably correlates better with progression of disability.[46]

CSF Evaluation

In MS patients, CNS synthesis of IgG is increased, whereas serum IgG levels are normal. IgG synthesis rate, or the so-called IgG index, both of which compare the amount of IgG in the CSF to that in blood as normalized to overall protein counts, are typically elevated. Electrophoretic studies of the CSF show that the IgG separates into a small number of discrete bands, which, when similar bands are not seen in the serum samples taken at the same time, are called *oligoclonal bands* (OCBs).[50] Oligoclonal banding (the presence of five or more oligoclonal bands) of IgG is present in 90% to 95% of patients with clinically definite, established MS but also may be seen in lower percentages of diseases that mimic MS or are quite different clinically.[50] Increasingly, with advances in MRI, CSF analysis is reserved only for patients with atypical clinical scenarios or individuals with possible MS in whom a CSF positive for OCBs may help to define a more definite diagnosis of MS. Although white blood cell counts are often slightly elevated in the CSF of MS patients, the presence of greater than 50×10^6/mL (50×10^9/L) mononuclear cells in the CSF usually indicates a diagnosis other than MS.[50]

Evoked Potentials

Evoked potentials may be helpful in establishing areas of demyelination that are clinically silent. Slowed conduction of visual, brainstem, and somatosensory potentials can be identified, although the sensitivity and specificity of these tests seem to be somewhat less than that seen with MRI or CSF evaluation. Newer diagnostic criteria allow only for the use of VEPs to aid in formal diagnosis.[43,44]

Blood Studies

A recent report has suggested that in CIS patients with abnormal brain MRIs and abnormal CSF consistent with MS, presence or absence of antimyelin antibodies in serum may be helpful in defining prognosis for further events consistent with clinically definite MS.[51] The utility of this test, if any, remains to be defined.

DIFFERENTIAL DIAGNOSIS

A number of disorders can mimic MS. Thus, most patients are screened with blood tests for rheumatologic, collagen-vascular, infectious, and sometimes inherited metabolic diseases. Magnetic resonance imaging may rule out tumors and cervical spondylosis. The use of MRI has led to evaluations for MS in many patients with little or no clinical history consistent with MS; while some of these patients may have MRI scans suggestive of MS (so-called RIS), most of these patients have nonspecific MRI scans with identifiable causes for their scan abnormalities, including age greater than 50 years, hypertension, and migraine.[52] There are many causes of nonspecific lesions seen in the subcortical white matter on a brain MRI, and use of established criteria for distinguishing MS lesions from other etiologies enhances diagnostic accuracy. Electromyography may help in diagnosing amyotrophic lateral sclerosis and neuropathies.

TREATMENT

Treatment of MS falls into three broad categories: symptomatic therapy, treatment of acute attacks, and disease-modifying therapies (DMTs) to alter the natural course of the disease. Symptomatic management of the disease is of utmost importance to maintain the patient's quality of life. Treatment of acute attacks will shorten the duration and possibly decrease the severity of the attack. Disease-modifying therapies that alter the course of the illness are most important to diminish progressive disability over time.

A number of different treatment modalities have been studied in the last 30 years, but many older trials had flawed designs. There are no universally accepted treatment algorithms, and treatments vary among clinicians and centers. Perhaps more importantly, treatment decisions frequently are based on the wishes and goals of individual patients. One potential algorithm for the immunotherapy of RRMS is shown in Figure 64–3.

CLINICAL CONTROVERSY

When patients initially show signs of RRMS, many practitioners begin treatment with IFN-β or glatiramer acetate (ABC-R medications). However, it is controversial which medication to use, and when to start. Most data support minimal, if any, differences in efficacy among the ABC-R medications. The role of natalizumab remains unclear, but under 10% of natalizumab prescriptions have been for patients who have never used the ABC-R medications. The introduction of fingolimod further complicates the issue. Most practitioners assist newly diagnosed patients in making the decision of which medication best fits their lifestyle and offers the maximum efficacy. In patients with severe depression, interferon therapy is contraindicated, and patients are encouraged to use glatiramer acetate.

■ TREATMENT OF ACUTE EXACERBATIONS

⑤ Mild acute exacerbations that do not produce functional decline may not require treatment. When functional ability is affected, the standard intervention is intravenous injection of high-dose corticosteroids. The American Academy of Neurology recommends that if treatment with steroids is warranted, it is best to use intravenous methylprednisolone.[53] The mechanism of action for corticosteroids in MS is unknown, but it is speculated that steroids improve recovery by decreasing edema in the area of demyelination.

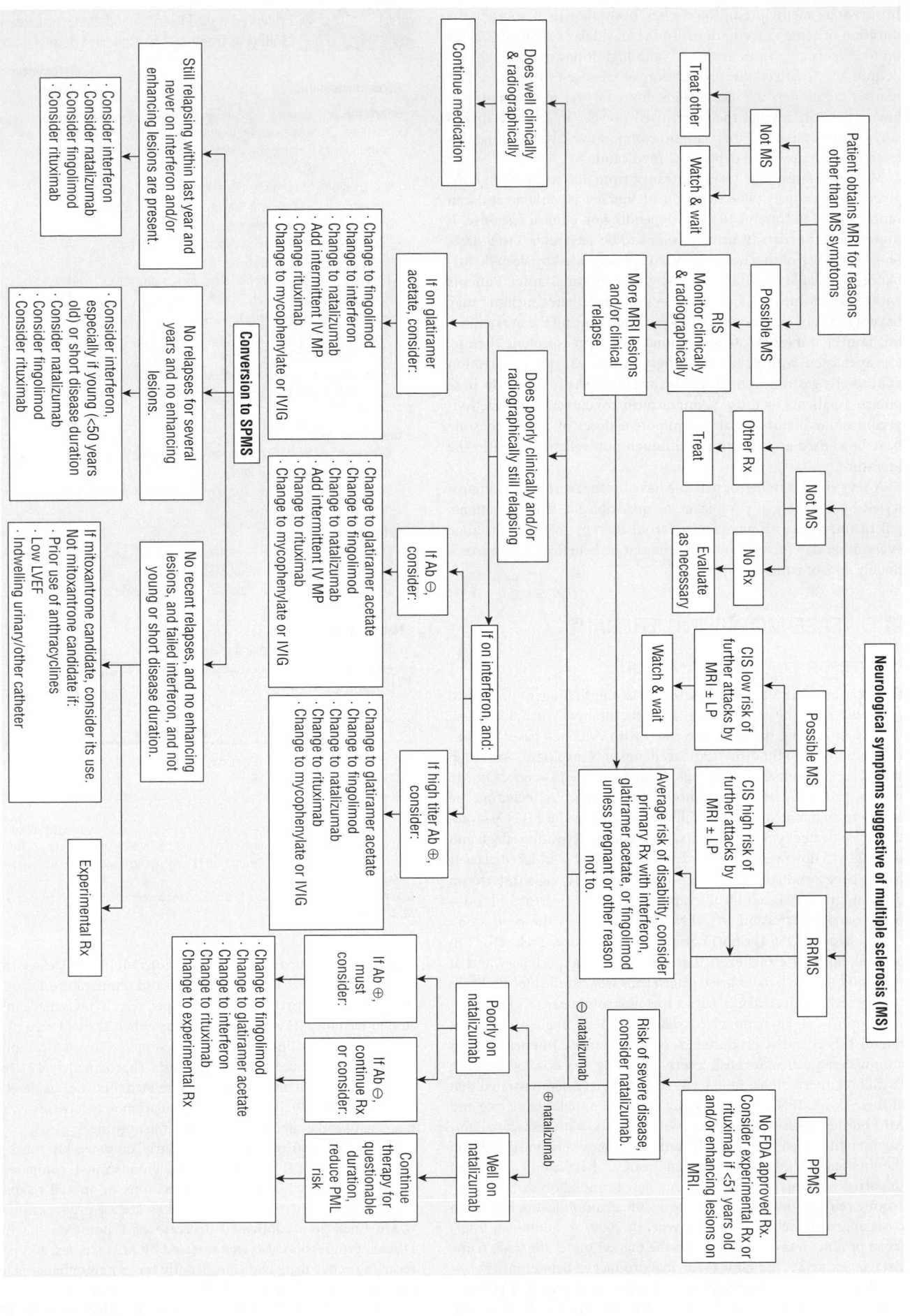

FIGURE 64-3. An algorithm for management of relapsing-remitting multiple sclerosis. (ABC-R, interferon β_{1a} [Avonex], interferon β_{1b} [Betaseron], glatiramer acetate [Copaxone], and interferon β_{1a} [Rebif]; IVIg, intravenous immunoglobulin.)

Intravenous methylprednisolone has been shown to shorten the duration of acute exacerbations, and it may delay repeat attacks for up to 2 years after optic neuritis,[53] although it has not been shown definitively to affect the progression of disease.[54] More recently, many practitioners are using high doses of oral methylprednisolone, especially mixing the lyophilized powder in flavored drinks such as smoothies, but there are no comparative data to define this as an equivalent way to deliver the medication.

Methylprednisolone doses can range from 500 to 1,000 mg/day, given intravenously. The duration of therapy is variable and can range from 3 to (rarely) 10 days, depending on clinical response. If improvement occurs, it usually begins to be seen after 3 to 5 days. Short-term use of this nature is often accompanied by sleep disturbance, a metallic taste, and, rarely, gastrointestinal upset. Patients with diabetes mellitus or a predilection to diabetes mellitus may have significant elevations of blood sugar, requiring the use of insulin. Longer durations of intravenous methylprednisolone therapy are associated with acne and fungal infections, mood alteration and, rarely, gastrointestinal hemorrhage (especially if used in hospitalized patients or those taking aspirin concurrently). If methylprednisolone is not available, equipotent doses of dexamethasone have been used as a substitute, although not well supported in the literature.

A very small number of patients have more severe attacks, manifested by hemiplegia, paraplegia, or quadriplegia. If these patients fail to improve with aggressive steroid therapy, plasma exchange every other day for seven treatments can be beneficial for approximately 40% of patients.

■ DISEASE-MODIFYING THERAPY

Interferon β_{1b} and Interferon β_{1a}

❻ Interferon (IFN)-β_{1b} (Betaseron) was the first agent proven to favorably alter the natural course of the illness.[55] In Table 64–2, disease-modifying therapies are listed with evidence-based recommendations from the American Academy of Neurology.[55] Although the exact mechanism of action is unknown, IFN-β_{1b}'s effect in MS may be caused by its immunomodulating properties, including the ability to augment suppressor cell function and reduce IFN-γ secretion by activated lymphocytes, its macrophage-activating effect, and its ability to downregulate the expression of IFN-γ-induced class II MHC gene products on antigen-presenting glial cells. Interferon also suppresses T-cell proliferation and may decrease blood—brain barrier permeability.[55] IFN-β also increases the production of regulatory CD56 (bright) natural killer cells and Treg cells.[56] In general, all interferons exert these actions in the periphery and at the blood—brain barrier level. Interferons work at the blood—brain barrier level by decreasing matrix metalloproteinases.

Interferon β_{1b} is a nonglycosylated synthetic analog of recombinant IFN-β and is produced in *Escherichia coli*. Interferon β_{1b} is administered subcutaneously every other day at a dose of 250 mcg (8 million international units). Clinical trials have demonstrated that at these doses, IFN-β_{1b} significantly reduces annual relapse rate and MRI burden of disease compared with placebo. With respect to clinical disability, however, no significant differences were noted between the interferon- and placebo-treated groups.[55] Betaseron is packaged in partially premixed syringes with a new formulation that does not require refrigeration and can be used with an autoinjector. Betaseron costs approximately $19,632 per year. In 2009, an additional interferon product was introduced into the market under the trade name Extavia. Extavia is the same medicinal product as Betaseron.

Interferon β_{1a} (Avonex and Rebif) is a natural-sequence glycosylated interferon produced in Chinese hamster ovary cells. Avonex is given as 30 mcg (6 million international units) intramuscularly once

TABLE 64-2	Evidenced-Based Recommendations for Disease Modifying Treatment of Multiple Sclerosis

Recommendations	Recommendation Grades[a]
Interferon β	
• Interferon β has been shown to reduce attack rates in patients with MS or those with CIS who are at high risk of developing MS	A-I
• It is appropriate to consider IFN-β for any patient with clinically definite MS or who already has RRMS or SPMS and is still experiencing relapses	A-I
• The effectiveness of IFN-β in patients with SPMS but without relapses is uncertain	U-I
• Route of administration of IFN-β products is probably not clinically important with regards to efficacy; however, the side effect profile does differ	B-II
• Rate of production of neutralizing antibodies is probably less with IFN-β_{1a} than with IFN-β_{1b}	B-I
• Presence of neutralizing antibodies may be associated with a reduction in the clinical effectiveness of IFN-β treatment	C-I
Glatiramer acetate	
• Glatiramer acetate has been shown to reduce the attack rate in patients with RRMS	A-I
• Treatment with glatiramer acetate may slow sustained disability progression in RRMS	C-I
Mitoxantrone	
• Mitoxantrone probably reduces the attack rate in patients with relapsing forms of MS	B-II, III
• Mitoxantrone may have a beneficial effect on disease progression in MS	C-II, III
Natalizumab	
• Natalizumab decreases clinical relapse rate, Gd – enhancing lesions, and new T2 lesions	A-I
• Natalizumab in RRMS positively changes measures of disease severity such as EDSS progression rate and changes lesions on MRI in RRMS	A-I

CIS, Clinically isolated syndrome; RCT, randomized controlled trial; RRMS, relapsing-remitting MS; SPMS, secondary-progressive MS.

[a]Strength of recommendations: A: established. B: probable. C: possible. U: inadequate data to support recommendation.

Quality of evidence: Class I, evidence from one or more prospective, randomized, controlled clinical trial; Class II, evidence from cohort or RCT not meeting criteria for class I; Class III, evidence from other controlled trials; Class IV, Evidence from uncontrolled studies, case reports, case series or expert opinion.

Reprinted with permission from Goodin et al.[55] and data from Goodin et al. Neurology 2008;71:766–773.

weekly. The prefilled syringes (33 mcg/0.5 mL, 4 per package) should be refrigerated, but can be kept at room temperature for 30 days. Avonex costs approximately $18,360 per year. Rebif is made in a very similar fashion as Avonex but given as either 22 or 44 mcg (0.5 mL) subcutaneously 3 times weekly. It is supplied in a 0.5-mL prefilled syringe with an autoinjector and costs approximately $21,163 per year. Rebif should also be kept refrigerated, but it is stable at room temperature for 30 days. A new formulation may have lower immunogenicity and a slightly better side-effect profile.[57]

When given 30 mcg intramuscularly once weekly for 2 years, patients receiving IFN-β_{1a} (Avonex) demonstrated, compared with placebo, statistically significant reductions in annual relapse rate (by approximately one-third) as well as disease progression, which was defined as a confirmed decrease of 1 point on the EDSS.[75] Disease progression also was assessed by MRI studies, and patients receiving active drug had significantly fewer new enhancing lesions compared with placebo-treated patients. Similar results were seen with higher dose (44 mcg), more frequent administration (3 times weekly), and subcutaneous injection of IFN-β_{1a} (Rebif).[55] Other studies reveal significant effects on slowing brain atrophy[58] and the progression of cognitive decline[59] in patients treated with Avonex. Taken together, these observations show that IFN-β possesses significant disease-modifying activity.

Side effects are similar with all the interferons. Baseline complete blood counts, platelet determinations, and liver function tests should be documented before starting therapy, at 1 month, then every 3 months for 1 year, and every 6 months thereafter. Small percentages of patients develop depressed cell counts and liver enzyme elevations that are usually transient and respond to discontinuation of therapy. Rare patients have developed true liver failure requiring liver transplant, and the package inserts for interferon β products have been altered, reflecting this risk. The most common adverse effects include injection-site redness, swelling, and, rarely, necrosis, as well as flu-like symptoms (e.g., fever, chills, myalgias). These symptoms can be mild or severe and are seen in most patients. The flu-like side effects typically occur for up to 24 hours after injection and typically abate within 1 to 3 months after starting the injections, but they persist in some patients. Injection-site reactions probably are worse with IFN-β_{1b}, can occur at any time, and can be lessened by using appropriate injection technique, including site rotation (thighs and buttocks), hydrocortisone cream, applying ice before and after the injection, or use of an autoinjector. Injecting the medications at body temperature (place under armpits) will decrease injection-site pain. Nonsteroidal antiinflammatory agents or acetaminophen taken before and at regular intervals for 24 hours after administration may alleviate the flu-like symptoms. Initiation of one-quarter or one-half the standard dose, and then increasing to full dosage over 1 to 2 months, also may be beneficial in reducing flu-like side effects.[60] Some authors suggest that, because of the transient immune activation that can occur following the introduction of IFN-β, a short burst of oral prednisone can alleviate some adverse effects.[60]

Less commonly reported side effects include shortness of breath, tachycardia, thyroid dysfunction, and depression. Clinicians must monitor patients carefully for signs of depression and treat accordingly. Although depression is a common finding in MS patients, all the interferons, especially IFN-β_{1b}, can produce depressive symptoms. Patients who develop depression should be monitored closely because of the risk for suicide. Other side effects usually are transient. Most patients will not feel better or have improvement in symptoms when taking interferons, and many will experience side effects; thus compliance can become a major issue. Finally, safety data on IFN-β in pregnancy and lactation are lacking. Abortifacient activity in primates has been noted, and until adequate safety data are available, women should be counseled as to appropriate contraception while using these products.

Although the adverse-effect profile of IFN-β_{1a} resembles that of IFN-β_{1b}, intramuscular IFN-β_{1a} (Avonex) may hold several advantages, including fewer local injection-site reactions and once-weekly administration versus subcutaneous injection every other day (or 3 days per week with Rebif).

Glatiramer Acetate (Copaxone)

Glatiramer acetate (Copaxone, formerly known as copolymer-1) is a synthetic polypeptide consisting of L-alanine, L-glutamic acid, L-lysine, and L-tyrosine. Although the precise mechanism of action of this compound is unknown, glatiramer acetate appears to mimic the antigenic properties of MBP.[61] This agent also may act by directly binding to MHC class II receptors and inhibiting binding of MBP peptides to T-cell receptor complexes.[61] Glatiramer acetate has demonstrated that it induces Th2 (antiinflammatory) lymphocytes in experimental allergic encephalomyelitis.[61] This is thought to contribute to "bystander" suppression at the site of the MS lesion and thereby reduce inflammation, demyelination, and axonal damage.[55]

Glatiramer acetate also may suppress T-cell activation, and recent studies suggest it may be associated with a neuroprotective effect by inducing brain-derived neurotrophic factor.[62]

Given as a daily 20-mg subcutaneous dose, glatiramer acetate appears to have a relatively mild adverse effect profile. Mild pain and pruritus at the injection site are the most frequent patient complaints. Approximately 10% of patients experience a one-time transient reaction consisting of chest tightness, flushing, and dyspnea beginning several minutes after injection and lasting usually no longer than 20 minutes. If patients have no history or evidence of coronary artery disease, they may be assured these reactions are almost always self-limited and benign. Several adverse effects that have been associated with the interferons, including flu-like symptoms and depression, do not appear to be provoked by glatiramer acetate. Multicenter trials with glatiramer acetate have demonstrated significant reductions in mean annual relapse rate (approximately 29%) that are comparable with the interferons.[55] An extension trial, completed after the original, pivotal 2-year study, suggests that glatiramer acetate may slow the progression of disability in patients with RRMS.[55] Glatiramer acetate also slows development of T_1 holes on brain MRIs,[63] and long-term uncontrolled data show that it remains safe and effective for individuals who continue to take it over 10 years.[64] The annual cost of glatiramer acetate is approximately $19,749 (20 mg/mL in 30 prefilled syringes). The product is stored in the refrigerator but can be kept at room temperature for up to 1 week.

CLINICAL CONTROVERSY

Because of the potential for progressive multifocal leukoencephalopathy (PML), controversy surrounds the proper selection of patients for natalizumab therapy. With the apparent superior efficacy of natalizumab compared to other disease-modifying therapies, many clinicians use natalizumab as a primary agent in selected individuals with RRMS who are identified with poor prognostic signs such as multiple early relapses, severe relapses with incomplete remission, and MRI markers of poor prognosis, such as high burden of disease on T_1 and T_2 images, or early signs of atrophy. Whether to restrict the use of natalizumab to a maximum number of months, or alter the dosing, in an effort to limit the risk of PML, remains unclear. Prior exposure to chemotherapy appears to increase risk of PML. The advent of a serology study for JC Virus exposure may alter clinicians' willingness to prescribe natalizumab as a first line agent or alter the duration that they prescribe it.

Natalizumab (Tysabri)

Natalizumab is a partially humanized monoclonal antibody directed at the cell surface adhesion molecule $\alpha_4\beta$-integrin (also known as very-late antigen 1, VLA-1). Natalizumab works by attaching to VLA-1 and blocking its interaction with its ligand on CNS endothelium vascular cell adhesion molecule (VCAM)-1. Thus, activated lymphocytes are denied entry past the blood—brain barrier. In a phase II study, compared to placebo, natalizumab significantly reduced the number of new gadolinium-enhancing lesions by more than 90%, and diminished relapses as well.[65] In a 2-year phase III trial (A Randomized, Placebo-Controlled Trial of Natalizumab for Relapsing Multiple Sclerosis [AFFIRM]), compared to placebo, annual relapse rate was reduced by more than 60%, gadolinium-enhancing lesions were lessened by more than 90%, and progression of disability was significantly delayed.[66] In a separate 2-year, phase III trial (The Safety and Efficacy of Natalizumab in Combination with

Interferon Beta-1a in Patients with Relapsing Remitting Multiple Sclerosis [SENTINEL]) in patients already taking IFN-β_{1a} (Avonex), those who had natalizumab added to IFN-β_{1a} had a relapse rate reduction of more than 50% and gadolinium-enhancing lesion reduction of 84% compared to patients who continued with IFN-β_{1a} alone.[67] In these trials, natalizumab was injected intravenously every 4 weeks and was relatively well tolerated, although approximately 1% of patients developed infusion reactions, and 6% developed neutralizing antibodies that diminished the efficacy of the drug.

On November 23, 2004, the FDA approved natalizumab, with the stipulation that the studies would continue, for use in relapsing MS in patients with inadequate response or intolerance to other MS therapies. In February 2005, Biogen and Elan voluntarily removed natalizumab from the market after receiving reports of two patients (one patient from the SENTINEL trial, and one patient in a Crohn's disease study), who both died after developing progressive multifocal leukoencephalopathy (PML), a rare brain infection most commonly seen in patients infected with human immunodeficiency virus.[68–70] One other patient who developed PML in the SENTINEL trial survived.[68–70] Further safety analysis did not identify other cases, and on March 9, 2006, an FDA panel reviewing the data suggested reapproval of natalizumab for use in relapsing patients who would be required to be placed in an ongoing safety registry (TOUCH). On June 5, 2006, the FDA reapproved use of natalizumab in the United States, with a black-box warning about PML. Since that time, over 71,000 patients around the world (roughly 50% in the United States) have been exposed to natalizumab for treatment of MS. As of September 2010, 68 cases of PML have been identified, all in patients using the medication for 12 months or longer. The incidence for developing PML is 1 in 1,000, though it tends to increase the longer a patient is on the drug. Plasma exchange (PLEX) has been utilized to help clear the drug more rapidly from the blood of affected patients.[91] An acute syndrome referred to as immune reconstitution inflammatory syndrome has been associated with acute neurological deterioration after PLEX, requiring the use of steroids.[72] Also in 2009, natalizumab has been approved for use in Crohn's disease.

Natalizumab is indicated as monotherapy, 300 mg every 4 weeks as an IV infusion. It is indicated for the relapsing forms of MS to delay the accumulation of physical disability and decrease the number of relapses in patients who have a documented inadequate response or intolerance to traditional MS therapies. The cost of natalizumab is approximately $31,200 annually (300 mg/15 mL), which does not include nursing and other fees.[73] Patients receiving natalizumab must be enrolled in the TOUCH program. In the future, patients' blood and CSF may be screened at baseline and every 6 months to assess the presence of JC and BK virus DNA.[74]

Fingolimod (Gilenya)

Approved September 21, 2010, fingolimod is the first oral DMT for MS. It has a unique mechanism of action as a sphingosine 1-phosphate receptor agonist. Fingolimod exhibits its immunosuppressant properties by sequestering circulating lymphocytes into secondary lymphoid organs and reduces the infiltration of T-lymphocytes and macrophages into the CNS. It may have neuroprotective effects. The agent is given daily at a dose of 0.5mg. In clinical trials it decreased annualized relapse rates by approximately 52% compared to interferon beta-1a. After 5 years of continuous fingolimod therapy, approximately 92% of patients were free of gadolinium enhancing lesions, though these data were with the 1.25 mg dose. Major side effects include pronounced first dose bradycardia and, rarely, bradyarrhythmia or atrioventricular block, infections, macular edema, a decrease in forced expiratory volume over 1 second, elevation of liver enzymes, and a sustained increase of approximately 1 to 2 mm Hg in systolic and diastolic blood pressure. Rare

cases of lymphoma have also been identified. The reversal of lymphopenia can take 2 to 4 weeks after discontinuation of the drug. Monitoring recommendations include baseline complete blood counts, liver function tests, ophthalmologic examinations, and electrocardiogram in patients with known heart problems. At the time of the first dose, baseline pulse and blood pressure must be taken, and the patient must be observed for 6 hours, although the monitoring setting may be individualized. The degree to which fingolimod's oral delivery may alter the likelihood of a patient using, or continuing to use, a self-injectable medication remains to be seen.

Mitoxantrone

7 Mitoxantrone (Novantrone), a member of the anthracenedione family, is approved by the FDA for reducing neurologic disability and the frequency of clinical relapses in patients with SPMS (chronic), PRMS, or worsening RRMS.[75] The MRI outcomes, however, were not as robust as those typically seen in the trials of relapsing patients alone.[76] Mitoxantrone is administered as a brief (5- to 15-minute) intravenous infusion dosed at 12 mg/m^2 every 3 months. An evaluation of left ventricular ejection fraction and electrocardiogram are required prior to administration of each dose and if signs or symptoms of congestive heart failure develop. The maximum allowable lifetime cumulative dose of mitoxantrone is 140 mg/m^2. Other potential side effects noted with this agent are nausea, alopecia, menstrual disorder, amenorrhea, upper respiratory tract infection, urinary tract infection, and leukemia. The role mitoxantrone will ultimately play in the treatment of MS remains unclear because potential cardiac toxicity limits its long-term use. More recent estimates also suggest the risk of leukemia may be as high as 1 in 145 patients, which has significantly decreased interest in its use for MS patients.[77] In addition, although patients with SPMS were included in the mitoxantrone in MS (MIMS—Effect of Mitoxantrone on MRI in Progressive MS) trial, resulting in FDA approval for use in SPMS, there was no substudy documenting slowing of progression specifically in this subgroup of patients.[75,76] Thus, support for use of mitoxantrone in this context is less strong.[55] The average wholesale cost of mitoxantrone is approximately $1,982 (average male) or $1,586 (average female) per infusion and will vary based on the patient's body surface area. Nursing, pharmacy, and technical fees must also be added to this estimate.

CLINICAL CONTROVERSY

Many RRMS patients have either been intolerant to, failed to respond to, or been unwilling to undergo the risk associated with all of the FDA-approved medications. There are some data supporting the use of a variety of agents which have been approved for other purposes, such as rituximab and mycophenylate. When to incorporate off-label uses of medications remains a controversy.

■ REMAINING QUESTIONS FOR DISEASE-MODIFYING THERAPY

8 Despite encouraging results from well-conducted clinical trials, several relevant issues remain. The most important question in the use of the DMTs is when to begin therapy. The Medical Advisory Board of the National Multiple Sclerosis Society has adopted recommendations regarding the use of the current MS DMTs (Table 64–3).[78]

Decisions about the use of any medication rest on determination of the severity of the illness, the efficacy of the medication, and the side effects and costs related to the therapy. Clearly,

TABLE 64-3 | **Disease Management Consensus Statement**

- Initiation of therapy with an IFN-β medication (Avonex, Betaseron, Rebif, Extavia) or glatiramer acetate is advised as soon as possible following a definite diagnosis of MS with active, relapsing disease, and can also be considered for selected patients with a first attack who are at high risk of MS.
- Natalizumab is FDA approved for patients who have had an inadequate response to, or are not able to tolerate other MS therapies.
- Mitoxantrone can be considered for patients with relapsing worsening disease or patients with secondary-progressive MS who are worsening, whether or not relapses are occurring.
- Patients' access to medication should not be limited by the frequency of relapses, age, or level of disability.
- Treatment is not to be stopped during evaluation for continuing treatment.
- Therapy is to be continued indefinitely, unless there is clear lack of benefit, intolerable side effects, new data that reveal other reasons for cessation, or better therapy becomes available.
- Interferon βs (Avonex, Betaseron, Rebif, Extavia), glatiramer acetate (Copaxone), mitoxantrone (Novantrone), and natalizumab (Tysabri), are all FDA approved for patients with MS and should be included in formularies and covered by third-party payers so that physicians and patients can determine the most appropriate agent on an individual basis.
- Movement from one immunomodulating drug to another should be permitted for medical reasons.
- None of these agents are approved for use in women trying to become pregnant, who are pregnant, or nursing mothers.

Data from Miller et al.[78] with permission.

these drugs slow the course of the illness but do not suppress it completely, and in some individuals, there is no apparent benefit. There is now, however, overwhelming evidence that the vast majority of untreated patients will have progressive disease over time. Pathologic data clearly show that even in acute lesions there is significant axonal damage that is essentially irreversible. MRI data show that 80% to 90% of all new enhancing lesions are asymptomatic, suggesting that a "quiet" clinical course does not necessarily mean there is not ongoing disease activity that ultimately will be reflected in cognitive problems and progressive spastic paraparesis.

Furthermore, it is now known that very early therapy is effective. In patients with CIS and two or more T_2 lesions on brain MRI (i.e., at high risk for developing clinically definite MS), placebo-controlled studies with all three of the interferon agents and glatiramer acetate have shown significant delay in a second attack and positive outcomes on a variety of MRI measures (BENEFIT = Betaseron in Newly Emerging Multiple Sclerosis for Initial Treatment; CHAMPS = Controlled High Risk Subjects Avonex Multiple Sclerosis Prevention Study; and ETOMS = Early Treatment of Multiple Sclerosis).[55,79] Thus, very early therapy is potentially warranted, and IFN-β_{1b}, IFN-β_{1a} (Avonex), and glatiramer acetate are approved by the FDA for use after CIS in those patients with abnormal MRIs consistent with demyelination, suggestive of high risk of further demyelinating events. The National Multiple Sclerosis Society recommends that patients with relapsing disease should be placed on Avonex, Betaseron (or Extavia), Copaxone, or Rebif (ABC-R) therapy immediately after the diagnosis.[78]

A second major issue is which drug to use in which patient. There has not been a single, randomized study comparing all four ABC-R drugs with one another in a similar patient population at the same time.[80] The pivotal placebo-controlled trials produced results that were more similar than different when comparing across trials, including a nearly identical one-third reduction in relapse rate for all four drugs over 2 years. A small number of studies have suggested higher dose, more frequent administration of interferon may be more efficacious than lower dose, less frequent administration,[81,82] but these differences appear modest. Other

studies argue against this,[83,84] and recent studies note no significant difference in outcomes between standard and double dose IFN-β_{1b} and glatiramer acetate,[85] and no difference between IFN-β_{1a} (Rebif) and glatiramer acetate.[86]

A concern with all three interferon products that further muddies our understanding of the clinical differences between the interferon products is the development of neutralizing antibodies. In clinical trials, 30% to 40% of patients receiving IFN-β_{1b} developed antibodies directed against the drug.[87] In these patients, the exacerbation rate was similar to that in placebo-treated patients. In patients on IFN-β_{1b}, neutralizing antibodies can occur first at 3 to 6 months and as late as 18 months. This product tends to be the most antigenic.[87] With IFN-β_{1a}, neutralizing antibodies were found in 22% of early trials of Avonex, but later studies reported that only 2% to 5% of treated patients developed antibodies; this decrease was caused by a formulation change of the drug making it the least antigenic.[84,87] Percentages for Rebif are intermediate, therefore moderately antigenic, at approximately 12% and can occur in the first 9 to 15 months of treatment, which is the same time frame for antibody production with Avonex.[55,87,88] The long-term clinical significance of these findings, however, is still not completely clear, although three recent studies have further confirmed the effect of neutralizing antibodies on relapses, MRI lesions, and progression of disability.[88–91] Whether these antibodies are truly cross-reactive between products is unknown, as is the duration during which antibodies can be detected. There are no general consensus guidelines regarding when to test for neutralizing antibodies, which assay to use, or what titer cutoff to apply to patients in clinical settings.[92] An important question is whether production of antibodies might be diminished with treatments such as corticosteroids. Another concern of practitioners is the relationship between active ingredients and varying excipients of interferon therapies and the production of neutralizing antibodies. Neutralizing antibodies are seen in approximately 6% of patients treated with natalizumab, and the antibodies seem to diminish efficacy.[67]

⑨ We now have experience for more than a decade with MS patients taking DMTs, yet continuing to have more relapses, more lesions on MRI, more disability, and ongoing slippage into SPMS.[93] There is no accepted definition of treatment inadequacy, although the Canadian Multiple Sclerosis Research Council has suggested a relatively simple approach that incorporates the elements of relapse rate, new MRI lesions, and change on the EDSS.[94] If a patient develops significant and persistent interferon antibodies, movement to a noninterferon (glatiramer acetate, natalizumab, fingolimod, mitoxantrone, or possibly rituximab[95]) is reasonable. When failing low-dose interferon, options include changing to a higher dose, more frequent administration of interferon, or changing to a noninterferon. A second option is addition of an immunosuppressant agent, such as monthly methylprednisolone,[96] azathioprine, methotrexate, or mycophenolate. As noted above, the addition of natalizumab to IFN-β_{1a} was effective, but produced rare cases of PML, and thus, this combination should not be used. The addition of a statin agent may worsen MS[97] although these results are not definitive.

■ SYMPTOMATIC MANAGEMENT

⑩ Many of the symptoms of MS do not require pharmacologic management or do not respond to it. This section addresses the primary symptoms in which pharmacologic management may be of benefit (Table 64–4).[30,94,98–100] See the preceding section on the treatment of acute exacerbations for a discussion of optic neuritis.

Gait Difficulties and Spasticity

Problems with gait can be caused by spasticity, weakness, ataxia, defective proprioception, or a combination of these factors. Spasticity

	Bladder	Sensory	
Spasticity	Symptoms	Symptoms	Fatigue
Baclofen	Propantheline	Carbamazepine	Amantadine
Dantrolene	Oxybutynin	Phenytoin	Antidepressants
Diazepam	Dicyclomine	Amitriptyline or	Modafinil
Tizanidine	DDAVP	other TCAs	Methylphenidate
Tiagabine	Self-catheterization	Gabapentin	Dextroamphetamine
Gabapentin	Imipramine or	Lamotrigine	
Pregabalin	amitriptyline	Pregabalin	
Botulinum toxin	Prazosin		
type A	Botulinum toxin		
Dalfampridine	type A		
	Solifenacin		
	Darifenacin		
	Trospium		
	Hyoscyamine		
	Fesoterodine		

TABLE 64-4 Treatment of Selected Primary Multiple Sclerosis Symptoms

DDAVP, desmopressin acetate; TCA, tricyclic antidepressant.
Data from Schapiro,[50] Freedman et al.,[94] Mitchell,[98] Goodman et al.,[99] Kinn and Larson.[100]

is amenable to pharmacologic intervention, whereas physical therapy may be required in treating gait disturbances owing to any of the other factors. Spasticity is encountered commonly and tends to affect the legs more markedly than the arms. Spasticity can result in falls; however, in the later stages of the disease, the increased muscle tone of a spastic limb often lends strength to patients with underlying weakness. Therefore, when using muscle relaxants, one must be careful not to decrease the tone to an extent that ambulation is actually hindered.[30,98] Baclofen (Lioresal), a γ-aminobutyric acid (GABA) analog, is the preferred agent and usually is started in dosages of 10 mg 3 times daily and titrated upward to achieve the desired response. Most patients achieve a satisfactory response with dosages between 40 and 80 mg/day; however, dosages higher than the recommended daily maximum of 80 mg are required by some patients.[30,98] A wearing-off is common, however, due to the relatively short duration of action. A longer-acting version of Lioresal is under study. Continuous intrathecal administration of baclofen may be an option for patients unable to tolerate or unresponsive to oral therapy. Baclofen should not be discontinued abruptly to avoid the possibility of seizures.[98] Small doses of diazepam (Valium) (e.g., 0.5–1 mg) often are added to baclofen in patients in whom optimal response has not been achieved.

Another effective agent with a different mechanism of action is tizanidine (Zanaflex). This short-acting, α-adrenergic agonist acts in the CNS to reduce spasticity by increasing presynaptic inhibition of motor neurons. It appears to have efficacy comparable with that of baclofen.[98] Dosage must be titrated slowly over 2 to 4 weeks, starting with 4 mg at bedtime, with adjustments based on clinical response. Effective tolerated dosages have ranged from 2 to 36 mg/day. Sedation, dizziness, and dry mouth are the most commonly reported adverse effects, but hypotension also can occur, as well as a rare but severe hepatotoxicity. Tizanidine can be added in small dosages to baclofen, sometimes resulting in better results and smaller doses of each drug.

In patients who are unable to tolerate baclofen or tizanidine, diazepam (Valium; 2–10 mg/day), clonazepam (Klonopin; 1–3 mg/day), or dantrolene sodium (Dantrium; 100–400 mg/day), may be considered as alternatives, but they generally are less effective than either baclofen or tizanidine. Mild spasticity also may respond to moderately high doses of gabapentin (Neurontin; 1,800–3,600 mg/day). Tiagabine (Gabitril 8–56 mg/day) may be useful in some patients with spasticity, but side effects can prohibit

its use. Pregabalin (Lyrica; 75–300 mg/day) has similar features and mechanism of actions as gabapentin, although pregabalin is approximately 3 times more potent and does not saturate the L-system transporter system in the gastrointestinal system, so it may prove useful in the treatment of spasticity in MS patients.

Botulinum toxin type A (Botox; dose depending on the muscles injected) has been shown to be effective in improving spasticity.[30] The amount of toxin required to exert an effect on spasticity is often too excessive to use safely in the larger muscles; therefore, its use is best limited to smaller areas of focal muscle spasm.

An alternative approach to gait disruption employs K^+ channel blockers such as 4-aminopyridine (4-AP). Recent studies have shown that 4-AP may modestly improve walking speed.[99] In early 2010, the FDA approved the use of a long-acting proprietary version of 4-AP, dalfampridine (Ampyra; 20mg/day), for use in the United States.

Tremor

Cerebellar symptoms such as tremor can be troubling and difficult to control. Medications that can be helpful include propranolol, primidone, and isoniazid.

Bowel and Bladder Symptoms

Patients commonly complain of incontinence, urgency, frequency, and nocturia, which are indications of a hyperreflexic bladder (i.e., inability to store urine). A number of anticholinergic agents, including oxybutynin chloride (Ditropan; 10–20 mg/day), tolterodine (Detrol; 2–4 mg/day), propantheline bromide (Pro-Banthine; 45–90 mg/day), hyoscyamine (Levsin; 0.75–1.5 mg/day), and dicyclomine hydrochloride (Bentyl; 30–80 mg/day) are used to treat this problem if symptoms are mild. Ditropan is now also available in an extended-release formulation (5 and 10 mg). In addition, tricyclic antidepressants, such as imipramine (Tofranil) and amitriptyline (Elavil), have been used for their anticholinergic properties. With all anticholinergic agents, great care must be used to avoid the problem of constipation, which is worsened by the patient's natural instinct to limit fluid intake (owing to the increasing urge to urinate). Newer medications include antimuscarinic agents such as trospium chloride (Sanctura; 40 mg/day), solifenacin succinate (Vesicare; 5–10 mg/day), darifenacin hydrobromide (Enablex; 7.5–15 mg/day), and fesoterodine (Toviaz; 4–8 mg/day). As an alternative, the synthetic antidiuretic hormone preparation desmopressin acetate (DDAVP; 0.2–0.6 mg/day) has been reported to be effective in the treatment of urgency and incontinence.[98] Use of DDAVP probably is best limited to bedtime so as to improve sleep and because there can be significant problems with hyponatremia and possible seizures if overused. Patients with significant sphincter dyssynergia may benefit from the oral use of α-adrenergic blockers such as prazosin (Minipress; 10–40 mg/day) or intramuscular use of botulinum toxin type A (Botox; dose depends on the muscles injected).

Intermittent self-catheterization with or without a concomitant anticholinergic agent is recommended in patients with large postvoid urine residual volumes (greater than 100 mL) or when the urinary problem is hyporeflexic in nature (failure to empty). Patients with large postvoid residual volumes are at risk for developing urinary tract infections (UTIs) and often are prescribed urinary acidifiers such as vitamin C or antiseptics such as methenamine mandelate to prevent infections. Antibiotics used for UTI prophylaxis include sulfamethoxazole/trimethoprim, cephalexin, cinoxacin, and nitrofurantoin.

Constipation is the most common bowel complaint. Many medications (narcotics, anticholinergics) in common use may worsen this problem, as may voluntary water restriction in those patients with urinary urgency and incontinence. Increases in dietary fiber and hydration may alleviate this problem, but in some instances laxatives or enemas may be necessary.

Major Depression

Major depression is common in patients with MS, and the risk of suicide may be increased markedly compared with healthy subjects.[101] Patients should be monitored closely for the development of major depressive symptomatology and treated accordingly (see Chapter 77). Interferon products and natalizumab should be used cautiously in patients with significant depression.

Sensory Symptoms

Numbness and paresthesia are frequent sensory complaints but usually do not require treatment. Some MS patients may develop acute or chronic pain syndromes[98] such as trigeminal neuralgia and painful dysesthesias, for which treatment is necessary. Carbamazepine (Tegretol; 400–1,200 mg/day) is the preferred agent for the treatment of trigeminal neuralgia. Other agents also commonly used for neuropathic pain include amitriptyline and related tricyclic antidepressants, gabapentin, pregabalin, and duloxetine.

Sexual Dysfunction

Sexual dysfunction in both men and women are common in MS, and counseling should be offered to both partners. Sildenafil citrate (Viagra), tadalafil (Cialis), and vardenafil (Levitra) are very effective for men with MS who have erectile dysfunction. Other options for men include alprostadil injection (Caverject) or intraurethral suppositories (MUSE). Viagra is currently being studied in females with MS and sexual dysfunction. In patients needing antidepressant therapy for whom sexual dysfunction is a concern, bupropion is preferable to selective serotonin reuptake inhibitors as it has a much lower incidence of sexual side effects.

Fatigue

Fatigue, one of the most common complaints in MS patients, can be severely disabling, but treatment is often overlooked. Typically present in the mid to late afternoon, it can increase with heat exposure, exertion, intercurrent infection, spasticity, weakness, and depression. Amantadine hydrochloride (100 mg twice daily) is used often and may offer significant relief.[30,94] Methylphenidate (Ritalin) and related products, and dextroamphetamine (Dexedrine) are used commonly for fatigue in MS. Modafinil (Provigil), at 100 mg twice daily, is also helpful for MS-related fatigue. In patients suffering from both depression and fatigue, a more activating antidepressant such as fluoxetine may be employed.

Cognition

Cognitive dysfunction is common in MS, affecting up to 50% or more of patients. It generally manifests itself as word finding difficulties and problems with concentration and short term memory. Cognitive dysfunction can be treated with stimulants or cholinesterase inhibitors.

■ COMPLEMENTARY AND ALTERNATIVE THERAPIES FOR MS

A large percentage of patients with MS use complementary and alternative medicine (CAM) instead of, or in addition to, disease-modifying and symptomatic therapies. Common CAM therapies include diet and dietary supplements, such as vitamins, minerals, and herbs. Antioxidant supplements vitamin A, C, E, α-lipoic acid, coenzyme Q10, grape seed, pine bark extracts, mangosteen and acai have suggestive evidence of benefiting MS patients. However,

for patients with MS, there is a theoretical risk involved with taking antioxidant supplements owing to their ability to stimulate the immune system (T cells and macrophages). Stimulating the immune system in patients with MS could be counterproductive, possibly worsening or exacerbating their disease, and may counteract the effects of immunomodulators. Other immune-stimulating supplements that should be used with caution are garlic, ginseng (Asian and Siberian), echinacea, cat's claw, astragalus, alfalfa, and stinging nettle. A few agents that may pose a problem in MS, but may have benefit when taken in moderation, are zinc, melatonin (for insomnia), and dehydroepiandrosterone.[102]

In general, there are insufficient data supporting the effectiveness and safety of CAM therapies for MS. However, for patients with MS who are willing to try new approaches with limited evidence, CAM may be a consideration in some cases. Healthcare providers can be a source of objective information regarding the use of CAM for MS and can assist their patients in making the best decision.[102]

■ INFLUENZA VACCINE RECOMMENDATIONS

A yearly flu shot is recommended for all patients with MS, including patients on any of the DMTs. The intranasal influenza vaccine, FluMist, which is a live, attenuated vaccine, is not recommended for patients with MS, however. As DMTs suppress the immune system, a patient taking one of these medications is at increased risk for developing an infection of the strain of virus given in the vaccine. Live virus vaccines are also more likely to cause an increase in MS disease activity than inactivated virus vaccines. Finally, it is unknown whether there are any direct interactions between DMTs and the intranasal influenza vaccine.[103] This information can likely be extrapolated to other vaccines, so if a patient is in need of a vaccination of any kind, "killed" virus vaccines are recommended.

Patients opting to take fingolimod who are varicella zoster virus antibody negative should consider receiving the varicella zoster virus immunization (even though it is a live attenuated vaccine) at least one month prior to beginning fingolimod. This should allow time to mount an antibody response prior to immunosuppression with fingolimod.

PHARMACOECONOMIC CONSIDERATIONS

As with many therapeutic decisions, economic cost, both to the individual and to society, must be considered. Currently, the annual cost of the DMTs is considerable. The *Red Book* average wholesale price (used for all products in this chapter) of each of the currently available interferons is between $18,300 and $21,200 per patient per year. Given this expense, it must be remembered that these therapies are not curative and that individual patients may experience variable results. Future investigations evaluating these therapeutic modalities clearly will need to address not only clinical but also economic and humanistic outcomes.

A recent cost-benefit analysis has identified that even more expensive therapies, such as natalizumab, may be cost-effective due to their ability to more effectively reduce the likelihood of relapses, thus resulting in lower treatment costs and hospitalization for acute relapses.[104]

EVALUATION OF THERAPEUTIC OUTCOMES

Response to treatment of acute exacerbations of MS is commonly seen within days. With respect to DMTs, it is important for the clinician to recognize that over the short term (days to weeks), little or no apparent benefit may be noted by either patient or clinician. Evaluation of therapeutic outcomes, such as decreased MS exacerbations and hospitalizations or perhaps slowed disease progression and disability (as measured using scales such as EDSS), must be conducted over a period of months to years. Patients should be provided with realistic goals and expectations of these treatment options and encouraged to participate in the evaluation of therapeutic response. Initially, it may be important to reevaluate patients at relatively short time intervals to monitor for adverse effects.

Safety monitoring of patients on interferon includes regular laboratory monitoring, patient observation, and questioning for adverse effects or changing disability, and regular neurologic examinations. Specific laboratory monitoring for individuals on interferon therapy should include a complete blood count, platelet count, and liver function tests. These should be completed at baseline, every 3 months for 1 year, and every 6 months thereafter. Glatiramer acetate requires no laboratory monitoring. In addition to counseling patients regarding the adverse effects associated with these drugs, pharmacists should actively encourage patients to comply with their prescribed regimens.

CONCLUSIONS

Multiple sclerosis is an inflammatory disease of the CNS that strikes young, genetically susceptible individuals living in high-risk geographic areas. Although the exact etiology of MS is unknown, it is likely that MS is an autoimmune disease triggered by an as yet undetermined environmental agent or agents. There is no cure, but quality of life can be improved through symptomatic management, and the disease course is partially suppressed by presently available DMTs.

ACKNOWLEDGMENT

The authors acknowledge the contributions of Michael Egeberg, PharmD, May Wong, PharmD, Nora Li, PharmD, and Joan Kaufman, illustrator, for their contributions to this chapter.

ABBREVIATIONS

4-AP: 4-aminopyridine

ABC-R: Avonex, Betaseron, Copaxone, and Rebif

CAM: complementary and alternative medicine

CIS: clinically isolated syndrome

CNS: central nervous system

CSF: cerebrospinal fluid

DDAVP: desmopressin

DMT: disease-modifying therapy

EBV: Epstein-Barr virus

EDSS: expanded disability status scale

FDA: Food and Drug Administration

GABA: γ-aminobutyric acid

HLA: human leukocyte antigen

IgG: immunoglobulin G

IL-2: interleukin-2

IL-10: interleukin-10

MHC: major histocompatibility complex

MBP: myelin basic protein

MRI: magnetic resonance imaging

MS: multiple sclerosis

MSFC: Multiple Sclerosis Functional Composite

OCBs: oligoclonal bands

PML: progressive multifocal leukoencephalopathy

PPMS: primary-progressive multiple sclerosis

PRMS: primary-relapsing multiple sclerosis

RIS: radiologically isolated syndrome

RRMS: relapsing-remitting multiple sclerosis

SPMS: secondary-progressive multiple sclerosis

TGF-β: transforming growth factor-β

UTI: urinary tract infection

VCAM: vascular cell adhesion molecule

VEP: visual evoked potential

VLA-1: very late antigen 1

REFERENCES

1. Ascherio A, Munger K. Epidemiology of multiple sclerosis: from risk factors to prevention. Semin Neurol 2008;28:17–28.
2. Goodin DS. The causal cascade to multiple sclerosis: a model for MS pathogenesis. PLoS One 2009;4:e4565.
3. Oksenberg JR, Baranzini SE, Sawcer S, Hauser SL. The genetics of multiple sclerosis: SNPs to pathways to pathogenesis. Nat Rev Genet 2008;9:516–526.
4. Ebers GC. Environmental factors and multiple sclerosis. Lancet Neurol 2008;7:268–277.
5. Healy BC, Ali EN, Guttmann CRG, et al. Smoking and disease progression in multiple sclerosis. Arch Neurol 2009;66:858–864.
6. Munger KL, Levin LI, Hollis BW. Serum 25-hydroxyvitamin D levels and risk of multiple sclerosis. JAMA 2006;296:2832–2838.
7. Zivadinov R, Weinstock-Guttman B, Hashmi K, et al. Smoking is associated with increased lesion volumes and brain atrophy in multiple sclerosis. Neurology 2009;73(7):504–510.
8. Frohman EM, Racke MK, Raine CS. Multiple sclerosis—The plaque and its pathogenesis. N Engl J Med 2006;354:942–955.
9. Levin LI, Munger KL, Rubertone MV, et al. Temporal relationship between elevation of Epstein-Barr virus antibody titers and initial onset of neurological symptoms in multiple sclerosis. JAMA 2005;293:2496–2500.
10. Sundstrom P, Nystrom M, Ruuth K, et al. Antibodies to specific EBNA-1 domains and HLA DRB1*1501 interact as risk factors for multiple sclerosis. J Neuroimmunol 2009;215(1–2):102–107.
11. Zivadinov R, Zorzon M, Weinstock-Guttman B, et al. Epstein-Barr virus is associated with grey matter atrophy in multiple sclerosis. J Neurol Neurosurg Psychiatry 2009;80(6):620–625.
12. Serafini B, Rosicarelli B, Franciotta D, et al. Dysregulated Epstein-Barr virus infection in the multiple sclerosis brain. J Exp Med 2007;204:2899–2912.
13. Willis SN, Stadelmann C, Rodig SJ, et al. Epstein-Barr virus infection is not a characteristic feature of multiple sclerosis brain. Brain 2009;132:3318–3328.
14. Willer CJ, Dyment DA, Risch, et al. Twin concordance and sibling recurrence rates in multiple sclerosis. Proc Natl Acad Sci U S A 2003;100:12877–12882.
15. Hafler DA, Compston A, Sawcer S, et al. Risk alleles for multiple sclerosis identified by a genomewide study. N Engl J Med 2007;357:851–862.
16. D'Netto MJ, Ward H, Morrison KM, et al. Risk alleles for multiple sclerosis in multiplex families. Neurology 2009;72:1984–1988.
17. Maier LM, Lowe CE, Cooper J, et al. IL2RA genetic heterogeneity in multiple sclerosis and type 1 diabetes susceptibility and soluble interleukin-2 receptor production. PLoS Genet 2009;5:e1000322.

18. Cree BA, Khan O, Bourdette D, et al. Clinical characteristics of African Americans versus Caucasian Americans with multiple sclerosis. Neurology 2004;63:2039–2045.

19. Cree BA, Al-Sabbagh A, Bennett R, et al. Response to interferon beta-1a treatment in African American multiple sclerosis patients. Arch Neurol 2005;62:1681–1683.

20. Reich D, Patterson N, DeJager PL, et al. A whole-genome admixture scan finds a candidate locus for multiple sclerosis susceptibility. Nat Genet 2005;37:1113–1118.

21. Trapp BD, Peterson J, Ransohoff RM, et al. Axonal transection in the lesions of multiple sclerosis. N Engl J Med 1998;338:278–285.

22. Truyen L, van Wuesberghe JHTM, Barkof F, et al. Accumulation of hypointense lesions ("black holes") on T_1 spin echo MRI correlates with disease progression in multiple sclerosis. Neurology 1996;47:1469–1476.

23. Pirko I, Lucchinetti CF, Sriram S, Bakshi R. Gray matter involvement in multiple sclerosis. Neurology 2007;68:634–642.

24. Zivadinov R, Minagar A. Evidence for gray matter pathology in multiple sclerosis: a neuroimaging approach. J Neurol Sci 2009;282:1–4.

25. Magliozzi R, Howell O, Vora A, et al. Meningeal B-cell follicles in secondary progressive multiple sclerosis associate with early onset of disease and severe cortical pathology. Brain 2007;130:1089–1104.

26. Reboldi A, Coisne C, Baumjohann D, et al. C-C chemokine receptor 6-regulated entry of T_H-17 cells into the CNS through the choroid plexus is required for the initiation of EAE. Nat Immunol 2009;10:514–523.

27. Zhou L, Chong MMW, Littman DR. Plasticity of CD4+ T-cell lineage differentiation. Immunity 2009;30:646–655.

28. Smolders J, Thewissen M, Peelen E, et al. Vitamin D status is positively correlated with regulatory T cell function in patients with multiple sclerosis. PLoS One 2009;4:e6635.

29. Owens GP, Bennett JL, Lassmann H, et al. Antibodies produced by clonally expanded plasma cells in multiple sclerosis cerebrospinal fluid. Ann Neurol 2009;65:639–649.

30. Schapiro RT. Managing symptoms of multiple sclerosis. Neurol Clin 2005;23:177–187.

31. Weinshenker BG. Natural history of multiple sclerosis. Ann Neurol 1994;36:S6–S11.

32. Confavreux C, Vukusic S. Natural history of multiple sclerosis: a unifying concept. Brain 2006;129(3):606–616.

33. Lebrun C, Bensa C, Debouverie M, et al. Association between clinical conversion to multiple sclerosis in radiologically isolated syndrome and magnetic resonance imaging, cerebrospinal fluid, and visual evoked potential: follow-up of 70 patients. Arch Neurol 2009;66:841–846.

34. Zivadinov R, Zorzon M. Is gadolinium enhancement predictive of the development of brain atrophy in multiple sclerosis? A review of the literature. J Neuroimag 2002;12:302–309.

35. Tremlett H, Paty D, Devonshire V. The natural history of primary progressive MS in British Columbia, Canada. Neurology 2005;65:1919–1923.

36. Hawker K, O'Connor P, Freedman MS, et al. Rituximab in patients with primary progressive multiple sclerosis: results of a randomized double-blind placebo-controlled multicenter trial. Ann Neurol 2009;66:460–471.

37. Kurtzke JF. Rating neurologic impairment in multiple sclerosis: An expanded disability status scale (EDSS). Neurology 1983;33:1444–1452.

38. Rudick RA, Cutter G, Reingold S. The multiple sclerosis functional composite: A new clinical outcome measure for multiple sclerosis trials. Mult Scler 2002;8:359–365.

39. Gordon-Lipkin E, Chodkowski B, Reich DS, et al. Retinal nerve fiber layer is associated with brain atrophy in multiple sclerosis. Neurology 2007;69:1603–1609.

40. Lee M, O'Brien P. Pregnancy and multiple sclerosis. J Neurol Neurosurg Psychiatry 2008;79:1308–1311.

41. Sadovnick AD, Eisen K, Ebers GC, Paty DW. Cause of death in patients attending multiple sclerosis clinics. Neurology 1991;41:1193–1196.

42. Swanson JW. Multiple sclerosis: Update in diagnosis and review of prognostic factors. Mayo Clin Proc 1989;64:577–586.

43. McDonald W, Compston A, Edan G, et al. Recommended diagnostic criteria for multiple sclerosis: Guidelines from the international panel on diagnosis of multiple sclerosis. Ann Neurol 2001;50:121–127.

44. Polman CH, Reingold SC, Edan G, et al. Diagnostic criteria for multiple sclerosis: 2005 revisions to the "McDonald Criteria." Ann Neurol 2005;58:840–846.

45. Frohman EM, Goodin DS, Calabresi PA, et al. The utility of MRI in suspected MS. Report of the Therapeutics and Technology Assessment Subcommittee of the American Academy of Neurology. Neurology 2003;61:1332–1338.

46. Fisher E, Rudick R, Simon J, et al. Eight-year follow-up study of brain atrophy in patients with MS. Neurology 2002;59:1412–1420.

47. Dalton C, Brex P, Miszkiel K, et al. New T_2 lesions enable an earlier diagnosis of multiple sclerosis in clinically isolated syndromes. Ann Neurol 2003;53:673–676.

48. Swanton JK, Rovira A, Tintore M, et al. MRI criteria for multiple sclerosis in patients presenting with clinically isolated syndromes: a multicentre retrospective study. Lancet Neurol 2007;6:677–686.

49. Lo CP, Kao HW, Chen SY, et al. Prediction of conversion from clinically isolated syndrome to clinically definite multiple sclerosis according to baseline MRI findings: a comparison of revised McDonald criteria and Swanton modified criteria. J Neurol Neurosurg Psychiatry 2009;80:1107–2209.

50. Olsson T. Cerebrospinal fluid. Ann Neurol 1994;36:S100–S102.

51. Berger T, Rubner P, Schautzer F, et al. Antimyelin antibodies as a predictor of clinically definite multiple sclerosis after a first demyelinating event. N Engl J Med 2003;349:139–145.

52. Carmosino MJ, Brousseau KM, Arciniegas DB, et al. Initial evaluations for multiple sclerosis in a university multiple sclerosis center: Outcomes and role of magnetic resonance imaging in referral. Arch Neurol 2005;62:585–590.

53. Kaufman DI, Trobe JD, Eggenberger ER, Whitaker JN. Practice parameter: The role of corticosteroids in the management of acute monosymptomatic optic neuritis. Report of the Quality Standards Subcommittee of the American Academy of Neurology. Neurology 2000;54:2039–2044.

54. Zivadinov R, Rudick RA, De Masi R, et al. Effects of IV methylprednisolone on brain atrophy in relapsing-remitting MS. Neurology 2001;57:1239–1247.

55. Goodin DS, Frohman EM, Garmany GP, et al. Disease-modifying therapies in multiple sclerosis: Report of the Therapeutics and Technology Assessment Subcommittee of the American Academy of Neurology and the Multiple Sclerosis Council for Clinical Practice Guidelines. Neurology 2002;58:169–178.

56. Vandebark AA, Huan J, Agotsch M, et al. Interferon-beta-1a increases CD56(bright) natural killer cells and CD4+CD25+ Foxp3 expression in subjects with multiple sclerosis. J Neuroimmunol 2009;215:125–128.

57. Giovannoni G, Barbarash O, Casset-Semanaz F, et al. Safety and immunogenicity of a new formulation of interferon beta-1a (Rebif New Formulation) in a Phase IIIb study in patients with relapsing multiple sclerosis: 96-week results. Mult Scler 2009;15:219–228.

58. Simon JH, Jacobs L, Campion M, et al. A longitudinal study of brain atrophy in relapsing MS. Neurology 1999;58:139–145.

59. Fischer JS, Priore RL, Jacobs LD, et al. Neuropsychological effects of interferon-β-la in relapsing multiple sclerosis. Ann Neurol 2000;48:885–892.

60. Frohman E, Phillips T, Kokel K, et al. Disease-modifying therapy in multiple sclerosis: Strategies for optimizing management. Neurology 2002;8:227–236.

61. Racke MK, Lovett-Racke AE, Karandikar NJ. The mechanism of action of glatiramer acetate treatment in multiple sclerosis. Neurology 2010;74(Suppl 1):S25–S30.

62. Azoulay D, Vachapova V, Shihman B, et al. Lower brain-derived neurotrophic factor in serum of relapsing remitting MS. Reversal by glatiramer acetate. J Neuroimmunol 2005;167:215–218.

63. Fillippi M, Rovaris M, Rocca MA, et al. Glatiramer acetate reduces the proportion of new MS lesions evolving into "black holes." Neurology 2001;57:731–733.

64. Ford CC, Johnson KP, Lisak RP, et al. A prospective open-label study of glatiramer acetate: over a decade of continuous use in multiple sclerosis patients. Mult Scler 2006;12:309–320.

65. Miller DH, Khan OA, Sheremata WA, et al. A controlled trial of natalizumab for relapsing multiple sclerosis. N Engl J Med 2003;348:15–23.

66. Polman CH, O'Conor PW, Havrdova E, et al. A randomized, placebo-controlled trial of natalizumab for relapsing multiple sclerosis (AFFIRM). N Engl J Med 2006;354:899–910.

67. Rudick RA, Stuart WH, Calabresi PA, et al. Natalizumab plus interferon beta-1a for relapsing multiple sclerosis (SENTINEL). N Engl J Med 2006;354:911–923.

68. Kleinschmidt-DeMasters BK, Tyler KL. Progressive multifocal leukoencephalopathy complicating treatment with natalizumab and interferon beta-1a for multiple-sclerosis. N Engl J Med 2005:353;369–374.

69. Langer-Gould A, Atlas SW, Green AJ, et al. Progressive multifocal leukoencephalopathy in a patient treated with natalizumab. N Engl J Med 2005;353:375–381.

70. Van Assche G, Van Ranst M, Sclot R, et al. Progressive multifocal leukoencephalopathy after natalizumab therapy for Crohn's disease. N Engl J Med 2005;353:362–368.

71. Khatri BO, Man S, Giovannoni G, et al. Effect of plasma exchange in accelerating natalizumab clearance and restoring leukocyte function. Neurology 2009;72:402–409.

72. Lindå H, von Heijne A, Major EO, et al. Progressive multifocal leukoencephalopathy after natalizumab monotherapy. N Engl J Med 2009;361:1081–1087.

73. Sweat B. Natalizumab update. Am J Health Syst Pharm 2007;64:705–716.

74. Sadiq SA, Puccio LM, Brydon EW. JCV detection in multiple sclerosis patients treated with natalizumab. J Neurol 2010;257:954–958.

75. Hartung HP, Gonsette R, Konig N, et al. Mitoxantrone in progressive multiple sclerosis, a placebo-controlled, double-blind, randomized, multicentre trial. Lancet 2002;360:2018–2025.

76. Krapf H, Morrissey SP, Zenker O, et al. Effect of mitoxantrone on MRI in progressive MS. Results of the MIMS trial. Neurology 2005;65:690–695.

77. Martinelli V, Bellantonio P, Bergamaschi R, et al. Incidence of acute leukaemia in multiple sclerosis patients treated with mitoxandrone: a multicentre retrospective Italian study. Neurology 2009;73:330–333.

78. Miller A, Lisak R, Bohen B, et al. National Multiple Sclerosis Society (NMSS). Disease Management Consensus Statement: Expert Opinion Paper. New York: National MS Society, June 20, 2007:1–8. http://www.nationalmssociety.org/docs/HOM/Exp_Consensus.pdf.

79. Freedman MS, Kappos L, Polman CH, et al. Betaseron in newly emerging multiple sclerosis for initial treatment (BENEFIT): clinical outcomes. Neurology 2006;(Suppl 2):A61.

80. Vartanian T. An examination of the results of the EVIDENCE, INCOMIN, and phase III studies of interferon beta products in the treatment of multiple sclerosis. Clin Ther 2003;1:105–118.

81. Durelli L, Verdun E, Bergui M, et al. Every-other-day interferon-β-1b versus once-weekly interferon-β-1a for multiple sclerosis: Results of a 2-year prospective randomized multicentre study (INCOMIN). Lancet 2002;359:1453–1460.

82. Panitch H, Goodin D, Francis G, et al. Randomized, comparative study of interferon-β-1a treatment regimens in MS. The EVIDENCE Trial. Neurology 2002;59:1496–1506.

83. Koch-Henriksen N, Sorensen PS, Christensen T, et al. A randomized study of two interferon-beta treatments in relapsing-remitting multiple sclerosis. Neurology 2006;66:1056–1060.

84. Clanet M, Radue E, Kappos L, et al. A randomized, double-blind, dose-comparison study of weekly interferon-β-1a in relapsing MS. Neurology 2002;59:1507–1517.

85. O'Connor P, Filippi M, Arnason B, et al. 250 mcg or 500 mcg interferon beta-1b versus 20 mg glatiramer acetate in relapsing-remitting multiple sclerosis: a prospective, randomised, multicentre study. Lancet Neurol 2009;8:889–897.

86. Mikol DD, Barkhof F, Chang P, et al. Comparison of subcutaneous interferon beta-1a with glatiramer acetate in patients with relapsing multiple sclerosis (the Rebif vs. Glatiramer Acetate in Relapsing MS Disease [REGARD] study): a multicentre, randomised, parallel, open-label trial. Lancet Neurol 2008;7:903–914.

87. Namaka M, Pollitt-Smith M, Gupta A, et al. The clinical importance of neutralizing antibodies in relapsing-remitting multiple sclerosis. Curr Med Res Opin 2006;22:223–239.

88. Bertolotto A. Neutralizing antibodies to interferon beta: Implications for the management of multiple sclerosis. Curr Opin Neurol 2004;17:241–246.

89. Francis GS, Rice GP, Alsop JC, et al. Interferon beta 1a in MS. results following development of neutralizing antibodies in PRISMS. Neurology 2005;65:48–55.

90. Kappos L, Clanet M, Sandberg-Wollheim M, et al. Neutralizing antibodies and efficacy of interferon beta-1a: A 4-year controlled study. Neurology 2005;65:40–47.

91. Giovannoni G, Goodman A. Neutralizing anti-IFN-beta antibodies: How much more evidence do we need to use them in practice? Neurology 2005;65:6–8.

92. Goodin DS, Frohman EM, Hurwitz B, et al. Neutralizing antibodies to interferon beta: Assessment of their clinical and radiographic impact: An evidence report. Neurology 2007;67:977–984.

93. Kappos L, Polman C, Pozzilli C, et al. Final analysis of the European multicenter trial on IFNβ-1b in secondary-progressive MS. Neurology 2001;57:1969–1975.

94. Freedman MS, Patry DG, Grand'Maison F, et al. Treatment optimization in multiple sclerosis. Can J Neurol Sci 2004;31:157–168.

95. Hauser SL, Waubant E, Arnold DL, et al. B-cell depletion with rituximab in relapsing-remitting multiple sclerosis. N Engl J Med 2008;358:676–688.

96. Sorensen PS, Mellgren SI, Svenningsson A, et al. NORdic trial of oral Methylprednisolone as add-on therapy to Interferon beta-1a for treatment of relapsing-remitting Multiple Sclerosis (NORMIMS study): a randomised, placebo-controlled trial. Lancet Neurol 2009;8:519–529.

97. Birnbaum G, Cree B, Altafullah I, et al. Combining beta interferon and atorvastatin may increase disease activity in multiple sclerosis. Neurology 2008;71:1390–1395.

98. Mitchell G. Update on multiple sclerosis therapy. Med Clin North Am 1993;77:231–249.

99. Goodman AD, Brown TR, Krupp LB, et al. Sustained-release oral fampridine in multiple sclerosis: a randomised, double-blind, controlled trial. Lancet 2009;373:732–738.

100. Kinn AC, Larsson PO. Desmopressin: A new principle for symptomatic treatment of urgency and incontinence in patients with multiple sclerosis. Scand J Urol Nephrol 1990;24:109–112.

101. Stenager EN, Stenager E, Koch Henriksen N, et al. Suicide and multiple sclerosis: An epidemiological investigation. J Neurol Neurosurg Psychiatry 1992;55:542–545.

102. Bowling AC. Complementary and Alternative Medicine in Multiple Sclerosis, 2nd ed. New York: Demos, 2007.

103. National MS Society. News Detail; 2009. http://nationalmssociety.org/news/news-detail/index.aspx?nid=2115.

104. Chiao E, Meyer K. Cost effectiveness and budget impact of natalizumab in patients with relapsing multiple sclerosis. Curr Med Res Opin 2009;25(6):1445–1454.

65

Epilepsy

SUSAN J. ROGERS AND JOSE E. CAVAZOS

KEY CONCEPTS

❶ Patient-specific treatment goals should be identified as early as possible.

❷ Accurate diagnosis and classification of seizure/syndrome type is critical to selection of appropriate pharmacotherapy.

❸ Patient characteristics such as age, comorbid conditions, ability to comply with the prescribed regimen, and presence or absence of insurance coverage can also influence the choice of antiepileptic drugs.

❹ Pharmacotherapy of epilepsy is highly individualized and requires titration of the dose to optimize antiepileptic drug therapy (maximal seizure control with minimal or no side effects). Approximately 50% to 70% of patients can be maintained on one antiepileptic drug.

❺ If the therapeutic goal is not achieved with monotherapy, a second drug can be added or a switch to an alternative single antiepileptic drug can be made. If a second antiepileptic drug is added it should have a different mechanism of action from the first, although there is no clear evidence in humans to support this.

❻ Some patients eventually can discontinue antiepileptic drug therapy. Several factors predict successful withdrawal of antiepileptic drugs.

❼ The appropriate use of antiepileptic drugs requires a thorough understanding of their clinical pharmacology, including mechanism of action, pharmacokinetics, adverse reactions, and drug interactions, as well as available dosage forms.

Epilepsy is a disorder that is best viewed as a symptom of disturbed electrical activity in the brain, which may have many etiologies. It is a collection of many different types of seizures that vary widely in severity, appearance, cause, consequence, and management. Seizures that are prolonged or repetitive can be life-threatening. Epilepsy is defined by the occurrence of at least two unprovoked seizures separated by 24 hours.[1] The effect epilepsy has on patients' lives can be significant and extremely frustrating. It is also important to recognize that seizures can be just one (albeit the most obvious) symptom of an epileptic disorder. Not

uncommonly, patients have other comorbid disorders, including depression, anxiety, and potentially neuroendocrine disturbances. Patients with epilepsy also may display neurodevelopmental delay, memory problems, and/or cognitive impairment. Although, by convention, the focus of drug treatment is on the abolition of seizures, clinicians must also try to address these common comorbidities.

EPIDEMIOLOGY

Each year, 120 per 100,000 people in the United States come to medical attention because of a newly recognized seizure.[1] At least 8% of the general population will have at least one seizure in a lifetime. However, it is common to have a seizure and not have epilepsy. The rate of recurrence of a first unprovoked seizure within 5 years ranges between 23% and 80%. Children with an idiopathic first seizure and a normal electroencephalogram (EEG) have a particularly favorable prognosis. Some seizures occur as single events resulting from withdrawal of central nervous system (CNS) depressants (e.g., alcohol, barbiturates, and other drugs) or during acute neurologic illnesses or systemic toxic conditions (e.g., uremia or eclampsia). Some patients will have seizures only associated with fever. These febrile seizures do not constitute epilepsy.[1]

The age-adjusted incidence of epilepsy is 44 per 100,000 person-years. Each year, approximately 125,000 new epilepsy cases occur in the United States; only 30% are in people younger than 18 years of age at the time of diagnosis. There is a bimodal distribution in the occurrence of the first seizure, with one peak occurring in newborn and young children and the second peak occurring in patients older than 65 years of age. The relatively high frequency of epilepsy in the elderly is now being recognized.

ETIOLOGY

Seizures occur because a group of cortical neurons discharge abnormally in synchrony. Anything that disrupts the normal homeostasis or stability of neurons can trigger hyperexcitability and seizures. Thousands of medical conditions can cause epilepsy, from genetic mutations to traumatic brain injury. A genetic predisposition to seizures has been observed in many forms of primary generalized epilepsy. Patients with mental retardation, cerebral palsy, head injury, or strokes are at an increased risk for seizures and epilepsy. The more profound the degree of mental retardation as measured by the intelligence quotient (IQ), the greater is the incidence of epilepsy. In the elderly, the onset of seizures is typically associated with focal neuronal injury induced by strokes, neurodegenerative disorders (e.g., Alzheimer's disease), and other conditions. In some cases, if an etiology of seizures can be identified and corrected, the patient may not require chronic antiepileptic drug (AED) treatment. Patients can also present with unprovoked seizures that do not have an identifiable cause, and thus by definition have idiopathic or cryptogenic epilepsy. *Idiopathic etiology* is the term used for suspected genetic cause, whereas *cryptogenic etiology* is used if no obvious cause is found for focal-onset seizures.

Many factors have been shown to precipitate seizures in susceptible individuals. Hyperventilation can precipitate absence seizures. Excessive sleep, sleep deprivation, sensory stimuli, emotional stress, and hormonal changes occurring around the time of menses, puberty, or pregnancy have been associated with the onset of or an increased frequency of seizures. A careful drug history should be obtained from patients presenting with seizures because theophylline, alcohol, high-dose phenothiazines, antidepressants (especially maprotiline or bupropion), and street drug use have been associated with provoking seizures. Perinatal injuries and small gestational weight at birth are also risk factors for the development of partial-onset seizures. Immunizations have not been associated with an increased risk of epilepsy.

PATHOPHYSIOLOGY

Seizures result from excessive excitation, or in the case of absence seizures, from disordered inhibition of a large population of cortical neurons.[2] This is reflected on EEG as a sharp wave or *spike*. Initially, a small number of neurons fire abnormally. Normal membrane conductances and inhibitory synaptic currents break down, and excess excitability spreads, either locally to produce a focal seizure or more widely to produce a generalized seizure. This onset propagates by physiologic pathways to involve adjacent or remote areas. The clinical manifestations depend on the site of the focus, the degree of irritability of the surrounding area of the brain, and the intensity of the impulse.[2]

There are multiple mechanisms that might contribute to synchronous hyperexcitability, including: (1) alterations in the distribution, number, type, and biophysical properties of ion channels in the neuronal membranes; (2) biochemical modifications of receptors; (3) modulation of second messaging systems and gene expression; (4) changes in extracellular ion concentrations; (5) alterations in neurotransmitter uptake and metabolism in glial cells; and (6) modifications in the ratio and function of inhibitory circuits. In addition, local neurotransmitter imbalances could be a potential mechanism for focal epileptogenesis. Transitory imbalances between the main neurotransmitters, glutamate (excitatory) and γ-aminobutyric-acid (GABA) (inhibitory), and neuromodulators (e.g., acetylcholine, norepinephrine, and serotonin) might play a role in precipitating seizures in susceptible patients.[2]

Control of abnormal neuronal activity with AEDs is accomplished by elevating the threshold of neurons to electrical or chemical stimuli or by limiting the propagation of the seizure discharge from its origin. Raising the threshold most likely involves stabilization of neuronal membranes, whereas limiting the propagation involves depression of synaptic transmission and reduction of nerve conduction.[2]

Prolonged seizures and continued exposure to glutamate can result in neuronal injury in vulnerable neuronal populations resulting in functional deficits, primarily in memory, and in permanent changes of wiring of the neuronal circuitry. Sprouting and reorganization of neuronal projections might lead to a chronic susceptibility to seizures, neuronal destruction, and brain damage. However, limited degree of neurogeneisis in the hippocampal pathways has been induced by epileptic seizures. The role of these newly born neurons is not well understood.

CLINICAL PRESENTATION

The International League Against Epilepsy has proposed two major schemes for the classification of seizures and epilepsies: the International Classification of Epileptic Seizures and the International Classification of the Epilepsies and Epilepsy Syndromes.[3,4] The International Classification of Epileptic Seizures (Table 65–1) combines the clinical description with certain electrophysiologic findings to classify epileptic seizures. Seizures are divided into two main pathophysiologic groups—partial seizures and generalized seizures—by EEG recordings and clinical symptomatology.

Partial (focal) seizures begin in one hemisphere of the brain and—unless they become secondarily generalized—result in an asymmetric motor manifestation. Partial seizures manifest as alterations in motor functions, sensory or somatosensory symptoms, or automatisms. Partial seizures with no loss of consciousness are classified as *simple partial* (SP). In some cases, patients will describe somatosensory symptoms as a "warning" prior to the development of a generalized tonic clonic (GTC) seizure. These warnings are, in fact, simple partial seizures and frequently are termed auras.

Partial seizures with an alteration of consciousness are described as *complex partial* (CP). With CP seizures, the patient can have automatisms, periods of memory loss, or aberrations of behavior. Some patients with CP epilepsy have been mistakenly diagnosed as having psychotic episodes. CP seizures also can progress to GTC seizures. Patients with CP seizures typically are amnestic to these events. A partial seizure that becomes generalized is referred to as a *secondarily generalized seizure*.

Generalized seizures have clinical manifestations that indicate involvement of both hemispheres. Motor manifestations are bilateral, and there is a loss of consciousness. Generalized seizures can be further subdivided by EEG and clinical manifestations. Generalized absence seizures are manifested by a sudden onset, interruption of ongoing activities, a blank stare, and possibly a brief upward rotation of the eyes. They generally occur in young children through adolescence. It is important to differentiate absence seizures from complex partial seizures.

TABLE 65–1	International Classification of Epileptic Seizures

I. Partial seizures (seizures begin locally)
  A. Simple (without impairment of consciousness)
    1. With motor symptoms
    2. With special sensory or somatosensory symptoms
    3. With psychic symptoms
  B. Complex (with impairment of consciousness)
    1. Simple partial onset followed by impairment of consciousness—with or without automatisms
    2. Impaired consciousness at onset—with or without automatisms
  C. Secondarily generalized (partial onset evolving to generalized tonic-clonic seizures)
II. Generalized seizures (bilaterally symmetrical and without local onset)
  A. Absence
  B. Myoclonic
  C. Clonic
  D. Tonic
  E. Tonic-clonic
  F. Atonic
  G. Infantile spasms
III. Unclassified seizures
IV. Status epilepticus

Data from Commission on the Classification and Terminology of the International League Against Epilepsy.[3,4]

With GTC seizures there is a sudden sharp tonic contraction of muscles followed by a period of rigidity and clonic movements. During the seizure, the patient may cry or moan, lose sphincter control, bite the tongue, or develop cyanosis. After the seizure, the patient may have altered consciousness, drowsiness, or confusion for a variable period of time (postictal period) and frequently goes into a deep sleep. Tonic and clonic seizures can also occur separately.

Brief shock-like muscular contractions of the face, trunk, and extremities are known as *myoclonic jerks*. They can be isolated events or rapidly repetitive. A sudden loss of muscle tone is known as an *atonic seizure*, which may present as a head drop, the dropping of a limb, or a slumping to the ground. These patients often wear protective head ware to prevent trauma.

The International Classification of Epilepsies and Epilepsy Syndromes adds components such as age of onset, intellectual development, findings on neurologic examination, and results of neuroimaging studies to define epilepsy syndromes more fully. Syndromes can include one or many different seizure types (e.g., Lennox-Gastaut syndrome). The syndromic approach includes seizure type(s) and possible etiologic classifications (e.g., idiopathic, symptomatic, or unknown). *Idiopathic* describes syndromes that are presumably genetic but also those in which no underlying etiology is documented or suspected. A family history of seizures is commonly present, and neurologic function is essentially normal except for the occurrence of seizures. *Symptomatic* cases involve evidence of brain damage or a known underlying cause. A *cryptogenic* syndrome is assumed to be symptomatic of an underlying condition that cannot be documented. Unknown or undetermined is used when no cause can be identified. This syndromic classification requires more information and is more important for prognostic determinations and response to treatment than for a classification based simply on seizure type.

CLINICAL PRESENTATION OF EPILEPSY

General

In most cases, the healthcare provider will not be in a position to witness a seizure. Many patients (particularly those with CP or GTC seizures) are amnestic to the actual seizure event. Obtaining an adequate history and description of the ictal event (including time course) from a witness is critically important. With treatment the typical clinical presentation of the seizure may change.

Symptoms

Symptoms of a specific seizure will depend on seizure type. Although seizures can vary between patients, they tend to be stereotyped within an individual.

- CP seizures can include somatosensory or focal motor features.
- CP seizures are associated with altered consciousness.
- Absence seizures can be almost nondetectable with only very brief (seconds) periods of altered consciousness.
- GTC seizures are major convulsive episodes and are always associated with a loss of consciousness.

Signs

Interictally (between seizure episodes), there are typically no objective or pathognomonic signs.

Laboratory Tests

There are currently no diagnostic laboratory tests for epilepsy. In some cases, particularly following GTC (or perhaps CP) seizures, serum prolactin levels can be transiently elevated.

Laboratory tests can be done to rule out treatable causes of seizures (e.g., hypoglycemia, altered electrolyte concentrations, infections, etc.) that do not represent epilepsy.

Other Diagnostic Tests

- EEG is very useful in the diagnosis of various seizure disorders.
- An epileptiform EEG is found in only approximately 50% of the patients who have epilepsy.
- A prolactin serum level obtained within 10 to 20 minutes of a tonic-clonic seizure can be useful in differentiating seizure activity from pseudoseizure activity but not from syncope.[5]
- Although magnetic resonance imaging (MRI) is very useful (especially imaging of the temporal lobes), a computed tomography (CT) scan typically is not helpful except in the initial evaluation for a brain tumor or cerebral bleeding.

TREATMENT

■ DESIRED OUTCOME

❶ The ideal goal of treatment for epilepsy is complete elimination of seizures and no side effects with an optimal quality of life (QOL). The best QOL is associated with a seizure-free state.[6] Often, however, a balance between efficacy and side effects must be accepted. With the older AEDs used as monotherapy, fewer than 50% of patients become seizure free.

Because therapy is continued for many years (often a lifetime), chronic side effects must be considered. If the patient is overly sedated or develops other significant side effects, some seizure control may have to be sacrificed to improve functioning. The patient should be involved in deciding what balance between frequency of seizures and the occurrence of side effects is most appropriate. The newer AEDs offer alternatives for balancing seizure frequency and drug side effects.

Providing optimal QOL also requires assessing all the concerns of patients with epilepsy, such as, issues about driving, economic security, forming relationships, safety, social isolation, social stigma, and so on. Patients with epilepsy can also have other neuropsychiatric comorbidities such as depression, anxiety, and sleep disturbances that need treatment.[7,8] Depression has been shown to have a significant impact on QOL in the patient with treatment-resistant epilepsy.[9]

■ GENERAL APPROACH TO TREATMENT

❷ The general approach to treatment involves assessment of seizure type and frequency, identification of treatment goals, development of a care plan, and a plan for follow-up evaluation. During the assessment phase, it is critical to establish an accurate diagnosis of the seizure type and classification in order to select the appropriate initial AEDs. Patient-specific treatment goals must be identified, and these can change over time. Despite appropriate AED treatment, approximately 30% to 35% of patients are refractory to treatment. In this setting, seizure freedom may not be obtained, and more obtainable goals should be established (e.g., decrease in the number of seizures and minimized drug adverse effects).

❸ Patient characteristics such as age, medical condition, ability to comply with a prescribed regimen, and insurance coverage also should be explored because these can influence AED choices or help to explain nonadherence to the regimen, a lack of response, or unexpected adverse effects.

Once the assessment is complete, for patients with new-onset seizures, the choice is whether to use drug therapy and, if so, which one. For a patient with long-standing epilepsy, adequacy of the current medication regimen must be evaluated. An AED should not be considered ineffective unless the patient has experienced unacceptable adverse effects with continued seizures.

❹ If a decision is made to start AED therapy, monotherapy is preferred, and approximately 50% to 70% of all patients with epilepsy can be maintained on one drug.[10,11] However, many of these patients are not seizure free. The percentage of patients who are seizure free on one drug varies by seizure type. After 12 months of treatment, the percentage who are seizure free is highest for those who have only GTC seizures (48%–55%), lowest for those who have only CP seizures (23%–26%), and intermediate for those with mixed seizure types (25%–32%).[11] Combining AEDs with different mechanisms of action to achieve freedom from seizures may be advantageous, although this approach is as yet unproven. Approximately 65% of patients can be expected to be maintained on one AED and be considered well controlled, although not necessarily seizure free.

❺ Of the 35% of patients with unsatisfactory control, 10% will be well controlled with a two-drug treatment. Of the remaining 25%, 20% will continue to have unsatisfactory control despite multiple drug treatment. There may be a genetic predisposition to epilepsy that is refractory to drug therapy. Some of these patients may become candidates for surgery or vagal nerve stimulator.

Once the care plan is established, an AED is selected. Patient education and assurance of patient understanding of the plan are essential. Detailed directions regarding titration, what to do in the event of a treatment-emergent side effect, and what to do if a seizure occurs must be provided to patients. Documentation of the assessment, care plan, and educational process is essential. Providing the patient with a seizure and side-effect diary will assist in the follow-up and evaluation phase. At the follow-up stage of treatment (which can be done in the hospital, clinic, pharmacy, or by phone), the treatment goals must be reviewed. If the goal has been achieved, new goals should be identified. For example, if the GTC seizures are now controlled, the goal may be to control partial seizures. If a patient fails to respond to the first AEDs, trials with other AEDs should be attempted as appropriate. Completion of the evaluation often requires a reassessment of the patient and development of a new care plan taking into account patient compliance, efficacy, and safety of the initial treatment.

Medication noncompliance can be the single most common reason for treatment failure. It is estimated that up to 60% of patients with epilepsy are noncompliant.[12] The rate of noncompliance is increased by the complexity of the drug regimen and by doses taken 3 and 4 times a day. Frequent uncontrolled seizures can also predispose a patient to noncompliance secondary to confusion over whether the drug was taken. Noncompliance is not influenced by age, sex, psychomotor development, or seizure type.[12]

Difference of opinion exists on the most appropriate time to initiate AED therapy. Treatment decisions vary depending on individual patient clinical characteristics and circumstances. Some clinicians start AED treatment after the first seizure, whereas others do not initiate treatment until a second, unprovoked seizure has occurred. Still others initiate prophylactic treatment following a CNS insult thought likely to cause epilepsy eventually (e.g., stroke or head trauma). Drug treatment may not be indicated when seizures have minimal impact on patients' lives or when there has been only a single seizure. If a patient presents after a single isolated seizure, one of three treatment decisions can be made: treat, possibly treat, or do not treat. These decisions are based on the probability of the patient having a second seizure (Table 65-2). For patients with no risk factors, the probability of a second seizure

TABLE 65-2 Recurrence Risk for Patients Experiencing One Unprovoked Seizure

Type of Patient	First-Year Risk (%)	Fifth-Year Risk (%)
Adults with single unproved seizure		34
No CNS insult	10	29
Influence of family history		
Sibling with seizure	29	46
No sibling with seizures	7	27
EEG patterns		
GSW on EEG	15	58
Normal EEG	9	26
Occurrence of previous seizure	10	39
Caused by an illness or childhood febrile seizure		
Remote symptomatic with Todd paresis	26	48
	41	75
Status epilepticus at onset	37	56
Prior acute seizure	60	80
Idiopathic	10	29

CNS, central nervous system; EEG, electroencephalogram; GSW, generalized spikes and waves. *Data from Leppik[13] and Gross-Tsur et al.[15]*

is less than 10% in the first year and approximately 24% by the end of 2 years. If risk factors are present, the recurrence rate can be as high as 80% after 5 years.[13] The decision on whether to start AED therapy often depends on patient-specific factors such as epilepsy syndrome, seizure etiology, presence of a neuroanatomic defect, and the EEG, as well as, the patient's lifestyle and preferences. Patients who have had two or more seizures generally should be started on AEDs.

■ WHEN TO STOP ANTIEPILEPTIC DRUGS

❻ The AEDs used to control seizures may not need to be given for a lifetime. Polypharmacy can be reduced, and some patients can discontinue AEDs altogether. The drug considered less appropriate for the seizure type (or the agent deemed most responsible for adverse effects) should be discontinued first. In some cases, decreasing the number of AEDs can decrease side effects and increase cognitive abilities. This improvement in cognition may be small, especially if the patient is on a drug that primarily affects psychomotor speed with less effect on higher-order cognitive functioning.

❼ Factors favoring successful withdrawal of AEDs include a seizure-free period of 2 to 4 years, complete seizure control within 1 year of onset, an onset of seizures after age 2 but before age 35, and a normal neurologic examination and EEG. Factors associated with a poor prognosis in discontinuing AEDs, despite a seizure-free interval, include a history of a high frequency of seizures, repeated episodes of status epilepticus, a combination of seizure types, and development of abnormal mental functioning. A 2-year seizure-free period is suggested for absence and rolandic epilepsy, whereas a 4-year seizure-free period is suggested for SP, CP, and absence seizures associated with tonic-clonic seizures. AED withdrawal generally is not suggested for patients with juvenile myoclonic epilepsy, absence with clonic-tonic-clonic seizures, or clonic-tonic-clonic seizures. The American Academy of Neurology (AAN) has issued guidelines for discontinuing AEDs in seizure-free patients.[14] After assessing the risks and benefits to both the patient and society, AED withdrawal can be considered in a patient meeting the following profile: seizure free for 2 to 5 years, a history of a single type of partial seizure or primary GTC seizures, a normal neurologic exam and normal IQ, and an EEG that has normalized with treatment. When these factors are present, the relapse rate is expected to be less than 32% for children and 39% for adults.

AED withdrawal should be done gradually, especially in patients with profound developmental disabilities. Some patients will have a recurrence of seizures as the AEDs are withdrawn. Sudden withdrawal is associated with the precipitation of status epilepticus. Withdrawal seizures are of particular concern for agents such as benzodiazepines and barbiturates. Seizure relapse has been reported to be more common if these AEDs are withdrawn over 1 to 3 months compared to over 6 months.

The risk of seizure relapse has been estimated at 10% to 70%. A meta-analysis determined that the relapse rate was 25% after 1 year and 29% after 2 years. Recurrence of seizures tends to occur early with at least one-half of the recurrences within 6 months of AED withdrawal and 60% to 90% within 1 year. Patients who relapse will generally become seizure free and in remission after AEDs are restarted although not necessarily immediately. The underlying epilepsy syndrome appears to determine prognosis for long-term remission.[15]

CLINICAL CONTROVERSY

It is not entirely clear which patients with epilepsy will require lifelong treatment. Although many clinicians feel that AED therapy is lifelong, others would argue that certain patients with idiopathic epilepsy and a normal neurologic examination and EEG are candidates for AED withdrawal following a prolonged period of seizure freedom (e.g., greater than 2–3 years). A large amount of the data supporting discontinuing AEDs has been obtained from children. Some adults will be reticent to discontinue AED therapy even if the clinician is in favor of it because of the fear of having a seizure and the consequences (e.g., loss of driver's license) that it would entail. The patient should agree and must be a willing participant in the plan to reduce or withdraw AED therapy.

■ NONPHARMACOLOGIC THERAPY

Nonpharmacologic therapy for epilepsy includes diet, surgery, and vagus nerve stimulation (VNS). A vagal nerve stimulator is an implanted medical device that is FDA approved for use as adjunctive therapy in reducing the frequency of seizures in adults and adolescents older than 12 years of age with partial-onset seizures that are refractory to AEDs. It is also used off-label in the treatment of refractory primary generalized epilepsy. The mechanisms of antiseizure actions of VNS are unknown. Human clinical studies have shown that VNS changes the cerebrospinal fluid (CSF) concentration of inhibitory and stimulatory neurotransmitters and activates specific areas of the brain that generate or regulate cortical seizure activity through increased blood flow. There is experimental evidence to suggest that the anticonvulsant effect of VNS is mediated by the locus coeruleus.[16]

The VNS device is relatively safe. It may also have a positive effect on mood and behavior, often independent of seizure reduction. The most common side effect associated with stimulation is hoarseness, voice alteration, increased cough, pharyngitis, dyspnea, dyspepsia, and nausea. Serious adverse effects reported include infection, nerve paralysis, hypoesthesia, facial paresis, left vocal cord paralysis, left facial paralysis, left recurrent laryngeal nerve injury, urinary retention, and low-grade fever. In the VNS studies, the percentage of patients who achieved a 50% or greater reduction in their seizure frequency (responders) ranged from 23% to 50%.

Surgery is the treatment of choice in selected patients with refractory focal epilepsy.[17] The success rate is beteen 80% and 90% in properly selected patients. Surgery reduces the risk of epilepsy-associated death, and it may also improve depression and anxiety in refractory epilepsy patients.[18,19] A recent systematic review/meta-analysis of published evidence of temporal lobe patients with pharmacoresistant epilepsy concluded that the combination of surgery with medical treatment is four-times as likely as medical treatment alone to achieve freedom from seizures.[20] A National Institutes of Health Consensus Conference identified three absolute requirements for surgery. They are (1) an absolute diagnosis of epilepsy, (2) failure on an adequate trial of drug therapy, and (3) definition of the electroclinical syndrome. A focus in the temporal lobe has the best chance for a positive outcome; however, extratemporal foci can be excised successfully in more than 75% of patients. The procedure is not without risk. Learning and memory can be impaired postoperatively, and general intellectual abilities are also affected in a small number of patients. Surgery may be particularly useful in children with intractable epilepsy. Patients may need to continue AED therapy for a period of time following successful epilepsy surgery, but dosage reduction may be achieveable.[17,21]

The ketogenic diet, devised in the 1920s, is high in fat and low in carbohydrates and protein, and it leads to acidosis and ketosis. Protein and calorie intake are set at levels that will meet requirements for growth. Most of the calories are provided in the form of heavy cream and butter. No sugar is allowed. Vitamins and minerals are supplemented. Medium-chain triglycerides can be substituted for the dietary fats. Fluids are also controlled. It requires strict control and parent compliance. Although some centers find the diet useful for refractory patients, others have found that it is poorly tolerated by patients. Long-term effects include kidney stones, increased bone fractures, and adverse effects on growth.[22] An international consensus statement has been published which offers recommendations for the clinical management of the patient with epilepsy using various forms of the ketogenic diet which may help with tolerability, including the use of the modified Atkins diet and the Low Glycemic Index Treatment.[23]

■ PHARMACOLOGIC THERAPY

Optimal management of epilepsy requires that AED treatment be individualized. Different patient groups (e.g., children, women of child-bearing potential, and the elderly) may be better suited to receive one AED than another by virtue not only of seizure type but also of susceptibility or relative risk for certain adverse effects. These issues are highlighted further below.

❼ Selection and optimization of AED therapy require not only an understanding of drug mechanism(s) of action and spectrum of clinical activity but also an appreciation of pharmacokinetic variability and patterns of drug-related adverse effects. An AED must be effective for the specific seizure type being treated. The drug treatments of first choice depend on the type of epilepsy, and drug-specific adverse effects and patient preferences. Ultimately, AED effectiveness is the result of the interaction of each of these factors. A suggested algorithm for a general approach to the treatment of epilepsy is shown in Figure 65–1.

Table 65–3 provides evidenced-based treatment recommendations by three professional/regulatory bodies.[24–28] In addition, recommendations from a U.S. panel of experts, which included more recent drug treatment data compared to the AAN-American Epilepsy Society (AES) recommendations are included.[29]

The mechanism of action of most AEDs can be categorized as (1) affecting ion channel kinetics, (2) augmenting inhibitory neurotransmission, or (3) modulating excitatory neurotransmission. Augmentation in inhibitory neurotransmission includes increasing CNS concentrations of GABA, whereas efforts to decrease excitatory neurotransmission are primarily focused on decreasing

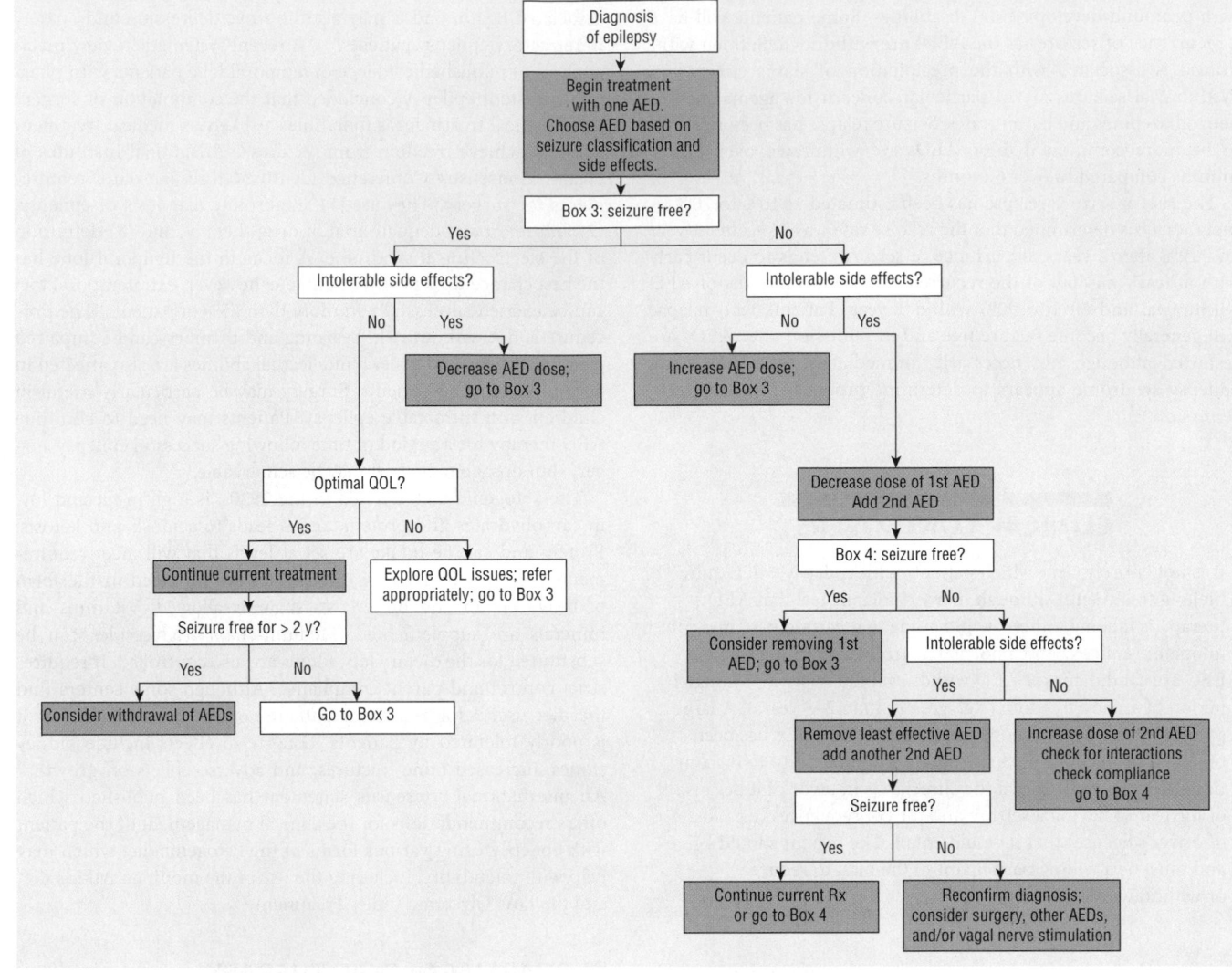

FIGURE 65-1. Algorithm for the treatment of epilepsy. (AED, antiepileptic drug; QOL, quality of life.)

(or antagonizing) glutamate and aspartate neurotransmission. AEDs that are effective against GTC and partial seizures probably reduce sustained repetitive firing of action potentials by delaying recovery of sodium channels from activation. Drugs that reduce corticothalamic T-type calcium currents are effective against generalized absence seizures. Myoclonic seizures respond to drugs that enhance $GABA_A$-receptor inhibition. In addition to mechanism of action, awareness of pharmacokinetic properties (Table 65–4), adverse effects (Table 65–5), AED-AED interactions (Table 65–6), and AED metabolic pathway as well as inducer or inhibitory effects on liver (Table 65–7) can aid in the optimization of AED therapy. Pharmacokinetic interactions are a common complicating factor in AED selection. Interactions can occur in any of the pharmacokinetic processes: absorption, distribution, metabolism or elimination. Caution should be used when AEDs are added to or withdrawn from a drug regimen.

Adverse effects of AEDs can be divided into acute and chronic (see Table 65–5). Acute effects can be dose/serum concentration—related or idiosyncratic. Concentration-dependent effects are common and troublesome but not usually life-threatening. Neurotoxic adverse effects are encountered commonly and can include sedation, dizziness, blurred or double vision, difficulty with concentration, and ataxia. In many cases these effects can be alleviated by decreasing the dose or avoided in some cases by titrating the dose

upward very slowly. Most idiosyncratic reactions are mild, but they can be more serious if the hypersensitivity involves one or more organ systems. Other idiosyncratic side effects including hepatitis or blood dyscrasias are serious but rare.

Acute organ failure, when it occurs, generally occurs within the first 6 months of AED therapy. Unfortunately, laboratory screening evaluations of blood and urine typically are not helpful in predicting or detecting the early stage of severe reactions and generally are not recommended in asymptomatic patients. An exception to this is in the screening of patients of Southeast Asian heritage for HLA-B*1502 antigen who are to receive carbamazepine and possibly phenytoin. There is a strong association between the presence of this antigen and Stevens—Johnson syndrome.[36] In any patient, laboratory assessment, including white blood cell counts and liver function tests, may be reasonable if the patient reports an unexplained illness (e.g., lethargy, vomiting, fever, or rash).[37] It is important to note that patients dosed and maintained within "therapeutic ranges" are also capable of experiencing toxicities to AEDs.[32] Another potential long-term adverse effect of AED treatment is osteomalacia and osteoporosis.[38,39] The bone disorders associated with AED use are a heterogeneous group of disorders, ranging from asymptomatic high-turnover disease, with findings of normal bone mineral density, to markedly decreased bone mineral density sufficient to warrant the diagnosis of osteoporosis. While the etiology of

TABLE 65-3 Drugs of Choice for Specific Seizure Disorders

Seizure Type	First-Line Drugs	Alternative Drugs[a]	Comments	Seizure Type	First-Line Drugs	Alternative Drugs[a]	Comments
Partial seizures (newly diagnosed)				U.K. guidelines[26,27]	Gabapentin		
U.S. guidelines[24,25]	*Adults & adolescents:*		*FDA approved:*		Lamotrigine		
	Carbamazepine		Carbamazepine		Levetiracetam		
	Gabapentin		Lacosamide		Oxcarbazepine		
	Oxcarbazepine		Phenobarbital		Tiagabine		
	Phenobarbital		Phenytoin	**Generalized seizures absence (newly diagnosed)**			
	Phenytoin		Topiramate				
	Topiramate		Valproic acid	U.S. guidelines[23,25]	Lamotrigine		*FDA approved:*
	Valproic acid						Ethosuximide
U.K. guidelines[26,27]	Carbamazepine						Valproic acid
	Lamotrigine			U.K. guidelines[26,27]	Lamotrigine		
	Oxcarbazepine			ILAE guidelines[28]	None	Ethosuximide	
	Topiramate					Lamotrigine	
	Valproic acid					Valproic acid	
ILAE guidelines[28]	*Adults:*	*Adults:*		U.S. Expert Panel 2005[32]	Ethosuximide	Lamotrigine	
	Carbamazepine	Gabapentin			Valproic acid		
	Phenytoin	Lamotrigine		**Primary generalized (tonic-clonic)**			
	Valproic acid	Oxcarbazepine					
		Phenobarbital					
		Topiramate		U.S. guidelines[24,25]	Topiramate		*FDA approved:*
	Children:	*Children:*					Lamotrigine
	Oxcarbazepine	Phenobarbital					Levetiracetam
		Phenytoin					Topiramate
		Topiramate		U.K. guidelines[26,27]	Lamotrigine		
		Valproic acid			Topiramate		
	Elderly:	*Elderly:*		ILAE guidelines[28]	None	*Adults:*	
	Gabapentin	Carbamazepine				Carbamazepine	
	Lamotrigine					Lamotrigine	
U.S. Expert Panel 2005[29]	Carbamazepine	Levetiracetam				Oxcarbazepine	
	Lamotrigine					Phenobarbital	
	Oxcarbazepine					Phenytoin	
Partial seizures (refractory monotherapy)						Topiramate	
						Valproic acid	
U.S. guidelines[24,25]	Lamotrigine		*FDA approved:*			*Children:*	
	Oxcarbazepine		Carbamazepine			Carbamazepine	
	Topiramate		Lamotrigine			Phenobarbital	
			Oxcarbazepine			Phenytoin	
			Phenobarbital			Topiramate	
			Phenytoin			Valproic acid	
			Topiramate			Lamotrigine	
			Valproic acid	U.S. Expert Panel 2005[29]	Valproic acid	Topiramate	
U.K. guidelines[26,27]	Lamotrigine			**Juvenile myoclonic epilepsy**			*FDA approved:*
	Oxcarbazepine						Levetiracetam (myoclonic seizures)
	Topiramate						
Partial seizures (refractory adjunct)				ILAE[28]	None	Clonazepam	
U.S. guidelines[24,25]	*Adults:*		*FDA approved:*			Lamotrigine	
	Gabapentin		Carbamazepine			Levetiracetam	
	Lamotrigine		Gabapentin			Topiramate	
	Levetiracetam		Lamotrigine			Valproic acid	
	Oxcarbazepine		Levetiracetam			Zonisamide	
	Tiagabine		Oxcarbazepine	U.S. Expert Panel 2005[29]	Valproic acid	Levetiracetam	
	Topiramate		Phenobarbital			Topiramate	
	Zonisamide		Phenytoin			Zonisamide	
	Children:		Pregabalin				
	Gabapentin		Tiagabine				
	Lamotrigine		Valproic acid				
	Oxcarbazepine		Vigabatrin				
	Topiramate		Zonisamide				

[a] Includes possibly effective drugs.
ILAE, International League Against Epilepsy.
Data from French et al.,[24,25] National Institute for Clinical Excellence,[26,27] Glauser et al.,[28] and Karceski et al.[29]

TABLE 65-4 Antiepileptic Drug Pharmacokinetic Data

AED	$t_{1/2}$ (h)	Time to steady state (days)	Unchanged (%)	V_D (L/kg)	Clinically Important Metabolite	Protein Binding (%)
Carbamazepine	12 M; 5–14 Co	21–28 for completion of auto-induction	<1	1–2	10,11-epoxide	40–90
Ethosuximide	A 60; C 30	6–12	10–20	0.67	No	0
Felbamate	16–22	5–7	50	0.73–0.82	No	~25
Gabapentin[a]	5–40[b]	1–2	100	0.65–1.04	No	0
Lacosamide	13	3	40	0.6	No	<15
Lamotrigine	25.4 M	3–15	0	1.28	No	40–50
Levetiracetam	7–10	2		0.7	No	<10
Oxcarbazepine	3–13	2		0.7	10-hydroxy-carbazepine	40
Phenobarbital	A 46–136; C 37–73	14–21	20–40	0.6	No	50
Phenytoin	A 10–34; C 5–14	7–28	<5	0.6–8.0	No	90
Pregabalin	A6–7[b]	1–2	90	0.5	No	0
Primidone	A 3.3–19; C 4.5–11	1–4	40	0.43–1.1	PB	80
Rufinamide	6–10	2	4	0.8–1.2	No	26–35
Tiagabine	5–13		Negligible		No	95
Topiramate	18–21	4–5	50–70	0.55–0.8 (male); 0.23–0.4 (female)	No	15
Valproic acid	A 8–20; C 7–14	1–3	<5	0.1–0.5	May contribute to toxicity	90–95 binding saturates
Vigabatrin	5–8	N/A	<2	0.8	No	0
Zonisamide	24–60	5–15		0.8–1.6	No	40–60

A, adult; AED, antiepileptic drug; C, child; Co, combination therapy; M, monotherapy; PB, phenobarbital; V_D, volume of distribution.

[a] The bioavailability of gabapentin is dose dependent.

[b] Half-life depends on renal function.

N/A= not applicable since effect depends on inhibiting enzyme.

Data from Faught,[30] Leppik,[31] and Patsalos et al.[32]

TABLE 65-5 Antiepileptic Drug Side Effects

Antiepileptic Drug	Acute Side Effects		Chronic Side Effects
	Concentration Dependent	**Idiosyncratic**	
Carbamazepine	Diplopia Dizziness Drowsiness Nausea Unsteadiness Lethargy	Blood dyscrasias Rash	Hyponatremia
Ethosuximide	Ataxia Drowsiness GI distress Unsteadiness Hiccoughs	Blood dyscrasias Rash	Behavior changes Headache
Felbamate	Anorexia Nausea Vomiting Insomnia Headache	Aplastic anemia Acute hepatic failure	Not established
Gabapentin	Dizziness Fatigue Somnolence Ataxia	Pedal edema	Weight gain
Lacosamide	Dizziness Headache Nausea Vomiting PR interval increase on ECG	Liver enzyme elevation	Not established
Lamotrigine	Diplopia Dizziness Unsteadiness Headache	Rash	Not established
Levetiracetam	Sedation Behavioral disturbance	Psychosis (rare)	Not established

(continued)

TABLE 65-5 Antiepileptic Drug Side Effects (continued)

Antiepileptic Drug	Acute Side Effects		Chronic Side Effects
	Concentration Dependent	**Idiosyncratic**	
Oxcarbazepine	Sedation Dizziness Ataxia Nausea	Rash	Hyponatremia
Phenobarbital	Ataxia Hyperactivity Headache Unsteadiness Sedation Nausea	Blood dyscrasias Rash	Behavior changes Connective tissue disorders Intellectual blunting Metabolic bone disease Mood change Sedation
Phenytoin	Ataxia Nystagmus Behavior changes Dizziness Headache Incoordination Sedation Lethargy Cognitive impairment Fatigue Visual blurring	Blood dyscrasias Rash Immunologic reaction	Behavior changes Cerebellar syndrome Connective tissue changes Skin thickening Folate deficiency Gingival hyperplasia Hirsutism Coarsening of facial features Acne Cognitive impairment Metabolic bone disease Sedation
Pregabalin	Dizziness Somnolence Blurred vision	Pedal edema Creatine kinase elevation Decrease platelets	Weight gain
Primidone	Behavior changes Headache Nausea Sedation Unsteadiness	Blood dyscrasias Rash	Behavior change Connective tissue disorders Cognitive impairment Sedation
Rufinamide	Dizzness Nausea Vomiting Somnolence	Multiorgan hypersensitivity Status epilepticus Leukopenia QT shortening	Not established
Tiagabine	Dizziness Fatigue Difficulties concentrating Nervousness Tremor Blurred vision Depression Weakness	Spike-wave stupor	Not established
Topiramate	Difficulties concentrating Psychomotor slowing Speech or language problems Somnolence, fatigue Dizziness Headache	Metabolic acidosis Acute angle glaucoma Oligohydrosis	Kidney stones Weight loss
Valproic acid	GI upset Sedation Unsteadiness Tremor Thrombocytopenia	Acute hepatic failure Acute pancreatitis Alopecia	Polycystic ovary–like syndrome Weight gain Hyperammonemia Menstual cycle irregularities
Vigabatrin	Permanent vision loss Fatigue Somnolence Weight gain Tremor Blurred vision	Abnormal MRI brain signal changes (infants with infantile spasms) Peripheral neuropathy Anemia	Permanent vision loss
Zonisamide	Sedation Dizziness Cognitive impairment Nausea	Rash Metabolic acidosis Oligohydrosis	Kidney stones Weight loss

Data from French et al.[24,25] Leppik,[31] Halford and Lapointe,[33] Cada et al.,[34] and Sabril [package insert].[35]

TABLE 65-6 Interactions between Antiepileptic Drugs

Antiepileptic Drug	Added Drug	Effect[a]	Antiepileptic Drug	Added Drug	Effect[a]
Carbamazepine (CBZ)	Felbamate	Incr. 10,11 epoxide	Pregabalin	No known interactions	
		Decr. CBZ	Primidone (PRM)	Carbamazepine	Decr. PRM
	Oxcarbazepine	Decr. CBZ			Incr. PB
	Phenobarbital	Decr. CBZ		Phenytoin	Decr. PRM
	Phenytoin	Decr. CBZ			Incr. PB
	Valproic acid	Incr. 10,11 epoxide		Valproic acid	Incr. PRM
Ethosuximide	Carbamazepine	Decr. ethosuximide			Incr. PB
	Phenobarbital	Decr. ethosuximide	Rufinamide (RUF)	Carbamazepine	Decr. RUF
	Phenytoin	Decr. ethosuximide		Phenobarbital	Decr. RUF
Felbamate (FBM)	Carbamazepine	Decr. FBM		Phenytoin	Decr. RUF
	Phenytoin	Decr. FBM		Primidone	Decr. RUF
	Valproic acid	Incr. FBM		Valproic acid	Incr. RUF
Gabapentin	No known interactions		Tiagabine (TGB)	Carbamazepine	Decr. TGB
Lacosamide (LAC)	Carbamazepine	Decr. LAC		Phenobarbital	Decr. TGB
	Phenobarbital	Decr. LAC		Phenytoin	Decr. TGB
	Phenytoin	Decr. LAC		Primidone	Decr. TGB
Lamotrigine (LTG)	Carbamazepine	Decr. LTG	Topiramate (TPM)	Carbamazepine	Decr. TPM
	Phenobarbital	Decr. LTG		Phenobarbital	Decr. TPM
	Phenytoin	Decr. LTG		Phenytoin	Decr. TPM
	Primidone	Decr. LTG		Primdione	Decr. TPM
	Valproic acid	Incr. LTG		Valproic acid	Decr. TPM
Levetiracetam (LEV)	Carbamazepine	Decr. LEV	Valproic acid (VPA)	Carbamazepine	Decr. VPA
	Phenobarbital	Decr. LEV		Felbamate	Incr. VPA
	Phenytoin	Decr. LEV		Lamotrigine	Decr. VPA (slight)
Oxcarbazepine	Carbamazepine	Decr. MHD[b]		Phenobarbital	Decr. VPA
	Phenobarbital	Decr. MHD[b]		Phenytoin	Decr. VPA
	Phenytoin	Decr. MHD[b]		Primidone	Decr. VPA
Phenobarbital (PB)	Felbamate	Incr. PB		Topiramate	Decr. VPA
	Oxcarbazepine	Incr. PB	Vigabatrin	No known interactions	
	Phenytoin	Incr. PB	Zonisamide (ZON)	Carbamazepine	Decr. ZON
	Valproic acid	Incr. PB		Phenobarbital	Decr. ZON
Phenytoin (PHT)	Carbamazepine	Incr. or decr. PHT		Phenytoin	Decr. ZON
	Felbamate	Incr. PHT		Primidone	Decr. ZON
	Methsuximide	Incr. PHT			
	Oxcarbazepine (>1,200 mg/d)	Incr. PHT			
	Phenobarbital	Incr. or decr. PHT			
	Topiramate	Incr. PHT			
	Valproic acid	Decr. Total PHT, then may incr. total PHT			
	Vigabatrin	Decr. PHT			

[a]Incr. = increased; Decr. = decreased.
[b]MHD = 10-mono-hydroxy-derivative.
Data from Patsalos et al.,[32] Halford and Lapointe,[33] and Cada et al.[34]

these osteopathies is uncertain, it has been hypothesized that certain drugs, including phenytoin, phenobarbital, carbamazepine, oxcarbazepine, felbamate, and valproic acid, may interfere with vitamin D metabolism. Whether the other AEDs cause these effects is unknown, however, current evidence suggests that lamotrigine does not. Common laboratory findings in these patients include elevated bone-specific alkaline phosphatase concentration, intact parathyroid hormone, and decreased serum calcium and 25-OH vitamin D concentrations. Patients receiving these drugs should receive supplemental vitamin D and calcium, as well as bone mineral density testing if other risk factors for osteoporosis are present.

The comparative effects of AEDs on cognition have been difficult to evaluate because of differences or inconsistencies in study design, seizure types studied, control for serum drug concentrations, and the neuropsychologic tests used. In general, there are not large differences between the older drugs, although the barbiturates phenobarbital and primidone appear to cause more cognitive impairment than other commonly used AEDs.[40,41] Phenytoin, particularly when serum concentrations are above the commonly accepted therapeutic range, may have a greater effect on motor function and

speed. Among the older AEDs, valproic acid may cause less impairment of cognition. Improvement in cognition has been reported in patients switched from phenytoin or phenobarbital to valproic acid. However, these improvements are subtle if patients are in the same relative area of the therapeutic range. Patients changed from polytherapy to monotherapy also may demonstrate improvement in cognition. Some of the newer agents are believed to cause fewer neurobehavioral or cognitive effects. Among the newer AEDs, gabapentin and lamotrigine have been shown in several studies to cause fewer cognitive impairments compared with older agents, such as carbamazepine.[42-44] Conversely, topiramate may cause substantial cognitive impairment, particularly when used at high doses or during rapid dose escalation.[44] In addition, these patients may not be fully aware of their deficits.[45,46] AED treatment itself may sometimes worsen seizures due to improper AED selection for a specific seizure type or syndrome or can represent a paradoxical toxic effect of the drug.[47]

Because most adult patients have localization-related (partial-onset) seizures, the most widely used AEDs traditionally have been carbamazepine, phenobarbital, phenytoin, and valproic acid.

TABLE 65-7 Antiepileptic Drugs Elimination Pathways and Major Effects on Hepatic Enzymes

Antiepileptic Drugs	Major Hepatic Enzymes	Renal Elimination (%)	Induced	Inhibited
Carbamazepine	CYP3A4; CYP1A2; CYP2C8	<1	CYP1A2; CYP2C; CYP3A; GT	None
Ethosuximide	CYP3A4	12–20	None	None
Felbamate	CYP3A4; CYP2E1; other	50	CYP3A4	CYP2C19; β-oxidation
Gabapentin	None	Almost completely	None	None
Lacosamide	CYP2C19	70	None	None
Lamotrigine	GT	10	GT	None
Levetiracetam	None (undergoes non-hepatic hydrolysis)	66	None	None
Oxcarbazepine (MHD is active oxcarbazepine metabolite)	Cytosolic system	1 (27 as MHD)	CYP3A4; CYP3A5; GT	CYP2C19
Phenobarbital	CYP2C9; other	25	CYP3A; CYP2C; GT	None
Phenytoin	CYP2C9; CYP2C19	5	CYP3A; CYP2C; GT	
Pregabalin	None	100	None	None
Rufinamide	Hydrolysis	2	CYP3A4 (weak)	CYP2E1 (weak)
Tiagabine	CYP3A4	2	None	None
Topiramate	Not known	70	CYP3A (dose dependent)	CYP2C19
Valproate	GT; β-oxidation	2	None	CYP2C9; GT epoxide hydrolase
Vigabatrin	None	Almost completely	CYP2C9	None
Zonisamide	CYP3A4	35	None	None

CYP, cytochrome P450 isoenzyme system; GT, glucuronyltransferase.
Data from Faught,[30] Leppik,[31] Patsalos et al.,[52] Halford and Lapointe,[53] Cada et al.,[34] and Sabril [package insert].[35]

For CP seizures, these AEDs have similar efficacy.[48,49] Of these, carbamazepine and phenytoin are the most commonly prescribed AEDs for partial seizures in the United States. This preference is largely based on data derived from two landmark trials conducted through the Veterans Administration (VA) Epilepsy Cooperative Study Group. In the first of these trials, patients with new-onset partial or generalized epilepsy were randomized to receive either carbamazepine, phenobarbital, phenytoin, or primidone.[48] After 3 years, patients who received either carbamazepine or phenytoin were equally likely and patients on phenobarbital or primidone were least likely to have remained on their originally assigned treatment. Thus, carbamazepine and phenytoin were considered the drugs of first choice in patients with new-onset partial or generalized seizures. Carbamazepine was associated with fewer side effects. A follow-up study using almost identical methods compared carbamazepine and valproic acid.[49] Carbamazepine- and valproic acid—treated groups had equal retention rates for tonic-clonic seizures. Carbamazepine was superior to valproic acid for efficacy in the treatment of partial seizures. Valproic acid caused slightly more adverse effects.

Based primarily on these trials, carbamazepine has been recognized as the AED of first choice for partial seizures. Several of the newer generation AEDs are now proving to be reasonable alternatives. The newer AEDs were first approved as adjunctive therapy for patients with refractory partial seizures. Monotherapy trials with several of these newer agents including lamotrigine, gabapentin, topiramate, oxcarbazepine and levetiracetam have now been completed.[50–52] Comparisons between lamotrigine and older agents including carbamazepine and phenytoin as initial monotherapy for partial seizures have been conducted in Europe, and the results suggest comparable effectiveness and perhaps better tolerability for lamotrigine, particularly in elderly patients. In a large, unblinded, randomized, controlled trial in hospital based outpatient clinics in the United Kingdom, lamotrigine was found to be clinically better than carbamazepine for time to treatment failure outcomes in newly diagnosed patients with partial seizures; lamotrigine was determined to be a cost effective alternative to carbamazepine. Other drugs studied in this trial were gabapentin, oxcarbazepine, and topiramate.[53] Results from a VA cooperative trial designed to compare gabapentin, lamotrigine, and carbamazepine in newly diagnosed elderly patients with partial seizures found that lamotrigine efficacy is comparable with that of both gabapentin and carbamazepine, and is better tolerated than carbamazepine but equal to gabapentin in this population.[54] Clinical data suggest that in newly diagnosed patients, oxcarbazepine is as effective as phenytoin, valproic acid, and immediate-release carbamazepine, with perhaps fewer adverse effects. Close examination of the conversion to monotherapy trials suggests that oxcarbazepine demonstrates efficacy even in patients who previously had an inadequate response to carbamazepine, in spite of their structural similarity. Lastly, levetiracetam in a one-year study was found to have equal efficacy and tolerability when studied against controlled-release carbamazepine.[55]

In addition, several monotherapy trials using an active control or pseudoplacebo design also have been conducted. Although these study designs provide evidence of efficacy for the newer drugs, because the comparison is between active drug and placebo in patients who continue to have seizures in spite of current treatment with standard AEDs, it is difficult to compare the efficacy of the newer drugs directly with the older AEDs. Generally speaking, the newer AEDs appear to have comparable efficacy to the older agents and are perhaps better tolerated.

To date, among the newer generation agents, lamotrigine, oxcarbazepine, and topiramate have received FDA approval for use as monotherapy in patients with partial seizures. Phenobarbital and primidone are also useful in partial seizures, but sedation and cognitive adverse effects limit their utility. Felbamate, which has monotherapy approval, is effective but has been associated with some significant side effects. Interpretation of monotherapy trials with the newer AEDs can be daunting owing to the unique study designs and specific patient populations employed. Withholding an effective AED (i.e., giving placebo) in patients with epilepsy is generally considered unethical. For more information the reader is referred to published reviews.[50]

Primarily generalized seizures such as absence seizures may respond differently pharmacologically than other seizure types. Phenytoin, phenobarbital, and carbamazepine, although effective in GTC and partial seizures, are ineffective for absence seizures, and in some cases, can precipitate an increase in seizure frequency. Absence seizures are best treated with ethosuximide, valproic acid, and perhaps lamotrigine. For levetiracetam, topiramate, and zonisamide, additional data are needed to confirm efficacy. Oxcarbazepine, gabapentin, and tiagabine do not appear to be effective in treating absence seizures, and can worsen this condition in some patients. If the patient has a combination of absence and other generalized or partial seizures, valproic acid or lamotrigine is the preferred first choice because they are effective for absence and other seizure types. If valproic acid is ineffective in treating a mixed seizure disorder that includes absence, ethosuximide could be used in combination with another AED.

The traditional treatment of tonic-clonic seizures is phenytoin; however, carbamazepine and valproic acid are increasingly used because these AEDs have a lower incidence of side effects with equal efficacy. Valproic acid generally is considered the drug of first choice for atonic seizures and for juvenile myoclonic epilepsy (JME). Lamotrigine and perhaps topiramate and zonisamide can be alternative agents for these seizure types. Levetiracetam has received FDA approval as adjunctive treatment of myoclonic seizures in patients with JME.

Results of a large, unblinded, randomized, controlled trial conducted in patients with new-onset generalized and unclassified epilepsy outpatients in the United Kingdom has helped to define the role of the newer generation drugs. These researchers found that for idiopathic generalized epilepsy, valproic acid was significantly better tolerated than topiramate and more efficacious than lamotrigine.[56]

Serum concentrations of the older AEDs should be viewed as a tool with which to optimize therapy for an individual patient, not as a therapeutic end point in itself. The serum concentration is a target that should be correlated with clinical response. The desired outcome is the cessation of seizures without side effects. Seizure control can occur before the "minimum" of the published therapeutic range is achieved, and side effects can appear before the "maximum" of the range is achieved. Some patients may need and tolerate concentrations beyond the maximum. The therapeutic range for AEDs can be different for different seizure types. Serum concentrations may need to be higher to control CP seizures than to control tonic-clonic seizures. Clinicians should define a therapeutic range for an individual patient above which there are side effects and below which the patient experiences seizures. Then serum levels can be useful to document lack of efficacy, loss of efficacy, noncompliance, and to determine how much room there is to increase a dose based on expected toxicity. Depending on the AED, serum levels can also be useful in patients with significant renal and/or hepatic disease, patients taking multiple drugs, and women who are pregnant or taking oral contraceptives (OCs). Therapeutic concentration ranges have not been clearly defined for some of the second generation AEDs.

THERAPEUTIC CONSIDERATIONS IN THE ELDERLY AND YOUNG

Use of AEDs in the elderly and young can pose special challenges.[32] Avoidance of AEDs that interact with other medications that the elderly are often taking is of upmost importance. Many of the AEDs are inducers or inhibitors of the CYP450 system, which can adversely affect the drug level of concomitantly administered drugs. Hypoalbuminemia is common in the elderly, and can make monitoring and adjustment of serum drug levels of highly albumin-bound AEDs, such as phenytoin, valproic acid, and tiagabine, problematic. The elderly also experience body mass changes, such as an increase in fat to lean body mass or decrease in body water, which can affect the volume of distribution of some drugs, and therefore possibly the elimination half-life. In addition, declining renal and/or hepatic function can occur in the elderly, which can require a lower dose of the AED. Lastly, the pharmacodynamic response to AEDs can change with aging such that elderly patients may be more sensitive to various neurocognitive adverse effects. Also, elderly patients' seizures may be controlled at relatively lower total serum concentrations.

For neonates and infants, an increase in the total body water to fat ratio and a decrease in serum albumin and α-acid glycoprotein can result in volume of distribution changes that can affect the elimination half-life of the AEDs. In addition, newborns up to the age of 2 to 3 years display decreased efficiency in renal elimination, with newborns being the most affected. Hepatic activity is also reduced in this population. However, by age 2 to 3 years, hepatic activity is more robust than that seen in adults. Therefore, children require higher doses of many of the AEDs than adults, whereas neonates and infants require lower doses. Lastly, rapidly changing and sometimes inconsistent metabolism in the patient groups above makes therapeutic drug monitoring especially important even though the definition of therapeutic blood level is less certain in these patients than in adults.

THERAPEUTIC CONSIDERATIONS IN WOMEN (AND MEN)

Many hormones influence brain electrical excitability, and estrogen and progesterone may interact in complex ways to alter neuronal excitability and protein synthesis.[57] Estrogen has a slight pro-convulsant effect, whereas progesterone exerts a mild anticonvulsant effect. Estrogen has a mild inhibitory effect on GABA receptors, potentiates excitatory glutaminergic activity, and can promote the development of kindling. Progesterone has the opposite effect and appears to potentiate GABA receptor activity and reduce neuronal discharge rates. AEDs, especially hepatic metabolizing enzyme inducers, increase the metabolism of these hormones and induce the production of sex hormone—binding globulin. This may lead to decreases in the unbound fraction of the hormone. Enzyme-inducing AEDs, including topiramate and oxcarbazepine at higher doses, can cause treatment failures in women taking OCs owing to induction of the metabolism of ethinyl estradiol and progestin. This may also be an issue with rufinamide, lamotrigine, and felbamate, all which have a small effect in decreasing the bioavailability of combination oral contraceptives (OCs). A supplemental form of birth control, in addition to OCs, is advised if breakthrough bleeding occurs. However medroxyprogesterone depot injection, copper intrauterine devices, and hormone-release intrauterine systems are not affected by AEDs. There are no data available on the efficacy of the emergency contraceptive pill in patients taking these AEDs, but it has been suggested that women use twice the normal dose of the postcoital pill.[58] Valproic acid, benzodiazepines, and most of the newer AEDs, such as gabapentin, levetiracetam, tiagabine, zonisamide, vigabatrin, and lacosamide, are not enzyme inducers and have not been implicated in reducing contraceptive effectiveness. Of note, OCs lower lamotrigine's serum level significantly and lower valproic acid's level about 20%.[32]

In some women, vulnerability to seizures is highest just before and during the menstrual flow (catamenial seizures) and at the time of ovulation. The increased susceptibility to seizures during those catamenial periods is associated with a slight increase of estrogen relative to progesterone. The risk of catamenial epilepsy is estimated at 12.5%, but it may be as high as 50% in women with epilepsy. This pattern of seizure exacerbation can also be related to progesterone withdrawal and changes in the estrogen-to-progesterone ratio. Conventional AEDs should be used as primary agents but intermittent supplementation with higher dose of AED or benzodiazepines should be considered. Acetazolamide also has been used during catamenial periods but with variable and limited success. Hormonal therapy with progestational agents, particularly cyclic natural progesterone therapy, may be effective. Reproductive endocrine disorders are common in women with epilepsy and include menstrual irregularity, infertility, sexual dysfunction, and possibly polycystic ovary syndrome (PCOS).[59] Potential mechanisms for these disturbances include disruption of the hypothalamic-pituitary-adrenal (HPA) axis via seizure discharges in limbic structures and/or AEDs.[62] AEDs, particularly the enzyme-inducing agents (e.g., carbamazepine, phenytoin, and phenobarbital), also may affect HPA function by altering the metabolism of the neuroactive sex hormones, including testosterone. Although a causal relationship has not yet been established, there is an apparent increased incidence of PCOS in women with epilepsy who are receiving valproic acid.[59]

During pregnancy there may be increased maternal seizures, pregnancy complications, and adverse fetal outcome.[60] Approximately 25% to 30% of pregnant women have increased seizures, whereas seizures decrease in a similar number. However, the risk of seizures is significantly less if the patient has been seizure free 12 months prior to the pregnancy.[61] Increased seizure frequency may result from either a direct effect on seizure threshold or a reduction in AED concentration. An increase in clearance has been reported for phenytoin, carbamazepine, phenobarbital, ethosuximide, lamotrigine, oxcarbazepine, levetiracetam, topiramate, and clorazepate during pregnancy. Protein binding may also be reduced. The altered disposition of AEDs can begin as early as the first 10 weeks of pregnancy, and may require up to 4 weeks postpartum to normalize (longer for carbamazepine and phenobarbital than for phenytoin).

Women with epilepsy have a higher incidence of adverse pregnancy outcomes. Although the risk of congenital malformations is 4% to 6% (twice as high as in nonepileptic women), more than 90% of pregnancies in epileptic mothers have satisfactory outcomes. Older data, much of which included AED polytherapy, indicated that barbiturates and phenytoin may cause congenital heart malformations, orofacial clefts, and other malformations. From these data the risk of neural tube defect with valproic acid and carbamazepine has been estimated to be 0.5% to 1%, respectively, and appears to be related to drug exposure during gestational days 0 to 28. Other adverse pregnancy outcomes associated with maternal seizures, but not necessarily caused by AEDs, are growth, psychomotor, and mental retardation. Women with epilepsy are also more likely to have miscarriages, and 10% to 20% of infants are born with low birth weight. Updated practice parameters are available to aid in the counseling and management of pregnant women with epilepsy.[62–64]

Some teratogenic effects may be prevented by adequate folate intake; therefore, prenatal vitamins with folic acid (0.4–5 mg/day) should be given to any woman of child-bearing potential who is taking AEDs.[60] Higher folate doses should be used in women with a history of a previous pregnancy with a neural tube defect or taking valproic acid. Higher AED doses and serum concentrations, polytherapy, and a family history of birth defects appear to increase the teratogenic risk of AEDs. Deciding on the most effective single-drug treatment prior to conception is vitally important. New AEDs are reported to be less teratogenic, and animal reproductive toxicology studies appear to be favorable. At present, clinical data are still limited, and more experience is needed before the true risk (or lack thereof) can be determined. However, multiple registries worldwide are collecting prospective data on pregnancy outcomes in users of newer and older AEDs. To date, results indicate that valproic acid mono- as well as polytherapy is associated with a significantly higher rate of fetal malformations compared to the other AEDs, especially at doses greater than 1,400 mg/day.[65,66] Some AEDs can cause neonatal hemorrhagic disorder, which can be prevented by administrating 10 mg/day vitamin K orally to the mother during the last month of pregnancy and/or administering parenteral vitamin K to the newborn at delivery.[64]

Most AEDs pass into the breast milk, and concentrations are measureable in breastfeeding infants. In general, the degree of protein binding of a given AED allows for prediction of its concentration in breast milk. AEDs with less protein binding accumulate more in breast milk. Treatment with AEDs is not necessarily a reason to discourage breastfeeding. In fact, an argument could be made that since AEDs should rarely be discontinued abruptly, breastfeeding is a reasonable way to allow for a downward titration of a medication that the baby was exposed to for the past 9 months. Infants born to women taking any AED (particularly barbiturates or benzodiazepines) should be closely observed for signs of excess sedation, irritability, or poor feeding.[60]

The perimenopausal period can be associated with worsening of seizures. At menopause, seizures often improve in frequency, particularly in women with a catamenial seizure pattern. The effect of hormone replacement therapy on seizure control is still unclear, but clinicians should monitor for seizure exacerbation in women receiving supplemental estrogen. Exacerbation of seizures has been noted in postmenopausal women on lamotrigine taking hormone replacement therapy.[67] Data suggest that men with epilepsy have reduced fertility, and that carbamazepine, oxcarbazepine, and valproic acid are associated with sperm abnormalities in these men. In addition, valproic acid seems to cause testicular atrophy resulting in reduced testosterone volume.[68]

■ CLINICAL CONSIDERATIONS WITH SPECIFIC DRUGS

Tables 65–4 through 65–8 list specific data (including pharmacokinetics, adverse effects, AED interactions, metabolism, and dosing) for each of the commonly used AEDs. Below we summarize the pharmacology, advantages and disadvantages, and perspectives on the place in therapy of each AED.

Carbamazepine

Pharmacology and Mechanism of Action The exact mechanism by which carbamazepine suppresses seizure spread is obscure, however, it is believed to act primarily by enhancing fast inactivation of voltage-gated sodium channels. In addition, interaction with voltage-gated calcium and potassium channels might also contribute to its activity.[69]

Pharmacokinetics The absorption of carbamazepine from immediate-release tablets is slow and erratic because of its low water solubility. There is also large variability in the peak-to-trough concentrations of up to 40%. There is no first-pass metabolism. Food, especially fat, may enhance the bioavailability of carbamazepine. Carbamazepine suspension is absorbed faster than the tablets.[70] Controlled-release (Tegretol-XR) and sustained-release (Carbatrol) preparations are also available, and they are bioequivalent in twice-daily (every 12 hours) dosing to immediate-release carbamazepine dosed 4 times daily (every 6 hours). Compared with immediate-release carbamazepine, both these formulations have lower peaks and higher troughs, which may decrease side effects and improve seizure control. Carbatrol can improve QOL measurements compared to the immediate-release product.[71] Patients should be told to take Tegretol-XR with food and that the casing will be excreted in the feces. It cannot be broken or crushed. Tegretol-XR and Carbatrol appear to be bioequivalent; however, there is less variability in the absorption of Carbatrol.[70]

Carbamazepine is a neutral and highly lipophilic drug that is highly protein bound to α_1-acid glycoprotein and albumin. The major metabolite is carbamazepine-10,11-epoxide, which has anticonvulsant activity in animals and humans.[70] The formation of the 10,11-epoxide is influenced by concurrent use of other enzyme-inducing or enzyme-inhibiting drugs; thus the 10,11-epoxide concentration may change with the administration of other drugs (e.g., valproate and felbamate) with no change in parent carbamazepine concentration.[70]

TABLE 65-8 Antiepileptic Drugs Dosing and Target Serum Concentration Ranges

	Trade Name	Usual Initial Dose	Usual Maximum Daily Dose	Target Serum Concentration Range
Barbiturates				
Phenobarbital	Various	1–3 mg/kg/day (10–20 mg/kg LD)	180–300 mg	10–40 mcg/mL (43–172 µmol/L)
Primidone	Mysoline	100–125 mg/day	750–2,000 mg	5–10 mcg/mL (23–46 µmol/L)
Benzodiazepines				
Clonazepam	Klonopin	1.5 mg/day	20 mg	20–70 ng/mL (0.06–0.22 µmol/L)
Diazepam	Valium	PO: 4–40 mg IV: 5–10 mg	PO: 4–40 mg IV: 5–30 mg	100–1,000 ng/mL (0.4–3.5 µmol/L)
Lorazepam	Ativan	PO: 2–6 mg IV: 0.05 mg/kg IM: 0.05 mg/kg	PO: 10 mg IV: 0.05 mg/kg	10–30 ng/mL (31–93 µmol/L)
Hydantoin				
Phenytoin	Dilantin	PO: 3–5 mg/kg (200–400 mg) (15–20 mg/kg LD)	PO: 500–600 mg	Total: 10–20 mcg/mL (40–79 µmol/L) Unbound: 0.5–3 mcg/mL (2–12 µmol/L)
Succinimide				
Ethosuximide	Zarontin	500 mg/day	500–2,000 mg	40–100 mcg/mL (282–708 µmol/L)
Other				
Carbamazepine	Tegretol	400 mg/day	400–2,400 mg	4–12 mcg/mL (17–51 µmol/L)
Felbamate	Felbatol	1,200 mg/day	3,600 mg	30–60 mcg/mL (126–252 µmol/L)
Gabapentin	Neurontin	900 mg/day	4,800 mg	2–20 mcg/mL (12–117 µmol/L)
Lacosamide	Vimpat	100 mg/day	400 mg	Not defined
Lamotrigine	Lamictal	25 mg every other day if on VPA; 25–50 mg/day if not on VPA	100–150 mg if on VPA; 300–500 mg if not on VPA	4–20 mcg/mL (16–78 µmol/L)
Levetiracetam	Keppra Keppra XR	500–1,000 mg/day	3,000–4,000 mg	12–46 mcg/mL (70–270 µmol/L)
Oxcarbazepine	Trileptal	300–600 mg/day	2,400–3,000 mg	3–35 mcg/mL (MHD) (12–139 µmol/L)
Pregabalin	Lyrica	150 mg/day	600 mg	Not defined
Rufinamide	Banzel	400–800 mg/day	3,200 mg	Not defined
Tiagabine	Gabitril	4–8 mg/day	80 mg	0.02–0.2 mcg/mL (0.05–0.5 µmol/L)
Topiramate	Topamax	25–50 mg/day	200–1,000 mg	5–20 mcg/mL (15–59 µmol/L)
Valproic acid	Depakene Depakene SR Depakote Depakote ER Depacon	15 mg/kg (500–1,000 mg)	60 mg/kg (3,000–5,000 mg)	50–100 mcg/mL (347–693 µmol/L)
Vigabatrin	Sabril	1,000 mg/day	3,000 mg	0.8–36 mcg/mL (6–279 µmol/L)
Zonisamide	Zonegran	100–200 mg/day	600 mg	10–40 mcg/mL (47–188 µmol/L)

IM, intramuscular; LD, loading does; MHD, 10-monohydroxy- derivative; PO, orally; VPA, valproic acid.
Data from Patsalos et al.,[32] Halford and Lapointe,[33] Cada et al.,[34] and Sabril [package insert].[35]

Carbamazepine induces its own metabolism (autoinduction), thereby decreasing its half-life after chronic therapy.[70] The presence of enzyme-inducing drugs reduces the half-life even more. The enzyme-induction effect begins within 3 to 5 days of starting therapy and takes 21 to 28 days to complete. Therefore, it is possible to achieve initial concentrations that are within the therapeutic range but have concentrations fall despite continued therapy and good compliance. Some patients who respond well to initial therapy may be labeled refractory or noncompliant if the autoinduction phenomenon is not considered. The autoinduction reverses rapidly if carbamazepine is discontinued. Carbamazepine also displays diurnal variation in its serum level with evening levels lower than morning levels.

Adverse Effects Carbamazepine side effects can parallel the rise and decline of serum concentrations daily. Neurosensory side effects (e.g., diplopia, blurred vision, nystagmus, ataxia, unsteadiness, dizziness, and headache) are the most common (35%–50% of patients). These side effects are more common during initiation of therapy and can dissipate with continued treatment. Carbamazepine can also cause nausea, which can be caused by a local effect of the drug on the GI tract, in which case food may help, or be caused by an effect on the brainstem, which may ultimately require discontinuation of the drug. Dosage manipulation, including the use of the controlled- or sustained-release preparations, should be tried

before the patient is considered to be intolerant of carbamazepine. Carbamazepine can cause hyponatremia, the incidence of which increases with age, however, its occurrence is lower than that seen with oxcarbazepine. Periodic determinations of serum sodium concentration are recommended, especially in the elderly.[70]

Leukopenia is the most common hematologic side effect, with an incidence as high as 10%. It usually is transient, even when the drug is continued, and can be caused by a redistribution of white blood cells (WBCs) rather than a decrease in their production. In about 2% of patients, leukopenia is persistent, but even patients with WBC counts of $3,000/mm^3$ ($3 \times 10^9/L$) or less do not seem to have an increased incidence of infection. A clinical guide is to continue carbamazepine therapy unless the WBC count drops to less than $2,500/mm^3$ ($2.5 \times 10^9/L$) and the absolute neutrophil count drops to less than $1,000/mm^3$ ($1 \times 10^9/L$).[70]

Drug Interactions Because of concentration-dependent efficacy and side effects, drug interactions with carbamazepine often are very significant. Drugs that inhibit CYP3A4 potentially may increase carbamazepine serum concentrations. Carbamazepine can induce the metabolism of other drugs.

Dosing and Administration The variable contributions of the 10,11-epoxide metabolite and free-carbamazepine concentrations have restricted a precise definition of the therapeutic range.

Loading doses of carbamazepine are indicated only for critically ill patients. During dosage titration, it must be remembered that carbamazepine clearance increases with time. Doses may be started at one-fourth to one-third the anticipated maintenance dose and increased every 2 to 3 weeks. Because of the auto- and heteroinduction of carbamazepine metabolism, it is necessary to administer the drug two to four times per day. Carbamazepine tablets should not be stored in places where they would be exposed to high heat and high humidity.[70]

Advantages Carbamazepine has been well studied. Oral solid and liquid dosage forms are available. The oral solid dosage form is available as an immediate-release tablet, as a sustained-release capsule, and a controlled-release tablet. The sustained- and controlled-release dosage forms allow for twice-daily dosing to reduce the peak-to-trough fluctuations. Compared with other first-generation AEDs, carbamazepine causes minimal cognitive impairment.

Disadvantages Carbamazepine has an active metabolite that can contribute to efficacy and toxicity. Other drugs can alter the concentration of this metabolite without changing the concentration of the parent carbamazepine. It induces its own metabolism, which complicates dosage titration. It also induces the metabolism of other medications, and other drugs may interact with it and/or its active metabolite. There is no parenteral formulation. There are clinically meaningful CNS side effects including sedation and nausea. One prospective study, however, found fewer side effects with the sustained-release formulation compared to the immediate-release formulation.[71] When ingested during the first trimester of pregnancy, carbamazepine has been associated with a 1% risk of spina bifida. Chronic carbamazepine use has also been associated with decreases in bone mineral density and 25-hydroxy(OH) vitamin D. The generic formulations of immediate-release tablets have been associated with breakthrough seizures when brands have been switched.

Place in Therapy Carbamazepine is considered a first-line therapy for patients with newly diagnosed partial seizures and for patients with primary generalized convulsive seizures who are not in an emergent situation.

Ethosuximide

Pharmacology and Mechanism of Action Ethosuximide is believed to exert its primary action through inhibition of T-type calcium channels.[69]

Pharmacokinetics Metabolism occurs in the liver by hydroxylation, and the metabolites are believed to be inactive. There is some evidence of nonlinear pharmacokinetics at higher concentrations.

Adverse Effects The most frequently reported side effects are nausea and vomiting (up to 40%), which may be minimized by administration of smaller doses and more frequent dosing.[72]

Drug Interactions Because ethosuximide is not protein bound, displacement interactions do not occur. Valproic acid may inhibit the metabolism of ethosuximide, but only if the metabolism of ethosuximide is near saturation.[73]

Dosing and Administration A loading dose is not required. Titration over 1 to 2 weeks to maintenance doses of 20 mg/kg per day usually results in therapeutic concentrations. Data suggest that patients can be managed successfully on once-a-day therapy; however, gastrointestinal (GI) distress appears to be dose related, and the total daily dose is usually divided into two equal doses.[70]

Advantages This drug is very effective in the treatment of absence seizures. It is generally well tolerated and has few pharmacokinetic interactions.

Disadvantages Ethosuximide has a very narrow spectrum of activity.

Place in Therapy Ethosuximide is still a first-line treatment for absence seizures.

Felbamate

Pharmacology and Mechanism of Action At therapeutic doses, felbamate appears to act by blocking N-methyl-D-aspartate (NMDA) synaptic responses and by modulating GABA$_A$ receptors. At higher doses it may modulate sodium channels and inhibit high-voltage activated calcium channels.[69]

Pharmacokinetics Felbamate is rapidly and well absorbed. The absorption is unaffected by food or antacids. Approximately 40% to 50% of a dose of felbamate is metabolized by hydroxylation and conjugation pathways in the liver, and the remainder is excreted unchanged in the urine. It displays linear pharmacokinetics.[74]

Adverse Effects The most frequently reported side effects prior to marketing were anorexia, weight loss, insomnia, nausea, and headache (sometimes severe). Anorexia and weight loss may be especially problematic in children and in patients with diminished caloric intake. After marketing, felbamate was found to be associated with aplastic anemia and acute liver failure. The onset was between 68 and 354 days of therapy. The approximate rate of occurrence of aplastic anemia is 1 in 3,000 and of hepatitis is 1 in 10,000. Data suggest a possible increased risk for aplastic anemia in patients, especially women, with a history of cytopenia, AED allergy or significant toxicity, viral infection, and/or immunologic problems.[24,25,75]

Drug Interactions Felbamate can induce or inhibit the metabolism of the older AEDs. Interactions between warfarin and felbamate have also been reported.[74]

Dosing and Administration The initial starting dose of felbamate is increased at 2-week intervals.

Advantages Felbamate has a broad spectrum of activity and a unique mechanism of action. It is approved for treating atonic seizures in patients with the Lennox—Gastaut syndrome and is also effective in treating patients with partial seizures.

Disadvantages The use of felbamate is limited by the association with aplastic anemia and hepatotoxicity, as well as multiple drug interactions.

Place in Therapy It should be reserved for patients not responding to other AEDs.

Gabapentin

Pharmacology and Mechanism of Action Gabapentin was designed to be a GABA agonist but does not react at the GABA receptor, alter GABA uptake, or interfere with GABA transaminase. Gabapentin appears to bind to an amino acid carrier protein and to act at a unique receptor. It inhibits high-voltage activated calcium channels.[69] It elevates human brain GABA levels, possibly via alterations in GABA synthesis or reversal of the neuronal GABA transporter, resulting in nonvesicular release of GABA.[76]

Pharmacokinetics Gabapentin is a substrate of the L-amino acid carrier protein in the gut (system L) and in the CNS.[77] This carrier protein transports the drug across the gut membrane by an active process. The binding of gabapentin to this system is saturable, and gabapentin therefore displays dose-dependent bioavailability that appears to vary considerably between individuals.[78] Food, including protein-rich meals, does not appear to interfere with gabapentin oral absorption.[79] Concentrations in human CSF are 5% to 35% of plasma levels, and tissue concentrations are approximately 80% of plasma levels.

Because gabapentin is eliminated exclusively by the kidneys, dosage adjustments are necessary in patients with significantly impaired renal function.[80]

Adverse Effects Fatigue, somnolence, dizziness, and ataxia are the most frequently reported side effects. Aggressive behavior has been reported in children.[81] The CNS effects of gabapentin are generally less than those of traditional AEDs. A withdrawal reaction characterized by anxiety, insomnia, nausea, sweating, and increased pain has also been reported with abrupt discontinuation in patients taking it for pain.

Drug Interactions Gabapentin does not induce or inhibit liver enzymes; therefore, drug interactions are not likely to occur. There is a 10% reduction in the clearance of gabapentin in patients taking cimetidine and a 20% reduction in the bioavailability if aluminum antacids are taken simultaneously with gabapentin. These interactions are unlikely to be clinically significant.

Dosing and Administration Typical starting doses of gabapentin are 300 mg at bedtime on the first day, increasing to 900 mg/day over 3 days. Faster titration rates (e.g., starting at 300–900 mg 3 times daily) have been well tolerated.[82] Data suggest gabapentin should be given at least 4 times a day when the total daily dose is 3,600 mg or greater.[73] It does not appear to be absorbed rectally. Patients with end-stage renal disease maintained on hemodialysis should receive an initial 300- to 400-mg dose with 200 to 300 mg gabapentin given after every 4 hours of hemodialysis.[80]

Advantages Gabapentin has multiple mechanisms of action and is mechanistically different from first-generation AEDs. It is not metabolized and is excreted unchanged by the kidney. It has a broad therapeutic index with minimal CNS adverse effects and few drug interactions. Doses can be escalated rapidly.

Disadvantages Gabapentin is absorbed by an active process that saturates at higher doses. This may require more frequent daily dosing for patients who need doses greater than 3,600 mg/day. Doses exceeding the 3,600 mg/day maximum listed in the package insert may be required in some patients to achieve seizure remission. There is no parenteral formulation.

Place in Therapy Gabapentin is a second-line agent for patients with partial seizures who have failed initial treatment. In addition, although monotherapy has no proven efficacy in previously diagnosed refractory patients, it may have a role in patients with less severe seizure disorders, such as new-onset partial epilepsy, particularly in the elderly. Gabapentin also has been shown to be useful for chronic pain and other nonepileptic conditions.

Lacosamide

Pharmacology and Mechanism of Action Lacosamide is a functionalized amino acid with unknown mechanism of action, but two mechanisms are suggested.[33] It selectively enhances slow inactivation of voltage-gated sodium channels, resulting in stabilization of hyperexcitable neuronal membranes and inhibition of repetitive neuronal firings. In addition, it binds to collapsin response mediator protein (CRMP-2), a phosphoprotein mainly expressed in the CNS, and it is involved in neuronal differentiation and control of axonal outgrowth. The role of CRMP-2 binding in seizure control is unknown.

Pharmacokinetics Lacosamide is rapidly and almost completely absorbed after oral administration, and food does not affect its bioavailability. There is a linear relationship between daily doses and serum concentrations up to 800 mg/day. No dosage adjustment is necessary in children or the elderly. Moderate hepatic and renal impairment have both been shown to increase systemic drug exposure up to approximately 40%.[33]

Adverse Effects The most frequent side effects of lacosamide are dose related, including dizziness, nausea, diplopia, abnormal coordination, ataxia, vomiting, and nystagmus. The drug can also cause a small increase in median PR interval (5–9 msec) on the ECG.

Drug Interactions The blood level of lacosamide is decreased by approximately 15% to 20% by enzyme-inducing AEDs.[33] It is a substrate of CYP2C19; however, there are no known drug interactions between lacosamide and drugs metabolized by CYP2C19. The drug does not appear to affect the serum concentration of OCs containing ethinyl estradiol and levonorgesterol.[33]

Dosing and Administration The starting dose is 100 mg/day in two divided doses, with dose increase by 100 mg/day every week until a daily dose of 200 to 400 mg has been reached. Studies have shown that a dose of 600 mg daily may be efficacious for some patients, but at the expense of more CNS side effects.

Advantages There is an intravenous form of lacosamide available for short-term replacement that appears to be safe, well tolerated, and easy to administer. It does not affect the serum level of other AEDs, and its serum level is minimally affected by enzyme-inducing AEDs. It has novel mechanism(s) of action.

Disadvantages Lacosamide is a controlled substance class V.

Place in Therapy It is a potent second-line agent that should be considered in those patients who have failed first-line AEDs.

Lamotrigine

Pharmacology and Mechanism of Action A primary mechanism of action for lamotrigine appears to be inhibition of voltage-dependent sodium channels; however, it also inhibits high voltage-activated calcium channels and attenuates release of glutamate and to a lesser extent, GABA and dopamine.[69]

Pharmacokinetics Lamotrigine is completely and rapidly absorbed, with a bioavailability of 98%. Food does not significantly affect absorption. It is also absorbed following rectal administration, but the bioavailability is approximately 50% of that of oral dosage forms. Lamotrigine clearance is higher in children and lower in the elderly compared with young adults. There are only modest differences in the pharmacokinetics of lamotrigine in the elderly versus younger subjects. Hepatic disease, depending on severity, can influence lamotrigine pharmacokinetics. Approximately 17% of a lamotrigine dose can be removed by hemodialysis, with the half-life being reduced to approximately 13 hours. For patients on dialysis, the half-life is much more prolonged between dialyses (57.4 hours).[84] The half-life is prolonged in patients with renal failure.

Adverse Effects The most frequently reported side effects of lamotrigine include diplopia, drowsiness, ataxia, and headache.[85] Adverse effects are more common when lamotrigine is given in combination with other AEDs (e.g., diplopia when given concomitantly with carbamazepine or tremor with valproic acid) compared with monotherapy, and they can be pharmacodynamic in nature. Lamotrigine can cause rash, which usually appears in the first 3 to 4 weeks of therapy. Patients who have developed a rash with another AED are more likely to develop a rash with lamotrigine.[86] The rash typically is generalized, erythematous, and morbilliform. However, a Stevens—Johnson reaction also has been reported. Some rashes, especially those which develop early, can necessitate the withdrawal of lamotrigine.[87] Risk factors for the emergence of more serious rashes appear to be concomitant use of valproic acid and situations where high initial doses or rapid dosage escalation is used. Data from several European monotherapy trials suggest that when dosed appropriately, the incidence of rash from lamotrigine is similar to that of older agents such as carbamazepine and phenytoin. The incidence is higher in children than in adults.

Drug Interactions Lamotrigine does not inhibit liver enzymes and has a low potential for pharmacokinetic interactions with other drugs. It has been found to decrease the bioavailability of the progesterone component (levonorgestrel) of a combination OC by 19%. The clinical relevance of this interaction has not been determined.[88]

Concomitant treatment with OCs can lead to a reduction in the serum concentrations of lamotrigine because of an induction of lamotrigine glucuronidation by ethinyl estradiol.[89] In addition lamotrigine serum levels can significantly increase during the week off OC treatment in some patients.[89]

Valproic acid substantially inhibits the metabolism of lamotrigine, with maximal inhibition occurring at valproic acid doses and serum concentrations of 500 mg/day and 40 to 50 mcg/mL (280–350 μmol/L), respectively.[85] A pharmacodynamic interaction can occur with concurrent carbamazepine therapy, causing an increase in CNS side effects.

Dosing and Administration In patients who are taking enzyme-inducing drugs, lamotrigine can be started more rapidly than in patients receiving valproic acid. The maintenance doses are also different. Managing dosing is critical owing to the relationship between rash, concomitant valproic acid treatment, and the dose escalation rate. Removal of inducers from a lamotrigine regimen may necessitate decreases in lamotrigine dose, whereas removal of valproic acid can necessitate an increase in the lamotrigine dose. A dispersible and oral disintegrating tablet are available for patients who cannot swallow an oral solid tablet.

Advantages Lamotrigine is potentially a broad-spectrum AED, having efficacy in partial seizures and several types of generalized seizures. Pediatric dosage forms are available as a chewable dispersable tablet and an oral disintegrating tablet. It neither induces nor inhibits the metabolism of other AEDs. Lamotrigine has linear pharmacokinetics and is not highly protein bound. It is generally well tolerated in both children and elderly patients and does not cause weight gain.

Disadvantages Lamotrigine is associated with rash, especially in patients who start at a high dose, have rapid dose escalation, and/or are taking concurrent valproic acid. Therefore, the initial doses must be low (especially if the patient is on valproic acid) and escalated slowly to maximize safety. There is no parenteral dosage form.

Place in Therapy Lamotrigine is useful as both adjunctive treatment in patients with partial seizures and as monotherapy. Lamotrigine monotherapy appears to have comparable effectiveness with more traditional AEDs such as carbamazepine and phenytoin. In addition, it may be a useful alternative for primary generalized seizure types such as absence and as adjunctive therapy for primary GTC seizures, the latter of which is an approved indication.

Levetiracetam

Pharmacology and Mechanism of Action Levetiracetam is chemically unrelated to other AEDs. Although the mechanism of action of levetiracetam has yet to be delineated, it is known that this drug is not active in the classic models used to test AEDs. The drug binds in the brain to the synaptic vesicle protein SV2A, which is believed to be important in its activity.[90] This agent may have a unique mechanism of action. Limited animal data suggest that levetiracetam may have *antiepileptogenic effects*, meaning that it may prevent the development of epilepsy under certain circumstances, however confirmation of this research is needed.[91]

Pharmacokinetics Absorption of levetiracetam is rapid and complete following oral administration, and it is not significantly affected by food or enteral nutrition formulas.[92] Renal elimination of unchanged parent drug accounts for the majority of clearance (66%), with the remainder being metabolized via nonhepatic enzymatic hydrolysis to inactive metabolites.[93] This pathway involves neither the CYP450 or UGT isozyme systems. Because it is eliminated renally, clinicians should anticipate age-related reductions in clearance in elderly patients. Conversely, levetiracetam clearance appears to be approximately 40% higher in children than in adults. In addition, patients with severe liver cirrhosis should initially receive one-half the recommended starting dose because of a 57% decrease in clearance.[94] Levetiracetam is excreted into breast milk in potentially clinically important amounts.[95] Data are sparse regarding serum concentration—effect relationships, so the role of therapeutic drug level monitoring remains unclear.

Adverse Effects Adverse effects appear to be modest, with sedation, fatigue, and coordination difficulties being the most common CNS effects. In children and young adults, agitation, irritability or somnolence/lethargy are the most frequently reported CNS side effects.[96] The mechanism underlying these effects is unknown. Formal studies evaluating the cognitive effects of this medication have not yet been conducted.

Drug Interactions Levetiracetam neither inhibits nor induces the CYP450, UGT, or epoxide hydrolase enzyme systems, and in vitro data predict a low potential for pharmacokinetic interactions. It does not appear to interact with other AEDs, warfarin, digoxin, or oral contraceptive drugs.[97,98]

Dosing and Administration Levetiracetam is available orally and parenterally, the latter for maintenance dosing only. The intravenous (IV) product has not been tested for intramuscular (IM) use, and therefore, should not be administered IM. Typically the initial dose is given twice daily, with dosage increments every 2 weeks. To minimize CNS side effects, dosing may be initiated at one-half this rate. The IV formulation should be given at the same frequency and dose as the oral product. Although not FDA approved, the oral dose of levetiracetam has been titrated up rapidly to 3,000 mg in 3 days in some intractable seizure patients with improvement seen after day 2.[99]

Advantages Levetiracetam is felt to have a novel, although unknown, mechanism of action. It has linear pharmacokinetics and is not metabolized by the cytochrome P450 system. No significant drug interactions, including with OCs, have been reported. Initial doses may be effective. The drug appears to be well tolerated, with transient sedation being the most troublesome adverse effect.

Disadvantages Dose adjustments are needed for patients with decreased renal function, and slower dose escalation may be needed to avoid CNS adverse effects. Behavioral problems can limit therapy in some patients.

Place in Therapy Levetiracetam is indicated for patients with partial seizures who have failed initial therapy. Its role as monotherapy for partial seizures remains to be clarified. It is approved for adjunctive treatment of myoclonic seizures in patients with JME and as adjunctive treatment of primarily generalized seizures in patients with idiopathic generalized epilepsy.

Oxcarbazepine

Pharmacology and Mechanism of Action Oxcarbazepine, which is structurally related to carbamazepine, is a prodrug that is rapidly converted to the active 10-monohydoxy derivative (MHD). The mechanism of action of oxcarbazepine is similar to that of carbamazepine. Oxcarbazepine and MHD block voltage-sensitive sodium channels, modulate the voltage-activated calcium currents, and increase potassium conductance. Interestingly, however, oxcarbazepine can display differing affinities for both sodium channels and Ca^{2+} channels compared with older drugs such as carbamazepine.[100] Whereas carbamazepine may modulate L-type Ca^{2+} channels, oxcarbazepine appears to modulate N- and P-type Ca^{2+} channels.[101] Whether these differences lead to differing patterns of clinical effectiveness is uncertain. It has no significant interactions with neurotransmitters or modulation of receptor sites.

Pharmacokinetics Oxcarbazepine is absorbed completely, and MHD is inactivated by glucuronide conjugation and eliminated by the kidneys.[102] Oxcarbazepine and its active metabolite do not undergo autoinduction. The relationship between dose and serum concentration is linear. Children 2 to 6 years of age need larger doses to achieve the same serum concentration, suggesting a more rapid clearance. The maximal drug concentration (C_{max}) and bio-availability of MHD in elderly volunteers were higher than in younger volunteers, and the elimination rate was slower, possibly reflecting decreased renal elimination. Patients with significant renal impairment may require a dosage reduction.

Adverse Effects Oxcarbazepine was marketed in more than 50 countries prior to approval in the United States. In U.S. clinical trials the most frequently reported adverse events were dizziness, nausea, headache, diarrhea, vomiting, upper respiratory tract infections, constipation, dyspepsia, ataxia, and nervousness. In comparative trials, oxcarbazepine generally caused fewer side effects than phenytoin, valproic acid, or carbamazepine. Dizziness may be more common in elderly patients than in young adults. CNS adverse effects appear to be far more common at doses greater than 1,200 mg/day. Hyponatremia, defined as a plasma sodium concentration of less than 125 mmol/L, has been reported in up to 25% of patients taking oxcarbazepine and occurs more often in elderly patients. Clinicians should be particularly watchful in patients receiving concomitant sodium-depleting drugs such as diuretics. Hyponatremia appears to occur less frequently in children. Clinicians should consider monitoring serum sodium levels following the initiation of oxcarbazepine, and they should instruct patients regarding the symptoms of hyponatremia. Approximately 25% to 30% of patients who develop a rash with carbamazepine will experience a similar reaction with oxcarbazepine.[24,25,75] The tolerability of oxcarbazepine has not been compared with that of extended-release formulations of carbamazepine that have lower peaks and potentially fewer side effects than immediate-release carbamazepine formulations.

Drug Interactions Oxcarbazepine decreases the bioavailability of ethinyl estradiol and levonorgestrel.[103] Women concurrently taking OCs should be counseled about the potential for contraceptive failure. Unlike carbamazepine, there are no interactions between cimetidine, erythromycin, or warfarin and oxcarbazepine. The administration of oxcarbazepine in doses greater than 1,200 mg with phenytoin has resulted in a 40% increase in the concentration of phenytoin, consistent with inhibition of CYP450 2C19. Oxcarbazepine treatment may modestly reduce lamotrigine serum concentrations, suggesting induction of UGT isozymes.[104]

The replacement of carbamazepine with oxcarbazepine may result in a drug interaction because an enzyme-inducing drug is being removed.

Dosing and Administration Doses and titration schedules differ regarding whether the drug is used for mono- or adjunctive therapy in adults vs children. Although not FDA approved, doses up to 60 mg/kg/day have been used in infants and children younger than 4 years of age to successfully control partial-onset seizures.[105] In patients being converted from carbamazepine, the typical maintenance dose of oxcarbazepine is 1.5 times the carbamazepine dose or less, if patients are on large doses of carbamazepine, due to autoinduction of carbamazepine but not oxcarbazepine.

Advantages The efficacy of oxcarbazepine is comparable with that of carbamazepine, phenytoin, and valproic acid. It may be better tolerated than phenytoin as monotherapy and therefore, less likely to be discontinued.[106] There is broad international experience with this drug.

Disadvantages About 30% of patients who have experienced a rash with carbamazepine have a cross-reaction with oxcarbazepine. There are more reports of hyponatremia with oxcarbazepine, especially in patients at risk. Replacing carbamazepine with oxcarbazepine can result in interactions owing to the removal of an enzyme inducer. Enzyme-inducing drugs can increase the clearance of MHD.

Place in Therapy Oxcarbazepine is indicated for use as monotherapy or adjunctive therapy in the treatment of partial seizures in adults and children as young as 4 years of age. It is also a potential first-line drug for patients with primary generalized convulsive seizures. Oxcarbazepine may also be effective in patients not demonstrating a response to carbamazepine.

Phenobarbital

Pharmacology and Mechanism of Action Phenobarbital may elevate seizure threshold by interacting with GABA receptors to facilitate intrinsic chloride channel function, by blocking high voltage-activated calcium channels, and by blocking α-amino-3-hydroxy-5-methylisoxazole-4-propionic acid (AMPA) and kainate receptors.[69]

Pharmacokinetics Phenobarbital is absorbed rapidly and completely regardless of whether it is given orally, intramuscularly, or rectally.[73] It penetrates the brain at a rate comparable with that of phenytoin, and peak concentrations are achieved 3 to 20 minutes after an IV dose.

Drugs affecting liver enzymes can alter phenobarbital metabolism, but phenobarbital clearance is not affected by liver blood flow. The elimination of phenobarbital is linear. Because tubular reabsorption of phenobarbital is pH dependent, the amount excreted renally can be increased by giving diuretics and urinary alkalinizers.[73] Clearance decreases in the elderly.[107]

Adverse Effects CNS side effects are the primary factors limiting the use of phenobarbital. Tolerance usually develops to initial complaints of fatigue, drowsiness, sedation, and depression. In children, paradoxically, the primary side effect is hyperactivity. It may also cause porphyria and rash, including serious rashes such as Stevens—Johnson syndrome.[108]

Drug Interactions Phenobarbital is a potent enzyme inducer and can increase the elimination of any drug metabolized by CYP450- or UGT-mediated metabolism. Cimetidine and chloramphenicol inhibit phenobarbital metabolism, necessitating a decrease in dose. Ethanol increases the metabolism of phenobarbital.[73]

Dosing and Administration In nonacute situations, phenobarbital should be started in low doses and titrated upward. The dose-concentration relationship is linear. Because the half-life of phenobarbital is long, doses can be given once daily, and bedtime dosing may minimize CNS depression.

Advantages Phenobarbital has linear and predictable pharmacokinetics. Multiple dosage forms (e.g., oral solid, oral liquid, IM, and IV) are available, and it is the most inexpensive AED.

Disadvantages Phenobarbital has significant side effects, including delayed intellectual development and hyperactivity in children and significant cognitive impairment in adults. It is an enzyme inducer and interacts with many other drugs metabolized by the cytochrome P450 system. Phenobarbital has a very long half-life, and dosage adjustments should not be made more often than every 2 to 3 weeks. The parenteral product contains 67% to 75% propylene glycol and 10% alcohol, which can result in significant respiratory depression and hypotension if infused too rapidly.

Place in Therapy Phenobarbital is the drug of choice for neonatal seizures but in other situations is reserved for patients who have failed therapy with other AEDs. It may be useful given IV in refractory status epilepticus.

Phenytoin

Pharmacology and Mechanism of Action The primary mechanism of action of phenytoin is believed to be its ability to inhibit voltage-dependent sodium channels.[69]

Pharmacokinetics The pharmacokinetics of phenytoin are complex. For a more in-depth understanding, the reader is referred to a more extensive review.[109] The oral absorption of phenytoin is almost complete. Dissolution is the rate-limiting step, and absorption may be saturable at higher doses, such as those used for oral loading. Absorption following IM administration of phenytoin is erratic and delayed, and IM injections are painful; however, IM absorption following fosphenytoin is rapid and well tolerated.

Phenytoin enters the brain rapidly and is redistributed to other body tissues, including breast milk and the placenta. Phenytoin competes for albumin sites with other highly protein-bound drugs. It is essential to know the patient's serum albumin level in interpreting the serum concentrations of phenytoin.[110] Patients with significant renal dysfunction will have altered phenytoin protein binding. Obesity increases the volume of distribution.

Phenytoin is metabolized in the liver by parahydroxylation. The major isoforms responsible for the metabolism of phenytoin are CYP2C9 and CYP2C19; the former displays polymorphism, which may affect the response to phenytoin.[69] Phenytoin displays Michaelis—Menton pharmacokinetics, and the metabolism of phenytoin saturates at doses used clinically. The clinical importance of this is that a small change in dose can result in a disproportionally large increase in serum concentrations, potentially leading to toxicity. In some patients the metabolism of phenytoin can saturate even at low serum concentrations within the therapeutic range. The long-held belief that the metabolism of phenytoin decreases with age in adults has recently been challenged.[111]

Adverse Effects When phenytoin is initiated, the CNS depressant effects include lethargy, fatigue, incoordination, blurred vision, higher cortical dysfunction, and drowsiness. These effects usually are transient and can be minimized by slow dosage titration. At very high concentrations of greater than 50 mcg/mL (200 μmol/L), phenytoin can exacerbate seizures.

It is unclear whether the chronic side effects of phenytoin are concentration or duration dependent. One of the more common chronic side effects is gingival hyperplasia. Good oral hygiene can minimize gingival hyperplasia and should be encouraged. Other chronic effects include vitamin D deficiency, osteomalacia, carbohydrate intolerance, immunologic disturbances, hypothyroidism, and peripheral neuropathy. Phenytoin is associated with rare hypersensitivity or idiosyncratic reactions resulting in rashes, Stevens—Johnson syndrome, pseudolymphoma, bone marrow suppression, lupus-like reactions, and hepatitis.[112]

Drug Interactions Phenytoin is associated with numerous drug interactions involving altered absorption, metabolism, and protein binding that can enhance or reduce its effects. It is an inducer of both CYP450 and UGT isozymes. The absorption of phenytoin can be increased or decreased with the administration of food depending on the composition of the meal. The bioavailability of phenytoin suspension can be decreased in patients receiving continuous enteral nutrient tube feedings. However, a single-dose study of simultaneous administration of enteral feeding found no difference in phenytoin bioavailability, suggesting that the mechanism was something other than physical contact.[109]

Phenytoin decreases folic acid absorption. Replacement of folic acid can reduce phenytoin concentration and result in loss of efficacy.[109]

Dosing and Administration Four oral dosage forms are available, and changing dosage forms can lead to changes in phenytoin serum concentrations. Whether or not a dosage form uses the parent drug or salt form should be considered when changing from one dosage form to another. One hundred milligrams of phenytoin acid is equal to 92 mg of phenytoin sodium. Phenytoin capsules are designated as immediate-release or extended-release. Only the extended-release capsules should be used in once-daily dosing.

Particle size rather than formulation may determine the rate of absorption.

If oral administration is not feasible, IV administration of phenytoin is preferred, as IM administration can cause tissue necrosis. Fosphenytoin is a prodrug for phenytoin and is available as a parenteral dosage form. Fosphenytoin is ordered in phenytoin equivalents (PE), the actual dose of phenytoin acid desired. It is very water-soluble and is converted rapidly to phenytoin systemically. Fosphenytoin can be given rapidly intravenously and intramuscularly with reliable absorption and minimal pain. It is significantly better tolerated than phenytoin.

Because of saturable absorption, an oral loading dose, such as 20 mg/kg, should be divided into four equal doses and given at 6-hour intervals. Subsequent dosage adjustments should be done cautiously owing to its nonlinear elimination. One author has suggested that if the serum concentration is less than 7 mcg/mL (28 μmol/L), the daily dose should be increased by 100 mg; if the serum concentration is between 7 and 12 mcg/mL (28 and 48 μmol/L), the daily dose can be increased by 50 mg; and if the serum concentration is greater than 12 mcg/mL (48 μmol/L), the daily dose can be increased by 30 mg or less. These increases are reported to result in less than 10% of patients achieving a phenytoin serum concentration greater than 25 mcg/mL (99 μmol/L).[113]

Advantages After more than 65 years, its risk-to-benefit ratio is well established. It is available in oral solid, oral liquid, extended-release oral solid, and parenteral (phenytoin and fosphenytoin) dosage forms, allowing flexibility in dosing and use in emergent situations. In some patients, the extended-release dosage form can be given once a day with good seizure control.

Disadvantages Phenytoin displays Michaels—Menton pharmacokinetics, meaning that the metabolism saturates at doses given clinically thus complicating dose titration. Also, phenytoin is an inducer of cytochrome P450 isozymes, is metabolized by cytochrome P450 enzymes, and is highly protein bound. Therefore, many drug interactions are associated with coadministration of this agent. It also has multiple significant adverse effects.

Place in Therapy Phenytoin has long been a first-line AED for primary generalized convulsive and partial seizures. However, its place in therapy may be reevaluated as more experience is gained with newer AEDs.

Pregabalin

Pharmacology and Mechanism of Action Pregabalin's mechanism of action is unknown, however, it is proposed that its binding to the subunit of the voltage-gated calcium channel may be responsible for a large part of its activity. This binding results in a decrease in the release of several excitatory neurotransmitters including glutamate, noradrenaline, substance P, and calcitonin gene-related peptide.[114]

Pharmacokinetics Pregabalin is a substrate of the L-amino acid carrier protein in the CNS. It does not display dose-dependent bioavailability. Food decreases the rate of absorption but not the bioavailability of the drug.[115]

Pregabalin is eliminated primarily by renal excretion as an unchanged drug, and therefore dosage adjustment is required in patients with significantly impaired renal function. In anuric patients, 50% of the dose is removed by 4 hours of hemodialysis.[115]

Adverse Effects Dizziness, somnolence, ataxia, blurred vision, and weight gain are the most frequently reported side effects. It is unknown if pregabalin causes aggressive behavior in children. A withdrawal reaction characterized by anxiety, nervousness, and irritability has been noted in patients being treated for generalized anxiety upon abrupt discontinuation of the drug.[116]

Drug Interactions Because pregabalin is predominantly excreted unchanged in the urine and undergoes negligible metabolism, drug interactions are unlikely.

Dosing and Administration Starting doses of pregabalin are divided into twice or thrice daily intervals. The manufacturer recommends that patients with end-stage renal disease maintained on hemodialysis receive a 25 to 75 mg daily dose with 25 to 75 mg given after every 4 hours of hemodialysis.

Advantages Pregabalin is somewhat more potent than gabapentin without the dose-limited GI absorption properties. It has minimal CNS side effects and no drug interactions.

Disadvantages It is a controlled substance class V. Like gabapentin it can cause weight gain and peripheral edema, especially as the dose is increased. There is no parenteral formulation available.

Place in Therapy Pregabalin is a second-line agent for patients with partial seizures who have failed initial treatment. It is also useful for chronic neuropathic pain and generalized anxiety disorder.[116]

Rufinamide

Pharmacology and Mechanism of Action Rufinamide is a triazole derivative structurally unlike any other AED. It suppresses neuronal hyperexcitability through prolongation of the inactivation phase of voltage-gated sodium channels.[117]

Pharmacokinetics Oral absorption is relatively slow with a t_{max} of 4 to 6 hours. At low doses (600 mg), the drug is relatively well absorbed (85%) when taken with food; however, the percentage of drug absorbed decreases with higher doses. Twice-daily dosing is recommended due to the slow absorption properties and the drug's short half-life (6–10 hours).[34] It is extensively metabolized with no active metabolites, with primary biotransformation by carboxylesterases. Although clinical data indicate that children and adults have similar pharmacokinetics, population pharmacokinetic modeling suggests that in the absence of interacting co-medication the drug may have a higher clearance in children.[117]

Adverse Effects The most common adverse effects include headache, dizziness, fatigue, somnolence, and nausea. These effects are dose dependent. Rufinamide may increase the incidence of convulsions in some patients, and may precipitate SE. Multiorgan hypersensitivity has occurred within 4 weeks of starting treatment in patients younger than 12 years of age.

Drug Interactions Rufinamide is a weak inhibitor of CYP2E1 and a weak inducer of CYP3A4; the later effect may be responsible for modestly lower levels of carbamazepine and triazolam when given concomitantly with rufinamide.[37] It may decrease the area under the curve of combination OCs containing ethinyl estradiol and norethindrone; however, it is not known if this is due to induction of CYP3A4 or uridine disphosphate glucuronosyl transferase (UDP-GT), or both. Rufinamide is responsible for a modest increase in the clearance of lamotrigine, phenobarbital, and phenytoin, and the effect is greater in children than adults. Carbamazepine, phenytoin, primidone, and phenobarbital significantly increase the clearance of rufinamide; however, it is believed this interaction is not entirely due to CYP450 enzyme induction. Valproic acid significantly decreases the clearance of rufinamide and elevates serum levels of rufinamide by 70%.

Dosing and Administration The initial dose of rufinamide is 400 to 800 mg/day given in divided doses with an increase in dose every other day until a maximum dose of 45 mg/kg/day or 3,200 mg/day (which ever is less) is obtained.

Advantages The drug is effective for seizures associated with Lennox—Gastaut syndrome without causing cognitive and psychiatric adverse effects. The dose can be rapidly escalated.

Disadvantages Drug interactions are common with rufinamide, and patients with Lennox—Gastaut are usually on multiple medications. It displays decreased absorption at higher doses and when taken on an empty stomach. The drug has caused convulsions and SE in some patients.

Place in Therapy As an adjunctive agent in controlling seizures in Lennox—Gastaut syndrome after patients have failed valproic acid, topiramate, and lamotrigine.

Tiagabine

Pharmacology and Mechanism of Action Tiagabine is a potent and specific inhibitor of GABA uptake into neuronal elements, thus, enhancing the action of GABA by decreasing its removal from the synaptic space.[118]

Pharmacokinetics Tiagabine is absorbed quickly and nearly completely after oral administration. There is a linear relationship between dose and serum concentrations. Children eliminate tiagabine slightly faster than adults. Hepatic impairment causes higher and more prolonged plasma concentrations of total and unbound drug. Renal dysfunction does not change its pharmacokinetics.[118] Tiagabine displays diurnal elimination, i.e., lower evening serum levels compared with morning levels.

Adverse Effects The most frequently reported adverse effects of tiagabine are dizziness, asthenia, nervousness, tremor, diarrhea, and depression. Adverse events usually are mild to moderate and transient, and most occur during dose titration.[119] CNS side effects can be diminished by taking tiagabine with food, thus slowing the absorption rate. It has increased the incidence of nonconvulsive SE in patients with chronic refractory partial epilepsy.[120] In addition, there are reports of SE or new onset seizures occurring in patients without a history of epilepsy.

Drug Interactions Food decreases the rate but not the extent of absorption. Tiagabine is displaced from protein by naproxen, salicylates, and valproate. However, tiagabine does not displace phenytoin, valproic acid, amitriptyline, tolbutamide, or warfarin.[118]

Dosing and Administration A clear dose-response has been demonstrated, and the minimal effective adult dose level is 30 mg/day. The initial dose is increased weekly.

Advantages Tiagabine has a known mechanism of action. It is the first drug marketed in the United States that acts only on GABA reuptake. It has linear pharmacokinetics and is not reported to interact with other drugs.

Disadvantages Initially high and rapid dosage escalation is associated with increased CNS side effects. Therefore, the drug must be started at a low dose and titrated gradually to response. Lower doses may be needed in patients with liver disease. Tiagabine is metabolized by CYP450 3A4 enzymes, and other drugs may alter its clearance. There is no parenteral formulation.

Place in Therapy Tiagabine is second-line therapy for patients with partial seizures who have failed initial therapy. It does not appear to have a role in primary generalized seizure types.

Topiramate

Pharmacology and Mechanism of Action Topiramate is a sulfamate-substituted monosaccharide with multiple modes of action involving voltage-dependent sodium channels, GABA-receptor subunits, high-voltage calcium channels, and kainate/AMPA subunits.[69] It also inhibits carbonic anhydrase, which likely is not a major mechanism of action.[69]

Pharmacokinetics Although generally considered to have linear absorption and elimination pharmacokinetics, a greater than proportional increase in both maximal peak concentration and area under the plasma concentration versus time curve has been observed and probably is explained by saturable binding to erythrocytes.[121] Approximately 50% of the dose is excreted renally unchanged; however, its metabolism is increased by approximately 50% when given with enzyme-inducing AEDs. Renal tubular reabsorption may be involved prominently in the renal handling of topiramate.[122]

Adverse Effects The main adverse events of topiramate are ataxia, impaired concentration, memory difficulties, attentional deficits, confusion, dizziness, fatigue, paresthesia, somnolence, and "thinking abnormally," which rarely has included psychosis. Most of these occurred during rapid titration and at higher doses.[123] Word-finding difficulties can be a problem with topiramate and can occur in a significant number of patients, especially patients with left posterior temporal lobe epilepsy or simple partial seizures.[124] Concomitant therapy with topiramate, valproic acid, or phenobarbital can cause cognitive dysfunction. Nephrolithiasis has occurred in 1.5% of patients receiving topiramate, which is 2 to 4 times the incidence in the general population. Patients should be encouraged to maintain adequate fluid intake in order to minimize this problem. Topiramate can cause metabolic acidosis at doses as low as 50 mg/day. Risk factors for this condition include renal disease, severe respiratory disorders, SE, diarrhea, surgery, and the ketogenic diet. Metabolic acidosis in part may explain the anorexia and weight loss seen with this drug.[75]

Drug Interactions Oral clearance of digoxin is slightly increased when topiramate is added. Topiramate coadministration can cause increased phenytoin serum concentrations in some patients. The variable response can be explained by the intersubject variability in the proportion of phenytoin clearance attributed to CYP2C19 metabolism and whether the patient is a homozygous or heterozygous carrier of the mutant allele responsible for the CYP2C9 and/or CYP2C19 "poor metabolizer" phenotype. Topiramate can modestly increase the oral clearance of valproic acid and increase formation of the 4-ene—valproic acid metabolite. However, the clinical significance of this interaction is unclear. Topiramate increases the clearance of ethinyl estradiol in a dose-dependant manner. Topiramate doses of less than 200 mg/day are unlikely to alter OC pharmacokinetics.[125]

Dosing and Administration Topiramate should be titrated slowly to avoid adverse events with dosage increments every 1 to 2 weeks. For patients on other AEDs, doses greater than 600 mg/day do not appear to lead to improved efficacy and can cause increased adverse effects; however, higher doses may prove beneficial to individual patients who tolerate them.[126]

Advantages Topiramate has multiple mechanisms of action and is a broad-spectrum AED. Elimination is primarily renal, but hepatic metabolism occurs, especially if given concomitantly with enzyme inducers. It has linear pharmacokinetics and few drug interactions.

Disadvantages With rapid dosage escalation, topiramate can compromise cognitive functioning, including impaired word finding and impair short-term memory. Therefore, initial doses should be low, and titration must be slow. Renal stones and weight loss have been associated with topiramate use. The dose should be decreased in patients with renal failure. There is no parenteral formulation.

Place in Therapy Topiramate is a first-line AED for partial seizures as an adjunct and/or monotherapy. It is also approved for the treatment of tonic-clonic seizures in primary generalized epilepsy.

Valproic Acid/Divalproex Sodium

Pharmacology and Mechanism of Action Alterations of the synthesis and degradation of GABA do not fully explain the antiseizure activity of valproic acid. Valproic acid may potentiate postsynaptic GABA responses, may have a direct membrane-stabilizing effect, and may affect potassium channels.[127]

Pharmacokinetics Valproic acid appears to be absorbed completely from available oral dosage forms when administered on an empty stomach.[127] However, the rate of absorption differs among preparations. Peak concentrations occur in 0.5 to 1 hour with the syrup, 1 to 3 hours with the capsule, and 2 to 6 hours with the enteric-coated tablet.[127] The extended-release formulation (Depakote-ER) is FDA approved for patients with migraine headache and epilepsy. The bioavailability of this formulation is approximately 15% less than that of enteric-coated divalproex sodium (Depakote).

Valproic acid is extensively bound to albumin, and this binding is saturable. Accordingly, the valproic acid free fraction will increase as the total serum concentration increases. Because of this saturable binding, measurement of unbound serum concentrations may be a better monitoring parameter than the total valproic acid serum concentration, especially at higher concentrations or in patients with hypoalbuminemia.[73]

The primary route of valproic acid metabolism is β-oxidation, although up to 40% of a dose may be excreted as the glucuronide. At least 10 metabolites of valproic acid have been identified. Some of these may have weak anticonvulsant activity, and at least one metabolite may be responsible for the hepatotoxicity reported. One of the lesser oxidative metabolites, 4-ene-VPA, causes hepatotoxicity in rats. The formation of this metabolite is increased when valproic acid is given with enzyme-inducing drugs.[127] Valproic acid displays diurnal elimination with lower evening serum levels occurring than morning levels. It crosses into the placenta and concentrations may be up to 5 times higher in cord serum blood than in the mother due to higher binding in the fetal compartment.[128]

Adverse Effects The most frequently reported side effects are gastrointestinal (up to 20%), including nausea, vomiting, anorexia, and weight gain. Pancreatitis is rare. GI complaints may be minimized, but not totally alleviated, with the enteric-coated formulation or by giving the drug with food. Alopecia and hair changes are temporary, and hair growth returns even with continued dosing. Weight gain can be significant for many patients and is associated with an increase in fasting insulin and leptin serum levels.[129] The increase in serum insulin is believed to be caused by the inhibition of metabolism of insulin by the liver.[130] This has led to the development of insulin resistance in obese male and female subjects.[127] Valproic acid causes minimal cognitive impairment.[127]

The most serious side effect reported with valproic acid is hepatotoxicity. Hyperammonemia is common (50%) but does not necessarily imply liver damage. Most liver failure deaths have occurred in patients who were younger than 2 years of age, had mental retardation, and received multiple AEDs. Hepatotoxicity occurred early in the course of therapy. Patients who complain of nausea, vomiting, lethargy, anorexia, and edema in the first 6 to 12 months of therapy should have liver function evaluated. Multiple AEDs can alter the metabolism of valproic acid, leading to increased formation of the potentially liver-toxic 4-ene-VPA. Valproic acid has been shown to alter carnitine metabolism, and it has been postulated that a deficiency of carnitine alters fatty acid oxidation that could lead to both liver toxicity and hyperammonemia.[131] However, valproic acid hepatotoxicity has occurred in a patient taking supplemental carnitine, and a prospective study demonstrated no effect on well-being when carnitine was added. Although carnitine can ameliorate hyperammonemia in part, it is expensive, and there are only limited data to support routine supplemental use in patients taking valproic acid.[132]

Thrombocytopenia and alterations in platelet aggregation occur in the patients receiving valproic acid, and these phenomena are related to serum concentration. These blood coagulopathies may occur more frequently in children than in adults.[133]

Drug Interactions Because it is highly protein bound, other highly protein-bound drugs (e.g., free fatty acids and aspirin) can displace valproic acid.

Valproic acid can inhibit specific CYP P450 isozymes, epoxide hydrolase, and UGT isozymes. The addition of valproic acid to phenobarbital results in a 30% to 50% decrease in phenobarbital clearance and significant toxicity if the dose of phenobarbital is not reduced. Data also suggest that combination OCs may increase the clearance of valproic acid and lower serum levels by 20%.[32] In addition, carbapenems, especially merepenem can lower valproic acid levels.[134]

Dosing and Administration Valproic acid in some patients may have a half-life long enough for once-daily dosing with enteric-coated divalproex, but more frequent dosing is the norm. Based on half-life data, twice-daily dosing is feasible with any valproic acid dosage form; however, children and patients taking enzyme inducers can require dosing 3 to 4 times daily.[73] The serum concentration—dose relationship is curvilinear (e.g., the concentration-dose ratio decreases with increasing dose) probably because of increasing free concentrations and a resulting increase in clearance.[73]

Valproic acid is available as a soft gelatin capsule, an enteric-coated tablet, a syrup, a "sprinkle capsule," an extended-release formulation designed for once-daily dosing, and an IV formulation for replacement of oral therapy or in situations where rapid loading is necessary.[127] This parenteral formulation must not be given intramuscularly because it can cause tissue necrosis. The sprinkle capsule, designed to be opened and mixed with food, has a slower rate of absorption, which results in fewer fluctuations in the peak-to-trough ratio. The syrup is absorbed more rapidly than any solid dosage form. The enteric-coated divalproex tablet is not sustained release. It must be metabolized in the gut to valproic acid. The enteric coating reduces GI distress. The enteric coating causes delayed absorption, although once the enteric coating dissolves, sodium divalproex has absorption, metabolism, and elimination rates similar to those of the gelatin capsule. If a patient is switched from Depakote to Depakote-ER, the dose should be increased by 14% to 20%. Depakote-ER may be given once daily.

Advantages Valproic acid is available in multiple dosage formulations. The IV formulation is especially well tolerated. It has a wide therapeutic index and is considered a broad-spectrum AED. It is also used in other neurologic or psychiatric disorders (e.g., migraine headache, bipolar disorder).

Disadvantages Some patients report significant weight gain with valproic acid, which may limit compliance. It has other side effects, such as alopecia, tremor, pancreatitis, PCOS, and thrombocytopenia. It has been associated with hepatic necrosis in young children. As an enzyme inhibitor, it is involved in multiple drug—drug interactions.

Place in Therapy Valproic acid is first-line therapy for primary generalized seizures, including myoclonic, atonic, and absence seizures. It can be used as both monotherapy and adjunctive therapy for partial seizures, and it can be very useful in patients with mixed seizure disorders.

Vigabatrin

Pharmacology and Mechanism of Action Vigabatrin is an amino acid that is a structural analog of GABA. It is a racemic mixture consisting of two enantiomers with only the S(+)-enantiomer active. Vigabatrin is a selective, irreversible inhibitor of GABA-transaminase, the enzyme that degrades GABA, thereby increasing GABA levels in the CNS.[135]

Pharmacokinetics Vigabatrin undergoes virtually no metabolism and is excreted unchanged in the urine.[32] It is rapidly absorbed from the GI tract, and food has no effect on its absorption. Serum vigabatrin levels are linearly related to dosage, but therapeutic levels are not related to duration of effect; duration of effect is directly related to regeneration of the enzyme which metabolizes GABA. Since vigabatrin undergoes virtually no metabolism and is excreted renally, dosage adjustment is necessary in renally impaired patients. Children have a higher vigabatrin clearance than adults and therefore require higher mg/kg doses.[32]

Adverse Effects Vigabatrin may aggravate seizures, particularly absence and myoclonic seizures in patients with generalized epilepsies. Patients with history of depression, psychosis, or behavioral disturbances may be at greater risk to develop psychiatric effects.[135] Vigabatrin causes progressive, irreversible, bilateral concentric visual field constriction in a high percentage of patients. It may also reduce visual acuity in a dose-related and life exposure—related manner. Vigabatrin is associated with weight gain and edema, peripheral neuropathy, somnolence, and fatigue.[35] In up to 11% of patients (up to age 3 years) treated with high doses of the drug for infantile spasms, magnetic resonance imaging (MRI) findings have been strongly suggestive of intramyelinic edema in select brain areas. These findings appear to be reversible, and their significance is unclear.[136]

Drug Interactions Vigabatrin induces CYP2C and therefore decreases phenytoin plasma levels by approximately 20%. One study noted at least a 10% increase in serum carbamazepine levels in the majority of patients started on adjunctive therapy with vigabatrin, which has not been supported in clinical trials.[35]

Dosing and Administration Vigabatrin's initial dose in adults for refractory complex partial seizures is 1,000 mg/day given in two divided doses with an increase by 500 mg/day weekly until 3,000 mg/day is reached. Initial dose in infants and children for infantile spasms is 50 mg/kg/day given in two divided doses with an increase by 25 to 50 mg/kg/day every 3 days to maximum dose of 150 mg/kg/day.

Advantages Vigabatrin has been widely studied and used in numerous countries throughout the world.

Disadvantages Adverse effects are sizeable and significant. It is available only through a restricted distribution program (SHARE program), which requires providers and patients to register. Vision should be checked at baseline and every 3 months for up to 3 to 6 months after drug discontinuation.

Place in Therapy Vigabatrin is a first-line agent for infantile spasms, particularly those with tuberous sclerosis as the etiology. It is a third-line adjunctive agent for refractory partial epilepsy.

Zonisamide

Pharmacology and Mechanism of Action Zonisamide, a synthetic 1,2-benzisoxazole derivative classified as a sulfonamide, is chemically different from other AEDs. It is a broad-spectrum AED believed to exert its antiepileptic effect by inhibition of slow sodium channels, by blockade of T-type Ca^{2+} channels, and possibly by inhibition of glutamate release. It also has a weak carbonic anhydrase inhibitory effect.[137]

Pharmacokinetics Zonisamide is well absorbed and reaches a maximum concentration in 2 to 5 hours. It is metabolized by CYP3A4 and to a much lesser extent by CYP2C19 and CYP3A5. Approximately 30% is excreted unchanged in the urine. Zonisamide is distributed to most tissues, but the drug is concentrated in the red blood cells. It crosses the placenta. The concentration in breast milk is similar to that in the plasma.[137]

Adverse Effects The most common adverse effects of zonisamide include somnolence, dizziness, anorexia, headache, nausea, agitation, word-finding difficulties, and irritability. Adverse effects may be more common during rapid dose escalation. Because it is structurally related to sulfonamides, hypersensitivity reactions can occur (0.02% of patients), and zonisamide should be used with caution (if at all) in patients with a confirmed allergy to sulfonamide compounds. A 2.6% incidence of symptomatic kidney stones has been reported in patients treated in the United States.[138] Because of reports of modest, reversible declines in renal function in some patients, monitoring of renal function may be advisable for certain patients. Oligohidrosis has been reported. In addition, modest weight loss has been reported with this agent.[24,25,75]

Drug Interactions Zonisamide does not inhibit or induce the cytochrome P450 system.

Dosing and Administration Zonisamide is given once or twice daily, however, once-daily dosing causes greater fluctuations in serum concentrations and perhaps more side effects. The dose should be increased every 2 weeks to response. Zonisamide is stable for 48 hours when mixed with water, apple juice, or pudding.

Advantages Zonisamide has multiple mechanisms of action and may be a broad-spectrum AED. There is broad international experience with this drug. It has a very long half-life, which is suitable for once- or twice-daily dosing. Patients may experience modest weight loss.

Disadvantages The dos of zonisamide should be titrated slowly to patient response. Renal stones and oligohidrosis have been reported. In addition, cognitive impairment can occur, especially if the dosage is escalated rapidly. It should be avoided in patients allergic to "sulfa drugs."

Place in Therapy Zonisamide is approved for the adjunctive treatment of partial seizures. Zonisamide is potentially effective in a variety of partial and primary generalized seizure types.

PHARMACOECONOMIC CONSIDERATIONS

CLINICAL CONTROVERSY

The place in therapy of the newer drugs is still being determined. The cost of the newer AEDs generally is much higher that that of the older drugs. Given that, in general, the efficacy of the newer drugs is comparable with that of the older agents, many clinicians (and patients) have been slow to adopt this newer generation of drugs. It is important to recognize that overall effectiveness encompasses both efficacy and tolerability assessments. Generally speaking, the newer generation of AEDs possess fewer adverse effects and seems to be better tolerated than older, far less expensive agents such as the barbiturates. Some may also have less costly long-term adverse effects such as effects on bone metabolism or the fetus, and they may cause fewer drug interactions, which require higher doses of drugs to avoid treatment failures. These differences may well justify the difference in cost, however, this needs to be determined on an individual basis.

The direct costs of epilepsy include the cost of the drug, treatment of adverse events, emergency room visits, drug levels, laboratory tests, physician visits, rehabilitation, and transportation. Indirect costs include the costs associated with time lost from work, the inability to get a job, decreased productivity, and mortality.

It is difficult to assess the cost of epilepsy to society. Pashko and coworkers, using a cohort of Pennsylvania Medicaid patients, estimated that the total direct cost of epilepsy is in excess of $10 billion annually, with the majority of the per-patient costs incurred for inpatient hospitalization (uncontrolled seizures or treatment-related toxicity).[139] Another study suggested that the direct costs of epilepsy made up approximately 37% of the total costs, with indirect costs accounting for the remainder.[140] This study also indicated that the costs were much less for a patient who is well controlled than for a patient who is poorly controlled. Drug costs in the Pashko study accounted for approximately 10% of the total costs of epilepsy. In a large retrospective trial involving Medicaid patients in Florida, New Jersey, and Iowa, it was determined that nonadherence in taking AEDs was associated with a significantly higher incidence of hospitalization and visits to the emergency room, which translated to a sizable increase in overall costs.[141] Providing the best QOL possible is a treatment goal for patients with epilepsy, while maintaining a balance between side effects and the number of seizures.[142] QOL takes into account all the concerns of patients with epilepsy, including their social and economic concerns. This can best be assessed by the patient. Complete seizure freedom leads to the best QOL. In one study, driving was listed as the most important concern by 28% of patients, followed by employment (21%), independence (9%), safety (6%), AED side effects (5%), seizure unpredictability (5%), and seizure avoidance (5%).[143] Assessment of QOL as a therapeutic outcome ultimately may be more meaningful than measuring blood levels of the AEDs. It is clear that the cheapest drug in epilepsy (e.g., phenobarbital) is not the best because of the number of side effects. Drug therapy that controls seizures, decreases side effects, improves the QOL, and reduces the use of other healthcare resources would be cost-effective. Because epilepsy treatment continues to be highly individualized, the drug or combination of drugs that controls seizures with the least number of side effects will be the drug of choice for that patient no matter how expensive the drug acquisition cost.

Because many patients with epilepsy require minimal variation in blood concentrations to prevent seizures and avoid side effects, generic prescribing for epilepsy remains controversial. Issues related to generic use have been clearly delineated in the literature.[144,145] A strong argument for the use of generic AEDs is that they will save huge amounts of money and should not cause harm, if patients are selected wisely, e.g., those who are newly diagnosed, or who are not fully controlled, or who are not seizure free on brand product. There is only one randomized study comparing brand name and generic drug products which involved Depakene versus generic valproic acid. This study found no difference between the products. However, substantial data continue to accumulate from large, retrospective, observational studies which indicate that generics may increase health care costs from emergency room visits and hospitalizations. In addition, utilization of multiple generics in the same patient may create problems. A recent retrospective trial studied patients being treated with multiple topiramate generics and reported an increase in hospitalizations and injuries, again supporting increased health care costs with use of generics.[146] What has yet to be determined is whether bioequivalence translates into therapeutic equivalence in the use of generic AEDs and whether there is a subset of patients where this is not true.

EVALUATION OF THERAPEUTIC OUTCOMES

A therapeutic range should be established for each patient to define concentrations that result in minimal side effects and optimal seizure control. This therapeutic plasma concentration range should be used to identify the appropriate patient-specific dose. Patients should be monitored long term for seizure control, comorbid conditions, social adjustment (including QOL assessments), drug interactions, compliance, and adverse effects. Periodic screening for comorbid neuropsychiatric disorders such as depression and anxiety is also important. Clinical response is more important than the serum drug concentrations.

Outcomes can be assessed by regular clinical monitoring, drug utilization review, and QOL assessments. Clinical monitoring involves identifying the number and type of seizures. Patients should record the severity and the frequency of seizures in a seizure diary. There should be a decrease in the number and/or severity of seizures. Patients and family should be questioned regularly to determine whether they are truly seizure free.

The treatment of epilepsy begins with a careful identification of the seizure type and selection of the most appropriate AED. Therapy should be initiated slowly, except in life-threatening situations, to avoid acute toxicity. Although most patients can be managed successfully on monotherapy, some patients' seizures remain uncontrolled despite the use of multiple AEDs. Some patients may be genetically refractory to AED therapy. The newer AEDs, as adjunctive therapy or monotherapy, offer additional opportunity to achieve complete seizure control. There is a continuing need for new AEDs and additional research in this area.

ABBREVIATIONS

AAN: American Academy of Neurology

AED: antiepileptic drug

AES: American Epilepsy Society

AMPA: α-amino-3-hydroxy-5-methylisoxazole-4-propionic acid

CNS: central nervous system

CP: complex partial

CSF: cerebral spinal fluid

CT: computed tomography

ECG: electrocardiogram

EEG: electroencephalogram

GABA: γ-aminobutyric-acid

GTC: generalized tonic-clonic

GI: gastrointestinal

HPA: hypothalamic-pituitary-adrenal

IM: intramuscular

ILAE: International League Against Epilepsy

IV: intravenous

IQ: intelligence quotient

JME: juvenile myoclonic epilepsy

MHD: mono-hydroxy-derivative

MRI: magnetic resonance imaging

NMDA: N-methyl-D-aspartate

OC: oral contraceptive

PCOS: polycystic ovary syndrome

QOL: quality of life

SE: status epilepticus

SP: simple partial

VNS: vagus nerve stimulation

WBC: white blood cell

REFERENCES

1. Sander JW. The epidemiology of epilepsy revisited. Curr Opin Neurol 2003;16:165–170.
2. Najm IM, Moddel G, Janigro D. Mechanisms of epileptogenesis and experimental models of seizures. In: Wyllie E, ed. The Treatment of Epilepsy, 4th ed. Philadelphia, PA: Lippincott Williams & Wilkins, 2006:91–102.
3. Commission on Classification and Terminology of the International League Against Epilepsy. Proposal for revised clinical and electroencephalographic classification of epileptic seizures. Epilepsia 1981;22:489–501.
4. Commission on Classification and Terminology of the International League Against Epilepsy. Proposal for revised classification of epilepsies and epileptic syndromes. Epilepsia 1989;30:389–399.
5. Chen DK, So YT, Fisher RS. Use of serum prolactin in diagnosing epileptic seizures. Report of the therapeutic and technology assessment subcommittee of the American Academy of Neurology. Neurology 2005;65:668–675.
6. Vickrey BG, Hays RD, Rausch R, et al. Quality of life of epilepsy surgery patients as compared with outpatients with hypertension, diabetes, heart disease, and/or depressive symptoms. Epilepsia 1994;35:597–607.
7. Schachter SC. Psychiatric comorbidity of epilepsy. In: Wyllie E, ed. The Treatment of Epilepsy, 4th ed. Philadelphia, PA: Lippincott Williams & Wilkins, 2006:1197–1200.
8. Bazil CW. Epilepsy and sleep disturbance. Epilepsy Behav 2003;4: S39–45.
9. Boylan LS, Flint LA, Labovitz DL, et al. Depression but not seizure frequency predicts quality of life in treatment-resistant epilepsy. Neurology 2004;62:258–261.
10. Brodie MJ, French JA. Management of epilepsy in adolescents and adults. Lancet 2000;356:323–328.
11. Mattson RH. Antiepileptic drug monotherapy in adults: Selection and use in new-onset epilepsy. In: Levy RH, Mattson RH, Meldrum BS, eds. Antiepileptic Drugs, 5th ed. Philadelphia, PA: Lippincott Williams & Wilkins, 2002:72–95.
12. Garnett WR. Antiepileptic drug treatment: Outcomes and adherence. Pharmacotherapy 2000;20:191S–199S.
13. Leppik IE. Contemporary Diagnosis and Management of the Patient with Epilepsy, 6th ed. Newton, PA: Handbooks in Health Care, 2006:66–76.
14. Quality Standards Subcommittee of the American Academy of Neurology. Practice parameter: A guideline for discontinuing antiepileptic drugs in seizure free patients [summary statement]. Neurology 1996;47:600–602.
15. Gross-Tsur V, O'Dell C, Shinnar S. Initiation and discontinuation of antiepileptic drugs. In: Wyllie E, ed. The Treatment of Epilepsy, 4th ed. Philadelphia, PA: Lippincott Williams & Wilkins, 2006:681–694.
16. Krahl SE, Clark KB, Smith DC, et al. Locus coeruleus lesions suppress the seizure-attenuating effects of vagus nerve stimulation. Epilepsia 1998;39:709–14.
17. Lachhwani DK, Wyllie E. Outcome and complications of epilepsy surgery. In: Wyllie E, ed. The Treatment of Epilepsy, 4th ed. Philadelphia, PA: Lippincott Williams & Wilkins, 2006:1176–1182.
18. Sperling MR, Harris A, Nei M, et al. Mortality after epilepsy surgery. Epilepsia 2005;46(Suppl 11):49–53.
19. Devinsky O, Barr WB, Vickrey BG, et al. Changes in depression and anxiety after resective surgery for epilepsy. Neurology 2005;65:1744–1749.
20. Schmidt D, Stavem K. Long-term seizure outcome of surgery versus no surgery for drug-resistant partial epilepsy: A review of controlled studies. Epilepsia 2009;50:1301–309.
21. Berg AT, Vickrey GB, Langfitt JT, et al. Reduction of AEDs in postsurgical patients who attain remission. Epilepsia 2006;47;64–71.
22. Groesbeck DK, Bluml RM, Kossoff EH. Long-term use of the ketogenic diet: Outcomes of 28 children with over 6 years diet duration. Neurology 2006;66(Suppl 2):A41.
23. Dossoff EH, Zupec-Kania BA, Amark PE, et al. Optimal clinical management of children receiving the ketogenic diet: Recommendations of the international ketogenic diet study group. Epilepsia 2009;50:304–17.

24. French JA, Kanner AM, Bautista J, et al. Efficacy and tolerability of the new antiepileptic drugs: I. Treatment of new onset epilepsy. Neurology 2004;62:1252–1260.

25. French JA, Kanner AM, Bautista J, et al. Efficacy and tolerability of the new antiepileptic drugs: II. Treatment of refractory epilepsy. Neurology 2004;62:1261–1273.

26. National Institute for Clinical Excellence. Newer Drugs for Epilepsy in Adults; 2006. http://www.nice.org.uk.

27. National Institute for Clinical Excellence. Newer Drugs for Epilepsy in Children; 2006. http://www.nice.org.uk.

28. Glauser T, Ben-Menachem E, Bourgeois B, et al. ILAE treatment guidelines: Evidenced-based analysis of antiepileptic drug efficacy and effectiveness as initial monotherapy for epileptic seizures and syndromes. Epilepsia 2006;47:1094–1120.

29. Karceski S, Morrell MJ, Carpenter D. Treatment of epilepsy in adults: Expert opinion. Epilepsy Behav 2005;7:S1–S64.

30. Faught E. Pharmacokinetic considerations in prescribing antiepileptic drugs. Epilepsia 2001;42(Suppl 4):19–23.

31. Leppik IE. Contemporary Diagnosis and Management of the Patient with Epilepsy, 6th ed. Newton, PA: Handbooks in Health Care, 2006:92–149.

32. Patsalos PN, Berry DJ, Bourgeois BFD, et al. Antiepileptic drugs-best practice guidelines for therapeutic drug monitoring: A position paper by the subcommission on therapeutic drug monitoring, ILAE Commission on Therapeutic Strategies. Epilepsia 2008;49:1239–76.

33. Halford JJ, Lapointe M. Clinical perspectives on lacosamide. Epilepsy Curr 2009;9:1–9.

34. Cada DJ, Levien TL, Baker DE. Rufinamide. Hosp Pharm 2009;44:412–22.

35. Sabril [package insert]. Deerfield, IL: Lundbeck Inc; August 2009.

36. Anderson GD. Pharmcokinetic, pharmacodynamic, and pharma-cogenetic targeted therapy of antiepileptic drugs. Ther Drug Monit 2008;30:173–80.

37. Harden CL. Therapeutic safety monitoring: What to look for and when to look for it. Epilepsia 2000;41(Suppl 8):S37–44.

38. Pack AM, Morrell MJ, McMahon DJ, et al. Bone health in young women with epilepsy after one year of antiepileptic drug monotherapy. Neurology 2008;70:1586–1593.

39. Lado F, Spiegel R, Masur JH, et al. Value of routine screening for bone demineralization in an urban population of patients with epilepsy. Epilepsy Res 2008;78:155–160.

40. Meador KJ, Gilliam FG, Kanner AM, Pellock JM. Cognitive and behav-ioral effects of antiepileptic drugs. Epilepsy Behav 2001;2:S1–S17.

41. Vermeulen J, Aldenkamp AP. Cognitive side-effects of chronic anti-epileptic drug treatment: A review of 25 years of research. Epilepsy Res 1995;22:65–95.

42. Meador KJ, Loring DW, Ray PG, et al. Differential cognitive effects of carbamazepine and gabapentin. Epilepsia 1999;40:1279–1285.

43. Meador KJ, Loring DW, Ray PG. Differential cognitive effects of carbamazepine and lamotrigine [abstract]. Neurology 2000; 54:A84.

44. Martin R, Kuzniecky R, Ho S, et al. Cognitive effects of topiramate, gabapentin and lamotrigine in healthy young adults. Neurology 1999;52:321–327.

45. Fritz N, Glogau S, Hoffman J, et al. Efficacy and cognitive side effects to tiagabine and topiramate in patients with epilepsy. Epilepsy Behav 2005;6:373–381.

46. Salinsky MC, Storzbach D, Spencer DC, et al. Effects of topiramate and gabapentin on cognitive abilities in healthy volunteers. Neurology 2005;64:792–798.

47. Sazgar M, Bourgeois B. Aggravation of epilepsy by antiepileptic drugs. Pediatr Neurol 2005;33:227–234.

48. Mattson RH, Cramer JA, Collins JF, et al. Comparison of car-bamazepine, phenobarbital, phenytoin, and primidone in partial and secondarily generalized tonic-clonic seizures. N Engl J Med 1985;313:145–151.

49. Mattson RH, Cramer JA, Collins JF, et al. A comparison of valproate with carbamazepine for the treatment of complex partial seizures and secondarily generalized tonic-clonic seizures in adults. N Engl J Med 1992;327:765–771.

50. Beydoun A, Kutluay E. Conversion to monotherapy: Clinical trials in patients with refractory partial seizures. Neurology 2003;60(Suppl 4):S13–S25.

51. French JA, Kanner AM, Bautista J, et al. Efficacy and tolerability of the new antiepileptic drugs: I. Treatment of new-onset epilepsy. Epilepsia 2004;45:401–409.

52. French JA, Kanner AM, Bautista J, et al. Efficacy and tolerability of the new antiepileptic drugs: II. Treatment of refractory epilepsy. Epilepsia 2004;45:410–423.

53. Marson AG, Al-Kharusi AM, Alwaidh M et al. The SANAD study of effectiveness of carbamazepine, gabapentin, lamotrigine, oxarba-zepine, or topiramate for treatment of partial epilepsy: an unblinded randomized controlled trial. Lancet 2007;369(9566):1000–1015.

54. Rowan AJ, Ramsay ER, Collins JF, et al. New onset geriatric epilepsy: A randomized study of gabapentin, lamotrigine, and carbamazepine. Neurology 2005;64:1868–1873.

55. Brodie MJ, Perucca E, Ryvlin P, et al. Comparison of levetiracetam and controlled-release carbamazepine in newly diagnosed epilepsy. Epilepsy 2007;68:402–408.

56. Marson AG, Al-Karusi AM, Alwaidh M, et al. The SANAD study of effectivenss of valproate, lamotrigine, or topiramate for generalized and unclassifiable epilepsy: An unblinded randomized controlled trial. Lancet 2007;369(9566):1016–1026.

57. Smith S, Wolley CS. Cellular and molecular effects of steroid hor-mones and CNS excitability. Cleve Clin J Med 2004;71:S5–S10.

58. Crawford PM. Managing epilepsy in women of childbearing age. Drug Saf 2009;32:293–307.

59. Morrell MJ, Montouris GD. Reproductive disturbances in patients with epilepsy. Cleve Clin J Med 2004;71:S19–S24.

60. Yerby MS, Kaplan P, Tran T. Risks and management of pregnancy in women with epilepsy. Cleve Clin J Med 2004;71:S25–S37.

61. Vajda FJ, Hitchcock A, Graham J et al. Seizure control in antiepileptic drug-treated pregnancy. Epilepsia 2008;49:172–176.

62. Harden CL, Hopp J, Ting TY et al. Management issues for women with epilepsy-Focus on pregnancy (an evidence-based review): 1. Obstetrical complications and change in seizure frequency. Epilepsia 2009;50:1229–1236.

63. Harden CL, Meador KJ, Pennell PB et al. Management issues for women with epilepsy-Focus on pregnancy (an evidence-based review): II. Teratogenesis and perinatal outcomes. Epilepsia 2009;50:1237–1246.

64. Harden CL, Pennell PB, Koppel BS et al. Management issues for women with epilepsy-Focus on pregnancy (an evidence-based review): III. Vitamin K, folic acid, blood levels, and breast-feeding. Epilepsia 2009;50:1247–1255.

65. Vajda FJE, Eadie MJ. Maternal valproate dosage and foetal malforma-tions. Acta Neurol Scand 2005:112:137–143.

66. Tomson T, Battino D. Teratogenicity of antiepileptic drugs: State of the art. Curr Opin Neurol 2005;18:135–140.

67. Harden CL, Herzog AG, Nikolov BG, et al. Hormone replacement therapy in women with epilepsy: A randomized, double-blind, pla-cebo-controlled study. Epilepsia 2006;47:1447–1451.

68. Isojaervi JIJ, Loefgren E, Juntunen KST, et al. Effect of epilepsy and antiepileptic drugs on male reproductive health. Neurology 2004;62:247–253.

69. Ferraro TN, Buono RJ. The relationship between the pharmacology of antiepileptic drugs and human gene variation: An overview. Epilepsy Behav 2005;7:18–36.

70. Garnett WR. Carbamazepine. In: Murphy J, ed. Clinical Pharmacokinetics, 2nd ed. Washington, DC: American Society of Health-Systems Pharmacists, 2004.

71. Ficker DM, Privitera M, Krauss G, et al. Improved tolerability and efficacy in epilepsy patients with extended-release carbamazepine. Neurology 2005;65:593–595.

72. Garnett WR. Ethosuximide. In: Murphy J, ed. Clinical Pharmacokinetics. Washington, DC: American Society of Health-Systems Pharmacists, 2004.

73. Garnett WR. Antiepileptics. In: Schumacher GE, ed. Therapeutic Drug Monitoring. Norwalk, CT: Appleton & Lange, 1995:345–395.

74. Pellock JM, Perhach JL, Sofia RD. Felbamate. In: Levy RH, Mattson RH, Meldrum BS, et al., eds. Antiepileptic Drugs, 5th ed. Philadelphia, PA: Lippincott Williams & Wilkins, 2002:301–318.

75. LaRoche SM, Helmers SL. The new antiepileptic drugs: Scientific review. JAMA 2004;291:605–614.

76. Taylor CP, Gee NS, Su TZ, et al. A summary of mechanistic hypothesis of gabapentin pharmacology. Epilepsy Res 1998;29:233–249.

77. Luer MS, Hamani C, Dujovny M, et al. Saturable transport of gabapentin at the blood—brain barrier. Neurol Res 1999;21:559–562.

78. Gidal BE, Radulovic LL, Kruger S, et al. Inter- and intrasubject variability in gabapentin (GBP) absorption and absolute bioavailability. Epilepsy Res 2000;40:123–127.

79. Gidal BE, Maly MM, Kowalski J, et al. Gabapentin absorption: Effect of mixing with foods of varying macronutrient content. Ann Pharmacother 1998;32:405–408.

80. Wong MO, Eldon MA, Keane WF, et al. Disposition of gabapentin in anuric subjects on hemodialysis. J Clin Pharmacol 1995;35:622–626.

81. Lee DO, Steingard RJ, Cesena M, et al. Behavioral side effects of gabapentin in children. Epilepsia 1996;37:87–90.

82. McLean MJ, Gidal BE. Gabapentin in the treatment of epilepsy: A dosing review. Clin Ther 2003;25:1382–1406.

83. Gidal BE, DeCerce J, Bockbrader HR, et al. Gabapentin bioavailability: Effect of dose and frequency of administration in adult patients with epilepsy. Epilepsy Res 1998;31:91–99.

84. Dickins M, Chen C. Lamotrigine: Chemistry, biotransformation, and pharmacokinetics. In: Levy RH, Mattson RH, Meldrum BS, et al., eds. Antiepileptic Drugs, 5th ed. Philadelphia, PA: Lippincott Williams & Wilkins, 2002:369–379.

85. Gilman JT. Lamotrigine: An antiepileptic agent for the treatment of partial seizures. Ann Pharmacother 1995;29:144–151.

86. Hirsch LJ, Weintraub DB, Buchsbaum R, et al. Predictors of lamotrigine-associated rash. Epilepsia 2006;47:318–322.

87. Messenheimer JA. Rash in adult and pediatric patients treated with lamotrigine. Can J Neurol Sci 1998;25:S14–S18.

88. Sidhu J, Bulsara S, Job S, Philipson R. A bi-directional pharmacokinetic interaction study of lamotrigine and the combined oral contraceptive pill in healthy subjects [abstract]. Epilepsia 2004;45(Suppl 7):330.

89. Christensen J, Petrenaite V, Atterman J, et al. Oral contraceptives induce lamotrigine metabolism: evidence from a double-blind, placebo-controlled trial. Epilepsia 2007;48:484–489.

90. Lynch BA, Lambeng N, Nocka K, et al. The synaptic vesicle protein SV2A in the binding site for the antiepileptic drug levetiracetam. Proc Natl Acad Sci U S A 2004;101:9861–9866.

91. Loscher W, Honack D, Rundfeldt C. Antiepileptogenic effects of the novel anticonvulsant levetiracetam (ucb LO59) in the kindling model of temporal lobe epilepsy. J Pharmacol Exp Ther 1998;284:474–479.

92. Fay MA, Sheth RD, Gidal BE. Oral absorption kinetics of levetiracetam: The effect of mixing with food or enteral nutrition. Clin Ther 2005;27:594–598.

93. Welty TE, Gidal BE, Ficker DM, Privitera MD. Levetiracetam: A different approach to the pharmacotherapy of epilepsy. Ann Pharmacother 2002;36:296–304.

94. Brockmoeller J, Thomsen T, Wittstock M, et al. Pharmacokinetics of levetiracetam in patients with moderate to severe liver cirrhosis (Child-Pugh classes A, B and C): Characterization by dynamic liver function tests. Clin Pharmacol Ther 2005;77:529–541.

95. Harden CL, Pennell PB, Koppel BS, et al. Practice parameter update: Management issues for women with epilepsy-focus on pregnancy (an evidence-based review): vitamin K, folic acid, blood levels, and breast-feeding. Neurology 2009;73:142–149.

96. Coppola G, Mangano S, Tortorella G, et al. Levetiracetam during 1-year follow-up in children, adolescents, and young adults with refractory epilepsy. Epilepsy Res 2004;59:35–42.

97. Perucca E, Gidal BE. Effects of antiepileptic comedication on levetiracetam pharmacokinetics: A pooled analysis of data from randomized adjunctive therapy trials. Epilepsy Res 2003;53:47–56.

98. Gidal BE, Baltes E, Otoul C, Perruca E. Effect of levetiracetam on the pharmacokinetics of adjunctive antiepileptic drugs: A pooled analysis of data from randomized clinic trials. Epilepsy Res 2005;64:1–11.

99. Stefan H, Wang-Tilz Y, Pauli E, et al. Onset of action of levetiracetam: A RCT trial using therapeutic intensive seizure analysis (TISA). Epilepsia 2006;47:516–522.

100. Ambrosio AF, Soares-Da-Silva P, Carvalho CM, Carvalho AP. Mechanisms of action of carbamazepine and its derivatives, oxcarbazepine, BIA 2–093 and BIA 2–024. Neurochem Res 2002;27:121–130.

101. Ambrosio AF, Silva AP, Malva JO, et al. Carbamazepine inhibits L-type Ca2+ channels in cultured rat hippocampal neurons stimulated with glutamate receptor agonists. Neuropharmacology 1999;38:1349–1359.

102. Lloyd P, Flesch G, Dieterle W. Clinical pharmacology and pharmacokinetics of oxcarbazepine. Epilepsia 1994;35:10–13.

103. Kalis MM, Huff NA. Oxcarbazepine, an antiepileptic agent. Clin Ther 2001;23:680–700.

104. May TW, Ramback B, Jurgens U. Influence of oxcarbazepine and methsuximide on lamotrigine concentrations in epileptic patients with and without valproic acid comedication: results of a retrospective study. Ther Drug Monit 1999;21:175–181.

105. Pina-Garza JE, Espinoza R, Nordli D, et al. Oxcarbazepine adjunctive therapy in infants and young children with partial seizures. Neurology 2005;65:1370–1375.

106. Muller M, Marson AG, Williamson PR. Oxcarbazepine versus phenytoin monotherapy for epilepsy. Cochrane Database Syst Rev 2006;2:CD003615.

107. Messina S, Battino D, Croci D, et al. Phenobarbital pharmacokinetics in old age: A case-matched evaluation based on therapeutic drug monitoring data. Epilepsia 2005;46:372–377.

108. Baulac M, Cramer JA, Mattson RH. Phenobarbital and other barbiturates: Adverse effects. In: Levy RH, Mattson RH, Meldrum BS, et al., eds. Antiepileptic Drugs, 5th ed. Philadelphia, PA: Lippincott Williams & Wilkins, 2002:528–540.

109. Tozer TN, Winter ME. Phenytoin. In: Evans WE, Schentag JJ, Jusko WJ, eds. Applied Pharmacokinetics, 3rd ed. Spokane, WA: Applied Therapeutics, 1992:25–1–44.

110. Anderson GD, Pak C, Doane KW, et al. Revised Winter-Tozer equation for normalized phenytoin concentrations in trauma and elderly patients with hypoalbuminemia. Ann Pharmacother 1997;31:279–284.

111. Ahn JE, Cloyd JC, Brundage RC, et al. Phenytoin half-life and clearance during maintenance therapy in adults and elderly patients with epilepsy. Neurology 2008;71:38–43.

112. Bruni J. Phenytoin and other hydantoins: Adverse effects. In: Levy RH, Mattson RH, Meldrum BS, et al., eds. Antiepileptic Drugs, 5th ed. Philadelphia, PA: Lippincott Williams & Wilkins, 2002:605–610.

113. Privitera MD. Clinical rules for phenytoin dosing. Ann Pharmacother 1993;27:1169–1173.

114. Ben-Menachem E. Pregabalin pharmacology and its relevance to clinical practice. Epilepsia 2004;45(Suppl 6):13–18.

115. Bialer M, Johannessen SI, Kupferberg HJ, et al. Progress report on new antiepileptic drugs: A summary of the seventh EILAT conference (EILAT VII). Epilepsy Res 2004;61:1–48.

116. Shneker BF, McAuley JW. Pregablin: A new neuromodulator with broad therapeutic indications. Ann Pharmacother 2005;39:2029–2037.

117. Perucca E, Cloyd J, Critchley D, et al. Rufinamide: Clinical pharmacokinetics and concentration-response relationships in patients with epilepsy. Epilepsia 2008;49:1123–1120.

118. Schachter SC. Tiagabine: Current status and potential clinical applications. Expert Opin Investig Drugs 1996;5:1377–1387.

119. Leppik IE. Tiagabine: The safety landscape. Epilepsia 1995;36:S10–S13.

120. Koepp MJ, Edwards M, Collins J, et al. Status epilepticus and tiagabine therapy revisited. Epilepsia 2005;46:1625–1632.

121. Gidal BE, Lensmeyer GL. Therapeutic drug monitoring of topiramate: Evaluation of the saturable distribution between erythrocytes and plasma in whole blood using an optimized HPLC method. Ther Drug Monit 1999;21:567–576.

122. Langtry HD, Gillis JC, Davis R. Topiramate: A review of its pharmacodynamic and pharmacokinetic properties and clinical efficacy in the management of epilepsy. Drugs 1997;54:752–773.

123. Shorvon SD. Safety of topiramate: Adverse events and relationship to dosing. Epilepsia 1996;37(Suppl 2):S18–S22.

124. Mula M, Trimble M, Thompson P, et al. Topiramate and word-finding difficulties in patients with epilepsy. Neurology 2003;60:1104–1107.

125. Gidal BE. Topiramate: Drug interactions. In: Levy RH, Mattson RH, Meldrum BS, et al., eds. Antiepileptic Drugs, 5th ed. Philadelphia, PA: Lippincott Williams & Wilkins, 2002:735–739.

126. Privitera M, Fincham R, Penry J, et al. Topiramate placebo-controlled dose-ranging trial in refractory partial epilepsy using 600-, 800-, and 1,000-mg daily dosages. Neurology 1996;46:1678–1683.

127. Davis R, Peters DH, McTavish D. Valproic acid: A reappraisal of its pharmacological properties and clinical efficacy in epilepsy. Drugs 1994;47:332–372.

128. Ornoy A. Valproic acid in pregnancy: How much are we endangering the embryo and fetus? Reproductive Toxicology 2009;28:1–10.

129. Greco R, Latini G, Chiarelli F, et al. Leptin, ghrelin, and adiponectin in antiepileptic patients treated with valproic acid. Neurology 2005;65;1808–1809.

130. Pylvaenen V, Pakarinen A, Knip M, Isojaervi J. Characterization of insulin secretion in valproate-treated patients with epilepsy. Epilepsia 2006;47:1460–1464.

131. Genton P, Gelissse P. Valproic acid: Adverse effects. In: Levy RH, Mattson RH, Meldrum BS, et al. Antiepileptic Drugs, 5th ed. Philadelphia, PA: Lippincott Williams & Wilkins, 2002:837–851.

132. Gidal BE, Inglese CM, Meyer JM, et al. Diet and valproate mediated transient hyperammonemia: Effect of l-carnitine supplementation in children with epilepsy. Pediatr Neurol 1997;16:301–305.

133. Gerstner T, Teich M, Bell N, et al. Valproate-associated coagulopathies are frequent and variable in children. Epilepsia 2006;47:1136–1143.

134. Comparison of carbapenem antibiotics. Pharmacist's Letter/Prescriber's Letter 2007;23(12):231205.

135. Ben-Menachem E, Dulac O, Chiron C. Vigabatrin. In: Engel J, Pedley TA. ed. Epilepsy: A Comprehensive Textbook, 2nd ed. Philadelphia: Lippincott Williams & Wilkins, PA, 2008:1683–1693.

136. Shorvon SD. Drug treatment of epilepsy in the century of the ILAE: The second 50 years, 1959–2009. Epilepsia 2009;50(Suppl 3): 93–130.

137. Welty TE. Zonisamide. In: Wyllie E., ed. The Treatment of Epilepsy, 4th ed. Philadelphia, PA: Lippincott Williams & Wilkins, 2006:891–899.

138. Lee BI. Zonisamide: Adverse effects. In: Levy RH, Mattson RH, Meldrum BS, et al., eds. Antiepileptic Drugs. Philadelphia, PA: Lippincott Williams & Wilkins, 2002:892–898.

139. Pashko S, McCord A, Sena MM. The cost of epilepsy and seizures in a cohort of Pennsylvania Medicaid patients. Med Interface 1993:84.

140. Begley CE, Annegers JF, Lairson DR, et al. Cost of epilepsy in the United States: A model based on incidence and prognosis. Epilepsia 1994;35:1230–1243.

141. Faught RE, Weiner JR, Gue'rin A. Impact of nonadherence to antiepileptic drugs on health care utilization and costs: Findings from the RANSOM study. Epilepsia 2009;50:501–509.

142. Gilliam F, Carter J, Vahle V. Tolerability of antiseizure medications. Neurology 2004;63(Suppl 4):S9–S12.

143. Gilliam F, Kuzniecky R, Faught E, et al. Patient-validated content of epilepsy-specific quality-of-life measurement. Epilepsia 1997;38:233–236.

144. Gidal BE, Tomson T. Debate: Substitution of generic drugs in epilepsy: Is there cause for concern? Epilepsia 2008;49(Suppl 9):56–62.

145. Privitera MD. Generic antiepileptic drugs: Current controversies and future directions. Epilepsy Curr 2008;8:113–117.

146. Duh MS, Paradis PE, Latre'mouille-Viau D, et al. The risks and costs of multiple-generic substitution of topiramate. Neurology 2009;72: 2122–2129.

CHAPTER **66**

Status Epilepticus

STEPHANIE J. PHELPS, COLLIN A. HOVINGA, AND JAMES W. WHELESS

KEY CONCEPTS

❶ Status epilepticus (SE) is a neurologic emergency that is associated with significant morbidity and mortality.

❷ Generalized convulsive status epilepticus (GCSE) is defined as any recurrent or continuous seizure activity lasting longer than 30 minutes in which the patient does not regain baseline mental status. Any seizure that does not stop within 5 minutes should be treated as impending SE.

❸ There are two types of status epilepticus, GCSE and nonconvulsive status epilepticus (NCSE). GCSE is the most common type.

❹ Most GCSE develops in patients with no history of epilepsy; however, a patient with preexisting epilepsy may experience GCSE as a result of acute anticonvulsant withdrawal, metabolic disorder, concurrent illness, or progression of neurologic disease.

❺ Although the pathophysiology of GCSE is unknown, experimental models have shown that there is a dramatic decrease in γ-aminobutyric acid–mediated inhibitory synaptic transmission and that glutamatergic excitatory synaptic transmission sustains the seizures.

❻ General treatment includes patient stabilization, adequate oxygenation, preservation of cardiorespiratory function, management of systemic complications, and aggressive assessment of underlying causes.

❼ The main purpose of treatment is to prevent or decrease morbidity and mortality of prolonged seizures. Pharmacologic treatment needs to be rapid and aimed at terminating both electrical and clinical seizures. The probability of poorer outcomes increases with increased length of electrographic seizure activity.

❽ Lorazepam is the preferred benzodiazepine in treatment of GCSE because of its long duration of action in the CNS.

❾ Currently, the hydantoins (phenytoin and fosphenytoin) are the long-acting anticonvulsants used most frequently. Either phenytoin or fosphenytoin should be given concurrently with benzodiazepines.

❿ The maximum rate of infusion for phenytoin and fosphenytoin in adults is 50 mg/min and 150 mg PE/min, respectively.

⓫ If GCSE is not controlled by two first-line agents (benzodiazepine plus hydantoin or phenobarbital), the GCSE is considered to be refractory. In these cases, newer anticonvulsants and/or pharmacologically induced coma should be used.

❶ Status epilepticus (SE) is a common neurologic emergency that is associated with brain damage and death. ❷ The traditional definition, provided by the International League Against Epilepsy Classification of Epileptic Seizures, defines SE as (1) any seizure lasting longer than 30 minutes whether or not consciousness is impaired or (2) recurrent seizures without an intervening period of consciousness between seizures.[1] Clinically, this definition has limited use, particularly in the case of generalized convulsive status epilepticus (GCSE), as the average seizure is less than 2 minutes; and only 40% of seizures lasting 10 to 29 minutes cease without treatment.[2,3] Pharmacoresistance[4] and mortality[3] significantly increase with increased seizure duration. Therefore, aggressive treatment of seizures lasting 5 minutes or more is strongly recommended. ❸ SE can present in several forms (Table 66–1), including GCSE and nonconvulsive status epilepticus (NCSE).[1]

NCSE occurs in approximately 25% of those with SE and is characterized by a fluctuating or continuous "twilight" state that produces altered consciousness and/or behavior (e.g., lethargy, decreased mental function). An altered electroencephalogram (EEG) is the most important diagnostic and management tool.[5] In most instances, a benzodiazepine and/or valproate remain drugs of choice for NCSE.[5] Although intravenous (IV) hydantoin or phenobarbital can be tried in patients who fail to respond, general anesthesia or barbiturate coma is not appropriate.[5] The reader is referred to a recent review for a more comprehensive discussion of NCSE and its pharmacologic management.[5]

GCSE is the most common and severe form of SE and is characterized by repeated primary or secondary generalized seizures that involve both hemispheres of the brain and are associated with a persistent postictal state.[4] This chapter will focus on the epidemiology, pathophysiology, presentation, and management of GCSE.

EPIDEMIOLOGY

It is difficult to determine the true incidence of GCSE. The worldwide and United States incidence is thought to range between 1.2 to 5 million and 100,000 to 152,000 cases each year, respectively.[4] GCSE has no predilection for gender or socioeconomic status but does occur more frequently in nonwhites across all ages.[6] Most episodes of GCSE occur in individuals with no history of epilepsy;

Learning objectives, review questions, and other resources can be found at **www.pharmacotherapyonline.com**.

TABLE 66-1 International Classification of Status Epilepticus

	Convulsive		Nonconvulsive	
International	**Traditional Terminology**	**International**	**Traditional Terminology**
Primary generalized SE • Tonic-clonic[a,b] • Tonic[c] • Clonic[c] • Myoclonic[b] • Erratic[d]	Grand mal, epilepticus convulsivus	Absence[c]	Petit mal, spike-and-wave stupor, spike-and-slow-wave or 3/s spike-and-wave, epileptic fugue, epilepsia minora continua, epileptic twilight, minor SE
Secondary generalized SE[a,b] • Tonic • Partial seizures with secondary generalization		Partial SE[a,b] Simple partial Somatomotor Dysphasic Other types Complex partial	Focal motor, focal sensory, epilepsia partialis continua, adversive SE Elementary Temporal lobe, psychomopartitor, epileptic fugue state, prolonged epileptic stupor, prolonged epileptic confusional state, continuous epileptic twilight state

SE, status epilepticus.
[a]Most common in older children.
[b]Most common in adolescents and adults.
[c]Most common in infants and young children.
[d]Most common in neonates.

TABLE 66-2 Etiology and Mortality for Pediatric and Adult Cases of Status Epilepticus

Etiology	Number of Cases (% Mortality) n = 200 Cases of Pediatric SE	Number of Cases (% Mortality) n = 512 Cases of Adult SE
Type I (no structural lesion)		
Infection	55 (5)	6 (35)
CNS infection	11 (0)	2 (20)
Metabolic	20 (5)	12 (36)
Low AED levels	16 (0)	24 (7)
Alcohol	0 (0)	13 (8)
Idiopathic	6 (0)	13 (18)
Type II (structural lesion)		
Anoxia/hypoxia	27 (13)	14 (65)
CNS tumor	3 (50)	5 (22)
CVA	5 (0)	26 (27)
Drug overdose	5 (0)	3 (23)
Hemorrhage	5 (11)	4 (35)
Trauma	13 (0)	3 (23)
Remote causes[a]	33 (5)	7 (13)

AED, antiepileptic drug; CVA, cerebrovascular accident; SE, status epilepticus.
Percentages do not add up to 100% because some patients had multiple etiologies.
[a]More than half of remote causes were congenital malformations and CVA in pediatric and adult patients, respectively.
Data from DeLorenzo et al.[6,8]

however, approximately 5% of adults and 10% to 25% of children with epilepsy will develop GCSE.[7] The incidence of GCSE is highest in those younger than 1 year of age and in those older than 60 years of age.

ETIOLOGY

Precipitating events for GCSE vary among studies and generally reflect different populations and referral patterns. ❹ Most episodes that occur in known epileptics occur because of acute anticonvulsant withdrawal, a metabolic disorder or concurrent illness, or progression of a preexisting neurologic disease. Common etiologies and mortality rates are shown in Table 66–2.[6,8] Precipitating events for GCSE are divided into those with and without neurologic structural lesions or those with a precipitating injury or insult. Cases with structural lesions or those with a specific neurologic insult are associated with a poor prognosis.

There are major differences in etiologies for pediatric and adult patients (see Table 66–2). During their first few weeks of life, infants who are born to addicted mothers can develop drug withdrawal seizures. Other neonates can develop GCSE because of a pyridoxine deficiency, which should resolve within hours following IV pyridoxine (100 mg). Acute encephalopathy and metabolic disorders are the major causes of GCSE in patients younger than 1 year of age. In young children, the cause is frequently a nonspecific illness such as fever and/or a viral illness. The most frequent precipitating events in adults are cerebrovascular disease, anticonvulsant withdrawal, and low anticonvulsant serum concentrations. Cerebrovascular disease is the leading cause in those who have their first seizures after age 60. A number of prescription, over-the-counter, and recreational drugs should be considered in anyone with

new-onset GCSE. Elevated anticonvulsant serum concentration or rapid anticonvulsant withdrawal can also precipitate GCSE.

MORBIDITY AND MORTALITY

GCSE is harmful to the brain and is associated with morbidity. However, whether the morbidity results from the underlying etiology or the GCSE itself remains to be determined. Most contend that the GCSE is responsible for the morbidity. Neuronal damage in animal models is evident following 30 to 60 minutes of GCSE regardless of the inducing stimulus, and most animals progress to develop epilepsy following a prolonged seizure. Interestingly, inhibiting the neuronal damage associated with seizures does not prevent the development of epilepsy, suggesting that the seizures themselves may be harmful. It is hard to establish a relationship between GCSE and long-term outcomes because it is difficult to weigh the effects of seizure type, etiology, duration, concurrent physiologic events, and therapy or lack thereof. It has been shown that patients with a history of prolonged febrile seizures who later developed epilepsy share similar histopathologic changes (i.e., hippocampal sclerosis) to those found in animal models of GCSE.[9,10] In these cases the period between the initial GCSE and the first epileptic seizure may be months to decades, suggesting a possible link between GCSE and the development of epilepsy. Importantly, studies of GCSE show that the currently available anticonvulsants do not reproducibly prevent the development of epilepsy following prolonged seizures.[9,11]

Patients who develop epilepsy following prolonged GCSE are less likely to experience remission of their seizures and may have decreased cognitive and memory function, mental retardation, or neurologic deficits.[4] Most studies have found that younger children, the elderly, and those with preexisting epilepsy have a higher propensity for sequelae. Unless accompanied by an underlying neurologic abnormality, fever-induced GCSE is less likely to be associated with sequelae.

The estimated mortality rate in the United States following GCSE ranges between 22,000 and 42,000 individuals per year.[8] Recent estimates suggest a mortality rate of up to 16% in children,[12] 20% in adults,[4] and 38% in the elderly.[6] When compared with other populations, neonates have a higher mortality and more neurologic sequelae.

Table 66–2 summarizes the etiology and corresponding mortality rates for GCSE.[6,8] Interestingly, the mortality associated with many etiologies is significantly greater in adults than in children. Unresponsive patients may die from GCSE, but more frequently they die from the acute illness that precipitated the GCSE. For example, patients with serious central nervous system (CNS) structural changes (e.g., hemorrhage, stroke) have a poor prognosis, whereas those (i.e., 80%–90%) with no structural lesion generally respond to IV phenytoin.

Two variables that affect outcome are the time between onset of GCSE and the initiation of treatment and the duration of the seizure. Mortality significantly increases with increased seizure duration (e.g., 2.6% for those with seizures 10–29 minutes vs 19% for those with seizures lasting >30 minutes).[2] Patients with GCSE lasting longer than 60 minutes have a higher mortality rate (32%) than those with seizures lasting less than 60 minutes (2.5%).[8] Mortality has decreased over the past decade and probably reflects a recognition of the need to initiate sequenced therapy immediately, and a greater understanding of the pathogenesis of GCSE.

PATHOGENESIS

Seizures occur when the excitatory neurotransmission overcomes inhibitory impulses in one or more brain regions (i.e., neural networks). Most seizures are brief (less than 5 minutes), largely because the brain's inhibitory mechanisms restore the balance of normal neurotransmission.[4] It is unknown why the mechanisms that control normal brain homeostasis fail. However, when seizures occur in close succession or the magnitude of the proconvulsant stimulus is severe, compensatory mechanisms can be overwhelmed and lead to GCSE.

❺ Although the exact cellular mechanisms responsible for the production of abnormal neural impulses are unknown, it appears that seizure initiation is caused by an imbalance between excitatory (e.g., glutamate, calcium, sodium, substance P, and neurokinin B) and inhibitory neurotransmission (e.g., γ-aminobutyric acid [GABA], adenosine, potassium, neuropeptide Y, opioid peptides, and galanin).[13] Seizure maintenance associated with GCSE is largely caused by glutamate acting on postsynaptic N-methyl-D-aspartate (NMDA) and α-amino-3-hydroxy-5-methyl-isoxazole-4-propionate (AMPA)/kainate receptors. Most of what is known about GCSE has focused on gated ion channels, with less known about receptor—second messenger systems (e.g., metabotropic glutamate receptors).[13]

During GCSE, glutamate activation of the NMDA and AMPA receptors causes opening of the gated calcium and sodium channels, which lead to neuronal depolarization. Sustained depolarization may maintain GCSE and eventually cause neuronal death through calcium-, free radical-, and kinase-mediated events.[9] Although drugs acting as NMDA and AMPA receptor antagonists seem attractive, it is likely that glutamate is not the sole mechanism for GCSE and that other mechanisms become increasingly important as the duration of seizures increases.

GABA$_A$ postsynaptic receptors control chloride channels to produce hyperpolarization (inhibition) of the postsynaptic cell membrane. These receptors have binding sites for GABA and select anticonvulsants (e.g., phenobarbital and benzodiazepines) and enhance GABA$_A$-mediated chloride inhibitory currents. It was previously thought that a decrease in presynaptic GABA led to prolonged seizures; however, it is currently held that GABA concentrations increase during the early phases of GCSE and continue to be elevated during late GCSE. Prolonged seizures lead to decreased inhibitory GABA$_A$-receptor density because of postsynaptic receptor endocytosis. Additionally, modification of GABA$_A$ receptors during SE may decrease response to both endogenous GABA and GABA agonists.[10] Clinically, the relative potencies of benzodiazepines and phenobarbital can be reduced up to tenfold if seizures persist for more than 30 minutes.[10] A similar phenomenon occurs with sodium channel antagonists (phenytoin); however, the magnitude of resistance is believed to be less.

PATHOPHYSIOLOGY

As GCSE continues, there are systemic alterations, progression of motor phenomena, and development of specific EEG findings.[14] Two distinct and predictable phases have been identified. Phase I occurs during the first 30 minutes of seizure activity, and phase II immediately follows. Although these systemic complications affect the prognosis of GCSE, a prolonged seizure can destroy neurons independent of these systemic events.[9] In fact, the systemic effects of induced seizures in animals can be blocked, but the damage to the neocortex, cerebellum, and hippocampus persists.

During phase I, each seizure produces marked increases in plasma epinephrine, norepinephrine, and steroid concentrations that can cause hypertension, tachycardia, and cardiac arrhythmias.[15] Within minutes, arterial systolic pressures can rise to above 200 mm Hg, and heart rate can increase by 83 beats per minute. Although blood pressure returns to normal within 60 minutes, mean arterial pressure does not fall below 60 mm Hg; hence, cerebral perfusion pressure is not compromised. In animals, cerebral blood flow is also increased, thereby protecting neurons from hypoxic injury.

Seizure-induced increases in sympathetic and parasympathetic stimulation of the heart, in the presence of a hypoxic myocardium, can result in ventricular arrhythmias. Autonomic neuron stimulation can cause a release of insulin and glucagon. Concurrently, circulating catecholamines cause an elevation of hepatic cyclic adenosine monophosphate, producing glycogenolysis. Although the patient can be hyperglycemic initially, serum glucose concentration begins to fall.

Seizure-induced muscular contractions and hypoxia cause lactic acid release, which can produce a severe acidosis that can be accompanied by hypotension and shock. Muscle contractions can be so severe that rhabdomyolysis with secondary hyperkalemia and acute tubular necrosis can occur. The airway can be obstructed, causing the patient to become cyanotic or hypoxic. Additionally, an increase in salivation and tracheal and pulmonary secretions can cause aspiration pneumonia. Although transient pleocytosis can develop, it should not be attributed to SE until infectious causes have been eliminated.

Between seizures, the EEG slows, and blood pressure normalizes. Although metabolic demands are increased, the brain is able to adequately compensate. During phase II (e.g., seizures exceed 30 minutes), the EEG ictal discharge and clonic motor activity become continuous, and the patient begins to decompensate. Despite elevated levels of catecholamines, the patient can become hypotensive. During this time, autoregulation of cerebral blood flow becomes dependent on mean arterial pressure and begins to fail. There continues to be an excessive consumption of oxygen and glucose; however, compensatory mechanisms are no longer able to keep up with demands.

During this time, the serum glucose concentration may be normal or decreased. Profound hypoglycemia, secondary to hyperinsulinemia, can occur in those with hepatic dysfunction or reduced glycogen stores. Hyperthermia and respiratory deterioration with hypoxia and ventilatory failure can develop. Metabolic and biochemical complications, including respiratory and metabolic acidosis, hyperkalemia, hyponatremia, and azotemia may develop. There is increased sweating and salivation.

CLINICAL PRESENTATION OF GCSE

Symptoms

- Impaired consciousness (e.g., lethargy to coma)
- Disorientation once GCSE is controlled
- Pain associated with injuries (e.g., tongue lacerations, shoulder dislocations, head trauma)

Early Signs

- Generalized convulsions
- Acute injuries or CNS insults that cause extensor or flexor posturing
- Hypothermia or fever suggestive of intercurrent illnesses (e.g., sepsis or meningitis)
- Incontinence
- Normal blood pressure or hypotension and respiratory compromise

Late Signs

- Clinical seizures may or may not be apparent
- Pulmonary edema with respiratory failure
- Cardiac failure (dysrhythmias, arrest, cardiogenic shock)
- Hypotension or hypertension
- Disseminated intravascular coagulation, multisystem organ failure
- Rhabdomyolysis
- Hyperpyremia

Initial Laboratory Tests

- Complete blood count (CBC) with differential
- Serum chemistry profile (e.g., electrolytes, calcium, magnesium, glucose, serum creatinine, alanine aminotransferase [ALT], aspartate aminotransferase [AST])
- Urine drug/alcohol screen
- Blood cultures
- Arterial blood gas to assess for metabolic and respiratory acidosis
- Serum drug concentration if previous anticonvulsant suspected or known

Other Diagnostic Tests

- Spinal tap if CNS infection suspected
- EEG should be obtained on presentation and once clinical seizures are controlled
- CT with and without contrast
- MRI
- Radiograph if indicated to diagnose fractures

CLINICAL PRESENTATION AND DIAGNOSIS

Accurate diagnosis requires observation, physical examination, laboratory assessment, EEG, and neurologic imaging. The nature and duration of the seizure should be obtained, and a diagnosis of GCSE should not be made until a clinician has observed at least one seizure. Most patients have an altered consciousness that ranges from obtunded to marked lethargy and somnolence with pronounced eyes-open unresponsiveness and waxy rigidity. Motor features can include muscle contractions, extensor or flexor posturing, and spasms. Over time, the clinical manifestations become less apparent. This has important ramifications in that seizures appear to have terminated without treatment or when an ineffective therapy is given.

In addition to an assessment of language and cognitive abilities, the physical and neurological examinations should assess motor, sensory, and reflex abnormalities, pupillary response, asymmetry, and posturing. The patient should also be examined for secondary injuries (e.g., tongue lacerations, shoulder dislocations, and head and facial trauma).

Laboratory tests are essential to the diagnosis of various etiologies. Hypoglycemia, hyponatremia, hypernatremia, hypomagnesemia, hypocalcemia, and renal failure all can cause seizures. A urine drug screen can help eliminate the possibility of illicit drug use or drug overdose. Serum drug concentration(s) should be obtained in those on chronic anticonvulsants, because high concentrations of certain medications can induce seizures, and low concentrations can reflect noncompliance or rapid drug withdrawal. A baseline serum concentration is necessary to determine whether a loading dose of a specific anticonvulsant is required. Assessment of other laboratory parameters (e.g., albumin, renal function, and hepatic function) that affect anticonvulsant dosing also can be useful. An EEG is a valuable diagnostic tool, particularly in those with prolonged GCSE in whom clinically apparent seizures are not always evident, but therapy should not be delayed while awaiting testing or results.

Once seizures have stopped, it is important to determine if the patient is febrile or has a systemic or CNS infection. Many physiologic consequences of GCSE (e.g., leukocytosis, pleocytosis, and hyperthermia) produce symptoms that can be confused with other conditions. If a CNS infection is suspected, empiric antibiotics should be started, and a spinal tap should be performed. Computed tomography (CT) or magnetic resonance imaging (MRI) should be obtained to eliminate vascular, neoplastic, or infectious etiologies.

TREATMENT

Various treatments are available for the management of GCSE. These range from abortion of impending SE with rescue medications to the use of pharmacological and nonpharmacological therapies for GCSE and refractory/resistant SE.

■ DESIRED OUTCOMES

The short-term desired outcomes of treatment of GCSE are (1) immediate termination of all clinical and electrical seizure activity, (2) no clinically significant adverse effects, and (3) lack of recurrent seizure activity. ❻ ❼ The long-term desired outcomes are to minimize or avoid the likelihood of pharmacoresistent epilepsy and/or the development of neurologic sequelae that significantly impact quality of life.

■ NONPHARMACOLOGIC THERAPY

Vital signs should be assessed, an adequate and protected airway should be established, ventilation should be maintained, and oxygen should be administered. Frequent arterial blood gas determinations should assess for metabolic acidosis, which should be treated with sodium bicarbonate if the pH is less than 7.2. Assisted ventilation should be used to correct respiratory acidosis.

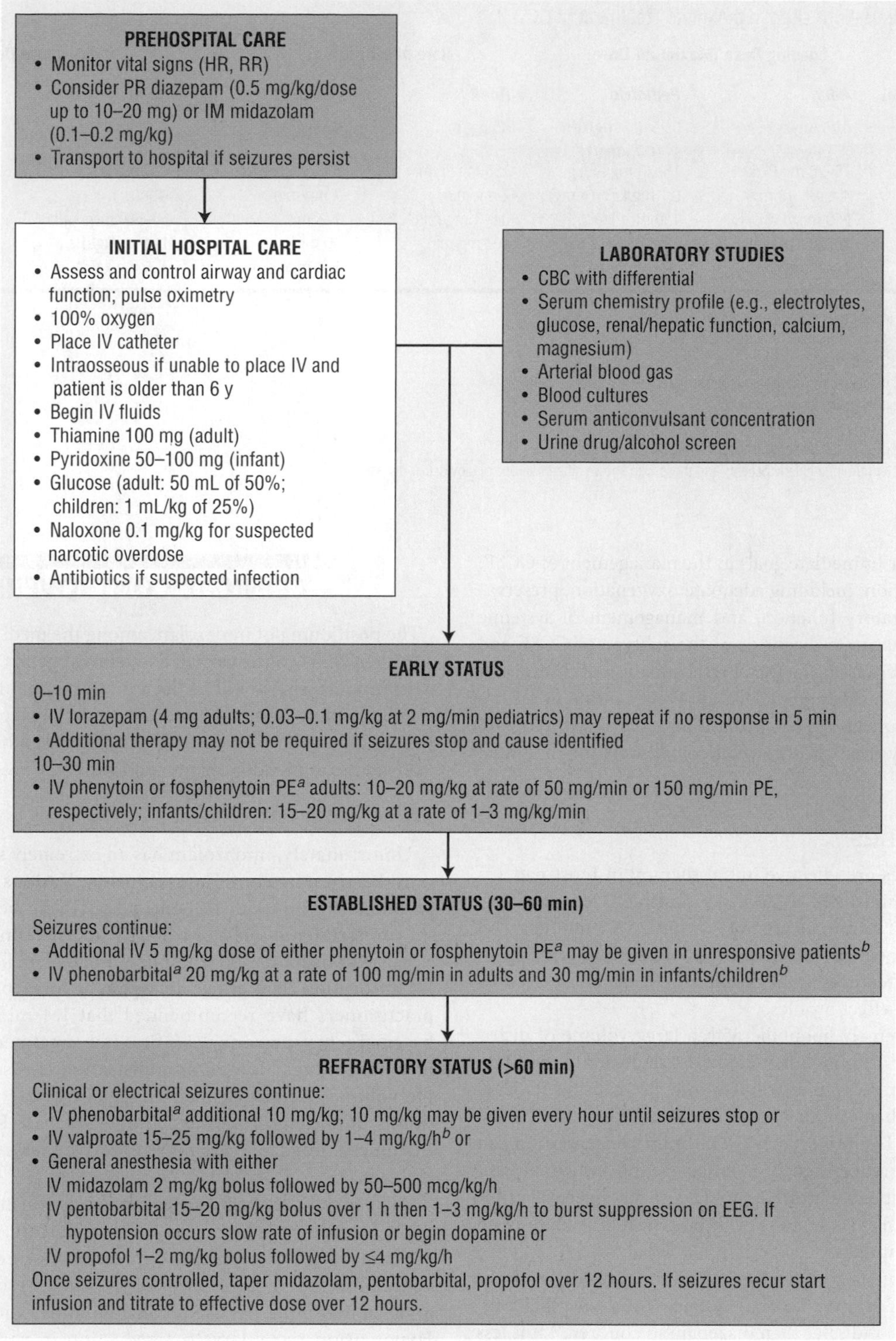

PREHOSPITAL CARE
- Monitor vital signs (HR, RR)
- Consider PR diazepam (0.5 mg/kg/dose up to 10–20 mg) or IM midazolam (0.1–0.2 mg/kg)
- Transport to hospital if seizures persist

INITIAL HOSPITAL CARE
- Assess and control airway and cardiac function; pulse oximetry
- 100% oxygen
- Place IV catheter
- Intraosseous if unable to place IV and patient is older than 6 y
- Begin IV fluids
- Thiamine 100 mg (adult)
- Pyridoxine 50–100 mg (infant)
- Glucose (adult: 50 mL of 50%; children: 1 mL/kg of 25%)
- Naloxone 0.1 mg/kg for suspected narcotic overdose
- Antibiotics if suspected infection

LABORATORY STUDIES
- CBC with differential
- Serum chemistry profile (e.g., electrolytes, glucose, renal/hepatic function, calcium, magnesium)
- Arterial blood gas
- Blood cultures
- Serum anticonvulsant concentration
- Urine drug/alcohol screen

EARLY STATUS
0–10 min
- IV lorazepam (4 mg adults; 0.03–0.1 mg/kg at 2 mg/min pediatrics) may repeat if no response in 5 min
- Additional therapy may not be required if seizures stop and cause identified
10–30 min
- IV phenytoin or fosphenytoin PE[a] adults: 10–20 mg/kg at rate of 50 mg/min or 150 mg/min PE, respectively; infants/children: 15–20 mg/kg at a rate of 1–3 mg/kg/min

ESTABLISHED STATUS (30–60 min)
Seizures continue:
- Additional IV 5 mg/kg dose of either phenytoin or fosphenytoin PE[a] may be given in unresponsive patients[b]
- IV phenobarbital[a] 20 mg/kg at a rate of 100 mg/min in adults and 30 mg/min in infants/children[b]

REFRACTORY STATUS (>60 min)
Clinical or electrical seizures continue:
- IV phenobarbital[a] additional 10 mg/kg; 10 mg/kg may be given every hour until seizures stop or
- IV valproate 15–25 mg/kg followed by 1–4 mg/kg/h[b] or
- General anesthesia with either
  IV midazolam 2 mg/kg bolus followed by 50–500 mcg/kg/h
  IV pentobarbital 15–20 mg/kg bolus over 1 h then 1–3 mg/kg/h to burst suppression on EEG. If hypotension occurs slow rate of infusion or begin dopamine or
  IV propofol 1–2 mg/kg bolus followed by ≤4 mg/kg/h
Once seizures controlled, taper midazolam, pentobarbital, propofol over 12 hours. If seizures recur start infusion and titrate to effective dose over 12 hours.

FIGURE 66-1. Algorithm for the treatment of GCSE. (CBC, complete blood count; EEG, electroencephalogram; GCSE, generalized convulsive status epilepticus; HR, heart rate; PR, per rectum; RR, respiratory rate.) [a]Because variability exists in dosing, monitor serum concentration. [b]If seizure is controlled, begin maintenance does and optimize using serum concentration monitoring.

Because electrical seizures may persist in the absence of clinical motor manifestations, an EEG should be performed in anyone who continues to have altered consciousness after clinical control of their seizures. Although hypoglycemia rarely causes GCSE, adults and children should receive 50 mL of a 50% dextrose solution, and 1 mL/kg of a 25% dextrose solution, respectively.[4,7] Because Wernicke encephalopathy can develop in alcoholics, adults should receive IV thiamine (100 mg) prior to glucose.[4] Serum glucose concentration should be determined to assess the need for further supplementation.

■ PHARMACOLOGIC THERAPY

When a seizure does not stop within 5 minutes, or when doubt exists regarding the diagnosis, patients should be treated as if they have GCSE. Figure 66–1 provides an algorithm for the treatment of GCSE.

TABLE 66-3 Medications Used in the Initial Treatment of GCSE

Anticonvulsant (Route)	Loading Dose (Maximum Dose)		Rate of Infusion		Maintenance Dose	
	Adult	Pediatric	Adult	Pediatric	Adult	Pediatric
Diazepam (IV bolus)	0.25 mg/kg[a,b,c] (40 mg)	0.25–0.5 mg/kg[a,c] (0.75 mg/kg)	<5 mg/min	<5 mg/min	Not used	Not used
Fosphenytoin IV	15–20 mg PE/kg	15–20 mg PE/kg	150 mg PE/min	3 mg PE/kg/min	4–5 mg PE/kg/d	5–10 mg PE/kg/d
Lorazepam (IV bolus)	4 mg[a,b,c] (8 mg)	0.1 mg/kg[a,c] (4 mg)	2 mg/min	2 mg/min	Not used	Not used
Midazolam IV	200 mcg/kg[a,d]	150 mcg/kg[a,d]	0.5–1 mg/min	2–3 min	50–500 mcg/kg/h[e]	60–120 mcg/kg/h[e]
Phenobarbital IV	10–20 mg/kg[e]	15–20 mg/kg[e]	100 mg/min	30 mg/min	1–4 mg/kg/d[e]	3–5 mg/kg/d[e]
Phenytoin IV	10–20 mg/kg[f]	10–20 mg/kg[f]	50 mg/min[g]	1–3 mg/kg/min	4–5 mg/kg/d[e]	5–10 mg/kg/d[e]

GCSE, generalized convulsive status epilepticus; PE, phenytoin equivalents.
[a]Doses can be repeated every 10 to 15 minutes until the maximum dosage is given.
[b]Initial doses in the elderly are 2 to 5 mg.
[c]Larger doses can be required if patients chronically on a benzodiazepine (e.g., clonazepam).
[d]Can be given by the intramuscular, rectal, or buccal routes.
[e]Titrate dose as needed.
[f]Administer additional loading dose based on serum concentration.
[g]The rate should not exceed 25 mg/min in elderly patients and those with known atherosclerotic cardiovascular disease.

❼ There are four immediate goals in the management of GCSE: (1) patient stabilization, including adequate oxygenation, preservation of cardiorespiratory function, and management of systemic complications; (2) accurate diagnosis of the subtype of GCSE and identification of precipitating factors; (3) termination of clinical and electrical seizures as early as possible; and (4) prevention of seizure recurrence. The benzodiazepines, hydantoins, and barbiturates are the most commonly used classes of anticonvulsants for the initial treatment of GCSE.

Benzodiazepines

The benzodiazepines are effective initial therapy in most patients and should be administered as soon as possible. Generally, one or two IV doses will terminate seizures within 2 to 3 minutes.[4] All benzodiazepines are equally effective; therefore, the preferred agent is determined by differences in the pharmacokinetic, pharmacoeconomic, and adverse-effect profiles.

Diazepam is extremely lipophilic with a large volume of distribution (1–2 L/kg).[15] Although it initially distributes into the brain within seconds, it rapidly redistributes into fat, causing its CNS half-life to be less than 1 hour and its duration of effect to be less than 30 minutes.[15] The rapid decrease in brain concentration can cause seizure recurrence; hence, a longer-acting anticonvulsant (e.g., phenytoin or phenobarbital) should also be given. The initial dose of diazepam (Table 66–3) can be repeated if there is no response within 5 minutes.[15]

❽ Most practitioners consider lorazepam the benzodiazepine of choice.[4,15] A recent Cochrane Database Review concluded that lorazepam is as effective and safer than diazepam in children.[16] It is less lipid soluble than diazepam and takes longer to achieve peak concentrations in the brain; however, its minimal redistribution into fat results in a longer duration of action in the CNS that can provide seizure protection for up to 24 hours.[4,15] It also has a higher-affinity binding to the benzodiazepine receptor than diazepam.

Initial lorazepam dosing (Table 66–3) can be repeated if the patient does not respond in 5 minutes.[4,15] Patients chronically on a benzodiazepine (e.g., clonazepam) might have developed tolerance and could require larger doses than other patients. Diazepam and lorazepam cause vein irritation and should be diluted with an equal volume of compatible diluent before administration. Diazepam and lorazepam contain propylene glycol, which can cause dysrhythmia and hypotension if administered too rapidly.[15] Because of slow and erratic absorption, they should not be given intramuscularly (IM).

CLINICAL CONTROVERSY

The positioning of midazolam among the medications used to treat GCSE is controversial. Some investigators recommend that midazolam should be the anticonvulsant of first choice and, therefore, should be used in lieu of lorazepam; others argue that it should be used after a hydantoin has failed; still others recommend it only for refractory GCSE.

Unfortunately, midazolam has an extremely short half-life and must be given by continuous infusion. Various routes of administration (e.g., buccal, IM, intranasal) have been used successfully to terminate seizures when IV access cannot be established. Because of its increased solubility, midazolam has a more reliable IM absorption than either diazepam or lorazepam. In fact, some practitioners have recommended that IM midazolam be given by emergency personnel as first-line treatment in the out-of-hospital setting.[17] Buccal administration is easily accomplished, the volume of fluid is small enough (e.g., 2–5 mL) that aspiration is unlikely. A recent Cochrane Database Review concluded that buccal midazolam is more effective than rectal diazepam in children.[16]

All benzodiazepines can impair consciousness and interfere with neurologic assessment. Although rare, brief (less than 1 minute) cardiorespiratory depression can necessitate assisted ventilation or require intubation. This is especially true if a benzodiazepine is used concomitantly with a barbiturate. Hypotension secondary to a reduction in vasomotor tone can occur following large doses.[4]

CLINICAL CONTROVERSY

The choice of long-acting anticonvulsant to give following the initial benzodiazepine is controversial. According to the Working Group on Status Epilepticus, phenytoin should be used in seizures that recur after treatment with a benzodiazepine.[15] Although this has been the practice for decades; no studies have documented the superiority of a hydantoin over other anticonvulsants. Thus, it is questionable if a hydantoin should be administered alone, in larger doses, or at all when seizures recur following benzodiazepine administration.

Phenytoin

❾ A hydantoin is the second-line agent in GCSE that is unresponsive to the benzodiazepines or in seizures that recur after successful treatment with a benzodiazepine.[4] Although it is effective in terminating seizures in 40% to 91% of patients,[15] it can be inferior to lorazepam, phenobarbital, or diazepam plus phenytoin at stopping GCSE within 20 minutes of their infusion.[18,19]

Phenytoin has a long half-life (20–36 hours) and causes less respiratory depression and sedation than the benzodiazepines or phenobarbital;[15] however, it cannot be delivered rapidly enough to be considered a first-line single agent. Injectable phenytoin should be diluted to less than or equal to 5 mg/mL in normal saline. Microcrystals will precipitate if it is mixed in a glucose-containing solution. The vehicle (40% propylene glycol) can cause administration-related hypotension and cardiac arrhythmias. These effects are more likely to occur if large loading doses are given to elderly individuals with preexisting cardiac disease or in critically ill patients with marginal blood pressure.[15] Vital signs and an ECG should be obtained during administration. The infusion rate should be slowed if the QT interval widens or if hypotension or arrhythmias develop.[15] **❿** The maximum rate of infusion is 50 mg/min in adults, 25 mg/min in the elderly, and 3 mg/kg/min in children weighing less than 50 kg (110 lb).[4]

Suggested IV loading doses are provided in Table 66–3.[15] A reduction in the loading dose is recommended for elderly patients,[15] and a larger loading dose is required in obese individuals.[20] If the patient has been on phenytoin prior to admission and the serum concentration is known, this should be considered in determining a loading dose. Although some advocate the administration of an additional 5 mg/kg in those with unresponsive GCSE, there is no evidence that this will be beneficial. This practice can cause concentrations to exceed the reference range and produce toxicity. Because phenytoin has poor lipid solubility and enters the brain slowly, it can take up to 60 minutes before the pharmacodynamic effect is apparent. This delay is important when considering administration of a second 5 mg/kg loading dose. Therapeutic serum concentrations, 10 to 20 mg/L (40–79 μmol/L), generally do not persist more than 24 hours; hence, maintenance doses (see Table 66–3) should be started within 12 to 24 hours of the loading dose.

Phenytoin has an alkaline pH, which may cause pain and burning during infusion; phlebitis can occur with chronic infusion, and tissue necrosis is likely on infiltration. IM administration is not recommended because absorption is delayed and erratic, and phenytoin can crystallize in tissue. Although oral loading doses have been used in patients not actively seizing, it may take 4 to 12 hours before adequate serum concentrations are obtained; thus, this practice is not recommended.

CLINICAL CONTROVERSY

The debate continues as to which hydantoin is preferred in GCSE. Although phenytoin has been used for decades, it is associated with a variety of problems related to its formulation. Conversely, fosphenytoin is associated with less infusion pain and IV-site complications and fewer hemodynamic effects than phenytoin. Although most practitioners believe that fosphenytoin is clearly a "better" formulation, many struggle with the advantages of fosphenytoin, given its cost.

Fosphenytoin

Fosphenytoin, a water-soluble phosphate ester, has no known pharmacologic activity.[21] It is converted rapidly (7–15 minutes) and completely (100%) to phenytoin by blood and tissue phosphatases after IV and IM dosing.[21] The conversion delay was a concern initially; however, this time is offset by high protein binding, saturable binding at high concentrations, and the rapid rate of infusion.[21] It does not contain propylene glycol and is compatible with most common IV fluids.

Nystagmus, dizziness, and ataxia are the most frequent adverse events and are attributed to phenytoin. The frequency of ECG or blood pressure changes is less than that for phenytoin. Nonallergic paresthesia and pruritus of the face and groin are unique to fosphenytoin and are related to dose and infusion rate, and rarely require discontinuation of fosphenytoin. These side effects typically subside within 5 to 10 minutes after the infusion.[21]

Fosphenytoin should be dosed using phenytoin equivalents (PE), thereby obviating the need for interconversion between phenytoin and fosphenytoin. The loading dose and rates of administration of fosphenytoin can be found in Table 66–3. Because of delays in achieving adequate phenytoin serum concentrations, a loading dose should not be given IM unless IV access is impossible. Continuous ECG, blood pressure, and respiratory status monitoring is recommended for all loading doses.

Fosphenytoin serum concentrations have no value. Serum phenytoin concentrations should be used for therapeutic drug monitoring, and the desired serum concentration range is the same as that for phenytoin. Fosphenytoin cross-reacts with some phenytoin immunoassays causing an overestimation of phenytoin concentration; hence, blood should not be obtained for at least 2 hours after IV and 4 hours after IM administration.[21]

CLINICAL CONTROVERSY

There are three different opinions regarding the use of phenobarbital in GCSE. Because barbiturates cause CNS and respiratory depression, as well as hypotension, most contend that phenobarbital should be the third-line agent when a benzodiazepine plus phenytoin has failed. Others suggest that the barbiturates are as safe and effective as other anticonvulsants and should be the drug of choice following a benzodiazepine. Still others support continuous-infusion midazolam as the third-line anticonvulsant before the barbiturates. Currently, most practitioners agree that phenobarbital is the long-acting anticonvulsant of choice in patients with hypersensitivity to the hydantoins or in those with cardiac conduction abnormalities.

Phenobarbital

Phenobarbital has biphasic distribution into body organs.[22] During phase I, the drug distributes into highly vascular organs, but it does not distribute into the brain. With the exception of fat, phenobarbital distributes throughout the body during phase II[22]; hence, lean body mass should be used in calculating doses in obese patients.[22] Although the highest brain concentrations occur 12 to 60 minutes after an IV dose,[22] seizures are controlled within minutes of the loading dose.[19] Despite two studies that found phenobarbital to be as effective as phenytoin, lorazepam, or diazepam plus phenytoin in patients with GCSE,[18] the Working Group on Status Epilepticus recommends that phenobarbital be given after a benzodiazepine plus phenytoin has failed.[15]

The loading and maintenance dose are given in Table 66–3. When necessary, larger loading doses (30 mg/kg) have been used in neonates without adverse effects. If the initial loading dose does not stop the seizures within 20 to 30 minutes, an additional 10 to 20 mg/kg can be given. If seizures continue, a third 10 mg/kg load can be given.[23] Phenobarbital exhibits first-order linear pharmacokinetics, and there is no maximum dose beyond which further doses are likely to be ineffective.[23] Once GCSE is controlled, the maintenance dose should be started within 12 to 24 hours.

Although injectable phenobarbital contains propylene glycol, it can be given more rapidly than phenytoin (see Table 66–3). It can be given IM, but its rate of absorption is too slow to be effective. Phenobarbital can depress consciousness and respiration. The risk of apnea and hypopnea can be more profound in patients treated initially with benzodiazepines.[4,15] If significant hypotension develops, the infusion should be slowed or stopped.[15]

■ TREATMENT OF REFRACTORY GCSE

⓫ When adequate doses of a benzodiazepine, hydantoin, or barbiturate have failed, the condition is termed *refractory*. Approximately 10% to 15% of patients will develop refractory GCSE, and approximately 30% whose seizures are "clinically" controlled will have persistent electrical manifestations after administration of these anticonvulsants. When a patient develops refractory GCSE, an intense search should be performed for an acute or progressive cause.

It should be remembered that the longer GCSE lasts, the harder it is to treat and that failure to treat aggressively early in the course of disease increases the likelihood of nonresponse.[15] While the goal is to stop electrical epileptiform activity, there is no consensus regarding the anticonvulsant of choice, sequencing of therapy, or treatment of refractory GCSE. Approaches used include the continuous infusion of a benzodiazepines, medically induced coma, valproate, lacosamide, levetiracetam, topiramate, propofol, or lidocaine. Doses for these agents can be found in Table 66–4. A meta-analysis compared midazolam, propofol, and pentobarbital in refractory GCSE.[25] Overall response rates were significantly greater in those treated with pentobarbital (92%) compared to midazolam (80%) and propofol (73%). Breakthrough seizures were more commonly observed with midazolam (51%) versus propofol (15%) and pentobarbital (12%). Although pentobarbital had a greater response rate, clinically significant hypotension was more common. Mortality rates were similar for the three drugs.

Benzodiazepines

Some advocated that anesthetic doses of midazolam should be the first-line agent in refractory GCSE.[25] Table 66–4 contains the loading and maintenance doses of midazolam. Most patients respond to these doses within an hour, but the continuous-infusion rate should be increased every 15 minutes in those who do not. Because tachyphylaxis can develop, frequent increases in the infusion rate can be necessary, and dosing should be guided by EEG response.

Once GCSE is terminated, dosages can be decreased by 1 mcg/kg/min every 2 hours. Successful discontinuation is enhanced by maintaining the patient's phenytoin and phenobarbital serum concentration(s) above 20 mg/L (79 μmol/L) and 40 mg/L (172 μmol/L), respectively. Because of midazolam's short half-life, patients can return to consciousness more rapidly than those receiving larger doses of more sedating anticonvulsants (e.g., phenytoin, phenobarbital). Generally, continuous-infusion midazolam has been well tolerated, with few cases of hypotension and respiratory depression. Hypotension and poikilothermia can occur and can require supportive therapies.

Large-dose continuous-infusion lorazepam also has been used successfully.[26] Unlike midazolam, lorazepam contains propylene glycol, which can accumulate during continuous infusions. Propylene glycol toxicity can cause a marked osmolar gap, metabolic acidosis, and renal toxicity.[27]

Medically Induced Coma

If there is an inadequate response to large doses of midazolam, anesthetizing the patient to suppress the cerebral ictal discharge is recommended.[15,24] Although it is likely that the patient is already being mechanically ventilated, intubation and respiratory support are mandatory during barbiturate coma. Because hypotension is a concern, it is essential that vital signs be monitored continuously. A short-acting barbiturate (usually either pentobarbital or thiopental) generally is preferred because it allows a more rapid reversal of coma.

Several sources note that the initial loading dose of pentobarbital is 5 mg/kg.[15] However, this dose is inadequate to achieve the serum concentrations (40 mg/L; 177 μmoL/L) necessary to induce an isoelectric EEG. Pentobarbital should be initiated with a loading dose of at least 10 to 20 mg/kg over 1 to 2 hours[24] (see Table 66–4). If hypotension occurs during the loading dose, the rate of administration should be slowed, or dopamine should be administered. The loading dose should be followed immediately by a continuous infusion.[15] Rates are typically begun at 1 mg/kg/h and titrated as needed up to a dose of 5 mg/kg/h. The maintenance infusion should be increased gradually until there is evidence of burst suppression on EEG (i.e., isoelectric EEG) or prohibitive adverse effects occur. Although the duration of barbiturate coma in most studies has been 2 to 3 days, it has been used safely for 53 days in

TABLE 66–4 Medications Used to Treat Refractory GCSE

Anticonvulsant (Route)	Loading Dose		Infusion Duration		Maintenance Dose	
	Adult	*Pediatric*	*Adult*	*Pediatric*	*Adult*	*Pediatric*
Lacosamide	200–300 mg	NA	3–5 min	NA	200 mg/d	NA
Levetiracetam IV	500–2,000 mg	15–70 mg/kg	33–66 mg/min	2–5 mg/kg/min	750–9,000 mg/d	20–60 mg/kg/d
Lidocaine IV	50–100 mg	1 mg/kg (max. dose = 3–5 mg/kg in first hour)	≤2 min	≤2 min	1.5–3.5 mg/kg/h	1.2–3 mg/kg/h
Midazolam IV	200 mcg/kg[a]	150 mcg/kg[a]	0.5–1 mg/min	0.5–1 mg/min	50–500 mcg/kg/h[b]	60–120 mcg/kg/h[b]
Pentobarbital IV	10–20 mg/kg	15–20 mg/kg	Over 1–2 h	Over 1–2 h	1–5 mg/kg/h[b]	1–5 mg/kg/h[b]
Propofol IV	2 mg/kg	3 mg/kg	Over 10 sec	Over 20–30 sec	5–10 mg/kg/h[b]	2–18 mg/kg/h[c]
Topiramate PO	300–1,600 mg	5–10 mg/kg	NA	NA	400–1,600 mg/d	5–10 mg/kg/d
Valproate IV	15–45 mg/kg	20–25 mg/kg	3 mg/kg/min	3 mg/kg/min	1–4 mg/kg/h[b]	1–4 mg/kg/h[b]

GCSE, generalized convulsive status epilepticus; NA, not available; PO, orally.
[a]Doses can be repeated twice every 10 to 15 minutes until the maximum dosage is given.
[b]Titrate dose as needed.
[c]Generally recommended not to exceed a dose of 4 mg/kg/h and a duration of 48 hours.

an 18-year-old patient.[28] To avoid complications (e.g., pneumonia, pulmonary edema), the pentobarbital should be discontinued as soon as possible. Twelve hours after a burst-suppression pattern is obtained, the rate of pentobarbital infusion should be titrated downward every 2 to 4 hours to enable the clinician to determine if the patient's GCSE is in remission. It is important to have other anticonvulsants at therapeutic amounts before pentobarbital is withdrawn so that the risk of seizure recurrence is minimized. Because pentobarbital is a potent hepatic enzyme inducer, doses of most concurrent anticonvulsants will need to be larger than usual maintenance doses. The patient will need to be monitored for side effects as deinduction occurs and anticonvulsant concentrations increase. This can take up to a month after pentobarbital's discontinuation.

Valproate

Although an IV dosage form has been approved by the FDA, it is not labeled for GCSE. A number of loading and continuous-infusion doses (see Table 66–4) have been used to treat GCSE in both adult and pediatric patients. Loading doses have ranged from 20 to 40 mg/kg.[25,29] Although the manufacturer originally recommended IV valproate be given no faster than 20 mg/min, much faster rates have been studied (40 mg/min; 2–10 mg/kg/min) and are used for administration of the loading dose.[25,29] The loading dose should be followed by a continuous or intermittent infusion. One study suggested the need to consider the effects of enzyme-inducing anticonvulsants when dosing and recommended that the continuous-infusion rate be determined by the presence of concurrent anticonvulsants (no inducers present, 1 mg/kg/h; one or more inducers [e.g., phenytoin, phenobarbital], 2 mg/kg/h; and inducers and pentobarbital coma, 4 mg/kg/h).[30]

In general, IV valproate has been well tolerated, with no cases of respiratory depression. Hemodynamic instability is extremely rare, but patients' vital signs should be monitored closely during the loading dose.

Propofol

Propofol is extremely lipid soluble, has a large volume of distribution, and has a very rapid onset of action. Its extremely short half-life promotes rapid awakening on drug discontinuation. Propofol's efficacy is comparable to midazolam for refractory GCSE.[24,31] Doses can be found in Table 66–4. Although controversial, it has been associated with progressive metabolic acidosis, hemodynamic instability, and bradyarrhythmias that maybe refractory to aggressive treatments.[32] Finally, a normal adult dose can provide over 1,000 calories (4186 J) per day as lipid at a cost to the patient that may exceed $800 per day.

Other Agents

In most reports, oral topiramate has been given in adults (300–1,600 mg/day) and in children (5–10 mg/kg/day).[13,25,33–36] Crushing the tablets and dissolving them in small amounts of water is necessary as no parenteral formulation is available. Doses as large as 25 mg/kg/day for 2 to 5 days have been used in children.[36] Response tends to be delayed hours to days. Because topiramate can induce metabolic acidosis and kidney stones, monitoring acid–base status and adequate hydration are recommended. Once seizures are controlled, doses should be tapered to a tolerable maintenance dose.

Oral doses of levetiracetam (750–9,000 mg/day) have been given in case series; however, doses larger than 3,000 mg/day do not add additional efficacy.[13,25,37] IV levetiracetam has begun to replace oral levetiracetam in refractory GCSE. Loading doses of up to 2,000 mg have been given to adults and up to 70 mg/kg in

children.[38–40] Levetiracetam is not hepatically metabolized and is minimally protein bound, which makes drug–drug interactions unlikely. There have been two case reports of lacosamide used in refractory GCSE and NCSE.[41,42] Like levetiracetam, its lack of effect on the metabolism on other medications make it attractive for use. Neither levetiracetam nor lacosamide has been associated with toxicities (respiratory depression, hypotension) noted with the older anticonvulsants.

Lidocaine has been used in refractory GCSE, but its use is not recommended unless other agents have failed.[43] It is administered IV and has a rapid onset of action. Table 66–4 gives the recommended initial loading and continuous-infusion doses. Although the reference serum concentration range for the antiarrhythmic effects of lidocaine is 2 to 6 mg/L (8.5–25.6 µmol/L), the reference range for GCSE has not been established. Serum lidocaine concentrations should be monitored to avoid drug accumulation and toxicity. CNS toxicity (e.g., fasciculations, visual disturbances, and tinnitus) can occur at concentrations between 6 and 8 mg/L (25.6 to 34.2 µmol/L); seizures and obtundation can develop when concentrations exceed 8 mg/L (34.2 µmol/L).

Halothane, isoflurane, ketamine, and other inhaled anesthetics can produce EEG suppression; however, these gases are difficult to deliver outside the operating room and require an anesthesiologist. No proven advantages have been shown over traditional anticonvulsants (e.g., barbiturate coma or continuous-infusion benzodiazepine), and these gases can increase intracranial pressure. If used, dosing is titrated to obtain EEG burst suppression. Finally, it is also prudent to validate that the patient does not have a low serum-magnesium concentration, because magnesium deficiency can lower the seizure threshold.

PHARMACOECONOMIC CONSIDERATIONS

The estimated reimbursement for treatment of GCSE varies greatly based on the age of the individual and the GCSE etiology. A population study showed that the median reimbursement for GCSE was $8,417.[44] Median reimbursements were significantly greater for those 17 to 45 years of age ($14,689), those with acute CNS injury ($16,919), and those withdrawing from alcohol or anticonvulsants ($11,239). Lowest median reimbursements were found in those 0 to 16 years of age ($6,140) and those with non-CNS injury ($6,669). For patients with lengths of stay shorter than 1 week, the average reimbursement was $7,000 but increased to $32,907 if the stay was longer than 1 week. For patients staying 1 month or more, reimbursements were more than $60,000. Compared with other acute disorders (myocardial infarction, congestive heart failure, and intracranial hemorrhage), reimbursements for GCSE are 1.6- to 1.9-fold greater.

A number of economic issues can have an impact on formulary considerations. Clearly, there are intra- and interclass differences in medication costs and in ancillary tests or technologies associated with select therapies. For example, the average wholesale prices for seven therapies initiated in a patient weighing 70 kg (154 lb) are:

- Diazepam (20 mg) plus generic phenytoin (1 g): $14.68
- Lorazepam alone (8 mg): $6.72
- Midazolam alone (0.25 mg/kg load, 0.1 mg/kg/h): $51.34
- Generic phenytoin (1 g) alone: $14.34
- Diazepam (20 mg) plus fosphenytoin PE (1 g): $154.14
- Phenobarbital (20 mg/kg) alone: $35.15
- IV valproate (25 mg/kg load, 1 mg/kg/h): $123.00

Although many practitioners have heralded the arrival of fosphenytoin as an important therapeutic advancement, it has created a fiscal and ethical dilemma for many institutions. Fosphenytoin is associated with less infusion pain and fewer IV-site complications and hemodynamic adverse effects than phenytoin; however, the cost of this agent ($149/g PE versus $14.47/g phenytoin) has caused many practitioners and administrators to struggle with the practical and ethical importance of the increased safety profile relative to the cost of the product to an institution. When evaluating the difference in cost of these two agents, it is important to remember that phenytoin requires the placement of two IV catheters because of its incompatibility with many solutions and medications that are given concurrently. Additionally, some practitioners are giving fosphenytoin intramuscularly in the emergency room for non-SE indications and thereby avoiding the placement of a catheter and use of an infusion device. Many institutions fail to consider the expense associated with a tissue infiltration of phenytoin, which can cause tissue necrosis that necessitates plastic surgery or amputation. The expense of a single multimillion-dollar lawsuit likely will offset the difference between phenytoin and fosphenytoin cost to several institutions.

There is little difference in expense if one advocates phenobarbital over midazolam as third-line therapy, but it might be argued that a patient who experiences phenobarbital-induced respiration depression ultimately may be more expensive to the healthcare system.

EVALUATION OF THERAPEUTIC OUTCOMES

Initial success is defined as termination of all clinical and electrical seizure activity, but ultimate success is measured by the patient's quality of life. The morbidity and mortality associated with GCSE are affected by the underlying etiology; however, these can be minimized by the rapid implementation of a rational therapeutic plan. An EEG is an extremely important tool that not only allows practitioners to determine when abnormal electrical activity has been aborted but also can assist in determining which anticonvulsant was effective. Because many of the anticonvulsants affect the cardiorespiratory system, it is imperative that vital signs (e.g., heart rate, respiratory rate, and blood pressure) be monitored during drug loading and infusion. Finally, it is imperative that the infusion site be assessed for any evidence of infiltration before and during administration of phenytoin. Information regarding the patient's past medical and drug history and imaging studies (e.g., MRI) also can help to determine if there is a defined etiology for the original episode of GCSE. This information then can be used to guide future medication therapy, as well as help in determining if the patient is at risk for a poor outcome.

CONCLUSION

Our understanding of the cellular basis, physiology, and neuropathology of GCSE continues to evolve. Over the past decade, research into an activated cascade of pathophysiologic changes in neurotransmission, GABAergic inhibition, and NMDA receptor channel—mediated events has enhanced our understanding of this disorder. Although anticonvulsants will continue to be the mainstay of therapy in terminating seizures, specific agents including antagonists of excitatory amino acid neurotransmitters (e.g., glutamate and calcium channel blockers) and agonists of inhibitory neurotransmitters (GABA) may help to block further neuronal damage beyond the epileptogenic focus. Likewise, additional trials investigating the role of newer anticonvulsants in GCSE are warranted.

ABBREVIATIONS

ALT: alanine aminotransferase

AMPA: α-amino-3-hydroxy-5-methyl-isoxazole-4-propionate

AST: aspartate aminotransferase

CBC: complete blood count

CNS: central nervous system

CT: computed tomography

ECG: electrocardiogram

EEG: electroencephalogram, electroencephalography

FDA: Food and Drug Administration

GABA: γ-aminobutyric acid

GCSE: generalized convulsive status epilepticus

MRI: magnetic resonance imaging

NCSE: nonconvulsive status epilepticus

NMDA: N-methyl-D-aspartate

SE: status epilepticus

REFERENCES

1. Commission on Classification of Terminology, International League Against Epilepsy. Proposal for revised clinical and electroencephalographic classification of epileptic seizures. Epilepsia 1981;22: 489–501.
2. DeLorenzo RJ, Garnett LK, Towne AR, et al. Comparison of status epilepticus with prolonged seizure episodes lasting from 10 to 29 minutes. Epilepsia 1999;40:164–169.
3. Jenssen S, Gracely EJ, Sperling MR. How long do most seizures last? A systematic comparison of seizures recorded in the epilepsy monitoring unit. Epilepsia 2006;47:1499–1503.
4. Lowenstein DH, Alldredge BK. Status epilepticus. N Engl J Med 1998;338:970–976.
5. Maganti R, Gerber P, Drees C, Chung S. Nonconvulsive status epilepticus. Epilepsy Behav 2008;12:572–586.
6. DeLorenzo RJ, Pellock JM, Towne AR, Boggs J. Epidemiology of status epilepticus. J Clin Neurophysiol 1995;12:316–325.
7. Shorvon S. The management of status epilepticus. J Neurol Neurosurg Psychiatry 2001;70(Suppl 2):II22–II27.
8. DeLorenzo RJ, Towne AR, Pellock JM, Ko D. Status epilepticus in children, adults, and the elderly. Epilepsia 1992;33:S15–S25.
9. Pitkanen A. Efficacy of current antiepileptics to prevent neurodegeneration in epilepsy models. Epilepsy Res 2002;50:141–160.
10. Wasterlain CG, Mazarati AM, Naylor D, et al. Short-term plasticity of hippocampal neuropeptides and neuronal circuitry in experimental status epilepticus. Epilepsia 2002;45(Suppl 5):20–29.
11. Temkin NR. Antiepileptogenesis and seizure prevention trials with anti-epileptic drugs: Meta-analysis of controlled trials. Epilepsia 2001;42:515–524.
12. Singh RK, Gaillard WD. Status epilepticus in children. Curr Neurol Neurosci Rep 2009;9:137–144.
13. Wasterlain CG, Chen JWY. Mechanistic and pharmacologic aspects of status epielpticus and its treatment with new antiepileptic drugs. Epilepsia 2008;49:63–73.
14. Lothman E. The biochemical basis and pathophysiology of status epilepticus. Neurology 1990;40:13–23.
15. Working Group on Status Epilepticus. Treatment of convulsive status epilepticus: Recommendations of the Epilepsy Foundation of America's Working Group on Status Epilepticus. JAMA 1993;270:854–859.
16. Appleton R, Macleod S, Martland T. Drug management for acute tonic-clonic convulsions including convulsive status epilepticus in children. Cochrane Database Syst Rev 2008;16:CD001905.
17. LeDuc TJ, Goellner WE, Sanadi NE. Out-of-hospital midazolam for status epilepticus. Ann Emerg Med 1996;28:377.

18. Shaner DM, McCurdy SA, Herring MO, Gabor AJ. Treatment of status epilepticus: A prospective comparison of diazepam and phenytoin versus phenobarbital and optional phenytoin. Neurology 1988;38:202–207.

19. Treiman DM, Meyers PD, Walton NY, et al. A comparison of four treatments for generalized convulsive status epilepticus. Veterans Affairs Status Epilepticus Cooperative Study Group. N Engl J Med 1998;339:792–798.

20. Abernethy DR, Greenblatt DJ. Phenytoin disposition in obesity: Determination of loading dose. Arch Neurol 1985;42:468–471.

21. Fischer JH, Patel TV, Fischer PA. Fosphenytoin: Clinical pharmacokinetics and comparative advantages in the acute treatment of seizures. Clin Pharmacokinet 2003;42:33–58.

22. Dodson WE, Rust RS. Phenobarbital: Absorption, distribution, and excretion. In: Levy R, Mattson R, Meldrum B, eds. Antiepileptic Drugs, 4th ed. New York: Raven Press, 1995:379–387.

23. Crawford TO, Mitchell WG, Fishman LS, Snodgrass SR. Very-high-dose phenobarbital for refractory status epilepticus in children. Neurology 1988;38:1035–1040.

24. Claassen J, Hirsch LJ, Emerson RG, Mayer SA. Treatment of refractory status epilepticus with pentobarbital, propofol, or midazolam: A systematic review. Epilepsia 2002;43:146–153.

25. Abend NS, Diugos DJ. Treatment of refractory status epilepticus: literature review and a proposed protocol. Pediatr Neurol 2008;38:377–390.

26. Labar DR, Ali A, Root J. High-dose IV lorazepam for the treatment of refractory status epilepticus. Neurology 1994;44:1400–1403.

27. Yaucher NE, Fish JT, Smith HW, Wells JA. Propylene glycol—associated renal toxicity from lorazepam infusion. Pharmacotherapy 2003;23:1094–1099.

28. Mirski MA, Williams MA, Hanlet DF. Prolonged pentobarbital and phenobarbital coma for refractory generalized status epilepticus. Crit Care Med 1995;23:400–404.

29. Wheless JW, Trieman DM. The role of the newer antiepileptic drugs in the treatment of generalized convulsive status epilepticus. Epilepsia 2008;49 (Suppl 9):74–78.

30. Hovinga CA, Chicella MF, Rose DF, et al. Use of IV valproate in three pediatric patients with nonconvulsive or convulsive status epilepticus. Ann Pharmacother 1999;33:579–584.

31. Brown LA, Levin GM. Role of propofol in refractory status epilepticus. Ann Pharmacother 1998;32:1053–1059.

32. Timpe EM, Eichner SF, Phelps SJ. Propofol-related infusion syndrome in critically ill pediatric patients: Coincidence, association, or causation? J Pediatr Pharmacol Ther 2006;11:17–42.

33. Kahriman M, Minecan D, Kutluay E, et al. Efficacy of topiramate in children with refractory status epilepticus. Epilepsia 2003;44:1353–1356.

34. Towne AR, Garnett LK, Waterhouse EJ, et al. The use of topiramate in refractory status epilepticus. Neurology 2003;60:332–334.

35. Blumkin L, Lerman-Sagie T, Houri T, et al. Pediatric refractory partial status epilepticus responsive to topiramate. J Child Neurol 2005;20:239–241.

36. Conway JM, Birnbaum AK, Kriel RL, Cloyd JC. Relative bioavailability of topiramate administered rectally. Epilepsy Res 2003;54:91–96.

37. Rossetti AO, Bromfield EB. Determinants of success in the use of oral levetiracetam in status epilepticus. Epilepsy Behav 2006;8:651–654.

38. Möddel G, Bunten S, Dobis C, et al. Intravenous levetiracetam: a new treatment alternative for refractory status epilepticus. J Neurol Neurosurg Psychiatry 2009;80:689–692.

39. Gallentine WB, Hunnicutt AS, Husain AM. Levetiracetam in children with refractory status epilepticus. Epilepsy Behav 2009;14:215–218.

40. Kirmani BF, Crisp ED, Kayani S, Rajab H. Role of intravenous levetiracetam in acute seizure management of children. Pediatr Neurol 2009;41:37–39.

41. Tilz C, Resch R, Hofer T, Eggers C. Successful treatment for refractory convulsive status epilepticus by parenteral lacosamide. Epilepsia 2010;51:316–317.

42. Kellinghaus C, Berning S, Besselmann M. Intravenous lacosamide as successful treatment for nonconvulsive status epilepticus after failure of first line therapy. Epilepsy Behav 2009;14:429–431.

43. Aggarwal P, Wali JP. Lidocaine in refractory status epilepticus: A forgotten drug in the emergency department. Am J Emerg Med 1993;2:243–244.

44. Penberthy LT, Towne A, Garnett LK, Perlin JB. Estimating the economic burden of status epileptic to the health care system. Seizure 2005;14:46–51.

67

Acute Management of the Brain Injury Patient

BRADLEY A. BOUCHER AND SHELLY D. TIMMONS

KEY CONCEPTS

❶ Cerebral ischemia is the key pathophysiologic event triggering secondary neuronal injury following severe traumatic brain injury (TBI). Intracellular accumulation of calcium is postulated to be a central pathophysiologic process in amplifying and perpetuating secondary neuronal injury via inhibition of cellular respiration and enzyme activation.

❷ *Guidelines for the Management of Severe Brain Injury*, published by the Brain Trauma Foundation/American Association of Neurological Surgeons, serve as the foundation on which clinical decisions in managing adult neurotrauma patients are based; comparable guidelines for infants, children, and adolescents have also been published.

❸ Correcting and preventing early hypotension (systolic blood pressure less than 90 mm Hg) and hypoxemia (Pao_2 less than 60 mm Hg [8.0 kPa]) are primary goals during the initial resuscitative and intensive care of severe TBI patients.

❹ The principal monitoring parameter for severe TBI patients within the intensive care environment is intracranial pressure (ICP). Cerebral perfusion pressure is also a critical monitoring parameter and should be maintained between 50 and 70 mm Hg (greater than 40 mm Hg in pediatric patients) through the use of fluids, vasopressors, and/or ICP normalization therapy.

❺ Nonspecific pharmacologic treatment in the management of intracranial hypertension should include analgesics, sedatives, antipyretics, and paralytics under selected circumstances.

❻ Specific pharmacologic treatment in the management of intracranial hypertension includes mannitol, furosemide, and high-dose pentobarbital. Neither routine use of corticosteroids nor aggressive hyperventilation (i.e., $Paco_2$ less than 25 mm Hg) should be used in the management of intracranial hypertension.

❼ Phenytoin (or alternatively carbamazepine) should be used to prevent seizures in TBI patients at high risk for the first 7 days after injury. Use of phenytoin for the prophylaxis of posttraumatic seizures usually should be discontinued after 7 days if no seizures are observed.

❽ Numerous investigational strategies (e.g., calcium antagonists, glutamate antagonists, antioxidants, free-radical scavengers, and progesterone) targeted at interrupting the pathophysiologic cascade of events occurring following severe TBI have been employed, but no proven therapeutic benefits have been identified.

Traumatic brain injury (TBI) is currently the leading cause of death and disability among children and young adults in the industrialized world.[1,2] A focus on TBI prevention, and improved acute care and rehabilitation must remain national priorties.[2] This chapter summarizes TBI epidemiology and pathophysiology, and highlights the major guidelines and systematic reviews of the literature pertaining to the management of severe TBI patients.

EPIDEMIOLOGY

It is estimated that approximately 1.4 million persons sustain a TBI each year in the United States.[1] Among these individuals, 235,000 require hospital admission and 50,000 die annually.[2] Importantly, over 5.3 million Americans currently live with disabilities as a result of their TBI, highlighting the enormous physical and emotional toll of this healthcare problem.[2] The economic effects of acute neurotrauma are also enormous, with estimates of spending on TBI patients requiring hospitalization of $60 billion in the United States in 2000.[3] Economic costs to society from lost productivity are also massive, especially considering the young age of many TBI patients.[4] Falls are the leading cause of TBI (28%) while motor vehicle accidents result in the greatest number of TBI-related hospitalizations and deaths overall.[2] Death rates from TBI are highest in patients 75 years of age or older.[2] TBI-related mortality in males has been reported to exceed that in females three-fold.[2] However, recent data suggest that female mortality may actually exceed the mortality rate in males in postmenopausal women.[5]

PRIMARY AND SECONDARY BRAIN INJURY PATHOPHYSIOLOGY

The neurologic sequelae of brain trauma can occur instantaneously as a consequence of the primary injury or can result from secondary injuries that follow within minutes, hours, or days.[1] Primary injury involves the external transfer of kinetic energy to various structural components of the brain (e.g., neurons, nerve synapses, glial cells, axons, and cerebral blood vessels). The biomechanical forces responsible for primary brain injury can be classified broadly as contact (e.g., blunt-object blow, penetrating-missile

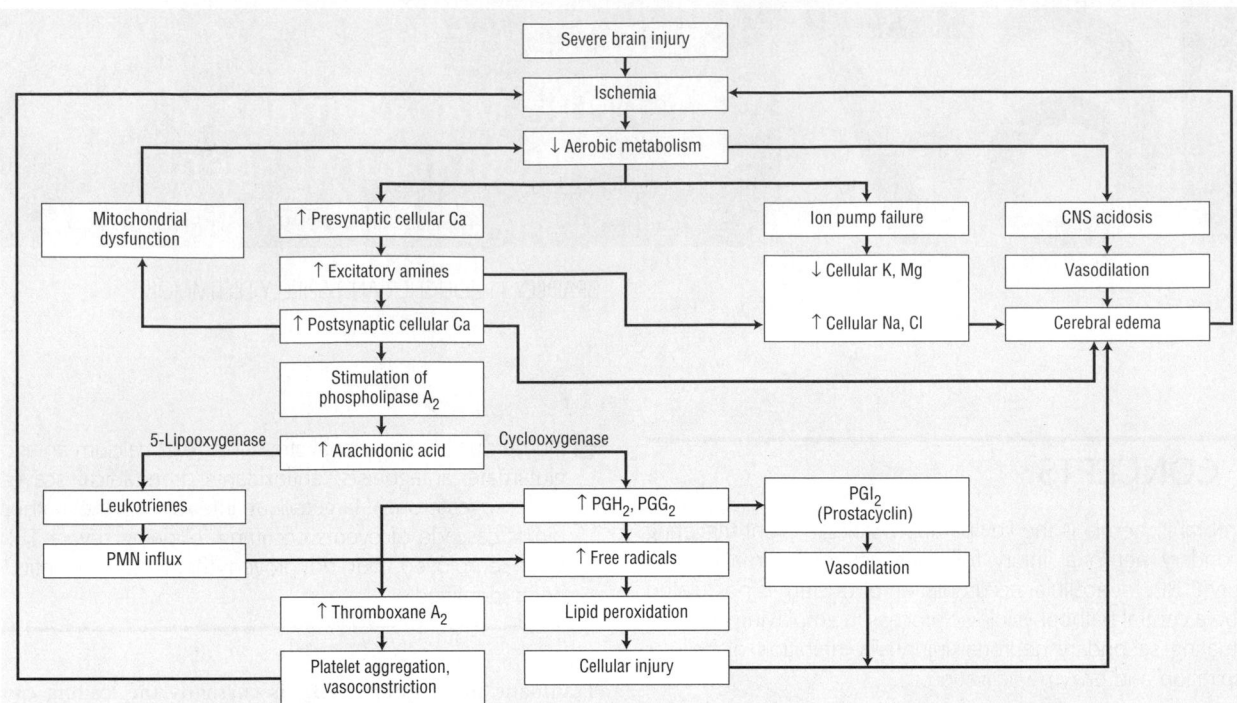

FIGURE 67-1. Schematic illustration of the cascade of biochemical events proposed to occur following severe neurotrauma (secondary brain injury). (Ca, calcium; CNS, central nervous system; K, potassium; Mg, magnesium; Na, sodium; Cl, chloride; PMN, polymorphonucleocyte; PG, prostaglandin.)

injuries) and acceleration/deceleration (e.g., instantaneous brain movements following motor vehicle accidents).[1] Primary injuries are categorized further as focal (e.g., contusions, hematomas) or diffuse.[4] The latter usually are associated with shearing or stretch forces, which primarily affect axons within the brain (i.e., diffuse axonal injury).[6] The type of primary injury (i.e., focal versus diffuse) is a major factor as to which of the secondary injury mechanisms discussed below will predominate following a TBI; however, many patients, especially those involved in high-speed accidents sustain both types of injury.[7]

❶ A complex sequence of pathophysiologic events precipitated by primary brain injury may seriously disrupt the normal central nervous system (CNS) balance between oxygen supply and demand.[7] Hypotension during the early posttraumatic period is a major contributor to this imbalance and a primary determinant of outcome.[1,6] The end result of this imbalance may be cerebral ischemia, the key pathophysiologic event triggering secondary injury.[7,8] Figure 67–1 is a simplified schematic of the processes that constitute secondary brain injury and their various interrelationships. The brain is particularly susceptible to ischemia because of its normally high resting energy requirement and its limited capacity to store oxygen, glucose, and adenosine triphosphate (ATP).[8] Ischemia following brain injury typically occurs in the first 6 to 24 hours following the insult.[9] Thereafter, patients can have hyperemia from days 1 to 3.[9] Vasospasm also can occur in approximately one fourth to one third of TBI patients.[6] These phenomena can result in imbalances in cerebral oxygen delivery (CDo_2) and consumption ($CMRo_2$), processes that are closely autoregulated under normal circumstances. Factors that can diminish cerebral oxygen supply following brain injury include cerebral edema, expanding mass lesions (e.g., epidural, subdural, and intracerebral hematomas), cerebral vasospasm, and loss of vasoregulatory control. Vasogenic cerebral edema can develop as a consequence of cerebral capillary endothelial damage and disruption of the blood-brain barrier.[7,8] Cytotoxic cerebral edema is a consequence of loss

of cell wall integrity that accompanies ischemia or hypoxia.[8] With cytotoxic and vasogenic edema comes expansion of the intracellular and extracellular fluid spaces, respectively. Elevated intracranial pressure (ICP) is the most detrimental consequence of cerebral edema formation and occurs as the brain tissue volume increases within the nondistensible skull. A significant increase in ICP may further compromise cerebral blood flow (CBF) and extend cytotoxic edema. Hence an increase in ICP can be self-perpetuating unless this cycle is reversed. Hypoxemia can further exacerbate local decreases in cerebral oxygen supply following acute respiratory failure and systemic hypotension. Metabolic demand also can increase following neurotrauma secondary to seizures, agitation, and temperature elevation.[8] Brain tissue affected by focal ischemia can have a dense core surrounded by a marginally viable region.[8] If adequate CBF is restored, the affected tissue may recover; however, sustained ischemia can result in further loss of cellular integrity and eventual cell death.

The two distinctive end points along the spectrum of secondary neuronal injury are (1) cellular necrosis characterized by cell membrane lysis, edema, and inflammation; and (2) apoptosis which leads to cell shrinkage and cell membrane dissolution.[7,8] Apoptosis which is also known as programmed cell death requires a cascade of intracellular events for completion of cell death.[7] The loss of ionic homeostasis is postulated to be a key event in fostering secondary brain injury following cerebral ischemia. Cellular influx of sodium, chloride, and water with a corresponding efflux of potassium and magnesium occurs secondary to cytotoxic edema and Na^+-K^+-ATPase pump dysfunction.[7,8] An influx of calcium into the presynaptic terminal ends of damaged neurons is mediated by N-type voltage-sensitive calcium channels. This influx is postulated to stimulate excessive release of the excitatory amines glutamate and aspartate from the affected neurons. These amines then accumulate in the neuronal synaptic cleft in the presence of cellular energy failure.[8] The result is ongoing stimulation of postsynaptic cells, which can result in an extension of neurotoxicity and cell death. Influx of calcium and additional sodium is stimulated by activation of ionophore receptors including the N-methyl-D-aspartate (NMDA) receptor.[7,8] Calcium influx and its intracellular accumulation initiate a number of events that amplify and perpetuate secondary neuronal injury. High intracellular concentrations of calcium result in mitochondrial dysfunction, which further inhibits cellular respiration, a process already affected by ischemic and/or hypoxic insults.[7] A second major deleterious effect of calcium is to stimulate activation of autodestructive enzymes, including phospholipases, endonucleases, and proteases, such as the caspase family of enzymes.[7,8] The effect of phospholipase A_2 stimulation includes formation of several arachidonic acid metabolites derived from membrane lipids: thromboxane A_2, prostaglandins, and leukotrienes.[7,8] The subsequent effects of these metabolites are lipid peroxidation and the formation of reactive oxygen species.[1,7,8] Recent data suggest that this event occurs very early after injury (e.g., before hospitalization), which may limit the effectiveness of exogenously administered antioxidants.[10]

Cell-mediated injury involving inflammatory mediators (e.g., proinflammatory cytokines) and nitric oxide activation is yet another possible mechanism involved in secondary neuronal injury.[7] Among the cell lines implicated are polymorphonuclear neutrophils, platelets, endothelial cells, and macrophages. Noteworthy is that limited data suggest that activation of some inflammatory mediators may actually be beneficial such that the relative balance of the mediators versus absolute concentrations may be the most significant pathophysiologic factor following TBI.[11] Stimulation of platelet aggregation, vasodilation, and vasoconstriction, intravascularly, also may occur. Lastly, data suggest that there may be a genetic vulnerability to the effects of TBI.[12,13] For example, preliminary evidence indicates that this may be related to faster recovery of aspartate uptake from the cerebral spinal fluid (CSF) and the CSF lactate/pyruvate ratio in TBI patients in the absence of the apolipoprotein E4 allele.[14] The latter is the same protein that has been associated with the deleterious effects of various types of Alzheimer disease.[14]

- A positive blood ethanol concentration and/or positive urine drug screen indicates that drug intoxication may be affecting the patient's mental status in addition to the TBI.
- Electrolyte disturbances can cause alterations in mental status, and their effects may interfere with assessment of neurological status relative to brain lesion.

Other Diagnostic Tests

- CT of the head is an important diagnostic tool for detecting the presence of mass lesions.

GCS, Glasgow Coma Scale; CSF, cerebrospinal fluid; TBI, traumatic brain injury; ABG, arterial blood gas; Pao$_2$, partial pressure of arterial blood oxygen; Paco$_2$, partial pressure of arterial blood carbon dioxide; CT, computed tomography.

CLINICAL PRESENTATION

The Glasgow Coma Scale (GCS) is the most widely used system to grade arousal and the functional capacity of the cerebral cortex.[6] The GCS defines the level of consciousness according to eye opening, motor response, and verbal response (Table 67–1). A GCS score of 15 corresponds to a normal neurologic examination. A GCS score of 3–8, 9–12, and 13–15 is consistent with severe, moderate, and mild brain injury, respectively.[6] The possibility of ethanol or drug intoxication, hypotension, hypoxia, postictal state, or hypothermia altering the neurologic examination always should be considered. Because narcotics and muscle relaxants affect the neurologic examination, they should not be administered until the initial examination is complete if at all possible. Simple, rapidly attainable clinical variables that are predictive of survival include patient age, GCS score (especially the motor score), pupillary reactivity, presence or absence of a hematoma, subarachnoid hemorrhage, midline shift, and appearance of the ventricular cisterns found on a computed tomographic (CT) scan of the head.[15]

CLINICAL PRESENTATION OF ACUTE BRAIN INJURY

General

- Level of consciousness on admission ranges from awake and alert to completely unresponsive (i.e., GCS 15 to 3, respectively).

Symptoms

- Posttraumatic amnesia (e.g., >1 hour), increasing dizziness, a moderate to severe headache, nausea/vomiting, limb weakness, or paresthesia may indicate more severe injury.

Signs

- CSF otorrhea or rhinorrhea, and seizures may indicate more severe injury.
- A rapid deterioration in mental status strongly suggests the presence of an expanding lesion within the skull.
- Severe TBI may be accompanied by significant alterations or instability in vital signs, including abnormal breathing patterns (e.g., apnea, Cheyne-Stokes respiration, tachypnea), hypertension, or bradycardia.

Laboratory Tests

- ABGs indicating hypoxia (i.e., decreased Pao$_2$) or hypercapnia (i.e., increased Paco$_2$) may indicate compromised ventilation.

TABLE 67-1	Glasgow Coma Scale
Response	**Score**
Eyes	
Open spontaneously	4
To verbal command	3
To pain	2
No response	1
Best motor response	
To verbal command	
Obeys	6
To painful stimulus (pressure to nailbeds)	
Localizes pain	5
Flexion, withdrawal	4
Flexion, abnormal (decorticate rigidity)	3
Extension (decerebrate rigidity)	2
No response	1
Best verbal response	
(arouse patient with painful stimulus if necessary)	
Oriented and converses	5
Disoriented and converses	4
Inappropriate words	3
Incomprehensible sounds	2
No response	1
Total	3–15

Data from the Lancet, Vol. 304, Teasdale G, Jennett B. Assessment of coma and impaired consciousness. A practical scale, 81–84, Copyright © 1974, with permission from Elsevier.

TREATMENT

General Traumatic Brain Injury Treatment Principles

❷ In July 1995, the Brain Trauma Foundation (BTF) published an extensive document entitled *Guidelines for the Management of Severe Brain Injury* as a joint initiative with the Guidelines Committee of the American Association of Neurological Surgeons (AANS) and the Joint Section on Neurotrauma and Critical Care of the AANS and the Congress of Neurological Surgeons, with subsequent revision in 2000.[16] A third revision was released in 2007.[17] This landmark publication constitutes the most widely accepted series of evidence-based standards, guidelines, and options for the care of severe TBI patients. As important are the data documenting that compliance with the BTF/AANS guidelines can result in improved outcomes relative to mortality rate, functional outcome scores, length of hospitalization, and cost.[18] Since then, guidelines addressing prehospital TBI management,[19] surgical management,[20] and management of penetrating brain injury have been published. Furthermore, TBI management guidelines for infants, children, and adolescents have been developed.[21] In addition, a series of systematic reviews addressing TBI management emanating from the Cochrane Library has been published.[22–27] These reviews have rigorously evaluated the literature for essentially all the major conventional TBI treatment strategies. The recommendations emanating from the published guidelines on TBI management and published systematic reviews will be highlighted throughout the remaining portion of this chapter. Until further clinical studies become available, recommendations from the published guidelines should serve as the foundation on which all clinical decisions in managing severe TBI are based. Nonetheless, it should be noted that the majority of the guidelines are based on class II evidence (primarily prospective clinical trials) and class III evidence (primarily retrospective clinical trials). Few class I evidence studies (i.e., prospective, randomized, controlled trials) are available for traumatic brain injury. The pharmacologic management of TBI is summarized in Table 67–2. Recommendations provided in this chapter pertain to adults and children unless specifically noted to the contrary.

■ DESIRED OUTCOMES

The overall goal in TBI management is not only reduction in morbidity and mortality but also optimization of long-term functional outcome for these patients. This requires careful attention to the following short-term therapeutic goals: (1) establishment of an adequate airway and maintenance of ventilation and circulation during the initial period of resuscitation and evaluation, (2) maintenance of balance between CDo_2 and $CMRo_2$, (3) prevention or attenuation of secondary neuronal injury, and (4) prevention and/or treatment of associated medical complications.

■ INITIAL RESUSCITATION

The first priority in the unconscious patient is the establishment of an airway, which ensures adequate oxygenation and prevents aspiration.[6,28] ❸ Thereafter, restoration of circulating blood volume and maintenance of systolic arterial pressure (SBP) greater than 90 mm Hg are of utmost importance.[1,17] In pediatric patients, the SBP goal should be greater than 70 mm Hg + (2 × age in years).[21] Correcting and preventing early hypotension (SBP less than 90 mm Hg) and hypoxia (Pao_2 less than 60 mm Hg [8.0 kPa]) are essential because these two factors are among the most powerful predictors of outcome.[17] Isotonic saline (0.9% normal saline)

TABLE 67–2 Pharmacologic Management of Traumatic Brain Injury

Hyperosmolar therapy
Mannitol is effective for control of increased intracranial pressure at doses of 0.25 g/kg to 1 g/kg body weight. (Evidence Level II)

Infection prophylaxis
Periprocedural antibiotics for intubation should be administered to reduce the incidence of pneumonia. (based largely on a single study). (Evidence Level II)
Routine prophylactic antibiotic use for ventricular catheter placement is not recommended to reduce infection. (Evidence Level III)

Deep venous thrombosis prophylaxis
Low molecular weight heparin or low dose unfractionated heparin should be used in combination with mechanical prophylaxis. However, there is an increased risk of expansion of intracranial hemorrhage. (Evidence Level III)

Anesthetics, analgesics, and sedatives
Prophylactic administration of barbiturates to reduce burst suppression (electroencephalogram is not recommended). (Evidence Level II)
High-dose barbiturate administration is recommended to control elevated ICP refractory to maximum standard medical and surgical treatment. Hemodynamic stability is essential before and after barbiturate therapy. (Evidence Level II)
Propofol is recommended for the control of ICP, but does not improve mortality or 6-month outcome. High-dose propofol can produce significant morbidity. (Evidence Level II)

Antiseizure prophylaxis
Prophylactic use of phenytoin or valproate is not recommended for preventing late PTS (greater than 7 days). (Evidence Level II)
Anticonvulsants are indicated to decrease the incidence of early PTS (within 7 days of injury) in high risk patients. (Evidence Level II)

Corticosteroids
The use of steroids is not recommended for improving outcome or reducing intracranial pressure. In patients with moderate or severe TBI, high-dose methylprednisolone is associated with increased mortality and is contraindicated. (Evidence Level II)

Evidence Level I. Good quality randomized controlled trial (RCT).
Evidence Level II. Moderate quality RCT; good quality cohort; good quality case-control.
Evidence Level III. Poor quality RCT; moderate or poor quality cohort; moderate or poor quality case control; case series, databases, or registries.
ICP, intracranial pressure; TBI, traumatic brain injury; PTS, posttraumatic seizures.
Data from Bratton et al.[17]

and lactated Ringer's solution have been traditionally used as initial resuscitation fluids of choice in TBI patients.[16] However, some clinicians believe that hypertonic saline (e.g., 3% or 7.5% saline) is beneficial in the resuscitation of TBI patients.[29] Clinical studies have yielded equivocal results relative to superiority over isotonic solutions.[1,30,31] Regardless, no clear consensus exists as to the optimal initial resuscitation fluid. While albumin therapy may be considered as an alternative to crystalloid fluid resuscitation, a retrospective analysis of 460 TBI patients revealed an increase in mortality (33.2%) compared with those patients receiving 0.9% normal saline.[32] Vasopressors and inotropic agents may be needed to maintain an adequate mean arterial pressure (MAP) if hypotension persists after adequate restoration of intravascular volume. Figure 67–2 is an algorithm summarizing treatment priorities in the initial management of acute TBI.

■ POSTRESUSCITATIVE CARE

Following successful resuscitation, priorities shift toward diagnostic evaluation of intracranial and extracranial injuries and emergent surgical intervention as needed. Evacuation of intracranial hematomas (i.e., epidural, subdural, and intracerebral hematomas) is essential to control ICP and improve outcome. Elevation of depressed skull fractures and débridement of penetrating wound tracts are other important emergent surgical procedures in TBI patients.

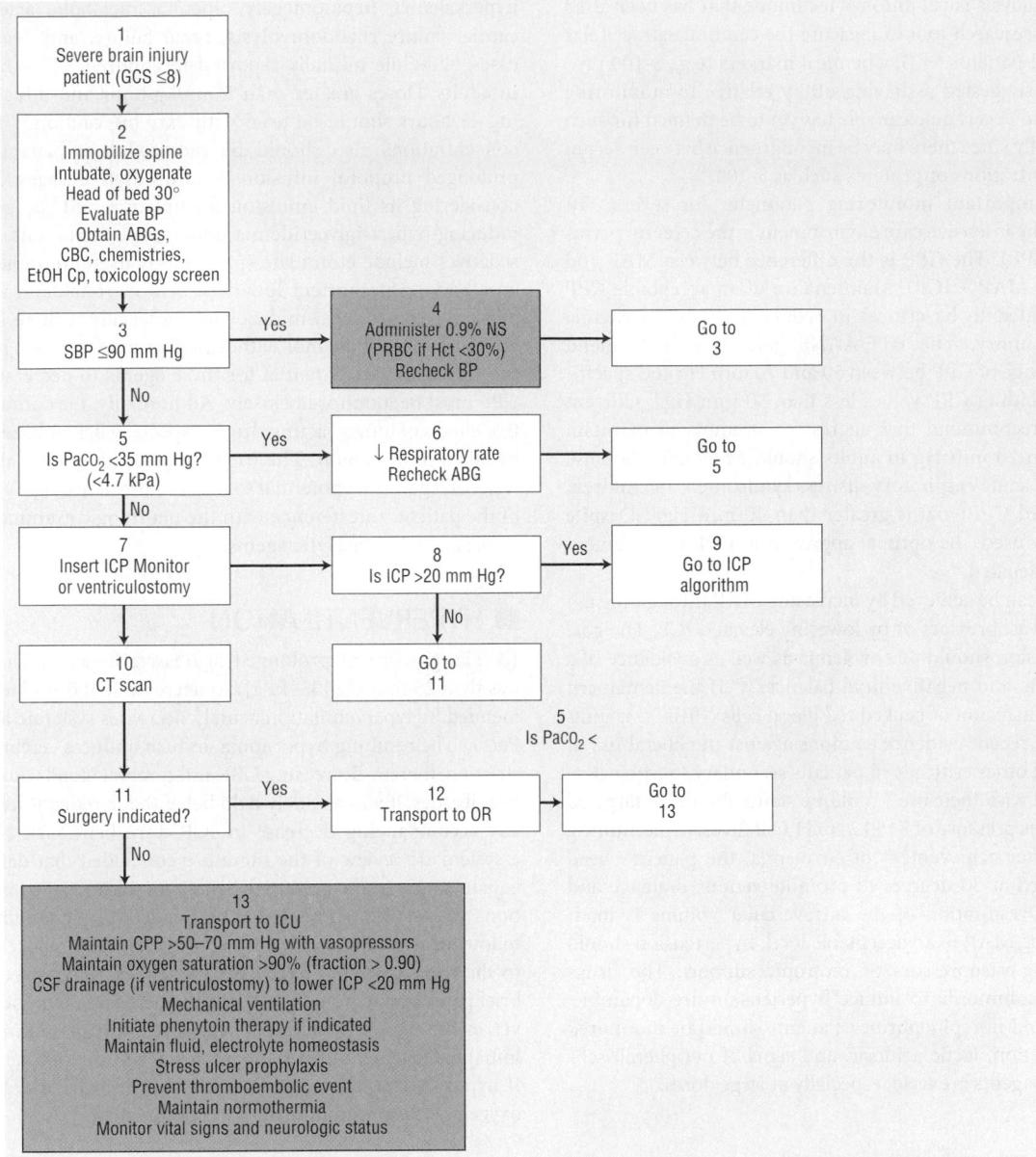

FIGURE 67-2. Algorithm for the acute management of the TBI patient. (GCS, Glasgow coma scale; BP, blood pressure; ABG, arterial blood gas; CBC, complete blood count; EtOH Cp, ethanol plasma concentration; SBP, systolic blood pressure; NS, normal saline; PRBC, packed red blood cells; Hct, hematocrit, $Paco_2$, partial pressure of arterial blood carbon dioxide; ICP, intracranial pressure; CT, computed tomography; OR, operating room; ICU, intensive care unit; CPP, cerebral perfusion pressure; CSF, cerebral spinal fluid.) *(Reprinted with permission from Boucher BA. Neurotrauma. In Carter BL, Angaran DM, Lake KD, Raebel MA, eds. Pharmacotherapy Self Assessment Program, 2nd ed. Critical Care Module. Kansas City, MO: American College of Clinical Pharmacy, 1995:220).*

Decompressive craniectomies (i.e., removal of variable amount of skull bone) with or without temporal or frontal lobectomy may be considered in patients with increases in ICP refractory to more conservative measures.[1] The beneficial effects of routine decompressive surgery in adult TBI patients to date are controversial.[33] Nonetheless, decompressive surgery in pediatric patients has generally yielded more favorable outcomes.[33] ❹ Continuous ICP monitoring (e.g., intraventricular catheter, intraparenchymal fiberoptic catheter) is indicated in salvageable patients with a GCS score of 3 to 8 after resuscitation with an abnormal admission CT scan, or in high-risk severe TBI patients with a normal CT scan who meet two of the following criteria: age older than 40 years, motor posturing, SBP less than 90 mm Hg.[17] Intraventricular catheters have a therapeutic advantage over the other alternatives but are associated with a higher complication rate and can be difficult to place in the

setting of the swollen brain. Specifically, CSF can be drained using this device as a means to lower ICP.[1] Continuous ICP monitoring is the only means to objectively evaluate the success of therapies used to decrease ICP. When the ICP exceeds 20 to 25 mm Hg, therapy should be initiated to decrease ICP below 20 mm Hg.[17,21] While used extensively in TBI patients and advocated within consensus guidelines, the need for a prospective, randomized, controlled trial to further define its value has recently been suggested.[34,35] Jugular venous oxygen saturation ($Sjvo_2$) monitoring is advocated by some practitioners for detection of global cerebral hypoxia (i.e., adequacy of CBF relative to $CMRo_2$), although it is technically difficult to achieve consistent results.[8,36] Hence its role remains confined predominantly to use in academic centers and for research.[8,36] The use of brain tissue oxygen monitoring may prove to be a superior alternative to $Sjvo_2$ to evaluate oxygen diffusion in TBI patients.[8,37]

Cerebral microdialysis is yet antoher technique that has been used successfully as a research tool to measure the cerebral extracellular chemistry of TBI patients.[8,38] Biochemical markers (e.g., S-100 protein) have been suggested as having utility relative to monitoring TBI patients.[39] However, no clear role has yet to be defined for such markers, especially since there may be incongruence between serum and brain concentrations of proteins such as S-100.[40]

❹ Another important monitoring parameter for severe TBI patients within the intensive care environment is the cerebral perfusion pressure (CPP). The CPP is the difference between MAP and ICP (i.e., CPP = MAP − ICP). Maintenance of an acceptable CPP has been postulated to be critical in reducing cerebral ischemia and secondary injury. The BTF/AANS guidelines recommend maintaining a range of CPP between 50 and 70 mm Hg and specifically indicate avoiding CPP values less than 50 mm Hg.[17] Current guidelines also recommend that aggressive attempts to maintain CPP greater than 70 mm Hg in adults should be avoided because of the risk of the acute respiratory distress syndrome.[17] In children, the recommended CPP goal is greater than 40 mm Hg.[21] Despite being commonly used, the optimal approach to CPP management continues to be debated.[41]

The goal CPP can be achieved by increasing MAP through the use of fluids and/or vasopressors or by lowering elevated ICP. The goal of volume expansion should be euvolemia as well as avoidance of a hypoosmolar state and negative fluid balance.[21,30] If the hematocrit is below 30%, transfusion of packed red blood cells (PRBCs) is indicated.[1] However, recent evidence cautions against the liberal use of blood in TBI and other critically ill patients secondary to worse outcomes associated with their use.[42] Volume status should be targeted to a central venous pressure of 7 to 12 cm H_2O if invasive monitoring is employed.[1] After achievement of euvolemia, the patient's head should be elevated at 30 degrees to promote venous drainage and decrease ICP. If restoration of the intravascular volume is inadequate in elevating MAP to an acceptable level, hypertension should be induced using vasopressors or inotropic support. The drugs employed most commonly to induce hypertension are dopamine, phenylephrine, and norepinephrine.[1] Patients should be monitored for renal dysfunction, lactic acidosis, and signs of peripheral ischemia when these agents are used, especially at large doses.

Treatment of Intracranial Hypertension

■ GENERAL PHARMACOLOGIC STRATEGIES

❺ The use of analgesics, sedatives, and paralytics has an important primary role in the management of intracranial hypertension (Fig. 67–3).[43] This is related directly to the association of pain, agitation, excessive muscle movement, and resisting mechanical ventilation with transient increases in ICP. Nonetheless, there have been no studies of the effect of sedation on outcome in patients with severe TBI.[17] Morphine sulfate is the most commonly used analgesic and sedative in this setting.[17] While fentanyl and sufentanil are gaining in popularity, their use may be associated with mild elevations in ICP.[17] Propofol has become the sedative of choice in TBI patients among many clinicians because of its ease of titration, rapidly reversible effects on discontinuation, and possible neuroprotective effects.[17] Although it is used for sedation in infants and children who are mechanically ventilated in the ICU setting, the Food and Drug Administration (FDA) requires that the manufacturer labeling contain specific information that propofol is not approved for sedation of pediatric patients admitted to an ICU. One of the biggest safety concerns with the use of propofol is the propofol infusion syndrome (PIS) characterized by

hyperkalemia, hepatomegaly, lipemia, metabolic acidosis, myocardial failure rhabdomyolysis, renal failure, and death in some cases.[17,44] While inititally reported in children, PIS can also occur in adults. Doses greater than 5 mg/kg/hour and infusion exceeding 48 hours should be used with extreme caution.[17] Triglyceride concentrations also should be monitored in patients receiving prolonged propofol infusions and/or high dosages of propofol considering its lipid emulsion formulation and the potential for inducing hypertriglyceridemia under these conditions. Alternative sedatives include etomidate (particularly useful in rapid-induction anesthesia), intermittent low-dose pentobarbital, and short-acting benzodiazepines (e.g., midazolam), especially if there is a reasonable suspicion of alcohol withdrawal as the underlying etiology of the agitation. The potential for these agents to decrease MAP and CPP must be monitored closely. Additionally, the cumulative sedative effects of longer-acting drugs, especially benzodiazepines, must be taken into account. The use of any sedative agent also must be weighed against its potential to obscure the neurologic examination of the patient. Interference with the neurologic examination is also associated with paralytic agents.

■ HYPERVENTILATION

❻ The practice of prolonged aggressive hyperventilation ($Paco_2$ less than 25 mm Hg [3.3 kPa]) to decrease ICP is no longer recommended.[17] Hyperventilation acutely decreases systemic and cerebral $Paco_2$. The resulting hypocapnia, in turn, induces cerebral vasoconstriction, thereby decreasing CBF and cerebral blood volume (CBV).[8] For decades, it was a widely held belief that a reduction in CBV and any accompanying decrease in ICP were beneficial. Nonetheless, a systematic review of the literature concluded that data are inadequate to ascertain potential benefit or harm from hyperventilation.[25] Hyperventilation should be avoided during the first 24 hours following acute TBI when CBF is often critically reduced according to the most current BTF/AANS guidelines.[17] Hyperventilation for brief periods may nonetheless be considered as a temporary maneuver in the setting of refractory intracranial hypertension or in the initial management of patients with signs of cerebral herniation.[17,21] If hypoventilation is performed, the use of $Sjvo_2$ or cerebral tissue oxygen perfusion monitoring is recommended.[17]

■ HYPOTHERMIA

While hypothermia has been discussed for nearly 50 years as a cerebral protective maneuver in TBI patients, a resurgence of interest has been fueled by the results of several preliminary studies in the early 1990s demonstrating trends in improvement in mortality and morbidity rates in severe TBI patients randomized to receive mild to moderate hypothermia. However, in the most extensive investigation to date, TBI patients randomized to receive hypothermia (n = 199) within 6 hours of injury (target body temperature 33°C [91.4°F]) and maintained for 48 hours did not have significantly improved outcomes at 6 months compared with a normothermia group of TBI patients (n = 196).[45] The BTF/AANS guidelines concur with these findings that prophylactic hypothermia is not significantly associated with decreased mortality when compared with normothermic controls.[17,46] A recent meta-analysis confirms these results, concluding that hypothermia is not beneficial in the management of TBI patients.[26] Nonetheless, the guidelines leave open the possibility that there may be a mortality benefit if this therapeutic maneuver is continued for more than 48 hours.[17,46] Depth of hypothermia, as well as the rate of rewarming after discontinuation of hypothermia, are additional factors that may affect outcomes with this therapeutic maneuver in TBI patients.[47,48] The mechanism underlying a protective effect of hypothermia is likely

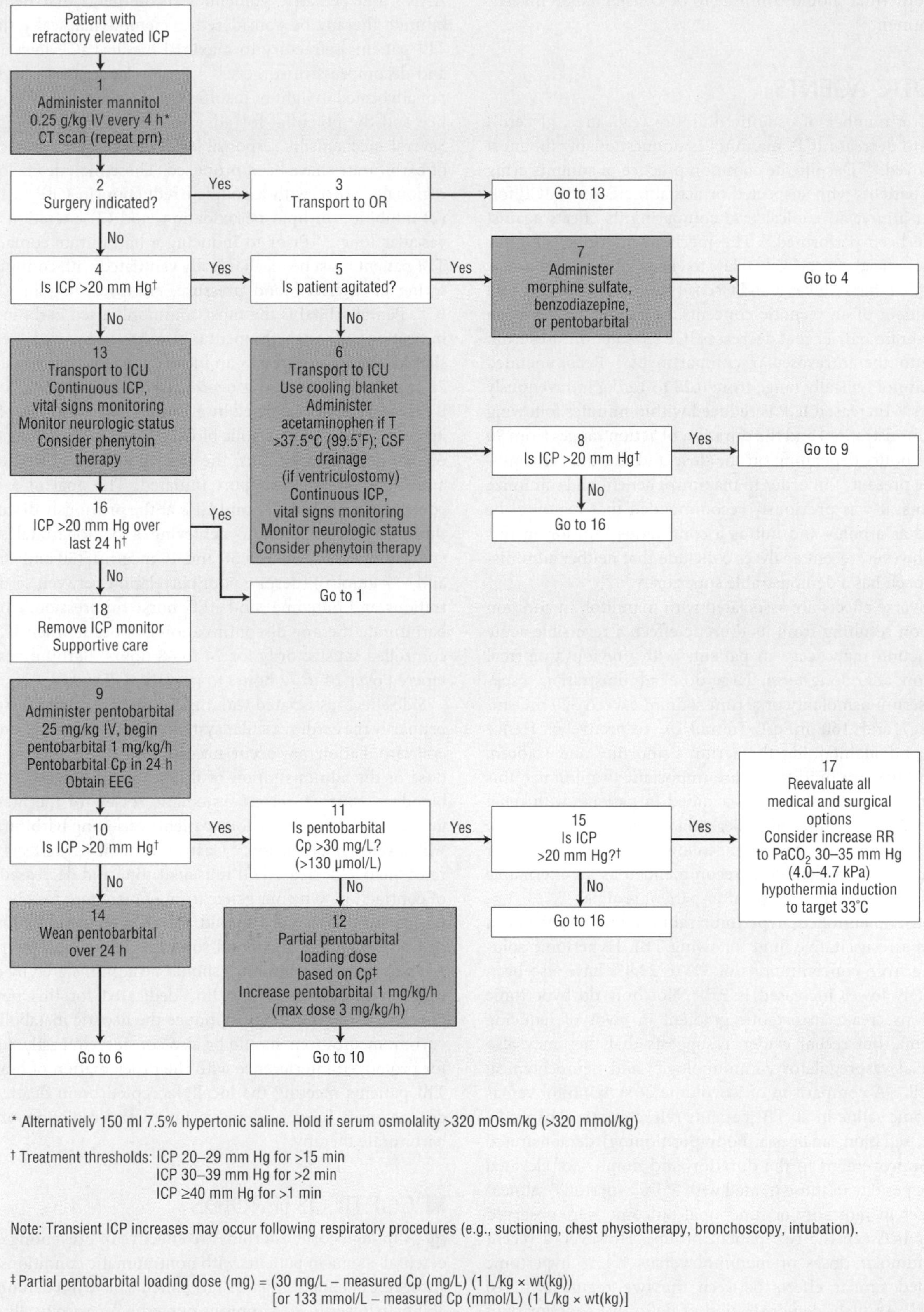

FIGURE 67-3. Algorithm for the management of increased ICP. (Cp, plasma concentration; CT, computed tomography; OR, operating room; ICP, intracranial pressure; ICU, intensive care unit; T, temperature; CSF, cerebral spinal fluid; EEG, electroencephalogram; RR, respiratory rate; Paco₂, partial pressure of arterial blood carbon dioxide.) *(Reprinted with permission from Boucher BA. Neurotrauma. In Carter BL, Angaran DM, Lake KD, Raebel MA, eds. Pharmacotherapy Self Assessment Program, 2nd ed. Critical Care Module. Kansas City, MO: American College of Clinical Pharmacy, 1995:224–225).*

multifactorial, although a reduction in CMR_{O_2} is offered most frequently as the basis of any therapeutic benefits. Potential side effects of hypothermia include coagulation disturbances, infectious complications, and cardiac arrhythmias.[46,47] An increase in ICP also may occur secondary to hypothermia-associated shivering that can be prevented with neuromuscular blocking agents. Unfortunately, these agents are also associated with potential adverse events. Considering these latter risks and equivocal data from clinical trials to date, hypothermia should continue to be considered an investigational treatment.[26]

OSMOTIC AGENTS

6 Although a number of osmotic diuretics (e.g., urea, glycerol) can be used to decrease ICP, mannitol is unquestionably the most widely employed.[1,17] Despite the common practice of administering mannitol to patients with suspected or actual increases in ICP following brain injury, no clinical trial comparing its effects against placebo have been performed.[27] The mechanisms responsible for mannitol's beneficial effects likely relate to (1) an immediate plasma-expanding effect that reduces blood viscosity and increases CBF and (2) establishment of an osmotic concentration gradient across an intact blood-brain barrier that decreases ICP as water diffuses from the brain into the intravascular compartment.[17] Recommended doses of mannitol typically range from 0.25 to 1 g/kg intravenously every 4 hours.[17] Increased ICP is reduced within minutes following mannitol administration, and the duration of action ranges from 90 minutes to 6 hours depending on the dose and the clinical conditions that are present.[17] In order to maximize benefit and minimize adverse events, it was previously recommended that mannitol be administered as a bolus and not as a continuous infusion in this setting.[1,16] However, recent analyses conclude that neither administration approach has a demonstrable superiority.[17,49]

Several adverse effects are associated with mannitol. In addition to hypotension resulting from its diuretic effect, a reversible acute renal dysfunction may occur in patients with previously normal renal function after long-term, large-dose administration, especially if the serum osmolality or serum sodium exceed 320 mOsm/kg (mmol/kg) and 160 mEq/L (mmol/L), respectively.[1] Hence monitoring and maintaining the serum osmolality and sodium, and replacing urinary fluid losses are important to minimize this adverse event. Mannitol should be avoided in patients with renal failure.[21] Acute exacerbation of underlying congestive heart failure and pulmonary edema also may occur following rapid intravascular volume expansion. Furosemide is recommended as an alternative diuretic for lowering ICP in these latter patient groups.

As previously mentioned, hypertonic saline solutions have been advocated as a resuscitative fluid following TBI. Hypertonic solutions ranging from concentrations of 3% to 23.4% have also been used to acutely lower increased ICP.[28,31] Not only do hypertonic saline solutions create an osmotic gradient in favor of reducing cerebral edema, but recent evidence suggests that they may also have beneficial vasoregulatory, immunologic, and neurochemical effects as well.[11] A comparison of isovolume 20% mannitol versus 7.5% hypertonic saline in 20 TBI patients refractory to nonspecific therapy (i.e., sedation, analgesia, body positioning) demonstrated significant improvement in the duration and number of elevated ICP episodes per day in those treated with 7.5% hypertonic saline.[50] No differences in mortality or functional outcome were observed in this study between the two patient groups. However, a recent study of equimolar doses of mannitol versus 7.45% hypertonic saline revealed similar effects between the two regimens in 20 TBI patients.[51] As such, demonstration of definitive superiority of hypertonic saline therapy compared with osmotic diuretics will require further investigation.

BARBITURATES

6 High-dose barbiturate therapy (i.e., *barbiturate coma*) has been used for decades in the management of increased ICP, despite a lack of evidence documenting beneficial effects on patient morbidity and mortality.[24] Nonetheless, based largely on beneficial outcomes observed in a randomized clinical trial published in 1988, BTF/

AANS and pediatric guidelines recommend that high-dose barbiturate therapy be considered in hemodynamically stable severe TBI patients refractory to maximal medical ICP-lowering therapy and decompressive surgery.[17,21] Prophylactic use of barbiturates is not advocated in light of insufficient evidence supporting this practice and the potential for adverse events (e.g., hypotension).[17,21,24] Several mechanisms responsible for the cerebral protective effects of barbiturates have been proposed. These include (1) lowering the regional $CMRo_2$ with a coupled reduction in CBF to these areas, (2) inhibition of lipid peroxidation, and (3) alteration of cerebral vascular tone.[1,43] Prior to inducing a barbiturate coma, the severe TBI patient must be mechanically ventilated with continuous monitoring of arterial blood pressure, electrocardiogram (ECG), and ICP. Pentobarbital is the most commonly used barbiturate for this indication, although thiopental also has been used. Pentobarbital should be administered as an intravenous loading infusion totaling 25 mg/kg (i.e., 10 mg/kg over 30 minutes and then 5 mg/kg per hour for 3 hours), followed by a maintenance infusion of 1 to 2 mg/kg per hour.[1,17] If the systolic blood pressure falls during the loading or maintenance infusions, the rate should be slowed temporarily and blood pressure support initiated. The goal of a barbiturate coma is to maintain ICP and CPP at the previously discussed target thresholds in addition to achieving a pentobarbital steady-state concentration of between 30 and 40 mcg/mL (30 and 40 mg/L; 133 and 177 µmol/L) (despite poor correlation between serum concentrations and outcome) and EEG burst suppression.[17] Initiation of barbiturate therapy discontinuation can occur when ICP has been controlled satisfactorily for 24 to 48 hours. Barbiturates should be tapered over 24 to 72 hours to prevent ICP spikes.

Side effects associated with high-dose barbiturate therapy involve primarily the cardiovascular system. Hypotension caused by peripheral vasodilation may occur, necessitating decreasing the barbiturate dose or the administration of fluids and vasopressors to maintain blood pressure. A recent systematic review of the literature suggested that one of every four patients receiving barbiturate therapy will develop hypotension.[24] Gastrointestinal (GI) effects of barbiturates include decreased GI muscular tone and decreased amplitude of contraction. On emergence from coma, there may be a period of GI hypermotility. Care should be taken to avoid extravasation of pentobarbital and thiopental solutions because severe tissue damage may occur. Barbiturates should be administered by continuous infusion through a central line dedicated for this purpose. The potential for barbiturates to induce the hepatic metabolism of concurrent medications should be also considered. Lastly, the potential for prolonged interference with the proclamation of brain death in TBI patients meeting the locally accepted brain death neurologic criteria must be considered prior to the initiation of high-dose barbiturate therapy.

CORTICOSTEROIDS

6 Although corticosteroids are effective in preventing or reducing cerebral edema in patients with nontraumatic conditions producing vasogenic edema, studies in TBI patients have not demonstrated the ability to lower ICP or improve outcome.[17,22] Specifically, use of corticosteroids following TBI has been associated with increased mortality and complications, including GI bleeding, glucose intolerance, electrolyte abnormalities, and infection. The largest investigation to date was known as the CRASH (Corticosteroid Randomization After Significant Head Injury) study.[52] In this study, 10,008 patients with a GCS score less than or equal to 14 were randomized to receive a 48-hour continuous infusion of methylprednisolone or placebo. Results of this study indicated a higher risk of death within 2 weeks of enrollment (relative risk 1.18) in those patients receiving corticosteroids compared with patients receiving placebo

$(P < 0.001)$.[52] Based on this and several other major randomized trials, the BTF/AANS adult and pediatric guidelines recommend that high-dose corticosteroids not be used in patients with moderate to severe TBI.[17,21]

Treatment and Prophylaxis of Complications

■ POSTTRAUMATIC SEIZURES

It is generally agreed that patients who have experienced one or more seizures following a moderate to severe TBI should receive anticonvulsant therapy to avoid increases in $CMRo_2$ that occur with the onset of subsequent seizures and to prevent the development of (sometimes subclinical) status epilepticus with associated increase in mortality. Initial therapy in these persons should consist of incremental intravenous doses of diazepam (5–40 mg for adults, 0.1–0.5 mg/kg for infants and children) or lorazepam (2–8 mg for adults, 0.03–0.1 mg/kg for infants and children) to terminate any active seizure activity followed by intravenous phenytoin to prevent seizure recurrence. Phenytoin dosing regimens for adults and pediatric patients include an intravenous loading dose of 15 to 20 and 10 to15 mg/kg, respectively, followed by a maintenance dose of 5 mg/kg/day. Alternatively, fosphenytoin, a water-soluble phosphate ester of phenytoin, can be administered intravenously or intramuscularly using the same doses, specified as phenytoin equivalents (PE). The merits of preventive anticonvulsant therapy in patients who have not had a seizure postinjury historically have been more controversial. Risk factors for early posttraumatic seizures (less than 7 days after injury) include a GCS score of less than 10, a cortical contusion, a depressed skull fracture, a subdural hematoma, an epidural hematoma, an intracerebral hematoma, a penetrating head wound, or a seizure within the first 24 hours of injury.[17] In a landmark randomized, placebo-controlled study, the incidence of early posttraumatic seizures in patients receiving placebo was 14.2% compared with 3.6% in patients receiving phenytoin ($P < 0.05$) without a significant increase in drug-related side effects.[53] ❼ A systematic review of the literature corroborated these findings, estimating an improved pooled relative risk for early seizure prevention of 0.34 (95% confidence interval, 0.21–0.54) in patients receiving anticonvulsants.[54] Thus it is recommended that phenytoin (or alternatively carbamazepine) should be used to prevent seizures in TBI patients at high risk for the first 7 days after injury.[17,21,55] Valproate therapy is not recommended based on a trend for higher mortality in a study comparing valproate-treated patients with those receiving phenytoin short-term therapy.[53] The benefits of prophylactic anticonvulsants beyond 7 days have not been demonstrated, and thus their use for this indication beyond 7 days is not recommended.[17,54] Unfortunately, despite reducing the incidence of early seizures following brain injury, no beneficial effects have been documented for anticonvulsants on patient mortality or long-term disability.[17,53,54] This is particularly disconcerting considering that the long-term risk of epilepsy after TBI has been documented to be increased up to 10 years or longer based on results of a recent population-based cohort study.[56]

CLINICAL CONTROVERSY

Persistant hyperglycemia may be an independent predictor of higher mortality in TBI patients. As such, tight glucose control may improve outcome in TBI patients. However, some authorities suggest that this practice is unproven and unsafe after brain injury

■ SUPPORTIVE CARE

While normalizing ICP and maintaining an adequate CPP are the highest priorities in preventing secondary injury following severe TBI, attention also must be given to preventing and/or treating systemic and extracranial complications.[17,21] This includes careful ongoing fluid and electrolyte management.[31] Common electrolyte disturbances in TBI patients that should be monitored and treated aggressively include hyponatremia, hypomagnesemia, hypokalemia, and hypophosphatemia. Aggressive nutritional support of the TBI patient is another important therapeutic consideration.[16,21] Evidence suggests that early feeding of TBI patients (i.e., by 7 days) may be associated with a trend toward better outcomes in terms of survival and disability.[17,57,58] Infectious complications commonly encountered in severe TBI patients include nosocomial pneumonia, sepsis, urinary tract infections, and meningitis.[1] Treatment of these potentially devastating infections should be aggressive, with careful attention being paid to antibiotic blood–brain barrier penetration for intracranial infections. Hyperthermia also should be avoided in TBI patients because patients with elevated temperatures have poorer outcomes than normothermic patients.[1,21,59] Hence aggressive maintenance of a core temperature of less than 37.5°C (99.5°F) using acetaminophen, nonsteroidal antiinflammatory drugs (NSAIDs), and cooling blankets is indicated for patients following severe TBI. Several experimental cooling techniques, including intravascular cooling for use in TBI patients refractory to conventional management strategies, were discussed in a recent review of this topic.[59] Other important therapeutic interventions include acute gastritis prophylaxis, and prevention of decubiti and contractures. Prevention of thromboembolic events is also an extremely important component of supportive care in TBI patients since the incidence of a deep venous thrombosis is higher in TBI patients compared with patients without brain injury.[1,60] This can be accomplished with the use of graduated compression stockings or intermittent pneumatic compression devices initially. Thereafter, systemic therapy (e.g., low-molecular-weight heparin) should generally be initiated within 2 to 3 days in combination with the mechanical devices until patients are ambulatory.[17,61] However, systemic anticoagulation must be used with caution in those patients with intracerebral hemorrhage, or in patients who may need to undergo craniotomy early in their course. Monitoring for a coagulopathy is important in any severe TBI patient since the incidence is high (greater than 30%), and coagulopathy is associated with a significantly longer ICU length of stay and an almost 10-fold increase in mortality based on data from a recent study.[62] Reversal of coagulopathy with recombinant factor VIIa in critically ill trauma patients with TBI is gaining in popularity among some physicians despite lacking an approved indication or large clinical trials demonstrating its safety and efficacy in TBI patients.[63,64]

CLINICAL CONTROVERSY

Off-label use of recombinant factor VII is advocated by some neurosurgeons for managing life-treatening intracranial hemorrhage in TBI patients. The potential for thromoembolic events using this procoagulant must be considered as part of any cost versus benefit analysis in these patients.

■ CLINICAL PATHWAYS/GUIDELINE IMPLEMENTATION

Use of clinical pathways and formal TBI management guidelines has been demonstrated to improve TBI patient outcomes and reduce institutional resource utilization as summarized in a current review.[65]

The magnitude of these improvements is revealed in a recent single center study in which patients with a good recovery or moderate disability increased from 50.3% to 61.5%, and charges for care were reduced by greater than $8,000.[18] Few practitioners would dispute the overall importance of integrating current evidence-based management guidelines into clinical practice as a means to optimize care and improve the functional outcome of TBI patients.[66]

■ INVESTIGATIONAL THERAPY

❽ The steady decrease in morbidity and mortality following severe neurotrauma over the last 30 years can be attributed largely to expeditious and aggressive management of events resulting in secondary injury (i.e., ischemia, hypoxia, increased ICP) using conventional treatment strategies. Numerous neuroprotective agents targeting specific pathophysiologic processes that are theorized to occur following severe TBI have been investigated over the last decade in an attempt to further enhance the prospects for a meaningful recovery. Prominent among these strategies have been attempts to modulate calcium influx through the administration of calcium antagonists[23,67,68] and glutamate antagonists including magnesium,[67,69–73] and the use of antioxidants/free-radical scavengers.[67] Inhibitors of inflammatory mediators also are under consideration as neuroprotective agents.[74] Unfortunately, none of these agents to date has demonstrated a significant reduction in morbidity or mortality following severe TBI in phase III clinical trials. Noteworthy is that a phase II pilot study recently demonstrated a decrease in mortality in 100 TBI patients randomized to receive a 3-day infusion of progesterone compared with placebo.[75] A follow-up, independently conducted, double-blinded clinical trial of progesterone in 159 TBI patients also improved outcome at 6 months postinjury,[76] prompting experts to call for a phase III trial of this promising pharmacologic strategy.[77] Other neuroprotective strategies use growth factors, including brain-derived neurotrophic factor and nerve growth factor,[78] that may have a future role in the management of TBI by promoting nerve cell regeneration and differentiation.[74] Such neurorestorative strategies can be classified as structural or functional. Lastly, there are miscellaneous agents including calpain inhibitors, inhibitors of caspases (enzymes involved in apoptosis) including erythropoietin and the antiinflammatory agent, minocycline, that are being considered as viable neuroprotective agents based on experimental TBI studies.[71,78,79] Despite generally negative clinical trial findings to date, the search is likely to continue for neuroprotective agents including those with multiple pathophysiologic targets that eventually may improve the long-term outcome in severe TBI patients.[80]

CLINICAL CONTROVERSY

A growing body of evidence from a small number of studies suggests that beta-blocker use may improve survival following TBI. Mechanistically, these benefits may be realized through reversal of a hyperadrenergic state often associated with TBI. A major concern with their use is the potential to reduce systemic blood pressure.

■ OTHER TREATMENT STRATEGIES

The concept of administering commercially available CNS active agents for nonapproved indications in TBI patients should presently be considered investigative therapy. One example is the use of CNS stimulants in the management and rehabilitation of TBI patients.

A comprehensive review of the use of methylphenidate relative to improving cognition following TBI was recently conducted. It was the opinion of the author that the literature does provide a degree of support for improvements in memory, attention, concentration, and mental processing in this patient subset, although results and study designs were highly variable for those investigations included in the analysis.[81] Another example is the use of Parkinson disease medications (e.g., amantadine, bromocriptine, carbidopa/levodopa) in severe TBI patients in an attempt to enhance dopamine release and inhibit reuptake within the injured region of the brain. A review of amantadine following TBI indicated that improved cognition and arousal were evident in the majority of patients studied.[82] Cholinergic agents such as donepezil have also undergone limited investigation in TBI patients.[83] Antidepressants represent yet another class of agents that has been studied in TBI patients.[83] While intuitively appealing, routine administration of psychostimulants to improve cognitive outcomes in TBI patients or drugs that enhance the biochemical milieu within the CNS following a TBI should be undertaken cautiously until large, well-controlled studies demonstrating beneficial effects are available. Additionally, the timing of administration of these drugs is controversial; the potential for cardiovascular side effects in the face of uncertain benefit would indicate that these drugs should be reserved for the postacute phase of treatment (i.e., weeks to months postinjury).

EVALUATION OF THERAPEUTIC OUTCOMES

The process for evaluation of therapeutic outcomes is summarized in Table 67–3. Patients with severe TBI require ICU monitoring initially with the goals of maintaining or reestablishing

TABLE 67-3	Evaluation of Therapeutic Outcomes
General	GCS: Record hourly initially, decrease frequency as neurologic status stabilizes
	Vital signs (BP, HR, RR, temperature): Record hourly initially, decrease frequency as neurologic status stabilizes
	Urine output: Record hourly initially, decrease frequency as neurologic status stabilizes
	Arterial oxygen saturation: Continuously while in intensive care unit
Risk of increased ICP	ICP: Record hourly, decrease frequency as ICP stabilizes <20 mm Hg (usually not until 48–72 hours postinjury at a minimum)
	CPP: Record hourly, decrease frequency as CPP stabilizes in the desired range[a]
Laboratory tests	Blood ethanol concentration and urine drug screen: On admission
	ABGs: Daily at a minimum while intubated, repeated as needed based on pulmonary instability requiring ventilator setting changes
	CBC: Daily while in intensive care unit
	Serum electrolytes (Na, K, Cl): Daily while in intensive care unit. Serum sodium and osmolality may be monitored as frequently as every six hours if osmotherapy (mannitol, furosemide, hypertonic saline) is being utilized
	Minerals (Mg, Ca, P): Daily initially until concentrations stable
Radiologic procedures	CT scan: Postresuscitation initially with repeat scan(s) as needed based on degree of neurologic instability (e.g., decrease in GCS) or initial CT appearance

GCS, Glasgow Coma Scale; BP, blood pressure; HR, heart rate; RR, respiratory rate; CSF, cerebrospinal fluid; TBI, traumatic brain injury; ICP, intracranial pressure; CPP, cerebral perfusion pressure; ABG, arterial blood gas; CBC, complete blood count; Na, sodium; K, potassium; Cl, chloride; Mg, magnesium; Ca, calcium; P, phosphorus; CT, computed tomography.
[a]Continuous monitoring mandated initially if technologically feasible.

neurologic and systemic homeostasis as well as readily detecting any neurologic deterioration. This requires frequent evaluation of the patient's neurologic status (e.g., GCS) and measurement of vital signs, urine output, and arterial oxygen saturation (as well as ICP in patients with an ICP monitor in place). Furthermore, careful attention must be paid to the potential for a variety of electrolyte, mineral, and acid-base disturbances, coagulopathies, and infections by obtaining various laboratory tests on a daily basis initially. The intensity of monitoring will be a function of the relative degree of neurologic and hemodynamic stability of the patient in the hours and days following the neurologic insult. Lastly, radiologic tests (e.g., CT scans) are essential not only for the initial diagnostic evaluation of TBI patients but also as means to evaluate the etiology for any subsequent neurologic deterioration as well.

ABBREVIATIONS

AANS: American Association of Neurological Surgeons

ABG: arterial blood gas

ATP: adenosine triphosphate

BTF: Brain Trauma Foundation

CBF: cerebral blood flow

CBV: cerebral blood volume

CDo_2: cerebral oxygen delivery

$CMRo_2$: cerebral oxygen consumption

CNS: central nervous system

CPP: cerebral perfusion pressure

CRASH: Corticosteroid Randomization After Significant Head Injury

CSF: cerebrospinal fluid

CT: computed tomography

FDA: Food and Drug Administration

ECG: electrocardiogram

GCS: Glasgow Coma Scale

GI: gastrointestinal

ICP: intracranial pressure

MAP: mean arterial pressure

NMDA: N-methyl-D-aspartate

NSAID: nonsteroidal antiinflammatory drug

PE: phenytoin equivalents

PIS: propofol infusion syndrome

PRBCs: packed red blood cells

SBP: systolic blood pressure

$Sjvo_2$: jugular venous oxygen saturation

TBI: traumatic brain injury

REFERENCES

1. Cohen SM, Marion DW. Traumatic brain injury. In: Fink MP, Abraham E, Vincent JL, et al., eds. Textbook of Critical Care. Philadelphia, PA: Elsevier Saunders, 2005:377–389.

2. Langlois JA, Rutland-Brown W, Thomas KE. Traumatic brain injury in the United States: emergency department visits, hospitalizations, and deaths. In: Centers for Disease Control and Prevention, National Center for Injury Prevention and Control. Atlanta, GA: CDC, 2006:1–55.

3. Finkelstein E, Corso P, Miller T. The Incidence and Economic Burden of Injuries in the United States. New York: Oxford University Press, 2006.

4. Ling GS, Marshall SA. Management of traumatic brain injury in the intensive care unit. Neurol Clin 2008;26:409–426, viii.

5. Ottochian M, Salim A, Berry C, et al. Severe traumatic brain injury: is there a gender difference in mortality? Am J Surg 2009;197:155–158.

6. Chang CWJ. Neurologic injury: pevention and initial care. In: Gabrielli A, Layon AJ, Yu M. eds. Civetta, Taylor, & Kirby's Critical Care. Philadelphia, PA: Wolters Kluwer/Lippincott Williams & Wilkins, 2007:1245–1260.

7. Clark RSB, Jenkins L, Lai YC, et al. Biochemical, cellular, and molecular mechanisms of neuronal death and secondary brain injury in critical care. In: Fink MP, Abraham E, Vincent JL, et al., eds. Textbook of Critical Care. Philadelphia, PA: Elsevier Saunders, 2005:263–273.

8. Manno EM, Rabinstein AA. Central nervous system. In: Gabrielli A, Layon AJ, Yu M. eds. Civetta, Taylor, & Kirby's Critical Care. Philadelphia: Wolters Kluwer/Lippincott Williams & Willkins; 2007:649–665.

9. Martin NA, Patwardhan RV, Alexander MJ, et al. Characterization of cerebral hemodynamic phases following severe head trauma: hypoperfusion, hyperemia, and vasospasm. J Neurosurg 1997;87:9–19.

10. Cristofori L, Tavazzi B, Gambin R, et al. Early onset of lipid peroxidation after human traumatic brain injury: a fatal limitation for the free radical scavenger pharmacological therapy? J Investig Med 2001;49:450–458.

11. Dutton RP, McCunn M. Traumatic brain injury. Curr Opin Crit Care 2003;9:503–509.

12. Waters RJ, Nicoll JA. Genetic influences on outcome following acute neurological insults. Curr Opin Crit Care 2005;11:105–110.

13. Jordan BD. Genetic influences on outcome following traumatic brain injury. Neurochem Res 2007;32:905–915.

14. Kerr ME, Ilyas Kamboh M, Yookyung K, et al. Relationship between apoE4 allele and excitatory amino acid levels after traumatic brain injury. Crit Care Med 2003;31:2371–2379.

15. Signorini DF, Andrews PJ, Jones PA, et al. Predicting survival using simple clinical variables: a case study in traumatic brain injury. J Neurol Neurosurg Psychiatry 1999;66:20–25.

16. Bullock R, Chesnut RM, Clifton GL, et al. Brain Trauma Foundation, Inc, American Association of Neurological Surgeons. Part 1: guidelines for the management of severe head injury. New York: Brain Trauma Foundation, Inc., 2000:1–165.

17. Bratton SL, Chestnut RM, Ghajar J, et al. Guidelines for the managment of severe head injury. The Brain Trauma Foundation. The American Association of Neurological Surgeons. The Joint Section on Neurotrauma and Critical Care. J Neurotrauma 2007;24(Suppl 1): S1–S106.

18. Fakhry SM, Trask AL, Waller MA, et al. Management of brain-injured patients by an evidence-based medicine protocol improves outcomes and decreases hospital charges. J Trauma 2004;56:492–499.

19. Gabriel EJ, Ghajar J, Jagoda A, et al. Guidelines for prehospital management of traumatic brain injury. J Neurotrauma 2002;19:111–174.

20. Bullock MR, Chesnut R, Ghajar J, et al. Guidelines for the surgical management of traumatic brain injury. Neurosurgery 2006;58(S2): 1–62.

21. Adelson PD, Bratton SL, Carney NA, et al. Guidelines for the acute medical management of severe traumatic brain injury in infants, children, and adolescents. Crit Care Med 2003;31:S417-SS491.

22. Alderson P, Roberts I. Corticosteroids for acute traumatic brain injury. Cochrane Database Syst Rev 2005:CD000196.

23. Langham J, Goldfrad C, Teasdale G, et al. Calcium channel blockers for acute traumatic brain injury. Cochrane Database Syst Rev 2003:CD000565.

24. Roberts I, Sydenham E. Barbiturates for acute traumatic brain injury. Cochrane Database Syst Rev 2000:CD000033.

25. Schierhout G, Roberts I. Hyperventilation therapy for acute traumatic brain injury. Cochrane Database Syst Rev 2000:CD000566.

26. Sydenham E, Roberts I, Alderson P. Hypothermia for traumatic head injury. Cochrane Database Syst Rev 2009:CD001048.

27. Wakai A, Roberts I, Schierhout G. Mannitol for acute traumatic brain injury. Cochrane Database Syst Rev 2007:CD001049.

28. Guha A. Management of traumatic brain injury: some current evidence and applications. Postgrad Med J 2004;80:650–653.

29. Bhardwaj A, Ulatowski JA. Hypertonic saline solutions in brain injury. Curr Opin Crit Care 2004;10:126–131.

30. Scalea TM. Does it matter how head-injury patients are resuscitated? In: Valadka AB, Andrews BT, eds. Neurotrauma. Evidence-Based Answers to Common Questions. New York: Thieme, 2005:3–7.

31. Rhoney DH, Parker D Jr. Considerations in fluids and electrolytes after traumatic brain injury. Nutr Clin Pract 2006;21:462–478.

32. Myburgh J, Cooper DJ, Finfer S, et al. Saline or albumin for fluid resuscitation in patients with traumatic brain injury. N Engl J Med 2007;357:874–884.

33. Sahuquillo J, Arikan F. Decompressive craniectomy for the treatment of refractory high intracranial pressure in traumatic brain injury. Cochrane Database Syst Rev 2006:CD003983.

34. Shafi S, Diaz-Arrastia R, Madden C, et al. Intracranial pressure monitoring in brain-injured patients is associated with worsening of survival. J Trauma 2008;64:335–340.

35. Smith M. Monitoring intracranial pressure in traumatic brain injury. Anesth Analg 2008;106:240–248.

36. Stocchetti N. Should I monitor jugular venous oxygen saturation? In: Valadka AB, Andrews BT, eds. Neurotrauma. Evidence-Based Answers to Common Questions. New York: Thieme, 2005:58–67.

37. Rosenthal G, Hemphill JC 3rd, Sorani M, et al. Brain tissue oxygen tension is more indicative of oxygen diffusion than oxygen delivery and metabolism in patients with traumatic brain injury. Crit Care Med 2008;36:1917–1924.

38. Hutchinson PJ. Microdialysis in traumatic brain injury–methodology and pathophysiology. Acta Neurochir Suppl 2005;95:441–445.

39. Korfias S, Stranjalis G, Boviatsis E, et al. Serum S-100B protein monitoring in patients with severe traumatic brain injury. Intensive Care Med 2007;33:255–260.

40. Kleindienst A, Ross Bullock M. A critical analysis of the role of the neurotrophic protein S100B in acute brain injury. J Neurotrauma 2006;23:1185–1200.

41. White H, Venkatesh B. Cerebral perfusion pressure in neurotrauma: a review. Anesth Analg 2008;107:979–988.

42. Salim A, Hadjizacharia P, DuBose J, et al. Role of anemia in traumatic brain injury. J Am Coll Surg 2008;207:398–406.

43. Maas AIR, Stocchetti N. Intensive care after neurosurgery. In: Fink MP, Abraham E, Vincent JL, et al., eds. Textbook of Critical Care. Philadelphia, PA: Elsevier Saunders, 2005.

44. Otterspoor LC, Kalkman CJ, Cremer OL. Update on the propofol infusion syndrome in ICU management of patients with head injury. Curr Opin Anaesthesiol 2008;21:544–551.

45. Clifton GL, Miller ER, Choi SC, et al. Lack of effect of induction of hypothermia after acute brain injury. N Engl J Med 2001;344:556–563.

46. Peterson K, Carson S, Carney N. Hypothermia treatment for traumatic brain injury: a systematic review and meta-analysis. J Neurotrauma 2008;25:62–71.

47. McIntyre LA, Fergusson DA, Hebert PC, et al. Prolonged therapeutic hypothermia after traumatic brain injury in adults: a systematic review. JAMA 2003;289:2992–2999.

48. Tokutomi T, Morimoto K, Miyagi T, et al. Optimal temperature for the management of severe traumatic brain injury: effect of hypothermia on intracranial pressure, systemic and intracranial hemodynamics, and metabolism. Neurosurgery 2003;52:102–111.

49. Roberts I, Schierhout G, Wakai A. Mannitol for acute traumatic brain injury. Cochrane Database Syst Rev 2003:CD001049.

50. Vialet R, Albanese J, Thomachot L, et al. Isovolume hypertonic solutes (sodium chloride or mannitol) in the treatment of refractory posttraumatic intracranial hypertension: 2 mL/kg 7.5% saline is more effective than 2 mL/kg 20% mannitol. Crit Care Med 2003;31:1683–1687.

51. Francony G, Fauvage B, Falcon D, et al. Equimolar doses of mannitol and hypertonic saline in the treatment of increased intracranial pressure. Crit Care Med 2008;36:795–800.

52. Roberts I, Yates D, Sandercock P, et al. Effect of intravenous corticosteroids on death within 14 days in 10008 adults with clinically significant head injury (MRC CRASH trial): randomised placebo-controlled trial. Lancet 2004;364.1321–1328.

53. Temkin NR. Preventing and treating posttraumatic seizures: the human experience. Epilepsia 2009;50(Suppl 2):10–13.

54. Schierhout G, Roberts I. Anti-epileptic drugs for preventing seizures following acute traumatic brain injury. Cochrane Database Syst Rev 2001:CD000173.

55. Chang BS, Lowenstein DH. Practice parameter: antiepileptic drug prophylaxis in severe traumatic brain injury: report of the Quality Standards Subcommittee of the American Academy of Neurology. Neurology 2003;60:10–16.

56. Christensen J, Pedersen MG, Pedersen CB, et al. Long-term risk of epilepsy after traumatic brain injury in children and young adults: a population-based cohort study. Lancet 2009;373:1105–1110.

57. Cook AM, Peppard A, Magnuson B. Nutrition considerations in traumatic brain injury. Nutr Clin Pract 2008;23:608–620.

58. Perel P, Yanagawa T, Bunn F, et al. Nutritional support for head-injured patients. Cochrane Database Syst Rev 2006:CD001530.

59. Thompson HJ, Tkacs NC, Saatman KE, et al. Hyperthermia following traumatic brain injury: a critical evaluation. Neurobiol Dis 2003;12:163–173.

60. Reiff DA, Haricharan RN, Bullington NM, et al. Traumatic brain injury is associated with the development of deep vein thrombosis independent of pharmacological prophylaxis. J Trauma 2009;66:1436–1440.

61. Macdonald RL. What is the safest way to prevent deep venous thrombosis and pulmonary embolism after head or spinal cord injury? How soon after surgery or injury can I anticoagulate my patients who develop deep venous thrombosis? In: Valadka AB, Andrews BT, eds. Neurotrauma. Evidence-Based Answers to Common Questions. New York: Thieme, 2005:43–49.

62. Talving P, Benfield R, Hadjizacharia P, et al. Coagulopathy in severe traumatic brain injury: a prospective study. J Trauma 2009;66:55–61.

63. Narayan RK, Maas AI, Marshall LF, et al. Recombinant factor VIIA in traumatic intracerebral hemorrhage: results of a dose-escalation clinical trial. Neurosurgery 2008;62:776–786.

64. Stein DM, Dutton RP, Kramer ME, et al. Reversal of coagulopathy in critically ill patients with traumatic brain injury: recombinant factor VIIa is more cost-effective than plasma. J Trauma 2009;66:63–72.

65. Marion DW. Evidenced-based guidelines for traumatic brain injuries. Prog Neurol Surg 2006;19:171–196.

66. Hartl R, Ghajar J. Does following the recommendations in the Guidelines for the Management of Severe Traumatic Brain Injury make a difference in patient outcome? In: Valadka AB, Andrews BT, eds. Neurotrauma. Evidence-Based Answers to Common Questions. New York: Thieme, 2005:120–123.

67. Farin A, Marshall LF. Why have therapeutic trials in head injury been unable to demonstrate benefits? In: Valadka AB, Andrews BT, eds. Neurotrauma. Evidence-Based Answers to Common Questions. New York: Thieme, 2005:124–131.

68. Vergouwen MD, Vermeulen M, Roos YB. Effect of nimodipine on outcome in patients with traumatic subarachnoid haemorrhage: a systematic review. Lancet Neurol 2006;5:1029–1032.

69. Arango MF, Mejia-Mantilla JH. Magnesium for acute traumatic brain injury. Cochrane Database Syst Rev 2006:CD005400.

70. Kalia LV, Kalia SK, Salter MW. NMDA receptors in clinical neurology: excitatory times ahead. Lancet Neurol 2008;7:742–755.

71. Schouten JW. Neuroprotection in traumatic brain injury: a complex struggle against the biology of nature. Curr Opin Crit Care 2007;13:134–142.

72. Temkin NR, Anderson GD, Winn HR, et al. Magnesium sulfate for neuroprotection after traumatic brain injury: a randomised controlled trial. Lancet Neurol 2007;6:29–38.

73. Willis C, Lybrand S, Bellamy N. Excitatory amino acid inhibitors for traumatic brain injury. Cochrane Database Syst Rev 2004:CD003986.

74. Doppenberg EM, Choi SC, Bullock R. Clinical trials in traumatic brain injury: lessons for the future. J Neurosurg Anesthesiol 2004;16:87–94.

75. Wright DW, Kellermann AL, Hertzberg VS, et al. ProTECT: a randomized clinical trial of progesterone for acute traumatic brain injury. Ann Emerg Med 2007;49:391–402.

76. Xiao G, Wei J, Yan W, et al. Improved outcomes from the administration of progesterone for patients with acute severe traumatic brain injury: a randomized controlled trial. Crit Care 2008;12:R61.

77. Vandromme M, Melton SM, Kerby JD. Progesterone in traumatic brain injury: time to move on to phase III trials. Crit Care 2008;12:153.

78. Jain KK. Neuroprotection in traumatic brain injury. Drug Discov Today 2008;13:1082–1089.

79. Wang KK, Larner SF, Robinson G, et al. Neuroprotection targets after traumatic brain injury. Curr Opin Neurol 2006;19:514–519.

80. Stoica B, Byrnes K, Faden AI. Multifunctional drug treatment in neurotrauma. Neurotherapeutics 2009;6:14–27.

81. Siddall OM. Use of methylphenidate in traumatic brain injury. Ann Pharmacother 2005;39:1309–1313.

82. Sawyer E, Mauro LS, Ohlinger MJ. Amantadine enhancement of arousal and cognition after traumatic brain injury. Ann Pharmacother 2008;42:247–252.

83. Tenovuo O. Pharmacological enhancement of cognitive and behavioral deficits after traumatic brain injury. Curr Opin Neurol 2006;19:528–533.

84. Teasdale G, Jennett B. Assessment of coma and impaired consciousness. A practical scale. Lancet 1974;2:81–84.

68

Parkinson's Disease

JACK J. CHEN, MERLIN V. NELSON, AND DAVID M. SWOPE

KEY CONCEPTS

❶ Thoughtful consideration for selection of initial therapy, management of drug dosing, and use of adjunctive therapies throughout the course of idiopathic Parkinson's disease (IPD) is necessary to optimize long-term therapeutic outcomes and minimize adverse effects.

❷ The optimal time to start drug therapy in IPD varies, but in general, treatment should be initiated when the disease begins to interfere with activities of daily living, employment, or quality of life. However, in the absence of functional impairment, rasagiline may be offered.

❸ Anticholinergic medication is useful for mild tremor-predominant IPD but should be used with caution in the elderly and in those with preexisting cognitive difficulties.

❹ As monotherapy, amantadine and monoamine oxidase type B (MAO-B) inhibitors provide benefits in early IPD, but the symptomatic effect is less than that of dopamine agonists and carbidopa/levodopa (L-dopa).

❺ Carbidopa/L-dopa is the most effective medication for symptomatic treatment and eventually all patients with IPD will require it.

❻ Most carbidopa/L-dopa–treated patients will develop motor complications (e.g., fluctuations and dyskinesias).

❼ MAO-B inhibitors and catechol-O-methyl-transferase inhibitors attenuate motor fluctuations in carbidopa/L-dopa–treated patients.

❽ Dopamine agonists are effective and, compared to L-dopa, associated with less risk of developing motor complications but more likely to cause psychiatric symptoms, such as hallucinations and impulse control disorders.

❾ Surgery is reserved for patients who require additional symptomatic relief or control of motor complications despite receiving medically optimized therapy.

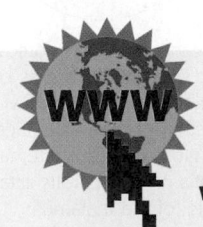

The complete chapter, learning objectives, and other resources can be found at **www.pharmacotherapyonline.com**.

The presence of tremor at rest, rigidity, bradykinesia, and postural instability (instability of balance) are considered the hallmark motor features of idiopathic Parkinson's disease (IPD). These clinical features of IPD were adeptly described in 1817 by James Parkinson.[1]

EPIDEMIOLOGY

Up to 1 million individuals in the United States have IPD. The approximate annual incidence of IPD (i.e., number of persons diagnosed with IPD per year) is age-dependent and ranges from 10 per 100,000 persons in the sixth decade of life (i.e., 50–59 years of age) to 120 per 100,000 persons in the ninth decade of life (i.e., 80–89 years of age).[2,3] Likewise, the prevalence of IPD also increases with age, affecting 1% of people older than age 65 years and 2.5% of those older than age 80 years. The usual age at time of diagnosis ranges between 55 and 65 years. A higher incidence is reported among males, with a male-to-female ratio of up to 2:1.

ETIOLOGY

The true etiology of IPD is unknown, but is likely the result of interactions between aging, genetic constitution, and environmental factors. In IPD, a key histopathologic feature is degeneration of dopaminergic neurons in the substantia nigra that project to the striatum (i.e., the nigrostriatal pathway).[4] Additionally, neuronal vulnerability in IPD extends beyond the nigrostriatal pathway and includes specific neurons in autonomic ganglia, basal ganglia, spinal cord, and neocortex.[5] In humans and primates, administration of the compound 1-methyl-4-phenyl-1,2,3,6-tetrahydropyridine (MPTP) results in a form of parkinsonism. The MPTP compound is converted by monoamine oxidase (MAO)-B to 1-methyl-4-phenylpyridinium ion (MPP+), a potent neurotoxin. MPP+ is toxic to neurons by inhibiting mitochondrial complex 1 of the electron transport chain, which results in the generation of excessive reactive oxygen species and cell death.[6] Several synthetic pesticides have a molecular structure similar to that of MPTP. Although IPD is sporadic, extensive epidemiologic research associates environmental factors, such as chronic exposure to pesticides and heavy metals (such as iron and manganese), rural living, and drinking well water, with a risk for lifetime development of IPD.[7-10] Interestingly, epidemiologic studies have consistently associated an inverse correlation between cigarette smoking and caffeine consumption for development of IPD.[11,12]

Intrinsically, the substantia nigra pars compacta (SNc) is a region characterized by high levels of oxidative stress because free radicals are generated from dopamine autooxidation mediated by MAO (Fig. 68–1). Several antioxidative molecules (e.g., glutathione) are present in the SNc to limit damage produced by free-radical attack,

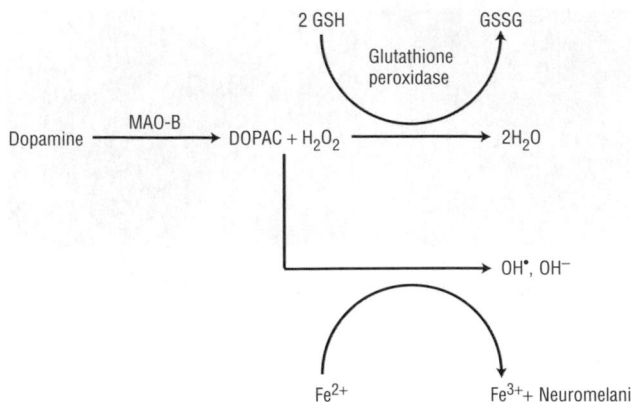

FIGURE 68-1. Dopamine metabolism results in hydrogen peroxide (H_2O_2) formation. If the glutathione system is deficient or excess hydrogen peroxide is present, hydrogen peroxide accepts an electron from ferrous iron (Fe^{2+}), forming ferric iron (Fe^{3+}) and the hydroxyl free radical ($OH^{\bullet}$). The hydroxyl free radical can cause lipid peroxidation, thereby damaging neuronal cell membranes. (DOPAC, 3,4-dihydroxyphenylacetic acid; GSH, glutathione; GSSG, glutathione disulfide; H_2O, water; OH, the hydroxide ion; MAO-B, monoamine oxidase B.)

but in IPD, such protection might be overwhelmed or impaired. Thus cellular damage from oxidant stress has long been discussed as an etiopathologic component of IPD.[13] The SNc is also rich in iron and copper, essential cofactors in the biosynthesis and metabolism of dopamine. The oxidation–reduction cycle of iron can also generate free radicals and toxic metabolites (Fig. 68-1). In addition, apoptosis (programmed cell death), excitotoxicity, inflammation, mitochondrial dysfunction, nitric oxide toxicity, proteosomal dysfunction, and autophagic cellular mechanisms are also implicated etiopathologic mechanisms in IPD.

Genetics may play a significant role, particularly if IPD begins before age 50 years.[14,15] More than a dozen gene mutations are associated with forms of parkinsonism. For example, autosomal dominant forms of parkinsonism are associated with mutations of the α-synuclein (*PARK1* and *PARK4*) and *leucine-rich repeat kinase 2* (*LRRK*) genes. Autosomal recessive forms are associated with mutations of *parkin (PARK2)* and *PTEN-induced putative kinase 1 (PINK1)* genes. Overall, these forms of genetically linked parkinsonisms constitute only a small percentage of total parkinsonism cases and their pathology and phenotypic aspects differ from that of IPD.

PATHOPHYSIOLOGY

In the SNc, the two hallmark histopathologic features of IPD are depigmentation of dopamine-producing neurons (i.e., loss of SNc neurons) and presence of Lewy bodies (neuronal cytoplasmic filamentous aggregates composed of the presynaptic protein α-synuclein) in the remaining SNc neurons. Lewy bodies appear in degenerating neurons in association with adjacent gliosis. Lewy pathology has been proposed to develop in a predictable anatomic distribution within the parkinsonian brain.[5] In the premotor stage of IPD, Lewy bodies are initially found in the medulla oblongata, locus coeruleus, raphe nuclei, and olfactory bulb. This may correlate with observations that anxiety, depression, and impaired olfaction is detectable in premotor stages of IPD. As IPD progresses, Lewy pathology ascends to the midbrain (particularly the SNc) and accounts for development of motor features. In advanced stages, Lewy pathology spreads to the cortex, and this may correlate with cognitive and additional behavior changes. The observation that Lewy pathology can spread into adjacent healthy neurons has given

rise to the postulate that prion-like propagation of α-synuclein aggregates may be occuring.

Pathologic findings reveal a correlation between the extent of nigrostriatal dopamine loss and the severity of certain IPD motor features (e.g., bradykinesia). The threshold for onset of clinically detectable IPD appears to be the loss of 70% to 80% of SNc neurons.[16] Functional neuroimaging studies suggest compensatory responses, such as upregulation of dopamine synthesis and downregulation of synaptic dopamine reuptake, occur as adaptive mechanisms beginning in the premotor stage of IPD. These adaptive responses may help to explain why the motor features are not clinically detectable until profound depletion (70%–80%) of SNc neurons has occurred.

Dopaminergic projections from the SNc to the striatum (putamen and caudate) synapse on two major populations of dopamine receptor-mediated efferent neurons (referred to as the direct and indirect pathways), which, in turn, mediate motor activity via a complex neuronal circuit involving the extrapyramidal system (Fig. 68-2). In IPD, the degeneration of the SNc neurons results in reduced activity within these two efferent pathways. The direct pathway involves activation of striatal dopamine$_1$ (D_1) dopamine receptors (which are coupled to adenylate cyclase) and stimulates

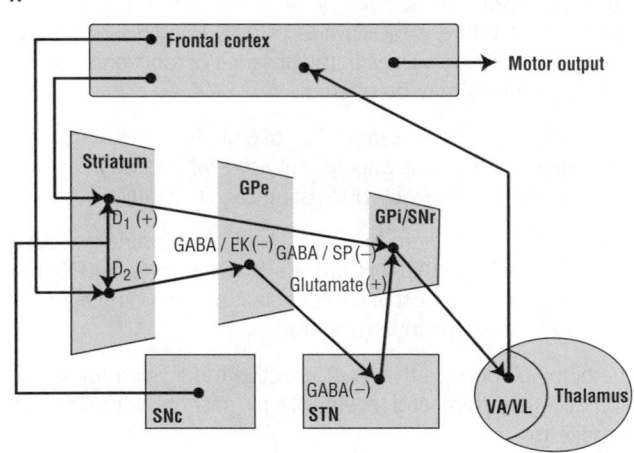

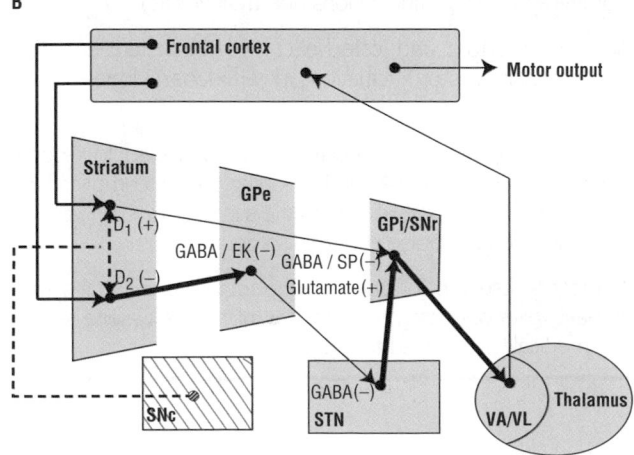

FIGURE 68-2. *A.* The normal balance of the basal ganglia–thalamocortical circuit. *B.* With nigrostriatal degeneration *(dashed line)*, there is loss of inhibition of the GPi by the direct pathway and activation of the GPi via the indirect pathway, resulting in decreased activation of the cortex. See text for details. (GPe, globus pallidus externa; GPi, globus pallidus interna; SNc, substantia nigra pars compacta; SNr, substantia nigra pars reticulata; STN, subthalamic nucleus; VA, ventroanterior nuclei of the thalamus; VL, ventrolateral nuclei of the thalamus.)

the inhibitory γ-aminobutyric acid (GABA)/substance P efferents to the globus pallidus interna (GPi) and substantia nigra pars reticulata. The GPi and substantia nigra pars reticulata efferents are inhibitory to the thalamus.[17] In IPD, the reduced activation of D_1 receptors results in greater inhibition of the thalamus. The indirect pathway involves activation of striatal dopamine$_2$ (D_2) dopamine receptors (which are coupled to a guanosine triphosphate-binding protein that opens potassium channels to hyperpolarize neurons, thereby reducing the excitability of the neuron).[17] Activation of striatal D_2 receptors inhibits GABA/enkephalin efferents (medium spiny neurons) to the globus pallidus externa. The globus pallidus externa projects GABA neurons to the subthalamic nucleus. Here, excitatory glutamatergic neurons project to the GPi. GPi output is inhibitory on the glutamatergic thalamic projections. In IPD, the reduced activation of D_2 receptors translates into greater inhibition of the thalamus. In IPD, restoring activity at the D_2 receptor appears to be of more importance than the D_1 receptor for mediating clinical improvements. Overall, loss of the presynaptic nigrostriatal dopamine neurons in IPD results in inhibition of thalamic activity and reduced activation of the motor cortex. Dopaminergic therapies help to restore motor activity.

In addition to dopamine, the synaptic organization of the basal ganglia also involves a variety of other neurotransmitters and neuromodulators, including acetylcholine, adenosine, enkephalins, GABA, glutamate, serotonin, and substance P. The potential role for drug modulation of these other neurotransmitters and receptor types is an active area of research and novel drug discovery for IPD.[18]

Atypical parkinsonian disorders, such as multiple system atrophy and progressive supranuclear palsy are characterized by damage to postsynaptic striatal neurons and dopamine receptors. Dopaminergic therapies provide less robust efficacy in atypical parkinsonism.

CLINICAL PRESENTATION

Although IPD is unmistakable in its advanced form, recognizing IPD during the early stages can be challenging. Clinically probable IPD can be diagnosed when at least two of the following are present: limb muscle rigidity, resting tremor (at 3–6 Hz and abolished by movement), or bradykinesia (Table 68–1).[19] Asymmetry in the presence or severity of these motor features is also a conspicuous finding. Overall, a diagnosis of IPD can be made with a high level of confidence in a patient who has resting tremor (along with bradykinesia and/or rigidity), prominent asymmetry, and a good response to dopaminergic therapy. For the diagnosis of IPD, other conditions must be reasonably excluded (Table 68–1). Medication-induced parkinsonism can mimic IPD, so it is important to establish if such medications have been used (especially drugs that block D_2 receptors, such as antipsychotics, metoclopramide, or phenothiazine antiemetics). Neurologic conditions that can be mistaken for IPD include atypical parkinsonisms (e.g., corticobasal ganglionic degeneration, forms of multiple system atrophy, progressive supranuclear palsy) and essential tremor. Because the management and prognosis of IPD differs from these other conditions, an accurate diagnosis is important. When the diagnosis is in doubt, referral to a movement disorders specialist is recommended.

PRESENTATION OF IDIOPATHIC PARKINSON'S DISEASE

General Features

- For clinically probable IPD, the patient exhibits at least two of the following: resting tremor, rigidity, or bradykinesia. Asymmetric onset and severity of these features is typical.

- Postural instability (difficulty with maintaining balance) is more common in advanced IPD.

Motor Symptoms

- The patient experiences decreased manual dexterity, difficulty arising from a seated position, diminished arm swing during ambulation, dysarthria (slurred speech), dysphagia (difficulty with swallowing), festinating gait (tendency to pass from a walking to a running pace), flexed posture (axial, upper/lower extremities), "freezing" at initiation of movement, hypomimia (reduced facial animation), hypophonia (reduced voice volume), and micrographia (diminution of handwritten letters/symbols) (Fig. 68–3).

Autonomic and Sensory Symptoms

- The patient experiences bladder and anal sphincter disturbances, constipation, diaphoresis, fatigue, olfactory disturbance, orthostatic blood pressure changes, pain, paresthesia, paroxysmal vascular flushing, seborrhea, sexual dysfunction, and sialorrhea (drooling).

Mental Status Changes

- The patient experiences anxiety, apathy, bradyphrenia (slowness of thought processes), confusional state, dementia, depression, hallucinosis/psychosis (typically drug induced), and sleep disorders (excessive daytime sleepiness, insomnia, obstructive sleep apnea, and rapid eye movement sleep behavior disorder).

Laboratory Tests

- No laboratory tests are available to diagnose IPD.

Other Diagnostic Tests

- Genetic testing is not routinely helpful.

- Neuroimaging may be useful for excluding other diagnoses.

- Medication history should be obtained to rule out drug-induced parkinsonism.

IPD develops insidiously and progressively worsens. Over many years, symptoms generally worsen to the point of severe disability, necessitating placement in a skilled nursing facility (especially with the development of dementia or frequent falling). However, in a subset of patients, clinical symptoms remain stable for many years.

Tremor of an upper extremity occurring at rest (and occasionally a postural tremor) is often the sole presenting complaint; however, only two-thirds of patients with IPD have tremor on diagnosis, and some never develop this sign. Tremor in IPD is present most commonly in the hands, sometimes with a characteristic pill-rolling motion. Less commonly, tremor may involve the jaw, legs, and toes. Like other motor features of IPD, resting tremor often begins unilaterally and becomes bilateral with disease progression. Stressful or emotional (either negative or positive) situations often increase the tremor amplitude and severity. Usually, volitional movement abolishes resting tremor, and tremor is absent during sleep. Although resting tremor is visibly noticeable in IPD and may cause social embarrassment for the patient, it often is the least physically disabling of the motor features.

Rigidity is the increased muscular resistance to passive range of motion and commonly affects the upper and lower extremities. If tremor is present in the affected extremity, the rigidity is associated with a cogwheel or ratchet-like quality upon examination. Facial muscles also are affected, resulting in hypomimia (masking of facial expressions) that may be erroneously interpreted as apathy, depression, or unfriendliness.

Bradykinesia refers to slowness of movement. Movement in IPD is often slow throughout an intended action, and difficulty with the

TABLE 68-1 Diagnostic Criteria for Idiopathic Parkinson's Disease and Differential Diagnosis

Idiopathic Parkinson's disease
  Clinically possible: Presence of one of the following: resting tremor, rigidity, or bradykinesia
  Clinically probable: Presence of at least two of the following: resting tremor, rigidity, or bradykinesia
  Clinically definite: Presence of at least two of the following: resting tremor, rigidity, or bradykinesia and a positive response to antiparkinsonian pharmacotherapy
Differential diagonsis
  Essential tremor
  Secondary parkinsonism
    Pharmacotoxicity (drug induced)
      Antiemetics (e.g., metoclopramide, prochlorperazine)
      Antipsychotics (e.g., phenothiazines, haloperidol, olanzapine, risperidone)
      Other drugs (α-methyldopa, cinnarizine, flunarizine, tetrabenazine)
    Environmental toxicity
      Carbon monoxide poisoning
      Manganese
      Methanol
      MPTP (1-methyl-4-phenyl-1,2,3,6-tetrahydropyridine)
      Organophosphates
    Infections
      Human immunodeficiency virus–associated parkinsonism
      Postencephalitic parkinsonism
      Subacute sclerosing panencephalitis
    Metabolic disorder
      Hypothyroidism
      Parathyroid abnormalities
    Neoplasms, strokes, traumatic lesions involving the nigrostriatal pathways
    Normal-pressure hydrocephalus
  Parkinsonism with other neuronal system degenerations
    Alzheimer with parkinsonism
    Corticobasal ganglionic degeneration
    Creutzfeldt-Jakob disease (CJD)
    Dementia with Lewy bodies
    Frontotemporal dementia
    Progressive supranuclear palsy
    Multiple-system atrophies
      Striatonigral degeneration
      Shy-Drager syndrome
      Olivopontocerebellar atrophy
    Familial (hereditary) parkinsonism
      Autosomal dominant
        α-Synuclein gene mutation (PARK1 and PARK4)
        Frontotemporal dementia parkinsonism (FTDP-17)
        Levodopa responsive dystonia
        Leucine-rich repeat kinase 2 (LRRK2) mutation
        Rapid-onset dystonia parkinsonism (DYT12)
        Spinocerebellar ataxias (SCA2, SCA3)
      Autosomal recessive
        Pantothenate kinase-associated neurodegeneration (PKAN)
        Niemann Pick type C
        Wilson disease
        Young-onset parkinsonism (DJ-1, parkin, PINK1)
      X-linked recessive
        Fragile X tremor/ataxia syndrome (FXTAS)
        Lubag (DYT3 or Filipino dystonia parkinsonism)
        Waisman syndrome (X-linked parkinsonism with mental retardation)

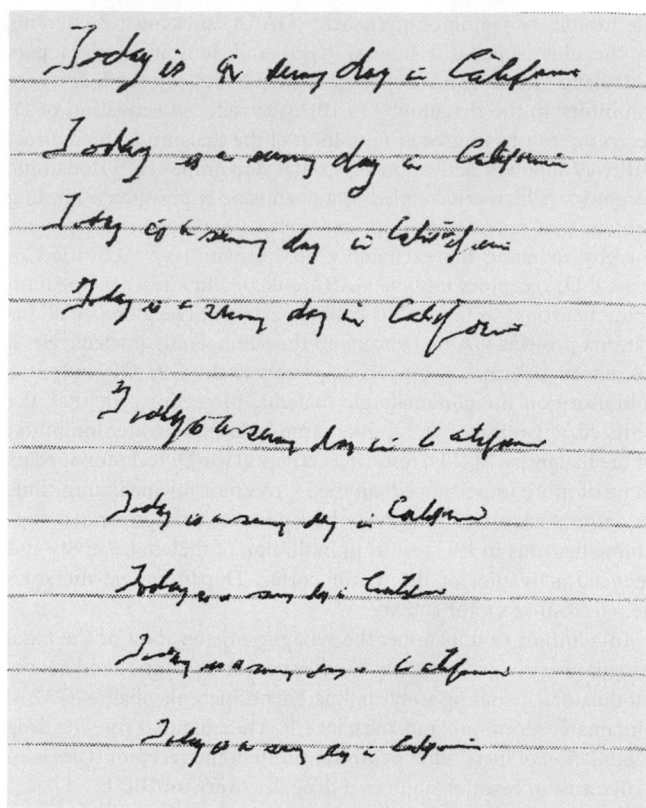

FIGURE 68-3. Example of micrographia in a patient with IPD. As the sentence, "Today is a sunny day in California" is repeatedly handwritten, progressive diminution of letter size occurs (micrographia). The height of each lined row is approximately 5/16 inches (8 mm). *(Courtesy of Jack J. Chen, PharmD, and David M. Swope, MD.)*

Postural instability, most common in advanced stages of IPD, is one of the most disabling problems of IPD because it increases the fall risk and is least amenable to pharmacotherapy. Testing for impaired postural responses by means of the pull test (in which a patient is unable to recover balance after sudden backward displacement at the shoulders) can help to identify the risk for falling. Many patients with impaired postural responses also have tendencies for propulsive gait (festination) and freezing, which also increases the risk of falling.

Although IPD is known predominantly as a disorder of motor capabilities, neuropsychiatric abnormalities also develop. Intellectual deterioration is not inevitable in IPD; however, some patients deteriorate in a manner indistinguishable from Alzheimer disease and other dementing conditions.[20] IPD patients are also at increased risk for anxiety and depression.[21] Although the disabilities of IPD may provoke depression in some instances, the underlying biochemical changes in the brain associated with IPD pathophysiology also predisposes for endogenous depression.

TREATMENT

■ DESIRED OUTCOMES

The goal in the management of IPD is to improve motor and nonmotor symptoms so that patients are able to maintain the best possible quality of life.[22] Specific objectives to consider when selecting an intervention include preservation of the ability to perform activities of daily living; improvement of mobility; minimization of adverse effects, treatment complications, putative disease modification; and improvement of nonmotor features such as

initiation of movement also occurs. A progressive slowing and decline in dexterity may impair tasks such as hand clapping, finger tapping, and handwriting (Fig. 68–3). Intermittent immobility (*freezing*) is another common characteristic. Freezing is especially likely to occur in situations such as when walking through a narrow doorway or initiating a turn. Patients also may experience a slow shuffling gait with difficulty halting their steps while in motion (festinating gait).

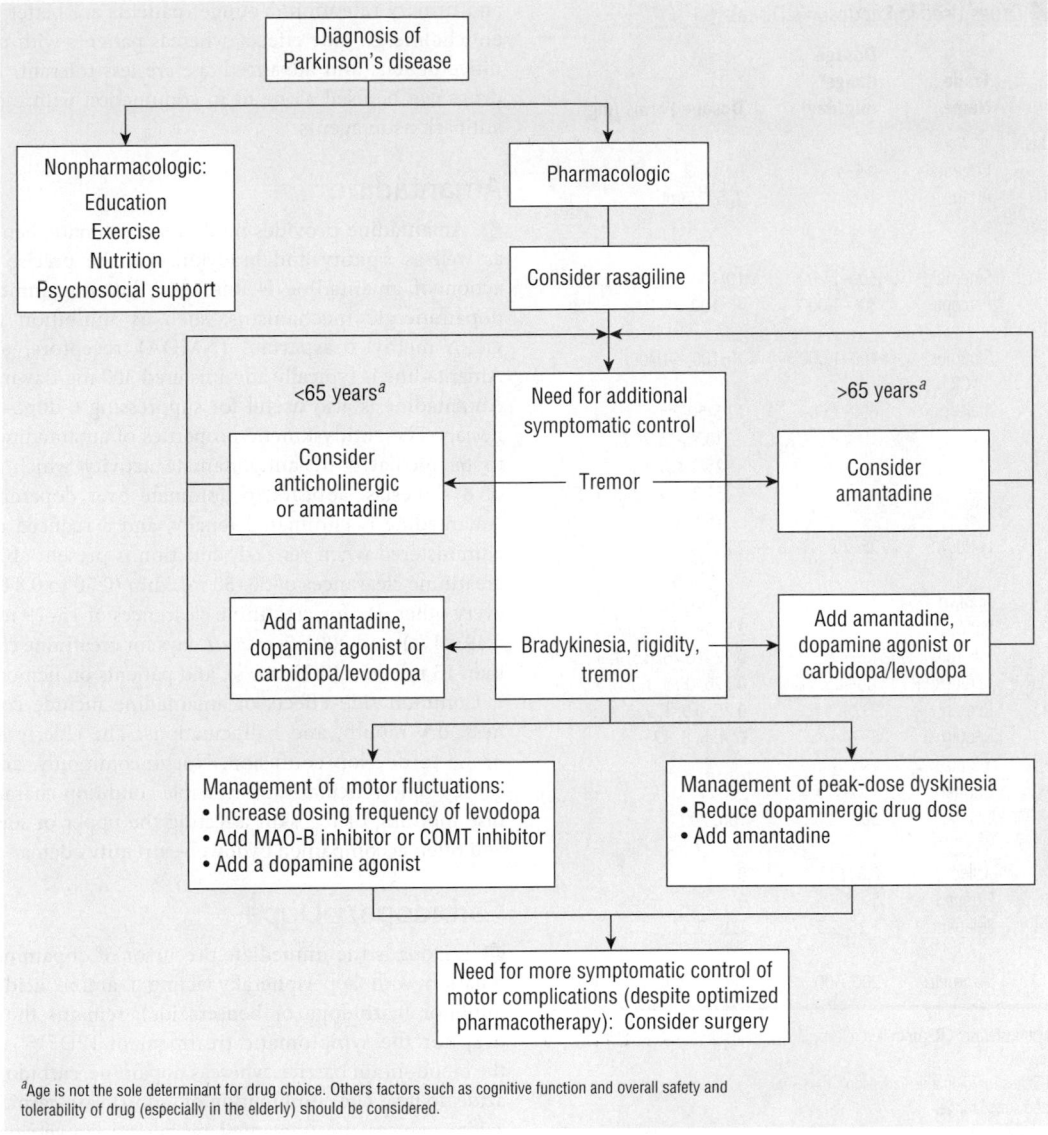

FIGURE 68-4. General approach to the management of early to advanced Parkinson's disease.

cognitive impairment, depression, fatigue, and sleep disorders. To accomplish some of these objectives, consultation with a specialist is helpful (e.g., movement disorders, physical therapy, psychiatry, and sleep medicine).

GENERAL APPROACH TO TREATMENT

❶ Once a correct diagnosis of IPD is made, nonpharmacologic and pharmacologic interventions must be considered. Figure 68–4 illustrates a general treatment approach for early and advanced IPD and Table 68–2 summarizes antiparkinsonian medications and mechanisms of action. Treatment guidelines and monographs are updated frequently to keep up with new information and changes in treatment paradigms.[23–28]

❷ In the absence of functional impairment, initial monotherapy may be initiated with an MAO-B inhibitor, such as rasagiline, with the addition of other therapeutic agents as IPD motor symptoms progressively worsen. Therapy with rasagiline in early stage PD has been demonstrated to slow the decline of motor function and is well tolerated. The definition of functional impairment is highly patient specific. Factors such as comorbid conditions, cognitive status, employment, lifestyle, and patients' desires must be considered when initiating pharmacotherapy.

In a "physiologically" young patient experiencing functional impairment, monotherapy with a dopamine agonist or rasagiline is preferred. For patients who are older, cognitively impaired, or experiencing moderately severe functional impairment, L-dopa (e.g., carbidopa/levodopa) is preferred. Ultimately, all patients will require the use of L-dopa (either as monotherapy or in combination with other agents). With the development of motor fluctuations, addition of a catechol-O-methyltransferase (COMT) inhibitor should be considered to extend L-dopa duration of activity, or if the patient is not already on an MAO-B inhibitor or dopamine agonist, addition of either one should be considered. For management of L-dopa induced peak-dose dyskinesias, the addition of amantadine should be considered. Surgery is considered only in patients who need more symptomatic control or who are experiencing severe motor complications despite pharmacologically optimized therapy.

The treatment plan evolves as the disease progresses and must include consideration of short-term symptomatic relief as well as long-term effects. Patient specific factors that guide selection of therapies include the "functional" age of the patient, patient's desired outcomes, cognitive status, severity of motor features, and response to any previous IPD therapies. Patient education should be communicated with realistic optimism. For example, it

TABLE 68-2 Drugs Used in Parkinson's Disease[a]

Generic Name	Trade Name	Dosage Range[b] (mg/day)	Dosage Forms (mg)
Anticholinergic drugs			
Benztropine	Cogentin	0.5–4	0.5, 1, 2
Trihexyphenidyl	Artane	1–6	2, 5, 2/5mL
Carbidopa/levodopa products			
Carbidopa/L-dopa	Sinemet	300–1,000[c]	10/100, 25/100, 25/250
Carbidopa/L-dopa ODT	Parcopa	300–1,000[c]	10/100, 25/100, 25/250
Carbidopa/L-dopa CR	Sinemet CR	400–1,000[c]	25/100, 50/200
Carbidopa/L-dopa/entacapone	Stalevo	600–1,600[d]	12.5/50/200, 18.75/75/200, 25/100/200, 31.25/125/200, 37.5/150/200, 50/200/200
Carbidopa	Lodosyn	25–75	25
Dopamine agonists			
Apomorphine	Apokyn	3–12	30/3 mL
Bromocriptine	Parlodel	15–40	2.5, 5
Pramipexole	Mirapex	1.5–4.5	0.125, 0.25, 0.5, 1, 1.5
Pramipexole ER	Mirapex ER	1.5–4.5	0.375, 0.75, 1.5, 3, 4.5
Ropinirole	Requip	9–24	0.25, 0.5; 1, 2, 3, 4, 5
Ropinirole XL	Requip XL	8–24	2, 4, 6, 8, 12
COMT inhibitors			
Entacapone	Comtan	200–1,600	200
Tolcapone	Tasmar	300–600	100, 200
MAO-B inhibitors			
Rasagiline	Azilect	0.5–1	0.5, 1
Selegiline	Eldepryl	5–10	5
Selegiline ODT	Zelapar	1.25–2.5	1.25, 2.5
Miscellaneous			
Amantadine	Symmetrel	200–300	100, 50/5 mL

COMT, catechol-*O*-methyltransferase; CR, controlled release; MAO, monoamine oxidase; ODT, orally disintegrating tablet.

[a]Marketed in the United States for idiopathic Parkinson's disease.
[b]Dosages may vary beyond stated range.
[c]Dosages expressed as L-dopa component.
[d]Dosages expressed as entacapone component.

should be explained that although there is no cure for IPD, modern medicine has many medications that can provide relief of symptoms. Nonpharmacologic interventions such as exercise should be encouraged, and attention to nonmotor features of IPD should not be neglected.

■ PHARMACOLOGIC THERAPY

Anticholinergic Medications

❸ Because dopamine provides negative feedback to acetylcholine neurons in the striatum, the degeneration of nigrostriatal dopamine neurons also results in a relative increase of striatal cholinergic interneuron activity. This increased cholinergic activity (caused by dopamine depletion) is believed to contribute to the tremor of IPD. The anticholinergic drugs (e.g., benztropine and trihexyphenidyl) are considered effective against tremor but no more so than dopaminergic agents.[23–25] Sometimes dystonic symptoms associated with IPD are also improved by anticholinergic agents. Use of anticholinergic agents is limited due to the development of intolerable side effects, necessitating dosage reduction or drug discontinuation. Common adverse effects include blurred vision, confusion, constipation, dry mouth, memory difficulty, sedation,

and urinary retention. Younger patients are better able to tolerate anticholinergic side effects, whereas patients with preexisting cognitive deficits and advanced age are less tolerant. Anticholinergic drugs can be used alone or in conjunction with L-dopa and other antiparkinson agents.

Amantadine

❹ Amantadine provides modest symptomatic benefit for tremor, as well as rigidity and bradykinesia. The precise mechanism of action of amantadine is unknown, but dopaminergic and nondopaminergic mechanisms, such as inhibition of glutamatergic *N*-methyl-D-aspartate (NMDA) receptors, are implicated. Amantadine is typically administered 300 mg/day in divided doses. Amantadine is also useful for suppressing L-dopa–induced dyskinesia.[27] The antidyskinetic properties of amantadine are presumed to be mediated by antiglutamate activity which, in the setting of dyskinesias, appears to dominate over dopaminergic activity. Amantadine is eliminated renally, and a reduced dose should be administered when renal dysfunction is present (100 mg/day with creatinine clearances of 30–50 mL/min (0.50 to 0.84 mL/s), 100 mg every other day for creatinine clearances of 15–29 mL/min (0.25 to 0.49 mL/s), and 200 mg every 7 days for creatinine clearances of less than 15 mL/min (0.25 mL/s), and patients on hemodialysis).

Common side effects of amantadine include confusion, dizziness, dry mouth, and hallucinations. The elderly are particularly prone to develop confusion. Not uncommonly, amantadine may cause livedo reticularis, a reversible condition characterized by diffuse mottling of the skin affecting the upper or lower extremities and often accompanied by lower-extremity edema.

Carbidopa/L-Dopa

❺ L-Dopa is the immediate precursor of dopamine and, in combination with a peripherally acting L-amino acid decarboxylase inhibitor (carbidopa or benserazide), remains the most effective drug for the symptomatic treatment of IPD.[23–25] L-Dopa crosses the blood–brain barrier, whereas dopamine, carbidopa, and benserazide do not. The combination of L-dopa with carbidopa or benserazide, reduces the unwanted peripheral conversion of L-dopa to dopamine. As a result, increased amounts of L-dopa are transported into the brain, and peripheral adverse effects of dopamine, such as nausea, are reduced. In the SNc, L-dopa is converted, via decarboxylation, to dopamine by the enzyme L-amino acid decarboxylase (Fig. 68–5). The converted dopamine is stored in the presynaptic SNc neurons until stimulated to be released into the synaptic cleft whereupon it binds to the D_1 and D_2 postsynaptic receptors. Dopamine activity is terminated primarily by reuptake back into the presynaptic neuron by means of a dopamine transporter. The enzymes MAO and COMT also inactivate dopamine.

❺ Regardless of what the initial therapeutic agent is, ultimately all patients with IPD will require L-dopa at some point. An initial maintenance L-dopa regimen of 300 mg/day (in divided doses and in combination with carbidopa or benserazide) often is adequate. With regard to carbidopa, about 75 mg/day is required to sufficiently inhibit the peripheral activity of L-amino acid decarboxylase, but some patients require more. Therefore, the usual initial maintenance carbidopa/L-dopa regimen is 25/100 mg 3 times daily. As the motor features of IPD become progressively more severe, use of higher dosages is required. There is no maximum allowable total daily L-dopa dose; however, the usual maximal dose needed by patients, even those with severe IPD, is 800 to 1,000 mg/day. Slow buildup of dose (e.g., increments of 100 mg L-dopa per week) can help to minimize treatment emergent side effects, such as nausea, postural hypotension, sedation, vivid dreaming, and vomiting.

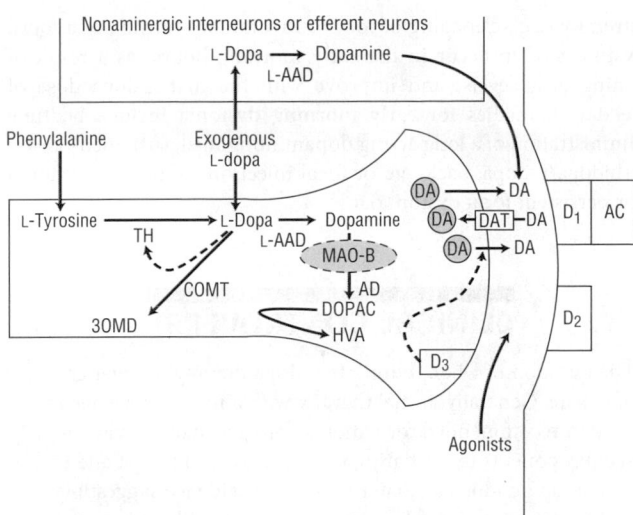

FIGURE 68-5. Dopamine metabolism in presynaptic dopamine neuron. (3OMD, 3-O-methyldopa; AC, adenylate cyclase; AD, aldehyde dehydrogenase; COMT, catechol-O-methyl transferase; D₁–D₃, dopamine receptors; DA, dopamine; DAT, dopamine transporter; DOPAC, 3,4-dihydroxyphenylacetic acid; HVA, homovanillic acid; L-AAD, L-aromatic amino acid decarboxylase; MAO-B, monoamine oxidase B; TH, tyrosine hydroxylase.)

TABLE 68-3	Common Motor Complications and Possible Initial Treatments
Effect	**Possible Treatments**
End-of-dose "wearing off" (motor fluctuation)	Increase frequency of carbidopa/L-dopa doses; add either COMT inhibitor or MAO-B inhibitor or dopamine agonist
"Delayed on" or "no on" response	Give carbidopa/L-dopa on empty stomach; use carbidopa/L-dopa ODT; avoid carbidopa/L-dopa CR; use apomorphine subcutaneous
Start hesitation ("freezing")	Increase carbidopa/L-dopa dose; add a dopamine agonist or MAO-B inhibitor; utilize physical therapy along with assistive walking devices or sensory cues (e.g., rhythmic commands, stepping over objects)
Peak-dose dyskinesia	Provide smaller doses of carbidopa/L-dopa; add amantadine

COMT, catechol-O-methyltransferase; CR, controlled release; MAO, monoamine oxidase; ODT, orally disintegrating tablet.

For patients with difficulty swallowing tablets, an orally disintegrating tablet preparation of carbidopa/L-dopa is available. Although this formulation rapidly dissolves on contact with saliva, the carbidopa/L-dopa does not undergo transmucosal absorption and must reach the proximal duodenum for absorption.

Pharmacokinetics There is marked intra- and intersubject variability in the time to peak plasma concentrations after oral L-dopa, and this may in part be attributed to differences in gastric emptying. L-Dopa is absorbed primarily in the proximal duodenum by a saturable large neutral amino acid transport system. Competition for this transporter by dietary or supplemental large neutral amino acids (e.g., leucine, phenylalanine) can interfere with L-dopa bioavailability.

L-Dopa is not bound to plasma proteins. Active transport across the blood–brain barrier occurs by the large neutral amino acid transporter system. Because large amounts of dietary large neutral amino acids may compete for transport across the blood–brain barrier and interfere with the clinical response to L-dopa, separation of L-dopa administration with high protein meals has been recommended. However, in patients with early IPD, this interaction is generally not significant. In advanced IPD, special diets involving protein restriction or redistribution may improve L-dopa responsiveness and are sometimes implemented. A metabolite of L-dopa, 3-O-methyldopa, also competes for transport, but it is not clear how this affects L-dopa clinical response.

When peripheral decarboxylation of L-dopa is inhibited by carbidopa or benserazide, 3-O-methylation (via COMT) becomes the predominant catabolic pathway. The elimination half-life of L-dopa is about 1 hour, and this is extended to about 1.5 hours with the addition of carbidopa or benserazide. With the addition of a COMT inhibitor such as entacapone to carbidopa/L-dopa, the elimination half-life is extended to about 2 to 2.5 hours.

❻ Motor Complications of L-Dopa Long-term L-dopa therapy is associated with a variety of motor complications, of which end-of-dose "wearing off" (motor fluctuations) and L-dopa peak-dose dyskinesias are the two most commonly encountered.[29] These motor complications can be disabling and challenging to manage. The approximate risk of developing either motor fluctuations or dyskinesia is 10% per year of L-dopa therapy.[30,31] However, motor complications can occur as early as 5 to 6 months after starting L-dopa therapy, especially if excessive doses are used initially.[32] Table 68-3 lists the motor complications associated with long-term treatment with L-dopa and suggested initial management strategies. Initiating therapy with the controlled-release form of carbidopa/L-dopa does not reduce the development of motor complications compared with standard-release carbidopa/L-dopa.[27]

❻ End-of-Dose Wearing Off. The terms "off" and "on" refer to periods of poor movement (i.e., return of tremor, rigidity, or slowness) and good movement, respectively. End-of-dose wearing off prior to a dose of medication is a common type of response fluctuation. This phenomenon is related to the increasing loss of neuronal storage capability for dopamine as well as the short half-life of L-dopa. Initially, exogenous L-dopa is taken up by the remaining SNc neurons, converted to dopamine, and stored in synaptic vesicles. With progressive loss of SNc neurons, storage capacity, and synthesis of endogenously derived dopamine, patients become more dependent on exogenous L-dopa. Hence the peripheral pharmacokinetic properties of L-dopa increasingly become the determinant of central dopamine synthesis. With advancing IPD, the duration of action of a single carbidopa/L-dopa dose progressively shortens, and in some cases may produce benefits for as little as 1 hour. As a result, carbidopa/L-dopa needs to be given more frequently so as to minimize daytime off episodes and to maximize on time. In addition to administering L-dopa doses more frequently, other options are available (see Table 68-3). In particular, the addition of the COMT inhibitor entacapone or the MAO-B inhibitor rasagiline extends the action of L-dopa, and either should be considered.[27] A controlled-release (CR) L-dopa product is available, but is not considered very effective for management of motor fluctuations.[27]

A dopamine agonist (e.g., pramipexole, ropinirole) also can be added to a carbidopa/L-dopa regimen in an attempt to minimize the occurrence of wearing off. For acute off episodes, a subcutaneously administered short-acting dopamine agonist, apomorphine, is available and possesses a rapid onset of effect (within 20 minutes). It is administered as needed.[33] Alternatively, chronic subcutaneous apomorphine infusion (not yet available in the United States) provides stable and continuous systemic and central drug concentrations and improves motor fluctuations and dyskinesias. Long-term therapy is limited by injection site skin reactions.[34] In addition, intraduodenal/jejunal L-dopa infusions produce constant and smoother stimulation of striatal dopamine receptors and thus stabilize response fluctuations. An infusible duodenal carbidopa/L-dopa gel (not yet available in the United States) has been demonstrated to be an effective and safe therapy, and, as with subcutaneous apomorphine infusion, would be considered a last-line pharmacologic therapy for patients with persistent, on/off fluctuations.[35] Although not commonly performed, sipping small amounts of carbidopa/L-dopa solution very frequently throughout the day is also a method for managing on/off fluctuations. A solution that is stable for 72 hours at room temperature can be prepared by adding 10 tablets of carbidopa/L-dopa 10/100 (or 25/100) mg and 2 g crystalline ascorbic acid to 1 L of water.[36]

Often, off episodes occur during the night, and patients will awaken in an off state (as a consequence of an overnight decline of drug levels). Bedtime administration of a dopamine agonist or a drug formulation that provides sustained drug levels overnight (e.g., carbidopa/L-dopa CR, ropinirole XL, pramipexole ER) can help reduce nocturnal off episodes and improve functioning upon awakening.

"Delayed-On" and "No-On" Response. "Delayed-on" or "no-on" (a delayed or absent onset of drug effect, respectively) responses to individual doses of carbidopa/L-dopa can be a result of delayed gastric emptying or decreased absorption in the duodenum. Chewing a tablet or crushing it and then drinking a full glass of water, or using the orally disintegrating tablet formulation on an empty stomach, can help mitigate effects of delayed gastric emptying. Additionally, subcutaneously administered apomorphine may be used as rescue therapy from delayed-on or no-on periods. A drug-free period ("drug holiday") has been investigated in an attempt to modify postsynaptic dopamine receptors and thus decrease unpredictable off states. Although not commonly performed because of discomfort (to the patient) and medical risks, when drug holidays are performed, it should be under close medical supervision.

Freezing. "Freezing," or a sudden, episodic inhibition of lower-extremity motor function, may occur and will interfere with ambulation and increase the risk of falls. Patients may report that their "feet suddenly feel stuck to the floor" during ambulation or that they have difficulty initiating steps (start hesitation) or turns (turn hesitation). Freezing often is exacerbated by anxiety or when perceived obstacles (e.g., doorways, turnstiles) are encountered. Although changes to the antiparkinson drug regimen may be attempted, improvements are unlikely. Physical therapy along with assistive walking devices and sensory cues are helpful.

Dyskinesias. Another complication of L-dopa therapy is "on" period dyskinesias (involuntary choreiform movements involving usually the neck, trunk, and lower/upper extremities). If patients report "shakiness," it is important to clarify if they are referring to tremor or dyskinesias. Dyskinesias usually are associated with peak striatal dopamine levels (peak-dose dyskinesia) and, simplistically, can be thought of as too much movement secondary to extension of the pharmacologic effect resulting in excessive striatal dopamine receptor stimulation. Less commonly, dyskinesias also can develop during the rise and fall of L-dopa effects (the dyskinesia–improvement–dyskinesia or diphasic pattern of response). In the case of peak-dose dyskinesias, use of lower individual doses of L-dopa is beneficial. With the lowering of the L-dopa dose, dyskinesias improve but at the cost of returning parkinsonian features, thereby necessitating an increase in dosage frequency or addition of another agent to counteract the effects of using a lower L-dopa dose. Glutamate overactivity may also be involved as suggested by the antidyskinesia effect of amantadine (NMDA receptor antagonist) and positive results of investigational studies of antiglutamate ligands in animal models.[37] For severe dyskinesias (despite pharmacologically optimized therapy), surgery should be considered.

"Off-Period" Dystonia. In IPD, dystonias (sustained muscle contractions) can occur and more commonly affect a distal lower extremity (e.g., clenching of toes or involuntary turning of a foot). Dystonias often occur in the early morning hours (as a result of waning drug levels) and improve with the first L-dopa dose of the day. Remedies for early morning dystonia include bedtime administration of a long acting dopamine agonist, sustained-release carbidopa/L-dopa, baclofen, or focal injections of botulinum toxin (for persistent focal dystonia).

CLINICAL CONTROVERSY

The question of when to initiate L-dopa therapy is a matter of debate. Generally, initial therapy with a non–L-dopa agent is often recommended for patients younger than 65 years of age. Proponents for initiating non–L-dopa agents first and then adding L-dopa at a later point, cite evidence suggesting that long-term L-dopa therapy is associated with an increased risk of motor complications that can be disabling and challenging to manage. Additionally, drugs such as rasagiline and dopamine agonists provide sufficient symptom control for mild to moderate IPD. The counterargument is that L-dopa is inexpensive, more effective, and the development of motor complications is an acceptable trade-off. Age alone should not be the major deciding factor, and ultimately, individualized considerations of a patient's disability should guide all interventions for IPD.

Monoamine Oxidase B Inhibitors

❹ Two selective MAO-B inhibitors, rasagiline and selegiline, are available in the United States for management of IPD. The selective inhibition of MAO-B in the brain interferes with the degradation of dopamine and results in prolonged dopaminergic activity. Both drugs contain a propargylamine moiety, which is essential for conferring irreversible inhibition of MAO-B. At therapeutic doses, these agents preferentially and irreversibly inhibit MAO-B over MAO-A.

A common concern with use of these agents is the potential for interactions with drugs that possess serotonergic activity. Concomitant use of MAO-B inhibitors with meperidine and other selected opioid analgesics is contraindicated because of a small risk of serotonin syndrome. However, concomitant use of other agents that enhance serotonin levels (e.g., antidepressants) is not contraindicated and can be used concomitantly when clinically warranted.

❹ ❼ Selegiline, also known as L-deprenyl, is marketed for extending L-dopa effects and is typically administered 5 mg twice daily. Selegiline is also available as an orally disintegrating tablet formulation administered 1.25 to 2.5 mg once daily. A transdermal formulation of selegiline is also available but is not indicated for IPD. As monotherapy in early IPD, conventional selegiline provides modest improvements in motor function.[23-25] In more advanced IPD, the adjunctive use of conventional selegiline can provide up to 1 hour of extended on time for patients with wearing off, although the data are inconsistent.[27] This inconsistent effect of conventional selegiline may be explained, in part, by poor and erratic bioavailability of the parent drug.

As an amphetamine pharmacophore, selegiline undergoes first-pass hepatic metabolism (predominantly via cytochrome P450 [CYP] 2B6 and 2C19) to end products of L-methamphetamine and L-amphetamine. Adverse effects of selegiline are minimal but can include insomnia (especially if administered at bedtime), hallucinations, and jitteriness. Selegiline also increases the peak effects of L-dopa and can worsen preexisting dyskinesias or psychiatric symptoms such as delusions. With the selegiline orally disintegrating tablet formulation, first-pass hepatic metabolism is bypassed as a consequence of transmucosal absorption of the drug. Hence, bioavailability characteristics of the parent drug are improved and formation of amphetamine metabolites is reduced. Thus, the selegiline orally disintegrating tablet formulation may provide an improved response relative to conventional selegiline.

4 7 Rasagiline is a second-generation, irreversible, selective MAO-B inhibitor administered at 0.5 or 1 mg once daily.[38] Rasagiline is effective as monotherapy in early IPD and also as add-on therapy for managing motor fluctuations in advanced IPD. In a large, placebo-controlled, 18-month, delayed-start clinical trial, patients initiated on rasagiline monotherapy early in IPD had less functional decline than did patients whose treatment was delayed for 9 months.[39] This suggests that earlier initiation with rasagiline (even before the onset of functional impairment) is associated with better long-term outcomes. For the management of patients with motor fluctuations, the efficacy of rasagiline appears similar to that of entacapone, offering approximately 1 hour of extra on time during the day.[40] Consequently, when an adjunctive agent is required for managing motor fluctuations, rasagiline is considered a first-line agent (as is entacapone).[27] Overall, rasagiline is well tolerated with minimal gastrointestinal or neuropsychiatric side effects. Rasagiline is metabolized by hepatic CYP1A2 to aminoindan, which is inactive and devoid of amphetamine-like properties.[38]

MAO-B inhibitors with a propargylamine molecular scaffolding have been investigated for neuroprotective properties (clinically referred to as disease modification). These agents inhibit the oxidative deamination of dopamine, which generates hydrogen peroxide and, ultimately, oxyradicals capable of damaging nigrostriatal neurons (see Fig. 68–1). Because MAO-B inhibition diverts dopamine catabolism to an alternate route that does not generate peroxide, MAO-B inhibitor therapy may spare neurons from oxidative stress. Additionally, MAO-B inhibitors have demonstrated antiapoptotic properties in laboratory experiments, further suggesting the possibility of disease modification. Clinical studies to demonstrate disease modification with selegiline have yielded inconclusive results, perhaps contributed in part by selegiline amphetamine metabolites as well as inadequate study methodology. However, results with rasagiline 1 mg/day from clinical studies utilizing methodology (i.e., delayed start) to demonstrate disease modification have been positive.[39,41]

CLINICAL CONTROVERSY

Great interest and debate surround the putative disease modifying effects of the MAO-B inhibitors. To date, only rasagiline has been shown to slow the rate of progression of motor impairment in patients with early IPD. A large clinical study demonstrated that earlier initiation of rasagiline is associated with better outcomes as compared to delaying therapy, and this was attributed to a disease modifying effect (as opposed to a symptomatic effect). Whether this is a class effect of MAO-B inhibitors is not known. However, selegiline is metabolized to amphetamine derivatives which have been demonstrated to neutralize neuroprotective effects in various preclinical studies. In a clinical study of the dopamine agonist pramipexole in patients with early IPD, no benefit of earlier initiation over delayed initation was observed.

COMT Inhibitors

7 Two COMT inhibitors, entacapone and tolcapone, have been developed to extend the effects of L-dopa and are indicated for managing wearing off.[27] Both reduce the peripheral conversion of L-dopa to dopamine, thus enhancing central L-dopa bioavailability. Consequently, in the absence of L-dopa, they have no effect on IPD symptoms. For patients with wearing off, these agents can decrease off-time significantly by increasing the L-dopa area under the curve by approximately 35%.[42] COMT inhibition is considered more effective than controlled-release carbidopa/L-dopa in providing consistent extension of L-dopa effect.[27] A triple-combination product of carbidopa/L-dopa/entacapone offers convenience for some patients (i.e., fewer tablets to administer).

Tolcapone inhibits both peripheral and central COMT. Its use is limited by reports of fatal hepatotoxicity, such that strict monitoring of hepatic function, especially during the first 6 months of therapy, is required. Because of the hepatotoxicity risk, tolcapone is reserved for patients with fluctuations that are not responding to other therapies.

Entacapone has a shorter half-life than tolcapone, and 200 mg needs to be given with each dose of carbidopa/L-dopa up to a maximum of 8 times per day. In clinical trials, both tolcapone and entacapone increased total daily on time by about 1 to 2 hours.[43,44] Dopaminergic adverse effects may occur and generally are manageable by reduction of the carbidopa/L-dopa dosage. With both agents, brownish-orange urinary discoloration may occur. Also, delayed onset of diarrhea (weeks to months later) can occur in up to 5% of patients. Unlike tolcapone, entacapone is not associated with hepatotoxicity and, if an adjunctive agent is needed for managing motor fluctuations, entacapone is considered one of the first choices.[27]

Dopamine Agonists

Dopamine agonists fall into two pharmacologic subtypes: ergot-derived agonists (bromocriptine) and the nonergot agonists (pramipexole, ropinirole). The nonergot dopamine agonists are safer than the ergot-derived agonists[45] and are useful as monotherapy in mild-moderate IPD, and also as adjuncts to L-dopa therapy in patients with motor fluctuations.[23–25,27] The dopamine agonists reduce the frequency of off periods and may allow reductions in L-dopa dosage.

8 Investigations comparing initial monotherapy with either L-dopa or a dopamine agonist in patients with IPD have revealed a significantly reduced risk of developing motor complications associated with dopamine agonists than with L-dopa.[46,47] Younger patients are more likely to develop motor complications; consequently, dopamine agonists are preferred over L-dopa. Older patients are more likely to experience intolerable side effects (e.g., hallucinations, orthostatic hypotension) from the dopamine agonists; consequently, carbidopa/L-dopa is preferred, particularly if cognitive problems or dementia is present. In terms of disease-modifying effects, the clinical data with dopamine agonists are inconclusive.[48–50]

Common adverse effects of dopamine agonists include nausea, confusion, hallucinations, light-headedness, lower-extremity edema, postural hypotension, sedation, and vivid dreaming. Less common but serious adverse effects include compulsive behaviors (e.g., pathologic gambling or shopping, hypersexuality), psychosis, and sleep attacks (sudden, unexpected episodes of sleep). Hallucinations and delusion can be managed using a stepwise approach (Table 68–4) that often involves the use of an atypical antipsychotic medication, such as clozapine or quetiapine.[21] The addition of a dopamine agonist to L-dopa therapy also can increase the frequency and severity of L-dopa induced dyskinesias, especially in patients with preexisting dyskinesias.

TABLE 68-4 Stepwise Approach to Management of Drug-Induced Hallucinosis and Psychosis in Parkinson's Disease

1. General measures such as evaluating for electrolyte disturbance (especially hypercalcemia or hyponatremia), hypoxemia, or infection (especially encephalitis, sepsis, or urinary tract infection).
2. Simplify the antiparkinsonian regimen as much as possible by discontinuing or reducing the dosage of medications with the highest risk-to-benefit ratio first.[a]
   a. Discontinue anticholinergics, including other nonparkinsonian medications with anticholinergic activity such as antihistamines or tricyclic antidepressants.
   b. Taper and discontinue amantadine.
   c. Discontinue monoamine oxidase-B inhibitor.
   d. Taper and discontinue dopamine agonist.
   e. Consider reduction of L-dopa (especially evening doses) and discontinuation of catechol-O-methyltransferase inhibitors.
3. Consider atypical antipsychotic medication if disruptive hallucinosis or psychosis persists.
   a. Quetiapine 12.5–25 mg at bedtime; gradually increase by 25 mg each week if necessary, until hallucinosis or psychosis improved or
   b. Clozapine 12.5–50 mg at bedtime; gradually increase by 25 mg each week if necessary until hallucinosis or psychosis improved (requires frequent monitoring for leukopenia).

[a]If dosage reduction or medication discontinuation is either infeasible or undesirable, go to step 3.

Initiation of a dopaminergic agonist is best performed by slow titration to minimize side effects. Pramipexole is initiated at a dose of 0.125 mg 3 times a day and increased every 5 to 7 days, as tolerated, to a maximum of 1.5 mg 3 times a day. An extended-release pramipexole formulation is also available for once-daily administration. Immediate-release ropinirole is initiated at 0.25 mg 3 times a day and increased by 0.25 mg 3 times a day on a weekly basis to a maximum of 24 mg/day. A controlled-release ropinirole formulation for once-daily administration is available.

Pramipexole is renally excreted with an 8- to 12-hour half-life. The initial dosage must be adjusted in renal insufficiency (0.125 mg twice daily for creatinine clearances of 35 to 59 mL/min [0.58 to 0.99 mL/s], 0.125 mg once daily for creatinine clearances of 15 to 34 mL/min [0.25 to 0.57 mL/s]). Ropinirole has a 6-hour half-life and is metabolized by CYP1A2. Potent inhibitors (e.g., fluoroquinolone antibiotics) and inducers (e.g., cigarette smoking) of this enzyme likely will lead to alterations in ropinirole clearance.

Apomorphine is an injectable nonergot dopamine agonist. It is an aporphine alkaloid originally derived from morphine but lacks narcotic properties.[33] Because of extensive hepatic first-pass metabolism, apomorphine is not suitable for oral administration and is administered subcutaneously. In some countries, apomorphine is also available for continuous subcutaneous infusion with minipumps. Apomorphine should not be injected intravenously. For patients with advanced IPD who are experiencing intermittent off episodes despite optimized therapy, administration of subcutaneous apomorphine effectively triggers an "on" response within 20 minutes.[33] The effective dose ranges from 2 to 6 mg per injection, with most patients requiring approximately 0.06 mg/kg. Sites of injection (abdomen, upper arm, and upper thigh) should be rotated to avoid development of subcutaneous nodules. The metabolic pathway of apomorphine remains unknown. Apomorphine elimination half-life is approximately 40 minutes, and the duration of benefit can be up to 100 minutes. Nausea and vomiting are common side effects, and prior to the initiation of apomorphine, patients should be premedicated with the antiemetic trimethobenzamide. Other side effects include dizziness, hallucinations, injection-site irritation, orthostatic hypotension, somnolence, and yawning. As a consequence of reports of severe hypotension and syncope, apomorphine is contraindicated with drugs in the serotonin (5HT₃)-receptor blocker class, including dolasetron, granisetron, and ondansetron.

SURGICAL THERAPY

9 Currently, surgery should be considered as an adjunct to pharmacotherapy when patients are experiencing frequent motor fluctuations or disabling dyskinesia or tremor despite an optimized medical regimen. There are several patient-selection criteria for surgery, including a diagnosis of L-dopa–responsive IPD. Anatomic targets include the thalamus, GPi, and the subthalamic nucleus. Bilateral, chronic, high-frequency electrical stimulation of a target site, also known as deep-brain stimulation (DBS), is the preferred surgical modality.[51]

In DBS surgery, a battery-powered neurostimulator (pacemaker-like device) is implanted subcutaneously below the clavicle and provides constant electrical stimulation, via electrode wires, to the targeted brain structure. Thalamic DBS is very effective for suppressing tremor (specifically arm tremor), but it does not significantly improve the other parkinsonian features (bradykinesia, rigidity, motor fluctuations, or dyskinesias). Although debatable, subthalamic nucleus DBS is favored over GPi DBS because it is considered more effective. Subthalamic nucleus DBS is associated with improvements in tremor, rigidity, bradykinesia, motor fluctuations, and dyskinesia, as well as lowering of antiparkinsonian medications. Problems with gait and postural instability do not improve significantly with DBS (or pharmacotherapy) and remain an unmet need; however, preliminary results for DBS of the pedunculopontine nucleus appear promising.[52]

DBS procedures require routine adjustment of the electrical stimulation parameters (e.g., voltage, frequency, and pulse width) to achieve optimal control while minimizing side effects. The electrical stimulation parameters (or "electrical dosage") are adjusted via a programmable handheld device to meet each patient's needs and are performed by physicians as well as other trained individuals, including nurse practitioners and clinical pharmacists.

In recent years, cell-based restorative procedures have appeared promising (implantation of dopamine producing cells such as human fetal mesencephalon tissue or retinal pigmented epithelial cells into the striatum) but have yielded disappointing clinical results.[53–54] Gene-based therapies are currently under investigation and remain highly experimental.[55]

PHARMACOECONOMIC CONSIDERATIONS

Pharmacoeconomic assessments in IPD are important. IPD places a high economic burden on society.[56] Based on an estimated 1 million cases of IPD in the United States, the direct costs associated with IPD are in the range of $4 to $8 billion per year. If indirect costs, such as lost productivity, are included, the economic burden of IPD significantly increases. Patient-specific factors that influence the cost of IPD include age of symptom onset; level of disability; presence of motor complications, falls, and dementia; and need for skilled nursing. For cost-effectiveness, the lowest dose that provides satisfactory symptomatic results should be used and, for patients already on carbidopa/L-dopa, optimization of the L-dopa regimen should be attempted before adding adjunctive agents. As the severity and level of disability increase, so do the costs associated with IPD. Likewise, the costs of treating patients with motor complications are considerably more than the costs of treating patients without motor complications. A similar trend applies for patients with hallucinations and psychosis who incur greater costs associated with nursing home placement. In more advanced

TABLE 68-5 Monitoring Parkinson's Disease Therapy

1. Monitor medication administration times. Educate the patient that immediate-release carbidopa/L-dopa is absorbed best on an empty stomach but is commonly taken with food to minimize nausea. Avoid administration of conventional selegiline in the late afternoon or evening to minimize insomnia.
2. Monitor to ensure that the patient and/or caregivers understand the prescribed medication regimen. For example, catechol-O-methyltransferase inhibitors work by enhancing the effect of L-dopa and that the patient should not discontinue medication without notifying the clinician.
3. Monitor and inquire specifically about dose-by-dose effects of medication, including response to doses of medication and the presence of dyskinesias, wearing-off effects, dizziness, nausea, or visual hallucinations. Offer suggestions to help alleviate these or encourage the patient to discuss with them with the clinician.
4. Monitor and inquire about concerns that caregivers may have about the patient, such as presence of abnormal behaviors, dyskinesias, falls, hallucinations, memory problems, mood changes, and sleep disorders.
5. Monitor for nonadherence and, if present, inquire for possible reasons (e.g., dosing convenience, financial issues, adverse effects) and offer suggestions.
6. Monitor for presence of drugs that can exacerbate idiopathic Parkinson's disease motor features (e.g., D_2 receptor blockers) or if the presence of an anticholinergic agent is causing cognitive impairment.

stages, the continued use of a dopamine agonist, MAO-B inhibitor, or COMT inhibitor can be a considerable expense for the patient, and the benefits must outweigh the potential risks or side effects. Pharmacologic treatments that delay disability or reduce the development of motor complications should be considered cost-effective in the long run.

EVALUATION OF THERAPEUTIC OUTCOMES

Table 68–5 lists the monitoring parameters for Parkinson's disease therapy. Patient and caregiver satisfaction is an important component of evaluating therapeutic outcomes. Toward this end, establishing appropriate treatment expectations is important and patients and caregivers should be educated that IPD is a neurodegenerative disease that progresses with time, and that some features will respond less well to pharmacotherapy (e.g., freezing, gait and postural instability). Patients and caregivers can participate in treatment by recording medication administration times as well as the duration of on and off times that can be reviewed at each visit. Periodic review of all medications that the patient is taking should be performed to identify use of medications (e.g., D_2-receptor blockers) that can exacerbate IPD motor features. If the patient reports memory problems, the medication profile should be screened for medications with anticholinergic properties and, if present, eliminated when possible. Assessment of the patient's general level of functioning, including activities of daily living and mobility, is important to determine when medication adjustments or physical therapy interventions are needed. Screening for anxiety or depressive disorders will help to determine if antidepressant or antianxiety therapy is needed. If falling is a problem, it is important to investigate whether falls are secondary to insufficient motor control or drug side effects such as dizziness and orthostatic hypotension. The former may necessitate an increase in dose of antiparkinson agents, and the latter a reduction in drug dosage. Physical therapy is also helpful for strengthening ambulation and balance skills to minimize falls. The patient should be questioned about any difficulties with their antiparkinson medications, including presence of adverse effects. Recommendations always should be made in view of the patient's perception of the severity of symptoms and effect on quality of life.

CONCLUSIONS

❶ Despite many advances in neuroscience, a definitive cause of IPD remains unknown. Each of the available therapies provide various degrees of symptomatic benefit, and the choice of agent is patient specific. The appropriate pharmacotherapy can significantly improve a patient's quality of life and functional status. The goal of management remains maintaining acceptable functional control with minimal treatment emergent complications. Thoughtful consideration for choice of initial and adjunctive therapy is critical for optimizing short- and long-term outcomes.

ABBREVIATIONS

COMT: catechol-O-methyl-transferase

CR: controlled release

DBS: deep-brain stimulation

GABA: γ-aminobutyric acid

GPi: globus pallidus interna

IPD: idiopathic Parkinson's disease

L-dopa: levodopa

MAO: monoamine oxidase

MPP+: 1-methyl-4-phenylpyridinium

MPTP: 1-methyl-4-phenyl-1,2,3,6-tetrahydropyridine

NMDA: N-methyl-D-aspartate

SNc: substantia nigra pars compacta

REFERENCES

1. Parkinson J. An essay on the shaking palsy. London: Sherwood, Neely, and Jones, 1817:1–66.
2. Van Den Eeden SK, Tanner CM, Bernstein AL, et al. Incidence of Parkinson's disease: Variation by age, gender, and race/ethnicity. Am J Epidemiol 2003;157:1015–1022.
3. Twelves D, Perkins KSM, Counsell C. Systematic review of incidence studies of Parkinson's disease. Mov Disord 2003;18:19–31.
4. Moore DJ, West AB, Dawson VL, et al. Molecular pathophysiology of Parkinson's disease. Annu Rev Neurosci 2005;28:57–87.
5. Braak H, Del Tredici K, Rub U, et al. Staging of brain pathology related to sporadic Parkinson's disease. Neurobiol Aging 2003;24:197–211.
6. Gerlach M, Riederer P, Przuntek H, et al. MPTP mechanisms of neurotoxicity and their implications for Parkinson's disease. Eur J Pharmacol 1991:208:273–286.
7. Migliore L, Coppedè F. Genetics, environmental factors and the emerging role of epigenetics in neurodegenerative diseases. Mutat Res 2009;667:82–97.
8. Tanner CM, Ross GW, Jewell SA, et al. Occupation and risk of parkinsonism: a multicenter case-control study. Arch Neurol 2009;66:1106–1113.
9. Dick FD, De Palma G, Ahmadi A, et al.; Geoparkinson study group. Environmental risk factors for Parkinson's disease and parkinsonism: the Geoparkinson study. Occup Environ Med 2007;64:666–672.
10. Firestone JA, Smith-Weller T, Franklin G, et al. Pesticides and risk of Parkinson's disease: a population-based case-control study. Arch Neurol 2005;62:91–95.
11. Di Monte DA. The environment and Parkinson's disease: Is the nigrostriatal system preferentially targeted by neurotoxins? Lancet Neurol 2003;2:531–533.
12. Logroscino G. The role of early life environmental risk factors in Parkinson's disease: What is the evidence? Environ Health Perspect 2005;113(9):1234–1238.
13. Jenner P. Oxidative stress in Parkinson's disease. Ann Neurol 2003;53(Suppl 3):S26–S38.

14. Hofer A, Gasser T. New aspects of genetic contributions to Parkinson's disease. J Mol Neurosci 2004;24:417–424.

15. Hardy J, Cai H, Cookson MR, et al. Genetics of Parkinson's disease and parkinsonism. Ann Neurol 2006;60:389–398.

16. Bernheimer H, Birkmayer W, Hornykiewicz O, et al. Brain dopamine and the syndromes of Parkinson's and Huntington: Clinical, morphological, and neurochemical correlations. J Neurol Sci 1973;20:415–455.

17. Smith Y, Bevan MD, Shink E, Bolam JP. Microcircuitry of the direct and indirect pathways of the basal ganglia. Neuroscience 1998;86:353–387.

18. Schapira AH, Bezard E, Brotchie J, et al. Novel pharmacological targets for the treatment of Parkinson's disease. Nat Rev Drug Discov 2006;5:845–854.

19. Gelb DJ, Oliver E, Gilman S. Diagnostic criteria for Parkinson's disease. Arch Neurol 1999;56:33–39.

20. Emre M. Dementia associated with Parkinson's disease. Lancet Neurol 2003;2:229–237.

21. Chen JJ. Anxiety, depression, and psychosis in Parkinson's disease: Unmet needs and treatment challenges. Neurol Clin 2004;22 (3 Suppl):S63–S90.

22. Chen JJ, Swope DM. Pharmacotherapy for Parkinson's disease. Pharmacotherapy 2007;27 (12 Pt 2):161S–173S.

23. Olanow CW, Stern MB, Sethi K. The scientific and clinical basis for the treatment of Parkinson's disease (2009). Neurology 2009;72 (21 Suppl 4):S1–136.

24. Management of Parkinson's disease: An evidence-based review. Mov Disord 2002;17 Suppl 4:S1–S166.

25. Miyasaki JM, Martin W, Suchowersky O, et al. Practice parameter: Initiation of treatment for Parkinson's disease: An evidence based review. Report of the Quality Standards Subcommittee of the American Academy of Neurology. Neurology 2002;58;11–17.

26. Suchowersky O, Gronseth G, Perlmutter J, et al. Quality Standards Subcommittee of the American Academy of Neurology. Practice Parameter: Neuroprotective strategies and alternative therapies for Parkinson's disease (an evidence-based review): Report of the Quality Standards Subcommittee of the American Academy of Neurology. Neurology 2006;66:976–982.

27. Pahwa R, Factor SA, Lyons KE, et al. Quality Standards Subcommittee of the American Academy of Neurology. Practice Parameter: Treatment of Parkinson's disease with motor fluctuations and dyskinesia (an evidence-based review): Report of the Quality Standards Subcommittee of the American Academy of Neurology. Neurology 2006;66:983–995.

28. Miyasaki JM, Shannon K, Voon V, et al. Quality Standards Subcommittee of the American Academy of Neurology. Practice Parameter: Evaluation and treatment of depression, psychosis, and dementia in Parkinson's disease (an evidence-based review): Report of the Quality Standards Subcommittee of the American Academy of Neurology. Neurology 2006;66:996–1002.

29. Hauser RA, McDermott MP, Messing S. Factors associated with the development of motor fluctuations and dyskinesias in Parkinson's disease. Arch Neurol 2006;63:1756–1760.

30. Stocchi F. Prevention and treatment of motor complications. Parkinsonism Relat Disord 2003;9(Suppl 2):S73–S81.

31. Pahwa R, Lyons KE. Options in the treatment of motor fluctuations and dyskinesias in Parkinson's disease: A brief review. Neurol Clin 2004;22(3 Suppl):S35–S52.

32. Parkinson Study Group. Levodopa and the progression of Parkinson's disease. N Engl J Med 2004;351:2498–2508.

33. Chen JJ, Obering C. Apomorphine in the management of motor fluctuations associated with Parkinson's disease. Clin Ther 2005;27;1710–1724.

34. Antonini A, Tolosa E. Apomorphine and levodopa infusion therapies for advanced Parkinson's disease: selection criteria and patient management. Expert Rev Neurother 2009;9:859–867.

35. Devos D; French DUODOPA Study Group. Patient profile, indications, efficacy and safety of duodenal levodopa infusion in advanced Parkinson's disease. Mov Disord 2009;24:993–1000.

36. Pappert EJ, Buhrfiend C, Lipton JW, et al. Levodopa stability in solution: Time course, environmental effects, and practical recommendations for clinical use. Mov Disord 1996;11:24–26.

37. Johnson KA, Conn PJ, Niswender CM. Glutamate receptors as therapeutic targets for Parkinson's disease. CNS Neurol Disord Drug Targets 2009;8:475–491.

38. Chen JJ, Swope DM, Dashtipour K. Comprehensive review of rasagiline, a second-generation monoamine oxidase inhibitor, for the treatment of Parkinson's disease. Clin Ther 2007;29:1825–1849.

39. Olanow CW, Rascol O, Hauser R; ADAGIO Study Investigators. A double-blind, delayed-start trial of rasagiline in Parkinson's disease. N Engl J Med 2009;361:1268–1278.

40. Rascol O, Brooks DJ, Melamed E, et al. Rasagiline as an adjunct to levodopa in patients with Parkinson's disease and motor fluctuations (LARGO, Lasting effect in Adjunct therapy with Rasagiline Given Once daily, study): A randomised, double-blind, parallel-group trial. Lancet 2005;365:947–954.

41. Parkinson Study Group. A controlled, randomized, delayed-start study of rasagiline in early Parkinson's disease. Arch Neurol 2004;61:561–566.

42. Ruottinen HM, Rinne UK. COMT inhibition in the treatment of Parkinson's disease. J Neurol 1998;245(suppl 3):25–34.

43. Holm KJ, Spencer CM. Entacapone: A review of its use in Parkinson's disease. Drugs 1999;58:159–177.

44. Keating GM, Lyseng-Williamson KA. Tolcapone. A review of its use in the management of Parkinson's disease. CNS Drugs 2005;19:165–184.

45. Zanettini R, Antonini A, Gatto G, et al. Valvular heart disease and the use of dopamine agonists for Parkinson's disease. N Engl J Med 2007;356:39–46.

46. Rascol O, Brooks DJ, Korczyn AD, et al. A five-year study of the incidence of dyskinesia in patients with early Parkinson's disease who were treated with ropinirole or levodopa. 056 Study Group. N Engl J Med 2000;342:1484–1491.

47. Parkinson Study Group. Pramipexole vs levodopa as initial treatment for Parkinson's disease: A 4-year randomized controlled trial. Arch Neurol 2004;61:1044–1053.

48. Parkinson Study Group. Dopamine transporter brain imaging to assess the effects of pramipexole vs levodopa on Parkinson's disease progression. JAMA 2002;287:1653–1661.

49. Whone AL, Watts RL, Stoessl AJ. Slower progression in early Parkinson's disease treated with ropinirole vs levodopa: The REAL-PET study. Ann Neurol 2003;54:93–101.

50. Schapira A, Albrecht S, Barone P, et al. Immediate vs. delayed-start pramipexole in early Parkinson's disease: the PROUD study. Parkinsonism Relat Disord 2009;15(Suppl 2):S81.

51. Kluger BM, Klepitskaya O, Okun MS. Surgical treatment of movement disorders. Neurol Clin 2009;27:633–677.

52. Stefani A, Lozano A, Peppe A, et al: Bilateral deep brain stimulation of the pedunculopontine and subthalamic nuclei in severe Parkinson's disease. Brain 2007;130 (Pt 6):1596–1607.

53. Olanow CW, Goetz CG, Kordower JH, et al. A double-blind controlled trial of bilateral fetal nigral transplantation in Parkinson's disease. Ann Neurol 2003;54:403–414.

54. Stover NP, Watts RL. Spheramine for treatment of Parkinson's disease. Neurotherapeutics 2008;5:252–259.

55. Isacson O, Kordower JH. Future of cell and gene therapies for Parkinson's disease. Ann Neurol 2008;64(Suppl 2):S122–138.

56. Dowding CH, Shenton CL, Salek SS. A review of the health-related quality of life and economic impact of Parkinson's disease. Drugs Aging 2006;23:693–721.

CHAPTER

69

Pain Management

TERRY J. BAUMANN, JENNIFER M. STRICKLAND, AND CHRIS M. HERNDON

KEY CONCEPTS

❶ It is important, whenever possible, to ask patients if they have pain, to identify the source of pain, and to assess the characteristics of the pain.

❷ Patients taking analgesics should be monitored for response and side effects, particularly sedation and constipation associated with the opioids.

❸ Oral analgesics are preferred over other dosage forms whenever feasible, but it is important to adjust the route of administration to the needs of the patient.

❹ Equianalgesic doses are useful as a guide when converting from one agent to another, but further dose titration usually is required to achieve treatment goals.

❺ Doses must be individualized for each patient and administered for an adequate duration of time. Around-the-clock regimens should be considered for acute and chronic pain. As-needed regimens should be used for breakthrough pain or when acute pain displays wide variability and/or has subsided greatly.

❻ For chronic pain that has a maladaptive inflammatory and/or neuropathic component, anticonvulsants, topical analgesics, tricyclic antidepressants, serotonin-norepinephrine reuptake inhibitors, and opioids should be considered.

❼ Whenever possible, a multidisciplinary approach and nonpharmacologic strategies should be used.

❽ Placebo therapy should not be used as an attempt to diagnose psychogenic pain.

Although the world is full of suffering, it is also full of the overcoming of it.

Helen Keller[1]

Humans have always known and sought relief from pain.[2] Today, pain's impact on society still is great, and indeed pain complaints remain a primary reason patients seek medical advice.[3]

Regrettably, many healthcare providers do not receive adequate training in this area, and new information is not widely disseminated

Learning objectives, review questions, and other resources can be found at
www.pharmacotherapyonline.com.

and/or understood. Clearly, pain management is enhanced when a multidisciplinary approach is applied. Thus, understanding the pathophysiology of pain therapy and maintaining a working knowledge of individual pain regimens are important key factors in addressing pain control.

DEFINITION

The accepted current definition of pain is: "an unpleasant sensory and emotional experience associated with actual or potential tissue damage or described in terms of such damage."[4] Pain often is so subjective, however, that many clinicians define pain as whatever the patient says it is. The best care is achieved when the patient comes first.

EPIDEMIOLOGY

Data from the National Health and Nutrition Examination Survey indicate that 1 in 4 Americans have suffered pain that lasts for more than 24 hours in the previous month and in those reporting pain, 42% state that it lasted more 1 year.[5] Seventy-six and a half million Americans report they are in chronic pain; this is more than the number of patients with heart disease, cancer, and diabetes combined.[6] The annual cost of pain to U.S. society can be estimated to be in the billions of dollars.[6,7] In 1 year, an estimated 25 million Americans will experience acute pain due to injury or surgery, and one-third of Americans will experience severe chronic pain at some point in their lives.[3] These numbers are expected to rise, as increasingly more Americans work beyond age 60 years and survive into their 80s.[7] The 106th Congress passed Title VI, Section 1603, of H.R. 3244 which declared a 10-year interval starting January 1, 2001, the "Decade of Pain Control and Research".[5] Unfortunately, despite much public attention, considerable focused education, and a number of consensus guidelines, pain often remains underestimated and undertreated.[3,5,8,9]

PATHOPHYSIOLOGY

The pathophysiology of pain involves a complex array of neural networks in the brain that are acted on by afferent stimuli to produce the experience we know as pain. In acute pain, this encounter is short lived; but in some situations, the changes may persist, and chronic pain develops.[10]

NOCICEPTIVE PAIN

Nociceptive pain typically is classified as either somatic (arising from skin, bone, joint, muscle, or connective tissue) or visceral (arising from internal organs such as the large intestine or pancreas).[11] Whereas somatic pain often presents as throbbing and well localized, visceral pain can manifest as pain feeling as if it is coming from other structures (referred) or as a more localized phenomenon.[11] We can think of nociception in terms of stimulation, transmission, perception, and modulation.[11]

Stimulation

The first step leading to the sensation of pain is stimulation of free nerve endings known as *nociceptors*. These receptors are found in both somatic and visceral structures. They distinguish between noxious and innocuous stimuli, and they are activated and sensitized by mechanical, thermal, and chemical impulses.[11] The underlying mechanism of these noxious stimuli (which in and of themselves may sensitize/stimulate the receptor) may be the release of bradykinins, hydrogen and potassium ions, prostaglandins, histamine, interleukins, tumor necrosis factor alfa, serotonin, and substance P (among others) that sensitize and/or activate the nociceptors.[12] Receptor activation leads to action potentials that are transmitted along afferent nerve fibers to the spinal cord (Fig. 69–1).[11]

Transmission

Nociceptive transmission takes place in $A\delta$ and C-afferent nerve fibers.[11] Stimulation of large-diameter, sparsely myelinated $A\delta$ fibers evokes sharp, well-localized pain, whereas stimulation of unmyelinated, small-diameter C fibers produces dull, aching, poorly localized pain.[11]

These afferent, nociceptive pain fibers synapse in various layers (laminae) of the spinal cord's dorsal horn, releasing a variety of neurotransmitters, including glutamate, substance P, and aspartate.[13] The complex array of events that influence pain can be explained in part by the interactions between neuroreceptors and neurotransmitters that take place in this synapse. For example, by stimulating

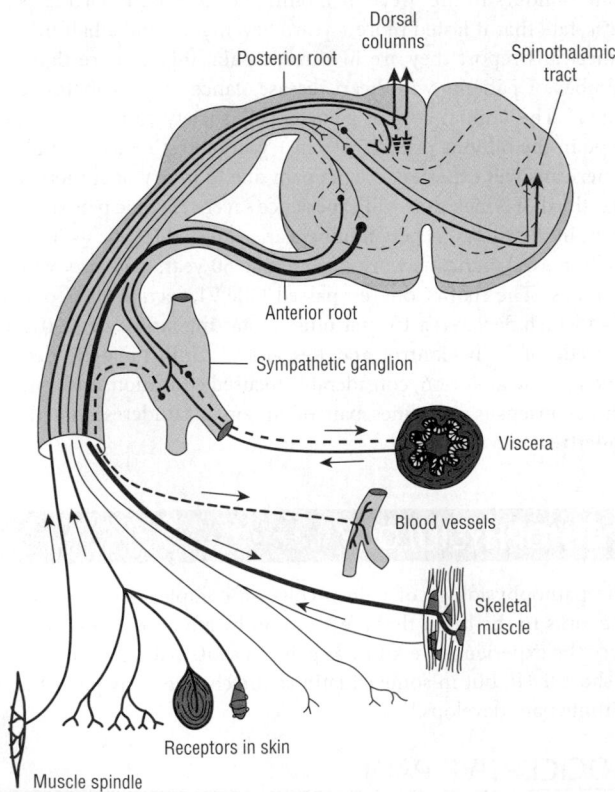

FIGURE 69-1. Schematic representation of nociceptive pain. *(Data modified from reference 69.)*

sensory myelinated fibers that intraconnect in the dorsal horn with pain fibers, nonnoxious stimuli can have an inhibitory effect on pain transmission (Fig. 69–1).[13] Functionally, the importance of the interplay between these different fibers and various neurotransmitters and neuroreceptors is evident in the analgesic response produced by topical irritants or transcutaneous electrical nerve stimulation. These pain-initiated processes reach the brain through a complex array of a number of ascending spinal cord pathways, which include the spinothalamic tract.[13] Information other than pain is also carried along these pathways. Thus, pain is influenced by many factors supplemental to nociception and precludes simple schematic representation. It is postulated that the thalamus acts as a relay station, as these pathways ascend and pass the impulses to central structures where pain can be processed further.[11]

Pain Perception

At this point in transmission, pain is thought to become a conscious experience that takes place in higher cortical structures. The brain may accommodate only a limited number of pain signals, and cognitive and behavioral functions can modify pain. Relaxation, distraction, meditation, and guided mental imagery may decrease pain by limiting the number of processed pain signals.[11] In contrast, a change in our neurobiochemical makeup that results in states such as depression or anxiety may worsen pain.

Modulation

The body modulates pain through a number of complex processes. One, known as the *endogenous opiate system*, consists of neurotransmitters (e.g., enkephalins, dynorphins, and β-endorphins) and receptors (e.g., μ, δ, and κ) that are found throughout the central nervous system (CNS).[14] Like exogenous opioids, endogenous opioids bind to opioid receptor sites and modulate the transmission of pain impulses.[11] Other receptor types also can influence this system. Blockade of N-methyl-D-aspartate (NMDA) receptors, found in the dorsal horn, may increase the μ-receptors' responsiveness to opiates.[14]

The CNS also contains a highly organized descending system for control of pain transmission. This system can inhibit synaptic pain transmission at the dorsal horn and originates in the brain.[11] Important neurotransmitters here include endogenous opioids, serotonin, norepinephrine, and γ-aminobutyric acid (GABA).[11]

Adaptive Inflammation

Inflammatory pain can be thought of as the body's shifting from preventing tissue damage to the promotion of healing (e.g., surgical wounds, traumatic injury).[10] As a result of the inflammatory process, the pain threshold is reduced and the injured area becomes more sensitive to pain.[10] This process decreases our contact with and movement of the injured area, thus promoting the progression of healing.[10] When this course of action outlives its functionality or when it is caused by diseases such as arthritis, it can move from an acute to a chronic problem (maladaptive inflammation).[10] According to McPherson[15]: "In response to tissue damage and inflammation, a significant alteration occurs in the chemical composition and properties of the neurons that innervate the inflamed tissues. These alterations reflect the nature and levels of the different proteins expressed by the sensory neurons. Altered production of these proteins may modify the phenotypes of the neurons, changing their transduction and transmission properties. Inflammatory pain is also associated with an increase in the excitability or responsiveness of neurons within the CNS, referred to as *central sensitization*. This phenomenon, like peripheral sensitization, is a major cause of hypersensitivity to pain after injury."

NEUROPATHIC AND FUNCTIONAL PAIN

Neuropathic and functional pain is distinctly different from nociceptive pain in that it becomes disengaged from noxious stimuli or healing[10] and often is described in terms of chronic pain. Neuropathic pain is a result of nerve damage, whereas functional pain can be thought of as abnormal operation of the nervous system.[10] A number of neuropathic pain syndromes (e.g., postherpetic neuralgia, diabetic neuropathy) and functional pain syndromes (e.g., fibromyalgia, irritable bowel syndrome, sympathetic induced pain, tension-type headaches, and some noncardiac chest pain)[10] exist. They often are underrecognized and difficult to treat.[11] In addition, the pain reported often is not evident by examining physical findings.[11]

The mechanism responsible for neuropathic and functional pain may be the nervous system's endogenous dynamic nature. Nerve damage or certain disease states may evoke changes seen in inflammatory pain, ectopic excitability, enhanced sensory transmission, nerve structure reorganization, and loss of modulatory pain inhibition.[10,15] Pain circuits rewire themselves both anatomically and biochemically.[16] This produces a mismatch between pain stimulation and inhibition, and a potential progressive increase in the discharge of dorsal horn neurons.[16]

Clinically, patients present with episodic or continuous pain transmission (often described as burning, tingling, shock like, or shooting), exaggerated painful response to normally noxious stimuli (hyperalgesia), and/or painful response to normally nonnoxious stimuli (allodynia).[3,16] This change over time may help to explain why this type of pain often manifests long after the actual nerve-related injury or when no actual injury is identified.

CLASSIFICATION OF PAIN

It is helpful in understanding pain to subdivide the presenting symptoms into acute pain, chronic pain, and cancer pain.

ACUTE PAIN

Acute pain can be a useful physiologic process, warning individuals of disease states and potentially harmful situations. Unfortunately, severe, unremitting, undertreated acute pain, when it outlives its biologic usefulness, can produce many deleterious effects. Aside from unnecessary suffering, untreated and undertreated acute pain has also been shown to increase one's risk for the development of chronic pain syndromes.[17] Acute pain is usually nociceptive in nature with common causes, including surgery, acute illness, trauma, labor, and medical procedures.[3]

CHRONIC PAIN

Under normal conditions, acute pain subsides quickly as the healing process decreases the pain-producing stimuli; however, in some instances, pain persists for months to years, leading to a chronic pain state with features quite different from those of acute pain (Table 69–1). This type of pain can be nociceptive, neuropathic/functional, or mixed.[3] Chronic pain can be classified as either being associated with cancer (cancer pain) or from noncancer etiologies (chronic noncancer pain). Chronic pain may result in changes to the receptors and nerve fibers in the nervous system, often making treatment even more difficult.[18]

CANCER PAIN

Pain associated with potentially life-threatening conditions is often called malignant pain or simply cancer pain.[3] This type of

TABLE 69-1 Characteristics of Acute and Chronic Pain

Characteristic	Acute Pain	Chronic Pain
Relief of pain	Highly desirable	Highly desirable
Dependence and tolerance to medication	Unusual	Common
Psychological component	Usually not present	Often a major problem
Organic cause	Common	May not be present
Environmental/family issues	Small	Significant
Insomnia	Unusual	Common component
Treatment goal	Cure	Functionality
Depression	Uncommon	Common

Data from Stimmel[2] and Jacobson and Mariano.[60]

pain includes both chronic and acute components and often has multiple etiologies. It is pain caused by the disease itself (e.g., tumor invasion, organ obstruction), treatment (e.g., chemotherapy, radiation, surgical incisions), or diagnostic procedures (e.g., biopsy).[3]

CLINICAL PRESENTATION

A patient-oriented approach is essential, and evaluation methods should not differ from those used in other medical conditions.[2] ❶ Therefore, a comprehensive history and physical examination are imperative to evaluate underlying diseases and possible other contributing factors.[2] This includes asking if the patient has pain and identifying the source of pain when possible, however, the absence of a discreet etiology should not preclude pain treatment.[2] A baseline characterization of pain can be obtained by assessing characteristics outlined in Table 69–2.[19]

Numerous validated scoring tools exist (e.g., numeric rating scale, visual analog scale, etc.),[3,20-22] however the tools need to be appropriate for the type of pain being evaluated, and can be inadequate if not used consistently, or used without clinical judgment. ❷ Proper patient assessment must include an evaluation of pain management. Pain intensity, pain relief, and medication side effects (e.g., opioid-induced sedation or constipation) must be assessed and reassessed on a regular basis. The timing and regularity of this assessment will depend on the type of pain and the medications administered. Postoperative pain and acute exacerbation of cancer pain may need to be assessed hourly, whereas chronic noncancer pain may require only daily or less frequent assessment. Pain intensity assessment is vital in acute pain, whereas functionality becomes more of an issue in chronic pain. Quality of life must be assessed on a regular basis in all patients. Many advocate using the four "A"s (analgesia, activity, aberrant drug behavior, and adverse effects) as key assessment measures for any patient with chronic pain.[23]

TABLE 69-2 Characteristics of Pain

Onset and duration	When did pain begin and how long has it been since the pain began?
Palliative factors	What makes the pain better?
Provocative factors	What makes the pain worse?
Quality	Describe the pain.
Location	Where is the pain?
Severity/intensity	How does this pain compare with other pain you have experienced?
Temporal factors	Does the intensity of the pain change with time?

Data from Twycross[19] and Berry et al.[3]

It is important to note that often objective signs are lacking for pain evaluation. Acute pain may result in increased sympathetic tone (e.g., hypertension, tachycardia, tachypnea); however, this response is usually diminished as acute pain progresses to chronic pain. The clinician must rely on the patient's description of their pain.[24]

CLINICAL PRESENTATION OF PAIN

Acute

General

☐ Obvious distress (e.g., trauma), infants may present with changes in feeding habits, increased fussiness. Those with dementia may exhibit changes in eating habits, increased agitation, calling out. Attention also must be given to mental/emotional factors that alter the pain threshold. Anxiety, depression, fatigue, anger, and fear in particular, are noted to lower this threshold, whereas rest, mood elevation, sympathy, diversion, and understanding raise the pain threshold.

Symptoms

☐ Can be described as sharp, dull, shock like, tingling, shooting, radiating, fluctuating in intensity, and varying in location (these occur in a timely relationship with an obvious noxious stimuli).

Signs

☐ Hypertension, tachycardia, diaphoresis, mydriasis, and pallor, but these signs are *not diagnostic*.

☐ In some cases there are no obvious signs.

☐ Comorbid conditions usually not present.

☐ Outcome of treatment generally predictable.

Laboratory Tests

☐ Pain is always subjective.

☐ There are *no* specific laboratory tests for pain.

☐ Pain is best diagnosed based on patient description and history.

Chronic

General

☐ Can appear to have no noticeable suffering. Attention also must be given to mental/emotional factors that alter the pain threshold. Anxiety, depression, fatigue, anger, and fear in particular, are noted to lower this threshold; whereas rest, mood elevation, sympathy, diversion, and understanding raise the pain threshold.

Symptoms

☐ Can be described as sharp, dull, shock-like, tingling, shooting, radiating, fluctuating in intensity, and varying in location (these often occur *without* a timely relationship with an obvious noxious stimuli).

☐ Over time, the pain stimulus may cause symptoms that completely change (e.g., sharp to dull, obvious to vague).

Signs

☐ Hypertension, tachycardia, diaphoresis, mydriasis, and pallor are seldom present.

☐ In most cases there are *no* obvious signs.

☐ Comorbid conditions often present (e.g., insomnia, depression, anxiety).

☐ Outcome of treatment often unpredictable.

Laboratory Tests

☐ Pain is always subjective.

☐ Pain is best diagnosed based on patient description and history.

☐ There are *no* specific laboratory tests for pain; however, history and/or diagnostic proof of past trauma (e.g., computed tomography) or present disease state (e.g., auto-antibodies) may be helpful in diagnosing etiology. General labs that may be considered include vitamin D levels, thyroid stimulating antibodies, and B_{12}.

Data from Twycross,[19] American Pain Society,[24] Turner et al.,[57] Hagen et al.,[58] Bernard et al.[59]

TREATMENT

■ NONPHARMACOLOGIC THERAPY

Various nonpharmacologic therapies have been found to be beneficial in the management of acute and chronic pain, including physical manipulation, application of heat or cold, massage, and exercise.[25]

Transcutaneous electrical nerve stimulation (TENS) has been used in managing both acute and chronic pain (e.g., surgical, traumatic, neuropathy, and musculoskeletal pain).[3] However, published evidence regarding long-term benefit is limited. As a result, routine use has not gained widespread acceptance.

Even though the cognitive, behavioral, and social aspects of pain are well established, psychological interventions for the treatment of acute pain are not used widely. Simple interventions (e.g., education or introductory information about sensations to expect after certain procedures) reduce patient distress and greatly reduce postprocedure suffering.[26] Other successful psychological techniques, including relaxation training, imagery, and hypnosis, have proven effective in the management of postprocedure pain and in cancer-related pain.[26,27] Moderate evidence demonstrates that cognitive behavioral therapy and biofeedback also may be useful nonpharmacologic tools in managing chronic pain.[28]

■ PHARMACOLOGIC TREATMENT

Many consider pharmacologic treatment to be the cornerstone of pain management.

Nonopioid Agents

Analgesia should be initiated with the most effective analgesic agent having the fewest side effects. Acetaminophen, acetylsalicylic acid (aspirin), and nonsteroidal antiinflammatory drugs (NSAIDs) often are preferred over opiates in the treatment of mild-to-moderate pain (Table 69–3). These drugs (with the exception of acetaminophen) prevent formation of prostaglandins produced in response to noxious stimuli, thereby decreasing the number of pain impulses received by the CNS.[24] NSAIDs may be particularly useful in the management of cancer-related bone pain.[27] Studies comparing the efficacy of these agents have been inconsistent. Therefore, the choice of a particular agent often depends on availability, cost, pharmacokinetics, pharmacologic characteristics, and the side-effect profile. Because of the large interpatient variability in response to individual NSAIDS, it is considered rational therapy to switch to another member of this class if there is inadequate response after a sufficient therapeutic trial of any single agent.[24] The duration of a sufficient trial has not been well defined; however, typically, a NSAID should be continued for a minimum of 1 month prior to evaluating the need to switch agents.

TABLE 69-3 Adult FDA-Approved Nonopioid Analgesics (Includes Only FDA-Approved Agents for Pain)

Class and Generic Name (Brand Name)	Approximate Half-Life (h)	Usual Dosage Range (mg)	Maximal Dose (mg/day)
Salicylates			
Acetylsalicylic acid[a]—aspirin (various)	0.25	325–1,000 every 4–6 h	4,000
Choline and magnesium trisalicylate (various)	9–17	1,000–1,500 every 12 h	3,000
		750 every 8 h (elderly)	
Diflunisal (Dolobid, various)	8–12	500–1,000 initial	1,500
		250–500 every 8–12 h	
Salsalate (various)	1	1,000 every 12 h or 500 every 6 hours	3,000
Para-aminophenol			
Acetaminophen[a] (Tylenol, various)	2–3	325–1,000 every 4–6 h	4,000[b]
Fenamates			
Meclofenamate (various)	0.8–3.3	50–100 every 4–6 h	400
Mefenamic acid (Ponstel)	2	Initial 500	1,000[c]
		250 every 6 h (max. 7 days)	
Pyranocarboxylic acid			
Etodolac (various) (immediate release)	7.3	200–400 every 6–8 h	1,000
			1,200 with extended-release product
Acetic acid			
Diclofenac potassium [Cataflam, various, Flector (patch)]	1.9	In some patients, initial 100, 50 three times per day	150[d]
		Patch available—to be applied twice daily to painful area (intact skin only)	
Propionic acids			
Ibuprofen[a] (Motrin, Caldolor, various)	2–2.5	200–400 every 4–6 h	3,200[e] 2,400[e] 1,200[f]
		Injectable, 400–800 every 6 h (infused over 30 min)	
Fenoprofen (Nalfon, various)	3	200 every 4–6 h	3,200
Ketoprofen (various)	2	25–50 every 6–8 h	300
			200 with extended-release product
Naproxen (Naprosyn, Anaprox, various)	12–17	500 initial	1,000[c]
		500 every 12 h or	
		250 every 6–8 h	
Naproxen sodium[a] (Aleve, various)	12–17	In some patients, 440 initial[f]	660[f]
		220 every 8–12 h[f]	
Pyrrolizine carboxylic acid			
Ketorolac—parenteral (various)	5–6	30[g]–60 (single IM dose only)	30[g]–60
		15[g]–30 (single IV dose only)	15[g]–30
		15[g]–30 every 6 h (IV dose)	60[g]–120
		(max. 5 days)	
Ketorolac—oral, indicated for continuation with parenteral only (various)	5–6	10 every 4–6 h (max. 5 days, which includes parenteral doses)	40
		In non-elderly patients, initial oral dose of 20	
Pyrazols			
Celecoxib (Celebrex)	11	Initial 400 followed by another 200 on first day, then 200 twice daily	400

[a]Available both as an over-the-counter preparation and as a prescription drug.
[b]Some experts believe 4,000 mg may be too high.
[c]Up to 1,250 mg on the first day.
[d]Up to 200 mg on the first day.
[e]Some individuals may respond better to 3,200 mg as opposed to 2,400 mg, although well-controlled trials show no better response; consider risk versus benefits when using 3,200 mg/day.
[f]Over-the-counter dose.
[g]Dose for elderly and those under 50 kg (110 lbs).
FDA, Food and Drug Administration; h, hours; IM, intramuscular; IV, intravenous; Nd, no data.
Data from American Pain Society,[24] Anonymous,[40,41] Watkins et al.,[61] and Caldolor.[65]

Opioid Agents

Opioids are often the next logical step in the management of acute pain and cancer-related chronic pain. They also may be an effective treatment option in the management of chronic noncancer pain; however, this continues to be somewhat controversial. Many times a trial of opioids is warranted, but such a trial should not be done without a complete assessment of the pain complaint, including an assessment of the patient's functionality and risk factors for opioid misuse and abuse.[29]

The classification of these agents, their equianalgesic doses, relative histamine-releasing characteristics, pharmacokinetics, and dosing guidelines are outlined in Tables 69–4 and 69–5. Opiate choice should be based on patient acceptance; analgesic effectiveness; and pharmacokinetic, pharmacodynamic, and side-effect profiles (Tables 69–4 and 69–6).

The pharmacologic activity of opioids depends on their affinity for opiate receptors.[14] Therapeutic activities and side effects range from those exhibited by the opiate agonists (e.g., morphine) to those seen with the opiate antagonists (e.g., naloxone). Partial

TABLE 69-4 Opioid Analgesics, Central Analgesics, Opioid Antagonist

Class and Generic Name (Brand Name)	Chemical Source	Relative Histamine Release	Route	Equianalgesic Dose in Adults (mg)	Approximate Onset (min)/ Half-Life (h)
Phenanthrenes (morphine-like agonists)					
Morphine (various)	Naturally occurring	+++	IM	10	10–20/2
			PO	30	
Hydromorphone (Dilaudid, various)	Semisynthetic	+	IM	1.5	10–20/2–3
			PO	7.5	
Oxymorphone (Numorphan, Opana)	Semisynthetic	+	IM	1	10–20/2–3
			PO	10	
Levorphanol (various)	Semisynthetic	+	IM	Variable	10–20/12–16
			PO	Variable	
Codeine (various)	Naturally occurring	+++	IM	15–30[a]	
			PO	15–30[a]	10–30/3
Hydrocodone (available as combination)	Semisynthetic	N/A	PO	5–10[a]	30–60/4
Oxycodone (various)	Semisynthetic	+	PO	15–30[b]	30–60/2–3
Phenylpiperidines (meperidine-like agonists)					
Meperidine (Demerol, various)	Synthetic	+++	IM	75	10–20/3–5
			PO	300[b]; not recommended	
Fentanyl (Sublimaze, Duragesic, various)	Synthetic	+	IM	0.1 25[c]	7–15/3–4
			Transdermal Buccal, transmucosal	Variable[d] Variable[d]	
Diphenylheptanes (methadone-like agonists)					
Methadone (Dolophine, various)	Synthetic	+	IM	Variable[e] (acute)	
			PO	Variable[e] (acute)	30–60/12–190
			IM	Variable[e] (chronic)	
			PO	Variable[e] (chronic)	
Propoxyphene (Darvon, various)	Synthetic	N/A	PO	65[a]	30–60/6–12
Agonist–antagonist derivatives					
Pentazocine (Talwin, various)	Synthetic	N/A	IM	Not recommended	
			PO	50[a]	15–30/2–3
Butorphanol (Stadol, various)	Synthetic	N/A	IM	2	10–20/3–4
			Intranasal	1[a] (one spray)	
Nalbuphine (Nubain, various)	Synthetic	N/A	IM	10	<15/5
Buprenorphine (Buprenex, various)	Synthetic	N/A	IM	0.3	10–20/2–3
Antagonist					
Naloxone (Narcan, various)	Synthetic	N/A	IV	0.4–2[f]	1–2 (IV), 2–5 (IM)/ 0.5–1.3
Central analgesics					
Tramadol (Ultram, various)	Synthetic	N/A	PO	50–100[a,g]	<60/5–7
Tapentadol (Nucynta)	Synthetic	N/A	PO	50–100[a,g]	Within 60/4

[a]Starting dose only (equianalgesia not shown).
[b]Starting doses lower (oxycodone 5–10 mg, meperidine 50–150 mg).
[c]Equivalent PO morphine dose = variable.
[d]For breakthrough pain only.
[e]The equianalgesic dose of methadone when compared with other opioids will decrease progressively the higher the previous opioid dose.
[f]Starting doses to be used in cases of opioid overdose.
[g]First day of dosing may administer second dose 1 hour after first dose.
IM, intramuscular; IV, intravenous; PO, oral.
Data from American Pain Society,[24] Gutstein and Akil,[30] McPherson,[32] Pasero et al.,[66] Anonymous,[40,41] Tapentadol,[46] Li.[52]

agonists and antagonists (e.g., pentazocine) compete with agonists for opiate receptor sites and, depending on the inherent agonist and antagonist properties, exhibit mixed agonist–antagonist activity. Mixed agonist–antagonist agents with analgesic activity appear to exhibit selectivity for analgesic receptor sites.[30] This may result in analgesia with fewer undesirable side effects. Efficacy and side effects also may further differ among agents because of receptor subtype variability.[31] This μ-receptor subtype variability may explain why some patients respond differently to certain opioids, specifically μ-receptor agonists.[31]

The effects of the opioid analgesics are relatively selective, and at normal therapeutic concentrations, these agents do not affect other sensory modalities,[30] such as sensitivity to touch, sight, or hearing; undesirable side effects may increase as the dose is escalated

(Table 69–6). Patients in severe pain may receive high doses of opioids with no unwanted side effects, but as the pain subsides, patients may not tolerate even very low doses.[30] Frequently, when opioids are administered, pain is not eliminated, but its unpleasantness is decreased.[30] Patients report that although their pain is still present, it no longer bothers them.

Opioids share related pharmacologic attributes and exert a profound effect on the CNS and gastrointestinal tract.[30] Mood changes, sedation, nausea, vomiting, decreased gastrointestinal motility, constipation, respiratory depression, dependence, and tolerance are evident in varying degrees with all agents.[3,30] Tolerance to side effects (except to constipation) often develops over time.[3] Some differences exist between the opioids in regards to incidence of side effects. Consideration of these differences assists in selection

TABLE 69-5	Dosing Guidelines	
Agent(s)	**Doses (Use Lowest Effective Dose, Titrate Up or Down Based on Patient Response, Opioid Tolerant Patients May Need Dose Modification)**	**Notes**
NSAIDs/ acetaminophen/ aspirin	Dose to maximum before switching to another agent (see Table 69–3)	Used in mild-to-moderate pain May use in conjunction with opioid agents to decrease doses of each Regular alcohol use and of acetaminophen may result in liver toxicity Care must be exercised to avoid overdose when combination products containing these agents are used
Morphine	PO 5–30 mg every 4 h[a] IM 5–20 mg every 4 h[a] IV 5–15 mg every 4 h[a] SR 15–30 mg every 12 h (may need to be every 8 h in some patients) Rectal 10–20 mg every 4 h[a]	Drug of choice in severe pain Use immediate-release product with SR product to control breakthrough pain in cancer patients Typical patient controlled analgesia IV dose is 1 mg with a 10 minute lock out interval Every-24-hour products available (Avinza should not exceed doses of 1,600 mg/day)
Hydromorphone	PO 2–4 mg every 4–6 h[a] IM 1–2 mg every 4–6 h[a] IV 0.5–2 mg every 4 h[a] Rectal 3 mg every 6–8 h[a]	Use in severe pain More potent than morphine; otherwise, no advantages Typical patient controlled analgesia IV dose is 0.2 mg with a 10 minute lock out interval. Every-24-hour product (Exalgo) available
Oxymorphone	IM 1–1.5 mg every 4–6 h[a] IV 0.5 mg every 4–6 h[a] PO immediate-release 5–10 mg every 4–6 h[a] PO extended-release 5–10 mg every 12 h[a]	Use in severe pain No advantages over morphine Use immediate-release product with controlled-release product to control breakthrough pain in cancer or chronic pain patients
Levorphanol	PO 2–3 mg every 6–8 h[a] (Levo-Dromoran) PO 2 mg every 3–6 h[a] (Levorphanol Tartrate) IM 1–2 mg every 6–8 h[a] IV 1 mg every 3–6 h[a]	Use in severe pain Extended half-life useful in cancer patients In chronic pain, wait 3 days between dosage adjustments
Codeine	PO 15–60 mg every 4–6 h[a] IM 15–60 mg every 4–6 h[a]	Use in mild to moderate pain Weak analgesic; use with NSAIDs, aspirin, or acetaminophen, analgesic prodrug
Hydrocodone	PO 5–10 mg every 4–6 h[a]	Use in moderate/severe pain Most effective when used with NSAIDs, aspirin, or acetaminophen Only available as combination product with other ingredients for pain and/or cough
Oxycodone	PO 5–15 mg every 4–6 h[a] Controlled release 10–20 mg every 12 h	Use in moderate/severe pain Most effective when used with NSAIDs, aspirin, or acetaminophen Use immediate-release product with controlled-release product to control breakthrough pain in cancer or chronic pain patients
Meperidine	IM 50–150 mg every 3–4 h[a] IV 5–10 mg every 5 min prn[a]	Use in severe pain Oral not recommended Do not use in renal failure May precipitate tremors, myoclonus, and seizures Monoamine oxidase inhibitors can induce hyperpyrexia and/or seizures or opioid overdose symptoms
Fentanyl	IV 25–50 mcg/h IM 50–100 mcg every 1–2 h[a] Transdermal 25 mcg/h every 72 h Transmucosal (Actiq Lozenge) 200 mcg may repeat × 1, 30 min after first dose is started, then titrate Transmucosal (Fentora Buccal Tablet) 100 mcg, may repeat × 1, 30 min after first dose is started, then titrate	Used in severe pain Do not use transdermal in acute pain Transmucosal for breakthrough cancer pain in patients already receiving or tolerant to opioids. Always start with lowest dose despite daily opioid intake
Methadone	PO 2.5–10 mg every 8–12 h[a] IM 2.5–10 mg every 8–12 h[a]	Effective in severe chronic pain Sedation can be major problem Some chronic pain patients can be dosed every 12 h Equianalgesic dose of methadone when compared with other opioids will decrease progressively the higher the previous opioid dose. Avoid dose titrations more frequently than weekly in chronic pain maintenance
Propoxyphene	PO 100 mg every 4 h[a] (napsylate) PO 65 mg every 4 h[a] (HCl) (maximum 600 mg daily of napsylate, 390 mg HCl)	Use in moderate pain Weak analgesic; most effective when used with NSAIDs, aspirin, or acetaminophen This drug is not recommended in the elderly Will cause carbamazepine levels to increase 100 mg of napsylate salt = 65 mg of HCl salt
Pentazocine	PO 50–100 mg every 3–4 h[b] (max. 600 mg daily, for those 50 mg tablet containing 0.5 mg of naloxone) PO 25 mg every 4 h[b] (max. 150 mg daily, for those 25 mg tablet containing 325 mg of acetaminophen)	Second-line agent for moderate-to-severe pain May precipitate withdrawal in opiate-dependent patients Parenteral doses not recommended
Butorphanol	IM 1–4 mg every 3–4 h[b] IV 0.5–2 mg every 3–4 h[b] Intranasal 1 mg (1 spray) every 3–4 h[b] If inadequate relief after initial spray, may repeat in other nostril × 1 in 60–90 min Max. 2 sprays (one per nostril) every 3–4 h[b]	Second-line agent for moderate-to-severe pain May precipitate withdrawal in opiate-dependent patients

(continued)

	Doses (Use Lowest Effective Dose, Titrate Up or Down Based on Patient Response, Opioid	
Agent(s)	**Tolerant Patients May Need Dose Modification)**	**Notes**
Nalbuphine	IM/IV 10 mg every 3–6 h[b] (max. 20 mg dose, 160 mg daily)	Second-line agent for moderate-to-severe pain
		May precipitate withdrawal in opiate-dependent patients
Buprenorphine	IM 0.3 mg every 6 h[b]	Second-line agent for moderate-to-severe pain
	Slow IV 0.3 mg every 6 h[b]	May precipitate withdrawal in opiate-dependent patients
		Transdermal delivery systems (5, 10, 20 micrograms/hour) available for every 7 day administration
	May repeat × 1, 30–60 min after initial dose	Naloxone may not be effective in reversing respiratory depression
Naloxone	IV 0.4–2 mg	When reversing opiate side effects in patients needing analgesia, dilute and titrate (0.1–0.2 mg every 2–3 min) so as not to reverse analgesia
Tramadol	PO 50–100 mg every 4–6 h[a]	Maximum dose for nonextended-release, 400 mg/24 h; maximum for extended release, 300 mg/24 h
	If rapid onset not required, start 25 mg/day and titrate over several days	Decrease dose in patient with renal impairment and in the elderly
	Extended release PO 100 mg every 24 h	
Tapentadol	PO 50–100 mg every 4–6 h[a]	First day of therapy may administer second dose after the first within 1 h
		Maximum dose first day 700 mg, max. dose thereafter 600 mg

TABLE 69-5 Dosing Guidelines (continued)

[a]May start with an around-the-clock regimen and switch to prn if/when the painful signal subsides or is episodic.
[b]May reach a ceiling analgesic effect.
IM, intramuscular; IV, intravenous; NSAID, nonsteroidal antiinflammatory drug; PO, oral; prn, as needed; SR, sustained release; HCL, hydrochloride
Data from American Pain Society,[24] Tapentadol,[46] and Anonymous.[40,41,68]

of the most appropriate agent. ❸ The route of administration depends on individual patient needs. In patients who have oral access, the oral route is preferred. However, the onset of analgesic effects for oral medications is approximately 45 minutes, and the peak effect usually occurs 1 to 2 hours after administration.[24] This delay must be a consideration when immediate relief is needed in the management of acute pain. Therefore, in some scenarios, such as acute severe pain (i.e., pain crisis) or when the patient is unable to take oral medications, alternative routes of therapy (e.g., intravenous) may be preferred. The relative potency, defined by the equianalgesic dose, of opioids differs greatly (Table 69–4). ❹ Equianalgesic dose tables are often based on single-dose studies without regard for patient variability and should be used only as a guide.[32] True opioid allergies are rare, but Table 69–4 also can be used when treating a patient who is allergic to opiates. Most reactions to opioids, such as itching or rash, are due to the associated histamine release from cutaneous mast cells, not a true allergic or immunoglobulin-E (IgE) or T-cell response.[33] Although caution is always advised, a decrease in potential cross-sensitivity is thought to exist when moving from one opioid structural class to another.[33] The classes are phenanthrenes (morphine-like agonists), phenylpiperidines (meperidine-like agonists), and diphenylheptanes (methadone-like agonists). When considering cross-sensitivity, the mixed agonist–antagonist class

acts much like the morphine-like agonists.[33] Reactions due to histamine release may be reduced by choosing agents shown to have less effect on histamine release. Morphine has been associated with the greatest histamine release, whereas agents such as oxycodone and fentanyl typically cause fewer histamine-related reactions (see Table 69–4).

❷ ❺ In the initial stages of acute pain, analgesics should be given around the clock. This should commence after administering a typical starting dose and titrating up or down, depending on the patient's degree of pain and demonstrated side effects (e.g., sedation).[24] As-needed schedules often produce wide swings in analgesic plasma concentrations thatcreate wide swings in pain and sedation. This may initiate a vicious cycle where increasing amounts of pain medications are needed for relief. ❺ As the painful state subsides and the need for medication decreases, as-needed schedules may be appropriate. As-needed schedules also may be useful in patients who present with pain that is intermittent or sporadic in nature (Fig. 69–2). When opioids are used in the management of persistent chronic pain, around-the-clock administration schedules should be utilized. As-needed or PRN opioids should be used in conjunction with around-the-clock regimens and when patients experience breakthrough pain. Breakthrough pain is a brief, transitory, exacerbation of moderate to severe pain typically occurring in patients with underlying persistent pain that may otherwise be controlled.[32]

Continuous intravenous and subcutaneous methods of opioid infusion are effective for some postoperative pain, but the probability of unwanted side effects is high, and this technique should be reserved for opioid tolerant patients.[24,34] An alternative method is patient-controlled analgesia (PCA). With this technique, patients can self-administer a preset dose of an intravenous opioid via a pump electronically interfaced with a timing device. Compared with traditional as-needed opioid dosing, PCA yields better pain control, improved patient satisfaction, and relatively few differences in side effects.[35]

Administration of opiates directly into the CNS (e.g., epidural and intrathecal/subarachnoid routes) has shown considerable promise in the control of acute, chronic noncancer, and cancer pain (Table 69–7)[30,36,37]; and is common in both large and small institutions throughout the United States. Because of reports of respiratory depression, pruritus, nausea, vomiting, urinary retention, and hypotension,[37] these methods of analgesia require careful monitoring and are best used by experienced practitioners.

TABLE 69-6 Major Adverse Effects of the Opioid Analgesics

Effect	**Manifestation**
Mood changes	Dysphoria, euphoria
Somnolence	Sedation, inability to concentrate
Stimulation of chemoreceptor trigger zone	Nausea, vomiting
Respiratory depression	Decreased respiratory rate
Decreased gastrointestinal motility	Constipation
Increase in sphincter tone	Biliary spasm, urinary retention (varies among agents)
Histamine release	Urticaria, pruritus, rarely exacerbation of asthma (varies among agents)
Tolerance	Larger doses for same effect
Dependence	Withdrawal symptoms upon abrupt discontinuation

Data from Stimmel[1] and Gutstein and Akil.[30]

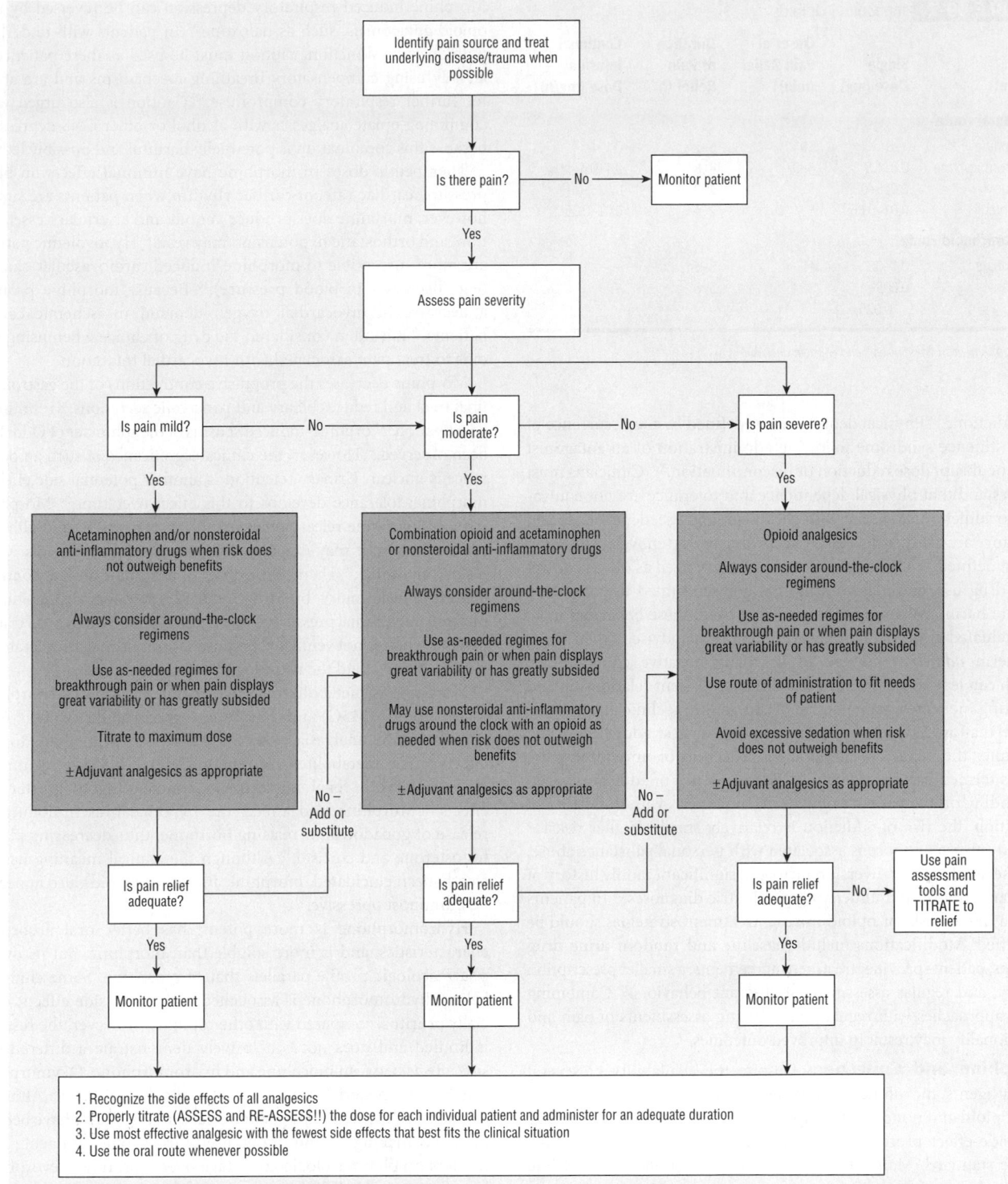

FIGURE 69-2. Algorithm for acute pain. *(Data modified from Omnicare, Inc., Acute Pain Pathway.)*

Respiratory depression is of concern and can occur within minutes with intrathecal fentanyl or manifest as late as 19 hours after a single dose of intrathecal morphine.[37] Guidelines mandate respiratory monitoring for at least 24 hours after a single dose of intrathecal or epidural morphine.[38] Naloxone is used to antagonize this effect. Analgesia and side effects are evident at lower doses when opioids are administered intrathecally instead of epidurally. Intrathecally, single morphine doses of 0.1 to 0.3 mg are common, whereas epidurally, doses of 1 to 6 mg are the norm.[30] These intrathecal and epidural opioids often are administered as a continuous-infusion and/or on a patient-controlled basis. When given simultaneously

with intrathecal or epidural local anesthetics such as bupivacaine, they have been proven safe and effective.[37] All agents administered directly into the CNS should be preservative free.

Tolerance, Dependence, Addiction, and Pseudoaddiction A barrier that consistently causes clinicians to misjudge and mistreat pain is the misunderstanding of opioid tolerance, physical dependence, addiction, and pseudoaddiction. Tolerance is the reduction of drug effect over time as a result of exposure to the drug.[39] It develops at different rates and with great patient variability. However, with stable disease, opioid use often stabilizes, and tolerance does not lead

TABLE 69-7 Intraspinal Opioids

Agent	Single Dose (mg)	Onset of Pain Relief (min)	Duration of Pain Relief (h)	Continual Infusion Dose (mg/h)
Epidural route				
Morphine	1–6	30	6–24	0.1–1
Hydromorphone	0.8–1.5	5–8	4–8	0.1–0.3
Fentanyl	0.025–0.1	5	2–8	0.025–0.1
Sufentanil	0.01–0.06	5	2–4	0.01–0.05
Subarachnoid route				
Morphine	0.1–0.3	15	8–34	–
Fentanyl	0.005–0.025	5	3–6	–

Data from American Pain Society[24] and Gutstein and Akil.[30]

to addiction.[39] "Physical dependence is defined by the occurrence of an abstinence syndrome following administration of an antagonist drug or abrupt dose reduction or discontinuation."[39] Clinicians must understand that physical dependence and tolerance are not equivalent to addiction; however, with chronic opioid use, dependence and tolerance are likely to develop.[24] According to Portenoy,[39] "Addiction is best defined as a behavioral pattern characterized as loss of control over drug use, compulsive drug use, and continued use of a drug despite harm." When opioids are being used, these behaviors must be evaluated continually. However, caution is advised when using the term *addiction* because of its many negative connotations, which can lead to a compromised clinician–patient relationship and resulting ineffective pain control.[24,39] In addition, clinicians must be aware that an individual's behaviors may suggest addiction, when in reality the behaviors noted are a reflection of unrelieved pain, this is termed pseudoaddiction.[24] The incidence of addiction varies depending on the patient population. In patients with no history of addiction, the risk of addiction is relatively small.[3] Higher risk for opioid misuse or abuse is associated with personal substance abuse, misuse, addiction or diversion history, a significant family history of substance abuse, and underlying psychiatric diagnoses.[29] In patients with a higher risk for opioid misuse, treatment strategies should be modified. Modifications include baseline and random urine drug screens, patient–provider treatment agreements, a smaller prescription supply, and regular assessment of aberrant behaviors.[29] Combining these approaches with regular and ongoing assessments of pain and functionality may result in improved outcomes.[29]

Morphine and Congeners Despite the availability of several newer agents, morphine remains the prototype opiate analgesic. As new opioid and nonopioid compounds are developed, their efficacy and side-effect profiles are typically compared against morphine as the standard. Many clinicians consider morphine the first-line agent when treating moderate-to-severe pain. Morphine can be given parenterally, orally, or rectally.

Side effects can be numerous, particularly when morphine is first initiated or when doses are significantly increased. Morphine causes nausea and vomiting through direct stimulation of the chemoreceptor trigger zone.[30] Opioid-induced nausea subsides over time.[3] Although euphoria and dysphoria have been reported, morphine's unpleasant effects are more prominent when administered to patients not experiencing pain.[30] As doses of morphine are increased, the respiratory center becomes less responsive to carbon dioxide, causing progressive respiratory depression.[30] This effect is less pronounced in patients being treated for severe or chronic pain.[3] Respiratory depression often manifests as a decrease in respiratory rate (although minute volume and tidal exchange also are affected) and is further compounded because the cough reflex is also depressed.[30]

Morphine-induced respiratory depression can be reversed by pure opioid antagonists, such as naloxone.[30] In patients with underlying pulmonary dysfunction, caution must be used as these patients are already using compensatory breathing mechanisms and are at risk for further respiratory compromise.[30] Caution is also urged when combining opiate analgesics with alcohol or other CNS depressants because this combination is potentially harmful and possibly lethal.[30]

Therapeutic doses of morphine have minimal effects on blood pressure, cardiac rate, or cardiac rhythm when patients are supine; however, morphine does produce venous and arteriolar vessel dilation, and orthostatic hypotension may result. Hypovolemic patients are more susceptible to morphine-induced cardiovascular changes (e.g., decreases in blood pressure).[30] Because morphine prompts a decrease in myocardial oxygen demand in ischemic cardiac patients,[30] it is often considered the drug of choice when using opioids to treat pain associated with myocardial infarction.

Morphine decreases the propulsive contractions of the gastrointestinal tract and reduces biliary and pancreatic secretions,[30] resulting in constipation. Morphine-induced spasms of the sphincter of Oddi have been observed.[30] However, the clinical significance of such an occurrence is unclear. Urinary retention is another potential side effect of morphine; tolerance develops to this effect over time.[30] Morphine-induced histamine release often manifests as pruritus, and although not seen often, it may exacerbate bronchospasm in patients with a history of asthma.[30] Therapeutic doses of morphine are not contraindicated in head injury, but drug-induced respiratory depression can increase intracranial pressure. Thus, caution is advised in head trauma patients who are not ventilated because morphine may exaggerate this pressure[30] and cloud the neurologic examination results.

Morphine is metabolized to two major metabolites, morphine-3-glucuronide (M3G) and morphine-6-glucuronide (M6G).[30] M6G contributes to analgesia, whereas M3G may contribute to side effects.[30] The metabolites are renally cleared and can accumulate in patients with renal impairment, contributing to greater side effects.[30] Morphine also affects the hypothalamus inhibiting the release of gonadotropin-relasing hormone, thus decreasing plasma testosterone and cortisol.[30] Although the clinical meaning has not clearly been elucidated, morphine and other opioids also appear to be immunosuppressive.[30]

Hydromorphone is more potent, has better oral absorption characteristics, and is more soluble than morphine, but its overall pharmacologic profile parallels that of morphine. Some clinicians believe hydromorphone is associated with fewer side effects, especially pruritus, compared with other opioids. However, the research is limited and does not conclusively demonstrate a difference in side effects between morphine and hydromorphone. Oxymorphone can be administered orally, rectally, and by injection. Although extended-release and immediate-release oral products have become available, making oxymorphone useful in chronic and acute pain, it offers no pharmacologic advantage over morphine. Levorphanol has an extended half-life, but its overall therapeutic effects are similar to the other agents in this class.

Codeine is a commonly used opiate in the treatment of mild-to-moderate pain. It often is combined with other analgesic products (e.g., acetaminophen). Unfortunately, it has the same propensity to produce side effects as morphine. Hydrocodone is another commonly prescribed opiate and is available for pain only in combination products with other analgesic agents (e.g., acetaminophen, ibuprofen). Its pharmacologic properties are similar to those of morphine. Oxycodone is a useful oral analgesic for moderate-to-severe pain. This is especially true when the product is used in combination with nonopioids. Although oxycodone shares basic morphine characteristics, the availability of an immediate-release and controlled-release oral dosage form also makes it very useful in persistent pain as well as acute pain.

Meperidine and Congeners (Phenylpiperidines) The prototype phenylpiperidine, meperidine, has a pharmacologic profile comparable with that of morphine; however, it is not as potent and has a shorter analgesic duration. Meperidine offers no analgesic advantage over morphine, has greater toxicity (CNS hyperirritability caused by its renally eliminated metabolite normeperidine),[40] and should be limited in use. In particular, avoid long-term usage, and use in patients at greatest risk for toxicity (e.g., elderly patients and those with renal dysfunction).

Fentanyl is a synthetic opioid structurally related to meperidine that is used often in anesthesiology as an adjunct to general anesthesia.[40] This agent is more potent and faster acting than meperidine (Table 69–4). It can be administered parenterally, transmucosally, and transdermally.

Methadone and Congeners Methadone has gained considerable popularity because of its oral efficacy, extended duration of action, and low cost. Although methadone is effective in acute pain,[41] it has gained particular prominence in treating cancer pain[36] and has increasingly been used in the management of chronic noncancer pain.[42] This despite the fact that, with repeated doses, the analgesic duration of action is prolonged,[41] it has an unpredictable half-life, it can cause excessive sedation, and it is difficult to titrate. Properties unique to methadone, compared with other opioids, include the D-isomer's ability to antagonize NMDA receptors, agonist effects at κ- and δ-opioid receptors, and blockade of serotonin and norepinephrine reuptake.[32,42] These properties may prove useful in the treatment of neuropathic and chronic pain or in patients with a maladaptive inflammatory component to their pain. However, few trials have thoroughly evaluated methadone's risks versus benefits.[29] Epidemiologic studies suggest a growing number of methadone related deaths, and cardiac arrhythmias have been associated with methadone, particularly at higher doses or when used concurrently with other agents that prolong QTc intervals.[29] The equianalgesic dose of methadone may decrease with higher doses of the previous opioid,[32] complicating conversions from other opioids to methadone.

CLIINICAL CONTROVERSY

Some clinicians believe that methadone should be tried before other opioids in many chronic pain conditions where an opioid is warranted because they believe that neuropathic pain is often a component. Other clinicians believe that sustained-released morphine or oxycodone are better first choices.

Propoxyphene usually is used in combination with acetaminophen for treatment of mild to moderate pain.[43] Propoxyphene is metabolized to norpropoxyphene, a potentially cardio-toxic metabolite.[30] Propoxyphene has been associated with medication injury in the elderly and its use is discouraged in these patients.[44] The U.S. Food and Drug Administration (FDA) has recently required more specific product labeling outlining this agent's possible risks and is requiring a new safety study to determine its risks versus its benefits.[43]

Opioid Agonist–Antagonist Derivatives Analgesic agents that stimulate the analgesic portion of opioid receptors while blocking or having no effect on the toxicity portion would be considered ideal. The agonist–antagonist derivatives were developed with this in mind. This analgesic class produces analgesia and has a ceiling effect on respiratory depression.[30] These agents also have a lower abuse potential than does morphine, but psychotomimetic responses (e.g., hallucinations and dysphoria, as seen with pentazocine), a ceiling analgesic effect, and a propensity to initiate withdrawal in opioid-dependent populations[30,40] have diminished their widespread clinical use.

Opioid Antagonists The pure opioid antagonist naloxone binds competitively to opioid receptors but does not produce an analgesic or opioid side-effect response. Therefore, it is used most often to reverse the toxic effects of agonist- and agonist–antagonist-derived opioids.

Central Analgesics

Tramadol and tapentadol are the only centrally acting analgesics currently available in the United States. Tramadol binds to μ-opiate receptors and inhibits norepinephrine and serotonin reuptake. Tapentadol also binds the μ-opiate receptor but inhibits largely norepinephrine reuptake. Tramadol is indicated for the relief of moderate to moderately severe pain, while tapentadol is indicated for moderate to severe acute pain.[41]

Both tramadol and tapentadol have side-effect profiles similar to that of the previously mentioned opioid analgesics (e.g., dizziness, nausea, somnolence, and constipation).[45,46] Tapentadol is a schedule II controlled substance, while tramadol is not scheduled.[46] Tapentadol has not been systematically evaluated in patients with seizure, and it should be used with caution in seizure patients.[41] Seizure risk may be elevated in patients taking tramadol.[41] Tramadol, may have a place in treating patients with chronic pain, especially neuropathic pain,[47] while tapentadol may be most useful in the management of acute pain.[41]

Adjuvant Analgesics

Adjuvant analgesics are pharmacologic agents with individual characteristics that make them useful in the management of pain but that typically are not classified as analgesics. Examples of adjuvant analgesics include antidepressants and anticonvulsants. ❻ Chronic pain that has a maladaptive inflammatory (e.g., low back pain) and/or neuropathic component (e.g., diabetic neuropathy) may require such agents (Table 69–8). Anticonvulsants (e.g., gabapentin, which may decrease neuronal excitability), tricyclic antidepressants, serotonin and norepinephrine reuptake inhibitor antidepressants (which block the reuptake of serotonin and norepinephrine, thus enhancing pain inhibition), and topically applied local anesthetics (which decrease nerve stimulation) all have been effective in managing chronic pain.[47]

In cancer patients, bone pain can be treated with radiopharmaceuticals. Both strontium-89 and samarium 153Sm lexidronam have been shown to provide pain relief.[41] Although antihistamines, amphetamines, and steroids have been used as adjuvant pain medications,[27] they have demonstrated only limited success as pain relievers.

Combination Therapy

The combination of opioid and nonopioid analgesics often results in analgesia superior to that produced by either agent alone.[26] This facilitates the use of lower doses and a more favorable side-effect profile, and, when needed, this approach is encouraged.

Regional Analgesia

Regional analgesia with properly administered local anesthetics can provide relief of both acute and chronic pain (Table 69–9).[3,37] These agents can be positioned by injection (e.g., in joints, in the epidural or intrathecal space, along nerve roots, or in a nerve plexus) or topically. Lidocaine in the form of a patch has proven effective in treating focal neuropathic pain.[47] Regional application of local

TABLE 69-8 Pharmacologic Management of Chronic Noncancer Pain

Type of Pain	Nonopioids	Opioids	Other Medications	Comments
Chronic low back pain	Acetaminophen	Short-term use for mild-to-moderate flare-ups	Tramadol, TCAs, AEDs	Acetaminophen first; tramadol or opioids in selected patients; AEDs or TCAs may be considered if neuropathic symptoms (evidence weak)
Fibromyalgia	Acetaminophen, NSAIDs	Long-term use not recommended	Tramadol, TCAs; AEDs, SNRIs	Acetaminophen considered first (evidence weak); TCAs, AEDs, SNRIs (stronger evidence); tramadol better alternative than opioids; NSAIDs only with other agents
Neuropathic pain	Acetaminophen or NSAIDs are rarely effective	Considered second-line therapy, are tried after AEDs and/or TCAs,	TCAs, AEDs, SNRIs, tramadol, topical (e.g., 5% lidocaine patch, capsaicin)	TCAs, SNRIs, AEDs, 5% lidocaine patch considered first line; tramadol, and opioids considered second-line agents; capsaicins considered third line

AED, antiepileptic drug; NSAIDs, nonsteroidal antiinflammatory drugs; SNRI, serotonin–norepinephrine reuptake inhibitor; TCA, tricyclic antidepressant.
Data from O'Connor and Dworkin,[47] Am J Manag Care,[63] Chou et al.,[64] and Herndon et al.[67]

anesthetics relieve pain by blocking nerve impulses.[41] High plasma concentrations can cause signs of CNS excitation and depression, including dizziness, tinnitus, drowsiness, disorientation, muscle twitching, seizures, and respiratory arrest.[40] Cardiovascular effects include myocardial depression, hypotension, decreased cardiac output, heart block, bradycardia, arrhythmias, and cardiac arrest.[41] Disadvantages of such methods include the need for skillful technical application, need for frequent administration, and highly specialized followup procedures.

■ SPECIAL CONSIDERATIONS IN ACUTE PAIN

❶ ❷ ❸ ❹ ❺ The World Health Organization (WHO) recommends a three-step ladder approach using the simplest dosage schedules and medications with the least amount of potential harm based on pain intensity ratings from mild, to moderate, to severe.[27] An acute pain algorithm outlining how to use these principles is given in Figure 69–2. The importance of reassessment and titration during this process cannot be overemphasized.

■ SPECIAL CONSIDERATIONS IN CANCER PAIN

Managing the pain of cancer encompasses both acute and chronic management techniques. **❼** Thus, pharmacologic treatment and psychological therapies are best combined with surgical methods, anesthetic procedures, and supportive care measures in a multidisciplinary approach to pain relief.[48,49] The goal is to provide patients with enough pain amelioration to tolerate diagnostic and therapeutic manipulation and permit the patient to function at a level that will allow freedom of movement and choice.[27] Assessment

TABLE 69-9 Local Anesthetics[a]

Agent (Brand Name)	Onset (min)	Duration (h)
Esters		
Procaine (Novocain, various)	2–5	0.25–1
Chloroprocaine (Nesacaine, various)	6–12	0.5
Tetracaine (Pontocaine)	≤15	2–3
Amides		
Mepivacaine (Polocaine, various)	3–5	0.75–1.5
Bupivacaine (Marcaine, various)	5	2–4
Lidocaine (Xylocaine, various)	<2	0.5–1
Prilocaine (Citanest)	<2	1–2
Ropivacaine[b] (Naropin)	10–30	0.5–6

[a]Unless otherwise indicated, values are for infiltrative anesthesia.
[b]Epidural administration.
Data from Anonymous.[40,41]

of the factors given in Table 69–2 also applies to cancer patients. Special attention must be given to continual reassessment of the painful state, adverse effects with medications, and aberrant behaviors. **❺** Individualization of therapy is always required.[27] Supportive care, in and outside the hospital, using programs such as hospice, is one of the cancer patient's greatest allies, not only in coping with pain but also in accepting the disease. The positive effect this has on the patient cannot be overstated. Pharmacologic management is the mainstay of therapy, and a typical progression of analgesic use in oncology patients is outlined in Figure 69–3.

■ SPECIAL CONSIDERATIONS IN CHRONIC NONCANCER PAIN

❼ The numerous etiologies that produce chronic noncancer pain make treatment complex, and overall management should be multidisciplinary. Evaluation objectives include establishing an accurate diagnosis, identifying iatrogenic factors, obtaining a comprehensive psychiatric and psychosocial assessment, paying special attention to family and social problems, and obtaining a description of factors that alleviate or exacerbate pain.[2] **❽** Given these objectives, placebos should never be used to diagnose pain.[4]

❼ In all cases of chronic noncancer pain, an integrated systematic approach (such as that often provided by pain clinics), with a strong emphasis on patient–clinician relationships, is essential. The goal is to improve or maintain the patient's level of functioning, decrease the rate of physical deterioration, decrease pain perception, improve the patient's sense of well-being, improve family and social relationships, and decrease dependency on drug therapy.[2] Patients and clinicians must realize that maximally effective treatment may take months or even years. During this time it may become necessary to use opioids for chronic noncancer pain patients. This has been a source of debate; however, recommendations exist when this modality becomes necessary that includes screening patients for risk of abuse, utilizing pain treatment "agreements," and distinctly outlining the treatment plan with patients.[29]

CLIINICAL CONTROVERSY

Many clinicians believe that some chronic painful conditions (e.g., osteoarthritis) should never be treated with opioids; whereas others believe that when other modalities are not effective or seem to pose more of a risk to that particular patient than does conventional therapy (e.g., NSAIDs), then opioids are necessary.

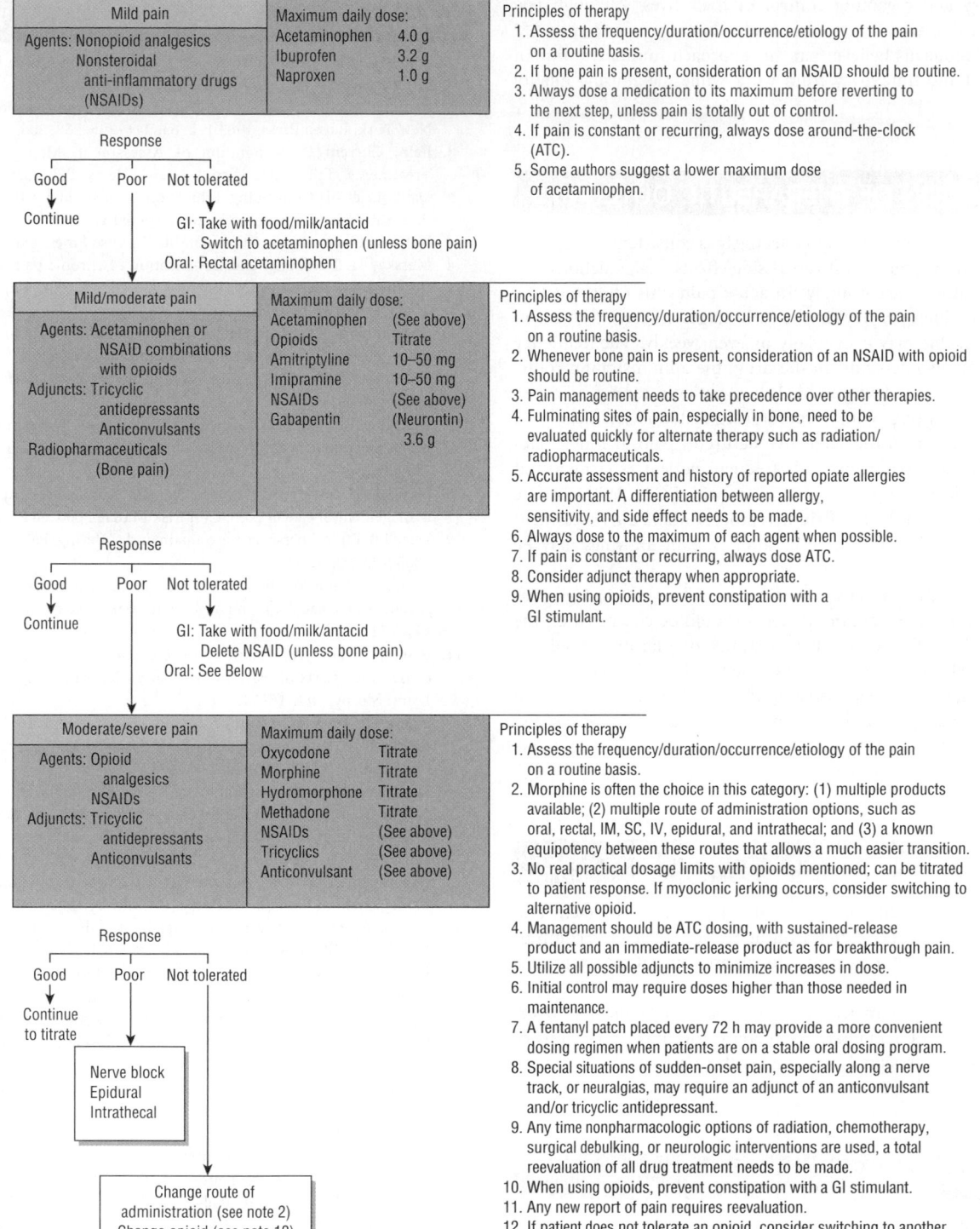

FIGURE 69-3. Algorithm for pain management in oncology patients. *(Data modified from the Kaiser Permanente Algorithm for Pain Management in Patients with Advanced Malignant Disease and reference 36.)*

■ SPECIAL POPULATIONS

The elderly and the young are at a higher risk for under-treatment because of inability to communicate or rate their pain. It is in these cases that parent or caregiver input becomes paramount to identify changes in behavior which might suggest pain (e.g., fussy, inconsolable, changes in eating patterns, crying out, or agitation). ❺ In addition, those living with chronic, debilitating, and life-threatening illnesses need specialized pain control and care that is palliative in nature.[50] Although care must be taken in these populations to ensure that proper individualized treatment

plans follow accepted guidelines,[50–53] the key concepts in pain management as outlined in this chapter are the guiding tenets in maximizing pain control.

PHARMACOECONOMIC CONSIDERATIONS

The *suffering* component of pain cannot be overemphasized. Swift relief from acute and cancer pain and well-planned treatment regimens in chronic noncancer pain will allow patients to concentrate on recovery and regaining control of their lives. Although few well-designed pharmacoeconomic studies have been performed,[54-56] most pain clinicians believe that this approach minimizes time in the hospital and time away from work while maximizing quality of life.

EVALUATION OF THERAPEUTIC OUTCOMES

② ⑤ The key to treating pain effectively is consistent monitoring for effectiveness (pain relief) versus side effects (e.g., sedation) and titrating treatment accordingly. In acute pain, this often must be done several times per day (in the early stages, hourly), whereas in chronic pain this may occur daily or even weekly. The frequency of evaluation also depends on the drug, the administration route, and other therapies being used. When patients cannot be asked about their pain (e.g., coma), monitoring agitation and heart rate is appropriate. Given the subjective nature of pain, the most successful therapies involve not only frequent patient assessment but also a large degree of patient control (as with PCA). With chronic pain, tools such as the Brief Pain Inventory, Initial Pain Assessment Inventory, McGill Pain Questionnaire, or pain drawings may be helpful.[3]

② All opioids can cause constipation. The best management of constipation is prevention. Patients should be counseled on the proper intake of fluids and fiber. A stimulating laxative should be added with chronic opioid use. As noted earlier, CNS depressants (e.g., alcohol, benzodiazepines) amplify CNS depression when used with opioid analgesics, and use of these combinations should be discouraged when possible. When the combinations are used, patients should be monitored closely.

CONCLUSIONS

Poor training of healthcare practitioners in pain assessment and management, improper patient education, and inadequate communication among healthcare professionals are some of the reasons for inadequate pain relief. The use of an integrated approach, incorporating the expertise of many disciplines, may well be the most overlooked principle of pain pharmacotherapy. It is the responsibility of all healthcare professionals who deal with pain to work together to ensure proper management.

ABBREVIATIONS

CNS: central nervous system

FDA: Food and Drug Administration

GABA: γ-aminobutyric acid

IM: intramuscular

IV: intravenous

M3G: morphine-3-glucuronide

M6G: morphine-6-glucuronide

NMDA: N-methyl-D-aspartate

NSAIDs: nonsteroidal antiinflammatory drugs

PCA: patient-controlled analgesia

PO: oral

TENS: transcutaneous electrical nerve stimulation

WHO: World Health Organization

REFERENCES

1. Selected quotes from Helen Keller. David Hawkins Quote Page. 1998, *http://www.river.org/~dhawk/keller-quotes.html*.

2. Stimmel B. Pain, Analgesia and Addiction: The Pharmacology of Pain. New York: Raven Press, 1983:1, 2, 63, 241–245, 259, 266.

3. Pain: Current Understanding of Assessment, Management, and Treatments. Editorial advisory board; Berry PH, Covington EC, Dahl JL, et al. Continuing Education Sponsored by the American Pain Society and supported by unrestricted education grant from the National Pharmaceutical Council, Inc. Release June 2006.

4. Merskey H. Taxonomy and classification of chronic pain syndromes. In: Benzon HT, Rathmell JP, Wu CL, et al., eds. Raj's Practical Management of Pain. Philadelphia, PA: Mosby, 2008:13–18.

5. Chartbook on Trends in Health to Americans with Special Feature on Pain. 2006;68–91. *www.cdc.gov/nchs/data/hus/hus06.pdf*.

6. Hahn KL. A decade of pain wasting away. Practical Pain Manag 2008;8:40–44.

7. Gallagher RM. Primary care and pain medicine: A community solution to the public health problem of chronic pain. Med Clin North Am 1999;83:555–583.

8. Mandala M, Moro C, Labianca R, et al. Optimizing use of opiates in the management of cancer pain. Clin Risk Manag 2006;2:447–453.

9. Ferrell B. Ethical perspectives on pain and suffering. Pain Manag Nurs 2005;6:83–90.

10. Woolf CJ. Pain: Moving from symptom control toward mechanism-specific pharmacologic management. Ann Intern Med 2004;140: 441–451.

11. Pasero C, Paice JA, McCaffery M. Basic mechanisms underlying the causes and effects of pain. In: McCaffery M, Pasero C, eds. Pain. St. Louis: Mosby, 1999:15–34.

12. Yaksh TL. A review of pain-processing pharmacology. In: Benzon HT, Rathmell JP, Wu CL, et al., eds. Raj's Practical Management of Pain. Philadelphia, PA: Mosby, 2008;135–149.

13. High KN. Pain pathways: peripheral, spinal, ascending, and descending pathways. In: Benzon HT, Rathmell JP, Wu CL, et al., eds. Raj's Practical Management of Pain. Philadelphia, PA: Mosby, 2008:119–134.

14. Cortazzo MH, Fishman SM. Major opioids and chronic opioid therapy. In: Benzon HT, Rathmell JP, Wu CL, et al., eds. Raj's Practical Management of Pain. Philadelphia, PA: Mosby, 2008:597–611.

15. McPherson ML. Chronic pain management: A disease-based approach. In: Chronic Illnesses: A Pharmacotherapy Self-Assessment Program. Kansas City, MO: American College of Clinical Pharmacy, 2005: 1–40.

16. Apkarian A. Pain and brain changes. In: Benzon HT, Rathmell JP, Wu CL, et al., eds. Raj's Practical Management of Pain. Philadelphia, PA: Mosby, 2008:151–173.

17. Hanley MA, Jensen MP, Smith DG, et al. Preamputation pain and acute pain predict chronic pain after lower extremity amputation. J Pain 2007;8:102–109.

18. Latremoliere A, Woolf CJ. Central sensitization: A generator or pain hypersensitivity by central neural plasticity. J Pain 2009;10:895–926.

19. Twycross RG. Pain and analgesics. Curr Med Res Opin 1978;5: 497–505.

20. National Institute of Health Pain Consortium. Pain Intensity Scales (last reviewed 1/17/2007). *http://painconsortium.nih.gov/pain_scales/index.html*.

21. Calmels P, Mick G, Perrouin-Verbe B, et al. Neuropathic pain in spinal cord injury: identification, classification, evaluation. Ann Phys Rehabil Med 2009;52:83–102.

22. Anderson KO. Assessment tools for the evaluation of pain in the oncology patient. Curr Pain Headache Rep 2007;11:259–264.

23. Passik SD, Kirsh KL. Protecting your practice: appropriate documentation for pain management. In: McCarbert BH, Passik SD, eds. Expert Guide to Pain Management. Philadelphia, PA: ACP Press, 2005:299–310.

24. American Pain Society. Principles of Analgesic Use in the Treatment of Acute Pain and Chronic Cancer Pain, 5th ed. Glenview, IL: American Pain Society, 2003.

25. Grobios M, Benny B, Chan KT. Yaksh TL. Physical medicine techniques in pain management. In: Benzon HT, Rathmell JP, Wu

CL, et al., eds. Raj's Practical Management of Pain. Philadelphia, PA: Mosby, 2008:135–149.

26. Clinical Practice Guideline. Acute Pain Management: Operative or Medical Procedures and Trauma. Publication No. 92–0032. Rockville, MD: Department of Health and Human Services, Public Health Service, Agency for Health Care Policy and Research [now called Agency for Healthcare Research and Quality], 1992.

27. Clinical Practice Guideline No. 9. Management of Cancer Pain. Publication No. 94–0592. Rockville, MD: Department of Health, Public Health Service, Agency for Health Care Policy and Research [now called Agency for Healthcare Research and Quality], 1994.

28. Turk D, Swanson K. Psychological interventions. In: Benzon HT, Rathmell JP, Wu CL, et al., eds. Raj's Practical Management of Pain. Philadelphia, PA: Mosby, 2008:739–755.

29. Chou R, Fanciullo GJ, Fine PG, et al. Clinical guidelines for the use of chronic opioid therapy in chronic noncancer pain. J Pain 2009;10:113–130.

30. Gutstein HB, Akil H. Opioid analgesics. In: Brunton LL, Lazo AS, Parker KL, eds. The Pharmacological Basis of Therapeutics, 11th ed. New York: McGraw-Hill, 2006:547–590.

31. Pasternak G. Molecular insights into [mu] opioid pharmacology: from the clinic to the bench. Clinical Journal of Pain 2010:26;S3–S9.

32. McPherson ML. Demystifying Opioid Conversion Calculations. A Guide For Effective Dosing. Bethesda, MD: American Society of Health-System Pharmacists, 2010.

33. Analgesic options for patients with allergic-type opioid reactions. Pharmacist's Lett/Prescriber's Lett 2006;22:220201.

34. American Society of Anesthesiologists Task Force on Acute Pain Management. Practice guidelines for acute pain management in the perioperative setting: An updated report by the American Society of Anesthesiolgists Task Force on Acute Pain Management. Anesthesiology 2004:100;1573–1581.

35. Momeni M, Crucitti M, DeKock M. Patient controlled analgesia in the management of postoperative pain. Drugs 2006;66:2321–2337.

36. Pain (PDQ) Health Professional Version, (Modified in 4/2010). http://www.cancer.gov/cancertopics/pdq/supportivecare/pain/Health Professional.

37. Melton S, Spencer S. Regional anesthesia techniques for acute pain management. In: Fishman SM, Ballantyne JC, Rathmell JP, eds. Bonica's Pain Management. Baltimore, MD, Philadelphia, PA: Wolters Kluwer Health/Lipincott Williams & Wilkins, 2010:723–754.

38. Horlocker TT, Burton AW, Connis RT, et al. Practice guidelines for the prevention, detection and management of respiratory depression associated with neuraxial opioid administration. Anesthesiology 2009;110:218–230.

39. Portenoy RK. Pain specialists and addiction medicine specialists unite to address critical issues. Am Pain Soc Bull 1999;9:2–13.

40. Anonymous. American Hospital Formulary Service. In: McVoy GK, ed. Drug Information. Bethesda, MD: American Society of Health-System Pharmacists, 2009.

41. Anonymous. Facts and Comparisons. Philadelphia, PA. Wolters Kluwer Health. Accessed August 2010.

42. Sandoval JA, Furlan AD, Mailis-Gagnon A. Oral methadone for chronic noncancer pain: A systematic literature review of reasons for administration, prescription patterns, effectiveness, and side effects. Clin J Pain 2005;21:503–512.

43. FDA website, 2009. http://www.fda.gov/NewsEvents/Newsroom/PressAnnouncements/ucm170769.htm.

44. Blackwell S, Montgomery M, Waldo D, et al. National study of medications associated with injury in elderly Medicare/Medicaid dual enrollees during 2003. J Am Pharm Assoc 2009;49:751–759.

45. Tramadol [package insert]. Raritan, NJ: Ortho-McNeil; 2007.

46. Tapentadol [package insert]. Raritan NJ: PriCara, Division of Ortho-McNeil-Janssen Pharmaceuticals, Inc; 2009.

47. O'Connor AB, Dworkin RH. Treatment of neuropathic pain: an overview of recent guidelines. Am J Med 2009;122:S22–S32.

48. Foley KM. The treatment of cancer pain. N Engl J Med 1985;313:84–95.

49. Gordon DB, Dahl JL, Miaskowski C, et al. American Pain Society recommendations for improving the quality of care and cancer pain management: American Pain Society Quality of Pain Task Force. Arch Int Med 2005;165:1574–1580.

50. Clinical Practice Guidelines for Quality Palliative Care, 2nd ed. National Consensus Project for Quality Palliative Care; 2009. www.nationalconcensusproject.org.

51. Clinical Practice Guideline, American Geriatrics Society Panel on Persistent Pain in Older Persons. The management of persistent pain in older persons. J Am Geriatr Soc 2009;57:1331–1346.

52. American Academy of Pediatrics and American Pain Society. The assessment and management of acute pain in infants, children and adolescents. Pediatrics 2001;108:793–797.

53. Lago P, Garetti E, Merazzi D, et al. Guidelines for procedural pain in the newborn. Acta Paediatr 2009;98:932–939.

54. Abernethy AP, Wheeler JL, Fortner BV. A health economic model of breakthrough pain. Am J Manag Care 2008;14:S129–S140.

55. Ritzwoller DP, Crounse L, Shetterly S, et al. The association of comorbidities, utilization, and costs for patients identified with low back pain. BMC Musculoskelet Disord 2006;7:72.

56. Rahimi SY, Vender JR, Macomson SD, et al. Postoperative pain management after craniontomy: Evaluation and cost analysis. Neurosurgery 2006;59:852–857.

57. Turner MK, Hooten WM, Schmidt JE, et al. Prevalence of clinical correlates of vitamin D inadequacy among patients with chronic pain. Pain Med 2008;9:979–984.

58. Hagen K, Bjoro T, Zwart J, et al. Do high TSH values protect against chronic musculoskeletal complaints? The Nord-Trondelag Health Study (HUNT). Pain 2005;113:416–421.

59. Bernard MA, Nakonezny PA, Kashner TM. The effect of vitamin B12 deficiency on older veterans and its relationship to health. J Am Geriatr Soc 1998;46:1199–1206.

60. Jacobson L, Mariano AJ. General considerations of chronic pain. In: Loeser JD, Butler SH, Chapman CR, et al., eds. Bonica's Management of Pain. Philadelphia, PA: Lippincott Williams & Wilkins, 2000: 241–254.

61. Watkins PB, Kaplowitz N, Slattery TJ, et al. Aminotransferase elevations in healthy adults receiving 4 grams of acetaminophen daily: A randomized controlled trial. JAMA 2006;296:87–93.

62. Li F. Pharmacologically induced histamine release: sorting out hypersensitivity reactions to opioids. Drug Therapy topics 2006:35 http://depts.washington.edu/druginfo/DTT/2006_Vol35_Files/V35N4.pdf.

63. Contemporary management strategies for fibromyalgia. Am J Manag Care 2009;15:S197–S218.

64. Chou R, Qaseem A, Snow V, et al. Diagnosis and treatment of low back pain: a joint clinical practice guideline from the American college of physicians and American pain society. Ann Intern Med 2007;147: 478–491.

65. Caldolor [package insert]. Nashville, TN: Cumberland Pharmaceuticals Inc.; 2009.

66. Pasero C, Portenoy RK, McCaffery M. Opioid analgesics. In: McCaffery M, Pasero C, eds. Pain. St. Louis, MO: Mosby, 1999:161–299.

67. Herndon CM, Hutchison RW, Berdine HJ, et al. Management of chronic nonmalignant pain with nonsteroidal anti-inflammatory drugs. Pharmacotherapy 2008;28:788–805.

68. Anonymous. Micromedex 2.0. Thomson Reuters. Accessed August 2010.

69. Byers MR, Bonica JJ. Peripheral pain mechanisms and nociceptor plasticity. In: Loeser JD, Butler SH, Chapman CR, et al, eds. Bonica's Management of Pain. Philadelphia, Lippincott Williams & Wilkins, 2000:26–72.

CHAPTER 70

Headache Disorders

DEBORAH S. MINOR

KEY CONCEPTS

❶ Acute migraine therapies should provide consistent, rapid relief and enable the patient to resume normal activities at home, school, or work.

❷ A stratified care approach, in which the selection of initial treatment is based on headache-related disability and symptom severity, is the preferred treatment strategy for the migraineur.

❸ Strict adherence to maximum daily and weekly doses of antimigraine medications is essential.

❹ Preventive therapy should be considered in the setting of recurring migraines that produce significant disability; frequent attacks requiring symptomatic medication more than twice per week; symptomatic therapies that are ineffective, contraindicated, or produce serious side effects; and uncommon migraine variants that cause profound disruption and/or risk of neurologic injury.

❺ The selection of an agent for migraine prophylaxis should be based on individual patient response, tolerability, convenience of the drug formulation, and comorbid conditions.

❻ Each prophylactic medication should be given an adequate therapeutic trial (usually 2–6 months) to judge its efficacy.

❼ A general wellness program and avoidance of migraine triggers should be included in the management plan.

❽ After an effective abortive agent and dose have been identified, subsequent treatments should begin with that same regimen.

Headache is one of the most common complaints encountered by healthcare practitioners and among the top three principal reasons given by adults 18 years of age and older for visiting emergency departments in the United States.[1] Headache can be symptomatic of a distinct pathologic process or can occur without an underlying cause. In 2004, the International Headache Society (IHS) updated its classification system and diagnostic criteria for headache disorders, cranial neuralgias, and facial pain[2] (Table 70–1). Designed to

facilitate headache diagnosis in clinical practice and research, the IHS classification provides more precise definitions and standardized nomenclature for both the primary (tension-type, migraine, and cluster headache) and secondary (symptomatic of organic disease) headache disorders. This chapter focuses on the management of the primary headache disorders.

Most recurrent headaches are the result of a benign chronic primary headache disorder.[3] Less often, headaches are symptomatic of a serious underlying medical condition, such as infection, cerebral hemorrhage, or brain mass lesion. The peak prevalence of tension-type and migraine headache, the most common of the primary headache disorders, occurs during the most productive years of life (20–55 years of age).[3] Despite the prevalence of these disorders and their associated disability, studies indicate that most headache sufferers do not seek appropriate medical care for their headaches.[4,5] An improved understanding of the diagnosis and pathophysiologic mechanisms of the primary headache disorders, particularly migraine, has led to the development of medications capable of providing rapid relief from moderate to severe attacks. However, a thorough evaluation of the headache history is essential to establish an accurate headache diagnosis and identify patients who can benefit from these specific therapeutic options.

MIGRAINE HEADACHE

EPIDEMIOLOGY

Results of the American Migraine Prevalence and Prevention Study indicate that 17.1% of women and 5.6% of men in the United States experience one or more migraine headaches per year.[5] The prevalence of migraine varies considerably by age and gender, but the epidemiologic profile has remained stable over the past 15 years.[5] Before the age of 12 years, migraine is more common in boys than in girls, but prevalence increases more rapidly in girls after puberty.[3] After age 12, females are two to three times more likely than males to suffer from migraine. Gender differences in migraine prevalence have been linked to menstruation, but these differences persist beyond menopause. Prevalence is highest in both men and women between the ages of 30 and 49 years.[5] The usual age of onset is 12 to 17 years of age for females and 5 to 11 years for males.[3] In the American Migraine Prevalence and Prevention Study, 93% of those with migraine reported some headache-related disability, and 54% were severely disabled or needed bed rest during an attack.[5] A number of neurologic and psychiatric disorders as well as cardiovascular diseases, including stroke, epilepsy, major depression, sleep apnea, and anxiety disorder, show increased comorbidity with migraine.[3,6] Whether this relationship is causal or representative of a common pathophysiologic mechanism is unknown. The economic burden of migraine is substantial; however, the indirect

TABLE 70-1 International Headache Society Classification System: Focus on Migraine Headache

Migraine
Migraine without aura
Migraine with aura
    Typical aura with migraine headache (aura lasting <1 hour)
    Typical aura with nonmigraine headache
    Typical aura without headache
    Familial hemiplegic migraine
    Sporadic hemiplegic migraine
    Basilar-type migraine
Childhood periodic syndromes that are commonly precursors of migraine
    Cyclical vomiting (self-limiting episodic condition)
    Abdominal migraine (episodic midline abdominal pain attacks lasting 1–72 hours)
    Benign paroxysmal vertigo of childhood (brief episodic vertigo)
Retinal migraine (repeated attacks of monocular visual disturbance)
Complications of migraine
    Chronic migraine (occurring on ≥15 days per month for >3 months)
    Status migrainous (debilitating attack lasting >72 hours)
    Persistent aura without infarction (symptoms persisting >1 week)
    Migrainous infarction (aura symptoms associated with an ischemic brain lesion)
    Migraine-triggered seizure
Probable migraine
    Probable migraine without aura
    Probable migraine with aura
    Probable chronic migraine
Tension-type headache
Cluster headache and other trigeminal autonomic cephalalgias
Other primary headaches
Headache attributed to head and/or neck trauma
Headache attributed to cranial or cervical vascular disorder
Headache attributed to nonvascular intracranial disorder
Headache attributed to a substance or its withdrawal
Headache attributed to infection
Headache attributed to disorder of homeostasis
Headache or facial pain attributed to disorder of cranium, neck, eyes, ears, nose, sinuses, teeth, mouth, or other facial or cranial structures
Headache attributed to psychiatric disorder
Cranial neuralgias and central causes of facial pain
Other headache, cranial neuralgia, central or primary facial pain

Adapted with permission from Headache Classification Committee of the International Headache Society. The international classification of headache disorders, 2nd ed. Cephalalgia 2004;24(Suppl 1):1–151.

costs from work-related disability far exceed the direct costs associated with treatment.[3]

ETIOLOGY AND PATHOPHYSIOLOGY

The etiologic and pathophysiologic mechanisms of migraine are not completely understood. According to earlier theories, the migraine aura was caused by intracerebral arterial vasoconstriction followed by reactive extracranial vasodilation and associated headache. Although studies of regional blood flow in the brain do not support this vascular hypothesis, the aura phase of migraine is associated with a reduction in cerebral blood flow that begins in the occipital region and moves across the cerebral cortex at a rate of 2 to 3 mm/min.[7,8] However, most clinicians now believe that the positive and negative symptoms of migraine are caused by neuronal dysfunction, not ischemia.[6–8] The neurologic changes of the aura parallel those that occur during cortical spreading depression, a neuronal event characterized by a wave of depressed electrical activity that advances across the brain cortex at a rate consistent with the spread of aura symptoms.[7] Migraine without aura is a neurobiologic disorder.[2] Migraine pain is believed to result from activity within the trigeminovascular system, a network of visceral afferent fibers that arises from the trigeminal ganglia and projects peripherally

to innervate the pain-sensitive intracranial extracerebral blood vessels, dura mater, and large venous sinuses[9] (Fig. 70-1). These fibers also project centrally, terminating in the trigeminal nucleus caudalis in the brainstem and upper cervical spinal cord, and thus provide a pathway for nociceptive transmission from meningeal blood vessels into higher centers of the central nervous system (CNS). Activation of trigeminal sensory nerves triggers the release of vasoactive neuropeptides, including calcitonin gene-related peptide (CGRP), neurokinin A, and substance P, from perivascular axons. The released neuropeptides interact with dural blood vessels to promote vasodilation and dural plasma extravasation, resulting in neurogenic inflammation.[6,7] Orthodromic conduction along trigeminovascular fibers transmits pain impulses to the trigeminal nucleus caudalis, where information is relayed further to higher cortical pain centers. Continued afferent input can result in sensitization of these central sensory neurons, producing a hyperalgesic state that responds to previously innocuous stimuli and maintains the headache.[7]

Despite recent advances in understanding of the pathophysiology of headache pain, there is still a considerable lack of knowledge regarding the mechanisms of attack initiation. Although the exact pathophysiology of migraine needs further elucidation, new neuroimaging techniques have provided insight into mechanisms. Previous vascular and neural theories of migraine development have merged into a combined theory of neurovascular mechanisms. Activity within the trigeminovascular system may be regulated in part by serotonergic neurons within the brainstem. Thus, the pathogenesis of migraine may be related to a defect or dysfunction in the activity of neuronal calcium channels mediating serotonin and excitatory neurotransmitter release in brainstem nuclei that modulate cerebral vascular tone and nociception.[7,9] This dysfunction may result in vasodilation of intracranial extracerebral blood vessels and consequent activation of the trigeminovascular system. Future research might further delineate the role of the brainstem as the "migraine generator."

Genetic factors seem to play an important role in susceptibility to migraine attacks. Studies in monozygotic twins suggest approximately 50% heritability of migraine with a multifactorial polygenic basis.[10] Although it is possible for any individual to experience a migraine attack, it is recurrence in the migraineur that is abnormal. Attack occurrence and frequency are governed by CNS sensitivity to migraine-specific triggers or environmental factors. Migraineurs appear to have a lowered threshold of response to specific environmental circumstances as a result of genetic factors that govern the balance of CNS excitation and inhibition at various levels.[10] Thus, trigger factors can be viewed as modulators of the genetic set point that predisposes to migraine headache. The hyperresponsiveness of the migrainous brain may be the result of an inherited abnormality in calcium and/or sodium channels and sodium/potassium pumps that regulate cortical excitability through the release of serotonin and other neurotransmitters.[6,10] Low levels of magnesium or dopamine, increased levels of excitatory amino acids such as glutamate, and alterations in levels of extracellular potassium also can affect the migraine threshold and initiate and propagate the phenomenon of cortical spreading depression.[11]

Serotonin (5-hydroxytryptamine [5-HT]) has long been implicated as an important mediator of migraine headache. Specific populations of 5-HT receptor subfamilies (5-HT$_1$ to 5-HT$_7$) appear to be involved in the pathophysiology and treatment of migraine headache.[7] Acute antimigraine drugs such as the ergot alkaloids and triptan derivatives are agonists of vascular and neuronal 5-HT$_1$ receptor subtypes, resulting in vasoconstriction of meningeal blood vessels and inhibition of vasoactive neuropeptide release and pain signal transmission.[7] Drugs used for

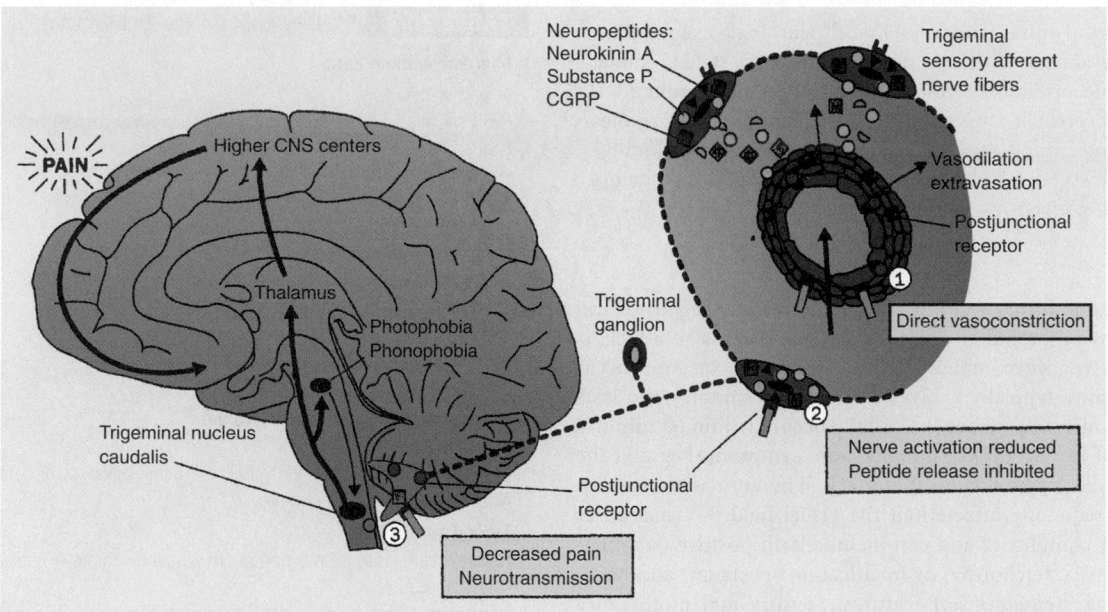

FIGURE 70-1. The pathophysiology of migraine headache. Vasodilation of intracranial extracerebral blood vessels (possibly the result of an imbalance in the brainstem) results in the activation of the perivascular trigeminal nerves that release vasoactive neuropeptides to promote neurogenic inflammation. Central pain transmission may activate other brainstem nuclei, resulting in associated symptoms (nausea, vomiting, photophobia, phonophobia). The antimigraine effects of the 5-HT$_{1B/1D}$ receptor agonists are highlighted at areas *1, 2,* and *3.* (CGRP, calcitonin gene-related peptide.) *(Reprinted from the Lancet, Vol. 351, Ferrari MD, Migraine, 1043–1051, Copyright © 1998, with permission from Elsevier.)*

migraine prophylaxis also modulate neurotransmitter systems. These actions and benefits in migraine management are consistent with the current understanding of migraine pathophysiology and neurovascular disorders.

CLINICAL PRESENTATION

The migraine attack has been divided into several phases. *Premonitory symptoms* are experienced by approximately 20% to 60% of migraineurs in the hours or days before the onset of headache.[2,7] The previously popular terms *prodrome* and *warning symptoms* should be avoided because these are often used mistakenly to include aura.[2] Premonitory symptoms vary widely among migraineurs but usually are consistent within an individual. Neurologic symptoms (e.g., phonophobia, photophobia, hyperosmia, and difficulty concentrating) are most common, but psychological (e.g., anxiety, depression, euphoria, irritability, drowsiness, hyperactivity, and restlessness), autonomic (e.g., polyuria, diarrhea, and constipation), and constitutional symptoms (e.g., stiff neck, yawning, thirst, food cravings, and anorexia) also are reported.[6–8]

CLINICAL PRESENTATION OF MIGRAINE HEADACHE

General

☐ Migraine is a common, recurrent, severe headache that interferes with normal functioning. It is a primary headache disorder divided into two major subtypes, migraine without aura and migraine with aura.

Symptoms

☐ Migraine is characterized by recurring episodes of throbbing head pain, frequently unilateral, that when untreated can last from 4 to 72 hours. Migraine headaches can be severe and associated with nausea, vomiting, and sensitivity to light, sound, and/or movement. Not all symptoms are present at every attack.

☐ In the headache evaluation, diagnostic alarms should be identified. These include: acute onset of the "first" or "worst" headache ever, accelerating pattern of headache following subacute onset, onset of headache after age 50 years, headache associated with systemic illness (e.g., fever, nausea, vomiting, stiff neck, and rash), headache with focal neurologic symptoms or papilledema, and new-onset headache in a patient with cancer or human immunodeficiency virus infection.

Signs

☐ A stable pattern, absence of daily headache, positive family history for migraine, normal neurologic examination, presence of food triggers, menstrual association, long-standing history, improvement with sleep, and subacute evolution are all signs of migraine headache. Aura can signal the migraine headache but is not required for diagnosis.

Laboratory Tests

☐ In selected circumstances and secondary headache presentation, serum chemistries, urine toxicology profiles, thyroid function tests, lyme studies, and other blood tests such as a complete blood count, antinuclear antibody titer, erythrocyte sedimentation rate, and antiphospholipid antibody titer can be considered.

Diagnostic Tests

☐ Perform a general medical and neurologic physical examination. Check for abnormalities: vital signs (fever, hypertension), funduscopy (papilledema, hemorrhage, and exudates), palpation and auscultation of the head and neck (sinus tenderness, hardened or tender temporal arteries, trigger points, temporomandibular joint tenderness, bruits, nuchal rigidity, and cervical spine tenderness), and neurologic examination (identify abnormalities or deficits in mental status, cranial nerves, deep tendon reflexes, motor strength, coordination, gait, and cerebellar function). Consider neuroimaging studies in patients with abnormal neurologic examination findings of unknown etiology and in those with additional risk factors warranting imaging.

The migraine *aura*, a complex of positive and negative focal neurologic symptoms that precedes or accompanies an attack, is experienced by approximately 31% of migraineurs on some occasions.[8] The aura typically evolves over 5 to 20 minutes and lasts less than 60 minutes. Headache usually occurs within 60 minutes of the end of the aura. Occasionally, aura symptoms begin at the onset of headache or during the attack. The aura is most often visual and frequently affects half the visual field.[2,8] Visual auras vary in their complexity and can include both positive (scintillations, photopsia, teichopsia, or fortification spectrum) and negative (scotoma, hemianopsia) features. Sensory and motor aura symptoms, such as paresthesias or numbness involving the arms and face, dysphasia or aphasia, weakness, and hemiparesis, also are reported.[7]

Of those with migraine in the United States, 14% experience more than four attacks per month, 63% experience one to four attacks per month, and 23% experience less than one attack per month.[5] Migraine *headache* can occur at any time of the day or night but occurs most often in the early morning hours on awakening. Pain is usually gradual in onset, peaking in intensity over a period of minutes to hours and lasting between 4 and 72 hours. Pain can occur anywhere in the face or head but most often involves the frontotemporal region. The headache is typically unilateral and throbbing or pulsating in nature; however, pain can be bilateral at onset or become generalized during the course of an attack.[2,7,12] Gastrointestinal symptoms almost invariably accompany the headache. During an attack, as many as 90% of migraineurs experience nausea, and emesis occurs in approximately one-third of patients.[7] Other systemic symptoms associated with the headache phase include anorexia, food cravings, constipation, diarrhea, abdominal cramps, nasal stuffiness, blurred vision, diaphoresis, facial pallor, and localized facial, scalp, or periorbital edema. Sensory hyperacuity, manifested as photophobia, phonophobia, or osmophobia, is reported frequently. Because headache pain usually is aggravated by physical activity, most migraineurs seek a dark, quiet room for rest and relief. Impaired concentration, depression, irritability, fatigue, or anxiety often accompany the headache. Once headache pain wanes, patients may experience a *resolution phase* characterized by feeling tired, exhausted, irritable, or listless. Impaired concentration may continue, as well as scalp tenderness or mood changes. Some patients experience depression and malaise, whereas others can feel unusually refreshed or euphoric.[7] The reader is referred to the IHS classification and recent reviews for descriptions of the classic migraine variants and other migraine subtypes[2,7,12,13] (see also Table 70–1).

Although headaches have many potential causes, most are considered to be primary headache disorders. A comprehensive headache history is the most important element in establishing the clinical diagnosis of migraine.[12] A thorough headache history always should be obtained, and information collected should include age at onset, attack frequency and timing, duration of attacks, precipitating or aggravating factors, ameliorating factors, description of neurologic symptoms, characteristics of the headache pain (quality, intensity, location, and radiation), associated signs and symptoms, treatment history, family and social history, and the impact of headaches on daily life.

TABLE 70-2 IHS Diagnostic Criteria for Migraine

Migraine without aura

At least five attacks

Headache attack lasts 4–72 hours (untreated or unsuccessfully treated)

Headache has at least two of the following characteristics:
- Unilateral location
- Pulsating quality
- Moderate or severe intensity
- Aggravation by or avoidance of routine physical activity (e.g., walking or climbing stairs)

During headache at least one of the following:
- Nausea, vomiting, or both
- Photophobia and phonophobia
- Not attributed to another disorder

Migraine with aura (classic migraine)

At least two attacks

Migraine aura fulfills criteria for typical aura, hemiplegic aura, or basilar-type aura

Not attributed to another disorder

Typical aura

Fully reversible visual, sensory, or speech symptoms (or any combination) but no motor weakness

Homonymous or bilateral visual symptoms including positive features (e.g., flickering lights, spot, lines) or negative features (e.g., loss of vision) or unilateral sensory symptoms including positive features (e.g., visual loss, pins and needles) or negative features (i.e., numbness), or any combination

At least one of the following:
- At least one symptom that develops gradually over a minimum of 5 minutes or different symptoms that occur in succession or both
- Each symptom lasts for at least 5 minutes and for no longer than 60 minutes
- Headache that meets criteria for migraine without aura begins during the aura or follows aura within 60 minutes

IHS, International Headache Society.

Adapted with permission from Headache Classification Committee of the International Headache Society. The international classification of headache disorders, 2nd ed. Cephalalgia 2004;24 (Suppl 1):1–151.

Secondary headache can be identified or excluded based on the headache history, as well as the results of general medical and neurologic examinations. Diagnostic and laboratory testing also can be warranted in the setting of suspicious headache features or an abnormal examination. The routine use of neuroimaging (computed tomography or magnetic resonance imaging) generally is not indicated in patients with migraine and a normal neurologic examination, but should be considered in patients with an unexplained abnormal neurologic examination or an atypical headache history.[8,12] Because migraine headaches usually begin by the second or third decade of life, headaches beginning after age 50 years suggest an organic etiology such as a mass lesion, cerebrovascular disease, or temporal arteritis. Table 70–2 lists the IHS diagnostic criteria for migraine with and without aura.[2]

TREATMENT

Migraines

■ DESIRED OUTCOME

Clinicians who care for migraineurs must appreciate the impact of this painful and debilitating disorder on the life of the patient, the patient's family, and the patient's employer. Treatment strategies must address both immediate and long-term goals. ❶ Acute migraine therapies should provide consistent, rapid relief and enable the patient to resume normal activities at home, school, or work. Recurrence of symptoms and treatment-related adverse

TABLE 70-3	Goals of Therapy in Migraine Management

Goals of long-term migraine treatment
Reduce migraine frequency, severity, and disability
Reduce reliance on poorly tolerated, ineffective, or unwanted acute pharmacotherapies
Improve quality of life
Prevent headache
Avoid escalation of headache medication use
Educate and enable patients to manage their disease
Reduce headache-related distress and psychological symptoms

Goals for acute migraine treatment
Treat migraine attacks rapidly and consistently without recurrence
Restore the patient's ability to function
Minimize the use of backup and rescue medications[a]
Optimize self-care for overall management
Be cost-effective in overall management
Cause minimal or no adverse effects

[a]Rescue medications are defined as medications used at home when other treatments fail that permit the patient to get relief without a visit to the physician's office or emergency department.
Data from Diamond and Cady[14] and Matchar et al.[15]

effects should be minimal. Ideally, patients should be able to manage their own headaches effectively without a medical visit. In addition, migraineurs should take an active role in the creation of a long-term formal management plan. An individualized approach to treatment can result in a reduction in attack frequency and severity, thus minimizing headache-related disability and emotional distress and improving the patient's quality of life. Goals of long-term and acute treatment of migraine are listed in Table 70–3.[14,15]

■ GENERAL APPROACH TO TREATMENT

Nonpharmacologic and pharmacologic interventions are available for the management of migraine headache; however, drug therapy remains the mainstay of treatment for most patients. Pharmacotherapeutic management of migraine can be acute (e.g., symptomatic or abortive) or preventive (e.g., prophylactic). When choosing acute or preventive therapies, the clinician should consider the patient's response to specific medications and their tolerability, as well as coexisting illnesses that can limit treatment choices. Abortive or acute therapies can be migraine-specific (e.g., ergots and triptans) or nonspecific (e.g., analgesics, antiemetics, nonsteroidal antiinflammatory drugs [NSAIDs], and corticosteroids) and are most effective at relieving pain and associated symptoms when administered at the onset of migraine[7,15–17] (Table 70–4). ❷ A stratified care approach in which the selection of initial treatment is based on headache-related disability and symptom severity is the preferred treatment strategy for the migraineur.[14,16] Because attack severity varies in individuals, patients may be advised to use nonspecific agents for mild to moderate headache not causing disability while reserving migraine-specific medications for more severe attacks. The absorption and efficacy of orally administered drugs can be compromised by gastric stasis or nausea and vomiting that accompany migraine.[16] Pretreatment with antiemetic agents or the use of nonoral treatment (e.g., suppositories, nasal sprays, or injections) is advisable when nausea and vomiting are severe.[7]

The frequent or excessive use of acute migraine medications can result in a pattern of increasing headache frequency and drug consumption known as *medication-overuse headache* (or *rebound headache*).[2,6,18] The syndrome appears to evolve as a self-sustaining headache-medication cycle in which the headache returns as the medication wears off, leading to the consumption of more drug for relief. The headache history often reflects the gradual onset of an atypical daily or near-daily headache with superimposed episodic migraine attacks. Medication overuse is one of the most common causes of chronic daily headache.[18] Agents most commonly implicated in this syndrome include simple and combination analgesics and opiates. Triptans are also implicated but only in men with a high frequency of headaches.[2,6,18] Discontinuation of the offending agent leads to a gradual decrease in headache frequency and severity and a return of the original headache characteristics. Although detoxification usually can be accomplished on an outpatient basis, hospitalization can be necessary for the control of refractory rebound headache and other withdrawal symptoms (e.g., nausea, vomiting, asthenia, restlessness, and agitation). ❸ Regulation of nociceptive systems and renewed responsiveness to therapy usually occur within 2 months following medication withdrawal.[2] Most experts recommend limiting use of acute migraine therapies to *2 or 3 days per week* to avoid the development of medication-misuse headache.[7]

Preventive migraine therapies are administered on a daily basis to reduce the frequency, severity, and duration of attacks and improve responsiveness to symptomatic migraine therapies[7,19–21] (Table 70–5). ❹ Preventive therapy should be considered in the setting of recurring migraines that produce significant disability despite acute therapy; frequent attacks occurring more than twice per week with the risk of developing medication overuse headache; symptomatic therapies that are ineffective, contraindicated, or produce serious side effects; uncommon migraine variants that cause profound disruption and/or risk of permanent neurologic injury (e.g., hemiplegic migraine, basilar migraine, and migraine with prolonged aura); and patient preference to limit the number of attacks.[7,17] Preventive therapy also may be administered preemptively or intermittently when headaches recur in a predictable pattern (e.g., exercise-induced migraine or menstrual migraine). The efficacy of the various agents used for migraine prophylaxis appears to be similar, but the quality of published data is limited for many commonly used drugs. Only propranolol, timolol, valproate, and topiramate are currently approved by the U.S. Food and Drug Administration (FDA) for the indication.[21,22] ❺ Thus the selection of an agent typically is based on its side-effect profile and the patient's comorbid conditions.[7] ❻ A therapeutic trial of 2 to 6 months is necessary to judge medication efficacy, but some reduction in attack frequency can be evident by the first month of therapy.[7,23] Drug therapy should be initiated with low doses and gradually increased until a therapeutic effect is achieved or side effects become intolerable. Drug doses for migraine prophylaxis are often lower than those necessary for other indications.[19] Overuse of acute headache medications will interfere with the effects of preventive treatment.[18,22] Prophylactic treatment usually is continued for at least 3 to 6 months after the frequency and severity of headaches have diminished and then is tapered gradually and discontinued.[7,19] Many migraineurs experience fewer and less severe attacks for lengthy periods following discontinuation of prophylactic medications or taper to a lower dose. Figures 70–2 and 70–3 identify treatment and management algorithms for migraine headache.

■ NONPHARMACOLOGIC THERAPY

Nonpharmacologic therapy of acute migraine headache is limited but can include application of ice to the head and periods of rest or sleep, usually in a dark, quiet environment. Preventive management of migraine should begin with the identification and avoidance of factors that consistently provoke migraine attacks in susceptible individuals[2,14,22,24] (Table 70–6). Changes in estrogen levels associated with menarche, menstruation, pregnancy, menopause, oral contraceptive use, and other hormone therapies can trigger, intensify, or alleviate migraine.[23] A headache diary

TABLE 70-4   Acute Migraine Therapies[a]

Medication	Dosage	Comments
Analgesics		
Acetaminophen	1,000 mg at onset; repeat every 4–6 hours as needed	Max. daily dose is 4 g
Acetaminophen 250 mg/aspirin 250 mg/ caffeine 65 mg	2 tablets at onset and every 6 hours	Available over-the-counter as Excedrin Migraine
Aspirin or acetaminophen with butalbital, caffeine	1–2 tablets every 4–6 hours	Limit dose to 4 tablets/day and usage to 2 days/week
Isometheptene 65 mg/dichloralphenazone 100 mg/acetaminophen 325 mg (Midrin)	2 capsules at onset; repeat 1 capsule every hour as needed	Max. of 6 capsules/day and 20 capsules/month
Nonsteroidal antiinflammatory drugs		
Aspirin	500–1,000 mg every 4–6 hours	Max. daily dose is 4 g
Ibuprofen	200–800 mg every 6 hours	Avoid doses >2.4 g/day
Naproxen sodium	550–825 mg at onset; can repeat 220 mg in 3–4 hours	Avoid doses >1.375 g/day
Diclofenac potassium	50–100 mg at onset; can repeat 50 mg in 8 hours	Avoid doses >150 mg/day
Ergotamine tartrate		
Oral tablet (1 mg) with caffeine 100 mg	2 mg at onset; then 1–2 mg every 30 minutes as needed	Max. dose is 6 mg/day or 10 mg/week; consider pretreatment with an antiemetic
Sublingual tablet (2 mg)		
Rectal suppository (2 mg) with caffeine 100 mg	Insert ½ to 1 suppository at onset; repeat after 1 hour as needed	Max. dose is 4 mg/day or 10 mg/week; consider pretreatment with an antiemetic
Dihydroergotamine		
Injection 1 mg/mL	0.25–1 mg at onset IM, IV or subcutaneous; repeat every hour as needed	Max. dose is 3 mg/day or 6 mg/week
Nasal spray	One spray (0.5 mg) in each nostril at onset; repeat sequence 15 minutes later (total dose is 2 mg or 4 sprays)	Max. dose is 3 mg/day; prime sprayer 4 times before using; do not tilt head back or inhale through nose while spraying; discard open ampules after 8 hours
Serotonin agonists (triptans)		
Sumatriptan Injection	6 mg subcutaneous at onset; can repeat after 1 hour if needed	Max. daily dose is 12 mg
Oral tablets	25, 50, 85 or 100 mg at onset; can repeat after 2 hours if needed	Optimal dose is 50–100 mg; max. daily dose is 200 mg; combination product with naproxen, 85 mg/500 mg
Nasal spray	5, 10, or 20 mg at onset; can repeat after 2 hours if needed	Optimal dose is 20 mg; max. daily dose is 40 mg; single-dose device delivering 5 or 20 mg; administer one spray in one nostril
Zolmitriptan		
Oral tablets	2.5 or 5 mg at onset as regular or orally disintegrating tablet; can repeat after 2 hours if needed	Optimal dose is 2.5 mg; max. dose is 10 mg/day Do not divide ODT dosage form
Nasal spray	5 mg (one spray) at onset; can repeat after 2 hours if needed	Max. daily dose is 10 mg/day
Naratriptan	1 or 2.5 mg at onset; can repeat after 4 hours if needed	Optimal dose is 2.5 mg; max. daily dose is 5 mg
Rizatriptan	5 or 10 mg at onset as regular or orally disintegrating tablet; can repeat after 2 hours if needed	Optimal dose is 10 mg; max. daily dose is 30 mg; onset of effect is similar with standard and orally disintegrating tablets; use 5-mg dose (15 mg/day max.) in patients receiving propranolol
Almotriptan	6.25 or 12.5 mg at onset; can repeat after 2 hours if needed	Optimal dose is 12.5 mg; max. daily dose is 25 mg
Frovatriptan	2.5 or 5 mg at onset; can repeat in 2 hours if needed	Optimal dose 2.5–5 mg; max. daily dose is 7.5 mg (3 tablets)
Eletriptan	20 or 40 mg at onset; can repeat after 2 hours if needed	Max. single dose is 40 mg; max. daily dose is 80 mg
Miscellaneous		
Butorphanol nasal spray	1 spray in 1 nostril (1 mg) at onset; repeat in 1 hour if needed	Limit to 4 sprays/day; consider use only when nonopioid therapies are ineffective or not tolerated
Metoclopramide	10 mg IV at onset	Useful for acute relief in the office or emergency department setting
Prochlorperazine	10 mg IV or IM at onset	Useful for acute relief in the office or emergency department setting

ODT, orally disintegrating tablet.
[a]Limit use of symptomatic medications to 2 or 3 days/week when possible to avoid medication-misuse headache.
Data from Silberstein,[7] Matchar et al.,[15] Smith,[16] and Bigal et al.[17]

that records the frequency, severity, and duration of attacks can facilitate identification of migraine triggers. **7** Patients also can benefit from adherence to a wellness program that includes regular sleep, exercise, and eating habits, smoking cessation, and limited caffeine intake. Behavioral interventions, such as relaxation therapy, biofeedback (often used in combination with relaxation therapy), and cognitive therapy, are preventive treatment options for patients who prefer nondrug therapy or when symptomatic therapies are poorly tolerated, contraindicated, or ineffective.[14,22]

TABLE 70-5	Prophylactic Migraine Therapies
Medication	**Dose**
β-Adrenergic antagonists	
Atenolol	25–100 mg/day
Metoprolol[a]	50–200 mg/day in divided doses
Nadolol	80–160 mg/day
Propranolol[a,b]	80–240 mg/day in divided doses
Timolol[b]	20–60 mg/day in divided doses
Antidepressants	
Amitriptyline	25–150 mg at bedtime
Doxepin	10–300 mg at bedtime
Nortriptyline	10–150 mg at bedtime
Protriptyline	5–60 mg at bedtime
Fluoxetine	10–80 mg/day
Venlafaxine[a]	75–225 mg/day
Gapapentin	900–2,400 mg/day in divided doses
Topiramate[b]	100 mg/day in divided doses
Valproic acid/divalproex sodium[b]	500–1,500 mg/day in divided doses
Verapamil[a]	240–480 mg/day in divided doses
Nonsteroidal antiinflammatory drugs[c]	
Ketoprofen[a]	150 mg/day in divided doses
Naproxen sodium[a]	550–1,100 mg/day in divided doses
Coenzyme Q10	300 mg/day in divided doses
Feverfew	10–100 mg/day in divided doses
Magesium gluconate	400–600 mg/day in divided doses
Petasites	150 mg/day in divided doses
Vitamin B$_2$	400 mg/day

[a]Sustained-release formulation available.
[b]FDA approved for prevention of migraine.
[c]Daily or prolonged use limited by potential toxicity.
Compiled from Silberstein,[7] Bigal,[19] Evans et al.,[20] and Rapoport and Bigal.[21]

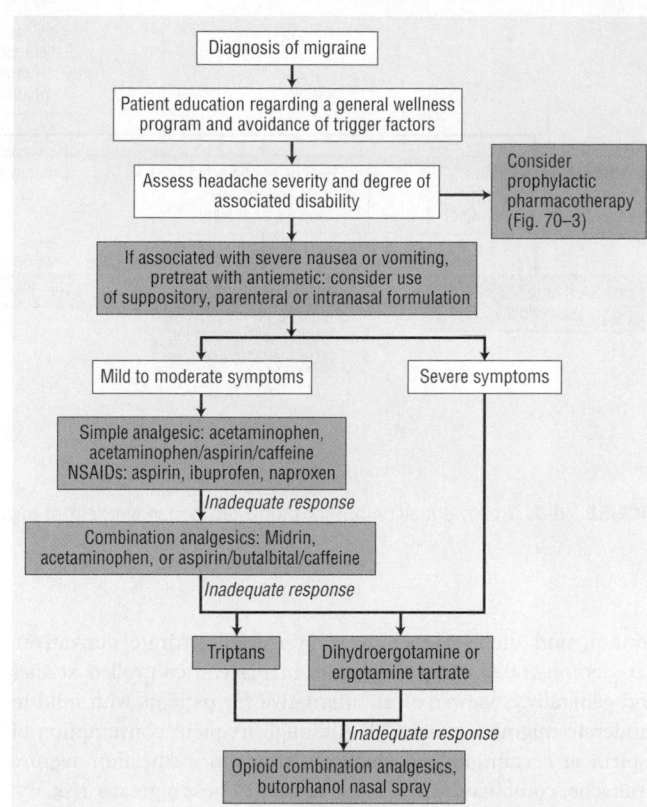

FIGURE 70-2. Treatment algorithm for migraine headaches.

■ PHARMACOLOGIC MANAGEMENT OF ACUTE MIGRAINE

Analgesics and NSAIDs

Simple analgesics and NSAIDs are effective medications for the management of many migraine attacks[7,14] (see Table 70–4). They offer a reasonable first-line choice for treatment of mild to moderate migraine attacks or severe attacks that have been responsive in the past to similar NSAIDs or nonopiate analgesics.[14] Of the NSAIDs, aspirin, ibuprofen, naproxen sodium, tolfenamic acid, and the combination of acetaminophen plus aspirin and caffeine have demonstrated the most consistent evidence of efficacy.[7,14] Evidence for other NSAIDs is either limited or inconsistent.[15] Acetaminophen alone is not generally recommended for migraine because the scientific support is not optimal.[7,15] Comparisons with other pharmacotherapeutic classes are limited.

NSAIDs appear to prevent neurogenically mediated inflammation in the trigeminovascular system through the inhibition of prostaglandin synthesis. Metoclopramide can speed the absorption of analgesics and alleviate migraine-related nausea and vomiting.[14] Suppository analgesic preparations are an option when nausea and vomiting are severe.[25] Acute NSAID therapy is associated with gastrointestinal (e.g., dyspepsia, nausea, vomiting, and diarrhea) and CNS side effects (e.g., somnolence, dizziness). NSAIDs should be used cautiously in patients with previous ulcer disease, renal disease, or hypersensitivity to aspirin.[15,26]

The over-the-counter combination of acetaminophen, aspirin, and caffeine was approved for the treatment of migraine in the United States because of its proven efficacy in relieving migraine pain and associated symptoms.[15,17] Aspirin and acetaminophen are also available in prescription combination products containing a short-acting barbiturate (butalbital) or narcotic (codeine, propoxyphene). No randomized, placebo-controlled studies support the efficacy of butalbital-containing products in the treatment of migraine. The use of butalbital-containing analgesics or narcotics should be limited because of concerns about overuse, medication-overuse headache, and withdrawal.[7,14,26] Midrin, a combination of acetaminophen, isometheptene mucate (a sympathomimetic

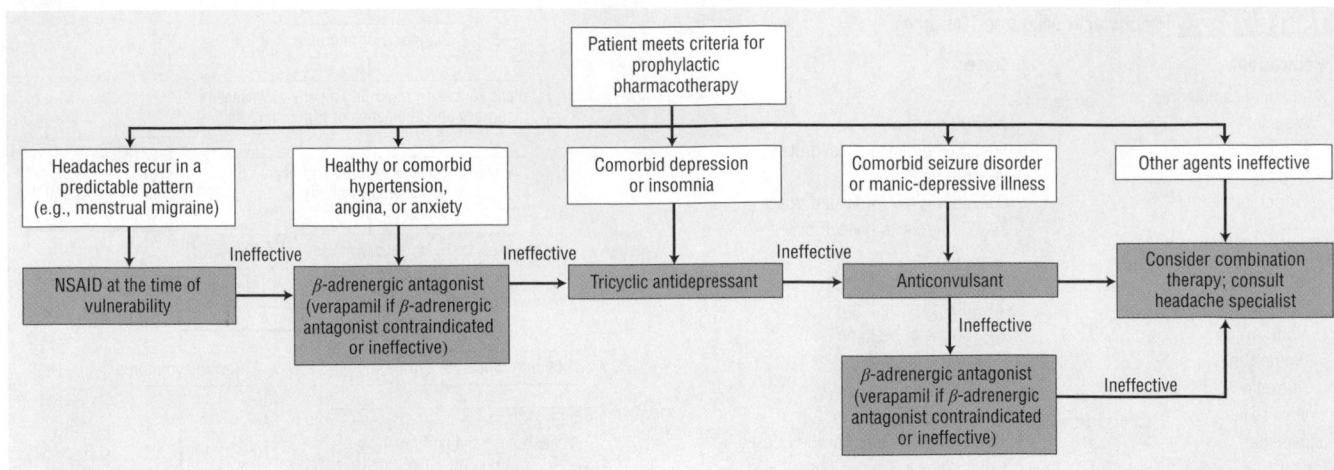

FIGURE 70-3. Treatment algorithm for prophylactic management of migraine headaches. (NSAID, nonsteroidal antiinflammatory drug.)

amine), and dichloralphenazone (a chloral hydrate derivative), has demonstrated modest benefits in placebo-controlled studies and generally is viewed as an alternative for patients with mild to moderate migraine attacks.[15,17] Although frequent consumption of aspirin or acetaminophen alone can result in medication-overuse headache, combination analgesics appear to pose a greater risk.[7,26]

Opiate Analgesics

Narcotic analgesic drugs (e.g., meperidine, butorphanol, oxycodone, and hydromorphone) are effective but generally should be reserved for patients with moderate to severe infrequent headaches in whom conventional therapies are contraindicated or as "rescue medication" after patients have failed to respond to conventional therapies.[7] Frequent use of narcotic analgesics can lead to the development of dependency and rebound headache.[26] The intranasal formulation of butorphanol, a synthetically derived opioid agonist-antagonist,

---

TABLE 70-6 Commonly Reported Triggers of Migraine

Food triggers
Alcohol
Caffeine/caffeine withdrawal
Chocolate
Fermented and pickled foods
Monosodium glutamate (e.g., in Chinese food, seasoned salt, and instant foods)
Nitrate-containing foods (e.g., processed meats)
Saccharin/aspartame (e.g., diet foods or diet sodas)
Tyramine-containing foods

Environmental triggers
Glare or flickering lights
High altitude
Loud noises
Strong smells and fumes
Tobacco smoke
Weather changes

Behavioral–physiologic triggers
Excess or insufficient sleep
Fatigue
Menstruation, menopause
Sexual activity
Skipped meals
Strenuous physical activity (e.g., prolonged overexertion)
Stress or post-stress

Data from Diamond and Cady,[14] Buse et al,[22] and Kelman.[24]

---

is a treatment option but should be reserved for use only as an alternative to frequent office or emergency department visits for injectable migraine therapies. Opioid therapy should be supervised closely.[16,17]

Antiemetics

Adjunctive antiemetic therapy is useful for combating the nausea and vomiting that accompany migraine headaches and the medications used to treat attacks (e.g., ergotamine tartrate). A single dose of an antiemetic, such as metoclopramide, chlorpromazine, or prochlorperazine, administered 15 to 30 minutes before ingestion of oral abortive migraine medications is often sufficient. Suppository preparations are available when nausea and vomiting are particularly prominent. Metoclopramide is also useful to reverse gastroparesis and improve absorption from the gastrointestinal tract during severe attacks.[15,16]

In addition to antiemetic effects, dopamine antagonist drugs also have been used successfully as monotherapy for the treatment of intractable headache (see Table 70–4). Prochlorperazine administered by the intravenous and intramuscular routes and intravenous metoclopramide provided more effective pain relief than placebo. Chlorpromazine also has provided relief of migraine headache when administered parenterally at doses of 12.5 to 37.5 mg. Domperidone has a possible role for preemptive treatment of migraine. The precise mechanism of action for these agents is unknown. The dopamine antagonists offer an alternative to the narcotic analgesics for the treatment of refractory migraine. Drowsiness and dizziness were reported occasionally and extrapyramidal side effects were reported infrequently in migraine trials.[15,25]

Miscellaneous Nonspecific Medications

Corticosteroids can be considered as rescue therapy for status migrainous (a severe, continuous migraine that can last up to 1 week).[7,15] Intravenous or intramuscular dexamethasone at a dose of 10 to 25 mg has also been used as an adjunct to abortive therapy.[25,27]

Limited studies suggest a role for intranasal lidocaine in the treatment of acute migraine headache.[15] Intranasal lidocaine, 1 to 4 drops of a 4% solution, provides rapid pain relief within 15 minutes of administration, but headache recurrence is common. Adverse effects generally are limited to local irritation, an unpleasant taste, and numbness of the throat.

Preliminary investigations of intramuscular droperidol have yielded favorable results in the treatment of acute migraine headache.[7] Future studies might establish a more defined role for this agent in migraine management.

Ergot Alkaloids and Derivatives

Ergotamine tartrate and dihydroergotamine are useful and can be considered for the treatment of moderate to severe migraine attacks (see Table 70–4). These drugs are nonselective 5-HT$_1$ receptor agonists that constrict intracranial blood vessels and inhibit the development of neurogenic inflammation in the trigeminovascular system.[7] Central inhibition of the trigeminovascular pathway is also reported as well as agonist activity at dopaminergic receptors. Venous and arterial constriction occur with therapeutic doses, but ergotamine tartrate exerts more potent arterial effects than dihydroergotamine.[14,17,26]

Ergotamine tartrate is available for oral, sublingual, and rectal administration. Oral and rectal preparations contain caffeine to enhance absorption and potentiate analgesia. Some patients respond preferentially to rectal dosing.[7,14] Dosage requirements should be titrated strictly to establish an effective but subnauseating dose for future attacks. Ergotamine is most effective when administered early in the migraine attack. Despite widespread clinical use since 1926, evidence supporting the efficacy of ergotamine in migraine is inconsistent.[7,14]

Dihydroergotamine is available for intranasal and parenteral administration by the intramuscular, subcutaneous, and intravenous routes.[7] Parenteral dihydroergotamine was viewed previously as inpatient or emergency department treatment for moderate to severe migraine or intractable headache, but patients can be trained to self-administer dihydroergotamine intramuscularly or subcutaneously. Clinical opinion suggests its use is relatively safe and effective when compared with other migraine therapies.[15]

Nausea and vomiting (resulting from stimulation of the chemoreceptor trigger zone) are among the most common adverse effects of the ergotamine derivatives. Pretreatment with an antiemetic agent should be considered with ergotamine and intravenous dihydroergotamine therapy. Other common side effects include abdominal pain, weakness, fatigue, paresthesias, muscle pain, diarrhea, and chest tightness. Rarely, symptoms of severe peripheral ischemia (ergotism), including cold, numb, painful extremities, continuous paresthesias, diminished peripheral pulses, and claudication can result from the vasoconstrictor effects of the ergot alkaloids. Gangrenous extremities, myocardial infarction, hepatic necrosis, and bowel and brain ischemia have also been reported. Dihydroergotamine is rarely associated with such side effects.[14,16,26] Triptans and ergot derivatives should not be used within 24 hours of each other.[26] Ergotamine derivatives are contraindicated in patients with renal or hepatic failure; coronary, cerebral, or peripheral vascular disease; uncontrolled hypertension; sepsis; and in women who are pregnant or nursing.[7,25] Dihydroergotamine does not appear to cause rebound headache, but dosage restrictions for ergotamine tartrate should be observed strictly to prevent this complication.[7]

Serotonin Receptor Agonists (Triptans)

Introduction of the serotonin receptor agonists, or triptans, represented a significant advance in migraine pharmacotherapy. The first member of this class, sumatriptan, and the second-generation agents zolmitriptan, naratriptan, rizatriptan, almotriptan, frovatriptan, and eletriptan are selective agonists of the 5-HT$_{1B}$ and 5-HT$_{1D}$ receptors. Relief of migraine headache is the result of three key actions: normalization of dilated intracranial arteries through enhanced vasoconstriction, peripheral neuronal inhibition, and inhibition of transmission through second-order neurons of the trigeminocervical complex.[14,26,28] These agents also display varying affinity for 5-HT$_{1A}$, 5-HT$_{1E}$, and 5-HT$_{1F}$ receptors. The triptans are appropriate first-line therapy for patients with mild to severe migraine and are used for rescue therapy when nonspecific medications are ineffective.[7]

Sumatriptan, the most extensively studied acute therapy, is available for subcutaneous, oral, and intranasal administration.[28] Subcutaneous sumatriptan is consistently superior to placebo in alleviating migraine headache and associated symptoms, with relief reported in 69% of patients at 1 hour (48%–49% pain-free) in a meta-analysis of placebo-controlled studies.[7] In addition to enhanced efficacy, subcutaneous sumatriptan has a more rapid onset of action when compared with the oral formulation.[7,28] The subcutaneous injection is packaged as an autoinjector device for self-administration by patients. Intranasal sumatriptan provides a faster onset of effect than the oral formulation and produces similar rates of response (relief in 61% of patients at 2 hours) in placebo-controlled studies.[7]

The second-generation triptans appear to offer an improved pharmacokinetic and pharmacodynamic profile compared with oral sumatriptan. In general, these agents have higher oral bioavailability and longer half-lives than oral sumatriptan, which theoretically could improve within-patient treatment consistency and reduce headache recurrence[7,16,28] (Table 70–7). Frovatriptan and naratriptan have the longest half-lives and a slower onset of action compared with other triptans. This may make them more suitable for patients that have migraine attacks of a slow onset and longer duration. Faster-acting triptans are better when a rapid onset is necessary. Despite the fact that oral absorption can be delayed during migraine attacks, most patients prefer oral formulations, primarily due to convenience.[7,16,28]

Results of placebo-controlled studies with each of the second-generation agents reveal somewhat comparable 2-hour response rates. Direct comparative clinical trials are necessary to determine their relative efficacy, but these are available for only a few of the triptans. A recent meta-analysis summarizes the efficacy and tolerability of the oral triptans across published and unpublished studies. At all marketed doses, the oral triptans are effective

TABLE 70-7	Pharmacokinetic Characteristics of Triptans			
Drug	**Half-Life (hours)**	**Time to Maximal Concentration (t_{max})**	**Bioavailability (%)**	**Elimination**
Almotriptan	3–4	1–3 hours	70	MAO-A, CYP3A4, CYP2D6
Eletriptan	5	1–1.25 hours	50	CYP3A4
Frovatriptan	25	2–4 hours	24–30	Mostly unchanged, CYP1A2
Naratriptan	5–6	2–3 hours	63–74	Largely unchanged, CYP450 (various isoenzymes)
Rizatriptan	2–3		40–45	MAO-A
Oral tablets		1–1.5 hours		
Disintegrating		1.6–2.5 hours		
Sumatriptan	2			MAO-A
SC injection		12–15 minutes	96	
Oral tablets		2.5 hours	14	
Nasal spray		1–2.5 hours	16	
Zolmitriptan	3		40	CYP1A2, MAO-A
Oral		2–2.5 hours		
Disintegrating		3 hours		
Nasal		4 hours		

CYP, cytochrome P450; MAO-A, monoamine oxidase type A.
Data from Silberstein,[7] Smith,[16] and Matthew and Loder.[28]

and well tolerated. Across studies for sumatriptan 100 mg, mean results were a 2-hour headache response of 59%, with 29% pain-free at 2 hours, 20% sustained pain-free, and 67% consistency. Compared with sumatriptan 100 mg, rizatriptan 10 mg showed better efficacy and consistency and similar tolerability; eletriptan 80 mg showed better efficacy, similar consistency, but lower tolerability; almotriptan 12.5 mg showed similar efficacy at 2 hours but better other results; naratriptan 2.5 mg and eletriptan 20 mg showed lower efficacy and better tolerability; and zolmitriptan 2.5 and 5 mg, eletriptan 40 mg, and rizatriptan 5 mg all showed similar results. Available data suggest lower efficacy for frovatriptan, although it has the longest half-life of the triptans.[7,17,28]

Clinical response to the triptans can vary considerably among individual patients. Individual responses cannot be predicted, and if one triptan fails, a patient can be switched successfully to another triptan.[7] ❽ After an effective agent and dose have been identified, subsequent treatments should begin with that same regimen. Combination therapy may also improve response rates and diminish migraine recurrence. A proprietary formulation of sumatriptan 85 mg plus naproxen 500 mg in a single tablet was more effective in clinical trials for headache relief and sustained pain-free response than either agent as monotherapy.[16,25]

Side effects to the triptans are common but usually mild to moderate in nature and of short duration. Adverse effects are consistent among the class and include paresthesias, fatigue, dizziness, flushing, warm sensations, and somnolence. Local side effects are reported with the subcutaneous (minor injection-site reactions) and intranasal (taste perversion, nasal discomfort) routes. Up to 15% of patients receiving a triptan consistently report "chest symptoms," including tightness, pressure, heaviness, or pain in the chest, neck, or throat. The mechanism of these symptoms is unknown, but a cardiac source of pain seems unlikely in most patients.[17,26] However, all triptans are partial agonists of human 5-HT coronary artery receptors in vitro, resulting in a small but significant vasoconstrictor response. Adverse cardiac events are rare with only isolated cases of myocardial infarction and coronary vasospasm with ischemia reported. Myocardial ischemia is unlikely in patients with normal coronary vasculature because 5-HT_{1B} receptors mediate less than 25% of the overall vasoconstrictor potential of the coronary vessels.[17] The triptans are contraindicated in patients with a history of ischemic heart disease (e.g., angina pectoris, Prinzmetal's angina, or previous myocardial infarction), uncontrolled hypertension, and cerebrovascular disease. Patients at risk for unrecognized coronary artery disease should use triptans with caution. Postmenopausal women, men older than 40 years of age, and patients with uncontrolled risk factors should receive a cardiovascular assessment prior to triptan use and have initial doses administered under medical supervision.[16,25] Triptans are also contraindicated in patients with hemiplegic and basilar migraine. The triptans should not be given within 24 hours of the ergotamine derivatives. Administration of sumatriptan, rizatriptan, and zolmitriptan within 2 weeks of therapy with monoamine oxidase inhibitors (MAOIs) is not recommended. Eletriptan should not be administered with cytochrome P450 3A4 inhibitors such as macrolide antibiotics, antifungals, and some antiviral therapies. Concomitant therapy with the selective serotonin reuptake inhibitors (SSRIs) or serotonin-norepinephrine reuptake inhibitors (SNRIs) (e.g., duloxetine, venlafaxine, mirtazepine, and sibutramine) can potentially cause serotonin syndrome. Regulatory agencies caution against concurrent administration although it appears the likelihood of CNS adverse events is extremely low. The potential risk of these combinations should be carefully considered and discussed with the patient.[16,26,29] Frequent use of the triptans has been associated with the development of medication-misuse headache.[14,15]

■ PROPHYLACTIC PHARMACOLOGIC THERAPY

β-Adrenergic Antagonists

β-Adrenergic antagonists are among the most widely used drugs for migraine prophylaxis. Propranolol, nadolol, timolol, atenolol, and metoprolol have proven efficacy in controlled clinical trials, reducing the frequency of attacks by 50% in 60% to 80% of patients[19] (see Table 70–5). Because the relative efficacy of the individual agents has not been established, selection of a β-blocker can be based on β-selectivity, convenience of the formulation, and tolerability. β-Blockers with intrinsic sympathomimetic activity are ineffective for migraine prophylaxis.[19] Although their precise mechanism of antimigraine action is unknown, β-blockers may raise the migraine threshold by modulating adrenergic or serotonergic neurotransmission in cortical or subcortical pathways. Though not first-line treatment for hypertension or anxiety, β-blockers may be useful along with other therapy in patients with comorbid anxiety, hypertension, or angina.[23] Side effects can include drowsiness, fatigue, sleep disturbances, vivid dreams, memory disturbance, depression, impotence, bradycardia, and hypotension. β-Blockers should be used with caution in patients with congestive heart failure, peripheral vascular disease, atrioventricular conduction disturbances, asthma, depression, and diabetes.[7,19,23]

Antidepressants

The beneficial effects of antidepressants in migraine are independent of their antidepressant activity and may be related to downregulation of central 5-HT_2 receptors, increased levels of synaptic norepinephrine, and enhanced endogenous opiod receptor actions.[30] Amitriptyline, the most widely studied antidepressant for migraine prophylaxis, has demonstrated efficacy in placebo-controlled and comparative studies.[19] Use of other antidepressants is based primarily on clinical and anecdotal experience (see Table 70–5). Other tricyclic antidepressants (TCAs) that have been used successfully for migraine prophylaxis include doxepin, nortriptyline, and protriptyline.[19] Anticholinergic side effects are common and limit use of these agents in patients with benign prostatic hyperplasia and glaucoma. Evening doses are preferred because of associated sedation. Increased appetite and weight gain can occur. Orthostatic hypotension and cardiac toxicity (slowed atrioventricular conduction) also are reported occasionally. The more favorable side-effect profile of nortriptyline and protriptyline could prove advantageous in patients who are particularly intolerant of the anticholinergic and sedative side effects of amitriptyline.[19]

SSRIs have not been studied extensively or proven consistently effective for the preventive treatment of migraine headaches.[19,23] Fluoxetine is the most studied SSRI for migraine prevention, but definitive benefit has not been demonstrated in a rigorous clinical study. Prospective data evaluating the other SSRIs (e.g., sertraline, paroxetine, fluvoxamine, and citalopram) are lacking.[7,19,30] These agents should not be considered as first- or second-line medications for the management of migraine, but they may be useful in patients with comorbid depression combined with, for example, an anticonvulsant for migraine prophylaxis.[23] A recent study suggests a possible benefit with venlafaxine, a SNRI.[20] Again, the potential risk of serotonin syndrome should be considered in patients using SSRIs or SNRIs along with a triptan.[16,29]

MAOIs, such as phenelzine, have been used in the management of refractory headache, but their complex adverse-effect profile limits their use to experienced prescribers. Strict adherence to a tyramine-free diet is necessary to avoid potentially life-threatening hypertensive crisis.[19,22] The reader is referred to Chapter 77 for dietary and concurrent medication restrictions for patients taking MAOIs.

Anticonvulsants

Anticonvulsant medications have emerged as important therapeutic options for migraine prophylaxis with valproate, divalproex, topiramate, and gabapentin all demonstrating efficacy. The beneficial effects of these agents are likely caused by multiple mechanisms of action, including enhancement of γ-aminobutyric acid (GABA)–mediated inhibition, modulation of the excitatory neurotransmitter glutamate, and inhibition of sodium and calcium ion channel activity.[21,30] Anticonvulsants are particularly useful in migraineurs with comorbid seizures, anxiety disorder, or manic-depressive illness.[19] The efficacy of valproic acid and divalproex sodium (a 1:1 molar combination of valproate sodium and valproic acid) has been demonstrated in multiple placebo-controlled studies. Nausea and vomiting, the most common early side effects, are self-limited and appear to be less common with divalproex sodium and gradual titration of doses. Alopecia, tremor, asthenia, somnolence, and weight gain are also common complaints.[7,17] The extended-release formulation of divalproex sodium is administered once daily and is better tolerated than the enteric-coated formulation.[20] Hepatotoxicity is the most serious side effect of valproate therapy, but the risk appears to be low in migraineurs (e.g., patients older than 10 years of age who are receiving monotherapy and have no underlying metabolic or neurologic disorder). Baseline liver function tests should be obtained, but routine follow-up studies are not necessary in asymptomatic adults on monotherapy.[7] Regular follow-up is necessary, however, for dosage adjustments and monitoring of effects.[19] Valproate is contraindicated in pregnant women (owing to potential teratogenicity) and patients with a history of pancreatitis or chronic liver disease. Although valproate level determinations can be useful for assessing compliance and toxicity, a recent study suggests that serum levels of less than 50 mcg/mL (346 μmol/L) (usual therapeutic level is 50–100 mcg/mL [346 to 693 μmol/L]) can provide similar benefit to higher levels. Doses of 500 to 1,000 mg per day are effective for many patients.[1]

Topiramate is the most extensively studied medication to date for migraine prophylaxis. Efficacy and improvements in health-related quality of life including daily work, home, and social activities have been demonstrated in several placebo-controlled studies.[19,22] To minimize adverse effects, topiramate should be initiated at a low dose, 25 mg, and titrated slowly up to a maximum daily dose of 200 mg. The target dose for migraine prevention is 100 mg daily for most patients. The benefits of topiramate are observed as early as two weeks after initiation of therapy, with significant reductions in migraine frequency within the first month. Approximately 50% of patients treated to target doses are responders (≥50% reduction in mean headache frequency). Treatment-emergent adverse events associated with topiramate include paresthesia, fatigue, anorexia, diarrhea, weight loss, hypesthesia, difficulty with memory, language problems, taste perversion, and nausea. Paresthesia is the most common adverse event, occurring in about half of patients at target doses. Weight loss, occurring in 9% to 12% of patients, is a unique adverse effect, as weight gain is a common reason to discontinue other preventive medications. Topiramate should be used with caution in patients with a history of kidney stones.[19,31]

A recent study suggests that gabapentin also may be an effective agent for migraine prevention in patients achieving a daily dose of 2,400 mg.[19] Somnolence and dizziness were the most commonly reported adverse events. Preliminary studies suggest a possible role for other anticonvulsants, including tiagabine, levetiracetam, and zonisamide; however, further clinical studies are needed to confirm their usefulness in migraine prophylaxis.[19,21]

Calcium Channel Blockers

The calcium channel blockers generally are considered second- or third-line options for preventive treatment when other drugs with established clinical benefit are ineffective or contraindicated. Verapamil is the most widely used calcium channel blocker for preventive treatment, but it provided only modest benefit in decreasing the frequency of attacks in two placebo-controlled studies.[7,19] The therapeutic effect of verapamil may not be noted for up to 8 weeks after initiation of therapy. Side effects of verapamil can include constipation, hypotension, bradycardia, atrioventricular block, and exacerbation of congestive heart failure. Evaluations of nifedipine, nimodipine, diltiazem, nisoldipine, nicardipine, and amlodipine have yielded equivocal results.[17,19,21]

NSAIDs

NSAIDs are modestly effective for reducing the frequency, severity, and duration of migraine attacks, but potential gastrointestinal and renal toxicity limit the daily or prolonged use of these agents.[17,20] Consequently, NSAIDs have been used intermittently to prevent headaches that recur in a predictable pattern, such as menstrual migraine. Administration of NSAIDs in the perimenstrual period can be beneficial in women with true menstrual migraine. NSAIDs should be initiated 1 to 2 days prior to the expected onset of headache and continued during the period of vulnerability.[23,31] If long-term NSAID therapy is initiated, monitoring of renal function and occult blood loss is necessary.

Miscellaneous Prophylactic Agents

A double-blind, placebo-controlled study demonstrated the efficacy of riboflavin (vitamin B$_2$) 400 mg daily in migraine prophylaxis. Riboflavin was well tolerated and associated with 50% or greater improvement in attack frequency in 54% of patients. However, the benefits of therapy became significant only after 3 months.[19,31] The angiotensin-converting enzyme inhibitor lisinopril and the angiotensin II receptor blocker candesartan provided effective migraine prophylaxis in recent double-blind, placebo-controlled, crossover studies of these agents.[31] Further research is needed to establish the safety and efficacy of the herbal medication feverfew (*Tanacetum parthenium*) because studies to date have yielded inconsistent and conflicting results.[19,31] At least two placebo-controlled studies have concluded that petasites, an extract from the plant *Petasites hybridus*, may be an effective preventive treatment for migraine.[19,31] Coenzyme Q10 was effective for migraine prevention and well tolerated in a small, randomized, double-blind, controlled study.[19,31]

Clinical trials evaluating various formulations of magnesium for migraine prevention have yielded mixed results. CNS levels of magnesium are known to be significantly low during migraine attacks. Magnesium supplementation may be particularly effective for prevention of menstrual migraine and in migraine patients with aura.[19,31] Localized injections of botulinum toxin type A have been used for various conditions and pain syndromes, including migraine headache. However, no consistent, statistically significant benefits have been found with migraine. The American Academy of Neurology concludes that botulinum toxin is probably ineffective.[31,32] Further study is needed to confirm the clinical utility and comparative efficacy of these miscellaneous agents for the prophylactic management of migraine.

PHARMACOECONOMIC CONSIDERATIONS

Although migraine is widely recognized as a disease that exacts an enormous toll on the sufferer, the direct and indirect costs associated with migraine headache impose a substantial burden on society as well. The direct medical costs associated with clinic visits for headache and migraine diagnosis and treatment are substantial, exceeding $1 billion per year. Migraine also results in high use of emergency rooms and urgent care centers.[1,3] Headache accounts for one third of all over-the-counter analgesic use in the United States, and gross sales from triptans alone total more than $1 billion per year. The indirect costs of the illness related to work absenteeism, decreased productivity, and impairment greatly exceed the direct cost of medical care.[3] Overall, the estimated lost productivity due to headache in the United States is $18 billion per year. The estimated indirect cost of migraine-specific related disability for American employers is approximately $13 billion each year.[3,19]

In 2004, only half of those surveyed with clear symptoms of migraine were diagnosed by a physician.[6] According to the American Migraine Prevalence and Prevention Study, although most episodic migraine sufferers take medications for their headaches, 21% used opioids or compounds containing barbiturates, and only 24% used a triptan.[6] Just 13% of this population were using medications specifically to prevent migraine, though 26% met criteria to be offered prophylaxis, and an additional 13% should be considered for treatment.[6] Because many migraineurs who receive inadequate care experience substantial levels of pain and disability, improvement in migraine diagnosis, care, and treatment potentially could result in lower direct and indirect costs of the disease.

Education of headache patients regarding required behavior changes and effective use of acute and prophylactic pharmacotherapy can be time-consuming, but it is also extremely cost-effective. Oversights can lead to decreased efficacy of medications resulting in repeat dosing and polypharmacy, decreased compliance, increased emergency visits, increased "doctor shopping," and, perhaps, increased use of expensive diagnostic procedures and inpatient services. Recent studies demonstrate that effective migraine treatment can reduce the functional disability and productivity loss associated with a migraine attack.[14,28] Patients with stratified care targeted to their needs had higher headache response rates, shorter disability times, less health service utilization, and less loss of productivity.[14]

SUMMARY

Acute and preventive pharmacotherapy for migraine should be individualized based on the individual patient response, tolerability of the available agents, and presence of comorbid conditions. Migraine management should be individualized on the basis of the patient's clinical presentation and medical history. Analgesics and NSAIDs can be considered the drugs of choice if effective for infrequent mild to moderate attacks. The triptans or dihydroergotamine can be used if initial therapies prove ineffective or as first-line therapy in moderate to severe migraine headache. Abortive therapy should be instituted early in the course of the attack to optimize efficacy and minimize migraine-related pain and disability. Preventive therapy should be considered in the setting of recurring migraines that produce significant disability, frequent attacks requiring symptomatic medication more than twice per week, symptomatic therapies that are ineffective, contraindicated, or produce serious side effects, and uncommon migraine variants that cause profound disruption and/or risk of neurologic injury. Efficacy of a prescribed prophylactic regimen should be reassessed periodically. A prolonged headache-free interval could allow for gradual dosage reduction and discontinuation of therapy.

TENSION-TYPE HEADACHE

EPIDEMIOLOGY

Tension-type headache is the most common type of primary headache, with an estimated 1-year prevalence ranging from 31% to 86%.[4,33] Prevalence peaks in the fourth decade and is higher among women. The incidence decreases with age.[33,34] Although an estimated 60% of tension-type headache sufferers experience some degree of functional impairment during their attacks, less than 15% of sufferers seek medical attention, likely because most have infrequent attacks. Infrequent episodic tension-type headache (defined as fewer than one episode per month) is experienced by 64% of sufferers, while 22% have frequent episodic tension-type headache (episodes on 1–14 days per month). The prevalence of chronic tension-type headache (≥15 days per month, perhaps without recognizable episodes) is estimated at 0.9% to 2.2%.[4,33] Risk factors associated with a poor outcome in tension-type headache include coexisting migraine, sleep problems, not being married and the presence of chronic tension-type headache.[34]

PATHOPHYSIOLOGY

Although tension-type headache is the most common type of headache, it is the least studied of the primary headache disorders, and there is limited understanding of key pathophysiologic concepts.[8] Some evidence supports that migraine and tension-type headaches represent a continuum of headache severity with similarities in mechanisms and pathophysiology.[8] However, more recently, tension-type headache has been recognized as a distinct disorder. The mechanism of pain in chronic tension-type headache is thought to originate from myofascial factors and peripheral sensitization of nociceptors. Central mechanisms also are involved.[8,33] Mental stress, nonphysiologic motor stress, a local myofascial release of irritants or a combination of these may be the initiating stimulus. Following activation of supraspinal pain perception structures, a self-limiting headache results in most individuals owing to central modulation of the incoming peripheral stimuli. Chronic tension-type headache can evolve from episodic tension-type headache in predisposed individuals due to a change in central circuits and nociceptive processing along the brainstem reflex pathway and subsequent sensitization of the CNS.[8,33,34] It is likely that other pathophysiologic mechanisms also contribute to the development of tension-type headache.

CLINICAL PRESENTATION

Premonitory symptoms and aura are absent with tension-type headache. The pain usually is mild to moderate in intensity and often is described as a dull, nonpulsatile tightness or pressure.[2,12] Bilateral pain is most common, but the location can vary (frontal and temporal pain are most common; occipital and parietal regions also may be affected).[2] The pain is classically described as having a "hatband" pattern. Associated symptoms generally are absent, but mild photophobia or phonophobia may be reported. The disability associated with tension-type headache typically is minor in comparison with migraine headache, and routine physical activity does not affect headache severity.[2,4] Palpation of the pericranial or cervical muscles can reveal tender spots or localized nodules in some patients.[2] Tension-type headache is classified as either episodic (infrequent or frequent) or chronic based on the frequency and duration of the attacks.[2]

TREATMENT

Tension-Type Headaches

■ GENERAL APPROACH TO TREATMENT

The vast majority of episodic tension-type headache sufferers self-medicate with over-the-counter medications and do not consult a healthcare professional. Although pharmacologic and nonpharmacologic treatments are available, simple analgesics and NSAIDs are the mainstay of acute therapy. Most agents used for tension-type headache have not been studied in controlled clinical trials.[35]

■ NONPHARMACOLOGIC THERAPY

Psychophysiologic therapy and physical therapy have been used in the management of tension-type headache. Behavioral therapies can consist of reassurance and counseling, stress management, relaxation training, and biofeedback. These therapies (alone or in combination) can result in a 35% to 50% reduction in headache activity.[36] Evidence supporting physical therapeutic options, such as heat or cold packs, ultrasound, electrical nerve stimulation, stretching, exercise, massage, acupuncture, manipulations, ergonomic instruction, and trigger point injections or occipital nerve blocks, is somewhat inconsistent. However, individual patients may benefit from selected modalities in reducing the frequency of tension-type headache or during an acute episode.[35]

■ PHARMACOLOGIC THERAPY

Simple analgesics (alone or in combination with caffeine) and NSAIDs are effective for the acute treatment of most mild to moderate tension-type headaches. Acetaminophen, aspirin, ibuprofen, naproxen, ketoprofen, and ketorolac have demonstrated efficacy in placebo-controlled and comparative studies.[35] Failure of over-the-counter agents can warrant therapy with prescription drugs. High-dose NSAIDs and the combination of aspirin or acetaminophen with butalbital or, rarely, codeine are effective options. Use of butalbital and codeine combinations should be avoided when possible owing to the high potential for overuse and dependency. As with migraine headache, acute medication should be taken for episodic tension-type headache no more than 9 days per month to prevent the development of chronic tension-type headache.[35] There is no evidence to support the efficacy of muscle relaxants in the management of episodic tension-type headache.[35] Preventive treatment is appropriate for most patients with chronic tension-type headache and should be considered in those with frequent episodic tension-type headache if frequency (>2 per week), duration (>3–4 hours), or severity results in medication overuse or substantial disability.[36] The principles of preventive treatment for tension-type headache are similar to those for migraine headache. TCAs are prescribed most often for prophylaxis, but other drugs also can be selected after consideration of comorbid medical conditions and respective side-effect profiles. SSRIs are not effective in patients with tension-type headache who do not have depression, however, limited studies support the use of the SNRIs mirtazapine and venlafaxine.[34,36] Injection of botulinum toxin into pericranial muscles has demonstrated inconsistent efficacy in the prophylaxis of tension-type headache and because of this, it is not recommended for use.[32,36]

CLUSTER HEADACHE

EPIDEMIOLOGY

Cluster headache, the most severe of the primary headache disorders, is characterized by attacks of severe, unilateral head pain that occur in series lasting for weeks or months (i.e., cluster periods) separated by remission periods usually lasting months or years.[2,37] Cluster headaches can be episodic or chronic.[2] Cluster headache is relatively uncommon among the primary headache disorders, but the exact prevalence is uncertain. The prevalence varies from 56 to 401 per 100,000.[37] Men are more likely than women to have cluster headache, and onset generally occurs after age 20.[37] Recent genetic epidemiological surveys support a predisposition for cluster headache can exist in certain families.[37,38]

PATHOPHYSIOLOGY

The etiologic and pathophysiologic mechanisms of cluster headache are not completely understood. The cyclic nature of attacks implicates a pathogenesis of hypothalamic dysfunction with resulting alterations in circadian rhythms.[8] Hypothalamus-regulated changes in cortisol, prolactin, testosterone, growth hormone, leuteinizing hormone, endorphin, and melatonin have been found during periods of cluster headache attack.[8,41] Neuroimaging studies performed during acute cluster headache attacks have demonstrated activation of the ipsilateral hypothalamic gray area, implicating the thalamus as a cluster generator.[8] Significant cranial autonomic activation occurs ipsilateral to the pain, through the same pathways that are activated during migraine.[8]

CLINICAL PRESENTATION

Attacks occur in cluster periods lasting 2 weeks to 3 months in most patients, followed by long pain-free intervals.[2,39] Periods of remission average 2 years in length but have been reported to be from 2 months to 20 years in duration. Approximately 10% of patients have chronic symptoms with attacks recurring for over 1 year without remission or with remission periods of less than 1 month.[2,39] Cluster headache attacks occur commonly at night and more commonly in the spring and fall.[39] Attacks occur suddenly, with pain peaking quickly after onset and generally lasting 15 to 180 minutes.[2] Auras are not present with cluster headaches. The pain is excruciating, penetrating, and of a boring intensity in orbital, supraorbital, and temporal unilateral locations.[2,39,40] The headache can be accompanied by conjunctival injection, lacrimation, nasal stuffiness, rhinorrhea, eyelid edema, facial sweating, miosis/ptosis, and restlessness or agitation. During the cluster period, attacks occur from once every other day to eight times per day.[2,39,40] Whereas migraine patients retreat to a quiet dark room, cluster headache patients generally sit and rock or pace about the room clutching their head.[39] There is a male preponderance in cluster headache, especially in the chronic form, and lifestyle habits such as smoking and consumption of alcohol or coffee are common.[40] Specific diagnostic criteria for cluster headaches are provided within the IHS classification system.[2]

TREATMENT

Cluster Headaches

As in migraine, therapy for cluster headaches involves both abortive and prophylactic therapy. Abortive therapy is directed at managing the acute attack. Prophylactic therapies are started early in the cluster period in an attempt to induce remission. Patients with chronic cluster headache can require prophylactic medications indefinitely.

■ ABORTIVE THERAPY

Oxygen

The standard acute treatment of cluster headache is inhalation of 100% oxygen by nonbreather facial mask at a rate of 7 to 10 L/min for 15 to 30 minutes.[41] Repeat administration can be necessary because of recurrence, as oxygen appears to merely delay, rather than abort, the attack in some patients.[41] No side effects have been reported with the use of oxygen, but caution should be used for those who smoke or have chronic obstructive pulmonary disease.

Ergotamine Derivatives

All forms of ergotamine have been used in cluster headaches, although no controlled clinical trials support their use.[41,42] In clinical use, intravenous dihydroergotamine results in the quickest response, and repeated administration for 3 to 7 days can break the cycle of frequent attacks.[41] Ergotamine tartrate also has provided effective relief of cluster headache attacks when administered sublingually or rectally, but the pharmacokinetics of these preparations frequently limit their clinical utility.[41] Dosing guidelines are similar to those for migraine headache therapy.

Triptans

The quick onset of subcutaneous and intranasal triptans make them safe and effective abortive agents for cluster headaches. Subcutaneous sumatriptan (6 mg) is the most effective agent. Nasal sprays are less effective but may be better tolerated in some patients. Adverse events reported in cluster headache patients are similar to those seen in migraineurs. Orally administered triptans have limited use in cluster attacks because of their relatively slow onset of action; oral zolmitriptan (10 mg), however, was beneficial in patients with episodic cluster headache with 60% experiencing mild or no pain at 30 minutes.[39,41,42]

■ PROPHYLACTIC THERAPY

Verapamil

Verapamil, the preferred calcium channel blocker for the prevention of cluster headaches, is effective in approximately 70% of patients.[41,42] The beneficial effects of verapamil often appear after 1 week of therapy. A typical suggested dosage range is from 360 to 720 mg/day, with some patients requiring up to 1,200 mg/day.[41,43]

Lithium

Lithium carbonate is effective for episodic and chronic cluster headache attacks and can be used in combination with verapamil. A positive response is seen in up to 78% of patients with chronic cluster headache, and in up to 63% of patients with episodic cluster headache.[41] The usual dose is 600 to 1,200 mg/day, with a suggested starting dose of 300 mg twice daily. Optimal plasma lithium levels for prevention of cluster headache have not been established, but trough values should not be more than 1.0 mEq/L (mmol/L).[41]

Initial side effects are mild and include tremor, lethargy, nausea, diarrhea, and abdominal discomfort. Thyroid and renal function must be monitored during lithium therapy. Lithium should be administered with caution to patients with significant renal or cardiovascular disease, dehydration, pregnancy, or concomitant diuretic or NSAID use.[39,41]

Ergotamine

Ergotamine, once commonly used, can be efficacious for prophylactic as well as abortive therapy of cluster headaches. A 2-mg bedtime dose is often beneficial for the prevention of nocturnal headache attacks. Daily use of 1 to 2 mg ergotamine alone or in combination with verapamil or lithium can provide effective headache prophylaxis in patients refractory to other agents with little risk of ergotism or rebound headache.[39,41] Although there is more literature on methysergide, a serotonergic agent related to ergotamine, as a prophylactic treatment for cluster headache, this agent is no longer available.[39]

Corticosteroids

Corticosteroids are useful for inducing remission.[39,41] Therapy is initiated with 40 to 60 mg/day prednisone and tapered over approximately 3 weeks. Relief appears within 1 to 2 days of initiating therapy. To avoid steroid-induced complications, long-term use is not recommended. Headaches can recur when therapy is tapered or discontinued.

Miscellaneous Agents

Other therapies that have been used in the acute management of cluster headache include intranasal lidocaine, hyperbaric oxygen, and subcutaneous octreotide. Limited studies or case reports also support the use of divalproex sodium, topiramate, gabapentin, intranasal civamide, intranasal capsaicin, tizanidine, baclofen, melatonin, transdermal clonidine, leuprolide, and intramuscular botulinum toxin for cluster prophylaxis. Neurosurgical intervention can be necessary for patients with chronic cluster headache that is resistant to all medical therapies.[41,42]

EVALUATION OF THERAPEUTIC OUTCOMES

Patients should be monitored for frequency, intensity, and duration of headaches, as well as any change in the headache pattern. To this end, migraineurs should be encouraged to keep a headache diary to document the frequency, severity, and duration of migraine attacks, as well as response to medication and potential trigger factors. Careful monitoring is essential to initiate the most appropriate pharmacotherapy, document therapeutic successes and failures, identify medication contraindications, and prevent or minimize adverse events. Patients using acute therapies should be monitored for frequency of use of prescription and over-the-counter medications to identify potential medication-misuse headache. Patient counseling is necessary to allow for proper medication use (e.g., self-injection with sumatriptan), to encourage early use of medications in the headache cycle, and to enhance patient compliance. Strict adherence to dosing guidelines should be stressed to minimize potential toxicity. Patterns of abortive medication use can be documented to establish the need for prophylactic therapy. Prophylactic therapies also should be monitored closely for adverse reactions, abortive therapy needs, adequate dosing, and compliance. Consultation with other healthcare practitioners should be encouraged when changes in headache patterns or medication use occur.

CONCLUSIONS

Although headache disorders such as migraine and cluster headaches appear to occur as a result of neuronal dysfunction, the precise etiology and nature of the dysfunction are unknown. Serotonergic neurotransmission and the trigeminovascular system appear to play important roles. A careful patient workup, including patient history, physical examination, and appropriate laboratory tests, should identify most headache patients with major disease. A variety of strategies can be helpful for managing migraine, tension-type, and cluster headaches. Management of primary headache disorders is directed at suppressing acute attacks and preventing recurrences. Continuing research will better define pathophysiologic mechanisms and aid the search for less toxic and more efficacious pharmacologic agents.

ABBREVIATIONS

5-HT: serotonin, 5-hydroxytryptamine

CGRP: calcitonin gene–related peptide

CNS: central nervous system

GABA: γ-aminobutyric acid

FDA: Food and Drug Administration

IHS: International Headache Society

MAOI: monoamine oxidase inhibitor

NSAID: nonsteroidal antiinflammatory drug

SNRI: serotonin-norepinephrine reuptake inhibitor

SSRI: selective serotonin reuptake inhibitor

TCA: tricyclic antidepressant

REFERENCES

1. National Center for Health Statistics. Health, United States, 2008 with chartbook. Hyattsville, MD, 2009:62–63.
2. Headache Classification Committee of the International Headache Society. The international classification of headache disorders, 2nd ed. Cephalalgia 2004;24(Suppl 1):1–151.
3. Lipton RB, Bigal ME. The epidemiology of migraine. Am J Med 2005;18(Suppl 1):S3–S10.
4. Lipton RB, Bigal ME, Steiner TJ, et al. Classification of primary headaches. Neurology 2004;63(3):427–435.
5. Lipton RB, Bigal ME, Diamond M, et al. Migraine prevalence, disease burden, and the need for preventive therapy. Neurology 2007;68:343–349.
6. Bigal ME, Ferrari M, Silberstein SD, et al. Migraine in the triptan era: lessons from epidemiology, pathophysiology, and clinical science. Headache 2009;49:S21–S33.
7. Silberstein SD. Migraine. Lancet 2004;363:381–391.
8. Schreiber CP. The pathophysiology of primary headache. Prim Care 2004;31:261–276.
9. Ferrari MD. Migraine. Lancet 1998;351:1043–1051.
1. Gardner KL. Genetics of migraine: An update. Headache 2006;46(Suppl 1):S19-S24.
11. Ramadan NM. Targeting therapy for migraine. Neurology 2005;64(Suppl 2):S4-S8.
12. Sadovsky R, Dodick DW. Identifying migraine in primary care settings. Am J Med 2005;118(Suppl 1):S11-S17.
13. Bajwa ZH, Sabahat A. Pathophysiology, clinical manifestations, and diagnosis of migraine in adults. UpToDate 2009;17.3;1–23. www.uptodate.com.
14. Diamond M, Cady R. Initiating and optimizing acute therapy for migraine: The role of patient-centered stratified care. Am J Med 2005;118(Suppl 1):S18-S27.
15. Matchar DB, Young WB, Rosenberg JA, et al. Evidence-Based Guidelines for Migraine Headache in the Primary Care Setting: Pharmacological Management of Acute Attacks. The U.S. Headache Consortium; 2000. www.aan.com/professionals/practice/guidelines.
16. Smith TR. The pharmacologic treatment of the acute migraine attack. Clin Fam Pract 2005;7(3):423–444.
17. Bigal ME, Lipton RB, Krymchantowski AV. The medical management of migraine. Am J Ther 2004;11(2):130–140.
18. Bigal ME, Lipton RB. Modifiable risk factors for migraine progression. Headache 2006;46:1334–1343.
19. Bigal ME, Lipton RB. The preventive treatment of migraine. Neurologist 2006;12(4):204–213.
20. Evans RW, Bigal ME, Grosberg B, Lipton RB. Target doses and titration schedules for migraine preventive medications. Headache 2006;46:160–164.
21. Rapoport AM, Bigal ME. Preventive migraine therapy: What is new. Neurol Sci 2004;25(Suppl 1):S177–S185.
22. Buse DC, Rupnow FT, Lipton RB. Assessing and managing all aspects of migraine: migraine attacks, migraine-related functional impairment, common comorbidites, and quality of life. Mayo Clin Proc 2009;84(5):422–435.
23. Silberstein SD, Dodick D, Freitag F, et al. Pharmacological approaches to managing migraine and associated comorbidities–clinical considerations for monotherapy versus polytherapy. Headache 2007;47:585–599.
24. Kelman L. The triggers or precipitants of the acute migraine attack. Cephalalgia 2007;27(5):394–402.
25. Bajwa ZH, Sabagat A. Acute treatment of migraine in adults. UpToDate 2009;17.3:1–24. www.uptodate.com.
26. Martin VT, Goldstein JA. Evaluating the safety and tolerability profile of acute treatments for migraine. Am J Med 2005;118(Suppl 1):S36-S44.
27. Colman I, Friedman BW, Brown MD, et al. Parenteral dexamethasone for acute severe migraine headache: meta-analysis of randomised controlled trials for preventing recurrence. BMJ 2008;336(7657):1359–1361.
28. Matthew NT, Loder EW. Evaluating the triptans. Am J Med 2005;118(Suppl 1):S28-S35.
29. Center for Drug Evaluation and Research. FDA Public Health Advisory: Drug Combination May Result in Serotonin Syndrome; 2006. www.fda.gov/cder/drug/advisory.
30. Matthew NT. Dynamic optimization of chronic migraine treatment. Neurology 2009;72(Suppl 1):S14-S20.
31. Bajwa ZH, Sabagat A. Preventive treatment of migraine in adults. UpToDate 2009;17.3:1–18. www.uptodate.com.
32. Naumann M, So Y, Argoff CE, et al. Assessment: botulinum neurotoxin in the treatment of autonomic disorders and pain (an evidence-based review): report of the Therapeutics and Technology Assessment Subcommittee of the American Academy of Neurology. Neurology 2008;70:1707–1714.
33. Taylor FR. Tension-type headache in adults: pathophysiology, clinical features, and diagnosis. UpToDate 2009;17.3:1–16. www.uptodate.com.
34. Bendtsen L, Jensen R. Tension-type headache: the most common, but also the most neglected, headache disorder. Curr Opin Neurol 2006;19(3):305–309.
35. Taylor FR. Tension-type headache in adults: acute treatment. UpToDate 2009;17.3:1–9. www.uptodate.com.
36. Taylor FR. Tension-type headache in adults: preventive treatment. UpToDate 2009;17.3:1–13. www.uptodate.com.
37. Russell MB. Epidemiology and genetics of cluster headache. Lancet Neurol 2004;3:279–83.
38. Broner SW, Cohen JM. Epidemiology of cluster headache. Curr Pain Headache Rep 2009;13:141–146.
39. Freitag FG. Cluster headache. Prim Care 2004;31:313–329.
40. Favier I, Haan J, Ferrari MD. Chronic cluster headache: A review. J Headache Pain 2005;6:3–9.
41. McGeeney, BE. Cluster headache pharmacotherapy. Am J Ther 2005;12(4):351–358.
42. 42. Tyagi A, Matharu M. Evidence base for the medical treatments used in cluster headache. Curr Pain Headache Rep 2009;13:168–178.
43. 43. Tfelt-Hansen P, Tfelt-Hansen J. Verapamil for cluster headache. Clinical pharmacology and possible mode of action. Headache 2009;49:117–125.

CHAPTER

71

Evaluation of Psychiatric Illness

MARK E. SCHNEIDERHAN, LEIGH ANNE NELSON, AND STUART MUNRO

KEY CONCEPTS

❶ Patients with psychiatric conditions are treated in all healthcare settings. All clinicians need to develop basic skills in psychiatric assessment to provide the best care for their patients.

❷ The *Diagnostic and Statistical Manual of Mental Disorders, Fourth Edition, Text Revision (DSM-IV-TR)* is the most widely accepted diagnostic reference. It, along with the *American Psychiatric Association Practice Guidelines for the Psychiatric Evaluation of Adults,* provides the clinician a standardized approach for the initial assessment and follow-up of patients with mental illness.

❸ At times, patients suffering from mental illness are challenging to assess, as their condition can prevent them from full cooperation. A range of strategies can be used to gather the needed information while maintaining the safety and comfort of both patient and clinician.

❹ A thorough medication history to identify all medications currently taken, as well as those previously taken, is a cornerstone of effective patient management. In addition, it must be determined whether there was an adequate trial (dose and duration) of current and prior medications for psychiatric illnesses.

❺ A baseline mental status examination, along with a specific target symptom list, is a critical tool in monitoring response to treatment.

❻ Several papers have been published in recent years recommending specific physical assessment and laboratory tests needed for the evaluation of patients with psychiatric conditions. Except for patients taking antipsychotics, no single standard exists, and testing is individualized based on the patient's age, medical history, current physical health, and cur-

rent medication use; and in consideration of the most recent expert opinion.

❼ Baseline and follow-up monitoring for metabolic disturbances should be instituted for all patients taking antipsychotics.

❶ Patients with mental illnesses are treated by clinicians from many disciplines and in all settings of healthcare, and they often receive the bulk of their care from nonpsychiatrists. Hence the need for good psychiatric assessment skills is not limited to mental health specialists. Along with traditional assessments used across all medical specialties (e.g., laboratory tests, medical history, and physical examination), psychiatric practitioners use additional strategies to manage their patients that are perhaps less objective in nature and less familiar to nonpsychiatric practitioners. This chapter provides a basic overview of appropriate assessment techniques used by clinicians to develop an individualized treatment plan for psychiatric patients. Readers needing greater depth than the materials provided in this chapter are referred to other sources.[1-6]

OVERVIEW OF THE DIAGNOSTIC AND STATISTICAL MANUAL OF MENTAL DISORDERS

❷ The *Diagnostic and Statistical Manual of Mental Disorders, Fourth Edition, Text Revision (DSM-IV-TR)* is the most widely accepted and most important diagnostic reference used in the care of the mentally ill. It provides a common language for practitioners to describe and diagnose psychiatric disorders.[7] Common language is essential because there is considerable overlap of symptoms across many diagnoses. The *Diagnostic and Statistical Manual of Mental Disorders, First Edition (DSM-I)* was introduced in 1952 and was the first manual on mental disorders to contain a description of diagnostic categories. The most recent edition, *DSM-IV-TR*, was released in 2000 and uses essentially the same diagnostic criteria sets as the *Diagnostic and Statistical Manual of Mental Disorders, Fourth Edition (DSM-IV).*[7] Its purpose is to correct factual errors in *DSM-IV* and update the text sections (e.g., associated features, prevalence, and differential diagnosis) with more contemporary data. A more significant rewriting of diagnostic criteria and introduction of new diagnoses will appear in *Diagnostic and Statistical Manual of Mental Disorders, Fifth Edition (DSM-V)*, which probably will not be available until May 2015.[7] The *DSM-IV-TR* contains many components that provide a comprehensive understanding of specific mental illnesses and assist in making an accurate diagnosis. For example, the multiaxial patient evaluation ensures that most factors that could contribute to, or complicate, the condition are considered during a patient assessment and throughout treatment planning. Axis I lists the principal psychiatric disorder (e.g., schizophrenia, etc), developmental disorders, or provisional diagnoses present in the patient. Mental retardation and personality disorders (e.g., antisocial, borderline, etc.) are listed on Axis II. Axis III lists existing physical disorders or conditions. Axis IV lists the severity of psychosocial stressors that might have contributed to a new or recurrent mental disorder or exacerbation of an existing condition. Stressors are rated on a scale of 1 (none) to 6 (catastrophic) and can be acute (lasting less than 6 months) or enduring (lasting longer than 6 months). Examples of stressors include difficulties with interpersonal relationships, parenting, occupation, living circumstances, finances, the legal system, and health. Axis V describes the global assessment of functioning (GAF), rated on a scale from 1 (persistent danger to self or others) to 90 (minimal or absent symptoms). A GAF rating is made based on the current level of functioning and can be used to describe the highest level of functioning achieved prior to the current evaluation. By documenting the baseline level of functioning, the GAF helps evaluate progress toward a patient's therapeutic goals.

DSM-IV-TR provides general information on all mental disorders recognized by the American Psychiatric Association (APA) and includes age of onset, clinical course, complications, predisposing factors, prevalence, and differential diagnoses. The specific diagnostic criteria for each mental illness and the number of symptoms required to establish a diagnosis are also listed. The *DSM-IV-TR* also includes decision trees for differential diagnosis and a glossary of technical terms. The *Clinical Interview Using DSM-IV* is a companion publication that provides extensive information on interviewing techniques helpful in establishing a specific *DSM-IV* diagnosis.[7]

Additional information besides the *DSM-IV-TR* diagnosis is required before a comprehensive treatment plan can be developed. The *American Psychiatric Association Practice Guidelines for Psychiatric Evaluation of Adults* (2nd edition) includes a full discussion of the domains needed for a thorough clinical evaluation. It also discusses issues of privacy, appropriate setting for assessment, and evaluations in special populations.[5]

In summary, the *DSM-IV-TR* and the APA practice guidelines allow clinicians to evaluate patients in a systematic manner, thereby creating better treatment plans and a more consistent evaluation of response.

THE CLINICAL INTERVIEW

The interview should be conducted in a quiet, nonstimulating, and comfortable area where the patient and the interviewer feel at ease.[6] The setting should be appropriate to the patient's level of acuity and the potential for risk to the patient and clinician. The interviewer should introduce himself or herself and explain what is about to happen in order to establish a trusting relationship. Generally, open-ended questions come first, followed by questions focused on more specific or personal data. Open-ended questions allow the patient to provide descriptions and other information in his or her own words. Even though more specific questions may then be necessary to fill in the gaps, beginning in this manner minimizes the risk of "leading" the patient. Patients can respond to specific questions and "yes" or "no" questions with answers they think the

interviewer wants to hear. The interviewer must be nonjudgmental about the information offered by the patient to develop trust and rapport and to ensure completeness and accuracy of the information. Whether a clinician takes notes or just listens during the interview is an individual decision, with the primary considerations being to make an accurate record of the content of the examination and assuring that the patient is comfortable with the note taking. Table 71–1 provides examples of questions useful for gathering information during the completion of the clinical interview.

TABLE 71-1 Examples of Interview Questions for Assessing Mental Illnesses

Mania
1. Do your thoughts go faster than you can say them?
2. Have you noticed a change in the amount of sleep that you require?
3. Have you spent a lot of money lately, and what did you spend it on?
4. Do you have a lot of extra energy?
(To assess hallucinations and delusions, see Schizophrenia section below.)

Depression
Do you cry without any reason?
Do you still enjoy the same hobbies/activities that you once did?
Has your weight changed recently?
Have you had changes in your energy level recently?
Do you have any guilty feelings?
Do you find it difficult to remember phone numbers, names of friends, appointments, and so on?
(To assess sleep and suicidal potential, see Sleep and Suicide sections below.)

Schizophrenia
Delusions
1. Do you feel that people plot against you?
2. Do you ever feel that you are watched or spied on?
3. Do you have any special abilities?
4. Does anyone ever try to mess with you or bother you?
5. Do others read your thoughts?
Hallucinations
1. Does the TV/radio ever tell you things?
2. Do you hear voices that other people don't hear?
3. What do they say? How many voices?
4. How often do they bother you?
5. Do the voices ever tell you to hurt yourself or someone else?
6. Have you ever heard your name called when there is no one there?
7. Have you ever seen anything strange that you can't explain?
8. Do you ever see things that bother you and no one else?
9. Do you want to act on what the voices say?
Thought broadcasting/insertion
1. If I stood by you, could I hear your thoughts?
2. Does your head ever act like a radio?
3. Do you feel that others can put thoughts in your head?

Insight
1. What reasons did your family give you for coming here?
2. What brought you here?
3. Do you consider yourself in need of help?
4. What does your medication do for you?

Sleep
1. Tell me about your sleep.
2. How many hours do you sleep each night at present?
3. How many hours do you usually sleep at night?
4. Do you sleep all through the night?
5. Is there a reason for your waking up?
6. Do you have trouble falling asleep?
7. How do you feel when you wake up?

Suicide potential
1. Do you feel your life is not worth living?
2. Do you ever think of hurting yourself?
3. Do you see things improving in the future?
4. Do you think you will try to hurt yourself now?
5. How would you do it?
6. Do you have the means to hurt yourself?

THE CHALLENGING PATIENT

❸ Patient assessments can be challenging when symptoms of the condition prevent effective engagement with the clinician. Excited patients may exhibit speech that is rapid and unorganized; whereas, depressed patients may respond with few words. Patients in the manic phases of bipolar disorder may not pause as they speak (pressured speech), making it difficult for the interviewer to interject. In all cases, the interviewer can regain control by politely redirecting the patient back toward the question. Psychotic patients may be paranoid and appear guarded or frightened by the questions. The best approach is to remain calm and respectful, use shorter or closed-ended questions, and seek only essential information until the patient is less paranoid. Patients can become agitated and occasionally violent. Often violence is preceded by increased psychomotor agitation as evidenced by pacing, speaking in a loud voice, or gripping the arms of the chair. When there is concern about safety, the interviewer should avoid any behavior that could be misconstrued as threatening, such as touching or unnecessary staring, and interview the patient in the presence of another healthcare provider. Both the patient and interviewer should have equal access to leave the room if either becomes too uncomfortable. If a patient becomes threatening to the interviewer, the interviewer should not hesitate to leave the room and call for help. If a patient describes suicidal thoughts, he or she should be further assessed using the questions outlined in Table 71–1, and depending on the results of further assessment should be directed to the appropriate type of care, including hospitalization for patients at immediate risk of harming themselves. A suicidal patient should never be left alone. Asking a patient about suicidal thoughts will not increase the risk. The risk is greater if these questions are never asked or signs of distress are ignored. Before any conclusions are made about a patient interview, the impact of culture on the patient's presentation should be considered. Something that sounds delusional in Western culture can be the norm in others. If a clinician is unclear whether culture of origin accounts for some of the patient's symptoms, he or she should consult with a family member or someone else familiar with the patient's culture of origin.

PSYCHIATRIC HISTORY

Both the patient's and the patient's family history of mental illness provide important information when formulating a diagnosis and treatment plan. Information should include the current and previous psychiatric diagnoses, the clinical presentation of each illness, time frame between episodes, level of functioning between episodes, length of each episode, total duration of illness, and treatment given during each episode as well as response to those treatments. Baseline functioning or the highest level of functioning achieved in the past few years is important because it helps to define a treatment goal. Information on the history of the current episode and reasons for presenting to the clinician also should be gathered. A family history should include a medication history of the immediate relatives because a family member's response to a given medication might predict an individual patient's response to that same medication.

SOCIAL HISTORY

A social history should include educational and occupational background, religion, marital status, substance-use patterns including tobacco, alcohol, and caffeine, and current living situation. By understanding a patient's living environment and social situation, strategies to foster treatment adherence, reduce stress, and increase social support can be developed. To probe this area initially, the clinician can ask patients to describe their social support network.

This can be followed by more specific questions such as "To whom are you closest?" or "In whom do you confide?"

MEDICATION HISTORY

❹ A thorough medication history is one of the most important contributions a clinician can make to treatment planning. The history should include medications for both psychiatric and medical conditions. It should list all medications taken by the patient, and report on how each was tolerated and the nature of the response to that drug or combination of drugs. All allergies must be noted. Because most psychiatric medications have a delay in the onset of effect, it is important to determine whether an adequate trial (dose and duration) was provided before the patient was deemed "nonresponsive" to that drug. If a patient has a history of nonadherence, specific causes such as cost, complicated dosing schedules, lack of insight, and adverse effects should be investigated.

MENTAL STATUS EXAMINATION

❺ The mental status examination (MSE) is a key patient assessment tool in psychiatry and is analogous to the physical examination in medicine. The MSE is completed through a direct patient interview and results in a description of current behavior, thoughts, perceptions, and functioning. The MSE provides an objective evaluation used in diagnosis, assessment of the course of the illness, and response to treatment. It is combined with other components of the patient workup (history of present illness, physical examination, appropriate laboratory tests, and medical and psychiatric history) to give a full picture of the presenting problem and factors contributing to the illness. The MSE has several components.[5–7]

Appearance and Attitude Toward Examiner

The appearance of the patient throughout the interview should be noted, including age, dress, grooming and hygiene, use of cosmetics, and facial expressions. A description of appearance also should include unusual physical characteristics and the general state of physical health. The interviewer should note whether the patient is cooperative, mute, hostile, paranoid, guarded, or withdrawn.

Activity

Motor activity may be excessive or diminished. Overactivity can include pacing; hand wringing; picking at clothing, skin, or hair; inability to sit still during the interview; and excessive hand gestures. Underactive patients move less than expected. Patients with rigid posture, an absence of movement, and failure to communicate may be catatonic, paranoid, or experiencing medication-induced adverse effects.

Speech and Language

The quantity, flow, and speed of speech and the amount of eye contact should be noted. The appropriateness and degree of eye contact varies significantly between cultures, and before poor eye contact is interpreted, the patient's cultural background should be considered. Speech should be assessed as to whether it proceeds logically in a goal-directed manner or whether the content is vague and poorly organized. Abnormal speech characteristics include thought blocking, whereby the person suddenly stops speaking without any obvious reason. Thought blocking usually occurs when a hallucination or delusion intrudes into the person's thinking or when upsetting issues are discussed. Circumstantial speech lacks a clear direction because of excess unnecessary information, but the circumstantial patient eventually will make his or her point. In tangential speech, however, the ultimate point is never made. *Perseveration* is repetition of an original answer to subsequent questions. *Flight of ideas* is overproductive, rapid speech during which the patient jumps rapidly from one idea to the next. *Mutism* is identified when the patient does not respond even though he or she is aware of the discussion.

Affect and Mood

Affect describes the patient's current emotional tone, as expressed through facial expression, body posture, and tone of voice, all of which can be objectively observed by the clinician. Mood describes feelings, which are subjectively reported by the patient. Change in facial expression and the presence of tears, flushing, sweating, or tremors should be noted. Affect can be described further by its range, appropriateness, intensity, and stability. For example, in schizophrenia or depression, the affect can be *flat*, whereby no change in expression occurs throughout the interview. In contrast, during a manic episode, the affect is very intense and often *excited*. *Blunted affect* denotes that the range of emotional expression is reduced, but not absent. An example of *inappropriate affect* is when a patient laughs in a situation that would be expected to produce sadness. A rapidly shifting affect from one extreme to the other is described as *labile*.

Thought and Perceptual Disturbances

A variety of thought disturbances can occur in mental illness. Many of these disturbances generally indicate the presence of psychosis or impaired reality testing. *Delusions* are fixed, false beliefs that are not based in reality or consistent with the patient's religion or culture. Delusions can be paranoid, somatic, or grandiose in nature. Delusions are often unshakable, and although the clinician can challenge the delusional thinking, one should not attempt to talk a patient out of a delusion. *Thought broadcasting* is the belief that one's thoughts are audible to others. *Hallucinations* are false sensory impressions or perceptions that occur in the absence of an external stimulus. Hallucinations can be auditory, visual, olfactory, tactile, or gustatory and can be continuous or intermittent. In contrast, *illusions* are visual misperceptions involving a misinterpretation of a real sensory stimulus. For example, a person who initially misperceives a curtain blown by the wind to be an intruder has experienced an illusion. This phenomenon does not always indicate a psychiatric illness and can be seen in persons without mental illness. Not all thought disturbances are indicative of psychosis. For example, the couplet of obsessions and compulsions can indicate the presence of obsessive-compulsive disorder, which is not considered to be a psychotic disorder. *Obsessions* are unwanted thoughts or ideas that intrude into a person's thinking. *Compulsions* are actions performed in response to the obsessions or to control anxiety associated with the obsession.

Evaluation of Cognition

The mental status exam assesses sensorium, attention, concentration, memory, and higher cognitive functions such as orientation and abstraction. The clinician should document whether the patient has received medications with sedative properties, because the outcome of the examination can be altered if central nervous system depressants were recently taken.

Sensorium, or level of consciousness, refers to the alertness of the patient, and if he or she is not fully alert, the amount of stimulation needed to awaken the patient. Attention and concentration can be assessed using serial subtraction by 7s ("serial 7s") or 3s, or by having a patient spell a five-letter word backward. General intelligence can be assessed loosely by asking factual information about current news items, recent presidents, or popular television shows or sporting events. *Memory* is the ability to recall past experiences and is classified as sensory stores (which lasts seconds), short-term

memory (the ability to recall newly acquired information after several minutes), working memory (i.e., immediate application of visual or auditory instructions), and long-term or remote memory (historical facts). Orientation to time, place, person, and situation assesses sensory stores and short-term memory. Asking a patient to recall three objects 5 minutes after they are learned is the definitive test for short-term memory. Deficits in short-term memory may be seen in depression and anxiety, but this finding is the hallmark feature of dementia. Asking the patient to do a certain task (e.g., pick up a pen with his or her right hand and then fold a piece of paper and pass it to the examiner) can assess the patient's working memory. Patients with cognitive deficits, such as those seen in dementias and schizophrenia, can exhibit deficits in working memory. Remote memory is assessed by asking patients to recall old facts about their lives, such as where they were born or where they went to school. Remote memory usually remains intact the longest in patients with intellectual decline, whereas the ability to create new memories is generally the first sign of a memory deficit. *Abstraction* is the ability to interpret information such as a proverb ("People in glass houses shouldn't throw stones") or identify similarities or differences between words (e.g., apple and orange). Abstraction is influenced by education, cultures and linguistic fluency; thus inability to abstract is not always a sign of a psychiatric disorder. Persons with schizophrenia often provide *concrete* (literal or superficial interpretations) or *bizarre* responses to probes of abstraction.

Insight and Judgment

Insight refers to patient awareness that he or she has a mental illness and the impact of that illness on his or her life. Patients typically demonstrate a lack of insight when they are psychotic. Patients with *poor* insight are often nonadherent with prescribed medications. Judgment is the ability to make decisions appropriate to the situation and can be impaired in a variety of mental illnesses. Judgment can be assessed by asking patients how they would handle either their current or a hypothetical situation. Both insight and judgment can be fluid. For example, intoxicated patients can demonstrate *poor* insight and judgment only to improve over several hours as their blood alcohol concentration decreases.

PHYSICAL EXAMINATION AND LABORATORY ASSESSMENT

There is no consensus about specific laboratory tests for diagnosing or evaluating mental illness.[2,5] The identification of biologic markers (e.g., pharmacogenomics) as diagnostic tools, predictors, or indicators of drug response is of great interest but currently of limited clinical usefulness. The most promising was the dexamethasone suppression test, proposed to be a marker for endogenous melancholic depression. However, its lack of sensitivity and specificity has limited its usefulness as a routine screening tool during a workup for depression.[2] Although there are no tests to definitively indicate that a patient has a specific mental illness (e.g., schizophrenia or bipolar disorder), laboratory tests are important to clarify the etiology of presenting symptoms.

Patients who present with psychiatric symptoms need a careful medical assessment because of overlapping symptoms.[1-3,6] A complete physical examination, along with a detailed medical and medication history, vital signs, weight and body mass index, a pregnancy test when indicated, and routine blood chemistry are commonly part of the workup of persons with mental illness. In most cases, a physical examination should be chaperoned.

Both medical illnesses and medications can cause the same psychiatric symptoms. The rapidity of onset of psychiatric symptoms is an important clue that a medical cause may be present. Most chronic mental illnesses have a prodromal period, whereas medically based psychiatric symptoms generally have a more rapid onset of symptoms. Patients older than 40 years of age at first presentation are more likely to have a medical cause for their psychiatric symptoms because major psychiatric illnesses such as schizophrenia and bipolar disorder usually first present in adolescence or early adulthood. Family history can provide additional clues. Patients with fluctuating levels of consciousness, disorientation, memory impairment, or visual, tactile, or olfactory hallucinations are more likely to have a medical basis for their presentation.

Patients with psychiatric illnesses, especially depression and anxiety disorders, often present with only physical complaints, leading to inappropriate care for medical problems that are not present or as serious as they may appear, while the root cause is ignored. In contrast, patients with severe persistent mental illness (e.g., schizophrenia) have increased risks for cardiovascular disease and are less likely to receive the same level of primary medical care compared to patients without mental illness.[8-10] Barriers to medical care include patient paranoia, ambivalence, and disorganization accounting for missed appointments; stigma toward mental illness; and poor communication between primary care and psychiatric clinicians.[11] Antipsychotic therapy can also cause or exacerbate medical conditions, such as diabetes mellitus, hyperlipidemia, or cardiac arrhythmias, necessitating an initial assessment and ongoing monitoring for these conditions while continuing treatment.[12,13]

6 General laboratory screening is useful for ruling out medical causes of psychiatric illnesses and medication monitoring. Urine drug screens and blood alcohol tests play an important role in identifying the contribution of substances of abuse to the presenting symptoms. Additional testing can include an electroencephalogram to evaluate for the presence of seizure activity or other neurologic conditions, computed tomography or magnetic resonance imaging to detect structural abnormalities, sedimentation rate and antinuclear antibodies for autoimmune disorders, a human immunodeficiency virus test, thyroid function tests, and vitamin B_{12} and folate concentrations for anemias.[2] Laboratory tests should be individualized to the age, medical/medication history, cooperativeness, and physical health of the patient, but extensive testing is usually unnecessary and not cost-effective.

Clinicians also use diagnostic tests to evaluate the relative safety of specific medications such as pregnancy monitoring with divalproex, renal status when using lithium, or an electrocardiogram when using a tricyclic antidepressant such as amitriptyline. Baseline information is often needed to help document future adverse effects from medications (e.g., lithium-induced hypothyroidism, clozapine-induced leukopenia, antipsychotic-induced diabetes mellitus). Serum concentration monitoring is recommended for medications with a narrow therapeutic index such as lithium, divalproex, and carbamazepine. Serum concentration monitoring can also be useful for assessing medication adherence when there is inadequate response. With the exceptions of lithium, divalproex, and clozapine, there is minimal data to support obtaining serum concentrations for optimizing medication efficacy in psychiatric disorders.

7 The 2004 expert consensus recommends that patients starting on newer antipsychotic agents should be screened for symptoms of metabolic syndrome including body weight (baseline, weeks 4, 8, and 12, then every 3 months (12 weeks), then annually), waist and hip measurements (baseline and annually), blood pressures (baseline, week 12, and annually), and fasting serum lipids and glucose (if possible at baseline, week 12, and annually for high-risk patients).[12-14] In 2007, it was reported that over 50% of patients on antipsychotics were not being monitored for diabetes and dyslipidemia.[15] Glucose and lipid monitoring continues to be underutilized for patients taking antipsychotics.

Although fasting serum results are preferred over random serum or capillary blood specimens, this should not be a barrier to adequate monitoring.[16] The clinician can employ random glucose, high-density lipoprotein cholesterol levels, or glycosylated hemoglobin A_{1c} if there is difficulty obtaining fasting serum levels.[13,15]

In summary, a range of assessments aid the clinician in making problem-focused workups to verify diagnoses and identifying underlying or potential drug-related problems[17] The MSE is the cornerstone of the psychiatric workup, although selective medical tests, a good medical, psychiatric, and medication history, and a thorough physical examination are also important.

PSYCHIATRIC RATING SCALES

Psychiatric rating scales are useful tools to provide an objective way of measuring subjective data (e.g., feelings, thoughts, and perceptions) and to screen or diagnose specific disorders. As there are so many types of scales to choose from, the clinician rater needs training and experience to select and use the most appropriate scale. Rating scales are used in a variety of settings, including research and patient care, and can serve an administrative purpose such as quality control.[4]

Drawbacks to the more frequent use of clinician-rated scales include the substantial time commitment for staff to administer the tests and the inability of some patients to tolerate these interviews, especially patients who are severely paranoid or agitated. In addition, repeated ratings are usually necessary to objectively describe longitudinal changes over a defined treatment period as opposed to a snapshot of a complex clinical situation.

Some rating scales are self-administered (patient-rated) and do not require a staff member to collect the data; thus they require minimal resources to administer and can provide valuable information, although some patients may be unable to self-administer a questionnaire for a variety of reasons, including limited literacy and severity of symptoms.

In contrast to symptom-based rating scales (e.g., Positive and Negative Syndrome Scale or Hamilton Depression scale), global rating scales, such as the Clinical Global Impression scale, assess the overall severity of illness based on a rater's clinical experience.[18-20] In general, these rating scales measure the presence or severity of symptoms and can assist in the diagnostic formulation.

Rating scales are also available to measure adverse side effects from psychiatric medications. Specific adverse side-effect measures can be used for specific categories of medications. Table 71–2 provides a summary of the most common rating scales used to assess and quantify the presence and severity of adverse effects.[21]

Sensitivity, specificity, reliability, and validity are important considerations when selecting a rating scale. *Sensitivity* refers to a test's ability to detect a symptom or illness, given that the symptom or illness is present. *Specificity* refers to a test's ability to determine that a symptom or illness is absent given that the person does not have the illness.

Reliability is the extent to which the score on the scale reflects the hypothetical "true" score and how much interference occurs from outside influences.[22] Reliability is reported by the correlation coefficient, which represents a chance correlation (zero) or perfect correlation (1). Rating scales with correlation coefficients of less than 0.7 are usually considered unreliable for clinical studies. Interrater reliability—agreement in rating scores among clinician raters—is important to achieve when multiple clinicians rate the same patient or population. Interrater reliability is established by having all raters independently rate individual patients at the same time to determine the correlation of their scores.

TABLE 71-2 Adverse Effects Measures

Rating Scale	Type	Scoring	Comments
Systematic Assessment for Treatment of Emergent Events–General Inquiry (SAFTEE-GI)	Structured interview and global assessment	Summary scores of number of events, average severity, and impairment	5–10 minutes to complete. Baseline and weekly evaluations. Easy to administer. The specific reported information might be more useful than an overall summary score
MED Watch	Global assessment	No scoring involved	Minutes to complete. The one-page form requires a narrative description of the problem or adverse reaction. Online submission: *www.fda.gov/medwatch/*
Abnormal Involuntary Movement Scale (AIMS)	Tardive dyskinesia (TD) assessment	12-item, 5-point severity scale. Items 1–4 orofacial movement; 5–7 extremity and truncal movement; 8-10 global severity; 11 and 12 problems with teeth or dentures (yes or no)	5–10 minutes to complete. Most commonly used. Diagnostic criteria: at least 3 months of antipsychotic treatment. Mild severity score (2) in two discrete areas or moderate severity (3) in one area (e.g., orofacial) indicates TD. Tremor is not counted
Dyskinesia Identification System: Condensed User Scale (DISCUS)	Tardive dyskinesia assessment	15-item, 5-point severity scale. Items 1, 2 face; 3 eyes; 4, 5 oral; 6–9 lingual; 10, 11 head/neck/trunk; 12, 13 upper limb; 14, 15 lower limb	5–10 minutes to complete. More descriptive criteria for scoring severity than the AIMS. Scoring based on three dimensions: frequency, detectability, and intensity. Tremor is not counted
Rating Scale for Extrapyramidal Side Effects (Simpson-Angus EPS Scale)	Drug-induced Parkinson and dystonia assessments	10-item, 5-point anchored severity scale. Mean score is obtained by adding all scores and dividing by 10. A mean score of 0.3 is the upper limit for no EPS	5–10 minutes to complete. Item domains include gait, arm dropping, shoulder shaking, elbow rigidity, wrist rigidity, leg pendulousness, head dropping, eye blinking, tremor, and salivation
Barnes Akathisia Scale (BAS)	Drug-induced akathisia	4 items including three 4-point anchored severity scored items and a 5-point global rating score item. Total score of 12 possible	10 minutes to complete. Items 1-3 (objective observation of restlessness, subjective awareness of restlessness, and subjective distress related to restlessness). Diagnostic criteria: requires both objective and subjective ratings of at least one in either two subjective items

EPS, extrapyramidal symptoms.
Data from Schooler and Chengappa[21] and Guy.[19]

Validity, in contrast, is the ability of a scale to measure what it was designed to measure. Various validity tests are performed on a rating scale to ensure that the scale assesses the appropriate aspects of the illness (content validity), the correlation with diagnoses or clinical change (concurrent validity), and the extent to which the scale measures symptom traits in contrast to a specific symptom (construct validity).

Psychiatric rating scales should not be confused with psychologic tests such as neuropsychologic and intellectual assessments and are best used as only one part of a comprehensive diagnostic plan. Tables 71-3, 71-4, and 71-5 describe commonly used patient-rated and clinician-rated scales for a variety of disease states.[18–20,23–26]

SYSTEMATIC MEASUREMENT OF COGNITIVE FUNCTION

Neuropsychiatric rating scales provide specific information such as the rate of change and severity of cognitive decline or improvement. They are useful in situations in which repeated measurements of a patient's mental status are needed because they allow the clinician to determine response to an intervention (e.g., medication) in a more systematic manner. In addition, some cognitive function measures are useful screens for Alzheimer disease and other causes of cognitive decline. A number of cognitive rating scales are available, the most common being the Mini-Mental Status Examination (MMSE).

The MMSE is a structured interview that globally assesses many cognitive domains, including orientation, visuospatial organization, memory, and reasoning to determine an overall score of cognitive function. The maximum score is 30, and a score of 23 or less is indicative of significant cognitive impairment. The MMSE takes 5 to 10 minutes to administer and is used routinely in the clinical setting.[27] Other examples of cognitive rating scales include the Blessed Information Memory Concentration test (BIMC), the Dementia Rating Scale (DRS-2), the Clock Drawing test (CDT), and Alzheimer's Disease Assessment Scale.[28–31]

Most of the rating scales involve a structured interview that requires clinician training to ensure accurate administration. Noise and distraction can affect the patient's performance ability; therefore, the interview should be conducted in a quiet area with adequate lighting. The interviewer should speak slowly and clearly to the patient when providing instructions or asking questions.

PSYCHOLOGICAL TESTING

Although most clinicians do not administer psychological testing, they can use the results to evaluate the role of medication in relationship to the diagnosis. Psychological testing alone cannot establish a firm diagnosis but can be a useful diagnostic tool when coupled with clinical judgment. Types of psychological testing include personality tests (e.g., Minnesota Multiphasic Personality Inventory-2), intelligence tests (e.g., Wechsler Adult Intelligence Scale–Revised, Wechsler Intelligence Scale for Children–Revised), projective tests (e.g. Rorschach), and neuropsychologic tests (e.g., Bender Visual Motor Gestalt Test).[3]

TABLE 71-3 Schizophrenia Rating Scales

Rating Scale	Type	Scoring	Comments
Brief Psychiatric Rating Scale (BPRS)	Clinician rated	18 items, 7-point severity scale: mildly ill ≃32, moderately ill ≃44, markedly ill ≃55, and severely ill ≃70 when correlated to the CGI	The anchored BPRS provides descriptions of each severity rating to increase the interrater reliability. The BPRS has four clusters of symptoms: thinking disturbance, anxious depression, withdrawal-retardation, and hostility-suspiciousness
Positive and Negative Syndrome Scale (PANSS)	Clinician rated	30-item scale, 7-point severity scale: mildly ill ≃57, moderately ill ≃75, markedly ill ≃95, and severely ill ≃116 when correlated to the CGI	Based on the 18-item BPRS for assessing the presence or absence of positive and negative symptoms, and psychopathology of schizophrenia
Clinical Global Impression (CGI) Scale CGI (S): Severity of Illness CGI (I): Global Improvement CGI: Efficacy Index	Clinician rated	Severity of illness and global improvement on 7-point rating scales. Efficacy index: 1–4 marked improvement; 5–8 moderate; 9–12 minimal; 13–16 unchanged/worse	Observational and non-symptom specific for assessing three global subsets: severity of illness, global improvement, and efficacy index measures both therapeutic and side effects

BPRS and PANSS data from Leucht et al.[18,20]

TABLE 71-4 Depression and Bipolar Disorder Rating Scales

Rating Scale	Type	Scoring	Comments
Hamilton Depression Scale (HAMD or HDRS)	Clinician rated	17-item scale; <6 = normal mood; 17–25 = moderate depression; >25 = severe depression	Used to screen patients for drug studies and to determine severity of symptoms and treatment outcome. HDRS is the standard to compare other depression rating scales against
Montgomery-Asberg Depression Rating Scale (MADRS)	Clinician rated	10-item, 7-point scale. For each item: 0 = no symptoms; 6 = severe symptoms	Differentiates between all the intermediate grades of depression. Decreases bias in patients with other medical illnesses and increased somatization (varied unexplained physical symptoms)
Beck Depression Inventory (BDI)	Patient rated	21-item scale; 0–9 = normal; 10–15 = mild depression; 16–19 = mild-moderate; 20–29 = moderate-severe; 30–63 = severe depression	The standard for depression self-rating scales and an objective measure of change in symptoms as a result of treatment
Zung Self-Rating Depression Scale (ZSDS)	Patient rated	20-item scale, 4-point severity; <50 = normal; 50–59 = minimal-mild; 60–69 = moderate-marked; ≥70 severe depression	Severity rated by frequency of occurrence of symptoms. May not be as sensitive in measuring changes in severity of symptoms
Patient Health Questionnaire (PHQ-9)	Patient rated	9-item, 4-point scale. For each DSM-IV depression criteria item: 0 = not at all; 3 = nearly every day. Score <10 = minimal depression symptoms	Commonly used in primary care to establish a diagnosis of depression and assess severity of depressive symptoms
Quick Inventory of Depressive Symptomatology (QIDS-C [Clinician] and QIDS-SR [Patient])	Clinician and patient rated	16-item scale; scores range from 0–27; 0–5 = none; 6–10 = mild; 11–15 = moderate; 16–20 = severe; 21–27 = very severe	Used to assess symptom severity and symptomatic change. QIDS-SR found to be as sensitive to symptom change as the HDRS. Has usefulness in both clinical and research settings
Young Mania Rating Scale (YMRS)	Clinician rated	11-item scale; 5-point severity; 13 = minimal; 20 = mild; 26 = moderate; 38 = severe	Used to screen patients for drug studies and to determine severity of symptoms and treatment outcome. YMRS is the standard to compare other mania rating scales against
Mood Disorder Questionnaire (MDQ)	Patient rated	15-item scale; score of ≥7 suggestive of bipolar spectrum disorder	Screens for a lifetime history of mania or hypomania. Does not assess severity of illness

TABLE 71-5 Anxiety Rating Scales

Rating Scale	Type	Scoring	Comments
Hamilton Anxiety Scale (HAM-A or HAM-AS or HAMRS)	Clinician rated	14 items, 5-point scales; scores of ≥18–20 for moderate anxiety	Consists of subscales to measure somatic and psychic anxiety
Self-Rating Anxiety Scale (Zung SAS)	Patient rated	20-item scale; 4-point intensity ratings	Correlates to the clinician-rated Anxiety Status Inventory (ASI); however, there is little information on the validity of either test
Sheehan Panic and Anticipatory Anxiety Scale (SPAAS)	Patient and clinician rated	3-part scale	Measures panic attacks, anticipatory anxiety, and limited symptom attacks
Yale-Brown Obsessive-Compulsive Scale (YBOCS)	Clinician rated	Semi-structured interview	Consists of several clusters of obsessions and compulsions. Used to assess baseline severity and change in treatment studies

CONCLUSIONS

Patient assessment is the basis from which a pharmaceutical care plan evolves. Problem identification and therapeutic monitoring cannot occur until a thorough assessment is completed. The initial assessment provides the basis for evaluating response to therapy throughout the course of treatment. Psychiatric assessment requires empathy and good listening skills on the part of the clinician because it is based primarily upon subjective interpretation and not objective tests. With careful data collection, clinicians can make substantial contributions to care that improve patient outcomes.

ACKNOWLEDGEMENTS

The authors are grateful to Patricia A. Marken, PharmD, FCCP, BCPP, Professor of Pharmacy Practice at the University of Missouri–Kansas City, College of Pharmacy, for her significant contributions to this chapter in previous editions.

ABBREVIATIONS

ADAS: Alzheimer's Disease Assessment Scale

AIMS: Abnormal Involuntary Movement Scale

APA: American Psychiatric Association

BAS: Barnes Akathisia Scale

BDI: Beck Depression Inventory

BIMC: Blessed Information Memory Concentration (test)

BPRS: Brief Psychiatric Rating Scale

CDT: Clock Drawing test

CGI (S): Clinical Global Impression Severity of Illness scale

CGI (I): Clincial Global Impression Global Improvement Scale

DISCUS: Dyskinesia Identification System: Condensed User Scale

DRS-2: Dementia Rating Scale

DSM-IV-TR: Diagnostic and Statistical Manual of Mental Disorders, Fourth Edition, Text Revision

EPS: extrapyramidal symptoms

GAF: Global Assessment of Functioning

HDRS: Hamilton Depression Rating Scale

MADRS: Montgomery-Asberg Rating Scale

MDQ: Mood Disorder Questionnaire

MMPI-2: Minnesota Multiphasic Personality Inventory-2

MMSE: Mini-Mental Status Examination

MSE: Mental Status Examination

MMSE: Mini-Mental Status Exam cognitive rating scale

PANSS: Positive and Negative Syndrome Scale

PHQ-9: Patient Health Questionnaire for assessment of depression

QIDS-C: Quick Inventory of Depressive Symptomatology-Clinician rating scale

QIDS-SR: Quick Inventory of Depressive Symptomatology-Subject rating scale

SAFTEE-GI: Systematic Assessment for Treatment Emergent Events-General Inquiry

SPAAS: Sheehan Panic and Anticipatory Anxiety Scale

YBOCS: Yale-Brown Obsessive-Compulsive Scale

YMRS: Young Mania Rating Scale

ZSDS: Zung Self-Rating Depression Scale

REFERENCES

1. Othmer E. Psychiatric interview, history, and mental status examination. In: Sadock BJ, Sadock VA, eds. Comprehensive Textbook of Psychiatry, Vol. 1, 8th ed. Philadelphia, PA: Lippincott Williams & Wilkins, 2005:794–826.

2. Guze BH, Love MJ, Deutsch SI. Medical assessment and laboratory testing in psychiatry. In: Sadock BJ, Sadock VA, eds. Comprehensive Textbook of Psychiatry, Vol. 1, 8th ed. Philadelphia, PA: Lippincott Williams & Wilkins, 2005:916–928.

3. Adams RL, Culbertson JL. Personality assessment: Adults and children. In: Sadock BJ, Sadock VA, eds. Comprehensive Textbook of Psychiatry, Vol. 1, 8th ed. Philadelphia, PA: Lippincott Williams & Wilkins, 2005:874–894.

4. Blacker D. Psychiatric rating scales. In: Sadock BJ, Sadock VA, eds. Comprehensive Textbook of Psychiatry, Vol. 1, 8th ed. Philadelphia. PA: Lippincott Williams & Wilkins, 2005:929–954.

5. McIntyre JS, Charles SC. Psychiatric evaluation of adults second edition. Am J Psychiatry 2006;163(Suppl)1:1–36.

6. Price P. Mental Status. In: Jones RM; Rospond RM, eds. Patient Assessment in Pharmacy Practice, 2nd ed. Philadelphia, PA: Lippincott Williams & Wilkins, 2008:368–413.

7. American Psychiatric Association. Diagnostic and Statistical Manual of Mental Disorders, Fourth Edition, Text Revision (DSM-IV-TR). Washington, DC: American Psychiatric Association, 2000.

8. Dickerson FB, Brown CH, Daumit DL, et al. Health status of individuals with serious mental illness. Schizophr Bull 2006;32:584–589.

9. Hennekens CH, Hennekens AR, Hollar D, Casey DE. Schizophrenia and increased risks of cardiovascular disease. Am Heart J 2005;150:1115–1121.

10. Cradock-O'Leary J, Young AS, Yano EM, et al. Use of general medical services by VA patients with psychiatric disorders. Psychiatr Serv 2002;53:874–878.

11. Bauer MS, Williford WO, McBride K, Shea NM. Perceived barriers to health care access in a treated population. Int J Psychiatry Med 2005;35:13–26.

12. American Diabetes Association, American Psychiatric Association, American Association of Clinical Endocrinologists, North American Association for the Study of Obesity. Consensus development conference on antipsychotic drugs and obesity and diabetes. Diabetes Care 2004;27:596–601.

13. Cohn TA, Sernyak MJ. Metabolic monitoring for patients treated with antipsychotic medications. Can J Psychiatry 2006;51:492–501.

14. Amiel JM, Mangurian CV, Ganguli R, Newcomer JW. Addressing cardiometabolic risk during treatment with antipsychotic medications. Curr Opin Psychiatry 2008;21:613–618.

15. Mackin P, Bishop DR, Watkinson H. A prospective study of monitoring practices for metabolic disease in antipsychotic treated community psychiatric patients [online exclusive article]. BMC Psychiatry 2007;7:28. http://www.biomedcentral.com/1471-244X/7/28.

16. Schneiderhan ME, Batscha C, Rosen C, Results of point-of-care glucose testing and basic metabolic screening in outpatients on antipsychotic agents. Pharmacother 2009;28(8):975–997.

17. Cipolle RJ, Strand LM, Morley PC. The Assessment. In: Pharmaceutical Care Practice: The Clinician's Guide, 2nd ed. New York: McGraw-Hill, 2004:152–161.

18. Leucht S, Kane JM, Kissling W, Hamann J, Etschel E, Engel R. Clinical implications of Brief Psychiatric Rating Scale scores. Br J Psych 2005;187:366–371.

19. Guy W. ECDEU (Early Clinical Drug Evaluation Unit) Assessment Manual for Psychopharmacology, rev. ed. DHEW (Department of Health, Education, and Welfare) Publication (ADM) 76–338. Washington, DC: U.S. Government Printing Office, 1976:158–169.

20. Leucht S, Kane JM, Kissling W, Hamann J, Etschel E, Engel RR. What does the PANSS mean? Schizophren Res 2005;79:231–238.

21. Schooler NR, Chengappa KNR. Adverse effect measures. In: Rush AJ, Pincus HA, First MB, et al., eds. Handbook of Psychiatric Measures, Vol. 11. Washington, DC: American Psychiatric Association, 2000:151–168.

22. Thompson C. Introduction. In: Thompson C, ed. The Instruments of Psychiatric Research. New York: Wiley, 1989:1–16.

23. Fankhauser MP, German ML. Understanding the use of behavioral rating scales in studies evaluating the efficacy of antianxiety and antidepressant drugs. Am J Hosp Pharm 1987;44:2087–2100.

24. Montgomery SA, Asberg M. A new depression scale designed to be sensitive to change. Br J Psychiatry 1979;134:382–389.

25. Sheehan DV. The Anxiety Disease. New York: Bantam, 1983:114–115.

26. Goodman WK, Price LH, Rasmussen SA, et al. The Yale-Brown Obsessive Compulsive Scale (Y-BOCS): II. Validity. Arch Gen Psychiatry 1989;46:1006–1011.

27. Folstein MF, Folstein SE, McHugh PR. "Mini-mental-state". A practical method for grading the cognitive state of patients for the clinician. J Psych Res 1975;12(3):189–198.

28. Blessed G, Tomlinson BE, Roth M. The association between quantitative measures of dementia and of senile change in the cerebral grey matter of elderly subjects. Br J Psychiatry 1968;114(512):797–811.

29. Mattis S. Mental status examination for organic mental syndrome in the elderly patient. In: Bellak L, Karasu TB, eds. Geriatric Psychiatry. New York: Grune & Stratton, 1976:77–101.

30. Sunderland T, Hill JL, Mellow AM, et al. Clock drawing in Alzheimer's disease: A novel measure of dementia severity. Am Geriatric Soc 1989;37:725–729.

31. Rosen WG, Mohs RC, Davis KL. A new rating scale for Alzheimer's disease. Am J Psychiatry 1984;141:1356–1364.

JULIE A. DOPHEIDE AND STEPHEN R. PLISZKA

CHAPTER 72

Childhood Disorders

KEY CONCEPTS

❶ Inattention and impulsivity caused by attention deficit/hyperactivity disorder (ADHD) begins before age 7 years and can continue into adolescence and adulthood, often requiring ongoing drug treatment.

❷ Stimulants are first-line treatment for ADHD because they are the most effective medications and have overall good tolerability. Atomoxetine, guanfacine extended release (XR), and bupropion are second-line alternatives for those unresponsive to or unable to tolerate stimulants. Clonidine and guanfacine can also be considered as adjuncts to stimulants to optimize treatment of oppositional symptoms or persistent insomnia.

❸ Coexisting disorders or symptoms such as anxiety, mood, and behavior dysregulation have an impact on drug selection for ADHD and can necessitate the use of additional agents.

❹ Tourette's disorder presents with both motor and vocal tics, which are present during childhood, plateau during adolescence, and can continue during adulthood with a fluctuating course.

❺ The decision to medicate patients with Tourette's disorder is based on the degree of concern perceived by the patient, symptom severity, and comorbid disorders.

❻ Individuals with Tourette's disorder are particularly sensitive to medication side effects, so medication dosing must be individualized carefully, and close monitoring is essential.

❼ Nondrug approaches to enuresis management, such as behavioral interventions and the use of bed-wetting alarms, are preferred because of lasting cure rates and avoidance of drug side effects.

❽ Desmopressin tablets are preferred over tricyclic antidepressants (TCAs) because of better safety and tolerability. Both desmopressin and TCAs have a rapid onset of effect (1–2 weeks); however, the relapse rate on drug discontinuation is high.

All neuropsychiatric disorders can first present during childhood.[1] Attention deficit/hyperactivity disorder (ADHD), Tourette's disorder, and enuresis are the focus of this chapter because, by definition, the onset of symptoms explicitly occurs during childhood.

Learning objectives, review questions, and other resources can be found at **www.pharmacotherapyonline.com**.

Treating children with psychotropic drugs requires a very different approach than treating adults. Children undergo neurologic, physiologic, and psychosocial changes throughout development. Age-related pharmacodynamic and pharmacokinetic differences can alter drug disposition and response. Well-defined diagnostic criteria guide drug selection;[1] however, comorbid disorders present treatment challenges.[2,3] Children may not be able to articulate symptom response or adverse effects of a medication. Psychotropic drug treatment of children is intended to control symptoms or behaviors that impair learning and development.[2,3]

The psychiatric assessment of a child requires obtaining information from the child, parents, caregivers, and teachers.

ATTENTION DEFICIT/HYPERACTIVITY DISORDER

A diagnosis of ADHD should be considered whenever a child presents with developmentally inappropriate inattention, impulsivity, and/or hyperactivity. Symptom presence and severity vary with the situation. It is unusual for a child to display signs of the disorder in all settings or even in the same setting at all times.[1]

CLINICAL PRESENTATION AND EPIDEMIOLOGY

❶ The onset of ADHD is typically by the age of 3 years and must occur by age 7 to meet the diagnostic criteria of the *Diagnostic and Statistical Manual of Mental Disorders* (Fourth Edition, Text Revision; *DSM-IV-TR*). However, recent studies in adults are challenging the age of onset criteria, suggesting little difference in functional impairment and response to methylphenidate in adults who meet onset criteria before age 7 and those who meet all criteria except age of onset.[5] ADHD occurs in 6% to 9% of children and is estimated to be present in 4% of adults.[3,4] In the United States, four boys are diagnosed with ADHD for every girl. This difference is likely because of higher rates of oppositional defiant disorder and conduct disorder in boys, compared with girls; thus, referrals for assessment are higher for boys. Symptoms can persist lifelong for both sexes, but hyperactivity is much less prominent in adolescence and adulthood.[3,6–8]

CLINICAL PRESENTATION OF ADHD

General
- Onset of symptoms must be before 7 years of age.

Symptoms
- Six or more of the symptoms must be present for 6 months; significant impairment must be seen in two or more settings

(e.g., home and school); symptoms must be documented by parent, teacher, and clinician.

- *Inattention*
  - Often fails to give close attention to details or makes careless mistakes in schoolwork or other activities
  - Often has difficulty sustaining attention
  - Often has difficulty organizing tasks and activities
  - Avoids tasks that require sustained mental effort
  - Often does not seem to listen when spoken to directly
  - Often does not follow through on instructions and fails to finish schoolwork, chores, or duties in the workplace
  - Is easily distracted by extraneous stimuli
  - Is often forgetful in daily activities
  - Loses things necessary for activities
- *Hyperactivity and impulsivity*
  - Often fidgets with hands or feet or squirms in seat
  - Often leaves seat when remaining seated is expected
  - Often runs about or climbs excessively at inappropriate times
  - Often has difficulty playing quietly
  - Often interrupts or intrudes on others

Data from American Psychiatric Association. Disorders usually First Evident in Infancy, Childhood or Adolescence. Diagnostic and Statistical Manual of Mental Disorders. 4th ed. Text rev. Washington, DC: American Psychiatric Association 2000:39–134.

Inattention and distractibility can be symptoms of an anxiety, mood, or psychotic disorder.[3,4,6] In some cases, other disorders coexist with ADHD; learning deficiencies and conduct or oppositional disorders are common comorbid conditions.[3,4,6] The presence of multiple comorbid conditions, particularly conduct or mood disorder, can increase the likelihood of ADHD chronicity into adulthood.[2,3,6,7]

Prescriptions for ADHD medication are increasing in all age groups, particularly in adolescents and young adults.[3,9] A National Poison Control Center study estimates that between 1998 and 2005, prescriptions for teenagers and preteenagers increased 133% for amphetamine products and 52% for methylphenidate products, 80% for both.[9]

ETIOLOGY AND PATHOPHYSIOLOGY

Both genetic and nongenetic factors are implicated in the pathogenesis. First-degree relatives of an individual with ADHD have a four- to eightfold increased chance of developing ADHD compared with the general population; monozygotic twins have up to a 90% concordance rate for ADHD.[3,10] Children with fetal alcohol syndrome, lead poisoning, and meningitis have a higher incidence of ADHD symptomatology.[3,4] ADHD is associated with a variety of environmental risks, including obstetric adversity, maternal smoking, and adverse parent–child relationships.[3,4] Dietary causes are unlikely.[3,4]

Although there are no definitive pathophysiologic markers for ADHD, imaging studies show subjects with ADHD have decreased total brain volume relative to controls in multiple brain regions (right prefrontal cortex, caudate nucleus, anterior cingulate gyrus, and cerebellum). Global thinning of the cortex has been observed in children with ADHD, and comparative studies show there is a delay

in cortical thickening in ADHD brains relative to age-matched controls.[3] These brain changes are thought to impair executive functioning necessary for prioritization of tasks, decision making, motor control, and an awareness of space and time.[3,11] Alterations in the "default mode" attention network have been found in adults with ADHD.[3] A lack of connectivity between the prefrontal cortex and precuneus (located in the midline of the parietal lobe) is associated with failure of suppression of the default mode network, causing lapses in attention and inhibitory control.[3]

Genetically mediated changes in serotonergic, cholinergic, and most notably dopaminergic function have been documented in children and adults with ADHD.[3,10,11] Deficits in the dopaminergic reward pathway in the ADHD brain impair the ability to delay gratification, resist distractions, regulate arousal, and attend to information or tasks that are dull or repetitive.[12] This dysfunction involves multiple dopaminergic receptors (D_2, D_3, D_4, and D_5) and dopamine active transporter protein (DAT), which is presynaptic.[11,12] Norepinephrine and epinephrine are agonists at dopaminergic receptors and are modulated by DAT as well.[13,14] Treatment with stimulants has been shown to improve the rate of cortical thickening, and pharmacotherapy can improve or normalize dopaminergic receptor function.[3,11] Those with demonstrated abnormalities in DAT seem to respond better to methylphenidate and atomoxetine.[13,14]

Effective treatments modulate dopamine and norepinephrine to improve executive functioning, regulate arousal, and sustain attention for improved performance. The clinical response associated with stimulants is not paradoxical and is not diagnostic for ADHD because stimulants can increase attention, decrease motor activity, and improve learning tasks in those with subclinical ADHD or in individuals with such problems from other sources (e.g., fatigue).[3,4,13]

TREATMENT

■ STIMULANTS

❷ ❸ Stimulants are considered first-line therapy in most cases of ADHD; however, comorbid conditions impact the drug selection process. Pharmacotherapy should be considered whenever a thorough diagnostic assessment results in a diagnosis of ADHD. Several studies demonstrate the superiority of stimulants over behavioral interventions in alleviating core symptoms of ADHD.[3,4,6] Emerging literature shows improvement in academic performance in medicated children with ADHD versus those unmedicated.[15,16,17] One National Institutes of Health (NIH) study of 594 fifth graders with ADHD showed those medicated (greater than 90% took stimulants) had 2.9 points higher math scores and 5.4 points higher reading scores compared with unmedicated children.[16] Another study involving 363 10- to 18-year-olds with ADHD showed medication improved but did not normalize cognition.[18]

Multimodal treatment, individualized to the specific needs of the child and family, is crucial for an overall positive therapeutic outcome.[4,16,19] Table 72–1 describes behavioral interventions for ADHD. Multimodal treatment includes parent training, family therapy, classroom interventions, and contingency management (e.g., rewards for good behavior).[4,6,7] Figure 72–1 provides an algorithm for drug selection in the treatment of ADHD.

Stimulants (e.g., methylphenidate, dexmethylphenidate, mixed amphetamine salts, and dextroamphetamine) are the most effective drug treatment options, with efficacy ranging from 70% to 96%.[3,4,6]

Methylphenidate and amphetamines block dopamine and norepinephrine reuptake; amphetamines also increase catecholamine release.[13] Both drugs inhibit monoamine oxidase (MAO), or

TABLE 72-1 Behavioral Interventions for ADHD

Technique	Description	Example
Positive reinforcement	Providing rewards or privileges contingent on the child's performance	Child completes an assignment and is permitted to play on the computer
Time-out	Removing access to positive reinforcement contingent on performance of unwanted or problem behavior	Child hits sibling impulsively and is required to sit for 5 minutes in the corner of the room
Response cost	Withdrawing rewards or privileges contingent on the performance of unwanted or problem behavior	Child loses free-time privileges for not completing homework
Token economy	Combining positive reinforcement and response cost. Child earns rewards and privileges contingent on performing desired behaviors and loses the rewards and privileges based on undesirable behavior	Child earns stars for completing assignments and loses stars for getting out of seat. The child cashes in the sum of stars at the end of the week for a prize

From Dopheide JA, Pliszka SR. Attention deficit hyperactivity disorder: An update. Pharmacotherapy 2009;29(6):656–679; Pliszka SR, Bernet W, Bukstein O, et al, for the American Academy of Child and Adolescent Psychiatry Work Group on Quality Issues. Practice parameter for the assessment and treatment of children and adolescents with attention deficit/hyperactivity disorder. J Am Acad Child Adolesc Psychiatry 2007;46:894–921; Jensen PS, Arnold LE, Swanson JM, et al. Three-year follow-up of the NIMH MTA study. J Am Acad Child Adolesc Psychiatry 2007;46:989–1002; and American Academy of Pediatrics. Clinical practice guideline: Treatment of the school-aged child with ADHD. Pediatrics 2001;108:1033–1044.

amphetamines, more potently than methylphenidate.[13] Because different stimulants work through slightly different mechanisms, the lack of response to one chemical class of stimulant (e.g., methylphenidate or dexmethylphenidate) does not preclude response to another class (e.g., dextroamphetamine or mixed amphetamine salts).[3,4,6]

Stimulant dosing should be titrated for maximum individual efficacy and minimum side effects (see Table 72–2).[3,4]

With immediate-release stimulants, most patients require a two or three times daily dosing schedule because of the short half-lives of these drugs (2–4 hours for methylphenidate and dexmethylphenidate and ~4–6 hours for dextroamphetamine or mixed

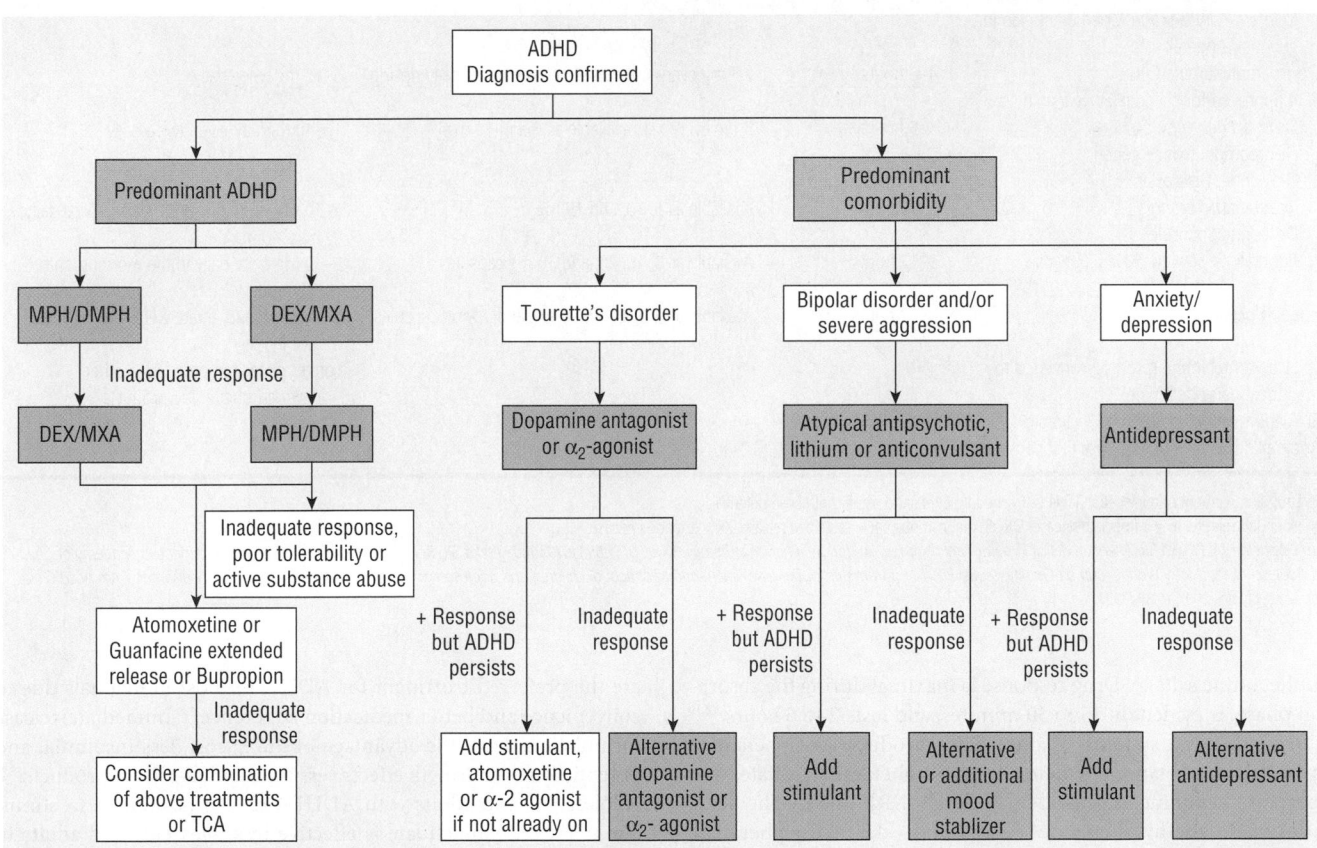

FIGURE 72-1. Algorithm for management of attention deficit/hyperactivity disorder (ADHD). Treat predominant disorder first, reassess, and consider alternative or adjunct medications for optimal symptom control. (DEX, dextroamphetamine; DMPH, dexmethylphenidate; MPH, methylphenidate; MXA, mixed amphetamine salts; TCA, tricyclic antidepressant.) (*Data from Dopheide JA, Pliszka SR. Attention deficit hyperactivity disorder: An update. Pharmacotherapy 2009;29(6):656–679; Pliszka SR, Bernet W, Bukstein O, et al, for the American Academy of Child and Adolescent Psychiatry Work Group on Quality Issues. Practice parameter for the assessment and treatment of children and adolescents with attention deficit/hyperactivity disorder. J Am Acad Child Adolesc Psychiatry 2007;46:894–921; Pliszka SR, Crismon ML, Hughes CW, et al. The Texas Children's Medication Algorithm project: Revision of the algorithm for pharmacotherapy of childhood attention-deficit/hyperactivity disorder. J Am Acad Child Adolesc Psychiatry 2006;45(6):642–657; Kowatch RA, DelBello MP. Pediatric bipolar disorder: Emerging diagnostic and treatment approaches. Child Adolesc Psych Clin N Am 2006;15:73–108; Dopheide JA. Recognizing and treating depression in children and adolescents. Am J Health Syst Pharm 2006;63:233–243; Kenny C, Kuo SH, Jimenez-Shahed J. Tourette's syndrome. Am Fam Physician 2008;77(5):651–660; and Muller-Vahl JT. The treatment of Tourette's syndrome: Current opinions. Expert Opin Pharmacother 2002;3:899–914.*)

TABLE 72-2 Stimulant Drugs Used in the Treatment of ADHD

Stimulant	Duration of Effect	Initial Dose and Available Strengths	Usual Dosing Range Maximum Dose
FDA approved for children ≥6years old			
Methylphenidate C-II[a]			
Short-acting IR	3–5 hours	5 mg two or three times daily; increase by 5–10 or 20 mg/day at weekly intervals	5–20 mg two or three times a day; max dose: 60 mg/day
Ritalin, methylin, generics			
Intermediate-acting	3–8 hours	SR, ER doses; corresponds to the IR dose	20–40 mg every A.M. or 40 mg every A.M. and 20 mg in the early afternoon; max dose: 60 mg/day
Ritalin SR			
Methylphenidate SR			
Metadate ER			
Methylin ER			
Long-acting	8–12 hours	20 mg every A.M.; available as 10, 20, and 30 mg	20–40 mg every A.M. and 20 mg in the early afternoon; max dose: 60 mg/day
Metadate CD 30% IR, 70% ER beads			
Ritalin LA 50% IR, 50% ER beads		20 mg every A.M.; available as 20, 30, and 40 mg	20–60 mg/day, given every A.M.; max dose: 60 mg/day
Concerta (OROS controlled-release delivery)			
ER inner compartments coated with IR methylphenidate		18 mg every A.M.; available as 18, 27, 36, and 54 mg; 90% bioavailability of IR	27–72 mg/day, given every A.M.; max dose: 72 mg/day
Daytrana methylphenidate transdermal system	12 hours when worn for 9 hours	10 mg (12.5 cm^2) applied to clean, dry area on hip each morning and removed after 9 hours	10 to 30 mg (12.5–37.5 cm^2) Drug active for 3 hours after patch removal
Dexmethylphenidate (Focalin) C-II	3–5 hours	2.5 mg every A.M. or twice daily; available as 2.5, 5, and 10 mg tablets	5–10 mg/day given twice a day; max initial dose: 7.5 mg/day; max dose: 20 mg/day
FDA approved for children ≥6 years old			
Focalin XR 50% IR, 50% ER beads	8–12 hours	5 mg every A.M.; available as 5, 10, and 20 mg capsules	5–20 mg/day, given every A.M. max dose: 20 mg/day
Mixed amphetamine salts C-II	4–6 hours	2.5 mg every A.M. once or twice daily dosing	10–40 mg/day (divided in two doses)
FDA approved for children ≥3 years old Short- to intermediate-acting Mixed amphetamine generics, Adderall			
Dextroamphetamine C-II	4–6 hours	2.5 mg every A.M. to two or three times daily dosing	5–15 mg twice daily
FDA approved for children ≥6 years old			
Short-acting	3–5 hours	5 mg every A.M.; available as 5 and 10 mg	10–40 mg/day given twice daily
Dextroamphetamine generics			
Dexedrine, Dextrostat			
Intermediate-acting	5–8 hours	Available as 5, 10, and 15 mg	5–30 mg every day or 5–15 mg twice daily; max: 40 mg/day
Dexedrine Spansule			
Adderall XR 50% IR, 50% ER beads	8–12 hours	Available as 5, 10, 20, and 30 mg capsules	5–30 mg once daily in the morning; max: 30 mg/day
Long-acting	8–12 hours	Available as 20, 30, 40, 50, 60, and 70 mg capsules	Start at low end, titrate weekly to response; give in A.M.
Lisdexamfetamine (prodrug converted to dextroamphetamine)			Longer onset compared with other dextroamphetamine products
FDA approved for children >6 years old			
Adderall XR 50% IR beads, 50% ER beads			

[a]The Drug Enforcement Administration label C-II, schedule II refers to significant abuse potential.
ER = extended release, IR = immediate release, OROS, oral osmotic, SR = sustained release, XR = extended release.
From Dopheide JA, Pliszka SR. Attention deficit hyperactivity disorder: An update. Pharmacotherapy 2009;29(6):656–679; and Pliszka SR, Bernet W, Bukstein O, et al, for the American Academy of Child and Adolescent Psychiatry Work Group on Quality Issues. Practice parameter for the assessment and treatment of children and adolescents with attention deficit/hyperactivity disorder. J Am Acad Child Adolesc Psychiatry 2007;46:894–921.

amphetamine salts).[3,4] Drug response is maximal during the absorption phase, is evident in 15 to 30 minutes, and lasts 2 to 6 hours.[3,4,19]

Drug delivery systems of once-daily products (amphetamine aspartate, amphetamine sulfate, dextroamphetamine sulfate, and dextroamphetamine saccharate [Adderall XR]; methylphenidate [Concerta]; methylphenidate [Daytrana]; dexmethylphenidate [Focalin XR]; methylphenidate [Metadate CD]; and methylphenidate long-acting [Ritalin LA]) provide 8 to 12 hours of symptom control.[3,4,6] Concerta uses an oral osmotic controlled-release delivery system, whereas other oral preparations use combinations of immediate-release and extended-release beads.[3,4] Concerta is a nondeformable tablet, and it should not be given to children with gastrointestinal (GI) narrowing because of the risk of obstruction. Methylphenidate transdermal system provides 12 hours of symptom control when worn for 9 hours.[4] Older wax-matrix sustained-release (SR) products (e.g., Ritalin SR) are less effective and infrequently used.[3,4] Once-daily stimulant formulations are the preferred treatment for ADHD in most individuals due to convenience and better medication adherence.[3,4] Immediate-release formulations have the advantage of lower cost, less insomnia, and potentially fewer growth effects versus extended-release products.[3,20] Adolescents and adults with ADHD are also responsive to stimulants.[21,22] Methylphenidate is effective in adolescents and adults in doses up to 1.5 mg/kg daily.[3,4,20] Lisdexamfetamine is a prodrug conjugated to an amino acid that requires cleavage during metabolism to the active dextroamphetamine. It has a longer onset of effect but may provide a smoother blood level compared with extended-release formulations. It is intended to pose less abuse potential.[3,4]

■ ADVERSE EFFECTS

The most common adverse effects of stimulants and their management strategies are listed in Table 72–3. Uncommon to rare but potentially serious adverse effects are discussed in the following sections.

TABLE 72-3	Stimulant Adverse Effects and Their Management
Adverse Effect	**Recommendation/Management Strategy**
Common	
Reduced appetite, weight loss	Give high-calorie meal when stimulant effects are low (at breakfast or at bedtime), or consider cyproheptadine at bedtime
Stomachache	Administer stimulant on a full stomach, lower dose if possible
Insomnia	Give dose earlier in the day; lower the last dose of the day or give it earlier; consider a sedating medication at bedtime (guanfacine, clonidine, melatonin, or cyproheptadine)
Headache	Divide dose, give with food, or give an analgesic (e.g., acetaminophen or ibuprofen)
Rebound symptoms	Consider longer-acting stimulant trial, atomoxetine, or antidepressant
Irritability/jitteriness	Assess for comorbid condition (e.g., bipolar disorder); reduce dosage; consider mood stabilizer or atypical antipsychotic
Uncommon to rare	
Dysphoria	Reduce dosage; reassess diagnosis; consider alternative therapy
Zombie-like state	Reduce dosage or change stimulant medication
Tics or abnormal movements	Reduce dosage; consider alternative medication
Hypertension, pulse fluctuations	Reduce dosage; change medication
Hallucinations	Discontinue stimulant; reassess diagnosis; mood stabilizer and/or antipsychotic may be needed

From Dopheide JA, Pliszka SR. Attention deficit hyperactivity disorder: An update. Pharmacotherapy 2009;29(6):656–679; and Pliszka SR, Bernet W, Bukstein O, et al, for the American Academy of Child and Adolescent Psychiatry Work Group on Quality Issues. Practice parameter for the assessment and treatment of children and adolescents with attention deficit/hyperactivity disorder. J Am Acad Child Adolesc Psychiatry 2007;46:894–921.

Psychiatric

The Food and Drug Administration (FDA) has added warnings to the labeling of all stimulants and atomoxetine. Hundreds of post-marketing reports of three broad categories of psychiatric adverse events have been associated with stimulants: psychosis or mania, aggression or violent behavior, and severe anxiety or panic attacks. All of these reactions require dose reduction or cessation of stimulant therapy and supportive treatment.[3,4]

Cardiac

A boxed warning for cardiovascular risks including sudden unexplained death has been added to ADHD stimulant drug labeling.[3] Clinical trial data show that children who take stimulants for ADHD can have an increased heart rate by ~5 beats/minute and/or increased blood pressure by 2 to 7 mm Hg.[23] A 10-year review showed a 20% increased risk for emergency department visits for cardiac symptoms in those taking either methylphenidate or amphetamine.[23] Of note, these individuals were more likely to have a coexisting anxiety disorder.

Stimulant products generally should not be used in pediatrics or adults with known structural cardiac abnormalities. The American Heart Association recommends careful screening of all children and adolescents prior to initiating pharmacologic therapy for ADHD, including a detailed patient and family history and physical examination. Ideally, a baseline electrocardiogram (ECG) should also be obtained, along with routine monitoring of pulse and blood pressure.[24] The FDA did not find the risk of sudden unexplained death to be greater in those taking stimulants than in the general population; therefore, no restriction in stimulant use has been recommended.[25]

Growth

Two reviews that analyzed approximately 32 studies indicated that stimulant treatment of ADHD can affect growth, but the effects are minimal or insignificant for most children. A study of 579 children showed a decrease of ~1 cm/year (~0.5 inch) in height over 1 to 3 years of continuous treatment with methylphenidate and a weight deficit of 3 kg (6.6 lbs) in the first year of treatment and 1.2 kg (2.6 lbs) in the second year of treatment.[3] Amphetamine products may be associated with more prominent growth effects than methylphenidate according to separate studies.[3] Proposed mechanisms of stimulant effects on growth include alterations in growth hormone or growth factor, decreased thyroxine secretion, and suppression of appetite leading to reduced caloric intake.[3,4,20]

In most cases, children should be given a drug-free trial every year.[4] Time off stimulant appears to lessen stimulant growth suppressant effects, but evidence is lacking to firmly determine the impact of drug holidays on growth.[3,4] Consideration must be given to the risks of negative effects on learning, socialization, and self-image while off stimulant therapy when determining the frequency and duration of the drug-free trial. Drug holidays are important because they provide time to reassess the need for continued treatment.[3,4] Drug dosage often varies from year to year, largely because of age-related pharmacokinetic changes. As a child develops, hepatic metabolism slows, and volume of distribution increases.

▪ NONSTIMULANTS

❷ Extended-release atomoxetine and guanfacine are second-line alternatives to the stimulants for treatment of ADHD in children and adolescents. Atomoxetine is also approved in adults. Their potential benefits relative to stimulants include no abuse potential, less potential for growth effects, and less sleep disturbance.[3,4] See Table 72–4 for dosing.

Atomoxetine is a selective norepinephrine reuptake inhibitor that should be taken in divided doses in the morning or late afternoon by children for improved tolerability. Adults can take it once daily, usually in the morning.[3,4] Placebo-controlled, short-term trials (6–12 weeks) have shown that atomoxetine is effective in reducing ADHD symptoms in children, teens, and adults, and 9-month continuation studies show ongoing benefit for responders. A controlled trial comparing atomoxetine, oral osmotic methylphenidate, and placebo over 6 weeks in 6- to 16-year-old patients showed that both drugs were significantly better than placebo at improving ADHD symptoms, but oral osmotic methylphenidate was superior to atomoxetine.[3,4]

Atomoxetine has a significantly slower onset of therapeutic effect than stimulants (2–4 weeks vs 1 hour with an effective stimulant dose). Atomoxetine is sometimes combined with a stimulant in partially responsive patients based on case series describing fewer late-day rebound effects and better sleep when atomoxetine is given in the evening; however, adverse effects are additive.[3,4,6]

Guanfacine and clonidine are central α_2-adrenergic agonists, acting both presynaptically to inhibit norepinephrine release and postsynaptically to increase blood flow in the prefrontal cortex. Increased blood flow in the prefrontal cortex has been shown to enhance working memory and executive functioning. Both interact with a multitude of neurotransmitter systems, including catecholamine, indolamine, α_2-receptors on parasympathetic neurons, opioids, imidazole, and amino acid systems.[13] Guanfacine has a longer elimination half-life (12–18 hours) compared with clonidine (2.5–4 hours), and its greater selectivity for the α_{2a}-receptor, compared with clonidine, imparts less sedation. Clonidine and immediate-release guanfacine are not as effective as stimulants for monotherapy treatment. They are prescribed frequently as

TABLE 72-4 Dosing and Adverse Effect Monitoring of Nonstimulant Drugs for ADHD

Drug	Dosing Range and Titration Schedule	Adverse Effect Monitoring
Antidepressants		
Atomoxetine (Strattera)	≤70 kg (≤154 lbs): start at 0.3–0.5 mg/kg every A.M. or twice daily, max: 1.4 mg/kg/day; ≥70 kg (≥154 lbs): start at 40 mg every A.M. or twice daily, max: 100 mg/day	Nausea, anorexia, ↑ blood pressure, ↑ pulse, insomnia, fatigue, sedation, severe liver injury, suicidality
Bupropion (Wellbutrin SR, XL)	50–300 mg/day; 3 mg/kg/day by end of week 1; can increase to 6 mg/kg/day or maximum of 300 mg/day as tolerated	Nausea, insomnia, rash, tics; dose-related risk of seizures
Tricyclic antidepressants: imipramine, desipramine, or nortriptyline	50–150 mg/day; start at 0.5–1 mg/kg/day; increase as tolerated to 2–3 mg/kg/day; max: 300 mg/day of desipramine (adults only) or 150 mg/day nortriptyline	Sedation, dizziness, constipation, heart block (check ECG), weight gain, overdose toxicity, rapid heartbeat
Antipsychotics		
Aripiprazole[a] (Abilify)	2–5 mg daily; can titrate weekly as tolerated to response (usual range: 5–20 mg/day)	Nausea, restlessness, insomnia extrapyramidal symptoms, dizziness, sedation
Haloperidol[a] (Haldol)	0.5–1 mg twice daily; can titrate every 3–4 days as tolerated to response (usual range: 0.5–5 mg/day)	Extrapyramidal symptoms, dizziness, ↑ prolactin, sedation
Olanzapine[a] (Zyprexa)	2.5–5 mg every day; can titrate every 3–4 days as tolerated to response (usual range: 7.5–15 mg/day)	Sedation, severe weight gain, restlessness, extrapyramidal symptom Diabetes, marked hyperlipidemia (never a first-line treatment)
Quetiapine[a] (Seroquel)	25–50 mg twice daily; can titrate every 3–4 days as tolerated to response (usual range: 200–600 mg/day)	Sedation, dizziness, weight gain, diabetes, hyperlipidemia
Risperidone[a] (Risperdal)	0.25–0.5 mg twice daily; can titrate every 3–4 days as tolerated to response (1–4 mg/day)	Extrapyramidal symptoms, dizziness, ↑ prolactin, hepatotoxicity, weight gain Diabetes, hyperlipidemia
Ziprasidone[a] (Geodon)	10–20 mg twice daily; can titrate every 3–4 days as tolerated to response (usual range: 40–120 mg/day)	Nausea, restlessness, insomnia extrapyramidal symptoms, sedation, QTc prolongation
Other		
Clonidine (Catapres)	0.05 mg two or four times daily; can increase as tolerated to 0.1–0.4 mg/day	Sedation, dizziness, heart block (check ECG), constipation
Guanfacine (Tenex) or guanfacine extended release (Intuniv)	0.5 once or twice daily; can increase as tolerated to 1–4 mg/day Give 1 mg in the A.M., titrate weekly to response	Same as above with potentially lower risk of sedation Effective dose higher in heavier children

ADHD = attention deficit/hyperactivity disorder, ECG = electrocardiogram; SR = sustained release, XL = extended-length.
[a]Short-term use (1–4 months) only for severe aggression associated with ADHD.
From Dopheide JA, Pliszka SR. Attention deficit hyperactivity disorder: An update. Pharmacotherapy 2009;29(6):656–679; Pliszka SR, Bernet W, Bukstein O, et al, for the American Academy of Child and Adolescent Psychiatry Work Group on Quality Issues. Practice parameter for the assessment and treatment of children and adolescents with attention deficit/hyperactivity disorder. J Am Acad Child Adolesc Psychiatry 2007;46:894–921; Schur SB, Sikich L, Findling RL, et al. Treatment recommendations for the use of antipsychotics for aggressive youth (TRAAY): 1. A review. J Am Acad Child Adolesc Psychiatry 2003;42:132–144; Pappadopulos E, Macintyre J, Crismon ML, et al. Treatment recommendations for the use of antipsychotics for aggressive youth (TRAAY): 2. J Am Acad Child Adolesc Psych 2003;42(2):145–161; and Correll CU. Assessing and maximizing the safety and tolerability of antipsychotics used in the treatment of children and adolescents. J Clin Psych 2008;69(Suppl 4):26–36.

adjuncts to reduce disruptive behavior, control aggression, or improve sleep.[3,4,6]

Extended-release guanfacine is approved for children and adolescents based on two large placebo-controlled trials involving over 300 patients each and long-term safety studies.[26,27] It appears at least as effective as other nonstimulants and is an acceptable second-line agent for children and adolescents unresponsive to or unable to tolerate stomach upset or insomnia with stimulant medications. Extended-release guanfacine is more sedating than stimulants or atomoxetine; therefore, sleepiness during the school day requires careful monitoring.

Bupropion, a monocyclic antidepressant, is a weak dopamine and norepinephrine reuptake inhibitor with no significant direct effect on serotonin or MAO. Its active metabolites augment noradrenergic and dopaminergic function. Investigations with bupropion in children demonstrated efficacy greater than placebo in two controlled trials and efficacy comparable with methylphenidate ($n = 15$ children) in another controlled trial.[3,4] Bupropion has less appetite suppression compared with stimulants but has a greater risk of seizures. It also may be effective in adults at antidepressant doses.[3,4,6,8]

Tricyclic antidepressants (TCAs) are last-line agents because they are the most dangerous in overdose and pose the greatest risk for cardiovascular side effects.[4,6] Imipramine and desipramine are the most systematically studied TCAs in the treatment of ADHD, although nortriptyline is also effective.[4,6] The onset of TCA clinical response occurs within the first 2 to 4 weeks.[4,6]

Variability in dosage requirements for atomoxetine, bupropion, and TCAs can be due to interpatient variability in plasma concentration achieved at a given dose. All are metabolized via cytochrome P450 (CYP) 2D6, and bioavailability and half-life can be 4 to 8 times greater in those taking a CYP2D6 inhibitor (e.g., bupropion, fluoxetine, or paroxetine) or in poor metabolizers. For example, atomoxetine's half-life is 5 hours in extensive metabolizers and 19 hours in poor metabolizers.[3,6] Bupropion is metabolized faster in prepubertal children, making twice daily dosing optimal for efficacy (even for bupropion SR).[6] Twice-daily dosing of atomoxetine is optimal in children and adolescents to improve tolerability.[3,6] Once-daily dosing of bupropion or atomoxetine is possible for most adults. If tolerance develops after months of therapy, a dosage adjustment can be necessary to compensate for age-related changes in distribution and metabolism.

❸ Lithium and anticonvulsants are used increasingly to control aggression and explosive behavior in patients with a diagnosis of ADHD. Some patients actually can have childhood-onset bipolar disorder or combined ADHD–bipolar disorder.[3,6] Lithium, valproate, and carbamazepine are effective for explosive behavior, aggression, and impulsivity, but they are not beneficial treatments for a child with the inattentive subtype of ADHD. Dosing starts in low divided doses with titration over 1 to 2 weeks to therapeutic response.[6,28]

Conventional antipsychotics improve symptoms of hyperactivity and impulsivity but can have negative effects on learning and cognitive functioning and can cause extrapyramidal side effects (e.g., dystonia and tardive dyskinesia) that limit their usefulness.[3,4,6,28] The atypical antipsychotics risperidone, olanzapine, quetiapine, ziprasidone, and aripiprazole have been used to control severe aggression in refractory cases of ADHD, particularly if conduct disorder or bipolar disorder coexists.[29,30] More studies are needed to clarify their place in therapy.[6,20,28–31]

If multiple drugs are started simultaneously, it is impossible to determine the impact of each drug. The predominance and urgency of symptoms guide the drug-selection process (see Fig. 72–1). For example, if a child presents as severely anxious or depressed with associated attentional problems, then an antidepressant should be initiated first with monitoring to determine if attentional symptoms improve.[3,4,6] When a child presents with severe ADHD and associated anxiety or depression, a stimulant should be initiated to treat the more severe ADHD. If ADHD symptoms improve significantly, but anxiety or depression persists, then an antidepressant can be added.[3,4,6] Careful monitoring is needed to detect drug interactions that lead to higher drug plasma levels and increased adverse effects.[6,28,32] Studies show that stimulants do not routinely make anxiety disorders worse, but they might not improve symptoms either.[3,4] In a child with epilepsy, methylphenidate is safe and effective; however, the child should be stabilized and seizure-free on an anticonvulsant prior to initiation of the stimulant.[33]

Adverse Effects

Possible adverse effects of atomoxetine, and their management, are similar to those of stimulants, including psychiatric and cardiac adverse effects (see Table 72–4). Atomoxetine has been associated with less growth suppression compared with stimulants, 0.44 cm over 2 years of treatment. It has a greater risk of fatigue, sedation, and dizziness compared with stimulants and bupropion. Unlike stimulants, atomoxetine labeling includes a bolded warning of potential for severe liver injury following reports in two patients. Also, it is the only FDA-approved ADHD medication with a labeled warning for new onset suicidality, 0.4% in atomoxetine treated patients versus 0% in patients receiving placebo.[3,4,6]

The most common side effects of clonidine and guanfacine are dose-dependent sedation, hypotension, and constipation.[3,4] Sedation usually subsides after 2 to 3 weeks of therapy.[3,4,6] Of concern are reports of bradycardia, syncope, rebound hypertension, heart block, and sudden death with clonidine.[6,34,35] Four children have died on the combination of methylphenidate and clonidine; however, complicating factors make it impossible to link the drug combination directly with the cause of death.[35] Overdoses, concurrent clonidine and stimulant administration, and missed doses of clonidine all add to the risk of adverse cardiovascular events.[32,33] Extended-release guanfacine appears to pose a lower risk of cardiac adverse effects according to available safety data.[26,27]

Bupropion's adverse effects include nausea, which can resolve over time or with slower dosage titration, and rash, which can require discontinuation of therapy if severe (see Table 72–4). Bupropion should not be used in children with a seizure or eating disorder because of unacceptable risk of seizures in these patients. Bupropion can cause or exacerbate tics.[3,4,6]

Possible central nervous system (CNS) adverse effects of TCAs include dizziness, aggressiveness, excitement, nightmares, insomnia, forgetfulness, and irritability. Similar to other antidepressants, TCAs carry a warning of the risk of new-onset suicidality in pediatric patients.[32] TCAs should be taken throughout the week and not just on school days. TCA-withdrawal effects are severe in children and include nausea, vomiting, and diarrhea.[32] Signs of CNS toxicity are confusion, impaired concentration, hallucinations, and delusions.

PHARMACOECONOMIC CONSIDERATIONS

A conservative annual cost of illness estimate for ADHD in 2005 dollars was calculated at $14,576 per child (range $12,000–$18,000). This estimate includes lost work for parents; the cost of special education, behavioral interventions, medications, and doctor and clinic visits; and the use of the juvenile justice system.[36] A large study found behavioral interventions were more expensive than immediate-release stimulant medication initially, but the long-term effects (e.g., lower rates of delinquency and substance abuse) lower costs. Atomoxetine was found most cost effective for those who could not take stimulants due to a lack of efficacy or poor tolerability.[37]

Once-daily stimulants are approximately 3 to 5 times as expensive as immediate-release formulations, but they can save money over time with improved adherence and symptom control. A retrospective analysis comparing immediate-release methylphenidate use patterns with oral osmotic methylphenidate use patterns in 5,939 patients over 34 months found that its use was associated with longer treatment periods, increased patient adherence, and fewer emergency room visits for injury, potentially decreasing overall costs.[38]

EVALUATION OF THERAPEUTIC OUTCOMES

Careful documentation of baseline symptoms and complaints over a 1-month predrug period is essential to the evaluation of therapeutic and adverse outcomes. Investigation regarding family history of psychiatric disorders and cardiac disease is essential to determine risk for related adverse drug reactions and to implement appropriate monitoring.[3,4] Baseline symptoms can be measured using videotapes, clinician rating scales (e.g., ADHD rating scale IV, Vanderbilt ADHD diagnostic scale), or both.[3,4] In addition, height, weight, and eating and sleeping patterns should be recorded at baseline and every 3 months.[3,4]

After the initiation and titration of any drug treatment, it is necessary that parents, teachers, and clinicians assess the overall functioning of the child using standardized rating scales to determine if significant therapeutic benefit justifies continuing medication.[3,4] Therapeutic effects of the stimulants include decreased motor activity and impulsivity and increased attention span.[3,4,13,15] This suggests that stimulants are indicated for ADHD symptoms and not for primary learning disorders. The benefits of drug therapy must outweigh the potential for adverse effects.[3,4,6,7]

Substance Abuse

ADHD itself is a known risk factor for the development of a substance use disorder.[3,7] A 3-year outcome study confirmed results of earlier studies by showing that children with ADHD as a whole were at least twice as likely to engage in substance abuse compared with non-ADHD controls.[3,7] Drug therapy was not associated with substance abuse in this study; however, drug therapy was associated with higher rates of delinquency at 36 months. Conduct disorder increased the risk of delinquency and substance abuse.[3,7]

Studies show nontreated or inadequately treated adolescents and adults with ADHD are at increased risk of substance abuse compared with those who are effectively treated with drug therapy.[3,39] Another study showed that children with later onset of methylphenidate initiation (ages 8–12 years) had greater substance use compared with those starting treatment earlier. It is possible that early treatment of ADHD has a protective effect toward the emergence of conduct disorder, which usually precedes antisocial personality disorder and increases the risk for delinquency and drug abuse.[3]

Atomoxetine and bupropion also require monitoring to detect changes in appetite, weight, and sleep patterns, as well as pulse or blood pressure. An adequate trial of atomoxetine or bupropion consists of 6 weeks at maximum tolerated doses unless response occurs at a lower dose.[3,4,6]

CLINICAL CONTROVERSY

The use of stimulants to treat ADHD in individualswith substance abuse disorders is controversial. A diagnosis of ADHD confers at least a twofold greater risk of adolescent and adult substance abuse.[2,3,4] The risk is greater if conduct disorder, antisocial personality, or bipolar disorder coexists.[3,4,7] Stimulant therapy does not increase the risk of substance abuse, and effective treatment of ADHD can facilitate functioning and reduce abuse. Regardless of the benefits, however, there is significant misuse or diversion of stimulant medications among older adolescents and young adults, necessitating vigilance among prescribers and careful risk-versus-benefit assessment.[7,9,39]

When guanfacine or clonidine is given, careful clinical monitoring for fatigue, dizziness, and autonomic changes (e.g., blood pressure and pulse) is recommended.[3,4] The American Heart Association has stated that electrocardiographic monitoring is not required for clonidine treatment in children, although many clinicians continue to assess for ECG changes.[33] When discontinuing treatment, clonidine and guanfacine should be withdrawn slowly (0.05 mg clonidine/0.5 mg guanfacine reductions every 3 days) to prevent rebound hypertension or behavioral dyscontrol.[3,4] A therapeutic trial requires 1 to 2 months to assess therapeutic response, although increased sleep usually occurs immediately.

The effects of TCAs on the ECG should be monitored carefully. Of more concern are reports of sudden death in children taking desipramine or imipramine.[6,32] Children and adolescents given TCAs should have pretreatment and follow-up ECGs to assess the effects of TCA therapy on cardiac rate and rhythm.[6,32]

CONCLUSION

In summary, the preferred first-line drug therapy for ADHD is either methylphenidate, dexmethylphenidate, mixed amphetamine salts, or dextroamphetamine. Extended-release atomoxetine and guanfacine are good options for those unresponsive to or unable to tolerate stimulants. Bupropion is a safer option than a TCA, but both are declining in use, given that FDA-approved treatments are better studied. All agents require careful cardiovascular monitoring. Mood stabilizers (e.g., lithium, divalproex, and carbamazepine) and atypical antipsychotics are adjuncts for control of aggression or comorbid bipolar disorder. Other agents require further investigation before their status in the treatment of ADHD can be fully determined.

TOURETTE'S DISORDER

EPIDEMIOLOGY AND CLINICAL PRESENTATION

Tourette's disorder, also known as Tourette Syndrome, is present in 0.7% to 1% of boys and 0.4% of girls.[40,41] The essential features of this CNS disorder are multiple motor and vocal tics that must be present for more than 1 year before the diagnosis of Tourette's disorder is made. A tic is a sudden, rapid, recurrent, nonrhythmic, stereotyped motor movement or vocalization.[40,41] The clinical

presentation can vary from barely noticeable to debilitating, and the type of tic expressed can change over time.[1,40,41]

CLINICAL PRESENTATION OF TOURETTE'S DISORDER

General
- Onset occurs before 18 years of age.

Symptoms
- Multiple motor or one or more vocal tics are present.
- Motor and vocal tics do not need to occur concurrently.
- Tics occur many times a day (usually in bouts) nearly every day or intermittently throughout a period of more than 1 year; during this time, there is never a tic-free period of more than 3 consecutive months.

Motor Tics
- Eye blinking, lip licking
- Facial twitching
- Shoulder shrugging
- Squatting, twirling

Vocal Tics
- Clicks, grunts
- Barking, yelping
- Throat clearing, echolalia
- Coprolalia, palilalia

Data from American Psychiatric Association.[1]

❹ Transient tic disorder is diagnosed if motor or vocal tics occur for less than 1 year, with chronic tic disorder diagnosed if motor or vocal tics are present for longer than 1 year.[40,41] Tics start by age 8 and are most prominent during childhood; 50% of children experience complete attenuation of symptoms by age 18. This natural history is thought to parallel the process of nigrostriatal innervation in the developing brain, implicating Tourette's disorder as a neurodevelopmental disorder.[1,40,41]

More than 90% of children with Tourette's disorder have coexisting conditions such as ADHD (75%), mood disorders (60%), obsessive-compulsive disorder (40%), other anxiety disorders, or a combination of comorbidities. Tourette's disorder itself does not cause diminished intellectual functioning; however, the severity of tics and associated illnesses can result in significant impairment in school functioning, sometimes necessitating special education classes.[40,41] A follow-up study in adults showed that the severity of vocal tics had a more negative impact on functioning than the severity of motor tics.[42]

ETIOLOGY AND PATHOPHYSIOLOGY

Tourette's disorder is inherited in a complex polygenic pattern. Symptoms and severity of the disorder vary from one generation to another.[40,41] The neurochemical pathophysiology involves an imbalance in the interaction of dopaminergic, serotonergic, γ-aminobutyric acid (GABA)-ergic, glutamatergic, cholinergic, noradrenergic, and opioid systems in multiple brain regions, most notably the basal ganglia and caudate nucleus. The imbalance can cause a lack of regulation of the brain's inhibitory mechanisms, resulting in tics and associated behavior disorders. This multisystem etiology best explains the success of a variety of treatments.[40,41]

TREATMENT

⑤ Whenever symptoms are severe enough to impair the child's ability to function, drug therapy should be initiated. Psychotherapy and behavioral treatment are useful adjuncts.[40]

The α-adrenergic antagonists clonidine and guanfacine are good first-line treatment for mild motor and vocal tics associated with Tourette's disorder.[40] Their milder side effect profile compared with dopaminergic blocking drugs and efficacy for anxiety and insomnia can be an advantage. In some patients, however, the response is limited to improvement in attention and behavior with no changes in the frequency of tics. Clonidine can be initiated at 0.05 mg at bedtime with weekly titration to response. The goal dose of clonidine is 0.1 mg three times daily to a maximum of 0.2 mg three times daily.[40] Guanfacine can be initiated at 0.5 mg at bedtime with a goal dose of 1 mg twice daily to a maximum of 1 mg three times daily. Case reports describe a positive response from the clonidine patch as well. The onset of therapeutic effects for both clonidine and guanfacine is slow, ranging from 2 weeks to a few months.[40,43]

Dopamine-blocking antipsychotic drugs (haloperidol, fluphenazine, pimozide, and risperidone) are the most effective drug treatment options for managing motor and vocal tics associated with Tourette's disorder, but they carry the risk of extrapyramidal side effects.[40,41,43] A controlled trial showed risperidone 3.8 mg/day was more effective than pimozide 2.9 mg/day and was associated with fewer extrapyramidal side effects.[44] A Cochrane database review of pimozide for Tourette's disorder showed it was slightly less effective than haloperidol but comparable in efficacy to risperidone.[45] Uncontrolled data show benefit from olanzapine, ziprasidone, and aripiprazole. All have sufficient dopamine type 2 (D_2) blockade to exert therapeutic benefit.[40,43,46]

Therapy with risperidone, pimozide, or haloperidol should be initiated at very low doses of 0.25 to 0.5 mg/day given at bedtime and then increased gradually. Gradual titration over 2 to 3 weeks helps minimize extrapyramidal and sedative effects while permitting careful assessment of response. Symptoms can regress within 48 to 72 hours after an effective dose is reached. Doses less than 5 mg/day are effective in controlling tics for most patients.[40,41,45,]

CLINICAL CONTROVERSY

The decision to treat Tourette's disorder with a D_2 receptor antagonist (atypical or conventional) rather than an α_2-agonist is controversial and can be challenging. The choice is usually based on whether high efficacy (D_2 antagonist) or milder adverse effect burden (α_2-agonist) is more desirable in an individual patient.[3,40,43]

■ COMORBIDITY

Pharmacotherapy of Tourette's disorder is challenging because of the common occurrence of coexisting disorders typically requiring medication combinations. Often the behavioral problems precede and are more disturbing than the involuntary movements, making them a treatment priority.[40–42]

■ TOURETTE'S AND ADHD

Pharmacotherapy with stimulants increases dopaminergic and noradrenergic activity, which has the potential to aggravate or precipitate tics, although short- and long-term studies in 71 children showed no worsening of tics with methylphenidate dosed up to 0.5 mg/kg/day.[3] Studies examining the comparative effects of methylphenidate and dextroamphetamine on tics in children found the majority experienced improvement in ADHD symptoms with acceptable effects on tics. Methylphenidate was better tolerated than dextroamphetamine.[3,40]

A double-blind, placebo-controlled trial compared methylphenidate or clonidine monotherapy to combination methylphenidate and clonidine in patients with ADHD and Tourette's disorder. Combination therapy demonstrated the greatest benefit in reducing symptoms of ADHD and tics ($P < 0.0001$).[3] Clonidine appeared most helpful for impulsivity and hyperactivity, whereas methylphenidate was most helpful for inattention. All treatments were well tolerated, but sedation was common (28%) in those receiving clonidine.[3] Patients and caregivers should be aware of the risks of using stimulants in children with Tourette's disorder (see ADHD section); careful monitoring is essential.[3,40]

A controlled trial of atomoxetine versus placebo in 117 children with ADHD and Tourette's disorder over 18 weeks showed treatment with atomoxetine 0.5 to 1.5 mg/kg/day improved symptoms of both, with overall good tolerability. Treatment-emergent nausea, decreased appetite, decreased body weight, and increased heart rate occurred significantly more often in those receiving atomoxetine compared with those receiving placebo.[3]

Clonidine or guanfacine alone are less effective alternatives to stimulants in the treatment of children with Tourette's disorder and ADHD. Guanfacine was administered to 34 children (mean age 10.4 years), with ADHD and tic disorder during an 8-week placebo-controlled trial at a dose of 1.5 to 3 mg/day. Tic severity decreased by 31% in the guanfacine group compared to 0% in the placebo group.[3] There was a mean improvement of 37% on the teacher-rated ADHD scale compared with 8% improvement with placebo. Because of its similarity to clonidine, guanfacine's cardiovascular effects warrant careful clinical monitoring.[3,4,6]

Results from these studies concur with the Texas Children's Medication Algorithm for ADHD, which recommends a stimulant (preferably methylphenidate) or atomoxetine as first-line treatment for ADHD in children with Tourette's disorder or chronic tics.[6]

■ TOURETTE'S AND ANXIETY OR MOOD DISORDERS

Therapeutic trials (6–12 weeks) of a selective serotonin reuptake inhibitor (SSRI) or clomipramine should be added to tic-specific therapy when obsessive-compulsive, anxiety, or depressive symptoms cause functional impairment in patients with Tourette's disorder.[3,40,41] Careful monitoring for behavioral activation, disinhibition, and motor restlessness is essential during SSRI or clomipramine therapy, because these symptoms can indicate increased risk for suicidal behavior or a switch to mania, requiring drug discontinuation.[3,32]

■ ADJUNCTIVE OR ALTERNATIVE TREATMENTS

For those who are unresponsive, partially responsive, or unable to tolerate dopamine antagonists or α_2-agonists, several adjuncts or alternative treatments are available. Clonazepam, topiramate, and baclofen appear to offer promise in relieving tics and associated symptoms.[40,43] Extensive clinical experience with the dopamine-depleting drug tetrabenazine shows improvement in motor and vocal tics, but controlled trials are needed.[40] Seven patients with antipsychotic-resistant tics and antibodies to caudate nucleus protein received single transfusions of immunoglobulin, which caused remission of motor and vocal tics for more than 6 months.[47] Botulinum toxin injected into the vocal cords has improved severe vocal tics in case reports, but it requires further study.[40] For truly severe and refractory cases, deep brain stimulation and even neurosurgery have been effective.[40] Nonpharmacologic interventions include support groups and "habit-reversal therapy."[48] Further information for patients, families, and educators is available on the Tourette's Syndrome Association website (http://www.tsa-usa.org).

■ ADVERSE EFFECTS

For clonidine and guanfacine, the most common adverse effect is sedation. Fortunately, tolerance usually develops to this effect over days to weeks. The most potentially serious side effects are cardiovascular (see the section on ADHD).[3,35] Other α_2-agonist side effects are dry mouth, constipation, headache, mood changes, and even a temporary worsening of tics in ~10% of patients.[3,43]

Atypical antipsychotics (e.g., risperidone, olanzapine, ziprasidone, and aripiprazole) pose similar adverse effect risks in children and adolescents compared with adults (see Table 72–4).[31,46] Available data show that children and adolescents are at higher risk for experiencing sedation, acute extrapyramidal side effects, hyperprolactinemia, withdrawal dyskinesia, and significant weight gain during treatment compared with adults. Risperidone is associated with more weight gain in youths than adults, and ziprasidone and aripiprazole do not seem to be as "weight neutral" in pediatric populations as in adults.[20,31] Ziprasidone carries a risk of QTc prolongation, although torsades de pointes has not been reported, and the clinical significance requires further study.[20,28,43]

❻ Adverse effects have been reported with haloperidol doses of 2 mg/day or greater. In one review of 24 patients treated with haloperidol for Tourette's disorder, 66.7% discontinued treatment because of intolerable side effects (e.g., dysphoria, akathisia, nervousness, sedation, dystonia, and cognitive dulling or feeling drugged).[49] Lowering the dose can alleviate side effects. An antiparkinsonian agent such as benztropine (at a starting dose of 0.5 mg orally twice daily) sometimes will reverse extrapyramidal side effects. Whether a patient with Tourette's disorder is developing a new tic or tardive dyskinesia can be difficult to determine.[3,40,43]

Pimozide is less likely to cause extrapyramidal side effects than haloperidol.[45] Anticholinergic side effects can occur in addition to drowsiness, and, occasionally, anxiety will occur. ECG changes, including T- and U-wave abnormalities and prolongation of the QTc interval, are found rarely with recommended therapeutic doses of pimozide for Tourette's disorder; however, drugs that inhibit CYP3A4 (e.g., clarithromycin and fluoxetine) should not be combined with pimozide because of the risk of excessively elevating pimozide blood levels, which can result in lethal QTc prolongation.[6,40]

PHARMACOECONOMIC CONSIDERATIONS

Haloperidol provides the most economic drug therapy because of high efficacy and low cost. Pimozide and atypical antipsychotics are more expensive than generic haloperidol, and they require ECG and metabolic monitoring, respectively. Although generic clonidine is inexpensive, delayed onset of effect and significantly lower efficacy substantially increase total costs of treatment.

EVALUATION OF THERAPEUTIC OUTCOMES

An adult outcome study involving 58 subjects with Tourette's disorder found that 40% were currently taking medication for their symptoms. The most frequently taken medications were antipsychotics (50%), antidepressants (36%), and clonidine (23%). Anticholinergic drugs, stimulants, and benzodiazepines were used by less than 10% of patients.[42] Evaluating therapeutic interventions

is challenging, as most patients can suppress their tics voluntarily for minutes to hours.[43] Also, numerous factors, such as stress, concentration, and relaxation, can affect tic frequency and severity. The use of regular videotaped assessments in conjunction with standardized rating scales (Yale Global Tic Severity Scale) is helpful in objectively evaluating symptoms, side effects, and overall drug response.[40–42]

❻ Individuals with Tourette's disorder are particularly sensitive to medication side effects, so medication dosing must be individualized with low starting doses and careful weekly titration to response, realizing that it can take 1 to 2 months for an adequate therapeutic trial. Children taking any dopamine-blocking medication should receive monitoring every 3 to 6 months for extrapyramidal effects and tardive dyskinesia with a standardized rating scale (e.g., Abnormal Involuntary Movement Scale [AIMS]).[31] Patients given pimozide or ziprasidone should receive baseline and follow-up ECGs.[31,43] Consult the ADHD section for additional monitoring recommendations for atypical antipsychotics.[40,42,43]

CONCLUSION

In summary, haloperidol, pimozide, and risperidone have the advantages of greatest efficacy and rapid onset in the treatment of Tourette's disorder. Ziprasidone, olanzapine, and aripiprazole show promise; however, comparison studies with haloperidol, pimozide, and risperidone are needed to determine their relative safety and efficacy. Clonidine and guanfacine have the advantage of causing no extrapyramidal side effects, but they are significantly less effective and require ongoing cardiovascular monitoring. Drug treatment must be highly individualized, considering comorbid disorders, side effect sensitivity, and drug interactions.

ENURESIS

The essential feature of enuresis is repeated involuntary or inappropriate voiding of urine by day or night that is not caused by a general medical condition.[1]

ETIOLOGY, PATHOPHYSIOLOGY, AND CLINICAL PRESENTATION

Medical causes of inappropriate voiding (e.g., diabetes mellitus, diabetes insipidus, seizure disorders, and urinary tract infections) should be ruled out.[50,51]

CLINICAL PRESENTATION OF ENURESIS

General

☐ Patients are 5 years old or older.

Symptoms

☐ Patients repeatedly void urine into bed and/or clothes involuntarily or intentionally.

☐ There is either a frequency of twice weekly for at least 3 consecutive months or the presence of clinically significant distress or impairment in social, academic (occupational), or other area of functioning.

Data from American Psychiatric Association. Diagnostic and Statistical Manual of Mental Disorders. 4th ed. Text rev. Washington, DC: American Psychiatric Association 2000:39–134.

Enuresis occurs in 12% to 25% of 4-year-olds, 7% to 10% of 8-year-olds, and 2% to 3% of 12-year-olds, with 1% to 3% continuing to experience enuresis in late teenage years.[50] After age 5 years, there is a 15% annual rate of spontaneous remission. The ratio of males to females with enuresis is 2:1.[50] Factors that predispose a child to enuresis include a positive family history, institutionalization, low socioeconomic status, reduced functional bladder capacity, delayed or lax toilet training, constipation, psychological factors, and developmental delay.[50] Some children with nocturnal enuresis lack the normal circadian variation in urine excretion rate, urine osmolality, and antidiuretic hormone (ADH) secretion. Nocturnal enuresis is not associated with a particular sleep stage, although children with enuresis can be more difficult to arouse.[50]

TREATMENT

The first steps in treating a child with enuresis are to educate the family about the high frequency of the problem, dispel any misconceptions, provide emotional support, and strongly discourage punishment.[51]

❼ Continence skills and various behavioral and conditioning methods remain the primary treatments for enuresis, and drug treatment remains a secondary approach.[50,51] Simple behavioral and physical interventions such as encouraging voiding at least once every 2 hours and having the child drink liberal fluids throughout the day with minimal fluids after 6 P.M. can decrease enuresis without any side effects or safety concerns.[51] Complex interventions, such as dry-bed training in combination with bed-wetting alarms, can be tried but require time and effort. There is insufficient evidence to support complex interventions without an alarm. After 3 to 4 months of using a bed-wetting alarm, enuresis is cured in two-thirds of children.[50,51]

Alarms are more effective than pharmacotherapy with longer lasting results, although medications work faster, within 2 weeks. Combining medications and alarms has been tried with mixed results.[50,51] Desmopressin tablets are preferred to TCAs (e.g., imipramine) because of greater efficacy and lower toxicity risk.[50,51] Oxybutynin and tolterodine may be effective adjuncts to desmopressin in partial responders, but they are not as effective as monotherapy.[50–52]

■ DESMOPRESSIN

❽ Desmopressin acetate, a synthetic analogue of the natural human ADH arginine vasopressin, is currently available in a nasal spray, which is no longer recommended, and a more widely used oral tablet for the treatment of nocturnal enuresis.[50,51] Desmopressin increases overnight urinary osmotic concentration by increasing water reabsorption and reducing the volume of urine entering the bladder.[50,51] It is effective in reducing the number of wet nights in 10% to 65% of children within 1 to 2 weeks, with cessation of bedwetting in up to 48% of children; however, up to 80% relapse upon discontinuation.[50,51]

In a 6-month, randomized, controlled trial comparing desmopressin (200–400 mcg), imipramine (25 mg), and combination desmopressin (200 mcg) and oxybutynin (5 mg) in 145 enuretic children (mean age 7.8 years), the combination produced the most rapid results, although the number of wet nights per month at 6 months was similar in the combination desmopressin/oxybutynin group (3.7 ± 5.4) compared with the desmopressin monotherapy group (4.0 ± 4.6). Both treatments were superior to imipramine (9.3 ± 8.3). The mean number of wet nights during the 2-week baseline period in all groups was 13. Tolerability was superior in the desmopressin groups compared with the imipramine group.[52]

Intranasal desmopressin should not be used because of the unacceptable risk of hyponatremia, which may cause seizures. Only the tablet form is approved by the FDA for primary nocturnal enuresis. For children 6 years of age or older, desmopressin tablets can be initiated at 200 mcg at bedtime. Approximately 1% of oral desmopressin is absorbed. Plasma concentrations reach a maximum approximately 45 minutes after administration. Effective dosages range from 200 to 600 mcg/day of oral desmopressin. The duration of action varies from 10 to 20 hours, and there is compensatory polyuria the following day when the drug wears off.[50,51]

■ TRICYCLIC ANTIDEPRESSANTS

❽ Imipramine is the most studied TCA, although desipramine, amitriptyline, and nortriptyline are also effective. Imipramine is effective in increasing dry nights for up to 60% of individuals, with cessation of bed-wetting in only ~20% of children.[50,51] The mechanism of action of TCAs in treating enuresis is unknown.[50,51] For children 6 years of age and older, the usual starting dose is 25 mg given 30 minutes before bedtime. Doses can be increased by 25 mg weekly until response is achieved. The usual effective dosing range is 1 to 2.5 mg/kg/night, and doses should not exceed 2.5 mg/kg/night. Most children respond within the first week.[50] Because of the risk of toxicity and death in overdose, the International Children's Continence Society recommends that TCA be used only when all other therapies have failed.[51]

■ ADVERSE EFFECTS

Desmopressin tablets can cause transient headache, chills, dizziness, nausea, and abdominal pain. Rarely, water intoxication, hyponatremia, and subsequent tonic-clonic seizures have been reported.[50,51] From 1972 to 2005, 151 postmarketing cases of hyponatremia were reported in children with nocturnal enuresis, of whom 145 were treated with intranasal desmopressin, and 6 received tablets. When desmopressin is administered, evening fluids should be restricted 1 hour before and 8 hours after drug administration. Desmopressin tablets should be stopped during acute illnesses that may lead to fluid or electrolyte imbalance. Prompt medical assessment is needed if headache, nausea, or vomiting develops, as these could be signs of hyponatremia. Concomitant medications that may lower sodium (e.g., antidepressants and oxcarbazepine) or illnesses that change hydration status (e.g., the flu) can increase the risk of hyponatremia.[50,51]

Adverse effects of TCAs are dose related and include sedation, dizziness, dry mouth, constipation, and weight gain, along with the risk of ECG changes, heart block, and lowering of the seizure threshold.[32,51]

PHARMACOECONOMIC CONSIDERATIONS

No pharmacoeconomic studies on enuresis are available. The use of a bed-wetting alarm provides the highest overall cure rate, and drugs are a secondary approach. Several types of reusable bed-wetting alarms are available, ranging from $30 to $170 per alarm, as opposed to $90 to $130 for a 30-day supply of desmopressin.[53] However, insurance companies commonly reimburse drug therapy, whereas most do not reimburse for alarms. Therapy with desmopressin is substantially more expensive than with TCAs because of higher cost.

EVALUATION OF THERAPEUTIC OUTCOMES

An accurate baseline of bed-wetting frequency must be established. A 50% or greater increase in dry nights is considered a therapeutic response. For example, if baseline dry nights are 2 out of 7 days per week, and drug treatment results in 4 or more dry nights per week, the drug is considered effective. If only one more dry night per week occurs, and the drug is at the low end of the dosing range, a dosage increase is needed.[50,51]

At least 1 week is needed to evaluate the efficacy of TCAs, and 2 weeks can be needed for evaluation of desmopressin. If drug treatment is ongoing for several months, particularly if enuresis has resolved, attempts to discontinue the drug every 3 to 6 months are recommended to assess for spontaneous remission. Slow tapering of the medication can decrease the frequency of relapse. Unfortunately, therapeutic drug efficacy does not extend beyond drug discontinuation.[50,51]

CONCLUSION

Initially, simple interventions such as lift and awaken can be implemented. A bed-wetting alarm in combination with complex behavioral interventions provides lasting cures for two-thirds of children. Drug therapy has the advantage of more rapid results, but relapse is high upon drug discontinuation.[50,51] Desmopressin tablets are preferred to imipramine because of better tolerability and safety.[47,48]

ABBREVIATIONS

ADH: Antidiuretic hormone

ADHD: Attention deficit/hyperactivity disorder

AIMS: Abnormal Involuntary Movement Scale

BMI: Body mass index

CNS: Central nervous system

DAT: Dopamine active transporter protein

D_1, D_2, D_3, D_4, D_5: Dopamine receptors

DSM-IV-TR: Diagnostic and Statistical Manual of Mental Disorders (Fourth Edition, Text Revision)

ECG: Electrocardiogram

FDA: Food and Drug Administration

GABA:γ-aminobutyric acid

MAO: Monoamine oxidase

MAOI: Monoamine oxidase inhibitor

OROS: Osmotically released oral delivery system

SSRI: Selective serotonin reuptake inhibitor

TCA: Tricyclic antidepressant

REFERENCES

1. American Psychiatric Association. Diagnostic and Statistical Manual of Mental Disorders. 4th ed. Text rev. Washington, DC: American Psychiatric Association 2000:39–134.
2. Barkley RA. Young adult outcome of hyperactive children: Adaptive functioning in major life activities. J Am Acad Child Adolescent Psychiatry 2006;45:192–202.
3. Dopheide JA, Pliszka SR. Attention deficit hyperactivity disorder: An update. Pharmacotherapy 2009;29(6):656–679.
4. Pliszka SR, Bernet W, Bukstein O, et al, for the American Academy of Child and Adolescent Psychiatry Work Group on Quality Issues. Practice parameter for the assessment and treatment of children and adolescents with attention deficit/hyperactivity disorder. J Am Acad Child Adolesc Psychiatry 2007;46:894–921.
5. Reinhardt MD, Benneti L, Victor MM, et al. Is age at onset criterion relevant for the response to methylphenidate in ADHD? J Clin Psych 2007;68:1109–1116.
6. Pliszka SR, Crismon ML, Hughes CW, et al. The Texas Children's Medication Algorithm project: Revision of the algorithm for pharmacotherapy of childhood attention-deficit/hyperactivity disorder. J Am Acad Child Adolesc Psychiatry 2006;45(6):642–657.
7. Jensen PS, Arnold LE, Swanson JM, et al. Three-year follow-up of the NIMH MTA study. J Am Acad Child Adolesc Psychiatry 2007;46:989–1002.
8. Weiss MD, Weiss JR. A guide to the treatment of adults with ADHD. J Clin Psychiatry 2004;65(Suppl 3):27–37.
9. Setlik J, Bond GR, Ho M. Adolescent prescription ADHD medication abuse is rising along with prescriptions for these medications. Pediatrics 2009;124(3):875–879.
10. Asherson P, Kuntsi J, Taylor E. Unraveling the complexity of ADHD: A behavioural genomic approach. Br J Psychiatry 2005;187:103–105.
11. Volkow ND, Wang GJ, Kollins SH. Evaluating dopamine reward pathway in ADHD. JAMA 2009;302(10):1084–1091.
12. Shaw P, Sharp WS, Morrison M, et al. Psychostimulant treatment and the developing cortex in ADHD. Am J Psych 2009;166:58–63.
13. Wilens TE. Mechanism of agents used for ADHD. J Clin Psychiatry 2006;67(Suppl 8):32–37.
14. Gilbert DL, Wang Z, Sallee FR, et al. Dopamine transporter genotype influences physiologic response to medication in ADHD. Brain 2006;129:2038–2046.
15. Semrud-Clikeman M, Pliszka S, Liotti M. Executive functioning in children with ADHD: Combined type with and without a stimulant medication history. Neuropsychology 2008;22:329–340.
16. Scheffler RM, Brown TT, Fulton BD, et al. Positive association between attention-deficit/hyperactivity disorder medication use and academic achievement during elementary school. Pediatrics 2009;123:1273–1279.
17. Biederman J, Seidman LJ, Carter RP, et al. Effects of stimulant medication on neuropsychological functioning in young adults with ADHD. J Clin Psych 2008;69:1150–1156.
18. Gualitieri CT, Johnson L. Medications do not necessarily normalize cognition in ADHD patients. J Atten Disord 2008;11:459–469.
19. American Academy of Pediatrics. Clinical practice guideline: Treatment of the school-aged child with ADHD. Pediatrics 2001;108:1033–1044.
20. Correll CU, Carlson HE. Endocrine and metabolic adverse effects of psychotropic medications in children and adolescents. J Am Acad Child Adolesc Psychiatry 2006;45(7):771–791.
21. Biederman J, Mick E, Surman C, et al. A randomized, placebo-controlled trial of OROS methylphenidate in adults with ADHD. Biol Psychiatry 2006;59:829–835.
22. Wilens TE, McBurnett K, Bukstein O, et al. Multisite controlled study of OROS methylphenidate in the treatment of adolescents with ADHD. Arch Ped Adolesc Med 2006;160:82–90.
23. Winterstein AG, Gerhard T, Shuster J, et al. Cardiac safety of methylphenidate versus amphetamine salts in the treatment of ADHD. Pediatrics 2009;124:e75–e80.
24. Vetter VL, Elia J, Erickson C, et al. Cardiovascular monitoring of children and adolescents with heart disease receiving stimulant drugs: A scientific statement from the American Heart Association Council on Cardiovascular Disease in the Young, Congenital Cardiac Defects Committee, and the Council on Cardiovascular Nursing. Circulation 2008;117:2407–2423.
25. U.S. Food and Drug Administration. Cardiovascular and psychiatric risk with drug treatments for ADHD. 2006. Available at: *http://www.fda.gov/ohrms/dockets/ac/06/slides/2006-4210s-index.htm*. Accessed July 12, 2009.
26. Biederman J, Melmed RD, Patel A, et al. A randomized, double-blind, placebo-controlled study of guanfacine extended release in children and adolescents with attention-deficit/hyperactivity disorder. Pediatrics 2008;121:e73–e84.
27. Sallee F, McGough J, Wigal T, et al. Long-term safety of guanfacine extended release in children and adolescents with attention-deficit hyperactivity disorder. J Child Adolesc Psychopharmacol 2009;19:215–226.
28. Kowatch RA, DelBello MP. Pediatric bipolar disorder: Emerging diagnostic and treatment approaches. Child Adolesc Psych Clin N Am 2006;15:73–108.

29. Schur SB, Sikich L, Findling RL, et al. Treatment recommendations for the use of antipsychotics for aggressive youth (TRAAY): 1. A review. J Am Acad Child Adolesc Psychiatry 2003;42:132–144.

30. Pappadopulos E, Macintyre J, Crismon ML, et al. Treatment recommendations for the use of antipsychotics for aggressive youth (TRAAY:.2. J Am Acad Child Adolesc Psych 2003;42(2):145–161.

31. Correll CU. Assessing and maximizing the safety and tolerability of antipsychotics used in the treatment of children and adolescents. J Clin Psych 2008;69(Suppl 4):26–36.

32. Dopheide JA. Recognizing and treating depression in children and adolescents. Am J Health Syst Pharm 2006;63:233–243.

33. Tan M, Appleton R. ADHD, methylphenidate, and epilepsy. Arch Dis Child 2005;90:57–59.

34. Hazell PL, Stuart JE. A randomized controlled trial of clonidine added to psychostimulant medication for hyperactive and aggressive children. J Am Acad Child Adolesc Psychiatry 2003;42:886–894.

35. Klein-Schwartz W. Trends and toxic effects from pediatric clonidine exposures. Arch Pediatr Adolesc Med 2002;156:392–396.

36. Pelham WE, Foster M, Robb JA. The economic impact of ADHD in children and adolescents. J Pediatric Psychology 2007;32(6):711–727.

37. Cottrell S, Tilden D, Robinson P, et al. A modeled economic evaluation comparing atomoxetine with stimulant therapy in the treatment of children with ADHD in the United Kingdom. Value Health 2008;11(3):376–388.

38. Kemner JE, Lage MJ. Effect of methylphenidate formulation on treatment patterns and use of emergency room services. Am J Health Syst Pharm 2006;63:317–322.

39. Upadhyaya HP, Rose K, O'Rourke K, et al. ADHD, medication treatment, and substance use patterns among adolescents and young adults. J Child Adolesc Psychopharmacol 2005;15(5):799–809.

40. Kenny C, Kuo SH, Jimenez-Shahed J. Tourette's syndrome. Am Fam Physician 2008;77(5):651–660.

41. Cavanna AE, Servo S, Monaco F, et al. The behavioral spectrum of Gilles de la Tourette syndrome. J Neuropsychiatry Clin Neurosci 2009;21(1):13–23.

42. Altman G, Staley JD, Wener P. Children with Tourette disorder: A follow-up study in adulthood. J Nerv Ment Dis 2009;197:305–310.

43. Muller-Vahl JT. The treatment of Tourette's syndrome: Current opinions. Expert Opin Pharmacother 2002;3:899–914.

44. Bruggeman R, van der Linden C, Buitelaar JK, et al. Risperidone versus pimozide in Tourette's disorder: A comparative double-blind parallel-group study. J Clin Psychiatry 2001;62:50–56.

45. Pringsheim T, Marras C. Pimozide for tics in Tourette's syndrome. Cochrane Database Syst Rev 2009;2:CD006996.

46. Budman C, Coffey B, Schechter R, et al. Aripiprazole in children and adolescents with Tourette disorder with and without explosive outbursts. J Child Adolesc Psychopharmacol 2008;18:509–515.

47. Zykov VP, Shcherbina E, Novikova EB, et al. Neuroimmune aspects of the pathogenesis of Tourette's syndrome and experience in the use of immunoglobulins in children. Neurosci Behav Physiol 2009;39: 635–638.

48. Wilhelm S, Deckersbach T, Coffey BJ, et al. Habit reversal versus supportive psychotherapy for Tourette's disorder: A randomized controlled trial. Am J Psychiatry 2003;160:1175–1177.

49. Silva RR, Munoz DM, Daniel W, et al. Causes of haloperidol discontinuation in patients with Tourette's disorder: Management and alternatives. J Clin Psychiatry 1998;57:129–135.

50. Fritz G, Rockney R, American Academy of Child and Adolescent Psychiatry Work Group. Practice parameter for the assessment and treatment of children and adolescents with enuresis. J Am Acad Child Adolesc Psychiatry 2004;43(12)1540–1550.

51. Robson, WLM. Evaluation and management of enuresis. New Engl J Med 2009;360:1429–1436.

52. Lee T, Suh HJ, Lee HJ, Lee JE. Comparison of effects of treatment of primary nocturnal enuresis with oxybutynin plus desmopressin alone or imipramine alone: A randomized controlled clinical trial. J Urol 2005;174:1084–1087.

53. Bed-wetting alarm prices. 2009. Available at: *http://www.bedwetting-store.com/Bedwetting_Alarms/alarm_group.htm*. Accessed September 29, 2009.

STEVEN C. STONER

KEY CONCEPTS

❶ Clinicians who specialize in the treatment of eating disorders feel that anorexia nervosa, bulimia nervosa, and eating disorders not otherwise specified should be commonly accepted as serious mental illnesses.

❷ Because the causes of eating disorders are complex, multidisciplinary treatment, including pharmacologic and nonpharmacologic interventions, are preferred to ensure a positive outcome. Although outpatient treatment is appropriate for the majority of patients, it is important to recognize the factors that indicate a need for inpatient treatment.

❸ Careful medical and psychiatric assessments are needed at baseline to determine the severity of illness and the complexity of comorbid conditions.

❹ In patients with anorexia nervosa, one goal is to achieve and maintain a body weight within 85% of the normal weight for age and height. If the patient is malnourished, oral refeeding with the daily caloric intake starting at 1,000 to 1,600 calories per day (4186 to 6697 J/day) and slowly titrating to 2,000 to 3,000 calories per day (8372 to 12,557 J/day) is preferred. Parenteral refeeding is a treatment of last resort.

❺ Antidepressants are considered to be ineffective for the core symptoms of anorexia nervosa and are reserved for patients with mood, anxiety, and obsessional symptoms that persist after weight has improved.

❻ Antidepressants can improve both mood and specific target symptoms in bulimia nervosa, but they remain adjunctive to nonpharmacologic treatments.

❼ Selective serotonin reuptake inhibitors are first-line agents when medications are indicated for bulimia nervosa. Compared with other antidepressant classes, they have improved tolerability and safety, although superior efficacy has not been studied. The dose of fluoxetine in bulimia nervosa is higher (60 mg/day) than the dose usually used in depression.

❽ An adequate drug therapy trial in bulimia nervosa is 4 to 8 weeks. If drug treatment fails, consider that the patient may be vomiting or using other purging methods affecting the absorption of the drug.

Learning objectives, review questions, and other resources can be found at **www.pharmacotherapyonline.com**.

❾ The optimal duration of antidepressant treatment for bulimia nervosa is unknown, but most clinicians continue them for 9 to 12 months in patients who respond and then reevaluate the need for ongoing medication management.

❶ The American Academy for Eating Disorders has taken the firm public stance that eating disorders are and should be classified as serious mental illnesses.[1] The spectrum of eating disorders encompasses several complex diseases, sharing the pathologic feature of overevaluation of body shape and weight. Eating disorders arise from the interaction between environmental, societal, developmental, psychosocial, genetic, and biologic factors. It is estimated that 5 to 10 million women and 1 million men in the United States alone have an eating disorder. The urbanization of society, social pressure, and obsession with perfection and being thin have led to an increasing prevalence of eating disorders, with the peak onset being between 16 and 20 years of age.[2-5] Anorexia nervosa, bulimia nervosa, and eating disorders not otherwise specified (EDNOS) are the primary disorders that have been identified.[6-10]

Despite an improved understanding of these cognitively and emotionally disabling and potentially fatal disorders, management remains difficult. Pharmacologic intervention is a small part of a comprehensive plan that emphasizes cognitive behavioral therapy (CBT) and psychotherapy.

EPIDEMIOLOGY

ANOREXIA NERVOSA

Anorexia nervosa occurs predominantly in girls and young women (90%) and usually presents in late adolescence (median onset 17 years of age), with new cases rarely diagnosed after age 40. The estimated prevalence of the disorder in the general population is 0.3% of females; however, a subthreshold level of symptoms is estimated to affect 0.37% to 1.3% of the population.[3,11-13] Longitudinal management of anorexia nervosa is difficult, even in cases where weight restoration is achieved. Rates of relapse requiring hospitalization within 1 year are estimated to exceed 30%.[14]

The promotion of the virtues of being thin is also a potentially negative environmental factor. Many websites, for example, inappropriately promote healthy lifestyle aspects of anorexia and being thin as a means of being in control, successful, and coping with life's pressures.[15]

BULIMIA NERVOSA

Bulimia nervosa also occurs predominantly in girls and young women (90%) and usually presents in adolescence or early adult life.[6]

Between 1% and 4.6% of adolescent and young adult females meet the diagnostic criteria for bulimia.[4,11,16,17]

EATING DISORDER NOT OTHERWISE SPECIFIED

EDNOS is also described in the American Psychiatric Association's *Diagnostic and Statistical Manual of Mental Disorders* (Fourth Edition, Text Revision; *DSM-IV-TR*).[4,16] Originally designed to capture eating disorder cases that did not meet diagnostic criteria of anorexia or bulimia, it has instead developed into a diagnosis of indifference. Its prevalence is estimated at 1% to 4.7% of the population, and up to 50% of patients with an eating disorder admitted to tertiary care settings are believed to have this condition.[11,18] These individuals present with symptoms characteristic of eating disorders but do not meet specific diagnostic criteria. Two examples of EDNOS are night eating syndrome (NES) and binge eating disorder (BED).

NES is most common in obesity clinic populations, often accompanied by depressive symptoms. The syndrome is defined by early morning anorexia, hyperphagia in the evening, nighttime insomnia, and subsequent early morning awakening.[10,19,20] NES affects an estimated 1.5% of the general population and 8.9% to 27% of patients in obesity clinics.[21-23] Patients with NES are reported to benefit from antidepressant therapy, most notably sertraline 50 to 200 mg daily.[10]

Although part of the EDNOS classification, BED continues to be classified as a research diagnosis. The diagnostic criteria for BED describe recurrent episodes of binge eating without compensatory behaviors (e.g., purging, excessive exercise, or fasting). BED typically presents later in life (older than 40 years of age), and approximately one-fourth of BED patients are male.[18,24]

ETIOLOGY AND PATHOPHYSIOLOGY

❷ The potential etiologic or exacerbating factors for eating disorders encompass physiologic, biochemical, developmental, genetic, psychosocial, and psychiatric phenomena. The biologic basis for eating disorders is difficult to delineate because it is unclear if the biologic changes are caused by or are a result of the aberrant eating behavior.

Abnormalities of the hypothalamic-pituitary-gonadal, hypothalamic-pituitary-adrenal, and hypothalamic-pituitary-thyroid axes are described as potential causes of anorexia nervosa. Amenorrhea is found in the majority of females with anorexia, providing support for the association with gonadotropin.[17] However, symptoms related to these abnormalities do not always correct with weight normalization, suggesting a primary biologic abnormality.[24]

The roles of serotonin, norepinephrine, and dopamine have been studied extensively, as these neurotransmitters have important functions in controlling eating behaviors. Dysfunctions in these systems are thought to be secondary to weight loss. Some aspects of serotonin function do remain abnormal after weight restoration, suggesting that other mechanisms are involved.[25,26] Another molecular genetic target of study is brain-derived neurotrophic factor (BDNF), which is also being studied in disease states such as depression.[27]

Strong genetic influences are present in anorexia and likely play a role in both bulimia and BED, independent of the presence of obesity.[28] Twin studies have shown concordance of ~55% and 35% in monozygotic twins and 5% and 30% in dizygotic twins for anorexia and bulimia, respectively. Genetic mutation studies have focused on polymorphisms of the serotonin 2A receptor, with mixed preliminary results.[24] One acquired hereditary abnormality being studied is the presence of low-function alleles associated with the serotonin transporter *(5-HTTLPR)* and serotonin 2A receptor gene *(−1438G/A)*, as findings suggest an association with poor treatment response.[29]

Emphasis is also placed on social stress and psychological and developmental issues related to dysfunctional family relationships triggering abnormal eating behavior.[4,17,18,30] Athletes are at risk for eating disorders, especially female gymnasts, ballet dancers, figure skaters, distance runners, swimmers, male wrestlers, and body builders.[31]

DIAGNOSTIC CRITERIA AND CLINICAL PRESENTATION

❸ Anorexia and bulimia occur together in ~30% to 64% of patients with eating disorders and may not be distinct diagnostic entities, but rather a continuum of symptoms. Thus, careful medical and psychiatric assessment at baseline is essential.[32-34] Many patients initially present with either anorexia or bulimia and alternate from one to the other. Figure 73–1 demonstrates similar and unique features of both disorders.

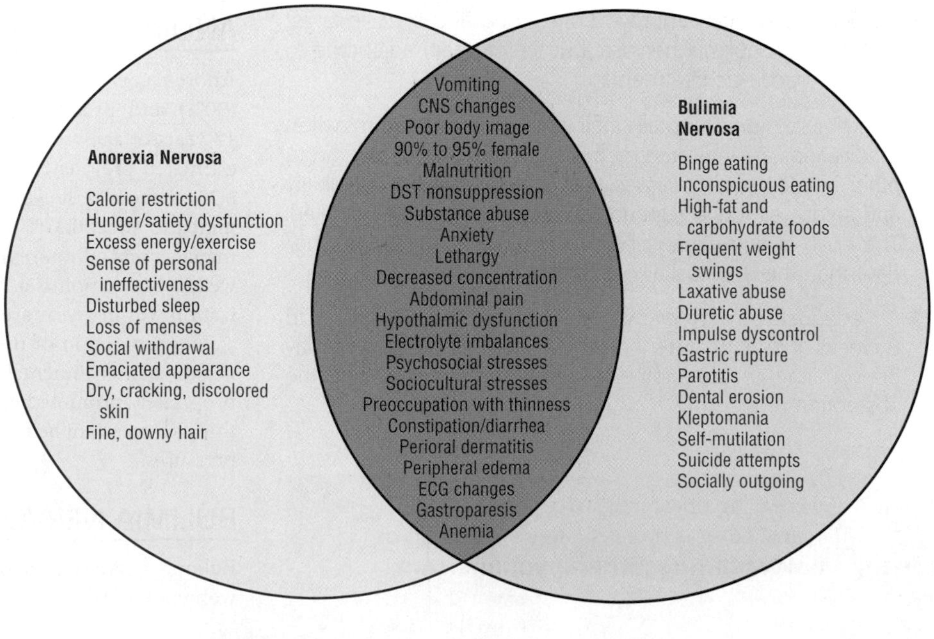

Anorexia Nervosa

Calorie restriction
Hunger/satiety dysfunction
Excess energy/exercise
Sense of personal
   ineffectiveness
Disturbed sleep
Loss of menses
Social withdrawal
Emaciated appearance
Dry, cracking, discolored
   skin
Fine, downy hair

Vomiting
CNS changes
Poor body image
90% to 95% female
Malnutrition
DST nonsuppression
Substance abuse
Anxiety
Lethargy
Decreased concentration
Abdominal pain
Hypothalmic dysfunction
Electrolyte imbalances
Psychosocial stresses
Sociocultural stresses
Preoccupation with thinness
Constipation/diarrhea
Perioral dermatitis
Peripheral edema
ECG changes
Gastroparesis
Anemia

Bulimia Nervosa

Binge eating
Inconspicuous eating
High-fat and
   carbohydrate foods
Frequent weight
   swings
Laxative abuse
Diuretic abuse
Impulse dyscontrol
Gastric rupture
Parotitis
Dental erosion
Kleptomania
Self-mutilation
Suicide attempts
Socially outgoing

FIGURE 73-1. Signs and symptoms of anorexia nervosa and bulimia nervosa. (DST, dexamethasone suppression test; ECG, electrocardiogram.)

The use of purging methods is not limited to bulimia. Self-induced vomiting is the most common form of purging behavior.[35] Laxative abuse is another form common in both anorexia and bulimia, used by an estimated 3% to 70% of patients.[35–37] Although ineffective as a weight-loss strategy, laxative abuse is often used in combination with other behaviors, including exercise, diuretics, enemas, and saunas. Within the diagnostic framework of anorexia, laxative abuse is most common in those identified with the purging subtype.[35] Psychiatric symptoms of depression, anxiety, and borderline personality disorder are also reported in those who abuse laxatives.[35–37]

Depression, schizophrenia, obsessive-compulsive disorder (OCD), and conversion disorders should be included in the differential diagnosis of anorexia and bulimia, as eating abnormalities can be a component of these illnesses. The salient differences are the overriding drive for thinness, disturbed body image, increased energy directed at losing weight, and binge eating episodes that are relatively specific for eating disorders. Most patients with eating disorders experience relief of psychiatric symptoms on refeeding.[18]

ANOREXIA NERVOSA

The core features of anorexia are refusal to maintain a minimal normal body weight (e.g., greater than 85% normal body weight or body mass index [BMI] greater than 17.5 kg/m²) and failure to make expected weight gains, intense fear and obsession about weight gain or being "fat," distorted body image, and amenorrhea for at least three consecutive cycles. Patients typically lack an appreciation for the degree of weight loss experienced or are preoccupied with the idea that a part of their body is too large, despite evidence to the contrary. The *DSM-IV-TR* further classifies anorexia nervosa as restricting type (failure to engage in binge eating or purging behavior) or binge eating/purging type, in which patients regularly participate in bingeing or purging.[16] The anorexic patient has difficulty sensing when he or she is full (satiety) and commonly complains of feeling bloated after eating. Patients also describe not feeling in control of various aspects of their life, particularly caloric intake. Anorexic patients often present with features of major depression, but these symptoms should initially be considered to be secondary to starvation and not a true mood disorder.

Several proposed changes for the not yet released fifth edition of *Diagnostic and Statistical Manual of Mental Disorders* are being considered. These include the potential elimination of the amenorrhea diagnostic component and elimination of the subclassifications of anorexia nervosa.[38]

CLINICAL CONTROVERSY

Many thought leaders believe the diagnostic criteria for anorexia nervosa are too complex and that some actual eating disorders do not fully meet the DSM-IV-TR criteria. Potential changes to the diagnostic criteria are being considered for the yet to be released DSM-V.

Psychiatric comorbidity is common, as up to 75% of patients have a primary mood disorder.[39] There is also a link between anorexia and personality disorders and anxiety disorders, such as social phobia and OCD.[40] The lifetime prevalence of OCD in patients with anorexia nervosa is reported to be as high as 40%;

the lifetime prevalence in the general population is 2.5%.[39–41] The impact that psychiatric comorbidity has on treatment outcomes of anorexia is unknown but is likely dependent upon the severity of the comorbidity itself. It is important to understand that deprivation of food may contribute to both mood and cognitive fluctuation.[42]

CLINICAL PRESENTATION OF ANOREXIA NERVOSA

General

- Patients refuse to maintain body weight and have distorted perceptions about their body.

Symptoms

- Patients have obsessions and fears about eating and gaining weight.
- They complain about feeling full even when they have eaten very little food.
- Denial of symptoms and low self-esteem are the norm. Patients often feel ineffective and have a lack of self-control.

Signs

- Weakness, lethgy, cachexia, amenorrhea, vomiting, restricted food intake, inappropriate exercise, delayed sexual development, edema, delayed gastric emptying, constipation, bradycardia, hypotension, osteoporosis, dry cracking skin, lanugo, callus on dorsum of hand, perioral dermatitis, erosion of dental enamel

Laboratory Abnormalities

- Hypokalemia, hypokalemic alkalosis, hypomagnesemia, leukopenia, QT interval prolongation, ST segment depression, U waves, hypercholesterolemia, anemia

Other Diagnostic Tests

- Nonspecific electroencephalogram (EEG) changes

BULIMIA NERVOSA

The core feature of bulimia nervosa is recurrent episodes of binge eating (an excessive intake of calorie-laden food over a short period of time). Persons with bulimia are overly sensitive about their weight and have a distorted body image. Most have normal weight, although they might fluctuate between being underweight and overweight. Patients lack control over their eating and participate in recurrent compensatory behavior to prevent weight gain. These behaviors may include self-induced vomiting; misuse of laxatives, diuretics, enemas, or other medications; strict dieting or fasting; or excessive exercise. To meet *DSM-IV-TR* criteria, the binges and compensatory behaviors must occur on average at least twice weekly for 3 months. Bulimia can further be differentiated by purging type (regularly engages in self-induced vomiting or the misuse of laxatives, diuretics, or enemas) or nonpurging type (uses other inappropriate compensatory behaviors, such as fasting or excessive exercise, but does not engage in purging activities).[16]

CLINICAL PRESENTATION OF BULIMIA NERVOSA

General

- Patients binge eat and stop when they have abdominal pain or self-induced vomiting or are interrupted by another person.

- They have a pattern of severe dieting followed by binge eating episodes.
- They are concerned about their body image but do not have the drive to thinness, which is characteristic of anorexia nervosa.

Symptoms

- Patients do not eat regular meals and do not feel satiety at the end of a meal.
- They may use laxatives for weight control.
- They have guilt, depression, and self-disparagement after binges.
- Social isolation can result from frequent bingeing.
- Chaotic and troubled personal relationships and substance abuse are common.

Signs

- Bingeing, vomiting, salivary gland inflammation, erosion of dental enamel, callus on dorsum of hand, perioral dermatitis, dental caries, parotid gland enlargement, abdominal pain, upper end of normal body weight or slightly overweight, frequent weight fluctuations, diminished masticatory ability

Laboratory Abnormalities

- Hypokalemia, hypochloremic metabolic acidosis, elevated serum amylase

Other Diagnostic Tests

- None

Under consideration for *DSM-V* is the potential standardization of the frequency of symptoms for bulimia and BED by reducing the requirement from two to one time per week for 3 consecutive months and also eliminating the subclassifications of bulimia nervosa.[38]

CLINICAL CONTROVERSY

Bulimia nervosa involves extensive binging and purging behaviors. New diagnostic considerations are being considered for DSM-V which would reduce the frequency of binging episodes necessary to establish the diagnosis of bulimia nervosa.

Patients typically binge and vomit at least once daily. Caloric intake varies, but patients can consume between 5,000 and 20,000 calories (20,929 and 83,716 J) during a single binge. Patients tend to consume foods that are easy to ingest, do not require much chewing or preparation, and are high in carbohydrates or fat. Binge eating is typically secretive and precipitated by a stressful event, followed by postbinge remorse. Binges often last less than 2 hours but can extend to more than 8 hours. To compensate for the excessive caloric intake, many patients fast for prolonged periods, exercise compulsively, purge, or abuse laxatives.

Psychiatric comorbidity includes depression (up to 80%), poor impulse control, and substance abuse. Approximately 30% to 37% of bulimic patients have a personal history of substance abuse.[43] Kleptomania and borderline and avoidant personality disorders are also frequently observed.[40,42,44] Patients also commonly steal laxatives and comfort items, such as candies and clothes.[17]

BINGE EATING DISORDER

Patients with binge eating disorder present with recurrent episodes of bingeing without the compensatory behaviors associated with anorexia or bulimia. It is estimated that 5% to 10% of patients seeking treatment for obesity have BED. Comorbid psychotic disorders are common and reported in >70% of BED patients.[45] Major depressive disorder and low self-esteem are common, although the self-deprecating focus on body image is less severe than in anorexia or bulimia.[22,41] Diagnostic criteria require that episodes of bingeing occur at least twice weekly over a period of 6 months.[16]

For the *DSM-V,* there may be standardization of frequency and time frame for compensatory behaviors as well as adding BED as a formal diagnosis.[38]

MEDICAL COMPLICATIONS OF EATING DISORDERS

The potential medical complications of eating disorders involve multiple organ systems. The type of medical complication encountered is dependent on the type and frequency of the eating disorder behavior. Cardiac complications may occur and can include wasted cardiac muscle, orthostatic hypotension, decreased cardiac output, arrhythmia, and QTc interval prolongation.[46] During caloric restoration, there is a potential risk for developing fatal cardiovascular collapse known as refeeding syndrome. This risk is reduced by the gradual versus rapid reintroduction of calories.

Metabolic (metabolic acidosis, metabolic alkalosis) and electrolyte disturbances (e.g., hypokalemia, hypomagnesemia, and hypocalcemia), and dehydration are often seen. Elevations in bicarbonate levels during periods of hypokalemia can be an indication that the patient is inducing vomiting or using dietary weight loss medications. Non-anion-gap acidosis has also been reported with the abuse of laxative agents. Additionally, both acute and chronic renal failure has been reported.

Gastrointestinal (GI), oropharyngeal, and dental complications are frequent, as are general complaints of lethargy and fatigue.

Hormonal changes related to the hypothalamic-pituitary-gonadal axis resulting from starvation are seen. These abnormalities include effects on estradiol, the gonadotropins (e.g., luteinizing hormone, follicle-stimulating hormone, and gonadotropin-releasing hormone), thyroid function, adrenal function, and growth hormone.[17,46] Specific to female athletes is the female athlete triad, defined by the development of irregular menses, osteoporosis, and disordered eating.[46,47] Osteopenia, osteoporosis, and infertility are potential long-term complications of suppressed estrogen. The restoration of weight, specifically in anorexia nervosa, reverses the bone loss, although estrogen supplementation does not appear to be effective.[48] In all cases, the preferred method to address these issues is the normalization of nutrition. The impact on female fertility is not well studied, although the ability to carry a pregnancy to term or to give birth to a child of average birth weight appears reduced.

Chronic starvation can contribute to brain atrophy. Decreases in white matter and cerebrospinal fluid volumes return to normal after a healthy weight is achieved, but gray matter loss can persist.[18,49,50] A thorough physical and laboratory evaluation, as described in Table 73–1, is essential to determine the severity of medical complications.[16,30,51]

TABLE 73-1	Physical and Laboratory Assessment of Eating Disorders
Evaluation	**Target Symptoms**
Pulse	Bradycardia
Blood pressure	Hypotension, orthostasis
Height/weight	Underweight for size and age/body mass index
Respiratory rate	Rapid if heart failure occurs during refeeding
Temperature	Hypothermia, cold intolerance
Electrocardiogram	ST depression, flat T waves, U waves, increased QT interval, atrioventricular block
GI	Hypoactive bowel sounds, gastritis, abdominal distention
Skin	Dryness, scaling, lanugo, hair loss, calluses on fingers and hands
Menses	Amenorrhea
Complete blood count	Leukopenia, anemias, thrombocytopenia
Electrolytes	Hypokalemia, hypomagnesemia, hypo- or hyperphosphatemia
pH	Metabolic alkalosis (acidosis if laxative abuse)
Amylase	Elevated; pancreatitis rare
Liver	Hypoalbuminemia, γ-glutamyl transferase if alcohol abuse
Thyroid	Low to low normal, but not true disease
Cortisol	Elevated with lack of suppression on dexamethasone suppression test
Bone density	Osteoporosis

From American Psychiatric Association. Diagnostic and Statistical Manual of Mental Disorders. 4th ed. Text revision. Washington, DC: American Psychiatric Press; 2000:583–596; American Psychiatric Association. Treatment of Patients with Eating Disorders, third edition. Am J Psychiatry 2006;163 (7 Suppl):4–54; and Halmi K. Eating disorders. In: Sadock BJ, Sadock VA, eds. Comprehensive Textbook of Psychiatry. 7th ed. Philadelphia: Lippincott Williams & Wilkins; 2000:1663–1676; National Collaborating Centre for Mental Health. Eating Disorders: Core Interventions in the Treatment and Management of Anorexia Nervosa, Bulimia Nervosa and Related Eating Disorders. London: British Psychological Society and Royal College of Psychiatrists; 2004:1–36.

TREATMENT

EATING DISORDERS

■ DESIRED OUTCOMES

The goals for patients with eating disorders are to reduce distorted body image; restore and maintain healthy body weight; establish normal eating patterns; improve psychologic, psychosocial, and physical problems; resolve contributory family problems; enhance compliance; and prevent relapse.[18] Specific to BED is the additional goal of weight loss.

■ ANOREXIA NERVOSA

The long-term prognosis of patients with anorexia nervosa is not clear, as studies focus only on patients receiving treatment. The course of the disorder most commonly consists of a single episode with subsequent return to normal weight, although patients can still experience issues with disturbed body image, disordered eating, and other psychiatric problems.[18] Some patients experience an unremitting course leading to death, whereas others suffer episodically. It is estimated that less than 50% of anorexic patients recover, and 20% remain chronically ill despite weight normalization, return of menses, and improved eating behaviors.[52] The prognosis is more favorable with longer follow-up care and younger age of onset, whereas a poorer prognosis is associated with chronic illness, lower initial weight, poor family relationships, obsessive-compulsive personality symptoms, and the presence of bulimia or purging behavior.[24,52–54] Long-term follow-up shows high mortality rates, with 5% to 10% of anorexic patients dying, most often the result of cardiac arrest or suicide.[16,52]

■ BULIMIA NERVOSA

The prognosis of bulimia nervosa, although not well studied, appears to be better than that of anorexia. Patients with milder presenting symptoms who are treated as outpatients tend to do better, whereas those with electrolyte imbalances, esophagitis, dental caries, and salivary gland enlargement have a more complicated course.[17] A 6-year follow-up study of patients who received intensive treatment found that 60% had a "good" response.[53] It is important to note that even in cases in which patients respond, they continue to exhibit symptoms that wax and wane. Total absence of symptoms is an uncommon outcome, and residual symptoms predispose the patient to relapse. The actual definition of recovery varies, as once-a-month binge–purge episodes are considered by some to be recovery if their episodes were previously more frequent, whereas other clinicians consider a patient recovered only when there is complete absence of these behaviors.[54]

■ GENERAL APPROACH TO TREATMENT

Treatment plans are individualized based on the severity of specific core features of the eating disorder and comorbid medical and psychiatric conditions. Psychiatrists, physician assistants, nurses, nutrition specialists, psychologists, and pharmacists play a role in the care of these complex patients. The absence of an adequate support system of family and friends can contribute to failed treatment. A critical first step is to determine the severity of illness, as that drives both the intensity and the setting for delivery of care. Hospitalization is based on the criteria outlined in Table 73–2 and is limited to only the most severely ill patients.[24,30,31] Medications are rarely indicated as a sole treatment for eating disorders, and many patients refuse medication, although they remain part of the comprehensive treatment strategy.[55–57] Comparative, double-blind, placebo-controlled trials are sparse, and most are limited by small sample sizes, ambivalent patient attitudes toward treatment, medical complications, and high dropout rates.[58]

TABLE 73-2	Criteria for Hospitalization of Patients with Eating Disorders

- Significant weight loss of 20% or more of normal weight, particularly if weight loss has been recent and rapid, severe starvation symptoms are present, or the patient has been ill for more than 2 years
- Reduced oral intake of food (sudden and persistent)
- Medical complications (e.g., edema) and metabolic abnormalities (e.g., hypoproteinemia) from bingeing, purging, and starvation (e.g., heart rate <40 bpm, blood pressure <90/60 mm Hg, glucose <60 mg/dL (<3.33 mmol/L), potassium <3 mEq/L (<3 mmol/L), or inability to maintain core temperature
- Co-occurring psychiatric symptoms, notably suicidal ideation, psychotic depression, or substance abuse and dependence
- Nonresponsive to outpatient treatment (after 3–4 months) and poor motivation to recover
- Demoralization or nonfunctional family
- Denial of severity of abnormal eating behaviors
- Continuous supervision required to prevent purging (vomiting or laxative abuse)

From American Psychiatric Association. Diagnostic and Statistical Manual of Mental Disorders. 4th ed. Text revision. Washington, DC: American Psychiatric Press; 2000:583–596; American Psychiatric Association. Treatment of Patients with Eating Disorders, third edition. Am J Psychiatry 2006;163(7 Suppl):4–54; Fairburn CG, Harrison PJ. Eating disorders. Lancet 2003;361:407–416; Halmi K. Eating disorders. In: Sadock BJ, Sadock VA, eds. Comprehensive Textbook of Psychiatry. 7th ed. Philadelphia: Lippincott Williams & Wilkins; 2000:1663–1676; Powers PS. Initial assessment and early treatment options for anorexia nervosa and bulimia nervosa. Psychiatr Clin North Am 1996;19:639–655; and National Collaborating Centre for Mental Health pages 1–36. Eating Disorders: Core Interventions in the Treatment and Management of Anorexia Nervosa, Bulimia Nervosa and Related Eating Disorders. London: British Psychological Society and Royal College of Psychiatrists; 2004:1–36.

■ ANOREXIA NERVOSA

Nonpharmacologic Treatments

CLINICAL CONTROVERSY

Cognitive behavioral therapy and other nonpharmacologic interventions are generally considered preferred first-line treatment options for anorexia nervosa. Controversy exists as to what level of symptomatology should be present to consider the initiation of pharmacologic therapy.

Evidence supports that nonpharmacologic treatments have the greatest likelihood of eliciting a response in anorexic patients.[18,55] This includes CBT, behavioral management, interpersonal psychotherapy, nutritional counseling, and family therapy.[18,30,59] Current guidelines suggest at least 6 months of psychotherapy.[59] CBT helps the patient overcome distorted thinking, including self-worth as measured by body image, feelings of being fat despite evidence to the contrary, and denial. CBT also teaches patients how to use strategies besides eating to cope. Interpersonal psychotherapy focuses on interpersonal relationships and functioning, whereas CBT provides positive reinforcement for weight gain.[39] The benefit of treatment based on an addiction model (12-step program) is not supported by the literature.[18,24] Many psychiatric symptoms in an acutely ill patient, such as depression and anxiety, diminish or disappear with weight restoration. Initial treatment is directed toward restoring a healthy weight (greater than 90% of normal weight for age-matched controls) and treating food phobias.[60] After achieving medical stability and appropriate weight, therapy can be redirected toward addressing ongoing interpersonal problems, weight maintenance, cognitive restructuring, and skill development for relapse prevention.[61] Oral refeeding, initially with liquid formulas if necessary, is the most common approach to weight restoration.

❹ In severe cases, nasogastric refeeding is preferred over Intravenous (IV) bolus dosing.[18] Total parenteral nutrition is reserved only for the management of severely malnourished patients and if other refeeding methods fail. The decision to administer total parenteral nutrition must be made carefully, because of the potentially devastating psychologic effect on patients who do not wish to gain weight.

Current clinical evidence suggests a controlled weight gain of 0.9 to 1.4 kg (2–3 lb) per week in inpatient settings and 0.2 to 0.5 kg (0.5–1 lb) per week in outpatient settings.[16,57,60] Recommendations vary; however, it is considered acceptable for patients to begin refeeding at 1,000 to 1,600 calories per day (4186 to 6697 J/day) (30–40 cal/kg/day [126–167 J/kg]) with slow titration upwards until they begin to demonstrate sustained weight gain.[18,59,62] This can require the intake of an additional 3,500 to 7,000 extra calories (14,650 to 29,301 J) per week.[59] Slow refeeding is important to minimize the risk of medical and psychologic consequences.[24]

Pharmacologic Therapy

Antidepressants Although many studies examine the role of antidepressants in the treatment of anorexia nervosa, they often have small sample sizes and large confidence intervals.[63] Antidepressants currently have no role in the acute treatment of anorexia, unless there is another clinical indication present.[18,24,55]

❺ Data suggest that medication is ineffective if a patient weighs less than 85% of his or her expected weight. Thus, antidepressants should be initiated only if depression, anxiety, obsessions, or compulsions persist after the target weight is achieved.[24,60,64] The duration of treatment when antidepressants are used in this manner is unclear, but one study showed benefit in treated patients for

1 year, and current guidelines suggest 9 to 12 months of therapy.[4,18,59] Antidepressants, along with psychotherapy, have been used to help maintain weight and prevent relapse, but data supporting this are limited.[65] Most clinicians prefer the selective serotonin reuptake inhibitor (SSRI) antidepressants because they are better tolerated and have greater cardiovascular safety than tricyclic antidepressants (TCAs) and monoamine oxidase inhibitors (MAOIs).[18,66] Because these patients are sensitive to anticholinergic and cardiovascular effects, if TCAs or MAOIs are used, low starting doses and slow titration toward an effective dose are appropriate. The risk of cardiotoxicity in a malnourished population must not be underestimated, and a baseline electrocardiogram (ECG) should be obtained before initiation of these agents.

Fluoxetine continues to be the most widely studied SSRI in anorexia. Most clinicians initiate at low doses, for example, 20 mg/day, and increase to a maximum of 60 mg/day based on response and tolerability.[62,63,65] Some clinical controversy exists regarding when antidepressant therapy should be initiated. During the starvation phases of anorexia, the majority of clinical trials suggest antidepressants are ineffective, and there is debate as to their effectiveness once weight restoration has occurred. Evidence from a 52-week, randomized, placebo-controlled clinical trial of 93 patients with the treatment arm receiving doses from 20 to 80 mg/day showed no difference between fluoxetine and placebo for time to relapse.[67]

Antipsychotics Typical antipsychotics were the first medications used to treat anorexia to reduce obsessive and paranoid thoughts about weight gain and anxiety and to promote weight gain.[68] However, there was little improvement, and the risks were considered to outweigh the benefits. Atypical antipsychotics have provided an additional alternative for treating anorexia. Most of the data are from case reports or small trials in both adolescents and adults using risperidone 0.5 to 1.5 mg daily, olanzapine 2.5 to 15 mg daily, and quetiapine 200 to 500 mg daily.[69–75] Improvement has been shown through weight increase and reduction of comorbid anxiety and depressive symptoms, but not all reports are favorable, and these agents require further study. Caution is urged in view of the report of increased QTc in an anorexic patient taking risperidone.[74] Optimal treatment duration is unknown, as most of the larger studies are less than or equal to 3 months in duration.

Miscellaneous Agents Metoclopramide can be helpful in reducing bloating, early satiety, and abdominal pain commonly found in anorexia, but it does not affect weight gain.[18] Low-dose, short-acting benzodiazepines (0.25 mg alprazolam or 0.5 mg lorazepam) given before meals are useful when severe anxiety limits eating.[18] Estrogen replacement has been used, but restoring menses through refeeding is a preferred approach to minimize bone density loss.

■ BULIMIA NERVOSA

Nonpharmacologic Therapy

The nondrug strategies used in bulimia are similar to those used with anorexia, and they are equally critical to success. CBT has the strongest evidence supporting its benefit in managing bulimia.[19,25] Current treatment guidelines suggest that CBT should consist of 16 to 20 sessions over a 4- to 5-month period.[59] Interpersonal psychotherapy also plays a role and has a moderate degree of evidence to support its use.[18,24] Nutritional counseling, planned meals, and self-monitoring can help interrupt the binge–purge cycle. Family therapy in bulimic patients is less critical than with anorexia, as these patients tend to be older. A recent study suggested that CBT-guided self-care was a more effective treatment approach in adolescents than family therapy, whereas other programs using self-help guides based on CBT have shown mixed results.[30,76] When such programs have been combined with medication, for example fluoxetine, enhanced response has been reported.[77,78] Data support the use of 12-step programs, but they should not be used as monotherapy.[18,24]

Pharmacologic Therapy

Antidepressants Antidepressants are used in the acute and maintenance phases of bulimia adjunctively with nonpharmacologic approaches. A wide array of antidepressants, including TCAs, MAOIs, trazodone, serotonin-norepinephrine reuptake inhibitors (SNRIs), and SSRIs, have been studied. Additionally, several reviews analyzing this body of literature have been published, although there continues to be limited placebo-controlled, randomized, double-blind clinical studies.[24,55] Antidepressants are reported to reduce depression, anxiety, obsessions, and impulsive behaviors such as binge eating and purging, and improve eating habits, although their impact on body dissatisfaction remains unclear. The presence of comorbid mood disorders is not necessary for an antidepressant response.[24,79,80]

The benefit appears to be more robust in the acute phase of the illness, as relapse despite continued antidepressant use is common in patients who are in or near remission.[24,30,57] Antidepressant response usually occurs in 6 to 8 weeks, and reduction in frequency of binge–purge behavior has been as high as 73% and as low as zero.[55] Abstinence rates (elimination of bingeing and purging behaviors) with short-term use range from zero to 68%. More data are needed to determine the long-term benefits of antidepressants for preventing relapse of bulimia symptoms. One trial evaluating the impact of fluoxetine versus placebo in the maintenance phase showed a better outcome in patients receiving fluoxetine 60 mg/day, although high dropout rates in both groups blurred the overall benefit.[81]

❼ SSRIs are the preferred agents because of their tolerability and because they have been studied in the largest number of patients. Fluoxetine remains the only medication with Food and Drug Administration (FDA) approval for bulimia. Tolerability is the primary criterion for selecting an antidepressant in the treatment of bulimia because of patients' heightened sensitivity to adverse effects and the lack of a clear difference in efficacy between the classes. Even though there is a suggestion that MAOIs produce the most robust effect, the risk of using these medications in impulsive patients limits their use.[57] SNRIs have shown promising results; however, the data supporting their use are limited to case reports.[82] Bupropion is not used in bulimic patients because of the increased risk of seizures.

Before initiating pharmacologic-based therapy, a careful baseline physical examination, ECG, and laboratory work-up are essential. Underlying ECG changes secondary to hypokalemia or bradycardia and atrioventricular block from starvation can be present. There is potential for fatal outcomes secondary to cardiac arrest or suicide. All antidepressants can cause seizures; thus, a careful risk–benefit assessment is warranted if the patient has predisposing factors such as a personal or family history of seizures, cerebrovascular disease, or alcohol or sedative-hypnotic withdrawal.

Doses in the treatment of bulimia nervosa are similar to those in patients treated for depression, though at the higher end of the range. Readers are referred to Chapter 78 for antidepressant dosing ranges. For fluoxetine, the higher end of the dosing range, 60 mg/day, can be necessary for response.[83] With other agents, most clinicians initially target the bottom to the middle of the dosing range and increase the dose if there is an inadequate response. Slow titration is needed to allow time to develop tolerance to adverse effects. If TCAs are used, serum concentration monitoring is recommended to ensure that absorption is not compromised by purging.

❽ The time for antidepressant onset of effect in bulimia is unclear. In the absence of data, the definition of a therapeutic trial from the depression literature (4–8 weeks at a therapeutic dose) should be used. Because the majority of subjects will not experience a complete remission, and there are few data on predictors of response

or whether switching to another class will improve response, a clear and specific target should be stated initially.[18]

❾ Optimal duration of treatment after response is poorly defined, although most clinicians treat for 9 months to 1 year and then reevaluate.

CLINICAL CONTROVERSY

Antidepressant therapy is the preferred treatment intervention for bulimia nervosa, however it is unclear whether long-term pharmacologic treatment reduces the risk of relapse compared to shorter duration treatment interventions of a year or less.

The evidence is mixed as to whether any early benefit is sustained; hence, the decision to continue treatment should be made based on both initial response and the maintenance of that benefit. If the symptoms return within a few months after antidepressant discontinuation, then the treatment might need to be reinitiated.

Figure 73–2 describes criteria for medication use in bulimia, but it must be noted that no evidence-based consensus for treatment has been endorsed, even with the recent guidelines, meta-analyses, and reviews of the literature.[4,18,24,55,57,59,66]

Mood Stabilizers (Lithium and Anticonvulsants) Because of the lack of evidence demonstrating their benefit, lithium and anticonvulsants are reserved for bulimic patients with a comorbid bipolar affective disorder.[18,84] Target serum concentrations and doses are similar to those used for patients with seizure or mood disorders. Lithium must be used cautiously, as fluid shifts related to purging and laxative abuse increase the risk of toxicity. The adverse effect of weight gain often makes mood stabilizers and anticonvulsants unacceptable to patients in the long term.

Miscellaneous Agents Low-dose benzodiazepines before meals can help reduce anxiety associated with refeeding, although long-term use is not warranted because of the risk of abuse and dependence. One double-blind trial with ondansetron has shown benefit, but there are insufficient data to recommend a specific role for this agent.[85] Antipsychotics and appetite suppressants do not play a role in managing central symptoms of bulimia.[24]

Nonpharmacologic versus Pharmacologic Approaches

The combination of pharmacologic and nonpharmacologic measures appears to produce the best chance for a positive outcome for patients with bulimia nervosa.[55] Antidepressants, specifically SSRIs, are the class of choice in bulimic patients, whereas other medications are reserved for patients with comorbid psychiatric conditions. Only in unusual circumstances should patients be treated with antidepressants alone. Evidence suggests the greatest benefit is during the acute phase of treatment, whereas data are mixed supporting their role in the prevention of relapse.

■ BINGE EATING DISORDER

As in anorexia and bulimia, CBT and interpersonal psychotherapy seem to be the most effective interventions.[24] Antidepressants, anticonvulsants, and appetite suppressants are the pharmacologic agents with the greatest promise in BED, but data are limited, trials are short in duration (20 weeks or less), and whether there is sustained benefit is unclear.[86] Although reports are mixed, antidepressants have demonstrated efficacy as monotherapy at reducing binge eating and improving depressed mood during the acute phases of

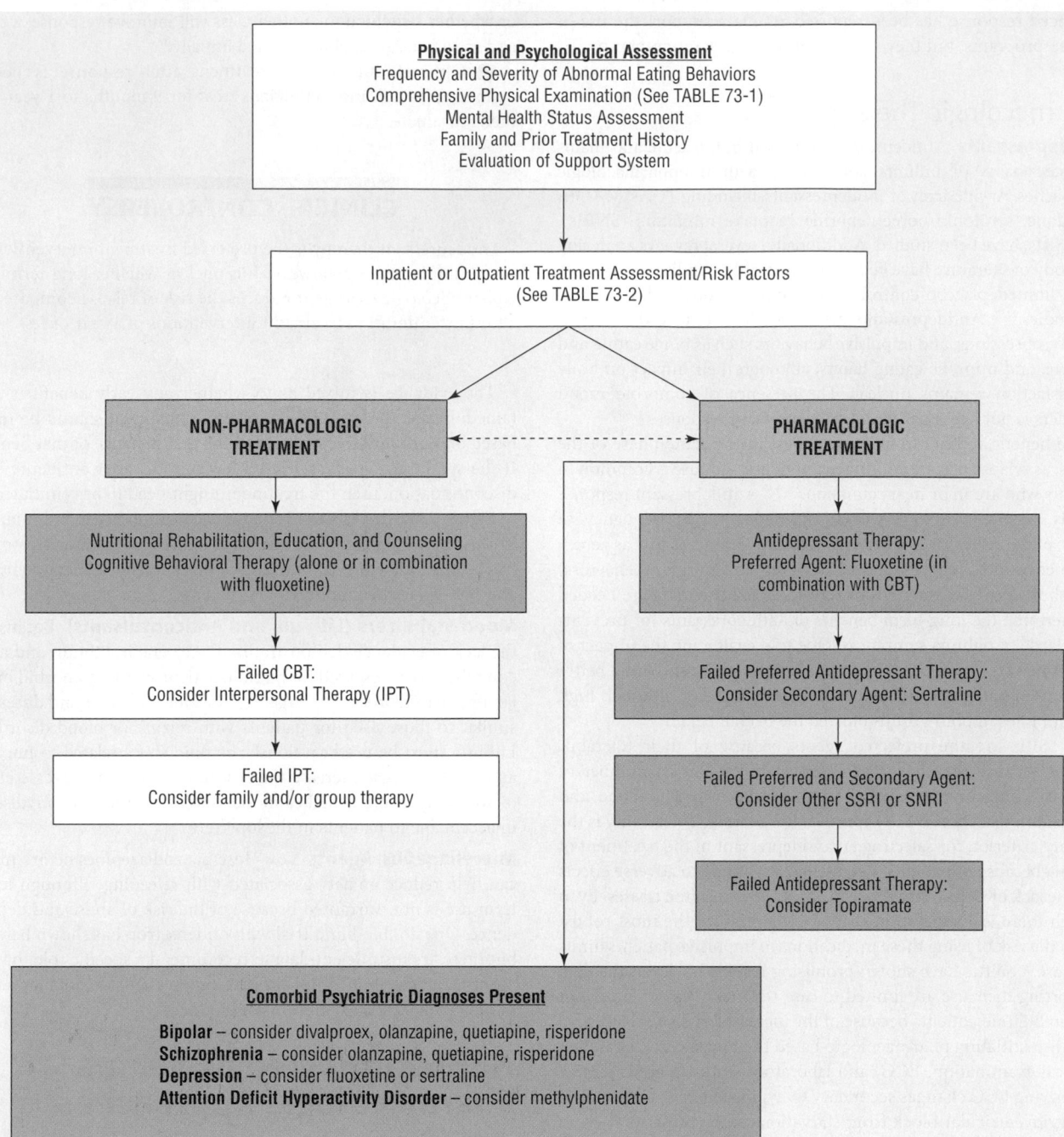

FIGURE 73-2. Bulimia nervosa treatment algorithm. (CBT, cognitive behavioral therapy; IPT, interpersonal pyschotherapy; SNRI, serotonin-norepineph-rine reuptake inhibitor; SSRI, selective serotonin reuptake inhibitor.)

the illness compared with placebo, but they can also be used in combination with CBT to augment response.[24,87–90] The majority of the data are with SSRIs given at antidepressant doses.[86] Topiramate 50 to 600 mg daily (a median dose 200 mg/day) has produced benefit in patients with impulse control disorder and because it promotes weight loss. Short-term data demonstrating superiority over placebo have been published, but data beyond 12 weeks' duration are lacking.[91] Sibutramine 10 to 15 mg/day has also demonstrated benefit in reducing weight and binge frequency in obese BED patients compared with placebo.[92] Orlistat 120 mg given three times daily, along with a calorie-restricted diet, has produced weight reduction in obese patients with BED.[93] Zonisamide (100–600 mg/day) has also displayed benefit at reducing binge eating frequency and promoting weight loss.[94]

In summary, the question of where BED fits on the diagnostic spectrum continues to be explored. Current literature suggests that three different types of pharmacologic agents (SSRIs, topiramate, and sibutramine) hold promise in the short term, but long-term data are lacking. As with other eating disorders, nonpharmacologic treatments are the key to a successful outcome.

PHARMACOECONOMIC CONSIDERATIONS

There are no formal evaluations of the economic impact of eating disorders on individual patients, on global healthcare costs, or on indirect costs such as unemployment, premature death, or disability payments. The chronic course, severe disability, and lack of improvement in up to one-third of patients suggest a significant cost impact. Clinicians should contribute to the appropriate use of resources by ensuring that medications are used in situations in which there is evidence demonstrating their benefit and that they are never used as the sole treatment modality. For example, antidepressants are started after normal weight is restored in anorexic patients and not to treat depressive symptoms in significantly malnourished patients. One study evaluating the relative costs of CBT alone, medication alone, or combination treatment in bulimia concluded that if overall effectiveness was the prime consideration, then CBT, with medication added if the response was inadequate, was the best approach. If cost-effectiveness was the basis for making treatment decisions, then antidepressants alone as a first step, followed by the addition of CBT when response is inadequate, is the preferred next intervention.[92]

EVALUATION OF THERAPEUTIC OUTCOMES

ANOREXIA NERVOSA

A combination of subjective and objective measures is used to assess patient response. A reduction in the frequency and severity of abnormal eating habits, normalized exercise patterns and laboratory tests, and a sustained weight close to age-matched normals are key indicators of response. A diary recording exercise frequency, menses, food intake, patterns of eating, and associated feelings while eating is a useful tool to track progress, especially in the outpatient setting. Weekly weigh-ins on the same scale, preferably at a clinician's office, help monitor progress early in treatment and reduce the focus on weight and anxiety caused by the variability found among different scales. Follow-up laboratory tests and ECGs are not part of routine monitoring unless the patient is restricting food intake, is purging, or continues to lose weight despite treatment. Inpatients require daily assessment of weight and caloric intake, vital signs, and urine output because of the more severe nature of their illness. They also can need monitoring of bathroom privileges early in their care. A healthy weight gain of no more than 0.2 to 0.5 kg (0.4 to 1.1 lb) per week toward a goal of 90% to 95% of normal weight or a BMI greater than 18.5 kg/m^2 is a critical sign of treatment success. A patient's use of coping skills and contingencies for dealing with stress other than manipulating food consumption also should be assessed. Antidepressants can assist in alleviation of persistent depression, anxiety, and obsessions, after weight restoration. Improvement in mood is expected to occur within 8 weeks. Patients receiving TCAs should be evaluated for dry mouth, constipation, hypotension, and sedation. Patients receiving SSRIs should be monitored for agitation, drug-induced anorexia, nausea, weight loss, and insomnia. The decision to use long-term medication must be based on specific and sustained improvement in the target symptoms, balanced against adverse effects.

BULIMIA NERVOSA

An individualized treatment and monitoring plan begins with a thorough assessment describing the baseline frequency and severity of treatment-responsive target symptoms and other associated findings. The assessment must be comprehensive, as a patient can hide his or her illness by shifting from one type of behavior to another (e.g., exercise to purging).

A comprehensive assessment includes a description of psychiatric symptoms, physical findings, frequency and severity of binge–purge episodes, laxative and ipecac use, exercise patterns, and laboratory and ECG abnormalities. Interpersonal and relationship problems should also be evaluated. Some findings indicating a more chronic

course of illness, such as salivary gland inflammation and erosion of dental enamel, can take months to reverse or might never normalize. Hence, these are not sensitive indicators of early treatment response. Data describing a patient's baseline level of functioning and previous response to treatment should be used to set goals in the current treatment plan.

Antidepressant response usually occurs within 4 to 8 weeks after the onset of treatment. If response does not occur, binge–purge behavior should be considered as a factor potentially contributing to the malabsorption of medication. If this behavior is not present, then every attempt should be made to maximize the dose. Serum concentration monitoring, when appropriate as with TCAs, should be done periodically (every 3–6 months if a patient is responding and tolerating the medication, or more frequently if clinically indicated). Evaluation of previously described adverse effects also should be part of the monitoring plan. If the patient responds, he or she should be followed for 6 to 12 months, then reassessed for the need for ongoing medication. If the patient relapses on medication discontinuation, then the medication should be restarted.

Ambulatory eating disorder patients present a particular challenge to clinicians. Impulsivity associated with bulimia nervosa can increase the risk for suicide. Prescriptions should be limited to small supplies. In addition, pharmacists should be alert to persons who make large or frequent purchases of laxatives or ipecac syrup, as this is an indicator of possible bulimic behaviors.

CONCLUSION

Our understanding of the pathophysiology and symptomatology of eating disorders has improved significantly over the past several years. Medication serves an adjunctive role to a variety of psychosocial therapies in anorexia nervosa, whereas it plays a more central role in bulimia nervosa and BED treatment. By gaining a greater understanding of the underlying physiologic changes and the psychosocial complications associated with eating disorders, treatment plans can be specifically designed for an individual patient with the goal of improving his or her quality of life.

ACKNOWLEDGMENTS

The author acknowledges the contributions of Patricia A. Marken, PharmD, and Roger W. Sommi, PharmD, authors of the Eating Disorders chapter (Chapter 66) in the seventh edition of *Pharmacotherapy: A Pathophysiologic Approach*.

ABBREVIATIONS

BDNF: Brain-derived neurotrophic factor

BED: Binge eating disorder

CBT: Cognitive behavioral therapy

DSM-IV-TR: Diagnostic and Statistical Manual of Mental Disorders (Fourth Edition, Text Revision)

ECG: Electrocardiogram

EDNOS: Eating disorder not otherwise specified

MAOI: Monoamine oxidase inhibitor

NES: Night eating syndrome

SSRI: Selective serotonin reuptake inhibitor

SNRI: Serotonin-norepinephrine reuptake inhibitor

TCA: Tricyclic antidepressant

REFERENCES

1. Klump KL, Bulik CM, Kaye WH, et al. Academy for Eating Disorders position paper: Eating disorders are serious mental illnesses. Int J Eat Disord 2009;42(2):97–103.

2. Bulik CM, Tozzi FC, Anderson C, et al. The relationship between eating disorders and components of perfectionism. Am J Psychiatry 2003;160:366–368.

3. McKnight investigators. Risk factors for the onset of eating disorders in adolescent girls: Results of the McKnight longitudinal risk factor study. Am J Psychiatry 2003;160:248–254.

4. Favaro A, Ferrara S, Santonastaso P. The spectrum of eating disorders in young women: A prevalence study in a general population sample. Psychosom Med 2003;65:701–708.

5. Striegel-Moore RH, Dohm FA, Kraemer HC, et al. Eating disorders in white and black women. Am J Psychiatry 2003;160:1326–1331.

6. Gull WW. Anorexia nervosa. Trans Clin Soc (Lond) 1874. In: Kaufman RM, Heifman M, eds. Evolution of Psychosomatic Concepts—Anorexia Nervosa: A Paradigm. New York: International Universities Press, 1964:22–28.

7. Lesegue C. De l'anorexic hysterique. Arch Gen Med 1873. In: Kaufman RM, Heifman M, eds. Evolution of Psychosomatic Concepts—Anorexia Nervosa: A Paradigm. New York: International Universities Press, 1964:385–395.

8. Russel G. Bulimia nervosa: An ominous variant of anorexia nervosa. Psychol Med 1979;9:429–448.

9. Striegel-Moore RH, Franko DL, May A, et al. Should night eating syndrome be included in the DSM? Int J Eat Disord 2006;39:544–549.

10. O'Reardon JP, Allison KC, Martino NS, et al. A randomized, placebo-controlled trial of sertraline in the treatment of night eating syndrome. Am J Psychiatry 2006;163:893–898.

11. Hoek H, van Hoeken D. Review of the prevalence and incidence of eating disorders. Int J Eat Disord 2003;34:383–386.

12. Bulik CM, Reba L, Siega-Riz AM, Reichborn-Kjennerud T. Anorexia nervosa: Definition, epidemiology, and cycle of risk. Int J Eat Disord 2005;37:52–59.

13. Wittchen HU, Nelson CB, Lachner G. Prevalence of mental disorders and psychosocial impairments in adolescents and young adults. Psychol Med 1998;28:109–126.

14. Pike KM. Long-term course of anorexia nervosa: Response, relapse, remission, and recovery. Clin Psychol Rev 1998;18:447–475.

15. Norris ML, Boydell KM, Pinhas L, Katzman DK. Ana and the Internet: A review of pro-anorexia websites. Int J Eat Disord 2006;39:443–447.

16. American Psychiatric Association. Diagnostic and Statistical Manual of Mental Disorders. 4th ed. Text revision. Washington, DC: American Psychiatric Press; 2000:583–596.

17. Sadock BJ, Sadock VA, eds. Kaplan and Sadock's Synopsis of Psychiatry: Behavioral Sciences/Clinical Psychiatry. 9th ed. Philadelphia: Lippincott Williams & Wilkins; 2003:739–750.

18. American Psychiatric Association. Treatment of Patients with Eating Disorders, third edition. Am J Psychiatry 2006;163(7 Suppl):4–54.

19. Stunkard A, Grace WJ, Wolff HG. The night eating syndrome: A pattern of food intake in certain obese patients. Am J Med 1955;19:79–86.

20. Birketvedt GS, Florholmen J, Sundsfjord J, et al. Behavioral and neuroendocrine characteristics of the night eating syndrome. JAMA 1999;282:657–663.

21. Gluck ME, Geliebter A, Satov T. Night eating syndrome is associated with depression, low self-esteem, reduced daytime hunger, and less weight loss in obese outpatients. Obes Res 2001;9:264–267.

22. Rand CS, MacGreggor AMC, Stunkard AJ. The night eating syndrome in the general population and among postoperative obesity surgery patients. Int J Eat Disord 1997;22:65–69.

23. Stunkard AJ, Berkowitz R, Wadden T, et al. Binge eating disorder and the night eating syndrome. Int J Obes Relat Metab Disord 1996;20:1–6.

24. Fairburn CG, Harrison PJ. Eating disorders. Lancet 2003;361:407–416.

25. Kaye WH. Neurobiology of anorexia and bulimia nervosa. Physiol Behav 2008;94:121–135.

26. Frank GK, Kaye WH, Meltzer CC, et al. Reduced 5-HT2 A receptor binding after recovery from anorexia nervosa. Biol Psychiatry 2002;52:896–906.

27. Ribases M, Gratacos M, Fernandez-Aranda F, et al. Association of BDNF with anorexia, bulimia, age of onset of weight loss in six European populations. Hum Mol Genet 2004;13(12):1205–1212.

28. Hudson JI, Lalonde JK, Berry JM, et al. Binge-eating disorder as a distinct familial phenotype in obese individuals. Arch Gen Psychiatry 2006;63:313–319.

29. Steiger H, Joober R, Gauvin L, et al. Serotonin-system polymorphisms (5-HTTLPR and -1438G/A) and responses of patients with bulimic syndromes to multimodal treatments. J Clin Psychiatry 2008;69:1565–1571.

30. Halmi K. Eating disorders. In: Sadock BJ, Sadock VA, eds. Comprehensive Textbook of Psychiatry. 7th ed. Philadelphia: Lippincott Williams & Wilkins; 2000:1663–1676.

31. Powers PS. Initial assessment and early treatment options for anorexia nervosa and bulimia nervosa. Psychiatr Clin North Am 1996;19:639–655.

32. Casper RC, Hedeker D, McClough JF. Personality dimensions in eating disorders and their relevance for subtyping. J Am Acad Child Adolesc Psychiatry 1992;31:830–840.

33. Eckert ED, Halmi KA, Marchi P, et al. Ten-year follow-up of anorexia nervosa: Clinical course and outcome. Psychol Med 1995;25:143–156.

34. Garner DM, Garfinkel PE, O'shaughnessy M. Validity of the distinction between bulimia with and without anorexia nervosa. Am J Psychiatry 1985;142:581–587.

35. Tozzi F, Thornton LM, Mitchell J, et al. Features associated with laxative abuse in individuals with eating disorders. Psychosom Med 2006;68:470–477.

36. Garner DM, Garner MV, Rosen LW. Anorexia nervosa "restrictors" who purge: Implications for subtyping anorexia nervosa. Int J Eat Disord 1993;13:171–185.

37. Shroff H, Reba L, Thornton LM, et al. Features associated with excessive exercise in women with eating disorders. Int J Eat Disord 2006;39:454–461.

38. Wilfley DE, Bishop ME, Wilson GT, Agras WS. Classification of eating disorders: Toward DSM-V. Int J Eat Disord 2009;40:S123–S129.

39. Halmi KA. Eating disorders: Anorexia nervosa, bulimia nervosa, and obesity. In: Hales RE, Yudofsky SC, eds. Essentials of Clinical Psychiatry. 3rd ed. Washington, DC: American Psychiatric Press; 1999:667–685.

40. Jordan J, Joyce PR, Carter FA, et al. Specific and nonspecific comorbidity in anorexia nervosa. Int J Eat Disord 2008;41:47–56.

41. Braun DL, Sunday SR, Halmi KA. Psychiatric comorbidity in patients with eating disorders. Psychol Med 1994;24:859–867.

42. Woodside BD, Staab R. Management of psychiatric comorbidity in anorexia nervosa and bulimia nervosa. CNS Drugs 2006;20(8):655–663.

43. Herzog DB, Keller MB, Sacks NR, et al. Psychiatric comorbidity in treatment seeking anorexics and bulimics. J Am Acad Child Adolesc Psychiatry 1992;31:810–818.

44. O'Brien KM, Vincent NK. Psychiatric comorbidity in anorexia and bulimia nervosa: Nature, prevalence, and causal relationships. Clin Psychol Rev 2003;23:53–74.

45. Grilo CM, White MA, Masheb RM. DSM-IV psychiatric disorder comorbidity and its correlates in binge eating disorder. Int J Eat Disord 2009;42(3):228–234.

46. Rome ES, Ammerman, S. Medical complications of eating disorders: An update. J Adolesc Health 2003;33:418–426.

47. Birch K. Female athlete triad. Br Med J 2005;330(7485):244–246.

48. Mehler PS, MacKenzie TD. Treatment outcomes of osteopenia and osteoporosis in anorexia nervosa: A systematic review of the literature. Int J Eat Disord 2009;42(3):195–201.

49. Kingston K, Szmukler G, Andrews D, et al. Neuropsychological and structural brain changes in anorexia nervosa before and after refeeding. Psychol Med 1996;26:15–28.

50. Lambe EK, Katzman DK, Mikulis DJ, et al. Cerebral gray matter volume deficits after weight recovery from anorexia nervosa. Arch Gen Psychiatry 1997;54:537–542.

51. Carney CP, Anderson AE. Eating disorders: Guide to medical evaluation and complications. Psychiatr Clin North Am 1996;19:657–679.

52. Steinhausen HC. The outcome of anorexia nervosa in the 20th century. Am J Psychiatry 2002;159(8):1284–1293.

53. Fichter MM, Quadfleig N. Six year course of bulimia nervosa. Int J Eat Disord 1997;22:361–384.

54. Herzog DB, Nussbaum KM, Marmor AK. Comorbidity and outcome in eating disorders. Psychiatr Clin North Am 1996;19:843–859.

55. Mitchell JE, deZwaan M, Roerig JL. Drug therapy for patients with eating disorders. Curr Drug Targets CNS Neurol Disord 2003;2:17–29.

56. Bacaltchuk J, Hay P. Antidepressants versus placebo for people with bulimia nervosa. Cochrane Database Syst Rev 2003;4:CD003391 [updated November 2005].

57. Nakash-Eisikovits O, Dierberger A, Westen D. A multidimensional meta-analysis of pharmacotherapy for bulimia nervosa: Summarizing the range of outcomes in controlled clinical trials. Harv Rev Psychiatry 2002;10:190–211.

58. Halmi KA, Agras WS, Crow S, et al. Predictors of treatment acceptance and completion in anorexia nervosa: Implications for future study designs. Arch Gen Psychiatry 2005;62:776–781.

59. National Collaborating Centre for Mental Health. Eating Disorders: Core Interventions in the Treatment and Management of Anorexia Nervosa, Bulimia Nervosa and Related Eating Disorders. London: British Psychological Society and Royal College of Psychiatrists; 2004:1–36.

60. Zerbe KJ. Multimodal treatment of severe eating disorders. Essent Psychopharmacol 2000;3:1–17.

61. Kleifield EI, Wagner S, Halmi KA. Cognitive-behavioral treatment of anorexia nervosa. Psychiatr Clin North Am 1996;19:715–737.

62. Yager J, Anderson AE. Anorexia nervosa. N Engl J Med 2005;353(14):1481–1488.

63. Bulik CM, Berkman ND, Brownley KA, et al. Anorexia nervosa treatment: A systematic review of randomized controlled trials. Int J Eat Disord 2007;40:310–320.

64. Berg C, Eriksson M, Lindberg G, Sodersten P. Selective serotonin reuptake inhibitors in anorexia. Lancet 1996;348:1459–1450.

65. Kaye WH, Nagata T, Weltzin TE, et al. Double-blind placebo-controlled administration of fluoxetine in restricting- and restricting-purging-type anorexia nervosa. Biol Psychiatry 2001;4:644–652.

66. Jimerson DC, Wolfe BE, Brotman AW, Metzger ED. Medication in the treatment of eating disorders. Psychiatr Clin North Am 1996;19:739–754.

67. Walsh BT, Kaplan AS, Attia E, et al. Fluoxetine after weight restoration in anorexia nervosa: A randomized controlled trial. JAMA 2006;295(22):2605–2612.

68. Dally PJ, Sargant W. A new treatment for anorexia nervosa. Br Med J 1960;1:1770–1773.

69. Powers PS, Santana CA, Bannon YS. Olanzapine in the treatment of anorexia nervosa: An open label trial. Int J Eat Disord 2002;32:146–154.

70. Barbarich N, McConaha C, Gaskill J, et al. An open trial of olanzapine in anorexia nervosa. J Clin Psychiatry 2004;65(11):1480–1482.

71. Malina A, Gaskill J, McConaha C, et al. Olanzapine treatment of anorexia nervosa: A retrospective study. Int J Eat Disord 2003;33:234–237.

72. Dunican KC, DelDotto D. The role of olanzapine in the treatment of anorexia nervosa. Ann Pharmacother 2007;41:111–115.

73. Mehler-Wex C, Romanos M, Kirchheiner J, Schulze UME. Atypical antipsychotics in severe anorexia nervosa in children and adolescents-review and case reports. Eur Eat Disorders Rev 2008;16:100–108.

74. Newman-Toker JJ. Risperidone in anorexia nervosa. J Am Acad Child Adolesc Psychiatry 2000;39:941–942.

75. Bissada H, Tasca GA, Barber AM, Bradwejn J. Olanzapine in the treatment of low body weight and obsessive thinking in women with anorexia nervosa: A randomized, double-blind, placebo-controlled trial. Am J Psychiatry 2008;165:1281–1288.

76. Schmidt U, Lee S, Beecham J, et al. A randomized controlled trial of family therapy and cognitive behavior therapy guided self-care for adolescents with bulimia nervosa and related disorders. Am J Psychiatry 2007; 164:591–598.

77. Mitchell JE, Fletcher L, Hanson K, et al. The relative efficacy of fluoxetine and manual-based self-help in the treatment of outpatients with bulimia nervosa. J Clin Psychiatry 2001;21:298–304.

78. Walsh BT, Fairburn CG, Mickley D, et al. Treatment of bulimia nervosa in a primary care setting. Am J Psychiatry 2004;161:556–561.

79. Mitchell JE, Groat R. A placebo-controlled, double-blind trial of amitriptyline in bulimia. J Clin Psychopharmacol 1984;4:186–193.

80. Hughes PL, Wells LA, Cunningham CJ, Ilstrup DM. Treating bulimia with desipramine: A double-blind, placebo controlled trial. Arch Gen Psychiatry 1986;43:182–186.

81. Romano SJ, Halmi KA, Sarkar NP, et al. A placebo-controlled study of fluoxetine in continued treatment of bulimia nervosa after successful fluoxetine treatment. Am J Psychiatry 2002;159:96–102.

82. Milano W, Siano C, Putrella C, Capasso A. Treatment of bulimia nervosa with fluvoxamine: A randomized controlled trial. Adv Ther 2005;22(3):278–283.

83. Fluoxetine Bulimia Nervosa Collaborative Study Group. Fluoxetine in the treatment of bulimia nervosa: A multicenter, placebo-controlled, double-blind trial. Arch Gen Psychiatry 1992;49:139–147.

84. McElroy SL, Kotwal R, Hudson JI, et al. Zonisamide in the treatment of binge eating disorder: An open-label, prospective trial. J Clin Psychiatry 2004;65(1):50–56.

85. Faris PL, Kim SW, Meller WH, et al. Effect of decreasing afferent vagal activity with ondansetron on the symptoms of bulimia nervosa: A randomized double-blind trial. Lancet 2000;355:792–797.

86. Carter WP, Hudson JI, Lalonde JK, et al. Pharmacologic treatment of binge eating disorder. Int J Eat Disord 2003;34:S74–S88.

87. Devlin MJ, Goldfein JA, Petkova E, et al. Cognitive behavioral therapy and fluoxetine as adjuncts to group behavioral therapy for binge eating disorder. Obes Res 2005;13(6):1077–1088.

88. Kaplan AS. Academy for Eating Disorders International Conference on Eating Disorders. Expert Opin Investig Drugs 2003;12:1441–1443.

89. McElroy SL, Casuto LS, Nelson EB, et al. Placebo-controlled trial of sertraline in the treatment of binge eating disorder. Am J Psychiatry 2000;157:1004–1006.

90. Hudson J, McElroy SL, Raymond NC, et al. Fluvoxamine in the treatment of binge eating disorder: A multicenter, placebo-controlled, double-blind trial. Am J Psychiatry 1998;155:1756–1762.

91. McElroy SL, Arnold LM, Shapira NA, et al. Topiramate in the treatment of binge eating disorder associated with obesity: A randomized, placebo-controlled trial. Am J Psychiatry 2003;160:255–261.

92. Appolinario JC, Gody-Matos A, Fontanelle LF, et al. An open trial of sibutramine in obese patients with BED. J Clin Psychiatry 2002;63:28–30.

93. Golay A, Laurent-Jaccard A, Habicht F, et al. Effect of orlistat in obese patients with binge eating disorder. Obes Res 2005;13(10):1701–1708.

94. Angras WS, Rossiter EM, Arnow B, et al. One-year follow-up of psychosocial and pharmacologic treatments for bulimia nervosa. J Clin Psychiatry 1994;55:179–183.

74

Substance-Related Disorders: Overview and Depressants, Stimulants, and Hallucinogens

PAUL L. DOERING

KEY CONCEPTS

❶ Problems related to abuse of chemical substances can occur acutely (e.g., respiratory arrest from using heroin) or after some length of time (e.g., dependence or withdrawal from continued use of an opiate).

❷ Pharmacotherapy of substance-related disorders is most often adjunctive to other modes of therapy such as counseling and intense psychotherapy.

❸ Withdrawal from certain classes of drugs (e.g., benzodiazepines or barbiturates) can be life-threatening, and steps must be taken to ensure that withdrawal is gradual and that it takes place in closely supervised settings.

❹ While there is much research focusing on drugs to treat the underlying addictive processes, to date the successes have been few. Prevention is the key. Because of their knowledge of pharmacology and the actions of drugs on the body, health professionals can play a key role in education of young people on the dangers of recreational drug use.

In 2001, the Schneider Institutes for Health Policy at Brandeis University[1] boldly declared that the abuse of alcohol, tobacco, and other drugs (ATOD) was the nation's number one health problem. Sadly, not much has changed since then to change their assessment. There are more deaths, illnesses, and disabilities from substance abuse than from any other preventable health condition. A recent report from the National Center on Addiction and Substance Abuse at Columbia University[2] found that for the year 2005 federal, state, and local government spending as a result of substance abuse and addiction was at least $467.7 billion.[2] A heavy smoker will stay 25% longer when hospitalized than a nonsmoker, and a problem drinker will stay four times as long as a nondrinker.[1] Of the more than 2 million deaths each year in the United States, approximately one in four is attributable to alcohol, illicit drug, or tobacco use.

In addition, one half to two thirds of homicides and serious crimes involve alcohol. Nearly one half of men arrested for homicide and assault test positive for an illegal drug.[1,2] ATOD abuse contributes to family problems, with one in four Americans reporting that alcohol has been a cause of trouble in the family, and alcohol abuse plays a part in one of three failed marriages.[1,2]

Learning objectives, review questions, and other resources can be found at
www.pharmacotherapyonline.com.

Since publication of the last edition of this textbook, a disturbing trend in drug abuse has continued: the use of medicinal drugs for nonmedicinal purposes. Between 1995 and 2002 there was a 163% increase in the number of emergency room visits tied to the abuse of prescription drugs, and these percentages continue to increase.[3] Prescription drugs now are a factor in one fourth of all overdose deaths reported in the United States. Central nervous system (CNS) agents, primarily analgesics (pain relievers), were involved in slightly less than one half (47%) of all drug-related suicide attempts that presented to emergency departments in 2005, including both prescription and over-the-counter (OTC) formulations. More than 56% of suicide-related emergency department visits included psychotherapeutic agents (e.g., benzodiazepines or antidepressants).[3]

This chapter and the next focus on the problems associated with the abuse of chemical substances and what clinicians can do to help deal with these problems.

KEY DEFINITIONS

The lack of a common vocabulary in substance abuse treatment and prevention leads to several problems. Wide arrays of terms are in common use, many without precise meaning. This lack of universal agreement on language hampers effective communication among professionals and leads to difficulties in formulating public policy and administering third-party reimbursement programs. The Liaison Committee on Pain and Addiction, a collaborative effort of the American Academy of Pain Medicine, the American Pain Society, and the American Society of Addiction Medicine has developed definitions related to the use of medications for the treatment of pain consistent with current understanding of relevant neurobiology, pharmacology, and appropriate clinical practice. The definitions have been approved by each of the three collaborating organizations. The following definitions resulted from this consensus development committee.[4]

- *Addiction* is a primary, chronic, neurobiologic disease, with genetic, psychosocial, and environmental factors influencing its development and manifestations. It is characterized by behaviors that include one or more of the following 5Cs: chronicity, impaired control over drug use, compulsive use, continued use despite harm, and craving.

- *Drug abuse* is a maladaptive pattern of substance use characterized by repeated adverse consequences related to the repeated use of the substance. Examples include failure to fulfill important obligations at work, school, or home; repeated use creating physical danger, such as driving under the influence; legal problems; and social or interpersonal problems such as arguments and fights.

- *Physical dependence* is a state of adaptation that is manifested by a drug class–specific withdrawal syndrome that can be produced by abrupt cessation, rapid dose reduction, decreasing blood level of the drug, and/or administration of an antagonist.

- *Tolerance* is a state of adaptation in which exposure to a drug induces changes that result in a diminution of one or more of the drug's effects over time.

EPIDEMIOLOGY

NATIONAL SURVEY ON DRUG USE AND HEALTH

The National Survey on Drug Use and Health (NSDUH)[5] is the primary source of statistical information on the use of illegal drugs by the U.S. population. Conducted by the federal government since 1971, the survey collects data from a representative sample of the population at their place of residence.

In 2008, the survey found that an estimated 20.1 million Americans aged 12 or older were current illicit drug users, meaning they had used an illicit drug during the month prior to the survey interview. An estimated 22.2 million Americans suffered from substance dependence or abuse because of drugs, alcohol, or both. The 2008 survey found that marijuana was the most commonly used illicit drug (15.2 million past month users). About 6.2 million Americans—2.5% of the population—said they abused prescription drugs in the past month in 2008, a decrease from 2.8% of the population in 2007, but still a monumental problem in our country.[5]

MONITORING THE FUTURE STUDY

Every year the Institute for Social Research at the University of Michigan conducts its Monitoring the Future Study, supported under a series of research grants from the National Institute on Drug Abuse.[6] A main purpose of this research is to study changes in the beliefs, attitudes, and behavior of young people in the United States.[6]

In 2009, 46,097 U.S. students in 8th, 10th, and 12th grades in 389 public and private secondary schools were surveyed.[6] Findings show that smoking marijuana is gaining popularity among U.S. teens, even though they have cut down on smoking cigarettes, binge drinking, and using methamphetamine.[6] Researchers postulate that the increase of smoking marijuana is partly attributable to the national debate over medical use of cannabis which may make the drugs seem safer to teenagers. In addition to marijuana, fewer teens also view prescription drugs and Ecstasy as dangerous, which may explain why more teens also are abusing prescription pain pills and attention-deficit drugs.[6]

Illicit or street drug use has shown considerable declines over the past decade or so, perhaps indicating a shift toward abuse of other prescription drugs. These include sedatives, tranquilizers, and narcotic drugs other than heroin (most of which are analgesics). As a result, they have become a much more important part of the nation's drug abuse problem.[6]

SUBSTANCE ABUSE EMERGENCIES: THE DAWN PROGRAM

Since the early 1970s, the Drug Abuse Warning Network (DAWN),[3] an ongoing national survey of hospital emergency departments (EDs), has collected information on patients seeking hospital emergency department treatment related to their use of an illegal drug or the nonmedical use of a legal drug. These data allow healthcare professionals to be better prepared to react to medical emergencies arising from illegal drug use and to target prevention and education programs to specific drug-using groups or populations.

Unfortunately, there is about a 2-year lag in the occurrences of ED visits and publication of the data and a limited number of metropolitan areas is surveyed.[3]

DAWN defines a *drug-related episode* as an ED visit that was induced by or related to the use of an illegal drug(s) or the nonmedical use of a legal drug for patients aged 6 to 97 years. In 2006, hospitals in the United States delivered a total of 113 million ED visits, and DAWN estimates that 1,742,887 ED visits were associated with drug misuse or abuse. Of those ED visits, some key findings include the following:

- 31% involved illicit drugs only
- 28% involved pharmaceuticals only
- 7% involved alcohol only in patients under the age of 21
- 13% involved illicit drugs with alcohol
- 10% involved alcohol with pharmaceuticals
- 8% involved illicit drugs with pharmaceuticals
- 3% involved illicit drugs with pharmaceuticals and alcohol

ECONOMIC IMPACT OF SUBSTANCE ABUSE

Substance abuse and addiction have an enormous impact on the economy. Over the years, the National Center on Addiction and Substance Abuse (CASA) at Columbia University has conducted studies aimed at quantifying the costs to local, state, and federal governments and agencies. The most recent figures[2] are based on 2005 spending because that was the most recent year for which data were available over the course of the latest study.

As noted earlier, substance abuse and addiction cost federal, state, and local governments at least $467.7 billion in 2005. The CASA report found that of $373.9 billion in federal and state spending, 95.6% ($357.4 billion) went to "shovel up the consequences and human wreckage of substance abuse and addiction";[2] only 1.9% went to prevention and treatment, 0.4% to research, 1.4% to taxation and regulation, and 0.7% to interdiction.

Of the $3.3 trillion total federal and state government spending, $373.9 billion—11.2%, more than $1 of every $10—was spent on tobacco, alcohol, illegal, and prescription drug abuse, addiction, and its consequences.[2]

For every $100 spent by state governments on substance abuse and addiction, the average spent on prevention, treatment, and research was $2.38. For each dollar in alcohol and tobacco taxes and liquor store revenues that federal and state governments collect, they spend $8.95 dealing with the consequences of substance abuse and addiction.[2]

ACUTE VERSUS CHRONIC PROBLEMS

❶ Misuse of chemical substances causes problems of two types: those that occur acutely and those that arise after continued use of a drug. Acute problems are usually predictable, given the pharmacology of the drug. Chronic abuse of chemical substances can cause a wide array of physical, psychological, and psychiatric morbities. The substance-induced disorders discussed here mainly include intoxication and withdrawal.

❶ The essential feature of substance dependence is the continued use of the substance despite adverse substance-related problems. The criteria for substance dependence are the same for each of the drugs or drug classes, varying only to fit the unique pharmacologic properties of each drug. Patients who take prescribed drugs for appropriate medical indications and in correct doses may still show tolerance, physical dependence, and withdrawal symptoms if the drug is stopped abruptly rather than being tapered. Tolerance and physical dependence are inevitable consequences of chronic treatment with opioids and certain other drugs, but by themselves, tolerance and physical dependence do not imply "addiction." To meet *Diagnostic and Statistical Manual of Mental Disorders, Fourth Edition, Text Revision (DSM-IV-TR)* criteria[7] for the diagnosis of substance dependence, at least three of the following must be present at any time in a 12-month period:

1. Tolerance

2. Withdrawal, indicated by the appearance of the characteristic withdrawal syndrome or the use of the same or related drug to relieve or avoid withdrawal symptoms

3. Substance is taken in larger amounts or over a longer period of time than was intended

4. Patient has a persistent desire or unsuccessful efforts to cut down or control substance use

5. Considerable time is spent in activities necessary to obtain the substance, use the substance, or recover from its effects

6. Social, occupational, or recreational activities are given up or reduced because of substance use

7. Substance use is continued despite knowledge of having a persistent or recurrent physical or psychologic problem caused or exacerbated by the substance

In 2008, an estimated 22.2 million persons (8.9% of the population aged 12 or older) were classified with substance dependence or abuse in the past year based on these criteria. Of these, 3.1 million were classified with dependence on or abuse of both alcohol and illicit drugs, 3.9 million were dependent on or abused illicit drugs but not alcohol, and 15.2 million were dependent on or abused alcohol but not illicit drugs.[5]

The characteristic feature of *substance abuse* is a maladaptive pattern of substance use indicated by repeated adverse consequences related to the repeated use of the substance.[7] Examples include failure to fulfill important obligations at work, school, or home; repeated use in situations in which it is physically dangerous, such as driving under the influence; legal problems; and social or interpersonal problems such as arguments and fights.[7] *Intoxication* refers to the development of a substance-specific syndrome after recent ingestion and presence in the body of a substance, and it is associated with maladaptive behavior during the waking state caused by the effect of the substance on the CNS. Examples include belligerence, mood lability, impaired judgment, and impaired social or occupational functioning. Evidence for recent intake of the substance can be obtained from the history, physical examination, or laboratory examination. The most common changes involve disturbances in perception, wakefulness, attention, thinking, judgment, motor behavior, and interpersonal behavior.

As with most illnesses, the course and prognosis of the disorders of substance use and dependence are variable. Untreated physical withdrawal from CNS depressants is potentially life-threatening, but withdrawal almost always can be managed successfully with proper medical care. Getting patients who are drug dependent to stop using drugs is very difficult, and many patients return to drug use even after treatment. As many as 75% of treated, substance-dependent patients will relapse at least once. Many patients, however, are able to obtain recovery with treatment and continued care in 12-step programs such as Alcoholics Anonymous or Narcotics Anonymous. Substance dependence or addiction can be viewed as a chronic illness that can be controlled successfully with treatment but cannot be cured and is associated with a high relapse rate. Without treatment, the course can progress to life-threatening severity, resulting from the effects of the drug, drug contaminants, or medical complications of use.[7] Recently, the definitions used in the *DSM-IV-TR* criteria have been criticized.[8] Although an in-depth discussion of the mechanism of drug addiction is beyond the scope of this chapter,

the interested reader is directed to a review article that presents the current understanding of the biology of drug addiction.[9]

DIVERSION OF PHARMACEUTICAL CONTROLLED SUBSTANCES

The nonmedical or recreational use of pharmaceutical controlled substances has dramatically increased in the United States in recent years, although there has been a slight downward trend when comparing 2007 to 2008. About 6.2 million Americans—2.5% of the population—said they abused prescription drugs in the past month in 2008. An estimated 4.7 million persons used pain relievers nonmedically in the past month in 2008, 1.8 million used tranquilizers, 904,000 used stimulants, and 234,000 used sedatives.[5]

In 2008 4.7 million teens reported they had abused a prescription drug at some time in their lives.[10,11] Family medicine cabinets were cited as the main source for obtaining prescription drugs. About 4 out of 10 (41%) teens agree that prescription drugs are much safer to use than illegal drugs. Furthermore, the same study concluded that 31% believe there is "nothing wrong" with using prescription medicines without a prescription "once in awhile."[10,11] From a supply standpoint for the first time, this year researchers asked 12- to 17-year olds how fast they can get prescription drugs, and found that 19% of teens (4.7 million) can get prescription drugs (in order to get high) in an hour; 35% (8.7 million) can get prescription drugs within a day.[11]

One of the main factors contributing to the nationwide increase in the diversion of pharmaceutical controlled substances has been the rise in the number of Internet sites that sell or facilitate the sale of these drugs for other than legitimate medical purposes.[12,13] So-called "prescription mills" remain a major source of diversion. The advent of rogue websites that cater to those who abuse pharmaceutical controlled substances has allowed the criminal operators of these sites to exploit the anonymity of the Internet to generate illicit sales of controlled substances, including prescriptions to an extent far exceeding those of any in-person prescription mill.[13] This is particularly evident when examining the data relating to the sales of hydrocodone, which is the most widely abused pharmaceutical controlled substance in the United States. According to data provided to the U.S. Drug Enforcement Administration (DEA)[13] in 2006 by registered distributors of controlled substances, 34 U.S. pharmacies supplying rogue Internet sites dispensed more than 98 million dosage units of hydrocodone. Hence, these pharmacies each dispensed an average of approximately 2.9 million dosage units of hydrocodone per pharmacy in a single year. By means of comparison, the average pharmacy in the United States dispenses approximately 88,000 dosage units of hydrocodone per year.[13]

For 5 years, CASA at Columbia University has been tracking the availability of controlled prescription drugs over the Internet. In an in-depth white paper on the subject of Internet diversion of prescription drugs, CASA referred to the Internet as a "Pharmaceutical Candy Store."[12] The disheartening results of this study helped Congress passed the Ryan Haight Act,[13] federal legislation that, effective April 13, 2009, made it illegal under federal law to "deliver, distribute, or dispense a controlled substance by means of the Internet, except as authorized by [the Controlled Substances Act]."

CNS DEPRESSANTS

BENZODIAZEPINES AND OTHER SEDATIVE-HYPNOTICS

Emergency department visits involving benzodiazepines clearly outnumber those involving any of the other types of psychotherapeutic agents. DAWN estimates that 195,625 ED visits associated with nonmedical use of pharmaceuticals involved benzodiazepines in 2006.[3] Alprazolam and clonazepam are the most frequent benzodiazepines seen in emergency department visits (65,236 visits and 33,557 visits, respectively). ED visits by patients taking diazepam and lorazepam were fewer (19,936 and 23,720, respectively).[3]

In clinical practice, the benzodiazepines largely have replaced the short-acting barbiturates and other nonbarbiturate sedative-hypnotics. Benzodiazepines with faster onset (e.g., diazepam) tend to be preferred by the recreational drug user because they are reinforcing. Flunitrazepam emerged in the mid-1990s as an illegal drug in the United States that was predominantly abused recreationally and associated with sexual assaults.[14]

PRESENTATION OF BENZODIAZEPINE INTOXICATION AND WITHDRAWAL

General

- The intoxicated patient may be in acute distress in overdoses or when benzodiazapines are combined with alcohol.

- Patients in withdrawal may also be in acute distress and should be treated with a benzodiazepine taper to prevent seizures.

Symptoms

- The patient may experience memory impairment, drowsiness, visual disturbances, confusion, and gastrointestinal disturbances. Patients may appear intoxicated, with slurred speech, poor coordination, swaying, and bloodshot eyes, with or without the odor of alcohol.[11–14]

Signs

- Hypotension or nystagmus may be observed, and urinary retention may occur.

Laboratory Tests

- Qualitative testing to confirm presence of benzodiazepines is useful for diagnostic purposes, but quantitative plasma concentrations are usually not clinically useful.

A dramatic drop in cases of flunitrazepam abuse followed the legal reclassification of the drug as a schedule I substance in Florida (and other states) in February 1997. The recent rise in alprazolam and clonazepam abuse/misuse coincides with the decreased use of flunitrazepam and represents a new trend in abuse of the benzodiazepines. Alprazolam (Xanax) has become particularly popular and is known on the street by its slang names, "Z-Bars," "Zandy bars," "footballs," and "Zannies," among others. Young people often take alprazolam or other benzodiazepines before going to the bar or dance club, ostensibly to lower the amount of alcoholic beverage needed to attain the desired level of intoxication. Unfortunately, this "pre-partying" is especially popular among women who do not like the taste of beer or find the caloric burden of drinking to be limiting. Sadly, whether taking intentionally or being given the drug without their knowledge or consent, these women become targets for sexual predators who know that the victim will have diminished recall of the events that take place. When a victim is unable to give precise details of what happened and when it happened, and is unable to identify the perpetrator, the chances of successful prosecution are greatly diminished.[14]

Because all benzodiazepines have abuse and dependence liability, patients cannot be switched from one benzodiazepine to another in hopes of decreasing a pattern of drug abuse or dependence behavior. Zolpidem, a nonbenzodiazepine, nonbarbiturate sedative, has been suggested to have little liability for physical dependence, but tolerance and withdrawal have been reported in association with its use as well.[15] Recent reports in the lay press have linked use of zolpidem to sleep walking, erratic driving, binge eating, and other similarly bizarre activities.

Benzodiazepines generally do not cause life-threatening respiratory depression (unless taken with other sedatives), as do the barbiturate-like drugs.[16] Long-term use of even therapeutic doses of benzodiazepines can cause physical dependence and withdrawal symptoms after abrupt discontinuation.[16] Occurrence of hallucinations or seizures would indicate severe physical withdrawal.

❷ Gradual tapering of dosage is also associated with less withdrawal and rebound anxiety than abrupt discontinuation. Dependence on sedative-hypnotics and benzodiazepines is summarized in Table 74–1. For additional information on benzodiazepine withdrawal, refer to Chapter 79.

TABLE 74-1	Dependence on Sedative-Hypnotics				
Generic Name	Common Trade Names	Oral Sedating Dose (mg)	Physical Dependence Daily Dose and Time Needed to Produce Dependence	Time Before Onset of Withdrawal (hours)	Peak Withdrawal Symptoms (days)[a]
Benzodiazepines					
Alprazolam	Xanax	0.25–8	8–16 mg × 42 days (est.)	8–24	2–3
Clorazepate	Tranxene	7.5–15	45–180 mg × 42–120 days (est.)	12–24	5–8
Diazepam	Valium	5–10	40–100 mg × 42–120 days	12–24	5–8
Flunitrazepam	Rohypnol	1–2	8–10 mg × 42 days (est.)	24–36	2–3
Barbiturates					
Amobarbital	Amytal	65–100	Same	8–12	2–5
Secobarbital	Seconal, Seco-8	100	800–2,200 mg × 35–37 days	6–12	2–3
Equal parts of secobarbitaland amobarbital	Tuinal	100	Same	6–12	2–3
Pentobarbital	Nembutal	100	Same	6–12	2–3
Nonbarbiturate sedative-hypnotics					
Chloral hydrate	Noctec	250	Exact dose unknown; 12 g/day chronically has led to delirium upon sudden withdrawal	6–12	2–3
Meprobamate	Equanil, Miltown, Meprotabs	400	1.6–3.2 g × 270 days	8–12	3–8

[a]Withdrawal symptoms are tremor, tachycardia, diaphoresis, nausea, vomiting, elevated blood pressure, delirium, seizures, and hallucinations.

γ-HYDROXYBUTYRATE

γ-Hydroxybutyrate (GHB) is a chemical compound structurally similar to the inhibitory brain neurotransmitter γ-aminobutyric acid. Primary groups using GHB include party and nightclub attendees. Like flunitrazepam, GHB is also characterized as a date rape drug.[14] Manifestations of acute GHB toxicity include coma, seizures, respiratory depression, and vomiting. Other documented effects of GHB include amnesia and hypotonia, abnormal sequence of rapid eye movement (REM) and non-REM sleep, and anesthesia. Doses greater than 50 mg/kg can decrease cardiac output and produce severe respiratory depression, seizure-like activity, and coma; coma and respiratory depression can be potentiated by concomitant use of alcohol. Treatment is restricted to nonspecific supportive care. Figure 74–1 shows a protocol recommended for treating suspected GHB overdose.

Until fairly recently, the majority of GHB sold on the streets was manufactured using inexpensive kits obtained over the Internet. The decreased Internet availability of kits to make GHB has been accompanied by an increased availability of chemical precursors to GHB as well as GHB analogs. Available in gyms and health food stores, these substances include γ-butyrolactone (GBL) and 1,4-butanediol.[17] GBL is converted in the body to GHB. Labels of marketed products can use unfamiliar synonyms to disguise the actual content. GBL is also known by the names 2(3H)-furanone dihydro, butyrolactone, 4-butyrolactone, dihydro-2(3H)-furanone, 4-butanolide, 2(3H)-furanone, dihydro, tetrahydro-2-furanone, and butyrolactone-γ.

GHB is being used and is being studied for a number of legitimate medical uses, including its use as an anesthetic, treatment of narcolepsy, and treatment of drug addiction. In fact, a pharmaceutical version of GHB (called by the alternate name of sodium oxybate [Xyrem]) was approved by the U.S. Food and Drug Administration (FDA) for cataplexy attacks in patients with narcolepsy in 2002. In November 2005, the FDA approved sodium oxybate for the treatment of excessive daytime sleepiness in patients with narcolepsy. Deaths from the pharmaceutical dosage forms have been reported.[18]

CARISOPRODOL

Carisoprodol is a prescription drug marketed since 1959 and used in primary care settings for the treatment of musculoskeletal conditions associated with muscle spasms and back pain. Its effectiveness for this use has been questioned.[19] It is marketed in the United States as Soma and in the U.K. as Carisoma as well as many generic versions. It is both structurally and pharmacologically related to meprobamate, a schedule IV substance. In fact, a substantial percentage of the drug is metabolized to meprobamate,[19] a drug with substantial barbiturate-like properties.

In legitimate medical practice carisoprodol is used as an adjunct to rest, physical therapy and other measures for relief of acute, painful musculoskeletal conditions.[19] The standard dosage for adults is 350 mg 3 times daily and at bedtime. Approximately 10.58 million prescriptions for carisoprodol were dispensed in 2008.

Skeletal muscle relaxant effects of carisoprodol may be related to its sedative properties.[19,20] Adverse effects are mostly related to

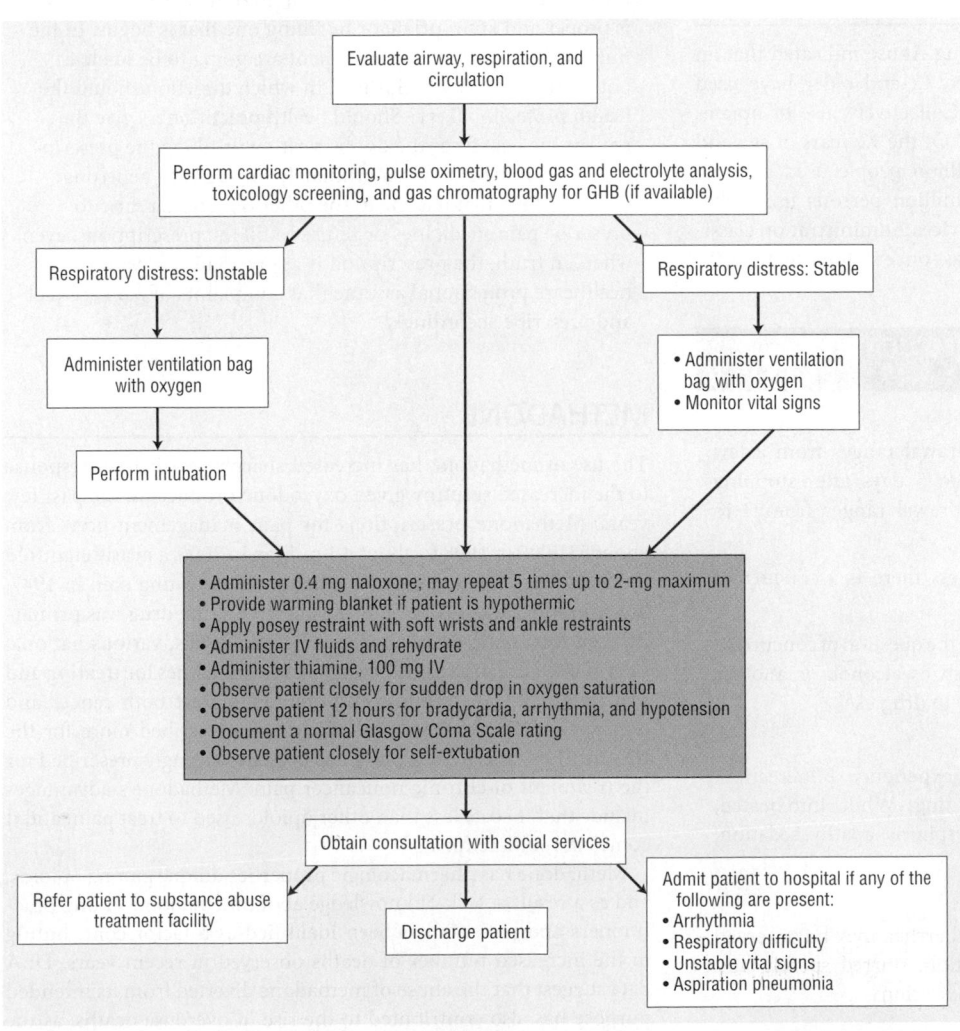

FIGURE 74-1. Protocol for treatment of suspected GHB (γ-hydroxybutyrate) overdose.

the CNS: drowsiness, dizziness, vertigo, ataxia, tremor, agitation, irritability, headache, depressive reactions, syncope, and insomnia. Carisoprodol may also adversely affect cardiovascular (tachycardia, postural hypotension, and facial flushing), gastrointestinal (nausea, vomiting, hiccup, and epigastric distress), and hematologic systems. It may cause idiosyncratic symptoms including extreme weakness, transient quadriplegia, ataxia, difficulty in speech, temporary loss of vision, double vision, dilated pupils, agitation, euphoria, confusion, and disorientation. Carisoprodol overdose has resulted in stupor, coma, shock, respiratory depression, and death.[20-22]

Data are clear that the diversion and abuse of carisoprodol have increased in the last decade.[18] According to 2007 NSDUH data, nonmedical use of carisoprodol by the U.S. population aged 12 and older was 1.1%, similar to or greater than the prevalence of abuse of other commonly abused schedule IV controlled drugs such as clonazepam (1.5%) and chlordiazepoxide (0.3%).[5] With prolonged abuse at high dosage, carisoprodol can lead to tolerance, dependence, and withdrawal symptoms in humans.[20]

According to the Diversion Drug Trends, published by the DEA on the trends in the diversion of controlled and noncontrolled pharmaceuticals,[19] carisoprodol continues to be one of the most commonly diverted drugs. Diversion and abuse of carisoprodol is prevalent throughout the country.

Ironically, carisoprodol is not controlled under the federal Controlled Substances Act of 1970. It is currently scheduled under state law in Alabama, Arizona, Arkansas, Florida, Georgia, Hawaii, Indiana, Kentucky, Louisiana, Massachusetts, Minnesota, Nevada, New Mexico, Oklahoma, Oregon, Texas, and West Virginia.

OPIATES

The National Household Survey on Drug Abuse indicated that an estimated 3,091,000 U.S. residents aged 12 and older have used heroin at least once in their lifetime. Collectively, use of opiates other than heroin is far more common. Of the 12 years of age and older population, an estimated 4.7 million people used narcotic pain relievers nonmedically, and 3.1 million persons used what Substance Abuse and Mental Health Services Administration classified as "OxyContin" nonmedically at least once in their lifetime.[23]

PRESENTATION OF OPIOID INTOXICATION AND WITHDRAWAL

General

- Onset of the acute phase of withdrawal ranges from a few hours after stopping heroin to 3 to 5 days after stopping methadone. The duration of withdrawal ranges from 3 to 14 days.

- Opioid withdrawal is not fatal unless there is a concurrent medical problem of major concern.

- The presence of delirium should raise the question of concurrent withdrawal from another drug, such as alcohol, or another cause of delirium possibly secondary to drug use.

Symptoms

- During withdrawal, patients can experience piloerection, insomnia, muscle aches, and yawning. While intoxicated, patients can experience euphoria, dysphoria, apathy, sedation, or attention impairment.

Signs

- Fever, lacrimation, diaphoresis, or diarrhea may be observed during withdrawal. Motor retardation, slurred speech, and miosis may be observed during intoxication.

Laboratory Tests

- Treatment is based more on clinical presentation because plasma opioid levels may not be clinically useful.

Other Diagnostic Tests

- Arterial blood gases, pulse oximetry, and pulmonary function tests are useful to assess respiratory depression.

By crushing controlled-release tablets, drug abusers can get the full 12-hour or more of narcotic effect almost immediately. Snorting or injecting the crushed tablet can lead to overdose and death. Abuse of this drug has caused a nationwide discussion on whether drugs of this nature should be more closely regulated. Various position statements and points of view on the benefits and risks have been expressed, but the limited space here precludes an exhaustive review of the issues. An excellent review of the appropriate use of opioid therapy for chronic pain has recently been published, and the interested reader is directed there for more information.[24]

CLINICAL CONTROVERSY

There is considerable debate about the appropriate use of prescribed opiates and how this might contribute to the overuse or abuse of these same drugs for nonmedicinal purposes. Not all decisions that physicians and other prescribers make are going to be correct. Likewise, pharmacists are going to make the wrong decision by either declining to fill a prescription that is proper and appropriate or by filling one that is bogus. In the final analysis, mistakes in judgment are going to be made in both directions. Given this fact, in which direction should the health professional err? Should health practitioners give the patient the benefit of the doubt, writing or filling the prescription, even if their decision ultimately turns out to be wrong? Or should the mandate be in the other direction: refuse to prescribe pain medicines or refuse to fill the prescriptions, even when, in truth, the prescription is appropriate and valid? Most healthcare professional assume that complaints of pain are real and prescribe accordingly.

METHADONE

The use of methadone has increased sharply, partially in response to the increased scrutiny given oxycodone products in the past few years. Methadone prescriptions for pain management grew from about 531,000 in 1998 to about 4.1 million in 2006, a nearly eightfold increase. The FDA approved methadone for treating pain in 1947, but from the early 1970s until the late 1990s, the drug was primarily used for treating addiction. In the mid-1990s, various national pain-related organizations began to issue guidelines for treating and managing pain, including using opioids to treat both cancer and noncancer pain. At first, methadone was prescribed more for the treatment of cancer pain, but it has been increasingly prescribed for the treatment of chronic noncancer pain. Methadone's advantages include that it costs less than other opioids used to treat pain, and it comes in multiple forms.[25]

Methadone has pharmacologic properties unique among opioids, and as a result, a lack of knowledge about methadone among practitioners and patients has been identified as a factor contributing to the increased number of deaths observed in recent years. DEA data suggest that the abuse of methadone diverted from its intended purpose has also contributed to the rise in overdose deaths, as the number of methadone drug items seized by law enforcement and analyzed in forensic laboratories increased 262%, from 2,865 in 2001 to 10,361 in 2007.[25]

To improve safety, in 2006, the FDA issued a Public Health Advisory[26] that included new labeling information regarding the use of methadone for pain and modified dosage instructions for those beginning pain management treatment with methadone. Methadone's elimination half-life (8–59 hours) is longer than its duration of analgesic action (4–8 hours). Healthcare professionals were reminded that methadone's peak respiratory depressant effects typically occur later, and persist longer than its peak analgesic effects. The FDA advised that during treatment initiation, methadone's full analgesic effect is usually not attained until 3 to 5 days of dosing.

Cross-tolerance between methadone and other opioids is incomplete. This incomplete cross-tolerance makes the conversion of patients on other opioids to methadone complex and does not eliminate the possibility of methadone overdose, even in patients tolerant to other opioids. Deaths have been reported during conversion from chronic, high-dose treatment with other opioid agonists to methadone. It is critical to understand the pharmacokinetics of methadone when converting patients from other opioids to methadone. Particular vigilance is necessary during treatment initiation, during conversion from one opioid to another, and during dose adjustments. Also, there are pharmacokinetic and pharmacodynamic drug interactions between methadone and many other drugs. Thus drugs administered concomitantly with methadone should be evaluated for interaction potential.[26]

DEXTROMETHORPHAN

Dextromethorphan abuse is one of the most common (and most dangerous) examples of OTC drug abuse.[27] Intoxication from consuming large doses of cough syrup is known on the street as "robodosing" or "robotripping." Handsful of cough and cold remedies are sometimes called "skittles" because they look similar to the popular fruit candy. Dextromethorphan creates a depressant and mild hallucinogenic effect when taken in large doses. Since the drug is available over the counter, it is easily procured by adolescents. Those who use the cough syrup to get high are sometimes called "syrup heads."[27]

Excessive doses are needed to induce effects that include hyperexcitability, lethargy, ataxia, slurred speech, diaphoresis, hypertension, nystagmus, and mydriasis. When taken at much higher doses, it acts as a dissociative anesthetic, similar to phencyclidine (PCP, "angel dust") and ketamine ("Special K"). These are the effects sought by those who use the drug to get high. At these high doses, dextromethorphan also is a CNS depressant.[27,28]

The recommended treatment for acute overdoses of dextromethorphan is naloxone. Although reports of its efficacy are mixed, it may be helpful in reversing the CNS depressant and neurologic effects.[28]

Dextromethorphan powder is available through the Internet and by home laboratory extraction from pharmaceutical products. Five deaths in the United States have been attributed to dextromethorphan powder sold over the Internet.[27]

CNS STIMULANTS

COCAINE

Cocaine is perhaps the most behaviorally reinforcing of all drugs of abuse. Clinicians estimate that approximately 10% of people who begin to use the drug recreationally will go on to serious, heavy use.

Once having tried cocaine, an individual cannot predict or control the extent to which he or she will continue to use the drug.

The most characteristic pharmacologic effect of cocaine is stimulation of the CNS. In the CNS, cocaine appears to mediate its effects primarily by blocking reuptake of catecholamine neurotransmitters such as norepinephrine and dopamine.

PRESENTATION OF COCAINE INTOXICATION AND WITHDRAWAL

General

  In overdoses, cocaine is a central nervous system and cardiac stimulant. Cocaine-elated deaths are often a result of cardiac arrest or seizures followed by respiratory arrest.

Symptoms

  Symptoms of intoxication include motor agitation, elation, euphoria, grandiosity, loquacity, hypervigilance, sweating or chills, nausea, and vomiting.

  Symptoms of withdrawal include fatigue, sleep disturbances, nightmares, depression, and changes in appetite.

  High doses of cocaine and/or prolonged use can trigger paranoia.

Signs

  Tachycardia, mydriasis, and either elevated or lowered blood pressure may be observed with overdose. Cardiac abnormalities (e.g., arrhythmias) and respiratory depression may be observed with overdose. Bradyarrhythmias, myocardial infarction, and tremors may be observed in acute withdrawal. Prolonged cocaine snorting can result in ulceration of the mucous membranes of the nose and can damage the nasal septum enough to cause it to collapse.

Laboratory Tests

  Qualitative drugs of abuse urine screening tests are useful, followed by confirmatory testing if necessary. Levels of the primary metabolite, benzoylecgonine, may help diagnose acute cocaine toxicity.

Other Diagnostic Tests

  Abnormal electroencephalograms may be observed with patients in acute withdrawal.

Cocaine is absorbed rapidly from virtually all sites of application. For many years, cocaine has been administered as the hydrochloride salt form, usually by inhalation, but also by injection. In the last 18 to 20 years, as the purity of cocaine hydrochloride obtained on the street declined, many users converted the cocaine hydrochloride to cocaine base, also known as "crack" or "rock." Smoking the drug leads to almost instant absorption and intense euphoria. Peak plasma concentrations of more than 900 ng/mL (3.0 μmol/L) have been achieved following inhalation of cocaine base vapors, compared with concentrations of only 150 to 200 ng/mL (0.49 to 0.66 μmol/L) achieved after inhalation of similar amounts of pure cocaine hydrochloride powder.[29]

The high from snorting can last 15 to 30 minutes, whereas that from smoking can last 5 to 10 minutes. Increased use can reduce the period of stimulation. An appreciable tolerance to the high can be developed, and many addicts report that they seek but fail to achieve as much pleasure as they did from their first exposure. Scientific evidence suggests that the powerful neuropsychologic reinforcing property of cocaine is responsible for an individual's continued use despite harmful physical and social consequences.

Recent research has helped clarify certain patterns of cocaine use, such as combining cocaine and alcohol. Such drug use would seem counterintuitive because cocaine is a CNS stimulant, and alcohol a CNS depressant. In the presence of alcohol, cocaine is metabolized to cocaethylene, a longer-acting but potent psychoactive compound compared to the parent drug.[30] The risk of death from cocaethylene is greater than from cocaine.[31] The cocaine-alcohol combination is one of the most commonly identified among individuals who come to hospital EDs with acute substance abuse problems.

Cocaine is metabolized and eliminated rapidly. The elimination half-life of cocaine is approximately 1 hour, and the duration of effect is very short.[29] The short duration of effect provides a powerful incentive for repeated use of the drug. Many users experience intense drug use cycling, sometimes lasting days, characterized by rapidly repeating doses of cocaine until their supply is exhausted. Laboratory monkeys, given a choice between food and cocaine around the clock for 8 days, consistently choose cocaine.

Complications of cocaine use frequently involve cardiovascular events.[32] Cocaine is a psychotomimetic drug, sometimes even at nontoxic doses. A kindling phenomenon has been described with cocaine in which neuronal function becomes altered with each dose of the drug. The psychosis is qualitatively very similar to a paranoid schizophrenic psychosis.[33] Although there is some controversy as to whether cocaine is associated with physical withdrawal on abrupt discontinuation, most clinicians feel that there is a characteristic syndrome of withdrawal effects, although they are not life-threatening.

AMPHETAMINE, METHAMPHETAMINE, AND OTHER STIMULANTS

According to the United Nations Office of Drugs and Crime, worldwide between 16 and 51 million people aged 15 to 64 used amphetamines-group substances at least once in 2007.[34] In the United States, people who reported that they had used methamphetamine in the previous month also dropped dramatically, from 529,000 people in 2007 to 314,000 in 2008.[3]

Street methamphetamine is referred to by many names, such as "speed," "meth," and "crank." Methamphetamine hydrochloride, clear chunky crystals resembling ice, can be inhaled by smoking. It is referred to as "ice," "crystal," and "glass" on the street.

The physiologic and psychologic effects of amphetamines and other stimulants are qualitatively similar to those of cocaine—they diminish fatigue, increase alertness, and suppress appetite. Pharmacologically, amphetamines increase the activity of catecholamine neurotransmitters (e.g., norepinephrine and dopamine) by increasing release and by inhibiting the degradative enzyme monoamine oxidase.[35] The longer duration of effect of methamphetamine has led to a shift away from cocaine and toward this longer-acting drug.

An analysis produced by the Rand Corporation[36] suggests that the economic cost of meth use in the United States reached $23.4 billion in 2005. Because of the difficulty in pinpointing the role of methamphetamine in crime, medical care and other factors, the RAND researchers gave a range of estimates, saying the overall toll may be as low as $16.2 billion or as high as $48.3 billion.[36]

These estimates include the burden of addiction, premature death, drug treatment, and many other costs associated with methamphetamine use. The RAND analysis found that nearly two thirds of the economic costs caused by methamphetamine use resulted from the burden of addiction and an estimated 900 premature deaths among users in 2005. For a sobering look at the methamphetamine epidemic in the United States the interested reader should view the full report.[36]

Methamphetamine is used orally, intranasally, rectally, by intravenous injection, and by smoking. Immediately after inhalation or intravenous injection, the methamphetamine user experiences an intense sensation, called a "rush" or "flash," that lasts only a few minutes and is described as extremely pleasurable.

PRESENTATION OF AMPHETAMINE INTOXICATION AND WITHDRAWAL

General

- Amphetamine intoxication is an acute condition that may result in death. Pharmacotherapy may be indicated for symptomatic control of seizures.

- Patients may experience withdrawal symptoms for several days, but are usually not in acute distress. Treatment is supportive in nature. Pharmacotherapy is not effective to treat the symptoms of amphetamine withdrawal.

Symptoms

- Depression, altered mental status, drug craving, dyssomnia, and fatigue are all symptoms of withdrawal.

- Amphetamine intoxication may present as increased wakefulness, increased physical activity, decreased appetite, increased respiration, hyperthermia, and euphoria. Other CNS effects include irritability, insomnia, confusion, tremors, convulsions, anxiety, paranoia, chest pain, and aggressiveness. Hyperthermia and convulsions can result in death.

Signs

- Patients with amphetamine intoxication may present with tachycardia, hypertension, or stroke.

Laboratory Tests

- A qualitative drug of abuse urine screening is used for diagnostic purposes. Confirmatory blood tests with gas chromatography and mass spectrophotometry may be used for verification.

Because methamphetamine elevates mood, people who experiment with it tend to use it with increasing frequency and in increasing doses, although this was not their original intent. The timing and intensity of the "rush" that accompanies the use of methamphetamine, which is a result of the release of high levels of dopamine in the brain, depends in part on the method of administration. Specifically, the effect is almost instantaneous when smoked or injected, whereas it takes approximately 5 minutes after snorting or 20 minutes after oral ingestion. Prolonged use of methamphetamine can result in a tolerance for the drug and increased use at higher dosage levels, creating dependence. Such continual use of the drug with little or no sleep may lead to an extremely irritable and paranoid state. Discontinuing use of methamphetamine often results in a state of depression, as well as fatigue, anergia, and some types of cognitive impairment that can last from 2 days to several months.

Both short- and long-term health effects have also been documented. Negative consequences of methamphetamine abuse range from anxiety and insomnia to convulsions, paranoia, and brain damage. Methamphetamine-induced caries, or "meth mouth" is a characteristic pattern of dental decay commonly observed in patients that smoke methamphetamine.[37]

In addition to the many direct effects on methamphetamine users are the indirect impacts on individuals and society. Flammable ingredients that include acetone, red phosphorous, ethyl alcohol, and lithium metal are used in methamphetamine cookers, often with disastrous results. Fires and explosions often ensue, resulting in severe burns and uncovering laboratories to local law enforcement.[38] Children of methamphetamine abusers are at high risk of neglect and abuse, and pregnant women's use of methamphetamine can cause growth retardation, premature birth, and developmental disorders in neonates. Within this particular group, effective treatment for methamphetamine dependence can be one of the most important strategies in reducing the spread of HIV and other associated communicable diseases.[38] Treatment for methamphetamine dependence is very difficult, and has a low success rate.[39]

The expanding global market is fed by an increase in clandestine manufacture of methamphetamine. Not only are there more laboratories in more countries, but their size and sophistication are also increasing. The number of clandestine methamphetamine laboratories seized nationwide by the DEA increased from 263 in 1994 to 1,815 in 2000, a 590% increase.[40] In 2008, state and local police agencies seized almost 6,783 clandestine laboratories in the United States. So-called "kitchen" laboratories are still discovered, but today clandestine laboratories with 100-kg capacities per week are also found. Initially the clandestine manufacture of methamphetamine was based primarily in the West and Southwest.[40] Today methamphetamine can be found in cities across the United States, although local law enforcement pressures have caused a decrease in "superlaboratories" capable of producing at least 10 pounds per production cycle.[41] Unfortunately, increased methamphetamine production by Mexican drug cartels has offset the decreased domestic production.

Methamphetamine is manufactured using the ephedrine or pseudoephedrine reduction method. In this process, ephedrine or pseudoephedrine is extracted from OTC cold and allergy tablets. Pharmacists should be wary of persons wishing to purchase large quantities of products containing nonprescription sympathomimetic products. As a precaution, federal legislation now mandates that pseudoephedrine-containing products be kept behind a counter, and suitable identification must be shown before they can be purchased.

ECSTASY AND OTHER METHAMPHETAMINE ANALOGS

Several dozen analogs of amphetamine and methamphetamine are mildly hallucinogenic. Two methamphetamine analogs of most concern are 3,4-methylenedioxyamphetamine and especially 3,4-methylenedioxymethamphetamine (MDMA or Ecstasy). Use of these compounds was particularly prevalent in the early 2000s. However, annual prevalence rates for ecstasy dropped considerably between 2000 and 2008, from 3.1% to 1.7% for 8th graders, from 5.4% to 2.9% for 10th graders, from 8.2% to 4.3% for 12th graders, from 9.1% to 3.7% among college students, and from 7.2% to 3.3% among young adults.[5]

The effects of MDMA usually last approximately 4 to 6 hours. Users of the drug say that it produces profoundly positive feelings, empathy for others, elimination of anxiety, and extreme relaxation. MDMA is also said to suppress the need to eat, drink, or sleep, enabling users to endure 2- to 3-day parties. Consequently, MDMA use sometimes results in severe dehydration or exhaustion. MDMA generally reduces inhibitions and creates a sense of euphoria, but it also can evoke anxiety and paranoia. Heavier doses generate depression, irrationality, and psychosis. Users claim they experience feelings of closeness with others and a desire to touch them.

MDMA use can result in a variety of acute psychiatric disturbances, including panic, anxiety, depression, and paranoid thinking.[37] Physical symptoms include muscle tension, nausea, blurred vision, faintness, chills, and sweating. MDMA also increases the heart rate and blood pressure. Other effects include hyperthermia, dehydration, vomiting, tremors, loss of control over body movements, insomnia, convulsions, rapid eye movements, and teeth and jaw clenching.

MDMA is perceived to be a harmless drug by many of its users, based in part on the fact that the risk of death is low compared with other drugs such as heroin and cocaine. However, mounting evidence points to neurotoxic effects of MDMA, involving a complex and incompletely understood mechanism. MDMA has been clearly shown to destroy serotonin-producing neurons in animals.[42] Doses of MDMA that produce neurotoxicity are only 2 or 3 times more than the minimum dose needed to produce a psychotropic response.

Researchers have found that heavy MDMA users have memory problems that persist for at least 2 weeks after they have stopped using the drug.[43] McCann and colleagues[44,45] conducted several studies to determine the effects of MDMA use on cognitive performance. MDMA users and controls were found to perform similarly on several cognitive tasks. However, MDMA subjects had significant performance deficits on a sustained-attention task requiring arithmetic calculations, a task requiring complex attention and incidental learning, a task requiring short-term memory, and a task of semantic recognition and verbal reasoning. The authors believe that their data provide further evidence that MDMA is neurotoxic to brain serotonin neurons in humans, and the behavioral data suggest that brain serotonin injury is associated with subtle but significant cognitive deficits.

Manufacturers of illicit drugs sometimes substitute other, potentially more dangerous substances for the one the buyer is expecting. Other suppliers produce products adulterated with chemical byproducts of the incomplete processing of active ingredients. One such chemical, *para*-methoxyamphetamine, is a drastically more potent hyperthermic agent than MDMA. Deaths from this chemical have been reported.[46]

HALLUCINOGENS

The drugs commonly classified as hallucinogens are lysergic acid diethylamide (LSD), psilocybin, dimethyltryptamine (DMT), mescaline, and other related compounds. LSD is one of the most potent mood-changing chemicals. It is manufactured from lysergic acid, which is found in ergot, a fungus that grows on rye and other grains.

Pharmacologically, LSD and related drugs stimulate both presynaptic (5-hydroxytryptamine [HT]$_{1A}$ and 5-HT$_{1B}$) and postsynaptic (5-HT$_2$) serotonin receptors in the brain, which functionally can cause either agonist or antagonist effects on serotonin activity.[48] Precisely how the hallucinogens exert their effects remains unclear. LSD is an extraordinarily potent compound, producing observable CNS effects at doses as low as 25 mcg.

LSD is sold on the street in tablets, capsules, and occasionally in liquid form. It is odorless, colorless, and tasteless and usually is taken by mouth. Often LSD is added to absorbent paper, such as blotter paper, and divided into small decorated squares, with each square representing one dose.

The effects of LSD are unpredictable. They depend on the amount taken; the user's personality, mood, and expectations; and the surroundings in which the drug is used. Usually the user feels the first effects of the drug 30 to 90 minutes after taking it. The physical effects include dilated pupils, higher body temperature, increased heart rate and blood pressure, sweating, loss of appetite, sleeplessness, dry mouth, and tremors.

Sensations and feelings change much more dramatically than the physical signs. The user can feel several different emotions at once or swing rapidly from one emotion to another. If taken in a large enough dose, the drug produces delusions and visual hallucinations. The user's sense of time and self changes. Sensations can seem to "cross over," giving the user the feeling of hearing colors and seeing sounds.

Many LSD users experience flashbacks, or recurrence of certain aspects of a person's experience, without the user having taken the drug again. A flashback occurs suddenly, often without warning, and can occur within a few days or more than a year after LSD use. Flashbacks usually occur in people who use hallucinogens chronically or have an underlying personality problem; however, otherwise healthy people who use LSD occasionally also can have flashbacks.

Most users of LSD voluntarily decrease or stop its use over time. LSD is not considered an addictive drug because it does not produce compulsive drug-seeking behavior. However, as with many of the addictive drugs, LSD use produces tolerance, so some users who take the drug repeatedly must take progressively higher doses to achieve the state of intoxication that they had achieved previously.

Psychologic symptoms of intoxication include a subjective intensification of perceptions, depersonalization, illusions, hallucinations, and synesthesias, the overflow of one sensory modality to another. LSD is the most potent and longest-acting hallucinogen; it is hundreds of times more potent than both psilocybin and mescaline. DMT is inactive when ingested orally but can be smoked, inhaled, or injected. There is cross-tolerance among LSD, psilocybin, and mescaline. There is no observable physical withdrawal syndrome after abrupt discontinuation of hallucinogenic drugs. Complications from hallucinogen use are primarily psychologic. Users sometimes experience prolonged episodes of panic—the so-called "bad trip." The flashbacks noted above are common, occurring in approximately 15% of users and occurring episodically up to several years after the last exposure to the drug. Flashbacks can occur spontaneously but are also triggered by other drugs, including marijuana, and by anxiety-provoking stimuli. Contrary to a widely held notion in the 1960s and early 1970s, there is no reliable evidence that hallucinogen use causes chromosome damage or genetic defects.

MARIJUANA

Marijuana, referred to as "reefer," "pot," "grass," or "weed," was the most commonly used illicit drug in 2008. Among persons aged 12 or older, the rate of past month marijuana use in 2008 (6.1%) was similar to the rate in 2007 (5.8%).[5] Of those, 54.5% used only marijuana, and 19.6% used marijuana and another illicit drug.[5] In 2008, marijuana was used by 75.7% of current illicit drug users and was the only drug used by 57.3% of them.[5] The rate of marijuana use for youth, while well off peak levels of the late 1990s, has edged up in the past year. According to the most recent Monitoring for the Future study, among 12th-graders 20.6% said they used it within the *past month*, compared with 19.4% in 2008 and 18.3% in 2006. Among 10th-graders, pot use in the past month rose to 15.9% this year from 13.8% in 2008. In the *past year*, the share of 8th-graders who smoked marijuana was 11.8%, compared with 10.9% in 2008. Tenth-graders' use was 26.7% this year and 23.9% in 2008. The percentage of 12th-graders was 32.8% compared with 32.4% in 2008.

Most users smoke marijuana in hand-rolled cigarettes (joints), while some use pipes or water pipes (bongs). Marijuana cigars called blunts have also become popular.[47] To make blunts, users slice open cigars and replace the tobacco with marijuana. Marijuana also is used to brew tea and is sometimes mixed into foods.

Marijuana's effects begin immediately after the drug enters the brain and last from 1 to 3 hours. If marijuana is consumed in food or drink, the short-term effects begin more slowly, usually in 30 minutes to 1 hour, and last longer, for as long as 4 hours. Smoking marijuana delivers several times more of its major active ingredient, delta-9-tetrahydrocannabinol (THC) into the blood than does eating or drinking the drug.[48]

Marijuana use impairs a person's ability to form memories, recall events, and shift attention from one thing to another. THC also disrupts coordination and balance by binding to receptors in the cerebellum and basal ganglia. Through its effects on the brain and body, marijuana intoxication can cause accidents. Studies show that approximately 6% to 11% of fatal accident victims test positive for THC. In many of these cases alcohol is detected as well.[49]

The principal psychoactive component of marijuana is THC. Hashish, the dried resin of the top of the plant, is much more potent than the plant itself. Increasingly sophisticated growing techniques have resulted in plants of greater potency. The average potency of marijuana increased in 2007 to the highest levels ever recorded, likely because of increased demand for higher-potency marijuana and improvements in cultivation techniques. According to University of Mississippi School of Pharmacy Potency Monitoring Project data, the average THC content in tested samples of marijuana in 2007 increased to the highest level ever recorded—9.64% in 2007, rising from 8.77% in 2006. The average THC content for hashish was 24.41% in 2008. Indoor cannabis cultivation is most prevalent in western states; however, indoor cultivation in eastern states, particularly Florida and Georgia, increased sharply in 2007.[40]

Marijuana has been used widely and is believed by many to be a relatively harmless, nonaddictive intoxicant. Chronic low doses of marijuana usually are not associated with significant physical withdrawal on abrupt discontinuation, but many chronic users exhibit compulsive drug-seeking and drug-use behaviors characteristic of addiction or dependence. Acutely, marijuana has many of the effects of alcohol—sedation, a decrease in reactivity and ability to perform complex tasks, and disinhibition. Chronic use is associated with all the risks of tobacco smoking, although marijuana smokers are commonly also tobacco smokers, and thus differentiation of effects is often difficult. Endocrine effects including amenorrhea, decreased testosterone production, and inhibition of spermatogenesis have been demonstrated. Marijuana is associated with an amotivational syndrome characterized by a behavioral pattern of apathy, dullness, impaired judgment, decreased concentration and memory, loss of interest in personal hygiene, and a general reduction of goal-directed behavior.[50]

Marijuana smoke is irritating to the lungs. Researchers have found that the daily use of one to three marijuana joints appears to produce approximately the same lung damage and potential cancer risk as smoking 5 times as many cigarettes.[51] The study results suggest that the way smokers inhale marijuana, in addition to its chemical composition, increases the adverse physical effects. The study findings refute the argument that marijuana is safer than tobacco because users smoke only a few joints a day.

Clearly, there is much more work to be done before the precise health and psychologic effects of marijuana use are well understood. In fact, many of these health issues remain the subject of much debate. Undoubtedly, opinions on its risks are polarized along the lines of proponents' views on what its legal status should be. This polarization of opinion has prevented the development of any consensus on what health information the medical profession should give to patients who are users or potential users of marijuana. There is conflicting evidence about many of the effects of marijuana use. Readers are referred to two excellent articles that attempt to summarize in a dispassionate way the evidence on the most probable adverse health and psychologic consequences of acute and chronic use of marijuana.[52,53]

CLINICAL CONTROVERSY

The mere mention of the words "medical marijuana" is bound to evoke strong emotions among laypersons and healthcare professionals alike. While the federal government continues to enforce laws that make possession and use of marijuana illegal, regardless of the intended purpose, at last count 13 of the U.S. states have legalized medical marijuana. While the safety and efficacy of marijuana to treat certain identifiable medical conditions has been confirmed, many other uses are supported by anecdote or limited clinical experience. However, the debate involves much more than whether cannabis works or not to treat illness. Instead, there are political, social, economic, and religious considerations that cloud the controversy over whether marijuana should be legalized for medical purposes. This debate is bound to continue for years to come.

INHALANTS

Inhalants are a diverse group of substances that include volatile solvents, gases, and nitrites that are sniffed, snorted, huffed, or bagged to produce intoxicating effects similar to those of alcohol. These substances are found in common household products such as glues, lighter fluid, cleaning fluids, paint products, nail polish remover, gasoline, rubber glue, waxes, and varnishes. Chemicals found in these products include toluene, benzene, methanol, methylene chloride, acetone, methylethyl ketone, methylbutyl ketone, trichloroethylene, and trichloroethane. The gas used as a propellant in canned whipped cream and in small metallic containers called "whippets" (used to make whipped cream) is nitrous oxide or "laughing gas."

Tiny cloth-covered ampules called "poppers" or "snappers" by abusers contain amyl nitrite, a medication used to dilate blood vessels. Butyl nitrite, sold as tape head cleaner and referred to as "rush," "locker room," or "climax," is often sniffed or huffed to get high.

Inhalants can be sniffed directly from an open container or huffed from a rag soaked in the substance and held to the face. Alternatively, the open container or soaked rag can be placed in a bag where the vapors can concentrate before being inhaled. Although inhalant abusers might prefer one particular substance because of taste or odor, a variety of substances can be used because of similar effects, availability, and cost. Once inhaled, the extensive capillary surface area of the lungs allows rapid absorption of the substance, and blood levels peak rapidly. Entry into the brain is fast, and the intoxicating effects are intense but short lived. Intoxication is often accompanied by headache and nausea, and users can experience hallucinations and delusions. The most serious physical risk of acute use is sudden death, usually from cardiac arrhythmias. Some users die from suffocation by plastic bags that contain the solvent. With chronic use, the drugs are toxic to virtually all organ systems. Psychologic impairment; impaired pulmonary, renal, and hepatic function; neuropathies; encephalopathy; and brain damage have all been observed.

Inhalants depress the CNS, producing decreased respiration and blood pressure. Users report distortion in perceptions of time and space. Many users experience headaches, nausea, slurred speech, and loss of motor coordination. A rash around the nose and mouth can be seen, and the abuser can start wheezing. An odor of paint or organic solvents on clothes, skin, and breath is sometimes a sign of inhalant abuse. Other indicators of inhalant abuse include slurred speech or staggering gait; red, glassy, watery eyes; and excitability or unpredictable behavior.

TREATMENT

Substance-Related Disorders

■ ACUTE DRUG INTOXICATIONS

Treatment of drug intoxication, summarized in Table 74–2, is primarily supportive. Vital functions are maintained while waiting for the drug to be eliminated. Whenever possible, drug therapy should be avoided because psychotropic drug therapy has the potential for worsening a toxic reaction to another psychoactive

TABLE 74-2	Pharmacologic Treatment of Substance Intoxication		
Drug Class	**Nonpharmacologic Therapy**	**Pharmacologic Therapy**	**Level of Evidence**[a,b]
Benzodiazepines	Support vital functions	Flumazenil 0.2 mg/min IV initially, repeat up to 3 mg max.	A1
Alcohol, barbiturates, and sedative-hypnotics (nonbenzodiazepines)	Support vital functions	None	B3
Opiates	Support vital functions	Naloxone 0.4–2 mg IV every 3 min	A1
Cocaine and other CNS stimulants	Monitor cardiac function	Lorazepam 2–4 mg IM every 30 min to 6 h as needed for agitation	B2
		Haloperidol 2–5 mg (or other antipsychotic agent) every 30 min to 6 h as needed for psychotic behavior	B3
Hallucinogens, marijuana, and inhalants	Reassurance; "talk-down therapy"; support vital functions	Lorazepam and/or haloperidol as above	B3
Phencyclidine	Minimize sensory input	Lorazepam and/or haloperidol as above	B3

[a]Strength of recommendations, evidence to support recommendation, A, good; B, moderate; C, poor.
[b]Quality of evidence: 1, evidence from more than 1 properly randomized, controlled trial; 2, evidence from more than one well-designed clinical trial with randomization, from cohort or case-controlled analytic studies or multiple time series; or dramatic results from uncontrolled experiments; 3, evidence from opinions of respected authorities, based on clinical experience, descriptive studies, or reports of expert communities.
Data from O'Brien,[16] Fudala et al.,[54] Smith and Seymour,[68] and Knapp et al.[69]

agent; however, when patients are agitated, combative, assaultive, hallucinating, or delusional, drug therapy may be required. Toxicology screens are useful in the evaluation and treatment process, but knowledge of the metabolism of the suspected drug and its excretion patterns is important for proper interpretation of test results. When toxicology screens are desired, blood or urine should be collected immediately upon the patient's arrival.

For alcohol and barbiturate intoxication, supportive treatment is the rule. For benzodiazepine intoxication, the benzodiazepine antagonist flumazenil can be used to reverse toxic effects. In the case of opiate intoxication, if the patient is unconscious and respiration is depressed, the opiate antagonist naloxone can be used to revive the patient. The usual dosage for naloxone in acute opiate toxicity is 0.4 to 2 mg intravenously, given approximately every 3 minutes as necessary. Although naloxone is effective in reversing opiate overdose, it also can precipitate physical withdrawal in physically dependent patients.

Intoxication with stimulants, including cocaine, is treated pharmacologically only if the patient is overtly psychotic and agitated.[55,56] Injectable benzodiazepines, usually lorazepam 2 to 4 mg intramuscularly every 30 minutes to 6 hours as necessary, can be used for agitation. As a backup to lorazepam, antipsychotic drugs can be used on a short-term basis, primarily in patients with psychotic symptoms, and usually at relatively low doses, such as haloperidol 2 to 5 mg intramuscularly every 30 minutes to 6 hours as necessary, followed by 5 to 15 mg orally per day in single or divided doses if the patient is still psychotic after initial treatment.[56]

A recent evidence-based guideline gives precise recommendations for treating the cardiovascular complications of cocaine abuse and provides insight into the epidemiology, pathophysiology, treatment, and prognosis of the cardiac effects of cocaine.[57] Seizures generally are treated supportively. Intravenous lorazepam or diazepam can be used if seizures progress to status epilepticus.[56]

Hallucinogen intoxication is treated in a manner similar to stimulant intoxication. Drug therapy often can be avoided because patients can respond to careful reassurance, or so-called talk-down therapy. When necessary, short-term antianxiety and/or antipsychotic drug therapy can be used, as described previously.

■ WITHDRAWAL

❸ Treatment of drug withdrawal is the primary indication for drug therapy in substance-related disorders. Goals of drug therapy include prevention of progression of withdrawal to life-threatening severity, and enabling the patient to be sufficiently comfortable and functional to participate in a behavioral treatment program and supportive drug therapy. The clinician should remember that withdrawal is usually part of a substance dependence disorder. In drug therapy for withdrawal, it is important to avoid reinforcing the patient's drug-seeking and drug-use behavior to the extent possible. Patients must be educated to deal with the stress of withdrawal without seeking drugs. A recent review on the management of drug and alcohol withdrawal has been published.[13] Treatment of drug withdrawal is summarized in Table 74–3.

■ CNS DEPRESSANT WITHDRAWAL

Benzodiazepines

❸ Treatment of benzodiazepine withdrawal is very similar to the treatment of alcohol withdrawal. The major difference in management is the length of treatment. The onset of withdrawal symptoms in patients physically dependent on the long-acting benzodiazepines can be delayed up to 7 days after discontinuation of the drug.[16] A common approach in detoxification of such patients is to initiate

TABLE 74-3 Treatment of Withdrawal from Some Common Drugs of Abuse

Drug or Drug Class	Pharmacologic Therapy	Level of Evidence[a,b]
Benzodiazepines		
Short to intermediate acting	Lorazepam 2 mg 3–4 times a day; taper over 5–7 days	A1
Long-acting	Lorazepam 2 mg 3–4 times a day; taper over additional 5–7 days	A1
Barbiturates	Pentobarbital tolerance test; initial detoxification at upper limit of tolerance test; decrease dosage by 100 mg every 2–3 days	B3
Opiates	Methadone 20–80 mg orally daily; taper by 5–10 mg daily or buprenorphine 4–32 mg orally daily, or clonidine 2 mcg/kg 3 times a day × 7 days; taper over additional 3 days	A1 (methadone and buprenorphine) B1 (clonidine)
Mixed-substance withdrawal		
Drugs are cross-tolerant	Detoxify according to treatment for longer-acting drug used	B3
Drugs are not cross-tolerant	Detoxify from one drug while maintaining second drug (cross-tolerant drugs), then detoxify from second drug	B3
CNS stimulants	Supportive treatment only; pharmacotherapy often not used; bromocriptine 2.5 mg 3 times a day or higher may be used for severe craving associated with cocaine withdrawal	B2

[a]Strength of recommendations, evidence to support recommendation, A, good; B, moderate; C, poor.
[b]Quality of evidence: 1, evidence from more than 1 properly randomized, controlled trial; 2, evidence from more than one well-designed clinical trial with randomization, from cohort or case-controlled analytic studies or multiple time series; or dramatic results from uncontrolled experiments; 3, evidence from opinions of respected authorities, based on clinical experience, descriptive studies, or reports of expert communities.
Data from O'Brien,[16] DHHS,[62] and Gorelick.[65]

treatment at usual dosages (chlordiazepoxide orally 50 mg 3 times a day; lorazepam orally 2 mg 3 times a day) and to maintain the initial dosage for 5 days, with gradual tapering over an additional 5 days. Detoxification in patients physically dependent on shorter-acting benzodiazepines is similar to treatment of alcohol withdrawal.

Among the benzodiazepines, alprazolam has been suggested to be more difficult to taper and discontinue than the other benzodiazepines. A longer, more gradual taper of the benzodiazepine used for detoxification can be needed. With all benzodiazepines, protracted minor abstinence symptoms—such as anxiety, insomnia, irritability, sensitivity to light and sound, and muscle spasms—can remain for several weeks in patients with a history of long exposure, even after the acute phase of benzodiazepine withdrawal is complete.

Barbiturates and Other Sedative-Hypnotic Drugs

❸ Although once used extensively, barbiturates and other nonbenzodiazepine sedating medications have been largely replaced by safer and more effective medications. Abuse problems with barbiturates resemble those seen with benzodiazepines in many ways. Withdrawal from barbiturates should be handled similarly to interventions for the abuse of alcohol and benzodiazepines.[16] Specific recommendations have been suggested for zolpidem withdrawal.[15]

Opiates

Opiate withdrawal syndrome is similar to a severe case of influenza. It is not life-threatening unless there is a concurrent life-threatening medical condition. Although most patients complain of symptoms of withdrawal such as cramping or insomnia, these symptoms are tolerable, and initiation of drug therapy can be avoided in many cases. Observable signs of withdrawal should be noted before initiation of drug therapy. Characteristic signs and symptoms of opiate withdrawal include pupillary dilatation, lacrimation, rhinorrhea, piloerection ("gooseflesh"), yawning, sneezing, anorexia, nausea, vomiting, and diarrhea. Seizures do not occur. Onset and duration of withdrawal symptoms and the time of peak occurrence depends on the half-life of the drug involved. Typically heroin withdrawal reaches a peak within 36 to 72 hours of discontinuation and can last for 7 to 10 days. For methadone, symptoms peak at 72 hours but can last for 2 weeks or more.[16]

In the past drug therapy for opioid withdrawal had typically been methadone, a synthetic opiate. Methadone is administered in decreasing doses over a period not exceeding 30 days (short-term detoxification) or 180 days (long-term detoxification). In 2009, a systematic review[58] including 1907 people from twenty trials was reported. The purpose of this report was to evaluate the effectiveness of tapered methadone compared with other detoxification treatments and placebo in managing opioid withdrawal on completion of detoxification and relapse rate. Comparing methadone versus any other pharmacological treatment (e.g., adrenergic agonists [11 studies], other opioid agonists [four studies], chlordiazepoxide [one study]) the authors found no clinical difference between the two treatments in terms of completion of treatment, relative risk (RR) 1.08 (95% CI, 0.95–1.24) and results at follow-up RR 1.17 (95% CI, 0.72–1.92). The studies included in this review confirm that slow tapering with temporary substitution of long acting opioids, can reduce withdrawal severity. Nevertheless the majority of patients relapsed to heroin use.[58]

Usually, opioid dependency is treated initially with detoxification. In the past, opioid-dependent patients relied on methadone or levo-alpha-acetylmethadol, but federal restrictions limited distribution of these drugs to a small number of methadone clinics. There were limited provisions for take-at-home dosing of methadone because of concern about the diversion of these drugs to illicit use.

■ USE OF BUPRENORPHINE IN OPIATE WITHDRAWAL AND MAINTENANCE

In 2002, buprenorphine was approved for opioid withdrawal. Prior to the passage of the federal Drug Addiction Treatment Act (DATA) of 2000,[59] office-based management of opioid dependence was illegal because existing federal laws prohibited physicians from prescribing narcotics for the sole purpose of maintaining a patient in a narcotic-addicted state.

The first of two formulations approved, Subutex, contains only buprenorphine and is intended for use at the beginning of treatment. The other, Suboxone, contains both buprenorphine and the opiate antagonist naloxone, and is intended to be used in maintenance treatment of opiate addiction. When buprenorphine with naloxone is administered sublingually, the naloxone component produces no clinically significant effect; however, after parenteral administration, naloxone-induced opioid antagonism occurs resulting in symptoms of withdrawal.[60,61]

To qualify, physicians must be board certified in addiction medicine/psychiatry or hold other special credentials, and physicians are required to obtain 8 hours of authorized training before they can prescribe medications for office-based treatment of opioid dependence.[60] DATA 2000, as amended in December 2006, specifies that an individual physician may have a maximum of 30 patients on opioid therapy at any one time for the first year. One year after the date on which a physician submitted the initial notification, the physician may submit a second notification of the need and intent to treat up to 100 patients.[60]

The goal of using buprenorphine for medically supervised withdrawal from opioids is to provide a transition from the state of physical dependence on opioids to an opioid-free state, while minimizing withdrawal symptoms (and avoiding side effects of buprenorphine).[61]

Medically supervised withdrawal with buprenorphine consists of an induction phase and a dose-reduction phase. Best practice guidelines collectively called Treatment Improvement Protocols (TIPs) are periodically issued for treatment of substance use disorders. TIP 40 (the guideline for the Use of Buprenorphine in the Treatment of Opioid Addiction),[62] provides consensus- and evidence-based guidance on the use of buprenorphine.

The statement recommends that patients dependent on short-acting opioids (e.g., hydromorphone, oxycodone, heroin) be inducted directly onto buprenorphine/naloxone tablets. The use of buprenorphine (either as buprenorphine monotherapy or buprenorphine/naloxone combination treatment) to taper off long-acting opioids should be considered only for those patients who have evidence of sustained medical and psychosocial stability, and should be undertaken in conjunction and in coordination with patients' overall opioid treatment programs. Induction protocols are shown in Figure 74–2.

Maintenance treatment with buprenorphine for opioid addiction consists of three phases: (1) induction, (2) stabilization, and (3) maintenance.[62] Induction is the first stage of buprenorphine treatment and involves helping patients begin the process of switching from the opioid of abuse to buprenorphine. The goal of the induction phase is to find the minimum dose of buprenorphine at which the patient discontinues or markedly diminishes use of other opioids and experiences no withdrawal symptoms, minimal or no side effects, and no craving for the drug of abuse. The consensus panel recommends that the buprenorphine/naloxone combination be used for induction treatment (and for stabilization and maintenance) for most patients. The consensus panel further recommends that initial induction doses be administered as observed treatment; further doses may be thereafter provided via prescription. To minimize the chances of precipitating withdrawal, patients who are transferring from long-acting opioids (e.g., methadone, sustained-release morphine, sustained-release oxycodone) to buprenorphine should be inducted using buprenorphine monotherapy, but switched to buprenorphine/naloxone soon thereafter.

The stabilization phase begins when a patient is experiencing no withdrawal symptoms, is experiencing minimal or no side effects, and no longer has uncontrollable cravings for opioid agonists. Dosage adjustments may be necessary during early stabilization, and frequent contact with the patient increases the likelihood of compliance. The longest period that a patient is on buprenorphine is the maintenance phase. This period may be indefinite. During the maintenance phase, attention must be focused on the psychosocial and family issues that have been identified during the course of treatment as contributing to a patient's addiction.[62]

Some other issues related to opioid abuse that need to be addressed during maintenance treatment include, but are not limited to, the following:[62]

- Psychiatric comorbidity
- Somatic consequences of drug use
- Family and support issues
- Structuring of time in prosocial activities

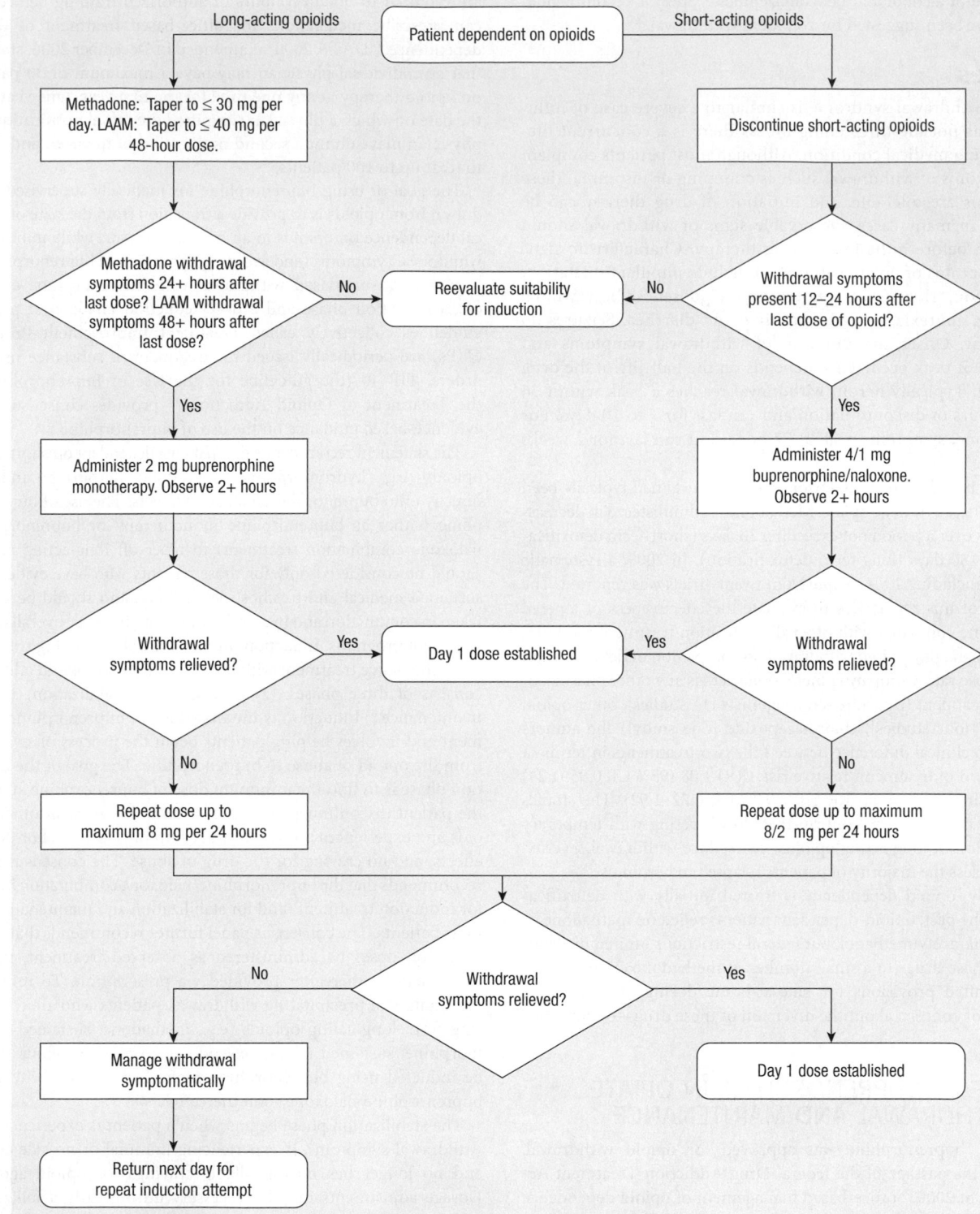

FIGURE 74-2. Determining the induction dose for days 1 to 2 of buprenorphine therapy. *(From reference 62.)*

- Employment and financial issues
- Legal consequences of drug use
- Other drug and alcohol abuse

A recent systematic review[63] evaluating the withdrawal component of buprenorphine treatment, including twenty-two studies involving 1,736 participants, was published. The major comparisons for buprenorphine were with methadone (5 studies) and clonidine or lofexidine (12 studies). Five studies compared different rates of buprenorphine dose reduction.

The authors concluded that severity of withdrawal is similar for withdrawal managed with buprenorphine and withdrawal managed with methadone, but withdrawal symptoms may resolve more quickly with buprenorphine. It appears that completion of withdrawal treatment may be more likely with buprenorphine relative to methadone (RR 1.18; 95% CI, 0.93–1.49; $P = 0.18$) but more studies are required to confirm this.[63]

A rapid detoxification technique has been developed that is designed to shorten detoxification by precipitating withdrawal through the administration of opioid antagonists such as naloxone or naltrexone.[64] This approach is thought to have the advantage of getting patients through detoxification rapidly, minimizing the risk of relapse, and initiating treatment more quickly with naltrexone maintenance combined with suitable psychosocial interventions. Ultrarapid detoxification represents a variant of this technique in which patients undergo opioid antagonist–precipitated withdrawal while under general anesthesia or heavy sedation. In the United States, there has been a rapid proliferation of programs offering ultrarapid detoxification, with some programs charging up to $15,000 per treatment.[64] Rapid detoxification remains unproven and controversial.

■ WITHDRAWAL FROM OTHER SUBSTANCES

Withdrawal from other drugs, including cocaine and other stimulants, is primarily supportive. However, pharmacotherapy recently has assumed a greater role in treating cocaine withdrawal and dependence. Bromocriptine, a dopamine antagonist at low dosages and an agonist at high dosages, is usually used in the treatment of parkinsonism and hyperprolactinemia and has been used to treat cocaine withdrawal symptoms and to reduce the craving for cocaine. Use of bromocriptine is based on the hypothesis that chronic use of cocaine causes dopamine depletion; therefore higher dosages should be used (i.e., 2.5 mg 3 times daily or higher). Despite initially promising pilot studies, recent evidence does not support the efficacy of bromocriptine to reduce cocaine use or craving.[65]

A more recent approach is the use of the cocaine vaccine that treats cocaine dependence. In the presence of the vaccine, the immune system forms antibodies that prevent cocaine from crossing the blood-brain barrier, blocking access to receptor sites in the brain. A recently published randomized, double-blind, placebo-controlled efficacy trial showed that a vaccine can prevent addicts from getting high by blocking the drug's effect on the brain, though it apparently does not blunt cravings for the drug.[66]

In this study, the vaccine had only limited success because it produced a suboptimal immune response in many patients. Those who reached the target antibody levels had significantly more cocaine-free urine samples than the others between the 9th and 16th weeks of the 6-month study, and 53% of them reduced their cocaine use by half, compared with only 23% in the group that was vaccinated but did not produce sufficient antibodies.[67]

■ SUBSTANCE DEPENDENCE

❷ The treatment of drug dependence is primarily behavioral. The patient generally is taught that complete abstinence is the only realistic alternative to a life of uncontrollable drug use and despair that ultimately will end in death, and that there is no intermediate, controllable level of drinking or use of another drug. There may be an extremely few individuals who can return to controllable levels of drinking alcohol, but it is impossible to predict who these individuals are. The prospect of life without alcohol or other drugs is incomprehensible to many patients. Entry into treatment often is facilitated by some type of leverage that the drug-dependent person associates with negative consequences, such as potential loss of job, divorce, legal problems, or deteriorating physical health. Early treatment is directed at penetrating the denial of a problem that is always present. The patient must be educated as to the disease of addiction, the effects of drugs, and the permanence of the condition.

As evidenced by the approval of the two buprenorphine products, there has been a trend toward outpatient treatment for drug dependence, caused in part by cost-containment efforts. Inpatient treatment programs can cost as much as $20,000 for a 4-week stay. When withdrawal symptoms are mild to moderate and there are no other medical indications for hospitalization, outpatient treatment can be an attractive alternative to inpatient treatment. One critical criterion for outpatient treatment is the patient's compliance with complete abstinence from the dependence-producing drug during the treatment experience.

Families must be involved in treatment. The course of the patient's illness often has a devastating effect on other family members. Severely depleted self-esteem, denial of the family member's addiction, feelings of responsibility for the family member's drug use, and other behaviors that parallel the addiction process are often present.

❹ Treatment must be a lifelong process. Aftercare, or what is now being called *continued care,* should include regular and frequent treatment in some form. Most drug-dependence treatment programs embrace a treatment approach based on the twelve steps to recovery. Among chemically dependent healthcare professionals, treatment that incorporates both 12-step and peer-led self-help groups can be most effective.

CONCLUSIONS

Substance use disorders remain one of the great public health issues of contemporary society. Dependence on drugs is a powerful emotional and political issue. Because we live in a chemically oriented society, everyone is affected in some way by drug abuse and drug dependence. Healthcare professionals must be particularly vigilant for problems associated with drug use, not only for our patients, but also for ourselves.

ABBREVIATIONS

ATOD: alcohol, tobacco, and other drugs

CASA: Center on Addiction and Substance Abuse

CNS: central nervous system

DATA: Drug Addiction Treatment Act

DAWN: Drug Abuse Warning Network

DEA: U.S. Drug Enforcement Administration

DMT: dimethyltryptamine

DSM-IV-TR: Diagnostic and Statistical Manual of Mental Disorders, Fourth Edition, Text Revision

GBL: γ-butyrolactone

GHB: γ-hydroxybutyrate

LSD: lysergic acid diethylamide

MDMA: 3,4-methylenedioxymethamphetamine

NSDUH: National Survey on Drug Use and Health

OTC: over-the-counter

PCP: Phencyclidine

REM: rapid eye movement

THC: delta-9-tetrahydrocannabinol

REFERENCES

1. Schneider Institute for Health Policy, Brandeis University. Substance Abuse: The Nation's Number One Health Problem. Key Indicators for Policy—Update. Princeton, NJ: Robert Wood Johnson Foundation, 2001:1–128.
2. National Center on Addiction and Substance Abuse at Columbia University. Shoveling Up II: The Impact of Substance Abuse on Federal, State and Local Budgets; May 2009.

3. Substance Abuse and Mental Health Services Administration, Office of Applied Studies. *Drug Abuse Warning Network, 2006: National Estimates of Drug-Related Emergency Department Visits.* DAWN Series D-30, DHHS Publication No. (SMA) 08-4339, Rockville, MD, 2008.

4. Savage SR, Joranson DE, Covington EC, et al. Definitions related to the medical use of opioids: Evolution towards universal agreement. J Pain Symptom Manage 2003;26:655–667.

5. Substance Abuse and Mental Health Services Administration. *Results from the 2008 National Survey on Drug Use and Health: National Findings.* Office of Applied Studies, NSDUH Series H-36, HHS Publication No. SMA 09-4434. Rockville, MD, 2009.

6. Johnston LD, O'Malley PM, Bachman JG, et al. Monitoring the Future national results on adolescent drug use: Overview of key findings. NIH Publication No. [yet to be assigned]. Bethesda, MD: National Institute on Drug Abuse, 2009.

7. American Psychiatric Association. Diagnostic and Statistical Manual of Mental Disorders, Fourth Edition, Text Revision. Washington, DC: American Psychiatric Association, 2000:191–198.

8. Heit HA, Gourlay DL. DSM-V and the definitions: time to get it right. Pain Med 2009;10:784–786.

9. Steven E, Hyman SE, Malenka RC, et al. Neural mechanisms of addiction: the role of reward-related learning and memory. Annu Rev Neurosci 2006;29:565–598.

10. The Partnership Attitude Tracking Study (PATS) Teens 2008 Report, Partnership for a Drug-Free America. February 26, 2009. *http://www. drugfree.org/Files/full_report_teens_2008.*

11. National Survey of American Attitudes on Substance Abuse XIV: Teens and Parents Conducted for The National Center on Addiction and Substance Abuse at Columbia University. August 2009. *http:// www.drugfree.org/Files/full_report_teens_2008.*

12. "You've Got Drugs!" V: Prescription Drug Pushers on the Internet. A CASAWhite Paper. July, 2008, National Center on Addiction and Substance Abuse at Columbia University, New York, NY.

13. Implementation of the Ryan Haight Online Pharmacy Consumer Protection Act of 2008. Department of Justice, Drug Enforcement Administration, 21 CFR Parts 1300, 1301, 1304, 1306, [Docket No. DEA-322I], RIN 1117–AB20, 15596 Federal Register/Vol. 74, No. 64/ Monday, April 6, 2009.

14. Bechtel LK, Holstege CP. Criminal poisoning: drug-facilitated sexual assault. Emerg Med Clin North Am 2007;25:499–525.

15. Victorri-Vigneau C, Dailly E, Veyrac G, Joillet P. Evidence of zolpidem abuse and dependence: results of the French Centre for Evaluation and Information on Pharmacodependence (CEIP) network survey. J Clin Pharmacol 2007;64:198–209.

16. O'Brien CP. Drug addiction and drug abuse. In: Brunton LL, Lazo JS, Parker KL, eds. Goodman and Gilman's The Pharmacological Basis of Therapeutics, 11th ed. New York: McGraw-Hill, 2006:614–615.

17. Wojtowicz JM, Yarema MC, Wax PM. Withdrawal from gamma-hydroxybutyrate, 1,4-butanediol and gamma-butyrolactone: a case report and systematic review. CJEM 2008;10(1):69–74.

18. Zvosec DL, Smith SW, Hall BJ. Three deaths associated with use of Xyrem. Sleep Med 2009;10:490–493.

19. Boothby LA, Doering PL, Hatton RC. Carisoprodol: A marginally effective skeletal muscle relaxant with serious abuse potential. Hosp Pharm 2003;38:337–345.

20. U.S. Department of Justice, Drug Enforcement Administration, Office of Diversion Control, Drugs and Chemicals of Concern: Carisoprodol. *http://www.deadiversion.usdoj.gov/drugs_concern/carisoprodol.htm.*

21. Bronstein C, Spyker D, Cantilena JR, et al. Annual Report of the American Association of Poison Control Centers' National Poison Data System (NPDS): 25th Annual Report. Clin Toxicol 2008;46: 927–1057.

22. Drugs Identified in Deceased Persons in Florida. 2008 Report. Florida Department of Law Enforcement, released June 2009. *http:// www.fdle.state.fl.us/Content/getdoc/a37959db-85e0-42f9-b6d6-cdef532f22f8/2008DrugReport.aspx.*

23. Substance Abuse and Mental Health Services Administration. Nonmedical uses of pain relievers: Characteristics of recent initiatives. The NSDUH Report, 2006;22:1–4. *http://www.oas.samhsa.gov/2k6/ pain/pain.pdf.*

24. Chou R, Fanciullo GJ, Fine PG, et al. Clinical guidelines for the use of chronic opioid therapy in chronic noncancer pain. J Pain 2009;10: 113–130.

25. Methadone-Associated Overdose Deaths; Factors Contributing to Increased Deaths and Efforts to Prevent Them. United States Government Accounting Office Report to Congressional Requesters. GAO-09-341; March 26, 2009. *http://www.gao.gov/new.items/d09341.pdf.*

26. U.S. Food and Drug Administration. Information for Healthcare Professionals: Methadone. Issued November 27, 2006. *http://www.fda;gov/ Drugs/DrugSafety/PostmarketDrugSafetyInformationforPatients and-Providers/ucm142841.htm.*

27. Doering PL, Boothby LA. Abuse of over-the-counter drugs. Drug Topics 2003;147:72.

28. Chyka PA, Erdman AR, Manoguerra AS, et al. American Assiciation of Poison Control Centers. Dextromethorphan poisoning: an evidence-based consensus guideline for out-of-hospital management. Clin Toxicol (Phila) 2007;45:662–677.

29. Carrera MR, Meijler MM, Janda KD. Cocaine pharmacology and current pharmacotherapies for its abuse. Bioorg Med Chem 2004;12: 5019–5030.

30. Laizure SC, Parker RB. Pharmacodynamic evaluation of the cardiovascular effects after the coadministration of cocaine and ethanol. Drug Metab Dispos 2009;37(2):310–314.

31. Farooq MU, Bhatt A, Patel M. Neurotoxic and cardiotoxic effects of cocaine and ethanol. J Med Toxicol. 2009;5:134–138.

32. Phillips K, Luk A, Soor GS, et al. Cocaine cardiotoxicity: a review of the pathophysiology, pathology, and treatment options. Am J Cardiovasc Drugs 2009;9:177–196.

33. Mahoney III JJ, Kalechstein AD, De La Garza II R, et al. Presence and persistence of psychotic symptoms in cocaine- versus methamphetamine-dependent participants. Am J Addict 2008;17:83–98.

34. World Drug Report 2009. United Nations Office on Drugs and Crime. United Nations, New York. *http://www.unodc.org/unodc/en/data-and-analysis/WDR-2009.html.*

35. King GR, Ellinwood EH. Amphetamines and other stimulants. In: Lowinson JH, Ruiz P, Millman RB, Langrod JG, eds. Substance Abuse: A Comprehensive Textbook, 4th ed. Baltimore, MD: Williams & Wilkins, 2005:277–302.

36. Nicosia N, Pacula RL, Kilmer B, et al. The economic cost of methamphetamine use in the United States, 2005. Rand Drug Policy Research Center, Monograph MG-829-MPF/NIDA. http://www.RAND.org/ pubs/mographs/2009/RAND_MG829.pdf.

37. Hamamoto DT, Rhodus NL. Methamphetamine abuse and dentistry. Oral Dis 2009;15:27–37.

38. Lineberry TW, Bostwick M. Methamphetamine abuse: A perfect storm of complications. Mayo Clin Proc 2006;81:77–84.

39. Shoptaw SJ, Kao U, Heinzerling K. Treatment for amphetamine withdrawal. Cochrane Database Syst Rev 2009:CD003021.

40. National Drug Intelligence Center. National Drug Threat Assessment 2009. United States Department of Justice; December 2008.

41. Dedel K, Scott MS. Clandestine Methamphetamine Labs, 2nd ed. Problem Oriented Guides for Police Series, Number 16; 2006. *http:// www.cops.usdoj.gov.*

42. Gouzoulis-Mayfrank E, Daumann J. Neurotoxicity of methylenedioxyamphetamines (MDMA; ecstasy) in humans: how strong is the evidence for persistent brain damage? Addiction 2006;101:348–361.

43. Indlekofer F, Piechatzek M, Daamen M. Reduced memory and attention performance in a population-based sample of young adults with a moderate lifetime use of cannabis, ecstasy and alcohol. J Psychopharmacol 2009;23(5):495–509.

44. McCann UD, Kuwabara H, Kumar A, et al. Persistent cognitive and dopamine transporter deficits in abstinent methamphetamine users. Synapse 2008;62:91–100.

45. McCann UD, Szabo Z, Vranesic M, et al. Positron emission tomographic studies of brain dopamine and serotonin transporters in abstinent (+/-)3,4-methylenedioxymethamphetamine ("ecstasy") users: relationship to cognitive performance. Psychopharmacology (Berl) 2008;200:439–450.

46. Lamberth PG, Ding GK, Nurmi LA. Fatal paramethoxy-amphetamine (PMA) poisoning in the Australian Capital Territory. Med J Aust 2008;188:426.

47. Kelly BC. Bongs and blunts: notes from a suburban marijuana subculture. J Ethn Subst Abuse 2005;4(3–4):81–97.

48. National Institute on Drug Abuse (NIDA) Research Report—Marijuana Abuse. NIH Publication No. 05-3859; 2005. *http://www.drugabuse.gov/PDF/RRMarijuana.pdf.*

49. Sewell RA, Poling J, Sofuoglu M. The effect of cannabis compared with alcohol on driving. Am J Addict 2009;18:185–193.

50. Cherek DR, Lane SD, Dougherty DM. Possible amotivational effects following marijuana smoking under laboratory conditions. Exp Clin Psychopharmacol 2002;10:26–38.

51. Williams M, Nowitz M, Weatherall M. Effects of cannabis on pulmonary structure, function and symptoms. Thorax 2007;62:1058–1063.

52. Kalant H. Adverse effects of cannabis on health: An update of the literature since 1966. Prog Neuropsychopharmacol Biol Psychiatry 2004;28:849–863.

53. Wang T, Collet JP, Shapiro S, et al. Adverse effects of medical cannabinoids: a systematic review. Evid Based Nurs 2009;12:16.7.

54. Fudala PJ, Greenstein RA, O'Brien CP. Alternative pharmacotherapies for opiate addiction. In: Lowinson JH, Ruiz P, Millman RB, Langrod JG, eds. Substance Abuse: A Comprehensive Textbook, 4th ed. Baltimore, MD: Williams & Wilkins, 2005:641–653.

55. Mathias S, Lubman DI, Hides L. Substance-induced psychosis: a diagnostic conundrum. J Clin Psychiatry 2008;69:358–367.

56. Carrera MR, Meijler MM, Janda KD. Cocaine pharmacology and current pharmacotherapies for its abuse. Bioorg Med Chem 2004;12:5019–5030.

57. McCord J, Jneid H, Hollander JE, et al. Management of cocaine-associated chest pain and myocardial infarction: a scientific statement from the American Heart Association Acute Cardiac Care Committee of the Council on Clinical Cardiology. Circulation 2008;117:1897–1907.

58. Amato L, Minozzi S, Ali R, et al. Methadone at tapered doses for the management of opioid withdrawal. Cochrane Database Syst Rev 2005:CD003409.

59. Drug Addiction Treatment Act of 2000 (DATA), Title XXXV of the Children's Health Act of 2000 (Pub L No. 106–310, 116 Stat 1222). *http://buprenorphine.samhsa.gov/fulllaw.html.*

60. CSAT Buprenorphine information center. The Center for Substance Abuse Treatment (CSAT), Substance Abuse and Mental Health Services Administration (SAMHSA). *http://buprenorphine.samhsa.gov/.*

61. Orman JS, Keating GM. Buprenorphine/naloxone: a review of its use in the treatment of opioid dependence. Drugs 2009;69:577–607.

62. TIP 40 Center for Substance Abuse Treatment. Clinical Guidelines for the Use of Buprenorphine in the Treatment of Opioid Addiction. Treatment Improvement Protocol (TIP) Series 40. DHHS Publication No. (SMA) 04-3939. Rockville, MD: Substance Abuse and Mental Health Services Administration, 2004. *http://www.ncbi.nlm.nih.gov/bookshelf/br.fcgi?book=hssamhsatip&part=A72248.*

63. Gowing L, Ali R, White JM. Buprenorphine for the management of opioid withdrawal. Cochrane Database Syst Rev 2009:CD002025.

64. Collins ED, Kleber HD, Whittington RA, Heitler NE. Anesthesia-assisted vs buprenorphine- or clonidine-assisted heroin detoxification and naltrexone induction: A randomized trial. JAMA 2005;294:903–913.

65. Gorelick DA, Wilkins JN. Bromocriptine treatment for cocaine addiction: Association with plasma prolactin levels. Drug Alcohol Depend 2006;81:189–195.

66. Orson FM, Kinsey BM, Singh RA, et al. Vaccines for cocaine abuse. Hum Vaccin 2009;5:194–199.

67. Martell BA, Orson FM, James Poling J, et al. Cocaine vaccine for the treatment of cocaine dependence in methadone-maintained patients. Arch Gen Psychiatry 2009;66:1116–1123.

68. Smith DE, Seymour RB. Benzodiazepines and other sedative-hypnotics. In: Galanter M, Kleber HD, eds. Textbook of Substance Abuse Treatment. Washington, DC: American Psychiatric Association, 1994:179–186.

69. Knapp CM, Ciraulo DA, Jaffe J. Opiates: Clinical aspects. In: Lowinson JH, Ruiz P, Millman RB, Langrod JG, eds. Substance Abuse: A Comprehensive Textbook, 4th ed. Baltimore, MD: Williams & Wilkins, 2005:180–195.

75

Substance-Related Disorders: Alcohol, Nicotine, and Caffeine

PAUL L. DOERING AND ROBIN MOORMAN LI

KEY CONCEPTS

❶ Tobacco is the number 1 preventable cause of death in the United States.

❷ Between 12 and 16 million Americans report current heavy alcohol use or alcohol abuse.

❸ Pharmacogenomics studies have identified genotypic and functional phenotypic variants that either serve to protect patients or predispose them toward alcohol dependence.

❹ Alcohol is a central nervous system depressant that shares many pharmacologic properties with the nonbenzodiazepine sedative hypnotics.

❺ The metabolism of alcohol is considered to follow zero-order pharmacokinetics, and this has important implications for the time course in which alcohol can exert its effects.

❻ Benzodiazepines are the treatment of choice for alcohol withdrawal.

❼ Disulfiram, naltrexone, and acamprosate are FDA-approved drug therapies for the treatment of alcohol dependence. The clinical utility of these agents to improve sustained abstinence remains controversial. Relapse is common.

❽ More than three quarters of smokers are nicotine dependent. Tobacco dependence is a chronic condition that requires repeated interventions.

❾ Use of nicotine replacement therapy along with behavioral counseling doubles cessation rates.

❿ Bupropion and varenicline are efficacious alone and in combination with nicotine replacement therapy for smoking cessation.

⓫ Special precautions are associated with the use of varenicline for smoking cessation.

⓬ Caffeine's pharmacologic actions are similar to those of other stimulant drugs. As such, abstinence from caffeine induces a distinct withdrawal syndrome that includes headache, drowsiness, and fatigue.

Learning objectives, review questions,
and other resources can be found at
www.pharmacotherapyonline.com.

KEY MEDICAL TERMS

Caffeinism: Caffeinism is the term coined to describe the clinical syndrome produced by acute or chronic overuse of caffeine.

Euphoria: A mood state characterized by an exaggerated, superficial sense of well-being, characterized by extreme happiness, sometimes more than is reasonable in a particular situation.

Intoxication: The development of a substance-specific syndrome after recent ingestion and presence in the body of a substance; and it is associated with maladaptive behavior during the waking state caused by the effect of the substance on the central nervous system.

Withdrawal: The development of a substance-specific physiologic syndrome after cessation of or reduction in intake of a substance that was used regularly.

❶ Alcohol, nicotine, and caffeine are considered by most to be socially acceptable drugs, yet they impose an enormous social and economic cost on our society. Approximately 443,000 deaths each year are attributable to tobacco use, making tobacco the number 1 preventable cause of death and disease in this country.[1,2] The three leading causes of death attributable to smoking include lung cancer, chronic obstructive pulmonary disease, and ischemic heart disease.[3]

❷ In 2008, heavy drinking was reported by 6.9% of the population aged 12 or older, or 17.3 million people.[4] More than one fifth (23.3%) of persons aged 12 or older participated in binge drinking at least once in the 30 days prior to the National Survey on Drug Use and Health in 2008. The World Health Organization estimates that there are approximately 2 billion people worldwide who consume alcoholic beverages, and 76.3 million with diagnosable alcohol-use disorders.[5] Long-term alcohol abuse often leads to chronic disease. A causal relationship between alcohol abuse and at least 60 types of chronic disease or injury have been established (e.g., esophageal cancer, liver cancer, and cirrhosis of the liver, epileptic seizures, homicide, and motor vehicle accidents) worldwide.[5] Nationally, according to the Drug Abuse Warning Network 2006 survey, 577,521 emergency department (ED) visits involved either alcohol in combination with another drug (all ages) or alcohol alone for patients under the age of 21. This is about one third (33%) of all drug misuse/abuse ED visits.[6]

❷ Worldwide, alcohol abuse leads to 1.8 million deaths annually.[5] Nationally, according to the Alcohol-Attributable Deaths Report 2001-2005, 79,646 U.S. citizens with medium and high average daily alcohol consumption die each year because of alcohol-related causes, including traffic collisions and cirrhosis of the liver.[7] Direct and indirect health and social costs of alcoholism to the nation are estimated to be $185 billion annually.[8]

Caffeine is currently the most widely used psychoactive substance in the world. In the United States, 80% to 90% of adults regularly consume behaviorally active doses of caffeine. Although research has shown that caffeine can cause a compulsive pattern of use, the prevalence of caffeine dependence and its clinical significance are difficult to determine.

ALCOHOL

EPIDEMIOLOGY OF ALCOHOL USE

Slightly more than half of Americans aged 12 or older reported being current drinkers of alcohol according to the National Survey on Drug Use and Health 2008 survey (51.6%).[4] This translates to an estimated 129 million people, which is similar to the 2007 estimate of 126.8 million people (51.1%). More than one fifth (23.3%) of persons aged 12 or older participated in binge drinking, defined as having five or more drinks on the same occasion, at least once in the 30 days prior to the survey.[4] This translates to about 58.1 million people. The rate in 2008 is the same as the rate in 2007 (23.3%). In 2008, heavy drinking was reported by 6.9% of the population aged 12 or older, meaning that they drank five or more drinks on the same occasion on at least five different days in the past month.[4]

THE DISEASE MODEL OF ADDICTION AS APPLIED TO ALCOHOLISM

The disease concept of addiction, using alcoholism as a model, states that addiction is a disease, and that individuals who suffer from the disease do not choose to contract the disease any more than someone who suffers from heart disease or diabetes mellitus chooses to contract that illness. A *disease* is defined as "any deviation from or interruption of the normal structure or function of any part, organ, or system (or combination thereof) of the body that is manifested by a characteristic set of symptoms and signs and whose etiology, pathology, and prognosis may be known or unknown."[9] Alcoholism, which is discussed as a prototype, meets all the definitional criteria. Diagnostic criteria for alcoholism do not specify frequency of drinking or amount of alcohol consumed. The key determinant is whether drinking is compulsive, out of control, and consequential when one drinks.

❸ It has long been recognized that alcoholism is heritable, as 50% to 60% of first-degree relatives of alcoholics become alcohol dependent themselves.[10] Past discussions have focused on whether this heritable risk is because of genetics, environment, or both. Recent research has identified several traits (or phenotypes), that attenuate one's risk of alcohol dependence. Initially based on data from preclinical studies, pharmacogenomics studies have identified genotypic and functional phenotypic variants that either serve to protect patients or predispose them toward alcohol dependence.[11] Large-scale pharmacoepidemiologic studies have further elucidated the environmental risk factors that are associated with either protective effects or predisposition toward alcoholism.[12] This is referred to as the "genome x" environment interaction effect. The known susceptibility genes, phenotypic characteristics, and environmental risk factors are summarized in Table 75–1.[11–15]

PHARMACOLOGY AND PHARMACOKINETICS OF ALCOHOL

Alcohol as a Drug

❹ Alcohol is a central nervous system (CNS) depressant that affects the CNS in a dose-dependent fashion, producing sedation that progresses to sleep, unconsciousness, coma, surgical anesthesia,

TABLE 75-1	Genotypic, Phenotypic, and Environmental Factors That Increase Alcohol Dependence Risk		
Susceptibility Genes	**Phenotype**	**Environment**

Regions on chromosomes 1 and 4 that code for the following receptors:
  GABA$_A$
  Serotonin 1b
  DRD4
  Tryptophan hydroxylase
  Neuropeptide Y
Gene that codes for:
  ALDH2
  5HTTLPR
	Personality traits that include:
	  Novelty seeking
	  Impulsivity
	  Aggression
	  Depression
	  Maximum number of alcoholic drinks consumed per day
		Religious background
		Urban residence (vs. rural)
		History of sexual abuse
		Being single
		Having deceased parents

ALDH2, aldehyde dehydrogenase 2; DRD4, type 4 dopamine receptor gene; GABA, gamma aminobutyric acid; 5HTTLPR, 5 hydroxytryptamine transporter.
Data from Bierut et al.,[11] Heath et al.,[12] Luo et al.,[13] Boothby and Doering,[14] and Krystal et al.[15]

and finally fatal respiratory depression and cardiovascular collapse. Alcohol affects endogenous opiates and several neurotransmitter systems in the brain, including γ-aminobutyric acid (GABA), glutamine, and dopamine. Alcohol is available in a variety of concentrations in various alcoholic beverages. There are approximately 14 g of alcohol in a 12-oz (355 mL) can of beer (approximately 5%), 4 oz (118 mL) of nonfortified wine (approximately 10%–14%), or one shot (1.5 oz [44 mL]) of 80-proof whiskey (40%). Full consumption of this amount will cause an increase in blood alcohol level of approximately 20 to 25 mg/dL (4.3 to 5.4 mmol/L) in a healthy 70-kg (154 lb) male, although this varies with the time frame over which the alcohol is consumed, the type of alcoholic beverage, whether food is consumed along with it, and many patient variables. The lethal dose of alcohol in humans is variable, but deaths generally occur when blood alcohol levels are greater than 400 to 500 mg/dL (87 to 109 mmol/L).[16]

CLINICAL CONTROVERSY

Moderate alcohol consumption has been suggested to improve health. The definition of moderate consumption is narrow: one drink or less per day for females, and two drinks or less per day for males. The major limitations of this research thus far are the observational study designs that cannot demonstrate cause and effect relationsips between alcohol consumption and positive health benefits.[18–21] Additional potential confounders in these studies include diet, exercise, disease states, other drug therapies known to promote or hinder cardiovascular health, and psychosocial factors such as stress management.

Pharmacokinetics

Absorption of alcohol begins in the stomach within 5 to 10 minutes of oral ingestion. The onset of clinical effects follows fairly rapidly. Peak serum concentrations of alcohol usually are achieved 30 to 90 minutes after finishing the last drink, although it is variable depending on the type of alcoholic beverage consumed, what and when the person last ate, and other factors.[17]

More than 90% of alcohol in the plasma is metabolized in the liver by three enzyme systems that operate within the hepatocyte. The remainder is excreted by the lungs and in urine and sweat. Alcohol is metabolized to acetaldehyde by alcohol dehydrogenase in the cell. In turn, acetaldehyde is metabolized to carbon dioxide and water by the enzyme aldehyde dehydrogenase. A second

TABLE 75-2 Specific Effects of Alcohol Related to BAC

BAC (%)ᵃ [mmol/L]	Effect
0.02–0.03 [4–8]	No loss of coordination, slight euphoria, and loss of shyness.
0.04–0.06 [9–14]	Feeling of well-being, relaxation, lower inhibitions, sensation of warmth. Euphoria. Some minor impairment of reasoning and memory, lowering of caution.
0.07–0.09 [15–21]	Slight impairment of balance, speech, vision, reaction time, and hearing. Euphoria. Judgment and self-control are reduced, and caution, reason, and memory are impaired. It is illegal to operate a motor vehicle in some states at this level.
0.10–0.125 [22–27]	Significant impairment of motor coordination and loss of good judgment. Speech can be slurred; balance, vision, reaction time, and hearing impaired. Euphoria. It is illegal to operate a motor vehicle at this level of intoxication.
0.13–0.15 [28–34]	Gross motor impairment and lack of physical control. Blurred vision and major loss of balance. Euphoria is reduced, and dysphoria is beginning to appear.
0.16–0.20 [35–43]	Dysphoria (anxiety, restlessness) predominates, nausea can appear. The drinker has the appearance of a "sloppy drunk."
0.25 [54]	Needs assistance in walking; total mental confusion. Dysphoria with nausea and some vomiting.
0.30 [65]	Loss of consciousness.
≥0.40 [>87]	Onset of coma, possible death caused by respiratory arrest.

BAC, blood alcohol concentration.
ᵃGrams of ethyl alcohol per 100 mL of whole blood.

pathway for oxidation of alcohol uses catalase, an enzyme located in the peroxisomes and microsomes. The third enzyme system, the microsomal alcohol oxidase system, has a role in the oxidation of alcohol to acetaldehyde. These last two mechanisms are of lesser importance than the alcohol dehydrogenase–aldehyde dehydrogenase system.[17]

❺ The metabolism of alcohol generally is said to follow zero-order pharmacokinetics.[17] This can, in fact, be an oversimplification because at very high or very low concentrations of alcohol the metabolism can follow first-order pharmacokinetics.[18] On average, the blood alcohol concentration (BAC) is lowered from 15 to 22.2 mg/dL (3.3 to 4.8 mmol/L) per hour in the nontolerant individual, assuming that the individual is in the postabsorptive state (Table 75–2). Alcohol has a volume of distribution of 0.6 to 0.8 L/kg, representing the total body water.[17]

CLINICAL INDICATORS OF CHRONIC ALCOHOL ABUSE

The CAGE questionnaire is a tool for detecting individuals more likely to be abusing alcohol and therefore at greater risk for alcohol withdrawal. CAGE is a mnemonic for four questions: (1) Do you ever feel the need to cut down on your alcohol use? (2) Have you ever been annoyed by others telling you that you drink too much? (3) Have you ever felt guilty about your drinking or something you did while drinking? (4) Do you ever have an "eye opener"? A positive response to two or more of these four questions suggests an increased likelihood of alcohol abuse with an average sensitivity of 0.71 (71%) and an average specificity of 0.90 (90%).[19]

Acute Effects of Alcohol

At lower serum concentrations, euphoria and disinhibition may be noted. Slurred speech, altered perception of the environment, impaired judgment, ataxia, incoordination, nystagmus, and hyperreflexia may occur. As plasma levels increase combative and destructive behavior may occur. With higher levels still, somnolence and respiratory depression may ensue. The typical effects of various BACs are shown in Table 75–2, although effects vary from individual to individual.

Alcohol Poisoning

Acute alcohol poisoning usually occurs with rapid consumption of large quantities of alcoholic beverages, because this type of drinking delivers a bolus of alcohol to the gastrointestinal (GI) tract. With sustained drinking of moderate amounts of alcohol, the user passes out before a toxic dose of alcohol can be ingested, and/or the person vomits to rid the stomach of its toxic reservoir. With rapid drinking as described, the person may fall asleep or pass out without vomiting, allowing continued alcohol absorption from the GI tract, while the patient sleeps, until fatal BACs are achieved.

Laboratory Studies

In the emergency room, a BAC should be ordered in any patient in whom alcohol ingestion is suspected, regardless of the presenting complaint. For clinical purposes, most laboratories report BAC in units of mg/dL or mmol/L. In legal cases, results are reported in percentage (grams of ethyl alcohol per 100 mL of whole blood). If the diagnosis is unclear, if the intoxication seems atypical, or when there is suspicion of multiple drug ingestions, a complete toxicologic screen to rule out the presence of other substances may be useful.

CLINICAL PRESENTATION OF ALCOHOL INTOXICATION AND WITHDRAWAL

General
- Acute alcohol detoxification and withdrawal after chronic alcohol abuse is a serious condition that can require hospitalization and adjunctive pharmacotherapy. If the BAC gets high enough, death is possible.

Symptoms
- The intoxicated patient can present with slurred speech and ataxia. The patient can be sedated or unconscious. As BACs decrease rapidly, nausea, vomiting, and hallucinations can ensue. Delirium and seizures are the most severe symptoms.

Signs
- The intoxicated patient can present with nystagmus.
- In withdrawal, the patient can present with tachycardia, diaphoresis, or hyperthermia.

Laboratory Tests
- In the emergency department, a BAC should be ordered when alcohol ingestion is suspected. Most laboratories report BAC in units of milligrams per deciliter. A whole blood alcohol level of 150 mg/dL (33 mmol/L) reported in the hospital corresponds to 0.15% BAC obtained by law enforcement.
- A complete toxicologic screen to rule out the presence of other substances can be useful.

Other Diagnostic Tests
- Differentiate acute alcohol intoxication from other medical illnesses (e.g., head trauma).
- Use computed tomography (CT) on any patient with focal neurologic findings, failure to improve, new-onset seizures, or mental status out of proportion to degree of intoxication.

TREATMENT

ALCOHOL-RELATED DISORDERS

Alcohol Withdrawal

Goals for alcohol-dependent persons trying to decrease or discontinue alcohol intake include: (1) the prevention and treatment of withdrawal symptoms (including seizures and delirium tremens) and medical or psychiatric complications, (2) long-term abstinence after detoxification, and (3) entry into ongoing medical and alcohol-dependence treatment.

■ PHARMACOLOGIC THERAPY

6 Symptom-triggered treatment with a benzodiazepine is the current standard of care in alcohol detoxification to manage and minimize symptoms and avoid progression to the more severe stages of withdrawal. A meta-analysis was performed to provide evidence-based recommendations on the pharmacologic management of alcohol withdrawal[20] and alcohol withdrawal delirium.[21] Trials comparing different benzodiazepines demonstrated that all appear similarly efficacious in reducing signs and symptoms of withdrawal.[20,21] Lorazepam is preferred by many clinicians because it can be administered intravenously, intramuscularly, or orally with predictable results. Another consideration in the choice of benzodiazepines is their potential for abuse during recovery. A Cochrane Review[22] of the effectiveness and safety of benzodiazepines in the treatment of alcohol withdrawal symptoms was published in 2005. According to this report: "the available data show that benzodiazepines are effective against alcohol withdrawal seizures when compared to placebo. However, there are no prominent differences between benzodiazepines and other drugs in success rates. Data on safety outcomes are sparse and fragmented. There is a need for larger, well-designed studies in this field."

Treatment Regimens

Symptom-Triggered Therapy With symptom-triggered therapy, medication is given only when the patient has symptoms. This approach results in treatment that is shorter, potentially avoiding over sedation and allowing the clinician to focus on specific therapy for alcohol dependence.[20,21] A typical regimen would include lorazepam 2 mg administered every hour as needed when a structured assessment scale—such as the Clinical Institute Withdrawal Assessment–Alcohol, Revised—indicates that symptoms are moderate to severe (Table 75–3).[23]

TABLE 75-3 Pharmacologic Agents Used in the Treatment of Alcohol Withdrawal					
Drug	Dose per Day (Unless Otherwise Stated)	Indication	Monitoring	Duration of Dosing	Level of Evidence[a]
Multivitamin	1 tablet	Malnutrition	Diet	At least until eating a balanced diet at caloric goal	B3
Thiamine	50–100 mg	Deficiency	CBC, WBC, nystagmus	Empiric × 5 days. More if evidence of deficiency	B2
Crystalloid fluids (typically D5-0.45 NS with 20 mEq of KCl per liter)	50–100 mL/hr	Dehydration	Weight, electrolytes, urine output, nystagmus if dextrose	Until intake and outputs stabilize and oral intake is adequate	A3
Clonidine oral	0.05–0.3 mg	Autonomic tone rebound and hyperactivity	Shaking, tremor, sweating, blood pressure	3 days or less	B2
Clonidine transdermal	TTS-1 to TTS-3	Autonomic tone rebound and hyperactivity	Shaking, tremor, sweating, blood pressure	1 week or less. One patch only	B3
Labetalol	20 mg IV every 2 hours as needed	Hypertensive urgencies and above	Blood pressure target	Individual doses as needed	B3
Antipsychotics, haloperidol	2.5 mg to 5 mg every four hours	Agitation unresponsive to benzodiazepines, hallucinations (tactile, visual, auditory, or otherwise) or delusions	Subjective response plus rating scale (CIWA-Ar or equivalent)	Individual doses as needed	B1
Antipsychotics, atypical Quetiapine Aripiprazole	25–200 mg 5–15 mg	Agitation unresponsive to benzodiazepines, hallucinations, or delusions in patients intolerant of conventional antipsychotics	Subjective response plus rating scale (CIWA-Ar or equivalent)	Individual doses as needed in addition to scheduled antipsychotic	C3
Benzodiazepines Lorazepam Chlordiazepoxide Clonazepam Diazepam	0.5–2 mg 5 mg–25 mg 0.5–2 mg 2.5–10 mg	Tremor, anxiety, diaphoresis, tachypnea, dysphoria, seizures	Subjective response plus rating scale (CIWA-Ar or equivalent)	Individual doses as needed Underdosing is more common than overdosing	A2
Alcohol oral		Prevent withdrawal	subjective signs of withdrawal	Wide variation	C3
Alcohol IV		Prevent withdrawal	subjective signs of withdrawal	Wide variation	C3

CBC, complete blood count; CIWA-Ar, Clinical Institute Withdrawal Assessment for Alcohol, revised; D5, dextrose 5%; KCl, potassium chloride; NS, normal saline; WBC, white blood cell count.
[a]Strength of recommendations, evidence to support recommendation: A, good; B, moderate; C, poor.
Quality of evidence: 1, evidence from more than 1 properly randomized, controlled trial; 2, evidence from more than 1 well-designed clinical trial with randomization, from cohort or case-controlled analytic studies or multiple time series; or dramatic results from uncontrolled experiments; 3, evidence from opinions of respected authorities, based on clinical experience, descriptive studies, or reports of expert communities.
Data from Mayo-Smith,[20] Mayo-Smith et al.[21]

Fixed-Schedule Therapy Over the years, benzodiazepines given regularly at a fixed dosing interval have been used for alcohol withdrawal. The major problem with this approach is underdosing of the benzodiazepine because of the phenomenon of cross-tolerance (see Table 75–3). Current guidelines take exception with this rigid approach, urging clinicians to allow for some degree of individualization within fixed-schedule therapy.[20,21]

Treatment of Alcohol Withdrawal Seizures

Alcohol withdrawal seizures do not require treatment with an anticonvulsant drug unless they progress to status epilepticus because seizures usually end before diazepam or another drug can be administered.[21,23] Phenytoin, which is not cross-tolerant to alcohol, does not prevent or treat withdrawal seizures, and without an intravenous loading dose, therapeutic blood levels of phenytoin are not reached until acute withdrawal is complete. Patients experiencing seizures should be treated supportively. An increase in the dosage and slowing of the tapering schedule of the benzodiazepine used in detoxification or a single injection of a benzodiazepine can be necessary to prevent further seizure activity. Patients with a history of withdrawal seizures can be predicted to experience an especially severe withdrawal syndrome. In such patients, a higher initial dosage of a benzodiazepine and a slower tapering period of 7 to 10 days are advisable.

Treatment of Nutritional Deficits and Electrolyte Abnormalities

Fluid status should be carefully assessed, and fluid, electrolyte, and vitamin abnormalities should be corrected. Hydration can be necessary in patients with vomiting, diarrhea, increased body temperature, or severe agitation. Alcoholics often have electrolyte imbalances because of inadequate nutrition and fluid volume related to antidiuretic hormone inhibition. Hypokalemia can be corrected with oral potassium supplementation as long as renal function is adequate. Hypophosphatemia is common but should be allowed to gradually correct with adequate nutrition if phosphorus levels are greater than 1 mg/dL (0.32 mmol/L). Hypomagnesemia is also common, but routine magnesium replacement for alcohol withdrawal is not recommended. Thiamine (vitamin B_1) is often depleted in alcoholics, particularly those with poor nutrition. Thiamine supplementation is standard because it can prevent the development of the Wernicke-Korsakoff syndrome (e.g., mental confusion, eye movement disorders, and ataxia [poor motor coordination]), which may not be reversible once it develops. An initial dose of 100 mg IV or IM is commonly used. In practice, thiamine is usually given 100 mg once daily orally, intravenously, or intramuscularly for 3 to 5 days.

It is not necessary for thiamine to be continued empirically for longer than 5 days (see Table 75–3).

Other nutritional deficits can also occur with chronic alcohol abuse primarily caused by poor eating habits. A multivitamin is usually given once daily. If clotting factors are abnormal because of decreased liver function and a relative inability to produce vitamin K–dependent clotting factors, then 2.5 to 25 mg of vitamin K can also be prescribed.

Alcohol hypoglycemia usually occurs in the absence of overt liver disease, and it is more likely if the patient is fasting or exercising or is sensitive to alcohol; it is less likely if the patient is obese. The alcohol directly interferes with hepatic gluconeogenesis but not glycogenolysis. The energy required for metabolism of alcohol is diverted away from the energy needed to take up lactate and pyruvate—substrates for gluconeogenesis. So, patients who drink alcohol can become hypoglycemic once glycogen stores are depleted. Neurologic symptoms of hypoglycemia can be confused with alcohol intoxication, and in the inpatient setting, blood glucose should be monitored regularly.

Treatment Settings

Alcohol withdrawal treatment can take place in hospitals, inpatient detoxification units, or outpatient settings. Inpatient treatment can be necessary when there are coexisting acute or chronic medical (including pregnancy), surgical, or psychiatric conditions that would complicate alcohol withdrawal. Only patients with mild to moderate symptoms should be considered for outpatient treatment, and it is a good idea to have a responsible, sober person available to help the patient monitor symptoms and administer medications. Patients with a strong craving for alcohol, those concurrently using other drugs, and those with a history of seizures or delirium tremens are not good candidates for outpatient treatment. Pharmacologic agents used in the treatment of alcohol withdrawal are summarized in Table 75–3.

PHARMACOLOGIC MANAGEMENT OF ALCOHOL DEPENDENCE

❼ In the United States, disulfiram, naltrexone, the once-monthly injectable extended-release naltrexone, and acamprosate are the only four drugs that are FDA-approved for the treatment of alcohol dependence. Disulfiram acts as a deterrent to the resumption of drinking, and naltrexone is a competitive opioid antagonist that has been shown to reduce cravings for alcohol. Acamprosate is a GABA-ergic agonist that modulates alcohol cravings (Table 75–4). Other drugs, including nalmefene, bupropion, various serotonergic

TABLE 75-4	Pharmacologic Agents Used in the Treatment of Alcohol Dependence					
Drug	**Dosage Range per Day**	**Indication**	**Monitoring**	**Duration of Dosing**	**Level of Evidence**[a]
Disulfiram	250 mg–500 mg	Deterrence	Facial flushing, liver enzymes	Indefinite	B2
Acamprosate	999 mg–1,998 mg and higher (333 mg tablets)	Craving	Patient-reported craving, renal function	Indefinite	A1
Naltrexone	50 mg–100 mg	Craving	Patient-reported craving	Indefinite	A1
Mood stabilizers (e.g., lamotrigine, topiramate, carbamazepine, valproic acid)	Seizure disorder doses	Craving	Patient-reported craving, plasma drug levels	Indefinite	B2
Antidepressants (e.g., clomipramine, bupropion, doxepin, maprotiline, fluoxetine)	Depression doses	Craving, depression, anxiety	Patient-reported craving	Indefinite	B2

[a]Strength of recommendations: A, B, C = good, moderate, and poor evidence to support recommendation, respectively.
Quality of evidence: 1, evidence from more than 1 properly randomized, controlled trial. 2, evidence from more than 1 well-designed clinical trial with randomization, from cohort or case-controlled analytic studies or multiple time series; or dramatic results from uncontrolled experiments. 3, evidence from opinions of respected authorities, based on clinical experience, descriptive studies, or reports of expert communities.
Data from Boothby and Doering,[14] Garbutt et al.[25,26]

agents (including selective serotonin reuptake inhibitors and vascular serotonin 5-HT$_3$ receptor antagonists), topiramate, and lithium also have been used either abroad or in the United States off-label for alcohol dependence. A recent meta-analysis[24] has been published with the primary objective of completing the efficacy profiles for acamprosate and naltrexone by contacting researchers when outcomes were missing and to compare them with each other. Naltrexone was found to have a significant effect on the maintenance of abstinence as well as the prevention of heavy drinking. Acamprosate was shown only to support abstinence; it did not influence alcohol consumption after the first drink. When the efficacy profiles of the two drugs were compared, acamprosate was found to be more effective in preventing a lapse, whereas naltrexone was better in preventing a lapse from becoming a relapse.

CLINICAL CONTROVERSY

The most difficult clinical problem in the treatment of alcohol-related illness is helping patients remain abstinent after alcohol detoxification. Acamprosate and naltrexone have been shown to be superior to nonpharmacologic therapy alone for maintenance of abstinence from alcohol; however, relapse during naltrexone and acamprosate therapy is still common. Disulfiram use has fallen out of favor. Studies have failed to prove it effective, and it is poorly tolerated. For this reason, most clinicians rarely recommend the use of disulfiram.

■ DISULFIRAM

Disulfiram deters a patient from drinking by producing an aversive reaction if the patient drinks. In the absence of alcohol, disulfiram has minimal effects. Disulfiram inhibits the liver enzyme aldehyde dehydrogenase in the biochemical pathway for alcohol metabolism, allowing acetaldehyde to accumulate. The resulting increase in acetaldehyde causes severe facial flushing, throbbing headache, nausea and vomiting, chest pain, palpitations, tachycardia, weakness, dizziness, blurred vision, confusion, and hypotension. Severe reactions including myocardial infarction, congestive heart failure, cardiac arrhythmia, respiratory depression, convulsions, and death can occur, particularly in vulnerable individuals. A recent review summarizes disulfiram's overall usefulness.[25]

■ NALTREXONE

Naltrexone, an opiate antagonist available in the United States since 1984 for the treatment of opioid dependence blocks the effects of exogenous opioids. In 1994, the FDA approved its use in the treatment of alcohol dependence. Naltrexone is thought to attenuate the reinforcing effects of alcohol, and those who consume alcohol while taking naltrexone report feeling less intoxicated and having less craving for alcohol.[25]

Short-term treatment (up to 12 weeks) with naltrexone decreases the chance of alcohol relapse by 36% versus placebo.[25] Naltrexone should not be given to patients currently dependent on opiates because it can precipitate a severe withdrawal syndrome. Naltrexone is associated with dose-related hepatotoxicity, but this generally occurs at doses higher than those recommended for treatment of alcohol dependence. Nevertheless, it is considered contraindicated in patients with hepatitis or liver failure, and liver function tests should be monitored monthly for the first 3 months and every 3 months thereafter.

Nausea is the most common side effect of naltrexone, occurring in approximately 10% of patients. Other side effects are headache, dizziness, nervousness, fatigue, insomnia, vomiting, anxiety, and somnolence. If dosed daily, naltrexone 50 mg per day is sufficient to effectively block μ-opioid receptors.

In April 2006, the FDA approved Vivitrol, a once-monthly intramuscular naltrexone formulation. The usual effective dose is 380 mg IM each month.[25,26] Extended release formulations reduce the likelihood of forgetting or choosing not to take medication, assuring that once the patient receives an injection, he or she will be "adherent" for the next month.[26]

■ ACAMPROSATE

Acamprosate is a glutamate modulator at the N-methyl-D-aspartate (NMDA) receptor that reduces alcohol craving. Acamprosate, approved in the United States in 2004, had been available in Europe for many years. Patients treated with acamprosate are more successful in maintaining abstinence from alcohol versus placebo. In addition, the combination of acamprosate and naltrexone has been shown to be more efficacious than acamprosate alone for the maintenance of abstinence from alcohol, when combined with psychosocial interventions. Acamprosate is well tolerated, with gastrointestinal adverse effects most common.[27] See Table 75-4 for dosing information for this and the other options used in treating alcohol dependence.

NICOTINE

Cigarette smoking is an enormous national health problem, and as healthcare professionals, we all must continue to work to help people to quit smoking. Clinical guidelines for tobacco use and dependence were released in 2000, which stressed the importance of healthcare professionals screening each patient for tobacco use.[28] In 2008, the clinical guidelines were updated, and many more patients are now counseled on the importance of smoking cessation. Telephone quit lines are now available in every state, and more patients are referred to smoking cessation counseling services. Additionally, more patients have access to FDA-approved medications for smoking cessation through private insurance or Medicaid compared to a decade ago.[28]

Despite this encouraging news, cigarette smoking continues to be the leading cause of preventable morbidity and mortality in the United States. When the CDC analyzed the data from the 2008 National Health Interview Survey (NHIS) it was found that the number of current smokers from the years 1998 to 2008 did decrease by 3.5%, but the proportion of current smokers from 2007 to 2008 did not change.[29] All healthcare providers should screen patients and utilize the clinical guidelines for tobacco use and dependence once a smoker is identified.[28]

EPIDEMIOLOGY OF TOBACCO USE

The National Survey on Drug Use and Health reported in 2007 that an estimated 28.6% (70.9 million) of the U.S. population 12 years of age and older used a tobacco product at least once in the month prior to being interviewed. Each day, about 1,000 persons younger than 18 years of age become regular smokers, and it is now estimated 20% (43.8 million) of high school students currently smoke on a regular basis.[30] In addition, 60 million Americans were current cigarette smokers, 13.3 million smoked cigars, 8.1 million used smokeless tobacco, and 2 million smoked pipes.[30] Data trends from the 2008 NHIS showed smoking prevalence did vary based on the level of education one had completed. The highest percentage of adults who admitted to smoking were adults who had earned a General Education Development certificate (41.3%). Those with a graduate level of education reported the lowest percentage of smoking (5.7%).[29]

The NHIS survey also found that 31.5% of adults currently living under the federal poverty level were current smokers in comparison with the 19.6% of smokers living above the federal poverty level.[29]

ECONOMIC IMPACT OF SMOKING

The direct healthcare expenditures associated with smoking total more than $96 billion per year, and the costs associated with lost productivity are estimated to be $97 billion. Smoking-attributable medical expenditures[31] in the adult Medicaid population total $22 billion, which is estimated as 11% of Medicaid program expenditures.[32] It has been calculated that if all Medicaid patients stopped smoking, the annual savings would reach $9.7 billion after 5 years.[28]

HEALTH RISKS OF SMOKING

Cigarette smoking substantially increases the risk of (1) cardiovascular diseases such as stroke, sudden death, and heart attack; (2) nonmalignant respiratory diseases including emphysema, asthma, chronic bronchitis, and chronic obstructive pulmonary disease; (3) lung cancer; and (4) other cancers.[33]

Exposure to environmental tobacco smoke (*passive exposure*) has been cited as the cause of 3,400 lung cancer deaths and 46,000 heart disease-related deaths in the United States every year.[34] Children who are exposed to environmental smoke have a higher risk of respiratory infection, asthma, and middle ear infections than those who are not exposed. Sudden infant death syndrome occurs more often in infants whose mothers smoked during pregnancy than in offspring of nonsmoking mothers.[34] The harmful effects of smoking on reproduction and pregnancy include reduced fertility and fetal growth, as well as increased risk of ectopic pregnancy and spontaneous abortion.[34]

PHARMACOLOGY OF NICOTINE

Nicotine is a ganglionic cholinergic agonist with pharmacologic effects that are highly dependent on dose. These effects include central and peripheral nervous system stimulation and depression, respiratory stimulation, skeletal muscle relaxation, catecholamine release by the adrenal medulla, peripheral vasoconstriction, and increased blood pressure, heart rate, cardiac output, and oxygen consumption. Cigarette smoking or low doses of nicotine produce an increased alertness and increased cognitive functioning by stimulating the cerebral cortex. At higher doses, nicotine stimulates the "reward" center in the limbic system of the brain.[35]

When nicotine is ingested a feeling of pleasure and relaxation can occur. Repetitive exposure to nicotine leads to neuroadaptation which builds tolerance to the initial effects. An accumulation of nicotine in the body leads to a more substantial withdrawal reaction if cessation is attempted.[36] Common symptoms experienced during withdrawal can include anxiety, difficulties concentrating, irritability, and strong cravings for tobacco. Onset of these withdrawal symptoms usually occurs within 24 hours and can last for days, weeks, or longer.[36]

CLINICAL PRESENTATION OF NICOTINE WITHDRAWAL

General

☐ The patient may experience anxiety but may not be in acute distress. Symptoms can wax and wane over time.

Symptoms

☐ The patient may complain of cravings, difficulty concentrating, frustration, irritability, and impatience. Hostility, insomnia, and restlessness can also occur.

Signs

☐ Increased skin temperature can be present.

TREATMENT

Nicotine Dependence

■ AGENCY FOR HEALTHCARE RESEARCH AND QUALITY CLINICAL PRACTICE GUIDELINE: TREATING TOBACCO USE AND DEPENDENCE

The Agency for Healthcare Research and Quality (AHRQ) periodically convenes expert panels to develop clinical guidelines for healthcare practitioners. Because of the widespread prevalence of smoking-related illnesses, its related morbidity and mortality, and the economic burden imposed, the agency convened a panel of experts in 1994 to develop guidelines on the treatment of tobacco addiction. The resultant guideline for smoking cessation was released in 1996. In May 2008, an updated version of the 1996 Smoking Cessation Clinical Practice Guideline was issued by AHRQ.[28]

The revised guideline suggests strategies for providing appropriate treatments for every patient. The panel reminds us that effective treatments for tobacco dependence now exist and that every patient should receive at least minimal treatment every time he or she visits a clinician (Figs. 75–1 and 75–2).

The guideline identified a number of key findings that clinicians should use:

1. Tobacco dependence is a chronic condition that often requires repeated intervention. However, effective treatments exist that can produce long-term or permanent abstinence.

2. Because effective tobacco dependence treatments are available, every patient who uses tobacco should be offered at least one of these treatments:
   • Patients willing to try to quit tobacco use should be provided with treatments that are identified as effective in the guideline.
   • Patients unwilling to try to quit tobacco use should be provided with a brief intervention that is designed to increase their motivation to quit.

3. It is essential that clinicians and healthcare delivery systems (including administrators, insurers, and purchasers) institutionalize the consistent identification, documentation, and treatment of every tobacco user who is seen in a healthcare setting.

4. Brief tobacco dependence treatment is effective, and every patient who uses tobacco should be offered at least brief treatment.

5. There is a strong dose-response relationship between the intensity of tobacco dependence counseling and its effectiveness. Treatments involving person-to-person contact (via individual, group, or proactive telephone counseling) are consistently effective, and their effectiveness increases with treatment intensity (e.g., minutes of contact).

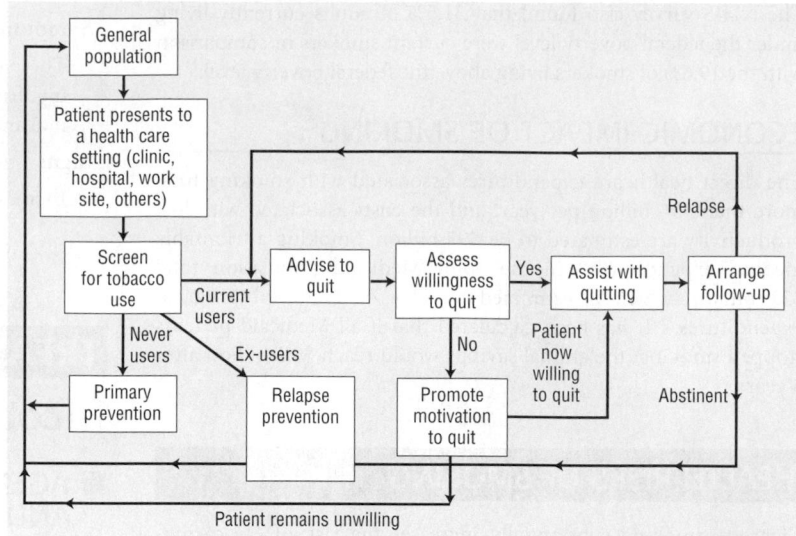

FIGURE 75-1. Model for treatment of tobacco use and dependence.

6. Three types of counseling and behavioral therapies were found to be especially effective and should be used with all patients who are attempting tobacco cessation:

- Provision of practical counseling (problem-solving/skills training)
- Provision of social support as part of treatment (intratreatment social support)
- Help in securing social support outside treatment (extratreatment social support)

❼ Numerous effective pharmacotherapy options for smoking cessation now exist (Table 75–5). Seven first-line pharmacotherapy options reliably increase long-term smoking abstinence rates: sustained-release (SR) bupropion, nicotine gum, nicotine inhaler, nicotine lozenge, nicotine nasal spray, nicotine patch, and varenicline. Combinations of these should be considered if a single agent has failed.

Two second-line pharmacotherapy options are considered efficacious and can be considered by clinicians if first-line options are not effective: clonidine and nortriptyline.

Tobacco-dependence treatments are both clinically effective and cost-effective relative to other medical and disease prevention interventions. As such, insurers and purchasers should ensure all insurance plans include as a reimbursed benefit the counseling and pharmacotherapeutic treatments that are identified as effective in this guideline, as well as clinician reimbursement for providing tobacco dependence treatment just as they are reimbursed for treating other chronic conditions.

■ OTHER FACTORS IMPORTANT TO THE SUCCESS OF A SMOKING-CESSATION STRATEGY

The AHRQ expert panel emphasized the importance of the type and intensity of the contact with the counselor to the success of the intervention. When interventions last for more than 10 minutes, the increase in cessation rates is much better than when interventions do not involve contact with a professional. Group and individual counseling is more effective than no intervention in increasing abstinence rates. Self-help materials (e.g., handouts, pamphlets, and brochures) without any direct physical contact are not effective.[37] Interventions are more successful when they include social support and training in general problem-solving skills, stress management, and relapse prevention. The number of treatment sessions offered is also important. Providing at least four or more sessions, longer than 10 minutes in length, and if possible providing treatments from multiple types of clinicians have proven higher success rates compared to less intensive interventions.[28] Although comprehensive behavioral interventions have been shown to be more effective in helping people quit smoking and remain abstinent, less intensive treatments are beneficial as well. Even minimal contacts lasting less than 3 minutes and simple advice to quit are more successful in increasing cessation rates than intervention involving no contact.[28]

❽ Counseling alone can be effective, but counseling efficacy is further augmented by the addition of pharmacotherapy. In a meta-analysis which included 111 trials with more than 43,000 participants using one or more of the five forms of nicotine replacement therapy (NRT) including nicotine gum, nasal spray, patches,

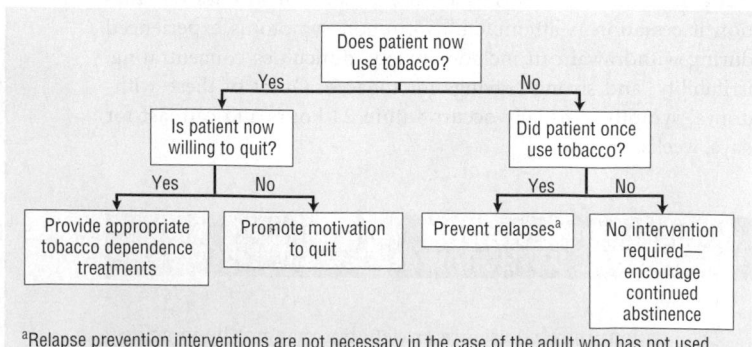

aRelapse prevention interventions are not necessary in the case of the adult who has not used tobacco for many years.

FIGURE 75-2. Algorithm for treating tobacco use.

lozenges, or inhaler, it was found the use of NRT led to a significant rate of cessation compared to the cessation rates with placebo.[38]

Although comprehensive programs are most effective, few smokers (10%–15%) seek formal assistance in quitting.[28]

■ PHARMACOLOGIC THERAPY FOR SMOKING CESSATION

All patients attempting to quit should be encouraged to use effective pharmacotherapy agents for smoking cessation except in the presence of special circumstances. Long-term smoking-cessation pharmacotherapy should be considered as a strategy to reduce the likelihood of relapse. As with other chronic diseases, the most effective treatment of tobacco dependence encompasses multiple modalities. Pharmacotherapy is a vital element of a multicomponent smoking cessation program that should also always include nonpharmacologic components. The clinician should encourage all patients initiating a quit attempt to use one or a combination of efficacious pharmacotherapy agents, although pharmacotherapy use requires special consideration with some patient groups (e.g., those with medical contraindications, those smoking fewer than 10 cigarettes a day, pregnant or breast-feeding women, and adolescent smokers). The role of pharmacotherapy in smoking cessation is summarized in Table 75–5.

■ NICOTINE-REPLACEMENT THERAPY

A Systematic Review of Nicotine Replacement Therapy

In 2009, a systematic review[38] of published studies was performed to determine the effectiveness of the different forms of NRT (e.g., chewing gum, transdermal patches, nasal spray, inhalers, and tablets) in achieving abstinence from cigarettes or a sustained reduction in the amount smoked. The review was also designed to determine whether the effect is influenced by the clinical setting in which the smoker is recruited and treated, the dosage and form of the NRT used, or the intensity of additional advice and support offered to the smoker; to determine whether combinations of NRT are more effective than one type alone; and to determine its effectiveness compared to other pharmacotherapy agents.

The review was limited to randomized trials in which NRT was compared to placebo or no treatment, or where different doses of NRT were compared. The main outcome measure was abstinence from smoking after at least 6 months of follow-up. For each trial, researchers used the most rigorous definition of abstinence, and confirmation with biochemical markers where available. The review includes 132 studies, 111 of which included a placebo or non–nicotine control arm. All of the commercially available forms of NRT were effective for smoking cessation. Use of NRT doubled the odds of quitting. Higher doses of nicotine patch can produce additional small increases in quit rates compared to lower doses. Only one study directly compared NRT to another pharmacotherapy, in which bupropion was significantly more effective than nicotine patch or placebo.[38]

In late 2009, the first head-to-head placebo-controlled trial comparing five smoking cessation pharmacotherapies with 1,504 smokers who had smoked at least 10 cigarettes per day for 6 months and who were interested in achieving cessation was published. Patients were randomized to receive SR bupropion, nicotine patch, nicotine lozenge, nicotine patch plus nicotine lozenge, bupropion plus nicotine lozenge, or placebo. The patients were required to use the assigned NRT plus attend six 10 to 20 minute individual counseling sessions. Two of the counseling sessions were held prior to beginning NRT, the second on the actual quit date. The other counseling sessions were then scheduled on weeks 1, 2, 4, and 8 from the quit date. Abstinence was confirmed by using blood tests to determine

TABLE 75-5	Pharmacologic Agents Used for Smoking Cessation				
Drug	Place in Therapy	Dosage Range	Duration	Comments/Monitoring Parameters	LOE[d]
Buproprion SR[a,b]	First-line	Titrate up to 150 mg orally twice daily.	3 to 6 months	Patients receiving both bupropion and a nicotine patch should be monitored for hypertension.	A1
Clonidine[b,c]	Second-line	Titrate to response; 0.2 to 0.75 mg per day	6 to 12 months	Monitor baseline electrolyte and lipid profiles, renal function, uric acid, complete blood count, and blood pressure	B2
Nicotine polacrilex (gum)[a]	First-line	Initial dose depends on smoking history: 2 to 4 mg every 1 to 8 hours	12 weeks (taper down over time)	Heart rate and blood pressure should be monitored periodically during nicotine replacement therapy.	A1
Nicotine inhaler[a]	First-line	24 to 64 mg per day (total daily dose)	3 to 6 months (taper down over time)	Heart rate and blood pressure should be monitored periodically during nicotine replacement therapy.	A1
Nicotine nasal spray[a]	First-line	8 to 40 mg per day (total daily dose)	14 weeks (taper down over time)	Heart rate and blood pressure should be monitored periodically during nicotine replacement therapy.	A1
Nicotine patch[a]	First-line	Initial dose depends on smoking history: 7 to 21 mg topically once daily	6 weeks (taper down over time)	Heart rate and blood pressure should be monitored periodically during nicotine replacement therapy.	A1
Nortriptyline[b,c]	Second-line	Titrate up to 75 to 100 mg orally daily	6 to 12 months	Dry mouth, blurred vision, and constipation are dose-dependent adverse effects.	B2
Varenicline[b]	First-line	Titrate up to 1 mg orally twice daily	3 to 6 months	Monitor renal function, especially in elderly patients. Nausea, headache, insomnia are dose-dependent adverse effects.	A1

LOE, level of evidence.

[a]Nicotine replacement therapies can be combined with each other and/or bupropion to increase long-term abstinence rates.

[b]Do not abruptly discontinue. Taper up initially, and taper off once therapy is complete.

[c]Clonidine and nortriptyline are not FDA-approved for smoking cessation.

[d]Strength of recommendations, evidence to support recommendation: A, good; B, moderate; C, poor.

Quality of evidence: 1, evidence from more than 1 properly randomized, controlled trial; 2, evidence from more than 1 well-designed clinical trial with randomization, from cohort or case-controlled analytic studies or multiple time series; or dramatic results from uncontrolled experiments; 3, evidence from opinions of respected authorities, based on clinical experience, descriptive studies, or reports of expert communities.

Data from U.S. Department of Health and Human Services.[28,34]

carbon monoxide. At 6 months it was found the quit rates were 40.1% for the nicotine patch plus nicotine lozenge, 34.4% for the nicotine patch, 33.5% for the nicotine lozenge, 33.2% for bupropion plus nicotine lozenge, 31.8% for bupropion alone, and 22.2% for placebo. It was postulated that the nicotine patch provided a stable blood level of nicotine in the blood to aid with withdrawal but the addition of the nicotine lozenge allowed for coverage during intense craving periods to decrease the chances of relapse.[39]

The AHRQ guidelines recommend use of NRT in the forms of transdermal nicotine patches, nicotine gum, nicotine sprays, nicotine inhalers, and nicotine lozenges.[28] Although cardiovascular disease is not an independent risk factor for acute myocardial events in patients taking NRT, NRT should be used with caution among particular cardiovascular patient groups: those in the immediate (within 2 weeks) post–myocardial infarction period, those with serious arrhythmias, and those with serious or worsening angina pectoris.[28]

Nicotine Gum

Clinicians should offer 4-mg rather than 2-mg nicotine gum to highly dependent smokers.[28] The 2-mg gum is recommended for patients smoking fewer than 25 cigarettes per day, whereas the 4-mg gum is recommended for patients smoking 25 or more cigarettes per day. Generally, the gum should be used for up to 12 weeks, no more than 24 pieces chewed per day. The dosage and duration of therapy should be tailored to meet the needs of each patient.

Nicotine gum currently is available exclusively as an over-the-counter medication and is packaged with important instructions on correct use, including chewing instructions. There is currently little evidence to suggest that combined use of the patch and gum increases abstinence beyond 24 weeks.

Gum should be chewed slowly until a peppery or minty taste emerges and then "parked" between cheek and gums to facilitate nicotine absorption through the oral mucosa. It should be chewed slowly and intermittently and parked for about 30 minutes or until the taste dissipates. Acidic beverages (e.g., coffee, juices, or soft drinks) interfere with the buccal absorption of nicotine, so eating and drinking anything except water should be avoided for 15 minutes before and during chewing. Patients often do not use enough gum to get the maximum benefit: they chew too few pieces per day, and they might not use the gum for a sufficient number of weeks. Instructions to chew the gum on a fixed schedule (at least one piece every 1–2 hours) for at least 1 to 3 months can be more beneficial than ad libitum use.

Nicotine Patch

9 The nicotine patch is available both as an over-the-counter medication and as a prescription drug and it approximately doubles long-term abstinence rates over those produced by placebo interventions.[38] Treatment of 8 weeks or less has been shown to be as efficacious as longer treatment periods. The 16- and 24-hour patches are of comparable efficacy.[33] Clinicians should consider starting treatment on a lower patch dose in patients smoking 10 or fewer cigarettes per day.[28]

A patch should be applied as soon as the patient wakes on the quit day and at the start of each day thereafter. The patient should place a new patch on a relatively hairless location, typically between the neck and waist. There are no restrictions on activity while using the patch. Patients who experience sleep disruption should remove the 24-hour patch prior to bedtime or use the 16-hour patch.

Nicotine Nasal Spray

Nicotine nasal spray more than doubles long-term abstinence rates when compared with a placebo spray. Nicotine nasal spray is available exclusively as a prescription medication. A dose of nicotine nasal spray consists of one 0.5-mg delivery to each nostril (1 mg total). Initial dosing should be one to two doses per hour, increasing as needed for symptom relief. The minimum recommended treatment is 8 doses per day, with a maximum limit of 40 doses per day (5 doses per hour). Each bottle contains approximately 100 doses. Recommended duration of therapy is 3 to 6 months. Patients should not sniff, swallow, or inhale through the nose while administering doses because this increases irritating effects.

Nicotine Lozenge

The nicotine lozenge is available as a 2-mg and a 4-mg dose. The 2-mg lozenge is recommended for patients who normally smoke their first cigarette later than 30 minutes after awakening, and the 4-mg lozenge is recommended for smokers who smoke within 30 minutes of waking. It is recommended that patients use at least nine lozenges daily the first 6 weeks of therapy. The duration of treatment is 12 weeks. It is recommended no more than 20 lozenges should be used in 1 day.[28] In comparison to the nicotine gum, nicotine release is more controlled and does not depend on the correct "chew and park" method required by the gum. The most common side effect of the lozenge is nausea. As with the nicotine gum, acidic beverages (e.g., coffee, juices, or soft drinks) interfere with the buccal absorption of nicotine, so eating and drinking anything except water should be avoided for 15 minutes before and during use of the lozenge.[28]

Instructing Patients in the Use of NRT

Compliance with NRT improves when the patient is presented a clear rationale for its use and a realistic expectation about the response. It should be explained to the patient that nicotine is responsible for addiction and that discontinuation of the nicotine causes craving for cigarettes, tension, irritability, sadness, problems with sleep, and difficulty concentrating. These are partly due to nicotine withdrawal. The patient should be told that using the patch results in less desire to smoke and provides an opportunity for a new nonsmoker to practice all the new nonsmoking skills without being burdened by craving. The patient should understand that with smoking, there are naturally peaks and valleys in the amount of nicotine in the bloodstream. With the patch there is a steady gradual rise in the blood nicotine concentration that levels off and remains constant for much of the day and then gradually decreases while the person is asleep. Maintaining an adequate blood level of nicotine lessens withdrawal symptoms.

A similar rationale can be used if patients are using gum. It should be emphasized that NRT is not a "magic bullet" and that the use of coping skills is essential for abstinence. The patch or the gum only buys time by reducing withdrawal symptoms and giving individuals a chance to figure out alternatives that they can use in place of smoking.[28]

CLINICAL CONTROVERSY

Some clinicians are hesitant to prescribe nicotine replacement therapy for smoking cessation during pregnancy because the safety and efficacy of nicotine replacement therapy has not been established in controlled clinical trials in this population. This logic is somewhat counterintuitive in that continued smoking exposes the unborn child to much higher levels of nicotine, and the harmful consequences of cigarette smoking during pregnancy are well documented.

Side Effects

Nicotine replacement products have relatively few side effects. Nausea and light-headedness are possible symptoms of nicotine overdose that warrant a reduction of the nicotine dose.

The most frequent side effect with the nicotine patch is skin irritation related to the adhesive or the medium containing nicotine and not to the nicotine itself. Approximately 50% of patients report skin irritation during the course of treatment with the patch. The patch site can be rotated to diminish this problem. The use of over-the-counter hydrocortisone cream (1%) or triamcinolone cream (0.5%) is recommended as a local treatment for patch-related skin irritations. Switching to a different brand of patch also can alleviate the problem because different products use different adhesives or media. The gum can be used instead of the patch when the skin irritation is severe. Less than 5% of patients were forced to discontinue therapy because of skin reactions.

Approximately 23% of patients using the patch report sleep disturbances, but the insomnia is hard to differentiate from the sleeplessness that often accompanies withdrawal itself, especially during the first few weeks of quitting.

Duration

Those who commit to quitting smoking using nicotine replacement should be told that treatment for up to three months is common.[40] However, some patients will experience severe withdrawal even beyond this time period so long term use of NRT might be indicated. Long term use of NRT has not been linked to any safety concerns and is supported by the 2008 updated U.S. Public Health Service Guidelines.[28]

Economic and Pharmacoeconomic Considerations

Most health insurers provide coverage for the chronic illnesses caused by smoking (e.g., chronic obstructive pulmonary disease, cancer, and myocardial infarction), yet few provide coverage for treating the nicotine addiction that caused those ailments.[28] The U.S. Public Health Service's Clinical Practice Guideline on Treating Tobacco Use and Dependence Update 2008 strongly encourages a comprehensive treatment plan for smoking cessation which includes both use of the recommended pharmacotherapy agents and extensive counseling. It has been shown if a comprehensive smoking cessation program is a paid or covered health benefit within the insurance plan an increased success rate for cessation is seen.[28] In 2006 it was estimated that 35% of Medicaid recipients smoked cigarettes but the current coverage of smoking cessation pharmacotherapy agents as well as counseling sessions are still very limited, and availability is inconsistent with the current federal clinical guidelines.[41] Accounting for direct healthcare expenditures and productivity losses (approximately $97 billion per year), the total economic burden of smoking is approximately $193 billion per year.[31] The CDC reports $203.9 billion was available to states from the years 2000 to 2009 from tobacco taxes and legal settlements. An investment of only 15% of these funds the states received on an annual basis would have funded every state tobacco control program. Unfortunately, it has been reported that states spent less than 3% on any tobacco prevention and cessation programs.[29] Expanding coverage of not only the pharmacotherapy agents available for smoking cessation but the reimbursement for counseling as recommended by the updated guidelines by the health insurers and by Medicaid programs is imperative to improve smoking abstinence rates.

■ NON-NICOTINE OPTIONS

Bupropion

🔟 Bupropion inhibits neuronal reuptake and potentiates the effects of norepinephrine and dopamine. Although its precise mechanism in smoking cessation is not well understood, dopamine has been associated with the rewarding effects of addictive substances. Withdrawal symptoms can be decreased by virtue of bupropion inhibition of norepinephrine uptake. The AHRQ panel concluded that SR bupropion is an efficacious smoking cessation treatment that patients should be encouraged to use.[28] Contraindications for bupropion use include current or past seizure disorders, a history of monoamine oxidase inhibitor use over the last 14 days, and a history of anorexia nervosa or bulimia. Along with multiple other precautions listed in the product labeling, current alcohol use, use of medications which lower seizure threshold (e.g., antidepressants, antipsychotics), and depression are possible concerns when using this medication.[28] In 2009, the FDA started requiring the manufacturers of Zyban (bupropion) and generic manufacturers to add new black box warnings and develop a medication guide highlighting the risk of serious neuropsychiatric symptoms in patients using this product. Possible symptoms include depressed mood, agitation, anxiety, hostility, changes in behavior, suicidal thoughts and behavior, and attempted suicide.[28]

A double-blind, placebo-controlled, randomized multicenter trial was conducted in which healthy smokers were randomized to receive either SR bupropion 150 mg twice daily or a placebo daily for 7 weeks and subsequently seen for counseling and follow-up for a total of 52 weeks. The primary end points were biochemically confirmed continuous abstinence at weeks 7 and 52. The authors specifically conducted this trial in the primary care setting to verify the general applicability of the results to the intended end users.[42] While similar studies have been performed in academic settings and have shown favorable results, the authors contend the real therapeutic potential or impact of a pharmacologic approach to smoking cessation must be evaluated by general practitioners in the primary care setting. They further assert that the approach should address healthy smokers and use continuous abstinence at week 52 as the most valid outcome measure. The results of this study showed bupropion was efficacious, with an absolute 25% of participants continuously abstinent at 1 year; it doubled the odds of continuous abstinence from week 4 to week 7 and from week 4 to week 52 compared with placebo.

A recent meta-analysis was conducted by the Cochrane Collaboration involving 49 trials utilizing bupropion for smoking cessation. Bupropion was shown to significantly increase the incidence of long-term cessation when used as a sole agent in 36 separate trials. Other trials which used bupropion as an add-on agent with NRT did not show additional benefit for improving cessation rates. The incidence of seizures was fairly low when considering 8,000 people were exposed to bupropion in these multiple studies and the rate of seizures was still less than the 1:10,000 estimated risk listed in the product safety information.[43]

🔟 For smoking cessation, the manufacturer recommends a dosage of 150 mg once daily for 3 days and then twice daily for 7 to 12 weeks or longer, with or without NRT. Patients are instructed to stop smoking during the second week of treatment and are encouraged to use counseling and support services along with the medication. For maintenance therapy, consider SR bupropion 150 mg twice daily for up to 6 months.[28]

Varenicline (Chantix)

⓫ Varenicline, a new and novel aid to smoking cessation, was approved by the FDA in 2006. It acts at sites in the nicotine-affected brain in two ways: by providing nicotine effects to ease withdrawal symptoms and by blocking the effects of nicotine from cigarettes if they resume smoking. Specifically, varenicline is a partial agonist that binds selectively to α_4-β_2-nicotinic acetylcholine receptors with a greater affinity than nicotine. When bound to the receptor, the drug blocks nicotine from binding and also evokes a response but to a lesser degree than nicotine. The stimulation of the receptor results in release of dopamine and thus provides a type of "reward" that can decrease craving and withdrawal symptoms.[44]

The recommended dosage for varenicline is 0.5 mg daily for 3 days, increase to 0.5 mg twice daily for 3 days, and then increase to 1 mg twice daily for a standard 12-week treatment. If abstinence has not been achieved after the 12-week treatment, then a second 12-week treatment may be prescribed.[44]

Varenicline is listed as a first-line agent in the updated clinical guidelines on treating tobacco use and dependence. Seven trials comparing varenicline with placebo, three of which also had a comparison with bupropion, were reviewed in a recent Cochrane Review meta-analysis. Varenicline caused a two- to three-fold increased likelihood of long-term smoking cessation compared with placebo. It was also found that varenicline's rate of cessation was greater than that of bupropion.[45]

Since 2006, when varenicline was approved by the FDA, alarming numbers of adverse effects including suicidal thoughts, erratic behavior, and aggressive behavior have been reported. The large number of reports led to the release of a Public Health Advisory by the FDA in February 2008.[46] The advisory stressed the importance of screening for any type of psychiatric illness or any behavior changes after starting varenicline. A boxed warning along with an update of the medication guide from the manufacturer was required by the FDA.[46] Specific warnings stress that patients should report any history of psychiatric illness and any changes in behavior or mood immediately to their prescribing practitioner. Impairment of the ability to drive or operate heavy machinery and the possibility of strange or vivid dreams are also stressed in the medication guide.[46]

■ SECOND-LINE MEDICATIONS

Second-line medications are pharmacotherapies for which there is evidence of efficacy for treating tobacco dependence, but which have a more limited role than first-line medications because (1) the FDA has not approved them for a tobacco-dependence treatment indication, and (2) there are more concerns about potential side effects than exist with first-line medications.[28] Second-line treatments should be considered for use on a case-by-case basis after first-line treatments have been used or considered.

Clonidine

Clonidine has been found to be efficacious as a smoking cessation treatment, although its only labeled indication is for treatment for hypertension. It can be used off-label as a second-line agent to treat tobacco dependence. A recent meta-analysis of six trials showed that clonidine increased smoking cessation rates by 11% (odds ratio [OR], 1.89; confidence interval [CI], 1.30–2.14). There was a high incidence of dose-dependent side effects, particularly dry mouth and sedation.[47] It should be noted that abrupt discontinuation of clonidine can result in symptoms such as nervousness, agitation, headache, and tremor, accompanied or followed by a rapid rise in blood pressure and elevated catecholamine levels.

Doses used in various clinical cessation trials have varied significantly, from 0.15 to 0.75 mg/day orally to 0.1 to 0.2 mg/day transdermally, without a clear dose-response relation to cessation. Initial dosing typically is 0.1 mg orally twice daily or 0.1 mg/day transdermally, increasing by 0.1 mg/day each week if needed. The duration also varied across the clinical trials, ranging from 3 weeks to 12 months. Most commonly reported side effects include dry mouth, drowsiness, dizziness, sedation, and constipation. Clonidine will lower blood pressure in most patients, thus blood pressure should be monitored.[28]

Nortriptyline

Nortriptyline is also considered to be efficacious as a second-line agent to treat tobacco dependence. It should be considered for smoking cessation under a clinician's direction in patients unable to use first-line medications because of contraindications and in patients who failed using first-line medications. Therapy is initiated 10 to 28 days before the quit date to allow nortriptyline to reach steady state at the target dose. Smoking cessation trials have initiated treatment at a dose of 25 mg/day, increasing gradually to a target dose of 75 to 100 mg/day. Duration of treatment used in smoking cessation trials has been approximately 12 weeks. Most commonly reported side effects include sedation, dry mouth, blurred vision, urinary retention, light-headedness, and tremor.[28]

Future Treatments

Work continues on the development of vaccines to be used in treating nicotine addiction. NicVAX (an experimental nicotine conjugate vaccine) is designed to cause the immune system to produce antibodies that bind to nicotine and prevent it from entering the brain. As a result, the positive stimulus in the brain that is normally caused by nicotine is no longer present, thereby taking away the physical motivation for smoking, consequently helping people to quit.[48,49]

Results from the phase II clinical studies on 301 patients who were smoking an average of 24 cigarettes a day showed the vaccine "induced the production of a long lasting antibody which helped in the prevention of a smoking relapse for up to 2 months in approximately 25% of the study participants."[50]

CLINICAL PRESENTATION OF EXCESSIVE CAFFEINE INTAKE

General

☐ The patient may not be in acute distress.

Symptoms

☐ The patient may complain of nausea, vomiting, diarrhea, and psychomotor agitation, and can appear restless, nervous, and excited.

Signs

☐ The patient can present with facial flushing, diuresis, and muscle twitching.

☐ Tachycardia or cardiac arrhythmias can also occur

Laboratory Tests

☐ Caffeine serum concentrations are rarely used clinically.

CAFFEINE

Caffeine is the most widely consumed behaviorally active substance in the world, generating an increased sense of well-being, happiness, energy, alertness, and sociability.[51] Caffeinism is the term coined to describe the clinical syndrome produced by acute or chronic overuse of caffeine. The syndrome usually is characterized by CNS and peripheral manifestations, most notably anxiety, psychomotor alterations, sleep disturbances, mood changes, and psychophysiologic complaints.[52]

As many as one in five adults consume doses of caffeine generally considered large enough to cause clinical symptoms.[51,52]

Pharmacologically, the risk of developing some meaningful clinical manifestations becomes high when intake exceeds 500 mg/day. This places 20% to 30% of North Americans at risk.[51] Caffeine has been proposed as a "model of drug abuse" despite the facts that its sale is largely unrestricted and that heavy consumption of caffeine-containing beverages is not considered to be drug abuse. An exhaustive review of caffeine dependence focused on the potential for abuse of caffeine and the nature of tolerance and withdrawal.[51] The information below represents a broad overview of these topics, and the reader interested in more detail is urged to consult the review by Juliano and Griffiths.[51]

EPIDEMIOLOGY OF CAFFEINE USE AND ABUSE

Caffeine is used by 80% of the population of the United States. In 1999 there were 108,000,000 coffee consumers in the United States spending approximately $9.2 billion in the retail sector and $8.7 billion in the food service sector every year.[53] The National Coffee Association found in 2001 that 52% of the adult population of the United States drinks coffee daily.[54] Newer market research data are available but are a closely protected proprietary secret. It is safe to say that in the 10 years since these data were freely available, coffee consumption has likely increased.

The majority of caffeine users progress to a pattern of frequent or daily consumption. Approximately one-fourth eventually begin consuming large quantities, exceeding 500 mg/day, and conservatively, 10% of all adults then progress to develop the syndrome of caffeinism. Mean daily consumption of caffeine in American children is surprisingly high. The Framingham Children's Study[57] investigated the amounts of caffeine consumed each day by children between the ages of 6 and 10 years (mean, 8.4 years for boys and 8.1 years for girls). Mean intake of caffeine was 16 ± 9.6 mg/day. Caffeinated soft drinks and chocolate furnished almost all of the caffeine.[55]

ENERGY DRINKS

In recent years a number of energy drinks containing caffeine, taurine, vitamins, and usually sugar have found their way onto the American market. Sold under brand names such as Red Bull, Monster Energy, Rockstar, and Full Throttle, these products are especially popular with adolescents and emerging adults, with sales exceeding half a million dollars in 2006.[56] This represents a more than 50% increase over 2005.[56] These products are generally marketed to enhance alertness or providing a short-term energy boost and do not constitute suitable sources of rehydration or restoration of electrolytes in association with athletic activity.[56]

Additionally, several manufacturers have marketed alcoholic beverages that have caffeine as an additional ingredient. Some may have other stimulant ingredients such as guarana, taurine, and ginseng. The Center for Science in the Public Interest has chosen to call these beverages "alcospeed."[57]

DIFFERENTIAL DIAGNOSIS

Caffeine intoxication is the only official diagnosis associated with caffeinism in the *Diagnostic and Statistical Manual of Mental Disorders, Fourth Edition, Text Revision (DSM-IV-TR)*.[9] Caffeine-induced anxiety can manifest as restlessness, nervousness, excitement, insomnia, diuresis, flushing, GI disturbance, muscle twitching, irritability, and jitteriness. If caffeine-induced insomnia requires specific treatment, caffeine-induced sleep disorder is an appropriate *DSM-IV-TR* diagnosis.[9]

Because excessive caffeine consumption is so widespread, a thorough history of caffeine use should be included in the routine assessment of all new patients in primary care medical settings. In this manner, the practitioner can use the information gathered to uncover high levels of caffeine intake and then use the information to pinpoint the cause of clinical signs and symptoms typical of caffeinism. Clinical manifestations of caffeinism almost always will lessen in intensity or disappear completely within 1 to 2 weeks after removing the drug.

PHARMACOLOGY OF CAFFEINE

Caffeine is rapidly and completely absorbed from the GI tract, reaching a peak blood level within 30 to 45 minutes of oral ingestion. It easily crosses the blood–brain barrier, and levels achieved in the brain are proportional to the dose administered.

The half-life of caffeine in humans is approximately 3.5 to 5 hours. Serious problems rarely result from overdoses of caffeine. In fact, the amount of caffeine needed to cause death in an average adult male is 5 to 10 g, the equivalent of 50 to 100 cups of regular brewed coffee. Thus the risk of overdose from dietary sources of caffeine is virtually nonexistent.

Caffeine increases the heart rate and force of contraction. It also has a strong diuretic effect. The key factor promoting caffeine use and dosage increases can be the drug's reinforcing effect on pleasure and reward centers of the brain. Caffeine's pharmacologic actions appear comparable (although less potent) in some aspects with those of other stimulants, such as amphetamines and cocaine.

CAFFEINE DEPENDENCE

Research has shown that abstinence from caffeine induces a distinct withdrawal syndrome. Evidence for the existence of a caffeine dependence syndrome was presented by Strain and associates.[58] In a structured psychiatric interview, subjects self-identified as having problems with caffeine use were evaluated for features of a *DSM-IV-TR* diagnosis of drug dependence. Those judged as caffeine dependent manifested at least three of four criteria (i.e., tolerance, withdrawal, persistent desire, or an unsuccessful attempt to reduce consumption and persistent use despite adverse psychologic or physical consequences). Of 99 people screened, 27 were evaluated by means of a structured psychiatric interview modified for the diagnosis of caffeine dependence; 16 of those subjects (59%) met the criteria. In a second phase of the study, 11 of the 16 caffeine-dependent individuals participated in a 2-day double-blind crossover study of caffeine deprivation. Nine showed evidence of caffeine withdrawal during the placebo phase, a finding that validated one of the criteria for the diagnosis of dependence.

CAFFEINE WITHDRAWAL

⓬ The frequency of the caffeine withdrawal syndrome is not well known, but it may be common. Withdrawal can occur when individuals who previously have been consuming caffeine on a regular basis suddenly discontinue its intake.[59] The syndrome can be characterized by the occurrence of headache, drowsiness, fatigue, and sometimes impaired psychomotor performance, difficulty concentrating, nausea, excessive yawning, and craving. These symptoms usually appear within 18 to 24 hours of discontinuation of intake, corresponding to the time required for the drug to leave the body.

The caffeine withdrawal headache is somewhat unique, starting with a sense of fullness in the head and progressing to throbbing and diffuse pain that is made worse by movement. The maximum intensity of the pain occurs 3 to 6 hours after beginning.

When caffeine is reintroduced, relief of withdrawal symptoms tends to occur within 30 to 60 minutes. At present, this appears to be the most effective "treatment" for the caffeine-withdrawal syndrome.

EFFECT ON SLEEP

Caffeine interferes with sleep in most nontolerant individuals.[51,52] Once tolerance has developed, people are much less likely to self-report sleep abnormalities, or they may sense that the insomnia has disappeared altogether. To illustrate, 53% of those consuming less than 250 mg/day agreed that caffeine before bedtime would prevent sleep, compared with 43% of those consuming 250 to 749 mg/day, and only 22% of those taking 750 mg/day or more. Even though the higher-level consumers denied that caffeine interferes with their sleep, studies done in the sleep laboratory confirm that caffeine consumers do have greater sleep latency, more frequent awakenings, and altered sleep architecture, and that these effects are dose related.

CAFFEINE DURING PREGNANCY

Over the years there has been much discussion on whether or not caffeine intake during pregnancy is harmful to the developing fetus. Results of research have been mixed, but in general, caffeine has not been shown to be a potent and consistent teratogen. Kuczkowski[60] recently published a review article highlighting the implications of caffeine intake in pregnancy, reviewing the latest evidence-based information available on this subject, and offering recommendations for practitioners providing peripartum care to expectant mothers who consume caffeine.

Based on the data reviewed, the author concluded that for the healthy pregnant adult, moderate daily caffeine intake at a dose level up to 400 mg/day (equivalent to 6 mg/kg body weight per day in a 65-kg [143 lb] person) is not associated with adverse effects such as general toxicity, cardiovascular effects, effects on bone status and calcium balance, changes in adult behavior, increased incidence of cancer, or effects on fertility. The study did not identify any significant positive associations between maternal caffeine consumption and cardiovascular malformations.

The March of Dimes advises women to limit their caffeine intake to less than 200 mg per day. This recommendation was prompted by the results of a study published in March 2008[61] reporting that pregnant women who consumed 200 mg or more of caffeine a day had double the risk of miscarriage compared with those who had no caffeine. Criticism of this study was swift to follow, and its conclusions have been called into question.

CAFFEINE AND HEADACHES

A recent Norwegian study[62] investigated the association between caffeine consumption and headache type and frequency in the general adult population. The results were based on cross-sectional data from 50,483 (55%) out of 92,566 invited participants aged greater than or equal to 20 years. A weak but significant association (OR, 1.16; 95% CI, 1.09–1.23) was found between high caffeine consumption and prevalence of infrequent headache. In contrast, headache greater than 14 days/month was less likely among individuals with high caffeine consumption compared to those with low caffeine consumption. The authors speculate that their results may indicate that high caffeine consumption changes chronic headache into infrequent headache due to the analgesic properties of caffeine. Alternatively, chronic headache sufferers tend to avoid intake of caffeine to not aggravate their headaches, whereas individuals with infrequent headache are less aware that high caffeine use can be a cause.

TREATMENT

Caffeinism

Caffeinism is treated by reducing or discontinuing the drug. It may be necessary to wean the patient off the drug gradually because going "cold turkey" can produce such serious symptoms that the drug must be restarted. Decaffeinated beverages can be substituted slowly for the caffeinated type. However, relapses are less likely to occur when the drug is discontinued all at once, probably because of the considerable self-discipline required to continue weaning the drug when one knows that an increase in dose will cause the symptoms to abate.

Patients with cardiovascular disease, especially arrhythmias, history of stroke or transient ischemic attacks should refrain totally. Patients with peptic ulcer disease, bipolar mood disorder, and schizophrenia should also be encouraged to avoid caffeine altogether.

The reader wishing more information about treatment of caffeine withdrawal should consult the systematic review by Juliano and Griffiths.[51] A review of research on coffee and its health effects has also been published and should be consulted for in-depth discussion of this issue.[63]

CONCLUSIONS

Use of alcohol, tobacco, and caffeine is so commonly accepted in our society that people take notice only when their use causes serious problems. When problems do occur, the human and economic costs are enormous. Healthcare professionals must be committed to helping people free themselves of the addictions that can occur with these common drugs.

ABBREVIATIONS

5-HT$_3$: serotonin-3

AHRQ: Agency for Healthcare Research and Quality

BAC: blood alcohol concentration

CNS: central nervous system

CT: computed tomography

DSM-IV-TR: *Diagnostic and Statistical Manual of Mental Disorders, Fourth Edition, Text Revision*

GABA: γ-aminobutyric acid

GI: gastrointestinal

NHIS: National Health Interview Survey

NMDA: *N*-methyl-D-aspartate

NRT: nicotine replacement therapy

NSDUH: National Survey on Drug Use and Health

SR: sustained release

REFERENCES

1. Centers for Disease Control and Prevention. State-specific smoking-attributable mortality and years of potential life lost—United States, 2000–2004. Morbidity and Mortality Weekly Report MMWR 2009;58(2):29–33.
2. Centers for Disease Control and Prevention. Health, United States, 2008. Hyattsville, MD: Centers for Disease Control and Prevention, National Center for Health Statistics, 2009.

3. Center for Disease Control and Prevention. The health consequences of smoking: A report from the surgeon general. Atlanta, GA: U.S. Department of Health and Human Services, CDC, 2004.

4. Substance Abuse and Mental Health Services Administration. Results from the 2008 National Survey on Drug Use and Health: National Findings (Office of Applied Studies, NSDUH Series H-36, HHS Publication No. SMA 09-4434). Rockville, MD; 2009. *http:// oas.samhsa.gov/nsduh/2k8nsduh/2k8Results.cfm#High.*

5. World Health Organization, Department of Mental Health and Substance Abuse. Geneva; 2004. Global Status Report on Alcohol 2004. *http://www.who.int/substance_abuse/publications/ global_status_report_ 2004_overview.pdf.*

6. Substance Abuse and Mental Health Services Administration, Office of Applied Studies. Drug Abuse Warning Network, 2006: National Estimates of Drug-Related Emergency Department Visits. DAWN Series D-30, DHHS Publication No. (SMA) 08-4339. Rockville, MD; 2008.

7. Alcohol-Related Disease Impact (ARDI) Dataset. National Center for Chronic Disease Prevention and Health Promotion, Alcohol and Public Health, Centers for Disease Control and Prevention. *https:// apps.nccd.cdc.gov/ardi/AboutARDIMethods.htm.*

8. Harwood, H. Updating Estimates of the Economic Costs of Alcohol Abuse in the United States: Estimates, Update Methods, and Data. Report prepared by The Lewin Group for the National Institute on Alcohol Abuse and Alcoholism; 2000. *http://pubs.niaaa.nih.gov/ publications/economic-2000/index.htm.*

9. Diagnostic and Statistical Manual of Mental Disorders, Fourth Edition, Text Revision. Washington DC: American Psychiatric Association, 2000:212–214.

10. Enoch MA. Genetic and environmental influences on the development of alcoholism – Resilience vs. risk. Ann N Y Acad Sci 2006;1094: 193–201.

11. Bierut LJ, Saccone NL, Rice JP, et al. Defining alcohol-related phenotypes in humans. The Collaborative Study on the Genetics of Alcoholism. Alcohol Res Health 2002;26:208–213.

12. Heath AC, Nelson EC, National Institute of Alcohol Abuse and Alcoholism. Effects of the interaction between genotype and environment. Research into the genetic epidemiology of alcohol dependence. Alcohol Res Health 2002;26:193–201.

13. Luo X, Kranzler HR, Zuo L, et al. Diplotype trend regression analysis of the ADH gene cluster and the ALDH2 gene: Multiple significant associations with alcohol dependence. Am J Hum Genet 2006;78:973–987.

14. Boothby LA, Doering PL. Health promotion and disease prevention. In: The Science and Practice of Pharmacotherapy. PSAP V, 2004. *http://www.accp.com/strp5b05.php.*

15. Krystal JH, Staley J, Mason G, et al. Gamma-aminobutyric acid type A receptors and alcoholism: Intoxication, dependence, vulnerability, and treatment. Arch Gen Psychiatry 2006;63:957–968.

16. Kugelberg FC, Jones AW. Interpreting results of ethanol analysis in postmortem specimens: a review of the literature. Forensic Sci Int 2007;165:10–29.

17. Samir Zakhari. Overview: How is alcohol metabolized by the body? Alcohol Res Health 2006; 29:245–254.

18. Norberg A, Jones AW, Hahn RG, Gabrielsson JL. Role of variability in explaining ethanol pharmacokinetics: Research and forensic applications. Clin Pharmacokinet 2003;42:1–31.

19. Dhalla S, Kopec JA. The CAGE questionnaire for alcohol misuse: a review of reliability and validity studies. Clin Invest Med 2007;30: 33–41.

20. Mayo-Smith MF. Pharmacological management of alcohol withdrawal. A meta-analysis and evidence-based practice guideline. American Society of Addiction Medicine Working Group on Pharmacological Management of Alcohol Withdrawal. JAMA 1997;278:144–151.

21. Mayo-Smith MF, Beecher LH, Fischer TL, et al. Working Group on the Management of Alcohol Withdrawal Delirium, Practice Guidelines Committee, American Society of Addiction Medicine. Management of alcohol withdrawal delirium. An evidence-based practice guideline [erratum Arch Intern Med 2004;164:2068]. Arch Intern Med 2004;164:1405–1412.

22. Ntais C, Pakos E, Kyzas P, Ioannidis JPA. Benzodiazepines for alcohol withdrawal. Cochrane Database Syst Rev 2005:CD005063.

23. Bråthen G, Ben-Menachem E, Brodtkorb E, et al. EFNS guideline on the diagnosis and management of alcohol-related seizures: report of an EFNS task force. EFNS Task Force on Diagnosis and Treatment of Alcohol-Related Seizures [erratum Eur J Neurol 2005;12:816.] Eur J Neurol 2005;12:575–581.

24. Rösner S, Leucht S, Lehert P, et al. Acamprosate supports abstinence, naltrexone prevents excessive drinking: evidence from a meta-analysis with unreported outcomes. J Psychopharmacol 2008;22:11–23.

25. Garbutt JC. The state of pharmacotherapy for the treatment of alcohol dependence. J Subst Abuse Treat. 2009;36(1):S15-S23; quiz S24–S25.

26. Garbutt JC, Kranzler HR, O'Malley SS, et al. Vivitrex Study Group. Efficacy and tolerability of long-acting injectable naltrexone for alcohol dependence: A randomized controlled trial [erratum JAMA 2005;293:1978 and JAMA 2005;293:2864]. JAMA 2005;293:1617–1625.

27. Boothby LA, Doering PL. Acamprosate for the treatment of alcohol dependence. Clin Ther 2005;27:695–714.

28. Fiore MC, Baily WC. Treating tobacco use and dependence. Clinical practice guidelines. Rockville, MD: U.S. Department of Health and Human Services, Public Health Service; 2000 (June); updated 2008 (May).

29. Centers for Disease Control and Prevention. Cigarette smoking among adults and trends in smoking cessation United States 2008. MMWR 2009. *http://www.cdc.gov/mmwr/preview/mmwrhtml/mm5844a2.htm.*

30. National Institutes on Drug Abuse InfoFacts: Cigarettes and other tobacco products; 2009. *http://www.nida.nih.gov/pdf/infofacts/ Tobacco09.pdf.*

31. Centers for Disease Control and Prevention. Fast Facts: Morbidity and mortality related to tobacco use; 2009. *http://www.cdc.gov/tobacco/ data_statistics/fact_sheets/fast_facts/index.htm#use.*

32. Armour BS, Finkelstein EA. State-level Medicaid expenditures attributable to smoking. Prev Chronic Dis 2009; 6:1–10.

33. Centers for Disease Control and Prevention. Smoking-attributable mortality, years of potential life lost, and productivity losses—United States, 2000-2004. MMWR 2008. *http://www.cdc.gov/mmwr/preview/ mmwrhtml/mm5745a3.htm.*

34. U.S. Department of Health and Human Services. The Health Consequences of Involuntary Exposure to Tobacco Smoke: A Report of the Surgeon General. Atlanta, GA: U.S. Department of Health and Human Services, Centers for Disease Control and Prevention, Coordinating Center for Health Promotion, National Center for Chronic Disease Prevention and Health Promotion, Office on Smoking and Health, 2006. *http://www.surgeongeneral.gov/library/ secondhandsmoke/report/citation.pdf.*

35. Balfour DJ. Neuroplasticity within the mesoaccumbens dopamine system and its role in tobacco dependence. Curr Drug Targets CNS Neurol Disord 2002;1:413–421.

36. Benowitz NL. Clinical pharmacology of nicotine implications for understanding, preventing, and treating tobacco addiction. Clin Pharmacol Ther 2008;83:531–541.

37. Ranney L, Melvin C. Systematic review: smoking cessation intervention strategies for adults and adults in special populations. Ann Intern Med 2006;145:845–856.

38. Perera S, Bullen C. Nicotine replacement therapy for smoking cessation [review]. Cochrane Collaboration 2009;4:1–163.

39. Piper ME, Smith SS. A randomized placebo-controlled clinical trial of 5 smoking cessation pharmacotherapies. Arch Gen Psychiatry 2009;66(11):1253–1262.

40. McRobbie H, Thornley S. The importance of treating tobacco dependence. Rev Esp Cardiol 2008;6:620–628.

41. Center for Disease Control and Prevention. MMWR State Medicaid Coverage for Tobacco–Dependence Treatments—United States; 2006. *http://www.cdc.gov/mmwr/preview/mmwrhtml/mm5705a2.htm.*

42. Fossati R, Apolone G. A double-blind placebo-controlled randomized trial of bupropion for smoking cessation in primary care. Arch Intern Med 2007;167(16):1791–1797.

43. Hughes JR, Stead LF. Antidepressants for smoking cessation. Cochrane Database Syst Rev 2007:CD000031.

44. Garrison G, Dugan S. Varenicline: A first line treatment option for smoking cessation. Clin Ther 2009;31:463–491.

45. Cahill K, Stead LF. Nicotine receptor partial agonist for smoking cessation. Cochrane Database Syst Rev 2008:CD006103.

46. FDA Public Health Advisory. Important Information on Chantix (varenicline); 2008. *www.fda.gov/drugs/drugsafety/publichealthadvisories/ucm051136.*

47. Gourlay SG, Stead LF, Benowitz NL. Clonidine for smoking cessation. Cochrane Database Syst Rev 2004:CD000058.

48. Cornuz J, Zwahlen S, et al. A vaccine against nicotine for smoking cessation: A randomized controlled trial. PLoS ONE 2008; 3:1–10.

49. National Institute on Drug Abuse Message from the director. Development of a nicotine vaccine; 2007. *http://www.drugabuse.gov/about/welcome/Messagenicvax.html.*

50. U.S. Department of Health and Human Services, National Institutes of Health, National Federal stimulus grant supports crucial study of anti-nicotine vaccine; 2009. *http://www.nih.gov/news/health/oct2009/nida-29.htm.*

51. Juliano LM, Griffiths RR. A critical review of caffeine withdrawal: empirical validation of symptoms and signs, incidence, severity, and associated features. Psychopharmacology 2004;176:1–29.

52. Hughes JR, Oliveto AH, Liguori A, et al. Endorsement of DSM-IV dependence criteria among caffeine users. Drug Alcohol Depend 1998;52:99–107.

53. Griffiths RR, Singer MR. Is caffeine a flavoring agent in cola soft drinks? Arch Fam Med 2000;9:727–734.

54. Gorman L. 2001 Specialty Coffee Market Research Report. Gourmet Retailer 2001;98-106. *http://www.gourmetretailer.com/gourmetretailer/images/pdf/coffee.pdf.*

55. Ellison RC, Singer MR, Moore LL, et al. Current caffeine intake of young children: Amount and sources. J Am Diet Assoc 1995;95:802–804.

56. Miller KE. Wired: energy drinks, jock identity, masculine norms, and risk taking. J Am Coll Health. 2008;56:481–489.

57. ALCOSPEED (Alcoholic Energy Drinks). Center for Science in the Public Interest. *http://www.cspinet.org/new/pdf/alcospeedfactsheet.pdf.*

58. Strain EC, Mumford GK, Silverman K, Griffiths RR. Caffeine dependence syndrome. Evidence from case histories and experimental evaluations. JAMA 1994;272:1043–1048.

59. Ozsungur S, Brenner D, El-Sohemy E. Fourteen well-described caffeine withdrawal symptoms factor into three clusters. Psychopharmacology 2009;201:541–548.

60. Kuczkowski KM. Caffeine in pregnancy. Arch Gynecol Obstet 2009;280:695–698.

61. Weng X, Odouli R, Li DK. Maternal caffeine consumption during pregnancy and the risk of miscarriage: a prospective cohort study. Am J Obstet Gynecol 2008;198:279.e1–279.e 8.

62. Hagen K, Thoresen K, Stovner LJ, Zwart JA. High dietary caffeine consumption is associated with a modest increase in headache prevalence: results from the Head-HUNT Study. J Headache Pain 2009;10:153–159.

63. Higdon J, Frei B. Coffee and health: A review of recent human research. Crit Rev Food Sci Nutr 2006;46:101–123.

76

Schizophrenia

M. LYNN CRISMON, TAMI R. ARGO, AND PETER F. BUCKLEY

KEY CONCEPTS

❶ The pathophysiology of schizophrenia may occur in one or more different neurotransmitter systems.

❷ The clinical presentation of schizophrenia is characterized by positive symptoms, negative symptoms, and impairment in cognitive functioning.

❸ Comprehensive care for individuals with schizophrenia must occur in the context of a multidisciplinary mental healthcare environment that offers psychotropic medication management and comprehensive psychosocial services.

❹ A thorough patient evaluation (e.g., history, mental status exam, physical exam, psychiatric diagnostic interview, and laboratory analysis) should occur to establish a diagnosis of schizophrenia and to identify potential co-occurring disorders, including substance abuse and general medical disorders.

❺ Given that it is challenging to differentiate among antipsychotics based upon efficacy, side-effect profiles become important in choosing an antipsychotic for an individual patient.

❻ Pharmacotherapy algorithms should emphasize monotherapies with antipsychotics of optimal efficacy: side-effect ratios and progress to medications with greater side-effect risks and then to combination regimens only in the most treatment-resistant patients.

❼ Adequate time on a given medication at a therapeutic dose is the most important variable in predicting medication response.

❽ Long-term, maintenance antipsychotic treatment is necessary for the vast majority of patients with schizophrenia in order to prevent relapse.

❾ Thorough patient and family psychoeducation should occur, including education about the illness, symptoms, prognosis, medication, psychosocial treatments, and methods to improve adaptive functioning.

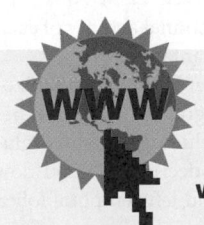

The complete chapter, learning objectives, and other resources can be found at **www.pharmacotherapyonline.com**.

❿ Pharmacotherapy decisions should be guided by systematic monitoring of patient symptoms, preferably with the use of brief symptom rating scales.

Schizophrenia is one of the most complex and challenging of psychiatric disorders. It represents a heterogeneous syndrome of disorganized and bizarre thoughts, delusions, hallucinations, inappropriate affect, and impaired psychosocial functioning. From the time that Kraepelin first described dementia praecox in 1896 until publication of the *Diagnostic and Statistical Manual of Mental Disorders, Fourth Edition, Text Revision (DSM-IV-TR)* in 2000, the description of this illness has continuously evolved.[1] Scientific advances that increase our knowledge of central nervous system (CNS) physiology, pathophysiology, and genetics will likely improve our understanding of schizophrenia in the future.

EPIDEMIOLOGY

According to the Epidemiologic Catchment Area Study, the lifetime prevalence of schizophrenia using strict diagnostic criteria ranges from 0.6% to 1.9%. If a broader definition is used, the lifetime rate rises to 2% to 3%.[2] The worldwide prevalence of schizophrenia is remarkably similar among most cultures. Schizophrenia most commonly has its onset in late adolescence or early adulthood and rarely occurs before adolescence or after the age of 40 years. Although the prevalence of schizophrenia is equal in males and females, the onset of illness tends to be earlier in males. Males most frequently have their first episode during their early 20s, whereas with females it is usually during their late 20s to early 30s.[1,3]

ETIOLOGY

Although the etiology of schizophrenia is unknown, research has demonstrated various abnormalities in brain structure and function.[4] However, these changes are not consistent among all individuals with schizophrenia The cause of schizophrenia is likely multifactorial; that is, multiple pathophysiologic abnormalities can play a role in producing the similar but varying clinical phenotypes we refer to as schizophrenia.

A neurodevelopmental model has been evoked as one possible explanation for the etiology of schizophrenia.[4] This model proposes that schizophrenia has its origins in some as yet unknown in utero disturbance, possibly occurring during the second trimester of pregnancy. Evidence for this is provided by the abnormal neuronal migration demonstrated in studies of schizophrenic brains. This "schizophrenic lesion" can result in abnormalities in cell shape, position, symmetry, connectivity, and functionally to the development of abnormal brain circuits.[4] Changes are consistent with a cell migration abnormality during the second trimester of pregnancy, and some studies associate upper respiratory infections during the second trimester of pregnancy with a higher incidence of schizophrenia.[5] Other studies show a relationship between obstetric complications or neonatal hypoxia and schizophrenia. Some studies associate low birth weight (less than 2.5 kg [5.5 lb]) with schizophrenia.[2] Maternal stress, perhaps related to the effects of circulating glucocorticoids in utero, may be a risk factor for schizophrenia. Maternal "stress" could derive from a variety of external and internal noxious events (malnutrition, infection, etc.). The resulting secondary "synaptic disorganization" associated with such insults is thought not to produce overt clinical manifestations of psychosis until adolescence or early adulthood because this is the corresponding time period of neuronal maturation.

Although studies have shown decreased cortical thickness and increased ventricular size in the brains of many patients with schizophrenia, this occurs in the absence of widespread gliosis.[4] One hypothesis is that obstetric complications and hypoxia, in combination with a genetic predisposition, could activate a glutamatergic cascade that results in increased neuronal pruning. It is hypothesized that this genetic predisposition may be related to genes controlling N-methyl-D-aspartate (NMDA) receptor activity. As a part of the normal neurodevelopmental process, pruning of dendrites occurs. In normal individuals, approximately 35% of the peak number of dendrites at 2 years of age are pruned by midadolescence. Some studies have shown a higher percentage of pruning in individuals with schizophrenia. Furthermore, synaptic pruning predominantly involves glutamatergic dendrites. Hypoxia or other prenatal insult can result in a decreased number of basal neurons from which to start, and glutamatergic activation can exaggerate the pruning process.[6]

Numerous studies have shown neuropsychologic abnormalities and impairment in reaching normal motor milestones and abnormal movements in young children who later develop schizophrenia.[3] Abnormalities in brain function occur long before the onset of psychotic symptomatology and provide empiric evidence for schizophrenia being a neurodevelopmental disorder.[4] However, the progressive clinical deterioration in many patients suggests that this illness can also have a neurodegenerative component. This is consistent with recent brain imaging studies that show deteriorative brain changes in patients with frequent relapses.[2,4,7] Schizophrenia may be neither neurodevelopmental or neurodegenerative in origin, but rather an illness exhibiting neurodegenerative propensity based on a vulnerable neurodevelopmental predisposition.[2,8,9]

GENETICS

Although a specific abnormality has not been discovered, evidence suggests a genetic basis for schizophrenia. Although the risk of developing schizophrenia is 0.6% to 1.9% in the U.S. population, the risk is approximately 10% if a first-degree relative has the illness and 3% if a second-degree relative has the illness.[2,10] If both parents have schizophrenia, the risk of producing a schizophrenic offspring increases to approximately 40%. Twin studies in dizygotic twins report that the risk of the second twin developing schizophrenia if one twin has the illness is between 12% and 14%. However, in monozygotic twins the risk increases to 48%.[10] Numerous adoption studies indicate that the risk for schizophrenia lies with the biologic parents, and change in the environment during the child's developmental stages does not alter this. If schizophrenia occurs in siblings, the onset of illness tends to occur at the same age in each, thus lessening the possibility of an environmental precipitant. A search for a genetic linkage in schizophrenia has been difficult, and any genetic etiologies in schizophrenia are likely heterogeneous, but

present with similar phenotypes. Potential loci have been identified on chromosomes 6, 8, 13, and 22.[10] The study of the genetics of schizophrenia has become increasingly molecular in focus.[2,11] Recent work has shown that polymorphism in the *VAL/MET* alleles of the catecholamine-O-methyl transferase gene can explain some of the frontal lobe functional deficits in a subset of individuals with schizophrenia.[10] Other recent studies have shown abnormalities in several genes that code for neurodevelopment and for trophic factors.[10–12] For example, dysbindin is a neurodevelopmental protein gene that is found on chromosome 6. Alleles associated with decreased dysbindin RNA in the dorsolateral prefrontal cortex have been reported in patients with schizophrenia and their families.[13] Another recent gene-wide linkage scan of a large pedigree showed increased signal at chromosome 8p, close to the gene that encodes for neuregulin—another neurodevelopmental gene.[14] Of particular excitement in the field has been the discovery of an overexpression of copy number variants (CNVs) in schizophrenia.[11,12,14] This work has fueled other new large-scale genetic studies that are ongoing in an attempt to replicate these findings.

PATHOPHYSIOLOGY

Computed axial tomography (CAT) scans and magnetic resonance imaging (MRI) studies show increased ventricular size, particularly in the third and lateral ventricles, in subtypes of schizophrenics. Recent studies also show a small decrease in brain size compared to matched controls. These changes appear to be consistent with brain asymmetry, the ventricular enlargement being most pronounced in the left temporal horn, and the decreased cortical size being most obvious in the left temporal lobe.[2,7] Not only does premorbid lower hippocampal volume predict onset of symptoms in high-risk individuals, these structural changes can progress throughout the course of the illness.[15] A reduction in medial temporal lobe volume has been reported in high-risk patients after they were scanned, indicating that some brain changes can be associated with the evolution of psychosis. In an extended analysis, high-risk subjects were compared with first-episode chronic schizophrenia and normal control groups according to hippocampal and amygdala volumes at baseline.[16] No difference in MRI volumes between the high-risk subjects and normal controls were observed, irrespective of whether the at-risk patients did or did not progress to overt psychosis. First-episode schizophrenia (but not other psychosis) groups had reduced (left) hippocampal volume. The implication that these changes occur during transition is intriguing and accords well with the notion of psychosis as a biologically toxic event. Changes in hippocampal volume may correspond with impairment in neuropsychologic testing.[2] Rather than a decrease in the number of neurons in affected brain areas, a decrease in axonal and dendritic communications between cells can result in a loss of connectivity that can be important with respect to neuronal adaptivity and CNS homeostasis.[2,4] These changes are likely consistent with the evidence for abnormal neuronal pruning.[4]

NEUROTRANSMITTER CHANGES

Four dopaminergic tracts are of primary interest. Table 76–1 outlines the origin, innervation, and primary functional activity of each tract, as well as the effects of dopamine (DA) antagonists.[6]

Evidence supports the presence of a DA-receptor defect in schizophrenia. Numerous positron emission tomography (PET) studies have shown regional brain abnormalities, including increased glucose metabolism in the caudate nucleus and decreased blood flow and glucose metabolism in the frontal lobe and left temporal lobe.[3] This can indicate dopaminergic hyperactivity in the head of the

TABLE 76-1 Dopaminergic Tracts and Effects of Dopamine Antagonists

Dopamine Tract	Origin	Innervation	Function	Dopamine Antagonist Effect
Nigrostriatal	Substantia nigra (A9 area)	Caudate nucleus Putamen	Extrapyramidal system, movement	Movement disorders
Mesolimbic	Midbrain ventral tegmentum (A10 area)	Limbic areas (e.g., amygdala, olfactory tubercle, septal nuclei) cingulate gyrus	Arousal, memory, stimulus processing, motivational behavior	Relief of psychosis
Mesocortical	Midbrain ventral tegmentum (A10 area)	Frontal and prefrontal lobe cortex	Cognition, communication, social function, response to stress	Relief of psychosis Akathisia
Tubero-infundibular	Hypothalamus	Pituitary gland	Regulates prolactin release	Increased prolactin concentrations

caudate nucleus and dopaminergic hypofunction in the frontotemporal regions. PET studies using dopamine-2 (D_2)-specific ligands suggest increased densities of D_2 receptors in the head of the caudate nucleus with decreased densities in the prefrontal cortex.[3,4] PET studies assessing dopamine-1 (D_1) function suggest that subpopulations of schizophrenics may have decreased densities of D_1 receptors in the caudate nucleus and the prefrontal cortex. Hypofrontality can be associated with lack of volition and cognitive dysfunction, core features of schizophrenia. It is unknown whether these changes represent a primary event or secondary processes related to other pathophysiologic abnormalities in schizophrenia. Because of the heterogeneity in the clinical presentation of schizophrenia, it has been suggested that the DA hypothesis can be more applicable to "neuroleptic-responsive psychosis," with multiple different etiologies possibly being responsible for causing schizophrenia.[2] Attempts have been made to develop relationships between these abnormal findings and behavioral symptoms present in schizophrenic patients. The positive symptoms are possibly more closely associated with DA-receptor hyperactivity in the mesocaudate, whereas negative symptoms and cognitive impairment are most closely related to DA-receptor hypofunction in the prefrontal cortex. Presynaptic D_1 receptors in the prefrontal cortex are thought to be involved in modulating glutamatergic activity, and this can be important with regard to working memory in individuals with schizophrenia.[2]

The glutamatergic system is one of the most widespread excitatory neurotransmitter systems in the brain. Alterations in its function, either hypo- or hyperactivity, can result in toxic neuronal reactions.[3] Dopaminergic innervation from the ventral striatum decreases the limbic system's inhibitory activity (perhaps through γ-aminobutyric acid [GABA] interneurons); thus, dopaminergic stimulation increases arousal. The corticostriatal glutamate pathways have the opposite effect, inhibiting dopaminergic function from the ventral striatum, therefore allowing the limbic system to have increased inhibitory activity. Descending glutamatergic tracts interact with dopaminergic tracts directly as well as through GABA interneurons. Glutamatergic deficiency produces symptoms similar to those of dopaminergic hyperactivity and possibly those seen in schizophrenia. Clinical support for this comes from the fact that phencyclidine, a potent psychotomimetic, is a noncompetitive antagonist at the NMDA receptor, a major glutamate receptor. Similarly, abuse of ketamine, a veterinary anesthetic, can resemble schizophrenia. Ketamine, a competitive antagonist at glutamatergic NMDA receptors, has been shown to lead to reduction in D_1 neurotransmission through glutamatergic inhibition of DA release.[17] It is proposed that schizophrenia may involve some in utero assault that leads to a developmental defect in NMDA receptor function—so-called NMDA hypofunction. This defect is proposed to have latent clinical expression with the psychotic manifestations from NMDA hypofunction not being seen until late adolescence or early adulthood. It has been shown that excess D_2 stimulation can impair NMDA transmission via GABAergic neurons. Thus the use of antipsychotic drugs may indirectly enhance glutamatergic transmission.[2]

Serotoninergic receptors are present on dopaminergic axons, and stimulation of these receptors decreases DA release, at least in the striatum.[6] Although somewhat more diffuse, the distribution of serotonergic neurons is similar to that of dopaminergic neurons, thus allowing these two neurotransmitter systems to innervate the same areas. In fact, 5-hydroxytryptamine$_2$ (serotonin-2; 5-HT$_2$) receptors and D_4 receptors have been found to be colocalized in the cortex.[2,6] Patients with schizophrenia with abnormal brain scans have higher whole-blood 5-HT concentrations, and these concentrations are correlated with increased ventricular size.[18] Second-generation antipsychotics (SGA), also known as atypical antipsychotics, with potent 5-HT$_2$ receptor antagonist effects reverse worsening of symptomatology induced by 5-HT agonists in patients with schizophrenia.[18]

❶ Schizophrenia is a complex disorder, and multiple etiologies likely exist. Based on current knowledge, it is naive to think that any currently proposed etiology can adequately explain the genesis of this complex disease. Molecular research involving genetically determined subtle changes in G proteins, protein metabolism, and other subcellular processes can eventually identify the biologic disturbances associated with schizophrenia.[2,4,8]

CLINICAL PRESENTATION

Schizophrenia is the most common functional psychosis, and great variability occurs in clinical presentation. Despite numerous attempts to portray a stereotype in movies and on television, the stereotypic schizophrenic essentially does not exist. Moreover, schizophrenia is not a "split personality." It is a chronic disorder of thought and affect with the individual having a significant disturbance in interpersonal relationships and ability to function in society.

The first psychotic episode can be sudden in onset with few premorbid symptoms, or commonly can be preceded by withdrawn, suspicious, peculiar behavior (schizoid). During acute psychotic episodes, the patient loses touch with reality, and in a sense, the brain creates a false reality to replace it. Acute psychotic symptoms can include hallucinations (especially hearing voices), delusions (fixed false beliefs), and ideas of influence (beliefs that one's actions are controlled by external influences). Thought processes are disconnected (loose associations), the patient may not be able to carry on logical conversation (alogia), and can have simultaneous contradictory thoughts (ambivalence). The patient's affect can be flat (no emotional expression), or it can be inappropriate and labile. The patient is often withdrawn and inwardly directed (autism). Uncooperativeness, hostility, and verbal or physical aggression can be seen because of the patient's misperception of reality. Self-care skills are impaired, and the patient is frequently dirty, unkempt, and in general has poor hygiene. Sleep and appetite are often disturbed. When the acute psychotic episode remits, the patient typically has residual features. This is an important point in differentiating schizophrenia from other psychotic disorders. Although residual symptoms and their severity vary, patients can have difficulty with anxiety management, suspiciousness, and lack of volition, motivation, insight, and judgment. Therefore, they often have difficulty living independently in the community. Because of poor anxiety management and suspiciousness, they are frequently withdrawn socially, and have difficulty forming close relationships with others. In addition, impaired volition and motivation contribute to poor self-care skills and make it difficult for the patient with schizophrenia to maintain employment.

Patients with schizophrenia frequently experience a lack of historicity, or difficulty in learning from their experiences. They can repeatedly make the same mistakes in social conduct and situations requiring judgment. They have difficulty understanding the importance of treatment, including medications, in maintaining their ability to function in society. Therefore, they tend to discontinue medications and other treatments, and this increases the risk of relapse and rehospitalization. The co-occurrence of substance abuse (predominantly alcohol or polysubstance—alcohol, cannabis, cocaine) in patients with schizophrenia is very common and is another frequent reason for relapse and hospitalization.[1,2] This effect can be caused by direct toxic effects of these drugs on the brain,[17] but is also caused by the medication nonadherence that is associated with substance abuse.

Although the course of schizophrenia is variable, the long-term prognosis for many patients is poor. It is marked by intermittent acute psychotic episodes and impaired psychosocial functioning between acute episodes, with most of the deterioration in psychosocial functioning occurring within 5 years after the first psychotic episode.[19,20] By late life, the patient can appear "burned out," that is, the patient ceases to have acute psychotic episodes, but residual symptoms persist. In a subpopulation of patients, probably 5% to 15%, psychotic symptoms are nearly continuous, and response to antipsychotics is poor.[19]

Schizophrenia is a chronic disorder, and the patient's history must be carefully assessed for dysfunction that has persisted for longer than 6 months. After their first episode, patients with schizophrenia rarely have a level of adaptive functioning as high as before the onset of the disorder. Table 76–2 summarizes the *DSM-IV-TR* criteria.[1]

TABLE 76-2 DSM-IV-TR Diagnostic Criteria for Schizophrenia

A. Characteristic symptoms: Two or more of the following, each persisting for a significant portion of at least a 1-month period:
 (1) Delusions
 (2) Hallucinations
 (3) Disorganized speech
 (4) Grossly disorganized or catatonic behavior
 (5) Negative symptoms
Note: Only one criterion A symptom is required if delusions are bizarre or if hallucinations consist of a voice keeping a running commentary on the person's behavior or two or more voices conversing with each other.
B. Social/occupational dysfunction: For a significant portion of the time since onset of the disorder, one or more major areas of functioning such as work, interpersonal relations, or self-care are significantly below the level prior to onset.
C. Duration: Continuous signs of the disorder for at least 6 months. This must include at least 1 month of symptoms fulfilling criterion A (unless successfully treated). This 6 months may include prodromal or residual symptoms.
D. Schizoaffective or mood disorder has been excluded.
E. Disorder is not due to a medical disorder or substance use.
F. If a history of a pervasive developmental disorder is present, there must be symptoms of hallucinations or delusions present for at least 1 month.

DSM-IV-TR, Diagnostic and Statistical Manual of Mental Disorders, 4th ed., text revision.
Reprinted with permission from the Diagnostic and Statistical Manual of Mental Disorders, Fourth Edition, Text Revision, (Copyright © 2000). American Psychiatric Association.

TABLE 76-3 Schizophrenia Symptom Clusters

Positive	Negative	Cognitive
Suspiciousness	Affective	Impaired attention
Unusual thought content	flattening	Impaired working memory
(delusions)	Alogia	Impaired executive function
Hallucinations	Anhedonia	
Conceptual disorganization	Avolition	

From American Psychiatric Association,[1] Lehman et al.,[19] and Velligan et al.[119]

❷ The *DSM-IV-TR* classifies the symptoms of schizophrenia into two categories: positive and negative. Recently greater emphasis has been placed on a third symptom category, cognitive dysfunction (Table 76–3).[19] The areas of cognition found to be abnormal in schizophrenia include attention, working memory, and executive function. Positive symptoms have traditionally attracted the most attention and are the ones most improved by antipsychotics. However, negative symptoms and impairment in cognition are more closely associated with poor psychosocial function. Along with these characteristic features of schizophrenia, many patients also have comorbid psychiatric and general medical disorders.[19,20] These include depression, anxiety disorders, substance abuse, and general medical disorders like respiratory disorders and metabolic disturbances. These comorbidities substantially complicate the clinical presentation and course of schizophrenia.

It has been suggested that symptom complexes can correlate with prognosis, cognitive functioning, structural abnormalities in the brain, and response to antipsychotic drugs. Negative symptoms and cognitive impairment can be more closely associated with prefrontal lobe dysfunction and positive symptoms with temporolimbic abnormalities. Many patients demonstrate both positive and negative symptoms. Patients with negative symptoms frequently have more antecedent cognitive dysfunction, poor premorbid adjustment, low level of educational achievement, and a poorer overall prognosis.[19]

TREATMENT

■ DESIRED OUTCOME

Pharmacotherapy is the mainstay of treatment in schizophrenia, and it is impossible in most patients to implement effective psychosocial rehabilitation programs in the absence of antipsychotic treatment.[19] **❸** A pharmacotherapeutic treatment plan should be developed that delineates drug-related aspects of therapy. Most deterioration in psychosocial functioning occurs during the first 5 years after the initial psychotic episode, and treatment should be particularly assertive during this period.[19,20] Explicit end points should be defined, including realistic goals for the target symptoms most likely to respond, and the relative time course for response.[19,20] Other goals include avoiding unwanted side effects, using the minimum effective dose, emphasizing adequate duration of treatment as a primary variable in determining response, and limiting augmentation medications to nonresponsive patients.

■ NONPHARMACOLOGIC THERAPY

Psychosocial rehabilitation programs oriented toward improving patients' adaptive functioning are the mainstay of nondrug treatment for schizophrenia. These programs can include case management, psychoeducation, targeted cognitive therapy, basic living skills, social skills training, basic education, work programs, supported housing, and financial support. In particular, programs aimed at employment and housing have been the more effective

TABLE 76-4	Psychotherapeutic Approaches to the Treatment of Schizophrenia

Individual	Group	Cognitive Behavioral
Supportive/counseling	Interactive/social	Cognitive behavioral therapy
Personal therapy		
Social skills therapies		Compliance therapy
Vocational sheltered employment rehabilitation therapies		

interventions and are considered "best practices." Programs that involve families in the care and life of the patient have been shown to decrease rehospitalization and improve functioning in the community. For particularly low-functioning patients, assertive intervention programs, referred to as *active community treatment* (ACT), are effective in improving patients' functional outcomes. ACT teams are available on a 24-hour basis and work in the patient's home and place of employment to provide comprehensive treatment, including medication, crisis intervention, daily living skills, and supported employment and housing.[19,20] Medication treatment cannot be successful without proper attention to these other aspects of care. People with schizophrenia need comprehensive care, with coordination of services across psychiatric, addiction, medical, social, and rehabilitative services. The level of coordination in the United States is often insufficient, and patients become at risk to "fall through the cracks." Recent national policy documents have called for greater coordination of care.[21,22] Additionally, emphasis is growing on the role that the person himself or herself plays in a recovery-based system of care, where the person's lifetime aspirations and goals become the center of care, rather than symptom reduction being the primary focus. This recovery-based approach recognizes the strengths and resilience of people with schizophrenia.[23] It also acknowledges how people with schizophrenia can also be a support to others who are coping with the illness.[24] It is important to frame clinical decision making in the context of a mutual process involving patient and clinician-rather than a unilateral "here's a prescription…please take these tablets" approach. Also, it is increasingly recognized that cognitive behavioral therapy can help some patients. A list of psychotherapeutic approaches to the treatment of schizophrenia is given in Table 76–4.

■ PHARMACOLOGIC THERAPY

Assessment Prior to Treatment

❹ The importance of initial accurate diagnostic assessment cannot be overemphasized. A thorough mental status examination, psychiatric diagnostic interview, physical and neurologic examination, complete family and social history, and laboratory workup must be performed to confirm the diagnosis and exclude general medical or substance-induced causes of psychosis. Laboratory tests, biologic markers, and commonly available brain imaging techniques do not assist in diagnosis or selection of medication. A pretreatment patient workup is important in not only excluding other pathology, but in serving as a baseline for monitoring potential medication-related side effects, and should include vital signs, complete blood count, electrolytes, hepatic function, renal function, electrocardiogram, fasting serum glucose, serum lipids, thyroid function, and urine drug screen.

SGAs (with the exception of clozapine) are first-line agents in the treatment of schizophrenia.[19,25] No absolute criterion distinguishes atypical (second generation) from typical (traditional, conventional, or first generation) antipsychotics, and no universally accepted

definition exists for an atypical antipsychotic.[18] Therefore, *second-generation antipsychotic* is a more appropriate term. Common to all definitions is the ability of the drug to produce antipsychotic response with few or no acutely occurring extrapyramidal side effects. Other attributes that have been ascribed to SGAs include enhanced efficacy, particularly for negative symptoms and cognition; absence or near absence of propensity to cause tardive dyskinesia; and lack of effect on serum prolactin.[18] To date, the only approved SGA that fulfills all of these criteria is clozapine.[18] Although early studies suggested that SGAs might have a superior effect on negative symptoms and cognition, this has not been confirmed in more recent studies.[2,19,25] The major advantage of atypical antipsychotics is their lower risk of neurologic side effects, particularly effects on movement. However, this is offset by increased risk of metabolic side effects with some SGAs, including weight gain, hyperlipidemias, and diabetes mellitus. ❺ Side-effect profiles differ among antipsychotics, and this information in combination with individual patient characteristics should be used in deciding which drug to use in an individual patient. Information from the algorithm (Fig. 76–1) and the adverse effects sections should be used in arriving at this decision.

Results from the Clinical Antipsychotic Trials of Intervention Effectiveness (CATIE) study indicate that olanzapine, compared with quetiapine, risperidone, ziprasidone, and the FGA perphenazine, has modest superiority in maintenance therapy when treatment persistence is the primary clinical outcome.[27] However, increased metabolic adverse effects occurred with olanzapine.

No known differences exist in efficacy between low- and high-potency FGAs. Previous patient or family history of response to an antipsychotic is helpful in the selection of an agent. Traditional dosage equivalents (expressed in "chlorpromazine equivalent dosages"—the equipotent dosage of any traditional FGA compared with 100 mg of chlorpromazine) can assist in determining the effective dosage range if the need arises to treat a patient with a different FGA. However, because SGAs differ in mechanism of action, the dose equivalents have little relevance when comparing dosages of SGAs. Table 76–5 lists antipsychotics and their usual dosage ranges.

■ PHARMACOTHERAPEUTIC ALGORITHM

❻ Figure 76–1 outlines a suggested pharmacotherapeutic algorithm for schizophrenia.[25,26,28] Stage 1 of the treatment algorithm applies to those patients experiencing their first episode of schizophrenia or to patients off of medications and re-entering treatment who do not have a history of nonresponse or nontolerance with antipsychotics. The clinician needs to evaluate the relative risk of extrapyramidal side effects (EPS) with FGAs versus the risk of metabolic side effects with different SGAs in making a decision for drug selection. The 2009 PORT recommendations do not recommend the use of olanzapine in first episode because of weight gain and metabolic side effects.[26] Stage 2 addresses pharmacotherapy in a patient who had inadequate clinical improvement with the antipsychotic used in stage 1. Stage 2 recommends an alternate antipsychotic monotherapy with the exception of clozapine.[25,26]

Because of safety concerns and the need for white blood cell (WBC) monitoring, it is recommended that patients be tried on two different monotherapy antipsychotic trials before proceeding to a trial of clozapine (stage 3).[25,26] Clozapine has superior efficacy in decreasing suicidal behavior, and it should be considered as a higher treatment option in the suicidal patient.[25,26] Clozapine can also be considered earlier in treatment in patients with a history of violence or comorbid substance abuse.[25,26]

Stage 4 of the treatment algorithm includes clozapine and augmentation with either a FGA, SGA, or electroconvulsive therapy (ECT).[25] Treatment algorithm recommendations after stage 3

Algorithm for the pharmacotherapy of schizophrenia

Choice of antipsychotic (AP) should be guided by considering the clinical characteristics of the patient and the efficacy and side effect profiles of available medication.

Forward stage(s) can be skipped depending on clinical picture or history of antipsychotic failures, and returning to an earlier stage may be justified by history of past response.

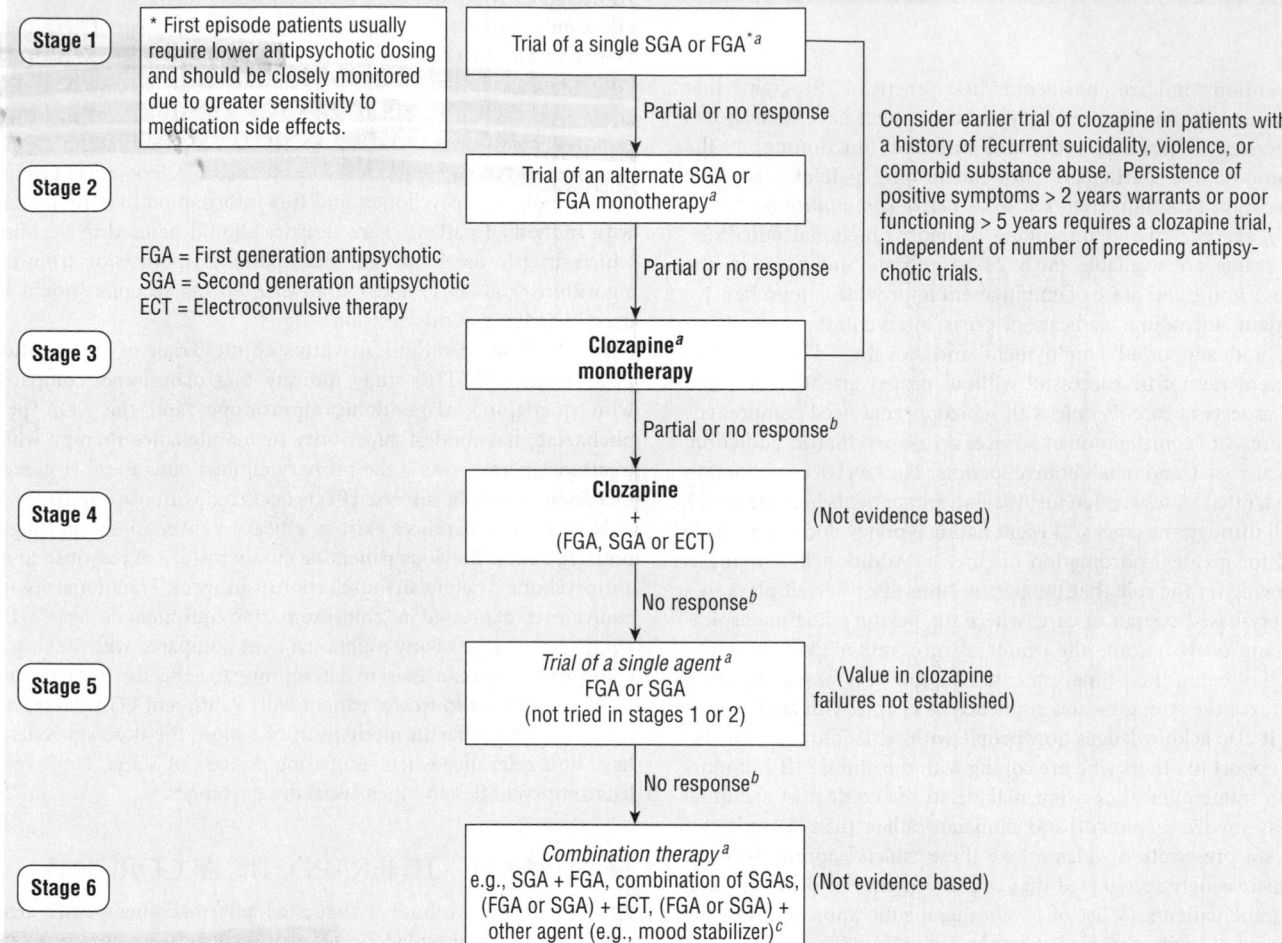

Stage 1

* First episode patients usually require lower antipsychotic dosing and should be closely monitored due to greater sensitivity to medication side effects.

Trial of a single SGA or FGA*ᵃ

Partial or no response

Consider earlier trial of clozapine in patients with a history of recurrent suicidality, violence, or comorbid substance abuse. Persistence of positive symptoms > 2 years warrants or poor functioning > 5 years requires a clozapine trial, independent of number of preceding antipsychotic trials.

Stage 2

Trial of an alternate SGA or FGA monotherapyᵃ

FGA = First generation antipsychotic
SGA = Second generation antipsychotic
ECT = Electroconvulsive therapy

Partial or no response

Stage 3

Clozapineᵃ monotherapy

Partial or no responseᵇ

Stage 4

Clozapine + (FGA, SGA or ECT)

(Not evidence based)

No responseᵇ

Stage 5

Trial of a single agent ᵃ FGA or SGA (not tried in stages 1 or 2)

(Value in clozapine failures not established)

No responseᵇ

Stage 6

Combination therapyᵃ e.g., SGA + FGA, combination of SGAs, (FGA or SGA) + ECT, (FGA or SGA) + other agent (e.g., mood stabilizer)ᶜ

(Not evidence based)

ᵃIf patient is inadequately adherent at any stage, the clinician should assess contributing factors and consider switching to long-acting monotherapy antipsychotic treatment,

ᵇA treatment refractory evaluation should be performed to reexamine diagnosis, substance abuse, medication adherence, and psychosocial stressors. cognitive behavioral therapy and other psychosocial augmentations should be considered.

ᶜWhenever a second medication is added to an antipsychotic (other than clozapine) for the purpose of improving psychotic symptoms, the patient is considered to be in stage 6.

FIGURE 76-1. Patient entry into the algorithm is determined by individual patient history, clinical presentation, and consideration of potential side-effect risk. Either first episode patients or patients who have been off of medications and are reentering treatment with no history of poor response to antipsychotics are entered at stage 1. Algorithm stages can be skipped if clinically appropriate, and one can go back stages if indicated. In general, inadequately responding patients should not remain in stages 1 or 2 longer than 12 weeks at therapeutic doses. Stage 3 should be at least 6 months. In stages 4, 5, and 6, a 12-week trial is recommended, and if there is greater than or equal to 20% improvement in positive symptoms at week 12, the medication trial warrants extension for an additional 12 weeks with dose titration as clinically warranted. The levels of evidence for algorithm recommendations are as follows: stage 1, level A for efficacy for both first-generation antipsychotics (FGAs) and second-generation antipsychotics (SGAs); stage 2, level A; stage 3, level A; stage 4, level C; stage 5, level C; stage 6, level C. Level A is supported by one or more randomized controlled trials. Level B is supported by large cohort studies, epidemiologic studies, and so on. Level C is supported only by case series, case reports, or expert opinion. *(Created based upon references 25, 26, 28.)*

TABLE 76-5 Available Antipsychotics: Doses and Dosage Forms

Generic Name	Trade Name	Traditional Equivalent Dose (mg)	Usual Dosage Range (mg/day)	Manufacturer's Maximum Dose (mg/day)[a]	Dosage Forms[b]
First-generation antipsychotics (traditional or typical antipsychotics)					
Chlorpromazine	Thorazine	100	100–800	2,000	T,L,LC,I,C-ER,S
Fluphenazine	Prolixin	2	2–20	40	T,L,LC,I,LAI
Haloperidol	Haldol	2	2–20	100	T,LC,I,LAI
Loxapine	Loxitane	10	10–80	250	C,LC
Molindone	Moban	10	10–100	225	T,LC
Perphenazine	Trilafon	10	10–64	64	T,LC,I
Thioridazine	Mellaril	100	100–800	800	T,LC
Thiothixene	Navane	4	4–40	60	C,LC
Trifluoperazine	Stelazine	5	5–40	80	T,LC,I
Second-generation antipsychotics (atypical antipsychotics)					
Aripiprazole	Abilify	NA	15–30	30	T,O,L
Asenapine	Saphris	NA	10–20	20	SL
Clozapine	Clozaril	NA	50–500	900	T,O
Iloperidone	Fanapt	NA	2–24	24	T
Olanzapine	Zyprexa	NA	10–20	20	T,I,O
Paliperidone	Invega	NA	3–9	12	ER
Paliperidone palmitate	Invega Sustenna	NA	39–234	234	LAI
Quetiapine	Seroquel	NA	250–500	800	T
Risperidone	Risperdal	NA	2–8	16	T,O,L
Risperidone	Risperdal Consta	NA	25–50 mg every 2 wk	50	LAI
Ziprasidone	Geodon	NA	40–160	200	C,I

[a]NA. This parameter does not apply to atypical antipsychotics.

[b]C, capsule; ER or SR, extended or sustained release; I, injection; L, liquid solution, elixir, or suspension; LC, liquid concentrate; LAI, long-acting injectable; O, orally disintegrating tablets; R, rectal suppositories; SL, sublingual tablet; T, tablet.

(i.e., clozapine monotherapy) are based more on anecdotal experiences and expert opinion than on empirical research.[25] In general, patients who experience poor improvement with clozapine do not respond well with other antipsychotic monotherapies (stage 5), thus the primary reason that clozapine augmentation is recommended at stage 4. Stage 6 combination pharmacotherapy interventions are not evidence based and should only be implemented with time limited, careful evaluation of a patient's symptom response and discontinuation of the combination if improvement does not occur.[25]

If partial or poor adherence contributes to inadequate clinical improvement, then long-acting injectable antipsychotics should be considered.[19,20,26] In addition to individuals who are identified as partially adherent, some patients may elect for long-acting injections instead of taking daily oral medication. A long-acting injectable antipsychotic can be substituted for an oral antipsychotic at any point in the algorithm where it is thought to be indicated.

The use of antipsychotic combinations is controversial, as limited evidence supports increased efficacy for combination antipsychotic treatment.

CLINICAL CONTROVERSY

Significant controversy exists regarding whether to use an FGA or an SGA as first-line treatment in schizophrenia. Although most studies have demonstrated a lower incidence of EPS with SGAs, weight gain and the risk of diabetes mellitus are significant adverse events with some of the SGAs, particularly olanzapine. Tension also exists between policy decision makers who are responsible for managing finite resources and clinicians who see clinical benefits of the SGAs in the patients they treat.

The use of antipsychotic combinations is controversial, as insufficient evidence exists to support their use. Regardless, combination antipsychotics are frequently used by clinicians, and testimonies attest to clinical benefits when a second SGA is added.

PREDICTORS OF RESPONSE

Obtaining a thorough medication history is important, and previous antipsychotic treatment should help guide the selection of drug therapy, in that either a good prior response favors the use of the same agent or a negative prior response suggests the selection of a dissimilar drug. Nonprescription and illicit drug use can influence psychiatric presentation and thus diagnosis or antipsychotic response. Amphetamines and other CNS stimulants, cocaine, corticosteroids, digitalis glycosides, indomethacin, marijuana, pentazocine, phencyclidine, and other drugs can induce psychosis in susceptible individuals or exacerbate psychosis in patients with preexisting psychiatric illness.[29] Patients with schizophrenia who continue to abuse alcohol or drugs usually have a poor response to medications and a poor prognosis. Alcohol, caffeine, and nicotine use potentially results in drug interactions.

Individual differences in patient response have been either proposed or identified, which can be clinically useful predictors of response.[19,20] Acute onset and short duration of illness, presence of acute stressors or precipitating factors, later age of onset, family history of affective illness, and good premorbid adjustment as reflected in stable interpersonal relationships or employment are all predictors of good response.[19,20]

Although controversial, affective symptoms can correlate with an overall good response. Negative symptoms and neuropsychologic deficits related to cognition and neurologic soft signs can correlate with poor antipsychotic response.[19,20] A patient's subjective response within the first 48 hours after being administered an FGA can be associated with drug responsiveness.[30] An initial dysphoric response, demonstrated by stating a dislike of the medication, or feeling worse or zombie-like, combined with anxiety or akathisia-like symptoms, is associated with poor drug response, adverse effects, and nonadherence.

The importance of developing a therapeutic alliance between the patient and the clinician cannot be underestimated. Patients who form positive therapeutic alliances are more likely to be adherent with all aspects of therapy, experience a better outcome at 2 years, and require smaller antipsychotic doses.

A certain minority of patients fail to benefit from antipsychotic therapy, and their psychosocial functioning can actually worsen. Unfortunately, no accepted method is available to identify these people before treatment.[19,26] Recent evidence suggests that pharmacogenetics can play a role in predicting treatment response, both with respect to symptom improvement and with liability to develop side effects.[30,31] However, insufficient information is available to recommend routine clinical testing.

■ INITIAL TREATMENT IN AN ACUTE PSYCHOTIC EPISODE

The goals during the first 7 days of treatment should be decreased agitation, hostility, combativeness, anxiety, tension, and aggression, and normalization of sleep and eating patterns. The usual recommendation is to initiate therapy and to titrate dose over the first few days to an average effective dose, unless the patient's physiologic status or history indicates that this dose can result in unacceptable adverse effects. Table 76–5 lists the usual dosage range, and an average dose is typically midrange. Because of increased sensitivity to side effects, particularly extrapyramidal side effects, in first-episode psychotic patients, typical dosing ranges are approximately 50% of the doses used in chronically ill individuals.[25] If "cheeking" of medication is suspected, liquid formulations and orally disintegrating tablets of different antipsychotics are available (see Table 76–5). If a patient has shown absolutely no improvement after 3 to 4 weeks at therapeutic doses, then an alternative antipsychotic should be considered (i.e., moving to the next treatment stage in the algorithm; see Fig. 76–1).[18,25]

Although some clinicians believe that larger daily doses are necessary in more severely symptomatic patients, data are not available to support this practice. Some symptoms, such as agitation, tension, aggression, and increased motor activity, can respond more quickly, but side effects can be more common with higher doses. However, interindividual differences in dosage and patient response do occur. In partial but inadequate responders who are tolerating the chosen antipsychotic, it may be reasonable to titrate above usual dose ranges. However, this tactic should be time-limited (i.e., 2–4 weeks), and if the patient does not achieve further improvement, the dose should either be decreased, or an alternative treatment strategy tried.[32] In general, rapid titration of antipsychotic dosage is not indicated.[32] However, intramuscular antipsychotic administration (e.g., aripiprazole 5.25–9.75 mg IM, haloperidol 2–5 mg IM, olanzapine 2.5–10 mg IM, or ziprasidone 10–20 mg IM) can be used to assist in calming a severely agitated patient. Agitation can be manifested as loud, physically or verbally threatening behavior, motor hyperactivity, or physical aggression. Although this technique can assist in calming an acutely agitated psychotic patient, it does not improve the extent of or time to remission, or the length of hospitalization. If haloperidol IM is used, the occurrence of EPS can eliminate some of the advantages of using an oral SGA. If the patient is receiving an antipsychotic within the usual therapeutic range, the use of lorazepam 2 mg IM as needed in combination with the maintenance antipsychotic is a rational alternative to an injectable antipsychotic. Hypotension, respiratory depression, and CNS depression are possible when injectable lorazepam and olanzapine are used concomitantly; thus this parenteral combination is not recommended.

■ STABILIZATION THERAPY

Improvement is usually a slow but steady process over 6 to 12 weeks or longer. During the first 2 to 3 weeks, goals should include increased socialization and improvement in self-care habits and mood. Improvement in formal thought disorder should follow and can take an additional 6 to 8 weeks to respond. Patients who are early in the course of their illness can experience a more rapid resolution of symptoms than individuals who are more chronically ill. In general, if a patient has no improvement with treatment after 3 to 4 weeks at therapeutic doses, or has achieved only a partial decrease in positive and negative symptoms within 12 weeks at adequate doses, then the next algorithm stage should be considered. In more chronically ill patients, symptoms can continue to improve for 3 to 6 months. During acute stabilization, usual labeled doses of SGAs are recommended (see Table 76–5); with FGAs, a range of 300 to 1,000 mg of chlorpromazine equivalents daily is recommended.[19,25] An optimum dose of the chosen drug should be estimated in the initial treatment plan. If the patient begins to show adequate response before or at this dosage, then the patient should remain at this dosage as long as symptoms continue to improve. ❼ In general, adequate time on a therapeutic antipsychotic dose is the most important factor in predicting medication response. However, if necessary, dose titration can continue within the therapeutic range every week or two as long as the patient has no side effects.

Before changing medications in a poorly responding patient, the following should be considered: Were the initial target symptoms indicative of schizophrenia or did they represent manifestations of a different diagnosis, a long-standing behavioral problem, a substance abuse disorder, or a general medical condition? Is the patient adherent with pharmacotherapy? Are the persistent symptoms poorly responsive to antipsychotics (e.g., impaired insight or judgment, or fixed delusions)? How does the patient's current status compare with response during previous exacerbations? Would this patient potentially benefit from a change to a different treatment stage (see Fig. 76–1)? Does this patient have a treatment-refractory schizophrenic illness?

The conclusion that a partially responding patient has achieved as much symptomatic improvement as possible is one that must be made with great care and after considering all possible treatment alternatives. However, treatment goals must be realistic. Medications are effective at decreasing many of the symptoms of schizophrenia (and are thus referred to as palliative), but they are not curative, and all symptoms may not abate. Although one should aim to achieve none to minimal residual positive symptoms with effective treatment, it is still unclear what a realistic goal is with regard to maximum improvement in negative symptoms.

It is important to screen patients for co-occurring mental disorders, and their presence can become more apparent during the stabilization or maintenance phases of schizophrenia treatment. Examples include substance abuse disorders, depression, obsessive-compulsive disorder, and panic disorder. As co-occurring disorders will limit symptom and functional improvement and increase the risk of relapse, it is critical that pharmacologic and nonpharmacologic interventions for the co-occurring disorder be implemented in combination with evidence-based treatment for schizophrenia.

■ MAINTENANCE TREATMENT

Maintenance drug therapy prevents relapse, as shown in numerous double-blind studies. The average relapse rate after 1 year is 18% to 32% with active drug (including some nonadherent patients) versus 60% to 80% for placebo.[19,33]

After treatment of the first psychotic episode in a schizophrenic patient, medication should be continued for at least 12 months after remission.[19,32] **8** Many schizophrenia experts recommend that patients with robust medication response be treated for at least 5 years. In chronically ill individuals, continuous or lifetime pharmacotherapy is necessary in the majority of patients to prevent relapse. This should be approached with the lowest effective dose of the antipsychotic that is likely to be tolerated by the patient.[19,32]

Antipsychotics should be tapered slowly before discontinuation. Abrupt discontinuation of antipsychotics, especially low-potency FGAs and clozapine, can result in withdrawal symptoms, felt to be a manifestation of rebound cholinergic outflow. Insomnia, nightmares, headaches, gastrointestinal symptoms (e.g., abdominal cramps, stomach pain, nausea, vomiting, and diarrhea), restlessness, increased salivation, and sweating are reported. When switching from one antipsychotic to another, it is often recommended to taper and discontinue the first antipsychotic over at least 1 to 2 weeks after the second antipsychotic is initiated.[19,32] Tapering may need to occur more slowly, especially with clozapine.[19,32]

Long-Acting Injectable Antipsychotics

Long-acting antipsychotics are recommended for patients who are unreliable in taking oral medication on a daily basis, and thus are not usually used as first-line therapy. Before a long-acting antipsychotic is initiated, it should be determined whether the patient's medication nonadherence is because of side effects. If so, an alternative medication with a more favorable side-effect profile should be considered before a long-acting injectable antipsychotic.

The patient's motivation for treatment is a major factor influencing outcome. Conversion from oral therapy to a long-acting injectable is most successful in patients who have been stabilized on oral therapy. The ideal patient for a long-acting injectable is the individual who does not like the daily reminder of oral medication or is unreliable in taking medications. Paliperidone palmitate is a long-acting injectable that has the advantage of once-monthly injections and easy conversion from oral to IM treatment. It has the disadvantage of being extremely expensive.[34] A long-acting formulation of olanzapine is under FDA review at the time of publication.

Conversion from an oral antipsychotic to a long-acting medication should start with stabilization on an oral dosage form of the same agent, for a short trial (3–7 days), to determine whether the patient tolerates the medication without significant side effects. With long-acting risperidone, measurable serum concentrations are not seen until approximately 3 weeks after single-dose administration. Thus, it is important that the oral antipsychotic be administered for at least 3 weeks after beginning the injections. Dose adjustments are recommended to be made no more often than once every 4 weeks.[32,35] The recommended starting dose with risperidone long-acting injection is 25 mg, and clinical experience suggests that titration to doses greater than or equal to 37.5 mg per injection may be necessary for maintenance treatment. Long-acting risperidone has demonstrated efficacy, with an optimum dose range between 25 and 50 mg given IM every 2 weeks. Doses above 50 mg every 2 weeks are not recommended, as research indicates no greater efficacy but more EPS.[25,35]

Paliperidone palmitate can be injected into either the deltoid or the gluteal muscle, and treatment is initiated with 234 mg on day 1 and 156 mg a week later. No overlap with oral drug is necessary. Monthly IM doses are then titrated according to response within a range of 39 to 234 mg.[34]

For fluphenazine decanoate, the simplest dosing conversion method recommends 1.2 times the oral fluphenazine daily dose for stabilized patients, rounding up to the nearest 12.5-mg interval, administered in weekly doses for the first 4 to 6 weeks; or 1.6 times the oral daily dose for more acutely ill patients.[36] Subsequently, fluphenazine decanoate can be administered once every 2 to 3 weeks. Oral fluphenazine can be overlapped for 1 week. For haloperidol decanoate, a factor of 10 to 15 times the oral haloperidol daily dose is commonly recommended, rounding up to the nearest 50-mg interval, administered in a once-monthly dose with an oral haloperidol overlap for the first month. A more assertive conversion method recommends 20 times the oral daily dose, but dividing the injection into consecutive doses of 100 to 200 mg every 3 to 7 days until the entire amount is given.[37] With this method, oral medication overlap is unnecessary. The haloperidol decanoate dose is decreased by 25% at both second and third month.

Injection site reactions have been reported with the haloperidol decanoate 100 mg/mL preparation, consisting of painful pruritic swelling at the injection site.[38] Acute EPS can be seen following injections of either fluphenazine or haloperidol decanoate. These effects are minimized with the use of risperidone microspheres. Both haloperidol and fluphenazine decanoate should be administered by a deep, "Z-tract" intramuscular method. Long-acting risperidone is injected by deep IM injection in the gluteus maximus, but Z-tracting is not necessary.

Methods to Enhance Patient Adherence

It is often a challenge for individuals with chronic illnesses to maintain high levels of medication adherence, and partial compliance is a reality in the treatment of all chronic illnesses.[39] Individuals with serious mental disorders have somewhat higher nonadherence rates than those with general medical disorders, with the following explanations provided: denial of illness, lack of insight, grandiosity or paranoia, no perceived need for medication, perceived lack of input into choice of medication or dosage, side effects, misperceived "allergies," or the number of medications prescribed or doses received daily. In fact, clinicians should expect partial compliance to be the norm with regard to medication-taking behavior. This should be approached in a nonjudgmental manner, with the clinician actively engaging the patient in care and using motivational interviewing techniques as mechanisms to enhance therapeutic alliance and patient adherence.

9 Education geared toward patients becoming more informed about their illness and the effectiveness and risks of treatment can help to increase adherence.[40] These programs should be staged so that patients initially receive basic information about their disorder and its symptoms and basic information about their medication and self-monitoring techniques. As the patient is capable of dealing with more complex information, more detailed information regarding schizophrenia, psychosocial treatments, and prognosis should be discussed. Patients and families should be taught self-monitoring techniques and when to report symptom exacerbation or medication side effects to the clinician.[40] Psychoeducation strategies should include motivational interview techniques in individual counseling as well as group activities.

Recent evidence suggests that cognitive behavioral therapy focusing on medication adherence can improve patient outcome.[41] This approach is called compliance therapy. Groups facilitated by trained individuals who have the illness can be more effective in enhancing awareness and acceptance of schizophrenia and necessary treatment than groups led only by professionals. Active involvement of family members further increases the likelihood of patient adherence with treatment. In addition to programs provided by community mental health centers, support groups operated by consumer groups such as the National Alliance on Mental Illness (NAMI) are available in most urban areas. Contact information for local NAMI chapters can be accessed at *www.nami.org*. In the hospital, self-medication administration can reinforce the patient's perception of their active role in their own treatment. When patients miss outpatient appointments, active outreach interventions must be implemented to enhance patient engagement in treatment.[19,40]

■ MANAGEMENT OF TREATMENT-RESISTANT SCHIZOPHRENIA

In general, "treatment resistant" describes a patient who has had inadequate symptom response from multiple antipsychotic trials.[19] Traditionally, treatment resistance has been defined as lack of improvement in positive symptoms, but it can be defined by poor improvement in negative symptoms, or even by medication intolerance. Between 10% and 30% of patients receive minimal symptomatic improvement after multiple FGA monotherapy trials.[19] An additional 30% to 60% of patients have partial but inadequate improvement in symptoms or unacceptable side effects associated with antipsychotic use.[19,25] In those patients failing two or more pharmacotherapy trials, a treatment refractory evaluation should be performed to reexamine diagnosis, substance abuse, medication adherence, and psychosocial stressors. Targeted cognitive behavioral therapy or other psychosocial augmentation strategies should be considered.[25]

Clozapine

Only clozapine has shown superiority over other antipsychotics in randomized clinical trials for the management of treatment-resistant schizophrenia. Most other SGAs have either not been studied in treatment-refractory patients or evaluated in small open trials. In a seminal study, clozapine was effective in approximately 30% of patients with treatment-resistant schizophrenia, compared with only 4% treated with a combination of chlorpromazine and benztropine.[42] The criteria for treatment-resistance require two treatment failures, and includes both FGAs and SGAs. Other treatment candidates for clozapine include those patients who cannot tolerate even conservative doses of other antipsychotics.

Symptomatic improvement with clozapine in the treatment-resistant patient often occurs slowly, and as many as 60% of patients may improve if clozapine is used for up to 6 months.[32] This, in combination with clozapine's adverse-effects profile, provides sufficient information to conclude that clozapine is not a panacea for schizophrenia. Polydipsia and hyponatremia (psychogenic water drinking) is a frequent problem among treatment-resistant patients, and clozapine reportedly decreases water drinking and increases serum sodium in such patients.[43]

Because of the risk of orthostatic hypotension, clozapine is usually titrated more slowly than other antipsychotics, particularly on an outpatient basis. If a 12.5-mg test dose does not produce hypotension, then clozapine 25 mg at bedtime is recommended, increased to 25 mg twice a day after 3 days, and then increased in 25- to 50-mg/day increments every 3 days until a dose of at least 300 mg/day is reached. Because high doses are associated with significantly increased side effects, including seizures, a clozapine serum concentration is recommended before exceeding 600 mg/day. If the clozapine serum concentration is less than 350 ng/mL (350 mcg/L; 1.07 µmol/L), then the dose should be increased as side effects allow to achieve this serum concentration.[27]

Augmentation and Combination Strategies

Little empirical evidence exists to guide treatment decisions for patients who do not respond to clozapine.[25,32,27] A small number of randomized trials have examined the efficacy of clozapine augmentation with SGAs, and the results have been more negative than positive (see Fig. 76–1).[25,27] Augmentation therapy involves the addition of a nonantipsychotic drug to an antipsychotic drug in a poorly or partially responsive patient, whereas combination treatment involves using two antipsychotics simultaneously. Several guidelines should be followed regarding augmentation: (a) augmentation should be used only in inadequately responding patients; (b) augmentation agents are rarely effective for schizophrenic symptoms when used alone; (c) augmentation responders usually improve rapidly; and (d) if augmentation does not improve symptomatology, the augmenting agent should be discontinued.[32]

Mood stabilizers are frequently used as an augmentation strategy. Lithium does not enhance antipsychotic effect but may improve labile affect and agitated behavior in selected patients.[44] Valproic acid and carbamazepine have also been used. A large placebo-controlled trial supports faster symptom improvement, but no difference in maintenance treatment, when divalproex was used in combination with either olanzapine or risperidone.[45] Enzyme induction with carbamazepine can cause a decrease in antipsychotic serum concentrations and potentially worsen psychotic symptoms in some patients.[19,32] The 2009 PORT recommendations do not endorse the use of mood stabilizer augmentation in treatment-resistant patients.[27]

Selective serotonin reuptake inhibitors (SSRIs), particularly fluoxetine and fluvoxamine, have reasonable evidence for improving negative symptoms when used as augmentation of FGAs. Potential benefits of combining SSRIs with SGAs require more study.[46] Consistently positive results have been reported when using SSRIs to treat obsessive-compulsive symptoms that worsen or arise during clozapine treatment.

Combining an FGA with an SGA and combining different SGAs have been suggested as intervention strategies for treatment-resistant patients. Pharmacodynamically, no rationale exists for explaining how combinations of antipsychotics would produce enhanced efficacy, and increased side effects, particularly increased EPS, metabolic effects, and hyperprolactinemia are possible results.[47] Clinically, no evidence exists to prove that antipsychotic combinations are superior to monotherapy, and the 2009 PORT recommendations do not support their use.[27] In general, a series of antipsychotic monotherapies, including clozapine, are preferred over antipsychotic combinations.[25,27,32] However, when clozapine fails to produce desired outcomes, a time-limited combination trial is sometimes recommended (see Fig. 76–1, stages 4 or 6).[19,25] Such antipsychotic combination treatment trials should be time limited (12 weeks) and the patient carefully evaluated with rating scales for changes in symptomatology. If no apparent improvement is observed, then one of the medications should be tapered and discontinued. However, if the patient has a partial response (greater than or equal to 20% improvement in positive symptoms) after 12 weeks with combination treatment in stages 4 or 6, medications should be titrated to doses at the upper end of the therapeutic range, and treatment should continue for an additional 12 weeks before a change in stage is considered.[32]

ANTIPSYCHOTIC DRUG MECHANISMS OF ACTION

The exact mechanism of action of antipsychotics is unknown. It has been suggested that antipsychotics be classified into three different categories: (a) typical or traditional (high D_2 antagonism and low 5-HT_{2A} antagonism); (b) atypical (moderate to high D_2 antagonism and high 5-HT_{2A} antagonism); and (c) atypical clozapine-like (low D_2 antagonism and high 5-HT_{2A} antagonism).[48,49] With the exception of aripiprazole, all current SGAs have a greater affinity for 5-HT_{2A} receptors than D_2 receptors.

Studies of antipsychotic receptor binding in humans have used PET scans to examine neurotransmitter receptor binding at steady-state, 12 hours post dose in small numbers of individuals. At least 60% to 65% D_2 receptor occupation is necessary to decrease positive psychotic symptoms, whereas blockade of approximately 77% or more of D_2 receptors is associated with EPS.[48,50] FGAs are dopamine receptor antagonists with high affinity for D_2 receptors. During chronic treatment with these agents, between 70% and 90% of D_2 receptors in the striatum are usually occupied. In contrast, during clozapine treatment only 38% to 47% of D_2 receptors are occupied, even with high doses. Newer SGAs have variable D_2 binding. With low-dose risperidone (2–5 mg/day), D_2 binding ranges from 60% to 79%, but with doses greater than 6 mg daily, binding commonly exceeds the 77% threshold associated with the development of EPS. Risperidone 2 mg/day produces 5-HT_{2A} binding greater than 70%, and with 4 mg/day it is nearly 100%.[48,51] Olanzapine 10 to 20 mg/day produces D_2 binding ranging from 71% to 80%, whereas at 30 to 40 mg/day, it ranges from 83% to 88%. At 5 mg/day, 5-HT_{2A} receptors are near saturation of binding.[48] Ziprasidone has the highest $5\text{-HT}_{2A}:D_2$ affinity ratio of any of the currently available antipsychotics. It is also a potent 5-HT_{1A} agonist.[52]

Quetiapine has the lowest D_2 binding. At doses of 300 to 600 mg/day, D_2 binding ranges from 0% to 27%. Even at quetiapine 800 mg/day, only 30% of D_2 receptors are occupied. At these same daily doses, 45% to 90% of 5-HT_{2A} receptors are occupied. However, when quetiapine D_2 binding is examined 2 to 3 hours post dose, 58% and 64% of receptors were occupied with 400 mg and 450 mg, respectively. Transient blockade of dopamine receptors may be adequate to produce antipsychotic effect, but long-term D_2 blockade is required for production of EPS and sustained hyperprolactinemia. Low D_2 binding, and thus atypicality, can be directly associated with how rapidly the antipsychotic disassociates from the D_2 receptor.[48,51] The availability of aripiprazole, a partial agonist at D_2 receptors, represents a further elaboration of the dopamine hypothesis of antipsychotic action.[49,53] It is proposed that aripiprazole works as a functional partial agonist. Aripiprazole is a rather weak 5-HT_{2A} antagonist but a potent 5-HT_{1A} agonist.[49,53]

Iloperidone has high affinity for D_2, D_3, and 5-HT_{2A} receptors, and moderate affinity for D_4, 5-HT_6, 5-HT_7, and α_1 receptors.[54] Asenapine has high affinity for 5-HT_{2A} and D_2 receptors as well as for α_1 and histamine-1 receptors. D_2 occupancy of approximately 80% is predicted to occur with a sublingual dose of 5 to 10 mg twice daily.[55] It is clear that the SGAs differ in their mechanisms of action and most likely in the manner in which they produce an atypical clinical profile.

The primary therapeutic effects of FGAs are thought to occur in the limbic system, including the ventral striatum, whereas EPS are thought to be related to DA blockade in the dorsal striatum. 5-HT_{2A} antagonism in combination with modest D_2 blockade leads to release of dopamine in the prefrontal cortex, and this is one explanation for the decrease in negative symptoms and improvement in cognition reported with atypical antipsychotics.

Antipsychotics vary in their effects on other neurotransmitter receptor systems.[48,49,51] Although the significance of these different mechanisms on efficacy is unclear, they do potentially explain differences in side-effect profiles. These differences in pharmacodynamic profiles point out that the SGAs are not all alike, and patients obtaining an inadequate clinical response (either efficacy or side effects) with one antipsychotic may have a superior response on an alternate drug. Thus serial SGA monotherapy trials should be tried in patients receiving a suboptimal clinical response (see Fig. 76–1).

PHARMACOKINETICS

As a class, antipsychotics are highly lipophilic and highly bound to membranes and plasma proteins. They distribute readily into most tissues with a high blood supply and can accumulate in tissues; therefore they have large volumes of distribution.[56] Most antipsychotics are largely metabolized, primarily through the cytochrome P450 (CYP) pathways in the liver, except for ziprasidone, which is largely metabolized by aldehyde oxidase. Fluphenazine, perphenazine, and risperidone are metabolized through CYP2D6, and thus are susceptible to polymorphic metabolism.[57] This is also one of the major pathways for the metabolism of iloperidone.[54] Thirty percent to 35% of Africans and Asians are slow to intermediate metabolizers, and approximately 0% to 5% of African Americans, 1% of Asians, and 0% to 5% of Caucasians are poor metabolizers.[57] In addition, some populations of patients, those from Ethiopian or Swedish descent in particular, may be ultra-rapid metabolizers. Polymorphism in CYP1A2 can potentially result in a decrease the metabolic rate of clozapine, and increased clozapine metabolic rate in smokers has been linked to a specific genotype.[57] The possibility of genetic polymorphism should be considered when dosing and monitoring the clinical effects of antipsychotics. Table 76–6 outlines the prominent metabolic pathways of selected antipsychotics.

Asenapine is unique in that it has less than 2% bioavailability after oral administration, but has a bioavailability of approximately 35% sublingually—the FDA approved route of administration. Eating and drinking within 10 minutes after sublingual administration will reduce bioavailability.[55]

Most antipsychotics have fairly long elimination half-lives, generally 24 hours or more, with the exception of quetiapine and ziprasidone, which have short half-lives.[53,56] Among the SGAs, only clozapine has an established therapeutic serum concentration, with efficacy being associated with a clozapine plasma concentration greater than 350 ng/mL (350 mcg/L; 1.07 μmol/L).[27] Whether a potential maximum therapeutic clozapine serum concentration exists is unknown. Clozapine serum concentration should be obtained before exceeding 600 mg daily; in patients who develop unusual or severe adverse side effects; in patients who are taking concomitant medications that can cause drug interactions; in patients who have age or pathophysiologic changes suggesting a change in pharmacokinetics; or for assessment of patient adherence.[32,33,56]

Long-acting risperidone is a suspension of drug in glycolic acid-lactate copolymer microspheres.[35] After IM injection the polymer is slowly hydrolyzed, and significant risperidone begins being released after about 3 weeks. The apparent β-phase half-life is 3 to 6 days.[35] With dosing every 2 weeks, steady-state risperidone concentrations are achieved after approximately 2 months. The apparent half-life with paliperidone palmitate after single dose administration ranges from 25 to 49 days.[34] The long-acting FGAs fluphenazine decanoate and haloperidol decanoate are esterified drugs formulated in sesame seed oil for deep intramuscular injection. Their absorption from the muscle and metabolism to the free base is sufficiently slow to cause absorption to be the rate-limiting step in determining their respective apparent half-lives.[36]

TABLE 76-6 Pharmacokinetic Parameters of Selected Antipsychotics

Drug	Bioavailability (%)	Half-Life (h)	Major Metabolic Pathways	Active Metabolites
Selected first-generation antipsychotics (FGAs)				
Chlorpromazine	10–30	8–35	FMO3, CYP3A4	7-hydroxy, others
Fluphenazine	20–50	14–24	CYP2D6	?
Fluphenazine decanoate		14.2 ± 2.2[a]days	CYP2D6	
Haloperidol	40–70	12–36	CYP1A2, CYP2D6, CYP3A4	Reduced haloperidol
Haloperidol decanoate		21 days	CYP1A2, CYP2D6, CYP3A4	Reduced haloperidol
Perphenazine	20–25	8.1–12.3	CYP2D6	7-OH-perphenazine
Second-generation antipsychotics (SGAs)				
Aripiprazole	87	48–68	CYP3A4, CYP2D6	Dehydroaripiprazole
Asenapine	<2% PO 35% SL Nonlinear	13–39	CYP1A2, UGT1A4	None known
Clozapine	12–81	11–105	CYP1A2, CYP3A4, CYP2C19	Desmethylclozapine
Iloperidone	96	18–33	CYP2D6, CYP3A4	P88
Olanzapine	80	20–70	CYP1A2, CYP3A4, FMO3	N-glucuronide; 2-OH-methyl; 4-N-oxide
Paliperidone ER	28	23	Renal unchanged (59%) Multiple pathways	None known
Paliperidone Palmitate		25–49 days	Renal unchanged (59%)Multiple pathways	None known
Quetiapine	9 ± 4	6.88	CYP3A4	7-OH-quetiapine
Risperidone	68	3–24	CYP2D6	9-OH-risperidone
Risperidone Consta		3–6 days	CYP2D6	9-OH-risperidone
Ziprasidone	59	4–10	Aldehyde oxidase, CYP3A4	None

[a]Based on multiple dose data. Single dose data indicate a β–half-life of 6–10 days.

Data from Citrome,[34,54,55] Harrison and Goa,[35] Ereshefsky et al.,[36,37] DeLeon et al.,[53] Mauri et al.,[56] Zhou, et al.,[57] Spina and de Leon.[111] and Urichuk, et al.[112]

■ ADVERSE EFFECTS

Table 76–7 presents the relative incidence of common categories of antipsychotic side effects. Side effects are discussed below with respect to organ system affected. A general approach to monitoring and assessing side effects requires prospective monitoring by clinicians, preferably using a thorough review of systems approach. Patient-oriented self-rated side-effect scales can be helpful, as many patients with schizophrenia do not readily complain of side effects.

With the variety of antipsychotics currently available, using an alternative medication should be considered in patients who complain of poorly tolerated side effects. Because medication side effects are one of the primary predictors of patient nonadherence, the clinician should take advantage of the treatment options currently available in an attempt to improve patient outcomes. As new antipsychotics become available, side effects and risks associated with different drugs should be reevaluated. As we learn more about relative side-effect risks (e.g., weight gain, glucose intolerance, QTc prolongation, acute EPS, and tardive dyskinesia), it will be necessary to regularly reconsider which antipsychotics should be considered first-line treatment alternatives.

Endocrine System

DA blockade in the tuberoinfundibular tract results in increased prolactin levels as DA is the major prolactin-inhibiting factor. Hyperprolactinemia may occur in up to 87% of patients treated with FGAs, risperidone or paliperidone. The major side effects associated with hyperprolactinemia are gynecomastia, galactorrhea, menstrual irregularities, decreased libido, and sexual dysfunction. Although not conclusive, chronic hyperprolactinemia has been associated with decreased bone density. Tolerance does

TABLE 76-7 Relative Side-Effect Incidence of Commonly Used Antipsychotics[a,b]

	Sedation	EPS	Anticholinergic	Orthostasis	Weight Gain	Prolactin
Aripiprazole	+	+	+	+	+	+
Asenapine	+	++	+/–	++	+	+
Chlorpromazine	++++	+++	+++	++++	++	+++
Clozapine	++++	+	++++	++++	++++	+
Fluphenazine	+	++++	+	+	+	++++
Haloperidol	+	++++	+	+	+	++++
Iloperidone	+	+/–	++	+++	++	+
Olanzapine	++	++	++	++	++++	+
Paliperidone	+	++	+	++	++	++++
Perphenazine	++	++++	++	+	+	++++
Quetiapine	++	+	+	++	++	+
Risperidone	+	++	+	++	++	++++
Thioridazine	++++	+++	++++	++++	+	+++
Thiothixene	+	++++	+	+	+	++++
Ziprasidone	++	++	+	+	+	+

EPS, extrapyramidal side effects; Relative side-effect risk: ±, negligible; +, low; ++, moderate; +++, moderately high; ++++, high.
[a]Side effects shown are relative risk based on doses within the recommended therapeutic range.
[b]Individual patient risk varies depending on patient-specific factors.

not appear to develop to antipsychotic induced hyperprolactinemia. Switching to aripiprazole or ziprasidone, which have minimal sustained effect on prolactin, is the most reasonable treatment option.[58]

Weight gain is frequently reported in both adults and children receiving antipsychotics.[58,59] Although the exact mechanism is uncertain, weight gain has been associated with antihistaminic effects, antimuscarinic effects, and blockade of 5-HT$_{2C}$ receptors including 5-HT$_{2c}$ receptor polymorphism. However, dietary factors and activity levels can play a significant role in this population, as does renourishment after a period of poor self-care. In particular, significant weight gain, as defined by greater than or equal to 7% of the baseline body weight, after 1 year of treatment has been seen in as many as is 80% of patients treated with olanzapine, 58% treated with risperidone, and 50% treated with quetiapine.[58] The risk of weight gain may be greater in patients with their first psychotic episode. Ziprasidone and aripiprazole both have been associated with minimal weight gain.

The clinical significance of weight gain during antipsychotic therapy is substantial. The risk of cardiovascular-related mortality is higher in individuals with schizophrenia,[58,60] and this is further aggravated by drug-related weight gain and the high prevalence of smoking. Additionally, obesity is a risk factor for diabetes mellitus.[58] Weight gain during treatment is a major reason for poor patient medication adherence, and patients commonly report weight gain as being a concern.[61]

Several different genetic variations have been correlated with predisposition for antipsychotic-associated weight gain. Recent meta-analysis of all genetic studies looking at the −759 C/T promoter region polymorphism of the 5-HT$_{2C}$ receptor gene confirmed an association of 5-HT$_{2C}$ in antipsychotic-induced weight gain.[62] Polymorphisms in leptin and leptin receptor genes have also been linked with clozapine and olanzapine-associated weight gain.[63,64] Alfa-2a-adrenergic receptor gene, G protein beta-3 subunit gene, and brain-derived neurotrophic factor (BDNF) gene have been genetic targets; however, results are inconsistent as to whether a relationship exists with these polymorphisms and antipsychotic-associated weight gain.[65–67]

A number of pharmacologic interventions have been attempted for antipsychotic-related weight gain, but in general these should be discouraged. Switching patients to antipsychotics less likely to cause weight gain, dietary restriction, exercise, and behavior modification programs are reported to be successful in small short-term studies.[68] An American Diabetes Association consensus task force recommends consideration of a change in antipsychotic if a patient gains more than 5% of baseline body weight after starting the drug.[69]

Schizophrenic patients have a higher prevalence of type 2 diabetes than the nonschizophrenic population. Beyond this, antipsychotics may adversely affect glucose levels in diabetic patients. The extent to which these effects are related to drug-induced weight increase is unclear.[58,69] Data collected from the FDA MedWatch Drug Surveillance System for clozapine, olanzapine, quetiapine, and risperidone indicate that nearly 60% of the new-onset diabetes reported occurred within the first 6 months of treatment initiation.[58,69] Olanzapine has the highest risk of new-onset diabetes followed by risperidone and then quetiapine. Although likely less than with the other SGAs, inadequate data are available to accurately estimate the risk with ziprasidone and aripiprazole.[58] Clozapine likely poses a risk at least as great as with olanzapine. The 2009 PORT recommendations do not recommend olanzapine as a first line antipsychotic option.[27] In March 2004, the FDA issued a safety alert requiring revisions in the labeling of all SGAs that describes the increased risk of diabetes mellitus in patients taking atypical antipsychotics.[70] Given the public health significance of diabetes,

clarifying the diabetogenic effect of SGAs is a major focus of current research. Moreover, designing care models and standards for managing diabetes in patients with schizophrenia is another major consideration.

CLINICAL CONTROVERSY

The relative risk of diabetes mellitus versus the risk of EPS associated with different antipsychotics makes individual antipsychotic choice challenging. This is particularly true given that olanzapine causes the most weight gain and appears to have the highest risk of precipitating diabetes mellitus (except for clozapine), but yet research does show some modest benefits with regard to efficacy.

Cardiovascular System

Orthostatic Hypotension Postural or orthostatic hypotension, defined as a greater than 20-mm Hg drop in systolic pressure, is caused by α-adrenergic blockade, and may occur in up top 75% of treated patients.[71] Antipsychotics with a greater risk should have their doses titrated over several days to decrease the risk of symptomatic hypotension. Antipsychotic combination treatment may result in a greater risk of orthostasis.[71] Orthostatic hypotension can occur in any patient, but diabetic patients with preexisting cardiovascular disease and the elderly seem particularly predisposed. Patients should be advised to slowly move to the standing position to allow for adaptation. Tolerance to this effect may occur within 2 to 3 months. If not, lower doses or a change to an antipsychotic with less α-blockade can be attempted.

Electrocardiographic Changes Among the antipsychotics, thioridazine, clozapine, iloperidone, and ziprasidone are most likely to cause electrocardiogram (ECG) changes. ECG changes include increased heart rate (through sinus tachycardia from anticholinergic effects, or reflex tachycardia from α-adrenergic blockade), flattened T waves, ST segment depression, and prolongation of QT and PR intervals. The most clinically important of these potential changes is prolongation of the QTc, which has been associated with ventricular arrhythmias, including torsades de pointes syndrome. Thioridazine has been shown to prolong the QTc on average approximately 20 milliseconds (msec) longer than haloperidol, risperidone, olanzapine, or quetiapine.[72] Thioridazine's effects on QTc prolongation is dose related, and has led to a black box warning in the FDA-approved product labeling. In the same study, ziprasidone prolonged the QTc approximately 10 msec longer or about one-half of the effect of thioridazine.[71] Widespread clinical use suggests that ziprasidone's effects on the ECG are not associated with clinical sequelae, unless the patient has baseline risk factors.[71] Iloperidone has a dose-related effect on QTc, with an average prolongation of about 9 msec at a dose of 20 to 24 mg/day.[54] Although the precise point at which QTc prolongation becomes clinically dangerous is unclear, it has been recommended to discontinue a medication associated with QTc prolongation if the interval consistently exceeds 500 msec.

Greater caution regarding antipsychotic choice and use is necessary in the elderly, in patients with preexisting cardiac or cerebrovascular disease, and in patients taking diuretics or medications that may prolong the QTc.[71] In patients older than 50 years of age, a pretreatment ECG is recommended, as are baseline serum potassium and magnesium levels. These factors should be considered in antipsychotic selection.

Sudden Cardiac Death A recent, large retrospective analysis found risk of sudden cardiac death with current use of FGAs and SGAs was twice that of nonusers of antipsychotics,[73,71] with risk increasing with escalated dose. Further meta-analysis has conferred a lack of evidence for differential effects on cardiovascular mortality favoring one class of antipsychotics over the other.[71,73] Further prospectively designed studies are needed to confirm a dose-dependent increase in cardiovascular sudden death with current antipsychotic use, and also to determine whether certain antipsychotics are associated with a greater risk than others.

Lipid Changes

Treatment with at least some SGAs and phenothiazines appears associated with elevations in serum triglycerides and cholesterol. Oxidation of apolipoprotein B lipoproteins and elevations in sterol regulatory element binding protein-controlled gene expression, are among the purported mechanisms by which these lipid changes occur during antipsychotic treatment.[74,75] Among the SGAs, less risk for change in serum lipid or cholesterol levels can occur with risperidone, ziprasidone, or aripiprazole.[58,60] In the CATIE trial, olanzapine was associated with greater and significant adverse effects on metabolic parameters, including lipids, blood glucose, and body weight versus the other study treatments, but these differences in tolerability did not affect discontinuation rates.[76]

The occurrence of weight gain, diabetes, and lipid abnormalities during antipsychotic therapy is consistent with the development of metabolic syndrome (i.e., syndrome X). Cohorts of patients with schizophrenia have shown elevated prevalence of metabolic syndrome as compared with general population cohorts. Prevalence rates of metabolic syndrome in U.S. populations range from 28% to 60%, with 40.9% reported in the prospectively designed CATIE trial.[77]

Metabolic syndrome consists of raised triglycerides (greater than or equal to 150 mg/dL [170 mmol/L]), low HDL cholesterol (less than or equal to 40 mg/dL [103 mmol/L] for males, l less than or equal to 50 mg/dL [1.29 mmol/L] for females), elevated fasting glucose (greater than or equal to 100 mg/dL [5.6 mmol/L]), blood pressure elevation (greater than or equal to 130/85 mm Hg), and weight gain (abdominal circumference greater than 102 cm [40 in] for males, greater than 88 cm [34 in] in females).[58,60] These abnormalities dictate an important role for general health screening and monitoring in patients with schizophrenia, and prompt intervention when such abnormalities occur. The propensity of individual antipsychotics to produce metabolic disturbances should be considered in the context of individual patient risk factors at the time of drug selection.

Autonomic Nervous System

Patients receiving antipsychotics or antipsychotics in combination with anticholinergics, can experience anticholinergic side effects (e.g., dry mouth, constipation, tachycardia, blurred vision, inhibition or impairment of ejaculation, urinary retention, or impaired memory). This is particularly so with low-potency FGAs, and the elderly are especially sensitive to these effects. Of the SGAs, clozapine and olanzapine have moderately high rates of causing anticholinergic effects. Constipation, caused by slowed peristaltic movement and decreased intestinal fluid content, should be closely monitored and treated, especially in the elderly. Paralytic ileus and necrotizing enterocolitis can also occur.

Central Nervous System

Extrapyramidal System

Dystonia. Dystonia is a state of abnormal tonicity, sometimes described simplistically as a severe "muscle spasm."[78,79] More accurately, they are prolonged tonic contractions, with a rapid onset,

TABLE 76-8	Agents Used to Treat Extrapyramidal Side Effects	
Generic Name	**Equivalent Dose (mg)**	**Daily Dosage Range (mg)**
Antimuscarinics		
Benztropine[a]	1	1–8[b]
Biperiden[a]	2	2–8
Trihexyphenidyl	2	2–15
Antihistaminic		
Diphenhydramine[a]	50	50–400
Dopamine agonist		
Amantadine	NA	100–400
Benzodiazepines		
Lorazepam[a]	NA	1–8
Diazepam	NA	2–20
Clonazepam	NA	2–8
β-Blockers		
Propranolol	NA	20–160

NA, not applicable
[a]Injectable dosage form can be given intramuscularly for relief of acute dystonia.
[b]Dosage can be titrated to 12 mg/day with careful monitoring; nonlinear pharmacokinetics have been reported.

usually within 24 to 96 hours of dosage initiation or dosage increase. They can be life-threatening, as in the case of pharyngeal-laryngeal dystonias, and can contribute to patient nonadherence. Types of dystonic reactions include trismus, glossospasm, tongue protrusion, pharyngeal-laryngeal dystonia, blepharospasm, oculogyric crisis, torticollis, and retrocollis. Dystonic reactions occur primarily with FGAs. Risk factors include younger patients (especially males), the use of high-potency agents, and high dosage. The overall incidence from the 1960s through the mid-1970s ranged from 2.3% to 10%, but as higher-potency traditional antipsychotics became more widely used, the rate increased to as high as 64%.

Intramuscular or intravenous anticholinergics (Table 76–8) or benzodiazepines are the treatments of choice for dystonia. Benztropine mesylate 2 mg or diphenhydramine 50 mg can be given intramuscularly or intravenously. Diazepam 5 to 10 mg by slow IV push or lorazepam 1 to 2 mg intramuscularly are treatment alternatives. Relief is typically seen within 15 to 20 minutes of an intramuscular injection and within 5 minutes of intravenous administration. The antipsychotic can be continued, with concomitant short-term use of oral anticholinergic agents. In general, prophylactic anticholinergic medications are not recommended routinely with all FGAs. However, prophylaxis is reasonable when using high-potency FGAs (e.g., haloperidol or fluphenazine) in young men, and in patients with a history of dystonia.[80] Dystonias can also be minimized by the use of lower initial FGA doses. Anticholinergics are good choices for prophylaxis, whereas amantadine has not been proven effective for this purpose. The risk of dystonia is greatly reduced with SGAs.

Akathisia. Akathisia is defined as the inability to sit still and as being functionally motor restless. The most accurate diagnosis is made by combining subjective complaints with objective symptoms (pacing, shifting, shuffling, or tapping feet). Subjectively, patients may describe a feeling of inner restlessness or disquiet or a compulsion to move or remain in constant motion. Akathisia occurs in 20% to 40% of patients treated with high-potency FGAs.[79,80] Akathisia is frequently accompanied by dysphoria.

Akathisia responds poorly to anticholinergics.[79,80] Traditionally, reduction in antipsychotic dosage has been considered the best intervention; however, this might not be a realistic goal in an acutely psychotic patient. A logical alternative is to switch to an antipsychotic with a lower risk of akathisia, or an antipsychotic previously used in the patient without adverse effect. Akathisia can occasionally occur with SGAs. Quetiapine and clozapine appear to have the lowest risk of producing akathisia.[79,80]

Benzodiazepines have been used for treatment of akathisia, but the high prevalence of co-occurring substance abuse in schizophrenia discourages their prescribing.[80] The β-blockers (e.g., propranolol in doses up to 160 mg daily, nadolol in doses up to 80 mg daily, and metoprolol in β_2-selective doses of 100 mg daily or less) are reported as effective.[80]

Pseudoparkinsonism. Pseudoparkinsonism, produced by D_2 blockade in the nigrostriatum, resembles idiopathic Parkinson disease. A patient with pseudoparkinsonism can present with any of four cardinal symptoms: (1) akinesia, bradykinesia, or decreased motor activity including difficulty initiating movement, as well as extreme slowness, mask-like facial expression, micrographia, slowed speech, and decreased arm swing; (2) tremor, known as pill-rolling type, that is predominant at rest and decreases with movement, usually involving the fingers and hands, although tremors can also be seen in the arms, legs, neck, head, and chin; (3) cogwheel rigidity, seen as the patient's limbs yielding in jerky, ratchet-like fashion when passively moved by the examiner; and (4) postural abnormalities and instability manifested as stooped posture, difficulty in maintaining stability when changing body position, and a gait that ranges from slow and shuffling to festinating. Fatigue and weakness can be noted, as well as oral abnormalities including dysphagia, dysarthria, and abnormal palmomental and glabellar reflexes. The overall incidence of pseudoparkinsonism from FGAs ranges from 15.4% to 36%, depending on the drug and dose. Akinesia alone can be seen in 59% of patients on high-potency FGAs. Other risk factors include increasing age and possibly female gender. The onset of symptoms is typically 1 to 2 weeks after initiation of antipsychotic therapy or a dose increase.

The efficacy of anticholinergic medications in treating symptoms of pseudoparkinsonism is well established.[79,80] Benztropine's long half-life allows once- to twice-daily dosing. Typical dosing is 1 to 2 mg twice a day up to a usual maximum dosage of 8 mg daily, although some patients will continue to respond to doses up to 12 mg. Trihexyphenidyl (2–5 mg 3 times a day), diphenhydramine (25–50 mg 3 times a day), and biperiden (2 mg 3 times a day) usually require thrice-daily administration. Diphenhydramine produces more sedation than the other agents. All of the anticholinergics have been abused for their euphoriant effects.[78] Symptoms typically begin to resolve within 3 to 4 days after initiation of treatment, but a minimum of at least 2 weeks of treatment is normally required for full response. Amantadine is generally as efficacious for pseudoparkinsonism as anticholinergics, with significantly less effect on memory function.[80] The need for prophylactic use of these agents against pseudoparkinsonism is less convincing than with dystonias, and is unnecessary when using SGAs.[80] The long-term treatment of pseudoparkinsonism with antiparkinsonism medication is somewhat controversial, and an attempt should be made to taper and discontinue these agents 6 weeks to 3 months after symptom resolution. If symptoms reappear, then switching to an SGA should be considered. The risk of pseudoparkinsonism with SGAs is low. When risperidone is used in doses greater than 6 mg/day, the risk of pseudoparkinsonism symptoms approaches that with FGAs. Quetiapine, aripiprazole, or clozapine are reasonable alternatives in a patient experiencing extrapyramidal side effects with other SGAs.[32,53,79,80]

Tardive Dyskinesia. Tardive dyskinesia is a syndrome characterized by abnormal involuntary movements occurring late in onset in relation to initiation of antipsychotic therapy. Tardive dyskinesia is sometimes irreversible and continues to be a controversial issue.

The classic description of tardive dyskinesia is the buccallingualmasticatory (BLM) syndrome, or orofacial movements. The onset of BLM movements is usually insidious. Typically, they are the first detectable signs of tardive dyskinesia and begin with mild forward, backward, or lateral movements of the tongue. As the disorder progresses, more obvious or frank BLM movements appear, including tongue thrusting, rolling, or fly-catching movements, and chewing or lateral jaw movements. Tardive dyskinesia symptoms can interfere with the patient's ability to chew, speak, or swallow. Further complications include oral ulcerations, inability to wear dentures, and inflammation and loosening of mandibular joints. Eating difficulties and malnutrition can be severe complications. Weight loss can be seen in patients with esophageal or respiratory manifestations but not in those with truncal movements. Facial movements include frequent blinking, brow arching, grimacing, upward deviation of the eyes, and lip smacking. Involvement of the extremities sometimes occurs, with the appearance of restless choreiform and distal athetosis of limbs including twisting, spreading, flexion and extension of fingers, toe tapping, and toe dorsiflexion. Unusual posture, hyperextension, pelvic thrusting, axial hyperkinesia ballismus, exaggerated lordosis, rocking, and swaying are occasionally observed. Among the differential diagnoses are withdrawal dyskinesias occurring after short-term use of antipsychotics, spontaneous orofacial dyskinesias in the elderly, orofacial dyskinesias in the edentulous, stereotypic movements in schizophrenics, Huntington disease, and congenital torsion dystonia. Orofacial movements are more common in older patients, whereas the truncal axial movements are classically reported in young adults. Movements can worsen with stress, decrease with sedation, and disappear during sleep. Concentration on motor tasks or attempts to suppress the movements can actually increase them.

Early signs of tardive dyskinesia can be reversible but if allowed to persist they can become irreversible, even with drug discontinuation. When the antipsychotic dose is decreased or tapered and discontinued, worsening of abnormal movements can occur, followed by possible slow improvement after months or years if the patient remains on lower doses or discontinues treatment. No standardized diagnostic criteria for tardive dyskinesia are available. Abnormal involuntary movements can be detected early through physical assessment and the use of rating scales. Available rating scales include the Abnormal Involuntary Movements Scale (AIMS) and the Dyskinesia Identification System: Condensed User Scale (DISCUS).[32,81] Neither scale is diagnostic in itself.

Risk factors include increasing age, the occurrence of acute EPS, poor antipsychotic drug response, diagnosis of organic mental disorder, diabetes mellitus, mood disorders, and possibly female gender.[78,79] Duration of antipsychotic therapy, daily dosage, and possibly total cumulative dosage are probably the most significant risk factors. Polymorphisms of the dopamine D_3 receptor, 5-HT$_{2C}$ receptor, and the superoxide dismutase-2 genes have all been implicated in varying the risk of TD with antipsychotic use.[82] Overall morbidity and mortality are greater in tardive dyskinesia patients.

With FGAs, the reported incidence of tardive dyskinesia ranges from 0.5% to 62%.[78,79] In a first episode of schizophrenia, the incidence is estimated at about 5% per year, with the overall prevalence ranging from 20% to 25% with long-term treatment. Among the elderly, the overall risk of tardive dyskinesia is higher.[78] Tardive dyskinesia is not always permanent, with remission of symptoms observed in 25% of patients after 5 years of continued treatment.[78]

The risk of tardive dyskinesia with SGAs is significantly lower.[79] A systematic review of 11 studies with SGAs lasting 1 year or more found an overall risk of tardive dyskinesia to be approximately 0.8% per year in nonelderly (<65 years) adults and 5.3% per year in the elderly (≥65 years). For individual agents, the annual incidence rates ranged from zero to 0.5% for olanzapine to 0.6% to 0.7% for risperidone or quetiapine. To date, there are no reports of tardive dyskinesia with clozapine monotherapy.

Prevention of tardive dyskinesia is important, as treatment of the movements once they occur is difficult. One of the more compelling arguments for the first-line use of SGAs is their lower risk of tardive dyskinesia.[25,32,83] (see Fig. 76–1). Regular neurologic examinations (AIMS or other scales) should be performed at baseline and at least quarterly to assess for early signs of tardive dyskinesia. At the first signs of tardive dyskinesia, the need for continuing antipsychotic treatment should be reassessed. In such situations, if the patient is taking an FGA and continuing treatment is indicated, the medication should be switched to an SGA.

Numerous drugs have been used in an attempt to treat tardive dyskinesia. In two controlled trials lasting 22 to 52 weeks, clozapine decreased abnormal involuntary movements.[78,84] Switching antipsychotic therapy to clozapine is a favored first-line pharmacotherapeutic strategy, particularly in patients with moderate to severe dyskinesias.[78,79,84]

Sedation and Cognition Chlorpromazine, thioridazine, mesoridazine, clozapine, olanzapine, and quetiapine are the most sedating antipsychotics. Administration of most or all of the daily dosage at bedtime can decrease daytime sedation and in some patients eliminate the need for hypnotic agents. Sedation occurs early in treatment and can decrease over time.[32] Oversedation can play a large role in cognitive, perceptual, and motor dysfunction. However, positive effects of medication on cognition are seen with chronic administration, evidenced by improvements in tasks involving visual-motor skills, attention to task, and working memory. Compared with FGAs, several studies have shown cognitive benefits of SGAs. However, results from the CATIE trial showed no differences in cognitive improvement between SGAs and the FGA perphenazine.[85] Comparative effects of different SGAs on cognition are as yet unclear, but available studies suggest that different SGAs can have effects on varying cognitive domains.[86] An algorithm-driven disease management program was shown to improve cognition over a 9-month period.[87]

Seizures An increased risk of drug-induced seizures occurs in all patients treated with antipsychotics. However, this risk is greater if the following predisposing factors are present: preexisting seizure disorder, history of drug-induced seizure, abnormal electroencephalogram (EEG), and preexisting CNS pathology or head trauma. Seizures are more closely associated with the use of higher doses, rapid dosage increases, and on initiation of treatment. When an isolated seizure occurs, a dosage decrease is first recommended; anticonvulsant therapy is not recommended. Although spontaneously occurring seizures have been reported with most antipsychotics, the highest potential risk for an antipsychotic-related seizure is with clozapine or chlorpromazine. If a change in antipsychotic therapy is required because of a drug-induced seizure, risperidone, molindone, thioridazine, haloperidol, pimozide, trifluoperazine, and fluphenazine are associated with the lowest potential.[80]

Thermoregulation Poikilothermia, the body temperature adjusting to the ambient temperature, can be a serious side effect of antipsychotic therapy in temperature extremes.[88] Hyperpyrexia can be a danger in hot weather or during exercise. Inhibition of sweating, a result of anticholinergic properties impairing the peripheral mechanisms of heat dissipation, can also contribute to this problem, which in its severest form can lead to heat stroke. Hypothermia is also a risk, particularly in the elderly (≥65 years) and in cold climates. All patients receiving antipsychotics should be educated about these potential problems. Thermoregulatory problems are reportedly more common with the use of low-potency FGAs and can occur with the more anticholinergic SGAs.

Neuroleptic Malignant Syndrome Neuroleptic malignant syndrome (NMS) occurs in 0.5% to 1% of patients receiving FGAs. The rate of NMS has diminished since the introduction of SGAs, and reliable current estimates of the incidence with SGAs are not available. NMS can occur more frequently in patients receiving high-potency FGAs, injectable or depot FGAs, and in patients who are dehydrated, with physical exhaustion, or organic mental disorders. Although less common, NMS has been reported with SGAs, including clozapine. The onset of symptoms varies from early in treatment to months later. It develops rapidly, over the course of 24 to 72 hours. NMS can occur after antipsychotic discontinuation, especially when depot agents are used. Possible mechanisms of NMS include disruption of the central thermoregulatory process or excess production of heat secondary to skeletal muscle contractions. The differential diagnosis includes heat stroke, lethal catatonia, anesthetic-associated malignant hyperthermia, anticholinergic toxicity, and monoamine oxidase inhibitor drug interactions. Cardinal signs and symptoms of NMS are body temperature exceeding 38°C (100.4°F), altered level of consciousness, autonomic dysfunction (tachycardia, labile blood pressure, diaphoresis, tachypnea, or urinary or fecal incontinence), and rigidity. Laboratory evaluation, although nonspecific, frequently shows leukocytosis with or without a left shift, increases in creatine kinase (CK), aspartate aminotransferase, alanine aminotransferase, lactate dehydrogenase, and myoglobinuria.[80]

Treatment should begin with antipsychotic discontinuation and supportive care. In many cases that alone is effective. The role of adjunctive agents is unclear, yet they are often used. The DA agonist bromocriptine reduces rigidity, fever, or CK in up to 94% of patients, whereas the use amantadine has been successful in up to 63% of patients. Dantrolene has been used as a skeletal muscle relaxant, with effects on temperature, heart rate, respiratory rate, and CK in up to 81% of patients.[80] Wide recognition and rapid antipsychotic discontinuation has drastically reduced mortality from 20% 25 years ago to 4% in the mid-1990s.

Many patients with schizophrenia, despite having had NMS, will require future antipsychotic pharmacotherapy. A review of antipsychotic rechallenges suggests that the risk of rechallenge is acceptable in most patients, provided that the patient is observed for an extended period of time (2 weeks or more is suggested) without antipsychotics, that there is careful monitoring and slow dose titration, and that the patient is maintained on the lowest possible dose.[80] A different antipsychotic, a SGA or a low potency FGA, should be used for rechallenge following an episode of NMS.

Psychiatric Side Effects Antipsychotic-induced akathisia, akinesia, and dysphoria can have unfortunate sequelae, resulting in what has been termed "behavioral toxicity."[30] Akinesia, characterized by "diminished spontaneity," results in symptoms of apathy and withdrawal, often mistaken for the negative symptoms of schizophrenia; these patients can actually appear depressed. Delirium and psychosis are reported with larger doses of FGAs or combinations of anticholinergics with FGAs. Chronic confusion and disorientation can occur in the elderly as a result of antipsychotic treatment.[89] Unfortunately, the link is not always made with antipsychotic therapy, and the patient is misdiagnosed with an delirium from a different etiology. This clinical presentation, called a *pseudodementia*, may be reversible on discontinuation of the antipsychotic.

Ophthalmologic Effects Anticholinergic effects of antipsychotics or concomitant antiparkinson medications can exacerbate narrow-angle (angle closure) glaucoma. Antipsychotics with low anticholinergic effects should be used in such individuals, and they should be appropriately monitored.[90]

Opaque deposits in the cornea and lens occur with chronic phenothiazine treatment, most frequently with chlorpromazine. Although visual acuity is not usually affected, periodic slit-lamp ophthalmologic examinations are frequently recommended in patients receiving long-term treatment with phenothiazines, as fully formed cataracts are a possibility.[90]

Because of cataract development and lenticular changes in animals, baseline and periodic eye examinations are recommended in the product labeling for quetiapine.[91] However, clinical use of quetiapine since marketing has not shown a significant risk of cataracts.[32,91] Retinitis pigmentosa can result from use of thioridazine doses greater than 800 mg daily. It is caused by melanin deposits and can result in permanent visual impairment or blindness.

Genitourinary System

Urinary hesitancy and retention is reported with low-potency FGAs and with clozapine. Anticholinergic effects cause smooth muscle slowing and paralyze the detrusor muscle of the bladder, requiring greater urine volume to evoke muscle contraction. Men with benign prostatic hypertrophy are especially prone to this effect.[92]

Urinary incontinence is thought to be caused by α-blockade, and among the SGAs, it appears to be particularly problematic with clozapine. The incidence has been reported to be as high as 44%, and it can be persistent in 25% of patients.[93]

Numerous mechanisms may result in sexual dysfunction, including dopaminergic blockade, hyperprolactinemia, histaminergic blockade (sedation), anticholinergic effects, and α-adrenergic blockade. Although inadequately studied, multiple mechanisms are likely responsible for sexual dysfunction. Unmedicated individuals with schizophrenia report decreased libido. Most but not all studies show a relationship between hyperprolactinemia and sexual dysfunction, including decreased libido, erectile dysfunction, difficulty achieving orgasm, and ejaculatory abnormalities. Although risperidone produces at least as much sexual dysfunction as FGAs, other SGAs, which have weak effects on prolactin, produce less sexual dysfunction. It is unclear whether hyperprolactinemia directly impairs sexual functioning, reflects high dopaminergic blockade from risperidone and FGAs, or is associated with other mechanisms of producing sexual dysfunction. Patients experiencing sexual dysfunction with FGAs or risperidone should be switched to an SGA with less effect on prolactin.[94]

Hematologic System

Transient leukopenia can occur during initial treatment with antipsychotics; however, it typically does not progress to clinically significant parameters.[95] The three antipsychotics with highest relative risk of neutropenic are in rank order clozapine, chlorpromazine, and olanzapine.[96] If the WBC count is less than 3,000/mm³ (3×10^9/L), or if the absolute neutrophil count (ANC) is less than 1,000/mm³ (1×10^9/L), the antipsychotic should be discontinued, and the WBC monitored closely until it returns to normal. Agranulocytosis reportedly occurs in 0.01% of patients receiving FGAs, and more frequently with chlorpromazine and thioridazine. The onset is usually within the first 8 weeks of therapy. Agranulocytosis can initially manifest as a local infection, with sore throat, leukoplakia, erythema, and ulcerations of the pharynx. These symptoms in any patient receiving antipsychotics should signal the immediate need for a WBC count. If either the WBC count or ANC falls below these parameters, the drug should be discontinued immediately and the patient monitored closely for the development of secondary infections. Isolated rare cases of thrombocytopenia and eosinophilia have been reported.

Agranulocytosis with clozapine significantly limits the usefulness of this agent. Data reveal that the risk of developing neutropenia or agranulocytosis with clozapine is approximately 3% and 0.8%, respectively.[96] Increasing age and female gender are associated with greater risk. The time period for greatest risk is between months 1 and 6 of treatment, and weekly WBC monitoring for the first 6 months of therapy is mandated in the FDA-approved product labeling. After the first 6 months, the labeling allows the frequency of WBC monitoring to be decreased to every 2 weeks for months 7

through 12, after which it can be decreased to monthly if all WBCs are normal. If the total WBC count drops to less than 2,000/mm³ (2×10^9/L), or the ANC is less than 1,000/mm³ (1×10^9/L), clozapine should be discontinued and the patient monitored closely. Granulocyte colony-stimulating factor filgrastim has been used in hope of hastening resolution or decreasing morbidity. In cases of moderate neutropenia (granulocytes 2,000–3,000/mm³ [2×10^9/L to 3×10^9/L], or ANC 1,000–1,500/mm³ [1×10^9/L to 1.5×10^9/L]), which occurs in up to 2% of patients, clozapine should be discontinued with daily monitoring of complete blood counts until values return to normal.

Dermatologic System

Allergic reactions are rare and usually occur within 8 weeks of initiating therapy, manifesting as maculopapular, erythematous, pruritic rashes that are evident on the face, neck, trunk, or extremities. Contact dermatitis, including the oral mucosa, can occur in patients or medical personnel. For patients, mixing the antipsychotic concentrate in a sufficient quantity of a nonacidic liquid and swallowing it quickly decreases problems in susceptible patients. Care should be taken in the handling and preparation of liquid FGAs.

Phenothiazine can absorb ultraviolet light, resulting in the formation of free radicals, which can have damaging effects on the skin. Both SGAs and FGAs cause photosensitivity. Erythema and severe sunburns can occur. Exposure to sunlight should be limited, and patients should be educated about the use of a maximally blocking sunscreen, hats, protective clothing, and sunglasses.[97,98]

Blue-gray or purplish skin coloration in areas exposed to sunlight occurs in patients receiving higher doses of low-potency phenothiazines during long-term administration, especially with chlorpromazine. It commonly occurs with concurrent corneal or lens pigmentation.

Miscellaneous Adverse Effects

A sometimes troubling side effect with clozapine is sialorrhea, which can occur in up to 54% of patients. The mechanism of clozapine-induced drooling is unclear. Although both anticholinergics and α-agonists have been used to treat clozapine related sialorrhea, research evidence is insufficient to make specific recommendations.[99]

■ TOXICITY WITH OVERDOSE

Acute overdose with antipsychotics rarely results in serious symptomatology. Mild intoxication manifests as sedation, hypotension, and miosis, whereas with severe intoxication, agitation and delirium can typically progress to motor retardation, seizures, cardiac arrhythmias, respiratory arrest, and coma. Dystonias and pseudoparkinsonism symptoms also occur. Supportive measures, gastric lavage, and activated charcoal are recommended. Induction of emesis can be difficult because of effects on the chemoreceptor trigger zone, and dialysis is ineffective because of the degree of drug-protein binding. Phenytoin or sodium bicarbonate are useful in the treatment of quinidine-like cardiac conduction effects on the QRS or QTc. Physostigmine is not generally recommended to reverse anticholinergic toxicity because of deleterious effects on arrhythmias and seizure threshold.[98]

■ USE IN PREGNANCY AND LACTATION

Minimal data exist regarding the effects of pregnancy on schizophrenia. However, disorganized thought processes, impaired cognition, and negative symptoms can have a detrimental effect on the functioning and self-care of the mother, and therefore adversely affect the fetus.[100] Currently available data assessing the risk of teratogenesis with antipsychotic agents are insufficient. Epidemiologic studies show a slightly increased risk of birth defects with low-potency FGAs. Haloperidol is the best studied of all antipsychotics, and no relationship between its use and teratogenicity has been found. A recent study has shown a greater than 2-fold elevated risk of preterm birth in women with schizophrenia taking FGAs as compared with unaffected mothers not taking antipsychotics.[101]

SGAs have increasing information available regarding safety in pregnancy; however, very few large studies and very few prospective studies have been performed to evaluate possible teratogenicity of SGAs. Definitive data are still lacking. Two prospectively designed nonrandomized, observational studies have reported no increased risk of teratogenic birth defects with SGA exposure.[102,103] One large registry data study performed in Sweden found a significant increased risk of cardiovascular defects with FGA or SGA exposure;[104] however, when stratifying by antipsychotic class, it was found that all defects were found in those exposed to FGAs, while no cardiovascular defects were reported with SGAs.[105]

Studies have shown differing results in regard to neonatal outcomes in infants exposed to SGAs in utero. Women with schizophrenia taking SGAs showed no significant risk of low birth weight (LBW), preterm birth, or infant considered small or large for gestational age (LGA) when compared to infants born to unaffected and unexposed mothers.[101] One prospectively designed study found a higher rate of LBW infants in mothers taking SGAs (10%) than in the reference group (2%),[102] while another recent prospective study reported higher rates of LGA infant births in women taking SGAs compared with those in the FGA and reference groups.[106]

Other potential interests in studying early and late exposure to antipsychotics include postnatal and gestational complications. Concern has been expressed regarding the use of clozapine in pregnancy.[107] The weight gain associated with olanzapine and clozapine and potential risk of gestational diabetes [108] should be considered in drug selection. Risk of neonatal EPS has been shown to be increased in those exposed in utero to FGAs, with effects in the infant lasting for 3 to 12 months after birth.[108] Other adverse neonatal outcomes reported in babies of mothers taking SGAs include respiratory complications and hypotonia.[108]

The risk of antipsychotic use must be weighed against the benefits of pharmacotherapy in pregnant women experiencing disorganized thoughts, delusions about change in body image or pregnancy, or who are unable to provide adequate prenatal care.[100]

Antipsychotics appear in breast milk with milk-to-plasma ratios of 0.5 to 1. However, 1 week after delivery, clozapine milk concentrations have been found to be as much as 279% of serum concentrations. Its use during breastfeeding is not recommended.[107] Overall, little is known about breast-feeding and the potential effects of antipsychotics on the neonate. Although not contraindicated, the lowest dosage should be used in the mother, and the infant should be carefully monitored.

■ DRUG INTERACTIONS

Most drug interactions occur because of pharmacodynamic or pharmacokinetic interactions. Common examples of pharmacodynamic interactions resulting in enhanced effect include the excess sedation that can occur when antipsychotics are used concomitantly with other medications that have sedative side effects. Additive antimuscarinic effects of antipsychotics used with other medications with antimuscarinic effects can result in urinary retention, constipation, blurred vision, or other anticholinergic side effects.[30,109] Both combined sedative and anticholinergic effects from multiple medications can result in impaired cognition,

particularly in the elderly and other patients predisposed to such problems.[109] Patients are more likely to experience symptomatic orthostatic hypotension when an antipsychotic is used with other medications that cause orthostasis. Although metoclopramide is prescribed for treating esophageal reflux, it is a DA antagonist, and patients are more likely to experience akathisia and other EPS if it is used concomitantly with antipsychotics.[72] Although some SSRIs can interact with antipsychotics through enzyme inhibition, they can also interact through pharmacodynamic mechanisms. $5\text{-}HT_2$ receptors are present on the presynaptic dopaminergic neuron, and their activation leads to decreased dopamine release from the presynaptic terminal. Increased availability of serotonin through SSRI effect can activate these receptors, decrease dopamine release, and add to the dopaminolytic effects of antipsychotics.[72] In the absence of enzyme inhibition, SSRIs can still precipitate akathisia or EPS when added to a patient stabilized on an antipsychotic. A potentially more dangerous interaction can occur when medications that slow myocardial conduction and thus prolong the QTc, are used in combination with antipsychotics that significantly prolong the QTc.[72] Medications that prolong the QTc should be monitored carefully in patients taking concomitant diuretics.[72] These effects can all increase the risk of clinically significant side effects.

Asenapine inhibits CYP2D6, and is the only SGA that has been shown to significantly affect the pharmacokinetics of other medications.[55] Table 76–6 lists the major pathways thought to be involved in the metabolism of SGAs. Risperidone is metabolized primarily by CYP2D6 to its active metabolite, 9-OH-risperidone (paliperidone), which is thought to have a similar pharmacodynamic profile.[72] CYP1A2 is the primary isoenzyme for metabolism of asenapine with CYP3A4 also being a significant pathway.[55]

Based on current information, inhibitors of CYP1A2 have the greatest potential for causing interactions with clozapine and olanzapine.[106] Examples include cimetidine, fluvoxamine, and fluoroquinolone antibiotics (e.g., ciprofloxacin) to varying degrees. To date, however, no serious inhibition interactions have been reported with olanzapine, which may be a result of olanzapine's wide therapeutic index. Carbamazepine has been reported to increase olanzapine elimination by as much as 50%.[110] Cigarette smoking is a potent inducer of CYP1A2, and one would expect lower mean olanzapine serum concentrations in smokers compared with nonsmokers.

Because of the risk of seizures with higher clozapine tissue concentrations, interactions which inhibit clozapine's metabolism are potentially significant. In particular, fluvoxamine increases clozapine serum concentrations by an average of two- to threefold and up to five-fold.[110,111] Fluoxetine and erythromycin can increase clozapine serum concentrations in some patients but to a lesser degree.[110,111] Mean clozapine serum concentrations are reported to be 32% lower in smokers compared with nonsmokers.[110] Carbamazepine can induce clozapine metabolism and lead to lower serum concentrations.[110]

A study with the potent CYP3A4 inhibitor ketoconazole showed minimal effects on ziprasidone single-dose pharmacokinetics, with only a 33% mean increase in the ziprasidone area under the time-versus-concentration curve.[72] These results are consistent with data suggesting that aldehyde oxidase is the major metabolic pathway for ziprasidone, with only 30% to 35% being metabolized by CYP3A4.[112]

Modest elevations of aripiprazole serum concentration occur in the presence of ketoconazole or quinidine, which inhibit CYP2D6 and 3A4, respectively. Carbamazepine has been reported to decrease aripiprazole serum concentrations.[53,111]

Since iloperidone is metabolized through CYP2D6 and 3A4, its clearance can be impaired by inhibitors of these pathways. Since iloperidone prolongs the QTc interval, these types of interactions have the potential to be clinically significant. For example, it is recommended that the iloperidone dose be decreased by 50% when used with CYP2D6 inhibitors such as fluoxetine or paroxetine.[54]

Table 76–9 summarizes potential antipsychotic drug interactions.

■ PHARMACOECONOMIC CONSIDERATIONS

It is estimated that approximately 80% of individuals suffering their first schizophrenic break will have recurrent episodes and significant lifetime psychosocial dysfunction. In 2004, the direct cost of treating schizophrenia in the United States was estimated to be

---

TABLE 76-9 Common Potential Drug Interactions with Antipsychotic Medications

Pharmacodynamic Drug Interactions with Antipsychotics

Mechanism of Interaction	Examples of Interacting Drugs or Other Substances			Clinical Effect
Muscarinic receptor blockade	*Anticholinergics* Benztropine Diphenhydramine Trihexyphenidyl			↑ Anticholinergic SE Blurred vision Constipation Impaired Cognition Urinary retention

Additive or synergistic sedation	*Sedatives*
	Benzodiazepines
	Concomitant AP
	Diphenhydramine
	Melatonin and melatonin
	  agonists
	Mirtazapine
	Trazodone
	TCAs
	Zaleplon
	Zolpidem
	Anticholinergics
	Benztropine
	Diphenhydramine
	Trihexyphenidyl
	Mirtazapine
				↑ Sedation
				Lethargy
				Impaired cognition Impaired psychomotor
				  activity
				↑ Risk of accidents

DA antagonist use for different indication	Metoclopramide			↑ EPS
Cardiovascular Interactions				
Additive effects on QTc	*TCA Antidepressants* Amitriptyline Clomipramine Imipramine	Procainamide Quinidine		↑ *Risk of ECG changes and dysrhythmias*
Electrolyte changes	Diuretics			
Stimulation of presynaptic 5-HT receptors on DA neuron	SSRIs			↑ *EPS*
Sympatholytics: αblockade–↓ NE release	Clonidine Methyldopa Prazosin			↑ Hypotension
↑ DA receptor binding	*Antipsychotics*			↑ SEs, particularly EPS

Pharmacokinetic Drug Interactions with Antipsychotics

Mechanism of Interaction	Examples of Interacting Drugs			Clinical Effect
Aripiprazole and Iloperidone				
Inhibition of AP metabolism (CYP2D6, CYP3A4)	*Antidepressants* Bupropion Clomipramine Doxepin Duloxetine Fluoxetine Fluvoxamine Paroxetine Sertraline *HIV Protease Inhibitors* Indinavir Nelfinavir Ritonavir	*Anti-infectives* Ciprofloxacin Clarithromycin Erythromycin Fluconazole Ketoconazole Itraconazole *Antipsychotics* Asenapine Chlorpromazine Haloperidol Perphenazine Thioridazine	*Miscellaneous* Amiodarone Chlorpheniramine Cimetidine Cocaine Diltiazem Diphenhydramine Cimetidine Grapefruit juice Haloperidol Hydroxyzine Methadone Quinidine Ticlopidine Verapamil	↑ AP effect ↑ SE
Induction of AP metabolism	*Antiepileptics* Carbamazepine Oxcarbazepine Phenobarbital Phenytoin	*Anti-infectives* Rifampin *Miscellaneous* Glucocorticoids Modafinil	*Herbals* St. John's wort	↓ AP effect

(continued)

TABLE 76-9 Common Potential Drug Interactions with Antipsychotic Medications (continued)

Pharmacokinetic Drug Interactions with Antipsychotics

Mechanism of Interaction	Examples of Interacting Drugs			Clinical Effect

Asenapine

Eating food or drinking liquids within 10 minutes of asenapine sublingual administration will decrease bioavailability.

Mechanism of Interaction	Examples of Interacting Drugs			Clinical Effect
Inhibition of AP metabolism (CYP1A2)	*Antidepressants* Fluvoxamine	*Anti-infectives* Ciprofloxacin Fluroquinolones	*Miscellaneous* Amidarone Cimetidine	↑ AP effect ↑ SE
Induction of AP metabolism	*Anti-infectives* Nafcillin	*Miscellaneous* Broccoli Brussel sprouts Chargrilled meat Smoking tobacco	*Miscellaneous* Insulin Modafinil Omeprazole	↓ AP effect

Clozapine

Mechanism of Interaction	Examples of Interacting Drugs			Clinical Effect
Inhibition of AP metabolism (CYP3A4, CYP1A2, CYP2C19)	*Antidepressants* Fluoxetine Fluvoxamine *HIV protease inhibitors* Indinavir Nelfinavir Ritonavir *Anticonvulsants* Felbamate Oxcarbazepine	*Anti-infectives* Ciprofloxacin Clarithromycin Erythromycin Fluconazole Ketoconazole Itraconazole Nafcillin	*Miscellaneous* Amidarone Diltiazem Cimetidine Grapefruit juice Haloperidol Modafinil Omeprazole Ticlopidine Topiramate Verapamil Cimetidine	↑ AP effect ↑ SE
Induction of AP metabolism	*Antiepileptics* Carbamazepine Phenobarbital Phenytion	*Anti-infectives* Rifampin *Miscellaneous* Glucocorticoids Insulin Modafinil Omeprazole	*Herbals* St. John's wort	↓ AP effect

Haloperidol

Mechanism of Interaction	Examples of Interacting Drugs			Clinical Effect
Inhibition of AP metabolism (CYP2D6, OP3A4, CYP1A2)	*Antidepressants* Bupropion Doxepin Duloxetine Fluoxetine Fluvoxamine Paroxetine Sertraline *HIV protease inhibitors* Indinavir Nelfinavir Ritonavir Sequinavir	*Anti-infectives* Ciprofloxacin Clarithromycin Erythromycin Fluoconazole Fluoroquinolones Ketoconazole Itraconazole *Antipsychotics* Chlorpromazine Perphenazine	*Miscellaneous* Amiodarone Chlorpheniramine Cimetidine Diltiazem Diphenhydramine Quinidine Diphenhydramine Cimetidine Grapefruit juice Hydroxyzine Methadone Quinidine Verapamil	↑ AP effect ↑ SE
Induction of AP metabolism	*Anticonvulsants* Carbamazepine Oxcarbazepine Phenobarbital Phenytoin	*Anti-infectives* Nafcillin Rifampin *Miscellaneous* Broccoli Brussel sprouts Chargrilled meat Glucocorticoids Insulin Modafinil Omeprazole Modafinil	*Herbals* St. John's wort Tobacco smoking	↓ AP effect

Iloperidone (See Aripiprazole)

Olanzapine

Mechanism of Interaction	Examples of Interacting Drugs			Clinical Effect
Inhibition of AP metabolism (CYP3A4 & CYP1A2)	*Antidepressants* Fluoxetine (norfluoxetine) Fluvoxamine *HIV Protease Inhibitors* Indinavir Nelfinavir Ritonavir	*Anti-infectives* Ciprofloxacin Clarithromycin Erythromycin Fluconazole Fluoroquinolones Ketoconazole Itraconazole	*Miscellaneous* Amiodarone Cimetidine Diltiazem Cimetidine Grapefruit juice Verapamil	↑ AP effect ↑ SE

(continued)

TABLE 76-9 Common Potential Drug Interactions with Antipsychotic Medications (continued)

Pharmacokinetic Drug Interactions with Antipsychotics

Mechanism of Interaction	Examples of Interacting Drugs			Clinical Effect
Induction of AP metabolism	*Aniepileptics* Carbamazepine Oxcarbazepine Phenobarbital Phenytoin *HIV protease inhibitors* Efavirenz Nivirapine	*Anti-infectives* Nafcillin Rifampin *Miscellaneous* Broccoli Brussel sprouts Chargrilled meat Glucocorticoids Insulin Modafinil Omeprazole	*Herbals* St. John's wort Smoking tobacco	↓ AP effect

Paliperidone

The bioavailability of paliperidone is significantly increased when it is taken with food. Although this could increase paliperidone effect, including adverse effects, the clinical significance is undetermined.

| *Quetiapine*
Inhibition of AP metabolism (CYP3A4) | *Antidepressants*
Fluoxetine (norfluoxetine)
Fluvoxamine
Nefazodone
HIV protease inhibitors
Indinavir
Nelfinavir
Ritonavir
Sequinavir | *Anti-infectives*
Ciprofloxacin
Clarithromycin
Erythromycin
Fluoconazole
Ketoconazole
Itraconazole | *Miscellaneous*
Amiodarone
Cimetidine
Diltiazem
Grapefruit juice
Verapamil | ↑ AP effect
↑ SE |
| Induction of AP metabolism | *Antiepileptics*
Carbamazepine
Oxcarbazepine
Phenobarbital
Phenytoin
HIV Protease Inhibitors
Efavirenz
Nivirapine | *Anti-infectives*
Rifampin
Miscellaneous
Glucocorticoids
Modafinil | *Herbals*
St. John's wort | ↓ AP effect |

Perphenazine and risperidone

Note: Because risperidone's metabolite formed through CYP2D6 metabolism is active (paliperidone), the clinical significance of metabolic drug interactions with risperidone is undetermined.

| Inhibition of AP metabolism (CYP2D6) | *Antidepressants*
Bupropion
Clomipramine
Doxepin
Duloxetine
Fluoxetine
Paroxetine
Sertraline

Antipsychotics
Chlorpromazine
Haloperidol (reduced haloperidol)
Perphenazine | *Miscellaneous*
Amiodarone
Cimetidine
Chlorpheniramine
Cocaine
Diphenhydramine
Cimetidine
Haloperidol
Hydroxyzine
Methadone
Quinidine | | ↑ AP effect
↑ SE |
| Induction of AP metabolism | Dexamethasone
Rifampin | | | ↓ AP effect |

Ziprasidone

The bioavailability of ziprasidone is increased twofold when it is taken with food. Consistent administration with food is recommended.

AP, antipsychotic; DA, dopamine; EPS, extrapyramidal symptoms; 5-HT, serotonin; SE, side effect; SSRI, serotonin selective reuptake inhibitor; TCAs, tricyclic antidepressants.
(Data from references 54, 55, 109–112, 122.)

nearly $23 billion and the total costs were over $62.6 billion.[113] The public mental healthcare sector provides the majority of services for individuals with schizophrenia. Mental healthcare costs for schizophrenia represent disproportionate expenditures for crisis intervention and hospitalization as compared with comprehensive outpatient services oriented toward maintaining remission and improving psychosocial functioning. The suboptimal or inadequate funding provided for efficient ambulatory mental health services further increases the demand for hospitalization, which diverts revenues that might be available for outpatient services. This has created a vicious revolving door cycle and is a major challenge facing public mental healthcare.

The advent of more expensive SGAs, accompanied by limited resources, has forced mental healthcare organizations to examine the outcomes and related economics of treating patients with SGAs compared with traditional, largely generic FGAs. Although several retrospective database studies found total mental healthcare cost advantages for SGAs versus FGAs, in the prospective effectiveness study, CATIE, total mental health costs were higher for SGAs than the FGA perphenazine, and these costs were driven by the higher acquisition costs of the SGAs.[114] Some studies have shown clozapine to result in lower overall mental healthcare costs, while others have shown no difference in costs compared with FGAs. Additionally, clozapine decreases suicidality more than comparator antipsychotics, and it is more effective in treatment-resistant schizophrenia.[115,116]

Despite mental health service utilization increasing 65% over the past decade, there has not been a corresponding decrease in the prevalence of mental disorders or in suicidality.[117] CATIE is the first prospective comparative effectiveness study to evaluate the clinical outcomes and costs associated with different treatments in schizophrenia. Until we have better information regarding the comparative effectiveness of different treatments and how to best implement these treatments, controversy regarding reimbursement for mental health services, including medication formulary decisions, will continue.

EVALUATION OF THERAPEUTIC OUTCOMES

Assessment of response has traditionally been done subjectively or empirically (a relative sense of how the clinician feels the patient is doing). A formal mental status examination (MSE) is used to structure the patient interview and focus on items related to appearance, mood, sensorium, intellectual functioning, and thought processes. However, the MSE is not specific for the measurement of drug response. ❿ Clinicians should be trained to use simple, standardized psychiatric rating scales to assist in objectively rating patient drug responses.[32,118] The Brief Psychiatric Rating Scale (BPRS) and the Positive and Negative Symptom Scale (PANSS) were developed for use in clinical trials as research tools to quantify symptoms and improvement seen with antipsychotic treatment.[118] Objectively, the use of a numeric indicator (e.g., 20%, 30%, or 40% reduction in BPRS score) has been used to quantify overall symptom reduction and classify patients according to different degrees of response. However, these types of rating scales are too long and unwieldy to be routinely used within the time constraints of most clinical practices. Symptom scales used in clinical practice must be sufficiently brief to be used during an ordinary clinic visit (e.g., 15–30 minutes) while measuring both

positive and negative symptoms, and being sufficiently representative of overall symptomatology. The four-item Positive Symptom Rating Scale and the Brief Negative Symptom Assessment are brief scales that meet such criteria (Table 76–10).[32,118] It is increasingly recognized that clinicians should be examining cognition as an outcome in treatment of schizophrenia. A brief cognition battery has been developed and validated, and it can be completed in 15 to 20 minutes.[119]

Similarly, the pharmacotherapeutic plan should include specific monitoring parameters for side effects. The plan should include how the potential side effect will be evaluated, and the frequency of assessment. Given the risk of weight gain, diabetes, and lipid abnormalities associated with many of the SGAs, a consensus task force led by the American Diabetes Association recommends the following baseline parameters before beginning antipsychotics: family history, weight, height, body mass index, waist circumference, blood pressure, fasting plasma glucose, and fasting lipid profile.[68] They also recommend follow-up monitoring of these parameters after beginning or changing SGAs. Weight should be monitored monthly for the first 3 months, and quarterly thereafter. The other parameters should be assessed at the end of 3 months and then annually. If normal, serum lipids can be monitored less often. Self-assessments can be a useful adjunct in treating the patient. Although the patient with schizophrenia may not always be accurate in evaluating symptom severity, the use of patient self-assessments increases patient engagement in care, enhances therapeutic alliance, and gives the clinician an opportunity to identify misconceptions the patient can have regarding symptoms associated with the illness, medication side effects, and the like.[118,120] Traditionally, clinicians have often accepted partial symptom response in schizophrenia as success, and have not been aggressive in attempting to achieve greater symptomatic remission. The advent of multiple different SGAs with varying, but overall favorable, side-effect profiles should encourage clinicians to be more assertive in attempting to achieve symptom remission. This is consistent with an increasing focus on remission as a goal of treatment and evolving recovery movements with an emphasis on consumerism in the care of the severely mentally ill.[21,22] A recent study showing how the Internet can be used to aid relapse prevention efforts gives us a glimpse of how consumerism may enhance and influence the care for schizophrenia in the future.[121]

TABLE 76-10 Brief Clinical Assessments for Monitoring Antipsychotic Response in Schizophrenia

4-Item Positive Symptom Rating Scale (PSRS)
Use each item's anchor points to rate the patient.

1. Suspiciousness	NA[a]	1	2	3	4	5	6	7
2. Unusual thought content	NA	1	2	3	4	5	6	7
3. Hallucinations	NA	1	2	3	4	5	6	7
4. Conceptual disorganization	NA	1	2	3	4	5	6	7
Each item is scored from 1 (not present) to 7 (extremely severe)							SCORE: _____

Brief Negative Symptom Assessment (BNSA)
Use each item's anchor points to rate the patient.

1. Prolonged time to respond	1	2	3	4	5	6
2. Emotion: Unchanging facial expression, blank, expressionless face	1	2	3	4	5	6
3. Reduced social drive	1	2	3	4	5	6
4. Poor grooming and hygiene	1	2	3	4	5	6
Each item is scored from 1 (normal) to 6 (severe)					SCORE: _____

[a] NA, not able to be assessed

To enhance consistency in ratings, the structured probes in the Administration Manual should be used each time the scales are used. The complete Administration Manual for the PSRS and the BNSA can be accessed from the appendices in the Texas Medication Algorithm Project Procedural Manual for Schizophrenia at the Texas Department of State Health Services Website http://www.dshs.state.tx.us/mhprograms/TIMA.shtm.

Argo TR, Crismon ML, Miller AL, et al. Schizophrenia Treatment Algorithms, Texas Medication Algorithm Project Procedural Manual. Austin, TX: Texas Department of State Health Services, 2008. 62 pps. Available at http://www.dshs.state.tx.us/mhprograms/TIMA.shtm. Copyrighted © by and reprinted with the express permission of the Texas Department of State Health Services.

CONCLUSIONS

Schizophrenia is a complex disease with multiple ramifications for patients and their families. Treatment issues remain clouded by the fact that the etiology of the illness is unknown. It is clear that no single treatment modality is adequate to properly manage a patient with schizophrenia. Antipsychotics are the bedrock of treatment. Antipsychotics are not a panacea and have multiple adverse effects that limit their effectiveness. However, when used within the context of multidisciplinary treatment, antipsychotics improve symptoms so that patients can appropriately participate in psychosocial rehabilitation programs. Scientific advances continue to expand our understanding of CNS physiology and the abnormalities present in schizophrenia. Advances in our understanding of the pathophysiology of schizophrenia should, in turn, result in the development of treatments that are more specific and more effective. In practice, it is mandatory that clinicians appropriately use their expanding armamentarium. It is important that clinicians appreciate the pharmacodynamic basis for treatment interventions so that they can effectively design and implement rational pharmacotherapeutic regimens. Finally, it is critical that clinicians more objectively evaluate individual patient response to medication so that treatment can be optimized. With these strategies, the gap between practice and science can be narrowed and patients' lives benefited.

ABBREVIATIONS

AIMS: Abnormal Involuntary Movement Scale

ANC: absolute neutrophil count

BDNF: brain-derived neurotrophic factor

BLM: buccal-lingual-masticatory

BPRS: Brief Psychiatric Rating Scale

CAT: computed axial tomography

CATIE: Clinical Antipsychotic Trials of Intervention Effectiveness study

CK: creatine kinase

CYP: cytochrome P450

CNS: central nervous system

D_1: dopamine-1 receptor

D_2: dopamine-2 receptor

DA: dopamine

DISCUS: Dyskinesia Identification System: Condensed User Scale

DSM-IV-TR: *Diagnostic and Statistical Manual of Mental Disorders, Fourth Edition, Text Revision*

ECG: electrocardiogram

ECT: electroconvulsive therapy

EEG: electroencephalogram

EPS: extrapyramidal side effect

FDA: U.S. Food and Drug Administration

FGA: first-generation antipsychotic

GABA: γ-aminobutyric acid

5-HT: serotonin

LFT: liver function test

MRI: magnetic resonance imaging

MSE: mental status examination

msec: millisecond

NAMI: National Alliance for the Mentally Ill

NMDA: *N*-methyl-D-aspartate

NMS: neuroleptic malignant syndrome

PANSS: Positive and Negative Symptom Scale

PET: positron emission tomography

SGA: second-generation antipsychotic

SSRI: selective serotonin reuptake inhibitor

WBC: white blood cell

REFERENCES

1. American Psychiatric Association. Schizophrenia and other psychotic disorders. In: Diagnostic and Statistical Manual of Mental Disorders, Fourth Edition, Text Revision. Washington, DC: American Psychiatric Association, 2000:297–319.
2. Os JV, Kapur S. Schizophrenia. Lancet 2009;374:635–645.
3. Jones P, Buckley P. Schizophrenia. London: Mosby, 2006.
4. Weinberger D. Schizophrenia as a neurodevelopmental disorder. In: Weinberger DR, Hirsch SR, eds. Schizophrenia. Oxford, UK: Blackwell Science, 2003:326–348.
5. Brown AS, Susser ES. In utero infection and adult schizophrenia. Ment Retard Dev Disabil Res Rev 2002;8:51–57.
6. Mahadik, SP, Evans DR. Is schizophrenia a metabolic brain disorder? Membrane phospholipid dysregulation and its therapeutic implications. Psychiatr Clin North Am 2003;26:41–63.
7. Ho BC, Andreasen NC, Nopoulos P, et al. Progressive structural brain abnormalities and their relationships to clinical outcome: A longitudinal magnetic resonance imaging study early in schizophrenia. Arch Gen Psychiatry 2003;60:585–594.
8. McClure RK, Lieverman JA. Neurodevelopmental and neurodegenerative hypothesis of schizophrenia: A review and critique. Curr Opin Psychiatry 2003;16(Suppl 2):S15–S28.
9. Buckley PF, Mahadik S, Evans D, Stirewalt E. Causes, course, and neurodevelopment of schizophrenia. Curr Psychosis Ther Rep 2003;1:41–49.
10. McDonald C, Murphy KC. The new genetics of schizophrenia. Psychiatr Clin North Am 2003;26:41–63.
11. The International Schizophrenia Consortium, Stone JL, O'Donovan MC, et al. Rare chromosomal deletions and duplications increase risk of schizophrenia. Nature 2008;455:237–241.
12. Stafansson H, Rujescu D, Cichon S, et al. Large recurrent microdeletions associated with schizophrenia. Nature 2008;455:232–236.
13. Weickert, CS Straub RE, McClintock BW, et al. Human dysbindin (DTNBP1) gene expression in normal brain and in schizophrenia prefrontal cortex and midbrain. Arch Gen Psychiatry 2004;61:544–555.
14. Suarez BK, Duan J, Sanders AR, et al. Genomewide linkage scan of 409 European-ancestry and African American families with schizophrenia: Suggestive evidence of linkage at 8p23.3-p21.2 and 11p13.1-q14.1 in the combined sample. Am J Hum Genet 2006;78:315–333.
15. Ke M, Zou R, Shen H, et al. Bilateral functional asymmetry disparity in positive and negative schizophrenia revealed by resting-state fMRI. Psychiatry Res 2010;182:30–39.
16. Velakoulis D, Wood SJ, Wong MT, et al. Hippocampal and amygdala volumes according to psychosis stage and diagnosis. A magnetic resonance imaging study of chronic schizophrenia, first-episode psychosis, and ultra-high risk individuals. Arch Gen Psychiatry 2006;63:139–149.
17. Narendran R, Frankle WG, Keefe R, et al. Altered prefrontal dopaminergic function in chronic recreational ketamine users. Am J Psychiatry 2005;162:2352–2359.
18. Meltzer HY. What's atypical about atypical antipsychotic drugs? Curr Opin Pharmacol 2004;4:53–57.
19. Lehman AF, Lieberman JA, Dixon LB, et al. American Psychiatric Association Practice Guidelines; Work Group on Schizophrenia. Practice guideline for the treatment of patients with schizophrenia, 2nd ed. Am J Psychiatry 2004;161(2 Suppl):1–56.
20. Castle DJ, Buckley PF. Schizophrenia. Oxford, UK: Oxford University Press, 2008.

21. President's New Freedom Commission on Mental Health. Achieving the Promise: Transforming Mental Health Care in America. Final Report. DHHS Pub. No. SMA-03-3832. Rockville, MD; 2003.

22. Improving the Quality of Health Care for Mental and Substance-Use Conditions: Quality Chasm Series. Committee on Crossing the Quality Chasm: Adaptation to Mental Health and Addictive Disorders. Rockville, MD: Institute of Medicine, National Academies Press; 2005.

23. Substance Abuse and Mental Health Services Administration National Consensus Statement on Mental Health Recovery Rockville, MD: U.S. Department of Health and Human Services; 2006.

24. Davidson L, Chinman M, Sells D, et al. Peer support among adults with mental illness: a report from the field. Schizophr Bull 2006;32:443–450.

25. Moore TA, Buchanan RW, Buckley PF, et al. The Texas Medication Algorithm Project antipsychotic algorithm for schizophrenia: 2006 update. J Clin Psychiatry 2007;68:1751–1762.

26. Buchanan RW, Kreyenbuhl J, Kelly DL, et al. The 2009 schizophrenia PORT psychopharmacological treatment recommendations and summary statements. Schizophr Bull 2010;36:71–93.

27. Lieberman JA, Stroup TS, McEvoy JP, et al. Effectiveness of antipsychotic drugs in patients with chronic schizophrenia. N Engl J Med 2005;353:1209–1223.

28. Alvarez-Jimenez M, Parker AG, Hetrick SE, et al. Preventing the second episode: a systematic review and meta-analysis of psychosocial and pharmacological trials in first-episode psychosis. Schizophrenia Bulletin 2009 Nov 9. [Epub ahead of print]

29. Green AL, Canuso CM, Brenner MJ, Wojcik JD. Detection and management of comorbidity in patients with schizophrenia. Psychiatr Clin North Am 2003;26:115–139.

30. Van Putten T, Marder SR. Behavioral toxicity of antipsychotic drugs. J Clin Psychiatry 1987;48(Suppl 9):13–19.

31. Miller D, Ellingrod V, Holman TL, et al. Clozapine-induced weight gain associated with 5HT2C receptor–759C/T polymorphism. Am J Med Genet B Neuropsychiatr Genet 2005;133:97–100.

32. Argo TR, Crismon ML, Miller AL, et al. Schizophrenia Treatment Algorithms, Texas Medication Algorithm Project Procedural Manual. Austin, TX: Texas Department of State Health Services; 2008. *http://www.dshs.state.tx.us/mhprograms/TIMA.shtm.*

33. Leucht S, Barnes TR, Kissling W, et al. Relapse prevention in schizophrenia with new-generation antipsychotics: A systematic review and exploratory meta-analysis of randomized, controlled trials. Am J Psychiatry 2003;160:1209–1222.

34. Citrome L. Paliperidone Palmitate – a review of the efficacy, safety and cost of a new second-generation depot antipsychotic medication. Int J Clin Pract 2010;64:216–239.

35. Harrison TS, Goa KL. Long-acting risperidone: A review of its use in schizophrenia. CNS Drugs 2004;18:113–132.

36. Ereshefsky L, Saklad SR, Jann MW, et al. Future of depot neuroleptic therapy: Pharmacokinetics and pharmacodynamic approaches. J Clin Psychiatry 1984;45(5 pt 2):50–59.

37. Ereshefsky L, Toney G, Saklad SR, Seidel DR. A loading dose strategy for converting from oral to depot haloperidol. Hosp Community Psychiatry 1993;44:1155–1161.

38. Hamann GL, Egan TM, Wells BG, et al. Injection site reactions after intramuscular administration of haloperidol decanoate 100 mg/mL. J Clin Psychiatry 1990;51:502–504.

39. Lindenmayer JP, Liu-Seifert H, Kulkarni PM, et al. Medication nonadherence and treatment outcomes in patients with schizophrenia or schizoaffective disorder with suboptimal prior response. J Clin Psychiatry 2009;70:990–996.

40. Rummel-Kluge C, Kissling W. Psychoeducation for patients with schizophrenia and their families. Expert Rev Neurother 2008;8:1067–1077.

41. O'Donnell C, Donohue G, Sharkey L, et al. Compliance therapy: A randomised controlled trial in schizophrenia. BMJ 2003;327:834.

42. Kane J, Honigfeld G, Singer J, et al. Clozapine for the treatment-resistant schizophrenic: A double-blind comparison with chlorpromazine. Arch Gen Psychiatry 1988;45:789–796.

43. Spears NM, Leadbetter RA, Shutty MS. Clozapine treatment in polydipsia and intermittent hyponatremia. J Clin Psychiatry 1996;57:123–128.

44. Leucht S, Kissling W, McGrath J. Lithium for schizophrenia revisited: A systematic review and meta-analysis of randomized controlled trials. J Clin Psychiatry 2004;65:177–186.

45. Casey DE, Daniel DG, Wassef AA, et al. Effect of divalproex combined with olanzapine or risperidone in patients with an acute exacerbation of schizophrenia. Neuropsychopharmacology 2003;28:182–192.

46. Silver H. Selective serotonin reuptake inhibitor augmentation in the treatment of negative symptoms of schizophrenia. Int Clin Psychopharmacol 2003;18:305–313.

47. Kapur S, Roy P, Daskalakis J, Remington G. Increased dopamine D_2 receptor occupancy and elevated prolactin level associated with addition of haloperidol to clozapine. Am J Psychiatry 2001;158:311–314.

48. Kapur S, Mamo D. Half a century of antipsychotics and still a central role for dopamine D_2 receptors. Prog Neuropsychopharmacol Biol Psychiatry 2003;27:1081–1090.

49. Meltzer L, Li Z, Kaneda Y, Ichikawa J. Serotonin receptors: Their key role in drugs to treat schizophrenia. Prog Neuropsychopharmacol Biol Psychiatry 2003;27:1159–1172.

50. Nyberg S, Eriksson B, Oxenstierna G, et al. Suggested minimal effective dose of risperidone based on PET measured D_2 and 5-HT_{2A} receptor occupancy in schizophrenic patients. Am J Psychiatry 1999;156:869–875.

51. Kapur S, Zipursky RB, Remington G. Clinical and theoretical implications of 5-HT_2 and D_2 receptor occupancy of clozapine, risperidone, and olanzapine in schizophrenia. Am J Psychiatry 1999;156:286–293.

52. Stahl SM, Shayegan DK. The psychopharmacology of ziprasidone: Receptor-binding properties and real-world psychiatric practice. J Clin Psychiatry 2003;64(Suppl 19):6–12.

53. De Leon A, Patel NC, Crismon ML. Aripiprazole: A comprehensive review of its pharmacology, clinical efficacy, and tolerability. Clin Ther 2004;26:649–666.

54. Citrome L. Iloperidone for schizophrenia: a review of the efficacy and safety profile for this newly commercialized second-generation antipsychotic. Int J Clin Pract 2009;63:1237–1248.

55. Citrome L. Asenapine for schizophrenia and bipolar disorder: a review of the efficacy and safety profile for this newly approved sublingually absorbed second-generation antipsychotic. Int J Clin Pract 2009;63:1762–1784.

56. Mauri MC, Volonteri LS, Colasanti A, et al. Clinical pharmacokinetics of atypical antipsychotics: a critical review of the relationship between plasma concentrations and clinical response. Clin Pharmacokinet 2007;46:359–388.

57. Zhou SF, Liu JP, Chowbay B. Polymorphism of human cytochrome P450 enzymes and its clinical impact. Drug Metabolism Reviews 2009;41:89–295.

58. Monteleone P, Martiadis V, Maj M. Management of schizophrenia with obesity, metabolic and endocrinological disorders. Psychiatr Clin North Am 2009;32:775–794.

59. Correll CU, Manu P, Olshanskiy, et al. Cardiometabolic risk of second-generation antipsychotic medications during first-time use in children and adolescents. JAMA 2009;302:1765–1773.

60. Meyer JM. Cardiovascular illness and hyperlipidemia in patients with schizophrenia. In: Meyer JM, Nasarallah HA, eds. Medical Illness and Schizophrenia. Washington, DC: American Psychiatric Press, 2003:53–80.

61. Weiden PJ, Ross R. Why do patients stop their antipsychotic medications? A guide for family and friends. J Psychiatr Pract 2002;8:413–416.

62. De Luca V, Mueller DJ, de Bartolomeis A, et al. Association of the HTR2C gene and antipsychotic induced weight gain: a meta-analysis. Int J Neuropsychopharmacol 2007;10(5):697–704.

63. Ellingrod VL, Bishop JR, Moline J, et al. Leptin and leptin receptor gene polymorphisms and increases in body mass index (BMI) from olanzapine treatment in persons with schizophrenia. Psychopharmacol Bull 2007;40(1):57–62.

64. Foster A, Miller del D, Buckley PF. Pharmacogenetics and schizophrenia. Psychiatr Clin North Am 2007;30(3):417–435.

65. Wang YC, Bai YM, Chen JY, et al. Polymorphism of the adrenergic receptor alpha 2a −1291C>G genetic variation and clozapine-induced weight gain. J Neural Transm 2005;112(11):1463–1468.

66. Bishop JR, Ellingrod VL, Moline J, Miller D. Pilot study of the G-protein beta3 subunit gene (C825T) polymorphism and clinical response to olanzapine or olanzapine-related weight gain in persons with schizophrenia. Med Sci Monit 2006;12(2):BR47–50.

67. Zhang XY, Zhou DF, Wu GY, et al. BDNF levels and genotype are associated with antipsychotic-induced weight gain in patients with chronic schizophrenia. Neuropsychopharmacology 2008;33(9):2200–2205.

68. American Diabetes Association. Consensus development conference on antipsychotic drugs and obesity and diabetes. Diabetes Care 2004;27:596–601.

69. Newcomer JW. Second-generation (atypical) antipsychotics and metabolic effects: A comprehensive literature review. CNS Drugs 2005;19(S1):1–93.

70. Zyprexa (olanzapine). MedWatch, U.S. Food and Drug Administration; 2004. *http://www.fda.gov/medwatch/SAFETY/2004/safety04.htm #zyprexa.*

71. Mackin P. Cardiac side effects of psychiatric drugs. Hum Psychopharmacol 2008;23:3–14.

72. Miller AL, Dassori A, Ereshefsky L, Crismon ML. Recent issues and developments in antipsychotic use. In: Dunner DL, Rosenbaum JF, eds. Psychiatric Clinics of North America Annual Review of Drug Therapy 2001. Philadelphia, PA: WB Saunders, 2001;8:209–235.

73. Weinmann S, Read J, Aderhold V. Influence of antipsychotics on mortality in schizophrenia: Systematic review. Schizophr Res 2009;113(1):1–11.

74. Fernø J, Raeder MB, Vik-Mo AO, et al. Antipsychotic drugs activate SREBP-regulated expression of lipid biosynthetic genes in cultured human glioma cells: a novel mechanism of action? Pharmacogenomics J 2005;5(5):298–304.

75. Sarandol A, Kirli S, Akkaya C, et al. Coronary artery disease risk factors in patients with schizophrenia: effects of short term antipsychotic treatment. J Psychopharmacol 2007;21(8):857–863.

76. Nasrallah HA. Metabolic findings from the CATIE trial and their relation to tolerability. CNS Spectr 2006;11(S7):32–39.

77. McEvoy JP, Meyer JM, Goff DC, et al. Prevalence of the metabolic syndrome in patients with schizophrenia: baseline results from the Clinical Antipsychotic Trials of Intervention Effectiveness (CATIE) schizophrenia trial and comparison with national estimates from NHANES III. Schizophr Res 2005;80(1):19–32.

78. Caplan JP, Epstein LA, Quinn DK, et al. Neuropsychiatric effects of prescription drug abuse. Neuropsychol Rev 2007;17:363–380.

79. Pierre JM. Extrapyramidal symptoms with atypical antipsychotics. Drug Saf 2005;28:191–208.

80. Haddad PM, Dursun SM. Neurological complications of psychiatric drugs: clinical features and management. Hum Psychopharmacol 2008;23:15–26.

81. Sprague RL, Kalachnik JE. Reliability, validity, and a total score cutoff for the Dyskinesia Identification System Condensed User Scale (DISCUS) with mentally ill and mentally retarded populations. Psychopharmacol Bull 1991;27:51–58.

82. Reynolds GP. The impact of pharmacogenetics on the development and use of antipsychotic drugs. Drug Discov Today 2007;12 (21–22):953–959.

83. Correll CU, Leucht S, Kane JM. Lower risk for tardive dyskinesia associated with second-generation antipsychotics: A systematic review of 1-year studies. Am J Psychiatry 2004;161:414–425.

84. Tamminga CA, Woerner MG. Clinical course and cellular pathology of tardive dyskinesia. In: Davis KL, Charney D, Coyle JT, Nemeroff C, eds. Neuropsychopharmacology: The Fifth Generation of Progress. Philadelphia, PA: Lippincott Williams & Wilkins, 2002:1831–1841.

85. Keefe RS, Bilder RM, Davis SM, et al. Neurocognitive effects of antipsychotic medications in patients with chronic schizophrenia in the CATIE trial. Arch Gen Psychiatry 2007;64:633–647.

86. Bilder RM, Goldman RS, Volavka J, et al. Neurocognitive effects of clozapine, risperidone, and haloperidol in patients with chronic schizophrenia or schizoaffective disorder. Am J Psychiatry 2002;159:1018–1028.

87. Miller AL, Crismon ML, Rush AJ, et al. The Texas Medication Algorithm Project: clinical results for schizophrenia. Schizophr Bull 2004;30:627–647.

88. Martin-Latry K, Goumy MP, Latry P, et al. Psychotropic drug use and the risk of heat-related hospitalization. European Psychiatry 2007;22:335–338.

89. Jackson N, Doherty J, Coulter S. Neuropsychiatric complications of commonly used palliative care drugs. Postgrad Med J 2008;84:121–126.

90. Li J, Tripathi RC, Tripathi BJ. Drug-induced ocular disorders. Drug Saf 2008;31:127–141.

91. Fraunfelder FW. Twice-yearly exams unnecessary for patients taking quetiapine. Am J Ophthalmol 2004;138:870–871.

92. Verhamme KM, Sturkenboom MC, Stricker BH, Bosch R. Drug-induced urinary retention: incidence, management, and prevention. Drug Saf 2008;31:373–388.

93. Tsakiri P, Oelke M, Michel MC. Drug-induced urinary incontinence. Drugs Aging 2008;25:541–549.

94. Knegtering H, van der Moolen AEGM, Castelein S, et al. What are the effects of antipsychotics on sexual dysfunctions and endocrine functioning? Psychoneuroendocrinology 2003;28(Suppl 2):109–123.

95. Hall RL, Smith AG, Ewards JG. Haematological safety of antipsychotic drugs. Expert Opin Drug Saf 2003;2:395–399.

96. Flanagan RJ, Dunk L. Haematological toxicity of drugs used in psychiatry. Hum Psychopharmacol 2008;23:27–41.

97. Meltzer HY, Fatemi SH. Treatment of schizophrenia. In: Schatzberg AF, Nemeroff CB, eds. Textbook of Psychopharmacology, 2nd ed. Washington, DC: American Psychiatric Press, 1998:747–774.

98. Perry PJ, Alexander B, Liskow B. Psychotropic Drug Handbook, 8th ed. Washington, DC: American Psychiatric Press, 2007:1–139.

99. Syed R, Au K, Cahill C, et al. Pharmacological interventions for clozapine-induced hypersalivation. Cochrane Database Syst Rev 2008;July 16(3):CD005579.

100. American Academy of Pediatrics Committee on Drugs. Use of psychoactive medication during pregnancy and possible effects on the fetus and newborn. Pediatrics 2000;105:880–887.

101. Lin HC, Chen IJ, Chen YH, et al. Maternal schizophrenia and pregnancy outcome: Does the use of antipsychotics make a difference? Schizophr Res 2010;116(1):55–60.

102. McKenna K, Koren G, Tetelbaum M, et al. Pregnancy outcome of women using atypical antipsychotic drugs: a prospective comparative study. J Clin Psychiatry 2005;66(4):444–449.

103. Coppola D, Russo LJ, Kwarta RF Jr, et al. Evaluating the postmarketing experience of risperidone use during pregnancy: pregnancy and neonatal outcomes. Drug Saf 2007;30(3):247–264.

104. Reis M, Källén B. Maternal use of antipsychotics in early pregnancy and delivery outcome. J Clin Psychopharmacol 2008;28(3):279–288.

105. Einarson A, Boskovic R. Use and safety of antipsychotic drugs during pregnancy. J Psychiatr Pract 2009;15(3):183–192.

106. Newham JJ, Thomas SH, MacRitchie K, et al. Birth weight of infants after maternal exposure to typical and atypical antipsychotics: prospective comparison study. Br J Psychiatry 2008;192(5):333–337.

107. Ernst CL, Goldberg JF. The reproductive safety profile of mood stabilizers, atypical antipsychotics, and broad-spectrum psychotropics. J Clin Psychiatry 2002;63(Suppl 4):42–55.

108. Gentile S. Antipsychotic therapy during early and late pregnancy. A systematic review. Schizophr Bull 2010;36(3):518–544.

109. Ereshefsky L. Drug-drug interactions with the use of psychotropic medications. CNS Spectrums 2009;14(8 Suppl):1–8.

110. DeVane CL, Markowitz JS. Antipsychotics. In: Levy RH, Thummel KE, Trager WF, et al. Metabolic Drug Interactions. Philadelphia, PA: Lippincott Williams & Wilkins, 2000:245–258.

111. Spina E, de Leon J. Metabolic drug interactions with newer antipsychotics: a comparative review. Basic Clin Pharmacol Toxicol 2007;100:4–22.

112. Urichuk L, Prior TI, Dursun, Baker G. Metabolism of atypical antipsychotics: involvement of cytochrome P450 enzymes and relevance for drug-drug interactions. Curr Drug Metabo 2008;9:410–418.

113. McEvoy JP. The costs of schizophrenia. J Clin Psychiatry 2007;68 (Suppl 14):4–7.

114. Rosenheck RA, Leslie DL, Sindelar J, et al. Cost-effectiveness of second-generation antipsychotics and perphenazine in a randomized trial of treatment for chronic schizophrenia. Am J Psychiatry 2006;163:2080–2089.

115. Hayhurst KP, Brown P, Lewis SW. The cost-effectiveness of clozapine: A controlled, population-based mirror-image study. J Psychopharmacol 2002;16:169–175.

116. Duggan A, Warner J, Knapp M, Kerwin R. Modeling the impact of clozapine on suicide in patients with treatment-resistant schizophrenia. Br J Psychiatry 2003;182:505–508.

117. Wang PS, Ulbricht CM, Schoenbaum M. Improving mental health treatments through comparative effectiveness research. Health Affairs 2009;28:783–791.

118. Miller AL, Chiles JA, Chiles JK, et al. The TMAP schizophrenia algorithms. J Clin Psychiatry 1999;60:649–657.

119. Velligan DI, DiCocco M, Bow-Thomas C, et al. A brief cognitive assessment (BCA) for use with schizophrenia patients in a community clinic. Schizophr Res 2004;71:273–283.

120. Toprac MG, Rush AJ, Conner TM, et al. The Texas Medication Algorithm Project patient and family education program: A consumer-guided initiative. J Clin Psychiatry 2000;61:477–486.

121. A. Spaniel F, Vohlidka P, Hrdlicka J, et al. ITAREPS: information technology aided relapse prevention programme in schizophrenia. Schizophr Res 2008;98(1–3):312–317.

122. Flockhart DA. Drug Interactions: Cytochrome P450 drug interaction table. *http://medicine.iupui.edu/clinpharm/ddis/table.asp.*

77

Major Depressive Disorder

CHRISTIAN J. TETER, JUDITH C. KANDO, AND BARBARA G. WELLS

KEY CONCEPTS

❶ Extensive treatment guidelines are available to assist in the treatment of major depressive disorder, including medication management. Clinicians treating individuals with major depressive disorder should be familiar with these guidelines.

❷ When evaluating a patient for the presence of depression, it is essential to rule out medical causes of depression and drug-induced depression.

❸ The goal of pharmacological treatment of depression is the resolution of current symptoms (i.e., remission) and the prevention of further episodes of depression (i.e., relapse or recurrence).

❹ When counseling patients with depression who are receiving antidepressant medications, the patient should be informed that adverse effects might occur immediately, while resolution of symptoms may take 2 to 4 weeks or longer. Adherence to the treatment plan is essential to a successful outcome, and tools to help increase medication adherence should be discussed with each patient.

❺ Antidepressants are generally considered equally efficacious in groups of patients with major depressive disorder. Therefore, other factors, such as age, side effects, and past history of response, are used to guide the selection of medication management.

❻ When determining if a patient has been nonresponsive to a particular pharmacotherapeutic intervention, it must be determined whether the patient has received an adequate dose for an adequate duration and whether the patient has been medication adherent.

❼ When evaluating response to an antidepressant, in addition to target signs and symptoms, the clinician must consider quality-of-life issues such as role, social, and occupational functioning. In addition, the tolerability of the agent should be assessed because the occurrence of side effects may lead to medication nonadherence, especially given the chronicity of the disease and need for long-term medication management.

Learning objectives, review questions, and other resources can be found at **www.pharmacotherapyonline.com**.

A diagnosis of major depressive disorder is given when an individual experiences one or more major depressive episodes without a history of manic, mixed, or hypomanic episodes. A major depressive episode is defined by the criteria listed in the *Diagnostic and Statistical Manual of Mental Disorders, Fourth Edition, Text Revision (DSM-IV-TR)*.[1] Depression is associated with significant functional disability, morbidity, and mortality.

Newer generations of antidepressants have provided pharmacological interventions that are effective and better tolerated than older agents like the tricyclic antidepressants (TCAs) and the monoamine oxidase inhibitors (MAOIs). In addition, substantial efforts have been undertaken to improve the ability of clinicians to recognize and appropriately treat the signs and symptoms of depression. This chapter focuses exclusively on the diagnosis and treatment of major depressive disorder.

❶ In the absence of well-accepted evidence-based medicine for the medication management of major depressive disorder, the reader is referred to the *Practice Guideline for the Treatment of Patients with Major Depressive Disorder, Second Edition*, which is available at *www.psych.org*. This extensive document is a practical guide to the management of depression based upon the best available data as well as clinical consensus.[2]

EPIDEMIOLOGY

The true prevalence of depressive disorders in the United States is unknown. The National Comorbidity Survey Replication found that 16.2% of the population studied had a history of major depressive disorder in their lifetime, and more than 6.6% had an episode within the past 12 months.[3] Women are at increased risk of depression from early adolescence until their mid-50s, with a lifetime rate that is 1.7 to 2.7 times greater than for men.[4] Although depression can occur at any age, adults 18 to 29 years of age experience the highest rates of major depression during any given year.[3] The estimated lifetime prevalence of major depression in individuals aged 65 to 80 recently was reported to be 20.4% in women and 9.6% in men.[5] Depressive disorders are common during adolescence, with comorbid substance abuse, suicide attempts, and deaths occurring frequently in these young patients.[6,7] Depressive disorders and suicide tend to occur within families. For example, approximately 8% to 18% of patients with major depression have at least one first-degree relative (father, mother, brother, or sister) with a history of depression, compared with 5.6% of the first-degree relatives of those without depression.[8] Furthermore, first-degree relatives of patients with depression are 1.5 to 3 times more likely to develop depression than normal controls.[1,8,9] A recent meta-analysis found that the heritability of liability for major depression was 37%, whereas the remaining 63% of the variance in liability was due to individual-specific environment.[10] Therefore major depressive disorder is relatively common, occurs

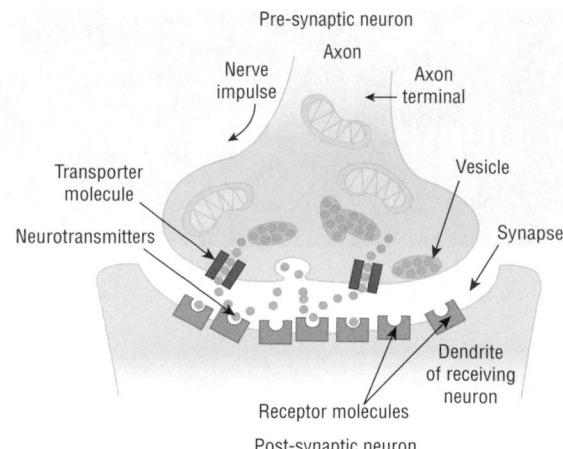

FIGURE 77-1. Monoamine neurotransmitter regulation at the neuronal level. Neurotransmitters (NTs) carry messages between cells. Each NT generally binds to a specific receptor, and this coupling initiates a cascade of events. NTs are reabsorbed back into nerve cells by reuptake pumps (i.e., transporter molecules) at which point they may be recycled for later use or broken down by enzymes. For their primary mechanism of action, most antidepressants are thought to inhibit the transporter molecules and allow more NT to remain in the synapse. *This figure was reproduced from the Mind Over Matter educational series, which is in the public domain and may be reproduced without permission. (Source: U.S. Department of Health and Human Services, National Institutes of Health, National Institute on Drug Abuse, Office of Science Policy and Communications, Science Policy Branch.)*

more frequently in women than men, and prevalence is influenced by both genetic and environmental factors.

ETIOLOGY

The etiology of depressive disorders is too complex to be totally explained by a single social, developmental, or biologic theory. Several factors appear to work together to cause or precipitate depressive disorders. The symptoms reported by patients with major depression consistently reflect changes in brain monoamine neurotransmitters, specifically norepinephrine (NE), serotonin (5-HT), and dopamine (DA).[11-13] Please see Figure 77–1 for a visual explanation as to how these monoamine neurotransmitters are regulated at the level of the neuron and within the synapse.

PATHOPHYSIOLOGY

Several years before the introduction of antidepressants, the cause of depression was linked to decreased brain levels of the neurotransmitters NE, 5-HT, and DA, although the actual cause remains unknown. This biogenic amine hypothesis evolved as a result of several observations made in the early 1950s. It was noted that the antihypertensive drug reserpine depleted neuronal storage granules of NE, 5-HT, and DA and produced clinically significant depression in 15% or more of patients.[14]

Although the reuptake blockade of monoamines (e.g., NE, DA, and 5-HT) occurs immediately upon administration of an antidepressant, the clinical antidepressant effects (i.e., measurable improvement) are generally delayed by weeks.[11,15] This delay may be the result of a cascade of events from receptor occupancy to gene transcription.[16] This delay in onset of action has caused researchers to focus on the adaptive changes induced by antidepressants.[12] Accordingly, theories that focus on adaptive (or chronic) changes in

amine receptor systems have emerged over the past decade. In the mid-1970s, it was recognized that chronic, but not acute, administration of antidepressants to animals caused desensitization of NE-stimulated cyclic adenosine monophosphate synthesis. In fact, for most antidepressants, downregulation of β-adrenergic receptors accompanies this desensitization.[17] Studies of many antidepressants have demonstrated that either desensitization or downregulation of NE receptors corresponds to a clinically relevant time course for antidepressant effects.[11] Other studies have revealed desensitization of pre-synaptic 5-HT$_{1A}$ autoreceptors following chronic administration of antidepressants.[18] Thus a theory based on changes in receptor sensitivity provides a cogent explanation of the delayed onset of therapeutic response of antidepressant drugs.[11] The dysregulation hypothesis incorporates the diversity of antidepressant activity with the adaptive changes occurring in receptor sensitization over several weeks. In this theory, emphasis is placed on a failure of homeostatic regulation of neurotransmitter systems rather than on absolute increases or decreases in their activities. According to this hypothesis, effective antidepressant agents restore efficient regulation to the dysregulated neurotransmitter system.[19]

It is apparent that no single neurotransmitter theory of depression is adequate. The 5-HT/NE link hypothesis maintains that both the serotonergic and noradrenergic systems are involved in an antidepressant response.[17] This hypothesis is also consistent with the rationale of the postsynaptic alteration theory of depression, which emphasizes the importance of β-adrenergic receptor downregulation for achieving an antidepressant effect.[17] Furthermore, both serotonergic and noradrenergic medications down-regulate β-adrenergic receptors, and there is a link between serotonin and norepinephrine.[17] This implies that medications that are effective in the treatment of depression act at both of these neurotransmitter systems.

Traditional explanations of the biologic basis of depressive disorders have focused largely on NE and 5-HT; however, most of the evidence that coalesced into the biogenic amine hypothesis of depression does not clearly distinguish between NE and DA. There is an abundance of evidence suggesting that dopamine transmission is decreased in depression and that agents that increase dopaminergic transmission have been found to be effective antidepressants.[20] Specifically, studies suggest that increased DA transmission in the mesolimbic pathway account for at least part of the mechanism of action of antidepressant medications.[20] The mechanisms by which antidepressant drugs alter DA transmission remain unclear, but may be mediated indirectly by primary actions at NE or 5-HT terminals. The complexity of the interaction between 5-HT, NE, and possibly DA is gaining greater appreciation, but a more in-depth understanding of the precise mechanism is needed.

More recent insight into the possible mechanisms underlying depressive disorders comes from studies on brain-derived neurotrophic factor (BDNF). BDNF is a growth factor protein that regulates the differentiation and survival of neurons. A growing body of evidence suggests this process might be disrupted in depressive disorders. More specifically, chronic stress and an associated increase in glucocorticoids such as cortisol may cause a disruption of BDNF expression in the hippocampus. This process may be prevented, or possibly even reversed, by antidepressant medications.[21] This is a relatively recent theory, which has not been firmly established. However, if proven valid, it demonstrates that antidepressants may help prevent deleterious effects of chronic stress and depressive symptoms.

BIOLOGIC MARKERS

Investigators continue to search for biologic or pharmacodynamic markers to assist in the diagnosis and treatment of depressed patients. Although no biologic marker has been discovered, several biologic abnormalities are present in many depressed patients. Approximately 45% to 60% of patients with major depression have a neuroendocrine abnormality, including hypersecretion of cortisol or a lack of cortisol suppression after dexamethasone administration (i.e., a positive dexamethasone suppression test). In fact, it has been suggested that the inability of the brain to suppress the hypothalamic-pituitary-adrenal (HPA) axis and the associated stress response could lead to the pathophysiology and symptoms of depression.[22] According to this theory, there is a disruption somewhere in the normal negative feedback system that controls cortisol levels (please see Figure 85–3 in the Adrenal Gland Disorders chapter for a visual display of this negative feedback system). There are many potential negative consequences of excess circulating cortisol, including disruption in BDNF expression as discussed above in the Pathophysiology section.

Unfortunately, the high rate of false-positive and false-negative results associated with neuroendocrine abnormalities in depressed patients limits the usefulness of testing for these markers, and has led to their relative lack of use in clinical practice. However, they still provide a clue as to the potential pathophysiology of depressive disorders, which may lead us to more effective treatment options.

CLINICAL PRESENTATION

❷ When a patient presents with depressive symptoms, it is necessary to investigate the possibility of a contributing medical or drug-induced etiology (Table 77–1). In fact, in the *DSM-IV-TR* there is a diagnostic category for both "Mood Disorder Due to a General Medical Condition" and "Substance-Induced Mood Disorder."[1] For example, up to 40% of patients with certain neurological disorders (e.g., stroke, Alzheimer's disease) develop depressive symptoms at some point during the course of their neurological illness.[1] Furthermore, individuals experiencing withdrawal from substances of abuse (e.g., cocaine) can present with depressive symptoms.[23] All depressed patients should have a complete physical examination, mental status examination, and basic laboratory workup, including a complete blood count with differential, thyroid function tests,

and electrolyte determinations to identify any potential medical problems. Lastly, a complete medication review should be performed because several medications may contribute to depressive symptoms (Table 77–1).[24] Once a medical condition or concomitant medication has been ruled out as the cause of the depressive symptoms, the patient should be evaluated for a major depressive disorder.

According to the *DSM-IV-TR*, a single major depressive episode is characterized by five or more of the symptoms described in Table 77–2. At least one of the symptoms is depressed mood (often an irritable mood in children or adolescents) or loss of interest or pleasure in nearly all activities.[1] These symptoms must have been present nearly every day for at least 2 weeks and must represent a change from the patient's previous level of functioning. The clinician must consider presenting symptoms, their duration, and the patient's current level of social, occupational, or other important areas of functioning. Significant stressors or life events may trigger depression in some individuals but not others; and there may be an important precipitant at the beginning of the disorder.[1] A patient diagnosed with major depressive disorder may have one or more recurrent episodes of major depression during their lifetime.

DEPRESSION RATING SCALES

Instruments to assess the severity of depressive symptoms can be used for both clinical and research purposes. For example, the Montgomery-Åsberg Depression Rating Scale (MADRS) is a clinician-administered scale that is commonly used in drug trials given its sensitivity to change.[25] Other depression rating scales are self-administered. For example, the Beck Depression Inventory (BDI) takes only 5 to 10 minutes to complete by the respondent.[26] For a more detailed explanation for both of these instruments, as well as other rating scales and evaluation approaches, please refer to Chapter 71.

EMOTIONAL SYMPTOMS

A major depressive episode is characterized by a persistent, diminished ability to experience pleasure. A loss of interest and pleasure in usual activities, hobbies, or work is common. Patients appear sad

---

TABLE 77-1 Common Medical Conditions, Substance Use Disorders, and Medications Associated with Depressive Symptoms

General medical conditions	Metabolic disorders	Substance use disorders (including *intoxication* and *withdrawal*)
Endocrine diseases	Electrolyte imbalance	Alcoholism
Hypothyroidism	Hypokalemia	Marijuana abuse and dependence
Addison or Cushing disease	Hyponatremia	Nicotine dependence
Deficiency states	Hepatic encephalopathy	Opiate abuse and dependence (e.g., heroin)
Pernicious anemia	Cardiovascular disease	Psychostimulant abuse and dependence (e.g., cocaine)
Wernicke encephalopathy	Coronary artery disease	**Drug therapy**
Severe anemia	Congestive heart failure	Antihypertensives
Infections	Myocardial infarction	Clonidine
AIDS	Neurologic disorders	Diuretics
Encephalitis	Alzheimer's disease	Guanethidine sulfate
Human immunodeficiency virus	Epilepsy	Hydralazine hydrochloride
Mononucleosis	Huntington disease	Methyldopa
Sexually transmitted diseases	Multiple sclerosis	Propranolol
Tuberculosis	Pain	Reserpine
Collagen disorder	Parkinson's disease	Hormonal therapy
Systemic lupus erythematosus	Poststroke	Oral contraceptives
	Malignant disease	Steroids/adrenocorticotropic hormone
		Acne therapy
		Isotretinoin
		Other
		Interferon-β_{1a}

Data from references 1, 23, and 24.

TABLE 77-2 DSM-IV-TR Criteria for Major Depressive Episode

A. Five (or more) of the following symptoms have been present during the same 2-week period and represent a change from previous functioning; at least one of the symptoms is either (1) depressed mood or (2) loss of interest or pleasure.

   Note: Do not include symptoms that are clearly due to a general medical condition or mood-incongruent delusions or hallucinations.

   1. Depressed mood most of the day nearly every day
   2. Markedly diminished interest or pleasure in all, or almost all, activities most of the day nearly every day
   3. Significant weight loss when not dieting or weight gain (e.g., a change of more than 5% of body weight in a month), or decrease or increase in appetite nearly every day
   4. Insomnia or hypersomnia nearly every day
   5. Psychomotor agitation or retardation nearly every day (observable by others, not merely subjective feelings of restlessness or being slowed down)
   6. Fatigue or loss of energy nearly every day
   7. Feelings of worthlessness or excessive or inappropriate guilt nearly every day
   8. Diminished ability to think or concentrate, or indecisiveness, nearly every day
   9. Recurrent thoughts of death (not just fear of dying), recurrent suicidal ideation without a specific plan, or a suicide attempt or a specific plan for committing suicide

B. The symptoms cause clinically significant distress or impairment in social, occupational, or other important areas of functioning.

C. The symptoms are not due to the direct physiological effects of a substance (e.g., a drug of abuse, a medication) or a general medical condition (e.g., hypothyroidism).

D. The symptoms are not better accounted for by bereavement (i.e., after the loss of a loved one), the symptoms persist for longer than 2 months or are characterized by marked functional impairment, morbid preoccupation with worthlessness, suicidal ideation, psychotic symptoms, or psychomotor retardation.

Reprinted with permission from the Diagnostic and Statistical Manual of Mental Disorders, Text Revision, Fourth Edition, (Copyright © 2000). American Psychiatric Association.

or depressed, and they are often pessimistic and believe that nothing will help them feel better. The presence of feelings of worthlessness or inappropriate guilt may identify patients at risk for suicide.[27] Anxiety symptoms are present in almost 90% of depressed outpatients. Patients often have guilt feelings that are unrealistic, and these may reach delusional proportions. Patients may feel that they deserve punishment and may view their present illness as a punishment. A patient suffering from major depression with psychotic features may hear voices (auditory hallucinations) saying that he or she is a bad person and that he or she should commit suicide. Depression with psychotic features may require hospitalization, especially if the patient becomes a danger to self or others.

PHYSICAL SYMPTOMS

Physical symptoms often motivate patients, especially the elderly, to seek medical attention. Chronic fatigue is a common complaint, with a decreased ability to perform normal daily tasks. Fatigue often appears worse in the morning and does not improve with rest. Complaints of pain, especially headache, often accompany fatigue.

Sleep disturbances generally present as frequent early morning awakening with difficulty returning to sleep. This may coexist with difficulty falling asleep and frequent nighttime awakening. Less frequently, depressed patients complain of increased sleep (hypersomnia), although they experience daytime exhaustion or fatigue.

Appetite disturbances, including complaints of decreased appetite, often result in substantial weight loss, especially in the elderly.[28] Some patients lose 2 pounds (0.9 kg) or more per week without dieting. Other patients, especially in the ambulatory setting, may overeat and gain weight, although they actually may not enjoy eating. They may crave specific foods. Some patients exhibit gastrointestinal

complaints, others cardiovascular complaints, especially palpitations. Patients frequently present with a loss of sexual interest or libido.[29]

INTELLECTUAL OR COGNITIVE SYMPTOMS

Intellectual or cognitive symptoms include a decreased ability to concentrate, slowed thinking, and a poor memory for recent events. Patients may appear confused and indecisive. Depression should be considered when cognitive symptoms are present in the elderly.[28]

PSYCHOMOTOR DISTURBANCES

Patients may appear noticeably slowed or retarded in physical movements, thought processes, and speech (psychomotor retardation). Conversely, depression may be accompanied by psychomotor agitation, manifesting as purposeless, restless motion (e.g., pacing, wringing of hands, or outbursts of shouting).

SUICIDE RISK EVALUATION AND MANAGEMENT

The Centers for Disease Control and Prevention lists suicide as the eleventh leading cause of death among Americans and the second leading cause of death among 25- to 34-year-olds. In 2006, there were 91 suicides per day in the United States.[30] All patients diagnosed with major depression should be assessed for suicidal thoughts. Factors associated with an increased risk for suicide include psychiatric and substance use disorders, adolescence and younger age adults, physical illness, recent stressful life event, childhood trauma, hopelessness, and male gender.[31] Those with a higher level of risk have high degrees of suicidal intent and describe more specific plans, in particular, those that are violent and irreversible.[31] It is important to remember that the risk of suicide in those recovering from major depression may increase as they develop the energy and capacity to act on a plan made earlier in a course of illness. Additionally, despite factors to help identify those at greatest risk, it remains very difficult to predict suicidality in any given individual. Therefore, when suicidal intent is suspected, it is important to ask, "Are you thinking about harming or killing yourself?" If the risk is significant, the patient must be referred immediately to an appropriate healthcare professional. Additionally, certain depression rating scales, such as the MADRS discussed above, include questions that target suicidality, which may help identify those patients at risk.

In September 2004, the FDA required manufacturers of antidepressants to add a boxed warning stating that antidepressants increase the risk of suicidal thinking and behavior in short-term studies in children and adolescents with depressive disorders. These risks have become a new source of concern among those treating their patients with antidepressants. In order to help deal with the confusion these risks have caused, experts have recommended[32] the following:

- It is especially important to closely monitor patients for suicidal ideation and behavior at the beginning of treatment and among younger patients.
- Discuss the possibility that adverse events may occur, including behavioral agitation or anger, and encourage patients to seek help should this occur.
- Deal with the subject of suicide directly.

It is important to note that there is little evidence to suggest that withholding antidepressant treatment decreases the risk of eventual suicide and may actually increase the risk. Furthermore, it may be that longer-term medication is needed for any protective effects against suicidality.[32]

In May 2007, the FDA released additional requests to the makers of antidepressants that the black box warning regarding suicidality be expanded to include warnings about the increased risk of suicidality (thinking and behavior) in young adults 18 to 24 years of age, during the initial stages of treatment.

TREATMENT

■ DESIRED OUTCOME

The goals of treatment are to reduce the symptoms of acute depression, facilitate the patient's return to a level of functioning like that before the onset of illness, and prevent further episodes of depression. Whether or not to hospitalize the patient is often the first decision that is made in consideration of the patient's risk of suicide, physical state of health, social support system, and presence of a psychotic depression.

■ GENERAL APPROACH TO TREATMENT

❸ There are three phases of treatment for patients with major depressive disorder: (1) the *acute* phase lasting from 6 to 10 weeks in which the goal is remission (i.e., absence of symptoms); (2) the *continuation* phase lasting 4 to 9 months after remission is achieved, in which the goal is to eliminate residual symptoms or prevent relapse (i.e., return of symptoms within 6 months of remission); and (3) the *maintenance* phase lasting at least 12 to 36 months in which the goal is to prevent recurrence (i.e., a separate episode of depression).[2,33] The risk of recurrence increases as the number of past episodes increase. The duration of antidepressant therapy depends on the risk of recurrence. Some investigators recommend lifelong maintenance therapy for persons at greatest risk for recurrence (persons younger 40 years of age with two or more prior episodes and persons of any age with three or more prior episodes).[2]

❹ Educating the patient and their support system (e.g., family and friends) regarding the delay in antidepressant effects and the importance of adherence should occur before and during the entire course of treatment. The treatment of major depressive disorder generally includes nonpharmacologic and pharmacologic strategies, which are discussed in further detail below.

■ NONPHARMACOLOGIC THERAPY

In addition to pharmacologic interventions, psychotherapy should be employed whenever the patient is able and willing to participate. Psychotherapy alone is not recommended for the acute treatment of patients with severe and/or psychotic major depressive disorder. However, if the depressive episode is mild to moderate in severity, psychotherapy may be the first-line therapy.[34] The effects of psychotherapy and antidepressant medications are considered to be additive. Combined treatment may be advantageous for patients with partial responses to either treatment alone and for those with a chronic course of illness. However, for uncomplicated, nonchronic major depressive disorder, combined treatment may provide no unique advantage.[34] Although not extensively evaluated, cognitive therapy, behavioral therapy, and interpersonal psychotherapy appear equally effective.[34] Maintenance psychotherapy as the sole treatment to prevent recurrence generally is not recommended. Often, medication alone may prevent a depressive recurrence during the maintenance phase.[34]

Electroconvulsive therapy (ECT) is a safe and effective treatment for certain severe mental illnesses, including major depressive disorder as well as other selected psychiatric illnesses. Patients with depression are candidates for ECT when a rapid response is needed, risks of other treatments outweigh potential benefits, there is a history of poor response to antidepressants and a history of good response to ECT, and the patient expresses a preference for ECT.[35] A course of ECT generally consists of either unilateral or bilateral ECT administered 2 to 3 times weekly for a total of 6 to 12 treatments. A rapid therapeutic response (10–14 days) has been reported. Although there are no absolute contraindications to the use of ECT, several conditions are associated with increased risk. These include increased intracranial pressure, cerebral lesions, recent myocardial infarction, recent intracerebral hemorrhage, bleeding, or otherwise unstable vascular condition. The use of an anesthetic as well as a nondepolarizing neuromuscular blocking agent decreases the morbidity associated with ECT.[35] Adverse effects of ECT include cognitive dysfunction, cardiovascular dysfunction, prolonged apnea, treatment-emergent mania, headache, nausea, and muscle aches. Cognitive changes associated with ECT include confusion immediately after the seizure and retrograde and anterograde memory disturbance. Most cognitive disturbances are transient, but some patients may report permanent loss of memory for events occurring over the months before, after, or during treatment.[35] Relapse rates during the year immediately following ECT are high unless maintenance antidepressant medication is prescribed. Guidelines developed by the American Psychiatric Association include indications and contraindications for the appropriate use of ECT, procedures for obtaining informed consent, and issues in administering ECT.[35]

Another nonpharmacologic treatment for depression is bright light therapy. Bright light therapy consists of the patient gazing into a 10,000-lux intensity light box, which is slanted downward toward the patients face for approximately 30 minutes/day. It has shown effectiveness for treating both the winter "blues," also known as seasonal affective disorder (SAD), and for adjunctive use in major depressive disorder with seasonal exacerbations.[2] Light therapy is well tolerated, with minor visual complaints being the most frequently reported event.[36] Consequently, anyone undergoing light therapy should receive baseline and periodic eye examinations. The combination of bright light therapy and an antidepressant may provide additional benefit beyond either approach alone.[2]

■ PHARMACOLOGIC THERAPY

Antidepressants can be classified in several ways, including by chemical structure and the presumed mechanism of antidepressant activity. Although the link between the presumed mechanism of drug action and antidepressant response is tenuous, this classification has the advantage of being based on established pharmacology and clearly explains some of the common, but expected, adverse effects. The knowledgeable clinician can use these facts to tailor treatment to individual patient needs and thereby optimize treatment outcome. Currently available antidepressants and initial dosages are shown in Table 77–3.

❺ Studies have found that antidepressants are of equivalent efficacy in groups of patients when administered in comparable doses. Because one cannot predict which antidepressant will be the most effective in an individual patient, the initial choice is made empirically. Factors that often influence the choice of an antidepressant include the patient's history of response, pharmacogenetics (history of familial antidepressant response), patient's concurrent medical history, presenting symptoms (e.g., fatigue as compared with psychomotor agitation), potential for drug–drug interactions, adverse events profile, patient preference, and drug cost.

Although the pathophysiology of major depression remains elusive, the clinician can now select from multiple approved drug therapies with different mechanisms of action.[2] Failure to respond to one antidepressant class or one antidepressant drug within a class

TABLE 77-3 Adult Dosages for Currently Available Antidepressant Medications[a]

Generic Name	Trade Name	Suggested Therapeutic Plasma Concentration ng/mL (nmol/L)	Initial Dose (mg/day)	Usual Dosage Range (mg/day)
Serotonin selective reuptake inhibitors				
Citalopram	Celexa		20	20–60
Escitalopram	Lexapro		10	10–20
Fluoxetine	Prozac		20	20–60
Fluvoxamine	Luvox		50	50–300
Paroxetine	Paxil		20	20–60
Sertraline	Zoloft		50	50–200
Serotonin/norepinephrine reuptake inhibitors				
Venlafaxine	Effexor		37.5–75	75–225
Desvenlafaxine	Pristiq		50	50
Duloxetine	Cymbalta		30	30–90
Aminoketone				
Bupropion	Wellbutrin		150	150–300
Triazolopyridines				
Nefazodone	Serzone		100	200–600
Trazodone	Desyrel		50	150–300
Tetracyclic				
Mirtazapine	Remeron		15	15–45
Tricyclics				
Tertiary amines				
Amitriptyline	Elavil	120–250 (433–903)[b]	25	100–300
Clomipramine	Anafranil		25	100–250
Doxepin	Sinequan		25	100–300
Imipramine	Tofranil	200–350 (713–1248)[c]	25	100–300
Secondary amines				
Desipramine	Norpramin	100–300 (375–1126)[c]	25	100–300
Nortriptyline	Pamelor	50–150 (190–570)	25	50–200
Monoamine oxidase inhibitors				
Phenelzine	Nardil		15	30–90
Selegeline (transdermal)	Emsam		6[d]	6–12[d]
Tranylcypromine	Parnate		10	20–60

[a]Doses listed are total daily doses; elderly patients are usually treated with approximately one-half of the dose listed.
[b]Parent drug plus metabolite.
[c]It has been suggested that combined imipramine + desipramine concentrations should fall between 150–240 ng/mL (535–900 nmol/L).
[d]Transdermal delivery system designed to deliver stated dose continuously over a 24-hour period.
Data from references 2, 15, 33, 42, and 67.

does not predict a failed response to another drug class or another drug within the class. Approximately 65% to 70% of patients with varying types of depression improve with drug therapy, compared with 30% to 40% who are well documented to improve with placebo.

MIXED SEROTONIN AND NOREPINEPHRINE REUPTAKE INHIBITORS

Although TCAs are effective in treating all depressive subtypes, their use has diminished greatly due to the availability of equally effective therapies that are much safer in overdose and better tolerated. All TCAs potentiate the activity of NE and 5-HT by blocking their reuptake. However, the potency and selectivity of TCAs for the inhibition of reuptake of NE and 5-HT vary greatly among these agents (Table 77–4). Because TCAs affect other receptor systems including the cholinergic, neurologic, and cardiovascular systems, adverse events are reported frequently during TCA therapy.[15]

Venlafaxine inhibits 5-HT reuptake at low doses, and NE reuptake at higher doses; thus, it is referred to as a *serotonin-norepinephrine reuptake inhibitor* (SNRI). The primary active metabolite of venlafaxine (i.e., desvenlafaxine) is also an SNRI and has been approved to treat depressive disorders. Duloxetine is an SNRI with both 5-HT and NE reuptake inhibition across all doses. Some studies suggest that the SNRIs may be associated with higher rates of response and remission than other antidepressants; however, most of these studies involved venlafaxine, and not all studies support this conclusion.[37]

SEROTONIN SELECTIVE REUPTAKE INHIBITORS

The efficacy of serotonin selective reuptake inhibitors (SSRIs) is superior to placebo and comparable to other classes of antidepressants in treating patients with major depression.[2,33] SSRIs are generally chosen as *first-line antidepressants* due to their safety in overdose and improved tolerability. Furthermore, the decision as to which SSRI to use *within* the class is typically based on the nuances of each medication, such as differences in drug interaction profile and other pharmacokinetic parameters (e.g., half-life), or due to cost considerations. These concepts will be discussed in greater detail later in this chapter.

TRIAZOLOPYRIDINES

Trazodone and nefazodone have dual actions on serotonergic neurons, acting as both 5-HT$_2$ antagonists and 5-HT reuptake inhibitors. They may also enhance 5-HT$_{1A}$-mediated neurotransmission.[15] Trazodone blocks α_1-adrenergic and histaminergic receptors leading to increased side effects (e.g., dizziness and sedation) that limit its use as an antidepressant. Recently, a longer-acting extended

TABLE 77-4 Relative Potencies of Norepinephrine and Serotonin Reuptake Blockade and Side-Effect Profile of Antidepressant Drugs

	Reuptake Antagonism		Anticholinergic Effects	Sedation	Orthostatic Hypotension	Seizures[a]	Conduction Abnormalities[a]
	Norepinephreine	*Serotonin*					
Serotonin selective reuptake inhibitors							
Citalopram	0	++++	0	+	0	++	0
Escitalopram	0	++++	0	0	0	0	0
Fluoxetine	0	+++	0	0	0	++	0
Fluvoxamine	0	++++	0	0	0	++	0
Paroxetine	0	++++	+	+	0	++	0
Sertraline	0	++++	0	0	0	++	0
Serotonin/norepinephrine reuptake inhibitors							
Venlafaxine[b] and desvenlafaxine	++++	++++	+	+	0	++	+
Duloxetine[c]	++++	++++	+	0	+	0	+
Aminoketone							
Bupropion[d]	+	0	+	0	0	++++	+
Triazolopyridines							
Nefazodone	0	++	0	+++	+++	++	+
Trazodone	0	++	0	++++	+++	++	+
Tetracyclic							
Mirtazapine	0	0	+	++	++	0	+
Tricyclics							
Tertiary amines							
Amitriptyline	++	++++	++++	++++	+++	+++	+++
Clomipramine	++	+++	++++	++++	++	++++	+++
Doxepin	++	++	+++	++++	++	+++	++
Imipramine	+++	+++	+++	+++	++++	+++	+++
Secondary amines							
Desipramine	++++	+	++	++	++	++	++
Nortriptyline	+++	++	++	++	+	++	++
Monoamine oxidase inhibitors							
Phenelzine	++	++	+	++	++	+	
Selegiline	0	0	0	+	++	0	0
Tranylcypromine	++	+	+	+	++	+	+

++++, high; +++, moderate; ++, low; +, very low; 0, absent.
[a]These are uncommon side effects of antidepressant drugs, particularly when used at normal therapeutic doses.
[b]Venlafaxine: primarily 5-HT at lower doses, NE at higher doses and DA at very high doses.
[c]Duloxetine: balanced 5-HT and NE reuptake inhibition.
[d]Bupropion: also blocks dopamine reuptake.
Data from references 15, 33, 37, 39, and 42.

release preparation of trazodone was approved by the FDA. However, its place in the treatment of major depressive disorder is yet to be determined. Nefazodone's use as an antidepressant has declined as well after reports of hepatic toxicity began to emerge. The FDA-approved nefazodone labeling includes a black box warning describing rare cases of liver failure.[38] The triazolopyridines are effective agents in treating major depression; however, they both carry risks that limit their usefulness as antidepressants.

■ AMINOKETONE

Bupropion has no appreciable effect on the reuptake of 5-HT, while having reuptake properties at both the norepinephrine and dopamine reuptake pumps.[18,39] These pharmacological properties make bupropion unique among all currently available antidepressants.

■ TETRACYCLIC

Mirtazapine enhances central noradrenergic and serotonergic activity through the antagonism of central presynaptic α_2-adrenergic autoreceptors and heteroreceptors.[40] Furthermore, it antagonizes 5-HT$_2$ and 5-HT$_3$ receptors as well as histamine receptors. The antagonism of 5-HT$_2$ and 5-HT$_3$ receptors has been linked to lower anxiety and gastrointestinal side effects, respectively. Blockade of histamine receptors is associated with the sedative properties of mirtazapine.[18]

■ MONOAMINE OXIDASE INHIBITORS

MAOIs increase the concentrations of NE, 5-HT, and DA within the neuronal synapse through inhibition of the MAO enzyme. Studies have demonstrated that similarly to TCAs, chronic therapy causes changes in receptor sensitivity (i.e., downregulation of β-adrenergic, α-adrenergic, and serotonergic receptors).[41] The MAOIs phenelzine and tranylcypromine are nonselective inhibitors of MAO-A and MAO-B. Recently, a selegeline transdermal patch was approved by the FDA for treatment of major depressive disorder that allows inhibition of MAO-A and MAO-B in the brain, yet has reduced effects on MAO-A in the gut[42] (see tyramine interactions with MAOIs below).

■ ST. JOHN'S WORT

Increasingly, consumers are choosing alternative forms of therapy, such as herbal medications including St. John's wort. Evaluations have found mixed results regarding the efficacy of the active ingredient in St. John's wort, hypericum, when compared with placebo and other antidepressants.[43] St. John's wort is available as an over-the-counter medication. Although this may allow certain advantages such as reduced cost of therapy and self-treatment, it also has the potential to result in circumvention of the healthcare system. St. John's wort has been found to have significant drug interactions with commonly used medications.[43] Perhaps most disconcerting is the fact that herbal medications are not regulated by the FDA, and manufacturers are not required to adhere to good manufacturing practices or provide proof of safety and/or efficacy. If St. John's wort is to be used, it should be administered under the guidance of a clinician trained in the treatment of depression, and a single-source product should be used continuously from a reputable and trusted manufacturer.

■ ADVERSE EFFECTS

Serotonin-Norepinephrine Reuptake Inhibitors

The adverse effects of antidepressant medications are summarized in Table 77–4. The TCAs affect several neurotransmitters and produce a wide range of pharmacologic actions, including several unwanted, but expected, adverse effects. The most commonly occurring side effects are dose-related and are associated with blockade of cholinergic receptors (anticholinergic effects) and include dry mouth, constipation, blurred vision, urinary retention, dizziness, tachycardia, memory impairment, and at higher doses, delirium).[41] Although some tolerance does develop to these adverse effects, they have the potential to impact patient adherence, particularly in the elderly and those receiving long-term maintenance therapy. Orthostatic hypotension is a common, dose-related, and potentially problematic adverse effect that has been attributed to the affinity of the TCAs for adrenergic receptors.[44] TCAs also cause cardiac conduction delays and may even induce heart block in patients with a preexisting conduction disorder. TCA overdose can produce severe arrhythmias.[44] Furthermore, the FDA released a warning in December 2009 that the desipramine prescribing information will be changed to reflect an increased risk of death in patients receiving desipramine who have a *family history* of sudden cardiac death, cardiac dysrhythmias, and cardiac conduction disturbances. More on this reaction can be found at the FDA's MedWatch website. Therefore, caution should be exercised when prescribing these agents, especially in higher doses, to patients with clinically significant cardiac disease, and to patients with a family history of a cardiac event. Additional adverse effects that may lead to TCA nonadherence include weight gain and sexual dysfunction.[45] Abrupt withdrawal of TCAs is often associated with symptoms suggestive of cholinergic rebound (e.g., dizziness, nausea, diarrhea, insomnia, and restlessness), especially if the daily dose exceeds 300 mg.[46] Therefore, the dose should be tapered over at least several days.

The most commonly reported adverse effects with venlafaxine are similar to those of SSRIs and may be dose related; they include nausea, sexual dysfunction, and activation.[2] Venlafaxine may also cause a dose-related increase in diastolic blood pressure, and baseline blood pressure is not a useful predictor of the occurrence of this phenomenon. Blood pressure should be monitored regularly during venlafaxine therapy, and dosage reduction or discontinuation may be necessary if sustained hypertension occurs.[47] Duloxetine was relatively well tolerated in short-term clinical trials; however, experience with long-term studies and in a larger population of patients will more clearly define the risks and benefits of this newly approved antidepressant. The most commonly reported adverse events were nausea, dry mouth, constipation, decreased appetite, insomnia, and increased sweating.[37,48]

Serotonin Selective Reuptake Inhibitors

The SSRIs include fluoxetine, citalopram, sertraline, paroxetine, escitalopram, and fluvoxamine. These drugs have a low affinity for histaminic, α_1-adrenergic, and muscarinic receptors, and therefore they produce fewer anticholinergic and cardiovascular adverse effects than the TCAs, and are not usually associated with significant weight gain.[49,50,51] The most common adverse effects, which

generally are mild and short lived, are gastrointestinal symptoms (i.e., nausea, vomiting, and diarrhea), sexual dysfunction in both males and females, headache, and insomnia.[50] A discontinuation or withdrawal syndrome may occur if SSRIs are abruptly discontinued. However, the longer the half-life of the drug and its active metabolite, the less likely a withdrawal syndrome will occur.[51,52] Although SSRIs are known to improve the anxiety symptoms associated with depression, a few patients experience an increase in anxiety symptoms or agitation early in treatment.

Triazolopyridines

Trazodone and nefazodone have minimal anticholinergic effects and 5-HT agonist side effects, but they can cause orthostatic hypotension. Sedation, cognitive slowing, and dizziness are the most frequent dose-limiting side effects associated with trazodone.[41] Common adverse effects associated with nefazodone include light-headedness, dizziness, orthostatic hypotension, somnolence, dry mouth, nausea, and asthenia (weakness). Due to the previously discussed potential for hepatic injury associated with nefazodone use treatment should not be initiated in individuals with active liver disease or with elevated baseline serum transaminases.[38] A rare but potentially serious adverse effect of trazodone is priapism, which is reported to occur in approximately 1 in 6,000 male patients. Some cases have required surgical intervention (1 in 23,000), and permanent impotence may result.[53] There have been no reports of priapism associated with nefazodone use in men, but there is a published case report of nefazodone-induced clitoral priapism.[54]

Aminoketone

Adverse effects associated with bupropion include nausea, vomiting, tremor, insomnia, dry mouth, and skin reactions. The occurrence of seizures in patients taking bupropion appears to be strongly dose related, and may be increased by predisposing factors such as history of head trauma and CNS tumor. Additionally, bupropion use is contraindicated in patients with eating disorders such as bulimia and anorexia, as these patients are prone to electrolyte abnormalities and are therefore at higher risk for seizure activity. At daily doses of 450 mg (the FDA-approved maximum dose) or less, the incidence of seizures is 0.4%.[55] Due to its pharmacological profile (i.e., pro-adrenergic) bupropion may cause activation or agitation in some patients.[18]

Tetracyclic

The most common adverse effects of mirtazapine are somnolence, weight gain, dry mouth, and constipation. Interestingly, side effects such as weight gain may be less with larger mirtazapine doses due to different mechanisms of action at different doses,[51] such as increased noradrenergic transmission as the dose is increased.

Monoamine Oxidase Inhibitors

The most common adverse effect of MAOIs is postural hypotension; this is more likely to occur with phenelzine than with tranylcypromine and may be minimized through divided dosage scheduling. Other common adverse effects include weight gain and sexual side effects (e.g., decreased libido, anorgasmia).[2] Phenelzine, the most frequently prescribed MAOI, has mild to moderate sedating effects, while tranylcypromine may exert a stimulating effect, and therefore insomnia can occur. In addition, fever, myoclonic jerking, and brisk deep tendon reflexes may occur.[56]

Hypertensive crisis, a potentially serious and life-threatening but rare adverse reaction, may occur when MAOIs are taken concurrently with certain foods, especially those high in tyramine

TABLE 77-5 Dietary Restrictions for Patients Taking Monoamine Oxidase Inhibitors[a]

Aged cheeses[b]
Sour cream[c]
Yogurt[c]
Cottage cheese[c]
American cheese[c]
Mild Swiss cheese[c]
Wine[d] (especially Chianti and sherry)
Beer
Herring (pickled, salted, dry)
Sardines
Snails
Anchovies
Canned, aged, or processed meats
Monosodium glutamate
Liver (chicken or beef, more than 2 days old)
Fermented foods
Canned figs
Raisins
Pods of broad beans (fava beans)
Yeast extract and other yeast products
Meat extract (marmite)
Soy sauce
Chocolate[e]
Coffee[e]
Ripe avocado
Sauerkraut
Licorice

[a]According to the FDA-approved Prescribing Information for the transdermal selegiline patch, patients receiving the 6 mg/24-hour dose are not required to modify their diet. However, patients receiving the 9 or 12 mg/24 hours are still required to follow the dietary restrictions similar to the other MAOIs.
[b]Clearly warrants absolute prohibition (e.g., English Stilton, blue, Camembert, cheddar).
[c]Up to 2 oz (59 mL) daily is acceptable.
[d]3 oz (89 mL) white wine or a single cocktail is acceptable.
[e]Up to 2 oz (59 mL) daily is acceptable; larger amounts of decaffeinated coffee are acceptable.
Recommended first-line drug and food interaction search engines: references 102 and 103.

(Table 77-5), or medications (Table 77-6). Ten milligrams of tyramine can cause a marked pressor effect, and 25 mg can result in a serious hypertensive crisis.[57] These incidents may culminate in cerebrovascular accident and death. Symptoms of hypertensive crisis include occipital headache, stiff neck, nausea, vomiting, sweating, and sharply elevated blood pressure. Hypertensive crises can be treated with antihypertensive agents such as captopril.[58]

TABLE 77-6 Medication Restrictions for Patients Taking Monoamine Oxidase Inhibitors

Amphetamines	Local anesthetics containing
Appetite suppressants	sympathomimetic vasoconstrictors
Asthma inhalants	Meperidine
Buspirone	Methyldopa
Carbamazepine	Methylphenidate
Cocaine	Other antidepressants[a]
Cyclobenzaprine	Other MAOIs
Decongestants (topical and systemic)	Reserpine
Dextromethorphan	Rizatriptan
Dopamine	Stimulants
Ephedrine	Sumatriptan
Epinephrine	Sympathomimetics
Guanethidine	Tryptophan
Levodopa	

[a]Tricyclic antidepressants may be used with caution by experienced clinicians in treatment-resistant populations.
Recommended first-line drug interaction search engines: references 102 and 103.

Education of patients taking MAOIs regarding dietary and medication restrictions is extremely important. Printed and verbal patient instructions should be provided. It is important that patients be instructed to consult a healthcare professional before taking any over-the-counter medications, including non-FDA approved items sold as herbal/dietary supplements. Patients should be taught to recognize the symptoms of hypertensive crisis and to seek immediate treatment should those symptoms occur.

CLINICAL CONTROVERSY

In recent years, numerous reports from the Food and Drug Administration warn healthcare providers of adverse effects associated with the use of the antidepressants in various populations. Many of these warnings have been accompanied by product labeling changes, including black box warnings. However, some of the warnings have not been unequivocally supported in the scientific literature. Therefore, the reader is encouraged to examine and understand these reports, and consider them within the context of the scientific literature.

PHARMACOKINETICS

The pharmacokinetics of the antidepressants are summarized in Table 77-7. Bioavailability is low (30%–70% for most TCAs) as a result of the first-pass hepatic effect, which shows great interindividual variation.[59] The TCAs have a large volume of distribution and concentrate in brain and cardiac tissue in laboratory animals. They are bound extensively and strongly to plasma albumin, erythrocytes, α_1-acid glycoprotein, and lipoprotein.[59] The major metabolic pathways are demethylation, aromatic and aliphatic hydroxylation, and glucuronide conjugation. Enterohepatic cycling has been described.[59,60] Metabolism of TCAs is linear within the usual dosage range. The elimination half-lives of the TCAs can vary greatly among individual patients.[59]

Venlafaxine is metabolized to an active metabolite, O-desmethylvenlafaxine, which contributes to the overall pharmacological effect,[61] and has received FDA approval as another option for the treatment of depressive disorders. Venlafaxine has the lowest plasma protein binding of any antidepressant (27%–30%), which reduces the likelihood of drug interactions via this mechanism. As might be expected, different formulations of venlafaxine with different pharmacokinetic profiles have lead to different adverse effect profiles. For example, venlafaxine extended-release, with its sustained plasma concentrations, has been associated with higher rates of sexual dysfunction among men (37%) as compared with the immediate-release formulation (6%).[61]

The diversity of SSRIs is evident not only in their chemical structures, but also in their pharmacokinetic profiles.[62,63] These unique pharmacokinetic attributes of each SSRI can be used to guide treatment. For example, the long half-life of fluoxetine and its active metabolite norfluoxetine may be beneficial in instances of partial nonadherence (e.g., missed doses). Conversely, caution must be taken to monitor for drug–drug interactions prior to combining another medication with fluoxetine. SSRIs are extensively distributed to the tissues, and all, with the possible exception of citalopram and sertraline, may have a nonlinear pattern of drug accumulation with long-term administration.[49,62] Therefore, the relationship between the dose and observed effect (e.g., side effect) may change over time for the non-linear SSRIs, and this needs to be considered during treatment.

Bupropion is metabolized to multiple active metabolites (see Table 77-7). There are currently three formulations of bupropion (immediate release, sustained release, and extended release), which

TABLE 77-7 Pharmacokinetic Properties of Antidepressants

Generic Name	Elimination Half-Life (h)[a]	Time of Peak Plasma Concentration (h)	Plasma Protein Binding (%)	Percentage Bioavailable	Clinically Important Metabolites
Serotonin selective reuptake inhibitors					
Citalopram	33	2–4	80	≥80	None
Escitalopram	27–32	5	56	80	None
Fluoxetine	4–6 days[b]	4–8	94	95	Norfluoxetine
Fluvoxamine	15–26	2–8	77	53	None
Paroxetine	24–31	5–7	95		None
Sertraline	27	6–8	99	36[c]	None
Serotonin/norepinephrine reuptake inhibitors					
Venlafaxine	5	2	27–30	45	O-Desmethylvenlafaxine
Desvenlafaxine	11	7.5	30	80	None
Duloxetine	12	6	90	50	None
Aminoketone					
Bupropion	10–21	3	82–88	[d]	Hydroxybupropion Threohydrobupropion Erythrohydrobupropion
Triazolopyridines					
Nefazodone	2–4	1	99	20	Meta-chlorophenylpiperazine
Trazodone	6–11	1–2	92	[d]	Meta-chlorophenylpiperazine
Tetracyclic					
Mirtazapine	20–40	2	85	50	None
Tricyclics					
Tertiary amines					
Amitriptyline	9–46	1–5	90–97	30–60	Nortriptyline
Clomipramine	20–24	2–6	97	36–62	Desmethylclomipramine
Doxepin	8–36	1–4	68–82	13–45	Desmethyldoxepin
Imipramine	6–34	1.5–3	63–96	22–77	Desipramine
Secondary amines					
Desipramine	11–46	3–6	73–92	33–51	2-Hydroxydesipramine
Nortriptyline	16–88	3–12	87–95	46–70	10-Hydroxynortriptyline

[a]Biologic half-life in slowest phase of elimination.
[b]4–6 days with chronic dosing; norfluoxetine, 4–16 days.
[c]Increases 30%–40% when taken with food.
[d]No data available.
Data from references 37, 63, 70, and 71.

are considered bioequivalent.[64] The bupropion peak plasma concentrations are lower for the sustained-release formulation of bupropion, and it is believed this may contribute to a lower seizure risk with that formulation.[65]

Mirtazapine undergoes extensive biotransformation to several metabolites[66] and is primarily eliminated in the urine (renal elimination). However, these metabolites are present at such low plasma concentrations as to minimally contribute to the overall pharmacologic profile of mirtazapine.

Altered Pharmacokinetics

Factors that influence TCA plasma concentrations include disease states, genetics, age, cigarette smoking, and concurrent drug administration. Hepatic disease may result in increased TCA plasma concentrations.[67] Renal failure does not alter nortriptyline metabolism, but the 10-hydroxy metabolite may accumulate, and protein binding may be diminished, with resulting enhanced sensitivity to the drug.[59] Clinicians should be alert to the possibility of higher-than-expected plasma concentrations of some TCAs in the elderly.

In patients with cirrhosis, the half-lives of fluoxetine and norfluoxetine increased to 7.6 and 12 days, respectively.[62] Patients with hepatic impairment had a twofold increase in plasma concentrations of paroxetine.[68] Similarly, in patients with mild stable cirrhosis, the half-life of sertraline was 2.5 times greater than in patients without liver disease.[69] Patients with renal impairment had a 2- to 4-fold increase in paroxetine plasma concentrations compared with normal volunteers.[68] Plasma concentrations of SSRIs in the elderly are reported to be greater than in younger patients.[62]

The clearance of venlafaxine, mirtazapine, and their metabolites may be reduced among patients with hepatic or renal disease,[70] and doses should be adjusted accordingly. Elderly patients may require a dose reduction with mirtazapine.[70]

Plasma Concentration and Clinical Response

Studies in acutely depressed patients have demonstrated a correlation between antidepressant effect and plasma concentrations for some TCAs. However, the patient's clinical response, not plasma concentration, dictates dosage adjustments. Some patients with plasma concentrations outside the suggested therapeutic plasma concentration range respond, whereas others are nonresponsive regardless of their plasma concentration. See Table 77–3 for a listing of suggested therapeutic plasma concentration ranges. There are four TCAs (nortriptyline, desipramine, imipramine, and amitriptyline) with evidence to support an association between plasma concentrations and clinical response. However, the best established therapeutic range is for nortriptyline (50–150 ng/mL [190–570 nmol/L]),[67] which appears to demonstrate a curvilinear plasma concentration-response relationship.

For the newer antidepressants, a correlation has not been established between plasma concentration and clinical response or adverse effects.

Plasma Concentration Monitoring

Because of interindividual variations in plasma concentrations achieved by a given dose, interpretation of plasma concentrations can be very difficult for the TCAs.[67] Although plasma level monitoring is not performed routinely, some indications include inadequate response, relapse, serious or persistent adverse effects, use of higher than standard doses, suspected toxicity, elderly patients, pregnant patients, cardiac disease, suspected nonadherence, suspected pharmacokinetic drug interactions, and when the manufacturer of the product changes. If plasma concentration monitoring is used to detect nonadherence, a cut-off as low as 30 ng/ml for the TCAs has been suggested to avoid confusion with low bioavailability or unusually rapid metabolism. Plasma concentrations should be obtained at steady state, usually after a minimum of 1 week at constant dosage. Sampling should be performed during the drug elimination phase, usually in the morning, 12 hours after the last dose. Samples collected in this manner are comparable for patients on once-, twice-, or thrice-daily regimens.[59]

■ DRUG INTERACTIONS

Serotonin-Norepinephrine Reuptake Inhibitors

Because the TCAs are metabolized in the liver through the cytochrome P450 system, they may interact with other drugs that modify hepatic enzyme activity or hepatic blood flow. TCAs are also extensively protein bound, which can cause drug interactions through displacement from protein-binding sites. Many commonly used medications can interact when given concurrently with TCAs. Due to their frequent co-administration, a common drug interaction occurs between the TCAs and certain SSRIs, such as paroxetine and fluoxetine. These drugs are known to inhibit cytochrome P450 (e.g., CYP 2D6) with the resultant increase in TCA plasma concentrations. Although MAOIs and TCAs may be coadministered safely in refractory patients with apparent increased efficacy compared with monotherapy, severe reactions (e.g., hypertensive crisis) and fatalities have occurred.[2,59] Therefore, this combination should be monitored extremely carefully. Lastly, the TCAs, SNRIs, and SSRIs can potentially be involved in a pharmacodynamic drug interaction known as the *serotonin syndrome (SS)*. This phenomenon will be described in further detail for SSRI drug interactions (i.e., the medications most commonly associated with this reaction) and within Table 77–8, which summarizes drug interactions for the newer-generation antidepressants.

Serotonin Selective Reuptake Inhibitors

Drug–drug interactions may occur when an SSRI is coadministered with another drug metabolized through the cytochrome P450 system. Two of the isoenzymes of the cytochrome P450 system, 2D6 and 3A4, are responsible for the metabolism of more than 80% of currently marketed drugs.[71] The ability of an SSRI, or any antidepressant, to inhibit or induce the activity of these enzymes will be a significant contributory factor in determining its capability to cause a pharmacokinetic drug interaction when administered concomitantly. Table 77–9 shows the cytochrome P450 enzyme inhibitory potential of the second- and third-generation antidepressant agents. In patients receiving a stable dose of any medication known to interact with SSRIs, if an SSRI is to be initiated, the starting dose should be low and titrated carefully to evaluate the potential importance of the interaction.

Certain pharmacodynamic drug interactions that may occur with SSRIs are concerning and require close monitoring. For example, the combination of an SSRI with another drug that augments serotonergic function (e.g., linezolid) can lead to SS, which is characterized by symptoms such as clonus, hyperthermia, and mental status changes.[72] However, these symptoms are not unanimously agreed upon (please see Clinical Controversy below for additional information). Therefore, a washout period of 2 to 5 weeks (depending on the half-life of the SSRI) may be necessary before the initiation of another serotonergic medication.

CLINICAL CONTROVERSY

Various criteria have been proposed for the diagnosis of SS. The typical triad of symptoms that has long been described includes mental status changes, autonomic instability, and neuromuscular abnormalities. However, SS has been identified in cases without all three of these symptoms being present. Therefore, alternative approaches to the well-accepted SS triad have been suggested. For example, it has been proposed[72] that the presence of any of the following symptom clusters is highly diagnostic of SS:

- Tremor + hyperreflexia
- Spontaneous clonus
- Muscle rigidity + temperature >38°C (100.4°F) + ocular clonus or inducible clonus
- Ocular clonus + agitation or diaphoresis
- Inducible clonus + agitation or diaphoresis

Other Agents

In contrast to the SSRIs that have potential for both pharmacokinetic and pharmacodynamic interactions, other newer-generation antidepressants such as venlafaxine, duloxetine, mirtazapine, and bupropion have drug interactions that are primarily pharmacodynamic. This may be partly explained by the relative lack of cytochrome P450 inhibition among these newer agents compared to SSRIs (see Table 77–9). As nefazodone use has been severely limited due to its potential to induce liver toxicity, and trazodone is primarily used as a non-FDA approved hypnotic at low doses, neither of these agents are likely to be involved in clinically significant drug interactions. However, it should be noted that nefazodone is a potent inhibitor of cytochrome P450 3A4.[71] Lastly, please refer to the MAOI adverse effects section above and Table 77–6 to read more about the hypertensive crisis that may result following the coadministration of MAOIs and other medications that increase the vasopressor response (e.g., amphetamines).

■ SPECIAL POPULATIONS

Elderly Patients

Depression in the elderly is a major public health problem. Many elderly depressed patients are inadequately treated, or depression is missed or mistaken for another disorder, such as dementia. In the elderly, depressed mood, the typical signature symptom of depression, may be less prominent than other depressive symptoms such as loss of appetite, cognitive impairment, sleeplessness, anergia, and loss of interest in and enjoyment of the normal pursuits of life.[73] Older adults may not recognize common symptoms associated with depression such as anhedonia (inability to experience pleasure), fatigue, and concentration difficulties. Somatic (physical) complaints are quite frequently the presenting symptoms in elderly depressed patients. Appropriate recognition and treatment of depression in the elderly is extremely important. In fact, individuals 65 years of age and older have a very high rate of suicidality.[74] Increased suicidal attempts present in the depressed elderly may

TABLE 77-8 Selected Drug Interactions of Newer-Generation Antidepressants

Antidepressant	Interacting Drug/Drug Class	Effect
Serotonin/norepinephrine reuptake inhibitors		
Venlafaxine and desvenlafaxine	MAOIs	Potential for hypertensive crisis, serotonin syndrome, delirium
	Sibutramine	Serotonin syndrome
	Triptans	Serotonin syndrome
Duloxetine	MAOIs	Potential for hypertensive crisis, serotonin syndrome, delirium
	Sibutramine	Serotonin syndrome
	Thioridazine	Thioridazine C_{max} increased; prolonged QTc interval
	Triptans	Serotonin syndrome
Serotonin selective reuptake inhibitors		
Citalopram and escitalopram	MAOIs	Potential for hypertensive crisis, serotonin syndrome, delirium
	Linezolid (*MAOI effects*)	Serotonin syndrome
	Sibutramine	Serotonin syndrome
	Triptans	Serotonin syndrome
Fluoxetine	Alprazolam	Increased plasma concentrations and half-life of alprazolam; increased psychomotor impairment
	Antipsychotics (e.g., haloperidol and risperidone)	Increased antipsychotic concentrations; increased extrapyramidal side effects
	β-Adrenergic blockers	Increased metoprolol serum concentrations; increased bradycardia; possible heart block
	Carbamazepine	Increased plasma concentrations of carbamazepine; symptoms of carbamazepine toxicity
	Linezolid (*MAOI effects*)	Serotonin syndrome
	MAOIs	Potential for hypertensive crisis, serotonin syndrome, delirium
	Phenytoin	Increased plasma concentrations of phenytoin; symptoms of phenytoin toxicity
	TCAs	Markedly increased TCA plasma concentrations; symptoms of TCA toxicity
	Sibutramine	Serotonin syndrome
	Triptans	Serotonin syndrome
	Thioridazine	Thioridazine C_{max} increased; prolonged QTc interval
Fluvoxamine	Alosetron	Increased alosetron AUC (6-fold) and half-life (3-fold)
	Alprazolam	Increased AUC of alprazolam by 96%, increased alprazolam half-life by 71%; increased psychomotor impairment
	β-Adrenergic blockers	Fivefold increase in propranolol serum concentration; bradycardia and hypotension
	Carbamazepine	Increased plasma concentrations of carbamazepine; symptoms of carbamazepine toxicity
	Clozapine	Increased clozapine serum concentrations; increased risk for seizures and orthostatic hypotension
	Diltiazem	Bradycardia
	MAOIs	Potential for hypertensive crisis, serotonin syndrome, delirium
	Methadone	Increased methadone plasma concentrations; symptoms of methadone toxicity
	Ramelteon	Increased AUC (190-fold) and C_{max} (70-fold)
	Sibutramine	Serotonin syndrome
	TCAs	Increased TCA plasma concentration; symptoms of TCA toxicity
	Theophylline and caffeine	Increased serum concentrations of theophylline or caffeine; symptoms of theophylline or caffeine toxicity
	Thioridazine	Thioridazine C_{max} increased; prolonged QTc interval
	Warfarin	Increased hypoprothrombinemic response to warfarin
Paroxetine	Antipsychotics (e.g., haloperidol, perphenazine and risperidone)	Increased antipsychotic concentrations; increased central nervous system and extrapyramidal side effects
	β-Adrenergic blockers	Increased metoprolol serum concentrations; increased bradycardia; possible heart block
	Linezolid (*MAOI effects*)	Serotonin syndrome
	MAOIs	Potential for hypertensive crisis, serotonin syndrome, delirium
	TCAs	Markedly increased TCA plasma concentrations; symptoms of TCA toxicity
	Sibutramine	Serotonin syndrome
	Triptans	Serotonin syndrome
	Thioridazine	Thioridazine C_{max} increased; prolonged QTc interval
Sertraline	Linezolid (*MAOI effects*)	Serotonin syndrome
	MAOIs	Potential for hypertensive crisis, serotonin syndrome, delirium
	Sibutramine	Serotonin syndrome
	Triptans	Serotonin syndrome
Tetracyclic		
Mirtazapine	Carbamazepine	Mirtazapine concentration decrease (60%)
	MAOIs	Theoretically central serotonin syndrome could occur
Aminoketone		
Bupropion	MAOIs	Potential for hypertensive crisis
	Medications that lower seizure threshold	Increased incidence of seizures

AUC, area under the curve, C_{max}, maximum concentration; MAOI, monoamine oxidase inhibitor.
Recommended first-line drug interaction search engines: references 102 and 103.

TABLE 77-9	Second- and Third-Generation Antidepressants and Cytochrome (CYP) P450 Enzyme Inhibitory Potential			
	CYP Enzyme			
Drug	*1A2*	*2C*	*2D6*	*3A4*
Buproprion	0	0	+	0
Citalopram	0	0	+	NA
Escitalopram	0	0	+	0
Fluoxetine	0	++	++++	++
Fluvoxamine	++++	++	0	+++
Mirtazapine	0	0	0	0
Nefazodone	0	0	0	++++
Paroxetine	0	0	++++	0
Sertraline	0	++	+	+
(des)Venlafaxine	0	0	0/+	0

++++, high; +++, moderate; ++, low; +, very low; 0, absent.
Data from references 49, 63, 70, and 71.

be due to access to firearms, diminished cognitive functioning, sleep disruptions, poor social interactions, and inattention among primary caregivers.[74]

Before initiating antidepressant treatment, a complete physical examination should be performed. In prescribing antidepressants, elderly patients may be either over- or undertreated. Overtreatment occurs when age-related pharmacokinetic and pharmacodynamic factors are overlooked. Undertreatment results from an overly conservative approach as a result of the patient's advanced age or concurrent medical problems. SSRIs are usually selected as first-choice antidepressants in the elderly, and this may enable the clinician to avoid some of the problematic adverse effects commonly associated with TCAs (e.g., sedative, anticholinergic, and cardiovascular-related side effects). Furthermore, there is evidence to suggest that the long-term use of antidepressants such as SSRIs in the elderly, administred with either psychotherapy or clinical management, may prevent a depressive relapse.[75] Bupropion and venlafaxine are often selected because of milder anticholinergic and less frequent cardiovascular side effects.[76] Mirtazapine has been shown to be an effective antidepressant in the elderly (at least 65 years of age) and better tolerated than SSRI paroxetine. Furthermore, secondary measures of anxiety and sleep were improved following mirtazapine administration.[77]

Pediatric Patients

Accumulating evidence indicates that childhood depression occurs quite commonly. Symptoms of depression in the young may vary from accepted diagnostic criteria and include several nonspecific symptoms such as boredom, anxiety, failing adjustment, and sleep disturbance.[78]

Data collected under controlled conditions that support the efficacy of antidepressants in children and adolescents are sparse, and no antidepressant, except fluoxetine, is FDA approved for the treatment of depression in patients younger than 18 years of age, although other antidepressants (e.g., sertraline) have been studied in this population.[79]

The use of antidepressants in children and adolsescents was complicated when, in March 2004, the FDA issued a black box warning in the product labeling for antidepressant medications warning clinicians and patients of the increased risk for suicidal ideation and behavior when antidepressants are used in this population. However, several retrospective longitudinal reviews of the use of antidepressants in children found no significant increase in the risk

of suicide attempts or deaths.[80-82] Furthermore, adolescents suffering from depression who remain untreated may successfully commit suicide.[83,84] Further study is needed to resolve this important clinical dilemma.

Several cases of sudden death have been reported in children and adolescents taking antidepressants, such as desipramine. A baseline electrocardiogram (ECG) is recommended before initiating treatment with a TCA in children and adolescents, and many clinicians recommend an additional ECG when steady-state plasma concentrations are achieved.[85]

The treatment of depression in children remains challenging, as depression can be difficult to diagnose and treat once identified. Antidepressants are used to treat depressed children and adolescents because no other definitive effective therapies are currently available. Also, demonstration of efficacy in this population, as well as in adults, is confounded by a high placebo response rate. However, the TCAs and several of the SSRIs remain viable treatment options when prescribed and monitored appropriately.

Pregnant and Lactating Patients

Approximately 14% of pregnant women develop a serious depression during pregnancy.[86] The data presented in several recent publications should be considered when making treatment decisions for pregnant women suffering from major depression.[86-88] The first evaluation looked at the risk of discontinuing antidepressant therapy in pregnant women suffering from depression and found a significant risk of relapse. In this study, women who discontinued antidepressant therapy were 5 times more likely to have a relapse during their pregnancy than were women who continued treatment.[88] Another study utilized population health data to determine whether exposure to SSRIs and depression in pregnant women differs from exposure to maternal depression alone. The authors found that prenatal exposure to SSRIs was associated with an increased risk of low birth weight and respiratory distress, and that this relationship remained after accounting for maternal illness severity.[86] A study by Chambers and colleagues reported a 6-fold greater likelihood of the occurrence of persistent pulmonary hypertension of newborn infants exposed to an SSRI after the 20th week of gestation.[87] A recent editorial on the use of antidepressants in pregnancy lists four therapeutic principles to guide the clinician in treating women during pregnancy: (1) Pregnancy does not protect against the occurrence of depression, and the likelihood of relapse is very high in untreated women with recurrent illness. (2) Maternal depression adversely affects child development, and prenatal depression may adversely affect the offspring. (3) When attempting to balance benefit and risk, transient postnatal behavioral abnormalities in the offspring of treated mothers must not be assumed to portend long-term compromise. (4) SSRIs, the most commonly used and best-tolerated treatment for depression, carry a small but significant risk for a serious medical consequence.[89]

In September 2009, the American Psychiatric Association and the American College of Obstetricians and Gynecologists released a report discussing the treatment of depression during pregnancy. One of the prominent conclusions of this report was that *both* antidepressant treatment and untreated depression have been associated with potential problems during pregnancy. However, studies to date have not been able to adequately control for all the necessary variables involved in birth outcomes (e.g., maternal depressive disorder) and more work needs to be done.[90]

In summary, the risks and benefits of drug therapy during pregnancy must always be weighed, and concerns about the risks of untreated depression during pregnancy should be considered. These include the possibility of low-birth-weight secondary to poor maternal weight gain, suicidality, potential for hospitalization, potential for marital discord, inability to engage in appropriate obstetric care, and difficulty caring for other children.[91] Several different approaches exist for dealing with pregnancy and antidepressant use. First, discontinuation of an antidepressant before conception is an option for women who are stable and appear likely to remain well while not taking antidepressant medication. Second, continuation of the antidepressant until conception may be reasonable. For those who have a history of depressive relapse after medication discontinuation, the antidepressant should be continued throughout pregnancy. Further evaluations of the newer antidepressant agents are needed to fully understand the risks associated with their use at various stages of the gestational period. Again, the risks of not treating depression in a pregnant woman should not be underestimated or minimized.

There is a great deal of uncertainty regarding long-term antidepressant exposure during breastfeeding due to the lack of data. However, sertraline and paroxetine both appear in relatively low concentrations in breast milk and in samples taken from infants.[92]

Relative Resistance and Treatment-Resistant Depression

The majority of "treatment-resistant" depressed patients are likely the result of inadequate therapy (relative resistance). This theory is supported by data from the National Institute of Mental Health (NIMH) Sequenced Treatment Alternatives to Relieve Depression (STAR*D) study, which is generally considered to be one of the premier antidepressant trials among patients with depressive disorders.[93] This study showed that one in three depressed patients who previously did not achieve remission using an antidepressant became symptom free with the help of an additional medication (e.g., bupropion SR) and one in four achieved remission after switching to a different antidepressant (e.g., venlafaxine XR).[93] Furthermore, patients can be switched to another medication within the same class. For example, patients in the STAR*D study not responding to an initial SSRI were shown to be as likely to respond to another SSRI as they were a medication from a different class.[94]

Although several different definitions for treatment-resistant depression have been proposed, the most widely accepted is depression which has not achieved remission even after two optimal antidepressant trails.[95] More than 40% of patients with major depressive disorder being treated with antidepressants meet these criteras.[95] Three pharmacologic approaches that have been used with success for treatment resistant depression include the following:

1. The current antidepressant may be stopped and a trial with another agent initiated (i.e., switching). For example, the STAR*D trial compared switching to mirtazapine (up to 60 mg/day) versus nortriptyline (up to 200 mg/day) after two consecutive failed medication treatments.[96] In the mirtazapine group, 12.3% of patients met the remission criterion of a score of 7 or less on the HAM-D, while 19.8% of nortriptyline patients met this criterion at the end of 14 weeks.

2. The current antidepressant can be augmented by the addition of another agent such as lithium, or another antidepressant can be added (i.e., combination antidepressant treatment). For example, the STAR*D trial evaluated the addition of lithium or T_3 (i.e., triiodothyronine) to current antidepressant treatment. After approximately 10 weeks, T_3 augmentation resulted in higher remission rates (24.7%) compared with lithium (15.9%). However, the differences between these two augmentation strategies were modest and not statistically significant.[95]

3. The use of atypical antipsychotic agents to augment the antidepressant response. In fact, aripiprazole was the first atypical antipsychotic to receive FDA approval for adjunctive

use in adults with major depressive disorder, and others will likely follow. Additionally, olanzapine *in combination* with fluoxetine (Symbyax) was approved for treatment resistant depression. Please refer to the FDA website for additional information on FDA approvals.

The American Psychiatric Association practice guideline for the treatment of patients with major depressive disorder offers guidance for managing patients who fail to respond. These guidelines advise that if patients fail to respond to medication after 6 to 8 weeks, a reappraisal of the treatment regimen should be considered.[2] Partial responders should consider changing the dose, augmenting the antidepressant, or adding psychotherapy or ECT. For those with no response, options include changing to a second antidepressant or the addition of psychotherapy or ECT. Comorbid medical or psychiatric conditions should be identified and treated because they may complicate treatment. Before changing a patient's treatment, the clinician is advised to evaluate the adequacy of the medication dosage and adherence with the prescribed regimen. A combination of two drugs should not be used when one drug will suffice.

❻ Issues to be addressed in assessing the patient who has not responded to treatment include the following:

1. Is the diagnosis correct?

2. Does the patient have a psychotic depression?

3. Has the patient received an adequate dose and adequate duration of treatment?

4. Do adverse effects preclude adequate dosing?

5. Has the patient adhered to the prescribed regimen?

6. Was a stepwise approach to treatment used?

7. Was treatment outcome adequately measured?

8. Is there a coexisting or preexisting medical or psychiatric disorder?

9. Are there other factors that interfere with treatment?

■ CLINICAL APPLICATION

A suggested algorithm for the management of uncomplicated major depressive disorder is shown in Figure 77–2. Recommended initial doses and dosage ranges are shown in Table 77–3. In elderly patients, as a general rule, dosing is initiated at one-half the initial dose administered to younger adults, and the dose is increased at a slower rate.

The usual initial adult dose of most TCAs is 25 mg at bedtime, and the dose may be increased by 25 to 50 mg every third day. The usual starting dose of venlafaxine is 75 mg/day and taken with food. Some patients may better tolerate a starting dose of 37.5 mg/day for a few days before beginning 75 mg/day. Depending on tolerability, the dose is then titrated to 150 mg/day. If needed, the dose may be further increased to 225 mg/day. Severely depressed patients may require doses as high as 375 mg/day. Both an immediate-release and extended-release formulation of venlafaxine are now available. Desvenlafaxine can be started and maintained at the same 50 mg dose, which may be an advantage compared with other antidepressants that need to be titrated up over time. Duloxetine can be started at 30 mg and titrated upward to 60 to 90 mg/day, given as a divided or single daily dose.

The recommended initial dose for the SSRIs citalopram, fluoxetine, and paroxetine is 20 mg and 10 mg for escitalopram. The initial dose for fluvoxamine and sertraline is 50 mg/day. The doses are titrated upwards depending on symptom response and adverse effects.

Bupropion is usually initiated at 75 mg twice daily, and this dose may be increased to 100 mg 3 times daily after a few days. Most patients will respond at 300 mg/day; however, an increase to

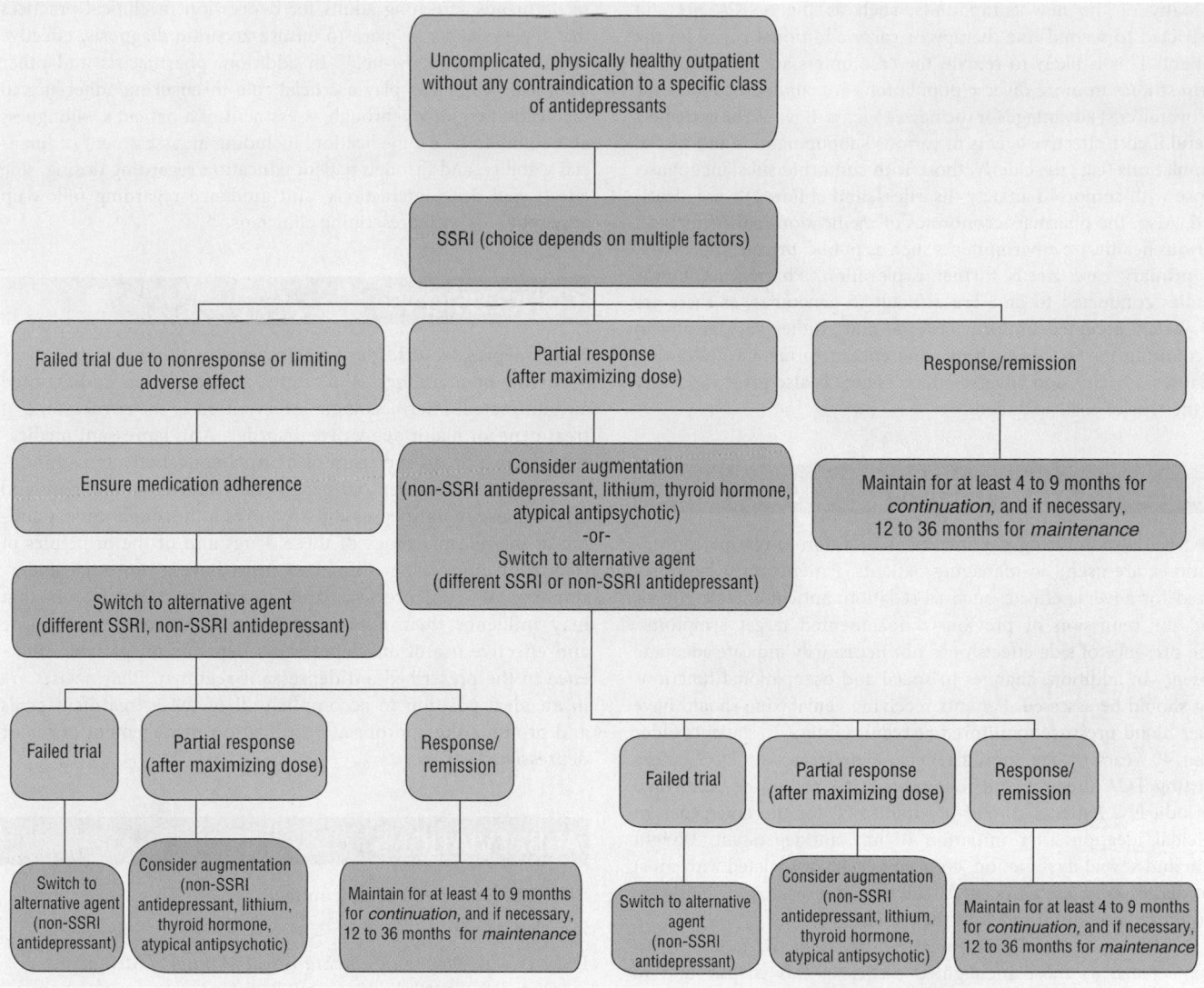

FIGURE 77-2. Algorithm for treatment of uncomplicated major depressive disorder. (SSRI, serotonin selective reuptake inhibitor.)

450 mg/day, given as 150 mg 3 times daily, may be considered in patients with no or partial response after several weeks of treatment at 300 mg/day. Additionally, both a 12-hour and 24-hour sustained-release formulation are available, allowing for less frequent dosing. The recommended starting dose of mirtazapine is 15 mg/day administered in a single dose at bedtime and the maximum recommended dose is 45 mg/day.

Caution is urged when switching from one antidepressant to another. It is important to remember that 3 to 4 weeks is usually required before a mood-elevating response is seen. A 6-week trial at a maximum dosage is considered an adequate trial.[2] It is crucial to counsel the patient about the expected lag time before the onset of clinical response. Patients uneducated in this regard often fail to adhere to their prescribed regimens.

■ PHARMACOECONOMIC CONSIDERATIONS

Cost of illness studies attempt to provide an estimation of the amount spent on a particular disease and to identify different components of the cost.[97] Ideally, direct, indirect, and intangible costs would be included. Direct costs include medical and nonmedical costs such as outpatient costs, inpatient costs, medication costs, transportation costs, and social services costs. Indirect costs include loss of productivity or reduced productivity. Intangible costs result

from a decreased quality of life for the depressed individual and his/her family. Intangible costs are often not considered in pharmacoeconomic models because an accurate quantification in monetary terms is difficult.[97] Most published studies do not include all of the relevant aspects necessary for credible economic analyses.[98] In addition, there is wide variability among studies with regard to cost inclusion and evaluation of treatment withdrawals, relapses, toxicity, and adverse effects.[98] When SSRIs were introduced, many managed care organizations restricted these medications to those who had failed treatment with the TCAs or who had been unable to tolerate these agents, with the belief that the SSRIs represented a more expensive approach to the treatment of depression. One of the major claims for SSRIs is the greater tolerability and safety profile in overdose when compared with TCAs.[99] Studies including the costs associated with hospitalization following TCA overdoses, as opposed to SSRI overdoses, indicate that overdoses with TCAs are significantly more expensive.[99] All of the randomized clinical trials evaluating total expenditure of SSRIs versus TCAs indicate a cost-advantage associated with SSRIs. This advantage may be due to greater tolerability. Recently, several of the SSRIs have lost patent exclusivity, and generic versions of these medications are available at substantially lower prices than the brand name versions. Due to this generic availability, the restrictions placed on SSRIs have been removed from most, if not all, organizations.

Many of the new compounds, such as the SNRIs, are still restricted to second-line therapy or carry additional copay for the patient. This is likely to remain the case unless additional longer-term studies in more diverse populations are conducted that show an overall cost advantage for the newer agents. It would be extremely useful if cost-effective agents in various subpopulations and special populations (e.g., the elderly, those with comorbid substance abuse, those with comorbid anxiety disorders, and children) were identified. Also, the pharmacoeconomics of medication management in various healthcare environments such as public, private, psychiatry, or primary care, needs further exploration. Pharmacoeconomic studies conducted to date are difficult to generalize, as there are no widely accepted uniform criteria, and studies vary greatly in accounting for factors such as adherence, treatment withdrawals, relapses, toxicity, and adverse effects. There is also great variability in the type of costs included.[98]

EVALUATION OF THERAPEUTIC OUTCOMES

❼ Several monitoring parameters, in addition to plasma concentrations, are useful in managing patients. Patients must be monitored for adverse effects, such as sedation, anticholinergic effects, and for remission of previously documented target symptoms. The presence of side effects does not necessarily indicate adequate dosage. In addition, changes in social and occupational functioning should be assessed. Patients receiving venlafaxine should have their blood pressure monitored at regular intervals. Patients older than 40 years of age should receive a pretreatment ECG before starting TCA therapy, and follow-up ECGs should be performed periodically. Patients should be monitored for the emergence of suicidal ideation after initiation of any antidepressant. Weight gain and sexual dysfunction, common events associated with most antidepressants, are associated with nonadherence and should be monitored and discussed with the patient.

In addition to the clinical interview, psychometric rating instruments (such as those highlighted earlier in this chapter and in Chapter 71) allow for rapid and reliable measurement of the nature and severity of depressive and associated symptoms. It is helpful to administer the rating scales prior to treatment, 6 to 8 weeks after initiation of therapy, and periodically thereafter. Interviewing a family member or friend (with the patient's permission) regarding symptoms and daily functioning also can assist in assessment of progress. Patients should be monitored at more frequent intervals early in treatment. Monitoring is then continued at regular intervals throughout the continuation and maintenance phases of treatment. Regular monitoring for reemergence of target symptoms should be continued for several months after antidepressant therapy is discontinued.

Finally, one useful set of criteria that can be used with a variety of psychometric scales was suggested by Mann.[33] Following these criteria, the following definitions are used: (1) *nonresponse* is less than 25% decrease in baseline symptoms, (2) *partial response* is a 26%–49% decrease in baseline symptoms, and (3) *partial remission or response* is greater than a 50% decrease in baseline symptoms. Consistent with other recommendations, *remission* is a return to baseline functioning with no symptoms present.[2]

COLLABORATIVE PRACTICE

Significant evidence exists to show that depression is common, chronic, and causes significant morbidity and mortality. Pharmacists, in conjunction with other healthcare providers, can play a crucial role in the screening, recognition, and treatment of this disorder. In fact, the U.S. Preventive Services Task Force recommends screening adults for depression in clinical practices that have systems in place to ensure accurate diagnosis, effective treatment, and follow-up.[100] In addition, pharmacists and other healthcare clinicians play a crucial role in ensuring adherence to medication regimens through assessment of a patient's willingness and ability to take a medication, including an assessment of financial viability, and through patient education regarding dosing, side effects and drug interactions, and guidance regarding follow-up appointments with prescribing clinicians.[101]

CONCLUSIONS

Major depressive disorder remains one of the most commonly occurring mental illnesses in adults, and it is often undiagnosed and untreated. Pharmacologic intervention is the cornerstone of treatment for major depressive disorder. Antidepressant medications have a broad spectrum of neurochemical effects and influence a variety of receptors peripherally and centrally. Safe and effective use of antidepressants requires a thorough understanding of the pharmacology of these drugs and of the principles of treatment monitoring. Clinicians must have a thorough understanding of antidepressant drug interactions and factors that may influence their pharmacokinetic parameters. Lastly, safe and effective use of antidepressants depends on patient adherence to the prescribed antidepressant regimen. Pharmacists are in an ideal position to accomplish all of these treatment goals and promote the appropriate medication management of major depressive disorder.

ABBREVIATIONS

BDNF: brain-derived neurotrophic factor

DA: dopamine

DSM-IV-TR: *Diagnostic and Statistical Manual of Mental Disorders, Fourth Edition, Text Revision*

ECG: electrocardiogram

ECT: electroconvulsive therapy

FDA: U.S. Food and Drug Administration

HPA: hypothalamic-pituitary-adrenal

5-HT: serotonin

LFT: liver function test

MAOI: monoamine oxidase inhibitor

NE: norepinephrine

REM: rapid eye movement

SAD: seasonal affective disorder

SNRI: serotonin-norepinephrine reuptake inhibitor

SS: serotonin syndrome

SSRI: serotonin selective reuptake inhibitor

TCA: tricyclic antidepressant

REFERENCES

1. American Psychiatric Association. Diagnostic and Statistical Manual of Mental Disorders, Fourth Edition, Text Revision. Washington, DC: American Psychiatric Association, 2000.
2. American Psychiatric Association. Practice guideline for the treatment of patients with major depressive disorder (revision). Am J Psychiatry 2000;157(Suppl):1–45.

3. Kessler RC, Berglund P, Demler O. The epidemiology of major depressive disorders: Results from the National Comorbidity Survey Replication (NCS-R). JAMA 2003;289:3095–3105.

4. Burt VK, Stein K. Epidemiology of depression throughout the female life cycle. J Clin Psychol 2002;63(Suppl 7):9–15.

5. Steffens DC, Skoog I, Norton MC, et al. Prevalence of depression and its treatment in an elderly population. The Cache County study. Arch Gen Psychiatry 2000;57:601–607.

6. Kessler RC, Walters EE. Epidemiology of DSM-III-R major depression and minor depression among adolescents and young adults in the National Comorbidity Survey. Depress Anxiety 1998;7:3–14.

7. Larsson B, Ivarsson T. Clinical characteristics of adolescent psychiatric inpatients who have attempted suicide. Eur Child Adolesc Psychiatry 1998;7:201–208.

8. Weissman MM, Gershon ES, Kidd KK, et al. Psychiatric disorders in the relatives of probands with affective disorder. Arch Gen Psychiatry 1984;41:13–21.

9. Warner V, Weissman MM, Mufson L, Wickramaratne PJ. Grandparents, parents, and grandchildren at high risk for depression: A three-generation study. J Am Acad Child Adolesc Psychiatry 1999;38:289–296.

10. Sullivan PF, Neale MC, Kendler KS. Genetic Epidemiology of Major Depression: Review and Meta-Analysis. Am J Psychiatry 2000;157:1552–1562.

11. Stahl SM. Blue genes and the mechanism of action of antidepressants. J Clin Psychiatry 2000;61:164–165.

12. Delgado PL. Depression: The case for a monoamine deficiency. J Clin Psychiatry 2000;61(Suppl 6):7–11.

13. Hirschfield RM. History and the evolution of the monoamine hypothesis of depression. J Clin Psychiatry 2000;61(Suppl 6):4–6.

14. Delgado PL, Moreno FA, Potter R, et al. Norepinephrine and serotonin in antidepressant action: Evidence from neurotransmitter depletion studies. In: Briley M, Montgomery SA, eds. Antidepressant Therapy at the Dawn of the Third Millennium. London: Marin Dunitz, 1997:141–163.

15. Baldessarini RJ. Drugs and the treatment of psychiatric disorders: Depression and anxiety disorders. In: Hardman JG, Limbrid LE, Goodman A, et al, eds. Goodman and Gilman's The Pharmacological Basis of Therapeutics, 10th ed. New York: McGraw-Hill, 2000: 447–484.

16. Stahl SM. Blue genes and the monoamine hypothesis of depression. J Clin Psychiatry 2000;61:77–78.

17. Feighner JP. Mechanism of action of antidepressant medications. J Clin Psychiatry 1999;60(Suppl 4):4–11.

18. Stahl S. Basic psychopharmacology of antidepressants, part 1: Antidepressants have seven distinct mechanisms of action. J Clin Psychiatry 1998;59(Suppl 4):5–14.

19. Siever LJ, Davis KL. Overview: Toward a dysregulation hypothesis of depression. Am J Psychiatry 1985;142:1017–1031.

20. Ordway GA, Klimek V, Mann JJ. Neurocircuitry of mood disorders. In: Neuropsychopharmacology: The Fifth Generation of Progress. Davis KL, Charney D, Coyle JT, Nemeroff C, eds. American College of Neuropsychopharmacology; 2002:1051–1064.

21. Berton and Nestler. New approaches to antidepressant drug discovery: beyond monoamines. Nat Rev Neuroscience 2006;7:137–151.

22. Thase M. Mood disorders. In: Neurobiology. Kaplan & Sadock's Comprehensive Textbook of Psychiatry. Sadock BJ, Sadock VA, eds. Philadelphia, PA: Lippincott Williams & Wilkins, 2004.

23. Sofuoglu M, Dudish-Poulsen S, Poling J, et al. The effect of individual cocaine withdrawal symptoms on outcomes in cocaine users. Addict Behav 2005;30:1125–1134.

24. Patten SB, Barbui C. Drug-induced depression: a systematic review to inform clinical practice. Psychother Psychosom 2004;73:207–215.

25. Montgomery SA, Asberg M. A new depression scale designed to be sensitive to change. Brit J Psychiatry 1979;134:382–389.

26. Beck AT, Ward CH, Mock J, Erbaugh J. An inventory for measuring depression. Arch Gen Psychiatry 1961;4:561–571.

27. McGirr A, Renaud J, Seguin M, et al. An examination of DSM-IV depressive symptoms and risk for suicide completion in major depressive disorder: A psychological autopsy study. J Affect Disord 2007;97:203–209.

28. Lebowitz BD, Pearson JL, Schneider LS, et al. Diagnosis and treatment of depression in late life: Consensus statement update. JAMA 1997;278:1186–1190.

29. Trivedi MH. The link between depression and physical symptoms. J Clin Psychiatry 2004;6(Suppl 1):12–16.

30. Centers for Disease Control and Prevention, National Center for Injury Prevention and Control. Suicide: Facts at a Glance; Summer 2009. http://www.cdc.gov/violenceprevention/pdf/Suicide-DataSheet-a.pdf.

31. Jacobs DG, Baldessarini RJ, Fawcett JA, et al. Practice guidelines for the assessment and treatment of patients with suicidal behaviors. Am J Psychiatry 2003;160(11 Suppl):1–60.

32. Fawcett JA, Baldessarini RJ, Coryell WH. Defining and managing suicidal risk in patients taking psychotropic medications. J Clin Psychiatry 2009;70(6):782–789.

33. Mann JJ. The medical management of depression. N Engl J Med 2005;353:1819–1834.

34. Blackburn IM, Moore RG. Controlled acute and follow-up trial of cognitive therapy and pharmacotherapy in outpatients with recurrent depression. Br J Psychiatry 1997;171:328–334.

35. Klapheke MM. Electroconvulsive therapy consultation: An update. Convuls Ther 1997;13:227–241.

36. Lafer B, Sachs GS, Labbate LA, et al. Side effects induced by bright light therapy. Am J Psychiatry 1994;151:1081–1083.

37. Stahl SM, Grady MM, Moret C, Briley M. SNRIs: Their pharmacology, clinical efficacy, and tolerability in comparison with other classes of antidepressants. CNS Spectrums 2005;10:732–747.

38. Ables AZ, Baughman III, OL. Antidepressants: update on new agents and indications. Am Fam Physician 2003;67:547–554.

39. Horst WD, Preskorn SH. Mechanism of action and clinical characteristics of three atypical antidepressants: Venlafaxine, nefazodone, bupropion. J Affect Disord 1998;51:237–254.

40. Gorman JM. Mirtazapine: Clinical overview. J Clin Psychiatry 1999;60(Suppl 17):9–13.

41. Bryant SG, Brown CS. Current concepts in clinical therapeutics: Major affective disorders, part 2. Clin Pharmacol 1986;5:385–395.

42. Patkar AA, Pae C-U, Masand PS. Transdermal selegiline: the new generation of monoamine oxidase inhibitors. CNS Spectrums 2006;11:363–375.

43. Cochrane Database of Systematic Reviews. St John's wort for depression. Cochrane Library, Cochrane Collaboration, 2006(3).

44. Nemeroff CB. The burden of severe depression: a review of diagnostic challenges and treatment alternatives. J Psychiatr Res 2007;41: 189–206.

45. Settle ED Jr. Antidepressant drugs: disturbing and potentially dangerous adverse effects. J Clin Psychiatry 1998;59(Suppl 16):25–30.

46. Haddad P. Antidepressant discontinuation reactions. In: Thompson C, chairperson. Discontinuation of antidepressant therapy: Emerging complications and their relevance [Academic Highlights]. J Clin Psychiatry 1998;59:541–548.

47. Feighner JP. Cardiovascular safety in depressed patients: Focus on venlafaxine. J Clin Psychiatry 1995;56:574–579.

48. Bauer M, Moller HJ, Schneider E. Duloxetine: a new selective and dual-acting antidepressant. Expert Opin Pharmacother 2006;7(4):421–427.

49. Preskorn SH. Clinically relevant pharmacology of selective serotonin reuptake inhibitors: An overview with emphasis on pharmacokinetics and effects on oxidative drug metabolism. Clin Pharmacokinet 1997;32(Suppl 1):1–21.

50. Goldstein BJ, Goodnick PJ. Selective serotonin reuptake inhibitors in the treatment of affective disorders: III. Tolerability, safety and pharmacoeconomics. J Psychopharmacol 1998;12(3 Suppl B):S55–S87.

51. Masand PS and Gupta S. Long-term side effects of newer-generation antidepressants: SSRIs, venlafaxine, nefazodone, buproprion, and mirtazapine. Ann Clin Psychiatry 2002;14:175–182.

52. Westenberg HG, Sander C. Tolerability and safety of fluvoxamine and other antidepressants. Int J Clin Pract 2006;60(4):482–491.

53. Aranoff GM. Trazodone associated with priapism. Lancet 1984;1:856.

54. Brodie-Meijer CC, Diemont WL, Buijs PJ. Nefazodone-induced clitoral priapism. Int Clin Psychopharmacol 1999;14:257–258.

55. Johnston JA, Lineberry CG, Ascher JA. A 102 center prospective study of seizures in association with bupropion. J Clin Psychiatry 1991;52:450–456.

56. Rabkin JG, Quitkin FM, McGrath P, et al. Adverse reactions to monoamine oxidase inhibitors: II. Treatment correlates and clinical management. J Clin Psychopharmacol 1985;5:2–9.

57. Neil JF, Licata SM, May SJ, Himmelhock JM. Dietary noncompliance during treatment with tranylcypromine. J Clin Psychiatry 1979;40:33–37.

58. Varon J, Marik PE. The diagnosis and management of hypertensive crises. Chest 2000;118:214–227.

59. Wells BG. Tricyclic antidepressants. In: Taylor WJ, Caviness MHD, eds. A Textbook for the Clinical Application of Therapeutic Drug Monitoring. Irving, TX, Abbott Laboratories, 1986:449–465.

60. Rudorfer MV, Potter WZ. Metabolism of tricyclic antidepressants. Cell Mol Neurobiol 1999;19:373–409.

61. Olver JS, Burrows GD, Norman TR. The treatment of depression with different formulations of venlafaxine: a comparative analysis. Human Psychopharmacology 2004;19:9–16.

62. DeVane CL. Metabolism and pharmacokinetics of the selective serotonin reuptake inhibitors. Cell Mol Neurobiol 1999;19:443–466.

63. Hemeryck A, Belpaire FM. Selective serotonin reuptake inhibitors and cytochrome P-450 mediated drug-drug interactions: an update. Curr Drug Metab 2002;3:13–37.

64. Jefferson JW, Pradko JF, Muir KT. Bupropion for major depressive disorder: Pharmacokinetic and formulation considerations. Clin Ther 2005;27:1685–1695.

65. Dunner DL, Zisook S, Billow AA, et al. A prospective safety surveillance study for bupropion sustained-release in the treatment of depression. J Clin Psychiatry 1998;59:366–373.

66. Timmer CJ, Sitsen JM, Delbressine LP. Clinical pharmacokinetics of mirtazapine. Clin Pharmacokinet 2000;38:461–474.

67. Watanabe MD, Winter ME. Tricyclic antidepressants: amitriptyline, desipramine, imipramine, and nortriptyline. In: Winter ME, ed. Basic Clinical Pharmacokinetics, 4th ed. Baltimore, MD: Lippincott Williams & Wilkins, 2004:423–437.

68. Krastev Z, Terzivoanov D, Vlahov V, et al. The pharmacokinetics of paroxetine in patients with liver cirrhosis. Acta Psychiatry Scand 1989;350(Suppl):91–92.

69. Demolis JL, Angebaud P, Grange JD, et al. Influence of liver cirrhosis on sertraline pharmacokinetics. Br J Clin Pharmacol 1996;42:394–397.

70. Kent JM. SNaRIs, NaSSAs, and NaRIs: new agents for the treatment of depression. Lancet 2000;355:911–918.

71. DeVane CL. Differential pharmacology of newer antidepressants. J Clin Psychiatry 1998;59(Suppl 20):85–93.

72. Boyer EW, Shannon M. Current concepts: the serotonin syndrome. N Engl J Med 2005;352:1112–1120.

73. Otong D. The art of prescribing. Antidepressants in late-life depression: prescribing principles. Perspect Psychiatr Care 2006;(2):149–153.

74. Turvey CL, Conwell Y, Jones MP, et al. Risk factors for late-life suicide. A prospective, community-based study. Am J Geriat Psychiatry 2002;10:398–406.

75. Reynolds CF 3rd, Dew MA, Pollock BG, et al. Maintenance treatment of major depression in old age. N Engl J Med 2006;354(11):1130–1138.

76. Kohn R, Epstein-Lubrow G. Course and outcomes of depression in the elderly Curr Pscyhiatr Rep 2006;8(1):34–40.

77. Schatzberg AF, Kremer C, Rodrigues HE, Murphy GM Jr; Mirtazapine vs. Paroxetine Study Group. Double-blind, randomized comparison of mirtazapine and paroxetine in elderly depressed patients. Am J Geriatr Psychiatry 2002;10:541–550.

78. Cosgrave E, McGorry P, Allen N, Jackson H. Depression in young people: A growing challenge for primary care. Aust Fam Physician 2000;29:123–127.

79. Wagner KD, Ambrosini P, Rynn M, et al. Efficacy of sertraline in the treatment of children and adolescents with major depressive disorder. JAMA 2003;290:1033–1041.

80. Olfson M, Marcus SC, Shaffer D. Antidepressant drug therapy and suicide in severely depressed children and adults: A case-control study. Arch Gen Psychiatry 2006;63(8):865–872.

81. Valuck RJ, Libby AM, Sills MR, et al. Antidepressant treatment and risk of suicide attempt by adolescents with major depressive disorder: a propensity-adjusted retrospective cohort study. CNS Drugs 2004;18(15):1119–1132.

82. Simon GE, Savarino J, Operskalski B, Wang PS. Suicide risk during antidepressant treatment. Am J Psychiatry 2006;163(1):41–47.

83. Hallfors DD, Waller MW, Ford CA, et al. Adolescent depression and suicide risk: association with sex and drug behavior. Am J Prev Med 2004;27(3):224–231.

84. Haavisto A, Sourander A, Ellila H, et al. Suicidal ideation and suicide attempts among child and adolescent psychiatric inpatients in Finland. J Affect Dsord 2003;76(1–3):211–221.

85. Leonard HL, Meyer HC, Swedo SE, et al. Electrocardiographic changes during desipramine and clomipramine treatment in children and adolescents. J Am Acad Child Adolesc Psychiatry 1995;34:1460–1468.

86. Oberlander TF, Warburton W, Misri S, et al. Neonatal outcomes after prenatal exposure to selective serotonin reuptake inhibitor antidepressants and maternal depression using population-based linked health data. Arch Gen Psychiatry 2006;63:898–906.

87. Chambers CD, Hernandex-Diaz S, Van Marter LJ, et al. Selective serotonin-reuptake inhibitors and risk of persistent pulmonary hypertension of the newborn. N Engl J Med 2006;354(6):579–587.

88. Cohen LS, Altshuler LL, Harlow BL, et al. Relapse of major depression during pregnancy in women who maintain or discontinue antidepressant treatment. JAMA 2006;295(5):499–507.

89. Rubinow, DR. Antidepressant treatment during pregnancy: between Scylla and Charybdis. Am J Psychiatry 2006;163(6):954–955.

90. Yonkers et al. The management of depression during pregnancy: a report from the American Psychiatric Association and the American College of Obstetricians and Gynecologists. General Hospital Psychiatry 2009;31:403–413.

91. Hendrick V, Altshuler L. Management of major depression during pregnancy. Am J Psychiatry 2002;159:1667–1673.

92. Freeman MP. Breastfeeding and antidepressants: clinical dilemmas and expert perspectives. J Clin Psychiatry 2009;70:291–292.

93. Sequenced Treatment Alternatives to Relieve Depression (STAR*D). http://www.edc.pitt.edu/stard.

94. Rush AJ, Trivedi MH, Wisniewski SR, et al. Bupropion-SR, sertraline, or venlafaxine-XR after failure of SSRIs for depression. N Engl J Med 2006;354:1231–1242.

95. Nierenberg AA, Fava M, Trivedi MH, et al. A comparison of lithium and T3 augmentation following two failed medication treatments for depression: A STAR*D Report. Am J Psychiatry 2006;163:1519–1530.

96. Fava M, Rush AJ, Wisniewski SR, et al. A comparison of mirtazapine and nortriptyline following two consecutive failed medication treatments for depressed outpatients: a STAR*D report. Am J Psychiatry 2006;163(7):1161–1172.

97. Luppa M, Heinrich S, Angermeyer MC, et al. Cost-of-illness studies of depression: A systematic review. J Affect Disord 2007;98:29–43.

98. Iqbal SU, Prashker M. Pharmacoeconomic evaluation of antidpressants. Pharmacoeconomics 2005;23(6):595–606.

99. Barbui C, Peercudani M, Hotopf M. Economic evaluation of antidepressive agents: A systematic critique of experimental and observational studies. J Clin Psychopharmacol 2003;23(2):145–154.

100. U.S. Preventive Services Task Force. Screening for Depression. May 2002. Agency for Healthcare Research and Quality. Rockville, MD. http://www.ahrq.gov/clinic/3rduspstf/depression/.

101. Finely P, Rens HR, Pont JT, et al. Impact of a collaborative pharmacy practice model on the treatment of depression in primary care. Am J Health Syst Pharm 2002;59:1518–1526.

102. Anonymous. Lexi-comp online™ interaction analysis. Lexi-Comp Online, Lexi-Comp, Inc. http://online.lexi.com.

103. Anonymous. Drug interactions. Thomson MICROMEDEX Healthcare Series. https://www.thomsonhc.com.

78

Bipolar Disorder

SHANNON J. DRAYTON

KEY CONCEPTS

❶ Bipolar disorder is a cyclic mental illness with recurrent mood episodes that occur over a person's lifetime. The symptoms, course, severity, and response to treatment differ among individuals.

❷ Bipolar disorder is likely caused by genetic factors, environmental triggers, and the dysregulation of neurotransmitters, neurohormones, and second messenger systems in the brain.

❸ The goal of therapy for bipolar disorder should be to improve functioning of the patient by reducing mood episodes. This is accomplished by maximizing the adherence to therapy and limiting adverse effects.

❹ Patients and family members should be educated about bipolar disorder and treatments. Long-term monitoring and adherence to treatment are major factors in obtaining stabilization of the disorder.

❺ Lithium and valproate are the mainstays of treatment for both acute mania and prophylaxis for recurrent manic and depressive episodes. Anticonvulsants, such as lamotrigine, carbamazepine, and oxcarbazepine, and second-generation antipsychotics, such as aripiprazole, olanzapine, risperidone, quetiapine, and ziprasidone are alternative or adjunctive treatments for bipolar disorder. Anticonvulsants may be more effective than lithium in several mood subtypes (e.g., mixed states and rapid cycling). The use of lithium, valproate, or quetiapine for acute bipolar depression should be considered as first-line treatment options.

❻ Baseline and follow-up laboratory tests are required for some medications to monitor for adverse effects.

❼ Some patients can be stabilized on one mood stabilizer, but others may require combination therapies or adjunctive agents during an acute mood episode. If possible, adjunctive agents should be tapered and discontinued when the acute mood episode remits and the patient is stabilized. Adjunctive agents may include benzodiazepines, additional mood stabilizers or antipsychotics, and/or antidepressants.

Learning objectives, review questions, and other resources can be found at **www.pharmacotherapyonline.com**.

❶ Bipolar disorder (previously known as manic-depressive illness) is one of the most common of the severe chronic psychiatric disorders. The cyclic mood disorder is characterized by recurrent fluctuations in mood, energy, and behavior encompassing the extremes of human experiences.[1–3] Bipolar disorder differs from recurrent major depression (or unipolar depression) in that a manic, hypomanic, or mixed episode occurs during the course of the illness.[1] Bipolar disorder is a lifelong illness with a variable course and requires both nonpharmacologic and pharmacologic treatments for mood stabilization.[1,2]

EPIDEMIOLOGY

The lifetime prevalence of bipolar I disorder (one or more manic or mixed episodes) is 0.4% to 1.6%; that for bipolar II disorder (recurrent major depressive episodes with hypomanic episodes) is approximately 0.5%.[1,2] A national comorbidity survey reported that the lifetime prevalence rate of a manic episode is 1.6% ± 0.3% for men and 1.7% ± 0.3% for women in the United States (~4 million people).[4] Bipolar I disorder occurs equally in men and women, whereas bipolar II disorder is more common in women.[1,2]

ETIOLOGY

❷ The exact etiology of bipolar disorder is unknown. Bipolar disorder is thought to be a complex genetic disease that is environmentally influenced and caused by a wide range of neurobiologic abnormalities. Stressful life events, alcohol or substance use, and changes in the sleep-wake cycle can elicit the expression of genetic or biologic vulnerabilities that cause dysregulation of neurotransmitters, neuroendocrine pathways, and second messenger systems.[3] Table 78–1 summarizes the etiologic theories of bipolar disorder.

PATHOPHYSIOLOGY

❷ Many theories have been proposed regarding the pathophysiology of mood disorders.[3] Family, twin, and adoption studies report an increased lifetime prevalence risk of having mood disorders among first-degree relatives of patients with bipolar disorder.[2,5] Genetic linkage studies suggest multiple gene loci can be involved in the heredity of mood disorders.[6–10] Neuroimaging studies have found neurochemical, anatomic, and functional abnormalities in bipolar patients.[10,11] Environmental or psychosocial stressors, nutritional deficiencies, infections, immunologic reactions, sleep deprivation, and disruption of circadian rhythms can cause dysregulation in neurotransmitters, hormones, endocrine function, neuropeptides, cations, intracellular second messengers, and signal transduction pathways.[1,2,10–17]

TABLE 78-1	Etiologic Theories of Bipolar Disorder

Genetic factors

80%–90% of patients with bipolar disorder have a biologic relative with a mood disorder (e.g., bipolar disorder, major depression, cyclothymia, or dysthymia).

First-degree relatives of bipolar patients have a 15%–35% lifetime risk of developing any mood disorder and a 5%–10% lifetime risk for developing bipolar disorder.

The concordance rate of mood disorders is 60%–80% for monozygotic twins and 14%–20% for dizygotic twins.

Linkage studies suggest that certain loci on genes and the X chromosome may contribute to genetic susceptibility of bipolar disorder.

Nongenetic factors

Perinatal insult

Head trauma

Environmental factors

Desynchronization of circadian or seasonal rhythms cause diurnal variations in mood and sleep patterns and can result in seasonal recurrences of mood episodes.

Changes in the sleep-wake cycle or light-dark cycle can precipitate episodes of mania or depression.

Bright light therapy can be used for the treatment of winter depression and can precipitate hypomania, mania, or mixed episodes.

Psychosocial or physical stressors

Stressful life events often precede mood episodes and can increase recurrence rates and prolong time to recovery from mood episodes.

Nutritional factors

Deficiency of essential amino acid precursors in the diet can cause a dysregulation of neurotransmitter activity (e.g., L-tryptophan deficiency causes a decrease in 5-HT and melatonin synthesis and activity).

Deficiency in essential fatty acids (e.g., omega-3 fatty acids) can cause a dysregulation of neurotransmitter activity.

Neurotransmitter/neuroendocrine/hormonal theories

Dysregulation between excitatory and inhibitory neurotransmitter systems; excitatory: NE, DA, glutamate, and aspartate; inhibitory: 5-HT and GABA.

Monoamine hypothesis

An excess of catecholamines (primarily NE and DA) cause mania.

Agents that decrease catecholamines are used for the treatment of mania (e.g., DA antagonists and α_2-adrenergic agonists).

Deficit of neurotransmitters (primarily NE, DA, and/or 5-HT) cause depression.

Agents that increase neurotransmitter activity are used for the treatment of depression (e.g., 5-HT and NE/DA reuptake inhibitors and MAOIs).

Dysregulation of amino acid neurotransmitters

Deficiency of GABA or excessive glutamate activity causes dysregulation of neurotransmitters (e.g., increased DA and NE activity).

Agents that increase GABA activity or decrease glutamate activity are used for the treatment of mania and for mood stabilization (e.g., benzodiazepines, lamotrigine, lithium, or valproic acid).

Cholinergic hypothesis

Deficiency of acetylcholine causes an imbalance in cholinergic-adrenergic activity and can increase the risk of manic episodes.

Agents that increase acetylcholine activity can decrease manic symptoms (e.g., use of cholinesterase inhibitors or augmentation of muscarinic cholinergic activity).

Increased central acetylcholine levels can increase the risk of depressive episodes.

Agents that decrease acetylcholine activity can alleviate depressive symptoms (i.e., anticholinergic agents).

Secondary messenger system dysregulation

Abnormal G protein functioning dysregulates adenylate cyclase activity, phosphoinositide responses, sodium/potassium/calcium channel exchange, and activity of phospholipases. Abnormal cyclic adenosine monophosphate and phosphoinositide secondary messenger system activity.

Abnormal protein kinase C activity and signaling pathways.

Hypothalamic-pituitary-thyroid axis dysregulation

Hyperthyroidism can precipitate manic-like symptoms.

Hypothyroidism can precipitate a depression and be a risk factor for rapid cycling; thyroid supplementation can be used for refractory rapid cycling and augmentation of antidepressants in unipolar depression.

Positive antithyroid antibody titers reported in patients with bipolar disorder.

Hormonal changes during the female life cycle can cause dysregulation of neurotransmitters (e.g., premenstrual, postpartum, and perimenopause).

Membrane and cation theories

Abnormal neuronal calcium and sodium activity and homeostasis cause neurotransmitter dysregulation.

Hypocalcemia has been associated with causing anxiety, mood irritability, mania, psychosis, and delirium.

Hypercalcemia has been associated with causing depression, stupor, and coma.

Extracellular and intracellular calcium concentrations may affect the synthesis and release of NE, DA, and 5-HT, as well as the excitability of neuronal firing.

Sensitization and kindling theories

Recurrences of mood episodes cause behavioral sensitivity and electrophysiologic kindling (similar to the amygdala-kindling models for seizures in animals) and can result in rapid or continuous mood cycling.

DA, dopamine; GABA, γ-aminobutyric acid; 5-HT, serotonin; MAOI, monoamine oxidase inhibitor; NE, norepinephrine.
Data from Goldberg and Harrow,[3] Kelso,[6] Lenox et al.,[7] Baron,[8] Bezchlibnyk and Young,[9] Goodnick,[10] Soares,[11] Manji et al.,[13] Gould and Manji,[14] Sobczak et al.,[15] Freeman et al.,[16] Ketter and Wang,[17] White,[18] Rasgon et al.,[19] and Mahmood and Silverstone.[20]

NEUROCHEMICAL THEORIES

The kindling and behavioral sensitization model postulates that psychosocial stressors can result in manic or depressive episodes because various brain networks are sensitized for exaggerated and spontaneous reactions secondary to neurotransmitter imbalances or dysregulation and voltage-gated ion channel abnormalities.[3,18] Dysregulation between neurotransmitters, neuropeptides, hormones, and secondary messenger systems can produce a cyclic rhythm disturbance in the central nervous system.[3,11,12,18] Abnormal calcium, potassium, and sodium homeostasis can alter neurotransmitter release and the secondary messenger system.[12,18] Hormonal changes during the menstrual cycle, postpartum period, and perimenopausal phase can contribute to mood dysregulation.[16,19]

The "permissive serotonin hypothesis" proposes that serotonin (5-hydroxytryptamine [5-HT]) plays a critical role in modulating brain activity (e.g., stabilization of the catecholamine system and inhibition of dopamine [DA] release), and is low in both mania and depression.[10] The hypothesis further states that the type of affective state that is expressed is determined secondarily by the level of norepinephrine (NE) (e.g., increased amounts of NE lead to mania, decreased amounts lead to depression). L-tryptophan or 5-HT deficiency and changes in the light-dark cycle may result in reduced melatonin secretion from the pineal gland that disrupts the sleep-wake cycle, alters circadian rhythms, and causes seasonal affective changes.[10,20]

The catecholamine hypothesis of mood disorders suggests that increased DA and NE activity contribute to hyperactivity and psychosis associated with the severe stages of mania, and reduced DA and NE activity causes depression.[3,10] A γ-aminobutyric acid (GABA) deficiency theory has been proposed for mania as it inhibits NE and DA activity.[3,10,12] Glutamate and aspartate, excitatory amino acid neurotransmitters, may be overactive and involved in causing manic episodes.[12] Cholinergic underactivity has been proposed to cause mania and overactivity of acetylcholine to cause depression.[10,12] Acetylcholine is an antagonist of the catecholamine system and contributes to the interaction between phosphatidylinositol and phosphatidylcholine secondary messenger systems.[12]

DIAGNOSTIC DIFFICULTY

Several medical, medication-induced, or substance-related causes of mania and depression have been identified (see Table 78–2 for causes of mania and Table 77–1 in Chapter 77 for causes of depression).[1,2] A complete medical, psychiatric, and medication history; physical examination; and laboratory testing are necessary to rule out any organic causes of mania or depression.[2] An accurate diagnosis is important because some psychiatric and neurologic disorders present with manic-like or depressive-like symptoms.[2,3] For example, attention-deficit/hyperactivity disorder and a manic episode have similar characteristics; thus individuals with bipolar disorder can be misdiagnosed and prescribed central nervous system stimulants.[5,21] Use of any substance that affects the central nervous system (e.g., alcohol, antidepressants, caffeine, central nervous system stimulants, hallucinogens, or marijuana) can worsen symptoms of mania or depression and decrease response to treatment.[2,10,22–24]

Another disease state that has a similar presentation to bipolar disorder is schizoaffective disorder. This disease is a mix between schizophrenia and bipolar disorder. Patients with schizoaffective disorder have mood episodes, but the distinguishing factor from bipolar disorder is that these patients experience psychosis even between mood episodes during periods of euthymia. Clinicians must rely on family members or others who know the patient well to determine if the patient is psychotic between mood episodes. It can be difficult for clinicians to obtain a full psychiatric history on patients, thus making schizoaffective disorder widely diagnosed. Schizoaffective disorder is treated with mood stabilizers and antipsychotics as maintenance therapy.

CLINICAL PRESENTATION

❶ The essential feature of bipolar spectrum disorders is a history of mania or hypomania that is not caused by any other medical condition, substance, or psychiatric disorder (see Table 78–2 for secondary causes of mania).[1,2] The *Diagnostic and Statistical Manual of Mental Disorders, Fourth Edition, Text Revision (DSM-IV-TR)* of the American Psychiatric Association (APA) details the present understanding of mood disorders.[1] Bipolar disorder is divided into four subtypes based on the identification of specific mood episodes: bipolar I, bipolar II, cyclothymic disorder, and bipolar disorder not otherwise specified. See Table 78–3 for a definition of mood

TABLE 78-2 Secondary Causes of Mania

Medical conditions that induce mania
- CNS disorders (brain tumor, strokes, head injuries, subdural hematoma, multiple sclerosis, systemic lupus erythematosus, temporal lobe seizures, Huntington disease)
- Infections (encephalitis, neurosyphilis, sepsis, human immunodeficiency virus)
- Electrolyte or metabolic abnormalities (calcium or sodium fluctuations, hyper- or hypoglycemia)
- Endocrine or hormonal dysregulation (Addison disease, Cushing disease, hyper- or hypothyroidism, menstrual-related or pregnancy-related or perimenopausal mood disorders)

Medications or drugs that induce mania
- Alcohol intoxication
- Drug withdrawal states (alcohol, α_2-adrenergic agonists, antidepressants, barbiturates, benzodiazepines, opiates)
- Antidepressants (MAOIs, TCAs, 5-HT and/or NE and/or DA reuptake inhibitors, 5-HT antagonists)
- DA-augmenting agents (CNS stimulants: amphetamines, cocaine, sympathomimetics; DA agonists, releasers, and reuptake inhibitors)
- Hallucinogens (LSD, PCP)
- Marijuana intoxication precipitates psychosis, paranoid thoughts, anxiety, and restlessness
- NE-augmenting agents (α_2-adrenergic antagonists, β-agonists, NE reuptake inhibitors)
- Steroids (anabolic, adrenocorticotropic hormone, corticosteroids)
- Thyroid preparations
- Xanthines (caffeine, theophylline)
- Over-the-counter weight loss agents and decongestants (ephedra, pseudoephedrine)
- Herbal products (St. John's wort)

Somatic therapies that induce mania
- Bright light therapy
- Sleep deprivation

CNS, central nervous system; DA, dopamine; 5-HT, serotonin; LSD, lysergic acid diethylamide; MAOI, monoamine oxidase inhibitor; NE, norepinephrine; PCP, phencyclidine; TCA, tricyclic antidepressant. *Data from American Psychiatric Association,[1] and Kaplan and Sadock.[90]*

TABLE 78-3 Mood Disorders Defined by Episodes

Disorder Subtype	Episode(s)[a]
Major depressive disorder, single episode	Major depressive episode
Major depressive disorder, recurrent	Two or more major depressive episodes
Bipolar disorder, type I[b]	Manic episode ± major depressive or mixed episode
Bipolar disorder, type II[c]	Major depressive episode + hypomanic episode
Dysthymic disorder	Chronic subsyndromal depressive episodes
Cyclothymic disorder[d]	Chronic fluctuations between subsyndromal depressive and hypomanic episodes (2 years for adults and 1 year for children and adolescents)
Bipolar disorder not otherwise specified	Mood states do not meet criteria for any specific bipolar disorder

[a]The length and severity of a mood episode and the interval between episodes varies from patient to patient. Manic episodes are usually briefer and end more abruptly than major depressive episodes. The average length of untreated manic episodes ranges from 4 to 13 months. Episodes can occur regularly (at the same time or season of the year) and often cluster at 12-month intervals. Women have more depressive episodes than manic episodes, whereas men have a more even distribution of episodes.
[b]For bipolar I disorder, 90% of individuals who experience a manic episode later have multiple recurrent major depressive, manic, hypomanic, or mixed episodes alternating with a normal mood state.
[c]Approximately 5%–15% of patients with bipolar II disorder will develop a manic episode over a 5-year period. If a manic or mixed episode develops in a patient with bipolar II disorder, the diagnosis is changed to bipolar I disorder.
[d]Patients with cyclothymic disorder have a 15%–50% risk of later developing a bipolar I or II disorder. *Data from American Psychiatric Association,[1] American Psychiatric Association,[2] and Goldberg and Harrow.[3]*

TABLE 78-4 Evaluation and Diagnosis of Mood Episodes

Diagnosis Episode	Impairment of Functioning or Need for Hospitalization[a]	DSM-IV-TR Criteria[b]
Major depressive	Yes	>2-Week period of either depressed mood or loss of interest or pleasure in normal activities, associated with at least five of the following symptoms: • Depressed, sad mood (adults); can be irritable mood in children • Decreased interest and pleasure in normal activities • Decreased appetite, weight loss • Insomnia or hypersomnia • Psychomotor retardation or agitation • Decreased energy or fatigue • Feelings of guilt or worthlessness • Impaired concentration and decision making • Suicidal thoughts or attempts
Manic	Yes	>1-Week period of abnormal and persistent elevated mood (expansive or irritable), associated with at least three of the following symptoms (four if the mood is only irritable): • Inflated self-esteem (grandiosity) • Decreased need for sleep • Increased talking (pressure of speech) • Racing thoughts (flight of ideas) • Distractible (poor attention) • Increased activity (either socially, at work, or sexually) or increased motor activity or agitation • Excessive involvement in activities that are pleasurable but have a high risk for serious consequences (buying sprees, sexual indiscretions, poor judgment in business ventures)
Hypomanic	No	At least 4 days of abnormal and persistent elevated mood (expansive or irritable); associated with at least three of the following symptoms (four if the mood is only irritable): • Inflated self-esteem (grandiosity) • Decreased need for sleep • Increased talking (pressure of speech) • Racing thoughts (flight of ideas) • Increased activity (either socially, at work, or sexually) or increased motor activity or agitation • Excessive involvement in activities that are pleasurable but have a high risk for serious consequences (buying sprees, sexual indiscretions, poor judgment in business ventures)
Mixed	Yes	Criteria for both a major depressive episode and manic episode (except for duration) occur nearly every day for at least a 1-week period
Rapid cycling	Yes	>4 Major depressive or manic episodes (manic, mixed, or hypomanic) in 12 months

[a]Impairment in social or occupational functioning; need for hospitalization because of potential self-harm, harm to others, or psychotic symptoms.
[b]The disorder is not caused by a medical condition (e.g., hypothyroidism) or substance-induced disorder (e.g., antidepressant treatment, medications, electroconvulsive therapy).
Reprinted with permission from American Psychiatric Association: Diagnostic and Statistical Manual of Mental Disorders, 4th ed., Text Revision. Washington, DC: American Psychiatric Association, 2000:345–401.

disorders by type of episode. The mood states are further separated into four subcategories to differentiate the current or most recent mood episode: major depressive, manic, hypomanic, or mixed. See Table 78–4 for the evaluation and diagnostic criteria of mood episodes. A new concept of "bipolar spectrum disorder" has been suggested that broadens the diagnosis to include dysthymia, cyclothymia, drug-induced hypomania, and recurrent unipolar depression.[3,25] Bipolar disorder is a cyclic mood disorder, and patients may sequentially experience different types of episodes with or without a period of normal mood (euthymia) between. Persons with bipolar disorder can have mood fluctuations that continue for months, or after one episode they can sometimes go years without recurrence of any type of mood episode. Comorbid psychiatric disorders associated with bipolar disorder include but are not limited to the following: alcohol and substance abuse, personality disorders, and anxiety disorders such as panic disorder, social anxiety disorder, and obsessive-compulsive disorder.[1–3,10,22,24,26]

MAJOR DEPRESSIVE EPISODE

Bipolar depression is often underdiagnosed and is frequently misdiagnosed as major depressive disorder.[2,27] Approximately 95% of patients with bipolar disorder experience episodes of depression during their lifetime.[1,3] Compared with manic episodes, depressive episodes are more frequent, longer lasting, and occur more

often in bipolar II than in bipolar I disorder.[3,28] Over a person's lifetime, depressive episodes can account for up to 80% of all mood episodes. Recurrent depressive episodes are more common in women compared to men.[3] In bipolar depression, patients have an increased suicide risk and often have mood lability, hypersomnia, low energy, psychomotor retardation, cognitive impairment, anhedonia, decreased sexual activity, slowed speech, carbohydrate craving, and weight gain (also called atypical depressive features).[3,28,29] Delusions, hallucinations, and suicide attempts are more common in bipolar depression than in unipolar depression.[3]

MANIC EPISODE

For a diagnosis of mania, the symptoms must last at least 1 week, the mood must be elevated (expansive or irritable), and there must be an impairment in functioning.[1] Acute mania usually begins abruptly, and symptoms escalate over several days. Common symptoms of mania include grandiosity, decreased need for sleep or food, pressured speech, flight of ideas (racing thoughts), distractibility, increased activity, poor judgment, and involvement in pleasurable activities with potentially negative consequences.[1] Patients with acute mania often have psychotic symptoms, thus some patients are incorrectly diagnosed as having schizophrenia.[10] Mania symptoms that can resemble paranoid schizophrenia are bizarre behavior, hallucinations, and paranoid or grandiose delusions. Seasonal changes, stressors, sleep deprivation, antidepressants, central nervous system stimulants, or bright light can precipitate a manic episode.

HYPOMANIC EPISODE

Hypomania is a less severe form of mania, and by definition does not cause a marked impairment in social or occupational functioning, and no delusions or hallucinations are present.[1,3] Patients with hypomania often do not seek treatment until they have a depressive episode, thus hypomania may not be recognized or reported.[2] Symptoms found in hypomanic episodes are similar to those of cocaine- or antidepressant-induced mood disorders; thus the differential diagnosis should rule out any substance-induced or medical conditions that present with elevated mood.[24] Hypomanic states should be closely monitored, because 5% to 15% of patients can rapidly switch to a manic episode.[3]

MIXED EPISODE

Bipolar "mixed episode" (previously known as mixed state, dysphoric mania, or depressive mania) is defined as the simultaneous occurrence of manic and depressive symptoms.[1,3] Mixed mood states occur in up to 40% of all episodes and are more common in younger and older patients and in females.[3] Mixed episodes are often difficult to diagnose and treat because of the fluctuating clinical presentation. Patients with mixed states often have comorbid alcohol and substance abuse, severe anxiety symptoms, a higher suicide rate, and a poorer prognosis.[3,24]

COURSE OF ILLNESS

❶ Bipolar disorder is frequently not recognized and treated for many years because of its fluctuating course and episodic mood states.[2,3,10] The onset of bipolar disorder is rare before puberty, but its incidence increases during late adolescence and into early adulthood (usually between the ages of 15 and 30 years).[1] The average age of onset of a first manic episode is 21 years for both men and women.[2] Bipolar disorder affects an estimated 1% of children and adolescents and is often harder to recognize, diagnose, and treat than in a typical adult patient.[1,2,23,30] Before the onset of mania, adolescents can exhibit irritability, hyperactivity, impulsivity, emotional lability, poor judgment, marked anxiety, insomnia, depression, and psychosis.[1,11,21] The first episode in females is more likely to be a major depressive episode, whereas males are more likely to first experience a manic episode.[1,2] Women are more likely to have mixed states, depressive episodes, and rapid cycling compared with men.[1,2] Onset of manic episodes after the age of 60 years is rare and is likely caused by a medical or neurologic condition (e.g., stroke, tumor, or dementia), medications, or substance use.[2]

The kindling theory is used to explain why bipolar disorder progresses over one's life and why preventative treatment is imperative. Episodes can become longer in duration and more frequent with aging.[2] Usually there is a period of normal functioning between episodes, but approximately 20% to 30% of patients with bipolar I disorder and 15% with bipolar II disorder have no period of euthymia because of mood lability, residual mood symptoms, or a direct switch to the opposite polarity.[1]

Rapid cycling (more than four mood episodes per year) is more common in females and occurs in approximately 10% to 20% of bipolar I and II disorder patients.[2,3,16,23] Frequent and severe episodes of depression appear to be the most common hallmark of rapid cycling. Use of alcohol, stimulants, antidepressants, sleep deprivation, hypothyroidism, and seasonal changes can play a role in rapid cycling.[3,23,31] Seasonal patterns of mania in the summer and depression during the winter have been observed. Rapid-cycling patients have a poorer long-term prognosis and often require combination therapies.[3]

Fluctuations in hormones and neurotransmitters during the luteal phase of the menstrual cycle, postpartum period, and during perimenopause (starting ~10 years before menopause) can precipitate mood changes and increase cycling.[1,16,19] Women with bipolar I disorder are at greater risk for relapse into mania or depression during the postpartum period.[2] If a severe mood episode occurs postpartum, there is an increased risk for recurrences during subsequent postpartum periods.[2]

Alcohol and substance abuse is common among patients with bipolar disorder and can have a significant impact on the age of onset, course of the illness, and response to treatment.[3,10,22] Alcohol and drug abuse or dependence has been reported in 46% and 41% of bipolar patients, respectively.[2,10] Patients with substance use disorders are more likely to have an earlier onset of their illness, mixed states, higher rates of relapse, a poorer response to treatment, comorbid personality disorders, increased suicide risk, and more psychiatric hospitalizations.[3] Bipolar patients often self-medicate with substances such as alcohol or cocaine during episodes, resulting in further impairment of judgment, poor impulse control, treatment nonadherence, and a worsening of the clinical course.[2,3,24]

More than one-half (55%–65%) of bipolar I patients have some degree of functional disability after the onset of their illness, and approximately 10% to 20% of bipolar patients have severe impairment in their psychosocial and occupational functioning.[2,3,32] In a 1-year longitudinal study in 258 bipolar patients, two-thirds had four or more mood episodes a year despite comprehensive pharmacologic treatment, and approximately 33.2% of the year was spent being depressed compared to 10.8% of the time in a manic phase.[32]

Compared with the general population, individuals with bipolar disorder have a 2.3-times higher mortality rate. Suicide attempts occur in up to 50% of patients with bipolar disorder, and approximately 10% to 19% of individuals with bipolar I disorder commit suicide.[1–3,29] Studies suggest patients with bipolar II disorder have more suicide attempts than bipolar I patients.[29] Suicidal ideation and attempts are most likely to occur in a depressive or mixed state and in patients with personality disorders, psychotic features, and/or a comorbid alcohol- and substance-use disorder.[2,3,33] Acutely manic or depressed patients can need hospitalization because they are suicidal, have violent or aggressive behavior, or lack appropriate judgment and insight.[2] Accidental deaths are more frequent during manic episodes when the person has grandiosity, hallucinations, or delusions that result in risk-taking behaviors.[2] In addition, bipolar patients have a higher mortality from endocrine, respiratory, and cardiovascular disease that can be related to higher rates of obesity, smoking, alcohol and substance abuse, infections, and lack of medical care.[2]

The best predictor for level of functioning during a person's lifetime is adherence with medication treatment. Medication discontinuation occurs in up to 50% of patients secondary to intolerance of drug-induced side effects.[34] Failure to recognize the disorder, reluctance to acknowledge it, or poor adherence with treatment are reasons an estimated two-thirds of patients with bipolar disorder do not receive appropriate treatment. Nonadherence with pharmacologic treatment and substance abuse are major factors in relapse and hospitalizations.[2,3]

TREATMENT

■ DESIRED OUTCOME

❸ The desired outcome for bipolar disorder is to prevent an acute manic, hypomanic, or depressive episode, to maintain good functioning, and to prevent further episodes of mania or depression.[2,3]

TABLE 78-5 General Principles for the Management of Bipolar Disorder

Goals of treatment

- Eliminate mood episode with complete remission of symptoms (i.e., acute treatment)
- Prevent recurrences or relapses of mood episodes (i.e., continuation phase treatment)
- Return to complete psychosocial functioning
- Maximize adherence with therapy
- Minimize adverse effects
- Use medications with the best tolerability and fewest drug interactions
- Treat comorbid substance use and abuse
- Eliminate alcohol, marijuana, cocaine, amphetamines, and hallucinogens
- Minimize nicotine use and stop caffeine intake at least 8 hours prior to bedtime
- Avoidance of stressors or substances that precipitate an acute episode

Monitor for

- Mood episodes: document symptoms on a daily mood chart (document life stressors, type of episode, length of episode, and treatment outcome); monthly and yearly life charts are valuable for documenting patterns of mood cycles
- Medication adherence (missing doses of medications is a primary reason for nonresponse and recurrence of episodes)
- Adverse effects, especially sedation and weight gain (manage rapidly and vigorously to avoid noncompliance)
- Suicidal ideation or attempts (suicide completion rates with bipolar I disorder are 10%–15%; suicide attempts are primarily associated with depressive episodes, mixed episodes with severe depression or presence of psychosis)

Data from American Psychiatric Association,[2] Goodnick,[10] and Suppes et al.[42]

The general principles and goals for the management of bipolar disorder are found in Table 78–5.

■ GENERAL APPROACH TO TREATMENT

❹ Treatment of bipolar disorder must be individualized because the clinical presentation, severity, and frequency of episodes vary widely among patients. Treatment approaches should include both nonpharmacologic and pharmacologic strategies.[3] Patients and family members should be educated about bipolar disorder (e.g., symptoms, causes, and course) and treatment options. Long-term adherence to treatment is the most important factor in achieving stabilization of the disorder.

❺ The treatment of bipolar disorder can vary depending on what type of episode the patient is experiencing. Once diagnosed with bipolar disorder, patients should remain on a mood stabilizer (e.g., lithium, valproate) for their lifetime. During acute episodes, medications can be added and then tapered once the patient is stabilized and euthymic. For example, when treating a patient for mania with psychotic features, the patient should be on a mood stabilizer and an antipsychotic. If the antipsychotic is the patient's maintenance therapy, the dose should be increased or perhaps the medication should be changed altogether if the patient goes into a manic episode. If treating a patient for a severe depressive episode, a clinician may need to maximize the dose of the mood stabilizer or add another medication (e.g., quetiapine).

Nonpharmacologic Therapy

The basics of nonpharmacologic approaches should address issues of adequate nutrition, sleep, exercise, and stress reduction.[3] Sleep deprivation, high stress, and deficiencies in dietary essential amino acids, fatty acids, vitamins, and minerals can exacerbate mood episodes and result in poorer outcomes.[3] Mood charting is an effective strategy in detecting early signs and symptoms of mania and depression. Another effective treatment is to combine medications with adjunctive psychoeducational programs, supportive counseling, insight-oriented psychotherapy (individual or group), couples or family therapy, cognitive behavioral therapy, and communication enhancement training.[2,3,10,35]

Most communities have self-help, support groups, and mental health organizations that provide information, educational materials, and counseling. For public information, individuals can contact the Depression and Bipolar Support Alliance at 800–826–3632 and *www.dbsalliance.org*; the National Alliance on Mental Illness (NAMI) at 800–950–6264 (help line) and *www.nami.org*; Mental Health America (National Mental Health Association) 800–969–6642 (resource center) and *www.nmha.org*; and the National Institute of Mental Health at 866–615–6464 and *www.nimh.nih.gov*.[2]

Several nonpharmacologic treatment strategies (e.g., electroconvulsive therapy [ECT], high-intensity bright light therapy, phase-advanced sleep schedule, and partial or complete sleep deprivation) have been used in the treatment of bipolar disorder.[2,3] The use of ECT for the treatment of severe episodes of mania, depression, psychotic features (e.g., hallucinations or delusions), mixed episodes, or rapid cycling should be considered for those patients who do not respond to medications.[2,3] Repetitive transcranial magnetic stimulation (rTMS) has been reported to be effective in bipolar disorder. Most data include the use of rTMS as augmentation in drug-resistant bipolar depression.[36] A small amount of data support the use of rTMS in treating mania and for maintenance treatment in bipolar depression.[37,38] Vagus nerve stimulation (VNS) may also have a role in treatment-resistant rapid-cycling bipolar disorder.[39] More studies are needed to assess the role of VNS in bipolar disorder.

Pharmacologic Therapy

❺ Pharmacotherapy is crucial for the acute and maintenance treatment of bipolar disorder and includes lithium, valproate, carbamazepine, lamotrigine, first- and second-generation antipsychotics, and adjunctive agents such as antidepressants and benzodiazepines. General treatment guidelines for the acute treatment of mood episodes in patients with bipolar I disorder are found in Table 78–6.

Product information, dosing and administration, and clinical use for agents used in the treatment of bipolar disorder are found in Table 78–7.

❺ The term *mood stabilizer* is often used to describe the class of medications used in the treatment of bipolar disorder, but this may not be accurate as some medications are more effective for acute mania, some for the depressive episode, and others for the maintenance phase.[40] Lithium, valproate (or divalproex sodium), extended-release carbamazepine, aripiprazole, olanzapine, quetiapine, risperidone, and ziprasidone are currently approved by the U.S. Food and Drug Administration (FDA) for the treatment of acute mania in bipolar disorder; only lithium, divalproex sodium, aripiprazole, olanzapine, and lamotrigine are approved for the maintenance treatment of bipolar disorder. Quetiapine is the only monotherapy antipsychotic that is FDA approved for bipolar depression. Lithium is the drug of choice for bipolar disorder with euphoric mania, whereas valproate has better efficacy for mixed states, irritable/dysphoric mania, and rapid cycling compared with lithium.[2]

Combination therapies (e.g., lithium plus valproate or carbamazepine; lithium or valproate plus SGA) can provide better acute response and long-term prevention of relapse and recurrence than monotherapy in some bipolar patients, particularly those with mixed states or rapid cycling.[2,40] The majority of patients hospitalized for an acute episode will be on combination therapy.

TABLE 78-6 Algorithm and Guidelines for the Acute Treatment of Mood Episodes in Patients with Bipolar I Disorder

Acute Manic or Mixed Episode		Acute Depressive Episode	
General guidelines		**General guidelines**	
Assess for secondary causes of mania or mixed states (e.g., alcohol or drug use)		Assess for secondary causes of depression (e.g., alcohol or drug use)	
Discontinue antidepressants		Taper off antipsychotics, benzodiazepines or sedative-hypnotic agents if possible	
Taper off stimulants and caffeine if possible			
Treat substance abuse		Treat substance abuse	
Encourage good nutrition (with regular protein and essential fatty acid intake), exercise, adequate sleep, stress reduction, and psychosocial therapy		Encourage good nutrition (with regular protein and essential fatty acid intake), exercise, adequate sleep, stress reduction, and psychosocial therapy	
Hypomania	**Mania**	**Mild to moderate depressive episode**	**Severe depressive episode**
First, optimize current mood stabilizer or initiate mood-stabilizing medication: lithium,[a] valproate,[a] carbamazepine,[a] or SGAs	**First**, two or three drug combinations: lithium,[a] valproate,[a] or SGA **plus** a benzodiazepine (lorazepam or clonazepam) and/or antipsychotic for short-term adjunctive treatment of agitation or insomnia; lorazepam is recommended for catatonia	**First**, initiate and/or optimize mood stabilizing medication: lithium[a] or quetiapine	**First**, optimize current mood stabilizer or initiate mood-stabilizing medication: lithium[a] or quetiapine
Consider adding a benzodiazepine (lorazepam or clonazepam) for short-term adjunctive treatment of agitation or insomnia if needed		Alternative anticonvulsants: lamotrigine[b] valproate,[a] antipsychotics: fluoxetine/olanzapine combination	Alternative fluoxetine/olanzapine combination
Alternative medication treatment options: oxcarbazepine	Do not combine antipsychotics		If psychosis is present, initiate an antipsychotic in combination with above
Second, if response is inadequate, consider a two-drug combination:	Alternative medication treatment options: carbamazepine[a]; if patient does not respond or tolerate, consider oxcarbazepine		Do not combine antipsychotics
• Lithium[a] **plus** an anticonvulsant or an SGA			Alternative anticonvulsants: lamotrigine[b] valproate,[a]
• Anticonvulsant **plus** an anticonvulsant or SGA	**Second**, if response is inadequate, consider a three-drug combination:		**Second**, if response is inadequate, consider carbamazepine[a] or adding antidepressant
	• Lithium[a] **plus** an anticonvulsant **plus** an antipsychotic		**Third**, if response is inadequate, consider a three drug combination:
	• Anticonvulsant **plus** an anticonvulsant **plus** an antipsychotic		• Lithium **plus** lamotrigine[b] **plus** an antidepressant
	Third, if response is inadequate, consider ECT for mania with psychosis or catatonia[d]; or add clozapine for treatment refractory illness		• Lithium **plus** quetiapine **plus** antidepressant
			Fourth, if response is inadequate, consider ECT for treatment-refractory illness and depression with psychosis or catatonia[d]

ECT, electroconvulsive therapy; MAOI, monoamine oxidase inhibitor; SNRI, serotonin-norepinephrine reuptake inhibitor; SGA, second-generation antipsychotic, SSRI, selective serotonin reuptake inhibitor; TCA, tricyclic antidepressant.

[a]Use standard therapeutic serum concentration ranges if clinically indicated; if partial response or breakthrough episode, adjust dose to achieve higher serum concentrations without causing intolerable adverse effects; valproate is preferred over lithium for mixed episodes and rapid cycling; lithium and/or lamotrigine is preferred over valproate for bipolar depression.

[b]Lamotrigine is not approved for the acute treatment of depression, and the dose must be started low and slowly titrated up to decrease adverse effects if used for maintenance therapy of bipolar I disorder. Lamotrigine may be initiated during acute treatment with plans to transition to this medication for long-term maintenance. A drug interaction and a severe dermatologic rash can occur when lamotrigine is combined with valproate (i.e., lamotrigine doses must be halved from standard dosing titration).

[c]Controversy exists concerning the use of antidepressants, and they are often considered third line in treating acute bipolar depression, except in patients with no recent history of severe acute mania or potentially in bipolar II patients.

[d]ECT is used for severe mania or depression during pregnancy and for mixed episodes; prior to treatment, anticonvulsants, lithium, and benzodiazepines should be tapered off to maximize therapy and minimize adverse effects.

Data from American Psychiatric Association,[2] CANMAT & ISBD,[41] and Suppes et al.[42]

Several guidelines and algorithms have been published regarding the treatment of bipolar disorder, and these are generally based on the best available data and the clinical consensus of experts. The Canadian Network for Mood and Anxiety Treatments (CANMAT) and International Society for Bipolar Disorders (ISBD) published updated treatment guidelines in 2009.[41] A new edition of *Practice Guideline for the Treatment of Patients with Bipolar Disorder* published by the APA is expected to be released in the near future.[2] The APA guidelines address the diagnosis, clinical course, epidemiology, and treatment strategies for adults but are not intended to be used as a standard of psychiatric care. The Texas Department of Mental Health and Mental Retardation has developed and implemented algorithms in the public mental health system to improve treatment outcomes with bipolar I disorder.[42] Several other states have also adopted and implemented programs similar to the Texas algorithm project. The Texas algorithm project data are in the process of being updated. The last updates posted are from 2007. In addition, an international task force of the World Federation of Societies of Biological Psychiatry (WFSBP) has published guidelines for the treatment of bipolar depression and mania.[43,44] The WFSBP mania

guidelines were updated in 2009, but bipolar depression (2002) and maintenance (2003) guidelines have yet to be updated.

Based on the CANMAT and ISBD guidelines and available research, an example treatment algorithm and guidelines for acute mood episodes in adult patients with bipolar I disorder are listed in Table 78–6.[41] Because newer anticonvulsants, SGAs, and combination therapies are under investigation for bipolar disorder, published guidelines, algorithms, and decision trees can quickly become out of date as new scientific knowledge evolves. Selection of treatments for acute mood episodes (e.g., manic or mixed, depressive, or rapid cycling) and for maintenance strategies to prevent relapses of mood episodes should be individualized. Treatment plans should be based on patient-specific characteristics, comorbid psychiatric and medical conditions, and avoidance of drug interactions and adverse effects.[2]

There are few controlled studies in children and adolescents with bipolar disorder, thus little is known about the long-term efficacy and safety of specific agents or for combination therapies in this population.[5,30] Lithium, valproic acid, and carbamazepine are all used in pediatric bipolar disorder. Lithium is the only medication

TABLE 78-7 Products, Dosage and Administration, and Clinical Use of Agents Used in the Treatment of Bipolar Disorder

Generic Name	Trade Name	Dosage and Administration	Clinical Use
Lithium salts: FDA approved for bipolar disorder			
Lithium carbonate[a,c]	Eskalith Eskalith CR Lithobid	900–2,400 mg/day in 2–4 divided doses, preferably with meals. There is wide variation in the dosage needed to achieve therapeutic response and trough serum lithium concentration (i.e., 0.6–1.2 mEq/L (mmol/L) for maintenance therapy and 1.0–1.2 mEq/L (mmol/L) for acute mood episodes taken 8–12 hours after the last dose).	Use alone or in combination with other drugs (e.g., valproate, carbamazepine, antipsychotics) for the acute treatment of mania and for maintenance treatment.
Lithium citrate[a,c]	Cibalith-S		
Anticonvulsants: FDA-approved for bipolar disorder			
Divalproex sodium[a]	Depakote Depakote ER	750–3,000 mg/day (20–60 mg/kg/day) given once daily or in divided doses for delayed-release divalproex or valproic acid. A loading dose of divalproex (20–30 mg/kg/day) can be given, then 20 mg/kg per day and titrated to a serum concentration of 50–125 mcg/mL (346–866 μmol/L) or clinical response.	Use alone or in combination with other drugs (e.g., lithium, carbamazepine, antipsychotics) for the acute treatment of mania and for maintenance treatment. Use caution when combining with lamotrigine because of potential drug interaction.
Valproic acid[a]	Stavzor		
Lamotrigine[c]	Lamictal	50–400 mg/day in divided doses. Dosage should be slowly increased (e.g., 25 mg/day for 2 wk, then 50 mg/day for wk 3 and 4, then 50-mg/day increments at weekly intervals up to 200 mg/day).	Use alone or in combination with other drugs (e.g., lithium, carbamazepine) for long-term maintenance treatment for bipolar I disorder.
Carbamazepine	Equetro[a]	200–1,800 mg/day in 2–4 divided doses. Dosage should be slowly increased according to response and adverse effects (e.g., 100–200 mg twice daily and increase by 200 mg/day at weekly intervals). Dose can be increased rapidly for inpatients. Extended-release tablets should be swallowed whole and not be broken or chewed.	Use alone or in combination with other medications (e.g., lithium, valproate, antipsychotics) for the acute and long-term maintenance treatment of mania or mixed episodes for bipolar I disorder. APA guidelines recommend reserving it for patients unable to tolerate or who have inadequate response to lithium or valproate.
Anticonvulsants: Not FDA approved for bipolar disorder			
Carbamazepine	Tegretol, Epitol Tegretol-XR Carbatrol	200–1,800 mg/day in 2–4 divided doses. Dosage should be slowly increased according to response and adverse effects (e.g., 100–200 mg twice daily and increase by 200 mg/day at weekly intervals). Dose can be increased rapidly for inpatients. Administer conventional tablets and suspension with meals. Extended-release tablets should be swallowed whole and not be broken or chewed. Carbatrol capsules can be opened and contents sprinkled over food.	Use alone or in combination with other medications (e.g., lithium, valproate, anti-psychotics) for the acute and long-term maintenance treatment of mania or mixed episodes for bipolar I disorder. APA guidelines recommend reserving it for patients unable to tolerate or who have inadequate response to lithium or valproate.
Valproic acid Valproate sodium	Depakene Depacon	750–3,000 mg/day (20–60 mg/kg/day) given once daily or in divided doses for delayed-release divalproex or valproic acid. A loading dose of divalproex (20–30 mg/kg/day) can be given, then 20 mg/kg/day and titrated to a serum concentration of 50–125 mcg/mL (346–866 μmol/L) or clinical response.	Use alone or in combination with other drugs (e.g., lithium, carbamazepine, antipsychotics) for the acute treatment of mania and for maintenance treatment. Use caution when combining with lamotrigine because of potential drug interaction.
Oxcarbazepine	Trileptal	300–1,200 mg/day in two divided doses. Dosage should be slowly adjusted up and down according to response and adverse effects (e.g., 150–300 mg twice daily and increase by 300–600 mg/day at weekly intervals). Dose can be increased rapidly for inpatients.	Use after patients have failed treatment with carbamazepine or have intolerable side effects. May have fewer adverse effects and be better tolerated than carbamazepine.
Atypical antipsychotics: FDA-approved for bipolar disorder			
Aripiprazole[a,c]	Abilify	10–30 mg/day once daily.	May be used in combination with lithium, valproate, or carbamazepine for the acute treatment of mania or mixed states (primarily with psychotic features) for bipolar I disorder.
Olanzapine[a,c]	Zyprexa Zyprexa Zydis	5–20 mg/day once daily or in divided doses.	
Olanzapine and Fluoxetine[b]	Symbyax	6–12 mg olanzapine and 25–50 mg fluoxetine daily.	
Quetiapine[a,c]	Seroquel	50–800 mg/day in divided doses or once daily when stabilized.	
Risperidone[a]	Risperdal Risperdal M-Tab	0.5–6 mg/day once daily or in divided doses.	
Ziprasidone[a]	Geodon	40–160 mg/day in divided doses. Administer with food.	
Benzodiazepines		Dosage should be slowly adjusted up and down according to response and adverse effects.	Use in combination with other medications (e.g., antipsychotics, lithium, valproate) for the acute treatment of mania or mixed episodes. Use as a short-term adjunctive sedative-hypnotic agent.

FDA approved agents may be used as monotherapy in various phases of the illness as noted by.[a,b,c]

[a]FDA approved for acute mania.

[b]FDA approved for acute bipolar depression.

[c]FDA approved for maintenance.

Data from American Psychiatric Association,[2] Goldberg and Harrow,[3] Goodnick,[10] Manji et al.,[12] White,[18] and CANMAT & ISBD.[41]

approved for children older than 12 years of age as a mood stabilizer.[45] Valproate data are limited. One double-blind, randomized, placebo-controlled trial of extended-release divalproex showed similar results to placebo for mania or mixed episodes in children and adolescents.[46] Risperidone and aripiprazole are FDA approved for pediatric bipolar mania. Olanzapine, quetiapine, and ziprasidone have support for their use by an FDA advisory panel for pediatric acute mania, but do not yet have FDA approval.[47] The advisory panel recommended that the FDA approve quetiapine in patients aged 10 to 17 years during a manic episode, olanzapine as a second-line therapy in young patients with manic or mixed episodes, and ziprasidone in patients aged 10 to 17 years as a second-line therapy in patients with manic or mixed episodes.[47] Long-term data are still needed for all of these agents. Published guidelines for treatment of bipolar disorder in children and adolescents include the *Practice Parameters for the Assessment and Treatment of Children and Adolescents with Bipolar Disorder* by the American Academy of Child and Adolescent Psychiatry.[5]

Specific Pharmacologic Therapies

Lithium Lithium was first used in 1949 as a treatment for mania and was approved in 1972 in the United States for the treatment of acute mania and for maintenance therapy. Despite numerous investigations into the biologic and clinical properties of lithium, there is no unified theory for its mechanism of action.[6,10,13,48] Chronic lithium administration may modulate gene expression and have neuroprotective effects. Lithium has unique pharmacokinetics because it is a monovalent cation. Lithium is rapidly absorbed, is widely distributed with no protein binding, is not metabolized, and is excreted unchanged in the urine and in other body fluids.[49] Lithium requires regular assessment of renal and thyroid functioning and lithium blood level monitoring to minimize adverse effects.[3]

Efficacy Lithium was the first established mood stabilizer, and is still considered a first-line agent for acute mania, acute bipolar depression, and continuation treatment of bipolar I and II disorders.[41] Early placebo-controlled studies with lithium reported up to a 78% response rate in aborting an acute manic or hypomanic episode, but more recent studies suggest a slower onset of action and a more moderate effectiveness when compared with other agents.[2,3,50] Lithium has displayed efficacy in acute mania trials similar to that of valproate, carbamazepine, risperidone, olanzapine, chlorpromazine, and other first-generation antipsychotics (FGAs).[2] In placebo-controlled studies in bipolar depression, lithium has been found to have efficacy, but there can be a 6- to 8-week delay for its antidepressant effects.[2] Lithium is more effective for pure or elated (classic) mania, and can be less effective for mania with psychotic features, mixed episodes, rapid or continuous cycling, alcohol and drug abuse, and in organic-induced mood states.[2,3,51]

Long-term lithium therapy is more effective in patients with fewer prior episodes, with a history of euthymia or good functioning between episodes, and with a family history of bipolar illness with a positive response to lithium. Lithium produces a prophylactic response in up to two-thirds of patients and reduces suicide risk by 8- to 10-fold.[2,50–52]

Patients maintained on standard serum concentrations of lithium (0.8–1.0 mEq/L [mmol/L]) may have fewer relapses than patients maintained on lower serum concentrations (0.4–0.6 mEq/L [mmol/L]).[2,3] Abrupt discontinuation or noncompliance with lithium therapy can increase the risk of relapse.[2,3] Discontinuation-induced refractoriness has been reported in approximately one-fifth of patients who previously were stabilized on lithium.[2,3]

Lithium augmentation of carbamazepine, lamotrigine, and valproate can improve treatment response in bipolar I disorder.[2,53]

Concomitant use of lithium with valproate or carbamazepine appears to be well tolerated but can increase the risk of sedation, weight gain, gastrointestinal complaints, and tremor.

Lithium is frequently combined with either FGAs or SGAs for treatment of euphoric acute mania with psychotic features. Case reports of neurotoxicity (e.g., delirium, cerebellar dysfunction, extrapyramidal symptoms, and severe tremors) have been published in elderly patients receiving lithium and FGAs.[49] Combining lithium with calcium channel blockers is not recommended because of reports of neurotoxicity and severe bradycardia with verapamil or diltiazem.[49] Acute neurotoxicity and delirium have been reported in patients receiving ECT with lithium (even at reduced dosages); therefore, lithium should be withdrawn and discontinued at least 2 days before ECT and should not be resumed until 2 to 3 days after the last treatment.

Adverse Effects Approximately 35% to 93% of patients treated with lithium will experience adverse effects. These are divided into those that occur early in therapy but are generally innocuous and transient, those that occur with long-term therapy and are usually not dose related, and toxic effects that occur with high serum concentrations.[2,49]

Initial side effects are often dose related and are worse at peak serum concentrations (1–2 hours postdose).[2] Standard approaches for minimizing adverse effects include lowering the dose, taking smaller doses with food, using extended-release products, and trying once-daily dosing at bedtime.[2] Gastrointestinal distress (e.g., nausea, vomiting, dyspepsia, and diarrhea) can be minimized by the standard approaches or by adding antacids or antidiarrheal agents.[2] Diarrhea can sometimes be managed by switching from tablet or capsule formulation to liquid formulation. Diarrhea produced by lithium is commonly an osmotic diarrhea, and therefore switching to a formulation that clears the gut quickly can ameliorate symptoms. Muscle weakness and lethargy develop in about 30% of patients, but these symptoms are usually transient. Polydipsia with polyuria and nocturia occurs in up to 70% of patients and can be managed by changing to once-daily bedtime dosing.

As many as 40% of patients complain of headache, memory impairment, confusion, poor concentration, and impaired motor performance.[10] A fine hand tremor can be evident in up to 50% of patients. Stress, concomitant use of antidepressants or antipsychotics, caffeine, sympathomimetics, and impending toxicity can exacerbate the tremor. Strategies to reduce the tremor include standard approaches (e.g., switch to long-acting preparation, lower dose if possible) or adding a β-adrenergic antagonist (e.g., propranolol 20–120 mg/day).

Lithium reduces the kidney's ability to concentrate urine and can cause a nephrogenic diabetes insipidus characterized by low urine specific gravity and a low osmolality polyuria (urine volumes greater than 3 L/day).[2,49] Lithium-induced nephrogenic diabetes insipidus is treated with loop diuretics, thiazide diuretics, or triamterene. If a thiazide diuretic is used (e.g., hydrochlorothiazide 50 mg/day), lithium doses should be decreased by 50%, and potassium levels should be monitored.[2] Amiloride, a potassium-sparing diuretic, has weaker natriuretic effects than thiazides and appears to be relatively safe with minimal effect on lithium clearance. Potassium supplements have been suggested as another treatment for lithium-induced polyuria.[10] Fluid restriction is not recommended because dehydration increases the risk of lithium toxicity. If edema occurs, treatment approaches include lowering sodium intake or using a diuretic (e.g., spironolactone); close monitoring for lithium toxicity is necessary because these treatments often increase lithium concentrations.

Patients on long-term lithium therapy have a 10% to 20% risk of developing morphologic renal changes (e.g., glomerular sclerosis, tubular atrophy, and interstitial nephritis) that is associated with impairment of water resorption and increased serum creatinine concentrations.[2] Lithium rarely causes nephrotoxicity if patients are maintained on the lowest effective dose, if once-daily dosing is used, if adequate hydration is maintained, and if toxicity is avoided.[10] Lithium should be avoided in patients with preexisting renal disease unless there is frequent monitoring.

Lithium is concentrated in the thyroid gland, interferes with thyroid hormone synthesis, and can induce the formation of thyroid antibodies.[49] Up to 30% of patients on maintenance lithium therapy develop transiently elevated thyroid-stimulating hormone concentrations, and 5% to 35% of patients develop a goiter and/or hypothyroidism.[2] Lithium-induced hypothyroidism is not dose-related, is observed 10 times more frequently in women (particularly in those with rapid cycling), and usually occurs after 6 to 18 months of therapy.[2] Hypothyroidism does not require discontinuation of lithium, because exogenous thyroid hormone (i.e., levothyroxine) can be added to the regimen. When lithium is discontinued, the need for exogenous thyroid hormone should be reassessed, because hypothyroidism can be reversible.

Lithium can cause a variety of benign and reversible cardiac effects, particularly T-wave flattening or inversion (in up to 30% of patients), atrioventricular block, and bradycardia.[2,10,49] Lithium rarely causes myocarditis, sinus node dysfunction, or sinoatrial block but can aggravate ventricular arrhythmias and atrial premature contractions. If a patient has significant preexisting cardiac disease, consultation with a cardiologist and an electrocardiogram is recommended at baseline and during lithium therapy.

Other late-appearing lithium side effects include benign reversible leukocytosis and a variety of dermatologic effects (e.g., acne and acneiform eruptions, alopecia, exacerbation of psoriasis, pruritic dermatitis, maculopapular rashes, and folliculitis).[3,12] Weight gain is common (~20% of patients gain >10 kg [22 lb]) and can be related to fluid retention, the consumption of high-calorie beverages as a result of polydipsia, or to a decreased metabolic rate because of hypothyroidism.[10,51] Decreased libido, sexual dysfunction, dry mouth, alterations in taste, changes in glucose tolerance, hypercalcemia, and hyperparathyroidism have been reported.[2,10,49] Severe neurologic disturbances such as coarse hand tremors, ataxia, slurred speech, myasthenia gravis, extrapyramidal syndrome, pseudotumor cerebri, and papilledema are occasionally observed.

Lithium is an extremely toxic drug if accidentally or intentionally taken in overdose. Lithium toxicity can occur with blood levels greater than 1.5 mEq/L (mmol/L), but elderly patients can have symptoms of toxicity at therapeutic levels.[2] Severe lithium intoxication occurs when concentrations are higher than 2.0 mEq/L (mmol/L), and there is a worsening in several key symptoms: *gastrointestinal* (e.g., vomiting, diarrhea, or incontinence); *coordination* (e.g., severe fine to coarse hand tremor, unstable gait, slurred speech, and muscle twitching); and *cognition* (e.g., poor concentration, drowsiness, disorientation, apathy, and coma).[2] Several reports of seizures, cardiac dysrhythmia, permanent neurologic impairments with ataxia and deficits in memory, and kidney damage with reduced glomerular filtration rate have been reported after lithium intoxication.[2]

Situations that predispose patients to lithium toxicity include sodium restriction, dehydration, vomiting, diarrhea, and drug interactions that decrease lithium clearance. Heavy exercise, sauna baths, hot weather, and fever can promote sodium loss. Patients should be cautioned to maintain adequate sodium and fluid intake (2.5–3 quarts [~2.5 to 3 L] per day of fluids) and to avoid the excessive use of coffee, tea, cola, and other caffeine-containing beverages and alcohol.

If lithium toxicity is suspected, the person should go to an emergency room to be monitored, and lithium should be discontinued.[2]

Gastric lavage and intravenous fluids can be needed, and the patient should be monitored for fluid balance, renal and electrolyte status, and neurologic changes. In cases of overdose with sustained-release lithium products, the development and duration of toxicity can be prolonged.[2] When lithium concentrations are above 3.5 to 4 mEq/L (mmol/L), intermittent hemodialysis (12 hours on and 12 hours off) can be started and continued until the lithium concentration is below 1 mEq/L (mmol/L) when taken 12 hours after the last dialysis. Hemodialysis is generally required when serum lithium levels are above 4 mEq/L (mmol/L) for patients on long-term treatment, and greater than 6 to 8 mEq/L (mmol/L) after acute poisoning.[2] Rebound increases in serum lithium concentrations can occur 5 to 8 hours after dialysis, thus repeat dialysis can be needed.[2]

Drug–Drug Interactions Thiazide diuretics, nonsteroidal anti-inflammatory drugs, cyclooxygenase-2 inhibitors, angiotensin-converting enzyme inhibitors, and salt-restricted diets can elevate lithium levels.[2] Neurotoxicity can occur when lithium is combined with carbamazepine, diltiazem, losartan, methyldopa, metronidazole, phenytoin, and verapamil.[2,49] Analgesics such as acetaminophen or aspirin and loop diuretics are less likely to interfere with lithium clearance. Caffeine and theophylline can enhance the renal elimination of lithium. Because lithium has no effect on hepatic metabolizing enzymes, it has fewer drug–drug interactions compared with carbamazepine, oxcarbazepine, and valproate.

Dosing and Administration Lithium dosing depends on the patient's age and weight, tolerance to adverse effects, and the acuity of the illness. Dosing is generally titrated up to achieve steady-state serum lithium concentrations of 0.6 to 1.2 mEq/L (mmol/L).[2] Lithium therapy is usually initiated with low to moderate doses (600 mg/day) for prophylaxis and higher doses (900–1,200 mg/day) for acute mania, using a 2- to 3-times daily dosing regimen.[2,49] Immediate-release lithium preparations should be given in two or three divided daily doses, whereas extended-release products can be given once or twice daily. In clinical practice many clinicians dose the immediate-release and extended-release preparations once daily. It can be best to initially begin a patient on divided dosing, but once stabilized many patients are able to switch to once daily dosing without decompensating.

Lithium levels are considered to be at steady state at approximately day 5, and serum samples should be drawn 12 hours postdose. Once a desired serum concentration has been achieved, levels should be drawn in 2 weeks and then if stable every 3 to 6 months or as clinically indicated. Maintenance lithium serum concentrations are usually measured every 3 months, but can be adjusted to every 6 months for stabilized patients, and every 1 to 2 months for patients with frequent mood episodes.[2] Lithium clearance rates increase by 50% to 100% during pregnancy and return to normal postpartum; thus lithium levels should be determined monthly during pregnancy and weekly the month before delivery. At delivery, rapid fluid changes can significantly increase lithium levels, thus a reduction to prepregnancy lithium doses and adequate hydration are recommended.[2]

The recommended guidelines for baseline and routine laboratory testing for lithium are listed in Table 78–8. The 12-hour postdose lithium serum concentration can be 12% to 33% higher with extended-release preparations and lower with regular-release tablets with divided dosage schedules. The dose should be adjusted based on the steady-state serum concentration drawn 12 hours (±30 minutes) after the last dose.[50] A therapeutic trial for outpatients should last a minimum of 4 to 6 weeks with lithium serum concentrations of 0.6 to 1.2 mEq/L (mmol/L). Acutely manic patients can require serum concentrations of 1 to 1.2 mEq/L (mmol/L), and some need up to 1.5 mEq/L (mmol/L) to achieve a therapeutic response. Although serum concentrations less than 0.6 mEq/L (mmol/L) are associated

TABLE 78-8 Guidelines for Baseline and Routine Laboratory Tests and Monitoring for Agents Used in the Treatment of Bipolar Disorder

	Baseline: Physical Examination & General Chemistry[a]	Hematologic Tests[b]		Metabolic Tests[c]		Liver Function Tests[d]		Renal Function Tests[e]		Thyroid Function Tests[f]		Serum Electrolytes[g]		Dermatologic[h]	
	Baseline	Baseline	6–12 mo	Baseline	6–12 mo	Baseline	6–12 mo	Baseline	6–12 mo	Baseline	6–12 mo	Baseline	6–12 mo	Baseline	3–6 mo
SGAs[i]	X			X	X										
Carbamazepine[j]	X	X	X			X	X	X				X	X	X	X
Lamotrigine[k]	X													X	X
Lithium[l]	X	X	X	X	X			X		X	X	X	X	X	X
Oxcarbazepine[m]	X											X	X		
Valproate[n]	X	X	X	X	X	X	X							X	X

[a]Screen for drug abuse and serum pregnancy.

[b]Complete blood cell count (CBC) with differential and platelets.

[c]Fasting glucose, serum lipids, weight.

[d]Lactate dehydrogenase, aspartate aminotransferase, alanine aminotransferase, total bilirubin, alkaline phosphatase.

[e]Serum creatinine, blood urea nitrogen, urinalysis, urine osmolality, specific gravity.

[f]Triiodothyronine, total thyroxine, thyroxine uptake, and thyroid-stimulating hormone.

[g]Serum sodium.

[h]Rashes, hair thinning, alopecia.

[i]Second-generation antipsychotics: Monitor for increased appetite with weight gain (primarily in patients with initial low or normal body mass index); monitor closely if rapid or significant weight gain occurs during early therapy; cases of hyperlipidemia and diabetes reported.

[j]Carbamazepine: Manufacturer recommends CBC and platelets (and possibly reticulocyte counts and serum iron) at baseline, and that subsequent monitoring be individualized by the clinician (e.g., CBC, platelet counts, and liver function tests every 2 weeks during the first 2 months of treatment, then every 3 months if normal). Monitor more closely if patient exhibits hematologic or hepatic abnormalities or if the patient is receiving a myelotoxic drug; discontinue if platelets are <100,000/mm³ (<100 × 10⁹/L), if white blood cell (WBC) count is <3,000/mm³ (<3 × 10⁹/L) or if there is evidence of bone marrow suppression or liver dysfunction. Serum electrolyte levels should be monitored in the elderly or those at risk for hyponatremia. Carbamazepine interferes with some pregnancy tests.

[k]Lamotrigine: If renal or hepatic impairment, monitor closely and adjust dosage according to manufacturer's guidelines. Serious dermatologic reactions have occurred within 2–8 weeks of initiating treatment and are more likely to occur in patients receiving concomitant valproate, with rapid dosage escalation, or using doses exceeding the recommended titration schedule.

[l]Lithium: Obtain baseline electrocardiogram for patients older than 40 years or if preexisting cardiac disease (benign, reversible T-wave depression can occur). Renal function tests should be obtained every 2–3 months during the first 6 months, then every 6–12 months; if impaired renal function, monitor 24-hour urine volume and creatinine every 3 months; if urine volume >3 L/day, monitor urinalysis, osmolality, and specific gravity every 3 months. Thyroid function tests should be obtained once or twice during the first 6 months, then every 6–12 months; monitor for signs and symptoms of hypothyroidism; if supplemental thyroid therapy is required, monitor thyroid function tests and adjust thyroid dose every 1–2 months until thyroid function indices are within normal range, then monitor every 3–6 months.

[m]Oxcarbazepine: Hyponatremia (serum sodium concentrations <125 mEq/L [mmol/L]) has been reported and occurs more frequently during the first 3 months of therapy; serum sodium concentrations should be monitored in patients receiving drugs that lower serum sodium concentrations (e.g., diuretics or drugs that cause inappropriate antidiuretic hormone secretion) or in patients with symptoms of hyponatremia (e.g., confusion, headache, lethargy, and malaise). Hypersensitivity reactions have occurred in approximately 25%–30% of patients with a history of carbamazepine hypersensitivity and requires immediate discontinuation.

[n]Valproate: Weight gain reported in patients with low or normal body mass index. Monitor platelets and liver function during first 3–6 months if evidence of increased bruising or bleeding. Monitor closely if patients exhibit hematologic or hepatic abnormalities or in patients receiving drugs that affect coagulation, such as aspirin or warfarin; discontinue if platelets are <100,000/mm³/L (<100 × 10⁹/L) or if prolonged bleeding time. Pancreatitis, hyperammonemic encephalopathy, polycystic ovary syndrome, increased testosterone, and menstrual irregularities have been reported; not recommended during first trimester of pregnancy due to risk of neural tube defects.

Data from American Psychiatric Association,[2] Goodnick,[10] McEvoy et al.,[49] McEvoy et al.,[54] McEvoy et al.,[58] McEvoy et al.,[60] and McEvoy et al.,[65] and American Diabetes Association et al.[67]

with higher rates of relapse, some patients can do well at 0.4 to 0.7 mEq/L (mmol/L).[2] For bipolar prophylaxis in elderly patients, serum concentrations of 0.4 to 0.6 mEq/L (mmol/L) are recommended because of increased sensitivity to adverse effects.[2]

Anticonvulsants

In the 1980s, anticonvulsants were investigated for manic-depressive illness as the disorder had similar characteristics to episodic neurologic disorders such as epilepsy and migraines. Divalproex sodium (also known as sodium valproate) was marketed in 1995 for the acute treatment of mania in adults and is now the most prescribed mood stabilizer in the United States. Divalproex sodium is FDA approved only for the treatment of acute manic or mixed episodes; however, it is commonly used in clinical practice as maintenance monotherapy for bipolar disorder. Valproate also has limited data supporting its use in acute bipolar depression. Carbamazepine is commonly used for both acute and maintenance therapy. The only formulation approved in the United States for bipolar disorder is extended-release carbamazepine, although other formulations can be used. Some data support the use of oxcarbazepine, a 10-keto analogue of carbamazepine, in the treatment of bipolar disorder; however, it is not approved for the treatment of bipolar disorder

in the United States. Valproate, carbamazepine, and oxcarbazepine each have a wide range of neurologic, gastrointestinal, electrolyte, and hematologic adverse effects that requires regular assessment and routine blood work.

Lamotrigine is FDA approved for the maintenance treatment of bipolar I disorder. Lamotrigine add-on or monotherapy has been used for treatment-refractory bipolar depression, but may not be supported by data from numerous clinical trials.[53] Lamotrigine is associated with hypersensitivity reactions and rare life-threatening skin rashes and requires slow dosage titration.[2]

Valproate Sodium and Valproic Acid The exact mechanism of action of valproic acid is not known. Valproic acid is a branched chain fatty acid and was originally used as an organic solvent before it was discovered in the 1960s to have anticonvulsant properties. Valproate has antimigraine, mood-stabilizing, and antiaggressive effects.[54] In 1995, the enteric-coated formulation divalproex sodium (valproate) was approved for the acute treatment of mania. Several controlled studies have shown valproate to be as effective as lithium and olanzapine in patients with pure mania, and it can be more effective than lithium in certain subtypes of bipolar disorder (e.g., rapid cycling, mixed states, bipolar disorder with comorbid substance abuse).[2,3,10,23,55] Placebo- and lithium-controlled and open studies report that valproate reduces or prevents recurrent manic, depressive, and mixed episodes.[2,3,10] Although valproate is not approved for bipolar disorder in children and adolescents, studies suggest that it is effective and well tolerated.[10,30]

Giving lithium, carbamazepine, antipsychotics, or benzodiazepines with valproate can augment its antimanic effects. The addition of valproate to lithium can have synergistic effects in treatment-refractory rapid cycling and mixed states, and the combination has demonstrated efficacy in maintenance therapy for bipolar I disorder.[23] Combinations of valproate and carbamazepine can have synergistic effects, but the potential drug interactions make blood level monitoring of both agents essential.[10] Adding adjunctive SGAs to valproate can be effective for breakthrough mania or if there is incomplete or partial response to monotherapy. Clozapine, olanzapine, and quetiapine can increase the risk of sedation and weight gain when combined with valproate. The combination of valproate and lamotrigine can be effective, but there is an increased risk of rashes, ataxia, tremor, sedation, and fatigue.[54,56]

Adverse Effects The most frequent dose-related adverse effects with valproate are gastrointestinal complaints (anorexia, nausea, indigestion, vomiting, mild diarrhea, and flatulence), fine hand tremors, and sedation.[2,10,54] The gastrointestinal complaints are usually transient, but giving the medication with food, using lower initial doses with gradual increases in doses, or switching to divalproex sodium extended-release tablets can minimize them.[2,10] Reduction of the dose or the addition of a β-blocker can alleviate tremors, and giving the total daily dose at bedtime can minimize daytime sedation.[2,10]

Other adverse effects of valproate include ataxia, lethargy, alopecia, changes in the texture or color of hair, pruritus, prolonged bleeding because of inhibition of platelet aggregation, transient increases in liver enzymes, and hyperammonemia.[10,54] Increased appetite and weight gain occurs in approximately 50% of patients on long-term valproate therapy. Thrombocytopenia can occur at higher doses, and patients should be monitored for bleeding and bruising. Lowering the valproate dose can restore platelet counts to normal levels.[2] Fatal necrotizing hepatitis is a rare idiosyncratic, non–dose-related adverse effect that has occurred in children with epilepsy receiving multiple anticonvulsants.[10,54] A life-threatening hemorrhagic pancreatitis has been reported in both children and adults.[2,10,54] An in-depth discussion of adverse effects can be found in Chapter 65.

Drug–Drug Interactions A summary of drug–drug interactions for valproate can be found in Chapter 65.

Dosing and Administration For healthy inpatient adults with acute mania, the initial starting dosage of valproate is typically 20 mg/kg/day in divided doses over 12 hours. The daily dose is adjusted by 250 to 500 mg every 1 to 3 days based on clinical response and tolerability. Maximum recommended dosing is 60 mg/kg/day (see Table 78–7).[2,10,54] For outpatients who are hypomanic or euthymic, or for elderly patients, the initial starting dose is generally lower (5–10 mg/kg/day in divided doses) and gradually titrated to avoid adverse effects. Once an optimal dose has been achieved, the total daily dose can be given twice daily or at bedtime if tolerated.[2,10,54] Extended-release divalproex can be administered once daily, but bioavailability can be 15% lower than immediate-release products, thus requiring slightly higher doses.[2] In clinical practice patients with bipolar disorder who are stable can be switched between formulations without having to change the dose. This is not the case for patients with seizure disorder.

Recommended baseline and routine laboratory tests for valproate are listed in Table 78–8. Although therapeutic serum concentrations of valproic acid have not been established in bipolar disorder, most clinicians use the anticonvulsant therapeutic serum range of

50 to 125 mcg/mL (345 to 866 μmol/L) taken 12 hours after the last dose.[2,10] In one study patients with valproate levels greater than 94.1 mcg/mL (651 μmol/L) had greater efficacy for bipolar mania.[57] Patients with cyclothymia or mild bipolar II disorder can have a therapeutic response to lower doses and blood levels, whereas some patients with a more severe form of bipolar disorder can require up to 150 mcg/mL (1,040 μmol/L). Serum valproic acid levels are most useful when assessing for compliance and toxicity.

CLINICAL CONTROVERSY

In the treatment of seizure disorders monitoring serum concentrations of valproic acid is controversial, and the same is true in bipolar disorder. Some clinicians feel that therapeutic blood level monitoring is essential for the appropriate treatment of bipolar disorder, whereas others feel that blood level monitoring is overused and, in many cases, unwarranted. Antiepileptic blood level monitoring should be viewed as a tool to be used as part of overall treatment optimization. Achievement of a specific "therapeutic" level should not be an absolute goal in and of itself.

Carbamazepine Carbamazepine, a dibenzazepine derivative, is structurally related to tricyclic antidepressants.[10] The precise mechanism of action of carbamazepine in affective disorders remains to be elucidated.[12] Carbamazepine is not a first-line agent for bipolar disorder, and is generally reserved for lithium-refractory patients, rapid cyclers, or for mixed states.[2,10] Carbamazepine has acute antimanic effects comparable to lithium and chlorpromazine, but its long-term effectiveness is unclear.[2,10] One comparison trial in hospitalized manic patients indicated that carbamazepine was less effective and needed more rescue adjunctive medications than valproate.[2] Other comparison studies with lithium have reported carbamazepine to be less effective than lithium for maintenance therapy.[2] In a double-blind, placebo-controlled crossover study and in an open study, carbamazepine showed efficacy in the treatment of bipolar depression.[2,10] Studies with treatment-refractory patients have reported that carbamazepine has both acute and long-term prophylactic effects.[3,10] A gradual loss of efficacy over time (similar to lithium and valproate) has been reported in some patients.[3,10]

The combination of carbamazepine with lithium, valproate, and antipsychotics is often used for treatment-resistant patients experiencing a manic episode.[10] Carbamazepine plus olanzapine was not found to be more effective than carbamazepine alone in the treatment of acute mania or mixed episodes.[41] Carbamazepine increases the hepatic metabolism of antidepressants, anticonvulsants, and antipsychotics; thus dosage increases can be necessary (see drug–drug interactions).[10,58] Calcium channel blockers (e.g., verapamil and diltiazem) increase carbamazepine blood levels; thus combination therapy should be closely monitored.[58] The combination of carbamazepine with nimodipine for treatment-refractory bipolar illness can have potential benefit.[59]

Adverse Effects A summary of adverse effects for carbamazepine can be found in Chapter 65. Acute overdoses of carbamazepine are potentially lethal, and serum levels above 15 mcg/mL (63 mmol/L) are associated with ataxia, choreiform movements, diplopia, nystagmus, cardiac conduction changes, seizures, and coma.[2] Gastric lavage, hemoperfusion, and symptomatic treatment are recommended for the management of carbamazepine toxicity.

Drug–Drug Interactions Carbamazepine significantly induces the hepatic cytochrome P450 isoenzyme 3A4 and to a lesser degree 1A2, 2C9/10, and 2D6, which increases the metabolism of many medications.[2,3,58] Women who receive carbamazepine require higher dosages of oral contraceptives or alternative contraceptive methods.[3]

Carbamazepine is metabolized to an active 10,11-epoxide metabolite, thus medications that inhibit 3A4 isoenzymes can result in carbamazepine toxicity (e.g., cimetidine, diltiazem, erythromycin, fluoxetine, fluvoxamine, isoniazid, itraconazole, ketoconazole, nefazodone, propoxyphene, and verapamil).[2,3,10,58] When carbamazepine is combined with valproate, the carbamazepine dose should be reduced because valproate displaces carbamazepine from protein-binding sites, thus increasing free levels.[3,10] Combining clozapine and carbamazepine is not recommended because of the possibility of bone marrow suppression with both agents.[10]

Dosing and Administration During an acute manic episode in most hospitalized patients, carbamazepine can be started at 400 to 600 mg/day in divided doses with meals and increased by 200 mg/day every 2 to 4 days up to 10 to 15 mg/kg per day. In outpatients the initial dose of carbamazepine should be lower and titrated gradually in order to avoid adverse effects. In clinical practice many patients are able to tolerate once daily dosing of carbamazepine once their mood episode has stabilized. The dose of carbamazepine should be gradually increased until response is achieved or there is evidence of toxicity. During the first month of therapy, serum concentrations of carbamazepine may be effected due to autoinduction of cytochrome P450 3A4 enzymes.[58]

Carbamazepine serum levels are usually obtained every 1 to 2 weeks during the first 2 months, and then every 3 to 6 months during maintenance therapy. Serum levels should be drawn 10 to 12 hours after the dose (trough levels) and at least 4 to 7 days after a dosage change. Although there is no correlation between carbamazepine serum concentration and degree of antimanic or antidepressant response, most clinicians attempt to maintain levels between 6 and 10 mcg/mL (25 and 42 mmol/L) (although some treatment-resistant patients can require serum concentrations of 12–14 mcg/mL [51–59 mmol/L]). Recommended baseline and routine laboratory tests for carbamazepine are listed in Table 78–8.

Oxcarbazepine Oxcarbazepine, a 10-keto analog of carbamazepine, blocks voltage-sensitive sodium channels, modulates voltage-activated calcium currents, and increases potassium conductance.[60] Initial trials suggested oxcarbazepine has mood-stabilizing effects similar to those of carbamazepine, with the advantages of milder adverse effects, no autoinduction of liver enzymes, and potentially fewer drug interactions.[2] There are currently less data supporting the use of oxcarbazepine than carbamazepine in the treatment of bipolar disorder. The APA treatment guidelines recommend the use of oxcarbazepine in any situation where one would use carbamazepine. However, many clinicians prefer to use oxcarbazepine only after a patient has failed treatment with carbamazepine or because of an adverse reaction or side effects. Genuine debate exists regarding drug interactions, side effects, and rates of hyponatremia with oxcarbazepine.

Adverse Effects Oxcarbazepine has dose-related adverse effects of dizziness, sedation, headache, ataxia, fatigue, vertigo, abnormal vision, diplopia, nausea, vomiting, and abdominal pain.[60] In one study, hyponatremia was reported to occur in patients taking oxcarbazepine and carbamazepine at rates of 29.9% and 13.5%, respectively.[61] Severe hyponatremia (sodium less than or equal to 128 mEq/L [mmol/L]) was reported by Dong and coworkers as 12.4% and 2.8% of patients for oxcarbazepine and carbamazepine, respectively.[61] An in-depth discussion of adverse effects can be found in Chapter 65.

Drug–Drug Interactions Oxcarbazepine, a cytochrome P450 2C19 enzyme inhibitor and a 3A3/4 enzyme inducer, has the potential for causing drug interactions.[60] Oxcarbazepine induces the metabolism of oral contraceptives, thus alternative contraceptive measures are required.[3,62]

Dosing and Administration Initial dosing is usually 150 to 300 mg twice daily, and daily doses can be increased by 300 to 600 mg every 3 to 6 days up to 1,200 mg/day in divided doses (with or without food).[60]

Lamotrigine Lamotrigine blocks voltage-sensitive sodium channels, modulates or decreases glutamate and aspartate release, and has antikindling properties.[3,12,53,56,63]

Efficacy The effectiveness of lamotrigine for the maintenance treatment of bipolar I disorder in adult patients was established in two multicenter double-blind, placebo-controlled studies.[2] Doses of 200 mg/day were more effective than lower doses, and there were no advantages to using 400 mg/day. Lamotrigine has both antidepressant and mood-stabilizing effects, it may have augmenting properties when combined with lithium or valproate, and has low rates of switching patients to mania.[56,64] Although lamotrigine is less effective for acute mania compared to standard mood stabilizers, it may be beneficial in the maintenance therapy of treatment-resistant bipolar I and II disorders, in rapid-cycling dysphoric mania, and in mixed states.[2,3,56] Lamotrigine seems to be most effective for the prevention of bipolar depression, therefore clinically it is often used in the treatment of patients with bipolar II. There are case reports of possible lamotrigine induced mania when added to lithium, carbamazepine, and valproate.[65] In each of the cases reported, the patients had depressive mood symptoms or rapid mood changes requiring additional therapy.[65]

Adverse Effects Common adverse effects include headache, nausea, dizziness, ataxia, diplopia, drowsiness, tremor, rash, and pruritus.[56,63] Approximately 10% of patients in premarketing clinical trials developed a maculopapular rash and required discontinuation of therapy.[56,63] Although most rashes are self-limiting and resolve with continued treatment, some cases progressed to life-threatening conditions such as Stevens-Johnson syndrome. The incidence of rash appears to be greatest with coadministration of valproate, with higher than recommended initial doses, and with rapid dose escalation.[63] Patients should be warned about the rash, and the need for discontinuing lamotrigine if the rash is diffuse, involves mucosal membranes, and is accompanied by a fever or sore throat. For an in-depth discussion of the adverse effects of lamotrigine, see Chapter 65.

Drug–Drug Interactions Valproate decreases the clearance of lamotrigine (i.e., more than doubles the half-life), and lamotrigine must be administered at a reduced dosage (approximately half the standard dose).[63] For an in-depth discussion of drug–drug interactions with lamotrigine, see Chapter 65.

Dosing and Administration For the maintenance treatment of bipolar disorder, the usual dosage range of lamotrigine is 50 to 300 mg/day. The target dose is generally 200 mg/day (100 mg/day in combination with valproate and 400 mg/day in combination with carbamazepine).[56,63] For patients not taking medications that affect lamotrigine's clearance, the dose is 25 mg/day for the first 2 weeks of therapy, 50 mg/day for weeks 3 and 4, 100 mg/day for week 5, and 200 mg/day for week 6 and beyond.[2,56,63] Patients who stop lamotrigine therapy for more than a few days should be restarted on the recommended dosage escalation titration schedule.

Antipsychotics

First-generation antipsychotics that block DA_2 receptors and SGAs that block both DA_2 and $5-HT_{2A}$ receptors are used to decrease DA activity in the treatment of mania and mixed states. First- and second-generation antipsychotics such as aripiprazole, haloperidol, olanzapine, quetiapine, risperidone, and ziprasidone are effective as monotherapy or adjunctive therapy in the treatment of acute mania.[66] Controlled studies in acute mania with lithium or valproate plus an antipsychotic suggest greater efficacy with combination therapies compared with any of these agents alone.[2,66] First-generation antipsychotics (e.g., chlorpromazine and haloperidol) are effective in up to 70% of patients with acute mania, particularly those with psychosis and psychomotor agitation. Second-generation antipsychotics have demonstrated similar efficacy for the treatment of acute mania associated with agitation, aggression, and psychosis.[2,66]

Treating acute bipolar depression is very challenging, and some antipsychotics may play a useful role. Quetiapine has four large randomized controlled trials supporting its use as a monotherapy treatment option for bipolar depression.[41] The fluoxetine/olanzapine combination also has efficacy data in treating bipolar depression.

Long-term safety of antipsychotics as monotherapy or as an adjunctive therapy for bipolar maintenance treatment still needs to be evaluated.[2,41,66] Risks versus benefits must be weighed due to the long-term adverse effects (e.g., obesity, type 2 diabetes, hyperlipidemia, hyperprolactinemia, and tardive dyskinesia) antipsychotics may cause.[66,68] Aripiprazole, olanzapine, and risperidone long-acting injection are effective monotherapy options for maintenance treatment in bipolar disorder.[41] Some data reported in abstract form support quetiapine for maintenance treatment. First-generation depot antipsychotics (e.g., haloperidol decanoate, fluphenazine decanoate) can have a place in maintenance treatment of bipolar disorder in patients who are noncompliant or treatment resistant.[2]

CLINICAL CONTROVERSY

The use of antipsychotics as long-term maintenance in bipolar disorder does not come without risk. For many years second-generation antipsychotics were considered a safer alternative to first-generation antipsychotics because they had a lower risk for causing movement disorders. However, the second-generation antipsychotics have other long-term risks associated with their use. Metabolic side effects should be considered when weighing risk/benefit ratio of various agents. The optimal management of weight gain and its consequences on physical and mental health is important. Clinicians must make prescribing decisions in collaboration with patients concerning the long-term treatment of bipolar disorder weighing the long-term risk of antipsychotics versus the traditional mood stabilizers (e.g., lithium or valproate).

Clozapine monotherapy has acute and long-term mood-stabilizing effects in refractory bipolar disorder, including conditions with mixed mania and rapid cycling, but requires regular white blood cell monitoring for agranulocytosis.[2,10,66]

Adverse Effects A summary of adverse effects for antipsychotics can be found in Chapter 76.

Drug–Drug Interactions A summary of drug interactions with antipsychotics can be found in Chapter 76.

Dosing and Administration For acute mania, higher initial doses of antipsychotics can be required (e.g., olanzapine 20 mg/day in hospitalized patients). Once acute mania is controlled (usually within 7–28 days), the antipsychotic can be gradually tapered and discontinued, and the patient maintained on the mood stabilizer alone.

Monitoring

6 Recommendations for baseline and routine laboratory testing for patients receiving carbamazepine, lamotrigine, lithium, oxcarbazepine, SGAs, and valproate are found in Table 78–8.

Alternative Medication Treatments

7 Benzodiazepines Weighing the risk to benefit ratio, high potency benzodiazepines such as clonazepam and lorazepam are commonly used as an alternative to or in combination with antipsychotics when patients are experiencing acute mania, agitation, anxiety, panic, and insomnia, or cannot take mood stabilizers (e.g., during the first trimester of pregnancy).[2,3,69,70] Lorazepam is available for intramuscular injection and is useful in the acute management of agitation. Benzodiazepines cause minimal adverse effects compared with antipsychotics, and at higher doses, rapidly sedate agitated patients.[3] Benzodiazepines can cause central nervous system depression, sedation, cognitive and motor impairment, dependence, and withdrawal reactions. When no longer required, benzodiazepines should be gradually tapered and discontinued to avoid withdrawal symptoms.

Antidepressants For many years antidepressants were recommended as adjunctive therapy for acute bipolar depression. Recent data from the Systematic Treatment Enhancement Program for Bipolar Disorder (STEP-BD) suggest that adjunctive antidepressants may be no better than placebo for acute bipolar depression when combined with mood stabilizers.[71] Controversy exists concerning the use of antidepressants, and many clinicians consider them third line in treating acute bipolar depression, except in patients with no history of severe and/or recent mania or potentially in bipolar II patients.[72] The concern of mood switching with the use of antidepressants is valid, although not common. Data show that the rates of mood switch with SSRIs is around 3.8%, similar to placebo when combined with mood stabilizers. The rate of mood switch with dual acting agents (e.g., TCAs or venlafaxine) is higher, and thus these agents should be used with caution.[72,73] It is very important that before initiating therapy with an antidepressant, the patient should be on a therapeutic dosage or blood level of a primary mood stabilizer.[2] Patients who have a history of mania after a depressive episode or who have frequent cycling should be treated cautiously with antidepressants.[2,3] In general, the antidepressant should be gradually withdrawn 2 to 6 months after remission, and the patient maintained on a mood-stabilizing agent.[28,74] For more information, see Chapter 77 for comparisons among antidepressants.

CLINICAL CONTROVERSY

The use of antidepressants in treating bipolar depression does not appear to have benefit over placebo according to recently published data from the Systematic Treatment Enhancement Program for Bipolar Disorder (STEP-BD). There are however meta-analysis data that show some utility of antidepressants. Antidepressants are no longer considered first line in treating bipolar depression, unless a patient has no recent or severe history of acute mania.

Calcium Channel Antagonists Calcium channel antagonists inactivate voltage-sensitive calcium channels, thus inhibiting neurotransmitter synthesis and release and neuronal signal transmission.[10,12] Verapamil, a nondihydropyridine, has demonstrated mood-stabilizing properties in some studies, but negative results were found in other trials.[2,3,10,75] Nimodipine, a dihydropyridine, can be more effective than verapamil for rapid-cycling bipolar disorder because of its anticonvulsant properties, high lipid solubility, and good penetration into the brain.[2,3,10,12,31,75] Calcium channel blockers are generally well tolerated, and the most common adverse effects are bradycardia and hypotension. These are seldom used in everyday clinical practice.

Newer Anticonvulsants Third-generation anticonvulsants have been investigated for treating bipolar disorder with the hope that a different mechanism of action would be beneficial for mood stabilization. Gabapentin, levetiracetam, tiagabine, topiramate, and zonasimide have negative or limited positive data supporting their use in bipolar disorder. Topiramate has been used as an add-on weight-reduction medication, but there are no randomized controlled trials supporting its use in bipolar disorder.[76]

Novel Agents and Dietary Intake Disturbances in 5-HT neurotransmission secondary to inadequate dietary L-tryptophan or abnormalities in tryptophan hydroxylase, 5-HT transporters, and 5-HT receptors was implicated in the pathophysiology of manic-depressive illness as early as 1958.[10] Low 5-HT activity may be a trait marker for bipolar disorder.[21] If available 5-HT is low, the synthesis and secretion of melatonin can be disrupted, thus causing circadian rhythm changes.[10] Acute tryptophan depletion has been shown to reverse the antidepressant effects of 5-HT reuptake inhibitors in depressed patients in remission, but may not negatively affect mood in lithium-stabilized bipolar patients.[77] Randomized controlled studies of L-tryptophan or 5-hydroxytryptophan have shown positive results in the acute treatment and prophylaxis of bipolar disorder.[10] Because 5-HT synthesis in the brain is dependent on dietary L-tryptophan intake, the importance of adequate and regular ingestion of animal-derived protein should be discussed with patients.[10]

A dietary deficiency in essential fatty acids (found in certain fish oils and flaxseed oil that contains α-linolenic acid) has been proposed as a potential cause of mood disorders.[78,79] Omega-3 fatty acids have been shown to suppress neuronal pathways and inhibit kindling processes by several mechanisms (e.g., inhibition of phosphatidylinositol and G-protein secondary messengers and blocking L-type calcium channels). Seafood and fish are rich dietary sources of omega-3 essential fatty acids, specifically docosahexaenoic acid and eicosapentaenoic acid.[79] Omega-3 fatty acids may have more antidepressant than antimanic effects.[80] Data reported by Keck and colleagues for bipolar depression and rapid cycling did not support the use of eicosapentaenoic acid.[81] The data supporting the use of omega-3 fatty acids is controversial and needs to be further evaluated.

Special Populations

The approach for treating bipolar disorder in special populations (e.g., comorbid medical or psychiatric disorders, pregnancy, or breastfeeding) can vary among clinicians. Patients with comorbid medical conditions or concomitant substance abuse, those older than 65 years of age, and pregnant patients can require different treatment approaches. Women have a high risk of relapse postpartum; therefore, prophylaxis with mood stabilizers is recommended immediately postpartum to decrease the risk of relapse.[82]

Prophylactic medications such as lithium or valproate can prevent postpartum episodes in women with bipolar disorder.[2] Pharmacotherapy during pregnancy is complicated, and the risk-to-benefit ratio must be weighed. Infants whose mothers took lithium during the first trimester of pregnancy may have a lower incidence of cardiovascular defects (particularly Ebstein anomaly) than was previously thought.[2,10] Current estimates of this malformation during the first trimester are estimated between 1:1,000 and 1:2,000.[82] Lithium freely crosses the placenta and is found in equal concentrations in maternal and fetal blood.[49] When lithium is used during pregnancy, it should be tapered down to the lowest effective dose necessary to decrease the risk of relapse. Lithium can cause "floppy" infant syndrome (e.g., low Apgar scores, lethargy, hypotonia, bradycardia, cyanosis, shallow respiration, and poor sucking), hypothyroidism, and nontoxic goiters. Milk concentrations of lithium range from 30% to 50% of the mother's serum concentration,

and serum concentrations in the nursing infant are 10% to 50% of the mother's; thus breastfeeding is usually discouraged.[2,11,83] If using lithium during pregnancy, dose adjustments and close monitoring of serum levels will be needed due to changes in glomerular filtration rates and renal perfusion rates during pregnancy and immediately after delivery.[84]

The use of anticonvulsants also poses a teratogenic risk when used during pregnancy. Neural tube defects cause the most concern for clinicians treating pregnant patients during their first trimester of pregnancy. Data from the North American Antiepileptic Drug Pregnancy Registry shows the risk of neural tube defects is about 1 in 1,500 for nonexposed babies.[85] Carbamazepine's risk of neural tube defects is estimated to be 0.5% to 1%.[12] Carbamazepine is excreted in breast milk (the milk-to-maternal plasma ratio of carbamazepine is ~0.4).[3] Craniofacial abnormalities, developmental delays, microcephaly, and other abnormalities are also of concern when using anticonvulsants. Data on lamotrigine show major malformation rates similar to the general population (2.9% vs 2%–3%, respectively), but data for lamotrigine is limited compared with some older anticonvulsants.[84] The International Lamotrigine Pregnancy Register reports 12 major congenital malformations from 414 first trimester exposures.[84] Valproate is usually not recommended during the first trimester of pregnancy because the risk of neural tube birth defects is about 1 in 20 exposed babies.[85] Australian registry data in patients with epilepsy show dose-related teratogenicity with doses greater than 1,100 mg/day of valproate.[86] Administration of folate can reduce the risk of neural tube defects; therefore the risks versus benefits of using valproate during pregnancy must be discussed with the patient.[10] Valproic acid is excreted into human breast milk in low concentrations (less than 1%–10% of the mother's serum level), so is considered to be compatible with breastfeeding.[3] One case report of thrombocytopenia and anemia from valproate exposure has been reported in a nursing infant. If the mother receives valproate during breastfeeding, mother and infant should have identical laboratory monitoring. Caution should be used when prescribing antipsychotics during pregnancy. There are far more data on the use of FGAs than SGAs during pregnancy. Some data are available for haloperidol and low-dose chlorpromazine, and these data show no elevated rate of physical malformations during first trimester exposure.[87] Higher doses of chlorpromazine used in treating psychiatric illness may be associated with neonatal withdrawal and extrapyramidal symptoms.[87] Data on other FGAs are limited. Data on the SGAs are more limited, but do not show an overall increased risk of fetal abnormalities.[87] Olanzapine, risperidone, and quetiapine comprise most of this data.[87] There are limited reports with clozapine, aripiprazole, and ziprasidone.[87] There is still a paucity of human data with antipsychotics and therefore risk-benefit ratio must be weighed.

Treatment of catatonia also varies from standard treatment in that mood stabilizers and antipsychotics have minimal effect. Catatonic features such as mutism, motor excitement, stereotypic movements, waxy flexibility, negativism, echopraxia, and echolalia are best treated with benzodiazepines, specifically lorazepam. The use of antipsychotics in catatonia should be minimized because of an increased risk of neuroleptic malignant syndrome. ECT is also a treatment option in this patient population.

PHARMACOECONOMIC CONSIDERATIONS

Bipolar disorder is one of the leading causes of chronic disability worldwide and shares characteristics of both major depressive disorder and schizophrenia.[3] Bipolar disorder is primarily treated in the public mental health sector, and a majority of patients receive lifelong disability coverage because of compromised functioning.[3]

The total cost to society for bipolar disorder is enormous and is exceeded only by the costs for treating individuals with schizophrenia.[10] It was estimated, more than a decade ago, that the total annual economic impact of bipolar disorder in the United States was approximately $45 billion per year.[88]

EVALUATION OF THERAPEUTIC OUTCOMES

The establishment and maintenance of a therapeutic alliance with a clinician is essential in monitoring a patient's psychiatric status and safety; enhancing treatment adherence; promoting good nutrition, sleep, and exercise; identifying stressors; recognizing new mood episodes; and minimizing adverse reactions and drug interactions.[2] Patients who have a partial response or nonresponse to established bipolar therapies should be reassessed for an accurate diagnosis, concomitant medical or psychiatric conditions, and medications or substances that exacerbate mood symptoms. Nonadherence to medication treatment, delusional symptoms, alcohol or substance abuse, rapid cycling, or mixed states are often associated with poorer treatment outcomes.

The evaluation of therapeutic outcomes for bipolar disorder requires regular monitoring by a clinician. More frequent office visits, telephone calls, and intensive outpatient programs are first-line strategies to prevent hospitalization during the acute treatment phase of a manic or depressive episode.[2] Patients (and family members if needed) should be actively involved with their treatment and help to monitor target symptoms, efficacy of treatment, treatment adherence, and adverse effects.[2]

Standardized rating scales for mania and depression are used to measure severity and changes in symptoms in clinical trials (e.g., Young Mania Rating Scale, brief bipolar disorder symptoms scale, Hamilton Rating Scale for Depression, and Montgomery-Åsberg Depression Rating Scale). Patient-rated life mood charts, a timeline of stressful life events, and a graphic display of sleep patterns are helpful in recognizing early symptoms of mood episodes and in documenting patterns and lengths of episodes.[2] A mood disorder questionnaire, a 13-item self-reported screening tool, was developed to differentiate bipolar disorder from other mood disorders (*www.dbsalliance.org/questionnaire/screening_intro.asp*).[2,25] Health-related quality of life scales such as the Short Form (SF)-36 and the Psychological General Well-Being Scale have been recommended to assess the quality of life in individuals with bipolar disorder.[89]

ABBREVIATIONS

APA: American Psychiatric Association

CANMAT: Canadian Network for Mood and Anxiety Treatments

DA: dopamine

DSM-IV-TR: *Diagnostic and Statistical Manual, Fourth Edition, Text Revision*

ECT: electroconvulsive therapy

FDA: U.S. Food and Drug Administration

FGAs: first-generation antipsychotics

GABA: γ-aminobutyric acid

5-HT: serotonin

ISBD: International Society for Bipolar Disorders

NAMI: National Alliance on Mental Illness

NE: norepinephrine

rTMS: repetitive transcranial magnetic stimulation

SGAs: second-generation antipsychotics

STEP-BD: Systematic Treatment Enhancement Program for Bipolar Disorder

VNS: vagus nerve stimulation

WFSBP: World Federation of Societies of Biological Psychiatry

REFERENCES

1. American Psychiatric Association: *Diagnostic and Statistical Manual of Mental Disorders, Fourth Edition, Text Revision.* Washington, DC: American Psychiatric Association, 2000:345–401.
2. American Psychiatric Association. Practice guideline for the treatment of patients with bipolar disorder (revision). Am J Psychiatry 2002;159:1–50.
3. Goldberg JF, Harrow M, eds. Bipolar Disorders: Clinical Course and Outcome. Washington, DC: American Psychiatric Press, 1999.
4. Kessler RC, McGonagle KA, Zhao S, et al. Lifetime and 12-month prevalence of DSM-III-R psychiatric disorders in the United States: Results from the national comorbidity survey. Arch Gen Psychiatry 1994;51:8–19.
5. Practice Parameters for the Assessment and Treatment of Children and Adolescents with Bipolar Disorder. J Am Acad Child Adolesc Psychiatry 2007;46:107–125.
6. Kelso JR. Arguments for the genetic basis of the bipolar spectrum. J Affect Disord 2003;73:183–197.
7. Lenox RH, Gould TD, Manji HK. Endophenotypes in bipolar disorder. Am J Med Genet 2002;114:391–406.
8. Baron M. Manic-depressive genes and the new millennium: Poised for discovery. Mol Psychiatry 2002;7:342–358.
9. Bezchlibnyk Y, Young LT. The neurobiology of bipolar disorder: Focus on signal transduction pathways and the regulation of gene expression. Can J Psychiatry 2002;47:135–148.
10. Goodnick PJ, ed. Mania: Clinical and Research Perspectives. Washington, DC: American Psychiatric Press, 1998.
11. Soares JC. Can brain imaging studies provide a "mood stabilizer signature?" Mol Psychiatry 2002;7(Suppl 1):S64–S70.
12. Manji HK, Bowden CL, Belmaker RH, eds. Bipolar Medications: Mechanisms of Action. Washington, DC: American Psychiatric Press, 2000.
13. Manji HK, Moore GJ, Chen G. Bipolar disorder: leads from the molecular and cellular mechanisms of action of mood stabilizers. Br J Psychiatry Suppl 2001;41:S107–S119.
14. Gould TD, Manji HK. Signaling networks in the pathophysiology and treatment of mood disorders. J Psychosom Res 2002;53:687–697.
15. Sobczak S, Honig A, van Duinen MA, Riedel WJ. Serotonergic dysfunction in bipolar disorders: A literature review of serotonergic challenge studies. Bipolar Disord 2002;4:347–356.
16. Freeman MP, Wosnitzer Smith K, Freeman SA, et al. The impact of reproductive events on the course of bipolar disorder in women. J Clin Psychiatry 2002;63:284–287.
17. Ketter TA, Wang PW. The emerging differential roles of GABAergic and antiglutamatergic agents in bipolar disorders. J Clin Psychiatry 2003;64(Suppl 3):15–20.
18. White HS. Mechanism of action of newer anticonvulsants. J Clin Psychiatry 2003;64(Suppl 8):5–8.
19. Rasgon N, Bauer M, Glenn T, et al. Menstrual cycle related mood changes in women with bipolar disorder. Bipolar Disord 2003;5:48–52.
20. Mahmood T, Silverstone T. Serotonin and bipolar disorder. J Affect Disord 2001;66:1–11.
21. Kim EY, Miklowitz DJ. Childhood mania, attention deficit hyperactivity disorder and conduct disorder: A critical review of diagnostic dilemmas. Bipolar Disord 2002;4:215–225.
22. Ostacher MJ, Perlis RH, Nierenberg AA, et al. Impact of substance use disorders on recovery from episodes of depression in bipolar disorder patients: prospective data from the systematic treatment enhancement program for bipolar disorder (STEP-BD). Am J Psych 2010;167:289–297.
23. Calabrese JR, Shelton MD, Rapport DJ, et al. Current research on rapid cycling bipolar disorder and its treatment. J Affect Disord 2001;67:241–255.

24. Sherwood Brown E, Suppes T, Adinoff B, Rajan Thomas N. Drug abuse and bipolar disorder: Comorbidity or misdiagnosis? J Affect Disord 2001;65:105–115.

25. Keck PE, Kessler RC, Ross R. Clinical and economic effects of unrecognized or inadequately treated bipolar disorder. J Psychiatr Pract 2008;14(Suppl 2):31–38.

26. Coryell W, Solomon DA, Fiedorowicz, et al. Anxiety and outcome in bipolar disorder. Am J Psychiatry 2009;166:1238–1243.

27. Bowden CL. Diagnosis and impact of bipolar depression. J Clin Psychiatry 2009:70(9):e32.

28. Sachs GS, Koslow CL, Ghaemi SN. The treatment of bipolar depression. Bipolar Disord 2000;2:256–260.

29. Abreu LN, Lafer B, Baca-Garcia E, Oquendo MA. Suicidal ideation and suicide attempts in bipolar disorder type I: an update for the clinician. Rev Bras Psiquiatr 2009;31(3):271–280.

30. Chang KD, Ketter TA. Special issues in the treatment of pediatric bipolar disorder. Expert Opin Pharmacother 2001;2:613–622.

31. Barrios C, Chaudhry TA, Goodnick PJ. Rapid cycling bipolar disorder. Expert Opin Pharmacother 2001;2:1963–1973.

32. Post RM, Denicoff KD, Leverich GS, et al. Morbidity in 258 bipolar outpatients followed for 1 year with daily prospective ratings on the NIMH life chart method. J Clin Psychiatry 2003;64:680–690.

33. Dalton EJ, Cate-Carter TD, Mundo E, et al. Suicide risk in bipolar patients: The role of comorbid substance use disorders. Bipolar Disord 2003;5:58–61.

34. Lingam R, Scott J. Treatment non-adherence in affective disorders. Acta Psychiatr Scand 2002;105:164–172.

35. Miklowitz DJ, Otto MW, Frank E, et al. Psychosocial treatments for bipolar depression; a 1-year randomized trail from the Systematic Treatment Enhancement Program. Arch Gen Psychiatry 2007;64: 419–427.

36. Dell'Osso B, Mundo E, D'Urso N, et al. Augmentative repetitive navigated transcranial magnetic stimulation (rTMS) in drug resistant bipolar depression. Bipolar Disord 2009;11:76–81.

37. Li X, Nahas Z, Anderson B, et al. Can left prefrontal rTMS be used as a maintenance treatment for bipolar depression? Depress Anxiety 2004;20:98–100.

38. Michael N, Erfurth A. Treatment of bipolar mania with right prefrontal rapid transcranial magnetic stimulation. J Affect Disord 2004;78:253–257.

39. Marangell LB, Suppes T, Zboyan HA, et al. A 1-year pilot study of vagus nerve stimulation in treatment-resistant rapid-cycling bipolar disorder. J Clin Psychiatry 2008;69:183–189.

40. Bauer MS, Mitchner L. What is a "mood stabilizer"? An evidence-based response. Am J Psychiatry 2004;161:3–18.

41. Canadian Network for Mood and Anxiety Treatments (CANMAT) and International Society for Bipolar Disorders (ISBD) collaborative update of CANMAT guidelines for the management of patients with bipolar disorder: update 2009. Bipolar Disord 2009;11:225–255.

42. Suppes T, Dennehy EB, Hirschfeld RM, et al. The Texas implementation of medication algorithms: update to the algorithms for treatment of bipolar I disorder. J Clin Psychiatry 2005;66:870–886.

43. Grunze H, Kasper S, Goodwin G, et al. World Federation of Societies of Biological Psychiatry (WFSBP) guidelines for biological treatment of bipolar disorders. Part I. Treatment of bipolar depression. World J Biol Psychiatry 2002;3:115–124.

44. Grunze H, Vieta E, Goodwin GM, et al. The World Federation of Societies of Biological Psychiatry (WFSBP) guidelines for the biological treatment of bipolar disorders: update 2009 on the treatment of acute mania. World J Biol Psychiatry 2009;10:85–116.

45. Madaan V, Chang KD. Pharmacotherapeutic strategies for pediatric bipolar disorder. Expert Opin Pharmacother 2007;8:1801–1819.

46. Wagner KD, Redden L, Kowatch RA, et al. A double-blind, randomized, placebo-controlled trial of divalproex extended-release in the treatment of bipolar disorder in children and adolescents. J Am Acad Child Adolesc Psychiatry 2009;48:519–532.

47. Kuehn BM. FDA panel OKs 3 antipsychotic drugs for pediatric use, cautions. JAMA 2009;302:833–834.

48. Shaldubina A, Agam G, Belmaker RH. The mechanism of lithium action: state of the art, ten years later. Prog Neuropsychopharmacol Biol Psychiatry 2001;25:855–866.

49. McEvoy GK, Miller J, Snow EK, et al. Lithium salts. AHFS Drug Information 2007. Bethesda, MD: American Society of Health-System Pharmacists, 2007:2566–2575.

50. Baldessarini RJ, Tondo L, Hennen J, Viguera AC. Is lithium still worth using? An update of selected recent research. Harv Rev Psychiatry 2002;10:59–75.

51. Goodwin FK. Rationale for long-term treatment of bipolar disorder and evidence for long-term lithium treatment. J Clin Psychiatry 2002;63(Suppl 10):5–12.

52. Baldessarini RJ, Tondo L, Hennen J. Lithium treatment and suicide risk in major affective disorders: Update and new findings. J Clin Psychiatry 2003;64(Suppl 5):44–52.

53. Calabrese JR, Huffman RF, White RL et al. Lamotrigine in the acute treatment of bipolar depression: results of five double-blind, placebo controlled clinical trials. Bipolar Disord 2008;10:323–333.

54. McEvoy GK, Miller J, Snow EK, et al. Valproate sodium, valproic acid, divalproex sodium. AHFS Drug Information 2007. Bethesda, MD: American Society of Health-System Pharmacists, 2007:2255–2262.

55. Macritchie K, Geddes JR, Scott J, et al. Valproate for acute mood episodes in bipolar disorder. Cochrane Database Syst Rev 2003;1:CD004052.

56. Malhi GS, Adams D, Berk M. Medicating mood with maintenance in mind: bipolar depression pharmacotherapy. Bipolar Disord 2009;11:55–76.

57. Allen MH, Hirschfeld RM, Wozniak PJ, et al. Linear relationship of valproate serum concentration to response and optimal serum levels for acute mania. Am J Psychiatry 2006;163:272–275.

58. McEvoy GK, Miller J, Snow EK, et al. Carbamazepine. AHFS Drug Information 2007. Bethesda, MD: American Society of Health-System Pharmacists, 2007:2220–2225.

59. Pazzaglia PJ, Post RM, Ketter TA, et al. Nimodipine monotherapy and carbamazepine augmentation in patients with refractory recurrent affective illness. J Clin Psychopharmacol 1998;18:404–413.

60. McEvoy GK, Miller J, Snow EK, et al. Oxcarbazepine. AHFS Drug Information 2007. Bethesda, MD: American Society of Health-System Pharmacists, 2007:2244–2246.

61. Dong Xiaoming, Leppik IE, White J, Rarick J. Hyponatremia from oxcarbazepine and carbamazepine. Neurology 2005;65:1976–1978.

62. Perucca E. Clinically relevant drug interactions with antiepileptic drugs. Br J Clin Pharmacol 2005;61:246–255.

63. McEvoy GK, Miller J, Snow EK, et al. Lamotrigine. AHFS Drug Information 2007. Bethesda, MD: American Society of Health-System Pharmacists, 2007:2233–2239.

64. Malhi GS, Mitchell PB, Salim S. Bipolar depression: Management options. CNS Drugs 2003;17:9–25.

65. Raskin S, Teitelbaum A, Zislin J, Durst R. Adjunctive lamotrigine as a possible mania inducer in bipolar patients. Am J Psychiatry 2006;163:159–160.

66. Tohen M, Vieta E. Antipsychotic agents in the treatment of bipolar mania. Bipolar Disord 2009;11:45–54.

67. American Diabetes Association, American Psychiatric Association, American Association of Clinical Endocrinologists, et al. Consensus development conference on antipsychotic drugs and obesity and diabetes. Diabetes Care 2004;27:596–601.

68. Marder SR, Essock SM, Miller AL, et al. Physical health monitoring of patients with schizophrenia. Am J Psychiatry 2004;161: 1334–1349.

69. McEvoy GK, Miller J, Snow EK, et al. Benzodiazepines. AHFS Drug Information 2007. Bethesda, MD: American Society of Health-System Pharmacists, 2007:2508–2518.

70. Alderfer BS, Allen MH. Treatment of agitation in bipolar disorder across the life cycle. J Clin Psychiatry 2003;64(Suppl 4):3–9.

71. Sachs GS, Nierenberg AA, Calabrese JR, et al. Effectiveness of adjunctive antidepressant treatment for bipolar disorder. N Engl J Med 2007;356:1711–1722.

72. Gigsman HJ, Geddes JR, Rendell JM, et al. Antidepressants for bipolar depression: a systematic review of randomized, controlled trials. Am J Psychiatry 2004;161:1537–1547.

73. Post RM, Altshuler LL, Leverich GS, et al. Mood switch in bipolar depression: comparison of adjunctive venlafaxine, bupropion, and sertraline. Br J Psychiatry 2006;189:124–131.

74. Sachs GS, Printz DJ, Kahn DA, et al. The expert consensus guideline series: Medication treatment of bipolar disorder 2000. Postgrad Med 2000;Spec No:1–104.

75. Levy NA, Janicak PG. Calcium channel antagonists for the treatment of bipolar disorder. Bipolar Disord 2000;2:108–119.

76. Aronne LJ, Segal KR. Weight gain in the treatment of mood disorders. J Clin Psychiatry 2003;64(Suppl 8):22–29.

77. Johnson L, El-Khoury A, Aberg-Wistedt A, et al. Tryptophan depletion in lithium-stabilized patients with affective disorder. Int J Neuropsychopharmacol 2001;4:329–336.

78. Noaghiul S, Hibbelm JR. Cross-national comparisons of seafood consumption and rates of bipolar disorders. Am J Psychiatry 2003;160:2222–2227.

79. Parker F, Gibson NA, Brotchie H, et al. Omega-3 fatty acids and mood disorders. Am J Psychiatry 2006;163:969–978.

80. Montgomery P and Richardson AJ. Omega-3 fatty acids for bipolar disorder. Cochrane Database Syst Rev 2008;2:CD005169.

81. Keck PE, Mintz J, McElroy SL, et al. Double-blind, randomized, placebo-controlled trials of ethyl-eicosapentaenoate in the treatment of bipolar depression and rapid cycling bipolar disorder. Biol Psychiatry 2006;60:1020–1022.

82. Yonkers KA, Wisner KL, Stowe Z, et al. Management of bipolar disorder during pregnancy and the postpartum period. Am J Psychiatry 2004;161:608–620.

83. Ernst CL, Goldberg JF. The reproductive safety profile of mood stabilizers, atypical antipsychotics, and broad-spectrum psychotropics. J Clin Psychiatry 2002;63(Suppl 4):42–55.

84. Dodd S, Berk M. The safety of medications for the treatment of bipolar disorder during pregnancy and the puerperium. Curr Drug Saf 2006;1:25–33.

85. US Food and Drug Administration. (2009, December 3). Information for Healthcare Professionals: Risk of Neural Tube Birth Defects following prenatal exposure to Valproate. *http://www.fda.gov/Drugs/Drug Safety/PostmarketDrugSafetyInformationforPatientsandProviders/ DrugSafetyInformationforHeathcareProfessionals/ucm192649.htm.*

86. Vajda FJE, Hitchcock A, Graham J, et al. The Australian register of antiepileptic drugs in pregnancy: the first 1002 pregnancies. Aust N Z J Obstet Gynaecol 2007;47:468–474.

87. Einarson A, Boskovic R. Use and safety of antipsychotic drugs during pregnancy. J Psychiatr Pract 2009;15:183–192.

88. Hirschfeld RMA, Vornik LA. Bipolar disorder–costs and comorbidity. Am J Manag Care 2005;11:S85–S90.

89. Namjoshi MA, Buesching DP. A review of the health-related quality of life literature in bipolar disorder. Qual Life Res 2001;10:105–115.

90. Kaplan HI, Sadock BJ. Synopsis of Psychiatry: Behavioral Sciences/ Clinical Psychiatry, 8th ed. Baltimore, MD: Lippincott Williams & Wilkins, 1998: 530.

SARAH T. MELTON AND CYNTHIA K. KIRKWOOD

CHAPTER

79

Anxiety Disorders I: Generalized Anxiety, Panic, and Social Anxiety Disorders

KEY CONCEPTS

❶ The long-term goal in generalized anxiety disorder (GAD) is remission with minimal or no anxiety symptoms and no functional impairment.

❷ Antidepressants are the agents of choice for the management of GAD.

❸ Antidepressants have a lag time of 2 to 4 weeks or longer before antianxiety effects occur in GAD.

❹ When monitoring the effectiveness of antidepressants in panic disorder, it is important to allow an adequate amount of time (8 to 12 weeks) to achieve full therapeutic response.

❺ Clonazepam and extended-release alprazolam are alternatives to immediate-release alprazolam for patients with panic disorder having breakthrough panic symptoms at the end of a dosing interval.

❻ The optimal duration of panic therapy is unknown; 12 to 24 months of pharmacotherapy is recommended before gradual drug discontinuation over 4 to 6 months is attempted.

❼ Social anxiety disorder (SAD) is a chronic long-term illness requiring extended therapy. After improvement, at least a 1-year medication maintenance period is recommended.

❽ The selective serotonin reuptake inhibitors or venlafaxine are considered first-line pharmacotherapy for SAD.

❾ An adequate trial of antidepressants in generalized social anxiety disorder lasts at least 8 weeks, and maximal benefit may not be seen until 12 weeks.

❿ The three principal domains in which improvement should be observed in generalized social anxiety disorder are symptoms, functionality, and well-being.

Anxiety is an emotional state commonly caused by the perception of real or perceived danger that threatens the security of an individual. It allows a person to prepare for or react to environmental changes. Everyone experiences a certain amount of nervousness and apprehension when faced with a stressful situation. This is an adaptive response and is transient in nature.

Learning objectives, review questions, and other resources can be found at **www.pharmacotherapyonline.com**.

Anxiety can produce uncomfortable and potentially debilitating psychologic (e.g., worry or feeling of threat) and physiologic arousal (e.g., tachycardia or shortness of breath) if it becomes excessive. Some individuals experience persistent, severe anxiety symptoms and possess irrational fears that significantly impair normal daily functioning. These persons often suffer from an anxiety disorder.[1]

Anxiety disorders are among the most frequent mental disorders encountered in clinical practice. Healthcare professionals often mistake anxiety disorders for physical illnesses, and only 23% of patients receive appropriate treatment.[2] Failure to diagnose and manage anxiety disorders results in negative outcomes including overuse of healthcare resources, increased morbidity, and mortality.[3] Individuals with anxiety disorders develop cardiovascular, cerebrovascular, gastrointestinal, and respiratory disorders at a significantly higher rate than the general population.[4]

To treat anxiety appropriately, the clinician must make a reliable diagnosis. It is essential that the distinction between short-term symptoms of anxiety and anxiety disorders be understood. Common or situational anxiety is a normal response to a stressful circumstance. Although symptoms can be severe, they are temporary and usually last no more than 2 or 3 weeks. Although short-term, as-needed treatment with an anxiolytic agent such as a benzodiazepine is common and can provide some symptomatic relief, prolonged drug therapy is not recommended.[5]

EPIDEMIOLOGY

Anxiety disorders, as a group, are the most commonly occurring psychiatric disorders. According to the National Comorbidity Survey Replication on the prevalence, severity, and comorbidity estimates of mental disorders in the United States, the most recent 1-year prevalence rate for anxiety disorders was 19.1% in persons aged 18 years and older. Specific phobias were the most common anxiety disorder, with a 12-month prevalence of 9.1%. The 1-year prevalence of generalized anxiety disorder (GAD) was 2.7%, that of panic disorder was 2.7%, and that of social anxiety disorder (SAD) was 7.1%.[6]

In general, anxiety disorders are a group of heterogeneous illnesses that develop before age 30 years and are more common in women, individuals with social issues, and those with a family history of anxiety and depression. Patients often develop another anxiety disorder, major depression, or substance abuse.[1–3] The clinical picture of mixed anxiety and depression is much more common than an isolated anxiety disorder.[2]

ETIOLOGY

The differential diagnosis of anxiety disorders includes medical and psychiatric illnesses and certain drugs.[2] Hypotheses on the etiology of anxiety disorders are based on interactions between a combination of

TABLE 79-1 Common Medical Illnesses Associated with Anxiety Symptoms

Cardiovascular
Angina, arrhythmias, cardiomyopathy, congestive heart failure, hypertension, ischemic heart disease, myocardial infarction

Endocrine and metabolic
Cushing's disease, diabetes, hyperparathyroidism, hyperthyroidism, hypothyroidism, hypoglycemia, hyponatremia, hyperkalemia, pheochromocytoma, vitamin B_{12} or folate deficiencies

Neurologic
Migraine, seizures, stroke, neoplasms, poor pain control

Respiratory system
Asthma, chronic obstructive pulmonary disease, pulmonary embolism, pneumonia

Others
Anemias, cancer, systemic lupus erythematosus, vestibular dysfunction

Data from Roy-Byrne et al.[2,4] and Rogers and Wolfe.[10]

TABLE 79-2 Drugs Associated with Anxiety Symptoms

Anticonvulsants: carbamazepine, phenytoin
Antidepressants: selective serotonin reuptake inhibitors, serotonin norepinephrine reuptake inhibitors, bupropion
Antihypertensives: clonidine, felodipine
Antibiotics: quinolones, isoniazid
Bronchodilators: albuterol, theophylline
Corticosteroids: prednisone
Dopa agonists: amantadine, levodopa
Herbals: ma huang, ginseng, ephedra
Illicit substances: ecstasy, marijuana
Nonsteroidal antiinflammatory drugs: ibuprofen, indomethacin
Stimulants: amphetamines, methylphenidate, nicotine, caffeine, cocaine
Sympathomimetics: pseudoephedrine, phenylephrine
Thyroid hormones: levothyroxine
Toxicity: anticholinergics, antihistamines, digoxin

Data from American Psychiatric Association[1] and Rogers and Wolfe.[10]

factors including vulnerability (e.g., genetic predisposition and early childhood adversity) and stress (e.g., occupational and traumatic experience). The vulnerability may be associated with genetic factors and neurobiological adaptations of the central nervous system (CNS).[7]

MEDICAL DISEASES ASSOCIATED WITH ANXIETY

Anxiety symptoms are an inherent part of the initial clinical presentation of several diseases, thus complicating the distinction between anxiety disorders and medical disorders.[2,4] Anxiety disorders are strongly and independently associated with chronic medical illness, low levels of physical health-related quality of life (QOL), and physical disability.[4] If anxiety symptoms are secondary to a medical illness, they usually will subside as the medical situation stabilizes. However, the knowledge that one has a physical illness can trigger anxious feelings and further complicate therapy. Persistent anxiety subsequent to a physical illness requires further assessment for an anxiety disorder. Common somatic symptoms of anxiety that frequently present in medical disorders include abdominal pain, palpitations, tachycardia, sweating, flushing, tremor, chest pain or tightness, and shortness of breath. Although less specific, symptoms of muscle tension, headache, and fatigue are also common manifestations of anxiety. Medical disorders most closely associated with anxiety are listed in Table 79–1.[2,4,8-10]

PSYCHIATRIC DISEASES ASSOCIATED WITH ANXIETY

Anxiety can be a presenting feature of several major psychiatric illnesses. Anxiety symptoms are extremely common in patients with mood disorders, schizophrenia, dementia, and substance use disorders. Most psychiatric patients will have two or more concurrent psychiatric disorders (comorbidity) within their lifetime.[6] It is important to diagnose and treat all comorbid psychiatric conditions in patients with anxiety disorders.

DRUG-INDUCED ANXIETY

Drugs are a common cause of anxiety symptoms (Table 79–2). Anxiety occurs during the use of CNS-stimulating drugs in a dose-dependent manner, but ingestion of minimal amounts can result in marked anxiety, including panic attacks, in some individuals. The onset of drug-induced anxiety is usually rapid after the initiation of therapy. A thorough medication history evaluating for a recent drug or dosage change is important to rule out a drug-induced etiology for the anxiety.

Anxiety occurs occasionally during the use of CNS depressants, especially in children and the elderly; however, anxiety complaints are more common as complications of drug withdrawal after the abrupt discontinuation of these agents.[8-10]

PATHOPHYSIOLOGY

Data from biochemical and neuroimaging studies indicate that the modulation of normal and pathologic anxiety states is associated with multiple regions of the brain and abnormal function in several neurotransmitter systems, including norepinephrine (NE), γ-aminobutyric acid (GABA), serotonin (5-HT), corticotrophin-releasing factor (CRF), and cholesystokinin.[11] Current neuroanatomic models of fear (i.e., the response to danger) and anxiety (i.e., the feeling of fear that is disproportionate to the actual threat) include some key brain areas. The amygdala, a temporal lobe structure, plays a critical role in the assessment of fear stimuli and learned response to fear.[11,12] The locus ceruleus (LC), located in the brain stem, is the primary NE-containing site, with widespread projections to areas responsible for implementing fear responses (e.g., vagus, lateral and paraventricular hypothalamus). The hippocampus is integral in the consolidation of traumatic memory and contextual fear conditioning. The hypothalamus is the principal area for integrating neuroendocrine and autonomic responses to a threat.[11,12]

NEUROCHEMICAL THEORIES

Noradrenergic Model

The basic premise of the noradrenergic theory is that the autonomic nervous system of anxious patients is hypersensitive and overreacts to various stimuli. Many anxious patients clearly display symptoms of peripheral autonomic hyperactivity. In response to threat or fearful situations, the LC serves as an alarm center, activating NE release and stimulating the sympathetic and parasympathetic nervous systems. Chronic central noradrenergic overactivity downregulates α_2-adrenoreceptors in patients with GAD. This receptor is hypersensitive in some patients with panic disorder.[11] By administering drugs that have a relatively specific effect on the LC, researchers have further explored the NE theory of anxiety and panic disorder. Drugs with anxiogenic effects (e.g., yohimbine [an α_2-adrenergic receptor antagonist]) stimulate LC firing and increase noradrenergic activity. NE in turn increases glutamate release (an excitatory neurotransmitter).[11] This produces subjective feelings of anxiety and can precipitate a panic attack in those with panic disorder, but not in normal volunteers.[11] Drugs with anxiolytic or antipanic effects (e.g., benzodiazepines and antidepressants) inhibit LC firing, decrease noradrenergic activity, and block the effects of anxiogenic drugs.[11]

GABA Receptor Model

There are two superfamilies of GABA protein receptors: $GABA_A$ and $GABA_B$. Drugs that reduce anxiety and produce sedation target the $GABA_A$ receptor. The $GABA_B$ receptor is a G-protein coupled receptor postulated to be involved in the presynaptic inhibition of GABA release.[11–13] $GABA_A$ receptors are ligand-gated ion channels composed of five protein subunits. Several classes of subunits (i.e., $\alpha_{1-6}, \beta_{1-3}, \gamma_{1-3}, \delta, \varepsilon, \theta, \pi, \rho, _{1-3}$) surround a central pore, and the receptor is connected to the cytoskeleton.[14] Benzodiazepine ligands enhance the inhibitory effects of GABA.[11,13] GABA, the major inhibitory neurotransmitter in the CNS, has a strong regulatory or inhibitory effect on the 5-HT, NE, and dopamine (DA) systems. When GABA binds to the $GABA_A$ receptor, neuronal excitability is reduced.

The specific role of the GABA receptors in anxiety disorders has not been established. The number of $GABA_A$ receptors can change with alterations in the environment (e.g., chronic stress), and the subunit expression can be altered by hormonal changes.[14] In patients with GAD, benzodiazepine binding in the left temporal lobe is reduced.[14] Abnormal sensitivity to antagonism of the benzodiazepine binding site and decreased binding was demonstrated in panic disorder.[11,14] This is consistent with the suggestion that panic disorder is secondary to a lack of central inhibition that results in uncontrolled elevations in anxiety during panic attacks.[13] Growth hormone response to baclofen in patients with generalized SAD suggests an abnormality of central $GABA_B$ receptor function.[15]

Serotonin Model

Although there are data suggesting that the 5-HT system is dysregulated in patients with anxiety disorders, definitive evidence that shows a clear abnormality in 5-HT function is lacking. 5-HT is primarily an inhibitory neurotransmitter that is used by neurons originating in the raphe nuclei of the brain stem and projecting diffusely throughout the brain (e.g., cortex, amygdala, hippocampus, and limbic system). Abnormalities in serotonergic functioning through release and uptake at the presynaptic autoreceptors ($5-HT_{1A/1D}$), the serotonin reuptake transporter (SERT) site, or effect of 5-HT at the postsynaptic receptors (e.g., $5-HT_{1A}$, $5-HT_{2A}$, and $5-HT_{2C}$) may play a role in anxiety disorders.[11,13] Preclinical models suggest that greater 5-HT function facilitates avoidance behavior; however, primate studies show that reducing 5-HT increases aggression.[11,13] It is postulated that greater 5-HT activity reduces NE activity in the LC, inhibits defense/escape response via the periaqueductal gray (PAG) region, and reduces hypothalamic release of CRF. The selective serotonin reuptake inhibitors (SSRIs) acutely increase 5-HT levels by blocking the SERT to increase the amount of 5-HT available postsynaptically, and are efficacious in blocking the manifestations of panic and anxiety.[11]

Low 5-HT activity may lead to a dysregulation of other neurotransmitters. NE and 5-HT systems are closely linked, and interactions between the two are reciprocal and vary. NE may act at presynaptic 5-HT terminals to decrease 5-HT release, and its activity at postsynaptic receptors can cause increased 5-HT release.

Buspirone is a selective $5-HT_{1A}$ partial agonist that is effective for GAD but not for panic disorder. Because the selective $5-HT_{1A}$ partial agonists reduce serotonergic activity, GAD symptoms may reflect excessive 5-HT transmission or overactivity of the stimulatory 5-HT pathways.[16] The comparable efficacy of the serotonin-norepinephrine reuptake inhibitor (SNRI), extended-release venlafaxine, at high and low dosages suggests that 5-HT (rather than NE) reuptake blockade contributes to the therapeutic effect in SAD.[17]

NEUROIMAGING STUDIES

Functional neuroimaging studies support the crucial role of the amygdala, anterior cingulate cortex (ACC) and insula in the pathophysiology of anxiety.[12] In GAD there is an abnormal increase in the brain's fear circuitry, as well as increased activity in the prefrontal cortex, which appears to have a compensatory role in reducing GAD symptoms.[18] Patients with panic have abnormalities of midbrain structures, including the PAG. Neuroimaging studies have shown activation of insula and upper brain stem (including the PAG), as well as deactivation of the ACC during experimental panic attacks.[19] Patients with SAD have greater activity than matched comparison subjects in the amygdala and insula, structures linked to negative emotional responses.[20] Both pharmacotherapy and psychotherapy decreased cerebral blood flow in the amygdala, hippocampus, and surrounding cortical areas in patients with SAD.[17]

CLINICAL PRESENTATION

The *Diagnostic and Statistical Manual of Mental Disorders, Fourth Edition, Text Revision* classifies anxiety disorders into several categories: GAD, panic disorder (with or without agoraphobia), agoraphobia, SAD, specific phobia, obsessive-compulsive disorder (OCD), posttraumatic stress disorder (PTSD), and acute stress disorder.[1] The characteristic features of these illnesses are anxiety and avoidance behavior. Anxiety symptoms must cause significant distress, and impairment in social, occupational, or other areas of functioning and should not be secondary to a drug or illicit substance or a general medical disorder, or occur solely as part of another psychiatric disorder.[1] OCD and PTSD are discussed in Chapter 80.

GENERALIZED ANXIETY DISORDER

The diagnostic criteria for GAD require persistent symptoms for most days for at least 6 months.[1] The essential feature of GAD is unrealistic or excessive anxiety and worry about a number of events or activities.[1] The anxiety or apprehensive expectation is accompanied by at least three psychologic or physiologic symptoms. Anxiety and worry are not confined to features of another psychiatric illness (e.g., having a panic attack, being embarrassed in public).[1]

CLINICAL PRESENTATION OF GENERALIZED ANXIETY DISORDER

Psychologic and Cognitive Symptoms

- Excessive anxiety
- Worries that are difficult to control
- Feeling keyed up or on edge
- Poor concentration or mind going blank

Physical Symptoms

- Restlessness
- Fatigue
- Muscle tension
- Sleep disturbance
- Irritability

Impairment

- Social, occupational, or other important functional areas
- Poor coping skills

Data from American Psychiatric Association[1] and Baldwin et al.[21]

The onset, course of illness, and comorbid conditions of GAD are important considerations. GAD has a gradual onset with an average age of 21 years; however, there is a bimodal distribution. Onset occurs earlier when GAD is the primary presentation and later when GAD is secondary. GAD can be exacerbated or precipitated in later life by severe psychologic stressors. Most patients present between the ages of 35 and 45 years, with women twice as likely to have GAD as men. GAD is the most common anxiety disorder in patients older than 55 years of age.[9] Tension surrounding life events also can play a role in the persistence of symptoms. The course of the illness is chronic (i.e., episodes can last for a decade or longer); there is a high percentage of relapse and low rates of recovery. The likelihood of remission at 2 years is 25%.[1] Patients report substantial interference with their lives and have a high probability of seeking treatment.[8] Lifetime comorbidity with another psychiatric disorder occurs in 90% of patients with GAD, with depression being found in over 60%.[8]

PANIC DISORDER

Panic disorder begins as a series of unexpected (spontaneous) panic attacks involving an intense, terrifying fear similar to that caused by life-threatening danger. The unexpected panic attacks are followed by at least 1 month of persistent concern about having another panic attack, worry about the possible consequences of the panic attack, or a significant behavioral change related to the attacks.[1] During an attack, patients describe at least four physiologic and physical symptoms. Panic attacks usually last no more than 20 to 30 minutes, with the peak intensity of symptoms within the first 10 minutes. Often patients seek help at a physician's office or emergency department, only to have their symptoms resolve before or on arrival. Because panic symptoms mimic those present in several medical conditions, patients often are misdiagnosed, and multiple referrals are common.[1]

CLINICAL PRESENTATION OF A PANIC ATTACK

Psychological Symptoms

- Depersonalization
- Derealization
- Fear of losing control, going crazy, or dying

Physical Symptoms

- Abdominal distress
- Chest pain or discomfort
- Chills
- Dizziness or light-headedness
- Feeling of choking
- Hot flushes
- Palpitations
- Nausea
- Paresthesias
- Shortness of breath
- Sweating
- Tachycardia
- Trembling or shaking

Data from American Psychiatric Association,[1] Baldwin et al.,[21] and Katon.[22]

Secondary to the panic attacks, up to 70% of patients develop agoraphobia.[22,23] Agoraphobia is anxiety about being in places or situations in which escape might be difficult or where help might not be available in the event of a panic attack.[1] As a result, patients often avoid specific situations (e.g., being in a crowd or flying) in which they fear a panic attack might occur.[1]

Complications of panic disorder include depression (10%–65% have major depressive disorder), alcohol abuse, and high use of health services and emergency rooms.[1] Patients with panic disorder have a high lifetime risk for suicide attempts compared with the general population.[22,23] The usual course is chronic but waxing and waning.

SOCIAL ANXIETY DISORDER

SAD is characterized by an intense, irrational, and persistent fear of being negatively evaluated or scrutinized in at least one social or performance situation. Exposure to the feared circumstance usually provokes an immediate situation-related panic attack. Blushing is the principal physical indicator and distinguishes SAD from other anxiety disorders. Adults with SAD usually recognize their fear is excessive and unreasonable; however, they are unable to overcome it without treatment. If necessary, the feared situation is avoided or endured with significant distress.[1] In individuals younger than 18 years of age, the duration of symptoms must be at least 6 months to meet the diagnostic criteria.[1]

CLINICAL PRESENTATION OF SOCIAL ANXIETY DISORDER

Fears of Being

- Scrutinized by others
- Embarrassed
- Humiliated

Some Feared Situations

- Eating or writing in front of others
- Interacting with authority figures
- Speaking in public
- Talking with strangers
- Use of public toilets

Physical Symptoms

- Blushing
- "Butterflies in the stomach"
- Diarrhea
- Sweating
- Tachycardia
- Trembling

Types

- Generalized: fear and avoidance extend to a wide range of social situations
- Nongeneralized: fear limited to one or two situations

Data from American Psychiatric Association,[1] Muller et al.,[17] and Schneier.[24]

The mean age of onset of SAD is during the mid-teens. Rates of SAD are slightly higher among women than men and more frequent in younger cohorts. It is a chronic disorder with a mean duration of 20 years.[1] People with SAD can be reluctant to seek professional help, despite the existence of beneficial treatments because consultation with a clinician is perceived as a feared social interaction.[17,24]

Differentiating SAD from other anxiety disorders can be difficult. Panic attacks occur in both SAD and panic disorder, but the distinction between the two is the rationale behind fear; fear of anxiety symptoms is characteristic of panic disorder, whereas fear of embarrassment from social interaction typifies SAD.[1] A majority of SAD patients eventually develop a concurrent mood, anxiety, or substance abuse disorder.[17,23]

SPECIFIC PHOBIA

Specific phobia is marked and persistent fear of a circumscribed object or situation (e.g., insects, or heights). Apart from contact with the feared object or situation, the patient is usually free of symptoms. Most persons simply avoid the feared object and adjust to certain restrictions on their activities.[1]

TREATMENT

Generalized Anxiety Disorder

■ DESIRED OUTCOME

The goals of therapy in the acute management of GAD are to reduce the severity and duration of the anxiety symptoms and to improve overall functioning. ❶ The long-term goal in GAD is remission with minimal or no anxiety symptoms, no functional impairment, and increased QOL.[25] Prevention of recurrence is another long-term consideration.

■ GENERAL APPROACH TO TREATMENT

Once GAD is diagnosed, a patient-oriented treatment plan, which usually consists of both psychotherapy and drug therapy, is developed. The plan depends on the severity and chronicity of symptoms, age, medication history, and comorbid medical and psychiatric conditions.[9,25] Factors such as anticipated adverse effects, history of prior response in the patient or family member, patient preference, and cost should be considered when treatment is initiated. Psychotherapy is the least invasive and safest treatment modality. Antianxiety medication is indicated for patients experiencing symptoms severe enough to produce functional disability. Table 79–3 lists drug choices for GAD, panic disorder, and SAD.

■ NONPHARMACOLOGIC THERAPY

Nonpharmacologic treatment modalities in GAD include psychoeducation, short-term counseling, stress management, psychotherapy, meditation, or exercise. Psychoeducation includes information on the etiology and management of GAD. Anxious patients should be instructed to avoid caffeine, nonprescription stimulants, diet pills, and excessive use of alcohol. Most patients with GAD require psychologic therapy, alone or in combination with antianxiety drugs, to overcome fears and to learn to manage their anxiety and worry.[5] Cognitive behavioral therapy (CBT) is the most effective psychologic therapy in GAD patients. CBT for GAD includes self-monitoring of worry, cognitive restructuring, relaxation training, and rehearsal of coping skills.[5] Psychotherapy or medication alone have comparable efficacy in acute treatment.[21] The relapse rate with CBT is less than with other types of psychologic modalities.[21] Controlled trials comparing the efficacy of combining drug and psychotherapy over long-term treatment are lacking.[21] Advantages of CBT over pharmacotherapy include patient preference and lack of troubling adverse effects. However, CBT is not widely available, requires specialized training, and entails weekly sessions for an extended time period (i.e., 12–20 weeks).[5]

■ PHARMACOLOGIC THERAPY

The benzodiazepines are the most effective, safe, and commonly prescribed drugs for the rapid relief of acute anxiety symptoms (Table 79–4). All benzodiazepines are equally effective anxiolytics, and consideration of pharmacokinetic properties and the patient's clinical situation will assist in the selection of the most appropriate agent.[5]

Because of the lack of dependency and tolerable adverse effect profile, antidepressants have emerged as the treatment of choice for the management of chronic anxiety, especially in the presence of comorbid depressive symptoms. Buspirone is an additional anxiolytic option (Table 79–5) in patients without comorbid depression or other anxiety disorders (e.g., panic disorder and SAD). Because of the high risk of adverse effects and toxicity, barbiturates, antipsychotics, antipsychotic-antidepressant combinations, and antihistamines generally are not indicated in the treatment of GAD.[3] The benzodiazepines are more effective in treating the somatic and autonomic symptoms of GAD as opposed to the psychic symptoms (e.g., apprehension and worry), which are reduced by antidepressants.[3]

TABLE 79-3	Drug Choices for Anxiety Disorders		
Anxiety Disorder	First Line Drugs	Second Line Drugs	Alternatives
Generalized anxiety	Duloxetine Escitalopram Paroxetine Sertraline Venlafaxine XR	Benzodiazepines Buspirone Imipramine	Hydroxyzine Pregabalin Quetiapine
Panic disorder	SSRIs Venlafaxine XR	Alprazolam Citalopram Clomipramine Clonazepam Imipramine	Phenelzine
Social anxiety disorder	Escitalopram Fluvoxamine CR Paroxetine Sertraline Venlafaxine XR	Clonazepam Citalopram	Clonazepam Gabapentin Mirtazapine Phenelzine Pregabalin

SSRI, selective serotonin reuptake inhibitor; XR, extended-release; CR, controlled-release.
Data from Bandelow et al.,[3] Davidson et al.,[8] Baldwin et al.,[21] Schneier,[24] and American Psychiatric Association.[26]

TABLE 79-4	Benzodiazepine Antianxiety Agents		
Generic Name	Brand Name	Approved Dosage Range (mg/day)[a]	Approximate Equivalent Dose (mg)
Alprazolam[b]	Niravam,[c] Xanax, Xanax XR	0.75–4 1–10[d]	0.5
Chlordiazepoxide[b]	Librium	25–400	10
Clonazepam[b]	Klonopin Klonopin Wafers[c]	1–4[d]	0.25
Clorazepate[b]	Tranxene Tranxene SD	7.5–60	7.5
Diazepam[b]	Valium	2–40	5
Lorazepam[b]	Ativan	0.5–10	1
Oxazepam[b]	Serax	30–120	15

XR, extended-release; SD, sustained-release.
[a]Elderly patients are usually treated with approximately one-half of the dose listed.
[b]Available generically.
[c]Orally disintegrating formulation.
[d]Panic disorder dose.
Equivalent doses from Chouinard.[27]

TABLE 79-5 Nonbenzodiazepine Antianxiety Agents for Generalized Anxiety Disorder

Generic Name	Trade Name	Starting Dose	Dosage Range (mg/day)[a]
Antidepressants			
Duloxetine[b]	Cymbalta	30 or 60 mg/day	60–120
Escitalopram[b]	Lexapro	10 mg/day	10–20
Imipramine[c]	Tofranil	50 mg/day	75–200
Paroxetine[b,c]	Paxil Pexeva	20 mg/day	20–50
Sertraline[c]	Zoloft	50 mg/day	50–200
Venlafaxine XR[b,c]	Effexor XR	37.5 or 75 mg/day	75–225[d]
Azapirone			
Buspirone[b,c]	BuSpar	7.5 mg twice per day	15–60[d]
Diphenylmethane			
Hydroxyzine[b,c,e]	Vistaril	25 or 50 mg 4 times daily	200–400
Anticonvulsant			
Pregabalin	Lyrica	50 mg 3 times daily	150–600
Atypical Antipsychotic			
Quetiapine XR	Seroquel XR	50 mg at bedtime	150–300

XR, extended-release
[a]Elderly patients are usually treated with approximately one-half of the dose listed.
[b]FDA approved for generalized anxiety disorder.
[c]Available generically.
[d]No dosage adjustment is required in elderly patients.
[e]FDA approved for anxiety and tension in children in divided daily doses of 50–100 mg.
Data from Bandelow et al,[3] Kavouss,[28] Gao et al,[29] Paxil package insert,[30] Cymbalta package insert,[31] Lexapro package insert,[32] Effexor XR package insert,[33] and Vistaril package insert.[34]

The most recent treatment guidelines from the World Federation of Societies of Biological Psychiatry and the British Association of Psychopharmacology are evidence-based.[3,21] A descriptive flowchart with recommendations based on levels of evidence from the International Psychopharmacology Algorithm Project for the psychosocial and pharmacologic management of GAD is shown in Figure 79–1.[8]

Alternative Drug Treatments

Hydroxyzine, pregabalin, and atypical antipsychotics are alternatives.[8,28,29] The antihistamine hydrozyzine was effective in studies conducted for as long as 12 weeks in patients with GAD. Hydrozyzine is commonly used in the primary care setting, but it is considered be to be a second-line agent because of adverse effects and lack of efficacy for comorbid disorders.[8] Pregabalin, which binds to the $\alpha_2\delta$ subunit of voltage-gated calcium channels to reduce nerve terminal calcium influx, acts on "hyperexcited" neurons. Pregabalin produced anxiolytic effects similar to lorazepam, alprazolam, and venlafaxine in acute efficacy trials.[28] Extended-release quetiapine 150 mg/day monotherapy was superior to placebo in 3 studies, and as effective as paroxetine 20 mg/day and escitalopram 10 mg/day but with an earlier onset of action.[29] In a 52-week treatment of GAD, extended-release quetiapine was superior to placebo in the prevention of anxiety relapse.[29] Quetiapine is not FDA approved for GAD, and the long-term risks and benefits of atypical antipsychotics in the treatment of GAD are unclear.[29] Analysis of data from pooled sample trials found kava-kava to be no more effective than placebo.[35] Because of reports of hepatotoxicity, kava-kava is not recommended as an anxiolytic.[35]

Special Populations

The management of anxiety in patients with substance abuse, pregnant women, children, elderly patients, and those patients with adherence problems requires special consideration in the choice of anxiolytic. Patients with GAD may misuse alcohol, cannabis, or other substances to manage anxiety. The symptoms of GAD are similar to those of withdrawal, and it is difficult to confirm the diagnosis of GAD until after abstinence is obtained. Benzodiazepine therapy should be avoided in this population.

There is evidence that maternal anxiety during pregnancy and the post-partum period potentially pose significant risk to the child. Clinical practice guidelines for anxiety disorders recommend use of fluoxetine, sertraline, or citalopram; however, perinatal syndromes (e.g., jitteriness, myoclonus, irritability) in the neonate and premature delivery have been reported.[21,36] Paroxetine (Category D) should be avoided in pregnant women because of risk of cardiovascular malformations.[30]

Cleft lip, cleft palate, and other teratogenic effects are associated with benzodiazepine use, but a causal relationship is inconclusive. Clinicians should avoid benzodiazepine use during the first trimester, use the lowest dosage for the shortest period of time, divide the total daily dosage into two or three doses to prevent high peak plasma levels, and use the agent as monotherapy.[8,36] Benzodiazepine risks during the third trimester include sedation, withdrawal symptoms, and "floppy" infant syndrome (e.g., hypotonia, low Apgar scores, hypothermia). Alprazolam should be avoided during pregnancy because of neonatal withdrawal. Should benzodiazepines be required during pregnancy, the preferred agents are clonazepam and lorazepam.[8] The antidepressants are favored for GAD during pregnancy based on safety considerations.[36] Diazepam and clonazepam should not be used in nursing mothers because infants can experience sedation, lethargy, and weight loss.[8]

There are few controlled clinical trials of drugs in children and adolescents with GAD. CBT alone or in conjunction with antidepressants can have long-term benefits.[8] Randomized controlled trials of fluovoxamine, fluoxetine, sertraline, and extended-release venlafaxine indicate short-term efficacy;[3,37,38] however, behavioral activation was reported with clonazepam.[3] No antidepressant is FDA-indicated for GAD in children or adolescents. Increased monitoring for behavioral activation with benzodiazepines and suicide-related adverse effects with antidepressants is necessary if these agents are prescribed.

Patients with hepatic disease are at risk for drug accumulation and subsequent complications. Duloxetine use should be avoided in patients with hepatic insufficiency.[31] Drug accumulation can result in the elderly secondary to a decreased capacity for oxidation and alterations in the volume of distribution. Therefore, intermediate- or short-acting benzodiazepines without active metabolites are preferred for chronic use. Elderly patients are also sensitive to the CNS adverse effects of benzodiazepines (regardless of half-life), and use is associated with a high frequency of falls and hip fractures. Venlafaxine, citalopram, duloxetine, and pregabalin showed efficacy in elderly patients with GAD.[3,39]

Antidepressant Therapy

❷ Antidepressants are considered first-line agents in the management of GAD. Extended-release venlafaxine, duloxetine, paroxetine, and escitalopram are FDA-approved antidepressants for GAD. Imipramine is considered when patients fail to respond to SSRIs or venlafaxine (see Table 79–5). ❸ The antianxiety response of antidepressants is delayed by 2 to 4 weeks or longer.[25] The pharmacokinetics and drug interactions of the antidepressants are reviewed in the chapter on depressive disorders (Chapter 77).

Efficacy Antidepressants are efficacious in the acute and long-term management of GAD. Data support the use of SSRIs

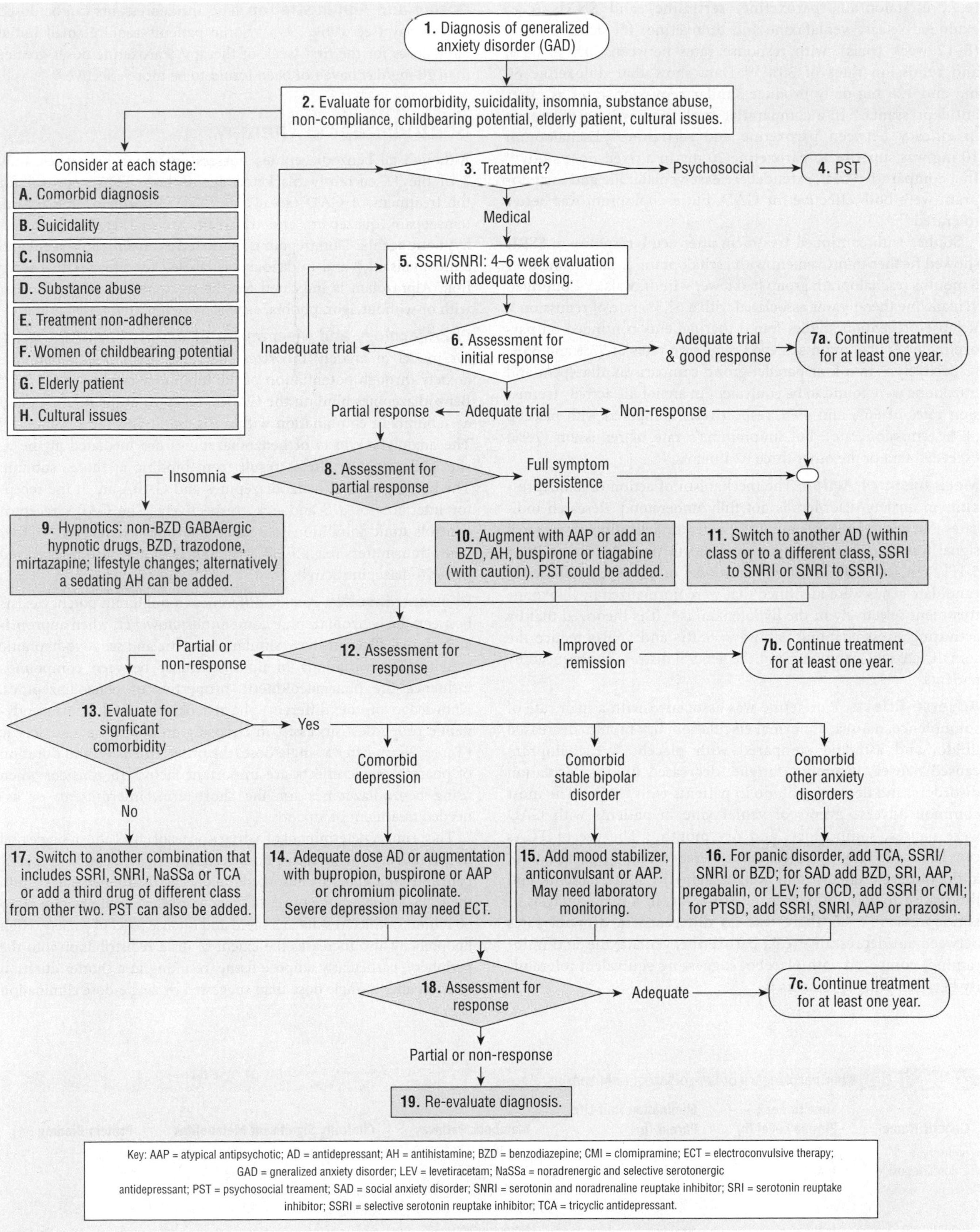

1. Diagnosis of generalized anxiety disorder (GAD)

2. Evaluate for comorbidity, suicidality, insomnia, substance abuse, non-compliance, childbearing potential, elderly patient, cultural issues.

Consider at each stage:

A. Comorbid diagnosis
B. Suicidality
C. Insomnia
D. Substance abuse
E. Treatment non-adherence
F. Women of childbearing potential
G. Elderly patient
H. Cultural issues

3. Treatment? → Psychosocial → **4.** PST

Medical

5. SSRI/SNRI: 4–6 week evaluation with adequate dosing.

Inadequate trial ← **6.** Assessment for initial response → Adequate trial & good response → **7a.** Continue treatment for at least one year.

Partial response ← Adequate trial → Non-response

Insomnia ← **8.** Assessment for partial response → Full symptom persistence

9. Hypnotics: non-BZD GABAergic hypnotic drugs, BZD, trazodone, mirtazapine; lifestyle changes; alternatively a sedating AH can be added.

10. Augment with AAP or add an BZD, AH, buspirone or tiagabine (with caution). PST could be added.

11. Switch to another AD (within class or to a different class, SSRI to SNRI or SNRI to SSRI).

Partial or non-response ← **12.** Assessment for response → Improved or remission → **7b.** Continue treatment for at least one year.

13. Evaluate for significant comorbidity → Yes

No

Comorbid depression

Comorbid stable bipolar disorder

Comorbid other anxiety disorders

17. Switch to another combination that includes SSRI, SNRI, NaSSa or TCA or add a third drug of different class from other two. PST can also be added.

14. Adequate dose AD or augmentation with bupropion, buspirone or AAP or chromium picolinate. Severe depression may need ECT.

15. Add mood stabilizer, anticonvulsant or AAP. May need laboratory monitoring.

16. For panic disorder, add TCA, SSRI/ SNRI or BZD; for SAD add BZD, SRI, AAP, pregabalin, or LEV; for OCD, add SSRI or CMI; for PTSD, add SSRI, SNRI, AAP or prazosin.

18. Assessment for response → Adequate → **7c.** Continue treatment for at least one year.

Partial or non-response

19. Re-evaluate diagnosis.

Key: AAP = atypical antipsychotic; AD = antidepressant; AH = antihistamine; BZD = benzodiazepine; CMI = clomipramine; ECT = electroconvulsive therapy; GAD = gneralized anxiety disorder; LEV = levetiracetam; NaSSa = noradrenergic and selective serotonergic antidepressant; PST = psychosocial treament; SAD = social anxiety disorder; SNRI = serotonin and noradrenaline reuptake inhibitor; SRI = serotonin reuptake inhibitor; SSRI = selective serotonin reuptake inhibitor; TCA = tricyclic antidepressant.

FIGURE 79-1. International Psychopharmacology Algorithm Project (IPAP) Generalized Anxiety Disorder (GAD) Algorithm Flowchart. Yellow, first-line treatment (Nodes 3-6); Green, second-line treatment (Nodes 8-12); Blue, third-line treatment, no comorbidity (Nodes 13-19); Orange, third-line treatment, with comorbidity (Nodes 14-16); Light green, assessment and evaluation. Levels of evidence used in development of the flowchart were: 1 = more than one placebo-controlled trial with sample sizes over 30; 2 = one placebo-controlled trial (or active versus active drug comparison) with sample size of 30 or greater; 3 = one or small (n < 30) placebo-controlled trial; 4 = case reports or open-label trials; and 5 = expert consensus without published evidence. *(Flowchart is used by permission of the International Psychopharmacology Algorithm Project, http://www.ipap.org.[8])*

(e.g., escitalopram, paroxetine, sertraline) and SNRIs (e.g., extended-release venlafaxine and duloxetine) for acute therapy (8–12 week trials), with response rates between 60% to 68%, and remission rates of 30%.[3,21] Data show that duloxetine 60 mg and 120 mg daily produce similar remission rates as other antidepressants.[39] In a comparative trial, there was no difference in efficacy between paroxetine and sertraline.[40] Escitalopram 10 mg was superior to paroxetine 20 mg in a fixed-dose study.[41] In a comparative trial, extended-release venlafaxine and escitalopram were both effective for GAD, but escitalopram was better tolerated.[42]

Studies with continued treatment after acute response to SSRIs showed further improvement with escitalopram or paroxetine over 6 months (escitalopram group had fewer withdrawals).[43] Continued venlafaxine therapy was associated with a 62.5% rate of remission.[44] Relapse-prevention studies found that patients continued on paroxetine or escitalopram achieved remission rates of 73% and 65%, respectively.[3,8] In a four parallel-group comparison, diazepam and trazodone were found to be equivalent in anxiolytic activity (remission rates of 66% and 69%, respectively) compared with placebo (47% remission rate), but imipramine's rate of remission (73%) exceeded that of the other three treatments.[37]

Mechanism of Action The mechanism of action of antidepressants in anxiety disorders is not fully understood. Research indicates that antidepressants modulate receptor activation of neuronal signal transduction pathways connected to the neurotransmitters 5-HT, DA, and NE. In an animal model of anxiety, a number of candidate genes were identified that were normalized by fluoxetine treatment selectively in the hypothalamus.[45] It is theorized that by activating stress-adapting pathways, SSRIs and SNRIs reduce the somatic anxiety symptoms and the general distress experienced by patients.

Adverse Effects Paroxetine was associated with a high rate of somnolence, nausea, abnormal ejaculation, dry mouth, decreased libido, and asthenia compared with placebo.[30] Escitalopram caused nausea, insomnia, fatigue, decreased libido, ejaculation disorders, and decreased libido in patients with GAD.[32] The most common adverse events of venlafaxine in patients with GAD were nausea, somnolence, and dry mouth.[33] The use of TCAs can be limited by troublesome adverse events (e.g., sedation, anticholinergic effects, and weight gain) in some patients and the risk of toxicity in overdose.[5] However, in a meta-analysis of antidepressant trials there was no difference in dropout rates between antidepressants (e.g., paroxetine, venlafaxine, and imipramine) compared with placebo, suggesting equivalent tolerability between antidepressants.[37]

Dosing and Administration The antidepressants can be dosed once a day (see Table 79–5). Some patients require small initial daily doses for the first week of therapy. Paroxetine doses greater than 20 mg/day have not been found to be more effective.[30]

Benzodiazepine Therapy

Although all benzodiazepines possess anxiolytic properties, only 7 of the 13 currently marketed agents have FDA approval for the treatment of GAD (see Table 79–4). Estazolam, flurazepam, temazepam, quazepam, and triazolam are marketed as sedative-hypnotic agents. Clonazepam is marketed as an antipanic agent and anticonvulsant,[46] and midazolam is labeled for preoperative sedation. Alprazolam is indicated for the treatment of panic disorder with or without agoraphobia, as well as GAD.[47]

Pharmacology and Mechanism of Action The GABA receptor model of anxiety theorizes that benzodiazepines ameliorate anxiety through potentiation of the inhibitory activity of GABA.[14] Benzodiazepines bind on the $GABA_A$ receptor at the α_1, α_2, α_3, and α_5 subunits in combination with a β subunit and the γ_2 subunit.[14] The anxiolytic effects of benzodiazepines are mediated at the α_2 site while sedative effects result from binding at the α_1 subunit. The binding sites of benzodiazepines and GABA are at the receptor interfaces of α/β and α/γ_2, respectively. The GABA receptor controls tonic inhibition to reduce neuronal excitability.[14] Other neurotransmitters (e.g., 5-HT, NE, and DA) may also be involved in benzodiazepine activity.

Pharmacokinetics A wide difference in milligram potency exists between the benzodiazepine compounds; however, when appropriately dosed, all agents have similar anxiolytic and sedative-hypnotic activity. The variations in lipid solubility between compounds influence the pharmacokinetic properties of benzodiazepines. Knowledge of the different pharmacokinetic and pharmacodynamic properties can assist in choosing an appropriate anxiolytic (Table 79–6). After a single dose, the onset, intensity, and duration of pharmacologic effects are important factors to consider when using benzodiazepines for the short-term, intermittent, or as-needed treatment of anxiety.

The primary determinant of a drug's onset of effect after a single oral dose is the rate of drug absorption. Because of high lipophilicity, diazepam and clorazepate are absorbed rapidly and distributed quickly into the CNS. Therefore the onset of anxiolytic effect occurs within 30 to 60 minutes, which results in a rapid and intense relief of anxiety. High lipophilicity also increases the extent of drug redistribution into the periphery, particularly adipose tissue, resulting in a shorter duration of effect after a single dose than suggested by single-dose elimination

TABLE 79-6 Pharmacokinetics of Benzodiazepine Antianxiety Agents

Generic Name	Time to Peak Plasma Level (h)	Elimination Half-Life, Parent (h)	Metabolic Pathway	Clinically Significant Metabolites	Protein Binding (%)
Alprazolam	1–2	12–15	Oxidation	–	80
Chlordiazepoxide	1–4	5–30	N-Dealkylation Oxidation	Desmethylchlordiazepoxide Demoxepam DMDZ[a]	96
Clonazepam	1–4	30–40	Nitroreduction	–	85
Clorazepate	1–2	Prodrug	Oxidation	DMDZ	97
Diazepam	0.5–2	20–80	Oxidation	DMDZ Oxazepam	98
Lorazepam	2–4	10–20	Conjugation	–	85
Oxazepam	2–4	5–20	Conjugation	–	97

[a]Desmethyldiazepam (DMDZ) half-life 50–100 h.
Data from Rosenbaum et al,[48] and Facts and Comparisons.[49]

half-life studies.[48] Clinically, patients perceive a rapid onset of action, but some experience an unpleasant feeling of drowsiness or loss of control. This "rush" can be euphoric and contribute to abuse.

Compared with diazepam, lorazepam and oxazepam are relatively less lipophilic and have a slower absorption and onset of effect. These benzodiazepines have smaller volumes of distribution and a resulting longer duration of action.[48]

Parenteral administration via the intramuscular route should be avoided with diazepam and chlordiazepoxide secondary to variability in the rate and extent of drug absorption. Intramuscular lorazepam provides rapid, reliable, and complete absorption.

After multiple dosing, the rate and extent of drug accumulation are functions of the drug's elimination half-life in relation to dosing intervals, clearance, and formation of active metabolites. Differences in clinical effects that occur during and after repeated dosages with the benzodiazepines are related in part to variability in metabolism and metabolite accumulation.[48]

The benzodiazepines undergo two primary metabolic processes, hepatic oxidation (catalyzed by cytochrome P450 3A4) and glucuronide conjugation. With the exception of lorazepam and oxazepam (which are conjugated only) and clonazepam (which undergoes nitroreduction), all benzodiazepines are oxidized first and then conjugated and excreted renally.[48] Diazepam's metabolism is also catalyzed by cytochrome P450 2C19. Oxidation can be impaired in patients with liver disease, in the elderly, and in those who simultaneously use drugs that inhibit oxidation resulting in higher levels of the parent drug and/or an active metabolite.

Many benzodiazepines are converted to desmethyldiazepam (DMDZ), an active metabolite with a long elimination half-life[48] (Table 79-6). DMDZ is further oxidized to oxazepam and then conjugated and excreted. After multiple dosing, accumulation of DMDZ is slow and extensive, providing a long-lasting antianxiety effect. If oxidation of DMDZ is impaired, the half-life is prolonged, and extensive drug accumulation can result with repeated dosing.

Clorazepate is a prodrug and possesses no anxiolytic effects until metabolized to DMDZ. Before absorption, clorazepate is metabolized rapidly in the stomach through a pH-dependent process under acidic conditions.

Benzodiazepines with shorter half-lives (e.g., alprazolam, lorazepam, and oxazepam) reach steady-state plasma concentrations rapidly, and drug accumulation after repeated dosing is minimal. Oxazepam and lorazepam have no active metabolites.

Benzodiazepine protein binding is extensive, especially for the drugs with a long elimination half-life. After a single dose of a benzodiazepine with a long elimination half-life, the expected duration of clinical activity may not parallel the drug's pharmacokinetic half-life because of drug redistribution.[48] After multiple dosing, drugs with long elimination half-lives and active metabolites require 1 to 2 weeks to reach steady state.

Efficacy Clinical trials of benzodiazepines show that 65% to 75% of patients with GAD have a marked to moderate response, with most of the improvement occurring in the first 2 weeks of therapy. Benzodiazepines are more effective on the somatic symptoms of anxiety and fail to obviate the cognitive or psychic symptoms (e.g., worry).[11,25] Up to 50% of patients fail to reach remission with benzodiazepine therapy, and rates of relapse exceed that of the antidepressants.[25]

Adverse Effects The most common adverse events associated with benzodiazepine therapy involve CNS depression. This is manifested clinically as drowsiness, sedation, psychomotor impairment, and ataxia.[25] A transient mild drowsiness is experienced commonly by patients during the first few days of treatment; however, tolerance often develops. Disorientation, depression, confusion, irritability, aggression, and excitement are reported.[25]

Impairment of memory and recall also can occur during benzodiazepine treatment. The memory loss induced by the benzodiazepines typically is limited to events occurring after drug ingestion (anterograde amnesia).[25,27,49] Anterograde amnesia is secondary to disordered consolidation processes that store information and is not impairment in the perception or retrieval of information.[2] Benzodiazepines with high affinity for binding to the benzodiazepine receptor (e.g., alprazolam) appear to possess a higher potential for amnesia.[27]

Abuse, Dependence, Withdrawal, and Tolerance Two serious complications of benzodiazepine therapy are the potential for abuse and development of physical dependence. Benzodiazepine abuse is rare in the general population of users; however, individuals with a history of multiple drug abuse (e.g., alcohol or sedatives) are at the greatest risk for becoming benzodiazepine abusers.[5]

Because of the chronicity of illness, persons with GAD and panic disorder are at high risk of developing benzodiazepine dependence. Benzodiazepine dependence is a physiologic phenomenon demonstrated by the appearance of a predictable abstinence syndrome (withdrawal symptoms) on abrupt discontinuation of therapy.[27] Withdrawal symptoms can result because of the sudden dissociation of a benzodiazepine from its receptor site. After abrupt discontinuation, an acute decrease in GABA neurotransmission results, producing a less inhibited CNS.

Benzodiazepine Discontinuation After benzodiazepine therapy is discontinued suddenly, several events can occur. Rebound anxiety represents an immediate but transient return of original symptoms having an increased intensity compared with baseline. Recurrence or relapse is the return of original symptoms with similar intensity as before treatment.

Withdrawal symptoms are the emergence of new symptoms and a worsening of preexisting symptoms after benzodiazepine discontinuation. Symptoms can persist for days to weeks and resolve gradually over months.

Common symptoms of benzodiazepine withdrawal include anxiety, insomnia, restlessness, muscle tension, and irritability. Less frequently occurring symptoms are nausea, malaise, coryza, blurred vision, diaphoresis, nightmares, depression, hyperreflexia, and ataxia. Tinnitus, confusion, paranoid delusions, hallucinations, and seizures occur rarely. Seizures can occur with both therapeutic and high doses of benzodiazepines with a short elimination half-life, usually within 3 days of drug discontinuation. They can occur approximately 1 week after discontinuation of agents with a long elimination half-life. High benzodiazepine doses, a long duration of therapy, and concurrent ingestion of drugs that lower the seizure threshold are risk factors for withdrawal seizures.

The onset of withdrawal symptoms in patients ingesting benzodiazepines with short elimination half-lives occurs much earlier (within 24–48 hours) than in those taking benzodiazepines with long elimination half-lives (within 3–8 days). Other factors associated with an increased incidence and severity of benzodiazepine withdrawal include high doses and long-term benzodiazepine therapy.

A strategy to minimize the severity of benzodiazepine withdrawal is a 25% per week reduction in dosage until 50% of the dose is reached, and then dosage reduction by one-eighth every 4 to 7 days.[27] If therapy exceeds 8 weeks, a slow dosage taper over 2 to 3 weeks is recommended; however, if the duration of treatment is 6 months, a taper over 4 to 8 weeks should ensue.[5] Long-term use of benzodiazepines (i.e., 1 year or longer) requires a 2- to 4-month slow taper.[5] Tapering will not eliminate the emergence of withdrawal symptoms entirely but will prevent severe withdrawal. Slow drug taper is extremely important for the drugs with a short elimination half-life, because some individuals have greater difficulty with discontinuation.

Withdrawal symptoms with short half-life benzodiazepines were no more severe than with longer half-life agents, therefore switching from a short- to long-acting benzodiazepine before gradual taper is not supported.[50,51] Adjunctive use of carbamazepine can help reduce withdrawal severity during the benzodiazepine taper.[50,51] Patients should avoid the intake of alcohol and stimulants during the withdrawal process. Although tolerance develops to the sedative, muscle relaxant, and anticonvulsant activities, the benzodiazepines do not appear to lose anxiolytic or antipanic efficacy. The anxiolytic efficacy of benzodiazepines in long-term clinical trials (greater than 6–8 months of chronic use) has not been reported.[5]

Drug Interactions Drug interactions with the benzodiazepines generally fall into two categories: pharmacodynamic and pharmacokinetic. Simultaneous use of alcohol and a benzodiazepine results in additive CNS depressant effects. In addition, concurrent use of a benzodiazepine and other drugs with CNS depressant properties (e.g., opioids, antipsychotics, and antihistamines) can potentiate the adverse sedative effects. When ingested alone in an overdose attempt, benzodiazepines are rarely life-threatening; however, the combination of benzodiazepines with alcohol or other CNS depressant agents is potentially fatal.

Concurrent use of medications that inhibit cytochrome P450 3A4 (e.g., ketoconazole, nefazodone, and ritonavir) can increase the blood levels of alprazolam and diazepam. Drugs that induce cytochrome P450 3A4 (e.g., carbamazepine, St. John's wort) can reduce benzodiazepine levels. Consult a drug interaction Website (e.g., *http://online.factsandcomparisons.com*) for further information.

Dosing and Administration Benzodiazepine dosage requirements vary widely among patients and must be individualized. Therapy should be initiated using low doses (e.g., alprazolam 0.25 mg 3 times a day or equivalent doses of other benzodiazepines) and titrated upward to relieve anxiety symptoms and avoid adverse events. After an initial treatment response is achieved, agents with long elimination half-lives can be dosed at bedtime. Dosage adjustments should be made weekly. Three to four weeks of a daily dose at the maximum dose constitutes an adequate clinical trial (see Table 79–4).[5]

The duration of benzodiazepine therapy for the acute management of anxiety should be limited to 2 to 4 weeks. In general, benzodiazepines should be used with a regular dosing regimen and not on an as-needed basis.[8] Only in the treatment of short-term distress (e.g., air travel, dental phobia) as-needed use may be justified.[3,8] Individuals with persistent symptoms should be managed with antidepressants because of the risk of dependence with continued benzodiazepine therapy.[25]

Patient education should include the anticipated length of drug therapy, potential side effects, and consequences of the ingestion of alcohol and other CNS depressants. Patients should understand that benzodiazepines provide symptomatic relief but do not solve underlying psychologic problems. Patients should be instructed not to decrease or discontinue benzodiazepine usage without contacting their prescriber.

Buspirone Therapy

Buspirone is a nonbenzodiazepine anxiolytic that lacks anticonvulsant, muscle relaxant, hypnotic, motor impairment, and dependence properties. It is considered to be a second-line agent for GAD because of inconsistent reports of efficacy (particularly long term), delayed onset of effect (i.e., 2 weeks or longer), and lack of efficacy for other potential concurrent depressive and anxiety disorders.[21,52] Unlike benzodiazepines, buspirone is effective for the psychic symptoms of anxiety.[52]

Pharmacology and Mechanism of Action Buspirone's anxiolytic mechanism of action is unknown. It is thought to exert its anxiolytic effect through partial agonist activity at the 5-HT$_{1A}$ presynaptic receptors, thus reducing the firing of 5-HT neurons.[52]

Pharmacokinetics After an oral dose, buspirone is absorbed rapidly and completely and undergoes extensive first-pass metabolism. The mean elimination half-life is 2.5 hours, and it must be dosed 2 to 3 times daily, which adversely affects adherence to the drug regimen.[25]

Adverse Effects Adverse events include dizziness, nausea, and headaches.[25]

Drug Interactions Drugs that inhibit cytochrome P450 3A4 (e.g., verapamil, itraconazole, fluvoxamine) can increase buspirone levels. Rifampin caused a 10-fold reduction in buspirone levels. Buspirone reportedly elevates blood pressure in patients taking a monoamine oxidase inhibitor (MAOI).

Dosing and Administration The dose of buspirone can be titrated in increments of 5 mg/day every 2 to 3 days as needed.[25] The onset of improvement in psychic symptoms precedes the relief of somatic symptoms; maximum therapeutic benefit might not be evident for 4 to 6 weeks.

Buspirone is a treatment option for patients with GAD, particularly for patients with uncomplicated GAD, in patients who fail other anxiolytic therapies, or in patients with substance abuse. It is not useful in clinical situations requiring immediate anxiolysis or for patients requiring as-needed anxiolytic therapy.[52] The use of benzodiazepines within the month previous to initiation of buspirone therapy was associated with reduced efficacy of buspirone because of its delayed onset in the reduction of somatic symptoms.[25]

■ PHARMACOECONOMIC CONSIDERATIONS

The total annual cost of anxiety disorders has been estimated to be between $42.3 billion and $46.6 billion, of which more than 75% can be attributed to morbidity, mortality, lost productivity, and other indirect costs.[53] The total cost estimate for anxiety disorders comprises more than 30% of the total expenditures for mental illnesses; the cost of anxiety drug therapy accounts for 53% of the drug expenditures for mental illnesses.[53]

GAD is associated with high rates of healthcare use and disability. The number of days missed from work increases when GAD is concurrent with one or more other psychiatric disorders. Patients with GAD tend to use family practitioners and gastroenterologists more frequently than healthy controls.[54] GAD ranks third among anxiety disorders in the rate of use of primary care physician time, and it is the leading cause of disability in the workplace in the United States.[54] Two decision analyses for GAD were published by researchers in the United Kingdom: venlafaxine was more cost-effective than diazepam,[55] and escitalopram was associated with higher treatment success and lower discontinuation rates and costs than paroxetine.[56]

CLINICAL CONTROVERSY

It is unclear if combining pharmacotherapy with CBT in patients with GAD confers greater overall efficacy than treatment with either approach alone. CBT is an option if patients fail consecutive antidepressant trials, however many patients lack access to CBT.

■ EVALUATION OF THERAPEUTIC OUTCOMES

Initially, anxious patients should be monitored once every 2 weeks[21] for a reduction in the frequency, duration, and severity of anxiety symptoms and improvement in functioning. The clinician should assess the patient for response to treatment by asking about specific target symptoms of anxiety and emergence of adverse events. Ideally, the patient should have no or minimal anxiety or depressive symptoms and no functional impairment. Use of an objective measurement of remission of GAD (e.g., Hamilton Rating Scale for Anxiety score less than or equal to 7 and a Sheehan Disability Scale score less than or equal to 1 on each item) can assist in the evaluation of drug response.[8,25] The definition of treatment resistance is defined as a poor, partial, or lack of response with at least two antidepressants from different classes. Treatment strategies for patients who do not achieve an appropriate response with a first-line agent include increasing the dose of the SSRI/SNRI; changing to a different agent in the same class; changing to a different agent of a different class; or augmentation of therapy.[5,8] At any point of nonresponse or loss of previous response, the clinician should assess for symptoms that may suggest a need for additional new medications, cause treatment nonadherence, or change management (e.g., suicidal thoughts, psychotic symptoms, substance abuse).[8] Once a patient has responded to pharmacotherapy, the regimen should be continued for at least 1 year.[8] Early discontinuation is associated with a greater risk of relapse.[8]

TREATMENT

Panic Disorder

■ DESIRED OUTCOME

The goal of therapy in panic disorder is remission. Patients should be free of panic attacks, have no or minimal anticipatory anxiety and agoraphobic avoidance, and no functional impairment.[26] Naturalistic studies indicate that after pharmacotherapy, over 50% of patients have occasional panic attacks, 40% experience agoraphobic avoidance, and most continue to take medications.[57]

■ GENERAL APPROACH TO TREATMENT

Therapeutic options include single or combined pharmacologic agents, concurrent psychotherapy, or psychotherapy followed by pharmacotherapy. Most patients without agoraphobic avoidance will improve with pharmacotherapy alone; however, if avoidance is present, CBT typically is initiated concurrently. With all effective drug therapies, resolution of agoraphobic avoidance tends to occur slowly. A meta-analysis of 11 randomized clinical trials comparing the use of SSRIs, TCAs, and CBT showed the effect on global anxiety and response to be similar among all treatments.[58]

In the most comprehensive study to date, efficacy of imipramine alone and CBT alone were equivalent in acute therapy for 3 months and during 6 months of maintenance therapy. Combined imipramine and CBT therapy was not significantly better than CBT or imipramine alone for acute therapy but was significantly better during maintenance. At 6 months after discontinuation, only patients previously treated with CBT maintained improvement (4% relapse) compared with a 25% relapse rate in patients previously treated with imipramine.[59] Adding psychosocial treatment to pharmacotherapy may improve long-term outcomes by reducing the likelihood of relapse when pharmacotherapy is stopped.[26]

■ NONPHARMACOLOGIC THERAPY

Patients should be educated to avoid substances that can precipitate panic attacks, including caffeine, nicotine, alcohol, drugs of abuse, and nonprescription stimulants.[1,26] Epidemiologic data suggest that daily smoking increases risk for panic attacks and may be a causal or exacerbating factor in some individuals with panic disorder.[57] Preliminary evidence suggests that aerobic exercise (e.g., walking for 60 minutes or running for 20–30 minutes 4 days/week) may benefit patients with panic disorder.[26] CBT is associated with short-term improvement in 80% to 90% of patients and 6-month improvement in 75% of patients. A course of CBT for panic disorder is 16 to 20 hours in length conducted over a period of 4 months.[60] Bibliotherapy (the use of self-help books), exercise, and Internet-based CBT are other options.[21,26]

■ PHARMACOLOGIC THERAPY

Panic disorder is treated effectively with several drugs including SSRIs, the TCA imipramine, and the benzodiazepines alprazolam and clonazepam[3,22,61] (Table 79–7). Alprazolam, clonazepam, sertraline, paroxetine, and venlafaxine are approved for this indication. SSRIs are the first-line agents because of their tolerability and efficacy in acute and long-term studies;[3,26,57] however, the benzodiazepines are the most commonly used drugs for panic disorder.[26] In a meta-analysis of the pharmacotherapy of panic disorder, the effect size of SSRIs and TCAs did not differ; however, the number of dropouts in the TCA group (31%) was significantly higher than in the SSRI group (18%).[57] A second meta-analysis comparing efficacy of benzodiazepines, TCAs, and SSRIs in panic disorder concluded that all treatments were equally efficacious with 50% to 80% of patients responding to treatment; however benzodiazepines were less effective for depression.[58] A long-term comparison study of SSRIs (e.g., citalopram, fluoxetine, fluvoxamine, paroxetine) found an equal overall response rate after 4 weeks of treatment. However, acute and long-term adverse effects differed between the drugs.[62] Five practice guidelines have been published.[3,22,26,60,63] An algorithm for the pharmacologic therapy of panic disorder appears in Figure 79–2.

TABLE 79-7	**Drugs Used in the Treatment of Panic Disorder**		
Class/Generic Name	**Brand Name**	**Starting Dose**	**Antipanic Dosage Range (mg)**
Selective serotonin reuptake inhibitors			
Citalopram[a]	Celexa	10 mg/day	20–60[b]
Escitalopram	Lexapro	5 mg/day	10–20[b]
Fluoxetine[a]	Prozac	5 mg/day	10–30[b]
Fluvoxamine[a]	Luvox	25 mg/day	100–300[b]
Paroxetine[a]	Paxil	10 mg/day	20–60[c]
	Pexeva		
	Paxil CR	12.5 mg/day	25–75[c]
Sertraline[a]	Zoloft	25 mg/day	50–200[c]
Serotonin norepinephrine reuptake inhibitor			
Venlafaxine XR[a]	Effexor XR	37.5 mg/day	75–225[c]
Benzodiazepines			
Alprazolam[a]	Xanax	0.25 mg 3 times a day	4–10[c]
	Xanax XR	0.5–1 mg/day	1–10[c]
Clonazepam[a]	Klonopin	0.25 mg once or twice per day	1–4[c]
Diazepam[a]	Valium	2–5 mg 3 times a day	5–20[b]
Lorazepam[a]	Ativan	0.5–1 mg 3 times a day	2–8[b]
Tricyclic antidepressant			
Imipramine[a]	Tofranil	10 mg/day	75–250[b]
Monoamine oxidase inhibitor			
Phenelzine	Nardil	15 mg/day	45–90[b]

[a]Available generically.
[b]Dosage used in clinical trials but not FDA approved.
[c]Dosage is FDA approved.
Data from Bandelow et al.[3] Katon,[22] and American Psychiatric Association.[26]

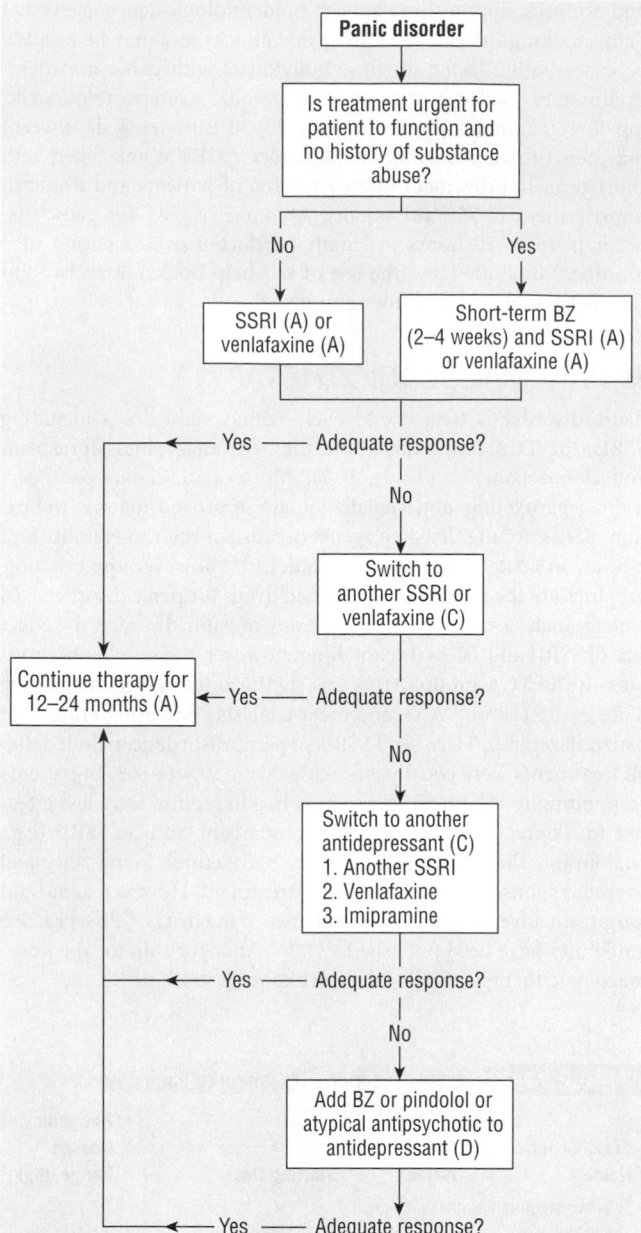

FIGURE 79-2. Algorithm for the pharmacotherapy of panic disorder. Strength of recommendations: A = directly based on category I evidence (i.e., meta-analysis of randomized controlled trials [RCT] or at least one RCT); B = directly based on category II evidence (i.e., at least one controlled study without randomization or one other type of quasi-experimental study); C = directly based on category III evidence (i.e., nonexperimental descriptive studies); D = directly based on category IV evidence (i.e., expert committee reports or opinions and/or clinical experience of respected authorities). (BZ, benzodiazepine; SSRI, selective serotonin reuptake inhibitor.) *(Data from APA[26] and NICE.[60])*

The efficacy of antidepressants was demonstrated in acute and long-term trials. Three 12-week, acute trials compared antidepressants. Escitalopram, but not citalopram, reduced the frequency of panic attacks although both improved QOL and reduced disease severity.[64] There was no difference in outcomes between paroxetine 40 to 60 mg and sertraline 50 to 150 mg daily.[65] Extended-release venlafaxine (75 mg or 150 mg) and paroxetine 40 mg achieved a 44% remission rate compared with that of placebo (24%).[66] Double-blind trials indicated that continuing sertraline, citalopram, or imipramine from 3 months to

1 year improved response rates.[22] Relapse prevention trials with fluoxetine, imipramine, paroxetine, sertraline, and extended-release venlafaxine resulted in reduced relapse rates compared with placebo.[21,26]

Benzodiazepines are considered second-line agents. Because of the risk of dependency, benzodiazepines should be used only after several trials of antidepressants have failed.[3,26] Because of potential emergence of depressive symptoms during treatment, benzodiazepines should not be used as monotherapy in a patient who is clinically depressed or has a history of depression. In patients whose illness is complicated by a history of alcohol or drug abuse, benzodiazepine use should be avoided.[26] Controlled trials have established that the short-term (4–6 weeks) addition of alprazolam or clonazepam to antidepressants produces a more rapid therapeutic response, with discontinuation of the benzodiazepine by week 7 of therapy.[63]

Alternative Drug Treatments

Buspirone, trazodone, bupropion, antipsychotics, antihistamines, and β-blockers are ineffective in panic disorder.[3,21,26] The majority of studies assessing the efficacy of MAOIs in treating panic disorder were open labeled and lacked adequate sample sizes. MAOIs are reserved for the most refractory or difficult patients.[21]

Special Populations

Elderly patients with panic disorder have fewer, less intense symptoms and avoidant behavior than younger patients.[67] Youth often present with fear that they are dying or being smothered, and agoraphobia can be manifested as a fear of leaving home.[68] CBT is effective in both populations. If pharmacotherapy is used, antidepressants, especially SSRIs, are preferred for management of panic disorder, and benzodiazepines are second-line agents because of potential problems with disinhibition in these two populations.

Antidepressant Therapy

Tricyclic Antidepressants

Efficacy Imipramine is the most studied TCA, alleviating panic attacks in 75% of patients with panic disorder. Imipramine effectively blocks panic attacks within at least 4 weeks; however, maximal improvement (including antiphobic response) does not occur until 8 to 12 weeks.[26]

Adverse Effects Up to 40% of patients experience stimulant-like side effects, including anxiety, insomnia, and jitteriness.[26] These side effects often affect patient compliance, prevent medication dosage increases, and interfere with the overall treatment outcome.

Other problems with TCA use in panic disorder are well documented and include anticholinergic effects, orthostatic hypotension, delayed onset of antipanic effects, and toxicity in overdose.[26] Approximately 25% of patients reportedly discontinue treatment because of side effects, especially weight gain.[26]

Dosing and Administration When using imipramine, treatment should be slowly increased by 10 mg every 2 to 4 days as tolerated.

Selective Serotonin Reuptake Inhibitors

Efficacy Clinical studies indicate that all SSRIs are effective in panic disorder.[21,26,57,58,69] The percentage of patients who become panic-free ranges between 60% and 80%.[26] ❹ The antipanic effect of SSRIs is delayed for at least 4 weeks, and some patients do not respond for 8 to 12 weeks.[26]

Adverse Effects Typical antidepressant doses of SSRIs can cause side effects of insomnia, jitteriness, restlessness, and agitation, and lead to drug discontinuation in patients with panic disorder. Transient gastrointestinal disturbances occur more frequently with SSRIs than with TCAs. Thus low initial SSRI doses should be prescribed.[26,58,69] Sleep disturbances, headaches, weight gain, and sexual dysfunction often are problematic.[26,57]

Dosing and Administration Low initial doses of SSRIs are recommended (see Table 79–7) to avoid stimulatory side effects (e.g., insomnia or nervousness), and should be maintained for the first week of therapy. Doses at the upper end of the dosing range can be necessary to achieve response.[60]

Serotonin Norepinephrine Reuptake Inhibitors

Efficacy Approximately 54% to 60% of patients were panic-free on extended-release venlafaxine 75 mg or 150 mg daily. The remission rates were 44% for both dosages in acute efficacy studies.[65]

Adverse Effects The most common adverse effects of extended-release venlafaxine in panic trials were nausea, somnolence, tremors, sweating, and abnormal sexual functioning.[33]

Dosing and Administration The dosage of venlafaxine can be increased at weekly intervals. A dose-response relationship was not evident in clinical trials.[33]

Benzodiazepines

Efficacy The high-potency benzodiazepines clonazepam and alprazolam are the preferred agents.[26,57] Diazepam and lorazepam are possibly effective in treating panic disorder when taken in sufficiently high doses.[26] Alprazolam is an ideal agent for patients who need rapid relief. Therapeutic response to benzodiazepines occurs in 1 to 2 weeks. Relapse rates of 50% or higher are common despite slow drug tapering.[51]

Adverse Effects Patient acceptance of benzodiazepines usually is not a problem, and except for sedation, side effects are reported rarely.

Dosing and Administration Doses of clonazepam can be increased by 0.25 or 0.5 mg every 3 days to 4 mg/day if needed.[46] Alprazolam can be slowly increased over several weeks to reach an ideal dose. ❺ The duration of action of immediate-release alprazolam can be as little as 4 to 6 hours with resulting breakthrough symptoms; use of the extended-release alprazolam or clonazepam will avoid this problem. Most patients require 3 to 6 mg/day of alprazolam, and some need higher doses to obtain a full therapeutic (antipanic and antiphobic) response.

Treatment Resistance Common reasons for treatment failures are comorbid psychiatric disorders, rapid dosage increases with resulting intolerable side effects, and underdosage.[26] All standard treatments should be tried before using augmentation strategies. In patients with a partial response to one agent, a low dose of another antipanic agent (e.g., a TCA, benzodiazepine, or an SSRI) can be added.[26]

Phases of Therapy

Acute Phase The main goal of therapy in the acute phase is reduction of symptoms (e.g., resolution of panic attacks, reduction in anxiety and phobic fears, resumption of the patient's usual activities).[21] The duration of this phase is generally 1 to 3 months depending on the choice of drug. Therapy should be altered if there is no response after 6 to 8 weeks of an adequate dose.

The guiding principle for SSRI and SNRI drugs in panic disorder is to start with low doses (approximately one-quarter to one-half of the starting doses for depression), use an adequate dose, and treat for about 12 weeks.[21] Side effects with the antidepressants, often from too high an initial dose, can prevent achievement of an optimal dosage, compromise treatment response, and contribute to patient nonadherence.

The duration of the acute phase with benzodiazepines is approximately 1 month because response is rapid. A regular dosing schedule rather than an as-needed schedule is preferred for patients with panic disorder who are taking benzodiazepines, where the goal is to prevent panic attacks rather than reduce symptoms once an attack has already occurred.[26]

Maintenance Phase and Discontinuation ❻ The optimal length of therapy is unknown; however, the total duration of therapy appears to be 12 to 24 months before drug discontinuation over 4 to 6 months is attempted.[26] The dose used in the acute phase is continued into the maintenance phase.[26] Citalopram, clomipramine, fluoxetine, sertraline, venlafaxine, and imipramine have been shown to maintain clinical effects for up to 1 year of treatment.[3,21] When drugs are discontinued too early, a high rate of relapse occurs; thus longer periods of treatment are associated with a more sustained response. Reinstitution of drug usually results in renewed clinical response.[26] Pharmacotherapy, even at long duration, might not prevent relapse, and many patients require long-term therapy.

The most important determinant of adherence with maintenance therapy is the tolerability of adverse events.[26] Some adverse events which are experienced short term become unbearable during long-term management (e.g., sexual dysfunction and weight gain). TCAs, SSRIs (except fluoxetine), and venlafaxine can be associated with discontinuation symptoms.

The primary risk of long-term benzodiazepine use is the development of dependency and withdrawal reactions on discontinuation. Abuse of benzodiazepines usually is confined to patients with a personal or family history of substance or alcohol use.[5,26,69] The approach to benzodiazepine discontinuation involves a slow and gradual tapering of the dose because withdrawal symptoms and rebound anxiety may occur during discontinuation. Benzodiazepines should be tapered over 2 to 4 months at rates no higher than 10% of the dose per week.[26]

Providing education about the disorder may relieve some of the symptoms of panic by helping the patient to realize that the symptoms are neither life-threatening nor uncommon. Patients should be informed regarding the lag time before a therapeutic response will occur and any problematic side effects. Many patients are reluctant to take drugs for fear that their illness will worsen or that they will become addicted. Adverse events are often perceived as a worsening of the illness and can contribute to nonadherence or prevent necessary dosage increases. Patients receiving benzodiazepines and antidepressants should be told not to decrease or discontinue therapy unless authorized by their clinician.[60]

■ PHARMACOECONOMIC CONSIDERATIONS

Patients with panic disorder have high rates of unemployment and receive welfare, disability benefits, and healthcare services.[3,26,57] They also have impaired emotional and physical health status and experience poor marital and social functioning.[21,22] Measures of QOL improved with imipramine, clonazepam, sertraline, and venlafaxine. Treatment with clomipramine, paroxetine, or fluoxetine improved work, social, and family responsibilities. Improvements in anxiety and phobic avoidance were significantly associated with QOL improvements.[21,22] In a cost-efficacy evaluation of individual and combined treatments for panic disorder, imipramine was the most cost-efficacious treatment option at the completion of the acute phase. CBT was the most cost-efficacious option at the end of maintenance treatment and 6 months after treatment termination.[70]

CLINICAL CONTROVERSY

The cognitive effects of benzodiazepines are a subject of debate. Benzodiazepines at higher doses can cause memory impairment. One meta-analysis reported that long-term benzodiazepine users performed worse than controls on domains of cognitive functioning. However, another review concluded that the literature does not provide evidence of long-term cognitive effects of benzodiazepines in patients with anxiety.

■ EVALUATION OF THERAPEUTIC OUTCOMES

During the first few weeks of the acute phase of therapy, patients with panic disorder should be seen every 1 to 2 weeks when starting a new medication, then every 2 to 4 weeks to adjust drug dosages based on improvement in panic symptoms and to monitor for adverse events.[60] After the dose is stabilized and symptoms have decreased, visits every 2 months should suffice.[60] The patient should be counseled to maintain a diary to record the date, time, frequency, duration, and intensity of panic episodes, level of anticipatory anxiety or agoraphobic avoidance, and the severity of distress and impairment related to panic disorder. Treatment outcomes can be assessed objectively by use of the Panic Disorder Severity Scale. Remission is defined as equal to or less than 3 with no or mild agoraphobic avoidance, anxiety, disability, or depressive symptoms. Treatment response is indicated by a 40% or greater reduction in overall score.[63]

At scheduled visits, the clinician can inquire about the level of disability experienced by the patient and have the patient complete the Sheehan Disability Scale (with a goal of less than or equal to 1 point on each item).[71] During drug discontinuation, the frequency of appointments should be increased to evaluate for emergence of potential withdrawal symptoms and monitor for relapse.

TREATMENT

Social Anxiety Disorder

■ DESIRED OUTCOME

The goals of therapy in the acute phase of treatment are to reduce physiologic symptoms of anxiety (e.g., tachycardia, flushing, and sweating), social anxiety, and phobic avoidance. The duration of this phase is 4 to 12 weeks, depending on the drug therapy.

The goals of therapy in the continuation phase (3–6 months) are to extend the therapeutic benefits, especially the patient's ability to participate in social activities, and improve QOL. Although the primary goal of treatment is to reduce anxiety symptoms to manageable levels, even modest reductions in avoidance and discomfort can be highly valued by patients.[24]

❼ At least a 1-year maintenance period is recommended to maintain improvement and decrease the rate of relapse.[17,63] Situations suggesting a possible need for long-term treatment include the presence of unresolved symptoms or comorbidity, an early onset of disease, and a prior history of relapse.[24] The long-term goal in the treatment of SAD is remission with the disappearance of the core symptoms of social anxiety, little or no anxiety, and no functional impairment or concurrent depressive symptoms.[71]

■ GENERAL APPROACH TO TREATMENT

Patients with generalized SAD should be treated aggressively. Obstacles to effective treatment include patient avoidance of therapy secondary to fear and shame, treatment directed toward somatic symptoms or concurrent conditions, and financial barriers.[17] Patients with SAD often respond more slowly and less completely than patients with other anxiety disorders. Therefore, it is important to set reasonable expectations for response to therapy. Consideration of current symptoms, prior treatments, concurrent conditions, and history of substance abuse guide treatment selection.

CBT and pharmacotherapy are effective in the treatment of SAD.[17,24,72,73] Pharmacotherapy is often the most practical choice because CBT might not be available outside of large urban areas. Acute treatment outcomes for CBT and pharmacotherapy are equal.[17,24] Drug therapy is superior in reducing subjective general anxiety acutely, although CBT has a greater likelihood of maintaining response after termination.[24,74]

There are no data to predict which patients will respond best to pharmacotherapy, CBT, or a combination[24] or maintain gains after discontinuing pharmacotherapy. The only significant indication of treatment response in pharmacotherapy is duration of treatment.[24] Some patients elect lifelong therapy, and many are reluctant to attempt drug discontinuation because of fear of relapse. Discontinuation of drug therapy after only 2 to 3 months resulted in higher rates of relapse than when therapy was continued for 5 to 12 months.[24] Data show that relapse rates after discontinuation of CBT are significantly less than those after discontinuation of effective pharmacotherapy.[17,24] Sertraline is the only medication approved for the long-term treatment of SAD, although paroxetine, escitalopram, and venlafaxine prevented relapse.[24,74,76]

■ NONPHARMACOLOGIC THERAPY

Patients should be educated about SAD and support groups. Self-help group programs that focus on effective communication can benefit people with public-speaking phobia.

CBT consists of exposure therapy, cognitive restructuring, relaxation training techniques, and social skills training.[24] Through CBT, patients learn to overcome anxiety in social situations and alter the beliefs and responses that maintain this anxiety. Therapy usually lasts several months and often is conducted in groups. In clinical trials, one-half to two-thirds of patients responded at 12 weeks.[24]

■ PHARMACOLOGIC THERAPY

Special Populations

SAD can present in children of preschool to elementary school age. If the disorder is not treated, it can persist into adulthood and increase the risk of depression and substance abuse. CBT and social skills training are effective nonpharmacologic therapies in children.[68,77] Placebo-controlled and open-label trials have provided evidence of efficacy of pharmacotherapy with an SSRI or SNRI in children 6 to 17 years of age.[68,77] Children and adolescents prescribed an SSRI or SNRI for social anxiety (or for other purposes) should be closely monitored for increased risk of suicidal ideation. Headache, nausea, drowsiness, insomnia, jitteriness, and stomach aches were reported in children receiving antidepressants.[68,77]

Benzodiazepines should be reserved as the last-line agents in children with SAD.[68,77] If prescribed, they should be used for the shortest time period possible. The adverse effects of benzodiazepines in children include drowsiness, oppositional behavior, disinhibition, and fatigue.

Approximately one-fifth of patients with SAD also suffer from an alcohol use disorder. Many people with SAD report that they use alcohol to cope with anxiety. Paroxetine significantly reduced social anxiety and the frequency and severity of alcohol use in patients with SAD and an alcohol use disorder.[78] MAOIs and benzodiazepines are not appropriate for patients with SAD and alcohol use disorder. SSRIs are the drugs of choice.

Antidepressant Therapy

❽ SSRIs and venlafaxine are beneficial for concurrent depression, and are safe when used in patients with substance abuse. Paroxetine, sertraline, extended-release venlafaxine, and extended-release fluvoxamine are approved for the treatment of generalized SAD, and are considered first-line agents because of efficacy and tolerability (Table 79–8). Controlled trials comparing different

TABLE 79-8	Drugs Used in the Treatment of Generalized Social Anxiety Disorder		
Class/Generic Name	**Brand Name**	**Starting Dose**	**Dosage Range (mg/day)**
Selective serotonin reuptake inhibitors			
Citalopram[a]	Celexa	20 mg/day	20–40[b]
Escitalopram	Lexapro	5 mg/day	10–20[b]
Fuvoxamine CR	Luvox CR	100 mg	100–300[c]
Paroxetine[a]	Paxil	10 mg/day	10–60[c]
Paroxetine CR	Paxil CR	12.5 mg/day	12.5–37.5[c]
Sertraline[a]	Zoloft	25–50 mg/day	50–200[c]
Serotonin-norepinephrine reuptake inhibitor			
Venlafaxine XR[a]	Effexor XR	75 mg/day	75–225[c]
Monoamine oxidase inhibitor			
Phenelzine	Nardil	15 mg at bedtime	60–90[b]
Alternative agents			
Buspirone[a,d]	BuSpar	10 mg twice per day	45–60[b]
Clonazepam[a,d]	Klonopin	0.25 mg/day	1–4[b]
Gabapentin[a]	Neurontin	100 mg 3 times a day	900–3,600[b]
Mirtazapine[a]	Remeron	15 mg at bedtime	30[b]
Pregabalin	Lyrica	100 mg 3 times a day	600[b]
Quetiapine	Seroquel	25 mg at bedtime	25–400[b]

XR, extended-release; CR, controlled-release.
[a]Available generically.
[b]Dosage used in clinical trials but not FDA approved.
[c]Dosage is FDA approved.
[d]Used as augmenting agent.
Data from Bandelow et al.,[3] Muller et al.,[17] Schneier,[24] Stein and Stein,[74] and Vaishnavi et al.[80]

SSRIs, or SSRIs and an SNRI, demonstrated equivalent efficacy between agents.[24,79] TCAs are not effective in SAD.[24] Evidence-based guidelines for the treatment of SAD were published by the World Federation of Societies of Biological Psychiatry, the British Association for Psychopharmacology, and the Canadian Psychiatric Association.[3,21,63] An algorithm for the pharmacotherapy of generalized SAD appears in Figure 79–3.

Selective Serotonin Reuptake Inhibitors

Efficacy The efficacy and safety of SSRIs in the treatment of SAD were established in large placebo-controlled trials.[81] Response rates to SSRIs ranged from 50% to 80%.[81]

Patients treated with paroxetine, sertraline, escitalopram, and fluvoxamine showed improvement in anxiety and avoidance symptoms and a decrease in disability.[24,79] SSRIs were well tolerated, and emergent adverse effects were similar to those of depression trials. The onset of effect was delayed 4 to 8 weeks, and maximum benefit was often not observed until 12 weeks or longer. Sertraline was effective in disabled patients suffering from the marked to severe form of generalized SAD.[81] Escitalopram was effective in the treatment of generalized social anxiety.[21,79] Limited data suggest that citalopram is also effective in treating SAD.[82] Mixed results have been reported for fluoxetine.[83]

Dosing and Administration SSRIs should be initiated at doses similar to those used for the treatment of depression and administered as a single daily dose (see Table 79–8). If the patient suffers from comorbid panic disorder, the SSRI dose should be started at one-fourth or one-half of the dose. After 24 weeks of therapy, measures of social anxiety were significantly better with escitalopram 20 mg compared with paroxetine 20 mg.[84] The dose response curve for SSRIs tends to be relatively flat, but individual patients can require higher doses. Increase the dose as tolerated in patients who have not responded after 4 weeks of therapy.[17,24] When discontinuing an SSRI, the dosage should be tapered monthly (i.e., decreasing sertraline by 50 mg or paroxetine by 10 mg) to reduce the risk of relapse and discontinuation symptoms. Escitalopram produced significantly fewer discontinuation symptoms compared with paroxetine in patients with SAD.[21]

Venlafaxine

Efficacy Extended-release venlafaxine was significantly better than placebo in improving social interaction, performance, avoidance factors, and some fear factors (e.g., public speaking).[85] Beneficial effects were seen by week 3. Venlafaxine was effective in patients who failed to respond to therapy with SSRIs.[17]

Adverse Effects Adverse effects included anorexia, dry mouth, nausea, insomnia, and sexual dysfunction.

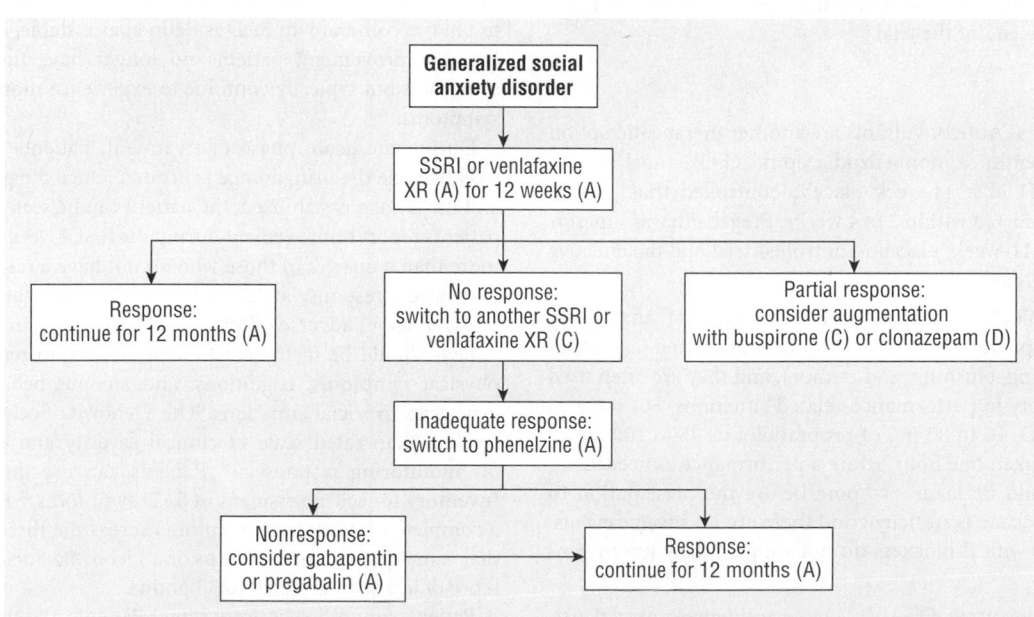

FIGURE 79-3. Algorithm for the pharmacotherapy of generalized social anxiety disorder. Strength of recommendations: A = directly based on category I evidence (i.e., meta-analysis of randomized controlled trials [RCT] or at least one RCT); B = directly based on category II evidence (i.e., at least one controlled study without randomization or one other type of quasi-experimental study); C = directly based on category III evidence (i.e., nonexperimental descriptive studies); D = directly based on category IV evidence (i.e., expert committee reports or opinions and/or clinical experience of respected authorities). (SSRI, selective serotonin reuptake inhibitor.) *(Data from Bandelow et al.,[3] and Stein and Stein.[74])*

Dosing and Administration Additional therapeutic benefits of venlafaxine above 75 mg/day were not shown.[85] Venlafaxine should be tapered slowly (i.e., decreasing by 37.5 mg/mo) to decrease the risk of relapse during discontinuation.

Mirtazapine Mirtazapine reduced social anxiety and improved QOL in women with SAD over 10 weeks.[86]

Alternative Agents

Benzodiazepines Benzodiazepines are commonly used in the treatment of patients who cannot tolerate or fail to respond to antidepressants.[24] Benzodiazepines are not considered first-line therapy for SAD because of concerns over the adverse effects, potential for dependence, the possibility of rebound anxiety, and ineffectiveness in the treatment of depression.[23,83] Clonazepam is the most extensively studied benzodiazepine for the treatment of generalized SAD.[24] Clonazepam improved fear and phobic avoidance, interpersonal sensitivity, fears of negative evaluation, and disability measures.[87] Adverse effects included sexual dysfunction, unsteadiness, dizziness, and poor concentration.[87]

If clonazepam is prescribed, the acute phase of therapy is about 1 month. Patients should be instructed not to decrease or discontinue clonazepam without consulting their clinician because of the risks of rebound anxiety and withdrawal symptoms. Patients on clonazepam for 6 months who were slowly tapered over 5 months maintained their treatment response.[17,24] Clonazepam should be gradually tapered at a rate not to exceed 0.25 mg every 2 weeks.[17,24]

CLINICAL CONTROVERSY

The role of benzodiazepines in the treatment of SAD is controversial. Some clinicians prescribe benzodiazepines in combination with an antidepressant in the acute management of SAD, then taper the benzodiazepine after 3 to 4 weeks. Recent data indicate that the addition of a benzodiazepine to an SSRI during the acute treatment of SAD does not provide more rapid response, although patients tended to have better outcomes at the end of the trial.

Anticonvulsants Anticonvulsants are another therapeutic option in SAD. Gabapentin, a nonbenzodiazepine GABA analog, was effective for SAD in a 14-week placebo-controlled trial.[17,24] The onset of effect occurred within 2 to 4 weeks. Pregabalin was superior to placebo in an 11-week, placebo-controlled trial and the effective dose was 600 mg/day.[88]

β-Blockers β-Blockers decrease the perception of anxiety by blunting the peripheral autonomic symptoms of arousal (e.g., rapid heart rate, sweating, blushing, and tremor), and they are often used to decrease anxiety in performance-related situations. For patients with specific SAD, 10 to 80 mg of propranolol or 25 to 100 mg of atenolol can be taken one hour before a performance as needed.[17,24] A test dose should be taken at home before the presentation to assure that β-blockade is sufficient and there are no adverse events. Controlled trials with β-blockers do not support daily use in generalized SAD.[17]

Treatment Resistance ❾ An adequate antidepressant trial usually consists of 8 to 12 weeks (at maximum dosages).[17,24] Subsequent options include a trial of a second SSRI or extended-release venlafaxine. Some patients experience clinical benefit during the first 4 weeks of therapy.[21,72] If nonresponsiveness continues, a trial of an alternative agent is warranted.

There are no data on the choice of treatments if antidepressants fail. Busprione[24,72] and clonazepam (in patients without a history of substance abuse) have been used as augmenting agents.[21] The combination of clonazepam and paroxetine over 10 weeks in a placebo-controlled trial did not lead to more rapid resolution of SAD symptoms.[87] However, the group that received the combination therapy had a higher response rate.

Atypical antipsychotics and MAOIs are options in treatment-resistant SAD. Quetiapine monotherapy showed a large effect size on the Social Phobia Inventory when compared with placebo.[80] Although phenelzine is effective in 77% of patients with SAD,[21,73] dietary restrictions, potential drug interactions, and adverse effects (e.g., weight gain and hypertensive crisis) have limited its use. If a patient is switched from another antidepressant to phenelzine, an appropriate washout period should be followed.

■ PHARMACOECONOMIC CONSIDERATIONS

Generalized SAD is associated with lower health-related QOL, a higher rate of lifetime suicide attempts, diminished educational and occupational attainment, and increased use of healthcare resources.[83] SAD was a significant, unrecognized impediment to efforts to reduce welfare reliance and achievement of economic self-sufficiency in women receiving welfare.[89]

Early intervention is important in the treatment of SAD. Patients treated with fluvoxamine, sertraline, paroxetine, or escitalopram showed a significantly greater improvement in functioning, disability, and QOL compared with placebo-treated patients.[24,80,90,91] In a relapse prevention study, patients treated with escitalopram experienced a better health-related QOL and more cost-effective therapy than placebo.[91] The acquisition cost of escitalopram was more than offset by a decrease in total costs of care.[91]

■ EVALUATION OF THERAPEUTIC OUTCOMES

❿ The pharmacotherapy of SAD can be monitored in three principal domains: SAD symptoms (e.g., fears and physical symptoms), functionality, and well-being or overall improvement.[17,24] Response to pharmacotherapy in SAD is defined as a stable, clinically meaningful improvement; patients no longer have the full range of symptoms but typically continue to experience more than minimal symptoms.[17,24]

During the acute phase of treatment, patients should be seen weekly while the drug dosage is titrated. Once the patient responds and the dosage is stabilized, the patient can be seen monthly. Many patients report improvement during the first 4 weeks of therapy, but more than a quarter of those who do not have a response at week 8 may have a response at 12 weeks. At each visit, the patient should be asked about adverse effects and improvement in symptoms. The patient should be instructed to keep a diary to record fear levels, physical symptoms, cognitions, and anxious behaviors in actual exposures to social situations. The Liebowitz Social Anxiety Scale is a clinician-rated scale of clinical severity and change in SAD for monitoring response.[17,24] Patients can use the Social Phobia Inventory for self-assessment of SAD symptoms.[24] Full remission is a complete resolution of symptoms across the three SAD domains that is maintained for 3 months or a Liebowitz Social Anxiety Scale score of less than or equal to 30 points.[71]

Patient counseling is important. Patients should be instructed about the gradual onset of effect, when to expect full therapeutic effects, and that long-term therapy is required. When drug therapy is discontinued, the dosage needs to be gradually decreased over several months, and the patient should be seen more frequently to monitor for signs and symptoms of relapse or withdrawal.

It is important to remember that although pharmacotherapy usually leads to improvement in social and occupational functioning, most patients do not achieve a full remission. Many patients require additional treatment, often in the form of CBT.

TREATMENT

Specific Phobia

Specific phobia is considered unresponsive to drug therapy, although highly responsive to CBT. The use of benzodiazepines or paroxetine in patients who failed CBT is supported by limited data. Benzodiazepines can be detrimental in patients with specific phobias treated with CBT.[21]

CONCLUSIONS

Anxiety disorders are common in the population and occur concurrently with other psychiatric disorders. The proper management of anxiety disorders begins with the correct diagnosis; not all patients should receive antianxiety agents. Nonpharmacologic interventions often are effective alone or when combined with drug therapy.

There are several subtypes of anxiety disorders, and the diagnosis determines the type of drug and nonpharmacologic intervention selected. Although benzodiazepines remain the drugs of choice for situational anxiety, antidepressants have emerged as first-line therapy for GAD, panic disorder, and SAD. Benzodiazepines are reserved for use in situations requiring immediate anxiety relief during the first 2 to 4 weeks of therapy with a long-term agent such as an antidepressant. Antidepressants, including SSRIs and SNRIs, and the benzodiazepines clonazepam and alprazolam, are used extensively in patients with GAD, panic disorder, and SAD.

The long-term goal of therapy for GAD, panic disorder, and SAD is remission of core anxiety symptoms with no impairment in functionality, minimal anxiety, and no depressive symptoms. Augmentation with atypical antipsychotics show some promise in treatment-resistant cases.

ABBREVIATIONS

ACC: anterior cingulated cortex

CBT: cognitive behavioral therapy

CNS: central nervous system

CRF: corticotrophin-releasing factor

DA: dopamine

DMDZ: desmethyldiazepam

GABA: γ-aminobutyric acid

GAD: generalized anxiety disorder

FDA: U.S. Food and Drug Administration

5-HT: serotonin

LC: locus ceruleus

MAOI: monoamine oxidase inhibitor

NE: norepinephrine

OCD: obsessive-compulsive disorder

PAG: periaqueductal gray matter

PTSD: posttraumatic stress disorder

QOL: quality of life

SAD: social anxiety disorder

SERT: serotonin reuptake transporter site

SNRI: serotonin-norepinephrine reuptake inhibitor

SSRI: selective serotonin reuptake inhibitor

TCA: tricyclic antidepressant

REFERENCES

1. American Psychiatric Association. Diagnostic and Statistical Manual of Mental Disorders, Fourth Edition, Text Revision. Washington, DC: American Psychiatric Association, 2000:429–484.
2. Roy-Byrne PP, Wagner A. Primary care perspectives on generalized anxiety disorder. J Clin Psychiatry 2004;(65 Suppl 13):20–26.
3. Bandelow B, Zohar J, Hollander E, et al. World Federation of Societies of Biological Psychiatry (WFSBP) guidelines for the pharmacological treatment of anxiety, obsessive-compulsive and post-traumatic stress disorders - first revision. World J Biol Psychiatry 2008;9(4):248–312.
4. Roy-Byrne PP, Davidson KW, Kessler RC, et al. Anxiety disorders and comorbid medical illness. Gen Hosp Psychiatry 2008;30:208–225.
5. Katzman MA. Current considerations in the treatment of generalized anxiety disorder. CNS Drugs 2009;23(2):103–120.
6. National Comorbidity Survey Replication (NCS-R) Lifetime and 12-month Prevalence Estimates. Data updated July 9, 2007. http://www.hcp.med.harvard.edu/ncs/index.php.
7. Smoller JW, Block SR, Young MM. Genetics of anxiety disorders: the complex road from DSM to DNA. Depress Anxiety 2009;26(11): 965–975.
8. Davidson JR, Zhang W, Connor KM, et al. A psychopharmacological treatment algorithm for generalized anxiety disorder (GAD). J Psychopharmacol 2010;24(1):3–26.
9. Baldwin DS, Polkinghorn C. Evidence-based pharmacotherapy of generalized anxiety disorder. Int J Neuropsychopharmacol 2005;8: 293–302.
10. Rogers MP, Wolfe DJ. Anxiety in the medical patient. Psychiatric Times 2007;24(3):1–4.
11. Martin EI, Ressler KJ, Binder E, et al. The neurobiology of anxiety disorders: Brain imaging, genetics, and psychoneuroendocrinology. Psychiatr Clin N Am 2009;32:549–575.
12. Damsa C, Losel M, Moussally J. Current status of brain imaging in anxiety disorders. Curr Opin Psychiatry 2009;22(1):96–110.
13. Matthew SJ, Price RB, Charney DS. Recent advances in the neurobiology of anxiety disorders: Implications for novel therapeutics. Am J Med Genet C Semin Med Genet 2008;148C(2):89–98.
14. Möhler H. GABAA receptor diversity and pharmacology. Cell Tissue Res 2006;326:505–516.
15. Condren RM, Lucey TV, Thakore JH. A preliminary study of baclofen-induced growth hormone release in generalised social phobia. Hum Psychopharmacol 2003;18:135–130.
16. Akimova E, Lanzenberger R, Kasper S. The serotonin-1A receptor in anxiety disorders. Biol Psychiatry 2009;66(7):627–635.
17. Muller JE, Koen LK, Seedat S, et al. Social anxiety disorder: Current treatment recommendations. CNS Drugs 2005;19(5):377–391.
18. Stein MB. Neurobiology of generalized anxiety disorder. J Clin Psychiatry 2009;70(Suppl 2):15–19.
19. Graeff FG, Del-Ben CM. Neurobiology of panic disorder: From animal models to brain neuroimaging. Neurosci Biobehav Rev 2008;32(7):1326–1335.
20. Etkin A, Wager TD. Functional neuroimaging of anxiety: A meta-analysis of emotional processing in PTSD, social anxiety disorder, and specific phobia. Am J Psychiatry 2007;164:1476–1488.
21. Baldwin DS, Anderson IM, Nutt DJ, et al. Evidence-based guidelines for the pharmacological treatment of anxiety disorders: Recommendations from the British Society for Psychopharmacology. J Psychopharmacology 2005;19:567–596.
22. Katon WJ. Panic disorder. N Engl J Med 2006;354:2360–2367.
23. Perugi G, Frare F, Toni C. Diagnosis and treatment of agoraphobia with panic disorder. CNS Drugs 2007;21(9):741–764.

24. Schneier FR. Social anxiety disorder. N Engl J Med 2006;355(10): 1029–1036.

25. Goodman WK. Selecting pharmacotherapy for generalized anxiety disorder. J Clin Psychiatry 2004;65(Suppl 13):8–13.

26. American Psychiatric Association. Practice guideline for the treatment of patients with panic disorder. Arlington, VA: American Psychiatric Association, 2009. *http://www.psychiatryonline.com/pracGuide/pracGuideTopic_9.aspx.*

27. Chouinard G. Issues in the clinical use of benzodiazepines: Potency, withdrawal and rebound. J Clin Psychiatry 2004;65(Suppl 5):7–12.

28. Kavoussi R. Pregabalin: From molecule to medicine. Eur Neuropsychopharmacol 2006;16:S128–S133.

29. Gao K, Sheehan DV, Calabrese JR. Atypical antipsychotics in primary generalized anxiety disorder or comorbid with mood disorders. Expert Rev Neurother 2009;9(8):1147–1158.

30. Paxil [package insert]. Research Triangle Park, NC: GlaxoSmithKline; August 2007.

31. Cymbalta [package insert]. Indianapolis, IN: Eli Lilly and Company; November 2009.

32. Lexapro [package insert]. St. Louis, MO: Forest Pharmaceuticals, Inc.; March 2009.

33. Effexor XR [package insert]. Philadelphia, PA: Wyeth Pharmaceuticals, Inc.; July 2009.

34. Vistaril [package insert]. New York: Pfizer Labs; December 2009.

35. Connor KM, Payne V, Davidson JRT. Kava in generalized anxiety disorder: Three placebo-controlled trials. Int Clin Psychopharmacol 2006;21:249–253.

36. Rubinchik SM, Kablinger AS, Gardener JS. Medications for panic disorder and generalized anxiety disorder during pregnancy. Prim Care Companion J Clin Psychiatry 2005;7:100–105.

37. Kapczinski F, Lima MS, Souza JS, et al. Antidepressants for generalized anxiety disorder. Cochrane Database Syst Rev 2003;2:CD003592.

38. Rynn MA, Riddle MA, Yeung PP, et al. Efficacy and safety of extended-release venlafaxine in the treatment of generalized anxiety disorder in children and adolescents: Two placebo controlled trials. Am J Psychiatry 2007;164:290–300.

39. Carter NJ, McCormack PL. Duloxetine: A review of its use in the treatment of generalized anxiety disorder. CNS Drugs 2009;23(6):523–541.

40. Ball SG, Kuhn A, Wall D, et al. Selective serotonin reuptake inhibitor treatment for generalized anxiety disorder: A double-blind, prospective comparison between paroxetine and sertraline. J Clin Psychiatry 2005;66:94–99.

41. Baldwin DS, Huuson AKT, Mehuylum E. Escitalopram and paroxetine in the treatment of generalized anxiety disorder. Br J Psychiatry 2006;189:264–272.

42. Korotzer BA, Gommoll C, Li D. Randomized placebo-controlled trial of escitalopram and venlafaxine XR in the treatment of generalized anxiety disorder. Depress Anxiety 2008;25(10):854–861.

43. Bielski RJ, Bose A, Chang CC. A double-blind comparison of escitalopram and paroxetine in the long-term treatment of generalized anxiety disorder. Ann Clin Psychiatry 2005;17:65–69.

44. Nimatoudis I, Zissis NP, Kogeorgos J, et al. Remission rates with venlafaxine extended release in Greek outpatients with generalized anxiety disorder. A double-blind, randomized, placebo-controlled study. Int Clin Psychopharmacol 2004;19(6):331–336.

45. David DJ, Samuels BA, Rainer Q, et al. Neurogenesis-dependent and -independent effects of fluoxetine in an animal model of anxiety/depression. Neuron 2009;62(4):479–493.

46. Klonopin [package insert]. Nutley, NJ: Roche Laboratories; May 2009.

47. Xanax XR [package insert]. New York, NY: Pfizer, Inc.; December 2005.

48. Rosenbaum JF, Arana GW, Hyman SE, et al. Handbook of Psychiatric Therapy, 5th ed. Philadelphia, PA: Lippincott Williams & Wilkins, 2005.

49. Benzodiazepines. Facts and Comparisons 4.0 Online. Wolters Kluwer Health, Inc.; 2009. *http://online.factsandcomparisons.com.*

50. Denis C, Fatseas M, Lavie E, et al. Pharmacological interventions for benzodiazepine mono-dependence in outpatient settings. Cochrane Database Syst Rev 2006;(3):CD005194.

51. Lader M, Tylee A, Donoghue J. Withdrawing benzodiazepines in primary care. CNS Drugs 2009;23(1):19–34.

52. Chessick C, Allen M, Thase M, et al. Azapirones for generalized anxiety disorder. Cochrane Database Syst Rev 2006;3:CD006115.

53. Devane CL, Chiao E, Franklin M, et al. Anxiety disorders in the 21st century: Status challenges, opportunities, and comorbidity with depression. Am J Manag Care 2005;11(12 Suppl):S344–S353.

54. Huffman DL, Dukes EM, Wittchen HU. Human and economic burden of generalized anxiety disorder. Depress Anxiety 2008;25(1):72–90.

55. Guest J, Russ J, Lenox-Smith A. Cost-effectiveness of venlafaxine XL compared with diazepam in treatment of generalized anxiety disorder in the United Kingdom. Eur J Health Econ 2005;6:136–145.

56. Jørgensen TR, Stein DJ, Despiegel N, et al. Cost-effectiveness analysis of escitalopram compared with paroxetine in the treatment of generalized anxiety disorder in the United Kingdom. Ann Pharmacotherapy 2006;40:1752–1758.

57. Royal Australian and New Zealand College of Psychiatrists Clinical Practice Guidelines Team for Panic Disorder and Agoraphobia. Australian and New Zealand clinical practice guidelines for the treatment of panic disorder and agoraphobia. Aust N Z J Psychiatry 2003;37:641–656.

58. Mitte K. A meta-analysis of the efficacy of psycho- and pharmacotherapy in panic disorder with and without agoraphobia. J Affect Disord 2005;88:27–45.

59. Raffa SD, Stoddard JA, White KS, et al. Relapse following combined treatment discontinuation in a placebo-controlled trial for panic disorder. J Nerv Ment Dis 2008;196(7):548–555.

60. National Institute for Clinical Excellence. The Management of Panic Disorder and Generalized Anxiety Disorder in Primary Care and Secondary Care: Clinical Guideline 22. London: National Collaborating Centre for Mental Health, December 2004.

61. Pollack MH. The pharmacotherapy of panic disorder. J Clin Psychiatry 2005;66(Suppl 4):23–27.

62. Dannon PN, Iancu I, Lowengrub K, et al. A naturalistic long-term comparison study of selective serotonin reuptake inhibitors in the treatment of panic disorder. Clin Neuropharmacol 2007;30(6):326–334.

63. Canadian Psychiatric Association. Clinical practice guidelines: Management of anxiety disorders. Can J Psychiatry 2006;51(8, Suppl 2): 9S–91S.

64. Bandelow B, Stein DJ, Dolberg OT, et al. Improvement of quality of life in panic disorder with escitalopram, citalopram, or placebo. Pharmacopsychiatry 2007;40(4):152–156.

65. Bandelow B, Behnke K, Lenior S, et al. Sertraline versus paroxetine in the treatment of panic disorder: An acute double-blind noninferiority trial. J Clin Psychiatry 2004;65:405–413.

66. Pollack MH, Lepola U, Koponen H, et al. A double-blind study of the efficacy of venlafaxine extended-release, paroxetine and placebo in the treatment of panic disorder. Depress Anxiety 2007;24:1–14.

67. Flint AJ, Gagnon N. Diagnosis and management of panic disorder in older adults. Drugs Aging 2003;20:881–891.

68. American Academy of Child and Adolescent Psychiatry. Practice parameter for the assessment and treatment of children and adolescents with anxiety disorders. J Am Acad Child Adolesc Psychiatry 2007;46(2):267–283.

69. Ferguson JM, Khan A, Mangano R, et al. Relapse prevention of panic disorder in adult outpatient responders to treatment with venlafaxine extended-release. J Clin Psychiatry 2007;68:58–68.

70. McHugh RK, Otto MW, Barlow DH, et al. Cost-efficacy and combined treatments for panic disorder. J Clin Psychiatry 2007;68(7):1038–1044.

71. Doyle AC, Pollack MH. Establishment of remission criteria for anxiety disorders. J Clin Psychiatry 2003;64(Suppl 15):40–45.

72. Blanco C, Muhammad SR, Schneier FR, et al. The evidence-based pharmacological treatment of social anxiety disorder. Int J Neuropsychopharmacol 2003;6:427–442.

73. Prasko J, Dockery C, Horacke J, et al. Moclobemide and cognitive behavioral therapy in the treatment of social phobia. A 6-month controlled study and 24-months follow up. Neuro Endocrinol Lett 2006;27(4):473–481.

74. Stein M, Stein DJ. Social anxiety disorder. Lancet 2008;371(9618): 1115–1125.

75. Van Amerigen M, Mancini C, Patterson B, et al. An evaluation of paroxetine in generalized social anxiety disorder. Expert Opin Pharmacother 2005;6(5):819–830.

76. Bech P, Lönn SL, Overø KF. Relapse prevention and residual symptoms: A closer analysis of placebo-controlled continuation studies with escitalopram in major depressive disorder, generalized anxiety disorder, social anxiety disorder, and obsessive-compulsive disorder. J Clin Psychiatry 2010;71(2):121–129.

77. Khan-Khalid S, Santibanez MP, McMicken C, Rynn MA. Social anxiety disorder in children and adolescents: Epidemiology, diagnosis, and treatment. Pediatr Drugs 2007;9(4):227–237.

78. Book SW, Thomas SE, Randall PK, Randall CL. Paroxetine reduces social anxiety in individuals with a co-occurring alcohol use disorder. J Anxiety Disord 2008;22(2):310–318.

79. Hansen RA, Gaynes BN, Gartlehner G, et al. Efficacy and tolerability of second-generation antidepressants in social anxiety disorder. Int Clin Psychopharmacol 2008;23(3):170–179.

80. Vaishnavi S, Alamy S, Zhang W, et al. Quetiapine as monotherapy for social anxiety disorder: a placebo-controlled study. Prog Neuropsychopharmacol Biol Psychiatry 2007;31(7):1464–1469.

81. Liebowitz MR, DeMartinis NA, Weihs K, et al. Efficacy of sertraline in severe generalized social anxiety disorder: Results of a double-blind, placebo-controlled study. J Clin Psychiatry 2003;64:785–792.

82. Schneier FR, Blanco C, Campeas R, et al. Citalopram treatment of social anxiety disorder with comorbid major depression. Depress Anxiety 2003;17:191–196.

83. Jörstad-Stein EC, Heimberg RG. Social phobia: An update on treatment. Psychiatr Clin North Am 2009;32(3):641–663.

84. Lader M, Stender K, Burger V, et al. Efficacy and tolerability of escitalopram in 12-and 24-week treatment of social anxiety disorder: Randomized, double-blind, placebo-controlled, fixed-dose study. Depress Anxiety 2004;19(4):241–248.

85. Stein MB, Pollack MH, Bystritsky A, et al. Efficacy of low and higher dose extended-release venlafaxine in generalized social anxiety disorder: A 6-month randomized controlled trial. Psychopharmacology (Berl) 2005;177(3):280–288.

86. Muehlbacher M, Nickel MK, Nickel C, et al. Mirtazapine treatment of social phobia in women—a randomized, double-blind, placebo-controlled study. J Clin Psychopharmacol 2005;25:580–583.

87. Seedat S, Stein MB. Double-blind, placebo-controlled assessment of combined clonazepam with paroxetine compared with paroxetine monotherapy for generalized social anxiety disorder. J Clin Psychiatry 2004;65(2):244–248.

88. Pande AC, Feltner DE, Jefferson JN, et al. Efficacy of the novel anxiolytic pregabalin in social anxiety disorder: A placebo-controlled, multicenter study. J Clin Psychopharmacol 2004;24: 141–149.

89. Tolman RM, Himle JH, Bybee D, et al. Impact of social anxiety disorder on employment among women receiving welfare benefits. Psychiatr Serv 2009;60:61–66.

90. Davidson J, Yaryura-Tobias J, Dupont R, et al. Fluvoxamine controlled-release formulation for the treatment of generalized social anxiety disorder. J Clin Psychopharmacol 2004;24:118–125.

91. Montgomery SA, Nil R, Durr-Pal N, et al. A 24-week randomized, double-blind, placebo controlled study of escitalopram for the prevention of generalized social anxiety disorder. J Clin Psychiatry 2005;66:1270–1278.

80

Anxiety Disorders II: Posttraumatic Stress Disorder and Obsessive-Compulsive Disorder

CYNTHIA K. KIRKWOOD, LISA B. PHIPPS, AND BARBARA G. WELLS

KEY CONCEPTS

❶ The short-term goal in posttraumatic stress disorder (PTSD) is reduction in core symptoms, while the long-term goal is remission.

❷ Cognitive behavioral therapy and eye movement desensitization and reprocessing are the most effective nonpharmacologic methods to reduce symptoms of PTSD.

❸ The selective serotonin reuptake inhibitors or venlafaxine are considered first-line treatment for PTSD.

❹ An adequate trial of selective serotonin reuptake inhibitors (SSRIs) in PTSD requires appropriate dosing, titration, and duration of treatment.

❺ PTSD compares with depression in the level of disability it imposes on patients.

❻ SSRIs are the drugs of choice for the treatment of obsessive-compulsive disorder (OCD).

❼ If an inadequate response to an SSRI for OCD occurs after 4 to 6 weeks at the maximum dose, switch to another SSRI.

❽ Medication taper can be considered after 1 to 2 years of treatment in patients with OCD.

Current world and local events (e.g., wars, terrorist attacks, earthquakes, kidnappings, interpersonal violence) have placed a renewed focus on posttraumatic stress disorder (PTSD). Initially diagnosed in veterans of war, PTSD is now acknowledged as a significant psychiatric illness in the civilian population and more recently among deployed service personnel of the Afghanistan and Iraq campaigns.[1,2] PTSD continues to be poorly recognized and diagnosed in clinical practice.[3] Because of its co-occurrence with other anxiety disorders, depression, and substance abuse, the overlapping symptoms can lead to diagnostic uncertainty. Advances in the science and treatment of PTSD can assist clinicians in all fields of healthcare to screen patients for a history of trauma and effectively manage PTSD if it is present.

Intrusive obsessive thoughts and compulsive ritualistic behaviors characterize obsessive-compulsive disorder (OCD). OCD can be severely debilitating and impair functioning in social, family, and

Learning objectives, review questions, and other resources can be found at **www.pharmacotherapyonline.com**.

work settings, with an overall decrease in quality of life (QOL).[4] OCD is associated with an increased risk of suicide, with 27% of patients reporting a previous history of suicide attempt.[5] Increased understanding of symptom dimensions and treatment response can improve QOL in patients suffering from OCD.

EPIDEMIOLOGY

The estimated lifetime prevalence of PTSD is 6.8% in the U.S. population.[6] Lifetime prevalence of OCD has been estimated at 1.6% in the general population and 2% to 4% in the pediatric population.[6,7]

PTSD is associated with the incidence of trauma. It is estimated that approximately 50% of men and 60% of women are exposed to a life-threatening traumatic event. Of these individuals 8.2% of men and 20% of women will develop PTSD.[8] Previous exposure to a trauma and the intensity of response to the event increase the risk of PTSD.[8] Men tend to be assaulted more frequently, but women have a higher rate of PTSD after assault. The incidence of PTSD is equal between men and women after rape (i.e., 50%) and natural disasters (i.e., less than 5%).[8] Genetic factors can increase vulnerability to PTSD if an individual is exposed to a traumatic event. Offspring of Holocaust survivors had a higher lifetime prevalence rate of PTSD compared with a control group.[8]

The epidemiology of OCD is influenced by age and gender. OCD typically begins early in life, with 20% of cases occurring in childhood, 29% in adolescence, and 49% of cases occurring by age 20.[1] Age of onset has a bimodal distribution with peaks around 10 and 21 years.[7] The onset of illness is earlier in men than in women.[1] Higher rates of other anxiety disorders are reported in first-degree relatives of patients with OCD.[9] Early age of onset has been associated with higher probabilities of comorbid impulse-control, somatoform, eating, and tic disorders.[10] Heredity is stronger when there is an early age of onset or comorbidity with tic disorders.[11]

ETIOLOGY

The exact etiologies of PTSD and OCD are not known. It is likely that abnormalities in several areas of brain functioning interact to cause these chronic anxiety disorders. Genetics may play a role in expression of PTSD and OCD, but environmental factors likely are also involved.

OCD has been characterized as a pediatric autoimmune neuropsychiatric disorder associated with streptococcal infections (PANDAS). In response to streptococcal infection, antibodies are produced in some individuals that temporally precipitate sudden onset or exacerbation of symptoms of OCD. Neuroimaging studies suggest that in these patients the antibodies produce inflammation of the basal ganglia. This leads to increased volumes of the caudate, putamen, and the globus pallidus, and subsequently to smaller caudate volumes potentially reflective of scarring or atrophy related to streptococcal infection.[12] Although most patients with OCD do not have a streptococcal etiology, an accurate medical history regarding onset of illness is imperative because specific treatment strategies are indicated.

PATHOPHYSIOLOGY

Research findings in the areas of neuroendocrinology, neurobiology, and neuroimaging have advanced a number of theories on the pathophysiology of anxiety disorders. Neuroendocrine changes in the hypothalamic-pituitary-adrenal (HPA) axis are implicated in the pathophysiology of PTSD.[8] As reviewed in the previous chapter (Chapter 79), data from neurochemical and neuroimaging studies indicate that the modulation of normal and pathologic anxiety states is associated with multiple regions of the brain (e.g., amygdala, hippocampus, thalamus, and prefrontal cortex).[8,13] Abnormal function in several neurotransmitter systems, including norepinephrine (NE), γ-aminobutyric acid (GABA), glutamate, dopamine (DA), and serotonin (5-HT) may affect the manifestations of anxiety disorders.[8,14]

NEUROENDOCRINE THEORIES

Neuroendocrine studies provide data that abnormalities occurring pretrauma, during trauma, and posttrauma contribute to PTSD.[8] Normally the immediate reaction to stress occurs as an automatic response from the amygdala to the sympathetic and parasympathetic systems and the HPA axis. The release of corticotropin-releasing factor (CRF) stimulates cortisol secretion from the adrenal gland. Both catecholamines and cortisol levels rise in tandem. Cortisol reduces the stress response by tempering the sympathetic reaction through negative feedback on the pituitary and hypothalamus.[8] These systems return to normal after a few hours.

Recent data implicate a role for the neuropeptides CRF and neuropeptide Y (NPY) in PTSD. Patients with PTSD have a hypersecretion of CRF but demonstrate subnormal levels of cortisol at the time of trauma and chronically.[8] Lower plasma cortisol concentrations were associated with greater severity of PTSD symptoms in nonmilitary patients.[14] Dysregulation of the HPA axis is postulated to be a risk factor for eventual development of PTSD.[8] Higher plasma concentrations of NPY were found in combat-exposed men who did not develop PTSD and could play a role in resiliency.[14]

NEUROCHEMICAL THEORIES

Several neurotransmitters may be involved in the pathophysiology of PTSD. 5-HT, NE, and glutamate are associated with the processing of emotional and somatic contents of memories in the amygdala. The cortex and hippocampus are involved in storing the facts and related cues of memory.[14] The noradrenergic theory posits that the autonomic nervous system of anxious patients is hypersensitive and overreacts to stimuli. The alarm center, the locus ceruleus, releases NE to stimulate the sympathetic and parasympathetic nervous systems. Hyperactive noradrenergic signaling in patients with PTSD is a consistent research finding and includes increased 24-hour catecholamine excretion.[14] Glutamate signaling abnormalities may result in distortion of amgydala-dependent emotional processing under stress.[14] Dysregulation of the processing of sensory input and memories may contribute to the dissociative and hypervigilant symptoms in PTSD. Abnormalities of GABA inhibition may lead to increased awareness or response to stress, as seen in PTSD.[14]

Both 5-HT and DA are implicated in the pathogenesis of OCD. Selective and potent serotonergic reuptake inhibitors have consistently been shown effective for symptoms of the illness.[15–18] A recent meta-analysis concluded that higher doses of selective serotonin reuptake inhibitors (SSRIs) were associated with improved efficacy in the treatment of OCD.[18] A Cochrane systematic review of 17 studies found that SSRIs were more effective than placebo in treating symptoms of OCD, and that SSRIs were similar to each other in efficacy.[17] DA dysregulation may contribute to some forms of OCD. Neurologic symptoms (e.g., tics) are part of the clinical presentation in some patients with OCD. Tourette's disorder, a disorder of DA function, is often a concurrent disease.[1] Augmentation with antipsychotic drugs may improve symptoms in patients with OCD who are partially or nonresponsive to SSRI monotherapy.[19–21]

NEUROIMAGING STUDIES

Neuroimaging studies suggest that certain areas of the brain are altered by psychologic trauma. In PTSD most functional neuroimaging studies have involved the amygdala, ventromedial prefrontal cortex (vmPFC), and hippocampus. Findings of increased activation of the amygdala after trauma-related imagery, sounds, or smells indicate that this structure plays a role in the persistence of traumatic memory.[13] Decreased amygdala activation is correlated with resilience to PTSD and response to cognitive behavioral therapy (CBT).[13] Hypofunctioning of the vmPFC is theorized to prevent extinction in patients with PTSD and is inversely correlated with severity of symptoms.[13,22] The most consistent findings are decreased hippocampal volumes and N-acetylaspartate levels in patients with PTSD.[13,22] In twin studies, the unaffected twin of patients with PTSD also demonstrated smaller hippocampi compared with twins without PTSD.[22] These findings suggest that lower hippocampal volumes in patients with PTSD are likely a precursor associated with vulnerability for subsequent development of PTSD.[23]

Neuroimaging studies of two models suggest that dysfunction in the cortical-striatal-thalamic circuits is responsible for impulsive behavior and inability to regulate socially acceptable behaviors.[24] Drugs that decrease hyperactivity in the cortical-striatal-thalamic circuits are theorized to decrease symptoms of OCD.[25]

CLINICAL PRESENTATION

The *Diagnostic and Statistical Manual of Mental Disorders, Fourth Edition, Text Revision* classifies anxiety disorders into several categories: generalized anxiety disorder, panic disorder (with or without agoraphobia), social anxiety disorder, specific phobia, OCD, PTSD, and acute stress disorder (ASD).[1] The characteristic features of these illnesses are anxiety and avoidance behavior. Generalized anxiety disorder, panic disorder, and social anxiety disorder are discussed in Chapter 79.

CLINICAL PRESENTATION OF POSTTRAUMATIC STRESS DISORDER

Re-Experiencing Symptoms

- Recurrent, intrusive distressing memories of the trauma
- Recurrent, disturbing dreams of the event
- Feeling that the traumatic event is recurring (e.g., dissociative flashbacks)
- Physiologic reaction to reminders of the trauma

Avoidance Symptoms

- Avoidance of conversations about the trauma
- Avoidance of thoughts or feelings about the trauma
- Avoidance of activities that are reminders of the event

- Avoidance of people or places that arouse recollections of the trauma
- Inability to recall an important aspect of the trauma
- Anhedonia
- Estrangement from others
- Restricted affect
- Sense of a foreshortened future (e.g., does not expect to have a career, marriage)

Hyperarousal Symptoms

- Decreased concentration
- Easily startled
- Hypervigilance
- Insomnia
- Irritability or anger outbursts

Subtypes

- Acute: duration of symptoms is less than 3 months
- Chronic: symptoms last for longer than 3 months
- With delayed onset: onset of symptoms is at least 6 months posttrauma

_____

Data from American Psychiatric Association[1] and Ballenger et al.[23]

POSTTRAUMATIC STRESS DISORDER

Exposure to a traumatic event is required for a diagnosis of PTSD.[1] The person must have witnessed, experienced, or have been confronted with a situation that involved definite or threatened death or serious injury, or possible harm to themselves or others. The patient's response to the trauma must include intense fear, helplessness, or horror.[1] Some examples of traumatic events include physical attacks by an intimate partner, road traffic accidents, military combat exposure, natural disasters, being held hostage, child sexual abuse, and witnessing a murder or injury of another.

The resulting PTSD symptoms include persistent reexperiencing of the traumatic event, avoidance of stimuli associated with the trauma, numbing of general responsiveness, and persistent symptoms of hyperarousal. Patients must have at least one reexperiencing symptom, at least three signs or symptoms of persistent avoidance of stimuli associated with the trauma, and at least two symptoms of increased arousal.[1] Symptoms from each category need to be present for longer than 1 month and cause significant distress or impairment in functioning. Most persons diagnosed with PTSD also meet criteria for another mental disorder.[1]

Anxiety and dissociative symptoms (e.g., sense of numbing or absence of emotional responsiveness, derealization, depersonalization, inability to recall important features of the event) emerging within 1 month after exposure to a traumatic stressor are classified as ASD. Symptoms of ASD are experienced during or immediately after the trauma, last for at least 2 days, and resolve within 4 weeks.[1]

The age of onset and course of PTSD are variable. PTSD can occur at any age. The presentation is not predictable because symptoms are related to the duration and intensity of the trauma, the presence of other psychiatric disorders, and how the patient deals with the trauma. Symptoms emerge soon after a traumatic event and either dissipate or chronically persist in survivors.[26] About 95% of patients who recover do so within a year, and 40% have persistent symptoms 6 years later. PTSD co-occurs with mood, anxiety, and substance use disorders. The course of illness is fluctuating, worsening with life stressors.[26]

OBSESSIVE-COMPULSIVE DISORDER

CLINICAL PRESENTATION OF OBSESSIVE-COMPULSIVE DISORDER

Obsessions

- Repetitive thoughts (e.g., feeling contaminated after touching an object, doubting whether the stove was turned off)
- Repetitive images (e.g., recurrent sexually explicit pictures)
- Repetitive impulses (e.g., need for symmetry or putting things in specific order, impulse to shout out obscenities in a church)

Compulsions

- Repetitive activities (e.g., hand washing, checking, ordering, need to ask, need to confess)
- Repetitive mental acts (e.g., counting, repeating words silently, praying)

_____

Data from American Psychiatric Association[1] and Jenike.[27]

Patients with OCD exhibit a great variety of symptoms on presentation to clinicians. The diversity and oddity of symptoms that manifest can obscure accurate diagnosis and delay appropriate treatment of the disorder. Patients can be secretive about symptoms and purposefully refuse to report symptoms.[27] Patients can present in a seemingly incongruous manner to nonpsychiatrists for other complaints—dermatologists for eczema or chapped skin, pediatricians for parental concerns over a child's compulsive hand washing, neurologists for tics, or dentists for gum lesions from compulsive teeth brushing.

The diagnostic criteria for OCD requires the presence of obsessions and/or compulsions (although most patients have both) that are severe enough to cause marked distress, to be time-consuming (occupy more than 1 hour per day), or to cause significant impairment in social or occupational functioning.[1] An obsession is a recurrent, persistent idea, thought, impulse, or image that is experienced as intrusive and inappropriate and produces marked anxiety. Common obsessions involve thoughts about contamination (e.g., concern with germs or dirt), repeated doubts, and needing to have things in a particular order.[1]

Individuals must recognize that their obsessions or compulsions are excessive or unreasonable. Obsessions must be acknowledged as products of the individual's own mind, and attempts must be made to ignore or suppress them. The obsessions produce marked feelings of anxiety and are not simply excessive worry about a real-life situation.[1]

A compulsion is defined as a repetitive behavior or mental act generally performed in response to an obsession. The most common compulsions involve washing and cleaning, counting, checking, and requesting or demanding assurances. Diagnostically, compulsive behavior is not pleasurable and is designed to prevent discomfort or the occurrence of a dreaded event that is often unknown. For example, many patients are obsessed with feelings of doubt (e.g., whether a door was left unlocked), causing them marked distress and leading to repetitive checking (or compulsive behaviors). These behaviors are usually performed according to certain rules or in a stereotyped fashion. Because patients recognize their compulsive behavior as silly or senseless, they become extremely adept at denying symptoms, disguising their rituals, and concealing their illness from friends and family.[1]

Patients with OCD often have concurrent depression, anxiety disorders, and alcohol abuse or dependence.[27] It is a chronic illness in most patients, with severity of symptoms varying in intensity over time. Many patients with OCD have significantly impaired QOL and ability to function. Irritable bowel syndrome has been associated with OCD, with one study reporting that approximately

35% of patients with OCD met criteria for irritable bowel syndrome compared with 2.5% of a control group.[28]

TREATMENT

Posttraumatic Stress Disorder

■ DESIRED OUTCOME

① The short-term goal of therapy in the management of PTSD is reduction in core symptoms (i.e., intrusive reexperiencing, avoidance, and hyperarousal). Patients should also have improvements in disability, concurrent psychiatric conditions, and QOL. The long-term goal in PTSD is remission.[29]

■ GENERAL APPROACH TO TREATMENT

In general, patients who seek treatment acutely after a trauma and are in intense distress should receive therapy based on their presenting symptoms (e.g., a nonbenzodiazepine hypnotic for difficulty sleeping). Short courses of trauma-focused cognitive behavioral therapy (TFCBT) can be helpful to prevent chronic PTSD in patients who present during the first 3 months of the event.[23] If symptoms (e.g., hyperarousal, avoidance, dissociation, sleep difficulties, or depressed mood) persist for 3 to 4 weeks and the patient experiences marked social, occupational, and/or interpersonal impairment, they can be treated with pharmacotherapy, psychotherapy, or both. Many patients with PTSD will improve substantially with pharmacotherapy but retain some symptoms. Treatment regimens usually combine psychoeducation, psychosocial support and/or treatment, and pharmacotherapy.[23]

■ NONPHARMACOLOGIC THERAPY

Psychotherapy can be used when a patient suffers from mild symptoms, in patients who prefer not to use medications, or in conjunction with drugs in patients with severe symptoms to improve response.[23] Patients who have experienced trauma should be educated that they can experience anxiety, depression, nightmares, and even flashbacks as a normal reaction to the event.[23] Brief courses of CBT in close proximity to the traumatic event resulted in lower rates of PTSD 3 and 6 months later.[23] Single-session critical incident stress debriefing was not shown to be effective in preventing development of PTSD and actually can cause harm.[23]

② Psychotherapies for treating PTSD include stress management, TFCBT and eye movement desensitization and reprocessing (EMDR), and psychoeducation.[30] Short-term reductions in symptoms can be achieved with stress management, group therapy, hypnosis, or psychodynamic therapy.[30] Cognitive and behavioral approaches are more effective than stress management or group therapy to reduce symptoms of PTSD.[31] Either TFCBT or EMDR can be used if symptoms are evident for longer than 3 months postevent.[32] Followup studies after a 3-month course of CBT demonstrated continued benefit for 3 to 12 months.[31] An 8-week comparison found EMDR more successful in maintaining improvements in PTSD scores than fluoxetine or placebo.[33] Psychoeducation includes information about the disease state, treatment options, and avoidance of excessive use of alcohol, nicotine, and other substances of abuse.

■ PHARMACOLOGIC THERAPY

③ Antidepressants are the major pharmacotherapeutic treatment for PTSD. In addition to their efficacy in PTSD, these agents are also effective for concurrent depression and anxiety disorders. SSRIs[34] or venlafaxine are the first-line pharmacotherapy of PTSD.[29] The tricyclic

| **TABLE 80-1** | Antidepressants Used in the Treatment of Posttraumatic Stress Disorder |||

Class/Generic Name	Starting Dose	Dosage Range (mg/day)
Selective serotonin reuptake inhibitors		
Citalopram[a]	20 mg/day	20–60[b]
Escitalopram	5 or 10 mg/day	10–20[b]
Fluoxetine[a]	10 mg/day	10–60[b]
Fluvoxamine[a]	50 mg/day	100–300[b]
Paroxetine[a]	10–20 mg/day	20–50[c]
Sertraline[a]	25 mg/day	50–200[c]
Other agents		
Amitriptyline[a]	25 or 50 mg/day	50–300[b]
Imipramine[a]	25 or 50 mg/day	50–300[b]
Mirtazapine[a]	15 mg/night	15–60[b]
Phenelzine	15 or 30 mg every night	15–90[b]
Venlafaxine extended-release[a]	37.5 mg/day	37.5–300[b]

[a]Available generically.
[b]Dosage used in clinical trials but not FDA approved.
[c]Dosage is FDA approved.
Date from Ballenger et al.[23] International Psychopharmacology Algorithm Project,[29] Paxil [package insert],[35] and Zoloft [package insert][36].

antidepressants (TCAs) and monoamine oxidase inhibitors (MAOIs) can also be effective, but they have less favorable side-effect profiles (Table 80–1). Sertraline and paroxetine are both approved for the acute treatment of PTSD,[35,36] and sertraline is approved for the long-term (i.e., 52 weeks) management of PTSD.[36] A number of drugs can be used as augmentation agents (e.g., antiadrenergic drugs and atypical antipsychotics).[29] Benzodiazepines are not effective for PTSD.[23,29] A number of treatment guidelines are published (see Stein et al., 2009 for review).[37] An algorithm from the International Psychopharmacology Algorithm Project for the treatment of PTSD appears in Figure 80–1.

Special Populations

Children who experience stress and trauma (e.g., sexual or physical abuse or loss of a parent) are predisposed to develop mood and anxiety disorders. SSRIs are the initial pharmacologic agents of choice in this patient population. Psychotherapy is also a treatment option (e.g., play therapy).[38]

Antidepressant Therapy

Selective Serotonin Reuptake Inhibitors SSRIs act pharmacologically to enhance serotonergic functioning. Large prospective studies documented the efficacy of sertraline and paroxetine in the acute management of PTSD. In a 12-week trial sertraline was effective across the spectrum of PTSD-specific, global, and functional outcome measures. Approximately 60% of the patients improved on symptom clusters of arousal and avoidance/numbing but not on reexperiencing.[39] Sixty percent of patients with PTSD receiving a paroxetine dose of 20 mg/day and 54% of patients receiving 40 mg/day responded; response was not related to dose.[40] In a flexible-dose trial, paroxetine significantly improved all three PTSD symptom clusters and disability compared with placebo at 12 weeks.[41] Fluoxetine showed efficacy in a placebo-controlled trial,[42] and fluvoxamine[43] and escitalopram[44] were efficacious in open trials in acute PTSD. In a comparison between sertraline and citalopram, PTSD symptoms improved significantly in both groups, but sertraline was significantly better in reducing avoidance/numbing than citalopram.[45] In general, SSRIs reduced the numbing symptoms of PTSD, whereas other drugs have not. Adverse reactions reported in patients with PTSD treated with SSRIs include gastrointestinal symptoms, sexual dysfunction, insomnia, and agitation. The results

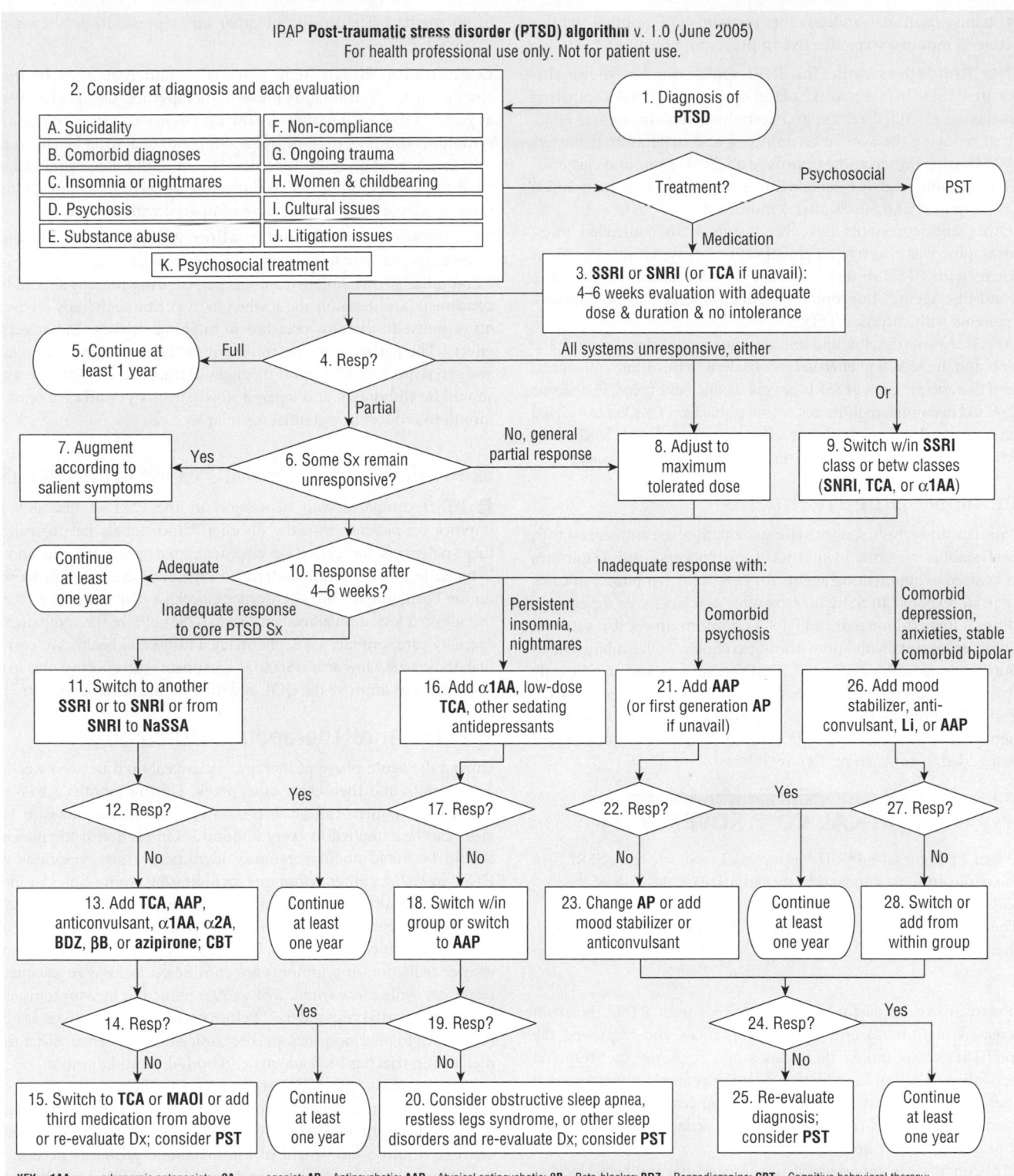

FIGURE 80-1. Algorithm for the pharmacotherapy of posttraumatic stress disorder. Levels of evidence (LOE): 1 = more than one adequately powered placebo-controlled trial (i.e., n = 30 per group or greater); 2 = one or more small placebo-controlled trials of monotherapy, combination or augmentation therapy; 3 = case series or open-label trials; 4 = either no published evidence, or presence of clinical consensus. LOE: Node 3 – LOE 1 (sertraline, paroxetine, fluoxetine); LOE 2 (mirtazapine, TCAs, MAOIs); LOE 3 (citalopram); LOE 4 (fluvoxamine); Node 7 – LOE 2 (prazosin, nefazodone, TCAs); LOE 3 (trazodone); Node 9 – LOE 4; Node 13 – Aggression, LOE 2 (prazosin, risperidone, olanzapine), Insomnia/nightmares, LOE 3 (trazodone), Anxiety/agitation, LOE 2 (risperidone), LOE 3 (olanzapine, buspirone), LOE 4 (tiagabine, β-blockers, α2-agonists); Node 15 – LOE 4; Node 16 – LOE 2, 3 (prazosin); LOE 4 (trazodone, TCAs, olanzapine, mirtazapine, quetiapine, zolpidem); Node 18 – LOE 4; Node 21 – LOE 2 (risperidone), LOE 3 (olanzapine, quetiapine) LOE 4 (SSRIs, anticonvulsants, antiadrenergics); Node 23 – LOE 4; Node 26 – LOE 4; Node 28 – LOE 4 (α1AA, α₁-adrenergic antagonist; α2A, α₂-agonist; AP, antipsychotic; AAP, atypical antipsychotic; βB, beta-blocker; BDZ, benzodiazepine; CBT, cognitive behavioral therapy; Dx, diagnosis; Li, lithium; MAOI, monoamine oxidase inhibitor; NaSSA, noradrenergic and selective serotonergic antidepressant; PST, psychosocial treatment; PTSD, posttraumatic stress disorder; Resp, response; SNRI, serotonin and norepinephrine reuptake inhibitor; SSRI, selective serotonin reuptake inhibitor; Sx, symptoms; TCA, tricyclic antidepressant.) *(Data from International Psychopharmacology Algorithm Project.29)*

of two long-term trials indicate that sertraline (12 months) and flu-oxetine (9 months) were effective in preventing relapse.[45,46]

Other Antidepressants The SNRI venlafaxine has shown efficacy in PTSD. In a 12-week, placebo-controlled trial comparing venlafaxine extended-release and sertraline, venlafaxine was effective in reducing the avoidance/numbing and hyperarousal clusters of PTSD, whereas sertraline improved all PTSD symptom clusters.[47] The remission rates for venlafaxine extended-release were 30.2% after 12 weeks[41] and 50.1% after 6 months.[48]

Other antidepressants have been studied in controlled trials. Mirtazapine was effective on global ratings of symptoms in 64% of patients with PTSD in doses up to 45 mg/day and is considered a second-line agent.[49] Bupropion sustained-release was not effective in patients with chronic PTSD.[50]

The TCAs amitriptyline and imipramine are considered second-line agents and the MAOI phenelzine is considered a third-line antidepressant if therapeutic trials of SSRIs or venlafaxine have failed. Phenelzine decreased insomnia, nightmares, and flashbacks. TCAs are associated with a higher burden of adverse effects compared with SSRIs (e.g., daytime drowsiness, toxicity in overdose, and poor compliance).[29]

Alternative Drug Treatments

Atypical antipsychotics, α_1-adrenergic antagonists, antidepressants, mood stabilizers, anticonvulsants, beta-blockers, and azapirones can be used as augmenting agents for persistent symptoms, in cases of partial response to SSRI therapy after 4–6 weeks, or for comorbidities.[29] Risperidone reduced PTSD symptoms in combat veterans on antidepressants with and without psychosis.[51] Olanzapine added adjunctively to SSRIs decreased PTSD symptoms and significantly improved sleep compared with placebo. Patients gained an average of 13.2 pounds (6 kg) over the course of the 8-week trial.[51] Quetiapine reduced core PTSD symptoms over a 8-week period when added to concurrent therapy.[52]

CLINICAL CONTROVERSY

When a patient with PTSD has a partial response to an SSRI the clinician must choose whether to increase the dose of the SSRI, augment with a second agent, or do both simultaneously. There are no published guidelines to direct clinicians with this therapeutic dilemma.

Prazosin can be useful in some patients with PTSD. Prazosin decreased nightmares and sleep disturbances and improved the core PTSD symptoms in daily doses of 1 to 4 mg. Its presumed mechanism of action is reduction of noradrenergic transmission.[53] Other options for persistent sleep disturbances with less evidence include trazodone, mirtazapine, low dose sedating TCAs, atypical antipsychotics, and zolpidem.[29]

Anticonvulsants, mood stabilizers, buspirone, and beta-blockers can assist in managing aggression.[29]

Dosage and Administration

Acute Phase PTSD symptoms respond slowly to pharmacotherapy, and some patients never experience full resolution. SSRIs should be started 3 to 4 weeks after exposure to a trauma in patients with no improvement in their acute stress response.[23] The initiation of an SSRI should be at a low dose with gradual titration upward toward antidepressant doses. ❶ Six to 12 weeks is an appropriate duration of antidepressant therapy to determine response.[29,54]

The dose of sertraline can be increased in weekly intervals by 50 mg/day up to a maximum dosage of 200 mg/day. Paroxetine can be increased by 10 mg/day in weekly intervals to a target dose

of 40 mg/day. The dosing of other antidepressants is shown in Table 80–1.

Continuation Phase Many patients are undergoing psychotherapy during the continuation phase of therapy, and dosages can vary as patients deal with past traumatic experiences. During this phase symptoms continue to improve, and the maximal drug benefit (i.e., improvement of disability) accrues.[54] Six-month relapse prevention trials in patients responsive to fluoxetine or sertraline indicate low rates of relapse with SSRI therapy compared with placebo.[54]

Maintenance and Discontinuation Patients with PTSD who respond to pharmacotherapy should continue treatment for at least 12 months.[29,54] If residual symptoms persist, drug therapy should be continued. The decision about when to discontinue therapy is based on response to therapy, presence of ongoing stresses, and adverse effects. The patient must be confident in the discontinuation plan and can require extra support throughout the process. Drug therapy should be withdrawn and tapered slowly over a period of at least 1 month to reduce the potential for relapse.

■ PHARMACOECONOMIC CONSIDERATIONS

❺ PTSD compares with depression in the level of disability it imposes on patients with the disorder.[55] Individuals fail to realize their potentials for career development, marriage, and education. Women in a healthcare maintenance organization with high scores on the Posttraumatic Stress Disorder Checklist had more than twice the adjusted total annual median cost ($1,283) of care (i.e., outpatient, specialty care, primary care, pharmacy and mental healthcare costs) than those with a low score ($609).[56] Treatment with effective pharmacotherapy can improve the QOL and functioning of these patients.[55]

Evaluation of Therapeutic Outcomes

During the acute phase of therapy, patients should be seen weekly for a month and then every other week. During months 3 to 6 of therapy, the patient can be seen monthly, and in months 6 to 12, visits can be extended to every 2 months. On each visit the patient should be asked about previously identified target symptoms of PTSD as well as other symptoms including insomnia, suicidal ideation, anger outbursts, irritability, psychosis, ongoing trauma, and disability. A remission in patients with PTSD is defined as a 70% or greater reduction in symptoms. Patients who have a 50% response or greater reduction in symptoms are considered to have an adequate response, while those with a 25% to 50% reduction in symptoms are considered partial responders.[29] Before deciding that a patient is not responsive to pharmacotherapy, the clinician should ensure that the medication trial has been adequate in both dose and duration.

Many patients with PTSD are sensitive to the adverse effects of drugs.[29] They should be monitored carefully for adverse reactions that can delay the escalation of drug dosages or cause the patient distress. Routine assessment of the metabolic profile is necessary if an atypical antipsychotic is used concurrently.[29] When pharmacotherapy is discontinued, patients should be seen more frequently and monitored carefully for signs of relapse or withdrawal.

TREATMENT

Obsessive-Compulsive Disorder

■ DESIRED OUTCOMES

Major goals of therapy for OCD include reduction in the frequency and severity of obsessive thoughts and time spent performing compulsive acts. Treatment for OCD generally does not completely eliminate obsessions or compulsions, but patients can feel remarkably improved with partial resolution of symptoms. Optimal treatment increases psychosocial and occupational functioning and improves overall QOL. Efforts should be made to minimize adverse drug events and prevent drug interactions.

■ GENERAL APPROACH TO TREATMENT

It is important at the outset of therapy to identify and document the specific target symptoms for pharmacotherapy. Rating scales can be used to measure symptom severity at baseline and during treatment to ascertain the degree of improvement. The Yale-Brown Obsessive-Compulsive Scale (YBOCS) is the most widely used clinician-administered scale. A QOL scale can assist the clinician in identifying other areas to target for treatment (e.g., depression and reduced physical well-being).[57]

The Food and Drug Administration (FDA) has approved five antidepressants for the management of OCD: clomipramine, fluoxetine, fluvoxamine, paroxetine, and sertraline. CBT and SSRIs are considered effective first-line treatment modalities.[58] Initial therapy may include CBT alone, SSRI monotherapy, or the combination of CBT and an SSRI, and is based on clinical judgment of symptom severity and patient preferences.[58] CBT alone can be used in cooperative patients who do not desire drug therapy, or those with mild anxiety or depressive symptoms. Patients unable to participate in CBT or with a prior history of medication therapy response should be treated with SSRI monotherapy. Combined CBT and SSRIs is recommended in patients with failure on an SSRI alone or in those with severe OCD. If a combination of CBT and an SSRI is unsuccessful, another SSRI should be tried before augmentation therapy. If there is no response or partial response to combined CBT and three adequate antidepressant trials (one of which is clomipramine), augmentation with another drug and more intensive CBT can be tried.[58] Augmentation with antipsychotics has proven efficacious in patients with partial response.[19–21,58]

CLINICAL CONTROVERSY

Patients with OCD who fail to respond to an initial trial of an SSRI are often switched to another SSRI. It is known that these patients are less likely to respond to venlafaxine.[58] There is a lack of data to predict the chance of response when switching to other medications such as mirtazapine or another SSRI.

Table 80–2 is a summary of key points from the treatment guidelines for OCD. Although some OCD symptoms can improve over the first few weeks of therapy, an adequate trial of any medication is considered to be 8 to 12 weeks at maximum tolerated dosage.

■ NONPHARMACOLOGIC TREATMENTS

A number of nonpharmacologic treatments are effective for OCD. CBT with behavioral techniques (e.g., exposure and response prevention [ERP], psychodynamic psychotherapy, and psychoanalysis) are the most common initial nonpharmacologic treatments of choice. Initially, 13-20 sessions are recommended. Clinicians can use motivational interviewing techniques to assist patients with treatment acceptance.[58]

Other options are transcranial magnetic stimulation (TMS), deep brain stimulation (DBS), and ablative neurosurgery. DBS is FDA-approved as a humanitarian device for severe, treatment-resistant OCD.[59] TMS and DBS should not be used alone as first-line

TABLE 80-2	Summary of Key Points in Treatment Guidelines for OCD	
Recommendation	**Level of Evidence**	**Comments**
First-line treatments		
CBT alone	I	13–20 sessions
SSRI alone	I	8–12 wk, at least 4–6 wk at maximum tolerated dose
CBT + SSRI	I	13–20 CBT sessions and 8–12 wk SSRI with 4–6 wk at maximum tolerated dose. If monotherapy with CBT or SSRI alone does not provide adequate response, combination therapy with CBT + SSRI should be tried before augmentation with another pharmacological agent
Second-line treatments		
Switch to another SSRI or clomipramine	I	
Augmentation with antipsychotic	II	
Third-line treatments		
Switch to another antipsychotic augmenting agent	II	
Augmentation of SSRI with clomipramine	III	
Maintenance and discontinuation phase		
After 1–2 years, gradual taper over several months	I	
Periodic CBT booster sessions for 3–6 months	II	

Levels of evidence:
[I] Recommended with substantial clinical confidence.
[II] Recommended with moderate clinical confidence.
[III] May be recommended on the basis of individual circumstances.
Data from American Psychiatric Association.[58]

treatments but may be added to CBT or used in refractory patients. Surgery should be reserved for rare cases.[58] Effects of ERP have been reported to last up to two years.[60]

■ PHARMACOLOGIC THERAPY

Practice Guidelines for the treatment of patients with OCD were published by the American Psychiatric Association.[58]

❻ SSRIs are considered to be the drugs of choice for OCD.[58] While not FDA approved, escitalopram has also shown efficacy in reduction of OCD symptoms.[61] Clomipramine, a TCA with strong 5-HT reuptake inhibition, is also FDA approved for the treatment of OCD. Clomipramine has an active metabolite, desmethylclomipramine, which inhibits norepinephrine reuptake.[62] Meta-analytic findings of greater efficacy of clomipramine than SSRIs are not consistent with comparative trial data.[58]

Alternative Drug Treatments

Recent studies have examined the use of ondansetron, dextroamphetamine, caffeine, and D-cycloserine as possible augmentation agents in refractory OCD patients with mixed results. A study of ondansetron found 9 of 14 patients with OCD responded to ondansetron augmentation therapy.[63] In a study of caffeine and dextroamphetamine augmentation, YBOCS score decreases ranged from 20% to 80% in the dextroamphetamine group and 27% to 89% in the caffeine group.[64] The number of exposure sessions necessary in patients treated with D-cycloserine was reduced compared with placebo initially.[65] These alternative treatments are reserved for refractory patients.[58]

Special Populations

Children and Adolescents OCD affecting children and adolescents is prevalent. There are symptom and treatment similarities and differences between OCD developing earlier in life and that which develops later. Younger patients exhibit poorer insight regarding obsessions, have more obsessions involving fear of harm and separation, and possess more rituals involving family members.[66] CBT provided in the group setting has been shown to be effective and is an alternative to individual CBT or medication treatment.[67] CBT weekly or daily and including family members has also been effective.[68] CBT and SSRI treatment are considered first-line for pediatric patients.[69]

Clomipramine, fluvoxamine, sertraline, paroxetine and fluoxetine are approved by the FDA for treatment of OCD in children and adolescents.[58] Childhood and adult OCD appear to respond similarly to drug therapy. SSRIs are effective and well tolerated in the treatment of OCD and are generally considered first-line agents.[58] Treatment with an SSRI produces a favorable response in 75% of children and adolescents with OCD. A combination of SSRI and CBT is preferred in most cases.[70] In children, the most commonly described side effects of SSRI therapy include nausea, headache, tremor, gastrointestinal complaints, drowsiness, akathisia, insomnia, disinhibition, and agitation.[70] The starting dose of clomimpramine in children is 25 mg daily in divided doses. The dose can be increased over the first 2 weeks up to 3 mg/kg or 100 mg, whichever is smaller. Over the next several weeks, the dose can be increased up to 3 mg/kg with a maximum of 200 mg daily.[62]

Hepatic and Renal Disease Clomipramine, fluoxetine, sertraline, paroxetine, fluvoxamine, and citalopram are extensively metabolized in the liver, and patients with significant liver disease should be prescribed these drugs cautiously and in lower doses than those used in healthy subjects. The pharmacokinetics of sertraline are not altered in patients with significant renal dysfunction, and dosage adjustment is not necessary in these patients.[36] Increased plasma concentrations of paroxetine occur in subjects with renal impairment.[35] The initial dose of paroxetine should be reduced in patients with severe renal impairment, and upward titration should occur more slowly.[35] No dosage adjustment is necessary for patients with renal impairment receiving clomipramine.[62]

Elderly Little information is available on treating OCD in the elderly. Case reports and anecdotal information suggest that the anti-obsessional drugs are likely to be equally effective in the elderly and in younger adults.[71] Selection of medication for an elderly person with OCD, however, should be based on history of response and adverse side-effect profile. Treatment should be initiated with low doses in elderly patients, and doses should be increased slowly, with vigilance for emergence of side effects.[58] Because of clomipramine's sedative and anticholinergic side effects, it is not usually chosen as first-line therapy for elderly OCD patients.[58] The safety of fluvoxamine has not been adequately studied in the elderly and patients with cardiovascular disease. Dosage should be reduced and titrated slowly during initiation of fluvoxamine therapy in elderly patients.

Sertraline plasma clearance in elderly patients was approximately 40% lower than in a group of younger individuals. Clearance of desmethylsertraline was also decreased in elderly men but not in elderly women.[36] In a multiple-dose study in the elderly, the minimal concentrations of paroxetine were 70% to 80% greater than in nonelderly subjects. The manufacturer recommends that the initial dose be reduced in the elderly (10 mg/day), and total daily doses should not exceed 40 mg.[35] The use of SSRIs in elderly patients is discussed in Chapter 77.

Pregnancy Risk-benefit analysis should be made by practitioners when deciding to use pharmacotherapy options during pregnancy.[58] The use of SSRIs in pregnancy and lactation is discussed in the chapter on depression (Chapter 77).

Antidepressant Therapy

Serotonergic Antidepressants The only potent 5-HT reuptake inhibitors consistently demonstrating efficacy in controlled trials are the TCA clomipramine and the SSRIs fluoxetine, fluvoxamine, paroxetine, and sertraline. Forty percent to 60% of patients with OCD respond to a serotonergic antidepressant. Improvement in symptoms is incomplete, and ranges from 20% to 40%. Most patients continue to have symptoms that limit their functioning.[27] Ten to 12 weeks constitute an adequate treatment period.[27]

Current evidence indicates that 5-HT is important for the anti-obsessional effects of medication. SSRIs and clomipramine inhibit 5-HT reuptake into the presynaptic neuron. Inhibiting reuptake of 5-HT makes more 5-HT available to postsynaptic receptors and reduces formation of the 5-HT metabolite 5-hydroxyindoleacetic acid. Although other antidepressants, such as imipramine and amitriptyline, inhibit 5-HT reuptake, they are less potent and selective than SSRIs. Prolonged exposure to increased amounts of 5-HT after chronic antidepressant treatment (2–3 weeks) leads to altered responsiveness of postsynaptic 5-HT receptors or presynaptic autoregulatory receptors that govern 5-HT release in specific brain regions. An improvement in obsessional symptoms may correlate with plasma concentrations of clomipramine but not desmethylclomipramine, the metabolite of clomipramine with less selectivity for 5-HT reuptake inhibition.

Most experts agree that SSRIs are better tolerated than clomipramine. SSRIs are less likely to cause cardiovascular, sedative, anticholinergic, and weight-gain side effects. Clomipramine is less likely than SSRIs to cause insomnia, akathisia, nausea, and diarrhea. Antidepressant side effects can be more severe when larger doses are used and with faster dose escalation. Tolerance to antidepressant adverse effects often develops over 6 to 8 weeks of treatment, and tolerance is more likely to develop to nausea, diarrhea, sedation, diminished libido and/or orgasm, anxiety, restlessness, insomnia, and anticholinergic side effects than to akathisia.[71]

Pharmacokinetics Clomipramine is rapidly absorbed following oral administration. Maximum plasma concentrations occur within 3 to 8 hours. It is highly protein-bound (greater than 90%) in the blood and has a half-life of 15 hours.[71] The drug is metabolized to desmethylclomipramine, which is pharmacologically active. The pharmacokinetics of SSRIs are discussed in Chapter 77.

Efficacy SSRIs are effective in the treatment of OCD. Well-designed trials comparing these medications with placebo, head-to-head comparative trials, and meta-analyses have established that fluoxetine, fluvoxamine, paroxetine, sertraline, citalopram, and escitalopram are equally effective and that clomipramine may be somewhat more effective.[15,61]

Other Antidepressants Venlafaxine, which acts as a serotonin and norepinephrine reuptake inhibitor, may be effective for OCD.[71]

Augmentation with Antipsychotics Augmentation of SSRI treatment with low doses of risperidone, quetiapine, or olanzapine may be helpful. Typical antipsychotics are generally not recommended because of an increased likelihood of extrapyramidal symptoms.[71,72] Risperidone, quetiapine, and olanzapine augmentation has the most evidence with response rates in the range of 40% to 50%.[19–21,58]

TABLE 80-3	Dosing of Serotonin Reuptake Inhibitors in the Treatment of Obsessive-compulsive Disorder		
Generic Name	Usual Initial Daily Dose (mg)	Usual Target Daily Dose (mg)	Usual Maximum Daily Dose (mg)
Citalopram[a,b]	20	40–60	80
Clomipramine[a]	25	100–250	250
Escitalopram[b]	10	20	40
Fluoxetine[a]	20	40–60	80
Fluvoxamine[a]	50	200	300
Paroxetine[a]	20	40–60	60
Sertraline[a]	50	200	200

[a]Available generically.
[b]Not FDA approved for treatment of obsessive-compulsive disorder. Optimal dosing guidelines are not well established.
Data from American Psychiatric Association Practice Guideline,[58] Paxil package insert,[35] Zoloft package insert,[36] and Anafranil package insert.[62]

Dosage and Administration Table 80–3 summarizes dosing guidelines for SSRIs and clomipramine. If there is inadequate response to an average dose, then it should be incrementally increased to the maximum dose within 5 to 9 weeks from the start of treatment. ❼ If there is an inadequate response after 4 to 6 weeks at the maximum dose, then another SSRI should be tried.[58] Eight to 12 weeks is considered an adequate trial before changing to another drug or augmenting with another agent.

Although the appropriate maintenance dose of antidepressants is unknown, it is notable that one investigator was successful in reducing the dose of clomipramine from a mean of 270 mg/day to 165 mg/day in the maintenance phase.[73]

■ PHARMACOECONOMIC CONSIDERATIONS

The annual outpatient direct cost for treatment of OCD in the United States in 1995 was $5.1 billion. In 1990, the total cost to the economy was $8 billion, which included expenditures for direct ($2.1 billion) and indirect costs. Direct costs included costs of hospitalization, outpatient professional services, and drugs. Indirect costs were costs associated with lost productivity, work loss, early retirement, and absenteeism. As OCD frequently has its onset in childhood or adolescence, loss of income over a lifetime is substantial.[74]

Another pharmacoeconomic consideration that impacts the provision of optimal treatment for patients with OCD relates to inability to pay for nonpharmacologic therapy. Although CBT has been shown to be a very effective modality, very often the patient cannot afford this therapy or does not have medical insurance that helps pay the associated costs.

■ EVALUATION OF THERAPEUTIC OUTCOMES

Target symptoms of OCD should be monitored closely. The degree of response can indicate a need to modify dosage, change drug, or augment therapy. Rating scales can be used to monitor symptom response to therapy for OCD (e.g., YBOCS) and changes in QOL. The clinician should inquire about and address problematic adverse effects (including the emergence of suicidal ideation) reported by the patient. Changes in social and occupational functioning should be assessed.

Patients older than 40 years of age should receive a pretreatment electrocardiogram before starting clomipramine. In patients with liver disease, baseline and periodic liver function tests are recommended when clomipramine is used. Patients receiving clomipramine who develop fever and sore throat should have leukocyte and differential white blood cell counts assessed to evaluate for agranulocytosis.

After patients have responded to the acute phase of treatment, treatment gains are maintained with maintenance-phase strategies.

❽ Monthly follow-up visits are recommended for at least 3 to 6 months, and a medication taper can be considered after 1 to 2 years of treatment. Medication should not be rapidly discontinued, and booster CBT sessions can reduce the risk of relapse when medication is withdrawn. The drug dosage can be decreased by 10% to 25% every 1 to 2 months with careful observation for symptom relapse.[58] Some patients require lifelong medication therapy.

CONCLUSIONS

The past decade has brought a renewed interest in the recognition and management of PTSD. Healthcare workers are sensitized to the devastating effects that PTSD can have on patient functioning and QOL. Adequately detecting and appropriately managing PTSD is important to improving the lives of patients who suffer from this illness. Data on the efficacy of SSRIs, SNRIs, and various augmenting agents support their use in achieving treatment remission. SSRIs are the first-line pharmacotherapy of PTSD and OCD. Research in OCD has resulted in new pharmacologic treatment strategies, especially with augmentation therapies.

ABBREVIATIONS

ASD: acute stress disorder

CBT: cognitive behavioral therapy

CRF: corticotrophin-releasing factor

DA: dopamine

DBS: deep brain stimulation

EMDR: eye movement desensitization and reprocessing

ERP: exposure and response prevention

FDA: U.S. Food and Drug Administration

5-HT: serotonin

GABA: γ-aminobutyric acid

HPA: hypothalamic-pituitary-adrenal

MAOI: monoamine oxidase inhibitor

NE: norepinephrine

NPY: neuropeptide Y

OCD: obsessive-compulsive disorder

PANDAS: pediatric autoimmune neuropsychiatric disorder associated with streptococcal infection

PTSD: posttraumatic stress disorder

QOL: quality of life

SNRI: serotonin-norepinephrine reuptake inhibitor

SSRI: selective serotonin reuptake inhibitor

TCA: tricyclic antidepressant

TFCBT: trauma-focused cognitive behavioral therapy

TMS: transcranial magnetic stimulation

vmPFC: ventromedial prefrontal cortex

YBOCS: Yale-Brown Obsessive Compulsive Scale

REFERENCES

1. American Psychiatric Association. Diagnostic and Statistical Manual of Mental Disorders, Fourth Edition, Text Revision. Washington, DC: American Psychiatric Association, 2000:429–484.

2. Hoge CW, Auchterlonie JL, Milliken CS. Mental health problems, use of mental health services, and attrition from military services after returning from Iraq or Afghanistan. JAMA 2006;295:1023–1032.

3. Lecrubier Y. Posttraumatic stress disorder in primary care: A hidden diagnosis. J Clin Psychiatry 2004;65(Suppl 1):49–54.

4. Eisen JL, Mancebo MA, Pinto A, et al. Impact of obsessive compulsive disorder on quality of life. Compr Psychiatry 2006;47:270–275.

5. Kamath P, Reddy YC, Kandavel T. Suicidal behavior in obsessive-compulsive disorder. J Clin Psychiatry 2007;68:1741–1750.

6. Kessler RC, Berglund P, Olga D, et al. Lifetime prevalence and age-of-onset distributions of DSM-IV disorders in the National Comorbidity Survey Replication. Arch Gen Psychiatry 2005;62:593–602.

7. Geller D. Obsessive-compulsive and spectrum disorders in children and adolescents. Psychiatr Clin North Am 2006;29:353–370.

8. Yehuda R. Risk and resilience in posttraumatic stress disorder. J Clin Psychiatry 2004;65(Suppl 1):29–36.

9. Grabe HJ, Ruhrmann S, Ettelt S, et al. Familiality of obsessive–compulsive disorder in nonclinical and clinical subjects. Am J Psychiatry 2006;163:1986–1992.

10. de Mathis MA, do Rosario MC, Diniz, JB, et al. Obsessive–compulsive disorder: Influence of age at onset on comorbidity patterns. European Psychiatry 2008;23:187–194.

11. Miguel EC, Leckman JF, Rauch S, et al. Obsessive–compulsive disorder phenotypes: Implications for genetic studies. Mol Psychiatry 2005;10:258–275.

12. Snider LA, Swedo SE. PANDAS: Current status and directions for research. Mol Psychiatry 2004;9:900–907.

13. Shin LM, Liberzon I. The neurobiology of fear, stress and anxiety disorders. Neuropsychopharmacology 2010;35:169–191.

14. Martin EI, Ressler KJ, Binder E, Nemeroff CB. The neurobiology of anxiety disorders: Brain imaging, genetics and psychoneuroendocrinology. Psychiatr Clin North Am 2009;32:549–575.

15. Rabinowitz I, Baruch Y, Barak Y. High-dose escitalopram for the treatment of obsessive-compulsive disorder. Int Clin Psychopharmacol 2008;23:49–53.

16. Koran LM, Aboujaoude E, Ward H, et al. Pulse-loaded intravenous clomipramine in treatment-resistant obsessive-compulsive disorder. J Clin Psychopharmacol 2006;26(1):79–83.

17. Soomro GM, Altman D, Rajagopal S, Oakley-Browne M. Selective serotonin re-uptake inhibitors (SSRIs) versus placebo for obsessive compulsive disorder (OCD). Cochrane Database Syst Rev 2008;(1):CD001765.

18. Bloch MH, McGuire J, Landeros-Weisengerger A, et al. Meta-analysis of the dose-response relationship of SSRIs in obsessive-compulsive disorder. Mol Psychiatry 2009 May 26 [Epub ahead of print]. doi:10.1038/mp.209.50.

19. Li X, May RS, Tolbert LC, et al. Risperidone and haloperidol augmentation of serotonin reuptake inhibitors in refractory obsessive-compulsive disorder: A crossover study. J Clin Psychiatry 2005;66:736–743.

20. Diniz J, Shavitt R, Pereira C, et al. Quetiapine versus clomipramine in the augmentation of selective serotonin reuptake inhibitors for the treatment of obsessive-compulsive disorder: A randomized, open-label trial. J Psychopharmacol 2010;24(3):297–307.

21. Vulink NC, Denys D, Fluitman SB, et al. Quetiapine augments the effect of citalopram in non-refractory obsessive-compulsive disorder: A randomized, double-blind, placebo-controlled study of 76 patients. J Clin Psychiatry 2009;70:1001–1008.

22. Rauch SL, Shin LM, Phelps EA. Neurocircuitry models of posttraumatic stress disorder and extinction: Human neuroimaging research—Past, present and future. Biol Psychiatry 2006;60:376–382.

23. Ballenger JC, Davidson JRT, Lecrubier Y, et al. Consensus statement update on posttraumatic stress disorder from the International Consensus Group on Depression and Anxiety. J Clin Psychiatry 2004;65(Suppl 1):55–62.

24. Friedlander L, Desrocher M. Neuroimaging studies of obsessive-compulsive disorder in adults and children. Clin Psychol Rev 2006;26:32–49.

25. Hollander E, Koran LM, Abramowitz JS. Obsessive-compulsive disorder: Strategies for optimal treatment. J Clin Psychiatry 2008;69:1647–1657.

26. Shalev AY. Posttraumatic stress disorder and stress-related disorders. Psychiatr Clin North Am 2009;32:687–704.

27. Jenike MA. Obsessive-compulsive disorder. N Engl J Med 2004;350:259–265.

28. Masand PS, Keuthen NJ, Gupta S, et al.. Prevalence of irritable bowel syndrome in obsessive-compulsive disorder. CNS Spectr 2006;11:21–25.

29. International Psychopharmacology Algorithm Project: Post-traumatic Stress Disorder, 2005. http://www.ipap.org/ptsd/index.htp.

30. Work Group on ASD and PTSD. Practice guideline for the treatment of patients with acute stress disorder and posttraumatic stress disorder. Am J Psychiatry 2004;161(11 Suppl):1–61.

31. Bisson J, Andrew M. Psychological treatment of post-traumatic stress disorder (PTSD). Cochrane Database Syst Rev 2005;2:CD003388. doi:10.1002/1465/14651858.CD003388.pub2.

32. National Institute for Clinical Excellence. Post-traumatic stress disorder (PTSD): The management of PTSD in adults and children in primary and secondary care. Clinical Guideline 26 March 2005. http://www.nice.org.uk/CG26/guidance/pdf/English.

33. van der Kolk BA, Spinazzola J, Blausteìn ME, et al. A randomized clinical trial of eye movement desensitization and reprocessing (EMDR), fluoxetine, and pill placebo in the treatment of posttraumatic stress disorder: Treatment effects and long-term maintenance. J Clin Psychiatry 2007;68:37–46.

34. Stein DJ, Ipser JC, Seedat S. Pharmacotherapy for post traumatic stress disorder (PTSD). Cochrane Database Syst Rev 2006;1:CD002795. doi:10.1002/1264/1858.CD002795.pub2.

35. Paxil [package insert]. Research Triangle Park, NC: GlaxoSmithKline; August 2009.

36. Zoloft [package insert]. New York, NY: Pfizer, Inc.; January 2009.

37. Stein DJ, Ipser J, McAnda N. Pharmacotherapy of posttraumatic stress disorder: A review of meta-analyses and treatment guidelines. CNS Spectr 2009;14:1(Suppl 1):25–31.

38. Ipser JC, Stein DJ, Hawkridge S, Hoppe L. Pharmacotherapy for anxiety disorders in children and adolescents. Cochrane Database Sys Rev 2009(3):CD005170. doi:10.1002/14651858.CD005170.pub2.

39. Brady K, Pearlstein T, Asnis GM, et al. Efficacy and safety of sertraline treatment of posttraumatic stress disorder: A randomized controlled trial. JAMA 2000;283:1837–1844.

40. Marshall RD, Beebe KL, Oldham M, Zaninelli R. Efficacy and safety of paroxetine treatment for chronic PTSD. A fixed-dose, placebo-controlled study. Am J Psychiatry 2001;158:1982–1988.

41. Tucker P, Zaninelli R, Yehuda R, et al. Paroxetine in the treatment of chronic posttraumatic stress disorder: Results of a placebo-controlled, flexible-dosage trial. J Clin Psychiatry 2001;62:860–868.

42. Martenyi F, Brown EB, Zhang H, et al. Fluoxetine versus placebo in posttraumatic stress disorder. J Clin Psychiatry 2002;63:199–206.

43. Tucker P, Smith KL, Marx B, et al. Fluvoxamine reduces physiologic reactivity to trauma scripts in posttraumatic stress disorder. J Clin Psychiatry 2000;20:367–372.

44. Robert S, Hamner MB, Ulmer HG, et al. Open-label trial of escitalopram in the treatment of posttraumatic stress disorder. J Clin Psychiatry 2006;67:1522–1526.

45. Tucker P, Potter-Kimball R, Wyatt DB, et al. Can physiologic assessment and side effects tease out differences in PTSD trials? A double-blind comparison of citalopram, sertraline, and placebo. Psychopharmacol Bull 2003;37:135–149.

46. Davidson JRT, Pearlstein T, Londborg P, et al. Efficacy of sertraline in preventing relapse of posttraumatic stress disorder: Results of a 28-week double-blind, placebo-controlled study. Am J Psychiatry 2001;158:1974–1981.

47. Davidson J, Rothbaum BO, Tucker P, et al. Venlafaxine extended release in posttraumatic stress disorder: A sertraline- and placebo-controlled study. J Clin Psychopharmacol 2006;26:259–267.

48. Davidson J, Baldwin D, Stein DJ, et al. Treatment of posttraumatic stress disorder with venlafaxine extended release: A 6-month randomized controlled trial. Arch Gen Psychiatry 2006;63:1158–1165.

49. Davidson JRT, Weisler RH, Butterfield MI, et al. Mirtazapine versus placebo in posttraumatic stress disorder: A pilot study. Biol Psychiatry 2003;53:188–191.

50. Becker ME, Hertzberg MA, Moore SD, et al. A placebo-controlled trial of bupropion SR in the treatment of chronic posttraumatic stress disorder. J Clin Psychopharmacol 2007;27:193–197.

51. Pae C, Lim H, Peindl K, et al. The atypical antipsychotics olanzapine and risperidone in the treatment of posttraumatic stress disorder: A meta-analysis of randomized, double-blind, placebo-controlled clinical trials. Inter Clin Psychopharmacol 2008;23:1–8.

52. Ahern EP, Mussey M, Johnson C, et al. Quetiapine as an adjunctive treatment for post-traumatic stress disorder: An 8-week open-label study. Int Clin Psychopharmacol 2006;21:29–33.

53. Raskind MA, Peskind ER, Kanter ED, et al. Reduction of nightmares and other PTSD symptoms in combat veterans by prazosin: A placebo controlled study. Am J Psychiatry 2003;160:371–373.

54. Davidson JRT. Pharmacologic treatment of acute and chronic stress following trauma. J Clin Psychiatry 2006;67(Suppl 2):34–39.

55. Seedat S, Lochner C, Vythilingum B, Stein DJ. Quality of life in posttraumatic stress disorder: Impact of drug treatment. Pharmacoeconomics 2006;24:989–998.

56. Walker EA, Katon W, Russo J, et al. Health care costs associated with posttraumatic stress disorder symptoms in women. Arch Gen Psychiatry 2003;60:369–374.

57. Rush A, First M, Blacker D, Handbook of Psychiatric Measures. 2nd Edition. Washington, DC: American Psychiatric Association, 2008. http://www.R2library.com/marc_frame.aspx? Resource ID = 1127.

58. American Psychiatric Association. Practice guideline for the treatment of patients with obsessive-compulsive disorder. Arlington, VA: American Psychiatric Association, 2007. http://www.psych.org/psych_pract/treatg/pg/prac_ guide.cfm.

59. Reclaim DBS [professional labeling]. Minneapolis: MN, Medtronics, Inc.; 2009.

60. Abramowitz J. The psychological treatment of obsessive-compulsive disorder. Can J Psychiatry 2006;51:407–416.

61. Dougherty DD, Jameson M, Deckersbach T, et al. Open-label study of high (30 mg) and moderate (20 mg) dose escitalopram for the treatment of obsessive-compulsive disorder. Inter Clin Psychopharmacol 2009;24:306–311.

62. Anafranil [package insert]. Hazelwood, MO: Mallinckrodt Inc.; May 2007.

63. Pallanti S, Bernardi S, Antonini S, et al. Ondansetron augmentation in treatment-resistant obsessive-compulsive disorder: A preliminary, single-blind, prospective study. CNS Drugs 2009;23:1047–1055.

64. Koran LM, Aboujaoude E, Gamel NN. Double-blind study of dextroamphetamine versus caffeine augmentation for treatment-resistant obsessive-compulsive disorder. J Clin Psychiatry 2009;70:1530–1535.

65. Kushner MG, Kim SW, Donahue C, et al. D-cycloserine augmented exposure therapy for obsessive-compulsive disorder. Biol Psychiatry 2007;62:835–838.

66. Geller DA. Obsessive-compulsive and spectrum disorders in children and adolescents. Psychiatr Clin North Am 2006;29:353–370.

67. Asbahr FR, Castillo AR, Ito LM, et al. Group cognitive-behavioral therapy versus sertraline for the treatment of children and adolescents with obsessive-compulsive disorder. J Am Acad Child Adolesc Psychiatry 2005;44:1128–1136.

68. Storch EA, Geffken GR, et al. Family-based cognitive-behavioral therapy for pediatric obsessive-compulsive disorder: Comparison of intensive and weekly approaches. J Am Acad Child Adolesc Psychiatry 2007;46:469–478.

69. Kalra SK, Swedo SE. Children with obsessive-compulsive disorder: Are they just "little adults"? J Clin Invest 2009;119:737–746.

70. Thomsen PH. Obsessive-compulsive disorder: Pharmacologic treatment. Eur Child Adolesc Psychiatry 2000;9(Suppl 1):176–184.

71. Denys D. Pharmacotherapy of obsessive-compulsive disorder and obsessive-compulsive spectrum disorders. Psychiatr Clin North Am 2006;29:553–584.

72. Blier P, Habib R, Flament MF. Pharmacotherapies in the management of obsessive-compulsive disorder. Can J Psychiatry 2006;51:417–430.

73. Mundo E, Bareggi SR, Pirola R, et al. Long-term therapy of obsessive-compulsive disorder: A double-blind controlled study. J Clin Psychiatry 1997;17:4–10.

74. Hollander E, Stein DJ, Kwon JH, et al. Psychosocial function and economic costs of obsessive-compulsive disorder. CNS Spectr 1997;2:16–25.

81

Sleep Disorders

JOHN M. DOPP AND BRADLEY G. PHILLIPS

KEY CONCEPTS

❶ Common causes of insomnia include concomitant psychiatric disorders, significant psychosocial stressors, excessive alcohol use, caffeine intake, and nicotine use.

❷ Good sleep hygiene, including relaxing before bedtime, exercising regularly, establishing a regular bedtime and wake-up time, and discontinuing alcohol, caffeine, and nicotine, alone and in combination with drug therapy, should be part of patient education and treatments for insomnia.

❸ Long-acting benzodiazepines should be avoided in the elderly.

❹ Benzodiazepine tolerance and dependence are avoided by using low-dose therapy for the shortest possible duration.

❺ Obstructive sleep apnea may be an independent risk factor for the development of hypertension. When hypertension is present, it is often refractory to drug therapy until sleep-disordered breathing is alleviated.

❻ Nasal continuous positive airway pressure is the first-line therapy for obstructive sleep apnea, and weight loss should be encouraged in all obese patients.

❼ Pharmacologic management of narcolepsy is focused on two primary areas: treatment of excessive daytime sleepiness and cataplexy.

❽ Short-acting benzodiazepine receptor agonists or melatonin taken at appropriate target bedtimes for east or west travel reduce jet lag and shorten sleep latency.

❾ Dopamine agonists are effective for restless legs syndrome and have replaced levodopa as first-line therapy.

Approximately 70 million Americans suffer with a sleep-related problem, and as many as 60% of those experience a chronic disorder.[1] In a study by the National Institute of Aging, of 9,000 patients age 65 years and older, more than 80% report a sleep-related disturbance.[1]

INTRODUCTION TO SLEEP

SLEEP CYCLES

Sleep is divided into two phases: nonrapid eye movement (NREM) sleep and rapid eye movement (REM) sleep. Humans typically experience four to six cycles of NREM and REM sleep, with each cycle lasting between 70 and 120 minutes.[2] There are four stages of NREM sleep. Healthy sleep will typically progress through the four stages of NREM sleep prior to the first REM period. From wakefulness, sleep typically progresses quickly through stages 1 and 2. Stage 1 of NREM sleep is the stage between wakefulness and sleep, and individuals describe this experience as being awake, being drowsy, or being asleep. During stages 3 and 4 NREM, both metabolic activity and brain waves slow. This slow-wave sleep occurs most frequently early in the sleep period. Stage 3 and stage 4 sleep are called *delta sleep*, as the sleep is characterized by high-amplitude slow activity known as delta waves (0.5–3 Hz). In this stage eye movements are absent, and muscle tone is atonic.[3]

REM sleep involves a dramatic physiologic change from NREM sleep, to a state in which the brain becomes electrically and metabolically activated.[2] REM occurs in bursts and is accompanied by a 62% to 173% increase in cerebral blood flow, generalized muscle atonia, bursts of bilateral rapid eye movements, poikilothermia, dreaming, and fluctuations in respiratory and cardiac rate.[2] REM cycles tend to lengthen in the later stages of the sleep cycle.[2]

CIRCADIAN RHYTHM

At birth human infants spend up to 20 hours a day sleeping. At 3 to 6 months of age there is a differentiation between REM and NREM sleep. By age 3 the ultradian sleep–wake rhythm changes to a circadian pattern. The suprachiasmatic nucleus of the brain serves as the biologic clock and paces the circadian rhythm. Although the length of a day is 24 hours, in environments devoid of light cues, the sleep–wake cycle lasts 24.2 hours.[3] In midlife, there is a gradual decline in sleep efficiency and sleep time.[2] The elderly have lighter and more fragmented sleep, with intermittent arousals, shifts in the sleep stages, and a gradual reduction of slow wave sleep.

NEUROCHEMISTRY

The neurochemistry of sleep is complex as sleep cannot be localized to either a specific area of the brain or a neurotransmitter. NREM sleep appears to be controlled by the basal forebrain, the area surrounding the solitary tract in the medulla and the dorsal raphe nucleus, which is primarily serotonergic.[3] Sleep is reduced when there are decreases in serotonin or destruction of the dorsal raphe nucleus in the brainstem, which contains most of the brain's serotonergic bodies. REM sleep appears to be turned on by cholinergic cells in the mesencephalic, medullary, and pontine gigantocellular regions. REM sleep appears to be turned off by the dorsal raphe nucleus, the locus coeruleus, and the nucleus parabrachialis lateralis, the latter two of which are primarily noradrenergic. The ascending reticular activating system and the posterior hypothalamus facilitate arousal and wakefulness.[4] Dopamine has an alerting effect; decreases in dopamine promote sleepiness.[5] Neurochemicals involved in wakefulness include norepinephrine and acetylcholine in the cortex and histamine and neuropeptides such as substance P and corticotropin-releasing factor in the hypothalamus.[5,6]

POLYSOMNOGRAPHY

Sleep is typically measured and observed in sleep laboratories using an electroencephalogram (EEG), electro-oculograms of each eye, electrocardiogram, electromyogram, air thermistors, abdominal and thoracic strain belts, and oxygen saturation monitor. This study is named polysomnography (PSG) and is used to assess and record variables that characterize sleep and aid in diagnosis of sleep disorders. Variables obtained during PSG include sleep onset, arousals, sleep stages, eye movements, leg and jaw movements, arrhythmias, airflow during sleep, respiratory effort, and oxygen desaturations.

CLASSIFICATION OF SLEEP DISORDERS

The *Diagnostic and Statistical Manual of Mental Disorders, Fourth Edition, Text Revision (DSM-IV-TR)* classifies sleep disorders into four categories based on etiology and requires a minimum of 1 month before a sleep disorder can be diagnosed.[7,8] Primary sleep disorders are those disorders in which there is no other etiology (mental disorder, substance-related disorder, or medical condition) responsible for the disorder. Primary sleep disorders appear to be based on an endogenous abnormality of the sleep–wake cycle, or circadian rhythm, and they are divided into dyssomnias (abnormality in the amount, quality, or timing of sleep) or parasomnias (abnormal behavioral or physiologic events associated with sleep, e.g., sleepwalking and REM behavior disorder). Dyssomnias include sleep disorders such as insomnia, narcolepsy, obstructive sleep apnea, and circadian rhythm disorders.

INSOMNIA

Insomnia is the most common complaint in general medical practice.[9] It causes distress, frequently because of a fear or a feeling of not being able to fall asleep at bedtime, and can impair work-related productivity because of daytime fatigue or drowsiness. Insomnia is subjectively characterized as a complaint of difficulty falling asleep, difficulty maintaining sleep, or experiencing nonrestorative sleep.[8] Insomnia lasting two or three nights because of jet lag, for example, is considered to be transient insomnia, whereas short-term insomnia usually resolves in less than 3 weeks. Insomnia, according to the *DSM-IV-TR*, is considered to be chronic when it lasts longer than 1 month.[8]

Epidemiology

Primary insomnia usually begins in early or middle adulthood and is rare in childhood or adolescence. More than 50% of the population complains of insomnia in their lifetime.[1] A 1-year prevalence study of insomnia in the United States reports that one third of the individuals surveyed complained of insomnia, and 17% reported that the symptoms were serious.[1] Conservative estimates of chronic

insomnia range from 9% to 12% in adulthood and up to 20% in the elderly.[1,10] Although young adults are more likely to complain that they have difficulty falling asleep, middle-aged and elderly adults are more likely to complain that they have middle-of-the-night awakening or early morning awakening. Women complain of insomnia twice as frequently as men. Individuals who are elderly, unemployed, separated, or widowed, and those with a lower socioeconomic status reported a significantly higher incidence of insomnia than the general population. Forty percent of individuals with insomnia also had a concurrent psychiatric disorder (anxiety, depression, or substance abuse).[9]

Despite the prevalence of insomnia, only 5% of individuals seek medical attention for management of their insomnia. Approximately 10% to 20% of those with insomnia use nonprescription drugs or alcohol to self-treat. Of the 3% of the population who are prescribed sedative–hypnotics for insomnia, 11% report use exceeding 1 year.[11]

Differential Diagnosis

Primary insomnia is considered to be an endogenous disorder caused by either a neurochemical or a structural disorder affecting the sleep–wake cycle. Individuals with primary insomnia can be light sleepers who are easily aroused by noise, temperature, or anxiety. Some studies suggest that primary insomnia is a "hyperarousal state," in that insomnia patients have increased metabolic rates compared with controls and thus take longer to fall asleep.[2] Comorbid insomnia is frequently a symptom or manifestation of another medical disorder. Evaluation of patients with a complaint of transient or short-term insomnia should focus on recent stressors, such as a separation, a death in the family, a job change, or college exams.

❶ Chronic insomnia is frequently comorbid with psychiatric or medical conditions. A complete diagnostic examination should be completed in these individuals and should include routine laboratory tests, physical and mental status examinations, as well as ruling out any medication- or substance-related causes.[12] Special consideration should also be given to other sleep disorders that can have a similar presentation, including restless legs syndrome, periodic limb movements of sleep, and sleep apnea. Common causes of insomnia are listed in Table 81–1.

TABLE 81-1	Common Etiologies of Insomnia
Situational	
Work or financial stress, major life events, interpersonal conflicts	
Jet lag or shift work	
Medical	
Cardiovascular (angina, arrhythmias, heart failure)	
Respiratory (asthma, sleep apnea)	
Chronic pain	
Endocrine disorders (diabetes, hyperthyroidism)	
Gastrointestinal (gastroesophageal reflux disease, ulcers)	
Neurologic (delirium, epilepsy, Parkinson disease)	
Pregnancy	
Psychiatric	
Mood disorders (depression, mania)	
Anxiety disorders (e.g., generalized anxiety disorder, obsessive-compulsive disorder)	
Substance abuse (alcohol or sedative-hypnotic withdrawal)	
Pharmacologically induced	
Anticonvulsants	
Central adrenergic blockers	
Diuretics	
Selective serotonin reuptake inhibitors	
Steroids	
Stimulants	

TREATMENT

Insomnia

Therapeutic management of insomnia is initially based on whether the individual has experienced a transient, short-term, or chronic sleep disturbance. Clinical history should assess the onset, duration, and frequency of the symptoms; effect on daytime functioning; sleep hygiene habits; and history of previous symptoms or treatment.[13] Management of all patients with insomnia should include identifying the cause of the insomnia, patient education on sleep hygiene, and stress management. Any unnecessary pharmacotherapy should be eliminated.[10] Transient insomnia, which occurs as a result of an acute stressor, is expected to resolve quickly and should be treated with good sleep hygiene and careful use of sedative-hypnotics.[14] Short-term insomnia, associated with situational, personal, or medical stress can be treated similarly.[13] Chronic insomnia requires careful assessment for possible underlying medical causes, nonpharmacologic techniques, and careful use of sedative-hypnotics.[12]

■ NONPHARMACOLOGIC THERAPY

❷ In many cases insomnia can be treated without sedative-hypnotics. Education about normal sleep and habits for good sleep hygiene are often sufficient interventions.[2] Nonpharmacologic interventions for insomnia frequently consist of short-term cognitive behavioral therapies, most commonly stimulus control therapy, sleep restriction, relaxation therapy, cognitive therapy, paradoxical intention, and education on good sleep hygiene (Table 81–2).[10,15,16] In patients age 55 and older, research indicates that cognitive behavioral therapy may be more effective than pharmacologic therapy at improving certain measures of insomnia.[17]

CLINICAL CONTROVERSY

Pharmacologic treatment is indicated for transient and short-term insomnia. Historically, the use of sedative hypnotic agents for greater than 1 month was frowned on and discouraged in fear of fostering drug dependence. Experts now agree that clinicians should encourage hypnotic therapy using the lowest effective dose for the shortest duration possible. However, long-term use of hypnotics is not contraindicated unless the patient has another contraindication (e.g., history of substance abuse, pregnancy, etc.).

■ PHARMACOLOGIC THERAPY

Miscellaneous Agents

Antihistamines exhibit sedating properties and are included in many over-the-counter sleep agents. They are effective in the treatment of mild insomnia and are generally safe.[13] Diphenhydramine and doxylamine are more sedating than pyrilamine. Increasing the dose of antihistamines will not produce a linear increase in response. The safety and efficacy of antihistamines over placebo have been documented in several studies. Antihistamines are considered to be less effective than benzodiazepines, and they have the disadvantages of anticholinergic side effects, which are especially troublesome in the elderly.[13,18]

Antidepressants are alternatives for patients with nonrestorative sleep who should not receive benzodiazepines, especially those who have depression, pain, or a risk of substance abuse. Using

TABLE 81-2 Nonpharmacologic Recommendations for Insomnia

Stimulus control procedures
1. Establish regular times to wake up and go to sleep (including weekends).
2. Sleep only as much as necessary to feel rested.
3. Go to bed only when sleepy. Avoid long periods of wakefulness in bed. Use the bed only for sleep or intimacy; do not read or watch television in bed.
4. Avoid trying to force sleep; if you do not fall asleep within 20–30 minutes, leave the bed and perform a relaxing activity (e.g., read, listen to music, or watch television) until drowsy. Repeat this as often as necessary.
5. Avoid daytime naps.
6. Schedule worry time during the day. Do not take your troubles to bed.

Sleep hygiene recommendations
1. Exercise routinely (three to four times weekly) but not close to bedtime because this can increase wakefulness.
2. Create a comfortable sleep environment by avoiding temperature extremes, loud noises, and illuminated clocks in the bedroom.
3. Discontinue or reduce the use of alcohol, caffeine, and nicotine.
4. Avoid drinking large quantities of liquids in the evening to prevent nighttime trips to the restroom.
5. Do something relaxing and enjoyable before bedtime.

antidepressants for insomnia without depression is common but not well studied, and the doses used for treating insomnia are not effective antidepressant doses.[18] Sedating antidepressants such as amitriptyline, doxepin, and nortriptyline are effective for inducing sleep continuity, although daytime sedation and side effects can be significant.[18] Anticholinergic activity, adrenergic blockage, and cardiac conduction prolongation can be problematic, especially in the elderly and in overdose situations.[18] Mirtazapine is a sedating antidepressant that may help patients sleep, but it may also cause daytime sedation and weight gain.

Trazodone in doses of 25 to 100 mg at bedtime is sedating and can improve sleep continuity.[11] Trazodone is popular for the treatment of insomnia in patients prone to substance abuse, as dependence is not a problem. Trazodone is frequently used in patients with selective serotonin reuptake inhibitor (SSRI) and bupropion-induced insomnia.[11] Caution should be used to avoid serotonin syndrome when used in these combinations. Other side effects include carryover sedation and α-adrenergic blockade. Orthostasis can occur at any age, but it is more dangerous in the elderly. Priapism is a rare but serious side effect.[19]

Ramelteon is a melatonin receptor agonist approved for the treatment of sleep onset insomnia. Ramelteon is selective for the MT1 and MT2 melatonin receptors that are thought to regulate the circadian rhythm and sleep onset. The recommended dose is 8 mg taken at bedtime to induce sleep. Although generally well tolerated, the most common adverse events reported are headache, dizziness, and somnolence. Ramelteon is not a controlled substance and can be a viable option for patients with a history of substance abuse.

Valerian is an herbal sleep remedy that has been studied for its sedative-hypnotic properties in patients with insomnia. The mechanism of action is not fully understood but may involve increasing concentrations of γ-aminobutyric acid (GABA). The recommended dose for insomnia ranges from 300 to 600 mg. An equivalent dose of dried herbal valerian root is 2 to 3 g soaked in 1 cup of hot water for 20 to 25 minutes.[20]

CLINICAL CONTROVERSY

The over-the-counter supplement melatonin is a popular treatment for insomnia. Although melatonin has demonstrated efficacy for inducing sleep, its use for the treatment of insomnia is not well supported by clinical studies. Further research is needed before melatonin can be recommended for the treatment of insomnia.

TABLE 81-3 Pharmacokinetics of Benzodiazepine Receptor Agonists

Generic Name (Brand Name)	t_{max}(Hours)[a]	Half-Life[b] (Hours)	Daily Dose Range (mg)	Metabolic Pathway	Clinically Significant Metabolites
Estazolam (ProSom)	2	12–15	1–2	Oxidation	–
Eszopiclone (Lunesta)	1–1.5	6	2–3	Oxidation Demethylation	–
Flurazepam (Dalmane)	1	8	15–30	Oxidation N-dealkylation	Hydroxyethylflurazepam, flurazepam aldehyde N-desalkylflurazepam[c]
Quazepam (Doral)	2	39	7.5–15	Oxidation, N-dealkylation	2-Oxo-quazepam, N-desalkylflurazepam[c]
Temazepam (Restoril)	1.5	10–15	15–30	Conjugation	–
Triazolam (Halcion)	1	2	0.125–0.25	Oxidation	–
Zaleplon (Sonata)	1	1	5–10	Oxidation	–
Zolpidem (Ambien)	1.6	2–2.6	5–10	Oxidation	–

[a]Time to peak plasma concentration.
[b]Half-life of parent drug.
[c]N-desalkylflurazepam, mean half-life 47 to 100 hours.

Benzodiazepine Receptor Agonists

The most commonly used treatments for insomnia have been the benzodiazepine receptor agonists. All benzodiazepine receptor agonists are effective as sedative-hypnotics and are FDA labeled for the treatment of insomnia (Table 81–3). The FDA recently required benzodiazepine receptor agonist labeling to include a caution regarding anaphylaxis, facial angioedema, and complex sleep behaviors (e.g., sleep driving, phone calls, sleep eating, etc.). The benzodiazepine receptor agonists consist of the newer nonbenzodiazepine GABA$_A$ agonists and the traditional benzodiazepines. All benzodiazepine receptor agonists bind to GABA$_A$ receptors in the brain, resulting in stimulatory effects on GABAergic transmission and hyperpolarization of neuronal membranes. Traditional benzodiazepines have sedative, anxiolytic, muscle relaxant, and anticonvulsant properties; newer nonbenzodiazepine GABA agonists possess only sedative properties.

Benzodiazepine Hypnotics

Benzodiazepines relieve insomnia by reducing sleep latency and increasing total sleep time. Benzodiazepines increase stage 2 sleep while decreasing REM, stage 3, and stage 4 sleep.[11] Benzodiazepine hypnotics should not be prescribed for individuals who are pregnant or who have untreated sleep apnea or a history of substance abuse. Patients should be instructed to avoid alcohol and other CNS depressants.

Pharmacokinetics The choice of a particular benzodiazepine can be based on its pharmacokinetic profile. When used as a single dose, extent of distribution and elimination half-life are important in predicting the duration of action. However, after multiple doses, the elimination half-life and formation of active metabolites determine the extent of drug accumulation and resultant clinical effects.[11] Advanced age, liver dysfunction, and drug interactions can prolong drug effects. The pharmacokinetic profiles of benzodiazepine receptor agonists are summarized in Table 81–3.

Adverse Effects Side effects are dose dependent and vary according to the pharmacokinetics of the individual benzodiazepine. High doses with long or intermediate elimination half-lives have a greater potential for producing daytime sedation, psychomotor incoordination, decreased concentration, and cognitive deficits. Tolerance to benzodiazepine hypnotic effects develops sooner with triazolam (after 2 weeks of continuous use) than with other benzodiazepine hypnotics.[11] Most traditional benzodiazepines maintain hypnotic efficacy for 1 month. However, tolerance can develop with time. Rapidly eliminated benzodiazepines have less potential for daytime sedation.[11]

Anterograde amnesia, an impairment of memory and recall of events occurring after the dose is taken, has been reported with most benzodiazepine receptor agonists.[11] Rebound insomnia, characterized by increased wakefulness beyond baseline amounts that last for 1 to 2 nights after abrupt discontinuation, occurs with benzodiazepine receptor agonists. Rebound insomnia occurs more frequently after high doses of triazolam, even when ingested intermittently.[11] The lowest effective dosage should be used to minimize rebound insomnia and avoid adverse effects on memory.

❸ Benzodiazepine half-lives are prolonged in older patients, increasing the potential for drug accumulation and the incidence of CNS side effects, including prolonged sedation and cognitive and psychomotor impairment. Benzodiazepine receptor agonists with long elimination half-lives are generally not first-line agents in these patients. There is an association between falls and hip fractures and the use of benzodiazepines with long elimination half-lives; thus flurazepam and quazepam should be avoided in elderly patients.[21]

Nonbenzodiazepine GABA$_A$ Agonists

Zolpidem, zaleplon, and eszopiclone are nonbenzodiazepine hypnotics that selectively bind to GABA$_A$ receptors and effectively induce sleepiness. Zolpidem, an imidazopyridine chemically unrelated to benzodiazepines or barbiturates, has a duration of action of 6 to 8 hours.[22] It is comparable in efficacy to benzodiazepine hypnotics and is effective for reducing sleep latency and nocturnal awakenings and increasing total sleep time. It does not appear to have significant effects on next-day psychomotor performance. A sustained release formulation of zolpidem is now available that is effective at increasing total sleep time and reducing wakefulness after sleep onset without significant carryover sedation.

The safety and efficacy of zolpidem for insomnia is similar to that of the benzodiazepines. Zolpidem is less disruptive of sleep stages than benzodiazepines. Adverse effects are dose related and can include drowsiness, amnesia, dizziness, headache, and gastrointestinal complaints.[22] Several cases of brief psychotic reactions have been reported in women, and recent reports of sleep-eating during zolpidem therapy have caused significant weight gain.[22] The recommended daily dose of zolpidem is 10 mg or 5 mg in elderly patients and those with hepatic impairment. The dosage can be increased to 20 mg per night.[22] Because food decreases its absorption, zolpidem should be taken on an empty stomach.[23]

Zaleplon is a pyrazolopyrimidine and has a rapid onset of action and a half-life of 1 hour, and it is metabolized to inactive metabolites.[24] It is effective for decreasing time to sleep onset but not for reducing nighttime awakening or for increasing total sleep time.[25] Because of its short half-life, zaleplon has no effect on next-day psychomotor performance and can be best used as a sleep aid for middle-of-the-night awakenings.[26] The recommended dose is 10 mg in adults and 5 mg in the elderly.[24] The most common adverse effects with zaleplon are dizziness, headache, and somnolence. There are two drug interactions of note: zaleplon plasma levels are increased when combined with cimetidine and decreased with rifampin.[22]

Eszopiclone is a pyrrolopyrazine hypnotic with a rapid onset of action and a half-life of 5 to 6 hours.[27] It is effective at reducing time to sleep onset, wake time after sleep onset, and number of awakenings, and increasing total sleep time and sleep quality. Eszopiclone's duration of action is up to 6 hours,[27] so it can be a better option for treatment of sleep maintenance insomnia or early morning awakenings than zaleplon. The most common adverse effects with eszopiclone are somnolence, unpleasant taste, headache, and dry mouth.[28] Eszopiclone is labeled for long-term use and may be taken nightly for up to 6 months.[28]

Other Considerations

In general, the nonbenzodiazepine hypnotics seem to be associated with less withdrawal, tolerance, and rebound insomnia than the benzodiazepine hypnotics. None of the nonbenzodiazepine $GABA_A$ agonists have significant active metabolites.

■ EVALUATION OF THERAPEUTIC OUTCOMES

An algorithm for the evaluation and treatment of sleep disorders is shown in Figure 81–1. Patients with short-term or chronic insomnia should be evaluated after 1 week of therapy to assess for drug efficacy, adverse effects, and adherence to nonpharmacologic recommendations.

Patients should be instructed to keep a sleep diary. The diary requires daily recording of bedtime, wake time, latency of sleep onset, number and duration of awakenings, medication ingestion, naps, and an index of sleep quality. For patients with chronic insomnia, possible medical, psychiatric, and pharmacologic causes should be identified and managed.[11] Patients with insomnia should receive education about possible medication side effects and their management. Prescriptions for benzodiazepine receptor agonists should be accompanied by printed information and verbal counseling on precautions.

❹ Clinicians should educate patients about the concepts of tolerance, withdrawal, and rebound insomnia. Tolerance and dependence can be avoided by using hypnotics at the lowest possible dose, intermittently, and for the shortest duration possible. Patients should receive instruction on the initiation of therapy about frequency of drug use and the expected duration of therapy, to help prevent development of dependence. Withdrawal symptoms can be diminished by tapering the dosage gradually.

SLEEP APNEA

Approximately 15 million Americans have sleep-disordered breathing.[29] The prevalence of sleep apnea in the U.S. adult population is 4% in males and 2% in females.[30] It appears to be more common in African Americans and less common in Asian populations. Sleep apnea also occurs in children and adolescents. It is characterized by repetitive episodes of cessation of breathing during sleep followed by blood oxygen desaturation and brief arousal from sleep to restart breathing. As a result, individuals with sleep apnea experience fragmented sleep, poor sleep architecture, and periods of apnea

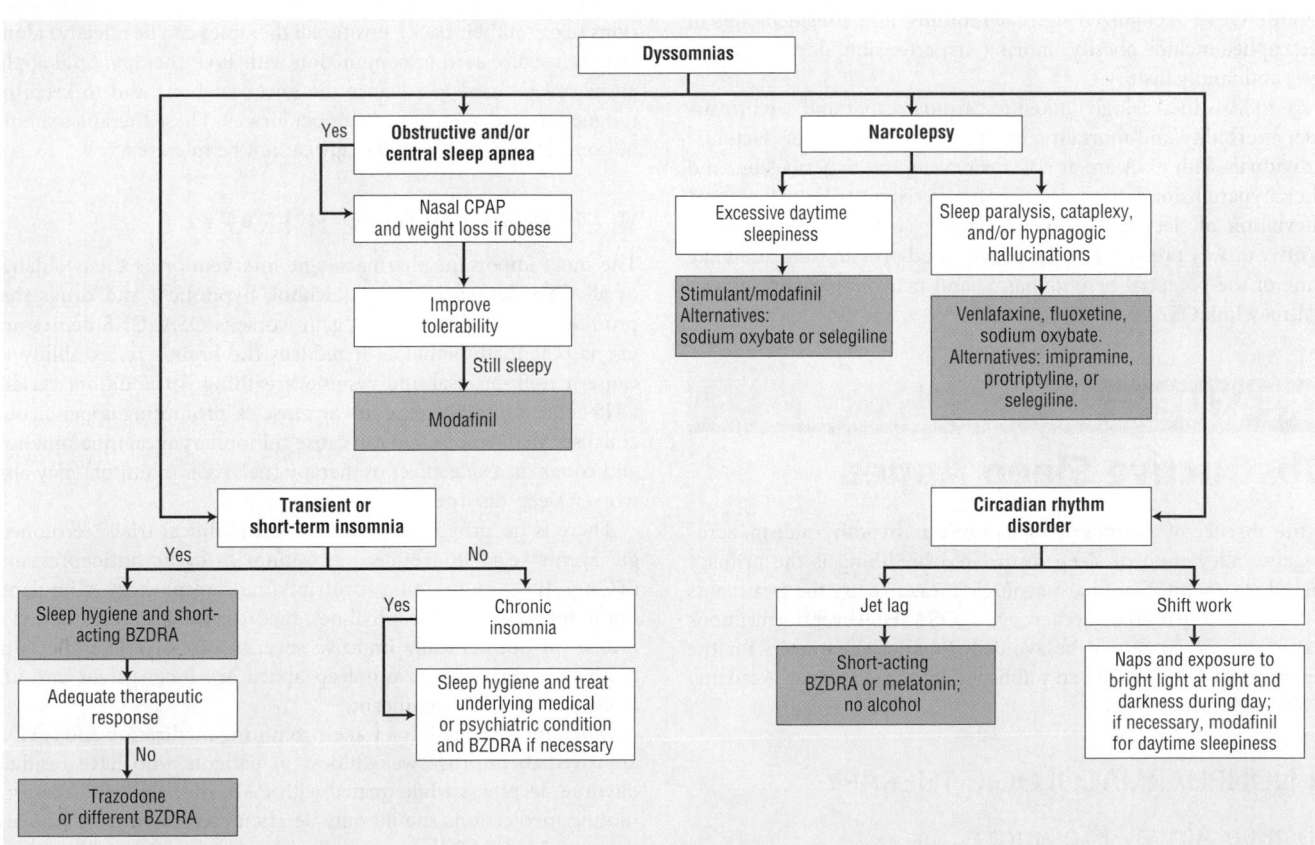

FIGURE 81-1. Algorithm for treatment of dyssomnias. (BZDRA, benzodiazepine receptor agonist; CPAP, continuous positive airway pressure.) *(Modified with permission from Jermaine DM. Sleep Disorders. In: Carter BL, Angaran DM, Lake KD, Raebel MA, eds. Pharmacotherapy Self-Assessment Program, 2nd ed. Neurology and Psychiatry. Kansas City: American College of Clinical Pharmacy, 1995;146–147.)*

and hypopnea. Polysomnography (PSG) is used to diagnose and quantify sleep apnea as central, obstructive, or mixed. Central sleep apnea (CSA) involves impairment of the respiratory drive, whereas obstructive sleep apnea (OSA) is caused by upper airway collapse and obstruction. Patients with mixed sleep apnea experience both central and obstructive sleep apnea. Severity of sleep apnea is determined by the number of apnea (total cessation of airflow) and hypopnea (partial airway closure with blood oxygen desaturation) episodes documented by PSG, and is expressed by calculating the respiratory disturbance index (RDI). Mild sleep apneics have an RDI of between 5 and 15 episodes per hour, moderate 15 to 30, whereas individuals with severe OSA can exhibit more than 30 episodes per hour.

Sleep apnea can affect behavior, cognitive abilities, and systemic disease.[31] Neurocognitive sequelae are important factors in motor vehicle accidents, loss of work-related productivity, and personality changes.[31,32] Alleviation of sleep disordered breathing can have a beneficial impact on both cardiovascular and neurobehavioral conditions.[33]

OBSTRUCTIVE SLEEP APNEA

OSA is characterized by partial or complete closure of the upper airway, posterior from the nasal septum to the epiglottis, during inspiration. The reason for the loss of upper airway patency is not fully understood and is likely caused by several competing factors. Anatomical factors including neck obesity, narrow airway, and fixed upper airway lesions (e.g., polyps, enlarged tonsils) can narrow the upper airway. Intraluminal negative pressure generated during each inspiration also promotes collapse of the upper airway that competes with dilating forces, primarily the pharyngeal dilator muscle. Acromegaly, amyloidosis, and hypothyroidism as well as neurologic conditions that impair upper airway muscle tone may cause OSA. The hallmarks of OSA are witnessed apneas, gasping, or both. Other recognized signs, symptoms, and considerations of sleep apnea include obesity, snoring, hypertension, daytime sleepiness, and family history.

❺ OSA is increasingly linked to cardiovascular and cerebrovascular morbidity and mortality, independent of other risk factors.[34] Individuals with OSA are at risk for developing hypertension, and when hypertension is present, it is often resistant to drug therapy.[35] Alleviation of sleep disordered breathing (with nasal continuous positive airway pressure) can improve blood pressure and attenuate some of the potential hemodynamic and neurohumoral responses that may link OSA to systemic disease.[36,37]

TREATMENT

Obstructive Sleep Apnea

In the absence of an underlying cause (e.g., hypothyroidism, acromegaly), alleviation of sleep disordered breathing is the primary goal of treatment. Nonpharmacologic measures are the treatments of choice. There is no drug therapy for OSA. However, medications that worsen sleep should be avoided. Practice parameters for the treatment of OSA have been published by the American Academy of Sleep Medicine.[38]

■ NONPHARMACOLOGIC THERAPY

Positive Airway Pressure

❻ Nasal positive airway pressure (PAP) during sleep is the standard treatment for most patients with OSA. PAP produces a positive pressure column in the upper airway using room air to maintain patency. A flexible tube connects the PAP machine to a mask that covers the nose.

PAP delivery may be continuous (CPAP) or bilevel, providing a reduced applied pressure during expiration. During PSG, the pressure setting is increased (up to 20 cm H_2O) until sleep-disordered breathing is eliminated. Barriers to PAP adherence, such as ill-fitted mask and nasal dryness, can be managed. PAP nonadherence for one night results in a complete reversal of the gains made in daytime alertness.[39] In the clinical setting, poor PAP adherence may impact blood pressure control and management in patients with OSA and hypertension.

Weight Reduction

Obesity can worsen sleep apnea, and weight management should be implemented for all overweight patients with OSA. OSA can itself predispose to weight gain and in obese patients with mild OSA weight loss alone can be effective.[40] Individuals who are morbidly obese and have severe OSA can undergo gastric stapling for weight loss.

Surgery

Surgical therapy (uvulopalatopharyngoplasty) opens the upper airway by removing the tonsils, trimming and reorienting the posterior and anterior tonsillar pillars, and removing the uvula and posterior portion of the palate. This is not a first-line option because it is invasive. In very severe cases tracheostomy can be necessary. This procedure can be indicated for select individuals that are morbidly obese, have severe facial skeletal deformity, experience severe drops in oxygen saturation (e.g., less than 70%), or have significant cardiac arrhythmias associated with their OSA.

Other Therapies

For individuals that experience OSA only during certain sleep positions (e.g., on their back), positional therapies can be effective alone but are usually used in conjunction with PAP therapy. Oral appliances can be used to advance the lower jawbone and to keep the tongue forward to enlarge the upper airway. These therapies should be considered when PAP therapy cannot be tolerated.[41]

■ PHARMACOLOGIC THERAPY

The most important pharmacologic intervention is the avoidance of all CNS depressants (e.g., alcohol, hypnotics) and drugs that promote weight gain. Weight gain worsens OSA. CNS depressant use is potentially lethal as it reduces the brain's reflex ability to cause a mini-arousal and resume breathing. In addition, certain CNS depressants can relax airway muscles, promoting upper airway collapse. Medications that can cause rhinopharyngeal inflammation and cough as a side effect of therapy (i.e., ACE inhibitor) may also worsen sleep-disordered breathing.

There is no drug therapy for OSA. In clinical trials, serotonergic agents (e.g., fluoxetine, paroxetine), tricyclic antidepressants (TCAs) (i.e., imipramine, protriptyline), respiratory stimulants (aminophylline and theophylline), medroxyprogesterone, and clonidine do not clinically improve severity of OSA. The effects of antihypertensive agents on sleep apnea are inconsistent and are likely not clinically significant.[34,42]

Modafinil (Provigil) is a wake-promoting medication and is FDA approved to improve wakefulness in patients who have residual daytime sleepiness while treated with PAP. Initiation of wake-promoting medications should only be attempted in patients who are using optimal PAP therapy to alleviate sleep-disordered breathing and are free of cardiovascular disease. In patients with concurrent rhinitis, nasal steroids are recommended for use along with PAP therapy.

■ EVALUATION OF THERAPEUTIC OUTCOMES

Individuals with sleep apnea should be evaluated after 1 to 3 months of treatment for improvement in alertness and daytime symptoms (improvement in memory and decreased irritability) and weight reduction. Individuals experiencing symptoms (e.g., daytime sleepiness, snoring, loss of blood pressure control) despite PAP therapy should have PSG repeated. Symptoms can recur if patients gain weight, requiring a higher pressure setting. Conversely, PAP pressure settings can be decreased if weight loss is achieved. Patient adherence to PAP therapy can be monitored by assessing the built-in compliance meter that measures the hours used at effective pressure.

CENTRAL SLEEP APNEA

CSA causes fragmented sleep and consequent daytime somnolence. However, unlike OSA, arousals from sleep are not required to initiate airflow. During PSG, there is an absence of airflow out of the mouth and nose with no activation of the inspiratory muscles. The prevalence of CSA is not well established and is less than OSA. CSA can be idiopathic but more commonly is caused by underlying autonomic nervous system lesions (e.g., cervical cordotomy), neurologic diseases (e.g., poliomyelitis, encephalitis, and myasthenia gravis), high altitudes, and congestive heart failure.[42] For these reasons, potential underlying causes for CSA should be evaluated and treated. For example, worsening CSA in heart failure patients can signal the need to optimize heart failure therapies.

A few medications have been studied in the setting of high altitude, heart failure, and idiopathic CSA, including acetazolamide, which induces a metabolic acidosis that stimulates respiratory drive, and theophylline, which improves severity of CSA but has no effect on clinical variables.[43,44] PAP therapy with or without supplemental oxygen also improves CSA. However, due to the lack of randomized trials there is no consensus on if and how CSA should be routinely managed, particularly in the setting of heart failure.

NARCOLEPSY

Narcolepsy is a severely debilitating neurologic disease that affects between 0.03% and 0.06% of adult Americans.[45] Despite the debilitating nature of the disease, it can be undiagnosed or misdiagnosed for years. It is equal or somewhat higher in men compared with women, and it has been noted in children and adolescents. However, it is commonly recognized in the second decade of life and increases in severity through the third and fourth decades.[45] Individuals with narcolepsy complain of excessive daytime sleepiness, and in the sleep laboratory, individuals with narcolepsy exhibit impairment of both the onset and the offset of REM and NREM sleep and have arousals and disturbed sleep during the night.

Four characteristic symptoms differentiate narcolepsy from other sleep disorders and are known as the *narcolepsy tetrad*: excessive daytime sleepiness, cataplexy, hypnagogic hallucinations, and sleep paralysis. Cataplexy, a sudden bilateral loss of muscle tone of varying severity and duration without the loss of consciousness, occurs in 70% to 80% of people with narcolepsy.[45] Patients can suffer subtle changes, such as jaw or head slumping, or severe weakness, such as knee buckling or collapsing to the ground. Cataplexy is often precipitated by situations characterized by high emotion (e.g., laughter, anger, excitement). Cataleptic episodes can be brief, lasting seconds, or can last for several minutes. Sleep paralysis is an episodic loss of voluntary muscle tone that occurs when the individual is falling asleep or waking. Individuals are conscious but not able to move or speak. Hallucinations while falling asleep (i.e., hypnagogic) and on awakening (i.e., hypnopompic)

are brief, dreamlike experiences that intrude into wakefulness. Nearly 70% of narcoleptics experience these hallucinations. Unfortunately, these symptoms sometimes lead to an incorrect diagnosis of mental illness.[45] Cataplexy, sleep paralysis, and hypnagogic hallucinations can be caused by REM sleep disturbances.[46]

The primary cause of narcolepsy is not known, and causes may include multiple external and internal factors. There can be a genetic component, as 3% of patients have a first-degree relative with the disorder.[46] Onset of disease occurs in adolescence or adulthood, but not at birth, suggesting that environmental influences might play a role. Molecular studies of human leukocyte antigen (HLA) have found a high prevalence of the HLA-DR2 and HLA-DQ6/DQB1 haplotypes in narcoleptics.[47] However, the HLA-DR2 haplotype is also common in the non-narcoleptic population and is not diagnostic.[46] The hypocretin-orexin neurotransmitter system has been implicated and can play a central role in narcolepsy. Neurons containing hypocretin-orexin are found in the lateral hypothalamus and project to various parts of the brain that are thought to regulate sleep. In 75% of narcoleptic patients, hypocretin-orexin is undetectable in cerebrospinal fluid.[47] Because narcoleptic patients have deficiencies in hypocretin-orexin–producing neurons,[48] an autoimmune process may be responsible for the destruction of hypocretin-producing cells.[49,50]

CLINICAL PRESENTATION OF NARCOLEPSY

Symptoms

- Patients may complain of excessive daytime sleepiness and disrupted nighttime sleep; often they have some accompanying REM sleep abnormality, sleep paralysis, cataplexy, and/or hallucinations.

Laboratory Tests

- Although not routinely tested, there is a high incidence of HLA haplotypes DR2 and HLA-DQ6/DQB1 in narcolepsy.

Other Diagnostic Tests

- Narcolepsy is definitively diagnosed using the multiple sleep latency test (nap test). The patient takes four to five naps in a day, and narcolepsy is diagnosed if the patient falls asleep quickly (within less than 5 minutes) and goes into REM sleep in two of those nap periods.

TREATMENT

Narcolepsy

Nonpharmacologic management of narcolepsy includes counseling the patient and family concerning the illness to alleviate misconceptions around the individual's behavior. Good sleep hygiene should be encouraged as well as two or more scheduled daytime naps. Daytime naps lasting 15 minutes each can help the individual with narcolepsy stay refreshed for several hours.

❼ Pharmacologic management of narcolepsy is focused on two primary areas: treatment of excessive daytime sleepiness (EDS) and cataplexy. Drug therapy for narcolepsy is summarized in Table 81–4.

Modafinil, a racemic compound unrelated to psychostimulants, is a recognized standard treatment for EDS.[51] Armodafinil is the active R-isomer of modafinil and is also FDA approved for treatment of EDS in narcolepsy. The precise mechanism of action of modafinil and armodafinil is not fully understood. Common adverse effects are usually mild and include headache, nausea,

TABLE 81-4 Drugs Used to Treat Narcolepsy[51]

Generic Name	Trade Name	Daily Dosage Range (mg)
Excessive daytime somnolence		
Dextroamphetamine	Dexedrine	5–60
Dextroamphetamine/ Amphetamine salts[a]	Adderall	5–60
Methamphetamine[b]	Desoxyn	5–15
Lisdexamfetamine	Vyvanse	20–70
Methylphenidate	Ritalin	30–80
Modafinil	Provigil	200–400
Armodafinil	Nuvigil	150–250
Sodium oxybate[c]	Xyrem	4.5–9 grams per night
Adjunct agents for cataplexy		
Fluoxetine	Prozac	20–80
Imipramine	Tofranil	50–250
Nortriptyline	Aventyl, Pamelor	50–200
Protriptyline	Vivactil	5–30
Venlafaxine	Effexor	37.5–225
Selegiline	Eldepryl	20–40

[a]Dextroamphetamine sulfate, dextroamphetamine saccharate, amphetamine aspartate, and amphetamine sulfate.
[b]Not available in some states.
[c]Also is effective at treating cataplexy.

nervousness, anxiety, and insomnia. The dose of modafinil is between 200 and 400 mg/day, and armodafinil doses are between 150 mg and 250 mg/day.[52] Although both of these agents are effective in treating EDS, they lack efficacy for the treatment of cataplectic symptoms.[53]

EDS can also be treated with stimulants to improve alertness and to increase daytime performance. Dextroamphetamine and methylphenidate also have FDA approval for the treatment of narcolepsy. Methamphetamine has also been used on an off-label basis. Methylphenidate and amphetamines have a fast onset of action and durations of 6 to 10 and 3 to 4 hours, respectively. The dose can range from 5 to 60 mg daily. Many clinicians prescribe both immediate-release and sustained-release stimulants to increase alertness throughout the day. Sustained-release stimulants are prescribed with scheduled administration times, and immediate release stimulants can be taken as needed when the patient requires alertness (e.g., driving, etc.).

Stimulants improve alertness, increase daytime performance, can elevate mood, and prevent sleep. Side effects can include insomnia, hypertension, palpitations, and irritability. Tolerance to long-term stimulant therapy can occur, necessitating dosage increases. Amphetamine use is associated with more likelihood of abuse and tolerance, especially when prescribed in high doses. Lisdexamfetamine is a new amphetamine prodrug rapidly absorbed and converted in the body to dextroamphetamine. Lisdexamfetamine has a longer duration of action and less risk of abuse since it is only active when taken orally.

The most effective treatments for cataplexy are TCAs, venlafaxine, and fluoxetine. The mechanism of antidepressants in relieving cataplexy, hypnagogic hallucinations, and sleep paralysis can be mediated through blockade of serotonin and norepinephrine reuptake in the locus coeruleus and raphe and subsequent suppression of REM sleep.[54] Imipramine, protriptyline, clomipramine, fluoxetine, and nortriptyline are effective in approximately 80% of patients. Selegiline improves hypersomnolence and cataplexy through REM suppression and an increase in REM latency. Methylphenidate and amphetamines alone are usually ineffective for cataplexy.

Sodium oxybate (γ-hydroxybutyrate, Xyrem) improves symptoms of EDS and decreases episodes of sleep paralysis, cataplexy, and hypnagogic hallucinations. Nightly administration of sodium oxybate changes sleep architecture to resemble normal sleep. It increases slow-wave sleep, decreases nighttime awakenings, and increases REM efficiency.[55] Sodium oxybate is available only as a liquid and is taken as two doses; one is taken at bedtime and the second dose is taken 2.5 to 4 hours later. Sodium oxybate is a potent sedative hypnotic and should not be used concomitantly with any other sedating medications. The most common side effects include nausea, somnolence, confusion, dizziness, and incontinence.

■ EVALUATION OF THERAPEUTIC OUTCOMES

The primary objective of pharmacologic treatment of narcolepsy is to reduce symptoms that adversely impact quality of life. The goal is to produce the fullest possible return of normal function for patients at work, school, home, and in social settings. Patients with narcolepsy should keep a diary of the frequency and severity of cataplexy, sleep paralysis, and sleep hallucinations. Patients should be evaluated regularly during medication titrations and then every 6 to 12 months to assess for adverse drug effects (e.g., sleep disturbances and cardiovascular abnormalities). The health care provider should consider the benefit-to-risk ratio for the individual patient, the cost of medication, the convenience of administration, and the cost of laboratory tests when selecting narcolepsy therapies.[51] One wake-promoting agent may work better than another in an individual patient. Thus, if one agent is not effective at adequate doses, a trial with another agent should be undertaken.

CIRCADIAN RHYTHM DISORDERS

The sleep–wake cycle is under the circadian control of oscillators and can be disrupted by misalignment between an individual's biologic clock and external demands on the sleep cycle. Circadian rhythm sleep disorders usually present with either insomnia or hypersomnia, depending on the individual's performance requirements. Two commonly occurring circadian rhythm sleep disorders are jet lag and shift work sleep problems.

JET LAG

Jet lag occurs when a person travels across time zones, and the external environmental time is mismatched with the internal circadian clock. Sleep disturbances typically last for 2 to 3 days but can last as long as 7 to 10 days if the time zone changes are greater than 8 hours. Compared with westward travel, eastward travel is associated with a longer duration of jet lag. Jet lag leads to increased incidence of gastrointestinal disturbances and a decrease in alertness and performance.

❽ Treatment of jet lag includes nonpharmacologic approaches alone or in combination with drug therapy. Jet lag can be minimized in coast-to-coast travel in the United States if the duration is less than 7 days and the normal sleep–wake cycle is observed. For travel lasting longer than 7 days, jet lag severity can be lessened by 1- to 2-hour adjustments in sleep and wake times prior to departure to the destination time zone. Short-acting benzodiazepine receptor agonists or 0.5 to 5 mg melatonin taken at appropriate target bedtimes for east or west travel reduce jet lag and shorten sleep latency.[56]

SHIFT WORK SLEEP DISORDER

Shift workers comprise approximately 20% of the workforce.[57] Night shift work causes a misalignment in the sleep–wake cycle and circadian rhythm that is associated with a decrease in alertness, performance, and quality of daytime sleep. More than 65% of workers on rotating shifts complain of insomnia, compared with only 20% who work one shift.[58] Shift workers ultimately are at risk of developing shift work sleep disorder (SWSD). SWSD is a complaint of insomnia or excessive sleepiness that occurs because of working shifts during normal sleep time.[7,57] Shift workers have a higher injury rate, divorce rate, occurrence of on-the-job sleepiness, and incidence of substance use. Shift workers may also be at increased risk of developing peptic ulcers, depression, breast cancer, and sleepiness-related accidents.[57,59,60] Night shift workers are usually in a state of permanent circadian misalignment because of the tendency to revert to conventional sleep schedules on their days off.[58]

Treatment for shift work sleep problems includes optimizing sleep hygiene, extending daytime sleep by sleeping in the afternoon, scheduling a 2- to 3-hour nap on days off from work, or switching to a day shift job. Short-acting benzodiazepine receptor agonists can consolidate sleep during day sleep periods and reduce lost sleep time. Modafinil is FDA approved to improve wakefulness in patients with excessive daytime sleepiness associated with SWSD. Scheduled exposure to bright lights at night and darkness in the daytime improves adaptation to night work and daytime sleep.[58] Melatonin has also been used successfully.

RESTLESS LEGS SYNDROME

Restless legs syndrome (RLS), or Ekbom syndrome, is characterized by paresthesias that are usually felt deep in the calf muscles but can also appear in the thighs and arms with the urge to keep limbs in motion. RLS occurs in both males and females, and it occurs more frequently in the elderly. It has been associated with chronic kidney disease, iron deficiency anemia, and pregnancy. Caffeine, stress, alcohol, and fatigue can worsen symptoms. Recent data suggest that RLS can be caused by iron deficiency in the substantia nigra in the CNS.[60] The diagnosis of RLS is based on patient- or partner-reported symptoms and specific diagnostic criteria. Criteria required to diagnose RLS include (1) an urge to move the limbs that is usually associated with uncomfortable and unpleasant sensations, (2) symptoms that begin or worsen during rest or inactivity, (3) symptoms that are exclusively present or worse in the evening or night, and (4) symptoms that are temporarily relieved by movement.[61] The discomfort returns when the person tries to sleep, resulting in insomnia.

❾ Dopamine agonists are effective for RLS and have replaced levodopa as first-line therapy.[62] Ropinirole and pramipexole are FDA approved for RLS.[62] Lower doses of dopamine agonists are used when treating RLS compared with Parkinson disease. Providers should caution patients that compulsive behaviors (e.g., gambling, shopping, eating, etc.) may emerge during therapy with dopamine agonists. Levodopa therapy is associated with a high incidence of symptom augmentation and, because of a short half-life, might not provide relief over the entire night. Augmentation is a worsening in symptom severity, increase in symptom distribution, or emergence of symptoms earlier in the evening. Sedative hypnotic agents can be effective in patients who have frequent awakenings from their RLS symptoms. Clonazepam at doses ranging from 0.5 mg to 2 mg has been most frequently studied; however, patients frequently experience carryover sedation because of its long duration of action. Shorter half-life sedative hypnotics (e.g., zolpidem, zaleplon, triazolam) can improve sleep and reduce daytime sleepiness without carryover sedation. Opiates such as methadone 5 to 20 mg, codeine 30 to 120 mg, and oxycodone 2.5 mg are very effective for patients with painful RLS. The potential for tolerance and dependence on opiate therapy should be considered. Gabapentin 300 to 900 mg near bedtime can also be considered for those with paresthetic or painful RLS symptoms.[63] Iron studies should be completed in patients with RLS and

iron supplementation initiated in those that are iron deficient. In patients with ferritin concentrations less than 50 to 75 mcg/L (ng/mL), iron supplementation improves RLS symptoms.[64] Patients with RLS or periodic limb movements of sleep should be evaluated regularly to monitor for excessive daytime somnolence, tolerance, efficacy, and adverse effects of the medication.

PERIODIC LEG MOVEMENTS OF SLEEP

RLS patients commonly have periodic limb movements during sleep, while approximately one-third of patients with PLMS have RLS.[62] PLMS are stereotypic, repetitive, periodic movements of the legs that occur during sleep every 20 to 40 seconds and last 10 minutes to several hours.[62] The movements usually involve the big toe, but the ankle, knee, and hip can also flex. They can be terminated by a violent kick or other body movement. Often patients will be unaware of these movements and only recognize consequent insufficient sleep and morning leg cramps. A bed partner can describe PLMS. PLMS is diagnosed in the sleep laboratory using electromyogram recordings. Bursts of muscle activity lasting 0.5 to 5 seconds that recur at least 40 times within 8 hours of sleep are diagnostic.[62]

PLMS can occur with RLS or alone because of systemic disease (e.g., renal failure) or drug therapy.[65] TCAs, SSRIs, dopaminergic antagonists, xanthines, nicotine, alcohol, and caffeine can all worsen PLMS. The treatment approach for PLMS is similar to that of RLS. If PLMS do not cause disruptions for the patient or bed partner or daytime symptoms, they might not require treatment. Symptomatic or problematic PLMS should be treated with dopaminergic medications to suppress limb movements or sedative hypnotics to reduce awakenings and consolidate sleep.

PARASOMNIAS

Parasomnias are abnormal behavior or physiologic events that either occur during sleep or are exaggerated by sleep. Many of these disorders are considered to be disorders of partial arousal from various sleep stages. Parasomnias can be categorized as disorders of arousal (sleepwalking, sleep terrors), sleep–wake transition disorders (sleeptalking), rhythmic movement disorder, REM parasomnias (REM-behavior disorder, nightmares), and miscellaneous parasomnias (enuresis, bruxism). Sleepwalking, sleep terrors, and sleeptalking predominantly occur during NREM sleep, whereas others (REM-behavior disorder) occur during REM sleep.

Sleepwalking and sleep terrors are found normally in children between the ages of 4 and 12 years and usually resolve in adolescence. These disorders are associated with psychopathology only if they persist into adulthood.[66] Sleep terrors can begin in adults between the ages of 20 and 30 years. Onset of sleepwalking in adults without a childhood history of sleepwalking should prompt a search for a neurologic or substance-use condition.[66] Sleepwalking and sleep terror disorder involve intrusions of wakefulness into NREM sleep during the first third of the night. In sleepwalking, individuals become ambulatory, are difficult to awaken, and are amnestic for the event. Sleep terrors involve intense fear and autonomic arousal. Individuals are difficult to awaken, inconsolable, and amnestic for the event.[66] Patients with REM-behavior disorder act out their dreams, often in a violent manner, and are at risk for injury.

Treatment of sleepwalking involves protecting the individual from harm by putting safety latches on doors and windows, removing hazardous objects from bedrooms, and covering glass doors with heavy curtains. In adult patients, benzodiazepines, SSRIs, or TCAs can be beneficial therapies for sleepwalking or other

NREM disorders of arousal.[67] Benzodiazepines can also be helpful in curtailing sleep terrors in adults.[66] Nightmares are anxiety-provoking dreams characterized by vivid recall. Treatment is directed at reducing stress, anxiety, and sleep deprivation. In extreme cases, low-dose benzodiazepines can be indicated. Clonazepam is the treatment of choice for REM behavior disorder. Melatonin (3–12 mg at bedtime) can also be an effective therapy for REM behavior disorder.[68]

PHARMACOECONOMIC CONSIDERATIONS

Despite the prevalence of sleep disorders, most cases go undiagnosed and untreated. In the United States, the direct and indirect costs of insomnia alone add over $100 billion to the national health care bill each year.[1,69] Improvements in recognition and treatment can decrease the economic burden and prevent progression to both medical and psychiatric disorders.

Quality of life can be improved by appropriate treatment. For example, treatment of OSA with PAP improves the number of years of good health by 5.5 quality-adjusted life years. Hypnotic therapy has also been found to markedly improve both the disorder and quality of life in shift workers.[70]

CONCLUSIONS

Disturbances of sleep affect approximately one third of the population. Patients with sleep disorders should be accurately identified and diagnosed. Patients can have one or more concomitant sleep disorders. Unrecognized and poorly treated sleep disorders can worsen severity of and ability to effectively treat underlying systemic diseases. Effective management of sleep disorders involves combined nonpharmacologic and pharmacologic treatment.

ABBREVIATIONS

CPAP: continuous positive airway pressure

CNS: central nervous system

CSA: central sleep apnea

DSM-IV-TR: Diagnostic and Statistical Manual of Mental Disorders, Fourth Edition, Text Revision

EDS: excessive daytime sleepiness

EEG: electroencephalogram

FDA: Food and Drug Administration

GABA: γ-aminobutyric acid

HLA: human leukocyte antigen

NREM: nonrapid eye movement (sleep)

OSA: obstructive sleep apnea

PAP: positive airway pressure

PLMS: periodic limb movement during sleep

PSG: polysomnography

RDI: respiratory disturbance index

REM: rapid eye movement (sleep)

RLS: restless legs syndrome

SSRI: selective serotonin reuptake inhibitor

SWSD: shift work sleep disorder

TCA: tricyclic antidepressant

REFERENCES

1. Walsh JK, Engelhardt CL. The direct economic costs of insomnia in the United States for 1995. Sleep 1999;22:S386–S393.
2. Neylan TC, Reynolds CF, Kupfer DJ. Sleep disorders. In: Yudofsky SC, Hales RE, eds. American Psychiatric Press Textbook of Neuropsychiatry, 3rd ed. Washington, DC: American Psychiatric Press, 2000:583–606.
3. Benca RM, Cirelli C, Rattenborg NC, Tononi G. Basic Science of Sleep. In: Sadock BJ, Sadock VA, eds. Kaplan and Sadock's Comprehensive Textbook of Psychiatry, 8th ed. Philadelphia, PA: Lippincott Williams & Wilkins, 2005:280–294.
4. Dagan Y, Abadi J. Sleep–wake disorder disability: A lifelong untreatable pathology of the circadian time structure. Chronobiol Int 2001;18:1019–1027.
5. Franken P. Long-term versus short-term processes regulating REM sleep. J Sleep Res 2002;11:17–28.
6. Stickgold R, Hobson JA, Fosse R, Fosse M. Sleep, learning and dreams: Off-line memory reprocessing. Science 2001;294:1052–1058.
7. American Sleep Disorders Association. International Classification of Sleep Disorders: Diagnostic and Coding Manual: Revised Addition. Rochester, MN: American Sleep Disorders Association, 1997.
8. American Psychiatric Association. Sleep disorders. In: Diagnostic and Statistical Manual of Mental Disorders, 4th ed., text revision. Washington, DC: American Psychiatric Press, 2000:597–644.
9. Shocat T, Umphress J, Isreal AG, Ancoli-Israel S. Insomnia in primary care patients. Sleep 1999;22(suppl 2):S359–S365.
10. Chesson AL, Anderson WM, Littner M, et al. Practice parameters for the nonpharmacologic treatment of chronic insomnia. Sleep 1999;8:1–6.
11. Kirkwood CK. Management of insomnia. J Am Pharm Assoc 1999;39:688–696.
12. Sateia MJ, Doghramji K, Hauri PJ, et al. Evaluation of chronic insomnia. Sleep 2000;23:1–39.
13. Lippmann S, Mazour I, Shabab H. Insomnia: Therapeutic approach. South Med J 2001;94:866–874.
14. Vaughn-McCall W. A psychiatric perspective on insomnia. J Clin Psychiatr 2001;62(suppl 10):27–32.
15. Espie C. Insomnia: Conceptual issues in the development, persistence and treatment of sleep disorders in adults. Annu Rev Psychol 2002;53:215–243.
16. Chesson A, Hartse K, McDowell-Anderson W. Practice parameters for the evaluation of chronic insomnia. Sleep 2000;23:1–5.
17. Sivertsen B, Omvik S, Pallesen S, et al. Cognitive behavioral therapy vs zopiclone for treatment of chronic primary insomnia in older adults: A randomized controlled trial. JAMA 2006;295:2851–2858.
18. Hauri PJ. Insomnia. Clin Chest Med 1998;19:157–168.
19. Jackson CW. Mood disorders. In: Mueller BA, ed. Pharmacotherapy Self Assessment Program (PSAP). Kansas City, MO: American College of Clinical Pharmacy, 2002:203–250.
20. Schulz V, Hansel R, Tyler VE. Rational Phytotherapy: A Physician's Guide to Herbal Medicine. Berlin: Springer; 1998:81.
21. Ancoli-Isreal S. Insomnia in the elderly: A review for the primary care practitioner. Sleep 2000;23:S23–S30.
22. Terzano MG, Rossi M, Palomba V, et al. New drugs for insomnia: Comparative tolerability of zopiclone, zolpidem and zaleplon. Drug Saf 2003;26:261–282.
23. Ambien, zolpidem [product information]. Bridgewater, NJ: Sanofi-Aventis; 2006.
24. Elie R, Ruteher E, Farr IK, et al. Sleep latency is shortened during 4 weeks of treatment with zaleplon, a novel nonbenzodiazepine hypnotic. J Clin Psychiatry 1999;60:536–544.
25. Walsh JK, Fry J, Erwin CS, et al. Efficacy and tolerability of 14-day administration of zaleplon 5 mg and 10 mg for the treatment of primary insomnia. Clin Drug Investig 1998;16:347–354.
26. Walsh JK, Pollack CP, Shark MMB, et al. Lack of residual sedation following middle-of-the-night zaleplon administration in sleep maintenance insomnia. Clin Neuropharmacol 2000;23:17–21.
27. Lunesta, eszopiclone [product information]. Marlborough, MA: Sepracor; 2005.

28. Krystal AD, Walsh JK, Laska E, et al. Sustained efficacy of eszopiclone over 6 months of nightly treatment: Results of a randomized, double-blind, placebo-controlled study in adults with chronic insomnia. Sleep 2003;26:793–797.

29. Young T, Peppard PE, Gottlieb DJ. Epidemiology of obstructive sleep apnea: A population health perspective. Am J Respir Crit Care Med 2002;165:1217–1239.

30. Young T, Palta M, Dempsey J, et al. The occurrence of sleep-disordered breathing among middle-aged adults. N Engl J Med 1993;328:1230–1235.

31. Peppard PE, Szklo-Coxe M, Hla KM, Young T. Longitudinal association of sleep-related breathing disorder and depression. Arch Intern Med 2006;166:1709–1715.

32. Young T, Finn L, Peppard PE, et al. Sleep disordered breathing and mortality: Eighteen-year follow-up of the Wisconsin sleep cohort. Sleep 2008;31:1071–1078.

33. Terán-Santos J, Jimenez-Gomez A, Cordero-Guevara J; for The Cooperative Group Burgos–Santander. The association between sleep apnea and the risk of traffic accidents. N Engl J Med 1999;340:847–851.

34. Somers VK, White DP, Amin R, et al. Sleep apnea and cardiovascular disease: An American Heart Association/American College of Cardiology Foundation scientific statement from the American Heart Association Council for High Blood Pressure Research Professional Education Committee, Council on Clinical Cardiology, Stroke Council, and Council on Cardiovascular Nursing. J Am Coll Cardiol 2008;52:686–717.

35. Goncalves SC, Martinez D, Gus M, et al. Obstructive sleep apnea and resistant hypertension: A case-control study. Chest 2007;132:1858–1862.

36. Becker HF, Jerrentrup A, Ploch T, et al. Effect of nasal continuous positive airway pressure treatment on blood pressure in patients with obstructive sleep apnea. Circulation 2003;107:68–73.

37. Kato M, Roberts-Thomson P, Phillips BG, et al. Impairment of endothelium dependent vasodilation of resistance vessels in patients with obstructive sleep apnea. Circulation 2000;102:2607–2610.

38. Morganthaler TI, Kapen S, Lee-Chiong T, et al. Practice parameters for the medical therapy of obstructive sleep apnea. Sleep 2006;29:1031–1035.

39. Kribbs NB, Pack AJ, Kline LR, et al. Effects of one night without nasal CPAP treatment on sleep and sleepiness in patients with obstructive sleep apnea. Am Rev Respir Dis 2003;147:1162–1168.

40. Peppard PE, Young T, Palta M, et al. Longitudinal study of moderate weight change and sleep-disordered breathing. JAMA 2000;284:3015–3021.

41. Ferguson KA, Cartwright R, Rogers R, et al. Oral appliances for snoring and obstructive sleep apnea: A review. Sleep 2006;29:244–262.

42. Grunstein RR, Hedner J, Grote L. Treatment options for sleep apnea. Drugs 2001;61:237–251.

43. Javaheri S. Acetazolamide improves central sleep apnea in heart failure: A double-blind, prospective study. Am J Respir Crit Care Med 2006;173:234–237.

44. Javaheri S, Parker TJ, Wexler L, et al. Effect of theophylline on sleep-disordered breathing in heart failure, N Engl J Med 1996;335:562–567.

45. Mitler M, Hayduk R. Benefits and risks of pharmacotherapy for narcolepsy. Drug Saf 2002;25:791–809.

46. Nakayama J, Miura M, Honda M, et al. Linkage of human narcolepsy with HLA association to chromosome 4p-13-q21. Genomics 2000;65:84–86.

47. Nishino S, Ripley B, Overeem S, et al. Low cerebrospinal fluid hypocretin (orexin) and altered energy homeostasis in human narcolepsy. Ann Neurol 2001;50:381–388.

48. Thannickal TC, Moore RY, Nienhuis R, et al. Reduced number of hypocretin neurons in human narcolepsy. Neuron 2000;27:469–474.

49. Lin L, Hungs M, Mignot E. Narcolepsy and the HLA region. J Neuroimmunol 2001;117:9–20.

50. Mignot E, Thorsby E. Narcolepsy and the HLA system (letter). N Engl J Med 2001;344:692.

51. Morgenthaler TI, Kapur VK, Brown T, et al. Practice parameters for the treatment of narcolepsy and other hypersomnias of central origin. Sleep 2007;30:1705–1711.

52. Robertson P, Hellriegel ET. Clinical pharmacokinetic profile of modafinil. Clin Pharmacokinet 2003;42:123–127.

53. Feldman N. Narcolepsy. South Med J 2003;96:277–287.

54. Rosenthal MS. Physiology and neurochemistry of sleep. Am J Pharm Educ 1998;62:204–208.

55. Mamelak M, Black J, Montplaisir J, et al. A pilot study of the effects of sodium oxybate on sleep architecture and daytime alertness in narcolepsy. Sleep 2004;27:1327–1334.

56. Herxheimer A, Petrie KJ, Cochrane Depression, Anxiety and Neurosis Group. Melatonin for the prevention and treatment of jet lag. [systematic review]. Cochrane Database Syst Rev 2005;4.

57. Drake CL, Roehrs T, Richardson G, et al. Shift work sleep disorder: Prevalence and consequences beyond that of symptomatic day workers. Sleep 2004;27:1453–1462.

58. Garbarino S, Nobili L, Beelke, M, et al. Sleep disorders and daytime sleepiness in state police shiftworkers. Arch Environ Health 2002;57:167–175.

59. Knutsson A. Health disorders of shift workers. Occup Med (Lond) 2003;53:103–108.

60. Connor JR, Boyer PJ, Menzies SL, et al. Neuropathological examination suggests impaired brain iron acquisition in restless legs syndrome. Neurology 2003;61:304–309.

61. Allen RP, Picchietti D, Hening W, et al. Restless legs syndrome: Diagnostic criteria, special considerations and epidemiology: A report from the Restless Legs Syndrome Diagnosis and Epidemiology workshop at the National Institutes of Health. Sleep Med 2003;4:101–119.

62. Hening WA, Allen RP, Earley CJ, et al.; Restless Legs Syndrome Task Force of the Standards of Practice Committee of the American Academy of Sleep Medicine. An update on the dopaminergic treatment of restless legs syndrome and periodic limb movement disorder. Sleep 2004;27:560–583.

63. Garcia-Borreguero D, Larrosa O, de la Llave Y, et al. Treatment of restless legs syndrome with gabapentin: A double-blind, cross-over study. Neurology 2002;59:1573–1575.

64. Wang J, O'Reilly B, Venkataraman R, et al. Efficacy of oral iron in patients with restless legs syndrome and low-normal ferritin: a randomized, double-blind, placebo-controlled study. Sleep Med 2009;10:973–975.

65. Montplaisir J, Nicolas A, Denesle R, Gomez-Mancilla B. Restless legs syndrome improved by pramipexole: A double-blind randomized trial. Neurology 1999;52:938–943.

66. Schenck CH, Mahowald MW. Parasomnias managing bizarre sleep-related behavior disorders. Postgrad Med 2000;107:145–156.

67. Mahowald MW. NREM sleep-arousal parasomnias. In: Kryger MH, Roth T, Dement WC, eds. Principles and Practice of Sleep Medicine, 4th ed. Philadelphia, PA: Elsevier Saunders; 2005:889–896.

68. Mahowald MW, Schenck CH. REM sleep parasomnias. In: Kryger MH, Roth T, Dement WC, eds. Principles and Practice of Sleep Medicine, 4th ed. Philadelphia, PA: Elsevier Saunders; 2005:897–916.

69. Fullerton DS. The economic impact of insomnia in managed care: A clearer picture emerges. Am J Manag Care 2006;12(suppl 8):S246–S252.

70. Leger D. Public health and insomnia: Economic impact. Sleep 2000;23(suppl 3):S69–S76.

71. Jermaine DM. Sleep disorders. In: Carter BL, Angaran DM, Lake KD, Raebel MA, eds. Pharmacotherapy Self-Assessment Program, 2nd ed. Psychiatry module. Kansas City: American College of Clinical Pharmacy; 1995:139–154.

CHAPTER 82

Disorders Associated with Intellectual Disabilities

NANCY BRAHM, JERRY MCKEE, AND DOUGLAS STEWART

KEY CONCEPTS

❶ Persons diagnosed with Down syndrome can be at increased risk for medical and psychiatric comorbidities.

❷ Develop treatment plans for persons with autism to increase social interactions, improve verbal and nonverbal communication, and minimize the occurrence or impact of ritualistic, repetitive behaviors and other related mood and behavioral problems (e.g., overactivity, irritability, self-injury).

❸ Differentiate between purported treatments for autism and effective treatments supported by evidence-based pharmacotherapy principles.

❹ Develop a structured teaching approach focusing on increasing social communication and integration with peers in persons with autism.

❺ Develop a psychopharmacologic treatment plan including monitoring of objective and measurable medication-responsive target behaviors and assessment of potential adverse effects.

❻ Differentiate between the four stages of Rett syndrome associated with developmental regression.

Intellectual disabilities (ID) can be identified in childhood or adolescence. Current criteria for a diagnosis are based on deficiencies in intellectual and adaptive functioning with an onset prior to 18 years of age.[1] This diagnosis is made regardless of the presence or absence of concomitant medical or psychiatric disorders. In the case of mild ID, deficiencies may not be initially apparent. Problems can be noted when the chronologic age of the child and the developmental milestones achieved by peers with similar backgrounds, cultures, and socioeconomic and psychosocial settings differ significantly.[1] These gaps widen as the individual ages.

Adaptive functioning deficits pose a number of challenges in treating those with an ID. This population can be 4 to 5 times more likely to experience mental health problems compared with the general population.[2] Until recently, little attention was given to this population and the need to evaluate them for psychiatric illnesses, leading to under-recognition of psychopathology. This oversight is a function of several factors, including limited population-specific training for clinicians and a general lack of clinical experience with patients with ID during training.[2] Additional barriers are individual deficits in expressive and receptive language, a lack of mental health screening initiatives, and limited diagnostic testing instruments specific to this population.[2]

Those with ID often have few social interactions and limited integration into the community. Stimulation and interaction with peers typically shapes behaviors in the general population. A different set of coping skills can develop in their absence. Self-talk is an example of a coping mechanism that can be misinterpreted for psychosis. Another potential problem for the clinician assessing persons with an ID is a significant gap between receptive and expressive language skills. If not readily recognized, intellectual capabilities can be overestimated, expectations falsely elevated, and coping skills can be inadequate, leading to anxiety-induced decompensation.[2]

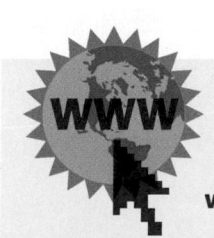

The complete chapter, learning objectives, and other resources can be found at **www.pharmacotherapyonline.com**.

SECTION 8

ENDOCRINOLOGIC DISORDERS

CHAPTER

83

Diabetes Mellitus

CURTIS L. TRIPLITT AND CHARLES A. REASNER

KEY CONCEPTS

❶ Diabetes mellitus (DM) is a group of metabolic disorders of fat, carbohydrate, and protein metabolism that results from defects in insulin secretion, insulin action (sensitivity), or both.

❷ The incidence of type 2 DM is increasing. This has been attributed in part to a Western-style diet, increasing obesity, sedentary lifestyle, and an increasing minority population.

❸ The two major classifications of DM are type 1 (insulin deficient) and type 2 (combined insulin resistance and relative deficiency in insulin secretion). They differ in clinical presentation, onset, etiology, and progression of disease. Both are associated with microvascular and macrovascular disease complications.

❹ Diagnosis of diabetes is made by four criteria: fasting plasma glucose ≥126 mg/dL; a 2-hour value from a 75-g oral glucose tolerance test ≥200 mg/dL; a casual plasma glucose level of ≥200 mg/dL with symptoms of diabetes; or a HbA$_{1c}$ ≥6.5%. The diagnosis should be confirmed by repeat testing if obvious hyperglycemia is not present.

❺ Goals of therapy in DM are directed toward attaining normoglycemia (or appropriate glycemic control based on the patient's comorbidities), reducing the onset and progression of retinopathy, nephropathy, and neuropathy complications, intensive therapy for associated cardiovascular risk factors, and improving quality and quantity of life.

❻ Metformin should be included in the therapy for all type 2 DM patients, if tolerated and not contraindicated, as it is the only

oral antihyperglycemic medication proven to reduce the risk of total mortality, according to the United Kingdom Prospective Diabetes Study (UKPDS).

❼ Intensive glycemic control is paramount for reduction of microvascular complications (neuropathy, retinopathy, and nephropathy) as evidenced by the Diabetes Control and Complications Trial (DCCT) in type 1 DM and the UKPDS in type 2 DM. The UKPDS also reported that control of hypertension in patients with diabetes will not only reduce the risk of retinopathy and nephropathy, but also reduce cardiovascular risk.

❽ Short-term (3–5 years), intensive glycemic control does not lower the risk of macrovascular events as reported by the Action in Diabetes and Vascular Disease, Action to Control Cardiovascular Risk in Diabetes, and Veterans Administration Diabetes Trial trials. Microvascular event reduction may be sustained, and macrovascular events reduced by improved early glycemic control, as evidenced by the UKPDS and DCCT follow-up studies. Significant reductions in macrovascular risk may take 15 to 20 years. This sustained reduction in microvascular risk and new reduction in macrovascular risk has been coined metabolic memory.

❾ Knowledge of the patient's quantitative and qualitative meal patterns, activity levels, pharmacokinetics of insulin preparations, and pharmacology of oral and injected antihyperglycemic agents are essential to individualize the treatment plan and optimize blood glucose control while minimizing risks for hypoglycemia and other adverse effects of pharmacologic therapies.

❿ Type 1 DM treatment necessitates insulin therapy. Currently, the basal-bolus insulin therapy or pump therapy in motivated individuals often leads to successful glycemic outcomes. Basal-bolus therapy includes a basal insulin for fasting and postabsorptive control, and rapid acting bolus insulin for mealtime coverage. Addition of mealtime pramlintide in patients with uncontrolled or erratic postprandial glycemia may be warranted.

⓫ Type 2 DM treatment often necessitates use of multiple therapeutic agents (combination therapy), including oral and/or injected antihyperglycemics and insulin to obtain glycemic goals due to the persistant reduction in β-cell function over time.

The complete chapter, learning objectives, and other resources can be found at **www.pharmacotherapyonline.com**.

Slowing, but not arresting, β-cell failure has been shown with thiazolidinediones and the GLP-1 agonist class of medications.

⑫ Aggressive management of cardiovascular disease risk factors in type 2 DM is necessary to reduce the risk for adverse cardiovascular events or death. Smoking cessation, use of antiplatelet therapy as a secondary prevention strategy and in select primary prevention situations, aggressive management of dyslipidemia: primary goal to lower low-density lipoprotein-cholesterol (<100 mg/dL) and secondarily to raise high-density lipoprotein-cholesterol to ≥40 mg/dL, and treatment of hypertension (again often requiring multiple drugs) to <130/80 mm Hg are vital.

⑬ Prevention strategies for type 1 DM have been unsuccessful. Prevention strategies for type 2 DM are established. Lifestyle changes, dietary restriction of fat, aerobic exercise for 30 minutes 5 times a week, and weight loss, form the backbone of successful prevention. No medication is currently FDA approved for prevention of diabetes, though several, including metformin, acarbose, pioglitazone, and rosiglitazone, have clinical trials demonstrating a delay of diabetes onset.

⑭ Patient education and ability to demonstrate self-care and adherence to therapeutic lifestyle and pharmacologic interventions are crucial to successful outcomes. Multidisciplinary teams of healthcare professionals including physicians (primary care, endocrinologists, ophthalmologists, and vascular surgeons), podiatrists, dietitians, nurses, pharmacists, social workers, behavioral health specialists, and certified diabetes educators are needed, as appropriate, to optimize these outcomes in persons with diabetes mellitus.

---

❶ Diabetes mellitus (DM) is a group of metabolic disorders characterized by hyperglycemia. It is associated with abnormalities in carbohydrate, fat, and protein metabolism and results in chronic complications including microvascular, macrovascular, and neuropathic disorders. Nearly 24 million Americans have DM, with as many as one-fourth of these patients being undiagnosed, and an additional 57 million potentially having pre-diabetes.[1] The economic burden of DM approximated $174 billion in 2007, including direct medical and treatment costs as well as indirect costs attributed to disability and mortality.[1] DM is the leading cause of blindness in adults aged 20 to 74 years, and the leading contributor to development of endstage renal disease. It also accounts for approximately 71,000 lower extremity amputations annually.[1] Finally, a cardiovascular event is responsible for two-thirds of deaths in individuals with type 2 DM.[1]

Optimal management of the patient with DM will reduce or prevent complications, and improve quality of life. Research and drug development efforts over the past several decades have provided valuable information that applies directly to improving outcomes in patients with DM and have expanded the therapeutic armamentarium. Additionally, interventions in an attempt to prevent complications and the onset of diabetes have been reported for type 1 and 2 DM.

EPIDEMIOLOGY

Type 1 DM is an autoimmune disorder developing in childhood or early adulthood, although some latent forms do occur. Type 1 DM idiopathic is a nonimmune form of diabetes frequently seen in minorities, especially Africans and Asians, with intermittent insulin requirements.[2] Type 1 DM accounts for 5% to 10% of all cases of DM and is likely initiated by the exposure of a genetically susceptible individual to an environmental agent.[3] Candidate genes and environmental factors are reportedly prevalent in the general population, but development of β-cell autoimmunity occurs in less than 10% of the genetically susceptible population and progresses to type 1 DM in less than 1% of the population.[4] The prevalence of β-cell autoimmunity appears proportional to the incidence of type 1 DM in various populations. For instance, the countries of Sweden, Sardinia, and Finland have the highest prevalence of islet cell antibody (3%–4.5%) and are associated with the highest incidence of type 1 DM; 22 to 35 per 100,000.[5] The prevalence of type 1 DM has been increasing over the last hundred years, but the cause of the increase is not fully understood.[6]

Markers of autoimmunity have been detected in 14% to 33% of persons with type 2 DM in some populations and manifest with early failure of oral agents and insulin dependence. This type of DM has also been referred to as latent autoimmune diabetes in adults (LADA).[5]

Maturity onset diabetes of youth (MODY), which can be due to one of at least six genetic defects, and endocrine disorders such as acromegaly and Cushing syndrome, can be secondary causes of DM.[7] These unusual etiologies, however, only account for 1% to 2% of the total cases of type 2 DM. See the section on other forms of diabetes mellitus later in this chapter for further discussion.

❷ The prevalence of type 2 DM is increasing. Type 2 DM accounts for as much as 90% of all cases of DM, and overall the prevalence of type 2 DM in the United States is about 10.7% in persons age 20 or older. Additionally, there is likely one person undiagnosed for every four persons currently diagnosed with the disease.[1] Multiple risk factors for the development of type 2 DM have been identified, including family history (i.e., parents or siblings with diabetes); obesity (i.e., ≥20% over ideal body weight, or body mass index [BMI] ≥25 kg/m²); habitual physical inactivity; race or ethnicity (see list below); previously identified impaired glucose tolerance, impaired fasting glucose, or HbA$_{1c}$ 5.7%–6.4% (see diagnosis of diabetes section); hypertension (≥140/90 mm Hg in adults); high-density lipoprotein (HDL) cholesterol ≤35 mg/dL and/or a triglyceride level ≥250 mg/dL; history of gestational diabetes mellitus (GDM) (see classification of diabetes section) or delivery of a baby weighing >9 pounds; history of vascular disease; presence of acanthosis nigricans; and polycystic ovary disease.[8] The prevalence of type 2 DM increases with age, it is more common in women than in men in the United States, and varies widely among various racial and ethnic populations, being especially increased in some groups of Native Americans, Hispanic American, Asian American, African American, and Pacific Island people[9] (Fig. 83–1). While the prevalence of type 2 DM increases with age (Fig. 83–2)[9], the disorder is increasingly being recognized in adolescence.

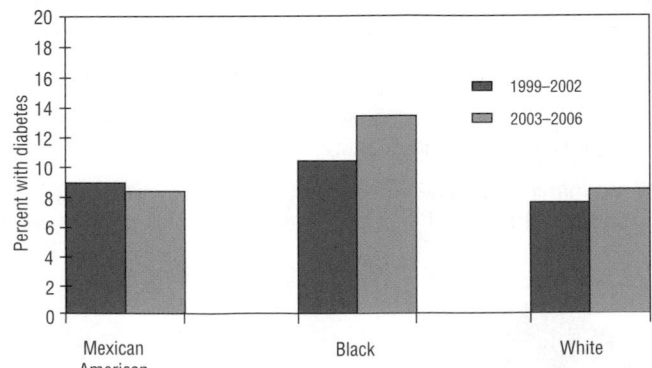

FIGURE 83-1. NHANES Prevalence of Diabetes by Race among Adults ≥20 Years of Age: United States, 1999–2002 and 2003–2006. *(Adapted from Cheung BMY, et al. Diabetes Prevalence and Therapeutic Target Achievement in the United States, 1999 to 2006. Am J Med 2009;122:443–453.)*

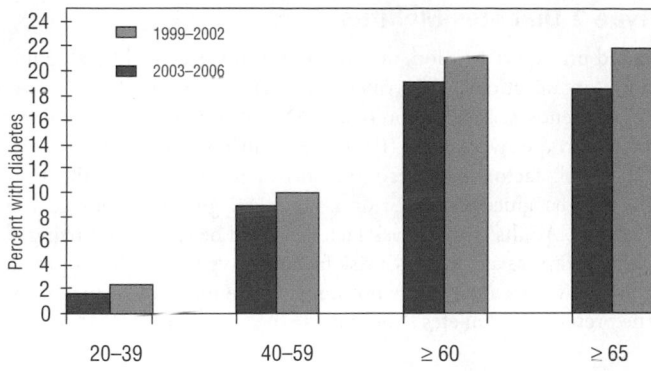

FIGURE 83-2. NHANES Prevalence of Diabetes by Age among Adults ≥20 Years of Age: United States, 1999–2002 and 2003–2006. *(Adapted from Cheung BMY, et al. Diabetes Prevalence and Therapeutic Target Achievement in the United States, 1999 to 2006. Am J Med 2009;122:443–453.)*

Much of the rise in adolescent type 2 DM is related to an increase in adiposity and sedentary lifestyle, in addition to an inheritable predisposition.[10] Most cases of type 2 DM do not have a well-known cause; therefore, it is uncertain whether it represents a few or many independent disorders manifesting as hyperglycemia.[11]

Gestational diabetes mellitus complicates roughly 7% of all pregnancies in the United States.[12] Most women will return to normoglycemia postpartum, but 30% to 50% will develop type 2 DM or glucose intolerance later in life.

PATHOGENESIS, DIAGNOSIS, AND CLASSIFICATION

CLASSIFICATION OF DIABETES

Diabetes is a metabolic disorder characterized by resistance to the action of insulin, insufficient insulin secretion, or both.[13] The clinical manifestation of these disorders is hyperglycemia. The vast majority of diabetic patients are classified into one of two broad categories: type 1 diabetes caused by an absolute deficiency of insulin, or type 2 diabetes defined by the presence of insulin resistance with an inadequate compensatory increase in insulin secretion. Women who develop diabetes due to the stress of pregnancy are classified as having gestational diabetes. Finally, uncommon types of diabetes caused by infections, drugs, endocrinopathies, pancreatic destruction, and known genetic defects are classified separately (Table 83–1).

TABLE 83-1	Etiologic Classification of Diabetes Mellitus

1. Type 1 diabetes[a] (β-cell destruction, usually leading to absolute insulin deficiency)
Immune mediated
Idiopathic

2. Type 2 diabetes[a] (may range from predominantly insulin resistance with relative insulin deficiency to a predominantly insulin secretory defect with insulin resistance)

3. Other specific types
Genetic defects of β-cell function
  Chromosome 20q, HNF-4α (MODY1)
  Chromosome 7p, glucokinase (MODY2)
  Chromosome 12q, HNF-1β (MODY3)
  Chromosome 13q, insulin promoter factor (MODY4)
  Chromosome 17q, HNF-1β (MODY5)
  Chromosome 2q, neurogenic differentiation 1/β-cell e-box transactivator 2 (MODY 6)
  Mitochondrial DNA
  Others
Genetic defects in insulin action
  Type A insulin resistance
  Leprechaunism
  Rabson-Mendenhall syndrome
  Lipoatrophic diabetes
  Others
Diseases of the exocrine pancreas
  Pancreatitis
  Trauma/pancreatectomy
  Neoplasia
  Cystic fibrosis
  Hemochromatosis
  Fibrocalculous pancreatopathy
  Others
Endocrinopathies
  Acromegaly
  Cushing syndrome
  Glucagonoma
  Pheochromocytoma
  Hyperthyroidism
  Somatostatinoma
  Aldosteronoma
  Others

Drug or chemical induced
  Vacor (pyriminil)
  Pentamidine
  Nicotinic acid
  Glucocorticoids
  Thyroid hormone
  Diazoxide
  β-Adrenergic agonists
  Thiazides
  Phenytoin
  α-Interferon
  Others
Infections
  Congenital rubella
  Cytomegalovirus
  Others
Uncommon forms of immune-mediated diabetes
  "Stiff-man" syndrome
  Anti-insulin receptor antibodies
  Others
Other genetic syndromes sometimes associated with diabetes
  Down syndrome
  Klinefelter syndrome
  Turner syndrome
  Wolfram syndrome
  Friedreich ataxia
  Huntington chorea
  Laurence-Moon-Bieldel syndrome
  Myotonic dystrophy
  Porphyria
  Prader-Willi syndrome
  Others

4. Gestational diabetes mellitus (GDM)

[a]Patients with any form of diabetes may require insulin treatment at some stage of their disease. Such use of insulin does not in itself classify the patient.
From Diabetes Care, Vol. 20, 1997; 1183-1197. Reproduced by permission of The American Diabetes Association.[13]

Type 1 Diabetes

❸ This form of diabetes results from autoimmune destruction of the β cells of the pancreas. Markers of immune destruction of the β cell are present at the time of diagnosis in 90% of individuals and include islet cell antibodies, antibodies to glutamic acid decarboxylase, and antibodies to insulin. While this form of diabetes usually occurs in children and adolescents, it can occur at any age. Younger individuals typically have a rapid rate of β-cell destruction and present with ketoacidosis, while adults often maintain sufficient insulin secretion to prevent ketoacidosis for many years, which is often referred to as latent autoimmune diabetes in adults.[5]

Type 2 Diabetes

❸ This form of diabetes is characterized by insulin resistance and a relative lack of insulin secretion, with progressively lower insulin secretion over time. Most individuals with type 2 diabetes exhibit abdominal obesity which itself causes insulin resistance. In addition, hypertension, dyslipidemia (high triglyceride levels and low HDL-cholesterol levels), and elevated inhibitor plasminogen activator-1 (PAI-1) levels, which contributes to a hypercoagulable state, are often present in these individuals. This clustering of abnormalities is referred to as the "insulin resistance syndrome" or the "metabolic syndrome." Because of these abnormalities, patients with type 2 diabetes are at increased risk of developing macrovascular complications. Type 2 diabetes has a strong genetic predisposition and is more common in all ethnic groups other than those of European ancestry. At this point the genetic cause of most cases of type 2 diabetes is not well defined.[14]

Gestational Diabetes Mellitus

Gestational diabetes mellitus is defined as glucose intolerance which is first recognized during pregnancy. Clinical detection is important, as therapy will reduce perinatal morbidity and mortality.

Other Specific Types of Diabetes

Genetic Defects Maturity onset diabetes of youth is characterized by impaired insulin secretion in respond to a glucose stimulus with minimal or no insulin resistance. Patients typically exhibit mild hyperglycemia at an early age, but diagnosis may be delayed, depending on the severity of presentation. The disease is inherited in an autosomal dominant pattern with at least six different loci identified to date (MODY 2 and 3 are most common). The production of mutant insulin molecules has been identified in a few families and results in mild glucose intolerance.

Several genetic mutations have been described in the insulin receptor and are associated with insulin resistance. Type A insulin resistance refers to the clinical syndrome of acanthosis nigricans, virilization in women, polycystic ovaries, and hyperinsulinemia. In contrast, type B insulin resistance is due to autoantibodies to the insulin receptor. Leprechaunism is a pediatric syndrome with specific facial features and severe insulin resistance due to a defect in the insulin-receptor gene. Lipoatrophic diabetes probably results from postreceptor defects in insulin signaling.

SCREENING

Type 1 Diabetes Mellitus

There is still a low prevalence of type 1 DM in the general population and due to the acuteness of symptoms in most individuals, screening for type 1 DM is not recommended.[8] Screening for islet autoantibody status in high-risk family members may be appropriate, but is recommended to be done in the context of ongoing clinical trials for the prevention of type 1 DM.

Type 2 Diabetes Mellitus

Based on expert opinion, and not uniformly accepted by all guidance organizations, the American Diabetes Association (ADA) recommends screening for type 2 DM at any age in individuals with who are overweight (BMI ≥25 kg/m²) and have at least one other risk factor. The recommended screening test is the fasting plasma glucose, HbA₁c, or 2-hour oral glucose tolerance test (OGTT). Adults without risk factors should be screened starting at age 45 years, as age itself is a risk factor for type 2 DM. The optimal time between screenings is not known. The index of suspicion for the presence of diabetes should guide the clinician.

Children and Adolescents

Despite a lack of clinical evidence to support widespread testing of children for type 2 DM, it is clear that more children and adolescents are developing type 2 DM. The ADA, by expert opinion, recommends that overweight (defined as BMI >85th percentile for age and sex, weight for height >85th percentile, or weight >120% of ideal [50th percentile] for height) youths with at least two of the following risk factors: a family history of type 2 diabetes in first- and second-degree relatives; Native Americans, African Americans, Hispanic Americans, and Asians/South Pacific Islanders; those with signs of insulin resistance or conditions associated with insulin resistance (acanthosis nigricans, hypertension, dyslipidemia, polycystic ovary syndrome, or small for gestational age birthweight); or maternal history of diabetes or gestational diabetes mellitus during the child's gestation be screened. Screening should be done every 3 years starting at 10 years of age or at the onset of puberty if it occurs at a younger age.[8]

Gestational Diabetes

Risk assessment for GDM should occur at the first prenatal visit. Women at high risk (positive family history, history of GDM or delivery of large-for-gestational–age infant, marked obesity, diagnosis of polycystic ovary syndrome, or member of a high-risk ethnic group) should be screened as soon as feasible. If the initial screening is negative they should undergo retesting at 24 to 28 weeks' gestation, as should all other pregnant women with the possible exception of low-risk primagravidas. Evaluation for GDM can be done in one of two ways. The one-step approach involves a 3-hour, 100 g-OGTT and may be cost-effective in high-risk patient populations. The two-step approach uses a screening test to measure plasma or serum glucose concentration 1 hour after a 50-g oral glucose load (glucose challenge test [GCT]), followed by a diagnostic 3-hour OGTT on the subset of women exceeding a glucose threshold of either ≥140 mg/dL (80% sensitive) or ≥130 mg/dL (90% sensitive). The diagnosis of GDM is based on the 100-g OGTT and at least two measured glucose values meeting or exceeding criteria. Criteria for diagnosis of GDM based on the OGTT are summarized in Table 83–2.

TABLE 83-2	Diagnosis of Gestational Diabetes Mellitus with a 100-g Glucose Load
100-g Glucose load	
Time	**Plasma Glucose**
Fasting	≥95 mg/dL (5.3 mmol/L)
1 hour	≥180 mg/dL (10.0 mmol/L)
2 hours	≥155 mg/dL (8.6 mmol/L)
3 hours	≥140 mg/dL (7.8 mmol/L)

Two or more values must be met or exceeded for a diagnosis of diabetes to be made. The test should be done in the morning after an 8- to 14-hour fast.

DIAGNOSIS OF DIABETES

❹ The diagnosis of diabetes requires the identification of a glycemic cut point, which discriminates normals from diabetic patients (Table 83–3). The cut points reflect the level of glucose above which microvascular complications have been shown to increase. Cross-sectional studies from Egypt, in Pima Indians, and in a representative sample from the United States have shown a consistent increase in the risk of developing retinopathy at a fasting glucose level above 99 to 116 mg/dL (5.5–6.4 mmol/L), at a 2-hour postprandial level above 125 to 185 mg/dL (6.9–10.3 mmol/L), and a hemoglobin A_{1c} (HbA$_{1c}$) above 5.9 to 6.0% (Fig. 83–3).[13,15,16]

TABLE 83-3	Criteria for the Diagnosis of Diabetes Mellitus[a]

1. HbA$_{1c}$ ≥6.5%. The test should be performed in a laboratory using a method that is National Glycohemoglobin Standardization Program (NGSP) certified and standardized to the DCCT assay.[a]

2. Fasting plasma glucose ≥126 mg/dL (7.0 mmol/L). Fasting is defined as no caloric intake for at least 8 hours.[a]

3. 2-hour plasma glucose ≥200 mg/dL (11.1 mmol/L) during an OGTT. The test should be performed as described by the World Health Organization, using a glucose load containing the equivalent of 75 g andydrous glucose dissolved in water.[a]

4. In a patient with classic symptoms of hyperglycemica or hyperglycemic crisis, a random plasma glucose concentration ≥200 mg/dL (11.1 mmol/L).

[a]In the absence of unequivocal hyperglycemia, criteria 1 to 3 should be confirmed by repeat testing.

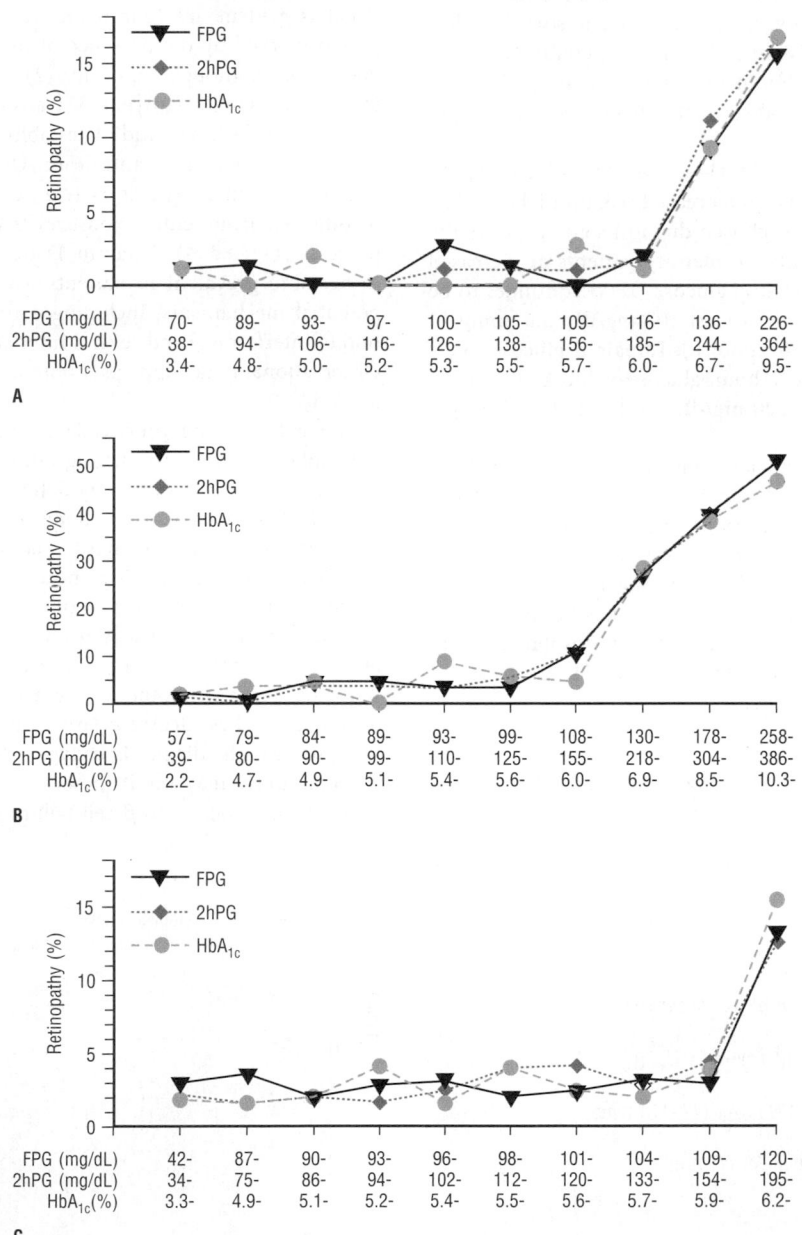

FIGURE 83-3. Prevalence of retinopathy by deciles of the distribution of fasting plasma glucose (FPG), 2-hour postprandial glucose (2-h PG), and hemoglobin A$_{1c}$ (HbA$_{1c}$) in *(A)* Pima Indians, *(B)* Egyptians, and *(C)* in 40- to 74-year old participants in National Health and Nutrition Examination Survey (NHANES) III.[8] The x-axis labels indicate the lower limit of each decile group. Note that these deciles and the prevalence rates of retinopathy differ considerably among the studies, especially the Egyptian study, in which diabetic subjects were oversampled. Retinopathy was ascertained by different methods in each study; therefore, the absolute prevalence rates are not comparable between studies, but their relationships with FPG, 2-h PG, and HbA$_{1c}$ are very similar within each population.

HbA$_{1c}$ ≥6.5% has been newly added as a fourth diagnostic criterion for diabetes mellitus. The HbA$_{1c}$ was not recommended in the past due to many nonstandardized assays. Most laboratories now use a method that is National Glycohemoglobin Standardization Program (NGSP) certified and standardized to the DCCT assay, which allows for cross-application of their results. If standardized, the HbA$_{1c}$ is logical for the diagnosis of diabetes as it measures glycemic exposure over the past 2 to 3 months, in contrast to a single-day, single-point glucose evaluation. In addition, patients do not have to be fasting. A HbA$_{1c}$ of 6.0% to 6.4% denotes a 10-fold increase in risk of diabetes, yet does not consistently identify patients with impaired fasting glucose or impaired glucose tolerance. In addition, there are slight race differences in normal HbA$_{1c}$ levels, so 6.5% was chosen to minimize these limitations. The ADA continues to recommend three other glucose criteria for the diagnosis of diabetes mellitus in nonpregnant adults (Table 83–3). It should be noted that a continuum of risk exists as glycemia increases, and sound clinical judgment as to the future risk of diabetes in the context of HbA$_{1c}$ and plasma glucose levels should be applied. If the patient has obvious hyperglycemia and diabetes, reconfirmation is no longer needed.

In addition, as shown in Table 83–4, the ADA added a HbA$_{1c}$ value of 5.7% to 6.4% to define an increased risk for diabetes. The HbA$_{1c}$ lower limit of 5.7% was chosen due to its good specificity, though it has a low sensitivity, to identify patients at increased risk for diabetes. Impaired fasting glucose (IFG) continues to be defined as a plasma glucose of at least 100 mg/dL (5.6 mmol/L) but less than 126 mg/dL (7.0 mmol/L). Impaired glucose tolerance (IGT), is defined as a 2-hour glucose value ≥140 mg/dL (7.8 mmol/L), but less than 200 mg/dL (11.0 mmol/L) during a 75 g-OGTT.

Serial measurements, at clinician-defined intervals, can help to identify patients moving toward diabetes, and those who are stable. Patients who have even minor increases in glucose or HbA$_{1c}$ values over time should be followed closely. Pathophysiologically, the fasting and postprandial glucose levels do not measure the same physiologic processes. The fasting glucose reflects hepatic glucose production, which is mainly determined by the insulin secretory capacity and glucagon released by the pancreas. The postprandial

glucose reflects uptake of glucose in peripheral tissues (muscle and fat) and depends on insulin sensitivity of these tissues. Also, the HbA$_{1c}$ measurement can be affected by several hemoglobinopathies, which necessitates the use of one of the plasma glucose criterion in these individuals.

PATHOGENESIS

Type 1 Diabetes Mellitus

Type 1 DM is characterized by an absolute deficiency of pancreatic β-cell function. Most often this is the result of an immune-mediated destruction of pancreatic β cells, but rare unknown or idiopathic processes may contribute. In immune mediated, a potential disruption of the T-helper 1/T-helper 2 balance may lead to higher T-helper 1 activity, with subsequent activation of the immune system and eventual destruction of pancreatic β cell. What is evident are four main features: (1) a long preclinical period marked by the presence of immune markers when β-cell destruction is thought to occur; (2) hyperglycemia when 80% to 90% of β cells are destroyed; (3) transient remission (the so-called "honeymoon" phase); and (4) established disease with associated risks for complications and death. Unknown is whether there is one or more inciting factors (e.g., cow's milk, or viral, dietary, or other environmental exposure) that initiate the autoimmune process[2] (Fig. 83–4). Vitamin D deficiency has been observed to be more prevalent in patients who develop type 1 DM, and potential mechanisms, including a role of vitamin D in reduction of interferon-γ and several interleukins, have been proposed. Observational data supports a potential role, but further study is needed.[17]

The autoimmune process is mediated by macrophages and T lymphocytes with circulating autoantibodies to various β-cell antigens. The most commonly detected antibody associated with type 1 DM is the islet cell antibody. The test for islet cell antibody, however, is difficult to standardize across laboratories. Other more readily measured circulating antibodies include insulin autoantibodies, antibodies directed against glutamic acid decarboxylase, insulin antibodies against islet tyrosine phosphatase, and several others. More than 90% of newly diagnosed persons with type 1 DM have one or another of these antibodies, as will 3.5% to 4% of unaffected first-degree relatives. Preclinical β-cell autoimmunity precedes the diagnosis of type 1 DM by up to 9 to 13 years. Autoimmunity may remit in some perhaps less-susceptible persons, or can progress to β-cell failure in others. These antibodies

TABLE 83-4	Categorization of Glucose Status

Fasting plasma glucose (FPG)
Normal
- FPG <100 mg/dL (5.6 mmol/L)
Impaired fasting glucose (IFG)
- 100–125 mg/dL (5.6–6.9 mmol/L)
Diabetes mellitus[a]
- FPG ≥126 mg/dL (7.0 mmol/L)
2-Hour postload plasma glucose (oral glucose tolerance test)
Normal
- Postload glucose <140 mg/dL (7.8 mmol/L)
Impaired glucose tolerance (IGT)
- 2-hour postload glucose 140–199 mg/dL (7.8–11.1 mmol/L)
Diabetes mellitus[a]
- 2-hour postload glucose ≥200 mg/dL (11.1 mmol/L)
HbA$_{1c}$
Normal
- HbA$_{1c}$ <5.7%
Increased risk of diabetes mellitus
- HbA$_{1c}$ 5.7% to 6.4%
Diabetes mellitus[a]
- HbA$_{1c}$ ≥6.5%

[a]Diagnosis to be confirmed if not unequivocal hyperglycemia (see Table 83–3).

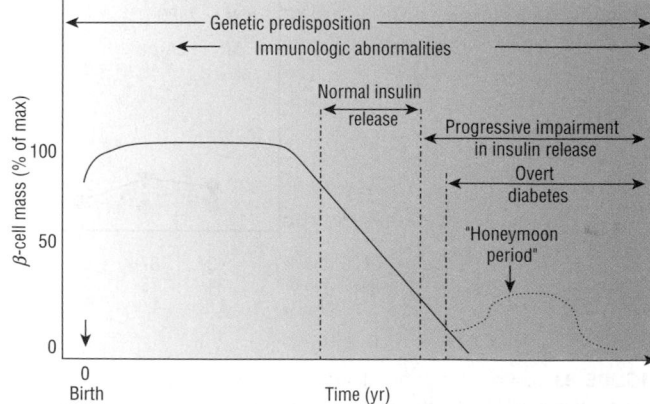

FIGURE 83-4. Scheme of the natural history of the β-cell defect in type 1 diabetes mellitus. *(Copyright © 2008 American Diabetes Association. From Medical Management of Type 1 Diabetes, Fifth Edition. Reprinted with permission from The American Diabetes Association.)*

are generally considered markers of disease rather than mediators of β-cell destruction. They have been used to identify individuals at risk for type 1 DM in evaluating disease prevention strategies. Other nonpancreatic autoimmune disorders are associated with type 1 DM, most commonly Hashimoto thyroiditis, but the extent of organ involvement can range from no other organs to polyglandular failure.[18]

There are strong genetic linkages to the *DQA* and *B* genes and certain human leukocyte antigens (HLAs) may be predisposing (*DR3* and *DR4*) or protective (*DRB1*04008-DQB1*0302* and *DRB1*0411-DQB1*0302*) on chromosome 6.[18] Other candidate gene regions have been identified on several other chromosomes as well. Because twin studies do not show 100% concordance, environmental factors such as infectious agents, chemical agents, and dietary agents are likely contributing factors in the expression of the disease.

Destruction of pancreatic β-cell function causes hyperglycemia due to an absolute deficiency of both insulin and amylin.[19] Insulin lowers blood glucose by a variety of mechanisms, including stimulation of tissue glucose uptake, suppression of glucose production by the liver, and suppression of free fatty acid (FFA) release from fat cells.[20] The suppression of free fatty acids plays an important role in glucose homeostasis. Increased levels of free fatty acids inhibit the uptake of glucose by muscle and stimulate hepatic gluconeogenesis.[21] Amylin, a glucoregulatory peptide hormone cosecreted with insulin, plays a role in lowering blood glucose by slowing gastric emptying, suppressing glucagon output from pancreatic alpha cells, and increasing satiety.[22] In type 1 DM, amylin production, due to β-cell destruction, is very low.

Type 2 Diabetes Mellitus

Normal Insulin Action In the fasting state 75% of total body glucose disposal takes place in non–insulin-dependent tissues: the brain and splanchnic tissues (liver and gastrointestinal tissues).[23] In fact, brain glucose uptake occurs at the same rate during fed and fasting periods and is not altered in type 2 diabetes.

The remaining 25% of glucose metabolism takes place in muscle, which is dependent on insulin.[24] In the fasting state approximately 85% of glucose production is derived from the liver, and the remaining amount is produced by the kidney.[24] Glucagon, produced by pancreatic α cells, is secreted in the fasting state to oppose the action of insulin and stimulate hepatic glucose production. Thus, glucagon prevents hypoglycemia or restores normoglycemia if hypoglycemia has occurred.[25] In the fed state, carbohydrate ingestion increases the plasma glucose concentration and stimulates insulin release from the pancreatic β cells. The resultant hyperinsulinemia (1) suppresses hepatic glucose production and (2) stimulates glucose uptake by peripheral tissues.[24] The majority (~80%–85%) of glucose that is taken up by peripheral tissues is disposed of in muscle, with only a small amount (~4%–5%) being metabolized by adipocytes. In the fed state, glucagon is suppressed.

Although fat tissue is responsible for only a small amount of total body glucose disposal, it plays a very important role in the maintenance of total body glucose homeostasis. Small increments in the plasma insulin concentration exert a potent antilipolytic effect, leading to a marked reduction in the plasma FFA level. The decline in plasma FFA concentration results in increased glucose uptake in muscle[24–28] and reduces hepatic glucose production.[29] Thus, a decrease in the plasma FFA concentration lowers plasma glucose by both decreasing its production and enhancing the uptake in muscle.

Type 2 diabetic individuals are characterized by (1) defects in insulin secretion; and (2) insulin resistance involving muscle, liver,

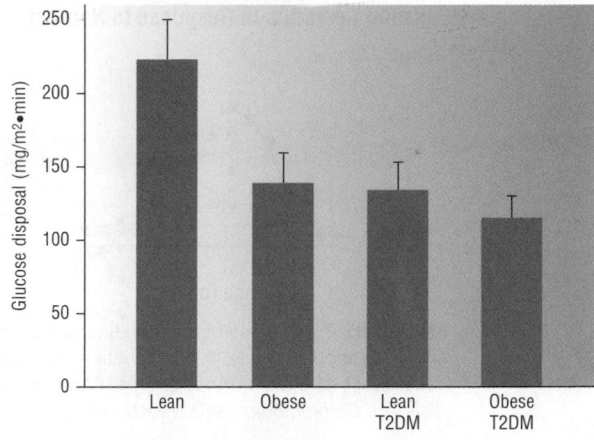

FIGURE 83-5. Whole body glucose disposal, a measure of insulin resistance, is reduced 40% to 50% in obese nondiabetic and lean type 2 diabetic individuals. Obese diabetic individuals are slightly more resistant than lean diabetic patients. *(From DeFronzo RA. Diabetes Reviews 1977;5:177–269.)*

and the adipocyte. Insulin resistance is present even in *lean* type 2 diabetic individuals (Fig. 83–5).

Impaired Insulin Secretion The pancreas in people with a normal-functioning β cell is able to adjust its secretion of insulin to maintain normal glucose tolerance. Thus, in nondiabetic individuals, insulin is increased in proportion to the severity of the insulin resistance and glucose tolerance remains normal. Impaired insulin secretion is a uniform finding in type 2 diabetic patients and the evolution of β-cell dysfunction has been well characterized in diverse ethnic populations.

The fasting plasma insulin concentration and oral glucose tolerance tests in 77 normal-weight type 2 diabetic patients and over 100 lean subjects with normal or impaired glucose tolerance were examined (Fig. 83–6). The relationship between the fasting plasma glucose concentration and the fasting plasma insulin concentration resembles an inverted U or horseshoe. As the fasting plasma glucose concentration rises from 80 to 140 mg/dL, the fasting plasma insulin concentration increases progressively, peaking

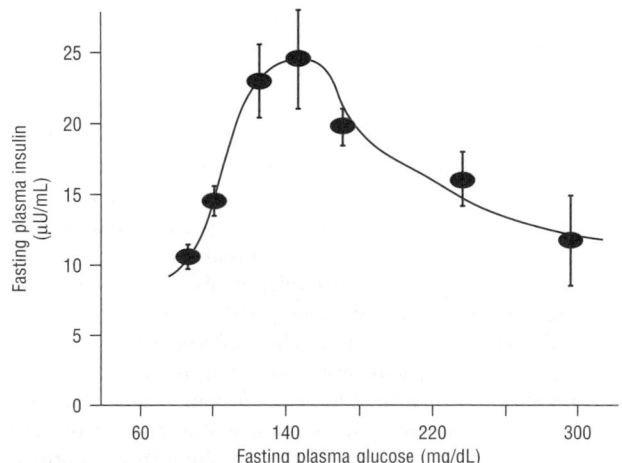

FIGURE 83-6. The relationship between fasting plasma insulin and fasting plasma glucose in 177 normal weight individuals. Plasma insulin and glucose increase together up to a fasting glucose of 140 mg/dL. When the fasting glucose exceeds 140 mg/dL, the β cell makes progressively less insulin, which leads to an overproduction of glucose by the liver and results in a progressive increase in fasting glucose. *(Reprinted from Med Clin N Am, Vol. 88., DeFronzo RA, Pathogenesis of type 2 diabetes mellitus, pages 787–835, Copyright © 2004, with permission from Elsevier.)*

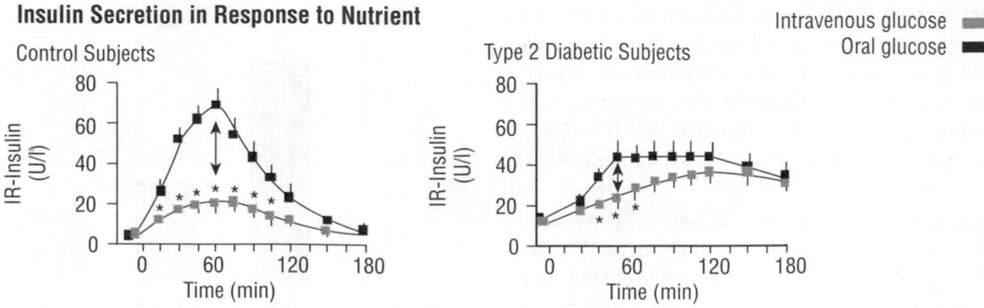

Insulin Secretion in Response to Nutrient

Control Subjects

Type 2 Diabetic Subjects

Intravenous glucose
Oral glucose

FIGURE 83-7. The loss of the incretin effect in type 2 diabetes mellitus. The plasma insulin responses to oral and intravenous glucose in nondiabetic subjects *(left)*, compared with patients with diabetes *(right)*. *(Adapted from Nauck M, Stockmann F, Ebert R, Creutzfeldt W. Reduced Incretin Effect in Type 2 (non-insulin dependent) diabetes. Diabetologia 1986;29:46–52.)*

at a value that is 2- to 2.5-fold greater than in normal weight nondiabetic controls. When the fasting plasma glucose concentration exceeds 140 mg/dL, the β cell is unable to maintain its elevated rate of insulin secretion and the fasting insulin concentration declines precipitously. This decrease in fasting insulin leads to an increase in hepatic glucose production overnight, which results in an elevated fasting plasma glucose concentration.[24]

In the type 2 diabetic patient, decreased postprandial insulin secretion is due to both impaired pancreatic beta cell function and a reduced stimulus for insulin secretion from gut hormones. The role gut hormones play in insulin secretion is best shown by comparing the insulin response to an oral glucose load versus an isoglycemic intraveneous glucose infusion. In nondiabetic control individuals 73% more insulin is released in response to an oral glucose load compared to reproducing the oral glucose load's plasma glucose curve by giving intravenous glucose (Fig. 83–7, left panel). This increased insulin secretion in response to an oral glucose stimulus is referred to as "the incretin effect" and suggests that gut-derived hormones when stimulated by glucose lead to an increase in pancreatic insulin secretion. In type 2 diabetic patients, this "incretin effect" is blunted with the increase in insulin secretion only being 50% of that seen in nondiabetic control individuals (Fig. 83–7). It is now known that two hormones, glucagon-like peptide 1 (GLP-1) and glucose-dependent insulinotropic polypeptide (GIP), are responsible for over 90% of the increased insulin secretion seen in response to an oral glucose load. Patients with type 2 diabetes remain sensitive to GLP-1 while they are often resistant to GIP.[25]

GLP-1 is secreted from the L-cells in the distal intestinal mucosa in response to mixed meals. Since GLP-1 levels rise within minutes of food ingestion neural signals initiated by food entry in the proximal gastrointestinal tract must simulate GLP-1 secretion. The insulinotropic action of GLP-1 is glucose dependent, and for GLP-1 to enhance insulin secretion, glucose concentrations must be higher than 90 mg/dL. In addition to stimulating insulin secretion, GLP-1 suppresses glucagon secretion, slows gastric emptying, and reduces food intake by increasing satiety. These effects of GLP-1 combine to limit postprandial glucose excursions. GIP is secreted by K-cells in the intestine and, like GLP, increases insulin secretion. However, GIP has no effect on glucagon secretion, gastric motility, or satiety. The half-life GLP-1 and GIP are short (<10 minutes). Both hormones are rapidly inactivated by removal of two N-terminal amino acids by the enzyme, dipeptidyl peptidase 4 (DPP-4). GLP-1 levels appears to decrease as glucose values increase from normal to type 2 DM.[25]

Site of Insulin Resistance in Type 2 Diabetes

Liver In type 2 diabetic subjects with mild to moderate fasting hyperglycemia (140–200 mg/dL, 7.8–1.1 mmol/L), basal

hepatic glucose production is increased by ~0.5 mg/kg/min. Consequently, during the overnight sleeping hours the liver of an 80-kg diabetic individual with modest fasting hyperglycemia adds an additional 35 g of glucose to the systemic circulation. This increase in fasting hepatic glucose production is the cause of fasting hyperglycemia.[24]

Following glucose ingestion, insulin is secreted into the portal vein and carried to the liver, where it suppresses glucagon secretion and reduces hepatic glucose output. Type 2 diabetic patients fail to suppress glucagon in response to a meal and may even have a paradoxical rise in glucagon levels. Thus, hepatic insulin resistance and hyperglucagonemia result in continued production of glucose by the liver. Therefore, type 2 diabetic patients have two sources of glucose in the postprandial state, one from the diet and one from continued glucose production from the liver. These sources of glucose in combination with a shortened gastric emptying time may result in marked hyperglycemia.

Peripheral (Muscle) Muscle is the major site of glucose disposal in man, and approximately 80% of total body glucose uptake occurs in skeletal muscle. In response to a physiologic increase in plasma insulin concentration, muscle glucose uptake increases linearly, reaching a plateau value of 10 mg/kg/min. In contrast, in lean type 2 diabetic subjects, the onset of insulin action is delayed for ~40 minutes, and the ability of insulin to stimulate leg glucose uptake is reduced by 50%. Impaired insulin signaling is a well established abnormality, with notable impairments at almost every step of activation due to insulin resistance, lipo- and glucotoxicity. The compensatory hyperinsulinemia required to overcome impaired insulin signaling (insulin resistance) can activate an alternative pathway through MAP kinase, which may be involved in atherosclerosis. Mitochondrial dysfunction may also play a role in muscle insulin resistance. Mitochondrial function and density appear to be lower in some studies of type 2 DM. This may result in less energy expenditure and an increased risk of dysfunction with high-fat diets.[24]

Peripheral (Adipocyte) In obese nondiabetic and diabetic humans, basal plasma FFA levels are increased and fail to suppress normally after glucose ingestion. FFAs are stored as triglycerides in adipocytes and serve as an important energy source during conditions of fasting. Insulin is a potent inhibitor of lipolysis, and restrains the release of FFAs from the adipocyte by inhibiting the hormone-sensitive lipase enzyme. It is now recognized that chronically elevated plasma FFA concentrations can lead to insulin resistance in muscle and liver, and impair insulin secretion. In addition to FFAs that circulate in plasma in increased amounts, type 2 diabetic and obese nondiabetic individuals have increased stores of triglycerides in muscle and liver, and the increased fat content correlates closely with the presence of insulin resistance in these tissues.

In summary, insulin resistance involving both muscle and liver is a characteristic feature of glucose intolerance in type 2 diabetic individuals. In the basal state, the liver represents a major site of insulin resistance, and this is reflected by overproduction of glucose. This accelerated rate of hepatic glucose output is the primary determinant of the elevated fasting plasma glucose concentration in type 2 diabetic individuals. In the fed state, both decreased muscle glucose uptake and impaired suppression of hepatic glucose production contribute to the insulin resistance. In obese individuals and in the majority (>80%) of type 2 diabetic subjects, there is an expanded fat cell mass and the adipocytes are resistant to the antilipolytic effects of insulin. Most obese and diabetic individuals are characterized by expanded visceral adiposity, discussed in detail later in the chapter, which is especially refractory to insulin effects and results in a high lipolytic rate. Not surprisingly, both type 2 diabetes and obesity are characterized by an elevation in the mean 24-hour plasma FFA concentration. Elevated plasma FFA levels, as well as increased triglyceride/fatty acyl CoA content in muscle, liver, and β cells, lead to the development of muscle/hepatic insulin resistance and impaired insulin secretion.

Cellular Mechanisms of Insulin Resistance

Insulin resistance and the components of the insulin resistance syndrome are described below.

Obesity and Insulin Resistance Weight gain leads to insulin resistance, and obese nondiabetic individuals have the same degree of insulin resistance as lean type 2 diabetic patients. In 1,146 nondiabetic, normotensive individuals, a progressive loss of insulin sensitivity when the BMI increased from 18 kg/m² to 38 kg/m² was documented. The increase in insulin resistance with weight gain is directly related to the amount of visceral adipose tissue. Subsets of obese, but metabolically normal patients do exist, as well as nonobese, but metabolically abnormal patients, so broad categorization of risk for a patient needs to be confirmed by further examination.

The term *visceral adipose tissue* (VAT) refers to fat cells located within the abdominal cavity and includes omental, mesenteric, retroperitoneal, and perinephric adipose tissue. VAT has been shown to correlate with insulin resistance and explain much of the variation in insulin resistance seen in a population of African Americans. Visceral adipose tissue represents 20% of fat in men and 6% of fat in women. This fat tissue has been shown to have a higher rate of lipolysis than subcutaneous fat, resulting in an increase in FFA production. These fatty acids are released into the portal circulation and drain into the liver, where they stimulate the production of very-low-density lipoproteins and decrease insulin sensitivity in peripheral tissues. VAT also produces a number of cytokines, such as TNF-α, interleukin 6, and resistin, which contribute to insulin resistance. These factors drain into the portal circulation and reduce insulin sensitivity in peripheral tissues.

The fat cell also has the capability of producing at least one hormone that improves insulin sensitivity: adiponectin. This factor is made in decreasing amounts as an individual becomes more obese.[24] In animal models, adiponectin decreases hepatic glucose production and increases fatty acid oxidation in muscle.[24]

The Metabolic Syndrome The association of insulin resistance with a clustering of cardiovascular risk factors including hyperinsulinemia, hypertension, abdominal obesity, dyslipidemia, and coagulation abnormalities has been referred to by a variety of names including "insulin resistance syndrome," "metabolic syndrome," "dysmetabolic syndrome," and "the deadly quartet," to name a few. Since the description of the "insulin resistance syndrome" by Reaven in 1988,[26] the number of associated factors has continued to

grow. Metabolic syndrome is a risk indicator, but not an absolute risk indicator, because it does not specifically account for all risk factors, such as age, sex, low-density lipoprotein cholesterol levels, or directly measure hypercoagulability of the proinflammatory condition. Patients with metabolic syndrome do have a higher risk for cardiovascular disease (CVD), and at least a 5-fold increase in their risk of type 2 DM.

The most recent definition of metabolic syndrome was adopted by multiple organizations in 2009 (Table 83–5).[27] Central obesity continues to be recognized as an important causative factor, but is no longer considered a prerequisite to having metabolic syndrome. Central obesity can be easily assessed using waist circumference, which is a good surrogate marker for VAT. It is imperative to measure the waist circumference correctly (just above hip bones and just below umbilicus, tape measure should be taught, but not tight), for accurate assessment. Ethnic group specific cut-points for waist circumference are pragmatic estimates taken from various data sources. As more complete data becomes available these values may be modified. Table 83–5 lists the ethnic specific values for waist circumference.

Prevalence. Regardless of the definition used, large numbers of adults in the United States have metabolic syndrome. The National Health and Nutrition Examination Survey (NHANES) 1999–2002 is the most scientifically rigorous sample of the U.S. population.[28] A total of 3,601 men and women aged >20 years were included in the survey. Using the NCEP definition (Table 83–5), the prevalence of metabolic syndrome was 33.7% of men and 35.4% of women. In a sample of 4,060 predominantly European adults from South Australia, metabolic syndrome was present in 19.4% of men and 14.4% of women using the ATP III definition.[29]

The impact of treating the clinical components of the metabolic syndrome in diabetes patients was demonstrated in the Steno-2 Study.[30] In this prospective study, 63 patients with diabetes and microalbuminuria were randomized to the usual therapy group and 67 patients were treated intensively. Intensive therapy consisted of diet and exercise and pharmacologic intervention aimed at reducing hyperglycemia, hypertension, dyslipidemia, microalbuminuria, and increased coagulopathy (aspirin therapy). Treatment goals for intensive therapy included a blood pressure <130/80 mm Hg, HbA_{lc} <6.5%, total cholesterol <175 mg/dL, and triglycerides <150 mg/dL. All patients in the intensive treatment group were given an aspirin and treated with an angiotensin-converting enzyme (ACE) inhibitor. Patients in the intensively treated group showed a 53% relative risk reduction in cardiovascular disease and a 61% relative risk reduction in nephropathy. In this small study, the magnitude of this reduction is greater than has been demonstrated with individual interventions, stressing the importance of targeting all the components of the metabolic syndrome. The study design did not allow conclusions regarding which interventions had the most impact.

CLINICAL PRESENTATION

The clinical presentations of type 1 DM and type 2 DM are very different. Autoimmune type 1 DM can occur at any age. Approximately 75% will develop the disorder before age 20 years, but the remaining 25%, including relatives of index patients, develop the disease as adults. Individuals with type 1 DM are often thin and are prone to develop diabetic ketoacidosis if insulin is withheld, or under conditions of severe stress with an excess of insulin counterregulatory hormones.[3] Twenty percent to 40% of patients with type 1 DM present with diabetic ketoacidosis after several days of polyuria, polydipsia, polyphagia, and weight loss.

TABLE 83-5 Defining of the Metabolic Syndrome

Defining the Metabolic Syndrome NCEP ATP III: Five Components of the Metabolic Syndrome (Individuals Having at Least Three Components Meet the Criteria for Diagnosis)

Risk Factor	Defining Level
Abdominal obesity	Waist circumference
Men	>102 cm (>40 in)
Women	>88 cm (>35 in)
Triglycerides	≥150 mg/dL
High-density lipoprotein C	
Men	<40 mg/dL
Women	<50 mg/dL
Blood pressure	≥130/≥85 mm Hg
Fasting glucose	≥110 mg/dL

2009 Statement of the International Diabetes Federation Task Force on Epidemiology and Prevention; National Heart, Lung, and Blood Institute; American Heart Association; World Heart Federation; International Atherosclerosis Society; and International Association for the Study of Obesity

Criteria for Clinical Diagnosis of the Metabolic Syndrome (Individuals having at least three components meet the criteria for diagnosis)

Measure	Categorical Cut Points
Elevated waist circumference[a]	Population- and country-specific definitions
Elevated triglycerides (drug treatment for elevated triglycerides is an alternate indicator)[b]	≥150 mg/dL (1.7 mmol/L)
Reduced HDL-C (drug treatment for reduced HDL-C is an alternate indicator)[b]	≤40 mg/dL (1.0 mmol/L) in males ≤50 mg/dL (1.3 mmol/L) in females
Elevated blood pressure Systolic ≥130 and/or diastolic ≥80 mm Hg (antihypertensive drug treatment in a patient with a history of hypertension is an alternate indicator)	
Elevated fasting glucose[c] (drug treatment of elevated glucose is an alternate indicator)	≥100 mg/dL

Current Recommended Waist Circumference Thresholds for Abdominal Obesity by Organization

Population	Organization (Reference)	Men (All values ≥)	Women (All values ≥)
Europid	IDF	94 cm	80 cm
Caucasian	WHO	94 cm (increased risk) 102 cm (still higher risk)	80 cm (increased risk) 88 cm (still higher risk)
Unites States	AHA/NHLBI (ATP III)	102 cm	88 cm
Canada	Health Canada	102 cm	88 cm
European	European European Cardiovascular Societies	102 cm	88 cm
Asia (including Japanese)	IDF	90 cm	80 cm
Asia	WHO	90 cm	80 cm
Japan	Japanese Obesity Society	85 cm	90 cm
China	Cooperative Task Force	85 cm	80 cm
Middle East	Mediterranean IDF	94 cm	80 cm
Sub-Saharan African	IDF	94 cm	80 cm
Ethnic Central and South American	IDF	90 cm	80 cm

HDL-C indicates high-density lipoprotein cholesterol.

[a]It is recommended that the IDF cut points be used for non-Europeans and either the IDF or AHA/NHLBI cut points used for people of European origin until more data are available.

[b]The most commonly used drugs for elevated triglycerides and reduced HDL-C are fibrates and nicotinic acid. A patient taking 1 of these drugs can be presumed to have high triglycerides and low HDL-C. High-dose −3 fatty acids presumes high triglycerides.

[c]Most patients with type 2 diabetes mellitus will have the metabolic syndrome by the proposed criteria.

Reproduced from Expert Panel on Detection.[124]

Reprinted with permission Circulation. 2009;120:1640–1645 © 2009 American Heart Association, Inc.

Occasionally, type 1 DM patients are diagnosed without multiple symptoms or diabetic ketoacidosis when they have blood tests drawn for other reasons. Because newly diagnosed patients with type 1 DM often have a small amount of residual pancreatic β-cell function, they may enter a "honeymoon" phase, when their blood glucose concentrations are relatively easy to control and small amounts of insulin are needed. Once this residual insulin secretion wanes, the patients are completely insulin deficient and tend to have more labile glycemia. Not all type 1 DM patients have complete insulin deficiency, and a small residual amount of insulin secretion is seen in some patients.

Patients with type 2 DM often present without symptoms, even though complications tell us that they may have been hyperglycemic for several years.[10] Often these patients are diagnosed secondary to unrelated blood testing. Lethargy, polyuria, nocturia, and polydipsia can be seen at diagnosis in type 2 diabetes, but significant weight loss at diagnosis is less common. Clinically, diabetes mellitus is a spectrum of diseases ranging from absolute insulin deficiency to relative insulin insulin deficiency, and patients can have normal to grossly abnormal insulin sensitivity. Classical clinical presentation characteristics should be used in conjuction with other definitive laboratory data to properly classify patients.

CLASSICAL CLINICAL PRESENTATION OF DIABETES MELLITUS[a]

Characteristic	Type 1 DM	Type 2 DM
Age	<30 years[b]	>30 years[b]
Onset	Abrupt	Gradual
Body habitus	Lean	Obese or history of obesity
Insulin resistance	Absent	Present
Autoantibodies	Often present	Rarely present
Symptoms	Symptomatic[c]	Often asymptomatic
Ketones at diagnosis	Present	Absent[d]
Need for insulin therapy	Immediate	Years after diagnosis
Acute complications	Diabetic ketoacidosis	Hyperosmolar hyperglycemic state
Microvascular complications at diagnosis	No	Common
Macrovascular complications at or before diagnosis	Rare	Common

[a]Clinical presentation can vary widely.

[b]Age of onset for type 1 DM is generally <20 years of age, but can present at any age. The prevalence of type 2 DM in children, adolescents, and young adults is increasing. This is especially true in ethnic and minority children.

[c]Type 1 may present acutely with symptoms of polyuria, nocturia, polydipsia, polyphagia, and weight loss.

[d]Type 2 children and adolescents are more likely to present with ketones, but after the acute phase may be treated with oral agents. Prolonged fasting can also produce ketones in individuals.

TREATMENT

Diabetes Mellitus

■ DESIRED OUTCOME

❺ The primary goals of DM management are to reduce the risk for microvascular and macrovascular disease complications, to ameliorate symptoms, to reduce mortality, and to improve quality of life.[8] Near-normal glycemia will reduce the risk for development of microvascular disease complications, but aggressive management of traditional cardiovascular risk factors (i.e., smoking cessation, treatment of dyslipidemia, intensive blood pressure control, and antiplatelet therapy) are needed to reduce the likelihood of development of macrovascular disease. Evidence-based guidelines, as published by the ADA, may help in the attainment of these goals (Table 83–6).[8]

Hyperglycemia not only increases the risk for microvascular disease, but contributes to poor wound healing, compromises white blood cell function, and leads to classic symptoms of DM. Diabetic ketoacidosis and hyperosmolar hyperglycemic state are severe manifestations of poor diabetes control, almost always requiring hospitalization. Reducing the potential for microvascular complications is targeted at adherence to therapeutic lifestyle intervention (i.e., diet and exercise programs) and drug-therapy regimens, as well as at maintaining blood pressure as near normal as possible.

■ GENERAL APPROACH TO TREATMENT

Appropriate care requires goal setting for glycemia, blood pressure, and lipid levels, regular monitoring for complications, dietary and exercise modifications, medications, appropriate self-monitoring of blood glucose (SMBG), and laboratory assessment of the aforementioned parameters.[8] Glucose control alone does not sufficiently reduce the risk of macrovascular complications in persons with DM.

■ GLYCEMIC GOAL SETTING AND HEMOGLOBIN A1C

Controlled clinical trials provide ample evidence that glycemic control is paramount in reducing microvascular complications in both type 1 DM[31] and type 2 DM.[32] HbA$_{1c}$ measurements are the gold standard for following long-term glycemic control for the previous 2 to 3 months.[33] Hemoglobinopathies, anemia, red cell membrane defects, transfusions, and any patient where the red blood cell lifespan is substantially increased or decreased can affect HbA$_{1c}$ measurements. Minimization of problems, such as sickle cell trait, and assurance of standardized results can be accomplished by ensuring the test is performed in a laboratory using a method that is National Glycohemoglobin Standardization Program (NGSP) certified and standardized to the DCCT assay. Other strategies such as measurement of fructosamine, which measures glycated plasma proteins and correlates to glucose control over the last 2 to 3 weeks, may be necessary to assess diabetes control in patients with altered red blood cell lifespan, though the fructosamine is less standardized, and not correlated to risk of complications.

The A1C-Derived Average Glucose study correlated multiple HbA$_{1c}$ and glucose readings to term a new phrase, estimated average glucose or eAG if abbreviated.[34] The eAG better correlates with HbA$_{1c}$ readings, and now is regularly reported below HbA$_{1c}$ values on laboratory results. For example, a HbA$_{1c}$ of 6% or 7%, correlates with an average glucose of 126 mg/dL or 154mg/dL, respectively, and online calculators and graphs are easily found.

Less stringent HbA$_{1c}$ goals (>7%) may be appropriate in patients with a history of severe hypoglycemia, limited life expectancy, advanced micro/macrovascular complications or comorbidities, at risk elderly, dementia, or in younger children. A HbA$_{1c}$ target of <7% is appropriate for others (Table 83–7), and lower values should be targeted if significant hypoglycemia, weight gain, and other adverse effects can be avoided.[8] New glycemic control recommendations for different age groups of type 1 DM patients are now recommended, based on the risk of hypoglycemia, the relatively low risk of complications prior to puberty, and psychological and/or developmental issues (Table 83–7).

■ MONITORING FOR COMPLICATIONS

The ADA recommends initiation of complications monitoring at the time of diagnosis of diabetes mellitus.[8] Current recommendations continue to advocate yearly dilated eye examinations in type 2 DM, and an initial dilated eye exam in the first 3 to 5 years in type 1 DM, then yearly thereafter. Less frequent testing (every 2–3 years) can be implemented upon the advice of an eye care specialist. The feet should be examined and the blood pressure assessed at each visit, with a distal polyneuropathy screen being performed yearly by simple tools, such as the 10-g force Semmes-Weinstein monofilament. A urine test for microalbumin once yearly from diagnosis is appropriate in type 2 DM, and initiated 5 years after diagnosis if the patient has type 1 DM. Yearly testing for lipid abnormalities, and more frequently if needed to achieve lipid goals, is recommended.

■ SELF-MONITORED BLOOD GLUCOSE AND CONTINUOUS GLUCOSE MONITORING

The advent of SMBG in the early 1980s revolutionized the treatment of DM, enabling patients to know their blood glucose

TABLE 83-6 Selected American Diabetes Association Evidence-Based Recommendations[a]

Recommendation Area	Specific Recommendation	Evidence Level[b]
Screening for diabetes	Screen overweight or obese at any age, those without risk factors should begin at 45 years.	B
	To screen for diabetes a FPG, 2-hour 75-g OGTT, or HbAl$_c$ are appropriate.	B
	Interval between screenings should be individualized based on risk, or every 3 years.	E
Monitoring	Home blood glucose monitoring is needed if on insulin.	A
	Subjects on other therapeutic interventions, including oral agents may need home blood glucose monitoring.	E
	Quarterly HbA$_{1c}$ in individuals not meeting glycemic goals, twice yearly in individuals meeting glycemic goals should be performed.	E
	In adults, measure fasting lipid profile at least annually.	E
	Perform an annual urine albumin excretion in type 1 diabetes with duration ≥5 years. Type 2 DM from diagnosis.	E
	All patients should be screened for polyneuropathy at diagnosis and at least annually thereafter.	B
	A dilated eye exam should be performed within 5 years of diagnosis in type 1 DM, and shortly after diagnosis in type 2 DM, with follow-up every year, or every 2–3 years as recommended by an eye specialist.	B
Glycemic goals	HbA$_{1c}$ goal for patients in general is <7%.	B
	HbA$_{1c}$ goal should be individualized, with <7% if achieved without significant hypoglycemia or adverse effects.	B
	Less stringent HbA$_{1c}$ goal may be appropriate in patients with a history of severe hypoglycemia, limited life expectancy, advanced micro/macrovascular complications or comorbidities, or in younger children.	C
Treatment		
Prevention of type 2 diabetes	Patients with IGT (A), IFG (E), or an A1C of 5.7–6.4% (E) should attempt weight loss (5%–10%), increasing physical activity.	See text
	Metformin may be considered in obese, <60-year-old patients at very high risk of diabetes, including "near" diabetes glucose or A1C, HTN, first-degree family history of diabetes.	E
Medical nutrition therapy	Weight loss is recommended for all insulin-resistant/overweight or obese individuals. Either low-carbohydrate or low-fat calorie restricted diets may work.	A
	In types 1 and 2 DM, intensive vs standard glucose control have not shown a significant reduction in CVD during randomized portions, but long-term follow-up of DCCT and UKPDS have shown targeting below A$_{1c}$ <7% may reduce long-term macrovascular disease.	B
	Saturated fat should be <7% of total calories.	A
	Monitoring carbohydrate intake by carbohydrate counting or exchanges is recommended.	A
	Glycemic index may give modest benefits over total carbohydrate intake.	B
Physical activity	150 minutes/week of moderate intensity exercise is recommended or 90 minutes of vigourous exercise/week.	A
	Resistance training of large muscle groups should be 3 × week.	A
Blood pressure	Systolic blood pressure should be treated to <130 mm Hg.	C
	Diastolic blood pressure should be treated to <80 mm Hg.	B
	Initial drug therapy should be with an ACE inhibitor or ARB.	C
Nephropathy	Type 1 DM with any degree of albuminuria-ACE inhibitor.	A
	Type 2 DM with microalbuminuria-ACE inhibitor or ARB.	A
	Type 2 DM with macroalbuminuria-angiotensin receptor blocker.	A
Dyslipidemia	The primary goal is an LDL <100 mg/dL.	A
	Statin therapy should be added to lifestyle, regardless of baseline lipid levels if patient has CVD, >40 years of age, and one other CVD risk fact.	A
	In patients with overt CVD, using a statin to acheive a LDL <70 mg/dL is an optional goal.	B
	Triglycerides should be lowered to <150 mg/dL.	C
	Raising HDL to >40 mg/dL in men and >50 mg/dL in women.	C
Antiplatelet	Use aspirin (75–162 mg daily) for secondary cardioprotection.	A
	Use aspirin (75–162 mg) for primary prevention in type 1 or 2 DM if the 10-year risk of CVD is >10%, or at least one additional risk factor is present.	C
	Clopidogrel (75 mg/day) is appropriate for patients with CVD and documented aspirin allergy.	B

[a]Based on American Diabetes Association Practice Recommendations[8]
[b]Evidence levels:
A = Clear evidence from well-conducted, generalizable, randomized controlled trials that are adequately powered.
B = Supportive evidence from well-conducted cohort studies or well-conducted case-control study.
C = Supportive evidence from poorly controlled or uncontrolled studies or conflicting evidence with weight of evidence supporting intervention.
E = Expert consensus or clinical experience.

concentration at any moment easily and relatively inexpensively. Frequent SMBG is necessary to achieve near-normal blood glucose concentrations and to assess for hypoglycemia and hyperglycemia, adjust prandial doses of insulin, and give corrective doses of insulin. This is particularly true in patients with type 1 DM, as most will be intensively managed with insulin.[33] The more intense the pharmacological regimen is, the more intense the SMBG needs to be (four or more times daily in patients on multiple insulin injections or pump therapy whether type 1 or type 2 DM). The optimal frequency of SMBG for patients with type 2 DM on oral agents is unresolved. Frequency of monitoring in type 2 DM should be

sufficient to facilitate reaching glucose goals and to test for hypoglycemia. The role of SMBG in improving glycemic control in type 2 DM patients is controversial, but has shown to reduce the HbA$_{1c}$ ~0.4% to no improvement.[35] What is clear is that patients must be empowered to change their therapeutic regimen (lifestyle and medications) in response to test results, or no meaningful glycemic improvement is likely to be effected.

Alternate site testing may improve adherence to SMBG recommendations, but only SMBG meters that can "sip" blood onto the strip will accommodate such testing. Alternate site glucose testing may be performed on alternative parts of the body, such as

TABLE 83-7 Glycemic Goals of Therapy by Organization and for Type 1 DM[R]

Biochemical index	ADA	ACE and AACE
Hemoglobin A$_{1c}$	<7%[a]	≤6.5%
Preprandial plasma glucose	70–130 mg/dL (3.9–7.2 mmol/L)	<110 mg/dL
Postprandial plasma glucose	<180 mg/dL[b] (<10 mmol/L)	<140 mg/dL

ADA plasma glucose and HbA$_{1c}$ goals for type 1 DM by age group[c]			
Values by age (years)	Plasma glucose goal Before meals	bedtime/overnight	A$_{1c}$
Toddlers and preschoolers (0–6)	100–180	110–200	<8.5% (but >7.5%)
School age (6–12)	90–180	100–180	<8.0%
Adolescents and young adults (13–19)	90–130	90–150	<7.5%

ADA, American Diabetes Association; ACE, American College of Endocrinology; AACE, American Association of Clinical Endocrinologists; DCCT, Diabetes Control and Complications Trial.

[a]Assay should be National Glycohemoglobin Standardization Program (NGSP) certified measurement and DCCT standardized. More stringent glycemic control may be appropriate if accomplished without significant hypoglycemia or adverse effects. Less stringent HbA$_{1c}$ goals may be appropriate in patients with a history of severe hypoglycemia, limited life expectancy, advanced micro/macrovascular complications or comorbidities, at-risk elderly, dementia, or in younger children.

[b]Postprandial glucose measurements should be made 1–2 hours after the beginning of the meal, generally the time of peak levels in patients with diabetes.

[c]Vulnerability to hypoglycemia and relatively low risk of complication prior to puberty considered. Adolescents and youg adults may have adult goals if without developmental and psychological issues, and if without excessive hypoglycemia.

the palm, forearm, thigh, and stomach. These areas tend to have less nerve endings and may be more comfortable for a patient, but several cautions must be observed. Alternate site glucose readings will lag behind fingertip capillary blood, as the capillary flow and density is often less in the alternate testing sites when compared with the fingertip. Alternate site testing is discouraged in any situation where immediate action will be needed based on the glucose reading, such as testing for hypoglycemia or in patients with hypoglycemia unawareness, wide fluctuations in SMBG, or when the blood glucose is know to be fluctuating, such as postprandially.

CLINICAL CONTROVERSY

SMBG improves glycemic control when insulin is used, but few well-conducted studies have shown significant glycemic reductions with increasing use of home blood glucose testing for type 2 DM patients not on insulin. The average HbA$_{1c}$ reduction with use of SMBG in type 2 DM patients not on insulin was 0.4%, though others have reported no glycemic improvement.[33] Patients must be empowered to change their therapeutic regimen (lifestyle and medications) in response to test results, or no meaningful glycemic improvement is likely to be effected, and thus the money spent on the strip is wasted.

Continuous glucose monitoring (CGM) may be useful in select patients. CGM measures interstitial glucose, which lags behind capillary SMBG, and the same cautions as alternate site testing should be followed. CGM can be useful in patients with frequent hypoglycemia or hypoglycemic unawareness, nocturnal hypoglycemia, for identification of fluctuating glucose patterns and/or previously unknown problems in patients with higher than expected HbA$_{1c}$ results. CGM still needs to be calibrated multiple times a day with SMBG readings to ensure accuracy, and a new sensor must be placed every 3 to 7 days. The ADA currently recommends that CGM can be considered in type 1 DM adults ≥25 years of age, and in others with the above issues noted.

■ NONPHARMACOLOGIC THERAPY

Diet

Medical nutrition therapy is recommended for all persons with DM and along with activity, is a cornerstone of treatment.[36] Paramount for all medical nutrition therapy is the attainment of optimal metabolic outcomes and the prevention and treatment of complications. For individuals with type 1 DM, the focus is on regulating insulin administration with a balanced diet to achieve and maintain a healthy body weight. A meal plan that is moderate in carbohydrates and low in saturated fat (<7% of total calories), with a focus on balanced meals is recommended. The amount (grams) and type (via the glycemic index, though controversial) of carbohydrates, whether accounted for by exchanges or carbohydrate counting, should be considered.[36] It is imperative that patients understand the connection between carbohydrate intake and glucose control. In addition, patients with type 2 DM often require caloric restriction to promote weight loss, and portion size and frequency are often issues. Rather than a set diabetic diet, advocate a diet using foods that are within the financial reach and cultural milieu of the patient. As most patients with type 2 DM are overweight or obese, bedtime and between-meal snacks are not needed if pharmacologic management is appropriate.

Activity

In general, most patients with DM can benefit from increased activity.[37] Aerobic exercise improves insulin sensitivity and glycemic control in the majority of individuals, and reduces cardiovascular risk factors, contributes to weight loss or maintenance, and improves well-being. The patient should choose an activity that she or he is likely to continue. Start exercise slowly in previously sedentary patients. It remains unclear which asymptomatic patients should be screened for CVD prior to the beginning of an exercise regimean. It may be reasonable in patients with long-standing disease (age >35 years, or >25 years old with DM ≥10 years), patients with multiple cardiovascular risk factors, presence of microvascular disease (especially renal disease), and patients with previous evidence of atherosclerotic disease should have a cardiovascular evaluation, probably including an electrocardiogram, with further workup related to CVD risk. In addition, several complications (uncontrolled hypertension, autonomic neuropathy, insensate feet, and retinopathy) may require restrictions on the activities recommended. Physical activity goals include at least 150 minutes/week of moderate (50%–70% maximal heart rate) intensity exercise. In addition, resistance training, in patients without retinal contraindications, is recommended for 30 minutes 3 times/week.

■ PHARMACOLOGIC THERAPY

Until 1995, only two options for pharmacologic treatment were available for patients with diabetes; sulfonylureas (for type 2 DM only) and insulin (for type 1 or 2). Since 1995, a number of new oral agents, injectables, and insulins have been introduced in the United States.

Currently, eight classes of oral agents are approved for the treatment of type 2 diabetes: α-glucosidase inhibitors, biguanides, meglitinides, peroxisome proliferator activated receptor γ agonists (which are also commonly identified as thiazolidinediones or glitazones), dipeptidyl peptidase 4 (DPP-4) inhibitors, dopamine agonists, bile acid sequestrants, and sulfonylureas. Oral antidiabetic agents are often grouped according to their glucose-lowering mechanism of action. Biguanides and thiazolidinediones are often categorized as insulin sensitizers due to their ability to reduce insulin resistance. Sulfonylureas and meglitinides are often categorized as insulin secretagogues because they enhance endogenous insulin release.

Diabetes treatment options continue to evolve, with newer oral agents and non-insulin injectables potentially altering future algorithms for the treatment of diabetes. The subsequent sections describe the current antidiabetic medications that are available to treat type 1 and type 2 diabetes mellitus.

Drug Class Information

Insulin _Pharmacology._ Insulin is an anabolic and anticatabolic hormone. It plays major roles in protein, carbohydrate, and fat metabolism. For a complete review of insulin action, the reader is referred to a diabetes physiology text.[38] Endogenously produced insulin is cleaved from the larger proinsulin peptide in the β cell to the active peptide of insulin and C-peptide, which can be used as a marker for endogenous insulin production. All commercially available insulin preparations contain only the active insulin peptide.

Characteristics. Characteristics that are commonly used to categorize insulins include source, strength, onset, and duration of action. Additionally, insulins may be characterized as analogs, defined as insulins that have had amino acids within the insulin molecule modified and/or "modifiers" added to impart particular physiochemical and pharmacokinetic advantages. Table 83–8 summarizes available insulin preparations.

U-100 and U-500, 100 units/mL and 500 units/mL, respectively, are the strengths of injectable insulin currently available in the United States. U-500 regular insulin is available for individuals that may require large doses of insulin to control their diabetes. In the United States, all other insulins are available only in U-100 strength. For some type 1 diabetes patients who require extremely low doses of insulin, dilution of U-100 insulin to obtain accurate insulin doses may be necessary. Diluents and empty bottles can be obtained from the manufacturers for dilution.

Historically, insulin came from either beef or pork sources. Beef insulin differs by three amino acids and pork by one amino acid when compared to human insulin. Manufacturers in the United States have discontinued production of beef and pork source

insulins as of December 2003, and now exclusively use recombinant DNA technology to manufacture insulin. Eli Lilly and Sanofi-Aventis currently use a non–disease-producing strain of _Escherichia coli_ for synthesis of insulin; whereas Novo Nordisk uses _Saccharomyces cerevisiae_, or bakers' yeast, for synthesis.

Purity of insulin refers to the amount of proinsulin and other impurities present in a given insulin product. Prior to 1980, most insulin contained enough impurities (300–10,000 ppm) to cause local reactions upon injection, as well as systemic adverse effects from antibody production. Modern technology has provided less expensive techniques to purify insulin. As a result, all insulin products contain ≤10 ppm of proinsulin, with purified preparations (all recombinant DNA human insulin and insulin analogs) containing <1 ppm of proinsulin.

Regular crystalline insulin naturally self-associates into a hexameric (six insulin molecules) structure when injected subcutaneously. Before absorption through a blood capillary can occur, the hexamer must dissociate first to dimers, and then to monomers. This principle is the premise for additives such as protamine and zinc described below, and modification of amino acids for insulin analogs. Lispro, aspart, and glulisine insulins dissociate rapidly to monomers, thus absorption is rapid. Lispro (B-28 lysine and B-29 proline human insulin; monomeric) insulin with two amino acids transposed, aspart (B-28 aspartic acid human insulin; mono- and dimeric) insulin with replacement of one amino acid, and glulisine (B-3 lysine and B-29 glutamic acid) are rapidly absorbed, peak faster, and have shorter durations of action when compared to regular insulin. Proteins tend to be insoluable near their isoelectric point, and glargine insulin uses this to prolong absorption. In comparison to human insulin, with an isoelectric point of 5.4, the analog glargine insulin (A-21 glycine, B-30a-arginine, B-30a L-arginine, and B-30b L-arginine human insulin) has an isoelectric point of 6.8. In the bottle, glargine is buffered to a pH of 4, a level at which it is completely soluble, resulting in a clear colorless solution. When injected into the neutral pH of the body, it rapidly forms microprecipitates that slowly dissolve into monomers and dimers which are then subsequently absorbed. The result is a long-acting, 24-hour duration insulin analog. Detemir, in contrast, attaches a C14 fatty acid (a 14 carbon fatty acid) at the B-29 position and removes the B-30 amino acid. This allows the fatty acid side chain to bind to interstitial albumin at the SQ injection site. Also, the formulation allows stronger hexamer (six molecules of insulin associated together) self associations, which prolong absorption. Once detemir dissociates from the interstitial albumin, it is free to enter a capillary, where it is again bound to albumin, which can further prolong action. It then travels to a site of action and interacts, after dissociation from albumin, with insulin receptors.

Insulin analogs are modified human insulin molecules, and safety is paramount for FDA approval. Key factors that should be considered in the approval process include local injection reactions, antigenicity, efficacy compared to human insulin, insulin receptor binding affinity, and insulin-like growth factor 1–receptor affinity (which is compared to that of human insulin to determine mitogenic potential).

Pharmacokinetics. Subcutaneous injection kinetics are dependent on onset, peak, and duration of action, and are summarized in Table 83–9. Absorption of insulin from a subcutaneous depot is dependent on several factors, including source of insulin, concentration of insulin, additives to the insulin preparations (e.g., zinc, protamine, etc), blood flow to the area (rubbing of injection area, increased skin temperature, and exercise in muscles near the injection site may enhance absorption), and injection site. Regular or NPH insulin is commonly injected in (from most

TABLE 83-8 Available Injectable and Insulin Preparations

Generic Name	Manufacturer	Analog[a]	Administration Options	Room Temperature[b] Expiration
Rapid-acting insulins				
Humalog (insulin lispro)	Lilly	Yes	Insulin pen 3-mL, vial, or 3-mL pen cartridge	28 days
NovoLog (insulin aspart)	Novo Nordisk	Yes	Insulin pen 3-mL, vial, or 3-mL pen cartridge	28 days
Apidra (insulin glulisine)	Sanofi-Aventis	Yes	Insulin pen 3-mL, vial, or 3-mL pen cartridge	28 days
Short-acting insulins				
Humulin R (regular) available in U-100 and U-500	Lilly	No	U-100, 10-mL vial U 500, 20-mL vial	28 days
Novolin R (regular)	Novo Nordisk	No	10-mL vial	30 days
Intermediate-acting insulins				
NPH				
Humulin N	Lilly	No	Vial, 3-mL prefilled pen	Vial: 28 days; pen: 14 days
Novolin N	Novo Nordisk	No	Vial	30 days
Long-acting insulins				
Lantus (insulin glargine)	Sanofi-Aventis	Yes	Vial, 3-mL pen, 3-mL pen cartridge	28 days
Levemir (insulin detemir)	Novo nordisk	Yes	Vial, 3-mL prefilled pen	42 days
Premixed insulins				
Premixed insulin analogs				
Humalog Mix 75/25 (75% neutral protamine lispro, 25% lispro)	Lilly	Yes	Vial, prefilled pen	Vial: 28 days; pen: 10 days
Novolog Mix 70/30 (70% aspart protamine suspension, 30% aspart)	Novo Nordisk	Yes	Vial, 3-mL prefilled pen	Vial: 28 days; others: 14 days
Humalog Mix 50/50 (50% neutral protamine lispro/ 50% lispro)	Lilly	Yes	Vial, 3-mL pen	Vial: 28 days; pen:10 days
NPH-regular combinations				
Humulin 70/30	Lilly	No	Vial, 3-mL prefilled pen	Vial: 28 days; pen: 10 days
Novolin 70/30	Novo Nordisk	No	Vial	30 days
Other injectables				
Glucagon like peptide-1 agonists	**(GLP-1 Agonists)**			
Byetta (exenatide)	Amylin/Lilly	No	5 mcg and 10 mcg pen, ~60 injections (doses)/pen	30 days (≤77°F)
Victoza (liraglutide)	Novo Nordisk	Yes	3-mL pen, can deliver 0.6 mg, 1.2 mg, or 1.8 mg dose	30 days
Amylinomimetic				
Symlin (pramlintide)	Amylin	Yes	5-mL vial, 1.5 mL pen: delivers 15, 30, 45, or 60 mcg dose; 2.7 mL pen: delivers 60 or 120 mcg dose	30 days

[a]All diabetes injectables available in the U.S. are now made by human recombinant DNA technology. An insulin analog is a modified human insulin molecule that imparts particular pharmacokinetic advantages.
[b]Room temperature defined as 59°–86°F. All products are good until expiration date on product if unopened and stored correctly.

rapid to slowest absorption): abdominal fat, posterior upper arms, lateral thigh area, and superior buttocks area. Insulin analogs, unlike regular or NPH insulin, appear to retain their kinetic profile at all sites of injection. U-500 regular insulin has a delayed onset, peak, and a longer duration of action when compared to U-100 insulin. Addition of protamine (NPH, NPL, and aspart protamine suspension) or excess zinc (historically lente or ultralente insulin) will delay onset, peak, and duration of the insulin's effect. Variability in absorption, inconsistent suspension of the insulin by the patient or healthcare provider when drawing up a

TABLE 83-9 Pharmacokinetics of Various Insulins Administered Subcutaneously

Type of Insulin	Onset (Hours)	Peak (Hours)	Duration (Hours)	Maximum Duration (Hours)	Appearance
Rapid acting					
Aspart	15–30 min	1–2	3–5	5–6	Clear
Lispro	15–30 min	1–2	3–4	4–6	Clear
Glulisine	15–30 min	1–2	3–4	5–6	Clear
Short-acting					
Regular	0.5–1.0	2–3	4–6	6–8	Clear
Intermediate acting[a]					
NPH	2–4	4–8	8–12	14–18	Cloudy
Long acting					
Detemir	2 hours	—[b]	14–24[c]	24	Clear
Glargine	4–5	—[b]	22–24[c]	24	Clear

[a]Lente and Ultralente insulin has been discontinued.
[b]Glargine is considered "flat" pharmacokinetically, and detemir has a slight peak, but both have exhibited peak effects during comparative testing, and these peak effects may necessitate changing therapy in a minority of type 1 DM patients.
[c]See text for further discussion.

dose, and inherent insulin action based on the pharmacokinetics of the products may all contribute to a labile glucose response. NPH and all suspension based insulins should be inverted or rolled gently at least 10 times to fully resuspend the insulin prior to each use.

As detemir insulin has a unique mechanism to prolong absorption, it should not be surprising that the pharmacokinetics are unique. Detemir insulin reported less intrapatient variability between injections (less "wobble" in insulin levels between injections) when compared with NPH or glargine insulin. This may be advantageous when variability in the insulin level may make a large difference in glycemic excursions, as in type 1 DM. It should be noted, at low dose (0.2 units/kg) the duration of action is approximately 14 to 16 hours, while at doses above 0.3units/kg, it is close to 24 hours. In type 1 DM, 30%–50% of patients may require twice daily use of detemir insulin to cover 24 hour basal insulin needs, but this is unlikely to be an issue in type 2 DM patients, as they tend to use more units per day to attain glycemic goals. Direct comparative data between glargine insulin and detemir insulin is difficult to interpret, as detemir insulin was allowed to be dosed twice daily. Equivalent glycemic control was attained with either insulin. It is possible that glargine insulin in a minority of type 1 DM patients may pharmacokinetically require twice daily dosing, but this is poorly documented in the literature.

The half-life of an intravenous (IV) injection of regular insulin is about 9 minutes. Thus the effective duration of action of a single IV injection is short, and changes in IV insulin rates will reach steady state in approximately 45 minutes. Intravenous pharmacokinetics of other soluble insulins (lispro, aspart, glulisine, and even glargine) are similar to IV regular insulin, but they have no advantages over IV regular insulin and are more expensive. For completeness, aspart and glulisine are both FDA approved for intravenous use.

Insulin is degraded in the liver, muscle, and kidney. Liver deactivation is 20% to 50% in a single passage. Approximately 15% to 20% of insulin metabolism occurs in the kidney. This may partially explain the lower insulin dosage requirements in patients with end-stage renal disease.

Currently, insulin must be injected to retain its glycemic lowering properties. Alternative absorption pathways, including pulmonary, topical, gastrointestinal, an even nasal are being explored. The first inhalation insulin was discontinued due to poor sales and subsequent reports of lung cancer, but Technosphere inhaled insulin (Afrezza) has been submitted to the FDA for review. The onset of action is similar to IV insulin, which is unique.

An educated patient in conjunction with a skilled practitioner can usually achieve excellent glycemic control with insulin therapy. Efficacy with insulin therapy is related to achieving glycemic control while minimizing the risk of potential side effects, specifically hypoglycemia and weight gain. Insulin is recommended in patients with extremely high fasting plasma glucose levels (>280–300 mg/dL) or HbA$_{1c}$, patients with ketonuria or ketonemia, symptomatic patients (weight loss with polyuria, polydipsia, and/or nocturia), gestational diabetes mellitus, pregnancy with diabetes, and if deemed appropriate by the clinician and patient.[39–42]

Microvascular Complications. Insulin has been shown to be as efficacious as any oral agent for treating DM. The United Kingdom Prospective Diabetes Study, which used sulfonylureas or insulin, showed equal efficacy in lowering the risk of microvascular events in newly diagnosed type 2 DM.[32] Similarly, in type 1 DM, the Diabetes Control and Complications Trial showed efficacy in reducing microvascular complications.[31]

Macrovascular Complications. The connection between high insulin levels (hyperinsulinemia), insulin resistance, and cardiovascular events incorrectly leads some clinicians to believe

that insulin therapy may cause macrovascular complications. The UKPDS and DCCT found no differences in macrovascular outcomes with intensive insulin therapy. One study, the Diabetes Mellitus, Insulin Glucose Infusion in Acute Myocardial Infarction study[43] reported reductions in mortality with insulin therapy. This group assessed the effect of an insulin-glucose infusion in type 2 DM patients who had experienced an acute myocardial infarction. Those randomized to insulin infusion followed by intensive insulin therapy lowered their absolute mortality risk by 11% over a mean follow-up period of approximately 3 years. This was most evident in subjects who were insulin-naïve or had a low cardiovascular risk prior to the acute myocardial infarction.[43] The importance of glycemic control in hospitalized patients is covered later in the chapter.

Adverse Effects. The most common adverse effects reported with insulin are hypoglycemia and weight gain. Hypoglycemia is more common in patients on intensive insulin therapy regimens versus those on less-intensive regimens. Also, patients with type 1 DM tend to have more hypoglycemic events compared to type 2 DM patients. In the UKPDS study, performed over 10 years, the percentage of diabetic patients that needed assistance (third-party or hospitalization) due to a hypoglycemic reaction was 2.3%. The UKPDS reported a rate of 36.5% for risk of any hypoglycemic event, including mild, self-treated events. In the DCCT, tighter control produced a risk three times higher for severe hypoglycemia compared to conventional therapy. Glycemic goals should incorporate hypoglycemic risk versus the benefit of lowering the glucose when HbA$_{1c}$ levels are near normal, especially in type 1 DM.

Minimization of risk for patients on insulin should include education about the signs and symptoms of hypoglycemia, proper treatment of hypoglycemia, and blood glucose monitoring. Blood glucose monitoring is essential for those on insulin, and is particularly of value in patients with hypoglycemia unawareness. Patients with hypoglycemia unawareness do not experience the normal sympathetic symptoms of hypoglycemia (tachycardia, tremulousness, and often, sweating). Initial hypoglycemia symptoms are neuroglycopenic in nature (confusion, agitation, loss of consciousness, and/or progression to coma). Patients with hypoglycemia unawareness should at least temporarily raise their glycemic goals (requiring a reduction in insulin dose) and check their blood glucose level prior to any activities that may be dangerous with a low blood sugar (e.g., driving and certain sports, among others). Proper treatment of hypoglycemia dictates ingestion of carbohydrates, with glucose being preferred. Unconsciousness is an indication for either IV glucose, or glucagon injection, which increases glycogenolysis in the liver. Glucagon use would be appropriate in any situation in which the patient does not have or cannot have ready IV access for glucose administration. Education for reconstitution and injection of glucagon is recommended for close friends and family of a patient who has recurrent neuroglycopenic events. The patient and close contacts should be informed that it can take 10 to 15 minutes for the injection to start raising glucose levels, and patients often vomit during this time. Proper positioning to avoid aspiration should be emphasized.

Weight gain is predominantly from increased truncal fat, and tends to be related to daily dose and plasma insulin levels present. Weight gain is undesirable in most type 2 DM patients, but may be seen as beneficial in underweight patients with type 1 DM. Weight gain appears to be related to intensive insulin therapy, and can be somewhat minimized by physiologic replacement of insulin.

Two forms of lipodystrophy, though much less common today in people with diabetes, still occur. Lipohypertrophy is caused by many injections into the same injection site. Due to insulin's anabolic actions, a raised fat mass is present at the injection site with resultant variable insulin absorption. Lipoatrophy, in contrast, is thought to be due to insulin antibodies or allergic type-reactions with destruction of fat at the site of injection. Injection away from the site with more purified insulin is recommended, though reports of lipoatrophy have been reported with most insulin preparations. Anecdotal evidence has shown that specially formulated cromolyn may help to stabilize the allergic type of reaction.

One large database associated glargine insulin with a higher risk of breast cancer, and possibly colon and pancreatic cancer, but other large database studies have shown no such association. Glargine in vitro has a higher affinity for IGF-1 than regular human insulin, which could theoretically explain the increased risk of cancer. However, in the observational, retrospective study, patients on glargine were older than patients on the comparator NPH insulin, which may explain the increased cancer rate observed. Supporting this premise, when glargine was used in intensive insulin therapy regimens in healthier populations, no such association was seen.

Drug–Drug Interactions. There are no significant drug–drug interactions with injected insulin, though other medications that may affect glucose control can be considered. Detemir does not have albumin binding interactions, as it occupies only a small percent of albumin binding sites. Table 83-10 lists common medications known to affect blood glucose levels.

Dosing and Administration. The dose of insulin for any person with altered glucose metabolism must be individualized. In type 1 DM, the average daily requirement for insulin is 0.5 to 0.6 units/kg, with approximately 50% being delivered as basal insulin, and the remaining 50% dedicated to meal coverage. During the honeymoon phase it may fall to 0.1 to 0.4 units/kg. During acute illness or with ketosis or states of relative insulin resistance, higher dosages

are warranted. In type 2 DM a higher dosage is required for those patients with significant insulin resistance. Dosages vary widely depending on underlying insulin resistance and concomitant oral insulin sensitizer use. Strategies on how to initiate and monitor insulin therapy will be described later in the therapeutics section.

Storage. It is recommended that unopened injectable insulin be refrigerated (36°–46°F) prior to use. The manufacturer's expiration date printed on the insulin is used for unopened, refrigerated insulin. Once the insulin is in use, the manufacturer-recommended expiration dates will vary based on the insulin and delivery device. Table 83–8 outlines manufacturer-recommended expiration dates for room temperature (59°–86°F) insulin. For financial reasons, patients may attempt to use insulins longer than their expiration dates, but careful attention must be paid to monitoring for glycemic control deterioration and signs of insulin decay (clumping, precipitates, discoloration, etc.) if this is attempted.

Glucagon-Like Peptide 1 Agonists

Exenatide Pharmacology. Exendin 4 is a 39-amino acid peptide isolated from the saliva of the Gila monster (Heloderma suspectum) and shares approximately 50% amino acid sequence with human glucagon-like peptide 1 (GLP-1). Exenatide is the synthetic version of naturally occuring exendin 4. Exenatide (Byetta) has been shown to bind to GLP-1 receptors in many parts of the body including the brain and pancreas. Exenatide and GLP-1 have common glucoregulatory actions. Exenatide enhances glucose dependent insulin secretion while suppressing inappropriately high postprandial glucagon secretion in the presence of elevated glucose concentrations, resulting in a reduction in hepatic glucose production. Exenatide increases satiety, which may result in weight loss, and slows gastric emptying so that the rate of glucose appearance into the plasma better matches the glucose disposition. The GLP-1 receptor activity is pharmacologic, and is approximately 3 to 4 times the normal peak physiologic GLP-1 activity. This is necessary to obtain gastric emptying and satiety effects, which are not seen at physiologic GLP-1 levels.

Pharmacokinetics. Exenatide concentrations are detectable in plasma within 10 to 15 minutes after subcutaneous injection, and the drug has a t_{max} of ~2 hours and a plasma half life of ~3.3 to 4.0 hours. Exenatide plasma concentrations increase in a dose-dependent manner and plasma exenatide concentrations are detectable for up to 10 hours postinjection, though pharmacodynamically, effects last for approximately 6 hours. Bioavailability of exenatide after injection in the abdomen, upper arm, or the thigh is similar. Elimination of exenatide is primarily by glomerular filtration with subsequent proteolytic degradation. When exenatide is administered to subjects with worsening degrees of renal insufficiency, there is a progressive prolongation of the half-life, and in dialysis patients, plasma clearance of exenatide is markedly reduced. The incidence of gastrointestinal side effects appears to be increased in individuals with impaired renal function, possibly due to higher plasma levels, thus caution is advised.

No significant differences in exenatide pharmacokinetics have been observed with obesity, race, gender, or advancing age (up to 73 years old).

Efficacy. The average HbA_{1c} reduction is approximately 0.9% with exenatide, though, similar to oral agents, it is dependent upon the baseline HbA_{1c} values. Three phase III trials reported similar HbA_{1c} reduction in patients on metformin, sulfonylureas, or both. It is recommended to lower the sulfonylurea dose only if GLP-1 agonists are started with near normal glucose levels. Sulfonylureas release insulin in a non-glucose dependent fashion and can cause occasional severe hypoglycemia. Exenatide significantly decreases postprandial glucose excursions, but has only a modest effect on

TABLE 83-10	Medications That May Affect Glycemic Control[a]	
Drug	**Effect on Glucose**	**Mechanism/Comment**
Angiotensin-converting enzyme inhibitors	Slight reduction	Improves insulin sensitivity
Alcohol	Reduction	Reduces hepatic glucose production
α-Interferon	Increase	Unclear
Atypical antipsychotics	Increase	Decrease insulin sensitivity; weight gain
Calcineurin inhibitors	Increase	Decrease insulin secretion
Diazoxide	Increase	Decreases insulin secretion, decreases peripheral glucose use
Diuretics (thiazides)	Increase	May increase insulin resistance
Glucocorticoids	Increase	Impairs insulin action
Fluoroquinolones	Increase/Decrease	Unclear, potential drug interaction with sulfonylureas or change in insulin secretion
Nicotinic acid	Increase	Impairs insulin action, increases insulin resistance
Oral contraceptives	Increase	Unclear
Pentamidine	Decrease, then increase	Toxic to β cells; initial release of stored insulin, then depletion
Phenytoin	Increase	Decreases insulin secretion
Protease inhibitors	Increase	Worsen insulin resistance
β-Blockers	May increase	Decreases insulin secretion
Ranolazine	Decrease	Improves oxidative glucose disposal
Salicylates	Decrease	Inhibition of I-κ-B kinase-β(IKK-beta) (only high doses, e.g., 4–6 g/day)
Sympathomimetics	Slight increase	Increased glycogenolysis and gluconeogenesis

[a]This list is not inclusive of all medications reported to cause glucose changes.

fasting plasma glucose values. If a patient has significant elevations in fasting plasma glucose levels, these should be corrected with other agents, and the exenatide added on. Exenatide may aid some patients' efforts to lose weight. The average weight loss in controlled trials was 1 to 2 kg over 30 weeks, without dietary advice being given to the patients, though long-term, open-label follow-up on 10 mcg BID shows continued and sustained weight loss for at least 3 years.[44] Approximately 84% of patients on exenatide lost some weight. Exenatide, through decreasing appetite and slowing gastric emptying, may reduce the number of calories a patient eats at a meal. If a patient does not decrease calorie intake, as exenatide does not increase caloric expenditure, no weight loss is likely to occur.

Microvascular Complications. Exenatide reduces the HbA_{1c} level, which has been shown to be related to the risk of microvascular complications.

Macrovascular Complications. No randomized clinical trials have examined the effect of exenatide on cardiovascular outcomes. Meta-analysis data reported a 30% (P = NS) reduction in the risk of cardiovascular events. Improvements in several cardiovascular risk factors have been reported. Plasma triglycerides (-37 ± 10 mg/dL) decreased, and plasma HDL cholesterol ($+4.5 \pm 0.4$ mg/dL) increased on open-label exenatide 10 mcg BID. Nonsignificant reductions in systolic and diastolic blood pressure were observed in the whole population, though a significant reduction was seen in subjects with above normal systolic blood pressure. The greatest improvement in cardiovascular risk factors was, in general, seen in subjects who had the greatest weight loss.[44]

Adverse Effects. The most common adverse effects associated with exenatide are gastrointestinal in nature. Nausea occurs in ~40% of subjects on 5 mcg, and ~45% to 50% of subjects on 10 mcg BID. Vomiting or diarrhea occurs in approximately 10% of patients placed on exenatide. Gastrointestinal adverse effects appear to decrease over time, but approximately 1 in 20 patients may have prolonged problems with one of the above side effects, possibly requiring discontinuation. As these adverse effects appear to be dose related, the patient should be started on a 5 mcg BID and titrated to 10 mcg BID only if the adverse effects are mostly gone. Also, when the patient is increased to the 10 mcg BID dose, these adverse effects may recur for a short period of time. Many episodes of nausea would be better characterized as stomach fullness, and patients should be instructed to eat slowly and stop eating when full, or risk nausea/vomiting. Also, weight loss appears not to be related to adverse effects, but rather to a reduction in calories consumed. Exenatide provides glucose-dependent insulin secretion, thus hypoglycemic rates when combined with metformin or a thiazolidinedione are not substantially increased, but when combined with a sulfonylurea or insulin, significant hypoglycemia may occur. Though exenatide reduces glucagon when the glucose is high, no suppression of counter-regulatory hormones has been noted during hypoglycemia. Exenatide antibodies can occur, but generally decrease over time and do not affect glycemic control. In approximately 5% of patients, titers may increase over time, resulting in a blunting of glycemic control in about half of these patients. Exenatide has been associated with the serious adverse effect of acute pancreatitis, but this has not been shown to be causal. Further study is needed, but several important points should be noted: (1) type 2 DM patients have many risk factors for pancreatitis such as gallstones, hypertriglyceridemia, obesity, and concomitant medication use; (2) GLP-1 agonists can mask initial signs of pancreatitis, as nausea, vomiting, and abdominal pain are common signs of pancreatitis; and (3) large database studies have not linked exenatide to a higher rate of acute pancreatitis. Clinically, do not use exenatide in a patient with a history of pancreatitis, and if a patient with abdominal pain, nausea, and/or vomiting presents it is best to discontinue

exenatide temporarily and clinically confirm that it is not a sign of a more serious underlying problem. Exenatide given twice daily does not change the risk of thyroid C-cell tumors in rats, and no signal for C-cell tumors has been reported in humans.

Drug Interactions. Exenatide delays gastric emptying, thus it can delay the absorption of other medications. Examples of medications that may be effected include oral pain medications and antibiotics dependent on concentration dependent killing. If rapid absorption of the medication is necessary, it is best to take the mediation one hour before, or at least 3 hours after the injection of exenatide. In addition, if the patient has gastroparesis, exenatide is not recommended.

Dosing and Administration. Exenatide dosing should be started with 5 mcg BID, and titrated to 10 mcg BID in 1 month or when tolerability allows and if warranted for glycemic control. Exenatide should be injected 0 to 60 minutes before the morning and evening meals. If the patient does not eat breakfast, they may take the first injection of the day at lunch. The peak effect of exenatide is at approximately 2 hours, so anecdotally the patient may get better appetite suppression if injected an hour prior to the meal. Storage and dosage availability information can be found in Table 83–8.

Liraglutide Pharmacology. Liraglutide (Victoza) is a GLP-1 receptor agonist. Liraglutide enhances glucose-dependent insulin secretion while suppressing inappropriately high glucagon secretion in the presence of elevated glucose concentrations, resulting in a reduction in hepatic glucose production. Liraglutide reduces food intake, which may result in weight loss, and slows gastric emptying so that the rate of glucose appearance into the plasma better matches the glucose disposition. During hypoglycemia, liraglutide does not stimulate insulin secretion and does not inhibit the release of the counterregulatory hormone glucagon. Liraglitide is produced through recombinant DNA technology, similar to the way insulin is made by the manufacturer, Novo Nordisk. Liraglitide has 97% amino acid sequence homology to endogenous GLP-1, with the only alteration being an arginine for lysine at position 34. A C-16 fatty acid (palmitic acid) is attached at position 26 (with a glutamic amino acid spacer to optimize GLP-1 receptor interaction) so that liraglutide can bind noncovalently to albumin, prolonging the half-life.

Pharmacokinetics. Self-association into a heptameric structure, and binding to albumin first in the interstitial space, then the blood, then the interstitial space around the GLP-1 receptor prolongs the half-life. In healthy individuals, the half-life is 13 hours, making it suitable for daily administration. Injection into the abdomen, upper arm, and thigh gave clinically similar pharmacokinetics, and the absolute bioavailability is approximately 50%. Maximum concentrations are reached approximately 8 to 12 hours after injection, and steady state is reached after approximately 3 days. Liraglutide has a mean apparent volume of distribution of 13 liters, and is extensively plasma protein bound (mostly to albumin as previously stated). The elimination half-life is 10 to 18 hours. Metabolism appears to be by degredation, similar to other large proteins, and several small minor metabolites (total of 3%–5% of the dose) may be found. The DPP-4 enzyme in vitro has been shown to slowly metabolize liraglutide, and this may be the case in vivo as well. The pharmacokinetics do not appear to be affected by age, race, and gender. Severe renal or mild to severe hepatic impairment may actually lower the AUC by approximately 25%, though the clinical significance of this on multiple dosing is not known.

Efficacy. The average HbA_{1c} reduction is approximately 1.1% with liraglutide, though, similar to oral agents, it is dependent on the baseline HbA_{1c} values. Phase III trials have been completed for monotherapy, metformin, sulfonylureas, both, or metformin plus rosiglitazone. HbA$_{lc}$ reduction with monotherapy 1.2 mg or 1.8 mg daily dose was significantly better than glimepiride 8 mg daily over 52 weeks. Liraglutide 1.2 mg (−0.9%) and 1.8 mg (−1.1%) daily sustained HbA$_{lc}$ reductions over 2 years, but glimepiride 8 mg daily (−0.6%) did not sustain the HbA$_{lc}$ reduction. Liraglutide consistently lowered the fasting plasma glucose level by approximately 25 to 40 mg/dL, and postprandial plasma glucose levels are reduced similarly. Due to the longer half-life, liraglutide can suppress glucagon overnight, which improves the fasting plasma glucose. Similar to exenatide, liraglutide treated patients may lose weight. The average weight loss in controlled trials was 1 to 3 kg over 26 weeks, and weight loss achieved appeared to be sustained through 2 years. Liraglutide, through decreasing appetite and slowing gastric emptying, may reduce the number of calories a patient eats at a meal.

Microvascular Complications. Liraglutide reduces the HbA$_{lc}$ level, which has been shown to be related to the risk of microvascular complications.

Macrovascular Complications. No published clinical trials have examined the effect of liraglutide on cardiovascular outcomes, though no signal of cardiovascular harm was noted upon FDA approval.

Adverse Effects. The most common adverse effects associated with liraglutide are gastrointestinal in nature. Nausea occurs in ~11% to 29% of subjects on 1.2 mg, and 14% to 40% of subjects on 1.8 mg daily. Vomiting may occur in approximately 5% of subjects, and diarrhea occurs in approximately 8% to 15% of patients placed on liraglutide. Gastrointestinal adverse effects appear to decrease over time, but approximately 5% to 10% of subjects withdrew due to gastrointestinal side effects. As these adverse effects appear to be dose releated, the patient should be titrated from 0.6 mg, to 1.2 mg, and to 1.8 mg as tolerated. Randomized trials did not allow for individualized titration, and likely had worse tolerability that can be obtained clinically by individualization of titration. Many episodes of nausea would be better characterized as stomach fullness, and patients should be instructed to eat slowly and stop eating when full, or risk nausea/vomiting. Liraglutide provides glucose-dependent insulin secretion, and hypoglycemic rates when combined with metformin ± a thiazolidinedione are not substantially increased, but when combined with a sulfonylurea or insulin, significant hypoglycemia may occur. When combined with a sulfonylurea, the rates of hypoglycemia were similar between addition of liraglutide or glargine insulin. Liraglutide antibodies can occur (4%–13%), but the rates are generally low and do not affect glycemic control or risk of side effects.

Liraglutide has been associated with the serious adverse event of acute pancreatitis, but this risk has not been shown to be causal. Further study is needed, but type 2 DM patients have many risk factors for pancreatitis such as gallstones, hypertriglyceridemia, obesity, and concommitant medication use. GLP-1 agonists can mask initial signs of pancreatitis, as nausea, vomiting, and abdominal pain are common signs of pancreatitis. Clinically, do not use liraglutide in a patient with a history of pancreatitis. If a patient with abdominal pain, nausea, and/or vomiting presents, it is best to discontinue liraglutide temporarily and proceed with an initial workup for pancreatitis.

A black box warning about thyroid C-cell tumors is listed on the package insert of liraglutide. Rodent models reported a higher risk of C-cell tumors of the thyroid, including medullary thyroid carcinoma. Medullary thyroid carcinoma, if not caught early, has high mortality rates, but rodents may simply be a poor model to study this effect as they express many more GLP-1 receptors on their thyroid than human beings. In addition, calcitonin, a marker used to screen for C-cell tumors, may increase by a non-clinically significant amount in select patients. No signal for C-cell tumors

in humans or non-human primates has been noted, and as clinical use increases, this will be reexamined. No monitoring is currently recommended, but liraglutide is contraindicated in patients with a personal or family history of medullary thyroid cancer, or if they have a history of multiple endocrine tumors.

Drug Interactions. Liraglutide delays gastric emptying, thus it can delay the absorption of other medications. Examples of medications that may be effected include oral pain medications and antibiotics dependent on threshold levels for efficacy. If rapid absorption of the medication is necessary, it is best to take the mediation 1 hour before, or at least 3 hours after the injection. Liraglutide may worsen gastroparesis and clinically it may not be prudent to use in this patient population.

Dosing and Administration. Dosing of liraglutide should be at 0.6 mg daily for ≥1 week, and then increased to 1.2 mg daily for ≥1 week. Patients may be maintained on the 1.2-mg dose, or increased to the maximum dose of 1.8 mg daily after ≥1 week. The 0.6-mg dose is considered a titration dose, and does not reduce the HbA$_{lc}$ substantially in the majority of patients. This titration is recommended to improve gastrointestinal tolerability, and titration should be individualized based on side effects and clinical response. Dosing is daily, and can be given independent of meals. As with exenatide, the reduction in insulin secretagogues may be necessary if the patient is near glycemic goal. Storage and dosage availability information can be found in Table 83–8.

Exenatide versus Liraglutide. In a head-to-head trial in type 2 DM subjects given metformin, sulfonylurea, or both over 26 weeks, liraglutide 1.8 mg daily lowered HbA$_{lc}$ (−1.1%) significantly more than exenatide 10 mcg BID (−0.8%). Liraglutide was better at reduction of fasting plasma glucose, but exenatide was slightly better at reduction of postprandial glucose. Both resulted in approximately 3-kg weight loss, and minor hypoglycemic events were slightly less frequent with liraglutide (26%) than with exenatide BID (34%). Nausea rates were similar for liraglutide (26%) and exenatide (28%), but the rate of persistence was lower with liraglutide, being below 10% by week 6, whereas exenatide did not reach this level until after week 22. No significant changes in calcitonin were noted and there were no reports of pancreatitis, but a small, significant increase in heart rate was noted with liraglutide (+3.3 beats per minute) versus exenatide (+0.7 beats per minute).[45]

Amylinomimetic

Pramlintide Pharmacology. Pramlintide (Symlin) is an antihyperglycemic agent used in patients currently treated with insulin. Pramlintide is a synthetic analog of amylin (amylinomimetic), a neurohormone co-secreted from the β cells with insulin. Amylin is very low or absent in type 1 DM, and lower than normal in type 2 DM patients requiring insulin therapy. Pramlintide is provided as a 37-amino acid polypeptide, which differs in amino acid sequence from human amylin by replacement positions 25 (alanine), 28 (serine), and 29 (serine) with proline. Pramlintide suppresses inappropriately high postprandial glucagon secretion, increases satiety, which may result in weight loss, and slows gastric emptying so that the rate of glucose appearance into the plasma better matches the glucose disposition.

Pharmacokinetics. The absolute bioavailability of pramlintide after subcutaneous injection is 30% to 40%. The t_{max} is approximately 20 minutes, but the C_{max} is dose dependent and appears to be linear. The $t_{1/2}$ is approximately 45 minutes, thus the pharmacodynamic duration of action is about 3 to 4 hours. Pramlintide does not extensively bind to albumin, and should not have significant binding interactions. Metabolism is primarily by the kidneys, and one active metabolite (2–37 pramlintide) has a similar half-life as the parent compound. No accumulation has been seen in renal insufficiency, but caution is advised. Injection into the arm may increase exposure and variability of absorption, so injection into the abdomen or thigh is recommended. Moderate to severe renal insufficiency does not affect exposure.

Efficacy. The average HbA_{1c} reduction is approximately 0.6% with pramlintide, though optimization of the insulin and pramlintide doses may result in further drops in HbA_{1c}. If the 120-mcg dose is used in type 2 DM patients on insulin, it may also result in 1.5-kg weight loss. In type 1 DM patients, the average reduction in HbA_{1c} was 0.4% to 0.5%. Prandial pramlintide added versus rapid-acting insulin in type 2 DM subjects uncontrolled on basal insulin reported similar efficacy, but with no weight gain, compared with ~5-kg weight gain with rapid-acting insulin. Pramlintide decreases prandial glucose excursions, but has little effect on the fasting plasma glucose concentration. When pramlintide is injected before the meal, gastric emptying may delay absorption of mealtime nutrients, necessitating delay of rapid-acting insulin. This may be overcome by injecting the meal-time insulin at the conclusion of the meal, or whenever the blood glucose starts to rise. The average weight loss in controlled trials was 1 to 2 kg, without dietary advice being given to the patients. Pramlintide, through decreasing appetite and slowing gastric emptying, may reduce the number of calories a patient eats at a meal.

Microvascular Complications. Pramlintide reduces the HbA_{1c} level, which has been shown to be related to the risk of microvascular complications.

Macrovascular Complications. No published clinical trials have examined the effect of pramlintide on cardiovascular outcomes.

Adverse Effects. The most common adverse effects associated with pramlintide are gastrointestinal in nature. Nausea occurs in ~20% of type 2 DM patients, and vomiting or anorexia occurs in approximately 10% of type 1 or type 2 DM patients. Nausea is more common in type 1 DM, occuring in ~40% to 50% of patients. The higher rate in type 1 DM related to gastrointestinal adverse effects appear to decrease over time and are dose releated, thus starting at a low dose and slowly titrating as tolerated is recommended. Pramlintide alone does not cause hypoglycemia, but it is indicated for use in patients on insulin, thus hypoglycemia can occur. The risk of severe hypoglycemia early in therapy is higher in type 1 DM than in type 2 DM patients. A 2-fold increase in severe hypoglycemic reactions in type 1 DM patients has been reported.

Drug Interactions. Pramlintide delays gastric emptying, thus it can delay the absorption of other medications. Examples of medications that may be effected include oral pain medications and antibiotics dependent on threshold levels for efficacy. If rapid absorption of the medication is necessary, it is best to take the mediation 1 hour before, or at least 3 hours after the injection of pramlintide.

Dosing and Administration. Pramlintide dosing varies in type 1 and type 2 DM. It is imperative that the prandial insulin dose, if used, be reduced 30% to 50% when pramlintide is started to minimize severe hypoglycemic reactions. Basal insulin may need to be adjusted only if the fasting plasma glucose is close to normal. In type 2 DM, the starting dose is 60 mcg prior to meals, and may be titrated to the maximally recommended 120-mcg dose as tolerated and warranted based on postprandial plasma glucose concentrations. In type 1 DM dosing starts at 15 mcg prior to meals, and can be titrated up in 15-mcg increments to a maximum of 60 mcg prior to each meal if tolerated and warranted. Snacks may or may not need to be covered with pramlintide (recommended if ≥250 kcal or ≥30 g of carbohydrate is eaten). Pramlintide in a vial allows individualization of titration at even smaller increments (by units) than

the package insert recommends, which may be useful in some type 1 DM patients. Each 2.5 units on a U-100 insulin syringe = 15 mcg of pramlintide. In addition, pramlintide has a pH of 4, and it is not recommended that pramlintide be mixed with any other insulin, thus this potentially adds additional injections a day. The addition of a pen device does help with the extra injections, but does not allow for smaller than recommended titrations. Storage information can be found in Table 83–8.

Sulfonylureas *Pharmacology.* The primary mechanism of action of sulfonylureas is enhancement of insulin secretion. Sulfonylureas bind to a specific sulfonylurea receptor (SUR) on pancreatic β cells. Binding closes an adenosine triphosphate–dependent K^+ channel, leading to decreased potassium efflux and subsequent depolarization of the membrane. Voltage-dependent Ca^{+2} channels open and allow an inward flux of Ca^{+2}. Increases in intracellular Ca^{+2} bind to calmodulin on insulin secretory granules, causing translocation of secretory granules of insulin to the cell surface and resultant exocytosis of the granule of insulin. Elevated secretion of insulin from the pancreas travels via the portal vein and subsequently suppresses hepatic glucose production.

Classification. Sulfonylureas are classified as first-generation and second-generation agents. The classification scheme is largely derived from differences in relative potency, relative potential for selective side effects, and differences in binding to serum proteins (i.e., risk for protein-binding displacement drug interactions). First-generation agents consist of acetohexamide, chlorpropamide, tolazamide, and tolbutamide. Each of these agents is lower in potency relative to the second-generation drugs: glimepiride, glipizide, and glyburide (Table 83–11). It is important to recognize that all sulfonylureas are equally effective at lowering blood glucose when administered in equipotent doses.

Pharmacokinetics. All sulfonylureas are metabolized in the liver; some to active, others to inactive metabolites (see Table 83–11). Cytochrome P450 (CYP450) 2C9 is involved with the hepatic metabolism of the majority of sulfonylureas. Agents with active metabolites or parent drug that are renally excreted require dosage adjustment or use with caution in patients with compromised renal function. The half-life of the sulfonylurea also relates directly to the risk for hypoglycemia. The hypoglycemic potential is therefore higher with chlorpropamide and glyburide. The long duration of effect of chlorpropamide may be particularly problematic in elderly individuals, whose renal function declines with age, and therefore it has great potential for accumulation, resulting in severe and protracted hypoglycemia. Individuals at high risk for hypoglycemia (e.g., elderly individuals and those with renal insufficiency or advanced liver disease) should be started at a very low dose of a sulfonylurea with a short half-life. Hypoglycemia on low-dose sulfonylureas may dictate a therapy without the risk of hypoglycemia, or a short-acting insulin secretagogue (nateglinide or repaglinide).

Efficacy. As mentioned earlier, when given in equipotent doses, all sulfonylureas are equally effective at lowering blood glucose. On average, HbA_{1c} will fall 1.5% to 2%, with fasting plasma glucose reductions of 60 to 70 mg/dL, but is dependent on baseline values. A majority of patients will not reach glycemic goals with sulfonylurea monotherapy. Patients who fail sulfonylurea usually fall into two groups: Those with low C-peptide levels and high (>250 mg/dL) fasting plasma glucose (FPG) levels. These patients are often primary failures on sulfonylureas (<30 mg/dL drop of FPG) and have significant glucose toxicity or slow-developing type 1 DM. The other group is those with a good initial response (>30 mg/dL drop of FPG), but which is insufficient to reach their glycemic goals. Over 75% of patients fall into the second group. Factors that portend a positive response include newly diagnosed patients with no indicators of type

TABLE 83-11 Oral Agents for the Treatment of Type 2 Diabetes Mellitus

Generic Name (Generic Version Available? Y = yes, N = no)	Brand	Dose (mg)	Recommended Starting Dosage (mg/day)		Equivalent Therapeutic Dose (mg)	Maximum Dose (mg/day)	Duration of Action	Metabolism or Therapeutic Notes
			Nonelderly	*Elderly*				
Sulfonylureas								
Acetohexamide (Y)	Dymelor	250, 500	250	125–250	500	1500	Up to 16 hours	Metabolized in liver; metabolite potency equal to parent compound; renally eliminated
Chlorpropamide (Y)	Diabinese	100, 250	250	100	250	500	Up to 72 hours	Metabolized in liver; also excreted unchanged renally
Tolazamide (Y)	Tolinase	100, 250, 500	100–250	100	250	1,000	Up to 24 hours	Metabolized in liver; metabolite less active than parent compound; renally eliminated
Tolbutamide (Y)	Orinase	250, 500	1,000–2,000	500–1,000	1,000	3,000	Up to 12 hours	Metabolized in liver to inactive metabolites that are renally excreted
Glipizide (Y)	Glucotrol	5, 10	5	2.5–5	5	40	Up to 20 hours	Metabolized in liver to inactive metabolites
Glipizide (Y)	Glucotrol XL	2.5, 5, 10, 20	5	2.5–5	5	20	24 hours	Slow-release form; do not cut tablet
Glyburide (Y)	DiaBeta Micronase	1.25, 2.5, 5	5	1.25–2.5	5	20	Up to 24 hours	Metabolized in liver; elimination 1/2 renal, 1/2 feces
Glyburide, micronized (Y)	Glynase	1.5, 3, 6	3	1.5–3	3	12	Up to 24 hours	Equal control, but better absorption from micronized preparation
Glimepiride (Y)	Amaryl	1, 2, 4	1–2	0.5–1	2	8	24 hours	Metabolized in liver to inactive metabolites
Short-acting insulin secretagogues								
Nateglinide (Y)	Starlix	60, 120	120 with meals	120 with meals	NA	120 mg 3 times a day	Up to 4 hours	Metabolized by cytochrome P450 (CYP450) 2C9 and 3A4 to weakly active metabolites; renally eliminated
Repaglinide (N)	Prandin	0.5, 1, 2	0.5–1 with meals	0.5–1 with meals	NA	16	Up to 4 hours	Caution with gemfibrozil or trimethoprim-potential hypoglycemia
Biguanides								
Metformin (Y)	Glucophage	500, 850, 1,000	500 mg twice a day	Assess renal function	NA	2550	Up to 24 hours	No metabolism; Renally secreted and excreted
Metformin ER (Y)	Glucophage XR	500, 750, 1,000 mg	500–1,000 mg with evening meal	Assess renal function	NA	2,550	Up to 24 hours	Take full dose with evening meal or may split dose; may consider trial if intolerant to immediate release
Thiazolidinediones								
Pioglitazone (N)	Actos	15, 30, 45	15	15	NA	45	24 hours	Metabolized by CYP 2C8 and 3A4; two metabolites have longer half-lives than parent compound

(continued)

TABLE 83-11 Oral Agents for the Treatment of Type 2 Diabetes Mellitus (continued)

Generic Name (Generic Version Available? Y = yes, N = no)	Brand	Dose (mg)	Recommended Starting Dosage (mg/day)		Equivalent Therapeutic Dose (mg)	Maximum Dose (mg/day)	Duration of Action	Metabolism or Therapeutic Notes
			Nonelderly	Elderly				
Rosiglitazone (N)	Avandia	2, 4, 8	2–4	2	NA	8 mg/day or 4 mg twice a day	24 hours	Metabolized by CYP2C8 and 2C9 to inactive metabolites that are renally excreted
α-Glucosidase inhibitors								
Acarbose (Y)	Precose	25, 50, 100	25 mg 1–3 times a day	25 mg 1–3 times a day	NA	25–100 mg 3 times a day	1–3 hours	Eliminated in bile
Miglitol (N)	Glyset	25, 50, 100	25 mg 1–3 times a day	25 mg 1–3 times a day	NA	25–100 mg 3 times a day	1–3 hours	Eliminated renally
Dipeptidyl peptidase 4 inhibitors (DPP-4 inhibitors)								
Sitagliptin (N)	Januvia	25, 50, 100	100 mg daily	25–100 mg daily based on renal function	NA	100 mg daily	24 hours	50 mg daily if creatinine clearance >30 to <50 mL/min; 25 mg if creatinine clearance <30 mL/min
Saxagliptin (N)	Onglyza	2.5, 5	5 mg daily	2.5–5 mg daily based on renal function	NA	5 mg daily	24 hours	2.5 mg daily if creatinine clearance <50 mL/min or if on strong inhibitors of CYP3A4/5
Bile Acid Sequestrants								
Colesevelam (N)	Welchol	625 mg tablet 1.875 g and 3.75 g oral suspension	6 tablets daily or 3 tablets BID 1.875 g BID or 3.75 g daily	6 tablets daily or 3 tablets BID 1.875 g BID or 3.75 g daily	NA	3.75 g/day	Not absorbed, local effect ~6 hours	Constipation may occur. Cautions: drug–drug absorption interactions, may increase triglycerides; contraindicated if TG >500 mg/dL
Dopamine agonist								
Bromocriptine mesylate (N)	Cycloset	0.8 mg tablets	1.6–4.8 mg daily	1.6–4.8 mg daily	NA	4.8 mg daily	4–5 hours	Take within 2 hours of rising with food. Significant nausea, other side effects, and drug–drug, drug–disease interactions may occur. See text for detailed information
Combination products								
Glyburide/ metformin (Y)	Glucovance	1.25/250 2.5/500 5/500	2.5–5/500 twice a day	1.25/250 twice a day; assess renal function	NA	20 of glyburide, 2,000 of metformin	Combination medication	Use as initial therapy: 1.25/250 mg twice a day
Glipizide/ metformin (Y)	Metaglip	2.5/250 2.5/500 5/500	2.5–5/500 twice a day	2.5/250; assess renal function	NA	20 of glipizide, 2,000 of metformin	Combination medication	Use as initial therapy: 2.5/250 mg twice a day
Rosiglitazone/ metformin (N)	Avandamet	1/500 2/500 4/500 2/1,000 4/1,000	1–2/500 twice a day	1/500 twice a day assess renal function	NA	8 of rosiglitazone; 2,000 of metformin	Combination medication	Past manufacturing problems, but recently reintroduced to market. May use as initial therapy

(continued)

TABLE 83-11 Oral Agents for the Treatment of Type 2 Diabetes Mellitus (continued)

Generic Name (Generic Version Available? Y = yes, N = no	Brand	Dose (mg)	Recommended Starting Dosage (mg/day)		Equivalent Therapeutic Dose (mg)	Maximum Dose (mg/day)	Duration of Action	Metabolism or Therapeutic Notes
			Nonelderly	Elderly				
Rosiglitazone/ glimepiride (N)	Avandaryl	4/1 4/2 4/4	4/1 or 4/2 once a day	4/1 daily	NA	8 mg of rosiglitazone, 8 mg of glimepiride	Combination medication	Recent labeling that it may increase cardiovascular events in patients with concomitant heart failure-caution
Pioglitazone/ metformin (N)	Actoplus Met	15/500 15/850	15/500 to 15/850 once or twice daily	15/500 daily to twice daily assess renal function	NA	45 mg of pioglitazone, 2,550 mg of metformin	Combination medication	
Pioglitazone/ glimepiride (N)	Duetact	30/2 30/4	30/2 or 30/4 daily	30/2 daily to avoid hypoglycemia	NA	45 mg pioglitazone, 8 mg glimepiride	Combination Medication	Maximum dose can not be given of either medication due to formulations available
Sitagliptin/ metformin (N)	Janumet	50/500 50/1,000	50/500 twice daily with meals up to 50/1000 twice daily with meals	Either given twice daily Assess Renal Function Prior to Use	NA	100 mg sitagliptin daily	Combination Medication	Follow renal precautions for metformin
Repaglinide/ metformin (N)	Prandimet	1/500 2/500	1/500 or 2/500 2 or 3 times daily with meals	1/500 or 2/500 2 or 3 times daily with meals Assess Renal Funciton Prior to Use	NA	10 mg repaglinied, 250 mg daily of metformin	Combination Medication	Follow renal precautions for metformin. Caution drug–drug interactions with repalginide

1 DM, high fasting C-peptide levels, and moderate fasting hyperglycemia (<250 mg/dL). If glycemic goals are met, a secondary failure rate of approximately 5% to 7% per year can be expected.

Microvascular Complications. Sulfonylureas showed a reduction of microvascular complications in type 2 DM patients in the UKPDS.[32] A more in-depth discussion follows later in the chapter.

Macrovascular Complications. The UKPDS reported no significant benefit or harm in newly diagnosed type 2 DM patients given sulfonylureas over 10 years. The University Group Diabetes Program study documented higher rates of coronary artery disease in type 2 patients given tolbutamide, when compared with patients given insulin or placebo, though this study has been widely criticized.[46,47] Some sulfonylureas bind to the SUR-2A receptor that is found in cardiac tissue. Binding to the SUR-2A receptor has been implicated in blocking ischemic preconditioning via K+ channel closure in the heart. Ischemic preconditioning is the premise that prior ischemia in cardiac tissue can provide greater tolerance of subsequent ischemia. Thus, patients with heart disease potentially have one compensatory mechanism to protect the heart from ischemia blocked. Conclusions are controversial and readers are referred to the pertinent articles for further discussion.[48–50]

Adverse Effects. The most common side effect of sulfonylureas is hypoglycemia. The pretreatment fasting plasma glucose is a strong predictor of hypoglycemic potential. The lower the FPG is upon initiation, the higher the potential for hypoglycemia. Also, in addition to the high-risk individuals outlined in the pharmacokinetics section, those who skip meals, exercise vigorously, or lose substantial amounts of weight are also more likely to experience hypoglycemia.

Hyponatremia (serum sodium <129 mEq/L) is reportedly associated with tolbutamide, but it is most common with chlorpropamide and occurs in as many as 5% of individuals treated. An increase in antidiuretic hormone secretion is the mechanism for hyponatremia. Risk factors include age >60 years, female gender, and concomitant use of thiazide diuretics.

Weight gain is common with sulfonylureas. In essence, patients who are no longer glycosuric and who do not reduce caloric intake with improvement of blood glucose will store excess calories. Other notable, although much less common, adverse effects of sulfonylureas are skin rash, hemolytic anemia, gastrointestinal upset, and cholestasis. Disulfiram-type reactions and flushing have been reported with tolbutamide and chlorpropamide when alcohol is consumed.

Drug Interactions. Several drugs are thought to interact with sulfonylureas, and Table 83–12 summarizes them by proposed mechanisms of action.[51] Drug interactions from protein-binding

TABLE 83-12 Drug Interactions with Sulfonylureas

Interaction	Drugs
Displacement from protein binding sites[a]	Warfarin, salicylates, phenylbutazone, sulfonamides
Alters hepatic metabolism (cytochrome P450)	Chloramphenicol, monoamine oxidase inhibitors, cimetidine, rifampin[b]
Altered renal excretion	Allopurinol, probenecid

[a]Many of these drug interactions may be metabolism-based.
[b]Inducer.
Reproduced from Gerich.[51]

changes should occur shortly after the interacting medication is given, as the concentration of free (thus active) sulfonylurea will acutely increase. First-generation sulfonylureas, which bind to proteins ionically, are more likely to cause drug–drug interactions than second-generation sulfonylureas, which bind nonionically.[52] The clinical importance of protein-binding interactions has been questioned, as the majority of these drug interactions have been found to be truly due to hepatic metabolism. Drugs that are inducers or inhibitors of CYP450 2C9 should be monitored carefully when used with a sulfonylurea. Additionally, other drugs known to alter blood glucose should be considered (see Table 83–10).

Dosing and Administration. The usual starting dose and maximum dose of sulfonylureas are summarized in Table 83–11. Lower dosages are recommended for most agents in elderly patients and those with compromised renal or hepatic function. The dosage should be titrated every 1 to 2 weeks (use a longer interval with chlorpropamide) to achieve glycemic goals. This is possible due to the rapid increase of insulin secretion in response to the sulfonylurea. Of note, immediate-release glipizide's maximal dose is 40 mg/day, but its maximal effective dose is about 10 to 15 mg/day. The maximal effective dose of sulfonylureas tends to be about 60% to 75% of their stated maximum dose.

Short-Acting Insulin Secretagogues ***Pharmacology.*** Though the binding site is adjacent to the binding site of sulfonylureas, nateglinide and repaglinide stimulate insulin secretion from the β cells of the pancreas, similarly to sulfonylureas. Repaglinide, a benzoic acid derivative, and nateglinide, a phenylalanine amino acid derivative, both require the presence of glucose to stimulate insulin secretion. As glucose levels diminish to normal, stimulated insulin secretion diminishes.

Pharmacokinetics. Both nateglinide and repaglinide are rapid-acting insulin secretagogues that are rapidly absorbed (~0.5–1 hour) and have a short half-life (1–1.5 hours). Nateglinide is highly protein-bound, primarily to albumin, but also to α_1-acid glycoprotein. Nateglinide is predominantly metabolized by CYP2C9 (70%) and CYP3A4 (30%) to less active metabolites. Glucuronide conjugation then allows rapid renal elimination. No dosage adjustment is needed in moderate to severe renal insufficiency. Repaglinide is highly protein bound, and is mainly metabolized by oxidative metabolism and glucuronidation. The CYP3A4 and 2C8 system have been show to be involved with metabolism. Approximately 90% of repaglinide is eliminated in the feces, with only 10% found in the urine. Moderate to severe renal insufficiency does not appear to affect repaglinide, but moderate to severe hepatic impairment may prolong exposure.

Efficacy. In monotherapy, both significantly reduce postprandial glucose excursions and reduce HbA$_{1c}$ levels. Repaglinide, dosed 4 mg 3 times a day, when compared with glyburide in diet-treated, drug-naïve patients reduced HbA$_{1c}$ levels less (1% vs 2.4%, from baseline, respectively).[53] Nateglinide, dosed 120 mg 3 times a day in a similar population reduced HbA$_{1c}$ values by 0.8%.[54] The lower efficacy of these agents versus sulfonylureas should be considered when patients are >1% above their HbA$_{1c}$ goal. These agents can be used to provide increased insulin secretion during meals, when it is needed, in patients close to glycemic goals. Also, it should be noted that addition of either agent to a sulfonylurea will not result in any improvement in glycemic parameters.

Adverse Effects. Hypoglycemia is the main side effect noted with both agents. Hypoglycemic risk appears to be less versus sulfonylureas. In part, this is due to the glucose-sensitive release of insulin. If the glucose concentration is normal, less glucose-stimulated release of insulin will occur. In two separate studies, nateglinide rates of hypoglycemia were 3% and repaglinide 15% versus glyburide and glipizide rates of 15% and 19%, respectively. Weight gain of 2 to 3 kg has been noted with repaglinide, whereas weight gain with nateglinide appears to be <1 kg.

Drug Interactions. Glycemic control and hypoglycemia should be closely monitored when glucuronidation inhibitors are given with repaglinide. Gemfibrozil, a medication used to treat hypertriglyceridemia in DM, more than doubles the half-life of repaglinide and has resulted in prolonged hypoglycemic reactions. Gemfibrozil is a potent glucuronidation inhibitor and CYP2C8 inhibitor. Trimethoprim, a CYP2C8 inhibitor, increased repaglinide levels by 60%. Nateglinide appears to be a weak inhibitor of CYP2C9 based on tolbutamide metabolism. Though no significant drug–drug interactions have been reported, caution should be used with strong CYP2C9 and CYP3A4 inhibitors.

Dosing and Administration. Nateglinide and repaglinide should be dosed prior to each meal (up to 30 minutes prior). The recommended starting dose for repaglinide is 0.5 mg in subjects with HbA$_{1c}$ <8% or treatment-naïve patients, increased weekly to a total maximum daily dose of 16 mg (see Table 83–11). The maximal effective dose of repaglinide is likely 2 mg with each meal, as a dose of 1 mg prior to each meal provides approximately 90% of the maximal glucose-lowering effect. Nateglinide should be dosed at 120 mg prior to meals, and does not require titration. A 60-mg dose is available, but the HbA$_{1c}$ decrement is small (0.3%–0.5%). If a meal is skipped, the medication can be skipped, and meals extremely low in carbohydrate content may not need a dose. Both agents may be used in patients with renal insufficiency, and may fit into therapy in patients in need of an insulin secretagogue but have hypoglycemia to sulfonylureas, mode to severe renal insufficiency, well-controlled diabetes, but with erratic meal schedules.

Biguanides ***Pharmacology.*** Metformin is the only biguanide available in the United States. Metformin has been used clinically for more than 50 years, and has been approved in the United States since 1995. Metformin enhances insulin sensitivity of both hepatic and peripheral (muscle) tissues. This allows for an increased uptake of glucose into these insulin-sensitive tissues. The exact mechanisms of how metformin accomplishes insulin sensitization are still being investigated, though adenosine 5′-monophosphate–activated protein kinase activity, tyrosine kinase activity enhancement, and glucose transporter 4 all play a part. Metformin has no direct effect on the β cells, though insulin levels are reduced, reflecting increases in insulin sensitivity.

Pharmacokinetics. Metformin has approximately 50% to 60% oral bioavailability, low lipid solubility, and a volume of distribution that approximates body water. Metformin is not metabolized and does not bind to plasma proteins. Metformin is eliminated by renal tubular secretion and glomerular filtration. The average half-life of metformin is 6 hours, though pharmacodynamically, metformin's antihyperglycemic effects last more than 24 hours.

Efficacy. Metformin consistently reduces HbA$_{1c}$ levels by 1.5% to 2.0%, fasting plasma glucose levels by 60 to 80 mg/dL, and retains the ability to reduce FPG levels when they are extremely high (>300 mg/dL). The sulfonylureas' ability to stimulate insulin release from β cells at extremely high glucose levels is often impaired, a concept commonly referred to as *glucose toxicity*. Metformin also has positive effects on several components of the insulin resistance syndrome. Metformin decreases plasma triglycerides and LDL-C by approximately 8% to 15%, as well increasing HDL-C very modestly (2%). Metformin reduces levels of PAI-1 and causes a modest reduction in weight (2–3 kg). In preliminary findings, metformin may also lower the risk of pancreatic, colon, and breast cancer in type 2 DM patients. Metformin, through adenosine 5′-monophosphate–activated protein kinase activity, may act as a growth inhibitor in some cancers and help to kill cancer "stem cells," which are resistant to chemotherapy.

Microvascular Complications. Metformin (n – 342) was compared with intensive glucose control with insulin or sulfonylureas in the UKPDS. No significant differences were seen between therapies with regard to reducing microvascular complications, but the power of the study is questionable.

❻ Macrovascular Complications. Metformin reduced macrovascular complications in obese subjects in the UKPDS.[55] Metformin significantly reduced all-cause mortality and risk of stroke versus intensive treatment with sulfonylureas or insulin. Metformin also reduced diabetes-related death and myocardial infarctions versus the conventional treatment arm of the UKPDS. It should be noted that the UKPDS had very few people on lipid-lowering therapy. Metformin is logical in overweight/obese patients, if tolerated and not contraindicated, as it is the only oral antihyperglycemic medication proven to reduce the risk of total mortality and is generic.

Adverse Effects. Metformin causes gastrointestinal side effects, including abdominal discomfort, stomach upset, and/or diarrhea in approximately 30% of patients. Anorexia and stomach fullness is likely part of the reason loss of weight is noted with metformin. These side effects are usually mild and can be minimized by slow titration. Gastrointestinal side effects also tend to be transient, lessening in severity over several weeks. If encountered, make sure patients are taking metformin with or right after meals, and reduce the dose to a point at which no gastrointestinal side effects are encountered. Increases in the dose may be tried again in several weeks. Anecdotally, extended-release metformin (Glucophage-XR) may lessen some of the GI side effects. Metallic taste, interference with vitamin B_{12} absorption, and hypoglycemia during intense exercise has been documented, but are clinically uncommon.

Metformin therapy rarely (3 cases per 100,000 patient-years) causes lactic acidosis. Any disease state that may increase lactic acid production or decrease lactic acid removal may predispose to lactic acidosis. Tissue hypoperfusion, such as that due to congestive heart failure, severe lung disease, hypoxic states, shock, or septicemia, via increased production of lactic acid; and severe liver disease or alcohol, via reduced removal of lactic acid in the liver, all increase the risk of lactic acidosis. The clinical presentation of lactic acidosis is often nonspecific flu-like symptoms, thus the diagnosis is usually made by laboratory confirmation of high lactic acid levels and acidosis. Metformin use in renal insufficiency, defined as a serum creatinine of 1.4 mg/dL in women and 1.5 mg/dL in men or greater, is contraindicated, as it is renally eliminated. Elderly patients, who often have reduced muscle mass, should have their glomerular filtration rate estimated by a 24 hour urine creatinine collection. If the estimated glomerular filtration rate is less than 60 mL/min, metformin should not be given. Though not recommended to be clinically implemented, recent evidence has reported that metformin may not accumulate in moderate to severe renal insufficiency, if a dose of 1,500 mg/day or less is used. Due to the risk of acute renal failure during intravenous dye procedures, metformin therapy should be withheld starting the day of the procedure and resumed in 2 to 3 days, after normal renal function has been documented.

Drug Interactions. Cimetidine competes for renal tubular secretion of metformin and concomitant administration leads to higher metformin serum concentrations. At least one case report of lactic acidosis with metformin therapy implicates cimetidine. Theoretically other cationic drugs may interact, but none have been reported to date.[56]

Dosing and Administration. Immediate-release metformin is usually dosed 500 mg twice a day with the largest meals to minimize gastrointestinal side effects. Metformin may be increased by 500 mg weekly until glycemic goals or 2,500 mg/day is achieved (see Table 83–11). Metformin 850 mg may be dosed daily, and

then increased every 1 to 2 weeks to the maximum dose of 850 mg 3 times a day (2,550 mg/day). Approximately 80% of the glycemic-lowering effect may be seen at 1,500 mg, and 2,000 mg/day is the maximal effective dose.

Extended-release metformin can be initiated at 500 mg a day with the evening meal and titrated weekly by 500 mg as tolerated to a single evening dose of 2,000 mg/day. Extended-release metformin 750 mg tablets may be titrated weekly to the maximum dose of 2,250 mg/day, though as stated above, 1,500 mg/day provides the majority of the glycemic-lowering effect. Twice daily to 3 times a day dosing of extended-release metformin may help to minimize gastrointestinal side effects and improve glycemic control.

Thiazolidinediones **Pharmacology.** Thiazolidinediones are also referred to as TZDs or glitazones. Pioglitazone (Actos) and rosiglitazone (Avandia) are the two currently approved thiazolidinediones for the treatment of type 2 DM (see Table 83–11). Thiazolidinediones work by binding to the peroxisome proliferator activator receptor-γ (PPAR-γ), which are primarily located on fat cells and vascular cells. The concentration of these receptors in the muscle is very low; thus this is unlikely to be the main site of action. Thiazolidinediones enhance insulin sensitivity at muscle, liver, and fat tissues indirectly. Thiazolidinediones cause preadipocytes to differentiate into mature fat cells in subcutaneous fat stores. Small fat cells are more sensitive to insulin and more able to store free fatty acids. The result is a flux of free fatty acids out of the plasma, visceral fat, and liver into subcutaneous fat, a less insulin-resistant storage tissue. Muscle intracellular fat products, which contribute to insulin resistance, also decline. TZDs also effect adipokines, (e.g., angiotensinogen, tissue necrosis factor-α, interleukin 6, plasminogen activator inhibitor 1) which can positively affect insulin sensitivity, endothelial function, and inflammation. Of particular note, adiponectin is reduced with obesity and/or diabetes, but is increased with TZD therapy, which improves endothelial function, insulin sensitivity, and has a potent antiinflammatory effect. Lastly, TZDs appear to improve mitochondrial function through a reduction in free fatty acids. Cyclin-dependent kinase 5 has also recently been purposed as an important activator of PPAR-γ.

Pharmacokinetics. Pioglitazone and rosiglitazone are well absorbed with or without food. Both are highly (>99%) bound to albumin. Pioglitazone is primarily metabolized by CYP2C8, a lesser extent by CYP3A4 (17%), and by hydroxylation/oxidation. The majority of pioglitazone is eliminated in the feces. Rosiglitazone is metabolized by CYP2C8, and to a lesser extent by CYP2C9, and also by N-demethylation and hydroxylation. Two-thirds is found in urine and one-third in feces. The half-lives of pioglitazone and rosiglitazone are 3 to 7 hours and 3 to 4 hours, respectively. Two active metabolites of pioglitazone with longer half-lives deliver the majority of activity at steady state. Pioglitazone requires no dosage adjustment in moderate to severe renal disease for pharmacokinetic reasons. Interestingly, with pioglitazone the AUC in women is 20% to 60% higher, which is not seen with rosiglitazone, but no dosage adjustment is recommended. Both medications have a duration of antihyperglycemic action of over 24 hours.

Efficacy. Pioglitazone and rosiglitazone, given for about 6 months, reduce HbA_{1c} values ~1.5% and reduce FPG levels by ~60 to 70 mg/dL at maximal doses. Glycemic-lowering onset is slow, and maximal glycemic-lowering effects may not be seen until 3 to 4 months of therapy. It is important to inform patients of this fact and that they should not stop therapy even if minimal glucose lowering is initially encountered. The efficacy of both drugs is dependent on sufficient insulinemia. If there is insufficient endogenous insulin production (β-cell function) or exogenous insulin delivery via injections, neither will lower glucose concentrations efficiently. Interestingly, patients who are more obese, or who gain weight on either medication tend to have a larger reduction in HbA₁c values. Pioglitazone consistently decreases plasma triglyceride levels by 10% to 20%, whereas rosiglitazone tends to have a neutral effect. LDL-C concentrations tend to increase with rosiglitazone 5% to 15%, but do not significantly increase with pioglitazone. Both appear to convert small, dense LDL particles, which have been shown to be highly atherogenic, to large, fluffy LDL particles that are less dense. Large, fluffy LDL particles may be less atherogenic, but any increase in LDL must be of concern. Both drugs increase HDL similarly, up to 3 to 9 mg/dL. Thiazolidinediones also affect several components of the insulin resistance syndrome. PAI-1 levels are decreased, and many other adipocytokines are affected, endothelial function improves, and blood pressure may decrease slightly.

Microvascular Complications.
Thiazolidinediones reduce HbA₁c levels, which have been shown to be related to the risk of microvascular complications.

Macrovascular Complications.
Macrovascular complications with thiazolidinediones are controversial. In PROactive, the prospective pioglitazone clinical trial in macrovascular events, pioglitazone 45 mg was added to standard therapy in patients who had experienced a macrovascular event or had peripheral vascular disease.[57] The two groups were well matched at baseline and the reported average observation time period was about 3 years. The primary endpoint (reduction in death, myocardial infarction, stroke, acute coronary syndrome, coronary revascularization, leg amputation, and leg revascularization) was reduced 10% (*P* = 0.095). The main secondary endpoint (all-cause mortality, nonfatal myocardial infarction, or stroke) was reduced 16% (*P* = 0.027). The seemingly dichotomous results relate to the inclusion of leg revascularization as a primary endpoint, which were increased in the pioglitazone group. Reasons for the increase are speculative, but may relate to more testing/inspection due to peripheral edema. Also of note, the pioglitazone group had 209 nonadjudicated admissions for heart failure occur versus 153 in the placebo group (*P* = 0.007), though fatal heart failure was not increased. Several published meta-analysis of rosiglitazone reported higher myocardial infarction (MI) rates with rosiglitazone, but none have reported a higher risk of mortality. A hazard ratio (HR) of 1.43 (95% confidence interval [CI], 1.03–1.98; *P* = 0.03) for the risk of an MI with rosiglitazone versus other oral agents was reported.[58] A prospective, multicenter, open-label noninferiority trial in 4,447 patients of rosiglitazone added to background metformin or sulfonylurea versus the active comparator metformin + sulfonylurea was recently reported (Rosiglitazone Evaluated for Cardiovascular Outcomes in Oral Agent Combination Therapy for Type 2 Diabetes [RECORD]). Rosiglitazone was noninferior to the comparator for all CV outcomes except for heart failure. A nonsignificant increase in risk for MI (HR, 1.14; 95% CI, 0.80–1.63) as well as a nonsignificant reduction in stroke (HR, 0.72; 95% CI, 0.49–1.05) was reported. On subset analysis, previous ischemic heart disease trended toward a higher risk (HR, 1.26; CI, 0.95–1.68; *P* = 0.055). Questions still linger about the study being underpowered and certain subsets of subjects taken off rosiglitazone when given insulin; but RECORD, the only study to look at CVD risk prospectively with rosiglitazone, was neutral.[59]

CLINICAL CONTROVERSY

At a minimum, antihyperglycemic drugs should be neutral on cardiovascular events, because the majority of people with diabetes die from CVD. Both pioglitazone and rosiglitazone, equally, can result in pulmonary edema and/or heart failure, and using them with insulin or in people with preexisting heart failure may increase the incidence. TZD-related congestive heart failure is not associated with a higher risk of mortality. Several

meta-analyse have reported an increased risk of MI with the use of rosiglitazone. In the randomized, prospective RECORD trial, rosiglitazone was noninferior to the comparator for all CV outcomes except for heart failure. In contrast, no study has shown an increased risk for MI with pioglitazone, and in PROactive, there was a significant 16% reduction in the combined endpoint of mortality, MI, and stroke. Overall, prospective evidence to date shows TZDs to be neutral on CVD risk except for heart failure, with a potential lowering of CVD risk with pioglitazone.

Adverse Effects.
Troglitazone, the first thiazolidinedione approved, caused idiosyncratic hepatotoxicity and had 28 deaths from liver failure, which prompted removal from the U.S. market in March 2000. Approximately 1.9% of patients placed on troglitazone had alanine aminotransferase (ALT) levels more than 3 times the upper limit of normal. The incidence, using these criteria for elevated liver enzymes, with pioglitazone (0.25%) and rosiglitazone (0.2%) has been low. No evidence of hepatotoxicity was reported in an analysis of more than 5,000 patients given rosiglitazone or pioglitazone.[60] Several case reports of hepatotoxicity with rosiglitazone or pioglitazone have been reported, but improvement in ALT was consistently noted when the drug was discontinued. Prior to therapy, it is recommended that an ALT be checked, and periodically after at the practitioner's discretion. Patients with ALT levels >2.5 times the upper limit of normal should not start either medication, and if the ALT is >3 times the upper limit of normal the medication should be discontinued.

Retention of fluid leads to many different possible side effects with rosiglitazone and pioglitazone. The etiology of the fluid retention has not been fully elucidated, but appears to include peripheral vasodilation and/or improved insulin sensitization at the kidney with a resultant increase in renal sodium and water retention. A reduction in plasma hemoglobin (2%–4%), attributed to a 10% increase in plasma volume, may result in a dilutional anemia which does not require treatment. Edema is also commonly (4%–5% in mono- or combination therapy) reported. When a thiazolidinedione is used in combination with insulin, the incidence of edema (~15%) is increased. Thiazolidinediones are contraindicated in patients with New York Heart Association Class III and IV heart failure, and great caution should be exercised when given to patients with Class I and II heart failure or other underlying cardiac disease, as pulmonary edema and heart failure have been reported. Edema tends to be dose related and if not severe, a reduction in the dose as well as use of diuretics, anecdotally hydrochlorothiazide with triamterene, amiloride, or spironolactone instead of loop diuretics, will allow the continuation of therapy in the majority of patients.[61] Rarely, thiazolidinediones have been reported to worsen macular edema of the eye.

Weight gain, which is also dose related, can be seen with both rosiglitazone and pioglitazone. Mechanistically, both fluid retention and fat accumulation play a part in explaining the weight gain. Thiazolidinediones, besides stimulating fat cell differentiation, also reduce leptin levels, which stimulate appetite and food intake. Average weight gain varies, but a 1.5- to 4-kg weight gain is not uncommon. Rarely, a patient will gain large amounts of weight in a short period of time, and this may necessitate discontinuation of therapy. Weight gain positively predicts a larger HbA₁c reduction, but must be balanced with the well-documented effects of long-term weight gain.

Thiazolidinediones have also been associated with an increased fracture rate in the upper and lower limbs in women and men, though women appear to have a higher risk. These fractures are not osteoporitic in the classic sense, and do not occur in common osteoporosis fracture sites such as spine or hip. Most occur in wrists, forearms, ankles, or feet. Versus comparative diabetes therapy, thiazolidinediones may increase the risk of a fracture by 25%. The underlying pathophysiology is speculative, but may relate to thiazolidinediones effect on the pluripotent stem cell and shunting of new cells to fat instead of osteocytes. It would be prudent to consider a patient's risk factors for fractures if a thiazolidinedione is being considered as antidiabetic therapy.

As a caution, premenopausal anovulatory patients may resume ovulation on thiazolidinediones. Adequate pregnancy and contraception precautions should be explained to all women capable of becoming pregnant, as both agents are pregnancy category C.

Drug Interactions. Significant drug interactions that can cause clinical sequelae have not been noted with either medication. Neither pioglitazone nor rosiglitazone appear to be inhibitors or inducers of CYP3A4/2C8 or CYP2C8/CYP2C9, respectively, though drugs that are strong inhibitors or inducers of these pathways (e.g., gemfibrozil or rifampin) may increase or decrease levels of active drug significantly.

Dosing and Administration. The recommended starting dosages of pioglitazone and of rosiglitazone are 15 to 30 mg once daily and 2 to 4 mg once daily, respectively. Dosages may be increased slowly based on therapeutic goals and side effects. The maximum dose and maximum effective dose of pioglitazone is 45 mg, and rosiglitazone is 8 mg once daily, though 4 mg twice a day may reduce HbA$_{1c}$ by 0.2% to 0.3% more versus 8 mg once daily.

α-Glucosidase Inhibitors Pharmacology. Currently, there are two α-glucosidase inhibitors available in the United States acarbose (Precose) and miglitol (Glyset). α-Glucosidase inhibitors competitively inhibit enzymes (maltase, isomaltase, sucrase, and glucoamylase) in the small intestine, delaying the breakdown of sucrose and complex carbohydrates.[62,63] They do not cause any malabsorption of these nutrients. The net effect from this action is to reduce the postprandial blood glucose rise.

Pharmacokinetics. The mechanism of action of α-glucosidase inhibitors is limited to the luminal side of the intestine. Some metabolites of acarbose are systemically absorbed and renally excreted, whereas the majority of miglitol is absorbed and renally excreted unchanged.

Efficacy. Postprandial glucose concentrations are reduced (40–50 mg/dL), while fasting glucose levels are relatively unchanged (~10% reduction). Efficacy on glycemic control is modest (average reductions in HbA$_{1c}$ of 0.3%–1%), affecting primarily postprandial glycemic excursions. Thus, patients near target HbA$_{1c}$ levels with near-normal fasting plasma glucose levels, but high postprandial levels, may be candidates for therapy.

Microvascular Complications. α-Glucosidase inhibitors modestly reduce HbA$_{1c}$ levels, which has been shown to be related to the risk of microvascular complications.

Macrovascular Complications. The STOP-NIDDM study, in subjects with impaired glucose tolerance, reported a significant reduction in the risk of cardiovascular events, though the total number of events were small.[64,65] No large cardiovascular study confirming these preliminary results has been done in prediabetes or diabetes patients.

Adverse Effects. The gastrointestinal side effects, such as flatulence, bloating, abdominal discomfort, and diarrhea, are very common and greatly limit the use of α-glucosidase inhibitors. Mechanistically, these side effects are caused by distal intestinal degradation of undigested carbohydrate by the microflora, which results in gas (CO_2 and methane) production. Microflora convert the carbohydrate to short-chain fatty acids which are mostly absorbed, thus there is not a large calorie loss. α-Glucosidase inhibitors should be initiated at a low dose and titrated slowly to reduce gastrointestinal intolerance. Beano, an α-glucosidase enzyme, may help to decrease gastrointestinal side effects, but may decrease efficacy slightly, and it is better to decrease carbohydrate or the dose of the α-glucosidase inhibitor.[66]

If a patient develops hypoglycemia within several hours of ingesting an α-glucosidase inhibitor, oral glucose is advised because the drug will inhibit the breakdown of more complex sugar molecules. Milk, with lactose sugar, may be used as an alternative when no glucose is available, as acarbose only slightly (10%) inhibits lactase.

Rarely, elevated serum aminotransferase levels have been reported with the highest doses of acarbose. It appeared to be dose and weight related, and is the premise for the weight-based maximum doses.

Dosing and Administration. Dosing for both miglitol and acarbose are similar. Initiate with a very low dose (25 mg with one meal a day); increase very gradually (over several months) to a maximum of 50 mg 3 times a day for patients ≤60 kg or 100 mg 3 times a day for patients >60 kg (see Table 83–11). Titration speed should be varied based on gastrointestinal side effects to the target dose. Both α-glucosidase inhibitors should be taken with the first bite of the meal so that drug may be present to inhibit enzyme activity. Only patients consuming a diet high in complex carbohydrates will have significant reductions in glucose levels. α-Glucosidase inhibitors are contraindicated in patients with short-bowel syndrome or inflammatory bowel disease, and neither should be administered in patients with serum creatinine >2 mg/dL, as this population has not been studied.

Dipeptidyl Peptidase 4 Inhibitors (DPP-4 Inhibitors)

Sitagliptin (Januvia) and saxagliptin (Onglyza) are the two DPP-4 inhibitors currently approved in the United States.

Pharmacology. DPP-4 inhibitors prolong the half-life of endogenously produced GLP-1 and glucose-dependent insulinotropic polypeptide (GIP) which is normally only minutes. GIP levels are normal in type 2 DM, and may contribute a minor amount of insulin secretion but have no effect on glucagon. It has clearly been shown that GLP-1 levels are deficient in type 2 DM. As these agents block nearly 100% of the DPP-4 enzyme activity for at least 12 hours, normal physiologic, nondiabetic GLP-1 levels are achieved. DPP-4 inhibitors significantly reduce the inappropriately elevated glucagon postprandially, though not back to nondiabetic levels, and improve insulin response to a high glucose level. Insulin levels tend to be unchanged with DPP-4 inhibitors, but glucose levels are reduced. This is an improvement in insulin secretion, as a nondiabetic person would decrease insulin secretion in response to the lower glucose readings. These drugs do not alter gastric emptying or have significant satiety effects.

Pharmacokinetics. Sitagliptin appears to have rapid absorption, with a t_{max} of approximately 1.5 hours. Absolute bioavailability after oral intake is approximately 87%. Only ~40% is bound to plasma proteins, and the volume of distribution is approximately 200 liters. The $t_{1/2}$ of sitagliptin is approximately 12 hours, and 79% of the dose of sitagliptin is excreted unchanged in the urine by active tubular secretion, though the organic anion transporter 3 or p-glycoprotein transport may be involved as well. Sitagliptin exposure is increased by approximately 2.3-, 3.8-, and 4.5-fold relative to healthy subjects for patients with moderate renal insufficiency (creatinine clearance [CL$_{cr}$] 30 to <50 mL/min), severe renal insufficiency (CL$_{cr}$ <30 mL/min), and ESRD (on dialysis), respectively. Though not a safety or adverse reaction issue, reduction of the dose based on renal function is appropriate, as only 100% of the enzyme can be inhibited, and long-term exposure to higher levels in humans has not been extensively studied. Pharmacodynamically, DPP-4 inhibition appeared to mirror directly the plasma concentration of sitagliptin. Doses of 50 mg produced at least 80% inhibition of DPP-4 enzyme activity at 12 hours, and 100 mg produced 80% inhibition of DPP-4 enzyme activity at 24 hours. Food had no effect on absorption kinetics of sitagliptin, and hepatic impairment, age, gender, or race had no effect on the pharmacokinetics.

The t_{max} increased about 20 minutes and the AUC increased about 27% when saxagliptin was administered with a high-fat meal, though saxagliptin may be given with or without meals. The oral bioavailability of saxagliptin is approximately 67%. Distribution is similar to the body water compartment. There is negligible protein binding, and one active metabolite, 5-hydroxy saxagliptin, which is half as potent a DPP-4 inhibitor as the parent compound, and contributes to activity. Metabolism is by the CYP3A4/5 system, and strong inhibitors or inducers will have an effect on activity. The half-life of saxagliptin and its active metabolite are 2.5 hours and 3.1 hours, respectively. Approximately 25% of the dose is found in feces representing unabsorbed drug and bile excretion. No accumulation was noted with saxagliptin or its active metabolite. Females have ~25% more exposure to 5-hydroxy saxagliptin, and exposure is increased 25% to 50% in elderly, likely due to renal clearance. The majority (75%) of saxagliptin and 5-hydroxy saxagliptin is renally eliminated, and some renal excretion is seen. In moderate (CL_{cr} 30–50 mL/min) or severe (CL_{cr} <30 mL/min) renal impairment, saxagliptin and its active metabolite exposure are increased 2.1- and 4.5-fold, respectively.

Efficacy. The average reduction in HbA_{1c} with sitagliptin or saxagliptin is approximately 0.7% to 1% at maximum dose. The HbA_{1c} decrement is dependent on the baseline value, with a larger reduction being seen with a higher baseline HbA_{1c}. As they are well tolerated, adjustment in the dose for adverse effects is unlikely.

Microvascular and Macrovascular Complications. HbA_{1c} levels are reduced, which has been related to a reduction in microvascular complications, but no outcome data are available to date.

Drug–Drug Interactions. Significant drug–drug interactions with sitaglitin are unlikely. Sitagliptin is metabolized approximately 20% by CYP450 3A4 with some CYP450 2C8 involvement, but is neither an inhibitor nor inducer of any CYP450 enzyme system. Sitagliptin is a p-glycoprotein substrate, but had negligible effects on digoxin and cyclosporine A, increasing the AUC by only 30%.

Saxagliptin is metabolized by CYP3A4/5, and is a substrate for p-glycoprotein substrate, but is neither an inhibitor nor inducer. Rifampin, an inducer, can decrease active levels by 50%. Moderate to strong inhibitors or inducers of CYP3A4/5, such as diltiazem or ketoconazole, can increase the AUC of saxagliptin by approximately 2-fold, with a corresponding decrease in the formation of the active metabolite 5-hydroxy saxagliptin. It is recommended that the dose of saxagliptin be limited to 2.5 mg daily if a stronger inhibitor is used.

Adverse Effects. Both drugs are very well tolerated, weight neutral, and do not cause gastrointestinal side effects. Mild hypoglycemia may occur, but in monotherapy or in combination with medication that have a low incidence of hypoglycemia, DPP-4 inhibitors do not increase the risk of hypoglycemia. Headache and nasopharyngitis, potentially related to the drug, may be slightly more common with DPP-4 inhibitors, but no significant increases in peripheral edema, hypertension, or cardiac outcomes have been noted to date.

Uticaria and/or facial edema may be seen in approximately 1% of patients, and discontinuation is warranted. Rare cases of Stevens-Johnson syndrome have been reported.

In regard to long-term safety, DPP-4 enzymes metabolize a wide variety of peptides (PYY, neuropeptide Y, growth hormone-releasing hormone, vasoactive intestinal polypeptide, and others) potentially affecting other regulatory systems. DPP-4 (also known as CD26) plays an important role for T-cell activation and theoretically the inhibition of DPP-4 could be associated with adverse immunologic reactions. Saxagliptin results in a dose-related reduction in absolute lymphocyte count. Approximately 1.5% of patients had a count less than 750 cells/microliter, and discontinuation/rechallenge was confirmed in some patients. The clinical relevance

is not known, but if prolonged infection is encountered, it is logical to measure lymphocyte counts and consider discontinuation.

Additionally DPP-8/9 inhibition in animals produced multiple toxicities. Sitagliptin is more selective for DPP-4 than DPP-8/9 (>2,600-fold). Saxagliptin and its active metabolite 5-hydroxy saxagliptin are more specific for DPP-4 than DPP-8 (400- and 950-fold) and DPP-9 (75- and 160-fold), respectively.

Dosing and Administration Sitagliptin is dosed orally at 100 mg daily unless renal insufficiency is present. The 50-mg dose is recommended if the creatinine clearance is 30 to less than 50 mL/min, or 25 mg if less than 30 mL/min. Equivalent serum creatinine levels are as follows: sitagliptin 50 mg daily in men, greater than 1.7 to 3.0 mg/dL, women, greater than 1.5 to 2.5 mg/dL; 25 mg daily in men, greater than 3.0 mg/dL, women, greater than 2.5 mg/dL. Saxagliptin is dosed orally 5 mg daily, unless the creatinine clearance is less than 50 mL/min, or strong CYP3A4/5 inhibitors are used, then the recommended daily dose is 2.5 mg. Because of their excellent tolerability profile and a fairly flat dose-response curve, these drugs should be maximally dosed, unless noted above.

Bile Acid Sequestrants Currently, the only bile acid sequestrant approved for the treatment of type 2 DM is colesevelam (Welchol).

Pharmacology. Colesevelam is a bile acid sequestrant which acts in the intestinal lumen to bind bile acid, decreasing the bile acid pool for reabsorption. Whether colesevelam's mechanism of action to lower plasma glucose levels is in the intestinal lumen, a systemic effect due to the intestinal lumen effect or some combination of these two is unknown.

Pharmacokinetics. Colesevelam is not absorbed from the intestinal lumen, thus there is not absorption, distribution, or metabolism.

Efficacy. HbA_{1c} reductions from baseline (~8.0%) were approximately 0.4% when a dose of 3.8 g/day was added to stable metformin, sulfonylureas, or insulin. The fasting plasma glucose was modestly reduced about 5 to 10 mg/dL. Colesevelam may also reduce LDL-C cholesterol. A 12% to 16% reduction in LDL-C was reported with type 2 DM and a baseline LDL-C concentrations of ~105 mg/dL. Triglycerides increased when combined with sulfonylureas or insulin, but not with metformin. Colesevelam is weight neutral. Pediatric patients (10–17 years of age) have been studied for cholesterol reduction, but not for type 2 DM.

Microvascular Complications. Bile acid sequestrants modestly reduce HbA_{1c} levels, which have been shown to be related to the risk of microvascular complications.

Macrovascular Complications. Though colesevelam lowers plasma glucose and LDL-C, it has not been proven to prevent cardiovascular morbidity or mortality.

Drug–Drug Interactions. There are multiple absorption related drug–drug interactions with colesevelam. Tables 83–13, 83–14, and 83–15 summarizes medications that may interact with colesevelam. It is recommended that medications suspected of an interaction should be moved at least 4 hours prior to dosing the colesvelam. Colesevelam has also been implicated in the malabsorption of fat-soluable vitamins (A, E, D, K). In addition to the obvious fat-soluble vitamin supplementation, this may have implications for associated conditions. Other drugs that are very fat soluble such as cyclosporine A, drugs that may be affected by a change in fat-soluble vitamin status such as warfarin and vitamin K, or conditions that may that may be potentially worsened by fat-soluble vitamin status such as some bleeding disorders or dermatologic conditions should be monitored.[67]

Adverse Effects. The most common side effects are gastrointestinal. Constipation (11%) and dyspepsia (8%) are more common with colesevelam than placebo. Because of the constipating effects of

TABLE 83-13	Drugs with Known Interactions

Levothyroxine
Glyburide
Oral contraceptives with ethinyl estradiol and norethindrone

colesevelam, it is not recommended in patients with gastroparesis, bowel obstruction, or a history of major gastrointestinal surgery. It also should not be used in patients with significant swallowing or esophageal issues, as it may worsen the underlying condition or cause obstruction. Colesevelam should be taken with a large amount of water to lower the risk of the above issues. Hypoglycemia rates were low, though caution with insulin or sulfonylureas is prudent.

Colesevelam, similar to all bile acid sequestrants, may raise triglyceride levels. The increase in triglycerides is proportional to baseline triglyceride levels, and colesevelam is contraindicated in patients with a triglyceride >500 mg/dL. Close monitoring is recommended if the baseline triglycerides greater than 300 mg/dL. Colesevelam is contraindicated in patients with a history of triglyceridemia induced pancreatitis, and prudent clinical judgement should be used in any patient with a history of pancreatitis and elevated triglycerides.

Dosing and Administration. Dosing for type 2 DM is six 625-mg tablets daily (total dose/day = 3.75 g), which may be split into 3 tablets 2 times a day if desired. A 3.75-g oral suspension packet, dosed daily, or a 1.875-g oral suspension packet dose twice daily is also available. Suspension packets must be diluted in a minimum of one-half to 1 cup of water. Take tablets and suspension with a large amount of water, if possible. All dosage forms should be administered with meals as colesevelam binds to bile released during the meal.

Dopamine Agonists Bromocriptine mesylate (Cycloset) is currently approved for the treatment of type 2 DM, but is not commercially available at the time this chapter was written.

Pharmacology. Bromocriptine is a dopamine agonist, but the exact mechanism of how bromocriptine improves glycemic control is unknown. In vertebrates, oscillations in neurotransmitters, including dopamine, can change the response to insulin, and animal and human data indicate that bromocriptine administered in the morning improves insulin sensitivity.

Pharmacokinetics. Bioavailability is 65% to 95% after an orally administered dose, bioavailability may be increased ~50% if given with a meal. Bromocriptine is highly protein bound, and has a volume of distribution of 61 liters. Only ~7% reaches the systemic circulation due to gastrointestinal-based metabolism and first-pass metabolism. Bromocriptine is extensively metabolized by the CYP3A4 pathway, and the majority (~95%) is excreted in the bile. The half-life is approximately 6 hours. Plasma exposure is increased in females by approximately 18% to 30%, but no dosage adjustment is currently recommended.

Efficacy. In clinical trials, bromocriptine mesylate reduced HbA_{1c} by a modest 0.1% to 0.4% from baseline (HbA_{1c} 8%–9%).

TABLE 83-14	Drugs with Postmarketing Reports or Narrow Therapeutic Indexes

Phenytoin
Warfarin
Digoxin
Fat-soluable vitamins (A, D, E, K)

TABLE 83-15	Drug that do not Likely Interact with Colesevelam

Cephalexin
Ciprofloxacin
Fenofibrate
Lovastatin
Metformin
Metoprolol
Pioglitazone
Quinidine
Repaglinide
Valproic acid
Verapamil

Microvascular and Macrovascular Complications. It is unclear what effect, if any, bromocriptine may have on outcomes, though no increase in cardiovascular event signal was detected from data presented to the FDA.

Drug–Drug Interactions. Bromocriptine is extensively metabolized by CYP3A4 and strong inhibitors or inducers may change bromocriptine levels. As bromocriptine is highly protein bound, it may increase the unbound fraction of other highly protein bound drugs. Several drug–drug and potential drug–disease interactions are present including antipsychotics in psychotic disorders as they decrease dopamine activity, atypical antipsychotics, as they may decrease the effectiveness of bromocriptine, and ergot-based therapy for migraines as bromocriptine may increase migraine and ergot related nausea and vomiting. There are case reports of hypertension and tachycardia when administered with sympathomimetic drugs in postpartum women, and bromocriptine should not be given to this group of potential patients. The effectiveness in other disease states where dopamine agonism may be indicated is unknown.

Adverse Effects. Adverse reactions leading to discontinuation occurred in 24% of bromocriptine patients compared to 9% in the placebo comparator group. Nausea, rhinitis, headache, asthenia, dizziness, constipation, and sinusitis all occurred in over 10% of subjects. Nausea occurred in 25% to 35% of patients, and vomiting, which tended to be more common in women, occurred in 5% to 6% of patients. Nausea, vomiting, fatigue, headache, and dizziness were common adverse events during the titration phase of phase 3 studies, and only 70% of completors could be titrated to the maximum dose. Orthostatic hypotension or syncope occurred in 2.2% and 1.4%, and 0.6% and 0.8% in the bromocriptine and placebo groups, respectively. No predisposing factors were identified, but caution should be exercised in patients with low, normal blood pressure. Somnolence was reported in 4.3% of patients on bromocriptine, compared with 1.3% in the placebo, and response to the drug should be ascertained prior to operating machinery or combining with other sedating medications. Psychiatric disorders including hallucinations and pathological gambling have been reported with other forms of bromocriptine, but were not seen in phase III trials.

Dosing and Administration. Bromocriptine is dosed with 0.8-mg tablets administered within 2 hours of waking from sleep daily. From 0.8 mg daily, the dose may be increased weekly based on response by 0.8-mg tablet increments, to a maximum of 4.8 mg daily (0.8 mg × 6 tablets, though it is unclear if another commercial dose could be made available). The minimal effective dose is 1.6 mg daily.

■ POTENTIAL FUTURE MEDICATIONS

Many medications for the treatment of diabetes are currently in late-phase development. No guarantee of FDA approval is given for any agent in development.

Exenatide Long-Acting-Release (Bydureon)

A once-weekly, long-acting injection preparation of the current twice-daily exenatide formulation is being developed. Exenatide is embedded in small beads of material similar to absorbable suture material. This allows for the embedded exenatide to be released over 1 week. Data out to 1 year has shown better FPG and HbA$_{1c}$ lowering than the current twice daily exenatide. Safety and side effects, with slightly less nausea with the weekly preparation, appears similar to twice daily exenatide.

Other Incretin Class Medications

Several other DPP-4 inhibitors may be approved, including alogliptin, dutogliptin, and linagliptin. There will likely be many DPP-4 inhibitors on the market soon. Taspoglutide, a once-weekly human analog GLP-1 agonist may also be approved in the next several years. Taspoglutide dosing is speculative, but will likely be 20 to 30 mg weekly.

Selective Sodium-dependent Glucose Cotransporter-2 Inhibitors (SGLT-2 Inhibitors)

SGLT-2 inhibitors works in the kidney to block the reabsorption of some glucose. Normally, all glucose is reabsorbed back into the systemic circulation from the kidney at normal glucose levels; about 10% through the SGLT-1 receptor, and 90% through the SGLT-2 receptor. Early data has shown approximately 50 to 80 grams of glucose per day may be allowed to pass into the urine with SGLT-2 inhibition. This lowers systemic glucose and allows weight loss. Glucose levels may be lowered in both type 1 and type 2 DM by this mechanism of action. Safety data has shown a slightly higher rate of genitourinary yeast infections to date. SGLT-1 is involved with glucose absorption in the gut, and selectivity is important, as inhibition of SGLT-1 may cause gastrointestinal toxicity. Dapagliflozin is currently the farthest in development, but several are being developed.

■ PIVOTAL TRIALS

Diabetes Control and Complications Trial

7 Much of the last century in diabetes care was dominated by the debate over whether glycemic control actually was causative in complications of DM. Animal studies and some human studies suggested that the worse the glycemia the greater the risk of complications. But "the glucose hypothesis" was not ultimately accepted as proven until the publication of the DCCT in 1993.[31] In this study, 1,441 patients with type 1 DM were divided into two groups: those without complications (726 subjects, primary prevention), and those with early microvascular complications (715 subjects, secondary prevention). These two groups were then again divided into two groups, one randomized to receive conventional therapy (one or two shots of insulin daily and infrequent SMBG with no attempt to change therapy based on home blood glucose readings), and the other to receive intensive therapy (3+ injections of insulin daily or insulin pump, with frequent SMBG and alteration of insulin therapy based on SMBG results, plus frequent contact with a health professional). After 6.5 years, mean follow-up with a difference in HbA$_{1c}$ between the two groups being ≈2% (≈9% vs ≈7%), retinopathy was decreased by 76% in the primary prevention cohort, with retinopathy progression reduced 54% in the secondary prevention group. Neuropathy was decreased by 60% in both groups combined. Microalbuminuria was decreased 39%, while macroproteinuria was reduced 54% with intensive therapy. Hypoglycemia was more common and weight gain greater with intensive therapy. A nonstatistically significant reduction in coronary events was seen in the intensively treated group as compared with the conventional

group. The DCCT revolutionized therapy of DM, demanding that stricter glycemic control be the goal.

United Kingdom Prospective Diabetes Study

The UKPDS was a landmark study for the care of patients with type 2 DM, confirming the importance of glycemic control for reducing the risk of microvascular complications.[32] More than 5,000 patients with newly diagnosed type 2 DM were entered into the study. Patients were followed for an average of 10 years. The major portion of the study assessed "conventional therapy" (no drug therapy unless the patient was symptomatic or had FPG >270 mg/dL), versus intensive therapy starting with either sulfonylureas or insulin, aimed at keeping the fasting plasma glucose <108 mg/dL. A subset of obese patients was studied using metformin as the primary therapeutic agent.

CLINICAL CONTROVERSY

Preservation of β-cell function, and thus arresting the progression of type 2 diabetes, is an important secondary goal after glycemic control. The UKPDS clearly showed that sulfonylureas, metformin, and insulin are ineffective in stopping the progressive β-cell failure. In animal models, TZDs, exenatide, and DPP-4 inhibitors have been able to arrest β-cell failure. In humans, durability of HbA$_{1c}$ reduction and β-cell function is improved with TZDs and GLP-1 agonists. These medications have shown to slow, through durable HbA$_{1c}$ reduction, but not to arrest the progressive β-cell decline in type 2 DM. Monotherapy with these medications will not likely succeed in fully arresting HbA$_{1c}$ deterioration over time, and only combination therapy, with drugs such as TZDs and GLP-1 agonists, may accomplish this, though long-term data are lacking.

Significant findings from the study include the following:

- Microvascular complications (predominantly the need for laser photocoagulation on retinal lesions) are reduced by 25% when median HbA$_{1c}$ is 7% as compared with 7.9%.[32]

- A continuous relationship exists between glycemia and microvascular complications, with a 35% reduction in risk for each 1% decrement in HbA$_{1c}$. No glycemic threshold for microvascular disease exists.[68]

- Glycemic control has minimal effect on macrovascular disease risk.[62] Excess macrovascular risk appears to be related to conventional risk factors such as dyslipidemia and hypertension.[69]

- Sulfonylureas and insulin therapy do not increase macrovascular disease risk.[32]

- Metformin reduces macrovascular risk in obese patients.[55]

- Vigorous blood pressure control reduces microvascular and macrovascular events.[69] There was no evidence for a threshold systolic blood pressure above 130 mm Hg for protection against complications. β-Blockers and ACE inhibitors appear to be equally efficacious.[70]

Long-Term Follow-Up of DCCT (EDIC) and UKPDS

At the conclusion of the DCCT and UKPDS trials, willing subjects continued to be followed over time to ascertain micro- and macrovascular outcomes. In the follow-up of the DCCT, called the Epidemiology of Diabetes Interventions and Complications (EDIC), several important points have been discovered. First, HbA$_{1c}$ levels between conventional and intensive groups converged to a HbA$_{1c}$ of approximately 8%. Despite similar HbA$_{1c}$ values, continued micro- and new macrovascular benefit was seen. Microvascular benefits were maintained for 10 to 15 years, and at 17 years of follow-up, a 57% (P = 0.02) reduction in death, first occurance of nonfatal MI and stroke was seen between the conventional and intensive groups.[71,72]

In the follow-up of the UKPDS, HbA$_{1c}$ (~8%) converged and values were not significantly different for the majority of the follow-up. After a mean follow-up of 8.5 years, a 24% (P = 0.001) reduction in microvascular complications (during the UKPDS, 25% reduction was reported) and a significant reduction in MI (15%; P = 0.014) and all-cause mortality (13%; P = 0.007) in the intensively treated group versus the conventional group was reported.[73] Early glycemic control may have long-standing benefits to patients over several decades, despite later glycemic control deterioration. This concept is being called metabolic memory or the legacy effect. These studies lay the framework for why early intensive glycemic control is important not only for short term, but also long-term prevention of complications.

ACCORD, ADVANCE, and VADT

The Action to Control Cardiovascular Risk in Diabetes (ACCORD),[74] Action in Diabetes and Vascular Disease (ADVANCE),[75] and Veterans Affairs Diabetes Trial (VADT)[76] were three trials that reported on the effects of glycemic control and macrovascular disease risk.

ACCORD randomized 10,251 high CVD risk subjects (CVD event or significant risk) with type 2 DM to intensive glycemic control (goal HbA$_{1c}$ <6%) or standard glycemic control (HbA$_{1c}$ 7.0%–7.9%). Multiple oral agents and/or insulin were allowed to achieve glycemic goals. Baseline HbA$_{1c}$ level was 8.1%, and the intensive glycemic group achieved a HbA$_{1c}$ of 6.4%, whereas standard glycemic control achieved a HbA$_{1c}$ of 7.5% when the study stopped after a mean follow-up period of 3.5 years. The study was stopped after an interim analysis reported an increase rate of mortality in the intensive arm (1.41 vs 1.14%/year; HR, 1.22; 95% CI, 1.01–1.46). Interestingly, the primary endpoint (myocardial, stroke, or cardiovascular death) was trending down due to a lower risk of nonfatal MI in the intensive therapy group. In addition, on subset analysis, individuals with a baseline HbA$_{1c}$ <8.0% or no previous CVD had a significant reduction in the primary outcome. Increased mortality could not be associated with a specific medication, hypoglycemia (higher in intensive group), lipid levels, or weight gain, though substantially increased in the intensive group. The dichotomous results have been hard to explain, though the ACCORD investigators reported that in the intensive group, it was subjects who could *not* attain intensive glycemic control goals who were at higher risk, not subjects who did achieve the goal. A 20% higher risk of death for each 1% above a HbA$_{1c}$ of 6% was reported.

ADVANCE randomized 11,140 subjects to intensive (≤6.5% HbA$_{1c}$) or standard therapy (investigator-driven goals). Extended-release gliclizide, a sulfonylurea available outside of the United States, was used as first-line therapy in the intensive group versus no gliclizide in the standard therapy group, though multiple other agents were needed in both groups. A baseline HbA$_{1c}$ was only 7.5%, and at the end of therapy, the intensive group versus standard group HbA$_{1c}$ was ~6.5% versus ~7.2%. ADVANCE reported a significant reduction in renal events, including new or worsening nephropathy (HR, 0.79; 95% CI, 0.66–0.93), but no difference in major macrovascular events (HR, 0.94; 95% CI, 0.84–1.06) with intensive versus standard therapy.

VADT randomized 1,791 subjects to intensive glycemic control (HbA$_{1c}$ goal <6.0%, and action required of >6.5%) versus nonintensive glycemic control (investigator determined). At entry, the HbA$_{1c}$ was the highest of the three trials (9.4%). Multiple medications including insulin were used to achieve glycemic control. The intensive group achieved a HbA$_{1c}$ of 6.9% versus 8.5% in the investigator

determined group. The primary endpoint of nonfatal MI, nonfatal stroke, CVD death, hospitalization for heart failure, and revascularization was not significantly different (HR, 0.88; 95% CI, 0.74–1.05) and mortality was unchanged.

These three trials should be viewed as confirmatory that short term (3–5 years) of intensive glycemic control do not positively affect the risk of macrovascular risk in type 2 DM. ACCORD reported that a subset of subjects that could not achieve intensive glycemic control may be at higher risk of death, but identifying these patients and implementing this recommendation into clinical practice may prove to be challenging. As previously mentioned in the EDIC and follow-up of the UKPDS, reduction of macrovascular events from improved glycemic control may take over a decade to come to fruition.

■ THERAPEUTICS

❽ Knowledge of the patient's quantitative and qualitative meal patterns, activity levels, pharmacokinetics of insulin preparations and other injectables, and pharmacology of oral and antidiabetic agents for type 2 DM are essential to individualize the treatment plan and optimize blood glucose control while minimizing risks for hypoglycemia and other adverse effects of pharmacologic therapies.

Type 1 Diabetes Mellitus

The choice of therapy for type 1 DM is simple: all patients need insulin. However, how that insulin is delivered to the patient is a matter of considerable practice difference among patients and clinicians. Historically, after the discovery of insulin by Banting and Best in 1921, frequent injections of regular insulin (initially the only insulin available) were given. Modifications of insulin led to longer-acting insulin suspensions and the use by many patients of one or two shots of longer-acting insulin each day. Because self-monitored blood glucose and HbA$_{1c}$ testing were not available at that time, patients and practitioners had no idea how well their patients' blood glucose concentrations were controlled, other than a vague sense from an indirect method, measurement of glucose in the urine. While the renal threshold for glucose is relatively predictable in young healthy subjects, it is highly variable in older patients and patients with renal disease. The advent of SMBG and HbA$_{1c}$ testing in the 1980s revolutionized the care of diabetes, enabling patients and practitioners to directly access blood glucose for assessment, and enabling the patient to make instantaneous changes in the insulin regimen if need be. Modern diabetes management would be impossible without these two tools.

Contemporary management of type 1 DM attempts to match carbohydrate intake with glucose-lowering processes, most commonly insulin, as well as with exercise. Attempts are made to allow the patient to live as normal a life as possible. Understanding the principles of glucose input and glucose egress from the blood will allow the practitioner and the patient great latitude in the management of patients with type 1 DM.

Simplistically speaking, one can break down normal insulin secretion into a relatively constant background level of insulin ("basal") for the fasting and postabsorptive period, and prandial spikes of insulin after eating ("bolus") (Fig. 83–8).[77] Insulin sensitivity and insulin secretion are not constant throughout the day, rendering the basal concept inaccurate. However, in most clinical situations, this approach provides a useful paradigm for understanding and applying insulin treatment for type 1 DM. The other basic principle to consider is that the timing of insulin onset, peak, and duration of effect must match meal patterns and exercise schedules to achieve near-normal blood glucose values throughout the day.

Historically, complexity of insulin regimens has usually been related to the number of injections of insulin administered per

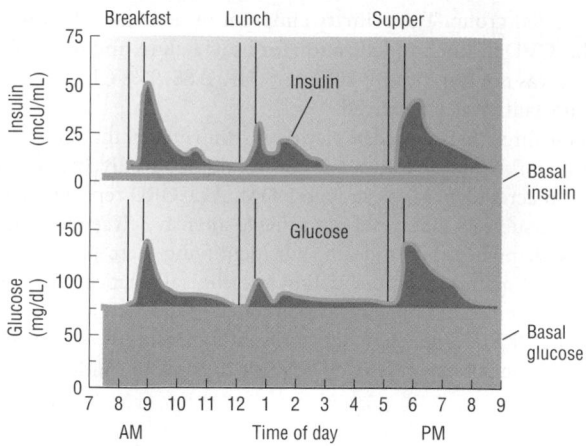

FIGURE 83-8. Relationship between insulin and glucose over the course of a day and how various insulin and amylinomimetic regimens could be given. (A, aspart; CS-II, continuous subcutaneous insulin infusion; D, detemir; G, glargine; GLU, glulisine; L, lispro; P, pramlintide; N, NPH; R, regular.)

Intensive insulin therapy regimens

	7AM (meal)	11 AM (meal)	5 PM (meal)	Bedtime
1. 2 doses,[a] R or rapid acting + N	R, L, A, GLU + N		R, L, A, GLU + N	
2. 3 doses, R or rapid acting + N	R, L, A, GLU + N	R, L, A, GLU	R, L, A, GLU + N	
3. 4 doses, R or rapid acting + N	R, L, A, GLU	R, L, A, GLU	R, L, A, GLU	N
4. 4 doses R or rapid acting + N	R, L, A, GLU + N	R, L, A, GLU	R, L, A, GLU	N
5. 4 doses,[b] R or rapid acting + long acting	R, L, A, GLU	R, L, A, GLU	R, L, A, GLU	G or D[b] (G may be given anytime every 24 hours)
6. CS-II pump	Bolus ←———— Adjusted basal	Bolus	Bolus ————→	
7. 3 doses pramlintide added to regimens above	P	P	P	

[a]Many clinicians may not consider this intensive insulin therapy
[b]May be given BID in type 1 DM = 5 doses

day. This is a reasonable classification. Clearly one injection of any insulin preparation daily will in no way mimic normal physiology, and therefore is unacceptable. Similarly, two injections of any insulin daily will fail to replicate normal insulin release patterns. Injection regimens that begin to approximate physiologic insulin release start with "split-mixed" injections of a morning dose of an intermediate acting insulin such as neutral protamine Hagedorn (NPH) and a "bolus" rapid-acting insulin or regular insulin before breakfast, and again before the evening meal. The presumption is made that the morning intermediate-acting insulin gives basal insulin for the day and covers the midday meal, the morning bolus insulin covers breakfast, the evening intermediate-acting insulin gives basal insulin for the rest of the day, and the evening bolus insulin covers the evening meal. If patients are very compulsive about consistency of timing of their injections and meals and intake of carbohydrate, such a strategy may be successful. However, most patients are not sufficiently predictable in their schedule and food intake to allow "tight" glucose control with such an approach.

The first modification that is frequently made to such a regimen is the movement of the evening NPH to bedtime (now three total injections per day) because the fasting glucose in the morning is too high. This approach improves glycemic control and reduces hypoglycemia, sufficiently intensifying the insulin therapy for some patients. However, many patients need a more intense approach that also allows greater flexibility in their lifestyle.

⑨ The basal-bolus concept is an attempt to replicate normal insulin physiology with a combination of intermediate- or long-acting insulin to give the basal component, and rapid-acting insulin to give the bolus component. Various strategies have been used for the former, including once- or twice-daily NPH or detemir, or once-daily insulin glargine. Most type 1 DM patients require two shots of all of the above insulins except insulin glargine. Insulin glargine or insulin detemir is a feasible basal insulin supplement for most patients with type 1 DM. The bolus insulin component is given before meals with regular insulin, insulin lispro, insulin aspart, or insulin glulisine. The rapid onset of action and short time course of rapid-acting insulin analogs more closely replicate normal physiology. This approach allows the patient to vary the amount of insulin injected, depending on the preprandial SMBG level, the anticipated activity (upcoming exercise may reduce insulin requirement), and anticipated carbohydrate intake. Most patients will have a prescribed dose of insulin preprandially that they vary by use of an "adjusted scale insulin" or "correction factor" to normalize a high plasma glucose reading in addition to the amount for the anticipated carbohydrate intake. A starting or empiric "correction factor" can be calculated to provide an approximate plasma glucose lowering (mg/dL) effect of 1 unit of short-acting insulin. Take 1,500 divided by the total daily insulin dose the patient currently uses. For rapid-acting insulins, some experts use 1,700 to 1,800 to account for the rapid reduction in glucose after injection. For example, if a patient is taking 45 units of basal insulin and 10 units of rapid-acting insulin at each of three meals, the total daily insulin dose equals 75 units. 1,500 divided by 75 is 20, thus each unit of insulin will lower the plasma glucose approximately 20 mg/dL. Follow-up SMBG data should be implemented to individualize the correction factor. Carbohydrate counting is a very effective tool for determining the amount of insulin to be injected preprandially. Although general algorithms for carbohydrate counting give rough guidelines, each patient will have to adjust the prescribed preprandial insulin dosage based on their response to different food items. An empiric estimate of how much carbohydrate (grams) 1 unit of rapid-acting insulin will cover is to take 500 divided by the total daily dose of insulin. If we add to the example above with a total daily insulin dose of 75 units, we would take 500 divided by 75, we find that empirically, 1 unit of rapid-acting insulin will cover approximately 7 g of carbohydrate. Follow-up SMBG data should be implemented to individualize this ratio.

In type 1 DM, approximately 50% of insulin replacement should be basal insulin, and the other 50% bolus insulin, split among the meals. If the patient's ratio is not near this recommendation, a reassessment of the regimen should be implemented. Empirically, patients may be begun on ≈0.6 units/kg/ day with basal insulin 50% of total dose and prandial insulin 20% of total dose prebreakfast, 15% prelunch, and 15% presupper. Type 1 DM patients generally require between 0.5 and 1 unit/kg/ day. The need for significantly higher amounts of insulin suggests the presence of insulin antibodies or insulin resistance (coexistent endocrinopathy or type 2 DM).

Obviously, insulin pump therapy (continuous subcutaneous insulin infusion [CSII], generally using a rapid-acting analog insulin) is the most sophisticated form of basal bolus insulin delivery system. CSII may be slightly more efficacious in achieving good glycemic control than multiple-dose insulin injections in a motivated patient. Extensive discussion of this mode of therapy is beyond the scope of this text. Nevertheless, the basic principles for implementation are the same. The one advantage of pump therapy is that the basal insulin dose may be varied, consistent with changes in insulin requirements throughout the day. In selected patients, this feature will allow greater glycemic control with CSII. However, insulin pumps require even greater attention to detail and frequency of SMBG than four injections daily.[78] In appropriately selected patients willing to pay sufficient attention to detail of SMBG and insulin administration, CSII can be a very useful form of therapy. CSII is a tool for diabetes control, and if the patient is not well controlled or unwilling to actively control the diabetes on injections, it is unlikely that the patient will have superior control on a pump.

Intensive therapy (basal bolus) to all adult patients with type 1 DM at the time of diagnosis is recommended to reinforce the importance of glycemic control from the outset rather than change strategies over time after lack of control. Occasional patients with an extended honeymoon period may need less intense therapy initially, but should be converted to basal bolus therapy at the onset of glycemic lability. For patients insisting on two injections daily, intermediate-acting insulin and a rapid-acting insulin or regular insulin (starting at 0.6 units/kg with two-thirds in the morning, two-thirds of the morning dose as intermediate acting insulin, and one-half of evening dose as intermediate-acting insulin) may be sufficient. Regardless of the regimen chosen, gross adjustments in the total insulin dose can be made based on HbA_{1c} measurements and symptoms such as polyuria, polydipsia, and weight gain or loss. Finer insulin adjustments can be determined on the basis of the results of frequent SMBG.

All patients receiving insulin should have extensive education in the recognition and treatment of hypoglycemia. Questioning about the recognition of hypoglycemia is warranted at each patient visit. Documentation of frequency of hypoglycemia, particularly that requiring assistance of another person, visit to an emergent or urgent care facility, or hospitalization, should be recorded. In type 1 DM, the development of hypoglycemia unawareness is common. It may result from progression of disease with autonomic neuropathy. Loss of adrenergic warning signs in such a situation is a relative contraindication to intensive insulin therapy. More commonly, type 1 DM patients have loss of warning signs because of a presumed lower set point for release of counterregulatory hormones as a result of frequent episodes of hypoglycemia ("hypoglycemia begets hypoglycemia"). In such situations, more normal hypoglycemia awareness may be restored by reduction or redistribution of the insulin dose to eliminate significant hypoglycemic episodes. Short-term treatment with theophylline will improve hypoglycemia awareness.[79] Other interventions that may help include coffee consumption or sympathomimetics. These therapies, other than possibly coffee, should not routinely be employed, but may be considered in refractory cases.

Children and pubescent adolescents, glycemic goals should be tempered with the risks of hypoglycemia. Table 83-7 lists glycemic goals for different age groups of type 1 DM patients. Therefore it is not unreasonable to use less intense management (two shots per day, premixed insulins) until the patient is postpubertal, if age specific goals can be maintained.[80]

Occasional patients have antibodies to injected insulin, but the significance of the antibodies is usually minimal. Human insulin therapy has not totally eliminated insulin allergies, although most patients have a local reaction that will dissipate over time. If mild reactions at the site of injection occur, assess the insulin injected. Many times the patient injects cold insulin, which causes vasodilation around the injection site. Anecdotally, a different source could be tried as well (yeast based if on E coli based, and vice versa). If the allergic reaction does not improve or is systemic, insulin desensitization can be carried out.[81] Protocols for desensitization are available from major insulin manufacturers. While more common in the animal insulin era, lipohypertrophy is still seen in some patients with long-standing type 1 DM. Such patients give their insulin injections in the same site to minimize discomfort. Because insulin absorption from an area of lipohypertrophy is unpredictable, avoidance of injections into these areas is mandatory.

Several common errors can occur in the therapy of patients with type 1 DM, causing erratic glucose fluctuations:

- Failure to take into account peaks of insulin action when using a peaking insulin and planning meals and/or activity. Eating should be planned around the peaks of the insulin.

- Random rotation of insulin injection sites. There is sufficient variability of insulin absorption from site to site that this practice alone may cause wide glucose swings. The most consistent absorption of insulin is from the abdominal wall. We try to get our patients to take all their injections in the abdomen. If the patient is unable or unwilling to follow this advice, then systematic site rotation is the next preferable option. The patient always gives the insulin injection in the same region of the body the same time of the day each day. For instance, the arms are always used every morning. Needless to say, the patient should not inject in a limb and then go out and exercise that limb, increasing blood flow and insulin absorption.

- Overinsulinization is a very common problem. The answer to all high blood glucose is not necessarily more insulin, as the patient may be insulinopenic, or may be "rebounding" from a previous low glucose and treating it with excessive amounts of carbohydrate. Fastidious SMBG, particularly during the night (or selected use of continuous glucose monitoring) will help sort this out. Also, practitioners sometimes do not adequately differentiate type 1 DM from type 2 DM when using insulin. Patients with type 1 DM are insulinopenic but have normal insulin sensitivity. Patients with type 2 DM have varying degrees of insulin resistance. Therefore, a 1 unit change in the dose of insulin for a patient with type 1 DM may have a dramatic effect on glucose concentrations, whereas in some patients with type 2 DM 10 to 20 times that amount of insulin may have little effect on glucose. Large changes in insulin dose in patients with type 1 DM are not usually indicated unless the patient's blood glucose control is very poor. Widely erratic SMBG results and/or weight gain often suggest overinsulinization.

- When in doubt, always double check the patient's technique for insulin dosing, insulin injection, and SMBG. Sometimes the simplest of errors results in miserable glycemic control.

Pramlintide in type 1 DM patients who continue to have erratic postprandial control despite implementation of the above strategies may be appropriate. It is imperative at initiation of therapy with pramlintide that each dose of prandial insulin (rapid-acting analog or regular insulin) be reduced by 30% to 50%, or severe hypoglycemic reactions may occur. Pramlintide should be judiciously titrated based on gastrointestinal adverse effects and postprandial glycemic goals. Anecdotally, due to delayed gastric emptying, injecting pramlintide prior to the meal and the rapid acting insulin after the meal may better match the appearance of the food with the postprandial increase in glucose. As pramlintide is not recommended for mixing, you are adding an additional prandial injection at each meal. A patient that is cognizant of the hypoglycemic risk, gastrointestinal side effects, and effective strategies to reduce both issues is needed.

Islet cell and whole pancreas transplantation are occasionally used in patients who require immunosuppressive therapy for other reasons, such as renal transplants.[82] There has been considerable interest in islet cell transplantation since investigators in Edmonton reported success without using glucocorticoids as immunosuppressive agents.[83] Some of these patients are able to stop insulin, though many require insulin secretion support from sulfonylureas or GLP-1 agonists.

Type 2 Diabetes Mellitus

Pharmacotherapy for type 2 DM has changed dramatically in the last few years with the addition of several new drug classes and recommendations to achieve more stringent glycemic control. Symptomatic patients may initially require treatment with insulin or combination oral therapy to reduce glucose toxicity (which may reduce β-cell insulin secretion and worsen insulin resistance). Patients with $HbA_{1c} \approx 7\%$ or less are usually treated with therapeutic lifestyle measures and an agent which will not cause hypoglycemia. Those with $HbA_{1c} > 7\%$ but <8.5% could be initially treated with single oral agents, or low dose combinations. Patients with higher initial HbA_{1c} may benefit from initial therapy with two oral agents, or even insulin.

❿ Depending on patient motivation and adherence to therapeutic lifestyle changes, most patients with HbA_{1c} greater than 9% to 10% will likely require therapy with two or more oral agents to reach glycemic goals. Treatment of type 2 DM often necessitates use of multiple therapeutic agents (combination therapy), to obtain glycemic goals.

The best initial oral therapy for patients with type 2 DM is widely debated. Based on the results of the UKPDS and safety record, obese patients (>120% ideal body weight) without contraindications should be started on metformin titrated to $\approx 2,000$ mg/day.[84] Near-normal weight patients may be better treated

with insulin secretagogues, though metformin will work in this population. Metformin is the only oral antihyperglycemic agent to ever report a reduction in total mortality. Despite this, long-term durability of HbA_{1c} reduction, due to the inability to stop progressive β-cell failure, is suboptimal with metformin, and patients over several years will often need additional therapy. An insulin secretagogue, such as a sulfonylurea, is often added second, though it has clearly been shown that sulfonylureas do not produce durable HbA_{1c} reductions. Better choices to sustain HbA_{1c} reductions would be a TZD or GLP-1 agonist. Goal-oriented therapy is what we should strive for, meaning the intervention should be in relation to the distance from the goal. When initial therapy is no longer keeping the patient at goal, if the HbA_{1c} is close to goal, one additional agent may be appropriate. If >1% to 1.5% above goal, it is unlikely any one oral agent will result in reaching the glycemic goal, and multiple oral agents or insulin therapy may be appropriate. Thiazolidinediones may be substituted in situations in which a patient is intolerant of, or has a contraindication to, metformin as an insulin sensitizer, understanding that thiazolidinediones should be used with caution in heart failure. Figure 83–9 is an algorithm developed by the Texas Diabetes Council for glycemic control. No algorithm can substitute for good clinical judgement, and algorithms for glycemic control start with the premise that the clinician will identify medication contraindications, adverse reactions, and comobidities that may be advantageous or harmful if the medication was taken.

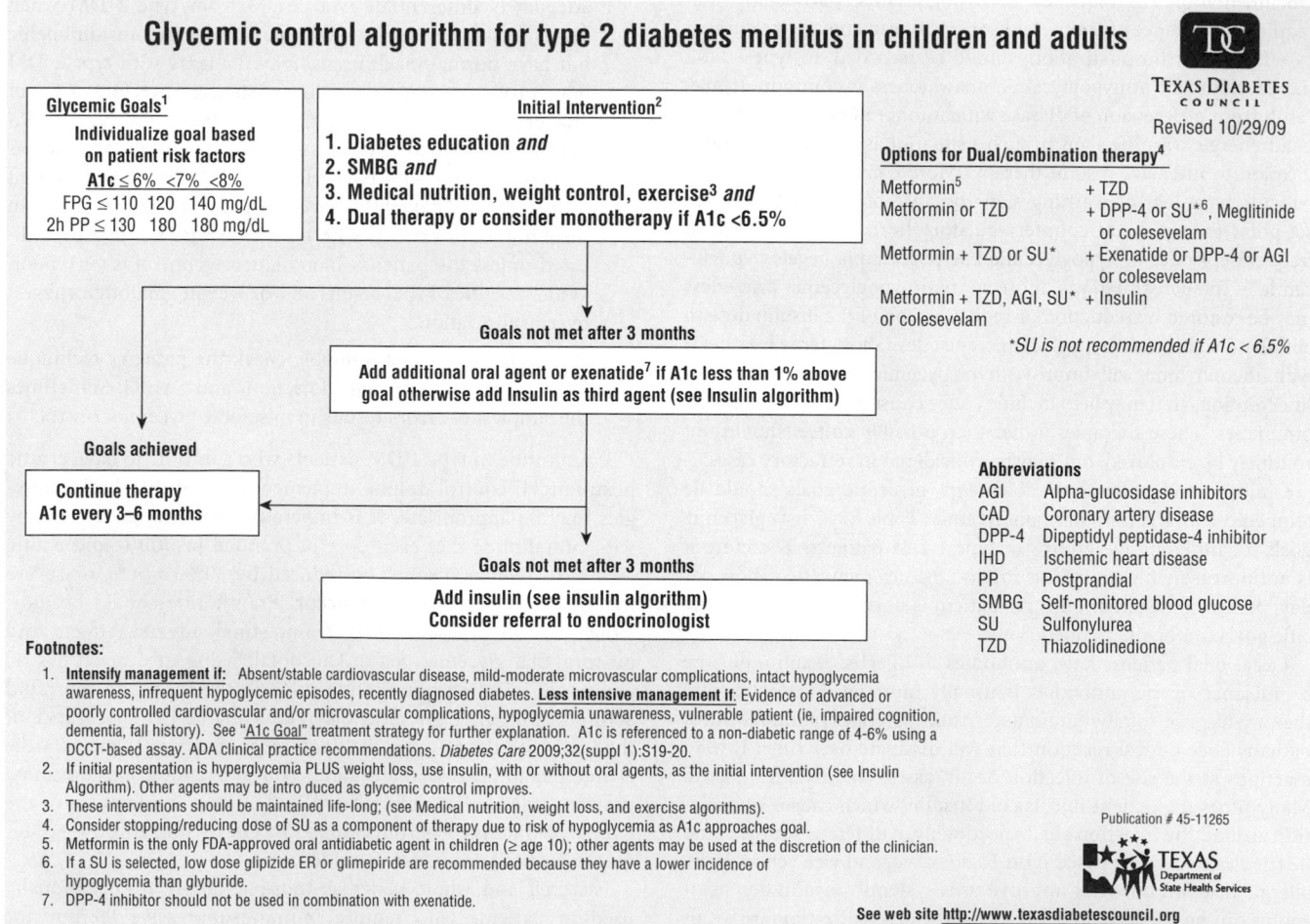

FIGURE 83-9. Glycemic control algorithm for type 2 DM in children and adults. See *www.texasdiabetescouncil.org* for current algorithms. *(Reprinted with permission from the Texas Diabetes Council.)*

We should also treat type 2 DM by matching therapy to the suspected underlying problem. Consider some simple questions to guide therapy: (1) How long has the patient had diabetes? The longer a patient has had diabetes, the more insulinopenic they likely are and the more likely that insulin therapy will be needed; (2) Fasting, postprandial, or both plasma glucose issue? Some drugs address postprandial better, whereas some address FPG better; (3) How far do we have to go to goal and what is the goal? Each oral agent has limits on HbA$_{1c}$ reduction, and the reduction is baseline HbA$_{1c}$ dependent; (4) Adverse effect profile? Contraindications, hypoglycemia potential, and tolerability are based on the current status of the patient; (5) Comorbidities? CVD, dementia, life expectancy, depression, osteoporosis, and other conditions where select medications may be poor choices and additionally those comorbidities may drive our HbA$_{1c}$ goal. Based on the ADVANCE, ACCORD, and VADT trials, a HbA$_{1c}$ goal may now be above 7% if certain comorbidities are present. See Figure 83–10 for HbA$_{1c}$ individualization based on comorbidities from the Texas Diabetes Council. Drugs such as metformin, TZDs, sulfonylureas, repaglinide, liraglutide, intermediate-acting insulins given at bedtime, and basal insulins control fasting plasma glucose more effectively. Exenatide, DPP-4 inhibitors, α-glucosidase inhibitors, nateglinide, and regular and rapid acting insulin better control postprandial glucose excursions. We can also guide therapy based on the risk of hypoglycemia. Metformin, TZDs, liraglutide, exenatide, DPP-4 inhibitors and α-glucosidase inhibitors have a low risk of hypoglycemia. Combining these agents will allow aggressive targeting of near-normal HbA$_{1c}$ levels while minimizing hypoglycemia and weight gain. Combining these agents early in the diagnosis of type 2 DM is logical to potentially realize the micro- and macrovascular reduction seen in the long-term follow-up of UKPDS.

Preserving β-cell function, thus arresting the progressive nature of type 2 DM, could be paradigm changing, but to date medications have only shown to slow, not arrest progression. In the UKPDS, insulin, metformin, or sulfonylureas did not halt β-cell failure. Thiazolidinediones and GLP-1 agonists (open label exenatide has shown durable HbA$_{1c}$ reduction to 3 years and liraglutide to 2 years) may potentially slow β-cell failure.[85,86] It appears unlikely any one drug class will arrest β-cell failure. Combination therapy with TZDs and GLP-1 agonists is logical as TZDs reduce apoptosis of β cells and GLP-1 agonists augment pancreatic function through insulin secretion in a glucose dependent manner and reduction of inappropriate glucagon, but long-term data is lacking. β-cell function is heavily damaged by the time type 2 DM is diagnosed, and it is possible that β-cell failure is inevitable by type 2 DM diagnosis. HbA$_{1c}$ reduction is dependent on baseline values, with higher reductions seen with higher values, but again, therapy should be goal oriented. Triple therapy is often with metformin, a sulfonylurea, and a TZD or DPP-4 inhibitor, but, a good alternative is to use metformin, a TZD, and a GLP-1 agonist, which can lower glucose levels and increase satiety, reducing the weight gain potential of a TZD, and still has a low risk of hypoglycemia. If the HbA$_{1c}$ is >8.5% to 9% on multiple therapies, insulin therapy should be considered. Sulfonylureas are often stopped when insulin is added and insulin sensitizers continued. This may be beneficial to decrease hypoglycemia, but continuing the sulfonylurea is permissible until multiple daily injections are started, at which time it should definitely be discontinued.

Virtually all patients with type 2 DM ultimately become relatively insulinopenic and will require insulin therapy. Insulin therapy for type 2 DM has changed dramatically in the last few years. Specifically, patients are often "transitioned" to insulin by using a bedtime injection of an intermediate- or long-acting insulin, and using oral agents primarily for control during the day.[87,88]

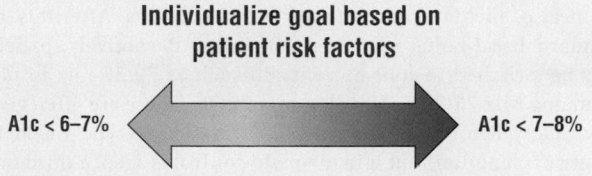

A1c Goals

Individualize goal based on patient risk factors

A1c < 6–7% ⟷ A1c < 7–8%

Intensify management if:
- Absent/stable cardiovascular disease
- Mild-moderate microvascular complications
- Intact hypoglycemia awareness
- Infrequent hypoglycemic episodes
- Recently diagnosed diabetes

Less intensive management if:
- Evidence of advanced or poorly controlled cardiovascular and/or microvascular complications
- Hypoglycemia unawareness
- Vulnerable patient (ie, impaired cognition, dementia, fall history)

A1c is referenced to a non-diabetic range of 4–6% using a DCCT-based assay. ADA clinical practice recommendations. *Diabetes Care* 2009;32(suppl 1):S19–20

See web site http://www.texasdiabetescouncil.org for latest version and disclaimer. Bibliography on back. TEXAS DIABETES COUNCIL

References

1. The action to control cardiovascular risk in diabetes study group. Effects of intensive glucose lowering in type 2 diabetes. N Engl J Med 2008;358:2545–2559.
2. The ADVANCE collaborative group. Intensive blood glucose control and vascular outcomes in patients with type 2 diabetes. N Engl J Med 2008;358:2560–2572.
3. The diabetes control and complications trial research group. The effect of intensive treatment of diabetes on the development and progression of long-term complications in insulin-dependent diabetes mellitus. N Engl J Med 1993;329:977–986.
4. The diabetes control and complications trial/epidemiology of diabetes interventions and complications (DCCT/EDIC) study research group. Intensive diabetes treatment and cardiovascular disease in patients with type 1 diabetes. N Engl J Med 2005;353:2643–2653.
5. Gæde P, Vedel P, Larsen N, Jensen GVH, Parving H-H, Pedersen O. Multifactorial intervention and cardiovascular disease in patients with type 2 diabetes. N Engl J Med 2003;348:383–393.
6. Gæde P, Lund-Anderson H, Parving H-H, Pedersen O. Effect of a multifactorial intervention on mortality in type 2 diabetes. N Engl J Med 2008;358:580–591.
7. Holman RR, Paul SK, Bethel MA, Matthews DR, Neil HAW. 10-Year follow-up of intensive glucose control in type 2 diabetes. N Engl J Med 2008;359:1577–1589.
8. Ohkubo Y, Kishikawa H, Araki E, et al. Intensive insulin therapy prevents the progression of diabetic microvascular complications in Japanese patients with non-insulin-dependent diabetes mellitus: a randomized prospective 6-year study. Diabetes Res Clin Pract 1995;28:103–117.
9. Reichard P, Bengt-Yngve N, Rosenqvist U. The effect of long-term intensified insulin treatment on the development of microvascular complications of diabetes mellitus. N Engl J Med 1993;329:304–309.
10. Shichiri M, Ohkubo Y, Kishikawa H, Wake N. Long term results of the Kumamoto Study on optimal diabetes control in type 2 diabetic patients. Diabetes Care 2000;23:Suppl 2:B21–B29.
11. UK prospective diabetes study (UKPDS) group. Intensive blood-glucose control with sulphonylureas or insulin compared with conventional treatment and risk of complications in patients with type 2 diabetes (UKPDS 33). Lancet 1998;352:837–853.
12. UK prospective diabetes study (UKPDS) group. Effect of intensive blood-glucose control with metformin on complications in overweight patients with type 2 diabetes (UKPDS 34). Lancet 1998;352:854–865.
13. The veterans affairs diabetes trial investigators. Glucose control and vascular complications in veterans with type 2 diabetes. N Engl J Med 2009;360:129–139.

FIGURE 83–10. A1C Goals. See *www.texasdiabetescouncil.org* for current algorithms. *(Reprinted with permission from the Texas Diabetes Council.)*

This strategy leads to less hyperinsulinemia during the day and is associated with less weight gain and has equal efficacy and a lower risk of hypoglycemia for up to 3 years when compared to starting prandial insulin or split-mix twice daily insulin.[89] Because most patients are insulin resistant, insulin sensitizers are commonly used with insulin therapy. Patients with type 2 DM are usually well buffered against hypoglycemia. Patients should be monitored for hypoglycemia by asking about nocturnal sweating, nightmares (both indicative of nocturnal hypoglycemia), palpitations, tremulousness, and neuroglycopenic symptoms, as well as SMBG. When bedtime insulin plus daytime oral medications fail to achieve glycemic goals, a conventional multiple daily dose insulin regimen while continuing the insulin sensitizers is often tried. This may mean adding an injection of bolus insulin with the largest meal of the day for a total of two injections. If this is unsuccessful, a bolus injection can be given with the second largest meal of the day, for a total of three injections. After this, the standard basal-bolus model is followed. Alternatively, patients may be switched to split mix insulin such as 70/30 mix insulin, Humalog Mix 75/25 or Novolog Mix 70/30. These are often given twice daily before the first and third meal (see type 1 DM for longer explanation) but if inadequate control is seen, a third dose of mix insulin may be given with the third meal of the day. This allows for better mealtime coverage, but can also increase the risk of hypoglycemia. Use of exenatide or pramlintide for prandial coverage can be considered. Exenatide should be injected twice daily before meals, whereas pramlintide can be given before each meal. Concerns and problems with insulin administration as addressed in the section on type 1 DM generally relate to the therapy of type 2 DM. However, patients with type 2 DM rarely

have hypoglycemia unawareness. Also, the variability of insulin resistance means that insulin doses may range from 0.7 to 2.5 units/kg or more. Figure 83–11 is an algorithm for insulin therapy options in type 2 diabetes developed by the Texas Diabetes Council. This algorithm gives most options for insulin therapy, but the choice of regimen should be individualized based on the discussion with the patient.

The availability of short-acting insulin secretagogues, rapid-acting insulin analogs, exenatide, DPP-4 inhibitors, and α-glucosidase inhibitors, all of which target postprandial glycemia, has reminded practitioners that glycemic control is a function of fasting and preprandial glycemia and postprandial glycemic excursions.[90] Therefore, postprandial glucose measurements may need more emphasis if the HbA_{1c} is near the glycemic goal. Currently, it remains controversial whether targeting after-meal glucose excursions will have more of an effect on complications risk than

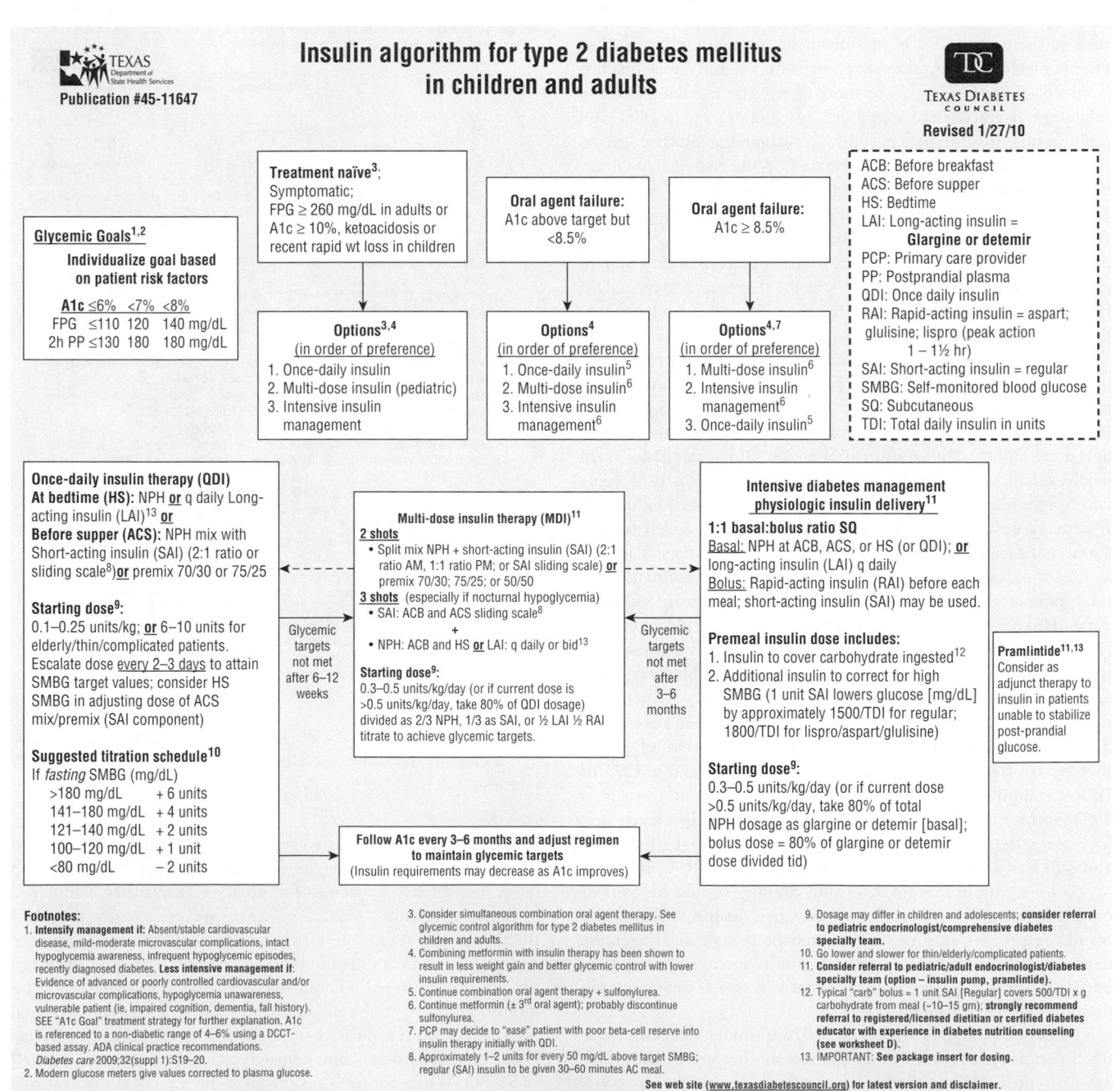

FIGURE 83-11. Insulin algorithm for type 2 DM in children and adults. See *www.texasdiabetescouncil.org* for current algorithms. (*Reprinted with permission from the Texas Diabetes Council.*)

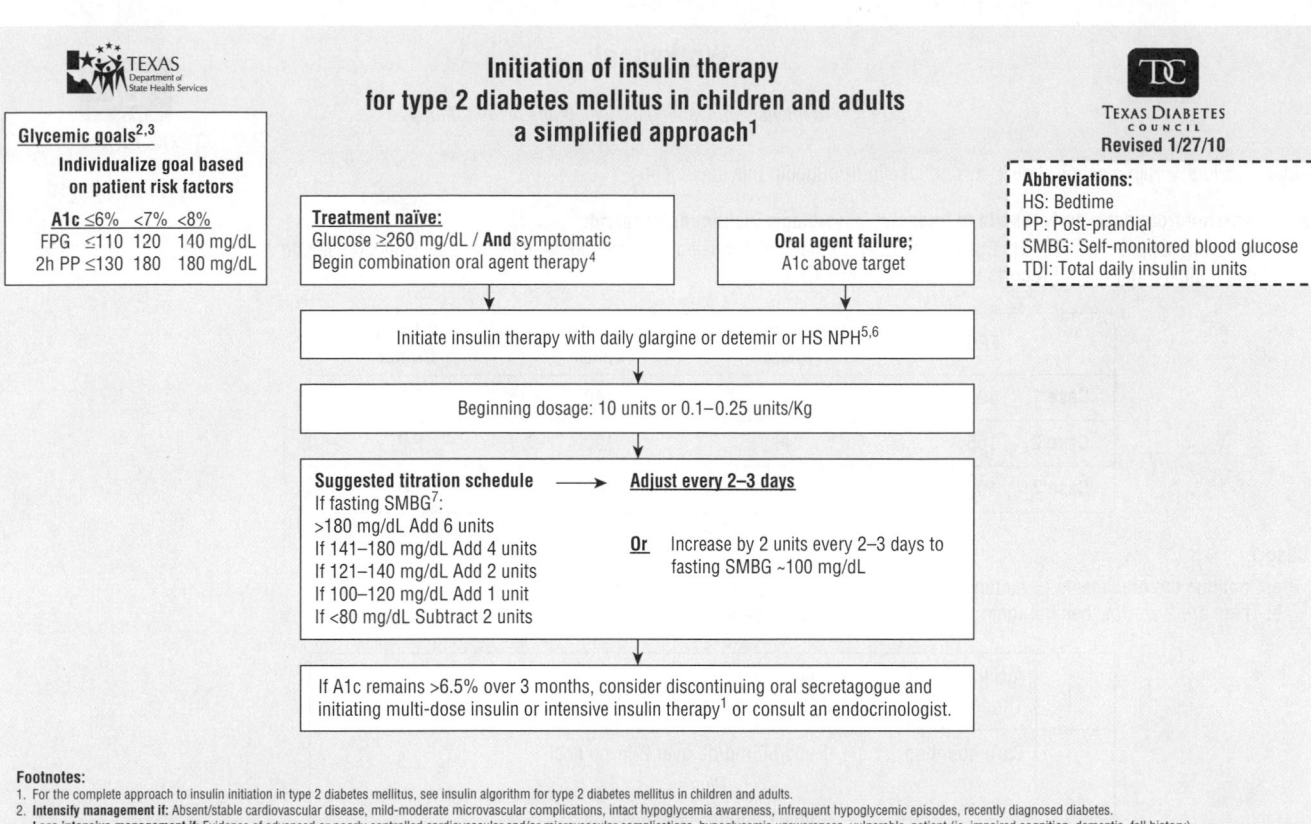

FIGURE 83-11. (continued)

more conventional strategies. Importantly, postprandial excursions proportionally contribute more than the FPG to the HbA_{1c} percentage when the HbA_{1c} nears goals, and thus will need to be targeted for optimal glycemic control in many patients. Most evidence is mostly in epidemiologic studies with post-glucose challenge glucose measurements in diabetes and nondiabetes subjects, not in prospective studies.[91]

■ SPECIAL POPULATIONS

Children and Adolescents with Type 2 DM

Type 2 DM is increasing in adolescence.[10] Obesity and physical inactivity seem to be particular culprits in the pathogenesis of this disease. Given the many years that the patient will have to live with diabetes, and recent evidence that the timeline for complications may mimic that of older adults, extraordinary efforts should be expended on lifestyle modification measures in an attempt to normalize glucose levels. Failing that strategy, the only labeled oral agent for use in children (10–16 years of age) is metformin, though sulfonylureas are also commonly used in therapy. Thiazolidinediones have not been studied in children, but studies to ascertain safety and efficacy are currently under way. Exenatide, as it potentially helps the child to lose weight, is also increasing, but the long-term effects of this therapeutic modality are unknown. Exenatide has been submitted to the FDA for approval in children. In adolescent females, the possibility of future pregnancy should be considered in the prescription of any drug regimen.

Elderly Patients with DM

Elderly patients with newly diagnosed DM (almost always type 2 DM) present a different therapeutic challenge. Consideration of the risks of hypoglycemia in this population and the probable life span should help determine if less stringent glycemic goals should be set. Thinner, older patients may primarily be treated with shorter-acting insulin secretagogues, low-dose sulfonylureas (preferably not long-acting ones), DPP-4 inhibitors, or α-glucosidase inhibitors. The risk for lactic acidosis, which increases with older age and the age-related decline in renal function, makes metformin therapy more problematic. In a patient whom weight gain or loss may not be unwelcome, thiazolidinediones or exenatide, respectively, may be considered, but falls risk and fracture risk must be considered with TZDs. DPP-4 inhibitors or α-glucosidase inhibitors may be advantageous due to low risk of hypoglycemia. Simple insulin regimens such as an injection of basal insulin daily may be appropriate for glycemic control in elderly patients with newly diagnosed DM.

Gestational DM and Pregnancy with Preexisting Diabetes

Gestational DM is diagnosed as previously described. Dietary therapy to minimize wide fluctuations in blood glucose is of paramount importance.[8,12] Intensive educational efforts are usually necessary. Pregnant women without DM maintain plasma glucose concentrations between 50 and 130 mg/dL. Frequent SMBG is needed to tell whether dietary interventions are successful. If

Worksheet

Advancing to intensive/physiologic basal: bolus insulin therapy

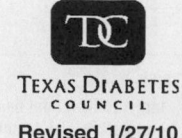

TEXAS DIABETES
COUNCIL
Revised 1/27/10

Note: "Analog" = Rapid acting (bolus) analog insulin throughout this document.

A. Conversion from once-daily insulin to intensive/physiologic insulin replacement:

Oral therapy failure: once-daily glargine was added to the oral regimen and titrated to 30 units per day. How do you add analog insulin if the patient reports the following SMBG values?

	FPG	2-hr pp Brkfst	2-hr pp Lunch	2-hr pp Dinner
Case 1	105	140	140	240
Case 2	105	140	190	240
Case 3	105	190	240	240

Case 1

a. Continue the oral agents (± sulfonylurea) and 30 units glargine or detemir (or NPH)
b. There are 2 approaches for adding analog (RAI) 10–15 minutes before a meal:

#1	Arbitrary start:	5 units
	Titrate:	Add 2 units every 2 days to reach 2-hr pp goal
#2	Carb-counting	1 unit/50 mg/dL over 2-hr pp goal
		Plus
		1 unit/15 grams carbohydrate
	Titrate:	Add 1 unit/50 mg/dL >2-hr pp goal every 2 days

Cases 2 and 3

As above, but add and titrate analog before each meal where the postprandial glucose is above goal. Also, <u>see part D, below</u> for more information on how to optimize the use of analog insulin. Re-evaluate each week to be certain that about half of the total daily dose is basal and half is bolus insulin.

B. Conversion from once-daily premix to intensive/physiologic insulin replacement:

Oral therapy failure: once-daily 70/30 premixed insulin was added and titrated to 30 units per day. The fasting glucose is at goal, but daytime control is poor. How do you convert to physiologic insulin therapy?

a. **Basal insulin dose:** The first step in the conversion is based on the total dose of intermediate-acting insulin. In this case, the person is taking 21 units of NPH or aspart-protamine insulin (70% x 30 units = 21 units). So, give 21 units basal glargine (use "unit-for-unit" conversion for once-daily intermediate regimens.) *Remember, do not stop oral agents (+ sulfonylurea) at this time.*

b. **Bolus insulin dose:** There are several ways to start the analog.
i. *See Case 1, page 2 (Arbitrary start or Carb-counting)*
ii. Begin with the previous dose of fast-acting insulin, divide it before meals and titrate every 2 days. In this case, the person was using 30 units of 70/30 or about 9 units of fast-acting insulin (30% x 30 units = 9 units). So give 3 units of analog before each meal and titrate every 2 days as per Case 1.

FIGURE 83-11. *(continued)*

fasting plasma glucose is >105 mg/dL, or 1-hour postprandial plasma glucose levels are >155 mg/dL, or if 2-hour postprandial plasma glucose levels are >130 mg/dL, insulin therapy is usually begun, but more aggressive use of medication is sometimes used by some clinicians. Goals during therapy are a preprandial goal of ≤95 mg/dL, and either a 1-hour postprandial plasma glucose levels ≤140 mg/dL, or 2-hour postprandial plasma glucose levels ≤120 mg/dL, and avoidance of ketones as much as possible. In patients who have preexisting type 1 or type 2 diabetes and become pregnant, premeal, bedtime, and overnight glucose should be 60 to 99mg/dL, with a peak postprandial of 100 to 129mg/dL. HbA₁c during pregnancy should be less than 6%. Titration of insulin and switching to more complicated regimens is guided by SMBG results. Use of basal insulins other than NPH is still debated, but with the ease of use of detemir or glargine insulin, their use in gestational DM will likely increase. In addition, pump therapy for the duration of the pregnancy is often instituted, as it can obtain excellent glycemic control and is quickly adjustable. Despite the

long-standing labeling of sulfonylureas as contraindicated in pregnancy, one randomized, open-label, controlled trial evaluated the efficacy of glyburide as compared to insulin initiated after 11 weeks' gestation.[92] Adequate control of blood glucose was achieved as compared to traditional insulin therapy, with less hypoglycemia in the glyburide group. No evidence of any difference in complications, specifically cord-serum insulin concentrations, incidence of macrosomia (birth weight ≥4,000 g), cesarean delivery, or neonatal hypoglycemia between regimens were noted. Glyburide was not detected in the cord serum of any infant. As the study limited enrollment beyond 11 weeks' gestation, no conclusions regarding teratogenicity can be made from this study. The ADA cites this study in a position paper and mentions its utility, but also warns that it is not a labeled use of the drug and suggests further studies are needed to establish its safety.[12] In addition, metformin has been studied in the treatment of GDM. Metformin crosses the placenta, but did not increase any complications associated with GDM when compared with insulin therapy, and patients

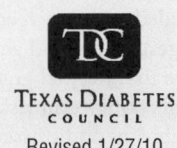

Revised 1/27/10

C. Conversion from twice-daily premix to intensive/physiologic insulin replacement:

Oral therapy failure in an 80 kg person: 70/30 premixed insulin was started and advanced to 60 units per day: 40 units before breakfast and 20 units before dinner. The fasting glucose was at goal, but wide glycemic excursions occurred at other times during the day and night. How do you convert this person to physiologic insulin therapy? There are several approaches. Use which ever method you want.

a. Start over and begin insulin at 0.5 units/kg. Give half as basal insulin and half as analog, divided before meals. In this case, the starting dose would be 40 units per day. Start giving 20 units glargine each morning and about 7 units analog before each meal. Titrate the basal and bolus insulins every 2 days to fasting and 2-hr postprandial goals.

b. Conversion based on current insulin usage:

Basal dose: The first step in the conversion is based on the 80% of the total dose of intermediate-acting insulin. In this case, the person is taking 42 units of NPH or aspart-protamine insulin (70% x 60 units = 42 units). When a person is taking multiple doses of intermediate-acting insulin, we give only 80% as glargine. So, give 34 units basal glargine (80% x 42 = ~34). Remember, *do not stop oral agents (+ sulfonylurea) at this time.*

Bolus insulin dose: There are several ways to start the analog.

i. *See Case 1, page 3 (Arbitrary start or Carb-counting)*

ii. Begin with the previous dose of fast-acting insulin, divide it before meals and titrate every 2 days. In this case, the person was using 60 units of 70/30 or 18 units of fast-acting insulin (30% x 60 units = 18 units). So, give 6 units of analog before each meal and titrate every 2 days as per Case 1.

c. **The "80%-80%"rule":** Similar to the above method, but yields an ideal ratio of basal:bolus insulin in one step. The dose of basal glargine will be 80% of the total intermediate insulin, and the analog will be 80% of the glargine dose, divided before meals.

    Basal dose: = 80% of total intermediate insulin

                = 80% x 42 units (70% x 60 = 42)

                = 34 units glargine

    Analog dose: = 80% of the glargine dose, divided TID

                = 80% x 34 units = 27 units

                = 27 units, divided tid = 9 units

                = 9 units aspart, glulisine or lispro before meals

Note: Total dose of insulin is conserved and an ideal ratio between basal and bolus will always result with the "80%–80%" method.

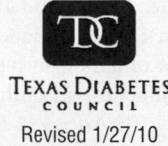

Revised 1/27/10

D. Optimizing analog insulin use

Tight control of blood glucose requires that the patient participates in the management of their diabetes. This includes monitoring their blood glucose and learning to count carbohydrates or "carb count." The following material explains how to calculate the dose of analog required to cover a meal and how to add extra analog to correct a hyperglycemic event.

a. Determining the dose of analog insulin to use before a meal

The "Rule of 500" is used to determine how many grams of carbohydrate 1 unit of analog insulin will cover. When this number is known, then the person can easily give the correct dose of analog by simply counting the grams of carbohydrate they intend to eat at the meal.

Specifically, 500 divided by the total daily insulin dose (500/TDI) yields the number of grams of carbohydrate that 1 unit of analog will cover. For example, if a person has established that they require about 50 units of insulin per day, then it follows that 1 unit of analog will cover 10 grams of carbohydrate (500/50 = 10). If the person carb counts 140 grams in the dinner meal, then the dose of analog will be 14 units given 10 minutes before eating.

b. Correcting for hyperglycemia

The "Rule of 1800" is used to determine how much insulin to use to bring a high glucose reading back to goal. Even with tight control, hyperglycemia occurs and people need to be able to correct this situation.

Specifically, 1800 divided by the total daily insulin dose yields a value indicating how much 1 unit of analog insulin will lower the blood glucose. Thus, if a person uses 90 units of insulin per day, then 1 unit of analog will reduce the blood glucose by 20 mg/dL (1800/90 = 20). *This augment dose of insulin can be used by itself to correct hyperglycemia, or added to the bolus dose if glucose is high before a meal.*

FIGURE 83-11. *(continued)*

preferred it overwhelmingly to insulin therapy. Further study is needed prior to recommending metformin in GDM. Patients with gestational DM should be evaluated 6 weeks after delivery to ensure that normal glucose tolerance has returned. Because these patients' long-term risk for the development of type 2 DM is considerable, periodic assessment after that is warranted.

■ SPECIAL SITUATIONS

Sick Days

Acute self-limited illness rarely presents a major problem for patients with type 2 DM, but can be a significant challenge for insulinopenic type 1 DM patients.[93] While caloric intake generally declines, insulin sensitivity also decreases, meaning that it may take greater amounts of insulin to control blood glucose concentrations. Patients need to be adept at frequent SMBG, checking urine ketones, use of short-acting insulin, and understanding that sugar intake in this situation is not "bad" but may be necessary to balance the glucose levels when extra insulin is needed during illness. We encourage patients to continue their usual insulin regimen and to use supplemental rapid-acting insulin based on SMBG results, with further additional insulin given if ketonuria develops. Sugar and electrolyte solutions, such as sports drinks, can be used to maintain hydration, to provide needed electrolytes if there are significant gastrointestinal or urinary losses, and to provide sugar to keep the patient from developing hypoglycemia because of the extra insulin that is usually needed. In contrast, type 2 patients may need to switch to sugar-free drinks if blood glucose levels are continually elevated. Most patients can be taught how to sufficiently manage sick days and avoid hospitalization.

Diabetic Ketoacidosis and Hyperosmolar Hyperglycemic State

Diabetic ketoacidosis and hyperosmolar hyperglycemic state are true diabetic emergencies.[94] A comprehensive discussion of their treatment is beyond the scope of this chapter. In patients with known diabetes, diabetic ketoacidosis is usually precipitated by insulin omission in type 1 DM, and intercurrent illness, particularly infection, in both type 1 and type 2 DM. However, patients with type 1 or type 2 DM (the latter being usually non-whites or Hispanics) may present at initial presentation. It is possible that some of the patients deemed to have type 2 DM actually have type 1 idiopathic DM. Patients with diabetic ketoacidosis may be alert, stuporous, or comatose at presentation. The hallmark diagnostic laboratory values include hyperglycemia, anion gap acidosis, and large ketonemia or ketonuria. Afflicted patients have fluid deficits of several liters and sodium and potassium deficits of several hundred milliequivalents. Restoration of intravascular volume acutely with normal saline, followed by hypotonic saline to replace free water, potassium supplements, and constant infusion insulin restore the patient's metabolic status relatively quickly. A flow sheet is often helpful in tracking the fluid and insulin therapies and laboratory parameters in these patients. Bicarbonate administration is generally not needed and may be harmful, especially in children. Treatment of the inciting medical condition is also vital. Hourly bedside monitoring of glucose and frequent monitoring (every 2–4 hours) of potassium is essential. Metabolic improvement is manifested by an increase in the serum bicarbonate or pH. Serum phosphorus usually starts high and plummets to lower-than-normal levels, though replacing phosphorus, while not unreasonable, is of questionable benefit in most patients. Fluid administration alone will reduce the glucose concentration, so a decrement in glucose values does not necessarily mean that the

patient's metabolic status is improving. Rare patients will require larger amounts of insulin than those usually given (5–10 units/h). We double the patient's insulin dose if the serum bicarbonate has not improved after the first 4 hours of insulin therapy. Constant infusion of a fixed dose of insulin and the administration of intravenous glucose when the blood glucose level decreases to <250 mg/dL is preferable to titration of the insulin infusion based on the glucose level. The latter strategy may delay clearance of the ketosis and prolong treatment. The insulin infusion should be continued until the urine ketones clear and the anion gap closes. Long-acting insulin should be given 1 to 3 hours prior to discontinuing the insulin infusion. Intramuscular regular insulin or subcutaneous insulin lispro or aspart given every 1 to 2 hours can be utilized rather than an insulin infusion in patients without hypoperfusion. Patients may develop hyperchloremic metabolic acidosis with treatment if they have been given large volumes of normal saline in the course of their treatment. Such a situation does not require any specific treatment.

Hyperosmolar hyperglycemic state usually occurs in older patients with type 2 DM, at times undiagnosed, or in younger patients with prolonged hyperglycemia and dehydration or significant renal insufficiency. Large ketonemia is usually not seen, as residual insulin secretion suppresses the production of ketones. Infection or another medical illness is the usual precipitant. Fluid deficits are usually greater and blood glucose concentrations higher (at times >1,000 mg/dL) in these patients than in patients with diabetic ketoacidosis. Blood glucose levels should be lowered very gradually with hypotonic fluids and low-dose insulin infusions (1–2 units/h). Rapid correction of the glucose levels, a drop greater than 75 to 100 mg/dL/h, is not recommended, as it can result in cerebral edema. This is especially true for children with diabetic ketoacidosis. Mortality is high with the hyperosmolar hyperglycemic state.

Hospitalization for Intercurrent Medical Illness

Patients on oral agents may need transient therapy with insulin to achieve adequate glycemic control. In patients requiring insulin, patients should receive scheduled doses of insulin with additional short-acting insulin. "Sliding-scale" insulin is to be discouraged, as it is notorious for not controlling glucose and for sometimes resulting in therapeutic misadventures, with wide swings in the blood glucose as the patient "bounces" from hypoglycemia to hyperglycemia.[95] In-hospital mortality is increased in many hyperglycemic conditions. At least one study documented a reduction in mortality in type 2 diabetes patients with acute MIs[96] who receive constant intravenous insulin during the acute phase of the event to maintain near-normal glucose concentrations. Similar mortality results have been documented in some intensive care unit settings using intravenous insulin and tight glucose control.[96,97] The American Diabetes Association and American Association of Clinical Endocrinologists released a joint consensus statement on inpatient glycemic control stating that glucose control measures should be implemented if the blood glucose is ≥180 mg/dL, and maintained between 140 and 180 mg/dL.[98] The Normoglycemia in Intensive Care Evaluation-Survival Using Glucose Algorithm Regulation trial, and several other negative trials, have resulted in this loosening of inpatient glycemic goals. Critically ill patients had a higher 90-day mortality when a goal of 81 to 108 mg/dL was targeted than when a blood glucose of ≤180 mg/dL (achieved 144 mg/dL) was targeted.[99] Many protocols for IV insulin infusion are currently available, and implementation for an inpatient setting should use a well-established protocol. It is prudent to stop metformin in all patients who arrive in acute care settings until full elucidation of the reason for presentation can be ascertained, as contraindications to metformin are prevalent in hospitalized patients.

Perioperative Management

Surgical patients may experience worsening of glycemia for reasons similar to those listed above for intercurrent medical illness.[100] Patients on oral agents may need transient therapy with insulin to control blood glucose. In patients requiring insulin, scheduled doses of insulin or continuous insulin infusions are preferred. For patients who can eat soon after surgery, the time-honored approach of giving one-half of the usual morning NPH insulin dose with dextrose 5% in water intravenously is acceptable, with resumption of scheduled insulin, perhaps at reduced doses, within the first day. For patients requiring more prolonged periods without oral nutrition and for major surgery, such as coronary artery bypass grafting and major abdominal surgery, constant infusion intravenous insulin is preferred. Use of intravenous insulin infusion has been shown to reduce deep sternal wound infections in patients after coronary artery bypass grafting, though there is no need to start the infusion during or before the procedure. Metformin should be discontinued temporarily after any major surgery until it is clear that the patient is hemodynamically stable and normal renal function is documented.

Reproductive-Age Women and Preconception Care for Women

An increasing prevalence of DM has been noted in reproductive-age women.[101,102] Prepregnancy planning is absolutely mandatory, as organogenesis is largely completed within 8 weeks, so good glycemic control should be obtained prior to conception. Unfortunately, major congenital malformations due to poor glucose control remain the leading cause of mortality and serious morbidity in infants of mothers with type 1 or type 2 diabetes. For women with diabetes mellitus controlled by lifestyle measures alone, conversion to insulin as soon as the pregnancy is confirmed is appropriate. For women with polycystic ovary disease who ovulate and become pregnant with insulin-sensitizer therapy such as metformin, conversion to insulin is recommended as soon as pregnancy is confirmed, but whether to continue the insulin sensitizer is a controversial topic. For example, in polycystic ovary disease insulin sensitizers are often needed to become pregnant, so some clinicians feel they should be continued. In Europe, metformin is sometimes used in pregnancy for type 2 DM, but the use is much lower in the United States. Metformin can cross the placenta, but this does not necessarily mean harm to the fetus. Patients previously treated with insulin may need intensification of their regimen to achieve therapeutic goals. Normal pregnancy is associated with a decrease in the blood glucose concentration as fuel is diverted to the fetus. Pregnant patients will be ingesting both meals and snacks daily. SMBG is generally intensified to try to reach glycemic targets and reduce fetal and maternal morbidity. Whether preprandial or postprandial glucose concentrations should be the target of therapy is hotly debated. Ketosis should be avoided, requiring urine monitoring for ketones in the morning and if the blood sugar is >200 mg/dL.

There has been some concern about the safety of insulin analogs in pregnancy, both for fetal development and advancement of microvascular complications. One study has shown no increase in retinopathy or progression of same with the use of insulin lispro in pregnancy.

■ SPECIAL TOPICS

Prevention of Diabetes Mellitus

⑫ Efforts to prevent type 1 DM with immunosuppressives,[103] niacinamide, injected insulin,[104] or oral insulin therapy[105] have been unsuccessful. The Diabetes Prevention Program[106] confirmed that modest weight loss in association with exercise can have a dramatic impact on insulin sensitivity and the conversion from impaired

glucose tolerance to type 2 diabetes. In this study approximately 2,000 individuals with impaired glucose tolerance were randomized to lifestyle changes (diet, exercise, and weight loss) versus usual care. The study, which was originally planned to be ongoing for 5 years, was stopped after 2.8 years because the results were so conclusive. The usual care group developed diabetes at the rate of 11% each year. The lifestyle arm developed diabetes at a rate of 5% per year, a 58% reduction in the risk of developing diabetes.[106] Surprisingly, a modest amount of diet and exercise yielded impressive results. The exercise program in the lifestyle group was walking 30 minutes 5 days each week. The mean weight loss over the 2.8-year study period was only 8 pounds. Similar results were seen in the Finnish Diabetes Study.[107] In the Diabetes Prevention Program[106] discussed above, approximately 1,000 of the study patients were randomized to metformin therapy. Metformin therapy reduced the risk of developing type 2 DM by 31% compared to usual care and resulted in a 4-pound weight loss.[106] Interestingly, young and overweight individuals on metformin had a greater reduction in the risk of developing diabetes than normal weight and older study patients.[106]

Metformin and acarbose[64] appear to mostly be treating early diabetes, because when the drugs were stopped, diabetes rates were close to the conversion rates for placebo. In contrast, the TRIPOD study[108] evaluated the ability of troglitazone to prevent the development of diabetes in women with a history of gestational diabetes. The rate of development of diabetes in the placebo arm of the study was approximately 12% per year, compared with about 5% in the treatment group. Total preservation of β-cell function was demonstrated over a 5-year period in women who had near-normal β-cell function at baseline and who initially responded to the drug.[108] The preservation of β-cell function was observed for at least 8 months after the drug had been discontinued. The DREAM trial evaluated rosiglitazone and/or ramipril treatment for the delay or prevention of type 2 DM in impaired glucose tolerant subjects.[109,110] Rosiglitazone 8 mg daily, over approximately 3 years, reduced the incidence of type 2 diabetes by 60%. In addition, a 37% nonsignificant increase in cardiovascular events was reported. Ramipril 15 mg daily did not significantly prevent the conversion to diabetes. It is possible that longer exposure could have made a difference, but the study was stopped prematurely. In contrast, valsartan, and angiotensin-receptor blocker (ARB), administered for 5 years was recently reported to reduce the risk of progression from impaired glucose tolerance to type 2 DM by 14%. The ACT Now trial used pioglitazone 45 mg daily in an IGT population and found an 81% reduction in the risk of development of diabetes over 3 years. It should be noted that no pharmacologic agents are currently FDA approved or recommended for prevention of type 2 diabetes, although the ADA recommends metformin in conjuction with lifestyle changes if the patient is younger, obese, has a family history of diabetes, dyslipidemia, hypertension, or a HbA$_{1c}$ >6%.[111] The next step is discussions with the FDA to decide how and if medications to prevent diabetes can be approved for this indication.

CLINICAL CONTROVERSY

Diabetes mellitus is associated with a substantially higher risk of morbidity and mortality. Pharmacologic prevention or delay of type 2 DM has been widely discussed since the release of the Diabetes Prevention Program results. Though lifestyle changes were effective, with a 58% lower relative risk of progression to diabetes, metformin 850 mg twice a day reduced the risk by 31%, and was essentially as effective as diet and exercise in young/obese subjects. Pioglitazone, rosiglitazone, acarbose, and even orlistat all have, to one extent or another, been able to delay the onset of type 2 DM. Despite these data, there are no FDA-approved drugs for the delay or prevention of diabetes. The ADA-recommended medications, in conjuction with lifestyle, for the delay or prevention of type 2 DM include metformin. It should be remembered that medications require monitoring and can have serious side effects. Many feel they are simply treating diabetes early, as there is considerable β-cell dysfunction documented in early impaired glucose tolerant subjects. Other than troglitazone, which is not on the market, no medication has clearly shown β-cell preservation. It is logical to try to use medications if they alter the decline of β-cell function, but this is currently off-label use and any attempt to use medication in these situations should be clearly and frankly discussed with the patient.

Patient Education

⓭ It is not satisfactory to give patients with DM brief instructions with a few pamphlets and expect them to manage their disease adequately.[112] Thinking that diabetes education is limited to one or two encounters is misguided; education is a lifetime exercise. Successful treatment of DM involves lifestyle changes for the patient (e.g., medical nutrition therapy, physical activity, self-monitoring of blood glucose and possibly of urine for ketones, recognition of hyper- and hypoglycemia, and taking prescribed medications). The American Association of Diabetes Educators (AADE) has developed the AADE7 self-care behaviors of healthy eating, being active, monitoring, taking medication, problem solving, reducing risk, and healthy coping, which is a good starting framework for patient discussions. The patient must be involved in the decision-making process and must learn as much about the disease and associated complications as possible. Emphasis should be placed on the evidence that indicates that complications can be prevented or minimized with glycemic control and management of risk factors for cardiovascular disease. Recognition of the need for proper patient education to empower them into self-care has generated programs for certification in diabetes education for pharmacists. Certified diabetes educators (CDEs) must document their patient education hours and sit for a certification examination that assesses the knowledge, tasks, and skills of an educator in order to become certified. An increasing number of nurses, pharmacists, dietitians, and physicians are becoming CDEs to document to the public that they meet a minimum standard for diabetes education, and to fulfill quality initiatives in meeting guidelines for education recognition. Being a CDE does not guarantee reimbursement of services, and CDEs who are not dietitians will often need to become part of a recognized program to obtain reimbursement. Currently the AADE and ADA have accreditation programs. **⓮**

■ TREATMENT OF CONCOMITANT CONDITIONS AND COMPLICATIONS

Retinopathy

Patients with established retinopathy should see an ophthalmologist or optometrist trained in diabetic eye disease. A dilated eye exam is required to fully evaluate diabetic eye disease. Early background retinopathy may reverse with improved glycemic control. More advanced retinopathy will not regress with improved glycemia, and may actually worsen with short-term improvements in glyce-

mia. Studies are under way to determine whether medical therapy independent of glucose control will prevent the development of advanced retinopathy. Laser photocoagulation has markedly improved sight preservation in diabetic patients.

Neuropathy

Peripheral neuropathy is the most common complication seen in type 2 DM patients in outpatient clinics.[113] Paresthesias, numbness, or pain may be the predominant symptom. The feet are involved far more often than the hands. Improved glycemic control may alleviate some of the symptoms. If neuropathy is painful, symptomatic therapy is empiric, including low-dose tricyclic antidepressants, anticonvulsants (gabapentin, pregabalin, carbamazepine, and maybe phenytoin), duloxetine, venlafaxine, topical capsaicin, and various pain medications, including tramadol and nonsteroidal antiinflammatory drugs. Recently, another anticonvulsant, topiramate, has shown promise in the reduction of symptoms, with the positive side effect of weight loss in type 2 diabetes patients, though tolerability is problematic. The numb variant of peripheral neuropathy is not treated with medication. Clinical manifestations of diabetic autonomic neuropathy include resting tachycardia, exercise intolerance, orthostatic hypotension, constipation, gastroparesis, erectile dysfunction, sudomotor dysfunction (anhidrosis, heat intolerance, gustatory sweating, and/or dry skin), impaired neurovascular function, and hypoglycemic autonomic failure. Gastroparesis can be a severe and debilitating complication of DM. Improved glycemic control, discontinuation of medications that slow gastric motility, and the use of metoclopramide (preferably for only a few weeks at a time) or erythromycin may be helpful. Gastric pacemakers as therapeutic hardware are rarely used, though available, and cisapride, removed from the market several years ago, is still available for compassionate use. Orthostatic hypotension may require pharmacologic management with mineralocorticoids or adrenergic agonist agents. In severe cases, supine hypertension is extreme, mandating that the patient sleep in a sitting or semirecumbent position. Patients with cardiac autonomic neuropathy are at a higher risk for silent MI and mortality. The hallmark of diabetic diarrhea is its nocturnal occurrence. Diabetic diarrhea frequently responds to a 10- to 14-day course of an antibiotic such as doxycycline or metronidazole. In more unresponsive cases, octreotide may be useful. Erectile dysfunction is common in diabetes, and initial treatment should include a trial of one of the oral medications currently available to treat erectile dysfunction. People with diabetes often require the highest doses of these medications to have an adequate response. Sudomotor dysfunction, as earlier defined, results in loss of sweating and resultant dry, cracked skin. Use of hydrating creams and ointments is needed.

Microalbuminuria and Nephropathy

Diabetes mellitus, particularly type 2 DM, is the biggest contributor statistically to the development of endstage renal disease in the United States.[114] The American Diabetes Association recommends a screening urinary analysis for albumin at diagnosis in persons with type 2 DM. Precise onset of type 2 DM can rarely be ascertained, and patients will often present at diagnosis with microvascular complications. In type 1 DM, microalbuminuria rarely occurs with short duration of disease or before puberty. Screening individuals with type 1 DM should begin with puberty and after 5 years' disease duration. There are three methods for assessing microalbuminuria: (1) measurement of the urine albumin:creatinine ratio in a random spot collection (preferably the first morning void); (2) 24-hour timed collection; and (3) timed (e.g., 4- or 10-hour overnight) collection. Microalbuminuria on a spot urine specimen is defined as a ratio of 30 to 300 mg/g albumin:creatinine. On timed collections, microalbuminuria is defined as 30 to 300 mg/24 hours or an albumin excretion rate of 20 to 200 mcg/min. Because of day-to-day variability, microalbuminuria should be confirmed on at least two of three samples over 3 to 6 months. Additionally, when assessing urine protein or albumin, conditions that may cause transient elevations in urinary albumin excretion should be excluded. These conditions include intense exercise, recent urinary tract infections, hypertension, short-term hyperglycemia, heart failure, and acute febrile illness.[114]

In type 2 DM, the presence of microalbuminuria is a strong risk factor for macrovascular disease and is frequently present at the time of diagnosis. Microalbuminuria is a weaker predictor for future kidney disease in type 2 versus type 1 DM.

Glucose and blood pressure control are most important for the prevention of nephropathy, and blood pressure control is the most important for retarding the progression of established nephropathy. ACE inhibitors and ARBs, considered first-line recommended treatment modalities, have shown efficacy in preventing the clinical progression of renal disease in patients with type 2 DM.[115-117] Diuretics frequently are necessary due to the volume-expanded state of the patient and are recommended second-line therapy. The American Diabetes Association and the National Kidney Foundation blood pressure goal of <130/80 mm Hg can be difficult to achieve. Three or more antihypertensives are often needed to treat to goal blood pressures.

Peripheral Vascular Disease and Foot Ulcers

Claudication and nonhealing foot ulcers are common in type 2 DM patients.[118] Smoking cessation, correction of lipid abnormalities, and antiplatelet therapy are important strategies in treating claudicants. Cilostazol may be useful for reducing intermittant claudication symptoms in select patients. Revascularization is successful in selected patients, though small vessel disease that cannot be bypassed is common in diabetes. Local débridement and appropriate footwear and foot care are vitally important in the early treatment of foot lesions. In more advanced lesions, topical treatments may be of benefit. Diabetic foot care is an excellent example of the adage, "an ounce of prevention is worth a pound of cure."

Coronary Heart Disease

⑪ The risk for coronary heart disease (CHD) is 2 to 4 times greater in diabetic patients than in nondiabetic individuals. CHD is the major source of mortality in patients with DM. Recent studies suggest that multiple risk factor intervention (lipids, hypertension, smoking cessation, and antiplatelet therapy)[8] will reduce the burden of excess macrovascular events. The ADA recommends aspirin therapy in all secondary prevention situations, and if allergic to aspirin, consider clopidogrel. Recent evidence in primary prevention studies of antiplatelet therapy in type 2 DM have not shown benefit. The ADA currently recommends that if the 10-year risk of CVD is at least 10%, or the patient is at your judgment high risk, or in women at least 50 years old or men at least 60 years old, primary prevention antiplatelet therapy can be considered. Epidemiologic data suggest that CHD prevention guidelines for type 2 DM apply equally to patients with type 1 DM.[8] β-Blocker therapy supplies an even greater protection from recurrent CHD events in diabetic patients than in nondiabetic subjects. Masking of hypoglycemic symptoms is a greater problem in type 1 DM patients than in patients with type 2 DM.

Lipids The Collaborative Atorvastatin Diabetes Study (CARDS) randomized diabetes subjects with no documented cardiovascular disease to atorvastatin 10 mg daily (n = 1,428) or placebo

(n = 1,410). The trial was stopped 2 years early (mean duration of follow-up was 3.9 years) after meeting the primary efficacy endpoint of major cardiovascular events, which were reduced by 37% (P = 0.001). All-cause death was reduced 27% (P = 0.059), and potentially could have had its significance influenced by the early stoppage of the trial.[119] The Heart Protection Study randomized 5,963 patients age >40 years with diabetes and total cholesterol >135 mg/dL. A significant 22% reduction (95% CI, 13–30) in the event rate for major cardiovascular events was seen with simvastatin 40 mg/day. This was evident even at lower LDL levels (<116 mg/dL), and suggests that ~30% to 40% reduction in LDL levels regardless of starting LDL levels may be appropriate.[120] The proper use of fibrates in diabetes continues to be controversial. The diabetic subgroup in the Veterans Administration HDL Intervention Trial (VA-HIT) of CHD patients with low HDL-C and low LDL-C showed approximately 22% reduction in CHD events in diabetic patients with known CHD when HDL-C was increased by approximately 6% by gemfibrozil.[121] The Fenofibrate Intervention and Event Lowering in Diabetes (FIELD) was conducted in 9,795 subjects (22% with previously documented CVD) with type 2 DM given fenofibrate 200 mg daily or placebo. A relative reduction of 11% (P = 0.16) was seen in any coronary event in conjunction with a slight increase in the risk of all-cause mortality (0.7%; P = 0.18). Reasons for this have been speculated on, including the increased use of statins in the placebo group, but continue to be controversial.[122] On subset analysis, only subjects without CVD had a significant reduction in CVD events. The lipid arm of the ACCORD[123] reported on 5,518 subjects randomized to fenofibrate or placebo given with low-dose simvastatin (~20 mg/day). Fenofibrate addition did not significantly lower cardiovascular events (0.92; 95% CI, 0.79–1.08). On subgroup analysis, women had a 30% higher risk of adverse cardiovascular outcomes, but this was not seen in the FIELD trial. In addition, the only subjects who had a lowering of CVD risk were subjects with high triglycerides combined with low HDL-C.

The National Cholesterol Education Program Adult Treatment Panel III (NCEP-ATP)[124] guidelines classify the presence of DM as a CHD risk equivalent, and therefore recommend that LDL-C be lowered to <100 mg/dL. An optional LDL goal in high-risk DM patients, such as those who already have CHD, has been updated to <70 mg/dL.[125] Unlike previous guidelines, more consideration is now given to HDL-C and triglycerides. The primary target is the treatment of LDL-C. After the LDL-C goal is reached (usually with a statin), via NCEP-ATP, triglycerides are possibly considered for pharmacologic management, assuming unresponsiveness to glycemic control efforts, weight management, and exercise. In such situations, a non–HDL-C goal is established (a surrogate for all apolipoprotein B–containing particles). The non–HDL-C goal for patients with DM is <130 mg/dL. Niacin or a fibrate can be added to reach that goal if triglycerides are 201 to 499 mg/dL. NCEP-ATP states that niacin or a fibrate can also be added if the LDL-C goal is reached, but if the patient has low HDL-C (<40 mg/dL), fibrates have very little, if any positive effect on HDL-C. Patients with marked hypertriglyceridemia (≥500 mg/dL) are at risk for pancreatitis. Efforts to reduce triglycerides with glycemic control, elimination of other secondary causes (including medications), and drug therapy (fibrate and/or niacin) are effective treatment strategies. The ADA also recommends similar LDL goals, but places raising HDL as the second priority (Table 83–16). The definitive role of pharmacologic therapy of HDL-C and/or hypertriglyceridemia in type 2 DM patients (beyond that seen with statin therapy) has yet to be proven in clinical trials, but is leaning heavily toward HDL-C being a very important second priority for the prevention of CVD.

TABLE 83-16	Classification of Lipid and Lipoprotein Levels in Adults[8,124,125]	
Parameter	Goal	Treatment (In Order of Preference)
LDL cholesterol	<100 mg/dL <70 mg/dL[a]	Lifestyle; HMG-CoA reductase inhibitors; cholesterol absorption inhibitor; niacin or fenofibrate
HDL cholesterol	Men >40 mg/dL Women >50 mg/dL	Lifestyle; nicotinic acid; fibric acid derivatives
Triglycerides	<150 mg/dL	Lifestyle; glycemic control; fibric acid derivatives; high-dose statins (in those with high LDL)

HDL, high-density lipoprotein; HMG-CoA, 3-hydroxy-3-methylglutaryl coenzyme A; LDL, low-density lipoprotein.
[a]May be optimal goal in patients with preexisting cardiovascular disease.

CLINICAL CONTROVERSY

The use of fibric acid derivatives and ezetimibe continues to be controversial in the treatment of dyslipidemia in diabetes patients. The FIELD trial using fenofibrate did not result in similar CVD reductions that have been documented in diabetes statin trials. The ACCORD lipid arm in type 2 DM patients added fenofibrate to low-dose simvastatin and did not lower the risk of CVD. The VA-HIT trial using gemfibrozil, though a subset, has shown a reduction in CVD outcomes. Fibric acid derivatives should be considered at least third-line therapy, unless triglycerides are high enough that LDL-C is not reported. It is reasonable to consider use of gemfibrozil as the first fibric acid derivative in diabetes subjects based on the FIELD and ACCORD data. If the drug–drug interaction of a statin with a fibric acid derivative is of paramount importance to the clinician, fenofibrate can be considered. Ezetimibe, and whether it can reduce CVD, continues to be controversial. Colesevelam, which does not have CVD outcomes in diabetes patients, may be a better choice as it will decrease LDL-C in conjuction with a statin, and has the added benefit of a modest reduction in HbA$_{1c}$. Neither should be considered until statin therapy is optimized.

Hypertension

The role of hypertension in increasing microvascular and macrovascular risk in patients with DM has been confirmed in the UKPDS[70] and Hypertension Optimization Treatment[126] trials. The American Diabetes Association recommends aggressive goals for blood pressure (<130/80 mm Hg) in patients with DM.[8] The ACCORD blood pressure arm studied type 2 DM patients, with a goal of achieving a systolic blood pressure of either <120 mm Hg (achieved 119 mm Hg) or <140 mm Hg (133 mm Hg achieved).[127] The lower pressure group did not have lower CVD or renal outcomes, but did lower the risk of stroke. ACE inhibitors and ARBs are generally recommended for initial therapy, as they have shown to be cardioprotective, and likely have special renal protection. Many patients require multiple agents, on average three agents, to obtain goals, so diuretics, calcium channel blockers, and β-blockers frequently are useful as second and third agents. African Americans need special consideration. African Americans receive renoprotection from ACE inhibitors or ARBs, but as a population may lower blood pressure slightly less with these agents. It is recommended that

combination therapy with a diuretic or calcium channel blocker be considered as first-line therapy. After initial therapy, which agent to add next is still controversial. Blood pressure goals are generally more difficult to achieve than glycemic goals or lipid goals in most diabetic patients.

CLINICAL CONTROVERSY

The systolic blood pressure target in diabetes may be in flux. Results of the ACCORD trial did not find improved cardiovascular or renal outcomes in patients who achieved a systolic blood pressure of ~120 mm Hg versus ~130 mm Hg. The lowering of the systolic blood pressure did lower the risk of stroke. Further analysis is warranted prior to drastic changes in blood pressure goals. Initial therapy choices for hypertension in diabetes mellitus usually includes ACE inhibitors or ARBs. In the diabetic subset of the ALLHAT, diuretics have shown equivalent cardiovascular protection to an ACE inhibitor. If ACE inhibitors and ARBs are not more cardioprotective, then why use them first line? Both have proven special renoprotective effects. If a clinician is meticulous in their yearly monitoring for microalbuminuria, it is possible that a diuretic or calcium channel blocker could be started as first-line therapy. As clinical inertia in yearly microalbuminuria screening is often documented, ACE inhibitors or ARBs are give first-line status. ACE inhibitors, ARBs, β-blockers, diuretics, or calcium channel blockers have all shown benefit in prevention of cardiovascular outcomes. Choice of monotherapy may not be important, as an average of two to three antihypertensive medications are needed to reach blood pressure goals.

Transplantation

Whole pancreas and islet cell transplantation are still relatively experimental procedures in patients with type 1 DM; those with endstage renal disease also receive kidney transplantation.[128]

PHARMACOECONOMIC CONSIDERATIONS

As described in the introduction, the direct and indirect costs of DM are substantial. Much of the indirect costs are related to loss of productivity due to the significant morbidity (hospitalizations, loss of vision, lower extremity amputations, kidney failure, and cardiovascular events) associated with the disease. For a disease that affects about 8% of the population, it is responsible for 11% to 12% of health expenditures (in 2007, direct $116 billion, indirect $58 billion[1]). With evidence from the DCCT and UKPDS to support intensive blood glucose control to reduce the risk of complications, the question of cost-effectiveness comes into play.

An economic model based on the DCCT approximates that 120,000 persons in the United States would meet criteria for intensive intervention. The cost of implementing intensive therapy over the lifetime of the population is estimated at $4 billion. The benefits of this strategy are net gains of 920,000 years of sight, 691,000 years free from endstage renal disease, and 678,000 years free from lower extremity amputations. The incremental cost per year of life gained is $28,661.[129] This is well within the limits of a cost-effective strategy and compares favorably to treatment of high blood pressure or hypercholesterolemia.

Economic analysis of intensive therapy for type 2 DM is more complex. Outcomes must also factor in the burden of CVD as the major cause of mortality. One model analyzed the health benefits and economics of treating type 2 DM with the goal of achieving normoglycemia, but using outcomes based on the DCCT trial results. Accounting for the prevalence of CVD in type 2 DM, an estimate of $16,002 incremental cost per quality-adjusted life-year gained was obtained. The limitation of this analysis is that while the UKDPS did demonstrate an improvement in diabetes-related outcomes, the overall efficacy on microvascular disease complications was not mirrored by the DCCT.

Two economic analyses were performed on data generated from the UKPDS, one assessing cost-effectiveness of an intensive blood glucose control policy in type 2 DM, and the other assessing improved blood pressure control in hypertensive patients with type 2 DM. In the first analysis, outcome was measured as the incremental cost per event-free year gained within the trial. Based on trial outcomes and assumptions, the incremental cost in the intensive treatment group per event-free year gained is $1,366. While intensive treatment costs were higher, the cost per event-free year gained appears cost-effective. The second analysis showed the incremental cost per extra year free from microvascular and macrovascular endpoints from intensive blood pressure control in a standard clinical practice model to be $1,498. The incremental cost per life-year gained was estimated at $619, again, demonstrating the cost-effectiveness of intensive intervention.[130,131]

EVALUATION OF THERAPEUTIC OUTCOMES

MONITORING OF THE PHARMACEUTICAL CARE PLAN

A comprehensive pharmaceutical care plan for the patient with DM will integrate considerations of goals to optimize blood glucose control and protocols to screen for, prevent, or manage microvascular and macrovascular complications. In terms of standards of care for persons with DM, one can review the document published by the American Diabetes Association that outlines initial and ongoing assessments for patients with DM.[8] The major performance measure by the National Committee for Quality Assurance (NCQA), such as Health Plan Employer Data and Information Set (HEDIS), should assess the ability to meet current standards of care and recognize the minimal treatment goals for glycemia, lipids, and hypertension, and provide targets for monitoring and adjusting pharmacotherapy as discussed in various sections above. Publicly reported quality measures continue to move closer to current guidelines, but lack the ability to differentiate reasons why a patient is not controlled. Glycemic control (tested minimally yearly; HbA_{1c} <8% is good control and HbA_{1c} >9% is poor control), lipid (percentage of patients with LDL <100 mg/dL), and hypertension (percentage of patients with blood pressure <130/80 mm Hg, but also with blood pressure <140/90) are NCQA-based measures. Glycemic control is paramount in managing type 1 or type 2 DM, but as readily identified from the above discussion, it requires frequent assessment and adjustment in diet, exercise, and pharmacologic therapies. The ADA also has clinical practice recommendations that are widely cited and followed.[8] Minimally, HbA_{1c} should be measured twice a year in patients meeting treatment goals on a stable therapeutic regimen. Quarterly assessments are recommended for those whose therapy has changed or who are not meeting glycemic goals. Fasting lipid profiles should be obtained as part of an initial assessment and thereafter at each follow-up visit if not at goal, annually if stable and at goal, or every 2 years if the lipid profile suggests low risk. Documenting regular frequency of foot exams (each visit), urine albumin assessment (annually), dilated ophthalmologic exams (yearly or more frequently with identified abnormalities), and office visits for follow-up are also important. Assessment for pneumococcal vaccine administration (and one time revaccination recommended in individuals at least 65 years old), annual administration of influenza vaccine, and routine assessment for and management of other cardiovascular risks (e.g., smoking and antiplatelet therapy) are components of preventive medicine strategies. The multiplicity of assessments for each patient visit are likely to be better facilitated utilizing an integrative computer program and electronic medical record, standardized progress note forms, or flow sheets, which assist the clinician in identifying whether the patient has met standards of care in the frequency of monitoring and achievement of defined targets of therapy.

ABBREVIATIONS

ACE: angiotensin-converting enzyme

ADA: American Diabetes Association

ALT: alanine aminotransferase

ARB: angiotensin-receptor blockers

BMI: body mass index

CDE: certified diabetes educator

CHD: coronary heart disease

CVD: cardiovascular disease

CSII: continuous subcutaneous insulin infusion

CYP450: cytochrome P450

DCCT: Diabetes Control and Complications Trial

DM: diabetes mellitus

FFA: free fatty acid

GCT: glucose challenge test

GDM: gestational diabetes mellitus

HbA_{1c}: hemoglobin A_{1c}

HDL-C: high-density lipoprotein cholesterol

IFG: impaired fasting glucose

IGT: impaired glucose tolerance

LADA: latent autoimmune diabetes in adults

LDL-C: low-density lipoprotein cholesterol

MODY: maturity onset diabetes of youth

NCEP-ATP: National Cholesterol Education Program Adult Treatment Panel

NHANES III: The Third National Health and Nutrition Evaluation Survey

NPH: neutral protamine Hagedorn

OGTT: oral glucose tolerance test

PAI-1: activator-1 plasminogen-inhibitor

PPAR-γ: peroxisome proliferator activator receptor-γ

SUR: sulfonylurea receptor

SMBG: self-monitoring of blood glucose

TZD: thiazolidinedione

UKPDS: United Kingdom Prospective Diabetes Study

VAT: visceral adipose tissue

REFERENCES

1. American Diabetes Association. Diabetes facts and figures. *http://www.diabetes.org/diabetes-basics/diabetes-statistics/*.
2. American Diabetes Association. Diagnosis and classification of diabetes mellitus. Diabetes Care 2010;33(Suppl 1):S62–S69.
3. Daneman D. Type 1 diabetes. Lancet 2006;367:847–858.

4. Raffel LJ, Scheuner MT, Rotter JI. Genetics of diabetes. In: Porte D Jr, Sherwin RS, eds. Ellenberg & Rifkin's Diabetes Mellitus, 5th ed. Stamford, CT: Appleton & Lange, 1997:401–454.

5. Bennett P, Rewers M, Knowler W. Epidemiology of diabetes mellitus. In: Porte D Jr, Sherwin RS, eds. Ellenberg & Rifkin's Diabetes Mellitus, 5th ed. Stamford, CT: Appleton & Lange, 1997:373–400.

6. Gale EA. The rise of childhood type 1 diabetes in the 20th century. Diabetes 2002;51:3353–3361.

7. Froguel P, Zouali H, Vionnet N, et al. Familial hyperglycemia due to mutations in glucokinase. Definition of a subtype of diabetes mellitus. N Engl J Med 1993;328:697–702.

8. American Diabetes Association. Standards for medical care in Diabetes–2010. Diabetes Care 2010;3(Suppl 1):S11–S61.

9. Cheung BMY, Ong KL, Cherny SS, et al. Diabetes prevalence and therapeutic target achievement in the United States, 1999 to 2006. Am J Med 2009;122:443–453.

10. American Diabetes Association. Type 2 diabetes in children and adolescents. Diabetes Care 2000;23:381–389.

11. Kahn SE, Porte D Jr. The pathophysiology of type II (non-insulin dependent) diabetes mellitus: Implications for treatment. In: Porte D Jr, Sherwin RS, eds. Ellenberg & Rifkin's Diabetes Mellitus, 5th ed. Stamford, CT: Appleton & Lange, 1997:487–512.

12. American Diabetes Association. Gestational diabetes mellitus. Diabetes Care 2004;27(Suppl 1):S88–S90.

13. Report of the expert committee on the diagnosis and classification of diabetes mellitus. Diabetes Care 1997;20:1183–1197.

14. van Tilburg J, van Haeften TW, Pearson P, Wijimenga C. Defining the genetic contribution of type 2 diabetes mellitus. J Med Genet 2001;38:569–578.

15. Engelgau MM, Thompson TJ, Herman WH, et al. Comparison of fasting and 2-hour glucose and HbA$_{1c}$ levels for diagnosing diabetes: diagnostic criteria and performance revisited. Diabetes Care 1997;20:785–791.

16. McCance DR, Hanson RL, Charles MA, et al. Comparison of tests for glycated haemoglobin and fasting and two hour plasma glucose concentrations as diagnostic methods for diabetes. BMJ 1994;308:1323–1328.

17. Zipitis CS, Akobeng AK Vitamin D supplementation in early childhood and risk of type 1 diabetes: a systematic review and meta-analysis. Arch Dis Child 2008;93:512–517.

18. Janeway CA. Immunology relevant to diabetes. In: Porte D Jr, Sherwin RS, eds. Ellenberg & Rifkin's Diabetes Mellitus, 5th ed. Stamford, CT: Appleton & Lange, 1997:287–300.

19. Edelman SV, Weyer C. Unresolved challenges with insulin therapy in type 1 and type 2 diabetes: potential benefit of replacing amylin, a second β-cell hormone. Diabetes Technol Ther 2002;4:175–189.

20. Cherrington AD. Banting Lecture 1997: Control of glucose uptake and release by the liver in vivo. Diabetes 1999;48:1198–1214.

21. McGarry JD. Banting Lecture 2001: Dysregulation of fatty acid metabolism in the etiology of type 2 diabetes. Diabetes 2002;51:7–18.

22. Nogid A, Pham DQ. Adjunctive therapy with pramlintide in patients with type 1 or type 2 diabetes mellitus. Pharmacotherapy 2006;26:1626–1640

23. DeFronzo RA. Pathogenesis of type 2 diabetes mellitus: Metabolic and molecular implications for identifying diabetes genes. Diabetes 1997;5:117–269.

24. DeFronzo RA. Pathogenesis of type 2 diabetes mellitus. Med Clin N Am 2004;88:787–835.

25. DeFronzo RA. From the triumvirate to the ominous octet: a new paradigm for the treatment of type 2 diabetes mellitus. Diabetes 2009;58:773–795.

26. Reaven GM. Role of insulin resistance in human disease. Diabetes 1988;37:1595–1607.

27. Alberti KGMM, Eckel RH, Grundy SM. et al. Harmonizing the metabolic syndrome. a joint interim statement of the International Diabetes Federation Task Force on Epidemiology and Prevention; National Heart, Lung, and Blood Institute; American Heart Association; World Heart Federation; International Atherosclerosis Society; and International Association for the Study of Obesity. Circulation 2009;120:1640–1645.

28. Ford ES. Prevalence of the metabolic syndrome defined by the International Diabetes Federation among adults in the U.S. Diabetes Care 2005;28:2745–2749.

29. Adams RJ, Appleton S, Wilson DH, et al. Population comparison of two clinical approaches to the metabolic syndrome: Implications of the new International Diabetes Federation consensus definition. Diabetes Care 2005;28:2777–2779.

30. Gaede P, Vedel P, Larsen N, et al. Multifactorial intervention and cardiovascular disease in patients with type 2 diabetes. N Engl J Med 2003;348:383–393.

31. Diabetes Control and Complications Trial Research Group. The effect of intensive treatment of diabetes on the development and progression of long-term complications in insulin-dependent diabetes mellitus. N Engl J Med 1993;329:977–986.

32. UK Prospective Diabetes Study Group. Intensive blood-glucose control with sulphonylureas or insulin compared with conventional treatment and risk of complications in patients with type 2 diabetes (UKPDS 33). Lancet 1998;352:837–853.

33. American Diabetes Association. Self-monitoring of blood glucose. Diabetes Care 1994;17:81–86.

34. Nathan DM, Kuenen J, Borg R. et al. Translating the A1C assay into estimated average glucose values. Diabetes Care 2008;31:1473–1478.

35. Welschen LMC, Bloemendal E, Nijpels G, et al. Self-monitoring of glucose in patients with type 2 diabetes who are not using insulin. Diabetes Care 2005;28:1510–1517.

36. American Diabetes Association. Nutrition recommendations and interventions for diabetes. Diabetes Care 2008;31(Suppl 1):S61–S78.

37. American Diabetes Association. Diabetes mellitus and exercise. Diabetes Care 2010;33(Suppl 1):S26–S27.

38. DeFronzo RA, Ferrannini E, Keen H, Zimmet P eds. International Textbook of Diabetes Mellitus, Vol. 1, 3rd ed. New York: John Wiley & Sons, 2004:277–302.

39. Dewitt DE, Dugdale DC. Using new insulin strategies in the outpatient treatment of diabetes: clinical applications. JAMA 2003;289:2265–2269.

40. DeWitt DE, Hirsch IB. Outpatient insulin therapy in type 1 and type 2 diabetes mellitus: scientific review. JAMA 2003;289:2254–2264.

41. Triplitt CL. How to initiate, titrate, and intensify insulin treatment in type 2 diabetes. US Pharm 2007;32:10–16.

42. Lepore M, Pampanelli S, Fanelli C, et al. Pharmacokinetics and pharmacodynamics of subcutaneous injection of long-acting human insulin analog glargine, NPH insulin, and ultralente human insulin and continuous subcutaneous infusion of insulin lispro. Diabetes 2000;49:2142–2148.

43. Malmberg K, for the DIGAMI Study Group. Prospective randomised study of intensive insulin treatment on long term survival after acute myocardial infarction in patients with diabetes mellitus. BMJ 1997;314:1512–1515.

44. Klonoff DC, Buse JB, Nielsen LL, et al. Exenatide effects on diabetes, obesity, cardiovascular risk factors and hepatic biomarkers in patients with type 2 diabetes treated for at least 3 years. Curr Med Res Opin 2008;24:275–286.

45. Buse JA, Rosenstock J, Schmidt WE, Montanya E, Blonde L. Liraglutide once a day versus exenatide twice a day for type 2 diabetes: a 26-week, randomized, parallel-group, multinational study, open-label trial (LEAD-6). Lancet 2009;374:39–47.

46. Schor S. The University Group Diabetes Program. A statistician looks at the mortality results. JAMA 1971;217:1673–1675.

47. Kilo C, Miller L, Williamson J. The crux of the UGDP. Spurious results and biologically inappropriate data analysis. Diabetologia 1980;18:179–185.

48. Brady PA, Jovanovic A. The sulfonylurea controversy: Much ado about nothing or cause for concern? J Am Coll Cardiol 2003;42:1022–1025.

49. Klamann A, Sarfert P, Lanhardt V, et al. Myocardial infarction in diabetic vs. non-diabetic subjects: survival and infarct size following therapy with sulfonylureas (glibenclamide). Eur Heart J 2000;21:220–229.

50. Riddle MC. Sulfonylureas differ in effects on ischemic preconditioning—is it time to retire glyburide? J Clin Endocrinol Metab 2003;88:528–530.

51. Gerich JE. Oral hypoglycemic agents. N Engl J Med 1989;321:1231–1245.

52. Triplitt C. Drug interactions of medications commonly used in diabetes. Diabetes Spectrum 2006;19:202–211.

53. Wolffenbuttel BH, Landgraf R, for the Dutch and German repaglinide study group. A 1-year multicenter randomized double-blind compari-

son of repaglinide and glyburide for the treatment of type 2 diabetes. Diabetes Care 1999;22:463–467.

54. Horton ES, Clinkingbeard C, Gatlin M, et al. Nateglinide alone and in combination with metformin improves glycemic control by reducing mealtime glucose levels in type 2 diabetes. Diabetes Care 2000;23:1660–1665.

55. UK Prospective Diabetes Study (UKPDS) Group. Effect of intensive blood-glucose control with metformin on complications in overweight patients with type 2 diabetes (UKPDS 34). Lancet 1998;352:854–865.

56. Dawson D, Conlon C. Case study: Metformin associated lactic acidosis: could orlistat be relevant? Diabetes Care 2003;26:2471–2472.

57. Dormandy JA, Charbonnel B, Eckland DJA et al. Secondary prevention of vascular events in patients with type 2 diabetes in the PROactive study prospective pioglitazone clinical trial in macrovascular events: a randomized controlled trial. Lancet 2005;366:1279–1289.

58. Nissen SE, Wolski K. The effect of rosiglitazone on the risk of myocardial infarction and death from cardiovascular causes. N Eng J Med 2007;356:1–15

59. Home PD, Pocock SJ, Beck-Nielsen H, et al. Rosiglitazone evaluated for cardiovascular outcomes in oral agent combination therapy for type 2 diabetes (RECORD): a multicentre, randomised, open-label trial. Lancet 2009;373:2125–2135.

60. Lebovitz HE, Kreider M, Freed MI. Evaluation of liver function in type 2 diabetic patients during clinical trials: evidence that rosiglitazone does not cause hepatic dysfunction. Diabetes Care 2002;25:815–821.

61. Nesto RW, Bell D, Bonow RO, et al. Thiazolidinedione use, fluid retention, and congestive heart failure. A consensus statement from the American Heart Association and the American Diabetes Association. Diabetes Care 2004;27:256–263.

62. Mooradian AD, Thurman JE. Drug therapy of postprandial hyperglycemia. Drugs 1999;57:19–29.

63. Campbell LK, Baker DE, Campbell RK. Miglitol: Assessment of its role in the treatment of patients with diabetes mellitus. Ann Pharmacother 2000;34:1291–1301.

64. Chiasson JL, Josse RG, Gomis R, et al. Acarbose for prevention of type 2 diabetes mellitus: The STOP-NIDDM randomized trial. Lancet 2002;359:2072–2077.

65. Chiasson JL, Josse RG, Gomis R, et al. Acarbose treatment and the risk of cardiovascular disease and hypertension in patients with impaired glucose tolerance: the STOP-NIDDM trial. JAMA 2003;290:486–494.

66. Lettieri JT, Dain B. Effects of beano on the tolerability and pharmacodynamics of acarbose. Clin Ther 1998;20:497–504.

67. Welchol [package insert]. Parsippany, NJ: Daiichi Sankyo; 2009.

68. Stratton IM, Adler AI, Neil HA. Association of glycaemia with macrovascular and microvascular complications of type 2 diabetes (UKPDS 35): Prospective observational study. BMJ 2000;321:405–412.

69. Adler AI, Stratton IM, Neil HA: Association of systolic blood pressure with macrovascular and microvascular complications of type 2 diabetes (UKPDS 36): Prospective observational study. BMJ 2000;321:412–419.

70. UK Prospective Diabetes Study Group. Efficacy of atenolol and captopril in reducing risk of macrovascular and microvascular complications in type 2 diabetes: UKPDS 39. BMJ 1998;317:713–720.

71. EDIC writing group. Sustained effect of intensive treatment of type 1 diabetes mellitus on development and progression of diabetic nephropathy: The Epidemiology of Diabetes Interventions and Complications of Study. JAMA 2003;290:2159–2167.

72. DCCT/EDIC Study Research Group. Intensive diabetes treatment and cardiovascular disease in patients with type 1 diabetes. N Engl J Med 2005;353:2643–2653.

73. Holman RR, Paul SK, Bethel MA, Mathews DR, Neil HAW. 10-year follow-up of intensive glucose control in type 2 diabetes. N Engl J Med 2008;359:1577–1589.

74. The Action to Control Cardiovascular Risk in Diabetes Study Group. Effects of intensive glucose lowering in type 2 diabetes. N Engl J Med 2008;358:2545–2559.

75. The ADVANCE Collaborative Group. Intensive blood glucose control and vascular outcomes in patients with type 2 diabetes. N Engl J Med 2008;358:2560–2572.

76. Duckworth W, Abraira C, Mortiz T, et al. Glucose control and vascular complications in veterans with type 2 diabetes. N Engl J Med 2009;360:1–11.

77. Strowig S, Raskin P. Intensive management of insulin-dependent diabetes mellitus. In: Porte D Jr, Sherwin RS, eds. Ellenberg & Rifkin's Diabetes Mellitus, 5th ed. Stamford, CT: Appleton & Lange, 1997:709–733.

78. Schade DS, Valentine V. To pump or not to pump. Diabetes Care 2002;25:2100–2102.

79. de Galan BE, Tack CJ, Lenders JW, et al. Theophylline improves hypoglycemia unawareness in type 1 diabetes. Diabetes 2002;51:790–796.

80. Rosenbloom AL, Schatz DA, Krischer JP, et al. Therapeutic controversy: Prevention and treatment of diabetes in children. J Clin Endocrinol Metab 2000;85:494–522.

81. Kelly DB, ed. Management of Type 1 Diabetes Mellitus, 3rd ed. Alexandria, VA: American Diabetes Association, 1998:211–222.

82. Halvorsen T, Levine F. Diabetes mellitus-cell transplantation and gene therapy approaches. Curr Mol Med 2001;1:273–286.

83. Shapiro AM, Ricordi C, Hering BJ, et al. International trial of the edmonton protocol for islet transplantation. N Engl J Med 2006;355:1318–1330.

84. DeFronzo RA. Pharmacologic therapy for type 2 diabetes mellitus. Ann Intern Med 1999;131:281–303.

85. Higa M, Zhou YT, Ravazzola M, et al. Troglitazone prevents mitochondrial alterations, beta cell destruction, and diabetes in obese prediabetic rats. Proc Natl Acad Sci U S A 1999;96:11513–11518.

86. Wang Q, Brubaker PL. Glucagon-like peptide-1 treatment delays the onset of diabetes in 8 week-old db/db mice. Diabetologia 2002;45:1263–1273.

87. Shank ML, Del Prato S, DeFronzo RA. Bedtime insulin/daytime glipizide. Effective therapy for sulfonylurea failures in NIDDM. Diabetes 1995;44:165–172.

88. Yki-Jarvinen H, Ryysy L, Nikkila K. Comparison of bedtime insulin regimens in patients with type 2 diabetes mellitus. A randomized, controlled trial. Ann Intern Med 1999;130:389–396.

89. Holman RR, Farmer AJ, Davies MJ, et al. Three-year efficacy of complex insulin regimens in type 2 diabetes. N Engl J Med 2009;361:1736–1747.

90. Bastyr EJ, Stuart CA, Brodows RG. Therapy focused on lowering postprandial glucose, not fasting glucose, may be superior for lowering HbA_{1c}. IOEZ Study Group. Diabetes Care 2000;23:1236–1241.

91. European Diabetes Epidemiology Group. Glucose tolerance and mortality. Comparison of WHO and American Diabetes Association diagnostic criteria. The DECODE study group. Diabetes Epidemiology: Collaborative analysis of diagnostic criteria in Europe. Lancet 1999;354:617–621.

92. Langer O, Conway DL, Berkus MD, et al. A comparison of glyburide and insulin in women with gestational diabetes mellitus. N Engl J Med 2000;343:1134–1138.

93. Laffel L. Sick-day management in type 1 diabetes. Endocrinol Metab Clin North Am 2000;29:707–723.

94. Kitabchi AE, Umpierrez GE, Miles JM, Fisher JN. Hyperglycemic crises in adult patients with diabetes. A consensus statement from the american diabetes association. Diabetes Care 2009;32:1335–1343.

95. Sawin CT. Action without benefit. The sliding scale of insulin use. Arch Intern Med 1997;157:489.

96. Malmberg K, Norhammar A, Wedel H. Glycometabolic state at admission: Important risk marker of mortality in conventionally treated patients with diabetes mellitus and acute myocardial infarction: Long-term results from the Diabetes and Insulin-Glucose Infusion in Acute Myocardial Infarction. Circulation 1999;99:2626–2632.

97. van den Berghe G, Wouters P, Weekers F, et al. Intensive insulin therapy in the critically ill patients. N Engl J Med 2001;345:1359–1367.

98. Moghissi ES, Korykowski MT, DiNardo M, et al. American association of clinical endocrinologists and american diabetes association consensus statement on inpatient glycemic control. Diabetes Care 2009;32:1119–1131.

99. The NICE-SUGAR Study Investigators. Intensive versus conventional glycemic control in critically ill patients. N Engl J Med 2009;360:1283–1297.

100. Montori VM, Bistrian BR, McMahon MM. Hyperglycemia in acutely ill patients. JAMA 2002;288:2167–2169.

101. American Diabetes Association. Preconception care of women with diabetes. Diabetes Care 2004;27(Suppl 1):S76–S78.

102. Ryan EA. Pregnancy in diabetes. Med Clin North Am 1998;82:823–845.

103. Schernthaner G. Progress in the immunointervention of type 1 diabetes mellitus. Horm Metab Res 1995;27:547–554.

104. Diabetes Prevention Trial-type 1 diabetes study group. Effects of insulin in relatives of patients with type 1 diabetes mellitus. N Engl J Med 2002;346:1685–1691.

105. Kakka R, Koda-Kimble MA. Can insulin therapy delay or prevent insulin-dependent diabetes mellitus? Pharmacotherapy 1997;17:38–44.

106. Diabetes Prevention Program Research Group. Reduction in the incidence of type 2 diabetes with lifestyle intervention or metformin. N Engl J Med 2002;346:393–403.

107. Tuomilehto J, Lindstrom J, Eriksson JG, et al, for the Finnish Diabetes Prevention Study Group. Prevention of type 2 diabetes mellitus by changes in lifestyle among subjects with impaired glucose tolerance. N Engl J Med 2001;344:1343–1350.

108. Buchanan TA, Xiang AH, Peters RK, et al. Preservation of pancreatic β-cell function and prevention of type 2 diabetes by pharmacological treatment of insulin resistance in high-risk Hispanic women. Diabetes 2002;51:2796–2803.

109. The Dream Trial Investigators. The effect of ramipril on the incidence of diabetes. N Engl J Med 2006;355:1551–1562.

110. The DREAM Trial Investigators. The effect of rosiglitazone on the frequency of diabetes in patients with impaired glucose tolerance or impaired fasting glucose. A randomised controlled trial. Lancet 2006;368:1096–1105.

111. Nathan DM, Davidson MB, Defronzo RA, et al. Impaired fasting glucose and impaired glucose tolerance. Implication for care. Diabetes Care 2007;30:753–759.

112. Funnell MM, Brown TL, Childs BP, et al. National standards diabetes self-management education. Diabetes Care 2010;33(Suppl 1):S89–S96.

113. Boulton AJ, Malik RA, Arezzo JC, Sosenko JM. Diabetic somatic neuropathies. Diabetes Care 2004;27:1458–1486.

114. American Diabetes Association. Diabetic nephropathy. Diabetes Care 2004;27(Suppl 1):S79–S83.

115. Lewis EJ, Hunsicker LG, Clarke WR, et al. Renoprotective effect of the angiotensin-receptor antagonist irbesartan in patients with nephropathy due to type 2 diabetes. N Engl J Med 2001;345:851–860.

116. Brenner BM, Cooper ME, deZeeuw D, et al. Effects of losartan on renal and cardiovascular outcomes in patients with type 2 diabetes and nephropathy. N Engl J Med 2001;345:861–869.

117. Parving HH, Lehnert H, Brochner-Mortensen J, et al. The effect of irbesartan on the development of diabetic nephropathy in patients with type 2 diabetes. N Engl J Med 2001;345:870–878.

118. Boulton AJM, Armstrong DG, Albert SF, et al. Comprehensive foot exam and risk assessment. Diabetes Care 2008;31:1679–1685.

119. Colhoun HM, Betteridge DJ, Durrington PN, et al. Primary prevention of cardiovascular disease with atorvastatin in type 2 diabetes in the collaborative atorvastatin diabetes study (CARDS): a multicentre, randomised placebo controlled trial. Lancet 2004;364:685–696.

120. Heart Protection Study Collaborative Group. MRC/BHF Heart Protection Study of cholesterol-lowering with simvastatin in 5963 people with diabetes: A randomised placebo-controlled trial. Lancet 2003;361:2005–2016.

121. Rubins HB, Robins SJ, Collins D, et al. Gemfibrozil for the secondary prevention of coronary heart disease in men with low levels of high-density lipoprotein cholesterol. Veterans Affairs High-Density Lipoprotein Cholesterol Intervention Trial Study Group. N Engl J Med 1999;341:410–418.

122. The FIELD study investigators. Effects of long-term fenofibrate therapy on cardiovascular events in 9795 people with type 2 diabetes mellitus (the FIELD study): randomised controlled trial. Lancet 2005;366:1849–1861.

123. The ACCORD Study Group. Effects of combination lipid therapy in type 2 diabetes. N Engl J Med 2010;362:1563–1574 (erratum 362:1748).

124. Expert Panel on Detection, Evaluation, and Treatment of High Blood Cholesterol in Adults. Executive Summary of the Third Report of the National Cholesterol Education Program (NCEP) Expert Panel on Detection, Evaluation, and Treatment of High Blood Cholesterol in Adults (Adult Treatment Panel III). JAMA 2001;285:2486–2496.

125. Grundy SM, Cleeman JI, Merz CN. Implications of recent clinical trials for the national cholesterol education program adult treatment panel III guidelines. Circulation 2004;110:227–239.

126. Hansson L, Zanchetti A, Carruthers SG. Effects of intensive blood-pressure lowering and low-dose aspirin in patients with hypertension: principal results of the Hypertension Optimal Treatment (HOT) randomised trial. HOT Study Group. Lancet 1998;351:1755–1762.

127. The ACCORD Study Group. Effects of intensive blood-pressure control in type 2 diabetes mellitus. N Engl J Med 2010;362:1628–1630.

128. Robertson RP, Davis C, Larsen J, et al. Pancreas and islet transplantation for patients with diabetes mellitus (technical review). Diabetes Care 2000;23:112–116.

129. Herman WH, Eastman RC. The effects on treatment on the direct costs of diabetes. Diabetes Care 1998;21(Suppl 3):C19–C24.

130. Gray A. Raikou M, McGuire A, et al. Cost effectiveness of an intensive blood glucose control policy in patient with type 2 diabetes: Economic analysis alongside randomized controlled trial (UKPDS 41). BMJ 2000;320:1373–1378.

131. Anonymous. Cost effectiveness analysis of improved blood pressure control in hypertensive patients with type 2 diabetes: UKPDS 40. BMJ 1998;317:720–726.

CHAPTER 84 Thyroid Disorders

JACQUELINE JONKLAAS AND ROBERT L. TALBERT

KEY CONCEPTS

1. The molecular biology of the thyroid hormones and their receptors has provided an in-depth understanding of the various mutations that give rise to hyper- and hypothyroidism.

2. Thyrotoxicosis is most commonly caused by Graves's disease, which is an autoimmune disorder in which thyroid-stimulating antibody (TSAb) directed against the thyrotropin receptor elicits the same biologic response as thyroid-stimulating hormone (TSH).

3. Hyperthyroidism may be treated with antithyroid drugs such as propylthiouracil (PTU) or methimazole (MMI), radioactive iodine (RAI: ^{131}I), or surgical removal of the thyroid gland; selection of the initial treatment approach is based on patient characteristics such as age, concurrent physiology (e.g., pregnancy), comorbidities (e.g., chronic obstructive lung disease), and convenience.

4. PTU and MMI reduce the synthesis of thyroid hormones and are similar in efficacy and adverse effects, but their dosing ranges differ by 10-fold.

5. Response to PTU and MMI is seen in 4 to 6 weeks with a maximal response in 4 to 6 months; treatment usually continues for 1 to 2 years, and therapy is monitored by clinical signs and symptoms and by measuring the serum concentrations of TSH and free thyroxine (T_4).

6. Many patients choose to have ablative therapy with ^{131}I rather than undergo repeated courses of PTU or MMI; most patients receiving RAI eventually become hypothyroid and require thyroid hormone supplementation.

7. Adjunctive therapy with β-blockers controls the adrenergic symptoms of thyrotoxicosis but does not correct the underlying disorder; iodine may also be used adjunctively in preparation for surgery and acutely for thyroid storm.

8. Hypothyroidism is most often due to an autoimmune disorder known as *Hashimoto's thyroiditis*, and the drug of choice for replacement therapy is levothyroxine.

9. Monitoring of levothyroxine replacement therapy is achieved by observing clinical signs and symptoms and by measuring the TSH (elevated for underreplacement, suppressed for overreplacement).

Learning objectives, review questions, and other resources can be found at **www.pharmacotherapyonline.com**.

Thyroid hormones affect the function of virtually every organ system. In the child, thyroid hormone is critical for normal growth and development. In the adult, the major role of thyroid hormone is to maintain metabolic stability. Substantial reservoirs of thyroid hormone in the thyroid gland and blood provide constant thyroid hormone availability. In addition, the hypothalamic–pituitary–thyroid axis is exquisitely sensitive to small changes in circulating thyroid hormone concentrations, and alterations in thyroid hormone secretion maintain peripheral free thyroid hormone levels within a narrow range. Patients seek medical attention for evaluation of symptoms due to abnormal thyroid hormone levels or because of diffuse or nodular thyroid enlargement.

THYROID HORMONE PHYSIOLOGY

THYROID HORMONE SYNTHESIS

1 The thyroid hormones thyroxine (T_4) and triiodothyronine (T_3) are formed on thyroglobulin, a large glycoprotein synthesized within the thyroid cell (Fig. 84–1). Because of the unique tertiary structure of this glycoprotein, iodinated tyrosine residues present in thyroglobulin are able to bind together to form active thyroid hormones.[1]

Iodide is actively transported through the basolateral membrane via a Na^+/I^- symporter from the extracellular space into the thyroid follicular cell against an electrochemical gradient, driven by the coupled transport of sodium.[2] Structurally related anions such as SCN^- (thiocyanate), ClO_4^- (perchlorate), and TcO_4^- (pertechnetate) are competitive inhibitors of iodine transport.[3] In addition,

3,5,3',5'-Thyroxine (T_4)

3,5,3'-Triiodothyronine (T_3)

3,3',5'-Triiodothyronine (reverse T_3, rT_3, T_3')

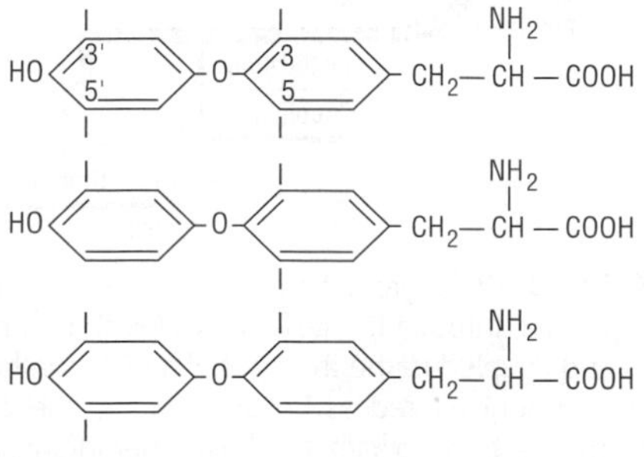

FIGURE 84-1. Structure of thyroid hormones.

TABLE 84-1	Thyroid Hormone Synthesis and Secretion Inhibitors
Mechanism of Action	**Substance**
Blocks iodide transport into the thyroid	Bromine
	Fluorine
	Lithium (?)
Impairs organification and coupling of thyroid hormones	Thionamides
	Sulfonylureas
	Sulfonamide (?)
	Salicylamide (?)
	Antipyrine (?)
Inhibits thyroid hormone secretion	Iodide (large doses), lithium

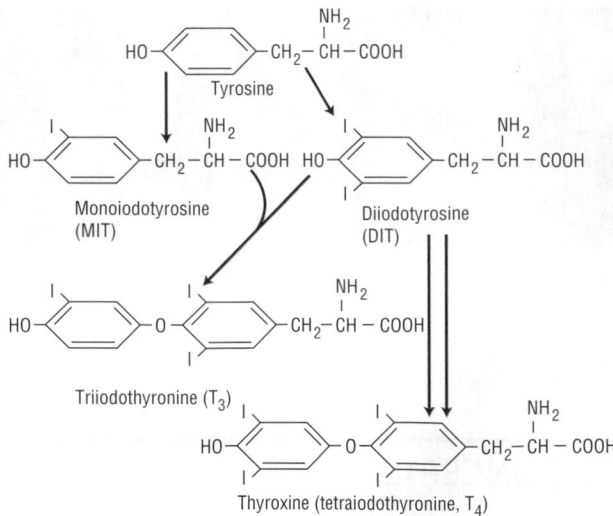

FIGURE 84-3. Scheme of coupling reactions. After tyrosine is iodinated to form monoiodotyrosine (MIT) or diiodotyrosine (DIT) (organification of the iodine), MIT and DIT combine to form triiodothyronine (T_3) or two molecules of DIT combine to form thyroxine T_4.

bromine, fluorine, and under certain circumstances lithium, block iodide transport into the thyroid (Table 84–1). Inorganic iodide that enters the thyroid follicular cell is ushered through the cell to the apical membrane, where it is transported into the follicular lumen by at least two efflux channels.[4,5] Located on the luminal side of the apical membrane, thyroid peroxidase oxidizes iodide and covalently binds the organified iodide to tyrosine residues of thyroglobulin (Fig. 84–2). It is interesting that although salivary glands and the gastric mucosa are able to actively transport iodide, they are unable to effectively incorporate iodide into proteins given the lack of similar oxidizing machinery. Similarly, when tyrosine molecules are iodinated on proteins other than thyroglobulin, they lack the proper tertiary structure needed to allow the formation of active thyroid hormones.

The iodinated tyrosine residues monoiodotyrosine (MIT) and diiodotyrosine (DIT) combine to form iodothyronines (Fig. 84–3). Thus, two molecules of DIT combine to form T_4, whereas MIT and DIT constitute T_3. In addition to its role in iodine organification, the hemoprotein thyroid peroxidase also catalyzes the formation of iodothyronines (coupling).

Iodine deficiency causes an increase in the ratio of MIT to DIT in thyroglobulin and leads to a relative increase in the production of T_3.[6] Because T_3 is more potent than T_4, the increase in T_3 production in iodine-depleted areas may be beneficial. The thionamide drugs

used to treat hyperthyroidism inhibit thyroid peroxidase and thus block thyroid hormone synthesis.

Thyroglobulin is stored in the follicular lumen and must reenter the cell, where the process of proteolysis liberates thyroid hormone into the bloodstream. Thyroid follicles active in hormone synthesis are identified histologically by columnar epithelial cells lining follicular lumens, which are depleted of colloid. Inactive follicles are lined by cuboidal epithelial cells and are replete with colloid. Both iodide and lithium block the release of preformed thyroid hormone, through poorly understood mechanisms.

T_4 and T_3 are transported in the bloodstream primarily by three proteins: thyroxine-binding globulin (TBG), transthyretin (TTR), and albumin.[7] It is estimated that 99.96% of circulating T_4 and 99.5% of T_3 are bound to these proteins. However, only the unbound (free) thyroid hormone is able to diffuse into the cell, elicit a biologic effect, and regulate thyroid-stimulating hormone (TSH; also known as *thyrotropin*) secretion from the pituitary. Multiple functions have been ascribed to these transport proteins, including (1) assuring minimal urinary loss of iodide, (2) providing a mechanism for uniform tissue distribution of free hormone, and (3) transport of hormone into the central nervous system.

Whereas T_4 is secreted solely from the thyroid gland, less than 20% of T_3 is produced in the thyroid. The majority of T_3 is formed from the breakdown of T_4 catalyzed by the enzyme 5′-monodeiodinase found in extrathyroidal peripheral tissues. Because the binding affinity of nuclear thyroid hormone receptors is 10 to 15 times higher for T_3 than T_4, the deiodinase enzymes play a pivotal role in determining overall metabolic activity. Three different monodeiodinase enzymes are present in the body.[8] Of the enzymes that catalyze 5′-monodeiodination, type I enzymes are present in peripheral tissues, whereas type II enzymes are found in the central nervous system, pituitary, and thyroid. Type III enzymes, found in the placenta, skin, and developing brain, inactivate T_4 and T_3 by deiodinating the inner ring at the 5 position. The principal characteristics of these enzymes are listed in Table 84–2. T_4 may also be acted on by the enzyme 5′-monodeiodinase to form reverse T_3, but this accounts for a small component of hormone metabolism. Polymorphisms in the deiodinase genes may prove to be of clinical significance. For example, a polymorphism in the type I deiodinase leading to increased activity seems to be associated with an increased circulating ratio of free T_3 to free

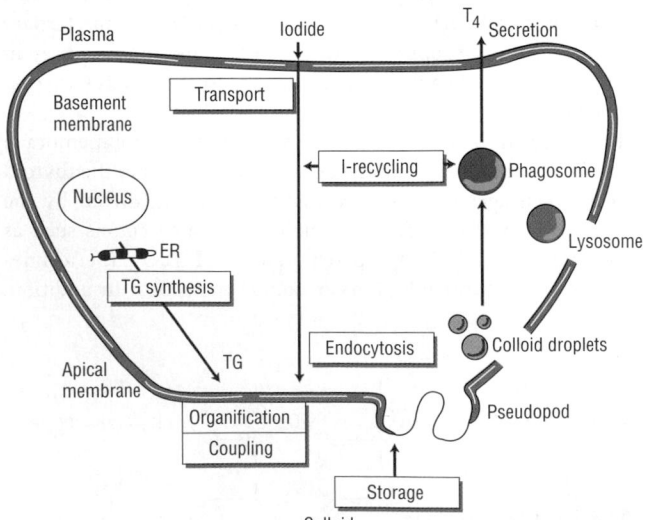

FIGURE 84-2. Thyroid hormone synthesis. Iodide is transported from the plasma, through the cell, to the apical membrane, where it is organified and coupled to the thyroglobulin (TG) synthesized within the thyroid cell. Hormone stored as colloid reenters the cell through endocytosis and moves back toward the basal membrane, where thyroxine (T_4) is secreted.

TABLE 84-2 Properties of Iodothyronine 5'-Deiodinase Isoforms

Property	Type I	Type II	Type III
Effect of propylthiouracil	Increase	Decrease	Increase
Tissue localization	Thyroid, liver, kidney	Pituitary, thyroid, CNS, brown adipose tissue	Placenta, developing brain, skin
Preferred substrate	$rT_3 > T_4 > T_3$	$T_4 > T_3$	T_3(sulfate)$> T_4$
Physiologic role	Extracellular T_3 production for peripheral tissue	Intracellular T_3 production, especially for brain in hypothyroidism or iodine deficiency	Inactivation of T_4 and T_3
Developmental expression	Expressed latest in development; predominant deiodinase in adult	Expressed second; especially high in brain and brown adipose tissue	Expressed first; high in developing brain; may be important for fetal thyroid hormone metabolism

rT_3, reverse T_3; T_3, triiodothyronine; T_4, thyroxine.

T_4.[9] Reverse T_3 has no known significant biologic activity. T_3 is removed from the body by deiodinative degradation and through the action of sulfotransferase enzyme systems converting to T_3 sulfate and 3,3-diiodothyronine sulfates, thus facilitating enterohepatic clearance. Thyronamines are derivatives of thyroid hormone that are present in very low concentrations in human serum. The most studied thyronamine, 3-iodothyronamine, can theoretically be made from thyroxine by decarboxylation and deiodination. Administration of pharmacologic amounts of 3-iodothyronamine to animals has profound effects on temperature regulation and cardiac function, and shifts fuel metabolism from carbohydrates to lipids. However, a possible physiological role for thyronamines has yet to be determined.[10]

The growth and function of the thyroid are stimulated by activation of the thyrotropin receptor by TSH.[11] The receptor belongs to the family of G-protein–coupled receptors. The thyrotropin receptor is coupled to the α subunit of the stimulatory guanine-nucleotide–binding protein ($G_s\alpha$), activating adenylate cyclase and increasing the accumulation of cyclic adenosine monophosphate. Through this mechanism, TSH stimulates the expression of thyroglobulin and thyroid peroxidase genes as well as increases apical iodide efflux. Somatic activating mutations in the receptor are commonly seen in autonomously functioning thyroid nodules.[12] Rarely, germline activating mutations of the TSH receptor have been reported in kindreds with Leclere syndrome, and thyrotoxicosis can result from germline activating mutations in G-protein signaling in McCune-Albright syndrome.[11,13-15] Conversely, thyrotropin resistance would result from point mutations that prevent TSH binding, leading to abnormalities in the thyrotropin receptor–adenylate cyclase system and congenital hypothyroidism.[16,17] Individuals with this abnormality have high levels of TSH but decreased thyroglobulin levels and a normal or small gland.

Thyroid hormone receptors regulate the transcription of target genes in the presence of physiologic concentrations of T_3.[18] Unlike most other nuclear receptors, thyroid hormone receptors also actively regulate gene expression in the absence of hormone, typically resulting in an opposite effect. Thyroid receptors translocate from the cytoplasm to the nucleus, interact in the nucleus with T_3, and target genes and other proteins required for basal and T_3-dependent gene transcription. Thyroid receptors exist in three isoforms, TRβ2, TRβ1, and TRα1, with variation in the expression of each in differing tissues. There is interest in developing thyroid hormone analogues that selectively activate specific TR isoforms. Such agents could theoretically have targeted desirable effects such as stimulating energy expenditure without having adverse effects on other tissues.[19]

The production of thyroid hormone is regulated in two main ways. First, thyroid hormone is regulated by TSH secreted by the anterior pituitary. The secretion of TSH is itself under negative feedback control by the circulating level of free thyroid hormone and the positive influence of hypothalamic thyrotropin-releasing hormone (TRH). Second, extrathyroidal deiodination of T_4 to T_3 is regulated by a variety of factors including nutrition, nonthyroidal hormones, ambient temperatures, drugs, and illness.

THYROTOXICOSIS

Thyrotoxicosis results when tissues are exposed to excessive levels of T_4, T_3, or both.[20] In the National Health and Nutrition Examination Survey III, 0.7% of those surveyed who were not taking thyroid medications and had no history of thyroid disease had subclinical hyperthyroidism (TSH <0.1 milli-international units/L; and T_4 normal), and 0.5% had "clinically significant" hyperthyroidism (TSH <0.1 milli-international units/L; and T_4 >13.2 mcg/dL).[21] The prevalence of suppressed TSH peaked for people aged 20 to 39, declined in those 40 to 79, and increased again in those 80 or older. Abnormal TSH levels were more common among women than among men.

CLINICAL PRESENTATION OF THYROTOXICOSIS

General

Signs and symptoms of hyperthyroidism affect multiple organ systems. Patients may have symptoms for an extended time period before the diagnosis of hyperthyroidism is made.

Symptoms

The typical clinical manifestations of thyrotoxicosis include nervousness, anxiety, palpitations, emotional lability, easy fatigability, menstrual disturbances, and heat intolerance. A cardinal sign is loss of weight concurrent with an increased appetite.

Signs

A variety of physical signs may be elicited including warm, smooth, moist skin, exophthalmos (in Graves's disease only), pretibial myxedema (in Graves's disease only), and unusually fine hair. Separation of the end of the fingernails from the nail beds (onycholysis) may be noted. Ocular signs that result from thyrotoxicosis include retraction of the eyelids and lagging of the upper lid behind the globe when the patient looks downward (lid lag). Physical signs of a hyperdynamic circulatory state are common and include tachycardia at rest, a widened pulse pressure, and a systolic ejection murmur. Gynecomastia is sometimes noted in men. Neuromuscular examination often reveals a fine tremor of the protruded tongue and outstretched hands. Deep tendon reflexes are generally hyperactive. Thyromegaly is usually present.

Diagnosis

Low TSH serum concentration. Elevated free and total T_3 and T_4 serum concentrations, particularly in more severe disease.

- Elevated radioactive iodine uptake (RAIU) by the thyroid gland when hormone is being overproduced; suppressed RAIU in thyrotoxicosis due to thyroid inflammation (thyroiditis)

Other tests

- Thyroid stimulating antibodies (TSAb)
- Thyroglobulin
- Thyrotropin receptor antibodies

For the elderly patient and for the patient with very severe disease, anorexia may be present as well. Elderly patients are also more likely to develop atrial fibrillation with thyrotoxicosis than younger patients. The frequency of bowel movements may increase, but frank diarrhea is unusual. Palpitations are a prominent and distressing symptom, particularly in the patient with preexisting heart disease. Proximal muscle weakness is common and is noted on climbing stairs or in getting up from a sitting position. Women may note their menses are becoming scanty and irregular. Extremely thyrotoxic (thyrotoxic storm) patients may have tachycardia, heart failure, psychosis, hyperpyrexia, and coma.[22]

DIFFERENTIAL DIAGNOSIS

If the clinical history and examination do not provide pathognomonic clues to the etiology of the patient's thyrotoxicosis, measurement of the radioactive iodine uptake (RAIU) is critical in the evaluation (Table 84-3). The normal 24-hour RAIU ranges from 10% to 30% with some regional variation that is due to differences in iodine intake. An elevated RAIU indicates true hyperthyroidism, that is, the patient's thyroid gland is actively overproducing T_4, T_3, or both. Conversely, a low RAIU in the absence of iodine excess indicates that high levels of thyroid hormone are not a consequence of thyroid gland hyperfunction but are likely due to thyroiditis or hormone ingestion. The importance of differentiating true hyperthyroidism from other causes of thyrotoxicosis lies in the widely different prognosis and treatment of the diseases in these two categories. Therapy of thyrotoxicosis associated with thyroid hyperfunction is mainly directed at decreasing the rate of thyroid hormone synthesis, secretion, or both. Such measures are ineffective in treating thyrotoxicosis that is not the result of true hyperthyroidism, because hormone synthesis and regulated hormone secretion are already at a minimum.

CAUSES OF THYROTOXICOSIS ASSOCIATED WITH ELEVATED RAIU

TSH-Induced Hyperthyroidism

To better understand these syndromes, we must first review TSH biosynthesis and secretion. TSH is synthesized in the anterior

TABLE 84-3 Differential Diagnosis of Thyrotoxicosis

Increased RAIU	Decreased RAIU
TSH-induced hyperthyroidism	Inflammatory thyroid disease
TSH-secreting tumors	Subacute thyroiditis
Selective pituitary resistance to T_4	Painless thyroiditis
Thyroid stimulators other than TSH[a]	Ectopic thyroid tissue
TSAb (Graves's disease)	Struma ovarii
hCG (trophoblastic diseases)	Metastatic follicular carcinoma
Thyroid autonomy	Exogenous sources of thyroid hormone
Toxic adenoma	Medication
Multinodular goiter	Food

hCG, human chorionic gonadotropin; RAIU, radioactive iodine uptake; TSAb, thyroid-stimulating antibodies; TSH, thyroid-stimulating hormone.

[a]The RAIU may be decreased if the patient has been recently exposed to excess iodine.

pituitary as separate α- and β-subunit precursors. The α subunits from luteinizing hormone (LH), follicle-stimulating hormone (FSH), human chorionic gonadotropin (hCG), and TSH are similar, whereas the β subunits are unique and confer immunologic and biologic specificity. Free β subunits are devoid of receptor binding and biologic activity and require combination with an α subunit to express their activity. Criteria for the diagnosis of TSH-induced hyperthyroidism include (1) evidence of peripheral hypermetabolism, (2) diffuse thyroid gland enlargement, (3) elevated free thyroid hormone levels, and (4) elevated or inappropriately "normal" serum immunoreactive TSH concentrations. Because the pituitary gland is extremely sensitive to even minimal elevations of free T_4, a "normal" or elevated TSH level in any thyrotoxic patient indicates the inappropriate production of TSH.

TSH-Secreting Pituitary Adenomas

TSH-secreting pituitary tumors occur sporadically and release biologically active hormone that is unresponsive to normal feedback control.[23] The mean age at diagnosis is around 40 years, with women being diagnosed more than men (8:7). These tumors may co-secrete prolactin or growth hormone; therefore the patients may present with amenorrhea/galactorrhea or signs of acromegaly. Most patients present with classic symptoms and signs of thyrotoxicosis. Visual-field defects may be present due to impingement of the optic chiasm by the tumor. Tumor growth and worsening visual-field defects have been reported following antithyroid therapy because lowering of thyroid hormone levels is associated with loss of feedback inhibition from high thyroid hormone levels.

Diagnosis of a TSH-secreting adenoma should be made by demonstrating lack of TSH response to TRH stimulation, inappropriate TSH levels, elevated α-subunit levels, and radiologic imaging; given the lack of routine availability of TRH, the other three criteria are essential. Note that some small tumors are not identified by MRI. Moreover, 10% of "normal" individuals may have incidental pituitary tumors or other benign focal lesions noted on pituitary imaging.

Transsphenoidal pituitary surgery is the treatment of choice for TSH-secreting adenomas. Pituitary gland irradiation is often given following surgery to prevent tumor recurrence. Bromocriptine and octreotide have been used to treat tumors, especially those that co-secrete prolactin.

Pituitary Resistance to Thyroid Hormone

Pituitary resistance to thyroid hormone (PRTH) refers to selective resistance of the pituitary thyrotrophs to thyroid hormone.[24] As nonpituitary tissues respond normally to thyroid hormone, patients experience the toxic peripheral effects of thyroid hormone excess. About twice as many women as men have been reported with this rare, probably familial syndrome. Multiple abnormalities have been reported in the initial 50 reported cases including schizophrenia (three patients), mental retardation (two patients), short fourth metacarpals (one patient), and Marfanoid habitus (one patient). About 90% of patients studied have an appropriate increase in TSH in response to TRH; conversely, the TSH will be suppressed by T_3 administration.

Patients with PRTH require treatment to reduce their elevated thyroid hormone levels. Determining the appropriate serum T_4 level is difficult because TSH cannot be used to evaluate adequacy of therapy. Any reduction in thyroid hormone carries the risk of inducing thyrotroph hyperplasia. Ideally, agents that suppress TSH secretion could be used to treat these individuals. Glucocorticoids, dopaminergic drugs, somatostatin and its analogs, and thyroid hormone analogs with reduced metabolic activity have all been tried; given the ability of retinoid X receptor ligands to inhibit TSH production, drugs like bexarotene may have therapeutic benefit in PRTH.[25]

THYROID STIMULATORS OTHER THAN TSH

Graves's Disease

❷ Graves's disease is an autoimmune syndrome that usually includes hyperthyroidism, diffuse thyroid enlargement, exophthalmos, and less commonly pretibial myxedema and thyroid acropachy (Fig. 84–4).[20,26,27] Graves's disease is the most common cause of hyperthyroidism, with a prevalence estimated to be 3 per 1,000 population in the United States. Hyperthyroidism results from the action of thyroid-stimulating antibodies (TSAb), which are directed against the thyrotropin receptor on the surface of the thyroid cell.[16,17] When these immunoglobulins bind to the receptor, they activate downstream G-protein signaling and adenylate cyclase in the same manner as TSH. Autoantibodies that react with orbital muscle and fibroblast tissue in the skin are responsible for the extrathyroidal manifestations of Graves's disease, and these autoantibodies are encoded by the same germline genes that encode for other autoantibodies for striated muscle and thyroid peroxidase.[28] Clinically, the extrathyroidal disorders may not appear at the same time that hyperthyroidism develops.

There is now compelling evidence that heredity predisposes the susceptible individual to development of clinically overt autoimmune thyroid disease in the setting of appropriate environmental and hormonal triggers. A role for gender in the emergence of Graves's disease is suggested by the fact that hyperthyroidism is approximately eight times more common in women than men. Other lines of evidence support a role for heredity. First, there is a well-recognized clustering of Graves's disease within some families. Twin studies in Graves's disease have revealed that a monozygotic twin has a 35% likelihood of ultimately developing the disease compared with a 3% likelihood for a dizygotic twin, resulting in estimation that the 79% of the predisposition to Graves's disease is genetic.[29] Second, the occurrence of other autoimmune diseases, including Hashimoto's thyroiditis, is also increased in families of patients with Graves's disease. Third, several studies have demonstrated an increased frequency of certain human leukocyte antigens (HLAs) for patients with Graves's disease. Differing HLA associations have been identified in the various ethnic groups studied. In whites, for example, the relative risk of Graves's disease in carriers of the HLA-DR3 haplotype is between 2.5 and 5, whereas lesser associations have been reported for HLA-B8 and the HLA-DQA*0501 allele.[30,31] As with other autoimmune conditions, certain polymorphisms of the T-cell immunoregulatory protein CTLA-4 have also been associated with Graves's disease. Despite these statistical associations, however, even detailed molecular genetic linkage studies have failed to identify specific genes responsible for the disease.[32]

The thyroid gland is diffusely enlarged in the majority of patients and is commonly 40 to 60 g (two to three times the normal size). The surface of the gland is either smooth or bosselated, and the consistency varies from soft to firm. For patients with severe disease, a thrill may be felt and a systolic bruit may be heard over the gland, reflecting the increased intraglandular vascularity typical of hyperplasia. Whereas the presence of any of the extrathyroidal manifestations of this syndrome, including exophthalmos, thyroid acropachy, or pretibial myxedema, in a thyrotoxic patient is pathognomonic of Graves's disease, most patients can be diagnosed on the basis of their history and examination of their diffuse goiter (see Fig. 84–4). An important clinical feature of Graves's disease is the occurrence of spontaneous remissions, albeit uncommon. The abnormalities in TSAb production may decrease or disappear over time in many patients.

The results of laboratory tests in thyrotoxic Graves's disease include an increase in the overall hormone production rate with a disproportionate increase in T_3 relative to T_4 (Table 84–4). In an occasional patient, the disproportionate overproduction of T_3 is

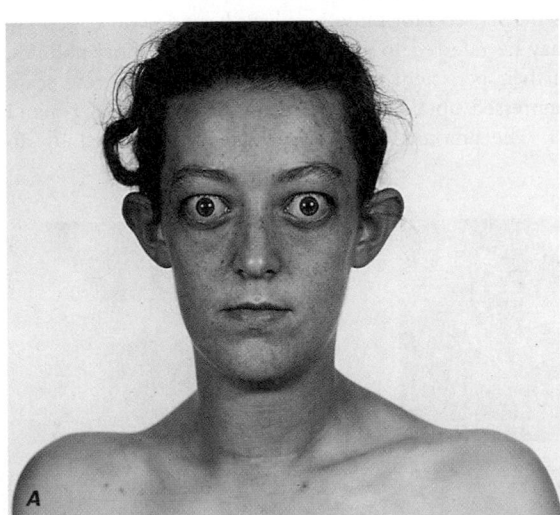

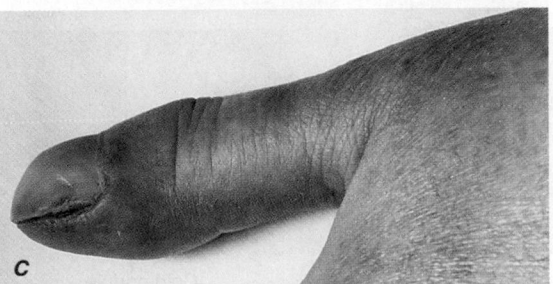

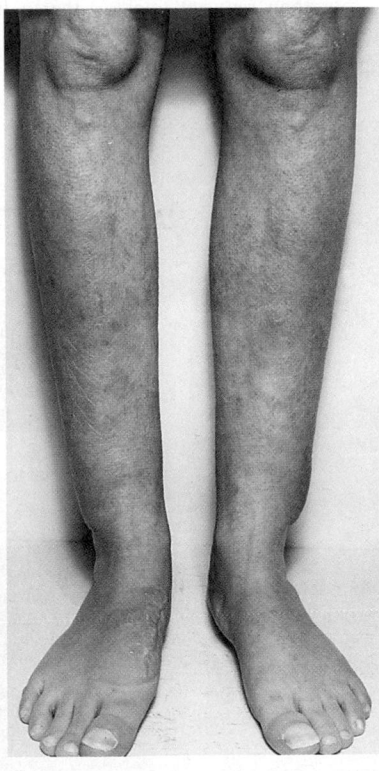

FIGURE 84-4. Features of Graves's disease. (A) Facial appearance in Graves's disease; lid retraction, periorbital edema, and proptosis are marked. (B) Thyroid dermopathy over the lateral aspects of the shins. (C) Thyroid acropachy. *(Reproduced with permission from Fauci AS, Kasper DL, Longo DL, Braunwald E, Havser SL, Jameson JL, Loscalzo J, eds. Harrison's Principles of Internal Medicine, 16th ed. New York: McGraw-Hill, 2005:2114.)*

TABLE 84-4	Thyroid Function Test Results in Different Thyroid Conditions					
	Total T₄	Free T₄	Total T₃	T₃ Resin Uptake	Free Thyroxine Index	TSH
Normal	4.5–1 0.9 mcg/dL	0.8–2.7 ng/dL	60–181 ng/dL	22–34%	1.0–4.3 units	0.5–4.7 milli- international units/L
Hyperthyroid	↑↑	↑↑	↑↑↑	↑	↑↑↑	↓↓
Hypothyroid	↓↓	↓↓	↓	↓↓	↓↓↓	↑↑
Increased TBG	↑	Normal	↑	↓	Normal	Normal

TBG, thyroid-binding globulin; TSH, thyroid-stimulating hormone.

exaggerated, with the result that only the serum T₃ concentration is increased (T₃ toxicosis). The saturation of TBG is increased due to the elevated levels of serum T₄ and T₃, which is reflected in elevated values for the T₃ resin uptake. As a result, the concentration of free T₄, free T₃, and the free T₄ and T₃ indices are increased to an even greater extent than are the measured serum total T₄ and T₃ concentrations. The TSH level will be undetectable due to negative feedback by elevated levels of thyroid hormone at the pituitary.

For the patient with manifest disease, measurement of the serum free T₄ concentration (or total T₄ and T₃ resin uptake), total T₃, and the TSH value will confirm the diagnosis of thyrotoxicosis. If the patient is not pregnant, a 24-hour RAIU should be obtained if there is any diagnostic uncertainty, e.g., recent onset of symptoms or other factors suggestive of thyroiditis. An increased RAIU documents that the thyroid gland is inappropriately utilizing the iodine to produce more thyroid hormone at a time when the patient is thyrotoxic.

Hypokalemic periodic paralysis is a rare complication of hyperthyroidism commonly observed in Asian and Hispanic populations.[33] It presents as recurrent proximal muscle flaccidity ranging from mild weakness to total paralysis. The paralysis may be asymmetric and usually involves muscle groups that are strenuously exercised before the attack. Cognition and sensory perception are spared, whereas deep tendon reflexes are markedly diminished commonly. Hypokalemia results from a sudden shift of potassium from extracellular to intracellular sites rather than reduced total body potassium. High carbohydrate loads and exercise provoke the attacks. Treatment includes correcting the hyperthyroid state, potassium administration, spironolactone to conserve potassium, and propranolol to minimize intracellular shifts.

Trophoblastic Diseases

Human chorionic gonadotropin is a stimulator of the TSH receptor and may cause hyperthyroidism.[34] The basis for the thyrotropic effect of hCG is the structural similarity of hCG to TSH (similar α subunits and unique β subunits). In hyperthyroid patients with very high hCG levels, serum TSH may be inappropriately detectable due to the weak cross-reactivity of hCG in the radioimmunoassay for TSH. For patients with hyperthyroidism caused by trophoblastic tumors, serum hCG levels usually exceed 300 units/mL and always exceed 100 units/mL. The mean peak hCG level in normal pregnancy is 50 units/mL. On a molar basis, hCG has only 1/10,000 the activity of pituitary TSH in mouse bioassays. Nevertheless, this thyrotropic activity may be very substantial for patients with trophoblastic tumors, whose serum hCG concentrations may reach 2,000 units/mL.

THYROID AUTONOMY

Toxic Adenoma

An autonomous thyroid nodule is a discrete thyroid mass whose function is independent of pituitary and TSH control.[35] The prevalence of toxic adenoma ranges from about 2% to 9% of thyrotoxic patients, and depends on iodine availability and geographic location. Toxic adenomas arise from gain-of-function somatic mutations of the TSH receptor or, less commonly, the $G_s\alpha$ protein; more than a dozen TSH receptor mutations have been described.[12] These nodules may be referred to as *toxic adenomas,* or "hot" nodules, because of their persistent uptake on a radioiodine thyroid scan, despite suppressed uptake in the surrounding nonnodular gland (Fig. 84–5). The amount of thyroid hormone produced by an

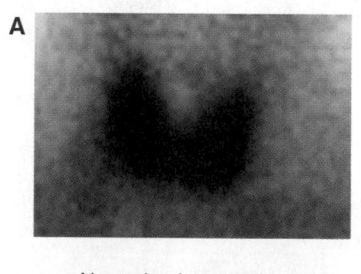

A
Normal to hyperactive

B
Hypoactive

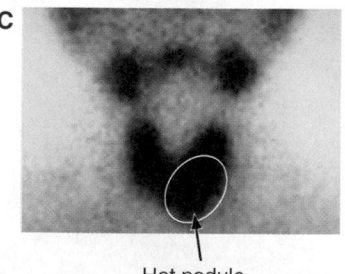

C
Hot nodule

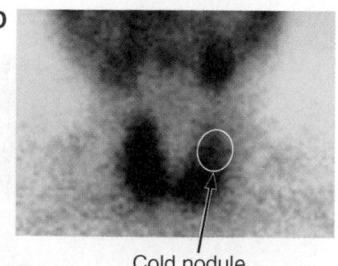

D
Cold nodule

FIGURE 84-5. Radioiodine thyroid scans. A. Normal or increased thyroid uptake of iodine-125 (¹²⁵I). (B) Thyroid with marked decrease in ¹²⁵I uptake in a large palpable mass. C. Increased ¹²⁵I uptake isolated to a single nodule, the "hot nodule." D. Decreased thyroid ¹²⁵I uptake in an isolated region, the "cold nodule." *(Reproduced with permission from Molina PE. Endocrine Physiology, 2nd ed. New York: McGraw-Hill, 2006:90. Images courtesy of Dr. Luis Linares, Memorial Medical Center, New Orleans, LA.)*

autonomous nodule is mass related. Therefore, hyperthyroidism usually occurs with larger nodules (i.e., those >3 cm in diameter). Older patients (>60 years) are more likely (up to 60%) to be thyrotoxic from autonomous nodules than are younger patients (12%). There are many reports of isolated elevation of serum T_3 for patients with autonomously functioning nodules. Therefore, if the T_4 level is normal, a T_3 level must be measured to rule out T_3 toxicosis. If autonomous function is suspected but the TSH is normal, the diagnosis can be confirmed by a failure of the autonomous nodule to decrease its iodine uptake during exogenous T_3 administration sufficient to suppress TSH. Surgical resection, thionamides, percutaneous ethanol injection, and radioactive iodine (RAI) ablation are treatment options, but since thionamides do not halt the proliferative process in the nodule, definitive therapies are recommended.[36] Ethanol ablation may be associated with pain and damage to surrounding extrathyroidal tissues, limiting its acceptance in the United States. It has been hypothesized that sublethal radiation doses received by the surrounding nonnodular thyroid tissue during RAI therapy of toxic nodules may lead to induction of thyroid cancer, and excess thyroid cancer mortality has recently been associated with RAI therapy of toxic nodular disease. Thus, an autonomously functioning nodule, if not large enough to cause thyrotoxicosis, can often be observed conservatively without therapy.

Multinodular Goiters

In multinodular goiters (MNGs; Plummer disease), follicles with autonomous function coexist with normal or even nonfunctioning follicles.[35] The pathogenesis of MNG is thought to be similar to that of toxic adenoma: diffuse hyperplasia caused by goitrogenic stimuli, leading to mutations and clonal expansion of benign neoplasms.[37] The functional status of the nodule(s) depends upon the nature of the underlying mutations, whether activating such as TSH receptor mutations or inhibitory such as ras mutations. Thyrotoxicosis in a MNG occurs when a sufficient mass of autonomous follicles generates enough thyroid hormone to exceed the needs of the patient. It is not surprising that this type of hyperthyroidism develops insidiously over a period of several years and predominantly affects older individuals with long-standing goiters. The patient's complaints of weight loss, depression, anxiety, and insomnia may be attributed to old age. Any unexplained chronic illness in an elderly patient presenting with a MNG calls for the exclusion of hidden thyrotoxicosis.[38] Third-generation TSH assays and T_3 suppression testing may be useful in detecting subclinical hyperthyroidism.[39]

A thyroid scan will show patchy areas of autonomously functioning thyroid tissue intermixed with hypofunctioning areas. When the patient is euthyroid, therapy is based upon the need to reduce goiter size due to mass-related symptoms such as dysphagia. Doses of thyroid hormone sufficient to suppress TSH levels may slow goiter growth or cause some degree of shrinkage, but in general, suppression therapy for nodular disease is inadequate to address mass effect.[40] The preferred treatment for toxic MNG is RAI or surgery. Surgery is usually selected for younger patients and patients in whom large goiters impinge on vital organs. Alternatively, percutaneous injection of 95% ethanol has also been used to destroy single or multinodular adenomas with a 5-year success rate approaching 80%.

CAUSES OF THYROTOXICOSIS ASSOCIATED WITH SUPPRESSED RAIU

Inflammatory Thyroid Disease

Subacute Thyroiditis Painful subacute (granulomatous or deQuervain) thyroiditis often develops after a viral syndrome, but rarely has a specific virus been identified in thyroid parenchyma.[41]

A genetic predisposition exists, with markedly higher risk for developing subacute thyroiditis for patients with HLA-Bw35. Systemic symptoms often accompany the syndrome, including fever, malaise, and myalgia, in addition to those symptoms due to thyrotoxicosis. Typically, patients complain of severe pain in the thyroid region, which often extends to the ear on the affected side.[42] With time, the pain may migrate from one side of the gland to the other. On physical examination, the thyroid gland is firm and exquisitely tender. Signs of thyrotoxicosis are present.

Thyroid function tests typically run a triphasic course. Initially, serum thyroxine levels are elevated due to release of preformed thyroid hormone from disrupted follicles. The 24-hour RAIU during this time is less than 2% due to thyroid inflammation and TSH suppression by the elevated thyroxine level. As the disease progresses, intrathyroidal hormone stores are depleted, and the patient may become mildly hypothyroid with an appropriately elevated TSH level. During the recovery phase, thyroid hormone stores are replenished, and serum TSH concentration gradually returns to normal. Recovery is generally complete within 2 to 6 months. Most patients remain euthyroid, and recurrences of painful thyroiditis are extremely rare. The patient with painful thyroiditis should be reassured that the disease is self-limited and is unlikely to recur. Thyrotoxic symptoms may be relieved with β-blockers. Aspirin (650 mg orally every 6 hours) will usually relieve the pain. Occasionally, prednisone (20 mg orally three times a day) must be used to suppress the inflammatory process. Antithyroid drugs are not indicated because they do not decrease the release of preformed thyroid hormone.

Painless Thyroiditis Since its description in 1975, painless (silent, lymphocytic) thyroiditis has been recognized as a common cause of thyrotoxicosis and may represent up to 15% of cases of thyrotoxicosis in North America.[43] In the setting of development of lymphocytic thyroiditis during the first 12 months after the end of pregnancy, the condition is also called *postpartum thyroiditis*.[44] The etiology is not fully understood and may be heterogeneous, but evidence indicates that autoimmunity underlies most cases. There is an increased frequency of HLA-DR3 and DR5 in patients with painless thyroiditis; nonendocrine autoimmune diseases are also more common. Histologically, diffuse lymphocytic infiltration is generally identified. The triphasic course of this illness mimics that of subacute thyroiditis. Most patients present with mild thyrotoxic symptoms. Lid retraction and lid lag are present, but exophthalmos is absent. The thyroid gland may be diffusely enlarged, but thyroid tenderness is absent.

The 24-hour RAIU will typically be suppressed to less than 2% during the thyrotoxic phase of painless thyroiditis. Antithyroglobulin and antithyroid peroxidase antibody levels are elevated in more than 50% of patients. Patients with mild hyperthyroidism and painless thyroiditis should be reassured that they have a self-limited disease, although patients with postpartum thyroiditis may experience recurrence of the disease with subsequent pregnancies. As with other thyrotoxic syndromes, adrenergic symptoms may be ameliorated with propranolol or metoprolol. Antithyroid drugs, which inhibit new hormone synthesis, are not indicated because they do not decrease the release of preformed thyroid hormone.

Ectopic Thyroid Tissue

Struma Ovarii Struma ovarii is a teratoma of the ovary that contains differentiated thyroid follicular cells and is capable of making thyroid hormone.[45] This extremely rare cause of thyrotoxicosis is suggested by the absence of thyroid enlargement in a thyrotoxic patient with a suppressed RAIU in the neck and no findings to suggest thyroiditis. The diagnosis is established by localizing functioning thyroid tissue in the ovary with whole-body radioactive iodine (^{131}I) scanning. Interestingly, struma ovarii without associated hyperthyroidism is much more common than struma ovarii associated with hyperthyroidism. Because the tissue is neoplastic and potentially malignant, combined surgical and radioiodine treatment of malignant struma ovarii for both monitoring and therapy of relapse is the recommended treatment.

Thyroid Cancer In widely metastatic differentiated papillary or follicular carcinomas with relatively well-preserved function, sufficient thyroid hormone can be synthesized and secreted to produce thyrotoxicosis.[46,47] In most instances, a previous diagnosis of thyroid malignancy has been made. The diagnosis can be confirmed by whole-body ^{131}I scanning. Treatment with ^{131}I is generally effective at ablating functioning thyroid metastases.

Exogenous Sources of Thyroid Hormone

Thyrotoxicosis factitia is produced by the ingestion of exogenous thyroid hormone.[48] Obesity is the most common nonthyroidal disorder for which thyroid hormone is inappropriately used, but thyroid hormone has been used for almost every conceivable problem from menstrual irregularities and infertility to hypercholesterolemia and baldness. There is little evidence to suggest that treatment with thyroid hormone is beneficial for such conditions in euthyroid individuals. Obviously, thyrotoxicosis factitia can also occur when too large a dose of thyroid hormone is employed for conditions in which it is likely to be beneficial, such as differentiated thyroid carcinoma. Rarely, thyrotoxicosis factitia is caused by the purposeful and secretive ingestion of thyroid hormone by disturbed patients (usually with a medical background) who wish to obtain attention or lose weight.

Thyrotoxicosis factitia should be suspected in a thyrotoxic patient without evidence of increased hormone production, thyroidal inflammation, or ectopic thyroid tissue. The RAIU uptake is at low levels because the patient's thyroid gland function is suppressed by the exogenous thyroid hormone.[49] Measurement of plasma thyroglobulin (TG) is a valuable laboratory aid in the diagnosis of thyrotoxicosis factitia. TG is normally secreted in small amounts by the thyroid gland; however, when thyroid hormone is taken orally, TG levels tend to be lower than the normal range. In other entities characterized by a low RAIU, such as thyroiditis, leakage of preformed thyroid hormone results in elevated TG levels. If a history of thyroid hormone ingestion is elicited or deduced, exogenous thyroid hormone should be withheld for between 4 and 6 weeks, and thyroid function tests repeated to document that the euthyroid state has been restored. Rarely, thyroid hormone analogues or metabolites may be the drug of abuse, specific detection of which may be difficult with standard thyroid hormone assays. For example, tiratricol [triiodothyroacetic acid (TRIAC)], an endogenous metabolite of T_3 that has been used for weight loss and paradoxically by body builders, will suppress TSH at high enough doses and may cross-react in many T_3 immunoassays; thus, thyrotoxicosis factitia due to tiratricol abuse may be misinterpreted as T_3 toxicosis.[50]

Amiodarone may induce thyrotoxicosis (2% to 3% of patients), overt hypothyroidism (5% of patients), subclinical hypothyroidism (25% of patients), or euthyroid hyperthyroxinema, depending upon the underlying thyroid pathology or lack thereof.[51] Because amiodarone contains 37% iodine by weight, approximately 6 mg/day of iodine is released for each 200 mg of amiodarone, 1,000 times greater than the recommended daily amount of iodine of 200 mcg/day. As a result of this iodine overload, iodine-exacerbated thyroid dysfunction commonly occurs among those patients with preexisting thyroid disease: thyrotoxicosis in patients with hyperthyroidism or euthyroid nodular autonomy

and hypothyroidism in patients with autoimmune thyroid disease. In contrast to hyperthyroidism with increased synthesis of thyroid hormone induced by amiodarone (type I), destructive thyroiditis with loss of TG and thyroid hormones also occurs (type II), typically among individuals with otherwise normal glands. The two types of amiodarone-induced thyrotoxicosis may be differentiated using color flow Doppler ultrasonography. Such distinction is critically important, given the therapeutic implications of the two syndromes: type I amiodarone-induced hyperthyroidism responds somewhat to thionamides, whereas type II may respond to glucocorticoids or iopanoic acid.[52-54] Unfortunately, however, the latter agent is no longer available. Obviously, RAI therapy is inappropriate in type I due to the drug-induced iodine excess, and in type II due to lack of increased hormone synthesis. The manifestations of amiodarone-induced thyrotoxicosis may be atypical symptoms such as ventricular tachycardia and exacerbation of underlying chronic obstructive pulmonary disease, both of which are even more significant given the severe underlying cardiac pathology that led to the use of the drug in the first place. Amiodarone also directly interferes with type I 5'-deiodinase, leading to reduced conversion of T_4 to T_3 and hyperthyroxinemia without thyrotoxicosis.

TREATMENT

Hyperthyroidism

■ DESIRED OUTCOMES

❸ Three common treatment modalities are used in the management of hyperthyroidism: surgery, antithyroid medications, and radioactive iodine (RAI) (Table 84–5). The overall therapeutic objectives are to eliminate the excess thyroid hormone and minimize the symptoms and long-term consequences of hyperthyroidism. Therapy must be individualized based on the type and severity of hyperthyroidism, patient age and gender, existence of nonthyroidal conditions, and response to previous therapy.[55,56] Clinical guidelines for the treatment of hyperthyroidism have been published by various groups.[57-59]

■ NONPHARMACOLOGIC THERAPY

Surgical removal of the hypersecreting thyroid gland became feasible in 1923 when Plummer discovered that iodine reduced the gland's vascularity, making this definitive procedure possible. Surgery should be considered for patients with a large thyroid gland (>80 g), severe ophthalmopathy, and a lack of remission on antithyroid drug treatment. In case of cosmetic or pressure symptoms, the choice in MNG stands between surgery, which is still the first choice, and radioiodine if uptake is adequate (hot). In addition to surgery, the solitary nodule, whether hot or cold, can be treated with percutaneous ethanol injection therapy. If hot, radioiodine is the therapy of choice.[60] Traditional preparation of the patient for thyroidectomy includes propylthiouracil (PTU) or methimazole (MMI) until the patient is biochemically euthyroid (usually 6 to 8 weeks), followed by the addition of iodides (500 mg/day) for 10 to 14 days before surgery to decrease the vascularity of the gland. Iodine supplementation in iodine-deficient areas of the country may lead to a greater reduction in remnant volume in nontoxic goiter.[61] Propranolol for several weeks preoperatively and 7 to 10 days after surgery has also been used to maintain a pulse rate of less than 90 beats/min. Combined pretreatment with propranolol and 10 to 14 days of potassium iodide also has been advocated.

TABLE 84-5 Treatments for Hyperthyroidism Caused by Graves's Disease

Treatment	Advantages	Disadvantages	Comment
Antithyroid drugs	Noninvasive Lower initial cost Low risk of permanent hypothyroidism Possible remissions due to immune effects	Low cure rate (30%–80%; average 40%–50%) Adverse drug reactions Drug compliance	First-line treatment in children, adolescents, and in pregnancy Initial treatment in severe cases or preoperative preparation
Radioactive iodine (^{131}I)	Cure of hyperthyroidism Most cost effective	Permanent hypothyroidism almost inevitable Might worsen ophthalmopathy Pregnancy must be deferred for 6–12 months; no breast-feeding Small potential risk of exacerbation of hyperthyroidism	Best treatment for toxic nodules and toxic multinodular goiter
Surgery	Rapid, effective treatment, especially in patients with large goiters	Most invasive Potential complications (recurrent laryngeal nerve damage, hypoparathyroidism) Most costly Permanent hypothyroidism Pain, scar	Potential in pregnancy if major side-effect from antithyroid drugs Useful when coexisting suspicious nodule present Option for patients who refuse radioiodine

The overall morbidity rate with surgery is 2.7%. Hyperthyroidism persists or recurs in 0.6% to 17.9% of patients after thyroidectomy for Graves's disease and is more common in children. The most common complications of surgery include hypothyroidism (up to about 49%), hypoparathyroidism (up to 3.9%), and vocal cord abnormalities (up to 5.4%). The frequent occurrence of hypothyroidism following surgery requires periodic follow-up for identification and treatment of these patients.[62,63]

■ PHARMACOLOGIC THERAPY

Antithyroid Medications

Thiourea Drugs ❹ Two drugs within this category, PTU and MMI, are approved for the treatment of hyperthyroidism in the United States.[64] They are classified as thioureylenes (thionamides), which incorporate an N—C—S =N group into their ring structures.

Mechanism of action. PTU and MMI share several mechanisms to inhibit the biosynthesis of thyroid hormone.[20] These drugs serve as preferential substrates for the iodinating intermediate of thyroid peroxidase and divert iodine away from potential iodination sites in TG. This prevents subsequent incorporation of iodine into iodotyrosines and ultimately iodothyronine ("organification"). Second, they inhibit coupling of monoiodotyrosine and diiodotyrosine to form T_4 and T_3. The coupling reaction may be more sensitive to these drugs than the iodination reaction. Experimentally, these drugs exhibit immunosuppressive effects, although the clinical relevance of this finding is unclear. For patients with Graves's disease, antithyroid drug treatment has been associated with lower TSAb titers and restoration of normal suppressor T-cell function. However, perchlorate, which has a different mechanism of action, also decreases TSAbs, suggesting that normalization of the thyroid hormone level may itself improve the abnormal immune function. PTU inhibits the peripheral conversion of T_4 to T_3. This effect is acutely dose-related and occurs within hours of PTU administration. MMI does not have this effect. Over time, depletion of stored hormone and lack of continuing synthesis of thyroid hormone results in the clinical effects of these drugs.

Pharmacokinetics. Both antithyroid drugs are well absorbed (80% to 95%) from the gastrointestinal tract, with peak serum concentrations about 1 hour after ingestion. The plasma half-life ranges of PTU and MMI are 1 to 2.5 hours and 6 to 9 hours, respectively, and are not appreciably affected by thyroid status. Urinary excretion is about 35% for PTU and less than 10% for MMI. These drugs are actively concentrated in the thyroid gland, which may account for the disparity between their relatively short plasma half-lives and the effectiveness of once daily dosing regimens even with PTU. Approximately 60% to 80% of PTU is bound to plasma albumin, whereas MMI is not protein bound. Methimazole readily crosses the placenta and appears in breast milk. Older studies suggested that PTU crosses the placental membranes only one tenth as well as MMI; however, these studies were done in the course of therapeutic abortion early in pregnancy. Newer studies show little difference between fetal concentrations of PTU and MMI, and both are associated with elevated TSH in about 20% and low T_4 in about 7% of the fetuses.[65]

❺ ***Dosing and monitoring.*** PTU is available as 50 mg tablets, and MMI as 5 and 10 mg tablets. MMI is approximately 10 times more potent than PTU. Initial therapy with PTU ranges from 300 to 600 mg daily, usually in three or four divided doses. MMI is given in two or three divided doses totaling 30 to 60 mg/day. Although the traditional recommendation is for divided doses, evidence exists that both drugs can be given as single daily doses. Patients with severe hyperthyroidism may require larger initial doses, and some may respond better at these larger doses if the dose is divided. The maximal blocking doses of PTU and MMI are 1,200 and 120 mg daily, respectively. Once the intrathyroidal pool of thyroid hormone is reduced and new hormone synthesis is sufficiently blocked, clinical improvement should ensue. Usually within 4 to 8 weeks of initiating therapy, symptoms will diminish and circulating thyroid hormone levels will return to normal. At this time the tapering regimen can be started. Changes in dose for each drug should be made on a monthly basis, because the endogenously produced T_4 will reach a new steady-state concentration in this interval. Typical ranges of daily maintenance doses for PTU and MMI are 50 to 300 mg and 5 to 30 mg, respectively.

If the objective of therapy is to induce a long-term remission, the patient should remain on continuous antithyroid drug therapy for 12 to 24 months. Antithyroid drug therapy induces permanent remission rates of 10% to 98%, with an overall average of about 40% to 50%.[66] This is much higher than the remission rate seen with propranolol alone, which is reported to range from 22% to 36%. Patient characteristics for a favorable outcome include older patients (>40 years), low ratio of T_4 to T_3 (<20), a small goiter (<50 g), short duration of disease (<6 months), no previous history of relapse with antithyroid drugs, duration of therapy 1 to 2 years or longer, and low TSAb titers at baseline or a reduction with treatment.[20] It is important that patients be followed every 6 to 12 months after remission occurs.

6 If a relapse occurs, alternate therapy with RAI is preferred to a second course of antithyroid drugs. Relapses seem to plateau after about 5 years and eventually 5% to 20% of patients will develop spontaneous hypothyroidism.

There has been interest in whether concurrent administration of T4 with thionamide therapy for thyrotoxicosis and subclinical hyperthyroidism can reduce autoantibodies directed toward the thyroid gland and improve remission rate. In a Japanese study, adjunctive treatment with thyroxine was associated with a 20-fold reduction in the recurrence rate of Graves's disease compared with the recurrence rate seen for patients treated with antithyroid drugs alone.[67] Attempts to reproduce these results in American and European patients with Graves's disease have failed to show any delay or reduction in the recurrence of Graves's disease with thyroxine administration.[68]

Adverse effects. Minor adverse reactions to PTU and MMI have an overall incidence of 5% to 25% depending on the dose and the drug, whereas major adverse effects occur in 1.5% to 4.6% of patients receiving these drugs.[64,69] Pruritic maculopapular rashes (sometimes associated with vasculitis based on skin biopsy), arthralgias, and fevers occur in up to 5% of patients and may occur at greater frequency with higher doses and in children. Rashes often disappear spontaneously but, if persistent, may be managed with antihistamines.

Perhaps one of the most common side effects is a benign transient leukopenia characterized by a white blood cell (WBC) count of less than 4,000/mm³. This condition occurs in up to 12% of adults and 25% of children, and sometimes can be confused with mild leukopenia seen in Graves's disease. This mild leukopenia is not a harbinger of the more serious adverse effect of agranulocytosis, so therapy can usually be continued. If a minor adverse reaction occurs with one antithyroid drug, the alternate thiourea may be tried, but cross-sensitivity occurs for about 50% of patients.[64]

Agranulocytosis is one of the serious adverse effects of thiourea drug therapy and is characterized by fever, malaise, gingivitis, oropharyngeal infection, and a granulocyte count less than 250/mm³.[64] These drugs are concentrated in granulocytes, and this reaction may represent a direct toxic effect rather than hypersensitivity. This toxic reaction has occurred with both thioureas, and the incidence varies from 0.5% to 6%. It is higher for patients over age 40 receiving a MMI dose greater than 40 mg/day or the equivalent dose of PTU, and is linked to HLA class II genes containing the DRB1*08032 allele.[70] Agranulocytosis usually develops in the first 3 months of therapy. Because the onset is sudden, routine monitoring is not recommended. Colony-stimulating factors have been used with some success to restore cell counts to normal, but it is unclear how effective this form of therapy is compared to routine supportive care.[71,72] Peripheral lymphocytes obtained from patients with PTU-induced agranulocytosis undergo transformation in the presence of other thioamides, suggesting that these severe reactions are immunologically mediated and patients should not receive other thionamides. Aplastic anemia has been reported with MMI and may be associated with an inhibitor to colony-forming units. Once antithyroid drugs are discontinued, clinical improvement is seen over several days to weeks. Patients should be counseled to discontinue therapy and contact their physician when flu-like symptoms such as fever, malaise, or sore throat develop.

Arthralgias and a lupus-like syndrome (sometimes in the absence of antinuclear antibodies) have been reported in 4% to 5% of patients. This generally occurs after 6 months of therapy. Uncommonly, polymyositis, presenting as proximal muscle weakness and elevated creatine phosphokinase, has been reported with PTU administration. Gastrointestinal intolerance is also reported to occur in 4% to 5% of patients. Patients receiving

interferon products for hepatitis C or other disorders may develop hyper- or hypothyroidism along with liver enzyme abnormalities.[73] Hypoprothrombinemia is a rare complication of thionamide therapy. Patients who have experienced a major adverse reaction to one thiourea drug should not be converted to the alternate drug because of cross-sensitivity.

Older reports suggested that congenital skin defects (aplasia cutis) may be caused by MMI and carbimazole, although a registry review from the Netherlands could not find an association between maternal use of these drugs and skin defects.[74] However, more recently, several serious congenital malformations including tracheoesophageal fistulas and choanal atresia have been observed with MMI and carbimazole but not PTU use during pregnancy.[75–77] Thus, in the past, PTU was considered the drug of choice throughout pregnancy for women with hyperthyroidism, because of concerns about the possible teratogenic effects of MMI. However, currently heightened concerns about the greater hepatoxicity of PTU than MMI have led to the recommendation that PTU no longer be considered a first-line drug, except during the first trimester of pregnancy.

Hepatoxicity can be seen with both MMI and PTU with a prevalence of approximately 1.3%. In mice, MMI undergoes epoxidation of the C-4,5 double bond by cytochrome P450 enzymes, and after being hydrolyzed, the resulting epoxide is decomposed to form N-methylthiourea, a proximate toxicant.[78,79] At moderate doses, some authors have found that initial enzyme elevations eventually normalize in most patients with continued therapy.[78] PTU-induced subclinical liver injury is common and is usually transient and asymptomatic.[80] Thus, it has generally been thought that therapy with PTU may be continued with caution in the absence of symptoms and hyperbilirubinemia. However, a 1997 literature review documented 49 cases of hepatoxicity. Twenty-eight cases were associated with PTU use, and 21 cases were associated with MMI use. The hepatoxicity was associated with seven deaths and three deaths in the PTU and MMI groups, respectively.[81] There did not appear to be a relationship between the dose or duration of thionamide treatment and outcome. During the past 20 years of PTU use in the United States, 22 adults developed severe hepatoxcitiy leading to nine deaths and five liver transplants. The risk of this complication was greater in children (1:2,000) than in adults (1:10,000). In light of such evidence, it was recommended by the American Thyroid Association and the United States and the Food and Drug Administration that PTU not be considered as first-line therapy in either adults or children.[81,82] One of three exceptions includes the first trimester of pregnancy, when the risk of MMI-induced embryopathy may exceed that of PTU-induced hepatotoxicity.

Iodides Iodide was the first form of drug therapy for Graves's disease. Its mechanism of action is to acutely block thyroid hormone release, inhibit thyroid hormone biosynthesis by interfering with intrathyroidal iodide utilization (the Wolff-Chaikoff effect), and decrease the size and vascularity of the gland. This early inhibitory effect provides symptom improvement within 2 to 7 days of initiating therapy, and serum T_4 and T_3 concentrations may be reduced for a few weeks. Despite the reduced release of T_4 and T_3, thyroid hormone synthesis continues at an accelerated rate, resulting in a gland rich in stored hormones. The normal and hyperfunctioning thyroid soon escapes from this inhibitory effect within 1 to 2 weeks by decreasing the active transfer of iodide into the gland. Iodides are often used as adjunctive therapy to prepare a patient with Graves's disease for surgery, to acutely inhibit thyroid hormone release and quickly attain the euthyroid state in severely thyrotoxic patients with cardiac decompensation, or to inhibit thyroid hormone release following radioactive iodine therapy. However, large doses of iodine may exacerbate hyperthyroidism or indeed precipitate hyperthyroidism in some previously euthyroid individuals (Jod-Basedow disease).[83] This Jod-Basedow phenomenon is most common in iodine-deficient areas, particularly for patients with preexisting nontoxic goiter. Iodide is contraindicated in toxic MNG.

Potassium iodide is available either as a saturated solution (SSKI), which contains 38 mg of iodide per drop, or as Lugol solution, which contains 6.3 mg of iodide per drop. The typical starting dose of SSKI is 3 to 10 drops daily (120 to 400 mg) in water or juice. There is no documented advantage to using doses in excess of 6 to 8 mg/day. When used to prepare a patient for surgery, it should be administered 7 to 14 days preoperatively. As an adjunct to RAI, SSKI should not be used before, but rather 3 to 7 days after RAI treatment, so that the radioactive iodide can concentrate in the thyroid. The most frequent toxic effect with iodide therapy is hypersensitivity reactions (skin rashes, drug fever, rhinitis, and conjunctivitis); salivary gland swelling; "iodism" (metallic taste, burning mouth and throat, sore teeth and gums, symptoms of a head cold, and sometimes stomach upset and diarrhea); and gynecomastia.

Other compounds containing organic iodide have also been used therapeutically for hyperthyroidism. These include various radiologic contrast media that share a triiodo- and monoaminobenzene ring with a propionic acid chain (e.g., iopanoic acid and sodium ipodate). The effect of these compounds is a result of the iodine content inhibiting thyroid hormone release as well as competitive inhibition of $5'$-monodeiodinase conversion related to their structures, which resemble thyroid analogs.[84] Unfortunately, these extremely useful agents are no longer available in the United States

Adrenergic Blockers ❼ Because many of the manifestations of hyperthyroidism are mediated by β-adrenergic receptors, β-blockers (especially propranolol) have been used widely to ameliorate thyrotoxic symptoms such as palpitations, anxiety, tremor, and heat intolerance. Although β-blockers are quite effective for symptom control, they have no effect on the urinary excretion of calcium, phosphorus, hydroxyproline, creatinine, or various amino acids, suggesting a lack of effect on peripheral thyrotoxicosis and protein metabolism. Furthermore, β-blockers do not reduce TSAb nor prevent thyroid storm. Propranolol and nadolol partially block the conversion of T_4 to T_3, but this contribution to the overall therapeutic effect is small in magnitude. Inhibition of conversion of T_4 to T_3 is mediated by d-propranolol, which is devoid of β-blocking activity, and l-propranolol, which is responsible for the antiadrenergic effects, has little effect on the conversion.

β-Blockers are usually used as adjunctive therapy with antithyroid drugs, RAI, or iodides when treating Graves's disease or toxic nodules; in preparation for surgery; or in thyroid storm. The only conditions for which β-blockers are primary therapy for thyrotoxicosis are those associated with thyroiditis. The dose of propranolol required to relieve adrenergic symptoms is variable, but an initial dose of 20 to 40 mg four times daily is effective (heart rate <90 beats/min) for most patients. Younger or more severely toxic patients may require as much as 240 to 480 mg/day because there seems to be an increased clearance rate for these patients. β-Blockers are contraindicated for patients with decompensated heart failure unless it is caused solely by tachycardia (high output). Nonselective agents and those lacking intrinsic sympathomimetic activity should be used with caution for patients with asthma and bronchospastic chronic obstructive lung disease. β-Blockers that are cardioselective and have intrinsic sympathomimetic activity may have a slight margin of safety in these situations. Other patients in whom contraindications exist are those with sinus bradycardia, those receiving monoamine oxidase inhibitors or tricyclic antidepressants, and those with spontaneous hypoglycemia. β-Blockers may also prolong gestation and labor during pregnancy. Other side effects include nausea, vomiting, anxiety, insomnia, light-headedness, bradycardia, and hematologic disturbances.

Antiadrenergic agents such as centrally acting sympatholytics and calcium channel antagonists may have some role in the symptomatic treatment of hyperthyroidism. These drugs might be useful when contraindications to β-blockade exist. When compared with nadolol 40 mg twice daily, clonidine 150 mcg twice daily reduced plasma catecholamines, whereas nadolol increased both epinephrine and norepinephrine after 1 week of treatment. Diltiazem 120 mg given every 8 hours reduced heart rate by 17%; fewer ventricular extrasystoles were noted after 10 days of therapy, and diltiazem has been shown to be comparable to propranolol in lowering heart rate and blood pressure.

Radioactive Iodine Although other radioisotopes have been used to ablate thyroid tissue, sodium iodide-131 (^{131}I) is considered to be the agent of choice for Graves's disease, toxic autonomous nodules, and toxic MNGs.[85,86] RAI is administered as a colorless and tasteless liquid that is well absorbed and concentrates in the thyroid. Sodium iodide-131 is a β- and γ-emitter with a tissue penetration of 2 mm and a half-life of 8 days. Other organs take up ^{131}I, but the thyroid gland is the only organ in which organification of the absorbed iodine takes place. Initially, RAI disrupts hormone synthesis by incorporating into thyroid hormones and TG. Over a period of weeks, follicles that have taken up RAI, and surrounding follicles develop evidence of cellular necrosis, breakdown of follicles, development of bizarre cell forms, nuclear pyknosis, and destruction of small vessels within the gland, leading to edema and fibrosis of the interstitial tissue. Predictors of successful treatment with RAI include higher ablative dose, female gender, lower free thyroxine levels at diagnosis, and absence of a palpable goiter.[87] Pregnancy is an absolute contraindication to the use of RAI since radiation will be delivered to the fetal tissue, including the fetal thyroid.

β-Blockers may be given any time without compromising RAI therapy, accounting for their role as a mainstay of adjunctive therapy to RAI treatment. If iodides are administered, they should be given 3 to 7 days after RAI to prevent interference with the uptake of RAI in the thyroid gland. Because thyroid hormone levels will transiently increase following RAI treatment due to release of preformed thyroid hormone, patients with cardiac disease and elderly patients are often treated with thionamides prior to RAI ablation. Occasionally, for patients with underlying cardiac disease, it may be necessary to reinstitute antithyroid drug therapy following radioactive iodine ablation. The standard practice is to withdraw the thionamide 4 to 6 days prior to RAI treatment and to reinstitute it 4 days after therapy is concluded. Administering antithyroid drug therapy following RAI treatment may result in a higher rate of posttreatment recurrence or persistent hyperthyroidism.[86] Pretreatment with PTU may lead to higher rates of treatment failure, but this does not appear to be the case with MMI pretreatment.[88,89] Use of lithium, as adjunctive therapy to RAI therapy, has multiple benefits of increasing the cure rate, shortening the time to cure, and preventing posttherapy increase in thyroid hormone levels.[90] Lithium is likely to achieve these effects by increasing RAI retention in the thyroid and inhibiting thyroid hormone release from the gland.

Corticosteroid administration will blunt and delay the rise in antibodies to the TSH receptor, TG, and thyroid peroxidase while reducing T_3 and T_4 concentrations following RAI. Bartalena and associates found no progression in ophthalmopathy for patients receiving prednisone after RAI compared with MMI (2% to 3% worsened) or no other treatment (5% with persistent worsening).[49] Theoretically, if shared thyroidal and orbital antigen is involved in the pathogenesis of Graves's ophthalmopathy, antigen released with RAI treatment could aggravate preexisting eye disease. Note also that thyroid ablation may decrease eye disease in the long term by removing the source of antigen, but it is unclear if RAI differs from surgery or thionamide for the risk of worsening eye disease.[91]

Destruction of the gland attenuates the hyperthyroid state, and hypothyroidism commonly occurs months to years following RAI.[92] The goal of therapy is to destroy overactive thyroid cells, and a single dose of 4,000 to 8,000 rad results in a euthyroid state in 60% of patients at 6 months or less. The remaining 40% become euthyroid within 1 year, requiring two or more doses. It is advisable that a second dose of RAI be given 6 months after the first RAI treatment if the patient remains hyperthyroid. Variables that predict an unsuccessful outcome of RAI include gender (men are less likely to develop hypothyroidism), race, the size of the thyroid (euthyroidism is less likely in large glands), severity of disease, and perhaps a higher level of TSAb. In a recent study predictors of successful treatment with RAI included higher ablative dose, female gender, lower free thyroxine levels at diagnosis, and absence of a palpable goiter.[93] The acute, short-term side effects of ^{131}I therapy are minimal and include mild thyroidal tenderness and dysphagia. Concern over increased risk of mutations and congenital defects now appears to be unfounded because long-term follow-up studies have not revealed increased risk for these complications.[94] In studies examining the risk of malignancies after RAI therapy, there seems to be a small but significant increase in the risk of cancer of the small bowel and thyroid.[94] Although RAI is very effective in the treatment of hyperthyroidism, long-term follow-up from Great Britain suggests that among patients with hyperthyroidism treated with RAI, mortality from all causes and mortality resulting from cardiovascular and cerebrovascular disease and fracture are increased.[95]

A common approach to Graves's hyperthyroidism is to administer a single dose of 5 to 15 mCi (80 to 200 μCi/g of tissue).[86] The optimal method for determining ^{131}I treatment doses for Graves's hyperthyroidism is unknown, and techniques have varied from a fixed dose to more elaborate calculations based on gland size, iodine uptake, and iodine turnover. In a trial of 88 patients with Graves's disease, no difference in outcome was seen among high or low, fixed or adjusted doses.[96] Thyroid glands estimated to weigh >80 g may require larger doses of RAI. Larger doses are likely to induce hypothyroidism and are seldom given outside the United States due to the imposition of stringent safety restrictions. For example, in the United Kingdom, a nursery school teacher is advised to stay out of school for 3 weeks following a 15 mCi dose of [131]I.[97]

EVALUATION OF THERAPEUTIC OUTCOMES: HYPERTHYROIDISM

After therapy (surgery, thionamides, or RAI) for hyperthyroidism has been initiated, patients should be evaluated on a monthly basis until they reach a euthyroid condition. Clinical signs of continuing thyrotoxicosis (tachycardia, weight loss, and heat intolerance, among others) or the development of hypothyroidism (bradycardia, weight gain, and lethargy, among others) should be noted. β-Blockers may be used to control symptoms of thyrotoxicosis until the definitive treatment has returned the patient to a euthyroid state. Once thyroxine replacement is initiated, the goal is to maintain both the free thyroxine level and the TSH concentration in the normal range. Once a stable dose of thyroxine is identified, the patient may be followed up every 6 to 12 months.

Finally, a common, potentially confusing clinical situation should be mentioned. Why are the TSH concentrations suppressed for some patients who are clinically hypothyroid and who have a low free T_4 level? For patients with long-standing hyperthyroidism, the pituitary thyrotrophs responsible for making TSH become atrophic. The average amount of time required for these cells to resume normal functioning is 6 to 8 weeks.[98] Therefore, if a thyrotoxic patient has his or her free T_4 concentration lowered rapidly, before the thyrotrophs resume normal function, a period of "transient central hypothyroidism" will be observed.

SPECIAL CONDITIONS

Graves's Disease And Pregnancy[99]

Inappropriate production of hCG is a cause of abnormal thyroid function tests during the first half of pregnancy, and hCG can cause either subclinical (normal T_4, suppressed TSH) or overt hyperthyroidism.[100,101] This is because the homology of hCG and TSH leads to hCG-mediated stimulation through the TSH receptor. A recent study showed that at hCG concentrations greater than 400,000 international units/L, TSH levels were invariably suppressed and free thyroxine levels were generally above the normal range. Most patients with hCG greater than 200,000 international units/L did not have symptoms of hyperthyroidism.[102] The variability of the thyrotropic potency of hCG is believed to depend on its carbohydrate composition.

Hyperthyroidism during pregnancy is almost solely caused by Graves's disease, with approximately 0.1% to 0.4% of pregnancies affected. Although the increased metabolic rate is usually well tolerated in pregnant women, two symptoms suggestive of hyperthyroidism during pregnancy are failure to gain weight despite good appetite and persistent tachycardia. There is no increase in maternal mortality or morbidity in well-controlled patients; however, postpartum thyroid storm has been reported in about 20% of untreated individuals. Fetal loss is also more common, due to the facts that spontaneous abortion and premature delivery are more common in untreated pregnant women, as are low-birth-weight infants and eclampsia. Transplacental passage of TSAb may occur, causing fetal as well as neonatal hyperthyroidism.[103] An uncommon cause of hyperthyroidism is molar pregnancy; women present with a large-for-dates uterus and evacuation of the uterus is the preferred management approach.[104]

Because RAI is contraindicated in pregnancy and surgery is usually not recommended (especially during the first trimester), antithyroid drug therapy is usually the treatment of choice. Methimazole readily crosses the placenta and appears in breast milk.

PTU is considered the drug of choice during the first trimester of pregnancy, with the lowest possible doses used to maintain the maternal T_4 level in the high-normal range.[82,87] During this period the risk of MMI-associated embryopathy is believed to outweigh that of PTU-associated hepatotoxicity. To prevent fetal goiter and suppression of fetal thyroid function, PTU is usually prescribed in daily doses of 300 mg or less and tapered to 50 to 150 mg daily after 4 to 6 weeks. PTU doses of less than 200 mg daily are unlikely to produce fetal goiter.[105] During the second and third trimesters, when the critical period of organogenesis is complete, MMI is thought to be the drug of choice because of the greater risk of hepatotoxicity with PTU.[82,87] Thionamide doses should be adjusted to maintain free T4 within 10% of the upper normal limit of the nonpregnant reference range.[99] During the last trimester, TSAbs fall spontaneously, and some patients will go into remission so that antithyroid drug doses may be reduced. A rebound in maternal hyperthyroidism occurs in about 10% of women and may require more intensive treatment postpartum than in the last trimester of pregnancy.[103] For example, a recent study of patients who were euthyroid after thionamide discontinuation and subsequently became pregnant showed a relative risk of a relapse of hyperthyroidism of 4.26 ocurring 4 to 8 months after delivery.[106]

Neonatal and Pediatric Hyperthyroidism

Following delivery, some babies of hyperthyroid mothers will be hyperthyroid due to placental transfer of TSAbs, which stimulates thyroid hormone production in utero and postpartum.[107,108] This is likely if the maternal TSAb titers were quite high. The disease is usually expressed 7 to 10 days postpartum and treatment with antithyroid drugs (PTU 5 to 10 mg/kg per day or MMI 0.5 to 1 mg/kg per day) may be needed for as long as 8 to 12 weeks until the antibody is cleared (immunoglobulin G half-life is about 2 weeks). Iodide (potassium iodide 1 drop per day or Lugol solution 1 to 3 drops per day) and sodium ipodate may be used for the first few days to acutely inhibit hormone release.

Childhood hyperthyroidism has classically been managed with either PTU or MMI. Long-term follow-up studies suggest that this form of therapy is quite acceptable, with 25% of a cohort experiencing remission every 2 years.[109] Again, current recommendations suggest use of MMI as a first-line agent in both adults and children.

Thyroid Storm

Thyroid storm is a life-threatening medical emergency characterized by decompensated thyrotoxicosis, high fever (often >103°F), tachycardia, tachypnea, dehydration, delirium, coma, nausea, vomiting, and diarrhea.[22] Although Graves's disease and less commonly toxic nodular goiter are usually the underlying thyrotoxic pathology, at least two cases of subacute thyroiditis leading to thyroid storm have been reported.[110-112] Precipitating factors for thyroid storm include infection, trauma, surgery, RAI treatment, and withdrawal from antithyroid drugs. Although the duration of clinical decompensation lasts for an average duration of 72 hours, symptoms may persist up to 8 days. With aggressive treatment, the mortality rate has been lowered to 20%. The following therapeutic measures should be instituted promptly: (1) suppression of thyroid hormone formation and secretion, (2) antiadrenergic therapy, (3) administration of corticosteroids, and (4) treatment of associated complications or coexisting factors that may have precipitated the storm. Specific agents used in thyroid storm are outlined in Table 84-6. PTU in large doses is generally the preferred thionamide because, in addition to interfering with the production of thyroid hormones, it also blocks the peripheral conversion of T_4 to T_3. A theoretical advantage of MMI is that it has a longer duration of action. If patients are unable to take medications orally, the tablets can be crushed into suspension and instilled by gastric or rectal tube[113] or given intravenously.[114] Iodides, which rapidly block the release of preformed thyroid hormone, should be administered after PTU is initiated to inhibit iodide utilization by the overactive gland. If iodide is administered

TABLE 84-6	Drug Dosages Used in the Management of Thyroid Storm
Drug	**Regimen**
Propylthiouracil	900–1,200 mg/day orally in four or six divided doses
Methimazole	90–120 mg/day orally in four or six divided doses
Sodium iodide	Up to 2 g/day IV in single or divided doses
Lugol's solution	5–10 drops three times a day in water or juice
Saturated solution of potassium iodide	1–2 drops three times a day in water or juice
Propranolol	40–80 mg every 6 h
Dexamethasone	5–20 mg/day orally or IV in divided doses
Prednisone	25–100 mg/day orally in divided doses
Methylprednisolone	20–80 mg/day IV in divided doses
Hydrocortisone	100–400 mg/day IV in divided doses

first, it could theoretically provide substrate for even higher levels of hormone.

Antiadrenergic therapy with the short-acting agent esmolol is preferred, both because it may be used in the patient with pulmonary disease or at risk for cardiac failure and because its effects may be rapidly reversed.[115] Corticosteroids are generally recommended, although there is no convincing evidence of adrenocortical insufficiency in thyroid storm, and the benefits derived from steroids may be caused by their antipyretic action and their effect of stabilizing blood pressure.[22] General supportive measures, including acetaminophen as an antipyretic (do not use aspirin or other nonsteroidal antiinflammatory agents because they may displace bound thyroid hormone), fluid and electrolyte replacement, sedatives, digitalis, antiarrhythmics, insulin, and antibiotics should be given as indicated. Plasmapheresis and peritoneal dialysis have been used to remove excess hormone (and to remove thyroid-stimulating immunoglobulins in Graves's disease) when the patient has not responded to more conservative measures, although these measures do not always work.[116]

HYPOTHYROIDISM

Hypothyroidism is defined as the clinical and biochemical syndrome resulting from decreased thyroid hormone production.[117] Overt hypothyroidism occurs in 1.5% to 2% of women and 0.2% of men, and its incidence increases with age. In the Third National Health and Nutrition Examination Survey, levels of serum TSH and total thyroxine (T_4) were measured in a representative sample of adolescents and adults (age 12 or older). Among 16,533 people who neither were taking thyroid medication nor reported histories of thyroid disease, 3.9% had subclinical hypothyroidism (serum TSH >4.5 milli-international units/L; and T_4 normal), and 0.2% had "clinically significant" hypothyroidism (TSH >4.5 milli-international units/L; and T_4 <4.5 mcg/dL).[21] The vast majority of patients have primary hypothyroidism due to thyroid gland failure due to chronic autoimmune thyroiditis. Special populations with higher risk of developing hypothyroidism include postpartum women, individuals with a family history of autoimmune thyroid disorders and patients with previous head and neck or thyroid irradiation or surgery, other autoimmune endocrine conditions (e.g., type 1 diabetes mellitus, adrenal insufficiency, and ovarian failure), some other nonendocrine autoimmune disorders (e.g., celiac disease, vitiligo, pernicious anemia, Sjögren' syndrome, and multiple sclerosis), primary pulmonary hypertension, and Down and Turner syndromes. Secondary hypothyroidism due to pituitary failure is uncommon but should be suspected in a patient with decreased levels of thyroxine and inappropriately normal or low TSH levels. Most patients with secondary hypothyroidism due to inadequate TSH production will have clinical signs of more generalized pituitary insufficiency, such as abnormal menses and decreased libido, or evidence of a pituitary adenoma, such as visual-field defects, galactorrhea, or acromegaloid features, but isolated TSH deficiency can be congenital or acquired as a result of autoimmune hypophysitis.[118] Generalized (peripheral and central) resistance to thyroid hormone is extremely rare.

Thyroid hormone is essential for normal growth and development during embryonic life. Uncorrected thyroid hormone deficiency during fetal and neonatal development results in mental retardation and/or cretinism. There is slowing of physical and mental activity, as well as of cardiovascular, gastrointestinal, and neuromuscular function.

A rise in the TSH level is the first evidence of primary hypothyroidism. Many patients will have a free T_4 level within the normal range (compensated hypothyroidism) and few, if any, symptoms of

CLINICAL PRESENTATION OF HYPOTHYROIDISM

General

☐ Hypothyroidism can lead to a variety of end-organ effects with a wide range of disease severity, from entirely asymptomatic individuals to patients in coma with multisystem failure. In the adult, manifestations of hypothyroidism are varied and nonspecific. In the child, thyroid hormone deficiency may manifest as growth or intellectual retardation.

Symptoms

☐ Common symptoms of hypothyroidism include dry skin, cold intolerance, weight gain, constipation, and weakness. Complaints of lethargy, depression, fatigue or loss of ambition and energy are also common but are less specific. Muscle cramps, myalgia, and stiffness are frequent complaints of hypothyroid patients. Menorrhagia and infertility may present commonly in women.

Signs

☐ Objective weakness is common, with proximal muscles being affected more than distal muscles. Slow relaxation of deep tendon reflexes is common. The most common signs of decreased levels of thyroid hormone include coarse skin and hair, cold or dry skin, periorbital puffiness, and bradycardia. Speech is often slow as well as hoarse. Reversible neurologic syndromes such as carpal tunnel syndrome, polyneuropathy, and cerebellar dysfunction may also occur. Galactorrhea may be found in women.

Diagnosis

☐ In primary hypothyroidism, TSH serum concentration should be elevated. In secondary hypothyroidism, TSH levels may be within or below the reference range; when TSH bioactivity is altered, the levels reported by immunoassay may even be elevated.

☐ Free and/or total T_4 and T_3 serum concentrations should be low.

Other tests

☐ Antithyroid peroxidase antibodies and anti-TG antibodies are likely to be elevated in autoimmune thyroiditis.

TABLE 84-7	Causes of Hypothyroidism
Primary Hypothyroidism	
Hashimoto's disease	
Iatrogenic hypothyroidism	
Others	
Iodine deficiency	
Enzyme defects	
Thyroid hypoplasia	
Goitrogens	
Secondary Hypothyroidism	
Pituitary disease	
Hypothalamic disease	

hypothyroidism. As the disease progresses, the free T_4 concentration will drop below the normal level. Interestingly, because of TSH stimulation, thyroidal production will shift toward greater amounts of T_3, and thus T_3 concentrations will often be maintained in the normal range in spite of a low T_4. The RAIU is not a useful test in the evaluation of a hypothyroid patient, as it may be low, normal, or even elevated.

CAUSES OF HYPOTHYROIDISM

Table 84–7 outlines the causes of hypothyroidism.

Chronic Autoimmune Thyroiditis

❽ Autoimmune thyroiditis (Hashimoto's disease) is the most common cause of spontaneous hypothyroidism in the adult.[119] Patients may present either with goitrous thyroid gland enlargement and mild hypothyroidism or with thyroid gland atrophy and more severe thyroid hormone deficiency. Both forms of autoimmune thyroiditis probably result from cell- and antibody-mediated thyroid injury. The bulk of evidence suggests that the presence of specific defects in suppressor T-lymphocyte function leads to the survival of a randomly mutating clone of helper T lymphocytes,

which are directed against normally occurring antigens on the thyroid membrane. Once these T lymphocytes interact with thyroid membrane antigen, B lymphocytes are stimulated to produce thyroid antibodies.[120]

Antithyroid peroxidase (antimicrosomal) antibodies are present in virtually all patients with Hashimoto's thyroiditis and appear to be directed against the enzyme thyroid peroxidase.[121] These antibodies are capable of fixing complement and inducing cytotoxic changes in thyroid cells. Antibodies that are capable of stimulating thyroid growth through interaction with the TSH receptor may occasionally be found particularly in goitrous hypothyroidism; conversely, antibodies that inhibit the trophic effects of TSH are present in the atrophic type.

Iatrogenic Hypothyroidism

Iatrogenic hypothyroidism follows exposure to excessive amounts of radiation (radioiodine or external radiation) or surgery. Hypothyroidism occurs within 3 months to a year after ^{131}I therapy in most patients treated for Graves's disease. Thereafter it occurs at a rate of approximately 2.5% each year. External radiation therapy to the region of the thyroid using doses of greater than 2,500 cGy for therapy of neck carcinoma also causes hypothyroidism. This effect is dose dependent, and more than 50% of patients who receive more than 4,000 cGy to the thyroid bed develop hypothyroidism. Total thyroidectomy causes hypothyroidism within 1 month.

Other Causes of Primary Hypothyroidism

Iodine deficiency, enzymatic defects within the thyroid gland, thyroid hypoplasia, and maternal ingestion of goitrogens during fetal development may cause cretinism. Early recognition and treatment of the resultant thyroid hormone deficiency is essential for optimal mental development.[122,123] Large-scale neonatal screening programs in North America, Europe, Japan, and Australia are now in place.[124] The frequency of congenital hypothyroidism in North America and Europe is 1 per 3,500 to 4,000 live births. In the United States, there are racial differences in the incidence of congenital hypothyroidism, with whites being affected seven times as frequently as blacks.

In the adult, hypothyroidism may rarely be caused by iodine deficiency and goitrogens. Rarely, iodine ingestion in the form of expectorants can lead to hypothyroidism. In sensitive persons (particularly those with autoimmune thyroiditis), the iodide blocks the synthesis of thyroid hormone, leading to an increased secretion of TSH and thyroid enlargement. Thus, both iodine excess and iodine deficiency can cause decreased secretion of thyroid hormone.

Causes of Secondary Hypothyroidism

Pituitary Disease TSH is required for normal thyroid secretion. Thyroid atrophy and decreased thyroid secretion follow pituitary failure. Pituitary insufficiency may be caused by destruction of

TABLE 84-8 Thyroid Preparations Used in the Treatment of Hypothyroidism

Drug/Dosage Form	Content	Relative Dose	Comments/Equivalency
Thyroid USP Armour Thyroid (T_4:T_3 ratio) 9.5 mcg:2.25 mcg, 19 mcg:4.5 mcg, 38 mcg:9 mcg, 57 mcg:13.5 mcg, 76 mcg:18 mcg, 114 mcg:27 mcg, 152 mcg:36 mcg,190 mcg:45 mcg tablets	Desiccated beef or pork thyroid gland	1 grain (equivalent to 60–100 mcg of T_4)	Unpredictable hormonal stability; inexpensive generic brands may not be bioequivalent.
Thyroglobulin Proloid 32 mg, 65 mg, 100 mg, 130 mg, 200 mg tablets	Partially purified pork thyroglobuin	1 grain	Standardized biologically to give T_4: T_3 ratio of 2.5:1; more expensive than thyroid extract; no clinical advantage.
Levothyroxine Synthroid, l evothroid, Levoxyl, Thyro-tabs, Unithroid and other generics 25, 50, 75, 88, 100, 112, 125, 137, 150, 175, 200, 300 mcg tablets; 200 and 500 mcg per vial injection	Synthetic T_4	50–60 mcg	Stable; predictable potency; generics are bioequivalent; when switching from natural thyroid to L- thyroxine, lower dose by 1/2 grain; variable absorption between products; half-life = 7 days, so daily dosing; considered to be drug of choice.
Liothyronine Cytomel 5, 25, and 50 mcg tablets	Synthetic T_3	15–37.5 mcg	Uniform absorption, rapid onset; half-life = 1.5 days, monitor TSH assays
Liotrix Thyrolar 1/4-, 1/2-, 1-, 2-, and 3-strength tablets	Synthetic T_4: T_3 in 4:1 ratio	50–60 mcg T_4 and 12.5–15 mcg T_3	Stable; predictable; expensive; lacks therapeutic rationale because T_4 is converted to T_3 peripherally.

TSH, thyroid-stimulating hormone.

thyrotrophs by either functioning or nonfunctioning pituitary tumors, surgical therapy, external pituitary radiation, postpartum pituitary necrosis (Sheehan syndrome), trauma, and infiltrative processes of the pituitary such as metastatic tumors, tuberculosis, histiocytosis, and autoimmune mechanisms.[125,126] In all these situations, TSH deficiency most often occurs in association with other pituitary hormone deficiencies. The identification of secondary hypothyroidism due to bexarotene use has led to recognition of the role of rexinoids, and retinoids to cause dysregulation of TSH production.[25,127]

For most hypothyroid patients with pituitary disease, serum TSH concentrations are generally low or normal. A serum TSH concentration in the normal range is clearly inappropriate if the patient's T_4 is low.

Note that pituitary enlargement in hypothyroidism does not invariably indicate the presence of a primary pituitary tumor. Pituitary enlargement is seen for patients with severe primary hypothyroidism due to compensatory hyperplasia and hypertrophy of the thyrotrophs.[128] With thyroid hormone replacement therapy, serum TSH concentrations decline, indicating that the TSH secretion is not autonomous, and the pituitary resumes a more normal configuration. These patients are easily separated from patients with primary pituitary failure by measuring a TSH level.

Hypothalamic Hypothyroidism TRH deficiency also causes a rare form of central hypothyroidism. In both adults and children it may occur as a result of cranial irradiation, trauma, infiltrative diseases, or neoplastic diseases.

TREATMENT

HYPOTHYROIDISM

■ PHARMACOLOGIC THERAPY

Desired Outcomes

The goals of therapy are to restore normal thyroid hormone concentrations in tissue, provide symptomatic relief, prevent neurologic deficits in newborns and children, and reverse the biochemical abnormalities of hypothyroidism.

General Approach

❾ Any of the commercially available thyroid preparations accomplish this goal (Table 84–8); however, levothyroxine (l-thyroxine, T4) is considered to be drug of choice for treatment of hypothyroidism. Other commercially available thyroid preparations can be obtained but are not considered preferred therapy. Available thyroid preparations are synthetic (levothyroxine, liothyronine, and liotrix) or natural (i.e. desiccated thyroid and TG) in origin. The availability of sensitive and specific assays for total and free hormone levels as well as TSH now allow definitive dose titration to allow adequate replacement without inadvertent overdose. The response of TSH to TRH had been advocated for use by some for "fine tuning" thyroid replacement, but this is not necessary if the third generation chemiluminometric assays for TSH, which have detection limits of about 0.01 milli-international units/L, are used. Moreover, TRH is no longer commercially available. Minimum clinical guidelines for the treatment of hypothyroidism have been published by the American Thyroid Association[59] and the American Association of Clinical Endocrinologists.[129]

Synthetic Thyroid Hormones

Levothyroxine (T_4; l-thyroxine) is the drug of choice for thyroid replacement and suppressive therapy because it is chemically stable, relatively inexpensive, and free of antigenicity and has uniform potency. Whereas T_3 and not T_4 is the biologically more active form of thyroid hormone, levothyroxine administration results in a pool of thyroid hormone that is readily and consistently converted to T_3; in this regard levothyroxine may be thought of as a prohormone. The ability of levothyroxine to achieve normal T_3 concentrations was illustrated in a study of recently athyreotic patients in whom levothyroxine monotherapy produced similar T_3 levels to those documented prior to the patient's thyroidectomy.[130] The half-life of levothyroxine is approximately 7 days. This long half-life is responsible for a stable pool of prohormone and the need for only once daily dosing with levothyroxine. Older studies with levothyroxine suggested that bioavailability was low and erratic; however, this product has been reformulated, and the average bioavailability is now approximately 80%.[131–133] Different levothyroxine preparations contain different excipients such as dyes and fillers. The bioavailability of Synthroid, Levoxine, and generic levothyroxine preparations were compared in a blinded, randomized, four-way crossover trial.[134] The study was sponsored by the manufacturers of Synthroid, who have challenged the authors' conclusions that the levothyroxine preparations are bioequivalent and should be interchangeable for the majority of patients. However, because the relationship between T_4 concentration and TSH is not linear, very small changes in T_4 concentration can lead to substantial changes in TSH, which is a more accurate reflection of hormone replacement status. Currently, the Food and Drug Administration mandates that levothyroxine bioequivalency testing be done for normal volunteers (600 mcg in the fasted state) and three baseline free thyroxine concentrations be used to correct for endogenous T_4 production. Bioequivalency is based on the area under the curve (AUC) and maximum concentration (Cmax) of T_4 out to 48 hours. Approximately 70% of the AUC is derived from endogenous production. TSH is not considered, and it is now very clear that T_4 is too insensitive as a measure of bioequivalency.[135,136] To avoid over- and undertreatment, once a product is selected, therapeutic interchange should be discouraged. Currently, there are several levothyroxine products available, and a number of permutations for interchange are available considering that there are AB1, AB2, AB3, and AB4 products available since no reference listed drug is mandated in bioequivalency testing.

The time to maximal absorption of levothyroxine is about 2 hours and this should be considered when T_4 concentrations is determined. Ingestion of levothyroxine with food can impair its absorption.[137] This can potentially affect the TSH concentration achieved if levothyroxine timing with respect to food is varied.[138] Mucosal diseases such as sprue, diabetic diarrhea, and ileal bypass surgery can also reduce absorption. Cholestyramine, calcium carbonate, sucralfate, aluminum hydroxide,[139] ferrous sulfate,[140] soybean formula,[141] dietary fiber supplements,[142] and espresso coffee[143] may also impair the absorption of levothyroxine from the gastrointestinal tract. Acid suppression with histamine blockers and proton pump inhibitors may also reduce levothyroxine absorption.[144] Drugs that increase nondeiodinative T_4 clearance include rifampin, carbamazepine, and possibly phenytoin. Selenium deficiency and amiodarone may block the conversion of T_4 to T_3.

Liothyronine (T_3) is chemically pure with known potency and has a shorter half-life of 1.5 days. Although it can be used diagnostically in the T_3-suppression test, T_3 has some clinical disadvantages, including a higher incidence of cardiac adverse effects, higher cost, and difficulty in monitoring with conventional laboratory tests. Liotrix is a combination of synthetic T_4 and T_3 in a 4:1 ratio that attempts to mimic natural hormonal secretion. It is chemically stable and pure and has a predictable potency. The major limitations to this product are high cost and lack of therapeutic rationale, because most T_3 is peripherally converted from T_4. In addition, the ratio of T_4:T_3 is much higher than the 14:1 molar ratio produced by the thyroid gland in humans.

Trials comparing levothyroxine alone to a combination of levothyroxine plus partial replacement with liothyronine (triiodothyronine) have generally shown that combinations of $T_4 + T_3$ are no better than T_4 alone.[145,146] Over 10 such trials with varying designs have been performed to date. In one trial of combination therapy Clyde, et al.[146] compared levothyroxine alone for treatment of primary hypothyroidism with combination therapy using levothyroxine plus liothyronine. These investigators demonstrated no beneficial changes in body weight, serum lipid levels, hypothyroid symptoms as measured by a health-related quality-of-life questionnaire, and standard measures of cognitive performance.[146] Two metaanalyses have also suggested no benefits.[147,148] However, a recent study, suggested that individuals harboring a specific deiodinase polymorphism may have a poorer psychological response to levothyroxine

therapy and a better response to combination therapy with both T_4 and T_3

Natural Thyroid Hormones

Desiccated thyroid is derived from hog, beef, or sheep thyroid gland. The United States Pharmacopeia, 23th ed., requires Thyroid USP to contain 38 mcg (±15%) of levothyroxine and 9 mcg (±10%) of liothyronine for each 65 mg (1 grain) of the labeled content of TG. Thyroglobulin USP should contain 36 mcg (±15%) of levothyroxine and 12 mcg (±10%) of liothyronine for each 65 mg (1 grain) of the labeled content of TG. Not all generic brands may be bioequivalent, and switching among brands for patients stabilized on one product should be discouraged. Thyroid USP, as an animal protein–derived product, may be antigenic in allergic or sensitive patients. Even though desiccated thyroid is inexpensive, its limitations preclude it from being considered as a drug of choice for hypothyroid patients. TG is a purified hog-gland extract, but it has no clinical advantages and is not widely used.

Dosing and Monitoring Recent studies suggest that the average maintenance dose of levothyroxine for most adults is about 125 mcg/day.[117] The replacement dose of levothyroxine is affected by body weight. Estimates of weight-based doses for replacement in hypothyroid patients include 1.6 mcg/kg/day and 1.7 mcg/kg/day.[149,150] There is, however, a wide range of replacement doses, necessitating individualized therapy and appropriate TSH monitoring to determine an adequate but not excessive dose.

In addition to alleviation of symptoms, the goal of treatment for patients with hypothyroidism is to maintain the patient's TSH within the normal range. Some clinicians are of the opinion that the traditional reference range of approximately 0.5 to 4.5 milli-international units/L includes at its upper end some individuals who have unrecognized thyroid disease.[151] Thus, some believe that the reference range should be modified downwards to 0.5 to 3.5 milli-international units/L or even 0.5 to 2.5 milli-international units/L.[152] If this premise is accepted, both the TSH values that trigger levothyroxine treatment and the TSH treatment goal could potentially be altered. There are cogent arguments on both sides of the issue. Those who would suggest maintaining current reference ranges believe that changes would result in the treatment with thyroid hormone of many individuals who would not necessarily benefit from treatment.[153] Those who favor narrowing the range suggest that additional patients would derive benefit from thyroid hormone treatment.[152] TSH reference ranges also differ for different populations, such as those who are pregnant, specific ethnic groups, and older individuals.

The required dose of levothyroxine is dependent on the patient's age[154] and the presence of associated disorders, as well as the severity and duration of hypothyroidism.[155] Most patients will require approximately 1.7 mcg/kg/day once they reach steady state for full replacement. Dose requirement may be better estimated based on ideal body weight, rather than actual body weight.[156] In young patients with long-standing disease and patients over age 45 without known cardiac disease, therapy should be initiated with 50 mcg daily of levothyroxine and increased to 100 mcg daily after 1 month. The recommended initial daily dose for older patients or those with known cardiac disease is 25 mcg per day titrated upward in increments of 25 mcg at monthly intervals to prevent stress on the cardiovascular system. Some patients may experience an exacerbation of angina with higher doses of thyroid hormone. Although the TSH is an indicator of under- or overreplacement, clinicians often fail to alter the dose of T_4 based on TSH clearly outside of the normal range.[157,158]

Patients with subclinical or mild hypothyroidism (seen more commonly for the elderly and women) have no or few signs or symptoms, normal serum T_3 and T_4 concentrations, and an elevated basal TSH concentration.[159,160] The prevalence of this disorder in the Third National Health and Nutrition Examination Survey (NHANES III) study was found to be 4.3%.[21] Although the treatment of subclinical hypothyroidism is controversial, patients presenting with marked elevations in TSH (>10 milli-international units/L) and high titers of thyroid peroxidase antibody (TPOAb) or prior treatment with ^{131}I may be most likely to benefit from treatment. Other patients who may improve with replacement include those with mild symptoms of hypothyroidism and depression. It should be noted that some studies find that only 1 of 4 treated patients experienced improvement.[161] Conservative treatment goals in this situation would be to maintain serum T_4 and T_3 levels in the normal range and reduce TSH to a value of 1 milli-international unit/L.

Once euthyroidism is attained, the daily maintenance dose of levothyroxine does not fluctuate greatly. As patients age, the dosing requirement may be reduced.[129] Third generation TSH assays improved the accuracy with which thyroid hormone replacement can be monitored. The TSH concentration is the most sensitive and specific monitoring parameter for adjustment of levothyroxine dose. Plasma TSH concentrations begin to fall within hours and are usually normalized within 2 weeks, but they may take up to 6 weeks for some patients, depending on the baseline value. TSH and T_4 concentrations are both used to monitor therapy, and they should be checked every 6 weeks until a euthyroid state is achieved. Laboratory assessment of thyroid function should be performed approximately 6 weeks after levothyroxine dose initiation or change. This time frame allows achievement of steady state, as the half-life of levothyroxine is approximately 1 week. Serum T_4 concentrations can be useful in detecting noncompliance, malabsorption, or changes in levothyroxine product bioequivalence. An elevated TSH concentration indicates insufficient replacement. The appropriate dose maintains the TSH concentration in the normal range. Thyroxine disposal is accelerated by nephritic syndrome, other severe systemic illnesses, and several antiseizure medications (phenobarbital, phenytoin, and carbamazepine) and rifampin. Pregnancy increases the thyroxine dose requirement for 75% of women, probably because of factors such as increased degradation by the placental deiodinase, increased T_4 pool size, and transfer of T_4 to the fetus. The etiology of hypothyroidism also affects the magnitude of the dosage increase.[162] Initiating postmenopausal hormone replacement therapy increases the dose needed in 35% of women, perhaps due to an increased circulating TBG level. Patient noncompliance with prescribed thyroxine, the most common cause of inadequate treatment, might be suspected for patients with a dose that is higher than expected, variable thyroid function test results that do not correlate well with prescribed doses, and an elevated serum thyrotropin concentration with serum free thyroxine at the upper end of the normal range, which can suggest improved compliance immediately before testing due to a lag in the thyrotropin response. The metabolism of other pharmacologic agents can be altered for patients with hypothyroidism. The mechanism might be decreased expression of hepatic enzymes involved in drug metabolism, as seen in hypothyroid rats. As a result, increased sensitivity to anesthetic and sedative agents, and higher serum levels of phenytoin have been reported. Hypothyroidism can also cause higher serum digoxin values, an effect attributed to a decreased volume of drug distribution. Conversely, hypothyroidism might decrease sensitivity to warfarin due to slowed metabolism of the vitamin K–dependent clotting factors, and restoration of euthyroidism can then increase the warfarin dose requirement.

For patients with central hypothyroidism caused by hypothalamic or pituitary failure, the serum TSH cannot be used to assess adequacy of replacement. Alleviation of the clinical syndrome and restoration of serum T_4 to the normal range are the only criteria available for estimating the appropriate replacement dose of levothyroxine. Concurrent use of dopamine, dopaminergic agents (bromocriptine), somatostatin or somatostatin analogs (octreotide), and corticosteroids suppresses TSH concentrations in individuals with primary hypothyroidism and may confound the interpretation of this monitoring parameter.[129]

TSH-suppressive levothyroxine therapy can be given to patients with nodular thyroid disease and diffuse goiter, to patients with a history of thyroid irradiation, and to patients with thyroid cancer. The rationale for suppression therapy is to reduce TSH secretion, which promotes growth and function in abnormal thyroid tissue. However, such management, other than for patients with thyroid cancer or with elevated TSH levels, is quite controversial. Some clinicians rarely recommend or use such therapy; others will recommend a trial of levothyroxine as suppressive therapy in some patients. The conclusions of three metaanalyses were that suppressive therapy for nodules was associated with a small decrease in nodule growth,[163] a statistically nonsignificant reduction in nodule growth,[164] and a significant reduction in nodule growth that was reduced with longer term treatment.[165] If suppressive therapy with levothyroxine is pursued, the age, gender, and menopausal status of the patient need to be considered, along with the risk of cardiac arrhythmias and reduced bone mineral density. Levothyroxine may be given in nontoxic MNG to suppress the TSH to low-normal levels of 0.5 to 1 milli-international unit/L if the baseline TSH is >1 milli-international unit/L. Goiter size and thyroid volume may be reduced with suppression therapy. Diffuse goiter associated with autoimmune thyroiditis may also be treated with levothyroxine to reduce goiter size and thyroid volume. Levothyroxine suppression therapy is of benefit to all but the lowest risk thyroid cancer patients and is generally used in the management of patients with differentiated thyroid cancer, with the TSH goal being influenced by the patient's thyroid cancer stage and other risk factors.[166] Current guidelines from the American Thyroid Association suggest suppressing the TSH to below 0.1 milli-international unit /L in higher risk patients, keeping TSH around the lower limit of normal (0.1 to 0.5 milli-international units/L) in low-risk patients.[167]

Adverse Effects Serious untoward effects are unusual if dosing is appropriate and the patient is carefully monitored during initial treatment. A cross-sectional study showed that of a population of 1,525 individuals taking levothyroxine, 40% actually had abnormal TSH values.[168] A recent study showed that 57% of individuals 65 years or older receiving thyroid hormone treatment had abnormal TSH values.[169] Both of these studies suggest failure to keep a patient's TSH at goal is common. Levothyroxine replacement in athyreotic hypothyroid patients restores systolic and diastolic left ventricular performance within 2 weeks, and the use of levothyroxine may increase the frequency of atrial premature beats but not necessarily ventricular premature beats. Excessive doses of thyroid hormone may lead to heart failure, angina pectoris, and myocardial infarction; rarely, the latter may be caused by coronary artery spasm. Allergic or idiosyncratic reactions can occur with the natural animal-derived products such as desiccated thyroid and TG, but these are extremely rare with the synthetic products used today. The 0.05 mg (50 mcg) Synthroid tablet is the least allergenic (due to a lack of dye and few excipients) and should be tried for the patient suspected to be allergic to thyroid hormone.

Hyperremodeling of cortical and trabecular bone due to hyperthyroidism leads to reduced bone density and may increase the risk of fracture. Compared with normal controls, excess exogenous thyroid hormone results in histomorphometric and biochemical changes similar to those observed in osteoporosis and untreated hyperthyroidism; however, at routinely used replacement doses, bone mineral density loss is less than that seen with untreated hyperthyroidism and only slightly greater than in controls.[170,171] The risk for this complication of therapy seems to be related to the dose of levothyroxine, patient age, and gender. Markers for bone turnover include urinary cross-linked *N*-telopeptides, pyridinoline of type I collagen, osteocalcin, and bone-specific alkaline phosphatase. When doses of levothyroxine are used to suppress TSH concentrations to below-normal values (less than 0.3 milli-international unit/L) in postmenopausal women, this adverse effect is more likely to be seen. Cortical bone is affected to a greater degree than trabecular bone at suppressive doses of levothyroxine. In contrast, it appears to be much less likely in men and in premenopausal women. Maintaining the TSH between 0.7 and 1.5 milli-international units/L does not alter bone mineral density in premenopausal women.

EVALUATION OF THERAPEUTIC OUTCOMES

HYPOTHYRODISM

Patients on optimal thyroid hormone replacement therapy should have TSH and free T_4 serum concentrations in the normal range. Those who are being treated for thyroid cancer should have TSH suppressed to low levels based on their risk stratification[167] and their TG should be undetectable. Given the half-life of 7 days of T_4, the appropriate monitoring interval is no more often than 4 weeks. The signs and symptoms of hypothyroidism should be improved or absent (see Clinical Presentation of Hypothyroidism above), although this may take several months for most to improve.

SPECIAL CONDITIONS

Myxedema Coma

Myxedema coma is a rare consequence of decompensated hypothyroidism.[172,173] Clinical features include hypothermia, advanced stages of hypothyroid symptoms, and altered sensorium ranging from delirium to coma. Mortality rates of 60% to 70% necessitate immediate and aggressive therapy. Traditionally, the initial treatment has been intravenous bolus levothyroxine 300 to 500 mcg. However, as deiodinase activity is markedly reduced, impairing T_4 to T_3 conversion, initial treatment with intravenous triiodothyronine or a combination of both hormones has also been advocated.[173] Glucocorticoid therapy with intravenous hydrocortisone 100 mg every 8 hours should be given until coexisting adrenal suppression is ruled out. Consciousness, lowered TSH concentrations, and normal vital signs are expected within 24 hours. Maintenance doses of levothyroxine are typically 75 to 100 mcg given intravenously until the patient stabilizes and oral therapy is begun. Supportive therapy must be instituted to maintain adequate ventilation, euglycemia, blood pressure, and body temperature. Any underlying disorder, such as sepsis or myocardial infarction, obviously must be diagnosed and treated.

Congenital Hypothyroidism[174]

In congenital hypothyroidism, full maintenance therapy should be instituted early to improve the prognosis for mental and physical development.[175] The average maintenance dose in infants and children depends on the age and weight of the child. Several studies demonstrate that aggressive therapy with levothyroxine is important for normal development, and current recommendations are for initiation of therapy within 45 days of birth at a dose of 10 to 15 mcg/kg/day.[124] This dose is used to keep T_4 concentrations at about 10 mcg/dL within 30 days of starting therapy and is associated with improved IQs in treated infants. The dose is progressively decreased to a typical adult dose as the child ages, the adult dose being given in the age range of 11 to 20 years.

Hypothyroidism in Pregnancy[99]

Hypothyroidism during pregnancy leads to an increased rate of stillbirths and possibly lower psychological scores in infants born of women who received inadequate replacement during pregnancy.[176] Thyroid hormone is necessary for fetal growth and must come from the maternal side during the first 2 months of gestation. Although liothyronine may cross the placental membrane slightly better than levothyroxine, the latter is considered the drug of choice. The objective of treatment is to decrease TSH to 1 unit/mL and maintain free T_4 concentrations in the normal range. Based on elevated TSH levels during pregnancy, it was found that the mean dose of levothyroxine had to be increased by 36 mcg/day to suppress TSH into the normal range. Increased production of binding proteins, a marginal decrease in free hormone concentration, modification of peripheral thyroid hormone metabolism, and increased thyroxine metabolism by the fetal–placental unit also contributes to increased thyroid hormone demand and the need for increased doses decreases after delivery.[100] Up to 60% of women need to have levothyroxine dose adjustment during pregnancy. Upward adjustment will be needed by the 8th week of pregnancy. The etiology of the hypothyroidism affects the magnitude of the required increase in levothyroxine dose.[162] After delivery the levothyroxine dose can be reduced based on T_4 concentrations and measurement of TSH, typically about 6 to 8 weeks after delivery.[99] Many patients can return to their prepregnancy dose requirement.

Effects of Hypothyroidism on Selected Medications

Hypothyroidism may affect the metabolism and clinical efficacy of several medications. Digitalis preparations have a decreased volume of distribution in the hypothyroid state, resulting in increased sensitivity to the digitalis effect. Therefore, many hypothyroid patients achieve a therapeutic effect at lower digitalis doses. Insulin degradation may be delayed in hypothyroidism, thereby requiring a lower insulin dose. Hypothyroidism delays the catabolism of clotting factors, and if a patient stabilized on warfarin is made euthyroid with levothyroxine, the patient may become excessively anticoagulated. Respiratory depressants such as barbiturates, phenothiazines, and opioid analgesics should be avoided, because increased sensitivity may increase carbon dioxide retention and precipitate myxedema coma.

RECOMBINANT TSH IN THYROID CANCER

Patients with previously treated differentiated (papillary, follicular, or their respective variants) thyroid carcinoma require lifelong monitoring for recurrent disease.[177,178] Two diagnostic tests that play a central role in the follow-up of these patients—serum TG measurement and radioiodine whole body scanning—are most accurate during TSH stimulation. Temporary discontinuation of thyroid hormone therapy was previously the sole effective approach for TSH-stimulated testing. However, hormone withdrawal is associated with the morbidity of hypothyroidism and occasional tumor progression. The introduction of recombinant TSH (rTSH)-stimulated testing offers an alternative therapy. Recent clinical trials have shown that the sensitivity of combined rTSH-stimulated radioiodine scanning and serum TG measurement has nearly equivalent sensitivity to testing after thyroid hormone withdrawal.[127,179] Furthermore, measurement of the rTSH-stimulated TG concentration is a more sensitive way to detect residual thyroid cancer or normal tissue than TG measurement on thyroid hormone therapy. Postthyroidectomy adjuvant radioiodine therapy can also be administered following rTSH, instead of thyroid hormone withdrawal, with equivalent rates of remnant ablation.[180] Patients for whom thyroid hormone withdrawal would be contraindicated may also be successfully treated with radioiodine following rTSH.[181] A recent study reporting short-term follow-up of 3.7 years on patients receiving their remnant ablation with rTSH showed that rates of residual and recurrent thyroid cancer did not differ between patients prepared for receiving radioiodine using rTSH versus withdrawal from levothyroxine.[182] Recently rTSH has also been used successfully to aid in the treatment of large, compressive goiters in individuals who are not surgical candidates. Radioiodine treatment, delivered following small doses of rTSH, can lead to improved radioiodine uptake and reduced goiter volume,[183] although this is not yet an approved use of rTSH.

NONTHYROIDAL ILLNESS

A wide variety of abnormalities of hypothalamic–pituitary–thyroid function, serum thyroid hormone binding, and extrathyroidal thyroid hormone metabolism occurs in patients with nonthyroidal illness.[13,14] These abnormalities frequently result in decreased serum T_3 concentrations and, with more severe nonthyroidal disease, lead to a decreased serum free T_4 concentration as well. Serum TSH concentrations are initially within the normal range but then tend to decrease with increasing severity of illness. The presence of coexisting primary hypothyroidism can be recognized for patients who have other illnesses by an elevation in the TSH concentration.

The degree and extent of the abnormality in thyroid function generally correlates with the severity of the nonthyroidal illness. These conditions are frequently referred to as the *euthyroid sick syndrome*. However, it is likely that these changes represent adaptive forms of hypothyroidism that serve to reduce the availability of thyroid hormones to lessen the catabolic impact of the nonthyroidal illness.

Decreased serum T_3 concentrations occur in patients with both acute and chronic illnesses. The fundamental cause of decreased serum T_3 concentrations in these situations is decreased extrathyroidal conversion of T_4 to T_3, normally mediated by T_4-5′-deiodinase. A circulating inhibitor of this enzyme, perhaps interleukin-6, is present in patients with nonthyroidal illness.[184] Serum total and free T_4 concentrations are usually normal in mild illness. The serum reverse T_3 concentration is characteristically high because the same enzyme, 5′-deiodinase, that is necessary to convert T_4 to T_3 is necessary to convert reverse T_3 to its breakdown products.

Low serum T_4 is seen in most critically ill patients.[185-187] This change is caused by diminished serum T_4 synthesis as well as impaired binding to serum transport proteins, resulting either from decreased serum concentrations of thyroid-binding globulin, thyroid-binding prealbumin, or albumin, or from inhibitors of T_4 binding. The free T_4 concentration is generally normal early in critical illness but also declines with more severe disease. This more severe degree of hypothyroidism, which occurs in severely ill patients, produces a greater reduction in thyroid hormone availability. The low serum T_4 concentrations for patients with nonthyroidal illness indicate a grave prognosis. In two studies, more than 60% of hospitalized patients with a low serum free T_4 index died. Although controversial, T_4 or T_3 supplementation has been of no benefit in this situation.[188]

To confuse matters, some patients with nonthyroidal illness have elevation of their serum T_4 concentration. Most commonly, this is seen in patients with psychiatric disorders during acute psychotic breaks. Thyroid hormone levels return to normal within 2 weeks after successful treatment of the underlying psychiatric disease.

The occurrence of these abnormalities requires that care be taken in diagnosing hypothyroidism or hyperthyroidism for patients who have nonthyroidal illnesses.

GOITROUS THYROID DISEASE

Endemic goiter is the major thyroid disease throughout the world, affecting more than 200 million people. Many goitrous glands contain one or more nodules. The introduction of iodide supplementation has eliminated goiter as a major medical problem in developed countries, though it continues to be a problem in developing countries whose geographic position makes them more susceptible to iodide deficiency. In 1924, Marine postulated that periods of iodide deficiency resulted in cyclic hyperplasia and involution of thyroid follicular cells with eventual development of nodular hyperplasia.[47,189] This hypothesis is still used to explain goiter formation today. Whatever the specific cause, the final common pathway appears to result from an inadequate thyroid hormone secretion with compensatory TSH secretion and eventual thyroid gland enlargement. The essential factor for the conversion of a hyperplastic iodine-deficiency goiter into a colloid goiter appears to be an acute reduction of TSH stimulation; therefore, any situation that would result in a cyclical increase and decrease in TSH secretion might eventually result in the production of a nodular goiter.

There has been an interest in the possibility that growth factors other than TSH play a role in the development of a goiter. Immunoglobulin fractions capable of stimulating thyroid growth have been found in patients with nontoxic goiter and Graves's disease. In these patients, thyroid growth–promoting immunoglobulin titers correlate with goiter size rather than with the thyroid hormone concentration.

Sporadic goiter is defined as a goiter occurring in a nonendemic goiter region. Although a number of known goitrogens and errors in thyroid hormone biosynthesis may cause goiter, the majority of cases of sporadic goiter have no known etiology.

Treatment of goiters can include a trial of thyroid hormone suppression in an effort to eliminate TSH as a possible stimulus for continued thyroid growth. Large, long-standing goiters seldom undergo significant reduction in size. If the patient is symptomatic (with dysphagia or dyspnea) or there is a question of malignant thyroid involvement, surgery is recommended.

PHARMACOECONOMIC CONSIDERATIONS

Although the initial expense of surgery would seem to make it the most expensive treatment option for hyperthyroidism, the relapse rates for thionamides and RAI are higher, and in longer-term follow-up there is not much difference between treatment options nor patients' opinions concerning treatment preferences as suggested by a 1998 study.[190] The cost proportion between the medical and surgical treatment in younger patients is 1:2.5 (1 = U.S.$1,126) before and 1:1.3 (1 = U.S. $2,284) after inclusion of the relapse costs. The proportion between the medical, surgical, and [131] I treatment in older patients is 1:2.5:1.6 (1 = U.S. $1,164) before and 1:1.6:1.4 (1 = U.S. $1,972) after inclusion of the relapse costs.

Multiple studies have addressed the role of thyroid supplementation in critically ill patients with cardiac disease, sepsis, pulmonary disease (e.g., acute respiratory distress syndrome), or severe infection, or with burn and trauma patients. In spite of a very large number of published studies, it is very difficult to form clear recommendations for treatment with thyroid hormone in the intensive care unit.[188]

CLINICAL CONTROVERSIES

Although the current FDA standards of bioavailability for thyroxine products suggest that several products are bioequivalent, the relationship between T_4 serum concentration and TSH response suggests that the products are not truly bioequivalent. New standards of bioequivalency may need to be developed for drug products like thyroxine.

Combination therapy of $T_4 + T_3$ for hypothyroidism generally offers no objective advantage over monotherapy, although subjective patient improvement or patient preference for combination therapy has been reported in a minority of studies. However, recent data suggest that patients with certain deiodinase polymorphisms may, in fact, derive a psychological benefit from combination therapy.

Multiple studies have addressed the role of thyroid supplementation for critically ill patients with cardiac disease, sepsis, pulmonary disease (e.g., acute respiratory distress syndrome), or severe infection or for patients with burn and trauma. In spite of a very large number of published studies, it is very difficult to form clear recommendations for treatment with thyroid hormone in the intensive care unit.

EVALUATION OF THERAPEUTIC OUTCOMES

Patients with idiopathic hypothyroidism and Hashimoto's thyroiditis on optimal thyroid hormone replacement therapy should have TSH and free T_4 serum concentrations in the normal range. Those who are being treated for thyroid cancer should have TSH suppressed to low levels, with the appropriate TSH concentration being determined based on the patient's risk of recurrence or progression, and TG should be undetectable. Given the half-life of T_4 of 7 days, the appropriate monitoring interval is no more often than 4 weeks. The signs and symptoms of hypothyroidism should be improved or absent (see Clinical Presentation of Hypothyroidism above), although this may take several months for most to improve.

ABBREVIATIONS

ClO_4^-: perchlorate

DIT: diiodotyrosine

FSH: follicle-stimulating hormone

$G_s\alpha$: the α subunit of the stimulatory guanine-nucleotide–binding protein

hCG: human chorionic gonadotropin

HLA: human leukocyte antigen

[131]I: sodium iodide 131

l-thyroxine: levothyroxine

LH: luteinizing hormone

MIT: monoiodotyrosine

MMI: methimazole

MNG: multinodular goiter

PRTH: pituitary resistance to thyroid hormone

PTU: propylthiouracil

RAI: radioactive iodine

RAIU: radioactive iodine uptake

rTSH: recombinant thyroid-stimulating hormone

SCN^-: thiocyanate

SSKI: saturated solution of potassium iodide

T_3: triiodothyronine

T_4: thyroxine

TBG: thyroid-binding globulin

TBPA: thyroid-binding prealbumin

TcO_4^-: pertechnetate

TG: thyroglobulin

TPOAb: thyroperoxidase antibodies

TRβ2, TRβ1, TRα1: thyroid hormone receptors

TRH: thyrotropin-releasing hormone

TSAb: thyroid-stimulating antibody

TSH: thyroid-stimulating hormone

REFERENCES

1. Nilsson M. Iodide handling by the thyroid epithelial cell. Exp Clin Endocrinol Diabetes 2001;109:13–17.
2. Dohan O, De la Vieja A, Paroder V, et al. The sodium/iodide symporter (NIS): characterization, regulation, and medical significance. Endocr Rev 2003;24:48–77.
3. Clewell RA, Merrill EA, Narayanan L, Gearhart JM, Robinson PJ. Evidence for competitive inhibition of iodide uptake by perchlorate and translocation of perchlorate into the thyroid. Int J Toxicol 2004;23:17–23.
4. Delange F, de Benoist B, Pretell E, Dunn JT. Iodine deficiency in the world: where do we stand at the turn of the century? Thyroid 2001;11:437–447.
5. Dunn JT, Dunn AD. Update on intrathyroidal iodine metabolism. Thyroid 2001;11:407–414.
6. Obregon MJ, Escobar del Rey F, Morreale de Escobar G. The effects of iodine deficiency on thyroid hormone deiodination. Thyroid 2005;15:917–929.
7. Schussler GC. The thyroxine-binding proteins. Thyroid 2000;10:141–149.
8. Bianco AC, Kim BW. Deiodinases: implications of the local control of thyroid hormone action. J Clin Invest 2006;116:2571–2579.
9. Panicker V, Cluett C, Shields B, et al. A common variation in deiodinase 1 gene DIO1 is associated with the relative levels of free thyroxine and triiodothyronine. J Clin Endocrinol Metab 2008;93:3075–3081.
10. Scanlan TS. Minireview: 3-Iodothyronamine (T1AM): a new player on the thyroid endocrine team? Endocrinol 2009;150:1108–1111.
11. Kopp P. The TSH receptor and its role in thyroid disease. Cell Mol Life Sci 2001;58:1301–1322.
12. Krohn K, Paschke R. Somatic mutations in thyroid nodular disease. Mol Genet Metab 2002;75:202–208.
13. Peeters RP, Debaveye Y, Fliers E, Visser TJ. Changes within the thyroid axis during critical illness. Crit Care Clin 2006;22:41–55, vi.
14. Peeters RP, van der Deure WM, Visser TJ. Genetic variation in thyroid hormone pathway genes; polymorphisms in the TSH receptor and the iodothyronine deiodinases. Eur J Endocrinol 2006;155:655–662.
15. Gillam MP, Kopp P. Genetic defects in thyroid hormone synthesis. Curr Opinion Pediatr 2001;13:364–372.
16. Ando T, Latif R, Davies TF. Thyrotropin receptor antibodies: new insights into their actions and clinical relevance. Best Pract Res Clin Endocrinol Metab 2005;19:33–52.
17. Davies TF, Ando T, Lin RY, Tomer Y, Latif R. Thyrotropin receptor-associated diseases: from adenomata to Graves's disease. J Clin Invest 2005;115:1972–1983.
18. Harvey CB, Williams GR. Mechanism of thyroid hormone action. Thyroid 2002;12:441–446.
19. Malm J, Farnegardh M, Grover GJ, Ladenson PW. Thyroid hormone antagonists: potential medical applications and structure activity relationships. Curr Med Chem 2009;16:3258–3266.
20. Cooper DS. Hyperthyroidism. Lancet 2003;362:459–468.

21. Hollowell JG, Staehling NW, Flanders WD, et al. Serum TSH, T(4), and thyroid antibodies in the United States population (1988 to 1994): National Health and Nutrition Examination Survey (NHANES III). J Clin Endocrinol Metab 2002;87:489–499.

22. Nayak B, Burman K. Thyrotoxicosis and thyroid storm. Endocrinol Metab Clin North Am 2006;35:663–686, vii.

23. Socin HV, Chanson P, Delemer B, et al. The changing spectrum of TSH-secreting pituitary adenomas: diagnosis and management in 43 patients. Eur J Endocrinol 2003;148:433–442.

24. Beck-Peccoz P, Persani L, Calebiro D, Bonomi M, Mannavola D, Campi I. Syndromes of hormone resistance in the hypothalamic-pituitary-thyroid axis. Best Pract Res Clin Endocrinol Metab 2006;20: 529–546.

25. Golden WM, Weber KB, Hernandez TL, Sherman SI, Woodmansee WW, Haugen BR. Single-dose rexinoid rapidly and specifically suppresses serum thyrotropin in normal subjects. J Clin Endocrinol Metab 2007;92:124–130.

26. Weetman AP. Controversy in thyroid disease. J Royal Coll Physicians London 2000;34:374–380.

27. Fung S, Malhotra R, Selva D. Thyroid orbitopathy. Australian Family Physician 2003;32:615–620.

28. Garrity JA, Bahn RS. Pathogenesis of Graves's ophthalmopathy: Implications for prediction, prevention, and treatment. Am J Ophthalmol 2006;142:147–153.

29. Brix TH, Kyvik KO, Christensen K, Hegedus L. Evidence for a major role of heredity in Graves's disease: a population-based study of two Danish twin cohorts. J Clin Endocrinol Metab 2001;86:930–934.

30. Ban Y, Concepcion ES, Villanueva R, Greenberg DA, Davies TF, Tomer Y. Analysis of immune regulatory genes in familial and sporadic Graves's disease. J Clin Endocrinol Metab 2004;89:4562–4568.

31. Ban Y, Davies TF, Greenberg DA, et al. Arginine at position 74 of the HLA-DR beta1 chain is associated with Graves's disease. Genes Immun 2004;5:203–208.

32. Taylor JC, Gough SC, Hunt PJ, et al. A genome-wide screen in 1119 relative pairs with autoimmune thyroid disease. J Clin Endocrinol Metab 2006;91:646–653.

33. Kung AW. Clinical review: Thyrotoxic periodic paralysis: a diagnostic challenge. J Clin Endocrinol Metab 2006;91:2490–2495.

34. Rodien P, Jordan N, Lefevre A, et al. Abnormal stimulation of the thyrotrophin receptor during gestation. Hum Reprod Update 2004;10: 95–105.

35. Siegel RD, Lee SL. Toxic nodular goiter. Toxic adenoma and toxic multinodular goiter. Endocrinol Metab Clin North Am 1998;27: 151–168.

36. Freitas JE. Therapeutic options in the management of toxic and non-toxic nodular goiter. Semin Nucl Med 2000;30:88–97.

37. Krohn K, Fuhrer D, Bayer Y, et al. Molecular pathogenesis of euthyroid and toxic multinodular goiter. Endocr Rev 2005;26:504–524.

38. Campbell AJ. Thyroid disorders in the elderly. Difficulties in diagnosis and treatment. Drugs 1986;31:455–461.

39. Papi G, Pearce EN, Braverman LE, Betterle C, Roti E. A clinical and therapeutic approach to thyrotoxicosis with thyroid-stimulating hormone suppression only. Am J Med 2005;118:349–361.

40. Sdano MT, Falciglia M, Welge JA, Steward DL. Efficacy of thyroid hormone suppression for benign thyroid nodules: Meta-analysis of randomized trials. Otolaryngol Head Neck Surg 2005;133:391–396.

41. Luotola K, Hyoty H, Salmi J, Miettinen A, Helin H, Pasternack A. Evaluation of infectious etiology in subacute thyroiditis—Lack of association with coxsackievirus infection. Apmis 1998;106:500–504.

42. Fatourechi V, Aniszewski JP, Fatourechi GZ, Atkinson EJ, Jacobsen SJ. Clinical features and outcome of subacute thyroiditis in an incidence cohort: Olmsted County, Minnesota, study. J Clin Endocrinol Metab 2003;88:2100–2105.

43. Pearce EN, Farwell AP, Braverman LE. Thyroiditis.[erratum appears in N Engl J Med 2003 Aug 7;349:620]. N Engl J Med 2003;348: 2646–2655.

44. Stagnaro-Green A. Postpartum thyroiditis. Best Pract Res Clin Endocrinol Metab 2004;18:303–316.

45. DeSimone CP, Lele SM, Modesitt SC. Malignant struma ovarii: a case report and analysis of cases reported in the literature with focus on survival and I131 therapy. Gynecol Oncol 2003;89:543–548.

46. Als C, Gedeon P, Rosler H, Minder C, Netzer P, Laissue JA. Survival analysis of 19 patients with toxic thyroid carcinoma. J Clin Endocrinol Metab 2002;87:4122–4127.

47. Delange F. Iodine deficiency in Europe and its consequences: an update. Eur J Nucl Med Mol Imaging 2002;29:S404–S416.

48. Meurisse M, Gollogly L, Degauque C, Fumal I, Defechereux T, Hamoir E. Iatrogenic thyrotoxicosis: Causal circumstances, pathophysiology, and principles of treatment-review of the literature. World J Surg 2000;24:1377–1385.

49. Bartalena L, Marcocci C, Bogazzi F, et al. Relation between therapy for hyperthyroidism and the course of Graves's ophthalmopathy. N Engl J Med 1998;338:73–78.

50. Ferner RE, Burnett A, Rawlins MD. Tri-iodothyroacetic acid abuse in a female body builder [letter]. Lancet 1986;1:383.

51. Basaria S, Cooper DS. Amiodarone and the thyroid. Am J Med 2005;118:706–714.

52. Bartalena L, Bogazzi F, Braverman LE, Martino E. Effects of amiodarone administration during pregnancy on neonatal thyroid function and subsequent neurodevelopment. J Endocrinol Invest 2001;24:116–130.

53. Bogazzi F, Bartalena L, Gasperi M, Braverman LE, Martino E. The various effects of amiodarone on thyroid function. Thyroid 2001;11: 511–519.

54. Martino E, Bartalena L, Bogazzi F, Braverman LE. The effects of amiodarone on the thyroid. Endocr Rev 2001;22:240–254.

55. Biondi B, Palmieri EA, Klain M, Schlumberger M, Filetti S, Lombardi G. Subclinical hyperthyroidism: Clinical features and treatment options. Eur J Endocrinol 2005;152:1–9.

56. Bartalena L, Tanda ML, Bogazzi F, Piantanida E, Lai A, Martino E. An update on the pharmacological management of hyperthyroidism due to Graves's disease. Expert Opinion on Pharmacotherapy 2005;6: 851–861.

57. Franklyn JA. Management guidelines for hyperthyroidism. Baillieres Clin Endocrinol & Metabolism 1997;11:561–571.

58. Surks MI Oe, Daniels GH, Sawin CT, Col NF, Cobin RH, Franklyn JA, Hershman JM, Burman KD, Denke MA, Gorman C, Cooper RS, Weissman NJ. Subclinical thyroid disease: scientific review and guidelines for diagnosis and management. JAMA 2004;291:228–238.

59. Singer PA, Cooper DS, Levy EG, et al. Treatment guidelines for patients with hyperthyroidism and hypothyroidism. Standards of Care Committee, American Thyroid Association. Jama 1995;273:808–812.

60. Hegedus L, Bonnema SJ, Bennedbaek FN. Management of simple nodular goiter: Current status and future perspectives. Endocr Rev 2003;24:102–132.

61. Carella C, Mazziotti G, Rotondi M, et al. Iodized salt improves the effectiveness of L-thyroxine therapy after surgery for nontoxic goitre: A prospective and randomized study. Clin Endocrinol 2002;57: 507–513.

62. Boger MS, Perrier ND. Advantages and disadvantages of surgical therapy and optimal extent of thyroidectomy for the treatment of hyperthyroidism. Surg Clin North Am 2004;84:849–874.

63. Zambudio AR, Rodriguez J, Riquelme J, Soria T, Canteras M, Parrilla P. Prospective study of postoperative complications after total thyroidectomy for multinodular goiters by surgeons with experience in endocrine surgery.[see comment]. Ann Surg 2004;240:18–25.

64. Cooper D. Drug therapy: Antithyroid drugs. N Engl J Med 2005;352:905–917.

65. Momotani N, Noh JY, Ishikawa N, Ito K. Effects of propylthiouracil and methimazole on fetal thyroid status in mothers with Graves's hyperthyroidism. Journal of Endocrinology and Metabolism 1997;82:3633–3636.

66. Raber W, Kmen E, Waldhausl W, Vierhapper H. Medical therapy of Graves's disease: Effect on remission rates of methimazole alone and in combination with triiodothyronine. Eur J Endocrinol 2000;142: 117–124.

67. Hashizume K, Ichikawa K, Sakurai A, et al. Administration of thyroxine in treated Graves's disease. Effects on the level of antibodies to thyroid-stimulating hormone receptors and on the risk of recurrence of hyperthyroidism. N Engl J Med 1991;324:947–953.

68. McIver B, Rae P, Beckett G, Wilkinson E, Gold A, Toft A. Lack of effect of thyroxine in patients with Graves's hyperthyroidism who are treated with an antithyroid drug. N Engl J Med 1996;334:220–224.

69. Bartalena L, Bogazzi F, Martino E. Adverse effects of thyroid hormone preparations and antithyroid drugs. Drug Safety 1996;15:53–63.

70. Tamai H, Sudo T, Kimura A, et al. Association between the DRB1*08032 histocompatibility antigen and methimazole-induced agranulocytosis in Japanese patients with Graves's disease. Annals of Internal Medicine 1996;124:490–494.

71. Tamai H, Mukuta T, Matsubayashi S, et al. Treatment of methimazole-induced agranulocytosis using recombinant human granulocyte colony-stimulating factor (rhG-CSF). J Clin Endocrinol Metab 1993;77:13561360.

72. Fukata S, Kuma K, Sugawara M. Granulocyte colony-stimulating factor (G-CSF) does not improve recovery from antithyroid drug-induced agranulocytosis: A prospective study. Thyroid 1999;9:29–31.

73. Monzani F, Caraccio N, Dardano A, Ferrannini E. Thyroid autoimmunity and dysfunction associated with type I interferon therapy. Clinical & Experimental Medicine 2004;3:199–210.

74. Van Dijke CP, Heydendael RJ, De Kleine MJ. Methimazole, carbimazole, and congenital skin defects. Annals of Internal Medicine 1987;106:60–61.

75. Di Gianantonio E, Schaefer C, Mastroiacovo PP, et al. Adverse effects of prenatal methimazole exposure. Teratology 2001;64:262–266.

76. Foulds N, Walpole I, Elmslie F, Mansour S. Carbimazole embryopathy: An emerging phenotype. American Journal of Medical Genetics Part A 2005;132A:130–135.

77. Clementi M, Di Gianantonio E, Pelo E, Mammi I, Basile RT, Tenconi R. Methimazole embryopathy: Delineation of the phenotype. American Journal of Medical Genetics 1999;83:43–46.

78. Gurlek A, Cobankara V, Bayraktar M. Liver tests in hyperthyroidism: Effect of antithyroid therapy. Journal of Clinical Gastroenterology 1997;24:180–183.

79. Mizutani T, Yoshida K, Murakami M, Shirai M, Kawazoe S. Evidence for the involvement of N-methylthiourea, a ring cleavage metabolite, in the hepatotoxicity of methimazole in glutathione-depleted mice: Structure-toxicity and metabolic studies. Chemical Research in Toxicology 2000;13:170–176.

80. Liaw YF, Huang MJ, Fan KD, Li KL, Wu SS, Chen TJ. Hepatic injury during propylthiouracil therapy in patients with hyperthyroidism. A cohort study. Annals of Internal Medicine 1993;118:424–428.

81. Williams KV, Nayak S, Becker D, Reyes J, Burmeister LA. Fifty years of experience with propylthiouracil-associated hepatotoxicity: What have we learned? J Clin Endocrinol Metab 1997;82:1727–1733.

82. Cooper DS, Rivkees SA. Putting propylthiouracil in perspective. J Clin Endocrinol Metab 2009;94:1881–1882.

83. Stanbury JB, Ermans AE, Bourdoux P, et al. Iodine-induced hyperthyroidism: Occurrence and epidemiology. Thyroid 1998;8:83–100.

84. Wolf J. Perchlorate and the thyroid gland. Pharmacological Reviews 1998;50:89–105.

85. Wartofsky L. Radioiodine therapy for Graves's disease: Case selection and restrictions recommended to patients in North America. Thyroid 1997;7:213–216.

86. Kaplan MM, Meier DA, Dworkin HJ. Treatment of hyperthyroidism with radioactive iodine. Endocrinol Metab Clin North Am 1998;27:205–223.

87. Bahn RS, Burch HS, Cooper DS, et al. The Role of Propylthiouracil in the Management of Graves's Disease in Adults: report of a meeting jointly sponsored by the American Thyroid Association and the Food and Drug Administration. Thyroid 2009;19:673–674.

88. Imseis RE, Vanmiddlesworth L, Massie JD, Bush AJ, Vanmiddlesworth NR. Pretreatment with propylthiouracil but not methimazole reduces the therapeutic efficacy of iodine-131 in hyperthyroidism. J Clin Endocrinol Metab 1998;83:685–687.

89. Santos RB, Romaldini JH, Ward LS. Propylthiouracil reduces the effectiveness of radioiodine treatment in hyperthyroid patients with Graves's disease. Thyroid 2004;14:525–530.

90. Bogazzi F, Giovannetti C, Fessehatsion R, et al. Impact of lithium on efficacy of radioactive iodine therapy for Graves's disease: A cohort study on cure rate, time to cure, and frequency of increased serum thyroxine after antithyroid drug withdrawal. J Clin Endocrinol Metab 2010;95:201–208.

91. Tallstedt L, Lundell G. Radioiodine treatment, ablation, and ophthalmopathy: A balanced perspective. Thyroid 1997;7:241–245.

92. Lazarus JH, Clarke S. Use of radioiodine in the management of hyperthyroidism in the UK: Development of guidelines. Thyroid 1997;7:229–231.

93. Boelaert K, Syed AA, Manji N, et al. Prediction of cure and risk of hypothyroidism in patients receiving 131I for hyperthyroidism. Clin Endocrinol 2009;70:129–138.

94. Franklyn JA, Maisonneuve P, Sheppard M, Betteridge J, Boyle P. Cancer incidence and mortality after radioiodine treatment for hyperthyroidism: A population-based cohort study. Lancet 1999;353: 2111–2115.

95. Franklyn JA, Maisonneuve P, Sheppard MC, Betteridge J, Boyle P. Mortality after the treatment of hyperthyroidism with radioactive iodine. N Engl J Med 1998;338:712–718.

96. Leslie WD, Ward L, Salamon EA, Ludwig S, Rowe RC, Cowden EA. A randomized comparison of radioiodine doses in Graves's hyperthyroidism. J Clin Endocrinol Metab 2003;88:978–983.

97. Franklyn JA. The management of hyperthyroidism. N Engl J Med 1994;330:1731–1738.

98. Uy HL, Reasner CA, Samuels MH. Pattern of recovery of the hypothalamic-pituitary-thyroid axis following radioactive iodine therapy in patients with Graves's disease. Am J Med 1995;99:173–179.

99. Chan GW, Mandel, S.J. Therapy Insight: Management of Graves's Disease During Pregnancy. Nat Clin Pract Endocrinol Metab 2007;3:470–478.

100. Glinoer D. Management of hypo- and hyperthyroidism during pregnancy. Growth Horm IGF Res 2003;13:S45-S54.

101. Lazarus JH, Kokandi A. Thyroid disease in relation to pregnancy: A decade of change. Clin Endocrinol 2000;53:265–278.

102. Lockwood CM, Grenache DG, Gronowski AM. Serum human chorionic gonadotropin concentrations greater than 400,000 IU/L are invariably associated with suppressed serum thyrotropin concentrations. Thyroid 2009;19:863–868.

103. Momotani N, Noh J, Ishikawa N, Ito K. Relationship between silent thyroiditis and recurrent Graves's disease in the postpartum period. J Clin Endocrinol Metab 1994;79:285–289.

104. Coukos G, Makrigiannakis A, Chung J, Randall TC, Rubin SC, Benjamin I. Complete hydatidiform mole. A disease with a changing profile. J Reprod Med 1999;44:698–704.

105. Momotani N, Yamashita R, Makino F, Noh JY, Ishikawa N, Ito K. Thyroid function in wholly breast-feeding infants whose mothers take high doses of propylthiouracil. Clin Endocrinol 2000;53:177–181.

106. Rotondi M, Cappelli C, Pirali B, et al. The effect of pregnancy on subsequent relapse from Graves's disease after a successful course of antithyroid drug therapy. J Clin Endocrinol Metab 2008;93:3985–3988.

107. Polak M, Le Gac I, Vuillard E, et al. Fetal and neonatal thyroid function in relation to maternal Graves's disease. Best Pract Res Clin Endocrinol Metab 2004;18:289–302.

108. Zimmerman D, Lteif AN. Thyrotoxicosis in children. Endocrinol Metab Clin North Am 1998;27:109–126.

109. Segni M, Leonardi E, Mazzoncini B, Pucarelli I, Pasquino AM. Special features of Graves's disease in early childhood. Thyroid 1999;9: 871–877.

110. Swinburne JL, Kreisman SH. A rare case of subacute thyroiditis causing thyroid storm. Thyroid 2007;17:73–76.

111. Sherman RG, Lasseter DH. Pharmacologic management of patients with diseases of the endocrine system. Dent Clin North Am 1996;40:727–752.

112. Sherman SI, Simonson L, Ladenson PW. Clinical and socioeconomic predispositions to complicated thyrotoxicosis: A predictable and preventable syndrome? Amer J Med 1996;101:192–198.

113. Zweig SB, Schlosser JR, Thomas SA, Levy CJ, Fleckman AM. Rectal administration of propylthiouracil in suppository form in patients with thyrotoxicosis and critical illness: Case report and review of literature. Endocr Pract 2006;12:43–47.

114. Hodak SP, Huang C, Clarke D, Burman KD, Jonklaas J, Janicic-Kharic N. Intravenous methimazole in the treatment of refractory hyperthyroidism. Thyroid 2006;16:691–695.

115. Duggal J, Singh S, Kuchinic P, Butler P, Arora R. Utility of esmolol in thyroid crisis. Can J Clin Pharmacol 2006;13:e292–e295.

116. Ozbey N, Kalayoglu-Besisik S, Gul N, Bozbora A, Sencer E, Molvalilar S. Therapeutic plasmapheresis in patients with severe hyperthyroidism

in whom antithyroid drugs are contraindicated. Int J Clin Pract 2004;58:554–558.

117. Roberts CG, Ladenson PW. Hypothyroidism. Lancet 2004;363: 793–803.

118. LaFranchi S. Thyroid hormone in hypopituitarism, Graves's disease, congenital hypothyroidism, and maternal thyroid disease during pregnancy. Growth Horm IGF Res 2006;16 Suppl A:S20–S24.

119. Roberts HJ. Aspartame disease: A possible cause for concomitant Graves's disease and pulmonary hypertension.[comment]. Texas Heart Inst J 2004;31:105–106.

120. Sinclair D. Clinical and laboratory aspects of thyroid autoantibodies. Ann Clin Biochem 2006;43:173–183.

121. Stassi G, De Maria R. Autoimmune thyroid disease: New models of cell death in autoimmunity. Nature Rev Immunol 2002;2:195–204.

122. Mitchell ML, Klein RZ. The sequelae of untreated maternal hypothyroidism. Eur J Endocrinol 2004;151.

123. Morreale de Escobar G, Obregon MJ, Escobar del Rey F. Role of thyroid hormone during early brain development. Eur J Endocrinol 2004;151.

124. Buyukgebiz A. Newborn screening for congenital hypothyroidism. J Pediatr Endocrinol Metab 2006;19:1291–1298.

125. Prabhakar VK, Shalet SM. Aetiology, diagnosis, and management of hypopituitarism in adult life. Postgrad Med J 2006;82:259–266.

126. Urban RJ. Hypopituitarism after acute brain injury. Growth Horm IGF Res 2006;16 (suppl A):S25–S29.

127. Sherman SI, Gopal J, Haugen BR, et al. Central hypothyroidism associated with retinoid X receptor-selective ligands. N Engl J Med 1999;340:1075–1079.

128. Joshi AS, Woolf PD. Pituitary hyperplasia secondary to primary hypothyroidism: A case report and review of the literature. Pituitary 2005;8:99–103.

129. Baskin HJ, Cobin RH, Duick DS, Gharib H, et al. American Association of Clinical Endocrinologists Medical Guidelines for Clinical Practice for Evalution and Treatment of Hyperthyroidism and Hypothyroidism. Endocr Pract 2002;8:457–469.

130. Jonklaas J, Davidson B, Bhagat S, Soldin SJ. Triiodothyronine levels in athyreotic individuals during levothyroxine therapy. JAMA 2008;299:769–77.

131. Blouin RA, Clifton GD, Adams MA, Foster TS, Flueck J. Biopharmaceutical comparison of two levothyroxine sodium products. Clin Pharm 1989;8:588–592.

132. Berg JA, Mayor GH. A study in normal human volunteers to compare the rate and extent of levothyroxine absorption from Synthroid and Levoxine. J Clinl Pharmacol 1992;32:1135–1140.

133. Gottwald R, Lorkowski G, Petersen G, Schnitzler M, Lucker PW. Bioequivalence of two commercially available levothyroxine-Na preparations in athyreotic patients. Methods Findings Exp Clin Pharmacol 1994;16:645–650.

134. Dong BJ, Hauck WW, Gambertoglio JG, et al. Bioequivalence of generic and brand-name levothyroxine products in the treatment of hypothyroidism. JAMA 1997;277:1205–1213.

135. Blakesley V, Awni W, Locke C, Ludden T, Granneman GR, Braverman LE. Are bioequivalence studies of levothyroxine sodium formulations in euthyroid volunteers reliable? Thyroid 2004;14:191–200.

136. Hennessey JV. Levothyroxine dosage and the limitations of current bioequivalence standards. Nat Clin Pract Endocrinol Metab 2006;2:474–475.

137. Wenzel KW. Bioavailability of levothyroxine preparations. Thyroid 2003;13:665.

138. Bach-Huynh TG, Nayak B, Loh J, Soldin S, Jonklaas J. Timing of levothyroxine administration affects serum thyrotropin concentration. J Clin Endocrinol Metab 2009;94:3905–3912.

139. Liel Y, Sperber AD, Shany S. Nonspecific intestinal adsorption of levothyroxine by aluminum hydroxide. Am J Med 1994;97: 363–365.

140. Shakir KM, Chute JP, Aprill BS, Lazarus AA. Ferrous sulfate-induced increase in requirement for thyroxine in a patient with primary hypothyroidism. South Med J 1997;90:637–639.

141. Jabbar MA, Larrea J, Shaw RA. Abnormal thyroid function tests in infants with congenital hypothyroidism: the influence of soy-based formula. J A Coll Nutr 1997;16:280–282.

142. Liel Y, Harman-Boehm I, Shany S. Evidence for a clinically important adverse effect of fiber-enriched diet on the bioavailability of levothyroxine in adult hypothyroid patients. J Clin Endocrinol Metab 1996;81:857–859.

143. Benvenga S, Bartolone L, Pappalardo MA, et al. Altered intestinal absorption of L-thyroxine caused by coffee. Thyroid 2008;18:293–301.

144. Sachmechi I, Reich DM, Aninyei M, Wibowo F, Gupta G, Kim PJ. Effect of proton pump inhibitors on serum thyroid-stimulating hormone level in euthyroid patients treated with levothyroxine for hypothyroidism. Endocrine Practice 2007;13:345–349.

145. Appelhof BC, Fliers E, Wekking EM, et al. Combined therapy with levothyroxine and liothyronine in two ratios, compared with levothyroxine monotherapy in primary hypothyroidism: A double-blind, randomized, controlled clinical trial. J Clin Endocrinol Metab 2005;90:2666–2674.

146. Clyde PW, Harari AE, Getka EJ, Shakir KM. Combined levothyroxine plus liothyronine compared with levothyroxine alone in primary hypothyroidism: A randomized controlled trial.[see comment]. JAMA 2003;290:2952–2958.

147. Grozinsky-Glasberg S, Fraser A, Nahshoni E, Weizman A, Leibovici L. Thyroxine-triiodothyronine combination therapy versus thyroxine monotherapy for clinical hypothyroidism: meta-analysis of randomized controlled trials. J Clin Endocrinol Metab 2006;91:2592–2599.

148. Escobar-Morreale HF, Botella-Carretero JI, Escobar del Rey F, Morreale de Escobar G. REVIEW: Treatment of hypothyroidism with combinations of levothyroxine plus liothyronine. J Clin Endocrinol Metab 2005;90:4946–4954.

149. Roti E, Minelli R, Gardini E, Braverman LE. The use and misuse of thyroid hormone. Endocr Rev 1993;14:401–423.

150. Burmeister LA, Goumaz MO, Mariash CN, Oppenheimer JH. Levothyroxine dose requirements for thyrotropin suppression in the treatment of differentiated thyroid cancer. J Clin Endocrinol Metab 1992;75:344–350.

151. Spencer CA, Hollowell JG, Kazarosyan M, Braverman LE. National Health and Nutrition Examination Survey III thyroid-stimulating hormone (TSH)-thyroperoxidase antibody relationships demonstrate that TSH upper reference limits may be skewed by occult thyroid dysfunction. J Clin Endocrinol Metab 2007;92:4236–4240.

152. Wartofsky L, Dickey RA. The evidence for a narrower thyrotropin reference range is compelling. J Clin Endocrinol Metab 2005;90: 5483–5488.

153. Surks MI, Goswami G, Daniels GH. The thyrotropin reference range should remain unchanged. J Clin Endocrinol Metab 2005;90: 5489–5496.

154. Sawin CT, Herman T, Molitch ME, London MH, Kramer SM. Aging and the thyroid. Decreased requirement for thyroid hormone in older hypothyroid patients. Am J Med 1983;75:206–209.

155. Kabadi UM. Influence of age on optimal daily levothyroxine dosage in patients with primary hypothyroidism grouped according to etiology. South Med J 1997;90:920–924.

156. Santini F, Pinchera A, Marsili A, et al. Lean body mass is a major determinant of levothyroxine dosage in the treatment of thyroid diseases. J Clin Endocrinol Metab 2005;90:124–127.

157. De Whalley P. Do abnormal thyroid stimulating hormone level values result in treatment changes? A study of patients on thyroxine in one general practice. Br J Gen Pract 1995;45:93–95.

158. Parle JV, Franklyn JA, Cross KW, Jones SR, Sheppard MC. Thyroxine prescription in the community: serum thyroid stimulating hormone level assays as an indicator of undertreatment or overtreatment.[see comment]. Br J Gen Pract 1993;43:107–109.

159. Garber JR, Hennessey JV, Liebermann JA, 3rd, Morris CM, Talbert RL. Clinical Upate. Managing the challenges of hypothyroidism. J Fam Pract 2006;55.

160. Vanderpump MP, Tunbridge WM. Epidemiology and prevention of clinical and subclinical hypothyroidism. Thyroid 2002;12:839–847.

161. Vanderpump M. Subclinical hypothyroidism: the case against treatment. Trends Endocrinol Metab 2003;14:262–266.

162. Loh JA, Wartofsky L, Jonklaas J, Burman KD. The magnitude of increased levothyroxine requirements in hypothyroid pregnant women depends upon the etiology of the hypothyroidism. Thyroid 2009;19:269–275.

163. Zelmanovitz F, Genro S, Gross JL. Suppressive therapy with levothy-roxine for solitary thyroid nodules: A double-blind controlled clinical study and cumulative meta-analyses. J Clin Endocrinol Metab 1998;83:3881–3885.

164. Castro MR, Caraballo PJ, Morris JC. Effectiveness of thyroid hormone suppressive therapy in benign solitary thyroid nodules: A meta-analysis. J Clin Endocrinol Metab 2002;87:4154–4159.

165. Sdano MT, Falciglia M, Welge JA, Steward DL. Efficacy of thyroid hormone suppression for benign thyroid nodules: Meta-analysis of randomized trials. Otolaryngol—Head Neck Surg 2005;133:391–396.

166. Jonklaas J, Sarlis NJ, Litofsky D, et al. Outcomes of patients with differentiated thyroid carcinoma following initial therapy. Thyroid 2006;16:1229–1242.

167. Cooper DS, Doherty GM, Duh QY, et al. Revised American Thyroid Association management guidelines for patients with thyroid nodules and differentiated thyroid cancer. Thyroid 2009;19:1167–1214.

168. Canaris GJ, Manowitz NR, Mayor G, Ridgway EC. The Colorado thyroid disease prevalence study. Arch Intern Med 2000;160:526–534.

169. Somwaru LL, Arnold AM, Joshi N, Fried LP, Cappola AR. High frequency of and factors associated with thyroid hormone over-replacement and under-replacement in men and women aged 65 and over. J Clin Endocrinol Metab 2009;94:1342–1345.

170. Vestergaard P, Mosekilde L. Hyperthyroidism, bone mineral, and fracture risk—A meta-analysis. Thyroid 2003;13:585–593.

171. Uzzan B, Campos J, Cucherat M, Nony P, Boissel JP, Perret GY. Effects on bone mass of long term treatment with thyroid hormones: A meta-analysis. J Clin Endocrinol Metab 1996;81:4278–4289.

172. Sarlis NJ, Gourgiotis L. Thyroid emergencies. Rev Endocr Metab Disord 2003;4:129–136.

173. Wartofsky L. Myxedema coma. Endocrinol Metab Clin North Am 2006;35:687–698, vii–viii.

174. American Academy of P, Rose SR, Section on E, et al. Update of newborn screening and therapy for congenital hypothyroidism. Pediatr 2006;117:2290–2303.

175. Rovet J, Daneman D. Congenital hypothyroidism: A review of current diagnostic and treatment practices in relation to neuropsychologic outcome. Paediatr Drugs 2003;5:141–149.

176. Haddow JE, Palomaki GE, Allan WC, et al. Maternal thyroid deficiency during pregnancy and subsequent neuropsychological development of the child.[see comment]. N Engl J Med 1999;341:549–555.

177. Sherman SI. Etiology, diagnosis, and treatment recommendations for central hypothyroidism associated with bexarotene therapy for cutaneous T-cell lymphoma. Clinl Lymphoma 2003;3:249–252.

178. Sherman SI. Thyroid carcinoma. Lancet 2003;361:501–511.

179. Haugen BR, Pacini F, Reiners C, et al. A comparison of recombinant human thyrotropin and thyroid hormone withdrawal for the detection of thyroid remnant or cancer. J Clin Endocrinol Metab 1999;84:3877–3885.

180. Pacini F, Ladenson PW, Schlumberger M, et al. Radioiodine ablation of thyroid remnants after preparation with recombinant human thyrotropin in differentiated thyroid carcinoma: Results of an international, randomized, controlled study. J Clin Endocrinol Metab 2006;91:926–932.

181. Robbins RJ, Driedger A, Magner J. Recombinant human thyrotropin-assisted radioiodine therapy for patients with metastatic thyroid cancer who could not elevate endogenous thyrotropin or be withdrawn from thyroxine. Thyroid 2006;16:1121–1130.

182. Elisei R, Schlumberger M, Driedger A, et al. Follow-up of low-risk differentiated thyroid cancer patients who underwent radioiodine ablation of postsurgical thyroid remnants after either recombinant human thyrotropin or thyroid hormone withdrawal. J Clin Endocrinol Metab 2009;94:4171–4179.

183. Fast S, Nielsen VE, Bonnema SJ, Hegedus L. Time to reconsider nonsurgical therapy of benign non-toxic multinodular goitre: Focus on recombinant human TSH augmented radioiodine therapy. Eur J Endocrinol 2009;160:517–528.

184. Torpy DJ, Tsigos C, Lotsikas AJ, Defensor R, Chrousos GP, Papanicolaou DA. Acute and delayed effects of a single-dose injection of interleukin-6 on thyroid function in healthy humans. Metab 1998;47:1289–1293.

185. Burman KD, Wartofsky L. Thyroid function in the intensive care unit setting. Crit Care Clin 2001;17:43–57.

186. Stathatos N, Levetan C, Burman KD, Wartofsky L. The controversy of the treatment of critically ill patients with thyroid hormone. Best Pract Res Clin Endocrinol Metab 2001;15:465–478.

187. Langton JE, Brent GA. Nonthyroidal illness syndrome: evaluation of thyroid function in sick patients. Endocrinol Metab Clin North Am 2002;31:159–172.

188. Stathatos N, Levetan C, Burman KD, Wartofsky L. The controversy of the treatment of critically ill patients with thyroid hormone. Best Pract Res Clin Endocrinol Metab 2001;15:465–478.

189. Simescu M, Varciu M, Nicolaescu E, et al. Iodized oil as a complement to iodized salt in schoolchildren in endemic goiter in Romania. Horm Res 2002;58:78–82.

190. Ljunggren JG, Torring O, Wallin G, et al. Quality of life aspects and costs in treatment of Graves's hyperthyroidism with antithyroid drugs, surgery, or radioiodine: results from a prospective, randomized study. Thyroid 1998;8:653–659.

85

Adrenal Gland Disorders

STEVEN M. SMITH AND JOHN G. GUMS

KEY CONCEPTS

❶ Glucocorticoid secretion from the adrenal cortex is stimulated by adrenocorticotropic hormone (ACTH) or corticotropin that is released from the anterior pituitary in response to the hypothalamic-mediated release of corticotropin-releasing hormone (CRH).

❷ To ensure the proper treatment of Cushing's syndrome, diagnostic procedures should (1) establish the presence of hypercortisolism and (2) discover the underlying etiology of the disease.

❸ The rationale for treating Cushing's syndrome is to reduce the morbidity and mortality resulting from disorders such as diabetes mellitus, cardiovascular disease, and electrolyte abnormalities.

❹ The treatment of choice for both ACTH-dependent and ACTH-independent Cushing's syndrome is surgery, whereas pharmacologic agents are reserved for adjunctive therapy, refractory cases, or inoperable disease.

❺ Pharmacologic agents that may be used to manage the patient with Cushing's syndrome include steroidogenesis inhibitors, adrenolytic agents, neuromodulators of ACTH release, and glucocorticoid-receptor blocking agents.

❻ Spironolactone, a competitive aldosterone receptor antagonist, is the drug of choice in bilateral adrenal hyperplasia (BAH)-dependent hyperaldosteronism.

❼ Addison's disease (primary adrenal insufficiency) is a deficiency in cortisol, aldosterone, and various androgens resulting from the loss of function of all regions of the adrenal cortex.

❽ Secondary adrenal insufficiency usually results from exogenous steroid use, leading to hypothalamic-pituitary-adrenal (HPA)-axis suppression followed by a decrease in ACTH release, and low levels of androgens and cortisol.

❾ Virilism results from the excessive secretion of androgens from the adrenal gland and often manifests as hirsutism in females.

Learning objectives, review questions, and other resources can be found at **www.pharmacotherapyonline.com**.

The adrenal glands were first characterized by Eustachius in 1563. After Addison identified a case of adrenal insufficiency in humans, adrenal anatomy and physiology flourished. Most of the work done in the early and mid-1900s centered on the glucocorticoid cortisol. With the discovery of aldosterone by Simpson and Tait in 1952, adrenal pharmacology turned toward the mineralocorticoid. Conn[1] followed with his classical description of primary aldosteronism in 1955, and numerous clinicians and investigators have continued to explore the variety of disease processes promoted through the adrenal gland.

PHYSIOLOGY, ANATOMY, AND BIOCHEMISTRY

The adrenal glands are located extraperitoneally to the upper poles of each kidney (Fig. 85–1). On average, each adrenal gland weighs 4 g and is 2 to 3 cm in width and 4 to 6 cm in length. The gland is fed by small arteries from the abdominal aorta and renal and phrenic arteries. Drainage of the adrenal gland occurs via the renal vein on the left and the inferior vena cava on the right.

The adrenal medulla occupies 10% of the total gland and is responsible for the secretion of catecholamines. The adrenal cortex accounts for the remaining 90% and is responsible for the secretion of three types of hormones (Fig. 85–2) from three separate zones.

The zona glomerulosa accounts for 15% of the total adrenal cortex and is responsible for mineralocorticoid production, of which aldosterone is the principal end product. Aldosterone maintains electrolyte and volume homeostasis by altering potassium and magnesium secretion and renal tubular sodium reabsorption. The zona fasciculata, the middle zone, makes up 60% of the cortex,

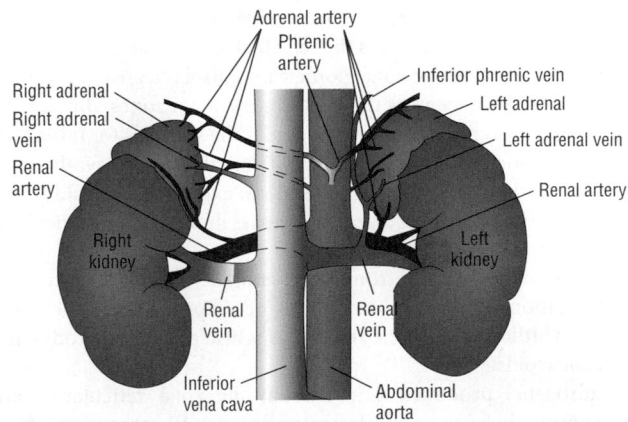

FIGURE 85-1. Anatomy of the adrenal gland.

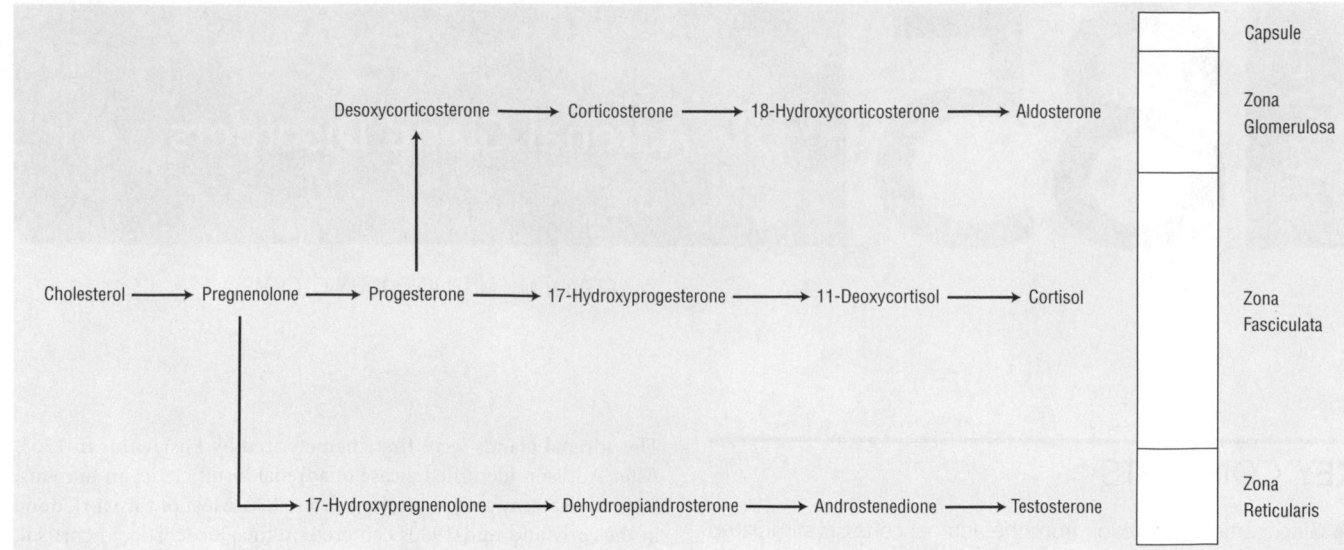

FIGURE 85-2. Hormone synthetic pathways in relation to the zones of the adrenal cortex.

is high in cholesterol, and is responsible for basal and stimulated glucocorticoid production. Glucocorticoids, mainly cortisol, are responsible for the regulation of fat, carbohydrate, and protein metabolism. The zona reticularis occupies 25% of the adrenal cortex, and is responsible for adrenal androgen production. The androgens, testosterone and estradiol, are the major end products and influence the reproductive system in addition to modulating primary and secondary sex characteristics.

HORMONE PRODUCTION AND METABOLISM

Adrenal steroid hormone synthesis begins with the conversion of cholesterol to pregnenolone by cytochrome P450 (CYP) enzymatic side-chain cleavage. Following this rate-limiting step, pregnenolone is converted to various 19- and 21-carbon steroids, depending on the enzymatic capabilities within each zone of the cortex. Androgenic properties predominate in the 19-carbon steroids, whereas mineralocorticoid and glucocorticoid properties manifest in the 21-carbon steroids.

Aldosterone production is initiated by the 21-hydroxylation of progesterone to form deoxycorticosterone. Subsequently, aldosterone synthase converts deoxycorticosterone to aldosterone through the intermediary, corticosterone. The zona glomerulosa preferentially produces aldosterone for three main reasons. First, the zona glomerulosa lacks 17α-hydroxylase activity and therefore can only convert pregnenolone to progesterone. Secondly, in contrast to the other zones, cells in the zona glomerulosa possess aldosterone synthase activity, which catalyzes the terminal steps in aldosterone synthesis. Lastly, cells of the zona glomerulosa display a greater number of angiotensin II receptors than cells of the other zones. Binding of angiotensin II to these receptors provides the stimulus for initiating the aldosterone biosynthesis cascade. Thus, aldosterone synthesis is a unique feature of the zona glomerulosa, explaining why aldosterone is not affected during disease processes limited to the fasciculata and/or reticularis.

Cortisol is produced from pregnenolone via four successive hydroxylations. These hydroxylations occur primarily in the zona fasiculata although the zona reticularis is also capable of producing glucocorticoids.

Androgens, produced primarily in the zona reticularis and less commonly in the zona fasiculata, have a 19-carbon structure and serve as precursors to more potent analogs produced in the periphery. The adrenal gland can synthesize estradiol and estrone from testosterone and androstenedione, respectively; however, these synthesized quantities are extremely small. The rates of production for the various steroids produced by the adrenal gland are listed in Table 85–1.

Glucocorticoid metabolism occurs in the liver and is responsible for converting inactive steroids to active metabolites, as well as modifying active steroids to less active or inactive metabolites. Most pharmaceutical steroid products are active; however, in the case of prednisone and cortisone, metabolism is necessary for conversion to the active prednisolone and cortisol, respectively.

Following metabolic conversion, glomerular filtration is primarily responsible for eliminating endogenously produced glucocorticoids. The half-life of cortisol is 70 to 120 minutes, whereas aldosterone exhibits extremely high intrinsic clearance and a corresponding half-life of only 15 minutes.

Metabolism and conversion of the various steroids can be altered by a variety of disease states and medicinal compounds. Drugs known to enhance steroid clearance include phenytoin, phenobarbital, rifampin, mitotane, and aminoglutethimide. Likewise, diseases

TABLE 85-1	Rates of Adrenal Production and Plasma Concentrations of Various Steroids	
Steroid	**24-Hour Secretion (mg)**	**Plasma Concentration (ng/dL)**
Aldosterone	0.15	2–9 (supine, normal-sodium diet)
Androstenedione	2.2–2.5	50–250
Corticosterone	1–4	2.4 ± 1.5 (female)
		4.2 ± 2.2 (male)
Cortisol	8–25	0–25 mcg/DL
11-Deoxycorticosterone	0.60	2–19
11-Deoxycortisol	0.40	12–158
Progesterone	0.0	<20 (female)[a]
		300–2,000 (female)[b]
		<20–140 (male)
Testosterone (total)	0.23 (female)	6–86 (female)
		270–1070 (male)

[a]Follicular phase of menstrual cycle.
[b]Luteal phase of menstrual cycle.
From Kratz A, Ferraro M, Sluss PM, Lewandrowski KB. Laboratory reference values. N Engl J Med 2004;351(15):1548–1563. Copyright © 2004 Massachusetts Medical Society. All rights reserved.

such as hyperthyroidism and renal disease (dexamethasone only) can enhance steroid clearance. In contrast, drugs such as estrogens and estrogen-containing oral contraceptives reduce steroid clearance. Similarly, liver disease, age, pregnancy, hypothyroidism, anorexia nervosa, protein-calorie malnutrition, and renal disease (prednisolone only) are associated with reduced steroid clearance.

Plasma glucocorticoids are bound to one of three plasma proteins in varying degrees. Corticosteroid-binding globulin (CBG), albumin, and α_1-glycoprotein are capable of binding glucocorticoids, with CBG being the principal binding protein. Steroid binding serves as a reservoir for steroids in their inactive state and ≥95% of cortisol is normally bound in this fashion. This binding prevents glucocorticoid activity at receptor-activating sites. Therefore, a final but important variable in altered plasma concentration of free (active) steroids is concentration of plasma proteins.

REGULATION OF HORMONE SECRETION

❶ Glucocorticoid secretion is regulated by the pituitary hormone, ACTH (also known as corticotropin). Under normal conditions, ACTH is released from the anterior pituitary in response to CRH, which is secreted by the median eminence of the hypothalamus (Fig. 85–3). Vasopressin and oxytocin have weak ACTH-releasing activity through binding to the inferior V_3 receptor. CRH, in combination with vasopressin and oxytocin, stimulates greater ACTH secretion than each hormone individually.

Additionally, histochemical studies have demonstrated that certain neurotransmitters have the unique ability to stimulate production of CRH or ACTH directly. Specifically, 5-hydroxytryptamine and norepinephrine have both been shown to increase levels of ACTH. After release, ACTH stimulates the adrenal gland to release cortisol and, to a lesser extent, aldosterone and androgens. The rising cortisol concentration inhibits the secretion of CRH and ACTH

through a negative-feedback mechanism. In addition, leptin, an adipocyte hormone, can have an inhibitory effect on HPA activity.

Adrenal androgens are regulated in a similar fashion to cortisol. When plasma androgen reaches sufficient concentrations, production is terminated via a negative feedback loop. Androgen release is increased during puberty and in women with hirsutism. Adrenal androgen release decreases with age and in fasting states, including anorexia nervosa.

In contrast to cortisol and adrenal androgens, regulation of aldosterone secretion is considerably more complex. The renin-angiotensin system regulates aldosterone secretion through both intrarenal and extrarenal mechanisms. Renin production and subsequent aldosterone secretion is stimulated by blood pressure lowering (due to volume depletion), erect posture, salt depletion, β-adrenergic stimulation, and central nervous system excitation (see Chap. 15). Renin production is inhibited by salt loading, angiotensin II, vasopressin, potassium, calcium, blood pressure increases, and a variety of drugs. The renin-mediated production of angiotensin II is the initial stimulus for aldosterone synthesis. Additionally, angiotensin II can be acted on by aminopeptidase and converted to angiotensin III. Angiotensin II and III are both capable of stimulating the zona glomerulosa to secrete aldosterone. Following aldosterone secretion, increases in renal sodium and water retention as well as blood pressure occur, thereby turning off the stimulus for renin release.

HYPERFUNCTION OF THE ADRENAL GLAND

CUSHING'S SYNDROME

In 1932, Cushing first described a syndrome of pituitary basophilism that attracted national attention. Until this time, no definitive diagnosis existed for patients with unexplained central obesity, cutaneous striae, osteoporosis, weakness, hypertension, diabetes mellitus, and congestion. Cushing emphasized that the disease was of a pituitary origin. Ten years later, Albright focused his attention on the sugar hormone, which he believed originated from the adrenal cortex.[2]

After the development of a method for measuring urinary steroids, Daughaday discovered elevated steroids in the urine of patients with Cushing's syndrome. Finally, the end product was identified, and Cushing's syndrome was correctly explained as an excess of cortisol in the plasma (hypercortisolism).

Etiology

Cushing's syndrome results from the effects of supraphysiologic levels of glucocorticoids originating either from exogenous administration or less commonly, from endogenous overproduction by the adrenal glands. Excess glucocorticoids are produced in response to overproduction of ACTH (ACTH-dependent) or by abnormal adrenocortical tissues regardless of ACTH stimulation (ACTH-independent). ACTH-dependent Cushing's syndrome (≈80% of all Cushing's cases) usually originates from overproduction of ACTH by the pituitary gland, which chronically stimulates the adrenal glands causing bilateral adrenal hyperplasia. Approximately 85% of these cases are caused by pituitary adenomas (Cushing's disease). Ectopic ACTH-secreting tumors and non-neoplastic corticotropin hypersecretion, possibly secondary to excess CRH production, account for the remainder of ACTH-dependent causes.[3] Ectopic ACTH syndrome refers to excessive ACTH production resulting from an endocrine or nonendocrine tumor, usually of the pancreas, thyroid, or lung. Small-cell carcinoma of the lung will lead to ectopic ACTH secretion in 0.5% to 2% of cases, whereas bronchial carcinoid tumors are usually the most common.[4] Distinguishing

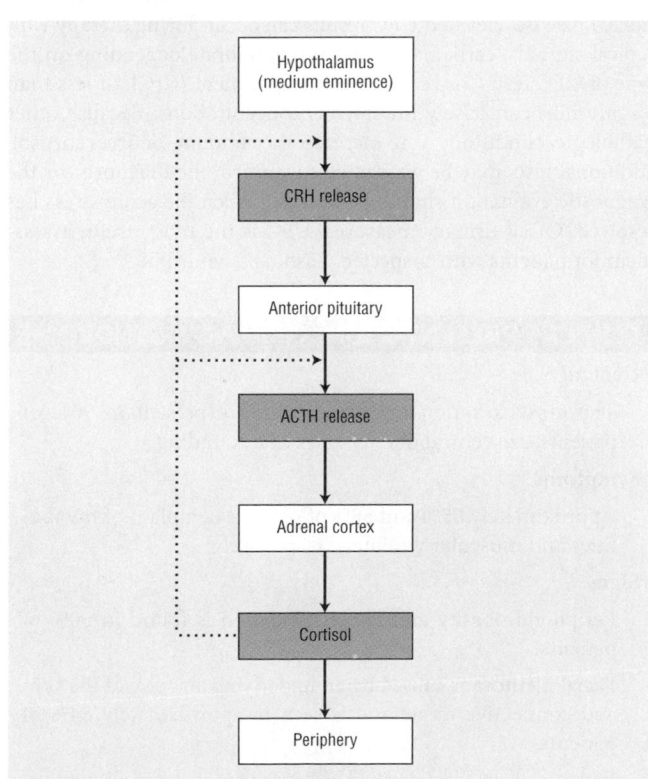

FIGURE 85–3. Negative feedback system involved in the regulation of cortisol secretion under normal conditions. (ACTH, adrenocorticotropic hormone; CRH, corticotropin-releasing hormone.)

TABLE 85-2 Various Etiologies of Cushing's Syndrome and Their Respective Differences

	Pituitary-Dependent	Ectopic ACTH Syndrome	Adrenal Adenoma	Adrenal Carcinoma
Course	Slow	Rapid	Slow	Rapid
Symptoms	Mild to moderate	Atypical	Mild to moderate	Severe
Dominant sex/age	Female/male	Male	None noted	Children
Virilization	+	+	+	+++
Abdominal mass	0	0	0	++
Plasma ACTH concentration	Slightly elevated	High	0	0
Dexamethasone suppression test	≥50% Suppression	No suppression	No suppression	No suppression
Iodocholesterol scan	Bilateral uptake	Bilateral uptake	Unilateral	None

ACTH, adrenocorticotropic hormone.

between the various etiologies requires a careful history and pertinent laboratory work (Table 85–2).

The remaining 20% of Cushing's syndrome cases are ACTH-independent and divided almost equally between adrenal adenomas and adrenal carcinomas, with rare cases caused by macronodular hyperplasia, primary pigmented nodular adrenal disease, and McCune-Albright syndrome.[3,5] The majority of adrenal cortex tumors are benign adenomas. Adrenal carcinoma is found more often in children than in adults with Cushing's syndrome.

Clinical Presentation

Patients with Cushing's syndrome commonly present (>90% of patients) with central obesity and facial rounding. In addition, approximately 50% of patients will exhibit some peripheral obesity and fat accumulation. Fat accumulation in the dorsocervical area (buffalo hump) can be associated with any major weight gain, whereas increased supraclavicular fat pads are more specific for Cushing's syndrome. Striae usually are present along the lower abdomen and take on a red to purple color. Traditionally, hypertensive complications have been major contributors to the morbidity and mortality of Cushing's syndrome. Hypertension is diagnosed in 75% to 85% of patients, with diastolic blood pressures greater than 119 mm Hg noted in over 20% of patients.[6] In addition, glucose intolerance is present in 60% of patients. Thus, many patients meet diagnostic criteria for the metabolic syndrome and have a corresponding increased risk of CHD and stroke. Screening for Cushing's syndrome in this population and in patients with uncontrolled diabetes mellitus has been suggested,[7,8] particularly when these conditions surface at an unusually early age.[9]

CLINICAL CONTROVERSY

Traditionally, obesity was used as screening tool because of its high prevalence in Cushing's syndrome. However, given the current epidemic of obesity, routine screening in all overweight and obese individuals may result in a high rate of false-positive tests.

Diagnosis

❷ The diagnosis of Cushing's syndrome involves two steps: (1) establishing the presence of hypercortisolism, which is relatively easy; and (2) differentiating between etiologies, which can be challenging (Fig. 85–4).[5,8,10] The presence of hypercortisolism can be established via the following tests: 24-hour urinary free cortisol (UFC), midnight plasma cortisol, late-night salivary cortisol, and/or the low-dose dexamethosone suppression test (DST) (using 1 mg dexamethasone for the overnight test or 0.5 mg/6 h for the classic 2-day study). However, because these tests cannot determine the etiology of Cushing's syndrome, other tests and procedures will be

subsequently employed. Such tests can include any of the following: plasma ACTH via IRMA or RIA; adrenal vein catheterization; metyrapone stimulation test; adrenal, chest, or abdominal CT; CRH stimulation test; IPSS; JVS; cavernous sinus sampling; and pituitary MRI. High-dose DST has been used in the past, but is no longer recommended due to its poor specificity and limited diagnostic value. Other possible tests and procedures include insulin-induced hypoglycemia, somatostatin receptor scintigraphy, the desmopressin stimulation test, the naloxone CRH stimulation test, the loperamide test, the hexarelin stimulation test, and radionuclide imaging.[5,6,8,10–15] Table 85–3 summarizes some of the tests used to diagnose Cushing's syndrome.

Elevated UFC concentrations are highly suggestive of Cushing's syndrome, especially values fourfold greater than the upper limit of normal.[3,12] In contrast to plasma measurements of cortisol, UFC measures only unbound cortisol. Consequently, the UFC test is unaffected by conditions and medications that alter CBG levels. Normal reference values for UFC are 20 to 90 mcg per 24-hour period. A two- to threefold increase in urine cortisol is not uncommon in the patient with hyperfunction of the adrenal gland. Starvation, hydration from water loading (greater than 5 liters per day), alcoholism, and acute stress are all capable of elevating urine cortisol concentrations. Likewise, elevated UFC results can occur during therapy with topical steroids, carbamazepine, and fenofibrate depending on the type of UFC test. Conversely, renal impairment (CrCL of less than 60 mL/min) can falsely lower UFC concentrations. Because other pathologic conditions can increase the amount of free cortisol, additional tests may be warranted to confirm the diagnosis, or the diagnostic evaluation should be repeated when the acute stress has resolved. Of all urinary measures, UFC is the most useful assessment for patients with suspected Cushing's syndrome.[8,12,14]

CLINICAL PRESENTATION: CUSHING'S SYNDROME

General

- The most common findings, which are present in 90% of patients, are central obesity and facial rounding.

Symptoms

- Approximately 65% and 58% of patients complain of myopathies and muscular weakness, respectively.

Signs

- Peripheral obesity and fat accumulation is found in 50% of patients.

- Facial plethora is caused by an underlying atrophy of the skin and connective tissue and is seen in approximately 84% of patients.

- Patients often are described as having moon faces with a buffalo hump.

- Hypertension is seen in 75% to 85% of patients.

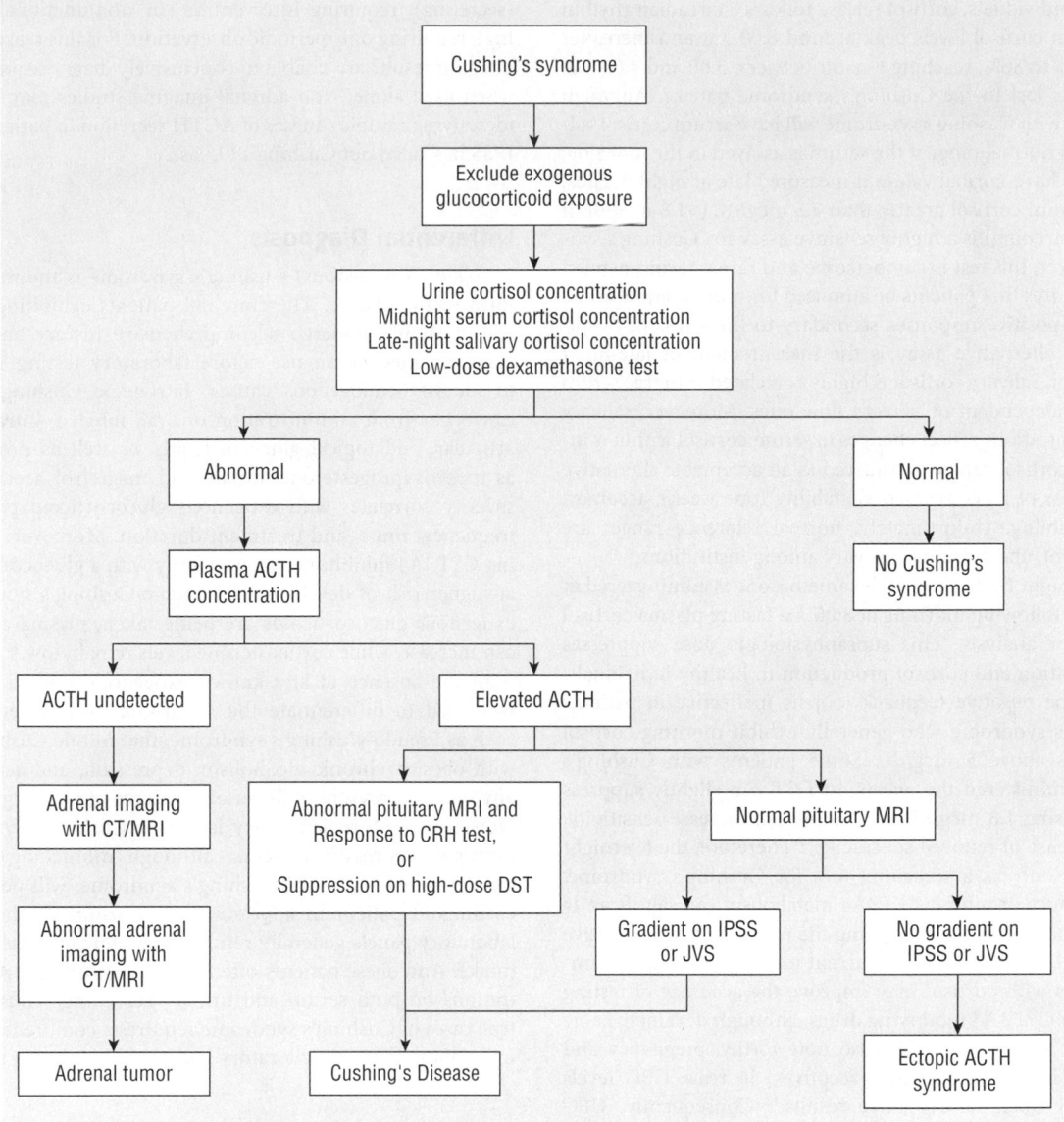

FIGURE 85-4. Algorithm for diagnosing Cushing's syndrome. (ACTH, adrenocorticotropic hormone.)

Psychiatric changes can occur in as many as 55% of patients.

Approximately 50% to 60% of patients will develop Cushing-induced osteoporosis. Of these, 40% will present with back pain and 20% will progress to compression fractures of the spine.

Gonadal dysfunction is common with amenorrhea seen in up to 75% of females.

Excess adrenal and ovary androgen secretion is responsible for 80% of females presenting with hirsutism.

Laboratory Tests

A midnight plasma cortisol, late-night salivary cortisol, 24-hour UFC, and/or low-dose DST will establish the presence of hypercortisolism.

Other Diagnostic Tests

The plasma ACTH test, metyrapone stimulation test, CRH stimulation test, or inferior petrosal sinus sampling will help determine the etiology.

TABLE 85-3	**Summary of Tests Used to Diagnose Cushing's Syndrome**			
Test	**Normal**	**Hyperplasia**	**Adenoma**	**Carcinoma**
Plasma				
Cortisol (mcg/dL, AM/PM)	5–25/5–15	↑/↑↑	↑↑/↑↑	↑↑↑/↑↑↑
After low-dose DST	↓	↔	↔	↔
After high-dose DST	↓	↓/↔	↔	↔
ACTH (pg/mL)	6–76	↑↑	↓	↓
Urine				
Cortisol (mcg/24 h)	20–90	↑↑	↑↑	↑↑↑
Saliva				
Cortisol (mcg/dL, PM)	Assay-dependent	↑↑	↑↑	↑↑↑

ACTH, adrenocorticotropic hormone; DST, dexamethasone suppression test.
From Kratz A, Ferraro M, Sluss PM, Lewandrowski KB. Laboratory reference values. N Engl J Med 2004;351(15):1548–1563. Copyright © 2004 Massachusetts Medical Society. All rights reserved.

In healthy individuals, cortisol release follows a circadian rhythm whereby serum cortisol levels peak around 8:00 AM and thereafter decline by 60% to 80%, reaching a nadir between 3:00 and 4:00 AM. This rhythm is lost in the Cushing's syndrome patient. Although many patients with Cushing's syndrome will have serum cortisol values in the high normal range if the serum is assayed in the morning, only 3.4% will have normal values if measured late at night.[16] Thus, a midnight serum cortisol greater than 7.5 mcg/dL (>1.8 mcg/dL if the patient is sleeping) is a highly sensitive assay for Cushing's syndrome. However, this test is cumbersome and rarely recommended because it requires that patients be admitted for more than 48 hours to avoid false-positive responses secondary to the stress of hospitalization. An alternative assay is the measurement of late-night salivary cortisol. Salivary cortisol is highly correlated with free serum cortisol and independent of salivary flow rates. Moreover, salivary cortisol concentrations reflect changes in serum cortisol within minutes. Salivary cortisol can be considered as an acceptable alternative to UFC because of its convenience, stability (one week), accuracy, and reproducibility. Unfortunately, normal reference ranges are assay-dependent, and cutoff points vary among institutions.[17,18]

In the overnight DST, 1 mg of dexamethasone is administered at 11:00 PM. The following morning at 8:00 AM fasting plasma cortisol is obtained for analysis. This supraphysiologic dose suppresses ACTH stimulation and cortisol production in healthy individuals. In contrast, the negative feedback loop is ineffective in patients with Cushing's syndrome who generally exhibit morning cortisol concentrations above 5 mcg/dL. Some patients with Cushing's symdrome administered the overnight DST can slightly suppress cortisol and using 1.8 mcg/dL as a cutoff can increase sensitivity, but at the expense of reduced specificity.[19] Therefore, the overnight DST is useful only as a screening tool for Cushing's syndrome. Drugs that induce or inhibit CYP3A4 metabolism can significantly alter dexamethasone levels, increasing the number of false-positive and false-negative DST tests. Concurrent measurements of dexamethasone levels with cortisol may improve the accuracy of testing for patients on CYP3A4 modifying drugs, although dexamethasone assays are not widely available. Also noteworthy, pregnancy and estrogen use (including oral contraceptives) increase CBG levels and frequently illicit false-positive results.[12] Consequently, UFC testing is preferred over DST in these patient populations.

The first test used to determine the etiology of Cushing's syndrome is the plasma ACTH test. Plasma ACTH concentrations can be measured via RIA or IRMA.[11] In ACTH-dependent Cushing's syndrome, ACTH can be normal or elevated. Very high levels of ACTH favor ectopic production. In contrast, ACTH values generally are low (less than 5 pg/mL) in ACTH-independent (adrenal) Cushing's syndrome. Furthermore, ACTH levels can appear artificially low in some ectopic ACTH-producing tumors because ACTH can be secreted as an active prohormone that is not detected by the assay.

IPSS offers the highest sensitivity and specificity of any test in differentiating the etiology of Cushing's syndrome. This technique requires catheterization of both petrosal sinuses with serial measurements of ACTH in each sinus and a peripheral vein after administration of CRH. A central-to-peripheral ACTH gradient is diagnostic for Cushing's disease whereas no gradient indicates ectopic ACTH production. Complications, such as venous thromboembolism, brain stem vascular damage, cost, and technical expertise can limit use of this test.[11] JVS uses the same concept as IPSS, is less invasive, and produces fewer complications; however, sensitivity is compromised.

Abnormal adrenal anatomy is effectively identified using high-resolution CT scanning and MRI.[20] Nodules as small as 1 to 1.5 cm on the adrenal cortex are easily identified by CT. With the use of thin-section scanning, nodules as small as 3 to 5 mm can be visualized.[21] Importantly, adrenal incendentalomas are prevalent in 5% to 10% of the general population. These masses may be functional

(secreting), requiring intervention, or nonfunctional (nonsecreting), requiring only periodic observation. For this reason, abnormal imaging results are unable to conclusively diagnose adrenal disease when used alone. Non-adrenal imaging studies may be useful for identifying ectopic sources of ACTH secretion in patients for whom IPSS has ruled out Cushing's disease.

Differential Diagnosis

Iatrogenic (exogenous) Cushing's syndrome is the most common form of the disease. Therefore, all patients exhibiting hypercortisolism should undergo a comprehensive history and evaluation assessing medication use before laboratory testing is performed to identify endogenous causes. Iatrogenic Cushing's syndrome can occur from administration of oral, inhaled, intranasal, intra-articular, and topical glucocorticoids, as well as progestins such as medroxyprogesterone acetate and megestrol acetate.[22] Disease severity correlates with exogenous glucocorticoid potency, dose, frequency, route, and treatment duration. Moreover, patients taking CYP3A4 inhibitors concomitantly with a glucocorticoid can be at higher risk of developing iatrogenic Cushing's syndrome.[23,24] If exogenous glucocorticoids are being taken, plasma cortisol levels can increase, while corticosterone levels remain low.[16]

In the absence of any known exogenous causes, the clinician will need to differentiate the syndrome from other syndromes, such as Pseudo-Cushing's syndrome, that mimic Cushing. Patients with obesity, chronic alcoholism, depression, and acute illness of any type can present with certain features of Cushing's syndrome. However, these patients may lack true Cushing's syndrome. For example, depressed patients, although mimicking the urinary steroid abnormalities of Cushing's syndrome, will not resemble a cushingoid patient in appearance. In chronic alcoholics, steroid laboratory panels generally return to baseline after ceasing alcohol intake. And obese patients often will have normal cortisol concentrations on both serum and urinary screening. Thus, identifying true cases of Cushing's syndrome requires a comprehensive history in combination with laboratory and possibly imaging assessment.

TREATMENT

❸ If left untreated, Cushing's syndrome is associated with high morbidity and mortality owing to associated disorders such as diabetes mellitus, cardiovascular disease, and electrolyte abnormalities. These disorders limit the survival of the patient with Cushing's syndrome to 4 to 5 years following initial diagnosis. The desired outcomes of treatment are to limit such detrimental outcomes and return the patient to a normal functional state by removing the source of hypercortisolism without causing any pituitary or adrenal deficiencies.

❹ The treatment of choice for both ACTH-dependent and ACTH-independent Cushing's syndrome is surgical resection of any offending tumors.[3,10] However, several secondary pharmacologic treatment plans are available, depending on the etiology of the disease (Table 85–4).[25,26] These pharmacologic options are generally used in preoperative patients or as adjunctive therapy in postoperative patients awaiting response. Rarely, monotherapy is used as a palliative treatment when surgery is not indicated.

■ PHARMACOLOGIC THERAPY

❺ Pharmacotherapy of Cushing's syndrome (dosing can be found in Table 85–4)[27] can be divided into four categories based on the anatomic site of action of the agent: (1) steroidogenesis inhibitors,

TABLE 85-4 Possible Treatment Plans in Cushing's Syndrome Based on Etiology

		Treatment			
				Dosing	
Etiology	Nondrug	Generic (Brand) Drug Name	Initial	Usual	Max
Ectopic ACTH syndrome	Surgery, chemotherapy, irradiation	Metyrapone (Metopirone) 250-mg capsules	0.5–1 g/day, divided every 4–6 h	1–2 g/day, divided every 4–6 h	6 g/day
		Aminoglutethimide (Cytadren) 250-mg tabs	0.5–1 g/day, divided two to four times a day for 2 weeks	1 g/day, divided every 6 h	2 g/day
Pituitary-dependent	Surgery, irradiation	Cyproheptadine (Periactin) 2 mg/5 mL syrup or 4-mg tabs	4 mg twice a day	24–32 mg/day, divided four times a day	32 mg/day
		Mitotane (Lysodren) 500-mg tabs	0.5–1 g/day, increased by 0.5–1 g/day every 1–4 weeks	1–4 g daily, with food to decrease GI effects	12 g/day
		Metyrapone	See above	See above	See above
Adrenal adenoma	Surgery, postoperative replacement	Ketoconazole (Nizoral) 200-mg tabs	200 mg once or twice a day	200–1200 mg/day, divided twice a day	1600 mg/day divided four times a day
Adrenal carcinoma	Surgery	Mitotane	See above	See above	See above

ACTH, adrenocorticotropic hormone.

(2) adrenolytic agents, (3) neuromodulators of ACTH release, and (4) glucocorticoid-receptor blocking agents.[25,26]

Steroidogenesis Inhibitors

As their name implies, steroidogenesis inhibitors block the production of cortisol. This class includes metyrapone, ketoconazole, etomidate, and aminoglutethimide. Metyrapone inhibits 11β-hydroxylase, the enzyme responsible for converting 11-deoxycortisol to cortisol. Following administration, a sudden decrease in cortisol levels occurs within hours and prompts a compensatory rise in plasma ACTH concentrations. As ACTH increases and blockage of cortisol synthesis persists, adrenal steroidogenesis efforts are shunted toward androgen production. Consequently, metyrapone is associated with significant androgenic side effects, including hirsutism and increased acne. In addition, metyrapone blocks aldosterone synthesis and causes the accumulation of aldosterone precursors, which exhibit weak mineralocorticoid activity. Blood pressure and electrolyte level variations can ensue, depending on the level of circulating 11-deoxycortisol and the degree of aldosterone inhibition. Additional adverse effects, including nausea, vomiting, vertigo, headache, dizziness, abdominal discomfort, and allergic rash, have been reported following administration, but are often signs of overtreatment.[25,26,28] Metyrapone is currently available through the manufacturer only for compassionate use.

The imidazole derivative antifungal, ketoconazole, effectively inhibits steroidogenesis via multiple mechanisms when used in large doses. In contrast to the quick onset of metyrapone, the benefits of ketoconazole therapy are achieved only after several weeks of therapy. In addition to lowering serum cortisol levels, ketoconazole exhibits anti-androgenic activity attributable to its inhibition of multiple CYP enzymes as well as 11β-hydroxylase and 17α-hydroxylase.[25] This activity may be beneficial in female patients with Cushing's syndrome, but can cause gynecomastia and decreased libido in males. Sustained therapy with ketoconazole also imparts beneficial effects on serum cholesterol profiles, including lowering total and LDL cholesterol levels. Ketoconazole induces a reversible elevation of hepatic transaminases in approximately 10% of patients.[29] Frequent liver function monitoring is recommended although progression to serious hepatotoxicity is rare. Additional common adverse effects include gastrointestinal discomfort and dermatologic reactions.

Ketoconazole may be used concomitantly with metyrapone to achieve synergistic reductions in cortisol levels. Because these drugs differ in their onset of action, coadministration allows for more complete suppression of cortisol synthesis. Moreover, the anti-androgenic actions of ketoconazole therapy may offset the androgenic potential of metyrapone, thus attenuating a major limitation of metyrapone therapy.

The anesthetic etomidate is an imidazole derivative similar to ketoconazole that inhibits 11β-hydroxylase.[25] Etomidate is available only in a parenteral formulation and is therefore limited to patients with acute hypercortisolemia requiring emergency treatment.

Initially, aminoglutethimide was used to treat refractory forms of epilepsy, but was later discovered to be a potent inhibitor of adrenal steroid synthesis. Aminoglutethimide inhibits the conversion of cholesterol to pregnenolone early in the steroid biosynthesis pathway, thereby inhibiting the production of cortisol, aldosterone, and androgens. Owing to these broad inhibitory actions, side effects, including severe sedation, nausea, ataxia, and skin rashes, limit the use of aminoglutethimide in many patients.[25,26] Moreover, because other steroidogenesis inhibitors offer greater efficacy combined with fewer side effects, aminoglutethimide has fallen out of favor in the treatment of Cushing's syndrome. If aminoglutethimide is used, it should be coadministered with another steroidogenesis inhibitor, usually metyrapone, secondary to high relapse rates with aminoglutethimide monotherapy.

Adrenolytic Agents

Mitotane is a cytotoxic drug that structurally resembles the insecticide dichlorodiphenyltrichloroethane (DDT). Mitotane inhibits the 11-hydroxylation of 11-desoxycortisol and 11-desoxycorticosterone in the cortex, resulting in a net inhibition of cortisol and corticosterone synthesis. Similar to ketoconazole, mitotane takes weeks to months to exert beneficial effects. Sustained cortisol suppression occurs in most patients and may persist following discontinuation of therapy in up to one third of patients. Because of its cytotoxic nature, mitotane degenerates cells within the zona fasciculata and reticularis, resulting in atrophy of the adrenal cortex. The zona glomerulosa is minimally affected during acute therapy but can become damaged following long-term treatment.[27,30]

Importantly, mitotane can induce significant neurological and gastrointestinal side effects and patients should be monitored carefully or hospitalized when initiating therapy. Nausea and diarrhea are common adverse effects that occur at doses greater than 2 g/day and can be avoided by gradually increasing the dose and/or administering the agent with food. Approximately 80% of patients treated with mitotane develop lethargy and somnolence, and other central nervous system adverse drug reactions occur in approximately 40% of patients. Furthermore, significant but reversible hypercholesterolemia and prolongation of bleeding times can result from mitotane use.[25,26] Mitotane increases production of corticosteroid binding globulin resulting in elevated plasma cortisol; thus, UFC and urinary steroid production should be monitored to assess response to therapy.[25] If necessary, steroid replacement therapy can be given. However, because mitotane also increases extraadrenal metabolism of exogenously administered corticosteroids, higher steroid replacement doses may be required.

Neuromodulatory Agents

Pituitary secretion of ACTH is normally mediated by various neurotransmitters, including serotonin, GABA, acetylcholine and the catecholamines. Although ACTH-secreting pituitary tumors (Cushing's disease) self-regulate ACTH production to some degree, these neurotransmitters are still capable of promoting pituitary ACTH production. Consequently, agents that target these neurotransmitters have been proposed for the treatment of Cushing's disease. Such agents include cyproheptadine, ritanserin, ketanserin, bromocriptine, cabergoline, valproic acid, octreotide, lanreotide, rosiglitazone, and tretinoin. However, none of these drugs have demonstrated consistent clinical efficacy in the treatment of Cushing's disease.

Cyproheptadine, a nonselective serotonin receptor antagonist and anticholinergic drug, can decrease ACTH secretion in some Cushing's disease patients. However, side effects, including sedation and weight gain, significantly limit the use of this drug. Likewise, selective serotonin type 2 receptor antagonists, including ritanserin and ketanserin, have demonstrated limited efficacy. Owing to their poor efficacy and high relapse rates, these drugs should be avoided except in nonsurgical candidates refractory to more conventional treatments.

Dopamine D_2 receptor agonists, including bromocriptine and cabergoline, initially reduce ACTH secretion in as many as half of all patients with Cushing's disease. This action occurs through activation of inhibitory D_2 receptors that are expressed in approximately 80% of pituitary adenomas.[31] Reductions in ACTH levels are often minor and rarely sustained with long-term bromocriptine therapy. Cabergoline exhibits a higher specificity and affinity for D_2 receptors as well as a prolonged half-life compared with bromocriptine, but long-term studies for cabergoline are lacking.

The somatostatin analogues, octreotide and lanreotide, generally are ineffective in reducing ACTH secretion in Cushing's disease. These two agents primarily target somatostatin receptor subtype 2 (sst_2), whereas pituitary adenomas predominantly express sst_5. Pasireotide, an investigational somatostatin analogue, exhibits a high affinity for both sst_2 and sst_5 and may show promise as a future treatment in Cushing's disease.

Glucocorticoid-Receptor Blocking Agents

Mifepristone (RU-486) is a potent progesterone- and glucocorticoid-receptor antagonist that inhibits dexamethasone suppression and increases endogenous cortisol and ACTH levels in normal subjects.[25,28] Limited clinical experience in Cushing's syndrome suggests that mifepristone is highly effective in reversing the manifestation of hypercortisolism. Though because of its novel site of action, mifepristone induces a compensatory rise in ACTH and cortisol levels. Consequently, efficacy and toxicity monitoring must rely on clinical signs rather than laboratory assessments. Given these monitoring challenges, mifepristone use remains investigational for the treatment of Cushing's syndrome.

Close monitoring of 24-hour UFC levels and serum cortisol levels are essential to detect treatment-induced adrenal insufficiency. Steroid secretion should be monitored with all of these drugs and steroid replacement given as needed. Whatever the choice, pharmacologic therapy in pituitary-dependent disease is mainly centered around patient stabilization prior to surgery or in patients waiting for potential response to other therapies.

◼ NONPHARMACOLOGIC THERAPY

Surgery

The treatment of choice for Cushing's disease is transsphenoidal resection of the pituitary microadenoma.[3,10,28,32] The advantages of this procedure include preservation of pituitary function, low complication rate, and high clinical improvement rate. The overall cure rate of histologically proven microadenomas approaches 90%, whereas remission rates for macroadenomas generally do not exceed 65%.

For persistent disease following transsphenoidal surgery or when tumor-specific surgery is not possible, several second-line treatment options are available and should be tailored toward the individual patient. In the case of persistent disease following transsphenoidal surgery, repeat surgery may be performed, although overall remission rates are lower with subsequent procedures. Alternatively, radiotherapy may be preferred for tumors invading the dura or cavernous sinus because these tumors respond poorly to surgical intervention.[33] Radiotherapy provides clinical improvement in approximately 50% of patients within 3 to 5 years, but increases the risk for pituitary-dependent hormone deficiencies (hypopituitarism).

Laparoscopic adrenalectomy is often preferred in patients with unilateral adrenal adenomas for whom transsphenoidal surgery and pituitary radiotherapy have failed or cannot be used.[3,10,28] Bilateral adrenalectomy rapidly reverses hypercortisolism. However, patients can develop Nelson syndrome, an aggressive pituitary tumor that secretes high quantities of ACTH, which causes hyperpigmentation. Because Nelson syndrome occurs in as many as 30% of bilateral adrenalectomy cases, patients should undergo regular MRI scans and ACTH level assessments. Additionally, these patients require lifelong glucocorticoid and mineralocorticoid supplementation.

Adrenal Adenoma

Surgical resection of benign adrenal adenoma is associated with relatively few side effects and a high cure rate (95%). The contralateral gland in the patient with adrenal adenoma is usually atrophic, therefore steroid replacement is needed both perioperatively and postoperatively. Table 85-5 outlines an approach to steroid replacement for three separate routes of hydrocortisone. Therapy should be continued for 6 to 12 months following surgery. Before replacement therapy is discontinued, recovery of the adrenal axis can be assessed by measuring the morning (8 AM) cortisol level. Cortisol levels should exceed 20 mcg/dL before discontinuing exogenous steroids.[22]

| TABLE 85-5 | Alternative Steroid Replacement Regimens in the Adrenal Adenoma Patient |

	Hydrocortisone Dose (mg)		
Time	IV	IM	PO
Operation day	300	50 before surgery and 50 after surgery	
Postoperative day 1	200	50 every 12 h	
Postoperative day 2	150	50 every 12 h	
Postoperative day 3	100	50 every 12 h	
Postoperative day 4		50 every 12 h	25 every 6 h
Postoperative day 5		25 every 12 h	25 every 6 h[a]
Postoperative day 7			25 every 6 h
Postoperative days 8–10			25 every 8 h
Postoperative days 11–20			25 every 12 h
Postoperative days 21+			20 at 8 AM
			10 at 4 PM

PO, orally.

[a]Add fludrocortisone 0.05–2 mg orally once daily starting on postoperative day 5. Adjust dose based on blood pressure, body weight, and serum electrolytes.

Adrenal Carcinoma

Unlike the benign adenoma patient, those with adrenal carcinoma have an unfavorable outcome with surgical resection.[10] Often the complete tumor cannot be excised, leaving the patient with some degree of symptomatology and extraadrenal involvement. Radiotherapy can be used if metastases are discovered. In the patient with adrenal carcinoma who is not a surgical candidate, the focus of treatment is on palliative pharmacologic intervention.

Mitotane may be used in inoperable functional and nonfunctional adrenal carcinoma or as adjuvant therapy in surgical patients with a high risk of relapse. However, mitotane induces tumor regression in less than 20% of patients.[34] Metyrapone, aminoglutethimide, and ketoconazole can be given to attempt control of steroid hypersecretion. 5-fluorouracil also has been used in combination therapy.

Ectopic ACTH Syndrome

In ectopic ACTH syndrome, ACTH-secreting tumors may exist in a variety of sites, including thymic, pulmonary, appendiceal, pancreatic, and thyroid tissues. Locating these sites is often difficult, but essential for determining an appropriate treatment strategy. Surgical resection is the most effective treatment option for these patients, but only approximately 10% to 30% of patients are cured following surgery due to high rates of metastatic disease or occult tumors. The remaining 70% to 90% receive postoperative medication.

Pharmacologic management with steroidogenesis inhibitors is effective in ectopic ACTH syndrome. Mitotane has been used in patients with ectopic ACTH syndrome; however, its side-effect profile generally limits its use. Mifapristone and somatostatin analogs also have been reported to reduce the clinical signs of ectopic ACTH syndrome.[35]

Additional tumor-directed therapy can include systemic chemotherapy, interferon α, chemoembolization, radiofrequency ablation, and radiation therapy.[33] If all else fails, bilateral adrenalectomy can prevent the downstream effects (e.g., steroidogenesis) of high levels of tumor ACTH secretion.

■ HYPERALDOSTERONISM

Excess aldosterone secretion is categorized as either primary or secondary hyperaldosteronism.[36–40] In primary aldosteronism (PA), the stimulation for aldosterone secretion arises from within the adrenal gland. Conversely, extraadrenal stimulation is classified as secondary aldosteronism.

Primary Aldosteronism

Etiology The most common causes of PA include BAH (65%) and aldosterone-producing adenoma (APA; otherwise known as Conn syndrome) (30%). Other rare causes include unilateral (primary) adrenal hyperplasia, adrenal cortex carcinoma, renin-responsive adrenocortical adenoma, and two forms of familial hyperaldosteronism (FH): FH type 1, or glucocorticoid-remediable aldosteronism (GRA) and FH type II.[36,37,39]

Clinical Presentation PA is present in approximately 10% of the general hypertensive population and is the leading cause of secondary hypertension. The disease is more common in women than men and diagnosis usually occurs between the third and sixth decade of life. Signs and symptoms can include arterial hypertension, which is often moderate to severe and resistant to pharmacologic intervention, as well as hypokalemia (10% to 40% of PA patients), muscle weakness, fatigue, and headache. These features are non-specific for PA and many patients are asymptomatic. Historically, hypokalemia was considered a requisite feature for PA diagnosis; however, normokalemia exists frequently in patients and should not obviate concern for PA.

TABLE 85-6 Differential Diagnosis of Primary Aldosteronism

Disease	Plasma Renin Concentration	Plasma Aldosterone Concentration	Blood Pressure
Primary aldosteronism	Low	High	High
Edematous disorders	High	High	Normal
Malignant hypertension	High	High	High
Congenital adrenal hyperplasia	Low	Low	High
Cushing's syndrome	Low to normal	Low to normal	High
Liddle syndrome	Low	Low	High
Bartter's syndrome	High	High	Low to normal
Licorice ingestion	Low	Low	High
Low-renin essential hypertension	Low	Low to normal	High

Diagnosis Diagnostic confirmation of PA is obtainable through screening, confirmatory tests, and subtype differentiation. As in Cushing's syndrome, discovery of the underlying etiology ensures proper treatment. Table 85–6 lists the various abnormalities that must be ruled out when suspicion of hyperaldosteronism is high.

CLINICAL PRESENTATION: PRIMARY ALDOSTERONISM

Symptoms

- Patients may complain of muscle weakness, fatigue, paresthesias, and headache.

Signs

- Hypertension
- Tetany/paralysis
- Polydipsia/nocturnal polyuria

Laboratory Tests

- A plasma-aldosterone–to–plasma-renin-activity ratio (PA:PRA), or aldosterone-to-renin ratio (ARR) greater than 20 is suggestive of primary aldosteronism
- Common laboratory findings include suppressed renin activity, elevated plasma aldosterone concentrations, hypernatremia (>142 mEq/L), hypokalemia, hypomagnesemia, elevated bicarbonate concentration (>31 mEq/L), and glucose intolerance

Confirmatory Tests

- Oral or intravenous saline loading, fludrocortisone suppression test (FST), and genetic testing

Initial diagnosis is made through proper screening of patients with suspected primary aldosteronism. Such patients include those with JNC stage two hypertension—appreciating that the prevalence of PA increases with hypertensive severity—and resistant hypertensives. Screening for primary aldosteronism is most often done by using the plasma-aldosterone-concentration–to–plasma-renin-activity ratio (PAC:PRA), otherwise known as the aldosterone-to-renin ratio (ARR). An elevated ARR is highly suggestive of PA; however, an optimal cutoff level remains undefined because testing conditions (posture, time, current drug therapy, recent dietary salt intake), patient characteristics, and variable levels of specificity and sensitivity among assays can significantly alter test results.[41] ARR cutoffs of 20 to 40 or 20 with an aldosterone level greater than 15 ng/dL are used most often.[38,42,43]

Following a positive ARR screening test, confirmatory testing must be performed to exclude any false-positive cases. Confirmatory tests include the oral sodium loading test, saline infusion test, FST, and the captopril challenge test. Although individual tests can vary in sensitivity, specificity and reliability, any test can be used depending on patient- and institution-specific considerations. FST generally is considered the most reliable, but requires hospitalization. Prior to performing these tests, potassium levels must be normalized and RAS-active agents should be temporarily discontinued, if possible. Positive tests indicate autonomous aldosterone secretion under inhibitory pressures and are diagnostic for PA. After diagnosis, patients with confirmed PA before age 20 or with a family history of PA or strokes before age 40 should undergo genetic testing to properly identify GRA.[41]

Differentiating between an APA and BAH is imperative to formulate a proper treatment plan. Most adenomas are singular and small (<1 cm) and occur more often in the left adrenal gland than the right. Patients with APA generally have more severe hypertension, more profound hypokalemia, and higher plasma and urinary aldosterone levels compared with patients with BAH. Adrenal venous sampling (AVS) provides the most accurate means of differentiating unilateral from bilateral forms of PA. However, AVS is expensive, invasive, and frequently unavailable. CT scanning can detect most adenomas, although an incidentaloma can occasionally cause confusion. If CT scanning is inconclusive, AVS is performed to characterize lateralization.[38,44-46]

The underlying abnormality in BAH remains a mystery, but some investigators believe that a hormone factor stimulates the zona glomerulosa, resulting in increased sensitivity to angiotensin II. In contrast to those with an APA, patients with BAH are able to maintain control of the renin-angiotensin system, with little effect following doses of ACTH.

Therapeutic Management

⑥ BAH-Dependent Aldosteronism. Aldosterone receptor antagonists are the treatment of choice in bilateral cases of primary aldosteronism. Spironolactone, a non-selective aldosterone receptor antagonist, competes with aldosterone for binding at the aldosterone receptor, thus preventing the negative downstream effects of aldosterone receptor activation. Additionally, spironolactone is capable of inhibiting aldosterone synthesis within the adrenal gland; however, the magnitude of this inhibition is relatively small and the effect only occurs at doses above those achieved with therapeutic doses.[47] Spironolactone is available in oral form, with most patients responding to doses between 25 and 400 mg/day. The clinician should wait 4 to 8 weeks before reassessing the patient for urinary electrolytes and blood pressure control. Adverse effects of spironolactone are dose-dependent and include gastrointestinal discomfort, impotence, gynecomastia, menstrual irregularities, and hyperkalemia. Gynecomastia and menstrual irregularities observed with spironolactone therapy arise from activity at androgen and progesterone receptors and inhibition of testosterone biosynthesis. Additionally, because salicylates increase the renal secretion of canrenone, the active metabolite, patients should be advised to avoid concomitant therapy with salicylates. In patients intolerant of spironolactone, alternative options include eplerenone and amiloride.[38,48-50]

Eplerenone is a selective aldosterone receptor antagonist with high affinity for the aldosterone receptor and low affinity for androgen and progesterone receptors. Consequently, eplerenone elicits fewer sex steroid-dependent effects while ostensibly maintaining similar efficacy to spironolactone; however, no significant comparative data exist between these two agents. Dosing starts at 50 mg daily, with titration to 50 mg twice a day.[48] Titration should occur at 4 to 8 week intervals. In addition, eplerenone is a substrate of

CYP3A4 and should not be taken with potent CYP3A4 inhibitors. Eplerenone has been proven effective in primary essential hypertension; however, its role in the management of hyperaldosteronism has not been established.[51]

Amiloride, a potassium-sparing diuretic, is dosed at 5 mg twice a day up to 30 mg/day if necessary. Amiloride is less effective than spironolactone and often requires additional therapy to adequately control blood pressure. Additional agents useful as second-line options include the calcium channel blockers, ACE inhibitors, and low-dose diuretics such as hydrochlorothiazide, although all lack outcome data evaluation in PA.[46,49]

Aldosterone synthase inhibitors, currently under development, may offer additional therapeutic options in the future.

APA-Dependent Aldosteronism. The treatment of choice for APA-dependent aldosteronism remains laparoscopic resection of the adenoma.[52] Nearly 100% of patients show blood pressure improvement while 30% to 72% are permanently cured.[50,53] Because APAs are small and often occur in multiples, resection should target the entire adrenal gland. In successful cases, blood pressure control is achieved in 1 to 3 months. Medical management can be efficacious in this population if surgery is contraindicated. However, medical management may be significantly more expensive than unilateral resection.

Glucocorticoid-Remediable Aldosteronism. Glucocorticoids are very effective in treating GRA.[37] Low doses are used (0.125 to 0.5 mg/day of dexamethasone or 2.5 to 5 mg/day of prednisone) because complete suppression of ACTH-stimulated aldosterone release is unnecessary. Spironolactone, eplerenone, and amiloride are alternative treatment options.[38]

Summary The diagnosis of PA is made through proper screening of suspected patients followed by confirmatory testing. Subsequent differentiation between the various etiologies ensures appropriate treatment (Fig. 85–5). Patients with APA can be distinguished from patients with BAH by CT scan, but adrenal venous sampling provides increased sensitivity and specificity. Treatment depends on the etiology with surgical resection in adenomas, and spironolactone, eplerenone, or amiloride plus second-line agents in patients with bilateral hyperplasia.

Secondary Aldosteronism

Secondary aldosteronism results from an appropriate response to excessive stimulation of the zona glomerulosa by an extraadrenal factor, usually the renin-angiotensin system. Excessive potassium intake can promote aldosterone secretion, as can oral contraceptive use, pregnancy (10 times normal by the third trimester), and menses. Congestive heart failure, cirrhosis, renal artery stenosis, and Bartter syndrome also can lead to elevated aldosterone concentrations.

Treatment of secondary aldosteronism is dictated by etiology. Control or correction of the extraadrenal stimulation of aldosterone secretion should resolve the disorder. Medical therapy with spironolactone is the mainstay of treatment until an exact etiology can be located.

HYPOFUNCTION OF THE ADRENAL GLAND

⑦ Primary adrenal insufficiency, or Addison's disease, most often involves the destruction of all regions of the adrenal cortex. Deficiencies arise in cortisol, aldosterone, and the various androgens and levels of CRH and ACTH increase in a compensatory manor. In developed countries, autoimmune dysfunction is responsible for most cases (80% to 90%), whereas tuberculosis predominates as

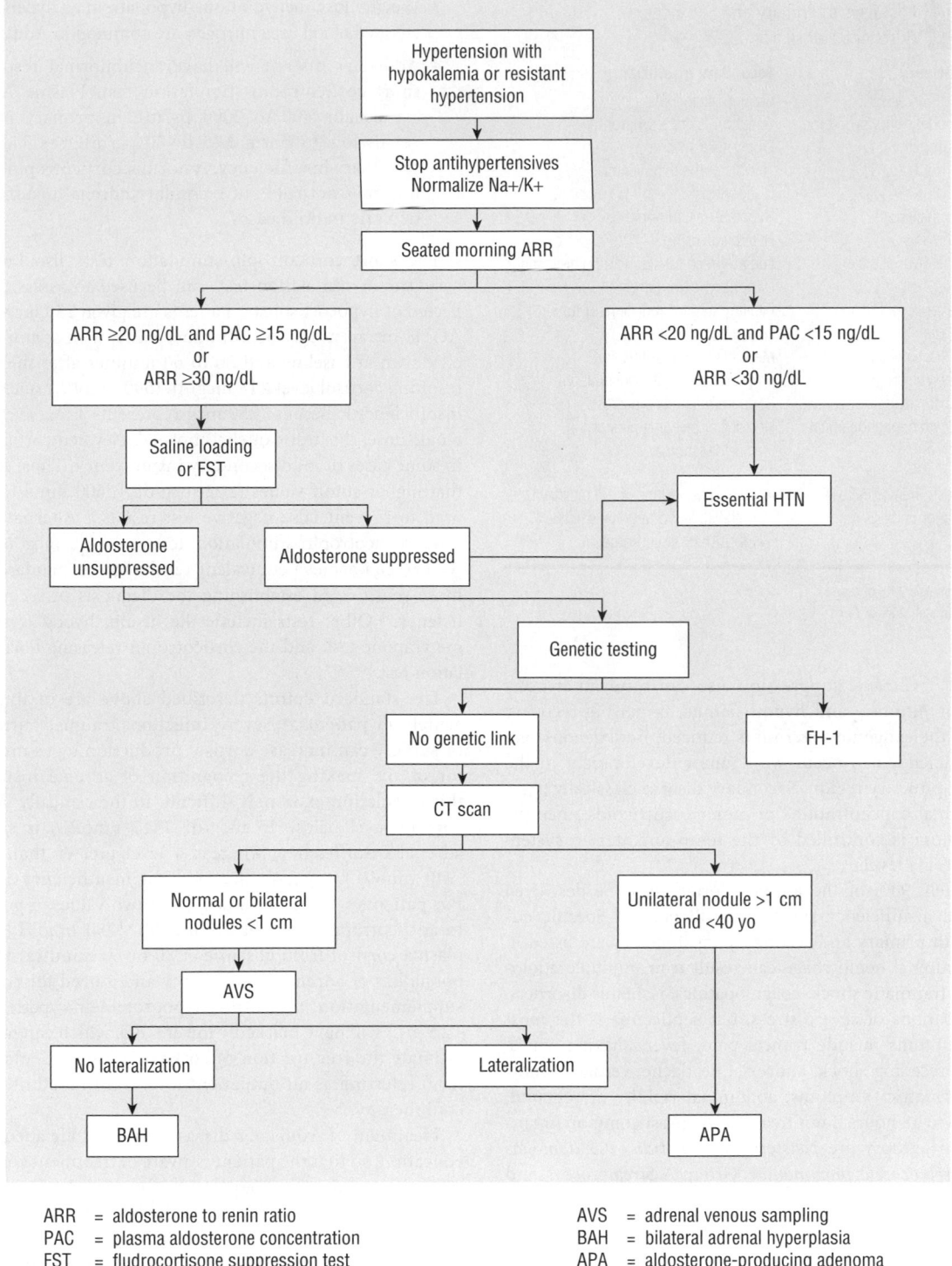

FIGURE 85-5. Algorithm for the diagnosis of primary aldosteronism.

ARR = aldosterone to renin ratio
PAC = plasma aldosterone concentration
FST = fludrocortisone suppression test
FH-1 = familial hyperaldosteronism type 1

AVS = adrenal venous sampling
BAH = bilateral adrenal hyperplasia
APA = aldosterone-producing adenoma

the cause in developing countries. Approximately 50% of patients with autoimmune etiologies present with one or more concomitant autoimmune disorders, usually involving other endocrine organs. Autoimmune thyroid disorders (e.g., Hashimoto's thyroiditis or Graves disease) are the most common, but the ovaries, pancreas, parathyroid gland and organs of the gastrointestinal system can also be affected. This polyglandular failure syndrome, termed autoimmune polyendocrine syndrome (APS), is associated with the idiopathic etiology only and has not been seen with adrenal insufficiency associated with tuberculosis or other invasive diseases. Medications that inhibit cortisol synthesis (ketoconazole), or

accelerate cortisol metabolism (phenytoin, rifampin, phenobarbital) can also cause primary adrenal insufficiency.[54]

❽ Secondary insufficiency is characterized by reduced glucocorticoid production secondary to decreased ACTH levels. Low levels of ACTH most commonly result from exogenous steroid use, leading to suppression of the HPA axis and decreased release of ACTH, resulting in impaired androgen and cortisol production. These effects occur with oral, inhaled, intranasal, and topical glucocorticoid administration.[55–57] Moreover, mirtazapine and progestins, such as medroxyprogesterone acetate and megestrol acetate, have been reported to induce secondary adrenal

TABLE 85-7 Etiologies of Primary and Secondary Adrenal Insufficiency

Primary Insufficiency	Secondary Insufficiency
Slow onset	Craniopharyngioma
Acquired immunodeficiency syndrome	Cure of Cushing's syndrome
Adrenomyeloneuropathy	Empty sella syndrome
Adrenoleukodystrophy	Tumors of the third ventricle
Amyloidosis	Histiocytosis
Autoimmune adrenalitis*a*	Hypothalamic tumors
Bilateral adrenalectomy	Hypopituitarism
Congenital adrenal hypoplasia	Long-term corticosteroid administration
Hemochromatosis	Lymphocytic hypophysitis
Isolated glucocorticoid deficiency	Pituitary surgery, radiation, or tumor
Metastatic neoplasia	Sarcoidosis
Systemic fungal, bacterial, or viral infections Tuberculosis*b*	Medications–progestins and glucocorticoid discontinuation
Medications–ketoconazole, etomidate, rifampin, phenytoin, phenobarbital	Postpartum pituitary necrosis
	Necrotic or bleeding pituitary macroadenoma
Fast onset	
Adrenal thrombosis, hemorrhage, sepsis, trauma, or necrosis	Head trauma, lesions of the pituitary stalk Pituitary or adrenal surgery for Cushing's syndrome

*a*Accounts for approximately 70% of cases.
*b*Accounts for approximately 20% of cases.

insufficiency.[58,59] Chronic suppression also can result in atrophy of the anterior pituitary and hypothalamus, impairing recovery of function if the exogenous steroid is reduced. Endogenous secondary insufficiency can occur with tumor development in the hypothalamic-pituitary region. Secondary disease classically presents with normal concentrations of mineralocorticoids since the zona glomerulosa is controlled by the renin-angiotensin system rather than ACTH levels.

Approximately 90% of the adrenal cortex must be destroyed before adrenal insufficiency symptoms will occur.[60] Specific etiologies for both primary and secondary insufficiency are listed in Table 85–7. Adrenal hemorrhage can result from multiple etiologies including traumatic shock, coagulopathies, ischemic disorders, and other situations of severe stress, but septicemia is the most common. Symptoms include truncal pain, fever, shaking, chills, hypotension preceding shock, anorexia, headache, vertigo, vomiting, rash, psychiatric symptoms, abdominal rigidity or rebound, and death in 6 to 48 hours if not treated. The most common organisms found on autopsy are *Neisseria meningitidis, Pseudomonas aeruginosa, Streptococcus pneumoniae*, Group A *Streptococcus*, and *Haemophilus influenzae*.[60,61]

ADDISON'S DISEASE

Distinguishing Addison's disease from secondary insufficiency is difficult; however, the following guidelines may be helpful:

1. Hyperpigmentation, commonly found in areas of skin exposed to increased friction, is seen only in Addison's disease because of excess secretion of ACTH and other proopiomelanocortin (POMC) peptides which induce melanocyte-stimulating hormone production. Secondary adrenal insufficiency is fundamentally characterized by deficient ACTH and POMC peptide secretion and a corresponding low level of melanocyte-stimulating hormone production. In fact, some patients with secondary insufficiency may exhibit pale-colored skin secondary to hypopigmentation.

2. Aldosterone secretion usually is preserved in secondary insufficiency.

3. Weight loss, dehydration, hyponatremia, hyperkalemia, and elevated blood urea nitrogen are common in Addison's disease.

4. Addison's disease will have an abnormal response to the short corticotropin-stimulation test. Plasma ACTH levels are usually 400 to 2000 pg/mL in primary insufficiency, versus low to normal (5 to 50 pg/mL; see Table 85–3) in secondary insufficiency. A normal corticotropin-stimulation test does not rule out secondary adrenal insufficiency, particularly in mild cases.

The short corticotropin-stimulation test, also known as the cosyntropin-stimulation test, can be used to assess patients suspected of hypocortisolism. Patients are given 250 mcg of synthetic ACTH intravenously or intramuscularly, with serum cortisol levels drawn at baseline and 30 to 60 minutes after the injection. A resulting cortisol level ≥18 mcg/dL (500 nmol/L) rules out adrenal insufficiency.[62] Because 250 mcg represents a massive supraphysiologic dose, this test can elicit normal, elevated cortisol responses in some cases of mild secondary insufficiency. Thus, some suggest that higher cutoff values (≥22 mcg/dL [≥600 nmol/L]) should be used to prevent false-negative test results.[63] Alternatively, a low-dose corticotropin-stimulation test, using 1 mcg of synethetic ACTH, can achieve equivalent results to the standard test and is more sensitive in establishing the diagnosis of secondary insufficiency.[64] Other tests include the insulin hypoglycemia test, the metyrapone test, and the corticotropin-releasing hormone stimulation test.[54,62,65]

The standard cutoffs described above are of limited use in acutely ill patients.[66] Severe infection, trauma, burns, illnesses, or surgery can increase cortisol production by as much as a factor of six, making the recognition of adrenal insufficiency in this population extremely difficult. In the critically ill, a random cortisol level below 15 mcg/dL (415 nmol/L) is suggestive of adrenal insufficiency, whereas a level greater than 34 mcg/dL (940 nmol/L) suggests that adrenal insufficiency is unlikely.[66] For patients who fall between these two values, a poor response to corticotropin (less than 9 mcg/dL [250 nmol/L] increase in plasma cortisol from baseline at 30 or 60 minutes) indicates the possibility of adrenal insufficiency and a need for corticosteroid supplementation.[66] A severe hypoproteinemic patient (albumin <2.5 g/L) will have markedly lower CBG, which can falsely underestimate the free fraction of cortisol. These patients can benefit from retesting as an outpatient to prevent indefinite glucocorticoid therapy.[54]

Treatment of Addison's disease must include adequate patient education, so that the patient is aware of treatment complications, expected outcome, consequences of missed doses, and drug side effects. The agents of choice are hydrocortisone, cortisone, and prednisone, administered twice daily with the treatment objective being the establishment of the lowest effective dose while mimicking the normal diurnal adrenal rhythm.[54] Usually a twice-daily dosing schedule is adequate with the dose depending on the agent used.

Endogenous cortisol production varies between 5 and 10 mg/m^2 per day.[67] Hence, the classic 12 to 15 mg/m^2 per day rule for cortisol supplementation can be excessive in most patients. Recommended starting doses to properly mimic endogenous cortisol production are 15 to 25 mg of hydrocortisone daily, which is roughly equal to 25 to 37.5 mg of cortisone acetate or 2.5 mg of prednisone.[54,65,67] The majority of the dose (67%) is given in the morning, whereas the remainder (33%) is given 6 to 8 hours later to duplicate the normal circadian rhythm of cortisol production. Since no laboratory test adequately determines the appropriateness of dosing, the patient's symptoms should be monitored every 6 to 8 weeks to assess proper glucocorticoid replacement.

In primary insufficiency, fludrocortisone acetate can be used to supplement mineralocorticoid loss. A dose of 0.05–0.2 mg by mouth once a day is adequate. If parenteral therapy is needed, 2 to 5 mg of deoxycorticosterone trimethylacetate in oil intramuscularly every 3 to 4 weeks can be substituted. Mineralocorticoid replacement attenuates the development of hyperkalemia, but may be unnecessary in all primary cases since glucocorticoids also contribute to mineralocorticoid binding. Adverse effects must be monitored closely. Symptoms include gastric upset, edema, hypertension, hypokalemia, insomnia, excitability, and diabetes mellitus. In addition, patient weight, blood pressure, and electrocardiogram should be monitored regularly.[65]

In women, the primary source of dehydroepiandrosterone (DHEA) and androgens is the adrenal cortex, specifically the zona reticularis. DHEA is converted to more potent androgens and estrogens in the periphery. Consequently, women with adrenal insufficiency can have decreased libido. DHEA, available as a dietary supplement, has been advocated as an option for female patients with adrenal insufficiency complaining of decreased libido and low energy.[68] However, clinical trial data for DHEA is conflicting, and a recent meta-analysis suggests no benefit for sexual well-being.[69] Given this limited efficacy and a lack of any standardization among the various commercial products, DHEA should not be used routinely in female patients to improve libido. DHEA may improve mood and well-being in select male and female patients who are already receiving optimal glucocorticoid and mineralocorticoid replacement.

Most adrenal crises occur secondary to glucocorticoid dose reduction or lack of stress-related dose adjustments. Patients receiving corticosteroid-replacement therapy should receive an additional 5 to 10 mg of hydrocortisone shortly before strenuous activities such as exercise.[65] Likewise, during times of severe physical stress such as febrile illnesses or injury, patients should be instructed to double their daily dose until recovery.[70,71] For major trauma, surgery, or in critically ill patients, larger doses are required. Parenteral therapy should be used for patients experiencing diarrhea or vomiting. In patients with concomitant, newly diagnosed, or uncontrolled hypothyroidism, thyroid replacement should take place only after adequate glucocorticoid replacement as euthyroidism can trigger an adrenal crisis by accelerating cortisol metabolism.[54]

The end point of therapy is difficult to assess in most patients, but a reduction in excess pigmentation is a good clinical marker. The development of features of Cushing's syndrome indicates excessive replacement. Treatment of secondary adrenal insufficiency is identical to primary disease treatment, except that mineralocorticoid replacement usually is unnecessary. Patient education is paramount with emphasis placed on the medication regimen and adrenal crisis prevention.

Acute Adrenal Insufficiency

Adrenal crisis, or Addisonian crisis, is characterized by an acute adrenocortical insufficiency. Adrenal crisis represents a true endocrine emergency. Anything that increases adrenal requirements dramatically can precipitate an adrenal crisis. Stressful situations, surgery, infection, and trauma all are potential triggering events, especially in the patient with some underlying adrenal or pituitary insufficiency. The most common cause of adrenal crisis is HPA-axis suppression brought on by chronic use of exogenous glucocorticoids and abrupt withdrawal.

Treatment of adrenal crisis involves the administration of parenteral glucocorticoids. Hydrocortisone is the agent of choice owing to its combined glucocorticoid and mineralocorticoid activity. Hydrocortisone is initially administered at a dose of 100 mg intravenously through rapid infusion, followed by a continuous infusion (usually 10 mg/hr) or intermittent bolus of 100 to 200 mg every 24 hours.[72] Intravenous administration is continued for 24 to 48 hours, at which time if the patient is stable, oral hydrocortisone can be administered at a dose of 50 mg every 6 to 8 hours, followed by tapering to the individual's chronic replacement needs. Fluid replacement often is required and can be accomplished with dextrose 5% in normal saline solution (D_5NS) at a rate to support blood pressure. During initial treatment for adrenal crisis, mineralocorticoid replacement generally is unnecessary because of hydrocortisone's mineralocorticoid activity (hydrocortisone 50 mg ≈ fludrocortisone 0.1 mg). If hyperkalemia is present after the hydrocortisone maintenance phase, additional mineralocorticoid supplementation can be achieved with 0.1 mg of fludrocortisone acetate daily.

Patients with adrenal insufficiency should be instructed to carry a card or wear a bracelet or necklace, such as MedicAlert, that contains information about their condition. Patients should also have easy access to injectable hydrocortisone or glucocorticoid suppositories in case of an emergency or during times of physical stress, such as febrile illness or injury.[65]

CLINICAL PRESENTATION: ADRENAL INSUFFICIENCY

Symptoms

- Patients commonly complain of weakness, weight loss, gastrointestinal symptoms, craving for salt, headaches, memory impairment, depression, and postural dizziness.

- Early symptoms of acute adrenal insufficiency also include myalgias, malaise, and anorexia. As the situation progresses, vomiting, fever, hypotension, and shock will develop.

Signs

- Increased pigmentation

- Hypotension (postural)

- Fever

- Decreased body hair

- Vitiligo

- Features of hypopituitarism (amenorrhea and cold intolerance)

Laboratory Tests

- The short corticotropin stimulation test can be used to assess patients suspected of hypercortisolism.

Other Diagnostic Tests

- Other tests include the insulin hypoglycemia test, the metyrapone test, and the corticotropin-releasing hormone stimulation test.

HYPOALDOSTERONISM

Hypoaldosteronism is rare and usually associated with low renin status (hyporeninemic hypoaldosteronism), diabetes, complete heart block, or severe postural hypotension, or it can occur postoperatively following tumor removal. Hypoaldosteronism can be part of a larger adrenal insufficiency or a standalone defect. In nonselective hypoaldosteronism, generalized adrenocortical insufficiency is the most likely etiology (see Addison's Disease). In selective hypoaldosteronism, insufficient aldosterone levels are precipitated by a specific defect in the stimulation of adrenal aldosterone secretion, with 21-hydroxylase deficiency being most common. Pseudohypoaldosteronism results from a defect in peripheral aldosterone action, whether from increased peripheral resistance or a reduced number of functional aldosterone receptors.

Laboratory analysis reveals hyponatremia, hyperkalemia, or both. Patients often will present with hyperchloremic metabolic acidosis. In most cases, the deficiency is in mineralocorticoid production and replacement with fludrocortisone in a dose of 0.1 to 0.3 mg is usually effective. Patients should be followed for blood pressure response as well as electrolyte status.

CONGENITAL ADRENAL HYPERPLASIA

Because many enzyme systems are needed to complete the complex cholesterol-to-cortisol pathway, enzyme deficiencies can lead to disruptions of the normal cascade of events (see Fig. 85–2). This group of enzyme disorders is collectively referred to as congenital adrenal hyperplasia because of the resultant chronic adrenal gland stimulation that occurs following enzyme deficiency.[73,74] The most frequent cause of congenital adrenal hyperplasia is steroid 21-hydroxylase deficiency, accounting for more than 90% of cases. Any enzyme deficiency is capable of affecting any one or all three of the steroid pathways. Therefore, treatment focuses on replacement of the deficient hormone, psychologic support, and surgical repair of the external genitalia in most female patients.[75] Six of the most common enzyme deficiencies are outlined briefly in Table 85–8.

ADRENAL VIRILISM

❾ Virilism, excessive secretion of androgens from the adrenal gland, commonly occurs as a result of congenital enzyme defects. Depending on the enzyme deficiency, patients accumulate excess levels of a variety of androgens, most notably testosterone. The condition affects females more often than males, with hirsutism being the dominant feature. Additional coexisting features can include voice deepening, acne, increased muscle mass, menstrual abnormalities, clitoral enlargement, redistribution of body fat and loss of female body contour, breast atrophy, and hair recession and crown balding.[76]

Treatment of virilism centers around suppression of the pituitary-adrenal axis with exogenous glucocorticoids. In adults, the usual steroids used are dexamethasone (0.25 to 0.5 mg), prednisone (2.5 to 5 mg), or hydrocortisone (10 to 20 mg).[77]

HIRSUTISM

Women presenting with hirsutism exhibit excess terminal hair growth in an androgen-dependent distribution. Such growth has obvious cosmetic consequences, but also can adversely affect quality-of-life and psychological well-being.[78] Most cases of hirsutism occur in women with some degree of excess androgen production. Androgen excess can be derived from either the ovaries or the adrenal glands, or rarely from pituitary disorders. Polycystic ovarian syndrome (PCOS) is responsible for most cases of ovarian excess and is the most common cause of hirsutism overall.[79] Congenital adrenal hyperplasia accounts for 5% of cases while adrenal and ovarian tumors cause hyperandrogenemia in 0.2% of women.

Cosmetic approaches generally are tried first, with repeated photoepilation offering the greatest long-term success.[79] If these approaches are unsuccessful, subsequent treatment should include pharmacologic intervention. Oral contraceptives are the treatment of choice in most hirsute women, particularly in those requiring concurrent contraception. If oral contraceptives are used, a progestin with low androgen activity (norethindrone, ethynodiol diacetate, or drospirenone) should be chosen. Antiandrogens, including spironolactone and finasteride, can supplement or replace oral contraceptive therapy in women who cannot or choose not to conceive. Antiandrogens can take 6 to 12 months to alleviate hirsutism and treatment should be continued for 2 years, followed by a slow dose reduction.[80] Glucocorticoids, such as dexamethasone, can be used if the androgen source is adrenal, but can induce cushingoid symptoms even in doses of 0.5 mg/day.

Gonadotropin-releasing hormone can be an effective adjunct or alternative to oral contraceptives if the source of androgen is ovarian. However, these products generally are not recommended due to excessive costs, injectible-only routes of administration, and adverse effects resulting from estrogen deficiency. Additionally, insulin sensitizers, such as metformin or thiazolidinediones, can show modest improvement in women with PCOS.

Eflornithine hydrochloride, an irreversible ornithine decarboxylase inhibitor, moderately reduces the rate of hair growth but does

TABLE 85–8	Congenital Adrenal Hyperplasia (CAH)		
Enzyme Deficiency (Disorder)	**Symptoms**	**Laboratory Tests**	**Comments**
21-Hydroxylase (nonvirilizing CAH)	Enlarged female genitalia and adrenal gland (caused by cholesterol)	All steroids are low in blood and urine	Poor prognosis for infants
17-Hydroxylase (nonvirilizing CAH)	Hypertension usually present	Low concentrations of cortisol and estrogens	Mineralocorticoid replacement not necessary
21-Hydroxylase (virilizing CAH)	Pubertal irregularities (acne, early pubic hair, voice lowering, and increased muscularity); mature normally with replacement	High progesterone, renin, 17-hydroxyprogesterone and ACTH; low cortisol, sodium, and aldosterone	Most common form of CAH (90% of total), incidence of 1:10,000; monitor growth velocity, bone age, renin, and 17-hydroxyprogesterone
11-Hydroxylase (virilizing CAH)	Hypertension secondary to high deoxycortisol and virilism from androgen excess; mistaken for Cushing, but no glucose intolerance	Low plasma cortisone and aldosterone; high ACTH and MSH concentrations	Second most common form of CAH (9% of total), incidence of 1:100,000; final step in biosynthesis of corticosterone and cortisol; found only in adrenal cortex
3-Hydroxysteroid dehydrogenase (mixed CAH)	Both cortisol and aldosterone deficiencies	Decreased aldosterone, cortisol, estrogens, and androgens; increased pregnenolone and cholesterol	Defect affects both adrenals and gonads
18-Hydroxysteroid dehydrogenase (corticosterone methyloxidase deficiency)	Hypotension	Restricted to zona glomerulosa; sole aldosterone defect; hyponatremia, hyperkalemia, increased renin	Mineralocorticoid replacement without glucocorticoid replacement

ACTH, adrenocorticotropic hormone; MSH, melanocyte-stimulating hormone.

not remove hair already present. The drug is available as a topical cream that is applied as a thin layer to the affected area twice daily, at least 8 hours apart. Reduction in unwanted hair can be noted within 6 to 8 weeks with a maximal effect at 8 to 24 weeks.[77,81] Skin irritation can occur that resolves on discontinuation.

PRINCIPLES OF GLUCOCORTICOID ADMINISTRATION

Originally, the term *glucocorticoid* was given to these agents to describe their glucose-regulating properties. However, carbohydrate metabolism is only one of the myriad of effects exhibited by steroids. The activity produced by these drugs is a function of the receptor activated (glucocorticoid versus mineralocorticoid) as well as the agent and dose prescribed.

The mechanism of action of glucocorticoids is complex and not fully known. The glucocorticoid enters the cell through passive diffusion and binds to its specific receptor. Between 5,000 and 100,000 receptors exist in each cell. Steroids exhibit various binding affinities to the vast number of receptors in almost every tissue and therefore elicit a wide variety of biologic effects.

Following receptor binding, a structural change occurs in the receptor, known as *activation*. After activation, the receptor-steroid complex binds to deoxyribonucleic acid sites in the cell called *glucocorticoid response elements* (GREs). This binding stimulates or inhibits transcription of nearby genes.

Pharmacokinetic properties of the glucocorticoids vary by agent and route of administration. In general, most orally-administered steroids are well absorbed. Water-soluble agents are more rapidly absorbed following intramuscular injection than are lipid-soluble agents. Intravenous administration is recommended when a quick onset of action is needed. A summary of these agents is provided in Table 85-9.

In addition to causing iatrogenic Cushing's syndrome, systemic steroids can lead to increased susceptibility to infection, osteoporosis, sodium retention with resultant edema, hypokalemia, hypomagnesemia, cataracts, peptic ulcer disease, seizures, and generalized suppression of the HPA-axis. Long-term complications tend to be insidious and less likely to respond to steroid withdrawal.

Suppression of the HPA-axis is a major concern whenever systemic steroids are tapered or withdrawn. Single doses of glucocorticoids can prevent the axis from responding to major stressors for several hours. In general, steroid administration at a high dose for long periods of time causes suppression of the axis. However, the possibility of suppression occurs any time the patient is exposed to supraphysiologic doses of a steroid.[22,82] Symptoms of steroid withdrawal resemble those seen in a patient with adrenocortical deficiency.

A variety of recommendations for steroid tapering are available.[22,83–85] In general, patients who have been on long-term steroid therapy will need to be gradually withdrawn toward physiologic doses over months. On average, the normal adult produces approximately 10 to 30 mg of cortisol per day with the peak concentration occurring around 8:00 AM. As the steroid or steroid-equivalent dose approaches the 20- to 30-mg level, the taper should be slowed and the patient checked for axis function. The primary modes to test HPA integrity are the ACTH test, either high- or low-dose, or a morning (8:00 AM) serum cortisol. A normal morning serum cortisol (>20 mcg/dL) or a normal ACTH test indicates that daily steroid maintenance therapy may be discontinued. If morning serum cortisol is between 3 and 20 mcg/dL, the ACTH- or CRH-stimulation test can be useful in the assessment of pituitary-adrenal function.[22] A morning cortisol less than 3 mcg/dL indicates axis suppression and the need for continued replacement therapy. Suppression can persist for up to a year in some patients. Caution should be used to prevent disease exacerbation during the steroid taper and to avoid the need for rebolusing the patient with another course of high-dose steroids.

Alternate day therapy (ADT) regimens have been promoted by some as a means to lessen the impact of prolonged steroid administration.[22,85] ADT theoretically minimizes the hypothalamic-pituitary suppression as well as some of the adverse effects seen with once-daily therapy. This hypothetical advantage may be especially pertinent in treating children and young adults, in whom growth suppression is a major concern. ADT is not recommended for initial management, but rather in the management of the stabilized patient who needs long-term therapy. The patient is exposed to "on" and "off" days, with the "on" day dose gradually increased corresponding with a dose-reduction in the "off" day dose over a period of 14 days. After two weeks, no medication is taken on "off" days. Not all patients will have equivalent disease control on ADT, and it should be avoided in certain indications.[22,85]

EVALUATION OF THERAPEUTIC OUTCOMES

Successful glucocorticoid therapy involves counseling and monitoring the patient, as well as recognizing complications of therapy (Table 85-10). The risk-to-benefit ratio of glucocorticoid administration should always be considered, especially with concurrent disease states such as hypertension, diabetes mellitus, peptic ulcer disease, and uncontrolled systemic infections.

TABLE 85-9	Relative Potencies of Glucocorticoids			
	Anti-Inflammatory	Equivalent Potency	Approximate Half-Life	Sodium-Retaining
Glucocorticoid	*Potency*	*(mg)*	*(min)*	*Potency*
Cortisone	0.8	25	30	2
Hydrocortisone	1	20	90	2
Prednisone	3.5	5	60	1
Prednisolone	4	5	200	1
Triamcinolone	5	4	300	0
Methylprednisolone	5	4	180	0
Betamethasone	25	0.6	100–300	0
Dexamethasone	30	0.75	100–300	0

TABLE 85-10 Factors in Successful Glucocorticoid Therapy

Monitoring	Glucose concentrations (serum and urine)
	Electrolytes (serum and urine)
	Ophthalmologic examinations
	Stool tests for occult blood loss
	Growth and development (children and adolescents)
Counseling	Take with food to minimize gastrointestinal discomfort
	Never discontinue medication on your own; check with your physician; gradual dose reduction is usually necessary
	Carry or wear medical identification indicating that you are on long-term glucocorticoid therapy
	Dosage increases can be necessary at times of increased stress (surgery or emergency treatments)
	Be aware of potential side effects (i.e., visual disturbances, bruising, and delayed wound healing)
	What to do if you miss a dose: If your dosing schedule is
	Every other day: Take as soon as possible if remembered that morning. If not remembered until later, skip that day. Take the next morning, then skip the following day.
	Every day: Take as soon as possible, but skip if almost time for the next dose. Never double doses.
Recognizing complications	Early in therapy and essentially unavoidable: insomnia, enhanced appetite, weight gain
	Common in patients with underlying risk factors: hypertension, diabetes mellitus, peptic ulcer disease
	Long-term intense treatment: cushingoid habitus, hypothalamic-pituitary-adrenal suppression, impaired wound healing
	Delayed and insidious: cataracts, atherosclerosis
	Rare and unpredictable: psychosis, glaucoma, pancreatitis

From United States Pharmacopeial Convention[87] and Barlow.[88]

ABBREVIATIONS

ACTH: adrenocorticotropic hormone

ADT: alternate day therapy

APA: aldosterone-producing adenoma

APS: autoimmune polyendocrine syndrome

ARR: aldosterone-to-renin ratio

AVS: adrenal venous sampling

BAH: bilateral adrenal hyperplasia

CBG: corticosteroid-binding globulin

CHD: coronary heart disease

CrCL: creatinine clearance

CRH: corticotropin-releasing hormone

CT: computed tomography

D_5NS: dextrose 5% in normal saline solution

DDT: dichlorodiphenyltrichloroethane

DST: dexamethasone suppression test

FH: familial hyperaldosteronism

FST: fludrocortisone suppression test

GRA: glucocorticoid-remediable aldosteronism

GRE: glucocorticoid response element

HPA: hypothalamic-pituitary-adrenal

IPSS: inferior petrosal sinus sampling

IRMA: immunoradiometric assay

JNC: Joint National Committee on Prevention, Detection, Evaluation, and Treatment of High Blood Pressure

JVS: jugular venous sampling

MRI: magnetic resonance imaging

PAC:PRA: plasma-aldosterone-concentration–to–plasma-renin-activity (ratio)

PA: primary aldosteronism

RIA: radioimmunoassay

RU-486: mifepristone

UFC: urine free cortisol

REFERENCES

1. Conn JW. Primary aldosteronism, a new clinical syndrome. J Lab Clin Med 1955;45:6–17.
2. Albright F. Cushing syndrome. Harvey Lect 1942–1943;38:123–186.
3. Newell-Price J, Bertagna X, Grossman AB, Nieman LK. Cushing's syndrome. Lancet 2006;367:1605–1617.
4. Isidori AM, Kaltsas GA, Pozza C, et al. The ectopic adrenocorticotropin syndrome: Clinical features, diagnosis, management, and long-term follow-up. J Clin Endocrinol Metab 2006;91:371–377.
5. Boscaro M, Barzon L, Sonino N. The diagnosis of Cushing's syndrome: Atypical presentations and laboratory shortcomings. Arch Intern Med 2000;160:3045–3053.
6. Williams GH, Dluhy RG. Disorders of the adrenal cortex. In: Fauci AS, Braunwald E, Kasper DL, et al., eds. Harrison's Principles of Internal Medicine, 17th ed. [electronic version]. 2008, AccessMedicine. *http://www.accessmedicine.com/content.aspx?aID=2900123.*
7. Catargi B, Rigalleau V, Poussin A, et al. Occult Cushing's syndrome in type-2 diabetes. J Clin Endocrinol Metab 2003;88:5808–5813.
8. Findling JW, Raff H. Screening and diagnosis of Cushing's syndrome. Endocrinol Metab Clin North Am 2005;34:385–402.
9. Nieman LK, Biller BMK, Findling JW, et al. The diagnosis of Cushing's syndrome: An Endocrine Society Clinical Practice Guideline. J Clin Endocrinol Metab 2008;93:1526–1540.
10. Nieman LK, Ilias I. Evaluation and treatment of Cushing's syndrome. Am J Med 2005;118:1340–1346.
11. Lindsay JR, Nieman LK. Differential diagnosis and imaging in Cushing's syndrome. Endocrinol Metab Clin North Am 2005;34:403–421.
12. Arnaldi G, Angeli A, Atkinson AB, et al. Diagnosis and complications of Cushing's syndrome: A consensus statement. J Clin Endocrinol Metab 2003;88:5593–5602.
13. Jackson RV, Hockings GI, Torpy DJ, et al. New diagnostic tests for Cushing's syndrome: Uses of naloxone, vasopressin and alprazolam. Clin Exp Pharmacol Physiol 1996;23:579–581.
14. Ambrosi B, Bochicchio D, Colombo P, et al. Loperamide to diagnose Cushing's syndrome. JAMA 1993;270:2301–2302.
15. Arvat E, Giordano R, Ramunni J, et al. Adrenocorticotropin and cortisol hyperresponsiveness to hexarelin in patients with Cushing's disease bearing a pituitary microadenoma, but not in those with macroadenoma. J Clin Endocrinol Metab 1998;83:4207–4211.
16. Newell-Price J, Trainer P, Besser M, Grossman A. The diagnosis and differential diagnosis of Cushing's syndrome and pseudo-Cushing's states. Endocr Rev 1998;19:647–672.
17. Papanicolaou DA, Mullen N, Kyrou I, Nieman LK. Nighttime salivary cortisol: A useful test for the diagnosis of Cushing's syndrome. J Clin Endocrinol Metab 2002;87:4515–4521.
18. Viardot A, Huber P, Puder JJ, et al. Reproducibility of nighttime salivary cortisol and its use in the diagnosis of hypercortisolism compared with urinary free cortisol and overnight dexamethasone suppression test. J Clin Endocrinol Metab 2005;90:5730–5736.
19. Findling JW, Raff H, Aron DC. The low-dose dexamethasone suppression test: A reevaluation in patients with Cushing's syndrome. J Clin Endocrinol Metab 2004;89:1222–1226.
20. Rockall AG, Babar SA, Sohaib SA, et al. CT and MR imaging of the adrenal glands in ACTH-independent Cushing's syndrome. RadioGraphics 2004;24:435–452.
21. Peppercorn PD, Reznek RH. State-of-the-art CT and MRI of the adrenal gland. Eur Radiol 1997;7:822–836.

22. Hopkins RL, Leinung MC. Exogenous Cushing's syndrome and glucocorticoid withdrawal. Endocrinol Metab Clin North Am 2005;34: 371–384.

23. Bolland MJ, Bagg W, Thomas MG, et al. Cushing's syndrome due to interaction between inhaled corticosteroids and itraconazole. Ann Pharmacother 2004;38:46–49.

24. Samaras K, Pett S, Gowers A, et al. Iatrogenic Cushing's syndrome with osteoporosis and secondary adrenal failure in human immunodeficiency virus-infected patients receiving inhaled corticosteroids and ritonavir-boosted protease inhibitors: Six cases. J Clin Endocrinol Metab 2005;90:4394–4398.

25. Nieman LK. Medical therapy of Cushing's disease. Pituitary 2002;5: 77–82.

26. Labeur M, Arzt E, Stalla GK, Paez-Pereda M. New perspectives in the treatment of Cushing's syndrome. Curr Drug Targets Immune Endocr Metabol Disord 2004;4:335–342.

27. McEvoy GK, ed. American Hospital Formulary Service (AHFS) Drug Information. Bethesda, MD: American Society of Health-System Pharmacists, 2005;15–16, 510–516, 1116–1118.

28. Utz AL, Swearingen B, Biller BM. Pituitary surgery and postoperative management in Cushing's disease. Endocrinol Metab Clin North Am 2005;34:459–478.

29. Dang CN, Trainer P. Pharmacological management of Cushing's syndrome: An update. Arq Ras Endocrinol Metab 2007;51:1339–1348.

30. Sonino N, Boscaro M. Medical therapy for Cushing's disease. Endocrinol Metab Clin North Am 1999;28:211–222.

31. Pivonello R, Ferone D, de Herder WW, et al. Dopamine receptor expression and function in corticotroph pituitary tumors. J Clin Endocrinol Metab 2004;89:2452–2462.

32. Semple PL, Vance ML, Findling J, Laws ER. Transsphenoidal surgery for Cushing's disease: Outcome in patients with a normal magnetic resonance imaging scan. Neurosurgery 2000;46:553–558.

33. Biller BMK, Grossman AB, Stewart PM, et al. Treatment of adrenocorticotropin-dependent Cushing's syndrome: A consensus statement. J Clin Endocrinol Metab 2008;93:2454–2462.

34. Veytsman I, Nieman L, Fojo T. Management of endocrine manifestations and the use of mitotane as a chemotherapeutic agent for adrenocortical carcinoma. J Clin Oncol 2009;27:4619–4629.

35. Morris D, Grossman A. The medical management of Cushing's syndrome. Ann N Y Acad Sci 2002;970:119–133.

36. Young WF. Minireview: Primary aldosteronism—Changing concepts in diagnosis and treatment. Endocrinology 2003;144:2208–2213.

37. Stowasser M, Gordon RD. Primary aldosteronism: From genesis to genetics. Trends Endocrinol Metab 2003;14:310–317.

38. Stowasser M, Gordon RD. Primary aldosteronism. Best Pract Res Clin Endocrinol Metab 2003;17:591–605.

39. Fardella CE, Mosso L. Primary aldosteronism. Clin Lab 2002;48:181–190.

40. Bope ET, Rakel RE, ed. Conn's Current Therapy 2005. Philadelphia, PA: Elsevier Saunders, 2005;745–747.

41. Funder JW, Carey RM, Fardella C, et al. Case detection, diagnosis, and treatment of patients with primary aldosteronism: An Endocrine Society clinical practice guideline. J Clin Endocrinol Metab. 2008;93:3266–3281.

42. Schwartz GL, Turner ST. Screening for primary aldosteronism in essential hypertension: Diagnostic accuracy of the ratio of plasma aldosterone concentration to plasma renin activity. Clin Chem 2005;51:386–394.

43. Stowasser M, Gordon RD, Gunasekera TG, et al. High rate of detection of primary aldosteronism, including surgically treatable forms, after "nonselective" screening of hypertensive patients. J Hypertens 2003;21:2149–2157.

44. Mulatero P, Dluhy RG, Giacchetti G, et al. Diagnosis of primary aldosteronism: From screening to subtype differentiation. Trends Endocrinol Metab 2005;16:114–119.

45. Young WF, Stanson AW, Thompson GB, et al. Role for adrenal venous sampling in primary aldosteronism. Surgery 2004;136:1227–1235.

46. Nwariaku FE, Miller BS, Auchus R, et al. Primary hyperaldosteronism: Effect of adrenal vein sampling on surgical outcome. Arch Surg 2006;141:497–502.

47. Ye P, Yamashita T, Pollock DM, Rainey WE. Contrasting effects of eplerenone and spironolactone on adrenal cell steroidogenesis. Horm Metab Res 2009;41:35–39.

48. Nishizaka MK, Calhoun DA. Primary aldosteronism: Diagnostic and therapeutic considerations. Curr Cardiol Rep 2005;7:412–417.

49. Young WF Jr. Primary aldosteronism: Management issues. Ann N Y Acad Sci 2002;970:61–76.

50. Young WF. Primary aldosteronism—Treatment options. Growth Horm IGF Res 2003;13:S102–S108.

51. Weinberger MH, White WB, Ruilope LM, et al. Effects of eplerenone versus losartan in patients with low-renin hypertension. Am Heart J 2005;150:426–433.

52. Meria P, Kempf BF, Hermieu JF, et al. Laparoscopic management of primary aldosteronism: Clinical experience with 212 cases. J Urol 2003;169:32–35.

53. Meyer A, Brabant G, Behrend M. Long-term follow-up after adrenalectomy for primary aldosteronism. World J Surg 2005;29:155–159.

54. Salvatori R. Adrenal insufficiency. JAMA 2005;294:2481–2488.

55. Levin C, Maibach HI. Topical corticosteroid-induced adrenocortical insufficiency: Clinical implications. Am J Clin Dermatol 2002;3: 141–147.

56. Bello CE, Garrett SD. Therapeutic issues in oral glucocorticoid use. Lippincotts Prim Care Pract 1999;3:333–341.

57. Sizonenko PC. Effects of inhaled or nasal glucocorticosteroids on adrenal function and growth. J Pediatr Endocrinol Metab 2002;15:5–26.

58. Goodman A, Cagliero E. Megestrol-induced clinical adrenal insufficiency. Eur J Gynaecol Oncol 2000;21:117–118.

59. Schule C, Baghai T, Bidlingmaier M, et al. Endocrinological effects of mirtazapine in healthy volunteers. Prog Neuropsychopharmacol Biol Psychiatry 2002;26:1253–1261.

60. Alevritis EM, Sarubbi FA, Jordan RM, Peiris AN. Infectious cause of adrenal insufficiency. South Med J 2003;96:888–890.

61. Torrey SP. Recognition and management of adrenal emergencies. Emerg Med Clin North Am 2005;23:687–702.

62. Dorin RI, Qualls CR, Crapo LM. Diagnosis of adrenal insufficiency. Ann Intern Med 2003;139:194–204.

63. Oelkers W. The role of high- and low-dose corticotropin tests in the diagnosis of secondary adrenal insufficiency. Eur J Endocrinol 1998;139:567–570.

64. Magnotti M, Shimshi M. Diagnosing adrenal insufficiency: Which test is best — the 1-mcg or the 250-mcg cosyntropin stimulation test? Endocr Pract 2008;14:233–238.

65. Arlt W, Allolio B. Adrenal insufficiency. Lancet 2003;361:1881–1893.

66. Cooper MS, Stewart PM. Corticosteroid insufficiency in acutely ill patients. N Engl J Med 2003;348:727–734.

67. Crown A, Lightman S. Why is the management of glucocorticoid deficiency still controversial: A review of the literature. Clin Endocrinol (Oxf) 2005;63:483–492.

68. Arlt W. Dehydroepiandrosterone replacement therapy. Semin Reprod Med 2004;22:379–388.

69. Alkatib AA, Cosma M, Elamin MB, et al. A systematic review and meta-analysis of randomized placebo-controlled trials of DHEA treatment effects on quality of life in women with adrenal insufficiency. J Clin Endocrinol Metab 2009;94:3676–3681.

70. Coursin DB, Wood KE. Corticosteroid supplementation for adrenal insufficiency. JAMA 2002;287:236–240.

71. Nieman LK, Turner MC. Addison's disease. Clin Dermatol 2006;24: 276–280.

72. Jacobi J. Corticosteroid replacement in critically ill patients. Crit Care Clin 2006;22:245–253.

73. Speiser PW, White PC. Congenital adrenal hyperplasia. N Engl J Med 2003;349:776–788.

74. Forest MG. Recent advances in the diagnosis and management of congenital adrenal hyperplasia due to 21-hydroxylase deficiency. Hum Reprod Update 2004;10:469–485.

75. Merke DP, Bornstein SR. Congenital adrenal hyperplasia. Lancet 2005;365:2125–2136.

76. Yildiz BO. Diagnosis of hyperandrogenism: Clinical criteria. Best Psract Res Clin Endocrinol Metab 2006;20:167–176.

77. Rosenfield RL. Hirsutism. N Engl J Med 2005;353:2578–2588.

78. Koulouri O, Conway GS. Management of hirsutism. BMJ 2009;338: 823–826.

79. Martin KA, Chang RJ, Ehrmann DA, et al. Evaluation and treatment of hirsutism in premenopausal women: An Endocrine Society

clinical practice guideline. J Clin Endocrinol Metab 2008;93: 1105–1120.

80. Azziz R. The evaluation and management of hirsutism. Obstet Gynecol, 2003;101:995–1007.

81. Moghetti P. Treatment of hirsutism and acne in hyperandrogenism. Best Pract Res Clin Endocrinol Metab 2006;20:221–234.

82. Henzen C, Suter A, Lerch E, et al. Suppression and recovery of adrenal response after short-term, high-dose glucocorticoid treatment. Lancet 2000;355:542–545.

83. Krasner AS. Glucocorticoid-induced adrenal insufficiency. JAMA 1999;282:671–676.

84. Kountz DS, Clark CL. Safely withdrawing patients from chronic glucocorticoid therapy. Am Fam Physician 1997;55:521–552.

85. Baxter JD. Advances in glucocorticoid therapy. Adv Intern Med 2000;45:317–349.

86. United States Pharmacopeial Convention Inc. USPDI. Advice for the patient: Drug Information in Lay Language, vol. II, 19th ed. Taunton, MA: Rand-McNally, 1999:612–616.

87. Barlow JE. Complications of therapy. In: Boumpas DT, moderator. Glucocorticoid therapy for immune mediated diseases: Basic and clinical correlates. Ann Intern Med 1993;119: 1198–1208.

86

Pituitary Gland Disorders

AMY HECK SHEEHAN, JACK A. YANOVSKI, AND KARIM ANTON CALIS

KEY CONCEPTS

❶ Pharmacologic therapy for acromegaly should be considered when surgery and irradiation are contraindicated, when there is poor likelihood of surgical success, when rapid control of symptoms is needed, or when other treatments have failed to normalize growth hormone (GH) and insulin-like growth factor 1 (IGF-1) concentrations.

❷ Pharmacotherapy for acromegaly using dopamine agonists provides advantages of oral dosing and reduced cost compared to somatostatin analogs and pegvisomant. However, dopamine agonists effectively normalize IGF-1 concentrations in only 10% of patients. Therefore, somatostatin analogs remain the mainstay of therapy.

❸ Blood glucose concentrations should be monitored frequently in the early stages of somatostatin analog therapy in all acromegalic patients.

❹ Pegvisomant appears to be the most effective agent for normalizing IGF-1 concentrations. However, further study is needed to determine the long-term safety and efficacy of this agent for the treatment of acromegaly.

❺ Recombinant GH is currently considered the mainstay of therapy for treatment of children with growth hormone-deficient (GHD) short stature. Prompt diagnosis of GHD and initiation of replacement therapy with recombinant GH is crucial for optimizing final adult heights.

❻ All GH products are generally considered to be equally efficacious. The recommended dose for treatment of GHD short stature in children is 0.3 mg/kg/wk.

❼ Pharmacologic agents that antagonize dopamine or increase the release of prolactin can induce hyperprolactinemia. Discontinuation of the offending medication and initiation of an appropriate therapeutic alternative usually normalize serum prolactin concentrations.

❽ Cabergoline appears to be more effective than bromocriptine for the medical management of prolactinomas and offers the advantage of less frequent dosing and decreased adverse events.

❾ Although preliminary data do not suggest cabergoline has significant teratogenic potential, cabergoline is not recommended for use during pregnancy, and patients receiving cabergoline who plan to become pregnant should discontinue the medication as soon as pregnancy is detected.

❿ Pharmacologic treatment of panhypopituitarism consists of glucocorticoids, thyroid hormone preparations, sex steroids, and recombinant GH, where appropriate, as lifelong replacement therapy.

Learning objectives, review questions, and other resources can be found at **www.pharmacotherapyonline.com**.

In the 1950s, Geoffrey Harris and his colleagues uncovered the physiologic importance of pituitary hormones and proposed the theory of neurohormonal regulation of the pituitary by the hypothalamus.[1] Today the pituitary gland is recognized for its essential role in body homeostasis, and for this reason it is often referred to as the "master gland." The hypothalamus and the pituitary gland are closely connected, and together they provide a means of communication between the brain and many of the body's endocrine organs. The hypothalamus uses nervous input and metabolic signals from the body to control the secretion of pituitary hormones that regulate growth, thyroid function, adrenal activity, reproduction, lactation, and fluid balance.

ANATOMY AND PHYSIOLOGY

The hypothalamus (Fig. 86–1) is a small region at the base of the brain that receives autonomic nervous input from different areas of the body to regulate limbic functions, food and water intake, body temperature, cardiovascular function, respiratory function, and diurnal rhythms. In addition, the hypothalamus controls the release of hormones from the anterior and posterior regions of the pituitary gland. Neurons in the hypothalamus produce vasopressin and oxytocin and make many hormone-releasing factors that stimulate or inhibit the release of trophic hormones. At the base of the hypothalamus, a projection known as the *median eminence* is rich with nerve axons and blood vessels and provides both chemical and physical connections between the hypothalamus and the pituitary gland.

The pituitary gland, also referred to as the *hypophysis*, is located at the base of the brain in a cavity of the sphenoid bone known as the *sella turcica*. The pituitary is separated from the brain by an extension of the dura mater known as the *diaphragma sella*. The pituitary is a very small gland, weighing between 0.4 and 1 g in adults. It is divided into two distinct regions, the anterior lobe, or adenohypophysis, and the posterior lobe, or the neurohypophysis (see Fig. 86–1).

The posterior pituitary gland secretes two major hormones: oxytocin and vasopressin (antidiuretic hormone) (Table 86–1).

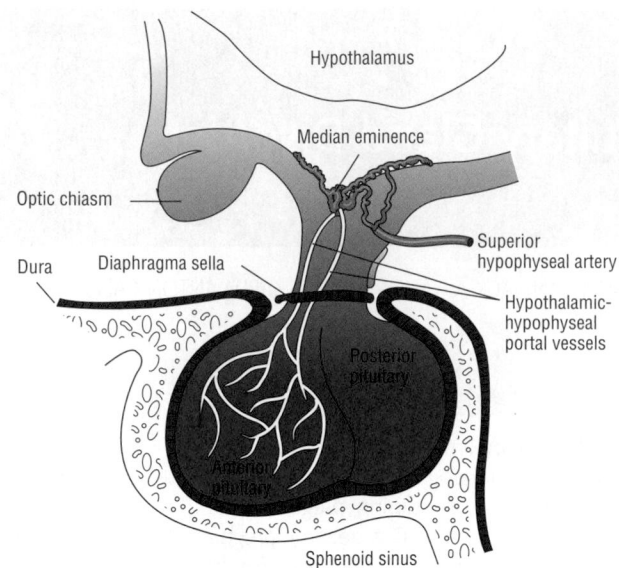

FIGURE 86-1. Pituitary gland.

Oxytocin release from the posterior pituitary causes contraction of the smooth muscles in the breast during lactation. It also plays a role in uterine contraction during parturition. Vasopressin is essential for proper fluid balance and acts on the renal collecting ducts to conserve water. Oxytocin and vasopressin are synthesized in the paraventricular and supraoptic nuclei of the hypothalamus. The posterior pituitary gland contains the terminal nerve endings of these two nuclei as well as specialized secretory granules that release hormones in response to appropriate signals. Loss of anterior pituitary function does not necessarily affect the release of vasopressin or oxytocin because these hormones actually are synthesized in the hypothalamus.

Unlike the posterior pituitary, the release of anterior pituitary hormones is not regulated by direct nervous stimulation but rather is controlled by specific hypothalamic-releasing and inhibitory hormones. The median eminence of the hypothalamus contains a large number of capillaries that converge to form a network of veins known as the *hypothalamic–hypophysial portal circulation*. Inhibiting and releasing hormones synthesized in the neurons of the hypothalamus reach the anterior pituitary via the hypothalamic–hypophysial portal vessels to control release of anterior pituitary hormones. Although there is a direct arterial blood supply to the anterior pituitary lobe, the hypothalamic–hypophysial portal vessels provide the primary blood supply (see Fig. 86–1). In contrast to the posterior pituitary, the anterior pituitary lobe is extremely vascular and has the highest rate of blood flow of all body organs.

The specialized secretory cells of the anterior pituitary lobe secrete six major polypeptide hormones (see Table 86–1). These include growth hormone (GH) or somatotropin, adrenocorticotropic hormone (ACTH) or corticotropin, thyroid-stimulating hormone (TSH) or thyrotropin, prolactin, follicle-stimulating hormone (FSH), and luteinizing hormone (LH). The release of these hormones is regulated primarily by hypothalamic-releasing and inhibiting hormones. Thyrotropin-releasing hormone (TRH) stimulates anterior pituitary release of TSH and prolactin, corticotropin-releasing hormone (CRH) stimulates anterior pituitary release of ACTH, growth hormone-releasing hormone (GHRH) stimulates anterior pituitary release of GH, and gonadotropin-releasing hormone (GnRH) stimulates anterior pituitary release of LH and FSH. Hypothalamic release of somatostatin inhibits release of GH, and hypothalamic release of dopamine (prolactin inhibitory hormone) inhibits the secretion of prolactin. Prolactin

differs from the other anterior lobe hormones in that an inhibiting factor, rather than a stimulating factor, is primarily responsible for controlling its secretion. In the absence of hypothalamic input, an excess of prolactin is produced, whereas a deficiency state of other anterior pituitary hormones results. Physiologic regulation and action of anterior and posterior pituitary hormones are summarized in Table 86–1.[2-4]

Destruction of the pituitary gland may result in secondary hypothyroidism, hypogonadism, adrenal insufficiency, GH deficiency, and hypoprolactinemia. The formation of certain types of pituitary tumors may result in pituitary hormone excess. Pituitary tumors may physically compress the pituitary and prevent the release of trophic hypothalamic factors that regulate pituitary hormones. In this chapter, the pathophysiology and role of pharmacotherapy in the treatment of acromegaly, short stature, hyperprolactinemia, and panhypopituitarism are discussed. (Also see Chapters 84, 85 and 87–91).

GROWTH HORMONE

GH has direct antiinsulin effects on lipid and carbohydrate metabolism. GH decreases utilization of glucose by peripheral tissues, increases lipolysis, and increases muscle mass. GH also stimulates gluconeogenesis in hepatocytes, impairs tissue glucose uptake, decreases insulin-receptor sensitivity, and impairs postreceptor insulin action. The growth-promoting effects of GH are largely mediated by insulin-like growth factors (IGFs) also known as *somatomedins*. GH stimulates the formation of insulin-like growth factor 1 (IGF-1) in the liver as well as in other peripheral tissues. This anabolic peptide acts as a direct stimulator of cell proliferation and growth. There are two types of insulin-like growth factors: IGF-1 and IGF-2. IGF-1 regulates growth to some extent before, and largely after, birth. In contrast, IGF-2 is thought to primarily regulate growth in utero.[5] GH is secreted by the anterior pituitary in a pulsatile fashion, with several short bursts that occur mostly at night. Because of the short half-life of GH in the plasma (~30 minutes), measurements of circulating GH concentrations throughout the waking hours usually are very low or undetectable. Daytime GH pulses are most likely to occur after meals, following exercise, or during periods of stress. The greatest amount of GH secretion occurs during the night within the first 1 to 2 hours of slow-wave sleep (stage III or IV). Secretion of GH is lowest during infancy, increases slightly during childhood, reaches its peak during adolescence, and then begins to gradually decline during the middle-age years.[3]

GROWTH HORMONE EXCESS

Acromegaly is a pathologic condition characterized by excessive production of GH. This is a rare disorder that affects approximately 50 to 70 adults per million.[6] Gigantism, which is even more rare than acromegaly, is the excess secretion of GH prior to epiphyseal closure in children.[7] Patients diagnosed with acromegaly are reported to have a 2- to 3-fold increase in mortality, usually related to cardiovascular, respiratory, or neoplastic disease.[8-10] Most patients are middle-aged at the time of diagnosis, and this disorder does not appear to affect one sex to a greater extent than the other. The most common cause of excess GH secretion in acromegaly is a GH-secreting pituitary adenoma, accounting for approximately 98% of all cases.[8] Rarely, acromegaly is caused by ectopic GH-secreting adenomas, GH cell hyperplasia, or excess GHRH secretion, or is one of the manifestations of multiple endocrine neoplasia syndrome type 1, McCune-Albright's syndrome, or the Carney complex, all very rare hypersecretory endocrinopathies.[8]

TABLE 86-1 Pituitary Hormones

Hormone	Stimulation	Inhibition	Physiologic Effects
Anterior pituitary hormones			
Growth hormone (GH)	*Physiologic*	*Physiologic*	Stimulates IGF-I production
	GH-releasing hormone	Somatostatin	IGF-I and GH promote growth
	Ghrelin	Elevated IGF-1	in all body tissues
	ADH	Growth hormone	
	GABA	Progesterone	
	Norepinephrine	Cortisol	
	Dopamine	Postprandial hyperglycemia	
	Serotonin	Elevated free fatty acids	
	Estrogen		
	Sleep		
	Stress		
	Exercise		
	Pharmacologic	*Pharmacologic*	
	α-Adrenergic agonists (e.g., clonidine)	Dopamine antagonists (e.g., phenothiazines)	
	β-Adrenergic antagonists (e.g., propranolol)	α-Adrenergic antagonists (e.g., phentolamine)	
	Dopamine agonists (e.g., bromocriptine)	β-Adrenergic agonists (e.g., isoproterenol)	
	GABA agonists (e.g., muscimol)	Serotonin antagonists (e.g., methysergide)	
Prolactin	*Physiologic*	*Physiologic*	
	TRH	Dopamine	Lactation
	VIP	GABA	
	Estrogen		
	Serotonin		
	Histamine		
	Endogenous opioids		
	Pregnancy and nursing		
	Pharmacologic	*Pharmacologic*	
	Dopamine antagonists (e.g., phenothiazines, haloperidol, methyldopa)	Dopamine agonists (e.g., L-dopa, bromocriptine, pergolide, cabergoline)	
	Opiates		
	Estrogens		
	H₂-antagonists (e.g., cimetidine)		
	MAO inhibitors		
Adrenocorticotropic hormone (ACTH)	CRH	Elevated cortisol	Glucocorticoid effects
			Pigmentation
Thyroid-stimulating hormone (TSH)	TRH	Thyroxine	Iodine uptake and thyroid
	Estrogens	Triiodothyronine	hormone synthesis
	Norepinephrine	Somatostatin	
	Serotonin	Glucocorticoids	
		Dopamine	
Luteinizing hormone (LH)	*Physiologic*		
	GnRH	Estradiol	Ovulation
	Pharmacologic	Testosterone	Maintains corpus luteum
	Clomiphene	Fasting	
Follicle-stimulating hormone (FSH)	*Physiologic*		
	GnRH	Estradiol	Ovarian follicle development
	Menopause	Inhibin	Stimulates estradiol and
	Ovarian disorders	Fasting	progesterone
	Pharmacologic		
	Clomiphene		
Posterior pituitary hormones			
Vasopressin (antidiuretic hormone [ADH])	Hyperosmolality	Hypervolemia	Acts on renal collecting ducts to
	Volume depletion	Hypoosmolality	prevent diuresis
Oxytocin	Parturition		Uterine contraction
	Suckling		Milk ejection

CRH, corticotropin-releasing hormone; GABA, γ-aminobutyric acid; GnRH, gonadotropin-releasing hormone; IGF-1, insulin-like growth factor-1; MAO, monoamine oxidase; TRH, thyrotropin-releasing hormone; VIP, vasoactive intestinal peptide.
Data from Amar and Weiss,[2] Cuttler,[3] and Molitch.[4]

The clinical signs and symptoms of acromegaly develop gradually over an extended period of time. In fact, because of the subtle and slowly developing changes in physical appearance caused by GH excess, most patients are not definitively diagnosed with acromegaly until 7 to 10 years after the presumed onset of excessive GH secretion.[9] Excessive secretion of GH and IGF-1 adversely affects several organ systems. Almost all acromegalic patients will present with physical signs and symptoms of soft-tissue overgrowth. Table 86–2 summarizes the classic clinical presentation of patients with acromegaly.[8-13] Some patients with acromegaly present with only a few of these classic signs and symptoms, making recognition of this disease extremely difficult.

TABLE 86-2 Clinical Presentation of Acromegaly

General
The patient will experience slow development of soft-tissue overgrowth affecting many body systems. Signs and symptoms may gradually progress over 7 to 10 years.

Symptoms
The patient may complain of symptoms related to local effects of the growth hormone (GH)-secreting tumor, such as headache and visual disturbances. Other symptoms related to elevated GH and insulin-like growth factor-1 (IGF-1) concentrations include excessive sweating, neuropathies, joint pain, and paresthesias.

Signs
The patient may exhibit coarsening of facial features, increased hand volume, increased ring size, increased shoe size, an enlarged tongue, and various dermatologic conditions.

Laboratory tests
The patient's GH concentration will be >1 mcg/L following an oral glucose tolerance test (OGTT) and IGF-1 serum concentrations will be elevated. Glucose intolerance may be present in up to 50% of patients.

Additional clinical sequelae
- Cardiovascular diseases such as hypertension, coronary heart disease, cardiomyopathy, and left ventricular hypertrophy are common in patients with acromegaly.
- Osteoarthritis and joint damage develops in up to 90% of acromegalic patients.
- Respiratory disorders and sleep apnea occur in up to 60% of acromegalic patients.
- Type 2 diabetes develops in approximately 25% of acromegalic patients.
- Patients with acromegaly may have an increased risk for development of esophageal, colon, and stomach cancer.

Data from Ben-Shlomo and Melmed,[8] Melmed,[9] Kauppinen-Makelin et al.,[10] Fatti et al.,[11] Vitale et al.,[12] and Webb et al.[13]

The diagnosis of acromegaly is based on a combination of diagnostic tests and clinical signs and symptoms. Random measures of plasma GH levels are not usually dependable because of the pulsatile pattern of release. The oral glucose tolerance test (OGTT) is commonly used as an important diagnostic tool. Postprandial hyperglycemia inhibits the secretion of GH for at least 1 to 2 hours. Therefore, an oral glucose load would be expected to suppress GH concentrations. However, patients with acromegaly continue to secrete GH during the OGTT. Because GH stimulates the production of IGF-1, serum IGF-1 concentrations can also be measured to aid in the diagnosis of acromegaly. Circulating IGF-1 is cleared from the body at a much slower rate than is GH, and measurements can be collected at any time of the day to identify patients with GH excess.[9] Current criteria for the diagnosis of acromegaly include failure of GH suppression <1 mcg/L following an OGTT in the presence of elevated IGF-1 serum concentrations.[14,15] With the development of more sensitive GH and IGF-1 assays, the cutoff value for diagnosis of acromegaly will likely decrease in the future. Insulin-like growth factor 1 binding protein 3 (IGFBP-3) also can be measured because it is positively regulated by GH and binds to circulating IGF-1 with high affinity. This test may be useful in monitoring response to therapy.[8] Computed tomography and magnetic resonance imaging of the pituitary are important diagnostic tests to confirm the presence of a pituitary adenoma.[9,14,15]

TREATMENT

Acromegaly

The primary treatment goals for patients diagnosed with acromegaly are to reduce GH and IGF-1 concentrations, improve the clinical signs and symptoms of the disease, and decrease mortality.[15–17] Many clinicians define biochemical control of acromegaly as suppression of GH concentrations to <1 mcg/L after a standard OGTT in the presence of normal IGF-1 serum concentrations.[16] The treatment of choice for most patients with acromegaly is transsphenoidal surgical resection of the GH-secreting adenoma.[9,15,16] Postsurgical cure rates have been reported to range from 50% to 90%, depending on the type of adenoma and the expertise of the neurosurgeon.[8,16,17] Complications of transsphenoidal surgery are relatively infrequent and include cerebrospinal fluid leak, meningitis, arachnoiditis, diabetes insipidus, and pituitary failure.[8] For patients who are poor surgical candidates, those who have not responded to surgical interventions, or others who refuse surgical treatment, radiation therapy may be considered. Radiation, however, may take several years to relieve the symptoms of acromegaly.

Because neither radiation therapy nor surgery will cure all patients with acromegaly, adjuvant drug therapy is often needed to control symptoms.[9,17,18]

■ PHARMACOLOGIC THERAPY

1 Drug therapy should be considered for acromegalic patients in whom surgery and irradiation are contraindicated, when there is poor likelihood of surgical success, when rapid control of symptoms is indicated, or when other treatments have failed to normalize GH and IGF-1 concentrations. Pharmacologic treatment options include dopamine agonists, somatostatin analogs, and the GH receptor antagonist pegvisomant. Dopamine agonists such as bromocriptine and cabergoline are effective in a small subset of patients and provide the advantages of oral dosing and reduced cost. Somatostatin analogs are more effective than dopamine agonists, reducing GH concentrations and normalizing IGF-1 in approximately 50% to 60% of patients. Pegvisomant, a GH receptor antagonist, is highly effective in normalizing IGF-1 concentrations in up to 97% of patients. However, additional long-term data are needed to establish the safety and efficacy of pegvisomant in the management of acromegaly.

■ DOPAMINE AGONISTS

2 In normal healthy adults, dopamine agonists cause an increase in GH production. However, when these agents are given to patients with acromegaly, there is a paradoxical decrease in GH production. Most clinical experience with the use of dopamine agonists in acromegaly is with bromocriptine. Other agents such as pergolide, cabergoline, and lisuride also have been used. Bromocriptine is a semisynthetic ergot alkaloid that acts as a dopamine-receptor agonist. Most trials assessing the efficacy of bromocriptine in the treatment of acromegaly were conducted in the 1970s and early 1980s. These studies determined that certain subsets of acromegalic patients have a favorable response to drug therapy with bromocriptine. These patients include individuals with high circulating concentrations of prolactin and patients who experience GH suppression following a single 2.5-mg dose of bromocriptine, known as a *bromocriptine challenge.*[19] A review evaluating 34 studies concluded that therapy with bromocriptine was effective in suppressing mean serum GH levels to <5 mcg/L in approximately 20% of patients.[20] Only 10% of patients experience normalization of IGF-1 concentrations with bromocriptine therapy, but >50% of patients treated with bromocriptine experience improvement in acromegalic symptoms.[9,21]

In the United States, bromocriptine is commercially available as 2.5-mg oral tablets and 5-mg oral capsules. In acromegalic patients, significant reductions in GH concentrations are observed within 1 to 2 hours of oral dosing. This effect persists for at least 4 to 5 hours. An overall clinical response in acromegalic patients typically occurs after 4 to 8 weeks of continuous bromocriptine therapy. For treatment of acromegaly, bromocriptine is initiated at a dose of 1.25 mg at bedtime and is increased by 1.25-mg increments every 3 to 4 days as needed.[19,20] Doses as high as 86 mg/day have been used for treatment of acromegaly, but clinical studies have shown that dosages >20 or 30 mg daily do not offer additional benefits in the suppression of GH.[20,21] When used for treatment of acromegaly, the duration of action of bromocriptine is shorter than that for treatment of hyperprolactinemia. Therefore, the total daily dose of bromocriptine should be divided into three or four doses.[19,21]

The most common adverse effects of bromocriptine therapy include central nervous system (CNS) symptoms such as headache, lightheadedness, dizziness, nervousness, and fatigue. Gastrointestinal effects such as nausea, abdominal pain, or diarrhea also are very common. Some patients may need to take bromocriptine with food to decrease the incidence of adverse gastrointestinal effects. Most adverse effects are seen early in the course of therapy and tend to decrease with continued treatment.[21] Bromocriptine may cause thickening of bronchial secretions and nasal congestion. Rare cases of psychiatric disturbances, pleural diseases, and an erythromelalgic syndrome (painful paroxysmal dilation of the blood vessels in the skin of the feet and lower extremities) have been reported with bromocriptine use. These conditions appear to be associated with higher doses and prolonged duration of therapy.[20,21]

Bromocriptine generally should be discontinued if a woman becomes pregnant while taking the drug. Surveillance of women who took bromocriptine throughout pregnancy does not suggest that bromocriptine is associated with an increased risk for birth defects.[21] If a woman becomes pregnant while taking bromocriptine, the risks and benefits of therapy should be fully considered. In most cases, the benefits of successful therapy outweigh the risks, and bromocriptine therapy should be continued if it is effective in improving symptoms and reducing elevated GH concentrations.

Other dopamine agonists that have been used to treat acromegaly include pergolide, cabergoline, lisuride, and quinagolide. Cabergoline may be especially useful in patients with pituitary tumors that secrete both prolactin and GH.[21,22] Quinagolide, a dopamine agonist available in Europe, has been shown to be more effective than both bromocriptine and cabergoline in normalizing GH and IGF-1 values in acromegalic patients.[19] Because of the potential cost advantages and convenience of oral administration, dopamine agonists are often considered for treatment of acromegaly prior to initiation of somatostatin analogs. However, the availability of long-acting somatostatin analogs has made these agents more attractive for first-line treatment of acromegaly.

■ SOMATOSTATIN ANALOGS

Octreotide and lanreotide are long-acting somatostatin analogs that are more potent in inhibiting GH secretion than endogenous somatostatin.[23,24] These agents also suppress the LH response to GnRH; decrease splanchnic blood flow; and inhibit secretion of insulin, vasoactive intestinal peptide (VIP), gastrin, secretin, motilin, serotonin, and pancreatic polypeptide.

Octreotide (Sandostatin) injection is commercially available in the United States for subcutaneous or intravenous administration. A long-acting intramuscular formulation of octreotide (Sandostatin LAR) is available for monthly administration. In addition to the treatment of acromegaly, octreotide has many other therapeutic uses, including the treatment of carcinoid tumors, vasoactive intestinal peptide-secreting tumors (VIPomas), gastrointestinal fistulas, variceal bleeding, diarrheal states, and irritable bowel syndrome.

The efficacy of octreotide for treatment of acromegaly has been determined by two major multicenter trials.[25,26] These studies determined that drug therapy with octreotide suppresses mean serum GH concentrations to <5 mcg/L and normalizes serum IGF-1 concentrations in 50% to 60% of acromegalic patients. Octreotide also is beneficial in reducing the clinical signs and symptoms of acromegaly. In a 6-month multicenter trial, 70% of patients experienced significant relief of headaches.[26] In some patients, relief of headache symptoms occurred within minutes of octreotide administration. In addition, middle-finger circumference was reduced significantly, and 50% to 75% of patients experienced improvement in symptoms of excessive perspiration, fatigue, joint pain, and cystic acne. Long-term follow-up of patients treated with octreotide LAR for up to 9 years showed octreotide therapy to be safe and effective for long-term use in acromegalic patients.[27] Octreotide also has been shown to improve the cardiovascular manifestations of acromegaly and to halt pituitary tumor growth, with some patients experiencing tumor regression.[25–28] Data from more recent studies indicate that shrinkage of pituitary tumor mass during octreotide therapy occurs in approximately 50% of patients.[29]

The pharmacodynamic effects of long-acting octreotide are similar to those of subcutaneously administered octreotide. Single monthly doses of long-acting octreotide have been shown to be at least as effective as daily doses of 300 or 600 mcg of subcutaneous octreotide administered in divided doses 3 times daily in normalizing IGF-1 levels and maintaining suppression of mean serum GH concentrations.[30] A large multicenter trial evaluating the efficacy of long-acting octreotide in acromegalic patients who previously had responded to subcutaneously administered octreotide reported suppression of GH concentrations to <5 mcg/L in 94% of patients and normalization of IGF-1 in 66% of patients following 1 year of therapy.[31]

Response to long-term therapy with octreotide is related to the presence and increased quantity of functioning somatostatin receptors located in the pituitary adenoma.[26] Identification of patients who most likely will respond to octreotide, prior to initiation of therapy, is important when considering the high cost of this medication and the inconvenience of subcutaneous or intramuscular drug administration. Suppression of serum GH concentrations after a single 50-mcg dose of octreotide has been used to predict a favorable long-term response to octreotide therapy.[32,33]

The initial dose of octreotide for treatment of acromegaly is 100 mcg administered every 8 hours.[18,20,24] Some clinicians recommend a starting dose of 50 mcg every 8 hours, then increasing the dose to 100 mcg every 8 hours after 1 week, to improve the patient's tolerance of adverse gastrointestinal effects. The dose can be increased by increments of 50 mcg every 1 to 2 weeks based on mean serum GH and IGF-1 concentrations. Patients who experience a significant rise in GH prior to the end of the 8-hour dosing interval may benefit from decreasing the dosing interval to every 4 to 6 hours. Although doses as high as 1,500 mcg/day have been used, doses >600 mcg daily generally do not offer additional benefits, and most patients are adequately managed with 100 to 200 mcg 3 times daily.[25,26] Patients who have been maintained on subcutaneous octreotide for at least 2 weeks and have shown response to therapy can be converted to the long-acting depot form of octreotide. The initial dose of long-acting octreotide is 20 mg administered intramuscularly in the gluteal region every 28 days. Steady-state serum concentrations are not obtained until after 3 months of therapy. Therefore, dosage adjustments for long-acting octreotide should not be considered until after this time. Some patients may require additional subcutaneous injections during the initial dose-titration phase in order to control symptoms. Long-acting octreotide doses >30 mg every 4 weeks have not been studied. A long-acting, intramuscular formulation of lanreotide (lanreotide LA) for twice monthly administration has been available in Europe for many years. Recently, a new formulation of lanreotide (Somatuline Depot) was approved for use in the United States for monthly deep subcutaneous administration. The efficacy of this preparation of lanreotide for the treatment of acromegaly has been evaluated in several prospective multicenter clinical trials involving treatment-experienced patients who were switched from intramuscular octreotide LAR or intramuscular lanreotide LA to monthly deep subcutaneous lanreotide.[34-36] These studies have determined that deep subcutaneous lanreotide suppresses mean serum GH concentrations to <5 mcg/L and normalizes serum IGF-1 concentrations in acromegalic patients to a similar extent as octreotide LAR and lanreotide LA. A 4-year follow-up of 23 patients treated with monthly deep subcutaneous lanreotide reported the drug to be well tolerated during long-term therapy with mean serum GH concentrations <5 mcg/L in 62% of patients and normalization of serum IGF-1 concentrations in 43% of patients.[37] Well-designed trials directly comparing the efficacy of intramuscular octreotide LAR to deep subcutaneous lanreotide are currently lacking. However, these two agents are generally regarded to have comparable efficacy.[16]

Lanreotide (Somatuline Depot) is commercially available in the United States as 60-mg, 90-mg, and 120-mg prefilled syringes. In contrast to octreotide LAR, lanreotide injection does not need to be reconstituted prior to administration. The initial recommended dose of lanreotide is 90 mg given by deep subcutaneous injection in the superior external quadrant of the buttock every 28 days. Injection sites should be alternated between the left and right side. The initial dose should be reduced to 60 mg every 28 days for patients with moderate or severe renal or hepatic impairment. After 3 months of therapy, the dose may then be titrated based on serum GH concentrations, serum IGF-1 concentrations, and control of clinical signs and symptoms of acromegaly.[36] Long-acting deep subcutaneous lanreotide injection in doses >120 mg every 28 days has not been studied.

The most common adverse effects of somatostatin analog therapy are gastrointestinal disturbances such as diarrhea, nausea, abdominal cramps, malabsorption of fat, and flatulence.[16,23] Gastrointestinal adverse effects occur in approximately 75% of patients but usually subside within 10 to 14 days of continued treatment.[23] Octreotide has been reported to cause injection-site pain (4%–31%), conduction abnormalities and arrhythmias (9%), biochemical hypothyroidism (2%–12%), biliary tract disorders (4%–50%), and abnormalities in glucose metabolism (2%–18%).[20,23] Lanreotide has been reported to cause injection-site reactions (9%), sinus bradycardia (3%), hypertension (5%), biliary tract disorders (20%), and abnormalities in glucose metabolism (7%).[36]

Somatostatin analogs also inhibit cholecystokinin release and gallbladder motility, predisposing patients to the development of cholelithiasis.[23] The development of gallstones is a long-term adverse effect of somatostatin analog therapy and is largely dependent on geographic factors, dietary habits, and length of therapy.[20,24] The incidence of gallstones in acromegalic patients receiving octreotide and lanreotide increases with length of therapy and has been reported to range from 20% to 50%.[24-26] However, most patients are asymptomatic, and the diagnosis of cholelithiasis usually is made following an ultrasonographic study that is not prompted by patient symptoms. It has been estimated that only 1% of patients will develop symptomatic gallstones during 1 year of octreotide treatment.[24] Because somatostatin analog-induced gallstones usually are present without clinical symptoms, prophylactic cholecystectomy or medical therapy with ursodeoxycholic acid for acromegalic patients with asymptomatic gallstones usually is not recommended.[9,16] A small number of studies have suggested that the incidence of gallstone development may be lower with long-acting octreotide compared to subcutaneous octreotide.[30,31] However, further studies are needed to confirm this observation.

❸ The effect of somatostatin analogs on glucose metabolism in patients with acromegaly is multifactorial. Decreases in serum GH concentrations induced by somatostatin analogs should result in decreased hepatic gluconeogenesis and increased insulin-receptor sensitivity. However, somatostatin analogs also decrease insulin secretion and increase IGFBP-1, which is known to inhibit the insulin-like effects of IGF-1. In addition, somatostatin analogs delay the gastrointestinal absorption of glucose, which may further alter glucose metabolism in acromegalic patients.[37] Small studies conducted in acromegalic patients receiving octreotide have reported improvement in insulin sensitivity as well as impaired insulin secretion.[38,39] Risk factors associated with worsening glucose tolerance included female sex and elevated baseline insulin values. Although somatostatin analogs appear to have a beneficial effect on glucose tolerance in most patients, glucose determinations should be obtained frequently in the early stages of therapy in all acromegalic patients.

■ GROWTH HORMONE RECEPTOR ANTAGONIST

❹ Pegvisomant (Somavert) is a genetically engineered GH derivative that binds to, but does not activate, GH receptors and inhibits IGF-1 production by the liver. This agent is different from other medications used in the management of acromegaly because it does not inhibit GH production; rather, it blocks the physiologic effects of GH on target tissues. Therefore, GH concentrations remain elevated during therapy, and response to treatment is evidenced by a reduction in IGF-1 concentrations. Unlike somatostatin analogs, the pharmacologic activity of pegvisomant does not depend on the presence and quantity of somatostatin receptors in the pituitary tumor.[40] Studies evaluating the clinical efficacy of pegvisomant in acromegalic patients have reported a dose-dependent normalization of IGF-1 concentrations in 54% to 89% of patients after 12 weeks of therapy and in 97% of patients after 1 year of therapy.[40,41] Significant improvements in the clinical signs and symptoms of acromegaly were reported and persisted throughout the 1-year treatment period.[41] Adverse effects include injection-site pain, gastrointestinal complaints such as nausea and diarrhea, and flu-like symptoms. Significant elevations in hepatic aminotransferase concentrations, which are generally reversible upon discontinuation of the drug, have been reported in approximately 25% of patients.[16,42] As a result, hepatic function tests should be monitored very closely during therapy as outlined in the product labeling, and the drug should be used with caution in patients with baseline elevations in hepatic aminotransferase concentrations. GH concentrations increased significantly during the first 6 months of therapy. Tumor growth has been reported in a small number of patients and there are theoretical concerns that persistently elevated GH concentrations may stimulate tumor growth or result in other unfavorable long-term effects.

Pegvisomant is commercially available in the United States for daily subcutaneous use. The first dose should be administered under the supervision of a physician as a 40-mg loading dose. Subsequent doses are self-administered by the patient starting at a dose of 10 mg daily. The dose can be adjusted in 5-mg increments based on serum IGF-1 concentrations every 4 to 6 weeks, up to a maximum daily dose of 30 mg.[43]

Based on the available data, pegvisomant appears to be among the most effective agents for normalizing IGF-1 serum concentrations. However, it is very expensive and further study is needed to determine the long-term safety and efficacy of pegvisomant in the treatment of acromegaly. Current guidelines for acromegaly management suggest pegvisomant therapy for patients who have failed to achieve normalization of IGF-1 serum concentrations with other treatments.[16]

COMBINATION THERAPY

Several small studies have suggested that combination therapy with octreotide and dopamine agonists (bromocriptine or cabergoline) or octreotide and pegvisomant may be more beneficial than monotherapy with either drug alone.[20,23,44] Because of the potential for additive adverse effects, combination therapy should be considered as a therapeutic option only for refractory patients who have not fully responded to monotherapy.[16]

PHARMACOECONOMIC CONSIDERATIONS

Cost-effectiveness comparisons of the various treatment options for patients with acromegaly have not been performed. Considering that approximately 40% of patients are not completely cured after transsphenoidal surgery, pharmacologic treatment often becomes necessary. Bromocriptine and cabergoline are available as oral dosage forms and are considerably less expensive than octreotide, lanreotide, and pegvisomant. However, these agents are not effective in the majority of patients. Long-acting octreotide and lanreotide offer a convenient method of once-monthly administration for acromegalic patients, and may result in improved patient compliance, quality of life, and overall disease management. Pegvisomant appears to be the most effective agent for normalizing IGF-1 concentrations and may be useful in patients who are intolerant to or have not responded to therapy with dopamine agonists or somatostatin analogs. However, pegvisomant is significantly more expensive than long-acting octreotide or lanreotide and requires daily subcutaneous injections. Long-term studies evaluating the safety of pegvisomant are needed to clearly define its role in the management of acromegaly. The drug therapy of choice for an acromegalic patient should be determined by careful consideration of several patient-specific factors, including clinical response, compliance, tolerability, and cost of therapy.

CLINICAL CONTROVERSY

Some clinicians advocate the use of somatostatin analogs prior to surgery in order to improve comorbidities that may complicate surgery. However, sufficient evidence is lacking.

CONCLUSIONS

Acromegaly is a chronic debilitating disease characterized by excess GH secretion most commonly caused by a GH-secreting pituitary adenoma. Transsphenoidal surgical resection of the adenoma is the current treatment of choice for most patients with acromegaly. Patients who are poor surgical candidates may receive radiation therapy or long-term pharmacologic therapy. Drug therapy options within the United States for acromegaly include dopamine agonists, somatostatin analogs, and pegvisomant. Figure 86–2 shows a treatment algorithm for the management of acromegaly.[9,16]

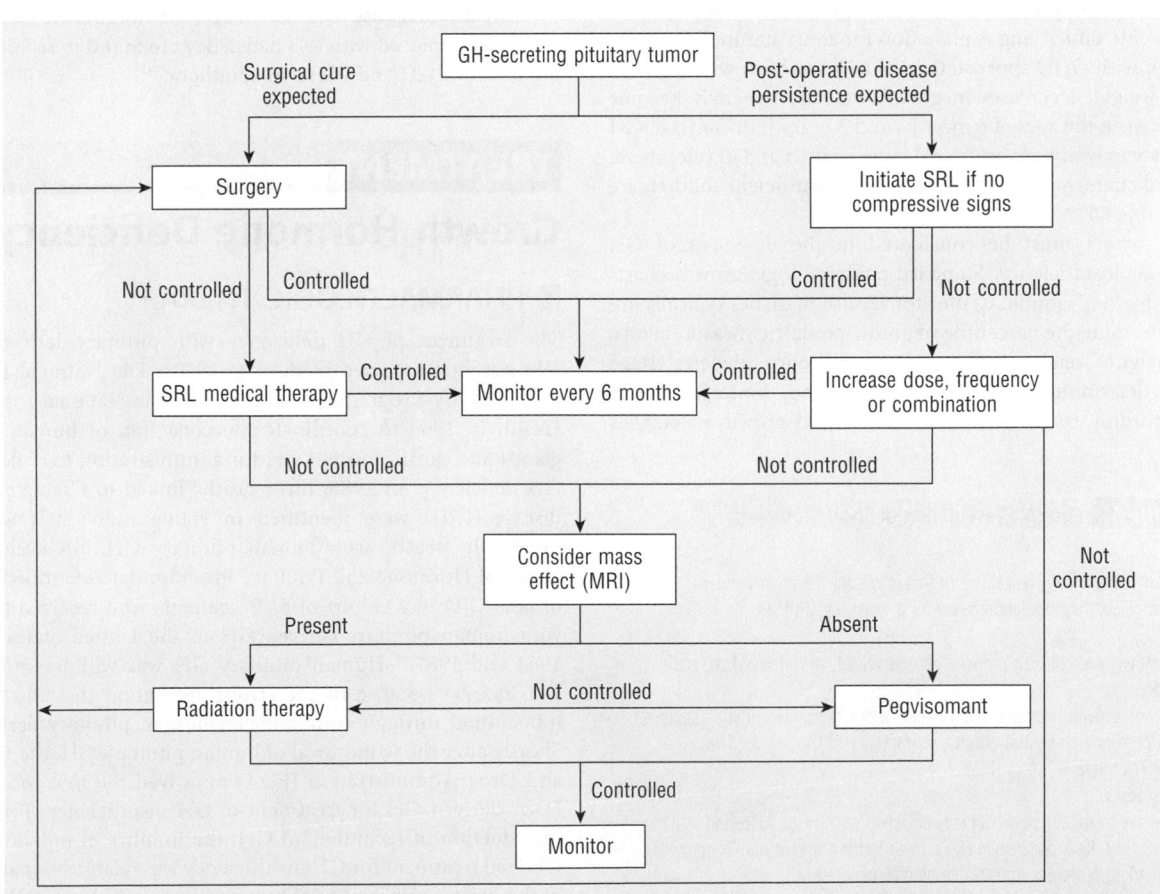

FIGURE 86-2. Treatment algorithm for acromegaly. (SRL, somatostatin analog ; MRI, magnetic resonance imaging.) *(Modified from Melmed S, Calao A, Barkan A, et al. Guidelines for Acromegaly Management: An Update. J Clin Endocrinol Metab 2009;94:1509–1517. Copyright 2009, The Endocrine Society.)*

GROWTH HORMONE DEFICIENCY

Short stature is a condition that is commonly defined by a physical height that is more than two standard deviations below the population mean and lower than the third percentile for height in a specific age group.[45–47] It has been estimated that more than 1.8 million children in the United States can be characterized as having short stature.[47] Short stature is a very broad term describing a condition that may be the result of many different causes. A true lack of GH is among the least common causes and is known as growth hormone-deficient (GHD) short stature. Absolute GH deficiency is a congenital disorder that can result from various genetic abnormalities, such as GHRH deficiency, GH gene deletion, and developmental disorders including pituitary aplasia or hypoplasia.[45,46] GH insufficiency is an acquired condition that can result secondary to hypothalamic or pituitary tumors, cranial irradiation, head trauma, pituitary infarction, and various types of CNS infections. In addition, psychosocial deprivation, hypothyroidism, poorly controlled diabetes mellitus, treatment of precocious puberty with LH-releasing hormone agonists, and pharmacologic agents such as glucocorticoids, methylphenidate, and dextroamphetamine may induce transient GH insufficiency.[45]

Short stature also occurs with several conditions that are not associated with a true GH deficiency or insufficiency. These conditions include intrauterine growth restriction; constitutional growth delay; malnutrition; malabsorption of nutrients associated with inflammatory bowel disease, celiac disease, and cystic fibrosis; chronic renal failure; skeletal and cartilage dysplasia; and genetic syndromes such as Turner syndrome.[45,46,48] In addition, many children are diagnosed with idiopathic or normal variant short stature. These patients have heights that are significantly lower than the third percentile but present with normal GH serum concentrations and no specific underlying explanation for short stature.[47]

Children with GHD short stature usually are born with an average birth weight. Decreases in growth velocity generally become evident between the ages of 6 months and 3 years.[45] In contrast, GH insufficiency may arise at any age during growth and development. The clinical characteristics of GHD or GH-insufficient children are listed in Table 86–3.[45,46]

Several factors must be considered in the diagnosis of GH deficiency or insufficiency. Standard epidemiologic growth charts developed by the National Center for Health Statistics typically are used to determine the percentile of anthropometric measurements, such as height, weight, and head circumference. Pubertal stage typically is determined using the Tanner method. Bone age is determined according to published standards, and growth velocity is calculated to determine the patient's height velocity percentile using standard growth-velocity charts.[45,46,48] GH deficiency is rarely seen in the absence of delayed skeletal maturation and decreased growth velocity. In addition, several different provocative stimuli that induce GH secretion may be used diagnostically to determine GH status. Common provocative pharmacologic GH stimuli include insulin-induced hypoglycemia, clonidine, L-dopa, arginine, glucagon, and GHRH.[46] A subnormal GH response during childhood is arbitrarily defined as a peak GH serum concentration <10 mcg/L during a 2-hour period after administration of one of these agents.[46] However, this maximum may be lower, depending on the specific assay and GH reference product used. For prepubertal and early pubertal patients (Tanner stage less than III), priming with sex hormones to improve the specificity of GH provocation tests is often considered. Some patients exhibit clinical signs of GH deficiency, subnormal growth velocity, and delayed bone age despite GH levels that are within normal limits after provocative testing. This makes diagnosis in this group of patients very difficult. Diagnosis based on GH stimulation tests becomes further complicated because of the paucity of data reporting the normal range of GH concentrations after provocative testing in healthy children and the fact that commercial GH and IGF-1 assays currently available may not be equivalent. Although a gold standard for diagnosis of GHD does not exist, treatment is generally recommended for children who have "idiopathic short stature" and pass GH provocative testing but have most of the following criteria: height greater than 2.25 standard deviations below the mean for age; subnormal growth velocity; delayed bone age; low serum IGF-1 and/or insulin-like growth factor binding protein 3 (IGFBP-3); and other clinical features consistent with GH deficiency.[49] Ultimately, careful consideration of multiple factors by a pediatric endocrinology specialist is required to correctly diagnose GH deficiency. Of note, more than half of children diagnosed with GH deficiency are found to secrete normal quantities of GH and IGF-1 in adulthood.[50]

TREATMENT

Growth Hormone Deficiency

■ PHARMACOLOGIC THERAPY

The treatment of GH deficiency with pituitary-derived human GH was first reported in the late 1950s. The National Hormone and Pituitary Program was founded by the National Institutes of Health in 1963 to coordinate the collection of human pituitary glands and purification of GH for administration to children with GH deficiency. In 1985, three deaths linked to Creutzfeldt-Jakob disease (CJD) were identified in young individuals who were previously treated with human pituitary GH. An evaluation of National Hormone and Pituitary Program data identified 26 cases of fatal CJD in a cohort of 6,107 patients who received treatment with human pituitary-derived GH in the United States between 1963 and 1985.[51] Human pituitary GH was withdrawn from the U.S. market because of the strong likelihood that the CJD was transmitted through contaminated human pituitary-derived GH. Shortly after the withdrawal of human pituitary GH, the U.S. Food and Drug Administration (FDA) approved the first recombinant DNA-derived GH for treatment of GH insufficiency. Prior to the introduction of recombinant GH, the number of individuals who received treatment for GH insufficiency was relatively small because of the limited availability of human pituitary tissue for GH extraction. Currently, with the widespread availability of recombinant GH products, a large number of children can receive GH replacement therapy at higher doses.

TABLE 86-3	Clinical Presentation of Short Stature

General
- The patient will have a physical height that is greater than two standard deviations below the population mean for a given age and sex.

Signs
- The patient will present with reduced growth velocity and delayed skeletal maturation.
- Children with growth hormone (GH)-deficient or GH-insufficient short stature may also present with central obesity, prominence of the forehead, and immaturity of the face.

Laboratory tests
- The patient will exhibit a peak GH concentration <10 mcg/L following a GH provocation test. Reduced insulin-like growth factor 1 and insulin-like growth factor 1 binding protein 3 concentrations may be present.
- Because GH deficiency may be accompanied by loss of other pituitary hormones, hypoglycemia and hypothyroidism may be noted.

Data from Hindmarsh and Brook[45] and American Association of Endocrinologists.[46]

CLINICAL CONTROVERSY

Most pediatric endocrinologists in the United States believe that GH therapy is appropriate treatment in certain patients with non-GHD short stature. However, given the high cost of therapy and small increases in height, use of GH in this patient population remains controversial.

■ RECOMBINANT GROWTH HORMONE

❺ Recombinant GH is currently considered the mainstay of therapy for treatment of GHD short stature. GH replacement therapy in children with documented GHD short stature produces a significant improvement in growth velocity within the first year of therapy and significantly improves final adult height.[52–55] The initial increase in growth velocity often is referred to as *catch-up growth*. Most of the initial studies evaluating the efficacy of GH therapy in GHD children were conducted for short periods of time in small numbers of patients, and, until recently, information about the long-term outcome of GH therapy was limited. Initial data suggested that final adult height is not substantially improved, with an average final adult height reported to be two standard deviations below the population mean.[56–59] Although these results were disappointing, it is important to note that a substantial percentage of patients included in these studies initially had received human pituitary GH in relatively low doses because of its limited availability. In addition, current GH dosing regimens with regard to frequency of administration have changed, making these data difficult to interpret and apply to patients who are receiving GH replacement therapy today. Recent studies evaluating the adult height of children who received only recombinant GH therapy with currently recommended dosing regimens suggest that current recombinant GH therapy has a greater impact on final adult height than previously reported.[52–55] These studies have reported average final adult heights ranging from 0.5 to 1.7 standard deviations below the population mean. Initiation of therapy at an early chronologic age, prior to the onset of puberty, is associated with a more favorable increase in final height.[46,53,54] Therefore, prompt diagnosis of GH deficiency and early initiation of replacement therapy with recombinant GH are crucial factors in optimizing the final adult height of children with GH deficiency.

Recombinant GH has been shown to increase the short-term growth rate in pediatric patients with chronic renal insufficiency, Turner syndrome, idiopathic short stature, Prader-Willi syndrome, short stature homeobox gene (SHOX) deficiency, Noonan syndrome, and children born small for gestational age (SGA), and is approved by the FDA for treatment of growth failure associated with these conditions. GH is also FDA approved for treatment of adult GH deficiency, short bowel syndrome in patients receiving specialized nutritional support, and acquired immunodeficiency syndrome wasting syndrome. When used in adult patients, the recommended dosage of recombinant GH is significantly lower than the dosage used in pediatric patients. Adult patients with GH deficiency during childhood must have the diagnosis of GH deficiency confirmed when they are adults. Long-term GH therapy in GHD adults significantly decreases body fat, increases muscle mass, and improves exercise capacity.[46] GH therapy in adults has been shown to improve the cardiac risk profile, bone mineral density, and psychological well-being.[60,61] In addition, GH currently is being investigated for a variety of disorders, including infertility, chronic fatigue, obesity, and natural aging.[46] Use of GH as an anabolic agent for management of acute catabolism is not recommended.[46]

The majority of short children in the United States do not have an identifiable medical cause for their condition, but with widespread availability of several recombinant GH formulations, many children have received GH therapy regardless of the underlying etiology of their short stature. The use of recombinant GH therapy in children with non-GHD short stature, also referred to as *idiopathic short stature*, has been studied by many investigators and was approved by the FDA in 2003.[62] However, the use of GH therapy in this patient population remains controversial. A meta-analysis of 38 clinical studies evaluating the efficacy of GH treatment in children with idiopathic short stature reported average increases in final adult height of 4 to 5 cm (1.6–2 inches) following a mean duration of therapy of 4.7 years.[63] This corresponded to an increase above the predicted final adult height of 0.56 to 0.63 standard deviations of the population mean. A more recently published randomized, double-blind, placebo-controlled trial with a mean GH treatment duration of 4.4 years reported an increase in final adult height of 3.7 cm (1.5 inches).[64] The slightly smaller height increase reported in the later study may be explained by the more stringent study design, lower mean GH doses, and GH treatment initiation at an older age (peripubertal) compared to the studies included in the meta-analysis.

❻ Ten different recombinant GH products currently are available for use in the United States (Genotropin, Humatrope, Norditropin, Nutropin, Nutropin AQ, Omnitrope, Saizen, Serostim, Tev-Tropin, and Zorbtive) Each of these products contains somatropin. Somatropin is composed of the same amino acid sequence as human pituitary GH. Recombinant GH formulations must be administered by intramuscular or subcutaneous injection. Nutropin AQ, Norditropin, and omnitrope are the only GH products available as liquid formulations. The remaining products are formulated as lyophilized powders for injection, and patients must be instructed regarding proper administration. A needle-free injection device (Tject) is available for use with Tev-Tropin. This device delivers a thin stream of recombinant GH that penetrates the stratum corneum and deposits into the subcutaneous tissue. This product may be particularly useful for patients who experience significant adverse effects from injections. The potency of GH products is expressed as international units per milligram (international units/mg), with 1 mg containing approximately 2.6 international units of GH. Direct comparisons between the different recombinant GH products have not been published. However, all GH products are generally considered to be equally efficacious. The recommended dose for treatment of GHD short stature in children is 0.3 mg/kg/week.[46] Recombinant GH can be administered daily or in equal doses 6 times per week, depending on the specific GH product used.[46] Dosing regimens with greater frequency of administration have been shown to provide more favorable short-term growth responses.[46] GH replacement therapy should be initiated as early as possible after diagnosis of GH insufficiency and continued until a desirable height is reached or growth velocity has decreased to <2.5 cm per year after the pubertal growth spurt. However, the suitable time point for discontinuation of therapy with growth-promoting doses remains controversial. Glucocorticoids may inhibit the growth-promoting effects of recombinant GH, and concomitant administration of androgens, estrogens, thyroid hormones, or anabolic steroids may accelerate epiphyseal closure and compromise final height.

Three large databases, the National Cooperative Growth Study, the Kabi International Growth Study, and the Australian and New Zealand growth database (OZGROW), have been developed to collect postmarketing adverse effect data or reports associated with recombinant GH. Development of these databases was prompted by the unexpected and tragic cases of CJD reported in patients treated with human pituitary GH. These databases are maintained by pharmaceutical companies that manufacture GH products.[65] Recombinant GH is generally well tolerated in children, and adverse effects are relatively uncommon.[65,66] A small number of patients may complain of injection-site pain or arthralgias. Idiopathic intracranial hypertension, also known as *pseudotumor cerebri*, has been reported in a very small number of children receiving GH therapy. This condition usually develops within the first 8 to 12 of weeks of treatment and presents with symptoms such as headache, blurred vision, diplopia, nausea, and vomiting.[65] The symptoms of idiopathic intracranial hypertension usually resolve after discontinuation of GH therapy, and long-term complications are rare. Cases of slipped capital femoral epiphysis have been reported in children with GH deficiency who are receiving GH therapy.[65] This condition is thought to occur as a result of the increased width of the femoral plate during GH treatment, but it also has been reported in GHD children who are not receiving GH replacement. Patients with this condition typically complain of hip or knee pain. Slipped capital femoral epiphysis can be managed by an orthopedic surgeon, and GH therapy does not need to be withdrawn. Because GH is known to cause decreased insulin sensitivity, hyperglycemia and diabetes mellitus may develop.[67] Patients who have specific predisposing risk factors for diabetes mellitus are at greatest risk for this adverse effect.[65–67] Glycosylated hemoglobin concentrations should be monitored in all patients receiving GH products.[46] GH may promote the growth of various types of neoplasms and increase tumor recurrence rates in patients with a history of malignancy.[46,65,66] For this reason, GH should not be administered to patients with an active malignant tumor or a history of recurrent tumor growth. In 1988, a Japanese report indicated that children receiving GH therapy were twice as likely to develop leukemia as children who were not receiving the hormone.[68] A more recent analysis of all collected reports of leukemia associated with GH therapy determined that these children had other leukemia risk factors (Fanconi's anemia, Bloom's syndrome, or history of cancer).[69] GH therapy in children without these risk factors does not appear to predispose children to develop leukemia.[65,66,69] Some patients may develop antibodies to recombinant GH. The development of antibodies during replacement therapy with recombinant GH products has been reported to be relatively low, affecting approximately 15% to 20% of patients.[70] More importantly, the presence of GH antibodies has not been shown to adversely affect growth response and appears to be clinically insignificant except in patients with GH gene deletions. Finally, recent postmarketing reports suggest an increased risk of death associated with long-term GH treatment in children with Prader-Willi syndrome who are severely obese or have severe respiratory impairment. GH treatment is contraindicated in patients with Prader-Willi syndrome who have any of these risk factors.

RECOMBINANT INSULIN-LIKE GROWTH FACTOR-1

Recombinant IGF-1 products, consisting of either IGF-1 alone (mecasermin [Increlex]) or IGF-1 in combination with IGFBP-3 (mecasermin rinfabate [Iplex]), have been recently approved by the FDA for the treatment of children with short stature due to severe primary IGF-1 deficiency (defined as children with height standard deviation score ≤−3.0 plus basal IGF-1 standard deviation score ≤−3.0, plus normal or elevated GH concentration) or GH gene deletion with neutralizing antibodies to GH. Recombinant IGF-1 products are not intended for use in subjects with secondary forms of IGF-1 deficiency, such as GH deficiency, malnutrition, hypothyroidism, or chronic treatment with pharmacologic doses of antiinflammatory steroids. Recombinant IGF-1 products have been shown to increase growth velocity in children with short stature who have low IGF-1 serum concentrations and resistance to GH.[71–74] However, the efficacy of these agents is less than that reported with GH products in patients with GH deficiency.

The recommended dose of mecasermin is 0.04 to 0.12 mg/kg administered by subcutaneous injection twice daily. Mecasermin rinfabate is administered by once-daily injections at a dose of 1 to 2 mg/kg. Because of the insulin-like effects of these products, patients should be monitored very closely for hypoglycemia, and the drug should be initiated at a dose at the lower end of the dosage range and administered with a meal or snack. The incidence of hypoglycemia may be less frequent with mecasermin rinfabate because of the longer half-life of the combination product.[71] Additional adverse effects experienced by patients receiving recombinant IGF-1 products include injection-site reactions, tonsillar/adenoidal hypertrophy, lymphoid hypertrophy, coarsening facial features, anaphylaxis, headache, dizziness, and arthralgia.[72,73,74] Intracranial hypertension has been reported in a small number of patients.[73] Additional studies are needed to elucidate the exact role of recombinant IGF-1 products in the management of short stature not caused by GH gene deletion or GH receptor defects.

EVALUATION OF THERAPEUTIC OUTCOMES

Appropriate monitoring of therapy for GHD and non-GHD short stature includes regular assessments of height, weight, growth velocity, serum alkaline phosphatase, and bone age every 6 to 12 months. Additional laboratory tests to monitor for potential adverse effects include serum glucose concentration and thyroid function. The dose of GH will periodically need to be increased as weight increases in growing children.

PHARMACOECONOMIC CONSIDERATIONS

The treatment of short stature with recombinant GH is expensive. Despite the prohibitive cost, recombinant GH remains the mainstay of therapy for children with GHD short stature. However, treatment of non-GHD short stature with recombinant GH is not widely accepted. The benefits in final adult height and increases in growth velocity, particularly in children with true GH deficiency, are associated with significant psychosocial benefits. Many clinicians believe that GH therapy can improve quality of life and should be made available to all children with short stature, regardless of whether or not they are GH deficient.[75] Until studies using recombinant GH more definitively demonstrate improvements in both final adult height and quality of life, the cost-effectiveness of GH, particularly for non-GHD short stature, remains uncertain.

CONCLUSIONS

GH deficiency during childhood results in short stature. Replacement with recombinant GH is considered the mainstay of therapy for patients with GHD short stature, but its use for treatment of non-GHD short stature remains controversial, albeit such treatment is FDA approved. Recombinant GH has proven to be safe for use in children and is associated with few adverse effects. The synthetic GHRH sermorelin and other GH-releasing peptides and preparations of IGF-1 may provide benefit for patients with non-GHD short stature. GH regimens can be particularly demanding and inconvenient for pediatric patients because they must be administered by subcutaneous injection. Knowledge of the long-term benefits and risks is critical to the development of rational, cost-effective treatments for patients with short stature.

PROLACTIN

PHYSIOLOGIC EFFECTS

Prolactin is secreted in a pulsatile fashion by the lactotroph cells of the anterior pituitary, with the highest peak concentrations observed during sleep.[4] The secretion of prolactin is regulated primarily by tonic hypothalamic inhibitory effects of dopamine. As described earlier in this chapter and as listed in Table 86–1, many factors can affect prolactin secretion. During pregnancy, prolactin serum concentrations rise substantially above normal. All other conditions characterized by excess prolactin serum concentrations, known as *hyperprolactinemia*, are considered pathologic.

HYPERPROLACTINEMIA

Hyperprolactinemia is a state of persistent serum prolactin elevation. Prolactin concentrations >20 mcg/L in women, and >25 mcg/L in men, observed on multiple occasions are generally considered indicative of hyperprolactinemia.[76,77] Hyperprolactinemia usually affects women of reproductive age.[76,78] The incidence of hyperprolactinemia in the general population is reported to be <1%.[77]

Hyperprolactinemia has several etiologies. The most common causes are benign prolactin-secreting pituitary tumors, known as *prolactinomas*, and various medications. Prolactinomas are classified according to size. Prolactin-secreting microadenomas are <10 mm in diameter and often do not increase in size.[4,77] In contrast, macroadenomas are tumors with a diameter >10 mm that continue to grow and can cause invasion of surrounding tissues.[4,77] In the presence of a prolactinoma, prolactin serum concentrations may remain normal or may be markedly elevated to thousands of micrograms per liter.

❼ Any pharmacologic agent that antagonizes dopamine or increases the release of prolactin can induce hyperprolactinemia (Table 86–4). Serotonin is a strong stimulator of prolactin secretion, and selective serotonin reuptake inhibitors (SSRIs) such as fluoxetine, paroxetine, sertraline, and fluvoxamine are the medications most frequently associated with hyperprolactinemia.[79] Prior to the increased use of SSRIs, antipsychotic medications with potent dopamine-receptor blockade, such as the phenothiazine derivatives

and haloperidol, were most often identified as the cause of drug-induced hyperprolactinemia.[86] Metoclopramide and domperidone, an antiemetic available in Europe, are potent dopamine-receptor antagonists reported to induce hyperprolactinemia.[79] Hormones such as estrogen and progesterone, commonly prescribed as oral contraceptives, can stimulate lactotroph growth to promote prolactin secretion and have been implicated in drug-induced hyperprolactinemia. Although the exact mechanism of action remains to be determined, the calcium channel-blocking agent verapamil has been associated with cases of hyperprolactinemia.[4,79] Methyldopa and reserpine, although not used frequently in clinical practice today, are antihypertensive agents that can stimulate prolactin secretion.[79] Prolactin concentrations may increase with administration of GnRH analogs such as leuprolide or goserelin.[79] Other medications rarely reported to cause hyperprolactinemia include H_2-receptor blocking agents, benzodiazepines, tricyclic antidepressants, dexfenfluramine, opioids, protease inhibitors, and monoamine oxidase inhibitors.[4,77,79] Prolactin levels do not typically rise to >150 mcg/L in cases of drug-induced hyperprolactinemia. Measurement of serum prolactin concentrations prior to the initiation of therapy with medications known to cause prolactin elevation may obviate the need for extensive examination of pituitary function and aid with the appropriate diagnosis of drug-induced hyperprolactinemia.

Less common etiologies include CNS lesions that physically compress the pituitary stalk and interrupt tonic hypothalamic dopamine secretion, resulting in hyperprolactinemia.[77] Increased TRH concentrations in hypothyroidism can stimulate prolactin secretion and cause hyperprolactinemia. During conditions of renal or hepatic compromise, the clearance of prolactin is decreased, resulting in elevated prolactin concentrations.[4] Despite vigorous diagnostic effort, the cause of hyperprolactinemia cannot always be determined. This is known as *idiopathic hyperprolactinemia* and most likely is a result of the presence of very small tumors that are not detected by standard imaging techniques.[76] It should be noted that many physiologic factors, such as stress (including the stress of phlebotomy), sleep, exercise, coitus, and eating, also can induce transiently elevated prolactin levels.[4,76] This emphasizes the importance of obtaining multiple prolactin measurements to confirm the diagnosis. Ideally, after an intravenous line is placed in the patient's arm, the patient should rest in a supine position or in a chair for 2 hours before prolactin samples are collected.

Elevated prolactin serum concentrations inhibit gonadotropin secretion and sex-steroid synthesis.[76] Because prolactin concentrations >60 mcg/L are associated with anovulation, women with hyperprolactinemia typically present with menstrual irregularities such as oligomenorrhea or amenorrhea and infertility.[7,76,77] In addition, approximately 40% to 80% of women with hyperprolactinemia will have galactorrhea.[76,77] The clinical presentation of patients with hyperprolactinemia is summarized in Table 86–5.[4,76,77]

The diagnosis of hyperprolactinemia, as defined by multiple prolactin serum concentrations >20 mcg/L in women and >25 mcg/L in men, is relatively simple. However, identifying the underlying cause of this abnormality may be more challenging. Patients with modest prolactin elevations should have multiple prolactin serum determinations to minimize the potential for detecting only transient increases in prolactin. A careful medication history is essential, and the presence of hypothyroidism, renal failure, or hepatic dysfunction should be evaluated. If the cause of hyperprolactinemia remains ambiguous, a computed tomography scan or magnetic resonance imaging study should be performed to determine the presence of a pituitary tumor.[76,77] If an underlying cause of elevated prolactin serum concentration is not determined, the hyperprolactinemia is considered to be idiopathic.

TABLE 86-4	Drug-Induced Hyperprolactinemia
Dopamine antagonists	
Antipsychotics	
Phenothiazines	
Metoclopramide	
Domperidone	
Prolactin stimulators	
Methyldopa	
Reserpine	
Selective serotonin reuptake inhibitors	
Dexfenfluramine	
Estrogens	
Progestins	
Protease inhibitors	
Gonadotropin-releasing hormone analogs	
Benzodiazepines	
Tricyclic antidepressants	
Monoamine oxidase inhibitors	
H_2-Receptor antagonists	
Opioids	
Other	
Verapamil	

Data from Molitch,[4] Mah and Webster,[77] Gillam et al.,[78] and Molitch.[79]

TABLE 86-5 Clinical Presentation of Hyperprolactinemia

General

Hyperprolactinemia most commonly affects women and is very rare in men.

Signs and symptoms

- The patient may complain of symptoms related to local effects of the prolactin-secreting tumor, such as headache and visual disturbances, that result from tumor compression of the optic chiasm.
- Female patients experience oligomenorrhea, amenorrhea, galactorrhea, infertility, decreased libido, hirsutism, and acne.
- Male patients experience decreased libido, erectile dysfunction, infertility, reduced muscle mass, galactorrhea, and gynecomastia.

Laboratory tests

Prolactin serum concentrations at rest will be >20 mcg/L on multiple occasions.

Additional clinical sequelae

- Prolonged suppression of estrogen in premenopausal women with hyperprolactinemia leads to decreases in bone mineral density and significant risk for development of osteoporosis.
- Risk for ischemic heart disease may be increased with untreated hyperprolactinemia.

Data from Molitch,[4] Schlechte,[76] and Mah and Webster.[77]

TREATMENT

Hyperprolactinemia

The treatment of hyperprolactinemia depends on the underlying cause of the abnormality. In cases of drug-induced hyperprolactinemia, discontinuation of the offending medication and initiation of an appropriate therapeutic alternative usually normalizes serum prolactin concentrations.[79] In cases for which an appropriate therapeutic alternative does not exist, medical therapy with dopamine agonists is warranted. Sex-steroid replacement also should be considered.[77] Treatment options for the management of prolactinomas include clinical observation, medical therapy with dopamine agonists, radiation therapy, and transsphenoidal surgical removal of the tumor.[4,76-78] Because prolactin-secreting microadenomas are very small and typically do not increase in size, treatment of these tumors is primarily directed toward alleviating symptoms.[76-78] The goal of therapy is to normalize prolactin serum concentrations and reestablish gonadotropin secretion to restore fertility and reduce the risk of osteoporosis. In patients with asymptomatic elevations in serum prolactin, observation and close follow up are appropriate.[76-78] For women with amenorrhea who do not wish to become pregnant, dopamine agonist therapy may not be necessary. In these patients, sex steroid replacement and close follow up may be sufficient.[76] Treatment goals are more aggressive in patients with prolactin-secreting macroadenomas because these tumors are larger and can cause invasion of local tissues with significant visual defects.[78] Therefore, in addition to normalizing prolactin concentrations, tumor shrinkage and correction of visual defects are primary goals of treatment.

Medical therapy with dopamine agonists usually is more effective than transsphenoidal surgery for both types of pituitary prolactinomas.[4,76-78] Postsurgical cure rates differ depending on tumor type and expertise of the neurosurgeon. Long-term cure rates are reported to be approximately 60% for microprolactinomas and only 25% for macroprolactinomas.[4] Transsphenoidal surgery for removal of prolactinomas usually is reserved for patients who are refractory to or cannot tolerate therapy with dopamine agonists and for patients with very large tumors that cause severe compression of adjacent tissues.[4,76-78] Radiation therapy may require several years for effective tumor shrinkage and reduction in serum prolactin concentrations and usually is used only in conjunction with surgery.[4]

PHARMACOLOGIC THERAPY

Medical therapy with dopamine agonists has proven to be very effective in normalizing prolactin serum concentrations, restoring menstruation, and reducing tumor size in approximately 80% to 90% of patients within 3 to 6 months of therapy.[4,77] Bromocriptine has been the mainstay of therapy since the 1970s. Cabergoline is a long-acting dopamine agonist that offers the advantage of less-frequent dosing. In recent years cabergoline has replaced bromocriptine as the agent of choice for the medical management of prolactinomas.

BROMOCRIPTINE

Bromocriptine was the first D_2-receptor agonist to be used in the treatment of hyperprolactinemia and has been the mainstay of therapy for over 20 years. It inhibits the release of prolactin by directly stimulating postsynaptic dopamine receptors in the hypothalamus. Hypothalamic release of dopamine (prolactin-inhibitory hormone) inhibits the release of prolactin. Decreases in serum prolactin concentrations occur within 2 hours of oral administration, with maximal suppression occurring after 8 hours and suppressive effects persisting for up to 24 hours. Medical therapy with bromocriptine normalizes prolactin serum concentrations, restores gonadotropin production, and shrinks tumor size in approximately 90% of patients with microprolactinomas and 70% of patients with macroprolactinomas.[78]

For the management of hyperprolactinemia, bromocriptine therapy typically is initiated at a dose of 1.25 to 2.5 mg once daily at bedtime to minimize adverse effects.[76,77] The dose can be gradually increased by 1.25-mg increments every week to obtain desirable serum prolactin concentrations. Usual therapeutic doses of bromocriptine range from 2.5 to 15 mg/day, although some patients may require doses as high as 40 mg/day.[77] Bromocriptine usually is administered in two or three divided doses, but once-daily dosing has also been shown to be effective.[78]

The most common adverse effects associated with bromocriptine therapy include CNS symptoms such as headache, lightheadedness, dizziness, nervousness, and fatigue. Gastrointestinal effects such as nausea, abdominal pain, and diarrhea also are common. Bromocriptine should be administered with food to decrease the incidence of adverse gastrointestinal effects. Although most of these adverse effects diminish with continued treatment, approximately 12% of patients will not tolerate the adverse effects associated with bromocriptine therapy.[78] Vaginal preparations of bromocriptine have been studied in an effort to decrease the incidence of adverse effects associated with oral dosage forms.[4,77,81]

Because most patients with hyperprolactinemia are women with a principal complaint of infertility, the safety of bromocriptine in pregnancy must be considered. One report of 100 pregnancies in women who received bromocriptine throughout gestation did not detect an increase in the risk for spontaneous abortion or incidence of congenital anomalies.[78] Although bromocriptine does not appear to be teratogenic, most clinicians discontinue therapy as soon as pregnancy is detected because the effects of in utero exposure to bromocriptine on gonadal function and fertility of the offspring remain unknown.[4,76-78] In patients with macroprolactinomas undergoing rapid tumor expansion, bromocriptine therapy may need to be continued throughout pregnancy.

PERGOLIDE

Pergolide is a dopamine-receptor agonist with affinity for both D_1- and D_2-receptors. This agent is 10 to 1,000 times more potent than bromocriptine on a per milligram basis. In the United States, pergolide was never FDA approved for treatment of hyperprolactinemia. However, it was used for many years as an effective alternative to bromocriptine in the management of patients with hyperprolactinemia and offered the advantage of once-daily dosing.[4,78] In 2007, pergolide was withdrawn from the U.S. market because of cases of cardiac valvulopathy.[82] Pathologic assessment suggested that the valvulopathy associated with pergolide appeared to be similar to that reported with other ergot alkaloids.

■ CABERGOLINE

❽ Cabergoline is a long-acting dopamine agonist with high selectivity and affinity for dopamine D_2-receptors. This agent is approved for treatment of hyperprolactinemia and has been shown to effectively reduce serum prolactin concentrations in 80% to 90% of hyperprolactinemic patients.[83-85] Cabergoline also effectively reduces tumor size in patients with both microprolactinomas and macroprolactinomas.[83-86] In a multicenter randomized trial comparing the efficacy of cabergoline and bromocriptine, serum prolactin levels were normalized in 83% of patients receiving cabergoline and 58% of patients receiving bromocriptine after 6 months of therapy.[87] Cabergoline also has proved effective in patients who are intolerant of or resistant to bromocriptine, and data suggest that cabergoline is as effective in men as in women with microprolactinomas and macroprolactinomas.[85,88,89]

Cabergoline is commercially available as 0.5-mg oral tablets. The initial dose of cabergoline for treatment of hyperprolactinemia is 0.5 mg once weekly or in divided doses twice weekly. This dose may be increased by 0.5-mg increments at 4-week intervals based on serum prolactin concentrations.[90] The usual dose is 1 to 2 mg weekly; doses >3 mg per week are infrequently required.[91] However, doses as high as 12 mg weekly have been used safely in patients with treatment-resistant prolactinomas.[92] Following oral administration, peak serum concentrations are obtained within 2 hours, and food does not affect absorption. Data from animal studies indicate that cabergoline is widely distributed to well-perfused organs, including the pituitary gland.[90] The elimination of cabergoline from the pituitary appears to be very slow; this rate may explain the long duration of action. Cabergoline is extensively metabolized in the liver by hydrolysis, and the dose should be reduced in patients with severe hepatic failure. This drug is eliminated primarily in the feces, and the elimination half-life ranges from 79 to 155 hours in hyperprolactinemic patients.[90]

The most common adverse effects reported with use of cabergoline are nausea, vomiting, headache, and dizziness.[78,90] These effects are similar to the adverse effects reported with bromocriptine and pergolide. However, in a large comparative study evaluating bromocriptine and cabergoline, fewer patients receiving cabergoline reported adverse effects than did patients receiving bromocriptine, and only 3% of the patients in the cabergoline group withdrew from the study because of adverse effects versus 12% of patients taking bromocriptine.[87] Other adverse events associated with use of cabergoline include gastrointestinal complaints, drowsiness, fatigue, paresthesias, dyspnea, suffocation sensation, and epistaxis.[78,90] As with other dopamine agonists, adverse events usually occur early in therapy and subside with continued treatment. However, in one study 15% to 20% of patients receiving cabergoline experienced a recurrence of early symptoms or an onset of new symptoms after several weeks of treatment.[87] Mild-to-moderate decreases in blood pressure have been observed in up to 50% of patients taking cabergoline; however, the incidence of symptomatic orthostatic hypotension has not been significant.[83,84,87] Transient increases in serum alkaline phosphatase, bilirubin, and aminotransferases have been reported in small numbers of patients receiving cabergoline.[87] Pleuropulmonary disease[78] and newly diagnosed cardiac

valve regurgitation[82] have been reported with cabergoline use at the larger doses used in the treatment of Parkinson's disease. Although symptomatic cardiac valve abnormalities have not been observed with cabergoline when administered in doses used for the treatment of prolactinomas, some clinicians have recommended routine echocardiography for patients receiving long-term cabergoline treatment for prolactinomas.[93,94]

❾ Use of cabergoline in pregnancy has not been extensively studied. However, several case reports of women who received cabergoline therapy during the first and second trimesters of pregnancy have not documented an increased risk of spontaneous abortion, congenital abnormalities, or tubal pregnancy.[90,91] However, prospective data in large numbers of pregnancies are lacking. Because of the long half-life and limited data on cabergoline use in pregnancy, current guidelines recommend that women receiving cabergoline therapy who plan to become pregnant should discontinue the medication as soon as pregnancy is detected.[91]

Other dopamine agonists that have been used in the treatment of hyperprolactinemia but are not commercially available in the United States include lisuride, terguride, metergoline, dihydroergocristine, and quinagolide.[78] Quinagolide, a D_2-receptor agonist used frequently in Europe, is dosed once daily. Quinagolide has been shown to be as effective as bromocriptine for the management of hyperprolactinemia and may be effective in the treatment of patients who are resistant to or intolerant of bromocriptine.[78]

■ EVALUATION OF THERAPEUTIC OUTCOMES

Prolactin serum concentrations should be monitored every 3 to 4 weeks after the initiation of any dopamine-agonist therapy to assess efficacy and appropriately titrate medication dosage.[76] In addition, symptoms such as headache, visual disturbances, menstrual cycles in women, and sexual function in men should be evaluated to assess clinical response to therapy. Once prolactin concentrations have normalized and clinical symptoms of hyperprolactinemia have resolved with dopamine-agonist therapy, prolactin serum concentrations should be monitored every 6 to 12 months. In patients receiving long-term treatment, the dose of the dopamine agonist can be gradually reduced or discontinued in some patients. For patients with microprolactinomas who have normal serum prolactin concentrations and at least a 50% reduction in tumor size, medical therapy may be withdrawn every 2 to 5 years to assess if remission has been achieved. In the case of macroprolactinomas, the dose of the dopamine agonist can be gradually reduced in some cases, but complete drug discontinuation should be attempted only if careful monitoring for renewed tumor growth can be ensured.[76,91,95]

■ PHARMACOECONOMIC CONSIDERATIONS

Medical therapy with dopamine agonists is more effective than transsphenoidal surgery or radiation for the management of hyperprolactinemia. Because most patients receive therapy for long periods, the medical management of hyperprolactinemia may result in considerable cost. Cabergoline has been shown to be more effective than bromocriptine and offers additional advantages such as a decreased incidence of adverse effects and improved patient compliance. Most clinicians agree that cabergoline is the most efficacious dopamine agonist currently available. However, the cost of cabergoline therapy is approximately 2 times greater than that of bromocriptine. Pharmacoeconomic studies are needed to assess whether the higher cost of cabergoline therapy is balanced by the potential added benefits.

■ CONCLUSIONS

Hyperprolactinemia is a common disorder that can have a significant impact on fertility. Hyperprolactinemia is most commonly caused by the presence of prolactin-secreting pituitary tumors and various medications that antagonize dopamine or increase the secretion of prolactin. Available treatment options for this disorder include medical therapy with dopamine agonists, radiation therapy, and transsphenoidal surgery. In most cases, medical therapy with dopamine agonists is considered the most effective treatment. Cabergoline has replaced bromocriptine as the mainstay of medical therapy because it appears to be better tolerated and more effective. However, because of limited data regarding the safety of cabergoline during pregnancy, bromocriptine remains the preferred agent when fertility is the primary purpose for treatment.

PANHYPOPITUITARISM

⑩ Panhypopituitarism is a condition of complete or partial loss of anterior and posterior pituitary function resulting in a complex disorder characterized by multiple pituitary hormone deficiencies. Patients with panhypopituitarism may have ACTH deficiency, gonadotropin deficiency, GH deficiency, hypothyroidism, and hyperprolactinemia. Panhypopituitarism can be classified as either primary or secondary depending on the etiology. Primary panhypopituitarism involves an abnormality within the secretory cells of the pituitary, whereas secondary panhypopituitarism is caused by a lack of proper external stimulation needed for normal release of pituitary hormones. Some of the most common causes of panhypopituitarism include primary pituitary tumors, ischemic necrosis of the pituitary, surgical trauma, irradiation, and various types of CNS infections. Pharmacologic treatment of panhypopituitarism is essential and consists of replacement of specific pituitary hormones after careful assessment of individual deficiencies. Replacement most often consists of glucocorticoids, thyroid hormone preparations, and sex steroids. Administration of recombinant GH also may be necessary. Patients with panhypopituitarism will need lifelong replacement therapy and constant monitoring of multiple homeostatic functions.

ABBREVIATIONS

ACTH: adrenocorticotropic hormone

CJD: Creutzfeldt-Jakob disease

CRH: corticotropin-releasing hormone

FSH: follicle-stimulating hormone

GH: growth hormone

GHD: growth hormone deficient

GHRH: growth hormone-releasing hormone

GnRH: gonadotropin-releasing hormone

IGF: insulin-like growth factor

IGFBP-3: insulin-like growth factor 1 binding protein 3

LH: luteinizing hormone

OGTT: oral glucose tolerance test

SGA: small for gestational age

SHOX: short stature homeobox-containing gene

SSRI: selective serotonin reuptake inhibitor

TRH: thyrotropin-releasing hormone

TSH: thyroid-stimulating hormone

VIP: vasoactive intestinal peptide

REFERENCES

1. Raisman G. An urge to explain the incomprehensible: Geoffrey Harris and the discovery of the neural control of the pituitary gland. Ann Rev Neurosci 1997;20:533–566.
2. Amar AP, Weiss MH. Pituitary anatomy and physiology. Neurosurg Clin North Am 2003;14:11–23.
3. Cuttler L. The regulation of growth hormone secretion. Endocrinol Metab Clin North Am 1996;25:541–571.
4. Molitch ME. Disorders of prolactin secretion. Endocrinol Metab Clin North Am 2001;30:585–610.
5. Le Roith D. Insulin-like growth factors. N Engl J Med 1997;336: 633–640.
6. Holdaway M, Rajasoorya C. Epidemiology of acromegaly. Pituitary 1999;2:29–41.
7. Eugster EA, Pescovitz OH. Gigantism. J Clin Endocrinol Metab 1999;84:4379–4384.
8. Ben-Shlomo A, Melmed S. Acromegaly. Endocrinol Metab Clin North Am 2001;30:565–583.
9. Melmed S. Acromegaly. N Engl J Med 2006;355:2558–2573.
10. Kauppinen-Makelin R, Sane T, Reunanen A, et al. A nationwide survey of mortality in acromegaly. J Clin Endocrinol Metab 2005;90: 4081–4086.
11. Fatti LM, Scacchi M, Pincelli AI, et al. Prevalence and pathogenesis of sleep apnea and lung disease in acromegaly. Pituitary 2001;4: 259–262.
12. Vitale G, Pivonello R, Galderisi M, et al. Cardiovascular complications in acromegaly: Methods of assessment. Pituitary 2001;4:251–257.
13. Webb SM, Casanueva F, Wass JA. Oncological complications of excess GH in acromegaly. Pituitary 2002;5:21–25.
14. Cordero RA, Barkan AL. Current diagnosis of acromegaly. Rev Endocr Metab Disord 2008;9:13–19.
15. Giustina A, Barkan A, Chanson P, et al. Guidelines for the treatment of growth hormone excess and growth hormone deficiency in adults. J Endocrinol Invest 2008;31:820–838.
16. Melmed S, Colao A, Barkan A, et al. Guidelines for acromegaly management: an update. J Clin Endocrinol Metab 2009;94:1509–1517.
17. Laws ER. Surgery for acromegaly: evolution of the techniques and outcomes. Rev Endocr Metab Disord 2008;9:67–70.
18. Melmed S. Acromegaly pathogensis and treatment. J Clin Invest 2009;119:3189–3202.
19. Colao A, Ferone D, Marzullo P, et al. Effect of different dopaminergic agents in the treatment of acromegaly. J Clin Endocrinol Metab 1997;82:518–523.
20. Jaffe CA, Barkan AL. Acromegaly recognition and treatment. Drugs 1994;47:425–445.
21. Orrego JJ, Barkan AL. Pituitary disorders. Drugs 2000;59:93–106.
22. Abs R, Verhelst J, Maiter D, et al. Cabergoline in the treatment of acromegaly: A study of 64 patients. J Clin Endocrinol Metab 1998;83: 374–378.
23. Felders RA, Hofland LJ, van Aken MO, et al. Medical therapy of acromegaly: efficacy and safety of somatostatin analogs. Drugs 2009;69:2207–2226.
24. Lamberts SE, Van der Lely A, de Herder WW, Hofland LJ. Drug therapy: Octreotide. N Engl J Med 1996;334:246–254.
25. Vance ML, Harris AG. Long-term treatment of 189 acromegalic patients with the somatostatin analog octreotide. Results of the international multicenter acromegaly study group. Arch Intern Med 1991;151:1573–1578.
26. Ezzat S, Snyder PJ, Young WF, et al. Octreotide treatment of acromegaly: A randomized, multicenter study. Ann Intern Med 1992;117: 211–218.
27. Cozzi R, Montini M, Attanasio R, et al. Primary treatment of acromegaly with ocretotide LAR: a long-term (up to nine years) prospective study of its efficacy in the control of disease activity and tumor shrinkage. J Clin Endocrinol Metab 2006;91:1397–1403.

28. Tolis, G, Angelopoulos NG, Katounda E, et al. Medical treatment of acromegaly: Comorbidities and their reversibility by somatostatin analogs. Neuroendocrinology 2006;83:249–257.

29. Melmed S, Sternberg R, Cook D, et al. A critical analysis of pituitary tumor shrinkage during primary medical therapy in acromegaly. J Clin Endocrinol Metab 2005;90:4405–4410.

30. McKeage K, Cheer S, Wagstaff AJ. Octreotide long-acting release (LAR): A review of its use in the management of acromegaly. Drugs 2003;63:2473–2499.

31. Lancranjan L, Brew Atkinson A, and the Sandostatin LAR Group. Results of European multicentre study with Sandostatin LAR in acromegaly patients. Pituitary 1999;1:105–114.

32. Gilbert JA, Miell JP, Chambers SM, et al. The nadir growth hormone after an octreotide test dose predicts the long-term efficacy of somatostatin analogue therapy in acromegaly. Clin Endocrinol 2005;62:742–747.

33. Coloa A, Ferone D, Lastoria S, et al. Prediction of efficacy of octreotide therapy in patients with acromegaly. J Clin Endocrinol Metab 1996;81:2356–2362.

34. Caron P, Bex M, Cullen DR, et al. One-year follow-up of patients with acromegaly treated with fixed or titrated doses of lanreotide Autogel. Clin Endocrinol 2004;60:734–740.

35. Alexopoulou O, Abrams P, Verhelst J, et al. Efficacy and tolerability of lanreotide Autogel therapy in acromegalic patients previously treated with octreotide LAR. Eur J Endocrinol 2004;151:317–324.

36. Croxtall JD, Scott LJ. Lanreotide Autogel: a review of its use in the management of acromegaly. Drugs 2008;68:711–723.

37. Ronchi CL, Boschetti M, Degli Uberti EC, et al. Efficacy of a slow-release formulation of lanreotide (Autogel 120) in patients with acromegaly previously treated with ocretotide long-acting release (LAR): an open, longitudinal, multicenter, study. Clin Endocrinol 2007;67:512–519.

38. Pereira AM, Biermasz NR, Roelfsema F, et al. Pharmacologic therapies for acromegaly: A review of their effects on glucose metabolism and insulin resistance. Treat Endocrinol 2005;4:43–53.

39. Baldelli R, Battista C, Leonetti F, et al. Glucose homeostasis in acromegaly: Effects of long-acting somatostatin analogues treatment. Clin Endocrinol 2003;59:492–499.

40. Trainer PJ, Drake WM, Katznelson L, et al. Treatment of acromegaly with the growth hormone-receptor antagonist Pegvisomant. N Engl J Med 2000;342:1171–1177.

41. Van Der Lely AJ, Hutson R, Trainer PJ, et al. Long-term treatment of acromegaly with pegvisomant, a growth hormone receptor antagonist. Lancet 2001;358:1754–1759.

42. Schreiber I, Buchfelder M, Droste M, et al. Treatment of acromegaly with the GH receptor antagonist pegvisomant in clinical practice: safety and efficacy evaluation from the German Pegvisomant observational study. Eur J Endocrinol 2007;156:75–82.

43. Somavert [prescribing information]. New York, NY: Pharmacia & Upjohn Company Division Pfizer Incorporated; 2009.

44. Neggers SJ, van Aken MO, Janssen JA, et al. Long-term efficacy and safety of combined treatment of somatostatin analogs and pegvisomant in acromegaly. J Clin Endocrinol Metab 2007;92:4598–4601.

45. Hindmarsh PC, Brook CGD. Short stature and growth hormone deficiency. Clin Endocrinol 1995;43:133–142.

46. American Association of Clinical Endocrinologists. Medical guidelines for clinical practice for growth hormone use in adults and children—2003 Update. Endocr Pract 2003;9:64–76.

47. Pasquino AM, Albanese A, Bozzola M, et al. Idiopathic short stature. J Pediatr Endocrinol Metab 2001;(Suppl 2):967–974.

48. Hindmarsh PC, Dattani MT. Use of growth hormone in children. Nat Clin Pract Endocrinol Metab 2006;2:260–268.

49. Wilson TA, Rose SR, Cohen P, et al. Update of guidelines for the use of growth hormone in children: The Lawson Wilkins Pediatric Endocrine Society Drug and Therapeutics Committee. J Pediatr 2003;143:415–421.

50. Tauber M, Moulin P, Pienkowski C, et al. Growth hormone (GH) retesting and auxological data in 131 GH-deficient patients after completion of treatment. J Clin Endocrinol Metab 1997;82:352–356.

51. Mills JL, Schonberger LB, Wysowski DK, et al. Long-term mortality in the United States cohort of pituitary-derived growth hormone recipients. J Pediatr 2004;144:430–436.

52. Blethen SL, Bapitista J, Kuntze J, et al. Adult height in growth hormone (GH)-deficient children treated with biosynthetic GH. J Clin Endocrinol Metab 1997;82:418–420.

53. August GP, Julius JR, Blethen SL. Adult height in children with growth hormone deficiency who are treated with biosynthetic growth hormone: The national cooperative growth study experience. Pediatrics 1998;102:512–516.

54. Frinkik JP, Baptista J. Adult height in growth hormone deficiency: Historical perspective and examples from the national cooperative growth study. Pediatrics 1999;104:1000–1004.

55. Thomas M, Massa G, Bourguignon JP, et al. Final height in children with idiopathic growth hormone deficiency treated with recombinant human growth hormone: The Belgian experience. Horm Res 2001;55:88–94.

56. Rikken B, Massa GG, Wit JM, and the Dutch Growth Hormone Working Group. Final height in a large cohort of Dutch patients with growth hormone deficiency treated with growth hormone. Horm Res 1995;43:136–137.

57. Chipman JJ, Hicks JR, Holcombe JH, Draper MW. Approaching final height in children treated for growth hormone deficiency. Horm Res 1995;43:129–131.

58. Serveri F. Final height in children with growth hormone deficiency. Horm Res 1995;43:138–140.

59. Coste J, Letrait M, Carel JC, et al. Long term results of growth hormone treatment in France in children of short stature: Population, register based study. BMJ 1997;315:708–713.

60. Bravenboer N, Holzmann PJ, ter Maaten JC, et al. Effect of long-term growth hormone treatment on bone mass and bone metabolism in growth hormone-deficient men. J Bon Miner Res 2005;20:1778–1784.

61. Rosilio M, Blum WF, Edwards DJ, et al. Long-term improvement of quality of life during growth hormone (GH) replacement therapy in adults with GH deficiency, as measured by questions on life satisfaction-hypopituitarism (QLS-H). J Clin Endocrinol Metab 2004;89:1684–1693.

62. Cohen P, Rogol AD, Deal CL, et al. Consensus statement on the diagnosis and treatment of children with idiopathic short stature: a summary of the Growth Hormone Research Society, the Lawson Wilkins Pediatric Endocrine Society, and the European Society for Paediatric Endocrinology Workshop. J Clin Endocrinol Metab 2008;93:4210–4217.

63. Finkelstein BS, Imperiale TF, Speroff T, et al. Effect of growth hormone therapy on height in children with idiopathic short stature. Arch Pediatr Adolesc Med 2002;156:230–240.

64. Werber E, LeschekS, Yanovski JA, et al. Effect of growth hormone treatment on adult height in peripubertal children with idiopathic short stature: A randomized, double-blind, placebo-controlled trial. J Clin Endocrinol Metab 2004;89:3140–3148.

65. Blethen SL, MacGillivray MH. A risk-benefit assessment of growth hormone use in children. Drug Saf 1997;17:303–316.

66. Bell J, Parker KL, Swinford RD, et al. Long-term safety of recombinant human growth hormone in children. J Clin Endocrinol Metab 2010;95:167–177.

67. Jeffcoate W. Growth hormone therapy and its relationship to insulin resistance, glucose intolerance and diabetes mellitus. Drug Saf 2002;25:199–212.

68. Wantanabe S, Tsunematsu Y, Fujimoto J, et al. Leukaemia in patients treated with growth hormone. Lancet 1988;1:1159–1160.

69. Ogilvy-Stuart A, Gleeson H. Cancer risk following growth hormone use in childhood: Implications for current practice. Drug Saf 2004;24:369–382.

70. Pirazzoli P, Cacciari E, Mandini M, et al. Follow-up of antibodies to growth hormone in 210 growth hormone-deficient children treated with different commercial preparations. Acta Paediatr 1995;84:1233–1236.

71. Backeljauw PF, Underwood LE, and the GHIS Collaborative Group. Therapy for 6.5–7.5 years with recombinant insulin-like growth factor I in children with growth hormone insensitivity syndrome: A clinical research center study. J Clin Endocrinol Metab 2001;86:1504–1510.

72. Collett-Solberg PF, Madhusmita M, and the Drug and Therapeutics Committee of the Lawson Wilkins Pediatric Endocrine Society. The role of recombinant human insulin-like growth factor-I in treating children with short stature. J Clin endocrinol Metab 2008;93:10–18.

73. Chernausek SD, Backeljauw PF, Frane J, et al. Long-term treatment with recombinant insulin-like growth factor (IGF)-1 in children with severe IGF-I deficiency due to growth hormone insensitivity. J Clin Endocrinol Metab 2007;992:902–910.

74. Rosenbloom AL. Insulin-like growth factor-I (rhIGF-I) therapy of short stature. J Pediatr Endocrinol Metab 2008;24:301–315.

75. Hardin DS, Woo J, Butsch R, et al. Current prescribing practices and opinions about growth hormone therapy: results of a nationwide survey of pediatric endocrinologists. Clin Endocrinol 2007;66: 85–94.

76. Schlechte JA. Prolactinoma. N Engl J Med 2003;349:2035–2041.

77. Mah PM, Webster J. Hyperprolactinemia: Etiology, diagnosis and management. Semin Reprod Med 2002;20:365–373.

78. Gillam MP, Molitch ME, Lombardi, et al. Advances in the treatment of prolactinomas. Endocr Rev 2006;27:485–534.

79. Molitch ME. Drugs and prolactin. Pituitary 2008;11:209–218.

80. Haddad PM, Wieck A. Antipsychotic-induced hyperprolactinemia: Mechanisms, clinical features and management. Drugs 2004;64: 2291–2314.

81. Darwish AM, Hafez E, El-Gelbali I, et al. Evaluation of a novel vaginal bromocriptine mesylate formulation: A pilot study. Fertil Steril 2005;83:1053–1055.

82. Schade R, Andersohn F, Suissa S, et al. Dopamine agonists and the risk of cardiac-valve regurgitation. N Engl J Med 2007;356:29–38.

83. Verhelst J, Abs R, Maiter D, et al. Cabergoline in the treatment of hyperprolactinemia: A study in 455 patients. J Clin Endocrinol Metab 1999;84:2518–2522.

84. Cannavo S, Curto L, Squadrito S, et al. Cabergoline: A first-choice treatment in patients with previously untreated prolactin-secreting pituitary adenoma. J Endocrinol Invest 1999;22:354–359.

85. Colao A, DiSarno A, Landi ML, et al. Macroprolactinoma shrinkage during cabergoline treatment is greater in naïve patients than in patients pretreated with other dopamine agonists: A prospective study in 110 patients. J Clin Endocrinol Metab 2000;85: 2247–2252.

86. Ferrari CI, Abs R, Bevan JS, et al. Treatment of macroprolactinoma with cabergoline: A study of 85 patients. Clin Endocrinol 1997;46:409–413.

87. Webster J, Piscitelli G, Polli A, et al. A comparison of cabergoline and bromocriptine in the treatment of hyperprolactinemic amenorrhea. N Engl J Med 1994;331:904–909.

88. DiSarno A, Landi ML, Cappabianca P, et al. Resistance to cabergoline as compared with bromocriptine in hyperprolactinemia: Prevalence, clinical definition, and therapeutic strategy. J Clin Endocrinol Metab 2001;86:5256–5261.

89. Colao A, Vitale G, Cappabianca P, et al. Outcome of cabergoline treatment in men with prolactinoma: Effects of a 24-month treatment on prolactin levels, tumor mass, recovery of pituitary function, and semen analysis. J Clin Endocrinol Metab 2004;89:1704–1711.

90. Rains CP, Bryson HM, Fitton A. Cabergoline: A review of its pharmacological properties and therapeutic potential in the treatment of hyperprolactinaemia and inhibition of lactation. Drugs 1995;49:255–279.

91. Casanueva FF, Molitch ME, Schlechte JA, et al. Guidelines of the Pituitary Society for the diagnosis and management of prolactinomas. Clin Endocrinol 2006;65:265–273.

92. Ono M, Miki N, Kawamata T, et al. Prospective study of high-dose cabergoline treatment of prolactinomas in 150 patients. J Clin Endocrinol Metab 2008;93:4721–4727.

93. Herring N, Szmigielski C, Becher H, et al. valvular heart disease and the use of cabergoline for the treatment of prolactinoma. Clin Endocrinol 2009;70:104–108.

94. Vallette S, Serri K, Rivera J, et al. Long-term cabergoline therapy is not associated with valvular heart disease in patients with prolactinomas. Pituitary 2009;12:153–157.

95. Colao A, DiSarno A, Cappabianca P, et al. Withdrawal of long-term cabergoline therapy for tumoral and nontumoral hyperprolactinemia. N Engl J Med 2003;349:2023–2033.

CHAPTER

87

Pregnancy and Lactation: Therapeutic Considerations

KRISTINA E. WARD AND BARBARA M. O'BRIEN

KEY CONCEPTS

❶ Physiologic changes modify drug pharmacokinetics during pregnancy, including changes in absorption, protein binding, distribution, and elimination, requiring individualized drug selection and dosing.

❷ Although drug-induced teratogenicity is a serious concern during pregnancy, most drugs required by pregnant women can be used safely. Informed selection of drug therapy is essential.

❸ Healthcare practitioners must know where to find and how to evaluate evidence related to the safety of drugs used during pregnancy and lactation.

❹ Pregnancy-influenced health issues, such as constipation, gastroesophageal reflux disease, and nausea/vomiting, can be treated safely and effectively with nonpharmacologic treatment or carefully selected drug therapy. Some acute and chronic illnesses pose additional risks during pregnancy, requiring treatment with appropriately selected and monitored drug therapies to avoid harm to the woman and the fetus.

❺ Understanding the physiology of lactation and pharmacokinetic factors affecting drug distribution, metabolism, and elimination can assist the clinician in selecting safe and effective medications during lactation.

Drug use in pregnancy and lactation is a topic often underemphasized in the education of health professionals. Drug use in pregnancy and lactation is a controversial and emotionally charged area because of medicolegal and ethical implications.

Clinicians are responsible for ensuring safe and effective therapy before conception, during pregnancy and parturition, and after

Learning objectives, review questions, and other resources can be found at **www.pharmacotherapyonline.com**.

delivery. Active patient participation is essential. Optimal treatments of illnesses during pregnancy sometimes differ from those used in the nonpregnant patient. Principles of drug use during lactation, although similar, are not the same as those applicable during pregnancy.

In many cases, medication dosing recommendations for acute or chronic illnesses in pregnant women are the same as for the general population. However, some cases require different dosing and selection of medications.

PHYSIOLOGY OF PREGNANCY

Fertilization and progression of pregnancy are complex, resulting in survival of only approximately 50% of embryos.[1] Because most losses occur early, usually in the first 2 weeks after fertilization, many women don't realize they were pregnant. Spontaneous loss of pregnancy later in gestation occurs in about 15% of pregnancies that survive the first 2 weeks after fertilization.[2]

Fertilization occurs when a sperm attaches to a receptor on the outer protein layer of the egg, the zona pellucida, and renders the egg nonresponsive to other sperm.[3] The attached sperm releases enzymes that cause the egg's chromosomes to mature, allowing the sperm to fully penetrate the zona pellucida and contact the egg's cell membrane. The membranes of the sperm and egg then combine to create a new, single cell called a zygote. Male and female chromosomes join in the zygote, fuse to create a single nucleus, and organize for cell division.[4]

Fertilization usually occurs in the fallopian tube.[4] The fertilized egg travels down the fallopian tube over 2 days, with cell division taking place. By day 3, the fertilized egg reaches the uterus. Cell division continues for another 2 to 3 days in the uterine cavity before implantation. Approximately 6 days after fertilization, the cell mass is termed a *blastocyst*. Human chorionic gonadotropin (hCG) now is produced in amounts detectable by commercial laboratories. Implantation begins with the blastocyst sloughing the zona pellucida to rest directly on the endometrium allowing initiation of growth into the endometrial wall. By day 10 postfertilization, the blastocyst is implanted under the endometrial surface and receives nutrition from maternal blood.[4] Now it is called an *embryo*.[4,5]

After the embryonic period (between weeks 2 and 8 postfertilization), the conceptus is renamed a *fetus*.[5] Most body structures are formed during the embryonic period, and they continue to grow and mature during the fetal period. The fetal period continues until the pregnancy reaches term, approximately 40 weeks after the last menstrual period.[6]

Gravidity is the number of times that a woman is pregnant.[5,7] A multiple birth is counted as a single pregnancy. *Parity* refers to the number of pregnancies exceeding 20 weeks' gestation and relates information regarding the outcome of each pregnancy. In sequence, the numbers reflect (1) term deliveries, (2) premature deliveries, (3) aborted and/or ectopic pregnancies, and (4) number of living children. A woman who has been pregnant four times; has experienced two term deliveries, one premature delivery, and one ectopic pregnancy; and has three living children would be designated G_4P_{2113}.

PREGNANCY DATING

Pregnancy lasts approximately 280 days (about 40 weeks or 9 months); the time period is measured from the first day of the last menstrual period to birth.[5,7] *Gestational age* refers to the age of the embryo or fetus beginning with the first day of the last menstrual period, which is about 2 weeks prior to fertilization. When calculating the estimated due date, add 7 days to the first day of the last menstrual period then subtract 3 months. Pregnancy is divided into three periods of 3 calendar months, each called a *trimester*.

PREGNANCY SIGNS AND SYMPTOMS

Early symptoms of pregnancy include fatigue and increased frequency of urination. At approximately 6 weeks' gestation, nausea and vomiting can occur. While commonly called *morning sickness*, it can happen at any time of the day. Nausea and vomiting usually resolve in 12 to 18 weeks' gestation. A pregnant woman can feel fetal movement in the lower abdomen at 16 to 20 weeks of gestation. Signs of pregnancy include cessation of menses, change in cervical mucus consistency, bluish discoloration of the vaginal mucosa, increased skin pigmentation, and anatomic breast changes.[5,7]

MATERNAL PHARMACOKINETIC CHANGES IN PREGNANCY

❶ Normal physiologic changes that occur during pregnancy may alter medication effects, resulting in the need to more closely monitor and, sometimes, adjust therapy. Physiologic changes begin in the first trimester and peak during the second trimester. For medications that can be monitored by blood or serum concentration measurements, monitoring should occur throughout pregnancy.

During pregnancy, maternal plasma volume, cardiac output, and glomerular filtration increase by 30% to 50% or higher, potentially lowering the concentration of renally cleared drugs.[8,9] As body fat increases during pregnancy, the volume of distribution of fat-soluble drugs may increase. Plasma albumin concentration decreases, which increases the volume of distribution of drugs that are highly protein bound. However, unbound drugs are more rapidly cleared by the liver and kidney during pregnancy, resulting in little change in concentration. Nausea and vomiting, as well as delayed gastric emptying, may alter the absorption of drugs. Likewise, a pregnancy-induced increase in gastric pH may affect the absorption of weak acids and bases. Higher levels of estrogen and progesterone alter liver enzyme activity and increase the elimination of some drugs but result in accumulation of others.

TRANSPLACENTAL DRUG TRANSFER

Although once thought to be a barrier to drug transfer, the placenta is the organ of exchange for a number of substances, including drugs, between the mother and fetus. Most drugs move from the maternal circulation to the fetal circulation by diffusion.[10] Certain chemical properties, such as lipid solubility, electrical charge, molecular weight, and degree of protein binding of medications, may influence the rate of transfer across the placenta.[10]

Drugs with molecular weights less than 500 Da readily cross the placenta, whereas larger molecules (600–1,000 Da) cross more slowly.[10] Drugs with molecular weights greater than 1,000 Da, such as insulin and heparin, do not cross the placenta in significant amounts.[10] Lipophilic drugs, such as opiates and antibiotics, cross the placenta more easily than do water-soluble drugs.[10] Maternal plasma albumin progressively decreases while fetal albumin increases during the course of pregnancy, which may result in higher concentrations of certain protein-bound drugs in the fetus.[10] Fetal pH is slightly more acidic than maternal pH, permitting weak bases to more easily cross the placenta. Once in the fetal circulation, the molecule becomes more ionized and less likely to diffuse back into the maternal circulation.[10]

DRUG SELECTION DURING PREGNANCY

❷ Although some drugs have the potential to cause teratogenic effects, most medications required by pregnant women can be used safely. There are many misconceptions about the association of medications and birth defects.

The baseline risk for congenital malformations is approximately 3% to 6%, with approximately 3% considered severe.[2] Medication exposure is estimated to account for less than 1% of all birth defects.[2] Genetic causes are responsible for 15% to 25%, other environmental issues (e.g., maternal conditions and infections) account for 10%, and the remaining 65% to 75% of congenital malformations result from unknown causes.[2]

Factors such as the stage of pregnancy during exposure, route of administration, and dose, can affect outcomes.[2,11] In the first 2 weeks following conception, exposure to a teratogen may result in an "all-or-nothing" effect, which could either destroy the embryo or cause no problems.[11] During organogenesis (18 to 60 days postconception), organ systems are developing, and teratogenic exposures may result in structural anomalies. For the remainder of the pregnancy, exposure to teratogens may result in growth retardation, central nervous system abnormalities, or death.[2] Examples of medications associated with teratogenic effects in the period of organogenesis include chemotherapy drugs (e.g., methotrexate, cyclophosphamide), sex hormones (e.g., diethylstilbestrol), lithium, retinoids, thalidomide, certain antiepileptic drugs, and coumarin derivatives. Other medications such as nonsteroidal antiinflammatory drugs and tetracycline derivatives are more likely to exhibit effects in the second or third trimester.

In summary, a small number of medications have the potential to cause congenital malformations, and many can be avoided during pregnancy. In situations where a drug may be teratogenic but is necessary for maternal care, considerations related to route of administration and dosing may lessen the risk.

METHODS OF DETERMINING DRUG SAFETY IN PREGNANCY

❸ When assessing the safety of using medications during pregnancy, an important consideration for the clinician is how to evaluate the quality of the evidence. Ideally, safety data from randomized, controlled trials is most desirable, but pregnant women are not usually eligible for participation in clinical trials. Other types of data commonly used to estimate the risk associated with medication use during pregnancy are animal studies, case reports, case-control studies, prospective cohort studies, historical cohort studies, and voluntary reporting systems.

Animal studies are a required component of drug testing, but extrapolation of the results to humans is not always valid.[12] Thalidomide was found to be safe in some animal models but proved to have teratogenic effects in human offspring.

Case reports are usually of limited value because a birth defect in the infant of a woman who used a medication during pregnancy may have occurred by chance.[12] Case-control studies identify an outcome (congenital anomaly), match subjects with and without that outcome, and report how often exposure to a suspected agent occurred. Recall bias is a concern in case-control studies, as women with an affected pregnancy may be more likely to remember drugs used during the pregnancy than those who had a normal outcome.

Cohort studies evaluate the intervention (use of a particular drug) in a group of persons and compare outcomes in a similar group of subjects without the intervention.[12,13] Prospective studies eliminate some of the problems with recall bias but require time and large numbers of participants. Despite these disadvantages, cohort studies are often used for evaluating the effects of a drug exposure on pregnancy outcomes.

Teratology information services provide pregnant women with information about potential exposures during pregnancy and follow these women throughout the pregnancy to assess the outcomes of the pregnancy.[12] The services may publish pooled data to facilitate information sharing about medications used during pregnancy. Some pharmaceutical companies have organized voluntary reporting systems (also called pregnancy registries) for drugs used during pregnancy.

RESOURCES

❸ Computerized databases (e.g., *www.motherisk.org*, LactMed [*www.toxnet.nlm.nih.gov*]), tertiary compendia, and textbooks with information from large cohorts of treated women offer valuable assistance. New information regarding drug use in pregnancy and lactation can be obtained from searches of the primary literature for cohort and case-control studies.

The Food and Drug Administration (FDA) developed risk categories (i.e., A, B, C, D, X, with A considered safe and X considered teratogenic) to guide clinicians regarding medication risk during pregnancy. The FDA ranks very few as safe during pregnancy (category A) because a controlled trial is required to establish safety; this implies that few drugs are safe. Because of multiple limitations of the risk categories, the FDA proposed a new system in 2008 to replace the risk categories with a fetal risk summary and lactation risk summary. Each section discusses clinical considerations and summarizes available data.[14]

In summary, drug safety information from product labeling may provide a rough estimate of risks for medication-related adverse fetal outcomes but must be used in conjunction with other information sources to make decisions about medication use in pregnant women.

GENERAL RECOMMENDATIONS FOR OPTIMIZING USE OF MEDICATIONS IN PREGNANCY

❷ Medications are necessary during pregnancy for treatment of acute and chronic conditions. Identifying patterns of medication use before conception, eliminating nonessential medications and discouraging self-medication, minimizing exposure to medications known to be harmful, and adjusting medication doses are all strategies to optimize the health of the mother while minimizing the risk to the fetus.

PRECONCEPTION PLANNING

Pregnancy outcomes are influenced by maternal health status, lifestyle, and history prior to conception.[15] More than 60% of pregnancies in the United States are unintended. Of women who receive prenatal care, 18% seek it after the first trimester.[16] The goal of preconception care is health promotion, evidence-based screening, and intervention in all women of reproductive age to ensure optimal health and improve pregnancy outcomes.[15]

The most common major congenital abnormalities are neural tube defects (NTDs), cleft palate and lip, and cardiac anomalies. Each year in the United States approximately 1 in 1,000 infants are born with NTDs.[17] Folic acid supplementation substantially reduces the incidence in offspring of women, including those with a history of NTDs.[16,17] Neural tube defects occur within the first month of conception because neural tube closure occurs during the first month of pregnancy. Folic acid supplementation is recommended throughout a woman's reproductive years since many pregnancies are unplanned and may not be recognized until after the first month. Dietary intake of folic acid is not sufficient. For all women of childbearing age, folic acid supplementation with 400 mcg/day is recommended.[16] For women at high risk or those who have a history of NTDs, folic acid 4 mg/day is recommended. Multivitamins should not be used to achieve folic acid doses higher than contained in the multivitamin product because of risk for vitamin A toxicity.

Use of alcohol and recreational drugs during pregnancy is associated with birth defects.[15] Of births in the United States in 2003, 10% of mothers smoked tobacco during pregnancy.[15] Smoking can cause preterm birth, low birth weight, and other adverse outcomes. In a systematic review of 72 trials of smoking cessation and perinatal outcomes, incidences of low birth weight and preterm birth were reduced, and birth weight increased by 54 g with smoking cessation.[18] Cognitive behavioral therapy and nicotine replacement therapy resulted in similar rates of smoking cessation; however, offering incentives and social support resulted in the highest rate of success. For women who cannot stop smoking with behavioral interventions alone, nicotine replacement therapies can be used with behavioral therapy. Use of nicotine replacement during pregnancy is controversial since its use is not supported by clinical trial data; however, nicotine replacement theoretically imparts less risk than exposure to the over 4,000 chemicals found in cigarettes.[19] Intermittent delivery formulations are recommended because most users ingest a smaller total daily dose than received from the topically applied patch.[20] If patches are necessary because of poor tolerability of other agents, they should be applied for 16 rather than 24 hours per day. The initial dose of the patch should be similar or higher than that used for nonpregnant women because of nicotine's rapid metabolism during pregnancy. Bupropion is an alternative to nicotine replacement for women who have not quit smoking with behavioral therapy because the risk of its use appears to be less than that of cigarette smoking. However, its efficacy for smoking cessation in pregnancy has not been determined. Bupropion use during pregnancy should be reported to the GlaxoSmithKline pregnancy registry. Varenicline's safety and effectiveness during pregnancy are unknown.

Prevention of infectious disease during pregnancy is important. Vaccination against *Rubella* and hepatitis B as part of preconception care reduces adverse pregnancy outcomes.[15] Influenza vaccination is generally offered to women who will be in their second or third trimester during influenza season. Women with comorbid conditions that increase risks of complications from influenza should receive vaccine regardless of time of gestation.

PREGNANCY-INFLUENCED ISSUES

④ Pregnancy causes or exacerbates conditions that pregnant women commonly experience, including constipation, gastroesophageal reflux, hemorrhoids, and nausea and vomiting. Gestational diabetes, gestational hypertension, and venous thromboembolism have the potential to cause adverse pregnancy consequences. Gestational thyrotoxicosis is usually self-limiting.

GASTROINTESTINAL TRACT

The prevalence of constipation during pregnancy ranges from 25% to 40%. Light physical exercise and increased intake of dietary fiber and fluid should be instituted first.[21] If additional treatment is needed, supplemental fiber and/or a stool softener is appropriate.[22] Osmotic laxatives (polyethylene glycol, lactulose, sorbitol, and magnesium and sodium salts) are acceptable treatments but should be reserved for occasional use only. Polyethylene glycol is considered by some the ideal laxative for use in pregnancy.[21,22] Senna and bisacodyl can be used occasionally. Castor oil and mineral oil should be avoided.

Gastroesophageal reflux disease occurs in up to 80% of pregnant women.[21] An algorithm starting with lifestyle and dietary modifications (e.g., small, frequent meals; alcohol and tobacco avoidance; food avoidance before bedtime; elevation of the head of the bed) should be used. If symptoms are not relieved, use of antacids (aluminum, calcium, or magnesium preparations) or sucralfate is acceptable. Sodium bicarbonate and magnesium trisilicate should be avoided. Evidence supports the use of ranitidine and cimetidine. Literature evaluating the use of famotidine and nizatidine is limited, but they are likely safe. If a patient is unresponsive to lifestyle changes and histamine-2 receptor blockers, metoclopramide is a viable option. Relatively few data are available on the use of proton pump inhibitors during pregnancy; use should be reserved for women with complicated or intractable gastroesophageal reflux.

The prevalence of hemorrhoids during pregnancy is believed to be higher than in the general population.[23] Therapy during pregnancy is conservative (i.e., high intake of dietary fiber, adequate oral fluid intake, and use of sitz baths) and may be helpful; however, there is a paucity of supporting data for all management options. Topical anesthetics, skin protectants, and astringents can be used. Other options for refractory hemorrhoids include rubber band ligation, sclerotherapy, and surgery.

Nausea and vomiting affect up to 90% of pregnant women, usually beginning during the fifth week of gestation and lasting through the first trimester; however, about 15% of women experience it throughout pregnancy.[21,24] Hyperemesis gravidarum (HEG; i.e., unrelenting vomiting causing weight loss of more than 5% prepregnancy weight and ketonuria) occurs in about 1% to 3% of women.[24] Dietary modifications, such as eating frequent, small, bland meals and avoiding fatty foods, may be helpful. Applying pressure at acupressure point P6 on the volar aspect of the wrist may be beneficial.

A number of pharmacotherapeutic approaches have been tried for treatment of nausea and vomiting. Multivitamins, pyridoxine (vitamin B$_6$), and antihistamines (including doxylamine) have shown efficacy.[21,24] Phenothiazines and metoclopramide are widely used and generally considered safe.[21,24] Evidence of safety and efficacy with ondansetron is limited, but ondansetron can be considered for HEG when other treatments fail. Corticosteroids are effective for HEG but are associated with a small increase in the risk of oral clefts when used during the first trimester.[21,24] Ginger has shown efficacy for hyperemesis in randomized, controlled trials and is probably safe.[21,24]

GESTATIONAL DIABETES

Gestational diabetes mellitus (GDM) is glucose intolerance first identified during pregnancy. It develops in about 4% of pregnant women, although the prevalence may range from 1% to 14%.[25] Screening for gestational diabetes is controversial.[25–27] The U.S. Preventative Services Task Force Independent Expert Panel concluded that there is a lack of evidence proving that screening for gestational diabetes decreases adverse maternal and fetal outcomes.[27] However, the American Diabetes Association recommends glucose testing for women with risk factors of gestational diabetes (e.g., obesity, history of the condition, glycosuria, or strong family history of diabetes) at the first prenatal visit.[25] If normal, testing should be repeated between weeks 24 and 28 of gestation. Pregnant women considered to have average risk should undergo testing for GDM between weeks 24 and 28 of gestation unless they are considered low risk. To meet criteria for low risk, a woman must fulfill *all* the following: (a) age younger than 25 years, (b) normal body weight, (c) no known diabetes in first-degree relatives, (d) no history of abnormal glucose tolerance, (e) no history of adverse obstetric outcomes, and (f) not a member of an ethnic group with a high prevalence of GDM (e.g., African Americans, Native Americans, Asian Americans, Hispanic Americans, Pacific Islanders). Initial screening for hyperglycemia in pregnancy is similar to that in the general population and is described in the American Diabetes Association practice guidelines.[25]

Dietary modification is considered first-line therapy for all women who have GDM, with additional caloric restriction for obese women.[26,28] Daily self-monitoring of blood glucose is required. Insulin therapy with recombinant human insulin should be initiated if the following levels are not achieved with dietary modification: fasting plasma glucose concentrations below 90–99 mg/dL (5.0–5.5 mmol/L), 1-hour postprandial plasma glucose concentration less than or equal to 140 mg/dL (7.8 mmol/L), or 2-hour postprandial plasma glucose concentration below 120–127 mg/dL (6.7–7.0 mmol/L).[26] Glyburide is an alternative because it minimally crosses the placenta.[26,28] Metformin may also be an alternative, but it crosses the placenta and is less well studied than insulin or glyburide.[28] There are data, though limited, supporting the use of postprandial over preprandial blood glucose monitoring in women requiring insulin treatment.[29] Recommended targets for self-monitored blood glucose are preprandial plasma glucose concentration between 80 and 110 mg/dL (4.4–6.1 mmol/L) and 2-hour postprandial plasma glucose concentration below 155 mg/dL (8.6 mmol/L).[30]

Evidence supporting dietary modification, self-monitored blood glucose, exercise, and pharmacologic interventions for women with GDM is largely based on one randomized clinical trial that showed reductions in perinatal morbidity (composite of death, nerve palsy, bone fracture, and shoulder dystocia) with nutritional education, blood glucose monitoring, and insulin treatment.[31,32]

HYPERTENSION

Approximately 10% of pregnancies are complicated by hypertension at some time during the pregnancy. Hypertension in pregnancy is divided into four categories: chronic hypertension (preexisting hypertension), gestational hypertension (hypertension without proteinuria), preeclampsia (hypertension with proteinuria), and preeclampsia superimposed on chronic hypertension.[33,34] Treatment of mild-to-moderate hypertension (defined as systolic blood pressure 140–169 mm Hg or diastolic blood pressure 90–109 mm Hg) reduces the risk of severe hypertension by 50%, but does not substantially affect fetal outcomes. However, severe hypertension (blood pressure greater than or equal to 160–170 mm Hg systolic or 110 mm Hg diastolic) can cause maternal complications, hospital admission, and potential premature delivery. Preeclampsia complicates 2%–8% of pregnancies and can cause poorer outcomes, including eclampsia (seizures in addition to preeclampsia), renal failure, coagulopathy, preterm delivery, and intrauterine growth restriction.[33]

Supplemental calcium 1–2 g/day decreases the relative risk of hypertension by 30% (range 14%–43%) and preeclampsia by 48% (range 31%–67%).[35] High-risk patients (those with the lowest initial calcium intake) benefited most; however, even women with adequate calcium intake at baseline had a 38% decrease in risk of preeclampsia. Therefore, 1 g/day of supplemental calcium is recommended for all pregnant women.

Nondrug managements center on activity restriction, psychosocial therapy, and biofeedback; however, no evidence indicates that any of these approaches improves pregnancy outcome, and prolonged bed rest may increase the risk of venous thromboembolic disease. Studies of antihypertensive drug therapy for mild-to-moderate hypertension (less than or equal to 160/110 mm Hg) in pregnancy have not conclusively shown a decrease in the risk of preeclampsia, neonatal death, preterm birth, or small-for-gestational-age babies. However, antihypertensives do prevent severe hypertension.[34,36] No evidence supports selection of one pharmacologic agent as first-line therapy. Commonly used drugs include methyldopa, labetalol, and calcium channel blockers.[36] Agents affecting the renin-angiotensin pathway (i.e., angiotensin-converting enzyme inhibitors, angiotensin receptor antagonists, and renin inhibitors) should probably be avoided throughout pregnancy.[36]

Drug therapy is indicated for women with blood pressure greater than or equal to 160/110 mm Hg. However, no consensus exists on when to initiate treatment, and recommendations vary from at least 140/90 mm Hg to 160/105 mm Hg.[36] As with mild-to-moderate hypertension in pregnancy, conclusive evidence supporting one antihypertensive agent over another is lacking, although agents to avoid include magnesium sulfate (unless indicated for eclampsia prevention), high-dose diazoxide, nimodipine, and chlorpromazine.[37]

Low-dose aspirin (75–81 mg/day) started after 12 weeks' gestation in women at risk for preeclampsia decreases the risk of its development by 17%, which corresponds to prevention of one preeclampsia case for every 72 at-risk women treated.[33,38] Low-dose aspirin also results in decreased rates of preterm birth (8% reduction) and fetal or neonatal death (14% reduction). In high-risk women (i.e., previous severe preeclampsia, renal disease, autoimmune disease, diabetes, and chronic hypertension), use of low-dose aspirin prevents one case for every 19 women treated. Features associated with moderate risk for preeclampsia include first pregnancy, adolescent maternal age, mild increase in blood pressure without proteinuria, abnormal uterine artery Doppler scan, family history of severe preeclampsia, and multiple fetuses; although some evidence refutes young maternal age as a risk factor.[33,38]

Preeclampsia may progress rapidly to eclampsia, a medical emergency, so signs and symptoms of preeclampsia must be monitored carefully. Eclampsia is the occurrence of seizures superimposed on preeclampsia.[33,39] Signs and symptoms of preeclampsia include blood pressure elevation; proteinuria; persistent severe headache; persistent new epigastric pain; visual changes; vomiting; hyperreflexia; sudden and severe swelling of hands, face, or feet; low platelet count; hemolytic anemia; increased serum creatinine; and elevated liver enzyme tests. The only cure for preeclampsia is delivery of the fetus. Treatment of hypertension in women with preeclampsia is the same as mentioned previously (e.g., methyldopa, labetalol, calcium channel blockers). Magnesium sulfate is recommended to prevent eclampsia as well as treat eclamptic seizures. Diazepam and phenytoin should be avoided.

THYROID ABNORMALITIES

During pregnancy, stimulation of the thyroid gland may occur because of hCG's structural similarity to serum TSH (thyrotropin).[40] In women with HEG, gestational transient thyrotoxicosis may result. Women are usually asymptomatic but may present with vomiting, increased serum free thyroxine, and decreased thyrotropin. Gestational transient thyrotoxicosis resolves as concentrations of hCG decline toward the end of the first trimester. Treatment with antithyroid medications is not usually needed. Nausea and vomiting can be treated as for patients without this pseudohyperthyroid state.

Postpartum thyroiditis occurs in approximately 4% of women within 1 to 4 months after childbirth because of increased thyroid hormone secretion.[41] Most cases resolve spontaneously; however, β-blockers (propranolol or labetalol) can provide symptomatic relief of adrenergic symptoms. Patients should be monitored since 2% to 5% of women go on to develop transient hypothyroidism 4 to 8 months postpartum; levothyroxine replacement is suggested for a total of 6 to 12 months. Up to 30% of women develop permanent hypothyroidism.

THROMBOEMBOLISM

Venous thromboembolism is estimated to occur in 0.06% to 0.13% of pregnancies; a five- to tenfold increase in risk over nonpregnant women.[42]

❹ Unfractionated heparin or adjusted-dose low-molecular weight heparin are recommended for treatment of acute thromboembolism during pregnancy, although low-molecular-weight heparin is preferred.[42] Treatment should be continued throughout pregnancy and for 6 weeks after delivery. Warfarin is not used because it causes nasal hypoplasia, stippled epiphyses, limb hypoplasia, and eye abnormalities; the risk period appears to be between 6 and 12 weeks' gestation. However, central nervous system anomalies are associated with second- and third-trimester exposure. Antepartum monitoring or anticoagulation plus postpartum anticoagulation is recommended for women with a single episode of thromboembolism and either (a) thrombophilia, (b) an idiopathic cause without thrombophilia, or (c) a pregnancy- or estrogen-related risk factor. Antepartum and postpartum anticoagulation should be given to women with two or more episodes of thromboembolism, women with antithrombin III deficiency, and women receiving long-term anticoagulation. Pregnant women with antiphospholipid antibodies and a history of pregnancy complications should receive antepartum aspirin in addition to unfractionated heparin or low-molecular-weight heparin.

Women with prosthetic heart valves should receive low-molecular-weight heparin or unfractionated heparin during pregnancy.[42] After a discussion of potential risks, a heparin product can be used until week 13 of gestation with subsequent substitution of warfarin until the middle of the third trimester when a heparin product should again be used. High-risk women with prosthetic heart valves (e.g., older-generation mitral valve, history of thromboembolism) may also receive low-dose aspirin (75–100 mg/day).

CONCLUSION

Women with pregnancy-influenced gastrointestinal issues can be treated safely with lifestyle modification or medications, many of them nonprescription. Gestational diabetes, hypertension, and thyrotoxicosis may or may not require drug therapy. Venous thromboembolism treatment or prevention usually requires therapy with a low-molecular-weight heparin or unfractionated heparin.

ACUTE CARE ISSUES IN PREGNANCY

❹ In some cases, the risks associated with the acute illness are magnified during pregnancy, and early screening and treatment become critical. In other cases, such as during treatment of certain sexually transmitted diseases, the urgency regarding treatment comes from an increased likelihood of infection leading to preterm labor. Occasionally, common acute care issues, such as migraine headache, improve during pregnancy.

URINARY TRACT INFECTION

❹ The most common infections in pregnant and nonpregnant women are urinary tract infections.[43] The incidence of asymptomatic bacteriuria ranges from 2% to 10% while estimates for acute cystitis range from 1% to 4%. Untreated, bacteriuria progresses to pyelonephritis in 20% to 40% of pregnant women compared with 1% to 2% of nonpregnant women. Complications of pyelonephritis include premature delivery, low infant birth weight, hypertension, anemia, bacteremia, and transient renal failure.[44] A urine culture is recommended to screen pregnant women for urinary tract infections between 12 and 16 weeks' gestation.[43] Use of other methods, such as dipsticks that measure nitrites or leukocyte esterase, requires high bacterial concentrations for a positive result, leading to false negatives and underdiagnosis.

Escherichia coli is the primary cause of infection in 80% to 90% of cases.[43] Other gram-negative rods, such as *Proteus mirabilis* and *Klebsiella pneumoniae*, as well as Group B *Streptococcus* (GBS) account for some infections. The presence of GBS in the urine indicates heavy colonization of the genitourinary tract, increasing the risk for GBS infection in the newborn.

To decrease the risk of pyelonephritis and its complications, treatment of asymptomatic bacteriuria is necessary.[44] β-Lactams are not known teratogens; however, the incidence of *E. coli* resistance to ampicillin and amoxicillin limits their use as single agents. Cephalexin is safe and effective. Nitrofurantoin is also safe and effective, but it is not active against *Proteus* species. It should not be used after week 37 in patients with glucose-6-phosphate dehydrogenase deficiency because of a theoretical risk for hemolytic anemia in the neonate; however, no cases are reported. Sulfa-containing drugs can contribute to the development of newborn kernicterus; use should be avoided during the last weeks of gestation. Trimethoprim is a folate antagonist and is relatively contraindicated during the first trimester because of associations with cardiovascular malformations. Regionally, increased rates of *E. coli* resistance to trimethoprim-sulfa may limit its use. Fluoroquinolones and tetracyclines are contraindicated. The optimal duration of therapy for asymptomatic bacteriuria in pregnancy has not been determined. Courses of 7 to 14 days are common, but shorter courses of 3 days may be sufficient.[43] Repeat urine cultures are recommended monthly for the remainder of gestation if asymptomatic bacteriuria is diagnosed.

Signs and symptoms of acute cystitis include urgency, frequency, hematuria, pyuria, and dysuria.[43] Treatment of acute cystitis is similar to that of asymptomatic bacteriuria. Using outcomes of cure rates, recurrent infection, incidence of preterm delivery or rupture of membranes, admission to neonatal intensive care, need for change of antibiotic, or incidence of prolonged fever, antibiotic treatment has demonstrated effectiveness in treating symptomatic urinary tract infections (including pyelonephritis) in pregnancy.[45] No specific treatment appeared superior to other commonly used treatments.

Patients with pyelonephritis usually present with bacteriuria and systemic symptoms of fever, flank pain, nausea, and vomiting.[43]

Hospitalization is the standard of care for pregnant women since many require intravenous hydration. Inpatient therapy has included parenteral administration of cephalosporins (e.g., cefazolin, ceftriaxone), ampicillin plus gentamicin, or ampicillin-sulbactam.[43,44] Switching to oral antibiotics can occur after the woman is afebrile for 48 hours. Outpatient antibiotic therapy can be considered after initial inpatient observation in women who are afebrile and less than 24 weeks' gestation. The total duration of antibiotic therapy for acute pyelonephritis is 10 to 14 days. Suppression therapy with nitrofurantoin 100 mg given nightly is recommended for the remainder of gestation because of the 20% recurrence rate.

SEXUALLY TRANSMITTED DISEASES

❹ Sexually transmitted diseases in pregnant women range from infections that may be transmitted across the placenta and infect the infant prenatally (e.g., syphilis) to organisms that may be transmitted during birth and cause neonatal infection (e.g., *Chlamydia trachomatis*, *Neisseria gonorrhoeae*, or herpes simplex virus) to infections that pose a threat for preterm labor (e.g., bacterial vaginosis). Screening is essential for early detection of most sexually transmitted diseases but may not be beneficial in other instances (e.g., bacterial vaginosis in low-risk patients). Sexual partners of women with certain infections (e.g., syphilis, *N. gonorrhoeae*, *C. trachomatis*) also require treatment to prevent recurrence of infection.

Syphilis

Serologic testing for syphilis should occur during the first prenatal visit.[46] For women who live in areas with a high prevalence of syphilis, are at high risk, have not been previously tested, or had positive serology in the first trimester, additional serologic testing during the third trimester and at delivery is recommended. With the exception of neurosyphilis, which is treated with aqueous penicillin G, the drug of choice for all stages of syphilis is benzathine penicillin G. Penicillin effectively prevents transmission to the fetus and treats the fetus, if already infected. For pregnant women, the dose and route of administration are determined by the stage of syphilis and do not differ from recommendations for nonpregnant patients. No alternatives for penicillin are acceptable for penicillin-allergic pregnant women; therefore, penicillin skin testing and desensitization are required.

Treatment during the second half of pregnancy may increase the risk for preterm labor and fetal distress because a Jarisch-Herxheimer reaction may occur; however, treatment should not be withheld or delayed.[46] All women should have serologic titers repeated at 28 to 32 weeks' gestation, at delivery, and as dictated by recommendations for the stage of disease.

Neisseria gonorrhoeae

Perinatal gonococcal infection results from exposure to the infected cervix during birth. Symptoms usually manifest within 2 to 5 days after delivery.[46] Milder manifestations include rhinitis, vaginitis, urethritis, and infection at the site of fetal monitoring. More severe presentations include ophthalmia neonatorum and sepsis.

Coinfection with *C. trachomatis* is common; treatment of most *N. gonorrhoeae* infections includes treatment for *C. trachomatis*.[46] Cotreatment regimens for presumptive or diagnosed *C. trachomatis* infection are described in the following section. Ceftriaxone 125 mg intramuscularly as a single dose or cefixime 400 mg orally in a single dose is the treatment of choice for *N. gonorrhoeae* cervical infection. Women with a cephalosporin allergy or intolerance should receive a single dose of spectinomycin 2 g intramuscularly. Quinolones and tetracyclines are contraindicated.

TABLE 87-1 Recommended Regimens for Treatment of Cervical Infections Due to Chlamydia in Pregnancy

First-line treatment
Azithromycin 1 g orally in a single dose or
Amoxicillin 500 mg orally three times daily for 7 days

Alternative regimens
Erythromycin base 500 mg orally four times per day for 7 days or
Erythromycin base 250 mg orally four times per day for 14 days
Erythromycin ethylsuccinate 800 mg orally four times per day for 7 days or
Erythromycin ethylsuccinate 400 mg orally four times per day for 14 days

Data from Centers for Disease Control and Prevention, Workowski KA, Berman SM Sexually transmitted diseases treatment guidelines, 2006. MMWR Recomm Rep 2006,55(RR-11):1–94.[46]

Chlamydia trachomatis

C. trachomatis infects the newborn through exposure to the infected cervix during delivery.[46] Perinatal infection most commonly causes conjunctivitis that develops 5 to 12 days postpartum. A subacute, afebrile pneumonia with an onset at ages 1 to 3 months may occur.

The treatment of choice for *C. trachomatis* cervicitis is azithromycin 1 g orally as a single dose or amoxicillin 500 mg three times daily for 7 days.[46] Erythromycin base or ethylsuccinate regimens are alternatives, but gastrointestinal intolerance and the required frequency of administration may limit patient acceptance. Erythromycin estolate increases the risk for hepatotoxicity and should be avoided (Table 87-1).

Genital Herpes

❹ Neonatal herpes often occurs in infants born to women lacking clinical evidence of genital herpes.[46] The risk of neonatal transmission is under 1% for women with a history of recurrent herpes at term, but is 30% to 50% for women who initially acquire genital herpes during the first half of their pregnancy. However, because recurrent herpes is more common than initial episodes during pregnancy, it remains the cause for most cases of neonatal transmission.

Prevention strategies include counseling uninfected women to avoid intercourse during the third trimester with partners having known or suspected genital herpes infection.[46,47] Women with no history of orolabial herpes should avoid receptive oral sex during the third trimester with partners who have orolabial herpes. Prevention of genital herpes transmission to pregnant women using antiviral agents has not been studied.

All women should be asked about symptoms of genital herpes at the time of delivery and should be examined for lesions.[46,47] Women who have no symptoms (including prodromal symptoms) or lesions proceed with vaginal childbirth; however, those with evidence of an outbreak undergo cesarean section to decrease the risk of neonatal transmission.

Maternal use of acyclovir during the first trimester has not demonstrated an increased risk for birth defects.[46] Valacyclovir is an alternative.[47] Safety data with famciclovir are limited. For initial or recurrent episodes, most women receive oral acyclovir therapy while intravenous acyclovir is reserved for severe infections. Women with an initial outbreak late in pregnancy may receive acyclovir, cesarean section, or a combination of the two. Acyclovir use during the last month of pregnancy may reduce the frequency of cesarean section because of fewer recurrences. In women seropositive for herpes simplex virus but who have not experienced an outbreak, no data suggest a treatment benefit.

Bacterial Vaginosis

Bacterial vaginosis results from the lack of normal vaginal flora (i.e., *Lactobacillus* species) and replacement with anaerobic bacteria, mycoplasmas, and *Gardnerella vaginalis*.[46] It is a risk factor for premature rupture of membranes, preterm labor, preterm birth, spontaneous abortion, and postpartum endometritis. Women with a history of preterm delivery should undergo screening for asymptomatic bacterial vaginosis at the first prenatal visit.

For symptomatic and asymptomatic women at high risk for preterm delivery, the recommended treatment regimen is metronidazole 500 mg orally twice daily for 7 days, metronidazole 250 mg orally three times daily for 7 days, or clindamycin 300 mg twice daily for 7 days. Conflicting data exist with regard to treating women at low risk for preterm labor. Vaginal preparations (e.g., metronidazole gel, clindamycin cream) have not demonstrated reductions in the risk of adverse pregnancy outcomes associated with bacterial vaginosis. Use of intravaginal clindamycin cream during the second half of pregnancy has caused low birth weight and neonatal infections.

HEADACHE

❹ Primary headaches (e.g., tension, migraine) in pregnant women are the most common types of headache.[48] Secondary headaches can also occur as a result of trauma, infection, preeclampsia, stroke, or cerebral venous thrombosis.

The majority of pregnant women with a history of migraine headaches experience symptom improvement during pregnancy. Eighteen percent to 86% of women improve, and the greatest improvements occur during the second and third trimesters.[48,49] Improvement is more likely in women who have migraine without aura and less likely in women with a history of menstrual migraine. Women with menstrual migraine are more likely to have postpartum recurrence.

Relaxation, stress management, and biofeedback are all effective nonpharmacologic treatment methods.[48,49] Acetaminophen (with or without codeine), codeine, or other narcotic analgesics can be used to treat headaches that do not respond to nonpharmacologic treatment. Aspirin should be avoided in the third trimester because it can cause narrowing of the ductus arteriosus, maternal and fetal bleeding, and decreased uterine contractility. Nonsteroidal antiinflammatory drugs (NSAIDs) are considered safe but are also contraindicated in the third trimester because of the potential for closure of the ductus arteriosus. Caffeine may be added to any of the foregoing treatments to improve response, but overuse may cause withdrawal headaches. Use of sumatriptan is controversial because of limited information about pregnancy outcomes with its use, but some clinicians recommend it for women who have not responded to other agents.[49] Ergotamine and dihydroergotamine are contraindicated. Metoclopramide can be used for patients who have migraine-associated nausea. Chronic, preventive treatment is reserved for women who have three to four severe episodes per month that are not responsive to other treatments. β-Blockers, such as propranolol, are commonly used but may be associated with side effects, including intrauterine growth retardation. Alternatives include calcium channel blockers and antidepressants.[48,49]

Tension headaches are less studied.[48,49] Most women report no change in the frequency or intensity of tension headaches. Tension headaches may be difficult to distinguish from secondary headaches. Primary treatments for tension headache are nonpharmacologic interventions, including exercise, biofeedback, and massage. Simple analgesics such as acetaminophen, ibuprofen, or caffeine are used if nonpharmacologic treatments fail. Opioids are rarely used.[48]

CHRONIC ILLNESSES IN PREGNANCY

❹ For the majority of women and their healthcare providers, pregnancy is a new consideration for a previously diagnosed health condition. Medications used to treat the chronic illness can often be used throughout the pregnancy and during breast-feeding.

ALLERGIC RHINITIS AND ASTHMA

❹ Asthma and rhinitis are common chronic illnesses in pregnancy. During pregnancy, asthma control may change and worsen maternal oxygenation resulting in significant health consequences in the mother and fetus. Rhinitis itself is unlikely to cause harm to the mother or fetus but may be associated with diminished quality of life.

Asthma affects approximately 8% of pregnancies.[50] During pregnancy almost equal proportions of patients have symptoms that worsen, improve, or remain unchanged.[51] Health consequences of untreated or poorly treated asthma include preterm labor, preeclampsia, intrauterine growth restriction, premature birth, low birth weight, and stillbirth; therefore, the treatment goal is symptom control.[51,52] Asthma is controlled when there are no daytime symptoms, limitations of activities, nocturnal symptoms, short-acting β_2-agonist use, or exacerbations, and there is normal pulmonary function.

Caring for patients with asthma should include (a) assessment and monitoring (including measures of pulmonary function), (b) identifying and controlling exposure to allergens and irritants (e.g., tobacco smoke), (c) patient education, and (d) a stepped approach to medication use.[51] The risks of medication use to the fetus are lower than the risks of untreated asthma.

Treatment recommendations are divided into six steps based on symptom control.[51,52] A short-acting β_2-agonist is recommended for all patients with asthma for quick relief of symptoms. For mild intermittent asthma, Step 1 recommends only a short-acting, inhaled β_2-agonist; albuterol is preferred during pregnancy.

Initiation of treatment for persistent asthma should begin with Step 2 unless the patient has severely uncontrolled asthma, in which case treatment may start at Step 3.[51,52] For persistent asthma, step-appropriate doses (low, medium, high) of inhaled corticosteroids form the foundation of the controller medication regimen. When possible, low-dose inhaled corticosteroids are the treatment of choice for women with mild persistent asthma. Budesonide is preferred during pregnancy, although other inhaled corticosteroids that were effective before pregnancy can be continued. Long-acting β_2-agonists are considered safe to use during pregnancy because of the similar pharmacologic and safety profiles compared with short-acting agents; use should follow the stepwise approach.[50–52] Cromolyn, leukotriene receptor antagonists, and theophylline are considered alternative treatments but are not preferred because they are less effective (cromolyn), there is less experience with them (leukotriene receptor antagonists), and there is more potential toxicity (theophylline) than with inhaled corticosteroids. For patients with the most severe disease, addition of systemic corticosteroids is recommended to gain control of symptoms.[51]

Allergic rhinitis may also improve, worsen, or remain the same during pregnancy.[53] Treatment strategies include avoidance of allergens, immunotherapy, and pharmacotherapy. Immunotherapy is not contraindicated in pregnancy, but dose increases during pregnancy are not advised to lessen risk for anaphylaxis.

First-line medications to treat allergic rhinitis during pregnancy include intranasal corticosteroids, nasal cromolyn, and first-generation antihistamines (e.g., chlorpheniramine, hydroxyzine).[53] Intranasal corticosteroids are the most effective treatment and have a low risk of systemic effect; beclomethasone and budesonide have been most widely studied.[53,54] Second-generation antihistamines (i.e., loratadine and cetirizine) do not appear to increase fetal risk but are less extensively studied than first-generation products. Oral decongestants, such as pseudoephedrine, may be associated with an increased risk for the rare birth defect gastroschisis. Use of an external nasal dilator, short-term topical oxymetazoline, or inhaled corticosteroids may be preferable to use of oral decongestants, especially during early pregnancy.

DERMATOLOGIC CONDITIONS

❹ Treatment of dermatologic conditions can often be delayed until after the delivery.[55] If treatment is required during gestation, topical agents considered to have minimal pregnancy risk include bacitracin, benzoyl peroxide, ciclopirox, clindamycin, erythromycin, metronidazole, mupirocin, permethrin, and terbinafine. Topical corticosteroids are generally considered safe for use but should be applied at the lowest possible dose for the shortest time. Systemic agents considered safe include acyclovir, amoxicillin, azithromycin, cephalosporins, cyproheptadine, dicloxacillin, diphenhydramine, erythromycin (except estolate), nystatin, and penicillins. Lidocaine and lidocaine with epinephrine can be used topically during pregnancy. Acitretin, fluorouracil, isotretinoin, methotrexate, and thalidomide should be avoided because of teratogenic potential.

DIABETES

❹ Poorly controlled diabetes can cause fetal malformations and fetal loss.[30] Women with diabetes should use effective contraception until optimal glycemic control is achieved before attempting pregnancy. Additionally, diabetic retinopathy may worsen, hypertension may develop, and renal function may deteriorate during pregnancy, requiring enhanced monitoring for these target-organ problems.[56]

For patients with both type 1 and type 2 diabetes, insulin is the drug treatment of choice.[56] However, glyburide and metformin may be alternatives.[26,28] Medical nutrition therapy and supervised physical activity programs should continue. Goals for self-monitored blood glucose are the same as for gestational diabetes.[30,56]

EPILEPSY

❹ Seizure frequency does not change for most pregnant women with epilepsy. Studies have demonstrated no frequency change in 54% to 80% of women with epilepsy, while decreased frequency ranges between 3% and 24% and increased frequency ranges from 14% to 32%.[57,58] Seizures may become more frequent because of changes in maternal hormones, sleep deprivation, and medication adherence problems (because of perceived teratogenic risk). Another potential cause is changes in free serum concentrations of antiepileptic drugs resulting from increased maternal volume of distribution, decreased protein binding from hypoalbuminemia, increased hepatic drug metabolism, and increased renal drug clearance. A woman's clinical condition and her free serum concentrations of antiepileptic drug should be the basis for dose adjustments.

The risks of untreated epilepsy to the fetus are considered to be greater than those associated with the antiepileptic drugs.[58] Major malformations are two to three times more likely to occur in children born to women taking antiepileptic drugs than to those who do not. Major malformations with valproic acid are dose related and range from 6.2% to 10.7%; use of valproic acid should be avoided if possible during pregnancy to minimize the risk of NTDs (e.g., spina bifida), facial clefts, and cognitive teratogenicity.[59,60] Rates of major malformation for monotherapy with antiepileptic drugs other than valproic acid range between 2.9% and 3.6%. Carbamazepine and lamotrigine appear to be safest based on available data. However, individual antiepileptic drugs are associated with malformations. Phenytoin, lamotrigine, and carbamazepine may cause cleft palate, while phenobarbital is associated with cardiac malformations. Polytherapy with antiepileptic drugs is associated with a greater rate of major malformation than monotherapy.[59,60]

When possible, antiepileptic drug monotherapy is recommended with medication regimen optimization occurring before conception.[59] Medication change solely to minimize teratogenic risk is not recommended. If drug withdrawal is planned, it should be attempted at least 6 months before attempting to conceive.[59] While vitamin K administration during the last month of gestation was previously recommended to decrease the risk of hemorrhagic complications in newborns, evidence to support this practice is lacking. The American Academy of Pediatrics recommends that all neonates receive vitamin K at delivery. All women taking antiepileptic drugs should receive folic acid supplementation; 4 to 5 mg daily starting before pregnancy and continuing through at least the first trimester.[58]

HUMAN IMMUNODEFICIENCY VIRUS INFECTION

❹ Pregnant women newly diagnosed with HIV, with or without prior treatment, should receive highly active antiretroviral therapy (HAART). The treatment regimen should be selected from those suggested for nonpregnant adults, with special consideration given to the teratogenic profile of each drug.[61] Women currently receiving antiretroviral treatment should be continued on their regimen when possible. If antiretroviral drugs are being used exclusively to prevent mother-to-child transmission, prophylaxis may be delayed until after the first trimester.

Zidovudine is the mainstay of antiretroviral therapy and is recommended for use during pregnancy, labor, and delivery, as well as during the postpartum period.[61] Lamivudine should be used along with zidovudine as the nucleoside reverse transcriptase inhibitor (NRTI) backbone of therapy when feasible. For HAART, two NRTIs plus either a nonnucleoside reverse transcriptase inhibitor (NNRTI) or a protease inhibitor is recommended; current guidelines recommend nevirapine or lopinavir/ritonavir. Efavirenz should be avoided during the first trimester and the entire pregnancy if possible. If therapy is discontinued during the first trimester, reintroduction of all medications should occur only when the ability to tolerate drug therapy is certain. All medications should be restarted at the same time to decrease risk of resistance. Zidovudine dosing recommendations during pregnancy are 300 mg twice daily or 200 mg three times a day. Intravenous zidovudine is recommended during labor, and the infant should receive the drug beginning 6 to 12 hours after birth and continuing for the first 6 weeks of life.

HYPERTENSION

❹ Treatment of stage 1 or 2 chronic hypertension (blood pressure 140–179 mm Hg systolic or 90–109 mmHg diastolic) during pregnancy is controversial because the physiologic drop in blood pressure during the first half of pregnancy may result in improved blood pressure control without drug treatment.[36,62] However, treatment may decrease uteroplacental blood flow and impair fetal development. Additionally, most of the increases in adverse fetal and maternal outcomes are caused by preeclampsia superimposed on chronic hypertension. Women should be monitored closely if treatment is discontinued, and therapy should be reinstituted if blood pressure exceeds 150 to 160 mm Hg systolic or 100 to 110 mm Hg diastolic or if target-organ damage occurs. Alternatively, antihypertensive drugs may be continued (except for angiotensin-converting enzyme inhibitors and angiotensin II receptor blockers) at the lowest effective dose. Use of diuretics (excluding spironolactone) is controversial but may be considered for chronic hypertension. Women with severe hypertension (blood pressure above 170 mmHg systolic or above 110 mmHg diastolic) should receive drug therapy to prevent occurrence of cerebrovascular hemorrhage or other target-organ damage.[37] Available evidence does not support superior efficacy of one agent versus another for blood pressure reduction.[34,36,37]

MENTAL HEALTH CONDITIONS

❹ Psychiatric illness affects approximately 500,000 pregnancies each year.[63,64] Anxiety disorders, including panic disorder, obsessive–compulsive disorder, generalized anxiety disorder, posttraumatic stress disorder, social anxiety disorder, and phobias, can cause adverse maternal and fetal outcomes such as spontaneous abortion, preterm delivery, prolonged labor, and fetal distress.[63]

Depression occurs in 10% to 16% of pregnant women.[63,64] Maternal depression is associated with greater risk for premature birth, low birth weight, and fetal growth restriction. In addition to the potential impact of maternal depression on obstetric complications, untreated depression may have long-term implications for normal infant development.[63] Up to 6.4% of Americans have bipolar disorder, with men and women equally affected, but the incidence in pregnancy is unknown. Patients with bipolar disorder may be more likely to relapse during pregnancy, especially with rapid discontinuation of drug therapy.[64]

Schizophrenia occurs in 1% to 2% of women, however the incidence in pregnancy is unknown.[63,64] Drug therapy is usually necessary, although some women refuse treatment because of concerns about teratogenicity or paranoid or delusional thinking. Maternal schizophrenia is associated with increased risk of perinatal death, low birth weight, small-for-gestational-age infants, cardiovascular malformations, preterm delivery, stillbirth, and infant death.[63]

Nonpharmacologic therapies may be tried in pregnant women with psychiatric illnesses who fail to respond or inadequately respond to drug therapy and in those who refuse drug therapy. Cognitive behavioral therapy and interpersonal psychotherapy have been shown beneficial in the treatment of anxiety disorders and depression.[64] Light therapy has also been effective for treatment of seasonal depression. Electroconvulsive therapy is considered safe and effective treatment of major depression, bipolar disorder, and schizophrenia.

Because most psychotropic medications are used to treat more than one condition, the reader should refer to other sources for information about treatment of specific mental health diagnoses. In general, monotherapy is preferred over polytherapy even if higher doses are required.[64]

Neither the selective serotonin reuptake inhibitors (SSRIs) nor the tricyclic antidepressants are considered major teratogens.[63] The SSRIs are the drugs of first choice for several mental health conditions in the general population and are widely used by pregnant women. Data suggest that paroxetine may cause a 1.5- to 2-fold increased risk of cardiac malformations; this finding has not been replicated for other SSRIs. About 1 two 2 newborns per 1,000 develop persistent pulmonary hypertension. Infants exposed to SSRIs in utero after 20 weeks' gestation developed persistent pulmonary hypertension at a rate 6 times greater than the background rate; this finding needs further confirmation.[65] Overall, the absolute risk of major malformations with SSRIs is small; approximately 2 in 1,000 births are affected.[63] Use of SSRIs late in pregnancy can precipitate neonatal withdrawal symptoms consisting of irritability and difficulty with feeding and breathing. There are concerns about adverse effects in infants born to women who use SSRIs during pregnancy. However, women who stop taking antidepressants are more likely to relapse, and this can also have implications for the well-being of the infant.

Studies completed over 30 years ago showed an increased risk of oral clefts with diazepam use during pregnancy; these findings were not confirmed in a subsequent study.[63] A recent meta-analysis found the absolute risk of oral cleft changed from 6 cases to 7 cases per 10,000 exposures (0.01%). Another large case-control study found no association between benzodiazepine use and congenital anomalies. Benzodiazepine use in the third trimester can cause infant sedation and withdrawal symptoms (i.e., restlessness, hypertonia, hyperreflexia, tremulousness, apnea, diarrhea, vomiting). "Floppy baby syndrome," consisting of low Apgar scores, hypothermia, poor muscle tone, feeding difficulties, and poor temperature adaptation, has also been described.

Mood stabilizers, such as lithium, lamotrigine, carbamazepine, and valproic acid, are often used to treat bipolar disorder.[63] The reader can find information related to the use of the seizure medications used for mood stabilization in the section on epilepsy.

Lithium's place in the treatment of bipolar disorder is controversial because of concerns about cardiovascular anomalies, especially Ebstein anomaly, in exposed infants.[63] A meta-analysis calculated that the relative risk for cardiac malformations was between 1.2 and 7.7 and for all congenital malformations was between 1.5 and 3. Stated differently, the risk for Ebstein anomaly after prenatal lithium exposure would rise from 1:20,000 to 1:1,000.[66] Other reported neonatal side effects include floppy baby syndrome, nephrogenic diabetes insipidus, hypoglycemia, cardiac arrhythmias, thyroid dysfunction, polyhydramnios, and premature delivery.[63,66] Lithium may cause lethargy, hypotonia, hypothermia, cyanosis, and changes in electrocardiogram in infants exposed through breast-feeding. If breastfeeding, the infant's lithium levels, thyroid function, and complete blood count should be monitored.

Chlorpromazine, haloperidol, and perphenazine have long histories of use during pregnancy, with no reported significant teratogenic effect.[63] Atypical antipsychotics are considered first-line treatment for schizophrenia because of their more favorable side-effect profiles and potential increased efficacy for treating negative symptoms compared with the older agents. However, use of atypical antipsychotics in pregnant women is controversial because of the limited data regarding teratogenic potential. Although olanzapine and clozapine have not been associated with increased risk for congenital malformations, they do cause weight gain and glucose intolerance, which have implications for poorer obstetric outcomes.[66] One study found a higher rate (10% vs. 2%) of low-birth-weight infants with olanzapine, clozapine, quetiapine, and risperidone compared with nonexposed infants.[63] At present, atypical antipsychotics do not appear to be safer than the typical agents.

THYROID DISORDERS

❹ Hypothyroidism affects 0.1 to 0.3% of pregnancies.[40] Untreated hypothyroidism increases the risk of preeclampsia, premature birth, miscarriage, and growth restriction; impaired neurological development in the fetus may also occur. Causes of hypothyroidism include autoimmune diseases (e.g., Hashimoto thyroiditis), iodine deficiency (uncommon in the United States), and thyroid dysfunction following surgery or ablative therapy for previous hyperthyroidism. Thyroid replacement therapy should be instituted with levothyroxine 0.1 to 0.15 mg/day in hypothyroid patients; the goal is to attain normal thyrotropin concentration. Women receiving thyroid replacement therapy before pregnancy may have an increased dosage requirement during pregnancy; any dose change should follow thyroid function testing. Laboratory follow-up of thyrotropin concentrations and free T_4 should occur every 8 weeks.

Hyperthyroidism affects approximately 0.2% of pregnancies and is associated with fetal death, low birth weight, intrauterine growth restriction, and preeclampsia.[40] Graves disease accounts for 95% of hyperthyroidism in pregnancy. Therapy includes the thioamides (initial doses are propylthiouracil 100–150 mg or methimazole 5–20 mg). Either agent is given three times daily with dose reduction after becoming euthyroid. Surgery is reserved for the most severe cases. The risks of uncontrolled hyperthyroidism outweigh the risks of the thioamides. Iodine-131 is contraindicated because of the risk of thyroid damage in the fetus. The goal of therapy is to attain free thyroxine concentrations near the upper limit of normal to allow for dose minimization and to limit fetal or neonatal hypothyroidism.

LABOR AND DELIVERY

Management of the pregnant woman during the perinatal period often requires drug therapy for pain and for potential complications.

PRETERM LABOR

Preterm labor occurs when there are cervical changes and uterine contractions between 20 and 37 weeks' gestation.[67,68] Preterm birth is the leading cause of infant morbidity and mortality in the United States, with an incidence of 12.8%. Risk factors for preterm delivery include previous preterm delivery, infections, multiple gestation, poverty, nonwhite race, maternal complication factors (e.g., smoking and use of illicit drugs or alcohol), and uterine functional causes (e.g., incompetent cervix); previous history and prior second trimester loss confer a higher risk.[67,68]

No adequate tests are available for monitoring and preventing preterm labor. Monitoring of uterine activity along with intensive surveillance does not minimize risk.[68] The presence of fetal fibronectin, a glycoprotein found in cervicovaginal secretions, indicates a high risk of preterm birth. Cervical shortening is also associated with preterm delivery. Fetal fibronectin determinations and cervical ultrasound have not helped to prevent preterm labor but have been useful for their negative predictive value.[68]

Tocolytic Therapy

The purposes of tocolytic therapy are threefold: (a) postpone delivery long enough to allow for the maximum effect of antenatal steroid administration; (b) allow for transportation of the mother to a facility equipped to deal with high-risk deliveries; and (c) prolongation of pregnancy when there are underlying, self-limited conditions that can cause labor, such as pyelonephritis or abdominal surgery, that are unlikely to cause recurrent preterm labor.[68–70] Tocolytics have not reduced the number of premature deliveries. The criteria for starting tocolysis are regular uterine contractions with cervical change. Tocolytic therapy should not be used in cases of intrauterine fetal demise, a lethal fetal anomaly, intrauterine infection, fetal distress, severe preeclampsia, vaginal bleeding, or maternal hemodynamic instability.

Four classes of tocolytics are available in the United States: β-agonists, magnesium, calcium channel blockers, and NSAIDs.[71] All four therapies have similar effectiveness in prolonging pregnancy from 48 hours to 1 week. However, this prolongation of pregnancy was not associated with a statistically significant reduction in overall rates of respiratory distress syndrome or neonatal death.

The β-agonists terbutaline and ritodrine have been used for tocolytic therapy.[69] Ritodrine is no longer available in the United States. Relative to other agents, β-agonists have a higher incidence of maternal side effects, including hyperkalemia, arrhythmias, hyperglycemia, hypotension, and pulmonary edema. Recommended terbutaline doses range from 250 to 500 mcg subcutaneously every 3 to 4 hours.[70]

Intravenous magnesium sulfate has been used for tocolysis; however, a Cochrane review does not support its effectiveness.[72] Heterogeneity of study designs and results along with small treatment arms in included studies may partially explain this finding;

however, its use remains controversial.[69] The incidence of cerebral palsy is increased in premature infants. In one study, intravenous magnesium use (6 g load followed by 2 g per hour continuous infusion) decreased the occurrence of moderate or severe cerebral palsy.[73] Although not the primary end point, the study suggests that women at risk for imminent delivery (up to 34 weeks' gestation) should receive intravenous magnesium. Maternal side effects are rare but can include pulmonary edema. At toxic levels, hypotension, muscle paralysis, tetany, cardiac arrest, and respiratory depression may occur.[70] Magnesium undergoes renal excretion; dose adjustment is required in women with impaired renal function.

CURRENT CONTROVERSY

Intravenous magnesium sulfate is commonly used in the United States for tocolysis. Some advocate cessation of its use because a Cochrane review found no difference in preterm delivery in the 48 hours after administration and an increase in perinatal death.[69,72]

Nifedipine is associated with fewer side effects than magnesium or β-agonist therapy.[69] Several studies have suggested that calcium channel blockers are superior to β-agonists for prolonging labor. One concern with the use of nifedipine is its hypotensive effect and corresponding change in uteroplacental blood flow. However, a meta-analysis showed reduced neonatal morbidity with calcium channel blocker use. With the initial diagnosis of preterm labor, 5 to 10 mg nifedipine can be administered sublingually every 15 to 20 minutes for three doses. After patient stabilization, if no evidence of continuing cervical dilation is seen, 10 to 20 mg nifedipine can be administered orally every 4 to 6 hours for preterm contractions.[70]

Nonsteroidal antiinflammatory drugs such as indomethacin have been used for tocolysis.[69,70] Oral or rectal doses of 50 to 100 mg, followed by an oral dose of 25 to 50 mg every 6 hours, have been used. An increased rate of premature constriction of the ductus arteriosus has been noted in infants with indomethacin use after 32 weeks' gestation and with use exceeding 48 hours.[69] Indomethacin may be used when tocolysis is needed despite treatment with magnesium for neuroprotection because other agents, such as calcium channel blockers, can cause hypotension when administered concurrently with magnesium.

Other Drug Therapies for Preterm Labor Prevention

Infection is a potential cause of preterm labor. Antibiotics have been used, in addition to tocolytics and corticosteroids, to improve the outcome of preterm labor; however, a Cochrane review showed no reduction in the incidence of preterm delivery but a trend toward increased neonatal mortality. Therefore, routine use of antibiotics is not recommended. However, if a patient experiences preterm premature rupture of membranes (PPROM) before 34 weeks' gestation, prophylactic antibiotics should be initiated. The combination of initial intravenous therapy (48 hours) with ampicillin and erythromycin, followed by 5 days of oral therapy with the same antibiotics, decreased the likelihood of chorioamnionitis and delivery for 3 weeks. Additionally, a reduction in major morbidities (i.e., death, respiratory distress syndrome, early sepsis, severe intraventricular hemorrhage, and necrotizing enterocolitis) was demonstrated.[74]

Progesterone administration in the setting of prior preterm birth is much debated. Two large randomized, controlled trials produced significant findings. First, the administration of intramuscular 17-alpha-hydroxyprogesterone weekly (250 mg) starting between weeks 16 and 20 and continued through week 36 in high-risk

women decreased the incidence of recurrent preterm birth.[75] The second study replicated the findings using vaginal progesterone suppositories (100 mg).[76] However, progesterone supplementation in women whose previous preterm birth occurred beyond 34 weeks produced similar rates of preterm delivery compared with placebo.[77] The American College of Obstetrics and Gynecology currently recommends that progesterone supplementation be limited to women with a singleton pregnancy and a previous history of spontaneous preterm birth.[78]

Antenatal Corticosteroids

❹ Use of antenatal corticosteroids for fetal lung maturation to prevent respiratory distress syndrome, intraventricular hemorrhage, and death in infants delivered prematurely is supported by a Cochrane review.[79] The current clinical recommendation is to administer betamethasone 12 mg intramuscularly every 24 hours for two doses or dexamethasone 6 mg intramuscularly every 12 hours for four doses to pregnant women between 26 and 34 weeks' gestation who are at risk for preterm delivery within the next 7 days. Benefits from antenatal corticosteroids are believed to begin within 24 hours.

Salvage ("rescue") treatment is administered to women who are at risk of delivering within 7 days but who have received a previous course of therapy. The incidence of respiratory distress syndrome was lower with the administration of rescue steroids compared with placebo (41.4% with betamethasone vs. 61.6% with placebo).[80]

GROUP B *STREPTOCOCCUS* INFECTION

❹ Maternal infection with group B *Streptococcus* (GBS) is associated with invasive disease in the newborn.[81,82] Women colonized with GBS have an increased risk for pregnancy loss, premature delivery, and transmission of the bacteria to the infant during delivery. Between 10% and 30% of pregnant women are colonized with GBS. The rate of invasive infection (defined as isolation of GBS from blood or other sterile body site excluding urine) in pregnant women is 0.12 per 1000 live births (range 0.11 to 0.14 per 1,000 births). The incidence of early-onset disease in neonates, although higher than in pregnant women, has declined steadily from 1.8 per 1,000 live births in 1990 to approximately 0.34 cases per 1,000 live births during 2003 to 2005. The consequences of neonatal infections include bacteremia, pneumonia, meningitis, and fatality in the newborn.[82] The case-fatality rate is approximately 4%.

Recommendations for prevention of GBS infection were updated in 2002.[82] Universal prenatal screening for GBS colonization is recommended. Antibiotics are given if the woman previously gave birth to an infant with invasive GBS disease or in the presence of GBS bacteriuria. All other pregnant women should have a vaginal/rectal culture at 35 to 37 weeks' gestation. If negative, antibiotics are not indicated. If a woman presents in labor and no screening information is available, antibiotics are given for fever greater than 100.4°F (38°C), membrane rupture at least 18 hours prior, or gestation under 37 weeks.

Penicillin G 5 million units given intravenously, followed by 2.5 million units given every 4 hours until delivery is the recommended treatment regimen.[82] Alternatively, ampicillin 2 g can be given intravenously, followed by 1 g every 4 hours. For women with penicillin allergy but not at risk for anaphylaxis, cefazolin 2 g intravenously, followed by 1 g every 8 hours, is recommended. In women at high risk for anaphylaxis, clindamycin 900 mg intravenously every 8 hours or erythromycin 500 mg intravenously every 6 hours is recommended. For penicillin-allergic women, GBS cultures should be sent for sensitivities. If resistant to clindamycin or erythromycin, vancomycin 1 g intravenously every 12 hours until delivery is appropriate.

CERVICAL RIPENING AND LABOR INDUCTION

Throughout gestation the cervix is closed and firm. During the last few weeks of pregnancy, the cervix softens and thins to facilitate labor.[83,84] This process is mediated by hormonal changes, including final mediation by prostaglandins E_2 and $F_2\alpha$, which increase collagenase activity in the cervix leading to thinning and dilation.

The rate of pregnancy induction ranges from 9.5% to 33.5%; the most common indications for induction are postdatism (beyond 42 weeks) and pregnancy-induced hypertension, which account for 80% of inductions.[83,84] Other reasons for induction include suspected fetal growth retardation, maternal hypertension, premature rupture of membranes with no active onset of labor, and social factors. Contraindications include placenta previa, oblique or transverse lie, pelvic structure abnormality, prolapsed umbilical cord, and active herpes. Concerns with induction of labor are ineffective labor and side effects, such as uterine hyperstimulation, that may adversely affect the infant and increase the likelihood of cesarean section.

Scoring systems have been used to determine the likelihood of successful labor induction. The Bishop scoring system is most commonly used and is based on five parameters: cervical dilation, cervical effacement (thinning), station of the baby's head, consistency of the cervix, and position of the cervix.[83,84] A Bishop score under 6 indicates the need for cervical ripening while a score above 8 corresponds to a likely successful vaginal delivery.

A number of nonpharmacologic methods are used for cervical ripening. Castor oil, hot baths, sexual intercourse, and nipple stimulation all have been suggested for labor induction.[83] Minimal evidence supports the efficacy of these methods. Use of a Foley catheter placed in an unfavorable cervix for ripening has been found as effective as prostaglandin E_2. Membrane stripping is safe and inexpensive.[83,84]

Prostaglandin E_2 analogs (e.g., dinoprostone [Prepidil gel, Cervidil vaginal insert]) are commonly used for cervical ripening. Prepidil 500 mcg is administered intracervically.[84] The dose may be repeated after 6 hours to a maximum of three doses in 24 hours. After administration, the patient remains supine for 30 minutes. Cervidil contains 10 mg dinoprostone with a slower, more constant release of medication than the gel. The insert is removed when labor begins or after 12 hours. Patients must be attached to a fetal heart rate monitor for the duration of Cervidil use and for 15 minutes after its removal.[83]

Misoprostol, a prostaglandin E_1 analog, is an effective and inexpensive drug for cervical ripening and labor induction.[84] Intravaginal administration of misoprostol is more effective than other prostaglandin agents and results in a shorter time to delivery. Oral misoprostol has been used successfully for cervical ripening and labor induction, but the evidence of safety is more extensive with intravaginal use. The most commonly encountered side effects are uterine hyperstimulation and meconium-stained amniotic fluid. Use of misoprostol is contraindicated in women with a previous uterine scar because of its association with uterine rupture, a catastrophic medical event.

CURRENT CONTROVERSY

Despite its efficacy and comparatively reasonable cost, some health systems have decided not to use misoprostol as an induction agent because of concerns about uterine rupture and lack of FDA indication for cervical ripening.[84]

Progesterone inhibits uterine contractions. Preliminary studies show that mifepristone, an antiprogesterone agent, compared with placebo results in a shorter time to delivery and fewer cesarean sections.[85] Limited information on fetal and maternal outcomes is available because of the small sample sizes.

Oxytocin is the most commonly used agent for labor induction after cervical ripening. By the end of pregnancy, the number of oxytocin receptors has increased by 300-fold.[83,84] A solution of 10 milliunits/mL is used for infusion. Oxytocin is effective in both low-dose (physiologic) and high-dose (pharmacologic) regimens.

LABOR ANALGESIA

In the first phase of labor, women perceive visceral pain caused by uterine contractions. Pain in the second phase of labor is associated with perineal stretching.[86]

Nonpharmacologic Approaches to Analgesia

Women who receive continuous support from nurses, midwives, childbirth educators, or doulas [laywomen trained in labor support], have fewer operative vaginal deliveries, cesarean deliveries, and requests for pain medication.[87] Warm water baths provide temporary pain relief but have not been shown to decrease the use of pharmacologic pain treatments. Intradermal injections of sterile water in the sacral area decrease back pain during labor for 45 to 120 minutes. However, requests for pain medication did not decrease in studies. Acupuncture has also been used for pain relief. Three randomized, controlled trials have shown that acupuncture decreases the need for analgesia, but more methodologically sound studies are needed. Use of audioanalgesia (music or white noise), relaxation and breathing techniques, application of heat and cold, aromatherapy, acupressure, and hypnosis have little to no evidence of effectiveness derived from randomized, controlled trials.

Pharmacologic Approaches to Labor Pain Management

The American College of Obstetricians and Gynecologists supports the concept that maternal request alone is a sufficient medical indication for labor analgesia.[88] The two main types of pharmacologic approaches in the United States are parenteral opioids and epidural analgesia.

Parenteral opioids are commonly used to alleviate labor pain.[89] In comparison with epidural analgesia, parenteral opioids have lower rates of oxytocin augmentation, result in shorter stages of labor, and require fewer instrumental deliveries.

Approximately 60% of women in the United States choose an epidural for pain relief during labor and report better pain relief than with other analgesic modalities.[89] With epidural analgesia, a catheter is introduced into the epidural space and an opioid and/or an anesthetic (e.g., fentanyl and/or bupivacaine) is administered. Combined spinal–epidural analgesia consists of injecting a single opioid bolus into the subarachnoid space to provide instant pain relief with additional use of a local anesthetic epidural. Patient-controlled epidural analgesia allows the patient to control the amount and timing of the anesthetic; it results in a lower total dose of local anesthetics used over the course of labor compared with continuous epidural infusions.[90]

Side effects of the regional anesthesia include hypotension, pruritus, and inability to void.[89] Epidural analgesia is associated with prolongation of the first and second stages of labor, higher numbers of instrumental deliveries, and maternal fever. A rare complication of epidural anesthesia is puncture of the subarachnoid space leading to a severe headache, which occurs in approximately 1% of women. Other complications include hypotension, nausea, vomiting, itching, and urinary retention. Low back pain has not been associated with the use of epidural analgesia.

POSTPARTUM HEMORRHAGE

The placenta is delivered after the delivery of the baby and is referred to as the third stage of labor. Postpartum hemorrhage is an obstetrical emergency and is a major cause of morbidity and mortality.[91] In the United States, the postpartum hemorrhage rate is approximately 1%–5% for vaginal deliveries.[92] The traditional definition of postpartum hemorrhage is more than 500 mL of blood within 24 hours of a vaginal delivery or 1,000 mL after a cesarean section; however, other definitions have also been suggested. Risk factors include retained placenta, failure to progress during the second stage of labor, placenta previa, placenta accreta, lacerations, instrumental delivery, large for gestational newborn, hypertensive disorders, induction of labor, augmentation of labor with oxytocin, prior history, obesity, and high parity.[93]

The most common cause of postpartum hemorrhage is uterine atony.[91,92] Initial management should include oxytocin. Early clamping and cutting of the umbilical cord as well as controlled traction of the cord also decrease the incidence.[91] Administration of a uterotonic medication (intramuscular oxytocin, ergotamine, or combination) before placental delivery and instituting active management of labor after all uncomplicated vaginal deliveries results in reduced maternal blood loss, fewer cases of postpartum hemorrhage, and less prolongation of the third stage of labor. Other uterotonic agents should be used if an inadequate response is attained with oxytocin alone. Methylergonovine, carboprost, misoprostol, and dinoprostone have all been used; less evidence is available for misoprostol and dinoprostone.

POSTPARTUM ISSUES

DRUG USE DURING LACTATION

❺ Most drugs transfer into breast milk, but breast-feeding may be continued in most circumstances. Healthcare providers should encourage breast-feeding women who require medications to continue breast-feeding whenever possible. Medications that are contraindicated or require the mother to pump and discard milk are few.

A wide variety of benefits (health, nutritional, immunologic, psychological, economic, developmental, and social) are imparted by breast-feeding to infants, mothers, and the family.[94,95] Women should breast-feed exclusively for 6 months and continue until at least 12 months of age while other foods are introduced.[95] Healthy People 2010 set a target of 75% of neonates being breast-fed at the time of birth and 50% of infants being breast-fed at 6 months of age.

Most drugs reach breast milk through passive diffusion, but other drug-related factors influence drug transfer from maternal circulation into breast milk, including (a) degree of protein binding in maternal plasma, (b) molecular weight, (c) lipid solubility (and corresponding fat content of milk), (d) maternal plasma concentration, (e) drug half-life, and (f) drug pH.[94,96] The degree of protein binding to maternal plasma proteins is one of the most significant factors affecting drug transfer to breast milk; highly bound medications transfer in low amounts. Low-molecular-weight drugs passively diffuse into breast milk, but larger molecules are not likely to transfer in large amounts. Higher lipid solubility of drugs also increases the likelihood of transfer. Colostrum is secreted in the first couple of days after birth and has high quantities of immunoglobulins, maternal lymphocytes, and maternal macrophages. Compared with mature milk, colostrum is lower in fat content, so highly lipid soluble drugs achieve higher concentrations in mature milk. The higher the concentration of drug in the mother's serum, the higher the concentration will be in the breast milk. As the drug is metabolized and

excreted by the mother, the mother's serum concentration drops, and drug in the breast milk may redistribute back into the mother's bloodstream. Maternal plasma pH is 7.4, while the pH of breast milk ranges between 6.8 and 7.[96] Weak bases are not ionized in the maternal circulation and easily transfer to breast milk. In the lower pH of breast milk, molecules become ionized and are less likely to diffuse back into maternal circulation ("ion trapping"). Likewise, drugs with longer half-lives are more likely to maintain higher levels in breast milk, resulting in greater exposure to the infant.

Infant-related factors may also influence the amount of drug ingested through breastfeeding.[94] Both the frequency of feedings and the amount of milk ingested are important considerations. Exclusively breast-fed infants are more likely to ingest larger amounts of drugs than older infants who receive other foods. Drugs unstable in gastric acid (aminoglycosides, omeprazole, heparin, insulin) are less likely to be absorbed by infants. Finally, infants may vary in their ability to metabolize and excrete ingested medication. Premature and full-term infants may not have full renal and liver function.

Strategies for reducing the risk to the infant include selection of medications that would be considered safe for use in the infant.[96] Drugs with shorter half-lives accumulate less, and those that are more protein bound do not cross into breast milk as well as those that are less protein bound. Drugs with lower oral bioavailability and lower lipid solubility are good choices. If the mother is using a once-daily medication, administration before the infant's longest sleep period may be advised to increase the interval to the next feeding. For medications taken multiple times per day, administration immediately after breast-feeding provides the longest interval for back diffusion of drug from the breast milk to the mother's serum. During short-term drug therapy, the mother can pump and discard milk to preserve her milk-producing capability if the medication is not considered compatible with breast-feeding.[94]

Industry-based research on transfer of drugs into breast milk is scarce.[94] Information from expert committees (e.g., American Academy of Pediatrics Committee on Drugs) and evidence-based textbooks or Web sites may be of assistance in providing reassurance regarding the safe use of medications in the lactating mother.

MASTITIS

Mastitis is inflammation in one breast.[97] It can be infectious or noninfectious; the most common cause is milk stasis. About 10% of women in the United States experience mastitis during the first 3 months postpartum. Signs and symptoms include breast tenderness, redness, warmth, and flulike symptoms.[98] Risk factors for developing mastitis include breast engorgement, plugged milk ducts, and cracked nipples.

Staphylococcus aureus is the most common bacterial cause of mastitis; *E. coli* and *Streptococcus* have also been implicated.[97,98] A 10- to 14-day course of antibiotics is usually given for treatment of mastitis; penicillinase-resistant penicillins (e.g., dicloxacillin, oxacillin) and cephalosporins (e.g., cephalexin) are frequently prescribed. Antiinflammatory drugs, such as ibuprofen, may provide some pain relief. Application of heat may also be helpful. Affected women should be counseled to continue breast-feeding from both breasts throughout treatment and to pump if breasts are not emptied completely with feedings.

POSTPARTUM DEPRESSION

Mood disorders in the postpartum period may include postpartum blues, postpartum depression, and postpartum psychosis.[99] Postpartum blues is common, usually affecting 15% to 85% of new mothers within the first 10 days of delivery, and generally does not require treatment. Symptoms include anxiety, anger, and sadness.

Postpartum psychosis is more severe but is rare, affecting less than 1% of new mothers.

Postpartum depression affects up to 15% of women.[99] Symptoms may develop during pregnancy or up to 6 months after delivery, although the strict definition for major depressive disorder after delivery specifies symptom occurrence within 1 month. Psychotherapy, including interpersonal psychotherapy, cognitive behavioral therapy, and group/family therapy, has been shown effective for treatment of postpartum depression.

In cases where pharmacotherapy is warranted, selection of medication with low transfer to breast milk is desirable. Sertraline is generally considered a first-line treatment because of its minimal transfer into breast milk and lack of reported adverse events in infants.[94,99] Paroxetine and nortriptyline are considered second-line.

CURRENT CONTROVERSY

Treatment of postpartum depression in the breast-feeding mother poses challenges since all antidepressants transfer into breast milk, and long-term effects on cognitive, behavioral, motor, and neurologic development are unknown.[99] Postpartum depression poses significant risks to both mother and infant. Benefits and risks of pharmacologic and nonpharmacologic therapy must be weighed in selecting treatments for women with postpartum depression.

RELACTATION

Adequate milk removal from the breast by breastfeeding or pumping is necessary to maintain or increase milk production.[100] Relactation is the process of increasing the breast milk supply for women who have failed lactogenesis II, who have inadequate milk production despite appropriate breastfeeding frequency or pumping, or who have weaned or never breast-fed after delivery. Lactation can also be induced in women who have not recently delivered a baby, such as adoptive mothers. The mainstay of therapy for this condition involves nipple stimulation either by the infant's nursing or by pumping of the breast with a mechanical pump or the hand.

Metoclopramide can be used for relactation if nonpharmacologic measures are ineffective because of its stimulation of prolactin secretion.[100] The most common dose is 10 mg orally three times daily for 7 to 14 days. Breast milk production can be increased up to 100% or more in women, although many of the studies have inadequate designs. Breast milk production may decrease after metoclopramide therapy is stopped, but production will continue if lactation has been established successfully.

CONCLUSION

Many women perceive a high inherent risk of birth defects with drug exposure during pregnancy. This perception, linked with a high rate of unplanned pregnancies, may create anxiety because of drug exposure prior to the discovery of pregnancy.

Some medications are considered safe for use in pregnancy because of frequent use with no apparent increase in the rate of congenital problems. In some cases, ensuring the health of the mother and the fetus will require selection or continuation of medications that have been associated with a higher risk of adverse effects to the fetus. In these instances, realistic information about the types and likelihood of adverse effects will aid the patient and her family in making decisions.

Healthcare providers who care for pregnant women must work in collaboration to seek, evaluate, and present the most contemporary and accurate information to their patients. Use of technology to access evidence-based resources, databases related to drug use in pregnancy, and primary and secondary literature may assist healthcare practitioners in accessing relevant medication information to manage drug therapy needs during pregnancy and lactation.

ACKNOWLEDGMENTS

The authors gratefully acknowledge the work of Denise L. Walbrandt Pigarelli, Connie K. Kraus, and Beth E. Potter, who served as authors in the 7th edition of *Pharmacotherapy: A Pathophysiologic Approach*.

ABBREVIATIONS

FDA: Food and Drug Administration

GBS: group B *Streptococcus*

GDM: gestational diabetes mellitus

HAART: highly active antiretroviral therapy

hCG: human chorionic gonadotropin

HEG: hyperemesis gravidarum

HIV: human immunodeficiency virus

NNRTI: nonnucleoside reverse transcriptase inhibitor

NRTI: nucleoside reverse transcriptase inhibitor

NSAIDs: nonsteroidal antiinflammatory drugs

NTDs: neural tube defects

PPROM: preterm premature rupture of the membranes

SSRIs: selective serotonin reuptake inhibitors

TSH: thyroid stimulating hormone

REFERENCES

1. Ord T. The scourge: Moral implications of natural embryo loss. Am J Bioeth 2008;8:12–9.
2. Brent RL. Environmental causes of human congenital malformations: The pediatrician's role in dealing with these complex clinical problems caused by a multiplicity of environmental and genetic factors. Pediatrics 2004;113(4 suppl):957–968.
3. Talbot P, Shur BD, Myles DG. Cell adhesion and fertilization: Steps in oocyte transport, sperm-zona pellucida interactions, and sperm-egg fusion. Biol Reprod 2003;68:1–9.
4. Cunningham FG, Leveno KJ, Bloom SL, et al. Implantation, embryogenesis, and placental development. In: Cunningham FG, Leveno KJ, Bloom SL, et al. Williams Obstetrics, Chap. 3, 22nd ed., *http://www.accessmedicine.com/content.aspx?aID=728347*.
5. Bernstein HB, Weinstein M. Normal pregnancy and prenatal care. In: DeCherney AH, Nathan L, eds. Current Diagnosis and Treatment Obstetrics and Gynecology, Chap. 9, 10th ed.: *http://www.accessmedicine.com/content.aspx?aID=2384287*.
6. Cunningham FG, Leveno KJ, Bloom SL, et al. Fetal growth and development. In: Cunningham FG, Leveno KJ, Bloom SL, et al. Williams Obstetrics, Chap. 4, 22nd ed.: *http://www.accessmedicine.com/content.aspx?aID=733548*.
7. Cunningham FG, Leveno KJ, Bloom SL, et al. Prenatal care. In: Cunningham FG, Leveno KJ, Bloom SL, et al. Williams Obstetrics, Chap. 8, 22nd ed.: *http://www.accessmedicine.com/content.aspx?aID=742204*.

8. McCarter-Spaulding DE. Medications in pregnancy and lactation. MCN Am J Matern Child Nurs 2005;30:10–17.

9. Kahn DA, Koos BJ. Maternal physiology during pregnancy. In: DeCherney AH, Nathan L, eds. Current Diagnosis and Treatment Obstetrics and Gynecology, Chap. 7, 10th ed.: *http://www. accessmedicine.com/content.aspx?aID=2383850.*

10. Syme MR, Paxton JW, Keelan JA. Drug transfer and metabolism by the human placenta. Clin Pharmacokinet 2004;43:487–514.

11. Polifka JE, Friedman JM. Medical genetics, I: Clinical teratology in the age of genomics. CMAJ 2002;167:265–273.

12. Irl C, Hasford J. Assessing the safety of drugs in pregnancy: The role of prospective cohort studies. Drug Saf 2000;22:169–177.

13. Schaefer C, Ornoy A, Clementi M, et al. Using observational cohort data for studying drug effects on pregnancy outcome—Methodological considerations. Reprod Toxicol 2008;26:36–41.

14. Content and format of labeling for human prescription drug and biological products: Requirements for pregnancy and lactation labeling (proposed rules). Federal Register 73:104 (May 29, 2008): 30831–30868.

15. Johnson K, Posner SF, Biermann J, et al. Recommendations to improve preconception health and health care—United States. A report of the CDC/ATSDR Preconception Care Work Group and the Select Panel on Preconception Care. MMWR Recomm Rep 2006;55(RR-6):1–23.

16. Korenbrot CC, Steinberg A, Bender C, Newberry S. Preconception care: A systematic review. Matern Child Health J 2002;6:75–88.

17. Folic acid for the prevention of neural tube defects: U.S. Preventive Services Task Force recommendation statement. Ann Intern Med 2009;150:626–631.

18. Lumley J, Chamberlain C, Dowswell T, et al. Interventions for promoting smoking cessation during pregnancy. Cochrane Database Syst Rev 2009(3):CD001055.

19. Coleman T. Recommendations for the use of pharmacological smoking cessation strategies in pregnant women. CNS Drugs 2007;21: 983–993.

20. Benowitz N, Dempsey D. Pharmacotherapy for smoking cessation during pregnancy. Nicotine Tob Res 2004;6(suppl 2):S189–202.

21. Keller J, Frederking D, Layer P. The spectrum and treatment of gastrointestinal disorders during pregnancy. Nat Clin Pract Gastroenterol Hepatol 2008;5:430–443.

22. Mahadevan U, Kane S. American gastroenterological association institute technical review on the use of gastrointestinal medications in pregnancy. Gastroenterology 2006;131:283–311.

23. Quijano CE, Abalos E. Conservative management of symptomatic and/or complicated haemorrhoids in pregnancy and the puerperium. Cochrane Database Syst Rev 2005(3):CD004077.

24. Badell ML, Ramin SM, Smith JA. Treatment options for nausea and vomiting during pregnancy. Pharmacotherapy 2006;26:1273–1287.

25. Diagnosis and classification of diabetes mellitus. Diabetes Care 2009;32(suppl 1):S62–67.

26. Serlin DC, Lash RW. Diagnosis and management of gestational diabetes mellitus. Am Fam Physician 2009;80:57–62.

27. Screening for gestational diabetes mellitus: U.S. Preventive Services Task Force recommendation statement. Ann Intern Med 2008;148: 759–765.

28. Metzger BE, Buchanan TA, Coustan DR, et al. Summary and recommendations of the Fifth International Workshop-Conference on Gestational Diabetes Mellitus. Diabetes Care 2007;30(suppl 2): S251–260.

29. de Veciana M, Major CA, Morgan MA, et al. Postprandial versus preprandial blood glucose monitoring in women with gestational diabetes mellitus requiring insulin therapy. N Engl J Med 1995;333:1237–1241.

30. Reece EA, Homko CJ. Prepregnancy care and the prevention of fetal malformations in the pregnancy complicated by diabetes. Clin Obstet Gynecol 2007;50:990–997.

31. Crowther CA, Hiller JE, Moss JR, et al. Effect of treatment of gestational diabetes mellitus on pregnancy outcomes. N Engl J Med 2005;352:2477–2486.

32. Alwan N, Tuffnell DJ, West J. Treatments for gestational diabetes. Cochrane Database Syst Rev 2009(3):CD003395.

33. Leeman L, Fontaine P. Hypertensive disorders of pregnancy. Am Fam Physician 2008;78:93–100.

34. Abalos E, Duley L, Steyn DW, Henderson-Smart DJ. Antihypertensive drug therapy for mild to moderate hypertension during pregnancy. Cochrane Database Syst Rev 2007(1):CD002252.

35. Hofmeyr GJ, Duley L, Atallah A. Dietary calcium supplementation for prevention of pre-eclampsia and related problems: A systematic review and commentary. BJOG 2007;114:933–943.

36. Podymow T, August P. Update on the use of antihypertensive drugs in pregnancy. Hypertension 2008;51:960–969.

37. Duley L, Henderson-Smart DJ, Meher S. Drugs for treatment of very high blood pressure during pregnancy. Cochrane Database Syst Rev 2006(3):CD001449.

38. Duley L, Henderson-Smart DJ, Meher S, King JF. Antiplatelet agents for preventing pre-eclampsia and its complications. Cochrane Database Syst Rev 2007(2):CD004659.

39. Duley L, Meher S, Abalos E. Management of pre-eclampsia. BMJ 2006;332:463–468.

40. Neale DM, Cootauco AC, Burrow G. Thyroid disease in pregnancy. Clin Perinatol 2007;34:543–557.

41. Casey BM, Leveno KJ. Thyroid disease in pregnancy. Obstet Gynecol 2006;108:1283–1292.

42. Bates SM, Greer IA, Pabinger I, et al. Venous thromboembolism, thrombophilia, antithrombotic therapy, and pregnancy: American College of Chest Physicians Evidence-Based Clinical Practice Guidelines, 8th ed. Chest 2008;133(6 suppl):844S–886S.

43. Mittal P, Wing DA. Urinary tract infections in pregnancy. Clin Perinatol 2005;32:749–764.

44. Schnarr J, Smaill F. Asymptomatic bacteriuria and symptomatic urinary tract infections in pregnancy. Eur J Clin Invest 2008;38(suppl 2): 50–57.

45. Vazquez JC, Villar J. Treatments for symptomatic urinary tract infections during pregnancy. Cochrane Database Syst Rev 2003(4):CD002256.

46. Workowski KA, Berman SM. Sexually transmitted diseases treatment guidelines, 2006. MMWR Recomm Rep 2006;55(RR-11):1–94.

47. ACOG Practice Bulletin. Clinical management guidelines for obstetrician-gynecologists. No. 82 June 2007. Management of herpes in pregnancy. Obstet Gynecol 2007;109:1489–1498.

48. Menon R, Bushnell CD. Headache and pregnancy. Neurologist 2008;14:108–119.

49. Martin SR, Foley MR. Approach to the pregnant patient with headache. Clin Obstet Gynecol 2005;48:2–11.

50. Schatz M, Dombrowski MP. Clinical practice: Asthma in pregnancy. N Engl J Med 2009;360:1862–1869.

51. Expert Panel Report 3 (EPR-3): Guidelines for the Diagnosis and Management of Asthma—Summary Report 2007. J Allergy Clin Immunol 2007;120(5 suppl):S94–138.

52. Global Strategy for Asthma Management and Prevention. Update from NHLB/WHO Workshop Report 1995. Global Initiative for Asthma (GINA), revised 2006: updated 2008.

53. Gilbert C, Mazzotta P, Loebstein R, Koren G. Fetal safety of drugs used in the treatment of allergic rhinitis: A critical review. Drug Saf 2005;28:707–719.

54. Piette V, Daures JP, Demoly P. Treating allergic rhinitis in pregnancy. Curr Allergy Asthma Rep 2006;6:232–238.

55. Leachman SA, Reed BR. The use of dermatologic drugs in pregnancy and lactation. Dermatol Clin 2006;24:167–197.

56. Preconception care of women with diabetes. Diabetes Care 2004;27(suppl 1):S76–78.

57. Harden CL, Hopp J, Ting TY, et al. Management issues for women with epilepsy-Focus on pregnancy (an evidence-based review), I: Obstetrical complications and change in seizure frequency: Report of the Quality Standards Subcommittee and Therapeutics and Technology Assessment Subcommittee of the American Academy of Neurology and the American Epilepsy Society. Epilepsia 2009;50:1229–1236.

58. Tomson T, Battino D. Pregnancy and epilepsy: What should we tell our patients? J Neurol 2009;256:856–862.

59. Harden CL, Sethi NK. Epileptic disorders in pregnancy: an overview. Curr Opin Obstet Gynecol 2008;20:557–562.

60. Harden CL, Meador KJ, Pennell PB, et al. Management issues for women with epilepsy-Focus on pregnancy (an evidence-based review), II: Teratogenesis and perinatal outcomes: Report of the

Quality Standards Subcommittee and Therapeutics and Technology Subcommittee of the American Academy of Neurology and the American Epilepsy Society. Epilepsia 2009;50:1237–1246.

61. Perinatal HIV Guidelines Working Group. Public Health Service Task Force Recommendations for Use of Antiretroviral Drugs in Pregnant HIV-Infected Women for Maternal Health and Interventions to Reduce Perinatal HIV Transmission in the United States. April 29, 2009:1–90, http://aidsinfo.nih.gov/contentfiles/perinatalgl.pdf.

62. Karthikeyan VJ, Lip GY. Hypertension in pregnancy: Pathophysiology and management strategies. Curr Pharm Des 2007;13:2567–2579.

63. ACOG Practice Bulletin: Clinical management guidelines for obstetrician-gynecologists number 92, April 2008 (replaces practice bulletin number 87, November 2007). Use of psychiatric medications during pregnancy and lactation. Obstet Gynecol 2008;111:1001–1020.

64. Van Mullem C, Tillett J. Psychiatric disorders in pregnancy. J Perinat Neonatal Nurs 2009;23:124–130.

65. Chambers CD, Hernandez-Diaz S, Van Marter LJ, et al. Selective serotonin-reuptake inhibitors and risk of persistent pulmonary hypertension of the newborn. N Engl J Med 2006;354:579–587.

66. Levey L, Ragan K, Hower-Hartley A, et al. Psychiatric disorders in pregnancy. Neurol Clin 2004;22:863–893.

67. Damus K. Prevention of preterm birth: A renewed national priority. Curr Opin Obstet Gynecol 2008;20:590–596.

68. Chandiramani M, Shennan A. Preterm labour: update on prediction and prevention strategies. Curr Opin Obstet Gynecol 2006;18: 618–624.

69. Giles W, Bisits A. Preterm labour: The present and future of tocolysis. Best Pract Res Clin Obstet Gynaecol 2007;21:857–868.

70. Weismiller DG. Preterm labor. Am Fam Physician 1999;59:593–602.

71. Haas DM, Imperiale TF, Kirkpatrick PR, et al. Tocolytic therapy: A meta-analysis and decision analysis. Obstet Gynecol 2009;113: 585–594.

72. Crowther CA, Hiller JE, Doyle LW. Magnesium sulphate for preventing preterm birth in threatened preterm labour. Cochrane Database Syst Rev 2002(4):CD001060.

73. Rouse DJ, Hirtz DG, Thom E, et al. A randomized, controlled trial of magnesium sulfate for the prevention of cerebral palsy. N Engl J Med 2008;359:895–905.

74. American College of Obstetricians and Gynecologists. Premature rupture of membranes. Practice Bulletin No. 80. Washington, DC: ACOG; 2007a.

75. Meis PJ, Connors N. Progesterone treatment to prevent preterm birth. Clin Obstet Gynecol 2004;47:784–795; discussion 881–882.

76. da Fonseca EB, Bittar RE, Carvalho MH, Zugaib M. Prophylactic administration of progesterone by vaginal suppository to reduce the incidence of spontaneous preterm birth in women at increased risk: A randomized placebo-controlled double-blind study. Am J Obstet Gynecol 2003;188:419–424.

77. Spong CY, Meis PJ, Thom EA, et al. Progesterone for prevention of recurrent preterm birth: Impact of gestational age at previous delivery. Am J Obstet Gynecol 2005;193(3 Pt 2):1127–1131.

78. ACOG Committee Opinion no. 419 October 2008 (replaces no. 291, November 2003). Use of progesterone to reduce preterm birth. Obstet Gynecol 2008;112:963–965.

79. Roberts D, Dalziel S. Antenatal corticosteroids for accelerating fetal lung maturation for women at risk of preterm birth. Cochrane Database Syst Rev 2006(3):CD004454.

80. Garite TJ, Kurtzman J, Maurel K, Clark R. Impact of a "rescue course" of antenatal corticosteroids: A multicenter randomized placebo-controlled trial. Am J Obstet Gynecol 2009;200:248 e1–9.

81. Phares CR, Lynfield R, Farley MM, et al. Epidemiology of invasive group B streptococcal disease in the United States, 1999–2005. JAMA 2008;299:2056–2065.

82. Schrag S, Gorwitz R, Fultz-Butts K, Schuchat A. Prevention of perinatal group B streptococcal disease. Revised guidelines from CDC. MMWR Recomm Rep 2002;51(RR-11):1–22.

83. Tenore JL. Methods for cervical ripening and induction of labor. Am Fam Physician 2003;67:2123–2128.

84. Sanchez-Ramos L. Induction of labor. Obstet Gynecol Clin North Am 2005;32:181–200.

85. Hapangama D, Neilson JP. Mifepristone for induction of labour. Cochrane Database Syst Rev 2009(3):CD002865.

86. Kuczkowski KM. Labor pain and its management with the combined spinal-epidural analgesia: What does an obstetrician need to know? Arch Gynecol Obstet 2007;275:183–185.

87. Simkin P, Bolding A. Update on nonpharmacologic approaches to relieve labor pain and prevent suffering. J Midwifery Womens Health 2004;49:489–504.

88. ACOG Committee Opinion no. 295: Pain relief during labor. Obstet Gynecol 2004;104:213.

89. Anim-Somuah M, Smyth R, Howell C. Epidural versus non-epidural or no analgesia in labour. Cochrane Database Syst Rev 2005(4):CD000331.

90. van der Vyver M, Halpern S, Joseph G. Patient-controlled epidural analgesia versus continuous infusion for labour analgesia: a meta-analysis. Br J Anaesth 2002;89:459–465.

91. Chong YS, Su LL, Arulkumaran S. Current strategies for the prevention of postpartum haemorrhage in the third stage of labour. Curr Opin Obstet Gynecol 2004;16:143–150.

92. Mousa HA, Alfirevic Z. Treatment for primary postpartum haemorrhage. Cochrane Database Syst Rev 2007(1):CD003249.

93. Sheiner E, Sarid L, Levy A, et al. Obstetric risk factors and outcome of pregnancies complicated with early postpartum hemorrhage: A population-based study. J Matern Fetal Neonatal Med 2005;18:149–154.

94. Ilett KF, Kristensen JH. Drug use and breastfeeding. Expert Opin Drug Saf 2005;4:745–768.

95. Gartner LM, Morton J, Lawrence RA, et al. Breastfeeding and the use of human milk. Pediatrics 2005;115:496–506.

96. Della-Giustina K, Chow G. Medications in pregnancy and lactation. Emerg Med Clin North Am 2003;21:585–613.

97. Jahanfar S, Ng CJ, Teng CL. Antibiotics for mastitis in breastfeeding women. Cochrane Database Syst Rev 2009(1):CD005458.

98. Walker M. Conquering common breast-feeding problems. J Perinat Neonatal Nurs 2008;22:267–274.

99. Pearlstein T, Howard M, Salisbury A, Zlotnick C. Postpartum depression. Am J Obstet Gynecol 2009;200:357–364.

100. Betzold CM. Galactagogues. J Midwifery Womens Health 2004;49: 151–154.

CHAPTER

88

Contraception

SARAH P. SHRADER, KELLY R. RAGUCCI, AND VANESSA A. DIAZ

KEY CONCEPTS

❶ The attitude of the patient and sexual partner toward contraceptive methods, efficacy rate, the reliability of the patient in using the method correctly (which may affect the effectiveness of the method), noncontraceptive benefits, and the patient's ability to pay must be considered when selecting a contraceptive method.

❷ Patient-specific factors (e.g., frequency of intercourse, age, smoking status, and concomitant diseases, or medications) must be evaluated when selecting a contraceptive method.

❸ Adverse effects or difficulties using the chosen method should be monitored carefully and managed in consideration of patient-specific factors.

❹ Accurate and timely counseling on the optimal use of the contraceptive method and strategies for minimizing sexually transmitted diseases must be provided to all patients when contraceptives are initiated and on an ongoing basis.

❺ Emergency contraception may prevent pregnancy after unprotected intercourse or when regular contraceptive methods have failed.

Unintended pregnancy is a significant public health problem. In the United States, approximately 62 million women are of childbearing age, and approximately 6 million become pregnant each year.[1] The most recent data reveal that 31% of pregnancies are unintended, with the highest rates occurring in women aged 25 to 44 years (38%).[1] About half of all unintended pregnancies end in abortion, and half also occurred in sexually active couples who claimed they used some method of contraception.[2] If the goal of contraception—for pregnancies to be planned and desired—is to be realized, education on the use and efficacy of contraceptive methods must be improved.

ETIOLOGY AND PATHOPHYSIOLOGY

Comprehension of the hormonal regulation of the normal menstrual cycle is essential to understanding contraception in women (Fig. 88–1). The cycle of menstruation begins with menarche, usually around age 12 years, and continues to occur in nonpregnant

Learning objectives, review questions, and other resources can be found at **www.pharmacotherapyonline.com**.

women until menopause, usually around age 50 years. Factors such as race, body weight, medical conditions, and family history can affect the menstrual cycle.[3,4] The cycle includes the vaginal discharge of sloughed endometrium called *menses*. The menstrual cycle comprises three phases: follicular (or preovulatory), ovulatory, and luteal (or postovulatory).

THE MENSTRUAL CYCLE

The first day of menses is referred to as *day 1 of the menstrual cycle* and marks the beginning of the follicular phase.[3,4] The follicular phase continues until ovulation, which typically occurs on day 14. The time after ovulation is referred to as the *luteal phase*, which lasts until the beginning of the next menstrual cycle. The median menstrual cycle length is 28 days, but it can range from 21 to 40 days. Generally, variation in length is greatest in the follicular phase, particularly in the years immediately after menarche and before menopause.[4]

The menstrual cycle is influenced by the hormonal relationships among the hypothalamus, anterior pituitary, and ovaries.[3] The hypothalamus secretes gonadotropin-releasing hormone (GnRH) in a pulsatile fashion.[3,4] These GnRH bursts stimulate the anterior pituitary to secrete bursts of gonadotropins, follicle-stimulating hormone (FSH), and luteinizing hormone (LH). FSH and LH direct events in the ovarian follicles that result in the production of a fertile ovum.

Follicular Phase

In the first 4 days of the menstrual cycle, FSH levels rise and allow the recruitment of a small group of follicles for continued growth and development (Fig. 88–1).[3,4] Between days 5 and 7, one follicle becomes dominant and later ruptures, releasing the oocyte. The dominant follicle develops increasing amounts of estradiol and inhibin, which cause a negative feedback on the hypothalamic secretion of GnRH and pituitary secretion of FSH, causing atresia of the remaining follicles recruited during the cycle.

Once the follicle has received FSH stimulation, it must receive continued FSH stimulation or it will die.[3,4] FSH allows the follicle to enlarge and synthesize estradiol, progesterone, and androgen. Estradiol stops the menstrual flow from the previous cycle, thickening the endometrial lining of the uterus to prepare it for embryonic implantation. Estrogen is responsible for increased production of thin, watery cervical mucus, which will enhance sperm transport during fertilization. FSH regulates the aromatase enzymes that convert androgens to estrogens in the follicle. If a follicle has insufficient aromatase, the follicle will not survive.

Ovulation

When estradiol levels remain elevated for a sustained period of time, the pituitary releases a midcycle LH surge (Fig. 88–1).[3,4] This LH surge stimulates the final stages of follicular maturation and

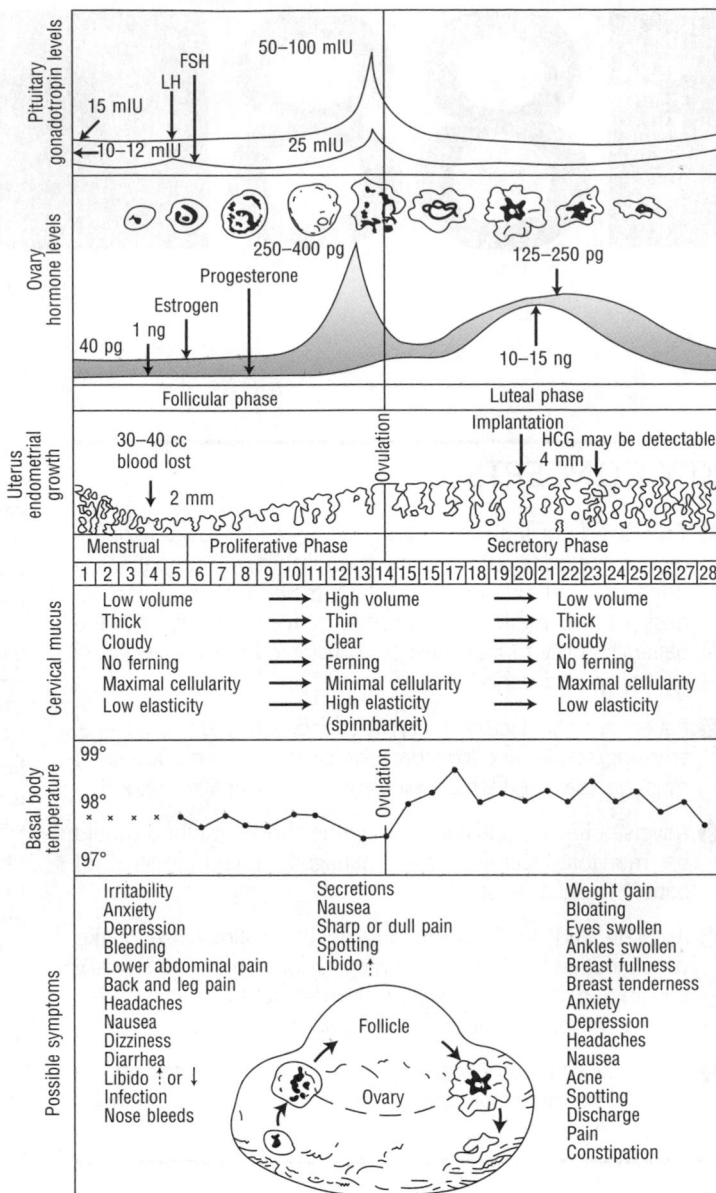

FIGURE 88-1. Menstrual cycle events, idealized 28-day cycle. (FSH, follicle-stimulating hormone; HCG, human chorionic gonadotropin, LH, luteinizing hormone.) *(From Hatcher et al.[4] This figure may be reproduced at no cost to the reader.)*

ovulation (follicular rupture and release of the oocyte). On average, ovulation occurs 24 to 36 hours after the estradiol peak and 10 to 16 hours after the LH peak. The LH surge, which occurs 28 to 32 hours before a follicle ruptures, is the most clinically useful predictor of approaching ovulation. After ovulation, the oocyte is released and travels to the fallopian tube, where it can be fertilized and transported to the uterus for embryonic implantation. Conception is most successful when intercourse takes place from 2 days before ovulation to the day of ovulation.

Luteal Phase

After rupture of the follicle and release of the ovum, the remaining luteinized follicles become the corpus luteum, which synthesizes androgen, estrogen, and progesterone (Fig. 88–1).[3,4] Progesterone helps to maintain the endometrial lining, which sustains the implanted embryo and maintains the pregnancy. It also inhibits GnRH and gonadotropin release, preventing the development of new follicles. If pregnancy occurs, human chorionic gonadotropin prevents regression of the corpus luteum and stimulates continued production of estrogen and progesterone secretion to maintain the pregnancy until the placenta is able to fulfill this role.

If fertilization or implantation does not occur, the corpus luteum degenerates, and progesterone production declines.[3,4] The life span of the corpus luteum depends on the continuous presence of small amounts of LH, and its average duration of function is 9 to 11 days. As progesterone levels decline, endometrial shedding (menstruation) occurs, and a new menstrual cycle begins. At the end of the luteal phase, when estrogen and progesterone levels are low, FSH levels start to rise, and follicular recruitment for the next cycle begins.

EPIDEMIOLOGY

Contraception implies the prevention of pregnancy following sexual intercourse by inhibiting viable sperm from coming into contact with a mature ovum (i.e., methods that act as barriers or prevent ovulation) or by preventing a fertilized ovum from implanting successfully in the endometrium (i.e., mechanisms that create an unfavorable uterine environment). These methods differ in their relative effectiveness, safety, and patient acceptability.[3-5]

The actual effectiveness of any contraceptive method is difficult to determine because many factors affect contraceptive failure.

A failure in patients who use the contraceptive agent properly is considered a method failure or perfect-use failure. It is also important to consider user failure or typical-use failure rates, which are usually higher because they take into account the user's ability to follow directions correctly and consistently.[3,4]

CLINICAL PRESENTATION

Most health maintenance annual visits should include assessment of and counseling about reproductive health. Clinicians may use this opportunity to provide contraception and educate patients on prevention of sexually transmitted diseases (STDs). Traditionally, hormonal contraception is provided subsequent to breast and pelvic examinations. However, the need for the physical examination may delay access to contraception, resulting in unintended pregnancies. In addition, requiring breast and pelvic examinations prior to prescription of hormonal contraception reinforces the incorrect perception that these methods of contraceptives are harmful. Therefore, the American Congress of Obstetrics and Gynecology (ACOG) and other national organizations allow provision of hormonal contraception after a simple medical history and blood pressure measurement.[6] Other preventive measures, such as pelvic and breast examinations, provision of the human papillomavirus vaccine, and screening for cervical neoplasia can be accomplished during routine annual office visits.[6–9]

TREATMENT

DESIRED OUTCOME

The obvious goal of treatment with all methods of contraception is to prevent pregnancy. However, many health benefits are associated with contraceptive methods, including prevention of STDs (with condoms), improvements in menstrual cycle regularity (with hormonal contraceptives), improvements in certain health conditions (with oral contraceptives [OCs]), and management of perimenopause.[3]

NONPHARMACOLOGIC THERAPY

Periodic Abstinence

1 **2** Motivated couples may use the abstinence (rhythm) method of contraception, avoiding sexual intercourse during the days of the menstrual cycle when conception is likely to occur. Physiologic changes, such as basal body temperature and cervical mucus are used during each cycle to determine the fertile period. The major drawbacks are the relatively high pregnancy rates and avoidance of intercourse for several days during each menstrual cycle.[3,4]

Barrier Techniques

1 **2** The effectiveness of barrier methods depends almost exclusively on motivation to use them consistently and correctly.[3,4] These methods include condoms, diaphragms, cervical caps, and sponges (Table 88–1). A major disadvantage is higher failure rates than most hormonal contraceptives; thus, provision of counseling and an advanced prescription for emergency contraception (EC) are recommended for all patients using barrier methods as their primary means of contraception.

Condoms create a mechanical barrier, preventing direct contact of the vagina with semen, genital lesions, and infectious secretions.[3,4] Most condoms in the United States are made of latex, which is impermeable to viruses. A small proportion are made

from lamb intestine, which is not impermeable to viruses. Synthetic condoms manufactured from polyurethane are another option, these condoms are latex-free and do protect against viruses. Condoms are used worldwide as protection from STDs including human immunodeficiency virus (HIV). When condoms are used in conjunction with any other barrier method, their effectiveness theoretically approaches 98%. Spillage of semen or perforation and tearing of the condom can occur, but proper use minimizes these problems.[4] Mineral oil–based vaginal drug formulations (e.g., Cleocin, Premarin, and Monistat), lotions, or lubricants can decrease the barrier strength of latex, thus making water-soluble lubricants (e.g., Astroglide, K-Y Jelly) preferable.[4] Condoms with spermicides are no longer recommended because they provide no additional protection against pregnancy or STDs and may increase vulnerability to HIV.[4]

The female condom (FC, formerly Reality brand) is a prelubricated, loose-fitting polyurethane sheath, closed at one end, with flexible rings at both ends.[3,4] Properly positioned, the ring at the closed end covers the cervix, and the sheath lines the walls of the vagina. The outer ring remains outside the vagina, covering the labia. The pregnancy rate is reported to be 21% in the first year of typical use. Male and female condoms should not be used together, as slippage and device displacement may occur.

The diaphragm, a reusable dome-shaped rubber cap with a flexible rim that is inserted vaginally, fits over the cervix in order to decrease access of sperm to the ovum. The diaphragm requires a prescription from a physician who has fitted the patient for the correct size.[3,4] Its effectiveness depends on its function as a barrier and on the spermicidal cream or jelly placed in the diaphragm before insertion. The diaphragm may be inserted up to 6 hours before intercourse and must be left in place for at least 6 hours afterward. However, leaving it in place for more than 24 hours is not recommended due to the potential for toxic shock syndrome. With subsequent acts of intercourse, the diaphragm should be left in place, and a condom should be used for additional protection.[3]

The cervical cap is a soft, deep cup with a firm round rim that is smaller than a diaphragm and fits over the cervix like a thimble.[3,4] Currently, two latex-free cervical caps are available by prescription in the United States: the FemCap and the Lea's Shield.[3] The FemCap is available in three sizes and should be filled with spermicide prior to insertion.[3,4] It is held in place against the cervix until the cap is removed. The Lea's Shield is available in only one size and is held in place by the vaginal wall; therefore, cervical size is not a factor.[3] Both caps can be inserted 6 hours prior to intercourse and should not be removed for at least 6 hours after intercourse. They may remain in place for multiple episodes of intercourse without adding more spermicide but should not be worn for more than 48 hours at a time to reduce the risk of toxic shock syndrome. Failure rates are higher than with other methods. Some studies have shown an increased risk of cervical dysplasia, so users must have a repeat Papanicolaou (Pap) smear 3 months after starting to use a cervical cap.[3] Diaphragms and cervical caps do not protect against some STDS including HIV, thus condoms should also be used.

PHARMACOLOGIC THERAPY

Spermicides

1 **2** Spermicides, most of which contain nonoxynol-9, are chemical surfactants that destroy sperm cell walls and act as barriers that prevent sperm from entering the cervical os.[4] They are available as creams, films, foams, gels, suppositories, sponges, and tablets.[3,4] Spermicides offer no protection against STDs. In fact, when used frequently (more than 2 times per day), nonoxynol-9 may increase the risk of transmission of HIV by causing small disruptions in the

TABLE 88-1 Comparison of Methods of Nonhormonal Contraception

Method	Absolute Contraindications	Advantages	Disadvantages	Percentage of Women with Pregnancy[a] Perfect Use	Typical Use
Condoms, male	Allergy to latex or rubber	Inexpensive STD protection, including HIV (latex only)	High user failure rate Poor acceptance Possibility of breakage Efficacy decreased by oil-based lubricants Possible allergic reactions to latex in either partner	2	15
Condoms, female	Allergy to polyurethane History of TSS	Can be inserted just before intercourse or ahead of time STD protection, including HIV	High user failure rate Dislike ring hanging outside vagina Cumbersome	5	21
Diaphragm with spermicide	Allergy to latex, rubber, or spermicide Recurrent UTIs History of TSS Abnormal gynecologic anatomy	Low cost Decreased incidence of cervical neoplasia Some protection against STDs	High user failure rate Decreased efficacy with increased frequency of intercourse Increased incidence of vaginal yeast UTIs, TSS Efficacy affected by oil-based lubricants Cervical irritation	6	16
Cervical cap (FemCap, Lea's Shield)	Allergy to spermicide History of TSS Abnormal gynecologic anatomy Abnormal Papanicolaou smear	Low cost Latex-free Some protection against STDs FemCap reusable for up to 2 years	High user failure rate Decreased efficacy with parity Cannot be used during menses	9	16[b]
Spermicides alone	Allergy to spermicide	Inexpensive	High user failure rate Must be reapplied before each act of intercourse May enhance HIV transmission No protection against STDs	18	29
Sponge (Today)	Allergy to spermicide Recurrent UTIs History of TSS Abnormal gynecologic anatomy	Inexpensive	High user failure rate Decreased efficacy with parity Cannot be used during menses No protection against STDs	9[c]	16[d]

HIV, human immunodeficiency virus; STD, sexually transmitted disease; TSS, toxic shock syndrome; UTI, urinary tract infection.
[a]Failure rates in the United States during first year of use.
[b]Failure rate with FemCap reported to be 29% per package insert.
[c]Failure rate with Today sponge reported to be 20% in parous women.
[d]Failure rate with Today sponge reported to be 32% in parous women.
Data from Hatcher and Nelson,[4] and Dickey.[5]

vaginal epithelium.[10,11] The World Health Organization (WHO) and the Centers for Disease Control and Prevention (CDC) do not promote products containing nonoxynol-9 for protection against STDs. Women at high risk for HIV infection or who are HIV infected should not use spermicides.[3,12,13]

Spermicide-Implanted Barrier Techniques

1 2 The vaginal contraceptive sponge (Today) contains 1 g of the spermicide nonoxynol-9.[4] It has a concave dimple on one side to fit over the cervix and a loop on the other side to facilitate removal. After being moistened with water, the sponge is inserted into the vagina up to 6 hours before intercourse. The sponge provides protection for 24 hours, regardless of the frequency of intercourse during this time. After intercourse, the sponge must be left in place for at least 6 hours before removal and should not be left in place for more than 24 to 30 hours to reduce the risk of toxic shock syndrome. Sponges should not be reused, after removal they should be discarded. The sponge comes in one size and is available over the counter (OTC).[4]

Hormonal Contraception

Hormonal contraceptives contain a combination of estrogen and progestin or a progestin alone. Oral contraceptive preparations first became available in the 1960s, but options have expanded to include a transdermal patch, a vaginal contraceptive ring, and long-acting injectable, implantable, and intrauterine contraceptives.

Combined hormonal contraceptives (CHCs) work primarily before fertilization to prevent conception. Progestins provide most of the contraceptive effect, by thickening cervical mucus to prevent sperm penetration, slowing tubal motility and delaying sperm transport, and inducing endometrial atrophy. Progestins block the LH surge, therefore inhibiting ovulation. Estrogens suppress FSH release from the pituitary, which may contribute to blocking the LH surge and preventing ovulation. However, the primary role of estrogen in hormonal contraceptives is to stabilize the endometrial lining and provide cycle control.[3–5]

Estrogens Two synthetic estrogens found in hormonal contraceptives available in the United States are ethinyl estradiol (EE) and mestranol. Mestranol, must be converted by the liver to EE before it is pharmacologically active and is 50% less potent than EE.[3–5] Most combined OCs, transdermal patch, and vaginal ring contain estrogen at doses of 20 to 50 mcg of EE.[4]

Progestins A variety of progestins are available in the United States and they vary in their progestational activity and differ with respect to inherent estrogenic, antiestrogenic, and androgenic effects.[3–5] Estrogenic and antiestrogenic properties are secondary to the extent of progestins' metabolism to estrogenic substances. Androgenic activity is dependent upon two variables: the presence of sex hormone (testosterone) binding globulin (SHBG-TBG) and the androgen:progesterone activity ratio. If the amount of SHBG-TBG is decreased, free testosterone levels increase and androgenic side effects are more prominent.[5]

Considerations with Combined Hormonal Contraceptive Use. ❶ When selecting a CHC, clinicians are challenged by weighing the benefits and risks associated with the many formulations available. The clinician must determine if the form of contraception is appropriate based upon the patient's lifestyle and potential adherence. A complete medical examination and Pap smear are not necessary before a CHC is prescribed. A medical history and blood pressure measurement should be obtained before prescribing a CHC, along with a discussion of the benefits, risks, and adverse effects with each patient.[3–5,14–16] For example, OCs are associated with noncontraceptive benefits, including relief from menstruation-related problems (e.g., decreased menstrual cramps, decreased ovulatory pain [mittelschmerz], and decreased menstrual blood loss), improvement in menstrual regularity and decreased iron deficiency anemia. Women who take combination OCs have a reduced risk of ovarian and endometrial cancer. There is a 50% reduction in risk in women who have used OCs for 5 years or more, and protection may persist for more than 10 years post-use. Combination OCs may also reduce the risk of ovarian cysts, ectopic pregnancy, pelvic inflammatory disease, endometriosis, uterine fibroids, and benign breast disease. The CHC transdermal patch and vaginal ring are other combined hormonal options that may be more convenient for women than taking a tablet each day.

❷ ❸ Adverse effects may hinder adherence and therefore efficacy, so they should be discussed prior to initiating a hormonal contraceptive agent (Table 88–2). Excessive or deficient amounts of estrogen and progestin are related to the most common adverse effects.[3–5] The CHC vaginal ring may be uncomfortable for some women and cause vaginal discharge. The CHC patch may cause irritation and now has information added to product labeling regarding the increased potential for thromboembolism.

An important concern regarding the use of CHCs is the lack of protection against STDs. Because of their high efficacy in preventing pregnancy, patients may choose not to use condoms. In addition to public health awareness, clinicians must encourage patients to use condoms for prevention of STDs. OCs have an extensive history of safety concerns, which traditionally were related to high dose estrogen tablets. To replace the traditional absolute and relative contraindications to the use of OCs, the WHO developed a graded list of precautions for clinicians to consider when initiating CHCs (Table 88–3).[4,12,13]

In addition to the WHO precautions, the ACOG provides information for clinicians to use when selecting CHCs for women with coexisting medical conditions.[17] Overall, the health risks associated with pregnancy, the specific health risks associated with CHCs and the noncontraceptive benefits of CHCs should be factored into risk-to-benefit considerations.

Women Older Than 35 Years. Use of CHC in women older than 35 years of age is controversial. Older women, especially women in their 40s retain a level of fertility even in the perimenopausal state and should use contraception to prevent pregnancy. Formulations with lower doses of estrogen (less than 30 mcg) have increased the use of CHCs in these women. In addition to the benefit of pregnancy prevention, they may improve or decrease the chance of developing perimenopausal and menopausal symptoms and increase bone mineral density (BMD). However, the benefits of using CHCs must be weighed against the risks in women older than 35. The increased risk of cardiovascular disease and venous thromboembolism (VTE) should be considered especially in perimenopausal women older than 40. Older data suggests an increased risk of myocardial infarction (MI) in older women using CHCs, although many women in

TABLE 88-2	Adverse Effects of Combined Hormonal Contraception and Their Management[a]
Adverse Effects	**Management**
Estrogen excess	
Nausea, breast tenderness, headaches, cyclic weight gain due to fluid retention	Decrease estrogen content in CHC Consider progestin-only methods or IUD
Dysmenorrhea, menorrhagia, uterine fibroid growth	Decrease estrogen content in CHC Consider extended-cycle or continuous regimen OC Consider progestin-only methods or IUD NSAIDs for dysmenorrhea
Estrogen deficiency	
Vasomotor symptoms, nervousness, decreased libido	Increase estrogen content in CHC
Early-cycle (days 1–9) breakthrough bleeding and spotting	Increase estrogen content in CHC
Absence of withdrawal bleeding (amenorrhea)	Exclude pregnancy Increase estrogen content in CHC if menses is desired Continue current CHC if amenorrhea acceptable
Progestin excess	
Increased appetite, weight gain, bloating, constipation	Decrease progestin content in CHC
Acne, oily skin, hirsutism	Decrease progestin content in CHC Choose less androgenic progestin in CHC
Depression, fatigue, irritability	Decrease progestin content in CHC
Progestin deficiency	
Dysmenorrhea, menorrhagia	Increase progestin content in CHC Consider extended-cycle or continuous regimen OC Consider progestin-only methods or IUD NSAIDs for dysmenorrhea
Late-cycle (days 10–21) breakthrough bleeding and spotting	Increase progestin content in CHC

CHC, combined hormonal contraceptive; IUD, intrauterine device; NSAID, nonsteroidal antiinflammatory drug; OC, oral contraceptive.

[a]CHC regimens should be continued for at least 3 months before adjustments are made based on adverse effects.

Data from Hatcher and Nelson,[4] and Dickey.[5]

these studies were current smokers and used older formulations containing higher doses (greater than 50 mcg) of estrogen. More recent data does not support the increased risk of cardiovascular disease when low dose formulations of CHCs are used in healthy, non-obese women. Other concerns include the increased risk of ischemic stroke in women with migraines and the increased risk of breast cancer in older women.[4,16–18]

The risks and benefits of using CHCs in women greater than 35 must be considered on an individual basis. The ACOG and WHO recommend that use of CHCs (with less than 50 mcg of estrogen) may be considered in healthy nonsmoking women. Furthermore, they recommend against the use of CHCs in women older than 35 with migraine (with or without aura), hypertension, dyslipidemia, current smoker, and type 1 or type 2 diabetes mellitus.[13,17]

Smoking. In early studies, OCs with 50 mcg EE or more were associated with MI in women who smoked cigarettes.[4,14,16,17] U.S. case-control studies have found that both nonsmoking and smoking women, regardless of age, taking OCs with less than 50 mcg EE did not have an increased risk of MI or stroke. However, these studies included few women older than 35 years who were smokers. European studies, with a higher population of older smoking women, demonstrated an increased risk of MI in this population.

TABLE 88-3 World Health Organization Precautions in the Provision of Combined Hormonal Contraceptives (CHCs)

Category 4: Refrain from providing CHCs to women with the following diagnoses
- Thrombophlebitis or thromboembolic disorder, or a history of these conditions
- Cerebrovascular disease, coronary artery disease, peripheral vascular disease
- Valvular heart disease with thrombogenic complications (e.g., pulmonary hypertension, atrial fibrillation, history of endocarditis)
- Diabetes with vascular involvement (e.g., nephropathy, retinopathy, neuropathy, other vascular disease or diabetes >20 years' duration)
- Migraine headaches with focal aura
- Uncontrolled hypertension (≥160 mm Hg systolic or ≥90 mm Hg diastolic)
- Major surgery with prolonged immobilization
- Thrombogenic mutations (e.g., factor V Leiden, protein C or S deficiency, antithrombin III deficiency, prothrombin deficiency)
- Breast cancer
- Acute or chronic hepatocellular disease with abnormal liver function, cirrhosis, hepatic adenomas, or hepatic carcinomas
- Age >35 years and currently smoking ≥15 cigarettes per day
- Known or suspected pregnancy
- Breastfeeding women <6 weeks postpartum

Category 3: Conditions may be adversely impacted by CHCs, and the risks generally outweigh the benefits; providers should exercise caution if combined CHCs are used in these situations, and patients should be carefully monitored for adverse effects
- Multiple risk factors for arterial cardiovascular disease
- Known hyperlipidemia
- Migraine headache without aura in women ≥35 years old
- History of hypertension (140–159 mm Hg systolic or 90–99 mm Hg diastolic)
- History of cancer, but no evidence of current disease for 5 years
- Cirrhosis, mild and compensated
- Symptomatic gallbladder disease
- Cholestatic jaundice with prior pill use
- Age >35 years and currently smoking <15 cigarettes per day
- Postpartum <21 days, not breastfeeding
- Breast-feeding women 6 weeks to 6 months postpartum
- Commonly used drugs that induce liver enzymes (rifampin, phenytoin, carbamazepine, barbiturates, primidone, topiramate) and reduce efficacy of CHC

Category 2: Some conditions may trigger potential concerns with CHCs, but benefits usually outweigh risks
- Family history of thromboembolism
- Superficial thrombophlebitis
- Uncomplicated valvular heart disease
- Diabetes without vascular disease
- Sickle cell disease

- Migraine headaches without aura in women <35 years old
- Hypertension during pregnancy, resolved postpartum
- Major surgery without prolonged immobilization
- Gallbladder disease (symptomatic and treated by cholecystectomy or asymptomatic)
- Cholestatic jaundice of pregnancy
- Undiagnosed breast mass
- Undiagnosed abnormal genital bleeding
- Cervical intraepithelial neoplasia or cervical cancer
- Obesity (body mass index ≥30 kg/m²)
- Age <35 years and currently smoking
- Breastfeeding women ≥6 months postpartum
- Age ≥40 years
- Drugs that may induce metabolism of CHC and reduce efficacy (griseofulvin, antiretroviral therapy)

Category 1: Do not restrict use of combined oral contraceptives for the following conditions
- Varicose veins
- History of gestational diabetes
- Nonmigrainous headaches
- Thyroid disease
- Thalassemia
- Iron deficiency anemia
- Depression
- Epilepsy
- Infectious diseases (HIV, schistosomiasis, tuberculosis, malaria)
- Minor surgery without immobilization
- Benign ovarian tumors
- Endometriosis
- Irregular or heavy vaginal bleeding, severe dysmenorrhea
- Sexually transmitted diseases
- Uterine fibroids
- Pelvic inflammatory disease
- Endometrial cancer
- Ovarian cancer
- History of pelvic surgery
- Trophoblast disease
- History of ectopic pregnancy
- Postabortion
- Postpartum women ≥21 weeks, not breastfeeding
- Menarche to 40 years of age
- Drug interactions with antibiotics other than rifampin and griseofulvin

CHC, combined hormonal contraception; HIV, human immunodeficiency virus.
Data from Hatcher and Nelson,[4] Dickey,[5] World Health Organization.[12,13]

Therefore, practitioners should prescribe CHC with caution, if at all, to women older than 35 years who smoke. The WHO precautions further state that smoking 15 or more cigarettes per day by women in this age group is a contraindication to CHC, and that the risks generally outweigh the benefits of CHC in those who smoke fewer than 15 cigarettes per day.[13] Progestin-only contraceptive methods should be considered for women in this group.

Hypertension. CHCs can cause small increases (i.e., 6–8 mm Hg) in blood pressure, regardless of estrogen dosage.[4,14,16,17] This has been documented in both normotensive and mildly hypertensive women given a 30 mcg EE OC. In case-control studies of women with hypertension, OCs have been associated with an increased risk of MI and stroke. Use of low dose CHC is acceptable in women younger than 35 years with well-controlled and frequently monitored hypertension. If a CHC-related increase in blood pressure occurs, discontinuing the CHC usually restores blood pressure to pretreatment values within 3 to 6 months.[4] Hypertensive women who have end-organ vascular disease or

who smoke should not use CHCs. Women with hypertension who are taking potassium-sparing diuretics, angiotensin-converting enzyme inhibitors, angiotensin-receptor blockers, or aldosterone antagonists may have increased serum potassium concentrations if they are also using an OC containing drospirenone, which has antialdosterone properties.[4]

Dyslipidemia. Generally, synthetic progestins adversely affect lipid metabolism by decreasing high-density lipoprotein (HDL) and increasing low-density lipoprotein (LDL).[4,16,17] Estrogens tend to have more beneficial effects by enhancing removal of LDL and increasing HDL levels. Estrogens may moderately increase triglycerides. As a net result, most low-dose CHCs have no significant impact on HDL, LDL, triglycerides, or total cholesterol. CHCs containing more androgenic progestins (e.g., levonorgestrel) may result in lower HDL levels in some patients. Although the lipid effects of CHCs theoretically can influence cardiovascular risk, the mechanism of increased cardiovascular disease in CHC users is believed to be due to thromboembolic and thrombotic changes, not atherosclerosis. Women with controlled dyslipidemia can use low dose CHCs, although periodic fasting lipid profiles are recommended. Women with uncontrolled dyslipidemia (LDL greater than 160 mg/dL [4.14 mmol/L], HDL less than 35 mg/dL [0.91 mmol/L], triglycerides greater than 250 mg/dL [2.83 mmol/L]) and additional risk factors (e.g., coronary artery disease, diabetes, hypertension, smoking, or positive family history) should use an alternative method of contraception.

Diabetes. Any effect of CHCs on carbohydrate and lipid metabolism is thought to be due to the progestin component.[4,17] However, with the exception of some levonorgestrel-containing products, formulations containing low doses of progestins do not significantly alter insulin, glucose, or glucagon release after a glucose load in healthy women or in those with a history of gestational diabetes. The new progestins are believed to have little, if any, effect on carbohydrate metabolism. CHCs do not appear to alter the hemoglobin A_{1c} values or accelerate the development of microvascular complications in women with type 1 diabetes. In the Nurses' Health Study, women who used OCs did not demonstrate any increased risk of developing type 2 diabetes.[17] Therefore, nonsmoking women younger than 35 years with diabetes but no associated vascular disease can safely use CHCs. Diabetic women with vascular disease (e.g., nephropathy, retinopathy, neuropathy, or other vascular disease or diabetes of more than 20 years' duration) should not use CHCs.

Migraine Headaches. Women with migraine headaches may experience a decreased or an increased frequency of migraine headaches when using CHCs.[4,14,16,17,19] Headaches may even occur during the hormone-free interval. Studies have demonstrated a higher risk of stroke in women experiencing migraine with aura compared to women with simple migraine. In population-based studies, the risk of stroke in women with migraines has been elevated twofold to threefold. However, given the low absolute risk of stroke in young women (age less than 35 years), the ACOG recommends considering CHCs in healthy, nonsmoking women with migraine headaches without aura.[17] Women of any age who have migraine with aura should not use CHC. Women who develop migraines (with or without aura) while receiving CHC should discontinue use and consider a progestin-only option.

Breast Cancer. Worldwide epidemiologic data from 54 studies in 25 countries (many of which studied high dose OCs) were collected to assess the relationship between OCs and breast cancer.[17] Overall, investigators noted a small increased risk of breast cancer associated with current or recent use, but OCs did not further increase risk in women with a history of benign breast disease or a family history of breast cancer. A more recent U.S.–based case-control study found no association between overall breast cancer and current or past OC use.[17] This study also found no association between depomedroxyprogesterone acetate (DMPA) and breast cancer. Although some studies have found differences in risk of breast cancer based on the presence of *BRCA1* and *BRCA2* mutations, the most recent cohort study found no association with low dose OCs and the presence of either mutation. The choice to use CHCs should not be affected by the presence of benign breast disease or a family history of breast cancer with either mutation. The WHO precautions state that women with a recent personal history of breast cancer should not use CHCs, but that CHCs can be considered in women without evidence of disease for 5 years.[13]

Thromboembolism. Estrogens increase hepatic production of factor VII, factor X, and fibrinogen in the coagulation cascade, therefore increasing the risk of thromboembolic events (deep vein thrombosis, pulmonary embolism). These risks are increased in women who have underlying hypercoagulable states (e.g., deficiencies in antithrombin III, protein C, and protein S; factor V Leiden mutations, prothrombin G2010 A mutations) or who have acquired conditions (e.g., obesity, pregnancy, immobility, trauma, surgery, and certain malignancies) that predispose them to coagulation abnormalities.[4,14,16,17,20] In U.S. case-control studies, the risk of VTE in women currently using low dose OCs (less than 50 mcg EE) was 4 times the risk in nonusers.[4,16,17] However, this risk is less than the risk of VTE incurred during pregnancy. OCs containing desogestrel have been associated with a 1.7 to 19 times higher risk of VTE than OCs containing levonorgestrel. Some clinicians argue that this difference reflects preferential prescribing of the newer, and perceived safer, progestin products for women at greater risk for VTE. Estrogen exposure in women using transdermal CHC may be greater than that in women taking OCs or using the vaginal ring over time, but the absolute risk of VTE in this population is unknown. Therefore, CHCs are contraindicated in women with a history of thromboembolic events and in those at risk due to prolonged immobilization with major surgery unless they are currently taking anticoagulants. Women with familial coagulopathies are at particular risk during pregnancy, given the risk of VTE and of fetal exposure to warfarin. CHCs reduce menstrual blood loss and are safe for use by women with appropriate anticoagulation. EC has not been associated with an increased risk of thromboembolic events.

Obesity. The prevalence of obesity continues to rise each year among all age groups including women of childbearing age. It has been hypothesized that women with increased body weight have increased basal metabolic rates and induction of hepatic enzymes, leading to increased hormonal clearance and decreased serum concentrations of hormonal contraceptives. In addition, women who are obese have more adipose tissue, increasing hormonal sequestration, and decreased free hormone serum concentrations resulting in lower efficacy.[4,17] In one recent case-control study, the odds ratio for pregnancy was 1.58 (CI, 1.11-2.24) and 1.72 (CI, 1.04-2.82) in women with a body mass index greater than 27 kg/m² or greater than 32 kg/m², respectively. The authors concluded that this association translates to an additional 2 to 4 pregnancies per 100 woman-years of use in overweight or obese users.[21] This decreased efficacy may be a particular issue with the low dose OCs. Along these same lines, ACOG recommends that the transdermal contraceptive patch should not be used as a first-line option in women weighing greater than 90 kg (198 lbs).[17] It is important to note, however, that the overall risk of decreased efficacy is relatively small when compared to the alternative of increased pregnancy rates when women do not use contraception. It should be noted that increased pregnancy rates have not been demonstrated in obese women using DMPA or the levonorgestrel IUD.

Obese women are also at risk of VTE. In a few population-based case-control studies, obesity (defined as a BMI greater than or equal to 30 kg/m²) was associated with an increased risk of VTE when all other factors, including age and estrogen dosage, were controlled. The mechanism to support the evidence is unclear. Women should be counseled on the risk and consider alternative contraceptive methods on an individual basis.

Systemic Lupus Erythematosus. Contraception is important in women with systemic lupus erythematosus (SLE) because the risks associated with pregnancy are high in this population. Historically, clinicians have thought that CHCs exacerbated the symptoms of SLE.[4,17,22] However, trials have shown that OCs do not increase the risk of flare among women with stable SLE and without antiphospholipid/anticardiolipin antibodies. Because 25% of women with SLE who become pregnant choose to terminate the pregnancy, effective contraception is essential for these patients. CHCs should be avoided in women with SLE and antiphospholipid antibodies or vascular complications; progestin-only contraceptives can be used in this situation.

Sickle Cell Disease. Two controlled trials have demonstrated a reduction in risk of vasoocclusive crises in women with sickle cell disease using DMPA as the method of contraception.[17] Theoretical concerns about the effects of CHCs on platelet activation and red cell deformity, for example, led clinicians to avoid their use in women with sickle cell disease. Because pregnancy carries such a high risk in this population, contraception with DMPA should be considered.

Oral Contraceptives ❶ ❷

With perfect-use, OCs have a 99% efficacy rate, but with typical-use up to 8% of users may become pregnant.[3-5] The OCs currently available are modifications of the original products introduced in the 1960s and contain significantly less estrogen and progestin.[3-5,14] High-dose formulations were associated with vascular and embolic events, cancers, and significant side effects, but reductions in hormone doses have been associated with fewer complications.

Monophasic OCs contain the same amounts of estrogen and progestin for 21 days, followed by 7-day placebo phase. Biphasic and triphasic pills contain variable amounts of estrogen and progestin for 21 days, also followed by a 7-day placebo phase. There are no published data demonstrating increased safety or significant differences in bleeding patterns with the multiphasic tablets compared to monophasic tablets.[3,4,14,23,24] Extended-cycle tablets and continuous combination regimens may offer some benefits for patients in terms of side effects and convenience. One particular extended-cycle OC increases the number of hormone-containing pills from 21 to 84 days, followed by a 7-day placebo phase, resulting in four menstrual cycles per year.[25] Another product provides hormone-containing tablets daily throughout the year.[15] Women taking extended-cycle and continuous-cycle tablets tend to have a decreased amount of bleeding over time, often leading to amenorrhea. Continuous combination regimens provide OCs for 21 days, then very-low-dose estrogen and progestin for an additional 4 to 7 days (during the traditional placebo phase).[26,27]

OCs containing newer progestins (desogestrel, drospirenone, gestodene, and norgestimate) are referred to as third-generation OCs. These progestins are potent progestational agents that have no estrogenic effects and are less androgenic compared with levonorgestrel on a weight basis. Therefore, these agents are thought to have improved side-effect profiles, such as improving mild to moderate acne.[3-5] Drospirenone also has antimineralocorticoid and antialdosterone activities, which may result in less weight gain compared to use of OCs containing levonorgestrel.[3-5] Few clinical trials have compared OCs and sample sizes are small, so the actual relevance of these differences in progestins remains unknown. A review by the Cochrane Library concluded that there was no evidence supporting a causal association between combination OCs or combination skin patches and weight gain.[28] Table 88–4 lists available OC products by brand name and specifies hormonal composition.

Progestin-only "minipills" (28 days of active hormone per cycle) are also available options.[3-5,14] Progestin-only oral contraceptives are less effective than combination OCs and are associated with irregular and unpredictable menstrual bleeding.[3-5] Minipills must be taken every day of the menstrual cycle at approximately the same time to maintain contraceptive efficacy. If a progestin-only oral contraceptive is taken more than 3 hours late, patients should use a backup method of contraception for 48 hours.[4] Minipills may not block ovulation (nearly 40% of women continue to ovulate normally), so the risk of ectopic pregnancy is higher with their use than with other hormonal contraceptives.

Initiating an Oral Contraceptive. ❹

Oral contraceptives may be initiated by several different methods, including on the first day of bleeding during the menstrual cycle, on the first Sunday after the menstrual cycle begins or on the fifth day after the menstrual cycle begins. The most popular method is to begin pills on the first Sunday after the menstrual cycle begins, as this may provide for weekends free of menstrual periods.[3,4,29] Women should be instructed to use a second method of contraception for at least 7 days after initiation for maximum effectiveness. It may be preferable to have women use additional contraception for the entire first cycle, due to user failure in the first month. In the "quick start" method for initiating OCs, the patient takes the first tablet on the day of her office visit.[3,4,29] Women should be instructed to use a second method of contraception for at least 7 days and informed that the menstrual period will be delayed until completion of the active tablets in the current OC pack. This method has been shown to be more successful in getting women to start OCs and to continue using OCs through the third cycle of use.

In the postpartum phase, there is concern about use of OCs because of the mother's hypercoagulability and the effects on lactation. The WHO precautions state that, in the first 21 days postpartum (when the risk of thrombosis is higher), estrogen-containing hormonal contraceptives should be avoided if possible (Table 88–3).[13] If contraception is required during this period, progestin-only oral contraceptives, injectable medroxyprogesterone acetate, and IUDs are acceptable choices. Although a review by the Cochrane Library indicated that existing randomized, controlled trials were insufficient to establish an effect of CHC, if any, on milk quality and quantity, the WHO recommends that women who are breastfeeding avoid CHCs in the first 6 weeks postpartum.[13,30] WHO precautions cite concerns about hormonal exposure in the newborn and diminished quality and quantity of breast milk due to early exposure to CHCs. Progestin-only oral contraceptives do not adversely affect milk production, so they can be used after 6 weeks postpartum. Once effective lactation has been established, particularly in women who are not exclusively breastfeeding, estrogen-containing hormonal contraceptives can be safely used.

Choice of Oral Contraceptive. ❶ ❷

Because all combined OCs are similarly effective in preventing pregnancy, the initial choice is based on the hormonal content and dose, preferred formulation, and coexisting medical conditions (Table 88–3).[13] In women without coexisting medical conditions, an OC containing 35 mcg or less of EE and less than 0.5 mg of norethindrone or an equivalent progestin is recommended (Table 88–4).[5] This strategy is based on evidence that complications and side effects from CHC (i.e., VTE, stroke, or MI) result from excessive hormonal content.[3-5,14] Adolescents, underweight women (less than 50 kg [110 lbs]), women older than 35 years, and those who are perimenopausal may have fewer side effects with OCs containing 20 to 25 mcg of EE. With nonadherence to OCs, the risk of pregnancy may be greater in women taking OCs containing less than 35 mcg of EE. Overweight and obese women may have higher contraceptive failure rates with low dose OCs and may benefit from pills containing at least 35 mcg of EE. Women with regular heavy menses initially may benefit from a 50 mcg EE OC because of their higher endometrial activity and women with regular light menses can be started on 20 mcg EE OCs. Women with oily skin, acne, or hirsutism should be given low androgenic OCs.[5]

Conventional regimens (21 days of active pills, 7 days of placebo) provide predictable menses. Because monophasic OCs may be easier to take, easier to identify/manage side effects, and easier to manipulate to alter the timing of the menstrual cycle, they are preferred over multiphasic OCs.[3-5] Extended-cycle OCs either eliminate or reduce the number of menstrual cycles per year, leading to less premenstrual symptoms and dysmenorrhea. Commercially available extended-cycle OCs are available, or monophasic 28 day OCs can be cycled by skipping the 7-day placebo phase. With continued use of extended-cycle OCs for 1 year, no significant changes adverse effects have been noted. However, long-term studies have not been performed to assess the risk of cancer, VTE, or changes

TABLE 88-4 Composition of Commonly Prescribed Oral Contraceptives[a]

Product	Estrogen	Micrograms[b]	Progestin	Milligrams[b]	Spotting and Breakthrough Bleeding
50 mcg estrogen					
Necon 1/50, Norinyl 1+50, Ortho-Novum 1/50	Mestranol	50	Norethindrone	1	10.6
Ovcon 50	Ethinyl estradiol	50	Norethindrone	1	11.9
Ovral, Ogestrel 0.5/50	Ethinyl estradiol	50	Norgestrel	0.5	4.5
Demulen 1/50, Zovia 1/50	Ethinyl estradiol	50	Ethynodiol diacetate	1	13.9
Sub-50 mcg estrogen monophasic					
Aviane, Lessina, Levlite, Lutera, Sronyx	Ethinyl estradiol	20	Levonorgestrel	0.1	26.5
Brevicon, Modicon, Necon 0.5/35, Nortrel 0.5/35	Ethinyl estradiol	35	Norethindrone	0.5	24.6
Demulen 1/35, Zovia 1/35, Kelnor	Ethinyl estradiol	37.4	Ethynodiol diacetate	1	37.4
Apri, Desogen, Ortho-Cept, Reclipsen, Solia	Ethinyl estradiol	30	Desogestrel	0.15	13.1
Levlen, Levora, Nordette, Portia	Ethinyl estradiol	30	Levonorgestrel	0.15	14
Junel 1/20, Junel Fe 1/20, Loestrin 1/20; Fe 1/20, Microgestin 1/20; Fe 1/20	Ethinyl estradiol	20	Norethindrone 1mg	1	26.5
Junel 1.5/30, Junel Fe 1.5/30, Loestrin Fe 1.5/30, Microgestin 1.5/30, Microgestin Fe 1.5/30	Ethinyl estradiol	30	Norethindrone acetate	1.5	25.2
Cryselle, Lo-Ovral, Low-Ogestrel	Ethinyl estradiol	30	Norgestrel	0.3	9.6
Necon 1/35, Norinyl 1+35, Norethin 1/35, Nortrel 1/35, Ortho-Novum 1/35	Ethinyl estradiol	35	Norethindrone	1	14.7
Ortho-Cyclen, Mononessa, Previfem, Sprintec	Ethinyl estradiol	35	Norgestimate	0.25	14.3
Ovcon-35, Balziva, Femcon Fe chewable, Zenchent	Ethinyl estradiol	35	Norethindrone	0.4	11
Yasmin	Ethinyl estradiol	30	Drospirenone	3	14.5
Sub-50 mcg estrogen monophasic extended cycle					
Loestrin-24 FE[c]	Ethinyl estradiol	20	Norethindrone	1	50[e]
Lybrel	Ethinyl estradiol	20	Levonorgestrel	0.09	52[e]
Seasonale, Jolessa, Quasense[d]	Ethinyl estradiol	30	Levonorgestrel	0.15	58.5[e]
Yaz[c]	Ethinyl estradiol	20	Drospirenone	3	52.5[e]
Beyaz[f]	Ethinyl estradiol	20	Drospirenone	3	52.5[e]
Sub-50 mcg estrogen multiphasic					
Cyclessa, Cesia, Velivet	Ethinyl estradiol	25 (7)	Desogestrel	0.1 (7)	11.1
		25 (7)		0.125 (7)	
		25 (7)		0.15 (7)	
Estrostep Fe, Tilia Fe, Tri-Legest Fe	Ethinyl estradiol	20 (5)	Norethindrone acetate	1 (5)	21.7
	Ethinyl estradiol	30 (7)	Norethindrone acetate	1 (7)	
	Ethinyl estradiol	35 (9)	Norethindrone acetate	1 (9)	
Kariva, Mircette	Ethinyl estradiol	20 (21)	Desogestrel	0.15 (21)	19.7
	Ethinyl estradiol	10 (5)	Desogestrel		
Gencept 10/11, Necon 10/11, Ortho-Novum 10/11	Ethinyl estradiol	35 (10)	Norethindrone	0.5 (10)	17.6
	Ethinyl estradiol	35 (11)	Norethindrone	1 (11)	
Ortho-Novum 7/7/7, Nortrel 7/7/7, Necon 7/7/7	Ethinyl estradiol	35 (7)	Norethindrone	0.5 (7)	14.5
	Ethinyl estradiol	35 (7)	Norethindrone	0.75 (7)	
	Ethinyl estradiol	35 (7)	Norethindrone	1 (7)	
Ortho Tri-Cyclen, Trinessa, Tri-Previfem, Tri-Sprintec	Ethinyl estradiol	35 (7)	Norgestimate	0.18 (7)	17.7
	Ethinyl estradiol	35 (7)	Norgestimate	0.215 (7)	
	Ethinyl estradiol	35 (7)	Norgestimate	0.25 (7)	
Ortho Tri-Cyclen Lo	Ethinyl estradiol	25 (7)	Norgestimate	0.18 (7)	11.5
	Ethinyl estradiol	25 (7)	Norgestimate	0.215 (7)	
	Ethinyl estradiol	25 (7)	Norgestimate	0.25 (7)	
Aranelle, Leena, Tri-Norinyl	Ethinyl estradiol	35 (7)	Norethindrone	0.5 (7)	25.5
	Ethinyl estradiol	35 (9)	Norethindrone	1 (9)	
	Ethinyl estradiol	35 (5)	Norethindrone	0.5 (5)	
Enpresse, Tri-Levlen, Triphasil, Trivora	Ethinyl estradiol	30 (6)	Levonorgestrel	0.05 (6)	
	Ethinyl estradiol	40 (5)	Levonorgestrel	0.075 (5)	
	Ethinyl estradiol	30 (10)	Levonorgestrel	0.125 (10)	
Sub-50 mcg estrogen multiphasic extended cycle					
Seasonique	Ethinyl estradiol	30 (84)	Levonorgestrel	0.15 (84)	42.5[e]
	Ethinyl estradiol	10 (7)	Levonorgestrel	0.15 (7)	
Progestin only					
Camila, Errin, Jolivette, Micronor, Nor-QD, Nora-BE	Ethinyl estradiol	–	Norethindrone	0.35	42.3

[a]28-day regimens (21-day active pills, then 7-day pill-free interval) unless otherwise noted.
[b]Number in parentheses refers to the number of days the dose is received in multiphasic oral contraceptives.
[c]28-day regimen (24-day active pills, then 4-day pill-free interval).
[d]91-day regimen (84-day active pills, then 7-day pill-free interval).
[e]Percentage reporting after 6–12 months of use.
[f]Contains folate supplementation (levomefolate calcium 0.451mg).
Data from Hatcher and Nelson,[4] Dickey,[5] and Anonymous.[14]

in fertility. Continuous combination regimens provide a shortened pill-free interval, from the traditional 7 days to 2 to 4 days. These regimens may be beneficial for women with symptoms such as dysmenorrhea or menstrual migraines.

Coexisting medical conditions and their impact on CHC use have been previously addressed. Women with migraine headaches, history of VTE, cardiovascular disease, cerebrovascular disease, and SLE with vascular disease are good candidates for progestin-only methods. In addition, women with a history of estrogen dependent cancer, smokers over the age of 35, and those who are postpartum and/or breastfeeding should use progestin-only or nonhormonal methods.[13,17]

Managing Oral Contraceptive Side Effects. ❸ Many symptoms occurring with early OC use (e.g., nausea, bloating, breakthrough bleeding) improve spontaneously by the third cycle of use after adjusting to the altered hormone levels.[3-5] Women should be counseled to continue their OC for 2 to 3 months before a change is made to adjust the hormonal content. However, a large majority of women who discontinue OCs do so because of the side effects. Patient education and early reevaluation within 3 to 6 months are necessary to identify and manage adverse effects, in an effort to improve adherence. A list of OC-related side effects and their management is given in Table 88-2.

If the patient has symptoms related to OC use, it is necessary to determine if the symptom indicates the presence or potential development of a serious illness (Table 88-5).[4,5] Patients should be instructed to immediately discontinue CHCs if they experience warning signs, described as ACHES (abdominal pain, chest pain, headaches, eye problems, and severe leg pain).[4]

Managing Oral Contraceptive Drug Interactions. ❸ The effectiveness of an OC is sometimes limited by drug interactions that interfere with gastrointestinal absorption, increase intestinal motility by altering gut bacteriologic flora, and alter the metabolism, excretion, or binding of the OC.[4,17,31] The lower the dose of hormone in the OC, the greater the risk that a drug interaction will compromise its efficacy. Women should be instructed to use an additional method of contraception if there is a possibility of a drug interaction altering the efficacy of the OC.[4] Although less well documented, these recommendations generally also apply to patients receiving transdermal and vaginal CHC products.

Of all antibiotics, rifampin is the one with a true documented pharmacokinetic interaction. Pharmacokinetic studies of other antibiotics have not shown any consistent interaction, but case reports of individual patients have shown a reduction in EE levels when OCs are taken with tetracyclines and penicillin derivatives.[31,32] The ACOG states that ampicillin, doxycycline, fluconazole, metronidazole, miconazole, fluoroquinolones, and tetracyclines do not decrease steroid levels in women taking OCs.[17] The Council on Scientific Affairs at the American Medical Association recommends that women taking rifampin should be counseled about the risk of OC failure and advised to use an additional nonhormonal contraceptive agent during the course of rifampin therapy. The council also recommends that women be informed about the small risk of interactions with other antibiotics, and, if desired, appropriate additional nonhormonal contraceptive agents should be considered. In addition, women who develop breakthrough bleeding during concomitant use of antibiotics and OCs (and other CHCs) should be advised to use an alternate method of contraception during the period of concomitant use.[31]

Women receiving certain anticonvulsants for a seizure disorder should be offered another form of contraception such as IUDs, injectable medroxyprogesterone, implants or nonhormonal options. Some anticonvulsants (mainly phenobarbital, carbamazepine, phenytoin) induce the metabolism of estrogen and progestin, inducing breakthrough bleeding and potentially reducing contraceptive efficacy. In addition, some anticonvulsants (e.g., phenytoin) are known teratogens.

Patient Instructions with Oral Contraceptives. ❹ Many women who take OCs are not educated properly on the appropriate use of these medications. Women should be given the package insert that accompanies all estrogen products and instructed to read it. The written patient information should be supplemented with verbal information describing the mechanism of the medication, both common and serious side effects and management of these side effects. Although several transient self-limiting side effects often occur, the patient should be aware of the danger signals that require immediate medical attention (Table 88-5). The benefits and risks should be discussed, including the fact that OCs provide no physical barrier to the transmission of STDs, including HIV. Detailed instructions on when to start taking the OC should be provided. Patients should be told the importance of routine daily administration to ensure consistent plasma concentrations and improve adherence and specific instructions should be given regarding what to do if a tablet is missed. The World Health Organization's Selected Practice Recommendations for Contraceptive Use was updated recently with regard to missed oral contraceptives.[33] In addition to when the tablet(s) is missed and how many are missed, the guidelines take into consideration whether the OC contains less than 30 mcg of EE. Limited evidence suggests that the risk of pregnancy is greater when 20 mcg tablets are missed than when 30 to 35 mcg tablets are missed. For instance, if a woman is taking a tablet containing 20 mcg EE and misses one dose or starts a pack 1 day late, she should take a tablet as soon as possible (two tablets on the same day) and then continue taking the rest of the tablets daily. No additional contraceptive protection is necessary. If, however, two or more tablets are missed or the pack is started 2 or more days late, the woman should follow the same instructions, but condoms should be used or she should abstain from sexual intercourse until she has taken active tablets for 7 days in a row. If missed tablets occur in the third week, she should finish the active tablets in the current pack and start a new pack the next day. She should not take the 7 inactive tablets. If the missed doses occur in the first week and unprotected intercourse has occurred, she should consider the use of emergency contraception. Instructions are similar for the 30 to 35 mcg tablets; however, no additional contraceptive protection is necessary unless three or more active tablets are missed or the woman starts a pack 3 or more days late. It should be noted that the

TABLE 88-5	Serious Symptoms That May Be Associated with Combined Hormonal Contraception
Serious Symptoms	**Possible Underlying Problem**
Blurred vision, diplopia, flashing lights, blindness, papilledema	Stroke, hypertension, temporary vascular problem of many possible sites, retinal artery thrombosis
Numbness, weakness, tingling in extremities, slurred speech	Hemorrhagic or thrombotic stroke
Migraine headaches	Vascular spasm, stroke
Breast mass, pain, or swelling	Breast cancer
Chest pain (radiating to left arm or neck), shortness of breath, coughing up blood	Pulmonary embolism, myocardial infarction
Abdominal pain, hepatic mass or tenderness, jaundice, pruritus	Gallbladder disease, hepatic adenoma, pancreatitis, thrombosis of abdominal artery or vein
Excessive spotting, breakthrough bleeding	Endometrial, cervical, or vaginal cancer
Severe leg pain (calf, thigh), tenderness, swelling, warmth	Deep-vein thrombosis

Data from Hatcher and Nelson,[4] and Dickey.[5]

Society of Obstetricians and Gynecologists of Canada also recently published guidelines in 2008 for missed doses.[34] These guidelines differ slightly and do not account for the estrogen content of the tablet. Instructions also may vary in package inserts, which can make for increased confusion with patients and providers. It may be prudent, when differing instructions exist, to recommend the more conservative of approaches when dealing with individual patient situations.

Discontinuing Oral Contraceptives and Return of Fertility.

The ACOG states that there is no evidence that OC use decreases subsequent fertility. The transdermal patch and vaginal ring CHCs also have similar effects on fertility. The average delay in ovulation after discontinuing OCs is 1 to 2 weeks; however, delayed ovulation is more common in women with a history of irregular menses. If amenorrhea does continue beyond 6 months, women should be counseled to see a gynecologist for further fertility workup.[3–5,17] Traditionally, women are counseled to allow two to three normal menstrual periods before becoming pregnant to permit the reestablishment of menses and ovulation. However, in several large cohort and case-control studies, infants conceived in the first month after discontinuation of an OC had no greater chance of miscarriage or being born with a birth defect than those born in the general population.

Transdermal Contraceptives ❶ ❷

A CHC is available as a transdermal patch (Ortho Evra), which includes 0.75 mg of EE and 6 mg of norelgestromin, the active metabolite of norgestimate.[3–5] Comparative trials have shown the transdermal patch to be as effective as combined OCs in patients weighing less than 90 kg (198 lbs). Of the 15 pregnancies reported in the clinical trials, five were among women weighing more than 90 kg (198 lbs); therefore, this product is not recommended as a first-line option for these women.[3,4,35] Some patients experience application-site reactions, but other side effects are similar to those experienced with OCs (e.g., breast discomfort, headache, and nausea).[3] A warning from the manufacturer states that women using the patch are exposed to approximately 60% more estrogen than from a typical OC containing 35 mcg of EE, but the mechanism is unclear. It is clear that there is increased estrogen exposure, but controversy exists correlating the increased exposure to increased risk of VTE, cardiovascular, and cerebrovascular events. Two epidemiologic studies present conflicting results. One trial indicates a higher incidence of VTE with the patch compared with a typical OC, whereas the other trial indicates there is no significant difference.[35–37] Currently, the U.S. Food and Drug Administration (FDA) is monitoring this risk because more consistent data are needed. The patch should be applied to the abdomen, buttocks, upper torso, or upper arm at the beginning of the menstrual cycle and replaced every week for 3 weeks (the fourth week is patch free).[3,4] The patch releases estrogen and progestin for 9 days. If the woman forgets to change her patch or restarts the active patches after the ninth day, a backup method should be used for 7 days. Approximately 5% of patches will need to be replaced because they become partly detached or fall off altogether, so single replacements are available. If the patch is detached for more than 24 hours, a new 4-week cycle should be started and a backup method used for 7 days.[3,4] Users have demonstrated greater adherence with the patch than with an OC, but whether this results in reduced pregnancy rates remains to be seen.[38] The benefits of adherence must be weighed against of the risk of increased estrogen exposure and possibility of VTE.

Vaginal Rings ❶ ❷

The vaginal contraceptive ring contains EE and etonogestrel (NuvaRing).[39] It is a 54-mm flexible ring, 4 mm in thickness.[3] Over a 3-week period, the ring releases approximately 15 mcg/day of EE and 120 mcg/day of etonogestrel. Comparative trials have shown the vaginal ring to be as effective as combined OCs. On the first cycle of use, the ring should be inserted on or before the fifth day of the menstrual cycle, remain in place for 3 weeks, then removed for 1 week to allow for withdrawal bleeding. The new ring

should be inserted on the same day of the week as it was during the last cycle, similar to starting a new OC pack on the same day of the week. A second method of contraception should be used if the ring has been expelled accidentally for more than 3 hours; if less than 3 hours, it should be washed and reinserted.[3,39]

❸ Side effects, precautions, and contraindications for use of the hormonal ring are similar to those for all CHCs. The most commonly reported reasons for discontinuation of use were device-related issues, such as foreign-body sensation, device expulsion, and vaginal symptoms. Cycle control with the vaginal ring appears to be equal or better than combined OCs, with a low incidence of breakthrough bleeding and spotting after the second cycle of use, presumably due to increased adherence and release of steady levels of estrogen and progestin.[40,41] Patient acceptability of the delivery system has been studied, and the majority of women do not complain of discomfort in general or during intercourse.[3] A potential concern is the possibility of increased VTE since etonogestrel, is a metabolite of desogestrel which may be associated with increased risk. A few cases of VTE have been reported in clinical trials, but currently there are no published data to support this concern.[3]

The ring should be inserted vaginally. In contrast to diaphragms and cervical caps, precise placement is not an issue because the hormones are absorbed anywhere in the vagina. Women should be in a comfortable position, and compress the ring between the thumb and index finger and push it into the vagina. There is no danger of inserting the ring too far because the cervix will prevent it from traveling up the genital tract. Removal of the ring is performed in a similar manner; pulling it out and discarding into the foil patch (the ring should not be flushed down the toilet).[39] Patients should be discouraged from douching, but other vaginal products, including antifungal creams and spermicides, can be used.[3,4,39]

Long-Acting Injectable and Implantable Contraceptives

Steroid hormones provide long-term contraception when injected or implanted into the skin. Progestins are used in existing injectable and implantable contraceptives.[3–5] Sustained progestin exposure blocks the LH surge, thus inhibiting ovulation. Should ovulation occur, progestins reduce ovum motility in the fallopian tubes. Even if fertilization occurs, progestins thin the endometrium, reducing the chance of implantation. Progestins also thicken the cervical mucus, producing a barrier to sperm penetration. These long-acting methods of contraception do not provide any protection from STDs.

❶ ❷ Women who particularly benefit from progestin-only methods are those who are breast-feeding, those who are intolerant to estrogens (i.e., have a history of estrogen-related headache, breast tenderness, or nausea) or those with concomitant medical conditions in which estrogen is not recommended (Table 88–3). Additionally, injectable and implantable contraceptives are beneficial for women with adherence issues. Pregnancy failure rates with long-acting progestin contraceptives are comparable to the rates with female sterilization.[3–5] Reports have stated an increased risk of ectopic pregnancies while using progestin-only methods, but no evidence supports this finding with use of the more recent injectable and implantable products.

Injectable Progestins. ❶ ❷

Medroxyprogesterone acetate is similar in structure to naturally occurring progesterone. DMPA (Depo-Provera) is administered every 3 months either by deep intramuscular injection in the gluteal or deltoid muscle or subcutaneously in the abdomen or thigh within 5 days of onset of menstrual bleeding.[42,43] With perfect use, the efficacy of DMPA is more than 99%; however, with typical use, 3% of women experience unintended pregnancy.[4] Although these injections may inhibit ovulation for up to 14 weeks, the dose should be repeated every 3 months (12 weeks) to ensure continuous contraception. The manufacturer recommends excluding pregnancy in women with a lapse of 13 or more weeks between injections for the intramuscular formulation or 14 or more weeks between injections for the subcutaneous formulation. Depo-Provera is available as a 150 mg/mL injection vial or prefilled syringe for IM injection and Depo-SubQ Provera 104 is available as a prefilled syringe.[42,43]

Although no adverse effects have been documented in infants exposed to DMPA through breast milk, the manufacturer recommends not initiating DMPA until 6 weeks postpartum in breastfeeding women. Women who are not breastfeeding but require contraception can receive DMPA immediately postpartum.[13,42] Women with sickle cell disease are good candidates for DMPA, as studies have demonstrated a reduction in sickle cell pain crises in women using DMPA.[13] In addition, women with seizure disorders may experience fewer seizures when taking DMPA for contraception.[4] The subcutaneous DMPA formulation is FDA approved for treatment of endometriosis-associated pain.[43] The incidence of *Candida* vulvovaginitis, ectopic pregnancy, and pelvic inflammatory disease, as well as endometrial and ovarian cancer, is decreased in women using DMPA for contraception compared with women using no contraception.[3,42]

Because return of fertility may be delayed after discontinuation of DMPA, it should not be recommended to women desiring pregnancy in the near future. The median time to conception from the first omitted dose is 10 months. Sixty-eight percent of women will be able to conceive within 12 months, 83% within 15 months, and 93% within 18 months of the last injection.[42,43]

❸ Menstrual irregularities are the most frequent adverse effects of both formulations of DMPA. In some cases, bleeding is severe enough to cause a significant drop in hemoglobin. Women who cannot tolerate prolonged bleeding may benefit from a short course of estrogen (e.g., 7 days of 2 mg estradiol or 1.25-mg conjugated estrogen given orally).[3,4] The incidence of irregular bleeding decreases from 30% in the first year to 10% thereafter. After 12 months of therapy, 55% of women report amenorrhea, with the incidence increasing to 68% after 2 years.[42,43] However, bleeding patterns beyond 1 year of use have not been established for the subcutaneous formulation.[43,44]

Other adverse effects, including breast tenderness, weight gain, and depression occur less commonly (less than 5%). However, weight gain averages 1 kg (2.2 lbs) annually and may not resolve until 6 to 8 months after the last injection.[42,43]

DMPA has been associated with short-term bone loss in younger women of reproductive age. This potential side effect may be due to lower ovarian estrogen production that occurs when gonadotropin secretion is suppressed.[17,45,46] Longitudinal studies of women over the age of 18 have shown significant declines in hip and/or spinal BMD when used for up to 2 years compared with those who did not use the medication. This effect appears to be partially reversible after discontinuation of treatment, and no studies have found evidence of osteoporosis or fractures in these users. The largest longitudinal study of adult women in the United States found that within 30 months following DMPA discontinuation, BMD of the spine and hip was similar to that of nonusers.[47] There is evidence from cross-sectional studies, however, to suggest that use of DMPA during adolescence before peak bone mass is achieved is detrimental in high-risk patients. Decreases in lumbar spine BMD of 1.5% and 3.1% in DMPA users after 1 and 2 years of use respectively have been demonstrated, compared with a 2.9% and 9.5% increase in controls over the same time periods. Because of these demonstrated effects on BMD, the FDA issued a black box warning for DMPA in 2004.[42,43] It states that DMPA should be continued for more than 2 years only if other contraceptive methods are inadequate. It also states that this loss seems to be greater with increasing duration of use and may not be completely reversible. Ultimately, it is unclear whether use of DMPA during adolescence or early adulthood will increase the risk

of fracture later in life or prevent them from achieving normal peak bone mass. What is clear is that clinicians should counsel patients on the benefits versus the risks of the medication and to make recommendations based upon available evidence. Patients should be encouraged to have an adequate daily intake of calcium and vitamin D and to exercise daily. Although controversial, some clinicians are recommending evaluations of BMD for those women on DMPA for greater than 2 years. However, ACOG does not currently recommend monitoring BMD solely in response to DMPA use.[45] This recommendation is based upon the fact that any observed short-term loss in BMD associated with DMPA use may be recovered and is unlikely to place a woman at risk of fracture during use or in later years.

Subdermal Progestin Implants. ❶ ❷ Implanon is a single 4-cm-long implant, containing 68 mg of etonogestrel, that is placed under the skin of the upper arm using a preloaded inserter.[48] Implanon releases etonogestrel at a rate of 60 mcg daily for the first month, then decreases to an average of 30 mcg daily at the end of the 3 years of recommended use. Etonogestrel suppresses ovulation in 97% of cycles. When ovulation is not suppressed, etonogestrel still is effective as the progestin thickens the cervical mucus and produces an atrophic endometrium. With perfect use, efficacy approaches 100% but may be reduced in women weighing more than 130% of their ideal body weight. Because only one rod is used, the difficulties experienced with insertion and removal hopefully will be avoided.

❹ The etonogestrel implant should be inserted between days 1 and 5 of the menstrual cycle in women who have not previously used hormonal contraception.[48] Women currently taking OCs can have the implant inserted within 7 days after taking the last active OC tablet. Women currently taking progestin-only oral contraceptives should have the implant inserted without skipping any days, on the same day that the progestin-only IUD is removed, or on the day that the DMPA injection is due. After removal, fertility returns within 30 days.

❸ The major adverse effect associated with Implanon is irregular menstrual bleeding, which led to discontinuation of the implant in 11% of patients in clinical trials.[48] Like the bleeding pattern seen with other progestins, some women (22%) became amenorrheic with continued use, but many continued to have prolonged bleeding and spotting (18%) and frequent bleeding (7%). Other adverse effects include headache, vaginitis, weight gain, acne, and breast and abdominal pain. The role of the progestin implant's influence on BMD has become an area of controversy since the FDA required an inclusion of a black box warning for DMPA. In theory, the etonogestrel implant system should not decrease BMD as much as DMPA because estrogen concentrations are not as consistently suppressed. Clinical trials have demonstrated no significant relationship between use of the hormonal implant and changes in BMD. In addition, there are no long-term data and no data demonstrating a correlation between the implant and fracture risk or an increase in osteoporosis.[49]

Implanon is a unique implantable contraceptive agent that provides enhanced adherence and prolonged efficacy. Therefore, it may be a good choice for women with a history of non-adherence, those who do not plan to have children for at least 3 years or those who have estrogen-related adverse effects or contraindications. Because fertility returns quickly after removal and Implanon does not affect bone health, it may be preferred over DMPA. Women should be counseled about the risk of irregular bleeding patterns so that patients will not request early removal of Implanon.

Intrauterine Devices

❶ ❷ The low-grade intrauterine inflammation and increased prostaglandin formation caused by IUDs and endometrial suppression caused specifically by the progestin-releasing IUD appear to be primarily spermicidal, although interference with implantation is a backup mechanism.[3,4,50,51] Efficacy rates with IUDs are greater than 99% with both perfect and typical use.[4] Although they are a very effective form of contraception and are increasing in popularity, the IUD still has several contraindications. Patients who should be excluded from use of IUDs include: current pregnancy, pelvic inflammatory disease (current or within past 3 months), STD (current), puerperal or postabortion sepsis, purulent cervicitis, undiagnosed abnormal vaginal bleeding, malignancy of genital tract, uterine anomalies or fibroids distorting uterine cavity, allergy to IUD component, Wilson's disease (for copper IUD). The risk of pelvic inflammatory disease among IUD users ranges from 1% to 2.5%. Because the increased risk of infection appears to be related to introduction of bacteria into the genital tract during IUD insertion, the risk is highest during the first 20 days after the procedure.[51,52] Two IUDs currently are marketed in the United States; all are T-shaped and are medicated, one with copper (ParaGard) and one with levonorgestrel (Mirena).[3,4]

❸ ParaGard provides better contraceptive effectiveness than previous copper devices and can be left in place for 10 years.[3,4] A disadvantage of ParaGard is increased menstrual blood flow and dysmenorrhea; average monthly blood loss among users increased by 35% in clinical trials. Mirena was released in the United States in 2001 and is becoming more widely used. It releases 20 mcg of levonorgestrel daily, but release decreases to 10 mcg daily over the 5 years of use.[3,4,50,51] Systemically absorbed levonorgestrel is minimal and considerably less than with OCs. The levonorgestrel IUD produces its effects locally via suppression of the endometrium, causing a reduction in menstrual blood loss. In contrast to the copper IUD, menstrual flow in users of the levonorgestrel IUD is decreased, and development of amenorrhea has been observed in 20% of users in the first year and 60% in the fifth year. A disadvantage of the levonorgestrel IUD is increased spotting in the first 6 months of use; women should be counseled that the spotting will decline gradually over time.[3,4,50,51]

IUDs should be considered because adherence is not an issue once inserted and result in immediate return of fertility once removed. The levonorgestrel IUD has many noncontraceptive benefits, specifically, it is a good choice for women with menorrhagia or dysmenorrhea because it reduces and may eliminate menstrual blood loss. IUDs, in general, are an alternative for women who cannot tolerate or have contraindications to estrogen-containing contraceptive agents. Recently, use in the adolescent and nulliparous population has been recommended in a select group of appropriate candidates due to the high contraceptive efficacy rate. It is important to adhere to the IUD contraindications and provide appropriate counseling to this population. Data to support wide use of this practice in this population are limited.[53]

CLINICAL CONTROVERSY

Use of IUDs is low in adolescents. Specifically in this group, patients and clinicians are concerned about the risk of pelvic inflammatory disease, infertility, and insertion complications. It is important to note there is limited evidence in adolescent and nulliparous women. However, it appears use in this population may be safe when used in appropriate candidates. Adolescent women need to be appropriately screened and counseled on STDs. In addition, these adolescent and nulliparous women have the highest risk of IUD expulsion and pain on insertion. Risks and benefits must be discussed with all patients prior to IUD insertion. The ACOG committee on adolescent healthcare endorses use of IUDs in adolescents who are appropriate candidates due to the high efficacy rates and the need to reduce pregnancy rates in adolescents.

Emergency Contraception

❺ EC is used to prevent unwanted pregnancy after unprotected sexual intercourse, including condom breakage, diaphragm dislodging, or sexual assault. Higher doses of combined estrogen and progestin or progestin-only containing products can be used.[3-5] Insertion of copper IUD is an option, although it is not an FDA approved or a widely used method of EC. Currently, a progestin-only formulation containing levonorgestrel (currently marketed as Plan B, Plan B One-Step, Next Choice) is approved specifically for EC in the United States.[3-5,54] Exact mechanisms of action of oral EC are being studied and vary according to the product used and the time a woman takes it in relation to her menstrual cycle.

Recent studies support that the primary mechanism of action of Plan B is inhibiting or delaying ovulation. Additional evidence suggests it may impair sperm transport and corpus luteum function, therefore inhibiting fertilization. The most recent data does not support that it may prevent the fertilized egg from implanting into the endometrium. Further research is ongoing in this area.[3,4,54-56] Pregnancy occurs when the fertilized egg is implanted into the endometrial lining. After intercourse, implantation of the fertilized egg typically takes approximately 5 days. Oral EC will not disrupt the fertilized egg after implantation has occurred.[3,4,54] The levonorgestrel-containing EC formulation is the regimen of choice due to availability, improved tolerability, and potentially increased efficacy rates. Plan B and Next Choice contain two tablets, each containing 0.75 mg of levonorgestrel. The first dose is taken within 72 hours of unprotected intercourse (although the sooner, the more effective); the second dose is taken 12 hours later.[3-5,54] One study found that 1.5 mg of levonorgestrel (two tablets of Plan B) taken as a single dose was as effective as taking the doses 12 hours apart and did not cause an increased incidence of adverse effects.[54,57] Due to this evidence, a new formulation (Plan B One-Step) containing 1 tablet of 1.5 mg of levonorgestrel taken within 72 hours of unprotected intercourse is currently being marketed and the older Plan B may be phased out.[58] Plan B was approved by the FDA in 2006 for OTC sales, as of 2009 it may be sold without a prescription to patients 17 years of age and older. It is sold only in pharmacies and must be stocked behind the counter. Patients must provide proof of age prior to purchasing the product. The manufacturer is continuing its efforts in gaining OTC status for increased provision to minors.[59]

❺ Despite the availability of progestin-only EC formulations, use of regular combined contraceptives for EC (i.e., Yuzpe method) still is permissible, although some studies suggest that they may not be as effective and may be associated with more adverse effects.[3,4,54] Specifically, the FDA has declared the following regimens containing the progestins norgestrel and levonorgestrel safe and effective methods of EC: Ovral and Ogestrel (two tablets per dose); Nordette, Levlen, Levora, Lo/Ovral, Low-Ogestrel, Cryselle, Jolessa, Enpresse, Portia, Seasonale, Seasonique, Triphasil, TriLevlen, or Trivora (four tablets per dose); and Alesse, Aviane, Lessina, Levlite, or Lutera (five tablets per dose).[3-5,43] Additionally, regular progestin-only oral contraceptives can be used as EC, but many tablets must be taken (i.e., Ovrette, 20 tablets per dose).[3,4,54] Patients should be counseled to take the appropriate number of tablets as soon as possible after unprotected sexual intercourse and to repeat the dose in 12 hours. Taking all the tablets at once as a single dose is not recommended when using combination oral contraceptives.

The efficacy of all EC regimens is improved when taken as soon as possible after unprotected intercourse (within the first 24 hours). EC is still effective when taken within 72 hours but begins to decline once that timeframe has elapsed.[3,4,54] However, one study suggests that EC may still be effective when used up to 120 hours after intercourse and should be considered in some women when use is delayed.[54,60] Determining the exact effectiveness rate is difficult;

however, the range has been reported to be between 59% and 94%. A meta-analysis of the literature has reported that EC may prevent an average of 75% of expected pregnancies when taken appropriately. It is recommended that women have an advanced prescription on hand or access to an OTC formulation to maximize the effectiveness of EC.[3,4,54]

Common adverse effects include nausea, vomiting, and irregular bleeding. Nausea and vomiting occur significantly less when progestin-only EC is administered. If the Yuzpe method is prescribed, antiemetics given 1 hour before the dose is taken may be warranted to prevent the increased amount of estrogen-induced gastrointestinal adverse effects. Many women will experience irregular bleeding regardless of which EC method is used, with the menstrual period usually occurring 1 week before or after the expected time. No current data regarding the safety of repeated use EC are available, but current consensus suggests the risks are low, and women can receive multiple regimens if warranted. Pharmacists and other healthcare providers have a key role in providing patient counseling regarding EC. Appropriate counseling should be provided regarding timing of the dose, common adverse effects, and use of a regular contraceptive method (backup barrier methods should be used after EC for at least 7 days).[54]

CLINICAL CONTROVERSY

Pharmacists who refuse to fill valid prescriptions for emergency contraception have been highly publicized in the media. Position statements published by the American Pharmaceutical Association and American College of Clinical Pharmacy support pharmacists' rights to decline filling a valid prescription if doing so conflicts with moral, ethical, or religious beliefs. However, it is the pharmacists' professional responsibility to refer the patient to another pharmacist who will fill the prescription in a timely, confidential, and nonjudgmental manner so that no harm is caused to the patient.

PHARMACOECONOMIC CONSIDERATIONS

About one third of all pregnancies in the United States are unintended.[1] Not all unintended pregnancies are unwanted; many are just "mistimed." The United States has a higher rate of induced abortions than most other industrialized western nations. Whatever method is used, preventing unintended pregnancy is highly cost-effective. With regard to the acquisition cost of reversible contraception, the most cost-effective barrier method is the male condom. However, reliable pharmacologic methods can also be cost-effective. Injectable, implantable, and IUD options may carry a higher initial cost but would be comparable or even less costly in the long run. OCs, the contraceptive patch, and the vaginal ring are actually the most expensive forms of reversible contraception yet are the most commonly utilized in this country. Overall, with regard to direct medical costs (e.g., method use, adverse effects, and unintended pregnancies) over 5 years, IUDs are the most cost-effective method of contraception, along with sterilization. All contraceptive options (barrier and pharmacologic) are more cost-effective than no method at all.[61]

EVALUATION OF THERAPEUTIC OUTCOMES

❹ Patients should receive both verbal and written instructions on the chosen method of contraception. Follow-up appointments can increase adherence and provide opportunities to address other health maintenance issues (e.g., self-breast examination, Pap smears, human papillomavirus vaccines, STD risk).[4]

Annual blood pressure monitoring is recommended for all users of CHC. When a patient with a history of glucose intolerance or diabetes mellitus begins or discontinues the use of CHC, glucose levels must be monitored closely for deterioration of the condition. Contraceptive users should also receive annual (more frequent if they are at risk for STDs) cytologic screening as well as annual examination for clinical problems related to CHC (e.g., breakthrough bleeding, weight gain, acne).

Women using Implanon should be monitored annually for menstrual cycle disturbances, weight gain, local inflammation, or infection at the implant site, acne, breast tenderness, headaches, and hair loss. Women using DMPA should be asked at 3-month follow-up visits about weight gain, menstrual cycle disturbances, and STD risks. Patients taking DMPA should be weighed, undergo blood pressure checks, and receive annual examinations as indicated based upon the age of the patient. Women using IUDs should be asked at 1- to 3-month follow-up visits about IUD placement (checking for IUD strings to assure the IUD is still in the proper position), changes in menstrual bleeding patterns, and symptoms and protection against STDs. Providers should check for proper IUD positioning and symptoms of upper genital tract infection.

Choosing a contraceptive method most suited to the patient's needs will reduce the chance of unintended pregnancy. A medical and sexual history and a thorough physical examination are essential when evaluating the various methods available. Understanding the risks and precautions associated with the methods available is essential for both patients and clinicians. Counseling about OTC availability of EC or advanced provision of EC prescription is warranted for all women of child-bearing age. Finally, providers should counsel women about healthy sexual practices and encourage use of male condoms in addition to other barrier or pharmacologic contraceptives when necessary to prevent STDs.

ABBREVIATIONS

ACOG: American College of Obstetrics and Gynecology

BMD: bone mineral density

BMI: body mass index

CDC: Centers for Disease Control and Prevention

CHC: combined hormonal contraception

DMPA: depot medroxyprogesterone acetate

EC: emergency contraception

EE: ethinyl estradiol

FDA: U.S. Food and Drug Administration

FSH: follicle-stimulating hormone

GnRH: gonadotropin-releasing hormone

HDL: high-density lipoprotein

HIV: human immunodeficiency virus

IUD: intrauterine device

LDL: low-density lipoprotein

LH: luteinizing hormone

MI: myocardial infarction

OC: oral contraceptive

OTC: over the counter

Pap: papanicolaou (smear)

SHBG-TBG: sex hormone (testosterone)-binding globulin

SLE: systemic lupus erythematosus

STD: sexually transmitted disease

VTE: venous thromboembolism

WHO: World Health Organization

REFERENCES

1. Chandra A, Martinez GM, Mosher WD, et al. Fertility, Family Planning, and Reproductive Health of U.S. Women: Data from the 2002 National Survey of Family Growth. National Center for Health Statistics. Vital Health Stat 23 (25);2005.

2. Get "In the Know": 20 Questions About Pregnancy, Contraception and Abortion; 2006. *http://www.guttmacher.org/in-the-know/index.html.*

3. Zieman M, Hatcher RA, Cwiak C, et al. A Pocket Guide to Managing Contraception. Tiger, GA: Bridging the Gap Foundation, 2007.

4. Hatcher RA, Nelson AL. Contraceptive Technology, 19th ed. New York: Ardent Media, 2007.

5. Dickey RP. Managing Contraceptive Pill Patients, 13th ed. Dallas, TX: EMIS Inc., 2007.

6. Stewart FH, Harper CC, Ellertson CE, et al. Clinical breast and pelvic examination requirements for hormonal contraception: Current practice versus evidence. JAMA 2001;285:2232–2239.

7. Steinbrook R. The potential of human papillomavirus vaccines. N Engl J Med 2006;354:1109–1112.

8. Centers for Disease Control and Prevention. HPV Vaccination; 2009. *http://www.cdc.gov/vaccines/vpd-vac/hpv/default.htm.*

9. Meckstroth KR. Physical examination before initiating hormonal contraception: What is necessary? Am Fam Physician 2006;74:32–33.

10. Roddy RE, Zekeng L, Ryan KA, et al. A controlled trial of nonoxynol 9 film to reduce male-to-female transmission of sexually transmitted diseases. N Engl J Med 1998;339:504–510.

11. Van Damme L, Ramjee G, Alary M, et al. Effectiveness of COL-1492, a nonoxynol-9 vaginal gel, on HIV-1 transmission in female sex workers: A randomised controlled trial. Lancet 2002;360:971–977.

12. World Health Organization. Medical Eligibility Criteria for Contraceptive Use, 3rd ed; 2004. *http://www.who.int/reproductive-health/publications/mec/index.htm.*

13. World Health Organization. Medical Eligibility Criteria for Contraceptive Use, 2008 update; 2008. *http://whqlibdoc.who.int/hq/2008/WHO_RHR_08.19_eng.pdf.*

14. Anonymous. Hormonal Contraception. Pharmacist's Letter/Prescriber's Letter 2007:23.

15. Lybrel [package insert]. Philadelphia, PA: Wyeth Pharmaceuticals Inc.; 2008. *http://www.wyeth.com/content/showlabeling.asp?id=489.*

16. Petitti DB. Combination estrogen-progestin oral contraceptives. N Engl J Med 2003;349:1443–1450.

17. Use of hormonal contraception in women with coexisting medical conditions. ACOG Practice Bulletin No 73. American College of Obstetricians and Gynecologists. Obstet Gynecol 2006;107:1453–1472.

18. Bhathena RK, Guillebauld J. Contraception for the older woman: an update. Climacteric 2006;9:264–276.

19. Curtis KM, Mohllajee AP, Peterson HB. Use of combined oral contraceptives among women with migraine and nonmigrainous headaches: a systematic review. Contraception 2006;73:189–194.

20. Sidney S, Petitti DB, Soff GA, et al. Venous thromboembolic disease in users of low-estrogen combined estrogen-progestin oral contraceptives. Contraception 2004;70:3–10.

21. Holt VL, Scholes D, Wicklund KG, et al. Body mass index, weight, and oral contraceptive failure risk. Obstet Gynecol 2005;105:46–52.

22. Petri M, Kim MY, Kalunian KC, et al. Combined oral contraceptives in women with systemic lupus erythematosus. N Engl J Med 2005;353:2550–2558.

23. Van Vliet HAAM, Grimes DA, Helmerhorst FM, Schulz KF. Biphasic versus monophasic oral contraceptives for contraception. Cochrane Database Syst Rev 2006;3:CD002032.

24. Van Vliet HAAM, Grimes DA, Helmerhorst FM, Schulz KF. Biphasic versus triphasic oral contraceptives for contraception. Cochrane Database Syst Rev 2006;3:CD003283.

25. Seasonique [package insert]. Pomona, NY: Duramed Pharmaceuticals, Inc.; 2008. *https://www.seasonique.com/docs/prescribing-information.pdf.*

26. Loestrin 24 Fe [package insert]. Rockaway, NJ: Warner Chilcott (US), LLC; 2009. *http://www.loestrin24.com/loestrin/pdf/pi_loestrin24_fe.pdf#page=1.*

27. Yaz [package insert]. Wayne, NJ: Bayer HealthCare Pharmaceuticals, Inc.; 2007. *http://www.yaz-us.com/index.jsp.*

28. Gallo MF, Lopez LM, Grimes DA, et al. Combination contraceptives: Effects on weight. Cochrane Database Syst Rev 2006;1:CD003987.

29. Lesnewski R, Prine L. Initiating hormonal contraception. Am Fam Physician 2006;71:105–112.

30. Truitt ST, Fraser AB, Grimes DA, et al. Combined hormonal versus nonhormonal versus progestin-only contraception in lactation. Cochrane Review Syst Rev 2003;3:CD003988.

31. Dickinson BD, Altman RD, Neilsen NH, Sterling ML. Drug interactions between oral contraceptives and antibiotics. Obstet Gynecol 2001;98:853–860.

32. Archer JS, Archer DF. Oral contraceptive efficacy and antibiotic interaction: A myth debunked. J Am Acad Dermatol 2002;46:917–923.

33. World Health Organization. Selected practice recommendations for contraceptive use, 2nd ed. Geneva: WHO, 2004.

34. Guilbert E, Black A, Dunn S, et al. Missed hormonal contraceptives: new recommendations. J Obstet Gynecol 2008;30:1050–1062.

35. Ortho Evra [package insert]. Raritan, NJ: Ortho-McNeil-Janssen Pharmaceuticals, Inc.; 2009. *http://www.myortho360.com/myortho360/shared/pi/OrthoEvraPI.pdf#zoom=100.*

36. Jick SS, Kaye JA, Russman S, Jick H. Risk of nonfatal venous thromboembolism in women using a contraceptive transdermal patch and oral contraceptives containing norgestimate and 35 mcg ethinyl estradiol. Contraception 2006;73:223–228.

37. Cole JA, Norman H, Doherty M, Walker AM. Venous thromboembolism, myocardial infarction, and stroke among transdermal contraceptive system users. Obstet Gynecol 2007;109:339–346.

38. Audet MC, Moreau M, Koltun WD, et al. Evaluation of contraceptive efficacy and cycle control of a transdermal contraceptive patch vs an oral contraceptive. A randomized controlled trial. JAMA 2001;285:2347–2354.

39. NuvaRing [package insert]. Roseland, NJ: Organon USA, Inc.; 2008. *http://www.spfiles.com/pinuvaring.pdf.*

40. Oddsson K, Leifels-Fischer B, Wiel-Masson D, et al. Superior cycle control with a contraceptive vaginal ring compared with an oral contraceptive containing 30 microg ethinyl estradiol and 150 microg levonogestrel : a randomized trial. Hum Reprod 2005;20:557–562.

41. Dieben T, Roumen F, Apter D. Efficacy, cycle control, and user acceptability of a novel combined contraceptive vaginal ring. Obstet Gynecol 2002;100:585–593.

42. Depo-Provera [package insert]. Kalamazoo, MI: Pharmacia & Upjohn Co.; 1999. *http://www.contracept.info/docs/depo-doctors.pdf.*

43. Depo-SubQ Provera 104 [package insert]. New York, NY: Pfizer, Inc; 2009. *http://media.pfizer.com/files/products/uspi_depo_subq_provera.pdf.*

44. Jain J, Jakimiuk AJ, Bode PR, et al. Contraceptive efficacy and safety of DMPA-SC. Contraception 2004;70:269–275.

45. Depot medroxyprogesterone acetate and bone effects. ACOG Practice Bulletin No. 415. American College of Obstetricians and Gynecologists. Obstet Gynecol 2008;112:727–730.

46. WHO statement on hormonal contraception and bone health; 2005. *http://www.who.int/reproductive-health/family_planning/docs hormonal_contraception_bone_health.pdf.*

47. Scholes D, LaCroix AZ, Ichikawa LE, et al. Injectable hormone contraception and bone density: results from a prospective study. Epidemiology 2002;13:581–587.

48. Implanon [package insert]. Kenilworth, NJ: Schering-Plough Corp.; 2009. *http://www.spfiles.com/piimplanon.pd.pdf.*

49. Hohmann H, Creinin MD. The contraceptive implant. Clin Obstet Gynecol 2007;50:907–917.

50. Jensen JT. Contraceptive and therapeutic effects of the levonorgestrel intrauterine system: An overview. Obstet Gynecol Surv 2005;60:604–612.

51. Intrauterine device. ACOG Practice Bulletin No. 59. American College of Obstetricians and Gynecologists. Obstet Gynecol 2005;105:223–232.

52. Mohllajee AP, Curtis KM, Peterson HB. Does insertion and use of intrauterine device increase the risk of pelvic inflammatory disease among women with sexually transmitted infection? A systematic review. Contraception 2006;73:145–153.

53. Intrauterine device and adolescents. ACOG Committee Opinion No. 392. American College of Obstetricians and Gynecologists. Obstet Gynecol 2007;110:1493–1495.

54. Emergency contraception. ACOG Practice Bulletin No. 69. American College of Obstetricians and Gynecologists. Obstet Gynecol 2005;106: 1443–1452.

55. International Consortium for Emergency Contraception Policy Statements; 2008. *www.cecinfo.org/publications/policy.htm.*

56. Novikova N, Weisberg E, Stanczyk FZ, et al. Effectiveness of levonorgestrel emergency contraception given before or after ovulation–a pilot study. Contraception 2007;75:112–118.

57. Von Hertzen H, Piaggo G, Ding J, et al. Low dose mifepristone and two regimens of levonorgestrel for emergency contraception: A WHO multicentre randomized trial. Lancet 2002;360:1803–1810.

58. Plan B One-Step [package insert]. Pomona, New York: Duramed Pharmaceuticals, Inc.; 2009.

59. U.S. Food and Drug Administration News and Events; 2009. *http://www.fda.gov/NewsEvents/Newsroom/PressAnnouncements/ ucm149568.htm.*

60. Rodrigues I, Grou F, Joly J. Effectiveness of emergency contraceptive pills between 72 and 120 hours after unprotected sexual intercourse. Am J Obstet Gynecol 2001;184:531–537.

61. Trussell J, Lalla AM, Doan QV, et al. Cost effectiveness of contraceptives in the United States. Contraception 2009;79:5–14.

89

Menstruation-Related Disorders

ELENA M. UMLAND, LARA CARSON WEINSTEIN, AND EDWARD M. BUCHANAN

KEY CONCEPTS

❶ Unrecognized pregnancy is the most common cause of amenorrhea. A urine pregnancy test should be one of the first steps in evaluating this disorder.

❷ For hypoestrogenic conditions associated with primary and secondary amenorrhea, estrogen (with a progestin) is provided.

❸ Causes of menorrhagia are either systemic disorders or specific uterine abnormalities.

❹ Pregnancy, including intrauterine pregnancy, ectopic pregnancy, and miscarriage, must be at the top of the differential diagnosis for any woman presenting with heavy menses.

❺ The reduction in menorrhagia-related blood loss with use of nonsteroidal antiinflammatory drugs and oral contraceptives is directly proportional to the amount of pretreatment blood loss.

❻ Intrauterine devices (IUDs) are considered therapeutic options in a variety of menstruation-related disorders. Guidelines from the American College of Obstetricians and Gynecologists indicate that both nulliparous and multiparous women at low risk of sexually transmitted diseases are good candidates for IUD use.

❼ Anovulatory bleeding is the standard terminology used to describe bleeding from the uterine endometrium as a result of a dysfunctioning menstrual system, specifically excluding an anatomic lesion of the uterus.

❽ Polycystic ovarian syndrome can present as a variety of menstruation disorders, including amenorrhea, menorrhagia, and anovulatory bleeding. Although its definition continues to evolve, it is generally considered a disorder of androgen excess that often includes polycystic ovarian morphology and ovulatory dysfunction.

❾ Metformin and thiazolidinedione use for anovulatory bleeding associated with PCOS is beneficial not only for anovulatory bleeding and fertility but also for improving glucose tolerance and other metabolic parameters that contribute to cardiovascular risk.

❿ The selective serotonin reuptake inhibitors are first-line pharmacologic treatment options for premenstrual dysphoric disorder.

Learning objectives, review questions,
and other resources can be found at
www.pharmacotherapyonline.com.

Problems related to the menstrual cycle are exceedingly common in women of reproductive age. This chapter discusses the most frequently encountered menstruation-related difficulties: amenorrhea, menorrhagia, anovulatory bleeding, dysmenorrhea, premenstrual syndrome (PMS), and premenstrual dysphoric disorder (PMDD). The need for effective treatments of these disorders stems from their impact on any or all of the following: a reduced quality of life, negative effects on reproductive health, and potential for long-term detrimental health effects, such as osteoporosis with amenorrhea and cardiovascular disease with polycystic ovary syndrome (PCOS).

AMENORRHEA

Amenorrhea is described as either primary or secondary in nature. Primary amenorrhea is the absence of menses by age 16 years in the presence of normal secondary sexual development or the absence of menses by age 14 in the absence of normal secondary sexual development. Secondary amenorrhea is the absence of menses for three cycles or for 6 months in a previously menstruating woman. There is a significant amount of overlap between the two. The initial evaluation of amenorrhea often is the same, regardless of age of onset, except in unusual clinical situations.[1]

EPIDEMIOLOGY

Primary amenorrhea occurs in less than 0.1% of the general population. Secondary amenorrhea, in comparison, has an incidence of 0.7% to 5% in the general population and occurs more frequently in women younger than 25 years with a history of menstrual irregularities and in those involved in competitive athletics.[2]

ETIOLOGY

❶ Unrecognized pregnancy is the most common cause of amenorrhea. A urine pregnancy test should be one of the first steps in evaluating this disorder. In organizing an approach to diagnosis and treatment, it is helpful to consider the organs involved in the menstrual cycle, which include the uterus, ovaries, anterior pituitary, and hypothalamus.

After excluding pregnancy, the most common causes of secondary amenorrhea are hypothalamic suppression, chronic anovulation, hyperprolactinemia, ovarian failure, and uterine disorders.[3]

PATHOPHYSIOLOGY

Each organ in the hypothalamic–pituitary–ovarian–uterine axis is of importance in determining amenorrhea's etiology and pathophysiology. Beginning with the uterus/outflow tract and progressing caudally will result in a comprehensive differential diagnosis.

TABLE 89-1 Pathophysiology of Selected Menstrual Bleeding Disorders

Organ System	Condition	Pathophysiology/Laboratory Findings
Amenorrhea		
Uterus	Asherman syndrome	Postcurettage/postsurgical uterine adhesions
	Congenital uterine abnormalities	Abnormal uterine development
Ovaries	Turner syndrome	Lack of ovarian follicles
	Gonadal dysgenesis	Other genetic abnormalities
	Premature ovarian failure	Early loss of follicles
	Chemotherapy/radiation	Gonadal toxins
Anterior pituitary	Pituitary prolactin-secreting adenoma	↑ Prolactin suppresses HPO axis
	Hypothyroidism	TRH causes ↑ prolactin, other abnormalities
	Medication (antipsychotics, verapamil)	↑ Prolactin suppresses HPO axis
Hypothalamus	"Functional" hypothalamic amenorrhea	↓ Pulsatile GnRH secretion in the absence of other abnormalities
	Eating disorder	↓ Pulsatile GnRH secretion, ↓ FSH and LH secondary to weight loss
	Exercise	↓ Pulsatile GnRH secretion, ↓ FSH and LH secondary to low body fat
	Anovulation/PCOS	Asynchronous gonadotropin and estrogen production, abnormal endometrial growth
Anovulatory bleeding		
Physiologic causes	Adolescence	Immaturity of the HPO axis; no LH surge
	Perimenopause	Declining ovarian function
Pathologic causes	Hyperandrogenic anovulation (PCOS)	Hyperandrogenism: high testosterone, high LH, hyperinsulinemia, and insulin resistance
	Hypothalamic dysfunction (physical or emotional stress, exercise, weight loss)	Suppression of pulsatile GnRH secretion and estrogen deficiency: low LH, low FSH
	Hyperprolactinemia (pituitary gland tumor, psychiatric medications)	High prolactin
	Hypothyroidism	High TSH
	Premature ovarian failure	High FSH
Menorrhagia		
Hematologic	von Willebrand's disease	Factor VII defect causing impaired platelet adhesion and increased bleeding time
	Idiopathic thrombocytopenic purpura	Decrease in circulating platelets, can be acute or chronic
Hepatic	Cirrhosis	Decreased estrogen metabolism, underlying coagulopathy
Endocrine	Hypothyroidism	Alterations in HPO axis
Uterine	Fibroids	Alteration of endometrium, changes in uterine contractility
	Adenomyosis	Alteration of endometrium, changes in uterine contractility
	Endometrial polyps	Alteration of endometrium
	Gynecologic cancers	Various dysplastic alterations of endometrium, uterus, cervix

FSH, follicle-stimulating hormone; GnRH, gonadotropin-releasing hormone; HPO, hypothalamic–pituitary–ovarian; LH, luteinizing hormone; PCOS, polycystic ovary disease; TSH, thyroid stimulating hormone; TRH, thyrotropin-releasing hormone.
Data from references 1–6.

Table 89–1 lists the pathophysiology of amenorrhea relative to the organ system(s) involved and the specific condition(s) that results in amenorrhea.

Uterus/Outflow Tract

For menstruation to occur, a uterus, functional endometrium, and patent vagina must be present. Several anatomic abnormalities may cause amenorrhea. If primary amenorrhea is the presenting symptom, a congenital anomaly such as imperforate hymen or uterine agenesis may be present and often discovered by physical examination. An acquired condition of the genital tract, such as Asherman syndrome or cervical stenosis, is more likely in secondary amenorrhea.

Ovaries

Normal ovarian function is critical for menstruation to occur. The ovaries must respond appropriately to follicle-stimulating hormone (FSH) and luteinizing hormone (LH) by secreting estrogen and progesterone in proper sequence to influence endometrial growth and shedding (Fig. 89–1).

Premature ovarian failure occurs when no viable follicles remain in the ovaries. This is because estrogen production is insufficient to stimulate endometrial growth in the absence of follicles. In a woman younger than 30 years, amenorrhea due to premature ovarian failure may be the result of genetic anomalies.[1]

The ovaries may play a role in amenorrhea through anovulation. Ovulation is required for the follicle (an estrogen-secreting body) to become a corpus luteum (a progesterone-secreting body). Without ovulation, the proper sequence of estrogen production, progesterone production, and estrogen/progesterone withdrawal will not occur. This can result in amenorrhea. Anovulation can occur secondary to thyroid disease, androgen excess (PCOS), or chronic illness.

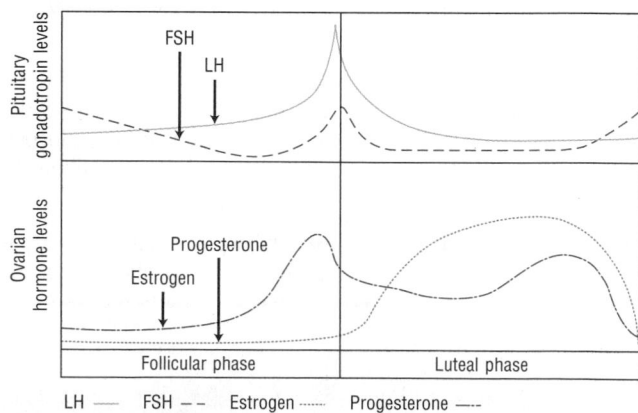

FIGURE 89-1. Summary of the normal menstrual cycle. (FSH, follicle-stimulating hormone; GnRH, gonadotropin-releasing hormone; LH, luteinizing hormone.)

Pituitary Gland

The anterior pituitary gland secretes FSH and LH in sequential fashion in response to hypothalamic stimulation and a complex ovarian feedback mechanism. Normal secretion of FSH and LH is altered by several endocrinologic and iatrogenic conditions, including thyroid disease, hyperprolactinemia, and dopaminergic drug administration.

Hypothalamus

The hypothalamus secretes cyclic gonadotropin-releasing hormone (GnRH), which causes the pituitary to produce FSH and LH. Disrupting this cyclic excretion will interrupt the hormonal cascade that results in normal menstruation. Anorexia nervosa, bulimia, intense exercise, and stress may cause hypothalamic amenorrhea.

CLINICAL PRESENTATION OF AMENORRHEA

General

- Although patients may be concerned about cessation of menses and implications for fertility, patients are generally not in acute distress.

Symptoms

- Patient will note cessation of menses.
- Patients may complain of infertility, vaginal dryness, or decreased libido.

Signs

- Cessation of menses for more than 6 months in women with established menstruation, absence of menses by age 16 years in the presence of normal secondary sexual development, or absence of menses by age 14 years in the absence of normal secondary sexual development
- Recent significant weight loss or weight gain
- Presence of acne, hirsutism, hair loss, or acanthosis nigrans may suggest androgen excess

Laboratory Tests

- Pregnancy test
- Thyroid-stimulating hormone
- Prolactin
- If PCOS is suspected, consider free or total testosterone, 17-hydroxyprogesterone, fasting glucose, fasting lipid panel
- If suspect premature ovarian failure, consider FSH, LH

Other Diagnostic Tests

- Progesterone challenge
- Pelvic ultrasound to evaluate for polycystic ovaries

TREATMENT

The treatment options for amenorrhea are as varied as its causes.

Desired Outcome

Therapeutic modalities for amenorrhea should ensure the occurrence of normal puberty and restore the menstrual cycle. Treatment goals include bone density preservation, bone loss prevention, and ovulation restoration, improving fertility as desired. Amenorrhea from hypoestrogenism may affect quality of life via hot flash induction (premature ovarian failure), dyspareunia, and, in prepubertal females, lack of secondary sexual characteristics and absence of menarche. Treatment is targeted at reversing these effects.

General Approach to Treatment

The overall success of any intervention to treat amenorrhea is dependent on proper identification of the disorder's underlying cause(s). Once the cause is identified, the appropriate intervention(s) can be made. For patients experiencing amenorrhea secondary to hypoestrogenic states, a diet rich in calcium and vitamin D is essential to avoid negative impact on bone health.

Nonpharmacologic Therapy

Nonpharmacologic therapy for amenorrhea varies depending on the underlying cause. Amenorrhea secondary to anorexia may respond to weight gain. In young women for whom excessive exercise is an underlying cause, reduction of exercise quantity and intensity are important.

Pharmacologic Therapy

❷ For hypoestrogenic conditions associated with primary or secondary amenorrhea, estrogen (with a progestin) is provided. It can be administered as an oral contraceptive (OC), conjugated equine estrogen, or estradiol patch. Estrogen therapy in this patient population reduces osteoporosis risk[7] and improves quality of life. Table 89–2 lists therapeutic agents for amenorrhea treatment, including recommended doses. Figure 89–2 illustrates a treatment algorithm for management of amenorrhea.

When hyperprolactinemia is the cause of amenorrhea, dopamine agonists, including bromocriptine and cabergoline aid in reducing prolactin concentrations and the resumption of menses. Bromocriptine requires multiple doses per day; cabergoline is dosed twice weekly. When compared with cabergoline, bromocriptine is less effective in normalizing prolactin levels and has a higher incidence of adverse events leading to treatment discontinuation.[10]

Amenorrhea related to PCOS-induced anovulation may respond to agents that reduce insulin resistance. Metformin and the thiazolidinediones for this purpose are discussed in the anovulatory bleeding section.

Progestins induce withdrawal bleeding in women with secondary amenorrhea. Several factors predict progesterone's efficacy for this purpose.[9] These factors include estrogen concentrations greater than or equal to 35 pg/mL (128 pmol/L) and endometrial thickness (greater initial thickness resulting in more withdrawal bleeding).

Progestin efficacy for secondary amenorrhea varies by formulation used. Progesterone in oil administered intramuscularly results in withdrawal bleeding in 70% of treated patients, whereas oral medroxyprogesterone acetate (MPA) induces withdrawal bleeding in 95% of treated patients.[9] Table 89–2 identifies the types and doses of progestins used for secondary amenorrhea treatment. Figure 89–2 illustrates when to consider progestin use for amenorrhea treatment.

Special Populations Amenorrhea in the adolescent population is of concern because this is the developmental time when peak bone mass is achieved. The cause of amenorrhea, whether primary or secondary, must be promptly identified in this population, as amenorrhea and its related hypoestrogenism negatively affect bone development. In addition to treating or eliminating amenorrhea's underlying cause, ensuring that the patient is receiving adequate amounts of calcium and vitamin D is imperative. Estrogen replacement, typically via an OC, is important.

Drug Class Information Table 89–3 identifies the significant pharmacologic properties, common adverse events, and clinically significant drug–drug and drug–food interactions of the agents used for amenorrhea management.

TABLE 89-2 Therapeutic Agents for Selected Menstrual Disorders

Specific Menstrual Disorder(s)	Agent(s)	Dose Recommended
Amenorrhea (primary or secondary)	CEE	0.625–1.25 mg by mouth daily on days 1–25 of the cycle[8]
	Ethinyl estradiol patch	50 mcg/24 hours[9]
	Combination OC	30–40 mcg formulations[7]
Amenorrhea (secondary)	Oral MPA	5–10 mg by mouth on days 14–25 of the cycle[8]
	Norethindrone	5 mg by mouth daily for 7–10 days[8]
	Micronized progesterone	400 mg by mouth daily for 7–10 days[8]
Amenorrhea related to hyperprolactinemia	Bromocriptine[3,10]	2.5 mg by mouth 2–3 times daily
	Cabergoline[3,10]	0.25 mg by mouth 2 times weekly (maximum 1 mg by mouth 2 times weekly)
Anovulatory bleeding	Combination OC	≤35 mcg ethinyl estradiol
Dysmenorrhea	Combination OC	Less than 35 mcg formulations + norgestrel or levonorgestrel[12]; use of extended-cycle formulations is beneficial for this indication
	Depo MPA[12]	150 mg intramuscularly every 12 weeks
	Levonorgestrel IUD[12,13,15]	20 mcg released daily
	NSAIDs (any are acceptable); the most commonly studied/cited are included in this table	Diclofenac 50 mg by mouth 3 times daily; ibuprofen 800 mg by mouth 3 times daily; mefenamic acid 500 mg by mouth as a loading dose, then 250 mg by mouth up to 4 times daily as needed[14]
		Naproxen 550-mg loading dose by mouth started 1–2 days prior to menses followed by 275 mg by mouth every 6–12 hours as needed[12]
	Celecoxib[12,13,16]	400 mg by mouth followed by 200 mg by mouth every 12 hours as needed during menses
Menorrhagia	Combination OC[18]	Optimal dose unknown
	Levonorgestrel IUD[17,18,19]	20 mcg released daily
	Oral MPA	5–10 mg by mouth on days 5–26 of the cycle or during the luteal phase[15,17]
	NSAIDs [17]	Doses as recommended for dysmenorrhea may be used; therapy should be initiated with the onset of menses[15]
	Tranexamic acid[17,20]	1,300 mg by mouth every 8 hours once heavy bleeding begins; dose for 4–7 days as needed per cycle.
PCOS-related amenorrhea and/or anovulatory bleeding	Depo MPA	150 mg intramuscularly every 12 weeks
	Combination OC[21,22]	≤30 mcg ethinyl estradiol with either desogestrel, norgestimate, or drospirenone
	Oral MPA	10 mg by mouth for 10 days[5]
	Metformin[5,22]	1,500–2,000 mg by mouth daily[22]
	Thiazolidinediones (pioglitazone, rosiglitazone)[5,22]	Pioglitazone 15–45 mg by mouth daily; rosiglitazone 4–8 mg by mouth daily
PMDD	Clomipramine[23]	25–75 mg by mouth daily taken either continuously or only during the luteal phase
	Drospirenone	3 mg (+ ≤30 mcg ethinyl estradiol) by mouth on days 1–21 of the menstrual cycle[24]
	Leuprolide	3.75 mg intramuscularly[23]
	SSRIs[25]	Citalopram 10–30 mg; escitalopram 10–20 mg[26]; fluoxetine 10–20 mg; fluvoxamine 50 mg; paroxetine 10–30 mg; sertraline 25–150 mg; all agents are given by mouth daily and can be dosed either continuously or during the luteal phase only[23]

CEE, conjugated equine estrogen; IUD, intrauterine device; MPA, medroxyprogesterone acetate; NSAID, nonsteroidal antiinflammatory drug; OC, oral contraceptive; PCOS, polycystic ovary syndrome; PMDD, premenstrual dysphoric disorder; SSRI, selective serotonin reuptake inhibitor.
Data from references 3, 5, 7–10, 12–17, 21–26.

PHARMACOECONOMIC CONSIDERATIONS

The largest price gap among agents used in amenorrhea management occurs when comparing the dopamine agonists bromocriptine and cabergoline in treating hyperprolactinemia. Cabergoline is slightly more effective, with fewer side effects and less frequent dosing, but its monthly cost is significantly greater than bromocriptine. Given this, it is reasonable to reserve its use for patients who are not successfully treated with bromocriptine or for whom bromocriptine's side effects are responsible for drug discontinuation.

EVALUATION OF THERAPEUTIC OUTCOMES

Table 89-4 lists the expected outcomes and specific monitoring parameters for treatment modalities used in amenorrhea management.

MENORRHAGIA

Menorrhagia is traditionally defined by menstrual blood loss greater than 80 mL per cycle. This definition has been questioned because of several factors, including difficulty quantifying menstrual loss

in clinical practice. Additionally, many women with "heavy menses" but blood loss less than 80 mL merit treatment consideration because of flow containment issues, unpredictably heavy flow days, or other associated symptoms.[20]

EPIDEMIOLOGY

Menorrhagia rates in healthy women range from 9% to 14%.[4]

ETIOLOGY

❸ Causes of menorrhagia are either systemic disorders or specific uterine abnormalities. **❹** Pregnancy, including intrauterine pregnancy, ectopic pregnancy, and miscarriage, must be at the top of the differential diagnosis for any woman presenting with heavy menses. In several studies of adolescents with acute menorrhagia, underlying bleeding disorders accounted for 3% to 13% of emergency room presentations. For example, von Willebrand's disease has an incidence of 1% in the general population;[29] its prevalence in women with menorrhagia may be as high as 20%.[30] Furthermore, 74% to 92% of women with von Willebrand's disease have menorrhagia.[6] Menorrhagia initially may present as heavy menses in the adolescent.[29] Hypothyroidism also may be

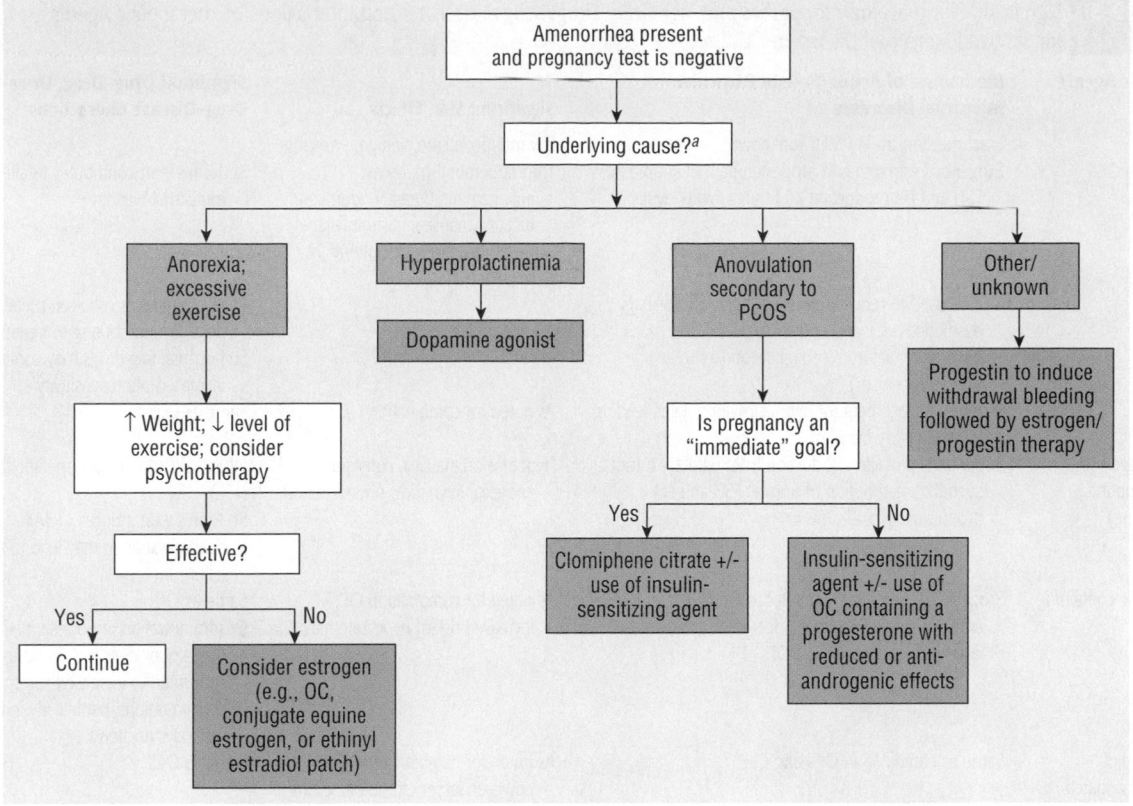

FIGURE 89-2. Treatment algorithm for amenorrhea. *a*Regardless of cause, adequate calcium and vitamin D intake must be ensured. (OC, oral contraceptive; PCOS, polycystic ovary syndrome.)

associated with heavy menses. Specific uterine causes of menorrhagia are more common in older childbearing women and include fibroids, adenomyosis, endometrial polyps, and gynecologic malignancies.

PATHOPHYSIOLOGY

Table 89–1 lists the pathophysiology of menorrhagia relative to the organ system(s) involved and the specific conditions that result in menorrhagia.

CLINICAL PRESENTATION OF MENORRHAGIA

General

☐ Patient may or may not be in acute distress.

Symptoms

☐ Patients may complain of heavy/prolonged menstrual flow. They also may have signs of fatigue and lightheadedness in cases of severe blood loss. These symptoms may or may not occur with dysmenorrhea.

Signs

☐ Orthostasis, tachycardia, and pallor may be noted, especially in cases of significant acute blood loss.

Laboratory Tests

☐ Complete blood count and ferritin levels; hemoglobin and hematocrit results may be low.

☐ If the history dictates, testing may be performed to identify coagulation disorder(s) as a cause.

Other Diagnostic Tests

☐ Pelvic ultrasound

☐ Pelvic magnetic resonance imaging

☐ Papanicolaou (Pap) smear

☐ Endometrial biopsy

☐ Hysteroscopy

☐ Sonohysterogram

TREATMENT

Initial treatment choice for menorrhagia is influenced by whether or not the woman desires to become pregnant.

Desired Outcome

Menorrhagia therapy should reduce menstrual blood flow, improve the patient's quality of life, and defer the need for surgical intervention. Table 89–2 lists the agents and their recommended dosing for menorrhagia management. Figure 89–3 presents an algorithm for menorrhagia treatment.

General Approach to Treatment

Several treatment options exist for menorrhagia. Initial and subsequent treatment options should be thoughtfully chosen in an effort to avoid surgery.

Nonpharmacologic Therapy

Nonpharmacologic interventions for menorrhagia include surgical procedures that are generally reserved for patients not responding

TABLE 89-3 Significant Pharmacologic Properties and Significant Drug–Drug and Drug–Food Interactions of Therapeutic Agents for Selected Menstrual Disorders

Therapeutic Agent/ Drug Class	Mechanism of Action/Role in Particular Menstrual Disorders	Significant Side Effects	Significant Drug–Drug, Drug–Food, Drug–Disease Interactions
Clomipramine	Exact mechanism in PMDD unknown	Dry mouth, fatigue, vertigo, sweating	
Combination OCs	Exogenous estrogen and progesterone that suppresses FSH and LH production and thus inhibits ovulation	Thromboembolism, breast enlargement, breast tenderness, bloating, nausea, gastrointestinal upset, headache, peripheral edema	St. John's wort contributes to altered menstrual bleeding
	Can be used to reduce menstrual flow (menorrhagia, dysmenorrhea), and control menstrual cycle (anovulatory bleeding secondary to hypoestrogenism)		Rifampin induces estrogen metabolism, possibly contributing to treatment failure Sulfa-containing drugs may contribute to increased photosensitivity
CEE	Estrogen replacement for hypoestrogenic states leading to anovulatory bleeding	As noted for combination OC	Same as OCs
Dopamine agonists (bromocriptine, cabergoline)	Suppresses prolactin production from pituitary tumors such that resumption of normal FSH and LH production occurs	Hypotension, nausea, constipation, anorexia, Raynaud's phenomenon	Inhibit CYP3A4 and are metabolized by CYP3A4 St. John's wort induces CP3A4; coadministration may lead to treatment failure
Drospirenone-containing OCs	Progesterone with antimineralocorticoid and antiandrogenic properties; decreases emotional lability associated with PMDD	As noted for combination OC; increased risk of hyperkalemia	Same as OCs Coadministration of potassium-sparing diuretics or diets high in potassium may contribute to increased serum potassium concentrations, particularly in women with renal dysfunction
Ethinyl estradiol transdermal patch	Same as combination OCs and CEE	As noted for combination OC; however, lesser effects on serum cholesterol concentrations because patch avoids first-pass metabolism	Same as OCs
Leuprolide	GnRH agent that contributes to suppression of FSH and LH and ultimately a reduction in estrogen and progesterone, inhibiting the normal menstrual cycle/ hormonal fluctuations	Hot flashes, night sweats, headache, nausea	
Levonorgestrel-containing IUD	Suppresses FSH and LH and ultimately estrogen and progesterone, inhibiting the usual growth of the endometrium	Irregular menses, amenorrhea	
MPA (oral and depot)	Suppresses FSH and LH and ultimately estrogen and progesterone, inhibiting the usual growth of the endometrium	Edema, anorexia, depression, insomnia, weight gain or loss, increase in serum total and LDL cholesterol, may reduce HDL cholesterol	
Metformin	Inhibits hepatic glucose production and increases sensitivity of tissues to insulin, thus reducing insulin resistance	Anorexia, nausea, vomiting, diarrhea, flatulence, lactic acidosis (rare)	IV contrast dye may increase the risk of lactic acidosis; stop metformin 1 day prior and restart when renal function is normal and stabilized following the IV dye
NSAIDs	Inhibits prostaglandin release that occurs with menses, thus reducing inflammatory response contributing to dysmenorrhea	Gastrointestinal upset, stomach ulcer, nausea, vomiting, heartburn, indigestion, rash, dizziness	
SSRIs	Exact mechanism in PMDD unknown	Sexual dysfunction (reduced libido, anorgasmia), insomnia, sedation, hypersomnia, nausea, diarrhea	
Thiazolidinediones	Increases peripheral tissue sensitivity to insulin, thus reducing insulin resistance	Weight gain, increase in total, LDL, and HDL cholesterol, edema, headache, fatigue, hepatic injury (rare)	
Tranexamic acid	Antifibrinolytic effects by reversibly blocking lysine binding sites on plasminogen, preventing fibrin degradation and a reduction in menstrual blood loss	Nausea, vomiting, diarrhea, dyspepsia	
Venlafaxine	Exact mechanism in PMDD unknown		

CEE, conjugated equine estrogen; FSH, follicle-stimulating hormone; GnRH, gonadotropin-releasing hormone; HDL, high-density lipoprotein; IUD, intrauterine device; LDL, low-density lipoprotein; LH, luteinizing hormone; MPA, medroxyprogesterone acetate; NSAID, nonsteroidal antiinflammatory drug; OC, oral contraceptive; PMDD, premenstrual dysphoric disorder; SSRI, selective serotonin reuptake inhibitor.

Data from references 7, 10, 11, 14, 15, 20, 23, 27, 28.

TABLE 89-4 Expected Outcome Measures for Select Menstrual Bleeding Disorders

Menstrual Disorder	Expected Outcome Measures: Specific Monitoring Parameters and Frequency of Monitoring
Amenorrhea	Patient should return after one month of treatment to evaluate whether menses has resumed. Menses should resume within 1–2 months of therapy.
	If amenorrhea has been long-standing and secondary to a hypoestrogenic condition, preservation/improvement of BMD is warranted. A baseline BMD test may be desirable; repeat test no sooner than 1–2 years.
	If amenorrhea is secondary to high prolactin levels, serum prolactin levels should be measured at baseline and weekly with dosage increases until response (resumption of menses) is observed; consider discontinuation of therapy after 6–12 months of menses and serum prolactin concentrations have normalized.
	In young women who have primary amenorrhea, normal breast development should occur over a time frame of several months of therapy.
Menorrhagia	Amount of blood lost with menses should be reduced (monitor decline in number of times feminine hygiene products such as pads and tampons require changing during menses) as observed within 1–2 menstrual cycles of therapy. Patient should return for evaluation after one full menstrual cycle of therapy.
	Hemoglobin/hematocrit should be measured at baseline and within 3 months of beginning therapy.
	Annual gynecologic examination should be performed in women receiving hormonal agents for treatment of menorrhagia. Serum lipid concentrations should be measured within 3–6 months of starting the hormonal regimen and repeated per national lipid guidelines as appropriate. Blood pressure should be measured at baseline and within 4–6 weeks of beginning any hormonal agents; repeat blood pressure measurements per national hypertension guidelines as appropriate.
Anovulatory bleeding	Patients should return for follow up within 1 week to evaluate alleviation of acute bleeding when present. Acute severe bleeding should decline within 10 days of therapy onset. Ovulation, if desired, can be measured via daily basal body temperature evaluation, use of home ovulation predictor kits, and serum FSH/LH measurements at the time of suspected ovulation. If resumption of ovulation is desired by women receiving metformin, it is important to be aware that metformin may contribute to resumption of ovulation after 3–6 months of therapy. In women with PCOS, baseline and repeat measurements of blood pressure, serum lipids, and blood glucose should be assessed per national guidelines to monitor for the development, presence, or progression of hypertension, hyperlipidemia, and diabetes.
	When OCs are used for control of abnormal uterine bleeding, improvement in the pattern of abnormal bleeding should occur within 1–2 menstrual cycles of therapy. Annual gynecologic examinations should be performed; serum lipid concentrations should be measured within 3–6 months of starting the OC and repeated per national lipid guidelines. Blood pressure should be measured at baseline and within 4–6 weeks of beginning any hormonal agents; repeat blood pressure measurements per national hypertension guidelines as appropriate.
Dysmenorrhea	Patient should return for evaluation of reduction in or absence of pelvic pain related to menses after 1–2 menstrual cycles of therapy. In addition, reduction in time lost from work/school and improved quality of life should be observed after a full 1–3 menstrual cycles of OC therapy.
	If NSAIDs are used, improvement in pain should be observed within hours of the dose.
PMDD	Reduction in or absence of initial symptoms and improved quality of life may be observed within 1–3 menstrual cycles of therapy. SSRIs have resulted in significant improvement after one cycle of treatment. If an OC containing drospirenone is used, serum potassium should be monitored within the first month of use if the woman is also receiving agents that predispose her to increased serum potassium concentrations. An annual gynecologic examination should be performed; serum lipid concentrations should be measured within 3–6 months of starting the OC and repeated per national lipid guidelines as appropriate. Blood pressure should be measured at baseline and within 4–6 weeks of beginning any hormonal agents; repeat blood pressure measurements per national hypertension guidelines as appropriate.

BMD, bone mineral density; FSH, follicle-stimulating hormone; LH, luteinizing hormone; NSAID, nonsteroidal antiinflammatory drug; OC, oral contraceptive; PCOS, polycystic ovary syndrome; PMDD, premenstrual dysphoric disorder; SSRI, selective serotonin reuptake inhibitor.

Data from references 4, 5, 27, 31–36.

to pharmacologic treatment. These interventions vary from conservative endometrial ablation to hysterectomy.[37]

Pharmacologic Therapy

Among the agents used to treat menorrhagia, the nonsteroidal antiinflammatory drugs (NSAIDs) have the advantage of administration only during menses. NSAID use is associated with a 20% to 50% reduction in blood loss in 75% of treated women.[15] In some patients, as much as an 80% reduction in blood loss has been observed.[15]

For women desiring to avoid pregnancy, OC use is beneficial for menorrhagia and should be considered. A 43% to 53% reduction in menstrual blood loss has been observed in 68% of menorrhagia patients treated with OCs containing greater than or equal to 35 mcg of estradiol.[15] ⑤ The reduction in menorrhagia-related blood loss with use of NSAIDs and OCs is directly proportional to the amount of pretreatment blood loss.[15]

Another menorrhagia treatment option is the levonorgestrel-releasing intrauterine device (IUD). This is a very effective treatment that consistently reduces menstrual flow by at least 90%.[15,38] In particular, an 86% reduction in blood loss has been observed after 3 months of use; as much as 97% after 12 months.[39] Its use has also resulted in postponing or cancelling scheduled endometrial ablation surgery or hysterectomy. Sixty percent of treated patients avoided hysterectomy when employing this treatment option.[38,40,41]

and its therapeutic efficacy is similar to endometrial ablation up to 2 years following treatment.[19]

Progesterone therapy either during the luteal phase of the menstrual cycle or for 21 days, starting on day 5 after onset of menses, results in a 32% to 50% reduction in menstrual blood loss.[15] However, progesterone use is not superior to other medical treatments, including the NSAIDs.[15]

Tranexamic acid was recently approved in the United States for primary menorrhagia treatment. Its use is associated with a significant 40% to 50% reduction in menstrual blood loss.[17]

Drug Treatments of First Choice For women who have menorrhagia associated with ovulatory cycles and do not desire hormonal therapy and/or contraception, NSAIDs during menses is a reasonable choice, in the absence of any contraindications or gastrointestinal illnesses such as peptic ulcer disease or gastroesophageal reflux disease. This choice is convenient (only taken during menses) and comparatively inexpensive. For women desiring contraception, it is reasonable to start with either an OC or the levonorgestrel-releasing IUD. Either choice is acceptable for both nulligravid and multiparous women who desire a long-term reversible form of contraception.[38] Given cost-effectiveness data, the levonorgestrel-releasing IUD is the best first-line choice for women desiring contraception.[42] Clinical trial data illustrate a higher failure rate with the OCs (62.5%) compared with the levonorgestrel-releasing IUD (34%) as the primary treatment method.[42]

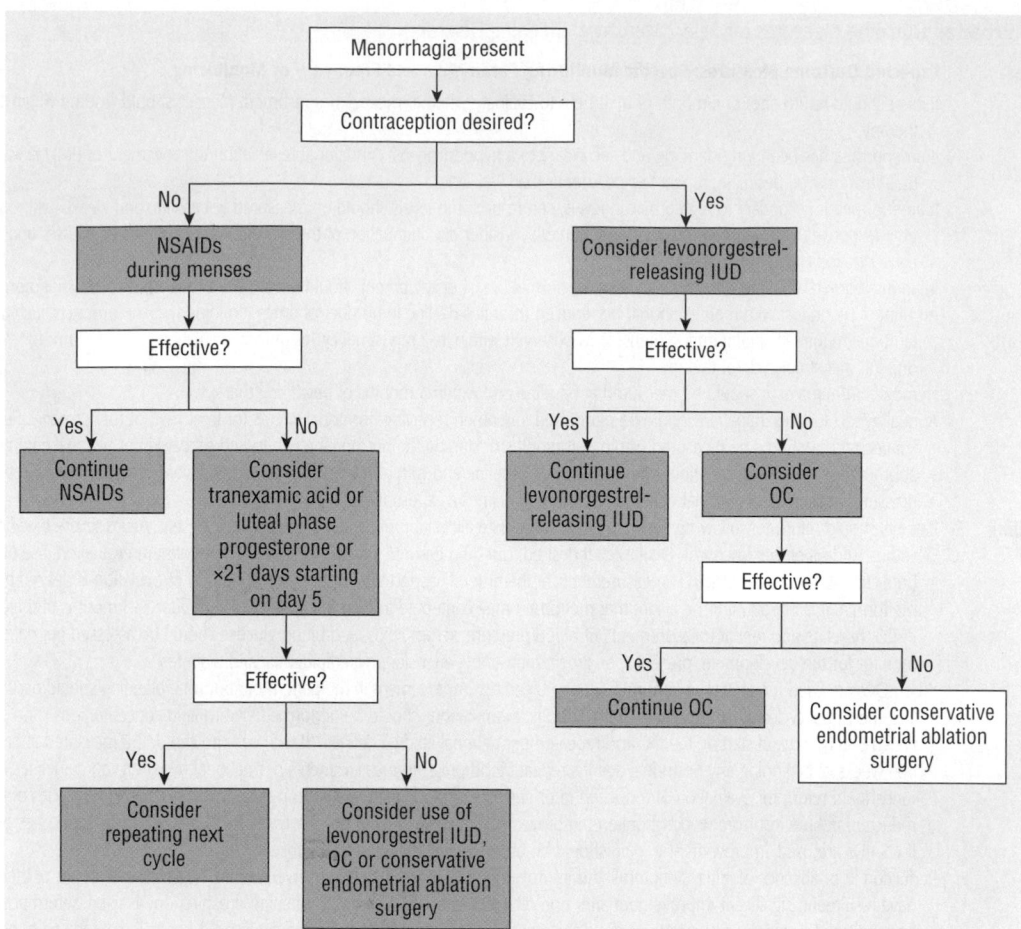

FIGURE 89-3. Treatment algorithm for menorrhagia. (IUD, intrauterine device; NSAIDs, nonsteroidal antiinflammatory drugs; OC, oral contraceptive.)

Alternative Drug Treatments Given their side effects, reduced efficacy compared with the first-line agents, and/or cost, use of oral progesterone and depot MPA should be reserved. Tranexamic acid is another treatment option. In comparison to luteal phase oral progesterone, tranexamic acid results in a significantly greater reduction in menstrual blood loss and greater relief of patient-reported symptoms.[15] Its use has been associated with a significant improvement in quality of life and high patient satisfaction following three cycles of use.[17,20]

Special Populations Although historically it was believed that IUD use should be avoided in nulliparous women, ❻ the American College of Obstetricians and Gynecologists (ACOG) indicate that both nulliparous and multiparous women at low risk of sexually transmitted diseases are good candidates for IUD use.[38] Therefore, any of the treatments discussed are options in any female presenting with menorrhagia. Dosage adjustment for tranexamic acid is recommended for reduced renal function. Women with serum creatinine between 1.4 and 2.8 mg/dL (124 and 248 μmol/L) should receive only 1,300 mg by mouth twice daily; women with serum creatinine between 2.9 and 5.7 mg/dL (256 and 504 μmol/L) should receive 1,300 mg by mouth once daily; those with serum creatinine above 5.7 mg/dL (504 μmol/L) should receive 650 mg by mouth once daily.

Drug Class Information Table 89–3 identifies the significant pharmacologic properties, common adverse events, and clinically significant drug–drug and drug–food interactions of the agents for menorrhagia management.

PHARMACOECONOMIC CONSIDERATIONS

The levonorgestrel-releasing IUD is the most cost-effective option when compared to surgical management and OCs in OC-naïve women and women who had received OCs with or without a response.[42]

EVALUATION OF THERAPEUTIC OUTCOMES

Table 89–4 illustrates the expected outcomes and specific monitoring parameters for the treatment modalities used in menorrhagia management.

ANOVULATORY BLEEDING

❼ Anovulatory bleeding is the standard terminology used to describe bleeding from the uterine endometrium as a result of a dysfunctioning menstrual system, specifically excluding an anatomic lesion of the uterus.[1,32] Anovulatory bleeding is also referred to as dysfunctional or irregular uterine bleeding.

EPIDEMIOLOGY

Anovulatory bleeding is the most common form of noncyclic uterine bleeding.[4] PCOS is the most common cause, with prevalence rates ranging from 5% to 10% in various reports, depending on the diagnostic criteria used (e.g., PCOS-NIH[43] or PCOS-Rotterdam[44]).[1,5,45,48] In fact, PCOS is the most common endocrine abnormality among U.S. women of reproductive age.[46] PCOS can present as a variety of menstruation disorders, including amenorrhea, menorrhagia, and/or anovulatory bleeding. Although its exact definition continues to evolve, it is a disorder of androgen excess that often includes polycystic ovarian morphology and ovulatory dysfunction. It is a significant risk factor for the metabolic syndrome, type 2 diabetes, dyslipidemia, hypertension, and possibly cardiovascular disease.[22,47,48] PCOS is a common cause of ovulation dysfunction in adult women.[22] Other common causes in adult women include hyperprolactinemia, hypothalamic amenorrhea, also known as hypogonadotropic hypogonadism, premature ovarian failure, and thyroid dysfunction.[1,32]

ETIOLOGY

When considering the etiology of anovulatory bleeding, the patient's age must be considered. All patients presenting with abnormal bleeding should be evaluated for pregnancy. Most adolescents will experience physiologic anovulatory cycles in the first few years following menarche because their hypothalamic–pituitary–gonadal axis is still maturing. However, if an adolescent has not developed regular menstrual cycles within 5 years of menarche, further evaluation for the cause, such as PCOS, should be considered.[49] Anovulatory cycles may "unmask" an underlying bleeding disorder. When irregular menses is associated with significant bleeding, an inherited bleeding disorder should be a considered cause, especially in adolescence.[6,32] Women experiencing anovulation in their reproductive years should be evaluated for pathologic causes, including PCOS, thyroid dysfunction, hyperprolactinemia, primary pituitary disease, premature ovarian failure, hypothalamic dysfunction, disordered eating, adrenal disease, and androgen-producing tumors. Women in their perimenopausal years may experience "physiologic" anovulatory cycles because of intermittently declining estrogen levels. Regardless of age, evaluation for endometrial hyperplasia and/or endometrial cancer should be considered when a woman experiences excessive bleeding with anovulatory cycles. When considering the etiology of anovulation, it is common for several conditions to coexist (e.g., PCOS and hypothyroidism), each contributing to the woman's constellation of symptoms. All common etiologies should be considered when beginning to evaluate anovulation.[1]

PATHOPHYSIOLOGY

Normal menstrual cycles occur through a complex interaction of the hypothalamus, pituitary gland, ovaries, and endometrium (Fig. 89–1). In an ovulatory cycle, the ovary produces a mature, estrogen-secreting follicle in response to FSH release from the pituitary. The endometrium proliferates under the influence of this estrogen production. At a critical level of estrogen concentration, the pituitary responds by producing an "LH surge," which creates a cascade of ovarian events, culminating in ovulation. Upon oocyte release, the follicle becomes a progesterone-producing corpus luteum. The endometrium "organizes" into secretory endometrium in the presence of adequate progesterone. If conception and implantation do not occur, corpus luteum involution causes a decline in estrogen and progesterone leading to predictable, organized menstrual flow as the endometrium sloughs.

If ovulation does not occur, progesterone is not produced, and the endometrium will continue to proliferate in an "unorganized" fashion under the influence of continued estrogen production. Eventually the endometrium will become so thick that it can no longer be supported by continued estrogen production. This results in unorganized, sporadic sloughing of the endometrium, characteristic of the unpredictable and heavy bleeding of anovulation. Anovulation has several etiologies. In adolescence, hypothalamic–pituitary axis

immaturity contributes to the absence of the LH surge required for ovulation. In the anorexic patient, the hypothalamus loses much of its pulsatile GnRH release, leading to low levels of FSH and LH, enough for estrogen production but not enough to induce ovulation.

CLINICAL PRESENTATION OF ANOVULATORY BLEEDING

General
- Patients may or may not be in acute distress.

Symptoms
- Irregular, heavy, or prolonged vaginal bleeding, perimenopausal symptoms (hot flashes, night sweats, vaginal dryness)

Signs
- Acne, hirsutism, obesity

Laboratory Tests
- If PCOS is suspected, consider free or total testosterone fasting glucose, fasting lipid panel
- If perimenopause is suspected, measure FSH
- Thyroid-stimulating hormone

Other Diagnostic Tests
- If the patient is older than 35 years, endometrial biopsy
- Pelvic ultrasound to evaluate for polycystic ovaries
- If perimenopause is suspected, measure FSH

TREATMENT

Optimizing anovulatory bleeding therapy depends on accurate identification of the disorder's cause(s). The treatment options for anovulatory bleeding are wide and varied.

Desired Outcome

Control of excessive bleeding in the short-term is paramount. Longer-term goals of therapy include restoring the natural cycle of orderly endometrial growth and shedding,[32,50] decreasing anovulation complications (e.g., osteopenia, infertility), and improving overall quality of life. Table 89–2 identifies the agents used to manage anovulatory bleeding and their recommended doses.

General Approach to Treatment

Although the appropriate primary treatment choice for anovulatory bleeding depends on the accurate diagnosis of its cause and identification of desired outcomes, additional treatment may be necessary to manage other signs and symptoms. Treatment to resolve anovulatory bleeding should be initiated and any underlying menorrhagia should be managed.

Nonpharmacologic Therapy

Nonpharmacologic treatment options for anovulatory bleeding depend on the underlying cause. In a woman of reproductive age with PCOS, weight loss may be beneficial.[22] In women who have completed childbearing or who have not responded to medical management, endometrial ablation or resection and hysterectomy are surgical options. Procedure choice involves shared decision making with the patient. In the short term, ablation results in less morbidity and shorter recovery periods. However, a significant number of women eventually undergo hysterectomy in the subsequent 5 years.[32]

Pharmacologic Therapy

Estrogen is the recommended treatment for managing acute severe bleeding episodes because it promotes endometrial stabilization.[50] Following its initial use to control acute bleeding episodes, therapy continuation may be necessary to prevent future occurrences. OC use fulfills this role and contributes to predictable menstrual cycles.

OCs prevent recurrent anovulatory bleeding by providing a progestin and suppressing ovarian hormones and adrenal androgen production. They also, indirectly, increase sex hormone–binding globulin (SHBG). SHBG binds androgens and reduces their circulating free concentrations. For women with high androgen levels and its related signs such as hirsutism (e.g., those with PCOS), OCs containing less than or equal to 35 mcg of ethinyl estradiol and a progesterone that exhibits minimal androgenic side effects (e.g., norgestimate and desogestrel) or with antiandrogenic effects (e.g., drospirenone) may be desirable.[22]

In women with contraindication(s) to estrogen or in whom the side effects are unacceptable, progesterone-only products are an option. They should be strongly considered for women experiencing menorrhagia associated with anovulatory bleeding.[51] In women with PCOS, depot and intermittent oral MPA provide endometrial protection through endometrial shedding.[5] If pregnancy is not a desired outcome of treatment, another progesterone option is placement of a levonorgestrel-containing IUD.[32,51]

Metformin and the thiazolidinediones, including pioglitazone and rosiglitazone, improve insulin sensitivity. In patients with PCOS, this contributes to reduced circulating androgen concentrations, increased ovulation rates,[5,52,53] and improved glucose tolerance.[5,22] These improvements occur due to the SHBG increase that occurs via increased insulin sensitivity. ❾ Metformin and thiazolidinedione use for anovulatory bleeding associated with PCOS is beneficial not only for anovulatory bleeding and fertility but also for improving glucose tolerance and other metabolic parameters that contribute to cardiovascular risk.[5,55] For women desiring pregnancy, metformin is pregnancy category B, and pioglitazone and rosiglitazone are category C.

CLINICAL CONTROVERSY

The overall role of metformin in treating PCOS, particularly its duration of therapy, remains controversial. For ovulation induction, data illustrate that metformin is highly effective in both clomiphene citrate–resistant patients and patients using it as initial therapy.[52,53] Its use throughout pregnancy has been associated with a reduction in early pregnancy loss rates.[54] The presence of dyslipidemia and hyperinsulinemia increases the long-term risk for developing cardiovascular disease in PCOS patients. Current research indicates that metformin should be considered to reduce cardiovascular risk in these women.[55] More research is needed to definitively identify the role(s) of metformin in PCOS.

If the treatment goal is improved fertility via ovulation induction, clomiphene citrate is an option. Treatment with 50 mg/day for 5 days can be initiated between menstrual cycle days 3 and 5. This often occurs after inducing withdrawal bleeding with a progesterone such as MPA 10 mg daily orally for 10 days. If ovulation does not occur with this dose of clomiphene, a dose of 100 mg/day is warranted. In rare instances, it may be increased by 50 mg increments up to 250 mg/day.

Drug Treatments of First Choice As with many menstruation-related disorders, there is not one universal treatment option of first choice for anovulatory bleeding. Rather, the treatment(s) chosen depends on accurate etiologic diagnosis as well as identification of the desired treatment outcome(s).

OCs are the first-choice treatment in women with anovulatory bleeding.[22] While controversial, the use of OCs containing ethinyl estradiol and a progesterone with minimal androgenic or antiandrogenic effects is effective for cycle control and minimizing the androgenic signs and symptoms of PCOS.[21,48]

CLINICAL CONTROVERSY

OCs are very effective for managing the acne and hirsutism that accompany PCOS; they also suppress ovarian androgen production and increase sex hormone binding globulin, thus reducing testosterone free concentrations. Controversy regarding their use in PCOS exists secondary to their potential adverse effects on insulin resistance, glucose tolerance, vascular reactivity, and coagulability.[22] Additional, longer-term clinical trials will identify whether the benefits of these agents outweigh the risks.

Relative to anovulation in women with PCOS, insulin-sensitizing agents, including metformin and the thiazolidinediones, improve ovulatory frequency and metabolic parameters. Clomiphene use may further assist in achieving ovulation induction.

More recent data supports even further the use of metformin compared with clomiphene for ovulation induction.[52,53] Metformin for ovulation induction[52] as well as its use throughout pregnancy[54] in women with PCOS has been associated with reduced miscarriage rates in this patient population.

Special Populations Anovulatory cycles are fairly common in the perimenarchal reproductive years. Ovulation typically is established 1 year or more following menarche. Anovulatory bleeding occurring in this population may be excessive. If excessive bleeding occurs, the patient should be evaluated for bleeding disorders. The prevalence of bleeding disorders, including von Willebrand disease, prothrombin deficiency, and idiopathic thrombocytopenia purpura, in this population ranges from 5% to 24%.[6]

If identified, the specific bleeding disorders should be treated. Acute severe bleeding can be managed with high-dose estrogen. OCs containing less than or equal to 35 mcg of ethinyl estradiol is a first-line treatment in adolescents with chronic anovulation.[50]

Drug Class Information Table 89–3 identifies the significant pharmacologic properties, common adverse events, and clinically significant drug–drug and drug–food interactions of agents used to treat anovulatory bleeding.

EVALUATION OF THERAPEUTIC OUTCOMES

Table 89–4 lists the expected outcomes and specific monitoring parameters for the treatment modalities used to manage anovulatory bleeding.

DYSMENORRHEA

Dysmenorrhea is one of the most commonly encountered gynecologic complaints. It is defined as crampy pelvic pain occurring with or just prior to menses. Primary dysmenorrhea implies pain in the setting of normal pelvic anatomy and physiology. Secondary dysmenorrhea is associated with underlying pelvic pathology.[14]

EPIDEMIOLOGY

Dysmenorrhea prevalence rates range from 16% to 90%.[33,34] Its presence may be associated with significant interference in work and school attendance. Risk factors include young age, heavy menses, nulliparity, early menarche, and cigarette smoking.[9,12]

ETIOLOGY

For most patients, dysmenorrhea is associated with normal ovulatory cycles and normal pelvic anatomy. This is referred to as primary, or functional, dysmenorrhea. However, in approximately 10% of the adolescents and young adults presenting with painful menses, an underlying anatomic or physiologic cause exists.[12]

PATHOPHYSIOLOGY

The most significant mechanism for primary dysmenorrhea is the release of prostaglandins and leukotrienes into the menstrual fluid, initiating an inflammatory response and possibly vasopressin-mediated vasoconstriction.[9,12,29] Causes of secondary dysmenorrhea include cervical stenosis, endometriosis, pelvic infections, pelvic congestion syndrome, uterine or cervical polyps, uterine fibroids, genital outflow tract obstructions, and pelvic adhesions.[12,34] Pregnancy and miscarriage must be considered in the presentation of dysmenorrhea.

CLINICAL PRESENTATION OF DYSMENORRHEA

General

  Patient may or may not be in acute distress, depending on the level of menstrual pain experienced.

Symptoms

  Patients complain of crampy pelvic pain beginning shortly before or at the onset of menses. Symptoms typically last from 1 to 3 days.

Laboratory Tests

  Pelvic examination should be performed to screen for sexually transmitted diseases as a cause of the pain in sexually active females.

  Gonorrhea, *Chlamydia* cultures or polymerase chain reaction, wet mount

Other Diagnostic Tests

  Pelvic ultrasound can be used to identify potential anatomic abnormalities such as masses/lesions or to detect ovarian cysts and endometriomas.

TREATMENT

Initial treatment choice is influenced by whether or not the woman desires pregnancy. Nonpharmacologic options have been studied and observed to be as effective as some existing pharmacologic options.

Desired Outcome

Medical management of dysmenorrhea should relieve the pelvic pain and result in reducing lost school and work days. Table 89–2 identifies the agents used to manage dysmenorrhea and their

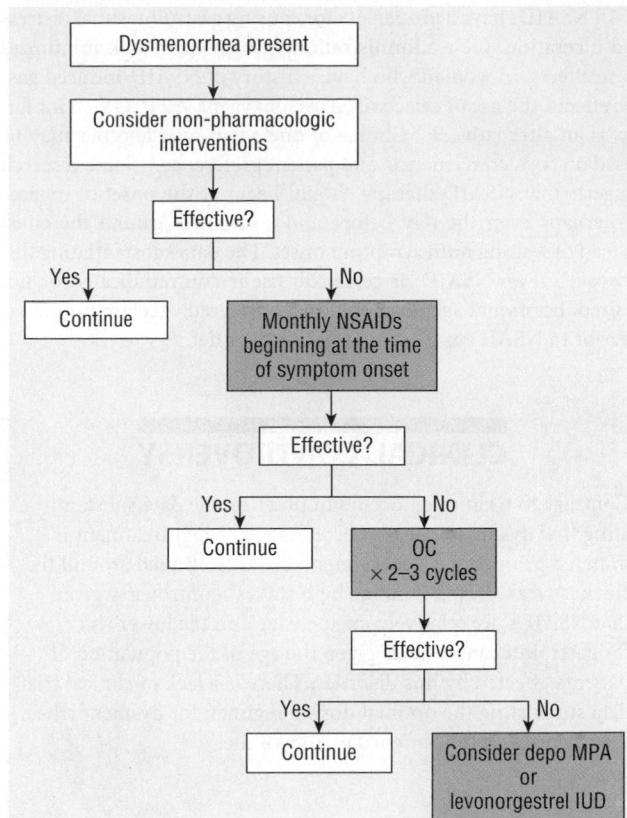

FIGURE 89-4. Treatment algorithm for dysmenorrhea. (IUD, intrauterine device; MPA, medroxyprogesterone acetate; NSAIDs, nonsteroidal antiinflammatory drugs; OC, oral contraceptive.)

recommended doses. Figure 89–4 shows a treatment algorithm for dysmenorrhea management.

General Approach to Treatment

A variety of effective treatment options for dysmenorrhea are available, including nonhormonal and hormonal pharmacologic options and noninvasive nonpharmacologic options. Treatment choice is influenced by the desire for contraception, the patient's level of sexual activity, potential for adverse effects, and cost.

Nonpharmacologic Therapy

Several nonpharmacologic interventions are used for managing dysmenorrhea. Among these, topical heat therapy, exercise, and a low-fat vegetarian diet have been shown to reduce dysmenorrhea intensity.[12,13,14,33] Dietary changes may shorten dysmenorrhea duration. Topical heat application via an abdominal patch worn for 12 consecutive hours/day is as effective as 400 mg of ibuprofen dosed 3 times daily.[56] Because topical heat, exercise, and dietary changes do not impart systemic effects, they are associated with little to no risk compared to the pharmacologic options. Nonpharmacologic options that are reserved for use following a failed trial of pharmacologic interventions include transcutaneous electric nerve stimulation, acupressure, and acupuncture.[14,33]

Pharmacologic Therapy

Given the role of prostaglandins in dysmenorrhea pathophysiology, NSAIDs are the initial treatment of choice. These agents do not differ in efficacy. The most commonly used agents are naproxen and ibuprofen.

All NSAIDs have a propensity for causing gastrointestinal distress and ulceration; their administration with food or milk minimizes these effects. In women who have a history of NSAID-induced gastric effects, the use of celecoxib, a cyclooxygenase 2 (COX-2) inhibitor, is an alternative.[12,16] Choice of one agent over another may be based on cost, convenience, and patient preference.[14] Some research suggests that NSAID therapy should begin at the onset of menses or perhaps even the day before and continued around the clock instead of waiting until symptom onset. The data substantiating this is weak.[33] If an NSAID or celecoxib use is contraindicated or not desired, hormonal agents should be considered. Acetaminophen is inferior to NSAID in treatment of this disorder.[14,33]

CLINICAL CONTROVERSY

Contrary to what often occurs in practice, the data substantiating that dysmenorrhea is best managed when treatment is initiated prior to the start of menses and continued around the clock is weak.[33] This is not a "high stakes" controversy given that NSAIDs are relatively inexpensive and the lower risk for gastrointestinal effects given the age of the population of patients affected by this disorder. There is a lack of clinical trial data supporting the optimal dosing regimen for dysmenorrhea, thus improving the patient's quality of life.

OCs improve dysmenorrhea by inhibiting endometrial tissue proliferation which reduces endometrial-derived prostaglandins that cause the pelvic pain.[12,13,33] Significant improvements in mild, moderate, and severe dysmenorrhea have been noted with OCs. Evidence supporting monophasic versus multiphasic OC regimens, however, is lacking. And while the use of extended-cycle OCs would be desirable for this purpose, data illustrating their superiority over traditional monthly OCs does not currently exist.

Depot MPA can be considered for dysmenorrhea treatment. Its efficacy is secondary to its ability to render most patients amenorrheic within 6 to 12 months of use.[14,33] Because the pelvic pain of dysmenorrhea is related to the prostaglandins released during menses, in the setting of amenorrhea the underlying cause of dysmenorrhea is removed.

Another progesterone product used for dysmenorrhea management is the levonorgestrel-releasing IUD. Observational data indicate its ability to reduce dysmenorrhea from 60% to 29% after 3 years of use.[12,14] As observed with depot MPA, this reduction likely is secondary to its effect in reducing menstrual flow.

Drug Treatments of First Choice Several factors influence the choice of first-line treatment for dysmenorrhea. If contraception is desired, then a hormonal option may be considered taking into account cost, adherence issues, and side effects. If contraception is not desired, then NSAID use would be desirable from cost and convenience standpoints. If NSAIDs are not tolerated, celecoxib could be recommended. In patients for whom OCs, NSAIDs, or celecoxib is not an option, topical heat should be considered.

Special Populations Dysmenorrhea is common in adolescent females. The treatment measures used for adult patients are also appropriate for adolescents. Although NSAIDs, topical heat, and OCs are among the top choices, use of the levonorgestrel IUD is also an option.[38]

Drug Class Information Table 89–3 identifies the significant pharmacologic properties, common adverse events, and clinically relevant drug–drug and drug–food interactions of agents used to treat dysmenorrhea.

PHARMACOECONOMIC CONSIDERATIONS

For women with third-party coverage for prescriptions, most OCs and the higher NSAID doses used for dysmenorrhea would be covered. For women without such coverage, the OC cost may be prohibitive. Generic forms of NSAIDs in over-the-counter strengths can be considered and are less expensive than marketed topical heat products, such as transdermal topical heat patches. Topical heat can be administered inexpensively via a reusable heating pad or hot water bottle. However, these products are not convenient to use.

EVALUATION OF THERAPEUTIC OUTCOMES

Table 89–4 lists the expected outcomes and specific monitoring parameters for the treatment modalities used in the management of dysmenorrhea.

PREMENSTRUAL SYNDROME AND PREMENSTRUAL DYSPHORIC DISORDER

PMS is a constellation of symptoms including mild mood disturbances and physical symptoms occurring prior to menses and resolving with menses initiation. It is distinct from PMDD.

EPIDEMIOLOGY

Up to 75% of menstruating women experience PMS symptoms.[57] However, a spectrum of premenstrual mood disturbances exists, and PMDD is the most severe. Approximately 3% to 8% of women have PMDD.[25,57]

ETIOLOGY AND PATHOPHYSIOLOGY

PMDD is a complex psychiatric disorder with multiple biological, psychological, and sociocultural determinants.[58] Although cyclic hormonal changes are in some way related to PMS and PMDD, the association is neither linear nor simple. When ovulation is suppressed medically or surgically, symptoms improve. Some evidence suggests that PMS and PMDD symptoms are related to low levels of the centrally active progesterone metabolite allopregnanolone in the luteal phase and/or lower cortical γ-aminobutyric acid levels in the follicular phase.[58] Women with PMS and PMDD may have enhanced sensitivity to progesterone.[35] Studies of the relationship between PMS and PMDD and testosterone levels are conflicting.[58] A number of studies suggest a link between PMS and PMDD and low serotonin levels.[35,58] Despite similar affective symptoms, hypothalamic–pituitary–adrenal (HPA) axis function in PMS and PMDD is distinct from that seen in major depressive disorder. Specifically, women with PMS show a decrease in stimulated HPA axis response, whereas this response is increased in women with major depressive disorder.[59] Although several cross-cultural studies suggest that PMS' physical symptoms are consistent across cultures, the negative affective symptoms are part of the negative "menstrual socialization" in Western culture.[1,58]

CLINICAL PRESENTATION OF PMDD

A summary of the American Psychiatric Association's criteria for PMDD is as follows:[1,58]

- Symptoms are temporally associated with the last week of the luteal phase and remit with onset of menses.

- At least five of the following symptoms are present: markedly depressed mood, marked anxiety, marked affective lability, marked anger or irritability, decreased interest in activities, fatigue, difficulty concentrating, changes in appetite, sleep disturbance, feelings of being overwhelmed, and physical symptoms, such as breast tenderness or bloating.

- One of the symptoms must be markedly depressed mood, anxiety, irritability, or affective lability.

- Symptoms interfere significantly with work and/or social relationships.

- Symptoms are not an exacerbation of another underlying psychiatric disorder.

- The criteria are confirmed prospectively by daily ratings over two menstrual cycles.

TREATMENT

Women experiencing PMS and PMDD symptoms miss significantly more work and school than do controls. They also report significant impairment of their ability to participate in social activities and hobbies and in their relationships with others.[60] Given this, the need for effective treatment modalities is clear.

Desired Outcome

PMS and PMDD interventions should alleviate the presenting symptoms and subsequently improve quality of life. Table 89–2 lists the various agents used in managing PMS and PMDD and their recommended dosing.

General Approach to Treatment

A treatment modality that is minimally invasive or without systemic effects is desired for initial therapy. Key to the successful choice of pharmacologic therapy for PMS and PMDD is having the patient chart her specific symptoms for at least 2 months.

Nonpharmacologic Therapy

Lifestyle interventions should be started and followed for 2 months while the patient charts her symptoms. Although these interventions lack significant supporting clinical trial data, anecdotal reports of efficacy exist. Some lifestyle changes for women with mild-to-moderate premenstrual symptoms include minimizing intake of caffeine, refined sugar, and sodium and increasing exercise.[23,57,61] Vitamin and mineral supplements, such as vitamin B_6 (50–100 mg daily) and calcium carbonate (1,200 mg daily), may help reduce the physical symptoms associated with PMS.[23,25] A clinical trial review concludes that the following options lack efficacy and safety data and should not be recommended: herbal medicines, homeopathic remedies, dietary supplements, relaxation, massage therapy, reflexology, chiropractic treatments, and biofeedback.[62]

Pharmacologic Therapy

If symptoms persist after 2 months of symptom charting and lifestyle modifications, pharmacologic therapy for PMDD management is warranted. Over the past decade, the selective serotonin reuptake inhibitors (SSRIs) have been studied significantly for this disorder.[26,63–65] Studies have revealed very positive results relative to most symptoms associated with PMDD. Other agents that have been studied and are alternatives include the selective serotonin–norepinephrine reuptake inhibitor venlafaxine, as well as OCs, tricyclic antidepressants, and GnRH agonists.

Drug Treatments of First Choice ❿ The first-line pharmacologic treatment options for PMDD are the SSRIs.[57] Among this class of agents, data support the use of citalopram, escitalopram, fluoxetine, fluvoxamine, paroxetine, and sertraline. Whether to dose these agents continuously or only during the luteal phase[63] and the optimal duration of treatment[66] are still not evident.

CLINICAL CONTROVERSY

Current evidence supports SSRIs as first-line PMDD treatment, either dosed continuously or during the luteal phase alone. Some evidence suggests that SSRI dosing at symptom onset also may be effective.[67] The bulk of studies include women over age 18 years and with treatment durations not longer than 3 to 6 months.[57] Contrary to the excitement surrounding luteal phase dosing, a recent meta-analysis found in favor of the continuous dosing regimen for efficacy.[65] Relapse rates appear to be higher with shorter-duration treatment (4 months vs 12 months).[66] The most effective dosing strategy[63] (continuous, luteal phase, or symptom onset), most efficacious treatments in the adolescent versus perimenopausal populations, and the optimal treatment duration[66] are not evident and warrant further investigation.

The SSRIs are efficacious in more than half of the treated patients compared to less than 30% of those receiving placebo.[23,64,67] A meta-analysis reports 50% or greater symptom reduction with SSRI treatment compared to baseline.[65] Improvement often occurs during the first cycle of use.[23]

Alternative Drug Treatments The tricyclic antidepressant clomipramine has been studied for PMDD treatment. In placebo-controlled trials, both continuous daily dosing and luteal phase administration proved effective.[23] Compared with the SSRIs, however, clomipramine is not well tolerated due to its side effects. Venlafaxine has been studied on a continuous daily basis[68] and during the luteal phase.[69] Both venlafaxine regimens resulted in significant symptom improvement (compared to placebo) in more than 60% of treated women.

If treatment with an SSRI or another antidepressant such as clomipramine is unsuccessful, hormonal treatment with a GnRH agonist, such as leuprolide, can be considered.[23] Leuprolide improves premenstrual emotional symptoms as well as some physical symptoms, such as bloating and breast tenderness. However, its cost, the need for intramuscular administration, and its hypoestrogenism side effects (e.g., vaginal dryness, hot flashes, and bone demineralization) limit its use.

The use of a monophasic OC containing 20 mcg of ethinyl estradiol and 3 mg of drospirenone, a progesterone with antiandrogenic effects, improves premenstrual symptoms in women with PMDD.[24] As with the SSRIs, optimal treatment duration is unknown, and superiority to other OCs has not been established.

Drug Class Information Table 89–3 lists the significant pharmacologic properties, common adverse events, and clinically relevant drug–drug and drug–food interactions of the agents used to treat PMDD.

PHARMACOECONOMIC CONSIDERATIONS

The SSRIs as first-line treatment options for PMDD management are comparably priced overall; however, a generic formulation of fluoxetine is available. Emerging data on the most appropriate dosing regimens may contribute even further to a reduction in the cost of managing this disorder.

EVALUATION OF THERAPEUTIC OUTCOMES

Table 89–4 lists the expected outcomes and specific monitoring parameters for the treatment modalities used in PMDD management.

CONCLUSIONS

Treatment success for the various menstruation-related disorders can be measured by the degree to which the care plan (1) relieves or reverses symptoms, (2) prevents or reverses the complications (e.g., osteoporosis, anemia, and infertility as noted with amenorrhea, menorrhagia, and anovulatory bleeding, respectively), and (3) minimizes side effects. The return of a regular menstrual cycle with minimal premenstrual symptoms or symptoms of dysmenorrhea is desirable. Depending on the desire for conception and subsequent therapy, this cycle may be ovulatory or anovulatory.

Once optimal therapy has been identified, the regimen can be continued as long as is deemed necessary. In amenorrhea, discontinuation of therapy may be warranted once menses resumes. In anovulatory bleeding, therapy may be discontinued once ovulatory menstrual cycles return. In menorrhagia, dysmenorrhea, and PMDD, optimal therapy may be continued until symptom resolution or until other health factors affect its continuation. For example, a woman taking OCs for menorrhagia or dysmenorrhea may discontinue them when she desires to become pregnant.

Symptom relief in dysmenorrhea should occur within hours of starting an NSAID or within the next menstrual cycle/menses if using OCs. Evaluate the patient for improvement of symptoms associated with amenorrhea, menorrhagia, anovulatory bleeding, or PMDD within one to two menstrual cycles. Ask patients at this visit about the type, frequency, and severity of current symptoms compared to their initial presenting symptoms. Refer patients with persistent symptoms for further medical evaluation to identify other underlying issues or complications.

Assess the effectiveness of therapy in resuming normal menstrual cycles with minimal related pain after an appropriate treatment interval (1–2 months). Assess improvement in quality of life measures such as physical, psychological, and social functioning and well-being. Evaluate the patient for adverse drug reactions, drug allergies, and drug interactions. Table 89–3 lists the common side effects that may occur and the monitoring required. Table 89–4 lists the specific expected outcome measures for each of the menstruation-related disorders discussed in this chapter.

ABBREVIATIONS

COX-2: cyclooxygenase 2

FSH: follicle-stimulating hormone

GnRH: gonadotropin-releasing hormone

HPA: hypothalamic–pituitary–adrenal axis

IUD: intrauterine device

LH: luteinizing hormone

MPA: medroxyprogesterone acetate

NSAID: nonsteroidal antiinflammatory drug

OC: oral contraceptive

PCOS: polycystic ovary syndrome

PMDD: premenstrual dysphoric disorder

PMS: premenstrual syndrome

SHBG: sex hormone–binding globulin

SSRI: selective serotonin reuptake inhibitor

REFERENCES

1. Speroff L, Fritz MA. Clinical Gynecologic Endocrinology and Infertility, 7th ed. Philadelphia. PA: Lippincott Williams & Wilkins, 2005:187–232, 401–463.
2. Lobo RA. Primary and secondary amenorrhea and precocious puberty: etiology, diagnostic evaluation, management. In: Comprehensive Gynecology, 5th ed. St. Louis, MO: Mosby, 2007:933–962.
3. Heiman DL. Amenorrhea. Prim Care Clin Office Pract 2009; 36:1–17.
4. Lobo RA. Abnormal uterine bleeding: ovulatory and anovulatory dysfunctional uterine bleeding, management of acute and chronic excessive bleeding. In: Comprehensive Gynecology, 5th ed. St. Louis, MO: Mosby, 2007:915–932.
5. Setji TL, Brown AJ. Polycystic ovarian syndrome: diagnosis and treatment. Am J Med 2007;120:128–132.
6. James AH, Kouides PA, Abdul-Kadir R, et al. Von Willebrand disease and other bleeding disorders in women: consensus on diagnosis and management from an international expert panel. Am J Obstet Gynecol 2009;201:12.e1–8.
7. Gordon CM, Nelson LM. Amenorrhea and bone health in adolescents and young women. Curr Opin Obstet Gynecol 2003;15:377–384.
8. Master-Hunter T, Heiman DL. Amenorrhea: Evaluation and treatment. Am Fam Physician 2006; 73:1374–1382.
9. Simon JA. Progestogens in the treatment of secondary amenorrhea. J Reprod Med 1999;44(2 Suppl):185–189.
10. Webster J, Piscitelli G, Polli A, et al. A comparison of cabergoline and bromocriptine in the treatment of hyperprolactinemic amenorrhea. N Engl J Med 1994;331:904–909.
11. Kvernmo T, Hartter S, Burger E. A review of the receptor-binding and pharmacokinetic properties of dopamine agonists. Clin Ther 2006;28:1065–1078.
12. Harel Z. Dysmenorrhea in adolescents and young adults. J Pediatr Adolesc Gynecol 2006;19:363–371.
13. French L. Dysmenorrhea in adolescents – diagnosis and treatment. Pediatr Drugs 2008;10(1):1–7.
14. French L. Dysmenorrhea. Am Fam Physician 2005;71:285–291.
15. Roy SN, Bhattacharya S. Benefits and risks of pharmacological agents used for the treatment of menorrhagia. Drug Saf 2004;27:75–90.
16. Daniels S, Robbins J, West CR, Nemeth MA. Celecoxib in the treatment of primary dysmenorrhea: results from two randomized, double-blind, active- and placebo-controlled, crossover studies. Clin Ther 2009;31(6):1192–1208.
17. Kadir RA. Menorrhagia: treatment options. Thrombosis Res 2009;123(Suppl 2):S21–S29.
18. Tasci Y, Caglar GS, Kayikcioglu F, et al. Treatment of menorrhagia with levonorgestrel releasing intrauterine system: effects on ovarian function and uterus. Arch Gynecol Obstet 2009;280:39–42.
19. Kaunitz AM, Meredith S, Inki P, et al. Levonorgestrel-releasing intrauterine system and endometrial ablation in heavy menstrual bleeding: a systematic review and meta-analysis. Obstet Gynecol 2009;113: 1104–1116.
20. Wellington K, Wagstaff AJ. Tranexemic acid: a review of its use in the management of menorrhagia. Drugs 2003;63(13):1417–1433.
21. Mathur R, Levin O, Azziz R. Use of ethinyl estradiol/drospirenone combination in patients with polycystic ovary syndrome. Ther Clin Risk Manag 2008;4(2):487–492.
22. Ehrmann, DA. Polycystic ovary syndrome. N Engl J Med 2005;352:1223–1236.
23. Grady-Weliky TA. Premenstrual dysphoric disorder. N Engl J Med 2003;348:433–438.
24. Lopez LM, Kaptein AA, Helmerhorst FM. Oral contraceptives containing drospirenone for premenstrual syndrome. Cochrane Database Syst Rev 2009; 2:CD006586.
25. Yonkers KA, O'Brien PMS, Eriksson E. Premenstrual syndrome. Lancet 2008;371:1200–1210.

26. Freeman EW, Sondheimer SJ, Sammel MD, et al. A preliminary study of luteal phase versus symptom-onset dosing with escitalopram for premenstrual dysphoric disorder. J Clin Psychiatry 2005;66:769–773.

27. Eng PM, Seeger JD, Loughlin J, et al. Serum potassium monitoring for users of ethinyl estradiol/drospirenone taking medications predisposing to hyperkalemia: physician compliance and survey of knowledge and attitudes. Contraception 2007;75:101–107.

28. Schurmann R, Blode H, Benda N, et al. Effect of drospirenone on serum potassium and drospirenone pharmacokinetics in women with normal or impaired renal function. J Clin Pharmacol 2006;46: 867–875.

29. Adams Hillard PJ, Deitch HR. Menstrual disorders in the college age female. Pediatr Clin North Am 2005;52:179–197.

30. James AH, Ragni MV, Picozzi VJ. Bleeding disorders in premenopausal women: (another) public health crisis for hematology? Hematology Am Soc Hematol Educ Program 2006;2006:474–485.

31. Warner PE, Critchley HO, Lumsden MA, et al. Menorrhagia I. Measured blood loss, clinical features, and outcome in women with heavy periods: A survey with follow-up data. Am J Obstet Gynecol 2004;190:1216–1223.

32. Casablanca Y. Management of dysfunctional uterine bleeding. Obstet Gynecol Clin N Am 2008;35:219–234.

33. Morrow C, Naumburg EH. Dysmenorrhea. Prim Care 2009;36(1):19–32.

34. Lentz GM. Primary and secondary dysmenorrhea, premenstrual syndrome, and premenstrual dysphoric disorder: etiology, diagnosis, management. In: Comprehensive Gynecology, 5th ed. St. Louis, MO: Mosby, 2007:900–914.

35. Dickerson LM, Mazyck PJ, Hunter MH. Premenstrual syndrome. Am Fam Physician 2003;67:1743–1752.

36. Warner PE, Critchley HO, Lumsden MA, et al. Menorrhagia II. Is the 80-mL blood loss criterion useful in management of complaint of menorrhagia? Am J Obstet Gynecol 2004;190:1224–1229.

37. Neuwirth RS. Cost effective management of heavy uterine bleeding: ablative methods versus hysterectomy. Curr Opin Obstet Gynecol 2001;13:407–410.

38. Intrauterine device. ACOG Practice Bulletin No. 59. American College of Obstetricians and Gynecologists. Obstet Gynecol 2005;105: 223–232.

39. ACOG Committee Opinion No. 337. Noncontraceptive uses of the levonorgestrel intrauterine system. Obstet Gynecol 2006;107: 1479–1482.

40. Hurskainen R, Paavonen J. Levonorgestrel-releasing intrauterine system in the treatment of heavy menstrual bleeding. Curr Opin Obstet Gynecol 2004;16:487–490.

41. Hurskainen R, Teperi J, Rissanen P, et al. Clinical outcomes and costs with the levonorgestrel-releasing intrauterine system or hysterectomy for treatment of menorrhagia: Randomized trial 5-year follow-up. JAMA 2004;291:1456–1463.

42. Blumenthal PD, Trussell J, Singh RH, et al. Cost-effectiveness of treatments for dysfunctional uterine bleeding in women who need contraception. Contraception 2006;74:249–258.

43. Zawadski JK, Dunaif A. Diagnostic criteria for polycystic ovary syndrome: Towards a rational approach. In: Dunaif A, Givens JR, Haseltine FP, eds. Polycystic Ovary Syndrome. Boston: Blackwell Scientific Publications, 1992;377–384.

44. Rotterdam ESHRE/ASRM-Sponsored PCOS Consensus Workshop Group. Revised 2003, consensus on diagnostic criteria and long-term health risks related to polycystic ovary syndrome. Fertil Steril 2004;81:19–25.

45. Carmina E, Azziz R. Diagnosis, phenotype and prevalence of polycystic ovary syndrome. Fertil Steril 2006;86(Suppl 1):S7–S8.

46. Azziz R, Woods KS, Reyna R, et al. The prevalence and features of the polycystic ovary syndrome in an unselected population. J Clin Endocrinol Metab 2004;89:2745–2749.

47. Azziz R, Carmina E, Didier D, et al. Position statement: Criteria for defining polycystic ovarian syndrome: An Androgen Excess Society Guideline. J Clin Endocrinol Metab 2006;91:4237–4245.

48. Costello MF, Shrestha B, Eden J, et al. Metformin versus oral contraceptive pills in polycystic ovary syndrome: a Cochran review. Human Reprod 2007;22(5):1200–1209.

49. Matytsina LA, Zoloto EV, Sinenko LV, et al. Dysfunctional uterine bleeding in adolescents: Concept of pathophysiology and management. Prim Care 2006;33:503–515.

50. Albers JR, Hull SK, Wesley RM. Abnormal uterine bleeding. Am Fam Phys 2004;69:1915–1926.

51. Ely JW, Kennedy CM, Clark EC, et al. Abnormal uterine bleeding: A management algorithm. J Am Board Fam Med 2006;19:590–602.

52. Palomba S, Orio F, Falbo A, et al. Prospective parallel randomized, double-blind, double-dummy controlled clinical trial comparing clomiphene citrate and metformin as the first-line treatment for ovulation induction in nonobese anovulatory women with polycystic ovary syndrome. J Clin Endocrinol Metab 2005;90:4068–4074.

53. Siebert TI, Kruger TF, Steyn DW, et al. Is the addition of metformin efficacious in the treatment of clomiphene citrate-resistant patients with polycystic ovary syndrome? A structured literature review. Fertil Steril 2006;86:1432–1437.

54. Khattab S, Mohsen IA, Foutouh IA, et al. Metformin reduces abortion in pregnant women with polycystic ovary syndrome. Gynecol Endocrinol 2006;22:680–684.

55. Banaszewska B, Duleba AJ, Spaczynski RZ, et al. Lipids in polycystic ovary syndrome: Role of hyperinsulinemia and effects of metformin. Am J Obstet Gynecol 2006;194:1266–1272.

56. Akin MD, Weingand KW, Hengehold DA, et al. Continuous low-level topical heat in the treatment of dysmenorrhea. Obstet Gynecol 2001;97:343–349.

57. Steiner M, Pearlstein T, Cohen LS, et al. Expert guidelines for the treatment of severe PMS, PMDD, and comorbidities: The role of SSRIs. J Womens Health 2006;15:57–69.

58. Ross LE, Steiner M. A biopsychosocial approach to premenstrual dysphoric disorder. Psychiatr Clin North Am 2003;26:529–546.

59. Roca CA, Schmidt PJ, Altemus M, et al. Differential menstrual cycle regulation of hypothalamic-pituitary-adrenal axis in women with premenstrual syndrome and controls. J Clin Endocrinol Metab 2003;88:3057–3063.

60. Mishell DR. Premenstrual disorders: Epidemiology and disease burden. Am J Manag Care 2005;11:S473–S479.

61. Jarvis CI, Lynch AM, Morin AK. Management strategies for premenstrual syndrome/premenstrual dysphoric disorder. Ann Pharmacother 2008;42:967–978.

62. Stevinson C, Ernst E. Complementary/alternative therapies for premenstrual syndrome: A systematic review of randomized clinical trials. Am J Obstet Gynecol 2001;185:227–235.

63. Steiner M, Hirschberg AL, Begeron R, et al. Luteal phase dosing with paroxetine controlled release (CR) in the treatment of premenstrual dysphoric disorder Am J Obstet Gynecol 2005;193:352–360.

64. Yonkers KA, Holthausen GA, Poschman K, et al. Symptom-onset treatment for women with premenstrual dysphoric disorder. J Clin Psychopharmacol 2006;26:198–202.

65. Shah NR, Jones JB, Aperi J, et al. Selective serotonin reuptake inhibitors for premenstrual syndrome and premenstrual dysphoric disorder – a meta-analysis. Obstet Gynecol 2008;111:1175–1182.

66. Freeman EW, Rickels K, Sammel MD, et al. Time to relapse after short- or long-term treatment of severe premenstrual syndrome with sertraline. Arch Gen Psychiatry 2009;66(5):537–544.

67. Kornstein SG, Pearlstein TB, Fayyad R, et al. Low-dose sertraline in the treatment of moderate-to-severe premenstrual syndrome: efficacy of 3 dosing strategies. J Clin Psychiatry 2006;67:124–132.

68. Freeman EW, Rickels K, Yonkers KA, et al. Venlafaxine in the treatment of premenstrual dysphoric disorder. Obstet Gynecol 2001;98(5 Pt 1):737–744.

69. Cohen LS, Soares CN, Lyster A, et al. Efficacy and tolerability of premenstrual use of venlafaxine (flexible dose) in the treatment of premenstrual dysphoric disorder. J Clin Psychopharmacol 2004;24:540–543.

CHAPTER 90

Endometriosis

DEBORAH A. STURPE

KEY CONCEPTS

❶ Endometriosis should be suspected in any woman of reproductive age, including adolescents, with recurring cyclic or acyclic pelvic pain and/or subfertility.

❷ The etiology of endometriosis is likely multifactorial; no single theory is satisfactory to explain all cases.

❸ No physical examination findings or laboratory tests are considered diagnostic for endometriosis. A definitive diagnosis can be made only via surgical visualization of lesions. Confirmation of diagnosis is not necessary in all cases.

❹ Treatment goals include improvement of painful symptoms and maintenance or improvement of fertility. Therapy is considered successful based on resolution of the patient's symptoms or achievement of pregnancy.

❺ All medical therapies are equally efficacious in treating endometriosis-related pain based on available evidence. The choice among agents is determined primarily by side effect profile, cost, and individual patient response.

❻ Endometriosis-related pain can be treated by medical or surgical therapy. Empirical medical therapy is likely more cost-effective and is recommended based on consensus guidelines.

❼ Endometriosis-related infertility is unresponsive to medical therapy. Conservative surgical therapy is the preferred treatment.

Endometriosis is a common cause of chronic pelvic pain in women and is associated with infertility. Characterized by the presence of endometrial tissue outside the uterus, endometriosis is a chronic, recurring disease.

❶ Endometriosis should be suspected in women, including adolescents, with subfertility, dysmenorrhea, dyspareunia, or chronic pelvic pain. Therapy is targeted at relieving symptoms and improving fertility.

Learning objectives, review questions, and other resources can be found at **www.pharmacotherapyonline.com**.

EPIDEMIOLOGY

The prevalence of endometriosis in the general population is estimated to be 5% to 10% of women.[1,2] Up to 70% of adult women and up to 50% of adolescents presenting with chronic pelvic pain may have endometriosis, and ~20% to 50% of women with infertility may have the disorder.[1,3–5] A genetic predisposition for endometriosis has been noted, as evidenced by disease rates that are up to seven times higher in primary relatives of affected women compared with the general population.[2]

CLINICAL CONTROVERSY

An association between endometriosis and ovarian cancer has been reported in the literature. Such reports often suggest that due to this association, aggressive treatment of endometriosis that includes surgical therapy should be recommended for many patients. However, this proposed association between endometriosis and cancer remains controversial. Consequently, data do not exist to enable evidence-based decision making in patients with endometriosis who may be at elevated risk for ovarian cancer.

ETIOLOGY

❷ The etiology of endometriosis is unknown. Multiple mechanisms for development of lesions are likely, including theories of retrograde menstrual flow, coelomic metaplasia, lymphatic and vascular spread, and immunologic abnormalities.[1,2,4] Involvement of immune system factors in the development and progression of endometriosis is recognized. Findings of abnormal B- and T-cell function, decreased apoptosis, and altered levels of prostanoids, cytokines, growth factors, interleukins, and aromatase in endometrial lesions and peritoneal fluid of affected women support this theory.[1,2,6]

PATHOPHYSIOLOGY

PAIN AND INFERTILITY

Endometriosis-associated pain is likely secondary to generation of local inflammation by the endometrial lesions, bleeding from the endometrial tissue, and irritation or compression of nerve fibers by endometrial implants.[5,7] Estrogen has been found to contribute to endometriosis pain due to its role in helping to produce endometrial tissue and in stimulating release of inflammatory substances.[2]

The exact mechanism by which endometriosis reduces fertility is unknown, but it may result from distorted pelvic anatomy, altered peritoneal function, and altered endometrial receptivity that impairs implantation.[8]

DISEASE STAGING

The severity of disease can be classified according to the American Association of Reproductive Medicine staging system (stage I, mild, to stage IV, severe), but clinical utility of this staging system is limited because findings do not correlate with painful symptoms, nor does the staging system predict pregnancy rates.[9,10] Staging may be useful, however, in guiding decisions regarding prognosis and treatment for infertility.[9]

CLINICAL PRESENTATION

Symptoms

□ The patient may be asymptomatic or complain of symptoms such as severe dysmenorrhea, deep dyspareunia, chronic pelvic pain (cyclic or acyclic), ovulation pain, cyclical or perimenstrual bowel and bladder complaints (e.g., GI disturbances, painful defecation, dysuria, and/or hematuria), chronic fatigue, or infertility.

Signs

□ Findings on physical examination are best observed during menstruation and may include pelvic tenderness, tender uterosacral ligaments, enlarged ovaries, or a fixed, retroverted uterus.

□ Findings on laparoscopic examination may range from a few small lesions located on the ovaries, serosal surfaces, or peritoneum to large cysts called endometriomas. Lesions are often described as: "powder burn" or "gunshot" lesions; dark brown, black, or blue lesions, nodules, and cysts; and "chocolate cysts" (endometriomas containing blood).

Diagnosis

□ Definitive diagnosis can be made only by direct surgical visualization of endometrial lesions; however, treatment guidelines allow for nondefinitive diagnosis in patients presenting with chronic pelvic pain provided that other causes of pain are ruled out and that pain responds to first-line empiric therapies.

Adapted from ESHRE guideline for the diagnosis and treatment of endometriosis. 2008. Available at: *http://guidelines.endometriosis.org.* Last accessed September 30, 2009; and Royal College of Obstetricians and Gynaecologists. The investigation and management of endometriosis. 2006. Available at: *http://www.rcog.org.uk/files/rcog-corp/uploaded-files/GT24InvestigationEndometriosis2006.pdf.* Last accessed September 30, 2009.

TREATMENT

The treatment of endometriosis varies depending on presenting symptoms, patient age, and desired outcome.

DESIRED OUTCOME

❹ Treatment goals for endometriosis depend on the patient's presentation. Only women with active symptoms (pelvic pain, infertility, or both) require therapy. Depending on the primary complaint, the goals of endometriosis treatment are (a) minimization or removal of endometrial deposits, (b) prevention of disease progression, (c) minimization of associated pain, and (d) prevention or correction of associated infertility.

GENERAL APPROACH TO TREATMENT

❺ The treatment of an asymptomatic patient with endometriosis consists of expectant management (watchful waiting) only because therapy is not indicated unless symptoms develop. For symptomatic patients, the foundation of therapy includes medical treatment, surgical treatment, or both. To date, no studies have directly compared medical and surgical treatment as first-line therapy. Furthermore, determining the optimal medical or surgical approach is difficult secondary to a paucity of well-designed, randomized, controlled trials. All commonly prescribed medical therapies relieve endometriosis-related pain by regressing lesions via induction of a pseudopregnancy or pseudomenopausal state but do not eradicate lesions or improve fertility. Therefore, the choice of initial therapy depends on multiple factors, such as the patient's primary complaint, the location and extent of disease, the desire for future fertility, the cost of therapy, contraindications to therapy, and potential side effects or complications of therapy.

❻ Guidelines recommend empirical treatment of chronic pelvic pain suspected to be secondary to endometriosis with combined hormonal contraceptives (CHCs) or progestins for at least 3 months.[9,10] Empiric therapy with a gonadotropin-releasing hormone (GnRH) agonist can also be considered in women, but it is less optimal due to greater expense and toxicity.[10] The duration of medical therapy is typically limited to 6 months for drugs with higher toxicity profiles (e.g., danazol and GnRH agonists), but CHCs and progestins may be continued indefinitely.[10] Conservative surgical therapy is recommended for treating painful symptoms in women who do not respond to, or have contraindications to, medical therapy or patients with other compelling reasons for surgery. Definitive treatment for endometriosis involves nonconservative surgical therapy via bilateral salpingo-oophorectomy, with or without hysterectomy. This therapy should be reserved for women not desiring future fertility who accept the potential complications of surgically induced menopause. A general treatment algorithm for endometriosis-related pain is shown in Figure 90–1.

❼ For women presenting with infertility as a primary complaint, first-line therapy involves surgical resection of endometrial lesions to restore normal anatomy, followed by watchful waiting.[8–10] Medical therapy alone is ineffective for endometriosis-related infertility and should be avoided.[9,10] For women in whom surgical intervention does not result in pregnancy, controlled ovarian stimulation with intrauterine insemination or in vitro fertilization may be recommended.[8–10] Pretreatment with a GnRH agonist for 3 to 6 months prior to in vitro fertilization cycles increases success rates.[9] Intrauterine insemination is preferred in women younger than age 35 with milder (stage I or II) disease, whereas in vitro fertilization is preferred in women over age 35 or those with more severe (stage III or IV) disease.[8]

NONPHARMACOLOGIC THERAPY: SURGERY

❸ Laparoscopy is used in endometriosis as both a diagnostic and a therapeutic tool, and guidelines recommend removal of visible lesions at the time of initial diagnosis.[9] Although a significant percentage of women will experience recurrence of painful symptoms after surgery, the use of adjunctive medical therapy postoperatively is no longer recommended due to the lack of documented efficacy at 12 and 24 months.[9,10] Conservative

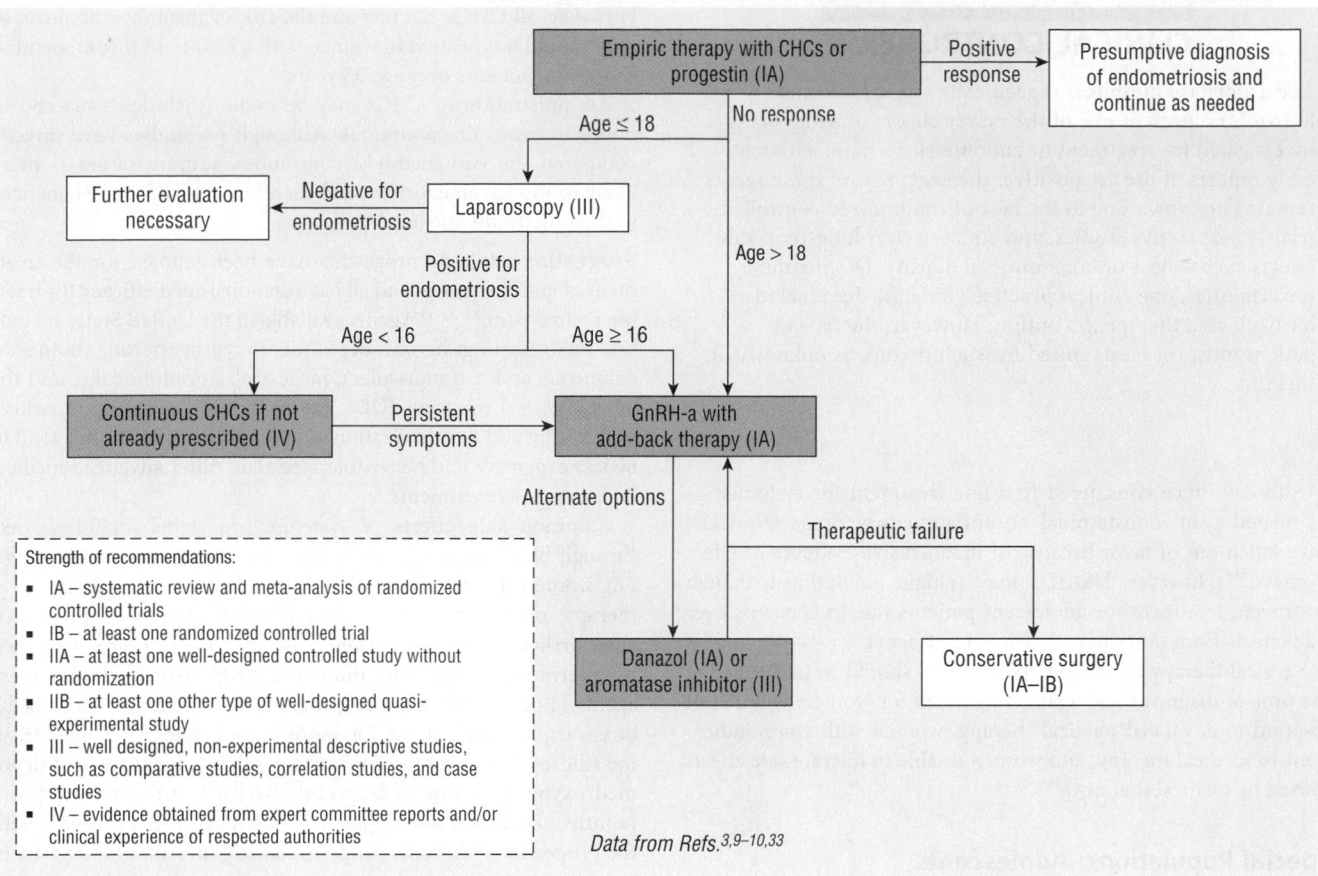

FIGURE 90-1. Treatment algorithm for cyclic/acyclic chronic pelvic pain and suspected endometriosis. CHC, combined hormonal contraceptive; GnRH-a, gonadotropin-releasing hormone agonist.

surgical therapy is also the primary treatment of endometriosis-associated infertility.

PHARMACOLOGIC THERAPY

Typically, pharmacologic therapy is the first choice for treatment of endometriosis-related pain to minimize risks from surgery. However, drug therapy will not treat endometriosis-related infertility.

Drug Treatments of First Choice

❺ First-line therapy for endometriosis-associated pain includes CHCs or progestins.[3,9,10] These two drug classes are considered as effective as, and less costly and toxic than, other endometriosis treatments. The choice of agent depends on patient characteristics, such as the desire for contraception, pain patterns, and contraindications. Long-term maintenance therapy with these agents may be considered for women achieving a good therapeutic response. A low-dose combined oral contraceptive administered cyclically was compared with a GnRH agonist in a randomized trial.[11] Both groups showed overall improvement in dyspareunia, nonmenstrual pain, and dysmenorrhea at 6 months. The rate of recurrent symptoms 6 months after cessation of therapy was equal between groups. Combined oral contraceptives can be administered on a continuous basis if desired. Studies on the efficacy of other formulations of CHCs (vaginal ring and transdermal patch) for treatment of endometriosis pain have not been conducted; however, the use of these agents in endometriosis is reasonable.

Systematic review has concluded that continuous therapy with oral progestins is no more or less effective than other therapies

for treatment of endometriosis-associated pain.[12] Two studies of subcutaneous depot medroxyprogesterone revealed statistically equivalent improvement in endometriosis-associated pain compared with the GnRH agonist leuprolide.[13,14] Studies examining the use of the levonorgestrel-releasing intrauterine device (IUD) also suggest efficacy in the treatment of endometriosis-associated pain, and this device is indicated in evidence-based practice guidelines.[9,10,15]

Alternative Drug Treatments

Adolescents (younger than 18 years) experiencing chronic pelvic pain despite therapy with first-line therapies should undergo evaluative laparoscopy prior to initiation of additional pharmacotherapy.[3]

In adolescents with endometriosis diagnosed by laparoscopy or in adults with chronic pelvic pain unresponsive to CHCs or progestins, advanced medical therapy for endometriosis pain may be considered.[3,9,10]

Agents that can be used as advanced medical therapy include danazol and GnRH agonists. Systematic reviews have concluded that both classes are effective choices, and neither class has been proven superior to the other.[16,17] The primary difference between treatments is the side effect profile and available dosage forms; therefore, the choice of agent depends on patient age, preference, and tolerance of side effects. Treatment should be continued for 6 months if relief is obtained.[9,10] For women treated with a GnRH agonist, add-back therapy with an estrogen and progestin combination should be recommended to minimize vasomotor side effects and bone mineral density loss.[9,10,18]

CLINICAL CONTROVERSY

The aromatase inhibitors (specifically anastrazole and letrozole) represent one of the newer classes of drugs being investigated for treatment of endometriosis pain. Although early reports of use are positive, the exact role of these agents remains unknown due to the lack of randomized controlled trials, comparative studies, and concern over long-term side effects such as loss of bone mineral density. Despite these uncertainties, one clinical practice guideline does include letrozole as a therapeutic option. However, the type of patient most (or least) suited for such therapy is unknown at this time.

Although once considered first-line treatment for endometriosis-related pain, nonsteroidal antiinflammatory drugs (NSAIDs) have fallen out of favor because of inconclusive evidence of effectiveness.[9,10] However, NSAIDs may remain an optional, though unproven, treatment for adolescent patients due to concerns over side effects from other non-first-line treatments.[3]

Surgical therapy for endometriosis pain should be performed at the time of diagnosis and again considered for women who do not respond to advanced medical therapy, women with contraindications to medical therapy, and women unable to tolerate side effects caused by medical therapy.[9,10]

Special Populations: Adolescents

④ Treatment goals for endometriosis in adolescent patients are pain control, minimization of disease progression, and preservation of fertility.[3,19] A treatment algorithm that includes therapy for adolescent patients is shown in Figure 90–1. Although progestins are likely to be well tolerated by the adolescent population, clinicians should be aware that efficacy has not been clearly established in this population, and concerns regarding long-term effects on bone mineral density and lipid profile are not clearly defined.[3,20] The effect of drugs on bone mineral density is of particular concern in young women who have not achieved peak bone mass; thus, add-back therapy should be considered for all adolescents receiving GnRH agonist therapy.[3,20] Danazol is not likely to be well tolerated by the adolescent population and generally is not recommended for use.[3,20]

Drug Class Information

When selecting therapy for endometriosis-related pain, the choice of drug within a class often depends on the strength of evidence for efficacy in endometriosis or specific patient factors.

Combined Hormonal Contraceptives CHCs treat the pain of endometriosis by decreasing menstrual flow and regressing endometrial implants through induction of an anovulatory and/or hypoestrogenic state.[3,21] Continuous therapy also can be used to suppress menstruation and induce a "pseudopregnancy"-like state.[3] Evidence-based guidelines consider combined oral contraceptives as effective as other medical therapies for relieving pain from endometriosis.[9,10] No evidence suggests that one combined oral contraceptive is superior to another. Additionally, although no specific studies have examined the efficacy of the contraceptive patch or vaginal ring in endometriosis, the effects of these agents likely are similar to those of the oral formulations.[3] Thus, the choice between CHCs should be guided by patient preference, likelihood of adherence, and cost. Side effects of CHCs typically are mild and may include nausea, bloating, headache, and breakthrough bleeding.

However, all CHCs can increase the risk of thromboembolism, so they should not be used in women with a history of thromboembolism or in smokers over age 35 years.

Administration of CHCs may be cyclic (includes a placebo or nondrug week) or continuous. Although no studies have directly compared the two methods, continuous administration is more likely to induce amenorrhea and therefore may be more beneficial in treating dysmenorrhea.[3,20]

Progestins Multiple progestins have been studied for the treatment of endometriosis, and all have demonstrated efficacy for treating related pain.[9,10,12–15] Agents available in the United States include oral medroxyprogesterone, depot medroxyprogesterone (both subcutaneous and intramuscular), megestrol, norethindrone, and the levonorgestrel-releasing IUD. The progestins treat endometriosis via atrophy and decidualization of endometrial tissue. They tend to be less expensive and better tolerated than other advanced medical endometriosis treatments.

Common side effects of systemic progestins include breakthrough bleeding, weight gain, fluid retention, and mood swings. For women desiring immediate future fertility after cessation of therapy, progestins may not be optimal secondary to prolonged amenorrhea and anovulation. Also of concern are unknown long-term effects on bone mineral density associated with these agents. Both depot medroxyprogesterone products carry black box warnings against use for more than 2 years.[22,23] However, in the studies that directly compared the subcutaneous form of depot medroxyprogesterone to leuprolide over a treatment period of 6 months, the extent and degree of bone loss were less severe with the progestin.[13,14] Specific progestin dosing information is given in Table 90–1.

Gonadotropin-Releasing Hormone Agonists GnRH agonists create a functional oophorectomy via inhibition of follicle-stimulating hormone (FSH) and luteinizing hormone (LH) secretion. This, in turn, diminishes endometrial implants. When first initiated, GnRH agonists create an initial gonadotropin flare prior to receptor downregulation that may cause a temporary increase in pain. Initiating therapy during the midluteal phase may minimize such effects.

Therapy with a GnRH agonist is superior to placebo and comparable to danazol for relief of endometriosis-associated pain.[16] Response rates are ~85% to 100% after 6 months of therapy, but recurrence rates at 5 years are 53%.[16,24–26] Although a GnRH agonist typically is taken for 6 months, one comparative study has shown equivalent efficacy and recurrence rates between 3 and 6 months of GnRH agonist therapy, and evidence-based guidelines therefore recommend 3 months of therapy as an option.[9,10,27] Therapy may also be extended beyond 6 months to maintain efficacy, although data regarding such extended usage are limited.

The three GnRH agonists currently available in the United States are goserelin, leuprolide, and nafarelin. These agents differ primarily by route of administration; therefore, the choice of therapy depends on patient preference. Specific dosing information for the GnRH agonists is given in Table 90–1.

Side effects are the primary limitation of GnRH agonist use. The pharmacologically induced hypoestrogenic environment results in bone loss and vasomotor symptoms such as hot flashes, vaginal dryness, and insomnia. Loss of bone mineral density is estimated at 4% to 6% over 6 months of GnRH agonist therapy and occurs at both the hip and spine, but this loss is partially to fully recoverable upon cessation of the drug.[28] Bone loss is progressive as use of the drugs is extended beyond 6 months; whether reversibility is maintained after such longer treatment periods is unknown.[29] Add-back therapy with estrogen and progestin combinations has been proven effective for treatment of vasomotor symptoms and

TABLE 90-1 Pharmacologic Therapy For Endometriosis-Associated Pain

Drug	Dose	Comments
CHCs		
Combined oral contraceptives (various)	One orally daily	Continuous administration may lessen dysmenorrhea
		Contraindicated in women with a history of thromboembolism; avoid in women older than 35 years who smoke
Contraceptive patch (Ortho-Evra)	One patch weekly	Continuous administration may lessen dysmenorrhea
		Contraceptive efficacy may be diminished in women >90 kg (198 lbs)
		Contraindicated in women with a history of thromboembolism; avoid in women older than 35 years who smoke
Contraceptive vaginal ring (Nuva Ring)	One ring monthly	Continuous administration may lessen dysmenorrhea
		Contraindicated in women with a history of thromboembolism; avoid in women older than 35 years who smoke
Progestins		
MPA	150 mg IM every 3 months	Generally well tolerated and less costly than GnRH-a or danazol
	120 mg sub-Q every 3 months	Black box warning to limit therapy to no more than 2 years' duration
		May delay return of fertility
LNG-IUS	One system inserted for up to 5 years	Additional benefit is long-term contraception
		May be difficult to insert in nulliparous women
GnRH-a		
Leuprolide	11.25 mg IM every 3 months	Vasomotor symptoms and bone loss may limit use
		Add-back therapy improves side effects and reduces bone loss
		Not preferred in younger adolescent patients secondary to bone loss
Goserelin	3.6 mg sub-Q monthly	Vasomotor symptoms and bone loss may limit use
		Add-back therapy improves side effects and reduces bone loss
		Not preferred in younger adolescent patients secondary to bone loss
Nafarelin	200 mcg (one spray) intranasally twice daily	Vasomotor symptoms and bone loss may limit use
		Add-back therapy improves side effects and reduces bone loss
		Not preferred in younger adolescent patients secondary to bone loss
Other		
Danazol	600–800 mg orally daily in divided doses	Androgenic side effects limit use; not preferred in adolescent patients secondary to side effect profile
NSAIDs		
Ibuprofen	400 mg orally every 4–6 hours	Use with caution in women with reactive airways disease, renal disease, or history of GI ulcer
Naproxen	250 mg orally every 6–8 hours	Use with caution in women with reactive airways disease, renal disease, or history of GI ulcer
Aromatase inhibitors		
Anastrazole	1 mg orally daily	Unknown efficacy compared with other therapies
		Add-back therapy may be necessary to prevent bone loss
		Reserve for failures to other therapeutic options
Letrozole	2.5 mg orally daily	Unknown efficacy compared with other therapies
		Add-back therapy may be necessary to prevent bone loss
		Reserve for failures to other therapeutic options

CHCs = combined hormonal contraceptives, GI = gastrointestinal, GnRH-a = gonadotropin-releasing hormone agonists, IM = intramuscular, LNG-IUS = levonorgestrel intrauterine system, MPA = medroxyprogesterone acetate, NSAIDs = nonsteroidal antiinflammatory drugs, sub-Q = subcutaneous

prevention of bone loss while maintaining GnRH agonist efficacy.[18] Add-back therapy dosing should approximate the low doses used for hormone replacement therapy. Thus, CHCs should not be prescribed for this purpose.

Women receiving GnRH agonist therapy should be encouraged to take supplemental calcium and to exercise. One small study suggests that women who exercise (walking and aerobic sessions) during 6 months of GnRH agonist therapy sustain similar bone mineral loss during therapy but have better recovery of bone mineral density after cessation of therapy compared with women who do not exercise.[30]

Danazol Danazol is a synthetic steroid analogue of 17-ethinyl testosterone. It induces anovulation, amenorrhea, and endometrial atrophy through pituitary suppression of the midcycle LH and FSH surge and induction of a high-androgen, low-estrogen environment. The drug also has immunosuppressive activity that may contribute to its efficacy. Formerly the "gold standard" of endometriosis treatment, the popularity of danazol has decreased with the development of agents with more favorable side effect profiles.

Danazol has proven effective as empirical as well as postoperative therapy. Symptomatic improvement has been reported in up to 80% to 90% of women using the drug, with the best results seen in women achieving amenorrhea.[31] A systematic review concluded that 6 months of danazol therapy is superior to placebo in relieving painful symptoms.[17]

The primary limitation of danazol therapy is the high occurrence of androgenic side effects, including weight gain, acne, hot flashes, decreased breast size, hirsutism, and increased low-density lipoprotein cholesterol. Use of vaginal danazol (200 mg/day) has been investigated in one small study, and this route of administration was effective in treatment of endometriosis pain while minimizing systemic side effects.[32] However, more data are needed before this strategy can be routinely recommended.

Danazol should not be initiated in women with hyperlipidemia or liver disease. Danazol is teratogenic, and barrier forms of contraception must be used. The dose of danazol ranges from 200 to 800 mg/day; most studies have used doses of 600 to 800 mg. Specific dosing information is given in Table 90–1.

Nonsteroidal Antiinflammatory Drugs NSAIDs are thought to treat the painful symptoms of endometriosis by interfering with prostaglandin production, but data are lacking to indicate the efficacy of this class of medications specifically in patients with endometriosis.[9,10] Long-term use of these agents may be limited by gastrointestinal or renal toxicity. They also may aggravate reactive airway disease and should be used with caution in such patients. Despite this uncertain risk-to-benefit ratio, some clinicians may still wish to try NSAIDs in patients unable to take other endometriosis therapies. NSAIDs commonly used for treatment of gynecologic pain are ibuprofen and naproxen.[31] Specific dosing information is listed in Table 90–1.

Aromatase Inhibitors Aromatase is a key enzyme in the biosynthesis of estrogen, and elevated levels of aromatase have been found in endometrial lesions compared with normal endometrium.[6,33] Thus, aromatase inhibitors are thought to treat endometriosis pain by direct inhibition of estrogen production. Data on efficacy of aromatase inhibitors in treating endometriosis pain are largely limited to case reports and nonrandomized, noncomparative studies, but there is evidence of efficacy for both letrozole and anastrazole, alone and in combination with GnRH agonists.[33]

Most information about the side effects of aromatase inhibitors comes from data in postmenopausal women. These side effects include hot flashes, vaginal dryness, and loss of bone mineral density. They have been minimized in the endometriosis population by use of add-back therapy.[6,33] Specific dosing information is listed in Table 90–1.

PHARMACOECONOMIC CONSIDERATIONS

6 Several cost considerations must be made when choosing endometriosis therapy. The cost of medical therapy must be weighed against the cost of surgical therapy, and the costs of each type of medical therapy must be weighed against another. Unfortunately, no recent data exist that explore the cost-effectiveness of the various treatment options. Generally, GnRH agonists and aromatase inhibitors are the most expensive agents, and CHCs and progestins are the least expensive.

EVALUATION OF THERAPEUTIC OUTCOMES

4 Monitoring of endometriosis therapy is focused on subjective relief of symptoms.[31] Although objective confirmation of lesion regression by laparotomy is feasible, the results typically are misleading because the number and size of lesions do not correlate well with symptoms.[31]

Endometriosis-related pain should be relieved within 2 months of initiating medical therapy. If symptoms persist, consideration should be given to different medical and/or surgical therapy. For endometriosis-related infertility, most experts recommend 6 months of watchful waiting after surgical intervention. If pregnancy is not achieved within that time, assisted reproductive techniques can be considered.

Careful monitoring of the patient for side effects to recommended drug therapy is important. Most of the monitoring can be accomplished by eliciting any subjective complaints from the patient at routine follow-up visits. However, certain drug therapies may require additional objective monitoring, such as fasting lipid profile and blood pressure measurements. The role of routine bone mineral density testing as a monitoring parameter for patients receiving GnRH agonists or aromatase inhibitors is not yet determined, especially because accuracy of bone mineral density results in predicting fracture risk in younger patients has not been well established, nor has a threshold of loss been established for discontinuation of therapy.

ABBREVIATIONS

CHCs: Combined hormonal contraceptives

FSH: Follicle-stimulating hormone

GnRH: Gonadotropin-releasing hormone

GnRH-a: Gonadotropin-releasing hormone agonist

IUD: Intrauterine device

LH: Luteinizing hormone

LNG-IUS: Levonorgestrel-releasing intrauterine system

NSAIDs: Nonsteroidal antiinflammatory drugs

Nulliparous: having never been pregnant

REFERENCES

1. Olive DL. Gonadotropin-releasing hormone agonists for endometriosis. N Engl J Med 2008;359:1136–1142.
2. Bulun SE. Endometriosis. N Engl J Med 2009;360:268–279.
3. American College of Obstetricians and Gynecologists. ACOG committee opinion: Endometriosis in adolescents. Obstet Gynecol 2005;105:921–927.
4. Farquhar C. Endometriosis. BMJ 2007;334:249–253.
5. Practice Committee of American Society for Reproductive Medicine. Treatment of pelvic pain associated with endometriosis. Ferti Steril 2008;90:S260–S269.
6. American College of Obstetricians and Gynecologists. ACOG committee opinion: Aromatase inhibitors in gynecologic practice. Obstet Gynecol 2008;112:405–407.
7. Evans S, Moalem-Taylor G, Tracey DJ. Pain and endometriosis. Pain 2007;132:S22–S25.
8. Practice Committee of the American Society for Reproductive Medicine. Endometriosis and infertility. Fertil Steril 2006;86:S156–S160.
9. ESHRE guideline for the diagnosis and treatment of endometriosis. 2008. Available at: *http://guidelines.endometriosis.org. Last accessed September 30, 2009.*
10. Royal College of Obstetricians and Gynaecologists. The investigation and management of endometriosis. 2006. Available at: *http://www.rcog.org.uk/files/rcog-corp/uploaded-files/GT24InvestigationEndometriosis2006.pdf. Last accessed September 30, 2009.*
11. Vercellini P, Trespidi L, Colombo A, et al. A gonadotropin-releasing hormone agonist versus a low-dose oral contraceptive for pelvic pain associated with endometriosis. Fertil Steril 1993;60:75–79.
12. Prentice A, Deary A, Bland ES. Progestagens and anti-progestagens for pain associated with endometriosis. Cochrane Database of Systematic Reviews 2009;3:CD002122.
13. Schlaff WD, Carson SA, Luciano A, et al. Subcutaneous injection of depot medroxyprogesterone acetate compared with leuprolide acetate in the treatment of endometriosis-associated pain. Fertil Steril 2006;85:314–325.
14. Crosignani PG, Luciano A, Ray A, Bergqvist A. Subcutaneous depot medroxyprogesterone acetate versus leuprolide acetate in the treatment of endometriosis-associated pain. Hum Reprod 2006;21:248–256.
15. Bahamondes L, Petta CA, Fernandes A, Monteiro I. Use of the levonorgestrel-releasing intrauterine system in women with endometriosis, chronic pelvic pain and dysmenorrhea. Contraception 2007;75:S134–S139.
16. Prentice A, Deary A, GoldbeckWood S, et al. Gonadotrophin-releasing hormone analogues for pain associated with endometriosis. Cochrane Database Syst Rev 2009;3:CD000346.
17. Selak V, Farquhar C, Prentice A, Singla AA. Danazol for pelvic pain associated with endometriosis. Cochrane Database Syst Rev 2009;3:CD000068.
18. Sagsveen M, Farmer JE, Prentice A, Breeze A. Gonadotrophin-releasing hormone analogues for endometriosis: Bone mineral density. Cochrane Database Syst Rev 2009;3:CD001297.
19. Attaran M, Gidwani GP. Adolescent endometriosis. Obstet Gynecol Clin North Am 2003;30:379–390.

20. Laufer MR. Current approaches to optimizing the treatment of endometriosis in adolescents. Gynecol Obstet Invest 2008;66:19–27.

21. Rice VM. Conventional medical therapies for endometriosis. Annals N Y Acad Sci 2002;955:343–352.

22. Depo-Provera package insert. Pharmacia and Upjohn Co. May 2006.

23. Depo-SubQ Provera 104 package insert. Pharmacia and Upjohn Co. June 2009.

24. Winkel CA, Scialli AR. Medical and surgical therapies for pain associated with endometriosis. J Women's Health Gend Based Med 2001;10:137–162.

25. Olive DL, Pritts EA. The treatment of endometriosis: A review of the evidence. Annals N Y Acad Sci 2002;955:360–372.

26. Bulletins-Gynecology AcoP. ACOG practice bulletin: Medical management of endometriosis. Int J Gynaecol Obstet 2000;71: 183–196.

27. Hornstein MD, Yuzpe AA, Burry KA, et al. Prospective randomized double-blind trial of 3 versus 6 months of nafarelin therapy for endometriosis associated pelvic pain. Fertil Steril 1995;63:955–962.

28. Surrey ES. Add-back therapy and gonadotropin-releasing hormone agonists in the treatment of patients with endometriosis: Can a consensus be reached? Fertil Steril 1999;71:420–424.

29. Hornstein MD, Surrey ES, Weisberg GW, Casino LA. Leuprolide acetate depot and hormonal add-back in endometriosis: A 12-month study. Obstet Gynecol 1998;91:16–24.

30. Bergstrom I, Freyschuss B, Jacobsson H, Landgren B. The effect of physical training on bone mineral density in women with endometriosis treated with GnRH analogs: A pilot study. Acta Obstet Gynecol Scand. 2005;84:380–383.

31. Mahutte NG, Arici A. Medical management of endometriosis-associated pain. Obstet Gynecol Clin North Am 2003;30:133–150.

32. Razzi S, Luisi S, Calonaci F, et al. Efficacy of vaginal danazol treatment in women with recurrent deeply infiltrating endometriosis. Fertil Steril 2007;88:789–794.

33. Patwardhan S, Nawathe A, Yates D, et al. Systematic review of the effects of aromatase inhibitors on pain associated with endometriosis. BJOG 2008;115:818–822.

91

Hormone Therapy in Women

SOPHIA N. KALANTARIDOU, DEVRA K. DANG,
SUSAN R. DAVIS, AND KARIM ANTON CALIS

KEY CONCEPTS

❶ The decision to use menopausal hormone therapy must be individualized and based on several parameters, including symptoms, osteoporosis risk, cardiovascular disease risk, breast cancer risk, and thromboembolism risk.

❷ The lowest effective dose of hormone therapy for the shortest duration needed for effective symptom control should be prescribed, weighing the potential benefits and risks for the individual woman.

❸ Hormone therapy is the most effective treatment option for alleviating vasomotor and vaginal symptoms of menopause.

❹ Osteoporosis prevention remains an indicated use of estrogen products; however, nonestrogen products, specifically bisphosphonates, are as effective as hormone therapy for preventing osteoporosis.

❺ Hormone therapy improves depressive symptoms in symptomatic menopausal women, most likely by relieving flushing and improving sleep. However, it may worsen quality of life in women without hot flushes.

❻ Cardiovascular disease, including coronary artery disease, stroke, and peripheral vascular disease, is the leading cause of death among women. Postmenopausal hormone therapy should not be used for reducing the risk of cardiovascular disease.

❼ Because of the increased risk of endometrial hyperplasia and endometrial cancer with estrogen monotherapy (unopposed estrogen), hormone therapy in women who have not undergone hysterectomy should include a progestogen in addition to the estrogen.

❽ Use of hormone therapy at doses lower than those prescribed historically is effective in the management of menopausal symptoms.

❾ Results from randomized trials of hormone therapy in postmenopausal women cannot be extrapolated to premenopausal women with ovarian dysfunction. Women with primary ovarian insufficiency need exogenous sex steroids to compensate for decreased production by their ovaries.

Learning objectives, review questions, and other resources can be found at **www.pharmacotherapyonline.com**.

MENOPAUSE AND PERIMENOPAUSAL AND POSTMENOPAUSAL HORMONE THERAPY

Menopause is the permanent cessation of menses following the loss of ovarian follicular activity.[1] By definition, it is a physiologic event that occurs after 12 consecutive months of amenorrhea, so the time of the final menses is determined retrospectively. Women who have undergone hysterectomy must rely on their symptoms to estimate the actual time of menopause.

EPIDEMIOLOGY

The median age at the onset of menopause in the United States is 51 years, whereas the average life expectancy for women is 81 years. Thus, American women can expect to be postmenopausal for more than one third of their lives. As the U.S. population ages, the number of women experiencing menopause is expected to rise. Although the age at menarche has declined steadily over centuries, probably as a result of improved nutrition, the age of onset for menopause appears to be relatively stable. Cigarette smokers, however, experience menopause 2 years earlier than nonsmokers on average. Women who have undergone hysterectomy are also more likely to have an earlier menopause despite preservation of their ovaries.

ETIOLOGY

Menopause refers to loss of ovarian function and subsequent hormonal deficiency. This can be due to the normal process of aging (i.e., natural menopause), surgery (total abdominal hysterectomy, bilateral oophorectomy), medications (e.g., chemotherapy), or pelvic irradiation.

PATHOPHYSIOLOGY

Characteristics of the human menstrual cycle throughout reproductive life are well described.[2] A woman is born with approximately two million primordial follicles in her ovaries. During a normal reproductive life span, she ovulates fewer than 500 times. The vast majority of follicles undergo atresia.

The hypothalamic–pituitary–ovarian axis dynamically controls reproductive physiology throughout the reproductive years. The pituitary is regulated by pulsatile secretion of gonadotropin-releasing hormone (GnRH) from the hypothalamus. Follicle-stimulating hormone (FSH) and luteinizing hormone (LH), produced by the pituitary in response to GnRH, regulate ovarian function. These gonadotropins also are influenced by negative feedback from estradiol and progesterone. Ovarian follicular activity is reflected by the circulating concentrations of sex steroids and by peptide hormones (e.g., inhibin and activin). The sex steroids include estradiol, produced by the dominant follicle; progesterone, produced by the corpus luteum after maturation of the dominant ovarian follicle; and androgens, primarily testosterone and androstenedione, secreted by the ovarian stroma. Sex steroids are important for the healthy functioning of many organs, including the bones, brain, skin, and reproductive and urogenital tracts. They act primarily by regulating gene expression.

Pathophysiologic changes associated with menopause are caused by loss of ovarian follicular activity.[1] Ovarian primordial follicle numbers decrease with advancing age, and at the time of the menopause, few follicles remain in the ovary. Hence, the postmenopausal ovary is no longer the primary site of estradiol or progesterone synthesis. The postmenopausal ovary secretes primarily androstenedione and testosterone. In contrast to the acute fall in circulating estrogen at the time of menopause, the decline in circulating androgens commences in the decade leading up to the average age of natural menopause and closely parallels increasing age.[3] Androgens are secreted by both the ovaries and the adrenal glands. Following menopause, direct ovarian androgen secretion appears to account for as much as 50% of testosterone production, with the adrenal gland being a less important source. Hypertrophy of the ovarian stroma may develop after menopause, probably secondary to high LH concentrations, thereby resulting in increased ovarian testosterone production. Alternatively, the ovaries may become fibrotic and a poor source of sex steroids.

No endocrine event clearly signals the time just prior to final menses.[4] Nonetheless, as women age, a progressive rise in circulating FSH[5] and a concomitant decline in ovarian inhibin[4] are observed. In women who continue to experience menstrual bleeding, FSH determinations on day 2 or 3 of the menstrual cycle are considered elevated when concentrations exceed 10 to 12 milli international units/mL (10 to 12 IU/L), an indication of diminished ovarian reserve. Clear elevations in serum FSH are seen in women approximately at age 40 years.[4] When ovarian function has ceased, serum FSH concentrations are greater than 40 milliinternational units/mL (40 IU/L).

CLINICAL PRESENTATION

The perimenopause is the period immediately prior to the menopause and the first year after menopause. The menopausal transition is the period of time when the endocrinologic, biologic, and clinical features of the approaching menopause commence.[4] The menopausal transition usually begins approximately 4 years prior to menopause and is characterized by menstrual cycle irregularity caused by increased frequency of anovulatory cycles. Vasomotor symptoms (hot flushes and night sweats), psychological symptoms (anxiety, mood swings, and depression), and disturbances of sexuality are increased markedly in the perimenopause. Menopause is characterized by a 10- to 15-fold increase in circulating FSH concentrations compared with concentrations of FSH in the follicular phase of the cycle, a fourfold to fivefold increase in LH, and a greater than 90% decrease in circulating estradiol concentrations.[4] During the perimenopause, FSH concentrations may rise to the postmenopausal range during some cycles but return to premenopausal levels during subsequent cycles. Thus, high concentrations of FSH should not be used to diagnose menopause in perimenopausal women. However, vasomotor symptoms in perimenopausal women may require treatment despite the presence of menstrual bleeding. Abnormal thyroid function and other conditions that may cause similar symptomatology should be excluded first. Dysfunctional uterine bleeding may occur during the perimenopausal years because of anovulatory cycles, but other gynecologic causes also should be considered. Treatment options for dysfunctional uterine bleeding include progestogens or low-dose oral contraceptives.

CLINICAL PRESENTATION AND DIAGNOSIS OF PERIMENOPAUSE AND MENOPAUSE

Symptoms

- Vasomotor symptoms (hot flushes and night sweats)
- Sleep disturbances
- Mood changes
- Sexual dysfunction
- Problems with concentration and memory
- Vaginal dryness and dyspareunia
- Arthralgia

Signs

- Perimenopause: Dysfunctional uterine bleeding as a result of anovulatory cycles (other gynecologic disorders should be excluded)
- Menopause: Signs of urogenital atrophy

Laboratory Tests

- Perimenopause: FSH on day 2 or 3 of the menstrual cycle greater than 10–12 milliinternational units/mL (10–12 IU/L)
- Menopause: FSH greater than 40 milliinternational units/mL (40 IU/L)

Other Relevant Diagnostic Tests

- Thyroid function tests
- Iron stores

TREATMENT

Treatment options for menopause include nonpharmacologic therapy for mild symptoms, and hormonal or nonhormonal therapy for moderate to severe symptoms.

■ DESIRED OUTCOMES

Menopause is a natural life event, not a disease. The goals of therapy for menopause are to relieve symptoms and improve quality of life while minimizing adverse effects.

■ GENERAL APPROACH TO TREATMENT

In women with mild vasomotor and/or vaginal symptoms, nonpharmacologic therapy can be considered. However, many women will require pharmacologic therapy for more severe symptoms. Figure 91–1 outlines a treatment algorithm for women requiring pharmacologic therapy. In the absence of contraindications, hormone therapy is appropriate mainly for women with hot flushes and vulvar or vaginal atrophy.[6] It is contraindicated in women with endometrial cancer, breast cancer, undiagnosed vaginal bleeding, coronary heart disease, thromboembolism (including recent spontaneous thrombosis or in the presence of a thrombophilia), stroke or transient ischemic attack, and active liver disease.[6] Relative contraindications include uterine leiomyoma, migraine headaches, and seizure disorder. In addition, oral estrogen should be avoided in women with hypertriglyceridemia, liver disease, and gallbladder disease. For these women, transdermal administration is a safer approach. The main reasons for discontinuing hormone therapy are side effects such as bleeding, breast tenderness, bloating, and "premenstrual-like symptoms." Reducing the dose or changing the regimen or the route of administration can minimize these effects.

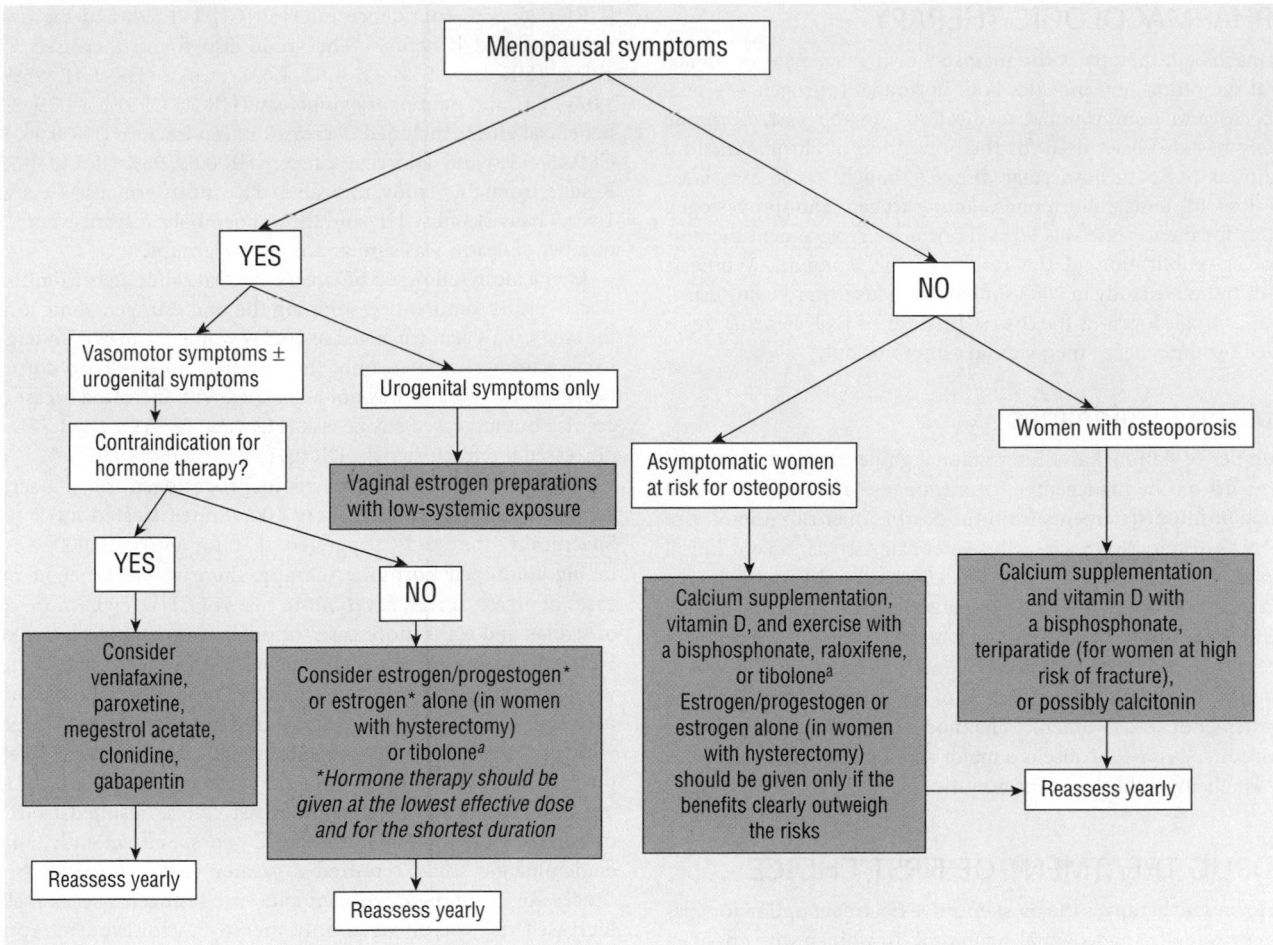

FIGURE 91-1. Algorithm for pharmacologic management of menopause symptoms. ªTibolone is currently not approved for use in the United States.

❶ The decision to use hormone therapy must be individualized and based on several parameters, including menopausal symptoms, osteoporosis risk, cardiovascular disease risk, breast cancer risk, and thromboembolism risk.

❷ Clinicians should prescribe the lowest effective dose of hormone therapy for the shortest duration needed for effective symptom control, weighing the potential benefits and risks for the individual woman. Recommendations should be specific to each woman's clinical profile and concerns. Approved indications of hormone therapy include treatment of vasomotor symptoms and urogenital atrophy and prevention of osteoporosis. Weighing risks and benefits, the Food and Drug Administration (FDA) determined that the indication for vasomotor symptoms (hot flushes and night sweats) should remain unchanged, but the other two indications for hormone therapy should be revised. For treatment of vasomotor symptoms, systemic hormone therapy remains the most effective pharmacologic intervention (see Fig. 91–1). For symptoms of urogenital atrophy, such as vaginal dryness, intravaginal products should be considered. In addition, although prevention of postmenopausal osteoporosis remains an indicated use of hormone therapy, consideration should be given to approved nonestrogen products, such as raloxifene and bisphosphonates (see Fig. 91–1).

Prior to initiating pharmacologic therapy, a complete medical history and physical examination should be performed. Medical history should include a personal or family history of cardiovascular disease and thrombotic problems. The physical examination should include a complete cardiovascular examination, clinical assessment of thyroid status, and breast and pelvic examinations. Papanicolaou cervical cytologic examination and screening mammography negative for malignancy are required before initiating hormone therapy. Thyroid function tests and lipoprotein lipid profile also are performed at the discretion of the clinician.

Each patient should be evaluated for the presence of indications (i.e., menopausal symptoms such as hot flushes or vaginal dryness) and possible contraindications. A thorough discussion of the risks and benefits of hormone therapy should be completed with the patient so that she can weigh the risks and benefits versus alternatives and make a rational decision about whether to use hormone therapy.

■ NONPHARMACOLOGIC THERAPY

In some women, menopausal symptoms can be managed effectively with lifestyle modifications, including wearing layered clothing that can be removed or added as necessary, lowering room temperature, decreasing intake of hot spicy foods, caffeine, and hot beverages, exercise, and other good general health practices. More recently, dietary supplements and nonpharmacologic therapies have been promoted as "complementary medicine" alternatives to hormone therapy. To date, little evidence supports the use of such nonprescription herbal products, which include various herbal remedies and soy-based supplements.

■ PHARMACOLOGIC THERAPY

Pharmacologic therapy is the mainstay of management of menopausal symptoms and includes both hormonal (estrogen +/- progestogen) and nonhormonal medications. In the past, hormone therapy has also been used for the prevention of chronic medical conditions (e.g., cardiovascular disease) thought to be associated with loss of female hormones, and estrogen and progestogen therapy for menopause was termed hormone replacement therapy. However, publication of the results of the landmark Women's Health Initiative study in 2002 shifted the focus toward using estrogen and progestogen at the lowest (instead of replacement) doses needed for the relief of menopausal symptoms only.

Published Guidelines

A number of national and international guidelines and consensus statements on the management of menopause are available. These include position statements from the North American Menopause Society, the Endocrine Society, the American Association of Clinical Endocrinologists, the Society of Obstetricians and Gynaecologists of Canada, the International Menopause Society, and the National Institutes of Health.[7-14] The United States Preventive Services Task Force also provides a recommendation statement on the use of hormone therapy for the prevention of chronic medical conditions in postmenopausal women.[15] The most current guidelines should be consulted, as menopause is a major area in women's health with new data being published continuously.

■ DRUG TREATMENT OF FIRST CHOICE

❸ Hormone therapy is the most effective treatment option for alleviating vasomotor and vaginal symptoms. In women with an intact uterus, hormone therapy consists of an estrogen plus a progestogen. In women who have undergone hysterectomy, estrogen therapy is given unopposed by a progestogen.

Hormone Therapy

Approved indications of postmenopausal hormone therapy include treatment of menopausal symptoms (e.g., hot flushes, night sweats, and urogenital atrophy) and osteoporosis prevention.[16] Much of what is known about the benefits and risks of hormone therapy in postmenopausal women comes from the landmark Women's Health Initiative (WHI) study. The WHI randomized controlled trial was a chronic disease prevention trial designed to evaluate the role of hormone therapy in reducing the risks of cardiovascular disease in older women and at the same time to investigate the effects on the risk of breast cancer.[17,18] The trial was conducted in a total of 68,132 mainly asymptomatic women who were an average 12 to 13 years postmenopausal (mean age 63 ± 7.11 years).[17,18] The continuous combined oral estrogen plus progestogen arm (conjugated equine estrogens 0.625 mg/day plus medroxyprogesterone acetate 2.5 mg/day) of the WHI trial was terminated early. This arm included 16,608 relatively healthy postmenopausal women aged 50 to 79 years at enrollment (mean age 63.2 years). The primary outcome was coronary heart disease (CHD) events, defined as nonfatal myocardial infarction and coronary artery disease death, with invasive breast cancer as the primary adverse outcome. The study also examined secondary outcomes, including stroke, thromboembolic disease, fractures, colon cancer, and endometrial cancer.[17] After a mean follow-up of 5.2 years (planned duration 8.5 years), the Data and Safety Monitoring Board recommended stopping this arm of the trial because of the occurrence of a prespecified level of invasive breast cancer. That is, women who received the active drug had an increased risk of invasive breast cancer (hazard ratio

[HR] 1.26, 95% confidence interval [CI] 1–1.59), and the overall risks exceeded benefits.[17] The study also found increased CHD events (HR 1.29, 95% CI 1.02–1.63), stroke (HR 1.41, 95% CI 1.07–1.85), and pulmonary embolism (HR 2.13, 95% CI 1.39–3.25). Beneficial effects included decreases in hip fracture (HR 0.66, 95% CI 0.45–0.98) and colorectal cancer (HR 0.63, 95% CI 0.43–0.92).[17] Results from this study indicated that short-term use (less than 1 year) has risks for CHD and thromboembolic disease events. The number of deaths was similar among the groups.

After a mean follow-up of 7 years, the Data and Safety Monitoring Board also recommended stopping the oral estrogen-alone arm of the study. This arm consisted of 10,739 women who had undergone hysterectomy. Estrogen-only therapy had no effect on coronary heart disease risk and was not associated with increased breast cancer risk but increased stroke risk (HR 1.39, [95% CI 1.1–1.77]) and decreased hip fracture risk (HR 0.61, 95% CI 0.41–0.91]).[18]

Among women in the estrogen plus progestogen arm, one serious adverse event occurred in every 100 women treated for 5 years. Specifically, the study suggested that for every 10,000 women taking combined hormone therapy, there would be eight more cases of breast cancer, seven more cases of CHD, eight more cases of stroke, and eight more cases of pulmonary embolism per year. However, six fewer colorectal cancers and five fewer hip fractures would be expected.[17,19] For the majority of women who had never used hormone therapy before enrolling in the study (6,280 treated with estrogen plus progestogen and 6,024 treated with placebo), the HR for breast cancer was 1.06 (95% CI 0.81–1.38), indicating that the burden of risk for breast cancer resulted from use of hormone therapy for more than 5 years. Subsequently, a large epidemiologic study reported a greater risk estimate of breast cancer for combined estrogen plus progestogen use as well as increased risk for estrogen-only therapy.[19] However, interpretation of these findings is limited by selection bias because the risk profiles of women who used hormone therapy were significantly different from those of nonusers.[19] It is unclear whether the type of estrogen compound or the dose, route, or administration method could be at least partly responsible for the risks observed in the WHI trial.

Regulatory authorities expressed major concerns about hormone therapy use following the publication of the results of the WHI trial,[16,20] and many women either stopped or become reluctant to use hormone therapy.[21] The WHI trial was conducted in older postmenopausal women. No randomized controlled clinical trials of the population of women normally targeted for hormone therapy (i.e., symptomatic perimenopausal or early postmenopausal women) have been reported. Although hormone therapy is not indicated for prevention of chronic diseases of aging, it remains the most effective treatment for vasomotor symptoms, impaired sleep quality, and urogenital symptoms of menopause.

Although it has been proposed that hormone therapy should be prescribed at the lowest possible dose for the shortest possible time,[16] evidence that new low-dose regimens are safer than traditionally prescribed doses is lacking. Weighing the risks and benefits, the FDA mandated the addition of new safety warnings to the labels of all systemic estrogens (regardless of route or dosage form), including estrogen-only and combined estrogen–progestogen products.[20] The labels caution that use of estrogen-containing hormone therapy regimens by postmenopausal women may be associated with an increased risk of myocardial infarction, stroke, breast cancer, and thromboembolism.[20]

Benefits of Hormone Therapy

Hormone therapy has been shown to relieve vasomotor symptoms, vaginal atrophy, prevent and treat osteoporosis, and reduce the risk of colon cancer.

Vasomotor Symptoms The major indication for postmenopausal hormone therapy is management of vasomotor symptoms. Most women with vasomotor symptoms require hormone treatment for fewer than 5 years, so the risks of therapy appear to be small.

Fewer than 25% of women experience a menopausal transition without symptoms, whereas more than 25% suffer severe menopausal symptoms, most commonly hot flushes and night sweats.[22]

Without treatment, hot flushes in most women typically disappear within 1 to 2 years, but in some untreated women hot flushes continue for more than 20 years.[23] Women with mild vasomotor symptoms often experience relief by lifestyle modification and at least 25% of women in clinical trials reported significant improvement of vasomotor symptoms when taking placebo. However, no therapy has been shown to be as effective as estrogen therapy in alleviating significant vasomotor symptoms. Estrogens diminish hot flushes in most women, and all types and routes of administration of estrogen are equally effective.[24] A dose-dependent relationship between estrogen administration and suppression of hot flushes is well established. Some women, especially younger women, may require a higher than average dose of estrogen to suppress symptoms. On the other hand, many women with hot flushes at the time of menopause require lower doses of estrogen.[24] Hormone therapy for menopausal symptoms can be stopped about 2 or 3 years after starting. If treatment can be tapered and stopped within 5 years, no evidence of increased risk of breast cancer is seen.[17]

Vaginal Atrophy Estrogen receptors have been demonstrated in the lower genitourinary tract, and at least 50% of postmenopausal women suffer symptoms of urogenital atrophy caused by estrogen deficiency.[25] Atrophy of the vaginal mucosa results in vaginal dryness and dyspareunia. Lower urinary tract symptoms include urethritis, recurrent urinary tract infection, urinary urgency, and frequency. Most women with significant vaginal dryness because of vaginal atrophy require local or systemic estrogen therapy for symptom relief. Such treatment also reduces the risk of recurrent urinary tract infections, possibly by modifying the vaginal flora.[26] Vaginal dryness and dyspareunia can be treated with an intravaginal estrogen cream, tablet, or ring. In clinical trials, vaginal estrogen appears to be better than systemic estrogen for relieving these symptoms and avoids high levels of circulating estrogen. Concomitant progestogen therapy generally is unnecessary if women are using low-dose micronized 17β-estradiol. However, regular use of conjugated equine estrogens (CEE) vaginal creams and other products that potentially promote endometrial proliferation in women with an intact uterus requires intermittent progestogen challenges (i.e., for 10 days every 12 weeks). This is an important caveat because vaginal atrophy requires long-term estrogen treatment.[26]

Urinary incontinence, which becomes more prevalent with increasing age, usually is not improved by estrogen therapy. In one large clinical trial, estrogen–progestogen therapy actually increased incontinence.[27]

Osteoporosis Prevention and Treatment Therapy directed at menopausal symptoms, such as hot flushes, often is short term. However, therapy directed at prevention of osteoporosis should be long term. For osteoporosis prevention, the advantages of hormone therapy must be weighed against the risks, including thrombosis and the increased incidence of cardiovascular disease and breast cancer;[17] and consideration should be given to approved nonestrogen alternatives.

Postmenopausal osteoporosis is a serious age-related disease that affects millions of women throughout the world. Menopause is accompanied by accelerated bone loss, and the central role of estrogen deficiency in postmenopausal osteoporosis is well established. Osteoporosis is characterized by reduced bone mass associated with architectural deterioration of the skeleton and increased risk for fracture.[8] Estrogen deficiency results in bone loss through its actions in accelerating bone turnover and uncoupling bone formation from resorption. It is important to recognize that bone loss commences 2 years before the final menstrual period.[28] Throughout menopause, the average loss of bone mineral density (BMD) is around 6.4% at the lumbar spine and 4%–5% at the femoral neck, with obese women experiencing less bone loss than nonobese women.[28] Annual bone mass decreases of 0.5% to 1% are seen after age 65 years.[29] An observational study of more than 9,000 postmenopausal women examined the relationship between endogenous estrogens and BMD, bone loss, fractures, and breast cancer.[30-33] Women with detectable serum estradiol concentrations (5–25 pg/mL [18–92 pmol/L]) had a 6% to 7% higher BMD at the total hip and spine compared with women with undetectable levels (less than 5 pg/mL [18 pmol/L]).[32] They also had significantly less bone loss at the hip than women with undetectable levels.[31] Women with undetectable serum estradiol concentrations had a relative risk of 2.5 for subsequent hip and vertebral fractures.[33] However, women with the highest estradiol serum concentrations had the greatest risk of developing breast cancer.[30]

The WHI randomized trial was the first study to demonstrate that hormone therapy reduces the risk of fractures at the hip, spine, and wrist in women not selected for having osteoporosis.[17,34] Hip and clinical vertebral fractures are reduced by 34%, and total osteoporotic fractures are reduced by 24%.[34] These findings are in agreement with observational data and several meta-analyses of the efficacy of hormone therapy for reducing fractures in postmenopausal women.[35] Estrogen therapy reduces bone turnover and increases bone density in postmenopausal women of all ages. The protective effect persists as long as the treatment is maintained. With cessation of therapy, postmenopausal bone loss resumes at the same rate as in untreated women. The standard bone-sparing daily estrogen dose is equivalent to 0.625 mg CEE.[36] However, lower doses of estrogen have been shown to increase bone mass to the same extent as standard-dose estrogen therapy.[37]

❹ Osteoporosis *prevention* remains an indicated use of estrogen products; however, nonestrogen products, specifically bisphosphonates, are as effective as hormone therapy for preventing osteoporosis. The FDA has withdrawn the "osteoporosis *treatment*" indication from estrogen products. Long-term hormone therapy is no longer an appropriate first-choice option for osteoporosis prevention because of the risks associated with its long-term use. Therefore, hormone therapy should be considered for osteoporosis prevention only in women at significant risk for osteoporosis who cannot take nonestrogen treatments such as bisphosphonates.

Bisphosphonates are analogs of pyrophosphate that inhibit bone resorption. Drugs in this class with FDA-approved indications for osteoporosis include alendronate, risedronate, ibandronate, and zoledronic acid. Bisphosphonates reduce the risk of both hip and vertebral fractures by 30% to 50%.[8] Bisphosphonates have no known impact on the incidence of cardiovascular disease or breast or endometrial cancer. A few trials have shown improved bone density over single therapy when a bisphosphonate is combined with estrogen or the selective estrogen receptor modulator raloxifene, but no fracture data are available as of this writing.[38] Some experts recommend cessation of bisphosphonate therapy after 5–10 years use because of accumulation in bone.[39]

General protective measures, such as regular weight-bearing exercise and avoidance of detrimental lifestyle habits such as smoking and alcohol abuse, are appropriate for all women. Some women require calcium supplementation to their dietary intake. Adequate vitamin D intake and/or supplementation is also needed. See Chap. 99 for a full discussion of osteoporosis prevention and treatment.

Colon Cancer Risk Reduction

Colorectal cancer is the fourth most common cancer and the second leading cause of cancer death in the United States (see Chap. 138). The estrogen–progestogen arm of the WHI study was the first randomized controlled trial to confirm that combined estrogen–progestogen therapy reduces colon cancer risk. Compared with placebo, six fewer colorectal cancers are reported per year in every 10,000 women taking hormone therapy.[17]

Quality of Life, Mood, Cognition, and Dementia

⑤ Hormone therapy improves depressive symptoms in symptomatic menopausal women, most probably by relieving flushing and improving sleep.[40] Women with vasomotor symptoms receiving hormone therapy have improved mental health and fewer depressive symptoms compared with women receiving placebo; however, hormone therapy may worsen quality of life in women without flushes.[41]

There is no evidence that hormone therapy improves quality of life or cognition in older, asymptomatic women.[40–44]

More than 33% of women 65 years and older will develop dementia during their lifetime.[45] Several observational studies have suggested that estrogen therapy may be protective against Alzheimer disease (see Chap. 63). The WHI Memory Study (an ancillary study of WHI trial) evaluated the effect of combined hormone therapy on dementia and cognition in 4,532 women 65 to 79 years old.[43] The study found that postmenopausal women 65 years and older taking estrogen plus progestogen therapy had twice the rate of dementia, including Alzheimer disease, than women taking placebo (HR 2.05, 95% CI 1.21–3.48).[43] In addition, estrogen plus progestogen therapy in these women did not prevent mild cognitive impairment, a cognitive and functional state between normal aging and dementia that frequently progresses to dementia.[43] The estrogen alone arm of the WHI trial showed similar findings.[46,47]

Hormone therapy does not improve quality of life in postmenopausal women who do not have vasomotor symptoms. Hormone therapy does not improve cognitive function compared with placebo and, more importantly, produces an increased risk (albeit small) of clinically meaningful cognitive decline among women 65 years and older taking hormone therapy.[41–44,46,47]

CLINICAL CONTROVERSY

Some clinicians believe that hormone therapy improves well-being and quality of life of postmenopausal women, whereas others believe that hormone therapy, at best, has no effect. Hormone therapy improves mood and well-being mainly in women with vasomotor symptoms and sleep disturbance.

Other Effects

Diabetes In healthy postmenopausal women, hormone therapy appears to have a beneficial effect on fasting glucose levels in women with elevated fasting insulin concentrations.[48] Also, in women with coronary artery disease, hormone therapy reduces the incidence of diabetes by 35%.[49] These findings provide important insights into the metabolic effects of hormone therapy but are insufficient to recommend the long-term use of hormone therapy in women with diabetes.

Body Weight A meta-analysis of randomized controlled trials showed that unopposed estrogen or estrogen combined with a progestogen has no effect on body weight, suggesting that hormone therapy does not cause weight gain in excess of that normally observed at the time of menopause.[50]

■ RISKS OF HORMONE THERAPY

The risks of hormone therapy include ovarian cancer, endometrial cancer, breast cancer, venous thromboembolism, gallbladder disease, and possibly cardiovascular disease in older women. The risks depend on the hormonal regimen used (estrogen only versus estrogen plus progestogen), the route of administration, dose, duration of therapy, age at treatment initiation, and the patient's other risk factors.

Cardiovascular Disease

⑥ Cardiovascular disease, including coronary artery disease, stroke, and peripheral vascular disease, is the leading cause of death among women. The American Heart Association recommends that post-menopausal hormone therapy should not be used for reducing the risk of coronary heart disease.[51]

In the previous decade, an expectation of coronary benefit had been a major reason for use of postmenopausal hormones because observational studies indicated that women who use hormone therapy have a 35% to 50% lower risk of coronary heart disease than nonusers.[52] In addition, previous studies have shown that estrogen exerts protective effects on the cardiovascular system, including lipid-lowering,[53] antioxidant,[54] and vasodilating effects.[54] Nevertheless, recent randomized clinical trials have provided no evidence of cardiovascular disease protection and even some evidence of harm with hormone therapy.[17,55–58]

The primary findings of the estrogen plus progestogen arm of the WHI trial showed an overall increase in the risk of CHD (HR 1.29, 95% CI 1.02–1.63) among healthy postmenopausal women 50 to 79 years old receiving combined estrogen–progestogen hormone therapy compared with those receiving placebo.[17] The primary findings of the estrogen-only arm of the WHI trial show no effect (either increase or decrease) on the risk of coronary heart disease in women taking estrogen alone.[18] Subgroup analyses performed in the years after the WHI was first published in 2002 and revealed that women who initiated hormone therapy 10 or more years after the time of menopause tended to have increased CHD risk compared with women who initiated therapy within 10 years of menopause.[59,60] Neither estrogen alone or estrogen plus progestogen were associated with a statistically significant effect on CHD in women aged 50–59 years, and hormone therapy was associated with reduced overall mortality, although this decrease was not statistically significant.[59]

More recently, new analyses from the WHI that included only adherent study participants found that the risk of CHD with estrogen plus progestogen use is increased in the first two years of treatment, even in women aged 50–59 years at study entry. However, the risk of CHD in women who initiated therapy within 10 years of menopause appears to decrease after six years of treatment.[60] It is important to remember that all of the above data from the WHI are from secondary analyses. In addition, the mean age of study participants was 63, while the average age of natural menopause is 51. Most women who commence estrogen or estrogen plus progestogen therapy do so within the first few years of becoming menopausal. It is still unclear how the cardiovascular effects of hormone therapy during perimenopause/early menopause and late menopause differ. There is a need for a long-term randomized controlled study of low-dose hormone therapy started around the time of menopause.[61] Hormone therapy should not be initiated or continued for the prevention of cardiovascular disease. Adherence to a healthful lifestyle (cessation of smoking, regular exercise, healthy diet, and body mass index less than 25 kg/m²) may prevent the onset of cardiovascular disease in postmenopausal women.[62,63]

In the estrogen plus progestogen arm of the WHI study, the increased risk for stroke and venous thromboembolism continued throughout the 5 years of therapy.[17] Increased risk was observed only for ischemic stroke and not for hemorrhagic stroke.[64] In the estrogen-alone arm of the study, a similar increased risk for stroke was observed.[18]

Breast Cancer

The WHI trial found that combined estrogen plus progestogen therapy has an increased risk of invasive breast cancer (HR 1.26, 95% CI 1.0–1.59) and a trend toward increasing risk with increasing duration of therapy.[17] The estrogen-only arm of the WHI trial found no increased risk for breast cancer during the 7-year follow-up period.[18] In the estrogen plus progestogen arm, the increased breast cancer risk did not appear until after 3 years of study participation.[17] The risk was seen only in women who initiated therapy within 5 years of the start of menopause but not in those who started therapy more than 5 years after menopause.[65] The breast cancers diagnosed in women in the hormone therapy group had similar histology and grade but were more likely to be in an advanced stage compared with women in the placebo group.[66] The risk of breast cancer returns to baseline rapidly after discontinuation of hormone therapy.[67] In an unselected postmenopausal population, the Million Women Study found that current use of hormone therapy increased breast cancer risk and breast cancer mortality (relative risk 1.66 and 1.22, respectively). Increased incidence was observed for estrogen-only use (relative risk 1.30), for estrogen plus progestogen (relative risk 2), and for tibolone (relative risk 1.45).[19]

For women in the United States, the lifetime risk of developing breast cancer is approximately one in eight,[68] and the greatest incidence occurs in women older than 60 years (see Chap. 136). In a collaborative re-analysis of data from 51 studies evaluating 52,705 women with breast cancer and 108,411 controls, less than 5 years of combined estrogen–progestogen therapy was associated with a 15% increase in breast cancer risk, and the risk increased with longer duration (relative risk 1.35 with 5 or more years of use).[69] However, 5 years after discontinuation of hormone therapy, the risk of breast cancer was no longer increased.[69]

Addition of progestogens to estrogen may increase breast cancer risk beyond that observed with estrogen alone.[70] The Iowa Women's Health Study showed that exposure to hormone therapy is associated with an increased risk of breast cancer that has a favorable prognosis.[71] These findings have been attributed to increased breast cancer screening in women taking hormone therapy. A study of the effects of hormone therapy in women with a family history of breast cancer found that those who were currently receiving hormone therapy had approximately the same increased relative risk as those who did not have a family history.[72] The overall mortality for women with a family history of breast cancer from all causes was reduced significantly among hormone therapy users.[72] These data suggest that hormone therapy use in women with a family history of breast cancer is not associated with a significantly increased incidence of the disease.

Sex steroid deficiency during menopause results in lipomatous involution of the breast, which is seen as decreased mammographic breast density and markedly improved radiotransparency of breast tissue. Thus, mammographic changes indicating breast cancer can be recognized more easily and earlier after the menopause. Conversely, combination hormone therapy results in increased mammographic breast density, and increased density on mammography has been associated with higher breast cancer risk.[73] Of note, increased mammographic density is not observed with estrogen-only therapy.[74]

Endometrial Cancer

The WHI trial suggests that combined hormone therapy does not increase endometrial cancer risk compared with placebo (HR 0.81, 95% CI 0.48–1.36).[75] Estrogen alone given to women with an intact uterus significantly increases uterine cancer risk.[76] The excess risk increases with dose and duration of estrogen (10 years of unopposed estrogen increases the risk 10-fold), is apparent within 2 years of the start of treatment, and persists for many years after estrogen replacement is discontinued.[76] Estrogen-induced endometrial cancer usually is of a low stage and grade at the time of diagnosis,[23] and it can be prevented almost entirely by progestogen coadministration. The sequential addition of progestogen to estrogen for at least 10 days of the treatment cycle or continuous combined estrogen–progestogen does not increase the risk of endometrial cancer.[77]

Lower doses of estrogen may be associated with a lower risk of endometrial hyperplasia.[78] Raloxifene does not result in endometrial hyperplasia, has no effect on endometrial thickness, is not associated with polyp formation, and has virtually no proliferative effect on the endometrium.[79] A 4-year trial of raloxifene in women with osteoporosis showed no increased risk of endometrial cancer.[80]

Ovarian Cancer

Lifetime risk of ovarian cancer is low (1.7%). The WHI trial suggests that combined hormone therapy may increase the risk of ovarian cancer (HR 1.58, 95% CI 0.77–3.24).[75] However, an observational study reported an increased risk of ovarian cancer in women taking postmenopausal estrogen-only therapy for more than 10 years (relative risk 1.8, 95% CI 1.1–3.0 and 3.2, 95% 1.7–5.7 for 10 to 19 years and 20 or more years, respectively) but no increased risk of ovarian cancer among women receiving combination estrogen–progestogen therapy.[81] A large prospective cohort study in Danish women found that use of hormone therapy was associated with an increased risk of ovarian cancer regardless of duration of use, formulation, dose of estrogen, progestogen type, hormone therapy regimen, and route of administration.[82]

Venous Thromboembolism

Venous thromboembolism, including thrombosis of the deep veins of the legs and embolism to the pulmonary arteries, is uncommon in the general population. The absolute risk of venous thromboembolism in nonhormone therapy users is approximately 1 in 10,000 women.[83] Women taking combined estrogen–progestogen hormone therapy have a twofold increased risk for thromboembolic events, with the highest risk occurring in the first year of use.[84] The absolute increase in risk is small, with 1.5 venous thromboembolic events per 10,000 women in 1 year.[84] Lower doses of estrogen are associated with a decreased risk for thromboembolism as compared with higher doses.[83] Oral administration of estrogen increases the risk of venous thromboembolism compared to the transdermal route.[85] Also, the norpregnane progestogens, unlike micronized progesterone and pregnane derivatives (e.g., medroxyprogesterone acetate), appear to be thrombogenic.

Currently, there is no indication for thrombophilia screening before initiating hormone therapy. However, hormone therapy should be avoided in women at high risk for thromboembolic events.

Gallbladder Disease

Gallbladder disease is a commonly cited complication of oral estrogen use. The WHI studies reported an increased risk for cholecystitis, cholelithiasis, and cholecystectomy among women taking oral estrogen or estrogen–progestogen therapy.[86] Transdermal estrogen is an alternative to oral therapy for women at high risk for cholelithiasis.

Estrogens

Estrogens are naturally occurring hormones or synthetic steroidal or nonsteroidal compounds with estrogenic activity. The primary accepted indication for estrogen-based hormone therapy is the relief of vasomotor symptoms, and the initial dose should be the lowest effective dose for symptom control.

Adverse Effects Common adverse effects of estrogen include nausea, headache, breast tenderness, and heavy bleeding. More serious adverse effects include increased risk for CHD, stroke, venous thromboembolism, breast cancer, and gallbladder disease.

Initiating therapy with low doses of estrogen often will minimize breast tenderness, unscheduled bleeding, and potentially other adverse effects. Transdermal estradiol is less likely than oral estrogen to cause nausea and headache. Also, transdermal estradiol is associated with a lower incidence of breast tenderness and deep vein thrombosis than is oral estrogen.[23,87,88] In many cases changing from one estrogen regimen to another can alleviate certain adverse effects. Lower dose estrogen therapy is also associated with less mastalgia.

Dose and Administration Various systemically administered estrogens (typically oral and transdermal) are suitable for replacement therapy (Tables 91–1 and 91–2). Estrogens can be administered orally, percutaneously (transdermal patches and topical products), intravaginally (creams, tablets, or rings), intramuscularly, and even subcutaneously in the form of implanted pellets. The choice of estrogen delivery (product, route, and method) should be determined in consultation with the patient to ensure acceptability and enhance adherence. In general, the oral and transdermal routes are used most frequently, with oral conjugated equine estrogens (CEEs) particularly popular in the United States. No evidence indicates that one estrogen compound is more effective than another in relieving menopausal symptoms or preventing osteoporosis.

Oral Estrogen Oral CEE has been available for more than 50 years. CEE is prepared from the urine of pregnant mares and is composed of estrone sulfate (50% to 60%) and multiple other equine estrogens such as equilin and 17α-dihydroequilin.[89]

Estradiol is the predominant and most active form of endogenous estrogens. A micronized form of estradiol (produced by a technique that yields extremely small particles of the pure hormone) is readily absorbed from the small intestines.[89] When given orally, estradiol is metabolized by the intestinal mucosa and the liver during the first hepatic passage, and only 10% reaches circulation as free estradiol. Metabolism of estrogen is partly mediated by the cytochrome P450 3A4 isoenzyme. Gut and liver metabolism converts a large proportion of estradiol to the less potent estrone. Thus, measurement of serum estradiol is not useful for monitoring oral estrogen replacement. The principal metabolites of micronized estradiol are estrone and estrone sulfate. Administration of estradiol via the oral route results in estrone concentrations that are three to six times those of estradiol. Ethinyl estradiol is a highly potent semisynthetic estrogen that has similar activity following administration by the oral or parenteral route.

Orally administered estrogens stimulate the synthesis of hepatic proteins and increase the circulating concentrations of sex hormone–binding globulin, which, in turn, may compromise the bioavailability of androgens and estrogens.

Other Routes Non-oral forms of estrogens (including transdermal, topical, and intravaginal) bypass the gastrointestinal tract and thereby avoid first-pass liver metabolism. These routes of estradiol delivery result in a more physiologic estradiol-to-estrone ratio (estradiol concentrations greater than estrone concentrations), as seen in the normal premenopausal state. Transdermal estrogen therapy also is less likely to affect sex hormone–binding globulin

TABLE 91-1	Systemic and Topical Estrogen Products[a,b,c]	
Estrogen	**Dosage Strength**	**Comments**
Oral estrogens		
Conjugated equine estrogens (Premarin)	0.3, 0.45, 0.625, 0.9, 1.25 mg	Orally administered estrogens stimulate synthesis
Synthetic conjugated estrogens (Cenestin, Enjuvia)	0.3, 0.45, 0.625, 0.9, 1.25 mg	of hepatic proteins and increase circulating
Esterified estrogens (Menest)	0.3, 0.625, 1.25, 2.5 mg	concentrations of sex hormone-binding globulin,
Estropipate (piperazine estrone sulfate) (Ogen, Ortho-Est, generics)	0.625, 1.25, 2.5, 5[d] mg	which, in turn, may compromise the bioavailability
Micronized 17β-estradiol (Estrace, generics)	0.5, 1,1.5[d], 2 mg	of androgens and estrogens
Estradiol acetate (Femtrace)	0.45, 0.9, 1.8 mg	
Transdermal estrogens[e]		
17β-estradiol transdermal patch (Alora, Climara, Esclim, Menostar, Vivelle, Vivelle Dot, generics)	14, 25, 37.5, 50, 60, 75,100 mcg per 24 h	Administered once or twice weekly depending on product
Topical estrogens[e]		
17β-estradiol topical emulsion (Estrasorb)	4.35 mg of estradiol hemihydrate per foil-laminated pouch	Single approved dose is 8.7 mg of estradiol hemihydrate per day (two pouches), which delivers 0.05 mg of estradiol per day. Apply to legs.
17β-estradiol topical gel (EsroGel, Elestrin, Divigel)	0.25 to 1 mg of estradiol per dose	Apply to either arm or thigh (depending on product) once daily
17β-estradiol transdermal spray (Evamist)	1.53 mg of estradiol per spray	1–3 sprays on inner surface of forearm once daily
Vaginal estrogens[e]		
Conjugated equine estrogens vaginal cream (Premarin)	0.625 mg conjugated equine estrogens per g	0.5–2 g per day
17β-estradiol vaginal cream (Estrace)	0.1 mg of estradiol per g	Maintenance dose is 1 g per day
17β-estradiol vaginal ring (Estring)	0.0075 mg per 24 h	Replaced every 90 days
Estradiol acetate vaginal ring (Femring)	0.05, 0.1 mg per 24 h	Replaced every 90 days
Estradiol hemihydrate vaginal tablet (Vagifem)	0.01, 0.025 mcg estradiol per tablet	Maintenance dose is 1 tablet twice weekly

[a]Systemic oral and transdermal estrogen and progestogen combination products are available in the United States.
[b]Systemic oral estrogen and androgen combination products are available in the United States.
[c]U.S. brand names.
[d]Not available in the United States.
[e]Women with elevated triglyceride concentrations or significant liver function abnormalities are candidates for non-oral estrogen therapy.

TABLE 91-2 Systemic Estrogen Products for Treatment of Menopausal Symptoms

Regimen	Standard Dose	Low Dose	Route	Frequency
Conjugated equine estrogens	0.625 mg	0.3 or 0.45 mg	Oral	Once daily
Synthetic conjugated estrogens	0.625 mg	0.3 mg	Oral	Once daily
Esterified estrogens	0.625 mg	0.3 mg	Oral	Once daily
Estropipate (piperazine estrone sulfate)	1.25 mg	0.625 mg	Oral	Once daily
Estradiol acetate	0.9 mg	0.45 mg	Oral	Once daily
Micronized 17β-estradiol	1–2 mg	0.25–0.5 mg	Oral	Once daily
Transdermal 17β-estradiol patch	50 mcg	25 mcg	Transdermal	Once or twice weekly
Implanted 17β-estradiol[a]	50–100 mg pellets	25 mg pellets	Pellets implanted subcutaneously	Every 6 months
17β-estradiol topical emulsion	2 pouches	–	Topical	Once daily
17β-estradiol topical gel	0.5–0.75 mg (depends on product)	Depends on product	Topical	Once daily
17β-estradiol transdermal spray	2–3 sprays	1 spray	Topical	Once daily
Estradiol acetate vaginal ring	12.4 mg ring (delivers 0.05 mg per day)	–	Intravaginally	Every 3 months

[a]Not available in the United States.

compared with oral therapy. These regimens produce little or no change in circulating lipids, coagulation parameters, or C-reactive protein levels.[90]

Transdermal estrogens share the advantages of other non-oral estrogen routes and have the added advantage of delivering estradiol to the general venous circulation at a continuous rate. Reactions at the application site occur in approximately 10% of women who use reservoir (alcohol-based) patches. The newer matrix systems (estrogen in adhesive) generally are better tolerated, and fewer than 5% of women experience skin reactions.[91] The incidence of skin irritation diminishes when the application site is rotated. Topical antiinflammatory products (e.g., hydrocortisone cream) can be applied for managing the rashes, and switching to another transdermal patch is often a viable option.

Topical preparations (gels, sprays, and emulsions) are convenient, but variability in drug absorption is common. This form of estrogen is also used for systemic therapy.

Estradiol pellets (implants) containing pure crystalline 17β-estradiol have been available for more than 50 years. They are inserted subcutaneously into the anterior abdominal wall or buttock. Pellets are difficult to remove and may continue to release estradiol for a long time after insertion. Implantation should not be repeated until serum estradiol concentrations have fallen to values similar to those at the midfollicular phase of the menstrual cycle. Estradiol pellets are not available in the United States.

Intravaginal creams, tablets, and rings are used for treatment of urogenital (vulval and vaginal) atrophy. However, this route of administration can have more than just a local effect. Systemic estrogen absorption is lower with vaginal tablets and rings (specifically Estring) compared with vaginal creams. Nonetheless, local application of the cream at low doses can reverse atrophic vaginal changes and avoid significant systemic exposure. Nonestrogen vaginal moisturizers and lubricants also may provide local symptom relief. These products can be used alone or in combination with locally-acting intravaginal estrogens. Intravaginal rings are a sustained-release delivery system composed of a biologically inert liquid polymer matrix with pure crystalline estradiol that can maintain adequate estradiol concentrations. One such intravaginal ring product (Femring) is designed to achieve systemic concentrations of estrogen and is indicated for treatment of moderate to severe vasomotor symptoms.

Progestogens

❼ Because of the increased risk of endometrial hyperplasia and endometrial cancer with estrogen monotherapy (unopposed estrogen), women who have not undergone hysterectomy should be treated concurrently with a progestogen in addition to the estrogen.[92]

Progestogens reduce nuclear estradiol receptor concentrations, suppress DNA synthesis, and decrease estrogen bioavailability by increasing the activity of endometrial 17-hydroxysteroid dehydrogenase, an enzyme responsible for converting estradiol to estrone.[76]

The first generation of progestogens included the C-19 androgenic progestogens norethindrone (also known as norethisterone), norgestrel, and levonorgestrel. More recent preparations have included the C-21 progestogens dydrogesterone and medroxyprogesterone acetate, which are less androgenic. Drospirenone, a synthetic progestogen analog of the potassium-sparing diuretic spironolactone, has both antiandrogenic and antialdosterone properties. Micronized progesterone also has become available for use in postmenopausal women. The most commonly used oral progestogens are medroxyprogesterone acetate, micronized progesterone, and norethindrone acetate. The latter now can be administered transdermally in the form of a combined estrogen–progestogen patch.

Adverse Effects Common adverse effects of progestogens include irritability, depression, and headache. Changing from a cyclic to a continuous-combined regimen or changing from one progestogen to another may decrease the incidence or severity of untoward effects. Adverse effects of progestogens are difficult to evaluate and can vary with the agent administered. Some women experience "premenstrual-like" symptoms, such as mood swings, bloating, fluid retention, and sleep disturbance. New methods and routes of progestogen delivery (e.g., by an intranasal spray or locally by an intrauterine device that releases levonorgestrel or a progesterone-containing bioadhesive vaginal gel) may be associated with fewer adverse effects. Women who are unable to tolerate a progestogen may be given unopposed estrogen if they are informed of the significant increased risk for endometrial cancer and have endometrial biopsy annually or whenever breakthrough vaginal bleeding occurs.

Dose and Administration Several progestogen regimens designed to prevent endometrial hyperplasia are available (Table 91–3). Progestogens must be taken for a sufficient period of time during each cycle. A minimum of 12 to 14 days of progestogen therapy each month is required for complete protection against estrogen-induced endometrial hyperplasia.[93] Of note, use of even low-dose estrogen, including some intravaginal preparations, requires progestogen coadministration for endometrial protection in women with an intact uterus.[94] However, rarely is progestogen administration needed in women who have undergone hysterectomy.

Methods of Combined Estrogen and Progestogen Administration

Four combination estrogen and progestogen regimens currently in use are continuous cyclic (sequential), continuous combined,

TABLE 91-3	Progestogen Doses for Endometrial Protection (Oral Cyclic Administration)
Progestogen	**Dose**
Dydrogesterone[a]	10–20 mg for 12–14 days per calendar month
Medroxyprogesterone acetate	5–10 mg for 12–14 days per calendar month
Micronized progesterone	200 mg for 12–14 days per calendar month
Norethindrone (norethisterone)[b]	0.7–1 mg for 12–14 days per calendar month
Norethindrone acetate	5 mg for 12–14 days per calendar month
Norgestrel[c]	0.15 mg for 12–14 days per calendar month
Levonorgestrel[d]	150 mcg for 12–14 days per calendar month

[a]Not available in the United States.
[b]In the United States, available in a progestogen-only oral dosage form as 0.35 mg tablets approved for prevention of pregnancy.
[c]Not available in a progestogen-only oral dosage form in the United States.
[d]In the United States, available in a progestogen-only oral dosage form as 75 mcg tablets approved for emergency contraception.

continuous long-cycle (or cyclic withdrawal), and intermittent combined (or continuous-pulsed) hormone therapy.[95] The latter two were introduced during the past decade. Sequential hormone therapy results in scheduled vaginal withdrawal bleeding but often is scant or completely absent in older women. For many women, scheduled withdrawal bleeding is one of the main reasons for avoiding or discontinuing hormone therapy. Because there is no physiologic need for bleeding, new hormone therapy regimens that reduce monthly bleeding (e.g., continuous long-cycle regimens) or prevent monthly bleeding (e.g., continuous combined and intermittent combined regimens) have been developed. Various hormone therapy regimens that combine an estrogen and a progestogen are available (Table 91–4).

Continuous Cyclic Estrogen–Progestogen (Sequential) Treatment Estrogen typically is administered continuously (daily). A progestogen is coadministered with the estrogen for at least 12 to 14 days of a 28-day cycle.[93] The progestogen causes scheduled withdrawal bleeding in approximately 90% of women. With this regimen, bleeding usually begins 1 to 2 days after the last

TABLE 91-4	Common Combination Postmenopausal Hormone Therapy Regimens
Regimen	**Doses**
Oral continuous-cyclic regimens	
CEE + MPA[a]	0.625 mg + 5 mg; 0.625 mg + 10 mg
Oral continuous-combined regimens	
CEE + MPA	0.625 mg + 2.5 mg; 0.625 mg + 5 mg; 0.45 mg + 2.5 mg; 0.3 mg + 1.5 mg/day
17β-Estradiol + NETA	1 mg + 0.1 mg; 1 mg + 0.25 mg; 1 mg + 0.5 mg/day
Ethinyl estradiol + NETA	1 mcg + 0.2 mg; 2.5 mcg + 0.5 mg; 5 mcg + 1 mg; 10 mcg + 1 mg/day
Transdermal continuous-cyclic regimens	
17β-Estradiol + NETA[a]	50 mcg + 0.14 mg; 50 mcg + 0.25 mg
Transdermal continuous-combined regimens	
17β-Estradiol + NETA	50 mcg + 0.14 mg; 50 mcg + 0.25 mg; 25 mcg + 0.125 mg

CEE, conjugated equine estrogens; MPA, medroxyprogesterone acetate; NETA, norethindrone acetate.
Other oral (drospirenone and norgestimate) and transdermal (levonorgestrel) progestogens also are available in combination with an estrogen.
[a]Estrogen alone for days 1–14, followed by estrogen–progestogen on days 15–28.

progestogen dose. Occasionally, bleeding begins during the latter phase of progestogen administration.

Continuous Combined Estrogen–Progestogen Treatment
Continuous combined estrogen–progestogen administration results in endometrial atrophy and the absence of vaginal bleeding. However, initially it causes unpredictable spotting or bleeding, which usually resolves within 6 to 12 months. Decreasing the estrogen dose or increasing the progestogen dose usually decreases or stops the spotting. Occasionally, a drug-free period of 1 or 2 weeks is useful to stop the bleeding.

Women who recently have undergone menopause have a higher risk for excessive, unpredictable bleeding while receiving continuous therapy; thus, this regimen is best reserved for women who are at least 2 years postmenopause. Continuous combined hormone therapy is more acceptable than traditional cyclic therapy.

Continuous Long-Cycle Estrogen–Progestogen Treatment
In order to decrease the incidence of uterine bleeding, a modified sequential regimen has been developed.[95] In the continuous long-cycle (or cyclic withdrawal) estrogen–progestogen regimen, estrogen is given daily, and progestogen is given six times per year, every other month for 12 to 14 days, resulting in six periods per year. Bleeding episodes may be heavier and last for more days than withdrawal bleeding with continuous cyclic regimens. The effect of continuous long-cycle estrogen–progestogen treatment on endometrial protection is unclear.

Intermittent Combined Estrogen–Progestogen Treatment
The intermittent combined estrogen–progestogen regimen, also called *continuous-pulsed estrogen–progestogen* or *pulsed-progestogen*, consists of 3 days of estrogen therapy alone, followed by 3 days of combined estrogen and progestogen, which is then repeated without interruption.[95] This regimen is designed to lower the incidence of uterine bleeding. It is based on the assumption that pulsed-progestogen administration will prevent down-regulation of progesterone receptors that can be produced by continuous combined regimens. The lower progestogen dose induces fewer side effects and can be better tolerated. The long-term effect of intermittent combined regimens in endometrial protection is undetermined.

Low-Dose Hormone Therapy

❽ Increasingly, it has become recognized that use of hormone therapy at doses lower than those prescribed historically is effective in the management of menopausal symptoms (see Table 91–2). The standard dose of estrogen previously believed to be effective in alleviating vasomotor symptoms is equivalent to 0.625 mg CEE,[36] but new evidence indicates that lower doses of estrogen also are effective in controlling postmenopausal symptoms and reducing bone loss.[96-99] The Women's Health, Osteoporosis, Progestin, Estrogen (HOPE) trial demonstrated equivalent symptom relief and bone density preservation without an increase in endometrial hyperplasia using lower doses of hormone therapy (CEE 0.45 mg/day and medroxyprogesterone acetate 1.5 mg/day).[97-99] Even ultralow doses of 17β-estradiol delivered by a vaginal ring (Estring) improved serum lipid profiles and prevented bone loss in elderly women.[100] Whether lower doses of estrogen will be safer (lower incidence of venous thromboembolism and breast cancer) remains to be proven. Nonetheless, evidence of harm associated with a standard dose of hormone therapy[17,18] has prompted many patients to either discontinue such therapy or taper to lower doses. In general, if adverse effects such as breast tenderness occur with initial doses, lowering the dose may resolve the problem and improve patient adherence. Alternatively, if vasomotor symptoms are not controlled adequately with a lower-dose regimen, increasing the estrogen dose may be a reasonable option.

CLINICAL CONTROVERSY

Although some clinicians believe that estrogen can be used safely at lower doses to treat postmenopausal women with severe and protracted vasomotor symptoms, others caution that such long-term therapy, even with lower doses of estrogen, may be associated with unacceptable risks.

Bioidentical Hormones Bioidentical hormone therapy has received much attention by patients, health care professionals, and the media since the initial publication of the WHI results. Bioidentical hormone therapy refers to the practice of using natural (e.g., estrone, estradiol, estriol progesterone, and testosterone), rather than synthetic, formulations of sex hormones. Often, these hormones are compounded to make a variety of topical formulations, in theory to individualize hormone therapy based on each patient's specific physiologic hormone levels as measured via salivary concentrations. This strategy is thought to reduce the risk of adverse effects. However, there is a paucity of evidence regarding both their efficacy and safety.[101] Bioidentical hormones appear to carry the same risks as traditional hormone therapy. Several major medical organizations, along with the FDA, have released statements that dissuade against the use of this treatment strategy.[102,103]

■ ALTERNATIVE DRUG TREATMENTS

In women who have contraindications to estrogen and progestogen use, prefer not to take estrogen and/or progestogen, or cannot tolerate estrogen and/or progestogen administration, a number of other medications may be considered, depending on the goals of therapy. These include the prescription medications testosterone, raloxifene, and tibolone (not currently available in the United States) as well as nonhormonal prescription medications (e.g., selective serotonin reuptake inhibitors). Some women prefer to use herbals and other natural therapies but the efficacy and safety of these methods have not been definitively established.

Alternatives to estrogen for treatment of hot flushes include tibolone, selective serotonin reuptake inhibitors (e.g., paroxetine, fluoxetine), dual serotonin and noradrenaline reuptake inhibitors (e.g., venlafaxine), medroxyprogesterone acetate, megestrol acetate, clonidine, and gabapentin (Table 91–5).[104] Progestogens alone may be an option for some women (e.g., those with a history of breast cancer or venous thrombosis), but weight gain, vaginal bleeding, and other adverse effects often limit their use. Tibolone and progestogens cannot be considered nonhormonal agents for treatment of hot flushes in women for whom hormone therapy is contraindicated. For this group of patients, selective serotonin reuptake

inhibitors and venlafaxine are considered by some to be a first-line therapy.[104,105] However, the efficacy of venlafaxine for treatment of hot flushes has not been shown to extend beyond 12 weeks.[106] Furthermore, in breast cancer patients, evidence suggests that selective serotonin reuptake inhibitors could interfere with metabolism of endocrine therapies, such as tamoxifen via cytochrome P450 2D6 inhibition.[107] Clonidine is often effective for symptom control, but its side effects (e.g. sedation, dry mouth, hypotension) are not always well tolerated by women.

Androgens

Pathophysiologic states affecting ovarian and adrenal function, along with aging, have been associated with androgen deficiency in women.[108] The therapeutic use of testosterone in women, although controversial, is becoming more widespread despite the lack of accurate clinical or biochemical findings of androgen deficiency.[108] Androgens have important biologic effects in women, acting both directly via androgen receptors in tissues, such as bone, skin fibroblasts, hair follicles, and sebaceous glands, and indirectly via the aromatization of testosterone to estrogen in the ovaries, bone, brain, adipose tissue, and other tissues.

Efficacy A cluster of symptoms that characterizes androgen insufficiency in women, manifested as diminished sense of well-being, persistent or unexplained fatigue, and sexual function changes such as decreased libido, decreased sexual receptivity, and decreased pleasure, has been reported.[108] However, studies designed to evaluate this have shown no relationships between serum total and free testosterone levels and either sexual function[109] or well-being[110] in women. Thus, as data supporting an androgen deficiency syndrome are lacking, in 2006 the American Endocrine Society recommended against making a diagnosis of androgen deficiency in women at the present time.[109] Several large randomized placebo-controlled clinical trials involving naturally[111,112] and surgically[113] postmenopausal women presenting with low libido demonstrate that testosterone therapy, with and without concurrent estrogen therapy, improves the quality of the sexual experience, with preliminary data that this may also apply to premenopausal women.[114]

Adverse Effects Absolute contraindications to androgen therapy include pregnancy or lactation and known or suspected androgen-dependent neoplasia. Relative contraindications include concurrent use of CEEs (for parenteral testosterone therapy), low sex hormone–binding globulin level (below the normal range for women) moderate to severe acne, clinical hirsutism, and androgenic alopecia.

Adverse effects from excessive dosage include virilization, fluid retention, and potentially adverse lipoprotein lipid effects, which are more likely with oral administration. There is no evidence that systemic transdermal testosterone is associated with increased

TABLE 91-5 Alternatives to Estrogen for Treatment of Hot Flushes

Drug	Dose (Oral)	Interval	Comments
Tibolone[a]	2.5–5 mg	Once daily	Tibolone is not recommended during the perimenopause because it may cause irregular bleeding
Venlafaxine	37.5–150 mg	Once daily	Side effects include dry mouth, decreased appetite, nausea, and constipation
Paroxetine	12.5–25 mg	Once daily	12.5 mg is an adequate, well-tolerated starting dose for most women; adverse effects include headache, nausea, and insomnia
Fluoxetine	20 mg	Once daily	Modest improvement seen in hot flushes
Megestrol acetate	20–40 mg	Once daily	Progesterone may be linked to breast cancer etiology; also, there is concern regarding the safety of progestational agents in women with preexisting breast cancer
Clonidine	0.1 mg	Once daily	Can be administered orally or transdermally; drowsiness and dry mouth can occur, especially with higher doses
Gabapentin	900 mg	Divided in 3 daily doses	Adverse effects include somnolence and dizziness; these symptoms often can be obviated with a gradual increase in dosing

[a]Not available in the United States.

TABLE 91-6	Androgen Regimens Used for Women		
Regimen	**Dose**	**Frequency**	**Route**
Methyltestosterone in combination with esterified estrogen	1.25–2.5 mg	Daily	Oral
Mixed testosterone esters	50–100 mg	Every 4–6 weeks	Intramuscular
Testosterone pellets	50 mg	Every 6 months	Subcutaneous (implanted)
Transdermal testosterone system[a]	150–300 mcg/day	Every 3–4 days	Transdermal patch
Nandrolone decanoate	50 mg	Every 8–12 weeks	Intramuscular

[a]Undergoing clinical trials in the United States.

cardiovascular morbidity or mortality[115] or of a significant change in the risk of invasive breast cancer.[116,117] However, further studies are required to determine the long term safety of testosterone in women.

Dose and Administration Testosterone is available as oral methyltestosterone in the United States and as testosterone implants in the United Kingdom. Of the available oral preparations, methyltestosterone in combination with esterified estrogen (either 0.625 mg esterified estrogen plus 1.25 mg methyltestosterone or 1.25 mg esterified estrogen plus 2.5 mg methyltestosterone) is the most widely studied.

Testosterone replacement for women is available in a variety of formulations (Table 91–6). Most of the earlier studies showing clinical improvement with testosterone therapy reported supraphysiologic levels. More recent studies using transdermal patch therapy have shown efficacy with free testosterone levels in the upper normal range for young women. The availability of testosterone regimens specifically designed for women has the potential to maintain testosterone levels within the normal range and help to clarify whether the apparent beneficial effects of testosterone therapy are physiologic or pharmacologic.[113,118] In general, testosterone treatment can be administered to postmenopausal women with and without concurrent estrogen therapy. At present, generalized use of testosterone is not recommended because the indications are inadequate, and evidence from long-term studies evaluating safety is lacking.[119]

Selective Estrogen Receptor Modulators

Selective estrogen receptor modulators (SERMs) are a group of nonsteroidal compounds that are chemically distinct from estradiol. They act as estrogen agonists in some tissues, such as bone, and as estrogen antagonists in other tissues, such as breast, through specific, high-affinity binding to the estrogen receptor.

Efficacy The ideal SERM would protect against osteoporosis and decrease the incidence of breast, endometrial, and colorectal cancer and coronary heart disease without exacerbating menopausal symptoms or increasing the risk of venous thromboembolism or gallbladder disease. To date, no SERM meets these ideals. Tamoxifen, the first-generation SERM (a nonsteroidal triphenylethylene derivative), has estrogen antagonist activity on the breast and estrogen-like agonist activity on bone and endometrium. The second generation of SERMs, most notably raloxifene (a nonsteroidal benzothiophene derivative), has become available for prevention of osteoporosis. Raloxifene does not alleviate, and may even exacerbate, vasomotor symptoms.

The Multiple Outcomes of Raloxifene Evaluation (MORE), a multicenter randomized, blinded, placebo-controlled trial, showed that raloxifene increases BMD in the spine and femoral neck and reduces the risk of vertebral fractures.[120] It has not been shown to decrease the risk of hip fractures. Raloxifene decreases bone loss in recently menopausal women without affecting the endometrium and has estrogen-like actions on lipid metabolism.[120] More importantly, the same study[121] and the Continuing Outcomes Relevant to Evista (CORE) trial[122] suggest that raloxifene use is associated

with a significantly lower incidence of breast cancer compared with placebo. This benefit is primarily due to a reduced risk of estrogen receptor–positive invasive breast cancers.[80,122] A prospective randomized double-blinded trial of 19,747 women at high risk for breast cancer (Study of Tamoxifen and Raloxifene [STAR]) showed that raloxifene is as effective as tamoxifen in reducing the risk of invasive breast cancer and has a lower risk of thromboembolic events.[123] A prospective randomized study (Raloxifene Use for the Heart [RUTH]) of 10,101 postmenopausal women (mean age 67.5 years) with coronary heart disease or multiple risk factors for coronary heart disease showed that raloxifene did not significantly affect the risk of coronary heart disease.[80] Raloxifene does not have a significant effect on cognitive function; however, there is a trend toward a smaller decline in verbal memory and attention scores among women receiving raloxifene.[124]

Adverse Effects Raloxifene is commonly associated with hot flushes and less often with leg cramps. Raloxifene use increases the risk of venous thromboembolism[80,120–122] and fatal stroke[80] to a degree similar to that of oral estrogen.

Dose and Administration Raloxifene is FDA-approved for the treatment and prevention of osteoporosis and for the reduction of the risk of invasive breast cancer in postmenopausal women with osteoporosis as well as postmenopausal women at high risk for invasive breast cancer. The dose is 60 mg orally once daily.

Tibolone

Tibolone is a gonadomimetic synthetic steroid in the norpregnane family with combined estrogenic, progestogenic, and androgenic activity.[125] Tibolone has been used for 2 decades in Europe for treatment of menopausal symptoms and prevention of osteoporosis but is currently not available in the United States. The hormonal effects of this synthetic steroid depend on its metabolism and activation in peripheral tissues. The parent compound has been described as a prodrug that is metabolized quickly in the gastrointestinal tract. It has several active metabolites, including a Δ4-isomer and 3α-OH and 3β-OH compounds.[125] The Δ4-isomer metabolite confers significant progestogenic and androgenic properties.

Efficacy Tibolone has beneficial effects on mood and libido and improves menopausal symptoms and vaginal atrophy. Tibolone protects against bone loss and significantly reduces the risk of vertebral fractures in postmenopausal women with osteoporosis.[126] It has also been shown to decrease the risk of breast cancer and colon cancer in older women (aged 60–85 years) in one randomized study.[127] It is also more effective than conventional hormone therapy for management of sexual dysfunction.[128]

Adverse Effects Tibolone use in elderly women has been reported to be associated with an increased risk of stroke.[126,127] Tibolone lowers concentrations of total cholesterol, triglycerides, and lipoprotein (a) but may decrease high-density lipoprotein (HDL) cholesterol.[89] The Million Women Study, an observational cohort study, found a greater risk of endometrial cancer (adjusted relative risk 1.79, 95% CI 1.43–2.25).[129] However, other randomized placebo-controlled studies have not shown an increased risk of endometrial cancer with tibolone and suggest that tibolone has an endometrial safety profile similar to continuous combined CEE and medroxyprogesterone acetate.[130]

The most commonly reported adverse effects of tibolone include weight gain and bloating.

Complementary and Alternative Medicine

Some women prefer to use natural remedies due to a belief that they are safer. Randomized, placebo-controlled trials of complementary and alternative therapies have been equivocal and have not established the safety and efficacy of herbal remedies, homeopathic treatments, or acupuncture for the prevention or treatment of hot flushes.

Phytoestrogens Phytoestrogens have physiologic effects in humans.[131] They are plant compounds with estrogen-like biologic activity and relatively weak estrogen receptor–binding properties. Epidemiologic studies suggest that consumption of a phytoestrogen-rich diet, which is common in traditional Asian societies, is associated with a lower risk of breast cancer.[131]

The biologic potencies of phytoestrogens vary. Most of these compounds are nonsteroidal and are less potent than synthetic estrogens. The three main classes of phytoestrogens are isoflavones, lignans, and coumestans, all of which are found in plants or their seeds.[131] The most commonly studied phytoestrogen is the isoflavone class. Genistein and daidzein are the most abundant active components of isoflavones. The concentration of isoflavones per gram of soy protein varies considerably among preparations. Also, a single plant often contains more than one class of phytoestrogen. Common food sources of phytoestrogens include soybeans (isoflavones), cereals, oilseeds such as flaxseed (lignans), and alfalfa sprouts (coumestans).

Mild estrogenic effects have been seen in postmenopausal women,[131] but current data suggest that phytoestrogen supplementation is no more effective than placebo in relieving hot flushes or other symptoms of menopause in postmenopausal women.[132]

Phytoestrogens decrease low-density lipoprotein (LDL) cholesterol and triglyceride concentrations with no significant change in HDL cholesterol concentrations.[133] Furthermore, phytoestrogens have the ability to inhibit LDL oxidation and normalize vascular reactivity in estrogen-deprived primates.[133] In addition, BMD may be improved by phytoestrogens.[131] Common adverse effects include constipation, bloating, and nausea.[134]

A recent meta-analysis reported that phytoestrogen use is not associated with increased rates of endometrial cancer, vaginal bleeding, and breast cancer.[134] Large, long-term studies are needed to further document the effects of phytoestrogens on the breast, bone, and endometrium. Furthermore, differences among classes of phytoestrogens must be identified clearly, including dosing and biologic activity, before phytoestrogens can be considered an alternative to conventional hormone therapy in postmenopausal women.

Other Herbal Products Black cohosh (*Cimicifuga racemosa* or *Acetaea racemosa*), a widely used herbal supplement, may not offer substantial benefits for relief of vasomotor symptoms as suggested by earlier trials.[135] This substance does not appear to have strong intrinsic estrogenic properties but may act through the serotonergic system. Black cohosh appears to be generally well tolerated, although hepatotoxicity has been reported. It is unclear if this is due to the herb itself or adulterations of commercially available products.[136] The long-term effects of black cohosh are unknown. Other herbals and alternative treatments that may be used by women include dong quai, red clover leaf (contains phytoestrogens), kava, and dehydroepiandrosterone. These have not been shown to be effective in the treatment of menopausal symptoms and may carry the risk of adverse events.[137] Complementary and alternative therapies should not be recommended to treat menopausal symptoms.

Pharmacoeconomic Considerations

Estrogens and progestogens used for postmenopausal hormone therapy are prescribed commonly in the United States, especially for the management of menopausal vasomotor symptoms. Even before publication of the WHI trial findings, only a fraction of women filled their hormone therapy prescriptions, and only 25% to 40% continued to take postmenopausal hormone therapy for more than 1 year.[138] This may be due to women's attitudes toward hormone therapy or a result of fear about adverse effects and associated risks. Hormone therapy use in the United States declined substantially after dissemination of the WHI trial results.[139]

Use of hormone therapy for the management of vasomotor symptoms is cost effective, and data supporting the use of nonhormonal alternatives are limited. The cost of hormone therapy varies depending on the route and method of delivery. Transdermal preparations are about twice as expensive as their equivalent oral preparations.[140] Women who have undergone hysterectomy use hormone therapy more frequently than do women with an intact uterus (58.7% vs 19.6%).[16]

EVALUATION OF THERAPEUTIC OUTCOMES

After the menopausal woman begins hormone therapy, a brief follow-up visit 6 weeks later may be useful to discuss patient concerns about hormone therapy and to evaluate the patient for symptom relief, adverse effects, and patterns of withdrawal bleeding. The FDA recommends that women who choose estrogen-based therapy should have yearly breast examinations, perform monthly breast self-examinations, and receive periodic mammograms (scheduled based on their age and risk factors). Also, women receiving hormone therapy should undergo annual monitoring, including a medical history, physical examination, pelvic examination, blood pressure measurement, and routine endometrial cancer surveillance, as indicated. Additional follow-up is determined based on the patient's initial response to therapy and the need for any modification of the regimen. An ultrasound, ideally transvaginal, and where indicated an endometrial biopsy should be performed in women taking cyclic hormone therapy if vaginal bleeding occurs at any time other than the expected time of withdrawal bleeding or when heavier or more prolonged withdrawal bleeding occurs. In women taking continuous combined hormone therapy, endometrial evaluation should be considered when irregular bleeding persists for more than 6 months after initiating therapy. However, there is no universal agreement that endovaginal ultrasonography is adequate for excluding endometrial pathology.

The main indication for hormone therapy is relief of menopausal symptoms, and hormone therapy should be used only as long as symptom control is necessary (typically 2–3 years). When hormone therapy is used under such conditions, the absolute risk of harm to an individual woman is very small.[17]

Many women have no difficulty abruptly stopping hormone therapy; others develop vasomotor symptoms after discontinuation. Although these symptoms usually are mild and resolve over a few months, in some women the symptoms are severe and intolerable. Few studies have addressed the appropriate method for discontinuing hormone therapy. There is no evidence that gradual discontinuation of hormone therapy reduces the recurrence of hot flushes compared with sudden discontinuation. Studies determining effective ways to reduce symptoms of estrogen withdrawal are needed.

BMD should be measured in women older than 65 years and in women younger than 65 years with risk factors for osteoporosis. Although bone densitometry has been shown to predict fractures, at present there are no guidelines for follow-up BMD testing. However, in women with significant bone loss, repeat testing should be performed as clinically indicated.

CONCLUSIONS

During the past decade, postmenopausal hormone therapy became one of the most frequently prescribed therapies in the United States. Menopause is a natural life event, not a disease. Therefore, the decision to use hormone therapy must be individualized based on the severity of menopausal symptoms, risk of osteoporosis, and consideration of factors such as cardiovascular disease, breast cancer, and thromboembolism (Table 91–7).

TABLE 91-7	Evidence-Based Hormone Therapy Guidelines for Menopausal Symptom Management	
Recommendation		**Recommendation Grade**[a]
In the absence of contraindications, estrogen-based postmenopausal hormone therapy should be used for treatment of moderate to severe vasomotor symptoms		A1
Systemic or vaginal estrogen therapy should be used for treatment of urogenital symptoms and vaginal atrophy		A1
Hormone therapy should be prescribed at the lowest effective dose and for the shortest duration		B2
Postmenopausal women taking estrogen-based therapy should be followed-up every year, taking into account findings from new clinical trials		A1
Postmenopausal women taking estrogen-based therapy should be informed about potential risks		A1
Safety and tolerability may vary substantially with the type and regimen of hormone therapy		B2
Breast cancer risk increases after use of continuous combined hormone therapy for longer than 5 years		A1
Breast cancer risk does not increase after long-term estrogen-only therapy (6.8 years) in postmenopausal women with hysterectomy		A1
Hormone therapy should not be used for primary or secondary prevention of coronary heart disease		A1
Oral hormone therapy increases risk of venous thromboembolism		A1
Non-oral hormone therapy may be safer for postmenopausal women at risk for venous thromboembolism who choose to take hormone therapy		B2
Oral hormone therapy increases risk of ischemic stroke		A1
Although hormone therapy decreases risk of osteoporotic fractures, it cannot be recommended as a first-line therapy for the treatment of osteoporosis		A1
Potential harm (cardiovascular disease, breast cancer, and thromboembolism) from long-term hormone therapy (use greater than 5 years) outweighs potential benefits		A1
Young women with primary ovarian insufficiency have severe menopausal symptoms and increased risk for osteoporosis and cardiovascular disease. Decisions on whether and how these young women must be treated should not be based on studies of hormone therapy in women older than 50 years.		B3

Quality of evidence: 1, evidence from more than one properly randomized controlled trial; 2, evidence from more than one well-designed clinical trial with randomization from cohort or case-controlled analytic studies or multiple time series, or dramatic results from uncontrolled experiments; 3, evidence from opinions of respected authorities based on clinical experience, descriptive studies, or reports of expert communities.
[a]Strength of recommendations: A, good evidence to support recommendation; B, moderate evidence to support recommendation; C, poor evidence to support recommendation.

Large prospective, randomized trials have shown that postmenopausal hormone therapy prescribed for disease prevention may cause more harm than good.[17,58] The WHI trial reported increased risk of cardiovascular disease, breast cancer, stroke, and thromboembolic disease among women using continuous combined therapy with CEE plus medroxyprogesterone acetate compared with placebo. In the estrogen-alone arm of the study, CEE had no effect on cardiovascular disease or breast cancer risk compared to placebo, but an increased risk of stroke and thromboembolic disease was noted in those who received estrogen. The WHI trial also demonstrated that quality of life and cognition were no better in the group receiving hormone therapy than in the placebo group, and that hormone therapy increases dementia risk in women 65 years or older.

Postmenopausal symptoms, such as hot flushes and vaginal dryness, remain a valid indication for hormone therapy in the absence of contraindications. For short-term use of hormone therapy for relief of menopausal symptoms, the benefits for many women outweigh the risks. For symptoms of genital atrophy alone, local estrogen and/or nonhormonal lubricants should be considered.

Long-term use of hormone therapy cannot be recommended routinely for osteoporosis prevention given the availability of alternative therapies, such as bisphosphonates and raloxifene. For long-term hormone therapy use, the potential harm (cardiovascular disease, breast cancer, and thromboembolism) outweighs the potential benefits. Hormone therapy should not be used for prevention of CHD. Women with cardiovascular risk factors (e.g., hypertension, lipid abnormalities) can benefit from reduction of these risk factors through interventions such as weight loss, lipid-lowering therapy, use of aspirin, and physical activity.

PRIMARY OVARIAN INSUFFICIENCY AND PREMENOPAUSAL HORMONE REPLACEMENT THERAPY

Primary ovarian insufficiency is a condition characterized by sex-steroid deficiency, amenorrhea, and infertility in women younger than 40 years.[141] Primary ovarian insufficiency was once considered irreversible and was described as "premature menopause" and the condition is still referred to as *premature ovarian failure*. However, primary ovarian insufficiency is not an early, natural menopause. Normal menopause results from ovarian follicle depletion, whereas primary ovarian insufficiency is characterized by intermittent ovarian function in half of affected women.[141] These women produce estrogen intermittently and may ovulate despite the presence of high gonadotropin concentrations. Pregnancies have occurred in 5% to 10% of women after the diagnosis of premature ovarian failure, even in women with no follicles observed on ovarian biopsy.

EPIDEMIOLOGY

The prevalence of primary ovarian insufficiency increases with increasing age, reaching approximately 1% of women by age 40 years.[142]

ETIOLOGY

A number of physiologic or metabolic abnormalities can lead to primary ovarian insufficiency (Table 91–8). In most cases, the etiology cannot be identified.

PATHOPHYSIOLOGY

Primary ovarian insufficiency may occur as a result of ovarian follicle dysfunction or ovarian follicle depletion and may present as either primary amenorrhea (absence of menses in a girl who

TABLE 91-8	Etiology of Primary Ovarian Insufficiency

Idiopathic: Karyotypically normal spontaneous primary ovarian insufficiency

Autoimmunity: (A) isolated autoimmune primary ovarian insufficiency or (B) as a component of an autoimmune polyglandular syndrome in association with Addison's disease, hypothyroidism, hypoparathyroidism, or mucocutaneous candidiasis

Iatrogenic: Chemotherapy, radiation, extensive ovarian surgery

X-chromosome abnormalities

Gonadotropin and gonadotropin-receptor abnormalities: Signal defects

Enzyme deficiencies: Cholesterol desmolase, 17α-hydroxylase, 17, 20-desmolase

Galactosemia

Blepharophimosis, ptosis, and epicanthus inversus syndrome type 1: Rare autosomal dominant syndrome in which primary ovarian insufficiency is the predominant syndrome

Perrault syndrome: Familial autosomal recessive primary ovarian insufficiency in association with deafness

has reached age 16 years) or secondary amenorrhea (cessation of menses in a woman previously menstruating for at least 6 months). Approximately 50% of women with primary ovarian insufficiency have documented ovarian follicle function.[141]

CLINICAL PRESENTATION

No characteristic menstrual pattern or history precedes primary ovarian insufficiency. Approximately 50% of patients with this condition have a history of oligomenorrhea or dysfunctional uterine bleeding (prodromal premature ovarian failure), and approximately 25% develop amenorrhea acutely. Some patients develop amenorrhea postpartum, whereas others experience amenorrhea after discontinuing oral contraceptives. Primary amenorrhea is not associated with symptoms of estrogen deficiency. In cases of secondary amenorrhea, symptoms may include hot flushes, night sweats, fatigue, and mood changes. Prodromal primary ovarian insufficiency may present with hot flushes even in women who menstruate regularly. Incomplete development of secondary sex characteristics may occur in women with primary amenorrhea, whereas these characteristics typically are normal in women with secondary amenorrhea. In general, women with primary ovarian insufficiency have normal fertility before the disorder develops.

Primary ovarian insufficiency is defined by the presence of at least 4 months of amenorrhea and at least two serum FSH concentrations measuring greater than 40 milliinternational units/mL (40 IU/L) (obtained at least 1 month apart) in women younger than 40 years. A complete history should be taken, considering other factors that can affect ovarian function such as prior ovarian surgery, chemotherapy, radiation, and autoimmune disorders. In patients with primary amenorrhea, particular attention should be paid to breast and pubic hair development according to Tanner stages. Short stature, stigmata of Turner syndrome, and other dysmorphic features of gonadal dysgenesis should be considered. Ideally, a pelvic examination is performed but is not always clinically appropriate. Alternatively, transabdominal ultrasonography can be performed in patients with primary amenorrhea to confirm the presence of normal anatomic structures. In the majority of cases, physical examination is completely normal. A karyotype should be performed in all patients experiencing primary ovarian insufficiency. Women with ovarian insufficiency and a karyotype containing a Y chromosome should undergo bilateral gonadectomy because of substantial risk for gonadal germ cell neoplasia.[141] Ovarian biopsy and antiovarian antibody testing are investigational procedures with no proven clinical benefit in primary ovarian insufficiency. As clinically indicated, the workup should include tests for the diagnosis of other possible associated autoimmune disorders, such as hypothyroidism, diabetes mellitus, and Addison's disease.

CLINICAL PRESENTATION OF PRIMARY OVARIAN INSUFFICIENCY

Symptoms

- Primary amenorrhea: No symptoms of estrogen deficiency
- Secondary amenorrhea: Vasomotor symptoms (hot flushes and night sweats), sleep disturbances, mood changes, sexual dysfunction, problems with concentration and memory, vaginal dryness, and dyspareunia

Signs

- Primary amenorrhea: Incomplete development of secondary sex characteristics
- Secondary amenorrhea: Normal development of secondary sex characteristics, signs of urogenital atrophy

Laboratory Tests

- FSH greater than 40 milliinternational units/mL (40 IU/L)
- Other relevant diagnostic tests (e.g., bone mineral density, ultrasound of the ovaries)
- Thyroid function tests, fasting glucose level, and adrenocorticotropic hormone stimulation test

In the majority of patients, ovarian insufficiency develops after the establishment of regular menses. Young women with primary ovarian insufficiency who develop ovarian dysfunction before they achieve peak adult bone mass sustain sex steroid deficiency for more years than do naturally menopausal women. This deficiency can result in a significantly higher risk for osteoporosis[143] and cardiovascular disease.[144,145] Importantly, a survey of more than 19,000 women between the ages of 25 and 100 years suggests that ovarian insufficiency occurring before age 40 years is associated with significantly increased mortality, with an age-adjusted odds ratio for all-cause mortality of 2.14 (95% CI 1.15–3.99).[146]

Young women find the diagnosis of primary ovarian insufficiency particularly traumatic and frequently need extensive emotional and psychological support. Although most of these women will, in fact, be infertile, it is important to emphasize that primary ovarian insufficiency can be transient and that spontaneous pregnancies have occurred even years after diagnosis.

TREATMENT

❾ Results from randomized trials of hormone therapy in postmenopausal women cannot be extrapolated to premenopausal women with ovarian dysfunction. Postmenopausal women who take hormone therapy prolong their exposure to estrogen beyond the average age of completion of their reproductive phase. In contrast, women with primary ovarian insufficiency need exogenous sex steroids to compensate for the decreased production by their ovaries. Importantly, 47% of young women with primary ovarian insufficiency have significantly reduced BMD within 1.5 years of their diagnosis despite taking standard hormone therapy.[143]

■ DESIRED OUTCOME

The goal of therapy in young women with primary ovarian insufficiency is to provide a hormone replacement regimen that maintains sex steroid status as effectively as the normal, functioning ovary.

■ GENERAL APPROACH TO TREATMENT

Hormone therapy with estrogen, progestogen, and testosterone is used and generally should be continued until the average age of natural menopause.

■ PHARMACOLOGIC THERAPY

Optimal hormone therapy depends on whether the patient has primary or secondary amenorrhea. Young women with primary amenorrhea in whom secondary sex characteristics have failed to develop initially should be given very low doses of estrogen in an attempt to mimic the gradual pubertal maturation process. A typical regimen is 0.3 mg CEE unopposed (i.e., no progestogen) daily for 6 months, with incremental dose increases at 6-month intervals until the required maintenance dose is achieved. Gradual dose escalation often results in optimal breast development and allows time for the young woman to adjust psychologically to her physical maturation. Cyclic progestogen therapy, given 12 to 14 days per month, should be instituted toward the end of the second year of treatment.

Women with secondary amenorrhea who have been estrogen deficient for 12 months or longer also should be given low-dose estrogen replacement initially to avoid adverse effects such as mastalgia and nausea. However, the dose can be titrated up to maintenance levels over a 6-month period, and progestogen therapy can be instituted with the initiation of estrogen therapy. Women with a brief history of secondary amenorrhea are less likely to experience undesired effects from hormone therapy if they are given a reduced dose for the first month of therapy, followed by a full dose from the second month onward.

An estrogen dose equivalent to at least 1.25 mg CEE (or 100 mcg transdermal estradiol) is needed to achieve adequate estrogen replacement in young women. A progestogen should be given for 12 to 14 days per calendar month to prevent endometrial hyperplasia (Table 91–9). Estrogens given in usual replacement doses do not suppress spontaneous follicular activity or ovulation. Because women with primary ovarian insufficiency can have spontaneous pregnancies, hormone therapy should produce regular, predictable menstrual flow patterns (i.e., only cyclic regimens should be used). Patients who miss an expected menses should be tested

for pregnancy and should discontinue hormone therapy. Because most young women negatively associate hormone therapy with menopause in older women, some clinicians prefer to prescribe oral contraceptives for hormone replacement in premenopausal women with hypogonadism. However, oral contraceptives may not inhibit ovulation or effectively prevent pregnancy in young women with elevated gonadotropin levels.

Women with primary ovarian insufficiency have testosterone deficiency.[147] In these young women, testosterone replacement, in addition to estrogen, may be important.[118] However, preliminary analysis of a prospective study at the National Institutes of Health suggests that long-term "physiologic" testosterone supplementation (150 mcg/day), in addition to standard hormone replacement, did not significantly improve BMD and sexual function in these young women.[148,149]

Importantly, all women with primary ovarian insufficiency should understand that hormone therapy generally should be continued until the average age of natural menopause and that long-term follow-up is necessary.

Pharmacoeconomic Considerations

Depending on the duration of therapy, the cost of therapy for primary ovarian insufficiency may be more or less than that associated with therapy for menopausal symptoms. The cost of therapy can be substantial for women who undergo fertility testing and treatment prior to receiving the diagnosis of primary ovarian insufficiency.

■ EVALUATION OF THERAPEUTIC OUTCOMES

Similar to the treatment of menopause, an assessment of the efficacy of hormone therapy, and its accompanying risks, should be performed on a regular basis. Young women with primary ovarian insufficiency should be monitored annually for their response to treatment, and their adherence with hormone therapy should be assessed regularly. Patients should be evaluated continuously for the presence of signs and symptoms of associated autoimmune endocrine disorders, such as hypothyroidism, adrenal insufficiency, and diabetes mellitus. Baseline BMD testing should be performed in all women with primary ovarian insufficiency. Mammography should be performed annually after age 40 years in accordance with accepted guidelines. Additional mammography screening in premenopausal women younger than 40 years who are receiving physiologic hormone therapy is not warranted. Other tests should be performed as clinically indicated.

CONCLUSIONS

Approximately 1% of women spontaneously develop ovarian insufficiency before age 40 years. Primary ovarian insufficiency is not an early natural menopause. Most affected women produce estrogen intermittently and may ovulate despite the presence of high gonadotropin concentrations. However, these women sustain sex steroid deficiency for more years than do naturally menopausal women, resulting in a significantly higher risk for osteoporosis and cardiovascular disease.

Women with primary ovarian insufficiency need exogenous sex steroids to compensate for the decreased production by their ovaries. Thus, premenopausal hormone therapy is required at least until these women reach the age of natural menopause.

The goal of therapy is to provide a hormone replacement regimen that maintains sex steroid status as effectively as the normal, functioning ovary. This usually requires the administration of estrogen at a dose greater than the standard dose given to older women experiencing natural menopause.

TABLE 91–9	Premenopausal Hormone Replacement Therapy for Young Women with Primary Ovarian Insufficiency		
Regimen	**Dose**	**Frequency**	**Route**
Estrogen therapy			
Conjugated equine estrogen	1.25 mg	Daily	Oral
Estropipate (piperazine estrone sulfate)	2.5 mg	Daily	Oral
Micronized 17β-estradiol	4 mg	Daily	Oral
Transdermal estrogen system	100 mcg/24 h	Once or twice weekly	Transdermal patch
Progestogen therapy			
Medroxyprogesterone acetate	10 mg	12–14 days[a]	Oral
Dydrogesterone[b]	20 mg	12–14 days[a]	Oral
Norethindrone acetate	10 mg	12–14 days[a]	Oral
Norethindrone (norethisterone)[b]	1 mg	12–14 days[a]	Oral
Micronized progesterone	200 mg	12–14 days[a]	Oral
Transdermal norethindrone[c]	250 mcg/24 h	Twice weekly for 14 days per calendar month	Transdermal patch

[a]Per calendar month.
[b]In the United States, available in a progestogen-only oral dosage form as 0.35 mg tablets approved for prevention of pregnancy.
[c]Available only in combination with estradiol.

Because women with primary ovarian insufficiency can have spontaneous pregnancies, hormone therapy should produce regular, predictable menstrual flow patterns. Patients who miss an expected menses should be tested for pregnancy and, if positive, the hormone therapy should be promptly discontinued.

Annual follow-up should include assessment of adherence with the prescribed hormone therapy regimen and evaluation for signs and symptoms of associated endocrine disorders.

ABBREVIATIONS

BMD: bone mineral density

CEE: conjugated equine estrogens

CHD: coronary heart disease

CORE: Continuing Outcomes Relevant to Evista

FDA: Food and Drug Administration

FSH: follicle-stimulating hormone

GnRH: gonadotropin-releasing hormone

HDL: high-density lipoprotein

HR: hazard ratio

LDL: low-density lipoprotein

LH: luteinizing hormone

MORE: Multiple Outcomes of Raloxifene Evaluation

NETA: norethindrone acetate

SERM: selective estrogen receptor modulator

WHI: Women's Health Initiative

REFERENCES

1. Richardson SJ, Senikas V, Nelson JF. Follicular depletion during the menopausal transition: Evidence for accelerated loss and ultimate exhaustion. J Clin Endocrinol Metab 1987;65:1231–1237.
2. Treloar AE, Boynton RE, Behn BG, Brown BW. Variation of the human menstrual cycle Through reproductive life. Int J Fertil 1967;12:77–126.
3. Zumoff B, Strain GW, Miller LK, Rosner W. Twenty-four-hour mean plasma testosterone concentration declines with age in normal premenopausal women. J Clin Endocrinol Metab 1995;80:1429–1430.
4. Burger HG. The endocrinology of the menopause. J Steroid Biochem Mol Biol 1999;69:31–35.
5. Lee SJ, Lenton EA, Sexton L, Cooke ID. The effect of age on the cyclical patterns of plasma LH, FSH, oestradiol and progesterone in women with regular menstrual cycles. Hum Reprod 1988;3:851–855.
6. Ettinger B, Barrett-Connor E, Hoq LA, et al. When is it appropriate to prescribe postmenopausal hormone therapy? Menopause 2006;13:404–410.
7. Endocrine Society scientific statement: postmenopausal hormone therapy. J Clin Endocrinol Metab 2010;95(suppl 1):S1–S66.
8. Management of osteoporosis in postmenopausal women: 2010 position statement of The North American Menopause Society. Menopause 2010;17:25–54;quiz55–56.
9. Aging, menopause, cardiovascular disease and HRT. International Menopause Society Consensus Statement. Climacteric 2009;12: 368–377.
10. Menopause and osteoporosis update 2009. The Society of Obstetricians and Gynaecologists of Canada clinical practice guideline. JOGC 2009;31:S1–S46.
11. Pines A, Sturdee DW, Birkhauser MH, et al. IMS updated recommendations on postmenopausal hormone therapy. Climacteric 2007;10:181–194.
12. The role of local vaginal estrogen for treatment of vaginal atrophy in postmenopausal women: 2007 position statement of The North American Menopause Society. Menopause 2007;14:355–369;quiz370–371.

13. Cobin RH, Futterweit W, Ginzburg SB, et al. American Association of Clinical Endocrinologists medical guidelines for clinical practice for the diagnosis and treatment of menopause. Endocr Pract 2006;12: 315–337.
14. National Institutes of Health State-of-the-Science Conference statement: Management of menopause-related symptoms. Ann Intern Med 2005;142:1003–1013.
15. Hormone therapy for the prevention of chronic conditions in postmenopausal women: Recommendations from the U.S. Preventive Services Task Force. Ann Intern Med 2005;142:855–860.
16. American College of Obstetricians and Gynecologists Women's Health Care Physicians. Executive summary. Hormone therapy. Obstet Gynecol 2004;104:1S–4S.
17. Rossouw JE, Anderson GL, Prentice RL, et al. Risks and benefits of estrogen plus progestin in healthy postmenopausal women: Principal results from the Women's Health Initiative randomized controlled trial. JAMA 2002;288:321–333.
18. Anderson GL, Limacher M, Assaf AR, et al. Effects of conjugated equine estrogen in postmenopausal women with hysterectomy: The Women's Health Initiative randomized controlled trial. JAMA 2004;291:1701–112.
19. Beral V. Breast cancer and hormone-replacement therapy in the Million Women Study. Lancet 2003;362:419–427.
20. Stephenson J. FDA orders estrogen safety warnings: agency offers guidance for HRT use. JAMA 2003;289:537–538.
21. Hersh AL, Stefanick ML, Stafford RS. National use of postmenopausal hormone therapy: annual trends and response to recent evidence. JAMA 2004;291:47–53.
22. Porter M, Penney GC, Russell D, et al. A population based survey of women's experience of the menopause. Br J Obstet Gynaecol 1996;103:1025–1028.
23. Barrett-Connor E. Hormone replacement therapy. BMJ 1998;317: 457–461.
24. Ettinger B. Vasomotor symptom relief versus unwanted effects: Role of estrogen dosage. Am J Med 2005;118 Suppl 12B:74–78.
25. Bachmann G. A new option for managing urogenital atrophy in postmenopausal women. Cont Obstet Gynecol 1997;42:13–28.
26. Davis S. Hormone replacement therapy. Indications, benefits and risk. Aust Fam Physician 1999;28:437–445.
27. Grady D, Brown JS, Vittinghoff E, et al. Postmenopausal hormones and incontinence: The Heart and Estrogen/Progestin Replacement Study. Obstet Gynecol 2001;97:116–120.
28. Sowers MR, Zheng H, Jannausch ML, et al. Amount of bone loss in relation to time around the final menstrual period and follicle-stimulating hormone staging of the transmenopause. J Clin Endocrinol Metab 2010;95:2155–2162.
29. Greenspan SL, Maitland LA, Myers ER, et al. Femoral bone loss progresses with age: A longitudinal study in women over age 65. J Bone Miner Res 1994;9:1959–1965.
30. Cauley JA, Lucas FL, Kuller LH, et al. Elevated serum estradiol and testosterone concentrations are associated with a high risk for breast cancer. Study of Osteoporotic Fractures Research Group. Ann Intern Med 1999;130:270–277.
31. Stone K, Bauer DC, Black DM, et al. Hormonal predictors of bone loss in elderly women: A prospective study. The Study of Osteoporotic Fractures Research Group. J Bone Miner Res 1998;13:1167–1174.
32. Ettinger B, Pressman A, Sklarin P, et al. Associations between low levels of serum estradiol, bone density, and fractures among elderly women: The study of osteoporotic fractures. J Clin Endocrinol Metab 1998;83:2239–2243.
33. Cummings SR, Browner WS, Bauer D, et al. Endogenous hormones and the risk of hip and vertebral fractures among older women. Study of Osteoporotic Fractures Research Group. N Engl J Med 1998;339:733–738.
34. Cauley JA, Robbins J, Chen Z, et al. Effects of estrogen plus progestin on risk of fracture and bone mineral density: The Women's Health Initiative randomized trial. JAMA 2003;290:1729–1738.
35. Wells G, Tugwell P, Shea B, et al. Meta-analyses of therapies for postmenopausal osteoporosis. V. Meta-analysis of the efficacy of hormone replacement therapy in treating and preventing osteoporosis in postmenopausal women. Endocr Rev 2002;23:529–539.

36. Lindsay R, Hart DM, Clark DM. The minimum effective dose of estrogen for prevention of postmenopausal bone loss. Obstet Gynecol 1984;63:759–763.

37. Langer RD. Efficacy, safety, and tolerability of low-dose hormone therapy in managing menopausal symptoms. J Am Board Fam Med 2009;22:563–573.

38. Lindsay R, Cosman F, Lobo RA, et al. Addition of alendronate to ongoing hormone replacement therapy in the treatment of osteoporosis: A randomized, controlled clinical trial. J Clin Endocrinol Metab 1999;84:3076–3081.

39. Watts NB, Diab DL. Long-term use of bisphosphonates in osteoporosis. J Clin Endocrinol Metab 2010;95:1555–1565.

40. Schmidt PJ, Nieman L, Danaceau MA, et al. Estrogen replacement in perimenopause-related depression: A preliminary report. Am J Obstet Gynecol 2000;183:414–420.

41. Hlatky MA, Boothroyd D, Vittinghoff E, et al. Quality-of-life and depressive symptoms in postmenopausal women after receiving hormone therapy: Results from the Heart and Estrogen/Progestin Replacement Study (HERS) trial. JAMA 2002;287:591–597.

42. Shumaker SA, Legault C, Rapp SR, et al. Estrogen plus progestin and the incidence of dementia and mild cognitive impairment in postmenopausal women: The Women's Health Initiative Memory Study: a randomized controlled trial. JAMA 2003;289:2651–662.

43. Rapp SR, Espeland MA, Shumaker SA, et al. Effect of estrogen plus progestin on global cognitive function in postmenopausal women: the Women's Health Initiative Memory Study: a randomized controlled trial. JAMA 2003;289:2663–2672.

44. Hays J, Ockene JK, Brunner RL, et al. Effects of estrogen plus progestin on health-related quality of life. N Engl J Med 2003;348:1839–1854.

45. Ott A, Breteler MM, van Harskamp F, et al. Incidence and risk of dementia. The Rotterdam Study. Am J Epidemiol 1998;147:574–580.

46. Shumaker SA, Legault C, Kuller L, et al. Conjugated equine estrogens and incidence of probable dementia and mild cognitive impairment in postmenopausal women: Women's Health Initiative Memory Study. JAMA 2004;291:2947–958.

47. Espeland MA, Rapp SR, Shumaker SA, et al. Conjugated equine estrogens and global cognitive function in postmenopausal women: Women's Health Initiative Memory Study. JAMA 2004;291:2959–968.

48. Espeland MA, Hogan PE, Fineberg SE, et al. Effect of postmenopausal hormone therapy on glucose and insulin concentrations. PEPI Investigators. Postmenopausal Estrogen/Progestin Interventions. Diabetes Care 1998;21:1589–1595.

49. Kanaya AM, Herrington D, Vittinghoff E, et al. Glycemic effects of postmenopausal hormone therapy: The Heart and Estrogen/progestin Replacement Study. A randomized, double-blind, placebo-controlled trial. Ann Intern Med 2003;138:1–9.

50. Norman RJ, Flight IH, Rees MC. Oestrogen and progestogen hormone replacement therapy for peri-menopausal and post-menopausal women: Weight and body fat distribution. Cochrane Database Syst Rev 2000:CD001018.

51. Mosca L, Collins P, Herrington DM, et al. Hormone replacement therapy and cardiovascular disease: A statement for healthcare professionals from the American Heart Association. Circulation 2001;104:499–503.

52. Grodstein F, Manson JE, Colditz GA, et al. A prospective, observational study of postmenopausal hormone therapy and primary prevention of cardiovascular disease. Ann Intern Med 2000;133:933–941.

53. Sack MN, Rader DJ, Cannon RO, 3rd. Oestrogen and inhibition of oxidation of low-density lipoproteins in postmenopausal women. Lancet 1994;343:269–270.

54. Koh KK, Jin DK, Yang SH, et al. Vascular effects of synthetic or natural progestagen combined with conjugated equine estrogen in healthy postmenopausal women. Circulation 2001;103:1961–1966.

55. Vickers MR, MacLennan AH, Lawton B, et al. Main morbidities recorded in the women's international study of long duration oestrogen after menopause (WISDOM): A randomised controlled trial of hormone replacement therapy in postmenopausal women. BMJ 2007;335:239.

56. Viscoli CM, Brass LM, Kernan WN, et al. A clinical trial of estrogen-replacement therapy after ischemic stroke. N Engl J Med 2001;345:1243–1249.

57. Herrington DM, Reboussin DM, Brosnihan KB, et al. Effects of estrogen replacement on the progression of coronary-artery atherosclerosis. N Engl J Med 2000;343:522–529.

58. Hulley S, Grady D, Bush T, et al. Randomized trial of estrogen plus progestin for secondary prevention of coronary heart disease in postmenopausal women. Heart and Estrogen/progestin Replacement Study (HERS) Research Group. JAMA 1998;280:605–613.

59. Rossouw JE, Prentice RL, Manson JE, et al. Postmenopausal hormone therapy and risk of cardiovascular disease by age and years since menopause. JAMA 2007;297:1465–1477.

60. Toh S, Hernandez-Diaz S, Logan R, et al. Coronary heart disease in postmenopausal recipients of estrogen plus progestin therapy: Does the increased risk ever disappear? A randomized trial. Ann Intern Med 2010;152:211–217.

61. Harman SM, Brinton EA, Cedars M, et al. KEEPS: The Kronos Early Estrogen Prevention Study. Climacteric 2005;8:3–12.

62. Stampfer MJ, Hu FB, Manson JE, et al. Primary prevention of coronary heart disease in women through diet and lifestyle. N Engl J Med 2000;343:16–22.

63. Hu FB, Stampfer MJ, Manson JE, et al. Trends in the incidence of coronary heart disease and changes in diet and lifestyle in women. N Engl J Med 2000;343:530–537.

64. Wassertheil-Smoller S, Hendrix SL, Limacher M, et al. Effect of estrogen plus progestin on stroke in postmenopausal women: The Women's Health Initiative: a randomized trial. JAMA 2003;289:2673–2684.

65. Prentice RL, Chlebowski RT, Stefanick ML, et al. Estrogen plus progestin therapy and breast cancer in recently postmenopausal women. Am J Epidemiol 2008;167:1207–1216.

66. Chlebowski RT, Hendrix SL, Langer RD, et al. Influence of estrogen plus progestin on breast cancer and mammography in healthy postmenopausal women: The Women's Health Initiative Randomized Trial. JAMA 2003;289:3243–3253.

67. Chlebowski RT, Kuller LH, Prentice RL, et al. Breast cancer after use of estrogen plus progestin in postmenopausal women. N Engl J Med 2009;360:573–587.

68. Swanson GM. Breast cancer risk estimation: A translational statistic for communication to the public. J Natl Cancer Inst 1993;85:848–849.

69. Breast cancer and hormone replacement therapy: Collaborative reanalysis of data from 51 epidemiological studies of 52,705 women with breast cancer and 108,411 women without breast cancer. Collaborative Group on Hormonal Factors in Breast Cancer. Lancet 1997;350:1047–1059.

70. Schairer C, Lubin J, Troisi R, et al. Menopausal estrogen and estrogen-progestin replacement therapy and breast cancer risk. JAMA 2000;283:485–491.

71. Gapstur SM, Morrow M, Sellers TA. Hormone replacement therapy and risk of breast cancer with a favorable histology: Results of the Iowa Women's Health Study. JAMA 1999;281:2091–2097.

72. Sellers TA, Mink PJ, Cerhan JR, et al. The role of hormone replacement therapy in the risk for breast cancer and total mortality in women with a family history of breast cancer. Ann Intern Med 1997;127:973–980.

73. McTiernan A, Martin CF, Peck JD, et al. Estrogen-plus-progestin use and mammographic density in postmenopausal women: Women's Health Initiative randomized trial. J Natl Cancer Inst 2005;97:1366–1376.

74. Stefanick ML, Anderson GL, Margolis KL, et al. Effects of conjugated equine estrogens on breast cancer and mammography screening in postmenopausal women with hysterectomy. JAMA 2006;295:1647–1657.

75. Anderson GL, Judd HL, Kaunitz AM, et al. Effects of estrogen plus progestin on gynecologic cancers and associated diagnostic procedures: The Women's Health Initiative randomized trial. JAMA 2003;290:1739–1748.

76. Casper RF. Estrogen with interrupted progestin HRT: A review of experimental and clinical studies. Maturitas 2000;34:97–108.

77. Pike MC, Peters RK, Cozen W, et al. Estrogen-progestin replacement therapy and endometrial cancer. J Natl Cancer Inst 1997;89:1110–1116.

78. Genant HK, Lucas J, Weiss S, et al. Low-dose esterified estrogen therapy: Effects on bone, plasma estradiol concentrations, endometrium, and lipid levels. Estratab/Osteoporosis Study Group. Arch Intern Med 1997;157:2609–2615.

79. Goldstein SR, Scheele WH, Rajagopalan SK, et al. A 12-month comparative study of raloxifene, estrogen, and placebo on the postmenopausal endometrium. Obstet Gynecol 2000;95:95–103.

80. Barrett-Connor E, Mosca L, Collins P, et al. Effects of raloxifene on cardiovascular events and breast cancer in postmenopausal women. N Engl J Med 2006;355:125–137.

81. Lacey JV, Jr., Mink PJ, Lubin JH, et al. Menopausal hormone replacement therapy and risk of ovarian cancer. JAMA 2002;288:334–341.

82. Morch LS, Lokkegaard E, Andreasen AH, et al. Hormone therapy and ovarian cancer. JAMA 2009;302:298–305.

83. Jick H, Derby LE, Myers MW, et al. Risk of hospital admission for idiopathic venous thromboembolism among users of postmenopausal oestrogens. Lancet 1996;348:981–983.

84. Nelson HD, Humphrey LL, Nygren P, et al. Postmenopausal hormone replacement therapy: Scientific review. JAMA 2002;288:872–881.

85. Canonico M, Oger E, Plu-Bureau G, et al. Hormone therapy and venous thromboembolism among postmenopausal women: impact of the route of estrogen administration and progestogens: the ESTHER study. Circulation 2007;115:840–845.

86. Cirillo DJ, Wallace RB, Rodabough RJ, et al. Effect of estrogen therapy on gallbladder disease. JAMA 2005;293:330–339.

87. Canonico M, Plu-Bureau G, Lowe GD, Scarabin PY. Hormone replacement therapy and risk of venous thromboembolism in postmenopausal women: Systematic review and meta-analysis. BMJ 2008;336:1227–1231.

88. Scarabin PY, Oger E, Plu-Bureau G. Differential association of oral and transdermal oestrogen-replacement therapy with venous thromboembolism risk. Lancet 2003;362:428–432.

89. Sturdee DW. Newer HRT regimens. Br J Obstet Gynaecol 1997;104:1109–1115.

90. Lowe GD, Upton MN, Rumley A, et al. Different effects of oral and transdermal hormone replacement therapies on factor IX, APC resistance, t-PA, PAI and C-reactive protein—a cross-sectional population survey. Thromb Haemost 2001;86:550–556.

91. Greendale GA, Lee NP, Arriola ER. The menopause. Lancet 1999;353:571–580.

92. Lethaby A, Farquhar C, Sarkis A, et al. Hormone replacement therapy in postmenopausal women: endometrial hyperplasia and irregular bleeding. Cochrane Database Syst Rev 2000:CD000402.

93. Effects of hormone replacement therapy on endometrial histology in postmenopausal women. The Postmenopausal Estrogen/Progestin Interventions (PEPI) Trial. The Writing Group for the PEPI Trial. JAMA 1996;275:370–375.

94. Cushing KL, Weiss NS, Voigt LF, et al. Risk of endometrial cancer in relation to use of low-dose, unopposed estrogens. Obstet Gynecol 1998;91:35–39.

95. Role of progestogen in hormone therapy for postmenopausal women: position statement of The North American Menopause Society. Menopause 2003;10:113–132.

96. Bachmann GA, Schaefers M, Uddin A, Utian WH. Lowest effective transdermal 17beta-estradiol dose for relief of hot flushes in postmenopausal women: a randomized controlled trial. Obstet Gynecol 2007;110:771–779.

97. Lindsay R, Gallagher JC, Kleerekoper M, Pickar JH. Effect of lower doses of conjugated equine estrogens with and without medroxyprogesterone acetate on bone in early postmenopausal women. JAMA 2002;287:2668–676.

98. Utian WH, Shoupe D, Bachmann G, et al. Relief of vasomotor symptoms and vaginal atrophy with lower doses of conjugated equine estrogens and medroxyprogesterone acetate. Fertil Steril 2001;75:1065–1079.

99. Pickar JH, Yeh I, Wheeler JE, et al. Endometrial effects of lower doses of conjugated equine estrogens and medroxyprogesterone acetate. Fertil Steril 2001;76:25–31.

100. Naessen T, Rodriguez-Macias K, Lithell H. Serum lipid profile improved by ultra-low doses of 17 beta-estradiol in elderly women. J Clin Endocrinol Metab 2001;86:2757–2762.

101. Boothby LA, Doering PL, Kipersztok S. Bioidentical hormone therapy: A review. Menopause 2004;11:356–367.

102. Bioidential hormones. The Endocine Society position statement. 2006. http://www.menopause.org/bioidenticalHT_Endosoc.pdf. Last accessed April 10, 2010.

103. Food and Drug Administration. Bio-identicals: sorting myths from facts. 2008, http://www.fda.gov/ForConsumers/ConsumerUpdates/ucm049311.htm.

104. Hickey M, Davis SR, Sturdee DW. Treatment of menopausal symptoms: What shall we do now? Lancet 2005;366:409–421.

105. Loprinzi CL, Kugler JW, Sloan JA, et al. Venlafaxine in management of hot flashes in survivors of breast cancer: a randomised controlled trial. Lancet 2000;356:2059–2063.

106. Evans ML, Pritts E, Vittinghoff E, et al. Management of postmenopausal hot flushes with venlafaxine hydrochloride: a randomized, controlled trial. Obstet Gynecol 2005;105:161–166.

107. Stearns V, Johnson MD, Rae JM, et al. Active tamoxifen metabolite plasma concentrations after coadministration of tamoxifen and the selective serotonin reuptake inhibitor paroxetine. J Natl Cancer Inst 2003;95:1758–1764.

108. The role of testosterone therapy in postmenopausal women: Position statement of The North American Menopause Society. Menopause 2005;12:496–511;quiz649.

109. Davis SR, Davison SL, Donath S, Bell RJ. Circulating androgen levels and self-reported sexual function in women. JAMA 2005;294:91–96.

110. Bell RJ, Donath S, Davison SL, Davis SR. Endogenous androgen levels and well-being: differences between premenopausal and postmenopausal women. Menopause 2006;13:65–71.

111. Shifren JL, Davis SR, Moreau M, et al. Testosterone patch for the treatment of hypoactive sexual desire disorder in naturally menopausal women: Results from the INTIMATE NM1 Study. Menopause 2006;13:770–779.

112. Davis SR, Moreau M, Kroll R, et al. Testosterone for low libido in postmenopausal women not taking estrogen. N Engl J Med 2008;359:2005–2017.

113. Shifren JL, Braunstein GD, Simon JA, et al. Transdermal testosterone treatment in women with impaired sexual function after oophorectomy. N Engl J Med 2000;343:682–688.

114. Davis S, Papalia MA, Norman RJ, et al. Safety and efficacy of a testosterone metered-dose transdermal spray for treating decreased sexual satisfaction in premenopausal women: A randomized trial. Ann Intern Med 2008;148:569–577.

115. van Staa TP, Sprafka JM. Study of adverse outcomes in women using testosterone therapy. Maturitas 2009;62:76–80.

116. Jick SS, Hagberg KW, Kaye JA, Jick H. Postmenopausal estrogen-containing hormone therapy and the risk of breast cancer. Obstet Gynecol 2009;113:74–80.

117. Davis SR, Wolfe R, Farrugia H, et al. The incidence of invasive breast cancer among women prescribed testosterone for low libido. J Sex Med 2009;6:1850–1856.

118. Kalantaridou SN, Calis KA, Mazer NA, et al. A pilot study of an investigational testosterone transdermal patch system in young women with spontaneous premature ovarian failure. J Clin Endocrinol Metab 2005;90:6549–6552.

119. Wierman ME, Basson R, Davis SR, et al. Androgen therapy in women: An Endocrine Society Clinical Practice guideline. J Clin Endocrinol Metab 2006;91:3697–3710.

120. Ettinger B, Black DM, Mitlak BH, et al. Reduction of vertebral fracture risk in postmenopausal women with osteoporosis treated with raloxifene: Results from a 3-year randomized clinical trial. Multiple Outcomes of Raloxifene Evaluation (MORE) Investigators. JAMA 1999;282:637–645.

121. Cummings SR, Eckert S, Krueger KA, et al. The effect of raloxifene on risk of breast cancer in postmenopausal women: results from the MORE randomized trial. Multiple Outcomes of Raloxifene Evaluation. JAMA 1999;281:2189–2197.

122. Martino S, Cauley JA, Barrett-Connor E, et al. Continuing outcomes relevant to Evista: breast cancer incidence in postmenopausal osteoporotic women in a randomized trial of raloxifene. J Natl Cancer Inst 2004;96:1751–1761.

123. Vogel VG, Costantino JP, Wickerham DL, et al. Effects of tamoxifen vs raloxifene on the risk of developing invasive breast cancer and other disease outcomes: the NSABP Study of Tamoxifen and Raloxifene (STAR) P-2 trial. JAMA 2006;295:2727–2741.

124. Yaffe K, Krueger K, Sarkar S, et al. Cognitive function in postmenopausal women treated with raloxifene. N Engl J Med 2001;344:1207–1213.

125. Kenemans P, Speroff L. Tibolone: clinical recommendations and practical guidelines. A report of the International Tibolone Consensus Group. Maturitas 2005;51:21–28.

126. Cummings SR. LIFT study is discontinued. BMJ 2006;332:667.

127. Cummings SR, Ettinger B, Delmas PD, et al. The effects of tibolone in older postmenopausal women. N Engl J Med 2008;359:697–708.

128. Nijland EA, Weijmar Schultz WC, Nathorst-Boos J, et al. Tibolone and transdermal E2/NETA for the treatment of female sexual dysfunction in naturally menopausal women: results of a randomized active-controlled trial. J Sex Med 2008;5:646–656.

129. Beral V, Bull D, Reeves G. Endometrial cancer and hormone-replacement therapy in the Million Women Study. Lancet 2005;365:1543–1551.

130. Langer RD, Landgren BM, Rymer J, Helmond FA. Effects of tibolone and continuous combined conjugated equine estrogen/medroxyprogesterone acetate on the endometrium and vaginal bleeding: Results of the OPAL study. Am J Obstet Gynecol 2006;195:1320–1327.

131. Murkies AL, Wilcox G, Davis SR. Clinical review 92: Phytoestrogens. J Clin Endocrinol Metab 1998;83:297–303.

132. Tice JA, Ettinger B, Ensrud K, et al. Phytoestrogen supplements for the treatment of hot flashes: The Isoflavone Clover Extract (ICE) Study: a randomized controlled trial. JAMA 2003;290:207–214.

133. Lissin LW, Cooke JP. Phytoestrogens and cardiovascular health. J Am Coll Cardiol 2000;35:1403–1410.

134. Tempfer CB, Froese G, Heinze G, et al. Side effects of phytoestrogens: A meta-analysis of randomized trials. Am J Med 2009;122:939–946.e9.

135. Newton KM, Reed SD, LaCroix AZ, et al. Treatment of vasomotor symptoms of menopause with black cohosh, multibotanicals, soy, hormone therapy, or placebo: A randomized trial. Ann Intern Med 2006;145:869–879.

136. National Institutes of Health Office of Dietary Supplements. Dietary supplements fact sheet: black cohosh. 2008, http://ods.od.nih.gov/factsheets/BlackCohosh_pf.asp.

137. Nedrow A, Miller J, Walker M, et al. Complementary and alternative therapies for the management of menopause-related symptoms: A systematic evidence review. Arch Intern Med 2006;166:1453–1465.

138. Ettinger B, Pressman A. Continuation of postmenopausal hormone replacement therapy in a large health maintenance organization: Transdermal matrix patch versus oral estrogen therapy. Am J Manag Care 1999;5:779–785.

139. Majumdar SR, Almasi EA, Stafford RS. Promotion and prescribing of hormone therapy after report of harm by the Women's Health Initiative. JAMA 2004;292:1983–1988.

140. Torgerson DJ, Reid DM. The pharmacoeconomics of hormone replacement therapy. Pharmacoeconomics 1999;16:9–16.

141. Kalantaridou SN, Davis SR, Nelson LM. Premature ovarian failure. Endocrinol Metab Clin North Am 1998;27:989–1006.

142. Coulam CB, Adamson SC, Annegers JF. Incidence of premature ovarian failure. Obstet Gynecol 1986;67:604–606.

143. Anasti JN, Kalantaridou SN, Kimzey LM, et al. Bone loss in young women with karyotypically normal spontaneous premature ovarian failure. Obstet Gynecol 1998;91:12–15.

144. Kalantaridou SN, Naka KK, Papanikolaou E, et al. Impaired endothelial function in young women with premature ovarian failure: Normalization with hormone therapy. J Clin Endocrinol Metab 2004;89:3907–3913.

145. van der Schouw YT, van der Graaf Y, Steyerberg EW, et al. Age at menopause as a risk factor for cardiovascular mortality. Lancet 1996;347:714–718.

146. Snowdon DA, Kane RL, Beeson WL, et al. Is early natural menopause a biologic marker of health and aging? Am J Public Health 1989;79:709–714.

147. Kalantaridou SN, Calis KA, Vanderhoof VH, et al. Testosterone deficiency in young women with 46,XX spontaneous premature ovarian failure. Fertil Steril 2006;86:1475–1482.

148. Popat VB, Kalantaridou SN, Vanderhoof VH, et al. Effect of long-term physiologic transdermal testosterone (150 mcg/day) replacement therapy on femoral neck bone density in women with spontaneous premature ovarian failure: Results of a 3-year double-blind placebo-controlled clinical trial. P1–349. Abstract presented at the Annual Meeting of the Endocrine Society, June 2–5, 2007. Toronto, Canada.

149. Kalantaridou SN, Vanderhoof VH, Calis KA, et al. Physiologic transdermal testosterone replacement (150 mcg/day) does not significantly improve sexual function in women with 46,XX spontaneous premature ovarian failure: A placebo-controlled randomized study. OR27-4. Abstract presented at the Annual Meeting of the Endocrine Society, June 2–5, 2007. Toronto, Canada.

CHAPTER

92

Erectile Dysfunction

MARY LEE

KEY CONCEPTS

❶ The incidence of erectile dysfunction is low in men younger than 40 years of age. The incidence increases as men age, likely as a result of concurrent medical conditions that impair the vascular, neurologic, psychogenic, and hormonal systems necessary for a normal penile erection.

❷ Many commonly used drugs have sympatholytic, anticholinergic, sedative, or antiandrogenic effects that may exacerbate or contribute to the development of erectile dysfunction. Clinicians should be familiar with these agents and be prepared to make adjustments in drug regimens to minimize adverse effects of these drugs on a patient's erectile function.

❸ The first step in clinical management of erectile dysfunction is to identify and, if possible, reverse the underlying causes. Risk factors for erectile dysfunction, including hypertension, diabetes mellitus, smoking, and chronic ethanol abuse, should be addressed and minimized.

❹ Specific treatments for erectile dysfunction include vacuum erection devices, pharmacologic treatments, psychotherapy, and surgery.

❺ The ideal treatment of erectile dysfunction should have a fast onset, be effective, be convenient to administer, be cost effective, have a low incidence of serious adverse effects, and be free of serious drug interactions.

❻ Specific treatment is first initiated with the least invasive forms of treatment, including vacuum erection devices or oral phosphodiesterase inhibitors, followed by intracavernosal injections or intraurethral inserts, and finally by surgical insertion of a penile prosthesis.

Learning objectives, review questions, and other resources can be found at
www.pharmacotherapyonline.com.

❼ Vacuum erection devices can have a slow onset of action (30 minutes) and are not discreet; therefore, they are most effective for a couple in a stable relationship.

❽ Although phosphodiesterase inhibitors are convenient and effective regardless of the etiology of erectile dysfunction, they fail in 30% to 40% of patients. Also, phosphodiesterase inhibitors are contraindicated in patients taking any dosage formulation of nitrate.

❾ Testosterone supplementation should be reserved for patients with primary or secondary hypogonadism who have erectile dysfunction as a consequence of a decreased libido. Testosterone supplementation should not be used by patients with erectile dysfunction who have normal serum testosterone levels.

❿ Although intracavernosal injections and intraurethral pellets of alprostadil are effective independent of the etiology of erectile dysfunction, they fail in one third of patients. To self-administer medication by these routes, patients require training to minimize administration-related adverse effects.

The National Institutes of Health Consensus Development Panel on Impotence defines erectile dysfunction as the failure to achieve a penile erection to allow for satisfactory sexual intercourse.[1] Patients may refer to it as impotence.

Erectile dysfunction must be distinguished from disorders of libido, ejaculatory disorders, and infertility, which are caused by different pathophysiologic mechanisms and are treated with alternative agents (Table 92–1). A patient may suffer from one or more disorders of sexual dysfunction. For example, an elderly man with primary hypogonadism may suffer from decreased libido and erectile dysfunction. Diagnosis of the type of sexual disorder that a patient has is a key to initiating the most appropriate treatment.

EPIDEMIOLOGY

❶ The incidence of erectile dysfunction is low in men younger than 40 years of age but increases as men age.[2–4] The Massachusetts Male Aging Study, a cross-sectional survey of a random sample of 1,290 men in the Boston area, was conducted during the period

TABLE 92-1	Types of Sexual Dysfunction in Men
Type of Dysfunction	**Definition**
Decreased libido	Decreased sexual drive or desire
Increased libido	Precocious puberty; inappropriate and excessive sexual drive or desire
Erectile dysfunction (impotence)	Failure to achieve a penile erection suitable for satisfactory sexual intercourse
Delayed ejaculation	Commonly referred to as "dry sex"; ejaculation is delayed or absent
Retrograde ejaculation	Ejaculate passes retrograde into the bladder, instead of toward the anterior urethra (antegrade) and out of the penis
Infertility	Sperm are insufficient in number, have abnormal morphology, or have inadequate motility, and fail to fertilize the ovum

from 1987 to 1989. The study reported an overall prevalence of 52% for any degree of erectile dysfunction in men aged 40 to 70 years, with an age-related increase in incidence ranging from 12.4% in men aged 40 to 49 years, up to 46.4% in men aged 60 to 69 years.[1,2] In the more recent Health Professional Follow-Up Study of more than 31,000 male health professionals aged 53 to 90 years, the prevalence of erectile dysfunction was 33%.[3] Interestingly, although the prevalence of erectile dysfunction increases with patient age, many patients fail to seek medical treatment.[4]

Erectile dysfunction is sometimes assumed to be a symptom of the aging process in men. However, more likely it results from concurrent medical conditions of the patient (e.g., hypertension, arteriosclerosis, hyperlipidemia, diabetes mellitus, or psychiatric disorders) or from medications that patients may be taking for these diseases.[2-5] For example, up to 50% of patients with diabetes mellitus develop erectile dysfunction, and medications such as β-blockers are associated with a high incidence of erectile dysfunction.

PHYSIOLOGY OF A NORMAL PENILE ERECTION

A normal penile erection requires full functioning of several physiologic systems: vascular, nervous, and hormonal. The patient also must be psychologically receptive to sexual stimuli.

VASCULAR SYSTEM

The penis comprises two corpora cavernosa on the dorsal side and one corpus spongiosum on the ventral side. The corpus spongiosum surrounds the urethra and forms the glans penis. The corpora are composed of multiple interconnected sinuses, which can fill with blood to produce an erection. The corpora cavernosa are encased by the tunica albuginea, a fibrous tissue membrane, which has limited distensibility. In the flaccid state, arterial flow into and venous outflow from the corpora are balanced. During the erectile phase, arterial blood flow increases and blood fills the sinusoids within the corpora, which causes penile swelling and elongation. The erection is prolonged by a decrease in venous outflow from the corpora, which is caused by compression of subtunical venules against the tunica albuginea by the swollen corpora (Fig. 92–1).

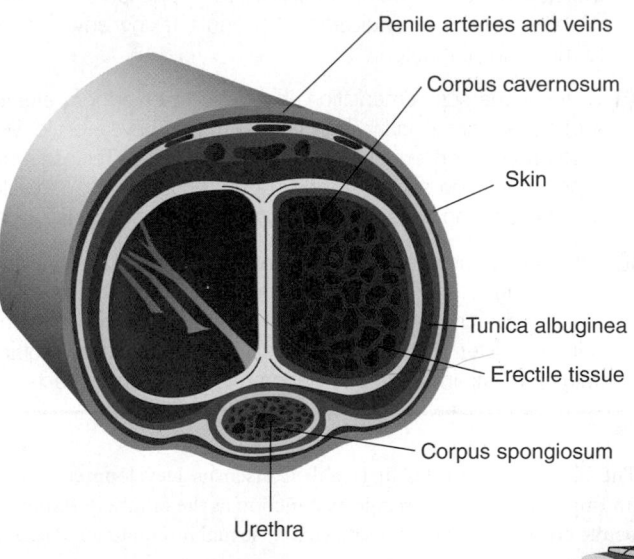

Penile arteries and veins

Corpus cavernosum

Skin

Tunica albuginea

Erectile tissue

Corpus spongiosum

Urethra

FIGURE 92-1. Microanatomy of and vascular changes in the penis in flaccid and erect states. In the flaccid state, arterial flow into and venous outflow from the corpora are balanced. During the erectile phase, arterial blood flow increases and blood fills the sinusoids within the corpora, causing penile swelling and elongation. The erection is prolonged by a decrease in venous outflow from the corpora, which is caused by compression of subtunical venules by the swollen corpora. *(From Walsh PC, ed. Campbell's Urology, 8th ed. Philadelphia, PA: WB Saunders, 2002:1595, 1697.)*

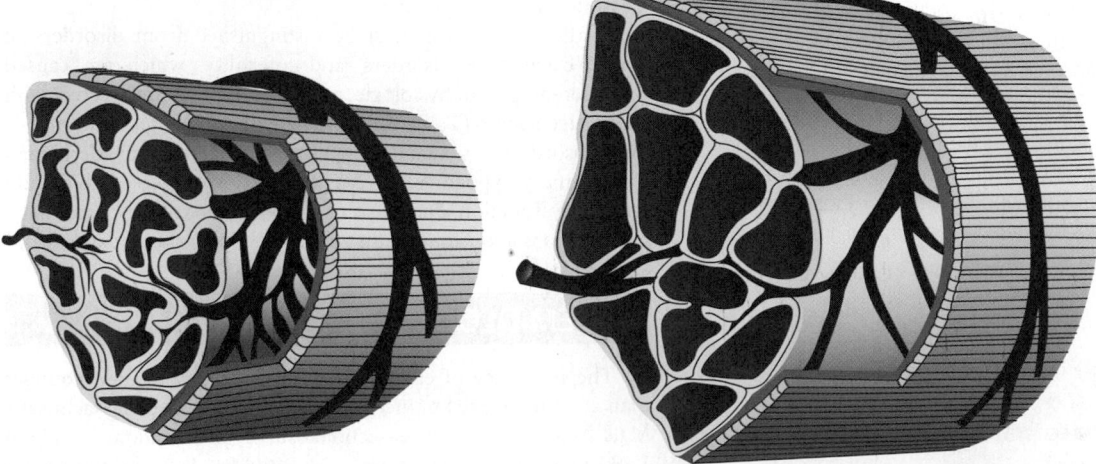

Flaccid State

Erectile Phase

Arterial flow into the corpora is enhanced by acetylcholine-mediated vasodilation. Acetylcholine indirectly enhances arterial flow to the corpora and increases sinusoidal filling of the corporal tissue. That is, acetylcholine is a coneurotransmitter, which works along with other nonpeptidinergic intracellular neurotransmitters—including cyclic guanosine monophosphate (cGMP), cyclic adenosine monophosphate (cAMP), or vasoactive intestinal polypeptide—to produce vasodilation. In effect, cGMP and cAMP are secondary messengers that direct desired effects in target tissues.[6]

Acetylcholine produces an erection probably through two different pathways. Through one pathway, in the presence of sexual stimulation to genital tissue, acetylcholine enhances the production of nitric oxide by endothelial cells and nonadrenergic–noncholinergic neurons. Nitric oxide enhances the activity of guanylate cyclase, which increases the conversion of cyclic guanosine triphosphate to cGMP. cGMP decreases intracellular calcium concentrations in smooth muscle cells of penile arteries and cavernosal sinuses. As a result, smooth muscle relaxation occurs, which enhances arterial blood flow to and blood filling of the corpora.[5] An erection results.

In an alternative pathway, acetylcholine or prostaglandin E enhances the activity of adenyl cyclase, which increases the conversion of cyclic adenosine triphosphate to cAMP, a potent muscle relaxant. Similar to cGMP, cAMP decreases intracellular calcium concentrations to produce smooth muscle relaxation in cells of the arteries and cavernosal sinuses. Arterial blood flow to and blood filling of the corpora are enhanced, and a penile erection results.[5]

NERVOUS SYSTEM AND PSYCHOGENIC STIMULI

Some erections are mediated by a sacral nerve reflex arc (e.g., erections can occur while the patient is sleeping). However, in the conscious patient, sensory sexual stimulation mediates erections via the central nervous system. That is, when a patient sees an attractive partner, hears sweet words, smells a particular scent, or tastes or touches a pleasant object, these situations can result in an erection. In this case, the patient's brain processes this information and the nervous impulse is carried down the spinal cord to peripheral cholinergic nerves that innervate the vascular supply to the corpora, resulting in an erection.

The medial preoptic area of the hypothalamus is thought to be that portion of the brain responsible for integrating external stimuli. Here dopamine exerts a proerectogenic effect, whereas, α_2-adrenergic stimulation causes the penis to become and/or remain flaccid. After moving down the spinal cord, nerve impulses travel to the penis by efferent peripheral nerves, including inhibitory sympathetic neurons (T11–L2), proerectogenic parasympathetic neurons (S2–S4), and proerectogenic somatic neurons (S2–S4).

In summary, acetylcholine produces an erection by working along with other coneurotransmitters, including cGMP and cAMP. Thus, an erection is mediated neurologically, maintained by arterial blood filling of the corpora, and sustained by occlusion of venous outflow from the corpora.

Detumescence, or the progression of an erect penis to a flaccid state, results from the actions of norepinephrine, which contracts vascular smooth muscle to decrease arterial inflow to the corpora and contracts sinusoidal tissue in the corpora. As a result, venous outflow from the corpora increases.

HORMONAL SYSTEM

Testosterone is principally produced by the testes at a daily rate of 4 to 8 mg. Production follows a circadian pattern with highest blood levels in the morning and lowest levels in the evening. Physiologically active (free) testosterone comprises only 2% of circulating blood levels. About 50% to 60% of testosterone in the bloodstream is tightly bound to sex hormone-binding globulin and is inactive. The rest of circulating testosterone is reversibly bound to albumin; this portion of testosterone is in equilibrium with the free fraction.

Testosterone stimulates libido (sexual drive) and increases muscle mass in males. In some target cells with 5-alpha reductase, testosterone is activated to dihydrotestosterone. Dihydrotestosterone, which is more potent than testosterone, stimulates prostate gland growth, increases facial and body hair, induces baldness, and causes acne. In adipose tissue, a small portion of testosterone is converted to estradiol which can lead to gynecomastia.

Beginning at age 40 years, men experience a gradual decrease in testicular production of testosterone, with an associated decrease in muscle mass and sexual function.[7] The Massachusetts Male Aging Study reported that 6% to 12% of elderly males had symptoms of hypogonadism.[8]

Within the normal physiologic serum total testosterone concentration range (normal, 300–1,100 ng/dL; 10.4–38.2 nmol/L), sexual drive is usually normal. However, because of variability in circulating levels of sex hormone binding globulin, a patient's serum concentration of testosterone should always be interpreted in the context of the patient's symptoms and physical exam findings. To confirm hypogonadism when the serum total testosterone concentration is equivocal, the clinician should obtain a serum free (bioavailable) testosterone level.

The relationship between erectile dysfunction and serum testosterone levels is complicated. Patients with normal serum testosterone levels may have erectile dysfunction, and patients with subnormal serum testosterone levels may have normal sexual function.[5] When a patient has hypogonadism and libido is decreased, a patient may not develop erections. In this case, erectile dysfunction is considered secondary to a decreased libido.

PATHOPHYSIOLOGY

Erectile dysfunction can result from any single abnormality or combination of abnormalities of the four systems necessary for a normal penile erection. Vascular, neurologic, or hormonal etiologies of erectile dysfunction are collectively referred to as *organic erectile dysfunction*. Approximately 80% of patients with erectile dysfunction have the organic type. Patients who do not respond to psychogenic stimuli have *psychogenic erectile dysfunction*.

Diseases that compromise vascular flow to the corpora cavernosum (e.g., peripheral vascular disease, arteriosclerosis, and essential hypertension) are associated with an increased incidence of erectile dysfunction. Diseases that impair nerve conduction to the brain (e.g., spinal cord injury or stroke) or conditions that impair peripheral nerve conduction to the penile vasculature (e.g., diabetes mellitus) can result in erectile dysfunction.

Diseases associated with hypogonadism, primary or secondary, result in subphysiologic levels of testosterone, which cause diminished sexual drive (decreased libido) and secondary erectile dysfunction. Primary hypogonadism can be associated with the normal aging process in men or surgical removal of the testes for treatment of prostate or testicular cancer. Secondary hypogonadism may result from hypothalamic or pituitary disorders of luteinizing hormone–releasing hormone or luteinizing hormone, respectively; or elevated prolactin levels, which can result from pituitary tumors or can occur in patients with chronic renal failure.

Patients must be in the proper mental frame of mind to be receptive to sexual stimuli. Patients who suffer from malaise, have

TABLE 92-2 Medication Classes That Can Cause Erectile Dysfunction

Drug Class	Proposed Mechanism by Which Drug Causes Erectile Dysfunction	Special Notes
Anticholinergic agents (antihistamines, antiparkinsonian agents, tricyclic antidepressants, phenothiazines)	Anticholinergic activity	• Second-generation nonsedating antihistamines (e.g., loratadine, fexofenadine, or cetirizine) are associated with less erectile dysfunction than first-generation agents • Selective serotonin reuptake inhibitor (SSRI) antidepressants cause less erectile dysfunction than tricyclic antidepressants. Of the SSRIs, paroxetine, sertraline, and fluoxetine cause erectile dysfunction more commonly than venlafaxine, nefazodone, trazodone, or mirtazapine. • Phenothiazines with less anticholinergic effect (e.g., chlorpromazine) can be substituted in some patients if erectile dysfunction is a problem
Dopamine antagonists (e.g., metoclopramide, phenothiazines)	Inhibit prolactin inhibitory factor, thereby increasing prolactin levels	• Increased prolactin levels inhibit testicular testosterone production; depressed libido results
Estrogens, antiandrogens (e.g., luteinizing hormone–releasing hormone superagonists, digoxin, spironolactone, ketoconazole, cimetidine)	Suppress testosterone-mediated stimulation of libido	• In the face of a decreased libido, a secondary erectile dysfunction develops because of diminished sexual drive
Central nervous system depressants (e.g., barbiturates, narcotics, benzodiazepines, short-term use of large doses of alcohol, anticonvulsants)	Suppress perception of psychogenic stimuli	
Agents that decrease penile blood flow (e.g., diuretics, peripheral β-adrenergic antagonists, or central sympatholytics [methyldopa, clonidine, guanethidine])	Reduce arteriolar flow to corpora	• Any diuretic that produces a significant decrease in intravascular volume can decrease penile arteriolar flow • Safer antihypertensives include angiotensin-converting enzyme inhibitors, postsynaptic α_1-adrenergic antagonists (terazosin, doxazosin), calcium channel blockers, and angiotensin II receptor antagonists
Miscellaneous • Finsteride, dutasteride • Lithium carbonate • Gemfibrozil • Interferon • Clofibrate • Monoamine oxidase inhibitors	Unknown mechanism	

From Thomas et al.[9] and Lee and Sharifi.[10]

reactive depression or performance anxiety, are sedated, have Alzheimer disease, have hypothyroidism, or have mental disorders, commonly complain of erectile dysfunction. In most studies, patients with psychogenic erectile dysfunction generally exhibit a higher response rate to various interventions than do patients with organic erectile dysfunction because the former have less severe disease.

Social habits of patients have been linked to erectile dysfunction. The vasoconstrictor effect of cigarette smoking may compromise blood flow to the corpora and decrease cavernosal filling. Excessive ethanol intake may lead to androgen deficiency, peripheral neuropathy, or chronic liver disease, all of which can contribute to erectile dysfunction.

❷ Medications may cause erectile dysfunction through similar pathophysiologic mechanisms (Table 92–2).[9-11] Medications are estimated to be responsible for approximately 10% to 25% of cases of erectile dysfunction.

CLINICAL PRESENTATION: ERECTILE DYSFUNCTION

General

☐ Men are affected emotionally in many different ways

☐ Depression

☐ Performance anxiety

☐ Marital difficulties and avoidance of sexual intimacy (patients are often brought to a physician by their partners)

☐ Nonadherence to medications patient believes are causing erectile dysfunction

Symptoms

☐ Erectile dysfunction or inability to have sexual intercourse

Signs

☐ If completing an International Index of Erectile Dysfunction survey, results are consistent with low satisfaction with the quality of erectile function.

☐ Medical history may identify concurrent medical illnesses, past surgical procedures that interfere with good vascular flow to the penis or damage nerve function to the corpora, or mental disorders associated with decreased reception of sexual stimuli.

☐ Medication history may reveal prescription or nonprescription medications that could cause erectile dysfunction.

☐ Physical examination may reveal signs of hypogonadism (e.g., gynecomastia, small testicles, decreased body hair or beard, decreased muscle mass), which may contribute to erectile dysfunction. The patient may have an abnormally curved penis when erect, decreased pulses in the pelvic region (suggesting impaired vascular flow to the penis), or decreased anal sphincter tone (suggesting impaired nerve function to the corpora). Men older than 50 years should undergo a digital rectal examination to determine whether an enlarged prostate is contributing to the patient's erectile dysfunction.

Laboratory Tests

☐ If patient has signs of hypogonadism and complains of decreased libido, a serum testosterone concentration may be below the normal range, which would be consistent with a hormonal cause of erectile dysfunction.

- If the patient has an enlarged prostate noted on digital rectal examination, a blood sample for prostate specific antigen should be obtained. If elevated, the patient should be evaluated for a prostate disorder, which could contribute to erectile dysfunction.

DIAGNOSIS

With the availability in the late 1990s of effective medications for erectile dysfunction independent of the etiology, diagnostic evaluation of erectile dysfunction became streamlined.[5,12] Key assessments include a description of the severity of erectile dysfunction, complete medical and surgical histories, review of concurrent medications, physical examination, and selected clinical laboratory tests.[12]

To assess the severity of erectile dysfunction, the patient should be asked about the quality of sexual intercourse for the last 4 weeks to 6 months. A self-administered standardized questionnaire, such as the International Index of Erectile Dysfunction (IIEF), is often used. It is administered before initiation of any treatment and repeated at regular intervals during treatment. It includes 15 questions about the quality of erectile function and satisfactoriness of sexual intercourse.[13] Questions include the following: How often were you able to maintain an erection? How difficult was it to sustain an erection? How satisfied are you with your sexual life? The physician should carefully assess the expectations for erectile function of the patient and the partner to ensure that expectations are reasonable. Shorter versions of the IIEF and other self-reporting questionnaires are also used in clinical practice.

A medical history should be obtained to identify concurrent medical illnesses (e.g., hypertension, atherosclerosis, hyperlipidemia, diabetes mellitus, depression) or surgical procedures (e.g., perineal or pelvic) that are risk factors for or are associated with organic or psychogenic erectile dysfunction. Underlying diseases that do not optimally respond to treatment should be addressed before specific treatment for erectile dysfunction is initiated. If the patient smokes cigarettes, drinks excessive amounts of ethanol, or uses recreational drugs, these social habits should be discontinued before specific treatment for erectile dysfunction is started.

A complete listing of the patient's prescription and nonprescription medications and dietary supplements should be reviewed by the clinician, who should identify drugs that may be contributing to erectile dysfunction. If possible, causative agents should be discontinued or the dose should be reduced.

A physical examination of the patient should include a check for hypogonadism (i.e., signs of gynecomastia, small testicles, and decreased beard or body hair). The penis should be evaluated for diseases associated with abnormal penile curvature (e.g., Peyronie disease), which are associated with erectile dysfunction. Femoral and lower extremity pulses should be assessed to provide an indication of vascular supply to the genitals. Anal sphincter tone and other genital reflexes should be checked for the integrity of the nerve supply to the penis. A digital rectal examination in patients 50 years or older is needed to rule out benign prostatic hyperplasia, which may contribute to erectile dysfunction.

Selected laboratory tests should be obtained to identify the presence of underlying diseases that could cause erectile dysfunction. They include a fasting serum blood glucose and lipid profile. Serum testosterone levels should be checked in patients older than 50 years and in younger patients who complain of decreased libido. At least two serial early morning serum testosterone levels are needed to confirm the presence of hypogonadism.[14,15]

Finally, erectile dysfunction is a potential marker for arteriosclerosis. Therefore, patients who present with erectile dysfunction should undergo a cardiovascular risk assessment to identify treatable medical conditions.[16,17]

TREATMENT

Erectile Dysfunction

■ DESIRED OUTCOMES

The goal of treatment is improvement in the quantity and quality of penile erections suitable for satisfactory intercourse. Simple as this may sound, healthcare providers must ensure that patients and their partners have reasonable expectations for any therapies that are initiated. Furthermore, only patients with erectile dysfunction should be treated. Patients who have normal sexual function should not seek—or be encouraged to seek—treatment in an effort to enhance sexual function or enable increased activity.[18]

■ GENERAL APPROACH TO TREATMENT

❸ The Second Princeton Consensus Conference is a widely accepted multidisciplinary approach to managing erectile dysfunction that maps out a stepwise treatment plan.[19-21] The first step in clinical management of erectile dysfunction is to identify and, if possible, reverse underlying causes. Risk factors for erectile dysfunction, including hypertension, diabetes mellitus, smoking, or chronic ethanol abuse, should be addressed and minimized. Patients should follow a heart-healthy lifestyle, which includes physical fitness, weight loss to achieve a normal body mass index, low cholesterol diets, no excessive ethanol intake, and no smoking.[22,23] In some cases, these types of interventions are sufficient to restore erectile function. However, if erectile dysfunction does not respond to these measures, specific treatment is indicated.

For patients with psychogenic erectile dysfunction, psychotherapy can be used as monotherapy or as an adjunct to specific treatments for the disorder. To enhance the relevance of psychotherapy, both the patient and the partner should be included in the counseling sessions. Treatment should be individualized and should address immediate factors that may be causing performance anxiety or depression. The effectiveness of psychotherapy is generally low, and long-term psychotherapy is often necessary.

❹ ❺ ❻ Specific treatments of erectile dysfunction include vacuum erection devices (VEDs), pharmacologic treatments, and surgery. The ideal treatment of this disorder should have a fast onset, be effective, be convenient to administer, be cost effective, have a low incidence of serious adverse effects, and be free of serious drug interactions (Table 92–3). Generally, when choosing from among treatment approaches, those that are least invasive are selected first; more invasive therapies are reserved for patients who do not respond to first-line agents.

The American Urological Association Guideline on the Management of Erectile Dysfunction clearly identifies oral phosphodiesterase inhibitors for first-line treatment. Vacuum erection devices, intracavernosal injection of erectogenic agents, or intraurethral prostaglandin inserts are second-line treatments; prescribing of a particular agent for a patient should be individualized. Surgical intervention should be reserved for patients who fail to respond to first- and second-line treatments.[24] A sample algorithm that guides selection of treatment is shown in Figure 92–2.

TABLE 92-3 Dosing Regimens for Selected Drug Treatments for Erectile Dysfunction

Route of Administration	Generic Name (Brand Name)	Dosage Form	Common Dosing Regimen
Oral	Yohimbine (Aphrodyne, Yocon, Yohimex)	5.4-mg tablet or capsule	5.4 mg 3 times per day
	Sildenafil (Viagra)	25-mg, 50-mg, 100-mg tablet	25–100 mg 1 h before intercourse
	Apomorphine (Uprima)[a]	10-mg sublingual tablet, 25-mg tablet and capsule	10–40 mg daily
	Fluoxymesterone (Halotestin)	2-mg, 5-mg, 10-mg, 50-mg tablet	5–20 mg daily
	Trazodone (Desyrel)	100-mg, 150-mg, 300-mg tablet	50–150 mg daily
	Vardenafil (Levitra)	2.5-mg, 5-mg, 10-mg, 20-mg tablet	5–10 mg 1 h before intercourse
	Tadalafil (Cialis)	5-mg, 10-mg, 20-mg tablet	5–20 mg before intercourse or 2.5–5 mg daily
Topical	Testosterone patch (Testoderm)	4 mg/patch, 6 mg/patch	4–6 mg/day; apply to scrotum
	Testosterone patch (Testoderm TTS)	4 mg/patch, 6 mg/patch	4–6 mg/day; apply to arm, buttock, back
	Testosterone patch (Androderm)	2.5 mg/patch	2.5–5 mg/day; apply to arm, back, abdomen, thigh
	Testosterone gel (AndroGel 1%)	5 g/pkt, 10 g/pkt 5 g/activiation	5–10 g/day; apply to shoulders, upper arms, abdomen
Intramuscular	Testosterone cypionate (Depo-Testosterone)	100 mg/mL, 200 mg/mL	200–400 mg every 2–4 wk
	Testosterone enanthate (Delatestryl)	100 mg/mL, 200 mg/mL	200–400 mg every 2–4 wk
Subcutaneous implant	Testosterone (Testopel)	75-mg pellet	150–450 mg every 3–4 mo
Intraurethral	Alprostadil (MUSE)	125-mcg, 250-mcg, 500-mcg, 1,000-mcg pellet	125–1,000 mcg 5–10 min before intercourse
Intracavernosal	Alprostadil (Caverject)	5-mcg, 10-mcg, 20-mcg injection	2.5–60 mcg 5–10 min before intercourse
	Alprostadil (Edex)	5-mcg, 20-mcg, 40-mcg injection	2.5–60 mcg 5–10 min before intercourse
	Papaverine[b]	30 mg/mL injection	Variable, usually used in combination with alprostadil and phentolamine
	Phentolamine[b]	2.5 mg/mL injection	Variable, usually used in combination with alprostadil and papaverine

[a]Not commercially available in the United States as a sublingual formulation; only available in United States as subcutaneous injection that is FDA approved for Parkinson's disease.
[b]Not FDA approved for this use.

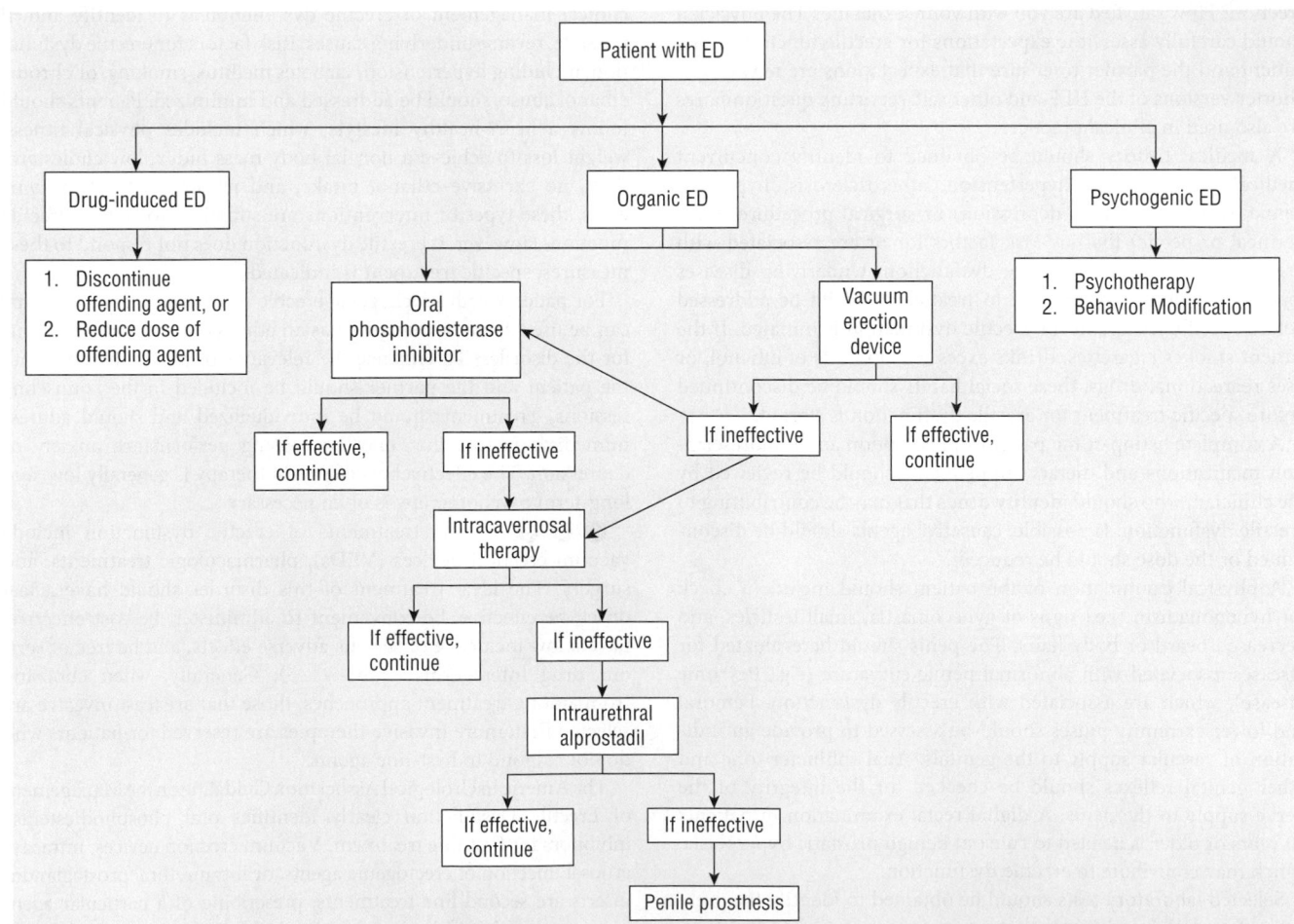

FIGURE 92-2. Algorithm for selecting treatment for erectile dysfunction. For organic erectile dysfunction (ED), oral agents are first-line therapy for younger patients, and vacuum erection devices are generally used first in older patients who are married or otherwise have a stable sexual relationship. These two approaches are sometimes used together in an effort to avoid surgical implantation of penile prostheses.

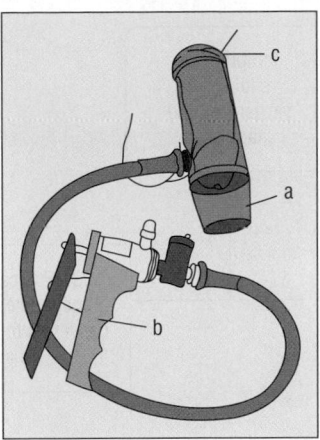

FIGURE 92-3. Technique for using a vacuum erection device with tension band or rubber constriction ring. The patient inserts his penis into the cylinder, which is then pushed up flush against his lower abdomen to create a vacuum chamber. The patient activates the pump to produce a vacuum pressure, which draws arteriolar blood into the corpora cavernosa. To prolong the erection, the patient can use constriction bands or tension rings, which are placed at the base of the penis, to keep the arteriolar blood in and reduce venous outflow from the penis. *(From http://kidney.niddk.nih.gov/kudiseases/pubs/impotence.)*

■ VACUUM ERECTION DEVICE

A VED has three parts: a pump, which generates a negative vacuum pressure; a cylinder, which is closed at one end and into which the penis is inserted; and tubing, which connects the pump to the cylinder. The patient inserts his penis into the open end of the cylinder, which is then pushed up flush against his lower abdomen to create a vacuum chamber. Then the patient activates the pump to produce a vacuum pressure, which draws arteriolar blood into the corpora cavernosa. To prolong the erection, the patient can use constriction bands or tension rings, which are placed at the base of the penis, to keep the arteriolar blood in and to reduce venous outflow from the penis. With the assistance of loading cones to protect the glans, these bands or rings can be rolled over the glans penis and up the erect penile shaft. Alternatively, they can be first threaded onto the plastic cylinder before the penis is inserted. Once the penis is erect, the band or ring can be rolled off the cylinder onto the base of the penis (Fig. 92–3).

❼ The onset of action of the VED is comparatively slow (30 minutes), which requires patience from both the patient and the sexual partner. VEDs are not discreet. That is, a patient's use of a VED is evident to the partner. For this reason, VEDs appear to work best in older patients who are married or who have stable sexual relationships. In this group, VEDs could be considered first-line therapy, and the overall satisfaction rate can be as high as 60% to 80%.[5,18] However, 6% to 11% of partners complain that the penis is cool to the touch or is discolored (bluish) in appearance, particularly when constriction bands are used.

VEDs may be used as second-line therapy in patients who do not respond to oral or injectable drug treatments for erectile dysfunction. The combination of a VED with intracavernosal or intraurethral alprostadil is associated with a higher efficacy rate than use of the VED alone. As a result, combination therapy sometimes is attempted before penile prosthesis surgery is considered in the patient who fails VED monotherapy.

VEDs are available with manual or battery-operated pumps. The latter offer greater convenience, particularly in patients with arthritis of the hands, who find manual pumps too difficult and tiring to operate. The American Urological Association recommends the use of commercially available VEDs by prescription only. These have safety mechanisms that minimize the likelihood of excessively high vacuum pressures which can cause penile discomfort and injury.[24]

Pain or injury from VEDs most often is caused by the constriction bands used to sustain an erection. Because these rings trap blood in the corpora and reduce arteriolar flow into the penis, the penile shaft may feel cold and numb. If the constriction bands are applied for longer than 30 to 60 minutes, the penile shaft may turn blue and hurt. Patients may complain that a hinge-like erection is produced in that the penis pivots on the rubber ring or tension band. Patients sometimes fail to ejaculate.

VEDs are contraindicated in patients with sickle cell disease. These patients are prone to priapism, which can be exacerbated by the use of constriction bands with VEDs. The devices also should be used cautiously by patients taking oral anticoagulants because warfarin, through a poorly understood and idiosyncratic mechanism, can cause priapism.

■ PHOSPHODIESTERASE INHIBITORS

Mechanism

In the presence of sexual stimulation, nitric oxide is released by neurons or endothelial cells in penile tissue, thereby enhancing the activity of guanylate cyclase, the enzyme responsible for conversion of guanylate triphosphate to cGMP (Fig. 92–4).[25] cGMP is a vasodilatory secondary messenger that upregulates the response to nitric oxide, increases smooth muscle relaxation, enhances arterial flow to the corpora cavernosa and enhances blood filling of cavernosal sinuses. Catabolism of cGMP is mediated by phosphodiesterase.

Three competitive, reversible inhibitors of the phosphodiesterase isoenzyme type 5 found in genital tissue are marketed for erectile dysfunction in the United States (Table 92–4). They act by decreasing catabolism of cGMP. However, phosphodiesterase isoenzyme type 5 is also found in peripheral vascular tissue, tracheal smooth muscle, and platelets. Inhibition of phosphodiesterase in these nongenital tissues can produce unwanted effects.

The three marketed phosphodiesterase inhibitors differ in their degree of selectivity in inhibiting other phosphodiesterase isoenzymes, pharmacokinetic profiles, drug–food interactions, and adverse effects (see Table 92–4).

Efficacy

Because of their apparent effectiveness, convenient route of administration, and comparatively low incidence of serious adverse effects, phosphodiesterase inhibitors are considered first-line therapy for erectile dysfunction, particularly in younger patients. They allow for discreet use. Although not based on direct comparison trials, all three commercially available phosphodiesterase inhibitors are considered to be equally effective.[26,27]

In the presence of sexual stimulation and in doses of 25 to 100 mg, sildenafil produces satisfactory erections in 56% to 82% of patients, independent of the etiology of erectile dysfunction. Similar results are documented in the product labeling for the other two agents in this class (65%–80% for vardenafil and 62%–77% for tadalafil). Response rates in the lower range for phosphodiesterase inhibitors have been documented in patients with diabetes mellitus or in patients after radical prostatectomy, probably due to neuropathy or surgery-related nerve damage, respectively.[24,25,28] The effectiveness of the drugs appears to be dose related.

❽ Approximately 30% to 40% of patients do not respond to phosphodiesterase inhibitors.[24] At least half of nonresponders can

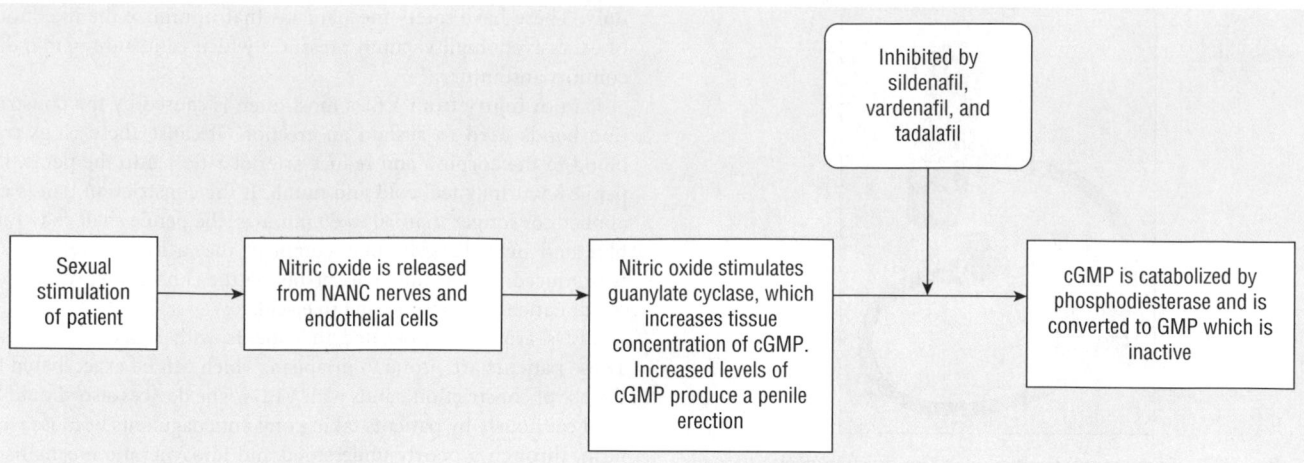

FIGURE 92-4. Mechanism of action of phosphodiesterase inhibitors. All inhibit catabolism of cGMP, a vasodilatory secondary messenger. (cGMP, cyclic guanosine monophosphate; NANC, nonadrenergic noncholinergic.)

benefit from education on proper use of the drugs, and this likely will prove true for the other agents used for erectile dysfunction. Education of patients should include the following points: (1) patients must engage in sexual stimulation (foreplay) for the best response; (2) sildenafil should be taken on an empty stomach, at least 2 hours before meals, for the fastest response, but the other two agents can be taken without regard to meals; (3) taking sildenafil or vardenafil with a fatty meal can decrease the absorption rate, but the absorption rate of tadalafil is not affected;[26] (4) patients who do not respond to the first dose should continue with the phosphodiesterase inhibitor for at least five to eight doses before failure is declared, as increasing success rates are reported with sequential dose administration;[27] (5) some patients require dosage titration up to 100 mg sildenafil, 20 mg vardenafil, or 20 mg tadalafil for a response;[27,28] (6) patients should avoid excessive alcohol intake, which can cause erectile dysfunction; and (7) involvement of the sexual partner can help improve the patient's response to treatment.

In addition, treatment of concomitant medical illnesses which contribute to erectile dysfunction (e.g., diabetes mellitus, hypertension, hypogonadism) should be optimized.[20]

The effectiveness of switching from one phosphodiesterase inhibitor to another when the patient does not respond to an initial agent is controversial. In two small studies, vardenafil was beneficial in patients who did not respond to sildenafil.[26,29] However, controlled clinical trials in larger patient groups are needed before this strategy is used as routine treatment.

The phosphodiesterase inhibitors should not be used by patients with normal erectile function. Also, according to Food and Drug Administration (FDA)–approved labeling, the drugs should not be used in combination with other forms of therapy for erectile dysfunction because prolonged erections (which may lead to priapism) may result.[30]

Long-term use of phosphodiesterase inhibitors is not associated with tachyphylaxis.[31,32]

TABLE 92-4 Pharmacodynamics and Pharmacokinetics of Phosphodiesterase Inhibitors

	Sildenafil (Viagra)[a]	Vardenafil (Levitra)[a]	Tadalafil (Cialis)[a]
Inhibits PDE-5	Yes	Yes	Yes
Inhibits PDE-6	Yes	Minimally	No
Inhibits PDE-11	No	No	Yes
Time to peak plasma level (h)	0.5–1	0.7–0.9	2
Fatty meal decreases rate of oral absorption?	Yes	Yes	No
Mean plasma half-life (h)	3.7	4.4–4.8	18
Percentage of dose excreted in feces	80	91–95	61
Percentage of dose excreted in urine	13	2–6	36
Duration (h)	4	4	24–36
Usual dose (mg) before intercourse	25–100	5–20	5–20
Daily dose (mg)	Not applicable	Not applicable	2.5–5
Dose (mg) in patients ≥65 y (mg)	25	5	5–20
Dose (mg) in moderate renal impairment	25–100	5–20	5
Dose (mg) in severe renal impairment	25	5–20	5
Dose (mg) in mild hepatic impairment	25–100	5–20	10
Dose (mg) in moderate hepatic impairment	25–100	5–10	10
Dose (mg) in severe hepatic impairment	25	Not evaluated	Not recommended
Dose in patients taking cytochrome P450 3A4 inhibitors[a]	25 mg	2.5–5 mg every 24–72 h	10 mg every 72 h

[a]Sildenafil doses should be decreased when any potent cytochrome P450 3A4 inhibitor (e.g., cimetidine, erythromycin, clarithromycin, ketoconazole, itraconazole, ritonavir, and saquinavir) is used. Vardenafil doses vary according to the agent used (2.5 mg every 72 hours for ritonavir; 2.5 mg every 24 hours for indinavir, ketoconazole 400 mg daily, and itraconazole 400 mg daily; and 5 mg every 24 hours for ketoconazole 200 mg daily, itraconazole 200 mg daily, and erythromycin). Tadalafil doses are reduced only when the drug is used with the most potent cytochrome P450 3A4 inhibitors (e.g., ketoconazole, ritonavir).
PDE, phosphodiesterase.

■ SELECTIVITY OF OTHER PHOSPHODIESTERASE ISOENZYMES

More than 25 different phosphodiesterase isoenzymes have been identified; however, the physiologic effects of stimulation and inhibition of some of these isoenzymes remain to be elucidated. Of note, phosphodiesterase isoenzyme type 6 is localized to the rods and cones of the eye. Inhibition of this isoenzyme has been associated with blurred vision and cyanopsia. Sildenafil is the most potent inhibitor of phosphodiesterase isoenzyme type 6, vardenafil is an intermediate inhibitor, and tadalafil is the least potent inhibitor.[26] Likewise, phosphodiesterase isoenzyme type 11 is localized to striated muscle. Inhibition of this isoenzyme has been associated with myalgia and muscle pain. Tadalafil exerts the greatest inhibitory activity against phosphodiesterase type 11.[6]

Pharmacokinetics and Drug–Food Interactions

Pharmacokinetic parameters of the phosphodiesterase inhibitors are listed in Table 92–4.

Vardenafil and sildenafil have similar pharmacokinetic profiles. Both drugs have a 1-hour onset of action and short duration of action. Oral absorption is significantly delayed when either drug is taken within 2 hours of a fatty meal. In contrast, tadalafil has a delayed onset of action of 2 hours, has a prolonged duration of action up to 36 hours, and food does not affect its rate of absorption. Thus, tadalafil offers greater spontaneity for patients, as one dose can last through an entire weekend and allow for multiple acts of sexual intercourse over multiple days with a single dose.[32]

The onset of action of these agents has undergone reexamination to assess how soon after drug administration patients can expect to have an erection suitable for intercourse. Although up to 50% of patients may develop an erection within 20 to 30 minutes of sildenafil 100 mg, vardenafil 20 mg, or tadalafil 20 mg, the rest of the patients may require a full hour to achieve an adequate erectile response.[33] Therefore, patients should be instructed to allow adequate time for the drug to work.

Concomitant ingestion of ethanol with phosphodiesterase inhibitors can result in orthostatic hypotension. Therefore, the manufacturer recommends that patients avoid ethanol when taking these medications.

All three phosphodiesterase inhibitors are hepatically catabolized principally by the cytochrome P450 3A4 microsomal isoenzyme and by other P450 isoenzymes (minor routes) and/or other hepatic enzymes. Sildenafil and vardenafil have active metabolites, which are excreted primarily in the feces (see Table 92–4).

Dosing

The usual oral doses of the phosphodiesterase inhibitors are listed in Table 92–4. Sildenafil and vardenafil should be taken on demand or at least 30 to 60 minutes before sexual intercourse. Tadalafil should be taken at least 2 hours before sexual intercourse. The durations of action for sildenafil and vardenafil are 4 to 5 hours, whereas the effects of tadalafil last for 36 hours. The agents vary as to whether doses must be adjusted for patients 65 years and older and those with compromised hepatic or renal function. Patients should be advised to take no more than the amount prescribed and to use only one dose per day (or less often in the case of some patients taking tadalafil). Doses greater than those recommended have been described in the published literature (e.g., tadalafil 100 mg); however, such dosing regimens have not consistently produced improved erectile responses.

For patients who do not respond to an adequate course of on-demand phosphodiesterase inhibitors for erectile dysfunction, daily low dosing of these agents may improve endothelial function in cavernosal tissue. That is, regular use of phosphodiesterase inhibitors may increase local concentrations of cGMP, which may lead to increased oxygen tension, improved blood flow, and reduced endothelial damage. A preliminary clinical trial of daily use of tadalafil 2.5 or 5 mg showed a 58% frequency of successful sexual intercourse compared with conventional on-demand use of tadalafil 5 to 20 mg, which produced a 21% frequency of success.[34,35] Other potential advantages of daily low dosing regimens include a lower potential for dose-related adverse effects, lower cost, and increased spontaneity of sexual intercourse. However, more extensive clinical study is needed to evaluate the benefit of daily dosing of phosphodiesterase inhibitors before the approach can be preferred to an on-demand regimen.

Adverse Effects

Most adverse effects of the phosphodiesterase inhibitors are mild or moderate and are self-limited, and patients often become tolerant to them with continued use.[36,37] The rates of drug discontinuation caused by adverse effects are low, ranging from 2.1% to 2.5%, and are similar for all three agents. In usual doses the most common adverse effects are headache (11%), facial flushing (12%), dyspepsia (5%), nasal congestion (3.4%), and dizziness (3%),[25] all of which result from vasodilation or smooth muscle relaxation secondary to inhibition of phosphodiesterase isoenzyme type 5 in extragenital tissues.[18]

Sildenafil and vardenafil produce an 8- to 10-mm Hg decrease in systolic and a 5 to 6 mm Hg decrease in diastolic blood pressure starting approximately 1 hour after a dose is taken and lasting for 4 hours. Most patients are asymptomatic as a result of these blood pressure changes, but some patients, particularly those taking multiple antihypertensives or nitrates or those with baseline hypotension, may develop clinical symptoms as a consequence of these peripheral vascular effects. Tadalafil does not produce decreases in blood pressure, but it must be used with caution in patients with cardiovascular disease because of the cardiac risk inherent to sexual activity. A management approach for such patients, developed based on an analysis of deaths in men who were using sildenafil and commonly referred to as the recommendations of the Princeton Consensus Guideline Conference II,[19] should be applied to all the phosphodiesterase inhibitors (Table 92–5).

Sildenafil and vardenafil cause increased sensitivity to light, blurred vision, or loss of blue–green color discrimination in 2% to 3% of patients. These effects result from inhibition of phosphodiesterase type 6 in the photoreceptor cells of in retinal rods and cones, particularly at doses larger than 100 mg. Visual adverse effects commonly occur at the time of peak serum concentrations. Although visual adverse effects are mild and reversible, caution regarding use is recommended for airplane pilots, who rely on green and blue lights for landing planes. Tadalafil has minimal to no inhibitory activity against type 6 phosphodiesterase, and no visual adverse effects have been reported.[38] Nevertheless, according to current product labeling, all phosphodiesterase inhibitors should be used cautiously in patients at risk for retinitis pigmentosa, a genetic disease associated with retinal phosphodiesterase deficiency.

Nonarteritic anterior ischemic optic neuropathy (NAION) is a sudden, unilateral, painless blindness, which may be irreversible. Isolated cases of NAION have been associated with phosphodiesterase inhibitor use.[39] Although a cause-and-effect relationship has not been definitively established, the blood pressure–lowering effects of these medications may decrease blood flow to the optic nerve and lead to sudden unilateral decrease in vision. Because NAION may lead to permanent vision loss, the FDA has required inclusion of warnings on the product labeling of phosphodiesterase inhibitors. Specifically, before receiving these agents, patients at risk

TABLE 92-5 Recommendations of the Second Princeton Consensus Conference for Cardiovascular Risk Stratification of Patients Being Considered for Phosphodiesterase Inhibitor Therapy

Risk Category	Description of Patient's Condition	Management Approach
Low risk	Has asymptomatic cardiovascular disease with < 3 risk factors for cardiovascular disease Has well-controlled hypertension Has mild, stable angina Has mild congestive heart failure (NYHA class I) Has mild valvular heart disease Had a myocardial infarction >6 weeks ago	Patient can be started on phosphodiesterase inhibitor
Intermediate risk	Has ≥3 risk factors for cardiovascular disease Has moderate, stable angina Had a recent myocardial infarction or stroke within the past 6 weeks Has moderate congestive heart failure (NYHA class II)	Patient should undergo complete cardiovascular workup and treadmill stress test to determine tolerance to increased myocardial energy consumption associated with increased sexual activity
High risk	Has unstable or symptomatic angina, despite treatment Has uncontrolled hypertension Has severe congestive heart failure (NYHA class III or IV) Had a recent myocardial infarction or stroke within past 2 weeks Has moderate or severe valvular heart disease Has high-risk cardiac arrhythmias Has obstructive hypertrophic cardiomyopathy	Phosphodiesterase inhibitor is contraindicated; sexual intercourse should be deferred

NYHA, New York Heart Association.
From Kostis et al.[21]

for NAION should be evaluated by an ophthalmologist. Patients at risk include a wide variety of patients: those with glaucoma, macular degeneration, diabetic retinopathy or hypertension, those who have undergone eye surgery or have experienced eye trauma, patients who are age 50 years or more, or smokers. A patient who experiences sudden vision loss while taking a phosphodiesterase inhibitor should be evaluated for NAION before continuing treatment.[40]

Tadalafil produces lower back and limb muscle pain, which occur in a dose-related fashion in 7% to 30% of patients treated with doses of 10 to 100 mg.[41] The mechanism for this is not known. It may be linked to inhibition of type 11 phosphodiesterase, a unique characteristic of tadalafil.

Vardenafil can cause prolongation of the QT interval. Therefore, it should be used cautiously in patients with this anomaly or in patients who are taking medications that prolong the QT interval (e.g., quinidine).

Priapism is a rare adverse effect of phosphodiesterase inhibitors, particularly sildenafil and vardenafil, which have shorter plasma half-lives than tadalafil. Priapism has been associated with excessive doses of the phosphodiesterase inhibitor or concomitant therapy involving other erectogenic drugs.

Drug Interactions

Patients taking organic nitrates may develop severe hypotension if they are taken with phosphodiesterase inhibitors as a result of two major factors: (1) organic nitrates on their own produce hypotension, and (2) organic nitrates are nitric oxide donors, which can stimulate the activity of guanylate cyclase and increase tissue levels of cGMP. For this reason, use of the three phosphodiesterase inhibitors is contraindicated in patients taking nitrates given by any route at scheduled times or intermittently.[19,42] Furthermore, nitrates should be withheld for 24 hours after sildenafil or vardenafil administration and for 48 hours after tadalafil administration.[19,42] Finally, if a patient who has taken a phosphodiesterase inhibitor requires medical treatment of angina, non–nitrate-containing agents (e.g., calcium channel blocker, β-adrenergic antagonist, morphine) should be used.

If severe hypotension occurs after exposure to nitrates and a phosphodiesterase inhibitor, the patient should be placed in a Trendelenburg position and aggressive fluid administration initiated. If severe hypotension continues, parenteral β-adrenergic agonists (e.g., dopamine) should be administered cautiously.

Interestingly, dietary sources of nitrates, nitrites, or L-arginine (a precursor for nitrates) do not interact with the phosphodiesterase inhibitors. This is because dietary sources do not increase circulating levels of nitric oxide in humans.

Sildenafil does not appear to interact with antihypertensive medications. In retrospective analyses of patients taking sildenafil in combination with α-adrenergic antagonists, β-adrenergic antagonists, diuretics, angiotensin-converting enzyme inhibitors, angiotensin receptor blockers, or calcium channel blockers, the incidence of hypotension was similar to that reported in patients taking sildenafil alone.[43,44] This finding was confirmed by a retrospective analysis of pooled data on more than 4,800 patients in 35 clinical trials.[30]

Small decreases in blood pressure with clinically symptomatic hypotension have been described in some patients taking sildenafil and tadalafil and immediate-release formulations of terazosin and doxazosin.[45] In contrast, concurrent administration of extended-release alfuzosin, silodosin, or tamsulosin, which produce lower peak serum concentrations than immediate-release formulations after administration or exhibit α_{1A}-adrenergic selectivity, show minimal or no decrease in blood pressure.[46–48] Package labeling for phosphodiesterase inhibitors include a caution about concomitant use of phosphodiesterase inhibitors and α-adrenergic antagonists.

Hepatic metabolism of all three phosphodiesterase inhibitors can be inhibited by enzyme inhibitors of CYP 3A4, including cimetidine, erythromycin, clarithromycin, ketoconazole, itraconazole, ritonavir, saquinavir, and grapefruit juice.[48–51] Lower starting doses should be used in these patients (see Table 92–4).

CLINICAL CONTROVERSY

Some clinicians believe that tachyphylaxis may develop with continuous use of sildenafil, but others believe that a lack of responsiveness may be due to worsening of underlying diseases that may contribute to the development of erectile dysfunction.[18] Positive treatment response despite continuous use of these agents for up to 6 years suggests that tachyphylaxis does not occur.[26,38]

TABLE 92-6	Comparison of Testosterone Replacement Regimens and Ideal Testosterone Replacement Regimen			
	Achieves Serum Testosterone Concentrations in Normal Range?	Produces Normal Circadian Pattern of Serum Testosterone Concentrations?	Produces Normal Pattern of Serum Concentrations of Androgen Metabolites?	Adverse Effects
Oral testosterone	No	No	No	Hyperlipidemia Sodium retention
Oral alkylated androgens	Yes	No	No	Hyperlipidemia Sodium retention Hepatotoxicity
Intramuscular testosterone cypionate or enanthate	Yes	No; produces supraphysiologic serum concentrations for several days after injection	No, excess testosterone is converted to estradiol	Mood swings Gynecomastia Polycythemia Hyperlipidemia
Transdermal nonscrotal skin patch	Yes	Yes, provided the patch is placed at night	Yes	Dermatitis due to permeation enhancers in formulation
Transdermal scrotal skin patch	Yes	Yes provided the patch is applied in the morning	No; 5α-reductase in scrotal skin metabolizes testosterone and increases serum concentrations of dihydrotestosterone	Dermatitis due to permeation enhancers in formulation
Transdermal gel	Yes	Yes	Yes	May be inadvertently transferred to others who rub up against the patient's skin treated area
Testosterone subcutaneous implant	Yes	No	No; produces elevated concentrations of dihydrotestosterone	Pellet may be extruded accidentally, resulting in loss of drug effect
Buccal system	Yes	No	No	Gum irritation, bitter taste

Data from Gore JL, Swerdloff RS, Rajfer J. Androgen deficiency in the etiology and treatment of erectile dysfunction. Urol Clin N Am 2005;32:457–468.

■ TESTOSTERONE REPLACEMENT REGIMENS

Mechanism

❾ Testosterone replacement regimens supply exogenous testosterone and restore serum testosterone levels to the normal range (300–1,100 ng/dL; 10.4–38.2 nmol/L). In so doing, testosterone replacement regimens correct symptoms of hypogonadism, which include malaise, loss of muscle strength, depressed mood, and decreased libido. Testosterone can directly stimulate androgen receptors in the central nervous system and is thought to be responsible for maintaining normal sexual drive. In addition, testosterone may stimulate nitric oxide synthase, thereby increasing cavernosal concentrations of nitric oxide, and enhancing the effects of phosphodiesterase type 5 in cavernosal tissue.[52]

Indications

Testosterone replacement regimens are indicated in symptomatic patients with primary or secondary hypogonadism, as confirmed by both the presence of a decreased libido and low serum concentrations of testosterone.[18] Serum testosterone concentrations typically are measured in the early morning because the secretion pattern of this hormone follows a circadian pattern, with highest serum concentrations in the morning hours. Simultaneous serum luteinizing hormone levels help to distinguish patients with primary hypogonadism, who have elevated luteinizing hormone levels, from those with secondary hypogonadism, who have decreased luteinizing hormone levels. Primary hypogonadism can be a characteristic of aging men who undergo andropause, in which the Leydig cells of the testes slowly and progressively decrease testosterone production.[52] Symptoms, including decreased libido, erectile dysfunction, gynecomastia, decreased muscle mass, increased body fat, and osteopenia, develop gradually over years.

Testosterone replacement regimens should never be administered to men with normal serum testosterone levels.

Efficacy

Testosterone replacement regimens restore muscle strength and sexual drive and improve mood in patients with hypogonadism. Improvements are generally observed within days or weeks of the start of testosterone replacement. Administration of testosterone will correct the serum testosterone level to the normal range. No additional benefit has been demonstrated for large doses of testosterone, which increase the serum testosterone level from the low end to the upper end of the normal range or to the above-normal range.[53] Testosterone replacement regimens do not directly correct erectile dysfunction; instead, they improve libido, thereby correcting secondary erectile dysfunction.[54]

Testosterone replacement regimens can be administered orally, parenterally, or transdermally (Table 92–6). Injectable testosterone replacement regimens are the preferred treatment for symptomatic patients with primary or secondary hypogonadism because they are effective, inexpensive, and not associated with the bioavailability problems or hepatotoxic adverse effects of oral androgens.[52] Although convenient for the patient, testosterone patches and gels are much more expensive than other forms of androgen replacement; therefore, they should be reserved for patients who refuse injectable testosterone.

In the ideal testosterone replacement regimen, the medication would mimic the normal circadian pattern of serum testosterone concentrations such that peak and trough concentrations occur in the early morning and late afternoon, respectively; produce serum concentrations in the normal range; produce serum concentrations of dihydrotestosterone and estradiol, which are metabolites of testosterone that mimic the normal physiologic pattern; and produce minimal adverse effects.[52] Table 92–6 compares commercially available testosterone replacement regimens for these characteristics and shows that an ideal regimen has yet to be identified.

Pharmacokinetics

Natural testosterone has poor oral bioavailability because of extensive first-pass hepatic metabolism; therefore, large doses must be taken. To improve oral bioavailability, alkylated derivatives were formulated. Of these derivatives, methyltestosterone and fluoxymesterone are more resistant to hepatic catabolism and can be taken in smaller daily doses, which are potentially safer. However, oral alkylated derivatives of testosterone are not metabolized to dihydrotestosterone or estradiol, and are associated with a higher incidence of serious hepatotoxicity and therefore are not preferred for management of hypogonadism.

An alternative to oral administration is the testosterone buccal system (Striant), which is applied to the gum above the upper incisor teeth twice per day. Over time it forms a gel from which testosterone is absorbed. One advantage of this route of administration is that the drug bypasses first-pass hepatic catabolism, which allows for increased bioavailability of testosterone.

Several testosterone esters have been formulated for intramuscular injection, with different durations of action (see Table 92–3). The shorter-acting testosterone propionate, which requires dosing 3 times per week, has been replaced with testosterone cypionate or enanthate, which can be dosed every 2, 4, or 6 weeks in most patients. An even longer-acting parenteral testosterone is available as a subcutaneous implant for dosing every 3 to 6 months. Although this schedule minimizes repeat visits to the clinician's office for dosing, the implant must be administered by a physician, and the implanted pellet may be extruded after administration. This extrusion has been reported in up to 8.5% of treated patients and results in loss of drug effect. These testosterone formulations produce suprapharmacologic patterns of serum testosterone during the dosing interval, which have been linked to mood swings in some patients.

Topical testosterone replacement regimens can be delivered as once-daily patches or gel. Testosterone patches increase serum testosterone levels into the normal range in 2 to 6 hours. Serum testosterone levels return to baseline 24 hours after patch administration. However, unlike oral or injectable supplements, transdermal testosterone patches applied at bedtime or testosterone gel applied each morning produce physiologic patterns of serum testosterone levels throughout the day. The clinical importance of this biochemical effect is unknown.[52]

The original Testoderm brand patch was formulated for scrotal application. Scrotal skin is thinner and has a richer vascular supply than does the skin on the arms or thighs. Therefore, application of Testoderm patches produces excellent absorption of the hormone. However, the patch can fall off when the scrotum becomes damp or moist, when the patient exercises, or if the scrotum is excessively hairy.

For improved convenience, Androderm and Testoderm TTS patches were formulated for application to the arms, buttocks, or back; Androderm can also be applied to the thighs. The addition of absorption enhancers and different adhesives has been linked to a higher incidence of contact dermatitis with Androderm patches compared with the original Testoderm scrotal patch.[55]

Testosterone gel 1% formulation (AndroGel) is applied in much larger doses (5 or 10 g each day) to the skin of the shoulders, upper arms, or abdomen. The hormone is absorbed quickly, within 30 minutes, but several hours may be required for complete absorption of the dose. For this reason, the patient should be reminded to wait at least 5 to 6 hours after application before showering. To prevent inadvertent transfer of testosterone gel to others, the patient should thoroughly wash his hands with soap and water after administration of a dose, and allow the application site to dry undisturbed for several minutes before dressing or covering it.

Dosing

Table 92–3 lists the usual doses for testosterone replacement regimens. Two to 3 months is considered an adequate treatment trial with a particular dose. Thus, a dose should not be increased until the patient has used one particular dose for at least this time period.[53] The serum testosterone level should return to the normal range and symptoms of androgen deficiency should be relieved with appropriate dosing.

Before initiating any testosterone replacement regimen in patients 40 years and older, patients should be screened for benign prostatic hyperplasia and prostate cancer. Both of these diseases are testosterone-dependent conditions and theoretically could be worsened by exogenous administration of testosterone. Prostate cancer is a contraindication to androgen supplementation. To screen for these conditions, a prostate-specific antigen serum concentration should be obtained and a digital rectal examination of the prostate performed. These tests are generally repeated at 1-year intervals after treatment is started.[52]

Adverse Effects

Testosterone replacement regimens can cause sodium retention, which can cause weight gain, or exacerbate hypertension, congestive heart failure, and edema. Gynecomastia can occur as a result of conversion of testosterone to estrogen in peripheral tissues. This has been reported most often in patients with liver cirrhosis.

Testosterone replacement regimens are contraindicated in patients with breast cancer and untreated prostate cancer.

Although serum lipoprotein perturbations may occur, testosterone replacement regimens have a neutral effect in that they decrease both total cholesterol and high-density lipoprotein cholesterol levels. No cases of cardiovascular disease have been reported with testosterone replacement regimens.

Large doses of parenteral testosterone can produce adverse metabolic effects. Thus, patients on long-term testosterone replacement regimens must undergo clinical laboratory testing for a serum testosterone level and hematocrit before starting treatment and every 6 to 12 months during treatment.[54] Repeated serum testosterone levels that exceed the normal range require a dosage reduction or increased interval between drug doses. If the hematocrit exceeds 55% (0.55), the testosterone replacement regimen should be withheld to avoid polycythemia and its consequences.

Oral alkylated testosterone replacement regimens have caused hepatotoxicity, ranging from mild elevations of hepatic transaminases to serious liver diseases, including peliosis hepatis (hemorrhagic liver cysts), hepatocellular and intrahepatic cholestasis, and benign or malignant tumors. For this reason, parenteral testosterone replacement regimens are preferred.

Topical testosterone patches may cause contact dermatitis, which responds well to topical corticosteroids. This adverse effect has been associated with the presence of permeation enhancers, which are added to patch formulations. If the dermatitis becomes problematic, an alternative is testosterone gel formulations, which are associated with a lower incidence of contact dermatitis compared with patches.

■ ALPROSTADIL

Mechanism

Alprostadil, also known as prostaglandin E_1, stimulates adenyl cyclase, resulting in increased production of cAMP, a secondary messenger that decreases the intracellular calcium concentration and causes smooth muscle relaxation of the arterial blood vessels and sinusoidal tissues in the corpora. This results in enhanced blood flow to and blood filling of the corpora.

Alprostadil is commercially available as an intracavernosal injection (Caverject and Edex) and as an intraurethral insert (medicated urethral system for erection [MUSE]).

Indications

Both commercially available formulations of alprostadil are FDA approved as monotherapy for management of erectile dysfunction. Alprostadil is more effective by the intracavernosal route than the intraurethral route.

The enhanced efficacy of the intracavernosal injection may be related to the excellent bioavailability of the drug when injected directly into the corpora cavernosum. In contrast, intraurethral alprostadil doses generally are several hundred times larger than intracavernosal doses. This is because intraurethral alprostadil must be absorbed from the urethra, through the corpus spongiosum, and into the corpus cavernosum, where it exerts its full proerectogenic effect.

Although several other agents, including papaverine, phentolamine, and atropine, have been used off-label for intracavernosal therapy, alprostadil is preferentially prescribed. This is because intracavernosal alprostadil has been FDA approved for erectile dysfunction, it does not require extemporaneous compounding, and it has a low potential for causing prolonged erections and priapism.

Both formulations of alprostadil are considered more invasive than VEDs or phosphodiesterase inhibitors. For this reason, intracavernosal alprostadil is generally prescribed after patients do not respond to or cannot use less invasive interventions. Intracavernosal alprostadil is preferred over intraurethral alprostadil because of its greater effectiveness. Intracavernosal alprostadil may be preferred in patients with diabetes mellitus, who are accustomed to injectable drug therapy and may have peripheral neuropathies, which decrease the patient's perception of pain upon injection. Intraurethral alprostadil is generally reserved as a treatment of last resort for patients who do not respond to other less invasive and more effective forms of therapy and who refuse surgery.

Intracavernosal Alprostadil

Efficacy The overall efficacy of intracavernosal alprostadil is 70% to 90%.[5] Three characteristics of intracavernosal alprostadil include the following:

1. The effectiveness of alprostadil is dose related over the range of 2.5 to 20 mcg. The mean duration of erection is directly related to the dose of alprostadil administered and ranges from 12 to 44 minutes.

2. A higher percentage of patients with psychogenic and neurogenic erectile dysfunction respond to alprostadil at a lower dose compared to patients with vasculogenic erectile dysfunction.

3. Tolerance does not appear to develop with continued use of intracavernosal alprostadil at home.

❿ Although 70% to 75% of patients respond to intracavernosal alprostadil, a high proportion of patients elect to discontinue its use over time. Depending on the study and the length of observation, 30% to 50% of patients voluntarily discontinue therapy, usually during the first 6 to 12 months. Common reasons for discontinuation include lack of perceived effectiveness; inconvenience of administration; an unnatural, nonspontaneous erection; needle phobia; loss of interest; and cost of therapy.[5,56]

Approximately one third of patients do not respond to usual doses of intracavernosal alprostadil. In these patients, intracavernosal alprostadil has been used successfully along with VEDs. Such combination therapy can be attempted by patients before transitioning to more invasive surgical procedures.[57,58] Alternatively, intracavernosal injections of synergistic combinations of vasoactive agents that act by different mechanisms have been used.[57] Intracavernosal drug combinations typically produce an erection that lasts longer than an erection produced by any one of the agents in the mixture. In addition, because of the low dosage of each agent in the combination,

fewer systemic and local fibrotic adverse effects develop compared with high-dose monotherapy. For example, when used in low-dose combination regimens, papaverine is less likely to induce hypotension and liver dysfunction, and phentolamine is less likely to induce tachycardia and hypotension.[58] However, as previously mentioned, such intracavernosal drug combinations are not commercially available and must be extemporaneously compounded.

Pharmacokinetics Intracavernosal injection should be administered into only one corpus cavernosum. From this injection site, the drug will reach the other corpus cavernosum through vascular communications between the two corpora. Alprostadil acts rapidly, with an onset of 5 to 15 minutes. The duration is directly related to the dose. Within the usual dosage range of 2.5 to 20 mcg, the duration of erection is no more than 1 hour. Higher doses are expected to exhibit a longer duration of action. Local enzymes in the corpora cavernosum quickly metabolize alprostadil. Any alprostadil that escapes into the systemic circulation is deactivated on first pass through the lungs.[5] Hence, the plasma half-life of alprostadil is approximately 1 minute, and the potential for systemic adverse effects is negligible. Dose modification is not necessary in patients with renal or hepatic disease.

Dosing The usual dose of intracavernosal alprostadil is 10 to 20 mcg, with a maximum recommended dose of 60 mcg. Doses greater than 60 mcg have not produced any greater improvement in penile erection but may cause hypotension or prolonged erections lasting more than 1 hour.[5] The dose should be administered 5 to 10 minutes before intercourse. The manufacturer recommends that patients be slowly titrated up to the minimally effective dosage to minimize the likelihood of hypotension. Under a physician's supervision, patients should be started with a 1.25-mcg dose, which can be increased in increments of 1.25 to 2.50 mcg at 30-minute intervals up to the lowest dose that produces a firm erection for 1 hour and does not produce adverse effects. In clinical practice, this process is rarely done because it is time consuming. Thus, many physicians start the patient on 10 mcg and move quickly up the dosage range to identify the best dose for the patient. To avoid adverse effects, patients should receive no more than one injection per day and not more than three injections per week.

Intracavernosal injections should be performed using a 0.5-inch, 27- or 30-gauge needle. A tuberculin syringe or a syringe prefilled with diluent as supplied by the manufacturer should be used to ensure precise measurement of doses. Patients with needle phobia, poor vision, or poor manual dexterity can use commercially available autoinjectors (e.g., PenInject) to facilitate administration of intracavernosal alprostadil.

Intracavernosal injections require that the patient or the sexual partner practice good aseptic technique (to avoid infection), have good manual skills and visual ability, and be comfortable with injection techniques. When practicing self-injection, the patient should use one hand to firmly hold the glans penis against his thigh to expose the lateral surface of the shaft. The injection should be made at right angles into one of the lateral surfaces of the proximal third of the penis. The injection should never be made into the dorsal or ventral surface of the penis. This will prevent inadvertent injection of the drug into arteries on the dorsal surface or the urethra on the ventral surface. After the injection, the penis should be massaged to help distribute the drug into the opposite corpus cavernosum. Injection sites should be rotated with each dose. Finally, manual pressure should be applied to the injection site for 5 minutes to reduce the likelihood of hematoma formation (Fig. 92–5).

Once the optimal dosage of intracavernosal alprostadil is established, the patient should return for routine medical followup every 3 to 6 months. Some patients subsequently require dosage adjustment, largely attributed to worsening of the underlying disease that is contributing to the erectile dysfunction.

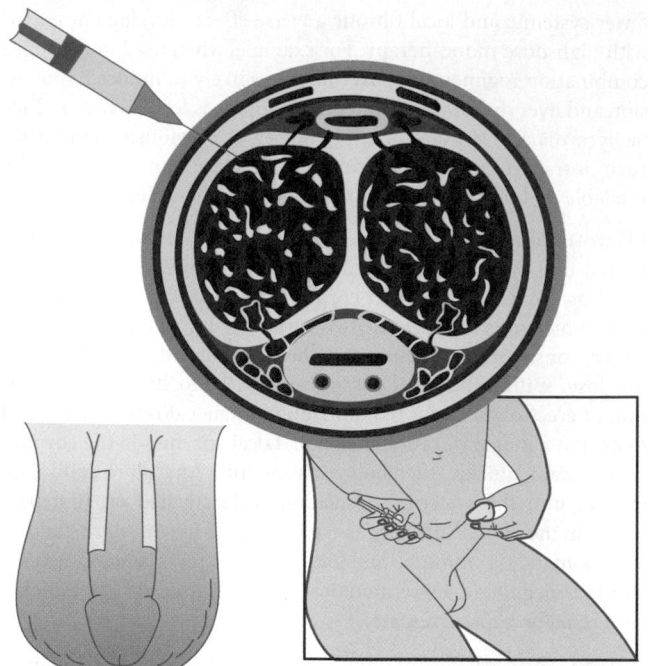

FIGURE 92-5. Technique for administration of intracavernosal injections. *(From Caverject [package insert]. New York, NY: Pfizer Inc; 1999. Data from http://media.pfizer.com/files/products/uspi_caverject_powder.pdf.)*

Adverse Effects Intracavernosal alprostadil is most commonly associated with local adverse effects, which occur most often during the first year of therapy. However, improved administration technique with continued use is believed to account for the lower frequency of adverse effects during subsequent treatment periods.

Intracavernosal injections are associated with several local adverse effects. Cavernosal plaques or areas of fibrosis at injection sites form in approximately 2% to 12% of patients. When they occur, the patient should suspend further injections until the plaques resolve. These plaques may cause penile curvature, similar to Peyronie disease, which makes sexual intercourse difficult or impossible. The cause of corporal fibrosis and plaque formation is unknown. This adverse effect may be caused by poor injection technique or by alprostadil itself. Although patients have developed corporal fibrosis, alprostadil may be less likely to cause this adverse effect compared to other intracavernosal drug combinations, such as phentolamine or papaverine. Unlike cavernosal fibrosis associated with large doses and repeated administration of papaverine, penile scarring secondary to alprostadil appears to be unpredictable.

Alprostadil causes penile pain in approximately 10% to 44% of patients. The pain has been described as a burning discomfort or dull pain near the injection site or during the erection, which generally does not persist after the penis becomes flaccid. The pain usually is mild, generally does not require discontinuation of therapy, and often abates even with continued treatment. However, 2% to 5% of patients discontinue taking alprostadil because of severe pain. The pain can be managed by oral analgesics (e.g., acetaminophen), if necessary. One investigator has recommended adding procaine to intracavernosal alprostadil, but this may mask the signs of more serious adverse effects of the drug or of penile injury during intercourse and is not recommended.[59] The mechanism of this adverse reaction is poorly understood. Alprostadil may intrinsically produce pain. Also, the pain may be a result of the pH of the parenteral solution. Alprostadil is acidic, and the commercially available Caverject formulation is buffered with sodium citrate, a weak base, to reduce pain on injection.

Priapism, a prolonged, painful erection lasting more than 1 hour, occurs in 1% to 15% of treated patients. It occurs most often during the dose titration period and is rare thereafter. Blood sludging in the corpora can lead to tissue hypoxia and cavernosal fibrosis and scarring. The risk for this complication is greatest for erections that persist beyond 4 hours. Patients are advised to seek medical attention immediately when drug-induced erections last more than 1 hour, as this is considered a urologic emergency. Its management includes supportive care, including analgesics for pain and sedatives for anxiety. In addition, needle aspiration of sludged blood in the corpora or intracavernosal injection of α-adrenergic agonists (e.g., phenylephrine) has been used. These procedures facilitate venous drainage of the corpora, allowing venous outflow to "catch up" with arterial inflow.

The likelihood of prolonged erections with intracavernosal alprostadil is dose related. Therefore, to prevent this adverse effect, the lowest effective dose should be used, and the dose should be titrated to ensure that the duration of the erection is no more than 1 hour.

Other local adverse effects include injection site hematomas and bruising. These effects are largely the result of poor injection technique. To minimize the risk of injection site hematomas, patients should be advised to apply pressure to the injection site for 5 minutes after each dose. Similarly, infection at the injection site has been reported. Meticulous aseptic technique is necessary to prevent this complication.

Intracavernosal alprostadil rarely causes systemic adverse effects, owing to the agent's local catabolism in cavernosal tissue and rapid deactivation in pulmonary tissue (if any of the drug escapes into the systemic circulation). However, large doses greater than 20 mcg are associated with dizziness and hypotension in some patients and is one reason why such large doses are not commonly used.

Intracavernosal injection therapy should be used cautiously by patients at risk for priapism, including patients with sickle cell disease or lymphoproliferative disorders. It should be used cautiously by patients who may develop bleeding complications secondary to injections, including patients with thrombocytopenia or those taking anticoagulants. It also should be used cautiously by patients who use poor-quality injection technique, including patients with psychiatric disorders, obese patients (who may not be able to reach or see the penile injection site), patients who are blind, and patients with severe arthritis.

Intraurethral Alprostadil

Efficacy ❿ Intraurethral alprostadil inserts are marketed as MUSE, which contains a medication pellet inside a prefilled urethral applicator. Multiple studies show this product has an overall effectiveness rate of 43% to 65%[5] compared with 70% to 90% for intracavernosal alprostadil. Its decreased effectiveness and inconvenient administration method have resulted in this product being considered a third-line treatment option for patients with erectile dysfunction. However, some patients respond to intraurethral alprostadil even though they did not respond to intracavernosal alprostadil.[60]

Intraurethral alprostadil has been combined with an adjustable penile constriction band to improve treatment response.[61]

Pharmacokinetics Following intraurethral instillation, alprostadil is absorbed quickly through the urethra, into the corpus spongiosum, and then into the corpora cavernosum. As much as 90% of each dose is absorbed by the urethra and corpus spongiosum in less than 10 minutes, with peak absorption occurring in 20 to 25 minutes. An estimated 20% of each dose is delivered to the corpora cavernosum. As with intracavernosal injections of alprostadil, any drug absorbed into the systemic circulation is rapidly metabolized on first pass through the lungs.

The onset after intraurethral insertion is similar to that of intracavernosal injection, 5 to 10 minutes.

Dosing The usual dose of intraurethral alprostadil is 125 to 1,000 mcg. The dose should be administered 5 to 10 minutes before sexual intercourse. No more than two doses per day are recommended. Before administration, the patient should be advised to empty his bladder, voiding completely.

Similar to intracavernosal injection treatments, intraurethral insertion of alprostadil requires good manual and visual skills to minimize the risk of urethral injuries. Intraurethral alprostadil is supplied in a prefilled intraurethral applicator. The patient should void first. With one hand the patient holds the glans penis, and with the other hand the patient inserts the intraurethral applicator 0.5 inch (1.3 cm) into the urethra. The drug pellet is then pushed into the urethra. The penis should be massaged to enhance drug dissolution in the urethral fluids and drug absorption (Fig. 92–6).

Adverse Effects The urethra can be injured because of improper administration technique. Injuries can lead to urethral stricture and difficulty voiding. Patients should receive complete education about optimal administration procedures before starting treatment.

Urethral pain has been reported in 24% to 32% of patients. Usually it is mild and does not require discontinuation of treatment. Female sexual partners may experience vaginal burning, itching, or pain, which probably is related to transfer of alprostadil from the man's urethra to the woman's vagina during intercourse.

Prolonged painful erections (priapism) have been rarely reported. Syncope and dizziness have been reported rarely (only 2%–3% of patients) and likely are related to use of excessively large doses.

CLINICAL CONTROVERSY

Although combinations of proerectogenic drugs (e.g., sildenafil plus alprostadil intracavernosal injection) may be used by some patients who do not respond to a single agent, such combinations are not recommended by the FDA and may lead to prolonged erections and priapism.

■ UNAPPROVED AGENTS

A variety of other commercially available and investigational agents have been used for management of erectile dysfunction. Although it is beyond the scope of this chapter to discuss all of them, some of the more commonly used agents are discussed here.

Trazodone

The mechanism by which trazodone produces an erection is not clear. It likely acts peripherally to antagonize α-adrenergic receptors. As a result, a predominant cholinergic effect results, which causes peripheral arteriolar vasodilation and relaxation of cavernosal tissues, enhancing blood filling of the corpora. Intracavernosal injection of trazodone in experimental studies supports this likely mechanism.[62]

Although some clinical trials suggested that trazodone 50 to 200 mg daily by mouth might be effective in the management of erectile dysfunction, these trials were generally poorly controlled, were nonrandomized, included small samples treated for short time periods, and did not include validated objective parameters of response.[62,63]

The adverse effects of trazodone, when used for erectile dysfunction, are similar to those reported with trazodone when used to treat depression and include dry mouth, sedation, and dizziness.

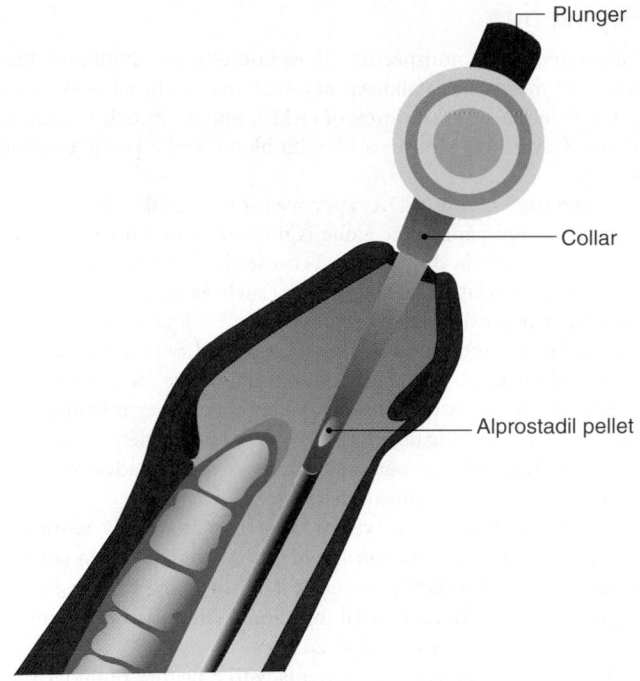

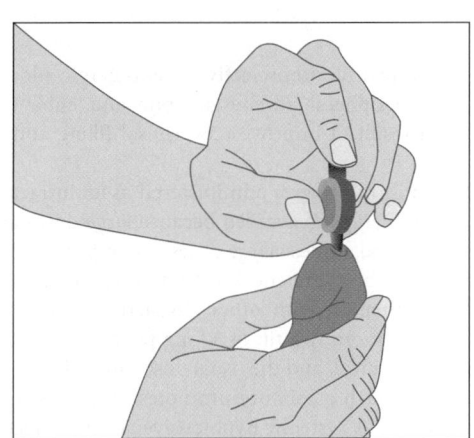

FIGURE 92-6. Technique for administration of intraurethral alprostadil with a medicated urethral system for erection applicator. *(From Muse [package insert]. Mountain View, CA: Vivus, Inc.; 2003. Data from http://www. vivus.com.)*

Yohimbine

Yohimbine, a tree-bark derivative also known as *yohimbe*, is widely used as an aphrodisiac. Yohimbine is a central α_2-adrenergic antagonistic that increases catecholamines and improves mood. Some investigators believe that yohimbine has peripheral proerectogenic effects. Yohimbine may reduce peripheral α-adrenergic tone, thereby permitting a predominant cholinergic tone, which could result in a vasodilatory response.[5,64] The usual oral dose is 5.4 mg 3 times per day.

A controlled clinical trial has shown that high-dose yohimbine (100 mg daily) is no more effective than placebo.[65] Based on a meta-analysis of published studies that came to the same conclusion, the American Urological Association has cautioned against the use of yohimbine.[24] In addition, yohimbine can cause many systemic adverse effects, including anxiety, insomnia, tachycardia, and hypertension.

Papaverine

Papaverine is a nonspecific phosphodiesterase inhibitor that decreases metabolic catabolism of cAMP in cavernosal tissue. As a result of enhanced tissue levels of cAMP, smooth muscle relaxation occurs. Cavernosal sinusoids fill with blood, and a penile erection results.

Papaverine is not FDA approved for erectile dysfunction. Intracavernosal papaverine alone is not commonly used for management of erectile dysfunction because the large doses required produce dose-related adverse effects, such as priapism, corporal fibrosis, hypotension, and hepatotoxicity.[58,66] Papaverine is more often administered in lower doses combined with phentolamine and/or alprostadil. A variety of formulas have been used, but no one mixture has been proven better than other mixtures (see Table 92–6). Combination formulations are considered safer and are associated with the potential for fewer serious adverse effects than high doses of any one of these agents.

A portion of each papaverine dose is systemically absorbed, and its prolonged plasma half-life of 1 hour contributes to adverse effects. The usual dose of papaverine is 7.5 to 60 mg when used as a single agent for intracavernosal injection. When used in combination, the dose decreases to 0.5 to 20 mg.

If treated with papaverine, patients with a history of underlying liver disease or alcohol abuse should undergo liver function testing at baseline and every 6 to 12 months during continued treatment.

Phentolamine

Phentolamine is a competitive nonselective α-adrenergic blocking agent. It reduces peripheral adrenergic tone and enhances cholinergic tone. As a result, it improves cavernosal filling and is proerectogenic.

Phentolamine has most often been administered as an intracavernosal injection. Monotherapy is avoided because large doses are required for an erection, and at these large doses systemic hypotensive adverse effects would be prevalent. Most often, phentolamine has been used in combination with other vasoactive agents for intracavernosal administration. A ratio of 30 mg papaverine to 0.5 to 1 mg phentolamine is typical, and the usual dose ranges from 0.1 to 1 mL of the mixture. Such a mixture promotes local effects of phentolamine and minimizes systemic hypotensive adverse effects.

Hypotension is the most common adverse effect of intracavernosal phentolamine. It is more common and more severe with large doses or in patients with poor injection technique who have injected into a vein (rather than the cavernosa). Prolonged erections have been reported in patients who used excessive doses of intracavernosal medications in combination.

■ PENILE PROSTHESES

Surgical insertion of a penile prosthesis is the most invasive treatment of erectile dysfunction. It is reserved for patients who do not respond to or who are not candidates for less invasive oral or injectable treatments.

Prosthesis insertion requires anesthesia and skilled urologists. Two prostheses are widely used: malleable and inflatable. Malleable or semirigid prostheses consist of two bendable rods that are inserted into the corpora cavernosa. The patient appears to have a permanent erection after the procedure; the patient is able to bend the penis into position at the time of intercourse.

The inflatable prosthesis has several mechanical parts. The inflatable prosthesis produces a more natural erection. The patient develops an erection only when the device is activated. Some newer advances in inflatable prosthesis technology have resulted in

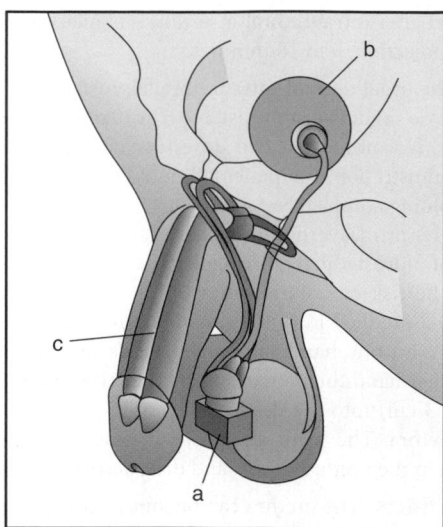

FIGURE 92-7. Example of surgically implanted penile prosthesis. (a, activation mechanism; b, reservoir with fluid for inflating prosthesis; c, inflatable rods in corpora.) (From http://kidney.niddk.nih.gov/kudiseases/pubs/impotence.)

devices with fewer mechanical parts. These devices can be placed during shorter surgical procedures and have a low 5-year mechanical failure rate (6%–10%) as compared with the original inflatable prostheses (Fig. 92–7).[67]

Penile prostheses provide penile rigidity suitable for vaginal intercourse and are associated with a greater than 90% patient satisfaction rate, which is generally higher than that observed with any other drug treatment or VED.[68] The surgical success rate after insertion is 82% to 98%.[5]

Adverse effects of prosthesis insertion can occur early or late after the surgical procedure. The most common early complication is infection. Late complications include mechanical failure of the prosthesis, particularly when an inflatable prosthesis has been inserted. With improved technology, the mechanical failure rate has decreased to 5%.[5] Other late complications include erosion of the rods through the penis or late-onset infection. Although some salvage procedures have been devised, in many cases the prosthesis requires removal.

EVALUATION OF THERAPEUTIC OUTCOMES

The primary therapeutic outcomes of specific treatments for erectile dysfunction include (1) improvement in the quantity and quality of penile erections suitable for intercourse and (2) avoidance of adverse drug reactions and drug interactions.

At baseline and after the patient has completed a clinical trial period of 1 to 3 weeks with a specific treatment for erectile dysfunction, the physician should conduct assessments to determine whether the quality and quantity of penile erections has improved. A patient's level of satisfaction is highly individualized, depending on his lifestyle and expectations. Therefore, a patient who has successful intercourse once per week might be completely satisfied, whereas another patient might judge this to be unsatisfactory. Patients with unrealistic expectations in this regard must be identified and counseled by clinicians to avoid adverse effects of excessive use of erectogenic agents.

Failure to improve the quality and quantity of penile erections suitable for intercourse after an appropriate clinical trial period with a specific treatment for erectile dysfunction occurs in a significant percentage of patients. In this case, physicians generally take the following steps in order:

1. Ensure that the patient has been prescribed a maximum tolerated dose and has an adequate clinical trial of a specific treatment before discarding it as ineffective.

2. Switch to another drug (see Fig. 92–4).

3. Reserve surgical treatment for patients who do not respond to drug treatment.

CONCLUSIONS

Erectile dysfunction is a common disorder of aging men. Its incidence is higher in patients with underlying medical disorders that compromise the vascular, neurologic, hormonal, or psychogenic systems necessary for a normal penile erection. Medications are common causes of erectile dysfunction. By correcting the underlying etiology, erectile dysfunction can often be reversed without the use of specific treatments.

When treatments of erectile dysfunction are needed, the least invasive forms of treatment should be used first because they produce the lowest incidence of serious adverse effects. VEDs or phosphodiesterase inhibitors are considered first-line treatments. If these treatments fail, intracavernosal alprostadil injection therapy can be initiated. If this treatment fails, the patient can attempt a combination of intracavernosal alprostadil plus VED, combination intracavernosal therapy, or intraurethral alprostadil. If this treatment fails, the patient may require insertion of a penile prosthesis.

Some insurance companies do not reimburse for drug treatments for erectile dysfunction, so cost is an important issue for some patients.

Clinicians should provide clear and simple advice. Patient confidentiality and privacy, which are extremely important to men with erectile dysfunction, should be maintained at all times.

ABBREVIATIONS

cAMP: cyclic adenosine monophosphate

cGMP: cyclic guanosine monophosphate

VED: vacuum erection device

REFERENCES

1. NIH Consensus Conference. NIH Consensus Development Panel on Impotence. Impotence. JAMA 1993;270:83–90.

2. Johannes CB, Aranjo AB, Feldman HA, et al. Incidence of erectile dysfunction in men 40–69 years old: Longitudinal results from the Massachusetts Male Aging Study. J Urol 2000;163:460–463.

3. Bacon CG, Mittleman MA, Kawach I, et al. Sexual function in men older than 50 years of age: Results from the Health Professionals Follow-up Study. Ann Intern Med 2003;139:161–168.

4. Lindau ST, Schumm LP, Laumann EO, et al. A study of sexuality and health among older adults in the United States. N Engl J Med 2007;357:762–774.

5. McVary KT. Erectile dysfunction. N Engl J Med 2007;357:2472–2481.

6. Carrier S. Pharmacology of phosphodiesterase inhibitors. Can J Urol 2003;10(Suppl 1):12–16.

7. Araujo AB, Esche GR, Kupelian V, et al. Prevalence of symptomatic androgen deficiency in men. J Clin Endocrinol Metab 2007;92:4241–4247.

8. Travison TG, Araujo AB, O'Donnell AB, et al. A population-level decline in serum testosterone levels in American men. J Clin Endocrinol Metab 2007;92:196–202.

9. Thomas A, Woodard C, Rovner ES, Wein AJ. Urologic complications of nonurologic medications. Urol Clin North Am 2003;30:123–131.

10. Lee M, Sharifi R. Sexual dysfunction in males. In Tisdale JE, Miller DA, eds. Drug-Induced Diseases: Prevention, Detection, and Management. Bethesda, MD: ASHP, 2005:455–467.

11. Balon R. SSRI-associated sexual dysfunction. Am J Psych 2006;163:1504–1509.

12. Lobo JR, Nehra A. Clinical evaluation of erectile dysfunction in the era of PDE-5 inhibitors. Urol Clin North Am 2005;32:447–455.

13. Rosen RC, Riley A, Wagner G, et al. The International Index of Erectile Function (IIEF): A multidimensional scale for assessment of erectile dysfunction. Urology 1997;49:822–830.

14. Buvat J, Lemaire A. Endocrine screening in 1,022 men with erectile dysfunction: Clinical significance and cost-effective strategy. J Urol 1997;158:1764–1767.

15. Zitzman M, Faber S, Nieschlag E. Association of specific symptoms and metabolic risks with serum testosterone in older men. J Clin Endocrinol Metab 2006;91:4335–4345.

16. Inman BA, St. Souver JL, Jacobson DJ, et al. A population-based longitudinal study of erectile dysfunction and future coronary artery disease. Mayo Clin Proceed 2009;84:108–113.

17. Nehra A. Erectile dysfunction and cardiovascular disease: efficacy and safety of phosphodiesterase type 5 inhibitors in men with both conditions. Mayo Clin Proceed 2009;84:139–148.

18. Burnett AL. Erectile dysfunction. J Urol 2006;175:S25–S31.

19. Rosen RC, Jackson G, Kostis JB. Erectile dysfunction and cardiac disease: Recommendations of the Second Princeton Conference. Curr Urol Rep 2006;7:490–496.

20. Rosen RC, Friedman M, Kostis JB. Lifestyle management of erectile dysfunction: The role of cardiovascular and concomitant risk factors. Am J Cardiol 2005;96(Suppl):76M–79M.

21. Kostis JB, Jackson G, Rosen R, et al. Sexual dysfunction and cardiac risk (the Second Princeton Consensus Conference). Am J Cardiol 2005;96:313–321.

22. Bacon CG, Mittleman MA, Kawachi I, et al. A prospective study of risk factors for erectile dysfunction. J Urol 2006;176:217–221.

23. Bacon CG, Mittleman MA, Kawachi I, et al. Sexual function in men older than 50 years of age: Results from the health professionals follow-up study. Ann Intern Med 2003;139:161–168.

24. American Urological Association Guideline on the Management of Erectile Dysfunction: Diagnosis and Treatment Recommendations; updated 2006. http://www.auanet.org/content/guidelines-and-quality-care/clinical-guidelines.cfm?sub=ed.

25. Jannini EA, Isidori AM, Gravina GL, et al. The Endotrial Study: a spontaneous, open label, randomized, multicenter cross-over study on the efficacy of sildenafil, tadalafil, and vardenafil in the treatment of erectile dysfunction. J Sex Med 2009;6:2547–2560.

26. Carson CC. PDE5 inhibitors: Are there differences? Can J Urol 2006;13(Suppl 1):34–39.

27. McCullough AR, Barada JH, Fawzy A, et al. Achieving treatment optimization with sildenafil citrate (Viagra) in patients with erectile dysfunction. Urology 2002;60(2 Suppl 2):28–38.

28. Guay AT. Optimizing response to phosphodiesterase therapy: Impact of risk-factor management. J Androl 2003;24(Suppl):S59–S62.

29. Brisson TE, Broderick GA, Thiel DD, et al. Vardenafil rescue rates of sildenafil nonresponders: Objective assessment of 327 patients with erectile dysfunction. Urology 2006;68:397–401.

30. Padma-Nathan H, Eardley I, Kloner RA, et al. A 4-year update on the safety of sildenafil citrate (Viagra). Urology 2002;60(Suppl 2B):67–90.

31. Carson CC. Long-term use of sildenafil. Expert Opin Pharmacother 2003;4:397–405.

32. Hellstrom WJ, Gittleman M, Karlin G, et al. Sustained efficacy and tolerability of vardenafil, a highly potent selective phosphodiesterase type 5 inhibitor in men without erectile dysfunction: results of a randomized, double-blind 26 week placebo-controlled pivotal trial. Urology 2003;61(4 suppl 1):8–14.

33. Shabsigh R, Seftel AD, Rosen RC, et al. Review of time of onset and duration of clinical efficacy of phosphodiesterase type 5 inhibitors in treatment of erectile dysfunction. Urology 2006;68:689–696.

34. Porst H, Giuliano F, Glina S. et al. Evaluation of the efficacy and safety of once-a-day dosing of tadalafil 5 mg and 10 mg in the treatment of erectile dysfunction: results of a multicenter, randomized, double-blind, placebo-controlled trial. Eur Urol 2006;50:351–359.

35. Donatucci CF, Wong DG, Giuliano F, et al. Efficacy and safety of tadalafil once daily: consideration for the practical application of a daily dosing option. Curr Med Res Opin 2008;24:3383–3392.

36. Hellstrom WJG, Kendirci M. Type 5 phosphodiesterase inhibitors: Curing erectile dysfunction. Eur Urol 2006;49:942–945.

37. Carson CC. Long-term use of sildenafil. Expert Opin Pharmacother 2003;4:397–405.

38. Carson CC, Rajfer J, Eardley I, et al. The efficacy and safety of tadalafil: an update. BJU Int 2004;93:1276–1281.

39. Laties A, Sharlip I. Ocular safety in patients using sildenafil citrate therapy for erectile dysfunction. J Sex Med 2006;3:12–27.

40. Wooltorton E. Visual loss with erectile dysfunction medication. CMAJ 2006;175:355

41. Gresser U, Gleiter CH. Erectile dysfunction: comparison of efficacy and side effects of the PDE-5 inhibitors sildenafil, vardenafil, and tadalafil-review of the literature. Eur J Med Res 2002;7:435–446.

42. Kloner RA, Hutter AM, Emmick JT. Time course of the interaction between tadalafil and nitrates. J Am Coll Cardiol 2003;42:1855–1860.

43. Tran D, Howles LG. Cardiovascular safety of sildenafil. Drug Saf 2003;26:453–460.

44. Kloner RA. Pharmacology and drug interaction effects of the phosphodiesterase 5 inhibitors: Focus on α blocker interactions. Am J Cardiol 2005;96(Suppl):42M-46M.

45. Kloner RA, Jackson G, Emmick JT, et al. Interaction between the phosphodiesterase 5 inhibitor, tadalafil, and 2 alpha-blockers, doxazosin and tamsulosin in healthy normotensive men. J Urol 2004;172:1935–1940.

46. Giuliano F, Kaplan SA, Cabanis MJ, Astruc B. Hemodynamic interaction study between the alpha$_1$ blocker alfuzosin and the phosphodiesterase-5 inhibitor tadalafil in middle-aged healthy male subjects. Urology 2006;67:1199–1204.

47. Carson CC. Combination of phosphodiesterase-5 inhibitors and α blockers in patients with benign prostatic hyperplasia: Treatments of lower urinary tract symptoms, erectile dysfunction, or both? BJU Int 2006;97(Suppl 2):39–43.

48. Ng C-F, Wong A, Cheng C-W, et al. Effect of vardenafil on blood pressure profile of patients with erectile dysfunction concomitantly treated with doxazosin gastrointestinal therapeutic system for benign prostatic hyperplasia. J Urol 2008;180:1042–1046.

49. Muirhead GJ, Wulff MB, Fielding H, et al. Pharmacokinetic interactions between sildenafil and saquinavir/ritonavir. Br J Clin Pharmacol 2000;50:99–107.

50. Sekar V, Lefebvre E, De Marez T, et al. Effect of repeated doses of darunavir plus low dose ritonavir on the pharmacokinetics of sildenafil in healthy male subjects: phase I randomized open-label, two way crossover study. Clin Drug Investig 2008;28:479–485.

51. Carson CC. Phosphodiesterase type 5 inhibitors: state of the therapeutic class. Urol Clin North Am 2007;34:507–515.

52. Gore JL, Swerdloff RS, Rajfer J. Androgen deficiency in the etiology and treatment of erectile dysfunction. Urol Clin North Am 2005;32:457–468.

53. Morales A, Tenover JL. Androgen deficiency in the aging male: When, who, and how to investigate and treat. Urol Clin North Am 2002;29:975–982.

54. Bolona ER, Uraga MV, Haddad RM, et al. Testosterone use in men with sexual dysfunction: a systematic review and meta-analysis of randomized placebo-controlled trials. Mayo Clin Proceed 2007;82:20–28.

55. Jordan WP. Allergy and topical irritation associated with transdermal testosterone administration: A comparison of scrotal and nonscrotal transdermal systems. Am J Contact Dermatol 1997;8:108–113.

56. Kendirci M, Tanriverdi O, Trost L, et al. Management of sildenafil treatment failures. Curr Opin Urol 2006;16:449–459.

57. Nehra A. Oral and non-oral combination therapy for erectile dysfunction. Rev Urol 2007;9:99–105.

58. Chen Y, Dai Y, Wang R. Treatment strategies for diabetic patients suffering from erectile dysfunction. Expert Opin Pharmacother 2008;9:257–260.

59. Albaugh J, Ferrans CE. Patient reported pain with initial intracavernosal injection. J Sex Med 2009;6:513–519.

60. Engel JD, McVary KT. Transurethral alprostadil as therapy for patients who withdrew from or failed prior intracavernous injection therapy. Urology 1998;51:687–692.

61. Jaffe JS, Antell MR, Greenstein M, et al. Use of intraurethral alprostadil in patients not responding to sildenafil citrate. Urology 2004;63:951–954.

62. Fink HA, MacDonald R, Rutks IR, Wilt TJ. Trazodone for erectile dysfunction: A systematic review and meta analysis. BJU Int 2003;92:441–446.

63. Vitezic D, Pelcic JM. Erectile dysfunction: Oral pharmacotherapy options. Int J Clin Pharmacol Ther 2002;40:393–403.

64. Tamier R, Mechanick JI. Dietary supplements and nutraceuticals in the management of andrologic disorders. Endocrinol Metab Clin North Am 2007;36:533–552.

65. Teloken C, Rhoden EL, Sogari P, et al. Therapeutic effects of high-dose yohimbine hydrochloride on organic erectile dysfunction. J Urol 1998;159:122–124.

66. Brown SL, Haas CA, Koehler M, et al. Hepatotoxicity related to intracavernous pharmacotherapy with papaverine. Urology 1998;52:844–847.

67. Henry GD, Wilson SK. Updates in inflatable penile prosthesis. Urol Clin North Am 2007;34:535–547.

68. Rajpurkar A, Dhabuwala CB. Comparison of satisfaction rates and erectile function in patients treated with sildenafil, intracavernous prostaglandin E1 and penile implant surgery for erectile dysfunction in urology practice. J Urol 2003;2003;170:159–163.

CHAPTER 93

Benign Prostatic Hyperplasia

MARY LEE

KEY CONCEPTS

❶ Although symptomatic benign prostatic hyperplasia (BPH) is rare in men younger than 50 years of age, it is very common in men 60 years and older because of androgen-driven growth in the size of the prostate. Symptoms commonly result from both static and dynamic factors.

❷ BPH symptoms may be exacerbated by medications, including antihistamines, phenothiazines, tricyclic antidepressants, and anticholinergic agents. In these cases, discontinuing the causative agent can relieve symptoms.

❸ Specific treatments for BPH include watchful waiting, drug therapy, and surgery.

❹ For patients with mild disease who are asymptomatic or have mildly bothersome symptoms and no complications of BPH disease, no specific treatment is indicated. These patients can be managed with watchful waiting. Watchful waiting includes behavior modification and return visits to the physician at 12-month intervals for assessment of worsening symptoms or signs of BPH.

❺ If symptoms progress to a moderate or severe level, drug therapy or surgery is indicated. Drug therapy with an α_1-adrenergic antagonist is an interim measure that relieves voiding symptoms. In select patients with prostates of at least 40 g, 5α-reductase inhibitors delay symptom progression and reduce the incidence of BPH-related complications.

❻ All α_1-adrenergic antagonists are equally effective in relieving BPH symptoms. Older second-generation immediate-release formulations of α_1-adrenergic antagonists (e.g., terazosin, doxazosin) can cause adverse cardiovascular effects, mainly first-dose syncope, orthostatic hypotension, and dizziness. For patients who can not tolerate hypotensive effects of the second-generation agents, the third-generation, pharmacologically uroselective agents (e.g., tamsulosin, silodosin) are good alternatives. An extended-release formulation of alfuzosin, a second-generation, functionally uroselective agent, has fewer cardiovascular adverse effects than immediate-release formulations of terazosin or doxazosin; however, whether extended-release doxazosin, alfuzosin, or silodosin have the same cardiovascular safety profile as tamsulosin is unclear.

❼ 5α-Reductase inhibitors are useful primarily for patients with large prostates greater than 40 g who wish to avoid surgery and can not tolerate the side effects of α_1-adrenergic antagonists. 5α-Reductase inhibitors have a slow onset of action, taking up to 6 months to exert maximal clinical effects, which is a disadvantage of their use. In addition, decreased libido, erectile dysfunction, and ejaculation disorders are common adverse effects, which may be troublesome problems in sexually active patients.

❽ Surgery is indicated for moderate to severe symptoms of BPH for patients who do not respond to or do not tolerate drug therapy or for patients with complications of BPH. It is the most effective mode of treatment in that it relieves symptoms in the greatest number of men with BPH. However, the two most widely used techniques, transurethral resection of the prostate and open prostatectomy, are associated with the highest rates of complications, including retrograde ejaculation and erectile dysfunction. Therefore, minimally invasive surgical procedures are often desired by patients. These relieve symptoms and are associated with a lower rate of adverse effects, but they have a higher reoperation rate than the gold standard procedures.

❾ Although widely used in Europe for treatment of BPH, phytotherapy should be avoided. Studies of these herbal medicines are inconclusive, and the purity of available products is questionable.

Benign prostatic hyperplasia (BPH) is the most common benign neoplasm of American men. A nearly ubiquitous condition among elderly men, BPH is of major societal concern, given the large number of men affected, the progressive nature of the condition, and the healthcare costs associated with it.

This chapter discusses BPH and its available treatments: watchful waiting, α_1-adrenergic antagonists, 5α-reductase inhibitors, and surgery. The limitations of phytotherapy are described.

EPIDEMIOLOGY

❶ According to the results of autopsy studies, approximately 80% of elderly men develop microscopic evidence of BPH. About half of the patients with microscopic changes develop an enlarged prostate gland, and as a result, they develop symptoms including difficulty emptying the contents from the urinary bladder. Approximately half of symptomatic patients eventually require treatment.

The peak incidence of clinical BPH occurs at 63 to 65 years of age. Symptomatic disease is uncommon in men younger than 50 years, but some urinary voiding symptoms are present by the time men turn 60 years of age. The Boston Area Normative Aging Study estimated that the cumulative incidence of clinical BPH was 78% for patients at age 80 years.[1] Similarly, the Baltimore Longitudinal Study of Aging projected that approximately 60% of men at least 60 years old develop clinical BPH.[2]

NORMAL PROSTATE PHYSIOLOGY

Located anterior to the rectum, the prostate is a small heart-shaped, chestnut-sized gland located below the urinary bladder. It surrounds the proximal urethra like a doughnut.

Soft, symmetric, and mobile on palpation, a normal prostate gland in an adult man weighs 15 to 20 g. Physical examination of the prostate must be done by digital rectal examination (i.e., the prostate is manually palpated by inserting a finger into the rectum). Thus, the prostate is examined through the rectal mucosa.

The prostate has two major functions: (1) to secrete fluids that make up a portion (20%–40%) of the ejaculate volume and (2) to provide secretions with antibacterial effect possibly related to its high concentration of zinc.[2]

At birth, the prostate is the size of a pea and weighs approximately 1 g. The prostate remains that size until the boy reaches puberty. At that time, the prostate undergoes its first growth spurt, growing to its normal adult size of 15 to 20 g by the time the young man is 25 to 30 years of age. The prostate remains this size until the patient reaches age 40 years, when a second growth spurt begins and continues for the rest of his lifetime. During this period, the prostate can quadruple in size or grow even larger.

The prostate gland comprises three types of tissue: epithelial tissue, stromal tissue, and the capsule. Epithelial tissue, also known as *glandular tissue*, produces prostatic secretions. These secretions are delivered into the urethra during ejaculation and contribute to the total ejaculate volume. Androgens stimulate epithelial tissue growth. Stromal tissue, also known as *smooth muscle tissue*, is embedded with α_1-adrenergic receptors. Stimulation of these receptors by norepinephrine causes smooth muscle contraction, which results in an extrinsic compression of the urethra, reduction of the urethral lumen, and decreased urinary bladder emptying. The normal prostate is composed of a higher amount of stromal tissue than epithelial tissue, as reflected by a stromal-to-epithelial tissue ratio of 2:1. This ratio is exaggerated to 5:1 for patients with BPH, which explains why α_1-adrenergic antagonists are quickly effective in symptomatic management and why 5α-reductase inhibitors reduce an enlarged prostate gland by only 25%.[2,3] The capsule, or outer shell of the prostate, is composed of fibrous connective tissue and smooth muscle, which also is embedded with α_1-adrenergic receptors. When stimulated with norepinephrine, the capsule contracts around the urethra (Fig. 93–1).

Testosterone is the principal testicular androgen in males, whereas androstenedione is the principal adrenal androgen. These two hormones are responsible for penile and scrotal enlargement, increased muscle mass, and maintenance of the normal male libido. These androgens are converted by 5α-reductase in target cells to dihydrotestosterone (DHT), an active metabolite. Two types of 5α-reductase exist. Type I enzyme is localized to sebaceous glands in the frontal scalp, liver, and skin. DHT produced at these target tissues causes acne and increased body and facial hair. Type II enzyme is localized to the prostate, genital tissue, and hair follicles of the scalp. In the prostate, DHT induces growth and enlargement of the gland.[3]

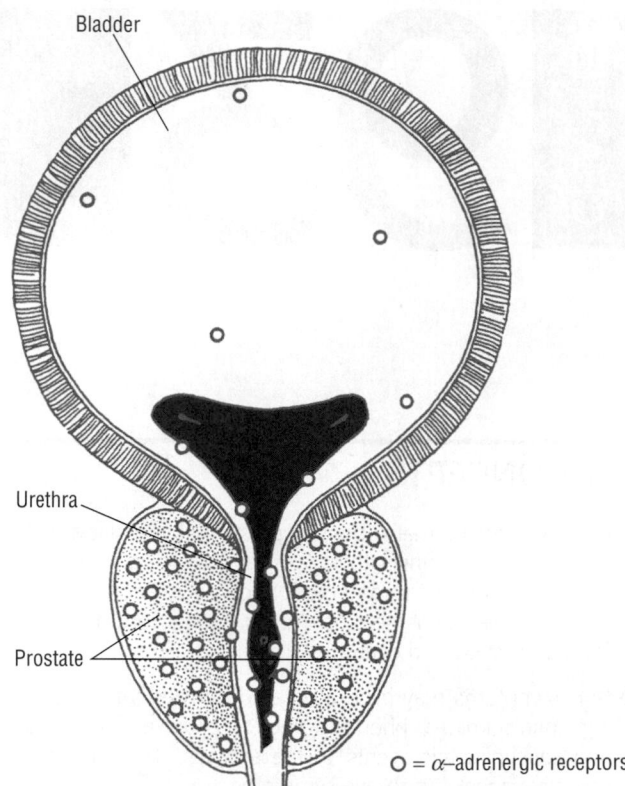

FIGURE 93-1. Representation of the anatomy of and α-adrenergic receptor distribution in the prostate, urethra, and bladder. *(Western Journal of Medicine 1994;161:501. Reproduced with permission from the BMJ Publishing Group.)*

In prostate cells, DHT has greater affinity for intraprostatic androgen receptors than testosterone, and DHT forms a more stable complex with the androgen receptor. Thus, DHT is considered a more potent androgen than testosterone in the prostate. Of note, despite the decrease in testicular androgen production in the aging male, intracellular DHT levels in the prostate remain normal, probably due to increased activity of intraprostatic 5α-reductase.[3]

Estrogen, a product of peripheral metabolism of androgens, is believed to stimulate the growth of the stromal portion of the prostate gland. Estrogens are produced when testosterone and androstenedione are converted by aromatase enzymes in peripheral adipose tissues. In addition, estrogens may induce the androgen receptor.[2] As men age, the ratio of serum levels of testosterone to estrogen decreases as a result of a decline in testosterone production by the testes and increased adipose tissue conversion of androgen to estrogen.

PATHOPHYSIOLOGY

Although the precise pathophysiologic mechanisms causing BPH remain unclear, the role of intraprostatic DHT and type II 5α-reductase in the development of BPH is evidenced by several observations:

- BPH does not develop in men who are castrated before puberty.

- Patients with type II 5α-reductase enzyme deficiency do not develop BPH.

- Castration causes an enlarged prostate to shrink.

- Administration of testosterone to orchiectomized dogs of advanced age produces BPH.

The pathogenesis of BPH is often described as resulting from both static and dynamic factors. Static factors relate to anatomic enlargement of the prostate gland, which produces a physical block at the bladder neck and thereby obstructs urinary outflow. Enlargement of the gland depends on androgen stimulation of epithelial tissue and estrogen stimulation of stromal tissue in the prostate. Dynamic factors relate to excessive α-adrenergic tone of the stromal component of the prostate gland, bladder neck, and posterior urethra, which results in contraction of the prostate gland around the urethra and narrowing of the urethral lumen.

Symptoms of BPH disease may result from static and/or dynamic factors, and this must be recognized when drug therapy is considered. For instance, some patients may present with obstructive voiding symptoms but have prostates of normal size. In these patients, dynamic factors likely are responsible for the symptoms. However, for patients with enlarged prostate glands, static and dynamic factors likely are working in concert to produce the observed symptoms. Moreover, the likelihood of developing moderate to severe voiding symptoms is directly related to the increasing size of the prostate gland.[4]

Static factors may be accentuated if the patient becomes stressed or is in pain. In these situations, increased α-adrenergic tone may precipitate excessive contraction of prostatic stromal tissue. When the stressful event resolves, voiding symptoms often improve.[2]

MEDICATION-RELATED SYMPTOMS

❷ Medications in several pharmacologic categories should be avoided for patients with BPH because they may exacerbate symptoms.[5] Testosterone replacement regimens, used to treat primary or secondary hypogonadism, deliver additional substrate that can be metabolized to DHT by the prostate. Although no cases of BPH have been reported because of exogenous testosterone administration, cautious use is advised for patients with prostatic enlargement. α-Adrenergic agonists, used as oral or intranasal decongestants (e.g., pseudoephedrine, ephedrine, or phenylephrine), can stimulate α-adrenergic receptors in the prostate, resulting in muscle contraction. By decreasing the caliber of the urethral lumen, bladder emptying may be compromised. Drugs with significant anticholinergic adverse effects (e.g., antihistamines, phenothiazines, tricyclic antidepressants, or anticholinergic drugs used as antispasmodics or to treat Parkinson disease) may decrease contractility of the urinary bladder detrusor muscle. For patients with BPH who have a narrowed urethral lumen, loss of effective detrusor contraction could result in acute urinary retention, particularly for patients with significantly enlarged prostate glands. Diuretics, particularly in large doses, can produce polyuria, which may present as urinary frequency, similar to that experienced by patients with BPH.

CLINICAL PRESENTATION

Patients with BPH can present with a variety of symptoms and signs of disease. All symptoms of BPH can be divided into two categories: obstructive and irritative.

Obstructive symptoms, also known as *prostatism* or *bladder outlet obstruction*, result when dynamic and/or static factors reduce bladder emptying. The force of the urinary stream becomes

---

CLINICAL PRESENTATION OF BENIGN PROSTATIC HYPERPLASIA

General

- Patient is in no acute distress unless he has moderate to severe symptoms or complications of BPH

Symptoms

- Urinary frequency, urgency, intermittency, nocturia, decreased force of stream, hesitancy, and straining

Signs

- Digital rectal examination reveals an enlarged prostate (>20 g) with no nodules or indurations; prostate is soft, symmetric, and mobile

Laboratory Tests

- Increased blood urea nitrogen (BUN) and serum creatinine with long-standing, untreated bladder outlet obstruction, elevated prostate-specific antigen (PSA) level

Other Diagnostic Tests

- Increased American Urological Association (AUA) Symptom Score, decreased urinary flow rate (<10 mL/s), and increased postvoid residual (PVR) urine volume

---

diminished, urinary flow rate decreases, and bladder emptying is incomplete and slow. Patients report urinary hesitancy and straining and a weak urine stream. Urine dribbles out of the penis, and the urinary bladder always feels full, even after patients have voided. Some patients state that they need to press on their bladder to force out the urine. In severe cases, patients may go into urinary retention when bladder emptying is not possible. In these cases, suprapubic pain can result from bladder overdistension.

Approximately 50% to 80% of patients have irritative voiding symptoms, which typically occur late in the disease course. Irritative voiding symptoms result from long-standing obstruction at the bladder neck. To compensate, the bladder muscle undergoes hypertrophy so that it can generate a greater contractile force to empty urine past the anatomic obstruction at the bladder neck. Although initially helpful, decompensation eventually occurs, and the hypertrophied bladder muscle is no longer able to generate adequate contractile force as it becomes hypersensitive and ineffective in storing urine. As a result, small amounts of urine irritate the bladder and initiate a bladder emptying response. Patients complain of urinary frequency and urgency. Bedwetting or clothes wetting occurs. Patients report waking up every 1 to 2 hours at night to void (nocturia), which significantly reduces quality of life.

Symptoms of BPH vary over time. Symptoms may improve, remain stable, or worsen spontaneously. Thus, BPH is not necessarily a progressive disease; in fact, some patients experience symptom regression. Between one and two thirds of men with mild disease stabilize or improve without treatment over 2.5 to 5 years.[2] However, other patients experience a slow progression of disease.

Collectively, obstructive and irritative voiding symptoms and their impact on a patient's quality of life are referred to as *lower urinary tract symptoms* (LUTS). However, LUTS is not pathognomonic for BPH and may be caused by other diseases, such as neurogenic bladder and urinary tract infection.[2]

Another presentation of BPH is silent prostatism. Patients have obstructive or irritative voiding symptoms but adapt to them and do not voluntarily complain about them. Such patients do not present for medical treatment until complications of BPH disease arise or a spouse brings in a symptomatic patient for medical care.

BPH can be a progressive disease, although the rate of progression is variable among patients.[2] When BPH progresses, it can produce complications that include the following:

- Acute, painful urinary retention, which can lead to acute renal failure
- Persistent gross hematuria when tissue growth exceeds its blood supply
- Overflow urinary incontinence or unstable bladder
- Recurrent urinary tract infection that results from urinary stasis
- Bladder diverticula
- Bladder stones
- Chronic renal failure from long-standing bladder outlet obstruction

Approximately 17% to 20% of patients with symptomatic BPH require treatment because of disease complications.[6] Older men with large prostates greater than 40 g are three times more likely to have severe symptoms or suffer from acute urinary retention and to require prostatectomy than patients with smaller prostates.[7,8] Thus, a serum PSA level of 1.4 ng/mL (1.4 mcg/L) has been used as a surrogate marker for an enlarged prostate gland to identify patients at risk for developing complications of BPH disease[6] and has been used to guide selection of the most appropriate treatment modality in some patients.[9,10]

DIAGNOSTIC EVALUATION

Because the obstructive and irritative voiding symptoms associated with BPH are not unique to the disease and can be presenting symptoms of other genitourinary tract disorders, including prostate or bladder cancer, neurogenic bladder, prostatic calculi, or urinary tract infection, the patient presenting with signs and symptoms of BPH must be thoroughly evaluated.

A careful medical history should be taken to ensure that a complete listing of symptoms is collected as well as to identify concomitant disorders that may be contributing to voiding symptoms. The medical history should be followed by a thorough medication history, including all prescription and nonprescription medications and dietary supplements that the patient is taking. Any drugs that could be causing or exacerbating the patient's symptoms should be identified. If possible, the suspected drugs should be discontinued or the dosing regimen modified to ameliorate the voiding symptoms.

The patient should undergo a physical examination, including a digital rectal examination, although the size of the prostate gland may not correspond to symptoms. BPH usually presents as an enlarged, soft, smooth, symmetric gland, greater than 20 g in size. Some patients have only a slightly enlarged gland and yet have bothersome or even serious voiding difficulties. Other patients have an intravesical enlargement of the prostate gland (i.e., the gland grows into the urinary bladder and produces a ball-valve blockage of the bladder neck). This type of prostate enlargement is not palpable on manual examination.

The patient's perception of the severity of BPH symptoms guides selection of a particular treatment modality in a patient. To evaluate the patient's perceptions objectively, validated instruments, such as the AUA Symptom Score, are commonly used. Using the AUA index, the patient rates the "bothersomeness" of seven obstructive and irritative voiding symptoms.[2,11] Each item is rated for severity on a scale from 0 to 5, such that 35 is the maximum score and is consistent with the most severe symptoms. In addition, the patient can complete a voiding diary in which he records the number of voids, the volume of each void, and voiding symptoms for several days. This information is used to evaluate symptom severity and to tailor recommendations for lifestyle modifications that may ameliorate symptoms.

The only clinical laboratory test that must be performed is a urinalysis. Because many of the voiding symptoms of BPH could be caused by other urologic disorders, a urinalysis can help screen for bladder cancer, stones, and infection. To screen for prostate cancer, another common cause of glandular enlargement, a PSA test should be performed for patients aged 40 years or more, with at least a 10-year life expectancy in whom the cost of the test will be outweighed by the potential benefit of diagnosing the disorder.[11]

Additional objective measures of bladder emptying should be performed if surgical treatment is being considered. Measures include peak and average urinary flow rate (normal is at least 10 mL/s). These measures are determined using a uroflowmeter, which checks the rate of urine flow out of the bladder. This is a quick noninvasive outpatient procedure in which the patient is instructed to drink water until his bladder feels full and then the patient's urinary flow is clocked during voiding. A low urinary flow rate (<10 to 12 mL/s) implies failure of bladder emptying or a functional disorder of the detrusor muscle. Thus, the degree of bladder outlet obstruction correlates poorly with peak urinary flow rate.[11]

Another objective measure is PVR urine volume (normal is 0 mL), which is assessed using a transabdominal ultrasound. A high PVR urine volume (>25 to 30 mL) implies failure of bladder emptying and a predisposition for urinary tract infections. Because of a weak correlation among voiding symptoms, prostate size, and urinary flow rate, most physicians use a combination of measures, including the patient's assessment of symptoms along with objective evaluation of urinary outflow and presence of complications of BPH to determine the need for treatment.

Many other tests can be performed if additional information is needed to assess the severity of BPH disease and its complications, to assist in the preoperative assessment of the patient, or to distinguish prostate enlargement due to BPH from that caused by prostate cancer. Tests include a serum BUN and creatinine, voiding cystometrogram, transrectal ultrasound of the prostate, intravenous pyelogram, renal ultrasound, and prostate biopsy.

TREATMENT

Benign Prostatic Hyperplasia

As a disease of symptoms, BPH is treated by relieving bothersome symptoms. Patients usually are stratified into three groups based on disease severity for the purposes of deciding a treatment approach (Table 93–1). However, literature about the natural history of BPH

TABLE 93-1	Categories of BPH Disease Severity Based on Symptoms and Signs	
Disease Severity	**AUA Symptom Score**	**Typical Symptoms and Signs**
Mild	≤7	Asymptomatic Peak urinary flow rate <10 mL/s Postvoid residual urine volume >25–50 mL
Moderate	8–19	All of the above signs plus obstructive voiding symptoms and irritative voiding symptoms (signs of detrusor instability)
Severe	≥20	All of the above plus one or more complications of BPH

AUA, American Urological Association; BPH, benign prostatic hyperplasia; BUN, blood urea nitrogen.

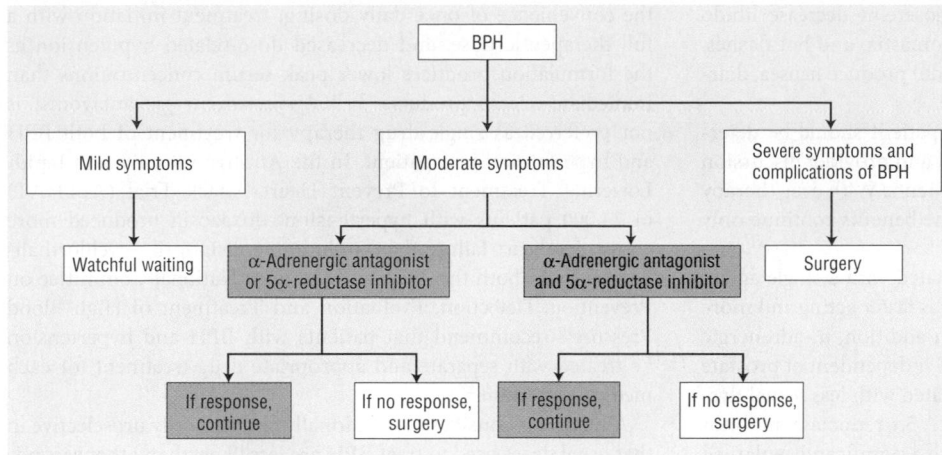

FIGURE 93-2. Management algorithm for benign prostatic hyperplasia (BPH).

and the significant risk of disease complications suggests that physicians also should consider preventing serious complications of BPH and decreasing the need for surgery as goals of treatment for select patients. This is a controversial topic complicated by many issues, including the variable costs of treatment options, the inability to clearly distinguish patients who experience spontaneous regression or disease stabilization from those in whom symptoms progress, and the potential benefit that may occur in a comparatively small number of treated patients.

The AUA Guidelines on Management of Benign Prostatic Hyperplasia is the principal tool used in the United States,[11] and the AUA recommendations are similar to the European[12] and Canadian Practice Guidelines (Fig. 93–2).[13]

❸ All patients should be encouraged to initiate and maintain a heart healthy lifestyle, including a low fat diet, high intake of plenty of fresh fruits and vegetables, regular physical exercise, and no smoking.[14] Specific treatment options include watchful waiting, pharmacologic therapy, and surgical intervention. Although phytotherapy is used by some patients alone or along with conventional medications for BPH, head-to-head comparisons with U.S. Food and Drug Administration (FDA)-approved treatments are lacking; consequently, such herbals can not be recommended at this time.

❹ Patients with mild disease are asymptomatic or have mildly bothersome symptoms and have no complications of BPH disease. For these patients, no specific treatment is indicated. These patients can be managed with watchful waiting, which entails having the patient return for reassessment at yearly intervals. At each return visit, the patient should complete a standardized, validated survey tool to assess severity of symptoms. Watchful waiting should be accompanied by patient education about the disease and behavior modification to avoid practices that exacerbate voiding symptoms. Behavior modification includes restricting fluids close to bedtime, minimizing caffeine and alcohol intake, frequent emptying of the bladder during waking hours (to avoid overflow incontinence and urgency), and avoiding drugs that could exacerbate voiding symptoms.[15] At each visit, physicians should assess the patient's risk of developing acute urinary retention by evaluating the patient's prostate size or using PSA as a surrogate marker of prostate enlargement.[11]

❺ If symptoms progress to the moderate or severe level, or the patient perceives his symptoms to be bothersome, the patient should be offered specific treatment. In these patients, watchful waiting delays—but does not decrease—the need for prostatectomy. In symptomatic patients, watchful waiting can lead to intractable urinary retention, increased PVR urine volumes, and significant voiding symptoms.[16] Recommended treatment options include drug therapy with an α_1-adrenergic antagonist or 5α-reductase

inhibitor, a combination of an α_1-adrenergic antagonist and a 5α-reductase inhibitor, or surgery.

Patients with serious complications of BPH should be offered surgical correction (transurethral or open prostatectomy, or a minimally invasive surgical procedure). Drug therapy is considered an interim measure for such patients because it only delays worsening of complications and the need for surgical intervention.[11,16]

■ PHARMACOLOGIC THERAPY

Drug therapy for BPH can be categorized into three types: agents that relax prostatic smooth muscle (reducing the dynamic factor), agents that interfere with testosterone's stimulatory effect on prostate gland enlargement (reducing the static factor), and combination therapy of an α_1-adrenergic antagonist and a 5α-reductase inhibitor (Table 93–2). Of the agents that relax prostatic smooth muscle, second- and third-generation α_1-adrenergic antagonists have been most widely used. These agents relax the intrinsic urethral sphincter and prostatic smooth muscle, thereby enhancing urinary outflow from the bladder. α_1-Adrenergic antagonists do not reduce prostate size. Of the agents that interfere with testosterone's stimulatory effect on prostate gland size, the only agents approved by the FDA are 5α-reductase inhibitors (e.g., finasteride, dutasteride). Other agents that interfere with androgen stimulation of the prostate have not been popular in the United States because of the many adverse effects associated with their use. The luteinizing hormone-releasing

TABLE 93-2 Medical Treatment Options for Benign Prostatic Hyperplasia

Category	Mechanism	Drug (Brand Name)
Reduces dynamic factor	Blocks α_1-adrenergic receptors in prostatic stromal tissue	Prazosin (Minipress) Alfuzosin (Uroxatral) Terazosin (Hytrin) Doxazosin (Cardura)
	Blocks α_{1A}-receptors in the prostate	Tamsulosin (Flomax) Silodosin (Rapaflo)
Reduce static factor	Blocks 5α-reductase enzyme	Finasteride (Proscar) Dutasteride (Avodart)
	Blocks dihydrotestosterone at its intracellular receptor	Bicalutamide (Casodex)[a] Flutamide (Eulexin)[a]
	Blocks pituitary release of luteinizing hormone	Leuprolide (Lupron)[a] Goserelin (Zoladex)[a]
	Blocks pituitary release of luteinizing hormone and blocks androgen receptor	Megestrol acetate (Megace)[a]

[a]Not FDA approved for treatment of benign prostatic hyperplasia.

hormone superagonists leuprolide and goserelin decrease libido and can cause erectile dysfunction, gynecomastia, and hot flashes. Antiandrogens (e.g., bicalutamide, flutamide) produce nausea, diarrhea, and hepatotoxicity.

Selection of a medical treatment for a patient should be determined on a case-by-case basis after patient and provider discussion of risks, benefits, and costs of various treatments. With drug therapy for BPH, patients must understand that the benefits continue only as long as the medication is taken.

If possible, drug therapy should be initiated with a single agent, usually an α_1-adrenergic antagonist, which is faster acting and more effective than a 5α-reductase inhibitor. In addition, α_1-adrenergic antagonists are effective in reducing LUTS independent of prostate size, have no effect on PSA, and are associated with less sexual dysfunction than are 5α-reductase inhibitors. A 5α-reductase inhibitor is a good first-choice agent for patients with a significantly enlarged prostate (>40 g) who can not tolerate the cardiovascular adverse effects of α_1-adrenergic antagonists. For patients at risk for developing complications of BPH, specifically patients with an enlarged prostate gland greater than 40 g[6,17] and an elevated PSA ≥1.4 ng/mL (1.4 mcg/L), combination drug therapy with an α_1-adrenergic antagonist and a 5α-reductase inhibitor is more beneficial than single drug therapy. The pharmacologic rationale for such a combination is that using two drugs with different mechanisms of action can be more effective than either drug alone. The clinical benefit of combination therapy is that it quickly relieves symptoms, delays disease progression and reduces the need for surgical intervention.

α-Adrenergic Antagonists

Three generations of α-adrenergic antagonists have been used to treat BPH. They all relax smooth muscle in the prostate and bladder neck. Because of their antagonism of presynaptic $\alpha2$-adrenergic receptors that results in tachycardia and arrhythmias, first-generation agents such as phenoxybenzamine have been replaced by the second-generation postsynaptic α_1-adrenergic antagonists and third-generation uroselective postsynaptic α_1-adrenergic antagonists.

❻ The second- and third-generation α_1-adrenergic antagonists are considered equally effective for treatment of BPH.[11,18,19] These agents generally improve the AUA Symptom Score by 30% to 40% within 2 to 6 weeks, depending on the need for up dose titration, increase urinary flow rate by 2 to 3 mL/s in 60% to 70% of treated patients, and reduce PVR urine volume. They have no effect on decreasing prostate volume. Finally, α_1-adrenergic antagonists do not reduce PSA levels, preserving the utility of this prostate cancer marker in this high-risk population.[11]

Second-generation agents include prazosin, terazosin, doxazosin, and alfuzosin. At the usual doses used to treat BPH, prazosin, terazosin, and doxazosin antagonize peripheral vascular α_1-adrenergic receptors in addition to those in the prostate. As a result, first-dose syncope, orthostatic hypotension, and dizziness are characteristic adverse effects. To improve tolerance to these adverse effects, therapy should start with a low dose of 1 mg daily and then should be slowly titrated up to a full therapeutic dose over several weeks.[20,21] Additive blood-pressure-lowering effects commonly occur when these agents are used with antihypertensive agents, which limit use of these agents for some patients. These agents differ in terms of duration of action and dosage formulation. Whereas prazosin requires dosing two to three times per day, terazosin, doxazosin, and alfuzosin offer more convenient once daily dosing. Because prazosin requires twice to thrice daily dosing and has significant cardiovascular adverse effects, it is not recommended in the current AUA guidelines for treatment of BPH.[11] Extended-release dosage formulations are available for doxazosin and alfuzosin. These offer the convenience of once daily dosing, treatment initiation with a full therapeutic dose, and decreased dose-related hypotension as the formulation produces lower peak serum concentrations than immediate-release products.[6,22–24] An α_1-adrenergic antagonist is not preferred as single-drug therapy for treatment of both BPH and hypertension in a patient. In the Antihypertensive and Lipid-Lowering Treatment to Prevent Heart Attack Trial (ALLHAT) of 24,000 patients with hypertension, doxazosin produced more congestive heart failure than amlodipine, lisinopril, or chlorthalidone.[25] Thus, both the AUA and the Joint National Committee on Prevention, Detection, Evaluation and Treatment of High Blood Pressure[26] recommend that patients with BPH and hypertension be treated with separate and appropriate drug treatment for each medical condition.[27]

Alfuzosin is considered functionally and clinically uroselective in that usual doses used to treat BPH are less likely than other second-generation agents to cause cardiovascular adverse effects in animal or human models.[23] This clinical observation has been seen more often with the once daily, extended-release formulation of alfuzosin, which is the only commercially available formulation in the United States, as compared with the immediate-release formulation that is dosed three times per day, which is available in Europe.[28] Its clinical uroselectivity has been postulated to be due to higher concentrations of alfuzosin achieved in the prostate versus serum after usual doses,[29] decreased blood–brain barrier penetration of alfuzosin,[23] absence of high peak serum levels with the extended-release formulation,[30] and fixed dosing schedule of the extended-release formulation. Extended-release alfuzosin dosing is FDA approved for 10 mg daily, with no dose titration increase.[28] This formulation is particularly convenient for physician prescribers and patients who are starting to take the medication.

Tamsulosin and silodosin are the only third-generation α_1-adrenergic antagonists available in the United States. They are an advance over second-generation agents in that they are selective for prostatic α_{1A}-adrenergic receptors, which comprise approximately 70% of the adrenergic receptors in the prostate gland.[31,32] Blockade of these receptors results in smooth muscle relaxation of the prostate and bladder neck without causing peripheral vascular smooth muscle relaxation. Tamsulosin and silodosin have low affinity for vascular α_{1B}-adrenergic receptors, which explains why hypotension is not a common adverse effect.

Tamsulosin's selectivity for α_{1A}-adrenergic receptors has multiple implications. Dose titration is minimal; therefore, patients can begin therapy with the lowest effective maintenance dose of 0.4 mg/day taken orally. Patients can be instructed to take the dose anytime during the day, unlike immediate-release formulations of terazosin and doxazosin, which should be taken at bedtime so that patients can sleep through the time when peak cardiovascular adverse effects are most likely to occur. However, for best oral absorption, tamsulosin should be taken on an empty stomach because food decreases the drug's bioavailability and reduces the peak serum concentration of the drug after dosing. The onset of peak action is quick, in the range of 1 week, and only a minority of patients will require uptitration to a higher daily dose. No decreases in blood pressure or increases in heart rate have been reported in normotensive patients, the elderly, subgroups of patients with well-controlled hypertension, or those with uncontrolled hypertension.[33] Thus, tamsulosin allows initiation of treatment with a therapeutic dose that is not limited by cardiovascular adverse effects, unlike immediate-release formulations of terazosin and doxazosin.[34] Finally, the addition of tamsulosin to select antihypertensive regimens of patients does not result in potentiation of the hypotensive effect of furosemide, enalapril, nifedipine, and atenolol.[35,36] Therefore, tamsulosin is a good choice, particularly for patients who can not tolerate hypotension; have severe coronary artery disease, volume depletion, cardiac

Drug	Half-life (h)	Usual Daily Dosage	Time to Peak Effect on BPH Symptoms[a]
TABLE 93-3 Dosing Schedule of α_1-Adrenergic Antagonists for Patients with Benign Prostatic Hyperplasia			
Prazosin (Minipress)	2–3	2–10 mg in two to three divided doses	2–6 weeks
Terazosin (Hytrin)	11–14	1–10 mg as a single dose; maximum 20 mg	2–6 weeks
Doxazosin (Cardura)	15–19	1–4 mg as a single dose; maximum 8 mg	2–6 weeks
Doxazosin GTS (Cardura XL)	15–19	4 or 8 mg as a single dose, maximum 8 mg	Several days
Alfuzosin (Uroxatral)	10	10 mg as a single dose	Several days
Tamsulosin (Flomax)	14–15	0.4 or 0.8 mg as a single dose	Several days
Silodosin (Rapaflo)	13	8 mg as a single dose	Several days

[a]Time to peak effect on benign prostatic hyperplasia (BPH) symptoms is dependent on the titration period to achieve full therapeutic daily doses.

arrhythmias, severe orthostasis, or liver failure; are taking multiple antihypertensives; or when the titration would be too complicated for the patient or produce an unacceptable delay in onset for a particular patient.

As compared with tamsulosin, silodosin requires dosage modification for patients with renal and hepatic impairment, has the potential for more drug interactions with inhibitors of CYP 3A4 (e.g., clarithromycin) and P-glycoprotein (e.g., cyclosporine), and has much less clinical experience with its use for patients with cardiovascular disease. For these reasons, tamsulosin is the preferred third-generation α_1-adrenergic antagonist in clinical practice.[32]

The usual doses of α_1-adrenergic antagonists are summarized in Table 93–3.

When using immediate-release formulations of the second-generation α_1-adrenergic antagonists terazosin and doxazosin, slow titration up to a therapeutic maintenance dose is necessary to minimize orthostatic hypotension and first-dose syncope. Conservatively, dosages should be increased in an orderly stepwise process, at 2- to 7-day intervals, depending on the patient's response to the medication. A faster titration schedule can be used as long as the patient does not develop orthostatic hypotension or dizziness. Two sample titration schedules for terazosin are as follows:

- **Schedule 1: Slow titration**
  Days 4 to 14: 2 mg at bedtime
  Weeks 2 to 6: 5 mg at bedtime
  Weeks 7 and on: 10 mg at bedtime

- **Schedule 2: Quicker titration**
  Days 1 to 3: 1 mg at bedtime
  Days 4 to 14: 2 mg at bedtime
  Weeks 2 to 3: 5 mg at bedtime
  Weeks 4 and on: 10 mg at bedtime

Patients should continue taking the drug as long as they continue to respond to it. Durable responses for 6 and 10 years have been reported for tamsulosin[37] and doxazosin,[38] respectively. If BPH symptoms worsen despite maximum tolerable drug doses, surgery should be considered.

With the exception of silodosin, no dosage adjustments are recommended for α_1-adrenergic antagonists for patients with renal failure. Because these drugs are hepatically catabolized, the lowest effective dose should be used for patients with hepatic dysfunction, and patients should be monitored carefully for adverse effects. With

the exception of silodosin, no specific dosing guidelines for this patient population are available. For silodosin, a reduced daily dose of 4 mg is recommended for patients with moderate renal impairment or those with hepatic dysfunction.

Approximately 10% to 12% of patients discontinue taking second-generation α_1-adrenergic antagonists because of adverse effects, especially those that affect the cardiovascular system (e.g., syncope, dizziness, hypotension).[39] Patients who tolerate hypotension poorly should avoid second-generation α_1-adrenergic antagonists. This includes patients with poorly controlled angina, serious cardiac arrhythmias, patients with reduced circulating volume, and patients taking multiple antihypertensives.[39] These patients are candidates for a third-generation α_1-adrenergic antagonist or finasteride, if drug therapy is deemed necessary. Whether extended-release alfuzosin or silodosin is a good choice remains to be elucidated in controlled comparison trials with tamsulosin.[40,41]

Tiredness and asthenia, ejaculatory dysfunction, flu-like symptoms, and nasal congestion are the most common dose-related adverse effects of tamsulosin and silodosin.[42] These adverse effects are extensions of their α-adrenergic antagonist activity and are unavoidable, but with proper education patients likely will not discontinue treatment.

Floppy iris syndrome has been associated with doxazosin, silodosin, and tamsulosin use, although the number of reported cases is highest with tamsulosin.[42,43] The mechanism for this adverse reaction is related to blockade of α_{1A}-adrenergic receptors in iris dilator muscles. As a result, during cataract surgery, papillary constriction occurs and the iris billows out (floppy iris), both of which complicate the procedure or can increase the likelihood of postoperative complications.[42–45] Patients who are taking α_1-adrenergic antagonists and who plan to undergo cataract surgery should inform their ophthalmologist that they are taking this medication so that appropriate measures can be taken during eye surgery, e.g., use of iris retractors, papillary expansion rings, or potent mydriatic agents.[43] Patients with severe sulfa allergy should avoid tamsulosin.

Caution is needed when CYP 3A4 inhibitors, e.g., cimetidine, diltiazem are used with α_1-adrenergic antagonists because a drug–drug interaction could lead to decreased metabolism of the latter agents. In contrast, concurrent use of potent CYP 3A4 stimulators, e.g., carbamazepine and phenytoin, may increase hepatic catabolism of α_1-adrenergic antagonists.

Phosphodiesterase inhibitors (e.g., sildenafil, vardenafil, tadalafil) may produce systemic hypotension if used in large doses along with α_1-adrenergic antagonists. The mechanisms for this interaction are related to the intrinsic vasodilatory effects of phosphodiesterase inhibitors and the higher susceptibility of elderly patients to venous pooling because of autonomic incompetence.[27,46] Therefore, package labeling for these drugs includes a caution to carefully monitor patients who are taking phosphodiesterase inhibitors with α_1-adrenergic antagonists.

CURRENT CONTROVERSY

Among the α_1-adrenergic antagonists, tamsulosin and extended-release alfuzosin have been associated with the highest and lowest incidences of ejaculatory dysfunction, respectively. Although some clinicians claim that this difference should be considered when selecting one agent over another, this adverse effect is of variable clinical significance. Some patients complain of decreased sexual satisfaction because of ejaculatory dysfunction, whereas other patients do not.

5α-Reductase Inhibitors

❼ Finasteride competitively inhibits type II 5α-reductase, suppresses intraprostatic DHT by 80% to 90%, and decreases serum DHT levels by 70%.[9] Dutasteride is a nonselective inhibitor of type I and II 5α-reductase. It more quickly and completely suppresses intraprostatic DHT production and decreases serum DHT levels by 90%.[47] However, direct comparison clinical trials show no advantages of these pharmacodynamic actions of dutasteride when compared with finasteride.[48] These agents are indicated for management of moderate to severe BPH disease for patients with enlarged prostate glands of at least 40 g.[48] For such patients, 5α-reductase inhibitors may slow disease progression and decrease the risk of disease complications, thereby decreasing the ultimate need for surgical intervention. When taken continuously for 6 years, finasteride has been shown to decrease the risk of acute urinary retention and prostatectomy.[49] For patients with severe disease, these agents generally can be used with a 6-month short course of an α₁-adrenergic antagonist, which will provide fast symptom relief until the 5α-reductase inhibitor starts to work. 5α-Reductase inhibitors may be preferred for patients with BPH and an enlarged prostate gland who have uncontrolled arrhythmias, have poorly controlled angina, are taking multiple antihypertensive agents, or are unable to tolerate hypotensive adverse effects of α₁-adrenergic antagonists.

5α-Reductase inhibitors reduce prostate size by 25%, increase peak urinary flow rate by 1.6 to 2.0 mL/s, improve voiding symptoms in approximately 30% of treated patients, and produce few serious adverse effects. Compared with α₁-adrenergic antagonists, 5α-reductase inhibitors have several disadvantages. 5α-Reductase inhibitors have a delayed peak onset of clinical effect, which is undesirable for patients with bothersome symptoms, and an adequate clinical trial is 6 to 12 months. In addition, the percentage of patients who experience objective improvement is less with 5α-reductase inhibitors than with α₁-adrenergic antagonists. 5α-Reductase inhibitors cause more sexual dysfunction than α₁-adrenergic receptor antagonists; therefore, physicians consider 5α-reductase inhibitors to be second-line agents for treatment of BPH in sexually active males (Table 93–4).[11]

Patients with BPH who have large prostate glands, PSA level less than 3 ng/mL (3 mcg/L) and are concerned about developing prostate cancer can be prescribed finasteride 5 mg daily for up to 7 years, which has been shown to reduce the 7-year prevalence of prostate cancer by 25% in the Prostate Cancer Prevention Trial.[50,51] However, in this study, finasteride was associated with a small increased risk of developing a higher-grade prostate cancer, which has a potential for invasiveness. Although originally thought to be an adverse effect of finasteride use, it is now thought that the higher incidence of prostate cancer is due to biopsy sampling bias. That is, since finasteride reduces the size of the prostate gland, this results in increased sensitivity of sampling biopsies to detect prostate cancer. The ongoing Reduction by Dutasteride in Prostate Cancer Events (REDUCE) trial should provide additional information on the value of 5α-reductase inhibitors in preventing prostate cancer.[52]

Finasteride is well absorbed from the gastrointestinal tract (95%), and its absorption is unaffected by food. Peak serum concentrations are reached 1 to 2 hours after the dose. Finasteride is highly protein bound. The liver extensively metabolizes finasteride to inactive metabolites, which are largely excreted in stool. The plasma half-life is 4.7 to 7.1 hours, but its biologic half-life probably is longer, as decreased serum DHT levels persist for up to 2 weeks after finasteride dosing is stopped.

For BPH, finasteride is given in doses of 5 mg by mouth daily. The dose can be taken with meals or on an empty stomach. No dosage adjustment is needed for patients with renal dysfunction. Although no dosage reduction is recommended for patients with hepatic insufficiency, patients should be monitored carefully. Maximal reductions in prostate volume or symptom improvement may not be evident for 12 months, but noticeable changes from baseline should occur after 6 months of continuous treatment. No clinically relevant drug interactions have been reported with 5α-reductase inhibitors.

Patients must continue to take 5α-reductase inhibitors as long as they respond. Durable responses to finasteride and dutasteride have been reported with continued treatment for 6 years[49] and 4 years,[48] respectively. Upon discontinuation of the drug, prostate size and voiding symptoms generally return to baseline.

5α-Reductase inhibitors can produce sexual dysfunction, and this has led to discontinuation of therapy in up to 12% of treated patients in one pooled analysis.[48] Ejaculation disorders (dry sex or delayed ejaculation) have been reported in 3% to 8% of treated patients.[53] These disorders, which are possible results of decreased prostatic secretion, are reversible with drug discontinuation.

Erectile dysfunction has been reported for 3% to 16% of patients.[48] It may be secondary to ejaculation disorders or may be due to drug-induced inhibition of nitric oxide synthase (which is needed to produce nitric oxide, a vasodilatory substance) in cavernosal tissue.[54] The role of 5α-reductase inhibitors in causing erectile dysfunction is not clear, as elderly men with BPH commonly develop erectile dysfunction as they age or have concurrent medical illnesses or concomitant drug therapies that may predispose to the development of sexual dysfunction.[53] Decreased libido has been reported in 2% to 10% of treated patients.[48]

Other minor adverse effects include nausea, abdominal pain, asthenia, dizziness, flatulence, headache, rash, muscle weakness, and gynecomastia.

5α-Reductase inhibitors are in FDA pregnancy category X, which means that they are contraindicated in pregnant females. Exposure of the male fetus to finasteride may produce pseudohermaphroditic offspring with ambiguous genitalia, similar to those of patients with a rare genetic deficiency of type II 5α-reductase. Because of this teratogenic effect, women who are pregnant or seeking to become pregnant should not handle 5α-reductase inhibitor tablets and should not have contact with semen from men being treated with 5α-reductase inhibitors. Women pharmacists of childbearing age should handle this product with rubber gloves if there is any chance that they are pregnant.

Usual doses of 5α-reductase inhibitors produce a median reduction of serum PSA levels by 50%. For this reason, PSA levels must

TABLE 93-4	Comparison of α₁-Adrenergic Antagonists and 5α-Reductase Inhibitors	
	α₁-Adrenergic Antagonists	**5α-Reductase Inhibitors**
Relaxes prostatic smooth muscle	Yes	No
Decreases prostate size	No	Yes
Halts disease progression	No	Yes
Peak onset	1–6 weeks	3–6 months
Efficacy	++	++ (for patients with enlarged prostates)
Frequency of dosing	1–2 times per day, depending on the agent and dosage formulation	Once per day
Decreases prostate-specific antigen	No	Yes
Sexual dysfunction adverse effects	+	++
Cardiovascular adverse effects	Yes	No

+ Motation is a quantitative assessment, for example 5α-reductase inhibitors cause more types of several dysfunction than α-adrenergic antagonists.

be measured before treatment begins, and the patient should have a digital rectal examination. After 6 months of therapy, the patient should have a repeat PSA. If the level does not decline by 50% and the patient has been adherent to the 5α-reductase inhibitor regimen, he should be evaluated for prostate cancer. Annually thereafter, the patient should have a PSA assay and digital rectal examination, and patients with an increase in PSA levels should be evaluated for prostate cancer or noncompliance to the prescribed regimen. To interpret a PSA level in a patient being treated with a 5α-reductase inhibitor, it is generally recommended that the actual measured level be doubled to get an estimate of the true level.[11,55]

CURRENT CONTROVERSY

Dutasteride is a nonselective 5α-reductase inhibitor that more quickly and effectively lowers intraprostatic DHT production and lowers plasma DHT levels than finasteride does. Whether these hormonal changes result in clinical advantages over finasteride remains to be elucidated.[47,48]

CURRENT CONTROVERSY

The combination of an α_1-adrenergic antagonist and 5α-reductase inhibitor can relieve LUTS, slow progression of BPH, and reduce the need for prostate surgery for patients with moderate to severe symptoms and a prostate of 40 g or larger. It may be possible to discontinue the α_1-adrenergic antagonist after the first several months; however, this potentially cost-saving measure requires further clinical study.

Combination Therapy

Combination therapy with an α_1-adrenergic antagonist and a 5α-reductase inhibitor is ideal for patients with severe symptoms, who also have an enlarged prostate gland of at least 40 g and PSA of at least 1.4 ng/mL (1.4 µg/L), a surrogate marker for an enlarged prostate gland.[6,11] Such patients appear to be at high risk for disease progression, as evidenced by symptom worsening and development of disease complications.[6] A regimen of finasteride and doxazosin for 5 years was shown to prevent symptom progression by 66%, decrease the risk of developing acute urinary retention by 81%, and decrease the need for prostate surgery by 67%.[6] In preliminary findings from a clinical trial of dutasteride versus tamsulosin versus the combination of dutasteride and tamsulosin for patients with large prostate glands (i.e., mean prostate volume of 55 ± 23 cc (55 ± 23 mL) and mean PSA of 4 ng/mL [4 mcg/L]), the combination drug regimen was more effective in reducing symptoms than dutasteride alone or tamsulosin alone. Whether the combination of dutasteride and tamsulosin prevents disease progression awaits long-term study results.[56] Although not proven by direct comparison trials, any combination of 5α-reductase inhibitor and α_1-adrenergic antagonist probably is similarly effective for patients with the aforementioned characteristics.[11] The disadvantages of a combination regimen include increased medication cost to the patient and an increased incidence of adverse drug effects (i.e., 18% to 27% of patients discontinued treatment due to hypotension).

Use of Anticholinergic Agents for Patients with BPH

Treatment with an α_1-adrenergic antagonist, 5α-reductase inhibitor, or surgery may improve urinary flow rate and bladder emptying;

however, the patient may still complain of irritative voiding symptoms (e.g., urinary frequency, urgency), which mimic those of overactive bladder syndrome. Oxybutynin and tolterodine have been used to relieve these symptoms. By blocking muscarinic receptors in the detrusor muscle, these agents can reduce uninhibited detrusor contractions, a sequela of prolonged bladder outlet obstruction from BPH. Thus, they can reduce urinary frequency and urgency. Because elderly patients are sensitive to the central nervous system adverse effects and dry mouth associated with anticholinergic agents, patients should be started on the lowest effective dose and then slowly titrated up.[57–59] Similarly in the presence of BPH, anticholinergic agents can rarely cause acute urinary retention. Therefore, prescribing anticholinergic agents should be done cautiously, and patients monitored closely.

■ SURGICAL INTERVENTION

❽ The gold standard for treatment of patients with complications of BPH is prostatectomy performed either transurethrally or as an open surgical procedure.[11,16] Surgical intervention is also used for patients with moderate to severe symptoms, who are not responsive to drug therapy, who are noncompliant with drug therapy, or who prefer surgical intervention. Surgical removal of the prostate offers the highest rate of symptom improvement, but it also has the highest complication rate.

With transurethral resection of the prostate (TURP), an endoscopic resectoscope inserted through the urethra is used to remove the inside core of the prostate. This enlarges the urethral opening at the bladder neck. TURP is performed only in men with enlarged prostates that are less than 50 g so that the resection can be completed in less than 1 hour. Often performed as outpatient surgery, this procedure produces on average a peak urinary flow rate increase of 125% and improvement of voiding symptoms by almost 90% in approximately 90% of patients.[16] A common complication of TURP is retrograde ejaculation, occurring in up to 75% of patients. Significant bleeding, urinary incontinence, and erectile dysfunction occur in smaller but significant numbers of patients (2% to 15%).[60,61] Approximately 2% to 10% and 12% to 15% of patients require second surgeries within 5 and 8 years, respectively.[60]

Men with larger prostates (>50 g) require an open surgical procedure (open prostatectomy), which can be performed retropubically or suprapubically. This necessitates hospitalization for at least a few days, anesthesia, and a longer recuperation time. Adverse effects of open prostatectomy include bleeding, urinary and soft-tissue infection, retrograde ejaculation in 77% of patients, erectile dysfunction in 16% to 33% of patients, and urinary incontinence in 2% of patients. The reoperation rate is 3% to 5% at 10 years.[11]

Transurethral incision of the prostate (TUIP) is an alternative surgical procedure for patients with moderate to severe voiding symptoms who have an enlarged prostate gland less than 30 g in size. In the short term TUIP is as effective as TURP but requires less operation time, causes less blood loss, and produces fewer adverse effects.[11] TUIP involves using an endoscopic resectoscope to make two or three incisions at the bladder neck to widen the opening. In limited long-term studies, the reoperation rate for TUIP is slightly higher than with TURP.

Minimally invasive surgical procedures are highly desirable by patients. The procedures are short (lasting minutes), have a lower potential to produce adverse effects, are less expensive than continuous drug therapy lasting years, and they may be particularly useful in debilitated patients who are poor surgical candidates. The ideal candidates have moderate to severe voiding symptoms with smaller sized prostate glands. These procedures typically use heat energy from microwaves, water, or laser to destroy prostate tissue.[11,62] Commonly used procedures include transurethral needle ablation of the prostate and transurethral microwave thermotherapy of the prostate.[63] A disadvantage of all minimally invasive surgical procedures is that the percentage of patients who may develop acute urinary retention in the immediate postoperative period and may require reoperation after an initial improvement in symptoms is higher than that of patients who undergo TURP or open prostatectomy.[64]

■ PHYTOTHERAPY

9 Although phytotherapy is widely used in Europe for the management of BPH, the published data on herbal agents are largely inconclusive and conflicting. Studies often lack placebo controls, which are essential for assessing treatments of BPH because spontaneous regression of symptoms can occur. Furthermore, because these agents are marketed under the Dietary Supplements Health and Education Act, their efficacy, safety, and quality are not regulated by the FDA. For these reasons, herbal products—including saw palmetto berry (*Serenoa repens*), stinging nettle (*Urtica dioica*), South African stargrass (*Hypoxis rooperi*), pumpkin seed (*Cucurbita pepo*), and African plum (*Pygeum africanum*)—are not recommended for treatment of BPH.[11,65–68] An excellent review on phytotherapy for BPH has been published.[68]

EVALUATION OF THERAPEUTIC OUTCOMES

The primary therapeutic outcome of BPH therapy is improvement of voiding symptoms with minimal treatment-related adverse effects. As a disease for which therapy is directed at the voiding symptoms that the patient finds most bothersome, assessment of outcomes depends on the patient's perceptions of the effectiveness of therapy. Use of a validated, standardized instrument, such as the AUA Symptom Score, for assessing patient's voiding symptoms is important in this process.[11]

For patients being considered for surgical treatment, objective measures of bladder emptying are useful and include the urinary flow rate and PVR urine volume (see Diagnostic Evaluation above).

Because this patient population is at high risk for prostate cancer, PSA should be measured and a digital rectal examination performed annually if the patient has a life expectancy of at least 10 years. For patients taking 5α-reductase inhibitors, a second PSA taken after 6 months of treatment should be compared with baseline measurements. If the patient is suspected of having developed renal impairment as a consequence of long-standing bladder outlet obstruction, then BUN and serum creatinine should be evaluated at regular intervals.

SUMMARY

An ubiquitous disease of aging men, symptomatic BPH requires medical attention to preserve the patient's quality of life and to prevent disease complications, many of which can be life threatening in this patient population. In men who have no or mildly bothersome symptoms, watchful waiting and behavior modification are the best treatment approach, as BPH remains stable or even regresses in approximately half of these men.

For patients with voiding symptoms that are moderate to severely bothersome, pharmacotherapy is indicated. An α₁-adrenergic antagonist is the agent of first choice. Second-generation agents include terazosin, doxazosin, and alfuzosin,

and third-generation agents include tamsulosin and silodosin. Immediate-release formulations of terazosin and doxazosin cause more cardiovascular adverse effects than do extended-release doxazosin or alfuzosin, tamsulosin, or silodosin. Whether extended-release doxazosin, extended-release alfuzosin, or silodosin are as well tolerated as tamsulosin for patients at risk for hypotension or hypotension-related morbidity remains to be elucidated. 5α-Reductase inhibitors are preferred drug treatment for patients with enlarged prostates who poorly tolerate the hypotensive adverse effects of α₁-adrenergic antagonists. However, 5α-reductase inhibitors have a slow onset of action. For patients who do not respond to monotherapy, combination drug therapy could be attempted. Such regimens have been found to be most effective for patients with enlarged prostates greater than 40 g. Alternatively, surgery is an option.

For patients who have complications of BPH, surgery is required. Although it has more adverse complications than does pharmacotherapy or watchful waiting, TURP is considered the gold standard.

ABBREVIATIONS

AUA: American Urological Association

BPH: benign prostatic hyperplasia

BUN: blood urea nitrogen

DHT: dihydrotestosterone

LUTS: lower urinary tract symptoms

PSA: prostate-specific antigen

PVR: postvoid residual

TUIP: transurethral incision of the prostate

TURP: transurethral resection of the prostate

REFERENCES

1. Glynn RJ, Campion EW, Bouchard GR, Silbert JE. The development of benign prostatic hyperplasia among volunteers in the normative aging study. Am J Epidemiol 1985;131:79–90.
2. Thorpe A, Neal D. Benign prostatic hyperplasia. Lancet 2003;361: 1359–1367.
3. Roehrborn CG. Pathology of benign prostatic hyperplasia. Int J Imp Res 2008;20:S11–S18.
4. St. Sauver JL, Jacobson DJ, Girman CJ, et al. Tracking of longitudinal changes in measures of benign prostatic hyperplasia in a population based cohort. J Urol 2006;175:1918–1922.
5. Selius BA, Subedi R. Urinary retention in adults: Diagnosis and initial management. Am Fam Physician 2008;77:643–650.
6. McConnell JD, Roehrborn CG, Bautista OM, et al. The long term effect of doxazosin, finasteride, and combination therapy on the clinical progression of benign prostatic hyperplasia. N Engl J Med 2003;349:2387–2398.
7. Trachtenberg J. Treatment of lower urinary tract symptoms suggestive of benign prostatic hyperplasia in relation to the patient's risk profile for progression. BJU Int 2005;95(suppl 4):6–11.
8. Marks LS, Roehrborn CG, Andriole GL. Prevention of benign prostatic hyperplasia disease. J Urol 2006;176:1299–1306.
9. Marks LS. Use of 5-α reductase inhibitors to prevent benign prostatic hyperplasia disease. Curr Urol Rep 2006;4:293–303.
10. Crawford ED. Management of lower urinary tract symptoms suggestive of benign prostatic hyperplasia: The central role of the patient risk profile. BJU Int 2005;95(suppl 4):1–5.
11. American Urological Association Practice Guidelines Committee. AUA guidelines on management of benign prostatic hyperplasia

(2003). Chapter 1: Diagnosis and treatment recommendations. J Urol 2003;170:530–547.

12. dela Rosette J, Alivizatos G, Madersbacher S, et al. European Association of Urology Guidelines on Benign Prostatic Hyperplasia, March 2004, *http://www.uroweb.org/fileadmin/tx eauguidelines/2.*

13. Nickel JC, Herschorn S, Corcos J, et al. Canadian guidelines for the management of benign prostatic hyperplasia. Can J Urol 2005;12: 2677–2683.

14. Moyad MA, Lowe FC. Educating patients about lifestyle modifications for prostate health. Am J Med 2008;121:S34–S42.

15. Ranjan P, Dalela D, Sankhwar S. Diet and benign prostatic hyperplasia: Implications for prevention. Urology 2006;68:470–476.

16. Wasson JH, Reda DJ, Bruskewitz RC, et al.; for the Veterans Affairs Cooperative Study Group on Transurethral Resection of the Prostate. A comparison of transurethral surgery with watchful waiting for moderate symptoms of benign prostatic hyperplasia. N Engl J Med 1995;332:75–79.

17. Kirby RS, Roehrborn C, Boyle P, et al. Efficacy and tolerability of doxazosin and finasteride alone or in combination in treatment of symptomatic benign prostatic hyperplasia—The Prospective European Doxazosin Combination Therapy (PREDICT) Trial. Urology 2003;61: 119–126.

18. Schwinn DA, Roehrborn CG. Alpha1-adrenoceptor subtypes and lower urinary tract symptoms. Int J Urol 2008;15:193–199.

19. Lowe F. Treatment of lower urinary tract symptoms suggestive of benign prostatic hyperplasia: Sexual function. BJU Int 2005;95 (suppl 4): 12–18.

20. Wilt TJ, MacDonald R, Rutks IR. Tamsulosin for benign prostatic hyperplasia. Cochrane Database Syst Rev 2003;1:CD002081.

21. Wilt TJ, Howe RW, Rutks IR, et al. Terazosin for benign prostatic hyperplasia. Cochrane Database Syst Rev 2002;4:CD003851.

22. Nickel JC, Sander S, Moon TD. A meta-analysis of the vascular-related safety profile and efficacy of alpha-adrenergic blockers for symptoms related to benign prostatic hyperplasia. Int J Clin Pract 2008;62: 1547–1559.

23. MacDonald R, Wilt TJ. Alfuzosin for treatment of lower urinary tract symptoms compatible with benign prostatic hyperplasia: A systematic review of efficacy and adverse effects. Urology 2005;66:780–788.

24. Goldsmith DR, Plosker GL. Doxazosin gastrointestinal therapeutic system. Drugs 2006;65:2037–2047.

25. Major cardiovascular events in hypertensive patients randomized to doxazosin vs chlorthalidone: The Antihypertensive and Lipid-Lowering Treatment to Prevent Heart Attack Trial (ALLHAT). ALLHAT Collaborative Research Group [erratum appear in JAMA 2002;288:2976]. JAMA 2000;283:1967–1975.

26. White WB, Moon T. Treatment of benign prostatic hyperplasia in hypertensive men. J Clin Hypertens 2005;7:212–217.

27. Kaplan SA, Neutel J. Vasodilatory factors in treatment of older men with symptomatic benign prostatic hyperplasia. Urology 2006;67: 225–231.

28. Elhilali MM. Alfuzosin: An α_1 receptor blocker for the treatment of lower urinary tract symptoms associated with benign prostatic hyperplasia. Expert Opin Pharmacother 2006;7:583–596.

29. Mottet N, Bressolle F, Delmas V, et al. Prostatic tissue distribution of alfuzosin in patients with benign prostatic hyperplasia following repeated oral administration. Eur Urol 2003;44:101–105.

30. Roehrborn CG for the ALFUS Study Group. Efficacy and safety of once daily alfuzosin in the treatment of lower urinary tract symptoms and clinical benign prostatic hyperplasia: A randomized, placebo-controlled trial. Urology 2001; 58:953–959.

31. Chapple CR. Pharmacotherapy for benign prostatic hyperplasia—The potential for α_1-adrenoceptor subtype-specific blockade. Br J Urol 1998;81(suppl):34–47.

32. Marks LS, Gittleman MC, Hill LA, et al. Rapid efficacy of the highly selective alpha (1A) adrenoceptor antagonist silodosin in men with signs and symptoms of benign prostatic hyperplasia: Pooled results of 2 phase 3 studies. J Urol 2009;181:2634–2640.

33. Chapple CR, Baert L, Thind P, et al. Tamsulosin 0.4 mg once daily: Tolerability in older and young patients with lower urinary tract symptoms suggestive of benign prostatic obstruction. The Europ Tamsulosin Study Group. Eur Urol 1997;32:462–470.

34. Djavan B, Chapple C, Milani S. State of the art on the efficacy and tolerability of alpha$_1$ adrenoceptor antagonists in patients with lower urinary tract symptoms suggestive of benign prostatic obstruction. Urology 2004;64:1081–1088.

35. Lowe FC. Coadministration of tamsulosin and three antihypertensive agents in patients with benign prostatic hyperplasia: Pharmacodynamic effect. Clin Ther 1997;19:730–742.

36. DeMey C. Cardiovascular effects of alpha blockers used for the treatment of symptomatic BPH. Impact on safety and well being. Eur Urol 2998;34(suppl 2):18–28.

37. Narayan P, Evans CP, Moon T. Long-term safety and efficacy of tamsulosin for the treatment of lower urinary tract symptoms associated with benign prostatic hyperplasia. J Urol 2003;170:498–502.

38. Dutkiewicz S. Long term treatment with doxazosin in men with benign prostatic hyperplasia: 10 year follow-up. Int Urol Nephrol 2004;36:169–173.

39. Nickel JC, Sander S, Moon TD. A meta-analysis of the vascular-related safety profile and efficacy of alpha adrenergic blockers for symptoms related to benign prostatic hyperplasia. Int J Clin Pract 2008;62: 1547–1559.

40. Hartung R, Matzkin H, Alcarez A, et al. Age, comorbidity and hypertensive co-medication do not affect cardiovascular tolerability of 10 mg alfuzosin once daily. J Urol 2006;175:624–628.

41. Michel MC, Chapple CR. Comparison of the cardiovascular effects of tamsulosin oral controlled absorption system (OCAS) and alfuzosin prolonged release (XL). Eur Urol 2006;49:501–508.

42. Oshika T, Ohashi Y, Inamura M, et al. Incidence of intraoperative floppy iris syndrome in patients on either systemic or topical α_1-adrenoceptor antagonist. Am J Ophthalmol 2007;143: 150–151.

43. Friedman AH. Tamsulosin and the intraoperative floppy iris syndrome. JAMA 2009;301:2044–2045.

44. Bell CM, Hatch WV, Fischer HD, et al. Association between tamsulosin and serious ophthalmic adverse events in older men following cataract surgery. JAMA 2009;301:1991–1996.

45. Lawrentschuk N, Bylsma GW. Intraoperative floppy iris syndrome and its relationship to tamsulosin: A urologist's guide. BJU Int 2006;97:2–4.

46. Nieminen T, Tammela TLJ, Koobi T, Kahonen M. The effects of tamsulosin and sildenafil in separate and combined regimens on detailed hemodynamics in patients with benign prostatic hyperplasia. J Urol 2006;175:2551–2556.

47. Anonymous. Dutasteride (Avodart) for benign prostatic hyperplasia. Med Lett Drugs Ther 2002;44:109–110.

48. Andriole GL, Kirby R. Safety and tolerability of the dual 5α-reductase inhibitor dutasteride in the treatment of benign prostatic hyperplasia. Eur Urol 2003;44:82–88.

49. Roehrborn CG, Bruskewitz R, Nickel JC, et al. Sustained decrease in incidence of acute urinary retention and surgery with finasteride for 6 years in men with benign prostatic hyperplasia. J Urol 2004;171: 1194–1198.

50. Thompson IM, Goodman PJ, Tangen CN, et al. The influence of finasteride on the development of prostate cancer. N Engl J Med 2003;349:215–224.

51. Kramer BS, Hagerty KL, Justman S, et al. Use of 5α-reductase inhibitors for prostate cancer chemoprevention. American Society of Clinical Oncology/American Cancer Society 2008 Clinical Practice Guideline. J Urol 2009;181:1642–1657.

52. Andriole GL, Roehrborn CG, Schulman C, et al. Effect of dutasteride on the detection of prostate cancer in men with benign prostatic hyperplasia. Urology 2004;64:537–543.

53. Rosen R, O'Leary M, Altwein J, et al. Ejaculatory disorders are frequent and bothersome in aging males with LUTS. A worldwide survey (MSAM-7) [abstract]. J Urol 2003;169(suppl 1):365.

54. Park KH, Kim SW, Kim KD, et al. Effects of androgens on the expression of nitric oxide synthase mRNA in rat corpus cavernosum. BJU Int 1999;83:327–333.

55. Andriole GL, Marberger M, Roehrborn CG. Clinical usefulness of serum prostate specific antigen for the detection of prostate cancer is preserved in men receiving the dual 5α reductase inhibitor dutasteride. J Urol 2006;175:1657–1662.

56. Roehrborn CG, Siami P, Baskin J et al. COMBAT Study Group. The effects of dutasteride, tamsulosin, and combination therapy in lower urinary tract symptoms in men with benign prostatic hyperplasia and prostate enlargement: 2 year results from the COMBAT study. J Urol 2008;179:616–621.

57. Rover ES, Kreder K, Sussman DO, et al. Effect of tolterodine extended release with or without tamsulosin on measures of urgency and patient reported outcomes in men with lower urinary tract symptoms. J Urol 2008;180:1034–1041.

58. Dmochowski R. Antimuscarinic therapy in men with lower urinary tract symptoms: What is the evidence? Curr Urol Rep 2006;7: 462–467.

59. Kaplan SA, Roehrborn CG, Rovner ES, et al. Tolterodine and tamsulosin for treatment of men with lower urinary tract symptoms and overactive bladder. JAMA 2006;296:2319–2328.

60. Rassweiler J, Teber D, Kuntz R, Hofmann R. Complications of transurethral resection of the prostate (TURP): Incidence, management, and prevention. Eur Urol 2006;50:969–980.

61. Kassabian VS. Sexual function in patients treated for benign prostatic hyperplasia. Lancet 2003;361:60–62.

62. Wei JT, Calhoun E, Jacobsen SJ. Urologic disease in America project: benign prostatic hyperplasia. J Urol 2005;173:1256–1261.

63. Lourenco T, Pickard R, Vale L, et al. Minimally invasive treatments for benign prostatic enlargement: systematic review of randomized controlled trials. Br Med J 2009; 2008:337,a1662.

64. Lourenco T, Armstrong N, N'Dow J, et al. Systematic review and economic modeling of effectiveness and cost utility of surgical treatments for men with benign prostatic enlargement. Health Tech Assessment 2008;12:1–167.

65. Debruyne F, Koch G, Boyle P, et al. Comparison of phytotherapeutic agent (Permixon) with an α-blocker (tamsulosin) in the treatment of benign prostatic hyperplasia: A 1-year randomized international study. Eur Urol 2002;41:497–507.

66. Gerber GS, Kuznetsov D, Johnson BC, et al. Randomized double blind controlled trial of saw palmetto in men with lower urinary tract symptoms. Urology 2001;58:960–964.

67. Avins AL, Bent S. Saw palmetto and lower urinary tract symptoms: What is the latest evidence? Curr Urol Rep 2006;7:260–265.

68. Bent S, Kane C, Shinohara K, et al. Saw palmetto for benign prostatic hyperplasia. N Engl J Med 2006;354:557–566.

ERIC S. ROVNER, JEAN WYMAN, THOMAS LACKNER, AND DAVID R.P. GUAY

KEY CONCEPTS

❶ In evaluating urinary incontinence, drug-induced or drug-aggravated etiologies must be ruled out.

❷ Accurate diagnosis and classification of urinary incontinence type are critical to the selection of appropriate pharmacotherapy.

❸ Nonpharmacologic, nonsurgical therapy is the cornerstone of management of several types of urinary incontinence, often should be the first therapy initiated, and should be continued even when drug therapy is initiated.

❹ Anticholinergic/antispasmodic agents are the pharmacologic therapies of choice for bladder overactivity (urge incontinence).

❺ Duloxetine (not approved for treatment of urinary incontinence in the United States), α-adrenergic receptor agonists, and topical (vaginal) estrogens (alone or together) are the pharmacologic therapies of choice in urethral underactivity (stress incontinence).

❻ Patient-specific treatment goals should be identified. They are not static and may change over time. Choice of therapy may be influenced by characteristics such as patient age, comorbidities, concurrent medications, and ability to adhere to the prescribed regimen. If therapeutic goals are not achieved with a given agent at optimal dosage, addition of a second agent or switching to an alternative single agent should be considered.

Urinary incontinence (UI) is defined as involuntary leakage of urine.[1] It is frequently accompanied by other bothersome lower urinary tract symptoms, such as urgency, increased daytime frequency, and nocturia. It is a common yet underdetected and underreported health problem that can significantly affect quality of life. Patients with UI may have depression as a result of the perceived lack of self-control, loss of independence, and lack of self-esteem, and they often curtail their activities for fear of an "accident." UI may also have serious medical and economic ramifications for untreated or undertreated patients, including perineal dermatitis, worsening of pressure ulcers, urinary tract infections, and falls.

Learning objectives, review questions, and other resources can be found at **www.pharmacotherapyonline.com**.

This chapter highlights the epidemiology, etiology, pathophysiology, and treatment of stress, urge, mixed, and overflow UI in men and women.

EPIDEMIOLOGY

Determining the true prevalence of UI is difficult because of problems with definition, reporting bias, and other methodologic issues.[2] Epidemiologic studies have not historically used a standard definition of the condition or a standard methodology for data recording, with some studies including "postvoid dribbling," while other studies specify "urinary leakage causing a social or hygienic problem." Many people suffer from UI, and the impact of this condition is substantial, crossing all racial, ethnic, and geographic boundaries. Compared with continent controls, patients with UI have an overall poorer quality of life.[3] Several studies have objectively shown that UI is associated with reduced levels of social and personal activities, increased psychological distress, and overall decreased quality of life as measured by numerous indices.[4,5] The condition can affect people of all age groups, but the peak incidence of UI, at least in women, appears to occur around the age of menopause, with a slight decrease in the age group 55 to 60 years, and then a steadily increasing prevalence after age 65 years.

One of the earliest comprehensive epidemiologic studies on UI was conducted by Diokno et al.[6] using a standardized survey questionnaire. The Medical, Epidemiologic, and Social Aspects of Aging survey found that the prevalence of UI in noninstitutionalized women 60 years of age and older was approximately 38%. Almost one third of those surveyed noted urine loss at least once weekly, and 16% noted UI daily. A publication from a National Institutes of Health working group conference estimated the median level of UI prevalence to be approximately 20% to 30% during young adult life, with a broad peak around middle age (30%–40% prevalence) and an increase in the elderly (30%–50% prevalence).[7]

In the United States, chronic UI is one of the most common reasons cited for institutionalization of the elderly, and the condition is frequently encountered in the nursing home setting.[8] Little is known about the basic differences in clinical and epidemiologic characteristics of incontinence across racial or ethnic groups. Some studies report a higher incidence of UI overall in white populations[9,10] as compared with African Americans, but differences in access to healthcare as well as cultural attitudes and mores may contribute to these differences.

Consistent across all studies of unselected, noninstitutionalized populations is that UI is at least half as common in men as in women.[11,12] Overall, the prevalence of UI in men has been estimated to be approximately 9%.[13] Unlike in women, the prevalence of UI in men increases with age across most studies, with the highest prevalence recorded in the oldest patient cohorts.[13]

ETIOLOGY AND PATHOPHYSIOLOGY

ANATOMY

The lower urinary tract consists of the bladder, urethra, urinary or urethral sphincter, and surrounding musculofascial structures, including connective tissue, nerves, and blood vessels. The urinary bladder is a hollow organ composed of smooth muscle and connective tissue located deep in the bony pelvis in men and women. The urethra is a hollow tube that acts as a conduit for urine flow out of the bladder. The interior surface of both the bladder and the urethra is lined by an epithelial cell layer termed the *transitional epithelium*, which is in constant contact with urine. Previously considered inert and inactive, transitional epithelium may play an active role in the pathophysiology of many lower urinary tract disorders, including interstitial cystitis and UI.[14] The urinary or urethral sphincter is a combination of smooth and striated muscle within and surrounding the most proximal portion of the urethra adjacent to the bladder in both men and women. This is a functional but not anatomic sphincter that includes a portion of the bladder neck or outlet as well as the proximal urethra.

URINARY CONTINENCE

To prevent incontinence during the bladder filling and storage phase of the micturition cycle, the urethra, or more accurately the urethral sphincter, must maintain adequate closure in order to resist the flow of urine from the bladder at all times until voluntary voiding is initiated. Urethral closure or resistance to flow is maintained to a large degree by the proximal (under involuntary control) and distal (under both voluntary and involuntary control) urinary sphincters, a combination of smooth and striated muscles within and external to the urethra. Variable contributions to urethral closure may also come from the urethral mucosa, submucosal spongy tissue, and the overall length of the urethra. During bladder filling and storage, the bladder accommodates increasing volumes of urine flowing in from the upper urinary tract without a significant increase in bladder (intravesical) pressure. The maintenance of a low intravesical pressure despite increasing volumes of urine is a unique property of the bladder and is termed *compliance*. In addition, bladder or detrusor smooth muscle activity is normally suppressed during the filling phase by centrally mediated neural reflexes. Normal bladder emptying occurs with opening of the urethra concomitant with a volitional bladder contraction. Bladder contraction occurs in a coordinated fashion, resulting in a rise in intravesical pressure. The rise in intravesical pressure is ideally of adequate magnitude and duration to empty the bladder to completion. Opening and funneling of the bladder outlet results in urine flow into the urethra until the bladder is emptied to near completion.

The primary motor input to the detrusor muscle of the bladder is along the pelvic nerves emanating from spinal cord segments S2 to S4. Parasympathetic impulses travel to the bladder along the efferent fibers of the pelvic nerves. The impulses pass through ganglia situated in the bladder wall before reaching their target. Acetylcholine appears to be the primary neurotransmitter at the neuromuscular junction in the human lower urinary tract. Both volitional and involuntary contractions of the detrusor muscle are mediated by activation of postsynaptic muscarinic receptors by acetylcholine. Of the five known subtypes of muscarinic receptors, the majority of bladder smooth muscle cholinergic receptors are of the M_2 variety. In humans, the ratio of M_2/M_3 receptor numbers is approximately 3:1. However, M_3 receptors are the subtype responsible for both emptying contractions of normal micturition as well as involuntary bladder contractions that may result in UI.[15] Thus most pharmacologic antimuscarinic therapy is primarily anti-M_3 based.

This description of the mechanisms of urinary continence is a bit simplistic. Many other neurohumoral pathways and mechanisms, both within and outside the urinary tract, may play substantial roles in urinary continence (and voiding dysfunction) and may be future therapeutic options for treatment of voiding dysfunction and UI. Examples include adrenergic, purinergic, serotoninergic, and dopaminergic pathways, tachykinin receptor antagonists, and calcium and potassium channel modulators.[15]

The bladder and urethra normally operate in unison during the bladder filling and storage phase, as well as the bladder emptying phase of the micturition cycle. The smooth and striated muscles of the bladder and urethra are organized during the micturition cycle by a number of reflexes coordinated at the pontine micturition center in the midbrain. Disturbances in the neural regulation of micturition at any level (brain, spinal cord, or pelvic nerves) often lead to characteristic changes in lower urinary tract function that may result in UI.[16]

Mechanisms of Urinary Incontinence

Simply stated, UI may occur as a result of abnormalities of only the urethra (including the bladder outlet and urinary sphincter) or only the bladder or as a combination of abnormalities in both.[17] Abnormalities may result in either overfunction or underfunction of the bladder and/or urethra, with resulting development of UI. Although this simple classification scheme excludes extremely rare causes of UI such as congenital ectopic ureters and urinary fistulas, it is useful for gaining a working understanding of the condition.

Urethral Underactivity (Stress Urinary Incontinence) Some patients characteristically note UI during exertional activities such as exercise, running, lifting, coughing, and sneezing. This implies that the compromised urethral sphincter is no longer able to resist the flow of urine from the bladder during periods of physical activity. In essence, increases in intraabdominal pressure during physical activity are transmitted to the bladder (an intraabdominal organ), compressing it and forcing urine through the weakened sphincter.

This type of UI is known as *stress urinary incontinence* (SUI). Although the exact etiology of urethral underactivity and SUI in women is incompletely understood, clearly identifiable risk factors include pregnancy, childbirth, menopause, cognitive impairment, obesity, and age.[18,19] The prevalence of SUI in women appears to peak during or after the onset of menopause. This implies that hormonal factors are important in maintaining continence.

In men, SUI is most commonly the result of prior lower urinary tract surgery or injury, with resulting compromise of the sphincter mechanism within and external to the urethra. Radical prostatectomy for treatment of adenocarcinoma of the prostate is probably the most common setting in which surgical manipulation leads to UI. Overall, SUI in the male is uncommon and, in the absence of prior prostate surgery, severe trauma, or neurologic illness, is extraordinarily rare. Transurethral resection of the prostate for benign prostatic hyperplasia (BPH; see Chap. 93) may lead to SUI in men.

Bladder Overactivity (Urge Urinary Incontinence) Bladder overactivity may occur during bladder filling and urine storage due to involuntary bladder (detrusor) contractions. Symptoms of bladder overactivity occur because the detrusor muscle is overactive and contracts inappropriately during the filling phase which, in the neurologically normal individual, results in a sense of urinary urgency. The terms *overactive bladder* and *detrusor overactivity* are distinct and should not be used interchangeably, as they frequently are. The International Continence Society defines overactive bladder as a symptom syndrome characterized by urinary urgency, with frequency and nocturia, with/without associated UI in the absence of a known pathologic condition that may result in similar symptoms (e.g., urinary tract infection, bladder cancer).[1] When UI occurs concomitantly with a sense of urinary urgency, it is termed urge urinary incontinence (UUI).[1] The latter is most commonly, although not invariably, associated with involuntary detrusor contractions.

Therefore, a diagnosis of overactive bladder does not require urodynamic testing for confirmation but is a diagnosis based on patient symptoms. Conversely, detrusor overactivity is a specific urodynamic diagnosis referring to the finding of involuntary detrusor contractions during the filling phase of a urodynamic study. Therefore, invasive urodynamic testing is required to make the diagnosis. Up to 40% of patients with overactive bladder do not demonstrate detrusor overactivity on urodynamic testing. The clinical significance of this finding is unknown. However, the effectiveness of pharmacologic therapy appears to be independent of the presence or absence of detrusor overactivity.[20] This distinction between overactive bladder (a symptom syndrome) and detrusor overactivity (a urodynamic diagnosis) is essential in fully understanding the patient population under study and the effects of pharmacologic therapy reported in the literature.

Symptoms characteristic of overactive bladder are urinary frequency and urgency, with or without urge incontinence. *Frequency* is defined as micturition more than eight times per day. *Urgency* is described as a sudden compelling desire to urinate that is difficult to delay.[1] People suffering from overactive bladder typically have to empty their bladder frequently, and, when they experience a sensation of urgency, they may leak urine if they are unable to reach the toilet quickly. Many patients have associated nocturia (>1 micturition per night) and/or nocturnal incontinence (enuresis). Nocturia and enuresis are particularly disruptive to sleep. For patients with incontinence, the amount of urine lost may be large, as the bladder may empty completely.

Most patients with overactive bladder and UUI have no identifiable underlying etiology and thus are classified as "idiopathic." Patients with a relevant neurologic condition and with urinary incontinence related to involuntary bladder contractions demonstrated on urodynamic testing are classified as having neurogenic detrusor overactivity. Clearly identifiable risk factors for UUI include normal aging, neurologic disease (including stroke, Parkinson's disease, multiple sclerosis, and spinal cord injury), and bladder outlet obstruction (e.g., due to BPH or prostate cancer).

The mechanism for overactive bladder and UUI must be either neurogenic or myogenic. The neurogenic hypothesis ascribes the condition to disease-related changes within the central or peripheral nervous systems.[21] The myogenic hypothesis states that overactive bladder and UUI result from changes within the smooth muscle of the bladder wall itself.[22] Precipitating factors, such as bladder outlet obstruction (BOO), can cause partial denervation of smooth muscle, leading to a state of decreased responsiveness to activation of intrinsic nerves but supersensitivity to contractile agonists and direct electrical activation and detrusor overactivity.[23] Indeed, overactive detrusor muscle from an individual with BOO may or may not be quite different as compared with the same muscle tissue from an individual with idiopathic or neurogenic detrusor overactivity in terms of many physiologic and anatomic characteristics (including receptor type[s] and density/densities, collagen content, and innervation).[24] A full discussion of these differences is beyond the scope of this chapter. Thus, in practice, UUI is difficult to categorize as either neurogenic or myogenic in origin, as these etiologies often seem to be interconnected and complementary.

Urethral Overactivity and/or Bladder Underactivity (Overflow Incontinence)

Overflow incontinence, the result of urethral overactivity and/or bladder underactivity, is an important but uncommon type of UI in both men and women. Overflow incontinence results when the bladder is filled to capacity at all times but is unable to empty, causing urine to leak from a distended bladder past a normal or even overactive outlet and sphincter.

In the setting of urethral overactivity, resistance to the flow of urine during volitional voiding is increased, resulting in functional or anatomic obstruction and incomplete bladder emptying. Clinically and practically, the most common causes of urethral overactivity in men are anatomic urethral obstruction, including that due to BPH and prostate cancer. In women, urethral overactivity is rare but may result from cystocele formation (with resultant kinking or obstruction of the urethra) or surgical overcorrection (iatrogenic obstruction) following anti-SUI surgery. In both men and women, overflow UI may be associated with systemic neurologic dysfunction or diseases, such as spinal cord injury or multiple sclerosis.

Bladder underactivity may result in overflow incontinence. Under certain circumstances, the detrusor muscle of the bladder may become progressively weakened and eventually lose the ability to voluntarily contract. In the absence of adequate contractility, the bladder is unable to empty completely, and large volumes of residual urine are left after micturition. Both myogenic and neurogenic factors have been implicated in producing the impaired contractility seen in this condition. Clinically, overflow incontinence is most commonly seen in the setting of long-term chronic bladder outlet obstruction in men, such as that due to BPH or prostate cancer, diabetes mellitus, or denervation due to radical pelvic surgery, such as abdominopelvic resection or radical hysterectomy.

Mixed Incontinence and Other Types of Urinary Incontinence

Various types of UI may coexist in the same patient. The combination of bladder overactivity and urethral underactivity is termed *mixed incontinence*. The diagnosis is often difficult because of the confusing array of presenting symptoms. Bladder overactivity may also coexist with impaired bladder contractility. This occurs most commonly in the elderly and is termed *detrusor hyperactivity with impaired contractility*.[25]

Functional incontinence is not caused by bladder- or urethra-specific factors. Rather, in patients with conditions such as dementia or cognitive or mobility deficits, the UI is linked to the primary disease process more than any extrinsic or intrinsic deficit of the lower urinary tract. An example of functional incontinence occurs in the postoperative orthopedic surgery patient. Following extensive orthopedic reconstructions such as total hip arthroplasty, patients are often immobile secondary to pain or traction. Therefore, patients may be unable to access toileting facilities in a reasonable amount of time and may become incontinent as a result. Treatment of this type of UI may involve simple interventions such as placing a urinal or commode at the bedside that allows for uncomplicated access to toileting.

Many localized or systemic illnesses may result in UI because of their effects on the lower urinary tract or the surrounding structures:

- Dementia/delirium
- Depression
- Urinary tract infection (cystitis)
- Postmenopausal atrophic urethritis or vaginitis
- Diabetes mellitus
- Neurologic disease (e.g., stroke, Parkinson's disease, multiple sclerosis, spinal cord injury)
- Pelvic malignancy
- Constipation
- Congenital malformations

❶ Many commonly used medications may precipitate or aggravate existing voiding dysfunction and UI (Table 94–1).

TABLE 94-1	Medications That Influence Lower Urinary Tract Function
Medication	**Effect**
Diuretics, acetylcholinesterase inhibitors	Polyuria, frequency, urgency
α-Receptor antagonists	Urethral relaxation and stress urinary incontinence in women
α-Receptor agonists	Urethral constriction and urinary retention in men
Calcium channel blockers	Urinary retention
Narcotic analgesics	Urinary retention from impaired contractility
Sedative hypnotics	Functional incontinence caused by delirium, immobility
Antipsychotic agents	Anticholinergic effects and urinary retention
Anticholinergics	Urinary retention
Antidepressants, tricyclic	Anticholinergic effects, α-antagonist effects
Alcohol	Polyuria, frequency, urgency, sedation, delirium
Angiotensin-converting enzyme inhibitors (ACEIs)	Cough as a result of ACEIs may aggravate stress urinary incontinence by increasing intraabdominal pressure

CLINICAL PRESENTATION

❷ UI may present in a number of ways, depending on the underlying pathophysiology. Generally, SUI is considered the most common type of UI and probably accounts for at least a portion of UI in more than half of all incontinent women. Some studies have found that mixed UI (SUI + UUI) is the most common type of UI.[6] However, the proportions of SUI versus UUI versus mixed UI vary considerably with age group and sex of patients studied, study methodology, and a variety of other factors. A complete medical history, including an assessment of symptoms and a physical examination, is essential for correctly classifying the type of incontinence and thereby assuring appropriate therapy.

CLINICAL PRESENTATION OF URINARY INCONTINENCE RELATED TO URETHRAL UNDERACTIVITY

General

☐ The patient usually notes UI during activities such as exercise, running, lifting, coughing, and sneezing. Occurs much more commonly in women (seen only in men with lower urinary tract surgery or injury compromising the sphincter).

Symptoms

☐ Urine leakage with physical activity (volume is proportional to activity level). No UI with physical inactivity, especially when supine (no nocturia). May develop urgency and frequency as a compensatory mechanism (or as a separate component of bladder overactivity).

Diagnostic Tests

☐ Observation of urethral meatus while patient coughs or strains.

CLINICAL PRESENTATION OF URINARY INCONTINENCE RELATED TO BLADDER OVERACTIVITY

General

☐ Can have bladder overactivity and UI without urgency if sensory input from the lower urinary tract is absent.

Symptoms

☐ Urinary frequency (>8 micturitions per day), urgency with or without urge incontinence; nocturia (≥1 micturition per night) and enuresis may be present.

Diagnostic Tests

☐ Urodynamic studies are the gold standard for diagnosis. Urinalysis and urine culture should be negative (rule out urinary tract infection as the cause of frequency).

CLINICAL PRESENTATION OF URINARY INCONTINENCE RELATED TO URETHRAL OVERACTIVITY AND/OR BLADDER UNDERACTIVITY

General

☐ Important but rare type of UI in both men and women. Urethral overactivity is usually due to prostatic enlargement (males) or cystocele formation or surgical overcorrection following stress incontinence surgery in women.

Symptoms

☐ Lower abdominal fullness, hesitancy, straining to void, decreased force of stream, interrupted stream, sense of incomplete bladder emptying. May have urinary frequency and urgency. Abdominal pain if acute urinary retention is present.

Signs

☐ Increased postvoid residual urine volume.

Diagnostic Tests

☐ Digital rectal examination or transrectal ultrasound to rule out prostatic enlargement. Renal function tests to rule out renal failure due to acute urinary retention.

URINE LEAKAGE

UI represents a spectrum of severity in terms of both volume of leakage and degree of bother to the patient. To carefully consider the level of patient discomfort when discussing urine leakage, the clinician must probe during the patient interview to accurately determine the precise nature of the problem.

Use of absorbent products, such as panty liners, pads, or briefs, is an obvious point of discussion, but the clinician must keep in mind that use of these products varies among patients. The number and type of pads may not relate to the amount or type of incontinence, as their use is a function of personal preference and hygiene. A high number of absorbent pads may be used every day by a patient with severe, high-volume UI or, alternatively, by a fastidiously hygienic patient with low-volume leakage who simply changes pads often to prevent wetness or odor. Nevertheless, a large number of pads that are described by the patient as "soaked" is indicative of high-volume urine loss.

Regardless of the volume of urine loss, the desire to seek evaluation and therapy for UI in all patients is almost always elective and contingent on the degree of bother to the individual patient. As with the use of absorbent products, patients differ with regard to the amount of urine loss they will tolerate before considering the condition bothersome enough to seek assistance.

SYMPTOMS

Under the best of circumstances, UI is difficult to categorize based on symptoms alone (Table 94–2).[26] In a study of patients who appeared to have SUI based on symptoms and patient history,

TABLE 94-2 Differentiating Bladder Overactivity from Urethral Underactivity

Symptoms	Bladder Overactivity	Urethral Underactivity
Urgency (strong, sudden desire to void)	Yes	Sometimes
Frequency with urgency	Yes	Rarely
Leaking during physical activity (e.g., coughing, sneezing, lifting)	No	Yes
Amount of urinary leakage with each episode of incontinence	Large if present	Usually small
Ability to reach the toilet in time following an urge to void	No or just barely	Yes
Nocturnal incontinence (presence of wet pads or undergarments in bed)	Yes	Rare
Nocturia (waking to pass urine at night)	Usually	Seldom

urodynamics showed that only 72% of patients had SUI as the sole cause of incontinence.[27]

Patients with urethral underactivity or SUI characteristically complain of urinary leakage with physical activity. Volume of leakage is proportional to the level of activity. They will often leak urine during periods of exercise, coughing, sneezing, lifting, or even when rising from a seated to a standing position. Patients with pure SUI will not have leakage when physically inactive, especially when they are supine. Often they will have little or no UI at night, will not awaken to void during the night (nocturia), will not wet the bed, and often do not even wear absorbent products during the night. Urinary urgency and frequency may be associated with SUI, either as a separate component caused by bladder overactivity (mixed incontinence) or as a compensatory mechanism wherein the patient with SUI learns to toilet frequently to prevent large-volume urine loss during physical activity.

Typical symptoms of bladder overactivity include frequency, urgency, and urge incontinence. Nocturia and nocturnal incontinence are often present. Urine leakage is unpredictable, and the volume loss may be large. Patients often wear protection both day and night. Urinary frequency can be affected by a number of factors unrelated to bladder overactivity, including excessive fluid intake (polydipsia) and bladder hypersensitivity states such as interstitial cystitis and urinary tract infection, and should be ruled out. In some patients, bladder overactivity manifests as UI without awareness in the absence of a sense of urinary urgency or frequency. *Urinary urgency*, a sensation of impending micturition, requires intact sensory input from the lower urinary tract. In patients with spinal cord injury, sensory neuropathies, and other neurologic diseases, a diminished ability to perceive or process sensory input from the lower urinary tract may result in bladder overactivity and UI without urgency or urinary frequency. When bladder contraction occurs without warning and sensation is absent, the condition is referred to as *reflex incontinence*.

Patients with overflow incontinence may present with lower abdominal fullness as well as considerable obstructive urinary symptoms, including hesitancy, straining to void, decreased force of urinary stream, interrupted stream, and a vague sense of incomplete bladder emptying. These patients may also have a significant component of urinary frequency and urgency. In patients with acute urinary retention and overflow incontinence, lower abdominal pain may be present. Although these symptoms are not specific for overflow incontinence, they may warrant further investigation, including an assessment of postvoid residual urine volume.

SIGNS

A presenting complaint of UI mandates a directed physical examination and a brief neurologic assessment. The workup ideally includes an abdominal examination to exclude a distended bladder, neurologic assessment of the perineum and lower extremities, pelvic examination in women (looking especially for evidence of prolapse or hormonal deficiency), and genital and prostate examination in men.

SUI can usually be objectively demonstrated by having the patient cough or strain during the examination and observing the urethral meatus for a sudden spurt of urine. In women, SUI may be associated with varying degrees of vaginal prolapse, including cystourethrocele (bladder and urethral prolapse), enterocele (small bowel prolapse), rectocele (rectal prolapse), and uterine prolapse. These conditions may have important implications for therapy in that treatment of the prolapse may result in improvement of urinary symptoms.

Perineal skin maceration, erythema, breakdown, and ulceration may be indicative of chronic, severe UI. Patients with chronic incontinence may manifest fungal infections of the skin of the perineum and upper thighs.

In both men and women, digital rectal examination provides an opportunity to check ambient rectal tone and the integrity of the sacral reflex arc (e.g., anal wink) as well as assess the patient's ability to perform a voluntary pelvic floor muscle contraction (i.e., Kegel exercise), which may be an important factor in deciding on appropriate therapy. In men, a digital examination of the prostate assesses for the presence of prostate cancer, inflammation, and BPH.

A targeted neurologic examination includes assessment of reflexes, rectal tone, and sensory or motor deficits in the lower extremities, which might be indicative of systemic or localized neurologic disease. Neurologic diseases have the potential to affect bladder and sphincter function and thus may have significant implications in the incontinent patient.

PRIOR MEDICAL OR SURGICAL ILLNESS

UI may present in the setting of concurrent, seemingly unrelated illnesses. New-onset UI may be the initial manifestation of systemic illnesses such as diabetes mellitus, metastatic malignancies, multiple sclerosis, and other neurologic illnesses. Central nervous system disease, or injury above the level of the pons, generally results in symptoms of bladder overactivity and UUI. Spinal cord injury or disease may manifest as bladder overactivity and UUI or as overflow incontinence, depending on the spinal level and completeness of the injury or disease.

Medications may have wide-ranging effects on lower urinary tract function (see Table 94-1). A thorough inquiry into the use of new medications in the setting of recent-onset UI may show a relationship.

Acute UI manifesting in the immediate postoperative setting may be secondary to a number of factors, including surgical manipulation and immobility, and to a number of medications, especially opioid analgesics. In the postoperative setting, acute urinary retention and overflow incontinence are commonly related to the administration of anesthetic agents and/or opioid analgesics in the perioperative period. These agents may have profound effects on bladder contractility that are completely reversible once the agents are metabolized and excreted.

Prior surgery may have effects on lower urinary tract function. UI following prostate surgery in men is highly suggestive of injury to the sphincter and resultant SUI. Pelvic surgery for benign and malignant conditions may result in denervation or injury to the lower urinary tract. This includes bowel surgery and gynecologic procedures. For example, new-onset total UI following gynecologic surgery suggests intraoperative bladder injury and subsequent development of a postoperative vesicovaginal fistula. Radiation therapy to the pelvis for malignant disease (e.g., prostate cancer or cervical cancer) may result in injury to the bladder or urethra and subsequent UI.

In women, UI may be related to several gynecologic factors, including childbirth, hormonal status, and prior gynecologic surgery. Pregnancy and childbirth, particularly vaginal delivery, are associated with SUI and pelvic prolapse. Significant SUI in the nulliparous woman is uncommon. UI that becomes progressive at or around menopause suggests a hormonal component that may be responsive to estrogen or hormone replacement therapy.

UI may present in the setting of other significant pelvic floor disorders, signs, and symptoms. Constipation, diarrhea, fecal incontinence, dyspareunia, sexual dysfunction, and pelvic pain may be related to UI. A history of gross hematuria in the setting of UI mandates further urologic investigation, including radiologic imaging of the upper urinary tract and cystoscopy. Acute dysuria with or without hematuria in the setting of UI suggests cystitis. Urinalysis and urine culture should be performed in these patients.

TREATMENT

Urinary Incontinence

■ NONPHARMACOLOGIC TREATMENT

❸ Nonpharmacologic treatment of UI is recommended as the first line of therapy at a primary care level. For patients in whom pharmacologic or surgical management is inappropriate or undesired, nondrug treatment is the only option. Examples of patients who fulfill these criteria include patients who are not medically fit for surgery, those who plan future pregnancies (which may adversely affect long-term surgical outcomes), those with overflow incontinence whose condition is not amenable to surgery or drug therapy, those with comorbid conditions that place them at high risk for adverse effects from drug therapy, those who are delaying surgery or do not want to undergo surgery, and those with mild to moderate symptoms who do not want to take medication.

For additional information on nonpharmacologic interventions for UI, readers are referred to comprehensive literature reviews and consensus opinions of treatment guidelines on nonpharmacologic interventions by multidisciplinary experts.[28] Table 94–3 summarizes the basic nondrug approaches.

Behavioral interventions are the first line of treatment for SUI, UUI, and mixed UI. Interventions include lifestyle modifications, toilet scheduling regimens, and pelvic floor muscle rehabilitation. Because the key to success with any type of behavioral intervention is motivation of patients or caregivers, these individuals must be active participants in developing a treatment plan. Regular follow-up is needed to help motivate patients and caregivers, provide reassurance and support, and monitor treatment outcomes.

■ PHARMACOLOGIC TREATMENT

Urge Urinary Incontinence

Pharmacotherapy is useful when UUI symptoms are not adequately controlled with nonpharmacologic therapies, particularly in patients with low functional bladder capacity, especially individuals who frequently attempt to toilet and are independent or require only limited assistance in toileting. In many cases, the combined use of pharmacotherapy with nonpharmacologic therapy produces a better response than either intervention alone.

❹ Anticholinergic/antispasmodic drugs have proved to be the most effective agents for suppressing premature detrusor contractions, enhancing bladder storage, and relieving UUI symptoms

and complications and constitute the pharmacotherapy of first choice for treatment of UUI (Tables 94–4 and 94–5).[29–48] Drugs with anticholinergic activity act by antagonizing muscarinic cholinergic receptors, through which efferent parasympathetic nerve impulses evoke detrusor contraction. Anticholinergics have been demonstrated to improve quality of life, with no significant differences between agents.[49] Women with mixed UI or UUI plus urethritis or vaginitis may benefit from a topical estrogen (alone or in combination with an anticholinergic drug). Patients with irritative symptoms of BPH that persist despite specific BPH treatment may benefit from anticholinergic therapy as well (caution is warranted because these agents may precipitate acute urinary retention).

Immediate-Release Oxybutynin Even though a substantial proportion of patients may discontinue oxybutynin immediate-release (IR) therapy because of its nonurinary antimuscarinic effects, oxybutynin IR remains the drug of first choice for treatment of UUI and the gold standard against which other drugs are compared. In addition to antimuscarinic effects (e.g., dry mouth, constipation, vision impairment, confusion, cognitive dysfunction, and tachycardia), oxybutynin IR is associated with orthostatic hypotension secondary to α-adrenergic receptor blockade as well as sedation and weight gain from histamine H_1-receptor blockade.[30,35,50–54] Furthermore, adverse effects jeopardize medication adherence and can prevent dose escalation to that needed for optimal benefit.

Emerging evidence suggests that the high incidence of adverse effects, especially dry mouth, with use of oxybutynin IR is largely due to the active metabolite N-desethyloxybutynin (DEO), which is generated during extensive first-pass metabolism in the liver and upper gastrointestinal tract.[55] The lower DEO plasma concentrations seen with long-acting forms of oxybutynin (which are due to reduced first-pass metabolism) compared with those of oxybutynin IR may explain the lesser propensity of the long-acting formulations to cause dry mouth and other anticholinergic adverse effects.

Another factor associated with the adverse effects of oxybutynin IR, especially in older patients, is the transient high peak serum oxybutynin plasma concentrations.[56] Oxybutynin IR is best tolerated when the dose is gradually escalated from no more than 2.5 mg twice daily to start, to 2.5 mg three times daily after 1 month, then further increased in increments of 2.5 mg/day every 1 to 2 months until the desired response or the maximum recommended or tolerated dose is attained. The optimal response usually requires no more than 5 mg three times daily (see Table 94–4).[30,57]

Adverse effects of oxybutynin IR can sometimes be managed by a dose reduction if this does not significantly compromise drug efficacy. Dry mouth can be relieved by use of sugarless hard candy, gum, or a saliva substitute. Constipation can be minimized by increasing the intake of water, dietary fiber, physical activity such as walking, or laxative therapy. The need for multiple daily dosing of oxybutynin IR can further jeopardize adherence, especially in people who take multiple medications or those who are cognitively impaired.

Extended-Release Oral Oxybutynin Because of the problems noted with oxybutynin IR, an extended-release (XL) formulation of oxybutynin was developed. It can be considered an alternative first-line therapy of UUI.[58]

Unlike oxybutynin IR, oxybutynin XL delivers a controlled amount of oxybutynin continuously throughout the gastrointestinal tract over a 24-hour period, reducing first-pass metabolism by cytochrome P450 (CYP) isoenzyme 3A4, which is present in higher concentrations in the upper portion of the small intestine than in the lower gastrointestinal tract.[58,59] This results in relative bioavailabilities of oxybutynin and DEO of 153% and 69%, respectively, for oxybutynin XL compared with oxybutynin IR.[60] The greater ratio of parent drug concentration to active metabolite concentration after

TABLE 94-3 Nonpharmacologic Management of Urinary Incontinence

Intervention	Description	Patient Characteristics
Lifestyle modifications	Self-management strategies targeted toward reducing or eliminating risk factors that cause or exacerbate urinary incontinence	Smoking cessation, weight reduction for obese patients with stress and urge incontinence, constipation prevention, caffeine reduction, fluid modification only for those with abnormally high fluid intake
Scheduling regimens		
Timed voiding	Toileting on a fixed schedule where interval does not change, typically every 2 hours during waking hours	Used for stress, urge, and mixed incontinence in patients with cognitive or physical impairments; used in patients without impairments who have infrequent voiding patterns
Habit retraining	Scheduled toiletings with adjustments of voiding intervals (longer or shorter) based on patient's voiding pattern	Used for institutionalized or homebound patients with cognitive or physical impairments; may be used in patients who have diuretic-induced incontinence
Prompted voiding	Scheduled toiletings that require prompts to void from a caregiver, typically every 2 hours; patient assisted in toileting only if response is positive; used in conjunction with operant conditioning techniques for rewarding patients for maintaining continence and appropriate toileting	Used for patients who are functionally able to use toilet or toilet substitute, able to feel urge sensation, and able to request toileting assistance appropriately; primarily used in institutional settings or in homebound patients with an available caregiver
Bladder training	Scheduled toiletings with progressive voiding intervals; includes teaching urge suppression strategies using relaxation and distraction techniques, self-monitoring, and use of reinforcement techniques; sometimes combined with drug therapy	Used for stress, urge, and mixed incontinence in patients who are cognitively intact, able to toilet, and motivated to comply with training program
Pelvic floor muscle rehabilitation		
Pelvic floor muscle exercises (e.g., Kegel exercises)	Regular practice of pelvic floor muscle contractions; may involve use of pelvic floor muscle contraction for prevention of stress leakage and urge inhibition	Used for stress, urge, and mixed incontinence in patients who can correctly contract pelvic floor muscles without using accessory muscles; requires cognitively intact and highly motivated patient
Biofeedback	Use of electronic or mechanical instruments to display visual or auditory information about neuromuscular or bladder activity; used to teach correct pelvic floor muscle contraction and/or urge inhibition; home trainers are available (e.g., Myself, DesChutes Medical Products, Bend, OR; Pathway MR-10 or MR-20, Prometheus Group, Dover, NH)	Used for stress, urge, and mixed incontinence in patients who have the capability to learn voluntary control through observation and are motivated; used in conjunction with pelvic floor muscle exercises
Vaginal weight training	Active retention of increasing vaginal weights (e.g., Step Free Weights, Medgo LLC, Venice, FL); typically used in combination with pelvic floor muscle exercises at least twice per day	Women with stress incontinence who are cognitively intact, can correctly contract pelvic floor muscles, able to stand, and have sufficient vaginal vault and introitus to retain cone, and are highly motivated; contraindicated in patients with moderate to severe pelvic organ prolapse
Acupuncture	Involves insertion of disposable sterile fine stainless steel needles into points on the skin that are thought to suppress or stimulate spinal and/or supraspinal reflexes to the bladder and/or urethra	Used for urge and mixed incontinence and urinary incontinence due to spinal cord injury
Nonimplantable electrical stimulation	Application of electrical current through vaginal, anal, surface, or fine needle electrodes; used to inhibit bladder overactivity and improve awareness, contractility, and efficacy of pelvic floor muscle contraction; hand-held stimulators for home use are available (e.g., Pathway, Prometheus Group, Dover, NH; Minnova, Empi, St. Paul, MN)	Used for stress, urge, and mixed incontinence in patients who are highly motivated; contraindicated in patients with diminished sensory perception; urinary retention, history of cardiac arrhythmia, cardiac pacemakers, implantable defibrillators, pregnant or attempting pregnancy; vaginal or anal electrodes are contraindicated in moderate or severe pelvic organ prolapse
Extracorporeal magnetic stimulation	Pulsed magnetic stimulation to pelvic floor musculature causing depolarization of motor neurons, thus inducing pelvic floor muscle contraction; stimulation is provided through a specially designed chair that contains a device for producing a pulsing magnetic field (e.g., Neotonus, Inc., Marietta, GA)	Used for treatment of stress, urge, and mixed incontinence; contraindicated in patients with demand cardiac pacemakers or metallic joint replacements; may be useful treatment option when other approaches fail or are not feasible
Antiincontinence devices		
Pessaries	Intravaginal devices designed to support the bladder neck, relieve minor to moderate pelvic organ prolapse, and change pressure transmission to the urethra (e.g., Cooper Surgical (Milex), Trumbull, CT; Mentor Corporation, Santa Barbara, CA)	Used for female stress incontinence and mild to moderate pelvic organ prolapse; in postmenopausal women, topical estrogen therapy is typically prescribed to prevent ulceration and breakdown of vaginal tissue; requires good manual dexterity to manipulate device
Bed or pant alarms	Sensor devices that respond to wetness; used to awaken or alert individuals via noise or vibrating mechanism (e.g., Nite Train-r, Koregon Enterprises, Inc., Beaverton, OR; Wet Call Alarm, AliMed, Dedham, MA)	Primarily used for nocturnal enuresis in children; system available for monitoring incontinence in home care and institutional environments
Urethral compression device (men only)	Penile clamp (e.g., Cunningham Incontinence Clamp, Bard Medical, Covington, GA; ActiCuf, GT Urological, Minneapolis, MN; Cook Continence, Cook Wound/Ostomy/Continence, Spencer, IN)	Used in male stress incontinence patients who are intact and have good manual dexterity
External collection devices (men only)	Condom catheter with leg bag	Used in men with urge, stress, and overflow incontinence and in those with functional impairments
Catheters	Disposable, intermittent urethral catheters and indwelling urethral and suprapubic catheters	Used for overflow incontinence; used in patients who are bed-bound or with significant mobility impairments and severe incontinence; those with terminal illness; those with sacral pressure ulcers until healing occurs

(continued)

TABLE 94-3 Nonpharmacologic Management of Urinary Incontinence (continued)

Intervention	Description	Patient Characteristics
Supportive interventions		
Toileting substitutes and other environmental modifications	Female and male urinals, bedside commodes, elevated toilet seats	Used for patients with mobility impairments that make reaching a toilet in timely fashion difficult
Absorbent products	Variety of reusable and disposable pads and pant systems; some products contain a polymer that absorbs and wicks urine away from the body	Used for all types of incontinence
Physical therapy	Gait and/or strength training	Used for frail elderly patients with mobility impairments that make reaching a toilet in timely fashion difficult

oxybutynin XL administration and, probably less importantly, the lower peak plasma drug concentration are believed to be the reasons for fewer dose- and concentration-dependent adverse effects and better patient tolerance with the XL preparation compared with oxybutynin IR.[61] Elimination of oxybutynin XL is not known to be altered in patients with renal or hepatic impairment or in geriatric patients (up to age 78 years).[58] The absence of an effect of advanced age on oxybutynin XL pharmacokinetics is unexpected because clearance of oxybutynin IR is significantly lower (by approximately 50%) in older patients compared with younger individuals.

Controlled studies have demonstrated that oxybutynin XL is significantly more effective than placebo and is as effective as oxybutynin IR in terms of reducing the mean number of UI episodes, restoring continence, decreasing the number of micturitions per day, and increasing urine volume voided per micturition.[34,35,50–52,62–64]

In short-term studies of up to 12 weeks' duration, oxybutynin XL was better tolerated than oxybutynin IR, with approximately 7% of patients discontinuing treatment because of adverse effects (compared with approximately 27% of those taking oxybutynin IR).[30,35,50,51,57,58] The rate and severity of adverse effects did not differ significantly between elderly persons (≥ 65 years old) and younger adults using the XL preparation. A 12-week study demonstrated the superiority of oxybutynin XL over tolterodine IR in reducing the mean number of weekly incontinence episodes and micturitions.[43]

In the Overactive Bladder: Performance of Extended-Release Agents (OPERA) trial, oxybutynin XL and tolterodine long-acting (LA) were equally effective in decreasing the mean number of incontinence episodes, but oxybutynin XL was superior in reducing weekly micturition frequency and achieving total dryness.[65]

TABLE 94-4 Pharmacotherapeutic Options in Patients with Urinary Incontinence

Type	Drug Class	Drug Therapy (Usual Dose)	Comments
Overactive bladder	Anticholinergic agents/ antispasmodics	Oxybutynin IR (2.5–5 mg two, three, or four times daily), oxybutynin XL (5–30 mg daily), oxybutynin TDS (3.9 mg/day) (apply one patch twice weekly), oxybutynin gel (1 sachet [100 mg] topically daily), tolterodine IR (1–2 mg twice daily), tolterodine LA (2–4 mg daily), trospium chloride extended release (60 mg daily), solifenacin (5–10 mg daily), darifenacin (7.5–15 mg daily), fesoterodine (4–8 mg daily)	Anticholinergics are first-line drug therapy (oxybutynin or tolterodine is preferred)
	Tricyclic antidepressants (TCAs)	Imipramine, doxepin, nortriptyline, or desipramine (25–100 mg at bedtime)	TCAs are generally reserved for patients with an additional indication (e.g., depression, neuropathic pain)
	Topical estrogen (only in women with urethritis or vaginitis)	Conjugated estrogen vaginal cream (0.5 g) three times per week for up to 8 months. Repeat course if symptom recurrence, or use estradiol vaginal insert/ring [2 mg (one ring)] and replace after 90 days if needed	Marginally effective for OAB; few adverse effects with vaginal cream and insert
Stress	Duloxetine[a]	40–80 mg/day (one or two doses)	Even though not FDA approved, duloxetine is first-line therapy; most adverse events diminish with time, so support patient during initial period of use
	α-Adrenergic agonists	Pseudoephedrine (15–60 mg three times daily) with food, water, or milk Phenylephrine (10 mg four times daily)	Pseudoephedrine and phenylephrine are alternative first-line therapies for women with no contraindication (notably hypertension); phenylpropanolamine was the preferred agent in the class until its removal from the U.S. market in 2000
	Estrogen	See estrogens (above). Works best if urethritis or vaginitis due to estrogen deficiency is present	Considered a less-effective alternative to α-adrenergic agonists and duloxetine. Combined α-adrenergic agonist and estrogen may be somewhat more effective than α-adrenergic agonist alone in postmenopausal women
	Imipramine	25–100 mg at bedtime	Imipramine is an optional therapy when first-line therapy is inadequate
Overflow (atonic bladder)	Cholinomimetics	Bethanechol (25–50 mg three or four times daily) on an empty stomach	Avoid use if patient has asthma or heart disease. Short-term use only. Never give IV or IM because of life-threatening cardiovascular and severe gastrointestinal reactions

IR, immediate-release; LA, long-acting; TDS, transdermal system; XL, extended-release.
[a]Not FDA-approved for this use. Doses provided are those best supported by clinical trials to date.

TABLE 94-5 Adverse Event Incidence Rates with First-Line Drugs for Bladder Overactivity[a]

Drug	Dry Mouth	Constipation	Dizziness	Vision Disturbance
Oxybutynin IR	85	40	32	20
Oxybutynin XL	35	7	5	2
Oxybutynin TDS	7	3	1	1
Oxybutynin gel	7	2	2	2
Tolterodine	61	13	6	8
Tolterodine LA	23	6	2	1
Trospium chloride IR	20	10	1	1
Trospium chloride XR	11	9	1	1
Solifenacin	11	5	2	4
Darifenacin	20	15	2	2
Fesoterodine	20	15	2	2

IR, immediate-release; LA, long-acting; TDS, transdermal system; XL, extended-release; XR, extended-release.

[a]All values constitute mean data, predominantly using product information from the manufacturers. Due to the absence of information regarding dizziness for oxybutynin IR in the product information, pooled data from references 52 and 69 have been used.

In another study that pooled results of two open-label studies, tolterodine LA was associated with significantly greater patient-perceived improvement in bladder control and fewer withdrawals due to adverse effects than oxybutynin XL. However, the treatments were similar in terms of patients' or physicians' perception of benefit over baseline and proportions of withdrawals due to lack of efficacy. However, the lack of blinding may have introduced patient and observer bias.[66]

Oxybutynin XL, available only in a tablet formulation, is administered once daily, with or without food, and should not be crushed or chewed (see Table 94–4). Like oxybutynin IR, the dosage does not require adjustment in patients of advanced age or in patients with renal or hepatic impairment. However, treatment should be initiated at the smallest recommended dosage in the elderly (5 mg once daily).[36,58] The maximum benefit of oxybutynin XL may not be realized for up to 4 weeks after starting therapy or after dose escalation. No known clinically relevant drug–drug interactions with either oxybutynin XL or oxybutynin IR have been identified. However, other drugs with anticholinergic activity may increase overall anticholinergic effects (i.e., produce an additive or synergistic pharmacodynamic interaction), as might be expected.[58] Another potential pharmacodynamic interaction involves the mutual antagonism of anticholinergic agents and cholinergic stimulants, such as the acetylcholinesterase inhibitors used to treat dementia.

Extended-Release Transdermal Oxybutynin The oxybutynin transdermal system (TDS), which delivers 3.9 mg/day, is applied twice weekly (every 3 or 4 days). Transdermal absorption of oxybutynin from this formulation bypasses first-pass hepatic and gut metabolism, resulting in similar plasma oxybutynin but lower plasma DEO concentrations compared with levels achieved after administration of an equivalent dose via the oral route.[55,67,68] No dosage adjustment of the TDS product for advancing age is necessary.[48]

Oxybutynin TDS is superior to placebo in reducing the number of incontinence episodes and micturitions and increasing the volume voided per micturition.[47,48] It is similar to oxybutynin IR in reducing the frequency of UUI episodes and improving patient-perceived urinary leakage.[69] Oxybutynin TDS and tolterodine LA are significantly superior to placebo and similar to each other in reducing the frequency of UUI episodes, increasing the volume voided per micturition, attaining complete continence, and improving quality of life.[47]

A combined analysis of two phase III studies demonstrated a significant decrease in the number of UUI episodes and urinary frequency and increase in the volume voided per micturition from baseline with oxybutynin TDS in a study population, half of whom were elderly. These results were similar to those achieved in other studies with younger adults.[70] A subgroup analysis of combined placebo-controlled and open-label studies found similar reductions in numbers of UUI episodes and daily micturitions in patients 65 years and older compared with younger adults.[71]

The most common adverse effects with the TDS formulation are pruritus (15%) and erythema (9%) at the application site. Dry mouth (7%), constipation (3%), dizziness (1%), and abnormal vision (1%) occur less frequently with the TDS formulation than with the IR formulation and with similar frequency compared with oxybutynin XL and tolterodine IR/LA.[43,48]

In a study population in which approximately half were elders, the incidences of total adverse events, dry mouth, constipation, abnormal vision, dizziness, and somnolence with oxybutynin TDS were similar to those observed in younger adults.[70] A subgroup analysis of combined placebo-controlled and open-label studies showed that the incidence of adverse events with oxybutynin TDS in patients 65 years and older was similar to that in younger adults. The rates of pruritus and overall treatment discontinuation were lower in elders compared with younger adults.[71]

Oxybutynin Gel. Oxybutyin, in a topical gel formulation applied once daily, delivers approximately 4 mg/day to the systemic circulation. It has the same indications as other oxybutynin products.[72] Transdermal absorption from this formulation has the same effects on oxybutynin and N-desethyloxybutynin plasma concentrations as seen with the TDS patch formulation.[73] No dosage adjustment is necessary for advanced age.[72] There is no clinical experience with the gel formulation in patients with renal or hepatic impairment but no dosage adjustment appears necessary in either pathophysiologic state.[72] Application of sunscreen 0.5 hours before or after application of the gel or showering 1 hour after application of the gel does not affect oxybutynin bioavailability.[72] In a phase III, 12-week, randomized, placebo-controlled study, recipients of the gel formulation (n = 389) exhibited significant reductions in urinary frequency and urge incontinence episodes and an increase in volume voided per micturition compared with placebo recipients (n = 400).[74] There are no data available comparing the gel formulation with an active control. The most common adverse events include pruritus (15%), erythema (9%), dermatitis (1.8%), and site reactions (5.4%) at the application site; xerostomia (7.5%); dizziness (1.5%); headache (1.5%); constipation (1.3%); and pruritus (1.3%).[72]

Immediate-Release Tolterodine Tolterodine is a competitive muscarinic receptor antagonist that can be considered first-line therapy for UI in patients with symptoms of urinary frequency, urgency, or urge incontinence.[37]

Controlled studies demonstrated that tolterodine was significantly more effective than placebo and as effective as oxybutynin IR in decreasing the mean daily number of micturitions and increasing the mean volume voided per micturition.[31,38–42,75,76] Although three controlled trials showed a significant decrease in the mean number of incontinence episodes per 24 hours compared with placebo, most other studies have not confirmed the finding, and the manufacturer's package insert does not claim a significant improvement in this parameter.[32,38–42,76] The only controlled study of the ability of tolterodine to restore urinary continence reported an insignificant effect size of 9% over placebo.[38]

Extended-Release Tolterodine In a controlled study of 1,529 adult outpatients with urinary frequency and UUI, tolterodine LA, an extended-release formulation of tolterodine, significantly decreased the mean number of weekly incontinence episodes (23% effect size over placebo and 7% effect size over tolterodine IR). Premature study withdrawal rates did not differ significantly between the two active treatments, but dry mouth was observed significantly less often in patients taking the LA formulation than among those receiving the IR formulation.[44]

Tolterodine LA was significantly superior to placebo and similar in elderly and young patient populations in reducing the frequencies of incontinence episodes and micturitions, increasing the volume voided per micturition and ability to complete tasks before voiding, and enhancing patient perception of benefit. Adverse effect types and frequencies were similar in the two age groups.[77]

A major consideration in using tolterodine is its pharmacokinetics, specifically its metabolism. The agent is predominantly eliminated by hepatic metabolism, which is partially under the control of genetic polymorphism.[37] The principal metabolic pathway in extensive metabolizers involves oxidation of the parent drug by CYP isoenzyme 2D6 to the active 5-hydroxymethyl metabolite (DD01), followed by further oxidation and dealkylation. In poor metabolizers who lack the CYP 2D6 (approximately 7% of the U.S. population), the principal metabolic pathway involves CYP 3A4, with dealkylation of the amino group, oxidation to a dealkylated hydroxy metabolite, and further oxidation to a dealkylated acid metabolite that undergoes glucuronidation. Because tolterodine is principally metabolized by CYP 3A4 in this case, its elimination may be impaired by inhibitors of this isoenzyme (e.g., fluoxetine, sertraline, fluvoxamine, macrolide antibiotics, azole antifungals, and grapefruit juice). For example, fluoxetine, an inhibitor of CYP 2D6 and 3A4, decreases the metabolism of tolterodine to DD01. The result is a mean 4.8-fold increase in the tolterodine area under the plasma concentration–time curve (AUC), mean 52% decrease in peak plasma concentration, and mean 20% decrease in the AUC of DD01.[37] Whether tolterodine significantly alters the pharmacokinetics of drugs metabolized by CYP 2D6 is unknown, so caution is advised with concurrent use with agents metabolized by CYP 2D6.

Single-dose interaction studies have demonstrated that concurrent administration of tolterodine LA with antacid leads to rapid release of drug (70% within 4 hours) and a mean 1.5-fold elevation in tolterodine peak plasma concentration compared with placebo. The same studies showed that the pharmacokinetics of oxybutynin XL were unaltered by concurrent antacid administration.[78] Another single-dose study showed that concurrent administration of tolterodine LA with omeprazole 20 mg once daily resulted in significantly increased peak plasma tolterodine concentrations compared with tolterodine LA given without prior omeprazole use. Conversely, no significant differences in peak plasma concentration of oxybutynin were evident when the XL formulation was administered with or without omeprazole. However, the AUCs of both agents were not significantly affected by omeprazole administration.[79] The clinical implication of this interaction is unclear. Whether a similar interaction exists with histamine H_2-receptor antagonists is unknown.

One of two phase I pharmacokinetic studies comparing tolterodine pharmacokinetics in healthy elderly volunteers (age 64–80 years) with those in healthy volunteers younger than 40 years found no significant differences in pharmacokinetic parameters between the groups. However, in the second phase I study, the mean serum concentrations of tolterodine and DD01 were 20% and 50% greater in elderly volunteers than in young healthy volunteers, respectively. Despite possibly altered pharmacokinetics in elderly individuals, no differences in the incidences and severity of adverse events between these age groups have been noted in clinical trials, so no dosage adjustment is recommended on the basis of age alone.[37]

Tolterodine elimination is diminished in patients with impaired hepatic function. Patients with hepatic cirrhosis who are extensive metabolizers exhibit a significantly higher mean AUC of DD01, higher serum tolterodine and DD01 concentrations, and longer terminal disposition half-life of tolterodine and DD01 than do healthy subjects who are extensive metabolizers. The tolterodine AUC is higher in cirrhotic patients who are poor metabolizers than in healthy people who are poor metabolizers.[37] If use of tolterodine cannot be avoided in patients with hepatic impairment or in those receiving inhibitors of CYP 3A4 (and possibly inhibitors of CYP 2D6), the initial dose should be reduced by 50% to tolterodine IR 1 mg twice daily or tolterodine LA 2 mg once daily.[37] No formal tolterodine dosage recommendation is possible based on available information for individuals who concurrently have hepatic impairment and are taking a CYP 3A4 and/or 2D6 inhibitor. Intuitively, the initial dose should not exceed 1 mg twice daily (IR) or 2 mg once daily (LA).

Elimination of tolterodine has not been evaluated in patients with impaired renal function; therefore, the drug should be used more cautiously in such individuals (i.e., starting dose of IR product is 1 mg twice daily with gradual dose escalation, if needed, to the usual maximum of 2 mg twice daily or a starting dose of the LA formulation is 2 mg once daily with gradual dose escalation, if needed, to the usual maximum of 4 mg once daily).[37]

Tolterodine is better tolerated than oxybutynin IR, with approximately 8% of patients discontinuing treatment prematurely (compared with approximately 27% of individuals taking oxybutynin IR).[30,32,38,39,41,50,79] The most common adverse effects of tolterodine are dry mouth, dyspepsia, headache, constipation, and dry eyes.[37]

Tolterodine, available only as a tablet formulation, can be taken with or without food. The LA product should not be crushed or chewed or taken less than 2 hours before or 4 hours after antacid administration. The maximum benefit from tolterodine may not be realized for up to 8 weeks after starting therapy or dose escalation.

Fesoterodine Fumarate Fesoterodine fumarate is a prodrug that is metabolized to the active metabolite, 5-hydroxymethyl tolterodine, by nonspecific plasma esterases. It is an alternative first-line therapy for UI in patients with symptoms of urinary frequency, urgency, or urge incontinence.[80] While both hepatic metabolism and renal excretion contribute to the elimination of the active metabolite, no dosage adjustment is necessary in patients with mild to moderate renal or hepatic impairment. The usual starting dose is 4 mg daily, increasing to 8 mg daily, as needed and tolerated. The dose of fesoterodine should not exceed 4 mg daily in the presence of severe renal impairment (creatinine clearance <30 mL/min [0.50 mL/s]) or in patients also taking potent CYP3A4 inhibitors. Fesoterodine has not been studied and is not recommended in patients with severe hepatic impairment.[80,81]

Placebo-controlled studies have demonstrated that fesoterodine 4 and 8 mg daily reduces the number of micturitions/day and the frequencies of incontinence episodes and urgency episodes per week, and the drug increases the number of continent days/week and volume voided/micturition. It also improves quality-of-life compared with placebo. Response is dose-related, with greater responses occurring with the 8 mg versus the 4 mg daily dose (exception: micturition frequency). In the only active comparator trial, fesoterodine 4 and 8 mg and tolterodine LA 4 mg (all given once daily) were all significantly superior to placebo in the majority of efficacy parameters. Fesoterodine and tolterodine were not compared statistically in the trial.

In a post hoc comparison, fesoterodine 8 mg daily was superior to tolterodine LA 4 mg daily in several efficacy parameters. Caution is warranted in interpreting the results of post hoc analyses, however.

The most common adverse effects of fesoterodine are dry mouth (27%), constipation (5.1%), dyspepsia (2%), and dry eyes (1.6%).[80] The most common adverse effects in the active comparator trial were dry mouth (3.8%, 21.7%, 16.9%); constipation (3.3%, 4.5%,

2.8%); and dry eyes (2.2%, 4.2%, <1%) in the fesoterodine 4 and 8 mg and tolterodine LA 4 mg recipients, respectively.[80,81]

At this time, fesoterodine does not appear to be a significant advance on existing anticholinergics in managing UUI.

Trospium Chloride Trospium chloride is a quaternary ammonium anticholinergic. It was approved in 2004 by the U.S. Food and Drug Administration (FDA) for the management of overactive bladder but has been available for many years in other countries. Trospium chloride has been comprehensively reviewed.[82] The data discussed here derive from that review, supplemented with detailed clinical trial data.

Preclinical studies have demonstrated that trospium chloride is an antimuscarinic agent in bladder and gastrointestinal tract tissues. It is poorly absorbed after oral administration (<10%), and food reduces bioavailability by 70% to 80%. It is principally cleared by the renal route (70%), with 80% of urinary excretion accounted for by the parent compound. The mean terminal disposition half-life in the presence of normal renal function is 10 to 12 hours. Advancing age and mild to moderate hepatic impairment do not affect trospium chloride pharmacokinetics to a clinically significant degree. In contrast, renal impairment does significantly reduce drug clearance. When creatinine clearance is less than 30 mL/min (0.50 mL/s), AUC is increased by a mean of 4.5-fold, peak plasma concentration by a mean of twofold, and terminal disposition half-life by a mean of two- to threefold.

Eleven published English-language studies on the efficacy/tolerability of trospium chloride for treatment of UUI are available. Except for the two trials (one published) described in the product information, clinical trials have emphasized cystometric, not clinical, endpoints.[83–92]

The paucity of clinical outcome data makes difficult the evaluation of trospium chloride compared with other approved anticholinergics. Although trospium chloride is statistically superior to placebo, the absolute differences in results between trospium chloride and placebo call into question the clinical relevance of such differences. In the four trials with active controls, results with trospium chloride were statistically equivalent to those with oxybutynin IR and tolterodine IR.[88–91] No comparative data with LA formulations of these two agents are available.

In a study involving a large proportion of elders (mean age, 63 years), the decreases in the number of UUI episodes and daily micturitions and increase in volume voided per micturition were significantly greater in trospium chloride recipients compared with placebo recipients.[92]

The expected anticholinergic adverse effects occur with trospium chloride as well. Of interest, the frequency of these events is increased in patients 75 years and older compared with younger subjects. This occurrence is believed to be pharmacodynamic (i.e., increased sensitivity) and not pharmacokinetic in nature. No data at present support the hypothesis that trospium chloride is less neurotoxic than nonquaternary ammonium anticholinergics (based on the hypothesis of reduced transit across the blood–brain barrier of trospium chloride due to its positive electrical charge on the quaternary nitrogen). Available drug–drug interaction data are clearly inadequate.

The usual dosage regimen is 20 mg twice daily. The drug should be taken on an empty stomach. Dosage reduction (by 50% of the daily dose) is recommended when creatinine clearance is less than 30 mL/min (0.50 mL/s). In patients 75 years and older, dose reduction to 20 mg once daily should be considered based upon tolerability. At this time, trospium chloride does not appear to be a significant advance over oxybutynin and tolterodine in managing UUI.

Extended-Release Trospium Chloride Like the immediate-release formulation, extended-release trospium chloride 60 mg daily is an alternative first-line therapy for treatment of overactive bladder with symptoms of UI, urgency, and urinary frequency.[93]

Because food decreases the bioavailability by 35% to 60%, extended-release trospium chloride must be taken on an empty stomach (1 hour before or 2 hours after meals).[93,94] Trospium is eliminated primarily unchanged in the urine. The pharmacokinetics of this version of trospium chloride in patients with mild to moderate renal impairment have not been studied, and it is not recommended in patients with severe renal impairment (creatinine clearance <30 mL/min [0.50 mL/s]).[93]

Extended-release trospium chloride was evaluated in two 12-week, randomized, controlled studies. In a Phase III study, extended-release trospium chloride 60 mg daily (n = 298) improved urinary frequency, urgency, and UI more than placebo did (n = 303).[95] In another phase III study, extended-release trospium chloride 60 mg daily (n = 267) improved the number of voids per day, number of UUI episodes per day, number of days with no UUI episodes, urgency severity, volume voided per micturition, and overactive bladder (OAB) Symptom Composite Score compared with placebo (n = 276).[96] There are no studies comparing extended-release trospium chloride with an active control.

The most common adverse effects with extended-release trospium chloride have been dry mouth (11%), constipation (9%), dizziness (2%), dry eyes (1.6%), flatulence (1.6%), nausea (1.4%), and abdominal pain (1.4%).[93]

At this time, extended-release trospium chloride does not appear to be a significant advance on trospium chloride or other existing anticholinergics in managing UUI.

Solifenacin Succinate Solifenacin succinate was approved by the FDA in late 2004 for treatment of overactive bladder with urge incontinence, urgency, and urinary frequency. Solifenacin succinate has been comprehensively reviewed.[97] The data discussed here derive from that review, supplemented with detailed clinical trial data.

Preclinical studies demonstrated that solifenacin is an antagonist at M_1, M_2, and M_3 muscarinic cholinergic receptors. Based on comparative ex vivo and animal studies with solifenacin and oxybutynin, solifenacin is believed to be a "uroselective" agent. The drug is well absorbed (mean absolute bioavailability, 88%), and food has no clinically relevant effect on absorption.[98,99] It is principally eliminated via metabolism and renal excretion of metabolites, with renal excretion of parent compound less than 10% of the dose. With a mean terminal disposition half-life of 50 to 60 hours, the drug can be dosed once daily.[100] Results of two placebo-controlled and two placebo- and active (tolterodine)-controlled clinical trials in UUI are available. Like oxybutynin and tolterodine, solifenacin significantly reduced the number of incontinence episodes, urge episodes, and micturitions per day and increased the volume voided per micturition in a dose-dependent fashion compared with placebo. In the active-controlled trials, solifenacin was statistically superior to tolterodine. However, neither of these two studies directly compared solifenacin and tolterodine.[101,102] Surprisingly, the effect of tolterodine in these trials was no better than that of placebo. A direct comparative trial of tolterodine ER demonstrated that the effect of solifenacin was significantly greater than that of tolterodine ER in terms of reducing the number of UUI episodes and pad usage and in improving patients' perception of their bladder condition.[103] An analysis of pooled data from two phase III studies showed that solifenacin recipients had significant improvement in five of 10 quality of life domains from baseline compared with placebo recipients.[104]

No comparative efficacy/tolerability data with oxybutynin are available. The effect sizes (solifenacin effect minus placebo effect) in these studies were similar to those noted with oxybutynin.

A retrospective analysis of pooled data from elders (mean age 72 years) in four phase III studies showed that compared with baseline, solifenacin recipients achieved a significantly greater decrease in number of UUI episodes, number of urgency episodes, and number of micturitions per day and a greater increase in the proportion of patients who became totally dry compared with placebo recipients.[105]

The recommended dose of solifenacin is 5 mg once daily. If the drug is well tolerated but the effectiveness is not optimal, the dose can be increased to 10 mg once daily. Little additional benefit is generally achieved with doses exceeding 5 mg daily. Solifenacin can be administered with or without food. For patients with creatinine clearance rates less than 30 mL/min (0.50 mL/s) or with moderate hepatic impairment (Child-Pugh class B), the daily dosage should not exceed 5 mg. If the patient has severe hepatic impairment (Child-Pugh class C), the drug should not be used. If the patient is receiving concurrent therapy with one or more potent CYP 3A4 inhibitors, the daily dose should not exceed 5 mg. In contrast to findings of preclinical studies, solifenacin behaves like a nonselective anticholinergic in humans, causing dry mouth, constipation, blurred vision, and other anticholinergic effects to a similar extent as tolterodine in clinical trials and oxybutynin in pharmacokinetic trials. At this time, solifenacin does not appear to be a significant advance over existing anticholinergics in managing UUI.

Darifenacin The data on darifenacin discussed here derive from a review,[106] supplemented with detailed clinical trial data.

Preclinical studies have demonstrated that darifenacin is an antagonist at M_1, M_3, and M_5 muscarinic cholinergic receptors. As with solifenacin, darifenacin is believed to be "uroselective" on the basis of preclinical data. The mean absolute bioavailabilities of the 7.5-, 15-, and 30-mg extended-release (ER) formulations are 15%, 19%, and 25%, respectively. Bioavailability is affected by formulation, CYP 2D6 genotype, dose, and race. Bioavailability is enhanced using an ER formulation (70%–110% higher than IR), in heterozygous CYP 2D6 extensive metabolizers and poor metabolizers (40%–90% higher than homozygous extensive metabolizers), and white race (56% higher than Japanese). Darifenacin is extensively metabolized, with cumulative urinary excretion of the parent compound less than 10%. The 2D6 and 3A4 isoenzymes of CYP are responsible for darifenacin metabolism. With a mean terminal disposition half-life of 3 to 5 hours (depending on CYP 2D6 metabolizer status), an ER formulation is needed to allow once-daily dosing. Results of four placebo-controlled clinical trials (one published) on UUI are available. Although a comparative study of darifenacin with oxybutynin IR showed that both agents significantly decreased the number of UUI episodes and their severity as well as urinary urgency and the number of micturitions compared with placebo, the active treatments were not directly compared.[107] A comparison with tolterodine IR and placebo showed that darifenacin 15 mg and 30 mg significantly decreased the number of UUI episodes from baseline after 2 weeks compared with placebo, but only the 30-mg daily dose continued to be superior to placebo after 12 weeks. Compared with placebo, tolterodine IR did not significantly decrease the number of UUI episodes from baseline at either time point. Darifenacin 30 mg once daily achieved a significantly greater decrease in the number of UUI episodes compared with tolterodine IR at both time points. At 12 weeks, both darifenacin and tolterodine IR produced significant improvements from baseline in the number of micturitions per day and volume voided per micturition compared with placebo.[108]

A large pooled subanalysis of patients 65 years and older from three phase III studies demonstrated that darifenacin produced a significant decrease in the number of UUI episodes, urgency episodes, and micturition frequency and an increase in volume voided

per micturition compared with placebo.[109] No comparative efficacy/tolerability data with anticholinergics other than tolterodine IR and oxybutynin IR are available.

The recommended daily dose of darifenacin is 7.5 to 15 mg once daily of the ER oral formulation. As with solifenacin, darifenacin behaves like a nonselective anticholinergic in humans, causing dry mouth, constipation, and other well-known anticholinergic adverse effects. Dry mouth was significantly more common with oxybutynin IR than either darifenacin or placebo.[110] In one study, the rates of treatment discontinuation and adverse events in elderly recipients of darifenacin were similar to those seen in other studies of darifenacin conducted in younger adults.[109] At this time, darifenacin does not appear to be a significant advance over existing anticholinergics in managing UUI.

CLINICAL CONTROVERSY

Should anticholinergic pharmacotherapy be used to treat UUI in patients with mild cognitive impairment or mild or moderate dementia?

Other Anticholinergics and Antispasmodics Other drugs for treatment of UUI are less effective, are no safer, or have not been adequately studied.[28,111] Thus their use is not recommended. Tricyclic antidepressants are generally no more effective than oxybutynin IR, and they exhibit a high incidence of bothersome and potentially serious adverse effects (e.g., orthostatic hypotension, cardiac conduction abnormalities, dizziness, and confusion). They are also potentially life threatening in overdose. Therefore, their use should be limited to individuals who have one or more additional medical indications for these agents (e.g., depression or neuropathic pain); patients with mixed UI (because of their effect of decreasing bladder contractility and increasing outlet resistance); and possibly those with nocturnal incontinence associated with altered sleep patterns.[28,111-114] Because of the lower incidence of adverse effects, desipramine and nortriptyline may be preferred over imipramine and doxepin. However, due to their lower anticholinergic activity, they may not be as effective.

CLINICAL CONTROVERSY

Which anticholinergic agent should be used as first-line pharmacotherapy of UUI (oxybutynin, tolterodine, trospium chloride, solifenacin, darifenacin, or fesoterodine) and which formulation of oxybutynin (oral IR, oral XL, TDS patch, or topical gel) or tolterodine (oral IR, oral LA) is unclear. Financial considerations currently favor generic oxybutynin IR, and this is the initial choice of many clinicians. Due to differences between agents in terms of adverse event rates, patient comorbidities may favor the use of more expensive branded agents.

Propantheline, a quaternary ammonium anticholinergic and potential treatment, produces a high incidence of adverse effects and is only modestly effective for UUI.[115-119] When used, propantheline appears to be best tolerated at a dose no more than 15 mg three times daily plus 60 mg at bedtime.[115]

Flavoxate is a tertiary amine that relaxes smooth muscle in vitro. Four controlled trials revealed that flavoxate is no more effective than placebo for treatment of UUI; therefore, flavoxate is not recommended.[28]

Dicyclomine hydrochloride, an anticholinergic agent that relaxes smooth muscle, produced minimal benefit as well as bothersome adverse effects in two small studies.[120,121]

Hyoscyamine, an anticholinergic and antispasmodic drug related to atropine, has been suggested for treatment of UUI, but data recommending its use are insufficient.[28]

In a meta-analysis, 50 randomized, controlled trials and three pooled analyses were examined for significant (with $P <0.05$) and nonsignificant (NS) differences. Adverse events were seen less frequently with use of LA products, as compared with IR formulations (oxybutynin: incidences of any AE, xerostomia, and moderate–severe or severe xerostomia; tolterodine: incidence of xerostomia). Of interest, the incidence of headache was higher with the use of LA versus IR formulations of tolterodine. The efficacy of LA tolterodine compared with the IR formulation favored the LA formulation for the parameters of number of micturitions and volume voided per micturition. However, the number of incontinence episodes and pad use were similar for the two formulations.[122]

For tolterodine IR, efficacy was similar for the 2 mg and 4 mg daily doses, while only xerostomia occurred more frequently with the 4 mg daily dose. With solifenacin, the only efficacy parameter different for the 5 mg and 10 mg daily doses was the percentage of patients with a 50% or greater reduction in incontinence episode frequency (10 mg > 5 mg). The 10 mg daily dose of solifenacin was associated with higher frequencies of study withdrawal due to adverse events, xerostomia, and constipation than was the 5 mg daily dose. For darifenacin, the 15 mg daily dose, as compared with the 7.5 mg daily dose, was associated with higher frequencies of study withdrawal due to adverse events, xerostomia, and constipation. Also, the 30 mg daily dose, as compared with the 15 mg daily dose, was associated with higher frequencies of xerostomia and constipation.[122]

For comparisons between drugs, only for oxybutynin versus tolterodine were the data adequate for meta-analysis. The IR products were similar in efficacy. Oxybutynin IR was associated with higher frequencies of any adverse event, study withdrawal due to adverse events, xerostomia of any grade, and moderate to severe or severe xerostomia, compared with tolterodine IR. Oxybutynin IR was also associated with higher frequencies of xerostomia and severe xerostomia than was tolterodine LA.[122]

Lastly, oral oxybutynin IR/tolterodine LA, as compared with the oxybutynin TDS (patch) formulation, produced similar reductions in the number of incontinence episodes. However, the oral agents were associated with higher frequencies of xerostomia and constipation, compared with the TDS (patch) formulation. In contrast, the TDS (patch) formulation was associated with higher frequencies of local (application site) reactions and study withdrawal due to adverse effects, compared with the oral agents.[122] The analysis predated the availability of the oxybutynin topical gel formulation.

In summary, the following can be concluded on the basis of available data. LA formulations are generally preferable over IR ones in terms of improved tolerability. Dose escalation of IR formulations may result in improved efficacy, albeit limited, at the cost of an increase in adverse event frequency/severity. The TDS (patch) route does not provide significant advantages over the oral route. No conclusion can be made currently with regard to the topical gel route.

Table 94–5 lists the adverse event frequencies for the most common events for oxybutynin, tolterodine, trospium chloride, solifenacin, darifenacin, and fesoterodine based on manufacturers' product information.

Botulinum Toxin A Enthusiasm is considerable for the application of botulinum toxin A for treatment of voiding dysfunction. Botulinum toxin is a naturally occurring powerful muscle relaxant produced by *Clostridium botulinum*.

Injected into smooth or striated muscle, botulinum toxin acts as a neurotoxin by temporarily paralyzing the muscle. The mechanism of action of the paralytic effect is generally ascribed to prevention of the release of the neurotransmitter acetylcholine into the synapse at the neuromuscular junction, although other pathways in neurotransduction may also be affected.

This compound is commercially produced for medical use in a number of conditions such as muscle spasticity, hyperhidrosis, and cosmetic reduction of skin wrinkles. It does not carry an FDA-approved indication in any lower urinary tract disorders, although many studies are ongoing. In the urinary tract, it can be used to treat overactive bladder (detrusor) muscle as well as external urethral sphincter spasticity. Botulinum toxin has been used successfully and safely in patients with neurogenic bladder dysfunction and nonneurogenic detrusor overactivity and overactive bladder.[123–125]

Botulinum toxin is delivered using a cystoscope equipped with a needle. The usual dosage is between 100 and 300 units per session. It is injected through the needle directly into the bladder muscle in 10 to 30 injections spaced over 5 to 10 minutes. The procedure is carried out as an outpatient procedure without general anesthesia. The duration of therapeutic effect varies, lasting usually from 4 to 8 months. Repeat injections are necessary to maintain the beneficial effects.

The adverse effects of botulinum toxin A when used in the urinary tract most frequently include dysuria, hematuria, urinary tract infection, and urinary retention. Urinary retention occurs in up to 20% of treated individuals and persists until the paralytic effects have worn off (up to 6 to 8 months). Therapeutic and adverse effects may not become evident for 3 to 7 days, presumably because this period of time is required for uptake of the toxin following injection.

Results of an open-label trial of intravesical botulinum toxin A in dimethylsulfoxide in 21 women with refractory idiopathic detrusor overactivity demonstrated a significant reduction in the frequency of incontinence episodes without any effect on postvoid residual urine volumes.[126] Much work remains to determine whether the intravesical (i.e., instillation into the bladder) route for botulinum toxin A administration is feasible for the treatment of OAB.

Catheterization Combined with Medications Patients with UUI and an elevated postvoid residual urine volume due to retention may require intermittent self-catheterization along with frequent voiding between catheterizations.

If intermittent catheterization is not possible, surgical placement of a suprapubic catheter may be necessary. Use of a chronic indwelling catheter should be avoided because of the increased occurrence of urinary tract infections and nephrolithiasis.

Regardless of catheterization status, patients may experience symptom relief with oxybutynin (IR, XL, or TDS formulations), tolterodine (IR or LA formulations), trospium chloride, solifenacin, fesoterodine, or darifenacin, as these agents relax the detrusor muscle and enhance bladder storage. Patients with UUI and symptoms of retention may also benefit from an α-adrenergic receptor antagonist that relaxes the internal bladder sphincter (e.g., prazosin, terazosin, doxazosin, tamsulosin, silodosin, and alfuzosin). Although theoretically of benefit, bethanecol, a cholinergic agonist, has not been demonstrated effective in improving bladder emptying in well-done trials. In addition, it causes numerous bothersome (e.g., muscle and abdominal cramping and diarrhea) and potentially life-threatening adverse effects and should not be used in patients with asthma or heart disease.[28]

Urethral Underactivity

❺ Urethral underactivity, or SUI, may be aggravated by agents with α-adrenergic receptor blocking activity, including prazosin, terazosin, doxazosin, tamsulosin, alfuzosin, silodosin, methyldopa, clonidine, guanfacine, guanadrel, and labetalol. The goal of therapy is to improve the urethral closure mechanism by stimulating α-adrenergic receptors in the smooth muscle of the bladder neck and proximal urethra, enhancing the supportive structures underlying the urethral epithelium, or enhancing the positive effects of serotonin and norepinephrine in the afferent and efferent pathways of the micturition reflex. There is no role for medications in the management of SUI after radical prostatectomy.[127]

Estrogens Local and systemic estrogens have been used extensively for the pharmacologic management of SUI since the 1940s. Estrogens are believed to work via several mechanisms, including enhancement of the proliferation of urethral epithelium, local circulation, and numbers and/or sensitivity of urogenital α-adrenergic receptors.[128] However, a trial has questioned whether estrogens exert a stimulatory effect on vaginal collagen production, at least over the short term.[129]

Open trials support the use of a variety of estrogens in the management of SUI: transdermal estradiol, conjugated estrogen vaginal cream, Estring, oral conjugated estrogen, oral quinestradol, oral estriol, intramuscular estrogens, estriol vaginal suppositories, and oral estradiol.[130] Variable effects of estrogen treatment on urodynamic parameters, such as maximum urethral closure pressure, functional urethral length, and pressure transmission ratio, have been noted in these studies. Progestogens have an antagonistic effect compared with estrogens, by reducing genitourinary tract muscle tone.

Results of four placebo-controlled comparative trials have not been as favorable, finding no significant clinical or urodynamic effects for oral estrogen compared with placebo.[131–134] In fact, observational studies have documented that estrogen use is associated with an increased risk of UI compared with that in nonusers.[135–138] Systemic estrogen therapy is associated with numerous adverse effects, including mastodynia, uterine bleeding, nausea, thromboembolism, cardiac and cerebrovascular ischemic events, and enhancement of the risk of certain cancers.[111] If estrogens are to be used for treatment of SUI, only topical products should be administered. Estrogen use is best justified when SUI exists with urethritis or vaginitis due to estrogen deficiency.

α-Adrenergic Receptor Agonists Numerous open trials have supported the use of a variety of α-adrenergic receptor agonists in SUI, including ephedrine, norfenefrine, phenylpropanolamine, and midodrine.[130] Phenylpropanolamine was withdrawn from the U.S. market in 2000 because of a risk for stroke in women using the agent.[139] Some patients may have leftover supplies of this agent or may obtain it from international sources. If so, individuals with the contraindications listed later in the chapter (especially coronary artery disease and/or cardiac arrhythmias) should be warned against self-treatment with this or other α-adrenergic receptor agonists.

Placebo-controlled comparative trials with phenylpropanolamine, norfenefrine, and norephedrine support the modest efficacy of these agents for treatment of mild or moderate SUI.[130,140] These agents have been found to variably affect maximum urethral closure pressure and functional urethral length.

Adverse effects include hypertension, headache, dry mouth, nausea, insomnia, and restlessness.[111] Contraindications to the use of these agents include the presence of hypertension, tachyarrhythmias, coronary artery disease, myocardial infarction, cor pulmonale, hyperthyroidism, renal failure, and narrow-angle glaucoma.

Usual doses for pseudoephedrine and phenylephrine are listed in Table 94–4.

Several studies have evaluated whether the clinical and urodynamic effects of a combination of estrogen and an α-adrenergic receptor agonist exceed those of the individual therapies in SUI.[141–145] In general, combination therapy has resulted in somewhat superior clinical and urodynamic responses compared with monotherapy,

including severity of complaints, amount of urine lost per episode, number of daily voluntary micturitions, number of leakage episodes per day, patient preference, pad use, maximum urethral closure pressure, functional urethral length, and pressure transmission ratio.

Duloxetine Duloxetine, a dual inhibitor of serotonin and norepinephrine reuptake, was approved in 2004 for treatment of depression and painful diabetic neuropathy.[146] Its use for treatment of SUI (for which the drug is approved in many countries but not in the United States) is based on studies in rats and cats demonstrating that central serotoninergic and noradrenergic regions are involved in ascending and descending control of urethral smooth muscle and the external urethral sphincter. These mechanisms facilitate the bladder-to-sympathetic reflex pathway, increasing urethral and external urethral sphincter muscle tone during the storage phase. Data documenting this control mechanism in humans are limited. The mean terminal disposition half-life, clearance, and volume of distribution of duloxetine in healthy volunteers are 10 to 12 hours, 114 to 119 L/h, and 1,787 to 1,943 L, respectively. The drug is extensively metabolized to inactive metabolites (via oxidation at the 4, 5, and/or 6 positions in the naphthyl ring, followed by further oxidation or via methylation) with elimination in the urine as conjugated metabolites. CYP 2D6 and 1A2 are involved in the ring oxidations. This involvement was demonstrated in studies of the interaction of duloxetine with the CYP 2D6 substrate desipramine (wherein desipramine's peak plasma concentration, AUC, and terminal disposition half-life were increased 1.7-, 2.9-, and 1.9-fold, respectively, and clearance fell by 66%) and the CYP 2D6 inhibitor paroxetine (wherein duloxetine's peak plasma concentration, AUC, and terminal disposition half-life increased 1.6-, 1.6-, and 1.3-fold, respectively, and clearance fell by 37%). Fluvoxamine, a CYP 1A2 inhibitor, increased duloxetine's peak plasma concentration, AUC, and terminal disposition half-life by over 5-fold, 2.5-fold, and 3-fold, respectively. Thus clinicians must be careful when prescribing duloxetine concurrently with CYP 2D6 and 1A2 substrates or inhibitors. The effect of advancing age on duloxetine pharmacokinetics is not clinically significant. Moderate hepatic dysfunction (Child-Pugh class B) significantly affects duloxetine disposition, increasing mean AUC and terminal disposition half-life by 5-fold and 3-fold, respectively, and reducing clearance 85% compared with controls. Mild or moderate renal impairment (creatinine clearance 30–80 mL/min [0.50–1.34 mL/s]) does not affect drug disposition. In severe renal impairment (hemodialysis patients), mean peak plasma concentration and AUC are both increased 100%, whereas metabolite concentrations are increased up to 900%.

Results of six large clinical trials with duloxetine in SUI have been published. All were double-blinded, randomized, placebo-controlled, and parallel group in design. Compared with placebo, duloxetine therapy produced significant reductions in incontinence episode frequency and number of micturitions per day, improvement in Incontinence quality of life questionnaire scores and patient self-assessment, and increase in mean micturition interval. Results were independent of baseline UI severity (severity based on incontinent episode frequency). Significant intergroup differences were seen by week 4. However, cure rates were generally not improved by duloxetine. When evaluating the absolute differences between treatments, the actual benefit of duloxetine was generally quite modest.

A randomized, placebo-controlled clinical trial evaluated the effects of duloxetine (80 mg daily), pelvic floor muscle training (PFMT), and the combination of both modalities on incontinent episode frequency, incontinence-related quality of life, pad use, and patient global impression of change. Sham PFMT was used in the placebo group. Results indicated that duloxetine plus PFMT were probably additive in effect and that combination therapy afforded greater improvement than either monotherapy.[147]

Although duloxetine is an encouraging development in the pharmacologic management of SUI, its adverse event profile may make adherence problematic. In the SUI trials, treatment-emergent adverse events occurred in 68% to 93% of duloxetine and 50% to 72% of placebo recipients. Premature study withdrawal rates (due to adverse events) were 12% to 33% for duloxetine and 2% to 8% for placebo. The frequencies of individual events in duloxetine recipients were nausea 9% to 46%, headache 7% to 27%, insomnia 13% to 14%, constipation 4% to 27%, dry mouth 4% to 22%, dizziness 8% to 16%, fatigue 10% to 18%, somnolence 8% to 13%, vomiting 6% to 13%, and diarrhea 4% to 6%. Of interest, the drug may be associated with small increases in blood pressure (like venlafaxine, another dual reuptake inhibitor) and withdrawal symptoms (sleep disturbances). Unfortunately, adherence to long-term therapy is quite poor due to a combination of adverse events and lack of efficacy.[148,149]

Despite these negatives, duloxetine is the first drug approved by a regulatory agency for treating SUI. Based on studies conducted to date, a dosage regimen of 40 to 80 mg/day (in one or two doses) appears reasonable. Initiating therapy with 40 mg daily for 2 weeks and then increasing to 80 mg daily (rather than initiating therapy with 80 mg daily) reduces the risks of nausea, dizziness, and premature drug discontinuation.[150] If the drug is to be stopped, it should be withdrawn slowly, reducing the dose by 50% for 2 weeks before discontinuation, unless the situation is potentially life-threatening.[150]

A double-blind, randomized, placebo-controlled clinical trial has recently demonstrated the benefit of venlafaxine 75 mg once daily for 12 weeks over placebo in terms of incontinence episode frequency, voiding interval, quality of life, and patient global impression of improvement.[151]

Overflow Incontinence

Overflow incontinence secondary to benign or malignant prostatic hyperplasia may be amenable to pharmacotherapy. For management of malignant prostatic disease, see Chapter 139. The pharmacotherapy of BPH is discussed in Chapter 93.

CLINICAL CONTROVERSY

The optimal approach to pharmacotherapy of SUI is unclear. Although not supported by evidence-based medicine, many clinicians initiate a trial of topical estrogen, followed by addition of an α-adrenergic receptor agonist in estrogen nonresponders unless contraindicated. Based on available data, duloxetine is the drug of choice for treatment of SUI, provided it is tolerated.

■ SURGICAL TREATMENT

Only rarely does surgery play a role in the initial management of UI.[152] In the absence of secondary complications from UI (e.g., skin breakdown or infection), the decision to surgically treat symptomatic UI should be based on the premise that the degree of bother or lifestyle compromise to the patient is great enough to warrant an elective operation, and that nonoperative therapy either is undesired or has been ineffective.

Successful application of surgery depends most on defining the underlying abnormalities responsible for UI (bladder vs urethra, underactivity vs overactivity). Once the underlying factors are determined, other considerations include renal function, sexual function, severity of leakage, history of abdominal or pelvic surgery, presence of concurrent abdominal or pelvic pathology requiring surgical correction, and finally the patient's suitability for, and willingness to accept the risks of, surgery.

When patients with uncomplicated SUI become dissatisfied with the initial management approaches of pelvic floor exercises, medications, and/or behavioral modification,[152] surgical treatment assumes the primary role.

Surgical correction of female SUI (urethral underactivity) is directed toward either (a) repositioning the urethra and/or creating a backboard of support, or otherwise stabilizing the urethra and bladder neck in a well-supported retropubic (intraabdominal) position that is receptive to changes in intraabdominal pressure; or (b) improving the sealing mechanism and/or creating compression or otherwise augmenting the urethral resistance provided by the intrinsic sphincteric unit, with (i.e., sling) or without (i.e., periurethral collagen and other injectables) urethral and bladder neck support. Midurethral synthetic slings have become the most common approach to the treatment of SUI in women in the United States. These can be inserted in outpatient procedures that have shorter convalescence periods and allow faster return to usual activities compared with many of the older procedures.

As noted previously, SUI in men is very rare in the absence of prior pelvic surgery, injury, or neurologic disease. In men, SUI can be treated in a number of ways. Collage or other bulking agents can be injected periurethrally and submucosally into the region of the external urinary sphincter. The goal of these injections is to improve the sealing effect of the poorly functioning sphincter mechanism. The vast majority of periurethral bulking injections in men are performed in a retrograde fashion under direct visualization through a cystoscope. This approach is less effective and far less durable than alternative surgical procedures, although it can be performed in the office setting without the need for general anesthesia. The artificial urinary sphincter is generally considered to be the gold standard for treatment of male SUI. Placement of the manually operated silicone device has been associated with very high long-term success and satisfaction rates.[153] Male slings placed through a perineal incision are a newer alternative to the artificial urinary sphincter. However, long-term efficacy and safety data are lacking.

Most patients with UUI are managed nonsurgically with a combination of behavioral modification, pelvic floor exercises, and pharmacologic therapy. Only rarely is surgery applied to the problem of UUI. Surgery for the treatment of UUI generally consists of implantation of a sacral nerve stimulator (neuromodulation) or augmentation (enlargement) cystoplasty. Posterior tibial nerve stimulation is a new office-based percutaneous treatment for UUI or OAB. Long-term efficacy and safety data are lacking. Additional information and a systematic review of these procedures are available.[154]

Few surgical treatments for bladder underactivity are effective. After an appropriate evaluation for reversible causes is performed, the most effective management of this condition is intermittent self-catheterization performed by the patient or a caregiver three or four times per day. Sacral nerve stimulation (neuromodulation) has shown some efficacy in this patient population, but success rates for detrusor underactivity (nonobstructive urinary retention) are inferior to those seen with urinary frequency and urgency. Proper patient selection for this therapy remains poorly defined. Alternative methods of management that are less satisfactory or more invasive include indwelling urethral or suprapubic catheters and urinary diversion.

Urethral overactivity is most commonly caused by anatomic obstruction. Anatomic obstruction in men is most often caused by benign prostatic enlargement (see Chap. 93).

Rarely, bladder outlet obstruction is caused by a functional obstruction at the level of the bladder neck. Hypertrophy of the smooth muscle fibers at the level of the bladder neck in men and women may result in obstruction to the flow of urine. In patients who do not respond to pharmacologic therapy with α-adrenergic receptor antagonists, endoscopic incision using the cystoscope is highly effective in treating this very uncommon condition.

EVALUATION OF THERAPEUTIC OUTCOMES

6 During long-term management of UI, patient-specific clinical signs and symptoms of most distress ("bother") to the individual must be monitored. A daily diary may be useful in this regard. Some of the short-form instruments used in incontinence research for measuring symptom impact and condition-specific quality of life can be used in clinical monitoring. In addition, quantitating the use of ancillary supplies, such as pads, may be useful. The goal of therapy is to minimize the signs and symptoms most bothersome to the patient, as well as the use of pads and other ancillary supplies or devices. Total elimination of UI signs and symptoms may not be possible, and patients and practitioners need to mutually establish realistic goals of therapy. Because the therapies for UI frequently have nuisance adverse effects (e.g., anticholinergic effects such as xerostomia, xerophthalmia, and constipation) that may compromise regimen adherence, the presence and severity of adverse effects must be carefully elicited at each visit to the healthcare practitioner. Emergence of adverse effects may necessitate drug dosage adjustment or use of alternative strategies (e.g., chewing sugarless gum, sucking on hard sugarless candy, or use of saliva substitutes in xerostomia) or even drug discontinuation.

ABBREVIATIONS

AUC: area under the plasma or serum concentration-versus-time curve

BPH: benign prostatic hyperplasia

CYP: cytochrome P450

DD01: 5-hydroxymethyl metabolite of tolterodine

DEO: *N*-desethyloxybutynin

ER: extended release

IR: immediate release

LA: long acting

NS: nonsignificant

OAB: overactive bladder

PFMT: pelvic floor muscle training

SUI: stress urinary incontinence

TDS: transdermal system

UI: urinary incontinence

UUI: urge urinary incontinence

XL: extended release

REFERENCES

1. Abrams P, Cardozo L, Fall M, et al. The standardization of terminology of lower urinary tract function: Report from the standardization subcommittee of the International Continence Society. Neurourol Urodyn 2002;21:167–178.
2. Arnold EP, Burgio K, Diokno AC, et al. Epidemiology and natural history of urinary incontinence (UI). In: Abrams P, Khoury S, Wein AJ, eds. Incontinence. Plymouth, United Kingdom: Plymbridge Distributors; 1999:199–226.
3. Simeonova Z, Milsom I, Kullendorff AM, et al. The prevalence of urinary incontinence and its influence on the quality of life in women from an urban Swedish population. Acta Obstet Gynecol Scand 1999;78:546–551.
4. Kobelt F, Kirchberger I, Malone-Lee J. Quality-of-life aspects of the overactive bladder and the effect of treatment with tolterodine. BJU Int 1999;83:583–590.
5. DuBeau CF, Kiely DK, Resnick NM. Quality of life impact of urge incontinence in older persons: A new measure and conceptual structure. J Am Geriatr Soc 1999;47:989–994.
6. Diokno AC, Brock BM, Brown MB, et al. Prevalence of urinary incontinence and other urological symptoms in the noninstitutionalized elderly. J Urol 1986;136:1022–1025.
7. Brown JS, Nyberg LM, Kusek JW, et al. Proceedings of the National Institute of Diabetes, Digestive and Kidney Diseases International Symposium on Epidemiologic Issues in Urinary Incontinence in Women. Am J Obstet Gynecol 2003;188:S77–S88.
8. Ouslander JG, Kane RL, Abrass IB. Urinary incontinence in elderly nursing home patients. JAMA 1982;248:1194–1198.
9. Bump RC. Racial comparisons and contrasts in urinary incontinence and pelvic organ prolapse. Obstet Gynecol 1993;81:421–425.
10. Burgio KL, Matthews KA, Engel BT. Prevalence, incidence and correlates of urinary incontinence in healthy, middle-aged women. J Urol 1991;146:1255–1259.
11. Fliegner JR, Glenning PP. Seven years experience in the evaluation and management of patients with urge incontinence of urine. Aust N Z J Obstet Gynecol 1979;19:42–44.
12. Breakwell SL, Walker SN. Differences in physical health, social interaction and personal adjustment between continent and incontinent homebound aged women. J Community Health Nurs 1988;5:19–31.
13. Malmsten UG, Milsom I, Molander U, Norlen LJ. Urinary incontinence and lower urinary tract symptoms: An epidemiological study of men aged 45–99 years. J Urol 1997;158:1733–1737.
14. Andersson K-E. Antimuscarinics for treatment of overactive bladder. Lancet Neurol 2004;3:46–53.
15. Andersson K-E, Wein AJ. Pharmacology of the lower urinary tract: basis for current and future treatments of urinary incontinence. Pharmacol Rev 2004;56:581–631.
16. Fowler C. Integrated control of the lower urinary tract—Clinical perspective. Br J Pharmacol 2006;147(suppl 2):s14–s24.
17. Blaivas JG, Heritz DM. Classification, diagnostic evaluation and treatment overview. In: Blaivas JG, ed. Topics in Clinical Urology—Evaluation and Treatment of Urinary Incontinence. New York: Igaku-Shoin: 1996:22–45.
18. Kuh D, Cardozo L, Hardy R. Urinary incontinence in middle-aged women: Childhood enuresis and other lifetime risk factors in a British prospective cohort. J Epidemiol Community Health 1999;53:453–458.
19. Groutz A, Gordon D, Keidar R, et al. Stress urinary incontinence: Prevalence among nulliparous compared with primiparous and grand multiparous premenopausal women. Neurourol Urodyn 1999;18:419–425.
20. Malone-Lee J, Henshaw DJ, Cummings K. Urodynamic verification of an overactive bladder is not a prerequisite for antimuscarinic response. Br J Urol Int 2003;92:415–417.
21. deGroat WC. A neurologic basis for the overactive bladder. Urology 1997;50(6A suppl):36–52.
22. Brading AF. A myogenic basis for the overactive bladder. Urology 1997;50(6A suppl):57–67.
23. Turner WH, Brading AF. Smooth muscle of the bladder in the normal and the diseased state: Pathology, diagnosis and treatment. Pharmacol Ther 1997;75:77–110.
24. Steers W. Pathophysiology of overactive bladder and urge urinary incontinence. Rev Urol 2002;4(suppl):S7–S18.
25. Resnick NM, Yalla S. Detrusor hyperactivity with impaired contractile function. An unrecognized but common cause of incontinence in the elderly patient. JAMA 1987;257:3076–3081.
26. Rovner ES, Wein AJ. Today's treatment of overactive bladder and urge incontinence. Womens Health Prim Care 2000;3:179–192.
27. James M, Jackson S, Shepard A, Abrams P. Pure stress leakage symptomatology: Is it safe to discount detrusor instability? Br J Obstet Gynaecol 1999;106:1255–1258.
28. Abrams P, Cardozo L, Khoury S, Wein A, eds. Incontinence. 4th ed. Plymouth, United Kingdom: Health Publications Ltd.; 2009.
29. Ouslander JG, Schnelle JF, Uman G, et al. Does oxybutynin add to the effectiveness of prompted voiding for urinary incontinence among nursing home residents? A placebo-controlled trial. J Am Geriatr Soc 1995;43:610–617.

30. Burgio KL, Locher JL, Goode PS, et al. Behavioral vs drug treatment for urge urinary incontinence in older women: A randomized controlled trial. JAMA 1998;280:1995–2000.

31. Drutz HP, Appell RA, Gleason D, et al. Clinical efficacy and safety of tolterodine compared to oxybutynin and placebo in patients with overactive bladder. Int Urogynecol 1999;10:283–289.

32. Abrams P, Freeman R, Anderstrom C, Mattiasson A. Tolterodine, a new antimuscarinic agent: As effective but better tolerated than oxybutynin in patients with an overactive bladder. Br J Urol 1998;81:801–810.

33. Tapp AJ, Cardozo LD, Versi E, Cooper D. The treatment of detrusor instability in post-menopausal women with oxybutynin chloride: A double blind placebo controlled study. Br J Obstet Gynaecol 1990;97:1063–1064.

34. Riva D, Casolati E. Oxybutynin chloride in the treatment of female idiopathic bladder instability. Clin Exp Obstet Gynecol 1984;11:37–42.

35. Schmidt RA; The Oxybutynin XL Study Group. Efficacy of controlled-release, once-a-day oxybutynin chloride for urge urinary incontinence. Jerusalem, International Continence Society, Sept. 14–17, 1998:188.

36. ALZA Corporation. Ditropan XL (oxybutynin chloride) extended-release tablets. Data on file. Palo Alto, CA: ALZA Corp.; 1999.

37. Pharmacia & Upjohn. Detrol (tolterodine) package insert. Kalamazoo, MI: Pharmacia & Upjohn; October 2005.

38. Pharmacia & Upjohn. Detrol (tolterodine). Data on file. Kalamazoo, MI: Pharmacia & Upjohn; 1998.

39. Appell RA. Clinical efficacy and safety of tolterodine in the treatment of overactive bladder: A pooled analysis. Urology 1997;50(suppl 6A):90–96.

40. Chancellor M, Freedman S, Mitcheson HD, et al. Tolterodine, an effective and well tolerated treatment for urge incontinence and other overactive bladder symptoms. Clin Drug Invest 2000;19:83–91.

41. Rentzhog L, Stanton SL, Cardozo L, et al. Efficacy and safety of tolterodine in patients with detrusor instability: A dose-ranging study. Br J Urol 1998;81:42–48.

42. Millard R, Tuttle J, Moore K, et al. Clinical efficacy and safety of tolterodine compared to placebo in detrusor overactivity. J Urol 1999;161:1551–1555.

43. Appell RA, Sand P, Dmochowski R, et al. Prospective randomized controlled trial of extended-release oxybutynin chloride and tolterodine tartrate in the treatment of overactive bladder: Results of the OBJECT study. Mayo Clin Proc 2001;76:358–363.

44. Van Kerrebroeck P, Kreder K, Jonas U, et al. Tolterodine once daily: Superior efficacy and tolerability in the treatment of the overactive bladder. Urology 2001;57:414–421.

45. Malone-Lee JG, Walsh JB, Maugourd M-F. Tolterodine: A safe and effective treatment for older patients with overactive bladder. J Am Geriatr Soc 2001;49:700–705.

46. Dmochowski RR, Sand PK, Zinner NR, et al. Comparative efficacy and safety of transdermal oxybutynin and oral tolterodine versus placebo in previously treated patients with urge and mixed urinary incontinence. Urology 2003;62:237–242.

47. Dmochowski RR, Davila GW, Zinner NR, et al. Efficacy and safety of transdermal oxybutynin in patients with urge and mixed urinary incontinence. J Urol 2002;168:580–586.

48. Watson Pharma, Oxytrol (oxybutynin transdermal system) package insert. Morristown, NJ: Watson Pharma; June 2005.

49. Khullar V, Chapple C, Gabriel Z, Dooley JA. The effects of antimuscarinics on health-related quality of life in overactive bladder: A systematic review and meta-analysis. Urology 2006;68(suppl 2A):38–48.

50. Nilsson CG, Lukkari E, Haarala M, et al. Comparison of a 10-mg controlled release oxybutynin tablet with a 5-mg oxybutynin tablet in urge incontinent patients. Neurourol Urodyn 1997;16:533–542.

51. Birns J, Malone Lee JG; and the Oxybutynin CR Study Group. Controlled-release oxybutynin maintains efficacy with a 43% reduction in side effects compared with conventional oxybutynin treatment. Neurourol Urodyn 1997;16:429–430.

52. Anderson RU, Mobley D, Blank B, et al. Once daily controlled versus immediate-release oxybutynin chloride for urge urinary incontinence. OROS Oxybutynin Study Group. J Urol 1999;161:1809–1812.

53. Katz IR, Sands LP, Bilker E, et al. Identification of medications that cause cognitive impairment in older people: The case of oxybutynin chloride. J Am Geriatr Soc 1998;46:8–13.

54. Kelleher CJ, Cardozo LD, Khullar S. A medium term analysis of the subjective efficacy of treatment for women with detrusor instability and low bladder compliance. Obstet Gynecol 1997;104:988–993.

55. Appell RA, Chancellor MB, Zobrist RH, et al. Pharmacokinetics, metabolism, and saliva output during transdermal and extended-release oxybutynin administration in healthy subjects. Mayo Clin Proc 2003;78:696–702.

56. Hughes KM, Lang JCT, Lazare R, et al. Measurement of oxybutynin and its N-desethyl metabolite in plasma and its application to pharmacokinetic studies in young, elderly and frail elderly volunteers. Xenobiotica 1992;22:859–869.

57. Amarenco G, Marquis P, McCarthy C, Richard F. Efficacy of oxybutynin on health related quality of life (HRQL) in 1701 women suffering from urinary urge incontinence (UUI). Eur Urol 1998;33(suppl 1):32–38.

58. Ortho-McNeil Pharmaceuticals. Ditropan XL (oxybutynin chloride) extended-release tablets package insert. Raritan, NJ: Ortho-McNeil Pharmaceuticals; June 2004.

59. Paine MF, Khalighi M, Fisher JM, et al. Characterisation of interintestinal and intraintestinal variations in human CYP3A-dependent metabolism. J Pharmacol Exp Ther 1997;283:1552–1562.

60. Gupta SK, Sathyan G. Pharmacokinetics of an oral once-a-day controlled-release oxybutynin formulation compared with immediate-release oxybutynin. J Clin Pharmacol 1999;39:289–296.

61. Buyse G, Waldeck K, Ver C, et al. Intravesical oxybutynin for neurogenic bladder: Less systemic side effects due to reduced first-pass metabolism. J Urol 1998;160:892–896.

62. Gleason DM, Susset J, White C. Evaluation of a new once-daily formulation of oxybutynin for the treatment of urinary urge incontinence. Urology 1999;54:420–423.

63. Susset JG, Gleason DM, White CF, et al. Open-label safety and dose conversion/determination of once-daily OROS oxybutynin chloride for urge urinary incontinence. J Urol 1998;159(suppl):36.

64. Moore KH, Hay DM, Imrie AE, et al. Oxybutynin hydrochloride (3 mg) in the treatment of women with idiopathic detrusor instability. Br J Urol 1990;66:479–485.

65. Diokno AC, Appell RA, Sand PK, et al. Prospective, randomized, double-blind study of the efficacy and tolerability of the extended-release formulations of oxybutynin and tolterodine for overactive bladder: Results of the OPERA trial. Mayo Clin Proc 2003;78:687–695.

66. Sussman D, Garely A. Treatment of overactive bladder with once-daily extended-release tolterodine or oxybutynin: The Antimuscarinic Clinical Effectiveness Trial (ACET). Curr Med Res Opin 2002;18:177–184.

67. Guay DRP. Clinical pharmacokinetics of drugs used to treat urge incontinence. Clin Pharmacokinet 2003;42:1243–1285.

68. Zobrist RH, Schmid B, Feick A, et al. Pharmacokinetics of the R- and S-enantiomers of oxybutynin and N-desethyloxybutynin following oral and transdermal administration of the racemate in healthy volunteers. Pharm Res 2001;18:1029–1034.

69. Davila GW, Daugherty CA, Sanders SW. A short-term, multicenter, randomized double-blind dose titration study of the efficacy and anticholinergic side effects of transdermal compared to immediate release oral oxybutynin treatment of patients with urge urinary incontinence. J Urol 2001;166:140–145.

70. Dmochowski RR, Nitti V, Staskin D, Luber K, Appell R, Davila GW. Transdermal oxybutynin in the treatment of adults with overactive bladder: Combined results of two randomized clinical trials. World J Urol 2005;23:263–270.

71. Davila GW, Dmochowski RR, Sanders SW. Influence of age on improvements in overactive bladder symptoms and adverse events during oxybutynin transdermal system treatment [abstract]. Obstet Gynecol 2002;99(suppl 1):103S–104S.

72. Watson Pharma. Gelnique (oxybutynin chloride 10% gel) package insert. Morristown, NJ: Watson Pharma; January 2009.

73. Caramelli KE, Staskin DR, Volinn W. Steady-state pharmacokinetics of an investigational oxybutynin gel in comparison with oxybutynin transdermal system. J Urol 2008;179(suppl):513–514 (abstract 1508).

74. Staskin DR, Dmochowski RR, Sand PK, et al. Efficacy and safety of oxybutynin chloride topical gel for overactive bladder: A randomized, double-blind, placebo controlled, multicenter study. J Urol 2009;181:1764–1772.

75. Leung HY, Yip SK, Cheon C, et al. A randomized trial of tolterodine and oxybutynin on tolerability and clinical efficacy for treating Chinese women with an overactive bladder. BJU Int 2002;90:375–380.

76. Malone-Lee J, Shaffu B, Anand C, Powell C. Tolterodine: Superior tolerability than and comparable efficacy to oxybutynin in individuals 50 years old or older with overactive bladder: A randomized controlled trial. J Urol 2001;165:1452–1456.

77. Zinner NR, Mattiason A, Stanton SL. Efficacy, safety, and tolerability of extended-release once-daily tolterodine treatment for overactive bladder in older versus younger patients. J Am Geriatr Soc 2002;50:799–807.

78. Dmochowski R, Sathyan G, Ye C, et al. The pH effect of drug release from extended-release formulations of oxybutynin and tolterodine. Proceedings of the Second International Consultation on Incontinence. Paris, France, July 2001.

79. Dmochowski R, Chen A, Sathyan G, MacDiarmid S, Gidwani S, Gupta S. Effect of the proton pump inhibitor omeprazole on the pharmacokinetics of extended-release formulations of oxybutynin and tolterodine. J Clin Pharmacol 2005;45:961–968.

80. Pfizer Laboratories, Toviaz (fesoterodine fumarate extended-release tablets) package insert. New York, NY: Pfizer; November 2008.

81. Guay DRP. Fesoterodine: A new antimuscarinic for overactive bladder. Aging Health 2009;5:599–613.

82. Guay DRP. Trospium chloride: An update on a quaternary anticholinergic for treatment of urge urinary incontinence. Ther Clin Risk Manage 2005;1:157–166.

83. Rudy D, Cline K, Harris R, Goldberg K, Dmochowski R. Multicenter phase III trial studying trospium chloride in patients with overactive bladder. Urology 2006;67:275–280.

84. Esprit Pharma. Sanctura (trospium chloride) tablets package insert. East Brunswick, NJ: Esprit Pharma; May 2004.

85. Cardozo L, Chapple CR, Toozs-Hobson P, et al. Efficacy of trospium chloride in patients with detrusor instability: A placebo-controlled, randomized, double-blind, multicentre clinical trial. BJU Int 2000;85:659–664.

86. Frohlich G, Bulitta M, Strosser W. Trospium chloride in patients with detrusor overactivity: Meta-analysis of placebo-controlled, randomized, double-blind, multi-center clinical trials on the efficacy and safety of 20 mg trospium chloride twice daily. Int J Clin Pharmacol Ther 2002;40:295–303.

87. Junemann K-P, Fusgen I. Placebo-controlled, randomized, double-blind, multicentre clinical trial on the efficacy and tolerability of 1 × 40 mg and 2 × 40 mg trospium chloride (Spasmo-Lyt®) daily for 3 weeks in patients with urge-syndrome [abstract]. Neurourol Urodyn 1999;18:375–376.

88. Hofner K, Ralph G, Wiedemann G, et al. Controlled, double-blind, multicenter clinical trial to investigate the long-term tolerability and efficacy of trospium chloride in patients with detrusor instability. World J Urol. 2003;20:392–399.

89. Madersbacher H, Stohrer M, Richter R, Burgdorfer H, Hachen HJ, Murtz G. Trospium chloride versus oxybutynin: A randomized, double-blind, multicentre trial in the treatment of detrusor hyperreflexia. Br J Urol 1995;75:452–456.

90. Junemann KP, Al-Shukri S. Efficacy and tolerability of trospium chloride and tolterodine in 234 patients with urge-syndrome: A double-blind, placebo-controlled, multicentre clinical trial [abstract]. Neurourol Urodyn 2000;19:488–490.

91. Halaska M, Ralph G, Wiedemann A, et al. Controlled, double-blind, multicentre clinical trial to investigate long-term tolerability and efficacy of trospium chloride in patients with detrusor instability. World J Urol 2003;20:392–399.

92. Zinner N, Gittelman M, Harris R, et al. Trospium chloride improves overactive bladder symptoms: A multicenter phase III trial. J Urol 2004;171:2311–2315.

93. Allergan, Sanctura XR (trospium chloride extended-release capsules) package insert. Irvine, CA: Allergan; September 2007.

94. DeMaagd G, Geibig JD. An overview of overactive bladder and its pharmacologic management with a focus on anticholinergic drugs. Pharmacol Ther 2006;31:462–474.

95. Staskin D, Sand P, Zinner N, et al. Once daily trospium chloride is effective and well tolerated for the treatment of overactive bladder: Results from a multicenter phase III trial. J Urol 2007;178:978–984.

96. Dmochowski R, Sand P, Zinner N, et al. Trospium 60 mg once daily (QD) for overactive bladder syndrome: Results from a placebo-controlled interventional study. Urology 2008;71:449–454.

97. Guay DRP. Drug forecast: Solifenacin: An investigational anticholinergic for overactive bladder. Consult Pharm 2004;19:437–444.

98. Kuipers ME, Krauwinkel WJ, Mulder H, Visser N. Solifenacin demonstrates high absolute bioavailability in healthy men. Drugs R D 2004;5:73–81.

99. Uchida T, Krauwinkel WJ, Mulder H, Smulders RA. Food does not affect the pharmacokinetics of solifenacin, a new muscarinic receptor antagonist: Results of a randomized crossover trial. Br J Clin Pharmacol 2004;58:4–7.

100. Smulders RA, Krauwinkel WJ, Swart PJ, Huang M. Pharmacokinetics and safety of solifenacin succinate in healthy young men. J Clin Pharmacol 2004;44:1023–1033.

101. Chapple CR, Arano P, Bosch JLHR, DeRidder D, Kraemer AEJL, Ridder AM. Solifenacin appears effective and well tolerated in patients with symptomatic idiopathic detrusor overactivity in a placebo- and tolterodine-controlled phase 2 dose-finding study. BJU Int 2004;93:71–77.

102. Chapple CR, Rechberger T, Al-Shukri S, et al. Randomized, double-blind placebo- and tolterodine-controlled trial of the once-daily antimuscarinic agent solifenacin in patients with symptomatic overactive bladder. BJU Int 2004;93:303–310.

103. Chapple CR, Martinez-Garcia R, Selvaggi L, et al. A comparison of the efficacy and tolerability of solifenacin succinate and extended release tolterodine at treating overactive bladder syndrome: Results of the STAR trial. Eur Urol 2005;48:464–470.

104. Kelleher CJ, Cardozo L, Chapple CR, Haab F, Ridder AM. Improved quality of life in patients with overactive bladder symptoms treated with solifenacin. BJU Int 2005;95:81–85.

105. Wagg A, Wyndaele JJ, Sieber P. Efficacy and tolerability of solifenacin in elderly subjects with overactive bladder syndrome: A pooled analysis. Am J Geriatr Pharmacother 2006;4:14–24.

106. Guay DRP. Drug forecast: Darifenacin: Another investigational anti-muscarinic for overactive bladder. Consult Pharm 2005;20:424–431.

107. Steers W, Corcos J, Foote F, Kralidis G. An investigation of dose titration with darifenacin, an M3-selective receptor antagonist. BJU Int 2005;95:580–586.

108. Foote J, Elhilali M. A multicenter, randomized, double-blind study of darifenacin versus tolterodine in the treatment of overactive bladder (OAB) [abstract]. Presented at the British Geriatrics Society meeting, Harrogate, UK, October 6–8, 2004:32.

109. Foote J, Glavind K, Kralidis G, Wyndaele JJ. Treatment of overactive bladder in the older patient: Pooled analysis of three phase III studies of darifenacin, an M3 selective receptor antagonist. Eur Urol 2005;48:471–477.

110. Zinner N, Tuttle J, Marks L. Efficacy and tolerability of darifenacin, a muscarinic M3 selective receptor antagonist (M3SRA), compared with oxybutynin in the treatment of overactive bladder (OAB). World J Urol 2005;23:248–252.

111. Owens RG, Karram MM. Comparative tolerability of drug therapies used to treat incontinence and enuresis. Drug Saf 1998;2:123–139.

112. Milner G, Hills NF. A double-blind assessment of antidepressants in the treatment of 212 enuretic patients. Med J Aust 1968;1:943–947.

113. Castleden CM, George CF, Renwick AG, Asher MJ. Imipramine—A possible alternative to current therapy for urinary incontinence in the elderly. J Urol 1981;125:318–320.

114. Lose G, Jorgenson L, Thuriedborg P. Doxepin in the treatment of female detrusor overactivity: A randomized double-blind crossover study. J Urol 1989;142:1024–1026.

115. Deguecker J. Drug treatment of urinary incontinence in the elderly: Controlled trial with vasopressin and propantheline bromide. Gerontol Clin 1965;7:311–317.

116. Zorzitto ML, Jewett MAS, Fernie GR, et al. Effectiveness of propantheline bromide in the treatment of geriatric patients with detrusor instability. Neurourol Urodyn 1986;5:133–140.

117. Blaivas JG, Labib AB, Michalik SJ, Zayed AAH. Cystometric response to propantheline in detrusor hyperreflexia: Therapeutic implications. J Urol 1980;124:259–262.

118. Holmes DM, Montz FJ, Stanton SL. Oxybutynin versus propantheline in the management of detrusor instability: A patient-regulated variable dose trial. Br J Obstet Gynaecol 1989;96:607–612.

119. Thuroff JW, Bunke B, Ebner A, et al. Randomized, double-blind, multicentre trial on treatment of frequency, urgency and incontinence related to detrusor hyperactivity: Oxybutynin versus propantheline versus placebo. J Urol 1991;145:813–817.

120. Beck RP, Arnusch D, King C. Results in treating 210 patients with detrusor overactivity incontinence of urine. Am J Obstet Gynecol 1976;125:593–596.

121. Castleden CM, Duffin HM, Millar AW. Dicyclomine hydrochloride in detrusor instability: A controlled clinical pilot study. J Clin Exp Gerontol 1987;9:265–270.

122. Novara G, Galfano A, Secco S, et al. A systematic review and meta-analysis of randomized controlled trials with antimuscarinic drugs for overactive bladder. Eur Urol 2008;54:740–764.

123. Brubaker L, Richter HE, Visco A, et al. Refractory idiopathic urge urinary incontinence and botulinum A injection. J Urol 2008;180:217–222.

124. Sahai A, Khan MS, Dasgupta P. Efficacy of botulinum toxin-A for treating idiopathic detrusor overactivity: Results from a single center, randomized, double-blind, placebo controlled trial. J Urol 2007;177:2231–2236.

125. Schmid DM, Roy S, Sulser T, et al. Prospects and limitations of treatment with botulinum neurotoxin type A for patients with refractory idiopathic detrusor overactivity. BJU Int 2008;102(suppl 1):7–10.

126. Petrou SP, Parker AS, Crook JE, et al. Botulinum A toxin/dimethylsulfoxide bladder instillations for women with refractory idiopathic detrusor overactivity: A phase I/II study. Mayo Clin Proc 2009;84:702–706.

127. Tsakiris P, de la Rosette JJ, Michel MC, et al. Pharmacologic treatment of male stress urinary incontinence: Systematic review of the literature and levels of evidence. Eur Urol 2008;53:53–59.

128. Schreiter F, Fuchs P, Stockamp K. Estrogenic sensitivity of α-receptors in the urethral musculature. Urol Int 1976;31:13–19.

129. Jackson S, James M, Abrams P. The effect of oestradiol on vaginal collagen metabolism in postmenopausal women with genuine stress incontinence. BJOG 2002;109:339–344.

130. Guay DRP. Incontinence. Clin Trends Pharm Pract 2002;(June):entire issue.

131. Samsioe G, Jansson I, Mellstrom D, Svanborg A. Occurrence, nature, and treatment of urinary incontinence in a 70-year-old female population. Maturitas 1985;7:335–342.

132. Wilson PD, Faragher B, Butler B, et al. Treatment with oral piperazine oestrone sulphate for genuine stress incontinence in postmenopausal women. Br J Obstet Gynaecol 1987;94:568–574.

133. Jackson S, Shepherd A, Brookes S, Abrams P. The effect of oestrogen supplementation on post-menopausal urinary stress incontinence: A double-blind placebo-controlled trial. Br J Obstet Gynaecol 1999;106:711–718.

134. Jackson S, Shepherd A, Brookes S, Abrams P. The effect of oestrogen supplementation on post-menopasual urinary stress incontinence: a double-blind placebo-controlled trial. Br J Obstet Gynecol. 1999;106:711–718.

135. Brown JS, Seeley DG, Fong J, et al. Urinary incontinence in older women: Who is at risk? Study of Osteoporotic Fractures Research Group. Obstet Gynecol 1996;87:715–721.

136. Thom DH, van den Eeden SK, Brown JS. Evaluation of parturition and other reproductive variables as risk factors for urinary incontinence in later life. Obstet Gynecol 1997;90:983–989.

137. Diokno AC, Brock BM, Herzog AR, Bromberg J. Medical correlates of urinary incontinence. Urology 1990;36:129–138.

138. Grady D, Brown JS, Vittinghoff E, et al., and HERS Research Group. Postmenopausal hormones and incontinence: The Heart & Estrogen/Progestin Replacement Study. Obstet Gynecol 2001;97:116–120.

139. Kernan WN, Viscoli CM, Brass LM, et al. Phenylpropanolamine and the risk of hemorrhagic stroke. N Engl J Med 2000;343:1826–1832.

140. Alhasso A, Glazener CM, Pickard R, N'dow J. Adrenergic drugs for urinary incontinence in adults. Cochrane Databse Syst Rev 2005;3:CD001842.

141. Ahlstrom K, Sandahl B, Sjoberg B, et al. Effect of combined treatment with phenylpropanolamine and estriol, compared with estriol treatment alone, in postmenopausal women with stress urinary incontinence. Gynecol Obstet Invest 1990;30:37–43.

142. Kinn A-C, Lindskog M. Estrogens and phenylpropanolamine in combination for stress urinary incontinence in postmenopausal women. Urology 1988;32:273–280.

143. Ek A, Andersson K-E, Gullberg B, Ulmsten U. Effects of oestradiol and combined norephedrine and oestradiol treatment on female stress incontinence. Zentralbl Gynakol 1980;102:839–844.

144. Kiesswetter H, Hennrich F, Englisch M. Clinical and urodynamic assessment of pharmacologic therapy of stress incontinence. Urol Int 1983;38:58–63.

145. Beisland HO, Fossberg E, Moer A, Sander S. Urethral sphincteric insufficiency in postmenopausal females: Treatment with phenylpropanolamine and estriol separately and in combination. Urol Int 1984;39:211–216.

146. Guay DRP. Duloxetine in the management of stress urinary incontinence. Am J Geriatr Pharmacother 2005;3:25–38.

147. Ghoneim GM, VanLeeuwen JS, Elser DM, et al. A randomized controlled trial of duloxetine alone, pelvic floor muscle training alone, combined treatment and no active treatment in women with stress urinary incontinence. J Urol 2005;173:1647–1653.

148. Vella M, Duckett J, Basu M. Duloxetine 1 year on: The long-term outcome of a cohort of women prescribed duloxetine. Int Urogynecol J 2008;19:961–964.

149. Bump RC, Voss S, Beardsworth A, et al. Long-term efficacy of duloxetine in women with stress urinary incontinence. Br J Urol Int 2008;102:214–218.

150. Bump R, Yalcin I, Voss S. The effect of duloxetine dose escalation and tapering on the incidence of adverse events (AE) in women with stress urinary incontinence (SUI) [abstract]. Neurourol Urodyn 2005;24:582.

151. Erdinc B, Gurates B, Celik H, et al. The efficacy of venlafaxine in the treatment of women with stress urinary incontinence. Arch Gynecol Obstet 2009;279:343–348.

152. Urinary Incontinence Guideline Panel. Urinary Incontinence in Adults: Clinical Practice Guideline. AHCPR Pub. No. 92-0038. Rockville, MD: Agency for Health Care Policy and Research, Public Health Service, U.S. Department of Health and Human Services; 1992.

153. Litwillwer SE, Kim KB, Fone PD, et al. Post-prostatectomy incontinence and the artificial urinary sphincter: A long-term study of patient satisfaction and criteria for success. J Urol 1996;156:1975–1980.

154. Abrams P, Cardozo L, Khoury S, Wein A, eds. Recommendations of the International Scientific Committee: Evaluation and treatment of urinary incontinence, pelvic organ prolapse, and faecal incontinence. In: Incontinence, 3rd ed. Plymouth, United Kingdom: Health Publications Ltd.; 2005:1589–1630.

CHAPTER

95

Function and Evaluation of the Immune System

PHILIP D. HALL, NICOLE WEIMERT PILCH, AND DANIEL H. ATCHLEY

KEY CONCEPTS

❶ Cells of the immune system are derived from the pluripotent stem cell. Hematopoiesis is a closely regulated to assure adequate amounts of each of the different types of blood cells. The development of the different kinds of cells or cell lineages depends on cell-to-cell interactions and hematopoietic growth factors.

❷ After activation, dendritic cells express higher concentrations of major histocompatibility complex class II molecules, B7-1, B7-2, CD40, ICAM-1, and LFA-3 molecules than other antigen-presenting cells. They also produce more IL-12. These differences may explain why in vitro dendritic cells are the most efficient antigen-presenting cell.

❸ A T lymphocyte expresses hundreds of T-cell receptors (TCRs). All the TCRs expressed on the surface of an individual T lymphocyte have the same antigen specificity.

❹ A B lymphocyte can simultaneously express membrane immunoglobulin as IgM (monomeric) or IgD with the same variable region (i.e., antigen-binding site). The B lymphocyte then can secrete different isotypes (e.g., IgM [pentamer], IgA, IgG, IgE) with the same variable region as the membrane immunoglobulin.

❺ A serum protein electrophoresis determines the total concentration of circulating immunoglobulins (i.e., IgG, IgA, IgM, IgD, and IgE). If one wishes to determine the concentration of the individual isotypes, one needs to order isotype quantification. The vast majority of clinical laboratories quantitate only IgG, IgM, and IgA because they are the most prevalent isotypes in the bloodstream. In patients with allergic disorders, quantification of IgE may be useful. Depending on the clinical laboratory, results may come back in IU/mL, kIU/L, or mg/L for IgE.

❻ An understanding of the mechanism by which immunomodulators act along with an understanding of the immune system allows a clinician to anticipate potential adverse effects. The benefit of manipulating the immune responses must be balanced with the potential consequences and long-term sequela of such manipulation.

The immune system is a complex network of barriers, organs, cellular elements, and molecules that interact to defend the body against invading pathogens. Actually, the *immune system* is composed of two distinct systems of immunity: innate immunity and adaptive immunity. In brief, innate immunity includes a series of nonspecific barriers (physical and chemical), along with cellular and molecular elements strategically predeployed and prepositioned to prevent and/or quickly neutralize infection. Working in concert with innate immunity is adaptive immunity. In contrast to innate immunity, adaptive immunity constantly evolves and adapts against invading pathogens. Its hallmarks include *diversity, memory, mobility, self vs non-self discrimination, redundancy, replication,* and *specificity.*[1] *Diversity* indicates the capability of the immune system to respond to many different pathogens or strains of pathogens. Immunological *memory* ensures a quicker and more vigorous response to a subsequent encounter with the same pathogen. *Mobility* of components of the immune system enables local reactions to provide systemic protection. *Discrimination of self vs non-self* helps prevent friendly-fire damage of the host by the immune system. *Redundancy* refers to the immune system's ability to produce components with similar biological effects from multiple cells lines, such as inflammatory cytokines. *Replication* of the cellular components of the immune system amplifies the immune response. *Specificity* describes the ability of the immune system to distinguish between dissimilar antigens.

MAJOR TISSUES AND ORGANS OF THE IMMUNE SYSTEM

While numerous cells of the immune system have the ability to migrate to most body tissues, some tissues and organs serve as key members of the immune system. These include primary and secondary lymphoid tissues and organs. *Primary lymphoid tissues*

Learning objectives, review questions, and other resources can be found at **www.pharmacotherapyonline.com**.

and organs provide an environment appropriate for the development and maturation of select cells of the immune system. It is here that these select cells of the immune system mature and become tolerant of self and competent to respond to foreign antigens. *Secondary lymphoid organs* provide an environment where various cells of the immune system interact with and respond to trapped foreign antigens.[2]

BONE MARROW

❶ Bone marrow is the predominant primary lymphoid tissue of the body because it is the source of all cellular elements of the blood (erythrocytes, leukocytes, and thrombocytes [i.e., platelets]). The few exceptions to this rule are mostly confined to fetal development when some blood cells are transiently produced in the yolk sac, liver, spleen, thymus, and lymph nodes.[3] Regardless of where they are formed, all blood cells arise from common self-renewing pluripotent stem cells via the process of *hematopoiesis* (Fig. 95–1). During hematopoiesis, pluripotent stem cells differentiate along particular myeloid and lymphoid lineages to produce the leukocytes of the immune system, erythrocytes, and thrombocytes.[4,5] Hematopoiesis

is controlled by soluble mediators called hematopoietic growth factors/cytokines or colony stimulating factors (CSFs) that are multifunctional and drive responses such as growth, survival, proliferation, differentiation, maturation, and functional activation.[6] The destiny of the leukocytes (if they survive the maturation process) is to become mature cells of the immune system directly from the bone marrow (all leukocytes except T lymphocytes), or to migrate out of the bone marrow to continue their maturation elsewhere (T lymphocytes). Selected hematopoietic growth factors are identified in Figure 95–1, and a more comprehensive list appears in Table 95–1. Currently, four human hematopoietic cytokines have one or more recombinant products that are FDA-approved for clinical use: erythropoietin (EPO); granulocyte colony-stimulating factor (G-CSF); granulocyte-macrophage colony-stimulating factor (GM-CSF); and interleukin 11 (IL-11).[7]

THYMUS

The thymus is a bi-lobed primary lymphoid organ located in the superior mediastinum between the aorta and the sternum. Its primary function is to produce mature T cells (thymus-dependent

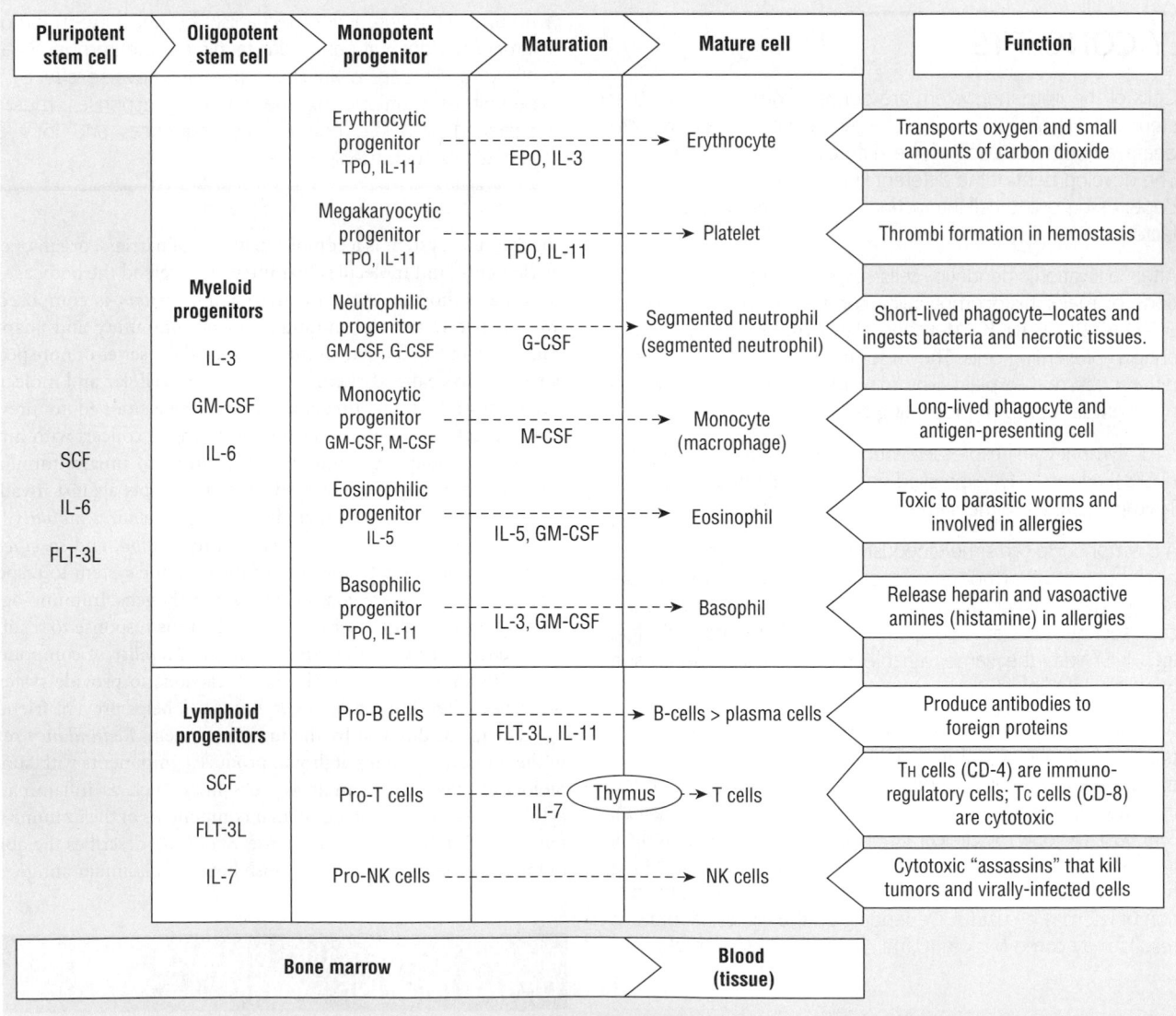

FIGURE 95-1. Basic model of hematopoiesis, outlining the various pathways blood cells take from their origin as bone marrow stem cells through stages in which they are progressively selected to become monopotent mature cells with specific functions. Selected hematopoietic growth factors include: EPO, erythropoietin; FTL-3L, fms-like tyrosine kinase ligand; GM-CSF, granulocyte-macrophage colony-stimulating factor; G-CSF, granulocyte colony-stimulating factor; IL, interleukin; M-CSF, macrophage colony-stimulating factor; SCF, stem cell factor; TPO, thrombopoietin.

TABLE 95-1	Hematopoietic Growth Factors or Colony Stimulating Factors	
Cytokine	**Sources**	**Principal Effects**
EPO	Kidney, liver	Erythrocyte production and maturation
GM-CSF	T lymphocytes, macrophages, bone marrow stromal cells	Maturation and activation of granulocytes, monocytes/macrophages, and eosinophils
G-CSF	Macrophages, bone marrow stromal cells	Maturation and activation of neutrophils
M-CSF	Macrophages, bone marrow stromal cells	Maturation and activation of monocytes/macrophages
TPO	Liver, kidney	Platelet production
SCF	Bone marrow stromal cells, constitutively	Stem cell and progenitor cells activation
FLT-3L	Bone marrow stromal cells	Early-acting growth factor
IL-3	T lymphocytes, macrophages,	Maturation and differentiation of hematopoietic and mast cells
IL-5	Activated T lymphocytes	Eosinophil production
IL-6	Activated T lymphocytes, bone marrow stromal cells	Progenitor cell stimulation
IL-7	Bone marrow stromal cells	T-cell maturation/survival
IL-11	Bone marrow stromal cells	Growth factor for B lymphocytes and megakaryocytes

EPO, erythropoietin; FLT-3L, fms-like tyrosine kinase ligand; GM-CSF, granulocyte-macrophage colony-stimulating factor; G-CSF, granulocyte colony-stimulating factor; IL. interleukin; M-CSF, macrophage colony-stimulating factor; SCF, stem cell factor; TPO, thrombopoietin.

lymphocytes), which are the leukocytes responsible for cell-mediated immunity, including cytotoxic actions and immunoregulation. Through an intricate multistep process called thymic education, T cells that respond appropriately and are beneficial to the immune system mature and leave the thymus. T cells that fail the thymic education test (99%) are eliminated via apoptosis.[1]

SPLEEN

The spleen is a slender elongated secondary lymphoid organ located in the upper left quadrant of the abdomen that receives blood from the splenic artery. Although it is not a vital organ, it functions as an immunological filter of the blood and destroys defective and old erythrocytes. It contains compartments designated as red pulp and white pulp and provides an environment for the interaction of its filtered debris from blood with antigen-presenting cells and lymphocytes responsible for cell-mediated responses (T cells) and lymphocytes responsible for antibody production (B cells). Red pulp serves as a site of red blood cell degradation, and the white pulp provides an environment for the interaction of B cells and T cells. The spleen sequesters many cellular elements (leukocytes, erythrocytes, and platelets) and can become dangerously congested in a condition termed *splenomegaly*.

LYMPH NODES

Lymph nodes are normally small BB-sized lymphoid organs widely distributed between the groin and the neck. While the spleen filters blood, lymph nodes act as immunological filters for interstitial lymphatic fluid from the body's tissues. Lymph nodes provide an environment for the interaction of filtered debris with antigen-presenting cells and other immune cells (T cells and B cells).[2] Lymph nodes may sequester activated immune cells (or tumor cells) and become inflamed and engorged causing lymphadenopathy.

TABLE 95-2	Functional Divisions of the Immune System	
	Innate	**Adaptive**
Exterior defenses	Skin, mucus, cilia, normal flora, saliva, low pH of the stomach, skin, genitourinary tract	None
Specificity	Limited and fixed	Extensive
Memory	None	Yes
Time to response	Hours	Days
Soluble factors	Lysozymes, complement, C-reactive protein, interferons, mannose-binding lectin, antimicrobial peptides[a]	Antibodies, cytokines
Cells	Neutrophils, monocytes, macrophages, natural killer cells, eosinophils	B lymphocytes, T lymphocytes

[a] Cathelicidins α-defensins, β-defensins.

MUCOSA-ASSOCIATED LYMPHOID TISSUE (MALT)

Mucosa-associated lymphoid tissue (MALT) is the most extensive component of human lymphoid tissue and is distributed along mucosal linings of the body.[8] MALT may consist of well-defined networks of primary lymphoid follicles and other associated immunocompetent cells (adenoids, appendix, intestinal Payer's patches, and tonsils), small solitary lymph nodes, or loosely organized clusters of lymphoid cells that are found in intestinal villi. The primary function of these tissues is to filter, trap, and remove pathogens that breach mucosal surfaces. In addition to neutralizing pathogens, MALT generates plasma cells (activated B cells) that secrete IgA antibodies.

As mentioned earlier, the immune system includes two functional divisions: (1) the *innate* or nonspecific which encodes evolutionary genes aimed at providing rapid responses against nonmammalian targets and (2) the *adaptive* or specific which utilizes cells which can genetically rearrange their DNA to create specific structures which bind individual antigens or proteins (Table 95–2).[9] Despite this simple separation, these divisions extensively interact.[10] Awareness of each component of the immune system and the consequences of disrupting homeostasis must be understood in order to appropriately dose, administer, and monitor the effect of medications given to manipulate immune responses.

METHODS TO DISTINGUISH SELF FROM NON-SELF

The immune system is designed to attack and destroy a broad spectrum of foreign antigens/pathogens. The immune system must however be able to distinguish self from non-self, termed *self-tolerance*, in order to avoid unleashing its components onto self-tissues.[11] The body employs many tactics to avoid attacking itself, and when self-tolerance fails this may lead to the development of an autoimmune disease.

INNATE IMMUNE SYSTEM

Physical Defense

Physical and chemical defenses are the most rudimentary form of innate immunity and the first line of defense against invading pathogens. The skin, the largest organ of the body, has the primary role of providing a physical defense. Alterations in the skin, such as burns or abrasions, allow an easy portal of entry for pathogens. The gastrointestinal tract also provides physical defense. The low pH of the stomach (pH 1–2) is inhospitable to most organisms. The rapid turnover of intestinal cells also limits systemic infection as cells including infected cells are sloughed frequently. Drugs, such as cell-cycle, phase-specific antineoplastics that disrupt the sloughing process, leave the patient at an increased risk for infections. Likewise, the respiratory tract has its forms of physical defense. The mucus coating the epithelial cells serves in part to prevent microorganisms from adhering to cell surfaces, and the cilia lining the epithelium of the lungs help to repel inhaled organisms. The combination of cilia, mucus, and reactive coughing provides a natural barrier to invasion via the respiratory tract. Other examples of mechanical or nonspecific defenses include normal urine flow, lysozymes in tears and saliva, and the normal flora in the throat, the lower gastrointestinal tract, and the genitourinary tract. Disruption of the normal physical defense system through mechanical ventilation, for example, places the host at substantial risk for penetration by a pathogenic organism.[12]

Innate Immune Response

If an infectious pathogen invades and is able to infiltrate through a host's physical defense system, innate immunity is employed to halt progression of the infection. Innate immunity is present from birth and utilizes a preexisting but limited repertoire of receptors to recognize and destroy pathogens. Innate immune cells include subgroups of leukocytes; specifically, monocytes/macrophages, neutrophils, basophils, mast cells and eosinophils. When stimulated by a foreign pathogen, mast cells and basophils secrete inflammatory mediators. Monocytes/macrophages, neutrophils, mast cells, and eosinophils act as phagocytes, which allow them to recognize, internalize, and destroy invading pathogens. This process may occur in two ways: opsonin-dependent or opsonin-independent phagocytosis. For opsonin-dependent phagocytosis, antibody (e.g., IgG), complement (e.g., C3b), or lectin (e.g., C-reactive protein) coat, or opsonize, the infectious pathogens. Once the pathogen is opsonized, the antibody, complement, or lectin binds to the receptors on the phagocyte (Fig. 95–2) and activates the phagocytic process. For opsonin-independent phagocytosis, innate leukocytes utilize pattern recognition receptors. Pattern recognition receptors recognize highly conserved

TABLE 95-3	Ligands for Pattern Recognition Receptors
Pathogen Ligand	**Type of Organism**
Lipoteichoic acid	Gram-positive organisms
Lipopolysaccharide	Gram-negative organisms
Mannose	Fungi, gram-positive, gram-negative
Double-stranded RNA	RNA viruses
Triacyl lipopeptides	Gram-positive, gram-negative
Peptidoglycans	Gram-positive
Bacterial flagella	Various

structures present on a large number of microorganisms. These highly conserved structures are essential for the microorganism's survival or pathogenicity. The pattern recognition receptors include the macrophage mannose receptor, macrophage scavenger receptor, and members of the toll-like receptor family. Pattern recognition receptors on the phagocytes directly recognize ligands (Table 95–3) on the surfaces of infectious pathogens leading to immediate phagocytosis of the pathogen (Fig. 95–2). Toll-like receptors are a family of pattern recognition receptors on the cell-surface of innate leukocytes. To date, 11 toll-like receptors have been identified in humans. They recognize a broad spectrum of antigens ranging from lipopolysaccharide and flagellin on bacteria to zymosan on yeast to double-stranded RNA from RNA viruses (Table 95–3). Binding of the ligand to the toll-like receptors allows the phagocyte to recognize and engulf the pathogen. This binding of toll-like receptors to its ligand also results in the secretion of chemokines, inflammatory cytokines, and antimicrobial peptides as well as the increased expression of co-stimulatory proteins (e.g., B7) and the major histocompatibility complex proteins by the phagocyte. This leads to the recruitment and activation of antigen-specific lymphocytes.[10,13,14] Other pattern recognition receptors that mediate phagocytosis include MARCO (macrophage receptor with collagenous structure), DC-SIGN (*D*endritic *C*ell-*S*pecific *I*ntercellular adhesion molecule-3-*G*rabbing *N*on-integrin), and dectin 1.

Cells of the Innate Immune System

Neutrophils, eosinophils, and basophils are considered granulocytes because of the presence of numerous cytoplasm granules in these cells that contain inflammatory mediators or digestive enzymes. Their names are derived from their staining characteristics; neutrophils are named because they stain a neutral pink. Neutrophils comprise the majority of leukocytes in the bloodstream. They are polymorphonuclear cells, often denoted as PMNs for this reason, which serve as the primary human defense against invasive bacteria. Neutrophils migrate from the bloodstream into infected or inflamed tissue in response to chemotactic factors, such as IL-8 and C3a and C5a, breakdown products of complement. In this migration, a process termed chemotaxis, neutrophils reach the site of inflammation and then recognize, adhere to, and phagocytose pathogens. Via the complement and antibody receptors located on its surface, neutrophils can recognize and engulf pathogens opsonized with complement or IgG (antibody). During phagocytosis, the engulfed pathogen is internalized within the phagocyte into a cytoplasmic lysosome. The neutrophil then releases its granular contents into lysosome and generates the release of oxidative metabolites that destroy the engulfed pathogens.[15] Neutrophils can also recognize pathogens via toll-like receptors.

Eosinophils are also granulocytic cells involved in innate immunity. They exhibit motility and migrate from the blood into the tissues. They play a less significant role in combating bacterial infections, but eosinophils play a major role against nonphagocytable multicellular

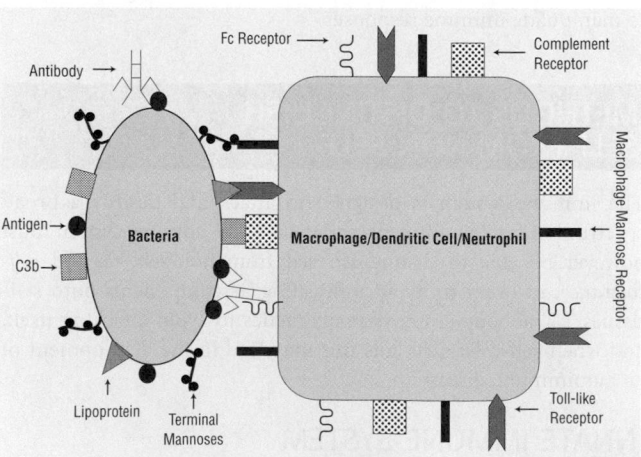

FIGURE 95-2. Phagocytosis of bacteria by macrophages, dendritic cells, and neutrophils. Macrophages, dendritic cells, and neutrophils recognize bacteria opsonized (coated) with antibody or complement (C3b). On the surface of macrophages, dendritic cells, and neutrophils reside receptors for antibody (Fc receptors) and complement (CR1, CR3, CR4). In addition, these cells may recognize the bacteria by pattern recognition receptors on the surface of macrophages, dendritic cells, and neutrophils. Pattern recognition receptors include toll-like receptors, scavenger receptors, and mannose receptors.

pathogens, such as parasites. After activation via high-affinity receptor for IgE (i.e., Fcε), eosinophils exocytose their granules causing the release of basic proteins or reactive oxygen species into the microenvironment, causing lysis of the parasite. In addition to Fcε receptors, eosinophils express lower levels of complement receptor 3 and Fcγ for IgG than neutrophils. The high affinity of eosinophils for IgE contribute to their role in the pathogenesis of allergic disorders (i.e., allergic asthma).[16]

Macrophages and monocytes are mononuclear cells capable of phagocytosis. Tissue macrophages arise from the migration of monocytes from the bloodstream into the tissues. Macrophages differ from monocytes by possessing an increased number of Fc and complement receptors. Macrophages are found within specific tissues such as the liver, spleen, gastrointestinal tract, lymph nodes, brain, and others. These specific types of macrophages are often called histiocytes, or referred to by a specialized name depending on the site where they are found (for example, Kupffer cells in the liver, osteoclasts in the bone, microglial cells in the central nervous system). The term reticuloendothelial system (RES) was commonly used to refer to macrophages found in reticular connective tissue, but the preferred nomenclature is now the mononuclear phagocyte system.[17]

Despite the first description in 1868 of Langerhans cells, a type of dendritic cell found in the skin, our current understanding of the biologic function of dendritic cells did not develop until the past decade. Before pathogen recognition, most dendritic cells are in an immature/resting state with limited ability to activate T lymphocytes, but they express numerous receptors (e.g., Fc receptors of IgG and IgE, macrophage mannose receptor, toll-like receptors) enabling rapid antigen recognition. Following antigen recognition and particle engulfment, dendritic cells become activated. This leads to a dramatic increase in their expression of the major histocompatibility complex (MHC) class II, B7, CD40, and adhesion molecules. Dendritic cells then begin to migrate through the tissues towards lymphoid organs (e.g., spleen, lymph nodes) to present antigen to T lymphocytes, causing activation of the adaptive immune system.[18]

❷ In addition to phagocytosing pathogens, macrophages and dendritic cells act as antigen-presenting cells (APCs) to stimulate the adaptive (specific) system. Macrophages and dendritic cells internalize the organism, digest it into small peptide fragments, and then combine these antigenic fragments together with MHC proteins. Once the APC has formed the antigen/MHC complex, the APC places the complex on its surface. This surface complex can then be recognized by the T-cell receptor on the surface of a T lymphocyte. The recognition of the antigen/MHC complex by the T-cell receptor is the first step in the activation of the T lymphocyte (Fig. 95–3). Other cells, B lymphocytes and mast cells, can also act as APCs (Fig. 95–4).[17–19]

Mast cells and basophils act primarily by releasing inflammatory mediators. Mast cells are tissue cells predominately associated with IgE-mediated inflammation. They are especially abundant in the skin, lungs, nasal mucosa, and connective tissue. Granules within the mast cells contain large amounts of preformed mediators that include histamine, heparin, and serotonin. Mast cells can also phagocytize, destroy, and present bacterial antigens to T lymphocytes.[18] Basophils are similar to mast cells because they contain granules filled with histamine, but they are typically found circulating in the blood and are not found in connective tissue. Like mast cells, basophils also express high-affinity IgE Fc receptors (Fcε). IgE- mediated anaphylaxis (type I hypersensitivity; Chap. 97) is caused by the stimulation of mast cell and/or basophil degranulation and the release of preformed mediators after allergen binds to IgE bound to the Fcε receptor on the surface of mast cells or basophils.[19]

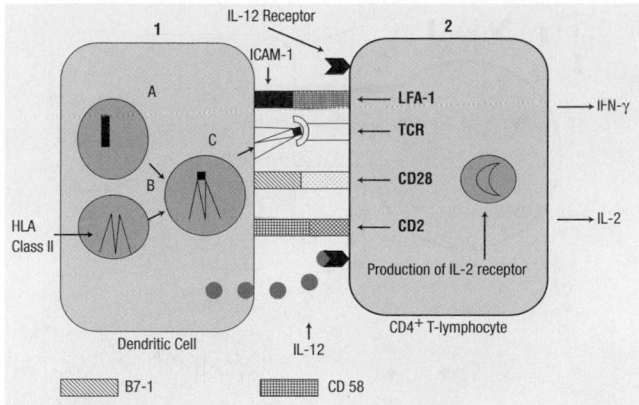

FIGURE 95-3. Induction of T-helper type 1 (TH₁) response. *1*. The antigen-presenting cell, in this case a dendritic cell, engulfs the pathogen by any of numerous cell surface receptors (see Fig. 95–2). After phagocytosis of the bacteria by the dendritic cell (A), the pathogen is digested into small peptides and become associated with major histocompatibility (MHC) class II within the endosome (B). Finally, the MHC class II plus peptide is expressed on the surface of the dendritic cell (C). The activated dendritic cell also secretes interleukin (IL)-12. *2*. Naïve CD4⁺ T-lymphocyte activation requires the T-cell receptor (TCR) to recognize the antigenic peptide in association with MHC class II as well as the B7-1 (CD80) binding to CD28. The binding of CD2-CD58 and LFA-1 (CD11a/CD18) allows adherence between the T lymphocyte and dendritic cell. Upon activation, the TH₁ CD4⁺ T lymphocyte secretes IL-2 and interferon (IFN)-γ and increases the production and expression of the IL-2 receptor. (ICAM, intercellular adhesion molecule.)

Soluble Mediators of the Innate Immune System

Soluble mediators of innate immunity include the complement system, mannose-binding lectin, antimicrobial peptides, and C-reactive protein (CRP).[9] The complement system consists of more than 30 proteins in the plasma and on cell surfaces that play a key role in immune defense. The four major functions of the complement system include (1) to lyse certain microorganisms and cells, (2) to stimulate the chemotaxis of phagocytic cells, (3) to coat or opsonize foreign pathogens which allows phagocytosis of the pathogen by leukocytes expressing complement receptors, and (4) to clear immune complexes. Complement factors (C3a, C5a) act as chemotactic factors for phagocytic cells.[20] Two different pathways stimulate the complement cascade. In the *classic pathway*, antibody binds to its target antigen and activates the first component of complement (C1), thereby initiating the complement cascade. The *alternative complement pathway* relies on the inability of microorganisms to clear spontaneously produced C3b, the active form of third complement protein, from their surface. Patients with hereditary deficiencies of complement have recurrent bacterial infections or immune complex disease because C3b plays a central role in opsonizing bacteria and clearing immune complexes. Both mannan-binding lectin and C-reactive protein are acute-phase reactants produced by the liver during the early stages of an infection. They bind to infectious pathogens that prompt the activation of the lectin or minor pathway of the complement system. Mannan-binding lectin binds to mannose-rich glycoconjugates on microorganisms while C-reactive protein binds to phosphorylcholine on bacterial surfaces.[9,20]

Chemokines play an essential role in linking the innate and adaptive immune response by orchestrating leukocyte trafficking. The chemokine system consists of a group of small polypeptides and their receptors. Chemokines possess four conserved cysteines. Based on the positions of the cysteines, almost all chemokines

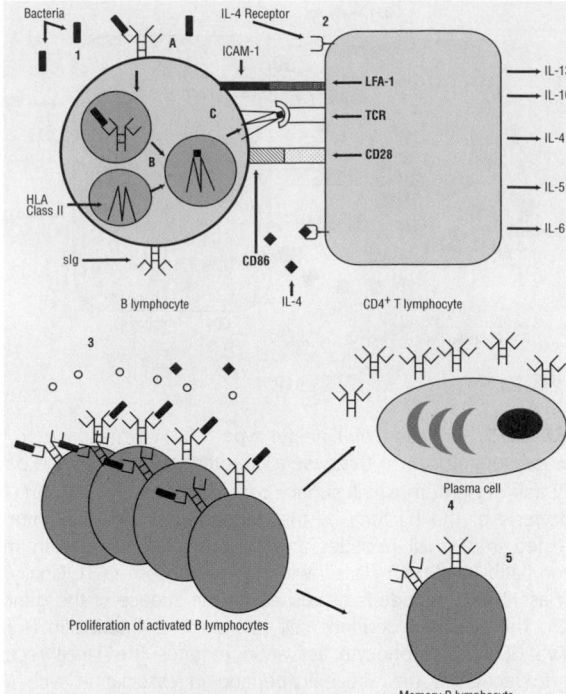

FIGURE 95-4. Induction of T-helper type 2 (TH₂) response. *1A.* A B lymphocyte recognizes invading bacteria via its surface immunoglobulin (sIg). *1B.* The bound bacteria are phagocytosed into an endosome, where the bacteria are broken down into small peptide fragments. *1C.* The small peptide fragments are placed within major histocompatibility complex (MHC) class II molecules and transported to the surface of the B lymphocyte for antigen presentation to a CD4⁺ T lymphocyte. *2.* CD4⁺ T-lymphocyte recognition requires antigen recognition within the MHC class II peptide groove by the T-cell receptor (TCR) and a secondary signal from B7-2 from the antigen-presenting cell, in this case a B lymphocyte, binding to CD28 on the T lymphocyte. When both signals are delivered, the CD4⁺ T lymphocyte becomes activated. In the TH₂ environment (see text), the naive CD4⁺ T lymphocyte develops into a TH₂ subtype and secretes interleukin (IL)-4, IL-5, IL-6, IL-10, and IL-13, which promote a TH₂ response. *3.* In the presence of these cytokines plus antigen binding to the sIg, the B lymphocyte becomes activated. The activated B lymphocyte becomes a plasma cell *(4)*, which produces and secretes immunoglobulin or becomes a memory B lymphocyte *(5)*. A minority of B lymphocytes become memory B lymphocytes.

fall into one of two categories: (1) CC group in which the conserved cysteines are contiguous or (2) CXC subgroup in which the cysteines are separated by some other amino acid ("X"). As with all ligand-receptor interactions, a cell can only respond to a chemokine if the cell possesses a receptor that recognizes the chemokine. Chemokine receptors are unique in that they traverse the membrane seven times. CC receptors (CCR) and CXC receptors (CXCR) bind CC ligands (CCL) and CXC ligands (CXCL), respectively (Table 95–4).

Binding of infectious pathogens to pattern recognition receptors stimulates the release of chemokines such as macrophage inflammatory protein (MIP)-1α, MIP-1β, MIP-3α, and IP-10 from macrophages and dendritic cells embedded in the tissues. These chemokines attract more immature dendritic cells to the site of inflammation/infection. Immature dendritic cells constitutively express CCR1, CCR5, and CCR6. The interaction between pattern recognition receptors on the dendritic cell to the infectious pathogen causes the activation and maturation of the dendritic cell. After activation, dendritic cells downregulate the expression of CCR1, CCR5, and CCR6 and upregulate the expression of CCR7. This switch in chemokine-receptor expression results in

TABLE 95-4	Common Chemokines	
Receptor	**Cell Expression**	**Ligand**
CCR1	Immature DC	MIP-1α, MIP-1β, MCP-2, RANTES
CCR3	Eosinophils, basophils	Eotaxin-1, eotaxin-2, eotaxin-3, MCP-4
CCR6	Immature DC	Exodus-1
CCR7	Activated DC	CCL21 (SLC), CCL19 (ELC)
CXCR1/2	Neutrophils	IL-8
CXCR3	Natural killer cells, activated T lymphocytes	IP-10

DC, dendritic cell; MCP, monocyte chemoattractant protein; RANTES, Regulated upon Activation Normal T lymphocyte Expressed and Secreted.

the antigen-loaded dendritic cell leaving the tissue and migrating toward the lymph nodes.[21]

Naturally occurring antimicrobial peptides include α-defensins, β-defensins, and cathelicidins. These peptides exhibit antibacterial, antifungal, and antiviral activity. Human antimicrobial peptides range in size from 29 to 37 amino acid residues in length. Neutrophils are rich source of both α- and β-defensins as well as cathelicidins. Other sources of the human antimicrobial peptides include keratinocytes, paneth cells of the intestinal and genital tracts, and epithelial cells of the pancreas and the kidney. These peptides can be induced at sites of inflammation or can be constitutively produced. The clinical interest in human antimicrobial peptides centers on their broad spectrum activity and their rapid onset of killing. They are believed to work by disrupting microbial membranes. An active area of research is how these peptides discriminate between microbial and host membranes.[22]

ADAPTIVE IMMUNE SYSTEM

Adaptive Immune Response: Antigen Recognition

The body will generally employ both the innate and adaptive immune responses to rapidly kill foreign pathogens.[9] The greatest difference between the innate and adaptive immune responses is in specificity and memory, characterized by antigen-specific receptors located on the surface of B and T lymphocytes.[11] The adaptive immune response also secretes cytokines to further amplify the innate immune response. The adaptive immune response can evolve with each subsequent infection whereas the innate response stays the same with each infection. During B- and T-lymphocyte development, an individual B or T lymphocyte rearranges its immunoglobulin and T-cell receptor genes, respectively, to produce a unique immunoglobulin or T-cell receptor, respectively. This DNA rearrangement generates enough B or T lymphocytes to recognize an estimated 10^{15} antigens.

The adaptive immune response can be divided into two major arms: humoral and cellular mediated. The humoral response is so denoted because it was discovered that the factors that provided the immune protection could be found in the "humor" or serum. B lymphocytes comprise the humoral arm. Activated B lymphocytes can differentiate into plasma cells that secrete immunoglobulin or memory B cells specific for each pathogen. T lymphocytes constitute the cell-mediated arm of the adaptive system. The immune protection provided by T lymphocytes cannot be transferred by serum alone. Rather, it is essential to actually have T lymphocytes present, thus the term cell-mediated immunity. T lymphocytes are specially tailored to defend against infections that are intracellular, such as viral infections, whereas

B lymphocytes secrete antibodies that can neutralize pathogens prior to their entry into host cells.

Adaptive Immune Response: Cells Which Mediate Antigen Recognition

The role of the T lymphocyte is to search and destroy pathogens that infect and replicate intracellularly. When these pathogens enter a cell they are no longer vulnerable to innate host defenses; therefore, it is critical that the T lymphocytes be able to distinguish which cells are infected and which cells are not. ❸ T lymphocytes do not recognize intact antigens, such as a bacterial cell wall. T lymphocytes only recognize processed antigens in association with MHC.

The *major histocompatibility complex*, a cluster of genes found on chromosome 6 in humans, is also known as the human leukocyte antigen (HLA) complex. The MHC is used by the immune system to distinguish self from non-self and provides a so-called immunologic "fingerprint." The genes from this complex encode for molecules that play a pivotal role in immune recognition and response. The MHC complex is divided into three different classes: I, II, and III. The molecules encoded by class I HLA genes include HLA-A, HLA-B, and HLA-C antigens. These molecules can be found on all nucleated cells within the body, as well as on platelets. Class I antigens are not found on mature red blood cells. Molecules encoded by class II HLA genes include HLA-DP, HLA-DQ, and HLA-DR. The expression of these molecules is more restricted and can be found primarily on cells of the immune system, namely antigen-presenting cells such as macrophages, dendritic cells, and B lymphocytes. The class III HLA antigens encode for soluble factors, complement, and tumor necrosis factors.[23] In order for a CD4+ T lymphocyte to become activated, CD4+ T lymphocyte must recognize the antigenic peptide in association with MHC class II (Figs. 95–3 and 95–4). CD8+ T lymphocytes recognize antigenic peptide in association with class I molecules. Class I molecules generally contain endogenous peptides from within the cell, such as those derived from viruses, while class II molecules contain exogenous peptides from antigen that has been phagocytosis and digested, such as bacterial peptides (Fig. 95–3). For it to destroy a virally infected cell, a CD8+ cytotoxic T lymphocyte requires two steps. First, its T-cell receptor must recognize the antigenic fragment, such as a viral protein, in association with MHC class I. The second step involves the co-stimulatory step of B7-CD28 binding. This process is further defined below. Because any cell can become infected, it is advantageous that the CD8+ cytotoxic T lymphocytes recognize the MHC class I molecule that is expressed on all cells except red blood cells. The ability of the MHC class I to present endogenous peptides allows the CD8+ cytotoxic T lymphocytes to constantly screen cells for infections.[23,24] Dendritic cells and macrophages demonstrate the unique capacity to direct exogenous antigens toward MHC class I molecules, a process termed cross-presentation.[25]

APCs (e.g., macrophages, dendritic cells) engulf the pathogen, digest it, and express its peptide fragments on their cell surface in association with their MHC. T lymphocytes use a specific antigen receptor, T-cell receptor (TCR), to propagate the immune response. The TCR is comprised of two chains with each chain having a variable and a constant region. The variation of the amino acid sequence within the variable domain of TCR gives the cell its unique antigen specificity. Linked to the TCR is a complex of single chains known as the CD3 complex.[9,19]

Naïve T lymphocytes, are cells that have not been previously exposed to an antigen specific for their TCR. These cells require two signals for activation. The first signal for activation involves the T lymphocyte recognizing both the processed antigen and the MHC molecule complex. The second signal involves the interaction of the B7-1 (CD80) or B7-2 (CD86) molecule on the APC with the CD28 molecule on the surface of the T lymphocyte (Figs. 95–3 and 95–4). Without the second signal, the naïve T lymphocyte becomes anergic or inactive. Memory T lymphocytes are less dependent on the second signal than are naïve T lymphocytes. CD28 is expressed on both resting and activated T lymphocytes while CTLA-4, a second ligand for B7 on T lymphocytes, is expressed only on activated T lymphocytes. CTLA-4 binding B7 transduces a negative signal so it plays a role in downregulating a T-lymphocyte response.[26] After the two activation signals, a message is sent through the TCR to the CD3 complex into the cell. Then a calcium influx occurs with subsequent activation of the T lymphocyte. Activated CD4+ T lymphocytes begin to express the high-affinity IL-2 receptor and to release multiple soluble factors (e.g., IL-2) to stimulate T lymphocytes and other cells of the immune system (Fig. 95–3). Autocrine stimulation by IL-2 leads to the proliferation of the activated T lymphocyte.

Cell surface markers delineate the functional activity of T-lymphocyte populations. All T lymphocytes express the CD3 protein. Typically, T lymphocytes are further divided into helper cells (CD4+), suppressor cells (CD8+), and cytotoxic cells (CD8+). Each of the subclasses appears to play a distinct role in the cell-mediated immune response. Naïve T lymphocytes express CD45RA, a high-molecular-weight isoform of CD45, while memory T lymphocytes express CD45RO, a lower-molecular-weight isoform of CD45.[27] The primary role of CD4+ cells is to stimulate other cells in the immune response. Functionally, CD4+ cells can be divided into TH_1 and TH_2. This functional system was first described in mice. TH_1 cells secrete IL-2 and γ-interferon and stimulate CD8+ cytotoxic cells, whereas TH_2 cells secrete IL-4, IL-5, and IL-10 and stimulate B-lymphocyte production of antibody.[28] Multiple factors determine whether a naïve CD4+ T lymphocyte develops into a TH_1 or a TH_2 cell. The cytokine microenvironment plays an important role in this development. IL-12 secreted by the APCs promotes TH_1, whereas IL-4 promotes TH_2 development. Other factors that promote TH_1 development include B7-1 (CD80), high-affinity of the TCR for the antigen, γ-interferon, and α-interferon. Factors that promote TH_2 development include B7-2 (CD86), low-affinity of the TCR for the antigen, IL-10, and IL-1.[29]

CD8+ T lymphocytes recognize antigen in association with MHC class I. CD8+ cytotoxic cells are instrumental in killing cells recognized as foreign, such as those that have become infected by a virus. CD8+ cytotoxic T lymphocytes also play an important beneficial role in the eradication of tumor cells, but moreover are responsible for rejection of transplanted organs.[19] Classically, a second type of CD8+ T lymphocytes was a suppressor cell. It is clear that some T lymphocytes help suppress the immune responses, but whether this subset is CD8+ is debatable. Emerging evidence is leading away from CD8+ T lymphocytes toward CD4+, CD25+ T lymphocytes in maintaining self-tolerance. The preferred term for these suppressive T lymphocytes is regulatory T lymphocytes.[30]

To fully activate the CD8+ cytotoxic T lymphocyte requires CD4+ T lymphocyte activation, namely the TH_1 subset, and its subsequent secretion of IL-2 (Fig. 95–5a). This model of CD8+ cytotoxic T lymphocyte activation requires the close proximity of two-antigen specific T lymphocytes. In addition, some CD8+ cytotoxic T-lymphocyte responses can occur in the absence of CD4+ T lymphocytes. New data suggests that CD4+ T-lymphocytes can activate/prime APCs through CD40. This interaction primes the APC (e.g., dendritic cell) to fully activate CD8+ cytotoxic T lymphocytes (Fig. 95–5b).[31] It is important to remember that the classification of CD4+ lymphocytes as T-helper lymphocytes and CD8+ lymphocytes as T-cytotoxic lymphocytes is not an

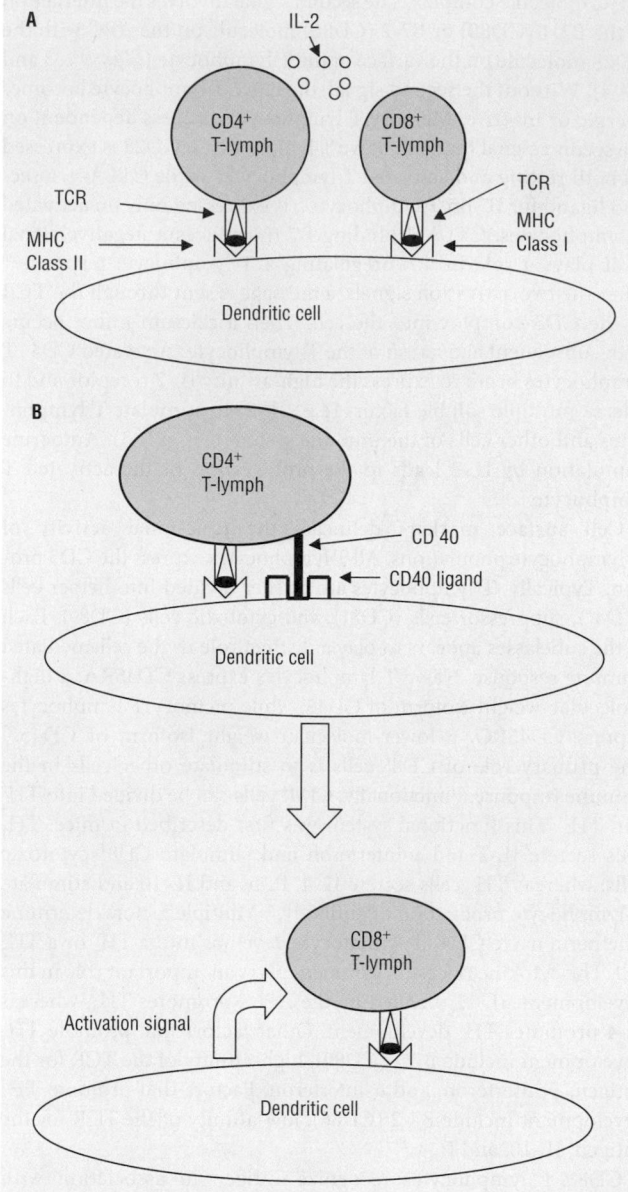

FIGURE 95-5. In the classic model of CD8+ T-lymphocyte activation *(A)*, CD4+ and CD8+ T lymphocytes recognize antigen on the same dendritic cell. In the presence of interleukin (IL)-2 from the activated CD4+ T lymphocyte and the recognition of antigen in association with major histocompatibility complex (MHC) class I, the CD8+ lymphocyte becomes activated. In the new model *(B)*, activated CD4+ T lymphocytes activate dendritic cells via CD40 ligand binding to CD40. The activated dendritic cell then migrates through the tissues to present antigen to CD8+ T lymphocytes. If recognition via the T-cell receptor (TCR) on the CD8+ T lymphocyte occurs, the dendritic cell can fully activate the CD8+ T lymphocyte without the presence of CD4+ T lymphocytes.

absolute. Some CD8+ T lymphocytes secrete cytokines similar to a T-helper lymphocyte, and some CD4+ T lymphocytes can act as cytotoxic cells.

Unlike neutrophils and macrophages, cytotoxic T lymphocytes are unable to ingest their targets. They destroy target cells by two different mechanisms: the *perforin system* and the *Fas ligand pathway*. After recognition by the cytotoxic T lymphocyte, cytoplasmic granules containing perforins and granzymes are rapidly oriented toward the target cell, and the contents of the granules are released into the intracellular space. Like the membrane attack complex formed after complement activation, perforins form a pore in

the target cell membrane. Besides a direct cytotoxic effect on the target cell, the pores produced by perforins allow the granzymes to penetrate into the target cell to induce apoptosis. The second mechanism of cytotoxicity involves the binding of Fas ligand on the cytotoxic T lymphocyte to the Fas receptor on the target cell. The Fas ligand is predominately expressed on CD8+ cytotoxic T lymphocytes and NK cells, and its expression increases after activation. After destroying that target cell by either mechanism, the cytotoxic T lymphocyte detaches from the target cell and attacks other targets.[32]

A B lymphocyte recognizes antigen via its antibody or immunoglobulin located on its cell surface (Fig. 95–4). The antibody on the surface can recognize an intact pathogen, such as bacteria, and present antigen to T lymphocytes (i.e., acting as APC). However, the major function of B lymphocytes is to produce antibody to bind to the invading pathogen, a process that first entails activation of the B lymphocyte. The activation of B lymphocytes also requires two steps: (1) recognition of antigen by the surface immunoglobulin and (2) the presence of B-lymphocyte growth factors (IL-4, -5, -6) secreted by activated CD4+ T lymphocytes. Once activated, the B lymphocyte becomes a plasma cell, a differentiated cell capable of producing and secreting antibody. A fraction of activated B lymphocytes do not differentiate into plasma cells, but rather form a pool of memory cells. The memory cells will respond to subsequent encounters with the pathogen, generating a quicker and more vigorous response to the pathogen. Some B lymphocytes can become activated without help from T lymphocytes, but these responses are generally weak and do not invoke memory.[9,19]

Natural killer (NK) cells, often referred to as large granular lymphocytes, are defined functionally by their ability to lyse target cells without prior sensitization and without restriction by MHC. Resting NK cells express the intermediate-affinity IL-2 receptor, CD122. Upon exposure to IL-2, NK cells exhibit greater cytotoxic activity against a wide variety of tumors. NK cells recognize target cells by two mechanisms. First, NK cells express an IgG Fc receptor, CD16 that allows recognition of IgG-coated cells. Second, NK cells express killer-activating and killer-inhibiting receptors. The killer-activating receptors recognize multiple targets on normal cells; however, the binding of MHC class I to the killer-inhibitor receptor blocks release of perforins and granzymes. Therefore, cells (e.g., tumor cells, virally infected cells) that downregulate MHC class I expression are susceptible to NK cell cytolysis. NK cells play important roles in the surveillance and the destruction of tumors and virally infected host cells, and in the regulation of hematopoiesis.[9,33]

Soluble Mediators of the Adaptive Immune Response

❹ When binding of a specific antigen to the surface immunoglobulin receptor of B lymphocytes occurs, the B lymphocyte matures into a plasma cell and produces large quantities of antibody that have the ability to bind to the inciting antigen. The secreted antibodies may be of five different isotypes. On primary exposure to the pathogen, the plasma cell will secrete IgM; then, eventually, there is a switch to predominately IgG. On second exposure, the memory B lymphocytes will predominately produce IgG. Isotype switching from IgM to IgG, IgA, or IgE is controlled by T lymphocytes.

An antibody or immunoglobulin is a glycoprotein comprised of two different chains, heavy and light (Fig. 95–6). The basic structure of every immunoglobulin consists of four peptide chains: two identical heavy chains and two identical light chains held together by disulfide bonds. The basic structure of the antibody is a Y-shaped figure. Each arm of the Y is formed by the linkage of

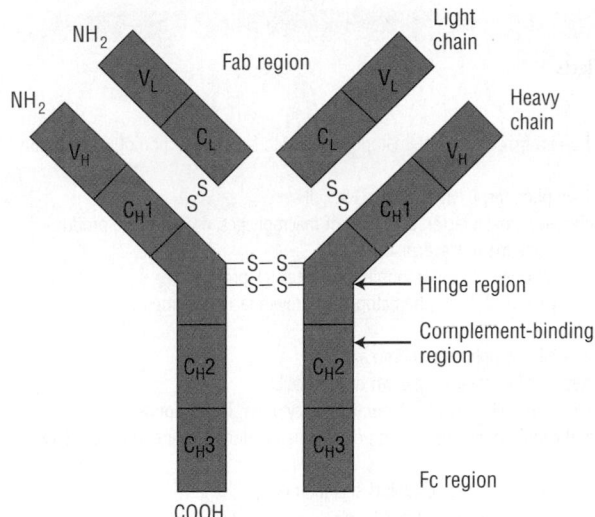

FIGURE 95-6. Schematic diagram of the structure of the immunoglobulin G (IgG) molecule. IgG molecule consists of two heavy (H) and two light (L) chains covalently linked by disulfide bonds. Each chain is composed of variable (V) and constant (C) regions. A light chain consists of one variable (V_L) and one constant (C_L) region. Heavy chains consist of one variable (V_H) and three or four constant (C_H) regions, depending on the isotype. The variable regions (V_L and V_H) compose the antigen-binding region of the IgG molecule, or fragment antigen binding (Fab). The constant regions provide the structure to the IgG molecule as well as binding the first component of complement (C_H2) and binding to Fc receptors via the Fc portion of the molecule (C_H3).

the end of the light chain to its heavy chain partner. These arms contain the portions described as the *fragments of antigen binding (Fab fragments)*. The stem of the Y contains the heavy chains which comprise the *fragment crystallizable (Fc fragment)* portion of the antibody. It is within the Fc portion that complement is activated once the antibody has bound its target. Likewise, it is the Fc portion of the antibody that is recognized by Fc receptors on the surface of phagocytes (Fig. 95–2). The amino acid composition of the same isotype is homogenous except in the variable regions of the light (V_L) and heavy chains (V_H). The variation in amino acid composition of the variable region gives the antibody its unique specificity (Fig. 95–6).

IgG, the most prevalent of the antibody classes, comprises approximately 80% of serum antibody. IgG is usually the second isotype of antibody to be produced in an initial humoral immune response. IgG is the only isotype of antibody that can cross the placenta. Therefore, early maternal humoral protection of neonates is primarily due to maternal IgG that crossed the placenta in utero.

Four different subclasses of IgG have been described: IgG1, IgG2, IgG3, and IgG4. These subclasses differ slightly in their constant amino acid sequences. IgG1 constitutes the majority (60%) of the subclasses. It appears that different subclasses recognize different types of antigen. IgG1 and IgG3 are principally responsible for recognition of protein antigens while IgG2 and IgG4 commonly bind to carbohydrate antigens. Another difference in the subclasses is the ability to activate complement with IgG3 and IgG1 being the most efficient, but IgG4 is unable to activate the complement system.

IgM can be found on the surface of B lymphocytes as a monomeric Y-shaped structure. In contrast, secreted IgM is a pentamer in which five of the monomers are joined together by a joining chain (J-chain). IgM is the first class of antibody to be produced on initial exposure to an antigen. Because the pentameric form of IgM has no Fc portions exposed, phagocytic cells cannot bind pathogens

opsonized by IgM. However, IgM is an excellent activator of the complement cascade by the classic pathway.

IgA is found primarily in the fluid secretions of the body: tears, saliva, nasal fluids; and also in the gastrointestinal, genitourinary, and respiratory tracts. IgA functions by preventing pathogens from adhering to and infecting the epithelial cells at these sites. IgA is also secreted in a nursing mother's breast milk as well as are IgG and IgM but in lower concentrations. In bodily secretions, IgA is in a dimeric form in which a J-chain and a secretory chain hold two monomers together. The dimeric form is resistant to proteolysis in mucosal secretions.

IgD is the least understood isotype. IgD is found on the surface of B lymphocytes at different stages of maturation and may be involved in the differentiation of these cells. The main function of circulating IgD has not yet been determined. However, mice treated with exogenous anti-IgD antibody display a marked increase in immunoreactivity and secretion of all types of immunoglobulins and several T-cell specific cytokines. High levels of anti-IgD autoantibodies of various subtypes have also been observed in most autoimmune diseases with frequencies of >50%, suggesting that IgD may play an important role in the etiology of these diseases.[34]

IgE is the least common of the serum antibody isotypes. Most of the IgE in the body is bound to the IgE Fc receptors on mast cells. When the IgE on the surface of mast cells binds antigen, it causes the release of various inflammatory substances (e.g., histamine) from the mast cell. The overall effect is the stimulation of inflammation. Asthma and hay fever are two examples of allergic reactions primarily due to antigen binding to IgE.[29]

Cytokines are soluble factors released or secreted by cells. These proteins affect the activity of other cells (paracrine) or the secreting cell itself (autocrine). For example, activated CD4+ T lymphocytes secrete IL-2 which activates itself as well as activating CD8+ T lymphocytes and NK cells. Research has shown that many cytokines (Table 95–5) have a broad spectrum of effects dependent on their concentration, the presence of other factors, and the target cell. New cytokine families and their roles in disease processes are being discovered daily. Cytokines provide communication between the divisions of the immune system. Cytokines produced from APCs generally promote chemotaxis of other cells and induce a state of inflammation.[35] Monocytes, as previously mentioned, use pattern recognition receptors, enabling the immune system to distinguish pathogenic proteins from nonpathogenic proteins through toll-like receptors stimulating T-lymphocyte activation.[35] Cytokines can also prevent activation or response of immunologic cells. For example, IL-10 is an anti-inflammatory cytokine that is produced in the respiratory tract to prevent IgE synthesis and activation of eosinophils when exposed to benign inhaled particles.[35] In vivo cytokines do not act alone but in combination with other cytokines. For example, activated CD4+ T lymphocytes secrete both IL-2 and interferon-γ which are synergistic in activating NK cells. As shown in Tables 95–1 and 95–5, cytokines are broadly classified as regulatory or hematopoietic growth factors.[19,36-40] This classification does not describe all their activities. Granulocyte macrophage-colony stimulating factor (granulocyte-macrophage colony-stimulating factor) released by activated T lymphocytes acts as a hematopoietic growth factor, but also activates granulocytes and macrophages to phagocytize foreign pathogens.

The division of the immune system into the two functional groups does not imply that the divisions do not interact. In order to generate a vigorous immune response, both soluble mediators (e.g., complement, antibody, and cytokines) and cells (e.g., neutrophils, macrophages, dendritic cells, T lymphocytes, and B lymphocytes) are needed. Generally, the innate system will respond first. Dendritic cells, macrophages and neutrophils in the tissues

TABLE 95-5 Cytokines

Cytokines	Sources	Principal Effects
Regulatory		
IL-1	Macrophages, fibroblasts, endothelial cells	Activation of T and B lymphocytes, hematopoietic growth factor, induction of inflammatory events
IL-2	CD4$^+$ T lymphocytes (TH$_1$ subset)	Activation of T lymphocytes, B lymphocytes, NK cells
IL-4	CD4$^+$ T lymphocytes (TH$_2$ subset), mast cells, basophils, eosinophils	B- and T-lymphocytes growth factor, activation of macrophages, promotes IgE production, proliferation of bone marrow precursors
IL-5	CD4$^+$ T lymphocytes (TH$_2$ subset), mast cells	Activation of B lymphocytes and eosinophils, promotes IgE production
IL-6	CD4$^+$ T lymphocytes (TH$_2$ subset), macrophages, mast cells, fibroblasts	T- and B-lymphocyte growth factor, hematopoietic growth factor, augments inflammation
IL-8	T lymphocytes, monocytes, endothelial cells, fibroblasts	Neutrophil, basophil, T-lymphocyte chemotaxis
IL-10	T and B lymphocytes, macrophages	Cytokine synthesis inhibitory factor, growth of mast cells
IL-12	Macrophages, neutrophils, dendritic cells	Induce TH$_1$ cells, ↑ NK cell activity, ↑ generation of cytotoxic T lymphocytes
IL-13	Activated T lymphocytes	Proliferation of B lymphocytes, suppression of proinflammatory cytokines, directs IgE isotype switching
IL-14	T lymphocytes	Induces B-lymphocyte proliferation, inhibits secretion of Igs
IL-15	Macrophages, fibroblasts, dendritic cells, epithelial cells	T-lymphocyte proliferation, activation of NK cells
IL-16	CD8$^+$ T lymphocytes, epithelial cells	Chemoattractant for CD4$^+$ T lymphocytes and eosinophils; stimulation of secondary cytokine secretion from and proliferation of CD4$^+$ T lymphocytes
IL-18	Macrophages	Induces IFN-γ production
IL-28, IL-29^a	Antigen-presenting cells, but proposed that all nucleated cells may produce	Alternative to IFN-α/IFN-β to provide immunity against viral infections by inhibiting viral replication
IL-31	Activated T lymphocytes	Involved in recruitment of polymorphonuclear cells, monocytes, and T cells to site of inflammation
IL-32	NK cells, T lymphocytes, epithelial cells	Induces proinflammatory cytokines including TNF-α and IL-8
TNF-α	Macrophages, NK cells, T and B lymphocytes, mast cells	Activation of neutrophils, endothelial cells, lymphocytes, liver cells to produce acute phase proteins
TNF-β	T lymphocytes	Tumoricidal
IFN-α	Monocytes, other cells	Antiviral, activation of NK cells and macrophages, upregulation of MHC class I
IFN-γ	T lymphocytes, NK cells	Activation of macrophages, NK cells, upregulation of MHC class I and II

IFN, interferon; Ig, immunoglobulin; IL, interleukin; MHC, major histocompatibility complex; NK, natural killer; TNF, tumor necrosis factor.
^{a}Also known as the new type III IFN-λ family.

will recognize pathogen via surface receptors (Fig. 95–2). In order to amplify the immune response, the antigen presenting cells will present antigen to CD4$^+$ T lymphocytes (Figs. 95–3 and 95–4). The activated CD4$^+$ T lymphocytes will then secrete cytokines to activate B lymphocytes, CD8$^+$ T lymphocytes, NK cells, macrophages, and neutrophils. The next section of the chapter discusses the evaluation of the immune system.

DISEASES OF THE IMMUNE SYSTEM

Although this chapter is not intended to detail the diseases of the immune system, it is necessary to review the terminology and provide specific examples of diseases of the immune system to understand the role of monitoring and possible intervention with pharmacotherapy. Diseases of the physical defense immune system are often not thought of as diseases of the immune system; however, the loss of normal physical defenses is the most common cause of impaired immunity resulting in infectious sequelae. For example, thick respiratory secretions secondary to altered chloride transport in cystic fibrosis leads to pathogen airway colonization. Primary immunodeficiency diseases are those characterized by either a genetic inability to produce components of the immune system (i.e., severe combined immunodeficiency or hypogammaglobulinemia) or acquired, as seen with HIV infection. Autoimmune diseases result from a dysregulation of a component or a combination of components of the immune system (e.g., rheumatoid arthritis, systemic lupus erythematosus).[41] Autoimmune diseases are often characterized by production of autoantibodies against a particular host structure that is critical

for normal function, or loss of tolerance or anergy to a ubiquitous antigen (i.e., gluten in celiac sprue).[41] Often medications that suppress the immune system are necessary to control symptoms and halt autoimmune disease progression. Exposure to immunosuppressant medications in the setting of autoimmune diseases or organ transplantation may reduce disease symptoms but at the cost of the host's ability to fight off infection or cancer. Exogenous regulation of the immune system must be done judiciously, and we must continue to discover new methods for the appropriate evaluation of immune responses.

EVALUATION OF THE IMMUNE SYSTEM'S FUNCTION

Assessment of a patient's immune function requires knowledge and understanding of multiple components including mechanical defenses, cell phenotypes and cell numbers, and soluble components. Recent developments in biotechnology have allowed for progress in further characterization of immune system components and their functions. This is important because the upregulation and downregulation of immune responses is necessary to treat various disease states. Therefore, pharmacotherapeutic considerations must balance the risk of disrupting normal immunologic homeostasis. Improvements in immune monitoring are necessary for the goal of patient-specific immunologic pharmacotherapy. Despite the technological advances, careful patient evaluations are required to accurately assess the structure and function of the immune system. Specific methods for assessment of patient immune status are discussed below.

TABLE 95-6	Examples of Alteration in Mechanical Immunodefenses That Result in Impaired Immune Status

Reduced gastric pH
  Achlorhydria
  Use of histamine-2 blockers and proton pump inhibitors
  Patients with acquired immunodeficiency syndrome
Break in skin barrier
Burns
  Surgical incision
  Penetrating trauma
  Vascular access devices
Impaired mucociliary function of the lungs
  Smoking
Impaired esophageal or epiglottal function
  Endotracheal intubation
  Stroke
  Recumbent position
Altered urine flow
  Urinary stones
  Anatomic deformities obstructing flow
  Bladder catheter
Anatomic alterations of the heart resulting in turbulent blood flow and endocarditis

TABLE 95-7	Leukocyte Counts in Adults		
Cell	**Absolute Count (Range)**[a]	**Percentage (Range)**[b]	
White blood cells	7,500 (4,500–11,000)	100	
Neutrophils	4,500 (2,300–7,700)	60 (50–70)	
Eosinophils	20 (0–45)	3 (0–5)	
Basophils	4 (0–20)	1 (0–2)	
Monocytes	30 (0–80)	4 (0–10)	
Lymphocytes	210 (160–240)	32 (28–39)	
T lymphocytes	140 (110–170)	72 (67–76)[b]	
CD4+	80 (70–110)	42 (38–46)[b]	
CD8+	70 (50–90)	35 (31–40)[b]	
B lymphocytes	30 (20–40)	13 (11–16)[b]	
Natural killer cells	30 (20–40)	14 (10–19)[b]	
CD4/CD8 ratio	1.2 (1.0–1.5)		

[a] Cell counts are expressed as cells/mm^3 or × 10^6/L.
[b] Percentage of lymphocyte subpopulations expressed as percentage of total lymphocyte population. For expression in SI units multiply each number by 0.01 to give the corresponding fraction.

INNATE IMMUNITY: EVALUATION OF MECHANICAL IMMUNODEFENSES

As discussed earlier, the mechanical aspects of host defense are extremely important in protection from infection; therefore, assessment of mechanical defenses is critical. Much of the assessment of mechanical immunodefense is accomplished by recognition of situations where such defense is compromised. Careful patient examination usually reveals the extent of compromise, and laboratory tests are generally not necessary for evaluation of this component. To assess the extent of compromise in mechanical immunodefenses, the clinician should carefully examine the patient and identify the specific types of risks present. Specific examples of altered mechanical defenses are listed in Table 95–6.

INNATE AND ADAPTIVE IMMUNITY: GROSS EVALUATION OF CELLULAR COMPONENTS

A major aspect of the assessment of immune function relates to the cells of the immune system. Assessment of cells in the clinical setting includes determination of cell type, cell number, and/or function. Generally, determination of the cell types and quantification of the cell numbers are performed first because of the ease of obtaining these results and the common correlation with the clinical situation.

To quickly screen cell numbers, a *white blood cell (WBC) count* with differential is performed. Normal cell counts are shown in Table 95–7.[42] This simple test often steers the differential diagnosis. In interpreting a WBC with differential, the clinician must consider several factors. A normal cell count does not mean that a leukocyte disorder does not exist. For example, in chronic granulomatous disease, a child has a normal neutrophil count, but the neutrophils are unable to destroy the bacteria. Second, a differential is reported as percentage of the WBC; therefore, one must also assess the absolute number as well as the percentage of white cell subtypes. For example, a patient admitted to the hospital with pneumonia has an elevated WBC (15,000 cells/mm^3 [15 × 10^9/L]) with a manual differential of 70% segs, 10% bands, 15% lymphocytes, and 5% monocytes. The WBC is predominately neutrophils; segs or mature neutrophils (70%) and bands or immature neutrophils (10%). The percentage of lymphocytes appears low at 15% (Table 95–7), but the absolute number of lymphocytes is actually normal, 2250 cells/mm^3 (15,000 cells/mm^3 × 0.15). A third factor to consider is that the majority of lymphocytes are in secondary lymphoid organs (e.g., lymph nodes, spleen), and changes in peripheral blood lymphocytes do not always mirror changes in the secondary lymphoid organs. Additionally, the majority of granulocytes, macrophages, and mast cells are also in the tissues, not the bloodstream.

Generally, the numbers of granulocytes (neutrophils, basophils, eosinophils) and monocytes are assessed by a WBC with differential. Increased WBC counts with immature neutrophils (bands, metamyelocytes, myelocytes, and promyelocytes) in the peripheral blood is called a "shift to the left," and is abnormal. It most often indicates a bacterial infection, but also can indicate trauma or leukemia. It has long been recognized that the lower the absolute neutrophil count, the greater the risk of infection. Drugs (e.g., chemotherapy) and diseases (e.g., collagen vascular disorders) may lower the neutrophil count and make the patient more susceptible to infections. Patients with a neutrophil count below 1,500 cells/mm^3 (1.5 × 10^9/L) are considered to have neutropenia. Functional analysis of these cell types is rarely done in routine clinical practice. Patients with suspected functional deficits in these cell types are generally referred to tertiary medical centers for evaluation and treatment.

A routine WBC with differential can determine the total lymphocyte count. Total lymphocyte count has been used as a measure of nutritional status, as this rapidly changes with nutrient loss or repletion. This is a relatively gross measure of a patient's immune status although it has been correlated to patient outcome and risk of infection.

Lymphocyte populations with different functions or in various stages of activation can be enumerated based on their cell surface markers. These cell surface markers are known as clusters of differentiation (CD). The CD is usually a protein or glycoprotein on the surface of the cell. CD followed by a number designates the marker. Hundreds of monoclonal antibodies have been designed to recognize these cell surface markers. Monoclonal antibodies can be labeled with a fluorescent marker. The labeled monoclonal antibodies are then incubated with the patient's cells. The antibodies will recognize and bind to the cells expressing the CD of interest, and the cells are then counted using flow cytometry. For flow cytometry, the cell suspension is put under pressure such that the cells flow past a laser in a stream of single cells. The laser will excite the fluorescently labeled antibodies bound to the lymphocytes. A light detector is able to count the labeled cell as the fluorescent tag emits light and determines the size of the cell based on its light

TABLE 95-8	Cluster of Differentiation (CD) Guide: Characterization of Human Leukocyte Antigens

CD	Predominant Cellular Distribution
CD3	All T lymphocytes
CD4	Helper T lymphocytes, either TH_1 or TH_2
CD5	T lymphocytes, B-lymphocyte subset
CD8	Cytotoxic/suppressor T lymphocytes
CD14	Monocytes, neutrophils
CD20	B lymphocytes
CD25	Activated T lymphocytes, B lymphocytes, interleukin-2 receptor α-chain (Tac)
CD33	Committed myeloid progenitor cells
CD34	Hematopoietic progenitor cells that include the stem cell
CD56	Natural killer cells
CD83	Dendritic cells

scatter. These evaluations are valuable for assessment of patients with immune deficiency states such as AIDS or leukemias, and for patients who have received organ transplants. For example, clinically quantification of CD3+ and CD4+ cells are used, for example, to monitor muromonab, a monoclonal antibody directed against the CD3 receptor. Also the number of CD4+ cells in HIV-positive patients correlates with the risk of and opportunistic infection and delineates the time to initiate antiviral therapy. Some of the more common CD antigens and their respective cellular distribution are listed in Table 95–8.[43] Flow cytometry can be used for leukocyte phenotyping, tumor cell phenotyping, as well as for some types of DNA analysis.

INNATE AND ADAPTIVE IMMUNITY: FUNCTIONAL EVALUATION

Counting the number of cells may help you estimate the function of the immune system, but several disease states exist in which there is an adequate number of cells but they are nonfunctional or they do not produce cytokines to communicate effectively. No single test exists to predict the function of the immune system with 100% accuracy. However, available tests can measure the viability of certain cell lines and communication between cells. Historically, the most common in vivo assay of lymphocyte function is the delayed hypersensitivity skin test. This test specifically evaluates the presence of delayed-type hypersensitivity or the presence of memory T lymphocytes. Specifically, a small amount of antigen, of which the patient is known to have been previously exposed, is administered. Under normal immunologic host conditions, exposure to this amount of antigen in the skin should produce lymphocytic infiltrate into the area within a few hours; followed by additional lymphocyte recruitment and phagocytes (e.g., macrophages, neutrophils) translocation. The maximal intensity of the inflammatory reaction occurs by 24 to 72 hours. This reaction is often referred to as type IV hypersensitivity (i.e., cell mediated; Chapter 97). A delayed-type hypersensitivity reaction is a test of cell-mediated immunity used to assess immunocompetency. The most common method to assess delayed-type hypersensitivity is to administer intradermally a panel of recall antigens. Commonly used antigens include *Candida albicans*, mumps, trichophyton, tetanus toxoid, and purified protein derivative of tuberculin (PPD).[44] Measurements in millimeters of induration at the site of injection should be taken 48 to 72 hours after placement of the antigens. A reaction is considered positive if the diameter of induration is 2 mm or greater. The degree of sensitivity correlates to the area of induration.[43] Reaction to even a single antigen indicates a functioning cell-mediated immunity. The majority of immunocompetent individuals will show a positive reaction to at least one of these antigens. Possible reasons for not mounting a response to these antigens include congenital T-lymphocyte deficiency, cancer, HIV, or immunosuppressive drug therapy.[44] No response is sometimes mounted because the individual being tested has not been previously exposed to a particular test antigen, although this is rare.

Global assessment of the in vivo immunologic response is also used commonly in solid organ transplantation during the diagnosis and assessment of acute rejection. For example, cellular rejection is detected on gross tissue biopsy by counting the number of lymphocytes present in the tissue and correlating their presence with other clinical findings, such as increasing serum creatinine in kidney transplant.

In vivo assessment of B-lymphocyte function involves immunizing the patient with a protein (e.g., tetanus toxoid) and a polysaccharide (e.g., pneumococcal polysaccharide vaccine) antigen to elicit and measure antibody responses after immunization. Two to 3 weeks after immunization, the patient's serum is tested for antibodies specific for the immunized antigen. This test measures B-lymphocyte responsiveness to the inoculated antigens but is reserved for patients who are suspected to have impaired B-lymphocyte function.[42]

A number of specific in vitro lymphocyte functional assays are used in the research setting. A few assays are performed at specialized clinical laboratories. One of these tests is the lymphocyte proliferation assay. In this assay, lymphocytes are obtained from a patient's peripheral blood and cultured in vitro. The cells are exposed to nonspecific mitogens such as pokeweed mitogen, phytohemagglutin, or concanavalin A. Then the cells are incubated in growth media containing tritium-labeled (^{3}H) thymidine, a nucleotide used in the synthesis of DNA. Normally in the presence of the mitogens, lymphocytes will be stimulated to proliferate. Proliferating lymphocytes will incorporate ^{3}H thymidine as they replicate DNA. The level of radioactivity of the cells can be measured on a β-scintillation counter and is proportional to the degree of proliferation. The patient sample needs to be compared to normal, healthy controls' lymphocytes. Patients with immune deficiencies (AIDS, cancer, etc.) have fewer active or less active lymphocytes, as detected by this test.

A modification of the lymphocyte proliferation assay can be used in allogeneic bone marrow transplantation to evaluate how closely a donor and host are "matched" in order to predict a patient's risk for developing graft-versus-host disease. A mixed lymphocyte culture (MLC) can be used to assess the potential of the donor cells to attack the host cells, graft-versus-host disease (Chap. 148). In this test, donor cells and host cells are incubated in vitro. The host lymphocytes are irradiated prior to the incubation so that they cannot proliferate. In vitro, ^{3}H thymidine is provided to the cells and uptake is measured. The degree of uptake correlates to level of proliferation of donor lymphocytes. If the cells are well matched, proliferation is minimal. If the cells are mismatched, proliferation will be noted with the level of proliferation predictive of the potential extent of graft-versus-host disease. With the introduction of DNA-based molecular typing of HLA antigens, the MLC is rarely used today. However, the MLC may play a role in selecting not completely histocompatible donors.[44]

The Cylex Immune Cell Function Assay was recently FDA approved as a novel test used to determine the magnitude of suppression of CD4+ cells.[45] Briefly, activity of CD4+ cells is measured by quantification of the amount of ATP produced and characterized as high, medium, or low.[46] Initial, retrospective experience has been reported in the solid organ transplant population. Although this assay is in its clinical infancy, it is one of the first functional assays aimed at assessing individual patient response to immunosuppressive therapy. This type of testing may allow for tailoring of immunosuppression.

More recently, evaluation of immune cell activity, such as factor forkhead box P3 (FOXP3) T-regulatory cell activity has been used to evaluate the incidence and severity of acute rejection based on elevated FOXP3 mRNA expression in urine and tissue cell samples. T-regulatory cells control autoimmune reactions; therefore, the presence of these cells in an allograft may indicate a level of "tolerance" to the donor tissue. Tolerance, basically, is a state in which the body knows that foreign tissue (e.g., kidney transplant) exists but does not attack it. Initial studies have evaluated biopsy samples from organ transplant recipient and correlated them with levels of FOXP3. Early evidence suggests that FOXP3 is present only during periods of inflammation, such as rejection, and potentially projects the allograft tissue.[47] In addition to the tests described above, a number of other tests and assays have been devised to evaluate the function of CD8+ T lymphocytes, NK cells, and monocytes/macrophages. Although these evaluations are not commonly performed, they may be helpful in some specific diseases and will likely be the way in which we monitor and detect immunologic events in the future. A thorough discussion of these tests is available.[48]

EVALUATION OF CYTOKINES AND CHEMOKINES

Often disease states involving the loss or upregulation of cytokines and chemokines are overlooked as diseases of the immune system. However, as we have just reviewed, cytokines and chemokines are essential components of both the innate and adaptive immune systems and provide the communication linking them together. Assays of humoral components may be either quantitative to determine the absolute concentration of the factor or qualitative to determine the function of the component.

IMMUNOGLOBULINS

Measurement of immunoglobulins is a direct measure of B-cell function. The most common evaluation of immunoglobulins is the estimation of total immunoglobulin. This is approximated by subtracting the albumin concentration from the total protein concentration in serum. This difference gives a gross estimation of the total immunoglobulin concentration. Actual determination of the total immunoglobulin concentration is done by serum protein electrophoresis (SPEP). Five separate zones are detected by this method: albumin, α_1-globulin, α_2-globulin, β-globulin, and γ-globulin.

❺ The γ-globulin fraction contains the five isotypes of immunoglobulin (i.e., IgG, IgA, IgM, IgE, and IgD). A normal total immunoglobulin or γ-globulin concentration ranges from 0.8 to 1.6 g/dL. This test is used to determine if patients have hypogammaglobulinemia (i.e., primary and secondary immunodeficiencies), a monoclonal peak (e.g., multiple myeloma, Waldenstrom macroglobulinemia), or

TABLE 95-9	Potential Indications for Measurement of Antigen-Specific Antibody
Environmental or drug allergy	
Exposure to or infection with bacteria	
Streptococci (ASO titer)	
Staphylococcus aureus (teichoic acid antibody)	
Neisseria gonorrhoeae	
Legionella pneumophila	
Exposure to or infection with viruses	
Human immunodeficiency virus	
Cytomegalovirus	
Epstein-Barr virus	
Hepatitis A, B, or C	
Rubella	
Exposure to or infection with other pathogens	
Syphilis	
Lyme disease	
Typhoid	
Chlamydia	
Immune disorders	
Rheumatoid factor antibody, rheumatoid arthritis	
Antinuclear antibodies, systemic lupus erythematosus	
Platelet-associated immunoglobulin G, idiopathic thrombocytopenic purpura	
Blood typing and crossmatching	
Transplantation	
Human leukocyte antigen (HLA) antibodies	

a polyclonal hypergammaglobulinemia (e.g., chronic inflammatory conditions such as systemic lupus erythematosus or chronic active hepatitis). Total immunoglobulin or γ-globulin concentrations cannot be used to measure antigen specific antibodies or specific isotypes, although other evaluations can.

In a patient suspected of having humoral immune deficiency or B-lymphocyte failure (i.e., primary and secondary hypogammaglobulinemia), specific immunoglobulin isotypes in the plasma should be measured.

There are many indications for the measurement of antigen-specific antibody. Some common indications are listed in Table 95–9. Methods to perform these measurements include enzyme-linked immunosorbent assay (ELISA), radioimmunoassay (RIA), and radioallergosorbent test (RAST) (Fig. 95–7). The most common reason to measure antigen-specific antibody is to determine whether or not a patient has been exposed to an infectious agent. Generally, IgM antibodies directed against the pathogen indicate an active or recent infection while IgG antibodies directed against the pathogen indicate prior exposure. This observation correlates with our understanding of B-lymphocyte responses in which plasma cells produce IgM initially in response to an infection, but later switches to IgG. Therefore, IgM antibodies will be

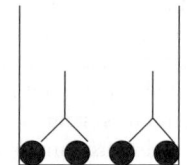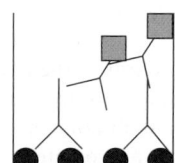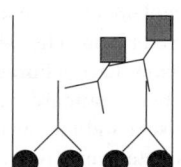

FIGURE 95-7. Enzyme-linked immunosorbent assay (ELISA). ELISA is a commonly used method for measuring concentrations of a wide variety of substances. To measure the concentration of antibodies to a particular antigen, the antigen is coated onto a solid phase, such as a microtiter plate or beads. If the purpose of the assay is to measure the concentration of antigen in solution, an antibody to the antigen is coated on the solid phase. The biologic fluid, often sera, is added to the wells. An enzyme-labeled anti-human antibody is added next. Finally, the chromogenic substrate for the enzyme is added. The intensity of the color as measured spectrophotometrically is proportional to the concentration of the antibody in the biologic fluid.

present during an active infection and shortly after recovery from the infection. IgG concentrations will increase at the end of the primary exposure, but predominate after a second exposure. IgG predominates after a second exposure because memory B lymphocytes predominately secrete IgG in the serum. Other uses of antigen-specific antibody include determining if a patient has had exposure and is likely to be protected from infection (e.g., hepatitis A virus) or to determine adequate response to vaccination (e.g., hepatitis B vaccine). Clinically, measurement of antihuman IgG antibodies is used pre- and post-solid organ transplant to detect and potentially predict allograft compatibility and treat antibody-mediated rejection.

Antigen-specific IgE is commonly measured in patients with allergies. Because the presence of antigen-specific IgE is related to clinical allergy, measurement of these antibodies can be helpful in diagnosing allergies and determining offending substances. A standard method for determination of allergen-specific IgE is the RAST. The basic technique involves adding the antigen of interest, which is bound to beads or disks, to the patient's serum. After precipitation and several washings, the antibody bound to the bead or disk is isolated. Finally, a radiolabeled antibody that binds to IgE is added. After further washings, the radiolabeled antibody bound to IgE, which is bound to the antigen on the bead or disk, is counted on a gamma counter.

Antigen skin testing is the preferred method to determine the presence of allergen-specific IgE. When it is produced, IgE binds to high-affinity IgE Fc receptors on basophils or mast cells. Contact of an allergen with the specific IgE on the basophil or mast cell surface causes activation of these cells and the release of inflammatory mediators (e.g., histamine). When this occurs systemically, it can cause anaphylaxis. When it occurs in a confined area such as the skin, erythema and induration are observed within a few minutes of allergen injection. This is the principle used for detection of penicillin allergy as well as for environmental or food allergies. A positive skin reaction ($\geq$5 mm of induration) within 15 to 20 minutes is indicative of the presence of allergen-specific IgE.

There are four subclasses of IgG: IgG1, IgG2, IgG3, and IgG4 that make up 65%, 20%, 10%, and 5% of total plasma IgG, respectively. Concentrations of the subclasses are often measured in patients with suspected primary and secondary hypogammaglobulinemia. IgG2 and IgG4 deficiencies are associated with chronic infections. IgG4 deficiencies are also associated with autoimmune disorders.

COMPLEMENT SYSTEM

The complement system consists of a group of over 30 different proteins involved in lysing and opsonizing invading pathogens as well as serving as chemotactic factors. Numbers following the letter C (e.g., C1, C2) name the various proteins of the complement system. A test for the global assessment of the complement system is the CH_{50}, the total hemolytic complement test. This test is based on the premise that complement is needed for a rabbit anti-sheep antibody to lyse sheep red blood cells. The source of the complement is the patient's serum. Each laboratory standardizes the test so normal ranges vary, but a standard curve is developed by adding titrated amounts of sera and measuring the amount of hemolysis. The hemolysis is determined with a spectrophotometer to measure the amount of hemoglobin released. The patient's serum is then tested, and the amount of serum that is needed to lyse 50% of the red blood cells is reported as the CH_{50}. This test does not provide an indication of the function of any specific complement component but is used as a screening test for any complement system defects. If a defect is found, individual complement proteins can then be evaluated by functional or immunochemical methods. Assessment of the complement system is important in

patients suspected of having humoral immune deficiencies (i.e., recurrent infections).[43]

Several disease states can alter complement concentrations. Low complement concentrations are frequently found during states of acute inflammation (e.g., systemic lupus erythematosus [SLE], rheumatoid arthritis, collagen vascular disorders, poststreptococcal glomerulonephritis, and subacute bacterial endocarditis). These states of apparent low complement concentrations are generally due to high rates of complement utilization or consumption that cannot be compensated for by increased complement synthesis.[20]

Since the liver is the primary source of several components of the complement system (i.e., C2, C3, C4, factors B and D), a global decrease in complement factors occurs in severe liver failure. Inherited complement deficiencies have been described in patients with SLE, autoimmune diseases, recurrent gonococcal and meningococcal infections, membranoproliferative glomerulonephritis, and hereditary angioedema.[20]

Clinically, the complement system has been used to diagnose and treat solid organ rejection. Antibody mediated or humoral rejection is evaluated by quantifying the amount of donor MHC specific antibody present in the recipient's serum. The presence of donor-specific antibodies is correlated with evidence of antibody mediated rejection on tissue samples. This is characterized by the presence of complement split products, namely C4d, which is present after complement-dependent antibody-mediated rejection. C4d covalently binds to the allograft tissue and can be stained for on biopsy samples. Unfortunately unless biopsy findings can be correlated with a clinical finding consistent with rejection, the presence of C4d and its prognosis on long-term allograft function are unknown.

CYTOKINES

Cytokines are an important means of communication among cells of the immune system and other organ systems. Multiple cytokines with overlapping and redundant functions have been identified. Methods to detect and measure cytokines in biological samples have been developed. For nearly all the currently identified cytokines, commercial kits are available to measure endogenous and exogenously administered cytokines. The most common and preferable methods to measure cytokines are ELISAs and RIAs. ELISAs and RIAs are easy to run and measure immunoactivity but not biologic activity (Fig. 95–7). Bioassays measure biologic activity, but are cumbersome and extremely variable. Using ELISA, we are able to measure only how much cytokine was produced by the cells in the culture. An ELISPOT is an enzyme-linked assay for detecting and enumerating cytokine-producing leukocytes.[49] In contrast to conventional ELISA, ELISPOT allows the user to detect absolute numbers and frequencies of cytokine secreting leukocytes.

We are still at the very early stages of interpreting the clinical relevance of endogenous cytokine concentrations. Not only is the immune system affected by cytokines such as IL-1, IL-6, TNF-α, but other systems (skeletal, endocrine, central nervous system) are also affected. Therefore, measurement of cytokine concentrations may be important in the evaluation of other systems as well as the immune system.

Administering cytokines in clinical practice may change not only the concentration of that particular cytokine, but also the resultant concentration of other cytokines. For example, systemic administration of GM-CSF to patients not only increases concentrations of GM-CSF but also of TNF-α, IL-6, IL-8, macrophage colony-stimulating factor and erythropoietin.[50,51] Secondary endogenous cytokine release should be taken into account when considering the therapeutic effects of these agents and when monitoring cytokine concentrations.

In the future, tissue concentrations as well as blood concentrations may be measured. For example, while many centers currently measure cyclosporine concentrations to estimate the potential for immunosuppressive effects, it may be advantageous to monitor IL-2 concentrations. One of the primary actions of cyclosporine is the inhibition of IL-2 production. Furthermore, perhaps it would be beneficial to measure tissue concentrations of IL-2 in the transplanted organ to get a better estimate of the extent of immunologic suppression.

SOLUBLE RECEPTORS AND RECEPTOR ANTAGONISTS

The inflammatory response is highly regulated. The activity of cytokines, their receptors, and their antagonists are in a delicate balance. Although cytokine receptors are typically thought of as being found on the target cell, soluble cytokine receptors can modulate the activity of cytokines in at least two ways: (1) acting as antiinflammatory agents by binding cytokines with high affinity, but without biological activity[52]; (2) augmenting cytokine activity by prolonging the cytokines plasma half- life and even maintaining agonist activity on cells that do not inherently respond to the cytokine.[53] Finally, antagonists to cytokine receptors have been identified.

Tumor necrosis factor-α (TNF-α) plays a central role in the inflammatory response by both increasing the expression of adhesion molecules in the tissues and by stimulating production of pro-inflammatory cytokines (e.g., IL-2, IL-8), prostaglandins, and nitric oxide. Soluble tumor necrosis factor receptors (sTNFRs) act primarily as inhibitors of TNF by preventing TNF from binding to the membrane-bound TNFRs, or by causing the cells to shed the receptor from the surface of the cell so that it can no longer serve as a signaling molecule.[54] Both monoclonal antibodies against TNF (e.g., infliximab) and sTNFRs (e.g., etanercept) have been shown to modulate the activity of TNF and are used clinically for the treatment of autoimmune diseases.

The best characterized receptor-binding antagonist is the interleukin-1 receptor antagonist (IL-1RA). IL-1RA blocks the binding of IL-1 to its receptor by competing for the same binding site, but IL-1RA does not possess agonist activity.[55] A recombinant IL-1RA, anakinra, is used clinically for the treatment of severe rheumatoid arthritis.[56]

Our developing understanding of soluble receptors and receptor antagonists allows us to better mimic natural mechanisms for minimizing the toxicity of exogenously administered cytokines (e.g., IL-1, IL-2, TNF-α, etc.) as well as immunomodulate various diseases (e.g., solid organ transplant rejection, collagen vascular disorders, sepsis, etc.)

MODULATION OF THE IMMUNE RESPONSE

6 Modulation of the immune response through administration of pharmacological agents or with blood product components does not come without a risk gained with the benefit. Providing supplementation to the immune system, for example during periods of sepsis with recombinant activated protein C (drotrecogin alfa) provides increased levels of protein C which decrease levels of pro-inflammatory IL-6 potentially limiting the effects of the immune reaction and preventing end organ damage at the cost of bleeding for over exposure to protein C. While TNF inhibitors interfering with the immune system to halt the damage of an autoimmune disorder may suppress symptoms, it places the patient at risk for opportunistic viral infections. Many of our newer biological agents directed at a pathway in the immune system are genetically engineered from animals and humanized to increase their biological effectiveness. As a result, these agents can serve as antigens to the

immune system and display variable effectiveness between and among patients over time. For example, an agent commonly used in solid organ transplantation is rabbit anti-thymocyte globulin, which is a polyclonal antibody directed against lymphocytes which given at the time of transplant or to treat rejection. Patients with previous exposure to this agent may have developed antibodies against the rabbit epitope of the drug. This results in either a decrease in the effectiveness of the drug, because it is bound by antibody or production of an immunologic reaction, commonly manifested by antibody-antigen complex deposition in the kidneys and joints producing high fevers and renal failure. Based on the very few examples presented here, one can understand why manipulation of the immune system must be carefully assessed and appropriate patient instruction given.

IMMUNOSUPPRESSION

Immunosuppression was first developed and used to allow transplantation of foreign tissues or to treat malignancies of the immune system. Today, the number of compounds and disease states in which the immune system is implicated is virtually unquantifiable. Therefore a thorough review of these drugs is beyond the scope of this chapter. These medications are usually very expensive and associated with potentially serious adverse effects. Immunosuppressants block critical steps of the immune response, and patients must be counseled on their risk of infection and the plan to monitor effectiveness of the immunosuppressant. Several key concepts and questions can be used to help clinicians discern the potential benefits and ramifications of administering any immunosuppressant. These include: (1) what is its mechanism of action, (2) what arm of the immune system does it effect, (3) when is its onset of action, (4) how was this compound derived and does it have the potential to stimulate antibody production if the patient is re-exposed, (5) is this compound's effect dose or duration related, (6) what type of infection is my patient at risk for and do I need to administer prophylactic medications, and (7) how do I monitor the biological effect of this compound?

IMMUNOPOTENTIATION

In an attempt to restore normal immune system function or to activate the immune system, immunopotentiators are often used. The best example of immunopotentiation of the immune system is the practice of immunizations. Active immunization with a vaccine or toxoid induces the host's immune system to confer protection against a pathogen (e.g., hepatitis A, hepatitis B, diphtheria toxoid, etc.). This process requires the uptake of the immunogenic epitope by antigen presenting cells followed by presentation to CD4$^+$ T lymphocytes and the subsequent development of either a cellular or humoral immune response.

In contrast to active immunization, passive immunity entails the administration of human immunoglobulin to provide short-term protection to individuals who will be or have been exposed to a pathogen. Intravenous immunoglobulin (IVIG) consists of >90% polyclonal IgG that is prepared from donated plasma. In patients with primary or secondary hypogammaglobulinemia, IVIG restores circulating IgG concentrations thus decreasing the incidence of infections in these patients. In addition to restoring IgG concentrations, IVIG can potentially immunomodulate the immune response. For example, in immune thrombocytopenic purpura, an autoantibody directed against the platelets leads to the destruction of the platelets by antibody-dependent cellular cytotoxicity. IVIG saturates the Fc receptors on phagocytic cells, thereby preventing the engulfment of autoantibody-opsonized platelets. IVIG can also contain anti-idiotype antibodies to immunomodulate an immune response. Anti-idiotype antibodies are directed against the idiotype or hypervariable region of a native antibody. After administration of IVIG, the anti-idiotypes bind to the hypervariable region of the autoantibody and prevent the autoantibody from opsonizing circulating platelets. In addition, the anti-idiotypes directed against the autoantibody can bind to the surface immunoglobulin on the B lymphocyte producing the autoantibody that leads to the destruction of the B lymphocyte.[57]

SUMMARY

Our understanding of the immune system has dramatically increased over the last decade. An immune response encompasses dynamic events involving both immunologic cells (e.g., phagocytes, lymphocytes) and soluble mediators (e.g., complement, cytokines, antibodies). A better understanding of the normal immune response allows us to investigate the pathophysiology of diseases in which the immune response is inappropriate. All clinicians need a basic understanding of the immune system and a familiarity with parameters to monitor immune system function in order to refine the development of immunologic treatments for diseases ranging from diabetes mellitus to collagen vascular disorders to cancer.

REFERENCES

1. Abbas AK, Lichtman AH. Maturation and selection of T-lymphocytes. In: Abbas AK, Lichtman AH. Basic Immunology. Philadelphia, PA: Saunders/Elsevier, 2009.
2. Abbas A, Lichtman A. Tissues of the immune system. In: Abbas AK, Lichtman AH. Basic Immunology. Philadelphia, PA: Saunders/Elsevier, 2009.
3. Blackburn ST. Hematologic and hemostatic systems. In: Blackburn ST. Maternal, Fetal, and Neonatal Physiology. St. Louis, MO: Saunders, 2007.
4. Marthur S, Schnexneider K, Hutchinson RE. Hematopoiesis. In: McPherson RA, Pincus MR. Clinical Diagnosis and Management by Laboratory Methods. Philadelphia, PA: Saunders, 2007.
5. McCance KL. Structure and function of the hematologic system. In: McCance KL, Huether SE. Pathophysiology, 5th ed. St Louis, MO: Elsevier Mosby, 2006.
6. Metcalf D. Hematopoietic cytokines. Blood 2008;111:485–491.
7. Barbour SY, Crawford J. Hematopoietic growth factors. In: Pazdur R, Wagman LD, Camphausen KA. Cancer Management: A Multidisciplinary Approach. London: CMPMedica Ltd, 2008.
8. Grethlein SJ. Mucosa-Associated Lymphoid Tissue; 2008. *http://emedicine.medscape.com/article/207891-overview*.
9. Delves PJ, Roitt IM. The immune system, first of two parts. N Engl J Med 2000;343:37–49.
10. Medzhitov R, Janeway C. Innate immunity. N Engl J Med 2000;343:338–344.
11. Chaplin DD. Overview of the human immune response. J Allergy Clin Immunol 2006;117:S430–S435.
12. Rennard SI, Romberger DJ. Host defenses and pathogenesis. Semin Respir Infect 2000;15:7–13.
13. Modlin RL. Mammalian toll-like receptors. Ann Allergy Asthma Immunol 2002;88:543–548.
14. Janeway CA, Medzhitov R. Innate immune recognition. Annu Rev Immunol 2002;20:197–216.
15. Witko-Sarsat V, Rieu P, Descamps-Latscha B, Lesavre P, Halbwachs Mecarelli L. Neutrophils: Molecules, functions, and pathophysiological aspects. Lab Invest 2000;80:617–653.
16. Rothenberg ME, Hogan SP. The eosinophil. Annu Rev Immunol 2006;24:147–174.
17. Aderem A, Underhill DM. Mechanisms of phagocytosis in macrophages. Annu Rev Immunol 1999;17:593–623.
18. Banchereau J, Steinman RM. Dendritic cells and the control of immunity. Nature 1998;392:245–252.
19. Delves PJ, Roitt IM. The immune system, second of two parts. N Engl J Med 2000;343:108–117.
20. Walport MJ. Complement, first of two parts. N Engl J Med 2001;344:1058–1066.
21. Luster AD. The role of chemokines in linking innate and adaptive immunity. Curr Opin Immunol 2002;14:129–135.
22. Izadpanah A, Gallo RL. Antimicrobial peptides. J Am Acad Dermatol 2005;52:381–390.
23. Klein J, Sato A. The HLA system, first of two parts. N Engl J Med 2000;343:702–709.
24. Klein J, Sato A. The HLA system, second of two parts. N Engl J Med 2000;343:782–786.
25. Hartgers FC, Figdor CG, Adema GJ. Towards a molecular understanding of dendritic cell immunobiology. Immunol Today 2000;21:542–545.
26. Reiser H, Stadecker MJ. Costimulatory B7 molecules in the pathogenesis of infectious and autoimmune diseases. N Engl J Med 1996;335:1396–1377.
27. Dutton RW, Bradley LM, Swain SL. T cell memory. Annu Rev Immunol 1998;16:201–223.
28. Farrar JD, Asnagli H, Murphy KM. T helper subset development: Role of instruction, selection and transcription. J Clin Invest 2002;109:431–435.
29. Constant SL, Bottomly K. Induction of TH1 and TH2 CD4+ T cell responses: The alternative approaches. Annu Rev Immunol 1997;15:297–322.
30. Bach JF. Regulatory T cells under scrutiny. Nat Rev Immunol 2003;3:189–198.
31. Lanzavecchia A. License to kill. Nature 19989:413–414.
32. Liu CC, Young LHY, Young JDE. Lymphocyte-mediated cytolysis and disease. N Engl J Med 1996;335:1651–1659.
33. Farag SS, Fehniger TA, Ruggeri L, Velardi A, Caligiuri MA. Natural killer cell receptors: new biology and insights into the graft-versus-leukemia effect. Blood 2002;100:1935–1947.
34. Preud'homme JL, Petit I, Barra A, Morel F, Lecron JC, Lelievre E. Structural and functional properties of membrane and secreted IgD. Mol Immunol 2000;15:871–887.
35. Steinke JW, Borigh L. Cytokines and chemokines. J Allergy Clin Immunol 2006;117:S441–S445.
36. Anonymous. Cytokines. In: Goldsby RA KT, Obsborne BA, Kuby J, eds. Immunology. New York: WH Freeman & Company, 2003:277–298.
37. Trinchieri G. Interleukin-12: A cytokine at the interface of inflammation and immunity. Adv Immunol 1998;70:83–243.
38. Wynn TA. IL-13 effector functions. Annu Rev Immunol 2003;21:425–456.
39. Kennedy MK, Park LS. Characterization of interleukin-15 (IL-15) and the IL-15 receptor complex. J Clin Immunol 1996;16:134–143.
40. Okamura H, Tsutsui J, Kashiwamura SI, Yoshimota T, Nakanishi K. Interleukin-18: A novel cytokine that augments both innate and acquired immunity. Adv Immunol 1998;70:281–312.
41. Lee SJ, Kavanaugh A. Autoimmunity, vasculitis, and autoantibodies. J Allergy Clin Immunol 2006;117:S445–S450.
42. Elliott MB. Interpretation of clinical laboratory test results. In: Boh LE, ed. Pharmacy Practice Manuel: A Guide to Clinical Experience. Baltimore, MD: Lippincott Williams & Wilkins, 2001:136–212.
43. Fleisher TA, Tomar RH. Introduction to diagnostic laboratory immunology. JAMA 1997;278:1823–1834.
44. Folds JD, Schmitz JL. Clinical and laboratory assessment of immunity. J Allergy Clin Immunol 2003;111:S702–S711.
45. United States Department of Health and Human Services. K013169; Cylex Immune Cell Function Assay, April 2002.
46. Zeevi A, Britz JA, Bentlejewski CA, et al. Monitoring immune function during tacrolimus tapering in small bowel transplant recipients. Transplant Immunol 2005;15:17–24.
47. Racusen LC. T-regulatory cells in human transplantation. Am J Transplant 2008;8:1359–1360.
48. Lowell C. Section II. Immunological laboratory tests. In: Parslow TG, Stites DP, Terr AI, Imboden JB, eds. Medical Immunology. New York: Lange Medical Books/McGraw-Hill Medical, 2001.

49. Helms T, Boehm BO, Asaad RJ, Trezza RP, Lehmann PV, TaryLehmann M. Direct visualization of cytokine-producing recall antigen-specific CD4 memory T cells in healthy individuals and HIV patients. J Immunol 2000;164:3723–3732.

50. Rabinowitz J, Petros W, Stuart A, Peters W. Characterization of endogenous cytokine concentrations after high-dose chemotherapy with autologous bone marrow support. Blood 1993;81: 2452–2459.

51. van Pelt L, Huisman M, Weening R, von dem Borne A, Roos D, van Oers R. A single dose of granulocyte-macrophage colony-stimulating factor induces systemic interleukin-8 release and neutrophil activation in healthy volunteers. Blood 1996;87:5305–5313.

52. Opal SM, DePalo VA. Anti-Inflammatory cytokines. Chest 2000;117:1162–1172.

53. Jones SA, Horiuchi S, Topley N, Yamamoto N, Fuller GM. The soluble interleukin 6 receptor: Mechanisms of production and implications in disease. FASEB J 2001;15:43–58.

54. Dinarello CA. Proinflammatory cytokines. Chest 2000;118:503–508.

55. Choy EH, Panayi GS. Cytokine pathways and joint inflammation in rheumatoid arthritis. N Engl J Med 2001;344:907–916.

56. Cohen S, Hurd E, Cush J, et al. Treatment of rheumatoid arthritis with anakinra, a recombinant human interleukin-1 receptor antagonist, in combination with methotrexate: Results of a twenty-four-week, multicenter, randomized, double-blind, placebo-controlled trial. Arthritis Rheum 2002;46:614–624.

57. Kazatchkine MD, Kaveri SV. Immunomodulation of autoimmune and inflammatory diseases with intravenous immune globulin. N Engl J Med 2001;345:747–755.

96

Systemic Lupus Erythematosus and Other Collagen-Vascular Diseases

JEFFREY C. DELAFUENTE AND KIMBERLY A. CAPPUZZO

KEY CONCEPTS

❶ Systemic lupus erythematosus (SLE) is a disease that predominantly occurs in women.

❷ The hallmark of SLE is the development of autoantibodies to cellular nuclear components, resulting in chronic inflammatory autoimmune disease. Symptoms and organ involvement depend on the nature of the autoantibodies.

❸ SLE has a wide spectrum of symptoms and organ system involvement, making therapy highly patient specific. In addition, the signs and symptoms will fluctuate over time.

❹ The wide spectrum of symptoms and organ system involvement makes pharmacotherapy difficult because therapy must be individualized based on each patient's disease activity.

❺ There is a paucity of quality evidence for the treatment of SLE except for lupus nephritis.

❻ Almost all classes of medications, including antiinflammatory and immunosuppressive agents, are reported to cause vasculitis in most major organ systems.

The collagen–vascular diseases are a heterogeneous group of diseases that can involve the musculoskeletal system, integument, and blood vessels. Each collagen–vascular disease has its own set of diagnostic criteria, although diagnosis can be difficult because of overlapping and nonspecific clinical presentations. The etiology of the various collagen–vascular diseases is often unknown, but the immune system usually is involved in the pathogenesis and manifestations of the disease. Therefore, pharmacotherapy usually includes antiinflammatory agents with or without immunosuppressive drugs.

Although the prevalence of other collagen–vascular diseases may be greater than that of systemic lupus erythematosus (SLE) (e.g., polymyalgia rheumatica), SLE is discussed most extensively in this chapter because it is a major collagen–vascular disease with numerous clinical manifestations, its pharmacotherapy can be complex, and a plethora of data is available on the therapy of SLE. As all the diseases discussed in this chapter have an immune-mediated pathogenesis, the therapeutic principles of SLE can be applied to other autoimmune collagen–vascular diseases. The collagen–vascular

diseases discussed include systemic sclerosis, polymyositis/dermatomyositis, polymyalgia rheumatica, and drug-induced vasculitis; these were chosen because they are seen in general practice.

SYSTEMIC LUPUS ERYTHEMATOSUS

SLE is a fluctuating multisystem disease with a diversity of clinical presentations. Abnormal immunologic function and formation of antibodies against "self-antigens" underlie the pathogenesis of SLE.

The term *lupus erythemateux* was first used in 1851 by Cazenave, a Frenchman who described an illness in a patient with manifestations occurring in the skin. It is not surprising that SLE was first recognized as a skin disorder because cutaneous manifestations constitute one of the most common clinical features of the disease. Further descriptions by Kaposi and Osler in the late 1800s led to the concept of a multisystem disease as it became recognized that patients developed complications in other organ systems.[1]

The hallmark of SLE is the development of autoantibodies to cellular nuclear components that leads to a chronic inflammatory autoimmune disease. Recognition of SLE as an autoimmune disease of multisystemic nature led the American College of Rheumatology to develop criteria for identifying lupus patients (Table 96–1). These criteria were developed in 1971, revised in 1982, and modified slightly in 1997. The criteria do not include all the clinical manifestations of the disease and are used primarily for distinguishing SLE from other collagen–vascular diseases.[2] If 4 or more of the 11 criteria are documented at any time in a patient's medical history, the diagnosis of SLE can be made with approximately 95% specificity and 85% sensitivity.[3] Although these criteria may be helpful, diagnosis requires additional serologic, immunopathologic, and clinical evaluations.

EPIDEMIOLOGY

❶ The incidence of SLE varies among ethnic groups with the annual incidence in adults ranging from 1.9 to 5.6 per 100,000 persons per year, with a prevalence of approximately 50 cases per 100,000 persons.[1,4,5] The disease occurs predominantly in women, with a reported female-to-male ratio approaching 10:1. Those afflicted with SLE are usually diagnosed between the ages of 15 and 45.[6,7] SLE is reported to be less prevalent in whites than in other ethnic groups, including blacks, Hispanics, Native Americans, and Asians.[6,7] Although the most typical SLE patient is a young adult woman, the disease can occur in people of any age or race and either gender.

ETIOLOGY

The etiology of abnormal autoantibody production and development of SLE is still unknown. Genetic, environmental, and hormonal factors all may play a role in loss of "self-tolerance"

TABLE 96-1 Revised Criteria for Classification of Systemic Lupus Erythematosus*

Criterion	Definition
Malar rash	Fixed erythema, flat or raised, over the malar eminences, tending to spare the nasolabial folds
Discoid rash	Erythematous raised patches with adherent keratotic scaling and follicular plugging; atrophic scarring may occur in older lesions
Photosensitivity	Skin rash as a result of unusual reaction to sunlight, by patient history or physician observations
Oral ulcers	Oral or nasopharyngeal ulceration, usually painless, observed by a physician
Arthritis	Nonerosive arthritis involving two or more peripheral joints, characterized by tenderness, swelling, or effusion
Serositis	Pleuritis–convincing history of pleuritic pain or rub heard by a physician or evidence of pleural effusion
	or
	Pericarditis–documented by electrocardiogram or rub or evidence of pericardial effusion
Renal disorder	Persistent proteinuria >0.5 g/day (500 mg/day) or >3+ if quantitation not performed
	or
	Cellular casts–may be red cell, hemoglobin, granular, tubular, or mixed
Neurologic disorder	Seizures–in the absence of offending drugs or known metabolic derangements, e.g., uremia, ketoacidosis, or electrolyte imbalance
	or
	Psychosis–in the absence of offending drugs or known metabolic derangements, e.g., uremia, ketoacidosis, or electrolyte imbalance
Hematologic disorder	Hemolytic anemia–with reticulocytosis
	or
	Leukopenia–fewer than 4,000 cells/mm³ (4×10^9/L) total on two or more occasions
	or
	Lymphopenia–fewer than 1,500 cells/mm³ (1.5×10^9/L) on two or more occasions
	or
	Thrombocytopenia–fewer than 100,000 /mm³ (100×10^9/L) in the absence of offending drugs
Immunologic disorder	Anti-DNA; antibody to native DNA in abnormal titer
	or
	Anti-Smith (Sm) antigen; presence of antibody to Sm nuclear antigen
	or
	Positive finding of antiphospholipid antibodies based on (1) an abnormal serum level of immunoglobulin (Ig)G or IgM anticardiolipin antibodies, (2) a positive test result for lupus anticoagulant using a standard method, or (3) a false-positive serologic test for syphilis known to be positive for at least 6 months and confirmed by *Treponema pallidum* immobilization or fluorescent treponemal antibody absorption test
Antinuclear	An abnormal titer of antinuclear antibody by immunofluorescence or an antibody equivalent assay at any point in time in the absence of drugs known to be associated with "drug-induced lupus" syndrome

*The proposed classification is based on 11 criteria. For the purpose of identifying patients in clinical studies, a person shall be said to have systemic lupus erythematosus if any 4 or more of the 11 criteria are present, serially or simultaneously, during any interval of observation.
From Tan EM, Cohen AS, Fries JF, et al. The 1982 revised criteria for the classification of systemic lupus erythematosus. Arthritis Rheum 1982;25:1274 and Hochberg MC. Updating the American College of Rheumatology Revised Criteria for the Classification of Systemic Lupus Erythematosus. Arthritis Rheum 1997;40;1725, with permission.

and expression of disease. A popular theory is that autoimmune disease such as SLE develops in genetically susceptible individuals after exposure to a triggering agent, possibly something in the environment.[7–9]

Genetic analysis shows that at least four susceptibility genes are required for the expression of lupus in humans.[9] Familial and twin studies indicate a genetic predisposition for the development of SLE. First-degree relatives of SLE patients are about 20 times more likely to develop SLE than the general population; more than 5% of cases are familial. The concordance rate among identical twins ranges from 24% to 58%, compared with 3% to 10% for nonidentical twins.[10] Multiple genes contribute to SLE susceptibility, and at least 100 genes have been linked to SLE in humans. Evidence indicates that major histocompatibility complex genes, particularly several human leukocyte antigen genes, may be important in lupus. However, nonmajor histocompatibility complex genes, such as immunoglobulin receptor genes and mannose-binding protein genes, also may contribute to disease susceptibility.[9,10] Environmental agents that may induce or activate SLE include sunlight (i.e., ultraviolet light), drugs, chemicals such as hydrazine (found in tobacco) and aromatic amines (found in hair dyes), diet, environmental estrogens, and infection with viruses or bacteria.[9] A number of viruses have been implicated as causative agents in genetically susceptible people with significant data identifying the Epstein Barr virus as a causative agent.[11,12] Additionally, androgen may inhibit and estrogen may enhance the expression of autoimmunity, and elevated circulating prolactin levels have been associated with lupus in males and females.[9,13]

PATHOPHYSIOLOGY

❷ SLE represents a clinical syndrome rather than a discrete disease with a unique pathogenesis. SLE has a large spectrum of symptoms and organ system involvement.[1] A major event in the development of SLE is excessive and abnormal autoantibody production and the formation of immune complexes. Patients may develop autoantibodies against multiple nuclear, cytoplasmic, and surface components of multiple types of cells in various organ systems in addition to soluble markers such as immunoglobulin G and coagulation factors; these autoantibodies account for the multiple-organ system involvement of the disease.[9]

Excessive autoantibody production results from hyperactive B lymphocytes. Multiple mechanisms likely lead to B-cell hyperactivity, including loss of immune self-tolerance and high antigenic load consisting of environmental and self-antigens presented to B cells by other B cells or specific antigen-presenting cells, a shift of T-helper type 1 cells to T-helper type 2 cells that further enhance B-cell antibody production, and defective B-cell suppression. Impairment in other immune regulatory processes involving T lymphocytes (suppressor T cells), cytokines (e.g., interleukins, interferon-γ, tumor necrosis factor-α, transforming growth factor-β), and natural killer cells also may be involved.[9,14]

Many autoantibodies are directed against nuclear constituents of the cell; collectively, they are called *antinuclear antibodies*. Several antinuclear antibodies are important because their presence or absence may aid in the diagnostic and clinical evaluation of patients with SLE. The SLE patient may have more than one antigen-specific antinuclear antibody in the patient's serum and tissues.[15] These are antibodies against such nuclear constituents as double-stranded, or native, DNA (dsDNA); single-stranded, or denatured, DNA (ssDNA); and RNA. Four RNA-associated antigens frequently occurring in SLE are the Smith (Sm) antigen, the small nuclear ribonucleoprotein (snRNP), the Ro (SS-A) antigen, and the La (SS-B) antigen.[12,16] Histone, a basic component of chromatin and nucleosomes, is another important nuclear component against which antinuclear antibodies are formed in lupus patients. Antibodies to dsDNA are highly specific for SLE and are present in 70% to 80% of patients.[12] Antibodies also may be directed against the phospholipid moiety of the prothrombin

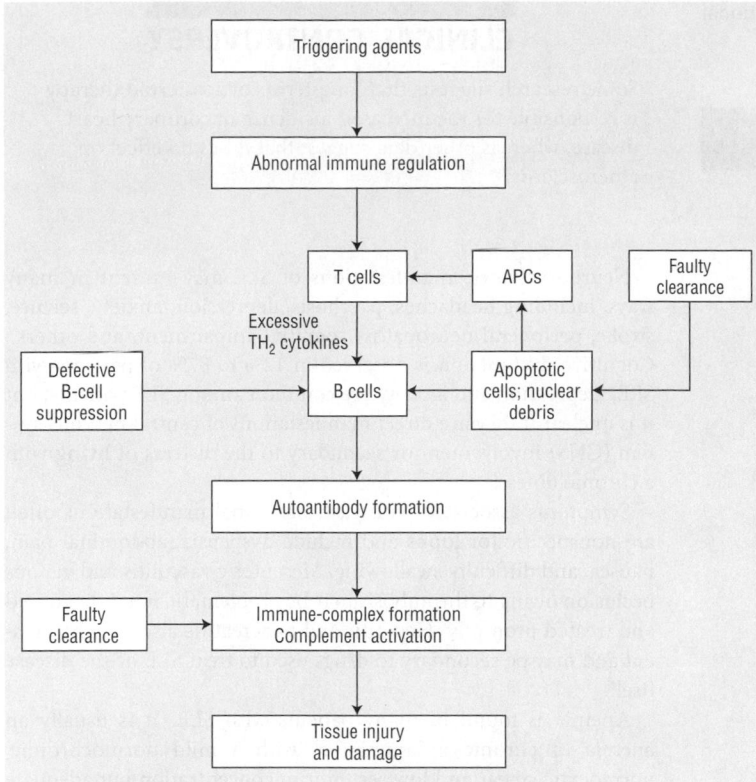

FIGURE 96-1. Pathogenesis of systemic lupus erythematosus (SLE). Environmental factors, such as infectious organisms, drugs, and chemicals, serve as triggering agents in genetically and hormonally susceptible individuals to induce a state of immune dysregulation. These abnormal immune responses lead to hyperactive T-helper type 2 lymphocyte and B-lymphocyte function. Suppressor T-lymphocyte function, cytokine production, faulty clearance mechanisms, and other immune regulatory mechanisms also are abnormal and fail to downregulate autoantibody formation from hyperactive B lymphocytes. The autoantibodies formed from this immune dysregulation become pathogenic, form immune complexes, and activate complement that leads to damage of host tissue. (APCs, antigen-presenting cells; TH_2, T-helper type 2.)

activator complex (lupus anticoagulant) and against cardiolipin. The lupus anticoagulant and anticardiolipin antibodies constitute the two main types in a group of autoantibodies called *antiphospholipid antibodies*.

These autoantibodies often are present many years before the diagnosis of SLE.[17] The appearance of these autoantibodies follows a predictable pattern, with accumulation of specific autoantibodies before the onset of clinical illness. For example, antinuclear, anti-La, anti-Ro, and antiphospholipid antibodies often precede the onset of SLE by many years, whereas anti-Sm and anti-snRNP antibodies appear only months before diagnosis, usually when clinical symptoms begin to manifest.

Immune dysregulation leading to B-cell hyperactivity and subsequent production of pathogenic autoantibodies, coupled with defective clearance of apoptotic cells, followed by immune-complex formation, complement activation, and defective clearance of immune complexes all lead to inflammatory reactions that ultimately result in tissue injury and damage. Figure 96–1 is an overview of the pathogenesis of SLE.[9]

CLINICAL PRESENTATION

❸ As mentioned previously, SLE is a multisystem disease. Below (see Clinical Presentation of Systemic Lupus Erythematosus) are many of the signs and symptoms and incidences for patients with SLE.[18] Although certain of these may be more common than others, each patient presents differently, and the course of the disease is highly unpredictable. Furthermore, SLE is not static, and most patients have fluctuations or flare-ups during the course of the disease.

Nonspecific signs and symptoms such as fatigue, fever, anorexia, and weight loss are seen frequently for patients with active disease. Musculoskeletal involvement (e.g., arthralgia, myalgia, and arthritis) is very common in SLE, with fever, malaise, or arthralgia frequently the chief complaint on initial presentation of the disease.[18] All major and minor joints may be affected, and the pattern of arthritis is often recurrent and of short duration, presenting mainly

as joint stiffness, pain, and sometimes inflammation. Objective evidence of musculoskeletal disease often is missing, although a few patients may present with deforming arthritis or subcutaneous nodules.

Manifestations in the skin are very common in lupus. The most well known of these is the butterfly rash, which occurs over the bridge of the nose and the malar eminences and is present in 50% of patients at some time during the disease.[18] The classic butterfly rash often is observed after sun exposure. In fact, photosensitivity is common to many SLE patients who present with cutaneous manifestations. Skin lesions characteristic of discoid lupus occur in up to 20% of patients with SLE and may occur without other clinical or serologic evidence of lupus.[18] Some individuals develop *subacute cutaneous lupus erythematosus* on exposure to sunlight.[18] Other cutaneous manifestations include vasculitis (which may be ulcerative), oral ulcers, Raynaud's phenomenon, and alopecia.[18]

Another common source of symptomatology in SLE is the pulmonary system, with manifestations such as pleurisy, coughing, and dyspnea. Pleurisy may present as pleuritic pain, a pleural rub, or a pleural effusion that usually is exudative in nature. Lupus pneumonitis may present acutely with fever, dyspnea, tachypnea, cough, rale, and patchy infiltrates or chronically with interstitial fibrosis. Pulmonary hypertension associated with SLE is more common than previously thought, which is likely a result of asymptomatic increases in pulmonary artery pressures being more common than symptomatic increases. Patients with SLE-associated pulmonary hypertension have a poor prognosis. Pulmonary embolism also should be ruled out for any SLE patient presenting with pleuritic chest pain and dyspnea.

Cardiac manifestations of SLE often present as pericarditis, myocarditis, electrocardiographic changes, or valvular heart disease, including the classic cardiac lesion of Libman-Sacks endocarditis (nonbacterial verrucous endocarditis).[19] Coronary artery disease (CAD) is being seen in SLE with increasing frequency as the life expectancy of SLE patients increases.[20] The development of heart disease in these patients is probably multifactorial, and traditional CAD risk factors are common for patients with SLE.

CLINICAL PRESENTATION OF SYSTEMIC LUPUS ERYTHEMATOSUS

Sign and/or Symptom	Incidence (%)
Musculoskeletal	
Arthritis and arthralgia	53 to 95
Constitutional	
Fatigue	81
Fever	41 to 86
Weight loss	31 to 71
Mucocutaneous	55 to 85
Butterfly rash	10 to 61
Photosensitivity	11 to 45
Raynaud's phenomenon	10 to 44
Discoid lesions	9 to 29
Central nervous system	13 to 59
Psychosis	5 to 37
Seizures	6 to 26
Pulmonary	
Pleuritis	31 to 57
Pleural effusion	12 to 40
Cardiovascular	
Pericarditis	2 to 45
Myocarditis	3 to 40
Heart murmur	1 to 44
Hypertension	23 to 46
Renal	13 to 65
Gastrointestinal	
Nausea	7 to 53
Abdominal pain	8 to 34
Bowel hemorrhage (vasculitis)	1 to 6
Hematologic	
Anemia	30 to 78
Leukopenia	35 to 66
Thrombocytopenia	7 to 30
Lymphadenopathy	10 to 59

Corticosteroid therapy and immunosuppressive therapy are also believed to be contributing factors in the development of these cardiac risk factors.[19] Although hypertension, obesity, and hyperlipidemia are common for SLE patients, these traditional risk factors do not account for the strikingly high cardiovascular event rate found in some recent studies.[21] Other SLE-related risk factors highlight the importance of autoimmunity and inflammation in the pathogenesis of accelerated atherosclerotic cardiovascular disease.[21,22] Additionally, two studies reported that long-term corticosteroid therapy was not associated with a significantly increased risk of accelerated atherosclerosis.[23,24] In fact, one of the studies[23] found that patients with higher mean daily doses of prednisone and more frequent use of other common therapies for SLE exhibited less plaque formation, which suggests that more aggressive control of disease activity actually may help to prevent CAD.[22,23]

CLINICAL CONTROVERSY

Some research suggests that long-term corticosteroid therapy is responsible for the increased incidence of coronary heart disease, whereas other data suggest that it has no effect on atherosclerosis.

Neuropsychiatric manifestations of SLE may present in many ways, including headaches, psychosis, depression, anxiety, seizure, stroke, peripheral neuropathy, cognitive impairment, and others.[4] Cognitive dysfunction is observed in 12% to 87% of patients with SLE. Depression and anxiety are common among SLE patients, but it is unclear if they are direct manifestations of central nervous system (CNS) involvement or secondary to the distress of living with a chronic illness.

Symptoms associated with gastrointestinal manifestations often are nonspecific for lupus and include dyspepsia, abdominal pain, nausea, and difficulty swallowing. Mesenteric vasculitis and venous occlusion owing to thrombosis may be problematic if not diagnosed and treated promptly. Hepatitis and pancreatitis also may be present and may be secondary to drugs used to treat SLE or the disease itself.

Anemia is found in many patients with SLE. It is usually an anemia of chronic inflammation, with a mild normochromic, normocytic smear and low serum iron concentration but adequate iron stores. Some patients may develop a hemolytic anemia with a positive Coombs test.[25] Leukopenia, usually mild, is a common finding for SLE patients. Both granulocytes and lymphocytes may be affected, but granulocytopenia is infrequent.[25] Thrombocytopenia may occur in SLE, often during disease exacerbation, but it is usually mild and does not increase bleeding tendency.[25] Another significant finding associated with SLE is the presence of antiphospholipid antibodies such as the lupus anticoagulant and anticardiolipin antibodies. Although the lupus anticoagulant is directed against the prothrombin activator complex, which implies potential bleeding complications, this is not the case. In fact, the presence of lupus anticoagulant, anticardiolipin, or other antiphospholipid antibodies may be associated with thrombosis, neurologic disease, thrombocytopenia, and fetal loss.[26]

Clinical evidence of renal involvement, such as a rising serum creatinine or proteinuria level, generally is associated with a poorer outcome compared with patients without renal involvement. Progression to end-stage renal disease is a major cause of morbidity and mortality in SLE. However, the extent and course of renal disease are quite variable, and many lupus nephritis patients do very well. The World Health Organization has classified lupus nephritis on the basis of histologic characteristics observed following renal biopsy. A revision of this system by the International Society of Nephrology and Renal Pathology Society recommends modifying the lupus nephritis classifications as minimal mesangial (class I), mesangial proliferative (class II), focal (class III), diffuse (class IV), membranous (class V), and advanced sclerosing (class VI).[27] Many patients progress from one form of nephritis to another during the course of the disease. Predictors of poorer outcome in lupus nephritis include African-American race, anemia, azotemia, poor initial response to immunosuppressive drugs, and flares of worsening renal function.[1]

DIAGNOSIS

As mentioned earlier, the diagnostic criteria listed in Table 96–1 should not be the primary means for diagnosing SLE, although many of the criteria may be valuable in the diagnostic process.

TABLE 96-2	Antinuclear Antibody Test: Patterns, Antigens, and Specificities	
Pattern	**Antigen**	**Disease**
Peripheral	dsDNA	SLE
Speckled	Acidic nuclear protein	Rheumatoid arthritis
	Ribonucleoprotein	SLE
	Extractable nuclear antigen	Scleroderma; mixed connective tissue disease
Homogeneous	dsDNA, ssDNA	Rheumatoid arthritis
	Histones	SLE; drug-induced lupus
Nucleolar	Nucleolar RNA	Progressive systemic sclerosis

ds, double-stranded; SLE, systemic lupus erythematosus; ss, single-stranded.

Epidemiologic characteristics, clinical signs and symptoms, and common laboratory abnormalities are all used in the diagnosis of SLE.

Once the disease is suspected, serologic tests may be helpful in making the diagnosis. A serologic test used extensively to aid in the diagnosis of SLE is the fluorescent antinuclear antibody (ANA) test. Nearly all SLE patients are ANA positive, but other diseases also can be associated with a positive test (Table 96–2). However, in other diseases, many of the positive ANA tests are of a lower titer. The pattern of immunofluorescence of the ANA test also may be of diagnostic value (Table 96–2), with a peripheral (also called *rim*) pattern being specific for SLE. Detecting antibodies to specific nuclear constituents also may be useful diagnostically. Antibodies to native DNA (dsDNA) and to Sm antigen are quite specific for and are considered diagnostic of SLE.[9,28,29]

PROGNOSIS

In earlier years, SLE was associated with a poor prognosis. For example, three decades ago 5-year survival was approximately 83% and 10-year survival was approximately 76%.[4] Today, as a result of improved treatment and improved diagnostic techniques that allow earlier diagnosis, the approximate 5-year survival rate is 96%, and the 15-year survival rate is 76%.[30] The natural course of SLE has changed dramatically not only because of improved therapies but also because of improvement in ability to manage patients with kidney disease (e.g., dialysis), infection, and CAD. However, complications of immunosuppressive treatment, CAD, and infection are still among the leading causes of death among SLE patients.[30]

TREATMENT

Systemic Lupus Erythematosus

❹ Desired treatment outcomes for the patient with SLE are twofold: (1) management of symptoms and induction of remission during times of disease flare and (2) maintenance of remission for as long as possible between disease flares. Figure 96–2 outlines an approach to the management of the patient with SLE. Because of the variability in clinical presentation of disease, treatment will vary accordingly and should be highly individualized. Optimal care of the patient with SLE will include education and support services in addition to the nonpharmacologic and pharmacologic

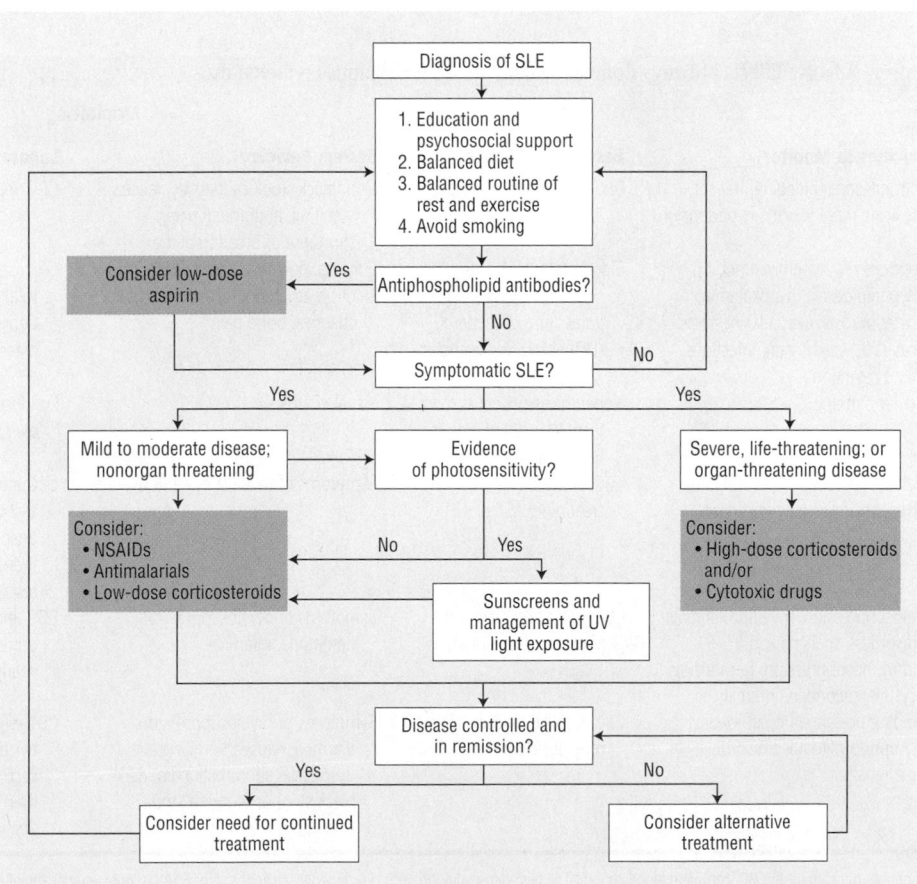

FIGURE 96-2. General approach to the management of SLE (NSAIDs, nonsteroidal antiinflammatory drugs; UV, ultraviolet).

treatments discussed below. Numerous lupus organizations exist throughout the world and can be located by contacting the Lupus Foundation of America (*http://www.lupus.org*), the Arthritis Foundation (*http://www.arthritis.org*), and Lupus Canada (*http://www.lupuscanada.org*).

■ NONPHARMACOLOGIC THERAPY

Several nonpharmacologic measures can be employed to manage symptoms and help maintain remission. Fatigue is a common symptom for patients with lupus. A balanced routine of rest and exercise, while avoiding overexertion, is essential in managing fatigue.[31] Avoidance of smoking may be particularly important because hydrazines in tobacco smoke may be an environmental trigger of lupus and likely contribute to accelerated CAD.[9] Smoking also has been associated with increased disease activity for SLE patients.[32] No specific dietary measures are known to clearly affect the clinical course of lupus. Many patients with SLE will need to limit exposure to sunlight and use sunscreens to block the possible exacerbating effects of ultraviolet light.[31] The amount of sunlight exposure limitation should be individualized.

■ PHARMACOLOGIC THERAPY

⑤ Drug therapy for SLE is often designed to suppress the immune response and inflammation. Except for lupus nephritis, large controlled clinical trials comparing treatment options for SLE are needed. Table 96–3 lists common agents and doses used to control SLE. In general, the choice of drug therapy depends on the extent and severity of disease. Table 96–4 describes select monitoring parameters and adverse events for many of the drugs used to treat collagen–vascular diseases.

TABLE 96-3 Drug Treatment of Systemic Lupus Erythematosus

Drug Class	Drug and Dose	Indication
NSAID	Various agents Antiinflammatory dose	Mild disease: fever, arthritis, skin rash, serositis
Antimalarial	Hydroxychloroquine 200–400 mg po daily Chloroquine 250–500 mg po daily	Mild disease: arthritis, skin rash, serositis
Corticosteroid	Prednisone 1–2 mg/kg/day po (or equivalent)	Initial control of severe disease
	<1 mg/kg/day (or equivalent)	Control of mild disease or maintenance after disease suppression with higher doses
	Methylprednisolone 500–1,000 mg IV daily for 3–6 days	Life-threatening disease
Cytotoxic	Cyclophosphamide 0.5–1 g/m² IV monthly for 6 months; then every 3 months for 2 years or for 1 year after remission Azathioprine 1–3 mg/kg po daily Cyclophosphamide 1–3 mg/kg po daily Mycophenolate mofetil 1–3 g po daily	Most commonly used in severe lupus nephritis; may be necessary for other severe disease manifestations

IV, intravenously; NSAID, nonsteroidal antiinflammatory drugs; po, orally.

Nonsteroidal Antiinflammatory Drugs

As discussed earlier, signs and symptoms such as fever, arthritis, and serositis are among the most common for patients with active disease. Therefore, for many patients with mild disease, initial

TABLE 96-4 Monitoring Adverse Effects of Drugs Commonly Used in Systemic Lupus Erythematosus

Drug	Toxicities to Monitor	Baseline Evaluation	Monitoring System Review	Monitoring Laboratory
Salicylates, NSAIDs	Gastrointestinal bleeding, hepatic toxicity, renal toxicity, hypertension	CBC, creatinine, urinalysis, AST, ALT	Dark/black stool, dyspepsia, nausea/vomiting, abdominal pain, shortness of breath, edema	CBC yearly, creatinine yearly
Corticosteroids	Hypertension, hyperglycemia, hyperlipidemia, hypokalemia, osteoporosis, avascular necrosis, cataract, weight gain, infections, fluid retention	Blood pressure, bone densitometry, glucose, potassium, cholesterol, (HDL, LDL), triglycerides	Polyuria, polydipsia, edema, shortness of breath, blood pressure, visual changes, bone pain	Glucose every 3–6 months, total cholesterol yearly, bone densitometry yearly to assess osteoporosis
Hydroxychloroquine	Macular damage	None unless patient is older than 40 years of age or has previous eye disease	Visual changes	Funduscopic and visual fields every 6–12 months
Azathioprine	Myelosuppression, hepatotoxicity, lymphoproliferative disorders	CBC, platelet count, creatinine, AST or ALT	Symptoms of myelosuppression	CBC and platelet count every 1–2 weeks with changes in dose (every 1–3 months thereafter), AST yearly, Pap test at regular intervals
Cyclophosphamide	Myelosuppression, myeloproliferative disorders, malignancy, immunosuppression, hemorrhagic cystitis, secondary infertility	CBC and differential and platelet count, urinalysis	Symptoms of myelosuppression, hematuria, infertility	CBC and urinalysis monthly, urine cytology and Pap test yearly for life
Mycophenolate mofetil	Myelosuppression, hepatotoxicity, lymphoproliferative disorders, malignancy	CBC, hepatic function tests, renal function tests	Symptoms of myelosuppression, diarrhea, nausea/vomiting, dyspepsia, abdominal pain, dark/black stool or blood in stool	CBC weekly during first month, twice monthly during the second and third months, then monthly through the first year

ALT, alanine transaminase; AST, aspartate transaminase; CBC, complete blood count; HDL, high-density lipoprotein; LDL, low-density lipoprotein; NSAIDs, nonsteroidal antiinflammatory drugs; Pap, papanicolaou.

Modified from American College of Rheumatology Ad Hoc Committee on Systemic Lupus Erythematosus Guidelines. Guidelines for referral and management of systemic lupus erythematosus in adults. Arthritis Rheum 1999;42:1790, with permission.

treatment with a nonsteroidal antiinflammatory drug (NSAID) is a logical choice. The choice of NSAIDs in SLE is empirical. The dose used should be adequate to provide antiinflammatory effects, although low-dose aspirin may be useful in the management of patients with antiphospholipid syndrome.[33]

Nonselective cyclooxygenase NSAIDs significantly increase the risk of gastric irritation and peptic ulceration. Coprescribing with a gastroprotective agent such as a proton pump inhibitor may be beneficial. Patients with SLE taking NSAIDs may experience a decline in renal function because of drug effects and not the underlying disease. NSAIDs can decrease renal blood flow and glomerular filtration rates and should be used cautiously for patients with nephritis. Awareness of this adverse effect is important because declining renal function may be attributed mistakenly to progression of lupus nephritis. Patients with SLE have a higher incidence of hepatotoxicity than do other patients taking traditional NSAIDs. The use of NSAIDs is also associated with aseptic meningitis in SLE patients.[34]

Antimalarial Drugs

Antimalarial agents such as chloroquine and hydroxychloroquine have been used successfully in the management of discoid lupus and SLE. A few controlled trials provide evidence for the role of antimalarial therapy in controlling disease exacerbations and as steroid-sparing agents.[35] In general, the manifestations of SLE that can be managed with antimalarials are cutaneous manifestations, arthralgia, fatigue, and fever.[1,31] Because these drugs are not effective immediately, they are best used in long-term management. Response to chloroquine occurs within 1 to 3 months, whereas the maximal effect of hydroxychloroquine may not occur for 6 to 12 months.[36] Hydroxychloroquine is probably safer than chloroquine and is considered the antimalarial of first choice.

The mechanism of action of the antimalarial drugs is uncertain. It has been proposed that antimalarials interfere with T-lymphocyte activation.[36] Other effects of antimalarials that may benefit patients with SLE include inhibition of cytokines, decreased sensitivity to ultraviolet light, antiinflammatory activity, antiplatelet effects, and antihyperlipidemic activity.[22,36]

Dosage and duration of therapy depend on patient response, tolerance of side effects, and development of retinal toxicity, which is a potentially irreversible adverse reaction associated with long-term therapy, especially with chloroquine. Current recommended doses of antimalarials in SLE are hydroxychloroquine 200 to 400 mg/day and chloroquine 250 to 500 mg/day. After 1 or 2 years of treatment, gradual tapering of dosage can be attempted. Some patients may require only 1 or 2 tablets per week to suppress cutaneous manifestations.[36]

Side effects of these drugs include CNS effects (e.g., headache, nervousness, insomnia, and others), rashes, dermatitis, pigmentary changes of the skin and hair, gastrointestinal disturbance (e.g., nausea), and reversible ocular toxicities such as cycloplegia and corneal deposits. Potentially serious retinal toxicity is uncommon when the currently recommended doses are used and is least common with hydroxychloroquine.[36] However, because of the possibility of permanent damage associated with the retinopathy, an ophthalmologic evaluation should be done at baseline and every 3 months when chloroquine is used and every 12 months when hydroxychloroquine is used.[36]

Corticosteroids

Corticosteroid therapy is commonplace in therapeutic regimens for SLE. Although evidence for improved survival with corticosteroid therapy is inadequate, these agents are known to suppress the clinical expression of disease and are considered by many to be a major factor in the improved prognosis in recent years. Most controlled trials of corticosteroid therapy have been conducted for patients with severe lupus nephritis, but evidence suggests that corticosteroids are also effective in the management of severe cases of CNS disease, pneumonitis, myositis, vasculitis, thrombocytopenia, and other clinical manifestations.[37]

A patient with the diagnosis of SLE does not automatically require corticosteroid therapy. Mild disease with such manifestations as fever, arthralgia, pleuritis, or skin manifestations may respond adequately to NSAIDs or antimalarials, but patients with clinical manifestations that are more serious or unresponsive to other drugs usually require corticosteroids.

The goal of treatment with corticosteroids in SLE is to suppress and maintain suppression of active disease with the lowest dose possible. For patients with mild disease, low-dose therapy (prednisone 10 to 20 mg/day) is adequate,[29,37] but for patients with more severe disease (severe hemolytic anemia or cardiac involvement), higher doses, such as prednisone 1 to 2 mg/kg daily, may be required. Once adequate suppression of disease is achieved, the dose should be tapered to the minimum amount required for continued disease suppression. When analyzing the need to treat with corticosteroids, the clinician should consider other conditions that may increase the risk of corticosteroid therapy, such as infection, hypertension, atherosclerotic disease, diabetes, obesity, osteoporosis, and psychiatric disease.

Steroid pulse therapy is the administration of short-term, high-dose intravenous corticosteroids with the goal of inducing remission in SLE patients with serious, life-threatening disease, such as severe active nephritis, CNS involvement, or hemolytic disease. A standard pulse regimen consists of intravenous methylprednisolone 500 to 1,000 mg for 3 to 6 consecutive days. Pulse therapy usually is followed by high-dose prednisone (1 to 1.5 mg/kg per day) therapy that is tapered to low-dose maintenance therapy.[37] Potential advantages of pulse therapy over high-dose oral steroids include a quicker response and avoidance of side effects associated with the longer duration of therapy required with oral steroids. Although generally well tolerated, methylprednisolone pulse therapy may result in significant adverse effects, including infection, gastrointestinal disturbances, rapid increases in blood pressure, arrhythmias, seizures, and sudden death. Furthermore, there are insufficient data from controlled clinical trials to clearly define the role of pulse steroids in the management of SLE. Thus pulse therapy represents an alternative mode of treatment for patients with life-threatening disease or disease unresponsive to other pharmacotherapy.

Cytotoxic Drugs

A considerable amount of literature exists describing the use of cytotoxic and immunosuppressive drugs in SLE, although few of these are reports of controlled clinical trials. Included in this category are the alkylating agent cyclophosphamide and the antimetabolite azathioprine. These agents, usually used in combination with corticosteroids, have been the mainstays of immunosuppressive therapy. Although both are known to suppress and stabilize extrarenal disease activity, much of the evaluation of these agents has focused on lupus nephritis, a major factor associated with morbidity and mortality in SLE.

Evidence supporting the use of cyclophosphamide in lupus nephritis has been collected over the last several decades. Controlled clinical trials have shown that cyclophosphamide improves long-term outcomes in lupus nephritis.[1,38,39] Based on controlled trials, combination prednisone and cyclophosphamide has become standard treatment for focal and diffuse proliferative lupus nephritis (World Health Organization classes III/IV) and is superior to prednisone alone.[38] No studies have evaluated cyclophosphamide in earlier stages of nephritis (World Health Organization classes II/III), and therefore, corticosteroids remain the treatment of choice for the initial treatment of nephritis.[40] Pulse intravenous cyclophosphamide plus prednisone is more effective at slowing progression to end-stage renal disease than either prednisone alone or prednisone plus azathioprine.[41] Cyclophosphamide plus corticosteroids, the current standard of care, decreases the risk of developing end-stage renal failure requiring dialysis and renal transplantation.[42,43] Intermittent pulse administration of intravenous cyclophosphamide is preferred over daily oral therapies because of reduced adverse effects. However, pulse cyclophosphamide plus prednisone is not always effective.

When used in combination with corticosteroids, cyclophosphamide is dosed at 1 to 3 mg/kg for oral therapy and 0.5 to 1 g/m² of body surface area for intravenous therapy. The most common route of cyclophosphamide administration is intravenous, although there is little evidence that this is better than oral administration.[44] Likewise, there is no evidence to suggest the optimal duration of treatment. Based on empirical experience, cyclophosphamide generally is dosed monthly for 6 to 7 months and then every 3 months for a period of either 2 years or for 1 year after the nephritis is in remission.[1,38,39] Of course, cyclophosphamide therapy is not without risk. Serious toxic effects include suppression of hematopoiesis, opportunistic infections, bladder complications (e.g., hemorrhagic cystitis and cancer), sterility, and teratogenesis. White blood cell counts must be monitored during cyclophosphamide therapy, and if the nadir is less than 1,500 cells/mm³ (1.5×10^9/L), the dose must be adjusted to keep the white cell count above 1,500 cells/mm³ (1.5×10^9/L).

Azathioprine can be used as a "steroid-sparing" agent, allowing for the reduction of corticosteroid doses.[29,42] Azathioprine has not been studied as extensively as cyclophosphamide for lupus nephritis. Data do not support the use of azathioprine as a part of an induction regimen; however, long-term maintenance azathioprine therapy may prevent renal flares after successful induction with cyclophosphamide.[39,42] Azathioprine is given orally in doses of 1 to 3 mg/kg per day, often in combination with corticosteroids for severe disease. Azathioprine generally is less toxic than cyclophosphamide, but adverse reactions may be serious and include myelosuppression, opportunistic infections including herpes zoster, cancer, hepatotoxicity, and ovarian failure.

Cyclophosphamide often is administered intravenously in intermittent pulse doses to minimize toxicity. To decrease the risk of bladder toxicity, patients should be well hydrated with oral or intravenous fluids, and urinary output should be monitored. Mesna may be used to prevent hemorrhagic cystitis. Mesna is dosed at 20% of the total cyclophosphamide dose and is administered immediately before cyclophosphamide therapy and 3, 6, and 9 hours after therapy.[45] Cyclophosphamide may be of benefit to some patients with other serious, refractory manifestations of lupus, including neurologic manifestations.[46]

Because of the adverse effects of cyclophosphamide, other approaches to treating lupus nephritis have been attempted. Mycophenolate mofetil is an immunosuppressive agent that is effective treatment for severe renal and nonrenal lupus refractory to conventional cytotoxic agents.[39,47] Mycophenolate mofetil has been investigated as an alternative to cyclophosphamide for induction of remission. In an open-label trial, mycophenolate mofetil was more effective than standard cyclophosphamide therapy, achieving a higher rate of complete and partial remissions.[43] Prednisone was used in both treatment arms. Mycophenolate mofetil was also better tolerated. In this study, mycophenolate mofetil was initially dosed at 500 mg twice daily and was increased to 750 mg twice daily after 2 weeks; the dose continued to be increased weekly to a maximum of 1,000 mg three times daily. A larger study with longer follow-up is needed before any definitive conclusion can be drawn about the superiority of mycophenolate mofetil as induction therapy. Patients with the most severe forms of lupus nephritis should receive the standard boluses of intravenous cyclophosphamide plus corticosteroid therapy, but mycophenolate mofetil plus corticosteroid therapy may be a reasonable option for patients with mild to moderate nephritis and good renal function.[48]

CLINICAL CONTROVERSY

The use of intravenous cyclophosphamide for lupus nephritis as the standard of care is being questioned as newer data suggest that mycophenolate mofetil may be just as effective for induction and maintenance therapy.

Alternatives to cyclophosphamide for maintenance therapy also have been studied. Following induction therapy with the standard cyclophosphamide protocol, patients were assigned to either intravenous cyclophosphamide (0.5 to 1 g/m² every 3 months), oral azathioprine (1 to 3 mg/kg per day) or oral mycophenolate mofetil (500 to 3,000 mg per day) with dose titrations. All groups received prednisone.[49] This open-label study showed that standard cyclophosphamide induction therapy followed by mycophenolate mofetil or azathioprine was more effective and better tolerated than standard cyclophosphamide bolus therapy. Although these data need to be interpreted cautiously because of study design limitations, azathioprine and mycophenolate mofetil are good options for maintenance therapy in lupus nephritis.[50]

Cytotoxic therapy is useful in combination with corticosteroids, allowing for lower steroid doses and improved efficacy compared with steroids alone. However, cytotoxic therapy must be monitored closely for adverse effects, and maximum response may take 6 months or longer for some patients. Monitoring for adverse events, such as infection, myelosuppression, and long-term malignancies is essential.

■ ALTERNATIVE AND EXPERIMENTAL TREATMENTS

As the pathogenesis of SLE continues to be elucidated, new and promising treatments are being developed. Many new therapeutic approaches are being studied in human clinical trials. Table 96-5 lists some agents currently available as well as new therapeutic agents in phase I, II, and III trials.[47,51]

■ SPECIAL POPULATIONS

Pregnancy

Pregnancy in SLE patients is associated with exacerbation of disease during pregnancy, exacerbation during the early postpartum

TABLE 96-5	Selected Experimental Agents for SLE
Treatment	**Possible Mechanism of Action**
Abatacept	Blocks interaction between T and B cells
Cyclosporine	Immunosuppressive
DHEA	Weak androgen; antiinflammatory
Eculizumab	Anticomplement (C_5)
Efalizumab	Anti-LFA-1 (T-cell adhesion molecule)
Epratuzumab	B-cell depletion
Infliximab	Tumor necrosis factor inhibitor
Rituximab	B-cell depletion
Sirolimus	Immunosuppression
Tacrolimus	Immunosuppression

DHEA, dehydroepiandrosterone; LFA-1, lymphocyte function antigen-1.

period, a greater incidence of spontaneous abortion, and a greater chance of developing preeclampsia or pregnancy-induced hypertension (particularly for patients with nephritis).

Exacerbation of lupus during pregnancy seems to be less likely if the disease is in remission at conception.[52,53] Disease exacerbations can be managed aggressively with corticosteroids, if needed, with little concern about harm to the fetus.[53] The decision to use other classes of drug therapy to control disease exacerbation should be highly individualized, although hydroxychloroquine is safe during pregnancy.[53,54] In fact, it may be safer to continue hydroxychloroquine during pregnancy than to discontinue it.[53] The decision to use cytotoxic drugs during pregnancy should be made with extreme caution because of potential harmful effects (e.g., teratogenesis, fetal loss) to the fetus.[55] Cyclosporine, methotrexate, and mycophenolate mofetil are contraindicated in pregnancy, but azathioprine can be used.[53] NSAIDs are generally safe in pregnancy but should be discontinued during the last weeks of pregnancy due to risk of premature closure of the ductus arteriosus.

Antiphospholipid antibodies may be associated with a greater likelihood of spontaneous abortion.[52,53] Corticosteroids, intravenous immunoglobulin, aspirin, and heparin, alone and in various combinations, have been used to try to improve fetal outcome.[29] Fetal survival increases with all these therapies, but there is some controversy about their use alone or in combination.[53,56] The optimal treatment regimen for pregnant patients with antiphospholipid antibodies is yet to be determined, although it has been recommended that women with antiphospholipid antibodies and no prior fetal losses should receive low-dose daily aspirin. High-risk women with a history of recurrent fetal loss should be treated with low-dose subcutaneous heparin with or without aspirin.[52,53] Low-molecular-weight heparin may be an effective alternative to low-dose heparin in the treatment of antiphospholipid syndrome-related pregnancy loss.

Although there is an increased chance of a high-risk pregnancy in women with SLE, appropriate planning and disease management will result in a high likelihood of a successful pregnancy and a healthy child.

Contraception

Estrogen-containing oral contraceptives have been avoided for women with SLE because of the link between estrogens and disease activity. Uncontrolled trials suggest that oral contraceptives exacerbate SLE, but this issue was only recently rigorously examined. There are good reasons to prescribe oral contraceptives in SLE: (1) outcomes of pregnancy are better when pregnancies are planned and conception occurs during disease remission, (2) women with very active disease or receiving teratogenic medications should use a very reliable method of birth control, and (3) estrogen-containing oral contraceptives may have a beneficial effect counteracting glucocorticoid-induced osteoporosis.[57]

The use of a combined oral contraceptive (ethinyl estradiol plus levonorgestrel), a progestin-only contraceptive (levonorgestrel), and an intrauterine device were compared for women with SLE.[58] This 12-month study showed comparable rates of disease flares and no clinically significant differences among all three groups during the trial. A placebo-controlled trial of ethinyl estradiol plus norethindrone also showed no difference in disease activity between the two groups over 12 months.[59] Neither of these two trials studied combined oral contraceptives in severe active SLE, leaving the issue of oral contraceptives for these patients unanswered. Because of the risk of thrombotic events for estrogen-treated women and the risk of thrombosis in SLE, antiphospholipid antibodies should be measured before oral contraceptives are started,

and oral contraceptives should probably be avoided if these antibodies are present.[57]

Antiphospholipid Syndrome and Thrombosis

As mentioned earlier, the presence of antiphospholipid antibodies may result in several clinical manifestations, including thrombosis.[26] There is no agreement on prophylaxis of patients with antiphospholipid antibodies without a history of thromboembolism.[56] For such patients, low-dose aspirin (81 to 325 mg/day) may be used prophylactically, although efficacy is controversial.[56] Patients with an acute thrombotic event should receive standard treatment with anticoagulants (e.g., heparin). Continued treatment with warfarin to prevent recurrence may require an international normalized ratio of 3 or greater for patients with antiphospholipid syndrome and recurrent thrombotic events.[29,56] However, there is no consensus on the intensity of anticoagulation or duration of secondary prophylaxis, but as recurrence is common, patients usually are treated with oral anticoagulants indefinitely.[29]

CLINICAL CONTROVERSY

The optimal dose of aspirin and the intensity of anticoagulation therapy have not been well established, and clinicians will use various strategies for prevention of thrombosis in the presence of antiphospholipid antibodies.

Drug-Induced Lupus

Up to 10% of SLE cases may be drug-induced.[60] More than 80 drugs have been implicated as causing drug-induced lupus (DIL), although the incidence for most of these drugs is low.[60,61] Procainamide and hydralazine are associated most commonly with DIL (Table 96-6). A consensus on diagnostic criteria for DIL does not exist. To meet criteria for DIL, a patient should have exposure to a suspected drug, no prior history of idiopathic SLE prior to the use of the drug, development of ANAs (usually antihistone antibodies) and at least one clinical feature of SLE, and

TABLE 96-6	Medications Implicated in Drug-Induced Lupus[a]	
Acebutolol	Interleukin 2	Pindolol
Amiodarone	**Isoniazid**	Primidone
Antitumor necrosis factor therapies	Labetalol	**Procainamide**
Atenolol	Lisinopril	Propranolol
Captopril	Lithium	Propylthiouracil
Carbamazepine	Lovastatin	**Quinidine**
Chlorpromazine	Mephenytoin	Reserpine
Ciprofloxacin	Methimazole	Simvastatin
Clobazam	**Methyldopa**	Streptomycin
Clonidine	Metoprolol	Sulfasalazine
Clozapine	**Minocycline**	Tetracycline
Diltiazem	Nifedipine	Thiazide diuretics
Ethosuximide	Oral contraceptives	Ticlopidine
Fluvastatin	Para-aminosalicylate	Timolol
Gold salts	Penicillamine	Tocainide
Griseofulvin	Penicillin	Valproate
Hydralazine	Phenytoin	Verapamil
Hydroxyurea	Phenylbutazone	Zafirlukast
Interferon (α, γ)	Phenelzine	

[a]Drugs in **boldface** represent those with best evidence of association.
Data from references 60 to 64.

rapid improvement of symptoms with a gradual decline in ANAs following drug discontinuation.[60–62] The epidemiologic characteristics of DIL are different from those of idiopathic SLE. In general, patients with procainamide- or hydralazine-induced lupus develop the disease much later in life compared with idiopathic SLE probably because most people who use these drugs are older. There is also an absence of female predominance when compared with idiopathic SLE.

Patients of the slow acetylator phenotype may have a greater risk for developing DIL, particularly with procainamide and hydralazine.[9,60] Procainamide-induced lupus can present as early as 1 month or even after years of therapy. Hydralazine-induced lupus is dose related, leading to the recommended maximum dose of 100 mg/day for men and 50 mg/day for women to minimize the risk of DIL.[63]

Musculoskeletal symptoms are the most common clinical manifestations, while renal manifestations and CNS involvement are rare. Other common features of DIL include fever, fatigue, pericarditis, pleurisy, and weight loss.[64] The classic malar rash is rare in DIL, and skin manifestations are generally less frequent than idiopathic SLE.[60] A positive ANA test is found in nearly all (>90%) hydralazine-induced cases and in 50% to 90% of procainamide-induced disease. The immunofluorescence pattern usually is homogeneous, and antibodies are primarily against ssDNA and not dsDNA as in idiopathic SLE. Antihistone antibodies are specific for DIL but might be found in only 20% of patients with idiopathic SLE.[60]

If signs and symptoms of SLE appear in a patient and are suspected to be drug related, the drug should be discontinued. If the lupus is drug induced, the clinical manifestations should disappear in days to weeks, although it may take up to 1 year or longer for symptoms and serologic abnormalities to resolve completely.[64] A NSAID might be useful in treating musculoskeletal manifestations. Other, more aggressive drug therapy should not be necessary unless manifestations are deemed more serious.

PHARMACOECONOMIC CONSIDERATIONS

Treating patients with SLE is costly, requiring frequent visits to physician offices for monitoring therapy and treating adverse reactions from therapy and hospitalization for disease exacerbation and adverse drug effects. Therefore, it is particularly important in the management of a potentially debilitating chronic disease such as SLE to achieve desired treatment outcomes in an optimal manner to minimize the impact on use of healthcare resources. Costs of treating patients with SLE are slightly higher in the United States compared with Canada and the United Kingdom, but outcomes are similar.[65] The estimated mean annual direct cost in the United States ranges between $10,000 and $14,000 with mediations contributing approximately 26% of direct costs.[66] Direct costs increase with more severe disease, longer disease duration, and worse mental and physical health status.[66]

Disability from lupus also greatly impacts patients' economic status. Indirect disease costs in terms of lost wages are high. In the first year following diagnosis the productivity cost is estimated at approximately $9,000.[66] Work disability ranges from approximately 15% to 51% over 3 to 15 years following diagnosis.[67]

SYSTEMIC SCLEROSIS

CLINICAL MANIFESTATIONS

Systemic sclerosis is characterized by alteration of the microvasculature and by massive deposition of collagen in the skin and internal organs. This disease can present as a spectrum of differing manifestations depending on affected areas and the extent of disease. Sclerosis of the skin is a hallmark for this disease, but other manifestations include a diffuse cutaneous (truncal) systemic sclerosis, with skin tightness and marked skin thickening involving most of the body. Internal organs can also be involved, such as the gastrointestinal tract, lung, kidney, or heart, and can result in death. *Scleroderma* refers to patients with only skin involvement. Disease that affects only the fingers and toes is referred to as *sclerodactyly*.

CLINICAL PRESENTATION OF SYSTEMIC SCLEROSIS

General
- Sclerosis of the skin

Symptoms
- Raynaud's phenomenon
- Dyspepsia
- Constipation
- Diarrhea
- Steatorrhea
- Esophageal dysmotility

Most patients with systemic sclerosis (>95%) have Raynaud's phenomenon, where the digits turn white, followed by a bluish color, which is then followed by reddening in response to an appropriate stimulus. The precipitating event is usually cold temperature or emotion. The pallor is caused by vasospasm, the bluish color is from ischemia, and the reddish color is caused by a reactive hyperemia. Raynaud's phenomenon is a common manifestation of other syndromes, and most patients with Raynaud's phenomenon do not have systemic sclerosis. Gastrointestinal symptoms related to dysphagia and gastroesophageal reflux disease or changes in bowel habits secondary to intestinal dysmotility are common particularly for patients with early disease. In recent years, the lung has emerged as a key target organ in systemic sclerosis. Over 90% of patients have evidence of interstitial lung disease upon autopsy, and 40% demonstrate restrictive changes via pulmonary function tests. Lung involvement is the leading cause of death, and survival is inversely related to the severity of restrictive lung disease.[68,69]

Survival rates are highly variable depending on the extent of disease presentation, organ involvement, and other factors. Systemic sclerosis has the highest mortality rate of all the connective tissue diseases, with a 5-year survival rate estimated as high as 90%[70] and a 10-year survival rate of approximately 55%.[68,69]

ETIOLOGY AND PREVALENCE

The cause of systemic sclerosis is unknown. Ninety-five percent of patients have identifiable autoantibodies. There are two major subsets of the disease: limited cutaneous and diffuse systemic sclerosis. Patients with limited cutaneous involvement often have the Calcinosis, Raynaud's phenomenon, Esophageal dysmotility, Sclerodactyly, and Telangiectasias (CREST) syndrome, whereas patients with diffuse systemic sclerosis have a more aggressive disease with renal, cardiac, or pulmonary involvement. The prevalence of the disease is estimated to be between 4 and 266 cases per 1 million persons.[68,70,71] The wide range may be a result of differences in diagnostic criteria, regional variation, or sample sizes used to estimate the prevalence.

TREATMENT

Systemic Sclerosis

Treatment is empirical because there are no well-controlled trials evaluating and comparing various forms of therapy. Available data are difficult to interpret because of the heterogeneity of the disease, spontaneous remissions that can occur, and lack of objective measures to assess changes in clinical status. D-penicillamine has been used for skin involvement, but data supporting its use remains controversial. Response appears to be best in younger patients, those able to tolerate long-term therapy, and in those with early diagnosis of the disease.[72] Additionally, there seems to be no therapeutic advantage of high-dose (750 to 1,000 mg/day) versus low-dose penicillamine (125 mg every other day) in the treatment of systemic sclerosis according to one multicenter placebo-controlled trial.[69] Response occurs over many months to years, and the drug is not always effective. The high incidence of severe adverse events and the increased dropout rates for D-penicillamine limit its usefulness. Methotrexate appears promising as an effective therapy for skin involvement.[70,73] Evidence from two recent randomized controlled trials suggests that oral or intravenous cyclophosphamide is beneficial for patients with early and progressive interstitial lung disease.[68] Modest improvement in lung function and health-related outcomes (dyspnea and skin thickening among others) were demonstrated after 1 year of cyclophosphamide therapy with or without subsequent treatment with azathioprine and prednisone.[68,74-76] Mycophenolate mofetil also has demonstrated modest benefit in multiple small studies, but controlled trials are lacking.[68,69] Antiinflammatory agents and corticosteroids have not been effective in systemic sclerosis.

Angiotensin-converting enzyme (ACE) inhibitors have improved survival dramatically for patients with renal involvement and improve outcomes for patients with disease-associated pulmonary hypertension or myocardial involvement.[68,69,77] Patients with sclerosis of the kidneys develop hypertension, leading to a renal crisis. For these patients, plasma renin activity and angiotensin concentrations can be more than twice normal. Renal involvement should be anticipated in all systemic sclerosis patients who develop hypertension. Patients with systemic sclerosis and hypertension should be treated and maintained with an ACE inhibitor regardless of renal involvement. ACE inhibitors should be used for patients on dialysis, and they have allowed some dialysis-dependent systemic sclerosis patients to discontinue dialysis.[69,77,78] Angiotensin receptor blockers are less effective than ACE inhibitors but may have an additive effect to ACE inhibitors in refractory cases.[78] Treatment of Raynaud's phenomenon requires patient education and sometimes drug therapy. Patients must maintain their peripheral extremity and core body temperatures. Wearing appropriate clothing in cold environments is essential. Reaching into a freezer with unprotected hands should be avoided. Drugs that can cause peripheral vasoconstriction, such as pseudoephedrine and β-blockers, should be avoided for patients with Raynaud's phenomenon or systemic sclerosis. Smoking causes cutaneous vasoconstriction and should be eliminated, and this includes passive smoke. When preventive measures are insufficient, aggressive oral vasodilator therapy is useful for decreasing the frequency and severity of Raynaud's phenomenon episodes and may limit peripheral vascular (ischemic) complications. Commonly used agents are calcium channel blockers (nifedipine) and angiotensin receptor blockers (losartan).[68,70,73] Although there are limited data, other agents that may be beneficial for Raynaud are selective serotonin reuptake inhibitors (fluoxetine), phosphodiesterase-5 inhibitors (sildenafil), and endothelin-1 receptor antagonists (bosentan).[68-70]

INFLAMMATORY MYOPATHIES

CLINICAL MANIFESTATIONS

The inflammatory myopathies are a heterogeneous group of relatively rare, chronic, inflammatory muscle diseases of unknown etiology. The major types of inflammatory myopathies are polymyositis (PM), dermatomyositis (DM), and inclusion body myositis (IBM). A fourth subtype, immune mediated necrotizing myopathy (NM), clinically resembles PM but has minimal inflammatory cell infiltrates on muscle biopsy.[79] DM is distinguished from PM by a typical rash, which is red, scaly, and plaque-like, over the knuckles, wrists, elbows, and knees and typically precedes or accompanies the onset of muscle weakness. A blue-purple discoloration on the upper eyelids with edema also can occur in DM. Patients with inflammatory myopathies generally present with progressive weakness. In DM, PM, and NM the heart (pericarditis leading to heart failure or arrhythmia) and lungs (interstitial lung disease) may be affected, and patients may present with dysphagia and/or dyspnea.[79,80] There is an increased risk of malignancy associated with PM, NM, and particularly DM.

An increased serum creatine kinase concentration and electromyography abnormalities are common. Other serum enzymes, such as the alanine transaminase, aspartate transaminase, and lactate dehydrogenase, also may be increased.[79,81] Muscle biopsies show either characteristic inflammatory cell infiltrates (PM, DM, and IBM) or necrotic muscle fibers (NM). ANAs are detected in 24% to 60% of DM, 16% to 40% of PM, and up to 20% of IBM patients. Some patients develop certain "myositis specific antibodies" as well.[79]

CLINICAL PRESENTATION OF POLYMYOSITIS AND DERMATOMYOSITIS

General

- Inflammation of skeletal muscle and skin

Symptoms

- Muscle weakness in shoulder and hip girdles and trunk
- Insidious onset
- Arthritis, Raynaud's phenomenon, and other symptoms of connective tissue diseases

---

TREATMENT

Inflammatory Myopathies

DM, PM, and NM patients usually respond to immunotherapies, while IBM patients usually do not.[79] A few small, randomized, double-blind, placebo-controlled trials evaluating the treatment of PM, DM, and IBM have been conducted, but evidence supporting use of drug therapy in large controlled trials is still lacking. It does appear that various immunotherapies may be helpful in both PM and DM. The goal of therapy is to increase muscle strength so as to improve function in activities of daily living (e.g., bathing, dressing, feeding, and toileting). Treatment consists of physical therapy during periods of remission and rest during periods of disease activity. Prednisone is the first line of drug therapy for PM and DM. Although the optimal dose of prednisone is not clear, most clinicians use prednisone at a starting dose of 60 to 100 mg/day or about 1 mg/kg per day as a single morning dose.[81] Higher prednisone doses of 1.5 mg/kg per day can be used if needed. The initial dose of prednisone is continued for at least 2 to 4 weeks or until maximum benefit is achieved or a remission is induced. The full effect of prednisone may not be evident for several months. After 4 months of treatment, approximately 85% of patients treated with prednisone will have normal muscle strength. The prednisone dose is tapered when muscle strength improves and serum creatine kinase concentrations decrease. If the patient is responding to prednisone and there are no serious side effects, the drug is tapered slowly over about 2 to 3 months and finally to a lower maintenance dose that may be alternate daily dosing if tolerated. The dose that maintains a good clinical response can be used as maintenance. Tapering too quickly can cause an exacerbation of disease activity. Monitoring serum creatine kinase concentrations is useful because they tend to increase several weeks before clinical symptoms become apparent. Some clinicians will treat patients with daily prednisone for 1 or more years, whereas others may use every-other-day therapy for many years.[79,81]

One complication from corticosteroid use is the development of a myopathy. Based on symptoms, it is difficult to know if increased muscle weakness is caused by the corticosteroid or to worsening disease status. Lowering the prednisone dose may be useful. If patients get better on a lower dose of prednisone, then most likely the muscle weakness was caused by the drug. It may take 2 to 8 weeks for this to become evident clinically. Use of serum creatine kinase concentration also may be helpful because this does not increase with steroid myopathy. It is possible that a steroid myopathy and worsening disease can coexist.

Although most patients with PM or DM improve with prednisone, some will not, and some will develop corticosteroid resistance. In these patients and in those in whom a complete response is not achieved, azathioprine may be used at a dose of 2 to 3 mg/kg per day as a single morning dose.[79] Clinical response may take 3 to 6 months. Another alternative is methotrexate at a dose of 7.5 to 20 mg once weekly. For patients resistant to these therapies, cyclophosphamide, cyclosporine, mycophenolate mofetil or rituximab can be tried.[79,80] Intravenous immunoglobulin (IVIG) at a dose of 2 g/kg every 1 to 2 months may be effective for patients with refractory disease not responding to prednisone/azathioprine therapy. Evidence from one randomized controlled trial for DM patients supports the use of IVIG in these patients.[80] Alternative therapies are often used in PM or DM, but there is no convincing evidence to support their use. These alternative therapies also may be beneficial for patients who can not take corticosteroids because of serious adverse effects.

POLYMYALGIA RHEUMATICA AND GIANT-CELL ARTERITIS

CLINICAL MANIFESTATIONS

Polymyalgia rheumatica (PMR) and giant-cell arteritis (GCA) are closely related diseases, and some experts consider them to be different phases of the same disease.[82,83]

PMR is a disease characterized by severe bilateral pain and aching in the shoulders, neck, and pelvic girdles with associated morning stiffness. Systemic symptoms such as low-grade fever, fatigue, and weight loss are frequently present.[84] GCA is a vasculitis of large- and medium-size vessels; it is the most common type of vasculitis in North America and Europe.[85] The most frequent symptom of GCA is headache, with bilateral pain usually in the temporal or occipital areas; signs of systemic inflammation are also usually present.[83,84,86] GCA was referred to

previously as *temporal arteritis* or *granulomatous arteritis*. Both PMR and GCA occur in people older than 50 years of age, and the incidence increases with age, peaking between ages 70 and 80 years.[83,84] Some patients go from exhibiting no symptoms to overt clinical manifestations overnight, whereas others have a gradual onset of symptoms over a number of weeks. The etiology is unknown.

TREATMENT

Polymyalgia Rheumatica and Giant-Cell Arteritis

The treatment of choice for both PMR and GCA is a corticosteroid, mainly prednisone.[83,84] Several different dosing regimens have been studied, but a recent systematic review of PMR treatment studies published in the primary literature concluded that a starting dose of 15 mg/day of prednisone appears effective in most PMR patients and that once initial remission (control of symptoms) was achieved, the prednisone dose should be tapered slowly based on clinical symptoms and laboratory parameters [e.g., erythrocyte sedimentation rate (ESR) and C-reactive protein (CRP) levels]. Additionally, once a stable prednisone maintenance dose of 10 mg/day was achieved, further dose reductions should be smaller than 1 mg per month (e.g., 1 mg every 2 months). The authors also concluded that despite the differences in starting doses and tapering protocols studied, prednisone doses between 10 and 20 mg/day appeared to control symptoms at PMR onset and generally allowed for corticosteroid therapy discontinuation for about half of patients after 2 years of treatment.[84] Usually the response to steroids is quite rapid, with complete or nearly complete symptom resolution within a few days. In fact, corticosteroid therapy is so effective that if improvement does not occur within a week, another diagnosis should be considered.[87] The prednisone should be tapered beginning 2 to 4 weeks following control of symptoms. The rate of tapering is based on clinical response. A taper of 2.5 mg/day at 2- to 4-week intervals to 10 mg/day followed by a slower tapering of 1 mg/day at monthly intervals has been suggested.[87,88] The lowest dose of prednisone that controls symptoms should be used for maintenance. Patients usually continue maintenance therapy for 1 to 3 years. Patients may experience a relapse when the prednisone is discontinued. For patients with GCA without visual or neurological symptoms but with systemic and inflammatory symptoms, daily prednisone doses of 40 to 60 mg (or 1 mg/kg/day) are generally used. Higher doses are recommended for patients with acute visual or neurological signs or symptoms (at least 80 mg/day or up to 2 mg/kg/day). In fact, it is common to hospitalize more acutely ill patients and start intravenous steroids such as methylprednisolone 250 mg every 6 hours for the first 3 to 5 days, then switch to high dose oral prednisone. High-dose prednisone is maintained for at least 4 to 6 weeks until systemic symptoms have diminished and laboratory markers of inflammation (ESR and CRP) have normalized. A slow taper should follow, and a maintenance dose of 7.5 to 10 mg/day is generally achieved in 6 to 12 months. Patients may require 1 to 5 years of steroid therapy.[83] Because these are diseases of the elderly, it is particularly important to use calcium and vitamin D supplements to prevent corticosteroid-induced osteoporosis. Prophylactic bisphosphonate therapy also should be considered. Unlike most other autoimmune diseases, other forms of immunosuppressive therapy are not as effective as corticosteroids in PMR and GCA.[86] However, there is evidence supporting methotrexate as a glucocorticoid-sparing agent when used to treat patients with

PMR in conjunction with prednisone.[84] Studies examining the role of methotrexate in treating patients with GCA have yielded conflicting results.[83]

CLINICAL PRESENTATION OF POLYMYALGIA RHEUMATICA AND GIANT-CELL ARTERITIS

General

☐ Aching and morning stiffness of neck, shoulder, and pelvic girdle musculature and torso.

Symptoms

☐ Pain and morning stiffness lasting 1 to 6 hours

☐ Fatigue, malaise, and weight loss usually present

☐ Anorexia

☐ Headache in GCA

Signs

☐ Low-grade fever

Laboratory Tests

☐ Erythrocyte sedimentation rate is generally >40 mm/h (11.1 μm/s) and often >100 mm/h (27.8 μm/s)

DRUG-INDUCED VASCULITIS

CLINICAL MANIFESTATIONS

Drugs are common causes of vasculitis, often occurring in the skin, but other organ involvement (kidney and lung in particular) can occur. The pathogenesis of inflammation of blood vessel walls caused by drugs is poorly understood. Even drugs used to treat inflammatory and immune-mediated disease, such as NSAIDs, sulfasalazine, and etanercept, can cause vasculitis.[89]

CLINICAL PRESENTATION OF DRUG-INDUCED VASCULITIS

General

☐ Signs and symptoms depend on organ involvement

Symptoms

☐ Rash

☐ Glomerulonephritis

☐ Hepatitis

☐ Fatigue

☐ Myalgia

☐ Arthralgia

Signs

☐ Fever

Long-term use of the offending agent is thought to be a risk factor for developing vasculitis, but length of use varies widely in case reports. Most classes of medications have been reported to cause vasculitis.[90] Although there are no specific diagnostic tests for drug-induced vasculitis, antineutrophil cytoplasmic autoantibodies have been identified in many cases of drug-induced vasculitis.[89,90] ESR and CRP are often elevated in drug-induced vasculitides; anemia may be present as well.[89]

TREATMENT

Drug-Induced Vasculitis

❻ The first step in therapy of drug-induced vasculitis is to discontinue the suspected inducing agent. This may be all that is necessary to abate symptoms in mild cases. For more serious cases, corticosteroids may be used, and where life-threatening organ involvement occurs, immunosuppressive therapy with agents such as cyclophosphamide or mycophenolate mofetil may be used. Following therapy, symptoms usually resolve within 1 to 4 weeks, except in cases of significant organ involvement.[89]

EVALUATION OF THERAPEUTIC OUTCOMES

The diversity of clinical features and disease severity associated with the collagen–vascular diseases leads to a number of possible clinical outcomes with a broad range of desired therapeutic outcomes. Achieving desired therapeutic outcomes for most of the collagen–vascular diseases is highly variable. Currently, it is not possible to predict which patients will have a satisfactory therapeutic response and which will have unrelenting progressive disease. These diseases often have fluctuating courses, necessitating frequent changes in drug therapy and drug doses.

Evaluation of drug therapy of several of the collagen–vascular diseases often only requires monitoring for resolution of symptoms such as rash or muscle pain. However, patients with life-threatening disease receiving aggressive pharmacotherapy may require intensive monitoring and evaluation of therapy. For example, the patient receiving cytotoxic drug therapy for severe lupus nephritis requires close monitoring of laboratory indices of renal function, as well as monitoring of symptomatology and laboratory indices for possible bone marrow suppression, infection, cystitis, or other potential adverse effects.

Evaluation of therapeutic outcomes also should include an awareness of the possibility of drug therapy mimicking signs and symptoms of disease, such as the lupus patient receiving NSAID therapy and presenting with renal insufficiency or the patient with PM receiving prednisone and presenting with an exacerbation of muscle weakness.

As patients live longer, as is the case with SLE, outcome measures other than mortality will be needed to assess the effect of treatment. Clinicians and researchers working with lupus patients have developed and continue to refine some of these alternative outcome measures. Three important domains for assessing lupus patients are disease activity, accumulated damage, and quality of life.[91] Table 96–7 lists several instruments useful for assessing patients with SLE.

TABLE 96-7	Instruments Used for Assessing Outcome Measures in Patients with Systemic Lupus Erythematosus
Outcome Domain	**Instrument**
Disease activity	Systemic Lupus Activity Measure (SLAM)/SLAM Revised (SLAM-R)
	Systemic Lupus Erythematosus Disease Activity Index (SLEDAI)
	European Community Lupus Activity Measure (ECLAM)
	British Isles Lupus Activity Group (BILAG)
	Lupus Activity Index (LAI)
Accumulated damage	Systemic Lupus International Collaborating Clinics/American College of Rheumatology (SLICC/ACR) damage index
Quality of life	Health Assessment Questionnaire (HAQ) functional ability index Medical Outcome Survey short form 36 (SF-36)
	Lupus Quality-of-Life Questionnaire (Lupus QoL)
	SLE Quality-of-Life Questionnaire (SLE QoL)

Data from reference 91.

CONCLUSION

SLE is a disease that affects multiple organ systems and consists of abnormal immunologic function and the development of auto-antibodies. The disease is quite variable in clinical presentation and progression. The cause of lupus is unknown, although several factors (e.g., genetics, environment, and hormones) may predispose an individual to the development of the disease. Although SLE was once thought to be rapidly fatal, today nearly 90% of patients survive 10 years.

Drug therapy is nonspecific and is aimed at suppressing the inflammation and abnormal immune response associated with active disease. Clinical trials with various agents often have been inadequate and contradictory, and the therapeutic management of lupus is not optimal. Nevertheless, drug therapy of recent years probably has contributed significantly to the improved survival of these patients. As the understanding of SLE progresses and advances in molecular biology occur, we can expect to see the development of more specific and optimal treatment and further improvement in survival.

Each of the collagen–vascular diseases has its own recommended form of therapy. For most of these diseases, there are few well-controlled clinical trials evaluating pharmacotherapy. Treatment of most of these diseases requires antiinflammatory or immuno-suppressive drugs. Monitoring therapeutic outcomes is essential because drugs and drug doses may need to be modified frequently.

ABBREVIATIONS

ACE: angiotensin-converting enzyme

ANA: antinuclear antibodies

CAD: coronary artery disease

CRP: C-reactive protein

DIL: drug-induced lupus

DM: dermatomyositis

DNA: deoxyribonucleic acid

dsDNA: double-stranded DNA

ESR: erythrocyte sedimentation rate

IVIG: intravenous immunoglobulin

NSAID: nonsteroidal antiinflammatory drug

PM: polymyositis

PMR: polymyalgia rheumatica

RNP: ribonucleoprotein

SLE: systemic lupus erythematosus

ssDNA: single-stranded DNA

RNA: ribonucleic acid

REFERENCES

1. Tassiulas JO, Boumpas DT. Clinical features and treatment of systemic lupus erythematosus. In: Firestein GS, Budd RC, Harris Jr ED, et al. eds. Kelly's Textbook of Rheumatology, 8th ed. Philadelphia, PA: Saunders Elsevier; 2009:1263–1300.
2. Tan EM, Cohen AS, Fries JF, et al. The 1982 revised criteria for the classification of systemic lupus erythematosus. Arthritis Rheum 1982;25:1271–1277.
3. Hochberg MC (for the Diagnostic and Therapeutic Criteria Committee of the American College of Rheumatology). Updating the American College of Rheumatology revised criteria for the classification of systemic lupus erythematosus [letter]. Arthritis Rheum 1997;40:1725.
4. Benseler SM, Silverman ED. Systemic lupus erythematosus. Pediatr Clin North Am 2005;52:443–467.
5. Bertsias G, Ioannidis JPA, Boletis J, et al. EULAR recommendations for the management of systemic lupus erythematosus. Report of a Task Force of the EULAR Standing Committee for International Clinical Studies Including Therapeutics. Ann Rheum Dis 2008;67:195–205.
6. D'Cruz DP. Systemic lupus erythematosus. BMJ 2006;332:890–894.
7. Lupus Foundation of America. Statistics about lupus, http://www.lupus.org/index.html.
8. Riemekasten G, Hahn BH. Key autoantigens in SLE. Rheumatol 2005;44:975–982.
9. Mok CC, Lau CS. Pathogenesis of systemic lupus erythematosus. J Clin Pathol 2003;56:481–490.
10. Perdriger A, Werner-Leyval S, Rollot-Elamrani K. The genetic basis for systemic lupus erythematosus. Joint Bone Spine 2003;70:103–108.
11. Doria A, Canova M, Tonon M, et al. Infections as triggers and complications of systemic lupus erythematosus. Autoimmun Rev 2008;8:24–28.
12. Rahman A, Isenberg DA. Systemic lupus erythematosus. New Engl J Med 2008;358:929–939.
13. McMurray RW, May W. Sex hormones and systemic lupus erythematosus. Arthritis Rheum 2003;48:2100–2110.
14. Lauwerys BR, Houssiau FA. Involvement of cytokines in the pathogenesis of systemic lupus erythematosus. Adv Exp Med Biol 2003;520:237–251.
15. Rahman A. Autoantibodies, lupus and the science of sabotage. Rheumatol (Oxford) 2004;43:1326–1336.
16. Shmerling RH. Autoantibodies in systemic lupus erythematosus: There before you know it. N Engl J Med 2003;349:1499–1500.
17. Arbuckle MR, McClain MT, Rubertone MV, et al. Development of auto-antibodies before the clinical onset of systemic lupus erythematosus. N Engl J Med 2003;349:1526–1533.
18. Powers DB. Systemic lupus erythematosus and discoid lupus erythematosus. Oral Maxillofacial Surg Clin N Am 2008;20:651–662.
19. Sitia S, Atzeni F, Sarzi-Puttini P, et al. Cardiovascular involvement in systemic autoimmune diseases. Autoimmun Rev 2009;8:281–286.
20. Hall FC, Dalbeth N. Disease modification and cardiovascular risk reduction: Two sides of the same coin? Rheumatol (Oxford) 2005;44:1473–1482.
21. Shattner A, Liang MH. The cardiovascular burden of lupus: A complex challenge. Arch Intern Med 2003;163:1507–1510.
22. Hahn BH. Systemic lupus erythematosus and accelerated atherosclerosis. N Engl J Med 2003;349:2379–2380.
23. Roman MJ, Shanker B, Davis A, et al. Prevalence and correlates of accelerated atherosclerosis in systemic lupus erythematosus. N Engl J Med 2003;349:2399–2406.
24. Asanuma Y, Oeser A, Shintani AK, et al. Premature coronary-artery atherosclerosis in systemic lupus erythematosus. N Engl J Med 2003;349:2407–2415.
25. Quismorio Jr. FP. Hematologic and lymphoid abnormalities in systemic lupus erythematosus. In: Wallace DJ, Hahn BH, eds. Dubois' Lupus Erythematosus 7th ed. Philadelphia, PA: Lippincott Williams & Wilkins; 2007:801–828.
26. Erkan D, Salmon JE, Lockshin MD. Antiphospholipid Syndrome. In: Firestein GS, Budd RC, Harris Jr ED, et al. eds. In: Kelly's Textbook of Rheumatol, 8th ed. Philadelphia, PA: Saunders Elsevier; 2009: 1301–1310.
27. Weening JJ, D'Agati VD, Schwartz MM, et al. The classification of glomerulonephritis in systemic lupus erythematosus revisited. J Am Soc Nephrol 2004;15:241–250.
28. Shmerling RH. Diagnostic tests for rheumatic disease: Clinical utility revisited. South Med J 2005;98:704–711.
29. Brasington RD Jr, Kahl LE, Ranganathan P, et al. Immunologic rheumatic disorders. J Allergy Clin Immunol 2003;111:S593–S601.
30. Ippolito A, Petri M. An update on mortality in systemic lupus erythematosus. Clin Exp Rheumatol 2008;26(suppl. 51):S72–S79.
31. Lupus: A Patient Care Guide for Nurses and Other Health Professionals, 3rd ed. Bethesda, MD: U.S. Department of Health and Human Services, National Institutes of Health, National Institute of Arthritis and Musculoskeletal and Skin Diseases; 2006:NIH Publication Number 06-4262.

32. Ghaussy NO, Sibbitt WL, Bankhurst AD, Qualls CR. Cigarette smoking and disease activity in systemic lupus erythematosus. J Rheumatol 2003;30:1215–1221.

33. Petri M. Clinical and management aspects of the antiphospholipid antibody syndrome. In: Wallace DJ, Hahn BH, eds. Dubois' Lupus Erythematosus 7th ed. Philadelphia, PA: Lippincott Williams & Wilkins; 2007:1262–1297.

34. Horizon AA, Wallace DJ. Risk:benefit ratio of nonsteroidal anti-inflammatory drugs in systemic lupus erythematosus. Expert Opin Drug Saf 2004;3:273–278.

35. Gordon DA, Klinkhoff AV. Second line agents. In: Harris ED Jr, Budd RC, Genovese MC, et al. eds. Kelley's Textbook of Rheumatol, 7th ed. Philadelphia, PA: Elsevier/Saunders; 2005:877–899.

36. Wallace DJ. Antimalarial Therapies. In: Wallace DJ, Hahn BH, eds. Dubois' Lupus Erythematosus 7th ed. Philadelphia, PA: Lippincott Williams & Wilkins; 2007:1152–1174.

37. Kirou KA, Boumpas DT. Systemic glucocorticoid therapy in systemic lupus erythematosus. In: Wallace DJ, Hahn BH, eds. Dubois' Lupus Erythematosus 7th ed. Philadelphia, PA: Lippincott Williams & Wilkins; 2007:1175–1197.

38. Tumlin JA. Lupus nephritis: Histology, diagnosis, and treatment. Bull NYU Hosp Jt Dis 2008;66:188–194.

39. Mok CC, Wong RWS, Lai KN. Treatment of severe proliferative lupus nephritis: The current state. Ann Rheum Dis 2003;62:799–804.

40. Bargman JM. How did cyclophosphamide become the drug of choice for lupus nephritis? Nephrol Dial Transplant 2009;24:381–384.

41. Ginzler EM, Dvorkina O. Newer therapeutic approaches for systemic lupus erythematosus. Rheum Dis Clin North Am 2005;315–328.

42. Houssiau FA, Ginzlet EM. Current treatment of lupus nephritis. Lupus 2008;17:426–430.

43. Ginzler EM, Dooley MA, Aranow C, et al. Mycophenolate mofetil or intravenous cyclophosphamide for lupus nephritis. N Engl J Med 2005;353:2219–2228.

44. Lai KN, Tang SCW, Mok CC. Treatment for lupus nephritis: A revisit. Nephrology 2005;10:180–188.

45. Davis JC, Klippel JH. Antimalarials and immunosuppressive therapies. In: Lahita RG, ed. Systemic Lupus Erythematosus, 4th ed. New York: Elsevier; 2004:1273–1293.

46. Gold R, Fontana A, Zierz S. Therapy of neurological disorders in systemic vasculitis. Semin Neurol 2003;23:207–214.

47. Karim MY, Pisoni CN, Khamashta MA. Update on immunotherapy for systemic lupus erythematosus—What's hot and what's not. Rhuematology 2009;48:332–341.

48. McCune WJ. Mycophenolate mofetil for lupus nephritis. N Engl J Med 2005;353:2282–2284.

49. Contreras G, Pardo V, Leclercq B, et al. Sequential therapies for proliferative lupus nephritis. N Engl J Med 2004;350:971–980.

50. Balow JE, Austin HA. Maintenance therapy for lupus nephritis—Something old, something new. N Engl J Med 2004;350:1044–1046.

51. Ferrera F, Filaci G, Rizzi M, et al. New therapies in SLE. Recent Pat Inflamm Allergy Drug Discov 2008;2:11–23.

52. Buyon JP. Updates on lupus and pregnancy. Bull NYU Hosp Jt Dis 2009;67:271–275.

53. Ruiz-Irastorza G, Khamashta MA. Managing lupus patients during pregnancy. Best Pract Res Clin Rheumatol 2009;23:575–582.

54. Costedoat-Chalumeau N, Amoura Z, Duhaut P, et al. Safety of hydroxychloroquine in pregnant patients with connective tissue diseases: A study of one hundred thirty-three cases compared with a control group. Arthritis Rheum 2003;48:3207–3211.

55. Petri M. Immunosuppressive drug use in pregnancy. Autoimmunity 2003;36:51–56.

56. Tuthill JI, Khamashta MA. Management of antiphospholipid syndrome. J Autoimmun 2009;33:92–98.

57. Bermas BL. Oral contraceptives in systemic lupus erythematosus—A tough pill to swallow? N Engl J Med 2005;353:2602–2604

58. Sanchez-Guerrero J, Uribe AG, Jimenez-Santana L, et al. A trial of contraceptive methods in women with systemic lupus erythematosus. N Engl J Med 2005;353:2539–2549.

59. Petri M, Kim MY, Kalunian KC, et al. Combined oral contraceptives in women with systemic lupus erythematosus. N Engl J Med 2005;353:2550–2558.

60. Antonov D, Kazandjieva J, Etugov D, Gospodinov D, Tsankov N. Drug-induced lupus erythematosus. Clin Dermatol 2004;22:157–166.

61. Rubin RL. Drug-induced lupus. Toxicology 2005;209:135–147.

62. Brogan BL, Olsen NJ. Drug-induced rheumatic syndromes. Curr Opin Rheumatol 2003;15:76–80.

63. Finks SW, Finks AL, Self TH. Hydralazine-induced lupus: Maintaining vigilance with increased use in patients with heart failure. South Med J 2006;99:18–22.

64. Sarzi-Puttini P, Atzeni F, Capsoni F, et al. Drug-induced lupus erythematosus. Autoimmunity 2005;37:507–518.

65. Clarke AE, Petri MA, Manzi S, et al. The systemic lupus erythematosus tri-nation study: Absence of a link between health resource use and health outcome. Rheumatol (Oxford) 2004;43:1016–1024.

66. Panopalis P, Yazdany J, Gillis JZ, et al. Health care costs and costs associated with changes in work productivity among persons with systemic lupus erythematosus. Arthritis Rheum 2008;59:1788–1795.

67. Scofield L, Reinlib L, Alarcon S, Cooper GS. Employment and disability issues in systemic lupus erythematosus: A review. Arthritis Rheum 2008;59:1475–1479.

68. Hinchcliff M, Varga J. Systemic sclerosis/scleroderma: A treatable multisystem disease. Am Fam Physician 2008;78:961–968.

69. Varga J. Systemic sclerosis: an update. Bull NYU Hosp Jt Dis 2008;66:198–202.

70. Bournia VKK, Vlachoyiannopoulos PG, Selmi C, Moutsopoulos HM, Gershwin ME. Recent advances in the treatment of systemic sclerosis. Clinic Rev Allerg Immunol 2009;36:176–200.

71. Mayers MD, Lacey JV Jr, Beebe-Dimmer J, et al. Prevalence, incidence, survival, and disease characteristics of systemic sclerosis in a large US population. Arthritis Rheum 2003;48:2246–2255.

72. Micromedex. Penicillamine, http://www.micromedex.com/products/hcs/.

73. Charles C, Clements P, Furst DE. Systemic sclerosis: Hypothesis-driven treatment strategies. Lancet 2006;367:1683–1691.

74. Tashkin DP, Elashoff R, Clements PJ, et al. Cyclophosphamide versus placebo in scleroderma lung disease. N Engl J Med 2006;354:2655–2666.

75. Hoyles RK, Ellis RW, Wellsbury J, et al. A multicenter, prospective, randomized, double-blind, placebo-controlled trial of corticosteroids and intravenous cyclophosphamide followed by oral azathioprine for the treatment of pulmonary fibrosis in scleroderma. Arthritis Rheum 2006;54:3962–3970.

76. Khanna D, Yan X, Tashkin DP, et al. Impact of oral cyclophosphamide on health-related quality of life in patients with active scleroderma lung disease: results from the scleroderma lung study. Arthritis Rheum 2007;56:1676–1684.

77. Lin ATH, Clements PJ, Furst DE. Update on disease-modifying anti-rheumatic drugs in the treatment of systemic sclerosis. Rheum Dis Clin North Am 2003;29:409–426.

78. Ong VH, Brough G, Denton CP. Management of systemic sclerosis. Clin Med 2005;5:214–219.

79. Amato AA, Barohn RJ. Evaluation and treatment of inflammatory myopathies. J Neurol Neurosurg Psychiatry 2009;80:1060–1068.

80. Wiendl H. Idiopathic inflammatory myopathies: current and future therapeutic options. Neurotherapeutics 2008;5:548–557.

81. Dalakas MC, Hohlfeld R. Polymyositis and dermatomyositis. Lancet 2003;362:971–982.

82. Weyand CM, Goronzy JJ. Giant-cell arteritis and polymyalgia rheumatica. Ann Intern Med 2003;139:505–515.

83. Kawasaki A, Purvin V. Giant cell arteritis: an updated review. Acta Ophthalmol 2009;87:13–32.

84. Hernández-Rodríguez J, Cid MC, López-Soto A, et al. Treatment of polymyalgia rheumatica: a systematic review. Arch Intern Med 2009;169:1839–1850.

85. Gonzalez-Gay MA, Vazquez-Rodriguez TR, Lopez-Diaz MJ, et al. Epidemiology of giant cell arteritis and polymyalgia rheumatica. Arthritis Rheum 2009;61:1454–1461.

86. Weyand CM, Goronzy JJ. Medium- and large-vessel vasculitis. N Engl J Med 2003;349:160–169.

87. Salvarani C, Cantini F, Hunder GG. Polymyalgia rheumatica and giant-cell arteritis. Lancet 2008;372:234–245.

88. Unwin B, Williams CM, Gillilans W. Polymyalgia rheumatica and giant cell arteritis. Am Fam Physician 2006;74:1547–1554.

89. Gao Y, Zhao M. Review article: Drug-induced anti-neutrophil cytoplasmic antibody-associated vasculitis. Nephrol 2009;14:33–41.

90. Wiik A. Drug-induced vasculitis. Curr Opin Rheumatol 2008;20:35–39.

91. Griffiths B, Mosca M, Gordon C. Assessment of patients with systemic lupus erythematosus and the use of lupus disease activity indices. Best Pract Res Clin Rheumatol 2005;19:685–708.

CHAPTER 97

Allergic and Pseudoallergic Drug Reactions

LYNNE M. SYLVIA AND JOSEPH T. DIPIRO

KEY CONCEPTS

❶ Hypersensitivity reactions are responsible for 6% to 10% of adverse reactions to medications. Although some reactions are relatively well defined, the majority are due to mechanisms that are either unknown or poorly understood.

❷ The following criteria suggest that a drug reaction may be immunologically mediated: (a) the reaction occurs in a small percentage of patients receiving the drug, (b) the observed reaction does not resemble the drug's pharmacologic effect, (c) the type of manifestation is similar to that seen with other allergic reactions (anaphylaxis, urticaria, serum sickness), (d) there is a lag time between first exposure of the drug and reaction, (e) the reaction is reproduced even by minute doses of the drug, (f) the reaction is reproduced by agents with similar chemical structures, (g) eosinophilia is present, or (h) the reaction resolves after the drug has been discontinued. Exceptions to each of these criteria are observed commonly.

❸ Anaphylaxis is an acute, life-threatening allergic reaction involving multiple organ systems that generally begins within 30 minutes but almost always within 2 hours after exposure to the inciting allergen. Anaphylaxis requires prompt treatment to restore respiratory and cardiovascular function. Epinephrine is administered as primary treatment to counteract bronchoconstriction and vasodilation. Intravenous fluids should be administered to restore intravascular volume.

❹ Factors that influence the likelihood of allergic drug reactions are the chemical composition of the drug, whether the drug contains proteins of nonhuman origin, the route of drug administration, and the sensitivity of the individual as determined by genetics, or environmental factors. For some drugs, genetic predisposition to specific HLA alleles has been identified as a risk factor for allergic-mediated skin reactions.

❺ Patients with a history of an immediate reaction to penicillin are advised not to receive cephalosporins if they can be avoided. Patients who have negative penicillin skin tests or experienced only mild cutaneous reactions, such as maculopapular rashes, have a low risk of serious reactions to cephalosporins.

❻ Less than 1% of patients receiving nonionic radiocontrast agents experience some type of adverse reaction. Of the variety of reactions reported, approximately 90% are allergic like, mostly urticarial, with severe reactions occurring as infrequently as 0.02%.

❼ Aspirin and other nonsteroidal anti-inflammatory drugs (NSAIDs) can produce two general types of reactions, urticaria/angioedema and rhinosinusitis/asthma, in susceptible patients. About 20% of asthmatics are sensitive to aspirin and other NSAIDs.

❽ Cross-reactivity between sulfonamide antibiotics and nonantibiotics is low. The low cross-reactive rate may be explained by differences in the chemical structures and reactive metabolites of the sulfonamide antibiotics and nonantibiotics.

❾ The basic principles of management of allergic reactions to drugs or biologic agents include (a) discontinuation of the medication or agent when possible, (b) treatment of the adverse clinical signs and symptoms, and (c) substitution, if necessary, of another agent.

❿ One of the most helpful tests to evaluate risk of penicillin allergy is the skin test. Skin testing can demonstrate the presence of penicillin-specific immunoglobulin E and predict a relatively high risk of immediate hypersensitivity reactions. Skin testing does not predict the risk of delayed reactions or most dermatologic reactions.

---

❶ *Allergic drug reactions, also known as hypersensitivity reactions,* result from an over-response of the immune system to the standard dose of a drug. The hyper-response of the immune system to the antigenic drug leads to host tissue damage manifesting as an organ-specific or generalized systemic reaction. Adverse drug effects not proven to be immune mediated but resembling allergic reactions in their clinical presentation are referred to as *allergic-like* or *pseudoallergic reactions.* Immunologically mediated adverse drug reactions account for 6% to 10% of all adverse drug reactions and even up to 15% by some estimates.[1,2] Examples of allergic drug reactions are anaphylaxis from β-lactam antibiotics, halothane hepatitis, Stevens Johnson syndrome from sulfonamides, allopurinol hypersensitivity syndrome and serum sickness from phenytoin.[3] Examples of pseudoallergic reactions are shock after radiocontrast media, aspirin-induced asthma, opiate-related urticaria, and flushing after vancomycin infusion.[3]

The true frequency of allergic drug reactions is difficult to determine because many reactions may not be reported, and others may be difficult to distinguish from nonallergic adverse events. Dermatologic reactions represent the most frequently recognized and reported form of allergic drug reaction.[4]

TABLE 97-1 Classification of Allergic Drug Reactions

Type	Descriptor	Characteristics	Typical Onset	Drug Causes
I	Anaphylactic (IgE mediated)	Allergen binds to IgE on basophils or mast cells, resulting in release of inflammatory medicators.	Within 30 min to <2 hours	Penicillin immediate reaction Blood products Polypeptide hormones Vaccines Dextran
II	Cytotoxic	Cell destruction occurs because of cell-associated antigen that initiates cytolysis by antigen-specific antibody (IgG or IgM). Most often involves blood elements.	Typically >72 h	Penicillin, quinidine, heparin, phenylbutazone, thiouracils, sulfonamides, methyldopa
III	Immune complex	Antigen–antibody complexes form and deposit on blood vessel walls and activate complement. Result is a serum sickness-like syndrome.	>72 h	May be caused by penicillins, sulfonamides, minocycline, hydantoins
IV	Cell-mediated (delayed)	Antigens cause activation of T lymphocytes, which release cytokines and recruit effector cells (e.g., macrophages, eosinophils).	>72 h	Tuberculin reaction Maculopapular rashes to a variety of drugs; Contact dermatitis Bullous exanthems Pustular exanthems

MECHANISMS OF ALLERGIC DRUG REACTIONS

Drugs can cause hypersensitivity reactions by a variety of immunologic mechanisms. Although some reactions are relatively well defined, most are due to mechanisms that are either unknown or poorly understood.[2,3]

❷ The following criteria suggest that a drug reaction may be immunologically mediated: (a) the observed reaction does not resemble the drug's pharmacologic effect, (b) there is a lag time between first exposure of the drug and reaction unless the recipient has been sensitized by prior exposure to the drug, which can lead to immediate reactions, (c) the reaction may occur even by minute doses of the drug, (d) the symptoms are characteristic of an allergic reaction (e.g., anaphylaxis, urticaria, serum sickness), (e) the reaction resolves after the drug has been discontinued, and (f) the reaction may be reproduced by agents with similar chemical structures.[2] Exceptions to each of these criteria are observed commonly. Many allergic reactions can be classified into one of four immunopathologic categories: type I, II, III, or IV (Table 97–1 and Fig. 97–1).[2,3]

EFFECTORS OF ALLERGIC DRUG REACTIONS

Allergic drug reactions can involve most of the major components of the innate and adaptive immune systems, including the cellular elements, immunoglobulins, complement, and cytokines. Most immunoglobulin isotypes have been implicated in immunologically mediated drug reactions. Immunoglobulin E (IgE) bound to basophils or mast cells mediates immediate (anaphylactic-type) reactions. IgG or IgM antibodies also may be involved in allergic reactions, resulting in destruction of cells and tissues. T lymphocytes have a major role in hypersensitivity reactions and are involved in all four types (I–IV) of the drug hypersensitivity reactions described by Coombs and Gell.[2,5,6]

CELLULAR ELEMENTS

A variety of cells are involved in drug hypersensitivity. Antigen-presenting cells (APCs) include macrophages, dendritic cells, and cutaneous Langerhan cells. APCs process the antigenic drug for subsequent recognition by T and B lymphocytes. Basophils and mast cells are instrumental in the development of immediate hypersensitivity reactions, whereas eosinophils are recruited in both immediate and nonimmediate reactions. Platelets and vascular endothelial cells are important because they also can release a number of inflammatory mediators.[7] Most cells of the body, including nerve cells, can become involved directly or indirectly in allergic drug reactions.

MEDIATORS OF ALLERGIC REACTIONS

The release of a number of preformed, pharmacologically active chemical mediators (e.g., histamine, heparin, proteases such as

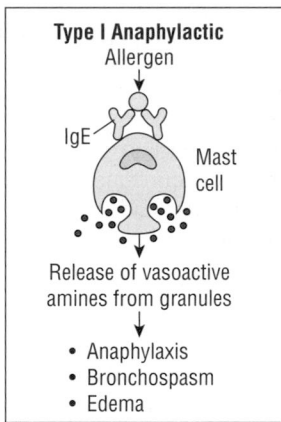
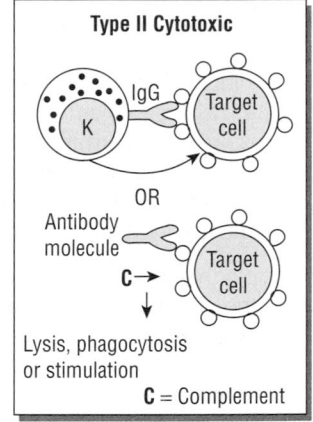
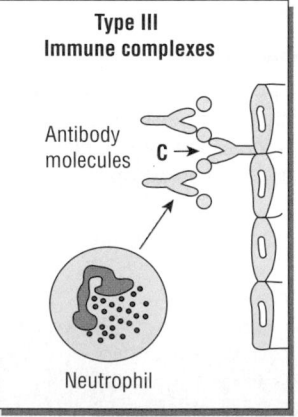
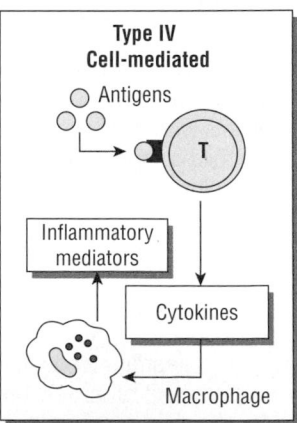

FIGURE 97-1. Types of hypersensitivity reactions.

tryptase and chymase, and a variety of other enzymes) is triggered when antigens cross-link IgE molecules on the surface of circulating basophils and tissue mast cells. Newly formed mediators include platelet-activating factor and arachidonic acid metabolites (e.g., prostaglandins, thromboxanes, and leukotrienes).

Histamine is a low-molecular-weight amine compound formed by decarboxylation of histidine and is stored in basophil and mast cell granules.[8] Release of histamine from these cells is triggered by antigen cross-linking IgE bound to specific receptors on the surface membranes of mast cells and basophils. The tissue effects of histamine are evident within 1 to 2 minutes, but it is rapidly metabolized within 10 to 15 minutes. The major effects of histamine on target tissues include increased capillary permeability, contraction of bronchial and vascular smooth muscle, and hypersecretion of mucus glands. Four classes of histamine receptors (H_1–H_4) are present to varying degrees in organs and tissues. H_1 receptors are most prominent in blood vessels and bronchial and intestinal smooth muscle.

Platelet-activating factor (PAF) is a glyceride-derived substance that is released by mast cells, alveolar macrophages, neutrophils, platelets, and other cells but not by basophils. It has potent bronchoconstrictor effects and causes platelet aggregation and lysis. It attracts neutrophils and causes their activation. PAF enhances vascular permeability and can cause pain, pruritus, and erythema.

The leukotrienes (LTs) are metabolites of arachidonic acid produced through the 5-lipoxygenase pathway that have potent effects on bronchial and vascular smooth muscle. Three important leukotrienes, LTC_4, LTD_4, and LTE_4, are produced by basophils or mast cells. These three substances are also referred to as *cysteinyl leukotrienes* and in older literature as *slow-reacting substances of anaphylaxis*. The LTs have more potent and longer-lasting bronchoconstrictor effects than histamine and can increase vascular permeability and cause arteriolar vasoconstriction followed by vasodilation. Their effects are slower in onset but longer lasting than those of histamine. Another product, LTB_4, is a potent chemoattractant, particularly for neutrophils. It is also produced by neutrophils, macrophages, and monocytes.

Prostaglandins (PGs) and thromboxanes are metabolites of arachidonic acid produced through the cyclooxygenase pathway. Some PGs have vasoconstrictive and/or bronchodilatory properties, whereas others are vasodilatory and/or bronchoconstrictive. PGD_2 is the major PG product of mast cells. It is a potent inhibitor of platelet aggregation and is a bronchoconstrictor. Thromboxanes cause platelet aggregation and are important regulators of coagulation.

The complement system consists of approximately 30 plasma proteins and is involved in hypersensitivity through a variety of immunologic responses, including enhancement of phagocytosis (opsonization of target cells), cell lysis, and generation of anaphylatoxins (C3a, C4a, and C5a), which can cause non–IgE-mediated activation of mast cells and release of inflammatory mediators.

CLASSIFICATION OF IMMUNOPATHOLOGIC DRUG REACTIONS

Immunologic mechanisms have been identified for some drug reactions, and many can be classified into one of four immunopathologic reactions, first described by Coombs and Gell. Small-molecular-weight molecules (<10 kDa) do not have the ability to serve as antigens on their own. With the exception of polypeptide compounds, most drugs are <1,000 Da. To become immunogenic, these small compounds must first covalently bind to carrier proteins in plasma or tissue. The combination of the drug bound to a carrier protein can be recognized as foreign by APCs and T

lymphocytes, culminating in an immune response. The more likely that large amounts of the drug become chemically bound to a protein, the greater the risk of producing an allergic reaction. Penicillin G (356 Da) is an example of a drug that binds covalently to serum proteins through amide or disulfide linkages. For drugs such as the sulfonamides, the parent compound first must be converted to a metabolite before it can combine with the macromolecule. The species that combines with the carrier macromolecule is referred to as a *hapten* or an *incomplete antigen*.[9] Some macromolecular drugs such as insulin are referred to as *complete antigens* because they are large enough to initiate an immune response without binding to another protein. Some small-molecular-weight drugs may cause an immune response through a non-hapten pathway.[5] Known as the p-i concept, this pathway involves a pharmacological interaction between the drug and the T-cell receptor that does not require the initial binding of the drug to a carrier protein or processing by APCs.[6]

TYPE I

Type I reactions require the presence of IgE specific for the drug or the portion of the drug that becomes a hapten. IgE specific for the drug allergen is produced on initial exposure to the drug. It then binds to basophils and mast cells through high-affinity receptors. On repeat exposure to the drug, two or more IgE molecules on the basophil or mast cell surface may bind to one multivalent antigen molecule (referred to as *cross-linking*; see Fig. 97–1), initiating an activation of the cell. Activation causes the extracellular release of granules with preformed inflammatory mediators, including histamine, heparin, proteases (tryptase in the mast cell), as well as generation of newly formed mediators, as previously discussed, such as LTs, PGs, thromboxanes, and PAF, among others.

Generation of a type I reaction can be evident as an immediate hypersensitivity reaction, or anaphylaxis. Immediate reactions may be limited to single organs, typically in the nasal mucosa (rhinitis), respiratory tract (acute asthma), skin, or gastrointestinal tract, or they can involve multiple organs simultaneously, termed *anaphylaxis*.

TYPE II

Type II immunopathologic reactions involve destruction of host cells (usually blood cells) through cytotoxic antibodies by one of two mechanisms (see Fig. 97–1). First, the drug binds to the cell as a hapten (e.g., the platelet or red blood cell). Antibodies (IgG or IgM) specific for the bound drug or to a component of the cell surface that has been altered by the drug then bind, initiating a cytolytic reaction. Cell destruction may be mediated by complement or by phagocytic cells that have antibody Fc receptors on their surfaces. Activation of complement near the cell surface can result in loss of cell membrane integrity and cell death. Alternatively, neutrophils, monocytes, or macrophages may bind to an antibody-coated cell through IgG Fc receptors on their cell surfaces, resulting in phagocytosis of the target cell. The process of enhancement of phagocytosis by antibody binding to cell surfaces or other particles is referred to as *opsonization*. In addition, cell-bound IgG may direct the non-phagocytic action of T cells or natural killer cells, which results in cell destruction by a process called *antibody-dependent cellular cytotoxicity*. This process can proceed in a nonspecific fashion as T cells bind to the target cell through IgG Fc receptors on the T-cell surface. Contact between the target and effector cells is necessary.

Cells commonly affected by these types of reactions include erythrocytes, leukocytes, and platelets, resulting in hemolytic anemia, agranulocytosis, or thrombocytopenia, respectively. This process may be initiated by drugs such as penicillin, quinidine, quinine, phenacetin, cephalosporins, and sulfonamides.

Another type of reaction that may affect the formed elements in blood is the "innocent bystander" reaction. With this type of reaction, antigen–antibody complexes formed in blood adhere nonspecifically to cells. Complement is then activated, resulting in cell lysis.

TYPE III

Type III immunologic reactions are caused by antigen–antibody complexes that are formed in blood. The complexes form with drug allergen and antibody in varying ratios and may deposit in tissues, resulting in local or disseminated inflammatory reactions. Antigen–antibody complex formation can result in platelet aggregation, complement activation, or macrophage activation. Chemotactic substances such as C4a also are produced. These substances cause the influx of neutrophils and result in the release of a number of toxic substances from the neutrophil (e.g., proteinases, collagenases, kinin-generating enzymes, and reactive oxygen and nitrogen substances), which can cause local tissue destruction.

Platelet aggregation may occur as a result of immune-complex formation, resulting in the formation of microthrombi and the release of vasoactive mediators. Also, insoluble complexes may be phagocytized by macrophages and activate these cells.

The formation of antigen–antibody complexes can lead to clinical syndromes such as the Arthus reaction. In this model, a high level of preformed specific IgG antibody combines with antigen to produce a localized edematous, erythematous reaction within 5 to 8 hours. The reaction involves local formation of insoluble antigen–antibody complexes, complement activation with release of C3a and C5a collectively referred to as *anaphylatoxins,* mast cell degranulation, and influx of polymorphonuclear cells.

TYPE IV

Type IV reactions are delayed hypersensitivity reactions that typically are demonstrated as dermatologic events mediated by T cells (CD4[+] or CD8[+]).[5,6] The Coombs and Gell classification of allergic drug reactions was developed prior to our understanding of the varied roles of T cells in the immune response. Four subclasses of type IV reactions (IVa–IVd) have been described.[5,6] In this subclassfication system, type IV reactions are differentiated based on the responding T cell (e.g., T helper type 1 cell, T helper type 2 cell, cytotoxic T cell), effector mechanism (e.g., recruitment of macrophages, eosinophils, or neutrophils) and clinical manifestations (e.g., contact dermatitis, bullous exanthems, maculopapular eruptions, pustular exanthems).[5,6] Type IV reactions require memory T cells specific for the antigen in question. On exposure to the antigen, the immune response is mediated by a specific subtype of T cell that orchestrates an inflammatory response through the secretion of cytokines and the recruitment of effector cells. These reactions are associated with a wide variety of adverse effects (e.g., contact dermatitis, maculopapular exanthemas, bullous exanthemas, eczema, or pustular exanthemas), and they also may be useful for diagnostic purposes. Examples of the latter include the purified protein derivative (PPD) antigen from *Mycobacterium tuberculosis* used in the tuberculin skin test and other recall skin test antigens, such as mumps. After intradermal injection, these antigens produce a local reaction (erythema and induration) within 48 to 72 hours. Delayed contact hypersensitivity also can be caused by a wide variety of chemicals and drugs.

OTHER ALLERGIC REACTIONS

The precise mechanism of many drug reactions is not known, although the reactions are believed to be immune mediated. Perhaps most common are the delayed dermatologic reactions that occur with a variety of drugs (especially penicillins and sulfonamides). These reactions may be evident as fixed drug eruptions, macropapular, morbilliform, or erythematous rashes; exfoliative dermatitis; photosensitivity reactions; or eczema. These reactions also may be manifest as late onset pruritus, urticaria, and angioedema.

A number of serious cutaneous adverse reactions, known as SCARs, may be the result of immunologic reactions. SCARs include drug rash with eosinophilia and systemic symptoms (DRESS) and the mucocutaneous disorders, Stevens Johnson syndrome (SJS) and toxic epidermal necrolysis (TEN). Drug-induced fever also may involve immunologic mechanisms. Other general types of reactions believed to be immune mediated in some cases include hepatic drug reactions (cholestatic or hepatocellular) and pulmonary reactions, for example, interstitial pneumonitis, which has been associated with nitrofurantoin.

ANAPHYLACTOID REACTIONS

Various drugs and other substances can produce anaphylactoid (anaphylaxis-like) reactions that are similar to anaphylaxis in clinical signs and symptoms. The substances causing these reactions can lead to the direct release or activation of inflammatory mediators from cells by a pharmacologic or physical effect rather than through cell-bound IgE. These reactions are the most severe form of pseudoallergy, but not all pseudoallergic reactions are anaphylactoid. Pseudoallergy refers to a wide array of reactions ranging from localized hives to life-threatening angioedema, hypotension, and anaphylaxis, all of which are explained by the nonimmunologic release or activation of inflammatory mediators. Drugs that can produce anaphylactoid reactions include vancomycin, opiates, iodinated radiocontrast agents, angiotensin-converting enzyme inhibitors, amphotericin B, and D-tubocurarine. The "red man syndrome" is a common example of a pseudoallergic reaction from vancomycin. If vancomycin is infused too rapidly, it can cause the direct release of histamine and other mediators from cutaneous mast cells, producing a typical clinical picture of itching, flushing, and hives, first around the neck and face and then progressing to the chest and other parts of the body usually beginning shortly after the infusion has begun. In some cases, the cutaneous manifestations of "red man syndrome" may be accompanied by hypotension, thereby constituting an anaphylactoid event. Most patients who have had "red man syndrome" will tolerate vancomycin if the rate of infusion is slowed. In rare cases, the severity of the reaction may preclude continued therapy with vancomycin. A number of other agents (including aspirin) may produce anaphylactoid reactions by altering the metabolism of inflammatory mediators such as PGs or kinins. Angioedema from angiotensin-converting enzyme inhibitors is a classic example of an anaphylactoid reaction. Although the mechanism by which this anaphylactic-like event occurs is not fully understood, inhibition of the breakdown of bradykinin and substance P by the angiotensin-converting enzyme inhibitor may explain the inflammation, increased vascular permeability and vasodilation.

CLINICAL MANIFESTATIONS OF ALLERGIC AND ALLERGIC-LIKE REACTIONS

ANAPHYLAXIS

❸ Anaphylaxis is an acute, life-threatening allergic reaction involving multiple organ systems that occurs in 10 to 20 per 100,000 population per year.[10,11] Approximately 1,500 deaths from anaphylaxis occur annually in the United States.[12] From 1.2% to 15% of the U.S. population may be at risk for anaphylactic reactions.[13]

Although many drugs may cause anaphylaxis (or anaphylactoid) reactions, the most commonly reported are penicillins, aspirin and other NSAIDs, and insulins.[10] In most patients, the initial signs and symptoms are referable to the skin (flushing, pruritus, urticaria, angioedema). The second most common symptoms are respiratory (tightness of the throat and chest, dysphagia, dysphonia and hoarseness, cough, stridor, shortness of breath, dyspnea, congestion, rhinorrhea, sneezing) followed by dizziness and gastrointestinal tract symptoms (nausea, crampy abdominal pain, vomiting, diarrhea).[14] Ten percent to 30% of patients develop hypotension. Additional cardiovascular effects include syncope, altered mental status, chest pain, and dysrhythmia.[11]

A consensus panel has constructed a definition of anaphylaxis as follows.[11,15] Anaphylaxis is highly likely when any one of the following three criteria are fulfilled:

1. Acute onset of an illness (minutes to several hours) with involvement of the skin, mucosal tissue, or both (e.g., generalized hives, pruritus or flushing, swollen lips/tongue/uvula) AND at least one of the following:
   - Respiratory compromise (e.g., dyspnea, wheeze/bronchospasm, stridor, reduced peak expiratory flow, hypoxemia)
   - Reduced blood pressure or associated symptoms of end-organ dysfunction (e.g., hypotonia, syncope, incontinence)

2. Two or more of the following that occur rapidly after exposure to a likely allergen (minutes to several hours):
   - Involvement of skin/mucosal tissue (as above)
   - Respiratory compromise (as above)
   - Reduced blood pressure or associated symptoms
   - Persistent gastrointestinal symptoms (e.g., crampy abdominal pain, vomiting)

3. Reduced blood pressure after exposure to known allergen (minutes to several hours)

The panel indicated that other presentations may indicate anaphylaxis and that the potential exists for false-positive results.

Anaphylactic reactions generally begin within 30 minutes but almost always within 2 hours of exposure to the inciting allergen. The risk of fatal anaphylaxis is greatest within the first few hours. After apparent recovery, anaphylaxis may recur 6 to 8 hours after antigen exposure. Because of the possibility of these "late-phase" reactions, patients should be observed for at least 12 hours after an anaphylactic reaction. Fatal anaphylaxis most often results from asphyxia due to airway obstruction either at the larynx or within the lungs. Cardiovascular collapse may occur as a result of asphyxia in some cases, whereas in others cases cardiovascular collapse may be the dominant manifestation from the release of mediators within the heart muscles and coronary blood vessels.

SERUM SICKNESS AND SERUM SICKNESS-LIKE DISEASE

Serum sickness is a clinical syndrome resulting from the effects of soluble circulating immune complexes that form under conditions of antigen excess. The reaction commonly results from the use of antisera containing foreign (donor) antigens such as equine serum in the form of antitoxins or antivenoms. The onset of serum sickness is usually 7 to 14 days after antigen administration. The onset may be more rapid with reexposure to the same agent in an individual with prior serum sickness. Fever, malaise, and lymphadenopathy are the most common clinical manifestations. Arthralgias, urticaria, and morbilliform skin eruption also may be present. A milder and more transient form of serum sickness is serum sickness-like disease (SSLD). The predominant feature of SSLD is a cutaneous eruption, either urticarial or maculopapular, that occurs within 5 to 21 days of drug administration.[16] As with serum sickness, the rash is usually preceded by a prodromal phase consisting of fever, malaise, lymphadenopathy, and arthralgias. SSLD has been associated with the administration of ciprofloxacin, bupropion, hydantoins, minocycline, sulfonamides, penicillins, and cephalosporins (especially cefaclor). SSLD is usually self-limiting after discontinuation of the causative agent, but it can sometimes progress to include vasculitis.

DRUG RASH WITH EOSINOPHILIA AND SYSTEMIC SYMPTOMS (DRESS)

Previously known by the term *drug hypersensitivity syndrome*, the triad of rash, eosinophilia and internal organ involvement is currently referred to as drug rash with eosinophilia and systemic symptoms (DRESS). Bocquet and colleagues[17] described the following criteria for a diagnosis of DRESS: (1) cutaneous drug eruption (usually a diffuse maculopapular rash accompanied by facial and neck edema); (2) hematologic abnormalities including eosinophilia greater than 1,500 cells/mm³ (1.5×10^9/L) or the presence of atypical lymphocytes; and (3) systemic involvement including adenopathies greater than 2 cm in diameter, hepatitis, interstitial nephritis, interstitial pneumonia or carditis.[17] Both the allopurinol hypersensitivity syndrome and anticonvulsant hypersensitivity syndrome are examples of DRESS.[18] Other drugs associated with DRESS include minocycline, dapsone, lamotrigine and the sulfonamides. The onset of DRESS is typically delayed ranging from 3 to 8 weeks after drug initiation, and there is a high degree of interpatient variability in the targeted organs and the severity of organ involvement.[17,18] The mortality rate associated with DRESS is 10% and it is largely attributed to systemic involvement of the liver, kidneys, or lungs.[18] Following discontinuation of the causative drug, the skin rash resolves and laboratory abnormalities normalize over a period of 4 to 8 weeks. Systemic corticosteroids (0.5–1 mg/kg/day prednisone or steroid equivalent) have been used in the treatment of DRESS based on the severity of organ involvement.

DRUG FEVER

Fever may occur in response to an inflammatory process or develop as a manifestation of a drug reaction. Drug fever occurs in as many as 10% of hospital inpatients.[19] Many drugs have been reported to cause fever, including acyclovir, heparin, methyldopa, procainamide, phenytoin, barbiturates, quinidine, and a variety of antibiotics (e.g., β-lactams, rifampin, sulfonamides, tetracycline, vancomycin). These drugs may affect the central nervous system directly to alter temperature regulation or stimulate the release of endogenous pyrogens (e.g., interleukin 1 and tumor necrosis factor) from white blood cells. Drugs also may cause fever as a result of their pharmacologic effects on tissues, for example, fever resulting from massive tumor cell destruction caused by chemotherapy. However, the mechanism of drug fever remains unknown for agents such as amphotericin B and radiographic contrast agents.

The temperature pattern of drug-induced fever is quite variable and therefore of little help in the diagnosis. It may be low grade and continuous or spiking and intermittent. A temporal relationship between drug administration and occurrence of fever has been noted for some medications. Generally, withdrawal of the causative agent results in prompt defervescence as soon as the drug is eliminated completely. Fever usually recurs on readministration of the causative agent.

DRUG-INDUCED AUTOIMMUNITY

Autoimmune diseases have been associated with drugs and may involve a variety of tissues and organs. A commonly recognized drug-related autoimmune disorder is systemic lupus erythematosus (SLE) induced by infliximab, etanercept, procainamide, hydralazine, quinidine, or isoniazid.[20] Exposure of susceptible persons to these agents appears to alter normal body proteins, RNA, or DNA in such a way as to make these components antigenic, leading to the formation of autoreactive antibodies and cells. Most patients treated with infliximab develop antinuclear antibodies, but only 2% of patients present with SLE symptoms. The most common clinical manifestations include arthralgias, myalgias, and polyarthritis. Facial rash, ulcers, and alopecia occur less frequently. Renal or pulmonary involvement also may occur. These reactions typically develop several months after beginning the drug and generally resolve soon after the drug is discontinued.[21]

Other syndromes believed to involve autoimmune mechanisms include drug-induced hemolytic anemia attributed to methyldopa, interstitial nephritis produced by methicillin, and hepatitis caused by phenytoin and halothane. Interstitial nephritis is characterized by fever, rash, and eosinophilia associated with proteinuria and hematuria. Hepatic damage due to drugs generally is manifested as either hepatocellular necrosis or cholestatic hepatitis. Drug-induced hepatitis has been associated with phenothiazines, sulfonamides, halothane, phenytoin, and isoniazid (see Chapter 45). Hepatocellular destruction is evidenced by elevations in serum transaminases. Hepatomegaly and jaundice sometimes may be evident. Cholestasis may be manifested by jaundice and elevations in serum alkaline phosphatase and sometimes by rash, fever, and eosinophilia.

VASCULITIS

Vasculitis is a clinicopathologic process characterized by inflammation and necrosis of blood vessel walls. The vasculitic process may be limited to the skin, or it may involve multiple organs, including the liver or kidney, joints, or central nervous system. Characteristically, cutaneous vasculitis is manifested by purpuric lesions that vary in size and number. Vasculitis also may be manifested as papules, nodules, ulcerations, or vesiculobullous lesions, generally occurring on the lower extremities but sometimes involving the upper extremities, including the hands. Drugs associated with vasculitis include allopurinol, β-lactam antibiotics, sulfonamides, thiazide diuretics, phenytoin, and vancomycin.

DERMATOLOGIC REACTIONS

A wide variety of dermatologic drug reactions have been reported to have an immunologic basis.[2,22] Cutaneous reactions are the most common manifestations of allergic drug reactions. Although most dermatologic reactions are mild and resolve promptly after discontinuing the drug, some such as SJS and TEN are serious or even life-threatening reactions. Both SJS and TEN are classified as progressive bullous or "blistering" disorders that constitute dermatologic emergencies.[23] They are considered severe variants of erythema multiforme. Similar to erythema multiforme, SJS and TEN are associated with the widespread development of a variety of skin lesions including macules, purpuric lesions and the target iris lesion. The target lesion is discrete, round, and identified by an area of central clearing surrounded by two concentric rings of edema and erythema. Unlike erythema multiforme, SJS and TEN are most commonly drug-induced rather than associated with recurrent herpes simplex viral infection, and they progress to include mucous membrane erosion and epidermal detachment.[23] Mucosal

membranes in the mouth, lips, nasal cavity, and conjunctivae are usually involved. As these syndromes progress, the erythematous lesions become more widespread on the face, trunk, and extremities, and many evolve into blisters. Within days after the onset of the lesions, full-thickness epidermal detachment occurs. SJS and TEN are often considered as a continuous spectrum of a disease, with TEN being the most severe form. The extent of epidermal detachment is used to distinguish between SJS and TEN (i.e., <10% detachment of body surface area with SJS; >30% detachment of body surface area with TEN). The term *SJS-TEN overlap* is used to describe cases in which epidermal detachment occurs on 10% to 30% of the body surface area.[23,24] Both SJS and TEN are associated with a number of long-term sequelae including permanent visual impairment, temporary nail loss, cutaneous scarring and irregular pigmentation. Being the more severe form, TEN is also more likely to be complicated by systemic organ involvement including acute kidney failure, neutropenia, and respiratory failure. A severity-of-illness scoring system known as SCORTEN has been developed to predict prognosis in patients with TEN.[25] SCORTEN uses seven independent risk factors based on an assessment within 24 hours of clinical presentation.

Cutaneous adverse reactions were reported to occur in 2.7% of hospitalized patients.[26] TEN is estimated to occur in 0.4 to 1.3 cases per 1 million people per year while SJS has been reported in 1 to 6 cases per 1 million people per year.[27,28] The mortality rates associated with SJS and TEN range from 1% to 5% and 10% to 70%, respectively.[28] Table 97–2 lists drugs and agents associated most commonly with cutaneous reactions.[22] In general, antimicrobials are implicated most frequently as the cause of cutaneous events with reaction rates ranging from 1% to 8%. The most likely offenders of SJS and TEN, determined in case-control studies, are the sulfonamides, particularly trimethoprim-sulfamethoxazole.[29] Other major offenders of SJS and TEN identified in these studies are allopurinol, the aminopenicillins, carbamazepine, chlormezanone, cephalosporins, the imidazole antifungals, lamotrigine, nevirapine, the oxicam NSAIDs, phenytoin, quinolones, and the tetracyclines.[29]

RESPIRATORY REACTIONS

Drugs may produce upper or lower respiratory tract reactions, including rhinitis and asthma. Respiratory tract manifestations may result from direct injury to the airways or may occur as a component of a systemic reaction (e.g., anaphylaxis). Asthma may be induced by aspirin and other NSAIDs or by sulfites used as preservatives in foods and medications. Other pulmonary drug reactions believed to be immunologic include acute infiltrative and chronic fibrotic pulmonary reactions. The latter is often caused by antineoplastic agents such as bleomycin. For a more detailed discussion of drug-induced pulmonary disease, see Chapter 36.

TABLE 97-2	Top 10 Drugs or Agents Reported to Cause Skin Reactions	
		Reactions per 1,000 Recipients
Amoxicillin		51.4
Trimethoprim–sulfamethoxazole		33.8
Ampicillin		33.2
Iopodate		27.8
Blood		21.6
Cephalosporins		21.1
Erythromycin		20.4
Dihydralazine hydrochloride		19.1
Penicillin G		18.5
Cyanocobalamin		17.9

Data from Roujeau JC, Stern RS. N Engl J Med 1994;331:1272–1285.

HEMATOLOGIC REACTIONS

Most formed elements and soluble components of the hematopoietic system may be affected by immunologic drug reactions. Eosinophilia is a common manifestation of drug hypersensitivity and may be the only presenting sign. Hemolytic anemia may result from hypersensitivity to drugs. Other hematologic reactions include thrombocytopenia, granulocytopenia, and agranulocytosis. For a detailed discussion of hematologic drug reactions, see Chapter 112.

FACTORS RELATED TO THE OCCURRENCE OR SEVERITY OF ALLERGIC DRUG REACTIONS

❹ Among the factors that influence the likelihood of allergic drug reactions are the degree to which the drug and its metabolites bind covalently to human proteins, how the drug is metabolized, whether the drug contains proteins of nonhuman origin (e.g., chimeric monoclonal antibodies, streptokinase) or antigenic excipients (e.g., peanut oil, FD&C dyes, sulfites, soybean emulsion), the route of exposure, and the sensitivity of the individual as determined by genetics, and environmental factors. Hypersensitivity can occur with any dose of a drug, but sensitization is more likely to occur with continuous dosing rather than single dosing. Once a patient has become sensitized, the severity of a reaction is often determined by the dose and the duration of exposure. The route of administration may also influence drug sensitivity. The topical route of drug administration appears to be the most likely to sensitize and predispose to drug reactions. The oral route is the safest, and the parenteral route is the most hazardous for administration of drugs in sensitive individuals. Relatively few cases of immediate hypersensitivity-associated deaths with oral β-lactam antimicrobials have been reported.

Individual host factors are important in determining drug sensitivity. A genetic predisposition for some types of allergic reactions has been identified. The presence of genetically determined human leukocytic antigen (HLA) alleles increases susceptibility to a number of drug hypersensitivity syndromes. In patients infected with the human immunodeficiency virus (HIV), hypersensitivity to abacavir has been associated with the presence of *HLA-B*5701*.[30] Severe immune-mediated cutaneous reactions to allopurinol including SJS and TEN have been associated with the presence of *HLA-B*5801* in Han Chinese.[31] In this same patient population, the presence of *HLA-B*1502* increases the risk of SJS and TEN with carbamazepine, phenytoin and fosphenytion.[32] Genetic factors can also influence the metabolic deactivation of drugs via phase 1 and 2 metabolism. For example, slow acetylators of procainamide and hydralazine are at increased risk for SLE. Genes also encode for the type of T cell receptor and the specific cytokines involved in the signaling of allergic drug reactions.

Drug allergies appear to develop with equal frequency in atopic and nonatopic individuals. In addition, patients with a history of drug allergy appear to be at increased risk for adverse reactions to other pharmacologic agents.[3] Age seems to be related to the risk of allergic reactions, as they occur less frequently in children. This may be related to immaturity of the immune system or decreased exposure. The presence of some concurrent diseases, particularly viral infections, predisposes to drug reactions. Examples include the higher rate of morbilliform rash when ampicillin is administered to patients with infectious mononucleosis, the higher rate of reactions to trimethoprim-sulfamethoxazole in HIV-infected patients and the relationship between infection with human herpes-virus 6 (HHV-6) and the development of drug rash with eosinophilia and systemic symptoms (DRESS).

DRUGS COMMONLY CAUSING ALLERGIC OR ALLERGIC-LIKE DRUG REACTIONS

β-LACTAM ANTIMICROBIALS

Allergy to β-lactam antibiotics is commonly reported by patients in healthcare settings.[33] Allergic reactions to penicillin occur in 0.7% to 8% of treatment courses but was as high as 15% in one retrospective report of hospitalized patients treated with penicillin.[34,35] Although most patients reporting penicillin allergy do not have allergy, a reported history is associated with a higher likelihood of positive skin test reactivity.[36] Only 10% to 20% of patients reporting penicillin allergy are found to be allergic by skin testing.[36] Patients with a history of immediate penicillin allergy who have a negative penicillin skin test are unlikely to react on subsequent courses of penicillins.[37]

The most common reactions to penicillin include urticaria, pruritus, and angioedema. All four of the major types of hypersensitivity reactions have been reported with penicillin, as well as some reactions that do not fit into these categories. A wide variety of idiopathic reactions occur, such as maculopapular eruptions, eosinophilia, SJS, and exfoliative dermatitis. Cutaneous reactions can occur in up to 4.4% of treatment courses of penicillin[38] and in up to 8% with aminopenicillins.[39] The incidence of ampicillin rash is close to 100% in patients with viral infections such as infectious mononucleosis.[40]

Some aspects of the mechanism of penicillin immunogenicity have been determined. Because benzylpenicillin is a relatively small molecule (356 Da), it must combine with macromolecules (presumably proteins) to elicit an immune response. Penicillin is rapidly hydrolyzed to a number of reactive metabolites that have the ability to covalently link to proteins. Of these metabolites, 95% is in the form of benzylpenicilloyl that binds covalently to the lysine residues of proteins such as albumin through an amide linkage involving the β-lactam ring (Fig. 97–2). This penicilloyl–protein conjugate is referred to as the *major antigenic determinant*. The other penicillin metabolites such as penilloate and penicilloate bind in lesser quantities to proteins. These are referred to as *minor antigenic determinants*. The terms *major* and *minor* refer to the relative proportions of these conjugates that are formed and not to the clinical severity of the reactions generated. Immediate hypersensitivity reactions may be mediated by IgE for both minor and major determinants. In fact, the minor antigenic determinants are more likely to cause life-threatening anaphylactic reactions.

In addition to the major and minor determinants, unique side chain determinants may mediate allergy to some penicillins. Both the aminopenicillins and piperacillin may cause hypersensitivity reactions via unique side chains on their structures.[41,42] Therefore, a patient may exhibit hypersensitivity to amoxicillin or piperacillin via a side chain determinant while exhibiting no reactivity to other penicillins. Careful history taking is needed to identify patients with high likelihood of side-chain specific reactions. Skin testing with dilute concentrations of amoxicillin, ampicillin, and piperacillin has been used to aid in the determination of side-chain specific reactions.[43–45]

Patients who are allergic to penicillins also may be sensitive to other β-lactams.[46,47] The exact incidence of cross-reactivity between cephalosporins and penicillins is not known but is believed to be low.[45,46] The risk was originally reported as 10% to 15% in the 1970s when cephalosporins were contaminated with trace amounts of penicillin. Current estimates of the cross-reactive risk between penicillin and the first- and second-generation cephalosporins are 5% to 7.5% and as low as 1% between penicillin and the third- and fourth-generation cephalosporins.[48] One percent to 8% of patients

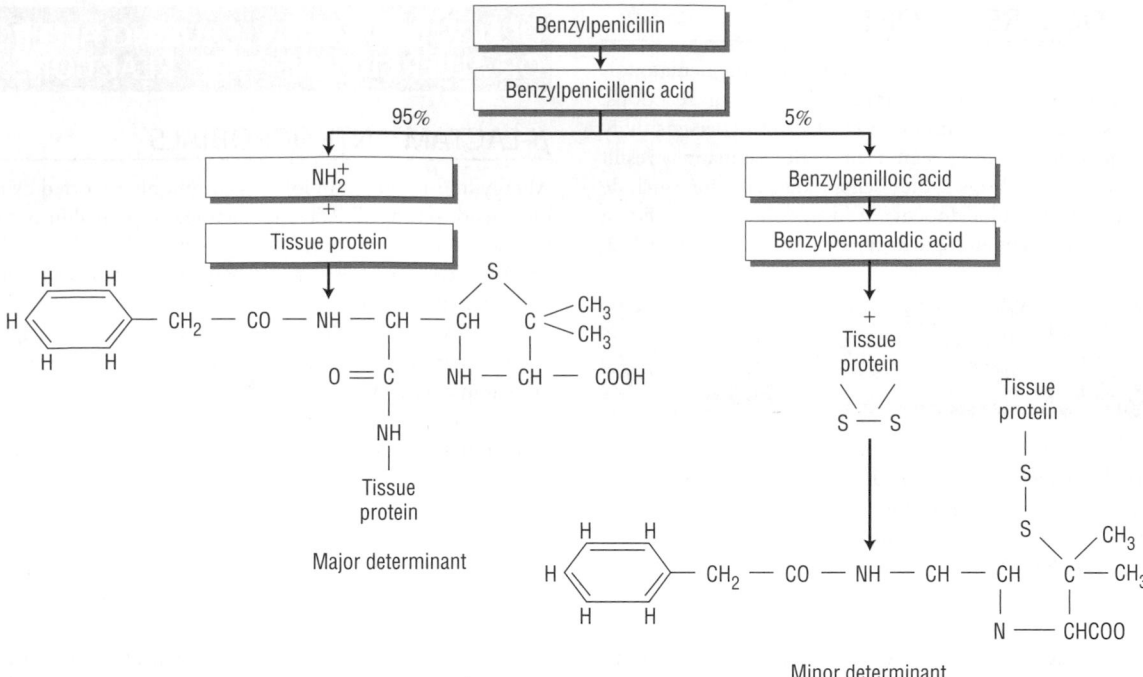

FIGURE 97-2. Formation of a benzylpenicilloyl hapten–protein complex.

with penicillin-specific IgE may develop an immediate-type hypersensitivity reaction to cephalosporins.[49] In contrast, patients with reported penicillin allergy and negative skin test are at no greater risk.[48]

❺ Cephalosporins should be avoided in patients with a history of hives or other immediate hypersensitivity reactions from penicillin, although some studies have suggested there is little risk of an allergic response to a cephalosporin even in a person with a positive skin test to penicillin. Based on the results of one meta-analysis, patients with penicillin allergy have the highest risk of cross-reactivity with the first generation cephalosporins (odds ratio [OR], 4.79; 95% confidence interval [CI], 3.71–6.17).[50] The odds of reacting to a second- and third-generation cephalosporin were 1.13 (95% CI, 0.61–2.12) and 0.45 (95% CI, 0.18–1.13), respectively.[50] The higher rate of cross-reactivity between penicillin and the first generation cephalosporins has been attributed to similarities in the R1 side chains of these agents.[45,46] The R1 side chain is connected to the opened β-lactam ring, thereby influencing the antigenicity of these agents. When assessing the potential for cross-reactivity between penicillins and cephalosporins, clinicians should evaluate the similarities in the R1 side chains of the agents.[45,46,50,51] Table 97–3 provides a list of penicillins and cephalosporins having similar side chains in the R1 position.

Cephalosporins can induce immune responses mediated by the core β-lactam structure or via unique side chain determinants.[46,48,50] In a patient with a cephalosporin allergy, skin testing with the major and minor determinants of penicillin can be used to identify the likelihood of reactivity to the core β-lactam ring. The risk of cross-reactivity between cephalosporins is considered to be higher than that between the penicillins and cephalosporins.[48] Cross-reactions may occur through identical R1 side chains. Of note, ceftazidime shares a common side chain with aztreonam.

The actual risk of a cross-reaction between the penicillins and the carbapenems appears to be much lower than originally described. The initial estimate of the cross-reactive risk was 47.4%, but current estimates range from 0.9% to 11%.[47] The initial estimate was based on the results of skin testing with penicillin and

nonstandardized carbapenem reagents. A number of retrospective studies reporting variable rates of cross-reactivity relied on self-reported histories as confirmation of penicillin allergy. Three recently published prospective studies used both skin testing methods and carbapenem challenge dosing to assess cross-reactive risk. In one of these studies, only 1 of 112 patients with skin test-confirmed penicillin allergy demonstrated a positive skin test to imipenem.[52] Challenge dosing with imipenem to a final dose of 500 mg was subsequently performed in 110 patients with negative imipenem skin tests; none of the 110 patients had a reaction. Results of two additional prospective studies, one of which was performed in children ages 3 to 14 years, suggest a low risk of cross-reactivity between penicillin and meropenem.[53,54] In both studies, only one patient with skin-test positivity to penicillin had a positive skin test to meropenem. Graded challenge dosing with meropenem was tolerated in 100% of the skin-test negative patients in both

TABLE 97-3	Chemical Similarities at the R1 Position (7 Position) of Commonly Used Penicillins and Cephalosporins

Similar Structure with Possibility of Cross-Sensitivity

Related	Related	Related
Penicillin G	Amoxicillin	Cefotaxime
Cephaloridine	Ampicillin	Ceftizoxime
Cephalothin	Cefaclor	Ceftriaxone
Cefoxitin	Cephalexin	Cefpodoxime
	Cephradine	Cefepime

Dissimilar Structure with Unlikely Cross-Reactivity

Not related	Not related
Cefazolin	Ceftazidime
Cefonicid	Cefamandole
Cefotetan	Cefixime
Cefuroxime	Ceftibuten
Cefoperazone	Cephapirin
Cefdinir	

studies. It is important to note that none of the skin-test negative patients were subsequently treated with full therapeutic regimens of the carbapenem. However, the high level of tolerability to challenge dosing suggests a low rate of cross-reactivity in skin-test negative patients. Based on these results, the routine practice of avoiding carbapenem use in patients with history of penicillin allergy should be reconsidered.[47]

Of the monobactams, aztreonam only weakly cross-reacts with penicillin and can be administered safely to most patients who are penicillin allergic.[47]

RADIOCONTRAST MEDIA

❻ Radiocontrast agents frequently cause reactions categorized as immediate (in ≤1 hour) or non-immediate (in 1–10 days) via both IgE-mediated and non-IgE–mediated mechanisms.[55] The frequency and severity of these reactions are influenced by the type of radiocontrast agent (ionic versus nonionic), and patient-specific factors such as history of atopy, asthma, or prior reaction to a radiocontrast agent. From <1% to >3% of patients receiving nonionic contrast media experienced an adverse reaction, with reports as high as 12.7% for mild reactions.[55,56] Delayed skin reactions, usually presenting as maculopapular exanthems, occur in 1% to 3% of patients over 5 to 7 days. Severe, immediate anaphylactic reactions occur in 0.01% to 0.04% of patients.[39] In addition, radiocontrast agents may cause dose-dependent toxic reactions that can produce renal impairment, cardiovascular effects, and arrhythmias.[57] The older, high-osmolar ionic agents that are now used less commonly have a greater frequency of reactions compared with the newer, low-osmolar agents.[55] The mechanism of reactions to radiocontrast agents is not clearly understood. Histamine release and mast cell triggering have been documented in severe immediate reactions, suggesting an IgE-mediated mechanism.[58] The older, high-osmolar radiocontrast agents can activate mast cells, basophils and the complement system directly (IgE-independent mechanism), resulting in the release of inflammatory mediators. The delayed-onset maculopapular rash appears to be T-cell mediated. The low-osmolar nonionic contrast agents appear to cause fewer anaphylactoid reactions.

The risk of anaphylactoid reactions to radiocontrast media is greater in women and in patients with a history of atopy or asthma.[55] Other recognized risk factors include a history of previous reaction, severe drug allergies, cardiac disease, and treatment with β-blockers.[56] Despite a common misconception, seafood allergy or iodine allergy does not predispose to radiocontrast media reactions. Neither skin tests nor oral tests are useful for predicting reactions to these agents. Although some regimens have been recommended to prevent the recurrence of immediate events in patients who have experienced reactions previously, the value of these preventive regimens has not been proven and their use remains controversial.[55,59] A commonly recommended regimen in high risk patients is oral prednisone (50 mg) 13, 7, and 1 hours before exposure with 50 mg of diphenhydramine given orally or intramuscularly 1 hour before exposure to prevent immediate reactions.[60] Ephedrine 25 mg orally has also been recommended 1 hour before the radiocontrast study as a component of the pretreatment regimen; however, ephedrine should not be used if the patient has history of unstable angina, hypertension or arrhythmia.[60] Other studies have examined the use of H_1- and H_2- antihistamines, clemastine, or cimetidine, respectively.[59]

INSULIN

Insulin is capable of producing allergic reactions through a variety of immunologic mechanisms. A protein molecule, insulin is a complete antigen. Allergic reactions have been reported with beef, pork, and recombinant human insulin, although the frequency of reactions with human insulin appears low. Reactions to insulin may involve the insulin molecule itself or other substances that have been added to insulin (e.g., protamine). Most patients have anti-insulin IgG antibodies after a few months of therapy.

Insulin reactions may be limited to the site of injection, or they may produce systemic reactions. Local reactions present most often as a wheal and flare at the injection site and may occur immediately after injection or up to 8 to 12 hours later. Generally, these reactions are mild, do not require treatment, and resolve with continued insulin administration. If a patient does not tolerate the local reaction well, antihistamines may be given or a different insulin source (or product of higher purity) may be substituted. Rarely, systemic reactions to insulin (e.g., urticaria or anaphylaxis) occur. IgE-mediated reactions to insulin allergy appear to be declining with greater use of human insulins.[61] Skin testing with various products can aid in selecting the type of insulin least likely to cause a systemic reaction. Human insulin appears to be least allergenic but occasionally may cause reactions. In some patients, insulin desensitization may be indicated.

ASPIRIN AND NONSTEROIDAL ANTIINFLAMMATORY DRUGS

❼ Aspirin and other NSAIDs can produce eight general types of reactions, four of which are related to cyclooxygenase inhibition.[62,63] These reactions can involve asthma and rhinitis, urticaria/angioedema, anaphylaxis and anaphylactoid reactions, aseptic meningitis, or pneumonitis. The two most prevalent aspirin sensitivity reactions are respiratory (asthma, rhinorrhea) and urticaria/angioedema. Approximately 9% to 20% of asthmatics are sensitive to aspirin and other NSAIDs.[62,64]

The rhinosinusitis/asthma syndrome typically develops in middle-aged patients who are nonatopic and have no history of aspirin intolerance. Women are 2.5 times more likely to develop aspirin-induced asthma than men.[65] It usually progresses from rhinitis to sinusitis with nasal polyps and steroid-dependent asthma. It is uncommon in children and young adults. However, children with asthma may be aspirin sensitive. Aspirin-sensitive asthma appears to be an inherited disorder characterized by overexpression of LTC_4 synthase in airways.[66] In aspirin-sensitive asthmatics, administration of aspirin and NSAIDs may provoke severe and sometimes fatal asthmatic attacks. The mechanism of aspirin sensitivity is not completely understood.

One suspected mechanism of aspirin and NSAID sensitivity is cyclooxygenase-1 blockade, which may facilitate depletion of prostaglandin E2 (PGE2) and production of alternative arachidonic acid metabolites (e.g., LTs).[62] PGE2 prevents mast cell degranulation, whereas LTs cause bronchoconstriction and increased mucus production. Increased LT production may also explain the development of angioedema and urticaria. This proported mechanism is supported by the observed correlation between the degree of cyclooxygenase-1 blockade and the risk of a sensitivity reaction; thus, agents such as acetaminophen, which minimally block cyclooxygenase 1, rarely cause reactions. Additional support is found in the clinical observation that LT-modifying drugs can reduce the severity of aspirin-induced asthma and urticaria.[62] It is also possible that aspirin and NSAIDs stimulate mast cells directly to release inflammatory mediators. Subjects with aspirin-induced asthma also have a marked increase in airway responsiveness to LTs.[67] Aspirin and the cyclooxygenase-2–selective inhibitors celecoxib and rofecoxib do not appear to be cross-reactive.[68–70]

In patients with aspirin sensitivity (asthma or urticaria), an oral challenge or provocation test can be performed to diagnose the condition. A number of different protocols to detect aspirin or NSAID sensitivity have been recommended, but the risk for anaphylaxis cannot be reliably predicted.[62,65] The challenge should be performed with great caution in a hospital setting with resuscitation equipment at hand. For patients with aspirin-induced asthma, desensitization is recommended. Aspirin desensitization has been shown to improve asthma symptom scores and lead to reductions in maintenance steroid doses. If desensitization is not performed, patients with aspirin sensitivity must avoid aspirin and the nonselective NSAIDs as the major preventive measure.

Aspirin and individual NSAIDs (e.g., ibuprofen, sulindac) can also cause IgE-mediated hypersensitivity. These reactions occur on re-exposure to the drug and may present as urticaria, bronchospasm or anaphylaxis with or without hypotension. A careful and complete allergy history may suggest true hypersensitivity to aspirin or an isolated NSAID. Such patients should be advised to avoid the specific NSAID and any structurally similar NSAIDs (e.g., all propionic acid derivatives, all indole acetic acid derivatives) because of the risk of cross-reactivity.

NSAIDs have been associated with pulmonary infiltrates and eosinophilia syndrome. Pulmonary infiltrates and eosinophilia syndrome is associated with fever, cough, dyspnea, infiltrates on chest roentgenogram, and a peripheral eosinophilia that develop 2 to 6 weeks after initiating treatment. Pulmonary infiltrates and eosinophilia syndrome occurs more frequently for naproxen compared with other NSAIDs and is noted to resolve rapidly after discontinuation of the offending agent.[71]

SULFONAMIDES

Sulfonamide drugs containing the sulfa (SO_2NH_2) moiety include antibiotics, thiazide and loop diuretics, oral hypoglycemics, and carbonic anhydrase inhibitors. Allergic reactions have been reported in 4.8% of 20,226 patients who received a sulfonamide antibiotic and in 2% of patients who received a nonantibiotic sulfonamide.[72] Although immediate IgE-mediated reactions such as anaphylaxis can occur, sulfonamides typically cause delayed cutaneous reactions, often beginning with fever and then followed by a rash (e.g., maculopapular or morbilliform eruptions). Infrequently, a seemingly benign maculopapular rash may progress to a mucocutaneous syndrome (e.g., SJS/toxic epidermal necrolysis).[1] Other reactions to sulfonamides may include hepatic, renal, or hematologic complications, which may be fatal. Immune-mediated sulfonamide reactions depend on the production of reactive metabolites in the liver.[73] Trimethoprim-sulfamethoxazole, considered the most highly reactive sulfonamide, contains an arylamine in the N4 position of its chemical structure allowing for the drug's metabolism to two highly reactive metabolites, a hydroxylamine and a nitroso-sulfonamide.[73,74] Structural differences between the sulfonamides antibiotics and non-antibiotics may influence the metabolic conversion and resultant reactivity of these compounds. Slow acetylator phenotype may also increase the risk for these reactions.[4]

❽ Cross-reactivity between sulfonamide antibiotics and non-antibiotics appears to be minimal, with cross-reactivity characterized as "highly unlikely."[75] In one study, about 10% of patients with history of allergy to an antibiotic sulfonamide subsequently reacted to a non-antibiotic sulfonamide (e.g., acetazolamide, loop diuretic, sulfonylurea, thiazide).[72] This low rate of cross-reactivity has been attributed in part to differences in the chemical structures of the antibiotic and non-antibiotic sulfonamides. The occurrence of allergic reactions after receipt of non-antibiotic sulfonamides has also been attributed to a predisposition to allergic reactions in the affected individuals rather than cross-reactivity with sulfonamide antibiotics.[72] In fact, in one study, cross-reactivity between

sulfonamide antibiotics and penicillin was higher than that between the antibiotic and nonantibiotic sulfonamides.[72]

Trimethoprim–sulfamethoxazole is used frequently for preventive or active treatment of *Pneumocystis jiroveci* pneumonia in patients with AIDS. Adverse reactions to trimethoprim–sulfamethoxazole occur much more frequently in human immunodeficiency virus (HIV)-positive patients.[76,77] Adverse effects to trimethoprim–sulfamethoxazole occur in 50% to 80% of AIDS patients compared with 10% of other immunocompromised patients.[77] Trimethoprim–sulfamethoxazole was associated with an adverse event rate of 26.3 per 100 person-years and hypersensitivity events at 22 per 100 person-years. Although reactions may include angioedema, SJS, and thrombocytopenia, most reactions to trimethoprim–sulfamethoxazole in HIV-infected patients are delayed and present as diffuse maculopapular rash with or without fever. The mechanism by which these allergic or allergic-like reactions occur in HIV-infected patients is unclear. It is unlikely that these reactions are IgG or IgE-mediated.[74,78] Theories support alterations in drug metabolism due to glutathione deficiency, a direct toxic or immunologic effect of the sulfonamide metabolites on body tissues, and increased expression of major histocompatibility complex proteins with increased recognition of the drug antigen by CD4 and CD8 cells.[74,78] The adverse event rate has been related to higher CD4+ T cell count >20 cells/mm³ ($>20 \times 10^6$/L), CD4/CD8 ratio <0.10 and treatment for less than 14 days.[77]

PHARMACEUTICAL EXCIPIENTS AND ADDITIVES

Pharmaceutical products contain a number of "inert" additives (e.g., dyes, fillers, buffers, and stabilizers) in addition to the therapeutic ingredients. These additives are not always inert and may cause adverse effects, including allergic reactions.

The azo dye tartrazine (FD&C Yellow No. 5) is associated with anaphylactoid reactions, acute bronchospasm, urticaria, rhinitis, and contact dermatitis.[79,80] Although the immunologic mechanisms are unclear, approximately 10% of aspirin-sensitive asthmatics are also intolerant to tartrazine,[81] suggesting a role for tartrazine as a cyclooxygenase inhibitor. As little as 0.85 mcg or as much as 25 mg tartrazine has provoked positive responses.[81]

Sulfites (including sulfur dioxide, sodium sulfite, sodium and potassium bisulfite, and sodium and potassium metabisulfite) are used commonly as antioxidants in pharmaceutical products and some foods. Many cases of adverse reactions associated with ingestion of sulfites (usually in foods) have been reported to the U.S. Food and Drug Administration (FDA),[82] including wheezing, dyspnea, chest tightness, urticaria, angioedema, flushing, weakness, nausea, anaphylaxis, and death.

IgE-mediated and nonimmunologic sulfite hypersensitivity has been demonstrated in children with a history of chronic asthma. Adverse reactions to sulfite-preserved injectables, such as gentamicin, metoclopramide, lidocaine, and doxycycline, have been reported. In contrast to reactions caused by foods, these reactions do not occur more frequently in steroid-dependent asthmatics and do not always coincide with a positive oral sulfite challenge.[83] Blunted bronchodilation may be observed in asthmatics following inhalation of sulfite-containing nebulizer solutions. Although many nebulizer solutions contain sulfites, metered-dose inhalers do not. Many aqueous epinephrine products also contain sulfites. The FDA labeling states that in emergency situations when sulfite-free preparations are not available, sulfite-containing epinephrine should not be withheld from a sulfite-intolerant individual because small subcutaneous doses of sulfites usually are well tolerated. However, an increased risk of anaphylaxis exists after subcutaneous injection in rare patients with a positive oral challenge to 5 to 10 mg sulfite.

Parabens (including methyl-, ethyl-, propyl-, and butylparaben) are used widely in pharmaceutical products as a biocidal agent. Most allergic reactions to parabens are observed after topical exposure.[84] Delayed hypersensitivity contact dermatitis occurs more often in individuals with preexisting dermatitis.[81] Immediate hypersensitivity after parenteral administration is rare. Although these agents are chemically related to benzoic acid and p-aminobenzoic acid, the evidence for cross-sensitivity is lacking.[81]

CANCER CHEMOTHERAPY AGENTS

Chemotherapy agents are implicated in hypersensitivity reactions in 5% to 15% of patients who receive them.[85] Up to 65% of patients receiving L-asparaginase experience immediate hypersensitivity reactions such as urticaria and anaphylaxis.[86]

The combination regimen of paclitaxel (or docetaxel) and carboplatin frequently is responsible for producing hypersensitivity reactions. Each agent precipitates a distinct reaction, allowing for differentiation between causative factors. Hypersensitivity reactions have been observed with paclitaxel and docetaxel as frequently as 34% of patients.[1,87,88] The reaction, typically occurring shortly after initiation of the first dose, is due to Cremophor EL, the polyoxyethylated castor oil vehicle for paclitaxel. Severe reactions are characterized by dyspnea, bronchospasm, urticaria, and hypotension. Minor reactions include flushing and rashes. In patients receiving a 3-hour infusion, the incidence of severe reactions is reduced to 1.3%, and the incidence of minor reactions is 42%.[89] To reduce the risk of hypersensitivity reaction, patients are routinely premedicated with corticosteroids and H_1- and H_2-receptor antagonists. A protein-bound formulation of paclitaxel (Abraxane) is available that avoids most of the hypersensitivity reactions.

Carboplatin hypersensitivity develops after six or more courses of carboplatin or its parent compound cisplatin.[90] Reactions typically develop shortly after completing the infusion or up to 3 days after therapy.[91] Symptoms of severe reaction include tachycardia, dyspnea, facial swelling, rigors, and hypotension. Mild reactions include itching, erythema, and facial flushing. Both skin testing with carboplatin and desensitization have been shown to be effective.[92,93]

Oxaliplatin hypersensitivity has been reported in as many as 12% of patients. Symptoms range from facial flushing to dyspnea. Management strategies include decreasing the rate of infusion and administration of corticosteroids and H_1- and H_2-receptor antagonists.[94] Desensitization has been successful in patients desiring to continue treatment after experiencing a hypersensitivity reaction.[95,96]

ANTICONVULSANTS

Many anticonvulsant drugs produce a variety of hypersensitivity reactions and pseudoallergic reactions. Drugs such as phenytoin, phenobarbital, carbamazepine, and lamotrigine can cause an "anti-convulsant hypersensitivity syndrome" characterized by fever, rash, lymphadenopathy, and internal organ involvement. Eosinophilia is frequently present and many reactions meet the definition of DRESS. Onset usually occurs several weeks into therapy.[97] In some cases, morbilliform rash develops into exfoliative dermatitis. The risk of cross-reactivity between the aromatic anticonvulsants (e.g., carbamazepine, phenobarbital, and phenytoin) ranges from 40% to 80%.[98] Oxcarbazepine, the 10-keto derivative of carbamazepine, has exhibited both in vitro and in vivo cross-reactivity with carbamazepine. A genetic marker for severe reactions to carbamazepine, phenytoin and fosphenytoin is the presence of the HLA-B*1502 allele.[32] This allele is found in 10% to 15% of patients from China, Thailand, Malaysia, Indonesia, the Philippines, and Taiwan. Concomitant use of valproate with lamotrigine significantly increases the risk of hypersensitivity as a result of reduced lamotrigine metabolism, leading to a prolonged elimination half-life.[99]

BIOLOGICS

Biologic agents (e.g., monoclonal antibodies, fusion proteins, recombinant proteins) are derived from living sources such as yeast, bacteria, animal cells, or mammalian cells.[100] Unlike nonbiologic agents, these large proteins can serve as complete antigens. Examples include recombinant insulin, erythropoietin, interferon-β, human growth hormone, infliximab, rituximab, and omalizumab. Immunologic reactions to these agents range from minor infusion or injection-site reactions to anaphylaxis. Depending on the agent, reactions can occur on first or subsequent exposure and the timing may be within 4 hours of drug administration or up to 14 days after an infusion.[100]

Factors influencing the antigenicity of biologic agents are patient-specific (e.g., atopy, congenital protein deficiency), production related (e.g., presence of contaminants or stabilizing agents, degree of protein glycosylation, presence of nonhuman protein sequences, storage temperature), and administration-related (e.g., route of administration, frequency of use, concurrent immunosuppressant use).[100] Of the monoclonal antibodies, reactions are most frequently observed with the murine-derived agents (0% human) and chimeric agents (75% human) as opposed to the humanized (>90% human) and human (100% human) agents. Some immune reactions to biologic agents result from the development of neutralizing antibodies that can prevent the protein from exerting its intended effect. Neutralizing antibodies have been shown to mediate reactions to interferon-β_{1b} and β_{1a}, infliximab, natalizumab, recombinant factor VIII, and recombinant factor IX.[100] Anti-infliximab antibodies, which occur in up to 60% of treated patients, are associated with higher frequency of infusion reactions and decreased therapeutic effect.[101] Concomitant administration of immunosuppressive agents such as prednisone or low dose methotrexate has been shown to decrease the incidence of antibody formation to infliximab.[100,101]

Delayed onset anaphylaxis, ranging from minutes to days post-injection, has been reported with omalizumab, a humanized monoclonal antibody targeted against IgE.[102,103] Omalizumab-treated patients require extended observation post-injection and are advised to carry an epinephrine auto-injector during and for 24 hours after drug administration.[102] Risk factors for this adverse event have not been identified. Inclusion of polysorbate 80 as a stabilizing agent in the formulation, and an alteration in the protein sequence via glycosylation, may influence the immunogenicity of omalizumab.[103]

Management of allergic or allergic-like reactions to biologic agents varies based on the culprit agent and the severity and nature of the reaction. Immediate management with epinephrine and permanent discontinuation of the drug may be warranted (e.g., omalizumab-induced anaphylaxis). Depending on the biologic agent, reactions may be managed by decreasing the infusion rate or lessened by pretreating with antihistamines and/or corticosteroids or administering concomitant steroid therapy.

TREATMENT

Allergic Reactions

❾ The basic principles for management of allergic reactions to drugs or biologic agents include (a) discontinuation of the medication or agent when possible, (b) treatment of the adverse clinical signs and symptoms, and (c) substitution, if necessary, of another agent.[104]

TABLE 97-4 Treatment of Anaphylaxis

1. Place patient in recumbent position and elevate lower extremities.
2. Monitor vital signs frequently (every 2–5 minutes) and stay with the patient.
3. Administer epinephrine 1:1,000 into nonoccluded site: (adults: 0.01 mL/kg up to a maximum of 0.2–0.5 mL every 5 minutes as needed, children: 0.01 mL/kg up to a maximum dose of 0.2–0.5 mL) subcutaneously or intramuscularly. If necessary, repeat every 5 minutes, up to 2 doses, then every 4 hours as needed.
4. Administer oxygen, usually 8–10 L/min; however, lower concentrations may be appropriate for patients with chronic obstructive pulmonary disease. Maintain airway with oropharyngeal airway device.
5. Administer the antihistamine diphenhydramine (Benadryl, adults 25–50 mg; children 1–2 mg/kg) usually given parenterally. Apply tourniquet proximal to site of antigen injection; remove every 10–15 minutes. Consider ranitidine 1 mg/kg diluted in D5W to a total volume of 20 mL given IV over 5 minutes.
6. If anaphylaxis is caused by an injection, administer aqueous epinephrine 1:1,000 into site of antigen injection; 0.15–0.3 mL into the injection site.
7. Treat hypotension with IV fluids or colloid replacement, and consider use of a vasopressor such as dopamine.
8. Treat bronchospasm resistant to epinephrine with nebulized albuterol 2.5–5 mg in 3 mL saline every 20 minutes for 3 doses; in children, 0.15 mg/kg via nebulizer every 20 minutes for 3 doses.
9. Give hydrocortisone, 5 mg/kg, or approximately 250 mg IV (prednisone 20 mg orally can be given in mild cases) to reduce the risk of recurring or protracted anaphylaxis. These doses can be repeated every six hours as required.
10. In refractory cases not responding to epinephrine because a β-adrenergic blocker is complicating management, glucagon 1 mg IV as a bolus may be useful. A continuous infusion of glucagon, 1–5 mg/h, may be given if required.

Reprinted and adapted from J Allergy Clin Immunol 1998;101:S465–S528. Joint Task Force on Practice Parameters for Allergy and Immunology. The diagnosis and management of anaphylaxis: an updated practice parameter. J Allergy Clin Immunol 2005;115:S483–S523.

■ ANAPHYLAXIS

Anaphylaxis requires prompt treatment to minimize the risk of serious morbidity or death. On presentation, attention should be given first to stopping the likely offending agent, if possible, and restoring respiratory and cardiovascular function. A protocol for treatment of anaphylaxis is presented in Table 97–4. Epinephrine is administered as primary treatment to counteract bronchoconstriction and vasodilation. Epinephrine should be administered intramuscularly in the lateral aspect of the thigh.[105] If blood pressure is not restored by epinephrine, crystalloid intravenous fluids should be administered to restore intravascular volume. Typically, 1 L of 0.9% sodium chloride or lactated Ringer solution is administered over 10 to 15 minutes. This can be repeated if the patient is still believed to be volume depleted. A maintenance intravenous fluid then is initiated. Intravenous fluids should be given early in the course of treatment in an attempt to prevent shock. An immediate priority is to establish and maintain an airway by the use of endotracheal intubation if necessary. When a patient with anaphylaxis is hypotensive, vasopressors may be needed in addition to crystalloids. Norepinephrine is the vasoconstrictor agent of choice for treatment of anaphylactic shock, although dopamine also may be useful. Patients in shock should remain supine with raised legs.[37]

Other agents may be required for treatment of anaphylactic reactions. Corticosteroids (hydrocortisone sodium succinate intravenously) can reduce the risk of late-phase reactions. In patients treated chronically with β-blockers, glucagon should be considered because its inotropic and chronotropic effects do not rely on β-receptor responsiveness.[60] Histamine (H₁) receptor blockers (e.g., diphenhydramine) can be administered to reduce some of the symptoms associated with anaphylaxis, but these agents are not effective as primary therapy. The combination of diphenhydramine and an H$_2$ receptor blocker (e.g., ranitidine) has been shown to be superior to diphenhydramine alone in the treatment of anaphylaxis.[60]

■ SKIN TESTING AND DRUG PROVOCATION TESTING

⑩ Identification of patients at high risk for allergic drug reactions requires careful history-taking with attention to the specific agent to which the patient reacted, a complete description of the reaction, and the time since last exposure to the culprit drug. The importance of accurate and complete history taking cannot be overstated. Although skin and oral provocation testing are used to assess reactive risk to some drugs, many of the testing procedures have not been validated. A drug provocation test, or DPT, involves the controlled administration of a drug for the purpose of diagnosing an immune response. DPTs can be used to evaluate sensitivity to aspirin.[106,107] When available, skin testing should be performed prior to a DPT due to the lesser risks incurred to the patient. For some drugs, skin testing can reliably demonstrate the presence of drug-specific IgE and predict a relatively high risk of immediate hypersensitivity reactions. Reliable skin test reagents are not available for most culprit drugs. Moreover, skin testing should not be performed in patients with history of severe mucocutaneous reactions (e.g., SJS, TEN) or other non-immediate reactions (e.g., serum sickness, vasculitis, hepatitis).

⑩ Skin testing can reduce the uncertainty of penicillin sensitivity and should be performed in all patients who have a history of an immediate allergy and require treatment with a β-lactam antibiotic. Penicillin skin testing in advance of need for penicillin treatment in patients with a history of penicillin allergy does not appear to induce sensitization.[108] Testing for the major penicillin determinant is accomplished with penicilloyl-polylysine (PPL; Pre-Pen), but this product is not currently available in the United States. If this agent is used alone, patients reacting only to minor determinants will be missed. At present, there is also no commercially available product that can be used to test for most of the minor determinants. Benzylpenicillin (at a concentration of 10,000 units/mL) has been used, but some reactive patients still will be missed. When commercially available β-lactams such as amoxicillin, penicillin G and ampicillin are used alone for skin testing, as many as 15% of patients with β-lactam allergies will be missed.[43] Skin testing with the major and minor determinants has been shown to facilitate the safe use of penicillin in up to 90% of patients with a history of immediate penicillin allergy.[109] Less than 1% of patients with a negative history, and up to 72% of patients with a convincing positive history of penicillin allergy have skin test positive reactivity.[110] In patients who report a history of penicillin allergy but are skin test negative, the risk of resensitization (i.e., conversion to a positive skin test) following a course of penicillin ranges from 1% to 28%.[46] The procedure for performing penicillin skin testing is given in Table 97–5.

A negative penicillin skin test indicates that the risk of life-threatening immediate reactions is extremely low with administration of penicillin or other β-lactams. Such patients are candidates for treatment with full therapeutic doses of a penicillin or a related β-lactam. Certain types of patients (e.g., those with dermatographism, taking antihistamines) may be unsuitable for skin testing because a false-positive or false-negative test may result. To prevent interference with skin testing, antihistamines should be discontinued at least one week prior to skin testing. Penicillin is the only drug for which the predictive value of skin testing has been well established. Although the negative predictive value is high, penicillin skin testing with the major and minor determinants does not identify those patients who are at risk for unique side chain-mediated reactions to β-lactams (e.g., third generation cephalosporins, piperacillin). Dilute concentrations of amoxicillin and piperacillin have been used to skin test

TABLE 97-5 Procedure for Performing Penicillin Skin Testing

A. Percutaneous (Prick) Skin Testing

Materials	Volume
Pre-Pen 6 × 10⁶ M (currently not commercially available in the United States)	1 drop
Penicillin G 10,000 units/mL	1 drop
β-Lactam drug 3 mg/mL	1 drop
0.03% albumin-saline control	1 drop
Histamine control (1 mg/mL)	1 drop

1. Place a drop of each test material on the volar surface of the forearm.
2. Prick the skin with a sharp needle inserted through the drop at a 45° angle, gently tenting the skin in an upward motion.
3. Interpret skin responses after 15 minutes.
4. A wheal at least 2 × 2 mm with erythema is considered positive.
5. If the prick test is nonreactive, proceed to the intradermal test.
6. If the histamine control is nonreactive, the test is considered uninterpretable.

B. Intradermal Skin Testing

Materials	Volume
Pre-Pen 6 × 10⁶ M (currently not commercially available in the United States)	0.02 mL
Penicillin G 10,000 units/mL	0.02 mL
β-Lactam drug 3 mg/mL	0.02 mL
0.03% albumin-saline control	0.02 mL
Histamine control (0.1 mg/mL)	0.02 mL

1. Inject 0.02–0.03 mL of each test material intradermally (amount sufficient to produce a small bleb).
2. Interpret skin responses after 15 minutes.
3. A wheal at least 6 × 6 mm with erythema and at least 3 mm greater than the negative control is considered positive.
4. If the histamine control is nonreactive, the test is considered uninterpretable.

Antihistamines may blunt the response and cause false-negative reactions.

From Sullivan TJ. Current Therapy in Allergy. St. Louis, MO: Mosby, 1985:57–61, with permission.

TABLE 97-6 Protocol for Oral Desensitization

Phenoxymethyl Penicillin

Step[a]	Concentration (units/mL)	Volume (mL)	Dose (units)	Cumulative Dose (units)
1	1,000	0.1	100	100
2	1,000	0.2	200	300
3	1,000	0.4	400	700
4	1,000	0.8	800	1,500
5	1,000	1.6	1,600	3,100
6	1,000	3.2	3,200	6,300
7	1,000	6.4	6,400	12,700
8	10,000	1.2	12,000	24,700
9	10,000	2.4	24,000	48,700
10	10,000	4.8	48,000	96,700
11	80,000	1.0	80,000	176,700
12	80,000	2.0	160,000	336,700
13	80,000	4.0	320,000	656,700
14	80,000	8.0	640,000	1,296,700
Observe for 30 min				
15	500,000	0.25	125,000	
16	500,000	0.5	250,000	
17	500,000	1.0	500,000	
18	500,000	2.25	1,125,000	

[a]The interval between steps is 15 min.

Reprinted from Immunol Allerg Clin North, Vol. 18, Weiss ME, Adkinson NF, Diagnostic Testing for Drug Hypersensivity, Immunol Allerg Clin North, 731–734, Copyright © 1998, with permission from Elsevier.

mild, transient allergic reactions either during the desensitization procedure or during penicillin therapy.[34] Patients who can take oral medication should undergo desensitization with oral drug. Once the desensitization protocol is begun, it should not be interrupted except for severe reactions. Antihistamines or epinephrine can be administered to treat reactions. In addition, if the patient completes the desensitization regimen and then undergoes full dose treatment, a lapse between doses of as few as 24 hours can allow for reemergence of sensitivity. Protocols for oral and intravenous penicillin desensitization are listed in Tables 97–6 and 97–7.

TABLE 97-7 Parenteral Desensitization Protocol

Injection No.	Benzylpenicillin Concentration (units)	Volume (mL)	Route
1[a,b]	100	0.1	ID
2	100	0.2	SC
3	100	0.4	SC
4	100	0.8	SC
5[b]	1,000	0.1	ID
6	1,000	0.3	SC
7	1,000	0.6	SC
8[b]	10,000	0.1	ID
9	10,000	0.2	SC
10	10,000	0.4	SC
11	10,000	0.8	SC
12[b]	100,000	0.1	ID
13	100,000	0.3	SC
14	100,000	0.6	SC
15[b]	1,000,000	0.1	ID
16	1,000,000	0.2	SC
17	1,000,000	0.2	IM
18	1,000,000	0.4	IM
19	Continuous IV infusion at 1,000,000 units/h		

[a]Administer doses at intervals of not less than 20 min.
[b]Observe and record skin wheal-and-flare response.
ID, intradermally; IM, intramuscularly; SC, subcutaneously.
Reprinted from Immunol Allerg Clin North, Vol. 18, Weiss ME, Adkinson NF, Diagnostic Testing for Drug Hypersensivity, Immunol Allerg Clin North, 731–734, Copyright © 1998, with permission from Elsevier.

for side chain mediated reactions.[43-45] The value of skin testing to predict the risk of allergic reactions to other antibiotics (e.g., sulfonamides, tetracyclines, fluoroquinolones) is largely unknown.

Skin testing is used to identify patients at risk for hypersensitivity reactions to carboplatin. The negative predictive value of intradermal skin testing with carboplatin has been shown to be 98% to 99% in patients who have received a number of treatment courses.[92]

■ DESENSITIZATION

For some patients with history of immediate penicillin or β-lactam allergy, no reasonable alternatives exist, and penicillin or a related β-lactam may be necessary for treatment of severe, life-threatening infection. In this situation, desensitization to the specific β-lactam required for treatment of the infection should be considered. Desensitization can reduce the risk of an IgE-mediated reaction such as anaphylaxis by rendering the mast cells less responsive to degranulation. Desensitization does not influence the likelihood of other types of reactions such as exfoliative dermatitis or SJS.

Desensitization should be performed by a physician experienced in the risks and management of severe allergic reactions in a hospital setting with resuscitation equipment available. The potential risks and benefits should be discussed with the patient. Desensitization should be performed with the specific β-lactam antibiotic that will be administered for treatment of the patient's infection. Prior to initiating the protocol, the patient should be stabilized and fluid, pulmonary, and cardiovascular function optimized. Premedications (antihistamines or corticosteroids) should not be used because these agents may mask the early signs of acute reactions and do not reliably reduce the severity of acute reactions. Approximately one third of patients who have undergone desensitization experience

Protocols for desensitization with other β-lactam antibiotics are also available.[111,112]

Skin tests to penicillin often become negative during and shortly after desensitization. The mechanism by which desensitization is protective is unclear. It does not appear that penicillin-specific IgE is neutralized or that IgG as "blocking antibody" is produced. One possible explanation is that basophils and mast cells attain some degree of tolerance on exposure to the antigen.

Although most reactions to trimethoprim-sulfamethoxazole in HIV-infected patients are not considered to be IgE mediated, the term *trimethoprim–sulfamethoxazole desensitization* is commonly recognized. The underlying mechanism by which desensitization to trimethoprim–sulfamethoxazole is achieved in these patients remains unknown. A number of protocols for trimethoprim–sulfamethoxazole desensitization are available, and many are also referred to as graded challenge protocols. Since these regimens have not been compared in controlled clinical trials, there is no preferred regimen. Desensitization of trimethoprim–sulfamethoxazole can be achieved within 2 days in most AIDS patients.[1,113] This can be accomplished by using the following schedule of oral doses (milligrams of sulfamethoxazole–trimethoprim): day 1: 9 AM, 4 and 0.8 mg; 11 AM, 8 and 1.6 mg; 1 PM, 20 and 4 mg; 5 PM, 40 and 8 mg; day 2: 9 AM, 80 and 16 mg; 3 PM, 160 and 32 mg; 9 PM, 200 and 40 mg; day 3: 9 AM, 400 and 80 mg, and 400 and 80 mg daily thereafter. With this desensitization regimen, the failure rate was associated with higher relative and absolute CD4 cell counts. Other investigators have described a 6-hour oral graded challenge in HIV-infected patients.[114] and a more gradual 9-day oral regimen.[115] Desensitization should not be attempted in any patient with history of an exfoliative reaction to trimethoprm-sulfamethoxazole.

Both rapid (over less than 4 hours) and traditional desensitization protocols are available for aspirin and clopidogrel.[116,117] Aspirin desensitization is more effective in patients with history of aspirin-induced asthma as compared to the angioedema/urticarial presentation.[65] A rapid 12-step protocol has been shown to be safe and effective for desensitizing patients to a variety of chemotherapeutic agents including carboplatin, cisplatin, oxaliplatin, paclitaxel, and rituximab.[93]

■ GRADED CHALLENGE

Also known as test dosing, a graded drug challenge involves the gradual introduction of a drug when there is a risk of reactivity. A graded drug challenge does not modify the immune response or allow for more rapid desensitization.[111] Instead, graded challenge is used when the risk of a severe reaction to a drug on re-exposure is low, no alternative drug is equally effective, and a reliable skin testing method is not available. A classic example is the gradual re-introduction of trimethoprim–sulfamethoxazole in a patient who had a mild maculopapular rash to the drug in the past. Graded challenge may also be used to test for cross-reactivity when the risk of a severe reaction is low (e.g., a patient with history of allergy to one cephalosporin who now requires a cephalosporin having a dissimilar R1 side chain).[111] Graded challenge protocols have been described for the slow introduction of furosemide in a patient with heart failure and history of sulfonamide allergy.[118] Challenge dosing is not recommended when there is history of a severe drug allergy (e.g., anaphylaxis, SJS, TEN). Premedications should not be used because they may mask signs of an early breakthrough allergic reaction. The starting dose is typically 1/10th to 1/100th of the therapeutic dose and the oral route of drug administration is preferred to limit the risk of a severe reaction.[111] If no reaction occurs to the initial dose, the dose may be increased in 2- to 5-fold increments and administered every 30 to 60 minutes until the full therapeutic dose is achieved.[45,111] There is no standard protocol for graded challenge

dosing; a therapeutic dose may be achieved over a matter of hours or days. Due to the risk of break-through allergic reactions, graded challenges should be performed in monitored settings.

ABBREVIATIONS

APC: antigen-presenting cell

DRESS: drug rash with eosinophilia and systemic symptoms

HLA: human leukocytic antigen

IgE: immunoglobulin E

LT: leukotriene

NSAID: nonsteroidal antiinflammatory drug

PAF: platelet-activating factor

PG: prostaglandin

PPD: purified protein derivative

SJS: Stevens Johnson syndrome

SLE: systemic lupus erythematosus

TEN: toxic epidermal necrolysis

REFERENCES

1. Gruchalla RS. Drug allergy. J Allerg Clin Immunol 2003;111: S548–S559.
2. Demoly P, Hillaire-Buys D. Classification and epidemiology of hypersensitivity drug reactions. Immunol Allergy Clin North Am 2004;24:345–356.
3. Adkinson NF. Drug allergy. In: Adkinson NF, Yunginger JW, Busse WW, Bochner BS, Holgate ST, Simous FER, eds. Middleton's Allergy: Principles and Practice, 6th ed. St. Louis, MO: Mosby, 2003.
4. Svensson CK, Cowen EW, Gaspari AA. Cutaneous drug reactions. Pharmacol Rev 2000;53:357–379.
5. Schnyder B, Pichler WJ. Mechanisms of drug allergy. Mayo Clin Proc 2009;84(3):268–272.
6. Posadas SJ, Pichler WJ. Delayed drug hypersensitivity reactions — new concepts. Clin Exp Allergy 2007;37:989–999.
7. Barnes PJ. Pathophysiology of allergic inflammation. In: Adkinson NF, Yunginger JW, Busse WW, Bochner BS, Holgate ST, Simous FER, eds. Middleton's Allergy: Principles and Practice, 6th ed. St. Louis, MO: Mosby, 2003.
8. MacGlashan D. Histamine: A mediator of inflammation. J Allerg Clin Immunol 2003;112:S53–S59.
9. Solensky R, Mendelson LM. Systemic reactions to antibiotics. Immunol Allergy Clin North Am 2001;21:679–697.
10. Tang AW. A practical guide to anaphylaxis. Am Fam Physician 2003;68:1325–1332.
11. Sampson HA, Munoz-Furlong A, Bock A, et al. Symposium on the definition and management of anaphylaxis: Summary report. J Allerg Clin Immunol 2005;115:584–591.
12. Matasar MJ, Neugut AI. Epidemiology of asthma. Curr Allergy Asthma Rep 2003;3:30–35.
13. Neuqut AI, Ghatak AT, Miller RL. Anaphylaxis in the United States: An investigation into its epidemiology. Ann Intern Med 2001;161: 15–21.
14. Kemp SF. Anaphylaxis: a review of causes and mechanisms. J Allergy Clin Immunol 2002;110:341–348.
15. Sampson HA, Munoz-Furlong A, Campbell RL, et al. Second symposium on the definition and management of anaphylaxis: Summary report—Second National Institute of Allergy and Infectious Diseases/ Food Allergy and Anaphylaxis Network Symposium. J Allerg Clin Immunol 2006;117:391–397.
16. Levenson DE, Arndt K, Stern RS Cutaneous manifestations of adverse drug reactions. Immunol Allergy Clin North Am 1991;11:493–516.
17. Bocquet H, Martine B, Roujeau JC. Drug-induced pseudolymphoma and drug hypersensitivity syndrome (drug rash with eosinophilia

and systemic symptoms; DRESS). Semin Cutan Med Surg 1996;15(4): 250–257.

18. Kano Y, Shiohara T. The variable clinical picture of drug-induced hypersensitivity syndrome/drug rash with eosinophilia and systemic symptoms in relation to the eliciting drug. Immunol Clin N Am 2009;29:481–501.

19. Johnson DH, Cuhna BA. Drug fever. Infect Dis Clin North Am 1996;10:85–91.

20. Rubin RL. Drug-induced lupus. Toxicology 2005;209:135–147.

21. Sarzi-Puttini P, Atzeni F, Capsoni F, Lubrano E, Doria A. Drug-induced lupus erythematosus. Autoimmunity 2005;38:507–518.

22. Roujeau JC, Stern RS. Severe adverse cutaneous reactions to drugs. N Engl J Med 1994;331:1272–1285.

23. Prendiville J. Stevens-Johnson syndrome and toxic epidermal necrolysis. Adv Dermatol 2002;18:151–173.

24. Bastuji-Garin S, Rzany B, Stern RS et al. Clinical classification of cases of TEN, SJS and erythema multiforme. Arch Dermatol 1993;129: 92–96.

25. Bastuji-Garin S, Fouchard N, Bertucci M, et al. SCORTEN: a severity of illness score for TEN. J Inves Dermatol 2000;115:149–153.

26. Hunziker T, Kunzi U, Braunschweig S, et al. Comprehensive hospital drug monitoring: Adverse drug reactions—A 20-year survey. Allergy 1997;52:388–393.

27. Wolf R, Orion E, Marcos B et al. Life-threatening acute adverse cutaneous reactions. Clin Dermatol 2005;2:171–181.

28. Letko E, Papiliodis DN, Papaliodis GN et al. Stevens-Johnson syndrome and toxic epidermal necrolysis: a review of the literature. Ann Allergy Clin Immunol 2005;94:419–436.

29. Mockenhaupt M, Viboud C, Dunant A et al. Stevens-Johnson syndrome and toxic epidermal necrolysis: assessment of medication risks with emphasis on recently marketed drugs. The EuroSCAR study. J Investig Dermatol 2008;128:35–55.

30. Mallal S, Phillips E, Carosi G et al. HLA-B*5701 screening for abacavir. N Engl J Med 2008;358:568–579.

31. Chia FL, Leong KP. Severe cutaneous adverse reactions to drugs. Curr Opin Allergy Clin Immunol 2007;7:304–309.

32. Man CBL, Kwan P, Baum L et al. Association between HLA-B* 1502 allele and antiepileptic drug-induced cutaneous reactions in Han Chinese. Epilepsia 2007;48:1015–1018.

33. Thethi AK, Van Dellen RG. Dilemmas and controversies in penicillin allergy. Immunol Allergy Clin North Am 2004;24:445–461.

34. Weiss ME, Adkinson NF. Immediate hypersensitivity reactions to penicillin and related antibiotics. Clin Allergy 1988;18:515–540.

35. Lee CE, Zembower TR, Fotis MA, et al. The incidence of antimicrobial allergies in hospitalized patients. Arch Intern Med 2000;160: 2819–2822.

36. Salkind AR, Cuddy PG, Foxworth JW. Is this patient allergic to penicillin? An evidence-based analysis of the likelihood of penicillin allergy. JAMA 2001;285:2498–2505.

37. Sicherer SH, Leung DYM. Advances in allergic skin disease, anaphylaxis, and hypersensitivity reactions to foods, drugs, and insect stings. J Allerg Clin Immunol 2004;114:118–124.

38. Hunziker T, Kunzi UP, Braunschweig S, et al. Comprehensive hospital drug monitoring (CHDM): Adverse skin reactions, a 20-year survey. Allergy 1997;52:388–393.

39. Bigby M. Rates of cutaneous reactions to drugs. Arch Dermatol 2001;137:765–770.

40. Pullen H, Wright N, Murdoch J. Hypersensitivity reactions to antibacterial drugs in infectious mononucleosis. Lancet 1967;1:1176–1178.

41. Romano A, Quaratino D, Papa G et al. Aminopenicillin allergy. Arch Dis Child 1997;76:513–517.

42. Romano A, DiFonso M, Viola M et al. Selective hypersensitivity to piperacillin. Allergy 2000;55:787.

43. Bousquet PJ, Co-Minh HB, Amoux B, Daures JP, Demoly P. Importance of mixture of minor determinants and benzylpenicilloyl poly-Llysine skin testing in the diagnosis of beta-lactam allergy. J Allerg Clin Immunol 2005;115:1314–1316.

44. Blanca M, Mayorga C, Torres MJ et al. Side chain specific reactions to beta-lactams: 14 years later. Clin Exp Allergy 2002;32:192–197.

45. Yates AB. Management of patients with history of allergy to beta-lactam antibiotics. Am J Med 2008;121:572–576.

46. Blanca M, Romano A, Torres MJ et al. Update on the evaluation of hypersensitivity reactions to betalactams. Allergy 2009;64:183–193.

47. Frumin J, Gallagher JC. Allergic cross-sensitivity between penicillin, carbapenem and monobactam antibiotics: what are the chances? Ann Pharmacother 2009;43:304–315.

48. Kelkar PS, Lu JT. Cephalosporin allergy. N Engl J Med 2001;345: 804–809.

49. Madaan A, Li JTC. Cephalosporin allergy. Immunol Clin North Am 2004;24:463–476.

50. Pichichero ME, Casey JR. Safe use of selected cephalosporins in penicillin-allergic patients: a meta-analysis. Otolaryngol Head Neck Surg 2007;136:340–347.

51. Pichichero ME. A review of evidence supporting the American Academy of Pediatrics recommendation for prescribing cephalosporin antibiotics in penicillin-allergic patients. Pediatrics 2005;115: 1048–1057.

52. Romano A, Viola M, Gueant-Rodriguez RM et al. Imipenem in patients with immediate hypersensitivity to penicillins. N Engl J Med 2006;354:2835–2837.

53. Romano A, Viola M, Gueant-Rodriguez RM et al. Brief communication: tolerability of meropenem in patients with IgE-mediated hypersensitivity to penicillins. Ann Intern Med 2007;146:266–269.

54. Atanaskovic-Markovic M, Gaeta F, Medjo B et al. Tolerability of meropenem in children with IgE-mediated hypersensitivity to penicillins. Allergy 2008;63:237–240.

55. Brocknow K. Immediate and delayed reactions to radiocontrast media: is there an allergic mechanism? Immunol Allergy Clin N Am 2009;29:453–468.

56. Christiansen C. X-ray contrast media—An overview. Toxicology 2005;209:185–187.

57. Idee JM, Pines E, Pringent P, Coror C. Allergy-like reactions to iodinated contrast agents. A critical analysis. Fundam Clin Pharmacol 2005;19:263–281.

58. Gueant-Rodriguez RM, Romano A, Barbaud A, Brucknow K, Gueant JL. Hypersensitivity reactions to iodinated contrast media. Curr Pharmaceut Design 2006;12:3359–3372.

59. Tramer MP, von Elm E, Loubeyre P, Hauser C. Pharmacologic prevention of serious anaphylactic reactions due to iodinated contrast media: Systematic review. BMJ 2006;333:663–664.

60. Lieberman P, Kemp SF, Oppenheimer J et al. The diagnosis and management of anaphylaxis: an updated practice parameter. J Allergy Clin Immunol 2005;115:S483–S523.

61. Heinzerling L, Raile K, Richlitz H et al. Insulin allergy: clinical manifestations and management strategies. Allergy 2008;63:148–155.

62. Stevenson DD, Simon RA, Zuraw BL. Sensitivity to aspirin and nonsteroidal anti-inflammatory drugs. In: Adkinson NF, Yunginger JW, Busse WW, Bochner BS, Holgate ST, Simous FER, eds. Middleton's Allergy: Principles and Practice, 6th ed. St. Louis, MO: Mosby, 2003.

63. Stevenson DD. Aspirin and NSAID sensitivity. Immunol Allergy Clin North Am 2004;24:491–505.

64. Babu KS, Salvi SS. Aspirin and asthma. Chest 2000;118:1470–1466.

65. Knowles SR, Drucker AM, Weber EA et al. Management options for patient with aspirin and nonsteroidal antiinflammatory drug sensitivity. Ann Pharmacother 2007;41:1191–1200.

66. Sanak M, Szczeklik A. Genetics of aspirin induced asthma. Thorax 2000;55(Suppl 2):S45–S47.

67. Lee TH. Mechanisms of aspirin sensitivity. Am Rev Respir Dis 1992;145:S34–S36.

68. Stevenson DD, Simon RA. Lack of cross-reactivity between rofecoxib and aspirin in aspirin-sensitive patients with asthma. J Allergy Clin Immunol 2001;108:47–51.

69. Woessner KM, Simon RA, Stevenson DD. The safety of celecoxib in patients with aspirin-sensitive asthma. Arthritis Rheum 2002;46: 2201–2206.

70. Gyllfors P, Bochenek G, Overholt J, et al. Biochemical and clinical evidence that aspirin-intolerant asthmatic subjects tolerate the cyclooxygenase 2-selective analgesic celecoxib. J Allerg Clin Immunol 2003;111:1116–1121.

71. Goodwin SD, Glenny RW. Nonsteroidal anti-inflammatory drug-associated pulmonary infiltrates with eosinophilia. Arch Intern Med 1992;152:1521–1524.

72. Strom BL, Schinnar R, Apter AJ, et al. Absence of cross-reactivity between sulfonamide antibiotics and sulfonamide nonantibiotics. N Engl J Med 2003;349:1628–1635.

73. Slatore CG, Tilles SA. Sulfonamide hypersensitivity. Immunol Allergy Clin North Am 2004;24:477–490.

74. Solensky R. Drug hypersensitivity. Med Clin N Am 2006;90:233–260.

75. Brackett CC, Singh H, Block JR. Likelihood and mechanisms of cross-allergenicity between sulfonamide antibiotics and other drugs containing a sulfonamide functional group. Pharmacotherapy 2004;24:856–870.

76. Temesgen Z, Beri G. HIV and drug allergy. Immunol Allergy Clin North Am 2004;24:521–531.

77. Davis CM, Shearer WT. Diagnosis and management of HIV drug hypersensitivity. J Allergy Clin Immunol 2008;121:826–832.

78. Dibbern DA, Montanaro A. Allergies to sulfonamide antibiotics and sulfur-containing drugs. Ann Allergy Asthma Immunol 2008;100:91–100.

79. Bhatia MS. Allergy to tartrazine in psychotropic drugs. J Clin Psychiatry 2000;61:473–476.

80. Ardern KD, Ram FS. Tartrazine exclusion for allergic asthma. Cochrane Database Syst Rev 2001;4:CD000460.

81. American Academy of Pediatrics Committee on Drugs. "Inactive" ingredients in pharmaceutical products. Pediatrics 1985;76:635–642.

82. Timbo B, Koehler KM, Wolyniak C, Klontz KC. Sulfites—A food and drug administration review of recalls and reported adverse events. J Food Protect 2004;67:1806–1811.

83. Campbell JR, Maestrello CL, Campbell RL. Allergic responses to metabisulfite in lidocaine anesthetic solution. Anesth Prog 2001;48:21–26.

84. Mowad CM. Allergic contact dermatitis caused by parabens: Two case reports and a review. Am J Contact Dermat 2000;11:53–56.

85. Weiss RB. Hypersensitivity reactions. Semin Oncol 1992;19:458–477.

86. Shepherd GM. Hypersensitivity reactions to chemotherapeutic drugs. Clin Rev Allergy Immunol 2003;24:253–262.

87. Markman M, Kennedy A, Webster K, et al. Combination chemotherapy with carboplatin and docetaxel in the treatment of cancers of the ovary and fallopian tube and primary carcinoma of the peritoneum. J Clin Oncol 2001;19:1901–1905.

88. Bookman MA, Kloth DD, Kover PE, et al. Intravenous prophylaxis for paclitaxel-related hypersensitivity reactions. Semin Oncol 1997;24:S19–13–S19–15.

89. Eisenhauer EA, ten Bokkel Huinink WW, Swenerton KD, et al. European-Canadian randomized trial of paclitaxel in relapsed ovarian cancer: High-dose versus low-dose and long versus short infusion. J Clin Oncol 1994;12:2654–2666.

90. Hendrick AM, Simmons D, Cantwell BMJ. Allergic reactions to carboplatin. Ann Oncol 1992;3:239–240.

91. Markman M, Kennedy A, Webster K, et al. Clinical features of hypersensitivity reactions to carboplatin. J Clin Oncol 1999;17:1141–1145.

92. Markman M, Zanotti K, Peterson G, et al. Expanded experience with an intradermal skin test to predict for the presence or absence of carboplatin hypersensitivity. J Clin Oncol 2003;21:4611–4614.

93. Castells MC, Tennant NM, Sloane DE et al. Hypersensitivity reactions to chemotherapy: outcomes and safety of rapid desensitization in 413 cases. J Allergy Clin Immunol 2008;122:574–580.

94. Saif MW. Hypersensitivity reactions associated with oxaliplatin. Expert Opin Drug Saf 2006;5:687–694.

95. Mis L, Fernando NH, Hurwitz HI, Morse MA. Successful desensitization to oxaliplatin. Anna Pharmacother 2005;39:966–969.

96. Gammon D, Bhargava P, McCormick MJ. Hypersensitivity reactions to oxaliplatin and the application of a desensitization protocol. Oncologist 2004;9:546–549.

97. Sullivan JR, Shear NH. The drug hypersensitivity syndrome: What is the pathogenesis? Arch Dermatol 2001;137:357–364.

98. Bohan KH, Mansuri TF, Wilson NM. Anticonvulsant hypersensitivity syndrome: implications for pharmaceutical care. Pharmacother 2007;27:1425–1439.

99. Schlienger RG, Knowles SR, Shear NH. Lamotrigine-associated anti-convulsant hypersensitivity syndrome. Neurology 1998;51:1172–1175.

100. Purcell RT, Lockey RF. Immunologic responses to therapeutic biologic agents. J Investig Allergol Clin Immunol 2008;18:335–342.

101. Kapetanovic MC, Larsson L, Truedsson L, et al. Predictors of infusion reactions during infliximab treatment in patients with arthritis. Arthritis Res Ther 2006;8:R131.

102. Limb SL, Starke PR, Lee CE, et al. Delayed onset and protracted progression of anaphylaxis after omalizumab administration in patients with asthma. J Allergy Clin Immunol 2007;120:1378–1381.

103. Cox L, Platts-Mills TAE, Finegold T, et al. American Academy of Allergy, Asthma and Immunology/American College of Allergy, Asthma and Immunology Joint Task Force Report on omalizumab-associated anaphylaxis. J Allergy Clin Immunol 2007;120:1373–1377.

104. Anderson JA. Allergic reactions to drugs and biologic agents. JAMA 1992;268:2845–2857.

105. Lieberman P. Use of epinephrine in the treatment of anaphylaxis. Curr Opin Allergy Clin Immunol 2003;3:313–318.

106. Weiss ME, Adkinson NF. Diagnostic testing for drug hypersensitivity. Immunol Allergy Clin North Am 1998;18:731–734.

107. Aberer W, Bircher A, Romaro A, et al. Drug provocation testing in the diagnosis of drug hypersensitivity reactions: General considerations. Allergy 2003;58:854–863.

108. Macy E, Mangat R, Burchetts RJ. Penicillin skin testing in advance of need: Multiyear follow-up in 568 test result-negative subjects exposed to oral penicillins. J Allerg Clin Immunol 2003;111:1111–1115.

109. Gadde J, Spence M, Wheeler B, Adkinson NF. Clinical experience with penicillin skin testing in a large inner-city STD clinic. JAMA 1993;270:2456–2463.

110. Kalogeromitros D, Rigopoulos D, Gregoriou S, et al. Penicillin hypersensitivity: Value of clinical history and skin testing in daily practice. Allerg Asthma Proc 2004;25:157–160.

111. Solensky R. Drug desensitization. Immunol Allergy Clin North Am 2004;24:425–443.

112. Tidwell BH, Cleary JD, Lorenz KR. Antimicrobial desensitization: a review of published protocols. Hosp Pharm 1997;32:1362–1369.

113. Caumes E, Guermonprez G, Lecomte C, et al. Efficacy and safety of desensitization with sulfamethoxazole and trimethoprim in 48 previously hypersensitive patients infected with human immunodeficiency virus. Arch Dermatol 1997;133:465–469.

114. Demoly P, Messaad D, Sahla H, et al. Six-hour trimethoprim-sulfa-methoxazole-graded challenge in HIV-infected patients. J Allerg Clin Immunol 1998;102:1033–1036.

115. Rich JD, Sullivan T, Greineder D, et al. Trimethoprim/sulfamethoxazole incremental dose regimen in human immunodeficiency virus-infected persons. Ann Allergy Asthma Immunol 1997;79:409–414.

116. Page NA, Schroeder WS. Rapid desensitization protocols for patient with cardiovascular disease and aspirin sensitivity in an era of dual antiplatelet therapy. Ann Pharmacother 2007;41:61–67.

117. Owen P, Garner J, Hergott L et al. Clopidogrel desensitization: case report and review of published protocols. Pharmacotherapy 2008;28:259–270.

118. Earl G, Davenport J, Narula J. Furosemide challenge in patients with heart failure and adverse reactions to sulfa-containing diuretics. Ann Intern Med 2003;138:358–359.

98

Solid-Organ Transplantation

HEATHER J. JOHNSON AND KRISTINE S. SCHONDER

KEY CONCEPTS

❶ A combination of two to four immunosuppressive drugs is used to target different levels of the immune cascade to prevent allograft rejection and allow lower doses of the individual agents to minimize their toxicity.

❷ Calcineurin inhibitors (CIs), such as cyclosporine and tacrolimus, which inhibit interleukin (IL)-2 and thus block T-cell activation are the backbone of immunosuppressive regimens. However, they are associated with significant adverse effects, namely, nephrotoxicity and neurotoxicity.

❸ Calcineurin inhibitor–induced nephrotoxicity is one of the most common side effects observed in transplant recipients and is the leading cause of renal dysfunction in nonrenal transplant patients. Therapeutic drug monitoring is used in an attempt to optimize the use of calcineurin inhibitors.

❹ Corticosteroids are a key component of immunosuppressive regimens because they block the initial steps in allograft rejection. However, the adverse effects associated with their long-term use have prompted the investigation of corticosteroid-free immunosuppressive protocols. Corticosteroids remain the cornerstone of the treatment of allograft rejection.

❺ Antiproliferative agents such as azathioprine and mycophenolate inhibit T-cell proliferation by altering purine synthesis to prevent acute rejection. Bone marrow suppression is the most significant adverse effect associated with these agents.

❻ Sirolimus and everolimus exert their activity by inhibiting the mTOR (mammalian target of rapamycin) receptor, which alters T-cell response to IL-2. The adverse effects associated with sirolimus include thrombocytopenia, anemia, and hyperlipidemia.

❼ Antibody preparations that target specific receptors on T cells are classified as depleting or nondepleting. Most lymphocyte-depleting antibodies are associated with significant infusion-related reactions.

❽ Long-term allograft and patient survival is limited by chronic rejection, cardiovascular disease, and long-term immunosuppressive complications such as malignancy.

Learning objectives, review questions, and other resources can be found at **www.pharmacotherapyonline.com**.

Solid-organ transplantation provides a lifesaving treatment for patients with end-stage cardiac, kidney, liver, lung, and intestinal disease. About 250 U.S. hospitals offer transplant services, and pharmacists are often an integral part of the transplant team. The Centers for Medicare and Medicaid Services regulations require that transplant programs have a multidisciplinary team including individuals with experience in pharmacology. While the regulations do not specifically state that each center must have a pharmacist, a pharmacist would certainly provide the desired expertise in transplant pharmacotherapy that the regulations mandate.[1]

With the success of transplantation, an increasing number of transplant recipients are in our communities. By the end of 2005 there were more than 160,000 people living with a solid-organ transplant in the United States.[1] In 2008, 27,963 solid-organ transplants were performed. Kidney transplants remain the most common; 10,551 were from cadaveric donors and 5,967 from living donors. The next most frequently transplanted organ was the liver, with 6,070 from cadaveric donors and 249 from living donors. Heart and pancreas (or combined kidney–pancreas) transplants account for over 2,100 and almost 1,300 transplants, respectively; over 1,900 lung transplants were performed as well.[1] While the demand for transplantation continues to grow, the number of cadaveric donors has remained relatively stable during the past decade. In 2008, more than 100,000 persons in the United States were waiting for a transplant (almost 70,000 people were awaiting a kidney, 16,000 a liver, and almost 3,000 were on the list for a heart transplant). Median waiting time for a cadaveric kidney is more than 3.5 years. For liver transplantation the median time to transplant is about 1 year, whereas for heart transplantation it is approximately 6 months. For heart, liver, and lung transplantation clinical status is an important factor affecting waiting times, with the sickest patients receiving priority for available organs.[1]

To increase the number of organs available for transplantation, several strategies have been employed in the past several years. The use of living donors for renal transplantation represents over one third of all kidney transplants, more than any other organ. Living-donor transplantation is also becoming increasingly important for those with end-stage liver and lung disease. Efforts to expand the cadaveric donor pool have included relaxation of age restrictions, development of better preservation solutions, use of "extended-criteria" and non–heart-beating donors, and the transplantation of one liver to more than one recipient, as well as the implantation of only a segment of a liver. Although very controversial, others advocate the creation of a regulated system for compensating individuals in a monetary fashion for the "donation" of a kidney.

Despite all these efforts, patients continue to die awaiting transplantation. In 2004, more than 7,000 people who were on transplantation waiting lists died. In all areas, efforts have been made to improve organ allocation by moving toward allocation based primarily on "medical necessity" versus time on the waiting list.

TABLE 98-1 Organ-Specific Patient and Graft Survival Rates[4]

Organ	Patient Survival (%)		Graft Survival (%)	
	1 Year	5 Years	1 Year	5 Years
Kidney				
Living donor	98.0	90.3	97.3	67.5
Deceased donor	94.8	80.6	90.0	80.2
Liver				
Living donor	90.6	76.1	84.1	68.6
Deceased donor	86.9	73.6	82.3	67.6
Heart	87.8	74.4	87.3	73.2

Although dialysis can be used for an extended period of time to partially replace the function of the kidneys, such options are not readily available for most liver and heart transplantation candidates. Left ventricular assist devices are now used commonly as a bridge to transplantation for many heart transplantation candidates, however, hepatocyte transplantation and artificial liver support remain investigational alternatives or bridges to liver transplantation.[2]

Patient and graft survival rates following transplantation have improved significantly over the past 30 years as a result of advances in pharmacotherapy, surgical techniques, organ preservation, and the postoperative management of patients (Table 98–1). In this chapter the epidemiology of end-stage kidney, liver, and heart disease is briefly reviewed, the pathophysiology of organ rejection is reviewed, the pharmacotherapeutic options for individualized immunosuppressive regimens are critiqued, and the unique complications of these regimens along with the therapeutic challenges they present are discussed.

EPIDEMIOLOGY AND ETIOLOGY

KIDNEY

Renal transplantation is the preferred long-term therapeutic option for most patients with end-stage renal disease because it provides patients with the greatest potential improvement in quality of life. Dialysis catheter-related infections, peritoneal dialysis-associated peritonitis, and scheduled dialysis treatments are avoided, and dietary restrictions are fewer. Patients who receive a renal transplant before the initiation of dialysis have markedly improved quality of life and prolonged life expectancy.[3] The use of living-donor transplantation has made this increasingly possible. Although the analysis of quality of life is complex, patients generally report improved quality of life following transplantation as compared with patients on maintenance dialysis.[4]

Diabetes mellitus, hypertension, and glomerulonephritis are the most common causes of end-stage renal disease leading to kidney transplantation and account for more than 70% of patients (see Chap. 52 and 53).[5] Patients with medical conditions such as unstable cardiac disease or recently diagnosed malignancy, for whom the risk of surgery or chronic immunosuppression would be greater than the risks associated with chronic dialysis, are generally excluded from consideration for transplantation.

CLINICAL CONTROVERSY

The life expectancy of patients infected with human immunodeficiency virus (HIV) has greatly improved in the recent decade, and more patients suffer end-stage organ failure due to co-infection with hepatitis or from HIV-nephropathy. Many clinicians do not consider patients infected with HIV to be appropriate candidates for transplantation because of the relative scarcity of available organs. Some centers consider transplantation of only live donor organs or extended-criteria organs.

LIVER

Noncholestatic cirrhosis (hepatitis C, alcoholic cirrhosis, hepatitis B, nonalcoholic steatohepatitis, and autoimmune hepatitis) is the primary cause of end-stage liver disease and more than 70% of liver transplant recipients have been diagnosed with one of these conditions.[1] Livers are allocated based on a United Network for Organ Sharing-adapted, Model for End-stage Liver Disease (MELD) score. This score, based on serum creatinine concentration, total serum bilirubin concentration, international normalized ratio, and etiology of cirrhosis, has been demonstrated to be a useful tool to predict impending mortality.

There are few absolute contraindications to liver transplantation. Patients should be free from active alcohol or substance abuse. Although hepatitis B and C can recur in the transplanted liver, these are not absolute contraindications to liver transplantation.[2,6]

HEART

Cardiac transplant candidates are typically patients with end-stage heart failure who have New York Heart Association class III or IV symptoms despite maximal medical management and have an expected 1-year mortality risk of 25% or greater without a transplant.[7,8] Idiopathic cardiomyopathy and ischemic heart disease account for heart failure in more than 90% of heart transplantation recipients.[1] Other etiologies include valvular disease, retransplantation for graft atherosclerosis or dysfunction, and congenital heart disease. Chapters 20 and 21 discuss the role of heart transplantation as a therapeutic option for patients with heart failure.

Absolute contraindications to orthotopic cardiac transplantation include the presence of an active infection (except in the case of an infected ventricular assist device, which is an indication for urgent transplantation) or the presence of other diseases (e.g. malignancy) that may limit survival and/or rehabilitation and severe, irreversible pulmonary hypertension.

PHYSIOLOGIC CONSEQUENCES OF TRANSPLANTATION

Transplantation is truly lifesaving for heart, liver, and lung transplantation recipients, whereas renal transplantation is associated with improved quality of life and survival when compared with dialysis.[9] Most heart transplantation patients return to New York Heart Association functional class I following transplantation. Although not all return to work, 89.9% of patients consider themselves to have no activity limitations at 1-year follow-up.[10] The specific physiologic consequences of kidney, liver, and heart transplantation are discussed next.

KIDNEY TRANSPLANTATION

The glomerular filtration rate of a successfully transplanted kidney may be near normal almost immediately after transplantation. In some patients, however, the concentration of standard biochemical indicators of renal function, such as serum creatinine and blood urea nitrogen, may remain elevated for several days. Standard formulas used to predict drug dosing rely on a stable serum creatinine and may be inaccurate immediately following transplantation (see Chap. 50).

Although the allograft is able to remove uremic toxins from the body, it may take several weeks for other physiologic complications of chronic renal failure, such as anemia, calcium and phosphate imbalance, and altered lipid profiles, to resolve. The renal production of erythropoietin and 1-hydroxylation of vitamin D may return toward normal early in the postoperative period. Because the onset of physiologic effects may be delayed, continuation of pretransplantation calcitriol, calcium supplementation, and/or phosphate binders may be warranted. The duration of therapy will depend on how rapidly kidney function improves. Patients should be monitored for hypophosphatemia and hypercalcemia.

Primary nonfunction of a renal allograft or delayed graft function (DGF) is characterized by the need for dialysis in the first postop week or the failure of the serum creatinine to fall by 30% of the pretransplantation value. The incidence of DGF in cadaveric renal transplantation ranges from 8% to 50% and results in a slower return of the kidney's excretory, metabolic, and synthetic functions. DGF is associated with prolonged hospital stays, higher costs, difficult management of immunosuppressive therapy, slower patient rehabilitation, and poor graft survival. Other early causes of renal dysfunction such as urethral obstruction or arterial or venous stenosis or thrombosis should be distinguished from DGF.

The primary cause of DGF is acute tubular necrosis (ATN). The incidence of ATN increases when kidneys are harvested from donors who recently experienced a cardiac arrest, from donors who were hypotensive or on vasopressors, or from older donors (age >55 years) and with prolonged periods of ischemia. While cyclosporine and tacrolimus have been implicated in the prolongation of ATN, a clear cause-and-effect relationship has not been established. Nonetheless, most clinicians will decrease calcineurin inhibitor doses in patients with ATN. DGF predisposes patients to acute rejection, possibly as a consequence of decreased calcineurin inhibitor levels and a resultant reduction in the level of immunosuppression.

LIVER TRANSPLANTATION

The physiologic consequences of liver transplantation are complex, involving changes in both metabolic and synthetic function. Postoperatively, the liver transplant recipient will likely have many fluid, electrolyte, and nutritional abnormalities. Biliary tract dysfunction may alter the absorption of fats and fat-soluble drugs.[11] Poor absorption of the lipid-soluble drug cyclosporine improves after successful liver transplantation and reestablishment of bile flow. Vitamin E deficiency and its neurologic complications in liver failure patients are reversed after successful liver transplantation. In stable adult liver transplant patients, the concentrations of retinol and tocopherol are similar to those seen in normal healthy subjects, indicating recovery of transplanted liver production and excretion of bile salts needed for fat-soluble vitamin absorption. Table 98–2 summarizes the effects of liver transplantation on metabolism and renal elimination that are seen in the immediate postoperative period. Most of these changes resolve as liver function normalizes.

The newly transplanted liver fails to function in 10% to 15% of recipients as the result of several different mechanisms. Early graft failure can result from preexisting disease in the donor, and even coagulation defects have been acquired through donor organs. The technical complexity of the operation can produce flaws in revascularization that also lead to graft nonfunction. Surgical complications include portal vein or hepatic artery thrombosis and bile duct leaks. Ischemic injury can also result in early graft dysfunction. While hyperacute rejection in liver transplantation rarely occurs, graft failure in the first 2 postoperative weeks may indicate antibody-mediated graft destruction.

TABLE 98-2	Perioperative Changes in Drug Disposition and Elimination Following Liver Transplantation	
	Result	**Comment**
Serum proteins		
↓ Albumin	↑ Free fraction of drugs usually bound to albumin	Diazepam, salicylic acid binding greater in liver transplant than chronic liver disease because of endogenous binding inhibitors (up to 45 days post-transplant)
↑ Alpha-1-Acid glycoprotein	Lower free fraction of drugs	Lidocaine
Metabolism/elimination		
Microsomal enzymes	↑ CYP2E1 activity	Increased drug metabolism (induction)
	↔ CYP2D6	Unaffected
	↓ CYP activity	Decreased drug elimination (inhibition)
Oxidation	Stable	
Conjugation	Normalizes after transplant	
Biliary function	↓ Absorption of lipophilic compounds	
	↑ Cyclosporine metabolites in blood	
Renal elimination	Elimination of gentamicin, vancomycin, cephalosporins less than predicted by serum creatinine	Renal elimination of metabolites limited

Adapted from reference 11.

HEART TRANSPLANTATION

The orthotopically transplanted heart is denervated and no longer responds to physiologic stimuli and pharmacologic agents in a normal manner (Table 98–3).[9] Patients, for example, do not experience angina. In situations requiring an increased heart rate such as exercise or hypotension, the denervated heart is unable to acutely increase heart rate but instead relies on increasing the stroke volume. Later in the course of exercise or hypotension, heart rate increases in response to circulating catecholamines. While the maximum exercise capacity of heart transplant recipients is below normal, most patients are able to resume normal lifestyles and reasonably vigorous activity levels. Partial reinnervation may occur over time, thereby facilitating more normal physiologic and pharmacologic responses and better exercise capacity.[10]

A number of autoregulatory, anatomic, and physiologic responses present in the normal heart are interrupted or blunted for the first 6 weeks after transplantation. The donor sinus node function may be impaired by preservation injury, direct surgical trauma at excision, the presence of long-acting antiarrhythmics (e.g., amiodarone) taken prior to transplant by the recipient, and a lack of "conditioning" responsiveness to catecholamines.[10] Consequently, the transplanted heart generally requires chronotropic support with either milrinone or pacing in the perioperative period to maintain a heart rate of 90 to 110 beats per minute and satisfactory hemodynamics (i.e., blood pressure, urine output, and tissue perfusion). Approximately 10% to 20% of transplant patients will have persistent chronotropic incompetence requiring either short courses of medications, such as terbutaline or theophylline, or permanent cardiac pacing.

Right ventricular function is frequently impaired, presumably as a result of preservation injury and elevated pulmonary vascular

TABLE 98-3 Altered Responses to Cardiac Drugs in the Denervated Transplanted Heart

Drug	Effect	Mechanism	Comment
Digitalis	Normal inotropic effect; minimal effect on AV node	Direct myocardial effect; denervation	
Atropine	No effect on AV node	Denervation	
Adrenaline/noradrenaline	Increased contractility; increased chronotropy	Denervation; hypersensitivity	Increased cardiac output mediated by increased heart rate
Isoproterenol	Normal increase in contractility; normal increase in chronotropy	No neuronal uptake	
Quinidine	No vagolytic effect	Denervation	
Verapamil	AV block	Direct effect	
Nifedipine	No reflex tachycardia	Denervation	
Hydralazine	No reflex tachycardia	Denervation	
β-Blocker	Increased antagonist effect	Denervation	Impaired heart rate response, use sparingly
Adenosine	Negative chronotropic effect	Hypersensitivity; effect on sinus node of denervated heart	Life-threatening asystole (>0.5 min) may occur if used to treat supraventricular arrhythmia or stress testing
Acetylcholine	Negative chronotropic effect	Hypersensitivity; effect on sinus node of denervated heart	

AV, atrioventricular.

Reproduced from Deng MC. Heart failure: Cardiac transplantation. Heart 2002;87:177–184 with permission from the BMJ Publishing Group Ltd.

resistance. A "restrictive" hemodynamic pattern may be present initially but usually improves in 6 weeks following transplantation. Donor–recipient size mismatch may contribute to early post-transplantation hemodynamic abnormalities characterized by higher right and left ventricular end-diastolic pressures. Supraventricular arrhythmias are usually transient and may result from overvigorous use of catecholamines or milrinone. If this type of arrhythmia occurs after the perioperative period, the astute clinician should consider the possibility of acute rejection.

Myocardial depression frequently occurs and generally requires inotropic support with agents such as dobutamine, milrinone, and epinephrine. On occasion, intra- or postoperative administration of vasodilators, including nitric oxide, and inotropic agents may be necessary to treat right-sided failure in the transplant patient; milrinone and isoproterenol are preferred in this setting.

Persistent abnormalities of diastolic function are often noted in the transplanted heart such that intracardiac pressures increase in an exaggerated fashion in response to exercise and/or volume infusion.[10] These abnormalities are due in part to denervation, but also to acute rejection or to the scarring secondary to previously treated rejection episodes, hypertension, or cardiac allograft vasculopathy.

Hypertension may occur following surgery secondary to the effect of elevated catecholamine levels and systemic vascular resistance as the residual effects of end-stage heart failure on the healthy heart. Systolic blood pressure should be maintained at 110 to 120 mm Hg to enhance cardiac function. In the acute post-transplantation period, intravenous nitroprusside or nitroglycerin may be needed, whereas oral angiotensin-converting enzyme inhibitors (ACEIs) and/or amlodipine are commonly used once the patient can ingest oral medications.

PATHOPHYSIOLOGY OF REJECTION

GENERAL CONCEPTS

Rejection of any transplanted organ is primarily mediated by activation of alloreactive T cells and antigen-presenting cells such as B lymphocytes, macrophages, and dendritic cells. Acute allograft rejection is caused primarily by the infiltration of T cells into the allograft, which triggers inflammatory and cytotoxic effects on the graft. Complex interactions between the allograft and cellular

cytokines, cell-to-cell interactions, CD4+ and CD8+ T cells, and B cells ultimately lead to chronic rejection and graft loss if adequate immunosuppression is not maintained.[12]

The sequence of events that underlies graft rejection is recognition, via MHC class I and II antigens, of the donor's histocompatibility differences by the recipient's immune system, recruitment of activated lymphocytes, initiation of immune effector mechanisms, and finally graft destruction. The specifics of this immune cascade of organ rejection are discussed in Chapter 95. The complex nature of cytokine interactions makes it very difficult to design drugs with exclusive actions (Fig. 98–1).

Rejection of the transplanted tissue can take place at any time following surgery and is classified clinically as hyperacute rejection, acute cellular rejection, and/or humoral or chronic rejection.[13]

Efforts are made to allocate well-matched, according to human leukocyte antigens (HLA)-A, -B, and -DR, kidneys to minimize rejection and enhance survival rates. However, the benefit of having no recipient donor mismatches may be negated by excessive cold ischemia time (>36 hours) and donor age older than 60 years. HLA tissue matching is not performed routinely before transplantation for livers and hearts because organ availability is more limited and the optimal cold ischemia time is shorter. However, if the potential recipient's blood is reactive against a panel of random donor blood samples (i.e., panel reactive antibody [PRA] >10% to 20%), a negative T-cell crossmatch is required prior to transplantation. Transplanted organs must be matched for ABO blood group compatibility with the recipient as ABO mismatching will result. Liver transplantation may be carried out in emergency situations across ABO blood groups, but survival is lower.

HYPERACUTE REJECTION

Hyperacute rejection may be evident within minutes of the transplantation procedure when preformed donor-specific antibodies are present in the recipient at the time of the transplant. Hyperacute rejection can also be induced by immunoglobulin G antibodies that bind to antigens on the vascular endothelium, such as class I MHC, ABO, and vascular endothelial cell antigens. Tissue damage can be mediated through antibody-dependent, cell-mediated cytotoxicity or through activation of the complement cascade. The ischemic damage to the microvasculature rapidly results in tissue necrosis.

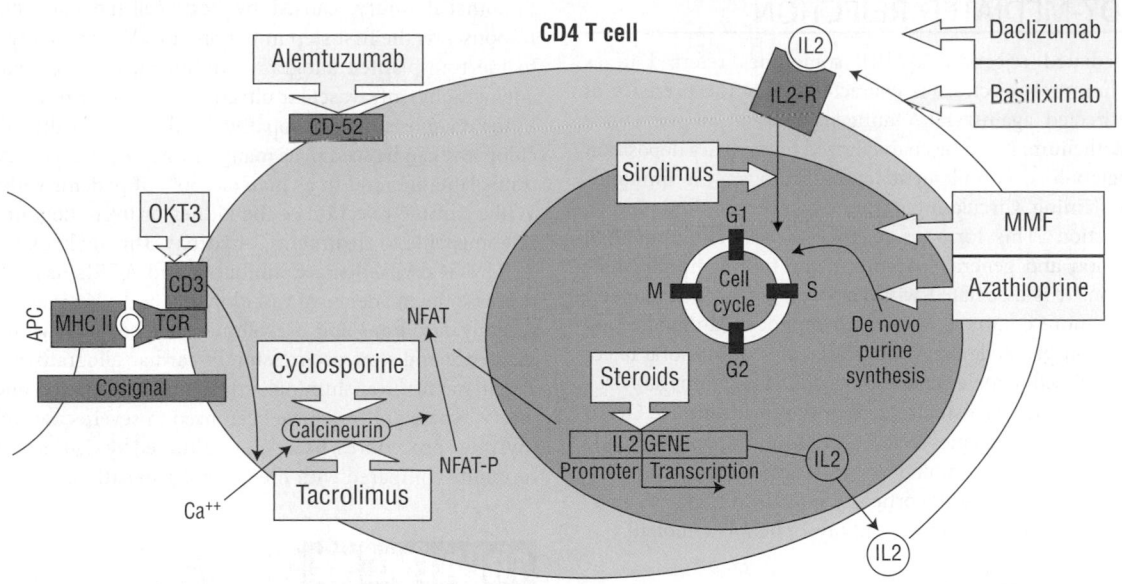

FIGURE 98-1. Stages of CD4 T-cell activation and cytokine production with identification of the sites of action of different immunosuppressive agents. Antigen major histocompatibility complex (MHC) II molecule complexes are responsible for initiating the activation of CD4 T cells. These MHC-peptide complexes are recognized by the T-cell recognition complex (TCR). A costimulatory signal initiates signal transduction with activation of second messengers, one of which is calcineurin. Calcineurin removes phosphates from the nuclear factors (NFAT-P) allowing them to enter the nucleus. These nuclear factors specifically bind to an interleukin (IL)-2 promoter gene facilitating IL-2 gene transcription. Interaction of IL-2 with the IL-2 receptor (IL-2R) on the cell membrane surface induces cell proliferation and production of cytokines specific to the T cell. (APC, antigen-presenting cells; MMF, mycophenolate mofetil.) (*Reprinted from Ann Thorac Surg, Vol. 77, Mueller XM, Drug immunosuppressive therapy for adult heart transplantation. Part I. Immune response to allograft and mechanism of action of immunosuppressants, pages 354–362, Copyright © 2004, with permission from Elsevier.*)

Hyperacute rejection has become uncommon in kidney and heart transplants. A positive crossmatch presents a serious risk for graft failure even if hyperacute rejection does not occur. A negative lymphocytotoxicity crossmatch does not entirely rule out the possibility of hyperacute rejection because non-MHC antigens on the vascular endothelium can serve as targets of donor-specific antibodies. Early graft dysfunction is treated with supportive care and retransplantation if possible. The reason for the rarity of hyperacute rejection in liver transplantation is not fully understood, but the local release of cytokines may alter the immunologic reaction in the liver.

ACUTE CELLULAR REJECTION

Acute rejection is most common in the first few months following transplantation but can occur at any time during the life of the allograft. Acute cellular rejection is mediated by alloreactive T-lymphocytes that appear in the circulation and infiltrate the allograft through the vascular endothelium. After the graft is infiltrated by lymphocytes, the cytotoxic cells specifically target and kill the functioning cells in the allograft. At the same time, local release of lymphokines attracts and stimulates macrophages to produce tissue damage through a delayed hypersensitivity–like mechanism. These immunologic and inflammatory events lead to nonspecific signs and symptoms including pain and tenderness over the graft site, fever, and lethargy.

Kidney

Acute rejection, which may affect up to 20% of patients during the first 6 months following transplantation, is evidenced by an abrupt rise in serum creatinine concentration of ≥30% over baseline. A specific histologic diagnosis can be obtained via biopsy of the allograft and is often used to guide therapy for rejection. A biopsy specimen with a diffuse lymphocytic infiltrate is consistent with acute cellular rejection. After the diagnosis of rejection has been confirmed, the potential risks and benefits of specific antirejection therapies must be evalu-

ated. Hypertension often worsens during an episode of rejection, and edema and weight gain are common as a result of sodium and fluid retention. Symptomatic azotemia may also develop in severe cases.

Liver

The liver is more likely to promote immunologic tolerance than the other vascularized organs. Approximately 18% of liver transplantation recipients will experience a rejection episode in the first post-transplant year. The clinical signs of acute cellular rejection include leukocytosis and a change in the color or quantity of bile for those who still have an external drainage tube in place. A serum bilirubin 50% over baseline or increases in hepatic transaminases to values more than three times the upper limit of normal, are sensitive markers of rejection. Although a liver biopsy provides definitive evidence of the diagnosis of rejection, a prompt response to antirejection medication has also proven useful as a means to differentiate rejection from other causes of hepatic dysfunction.

Heart

More than 60% of heart transplantation recipients will experience at least one episode of acute rejection during the first year, with 90% of all rejections occurring within the first 6 months.[14] Because rejection of the cardiac allograft is not necessarily accompanied by overt clinical signs or symptoms and because the incidence of acute rejection is highest during this time period, endomyocardial biopsies are often performed at regularly scheduled intervals following transplantation.[15] A typical biopsy schedule would be weekly for the first postoperative month, biweekly for the next 2 months, and monthly to bimonthly through the remainder of the first post-transplant year. Nonspecific symptoms, including low-grade fever, malaise, mild reduction in exercise capacity, heart failure, or atrial arrhythmias may also be evident and if present are reflective of a more severe rejection episode.

ANTIBODY-MEDIATED REJECTION

Antibody-mediated rejection (AMR), sometimes referred to as vascular or humoral rejection, is characterized by the presence of antibodies directed against HLA antigens present on the donor vascular endothelium. It can be characterized by capillary deposition of immunoglobulins, complement, and fibrinogen on immuno-fluorescence staining. Circulating immune complexes often precede humoral rejection. This form of rejection is less common than cellular rejection and generally occurs in the first 3 months after transplantation. It is associated with an increased fatality rate and appears to be more common when antilymphocyte antibodies are used for rejection prophylaxis. An increased risk of humoral rejection is associated with female gender, elevated PRA, cytomegalovirus seropositivity, a positive crossmatch, and prior sensitization to OKT3 (muromonab CD3).[16] Strategies to reverse humoral rejection include plasmapheresis, often in combination with intravenous immuno-globulin, high-dose intravenous corticosteroids, antithymocyte glob-ulin, cyclophosphamide, rituximab, and mycophenolate mofetil.

CHRONIC REJECTION

Chronic rejection is a major cause of graft loss. It presents as a slow and indolent form of acute cellular rejection, in which the involvement of the humoral immune system and antibodies against the vascular endothelium appear to play a role. Persistent perivascular and inter-stitial inflammation is a common finding in kidney, liver, and heart transplantation. As a result of the complex interaction of multiple drugs and diseases over time, it is difficult to delineate the true nature of chronic rejection. Unlike acute rejection, chronic rejection is not reversible with any immunosuppressive agents currently available.

Kidney

Advances in the management of acute rejection during the last decade have increased the duration of functioning grafts from living and cadaveric donors by more than 70%.[17] Chronic allograft neph-ropathy remains the most common cause of graft loss in the late post-transplantation period (>1 year). The histopathologic char-acteristics of chronic allograft nephropathy include vascular inti-mal hyperplasia, tubular atrophy, interstitial fibrosis, and chronic glomerulopathy. Structural changes are seen in as many as 40% of kidney transplantation patients 1 year after transplantation and may present as early as 3 months.[18] Hypertension, proteinuria, and a progressive decline in renal function represent the classic clinical triad of chronic allograft nephropathy. Factors that contribute to the development of chronic allograft nephropathy include calcineu-rin inhibitor nephrotoxicity, polyomavirus infection, hypertension, donor-related factors including ischemia time and undetected kidney disease in the donor kidney, and recurrence of the primary kidney disease in the recipient.

Liver

Approximately 3 to 5% of transplant livers are affected by chronic rejection, which is characterized by an obliterative arteriopathy and the gradual loss of bile ducts, often referred to as the vanishing bile duct syndrome. Initially patients experience an asymptomatic rise in the alkaline phosphatase and γ-glutamyl transpeptidase. As levels of bilirubin increase, patients become jaundiced and may experi-ence itching.

Heart

Cardiac allograft vasculopathy, characterized by accelerated intimal thickening or development of atherosclerotic plaques, is the leading cause of graft failure and death in heart transplant recipients.[19]

Endothelial injury, caused by both cell-mediated and humoral responses, is the first step in the process. Vasculopathy is restricted to the transplanted allograft. Routine surveillance with coronary angiography, intravascular ultrasound, or other procedures can aid in the diagnosis of vasculopathy. Evidence of cardiac allograft vas-culopathy can be seen in as many as 14% of patients within 1 year of transplantation and in as many as 50% of patients within 5 years.[19] While chronic rejection of the kidney or liver allograft is generally not amenable to treatment, 3-hydroxy-3-methylglutaryl-coenzyme A (HMGCoA) reductase inhibitors and ACEIs have been used to decrease the incidence of vasculopathy in the heart allograft.[19] More recently, sirolimus and everolimus have been shown to reduce the incidence and slow progression of cardiac allograft vasculopathy.[19] Percutaneous transluminal coronary angioplasty and coronary artery bypass grafting have been used in severe cases of vasculopa-thy; these procedures, however, are limited by significantly increased mortality compared with the general population.[19]

TREATMENT

Immunosuppression

■ DESIRED OUTCOME

Immediately following surgery, the primary goal of therapy is to prevent hyperacute and acute rejection. The high doses of immu-nosuppressants required to achieve this goal, if maintained long term, may result in serious complications such as nephrotoxicity, infection, thrombocytopenia, and drug-induced diabetes. Therefore rapid dosage reductions are frequently used to minimize these effects. Transplant immunosuppression must be balanced to opti-mize both graft and patient survival.

■ GENERAL APPROACH TO TREATMENT

❶ A multidrug approach is rational from an immunomechanistic viewpoint because the many agents have overlapping and poten-tially synergistic mechanisms of action. Furthermore, the use of a multidrug immunosuppression regimen may allow the use of lower doses of individual agents, thus reducing the severity of dose-related adverse effects (Fig. 98–2). The protocols and individual drug regimens tend to be medical center specific. Although induction therapy may not be uniformly used, in almost every setting, patients receive IV methylprednisolone intraoperatively. Patients may also receive a descending dose of methylprednisolone over the first 5 to 7 postoperative days before beginning oral prednisone. Protocols generally combine a drug from two or three of the following classes: calcineurin inhibitors, antimetabolites or proliferation signal inhibi-tors, and corticosteroids.

If rejection is suspected, a biopsy can be done for definitive diag-nosis or the patient may be empirically treated for rejection. Empiric treatment generally involves administration of high-dose corticos-teroids, usually 500 to 1,000 mg of methylprednisolone intrave-nously for one to three doses. If signs and symptoms of rejection are resolved with empiric therapy, the maintenance immunosuppressive regimen is generally modified to provide a greater level of overall immunosuppression. If rejection is confirmed by biopsy, treatment may be based on the severity of rejection with polyclonal and mono-clonal antibodies being reserved for moderate to severe rejections or those that have not responded to a course of corticosteroids.

Induction Therapy

Induction therapy involves the use of a high level of immunosuppres-sion, at the time of transplantation, with or without the immediate

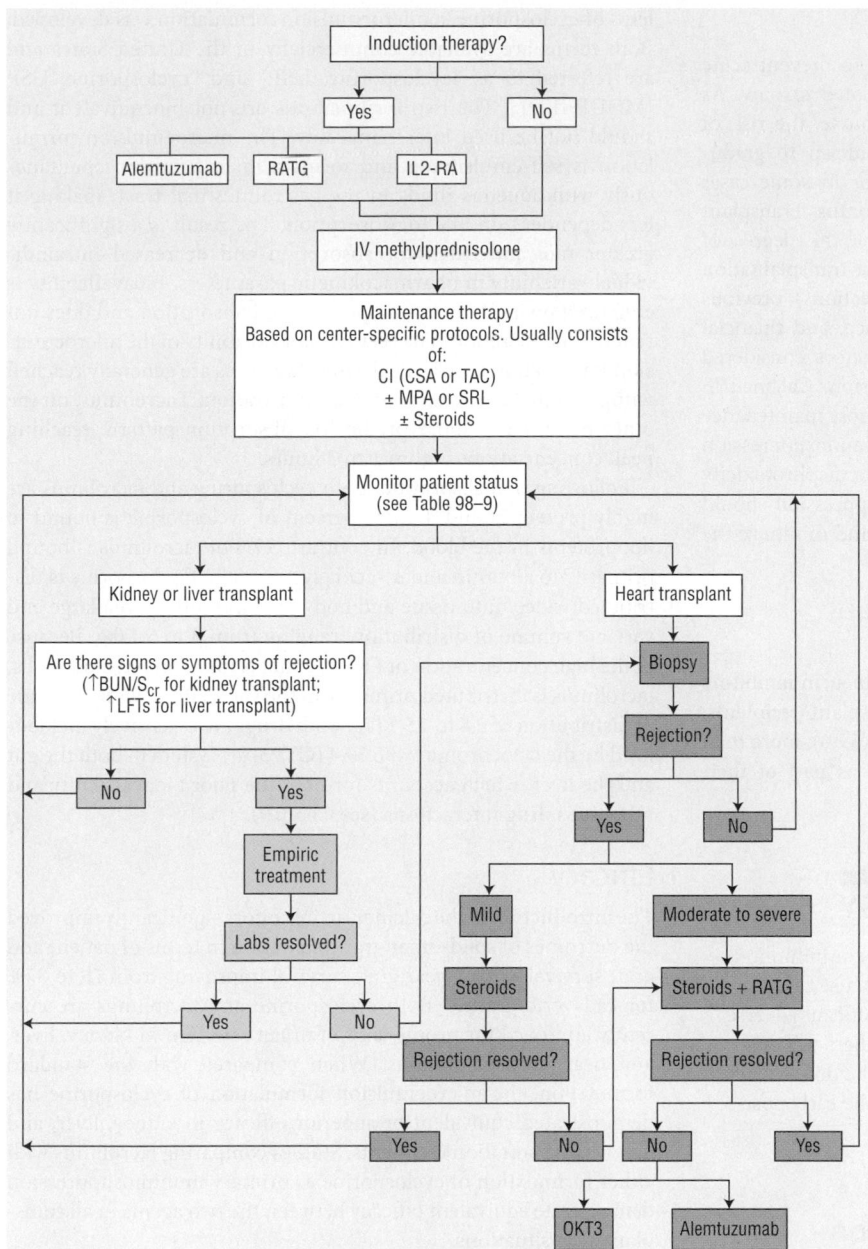

FIGURE 98-2. General approach to solid-organ transplant immunosuppression. (BUN, blood urea nitrogen; CI, calcineurin inhibitor; CSA, cyclosporine; IL2RA, interleukin-2 receptor antagonist; LFTs, liver function tests; MPA, mycophenolic acid; OKT3, muromonab CD3; RATG, rabbit antithymocyte immunoglobulin; S_{cr}, serum creatinine; SRL, sirolimus; TAC, tacrolimus.)

introduction of cyclosporine or tacrolimus (see Fig. 98–2). Induction therapy consists of one of two perioperative immunosuppressive strategies: (a) the provision of a highly intense level of immunosuppression, often on the basis of patient-specific risk factors such as age and race, or (b) the use of antibody therapy to provide enough immunosuppression to delay the initiation of therapy with the nephrotoxic calcineurin inhibitors. The rationale for delayed calcineurin inhibitor administration varies slightly depending on the type of transplant. In renal transplantation, the newly transplanted kidney is very susceptible to nephrotoxic injury, whereas in liver and heart transplantation, the idea is to protect patients with preexisting renal insufficiency from further insults during the perioperative period. Additionally, calcineurin inhibitor dosage adjustment to maintain target concentrations may be difficult in the perioperative period secondary to fluctuation of gastrointestinal motility and enteral intake.

Acute Rejection

The primary goal of acute rejection therapy is to minimize the intensity of the immune response and prevent irreversible injury to the allograft. The available options include (a) increasing the doses of current immunosuppressive drugs, (b) "pulse" corticosteroids with subsequent dose taper, (c) addition of another immunosuppressant indefinitely, or (d) short-term treatment with a polyclonal or monoclonal antibody. The treatment of acute rejection almost always begins with "pulse" corticosteroid therapy for several days (oral or intravenously). Recent data in renal transplantation indicate, however, that African Americans do not respond as well to corticosteroids; thus antithymocyte globulin may be preferable for this patient population.[20]

Cytolytic agents are often reserved for those with corticosteroid-resistant rejection, signs of hemodynamic compromise (heart), or more severe rejections. Other innovative forms of therapy for persistent or intractable rejection have been investigated, including mycophenolate mofetil, tacrolimus, low-dose methotrexate, sirolimus, total lymphoid irradiation, and plasmapheresis and intravenous immunoglobulin. Prophylactic agents such as valganciclovir, nystatin, trimethoprim-sulfamethoxazole, H_2-receptor antagonists or proton-pump inhibitors, and/or antacids may be added to minimize adverse effects associated with these intensive immunosuppression regimens.

Maintenance Therapy

The goal of maintenance immunosuppression is to prevent acute and chronic rejection while minimizing drug-related toxicity. As patients progress through the post-transplant course, the risk of acute rejection decreases, thus allowing the clinician to gradually reduce the doses of immunosuppressants or in some cases totally withdraw them over a period of 6 to 12 months. Transplant organ and type (cadaveric versus living-donor), the degree of HLA mismatch, time after transplantation, post-transplantation complications (including the number of acute rejections), previous immunosuppressive adverse reactions, compliance, and financial considerations are among the patient-specific factors considered in individualizing maintenance immunosuppression. Calcineurin inhibitors are generally a central component in most maintenance regimens, although calcineurin inhibitor–free immunosuppression remains a future goal because of the significant nephrotoxicity associated with these agents. Ideally, immunosuppression should be optimized to prevent acute rejection episodes and minimize the occurrence of chronic rejection.

■ CALCINEURIN INHIBITORS

❷ Cyclosporine and tacrolimus are the two calcineurin inhibitors (CIs) currently used for most solid-organ transplant recipients. With the exception of heart transplant recipients (59%), more than 80% of transplant recipients receive tacrolimus as part of their immunosuppressive regimen.[1]

CLINICAL CONTROVERSY

Although calcineurin inhibitors are the mainstay of immunosuppressive protocols, some clinicians attempt to use calcineurin inhibitor–sparing protocols to avoid the significant adverse effects associated with calcineurin inhibitors. Others will delay the initiation of calcineurin inhibitors to avoid the dose-related adverse effects associated with their use during the early post-transplantation period.

Pharmacology/Mechanism of Action

Calcineurin inhibitors block T-cell proliferation by inhibiting the production of IL-2 and other cytokines by T cells (see Fig. 98–1). Cyclosporine and tacrolimus bind to unique cytoplasmic immunophilins cyclophilin and FK-binding protein-12 (FKBP12), respectively. The drug–immunophilin complex inhibits the action of calcineurin, an enzyme that activates the nuclear factor of activated T cells, which is, in turn, responsible for the transcription of several key cytokines necessary for T-cell activity, including IL-2. IL-2 is a potent growth factor for T cells and ultimately is responsible for activation and clonal expansion.

Pharmacokinetics

The calcineurin inhibitors are highly lipophilic compounds, with variable but generally low bioavailability of approximately 30% (range: 5% to 60%). Unlike tacrolimus, cyclosporine depends on bile for intestinal absorption, which lends to more interpatient and intrapatient variability. Liver recipients with a T-tube for diversion of bile may thus experience incomplete and erratic absorption of cyclosporine.

Because of the significant variability in absorption of cyclosporine, peak concentrations are reached within 2 to 6 hours of oral administration. To overcome the pharmacokinetic problems of cyclosporine, a microemulsion formulation was developed. Both forms are available commercially in the United States and are referred to as "cyclosporine, USP" and "cyclosporine, USP [MODIFIED]." The two formulations are not bioequivalent and should not be used interchangeably. The microemulsion formulation is self-emulsifying and forms a microemulsion spontaneously with aqueous fluids in the gastrointestinal tract, making it less dependent on bile for absorption. The result is a significantly greater rate and extent of absorption and decreased intraindividual variability in pharmacokinetic parameters. Bioavailability is enhanced owing to better dispersion and absorption and does not require bile excretion. The relative bioavailability of the microemulsion formulation is 60%. Peak concentrations are generally reached within 1.5 to 2 hours after oral administration. Tacrolimus, on the other hand, has a more predictable absorption pattern, reaching peak concentrations within 1 to 3 hours.

Following oral absorption, both cyclosporine and tacrolimus are highly protein bound. Ninety percent of cyclosporine is bound to lipoproteins in the blood. In contrast, 99% of tacrolimus is bound primarily to albumin and α_1-acid glycoprotein. Cyclosporine is distributed widely into tissue and body fluids, resulting in a large and variable volume of distribution, ranging from 3 to 5 L/kg. Because of the high concentration of FKBP12 that is found in red blood cells, tacrolimus is distributed primarily in the vasculature, with a volume of distribution of 0.8 to 1.9 L/kg. Both drugs are extensively metabolized by the cytochrome P450 3A4 (CYP3A4) system in both the gut and the liver, which accounts for both the poor bioavailability and numerous drug interactions (see Chap. 9).

Efficacy

The introduction of the calcineurin inhibitors significantly improved the outcomes of solid-organ transplantation in terms of patient and graft survival, with 1-year graft survival improving from 75 to 87% for cadaveric grafts.[17] Both cyclosporine and tacrolimus are currently approved for prophylaxis of organ rejection in kidney, liver, and heart transplantations. When compared with the standard formulation, the microemulsion formulation of cyclosporine has demonstrated equivalent or superior efficacy in kidney, liver, and heart transplantation recipients. Studies comparing tacrolimus with either formulation of cyclosporine as primary immunosuppression demonstrate equivalent efficacy between the two agents in all transplantation situations.

Monotherapy with calcineurin inhibitors has been described.[21] The avoidance of long-term corticosteroids is the primary advantage of calcineurin inhibitor monotherapy, whereas the primary disadvantage is the higher incidence of rejection. As a result, calcineurin inhibitors are rarely used as monotherapy.

Adverse Effects

Table 98–4 summarizes the adverse effects of calcineurin inhibitors, cyclosporine and tacrolimus, and other immunosuppressants. The nephrotoxic potential of both drugs is equal and is often related to the dose and duration of exposure. Neurotoxicity typically manifests as tremors, headache, and peripheral neuropathy; occasionally, however, seizures have been observed. Tacrolimus may be associated with an increased occurrence of neurologic complications compared with cyclosporine.

Cyclosporine appears to have a greater propensity to cause or worsen hypertension and hyperlipidemia compared with tacrolimus.[22-25] On the other hand, hyperglycemia is more common with tacrolimus than with cyclosporine but is often reversible when doses of tacrolimus and/or corticosteroids are reduced.[23] Cyclosporine is associated with cosmetic effects, such as hirsutism and gingival hyperplasia, which may be managed by converting

TABLE 98-4	Comparison of Common Adverse Effects of Maintenance Immunosuppressants					
AZA	**MMF**	**SIR**	**Steroids**	**CSA**	**TAC**
Nausea, vomiting	Diarrhea, nausea	Hyperlipidemia	GI bleeding	Hyperlipidemia	Diarrhea, nausea
Thrombocytopenia	Leukopenia	Thrombocytopenia	Hyperlipidemia	Nephrotoxicity	Hepatotoxicity
Leukopenia		Leukopenia	Leukocytosis	Tremor	Nephrotoxicity
			Hypertension	Hypertension	Tremor, headache
			Hyperglycemia	Hyperglycemia	Hypertension
			Weight gain	Gingival hyperplasia	Hyperglycemia
			Mood changes	Hirsutism	Hyperkalemia, hypomagnesemia

AZA, azathioprine; CSA, cyclosporine; MMF, mycophenolate mofetil; SIR, sirolimus; TAC, tacrolimus.

from cyclosporine to tacrolimus or by proper hygiene in patients who cannot be switched to tacrolimus. Tacrolimus, in contrast, has been reported to cause alopecia, which is usually self-limiting and reversible.

Calcineurin Inhibitor Nephrotoxicity

❸ Two types of nephrotoxicity can occur with calcineurin inhibitors. Acute nephrotoxicity is frequently seen early and is dose dependent and reversible, but chronic nephropathy is more common. Clinical manifestations of calcineurin inhibitor nephrotoxicity include elevated serum creatinine and blood urea nitrogen levels, hyperkalemia, hyperuricemia, mild proteinuria, and a decreased fractional excretion of sodium. Calcineurin inhibitor nephrotoxicity is recognized as the leading cause of renal dysfunction following nonrenal solid-organ transplant.

The predominant mechanism for calcineurin inhibitor nephrotoxicity is renal vasoconstriction, primarily of the afferent arteriole, resulting in increased renal vascular resistance, decreased renal blood flow by up to 40%, reduced glomerular filtration rate by up to 30%, and increased proximal tubular sodium reabsorption with a reduction in urinary sodium and potassium excretion. A number of other mechanisms have been implicated, including changes in the renin–angiotensin–aldosterone system, prostaglandin synthesis, nitrous oxide production, sympathetic nervous system activation, and calcium handling.[26]

Measures to reduce calcineurin inhibitor nephrotoxicity include delaying administration immediately postoperatively in patients at high risk for nephrotoxicity (using alternative induction protocols including an IL-2 receptor antagonist or antilymphocyte globulin), monitoring calcineurin inhibitor trough blood levels and reducing the calcineurin inhibitor dosage if the vasoconstrictive effects are problematic, and avoiding other nephrotoxins (e.g., aminoglycosides, amphotericin B, and nonsteroidal antiinflammatory agents) when possible. Currently, no proven therapies consistently prevent or reverse the nephrotoxic effects of calcineurin inhibitors.

In patients who have received a kidney transplant, it is often difficult to differentiate calcineurin inhibitor nephrotoxicity from renal allograft rejection. Because the clinical features of acute renal allograft rejection and calcineurin inhibitor nephrotoxicity may overlap considerably, a renal biopsy is necessary to differentiate the two (Table 98-5). However, differentiating between chronic renal allograft rejection and calcineurin inhibitor nephrotoxicity may be more difficult because, in addition to clinical signs and symptoms, biopsy findings may also be similar.

Drug–Drug and Drug–Food Interactions

Drug interactions occur frequently with the calcineurin inhibitors because they are substrates for CYP3A4 and P-glycoprotein.[27–29] The most commonly administered drugs that are known to significantly alter cyclosporine and tacrolimus levels are highlighted in Table 98-6. Inhibitors of CYP3A4, such as diltiazem or erythromycin, can increase drug concentrations up to 82%, whereas drugs that induce CYP3A4 activity, such as phenytoin or rifampin, can decrease drug concentrations by 50%.[22] Some have taken advantage of these interactions by routinely prescribing CYP3A4 inhibitors to reduce the dosage and cost of calcineurin inhibitor therapy while maintaining the same therapeutic concentrations. This strategy seems more beneficial with cyclosporine than with tacrolimus.[30–32] While in vitro data suggest that drugs that increase the pH of the GI tract, such as magnesium-, aluminum-, or calcium-containing antacids, sodium bicarbonate, and magnesium oxide, can cause a pH-mediated degradation of tacrolimus by physically adsorbing tacrolimus in the GI tract, this has not been borne out in clinical studies.[33] Some clinicians suggest separating such compounds from tacrolimus administration by at least 2 hours to avoid any potential interaction.

Cyclosporine, and to a lesser extent, tacrolimus, are inhibitors of CYP3A4.[34] The inhibitory effects of cyclosporine and tacrolimus on CYP3A4 can be seen with weaker substrates, such as the HMG-CoA reductase inhibitors ("statins"). Concomitant administration of a calcineurin inhibitor with an HMG-CoA reductase inhibitor results in an increase in the HMG-CoA reductase inhibitor levels, which increases the risk of HMG-CoA reductase inhibitor adverse effects, most notably myopathy.[35] Patients should be monitored for clinical signs of myopathy when receiving HMG-CoA reductase inhibitors in combination with cyclosporine and tacrolimus.

TABLE 98-5	Differential Diagnosis of Acute Rejection and Cyclosporine or Tacrolimus Nephrotoxicity	
	Nephrotoxicity in Renal Transplant Recipients	
	Acute Rejection	**CSA or TAC Nephrotoxicity**
History	Often <4 weeks postoperatively	Often >6 weeks postoperatively
Clinical presentation	Fever	Afebrile
	Hypertension	Hypertension
	Weight gain	Graft nontender
	Graft swelling/tenderness	Good urine output
	Decreased daily urine volume	
Laboratory biopsy	Rapid rise in serum Cr (0.3 mg/dL/day [27 micromol/L/day])	Gradual rise in serum Cr (>0.15 mg/dL/day [>13 micromol/L/day])
	Normal CSA or TAC concentration	Elevated CSA or TAC concentration
	Interstitial lymphocytic infiltrates	Interstitial fibrosis, tubular atrophy, glomerular thrombosis, arterial inflammation

Cr, creatinine; CSA, cyclosporine; TAC, tacrolimus.

TABLE 98-6 Effect of Concomitant Drug Administration on Cyclosporine, Tacrolimus, and Sirolimus

Cyclosporine Levels		Tacrolimus Levels		Sirolimus Levels	
Increase	*Decrease*	*Increase*	*Decrease*	*Increase*	*Decrease*
Ketoconazole	Rifampicin	Ketoconazole	Rifampin	Ketoconazole	Rifampin
Fluconazole	Phenytoin	Fluconazole	Dexamethasone	Fluconazole	Phenytoin
Itraconazole	Phenobarbital	Itraconazole	Phenytoin	Itraconazole	
Voriconazole	Carbamazepine	Voriconazole		Voriconazole	
Erythromycin	Sulfadimidine	Erythromycin		Erythromycin	
Levofloxacin	Trimethoprim	Levofloxacin		Clarithromycin	
Diltiazem	Mycophenolic	Diltiazem		Diltiazem	
Verapamil	Acid (vs TAC)	Verapamil		Verapamil	
Danazol		Danazol		Atorvastatin	
Nicardipine		Cimetidine		Cyclosporine	
Metoclopramide		Omeprazole		Protease inhibitors	
Methylprednisolone		Clotrimazole			
Norethisterone		Nefazodone			
Sirolimus		Corticosteroids			
Tacrolimus		Cyclosporine			
Protease inhibitors		Basiliximab			
		Protease inhibitors			

Adapted from references 27, 28, 29, and 40.

Consistency in administration of the calcineurin inhibitors with regard to meals and food intake is important to sustain an effective concentration time profile. High-fat meals can enhance both plasma clearance and the volume of distribution of cyclosporine by more than 60%.[36] Food reduces the rate and extent of tacrolimus absorption, and a high-fat meal may further delay gastric emptying and reduce the maximum achieved serum concentration (C_{max}), and the area under the concentration–time curve (AUC).[31] Furocoumarins, such as quercetin, naringin, and bergamottin, found in grapefruit juice, are potent inhibitors of CYP3A4 and have increased both cyclosporine and tacrolimus concentrations significantly. The AUC and C_{max} of cyclosporine have been reported to be increased by more than 55% and 35%, respectively.[37]

Dosing and Administration

Initial oral cyclosporine doses range from 8 to 18 mg/kg per day administered every 12 hours. Higher doses of cyclosporine are used more commonly in two-drug regimens, whereas lower doses are part of triple-drug regimens. Oral tacrolimus doses range from 0.1 to 0.3 mg/kg per day given every 12 hours. If oral administration is not possible, both drugs can be administered intravenously at one third the oral dosage, to account for first-pass metabolism. A once-daily formulation of tacrolimus is currently available in Canada and Europe. After mg:mg conversion based on total daily dose, about one third of patients required downward dose adjustments on the basis of 24-trough concentrations.[38] The usual intravenous dose of cyclosporine is 2 to 5 mg/kg per day, given as a continuous infusion or as single or twice-daily injection. Intravenous tacrolimus doses range from 0.05 to 0.1 mg/kg per day and must be administered by continuous infusion. Children require higher doses to maintain therapeutic drug concentrations, up to 14 to 18 mg/kg per day for cyclosporine and 0.3 mg/kg per day for tacrolimus.

Therapeutic Drug Monitoring

Calcineurin inhibitor serum concentrations are measured routinely in an attempt to optimize therapy (Table 98–7). The most common and practical method for monitoring calcineurin inhibitors is by measuring trough blood concentrations. Radioimmunoassay (RIA) and fluorescence polarization immunoassay are the most commonly used methods to measure cyclosporine concentrations. Tacrolimus concentrations are most commonly measured by microparticle

enzyme immunoassays or enzyme-linked immunoassays. Both drugs can be measured by high-performance liquid chromatography (HPLC), which is recognized as the reference procedure.[36] Therapeutic target ranges are assay specific because some quantitate parent plus metabolite concentration, while others only measure the parent compound. Thus, the target concentrations will be lower for the specific assays (HPLC) compared with nonspecific assays (RIA and microparticle enzyme immunoassays) by approximately 20% to 25%. The specific goal level for both drugs is dependent on transplant type, time after transplantation, concomitant immunosuppression, and transplantation center. One review of the role of tacrolimus in renal transplantation suggests that target 12-hour whole blood concentrations for tacrolimus are 15 to 20 ng/mL (15 to 20 µg/L; 18.6 to 24.8 nmol/L) (0 to 1 month after transplantation), 10 to 15 ng/mL (10 to 15 µg/L; 12.4 to 18.6 nmol/L) (1 to 3 months after transplantation), and 5 to 12 ng/mL (5 to 12 µg/L; 6.2 to 14.9 nmol/L) (>3 months after transplantation).[24] Serum drug concentrations should be measured frequently (daily or three times per week) following initiation of the drug and during the stabilization period after transplantation. As the time increases after transplantation, serum concentrations are measured less frequently, usually monthly.

Studies have revealed lack of predictive value of trough cyclosporine concentrations and rejection.[39] Alternative strategies, including AUC and peak concentration, have been suggested to better correlate with rejection.[36,39] Limited sampling techniques using two to five blood samples within the first 4 hours after an oral dose have been used. AUC levels > 4,400 mcg/L (> 3361 nmol/L) per hour correlate with a reduction in rejection.[36,39] Some transplantation

TABLE 98-7 Therapeutic Concentrations of Immunosuppressants by Various Methods

Drug	Sampling Medium	Concentrations (ng/mL or mcg/L)	
		HPLC	RIA
Cyclosporine	Whole blood	100–300	375–400
	Plasma	75–100	150–250
Tacrolimus	Whole blood	8–13	5–20
	Plasma		0.2–0.8
Sirolimus (with CIs)	Whole blood	10–15	15–20
Sirolimus (without CIs)	Whole blood	15–25	20–30

CIs, calcineurin inhibitors; HPLC, high performance liquid chromatography; RIA, radioimmunoassay.

centers have adopted this strategy to manage cyclosporine levels because of the convenience of a single blood sample. The suggested therapeutic range for C_2 cyclosporine levels is 1,500 to 2,000 ng/mL (1,500 to 2,000 μg/L; 1248 to 1664 nmol/L) for the first few months after transplant and 700 to 900 ng/mL (700 to 900 μg/L; 582 to 749 nmol/L) after 6 to 12 months.[39] The predictive value of trough concentrations and rejection is also being questioned with tacrolimus. As a result, pharmacokinetic profiling with AUC and peak concentrations to determine alternative monitoring strategies are also being explored with tacrolimus.[39]

■ CORTICOSTEROIDS

❹ Corticosteroids have been used since the beginning of the modern transplantation era. Despite their many adverse events, they continue to be a cornerstone of immunosuppression regimens in many transplant centers, with 40 to 70% of liver and kidney transplant patients, respectively, receiving corticosteroids at the time of hospital discharge.[1] The most commonly used corticosteroids in transplantation are methylprednisolone and prednisone.

Pharmacology/Mechanism of Action

Corticosteroids block cytokine activation by binding to corticosteroid response elements, thereby inhibiting IL-1, IL-2, IL-3, IL-6, γ-interferon, and tumor necrosis factor-α synthesis (see Fig. 98–1). Additionally, corticosteroids interfere with cell migration, recognition, and cytotoxic effector mechanisms.[40]

Pharmacokinetics

Prednisone is converted to active prednisolone in the body and has multiple effects on the immune system. Prednisone is very well absorbed from the GI tract and has a long biologic half-life, permitting daily administration.

Efficacy

Animal models of transplantation in the 1950s and 1960s used corticosteroids empirically in combination with azathioprine. Corticosteroids subsequently became a part of the immunosuppressive regimens used in the first human transplantations[41] and continue to be used in immunosuppressive protocols today. The efficacy of corticosteroids is irrefutable based on the decades of clinical experience. Systematic studies comparing corticosteroid-free immunosuppressive agent combinations with conventional therapy are difficult to perform because of the hundreds of potential combinations that now exist. However, recent studies of corticosteroid-free immunosuppressive agent combinations with newer, more specific immunosuppressants suggest that corticosteroids may in the future have less of a role in maintenance immunosuppression.[21,22]

Adverse Effects

Adverse effects of prednisone that occur in more than 10% of patients include increased appetite, insomnia, indigestion (bitter taste), and mood changes. Side effects that occur less often but which are seen with high doses or prolonged therapy include cataracts, hyperglycemia, hirsutism, bruising, acne, sodium and water retention, hypertension, bone growth suppression, and ulcerative esophagitis (see Table 98–4).

Drug–Drug and Drug–Food Interactions

Barbiturates, phenytoin, and rifampin induce hepatic metabolism of prednisone and thus decrease the effectiveness of prednisone. Prednisone decreases the effectiveness of vaccines and toxoids.[40]

Dosing and Administration

An intravenous corticosteroid, commonly high-dose methylprednisolone, is given at the time of transplantation. The dose of methylprednisolone is tapered rapidly and discontinued within days, and oral prednisone is initiated. Prednisone doses are tapered progressively over time, depending on the type of additional immunosuppression and organ function. It is preferable to administer corticosteroids between 7 AM and 8 AM to mimic the body's diurnal release of cortisol. While conversion to alternate-day regimens or complete withdrawal of prednisone in patients with stable posttransplantation courses has been used with success in some transplantation centers, corticosteroids are often continued for the entire life of the functional graft. The adverse effects of corticosteroids are summarized in Table 98–4.

The first-line therapy for the treatment of acute graft rejection is high-dose intravenous methylprednisolone (250 to 1,000 mg) daily for 3 days or oral prednisone (200 mg). Doses of oral prednisone are then tapered over 5 days to 20 mg/day. Prednisone should be taken with food to minimize GI upset. It is becoming a frequent practice to taper prednisone, with the goal of discontinuation over a period of months. Corticosteroids should never be discontinued abruptly; tapering should be gradual because of suppression of the hypothalamic–pituitary–adrenal axis. Corticosteroids slow the growth rates in children, prompting clinicians to use alternate-day dosing or to withhold corticosteroids until rejection occurs.

■ ANTIMETABOLITES

❺ Antimetabolites have been used since the early days of transplantation because they prevent proliferation of lymphocytes. Azathioprine, long considered a part of the "gold standard" regimen with cyclosporine and corticosteroids, has largely been supplanted by mycophenolic acid derivatives as they are more specific in their effects on lymphocytes and have fewer side effects.

Mycophenolate

Mycophenolic acid (MPA) was first isolated from the *Penicillium glaucum* mold. Two formulations of MPA are currently available in the United States: mycophenolate mofetil is the morpholinoethyl ester of MPA, whereas mycophenolate sodium is available as an enteric-coated formulation of the sodium salt of MPA.

Pharmacology/Mechanism of Action The immunosuppressive effect of MPA is exerted through noncompetitive binding to inosine monophosphate dehydrogenase, the key enzyme responsible for guanosine nucleotide synthesis via the de novo pathway. Inhibition of inosine monophosphate dehydrogenase results in decreased nucleotide synthesis and diminished DNA polymerase activity, ultimately reducing lymphocyte proliferation.[42] The actions of MPA are more specific for T and B cells, which use only the de novo pathway for nucleotide synthesis (see Fig. 98–1). Other cells within the body have a salvage pathway by which they can synthesize nucleotides, making them less susceptible to the actions of MPA and thereby reducing, but not eliminating, the potential for the hematologic adverse effects seen with azathioprine. In addition to decreasing lymphocyte proliferation, MPA may also downregulate activation of lymphocytes.[43]

Pharmacokinetics Because MPA is unstable in an acidic environment, mycophenolate mofetil acts as a prodrug that is readily absorbed from the GI tract, after which it is rapidly and completely converted to MPA by first-pass metabolism. The enteric coating of mycophenolate sodium protects MPA from the acidic gastric pH and allows for MPA to be released directly into the small intestine for absorption. The absolute bioavailability of MPA when delivered from mycophenolate mofetil and mycophenolate sodium is 94% and 72%, respectively. Peak concentrations of MPA are reached within 1 hour following administration of either preparation.

A total of 97% of MPA is bound to albumin in the blood. MPA is eliminated by the kidney and also undergoes glucuronidation in the liver to an inactive glucuronide metabolite (MPAG) that is excreted in the bile and urine. Enterohepatic cycling of MPAG can lead to deconjugation, thereby recirculating MPA into the bloodstream. The half-life of MPA is 18 hours.

Efficacy Currently, mycophenolate mofetil is approved for use in kidney, liver, and heart transplantations. Mycophenolate sodium was approved in 2004 for use in kidney transplantations only. Early studies comparing mycophenolate to azathioprine in patients receiving cyclosporine and corticosteroids demonstrated a statistically significant improvement in patient and graft survival at 1 and 3 years.[44] Subsequent studies have confirmed the efficacy of mycophenolate combined with tacrolimus. Mycophenolate has also demonstrated efficacy in the treatment of acute rejection.[45]

Mycophenolic acid derivatives are a key component of calcineurin inhibitor–sparing protocols. Although mycophenolate monotherapy has been investigated, patients experienced an unacceptable increase in rejection. Combination of mycophenolate with sirolimus, on the other hand, resulted in improved renal function with no change in acute rejection and patient and graft survival.[44]

Adverse Effects Unlike cyclosporine and tacrolimus, MPA is not associated with nephrotoxicity, neurotoxicity, or hypertension. The most common side effects are related to the GI tract, including nausea, vomiting, diarrhea, and abdominal pain (see Table 98–4), which occur with similar frequency during intravenous and oral therapy. Strategies to reduce GI symptoms include dose reduction, division of the total daily dose into three or four doses, administration with food, or titration upward from lower doses during initial therapy. Mycophenolate also has hematologic effects, such as leukopenia and anemia, particularly with higher doses. Recently, the rare but serious adverse events of progressive multifocal leukoencephalopathy (PML) and pure red cell aplasia have been reported. Because peripheral intravenous mycophenolate administration is associated with local edema and inflammation, central venous administration may be the preferred route.

Drug–Drug and Drug–Food Interactions Food has no effect on MPA AUC, but it delays the absorption and decreases MPA C_{max} by 40% and 33% when mycophenolate mofetil and mycophenolate sodium, respectively, are administered. Administration with aluminum- and magnesium-containing antacids or cholestyramine significantly decreases the AUC of MPA and should be avoided.[42] It has been suggested that administration of iron may produce similar results, but this has not been tested.

Acyclovir, commonly used in renal transplant recipients for the treatment and prevention of viral infections, competes with MPAG for renal tubular secretion. AUCs of both entities are increased with concomitant acyclovir and mycophenolate administration. No pharmacokinetic interaction with other antiviral agents has been demonstrated, but, there is potential for additive pharmacodynamic effects such as bone marrow suppression.

Decreased MPA trough concentrations have been reported when mycophenolate is administered with cyclosporine compared with those achieved when mycophenolate is given with tacrolimus or sirolimus. This interaction is most likely a result of cyclosporine interference with the enterohepatic recycling of MPAG, which results in decreased MPA concentrations.[46] To achieve equivalent MPA and MPAG serum concentrations, it may be necessary to administer higher doses of mycophenolate with cyclosporine compared to tacrolimus.

Dosing and Administration Mycophenolate mofetil is currently available in both oral and intravenous formulations. Although intravenous administration of equal doses closely mimics oral administration, the two cannot be considered bioequivalent.

Mycophenolate sodium is only available as an oral formulation. To optimize immunosuppression and minimize adverse effects, mycophenolate is administered in two divided doses given every 12 hours. The total daily dose for kidney and liver transplants is 2 g/day for mycophenolate mofetil and 1.44 g/day for mycophenolate sodium. A higher level of immunosuppression is required for heart transplants; thus for these patients a total daily dose of 3 g/day for mycophenolate mofetil and 2.16 g/day for mycophenolate sodium is recommended. The recommended pediatric dose is 600 mg/m² for mycophenolate mofetil and 400 mg/m² for mycophenolate sodium, in two divided doses.

While an increasing body of literature exists, the routine therapeutic drug monitoring of mycophenolic acid remains controversial. Plasma appears to be the most appropriate medium in which to measure MPA for therapeutic drug monitoring. Numerous studies have demonstrated a relationship between plasma MPA concentrations and improved clinical outcomes in patients receiving concomitant CIs and corticosteroids. Patients with trough MPA levels between 1.0 and 3.5 mcg/mL (1.0–3.5 mg/L; 3.1 to 10.9 micromol/L) experienced fewer significant complications. Free (fMPA) concentrations as opposed to total MPA concentrations have been suggested as the relevant measure, especially in patients with liver disease, hypoalbuminemia, and severe infection.[47] Trough concentrations may not be accurate in predicting total drug exposure during a 12-hour interval and thus AUC monitoring has been proposed as the most appropriate measure of MPA drug exposure to predict therapeutic outcomes.[47] Better outcomes are associated with MPA AUC levels of greater than 42.8 mcg/mL (42.8 mg/L; 134 micromol/L) per hour (by HPLC),[48] although a reference range of 30 to 60 mcg/mL (30 to 60 mg/L; 94 to 188 micromol/L) per hour has been proposed.[49] The correlation between MPA AUC levels and adverse effects is low. Further studies are required to determine the best means to evaluate MPA levels, the acceptable targets for each, and the appropriate strategy to monitor MPA levels.[48,49]

Azathioprine

Azathioprine, a prodrug for 6-mercaptopurine (6-MP), has been used as an immunosuppressant in combination with corticosteroids since the earliest days of the modern transplantation era. It is associated with substantial toxicities, however, and its use has dramatically declined with the availability of newer immunosuppressants.

Pharmacology/Mechanism of Action Azathioprine is an inactive compound that is converted rapidly to 6-MP in the blood and is subsequently metabolized by three different enzymes. Xanthine oxidase, found in the liver and GI tract, converts 6-MP to the inactive final end product, 6-thiouric acid. Thiopurine S-methyltransferase, found in hematopoietic tissues and red blood cells, methylates 6-MP to an inactive product, 6-methylmercaptopurine. Finally, hypoxanthine-guanine phosphoribosyltransferase is the first step responsible for converting 6-MP to 6-thioguanine nucleotides (6-TGNs), the active metabolites, which are incorporated into nucleic acids, ultimately disrupting both the salvage and de novo pathways of DNA, RNA, and protein synthesis. This process is toxic to the cell and renders the cell unable to proliferate (see Fig. 98–1). Eventually, 6-TGNs are catabolized by xanthine oxidase and thiopurine S-methyltransferase to inactive products.[50]

Pharmacokinetics Oral bioavailability of azathioprine is approximately 40%. Metabolism of 6-MP is primarily by xanthine oxidase to inactive metabolites, which are excreted by the kidneys. The half-life of azathioprine, the parent compound, is very short, approximately 12 minutes. The half-life of 6-MP is longer, ranging from 0.7 to 3 hours. However, it is the activity of the 6-TGNs that determines the pharmacodynamic half-life of the drug. The half-life of 6-TGNs has been estimated to be 9 days.[50]

Adverse Effects Dose-limiting adverse effects of azathioprine are often hematologic (see Table 98–4). Leukopenia, anemia, and thrombocytopenia can occur within the first few weeks of therapy and can be managed by dose reduction or discontinuation of azathioprine. Other common adverse effects include nausea and vomiting, which can be minimized by taking azathioprine with food. Alopecia, hepatotoxicity, and pancreatitis are less common adverse effects of azathioprine and are reversible on dose reduction or discontinuation.

Drug–Drug and Drug–Food Interactions The xanthine oxidase inhibitor allopurinol can increase azathioprine and 6-MP concentrations by as much as fourfold. The metabolic pathways shift to favor production of 6-TGNs, which ultimately results in increased bone marrow suppression and pancytopenia. Doses of azathioprine should be reduced by 50% to 75% when allopurinol is added. Additional clinically significant drug interactions include other bone marrow–suppressing agents such as ganciclovir, trimethoprim-sulfamethoxazole, and sirolimus, and other drugs that irritate the GI tract.

Dosing and Administration Initial doses of azathioprine are 3 to 5 mg/kg per day intravenously or orally. Individualization to maintain the white blood cell count between 3,500 and 6,000 cells/mm (3.5 and 6.0×10^9/L) may be accomplished in some with doses as low as 0.25 mg/kg per day.[2] Patients are often instructed to take azathioprine in the evening when initiating or titrating therapy to allow for dose adjustments based on morning determinations of their white blood cell count.

■ MAMMALIAN TARGET OF RAPAMYCIN INHIBITORS

6 Two mammalian target of rapamycin (mTOR) inhibitors have been approved in the United States for use in transplantation. Sirolimus, also known as rapamycin, is an immunosuppressive macrolide antibiotic that is structurally similar to tacrolimus, and is effective in reducing the risk of acute rejection. Sirolimus is thought to have potential to reduce chronic rejection, but this remains to be proven. Everolimus was approved in 2009.

Pharmacology/Mechanism of Action Sirolimus and everolimus both bind to FKBP12, forming a complex that binds to mTOR, which inhibits the response to cytokines (see Fig. 98–1). IL-2 stimulates mTOR to activate kinases that ultimately advance the cell cycle from G1 to the S phase. Thus they reduce T-cell proliferation by inhibiting the cellular response to IL-2 and progression of the cell cycle. To this end, this class is also referred to as proliferation signal inhibitors.[51,52]

Pharmacokinetics Bioavailability after oral administration is low for both, only 15–16%, with peak concentrations being reached within 1 to 2 hours for sirolimus and 0.5–4 hours for everolimus.[51,52] Both have large volumes of distribution, 5.6–16.7 L/kg for sirolimus and about 110 L for everolimus. Both are metabolized primarily by CYP3A4 both in the gut and in the liver. Likewise, both are also substrates for P-glycoprotein. The half-life for sirolimus is reported to be 60 hours but can be as long as 110 hours in patients with liver dysfunction, while that of everolimus is much shorter, 18–35 hours.[51,52]

Efficacy Sirolimus is only approved for the prevention of rejection in kidney transplant recipients when given in combination with corticosteroids and cyclosporine or after withdrawal of cyclosporine

in patients with low to moderate immunologic risk. Sirolimus has also been demonstrated to be effective in combination with tacrolimus or mycophenolate in kidney transplants, with patient survival rates >99% and graft survival rates >96%.[51] Combination therapy with sirolimus and mycophenolate can be used to avoid the use of calcineurin inhibitors and decrease the risk of nephrotoxicity. Everolimus was approved for use in renal transplantation in combination with basiliximab, cyclosporine, and corticosteroids.

Two Phase III trials evaluated the use of sirolimus in kidney transplants. All patients in both studies received cyclosporine and corticosteroids and were randomly assigned to one of three groups: (a) sirolimus in a fixed dose—a 6-mg loading dose followed by 2 mg daily; (b) a 15-mg loading dose followed by 5 mg daily; or (c) azathioprine in the U.S. trial or placebo in the global trial. The results of both studies showed similar patient and graft survival in all groups at 12 months but lower rates of acute rejection in the sirolimus arms compared with azathioprine and placebo.[51]

Early cyclosporine withdrawal has been studied in patients receiving sirolimus-based immunosuppressive protocols. Patients receiving sirolimus who did not have a recent or severe rejection episode and adequate renal function 3 months after transplant were enrolled. Patients were randomly assigned to continue triple-drug therapy with sirolimus (adjusted to trough concentrations of greater than 5 ng/mL), cyclosporine, and corticosteroids or double-drug therapy with sirolimus (adjusted to trough concentrations of 20 to 30 ng/mL) and corticosteroids. Rejection occurred in 5.6% of patients after discontinuation of cyclosporine, with no difference in graft survival. Long-term follow-up (2 years) showed improved renal function and blood pressure without an increase in acute rejection or graft loss in patients who discontinued cyclosporine.[51]

Everolimus in combination with reduced doses of cyclosporine (target 100–200ng/ml for the first month post transplant) and steroids was comparable to mycophenolic acid (1.44 g/day) in combination with standard cyclosporine doses (target 100–200 ng/mL in the first month) and steroids in terms of biopsy-proved rejection, graft loss, or death. There was no difference in estimated GFR at 12 months. Similarly, a trial of high-dose everolimus/low-dose CSA (target 8—12 ng/mL vs. 3—8 ng/mL) showed no difference in 6- and 12-month GFR between the two groups despite differences in CSA exposure.[53]

Currently, because the safety and efficacy of sirolimus and everolimus have not been established in liver or lung transplants, it is recommended that their use be avoided in these populations immediately following transplant. In contrast, limited data on the use of sirolimus in heart transplantation indicate benefit in reversing acute rejection in patients who do not respond to antilymphocyte therapy.[51] Furthermore, mTOR inhibitors may slow the progression of vasculopathy, which may have an impact on chronic rejection and long-term patient survival after heart transplantation.[19]

Adverse Effects Both everolimus and sirolimus are associated with dose-related myelosuppression. Thrombocytopenia is usually seen within the first 2 weeks of sirolimus therapy but generally improves with continued treatment; leukopenia and anemia are also typically transient.[51,52] Sirolimus trough serum concentrations greater than 15 ng/mL have been correlated with thrombocytopenia and leukopenia.[51] Hypercholesterolemia and hypertriglyceridemia are also common in patients receiving everolimus or sirolimus. It is postulated that the mechanism of this adverse effect is related to an overproduction of lipoproteins or inhibition of lipoprotein lipase. Peak cholesterol and triglyceride levels are often seen within 3 months of sirolimus initiation but usually decrease after 1 year of therapy and can be managed by reducing the dose, discontinuing sirolimus, or initiating therapy with an HMG-CoA reductase inhibitor or fibric acid derivative. One study suggests that the dyslipidemia associated with sirolimus is not a major risk factor for early cardiovascular complications following kidney transplantation.[54] Delayed wound healing and dehiscence could be a result of inhibition of smooth muscle proliferation and intimal thickening.[51] Mouth ulcers also have been reported with sirolimus, more commonly with the oral solution, possibly as a direct effect of the drug or secondary to activation of herpes simplex virus.[55] Reversible interstitial pneumonitis has been described in kidney, liver, and heart–lung transplantation recipients.[51] Other adverse effects reported with sirolimus include increased liver enzymes, hypertension, rash, acne, diarrhea, and arthralgia (see Table 98–4).

Drug–Drug and Drug–Food Interactions The major metabolic pathway for everolimus and sirolimus is CYP3A4; thus, the drug interactions mediated by induction or inhibition of the CYP3A4 enzyme system are similar to those seen with cyclosporine and tacrolimus (see Table 98–5). Administration of the microemulsion formulation of cyclosporine with sirolimus significantly increases the AUC and trough sirolimus levels. The same is not seen with the standard formulation of cyclosporine. Conversely, cyclosporine concentrations and AUC are also increased when it is given concomitantly with sirolimus. The mechanism is proposed to be competitive binding to CYP3A4 and P-glycoprotein.[51,52] It is recommended that patients separate the dose of sirolimus and cyclosporine by 4 hours to minimize the interaction.[51] Concomitant administration of tacrolimus does not affect sirolimus levels.[51] Although everolimus AUC was increased by the administration of a single dose of cyclosporine modified, no specific recommendations for dose timing are given. It should be expected, however, that any changes in CSA dose may also necessitate a modification of everolimus dose and increased therapeutic drug monitoring is indicated.[52]

As with cyclosporine and tacrolimus, grapefruit juice increases sirolimus levels. Administration of sirolimus with a high-fat meal is associated with a delayed rate of absorption, decreased C_{max}, and increased AUC, indicating an increased drug exposure, whereas the half-life remains unchanged.[51] Conversely, administration of everolimus with a high-fat meal decreases both C_{max} and AUC.[52]

Dosing and Administration A fixed sirolimus dosing regimen is approved for concomitant use with cyclosporine that includes a loading dose of 6 or 15 mg followed by 2 or 5 mg daily, respectively. Therapeutic monitoring of sirolimus is advocated using wholeblood concentrations measured by HPLC, which is specific for the parent compound (see Table 98–7). For everolimus a starting dose of 0.75 mg twice daily is indicated in regimens that contain cyclosporine, corticosteroids, and basiliximab. Target concentrations are 3—8 ng/ml.

Antibody Agents

❼ Both polyclonal and monoclonal antibody preparations are used in transplantation. These agents can also be differentiated by their level of specificity, that is, particular receptor(s), or their downstream affects. In the following text the agents are discussed as those that deplete lymphocytic cell lines (depleting antibodies) and those that generally bind to specific receptors but do not result in depletion of the cell to which they bind.

■ DEPLETING ANTIBODIES

Antithymocyte Globulin

Two antithymocyte globulins are available in the United States: ATG (Atgam, Pfizer, New York, NY), an equine polyclonal antibody, and RATG (Thymoglobulin, Genzyme, Cambridge, MA), a rabbit polyclonal antibody. The rabbit preparation is less immunogenic and

may have other advantages over the equine preparation. Both ATG and RATG are often used as induction therapy to prevent acute rejection. In 2006 40–60% of kidney transplant recipients received RATG induction, for example.[1]

Pharmacology/Mechanism of Action Because of their polyclonal antibody nature, both ATG and RATG exert their immunosuppressive effect by binding to a wide array of lymphocyte receptors (CD2, CD3, CD4, CD8, CD25, and CD45). Binding of ATG or RATG to the various receptors results in complementmediated lysis and subsequent lymphocyte depletion. While T cells are the major lymphocytic target for the compounds, other blood cell components such as B cells and other leukocytes are also affected (see Fig. 98–1). Damaged T cells are subsequently removed by the spleen, liver, and lungs.

Pharmacokinetics ATG is poorly distributed into lymphoid tissue and binds primarily to circulating lymphocytes, granulocytes, and platelets. The terminal half-life of ATG is 5.7 days. RATG has a volume of distribution of 0.12 L/kg, and its terminal half-life in renal transplant recipients is significantly longer than ATG at 30 days.[56] Peak plasma concentrations are reached after 5 to 7 days of ATG or RATG infusions. Antiequine antibodies can form in up to 78% of patients who are receiving ATG therapy. Similarly, antirabbit antibodies have been reported in up to 68% of patients who are receiving RATG therapy. The effects of preformed antibodies on the efficacy and safety of these preparations have not been studied adequately.

Efficacy ATG and RATG are used most commonly for the treatment of acute allograft rejection or as induction therapy to prevent acute rejection. ATG is currently approved for both indications in kidney transplants. RATG is approved only for the treatment of acute allograft rejection in kidney transplantations. Both drugs have been studied extensively for both indications.

Use of RATG as part of quadruple therapy in liver transplantation is associated with similar rates of patient and graft survival and acute rejection compared with dual therapy. In kidney transplant RATG was associated with improved graft survival at 5 years as compared with equine ATG. Quadruple-drug therapy results in similar rates of patient and graft survival and malignancy in heart transplantations, but a significantly lower rate of acute rejection and infection episodes is seen at 1 year compared with triple-drug therapy. Cytomegalovirus (CMV) is an adverse effect of this strategy, but recent data indicate that routine prophylaxis is successful in this setting.[57]

Adverse Effects Most adverse effects reported with ATG and RATG are related to the lack of specificity for T cells owing to their polyclonal nature. Dose-limiting myelosuppression (leukopenia, anemia, and thrombocytopenia) occurs frequently. Other adverse effects include anaphylaxis, hypotension, hypertension, tachycardia, dyspnea, urticaria, and rash. Serum sickness is seen more frequently with ATG than with RATG. Nephrotoxicity has been reported but is rare in the absence of serum sickness. Infusion-related febrile reactions are most common with the first few doses and can be managed by premedicating the patient with acetaminophen, diphenhydramine, and corticosteroids. Finally, as with any immunosuppressive agent, ATG and RATG are associated with an increased risk of infections, particularly viral infections, and malignancy.

Drug–Drug and Drug–Food Interactions Administration of ATG or RATG can interfere with the immune response to live vaccines, such as varicella vaccine. If a live vaccine is administered within 2 months of receiving one of these immunoglobulins, protection may not be conferred.

Dosing and Administration ATG doses range from 10 to 30 mg/kg per day as a single dose for 7 to 14 days. RATG is a more potent compound and is administered at doses of 1 to 1.5 mg/kg per day as a single dose for 7 to 14 days for acute rejection or for 5 to 10 days for induction of immunosuppression. Although literature reports now support peripheral administration of both agents, it is recommended that both ATG and RATG be administered through a central line or through a high-flow vein with an in-line 0.22-micron filter over at least 4 hours to minimize phlebitis and thrombosis whenever possible.[57,58]

Muromonab-CD3

Pharmacology/Mechanism of Action OKT3 is a murine monoclonal antibody to the CD3 receptor on mature human T cells (see Fig. 98–1). Administration of OKT3 results in both T-cell depletion and functional alteration. Cells reappear after a few days but bear no CD3 receptors. After cessation of OKT3 therapy, T-cell function normalizes in a week.[59]

Pharmacokinetics OKT3 has a volume of distribution of 6.5 L and half-life of about 18 hours. Concentrations above 0.9 mcg/mL (0.9 mg/L) are considered therapeutic. An OKT3 concentration of 0.8 mcg/mL (0.9 mg/L) or greater in combination with a CD3+ T-cell count of <25 cells/mL (<25 × 10⁶/L) is also a reasonable therapeutic target. If CD3 levels begin to rise, this may signify the presence of antimurine antibodies antagonizing the actions of OKT3. Administration of mycophenolate mofetil has been suggested to reduce the formation of antimurine antibodies during OKT3 administration. Although T-cell depletion is achieved within minutes of administration, resolution of rejection takes 3 to 4 days.

Efficacy OKT3 has been used as induction therapy at doses of 5 mg/day for 7 to 14 days. OKT3 can be used safely and successfully as an acute rejection therapy in patients who have undergone previous OKT3 induction.[59] Specifically, these studies confirm that the presence of low anti-OKT3 antibody titers (≤1:100) does not preclude successful retreatment with OKT3 for rejection. Aside from intestinal transplantation, OKT3 is usually reserved for treatment of corticosteroid-resistant rejection.

Adverse Effects OKT3 administration is associated with a cytokine release syndrome including fever, chills, rigors, pruritus, and alterations in blood pressure, which is most common with the first dose. Methylprednisolone, acetaminophen, and diphenhydramine are commonly administered as premedications to prevent or minimize the severity of this syndrome. Other adverse effects include capillary leak syndrome and pulmonary edema, especially in fluid-overloaded patients. Aseptic meningitis, another potential complication of OKT3 therapy, warrants discontinuation of OKT3. Other adverse effects include encephalopathy, nephrotoxicity, infection, and post-transplantation lymphoproliferative disorder.[40]

Drug-Drug and Drug-Food Interactions No drug or food interactions have been reported with OKT3.

Dosing and Administration OKT3 should be filtered with a 0.2- to 0.22-micron filter and then administered as an intravenous push over 1 minute. The dose of OKT3 is usually 5 mg/day for 5 to 14 days.[59] Vital signs should be assessed frequently during the first few doses, and it is advisable to have a physician present for the first dose. A high proportion of patients treated with OKT3 form antibodies to one of the components of OKT3 and may not be able to receive or adequately respond to retreatment.[59] The dosages of other immunosuppressant drugs may be decreased to avoid over-immunosuppression during OKT3 therapy.

Alemtuzumab

Alemtuzumab is approved for use in B-cell chronic lymphocytic leukemia. However, its effects on depleting both T and B lymphocytes make it useful in solid-organ transplants. While alemtuzumab is not FDA approved for solid organ transplantation, it is increasingly recognized as a viable therapeutic option. In 2006 10% of kidney transplant patients received alemtuzumab at the time of transplant.[1]

Pharmacology/Mechanism of Action Alemtuzumab is a humanized monoclonal antibody against the CD52 surface antigen found on both T and B lymphocytes, as well as macrophages, monocytes, eosinophils, and natural killer cells. When alemtuzumab binds to the CD52 surface antigen, antibody-dependent lysis occurs, which removes both T and B lymphocytes from the blood, bone marrow, and organs, resulting in complete lymphocyte depletion.[60]

Pharmacokinetics The pharmacokinetics of alemtuzumab in solid-organ transplantation patients have not been investigated. Data from patients with B-cell chronic lymphocytic leukemia indicate that the volume of distribution of alemtuzumab after repeated dosing is 0.18 L/kg. The mean half-life after the first 30 mg dose was 11 hours, but increased to 6 days after 12 weeks of therapy. The extrapolation of these data to solid-organ transplantation is difficult because of the differences in dosing strategies (single or double doses in solid-organ transplantation versus weekly to thrice weekly dosing in B-cell chronic lymphocytic leukemia). One or two doses of alemtuzumab result in complete and prolonged lymphocyte depletion. Following administration, B lymphocyte counts return to normal within 3 to 12 months. T lymphocytes, however, remain depressed for as long as 3 years following administration.[60,61]

Efficacy Recent data suggest that alemtuzumab is effective as induction therapy for the prevention of acute rejection in kidney, liver, pancreas, intestinal, and lung transplants.[60] Additionally, alemtuzumab has been used to successfully treat acute rejection following transplantation and is effective for corticosteroid- and antibody-resistant rejection.[61,62] The most promising role of alemtuzumab in solid-organ transplantation is its use in corticosteroid-sparing protocols, which allow for calcineurin inhibitor monotherapy following transplantation. Tacrolimus appears to be the optimal calcineurin inhibitor to use for monotherapy immunosuppression in patients who receive alemtuzumab induction.

Adverse Effects Adverse effects of alemtuzumab are primarily infusion related, hematologic, and infectious. Infusion-related reactions include rigors, hypotension, fever, shortness of breath, bronchospasms, and chills. The potential for developing these reactions can be reduced by administering premedications such as acetaminophen, corticosteroids and diphenhydramine or by administering smaller doses and escalating the dose gradually. Hematologic effects include pancytopenia, neutropenia, thrombocytopenia, and lymphopenia.

Drug–Drug and Drug–Food Interactions No drug or food interactions have been reported with alemtuzumab.

Dosing and Administration Several dosing regimens have been proposed for alemtuzumab in solid-organ transplantation. The most common dosing strategy for alemtuzumab is 30 mg as a single dose; some centers administer a second dose 1 to 5 days after transplantation.[60] Other studied dosing strategies include 0.3 mg/kg per dose, as a single- or multiple-dose regimen, and, finally, two 20-mg doses given on the day of transplantation and the first postoperative day.[62]

◼ NONDEPLETING ANTIBODIES

Interleukin-2 Receptor Antagonists

Basiliximab, a chimeric monoclonal antibody (25% murine) is the only available IL-2 receptor antagonist in the United States. Daclizumab, a humanized monoclonal antibody (90% human, 10% murine) was withdrawn in 2009. Daclizumab contains a greater proportion of human sequences, making it theoretically less immunogenic. The percentage of murine component determines the antibody's affinity for the epitope. Consequently, the chimeric antibody basiliximab has a higher affinity than daclizumab.[63]

Pharmacology/Mechanism of Action Both basiliximab and daclizumab exert their immunosuppressive effect by specifically binding to the α-chain (CD25) on the surface of activated T lymphocytes (see Fig. 98–1). Binding of either basiliximab or daclizumab to the IL-2 receptor prevents IL-2-mediated activation and proliferation of T cells, a critical step in clonal expansion of T cells and the development of allograft rejection. Saturation of the IL-2 receptor occurs rapidly and confers an immunosuppressive effect immediately.[63]

Pharmacokinetics Most of the pharmacokinetic data available for both basiliximab and daclizumab are in renal transplantation patients. Caution must be used when extrapolating these data to nonrenal transplantation recipients. The volume of distribution is approximately 5.3 L for daclizumab and 8 L for basiliximab. Basiliximab and daclizumab saturate CD25 in vivo at serum concentrations of 0.2 and 1 mg/L or greater, respectively.[64] The terminal half-life of daclizumab is about 20 days in renal transplantation patients compared with 3 to 4 days in bone marrow transplant recipients. Basiliximab has a shorter half-life of approximately 7 days in renal transplant recipients. Clearance of both drugs is increased in patients who have received a liver transplant, primarily as a consequence of drainage of ascites. It is recommended that patients with greater than 10 L of ascites receive an additional dose of basiliximab on postoperative day 8.[65] Therapeutic concentrations of daclizumab range from 5 to 10 mg/L.

Efficacy Both basiliximab and daclizumab are approved for use in kidney transplantation in combination with cyclosporine and corticosteroids, although induction therapy has also been studied extensively in liver and heart transplantation recipients. In 2006 28% of kidney and heart transplant recipients received an IL-2 receptor antagonist at the time of transplant.[1] A meta-analysis of daclizumab and basiliximab in renal transplantation concluded that IL-2 receptor antagonists reduced the risk of rejection significantly with no increases in graft loss, infectious complications, malignancy, or death.[66] Similar results were seen in liver and heart transplantation.[65]

IL-2 receptor antagonists offer a reasonable addition to calcineurin inhibitor– or corticosteroid-sparing protocols. While calcineurin inhibitor therapy can not be completely avoided in most cases,[64] IL-2 receptor antagonists allow for delayed use or reduced doses of calcineurin inhibitors, thus minimizing the risk of nephrotoxicity in the early post-transplantation period. Similar rates of rejection and corticosteroid-resistant rejection were seen in patients with DGF who received an IL-2 receptor antagonist in conjunction with lower tacrolimus doses compared with patients without DGF who received standard tacrolimus doses and no IL-2 receptor inhibitor induction.[63]

Adverse Effects Few adverse effects have been reported with basiliximab and daclizumab. In contrast to lymphocyte-depleting agents, basiliximab and daclizumab have not been associated with infusion-related reactions. However, since the marketing of basiliximab, an increased number of hypersensitivity reactions have been reported. Of note, only one patient developed anti-idiotypic antibodies to the murine portion during clinical trials.[65] The manufacturer of basiliximab reported an increase in mortality in a placebo-controlled trial, which was associated with an increase in severe infections. No increased risk of malignancy has been reported.

Drug–Drug and Drug–Food Interactions Reports of increased cyclosporine and tacrolimus levels in patients receiving concomitant basiliximab were recently published.[63,64] Both authors hypothesized a potential interaction with the cytochrome P450. No drug interactions have been reported with daclizumab.

Dosing and Administration Basiliximab is administered as two 20-mg intravenous doses, intraoperatively and again on postoperative day 4. Basiliximab is compatible with both 0.9% sodium chloride and 5% dextrose and can be administered either centrally or peripherally over 20 to 30 minutes in a volume of 50 mL. This regimen results in saturation of the IL-2 receptor for 30 to 45 days. The approved daclizumab dosing regimen for renal transplantation is 1 mg/kg every 2 weeks from the time of transplant for a total of 5 doses. Daclizumab should be diluted in 50 mL of sterile 0.9% sodium chloride and administered peripherally or centrally over 15 minutes. This regimen saturates the IL-2 receptors for approximately 90 to 120 days after renal transplantation.[64] Alternative dosing regimens have been proposed for daclizumab in combination with tacrolimus, mycophenolate, and corticosteroids: 1 mg/kg every 2 weeks for 5 doses, 2 mg/kg every 2 weeks for 2 doses, or 2 mg/kg on day 0 followed by 1 mg/kg on day 5.[64,67]

Investigational Agents

Belatacept Belatacept, derived from abatacept, is a selective costimulation blocker that binds costimulatory ligands (CD80 and CD86) on antigen presenting cells. This prevents interaction of CD80 and 86 with CD28 on T cells thus inhibiting T-cell activation. Belatacept is still in the investigational phase of development.[68]

In a phase II evaluation of two dosing strategies of belatacept versus cyclosporine in combination with basiliximab, mycophenolate mofetil, and corticosteroids in 218 renal transplant patients there was no difference in the rates of acute cellular rejection at 6 months. However, in patients treated with belatacept, GFR as measured by iohexol clearance was significantly higher than cyclosporine-treated patients at 12 months. Chronic allograft nephropathy as detected by protocol biopsy was also significantly lower in the belatacept groups. Belatacept has been well tolerated. At 12-month follow-up no adverse effects were reported in greater number in the belatacept groups. Cyclosporine–treated patients experienced more hypertension and hyperlipidemia.[68]

Belatacept was administered by intermittent intravenous infusion. While this improves compliance in some patients, the inability to reverse immunosuppression in patients with life-threatening infections may hinder acceptance.[68] Ongoing trials will define dosing strategies and place in transplant therapy, if any, for belatacept.

Bortezomib Bortezomib, a proteosomal inhibitor that is FDA approved for the treatment of multiple myeloma, has recently been used in the treatment of AMR. Everly and colleagues reported the use of bortezomib in six renal transplant recipients with AMR and concurrent ACR. In this small series rejection was reversed, donor-specific antibody levels decreased, and renal allograft function improved. All patients received four doses of intravenous bortezomib 1.3mg/m². Side effects included gastrointestinal, thrombocytopenia, and paresthesias.[69] Bortezomib may also be effective in preventing the development of AMR. Trivedi and colleagues used four doses of bortezomib 1.3 mg/ m² in a group of patients with elevated anti-HLA antibody levels in the absence of acute rejection after transplantation. Patients also received methylprednisolone and treatment with plasmapheresis. Antibody elevations resolved in 9 of 11 patients in 14 to 87 days. The incidence of rejection was not reported.[70]

Rituximab Rituximab is a humanized monoclonal antibody against the CD20 receptor found on B cells. While it is FDA approved for non-Hodgkin lymphoma and rheumatoid arthritis, it has also been used in various aspects of transplant medicine, including treatment of AMR and suppression of alloantibodies prior to transplantation.[71] The optimal dose of rituximab in transplantation has not been defined.

TABLE 98-8	Factors Negatively Affecting Allograft and Patient Survival		
	Kidney	**Liver**	**Heart**
Donor factors	Decreased HLA matching Increased age Increased serum creatine Cardiac instability Prolonged ischemia time History of hypertension	Size mismatch Age (youngest, oldest)	Size mismatch Increased age Prolonged ischemia time
Recipient factors	Age <15, >50 years Retransplantation African race Elevated PRA Multiparous women Poor drug compliance	Increased age Retransplantation African race ICU pretransplant ABO blood type Poor drug compliance	Age <5, >60 years ICU pretransplant Mechanical ventilation LVAD IABP Poor drug compliance

HLA, human leukocyte antigens; IABP, intraaortic balloon pump; LVAD, left ventricular assist device; PRA, panel of reactive antibodies.

EVALUATION OF THERAPEUTIC OUTCOMES

❽ The success of transplantation can be measured in terms of length of graft and patient survival or quality of life. Several donor and recipient factors that have an impact on graft and patient survival have been identified (Table 98–8). The greatest risk to short-term graft survival is acute rejection. Routine surveillance of appropriate biochemical markers and serum drug concentrations are essential to minimize the potential for acute rejection. These parameters should be assessed daily to weekly for the first 1 to 3 months after transplantation. Monitoring should include complete blood counts, serum electrolyte concentrations, serum creatinine and blood urea nitrogen concentrations, and the appropriate serum drug concentrations. Liver function tests should also be evaluated using the same schedule in liver transplantation recipients. Routine biopsies are necessary to monitor for acute rejection in heart transplantation recipients. As the time after transplantation increases, the frequency of monitoring decreases. Once 3 months have elapsed after transplantation, monitoring of these parameters can be reduced to biweekly or monthly for most patients.

Long-term graft survival is limited by chronic rejection. Overall survival rates for solid-organ transplantations are described in terms of half-life, or the time after transplantation at which only 50% of transplanted organs are still functioning. Estimated half-lives for kidneys are 26.9 years for HLA-identical grafts and 12.2 and 10.8 years, respectively, for grafts from a sibling or parent who are 1-haplotype matches. The estimated half-life for HLA-matched grafts was 17.3 years while a markedly lower value of 7.8 years has been noted with mismatched kidneys.[17] The overall median patient survival time for heart transplantation recipients is 9.8 years, but in these patients surviving the first year after transplantation, the median survival increases to 12 years.[1] The highest rate of mortality occurs within the first year after liver transplantation due to the risks of surgery and early postoperative complications. Table 98–9 depicts a typical post-transplantation laboratory monitoring plan.

ECONOMIC CONSIDERATIONS

Renal transplant has been shown to be the most cost-effective means of chronic renal replacement therapy.[72] The degree to which patients remain eligible for Medicare coverage after transplantation impacts kidney allograft survival, presumably secondary to effects on medication availability and compliance. Lifetime extension of Medicare-covered immunosuppression has been associated with improved allograft survival in low-income recipients, with a relative reduction in graft failure rates of 21–27%. In patients who do not otherwise qualify due to age or disability, Medicare currently only provides coverage for immunosuppression for the first 3 years after transplant.[73] Noncompliance has been associated with a sevenfold increased risk of graft failure.[74]

The assessment of the economic impact of liver and heart transplantation is complex. Unlike renal transplantation, liver and heart transplantation is lifesaving. However, there are factors that impact the overall cost of liver transplant that may impact patient selection. Patients awaiting transplant at home, for example, cost less than those who were hospitalized ($114,000 vs $154,000 and $211,000 for ward and ICU care, respectively). Malnutrition and renal impairment have also been shown to increase costs associated with liver transplant by 38% and 39%, respectively.[75] It has been estimated that the total charges for a given heart transplant were approximately $300,000 for the first year, with an additional $20,000 per year of follow-up. If cardiac-assist devices become a viable long-term therapeutic option for end-stage heart failure (estimates of $100,000–$500,000 per year), this will have a significant therapeutic as well as economic impact.[76]

TABLE 98-9	Laboratory Monitoring after Transplantation as a Function of Time Post-Transplant				
	1–2 Weeks	**1 Month**	**2–4 Months**	**4–12 Months**	**>12 Months**
SCr/BUN	Daily	1–2 times per week	Every 1–2 weeks	Monthly	Every 1–2 months
Chemistries[a]	Daily	1–2 times per week	Every 1–2 weeks	Monthly	Every 1–2 months
Liver function tests[b]					
Kidney or heart recipient	Once	Once	Monthly	Every 1–3 months	Every 1–3 months
Liver recipient	Daily	1–3 times per week	Every 1–2 weeks	Monthly	Every 1–2 months
Immunosuppressant level	Daily	1–2 times per week	Every 1–2 weeks	Monthly	Every 1–2 months
Complete blood count[c]	Daily	1–2 times per week	Every 1–2 weeks	Monthly	Every 1–2 months
Lipid panel[d]	Once	Every 3 months	Every 3 months	Every 3 months	Every 3 months
HbA_{1c}	Once	Every 3 months	Every 3 months	Every 3 months	Every 3 months

BUN, blood urea nitrogen; HbA_{1c}, hemoglobin A1c; SCr infusion, serum creatinine.
[a]Chemistries include sodium, potassium, chloride, CO_2 content, magnesium, calcium, phosphorus, and blood glucose.
[b]Liver function tests include total bilirubin, aspartate transaminase (AST), alanine transaminase (ALT), gamma glutamyl transpeptidase (GGTP), alkaline phosphatase.
[c]Complete blood count includes white blood cells (WBC), red blood cells (RBC), platelets, and/or differential.
[d]Lipid panel includes total cholesterol, low-density lipoprotein (LDL), high-density lipoprotein (HDL), triglyceride, and/or very low-density lipoprotein (VLDL).

CLINICAL CONTROVERSY

Generic formulations of cyclosporine, mycophenolate mofetil, and tacrolimus are AB rated by the FDA for bioequivalence, based on studies in normal volunteers as opposed to transplant patients. The narrow therapeutic window of these drugs warrants increased monitoring for efficacy and toxicity when switching formulations. While some clinicians may prefer to maintain patients on the innovator product to avoid additional monitoring, it may not be economically feasible for the patient. Patients should be advised to work with their pharmacist and inform the transplant center when they change product manufacturers.

GENERIC SUBSTITUTION

In recent years a number of generic versions of immunosuppressants have entered the market. While generic versions of corticosteroids and azathioprine have long been in the marketplace, there are now generic versions of cyclosporine, USP [MODIFIED], tacrolimus, and mycophenolate mofetil, the latter being considered narrow therapeutic index drugs. While these formulations have demonstrated bioequivalence to the innovator product in healthy individuals, bioequivalence testing in transplant patients is not required for approval.[77]

Although there would be no differences in the action of the molecule once absorbed into the systemic circulation, several potential differences in absorption could result in variability not seen in healthy volunteers. The presence of diabetes may delay gastric emptying, whereas cystic fibrosis may lead to differences in tacrolimus or cyclosporine secondary to fat malabsorption. None of these generic formulations have been studied in pediatric patients.[78,79]

As generic medications may offer a significant cost advantage compared with the innovator product, their use will increase over time. Much of the concern with generic substitution for immunosuppressant and other narrow therapeutic index medications relates to the potential for unmonitored changes in formulations. Systems that alert patients and prescribers to changes in formulation (e.g., labels on medications, direct notification to physicians) could trigger clinicians to more closely monitor patients for efficacy and toxicity as well as heightened therapeutic drug monitoring during a switch. However, the extent to which increased monitoring could offset cost savings associated with generic substitution has not been fully delineated.

IMMUNOSUPPRESSION-RELATED COMPLICATIONS

Comorbidities such as cardiovascular disease and malignancy, recurrent disease, drug toxicities (namely nephrotoxicity), and chronic rejection are the primary causes of mortality in patients who have a functioning graft 5 or more years after transplantation.[1]

CARDIOVASCULAR DISEASE

Cardiovascular disease is a leading cause of morbidity and mortality in transplant patients.[80] Preexisting cardiovascular disease, which is common in end-stage organ failure, is not reversed with transplantation. Additionally, hypertension, hyperlipidemia, and diabetes are common complications in transplantation recipients and are independent risk factors that contribute significantly to cardiovascular disease. Chronic rejection has been linked to hypertension and hyperlipidemia.[81,82]

HYPERTENSION

Corticosteroids, cyclosporine, tacrolimus, and impaired kidney graft function may cause post-transplantation hypertension. The primary mechanism of calcineurin inhibitor–associated hypertension in heart transplantation recipients may be related to the calcineurin inhibitor–induced stimulation of intact renal sympathetic nerves and the absence of reflex cardiac inhibition of the sympathetic nervous system, but a number of other mechanisms, including decreased prostacyclin and nitric oxide production have also been proposed.[39,83,84] In addition to the propensity to cause peripheral vasoconstriction, calcineurin inhibitors promote sodium retention, resulting in extracellular fluid volume expansion. Tacrolimus appears to have less potential to induce hypertension following transplantation than cyclosporine.[24,85]

Calcium channel blockers have traditionally been the first-line agents to treat hypertension after transplantation.[86] Calcium channel blockers may ameliorate the nephrotoxic effects of cyclosporine, improve renal hemodynamics, decrease the incidence of DGF and the development of allograft atherosclerosis, and provide some immunosuppression. Calcium channel blockers, however, may also contribute to gingival hyperplasia that is often associated with cyclosporine-based immunosuppression.[81]

ACEIs and angiotensin II receptor blockers have traditionally been avoided in kidney transplantation recipients, especially in the perioperative phase, because of the potential for hyperkalemia and their potentially negative influence on glomerular filtration rate. ACEIs and angiotensin II receptor blockers are now considered to be an equivalent alternative to calcium channel blockers for the treatment of hypertension in all transplant recipients. When ACEIs or angiotensin II receptor blockers are used in patients after transplantation, serum creatinine and potassium levels should be monitored closely. If the increase in serum creatinine is greater than 30% within 1 to 2 weeks after initiating ACEIs or angiotensin II receptor blockers, other alternatives must be considered (see Chap. 19).

Multiple antihypertensive agents are usually necessary to achieve the goal blood pressure in transplant recipients; consequently, the addition of a β-blocker, diuretic, or centrally acting antihypertensive is usually necessary. Beta-Blockers are generally considered to be second-line therapy in solid-organ transplantation recipients because of the potential to worsen metabolic disturbances caused by immunosuppressants, such as hyperkalemia and dyslipidemia. Calcineurin inhibitor–induced hypertension is often salt-sensitive, making it very responsive to diuretics. Central-acting agents (e.g., clonidine) are used often as adjunctive therapy in transplantation recipients who are unable to achieve blood pressure control with calcium channel blockers or ACEIs.

HYPERLIPIDEMIA

Hyperlipidemia may be exacerbated by corticosteroids, calcineurin inhibitors, sirolimus, diuretics, and β-blockers.[82,87] Corticosteroids promote insulin resistance and a decrease in lipoprotein lipase activity, as well as excessive triglyceride production. The mechanism of calcineurin inhibitor–induced hyperlipidemia is not well understood. Calcineurin inhibitors may decrease the activity of the low-density lipoprotein (LDL) receptor or lipoprotein lipase, altering LDL catabolism.[82] Tacrolimus appears to have less potential than cyclosporine to induce hyperlipidemia.[22,23,25,82] It is controversial whether the management of hyperlipidemia in transplant recipients should be more aggressive than current guidelines for the general population established by the National Cholesterol Education Program.[88] Aggressive lipid lowering may not only arrest the progress or prevent the complications of atherosclerosis but may also promote graft survival in the kidney and heart transplant recipients.

For most patients, the combination of dietary intervention and an HMG-CoA reductase inhibitor should be considered the treatment of choice. HMG-CoA reductase inhibitors are highly effective in the treatment of hyperlipidemia, especially increased LDL, in transplantation patients. HMG-CoA reductase inhibitors as a class also have immunomodulatory effects on MHC expression and T-cell activation and reduce cardiac allograft rejection.[82,89]

HMG-CoA reductase inhibitors should be used with caution in transplantation recipients because of several reports of rhabdomyolysis when these agents are combined with calcineurin inhibitors.[35,89] Safety measures include using low HMG-CoA reductase inhibitor doses and avoiding inappropriately high cyclosporine or tacrolimus concentrations. The concurrent use of medications known to increase the risk of myopathy (such as gemfibrozil) should be avoided.[82] Patients should be informed of the signs and symptoms of rhabdomyolysis. Baseline and follow-up creatine phosphokinase measurements (every 6 months) have been used to identify patients who develop subclinical rhabdomyolysis when cholesterol-lowering therapy is used. Pravastatin may be preferred as a result of its lower interactive potential with calcineurin inhibitors because it is not metabolized by CYP3A4. The potential for hepatotoxicity from HMG-CoA reductase inhibitors warrants close monitoring of liver function in all transplantation recipients.[87]

Bile acid–binding resins may be used to lower cholesterol in transplant patients, but adequate doses are difficult to achieve without the development of GI adverse effects. Because the absorption of cyclosporine is dependent on the presence of bile in the GI tract, patients should be instructed to separate dosing of bile acid–binding resins and cyclosporine by at least 2 hours. Bile acid–binding resins should also be separated from other immunosuppressants by at least 2 hours to avoid physical adsorption in the GI tract. For transplant patients who have hypertriglyceridemia refractory to dietary intervention, fish oil and fibric acid derivatives are well-tolerated, effective alternatives (see Chap. 28). Fibric acid derivatives are most effective in lowering serum triglyceride concentrations.

New-Onset Diabetes after Transplantation

Corticosteroids and calcineurin inhibitors can impair glucose control in previously diabetic patients, as well as cause new-onset diabetes after transplantation (NODAT) in 4% to 20% of patients. Corticosteroids induce insulin resistance and impair peripheral glucose uptake, whereas calcineurin inhibitors appear to inhibit insulin production.[82] Tacrolimus seems to be more diabetogenic than cyclosporine, although recent studies have failed to show a statistical difference.[22] Other possible risk factors that have been identified for NODAT include African American or Hispanic ethnicity, age >40 years, family history, and weight, as well as CMV and Hepatitis C virus infection.[82]

Up to 40% of patients with NODAT will require insulin therapy.[81] In diabetic patients who can be managed with an oral hypoglycemic agent, glipizide, which is metabolized extensively by the liver, may be preferred over renally eliminated agents such as glyburide. Metformin should be used with extreme caution because of the risk of accumulation and lactic acidosis in those with moderate renal impairment. Regardless of therapy, frequent blood glucose monitoring is imperative in the early postoperative phase both to improve glucose control and to identify those with NODAT. Changes in renal function secondary to calcineurin inhibitor nephrotoxicity or DGF or acute rejection in kidney transplant recipients affects the elimination of many hypoglycemic agents, including insulin, and may result in hyper- or hypoglycemia. Dose changes of immunosuppressant drugs also affect glycemic control. Tapering of immunosuppressive medications may result in reduced insulin requirements, whereas corticosteroid pulses for the treatment of rejection may result in increased insulin requirements.

INFECTION

Increased risk of infection is a natural consequence of therapeutic immunosuppression. Many infections, including cytomegalovirus and fungal infections, in solid organ transplant recipients are reviewed in Chapter 131.[90]

Polyomavirus-associated nephropathy (PVAN) is an important cause of renal dysfunction in kidney transplant recipients. The specific polyomavirus that infects kidney allografts is the BK virus. Primary infection with BK virus occurs in childhood as an asymptomatic infection in 50% to 90% of the general population. The precise mechanism of transmission is not clear but is suspected to be via the oral or respiratory routes. The virus then remains latent primarily in the genitourinary tract. Reactivation of BK virus is limited to people with compromised immune function and is most common in kidney transplant recipients. Reactivation can be detected as the presence of BK virus in the urine of approximately 30% to 40% of kidney transplant recipients, although it does not progress to nephropathy in the majority of patients. However, BK viremia if it develops has been noted to progress to allograft nephropathy in 50% of patients.[91] The development of BK virus nephropathy results in graft loss in about 46% of affected patients.[91]

It has been recommended that all kidney transplant recipients be screened for urinary BK virus replication at least every 3 months during the first 2 years post-transplant or in the event of any renal dysfunction or allograft biopsy. If positive, the result should be confirmed within 4 weeks by quantitative assay in plasma or urine. PVAN is definitively diagnosed by kidney allograft biopsy but may be mistaken for acute rejection if the pathologist does not recognize the presence of BK virus inclusions in renal tubular cells. Differentiation between the two is very important as treatment of acute rejection with increased immunosuppression can worsen BK virus nephropathy. The mainstay of treatment is a reduction in immunosuppression, which should be instituted when BK viremia is detected. The risks of acute rejection resulting from decreased immunosuppression must be weighed against the potential benefits of resolving BK viremia. Cidofovir, a potent nephrotoxic antiviral used for the treatment of CMV retinitis, has also been used for the treatment of BK virus in very low doses (0.25–0.33 mg/kg) without probenicid administered every 2 to 3 weeks.[92]

Hepatitis C recurs almost universally following liver transplantation, resulting in chronic hepatitis or cirrhosis in 90% of patients by 5 years. These patients tend to experience a much more aggressive course than that observed in immunocompetent patients. While short-term survival is not affected, hepatitis C virus infection recurrence results in the need for retransplantation in more than 10% of patients originally transplanted for hepatitis C virus. Pegylated interferons as monotherapy or in combination with ribavirin have been used after liver transplantation, in both the acute and chronic phases of hepatitis C virus infection and as prophylactic or preemptive therapy. Although some patients do achieve sustained viral responses, the rates are generally lower than for immunocompetent patients, 10% to 30% versus 30% to 70%, respectively, for combination therapy. Preexisting anemia and renal dysfunction make it difficult to maintain ribavirin at effective doses. Combination of immunosuppressive drugs and interferon may result in dose-limiting neutropenia. Administration of hematopoietic growth factors may be needed to allow administration of adequate doses of interferons and ribavirin. Even with these adjunctive therapies high rates of therapy discontinuation are still reported.[93,94]

In the absence of preventative therapy, hepatitis B recurs in approximately 80% of patients. Initial studies with short-term intravenous administration of hepatitis B immunoglobulin (HBIg) showed equally high rates of recurrence upon discontinuation of therapy. However, strategies that employ the long-term administration of HBIg with or without antiviral therapy report much lower recurrence rates, 15% to 30% and 20% to 40%, for nonreplicative and replicative hepatitis B virus, respectively. Common strategies include intravenous HBIg 10,000 units during the anhepatic phase followed by 10,000 units daily for 6 days. Antihepatitis B surface titer should be monitored weekly to ensure adequate levels for protection as well as to optimize HBIg use. HBIg has been typically dosed to maintain titers >100 to 500 international units/L. Long-term HBIg therapy is extremely costly, estimated at $100,000 for the first postoperative year and $50,000 for each subsequent year. Combination therapy with antiviral agents appears to be synergistic and is the current standard. Lamivudine resistance is a concern with long-term utilization both pre- and post-transplant. The role of newer antiviral agents, including adefovir, entecavir, and tenofovir, remains to be defined. Other strategies that have been investigated and show promise include pretransplant viral load reduction and reduced-dose HBIg. Treatment for active hepatitis B virus graft infection should include HBIg, antiviral therapy, and concomitant reduction in immunosuppression.[94]

MALIGNANCY

Although advances in immunosuppression have decreased the incidence of acute rejection and increased patient survival, they have also increased the patient's lifetime exposure to immunosuppression. While the precise mechanism is unclear, post-transplantation malignancy seems to be related to the overall level of immunosuppression, as evidenced by a difference in the rates of malignancy associated with quadruple versus triple versus dual immunosuppressant regimens. The risk of de novo malignancy in transplantation recipients is increased three- to fivefold over the general population. The age-adjusted incidence of lung, breast, colon, and prostate cancers was doubled in renal transplant recipients. A number of cancers that are uncommon in the general population occur with much higher prevalence in transplantation recipients: post-transplantation lymphomas and lymphoproliferative disorders (PTLDs), Kaposi sarcoma, renal carcinoma, in situ carcinomas of the uterine cervix, hepatobiliary tumors, and anogenital carcinomas. Skin cancers are the most common tumors. Factors that may predispose transplant recipients to skin cancers include copious sun exposure and therapy with azathioprine.[95] While too early to definitively assess the impact of mycophenolic acid derivatives on malignancy, one analysis showed a lower risk of PTLD with MMF compared with AZA. Inhibitors of mTOR have a theoretical benefit in terms of the development of malignancy. In addition to immunosuppressive properties, mTOR inhibitors also have antiproliferative effects. In fact, a decreased incidence of malignancy was reported in patients receiving mTOR inhibitors versus CNIs, and conversion to PSIs from CNIs can result in regression of Kaposi sarcoma.[95]

PTLD encompasses a broad spectrum of disorders, ranging from benign polyclonal hyperplasias to malignant monoclonal lymphomas. Factors that predispose patients to PTLD include Epstein-Barr virus seronegativity at transplantation and intense immunosuppression, particularly with OKT3 and antithymocyte globulin. Nonrenal transplantation recipients are more likely to develop PTLD secondary to the heavy immunosuppression used to reverse rejection. Administration of ganciclovir or acyclovir preemptively during antilymphocyte therapy may decrease the risk of eventual PTLD. Treatment of life-threatening PTLD generally includes severe reduction or cessation of immunosuppression. Other options include systemic chemotherapy or rituximab.[96]

Post-transplantation malignancies appear an average of 5 years after transplantation and increase with the length of follow-up. As many as 72% of patients surviving greater than 20 years may be affected. Malignancy accounts for 11.8% of deaths after cardiac transplantation and is the single most common cause of death in the sixth to the tenth post-transplant years.[95]

CONCLUSIONS

Transplantation is a lifesaving therapy for several types of end-organ failure. Advances in the understanding of transplant immunology have produced an unprecedented number of choices in terms of immunosuppression. The increasing number of effective immunosuppressive medications and therapies offers clinicians diverse ways to prevent allograft rejection in a patient-specific manner. However, the vast array and efficacy of currently available immunosuppressive agents make it increasingly difficult to evaluate their long-term efficacy. Clinicians must be keenly aware of the adverse effects of immunosuppressive medications and their treatment in order to optimize the care of the transplanted patient.

ABBREVIATIONS

6-MP: 6-mercaptopurine

ACEI: angiotensin-converting enzyme inhibitor

ACR: acute cellular rejection

AMR: antibody-mediated rejection

ATG: antithymocyte globulin

ATN: acute tubular necrosis

AUC: area under the concentration curve

C_2: concentration 2 hours after dose

C_{max}: peak concentration

CMV: cytomegalovirus

CYP: cytochrome P450 liver enzyme system

DGF: delayed graft function

FKBP: FK-binding protein

GI: gastrointestinal

HBIg: hepatitis B immunoglobulin

HIV: human immunodeficiency virus

HLA: human leukocyte antigen

HPLC: high-performance liquid chromatography

IL: interleukin

LDL: low-density lipoprotein

MELD: model for end-stage liver disease

MHC: major histocompatibility complex

MPA: mycophenolic acid

MPAG: mycophenolic acid glucuronide

mTOR: mammalian target of rapamycin

NODAT: new-onset diabetes after transplantation

OKT3: muromonab-CD3

PML: progressive multifocal leukoencephalopathy

PRA: panel of reactive antibodies

PSI: proliferation signal inhibitor

PTLD: post-transplantation lymphoproliferative disorder

PVAN: polyomavirus associated nephropathy

RIA: radioimmunoassay

t_{max}: time to peak concentration

REFERENCES

1. 2007 Annual Report of the U.S. Organ Procurement and Transplantation Network and the Scientific Registry of Transplant Recipients: Transplant Data 1996–2006. Rockville, MD: Department of Health and Human Services, Health Resources and Services Administration, Healthcare Systems Bureau, Division of Transplantation; Richmond, VA: United Network for Organ Sharing; Ann Arbor, MI: University Renal Research and Education Association; 2007.

2. Wiesner RH, Rakela J, Ishitani MB, et al. Recent advances in liver transplantation. Mayo Clin Proc 2003;78:197–210.

3. Wolfe RA, Ashby VB, Milford EL, et al. Comparison of mortality in all patients on dialysis, patients on dialysis awaiting transplantation and recipients of a first cadaveric transplant. N Engl J Med 1999;341:1725–1730.

4. Pablo R, Ortega F, Baltar JM, et al. Health-related quality of life (HRQOL) of kidney transplanted patients: Variables that influence it. Clin Transplant 2000;14:199–207.

5. U.S. Renal Data System, USRDS 2008 Annual Data Report: Atlas of Chronic Kidney Disease and End-Stage Renal Disease in the United States. Bethesda, MD: National Institutes of Health, National Institute of Diabetes and Digestive and Kidney Diseases; 2008.

6. Saab S, Wang V. Recurrent hepatitis C following liver transplant: Diagnosis, natural history and therapeutic options. J Clin Gastroenterol 2003;37:155–163.

7. Keck BM, Bennett LE, Rosendale J, et al. Worldwide Thoracic Organ Transplantation: A report from the UNOS/ISHLT International Registry for Thoracic Organ Transplantation. In: Cecka JM, Terasaki PI, eds. Clinical Transplants 1999. Los Angeles: UCLA Immunogenetics Center; 1999:35–49.

8. Kavanagh R, Yacoub MH, Kennedy J, et al. Return to work after heart transplantation: 12-year follow-up. J Heart Lung Transplant 1999;18:846–851.

9. Deng MC. Heart failure: Cardiac transplantation. Heart 2002;87:177–184.

10. Braith RW, Edwards DG. Exercise following heart transplantation. Sports Med 2000;30:171–192.

11. Venkataramanan R, Habucky K, Burckart GJ, et al. Clinical pharmacokinetics in organ transplant patients. Clin Pharmacokinet 1989;16:134–161.

12. LeMoine A, Goldman M, Abramowicz D. Multiple pathways to allograft rejection. Transplantation 2002;73:1373–1381.

13. Mueller XM. Drug immunosuppressive therapy for adult heart transplantation, I: Immune response to allograft and mechanism of action of immunosuppressants. Ann Thorac Surg 2004;77:354–362.

14. Taylor DO, Edwards LB, Boucek MM, et al. Registry of the international society for heart and lung transplantation: Twenty-second official adult heart transplant report—2005. J Heart Lung Transplant 2005;24:945–955.

15. Stewart S, Winters GL, Fishbein MC, et al. Revision of the 1990 working formulation for the standardization of nomenclature in the diagnosis of heart rejection. J Heart Lung Transplant 2005;24:1710–1720.

16. Michaels PJ, Espejo ML, Kobashigawa J, et al. Humoral rejection in cardiac transplantation: Risk factors, hemodynamic consequences and relationship to transplant coronary artery disease. J Heart Lung Transplant 2003;22:58–69.

17. Hariharan S, Johnson CP, Bresnahan BA, et al. Improved graft survival after renal transplantation in the U.S., 1988 to 1996. N Engl J Med 2000;342:605–612.

18. Merville P. Combating chronic renal allograft dysfunction: Optimizing immunosuppressive regimens. Drugs 2005;65:615–631.

19. Schmauss D, Weis M. Cardiac allograft vasculopathy: Recent developments. Circulation 2008;117;2131–2141.

20. Vasquez EM, Benedetti E, Pollak R. Ethnic differences in clinical response to corticosteroid treatment of acute allograft rejection. Transplantation 2001;71:229–233.

21. Augustine JJ, Hricik DE. Steroid sparing in kidney transplantation: Changing paradigms, improving outcomes, and remaining questions. Clin J Am Soc Nephrol 2006;1:1080–1089.

22. Scott LJ, McKeage K, Keam SJ, Plosker GL. Tacrolimus: A further update of its use in the management of organ transplantation. Drugs 2003;63:1247–1297.

23. Bowman LJ, Brennan DC. The role of tacrolimus in renal transplantation. Expert Opin Pharmacother 2008;9:635–643.

24. Keogh A. Calcineurin inhibitors in heart transplantation. J Heart Lung Transplant 2004;23:S203–S206.

25. Jose M. Calcineurin inhibitors in renal transplantation: Adverse effects. Nephrology 2007;12:S66–S74.

26. Bobadilla MA, Gamba G. New insights into the pathophysiology of cyclosporine nephrotoxicity: A role of aldosterone. Am J Physiol Renal Physiol 2007;293:F2–F9.

27. Spriet I, Meersseman W, deHoon J, von Winckelmann S, Wilmer A, Willems L. Mini-series, II: Clinical aspects. Clinically relevant CYP450-mediated drug interactions in the ICU. Intensive Care Med 2009;35:603–612.

28. Bernardo JF, McCauley J. Drug therapy in transplant recipients: Special considerations in the elderly with comorbid conditions. Drugs Aging 2004;21:323–348.

29. Staatz CE, Tett SE. Clinical pharmacokinetics and pharmacodynamics of tacrolimus in solid organ transplantation. Clin Pharmacokinet 2004;43:623–653.

30. Jones TE. The use of other drugs to allow a lower dosage of cyclosporine to be used: Therapeutic and pharmacoeconomic considerations. Clin Pharmacokinet 1999;32:357–367.

31. Kothari J, Nash M, Zaltzman J et al. Diltiazem use in tacrolimus-treated renal transplant recipients. J Clin Pharm Therap 2004;29:425–430.

32. Kumana CR, Tong MKL, Li CS et al. Diltiazem co-treatment in renal transplant patients receiving microemulsion cyclosporin. Br J Clin Pharmacol 2003;56:670–678.

33. Chisholm MA, Mulloy LL, Jagadeesan M et al. Coadministration of tacrolimus with anti-acid drugs. Transplantation 2003;76:665–666.

34. Christians U, Jacobsen W, Benet LZ, Lampen A. Mechanisms of clinically relevant drug interactions associated with tacrolimus. Clin Pharmacokinet 2002;41:813–851.

35. Asberg A. Interactions between cyclosporine and lipid-lowering drugs: Implications for organ transplant recipients. Drugs 2003;63:367–378.

36. Schiff J, Cole E, Cantarovich M. Therapeutic monitoring of calcineurin inhibitors for the nephrologist. Clin J Am Soc Nephrol 2007;2:374–384.

37. Nowack R. Cytochrome P450 enzyme, and transport protein mediated herb–drug interactions in renal transplant patients: Grapefruit juice, St. John's Wort—and beyond! Nephrology 2008;13:337–347.

38. Cross SA and Perry CM. Tacrolimus once-daily formulation: In the prophylaxis of transplant rejection in renal or liver allograft recipients. Drugs 2007;67:1931–1943.

39. Kuypers DRJ. Immunosuppressive drug monitoring—What to use in clinical practice today to improve renal graft outcome. Transpl Intl 2005;18:140–150.

40. Bush WW. Overview of transplantation immunology and the pharmacotherapy of adult solid organ transplant recipients: Focus on immunosuppression. AACN Clin Issues 1999;10:253–269.

41. Halloran PF. Immunosuppressive drugs for kidney transplantation. N Engl J Med 2004;351:2715–2729.

42. Shaw LM, Figurski M, Milone MC, et al. Therapeutic drug monitoring of mycophenolic acid. Clin J Am Soc Nephrol 2007;2:1062–1072.

43. Weigel G, Griesmacher A, Karimi A, et al. Effect of mycophenolate mofetil therapy on lymphocyte activation in heart transplant recipients. J Heart Lung Transplant 2002;21:1074–1079.

44. Ciancio G, Miller J, Gonwa TJ. Review of major clinical trials with mycophenolate mofetil in renal transplantation. Transplantation 2005;80(2S):S191–S200.

45. Shah S, Collett D, Johnson R, et al. Long-term graft outcome with mycophenolate mofetil and azathioprine: A paired kidney analysis. Transplantation 2006;82:1634–1639.

46. Kuypers DR. Influence of interactions between immunosuppressive drugs on therapeutic drug monitoring. Ann Transplant 2008;13:11–18.

47. Elbarbary FA, Shoker AS. Therapeutic drug measurement of mycophenolic acid derivatives in transplant patients. Clinical Biochemistry 2007;40:752–764.

48. Cox VC, Ensom MHH. Mycophenolate mofetil for solid organ transplantation: Does the evidence support the need for clinical pharmacokinetic monitoring? Ther Drug Monit 2003;25:137–157.

49. Shaw LM, Korecka M, Venkataramanan R, et al. Mycophenolic acid pharmacodynamics and pharmacokinetics provide a basis for rational monitoring strategies. Am J Transplant 2003;3:534–542.

50. Lancaster DL, Patel N, Lennard L, Lilleyman JS. 6-Thioguanine in children with acute lymphoblastic leukemia: Influence of food on parent drug pharmacokinetics and 6-thioquanine nucleotide concentrations. Br J Clin Pharmacol 2001;51:531–539.

51. Augustine JJ, Bodziak KA, Hricik DE. Use of sirolimus in solid organ transplantation. Drugs 2007;67:369–391.

52. Monchaud C, Marquet P. Pharmacokinetic optimization of immunosuppressive therapy in thoracic transplantation: part II. Clin Pharmacokinet. 2009;48:489–516.

53. Salvadori M, Scolari MP, Bertoni E, et al. Everolimus with very-low exposure cyclosporine A in de novo kidney transplantation: a multicenter, randomized, controlled trial. Transplantation. 2009;88: 1194–1202.

54. Chueh SCJ, Kahan BD. Dyslipidemia in renal transplant recipients treated with a sirolimus and cyclosporine-based immunosuppressive regimen: Incidence, risk factors, progression, and prognosis. Transplantation 2003;76:375–382.

55. van Gelder T, ter Meulen CG, Hené R, et al. Oral ulcers in kidney transplant recipients treated with sirolimus and mycophenolate mofetil. Transplantation 2003;75:788–791.

56. Bunn D, Lea CK, Bevan DJ, et al. The pharmacokinetics of anti-thymocyte globulin (ATG) following intravenous infusion in man. Clin Nephrol 1996;45:29–32.

57. Webster AC, Pankhurst T, Rinaldi F, Chapman JR, Craig JC. Monoclonal and polyclonal antibody therapy for treating acute rejection in kidney transplant recipients: A systematic review of randomized trial data. Transplantation 2006;81:953–965.

58. Hardinger KL. Rabbit antithymocyte globulin induction therapy in adult renal transplantation. Pharmacotherapy 2006;26:1771–1783.

59. Wilde MI, Goa KL. Muromonab-CD3: A reappraisal of it pharmacology and use as prophylaxis of solid organ transplant rejection. Drugs 1996;51:865–894.

60. Morris PJ, Russell NK. Alemtuzumab (Campath-1H): A systematic review in organ transplantation. Transplantation 2006;81:1361–1367.

61. Bloom DD, Hu H, Fechner JH, Knechtle SJ. T-lymphocyte alloresponses of Campath-1H-treated kidney transplant patients. Transplantation 2006;81:81–87.

62. Tan HP, Smaldone MC, Shapiro R. Immunosuppressive preconditioning or induction regimens: Evidence to date. Drugs 2006;66: 1535–1545.

63. Chapman TM, Keating GM. Basiliximab: A review of it use as induction therapy in renal transplantation. Drugs 2003;63:2803–2835.

64. Mottershead M, Neuberger J. Daclizumab. Expert Opin Biol Thera 2007;7:1583–1596.

65. Ramirez CB, Marino IR. The role of basiliximab induction therapy in organ transplantation. Exper Opin Biol Ther 2007;7:137–148.

66. Adu D, Cockwell P, Ives NJ, et al. Interleukin-2 receptor monoclonal antibodies in renal transplantation: Meta-analysis of randomized trials. BMJ 2003;326:789–794.

67. Stratta RJ, Alloway RR, Lo A, Hodge E. Two-dose daclizumab regimen in simultaneous kidney-pancreas transplant recipients: Primary end point analysis of a multicenter, randomized study. Transplantation 2003;75:1260–1266.

68. Gahdhi AM, Fazli U, Rodina V, et al. Costimulation targeting therapies in organ transplantation. Curr Opin Organ Transplant 2008;13:622–626.

69. Everly MJ, Everly JJ, Susskind B, et al. Bortezomib provides effective therapy for antibody- and cell-mediated acute rejection. Transplantation 2008;86:1754–1761.

70. Trivedi HL, Terasaki P, Feroz A, et al. Abrogation of anti-HLA antibodies via proteasome inhibition. Transplantation 2009;87:1555–1561.

71. Becker YT, Milagros SP, Sollinger HW. The emerging role of rituximab in organ transplantation. Transplant International 2006;19:621–628.

72. Howard K, Salkeld F, White S, et al. The cost-effectiveness of increasing kidney transplantation and home-based dialysis. Nephrology 2009;14:123–132.

73. Woodward RS, Page TF, Soares R, et al. Income-related disparities in kidney transplant graft failures are eliminated by Medicare's immunosuppression coverage. AM J Transplant 2008;8:2636–2646.

74. Butler JA, Roderick R, Mullee M, et al. Frequency and impact of nonadherence to immunosuppressant after renal transplantation: A systematic review. Transplantation 2004;77:769–778.

75. O'Grady JG. Clinical economics review: Liver transplantation. Aliment Pharmacol Ther 1997;11:445–451.

76. Evans RW. Economic impact of mechanical cardiac assistance. Prog Cardiovasc Dis 2000;43:81–94.

77. Christians U, Klawitter J, Clavijo CF. Bioequivalence testing of immunosuppressants: Concepts and misconceptions. Kidney International 2010;77:S1–S7.

78. Uber PA, Ross HJ, Zuckermann AO, et al. Generic drug immunosuppression in thoracic transplantation: An ISHLT educational advisory. J Heart Lung Transplant 2009;28:655–660.

79. Alloway RR, Isaacs R, Lake K, et al. Report for the American Society of Transplantation conference on immunosuppressive drugs and the use of generic immunosuppressants. Am J Transplant 2003;10:1211–1215.

80. Bostom AD, Brown RS, Chavers BM, et al. Prevention of post-transplant cardiovascular disease: Report and recommendations of an ad hoc group. Am J Transplant 2002;2:491–500.

81. Zhang R, Leslie B, Boudreaux P, et al. Hypertension after kidney transplantation: Impact, pathogenesis and therapy. Am J Med Sci 2003;325:202–208.

82. Subramanian S, Trence DL. Immunosuppressive agents: Effects on glucose and lipid metabolism. Endocrinol Metab Clin N Am 2007;36:891–905.

83. Textor SC, Taler SJ, Canzanello VJ, Schwartz L. Cyclosporine, blood pressure and atherosclerosis. Cardiol Rev 1997;5:141–151.

84. Ventura HO, Malik FS, Mehra MR, et al. Mechanisms of hypertension in cardiac transplantation and the role of cyclosporine. Curr Opin Cardiol 1997;12:375–381.

85. Chobanian AV, Bakris GL, Black HR, et al. The seventh report of the Joint National Committee on Prevention, Detection, Evaluation, and Treatment of High Blood Pressure: The JNC 7 report. JAMA 2003:289;2560–2572.

86. Tylicki L, Habicht A, Watchinger B, Hörl WH. Treatment of hypertension in renal transplant recipients. Curr Opin Urol 2003;13:91–98.

87. Kasiske B, Cosio FG, Beto J, et al. Clinical practice guidelines for managing dyslipidemias in kidney transplant patients: A report from the Managing Dyslipidemias in Chronic Kidney Disease Work Group of the National Kidney Foundation Kidney Disease Outcomes Quality Initiative. Am J Transplant 2004;4(suppl 7):13–53.

88. Grundy SM, Cleeman JI, Bairey Merz CN, et al. Implications of recent clinical trials for the national cholesterol education program adult treatment panel III guidelines. Circulation 2004;110–227–239.

89. Gazi IF, Liperopoulous EN, Athyros VG, et al. Statins and solid organ transplantation. Current Pharm Des 2006;12:4771–4783.

90. Fishman JA. Infection in solid-organ transplant recipients. N Eng J Med 2007;357:2601–2614.

91. Hirsch HH, Brennan DC, Drachenberg CB, et al. Polyomavirus-associated nephropathy in renal transplantation: Interdisciplinary analyses and recommendations. Transplantation 2005;79:1277–1286.

92. de Bruyn G, Limaye AP. BK-virus associated nephropathy in kidney transplant recipients. Rev Med Virol 2004;14:193–205.

93. Fredrick RT, Hassanein TI. Role of growth factors in the treatment of patients with HIV/HCV coinfection and patients with recurrent hepatitis C following liver transplantation. J Clin Gastroenterol 2005;39:S14–S22.

94. Roche B, Samuel D. Treatment of hepatitis B and C after liver transplantation, II: Hepatitis C. Transpl Int 2005;17:759–766.

95. Dantal J, Pohanka E. Malignancies in renal transplantation: An unmet medical need. Nephrol Dial Transplant 2007;22:i4–i10.

96. Lee JJ, Lam MSH, Rosenberg A. Role of chemotherapy and rituximab for treatment of posttransplant lymphoproliferative disorder in solid organ transplantation. Ann Pharmacother 2007;41:1648–1659.

CHAPTER

99

Osteoporosis and Other Metabolic Bone Diseases

MARY BETH O'CONNELL AND SHERYL F. VONDRACEK

KEY CONCEPTS

❶ Perimenopausal and postmenopausal women, men older than age 50 years, and those with potential disease- or medication-induced bone loss should be assessed for osteoporosis. Patients with early-onset or severe osteoporosis should be evaluated for secondary causes of bone loss.

❷ Inadequate vitamin D concentrations, which sometimes cause osteomalacia, can be insidious and coexist with osteoporosis. A serum 25(OH) vitamin D concentration should be obtained in patients with osteoporosis, at high risk for low vitamin D concentrations, or with symptoms suggestive of inadequate vitamin D such as unexplained muscle weakness, falls, or pain.

❸ Osteoporosis in men is often secondary to certain diseases and medications and responds well to a bone-healthy lifestyle, bisphosphonate or teriparatide therapy, and in some cases, testosterone replacement.

❹ Estimation of an adult person's 10-year probability of developing an osteoporotic fracture can be estimated with the FRAX tool. Central bone densitometry can determine bone mass, predict fracture risk, and influence patient and provider treatment decisions. Portable equipment can be used for screening in the community to determine the need for further testing.

❺ All people, regardless of age, should incorporate a bone-healthy lifestyle beginning at birth and continuing throughout life, that emphasizes regular exercise, nutritious diet, tobacco avoidance, minimal alcohol use, and fall prevention to prevent and treat osteoporosis.

❻ The adequate intake for calcium in American adults is 1,000 to 1,200 mg of elemental calcium daily in divided doses from diet or supplements. The adequate intake for American

adults is 400 to 1,000 units (seniors 800–1,000 units) of vitamin D daily, mainly from supplements, with some experts recommending higher doses.

❼ Bisphosphonates decrease vertebral, hip, and nonvertebral fractures and are considered the medication of choice for osteoporosis treatment. Adherence with bisphosphonates is frequently suboptimal, which has been associated with less fracture prevention. Assessment of correct administration should be frequently conducted with repeat patient education as needed.

❽ Raloxifene is an alternative treatment option to prevent vertebral fractures, particularly in women who cannot tolerate, should not, or will not take bisphosphonates. Raloxifene also decreases invasive breast cancer risk. Postmenopausal women at high risk for breast cancer might choose this medication to obtain dual benefits.

❾ Healthcare providers can have an important role in prevention and treatment of osteoporosis by conducting osteoporosis assessments at health fairs and community pharmacies, identifying and resolving disease and medication-induced bone loss/osteoporosis, ensuring medications are taken accurately, identifying and resolving medication-related problems resulting in suboptimal adherence, and encouraging secondary fracture prevention in patients with past hip or vertebral fractures.

❿ Patients taking long-term oral glucocorticoids need to be identified and started on a bone-healthy lifestyle with higher intakes of calcium and vitamin D and usually bisphosphonate therapy to prevent or treat osteoporosis.

Learning objectives, review questions, and other resources can be found at
www.pharmacotherapyonline.com.

❶ Osteoporosis is a major public health threat for an estimated 44 million Americans or 55% of the people 50 years of age and older.[1] Low bone density (sometimes referred to as osteopenia) is estimated in 34 million Americans[1] and in 37% to 50% of white women.[2] In the United States, 8 million women and 2 million men are estimated to have osteoporosis. Osteoporosis is a bone disorder characterized by low bone density, impaired bone architecture, and compromised bone strength predisposing a person to increased fracture risk.[3] The development of osteoporosis and osteoporotic fractures is

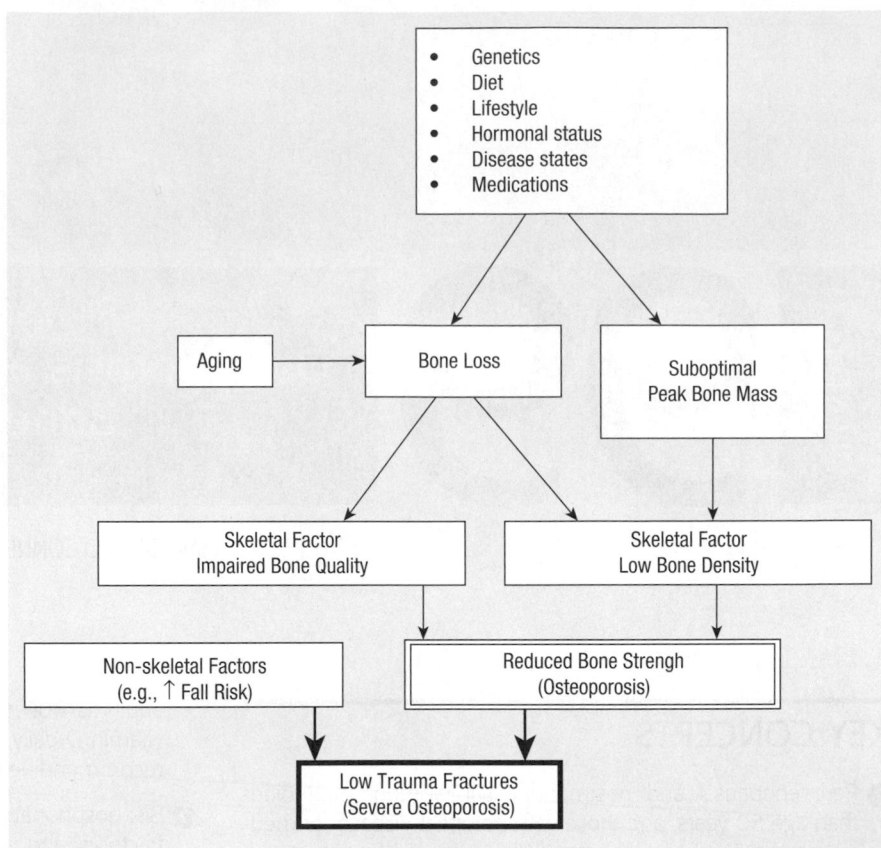

FIGURE 99-1. Etiology of osteoporosis and osteoporotic fractures.

multifactorial, beginning with genetics and lifestyles unhealthy for bone growth and maintenance, along with other skeletal factors, which lead to compromised bone strength, and nonskeletal factors that lead to falls (Fig. 99–1). Everyone must take an active role in educating people of all ages as well as other healthcare providers on healthy bone lifestyle habits and osteoporosis prevention and treatment options.

EPIDEMIOLOGY

❶ Osteopenia, osteoporosis, and osteoporotic fractures are very common and affect all ethnic groups. Osteopenia is estimated to occur in 50% of Asian, 47% of Hispanic, 45% of Native American, 40% of white, and 28% of black women.[4] Osteoporosis affects 12% of Native American, 10% of Asian, 10% of Hispanic, 7% of white, and 4% of black women. Disease prevalence greatly increases with age; from 4% in women 50 to 59 years of age to 44% to 52% in women 80 years of age and older.[2] White and Hispanic women have the highest fragility fracture rate followed by Native American, African American, and Asian women when the data are adjusted for weight, bone mineral density (BMD), and other factors.[4] About 8 to 13 million men aged 50 years and older (i.e., 28%–47%) have osteopenia, with an osteoporosis prevalence of 6% to 13%.[5,6] Although osteoporosis is a common finding in seniors with fractures, up to 50% of fragility fractures occur in patients with normal bone mass or osteopenia.[2]

Low trauma (fragility) wrist and vertebral fractures are common throughout adulthood, and hip fractures are more common in seniors. Fracture incidence was estimated to be 2 million (71% in women, 29% in men) in 2005, with an estimated total medical cost of $17 billion.[7] Fractures in women accounted for 75% of the costs and in seniors 87% of the costs. Hip fractures represented 72% of these costs. Forecasting predicts 3 million fractures at a cost

of $25 billion in 2025. Newer information is beginning to suggest that fracture incidence might be decreasing for both sexes,[8] with the hypothesis related to better efforts at osteoporosis prevention (e.g., improved risk factor identification, diagnosis, and bone-healthy lifestyle education) and use of prescription antiosteoporotic medications. In a woman's lifetime, she has a 17% likelihood of a hip fracture, 15.6% likelihood of a vertebral fracture, and 16% likelihood of a forearm fracture.[2] In a man's lifetime, osteoporotic fracture risk is 15%.[6]

BONE PHYSIOLOGY

The skeleton comprises two types of bone.[9] Cortical bone makes up the majority of the skeleton (80%) and is found mostly in the long bones (e.g., forearm and hip). Trabecular bone is found mostly in the vertebrae and ends of long bones. It is 10 times more metabolically active compared with cortical bone, having a much higher bone turnover rate because of its large surface area and honeycomb-like shape.

Bone is made of collagen and mineral components.[9] The collagen component gives bone its flexibility and energy-absorbing capability. The mineral component gives bone its stiffness and strength. The correct balance of these substances is needed for bone to adequately accommodate stress and strain and resist fractures. Imbalances can impair bone quality and lead to reduced bone strength.

Bone strength reflects the integration of bone quality and BMD (bone mass). Bone mass increases rapidly throughout childhood and adolescence. Ninety-five percent of peak bone mass is attained by age 18 to 20 years, with small gains until approximately age 30 years.[10] Peak bone mass is highly dependent on genetic factors that account for approximately 60% to 80% of the variability.[11] The remaining 20% to 40% is influenced by modifiable factors such as nutritional intake (e.g., calcium, vitamin D, and protein), exercise,

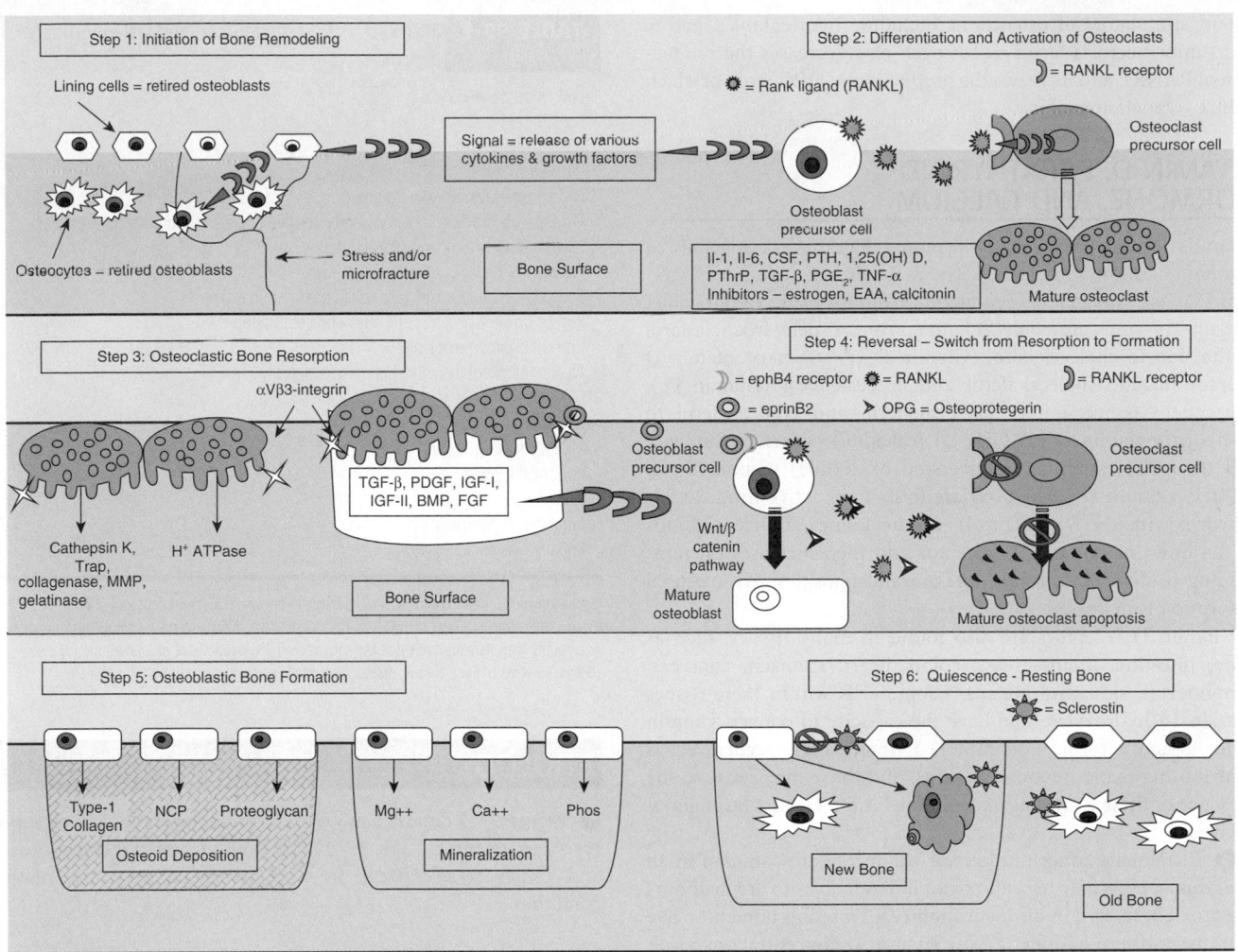

FIGURE 99-2. Bone remodeling cycle.[9,12–16] (1,25(OH) D, calcitriol/1α,25dihydroxyvitamin D; BMP, bone morphogenetic protein; Ca, calcium; CSF, colony-stimulating factors; EAA, estrogen agonist/antagonist; FGF, fibroblast growth factor; IGF, insulin-like growth factor; Il, interleukin; Mg, magnesium; MMP, matrix metalloproteinases; NCP, noncollagenous proteins; OPG, osteoprotegerin; PDGF, platelet-derived growth factor; PG, prostaglandin; Phos, phosphorous; PTH, parathyroid hormone; PTHrP, parathyroid hormone-related protein; TGF, transforming growth factor; TNF, tumor necrosis factor; Trap, tartrate-resistant acid phosphate.)

adverse lifestyle practices (e.g., smoking), hormonal status, and certain diseases and medications. Optimizing peak bone mass is important for preventing osteoporosis. The higher the peak bone mass, the more bone one can lose before being at an increased fracture risk.

Bone remodeling is a dynamic process that occurs continuously throughout life Figure 99–2.[9,12–16] One to two million tiny sections of bone are in the process of remodeling at any given time. The complete physiology of bone remodeling is not fully known but appears to begin with signals from lining cells or osteocytes (bone communication cells) that are triggered by stress, microfractures, biofeedback systems, and potentially certain diseases and medications (see Fig. 99–2, step 1).[17] Many cytokines, growth factors, and hormones influence each remodeling step. A major stimulus for hematopoietic stem cell (monocyte–macrophage lineage) differentiation to become mature osteoclasts (bone resorbing cells) is the receptor activator of nuclear factor kappa B ligand (RANKL), which is emitted from the osteoblast (bone-forming cells) in step 2 and binds to its receptor RANK on the surface of osteoclast precursors. RANKL also stimulates mature osteoclast activation and bone adherence via integrins to resorb bone. Proteinases are secreted to resorb the protein matrix, and hydrogen ions are secreted to dissolve the mineralized component (step 3). After bone is resorbed and a cavity is created, additional cytokines and growth factors,

some working through Wnt/β-catenin pathways, are released that first mature osteoblasts from mesenchymal stem cells and then stimulate bone formation (step 4). Osteoclasts also produce ephrinB2 that adheres to ephB4 receptors on osteoblasts and osteoblast precursors to stimulate osteoblast differentiation and activity. Mature osteoblasts produce osteoprotegerin (OPG) that binds (step 4) to RANKL, thereby stopping bone resorption.

Bone formation occurs over two phases.[9,13,16] First, osteoblasts fill the resorption cavity with osteoid, and then mineralization occurs (step 5). Once bone formation is complete, mature osteoblasts undergo apoptosis or become lining cells or osteocytes (step 6). Osteocytes produce sclerostin, which inhibits Wnt signaling and bone formation. Quiescence is the phase when bone is at rest until another remodeling cycle is initiated at that site.

With the mapping of the genome, exploration into genetic control of bone physiology and pathophysiology is being explored.[18] Nine genes have been mapped to BMD regulation and four genes to fracture risk. Genetic modulation is in its infancy for osteoporosis prevention and treatment but might lead to new medications.

Estrogen has many positive effects on the bone remodeling process, with most of its actions helping to maintain a normal bone resorption rate.[12,19] Estrogen suppresses the proliferation and differentiation of osteoclasts and increases osteoclast apoptosis. Estrogen decreases the production of several cytokines that are potent stimulators of osteoclasts, including interleukins 1 and 6, and tumor necrosis factor-α. Estrogen also decreases the production of RANKL and increases the production of OPG, both of which reduce osteoclastogenesis.[20]

VITAMIN D, PARATHYROID HORMONE, AND CALCIUM

Vitamin D and parathyroid hormone (PTH) work together to maintain calcium homeostasis. The most abundant source of vitamin D is the endogenous production from exposure to ultraviolet B light. The sun's ultraviolet B light converts 7-dehydrocholesterol in the skin to cholecalciferol (vitamin D_3).[21,22] Dietary vitamin D sources include cholecalciferol and ergocalciferol (vitamin D_2). Subsequent conversion of cholecalciferol and ergocalciferol to 25-hydroxyvitamin D [25(OH) D] (calcidiol) occurs in the liver, and then PTH stimulates conversion of 25(OH) vitamin D via 25(OH) vitamin D-1α-hydroxylase to its final active form, 1α,25-dihydroxyvitamin D (calcitriol), in the kidney. Calcitriol binds to the intestinal vitamin D receptor and then increases calcium-binding protein. As a result, calcium and phosphorous intestinal absorption is increased.

Vitamin D receptors are also found in many tissues, such as bone, intestine, brain, breast, colon, heart, stomach, pancreas, lymphocytes, skin, and gonads.[22] Some cells within these tissues contain 1α-hydroxylase and have the capacity to convert vitamin D to its active form.[21] Vitamin D is increasingly recognized as contributing many nonbone benefits, and those may relate to the presence of these conversion capabilities and receptors throughout the body.

❷ Inadequate concentrations of vitamin D are common in all age groups, especially in seniors and individuals who are malnourished or obese, live in an institution (e.g., nursing home), or live in more northern latitudes.[22] Low vitamin D concentrations result from insufficient intake, dietary fat malabsorption, decreased sun exposure, decreased skin production, or decreased liver and renal metabolism. Endogenous synthesis of vitamin D can be decreased by factors that affect exposure to or decrease skin penetration of ultraviolet B light. Sunscreen use, full body coverage with clothing (e.g., women wearing veiled, full-length dresses), and darkly pigmented skin can all cause a decrease in vitamin D production. Seasonal variations in vitamin D concentrations are also seen with nadirs in late winter and peaks in late summer.[22]

Calcium absorption under normal conditions is approximately 30% to 40%, decreasing to 10% to 15% with low vitamin D concentrations.[23,24] Calcium absorption is predominantly an active rate-limited process controlled by many hormones such as vitamin D and estrogen. Less than 15% is absorbed through passive diffusion, which is not rate limited.[25,26] A calcium transporter is required to bring calcium from the gut into the tissue wall. There it binds to calbindin to be transported across the enterocyte and is extruded into the circulation via Ca^{2+} adenosinetriphosphatase (ATPase) and the sodium/calcium exchanger (NCX). When the calcium sensing receptor (CaSR) on parathyroid cells senses low serum calcium, PTH production increases. PTH then increases calcitriol production and calcium reabsorption by the kidney. Calcium absorption increases as 25(OH) vitamin D concentrations increase until 29 to 32 ng/mL (72–80 nmol/L) when the effect plateaus; this observation provides the rationale for the cutoff point for vitamin D sufficiency at around 30 ng/mL (75 nmol/L).[22,27] Sometimes the increased fractional calcium absorption is insufficient to maintain normal serum calcium, and thus bone resorption is needed for correction. Together, PTH and calcitriol increase osteoclast activity, thereby releasing calcium from bone to restore calcium homeostasis.

TABLE 99-1	Risk Factors for Osteoporosis and Osteoporotic Fractures[2,3,28]

Low bone mineral density[a]
Female sex[a]
Advanced age[a]
Race/ethnicity[a]
History of a previous low-trauma (fragility) fracture as an adult[a]
Osteoporotic fracture in a first-degree relative (especially parental hip fracture[a])
Low body weight or body mass index[a]
Premature menopause (before 45 years old)[b]
Secondary osteoporosis[b] (especially rheumatoid arthritis[a])
Past or present systemic oral glucocorticoid therapy[a]
Current cigarette smoking[a]
Alcohol intake of three or more drinks per day[a]
Low calcium intake
Low physical activity
Minimal sun exposure
Poor health/frailty
Recent falls
Cognitive impairment
Impaired vision

[a]Factors included in the World Health Organization fracture risk assessment tool (FRAX).
[b]Secondary causes included in the FRAX tool question are diabetes type 1, osteogenesis imperfecta as an adult, long-standing untreated hyperthyroidism, hypogonadism, premature menopause (before 45 years of age), chronic malnutrition, malabsorption, and chronic liver disease.

ETIOLOGY

❶ Figure 99–1 depicts a model describing the etiology of osteoporosis and fractures. Table 99–1[2,3,28] lists risk factors for osteoporosis, and Tables 99–2[2,5,29,30] and 99–3[31,32] list secondary causes of this condition.

LOW BONE DENSITY

BMD is a major predictor of fracture risk. Every standard deviation decrease in BMD in women represents a 10% to 12% decrease in bone mass and a 1.5- to 2.6-fold increase in fracture risk.[2] Low BMD can occur as a result of bone loss or failure to reach a normal peak bone mass.

Bone loss occurs when bone resorption exceeds bone formation, usually from high bone turnover; when the number or depth of bone resorption sites greatly exceeds the rate and ability of osteoblasts to form new bone. Women and men begin to lose a small amount of bone mass starting in the third to fourth decade of life as a consequence of a slight reduction in bone formation.[33] During perimenopause and for up to 4 years after menopause, women can experience an accelerated rate of bone loss because of the drop in circulating estrogen and subsequent increase in bone resorption.[2,20] The rate and duration of loss can vary greatly, with up to 2% to 5% of bone density lost per year, and can differ depending on the skeletal site measured. Seniors steadily lose bone mass at approximately 0.5% to 1.5% per year as a consequence of an accelerated rate of bone remodeling combined with reduced bone formation.[2,16]

The major factors (see Tables 99–1, 99–2, and 99–3) influencing bone losses are hormonal status, exercise, aging, nutrition, lifestyle, disease states, medications, and some genetic influences. Nonhormonal risk factors are similar between women and men.

IMPAIRED BONE QUALITY

In addition to BMD, the strength of bone is highly affected by the quality of the bone's material properties and its structure.[33] For example, accelerated bone turnover can result in bone loss but can also impair bone quality and the structural integrity of bone by

TABLE 99-2 Select Medical Conditions Associated with Osteoporosis in Children and Adults[2,5,29,30]

Endocrine/hormonal
Primary or secondary ovarian failure
Testosterone deficiency
Hyperthyroidism
Cushing's disease
Growth hormone deficiency (in children)
Primary hyperparathyroidism
Type 1 diabetes

Gastrointestinal
Nutritional disorders (e.g., anorexia nervosa)
Malabsorptive states (chronic pancreatitis)
Crohn's or celiac disease
Chronic liver disease (e.g., primary biliary cirrhosis)
Gastrectomy or Billroth I

Inflammatory disorders
Rheumatoid arthritis
Ankylosing spondylitis

Chronic illness
Cystic fibrosis (malabsorption)
Chronic kidney disease
Malignancies (multiple myeloma, lymphoma, leukemia)
Human immunodeficiency virus infection/acquired immunodeficiency syndrome
Organ transplant

Disuse/immobility
Muscular dystrophy
Chronic obstructive pulmonary disease
Multiple sclerosis
Stroke/cerebrovascular accident

Genetic
Osteogenesis imperfecta
Turner syndrome
Down syndrome
Marfan syndrome
Klinefelter's syndrome
Cystic fibrosis
Hemochromatosis
Hyphophosphatasia

increasing the quantity of immature bone that is not yet adequately mineralized. Also, bone loss resulting in thinning of trabeculae—as seen in men with aging—is less damaging to the quality of bone structure compared with bone loss that results in damage to trabecular crosslinks, which results in decreased bone strength/quality, as seen in women.[34] Bone quality assessment is important because changes in bone quality affect bone strength much more than bone mass changes. Future osteoporosis diagnostic testing will assess both bone quality and density.

FALLS

Although up to 50% of vertebral fractures can occur spontaneously with minimal to no trauma, most wrist fractures and greater than 90% of hip fractures result from a fall from standing height or less.[2] One third to one half of all seniors fall each year, and 50% fall more than once. Up to 5% of all falls will result in a fracture. According to 2006 statistics, 2.1 million seniors were treated in the emergency department and 600,000 hospitalized for fall-related injuries, incurring costs of about $20 billion.[35] Close to 17,000 seniors died in 2006 due to a fall-related injury.[36]

PATHOPHYSIOLOGY

Osteoporosis pathophysiology depends on sex, age, genetics,[18] and presence of secondary causes.

POSTMENOPAUSAL OSTEOPOROSIS

The accelerated bone loss during perimenopause and postmenopause results from enhanced resorption, mainly as a result of the loss in ovarian hormone production, specifically estrogen. Estrogen deficiency increases proliferation, differentiation, and activation of new osteoclasts and prolongs survival of mature osteoclasts.[12,19] Interleukins, prostaglandin E_2, tumor necrosis factor α, and interferon γ also increase, resulting in more RANKL and less OPG. Loss of estrogen also increases calcium excretion and decreases

TABLE 99-3 Selected Medications Associated with Increased Bone Loss and/or Fracture Risk[31,32]

Medications	Comments
AIDS/HIV medications	
Nucleoside reverse transcriptase inhibitors (antiretroviral therapy, ART) (zidovudine, didanosine, lamivudine)	↓ BMD (ART > PI), no fracture data; increased osteoclast activity and decreased osteoblast activity
Protease inhibitors (PI) (nelfinavir, indinivir, saquinavir, ritonavir, lopinavir)	
Anticonvulsant therapy (phenytoin, carbamazepine, phenobarbital, valproic acid)	↓ BMD and ↑ fracture risk; increased vitamin D metabolism leading to low 25(OH) vitamin D concentrations
Aromatase inhibitors (e.g., letrozole, anastrozole)	↓ BMD and ↑ fracture risk; reduced estrogen concentrations
Furosemide	↑ fracture risk; increased calcium renal elimination
Glucocorticoids (long-term oral therapy)	↓ BMD and ↑ fracture risk; dose and duration dependent; see special populations section
Gonadotropin-releasing hormone (GnRH) agonists or analogs (e.g., leuprolide, goserelin)	↓ BMD and ↑ fracture risk; decreased sex hormone production
Heparin (unfractionated, UFH) or low molecular weight heparin (LMWH)	↓ BMD and ↑ fracture risk (UFH >>> LMWH) with long-term use (e.g., >6 mo); decreased osteoblast function and increased osteoclast function
Medroxyprogesterone acetate depot administration (DMPA)	↓ BMD, no fracture data; possible BMD recovery with discontinuation; central DXA monitoring of BMD recommended with ≥2 years of use; decreased estrogen concentrations
Proton pump inhibitor therapy (long-term therapy)	↑ vertebral and hip fracture risk; possible calcium malabsorption secondary to acid suppression for carbonate salts
Selective serotonin reuptake inhibitors	↑ hip fracture risk; decreased osteoblast activity
Thiazolidinediones (TZDs) (pioglitazone, rosiglitazone)	↓ BMD and ↑ fracture risk; risk may be greater in women than men; decreased osteoblast function
Thyroid—excessive supplementation	↓ BMD and ↑ fracture risk (> in men); risk increases with TSH concentration <0.1 µIU/mL (<0.1 mIU/L); possible increase in bone resorption
Vitamin A—excessive intake (≥1.5 mg of retinol form)	↓ BMD and ↑ fracture risk; decreased osteoblast activity and increased osteoclast activity

BMD, bone mineral density; TSH, thyroid-stimulating hormone; DXA, dual-energy x-ray absorptiometry.

calcium gut absorption. The number of remodeling sites increases, and resorption pits are deeper and inadequately filled by normal osteoblastic function. Significant bone density is lost and bone architecture is compromised. Trabecular bone is most susceptible, leading to vertebral and wrist fractures.

MALE OSTEOPOROSIS

❸ Bone physiology of men is under both estrogen and androgen control and influenced by similar hormones and cytokines as female bone.[12] Men are at a lower risk for developing osteoporosis and osteoporotic fractures because of larger bone size, greater peak bone mass, increase in bone width with aging, and fewer falls.[34,37] Men also do not undergo a period of accelerated bone resorption similar to menopause. However, men have a higher mortality rate after fractures.

The etiology of male osteoporosis tends to be multifactorial with secondary causes (see Tables 99–2 and 99–3) and aging being the most common contributing factors.[6,37] In young and middle-age men, a secondary cause for bone loss is usually identified, with hypogonadism being the most common. Idiopathic osteoporosis (no known cause) can occur.

AGE-RELATED OSTEOPOROSIS

Age-related osteoporosis occurs in seniors, mainly as a result of hormone, calcium, and vitamin D deficiencies leading to an accelerated bone turnover rate in combination with reduced osteoblast bone formation.[16] Hip fracture risk rises dramatically in seniors as a consequence of the cumulative loss of cortical and trabecular bone and an increased risk for falls.

SECONDARY CAUSES OF OSTEOPOROSIS

❶ A secondary cause (see Tables 99–2 and 99–3) is identified in more than half of premenopausal and perimenopausal women, about one third of postmenopausal women, and more than two thirds of men.[2,6,29–31] The most common secondary cause for osteoporosis is glucocorticoid therapy, which is discussed later in the Glucocorticoid-Induced Osteoporosis section.

CLINICAL PRESENTATION

Table 99–4 outlines the clinical presentation of osteoporosis.

Osteoporosis is diagnosed by BMD measurement or presence of a fragility (i.e., low trauma) fracture. Two thirds of patients with a vertebral fracture are asymptomatic or attribute mild lower back pain to "old age." The other third present with moderate to severe back pain that radiates down their leg after a new vertebral fracture. The pain usually subsides significantly after 2 to 4 weeks; however, residual chronic lower back pain may persist. Multiple vertebral fractures decrease height and sometimes curve the spine (kyphosis or lordosis) with or without significant back pain. Patients who have experienced a nonvertebral fracture frequently present with severe pain, swelling, and reduced function and mobility at the fracture site.

CONSEQUENCES OF OSTEOPOROSIS

A fragility fracture is defined as one that occurs as a result of a fall from standing height or less or with minimal to no trauma. Fractures of the vertebrae, hip, forearm, or humerus are considered major osteoporotic fractures.[28] Fractures of the face, skull, fingers, and toes are typically not considered osteoporosis-related. Osteoporotic fractures can lead to increased morbidity and mortality

TABLE 99–4	Clinical Presentation of Osteoporosis

General
- Many patients are unaware they have osteoporosis and present only after fracture
- Fractures can occur after bending, lifting, or falling, or independently of any activity

Symptoms
- Pain
- Immobility
- Depression, fear, and low self-esteem from physical limitations and deformities
- Two thirds of vertebral fractures are asymptomatic

Signs
- Shortened stature (loss of more than 1.5 inches [3.8 cm]), kyphosis, or lordosis
- Vertebral, hip, wrist, or forearm fracture
- Low bone density on radiography

Laboratory tests
- Routine tests to detect a possible secondary cause: complete blood count, creatinine, calcium, phosphorous, alkaline phosphatase, albumin, and thyroid-stimulating hormone. Free testosterone, 25(OH) vitamin D, and 24-hour urine concentrations of calcium and phosphorous are frequently assessed
- Urine or serum biomarkers (e.g., NTX, osteocalcin) are sometimes used, especially to determine if high bone turnover exists
- Additional testing might be necessary if the patient's history, physical examination, or the initial laboratory or diagnostic tests suggest a specific secondary cause

Other diagnostic tests
- Spine and hip bone density measurement using dual-energy x-ray absorptiometry (DXA)
- Vertebral fracture assessment (VFA) with DXA technology
- Radiograph (routine lateral thoracolumbar x-ray) to confirm vertebral fracture

NTX, N-terminal crosslinking telopeptide of type 1 collagen.

and decreased quality of life. Depression is common because of fear, pain, loss of self-esteem from physical deformity, and loss of independence and mobility.

Symptomatic vertebral fractures can cause significant pain, physical deformity, and adverse health consequences. Patients with severe kyphosis can experience respiratory problems as a result of compression of the thoracic region and gastrointestinal complications, such as poor nutrition, from intraabdominal compression. Women and men who suffer a symptomatic vertebral fracture have a lower survival rate compared with those without a fracture history.[3]

Wrist fractures occur more commonly in younger postmenopausal women and are frequently a result of a fall on an outstretched hand. Negative outcomes include prolonged pain and weakness, and decreased advanced (instrumental) activities of daily living (such as cooking and shopping).

Hip fractures are associated with the greatest increase in morbidity and mortality. In 2006, hip fractures resulted in approximately 330,000 hospital admissions.[38] Nearly 90% of these were in seniors. After a hip fracture, only 50% of patients regain their ability to perform basic activities of daily living, while 20% become nonambulatory.[39,40] Overall, 3% to 54% of patients die during the initial hospitalization for hip fracture, and 14% to 36% die within 1 year either from complications of the hip fracture or other comorbid disease processes. Men have a twofold higher 1-year mortality rate after hip fracture than women.

Once a low-trauma fracture has occurred, the risk for subsequent fractures goes up exponentially. In subjects with one clinical vertebral fracture, the chance of experiencing any new fracture was 2.8-fold higher, and with two or more vertebral fractures it was 12-fold higher, than for subjects who did not have baseline fractures.[41]

PATIENT ASSESSMENT

Bone pain, postural changes (i.e., kyphosis), and loss of height are simple useful physical examination findings. A height loss greater than 1.5 inches (3.8 cm) from the tallest mature height is considered significant and warrants further investigation. Height should be routinely measured using a wall-mounted stadiometer. Proper technique is essential, as can be seen at the National Institutes of Health Web site.[42] A spine radiograph can be obtained to confirm the presence of vertebral fractures. Low bone density or osteopenia reported on routine radiographs is a sign of significant bone loss and requires further evaluation for osteoporosis. In addition to physical examination and laboratory studies (see Table 99–4), patients can be assessed with risk factor assessments, osteoporosis questionnaires, peripheral and central dual-energy x-ray absorptiometry (DXA), and biomarkers.[5]

RISK FACTOR ASSESSMENT

❹ The aim of an initial osteoporosis risk assessment (see Table 99–1) is to identify those patients who are at highest risk for low bone density and who would benefit from further evaluation. Many risk factors for osteoporosis have been identified and are similar for both sexes. The majority of risk factors are predictors of either low BMD (e.g., female sex, ethnicity) or an increased fracture/fall risk (e.g., cognitive impairment, previous falls). The most important risk factors are those associated with fracture risk independent of BMD and fall risk. These major risk factors, in combination with BMD, are used to determine which patients are at greatest risk for fracturing and would benefit most from pharmacologic intervention.

A fracture prediction model used for treatment risk stratification was developed by the World Health Organization (WHO).[5,28,43] The WHO model for the United States uses the following risk factors: age, race/ethnicity, sex, previous fragility fracture, parent history of hip fracture, body mass index, glucocorticoid use (ever), current smoking, alcohol use of three or more drinks per day, rheumatoid arthritis, and select secondary causes with femoral neck BMD data optional to predict an individual's percent probability of fracturing in the next 10 years. Other osteoporosis risk assessment tools exist but are usually just used in research versus patient care.[5]

SCREENING USING PERIPHERAL BONE MINERAL DENSITY DEVICES

Peripheral bone density devices that utilize x-ray absorptiometry or quantitative ultrasonometry are helpful as screening tools to determine which patients require further evaluation with central DXA.[44] They should not be used for diagnosis or for monitoring response to therapy. Peripheral DXA of the forearm, heel, and finger uses a low amount of radiation. Heel quantitative ultrasonometry uses sound waves without radiation or need for specialty training.

Because peripheral devices are considerably less expensive than central DXA, easy to use, portable, fast (<5 minutes), and can predict general fracture risk, they are very popular for screening patients at health fairs, community pharmacies, and clinics. No guidelines specifically address who should undergo peripheral bone density screening.[45] However, the best population to screen is younger postmenopausal women without major risk factors for osteoporosis because a low peripheral BMD value in this population would support the need for further testing. The specific peripheral T-score threshold for referral is not universally defined and varies by device.[46] Healthy premenopausal women and patients already identified as being at high risk for osteoporosis based on risk factors, fragility fracture, or secondary causes for osteoporosis, should not be screened but rather referred to a physician for central DXA testing.

CENTRAL DUAL-ENERGY X-RAY ABSORPTIOMETRY

❹ BMD measurements at the hip or spine can be used to assess fracture risk, establish the diagnosis and severity of osteoporosis, and sometimes confirm osteoporosis as causative for low-trauma fractures.[2,5,44] Central DXA is considered the gold standard for measuring BMD because of its high precision, short scan times, low radiation dose (comparable to the average daily dose from natural background), and stable calibration. Measurement of lumbar spine, proximal femur, and total hip BMD is recommended with the lowest BMD value used for diagnosis. Newer methods, such as micromagnetic resonance imaging, are undergoing investigation to provide measurements of bone quality in addition to bone density.[44]

Several consensus guidelines or position statements are available that discuss which patients should undergo central DXA testing.[2,3,5,46] Most are consistent in recommending central BMD testing for all women aged 65 years or older, men aged 70 years or older, postmenopausal women younger than 65 years of age and men 50 to 69 years old with risk factors for fracture, and patients with an identified secondary cause for bone loss. Patients with a fragility fracture do not need a DXA for an osteoporosis diagnosis, but the results are helpful for determining the severity of osteoporosis and as a baseline for monitoring response to therapy. The DXA results can also help patients make decisions about the need for lifestyle changes and prescription osteoporosis medications. In the absence of a suspected or known secondary cause for osteoporosis or a history of a low-trauma fracture, central BMD testing is not recommended for children, premenopausal women, or men under 50 years of age.

A central DXA BMD report provides the actual bone density value, T-score, and Z-score. The actual bone density value (g/cm^2) is most useful for serial monitoring of therapy response, which is typically performed 1 to 2 years after medication initiation. The T-score is used for diagnosis and is a comparison of the patient's measured BMD to the mean BMD of a healthy, young (20- to 29-year-old), sex-matched white reference population. The T-score is the number of standard deviations from the mean of the reference population. Ethnic-specific reference databases are not recommended at this time. The Z-score is similar but compares the patient's BMD to the mean BMD for a healthy sex- and age-matched population. Patient-reported ethnicity should be used for the Z-score if available. The Z-score is sometimes helpful in determining whether a secondary cause for osteoporosis is present and is used for diagnosis in children, premenopausal women, and men younger than 50 years of age.

Using the spine DXA image, an assessment of morphometric vertebral fractures, the vertebral fracture assessment (VFA), can be calculated.[47] Initially a research tool, this analysis of T4 to L4 vertebrae after a DXA is increasing in utilization, especially for seniors. Each vertebra is assessed for compression (wedge, biconcave, and crush) and described as normal or mild, moderate, and severe compression. This result becomes important for treatment decisions in patients with low bone mass

LABORATORY TESTS

Laboratory testing (see Table 99–4) is used to identify secondary causes of bone loss. If a preliminary investigation indicates a possible secondary cause, additional testing might be needed.

❷ Serum 25(OH) vitamin D is the best indicator of total body vitamin D status. Data suggest that serum 25(OH) vitamin D concentrations of at least 75 nmol/L or 30 ng/mL (1 ng/mL = 2.5 nmol/L) are necessary to maximize intestinal calcium absorption, minimize secondary hyperparathyroidism, and reduce fracture risk.[21,22] Although still highly debated, most experts believe that the goal 25(OH) vitamin D concentration should be 30 to 100 ng/mL (75–250 nmol/L); concentrations between 20 and 29 ng/mL (50–72 nmol/L) are insufficient for optimal health, and concentrations below 20 ng/mL (50 nmol/L) would constitute deficiency.[48,49] Osteomalacia or severe vitamin D deficiency, which is discussed later under the Other Metabolic Bone Disorders section, can occur at concentrations less than 10 ng/mL (25 nmol/L).[50]

Because vitamin D assays are fairly expensive and large interlab assay variability exists, routine vitamin D screening cannot be recommended at this time. However, a 25(OH) vitamin D concentration should be considered in anyone at higher risk for low vitamin D (e.g., seniors, patients who are obese or who have minimal sun exposure, insufficient vitamin D intake, dark pigmented skin, or certain medical conditions, or are on medications known to affect vitamin D metabolism), and patients with low bone density, history of a low-trauma fracture or frequent falls, or history of unexplained muscle weakness and/or bone pain.

BONE TURNOVER MARKERS

Urine and serum bone turnover markers are either enzymes or proteins produced during bone formation or breakdown.[51,52] Bone-specific alkaline phosphatase, osteocalcin, and procollagen type 1 propeptides are examples of bone formation markers. Hydroxypyridinium crosslinks of collagen pyridinoline and deoxy-pyridinoline, C-terminal crosslinking telopeptide of type 1 collagen, and N-terminal crosslinking telopeptide of type 1 collagen are examples of bone resorption markers. Increased concentrations of bone resorption markers (≥ 2 standard deviations above the premenopausal range) have been shown in some studies to predict fracture risk; however, results have been inconsistent. Although not diagnostic, these tests might be helpful in identifying accelerated bone turnover and increased fracture risk or in monitoring response to therapy.

DIAGNOSIS OF OSTEOPOROSIS

The diagnosis of osteoporosis is based on a low-trauma fracture or central hip and/or spine DXA using WHO T-score thresholds. Osteopenia or low bone mass is a T-score between −1 and −2.5, and osteoporosis is a T-score at or below −2.5.[2,3,5,46] Although these definitions are based on data from postmenopausal white women, they are applied to perimenopausal women, men age 50 years and older, and other race/ethnic groups. The diagnosis of osteoporosis in children, premenopausal women, and men under 50 years of age should be based on a Z-score at or below −2.0 in combination with other risk factors or fracture.[46]

PREVENTION AND TREATMENT

Osteoporosis

The foundation for osteoporosis prevention and treatment is a bone healthy lifestyle beginning at birth and continuing throughout life. Supplements and medications are used when lifestyle habits are suboptimal and/or osteoporosis has developed.

DESIRED OUTCOMES

The primary goal of osteoporosis management should be prevention. Optimizing skeletal development and peak bone mass accrual in childhood, adolescence, and early adulthood will ultimately reduce the future incidence of osteoporosis. Once low bone mass or osteoporosis develops, the objective is to stabilize or improve bone mass and strength and prevent fractures. In patients who have already suffered osteoporotic fractures, reducing pain and deformity, improving functional capacity, improving quality of life, and reducing future falls and fractures are the main goals.

GENERAL APPROACH TO PREVENTION AND TREATMENT

⑤ A bone-healthy lifestyle should begin at birth and continue throughout life. Insuring adequate intakes of calcium and vitamin D along with other bone-healthy lifestyle practices are the first steps in prevention and treatment. Recent guidelines/position statements recommend considering prescription therapy in any postmenopausal woman or man age 50 years and older presenting with one of the following scenarios: a hip or vertebral fracture; T-score of −2.5 or lower; or low bone mass (T-score between −1.0 and −2.5) with a secondary cause associated with a high risk for fracture, a history of prior fracture, a 10-year probability of hip fracture of 3% or more, or a 10-year probability of any major osteoporosis-related fracture of 20% or more.[2,3] Figure 99–3 provides an osteoporosis management algorithm for postmenopausal women and men 50 years and older that incorporates both nonpharmacologic and pharmacologic approaches.

NONPHARMACOLOGIC THERAPY

④ Nonpharmacologic therapy, referred to as a bone-healthy lifestyle, includes a nutritious diet, smoking cessation, minimal alcohol intake, exercise, and fall prevention. Consumers might opt for self-care and use the Internet for decisions about osteoporosis management, especially regarding options that are natural or available without a prescription. Since Internet information can be wrong or misleading,[53] consumers should discuss nonprescription medication choices with a healthcare professional.

Diet

Overall, a diet well balanced in nutrients and minerals and limited in alcohol, caffeine, and carbonated cola beverages[54] is important for bone health.

Calcium ⑤ ⑥ Data clearly indicate that adequate calcium intake is necessary for the development of bone mass during growth and for its maintenance throughout life.[2,55] Adequate calcium intake is an essential component of all osteoporosis prevention and treatment strategies.

Table 99–5 summarizes the recommended intakes for calcium based on age.[56–59] Achieving daily calcium requirements from calcium-containing foods,[57,60] which also contain other essential nutrients, is preferred. Milk and other dairy products have the highest amount of calcium per serving and are available in low-fat options. Some food sources are absorbed well but have low elemental calcium content (e.g., broccoli). Other foods contain oxalic acid (e.g., spinach) or phytic acid (e.g., wheat bran) that bind calcium contained in the food, decreasing its absorption.[57] For example, to get the same amount of calcium in one 8-ounce (~240 mL) glass of milk, one would need to eat 2.25 cups (~530 mL) of cooked broccoli or 8 cups (~1900 mL) of cooked spinach.

People should be encouraged to evaluate their food and beverage intake to determine if they are receiving adequate intakes.

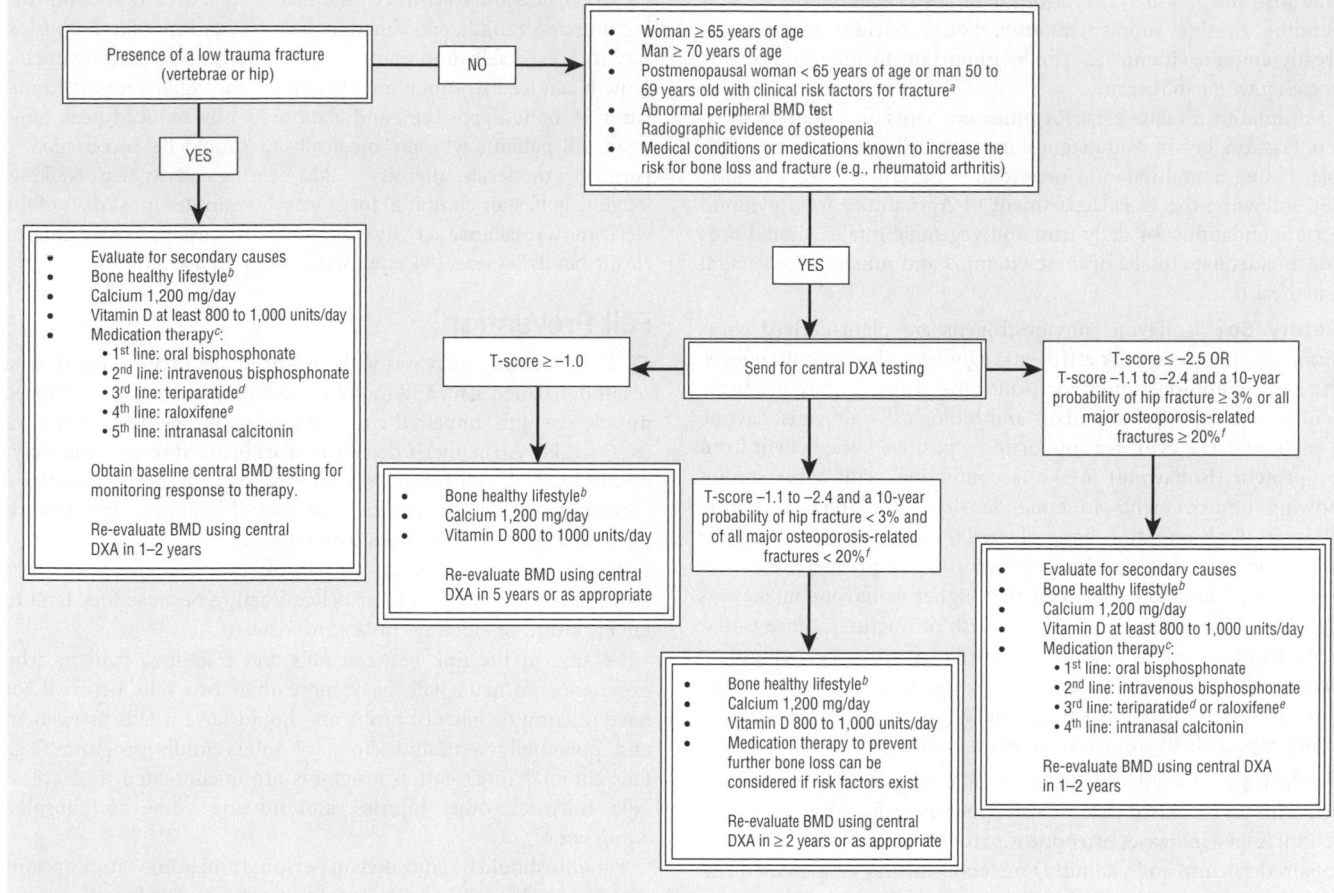

FIGURE 99-3. Algorithm for the management of osteoporosis in postmenopausal women and men aged 50 and older.[2,3]

To calculate the amount of calcium in a serving of food, consumers can add a zero to the percentage of the daily value listed on food labels. For example, a serving of milk (8 oz. [~240 mL]) has 30% of the daily value of calcium. This translates to 300 mg calcium per serving.

Approximately 25% of the U.S. population has some level of lactose intolerance, with the incidence in Asian (80%) and African American (50%) populations being much higher than in whites (10%).[57] Lactose-intolerant patients have several options, including products containing lactase (Lactaid), lactose-reduced milk, lactose-free milk, calcium-fortified soy milk, certain aged cheeses, or yogurt with active cultures along with other nondairy calcium-fortified products (e.g., orange juice, breakfast cereals, and energy bars).

Vitamin D ⑤ ⑥ Table 99–5 lists the recommended adequate intakes for Vitamin D.[3,56,58] The three main sources of vitamin D are sunlight, diet, and supplements. Websites can be used to identify the few foods high in vitamin D.[61] To calculate the amount of vitamin D in a serving of food, multiply the % daily value of vitamin D listed on the food label by 4 (e.g., 20% vitamin D = 80 units). Because few foods are naturally high or fortified with vitamin D, most people, especially seniors, require supplementation.

Other Nutrients and Minerals Vitamin K is a cofactor for carboxylation (activation) of proteins, such as osteocalcin, which are involved in bone formation. Several studies have demonstrated that vitamin K deficiency can contribute to bone loss and an increased risk for fractures.[62,63] Studies evaluating the benefits of vitamin K supplementation are conflicting, with some demonstrating reduced

TABLE 99-5	Calcium and Vitamin D Recommended Daily Intakes[56–59]	
Group and Ages	**Elemental Calcium (mg)[a,b]**	**Vitamin D (units)[b]**
Infants		
Birth to 6 months	210	400[c]
6–12 months	270	400[c]
Children/Adolescents		
1–3 years	500	400[c]
4–8 years	800	400[c]
9–18 years	1,300	400[c]
Adults		
19–49 years	1,000	400 – 800[d]
≥50 years	1,200	800 – 1,000[d]

[a]Recommendations from the U.S. Institute of Medicine of the National Academy of Sciences. Most experts feel the vitamin D dose for 19–49 years old is too low. New Institute of Medicine recommendations were due in 2010 after this chapter was prepared.
[b]U.S. Institute of Medicine of the National Academies recommends not to exceed more than 2,500 mg/day elemental calcium or 2,000 units/day of vitamin D (controversial).[56]
[c]2008 recommendations from the American Academy of Pediatrics.[58]
[d]2008 recommendations from the National Osteoporosis Foundation.[59]

bone loss and fracture risk. More data are needed before recommending routine supplementation. Some calcium supplements already contain vitamin K. This is important to note for patients receiving warfarin therapy.

Minimal to no data exist for other nutrients and minerals such as potassium, boron, and magnesium.[55,64] Until more data are available, taking a multivitamin once daily and consuming a healthy diet, following the U.S. Department of Agriculture food pyramid recommendations for daily fruit and vegetable intake, should provide an adequate intake of these vitamins and minerals for general bone health.

Dietary Soy Isoflavone phytoestrogens are plant-derived compounds that possess weak estrogenic agonist and antagonist effects. The most common source for isoflavone is dietary soy products. Genistein is the most abundant and biologically active isoflavone in soybeans. The evidence supporting a positive bone benefit from soy protein (isoflavone) intake is conflicting, with some studies showing improvements in bone density with larger isoflavone intakes.[2,65] Only one study has evaluated the association between soy intake and fracture risk. This population-based prospective cohort study from China demonstrated that higher isoflavone intake was associated with a significantly lower risk of fractures. Since isoflavones from soy foods appear safe, patients can be encouraged to increase their intake, but true benefits on fracture are not clear. More information is needed on the safety of isoflavone supplements, especially in women with breast cancer.

Alcohol ❺ Alcohol consumption in moderation is not associated with an increased risk for osteoporosis or fractures. Excessive alcohol intake increases osteoporosis risk because of poor nutrition, impaired calcium and vitamin D metabolism, and an increased risk for falls.[2] According to 2005 dietary guidelines, alcohol consumption should not exceed one drink per day for women and two drinks per day for men.[66]

Caffeine ❺ Although results are conflicting, excessive caffeine consumption is associated with increased calcium excretion, increased rates of bone loss, and a modestly increased risk for fracture.[67] Ideally, caffeine consumption should be limited to two servings or less per day. Moderate caffeine intake (two to four servings per day) should not be a concern if adequate calcium intake is achieved daily.

Carbonated Beverages ❺ Consumption of cola beverages, even without caffeine, is associated with decreased BMD and increased fracture risk; however, data are conflicting.[54] The phosphoric acid content of cola beverages is thought to contribute to bone loss by altering calcium balance. This effect is compounded by decreased milk consumption and consequent reductions in calcium intake with the increase in carbonated beverage intake seen in the United States.[55]

Smoking Cessation

❺ Counseling patients of all ages on smoking cessation can help to optimize peak bone mass, minimize bone loss, and ultimately reduce fracture risk. Cigarette smoking is an independent risk factor for osteoporosis and is associated with up to an 80% increased relative risk for hip fracture.[2,68] The effect is dose and duration dependent. A decrease in sex hormone concentrations, reduced intestinal calcium absorption, a direct toxic effect on osteoblasts, and detrimental effects of smoking on neurovascular function have been implicated for the negative bone effects.

Exercise

❺ Physical activity or exercise is an important nonpharmacologic approach to preventing osteoporotic fractures. Exercise can decrease the risk of falls and fractures by stabilizing bone density and improving muscle strength, coordination, balance, and mobility.[2] Physical activity is especially important early in life as lack of exercise during growth can lead to suboptimal loading/straining, decreased stimulation of bone deposition, and a subsequently reduced peak bone mass. All patients who are medically fit should be encouraged to perform a moderate-intensity weight-bearing activity (e.g., walking, jogging, golf, stair climbing) for at least 30 minutes most days of the week and a resistance activity (e.g., weight machines, free weights, or elastic bands) at least twice per week for 20 to 30 minutes.[3]

Fall Prevention

❺ Risk of falling increases with advanced age predominantly as a result of balance, gait, and mobility problems, poor vision, reduced muscle strength, impaired cognition, multiple medical conditions (e.g., stroke, Alzheimer's dementia, Parkinson disease), and polypharmacy.[2,69] Psychoactive medications such as benzodiazepines, antidepressants, antipsychotics, sedative–hypnotics, and opioids have been strongly associated with falls.

The ability to adapt to falls also decreases with aging. Seniors are more likely to sustain a hip or pelvic fracture because they tend to fall backward or sideways instead of forward.

Because of the link between falls and fractures, patients who experience an acute fall, have more than two falls per year, or have walking or balance problems should have a falls assessment and potentially a multidisciplinary intervention program (e.g., falls clinic).[69] Intervention programs are documented to decrease falls, fractures, other injuries, and nursing home and hospital admissions.[70]

Patients should be educated on personal and home safety options to decrease falls.[2,69] Websites provide great patient education materials with solutions for commonly observed safety problems.[71–73] Medication profiles should also be reviewed for any unnecessary medications that can affect cognition and balance and potentially increase fall risk. Consideration should be given to replacing high-risk medications with safer alternatives. Adequate vitamin D intake has been associated with reduced falls.[74,75] Maintenance of a regular individualized exercise program, such as tai chi, should be recommended to improve body strength, balance, and agility.

Other recommendations include resolving vision, blood pressure, heart rate/rhythm, and foot problems and using proper footwear.

External hip protectors are specialized undergarments designed to pad the area surrounding the hip, decreasing the force of impact from a sideways fall. Conflicting results and poor adherence limit their use.[2]

■ PHARMACOLOGIC THERAPY

Because nonpharmacologic interventions alone are frequently insufficient to prevent or treat osteoporosis, medication therapy is often necessary. Table 99–6[2,3,5,76] describes fracture and BMD effects, and Table 99–7 describes important aspects of common osteoporosis medications. These medications should always be combined with a bone-healthy lifestyle.

■ MEDICATION

Treatments of First Choice

Combined with adequate calcium and vitamin D intakes, bisphosphonates are the prescription medication of choice, with teriparatide, denosumab, raloxifene, and calcitonin considered alternative agents.[2,3] Duration of bisphosphonate therapy has not been defined, but safety data exist for periods of 7 to 10 years. Short-term (18–24 months) teriparatide is usually reserved for

TABLE 99-6 Fracture and Bone Mineral Density Effects of Antiosteoporosis Medications from Pivotal Fracture Trials in Postmenopausal Women[a,3,5,76]

Medication	Vertebral Fracture	Nonvertebral Fracture	Hip Fracture	% Change in Spine BMD[b]	% Change in Hip BMD[b,c]
Bisphosphonates	41%–70% ↓	25%–39% ↓[d]	40%–51% ↓[e]	4.3–6.7% ↑	2.8–6.0% ↑
Calcitonin	33% ↓	↔	↔	0.7% ↑ (NS)	↔
Denosumab	68% ↓	20% ↓	40% ↓	9.2% ↑	6.0% ↑
Estrogen with or without progestogen	33%–40% ↓	13%–27% ↓	34% ↓	3.5–7% ↑[f]	1.7–4.1% ↑[f]
Raloxifene	30% ↓	↔	↔	2.6% ↑	2.1% ↑
Teriparatide	65% ↓	53% ↓	↔	8.6% ↑	3.6% ↑

%, percent; BMD, bone mineral density; ↓, decrease; ↑, increase; ↔, no significant change; NS, not significant.
[a]No head to head fracture studies, clinical trials with different patient samples and study designs, data should only be used for relative between-class comparisons.
[b]Relative to placebo.
[c]Total hip (alendronate, ibandronate, zoledronic acid, denosumab, teriparatide) or femoral neck (risedronate, raloxifene).
[d]Risedronate and zoledronic acid only; nonvertebral fracture reductions with ibandronate and alendronate were not significant.
[e]Alendronate, risedronate, and zoledronic acid only; hip fracture data not reported with ibandronate.
[f]Data obtained from nonpivotal fracture trials.

TABLE 99-7 Medications Used to Prevent and Treat Osteoporosis

Drug	Adult Dosage	Pharmacokinetics	Adverse Effects	Drug Interactions
Antiresorption Medications				
Calcium	200–1,300 mg/day to achieve adequate intake (see Table 99-5); divided doses	Absorption—predominantly active transport with some passive diffusion; fractional absorption 10%–60%; calcium carbonate absorption improved if given with food; fecal elimination for the unabsorbed and renal elimination for the absorbed calcium	Constipation, gas, upset stomach, rare kidney stones; potential concern about doses >1,500 mg daily	• Carbonate products – decreased absorption with proton pump inhibitors • Decrease absorption of iron, tetracycline, quinolones, alendronate, risedronate, etidronate, phenytoin, and fluoride when given concomitantly • Antagonist of verapamil • Induce hypercalcemia with thiazide diuretics • Fiber laxatives, oxalates, phytates, and sulfates can decrease calcium absorption if given concomitantly
Vitamin D D₃ (cholecalciferol)	400–1,000 units/day to achieve adequate intake (see Table 99-5); if low 25(OH) vitamin D concentrations, malabsorption or multiple anticonvulsants might require higher doses (>2,000 units daily)	Hepatic metabolism to 25(OH) vitamin D and then renal metabolism to 1,25 (OH) vitamin D, the active moiety for bone effects; other active and inactive metabolites	Hypercalcemia, (weakness, headache, somnolence, nausea, cardiac rhythm disturbance), hypercalciuria	• Phenytoin, barbiturates, carbamazepine, rifampin increase vitamin D metabolism • Cholestyramine, colestipol, orlistat, or mineral oil decrease vitamin D absorption • May induce hypercalcemia with thiazide diuretics in hypoparathyroid patients
D₂ (ergocalciferol)	For vitamin D deficiency, 50,000 units once to twice weekly for 8–12 weeks; repeat as needed until therapeutic concentrations; occasionally 50,000 units monthly for maintenance			
1,25(OH) vitamin D (calcitriol, Rocaltrol po, Calcijex iv)	0.25–0.5 mcg orally or 1–2 mcg/mL intravenously daily for renal osteodystrophy, hypoparathyroidism, or refractory rickets			
Bisphosphonates Alendronate (generic, Fosamax)	5 mg daily, 35 mg weekly (prevention) 10 mg daily or 70 mg tablet, 70 mg tablet with vitamin D 2,800 or 5,600 units, or 75 mL liquid weekly (treatment)	Poorly absorbed (<1%), decreasing to zero with food or beverage intake; long bone t₁/₂ (2–10 years); renal elimination (of absorbed) and fecal elimination (unabsorbed)	Common: nausea/dyspepsia (oral); transient flu-like illness (injectables) Rare: GI perforation, ulceration, and/or bleeding (oral); musculoskeletal pain; osteonecrosis of the jaw; atypical fractures	• Do not coadminister with any other medication or supplements (including calcium and vitamin D)
Risedronate (Actonel)	5 mg daily, 35 mg weekly, 75 mg for 2 days monthly, 150 mg monthly			
Ibandronate (Boniva)	150 mg monthly, 3 mg intravenous quarterly			

(continued)

TABLE 99-7	Medications Used to Prevent and Treat Osteoporosis (continued)			
Drug	**Adult Dosage**	**Pharmacokinetics**	**Adverse Effects**	**Drug Interactions**
Antiresorption Medications				
Zoledronic acid (Reclast)	5 mg intravenous infusion yearly (treatment), 5 mg intravenous infusion every 2 year (prevention)			
Estrogen Agonist/Antagonist				
Raloxifene (Evista)	60 mg daily	Hepatic metabolism	Hot flushes, leg cramps, venous thromboembolism, peripheral edema, rare cataracts, and gallbladder disease; black-box warning for fatal stroke	None
Bazedoxifene[a] (Viviant, Conbriza)	20 or 40 mg daily			
Bazedoxifene with conjugated equine estrogens[a] (Aprela)	20 or 40 mg daily plus 0.45 or 0.625 mg daily			
Lasofoxifene (Fablyn)[a]	0.25–0.5 mg daily			
Calcitonin (Miacalcin)	200 units intranasally daily, alternating nares every other day	Renal elimination 3% nasal availability	Rhinitis, epistaxis	None
Denosumab (Prolia)	60 mcg subcutaneously every 6 months	T_{max} = 10 days, $t_{1/2}$ = 25.4 days	Back, extremity, and musculoskeletal pain; hypercholesterolemia, cystitis, serious infection, skin problems, osteonecrosis of the jaw, and bone turnover suppression	None
Formation Medications				
Teriparatide (PTH 1–34 units) (Forteo)	20 mcg subcutaneously daily for up to 2 years	95% bioavailability T_{max} ~30 minutes $t_{1/2}$ ~60 minutes Hepatic metabolism	Pain at injection site, nausea, headache, dizziness, leg cramps, rare increase in uric acid, slightly increased calcium	None

T_{max}, time to maximum concentration; $t_{1/2}$, half-life; GI, gastrointestinal; im, intramuscular
[a]Investigational product

severe osteoporosis and then followed by bisphosphonate therapy. The algorithm (see Fig. 99–3) helps determine for whom medication therapy should be used. Osteoporosis prescription medications in children, pre- and perimenopausal women, and men younger than 50 years old are controversial and undergoing further investigation.

Published Guidelines and Treatment Protocols

The 2008 National Osteoporosis Foundation's clinician's guide and the 2010 North American Menopause Society's position statement provide guidance on osteoporosis prevention and treatment strategies.[2,3] Some additional subspecialty guidelines exist (e.g., osteoporosis and gastrointestinal [GI] diseases[77]) but will not be covered here. Applying the National Osteoporosis Foundation's guidelines to a large clinical database, researchers found that about 72% of women ≥65 years old and 93% of women ≥75 years old would be eligible for treatment.[78] Even with guidelines and algorithms, many patients are not being evaluated nor receiving appropriate osteoporosis therapy, even after a hip fracture.[5]

Antiresorptive Therapies

Antiresorptive therapies include calcium, vitamin D, bisphosphonates, estrogen agonists antagonists (known previously as selective estrogen receptor modulators or SERMs), calcitonin, denosumab, estrogen, and testosterone.

Calcium Supplementation ⑤ ⑥ Calcium imbalance can result from inadequate dietary intake, decreased fractional calcium absorption, or enhanced calcium excretion. Adequate calcium intake (see Table 99–5) is considered the standard for osteoporosis prevention and treatment and should be combined with vitamin D and osteoporosis medications when needed.[56,57] Supplemental calcium intake will be needed in the majority of people with or at risk for osteoporosis as survey data indicate that the average U.S. female and male diet contains only 660 and 797 mg calcium per day, respectively.[2,57]

Efficacy. Although calcium increases BMD, fracture prevention is minimal. Almost all trials and observational studies showed the children and adults with the higher calcium intakes had greater increases or maintenance of BMD compared to BMD losses with placebo.[55] Calcium's BMD effects are less than other antiresorptive and formation osteoporosis medications. Fracture prevention is only documented with concomitant vitamin D therapy. Some data support other calcium benefits such as decreased blood pressure, cholesterol, and colorectal cancer risk.[79]

Adverse Events/Precautions. Calcium's most common adverse reaction, constipation, can first be treated with increased water intake, dietary fiber, and exercise. If still unresolved, smaller and more frequent administration or lower total daily dose can be tried. Calcium carbonate can create gas and cause stomach upset, which might resolve with calcium citrate, a product with fewer GI side effects. While the upper tolerable limit for calcium is 2,500 mg/day, consistently exceeding daily recommended intakes does not provide additional benefits and might increase certain patients' risk for heart disease.[80] Therefore, average daily calcium dietary intake needs to be known to calculate correct safe supplementatal dose.

Calcium rarely causes kidney stones. Some patients with a history of kidney stones can still ingest adequate amounts of calcium depending on the type of stones and/or will require increased fluid intake and decreased salt intake with their calcium supplementation.

Administration. Most children and adults of all ethnic backgrounds do not ingest sufficient dietary calcium and therefore require supplements. To ensure adequate calcium absorption, 25(OH) vitamin D concentrations should be maintained in the normal range (30 – 100 ng/mL [75 – 250 nmol/L]).[22] Because fractional calcium absorption is dose limited, maximum single doses of 500 to 600 mg or less of elemental calcium are recommended. Calcium carbonate is the salt of choice as it contains the highest amount of elemental calcium (40%) and is the least expensive. Calcium carbonate should be taken with meals to enhance absorption. Calcium citrate absorption (21% calcium) is acid-independent and need not be administered with meals. Although tricalcium phosphate contains 38% calcium, calcium-phosphate complexes could limit overall calcium absorption. This product might be helpful in patients with hypophosphatemia that cannot be resolved with increased dietary intake. Disintegration and dissolution rates vary significantly between products and lots. Products labeled "USP Verified" for "United States Pharmacopeia," which guarantees the identity, strength, purity, and quality of the product, should be recommended when possible. Oyster shell (other than the OsCal brand) or coral calcium should not be recommended because of concerns for high concentrations of lead and other heavy metals. Some calcium products come in alternative dosage forms (e.g., chews, dissolvable tablet, liquid), which can be beneficial for select patients (e.g., swallowing problems).

"Bone designer" nonprescription products continue to be developed by combining calcium and vitamin D with other nutrients, some of which are associated with bone physiology (e.g., magnesium, manganese, boron, vitamin K).[55,64] Newer products contain genistein, phytosterols, and aspirin. Minimal BMD and no fracture data exist for these combination products. Because product labeling is confusing, patients might not realize they need four to six tablets per day to obtain adequate calcium intakes. These products are also more expensive. Combining too many vitamins and supplements might lead to upper-tolerable nutrient limits being exceeded and a concern for toxicities.

Vitamin D Supplementation ❺ ❻ Vitamin D intake is critical for the prevention and treatment of osteoporosis because it maximizes intestinal calcium absorption. Given its safety, low cost, and other benefits of vitamin D, no patient should have an inadequate intake.

Efficacy. Data show that higher dose vitamin D supplementation is needed for fracture and fall prevention. Based on a meta-analysis, higher doses of vitamin D (>400 units daily) decreased nonvertebral and hip fractures by approximately 20%.[81] These results are consist with a previous meta-analysis showing doses of 700 to 800 units reduced fractures, but doses of 400 units per day did not.[82] Some but not all studies support vitamin D decreasing falls.[74,75] Conflicting results between studies are thought to be a result of differences in vitamin D dosing, concomitant calcium administration, adherence, and baseline vitamin D status of subjects.

Vitamin D has other potential nonskeletal benefits. Improvement in muscle strength and cardiovascular function, decreased cancer risk (e.g., breast, colon, and prostate cancers), and positive immunomodulatory effects (e.g., multiple sclerosis, type 1 diabetes, rheumatoid arthritis) have been proposed.[21]

Administration. Seniors and patients being treated for osteoporosis should take at minimum 800 to 1,000 units of vitamin D through food and supplementation with a goal to maintain their 25(OH) vitamin D concentration within the sufficient range (i.e., ≥30 ng/mL [≥ 75 nmol/L]).[2,3] Several experts believe higher doses (i.e., up to 4,000 units of vitamin D daily) should be recommended, especially in certain populations.[27] In one Canadian study, 1,000 units vitamin D daily only resulted in 35% of seniors in the therapeutic range (> 30 ng/mL [>75 nmol/L]), whereas 4,000 units per day resulted in 88% in the therapeutic range.[83] In another study, 3,800 units were required to achieve and maintain therapeutic ranges when patients' initial 25(OH) vitamin D concentration was at least 22 ng/mL [55 nmol/L]); 5,000 units were required for those with a 25(OH) vitamin D concentration less than 22 ng/mL (55 nmol/L).[84]

Whether cholecalciferol (vitamin D_3) is more efficient than ergocalciferol (vitamin D_2) at raising 25(OH) vitamin D concentrations is controversial, with data supporting both arguments.[22,85] Usual supplementation is with daily nonprescription cholecalciferol vitamin D products. However, higher-dose prescription ergocalciferol regimens administered weekly, monthly, or quarterly are used for replacement and maintenance therapy.[22] Approximately 100 units vitamin D_3 daily will raise the 25(OH) vitamin D concentration by 1 ng/mL (2.5 nmol/L). More than one multivitamin or large doses of cod liver oil daily are no longer advocated because of the risk of hypervitaminosis A, which can increase bone loss. Because the half-life of vitamin D is about 1 month, approximately 3 months of therapy are required before a new steady state is achieved and a repeat 25(OH) vitamin D concentration can be obtained.

Individuals with deficient concentrations of vitamin D are at risk for osteomalacia. Their management is discussed in Other Metabolic Bone Diseases later in the chapter. In patients with disorders affecting vitamin D absorption (e.g., celiac disease, cystic fibrosis, or Crohn's disease), higher doses and more frequent monitoring are required. In patients with severe hepatic or renal disease, the activated form of vitamin D (calcitriol) might be more appropriate. However, new information with regard to vitamin D's nonbone effects suggests replacement with both cholecalciferol and calcitriol might be needed.[21]

CLINICAL CONTROVERSY

Some experts believe that the upper tolerable limit for vitamin D should be raised and that the recommended daily allowance for vitamin D should be at least 2,000 units per day. In one study, up to 4,000 units vitamin D daily was needed for approximately 90% of the sample to maintain 25(OH) vitamin D concentrations at ≥30 ng/mL (≥75 nmol/L).[83,84] Some suggest daily doses less than 10,000 units would be safe.[21] The dietary reference intakes are currently being reevaluated by the Institute of Medicine of the National Academy of Sciences.

Bisphosphonates ❼ Bisphosphonates mimic pyrophosphate, an endogenous bone resorption inhibitor.[86] Bisphosphonate antiresorptive activity results from blocking prenylation and inhibiting guanosine triphosphatase-signaling proteins, which lead to decreased osteoclast maturation, number, recruitment, bone adhesion, and life span. Their various R2 side chains produce different bone binding, persistence, and affinities; however, the

resulting clinical significances are not known. All bisphosphonates become incorporated into bone, giving them long biologic half-lives of up to 10 years. Alendronate, risedronate, and intravenous zoledronic acid are FDA-indicated for postmenopausal, male, and glucocorticoid-induced osteoporosis (see Table 99–7). Intravenous and oral ibandronate are indicated only for postmenopausal osteoporosis.

Efficacy. Of the antiresorptive agents, bisphosphonates consistently provide some of the higher fracture risk reductions and BMD increases (see Table 99–6).[2,3,5,76,87] Fracture clinical trial data only exist for daily oral bisphosphonate and annual intravenous therapy, not weekly, monthly, or quarterly regimens. Although hip fracture reduction was not seen with daily oral ibandronate, the hip fracture incidence in the placebo group was low, suggesting the study might have been underpowered. Fracture reductions are demonstrated as early as 6 months, with the greatest fracture reduction seen in patients with lower initial BMD and in those with the greatest BMD changes with therapy. Although comparative fracture prevention trials do not exist, no differences between oral bisphosphonates and fractures were found based on claims data.[88] Annual intravenous zoledronic acid has documented both secondary fracture prevention and a decrease in mortality in the treated group.[89] Zoledronic acid has also been documented to decrease bone loss and fractures for patients receiving certain chemotherapy.[90]

BMD increases with bisphosphonates are dose dependent and greatest in the first 6 to 12 months of therapy. Small increases continue over time at the lumbar spine, but plateau after 2 to 5 years at the hip. After discontinuation, the increased BMD is sustained for a prolonged period of time that varies depending on the bisphosphonate used.[91] Weekly alendronate, weekly and monthly risedronate, and monthly oral and quarterly intravenous ibandronate therapy produce equivalent BMD changes to their respective daily regimens. Weekly alendronate therapy increases BMD more than weekly risedronate therapy[92]; however, no evidence indicates that this difference would equate to greater fracture efficacy. Weekly alendronate and monthly ibandronate produced similar BMD effects.[93]

The BMD increases with alendronate, risedronate, and zoledronic acid in men are similar to those in postmenopausal women.[37] Because of a lack of fracture data from pivotal trials in men, bisphosphonates are only FDA indicated to increase BMD, not to reduce fracture risk in men. Pooled analysis of risedronate studies did document fracture prevention in men, and alendronate has been shown to decrease radiographic but not clinical vertebral fractures.[94,95]

CLINICAL CONTROVERSY

Women without evidence of a low-trauma fracture and who have responded well to bisphosphonate therapy—for example, those with BMD increasing into the osteopenic range (e.g., T-score > –2)—are being considered for a "drug holiday."[91] Patients are taken off their bisphosphonate therapy and followed serially with bone turnover markers and central DXA BMD. The FLEX study demonstrated prolonged suppression of bone turnover and maintenance of BMD in selected postmenopausal women after 5 years off of alendronate therapy. Data with risedronate after 1 year of discontinuation indicated a continued fracture benefit despite significant increases in bone turnover markers and decreases in BMD.[2,91] No data about effects after discontinuation with the other bisphosphonates are available. Guidelines for the duration and monitoring of such a drug holiday and the impact of this practice on fracture risk are not yet available.

Adverse Events/Precautions. If oral bisphosphonates are prescribed correctly and the patient takes them correctly, their adverse effects are minimal.[96,97] Patients with creatinine clearances less than 30 to 35 mL/min (0.50–0.58 mL/s), who have serious GI conditions (abnormalities of the esophagus that delay emptying, such as stricture or achalasia), or who are pregnant should not take bisphosphonates. Some experts suggest bisphosphonates can be used in select patients with decreased renal function (see Chapters 52 and 53 on Chronic Kidney Disease).[98]

Weekly and monthly therapies have similar common but less serious GI effects (perforation, ulceration, GI bleeding) than daily therapy. The GI event rates were not increased with concomitant nonsteroidal anti-inflammatory medication use. If GI adverse events occur, switching to a different bisphosphonate might resolve the problem. Patients should be encouraged to discuss GI complaints with a healthcare provider. Intravenous ibandronate and zoledronic acid can be used for patients with GI contraindications or intolerances to oral bisphosphonates. Other common bisphosphonate adverse effects include injection reactions and musculoskeletal pain. Local injection-site reactions and acute phase reactions (e.g., fever, flulike symptoms) can occur but usually diminish with subsequent injections. If severe musculoskeletal pain occurs, the medication can be discontinued for a short term or permanently.

Rare adverse effects include osteonecrosis of the jaw and subtrochanteric femoral (atypical) fractures.[96,97,99] Osteonecrosis of the jaw (ONJ; black box warning) occurs more commonly in patients with cancer, chemotherapy, radiation, and or glucocorticoid therapy receiving higher-dose intravenous bisphosphonate therapy. With oral therapy, about 1 in 100,000 patients might get ONJ.[99] When possible, major dental work should be completed before bisphosphonate initiation. For patients already on therapy, some practitioners withhold bisphosphonate therapy during and after major dental procedures, but no data exist to support any beneficial effect of such practice. For patients with rare and unusual bone fractures while on long-term bisphosphonates, a metabolic bone disease workup should be conducted.

Administration. Before bisphosphonates are used, and especially before intravenous administration, the patient's serum calcium concentrations must be normal. Because bioavailability is very poor for bisphosphonates (<1% to 5%) and to minimize GI side effects, each oral dose should be taken with at least 6 ounces of plain tap water (not coffee, juice, mineral water, or milk) at least 30 (60 for ibandronate) minutes before consuming any food, supplements (including calcium and vitamin D), or medications. The weekly, raspberry-flavored, oral solution needs to be taken with only 2 ounces (~60 mL) of water and can be used for patients with swallowing difficulties (e.g., after stroke, tube feeding). The patient should also remain upright (i.e., either sitting or standing) for at least 30 minutes after alendronate and risedronate and 1 hour after ibandronate administration. A patient who misses a weekly dose can take it the next day. If more than 1 day has lapsed, that dose is skipped until the next scheduled ingestion. If a patient misses a monthly dose, it can be taken up to 7 days before the next administration.

The intravenous products need to be administered by a healthcare provider. The quarterly ibandronate injection comes as a prefilled syringe (3 mg/mL) kit with a butterfly needle. The injection is given intravenously over 15 to 30 seconds. The injection can also be diluted with dextrose 5% in water or normal saline and used with a syringe pump. Once-yearly administration of zoledronic acid should be infused over at least 15 minutes with a pump. Acetaminophen or ibuprofen can be given to decrease acute phase reactions.

Although these medications are effective, adherence is poor and results in decreased effectiveness.[100–102] Although most patients prefer once-weekly or once-monthly bisphosphonate administration to daily therapy, adherence is still a problem. Even after a hip fracture, bisphosphonate persistence is suboptimal.[103] For patients with adherence issues, the monthly e-mails or postcards sent by the ibandronate manufacturer might be helpful. Intravenous ibandronate and zoledronic acid could be used as replacements if cost is not an issue. Weekly alendronate plus vitamin D can potentially help to ensure better adherence with vitamin D intake.

Mixed Estrogen Agonists/Antagonists ⑧ Raloxifene, a second-generation mixed estrogen agonist/antagonist (EAA) approved for prevention and treatment of postmenopausal osteoporosis, has estrogenic agonist actions in bone but antagonist actions in breast and uterine tissue (see Table 99–7). Bazedoxifene with and without conjugated equine estrogens[89] and lasofoxifene[104] are newer second-generation EAAs that might be approved soon.

Efficacy. Raloxifene decreases vertebral fractures and increases spine and hip BMD, but to a lesser extent than bisphosphonates (see Table 99–6).[2,3,76,105] Eight-year data support long-term effects and safety in postmenopausal women. After raloxifene discontinuation, the medication effect is lost, with bone loss returning to age- or disease-related rates. For women with severe osteoporosis, particularly when hip fracture risk reduction is desired, a bisphosphonate might be a better choice. Since estradiol is important for bone health in men, some preliminary data have documented benefits of raloxifene in men with hypogonadism and prostate cancer.[37]

Raloxifene has additional benefits that might influence its selection. Raloxifene has an FDA-approved indication for invasive breast cancer risk reduction.[2,105] Thus in a subset of women, this additional benefit might warrant raloxifene use for dual osteoporosis and breast cancer prevention.

Some of the investigational EAAs have also documented breast cancer risk prevention. Raloxifene causes some positive lipid effects (decreased total and low-density lipoprotein cholesterol, neutral effect on high-density lipoprotein cholesterol, slightly increased triglycerides). However, no reduction in cardiovascular effects was demonstrated in the RUTH (Raloxifene Use for the Heart) or MORE-CORE (Multiple Outcomes with Raloxifene study and its continuation) trials.[105]

Adverse Events/Precautions. Hot flushes occur with a greater likelihood in women recently finishing menopause or discontinuing estrogen therapy.[105] Raloxifene rarely causes endometrial bleeding. Raloxifene is contraindicated for women with an active or past history of venous thromboembolic event. Therapy should be stopped if a patient anticipates extended immobility.

In large trials, no change in overall death, cardiovascular death, or overall stroke incidence was seen; however, a slight increase in fatal stroke was documented, resulting in a black box warning.[2,105] Women at high risk for a stroke (e.g., Framingham stroke risk score ≥13)[106] or coronary events and those with known coronary artery disease, peripheral vascular disease, atrial fibrillation, or a prior history of cerebrovascular events might not be good candidates for this medication.

Administration. Similar to bisphosphonates, adherence and persistence problems exist.[102]

Calcitonin Calcitonin is an endogenous hormone released from the thyroid gland when serum calcium is elevated.[107] The prescription product contains salmon calcitonin, which is more potent and longer lasting than the mammalian form. Calcitonin is FDA indicated for osteoporosis treatment for women who are at least 5 years past menopause (see Table 99–7). Because efficacy is less robust than the other antiresorptive therapies, calcitonin is reserved as third-line treatment. Intermittent nasal regimens and an oral product are being explored.

Efficacy. Only vertebral fractures have been documented to decrease with intranasal calcitonin therapy (see Table 99–6).[2,76,107] Calcitonin does not consistently affect hip BMD and does not decrease hip fracture risk.

Calcitonin might provide pain relief to some patients with acute vertebral fractures, about a 2.5-point change on a visual analog scale.[107] If used, calcitonin should be prescribed for short-term (4 weeks) treatment and should not be used in place of other more effective and less expensive analgesics nor should it preclude the use of more appropriate osteoporosis therapy.

Administration. Subcutaneous administration with 100 units daily is available but rarely used because of more adverse effects and costs.

Denosumab Therapy Recently approved; see investigational agents, Tables 99–6 and 99–7, Figure 99–3, and addendum.

Estrogen Therapy Although estrogens are FDA indicated for prevention of osteoporosis, they should only be used short-term in women who need estrogen therapy for the management of menopausal symptoms as the risks of estrogen therapy outweigh the bone benefits.[2,76,108] Even though the Women's Health Initiative trials only assessed one dose of conjugated equine estrogens, most clinicians extrapolate the results to all postmenopausal estrogen therapies until data indicate otherwise.

Efficacy. Hormone therapy (HT)—that is, estrogen with (EPT) or without (ET) a progestogen—significantly decreases fracture risk (see Table 99–6).[2,108] Increases in BMD are less than with bisphosphonates, denosumab, or teriparatide, but greater than with raloxifene and calcitonin. Oral and transdermal estrogens at equivalent doses and continuous or cyclic HT regimens have similar BMD effects. Effect on BMD is dose dependent, with some benefit seen with lower estrogen doses; however, fracture risk reduction has not been demonstrated with the lower doses. When HT is discontinued, bone loss accelerates and fracture protection is lost.

Adverse Events/Precautions/Administration. The lowest effective HT dose that prevents and controls menopausal symptoms is used and discontinued as soon as possible.[108] A complete discussion of adverse events, precautions, and administration for all ET and estrogen and progestogen combination products can be found in Chapter 91.

Testosterone Decreased testosterone concentrations are seen with certain gonadal diseases, eating disorders, glucocorticoid therapy, oophorectomy, menopause, and andropause.

Efficacy. A few studies of testosterone or methyltestosterone replacement in men and women, respectively, have demonstrated increases in BMD, but no data on fracture prevention exist.[34,109] Adding alendronate to testosterone therapy in hypogonadal men improved BMD benefits. Testosterone replacement should not be used solely for the prevention or treatment of osteoporosis, but it might be beneficial to reduce bone loss in patients needing therapy for hypogonadal symptoms or for women with low libido.

Adverse Events/Precaution/Administration. Patients and partners of those using testosterone gel products should be evaluated frequently for adverse events.

Anabolic Therapies

Currently teriparatide is the only available medication that increases bone formation.

Teriparatide Teriparatide is a recombinant product representing the first 34 amino acids in human PTH (see Table 99–7). Teriparatide increases bone formation, the bone remodeling rate, and osteoblast number and activity. Both bone mass and

architecture are improved. Teriparatide is FDA indicated for post-menopausal women, men, and patients on glucocorticoids who are at high risk for fracture. For example, patients who have a history of osteoporotic fracture, multiple risk factors for fracture, very low bone density (e.g., T-score < −3.5), or have failed or are intolerant of previous bisphosphonate therapy could be candidates for PTH therapy. Human PTH (1–31), oral PTH, intranasal PTH, and once-weekly subcutaneous teriparatide administration are being investigated.

Efficacy. Teriparatide reduces vertebral and nonvertebral fracture risk in postmenopausal women (see Table 99–6); however, no fracture data are available in men or for patients taking glucocorticoids.[2,110] Lumbar spine BMD increases are greater than other osteoporosis medications. Although wrist BMD is decreased, wrist fractures are not increased. Discontinuation of teriparatide therapy results in a decrease in BMD, which can be alleviated with subsequent antiresorptive therapy.

Using a second course of teriparatide is controversial. Some advocate no second course.[111] One study found that a second course of teriparatide increased BMD but not to the extent with the first course.[112]

Adverse Events/Precautions. Transient hypercalcemia rarely occurs. A trough serum calcium concentration is recommended 1 month after initiation of therapy. If high (>10.6 mg/mL [>2.65 mmol/L]), calcium intake should be decreased.

Because of an increased incidence of osteosarcoma in rats, teriparatide contains a black box warning against use in patients at increased baseline risk for osteosarcoma (e.g., Paget's bone disease, unexplained elevations of alkaline phosphatase, pediatric patients, young adults with open epiphyses, or patients with prior radiation therapy involving the skeleton).[110] In addition, teriparatide should not be used in patients with hypercalcemia, metabolic bone diseases other than osteoporosis, metastatic or skeletal cancers, or premenopausal women of child-bearing potential.

Administration. Teriparatide is commercially available as a pre-filled "pen" delivery device. The pen must be kept refrigerated and can be used immediately after removing from the refrigerator. The subcutaneous injection is delivered to the thigh or abdominal area with site rotation. The administration of the first dose should take place with the patient either sitting or lying down in case orthostatic hypotension occurs. The pen must be discarded 28 days after the initial injection. The patient should be reeducated on correct use with each pen refill.

Teriparatide is the most expensive osteoporosis therapy. Prior authorization may be required. Special arrangements need to be made when patients travel, especially on airplanes.

Combination Therapy

Combination antiresorptive and anabolic therapies have been evaluated with conflicting results.[2,110] Greater increases in BMD have sometimes been demonstrated when a less potent antiresorptive agent, raloxifene or HT, was used with PTH, whereas a blunting of the BMD effect has been seen when combined with alendronate. The effects of other bisphosphonates in combination with PTH might be different as some newer literature is beginning to reveal. This therapeutic issue is still being explored.[113]

Because there is no clear benefit (no documented increased fracture prevention) and there is potential for increased cost, adverse effects, and nonadherence, combination therapy is not recommended.

Investigational Therapies

Besides the aforementioned investigational products, new medication classes are also being developed.

RANKL Inhibitors Denosumab is a fully human monoclonal antibody that binds to RANKL, blocking its ability to bind to its receptor activator of nuclear factor kappa B (RANK) on the surface of osteoclast precursor cells and mature osteoclasts (see Table 99–7). Denosumab inhibits osteoclastogenesis and increases osteoclast apoptosis.

Denosumab was recently approved for select postmenopausal women (see Figure 99–3) and is still being evaluated for chemotherapy-induced osteoporosis. Denosumab 60 mg subcutaneous injection every 6 months for 3 years significantly decreased vertebral fractures by 68%, nonvertebral fractures by 20%, and hip fractures by 40% in postmenopausal women.[89] The same dose improved BMD and decreased new vertebral fractures without significant changes in nonvertebral or clinical vertebral fractures in men receiving androgen deprivation therapy.[114] The BMD effects are at least similar to weekly alendronate and can increase BMD in patients with prior alendronate therapy; however, these studies did not evaluate any fracture outcomes.[115] Activity appears to dissipate upon medication discontinuation.

Adverse effects include back, extremity, and musculoskeletal pain, hypercholesterolemia, cystitis, decreased serum calcium, and skin problems, which were generally similar to placebo or weekly alendronate. Rare, serious adverse effects include serious infections, osteonecrosis of the jaw, and bone turnover suppression.

Other Investigational Medication Classes Additional new classes of medications are beginning to show promise.[13]

Although injectable OPG, a competitive inhibitor of RANKL, blocked osteoclastic differentiation and decreased bone resorption biomarkers in phases I and II, further development has ceased. However, agents to enhance endogenous OPG, decrease RANKL production, or block RANKL binding to receptor activator of nuclear factor kappa B are being developed.

Agents to block osteoclast attachment ($\alpha v \beta_3$ integrin receptor antagonists), inhibit bone matrix degradation (cathepsin K inhibitors, e.g., odanacatib and relacatib), or change osteoclast and osteocyte cell structure (antisclerostin monoclonal antibodies) are in phase I, II, and III clinical trials.

Strontium ranelate and tibolone are approved in Europe, and the latter agent is approved in Canada. Most likely, these two medications will not be marketed in the United States.

◼ VERTEBROPLASTY AND KYPHOPLASTY

Sometimes patients with debilitating pain between 6 and 52 weeks after a vertebral fracture might undergo vertebroplasty or kyphoplasty during which bone cement is injected into the fractured vertebral space.[116] The procedure stabilizes the damaged vertebrae and reduces pain in 70% to 95% of patients. However, not all studies have documented benefit of this procedure, and concerns about long-term outcomes are surfacing.[117] Adverse events are uncommon but include cement leakage into the spinal column, which can result in complicating nerve damage, and vertebral fracturing around the cement.[118]

SPECIAL POPULATIONS

❾ Osteoporosis is a particular threat to all age groups and in some subgroups because of genetic abnormalities, diseases, and medications.

CHILDREN

Although rare, osteoporosis in children and adolescents can lead to significant pain, deformity, and chronic disability. Secondary causes are the main contributors to osteoporosis in children (Tables 99–2 and 99–3).[119] Idiopathic juvenile osteoporosis is a condition that can develop in previously healthy children (mostly between 8 and 12 years of age) and is only diagnosed after the exclusion of all other possible causes of osteoporosis. It can spontaneously resolve after 3 to 5 years, but sequelae can persist into adulthood. Although the pathogenesis is unknown, reduced osteoblastic bone formation mainly in trabecular regions appears to play a primary role.

The diagnosis and treatment of osteoporosis in children and adolescents is challenging. No guidelines or consensus recommendations exist. The International Society for Clinical Densitometry's official position is that the diagnosis of osteoporosis in children (<20 years of age) requires the presence of a clinically significant fracture history (long bone fracture of the lower extremity, vertebral compression fracture, or two or more long bone fractures of the upper extremities) in combination with low bone mass.[120] Low bone mass is defined as a Z-score below a −2.0 (adjusted for body size and ethnicity/race) using central DXA of the spine or total body.

After correcting any underlying causes and instituting a bone-healthy lifestyle, pharmacologic treatment should be considered for children with low bone mass and low trauma fractures.[121] Several small studies, mostly evaluating the intravenous bisphosphonate pamidronate or oral alendronate, have demonstrated increases in BMD. No studies have demonstrated fracture efficacy in this population. The optimal medication, dose, and duration of therapy are unknown, and more safety data are needed. A major concern with bisphosphonates is their effect on longitudinal bone growth and modeling; however, fracture healing, skeletal growth/maturation, or the appearance of growth plates does not appear to be impaired. Teriparatide cannot be used in children as it has a black box warning indicating an increased risk for osteosarcoma.

PREMENOPAUSAL WOMEN

Clinically significant bone loss and fractures in healthy premenopausal women are rare.[122] Approximately 15% of healthy premenopausal women will have low BMD as a normal variation of peak bone mass. Low peak bone mass is a major risk factor for postmenopausal osteoporosis and fractures but thus far is not a predictor of an increased risk for fractures in the premenopausal years. This might be a result of better bone architecture contributing to better bone strength in younger women.

Routine bone density screening and testing are not cost effective and should not be performed in healthy premenopausal women. No evidence supports that identifying low bone density in healthy premenopausal women results in improved bone-healthy lifestyle practices nor does any evidence exist to support that pharmacologic treatment will reduce future fracture risk in this population.

Most premenopausal women with osteoporosis (Z-score < −2.0) or a history of low trauma fracture have an identifiable secondary cause (see Tables 99–2 and 99–3). Therefore, premenopausal women presenting with a history of low-trauma fracture or with a suspected secondary cause for osteoporosis should undergo central DXA testing; if BMD is low, the patient should be considered for pharmacologic therapy. Women with an unidentified cause for osteoporosis and no history of fracture should be treated with a bone-healthy lifestyle and watchful waiting.

Pharmacologic therapy for osteoporosis should be used with caution in premenopausal women as efficacy and safety have not been adequately demonstrated. The oral bisphosphonates, intravenous ibandronate, calcitonin, and teriparatide are in pregnancy category C. Zoledronic acid is in pregnancy category D. Raloxifene is in pregnancy category X.

Bisphosphonates are incorporated into the bone matrix and slowly released over time. A theoretical concern is a risk for fetal harm with pregnancies that occur during and after therapy has been stopped. While limited case reports have documented healthy infants after bisphosphonate use, more safety data are needed.

THE "OLDER" SENIOR

Osteoporosis and adverse outcomes from fractures increase with age.[16,39] Age is an independent risk factor for osteoporosis and osteoporotic fractures, with the prevalence increasing dramatically with age. Seniors are living longer. The average additional life span for an 85-year-old was 6.8 years in 2003 and it is estimated that the number of people in the United States age 85 years and older will increase from 5.1 million in 2004 to 7.3 million by 2020. The number of "older" seniors with osteoporosis is on the rise, yet the condition is vastly underdiagnosed and undertreated in this population.

Central DXA BMD testing is cost-effective in the older senior. If central DXA testing is not feasible (e.g., patient is institutionalized), heel or forearm testing using a portable quantitative ultrasound or peripheral DXA device can be used for risk stratification. Alternatively, calculation of the 10-year probability for hip or major osteoporotic fracture using FRAX can possibly be used.

Older seniors should practice a bone-healthy lifestyle, ingest adequate calcium and vitamin D, and implement measures to prevent falls. When deciding whether or not to use prescription medications in older seniors, the following factors need to be taken into consideration: remaining life span, ability to take and afford medications, cognitive function, GI disorders, polypharmacy, desire to avoid additional medications, and regimen complexity. Although efficacy and safety data are limited in the older senior, evidence consistently shows that those at highest risk for fracture benefit most from pharmacologic therapy.

GLUCOCORTICOID-INDUCED OSTEOPOROSIS

❿ Glucocorticoids are the most common secondary cause of osteoporosis and the third most common cause of osteoporosis overall.[32] Approximately 30% to 50% of patients taking chronic oral glucocorticoids will experience a fracture. Bone losses are rapid, with the greatest decrease occurring in the first 6 to 12 months of therapy. Low to medium doses of inhaled glucocorticoids have no appreciable effect on bone density and fracture risk. The impact of long-term, high-dose inhaled glucocorticoids needs further evaluation.

The pathophysiology of glucocorticoid-induced osteoporosis (GIO) is multifactorial. Glucocorticoids decrease bone formation through decreased proliferation and differentiation, and enhanced apoptosis of osteoblasts.[12,32] They can interfere with the bone's natural repair mechanism through increased apoptosis of osteocytes, the bone's communication cells. Glucocorticoids increase bone resorption by increasing RANKL and decreasing OPG. They can reduce estrogen and testosterone concentrations and create a negative calcium balance by decreasing calcium absorption and increasing urinary calcium excretion. The underlying disease processes might also contribute negatively to bone metabolism.

The 2001 American College of Rheumatology guidelines provide direction and are being updated.[123] A baseline BMD using central DXA is recommended for all patients starting on 5 mg or more daily of prednisone equivalent for at least 6 months. BMD testing should also be considered at baseline in patients being started on shorter durations of systemic glucocorticoids if they are at high risk for low bone mass and fractures based on risk factors (e.g., age >65 years, postmenopausal, current smoker, and personal history of a low trauma fracture as an adult). Because of the rapid loss of bone that can occur with oral glucocorticoid therapy, central DXA can be repeated every 6 to 12 months if needed. Patients using high-dose inhaled corticosteroids should be evaluated for low bone mass or osteoporosis.

In addition to a bone-healthy lifestyle, pharmacologic therapy is required.[123,124] All patients starting or receiving long-term systemic glucocorticoid therapy should ingest 1,500 mg elemental calcium and 800 to 1,200 units of vitamin D daily and practice a bone-healthy lifestyle. Oral alendronate and risedronate and intravenous zoledronic acid have documented efficacy and are FDA indicated for GIO. The guidelines recommend all patients newly starting on systemic glucocorticoids (≥5 mg/day of prednisone equivalent) for an anticipated duration of at least 3 months should receive preventive bisphosphonate therapy.

Zoledronic acid is approved for patients with an anticipated steroid duration of at least 1 year. A more conservative approach might be considered in premenopausal women of child-bearing potential.

Bisphosphonate therapy is also recommended for patients starting or receiving long-term glucocorticoid therapy with documented low bone density (T-score < −1.0) or evidence of a low-trauma fracture.

Teriparatide is the only anabolic therapy commercially available that increases bone formation. Teriparatide can be used if bisphosphonates are not tolerated or are contraindicated.

Testosterone replacement therapy may be considered in men, and high-dose hormonal oral contraceptives for premenopausal women with documented hypogonadism.

TRANSPLANTATION OSTEOPOROSIS

Patients undergoing solid-organ transplantation (e.g., kidney, lung, heart, and liver) have a high risk for osteoporosis and osteoporotic fractures.[125] Prior to transplantation, many patients have osteoporosis or low BMD because of osteoporosis risk factors (see Table 99–1) and negative bone effects from their underlying diseases (e.g., alcoholism, cachexia, impaired liver or kidney function, hypogonadism, and deconditioning) and medications (see Tables 99–2 and 99–3). After transplantation, bone loss and fracture risk increase dramatically within the first 6 to 12 months, mainly as a consequence of high-dose systemic glucocorticoid exposure and the use of calcineurin inhibitors (e.g., cyclosporine). Sometimes bone loss slows or improves within 1 year of transplant.

Before transplantation, patients should be evaluated for metabolic bone disease with lab tests and physical examination for secondary causes (see Tables 99–2 and 99–3), radiographs for vertebral fractures, and central DXA.[125] Regardless of BMD results, patients should be counseled on a bone-healthy lifestyle and instructed to take 1,000 to 1,200 mg of elemental calcium and 800 to 1,000 units of vitamin D daily to maintain sufficient concentrations. Calcitriol (1,25-dihydroxyvitamin D) at a dose of 0.5 mcg daily might be needed for renal and/or liver dysfunction. Pretransplant patients with osteoporosis or a low trauma fracture, except patients with end-stage renal disease awaiting kidney transplantation, should be started on bisphosphonate therapy. In patients with normal BMD prior to transplant, short-term bisphosphonate therapy (6 – 12 months) can be used to prevent bone loss after transplant. PTH has not been studied in the transplant population and is contraindicated in kidney transplant patients with secondary hyperparathyroidism. Testosterone replacement might be considered for men, and high-dose hormonal oral contraceptives are options for premenopausal women with hypogonadism. Central DXA can be repeated as early as 6 to 12 months to evaluate bone loss and the effects of treatment.

CHRONIC KIDNEY DISEASE

Chronic kidney disease is defined as kidney damage for at least 3 months with or without a decrease in glomerular filtration rate (GFR) or a GFR less than 60 mL/min/1.73 m^2 (0.58 mL/s/m^2) for at least 3 months with or without kidney damage. In patients with a creatinine clearance (CrCl) greater than 30 mL/min (0.50 mL/s), osteoporosis can be managed routinely (see Fig. 99–3). As noted in FDA-approved product labeling, bisphosphonates are not recommended for patients with CrCl less than 30 or 35 mL/min (0.50 or 0.58 mL/s) because of potential drug accumulation. Newer data suggest that differences in the origin of chronic kidney disease, either intrinsic kidney damage or aging, might influence safety of these medications in those with age-related chronic kidney disease.

Based on large retrospective or pooled studies, oral bisphosphonates (CrCl as low as 15 mL/min [0.25 mL/s]), raloxifene (CrCl <45 mL/min [0.75 mL/s]), and teriparatide (CrCl as low as 30 – 49 mL/min [0.50 – 0.82 mL/s]) appear safe and efficacious in patients with age-related declines in renal function.[126,127] Some experts recommend decreasing dose by 50% or extending the dosing interval, and using the agent for less than 3 years.[98]

Renal osteodystrophy describes a constellation of metabolic bone disorders that develop in patients with stages 4 and 5 chronic kidney disease (GFR <30 mL/min/1.73 m^2 [<0.29 mL/s/m^2]) as a consequence of intrinsic kidney damage. Bone biopsy might be necessary to differentiate the different types of renal osteodystrophy from osteoporosis in this population. Antiresorptive therapies would be appropriate for the management of osteoporosis; however, they are contraindicated in patients with osteomalacia or adynamic bone and may be ineffective for osteitis fibrosa cystica.[126]

GASTROINTESTINAL DISEASES

The three most common gastrointestinal disorders associated with increased osteoporosis risk are inflammatory bowel disease, celiac disease, and postgastrectomy states.[77] Impaired absorption of key nutrients and minerals, chronic systemic glucocorticoid use, and increased levels of inflammatory cytokines are implicated.[128] The role of proinflammatory cytokines needs further investigation.

The prevalence of osteoporosis in patients with inflammatory bowel disease (e.g., Crohn's disease or ulcerative colitis) ranges from 17% to 41%, and the relative risk for fracture is approximately 40% higher than that for the general population.[77,128] When glucocorticoids are used, the GIO prevention and treatment guidelines should be followed.[123]

Celiac disease is an inherited autoimmune disorder in which the ingestion of the protein gluten triggers an immune reaction that damages the mucosal lining of the small intestine and leads to impaired nutrient absorption.[129] Approximately 1% of the population has celiac disease, with women having twice the incidence of men. Low bone density is seen in up to 70% of patients with celiac disease. Long-term fracture risk is estimated to be double that of the general population.[77] Impaired nutrient absorption, especially calcium and vitamin D, plays a central role in the bone loss, requiring 25(OH) vitamin D monitoring. Celiac disease management requires a gluten-free diet, which can significantly increase BMD by approximately 5% within 1 year.[77,130]

Patients undergoing total or partial gastrectomy are at high risk for osteoporosis. The incidence of osteoporosis may be as high as 32% to 42% with a 30-year cumulative risk for fracture of 72% in women and 48% in men.[77] Although the pathophysiology of bone disease in postgastrectomy is unknown, reduced nutritional intake of protein might play a role. Bone density evaluation using central DXA should be considered in all patients who are more than 10 years postgastrectomy.

PHARMACOECONOMIC CONSIDERATIONS

The estimated burden for fractures in 2005 was $17 billion and is expected to increase to $25 billion by 2025.[7] Consequently, determining who should be screened and treated for osteoporosis and fracture prevention is important. Various studies use different assumptions in their models.

Pharmacoeconomic considerations were used to determine 3% as the 10-year probability of hip fracture as a decision point in the NOF guidelines for which patients with low bone mass to treat.[131] The value of $60,000 per quality-adjusted life-year was the cut point for cost-effectiveness. Sensitivity analysis was conducted for age, sex, and race/ethnicity, yielding similar results.

Preventing osteoporosis in postmenopausal women with normal or osteopenic BMD is not cost-effective.[132] However, screening older women and only using a bisphosphonate for those with osteoporosis is cost-effective.[133] The cost per quality-adjusted life-year decreased from $40,100 for women 65 to 74 years old to a cost savings for women 85 years and older.

For men, screening and treating men after the age of 65 years with a low-trauma fracture and screening and treating men 80- to 85-years-old without a previous fracture were cost-effective when therapy costs were assumed to be $1,000 annually.[134] With generic medications, screening at a lower older age in men might be warranted based on cost savings. In a different senior study, bisphosphonates were found to produce the greatest gain in quality-adjusted life-years at the lowest cost (i.e., 0.0637; $4,200), followed by PTH (0.0574; $6,833), calcitonin (0.0348; $5,761), and raloxifene (0.0339; $5,676).[135]

EVALUATION OF THERAPEUTIC OUTCOMES

Besides monitoring for efficacy and safety, adherence evaluation should also be conducted.

MONITORING OF THE PHARMACEUTICAL CARE PLAN

Central DXA BMD measurements can be obtained every 1 to 2 years for monitoring bone loss and every 2 years for assessing treatment response.[5] In patients with conditions associated with higher rates of bone loss (e.g., glucocorticoid use), more frequent monitoring might be warranted.

To minimize test variability, BMD testing should be performed on the same DXA machine. A negative change in absolute BMD that exceeds the precision error of the machine at that site (approximately 3% for spine and 4% for hip) is considered a clinically significant BMD loss and warrants further investigation. Because changes in BMD do not entirely explain changes in fracture risk, many experts believe that decisions on whether or not to continue a particular therapy should not be based solely on BMD response.

Biochemical markers of bone turnover have been evaluated for use in monitoring early responses to medications, especially for identifying therapy nonresponders or possibly promoting adherence.[51,52] Bone resorption markers, with the first or second morning void for urinary N-terminal crosslinking telopeptide of type 1 collagen or morning for serum C-terminal crosslinking telopeptide of type 1 collagen, are typically performed after an overnight fast at baseline and repeated after 3 to 6 months of therapy. These parameters will decrease with effective therapy. Circadian variability, seasonal variations, food intake, and recent exercise can all impact results. Because no consensus on result interpretation and high test variability exist, these tests are not yet considered routine.

PHARMACY SERVICES

❾ Pharmacists play an important role in screening and monitoring for osteoporosis. Community pharmacy screenings with ultrasonography identify patients who are at risk, and consultations with a pharmacist or other healthcare professional can increase lifestyle changes, medication use, and DXA referrals. This practice has been financially sustainable in the community pharmacy setting.[136] Since adherence is strongly linked to fracture prevention,[100,101] pharmacists should help identify and resolve medication-related problems that are affecting adherence for patients taking antiosteoporotic medications.

Pharmacists can also increase use of these medications after a low-trauma fracture by using databases to identify undertreated patients. They can increase diagnostic testing and osteoporosis prevention/treatment, and identify and resolve medication and disease causes of bone loss, especially in special patient populations at greater risk.

OTHER METABOLIC BONE DISORDERS

Because of increased interest in bone diseases and newer medications, better therapies are being explored and developed for other bone diseases.

OSTEOMALACIA

Osteomalacia, meaning "soft bones," is a condition seen in adults in which the bone is significantly undermineralized. Rickets is the childhood equivalent of osteomalacia. The most common cause of osteomalacia is severe, prolonged vitamin D deficiency. Disorders that cause hypophosphatemia and, rarely, medications such as long-term anticonvulsant therapy can also cause osteomalacia.[50]

Patients with osteomalacia present with pathologic fractures and/or deep bone pain, proximal muscle weakness, or no obvious symptoms but low BMD. Patients with osteomalacia will have an extremely low 25(OH) vitamin D concentration (<10 ng/mL [<25 nmol/L]) and might have an elevated bone-specific alkaline phosphate and hypocalcemia. The treatment of osteomalacia caused by vitamin D deficiency is high-dose vitamin D replacement therapy. Prescription oral ergocalciferol 50,000 units once to twice weekly for at least 8 weeks is a regimen that is frequently used to raise vitamin D concentrations into the sufficient range. Other high-dose oral and intramuscular vitamin D regimens have also been used. Once 25(OH) vitamin D concentrations are greater than 30 ng/mL (75 nmol/L), chronic maintenance vitamin D therapy can be instituted. Oral ergocalciferol 50,000 units once or twice a month or nonprescription cholecalciferol at least 1,000 units up 2,000 units once daily are reasonable maintenance options.

PAGET'S DISEASE

Unlike osteoporosis, which is a systemic disorder affecting the entire skeleton, Paget's disease is a disorder of bone remodeling in discrete sections of bone. The main areas affected are the skull, spine, pelvis, femur, and tibia.[137] In this condition, the osteoclasts are abnormally large and have heightened activity, increasing the bone turnover rate and affecting both bone resorption and formation. The accelerated bone formation does not allow for proper layering of collagen, leading to disorganized or woven bone. The disease is usually asymptomatic; however, patients can experience bone pain, headaches with skull involvement, fractures, skeletal deformities, and, rarely, malignant transformation into osteosarcoma.

Paget's disease tends to occur in adults 50 years and older, with a slight predominance in men and patients of north European ancestry.[137] The disease affects approximately 1% to 2% of adults. Various environmental and genetic factors cause Paget's disease, with viral causes a controversial pathogenesis. Paget's disease is typically discovered because of an unexplained elevation in serum alkaline phosphatase or classic bone findings on routine x-ray films.

Bisphosphonates are the medication of choice for managing Paget's disease because they work directly on osteoclasts to slow down bone turnover, allowing more time for proper bone formation.[137,138] Six bisphosphonates are FDA indicated for the treatment of Paget's disease. Calcium and vitamin D deficiencies need to be corrected before beginning bisphosphonate therapy. The most commonly used regimens are risedronate 30-mg tablet orally once daily for 2 months; pamidronate 60-mg intravenous infusion over 4 hours for 3 consecutive days; alendronate 40-mg tablet orally once daily for 6 months, and a one-time intravenous infusion of 5-mg zoledronic acid.

Zoledronic acid and risedronate regimens were compared in a head-to-head study, with zoledronic acid demonstrating a superior and more rapid and sustained therapeutic response.[139] Demonstrated efficacy and convenience make zoledronic acid a good initial choice for most patients. Relapse after treatment is common (e.g., 28% in 5 years). Therapy can be repeated if symptoms return or serum alkaline phosphatase increases by 25% or more.

Subcutaneous or intramuscular salmon calcitonin is an approved option if bisphosphonate therapy is contraindicated. Analgesics, anti-inflammatory medications, and some forms of alternative healing might be needed to treat the pain symptoms.

CONCLUSIONS

Osteoporosis is a public health priority, as the prevalence of both the disease and fracture incidence is expected to increase in the next 10 to 20 years because of the increasing age of the population in many countries. Osteoporosis prevention begins at birth and continues throughout life by practicing a bone-healthy lifestyle (adequate calcium and vitamin D intake, exercise, no smoking, minimal alcohol use, and fall prevention). Generally osteoporosis occurs in postmenopausal women and senior men; however, the disease can occur in all ages as a result of secondary causes such as genetics, diseases, and medications. Portable ultrasonography machines can screen for osteoporosis but central bone densitometry (DXA) is used for diagnosis and monitoring.

Bisphosphonates are the medication class of choice because they decrease hip, nonvertebral, and vertebral fractures, are relatively safe, and are affordable. Teriparatide is the only medication that can build bone; however, cost and subcutaneous administration limit its use. Although medications decrease fracture risk, prescribing of antiosteoporotic and preventive medications and adherence to such therapy is low. Suboptimal medication adherence is documented to decrease fracture prevention outcomes.

As osteoporosis management becomes more streamlined for postmenopausal women, practitioners are not only identifying other special populations at risk for osteoporosis (e.g., men, transplantation patients, glucocorticoid therapy, cancer therapies) but determining the best strategies for osteoporosis prevention and treatment. New agents and medication classes to prevent and treat osteoporosis show promise.

Other bone disorders, especially those related to vitamin D insufficiency and deficiency can be improved or eliminated with appropriate medications. Since most people are low in vitamin D, patients at risk for or with symptoms of bone disorders should have a 25(OH) vitamin D level drawn, with appropriate replenishment and maintenance vitamin D therapy instituted.

ADDENDUM

Denosumab was approved after this chapter was completed. Additional information includes serum calcium needs to be normal and major dental work should be completed before use. The product is a refrigerated prefilled pen that can be at room temperature up to 14 days before administration. Also available is a single use vial. Injection can be given in the upper arm, upper thigh, and abdomen.

Because of concerns about serious side effects, a medication guide, as part of the Risk Evaluation and Mitigation Strategy (REMS), is given to the patients. All providers are encouraged to participate in the an optional Postmarketing Active Surveillance Program to evaluate adverse effects. The prescriber can delegate this monitoring to other healthcare professionals, which could be a pharmacist including pharmacists.

ABBREVIATIONS

25(OH) vitamin D: calcidiol/25-hydroxyvitamin D

BMD: bone mineral density

DXA: dual-energy x-ray absorptiometry

EAA: estrogen agonist antagonist

EPT: estrogen progestogen therapy

ET: estrogen therapy

FRAX: World Health Organization fracture risk assessment tool

GFR: glomerular filtration rate

GI: gastrointestinal

GIO: glucocorticoid-induced osteoporosis

HT: hormone therapy (estrogen with or without a progestogen)

OPG: osteoprotegerin

PTH: parathyroid hormone

RANKL: receptor activator of nuclear factor-kappa B ligand

WHO: World Health Organization

REFERENCES

1. National Osteoporosis Foundation. Fast facts on osteoporosis, *nof.org/osteoporosis/diseasefacts.htm*.

2. The North American Menopause Society. Management of osteoporosis in postmenopausal women: 2010 position statement of the North American Menopause Society. Menopause 2010;17:25–54.

3. National Osteoporosis Foundation. Clinician's guide to prevention and treatment of osteoporosis. 2010, *www.nof.org/professionals/NOF_ClinicanGuide2009_v7.pdf*.

4. Barrett-Connor E, Siris ES, Wehren LE, et al. Osteoporosis and fracture risk in women of different ethnic groups. J Bone Miner Res 2005;20:185–194.

5. Lim LS, Hoeksema LJ, Sherin K. Screening for osteoporosis in the adult U.S. population: ACPM position statement on preventive practice. Am J Prev Med 2009;36:366–375.

6. Briot K, Cortet B, Tremollieres F, et al. Male osteoporosis: Diagnosis and fracture risk evaluation. Joint Bone Spine 2009;76:129–133.

7. Burge R, Dawson-Hughes B, Solomon DH, et al. Incidence and economic burden of osteoporosis-related fractures in the United States, 2005–2025. J Bone Miner Res 2007;22:465–475.

8. Leslie WD, O'Donnell S, Jean S, et al. Trends in hip fracture rates in Canada. JAMA 2009;302:883–889.

9. Clarke B. Normal bone anatomy and physiology. Clin J Am Soc Nephrol 2008;3(suppl 3):S131–139.

10. Cohen A, Shane E. Treatment of premenopausal women with low bone mineral density. Curr Osteoporos Rep 2008;6:39–46.

11. Lewiecki EM. Premenopausal bone health assessment. Curr Rheumatol Rep 2005;7:46–52.

12. Imai Y, Kondoh S, Kouzmenko A, et al. Regulation of bone metabolism by nuclear receptors. Mol Cell Endocrinol 2009;310:3–10.

13. Martin TJ, Sims NA, Ng KW. Regulatory pathways revealing new approaches to the development of anabolic drugs for osteoporosis. Osteoporos Int 2008;19:1125–1138.

14. Leibbrandt A, Penninger JM. RANK/RANKL: Regulators of immune responses and bone physiology. Ann N Y Acad Sci 2008;1143: 123–150.

15. Yavropoulou MP, Yovos JG. Osteoclastogenesis—current knowledge and future perspectives. J Musculoskelet Neuronal Interact 2008;8:204–216.

16. Duque G, Troen BR. Understanding the mechanisms of senile osteoporosis: New facts for a major geriatric syndrome. J Am Geriatr Soc 2008;56:935–941.

17. Vondracek SF, Chen JT, Csako G. Osteoporosis pathophysiology and new drug development. Clin Rev Bone Miner Metab 2004;2:293–313.

18. Richards JB, Kavvoura FK, Rivadeneira F, et al. Collaborative meta-analysis: Associations of 150 candidate genes with osteoporosis and osteoporotic fracture. Ann Intern Med 2009;151:528–537.

19. Sipos W, Pietschmann P, Rauner M, et al. Pathophysiology of osteoporosis. Wien Med Wochenschr 2009;159:230–234.

20. Drake MT, Khosla S. Role of sex steroids in the pathogenesis of osteoporosis. In: Primer on the Metabolic Bone Diseases and Disorders of Mineral Metabolism. Washington, DC: American Society of Bone Mineral Metabolism; 2008:208–213.

21. Heaney RP. Vitamin D in health and disease. Clin J Am Soc Nephrol 2008;3:1535–1541.

22. Holick MF, Chen TC. Vitamin D deficiency: A worldwide problem with health consequences. Am J Clin Nutr 2008;87:1080S–1086S.

23. Holick MF. High prevalence of vitamin D inadequacy and implications for health. Mayo Clin Proc 2006;81:353–373.

24. Heaney RP. Vitamin D and calcium interactions: Functional outcomes. Am J Clin Nutr 2008;88:541S–544S.

25. Bronner F. Recent developments in intestinal calcium absorption. Nutr Rev 2009;67:109–113.

26. Khanal RC, Nemere I. Regulation of intestinal calcium transport. Annu Rev Nutr 2008;28:179–196.

27. Hanley DA, Davison KS. Vitamin D insufficiency in North America. J Nutr 2005;135:332–337.

28. Kanis JA. FRAX WHO fracture risk assessment tool, www.shef.ac.uk/FRAX.

29. Serota AC, Lane JM. Osteoporosis (secondary). 2009, eMedicine. medscape.com/article/311449–overview.

30. Kelman A, Lane NE. The management of secondary osteoporosis. Best Prac Res Clin Rheumatol 2005;19:1021–1037.

31. Borgelt LM, Vondracek SF. Osteoporosis and osteomalacia. In: Tisdale JE, Miller DA, eds. Drug-induced diseases: Prevention, detection and management, 2nd ed. Bethesda, MD: American Society of Health-Systems Pharmacists; 2010:991–1004.

32. Caplan L, Saag KG. Glucocorticoids and the risk of osteoporosis. Expert Opin Drug Saf 2009;8:33–47.

33. Seeman E, Delmas PD. Bone quality—The material and structural basis of bone strength and fragility. N Engl J Med 2006;354: 2250–2261.

34. Tuck SP, Francis RM. Testosterone, bone and osteoporosis. Front Horm Res 2009;37:123–132.

35. Healthcare Costs and Utilization Project. Emergency visits for injurious falls among the elderly, 2006. Statistical brief #80. 2009, www.hcup-us.ahrq.gov/reports/statbriefs/sb80.jsp.

36. Centers for Disease Control and Prevention National Center for Injury Prevention and Control. WISQARS injury mortality reports, 1999–2006. http://webappa.cdc.gov/sasweb/ncipc/mortrate10_sy.html.

37. Khosla S. Update in male osteoporosis. J Clin Endocrinol Metab 2010;95:3–10.

38. Centers for Disease Control and Prevention National Center for Health Statistics. Health data interactive, www.cdc.gov/nchs/hdi.htm.

39. Vondracek SF, Linnebur SA. Diagnosis and management of osteoporosis in the older senior. Clin Interv Aging 2009;4:121–136.

40. Auron-Gomez M, Michota F. Medical management of hip fracture. Clin Geriatr Med 2008;24:701–719, ix.

41. Klotzbuecher CM, Ross PD, Landsman PB, et al. Patients with prior fractures have an increased risk of future fractures: A summary of the literature and statistical synthesis. J Bone Miner Res 2000;15: 721–739.

42. Health 24. Measure your height, www.health24.com/dietnfood/Great_diet_guides/15-3089-3242.asp.

43. Kanis JA, Oden A, Johnell O, et al. The use of clinical risk factors enhances the performance of BMD in the prediction of hip and osteoporotic fractures in men and women. Osteoporos Int 2007;18: 1033–1046.

44. Griffith JF, Genant HK. Bone mass and architecture determination: State of the art. Best Pract Res Clin Endocrinol Metab 2008;22: 737–764.

45. Raisz LG. Clinical practice. Screening for osteoporosis. N Engl J Med 2005;353:164–171.

46. The International Society for Clinical Densitometry. 2007 official positions of the International Society for Clinical Densitometry, www.iscd.org/Visitors/pdfs/ISCD2007OfficialPositions-Adult.pdf.

47. van Brussel MS, Lems WF. Clinical relevance of diagnosing vertebral fractures by vertebral fracture assessment. Curr Osteoporos Rep 2009;7:103–106.

48. Stechschulte SA, Kirsner RS, Federman DG. Vitamin D: Bone and beyond, rationale and recommendations for supplementation. Am J Med 2009;122:793–802.

49. Holick MF. Vitamin D deficiency. N Engl J Med 2007;357:266–281.

50. Lips P, van Schoor NM, Bravenboer N. Vitamin D related disorders. In: Roden C, ed. Primer on the Metabolic Bone Diseases and Disorders of Mineral Metabolism, 7th ed. Washington, DC: American Society of Bone Mineral Metabolism; 2008.

51. Brown JP, Albert C, Nassar BA, et al. Bone turnover markers in the management of postmenopausal osteoporosis. Clin Biochem 2009;42:929–942.

52. Singer FR, Eyre DR. Using biochemical markers of bone turnover in clinical practice. Cleve Clin J Med 2008;75:739–750.

53. Whelan AM, Jurgens TM, Bowles SK, et al. Efficacy of natural health products in treating osteoporosis: What is the quality of internet patient advice? Ann Pharmacother 2009;43:899–907.

54. Tucker KL, Morita K, Qiao N, et al. Colas, but not other carbonated beverages, are associated with low bone mineral density in older women: The Framingham osteoporosis study. Am J Clin Nutr 2006;84:936–942.

55. Heaney RP. Dairy and bone health. J Am Coll Nutr 2009;28(suppl 1): 82S–90S.

56. Standing Committee on the Scientific Evaluation of Dietary Reference Intakes FaNB Institute of Medicine. Dietary Reference Intakes for Calcium, Phosphorous, Magnesium, Vitamin D, and Fluoride. Washington, DC: National Academy Press; 1997.

57. National Institute of Health Office of Dietary Supplements. Dietary supplement fact sheet: Calcium. 2009, ods.od.nih.gov/factsheets/calcium.asp.

58. Wagner CL, Greer FR. Prevention of rickets and vitamin D deficiency in infants, children, and adolescents. Pediatrics 2008;122:1142–1152.

59. National Osteoporosis Foundation. Vitamin D and bone health. 2008, www.nof.org/prevention/vitaminD.htm.

60. United States Department of Agriculture. USDA national nutrient database for standard reference, release 17 calcium, ca (mg) content of selected foods per common measure, sorted by nutrient content. www.nal.usda.gov/fnic/foodcomp/Data/SR17/wtrank/sr17w301.pdf.

61. United States Department of Agriculture. USDA national nutrient database for standard reference, release 22. Vitamin D (IU) content of selected foods per common measure, sorted by nutrient content. www.ars.usda.gov/SP2UserFiles/Place/12354500/Data/SR22/nutrlist/sr22w324.pdf.

62. Cheung AM, Tile L, Lee Y, et al. Vitamin K supplementation in postmenopausal women with osteopenia (ECKO trial): A randomized controlled trial. PLoS Med 2008;5:e196.

63. Gundberg CM. Vitamin K and bone: Past, present, and future. J Bone Miner Res 2009;24:980–982.

64. O'Neill CK, Evans E. Beyond calcium and vitamin D. Is there a role for other vitamins, minerals, and nutrients in osteoporosis? Clin Rev Bone Miner Metab 2004;2:325–339.

65. Atmaca A, Kleerekoper M, Bayraktar M, et al. Soy isoflavones in the management of postmenopausal osteoporosis. Menopause 2008;15:748–757.

66. United States Department of Agriculture. Dietary guidelines for Americans 2005. Alcoholic beverages. 2005, *www.health.gov/ DIETARYGUIDELINES/dga2005/document/html/chapter9.htm.*

67. Hallstrom H, Wolk A, Glynn A, et al. Coffee, tea and caffeine consumption in relation to osteoporotic fracture risk in a cohort of Swedish women. Osteoporos Int 2006;17:1055–1064.

68. Wong PK, Christie JJ, Wark JD. The effects of smoking on bone health. Clin Sci (Lond) 2007;113:233–241.

69. American Geriatrics Society and British Geriatric Society. AGS/BGS clinical practice guideline: Prevention of falls in older persons. 2009, *www.americangeriatrics.org/education/prevention_of_falls.shtml.*

70. Beswick AD, Rees K, Dieppe P, et al. Complex interventions to improve physical function and maintain independent living in elderly people: A systematic review and meta-analysis. Lancet 2008;371:725–735.

71. Centers for Disease Control and Prevention. Home and recreational safety: Falls among older adults: Brochures and posters. 2009, *www. cdc.gov/HomeandRecreationalSafety/Falls/fallsmaterial.html.*

72. Department of Health and Human Services Centers for Disease Control and Prevention and National Center for Injury Prevention and Control. Check for safety, a home fall prevention checklist for older adults. *www.cdc.gov/ncipc/pub-res/toolkit/CheckListForSafety.htm.*

73. National Council on Aging. Fall prevention, *www.healthyaging programs.org/content.asp?sectionid=69.*

74. Bischoff-Ferrari HA, Dawson-Hughes B, Staehelin HB, et al. Fall prevention with supplemental and active forms of vitamin D: A meta-analysis of randomized controlled trials. BMJ 2009;339:b3692.

75. Broe KE, Chen TC, Weinberg J, et al. A higher dose of vitamin d reduces the risk of falls in nursing home residents: A randomized, multiple-dose study. J Am Geriatr Soc 2007;55:234–239.

76. MacLean C, Newberry S, Maglione M, et al. Systematic review: Comparative effectiveness of treatments to prevent fractures in men and women with low bone density or osteoporosis. Ann Intern Med 2008;148:197–213.

77. Bernstein CN, Leslie WD, Leboff MS. AGA technical review on osteoporosis in gastrointestinal diseases. Gastroenterology 2003;124:795–841.

78. Donaldson MG, Cawthon PM, Lui LY, et al. Estimates of the proportion of older white women who would be recommended for pharmacologic treatment by the new U.S. National Osteoporosis Foundation Guidelines. J Bone Miner Res 2009;24:675–680.

79. Meacham S, Grayscott D, Chen JJ, et al. Review of the dietary reference intake for calcium: Where do we go from here? Crit Rev Food Sci Nutr 2008;48:378–384.

80. Bolland MJ, Avenell A, Baron JA, et al. Effect of calcium supplements on risk of myocardial infarction and cardiovascular events: meta-analysis. BMJ 2010;341:c3691.

81. Bischoff-Ferrari HA, Willett WC, Wong JB, et al. Prevention of nonvertebral fractures with oral vitamin D and dose dependency: A meta-analysis of randomized controlled trials. Arch Intern Med 2009;169:551–561.

82. Bischoff-Ferrari HA, Willett WC, Wong JB, et al. Fracture prevention with vitamin D supplementation: A meta-analysis of randomized controlled trials. JAMA 2005;293:2257–2264.

83. Vieth R, Chan PC, MacFarlane GD. Efficacy and safety of vitamin D3 intake exceeding the lowest observed adverse effect level. Am J Clin Nutr 2001;73:288–294.

84. Aloia JF, Patel M, Dimaano R, et al. Vitamin D intake to attain a desired serum 25-hydroxyvitamin D concentration. Am J Clin Nutr 2008;87:1952–1958.

85. Holick MF, Biancuzzo RM, Chen TC, et al. Vitamin D2 is as effective as vitamin D3 in maintaining circulating concentrations of 25-hydroxyvitamin D. J Clin Endocrinol Metab 2008;93:677–681.

86. Russell RG, Watts NB, Ebetino FH, et al. Mechanisms of action of bisphosphonates: Similarities and differences and their potential influence on clinical efficacy. Osteoporos Int 2008;19:733–759.

87. Bilezikian JP. Efficacy of bisphosphonates in reducing fracture risk in postmenopausal osteoporosis. Am J Med 2009;122:S14–21.

88. Harris ST, Reginster JY, Harley C, et al. Risk of fracture in women treated with monthly oral ibandronate or weekly bisphosphonates: The evaluation of ibandronate efficacy (VIBE) database fracture study. Bone 2009;44:758–765.

89. Silverman SL. New therapies for osteoporosis: Zoledronic acid, bazedoxifene, and denosumab. Curr Osteoporos Rep 2009;7:91–95.

90. Doggrell SA. Clinical efficacy and safety of zoledronic acid in prostate and breast cancer. Expert Rev Anticancer Ther 2009;9:1211–1218.

91. Geusens P. Bisphosphonates for postmenopausal osteoporosis: Determining duration of treatment. Curr Osteoporos Rep 2009;7:12–17.

92. Reid DM, Hosking D, Kendler D, et al. A comparison of the effect of alendronate and risedronate on bone mineral density in postmenopausal women with osteoporosis: 24-month results from facts-international. Int J Clin Pract 2008;62:575–584.

93. Emkey R, Delmas PD, Bolognese M, et al. Efficacy and tolerability of once-monthly oral ibandronate (150 mg) and once-weekly oral alendronate (70 mg): Additional results from the monthly oral therapy with ibandronate for osteoporosis intervention (MOTION) study. Clin Ther 2009;31:751–761.

94. Zhong ZM, Chen JT. Anti-fracture efficacy of risedronic acid in men: A meta-analysis of randomized controlled trials. Clin Drug Investig 2009;29:349–357.

95. Ebeling PR. Clinical practice. Osteoporosis in men. N Engl J Med 2008;358:1474–1482.

96. Kennel KA, Drake MT. Adverse effects of bisphosphonates: Implications for osteoporosis management. Mayo Clin Proc 2009;84:632–637; quiz 638.

97. Recker RR, Lewiecki EM, Miller PD, et al. Safety of bisphosphonates in the treatment of osteoporosis. Am J Med 2009;122:S22–32.

98. Miller PD. Diagnosis and treatment of osteoporosis in chronic renal disease. Semin Nephrol 2009;29:144–155.

99. Khan AA, Sandor GK, Dore E, et al. Bisphosphonate associated osteonecrosis of the jaw. J Rheumatol 2009;36:478–490.

100. Rabenda V, Hiligsmann M, Reginster JY. Poor adherence to oral bisphosphonate treatment and its consequences: A review of the evidence. Expert Opin Pharmacother 2009;10:2303–2315.

101. Siris ES, Selby PL, Saag KG, et al. Impact of osteoporosis treatment adherence on fracture rates in North America and Europe. Am J Med 2009;122:S3–13.

102. Weycker D, Macarios D, Edelsberg J, et al. Compliance with drug therapy for postmenopausal osteoporosis. Osteoporos Int 2006;17:1645–1652.

103. Rabenda V, Vanoverloop J, Fabri V, et al. Low incidence of anti-osteoporosis treatment after hip fracture. J Bone Joint Surg Am 2008;90:2142–2148.

104. Gennari L. Lasofoxifene, a new selective estrogen receptor modulator for the treatment of osteoporosis and vaginal atrophy. Expert Opin Pharmacother 2009;10:2209–2220.

105. Goldstein SR, Duvernoy CS, Calaf J, et al. Raloxifene use in clinical practice: Efficacy and safety. Menopause 2009;16:413–421.

106. Barrett-Connor E, Cox DA, Song J, et al. Raloxifene and risk for stroke based on the Framingham stroke risk score. Am J Med 2009;122:754–761.

107. Chesnut CH, 3rd, Azria M, Silverman S, et al. Salmon calcitonin: A review of current and future therapeutic indications. Osteoporos Int 2008;19:479–491.

108. Practice Committee of the American Society for Reproductive Medicine. Estrogen and progestogen therapy in postmenopausal women. Fertil Steril 2008;90:S88–102.

109. Clarke BL, Khosla S. Androgens and bone. Steroids 2009;74:296–305.

110. File E, Deal C. Clinical update on teriparatide. Curr Rheumatol Rep 2009;11:169–176.

111. Finkelstein JS, Wyland JJ, Leder BZ, et al. Effects of teriparatide retreatment in osteoporotic men and women. J Clin Endocrinol Metab 2009;94:2495–2501.

112. Cosman F, Nieves JW, Zion M, et al. Retreatment with teriparatide one year after the first teriparatide course in patients on continued long-term alendronate. J Bone Miner Res 2009;24:1110–1115.

113. Cosman F, Wermers RA, Recknor C, et al. Effects of teriparatide in postmenopausal women with osteoporosis on prior alendronate or raloxifene: Differences between stopping and continuing the antiresorptive agent. J Clin Endocrinol Metab 2009;94:3772–3780.

114. Smith MR, Egerdie B, Hernandez Toriz N, et al. Denosumab in men receiving androgen-deprivation therapy for prostate cancer. N Engl J Med 2009;361:745–755.

115. Kendler DL, Roux C, Benhamou CL, et al. Effects of denosumab on bone mineral density and bone turnover in postmenopausal women transitioning from alendronate therapy. J Bone Miner Res 2010;25:72–81.

116. McGirt MJ, Parker SL, Wolinsky JP, et al. Vertebroplasty and kyphoplasty for the treatment of vertebral compression fractures: An evidenced-based review of the literature. Spine J 2009;9:501–508.

117. Kallmes DF, Comstock BA, Heagerty PJ, et al. A randomized trial of vertebroplasty for osteoporotic spinal fractures. N Engl J Med 2009;361:569–579.

118. Lee MJ, Dumonski M, Cahill P, et al. Percutaneous treatment of vertebral compression fractures: A meta-analysis of complications. Spine 2009;34:1228–1232.

119. Rauch F, Bishop N. Juvenile osteoporosis. In: Primer on the Metabolic Bone Diseases and Disorders of Mineral Metabolism, 7th ed. Washington, DC: American Society of Bone Mineral Research; 2008.

120. The International Society for Clinical Densitometry. 2007 pediatric official positions of the International Society for Clinical Densitometry. 2007, www.iscd.org/Visitors/pdfs/ISCD2007OfficialPositions-Pediatric.pdf.

121. Bachrach LK, Ward LM. Clinical review, I: Bisphosphonate use in childhood osteoporosis. J Clin Endocrinol Metab 2009;94:400–409.

122. Vondracek SF, Hansen LB, McDermott MT. Osteoporosis risk in premenopausal women. Pharmacotherapy 2009;29:305–317.

123. Recommendations for the prevention and treatment of glucocorticoid-induced osteoporosis: 2001 update. American College of Rheumatology ad hoc committee on glucocorticoid-induced osteoporosis. Arthritis Rheum 2001;44:1496–1503.

124. van Brussel MS, Bultink IE, Lems WF. Prevention of glucocorticoid-induced osteoporosis. Expert Opin Pharmacother 2009;10:997–1005.

125. Stein E, Ebeling P, Shane E. Post-transplantation osteoporosis. Endocrinol Metab Clin North Am 2007;36:937–963, viii.

126. Toussaint ND, Elder GJ, Kerr PG. Bisphosphonates in chronic kidney disease: Balancing potential benefits and adverse effects on bone and soft tissue. Clin J Am Soc Nephrol 2009;4:221–233.

127. Ishani A, Blackwell T, Jamal SA, et al. The effect of raloxifene treatment in postmenopausal women with CKD. J Am Soc Nephrol 2008;19:1430–1438.

128. Ali T, Lam D, Bronze MS, et al. Osteoporosis in inflammatory bowel disease. Am J Med 2009;122:599–604.

129. Green PH, Cellier C. Celiac disease. N Engl J Med 2007;357:1731–1743.

130. Bianchi ML, Bardella MT. Bone in celiac disease. Osteoporos Int 2008;19:1705–1716.

131. Tosteson AN, Melton LJ, 3rd, Dawson-Hughes B, et al. Cost-effective osteoporosis treatment thresholds: The United States perspective. Osteoporos Int 2008;19:437–447.

132. Schousboe JT, Nyman JA, Kane RL, et al. Cost-effectiveness of alendronate therapy for osteopenic postmenopausal women. Ann Intern Med 2005;142:734–741.

133. Schousboe JT, Ensrud KE, Nyman JA, et al. Universal bone densitometry screening combined with alendronate therapy for those diagnosed with osteoporosis is highly cost-effective for elderly women. J Am Geriatr Soc 2005;53:1697–1704.

134. Schousboe JT, Taylor BC, Fink HA, et al. Cost-effectiveness of bone densitometry followed by treatment of osteoporosis in older men. JAMA 2007;298:629–637.

135. Pfister AK, Welch CA, Lester MD, et al. Cost-effectiveness strategies to treat osteoporosis in elderly women. South Med J 2006;99:123–131.

136. Liu Y, Nevins JC, Carruthers KM, Doucette WR, McDonough RP, Pan X. Osteoporosis risk screening for women in a community pharmacy. J Am Pharm Assoc (2003) 2007;47:521–526.

137. Ralston SH, Langston AL, Reid IR. Pathogenesis and management of Paget's disease of bone. Lancet 2008;372:155–163.

138. Silverman SL. Paget's disease of bone: Therapeutic options. J Clin Rheumatol 2008;14:299–305.

139. Reid IR, Miller P, Lyles K, et al. Comparison of a single infusion of zoledronic acid with risedronate for Paget's disease. N Engl J Med 2005;353:898–908.

CHAPTER 100

Rheumatoid Arthritis

ARTHUR A. SCHUNA

KEY CONCEPTS

❶ Rheumatoid arthritis (RA) is a systemic disease characterized by symmetrical inflammation of joints yet may involve other organ systems.

❷ Control of inflammation is the key to slowing or preventing disease progression as well as managing symptoms.

❸ Drug therapy should be only part of a comprehensive program for patient management which would also include physical therapy, exercise, and rest. Assistive devices and orthopedic surgery may be necessary in some patients.

❹ Disease-modifying antirheumatic drugs (DMARDs) or biologic agents should be started within 3 months of the diagnosis of RA.

❺ Nonsteroidal antiinflammatory drugs and/or corticosteroids should be considered adjunctive therapy early in the course of treatment and as needed if symptoms are not adequately controlled with DMARDs.

❻ When DMARDs used singly are ineffective or not adequately effective, combination therapy with two or more DMARDs or a DMARD plus biologic agent may be used to induce a response.

❼ Patients require careful monitoring for toxicity and therapeutic benefit for the duration of treatment.

Rheumatoid arthritis (RA) is the most common systemic inflammatory disease characterized by symmetrical joint involvement. Extraarticular involvement, including rheumatoid nodules, vasculitis, eye inflammation, neurologic dysfunction, cardiopulmonary disease, lymphadenopathy, and splenomegaly, can be manifestations of the disease. Although the usual disease course is chronic, some patients will enter a remission spontaneously.

EPIDEMIOLOGY

Rheumatoid arthritis is estimated to have a prevalence of 1% and does not have any racial predilections. It can occur at any age, with increasing prevalence up to the seventh decade of life. The disease is 3 times more common in women. In people ages 15 to 45 years, women predominate by a ratio of 6:1; the sex ratio is approximately equal among patients in the first decade of life and in those older than age 60 years.

Epidemiologic data suggest that a genetic predisposition and exposure to unknown environmental factors may be necessary for expression of the disease. The major histocompatibility complex molecules, located on T lymphocytes, appear to have an important role in most patients with RA. These molecules can be characterized using human lymphocyte antigen (HLA) typing. A majority of patients with RA have HLA-DR4, HLA-DR1, or both antigens in the major histocompatibility complex region. Patients with HLA-DR4 antigen are 3.5 times more likely to develop RA than those patients who have other HLA-DR antigens.[1] Although the major histocompatibility complex region is important, it is not the sole determinant, because patients can have the disease without these HLA types. Rheumatoid arthritis is 6 times more common among dizygotic twins and nontwin children of parents with rheumatoid factor-positive, erosive rheumatoid arthritis when compared with children whose parents do not have the disease. If one of a pair of monozygotic twins is affected, the other twin has a 30 times greater risk of developing the disease.[2,3]

PATHOPHYSIOLOGY

❶ Chronic inflammation of the synovial tissue lining the joint capsule results in the proliferation of this tissue. The inflamed, proliferating synovium characteristic of rheumatoid arthritis is called *pannus*. This pannus invades the cartilage and eventually the bone surface, producing erosions of bone and cartilage and leading to destruction of the joint. The factors that initiate the inflammatory process are unknown.

The immune system is a complex network of checks and balances designed to discriminate self from non-self (foreign) tissues. It helps rid the body of infectious agents, tumor cells, and products associated with the breakdown of cells. In rheumatoid arthritis, this system no longer can differentiate self from non-self tissues and attacks the synovial tissue and other connective tissues.

The immune system has both humoral and cell-mediated functions (Fig. 100–1). The humoral component is necessary for the formation of antibodies. These antibodies are produced by plasma cells, which are derived from B lymphocytes. Most patients with RA form antibodies called *rheumatoid factors*. Rheumatoid factors have not been identified as pathogenic, nor does the quantity of these circulating antibodies always correlate with disease activity. Seropositive patients tend to have a more aggressive course of their illness than do seronegative patients. Immunoglobulins can activate the complement system. The complement system amplifies the immune response by encouraging chemotaxis, phagocytosis, and

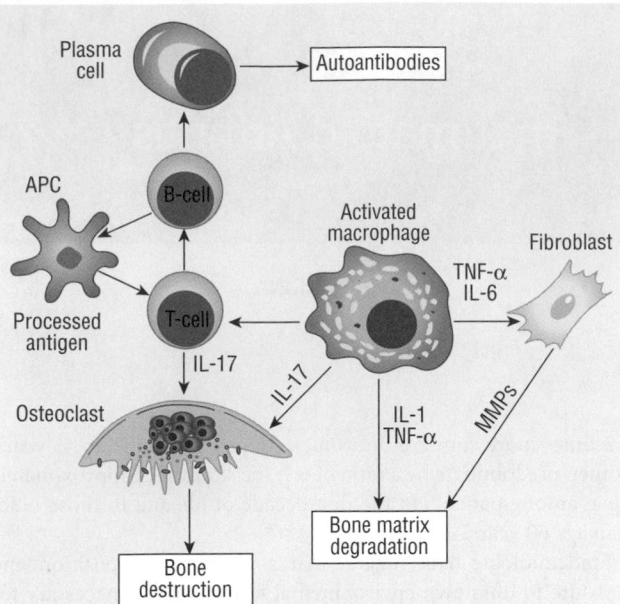

FIGURE 100-1. Pathogenesis of the inflammatory response. Antigen-presenting cells process and present antigens to T cells which may stimulate B cells to produce antibodies and osteoclasts to destroy and remove bone. Macrophages stimulated by the immune response can stimulate T cells and osteoclasts to promote inflammation. They also can stimulate fibroblasts which produce matrix metalloproteinases to degrade the bone matrix and produce proinflammatory cytokines. Activated T cells and macrophages release factors that promote tissue destruction, increase blood flow, and result in cellular invasion of synovial tissue and joint fluid. (APC, antigen-presenting cell; MMP, matrix metalloproteinase; IL, interleukin; TNF-α, tumor necrosis factor α.)

the release of lymphokines by mononuclear cells, which are then presented to T lymphocytes. The processed antigen is recognized by major histocompatibility complex proteins on the lymphocyte, which activates it to stimulate the production of T and B cells. The proinflammatory cytokines tumor necrosis factor (TNF), interleukin (IL)-1 and IL-6 are key substances in the initiation and continuance of rheumatoid inflammation. Lymphocytes may be either B cells (derived from bone marrow) or T cells (derived from thymus tissue). T cells may be either CD4+ (T-helper) or CD8+ (cytotoxic or killer) T cells. There are two subtypes of T-helper cells: TH$_1$, which promote inflammation by producing interferon-γ, tumor necrosis factor, and IL-2; and TH$_2$, which produce the antiinflammatory cytokines IL-4, IL-5, and IL-10. In addition to TH$_1$-TH$_2$, a third type of T cell has been identified known as TH$_{17}$. It can produce IL-17. IL-17 can induce proinflammatory cytokines in fibroblasts and synoviocytes and stimulate the release of matrix metalloproteinases and other cytotoxic substances which leads to cartilage destruction. CD8+ killer T cells have a regulatory effect on the immune process by suppressing activity of CD4+ cells through release of antiinflammatory cytokines and promoting apoptosis (cell death). Activated T cells produce cytotoxins, which are directly toxic to tissues, and cytokines, which stimulate further activation of inflammatory processes and attract cells to areas of inflammation. Macrophages are stimulated to release prostaglandins and cytotoxins.[4–6] T-cell activation requires both stimulation by proinflammatory cytokines as well as interaction between cell surface receptors, called co-stimulation. One of these costimulation interactions is between CD28 and CD80/86. The binding of the CD80/86 receptor by abatacept has proved to be an effective treatment for RA but preventing costimulation interactions between T cells.[7]

Although it has been suggested that T cells play a key role in the pathogenesis of RA, B cells clearly have an equally important role. Evidence for this importance may be found in the effectiveness of B-cell depletion using rituximab in controlling rheumatoid inflammation. Activated B cells produce plasma cells, which form antibodies. These antibodies in combination with complement result in the accumulation of polymorphonuclear leukocytes, which release cytotoxins, oxygen free radicals, and hydroxyl radicals that promote cellular damage to synovium and bone. The benefits of B-cell depletion occur even though antibody formation is not suppressed with rituximab therapy suggesting other mechanisms play a role in reducing RA activity. B cells produce cytokines that may alter the function of other immune cells, and they also have the ability to process antigens and act as antigen-presenting cells, which interact with T cells to activate the immune process.[8–11]

In the synovial membrane, CD4+ T cells are abundant and communicate with macrophages, osteoclasts, fibroblasts and chondrocytes either through direct cell–cell interactions using cell surface receptors or through proinflammatory cytokines such as TNF-α, IL-1, and IL-6. These cells produce metalloproteinases and other cytotoxic substances, which lead to the erosion of bone and cartilage. They also release substances promoting growth of blood vessels and adhesion molecules, which assists in proinflammatory cell trafficking and attachment of fibroblasts to cartilage and eventual synovial invasion and destruction.[12–14]

Vasoactive substances also play a role in the inflammatory process. Histamine, kinins, and prostaglandins are released at the site of inflammation. These substances increase both blood flow to the site of inflammation and the permeability of blood vessels. These substances cause the edema, warmth, erythema, and pain associated with joint inflammation and make it easier for granulocytes to pass from blood vessels to the site of inflammation.

CLINICAL PRESENTATION OF RHEUMATOID ARTHRITIS

Symptoms

Joint pain and stiffness of more than 6 weeks' duration. May also experience fatigue, weakness, low-grade fever, loss of appetite. Muscle pain and afternoon fatigue may also be present. Joint deformity is generally seen late in the disease.

Signs

Tenderness with warmth and swelling over affected joints usually involving hands and feet. Distribution of joint involvement is frequently symmetrical. Rheumatoid nodules may also be present.

Laboratory Tests

Rheumatoid factor (RF) detectable in 60% to 70%.

Anticyclic citrullinated peptide (anti-CCP) antibodies have similar sensitivity to RF (50%–85%) but are more specific (90%–95%) and are present earlier in the disease.

Elevated erythrocyte sedimentation rate and C-reactive protein are markers for inflammation.

Normocytic normochromic anemia is common as is thrombocytosis.

Other Diagnostic Tests

Joint fluid aspiration may show increased white blood cell counts without infection, crystals.

Joint radiographs may show periarticular osteoporosis, joint space narrowing, or erosions.

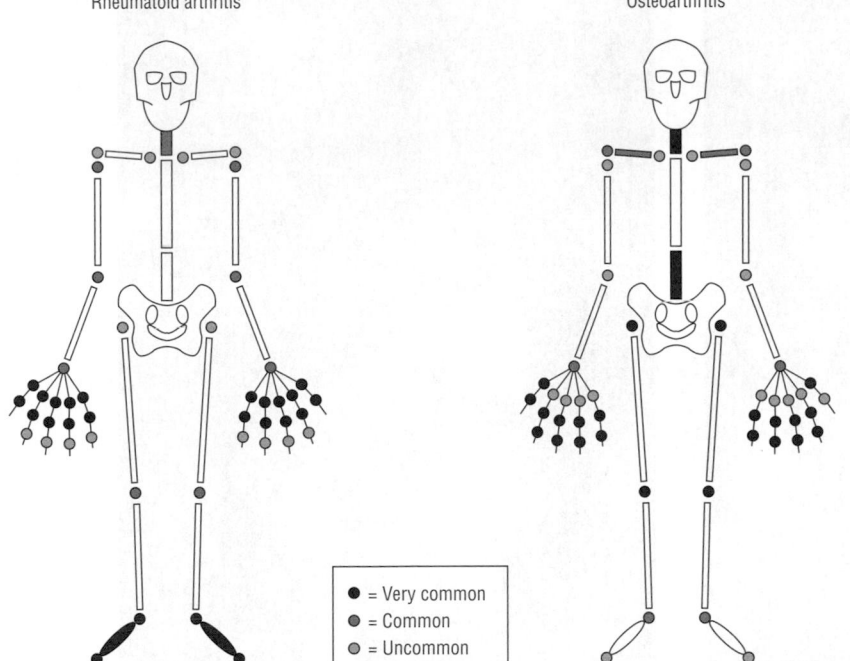

Rheumatoid arthritis   Osteoarthritis

● = Very common
● = Common
● = Uncommon

FIGURE 100-2. Patterns of joint involvement in rheumatoid arthritis and osteoarthritis.

The end results of the chronic inflammatory changes are variable. Loss of cartilage may result in a loss of the joint space. The formation of chronic granulation or scar tissue can lead to loss of joint motion or bony fusion (called *ankylosis*). Laxity of tendon structures can result in a loss of support to the affected joint, leading to instability or subluxation. Tendon contractures also may occur, leading to chronic deformity.[12,15]

The symptoms of RA usually develop insidiously over the course of several weeks to months. Prodromal symptoms include fatigue, weakness, low-grade fever, loss of appetite, and joint pain. Stiffness and muscle aches (myalgias) may precede the development of joint swelling (synovitis). Fatigue may be more of a problem in the afternoon. During disease flares, the onset of fatigue begins earlier in the day and subsides as disease activity lessens. Most commonly, joint involvement tends to be symmetrical; however, early in the disease some patients present with an asymmetrical pattern involving one or a few joints that eventually develops into the more classic presentation. Approximately 20% of patients develop an abrupt onset of their illness with fevers, polyarthritis, and constitutional symptoms (e.g., depression, anxiety, fatigue, anorexia, and weight loss).[2,3]

No single test or physical finding can be used to make the diagnosis of RA. In early disease the diagnosis can be particularly challenging given that radiographic findings are usually not found and rheumatoid factor test can be undetectable. Duration of joint pain and swelling and morning stiffness lasting more than 1 hour and involvement of three or more joints are important early predictors of the development of persistent erosive rheumatoid arthritis.[16]

JOINT INVOLVEMENT

The joints affected most frequently by rheumatoid arthritis are the small joints of the hands, wrists, and feet (Fig. 100–2). In addition, elbows, shoulders, hips, knees, and ankles may be involved. Patients usually experience joint stiffness that typically is worse in the morning. The duration of stiffness tends to be correlated directly with disease activity, usually exceeds 30 minutes, and may persist all day. Chronic inflammation with lack of an adequate exercise program results in loss of range of motion, atrophy of muscles, weakness, and deformity (Figs. 100–3 and 100–4).

On examination, the swelling of the joints may be visible or may be apparent only by palpation. The swelling feels soft and spongy because it is caused by proliferation of soft tissues or fluid accumulation within the joint capsule. The swollen joint may appear erythematous and feel warmer than nearby skin surfaces, especially early in the course of the disease. In contrast, the swelling associated with osteoarthritis usually is bony (caused by osteophytes) and infrequently is associated with signs of inflammation.

Involvement of the hands and wrists is common in RA. Hand involvement is manifested by pain, swelling, tenderness, and grip weakness during the acute phase and by subluxation, instability, deformity, and muscle atrophy in the chronic phase of the disease. Functional difficulties with clasp, grasp, and pinch alter both strength and fine motor movement.

Deformity of the hand may be seen with chronic inflammation. These changes may alter the mechanics of hand function reducing grip strength and making it difficult to perform usual daily activity.

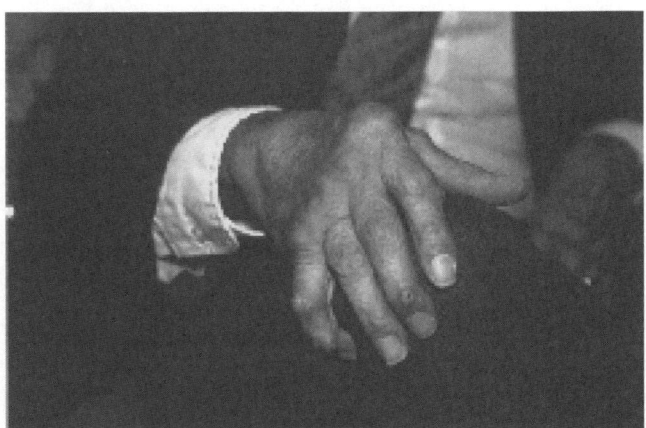

FIGURE 100-3. Deformities of rheumatoid arthritis, with marked ulnar deviation, swan-neck deformity, active synovitis, and nodules. *(Reproduced with permission from Brunicardi FC, Anderson DK, Billiar TR, Dunn DL, Hunter JG, Matthews JB, Pollock RE, Schwartz SI. Schwartz's Principles of Surgery, 8th ed. New York: McGraw-Hill, 2005.)*

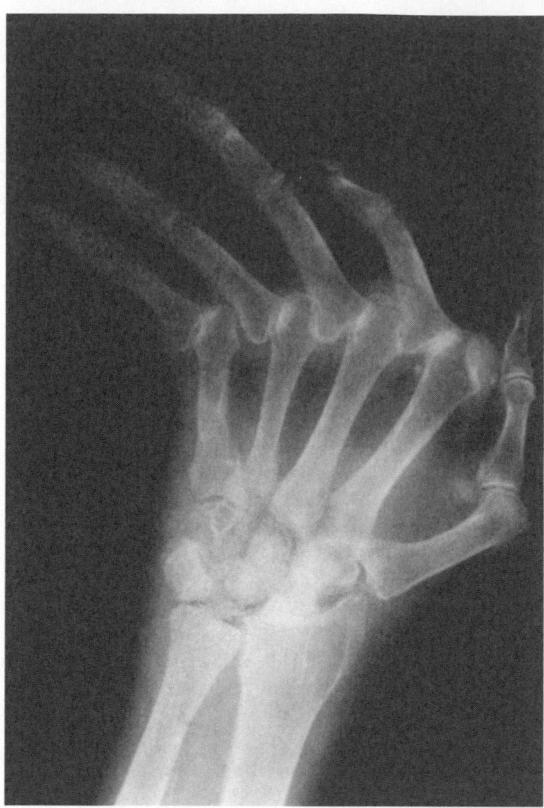 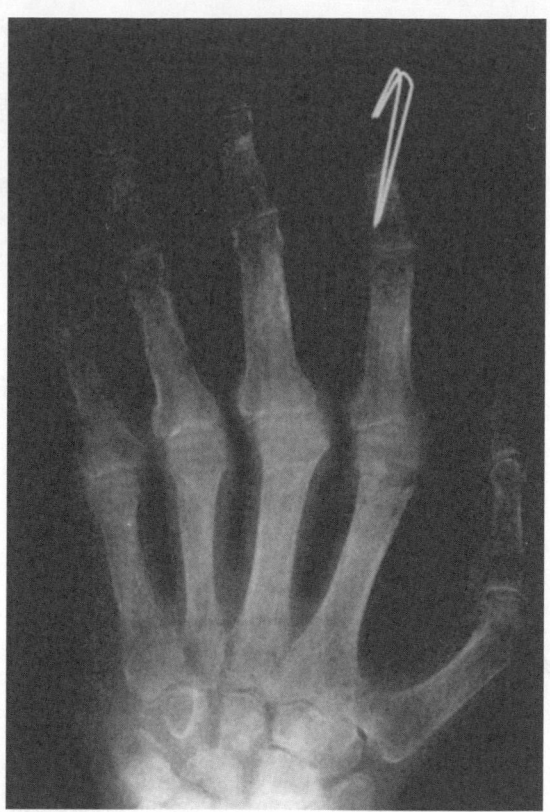

A   B

FIGURE 100-4. *A*. Preoperative view of metacarpophalangeal joints in rheumatoid arthritis. *B*. Following resection arthroplasty. *(Reproduced with permission from Skinner H, ed. Current Diagnosis & Treatment in Orthopedics, 4th ed. New York: McGraw-Hill, 2006:592.)*

Pain in the elbow and shoulder may be the result of true joint inflammation or inflammation of soft-tissue structures such as tendons (tendonitis) or the bursa (bursitis). The knee also can be involved, with loss of cartilage, instability, and joint pain. Synovitis of the knee may cause the formation of a cyst behind the knee called a *popliteal* or *Baker cyst*. These cysts may become painful as they get tense, or they may rupture, producing a clinical picture similar to thrombophlebitis secondary to the release of inflammatory components into the area of the calf muscle (pseudothrombophlebitis syndrome). Chronic joint pain leads to muscle atrophy, which can result in a laxity of the ligamentous structures that support the knee, causing instability. Maintenance of an adequate range of motion of the knee is essential to normal gait.

Foot and ankle involvement in RA is common. The metatarsophalangeal joints are involved frequently in RA, making walking difficult. Subluxation of the metatarsal heads leads to "cock-up" or hammer toe deformities. Subluxation also may cause a flexion deformity at the proximal interphalangeal joint of the toe, leading to pressure necrosis of the skin over the joint secondary to irritation caused by shoes. Hallux valgus (lateral deviation of the digit) and bunion or callus formation may occur at the great toe. A widening of the foot occurs commonly with long-standing disease.

Involvement of the spine usually occurs in the cervical vertebrae; lumbar vertebral involvement is rare. Involvement of the first and second cervical vertebrae (C1–C2) can lead to instability of this joint. Patients with this problem are at a greater risk for spinal cord compression, although this complication is rare.

The temporomandibular joint (jaw) can be affected, resulting in malocclusion and difficulty in chewing food. Inflammation of cartilage in the chest can lead to chest wall pain. Hip pain may occur as a result of destructive changes in the hip joint, soft-tissue inflammation (e.g., bursitis), or referred pain from nerve entrapment at the lumbar vertebrae.

EXTRAARTICULAR INVOLVEMENT

Although joint involvement in RA is a hallmark finding in rheumatoid arthritis, it is important to recognize that, as a systemic disease, other organ systems are often involved.

Rheumatoid Nodules

Rheumatoid nodules occur in 20% of patients with RA. These nodules are seen most commonly on the extensor surfaces of the elbows, forearms, and hands but also may be seen on the feet and at other pressure points. They also may develop in the lung or pleural lining of the lung and, rarely, in the meninges. Rheumatoid nodules usually are asymptomatic and do not require any special intervention. Nodules are observed more commonly in patients with erosive disease.[17]

Vasculitis

Vasculitis usually is seen in patients with long-standing RA. Vasculitis may result in a wide variety of clinical presentations. Invasion of blood vessel walls by inflammatory cells results in an obliteration of the vessel, producing infarction of tissue distal to the area of involvement. Most commonly, small-vessel vasculitis produces infarcts near the ends of the fingers or toes, especially around the nail beds. These infarcts are usually of little consequence.

Vasculitis also may cause the breakdown of skin, especially in the lower extremities, producing ulcers that may be indistinguishable in appearance from stasis ulcers. However, these ulcers do not heal with the usual modes of treatment used for stasis ulcers.

Involvement of larger vessels with vasculitis can result in life-threatening complications. Infarction of vessels supplying blood to nerves can cause irreversible motor deficits. Involvement of vessels supplying other organ systems can lead to visceral involvement and a polyarteritis nodosa-like illness. Aggressive treatment of the inflammatory process is necessary in these patients. Fortunately, the more serious vasculitic picture is seen rarely.

Pulmonary Complications

Rheumatoid arthritis may involve the pleura of the lung, which is often asymptomatic, although pleural effusions may result. Pulmonary fibrosis also may develop as a result of rheumatoid involvement; smoking appears to increase the risk of this complication. Rheumatoid nodules may develop in lung tissue and appear similar to neoplasms on chest radiographs. Interstitial pneumonitis and arteritis are rare, potentially life-threatening complications of RA.

Ocular Manifestations

Ocular manifestations include keratoconjunctivitis sicca and inflammation of the sclera, episclera, and cornea. Atrophy of the lacrimal duct may result in a decrease in tear formation, causing dry and itchy eyes, termed *keratoconjunctivitis sicca*. When this is observed in association with RA, it is referred to as *Sjögren's syndrome*. Artificial tears may be used to relieve symptoms. The salivary glands may also be involved in Sjögren's syndrome, resulting in dry mouth (xerostomia). Inflammation of the superficial layers of the sclera (episcleritis) is generally self-limiting. Involvement of deeper tissues (scleritis) usually results in a more serious, painful, and chronic inflammation. Rheumatoid nodules may develop on the sclera.

Cardiac Involvement

The heart is sometimes affected by RA. Rheumatoid arthritis is associated with an increased risk of cardiovascular mortality. This risk appears to be higher in those with more active inflammation and is reduced with treatment, particularly with methotrexate.[18,19] Pericarditis may occur, resulting in the accumulation of fluid. Although many patients show evidence of previous pericarditis at autopsy, the development of clinically evident pericarditis with tamponade is a rare complication. Cardiac conduction abnormalities and aortic valve incompetence, caused by aortic root dilation, may occur. Myocarditis is a rare complication of RA.

Felty's Syndrome

Rheumatoid arthritis in association with splenomegaly and neutropenia is known as *Felty's syndrome*. Thrombocytopenia also may be a manifestation of the syndrome. Patients with Felty's syndrome and severe leukopenia are more susceptible to infection. The decrease in granulocytes appears to be mediated by the immune system because splenectomy does not result in improvement of the patient.[17]

Other Complications

Lymphadenopathy may occur in patients with RA, particularly in nodes proximal to more actively involved joints. Renal involvement is rare but can be associated with treatment, including nonsteroidal antiinflammatory drugs (NSAIDs), gold salts, and penicillamine. Amyloidosis is a rare complication of longstanding RA. It appears to be more common in Europe than in the United States.

LABORATORY FINDINGS

Hematologic tests often reveal a mild to moderate anemia with normocytic, normochromic indices. The hematocrit may fall as low as 30%. The anemia is usually inversely related to inflammatory disease activity and is referred to as an *anemia of chronic disease*. This type of anemia does not respond to iron therapy and can present a diagnostic dilemma because NSAIDs may induce gastritis and chronic blood loss, leading to iron-deficiency anemia. Laboratory tests useful in differentiating these anemias include stool guaiac (or other stool tests for occult blood), serum iron-to-iron-binding capacity ratio (decreased in iron deficiency), ferritin (decreased in iron deficiency), and mean corpuscular volume (more likely to be decreased in iron deficiency). Other causes of anemia also must be considered in the differential diagnosis (see Chapters 109 and 111).

Thrombocytosis is another common hematologic finding with active RA. Platelet counts rise and fall in direct correlation with disease activity in many patients. Thrombocytopenia may result from toxicity of immunosuppressive therapy. Thrombocytopenia also may be observed in Felty's syndrome or vasculitis.

Although leukopenia is associated with Felty's syndrome, it also may result from toxicity of methotrexate, gold, sulfasalazine, penicillamine, and immunosuppressive drugs. Leukocytosis is seen commonly as a result of corticosteroid treatment.

The erythrocyte sedimentation rate is usually elevated in patients with RA and other inflammatory diseases. This test is very nonspecific, and although the erythrocyte sedimentation rate usually falls as patients respond to therapy, there is a large variability among patients in response to treatment. C-reactive protein is another nonspecific marker for inflammatory arthritis when it is elevated. This protein is produced by the liver in response to certain cytokines.

Rheumatoid factor is present in 60% to 70% of patients with RA. The usual laboratory test for rheumatoid factor is an antibody specific for immunoglobulin (Ig)M rheumatoid factor. Patients with RA and a negative test for rheumatoid factor may have IgG or IgA rheumatoid factors, but tests for these are not routinely available. Rheumatoid factor tests may be reported positive at a specific serum dilution. Serum is diluted to a standard series of dilutions; the greatest dilution that yields a positive test result will be reported (e.g., rheumatoid factor positive at 1:640). Some laboratories quantify rheumatoid factor rather than using titers. Higher dilutional titers or serum concentrations of rheumatoid factors usually indicate a more severe disease, but like the erythrocyte sedimentation rate, the large interpatient variability makes this test unreliable as a means of assessing patient progress. Rheumatoid factor may be positive in patients without RA (Table 100–1).

Anticyclic citrullinated peptide antibody has similar sensitivity for RA, being found in 50% to 85% of patients with the disease, but is

TABLE 100-1	Diseases Associated with a Positive Rheumatoid Factor

Rheumatic diseases
   Rheumatoid arthritis
   Sjögren's syndrome (with or without arthritis)
   Systemic lupus erythematosus
   Progressive systemic sclerosis
   Polymyositis/dermatomyositis
Infectious diseases
   Bacterial endocarditis
   Tuberculosis
   Syphilis
   Infectious mononucleosis
   Infectious hepatitis
   Leprosy
Other causes
   Aging
   Interstitial pulmonary fibrosis
   Cirrhosis of the liver
   Chronic active hepatitis
   Sarcoidosis

more specific (90%–95%) and is detectable very early in the disease. Many rheumatologists will do both tests in evaluating new patients.

Antinuclear antibodies are detected in 25% of patients with RA. These antibodies usually have a diffuse pattern of immunofluorescence. Tests for antibodies to double-stranded DNA (usually positive in systemic lupus erythematosus) are negative. Serum complement is usually normal, although complement concentrations of joint fluid often are depressed from consumption secondary to the inflammatory process. In patients with vasculitis, serum complement concentrations may be low.[20,21]

Synovial fluid usually is turbid because of the large number of leukocytes in inflammatory fluid. White cell counts of 5,000 to 50,000/mm³ (5×10^9 to 50×10^9/L) are not uncommon in inflamed joints. The fluid is usually less viscous than that in normal joints or in fluid associated with osteoarthritis. Glucose concentrations of joint fluid are normal or low compared with those in serum drawn at the same time as synovial aspirates. The decrease is not as profound as the decrease associated with joint infection or systemic lupus erythematosus.

Early radiographic manifestations of RA include soft-tissue swelling and osteoporosis near the joint (periarticular osteoporosis). Joint space narrowing occurs as a result of cartilage degradation. Erosions tend to occur later in the course of the disease and usually are seen first in the metacarpophalangeal and proximal interphalangeal joints of the hands and the metatarsophalangeal joints of the feet. Periodic joint radiographs are a useful way of evaluating disease progression.

Seronegative Inflammatory Arthritis

Although RA may have a negative rheumatoid factor titer, a number of other systemic inflammatory arthritic conditions exist including psoriatic arthritis, reactive arthritis, ankylosing spondylitis, and arthritis associated with inflammatory bowel disease. These conditions often tend to be less aggressive than what is typically seen with RA. Detailed discussion about these conditions is beyond the scope of this chapter, but further information may be found elsewhere.[2] Management principles are similar to those for RA.

TREATMENT

Rheumatoid Arthritis

■ DESIRED OUTCOME

❷ The primary objective is to improve or maintain functional status, thereby improving quality of life. Treatment of RA is a multifaceted approach that includes pharmacologic and nonpharmacologic therapies. Recent emphasis has been placed on aggressive treatment early in the disease course. The ultimate goal is to achieve complete disease remission, although this goal may not be possible to achieve in some patients. Additional goals of treatment include controlling disease activity and joint pain, maintaining the ability to function in daily activities or work, improving the quality of life, and slowing destructive joint changes.

■ NONPHARMACOLOGIC THERAPY

❸ Rest, occupational therapy, physical therapy, use of assistive devices, weight reduction, and surgery are the most useful types of nonpharmacologic therapy used in patients with RA. Rest is an essential component of a nonpharmacologic treatment plan. It relieves stress on inflamed joints and prevents further joint destruction. Rest also aids in alleviation of pain. Too much rest and

immobility, however, may lead to decreased range of motion and, ultimately, muscle atrophy, and contractures.

Occupational and physical therapy can provide the patient with skills and exercises necessary to increase or maintain mobility. These disciplines also may provide patients with supportive and adaptive devices such as canes, walkers, and splints.

Other nonpharmacologic therapeutic options include weight loss and surgery. Weight reduction helps to alleviate inflamed joint stress. This should be instituted and monitored with close supervision of a healthcare professional. Tenosynovectomy, tendon repair, and joint replacements are surgical options for patients with RA. Such management is reserved for patients with severe disease.[22-24]

■ PHARMACOLOGIC THERAPY

❹ ❺ A disease-modifying antirheumatic drug (DMARD) should be started within the first 3 months of symptom onset (Fig. 100–5).[22] Early introduction of DMARDs results in a more favorable outcome.[25-30] NSAIDs and/or corticosteroids may be used for symptomatic relief if needed. They provide relatively rapid improvement in symptoms compared with DMARDs, which may take weeks to months before benefit is seen; however, NSAIDs have no impact on disease progression and the long-term complication risk of corticosteroids make them less desirable.[28]

Early treatment with DMARDs can reduce mortality. Patients with RA have increased mortality compared to people without the disease. In one trial, methotrexate reduced risk of mortality.[18] Early treatment with DMARDs in patients followed for up to 10 years had mortality rates similar to patients without the disease.[31]

DMARDs including biologic agents should be used in all patients except those with limited disease. DMARDs commonly used include methotrexate, hydroxychloroquine, sulfasalazine, and leflunomide. The biologic agents that have disease-modifying activity include the anti-TNF drugs (etanercept, infliximab, adalimumab, certolizumab, golimumab), the costimulation modulator abatacept, and rituximab, which depletes peripheral B cells. Less frequently used are the IL-1 receptor antagonist anakinra, azathioprine, D-penicillamine, gold (including auranofin), minocycline, cyclosporine, and cyclophosphamide. This is due to either less efficacy, high toxicity, or both. The order in which the first-line agents are used is not clearly defined, although methotrexate is often chosen because long-term data suggests superior outcomes with methotrexate than with other DMARDs and a lower cost than biologic agents. Leflunomide appears to have similar long-term efficacy as that of methotrexate.[32]

The biologics have proven effective for patients who fail treatment with other DMARDs. Infliximab should be given in combination with methotrexate to prevent development of antibodies that may reduce drug efficacy or induce allergic reactions. Methotrexate

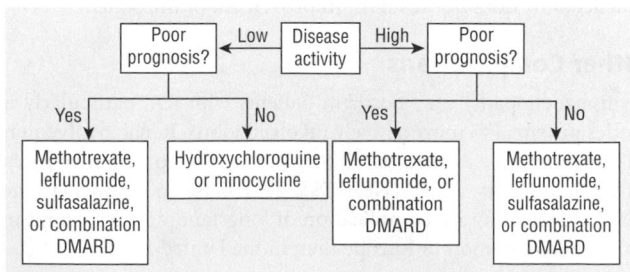

FIGURE 100-5. Algorithm for treatment of rheumatoid arthritis using non-biologic DMARDs. Poor prognosis is defined as limitation in function, extra-articular findings (rheumatoid nodules, vasculitis, Felty syndrome, Sjogren syndrome, rheumatoid lung findings, erosions on radiograph). (DMARD, disease-modifying antirheumatic drug; MTX, methotrexate; NSAID, nonsteroidal antiinflammatory drug.)

in combination with other biologics is more effective than biologic monotherapy and the combination is frequently used.[23]

❻ Combination therapy with two or more DMARDs may be effective when single-DMARD treatment is unsuccessful.[28,33–39] One study suggests that the initial combination therapy with either methotrexate, sulfasalazine plus prednisone, or infliximab plus methotrexate were superior to more conventional sequential monotherapy or step-up combinations of DMARDs in early rheumatoid arthritis.[35] For patients with moderate to high disease activity, the American College of Rheumatology recommendations for nonbiologic and biologic DMARDs are dual DMARD combinations of methotrexate plus hydroxychloroquine, methotrexate plus leflunomide, or methotrexate plus sulfasalazine. They also recommend the triple combination of sulfasalazine, hydroxychloroquine, and methotrexate.[23]

Corticosteroids can be used in various ways. They are valuable in controlling symptoms before the onset of action of DMARDs. A burst of corticosteroids can be used in acute flares. Continuous low doses may be adjuncts when DMARDs do not provide adequate disease control. Corticosteroids may be injected into joints and soft tissues to control local inflammation. Corticosteroids seldom should be used as monotherapy. There are data to suggest they have disease-modifying activity;[35,36,40] however, it is preferable to avoid chronic use when possible to avoid long-term complications. NSAIDs and DMARDs have steroid-sparing properties that permit reductions of corticosteroid doses.

As immunosuppression may reduce the ability to mount an antibody response, the need for immunizations should be assessed, and these should be administered if needed before nonbiologic or biologic DMARDs are started.[23] Postvaccination antibody titers seem to be only minimally affected by conventional DMARDs and TNF antagonists. Rituximab and abatacept seem to reduce the ability to develop antibodies after vaccination. Live vaccines are not recommended for patients taking biologic DMARDs.[41]

The American College of Rheumatology published recommendations for use of nonbiologic and biologic DMARDs in 2008. These recommendations are not intended to be prescriptive but provide guidance for treatment choice. Recommendations are given based on disease duration, degree of disease activity, and likely prognosis. The recommendations take into account barriers to treatment, including cost and insurance restrictions, by suggesting treatment options with and without expensive biologic treatments. Simplified algorithms summarizing these treatment recommendations are provided in Figures 100–5 and 100–6. For more details, see the published recommendation.[23]

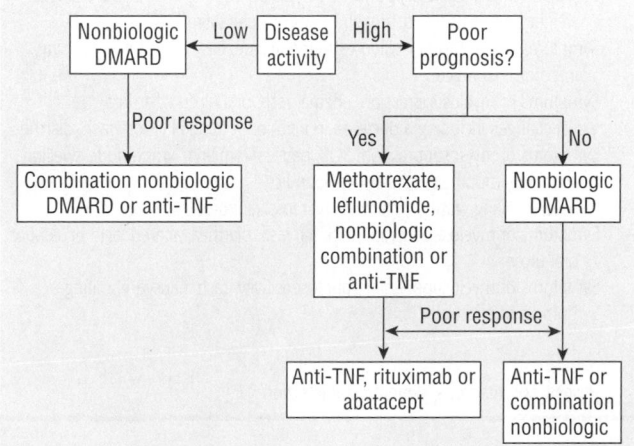

FIGURE 100–6. Algorithm for treatment of rheumatoid arthritis using biologic agents.

❼ Tables 100–2, 100–3, and 100–4 provide monitoring parameters and dosing guidelines for DMARDs and NSAIDs used in rheumatoid arthritis.

Nonsteroidal Antiinflammatory Drugs

NSAIDs should seldom be used as monotherapy for rheumatoid arthritis because they do not alter the course of the disease; instead, they should be viewed as adjuncts to DMARD treatment. NSAIDs possess both analgesic and antiinflammatory properties and reduce stiffness associated with RA. NSAIDs mainly inhibit prostaglandin synthesis, which is only a small portion of the inflammatory cascade. For details on these agents see Chapter 101, Osteoarthritis.

Methotrexate

Methotrexate is now considered the nonbiologic DMARD of choice by many rheumatologists for treating RA. In psoriatic arthritis it not only treats the joint symptoms but also improves the skin disease for most patients. Methotrexate is contraindicated in pregnant and nursing women. It is also contraindicated in patients with chronic liver disease, immunodeficiency, pleural or peritoneal effusions, leukopenia, thrombocytopenia, preexisting blood disorders, and a creatinine clearance of less than 40 mL/min.

Absorption of methotrexate is variable and averages approximately 70% of an oral dose. Methotrexate is 35% to 50% bound to albumin; it may be displaced by highly protein-bound drugs such as NSAIDs, but the clinical importance of this interaction in the relatively low doses of methotrexate used in RA is unknown. Methotrexate is extensively metabolized intracellularly to polyglutamated derivatives. It is excreted by the kidney, 80% unchanged, by glomerular filtration and active transport. Some methotrexate may be reabsorbed, but this transport process may be saturated even with low doses, resulting in increased renal clearance.

Methotrexate inhibits cytokine production, inhibits purine biosynthesis, and may stimulate release of adenosine, all of which may lead to its antiinflammatory properties. The drug has a fairly rapid onset of action; results may be seen as early as 2 to 3 weeks after starting therapy. Some 45% to 67% of patients remain on methotrexate therapy in studies ranging from 5 to 7 years.[42,43] Methotrexate may be given intramuscularly, subcutaneously, or orally. Doses greater than 15 mg per week generally are given parenterally because of decreased oral bioavailability of larger doses.

The toxicities of methotrexate therapy are mainly gastrointestinal, hematologic, pulmonary, and hepatic. Stomatitis occurs in 3% to 10% of patients and may be painful or painless. Diarrhea, nausea, and vomiting may occur in up to 10% of patients. The most common hematologic toxicity is thrombocytopenia in 1% to 3% of patients. Leukopenia also may occur, but in a smaller number of patients. Although pulmonary fibrosis and pneumonitis can be severe adverse effects, they are rare.

Elevated liver enzymes may occur in up to 15% of patients; cirrhosis is rare. Liver function tests, aspartate aminotransferase or alanine aminotransferase, should be performed periodically. Methotrexate should be discontinued if these test values show sustained results greater than twice the upper limits of normal. An albumin blood level also should be checked periodically as a sign of liver toxicity because some patients may not have liver inflammation manifested by aspartate aminotransferase or alanine aminotransferase elevation. Liver biopsy is now recommended before beginning methotrexate therapy only for patients with a history of excessive alcohol use, ongoing hepatitis B or C infection, or recurring elevation of aspartate aminotransferase. Biopsies dur-

TABLE 100-2 Usual Doses and Monitoring Parameters for Antirheumatic Drugs

Drug	Usual Dose	Initial	Maintenance
Nonsteroidal anti-inflammatory drugs	See Table 101–2 in Chap. 101	S_{cr} or BUN, CBC q 2–4 wk p starting therapy × 1–2 mo salicylates: serum salicylate levels if therapeutic dose and no response	Same as initial plus stool guaiac q 6–12 mo
Methotrexate	Oral or IM: 7.5–15 mg q wk	Baseline: AST, ALT, alk phos, alb, t. bili, hep B & C studies, CBC w/plt, S_{cr}	CBC w/plt, AST, alb q 1–2 mo
Leflunomide	Oral: 100 mg daily for 3 days then 10–20 mg daily or 10–20 mg daily without loading dose	Baseline: ALT, CBC with platelets	CBC with platelets and ALT monthly initially and then every 6–8 wk
Hydroxychloroquine	Oral: 200–300 mg bid, after 1–2 mo may to 200 mg bid or daily	Baseline: color fundus photography and automated central perimetric analysis	Ophthalmoscopy q 9–12 mo and Amsler grid at home q 2 wk
Sulfasalazine	Oral: 500 mg bid, then ? to 1 g bid max	Baseline: CBC w/plt, then q week × 1 month	Same as initial–q 1–2 mo
Minocycline	Oral 100–200 mg daily	None	None
Etanercept	50 mg SC weekly	Tuberculin skin test	None
Infliximab	3 mg/kg IV at 0, 2, 6 weeks then q 8 weeks	Tuberculin skin test	None
Adalimumab	40 mg SC q 2 weeks	Tuberculin skin test	None
Rituximab	1,000 mg twice, 2 weeks apart	None	None
Abatacept	<60 kg (<132 lbs)–500 mg 60–100 kg (132–220 lbs)–750 mg >100 kg (>220 lbs)–1,000 mg	None	None
Tocilizumab	4–8 mg/kg q 4 weeks	AST/ALT, CBC w/plt, lipids	AST/ALT, CBC w/plt, lipids q 4–8 weeks
Anakinra	100 mg SC daily	Neutrophil count	Neutrophil count monthly for 3 months then quarterly up to 1 year
Auranofin	Oral: 3 mg daily to bid	Baseline: UA, CBC w/plt	Same as initial–q 1–2 mo
Gold thiomalate	IM: 10 mg test dose, then weekly dosing 25–50 mg, after response may ↑ dosing interval	Baseline & until stable: UA, CBC w/plt preinjection	Same as initial–every other dose
Azathioprine	Oral: 50–150 mg daily	CBC w/plt, AST q 2 weeks × 1–2 months	Same as initial–q 1–2 mo
D-Penicillamine	Oral: 125–250 mg daily, may ↑ by 125–250 mg q 1–2 months, max 750 mg daily	Baseline: UA, CBC w/plt, then q week × 1 month	Same as initial–q 1–2 mo, but q 2 wk if dose change
Cyclophosphamide	Oral: 1–2 mg/kg/day	UA, CBC w/plt q week × 1 month	Same as initial–q 2–4 wk
Cyclosporine	Oral: 2.5 mg/kg/day	S_{cr}, blood pressure q month	Same as initial
Corticosteroids	Oral, IV, IM, IA, and soft-tissue injections: variable	Glucose, blood pressure q 3–6 months	Same as initial

alb, albumin; alk phos, alkaline phosphatase; ALT, alanine aminotransferase; AST, aspartate aminotransferase; BUN, blood urea nitrogen; CBC, complete blood count; hep, hepatitis; IA, intraarticular; IM, intramuscular; IV, intravenous; p, after; plt, platelet; q, every; S_{cr}, serum creatinine; t. bili, total bilirubin; UA, urinalysis.

ing methotrexate therapy are recommended only for patients who develop consistently abnormal liver function tests.[22]

Because the drug is teratogenic, patients should use contraception to avoid pregnancy and discontinue the drug if conception is planned.

Because it is a folic acid antagonist, methotrexate can induce a folic acid deficiency. This deficiency is thought to be partly responsible for methotrexate toxicity, and supplementation with folic acid does alleviate some adverse effects. Addition of folic acid to a methotrexate regimen for RA does not compromise drug efficacy.[22,23,44–47]

TABLE 100-3 Clinical Monitoring of Drug Therapy in Rheumatoid Arthritis

Drug	Toxicities Requiring Monitoring	Symptoms to Inquire About[a]
NSAIDs and salicylates	GI ulceration and bleeding, renal damage	Blood in stool, black stool, dyspepsia, nausea/vomiting, weakness, dizziness, abdominal pain, edema, weight gain, SOBC
Corticosteroids	Hypertension, hyperglycemia, osteoporosis[b]	Blood pressure if available, polyuria, polydipsia, edema, SOB, visual changes, weight gain, headaches, broken bones or bone pain
Azathioprine	Myelosuppression, hepatotoxicity, lymphoproliferative disorders	Symptoms of myelosuppression (extreme fatigue, easy bleeding or bruising, infection), jaundice
Gold (intramuscular or oral)	Myelosuppression, proteinuria, rash, stomatitis	Symptoms of myelosuppression, edema, rash, oral ulcers, diarrhea
Hydroxychloroquine	Macular damage, rash, diarrhea	Visual changes including a decrease in night or peripheral vision, rash, diarrhea
Methotrexate	Myelosuppression, hepatic fibrosis, cirrhosis, pulmonary infiltrates or fibrosis, stomatitis, rash	Symptoms of myelosuppression, SOB, nausea/vomiting, lymph node swelling, coughing, mouth sores, diarrhea, jaundice
Leflunomide	Hepatitis, GI distress, alopecia	Nausea/vomiting, gastritis, diarrhea, hair loss, jaundice
Penicillamine	Myelosuppression, proteinuria, stomatitis, rash, dysgeusia	Symptoms of myelosuppression, edema, rash, diarrhea, altered taste perception, oral ulcers
Sulfasalazine	Melosuppression, rash	Symptoms of myelosuppression, photosensitivity, rash, nausea/vomiting
Etanercept, adalimumab, golimumab, certolizumab, tocilizumab, anakinra	Local injection-site reactions, infection	Symptoms of infection
Infliximab, rituximab, abatacept	Immune reactions, infection	Postinfusion reactions, symptoms of infection

GI, gastrointestinal; NSAIDs, nonsteroidal antiinflammatory drugs; SOB, shortness of breath.
[a]Altered immune function increases infection which should be considered particularly in those patients taking azathioprine, methotrexate, and corticosteroids or other drugs as a symptom of myelosuppression.
[b]Osteoporosis is unlikely to manifest itself early in treatment, but all patients should be taking appropriate steps to prevent bone loss.
From American College of Rheumatology Ad Hoc Committee on Clinical Guidelines. Guidelines for monitoring drug therapy in rheumatoid arthritis. Arthritis Rheum 1996;39:723–731.

TABLE 100-4 Dosage Regimens for Nonsteroidal Antiinflammatory Drugs

| Drug | Adult | Recommended Antiinflammatory Total Daily Dosage | |
		Children	Dosing Schedule
Aspirin	2.6–5.2 g	60–100 mg/kg	Four times daily
Celecoxib	200–400 mg	–	Daily to twice daily
Diclotenac	150–200 mg		Three times per day to 4 times daily
			Extended release twice daily
Diflunisal	0.5–1.5 g	–	Twice daily
Etodolac	0.2–1.2 g (max. 20 mg/kg)	–	Twice daily to 4 times daily
Fenoprofen	0.9–3.0 g	–	Four times daily
Flurbiprofen	200–300 mg	–	Twice daily to 4 times daily
Ibuprofen	1.2–3.2 g	20–40 mg/kg	Three times per day to 4 times daily
Indomethacin	50–200 mg	2–4 mg/kg (max. 200 mg)	Twice daily to 4 times daily
			Extended release daily
Meclofenamate	200–400 mg	–	Three times per day to 4 times per day
Meloxicam	7.5–15 mg	–	Daily
Nabumetone	1–2 g	–	Daily to twice daily
Naproxen	0.5–1.0 g	10 mg/kg	Twice daily
			Extended release–daily
Naproxen sodium	0.55–1.1 g	–	Twice daily
Nonacetylated salicylates	1.2–4.8 g	–	Twice daily to 6 times per day
Oxaprozin	0.6–1.8 g (max. 26 mg/kg)	–	Daily to 3 times a day
Piroxicam	10–20 mg	–	Daily
Sulindac	300–400 mg	–	Twice daily
Tolmetin	0.6–1.8 g	15–30 mg/kg	Twice daily to 4 times daily

Leflunomide

Leflunomide is a DMARD that inhibits pyrimidine synthesis, leading to a decrease in lymphocyte proliferation and modulation of inflammation. It is given as a loading dose of 100 mg daily for 3 days, followed by a maintenance dose of 20 mg daily. Lower doses may be used if patients have gastrointestinal intolerance, complain of hair loss, or have other signs of dose-related toxicity. The loading dose allows the patient to achieve a more rapid therapeutic response, usually within the first month. The long elimination half-life of the drug (14–16 days) would require the patient to take the drug for several months to achieve steady state without a loading dose. Some rheumatologists prefer to begin with maintenance dosing as the loading dose may put the patient at increased risk for toxicity.

Leflunomide has efficacy similar to methotrexate for treating RA. The drug may cause liver toxicity and is contraindicated in patients with preexisting liver disease. Patients taking the drug should have alanine aminotransferase monitored monthly initially and periodically thereafter as long as they continue treatment. Leflunomide may cause bone marrow toxicity and complete blood count with platelets is recommended monthly for 6 months and then every 6 to 8 weeks thereafter.

The drug is teratogenic, and appropriate contraceptive measures are recommended to avoid pregnancy for all sexually active male and female patients who are taking leflunomide. If conception is desired, leflunomide must be discontinued. Because leflunomide undergoes enterohepatic circulation, the drug takes many months to drop to a plasma concentration considered safe during pregnancy (<0.02 μg/mL [<0.02 mg/L; 74 nmol/L]). Cholestyramine may be used to rapidly clear the drug from plasma. In addition to pregnancy, cholestyramine use may be warranted to rapidly clear the drug in the event of severe toxicity.[32,48–51]

Hydroxychloroquine

The pharmacokinetics of hydroxychloroquine are poorly understood. It is well absorbed orally and widely distributed to body tissues. Hydroxychloroquine is partially metabolized in the liver and is excreted by the kidney. The onset of action of hydroxychloroquine may be delayed up to 6 weeks, but the drug is considered a therapeutic failure only when 6 months of therapy without a response has elapsed.

The main advantage of hydroxychloroquine is the lack of myelosuppressive, hepatic, and renal toxicities that may be seen with other DMARDs, which simplifies monitoring. Short-term toxicities of hydroxychloroquine include gastrointestinal effects such as nausea, vomiting, and diarrhea, which can be managed by taking doses with food. Ocular toxicity includes accommodation defects, benign corneal deposits, blurred vision, scotomas (small areas of decreased or absent vision in the visual field), and night blindness. Although the risk of true retinopathy with hydroxychloroquine approaches zero, preretinopathy may occur in 2.7% of patients. All patients must understand the importance of adhering to hydroxychloroquine monitoring guidelines, as delineated in Table 100–2. Any visual change must be reported immediately. Dermatologic toxicities include rash, alopecia, and increased skin pigmentation; neurologic adverse effects such as headache, vertigo, and insomnia usually are mild.[38,52,53]

Sulfasalazine

Sulfasalazine, a prodrug, is cleaved by bacteria in the colon into sulfapyridine and 5-aminosalicylic acid. It is believed that the sulfapyridine moiety is responsible for the agent's antirheumatic properties, although the exact mechanism of action is unknown. Once the colonic bacteria have cleaved sulfasalazine, sulfapyridine and 5-aminosalicylic acid are absorbed rapidly from the gastrointestinal tract. Sulfapyridine distributes rapidly throughout the body, but higher concentrations are found in certain tissues such as serous fluid, liver, and intestines. Both sulfasalazine and its metabolites are excreted in the urine. Antirheumatic effects should be seen in 2 months.

Use of sulfasalazine is often limited by its adverse effects. Gastrointestinal adverse effects such as nausea, vomiting, diarrhea, and anorexia are the most common. These can be minimized by initiating therapy with low doses and titrating gradually to higher doses, dividing the dose more evenly throughout the day, or using enteric-coated preparations. Rash, urticaria, and serum sickness-like reactions can be managed with antihistamines and, if indicated, corticosteroids. If a hypersensitivity reaction occurs, therapy should be stopped immediately and another DMARD substituted. Sulfasalazine is associated with leukopenia, alopecia, stomatitis, and elevated hepatic enzymes. It also may cause the patient's urine and skin to turn a yellow-orange color, which is of no clinical consequence however; patients should be educated about this to avoid premature discontinuance.

Sulfasalazine's absorption can be decreased when antibiotics are used that destroy the colonic bacteria. Sulfasalazine also binds iron supplements in the gastrointestinal tract that can lead to a decreased absorption of sulfasalazine. The administration of these two agents should be separated temporally to avoid this interaction. Sulfasalazine can potentiate warfarin's effects by displacing it from protein-binding sites. Close monitoring of the patient's international normalized ratio is indicated.[54,55]

Minocycline

The tetracycline derivative minocycline has been suggested as a treatment alternative for patients with RA who have low disease activity and without features of poor prognosis. A meta-analysis of 10 clinical trials using tetracyclines for more than 3 months found mild reductions in tender and swollen joint counts and erythrocyte sedimentation rate but no effect on erosion progression; however, the number of patients and treatment duration in the 2 trials that looked at erosions were limited.[56]

The dose of minocycline in RA is 100–200 mg daily.[56]

Adverse effects are uncommon and were reported no more frequently than placebo control groups.[56]

Other Disease-Modifying Antirheumatic Drugs

Gold salts, azathioprine, D-penicillamine, cyclosporine, and cyclophosphamide have all been used to treat RA. Although these drugs can be effective and they may be of value in certain clinical settings, they are used less frequently today because of toxicity, lack of long-term benefit, or both. Tables 100–2 and 100–3 provide dosing information and toxicity information.

Biologic Agents

Biologic agents are genetically engineered protein molecules that block the proinflammatory cytokines TNF-α (infliximab, etanercept, adalimumab, golimumab, and certolizumab), IL-1 (anakinra), and IL-6 (tocilizumab), deplete peripheral B cells (rituximab), or bind to CD80/86 on T cells to prevent the costimulation needed to fully activate T cells (abatacept). These drugs may be effective when other DMARDs fail to achieve adequate responses but are considerably more expensive to use. Other than anakinra and tocilizumab, these agents have no toxicity that requires laboratory monitoring, but they do carry a small increased risk for infection. There is an increased incidence of tuberculosis in patients treated with these agents. Tuberculin skin testing is recommended prior to treatment with these drugs so that latent tuberculosis can be detected.[57–60] Patients with a history of significant tuberculosis exposure or recurrent infection may not be good candidates for these drugs. Those who develop infections while on biologic agents should at least temporarily discontinue them until the infection is cured. Live vaccines should not be given to patients taking biologic agents.

TNF-α Inhibitors

Congestive heart failure (CHF) is a relative contraindication for anti-TNF agents. Increased cardiac mortality has been seen in patients treated with infliximab and etanercept-associated heart failure exacerbations have been documented.[51,61–63] Patients with a history of uncompensated CHF or recent hospital admissions for CHF should not use anti–TNF-α therapy. Patients whose CHF worsens while taking anti–TNF-α therapy should discontinue the drug.

Anti–TNF-α therapy has been reported to induce a multiple sclerosis-like illness or exacerbate multiple sclerosis in patients with the disease. Patients with neurologic symptoms suggestive of multiple sclerosis should discontinue therapy. TNF inhibitors may predispose patients to increased cancer risk, especially lymphoproliferative cancer, as TNF plays a role in ridding the body of cancer cells. The U.S. Food and Drug Administration (FDA) added a black box warning to product labeling for anti-TNF drugs alerting prescribers of increased lymphoproliferative and other cancers in children and adolescents treated with these drugs.[64]

Etanercept Etanercept is a fusion protein consisting of two p75-soluble TNF receptors linked to an Fc fragment of human IgG_1. The drug binds to TNF, making it biologically inactive and preventing it from interacting with the cell-surface TNF receptors that would lead to cell activation.

The drug is given by subcutaneous injection, 50 mg once weekly or 25 mg twice weekly, usually through self-injections or administration by a caregiver. Aside from local injection-site reactions, adverse effects are rare. There are case reports of pancytopenia and neurologic demyelinating syndromes like multiple sclerosis associated with use of etanercept, but these are rare. No laboratory monitoring is required. Clinical trials have used etanercept in patients who failed DMARDs. Response was seen in 60% to 75% of patients. The drug has also been FDA approved for the treatment of juvenile rheumatoid arthritis, ankylosing spondylitis, psoriatic arthritis, and moderate to severe psoriasis. Clinical trials have shown that it slows erosive disease progression to a greater degree than oral methotrexate therapy.[65–70]

Infliximab Infliximab is a chimeric antibody combining portions of mouse and human IgG_1. An anti-TNF antibody was created by exposing mice to human TNF. The binding portion of that antibody was fused to a human constant-region IgG_1 to reduce the antigenicity of the foreign protein. This antibody, when injected in humans, binds to TNF and prevents its interaction with TNF receptors on inflammatory cells.

Infliximab is given by intravenous infusion at a dose of 3 mg/kg at 0, 2, and 6 weeks and then every 8 weeks. To prevent the formation of antibodies to this foreign protein, methotrexate should be given orally in doses typically used to treat RA for as long as the patient continues on infliximab. Antibodies develop in 7% to 15% of patients, which leads to a greater risk of infusion reactions and also may reduce the efficacy of the drug. Loss of response may be seen in patients with RA who have good initial response requiring increased doses or shorter intervals between doses to maintain response. Infusion reactions may occur in any patient treated with the drug. Both acute (within 24 hours of infusion) and delayed (24 hours to 14 days) reactions following infusion have been identified. An acute infusion reaction with symptoms including fever, chills, pruritus, and rash may occur during infusion or within 1 to 2 hours after giving the drug. Treatment includes slowing infusion rates and administering acetaminophen, diphenhydramine, or corticosteroids, depending on the severity of symptoms. Fortunately these reactions are rarely severe or anaphylactic in nature.[71] The drug may increase risk of infection. Autoantibodies and lupus-like syndrome also have been reported. In clinical trials, the combination of methotrexate plus infliximab halted progression of joint damage in patients and was superior to methotrexate monotherapy.[72–74] In addition to rheumatoid arthritis, infliximab is indicated for the treatment of psoriatic arthritis and ankylosing spondylitis.[72,75]

Adalimumab Adalimumab is a human IgG_1 antibody to TNF. Because it has no foreign protein components, it is less antigenic than infliximab. The drug is provided as either premixed syringes or injection pens containing 40 mg, which is administered by subcutaneous injection every 14 days. It has similar response rates to those seen with the other TNF inhibitors. Local injection-site reactions were the most common adverse reactions noted in clinical trials. It has the same precautions regarding tuberculosis and other infections as the other biologics.[76–80]

Golimumab Golimumab is a human antibody to TNF-α. In addition to RA, this agent is also indicated for treatment of psoriatic arthritis and ankylosing spondylitis. The drug is available as an injection pen, through which doses of 50 mg is given monthly by subcutaneous injection. Precautions are similar to other TNF-α inhibitors.

Certolizumab Certolizumab is a humanized antibody specific for human TNF-α. For RA, dosing recommendations are for 400 mg (2 doses of 200 mg) given by subcutaneous injection at weeks 0, 2, and 4 followed by 200 mg every 2 weeks. Precautions and side effects are similar to other TNF-α inhibitors.

Abatacept Abatacept is a costimulation modulator approved for the treatment of RA in patients with moderate to severe disease who fail to achieve an adequate response from one or more DMARDs. By binding to CD80/CD86 receptors on antigen-presenting cells, abatacept inhibits interactions between the antigen-presenting cells and T cells, preventing the T cell from activating to promote the inflammatory process, which results in reductions in cytokines, T-cell proliferation, and other consequences of T-cell activation. Abatacept is a fusion protein made using the extracellular domain of human cytotoxic T-lymphocyte antigen 4 (the binding portion of the drug) and a fragment of the Fc domain of human IgG modified to prevent complement fixation. The drug is given by intravenous infusion based on patient weight (<60 kg [<132 lb]: 500 mg; 60–100 kg [132–220 lb]: 750 mg; >100 kg [>220 lb]: 1,000 mg) every 2 weeks for two doses after the initial dose and then every 4 weeks. The adverse effects include headache, nasopharyngitis, dizziness, cough, back pain, hypertension, dyspepsia, urinary tract infection, rash, and extremity pain reported more frequently than placebo in clinical trials. Infusion reactions were 50% more likely with abatacept than with placebo and there was a slightly higher rate of serious infections with active treatment.[81–83] In patients who failed to achieve adequate responses with TNF-α inhibitors, half had a clinical response to abatacept.[84] Live vaccines should not be given to patients during and for 3 months after the completion of abatacept therapy.[84]

Rituximab Rituximab is a monoclonal chimeric antibody consisting of mostly human protein with the antigen-binding region derived from a mouse antibody to CD20 protein found on the cell surface of mature B lymphocytes. The binding of rituximab to B cells results in nearly complete depletion of peripheral B cells, with a gradual recovery over several months. The prolonged effect on B cells results in a duration of action that allows for intermittent therapy which varies based on reactivation of arthritis symptoms. Rituximab is useful in patients who failed methotrexate or TNF inhibitors.[85–89] Two infusions of 1,000 mg are given 2 weeks apart. Methylprednisolone 100 mg should be given 30 minutes prior to rituximab to reduce the incidence and severity of infusion reactions. Acetaminophen and antihistamines may also be of benefit in patients who have a history of reactions. Methotrexate should be given concurrently in the usual doses used for RA, as the combination has proved to provide the best therapeutic outcomes. Duration of benefit is variable after a course of rituximab and patients will need retreatment with reactivation of their disease. The drug is currently FDA approved for TNF inhibitor treatment failures. Live vaccines should not be given to patients given rituximab.

Tocilizumab IL-6 is a major cytokine believed to have a role in promoting inflammation in RA. Tocilizumab attaches to IL-6 receptors, which prevents the cytokine from interacting with cells. In clinical trials, 4 to 8 mg/kg was given intravenously every 4 weeks. It has been used as monotherapy or in combination with methotrexate. Infusion reactions and increased infection risk have been reported. Additionally, increased plasma lipids have been reported in tocilizumab-treated patients.

Anakinra Anakinra is a naturally occurring IL-1 receptor antagonist. Results of clinical trials suggest it to be less effective than other biologic DMARDs.[90] The American College of Rheumatology did not include anakinra in their RA treatment recommendations due to limited use of this drug, but some patients could benefit from treatment with this drug.[23]

Treatment Strategies for Patients with Suboptimal Response to Biologics

TNF-α antagonists are generally the first biologic agents chosen for use in patients with RA. Approximately 30% of patients discontinue treatment with these drugs because of lack of efficacy or adverse effects.

In such situations, addition of a nonbiologic DMARD may be beneficial if the patient is not already taking one. Dose escalation or decreased interval between infusions may be useful for those patients taking infliximab. Higher doses of other TNF-α inhibitors have not been demonstrated to be effective. Choosing an alternative TNF-α inhibitor may be beneficial for some patients. Treatment with rituximab or abatacept may also prove to be effective in TNF-α treatment failures. Combination biologic DMARD therapy is not recommended because of the increased risk for infection.[91]

Corticosteroids

Corticosteroids are used in RA for their antiinflammatory and immunosuppressive properties. They interfere with antigen presentation to T lymphocytes, inhibit prostaglandin and leukotriene synthesis, and inhibit neutrophil and monocyte superoxide radical generation. Corticosteroids also impair cell migration and cause redistribution of monocytes, lymphocytes, and neutrophils, thus blunting the inflammatory and autoimmune responses.

Oral corticosteroids are absorbed rapidly and completely from the gastrointestinal tract. They are metabolized and inactivated primarily by the liver and excreted in the urine. The elimination half-life of most corticosteroids is sufficiently long that once-daily dosing is possible.

Oral corticosteroids can be used in several ways. They can be used in bridging therapy, continuous low-dose therapy, and short-term, high-dose bursts to control flares. Oral steroids (e.g., prednisone, methylprednisolone) can be used to control pain and synovitis while DMARDs are taking effect. This is termed *bridging therapy* and is often used in patients with debilitating symptoms when DMARD therapy is initiated. Patients with difficult-to-control disease may be placed on low-dose, long-term corticosteroid therapy to control their symptoms. Prednisone doses below 7.5 mg daily are well tolerated but are not devoid of the long-term adverse effects associated with corticosteroids. The lowest dose of corticosteroid that controls symptoms should be used to reduce adverse effects. Alternate-day dosing of low-dose oral corticosteroids usually is ineffective in RA; symptoms usually flare on days without medication. High-dose corticosteroid bursts often are used to suppress disease flares. High doses are sustained for several days until symptoms are controlled, followed by a taper to the lowest effective dose.

Corticosteroids also may be delivered by injection. The intramuscular route may be preferable in patients with adherence problems for short-term therapy. Long-acting depot forms of corticosteroids include triamcinolone acetonide, triamcinolone hexacetonide, and methylprednisolone acetate. This provides the patient with 2 to 6 weeks of symptomatic control. The depot effect provides a physiologic taper, avoiding withdrawal reaction associated with hypothalamic–pituitary axis suppression. Intravenous corticosteroids may be used to provide the patient with large amounts of drug during a steroid burst to control severe symptoms. Intraarticular injections of depot forms of corticosteroids can be useful in treating synovitis and pain when a small number of joints are affected. The onset and duration of symptomatic relief are similar to those of intramuscular injection. The intraarticular route often is preferred because it is associated with the fewest number of systemic adverse effects. If efficacious, intraarticular injections may be repeated every 3 months. No one joint should be injected more than 2 to 3 times per year because of the risk of accelerated joint destruction and atrophy of tendons. Soft tissues such as tendons and bursae also may be injected. This may help control the pain and inflammation associated with these structures. The onset and duration of symptomatic relief are similar to those of intramuscular and intraarticular injections.

The major limitation to the long-term use of corticosteroids is adverse effects. They include hypothalamic-pituitary–adrenal suppression, Cushing's syndrome, osteoporosis, myopathies, glaucoma, cataracts, gastritis, hypertension, hirsutism, electrolyte imbalances, glucose intolerance, skin atrophy, and increased susceptibility to infections. To minimize these effects, use the lowest effective corticosteroid dose and limit the duration of use. Prednisolone 7.5 mg daily results in an average of 9.5% loss of bone density from the spine. Corticosteroids double the risk for osteoporosis in patients.[92] Patients on long-term therapy should be given calcium and vitamin D to minimize bone loss. Alendronate is effective in preventing bone loss in corticosteroid-treated patients and should be considered prophylactically for patients when long-term corticosteroid therapy is anticipated, particularly for patients who are at high risk of bone loss (e.g., postmenopausal women, elderly).[93-96] There is no evidence that corticosteroids alone increase the risk of gastrointestinal ulcerations, although they often have been implicated. Consequently, gastrointestinal protective measures usually are not indicated.[97-99]

■ PHARMACOECONOMIC CONSIDERATIONS

The total cost of treating a patient with RA is estimated to be between $11,500 and $17,000 annually (2008 dollars). Of this, drugs account for roughly 10% of the total, excluding monitoring costs. These costs are approximately three times the cost of medical care for patients of similar age and gender without RA. However, if biologic agents are used, the cost of this drug therapy alone may be $12,000 or more annually. The costs must be balanced against the high cost of disability on earning potential in these patients. Men with RA have average annual wages 50% lower than those of men of similar age without RA. In women with the disease, average annual wages are only 25% of the wages of those women without the disease. The costs of disability make treatment worth the price if disability can be prevented or delayed and patients can continue to function as productive members of society.[100]

CLINICAL CONTROVERSIES

1. The order of DMARD or biologic agent choice is not clearly defined. No direct comparative studies exist for biologics to guide in the determination of optimal treatment order.

2. Should combination DMARD be tried before biologic agents?

3. Even the best therapy available today does not completely eliminate all signs and symptoms of disease for most patients. How much treatment is enough?

4. Some patients show evidence of disease progression in spite of apparent control of clinical symptoms. How can these patients be identified and treatment course changed before progression occurs?

EVALUATION OF THERAPEUTIC OUTCOMES

The evaluation of therapeutic outcomes is based primarily on improvements of clinical signs and symptoms of RA. Clinical signs of improvement include a reduction in joint swelling, decreased warmth over actively involved joints, and decreased tenderness to joint palpation. Improvement in RA symptoms includes reduction in perceived joint pain and morning stiffness, longer time to onset of afternoon fatigue, and improvement in ability to perform activities of daily living. Improvement of activities of daily living may be assessed objectively using a Health Assessment Questionnaire score. Joint radiographs may be of some benefit in assessing the progression of the disease and should show little or no evidence of disease progression if treatment is effective.

Laboratory monitoring is of little value in monitoring individual patient response to therapy. Tables 100–2 and 100–3 provide monitoring of drug toxicity information. Routine monitoring of patients is essential to the safe use of these drugs. In addition, patients should be questioned about symptoms of the adverse effects outlined in the drug section of this chapter.

CONCLUSIONS

Rheumatoid arthritis is the most common inflammatory arthritis, affecting approximately 1% of the population. The disease is characterized by symmetrical swelling and stiffness of the involved joints. The stiffness is usually more prominent in the morning. Extraarticular features of RA include rheumatoid nodules, vasculitis, and ocular, cardiac, and pulmonary complications. The course of the disease is highly variable. Treatment is aimed at relieving pain and inflammation and maintaining and preserving joint function. Nondrug therapy, including exercise and adequate rest periods, should also be used early in the course of treatment. Early use of a DMARD or biologic agent results in better patient outcomes. Methotrexate, sulfasalazine, and hydroxychloroquine are often considered for initial therapy. Biologics have also been shown to be effective in these patients but may be considered second choice because of cost considerations; however, they are effective in patients who fail to achieve adequate response from nonbiologic DMARDs. Combination DMARDs or biologics may be considered in those who fail adequate trials of single-agent therapy. Corticosteroids and NSAIDs may be useful adjuncts for treatment, but because of adverse effects and limited impact on long-term outcomes, they should not be considered as sole treatment for most patients.

ABBREVIATIONS

CHF: congestive heart failure

DMARD: disease-modifying antirheumatic drug

HLA: human lymphocyte antigen

Ig: immunoglobulin

IL: interleukin

NSAID: nonsteroidal antiinflammatory drug

RA: rheumatoid arthritis

TNF-α: tumor necrosis factor α

REFERENCES

1. Smith JB, Haynes MK. Rheumatoid arthritis—A molecular understanding. Ann Intern Med 2002;136(12):908–922.
2. Klippel JH CL, Stone JH, Crofford LJ, White PH, eds. Primer on the Rheumatic Diseases, 13th ed. Atlanta, GA: Arthritis Foundation, 2008.
3. Harris ED, Firestein GS. The clinical features of rheumatoid arthritis. In: Firestein GS, Budd RC, Harris ED, et al., eds. Kelley's Textbook of Rheumatology, 8th ed; MDConsult, 2008. http://www.mdconsult.com.
4. Jiang H, Chess L. Regulation of immune response by T cells. N Engl J Med 2006;354:1166–1176.
5. Brennan FM, McInnes IB. Evidence that cytokines play a role in rheumatoid arthritis. J Clin Invest 2008;118:3537–3545.
6. Moissec P, Korn T, Kuchroo VK. Interleukin-17 and type 17 helper T cells. N Engl J Med 2009;361:888–898.
7. Isaacs JD. Therapeutic t-cell manipulation in rheumatoid arthritis: past, present and future. Rheumatology 2008;49:1461–1468.
8. Tsokos GC. B cells, be gone—B-cell depletion in the treatment of rheumatoid arthritis. N Engl J Med 2004;350(25):2546–2548.
9. Weinstein E, Peeva E, Putterman C, Diamond B. B-cell biology. Rheum Dis Clin North Am 2004;30(1):159–174.
10. Carter RH. B cells in health and disease. Mayo Clin Proc 2006;81:377–384.
11. Youinou P, Taher TE, Pers J-O, Mageed RA, Renaudineau Y. B lymphocyte cytokines and rheumatoid autoimmune disease. Arthritis Rheum 2009;60:1873–1880.
12. Choy EH, Panayi GS. Cytokine pathways and joint inflammation in rheumatoid arthritis. N Engl J Med 2001;344(12):907–916.
13. Arend WP. Physiology of cytokine pathways in rheumatoid arthritis. Arthritis Care Res 2001;45:101–106.
14. Huber LC, Distler O, Tarner I, Gay RE, Gay S, Pap T. Synovial fibroblasts: key players in rheumatoid arthritis. Rheumatology 2006;45:669–675.
15. Firestein GS. Etiology and pathogenesis of rheumatoid arthritis. In: Firestein GS, Budd RC, Harris ED, et al., eds. Kelley's Textbook of Rheumatology, 8th ed; MDConsult, 2008. http://www.mdconsult.com.
16. Visser H. Early diagnosis of rheumatoid arthritis. Best Pract Res Clin Rheumatol 2005;19(1):55–72.
17. Hard ER. Extraarticular manifestations of rheumatoid arthritis. Semin Arthritis Rheum 1979;8:151–176.
18. Choi HK, Hernan MA, Seeger JD, et al. Methotrexate and mortality in patients with rheumatoid arthritis: A prospective study. Lancet 2002;359:1173–1177.
19. Wallberg-Jonsson S, Johansson H, Ohman ML, Rantapaa-Dahlqvist S. Extent of inflammation predicts cardiovascular disease and overall mortality in seropositive rheumatoid arthritis. A retrospective cohort study from disease onset. J Rheumatol 1999;26(12):2562–2571.
20. Colglazier CL, Sutej PG. Laboratory testing in rheumatic diseases: A practical review. South Med J 2005;98(2):185–191.
21. Shmerling RH. Diagnostic tests for rheumatic disease: Clinical utility revisited. South Med J 2005;98(7):704–711.
22. American College of Rheumatology Subcommittee on Rheumatoid Arthritis G. Guidelines for the management of rheumatoid arthritis: 2002 Update. Arthritis Rheum 2002;46(2):328–346.
23. Saag KG, Teng GG, Patkar NM, Anuntiyo J, et al. American College of Rheumatology 2008 recommendations for the use of nonbiologic and biologic disease-modifying antirheumatic drugs in rheumatoid arthritis. Arthritis Rheum 2008;59:762–784.
24. Genovese MC. The treatment of rheumatoid arthritis. In: Firestein GS, Budd RC, Harris ED, et al., eds. Kelley's Textbook of Rheumatology, 8th ed; MDConsult, 2008. http://www.mdconsult.com.
25. Mottonen T, Hannonen P, Korpela M, et al. Delay to institution of therapy and induction of remission using single-drug or combination-disease-modifying antirheumatic drug therapy in early rheumatoid arthritis. Arthritis Rheum 2002;46(4):894–898.
26. Tsakonas E, Fitzgerald AA, Fitzcharles MA, et al. Consequences of delayed therapy with second-line agents in rheumatoid arthritis: A 3-year followup on the Hydroxychloroquine in Early Rheumatoid Arthritis (HERA) study. J Rheumatol 2000;27(3):623–629.
27. Verstappen SM, Jacobs JW, Bijlsma JW, et al. Five-year followup of rheumatoid arthritis patients after early treatment with disease-modifying antirheumatic drugs versus treatment according to the pyramid approach in the first year. Arthritis Rheum 2003;48(7):1797–1807.
28. Goldbach-Mansky R, Lipsky PE. New concepts in the treatment of rheumatoid arthritis. Annu Rev Med 2003;54:197–216.
29. O'Dell JR. Therapeutic strategies for rheumatoid arthritis. N Engl J Med 2004;350(25):2591–2602.
30. Quinn MA, Cox S. The evidence for early intervention. Rheum Dis Clin N Am 2005;31:575–589.
31. Kroot EJ, VanLeeuwen MA, VanRijswijk MH, et al. No increased mortality in patients with rheumatoid arthritis: Up to 10 years of follow up from disease onset. Ann Rheum Dis 2000;59:954–958.
32. Kalden JR, Schattenkirchner M, Sorensen H, et al. The efficacy and safety of leflunomide in patients with active rheumatoid arthritis: A five-year followup study. Arthritis Rheum 2003;48(6):1513–1520.
33. Bingham S, Emery P. Combination therapy in rheumatoid arthritis. Springer Semin Immunopathol 2001;23(1-2):165–183.
34. Dougados M, Combe B, Cantagrel A, et al. Combination therapy in early rheumatoid arthritis: A randomised, controlled, double blind 52 week clinical trial of sulphasalazine and methotrexate compared with the single components. Ann Rheum Dis 1999;58(4):220–225.
35. Goekoop-Reuterman YP, deVries-Bouwstra JK, Allaart CF, et al. Comparison of treatment strategies in early rheumatoid arthritis: A randomized trial. Ann Intern Med 2007;146:406–415.
36. O'Dell JR. Combinations of conventional disease-modifying antirheumatic drugs. Rheum Dis Clin North Am 2001;27(2):415–426, x.
37. Pincus T, O'Dell JR, Kremer JM. Combination therapy with multiple disease-modifying antirheumatic drugs in rheumatoid arthritis: A preventive strategy. Ann Intern Med 1999;131(10):768–774.
38. Kremer JM. Rational use of new and existing disease-modifying agents in rheumatoid arthritis. Ann Intern Med 2001;134(8):695–706.
39. Goekoop-Ruitermann YPM, deVries-Bouwstra JK, Allaart CF, va Zeben D, et al. Comparison of treatment strategies in early rheumatoid arthritis: A randomized trial. Ann Intern Med 2007;146:406–415.
40. Bijlsma JW, Van Everdingen AA, Huisman M, De Nijs RN, Jacobs JW. Glucocorticoids in rheumatoid arthritis: Effects on erosions and bone. Ann N Y Acad Sci 2002;966:82–90.
41. Glick T, Müller-Ladner U. Vaccination in patients with chronic rheumatic or autoimmune diseases. Clin Infect Dis 2008;46:1459–1465.
42. Pincus T, Ferraccioli G, Sokka T, et al. Evidence from clinical trials and long-term observational studies that disease-modifying anti-rheumatic drugs slow radiographic progression in rheumatoid arthritis: Updating a 1983 review. Rheumatology 2002;41(12):1346–1356.
43. Wolfe F, Hawley DJ, Cathey MA. Termination of slow acting antirheumatic therapy in rheumatoid arthritis: A 14-year prospective evaluation of 1017 consecutive starts. J Rheumatol 1990;17:994–1002.
44. Kremer JM. Methotrexate and emerging therapies. Rheum Dis Clin North Am 1998;24(3):651–658.
45. O'Dell JR. Methotrexate use in rheumatoid arthritis. Rheum Dis Clin North Am 1997;23(4):779–796.
46. Borchers AT, Keen CL, Cheema GS, Gershwin ME. The use of methotrexate in rheumatoid arthritis. Semin Arthritis Rheum 2004;34(1):465–483.

47. Suarez-Almazor ME, Belseck E, Shea BJ, Tugwell P, Wells G. Methotrexate for treating rheumatoid arthritis. Cochrane Database Syst Rev 1998(2):CD000959.

48. Prakash A, Jarvis B. Leflunomide: A review of its use in active rheumatoid arthritis. Drugs 1999;58(6):1137–1164.

49. Strand V, Cohen S, Schiff M, et al. Treatment of active rheumatoid arthritis with leflunomide compared with placebo and methotrexate. Leflunomide Rheumatoid Arthritis Investigators Group. Arch Intern Med 1999;159(21):2542–2550.

50. Osiri M, Shea BJ, Robinson V, et al. Leflunomide for treating rheumatoid arthritis. Cochrane Database Syst Rev 2003(1):CD002047.

51. Cush JJ. Safety overview of new disease-modifying antirheumatic drugs. Rheum Dis Clin North Am 2004;30(2):237–255, v.

52. Maturi RK, Folk JC, Nichols B, Oetting TT, Kardon RH. Hydroxychloroquine retinopathy. Arch Ophthalmol 1999;117(9):1262–1263.

53. Suarez-Almazor ME, Belseck E, Shea B, Homik J, Wells G, Tugwell P. Antimalarials for treating rheumatoid arthritis. Cochrane Database Syst Rev 2000(4):CD000959.

54. Weinblatt ME, Reda D, Henderson W, et al. Sulfasalazine treatment for rheumatoid arthritis: A metaanalysis of 15 randomized trials. J Rheumatol 1999;26(10):2123–2130.

55. Rains CP, Noble S, Faulds D. Sulfasalazine: A review of its pharmacological properties and therapeutic efficacy in the treatment of rheumatoid arthritis. Drugs 1995;50:137–156.

56. Stone M, Fortin PR, Pacheco-Tena C, Inman RD. Should tetracycline treatment be used more extensively for rheumatoid arthritis? Metaanalysis demonstrates clinical benefit with reduction in disease activity. J Rheumatol 2003;30:2112–2122.

57. Gomez-Reino JJ, Carmona L, Valverde VR, Mola EM, Montero MD. Treatment of rheumatoid arthritis with tumor necrosis factor inhibitors may predispose to significant increase in tuberculosis risk: A multicenter active-surveillance report. Arthritis Rheum 2003;48(8):2122–2127.

58. Keane J, Gershon S, Wise RP, et al. Tuberculosis associated with infliximab, a tumor necrosis factor alpha-neutralizing agent. N Engl J Med 2001;345(15):1098–1104.

59. Myers A, Clark J, Foster H. Tuberculosis and treatment with infliximab. N Engl J Med 2002;346(8):623–626.

60. Weisman MH. What are the risks of biologic therapy in rheumatoid arthritis? An update on safety. J Rheumatol Suppl 2002;65:33–38.

61. Chung ES, Packer M, Lo KH, Fasanmade AA, Willerson JT. Randomized, double-blind, placebo-controlled, pilot trial of infliximab, a chimeric monoclonal antibody to tumor necrosis factor-alpha in patients with moderate-to-severe heart failure: Results of the anti-TNF Therapy Against Congestive Heart Failure (ATTACH) trial. Circulation 2003;107(25):3133–3140.

62. Kwon HJ, Cote TR, Cuffe MS, Kramer JM, Braun MM. Case reports of heart failure after therapy with a tumor necrosis factor antagonist. Ann Intern Med 2003;138(10):807–811.

63. Scott DL, Kingsley MB. Tumor necrosis factor inhibitors for rheumatoid arthritis. N Engl J Med 2006;355:704-712

64. Food and Drug Administration. Information for Healthcare Professionals: Tumor Necrosis Factor (TNF) Blockers (marketed as Remicade, Enbrel, Humira, Cimzia, and Simponi). FDA Alert August 4, 2009. *http://www.fda.gov/Drugs/DrugSafety/Postmarket DrugSafetyInformationforPatientsandProviders/DrugSafety InformationforHeathcareProfessionals/ucm174474.htm.*

65. Bathon JM, Martin RW, Fleischmann RM, et al. A comparison of etanercept and methotrexate in patients with early rheumatoid arthritis [erratum N Engl J Med 2001;344(3):240]. N Engl J Med 2000;343(22):1586–1593.

66. Genovese MC, Bathon JM, Martin RW, et al. Etanercept versus methotrexate in patients with early rheumatoid arthritis: Two-year radio-graphic and clinical outcomes. Arthritis Rheum 2002;46(6):1443–1450.

67. Moreland LW, Schiff MH, Baumgartner SW, et al. Etanercept therapy in rheumatoid arthritis. A randomized, controlled trial. Ann Intern Med 1999;130(6):478–486.

68. Genovese MC, Kremer JM. Treatment of rheumatoid arthritis with etanercept. Rheum Dis Clin North Am 2004;30(2):311–328, vi–vii.

69. Nanda S, Bathon JM. Etanercept: A clinical review of current and emerging indications. Expert Opin Pharmacother 2004;5(5):1175–1186.

70. Blumenauer B, Judd MG, Cranney A, et al. Etanercept for the treatment of rheumatoid arthritis. Cochrane Database Syst Rev 2003(3):CD004525.

71. Cheifitz A, Mayer L. Monoclonal antibodies, immunogenicity, and associated infusion reactions. Mt Sinai J Med 2005;72:250–256.

72. Blumenauer B, Judd M, Wells G, et al. Infliximab for the treatment of rheumatoid arthritis. Cochrane Database Syst Rev 2002(3):CD003785.

73. Maini R, St Clair EW, Breedveld F, et al. Infliximab (chimeric anti-tumour necrosis factor alpha monoclonal antibody) versus placebo in rheumatoid arthritis patients receiving concomitant methotrexate: A randomised phase III trial. ATTRACT Study Group. Lancet 1999;354(9194):1932–1939.

74. Lipsky PE, van der Heijde DM, St Clair EW, et al. Infliximab and methotrexate in the treatment of rheumatoid arthritis. Anti-Tumor Necrosis Factor Trial in Rheumatoid Arthritis with Concomitant Therapy Study Group. N Engl J Med 2000;343(22):1594–1602.

75. Maini SR. Infliximab treatment of rheumatoid arthritis. Rheum Dis Clin North Am 2004;30(2):329–347, vii.

76. Navarro-Sarabia F, Ariza-Ariza R, Hernandez-Cruz B, Villanueva I. Adalimumab for treating rheumatoid arthritis. Cochrane Database Syst Rev 2005(3):CD005113.

77. den Broeder A, van de Putte L, Rau R, et al. A single dose, placebo controlled study of the fully human anti-tumor necrosis factor-alpha antibody adalimumab (D2E7) in patients with rheumatoid arthritis. J Rheumatol 2002;29(11):2288–2298.

78. Weinblatt ME, Keystone EC, Furst DE, et al. Adalimumab, a fully human anti-tumor necrosis factor alpha monoclonal antibody, for the treatment of rheumatoid arthritis in patients taking concomitant methotrexate: The ARMADA trial [erratum Arthritis Rheum 2003;48(3):855]. Arthritis Rheum 2003;48(1):35–45.

79. Bang LM, Keating GM. Adalimumab: A review of its use in rheumatoid arthritis. BioDrugs 2004;18(2):121–139.

80. Keystone E, Haraoui B. Adalimumab therapy in rheumatoid arthritis. Rheum Dis Clin North Am 2004;30(2):349–364, vii.

81. Maxwell L, Singh JA. Abatacept for rheumatoid arthritis. Cochrane Database Syst Rev 2009(4):CD007277.

82. Hervey PS, Keam SJ. Abatacept. BioDrugs 2006;20(1):53–61; discussion 62.

83. Genovese MC, Becker JC, Schiff M, et al. Abatacept for rheumatoid arthritis refractory to tumor necrosis factor alpha inhibition. N Engl J Med 2005;353(11):1114–1123.

84. Orencia [package insert]. Princeton, NJ: Bristol-Meyers Squibb; August 2009. *http://packageinserts.bms.com/pi/pi_orencia.pdf.*

85. Cohen SB, Emery P, Greenwald MW, et al. Rituximab for rheumatoid arthritis refractory to anti-tumor necrosis factor therapy: Results of a multicenter, randomized, double-blind, placebo-controlled, phase III trial evaluating primary efficacy and safety at twenty-four weeks. Arthritis Rheum 2006;54(9):2793–2806.

86. De Vita S, Quartuccio L. Treatment of rheumatoid arthritis with rituximab: An update and possible indications. Autoimmun Rev 2006;5(7):443–448.

87. Emery P, Fleischmann R, Filipowicz-Sosnowska A, et al. The efficacy and safety of rituximab in patients with active rheumatoid arthritis despite methotrexate treatment: Results of a phase IIB randomized, double-blind, placebo-controlled, dose-ranging trial. Arthritis Rheum 2006;54(5):1390–1400.

88. Smolen JS, Emery P, Keystone EC, et al. Consensus statement on the use of rituximab in patients with rheumatoid arthritis. Ann Rheum Dis 2007;66:143–150.

89. Schuna, AA. Rituximab for the treatment of rheumatoid arthritis. Pharmacotherapy 2007;27:1702–1710.

90. Mertens M, Singh JA. Anakinra for rheumatoid arthritis. Cochrane Database Syst Rev 2009(1): CD005121.

91. Lutt JR, Deodhar A. Rheumatoid arthritis: Strategies in the management of patients showing an inadequate response to TNFα antagonists. Drugs 2008;68:591–606.

92. DaSilva JAP, Jacogs JWG, Kirwan JR, et al. Safety of low dose glucocorticoid treatment in rheumatoid arthritis: published evidence and prospective trial data. Ann Rheum Dis 2006;65: 285–293.

93. Adachi JD, Saag KG, Delmas PD, et al. Two-year effects of alendronate on bone mineral density and vertebral fracture in patients receiving glucocorticoids: A randomized, double-blind, placebo-controlled extension trial. Arthritis Rheum 2001;44(1):202–211.

94. McIlwain HH. Glucocorticoid-induced osteoporosis: Pathogenesis, diagnosis, and management. Prev Med 2003;36(2):243–249.

95. da Silva JAP, Jacobs JWG, Kirwan JR, Boers M, et al. Safety of low dose glucocorticoid treatment in rheumatoid arthritis: published evidence and prospective trial data. Ann Rheum Dis 2006;65: 285–293.

96. American College of Rheumatology Ad Hoc Committee on Glucocorticoid-Induced Osteoporosis. Recommendations for the prevention and treatment of glucocorticoid-induced osteoporosis. Arthritis Rheum 2001;44:1496–1503.

97. Morand EF. Corticosteroids in the treatment of rheumatologic diseases. Curr Opin Rheumatol 1998;10(3):179–183.

98. Bijlsma JWJ, Saag KG, Buttgereit F, da Silva JAP. Developments in glucocorticoid therapy. Rheum Dis Clin N Am 2005;31:1–17.

99. Criswell LA, Saag KG, Sems KM, et al. Moderate-term, low-dose corticosteroids for rheumatoid arthritis. Cochrane Database Syst Rev 1998(3):CD001158.

100. Gabriel SE, Coyle D, Moreland LW. A clinical and economic review of disease-modifying antirheumatic drugs. Pharmacoeconomics 2001; 19(7): 715–728.

CHAPTER 101

Osteoarthritis

LUCINDA M. BUYS AND MARY ELIZABETH ELLIOTT

KEY CONCEPTS

❶ Millions of Americans have osteoarthritis (OA). OA prevalence increases with age; women more commonly affected than men.

❷ Contributors to OA are systemic (e.g., age, gender, genetics, hormonal status, obesity, and occupational or recreational activity) and/or local (e.g., injury, overloading of joints, muscle weakness, or joint deformity).

❸ OA is primarily a disease of cartilage that reflects a failure of the chondrocyte to maintain proper balance between cartilage formation and destruction. This leads to loss of cartilage in the joint, local inflammation, pathologic changes in underlying bone, and further damage to cartilage triggered by the affected bone.

❹ The most common symptom associated with OA is pain, which leads to decreased function and range of motion. Pain relief is the primary objective of medication therapy.

❺ Manifestations of OA are local, affecting one or a few joints, usually the knees, hips, and hands. Osteophytes (bony proliferation of affected joints) are often found, in contrast to the soft-tissue swelling of rheumatoid arthritis.

❻ Nonpharmacologic therapy is the foundation of the pharmaceutical care plan and should be initiated before or concurrently with pharmacologic therapy.

❼ Based upon efficacy, safety, and cost considerations, scheduled acetaminophen, up to 4 g/day, should be tried initially for pain relief in OA. If this fails, a nonsteroidal antiinflammatory drug (NSAID) may be tried, if there are no contraindications.

❽ NSAIDs are associated with gastrointestinal (GI), renal, cardiovascular, liver, and central nervous system toxicity. Monitoring with complete blood count, serum creatinine, hepatic transaminase levels, and blood pressure readings can be valuable in detecting potential toxicity.

❾ Strategies to reduce NSAID-induced GI toxicity include the use of nonacetylated salicylates, cyclooxygenase-2 (COX-2])–selective inhibitors, or the addition of misoprostol or a proton pump inhibitor. COX-2–selective inhibitors vary in their ability to prevent GI toxicity, and concomitant use of aspirin largely negates the gastroprotective effect of COX-2–selective inhibitors.

❿ COX-2–selective inhibitors can increase the risk of cardiovascular events. This may be a class effect, but the extent of this risk varies among COX-2–selective inhibitors, and traditional NSAIDs may also pose risks. This hazard, in addition to the GI toxicity possible with all NSAIDs, underscores the importance of using NSAIDs only as needed and after assessing the individual patient's risk. New guidelines to reduce GI and cardiovascular risk for those who require treatment with NSAIDs have been developed.

⓫ Other agents useful in treating OA include topical NSAIDs or capsaicin, glucosamine and chondroitin in combination, and intraarticular injections of corticosteroids or hyaluronic acid.

Osteoarthritis (OA) is the most common joint disease and is one of the 10 most disabling conditions in the United States and other developed nations.[1,2] Approximately 15% of the population is affected by OA, including 50% of those over 65 and 85% of those aged at least 75. The progressive destruction of articular cartilage has long been appreciated in OA, but OA involves the entire diarthrodial joint, including articular cartilage, synovium, capsule, and subchondral bone, with surrounding ligaments and muscles also playing important roles. Changes in structure and function of these tissues produce clinical OA, characterized by joint pain and tenderness, with decreased range of motion, weakness, joint instability, and disability. Knee OA alone is as important a contributor to disability as cardiovascular disease and more important than other comorbidities in this respect.

This chapter will review the epidemiology, etiology, pathogenesis, and diagnosis of OA. It then will focus on pharmacologic and nonpharmacologic treatments currently in use for OA, as well as investigational agents. Because millions of persons take medications for OA, the overall risks posed by these medications require serious consideration, particularly by clinicians who treat or advise patients on drug therapy for OA. This chapter examines the risks and benefits of OA treatments, with emphasis on those individuals who have the highest risk for adverse events, to help clinicians maximize benefit and reduce risks to their patients with OA.

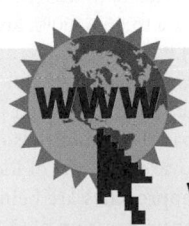

The complete chapter, learning objectives, and other resources can be found at **www.pharmacotherapyonline.com**.

EPIDEMIOLOGY

OA is the leading cause of disability in the United States.[1,3] The prevalence of arthritis-related disability is expected to increase to 11.6 million in the United States by 2020. The annual cost attributed to OA (medical care and lost wages) is estimated at $65 million in the United States.[4]

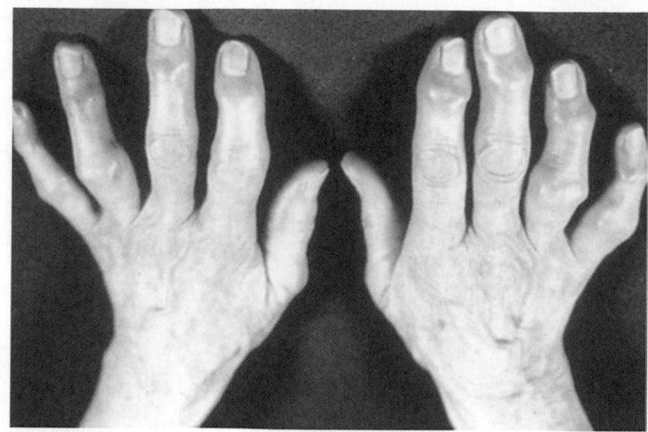

FIGURE 101-1. Heberden nodes (distal interphalangeal joint) noted on all fingers and Bouchard nodes (proximal interphalangeal joint) noted on most fingers. *(From Johnson BE. Arthritis: Osteoarthritis, Gout and Rheumatoid Arthritis. In: South-Paul JE, Matheny SC, Lewis EL, eds. Current Diagnosis and Treatment in Family Medicine. New York: McGraw-Hill; 2004:266, 267.)*

PREVALENCE BY AGE, SEX, AND RACE

❶ Prevalence estimates for OA vary with age, gender, genetics, ethnic group, the specific joint involved, and methods used for diagnosis or ascertainment. Prevalence of OA increases with age. In the United States, for persons age 25 to 74, prevalence is estimated at 12%, with 60% to 70% of those over age 70 affected.[1,5] Prevalence for symptomatic knee OA is 5% for all persons over age 25, but 12% for those over 55. [1] Prevalence of symptomatic hip OA is 4%, leading to about 200,000 total hip replacements per year in the United States. Radiologically confirmed hip OA shows clear trends through all age groups, affecting 1.6% of those between ages 30 to 39, up to a prevalence of 14% in those over 85 years of age.[6] Hand OA is found in 5% of those age 40, but in 65% of those over 80 years of age.[7]

Prevalence of hip OA is 9% in white populations, but is only 4% for Asian, black, and Indian populations. Before age 50, men are more likely to have OA than women, attributed to higher rates of sports and other injuries.[4] Women exhibit a higher prevalence of hip and knee OA than men, and are at especially greater risk of hand OA, with 26% of women and 13% of men over age 70 affected.[7] Women are also more likely to have inflammatory OA of the proximal and distal interphalangeal joints of the hands, giving rise to the formation of Bouchard and Heberden nodes, respectively (Fig. 101–1).

INCIDENCE

Using a population database of approximately 4 million persons, a recent Canadian study estimated the annual incidence rate of physician-diagnosed OA in men to be 11.6 per 1000 in the period 2003 to 2004, similar to the rate of 11.3 per 1000 estimated for 1996 to 1997.[8] For women, the incidence rate significantly increased from 14.7 to 16.7 per 1000 from the period 1996 to 1997 to the period 2003 to 2004. Some of the increase observed for women could have resulted from the aging of the population and with women's longer life expectancy.

ETIOLOGY

❷ The etiology of OA is multifactorial. Many patients have more than one risk factor for the development of OA. The most common risk factors for the development of OA include obesity, occupation, participation in certain sports, history of joint trauma, and a genetic predisposition. Patients with osteoporosis are also less likely to have OA, possibly due to the opposite influences of body weight on bone strength and OA risk.

OBESITY

The most important preventable risk factor for OA of the knee, hip, and hand is obesity, a particularly concerning fact given the increasing prevalence of obesity in the United States and many other countries.[1] Obesity often precedes OA and contributes to its development, rather than occurring as a result of inactivity from joint pain. In a three-decade Framingham Study, the highest quintile of body mass was associated with a higher relative risk of knee OA (relative risk of 1.5 to 1.9 for men and 2.1 to 3.2 for women).[9] Another study of 1,108 men in their twenties showed that a high body mass index was associated with later development of knee OA.[10] The risk of developing OA increases by approximately 10% with each additional kilogram of weight, and in obese persons without OA, weight loss of even 5 kg (11 lbs) decreases the risk of future knee OA by half.[9] In addition to being a risk factor for OA, obesity is also a predictor for eventual prosthetic joint replacement.

OCCUPATION, SPORTS, AND TRAUMA

OA risk is increased for those in occupations requiring prolonged standing, kneeling, squatting, lifting or moving of heavy objects, such as shipbuilding, mining, some types of factory work, carpentry, and farming.[3] Repetitive motion also contributes to hand OA, with the dominant hand usually affected.[7] Risk for OA depends on the type and intensity of physical activity. OA is associated with participation in activities such as wrestling, boxing, baseball pitching, cycling, and football, although recreational participants may not have the increased risk seen in the professional athlete. Recreational exercise (walking, jogging) by middle-aged persons did not increase or decrease risk of knee OA over 9 years of follow-up.[11]

Sports or traumatic injury to articular cartilage greatly increases OA risk.[12] Meniscal damage also increases the risk of knee OA because of the loss of proper load bearing and shock absorption, increased focal load on cartilage and on subchondral bone. Quadriceps muscle weakness also increases the risk for knee OA, as these muscles are important in maintaining joint stability.[1,4] Knee malalignment does appear to increases OA risk, but this is still under debate.[4,13,14] Knee malalignment does increase risk for faster progression of OA.[13]

Age at injury does matter, because older individuals who damage ligaments tend to develop OA more rapidly than young people with a similar injury. However, trauma that occurs early in life is significant: The incidence of knee OA by age 65 years was more than doubled for men who sustained a knee injury in adolescence compared with those who had not.[15]

GENETIC FACTORS

OA is a disease in which many genes play a role. Genetic links have been shown with OA of the first metatarsophalangeal joint and with generalized OA. Heberden nodes are 10 times more prevalent in women than in men, for example, with a twofold higher risk if the woman's mother had them. Twin studies indicate that OA can be attributed substantially to genetic factors (39% to 65%, 60%, and 70% for hand, hip, and spine OA, respectively).[16]

Genome-wide linkage studies (GWAS) (associating OA with a specific region out of the total human genome) have been used to search for the genetic basis for OA.[17] Studies based on hundreds of pedigrees from numerous countries have uncovered dozens of loci that include OA-related genes. Several other approaches are being use to link genetic influences to development or progression of OA.

Twin studies as noted above have provided clues. In other twin studies of OA progression, radiographic measurements over 2 years showed that the increased risk for a sibling having radiographic progression if the proband had progression was threefold for joint space narrowing and 1.5-fold for osteophyte progression.[18]

Using linkage analysis and other methods, genetic associations to OA include genes related to inflammation (e.g. IL1, IL-10), Wnt signaling (FRZB, LRP5), bone morphogenetic proteins (*BMP2*, *BMP5*, and *GDF5*), and proteases or their inhibitors (*ADAM12*, *TNA*, *AACT*).[17] At present, for most genes that have been identified by any method as being linked to OA, the associations have been weak or modest, even if replicable. However, recent work has shown that the risk of developing OA may be substantially determined by a combination of modest genetic differences.[19] There are now large cohorts of people with OA of the hip, knee, or multiple joints whose participation can identify specific genes important in influencing progression of OA or which identify persons at high risk for developing OA. Prospective studies are investigating factors affecting incidence and progression of knee OA including the Osteoarthritis Initiative, a multicenter, 4-year observational study of men and women, funded by the U.S. National Institutes of Health.

In addition to the importance of chromosomal DNA in OA, recent work has shown that mitochondrial DNA (inherited through the maternal route) may be important.[20] Of specific human mitochondrial DNA haplogroups, the J haplogroup was associated with a 54% reduced risk of developing OA and a 65% reduced risk of severe progression of OA, whereas haplogroup U had an 80% higher risk for severe OA progression. Given that mitochondrial DNA is important in oxidative respiration and that defects in mitochondrial respiration have been seen in OA chondrocytes, it may be that not only chromosomal DNA is important in OA, but mitochondrial DNA is as well.

PATHOPHYSIOLOGY

OA falls into two major etiologic classes. *Primary (idiopathic) OA*, the most common type, has no identifiable cause. Subclasses of primary OA are *localized OA*, involving one or two sites, and *generalized OA*, affecting three or more sites. *Erosive OA* is used to describe the presence of erosion and marked proliferation in the proximal and distal interphalangeal joints of the hands. *Secondary OA* is that associated with a known cause such as rheumatoid or another inflammatory arthritis, trauma, metabolic or endocrine disorders, and congenital factors.[3,4]

Although OA was previously considered a wear-and-tear disease, increased knowledge of articular cartilage has led to a more dynamic understanding of OA. Some changes in the OA joint may reflect compensatory processes to maintain function in the face of ongoing joint destruction. Not only biomechanical forces but also inflammatory, biochemical, and immunologic factors are involved. Understanding the biology and function of normal cartilage aids in understanding OA and is summarized below.

NORMAL CARTILAGE

Function, Structure, and Composition of Cartilage

Articular cartilage possesses viscoelastic properties that provide lubrication with motion, shock absorbency during rapid movements, and load support. In synovial joints, articular cartilage is found between the synovial cavity on one side and a narrow layer of calcified tissue overlying subchondral bone on the other side (Fig. 101–2).[21] The layer of cartilage is narrow with human medial femoral articular cartilage being approximately 2 to 3 mm thick. Despite this, healthy articular cartilage in weight-bearing joints withstands millions of cycles of loading and unloading each year. Cartilage is easily compressed, losing up to 40% of its original height when a load is applied. Compression increases the area of contact and disperses force more evenly to underlying bone, tendons, ligaments, and muscles. In addition, cartilage is almost frictionless, and together with its compressibility, this enables smooth movement in the joint, distributes load across joint tissues to prevent damage, and stabilizes the joint.

Strength, a low coefficient of friction, and compressibility of cartilage derive from its unique structure. Cartilage is composed of a complex, hydrophilic, extracellular matrix (ECM). It is approximately 75% to 85% water and 2% to 5% chondrocytes (the only cells in cartilage), and it contains collagen proteins, smaller amounts of several other proteins, proteoglycans, and long hyaluronic acid molecules.[21] The two major structural components in articular cartilage are type II collagen and aggrecans.[22] Type II collagen has a tightly woven triple helical structure, which provides the tensile strength of cartilage. Aggrecan is a proteoglycan linked with hyaluronic acid, providing the long aggrecan molecules a high negative charge. These are squeezed together by surrounding fibrils of type II collagen. The strong electrostatic repulsion of proteoglycans held in close proximity gives cartilage the ability to withstand further compression. Within the cartilage ECM are the chondrocytes, responsible for laying down all the components of cartilage.

Normal cartilage turnover helps repair and restore cartilage and thus respond to the usual demands put on cartilage by loading and physical activity. In healthy adult cartilage, chondrocyte metabolism is slow, with a dynamic balance between anabolic processes. This metabolism is promoted by growth factors, including bone morphogenetic protein 2, insulin-like growth factor-1, transforming growth factor, by catabolism and proteolysis stimulated by matrix metalloproteinases (MMPs), tumor necrosis factor-α (TNF-α, interleukin-1, and other cytokines. Tissue inhibitors

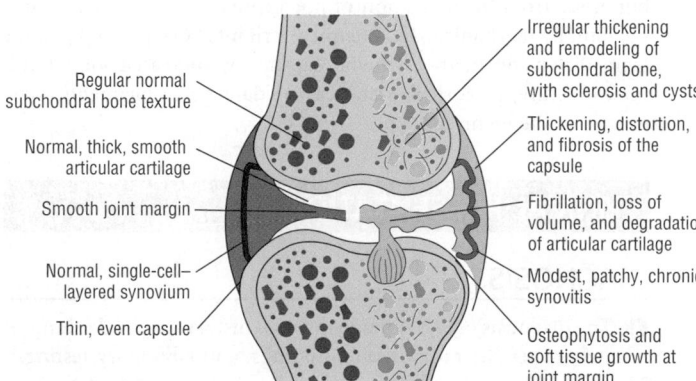

FIGURE 101-2. Characteristics of osteoarthritis in the diarthrodial joint. *(Courtesy of Dr. D. Gotlieb.)*

of metalloproteinase (TIMP) also contribute to the balance by restraining the catabolic actions of MMPs. If cartilage is injured, chondrocytes react by removing the damaged areas and increasing synthesis of matrix constituents to repair and restore cartilage.

Another component supporting healthy joints are the joint protective mechanisms, such as muscles bridging the joint, sensory receptors in feedback loops to regulate muscle and tendon function, supporting ligaments, and subchondral bone that has shock-absorbent properties.

Finally, it is important to note that adult articular cartilage is avascular, with chondrocytes nourished by synovial fluid. With movement and cyclic loading and unloading of joints, nutrients flow into the cartilage, whereas immobilization reduces nutrient supply. This is one of the reasons that normal physical activity is beneficial for joint health.

OSTEOARTHRITIC CARTILAGE

❸ Important contributors to the development of OA are local mechanical influences, genetic factors, inflammation, and aberrant chondrocyte function leading to loss of articular cartilage. At a molecular level, OA pathophysiology involves the interplay of dozens, if not hundreds, of extracellular and intracellular molecules with roles including chondrocyte regulation, phenotypic changes, proteolytic degradation of cartilage components, and interactions between articular cartilage, underlying subchondral bone, and the joint synovium.

OA most commonly begins with damage to articular cartilage, through trauma or other injury, excess joint loading from obesity or other reasons, or instability or injury of the joint that causes abnormal loading. In response to cartilage damage, chondrocyte activity increases in an attempt to remove and repair the damage. Depending on the degree of damage, the balance between breakdown and resynthesis of cartilage can be lost, and a vicious cycle of increasing breakdown can lead to further cartilage loss.[1,12,22,23] Destruction of aggrecans by the proteolytic enzyme (ADAMTS-5) is considered to play a key role. Recent work suggests the involvement of a collagen receptor, named *DDR-2*, located on the chondrocyte cell surface.[24] In healthy cartilage, DDR-2 is inactive, masked from contact with collagen by aggrecans. Damage to cartilage triggers aggrecans destruction, thus exposing DDR-2 to collagen. The active DDR-2 then increases activity of MMP-13, which destroys collagen. Collagen breakdown products then further stimulate DDR-2, with a vicious circle in which more collagen is destroyed and cartilage.

Other mechanisms contribute to the initiation and perpetuation of cartilage loss. Further insights into the complex process have been gained by research showing the following:

1. Expression of hundreds of specific genes are affected by acute experimental injury of human cartilage tissue, that is, injury alters the chondrocyte phenotype.[25]

2. Within different regions of human OA cartilage obtained at surgery, chondrocyte gene expression from the most damaged areas of cartilage is different from that from less damaged or normal areas.[26]

3. Comparative proteomics of articular cartilage from normal persons compared with those with OA showed different expression.[27]

Finally, some of the changes seen soon after acute cartilage damage are the same changes that have been seen in OA as compared with normal cartilage. Such studies should provide valuable clues to explain the mechanism of cartilage loss and potentially identify targets for drug development.

In addition to changes taking place in OA cartilage, there is also a role in OA for the subchondral bone adjacent to articular cartilage.

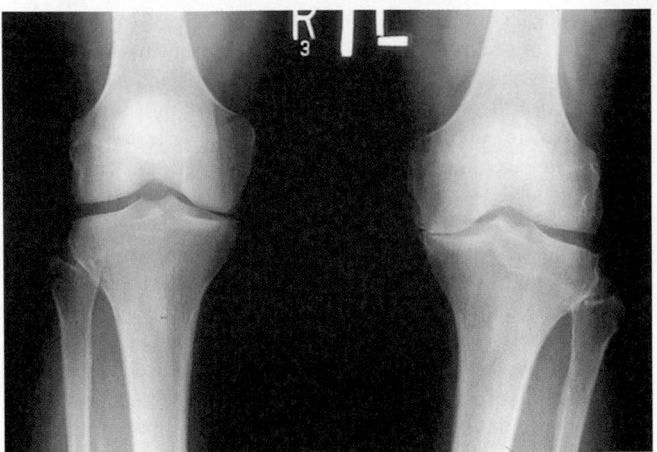

FIGURE 101-3. Plain x-ray films of the knee demonstrating joint space narrowing. *(From Johnson BE. Arthritis: Osteoarthritis, Gout and Rheumatoid Arthritis. In: South-Paul JE, Matheny SC, Lewis EL, eds. Current Diagnosis and Treatment in Family Medicine. New York: McGraw-Hill; 2004:267.)*

Subchondral bone undergoes pathologic changes that may precede, coincide with, or follow damage to the articular cartilage. This damage to subchondral bone may play an essential role in allowing damage to articular cartilage to progress.[28] In OA, subchondral bone releases vasoactive peptides and MMPs. Neovascularization and subsequent increased permeability of the adjacent cartilage occur and contributes further to cartilage loss.

Substantial loss of cartilage causes joint space narrowing and leads to a painful, deformed joint (Fig. 101-3). Furthermore, the remaining cartilage softens and develops fibrillations (vertical clefts into the cartilage), and there is splitting, further loss of cartilage, and exposure of underlying bone.[2] As cartilage is destroyed and the adjacent subchondral bone undergoes pathologic changes, cartilage is eroded completely, leaving denuded subchondral bone, which becomes dense, smooth, and glistening (eburnation). A more brittle, stiffer bone results, with decreased weight-bearing ability and development of sclerosis and microfractures. New bone formations, or osteophytes, also appear at joint margins distant from cartilage destruction and are thought to arise from local and humoral factors. There is direct evidence that osteophytes can help stabilize osteoarthritic joints.[29]

Accompanying the changes in cartilage and subchondral bone, local inflammatory changes and pathologic changes can occur in the joint capsule and synovium. Infiltration of the synovium with T cells with T-helper type 1 phenotype occurs, as well as the appearance of immune complexes.[16] Contributors to this inflammation may include crystals or cartilage shards in synovial fluid. With increased levels of interleukin-1, prostaglandin E$_2$, TNF-α, and nitric oxide observed in synovial fluid, these agents could also play a role.[29,30] With inflammatory changes in the synovium, effusions and synovial thickening occur.

❹ The pain of OA is not related to the destruction of cartilage but arises from the activation of nociceptive nerve endings within the joint by mechanical and chemical irritants.[1] OA pain may result from distension of the synovial capsule by increased joint fluid, microfracture, periosteal irritation, or damage to ligaments, synovium, or the meniscus.

CLINICAL PRESENTATION

DIAGNOSIS

❺ The diagnosis of OA is made through history, physical examination, characteristic radiographic findings, and laboratory testing.[3,4] The major diagnostic goals are (1) to discriminate between primary and secondary OA and (2) to clarify the joints involved, severity of joint involvement, and response to prior therapies, providing a basis for a treatment plan. The American College of Rheumatology has published traditional diagnostic criteria and "decision trees" for OA diagnosis.[31] As for all guidelines, the authors stress these are for assisting the clinician rather than replacing clinical judgment. For example, traditional criteria are as follows: (1) For hip OA, a patient must have pain in the hip and at least two of the following three: an erythrocyte sedimentation rate <20 mm/h (<5.6 μm/s), femoral or acetabular osteophytes on radiography, or joint space narrowing on radiography. This provides a sensitivity of 89% and a specificity of 91%. (2) For knee OA, a patient must have pain at the knee and osteophytes on radiography plus one of the following: age older than 50 years, morning stiffness no more than 30 minutes, crepitus on motion, bony enlargement, bony tenderness, or palpable warmth. This provides a sensitivity of 95% and a specificity of 69%. The addition of laboratory or radiographic data further improves accuracy of diagnosis. Criteria for hand OA have also been published.[32]

CLINICAL PRESENTATION OF OSTEOARTHRITIS

Age
- Usually elderly

Gender
- Age <45 more common in men
- Age >45 more common in women

Symptoms
- Pain
- Deep, aching character
- Pain on motion
- Pain with motion early in disease
- Pain with rest late in disease
- Stiffness in affected joints
- Resolves with motion, recurs with rest ("gelling" phenomenon)
- Usually duration <30 minutes
- Often related to weather
- Limited joint motion
- May result in limitations activities of daily living
- Instability of weight-bearing joints

Signs, history, and physical examination
- Monarticular or oligoarticular; asymmetrical involvement
- Hands
- Distal interphalangeal joints
- Heberden nodes (osteophytes or bony enlargements) (Fig. 101–1)
- Proximal interphalangeal joints
- Bouchard's nodes (osteophytes)
- First carpometacarpal joint
- Osteophytes give characteristic square appearance of the hand (shelf sign)
- Knees
- Patellofemoral compartment involvement
- Pain related to climbing stairs
- Medial compartment involvement
- Genu varum (bowlegged deformity)
- Lateral compartment involvement

- Genu valgum (knock-kneed deformity)
- Transient joint effusions
- Typically noninflammatory synovial fluid (WBC <2000/mm³ [<2 × 10⁹/L])
- Hips
- Groin pain during weight-bearing activities
- Stiffness, especially after inactivity
- Limited joint motion
- Spine
- L3 and L4 involvement is most common in the lumbar spine
- Signs and symptoms of nerve root compression
- Radicular pain
- Paresthesias
- Loss of reflexes
- Muscle weakness associated with the affected nerve root
- Feet
- Typically involves the first metatarsophalangeal joint
- Other sites, less commonly involved
- Shoulder, elbow, acromioclavicular, sternoclavicular, and temporomandibular joints

Observation on joint examination
- Bony proliferation or occasional synovitis
- Local tenderness
- Crepitus
- Muscle atrophy
- Limited motion with passive/active movement
- Deformity

Radiologic evaluation
- Early mild OA
- Radiographic changes often absent
- Progression of OA
- Joint space narrowing
- Subchondral bone sclerosis
- Marginal osteophytes
- Late OA
- Abnormal alignment of joints
- Effusions

Characteristics of synovial fluid
- High viscosity
- Mild leukocytosis (<2000 WBC/mm³ [<2 × 10⁹/L])

Laboratory values
- No specific test
- Erythrocyte sedimentation rate and hematologic and chemistry survey are normal

PROGNOSIS

The prognosis for patients with primary OA is variable and depends on the joint involved. If a weight-bearing joint or the spine is involved, considerable morbidity and disability are possible. In the case of secondary OA, the prognosis depends on the underlying cause. Treatment of OA may relieve pain or improve function but does not reverse preexisting damage to the articular cartilage.

TREATMENT

Osteoarthritis

■ DESIRED OUTCOME

Management of the patient with OA begins with a diagnosis based on a careful history, physical examination, radiographic findings, and an assessment of the extent of joint involvement. Treatment should be tailored to each individual. Goals are (1) to educate the patient, family members, and caregivers; (2) to relieve pain and stiffness; (3) to maintain or improve joint mobility; (4) to limit functional impairment; and (5) to maintain or improve quality of life.[3,33–36]

General Approach to Treatment

Treatment for each OA patient depends on the distribution and severity of joint involvement, comorbid disease states, concomitant medications, and allergies (Fig. 101–4). Management for all individuals with OA should begin with patient education, physical and/or occupational therapy, and weight loss or assistive devices if appropriate.[3,34–36]

The primary objective of medication is to alleviate pain.[3,34–37] Scheduled acetaminophen, up to 4 g/day, should be tried initially. If this is ineffective, nonsteroidal antiinflammatory drugs (NSAIDs) are prescribed, or possibly a cyclooxygenase-2 (COX-2)–selective inhibitor (celecoxib) if warranted. Application of capsaicin or topical NSAID creams over specific joints can be helpful adjuncts for pain control. Joint aspiration followed by glucocorticoid can relieve pain and is offered concomitantly with oral analgesics or after their lack of efficacy, depending on the practitioner's preference. Opioid analgesics are a final medication to prescribe if other therapies are unsuccessful. When symptoms are intractable or there is significant loss of function, joint replacement may be appropriate if the patient is a surgical candidate.

Finally, for patients interested in clinical trials, investigational strategies with oral doxycycline, MMP inhibitors, disease-modifying OA drugs, or cartilage transplantations may be considered.

For management of patients with OA, the Third Canadian Consensus Conference Group recently summarized evidence-based recommendations (Table 101–1).[38] As with all guidelines, these are for assisting the clinician rather than replacing the clinician's judgment based on the patient's characteristics. The American College of Rheumatology, as well as others, recommends acetaminophen as the drug of first choice.[36,39,40] For patients with risk factors for GI complications, selection of a nonselective NSAID plus a proton pump inhibitor (PPI) or a COX-2–selective inhibitor plus a PPI is supported by much recent evidence, as described in this chapter.

■ NONPHARMACOLOGIC THERAPY

❻ The first step in OA treatment is patient education about the disease process, the extent of OA, the prognosis, and treatment options. Education is paramount in that OA is often seen as a wear-and-tear disease, an inevitable consequence of aging for which nothing helps. Even worse, patients may resort to the use of alternative but unproven medications or quackery. Patients should be warned about these and encouraged to access information from local or national units of the Arthritis Foundation.[41] The Arthritis Foundation provides literature about OA and OA medications and information about local clinics and agencies offering physical and economic assistance. The Arthritis Foundation also sponsors support groups and public education programs.

The benefits of patient education have been documented in a variety of programs. These programs are provided across a wide spectrum of delivery methods: from trained volunteers using telephone calls to group sessions for patient support to one-on-one educational sessions with physical therapists or nurse educators. While nearly all of these delivery methods are effective, cost of delivery is highly variable. Long-term cost-effectiveness is very important for sustainability of these patient education programs.

Diet

Excess weight increases the biomechanical load on weight-bearing joints and is the single best predictor of need for eventual joint replacement.[10,42–44] Even a 5 kg (11 lb) weight loss can decrease the load on a weight-bearing joint. Weight loss is associated with decreased symptoms and disability, although results are variable.[42,44,45] At least one randomized, controlled trial has demonstrated improvement in pain and self-reported physical function using a combination of modest weight loss (5%) and exercise.[46] There is a large weight-loss trial under way, The Intensive Diet and Exercise for Arthritis trial (IDEA), that will address weight-related joint loading and inflammatory biomarkers.[47] Although weight loss requires a motivated patient, it should be encouraged and supported for all overweight patients with OA.

Physical and Occupational Therapy

Physical therapy—with heat or cold treatments and an exercise program—helps to maintain and restore joint range of motion and to reduce pain and muscle spasms. Warm baths or warm water soaks may decrease pain and stiffness. Heating pads should be used with caution, especially in the elderly. Patients should be warned not to fall asleep on the heat source or to lie on it for more than brief periods to avoid burns.

Exercise programs and quadriceps strengthening can improve physical functioning and can decrease disability, pain, and analgesic use by OA patients.[46,48] Isometric exercise is preferred over isotonic exercise because the latter can aggravate affected joints. Exercises should be taught and then observed before the patient exercises at home, ideally three to four times daily. The patient should be instructed to decrease the number of repetitions if severe pain develops with exercise.

The decision about whether to encourage walking should be made on an individual basis. With weak or deconditioned muscles, the load is transmitted excessively to the joints; so weight-bearing activities can exacerbate symptoms. However, avoidance of activity by those with hip or knee OA leads to further deconditioning or weight gain. A program of patient education, muscle stretching and strengthening, and supervised walking can improve physical function and decrease pain for patients with knee OA.[48] Referral to the physical and/or occupational therapist is especially helpful for patients with functional disabilities. The therapist can assess muscle strength and joint stability and recommend exercises and methods of protecting the affected joint from excessive forces. The therapist can also provide assistive and orthotic devices, such as canes, walkers, braces, heel cups, splints, or insoles for use during exercise or daily activities.

Surgery

Surgery can be recommended for OA patients with functional disability and/or severe pain unresponsive to conservative therapy. Criteria for total joint replacement (arthroplasty) of the knee were developed at an National Institutes of Health consensus conference.[49] Likewise, criteria for total hip replacement, as well as a summary of clinical outcomes resulting from this procedure have

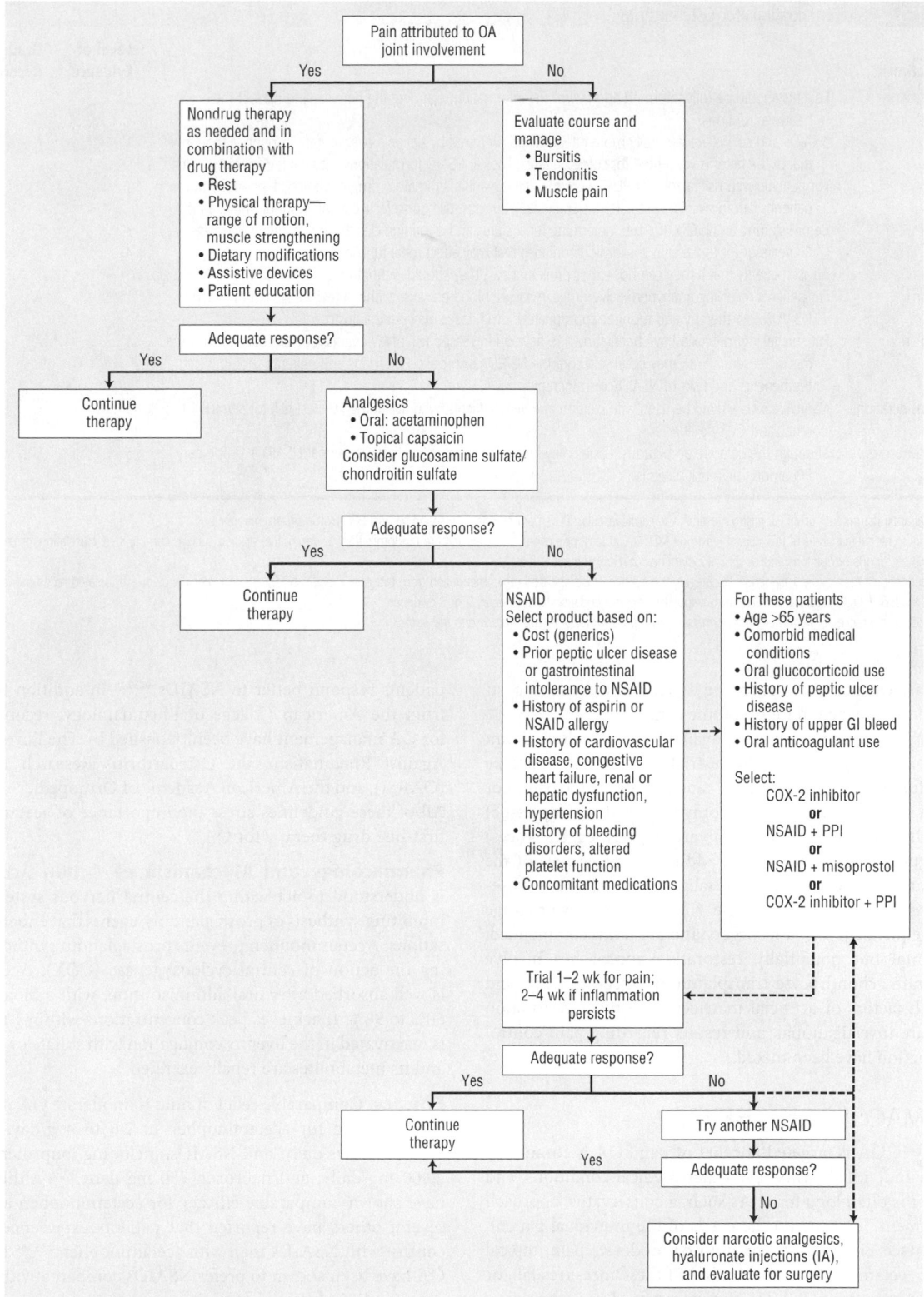

FIGURE 101-4. Treatment algorithm for osteoarthritis. (COX, cyclooxygenase; GI, gastrointestinal; IA, intraarticular; NSAID, nonsteroidal antiinflammatory drug; OA, osteoarthritis; PPI, proton pump inhibitor.)

been published.[50] These hip and knee replacement recommendations have been based on critical review of the literature as well as on expert opinion. For patients with advanced disease, a partial or total arthroplasty can relieve pain and improve motion, with the best outcomes after total hip or knee arthroplasty. Total joint arthroplasty is responsible for a large portion of the direct medical costs associated with OA in the United States.

Recently, the cost-effectiveness of total knee arthroplasty has been evaluated for a Medicare-age population.[51] Calculations were based on Medicare claims data and costs and outcomes data. Cost projections were calculated for lifetime costs as well as quality-adjusted life expectancy (QALE) for different risk populations and across low-volume to high-volume hospitals. Although total knee arthroplasty was found to be cost-effective across hospital settings

TABLE 101-1 Recommendations for Osteoarthritis[a]

Recommendation		Level of Evidence	Grade of Recommendation
1. Patient-physician communication	Patients should be fully informed about evolving information regarding the benefits and risks of their treatment options.	3	C
2. Indications	NSAIDs and coxibs are generally more effective and preferred by patients over acetaminophen, although a trial of the latter is warranted for some patients. Topical NSAID formulations may confer benefit in knee OA	1	A
3. GI toxicity	For patients with risk factors for PUB, a coxib is still the antiinflammatory drug of choice, depending on the patient's cardiovascular risks. High-risk patients who must use nonselective NSAIDs should have a PPI.	1	A
4. Renal	Before starting an NSAID or coxib, determine renal status and creatinine clearance for patients over age 65 years or for those with comorbid conditions that may affect renal function.	3	C
	Advise patients that if they can not eat or drink that day, they should withhold that day's dose of NSAID/coxib.	4	D
5. Hypertension	For patients receiving antihypertensive drugs, measure blood pressure within a few weeks after initiating NSAID/coxib therapy and monitor appropriately; drug doses may need adjustment.	1	A
6. Cardiovascular	Patients taking rofecoxib have been shown to have an increased risk of CV events. Current data suggest that this increased CV risk may be an effect of the NSAID/coxib class. Physicians and patients should weigh the benefits and risks of NSAID/coxib therapy.	1	A
7. Geriatric consideration	NSAIDs/coxibs should be used with caution in elderly patients, who are at the greatest risk for serious GI, renal, and CV side effects.	3	C
8. Pharmacoeconomics	Although the data are ambiguous, coxibs may be more cost-effective than traditional NSAID + proprietary PPI among high-risk patients.	3	C

NSAID, nonsteroidal antiinflammatory drug; GI, gastrointestinal; CV, cardiovascular; PUB, perforations, ulcers, and bleeds; PPI, proton pump inhibitor.
Categories of evidence: 1A, metaanalysis of RCT; 1B, at least one RCT; 2A, at least one controlled study without randomization; 3, descriptive studies, such as comparative, correlation, or case-control studies; 4, expert committee reports or opinions and/or clinical experience of respected authorities.
Grades of recommendations: A, category 1 evidence; B, category 2 evidence or extrapolated recommendation from category 1 evidence; C, category 3 evidence or extrapolated recommendation from category 1 or 2 evidence; D, Category 4 evidence or extrapolated recommendation from category 2 or 3 evidence.
From Table 4, p. 153, of reference 38. Reprinted with permission from the Journal of Rheumatology and the author.

and patient risk category, the procedure was found to be most cost-effective when performed in high-volume centers.

Other surgical options are also available. Arthrodesis (joint fusion) can reduce pain but will restrict motion and may be appropriate for smaller joints that are causing intractable pain. For patients with mild knee OA, an osteotomy (removal of bony tissue) may correct the misalignment of genu varum ("bowlegged" knees) or genu valgum ("knock-knees"). In addition, osteotomies of the pelvis or femur can ameliorate joint misalignment in hip OA, subsequently slowing progression of disease. Knee arthroscopy or lavage appear to be equivalent to sham surgery and are not recommended.[39] Experimental but potentially restorative approaches involve soft-tissue grafts, chondrocyte transplantation, gene therapy, and use of growth factors or artificial matrices.[52] Cartilage-restoration approaches are investigational, and results regarding pain control and joint function have been mixed.

■ PHARMACOLOGIC THERAPY

Drug therapy in OA is targeted at relief of pain. OA is commonly seen in older individuals who have other medical conditions, and OA treatment is often long term. As such, a conservative approach to drug treatment, focusing on the needs of the individual patient, is warranted (see Fig. 101-3). For mild or moderate pain, topical analgesics or acetaminophen can be used. If these measures fail, or if there is inflammation, NSAIDs may be useful. Even when drug therapy is initiated, appropriate nondrug therapies should be continued and reinforced. Nondrug modalities are the cornerstone of OA management and may provide as much relief as drug therapy.

Acetaminophen

Place in Therapy ❼ The American College of Rheumatology as well others recommend acetaminophen as first-line drug therapy for pain management in OA because of its relative safety, efficacy, and lower cost compared with NSAIDs.[36,39,40] Pain relief with acetaminophen has been reported as similar to that obtained with aspirin, naproxen, ibuprofen, and other NSAIDs, although many

patients respond better to NSAIDs.[36,39,40] In addition to guidelines from the American College of Rheumatology, recommendations for OA management have been published by The European League Against Rheumatism, the Osteoarthritis Research International (OARSI), and the American Academy of Orthopedic Surgeons.[36,39,40] All of these guidelines stress the importance of acetaminophen as first-line drug therapy for OA.

Pharmacology and Mechanism of Action Acetaminophen is understood to act within the central nervous system (CNS) by inhibiting synthesis of prostaglandins, agents that enhance pain sensations. Acetaminophen prevents prostaglandin synthesis by blocking the action of central cyclooxygenase (COX). Acetaminophen is well absorbed after oral administration, with a bioavailability of 60% to 98%. It achieves peak concentrations within 1 to 2 hours, it is inactivated in the liver by conjugation with sulfate or glucuronide, and its metabolites are renally excreted.

Efficacy Comparable relief of mild to moderate OA pain has been demonstrated for acetaminophen at 2.6 to 4 g/day, aspirin 650 mg four times daily, and NSAIDs, including ibuprofen at 1,200 or 2,400 mg daily, and naproxen 750 mg daily.[40,53] Although studies have shown comparable efficacy for acetaminophen and NSAIDs, several others have reported that patients experience better pain control with NSAIDs than with acetaminophen.[40,53,54] Patients with OA have been shown to prefer NSAIDs compared with acetaminophen in clinical trials, but when queried using a questionnaire that included considerations of side effects, NSAIDs were less preferred by patients.[55]

Adverse Effects Although acetaminophen is one of the safest analgesics, its use carries some risks, primarily hepatotoxicity and possibly renal toxicity with long-term use.[33,56] Serious hepatotoxicity, including fatalities, have been well documented with acetaminophen overdose (see Chap. 14 for treatment of acetaminophen overdose). Continued reports of serious hepatotoxicity, including fatalities from unintentional overdose, have led to labeling revisions of all nonprescription acetaminophen containing analgesics.[57] Unintentional overdoses of acetaminophen are due to a variety of circumstances including narrow therapeutic window at the maximum dose (4 g/day), interpatient differences in sensitivity to liver injury from acetaminophen, a wide array of nonprescription and prescription products that contain acetaminophen, which may be hard for patients to identify on the label, and consumers' lack knowledge about the association of acetaminophen and liver injury.

In a study of normal, healthy volunteers administered acetaminophen 4 g/day (1 g every 6 hours), alone or with concomitant opioid therapy, for 14 days, elevations of alanine aminotransferase at levels above three times the upper limits of normal were found in 31% to 44% of patients, depending on treatment group.[58] None of these participants had clinical symptoms of acute liver disease. Although the results of this study are not robust enough to alter the current standard dosing recommendations, it serves as an important reminder that the maximum dose of acetaminophen should be not be exceeded in any patient population and that chronic use of the maximum daily dose of 4 g/day can affect the liver. Acetaminophen should be used cautiously for patients with liver disease or for those who abuse alcohol. Acute liver failure has been reported for patients taking less than 4 g/daily.[59] The most common risk factor for liver failure for these patients was chronic alcohol intake. The FDA has recommended that chronic alcohol users (three or more drinks daily) should be warned regarding an increased risk of liver damage or GI bleeding with acetaminophen. Other individuals do not appear to be at increased risk of GI bleeding.

The National Kidney Foundation strongly discourages the use of nonprescription combination analgesic products (e.g., acetaminophen and NSAIDs) because this is associated with an increased prevalence of renal failure.[56]

Drug–Drug Interactions and Drug–Food Interactions Drug interactions with acetaminophen can occur; for example, isoniazid can increase the risk of hepatotoxicity. Chronic ingestion of maximal doses of acetaminophen may intensify the anticoagulant effect for patients taking warfarin; such individuals may need closer monitoring. Although food decreases the maximum serum concentration of acetaminophen by approximately half, the overall efficacy is unchanged.

Dosing and Administration When used for chronic OA, acetaminophen should be administered in a scheduled manner. It may be taken with or without food. Acetaminophen can be taken at 325 to 650 mg every 4 to 6 hours, but the total dose must not exceed 4 g daily (see Adverse Effects above). New labeling requirements will warn patients about potential toxicity if they inadvertently ingest

more than the recommended dose when using multiple products containing acetaminophen. If acetaminophen is used in the setting of chronic alcohol intake or in those with underlying liver disease, the duration should be limited, and the dose should not exceed 2 g daily

Nonsteroidal Antiinflammatory Drugs

Place in Therapy The American College of Rheumatology, the Third Canadian Consensus Conference Group, the Osteoarthritis Research Society International, and other organizations recommend consideration of NSAIDs for OA patients in whom acetaminophen is ineffective. Nonselective NSAIDS and COX-2–selective NSAIDS are superior to acetaminophen for improving symptoms and functional limitations.[60] Nonselective NSAIDs and COX-2–selective NSAIDs all display comparable analgesic and antiinflammatory efficacy and are similarly beneficial in OA (Table 101–2).[60-62]

Pharmacology and Mechanism of Action Blockade of prostaglandin synthesis by inhibiting COX enzymes (COX-1 and COX-2) accounts for NSAIDs' ability to relieve pain and inflammation (Fig. 101–5).[60,63-65] Because nonspecific NSAIDs and COX-2–selective inhibitors have similar efficacy, drug selection often depends on toxicity and cost. There is increasing concern regarding safety of all nonselective and COX-2–selective NSAIDs, particularly in the GI and cardiovascular areas. The next section will review the differences between nonspecific NSAIDs and COX-2–selective inhibitors.

Nonspecific NSAIDs and COX-2–Selective Inhibitors The COX-1 enzyme participates in "housekeeping" or routine physiologic functions such as generation of gastroprotective prostaglandins to promote gastric blood flow and bicarbonate generation (see Fig. 101–5).[60,64] COX-1 is expressed constitutively not only in gastric mucosa but also in vascular endothelial cells, platelets, and renal collecting tubules so that COX-1–generated prostaglandins and thromboxane also participate in hemostasis and renal blood flow. In contrast, the COX-2 enzyme is not as widely expressed in most body tissues but is rapidly induced by inflammatory mediators, local injury, and cytokines including interleukins, interferon, and TNF. Prostaglandins made by COX-2 contribute to pain sensations in OA and other conditions. Prostaglandins made by the COX-2 enzyme, including prostacyclin (prostaglandin I_2) are also implicated in some physiologic processes, including renal function, tissue repair, reproduction, and development.

Nonspecific NSAIDs block both COX-1 and COX-2 enzymes. COX-1 blockade with nonspecific NSAIDs can lead to GI ulcers and increased bleeding risk by inhibiting platelet aggregation.[60,64,65] COX-2–selective agents ("coxibs") were developed to exploit these agents' ability to reduce prostaglandins, inflammation, and pain, without blocking effects of COX-1. These agents are efficacious in relieving OA and other pain, and some do have improved GI safety. Celecoxib was the first COX-2–selective agent marketed and has been widely used for pain relief in OA and other conditions.[60,62] Rofecoxib was withdrawn from the worldwide market over concern about increased cardiovascular risk. Valdecoxib was withdrawn due to concerns about cardiovascular safety and about serious skin reactions, including deaths. Lumiracoxib and etoricoxib are not FDA approved but are marketed in several other countries; lumiracoxib has been withdrawn from the market in the United Kingdom and Australia.

It is now appreciated that the COX-2 enzyme may play an important physiologic role in normal hemostasis. The COX-2 enzyme, found in blood vessel endothelial cells, leads to production of prostaglandin I_2 (prostacyclin), which has antithrombotic effects. The COX-1 found in platelets forms thromboxane A_2 a prothrombotic molecule. Thus, blocking COX-2 alone could upset the hemostatic

TABLE 101-2 Medications Commonly Used in the Treatment of Osteoarthritis

Medication	Dosage and Frequency	Maximum Dosage (mg/day)
Oral analgesics		
Acetaminophen	325–650 mg every 4–6 hours or 1 g 3–4 times/day	4,000
Tramadol	50–100 mg every 4–6 hours	400
Acetaminophen/codeine	300 to 1000 mg/15 to 60 mg every 4 hours as needed	4,000 mg/360mg[a]
Acetaminophen/oxycodone	325 to 650 mg/2.5 to 10 mg every 6 hours as needed	4,000 mg/40mg[a]
Topical analgesics		
Capsaicin 0.025% or 0.075%	Apply to affected joint 3–4 times per day	
Nutritional supplements		
Glucosamine HCl/chondroitin sulfate	500mg/400 mg 3 times/day	1,500/1,200
Nonsteroidal antiinflammatory drugs (NSAIDs)		
Carboxylic acids		
Acetylated salicylates		
Aspirin, plain, buffered, or enteric coated	325–650 mg every 4–6 hours for pain; antiinflammatory doses start at 3,600 mg/day in divided doses	3,600[b]
Nonacetylated salicylates		
Salsalate	500–1,000 mg 2–3 times a day	3,000[b]
Diflunisal	500–1,000 mg 2 times a day	1,500
Choline salicylate[c]	500–1,000 mg 2–3 times a day	3,000[c]
Choline magnesium salicylate	500–1,000 mg 2–3 times a day	3,000[c]
Acetic acids		
Etodolac	800–1200 mg/day in divided doses	1,200
Diclofenac	100–150 mg/day in divided doses	200
Indomethacin	25 mg 2–3 times a day; 75 mg SR once daily	200; 150
Ketorolac[d]	10 mg every 4–6 hours	40
Nabumetone[e]	500–1,000 mg 1–2 times a day	2,000
Propionic acids		
Fenoprofen	300–600 mg 3–4 times a day	3,200
Flurbiprofen	200–300 mg/day in 2–4 divided doses	300
Ibuprofen	1,200–3,200 mg/day in 3–4 divided doses	3,200
Ketoprofen	150–300 mg/day in 3–4 divided doses	300
Naproxen	250–500 mg twice a day	1,500
Naproxen sodium	275–550 mg twice a day	1,375
Oxaprozin	600–1,200 mg daily	1,800
Fenamates		
Meclofenamate	200–400 mg/day in 3–4 divided doses	400
Mefenamic acid[f]	250 mg every 6 hours	1,000
Oxicams		
Piroxicam	10–20 mg daily	20
Meloxicam	7.5 mg daily	15
Coxibs		
Celecoxib	100 mg twice daily or 200 mg daily	200 (400 for RA)

[a]Maximum dosage in combination product limited by acetaminophen maximum of 4,000 mg/d.
[b]Monitor serum salicylate levels over 3 to 3.6 g/day.
[c]Only available as a liquid; 870 mg salicylate/5 mL.
[d]Not approved for treatment of OA for more than 5 days.
[e]Nonorganic acid but metabolite is an acetic acid.
[f]Not approved for treatment of OA.
RA, rheumatoid arthritis; SR, sustained release.

balance, in favor of thromboxane A_2, with prothrombotic events possible.[64-66] Whether the "prothrombotic imbalance" explanation causes the increased cardiovascular risk seen with COX-2–selective inhibitors remains unknown.[64-66] Celecoxib carries a black-box warning for cardiovascular and GI risks, as do other NSAIDs at this time.

Pharmacokinetics

The various NSAIDs exhibit several pharmacokinetic similarities, including high oral availability, high protein binding, and absorption as active drugs (except for sulindac and nabumetone, which require hepatic conversion for activity). The most important difference in NSAIDs is a serum half-life ranging from 1 hour for tolmetin to 50 hours for piroxicam, impacting the frequency of dosing and, potentially, compliance with therapy.[54] Elimination of NSAIDs largely depends on hepatic inactivation, with a small fraction of active drug being renally excreted. NSAIDs penetrate joint fluid, reaching approximately 60% of blood levels.

Efficacy

Prescription-strength NSAIDs are often prescribed for OA patients after treatment with acetaminophen proves ineffective or for patients with inflammatory OA. All NSAIDs and aspirin have similar analgesic and antiinflammatory effects, but these agents are only modestly more effective than acetaminophen.[60-62] In evaluating efficacy in OA studies, commonly used end points include pain on the visual analog scale (0 to 100) and the patient's global assessment of disease activity and functional status, using the Western Ontario and McMaster Universities Osteoarthritis Index questionnaire.[67] Effect size for NSAID treatment of OA is estimated at 0.32 (95% CI, 0.24-0.39) in comparison with that for acetaminophen at 0.21 (95% CI, 0.02-0.41). Because of differences among study designs and

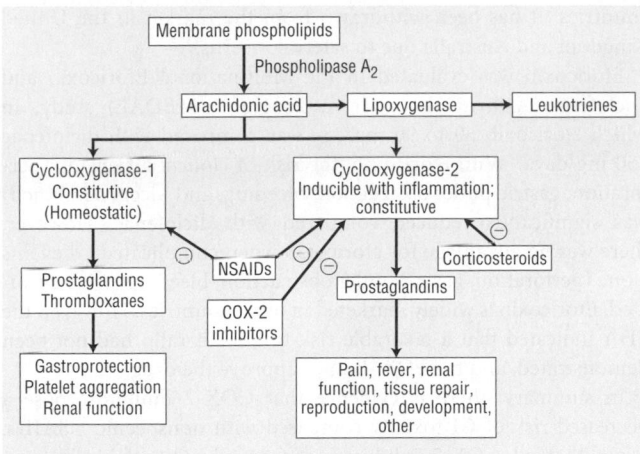

FIGURE 101-5. Pathway of synthesis for prostaglandins and leukotrienes. COX-1 and COX-2 are cyclooxygenase-1 and cyclooxygenase-2 enzymes, respectively. The minus (−) sign indicates inhibitory influence. Prostaglandins include PGE_2 and PGI_2; the latter is also known as prostacyclin.

patient populations, comparisons among efficacies of treatments are best made within the same study.

There is no definitive evidence to support superior efficacy for any NSAID.[60-62] However, individual patient response does differ among NSAIDs. The prescriber often relies on personal experience in choosing an NSAID. To assess efficacy in the individual patient, a trial that is adequate in time (2 to 3 weeks) and dose is needed. If the first trial fails, another NSAID in the same or another chemical class can be tried until an effective agent is found (see Table 101–2). Patients must understand this approach, appreciate the importance of adherence to medication therapy throughout this trial period, and actively participate in assessment of drug efficacy. Combining two NSAIDs increases adverse effects without providing additional benefit.

COX-2–selective inhibitors demonstrate similar analgesic benefits to traditional NSAIDs and to each other.[60-62] Celecoxib, lumiracoxib, and etoricoxib provided significant relief in OA compared with placebo and showed efficacy similar to other comparator NSAIDs. The newer COX-2–selective inhibitors have also been compared with older COX-2–selective inhibitors: Etoricoxib 30 mg/day and lumiracoxib 100 to 200 mg/day were similarly efficacious as celecoxib 200 mg/day and superior to placebo for OA.

Given that no proven efficacy differences exist among all traditional and COX-2–selective NSAIDs in OA, it is especially important that potential toxicities of these agents be rigorously examined. These safety issues are reviewed below.

Adverse Effects

Gastrointestinal Effects of Nonselective NSAIDs ❽ The

most common adverse effects of NSAIDs involve the GI tract, contributing to many treatment failures.[3,68-70] Minor complaints—nausea, dyspepsia, anorexia, abdominal pain, flatulence, and diarrhea—affect 10% to 60% of patients. To minimize these symptoms, NSAIDs should be taken with food or milk, except for enteric-coated products, which should *not* be taken with milk or antacids.

All NSAIDs have the potential to cause GI bleeding. [38,68] Un-ionized NSAIDs enter gastric mucosal cells, release hydrogen ions, and are concentrated ("ion trapped") within cells, resulting in cell death or damage. Gastric mucosal injury can also result from NSAID inhibition of gastroprotective prostaglandins.

The most common sites of GI injury are the gastric and duodenal mucosae. [68,69,71] The incidence of gastric ulcers with NSAID use is approximately 11% to 13%, and that for duodenal ulcers is 7% to 10%. Serious GI complications are associated with NSAIDs,

including perforations, gastric outlet obstruction, and bleeding. These important GI complications occur in 1.5% to 4% of patients per year. NSAIDs are so widely used that these small percentages translate into substantial morbidity and mortality. Moreover, the risk increases to 9% per year for patients with the risk factors of advanced age, history of peptic ulcer or GI bleeding, or cardiovascular disease. Consequently, about 16,500 deaths and 103,000 hospitalizations in the United States are associated annually with NSAID use in rheumatoid arthritis or OA patients.[4] A recent review that included a total of 1.3 million patients taking traditional NSAIDS for at least 2 months showed that 1 in 5 developed endoscopically evident ulcers, 1 in 70 had ulcer symptoms, 1 in 150 developed a GI tract perforation, and 1 in 1,200 died.[38]

A key part of the clinician's decision regarding starting NSAID therapy for an OA patient is the patient's risk for GI toxicity. [3,68-71] Increased GI risk is seen for those with a history of complicated ulcer [relative risk (RR) 13.5], use of multiple NSAIDs, including aspirin (RR = 9), use of high-dose NSAID (RR = 7), use of anticoagulant (RR = 6.4), age older than 70 years (RR = 5.6), and concomitant use of corticosteroids (RR = 2.2).[38]

Medications are available for the treatment or prevention of ulcers in high-risk patients. [32,69,70,72] Misoprostol protects against both gastric and duodenal NSAID-induced ulcers, and more importantly, their associated serious GI complications (perforations, gastric outlet obstruction, and bleeding). Unfortunately, misoprostol frequently causes diarrhea and abdominal cramps. Because of its abortifacient properties, misoprostol is contraindicated in pregnancy and in women of childbearing age who are not maintaining adequate contraception. It must be dispensed in its original container, which carries a warning for these individuals. Misoprostol is also available in a combination product with diclofenac, which bears the same restrictions as misoprostol alone.

Other agents have been evaluated in attempts to prevent NSAID-induced gastropathy. PPIs are effective, although neither sucralfate or H_2 antagonists have been shown to be protective.

Recently, Canadian consensus guidelines were developed to recommend gastroprotection for those on NSAID therapy.[70] The multidisciplinary group focused on four areas: Benefits of traditional NSAIDs, aspirin, and COX-2 inhibitors; harms of traditional NSAIDs, aspirin, and COX-2 inhibitors; reducing harms of traditional NSAIDs, aspirin, and COX-2 inhibitors; and economic considerations. Recommendations were made for patients at low GI and cardiovascular risk, low GI risk and high cardiovascular risk, high GI risk and low cardiovascular risk, and for those with high GI and cardiovascular risk (Fig. 101–6).

Gastrointestinal Effects of COX-2–Selective Inhibitors Celecoxib, rofecoxib, and all COX-2–selective inhibitors studied to date have demonstrated fewer endoscopically observed ulcers compared with traditional NSAIDs. Such ulcers are relatively common with NSAIDs and are often asymptomatic. Data regarding the rare but serious GI complications of perforation, obstruction, or bleeding are more difficult to obtain as very large numbers of patients are required for such studies.

In the Celecoxib Long-Term Arthritis Safety Study (CLASS) study, there was a reduced risk of ulcer complications and symptomatic ulcers for 400 mg daily celecoxib compared with nonselective NSAID combined at the 6-month point but not at one year. Celecoxib also did not decrease the risk of ulcer complications alone (perforation, obstruction, bleeding), and there was no gastroprotection by celecoxib in those taking aspirin. In the Successive Celecoxib Efficacy and Safety Study I (SUCCESS-I), however, celecoxib significantly reduced the risk of GI complications and of combined GI complications and symptomatic ulcers over 12 weeks, in comparison with nonselective NSAIDs.[73] Celecoxib did not reduce GI events in those taking aspirin.

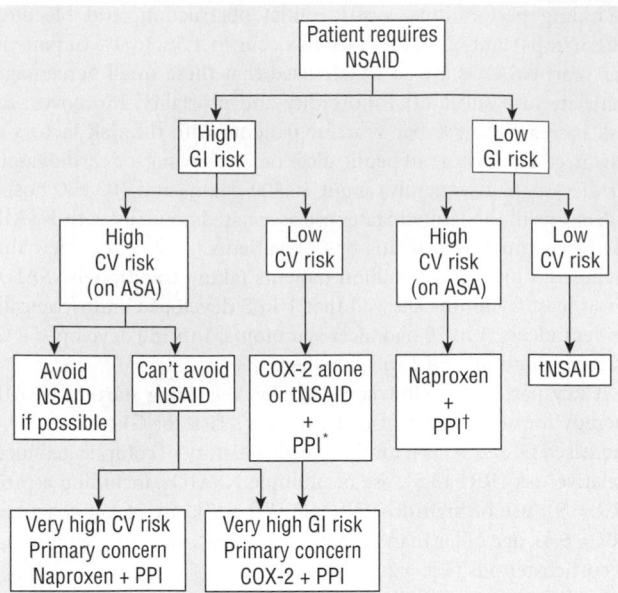

FIGURE 101-6. Algorithm for the use of long-term NSAID therapy and gastroprotective agents according to a patient's gastrointestinal and cardiovascular risk. *In high-risk patients, a COX-2 inhibitor and a tNSAID plus proton pump inhibitor (PPI) show similar reductions of rebleeding rates, but these reductions may be incomplete. †In general, most patients on acetylsalicylic acid plus naproxen would need the addition of a PPI. However, for some patients at very low GI risk, naproxen alone may be appropriate. *(Rostom A, Moayyedi P, Hunt R; Canadian Association of Gastroenterology Consensus Group. Canadian consensus guidelines on long-term nonsteroidal anti-inflammatory drug therapy and the need for gastroprotection: benefits versus risks. Aliment Pharmacol Ther. 2009 Mar 1;29(5):481. Wiley-Blackwell Publishers.)*

A systematic review of eight studies, three of which focused on celecoxib, demonstrated a 58% reduced risk for celecoxib compared with nonselective NSAID for ulcer complications and a 59% reduced risk for celecoxib compared with nonselective NSAID for ulcer complications combined with symptomatic ulcers.[60] Celecoxib use was also found to have significantly fewer GI symptoms of dyspepsia, nausea, diarrhea, and abdominal pain). Celecoxib users did have a modest (26%) but significant increased risk of "GI symptoms" compared with placebo.[73]

In addition and in celecoxib's favor, its use was associated with decreased outpatient physician claims for upper GI symptoms compared with other prescription nonspecific NSAIDs. Celecoxib was also comparable to a combination of diclofenac and omeprazole in reducing the risk of recurrent GI bleeding for patients who had a prior GI bleed.[74] Celecoxib remains on the market and is an alternative to traditional NSAIDs for those at high risk for GI toxicity.

GI safety for rofecoxib was evaluated in the Vioxx Gastrointestinal Outcomes Research (VIGOR) study, where patients were randomized to receive rofecoxib 50 mg daily or naproxen 500 mg twice daily; use of concomitant aspirin was prohibited. Those randomized to rofecoxib experienced a 50% lower risk of serious GI events.[75,76] These findings led to its approval by the FDA, but rofecoxib was withdrawn from the worldwide market in 2004 because of increased risk of cardiovascular events, as discussed in the section on cardiovascular risk.[76]

Lumiracoxib was evaluated in the Therapeutic Arthritis Research and Gastrointestinal Event Trial (TARGET).[77] With lumiracoxib, there was a significant 66% reduction in the risk of ulcer complications (perforation, gastric outlet obstruction, bleeding) compared with naproxen. However, in those taking aspirin, there was no protective effect of lumiracoxib. As mentioned earlier, lumiracoxib did not receive FDA approval but has been widely marketed in other

countries. It has been withdrawn from the market in the United Kingdom and Australia due to safety concerns.

Etoricoxib was evaluated in the Multinational Etoricoxib and Diclofenac Arthritis Long-Term Program (MEDAL) study, in which etoricoxib 60 to 90 mg/day was compared with diclofenac 150 mg/day.[78] With etoricoxib, the risk of *clinical* GI events (perforation, gastric outlet obstruction, bleeding, and ulcers combined) was significantly reduced compared with diclofenac. However, there was no advantage for etoricoxib when complicated GI events alone (perforation, gastric outlet obstruction, bleeding) were evaluated. Etoricoxib is widely marketed in other countries. However, the FDA indicated that a favorable risk-to-benefit ratio had not been demonstrated, and the FDA did not approve the drug.

In summary, there is evidence that COX-2 inhibitors pose a decreased risk of GI toxicity compared with nonspecific NSAIDs. Proof that all COX-2 inhibitors are equally GI safe is lacking; this may reflect intrinsic differences among agents, result from differences in study design, patient population, or concomitant medication use. All COX-2–selective inhibitors decrease the risk of endoscopic ulcers and reduce GI symptoms such as dyspepsia and nausea. Celecoxib decreased the risk of ulcer complications as well as symptomatic ulcers. Lumiracoxib also reduced the risk ulcer complications as well as symptomatic ulcers. Etoricoxib did reduce clinical GI events, but it was not proven to decrease the risk of ulcer complications. No COX-2–selective inhibitor has been proven to reduce the risk of ulcer complications for those patients taking aspirin. This is an important limitation because many of the same patients who are in need of OA pain relief also need cardioprotective aspirin.

Finally, aside from using a COX-2 inhibitor or using a nonspecific NSAID with a PPI for gastroprotection, the combination of celecoxib with a PPI has also been studied. For patients at very high GI risk, who had experienced a prior GI bleed, the combination of a PPI with celecoxib substantially decreased the risk of future bleeding ulcers compared with celecoxib alone.[74]

Cardiovascular Risk of COX-2 Inhibitors and Traditional NSAIDs
In 2004, rofecoxib was withdrawn from the market after analysis of the Adenomatous Polyp Prevention on Vioxx (APPROVe) trial, where rofecoxib doubled the risk of cardiovascular events compared with placebo.[76] Celecoxib use in the Adenoma Prevention with Celecoxib (APC) trial also increased cardiovascular risk.[79] These observations raised questions about the cardiovascular safety of all COX-2–selective NSAIDs and even traditional NSAIDs. The FDA formulated regulations and new labeling on all NSAIDs, and these events prompted metaanalyses of randomized controlled trials of COX-2–selective inhibitors and of NSAIDs.[80–83] Case control and cohort studies of patients using these agents have also examined cardiovascular risks involved with their use.[81,82]

The increased cardiovascular risk posed by rofecoxib was clearly demonstrated in the APPROVe trial, and the VIGOR trial also showed this risk.[38] The cardiovascular risk of celecoxib, particularly when used at the approved dose for OA (200 mg daily) is much less certain. In the CLASS study, a small but insignificant increase risk in cardiovascular risk was shown at a dose of 400 mg/day, and the APC trial showed a significantly increased risk with a dose greater than 400 mg/day. However, the Alzheimer Disease Antiinflammatory Prevention Trial (ADAPT) study, using 200 mg twice daily, did not show increased cardiovascular risk.[82]

The cardiovascular safety of lumiracoxib was evaluated in the TARGET study.[77] Cardiovascular risk with lumiracoxib showed a nonsignificant increase relative to ibuprofen, but not in comparison to naproxen, and this increase was only seen in those not taking aspirin. The cardiovascular safety of etoricoxib was evaluated in the MEDAL study.[80] Etoricoxib (60 or 90 mg daily) and diclofenac (150 mg daily) were compared, and very similar event rates for thrombotic cardiovascular events occurred for the etoricoxib group and for the diclofenac group. Both studies had drawbacks. TARGET had few events (50 and 59 in the two groups). For the MEDAL study, diclofenac was not an ideal comparator to show that etoricoxib had no increased risk relative to nonselective NSAIDs, as it also possessed come COX-2 activity.

Other studies on coxibs including cardiovascular events and a metaanalysis of 138 randomized controlled trials including 145,373 patients were carried out.[81] Studies were analyzed for MI, stroke, or cardiovascular death, as well as a combined end point for all three ("cardiovascular events"). Coxibs as a whole, compared with placebo, increased the risk for cardiovascular events, RR of 1.42 (1.13-1.78). There was no increased risk for strokes alone, and increased risk was primarily due to myocardial infarction (MI), with a RR of 1.86 (1.33-2.59). This increased risk was spread across the class of COX-2–selective inhibitors, but most information came from trials of celecoxib and rofecoxib. For celecoxib, there was a significant trend for increased cardiovascular risk with higher daily doses (at or above 400 mg/day). In comparing coxibs with traditional NSAIDs, coxibs were associated with significantly more cardiovascular events than naproxen, RR = 1.57 (1.21–2.03), again primarily due to MIs, RR = 2.04 (1.41–2.96).

The same work also included metaanalyses of NSAIDs compared with placebo. Traditional NSAIDs showed increased cardiovascular events with diclofenac [RR = 1.63 (1.12-2.37)] and an insignificant increase with ibuprofen [RR = 1.51 (0.96-2.37)], but no increased risk with naproxen. A drawback in this work was that with the number of cardiovascular events in the metaanalyses, it was not possible to statistically differentiate the risk of one coxib compared with another. However, no heterogeneity was seen among the coxibs studied, which suggests a class effect.

Further insights into the cardiovascular risk of celecoxib was obtained from a pooled analysis of 7,950 patients in six placebo-controlled trials using three dose regimens of celecoxib (Cross Trial Safety Analysis).[82] Although the analysis was limited to conditions other than arthritis, it provides insight on the relationship between celecoxib dose and events and the importance of underlying cardiovascular risk. For the composite end point of cardiovascular death, MI, stroke, heart failure, or thromboembolic events, for all dose regimens, the overall hazard ratio for celecoxib compared with placebo was 1.6 (95% CI, 1.1-2.3). The hazard ratios with different doses were 3.1 (95% CI, 1.5-6.1) for 400 mg twice daily, 1.8 (95% CI, 1.1-3.1) for the 200 mg twice daily dosing, and the lowest risk, 1.1 (95% CI, 0.6-2.0) for 400 mg once daily dosing. In the study, patients were also stratified at baseline into three cardiovascular risk groups. The overall event rate increased when comparing the groups with low, intermediate, and highest baseline risk. When adjusted for baseline cardiovascular risk, there was a highly significant trend for increased risk, again increasing with dose. The adverse effect of dose was highest in those classified as high risk at baseline. Whether patients used or did not aspirin, celecoxib was associated with increased risk.

In addition to controlled trials, analysis of cohort or case control studies can also contribute to information about risk, but such studies have confounders and do not necessarily produce consistent findings. In a systematic review of observational studies of COX-2 inhibitors and traditional NSAIDs, including approximately 1 million patients, risk for cardiovascular events were calculated in comparison with nonusers or those with remote use of NSAIDs.[83] The summary RR was 1.33 (95% CI, 1.00-1.79) for rofecoxib 25 mg/day and 2.19 (95% CI, 1.64 to 2.91) with more than 25 mg/day, with risk apparent within the first month of treatment. Celecoxib summary RR was 1.06 (95% CI, 0.91-1.23), but there was much variation in risk among studies. Other summary RRs examined were for naproxen at 0.97 (95% CI, 0.87-1.07), piroxicam at 1.06 (95% CI, 0.70-1.59), and ibuprofen at 1.07 (95% CI, 0.97-1.18). Diclofenac,

however, showed an increased summary RR of 1.40 (CI, 1.16-1.70), which is concerning.[83]

Taken together, the above data, both from controlled trials and from observational studies, confirm the increased cardiovascular risk seen with rofecoxib. Celecoxib 200 mg/day or even 400 mg/day does not appear to increase risk, but cardiovascular risk is likely increased with doses above 400 mg/day. In addition, , the risk of taking higher doses of celecoxib is greater for those with high cardiovascular risk than for those with low cardiovascular risk. Although studies with lumiracoxib and ctoricoxib are somewhat reassuring and do not point to substantially increased cardiovascular risk, further work is needed on this issue. The balance of the evidence also suggests that, for the traditional NSAIDs that have been examined, with the exception of diclofenac, there is no significant or substantial increase in risk.

These differences may depend on the degree of selectivity of specific COX-2 inhibitors for COX-2 versus COX-1 enzymes. COX-2 selectivity is relative: Some traditional NSAIDs, such as diclofenac, possess some COX-2 selectivity, and even among the formally labeled COX-2 inhibitors, COX-2 selectivity varies. Interestingly, rofecoxib is more COX-2 selective than celecoxib. It is possible that rofecoxib's greater selectivity is responsible both for better GI protection *and* for increased cardiovascular risk. Such a connection is plausible, given the effects of COX-1 and COX-2 enzymes on the formation of thromboxane A_2 and prostacyclin. A highly selective COX-2 inhibitor may tilt the balance in favor of thromboxane A_2, thus promoting platelet aggregation (beneficial for preventing GI bleeding, but posing a prothrombotic risk to the cardiovascular system).

Key issues for any future coxib development will be their degree of gastroprotection and what, if any, cardiovascular risk they pose. Further study will be needed to determine if one or more of these agents will be safe for the cardiovascular system and also gastroprotective, or whether the degree of gastroprotection is inextricably linked to the extent of cardiovascular risk for all COX-2–selective inhibitors.

CLINICAL CONTROVERSY

There is continuing controversy surrounding the clinically meaningful gastroprotective effects of COX-2 inhibitors and the cardiovascular risks they may pose. Are all COX-2 inhibitors GI protective? Do they all pose cardiovascular risk? Furthermore, while the gastrointestinal complications associated with traditional NSAIDs are well recognized, the cardiovascular risks posed by these agents are somewhat less clear. Some clinicians have applied the cardiovascular risk data regarding all NSAIDs (COX-1 and COX-2 selective) to practice with complete avoidance of all NSAIDs. Questions still remain regarding the relative safety of short courses of low-dose NSAIDs for cardiac patients with unrelieved OA pain.

Considerations for Patients at Risk for Both GI and Cardiovascular Events ❾ Several American and international organizations have recommended strategies for NSAID use among patients at high risk for GI or cardiovascular events. Evidence-based Canadian consensus guidelines on long-term NSAID therapy, considering both GI and cardiovascular risk, were recently developed (Fig 101–7).[70] The recommendations presupposed use of cardioprotective aspirin in those with increased cardiovascular risk. For those without increased GI or cardiovascular risk, a nonspecific NSAID was recommended. For patients with low GI risk but high cardiovascular risk, naproxen may be safer than other NSAIDs. For those with increased GI risk but without increased cardiovascular risk, a COX-2–selective inhibitor, combined with a PPI, is probably

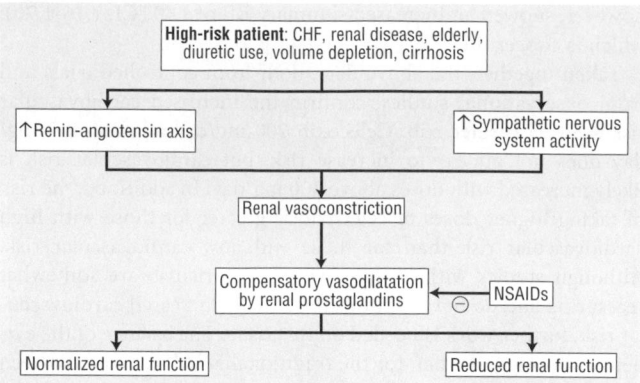

FIGURE 101-7. Mechanisms implicated in NSAID-induced renal injury. The minus (−) sign indicates inhibitory influence (CHF, congestive heart failure; NSAIDs, nonsteroidal antiinflammatory drugs).

safest from the GI perspective. For those patients who are at high GI and cardiovascular risk, careful consideration of which risk is most concerning is needed. If GI safety is paramount, a COX-2 inhibitor plus a PPI is recommended. If cardiovascular risk is the most concerning, naproxen plus a PPI would be preferred.

Other Toxicities Associated with NSAIDs ⑩ NSAIDs

may cause kidney diseases, including acute renal insufficiency, tubulointerstitial nephropathy, hyperkalemia, and renal papillary necrosis.[84-86] Clinical features of these NSAID-induced renal syndromes include increased serum creatinine and blood urea nitrogen, hyperkalemia, elevated blood pressure, peripheral edema, and weight gain. Mechanisms of NSAID injury include direct toxicity and inhibition of local prostaglandins that promote vasodilation of renal blood vessels and preserve renal blood flow. Patients at high risk are those with conditions associated with decreased renal blood flow or taking certain medications. Examples are those with chronic renal insufficiency, congestive heart failure, severe hepatic disease, and nephrotic syndrome, those of advanced age, or those taking diuretics, angiotensin-converting enzyme inhibitors, cyclosporine, or aminoglycosides (Fig. 101–7).

Close monitoring is advisable for high-risk patients taking an NSAID, with monitoring of serum creatinine at baseline and within 3 to 7 days of drug initiation. For those with impaired renal function, the National Kidney Foundation recommends acetaminophen over NSAIDs, although acetaminophen may pose risks also, as discussed above.

Coxibs can also pose renal risks, and there is neither evidence nor rationale why this class of drugs would be safer than nonspecific NSAIDs. In a metaanalysis of randomized trials of NSAIDs including more than 100,000 patients, rofecoxib was shown to significantly increase risk of renal toxicity in comparison to placebo, celecoxib, and nonspecific NSAIDs.[86] Although rofecoxib is now off the market, this study provides an important caution as new coxibs are approved: Renal safety of coxibs may differ substantially. Keeping in mind that many OA patients may not be as healthy as trial participants, it is prudent to prescribe all coxibs and other NSAIDs with caution for patients who are at increased risk for renal dysfunction.

Coxibs and NSAIDs uncommonly cause drug-induced hepatitis; the two NSAIDs most frequently implicated are diclofenac and sulindac. Patient monitoring should include periodic liver enzymes (aspartate aminotransferase and alanine aminotransferase), with cessation of therapy if these values exceed two to three times the normal range. In a pooled analysis of 41 studies including celecoxib, there was a low rate of serious, hepatic-related adverse events with celecoxib (1.11%), with no significant difference from naproxen or ibuprofen, but a significantly higher incidence with diclofenac (4.24%).[87]

Other toxic effects of NSAIDs include hypersensitivity reactions, rash, and CNS complaints of drowsiness, dizziness, headaches, depression, confusion, and tinnitus.[54] Although NSAIDs are generally avoided for patients with asthma who are aspirin-intolerant, studies indicate that celecoxib is well tolerated in aspirin-sensitive asthma, providing a viable option for these patients.[88] Celecoxib is a sulfonamide and is thus contraindicated for those with sulfa allergies. However, some patients with sulfa allergies have shown no reaction to celecoxib, and in a metaanalysis including more than 11,000 patients, allergic reactions for those who did have sulfonamide allergies were similar in those taking celecoxib compared with those taking other NSAIDs.

All nonspecific NSAIDs inhibit COX-1–dependent thromboxane production in platelets and thus increase bleeding risk. Importantly, aspirin inhibition is irreversible, and bleeding time requires 5 to 7 days to normalize after cessation of therapy, as new platelets enter the circulation. Other nonspecific NSAIDs inhibit thromboxane formation reversibly, with normalization of platelet function 1 to 3 days after the drug is stopped. The nonacetylated salicylate products and nabumetone, which have partial COX-2 selectivity, may be preferable to nonspecific NSAIDs.[54] COX-2–selective inhibitors do not block thromboxane synthesis and should pose even less bleeding risk. However, because warfarin and celecoxib are metabolized by the cytochrome P450 isoenzyme CYP2C9, patients receiving warfarin and COX-2 inhibitors should be followed closely.

Finally, NSAIDs should be used only with great caution and only if definitely necessary during pregnancy because of the risk to the fetus posed by the bleeding problems. In late pregnancy, all NSAIDs should be avoided because they may enhance premature closure of the ductus arteriosus. Many NSAIDs, including naproxen, diclofenac, and celecoxib have a pregnancy risk factor of C/D (third trimester), and ibuprofen is listed as category D throughout pregnancy. Acetaminophen has a pregnancy risk factor of B.

Drug–Drug and Drug–Food Interactions

Important drug interactions with NSAIDs can be pharmacokinetic or pharmacodynamic in origin and have been reviewed.[54,89] The most potentially serious interactions include the use of NSAIDs with lithium, warfarin, other agents that increase bleeding risk, oral hypoglycemics, methotrexate, antihypertensives, angiotensin-converting enzyme inhibitors, β-blockers, and diuretics. Anticipation and careful monitoring often can prevent serious events when these drugs are used together. In addition, there are probable drug interactions with tacrolimus for ibuprofen, naproxen, diclofenac, and possibly other NSAIDs.

Another drug interaction has been noted for those taking some NSAIDs and cardioprotective doses of aspirin. Ibuprofen, used at doses of 400 mg or more, may block aspirin's antiplatelet effect if it is taken prior to aspirin. Patients are advised to take a single dose of ibuprofen at least 30 minutes after taking aspirin, or they should take their aspirin at least 8 hours after taking ibuprofen.[90] It is possible that other nonselective NSAIDs, such as naproxen, also may cause such interactions. Acetaminophen does not appear to interfere with the antiplatelet effect of aspirin.

Specific drug interactions are also seen with coxibs. Celecoxib metabolism is primarily via CYP2C9.[89] In clinical studies, increased celecoxib levels were seen with fluconazole administration. Cytochrome P450 inducers such as rifampin, carbamazepine, and phenytoin have the potential to reduce celecoxib levels. However, no clinically significant interactions have been documented with celecoxib and methotrexate, glyburide, ketoconazole, phenytoin, or tolbutamide. Because celecoxib inhibits CYP2D6, it has the potential to increase concentrations of a variety of agents, including antidepressants. Celecoxib increases lithium levels, as do other NSAIDs; thus, caution is needed when using coxibs or NSAIDs with lithium.

Dosing and Administration Administration of NSAIDs must be tailored to the individual patient with OA. For the OA patient who has failed an adequate trial of acetaminophen, trial with an NSAID is warranted, if no contraindications exist. Selection of an NSAID depends on the prescriber's experience, medication cost, patient preference, allergies, toxicities, and adherence issues. Individual patient response differs among NSAIDs (see Table 101–2), so if an inadequate response is obtained with one NSAID, another NSAID may yet provide benefit.[40,54,91]

Topical Therapies

⓫ Topical products can be used alone or in combination with oral analgesics or NSAIDs. Capsaicin, isolated from hot peppers, releases and ultimately depletes substance P from afferent nociceptive nerve fibers. Substance P has been implicated in the transmission of pain in arthritis, and capsaicin cream has been shown in four placebo-controlled studies to provide pain relief in OA when applied over affected joints.[40,92] Data comparing topical capsaicin to other effective pharmacologic treatments for OA is lacking.

Adverse events associated with capsaicin are primarily local, with one in three patients experiencing burning, stinging, and/or erythema that usually subsides with repeated application. Some patients may experience coughing associated with application. Capsaicin is a nonprescription product available as a cream, gel, or lotion in concentrations ranging from 0.025% to 0.075%.

To be effective, capsaicin must be used regularly, and it may take up to 2 weeks to take effect. Although use is recommended four times a day, a twice-daily application may enhance long-term adherence and still provide adequate pain relief.[92] Patients should be warned not to get the cream in their eyes or mouth and to wash their hands after application. When patients were queried using an electronic questionnaire that considered possible toxicities of treatments, as well as route of administration and cost, capsaicin was the most preferred by patients, even when it was portrayed as being less effective than NSAIDs.[55]

Topical NSAIDs can be used to achieve NSAID efficacy for the treatment of OA, while avoiding the serious adverse effects associated with systemic NSAID therapy. The mechanism of action of topical NSAIDs is thought to be primarily by local inhibition of COX-2 enzymes, although it is unclear if there are other factors that contribute to the beneficial effects of these agents. There tends to be high placebo response rates associated with topical therapy in general, as the act of rubbing itself may desensitize local nerve endings and activate pain-gating mechanisms, but active topical NSAID therapy is consistently superior to placebo.[93]

Topical NSAIDs are commonly associated with dermatologic adverse effects at the application site including pruritus, burning, pain, and rash with serious adverse events being rare. It is unclear if topical NSAIDs are associated with significant cardiovascular or gastrointestinal adverse events, although current data suggest relative safety.[94] Treatment with topical NSAIDs can be considered when first-line agents fail, are contraindicated, or are poorly tolerated. Recent treatment guidelines from the American Academy of Orthopedic Surgeons recommends topical NSAIDs as acceptable first-line therapy, although OARSI and ACR continue to recommend these agents as second line.[36,39,40]

The only FDA-approved topical NSAID for OA is diclofenac gel 1%. Other topical NSAIDs—including ibuprofen, ketoprofen, and indomethacin—are available as extemporaneously compounded products or as nonprescription products. It is important to note that many variables influence the extent and rate of absorption of topical drugs including the vehicle of the formulation, the molecular weight of the drug, and the hydrophilicity of the drug.[94] Care should be taken to choose a topical NSAID with a reliable delivery system.

Topical diclofenac 1% gel is applied four times daily using the dose measuring cards provided by the manufacturer. Patients should not exceed the recommended dose. Patients should avoid oral NSAIDs while using topical products to minimize potential for additive adverse effects. Care should be taken to avoid contact with the eyes or open wounds.

Although not well studied in a controlled setting, the use of topical rubefacients, containing methylsalicylate, trolamine salicylate, and other salicylates, may have modest, short-term efficacy in the treatment of acute pain associated with musculoskeletal conditions, including OA.[95] These agents act by providing topical counterirritation to the affected joint area rather than by local inhibition of COX-2 enzymes. Chronic OA pain may respond less favorably than acute pain. Clinically significant adverse events are local skin reactions that occur rarely. There are no reports of systemic toxicity associated with topical rubefacients.

Glucosamine and Chondroitin

Interest in chondroitin and glucosamine was spurred initially by anecdotal reports of benefit in animals and humans and by the ability of these substances to stimulate proteoglycan synthesis from articular cartilage in vitro. The excellent safety profile of these agents makes them especially appealing for use in those at high risk for adverse events, such as elderly patients, and in those with multiple morbidities. Over the last several years, enthusiasm for these agents has waned as additional data has become available to the point that two recent evidence-based guidelines recommend against the use of glucosamine and chondroitin for the treatment of knee OA.[39,96]

Numerous trials have been conducted with suboptimal study designs, and this has led to a variable response to glucosamine and/or chondroitin.[96] Study design flaws have included small sample size, wide intersubject heterogeneity, industry sponsorship, lack of clinically important end points, as well as lack of data related to intention-to-treat analysis. Conducting a metaanalysis of these type glucosamine and chondroitin trials does not necessarily solve the initial trial design issues. In contrast to the early reports of suboptimally designed studies, a large, well-controlled National Institutes of Health–sponsored study demonstrated no significant clinical response to glucosamine therapy alone, chondroitin therapy alone, or combination glucosamine–chondroitin therapy when compared with placebo across all patients.[97] This trial provides the highest quality evidence available on the efficacy of glucosamine and chondroitin to date. However, subgroup analyses for patients with moderate to severe knee pain showed a response to combination glucosamine–chondroitin therapy superior to placebo, although this finding did not reach the predetermined threshold for pain reduction. The safety of the glucosamine and chondroitin therapy was similar to that of placebo.

The exact role of glucosamine, chondroitin, or a combination of the two products is still unclear. Because of the relative safety of these agents, many clinicians consider a trial of glucosamine–chondroitin reasonable for patients with moderate to severe knee OA considering the adverse effects associated with traditional OA treatments. Dosing should be at least 1,500 mg/day of glucosamine and 1,200 mg/day of chondroitin. The glucosamine component should be the sulfate salt rather than the hydrochloride salt, as nearly all positive efficacy studies used the better-absorbed sulfate salt. Glucosamine-related adverse events are generally mild and include gastrointestinal symptoms (gas, bloating, cramps). If made from shellfish, however, glucosamine should not be used for patients with shellfish allergies. The initial concerns regarding glucosamine-induced hyperglycemia had likely been overstated since later safety data in both healthy subjects and those with type 2 diabetes mellitus did not show significant elevations in blood glucose. Chondroitin is extremely well tolerated with the most common adverse effect being nausea. Depending on the source of chondroitin (cattle, pig, or shark), this compound could also pose risk to persons who are allergic to shark.

Because glucosamine and chondroitin are marketed in the United States as dietary supplements, neither the products nor their purity is adequately regulated by the FDA. The potential consequences related to the lack of regulatory oversight for these products can affect both efficacy and safety. Products containing less than labeled doses can compromise efficacy, while those containing ingredients not included on the labeling can compromise safety. A variety of brand name and generic products are available.

CLINICAL CONTROVERSY

The role of herbal and supplement therapies in the treatment of OA is a source of continuing controversy. A variety of herbal therapies—including ginger, devil's claw, methylsulfonylmethane, flavonoids, willow bark, fish oils, avocado/soybean unsaponifiables, and *Boswellia serrata*—have been purported to have efficacy in the treatment of pain associated with OA. Many patients encounter advertising and other publications in the lay media extolling the benefits of these products. Unfortunately, the lack of scientific trials evaluating these agents makes it difficult to determine their role in therapy. Until additional efficacy and safety information becomes available, recommendations regarding the routine use of these products should be tempered by known drug safety data (if available) and other related safety issues. Costs of therapy, delays in seeking treatments known to be effective, and potential exposure to products produced without standard manufacturing processes can also lead to poor outcomes for patients.

Corticosteroids

Intraarticular glucocorticoid injections can provide excellent pain relief, particularly when a joint effusion is present.[40,98] Aspiration of the effusion and injection of glucocorticoid are carried out aseptically, with examination of the aspirate recommended to exclude crystalline arthritis or infection. (This incidence is low, however—approximately 1 in 50,000 procedures.) After injection, the patient should minimize activity and stress on the joint for several days. Initial pain relief may be seen within 24 to 72 hours after injection, with peak pain relief about 7 to 10 days after injection and lasting up to 4 to 8 weeks.

Several randomized, placebo-controlled, double-blind studies have shown that intraarticular corticosteroids are superior to placebo in alleviating knee pain and stiffness caused by OA.[98] The branched esters of triamcinolone and methylprednisolone are preferred by practitioners because of the reduced solubility that allows the agents to remain in the joint space longer. There is no evidence of a clinically superior corticosteroid for intraarticular use, with equipotent doses of methylprednisolone acetate and triamcinolone hexacetonide having similar efficacy.[99] Average doses for injection of large joints in adults are 10 to 20 mg of triamcinolone hexacetonide or 20 to 40 mg of methylprednisolone acetate. This therapy is generally limited to three or four injections per year due to the potential systemic effects of corticosteroids and because the need for more frequent injections indicates little response to the therapy.

Adverse events associated with intraarticular injection of corticosteroids can be local or systemic in nature. Systemic adverse events are the same as with any other systemic corticosteroid and

can include hyperglycemia, edema, elevated blood pressure, dyspepsia, and, rarely, adrenal suppression with continuous, repeated injections. Hyperglycemia may occur in patients with stable diabetes mellitus as well as those without history of abnormal glycemic control.[39] Local adverse effects can include infection in the affected joint, osteonecrosis, tendon rupture, and skin atrophy at the injection site. It has long been thought that intraarticular corticosteroids can hasten cartilage loss, but the potential risk of cartilage destruction with steroid injections has not been substantiated. The rate of cartilage loss tends to be similar between treated and control groups.

Systemic corticosteroid therapy is not recommended in OA, given the lack of proven benefit and the well-known adverse effects with long-term use.

Hyaluronate Injections

Agents containing hyaluronic acid (HA; sodium hyaluronate) are available for intraarticular injection for treatment of knee OA.[100] High-molecular-weight HA is an important constituent of synovial fluid. Endogenous HA may also have antiinflammatory effects. Because the concentration and molecular size of synovial HA decreases in OA, administration of exogenous HA products have been studied, with the theory that this could reconstitute synovial fluid and reduce symptoms. In fact, HA injections temporarily and modestly increase viscosity. HA injections appear to have positive effects on pain and function compared with placebo, although most studies were short term and poorly controlled, and placebo injections also reduced OA pain dramatically. When evaluating pain score improvements, it is essential to determine if score improvement corresponds to clinically meaningful improvement for patients. Extensive evaluation of the literature has revealed potential publication bias of HA studies including bias related to high levels of industry sponsorship as well as a substantial number of studies with unpublished data.[96] Most HA products are injected once weekly for either 3 or 5 weeks, depending on the specific agent administered. There are six commercially available preparations: Hyalgan, Euflexxa (20 mg sodium hylaronate/2 mL), Supartz (25 mg sodium hylaronate/2.5 mL), Synvisc (16 mg hylan polymers/ 2 mL), Synvisc-One (48 mg hylan polymers/6 mL), and Orthovisc (30 mg hyaluronan/2 mL). Hyalgan and Supartz are administered weekly for five injections, whereas Synvisc, Euflexxa, and Orthovisc are administered weekly for three injections. Synvisc-One is administered as single one time dose with efficacy up to 26 weeks. Injections are generally well tolerated, although acute joint swelling, effusion, and stiffness can occur as well as local skin reactions, including rash, ecchymoses and pruritus have been reported. Rarely, systemic adverse events including hypersensitivity reactions have occurred.

HA injections may be beneficial for patients with knee OA unresponsive to other therapies. HA products have not been shown to benefit patients with hip OA.[101] These agents are expensive because the treatment includes both drug costs and administration costs. As a result, HA injections are often used after more effective and less expensive therapies have demonstrated a lack of efficacy.

Opioid Analgesics

Low-dose opioid analgesics can be useful for patients who experience no pain relief with acetaminophen, NSAIDs, intraarticular injections, or topical therapy. For patients with underlying diseases that limit the use of nonopioid analgesics, opioid analgesics can effectively relieve pain. A common clinical scenario may include the patient who cannot take NSAIDs because of renal failure or cardiovascular disease. Patients in whom all other treatment options have failed and who are at high surgical risk, precluding joint arthroplasty are also candidates for opioid therapy. As many patients with OA are elderly, it is important to carefully use opioids to promote safety. The following recommendations have been suggested to optimize opioid therapy: (1) use the least invasive route of administration, (2) initiate one agent at a time, at a low dose, (3) allow a sufficiently long interval between dose increases to allow an assessment of efficacy and safety, (4) use a long-acting preparation, (5) therapy should be constantly monitored and adjusted if necessary, (6) changing opioids may be necessary.[102]

Sustained-release (SR) compounds usually offer better pain control throughout the day, and are used when immediate-release (IR) opioids do not provide a sufficient duration of pain control. A variety of immediate and sustained-release opioid compounds have been studied including oxycodone IR and SR, morphine IR and SR, hydromorphone and fentanyl transdermal patch.[102]

Adverse effects are common in opioid-treated OA patients. More than 75% of patients in clinical trials experience at least one typical opioid-related (nausea, somnolence, constipation, and dizziness) adverse effect. Although this is not an unexpected finding, it serves as a reminder to use opioids cautiously in elderly patients who may be more susceptible to adverse effects.

If pain is intolerable and limits activities of daily living, and the patient has sufficiently good cardiopulmonary health to undergo major surgery, joint replacement may be preferable to continued reliance on opioids.

Tramadol

Tramadol, an analgesic with affinity for the μ-opioid receptor, as well as weak inhibition of the reuptake of norepinephrine and serotonin neurotransmitter has modest analgesic effects (with or without acetaminophen) for patients with OA when compared with placebo.[103] Tramadol is also modestly effective as add-on therapy for patients taking concomitant NSAIDs or COX-2–selective inhibitors.[104] As with opioid analgesics, tramadol may be helpful for patients who cannot take NSAIDs or COX-2–selective inhibitors. Tramadol should be initiated at a lower dose (100 mg per day) and may be titrated as needed for pain control to a dose of 200 mg per day. Tramadol is available in a combination tablet with acetaminophen and as a sustained-release tablet.

Opioid-like adverse effects such as nausea, vomiting, dizziness, constipation, headache, and somnolence are common with tramadol. These occur in 60% to 70% of treated patients, and 40% discontinue tramadol because of an adverse effect.[103] Although the frequency of adverse effects is high, the severity of adverse effects is less than with NSAIDs, as tramadol use is not associated with life-threatening gastrointestinal bleeding or renal failure.

Considerations for Future Therapeutic Options

Strategies aimed at expanding therapeutic options are concentrated on an array of disease-modifying drugs targeted at preventing, retarding, or reversing damage to articular cartilage. Thus far, OA is a progressive disease that can only be treated symptomatically. Because of this, clinicians are very interested in nonpharmacologic measures and pharmacologic therapy that can slow the progression of damage to the articular cartilage. Current approaches to slow progression of OA are directed at 3 different tissue specific targets: (1) cartilage, (2) synovial membrane, and (3) subchondral bone. One modality being explored in the preclinical stage is that of autologous chondrocyte transplantation (ACT) using mesenchymal stem cells, a treatment aimed at restoring cartilage lost or damaged by OA.

Therapies directed at preserving cartilage include enzyme inhibitors of MMPs, inhibitors of inducible nitric oxide synthase, inhibitors of eicosanoids, and nerve growth factor inhibitors.[105] Several of these investigational agents have progressed from testing in animal

models to clinical trials in humans. Doxycycline, as a tissue inhibitor of metalloproteinases potentially decreases cartilage destruction. In knee OA, doxycycline has been shown to delay loss of articular cartilage (joint space narrowing) in humans when compared with placebo.[106] Ongoing phase III clinical trials with licofelone, a lipoxygenase/cyclooxygenase inhibitor (LOX/COX) have demonstrated some encouraging preliminary data in delaying progression of OA.[107] Combined LOX/COX inhibitor may decrease the production of proinflammatory leukotrienes associated with the progression of OA. An agent targeted toward maintaining synovial membrane integrity is diacerein, an interleukin-1β inhibitor. In a metaanalysis including a total of 2,069 OA patients, this agent decreased pain to a modest but statistically significant extent compared with placebo. In long-term studies, diacerein appeared to show a significant slowing of progression of joint space narrowing at the hip, but not at the knee.[108]

Slowing the progression of OA may also be achieved by attempts to modify or repair bony changes associated with OA. Current strategies being evaluated in humans include the use of bisphosphonates, calcitonin, selective estrogen receptor modulators, parathyroid hormone, strontium, and MMP-13 inhibitors. The definitive role of these agents in modifying bone resorption as a strategy to delay the progression of bone damage associated with OA is yet to be determined. Aside from agents that may prevent disease progression, attempts to find new agents or methods to treat symptoms of OA are being made. There is recent interest in the potential of COX-inhibiting nitric oxide-donor compounds (CINODs) to relieve OA pain while sparing GI adverse effects.[45,109] Published clinical data on the CINOD, Naproxinod, has shown that it provided some improvement in GI tolerance, and was similarly efficacious as naproxen for pain control in OA patients. naproxinod may also have advantages with regard to blood pressure, as it provided a small decrease in blood pressure of treated subjects, whereas comparator NSAIDs caused a small increase in blood pressure. Another agent being studied is avocado/soy unsaponifiables (ASUs). A recent metaanalysis including a total of 664 participants with knee or hip OA showed that subjects randomized to ASU demonstrated a modest but significant improvement in pain.[45] It is theorized that the oily fractions of avocado unsaponifiables decrease production of nitric oxide and stimulate production of plasminogen activator inhibitor-1 that can decrease MMPs.

In addition to pharmacologic agents, acupuncture has been examined in OA. In a systematic analysis of 18 randomized, controlled trials of manual or electroacupuncture, 10 showed positive effects for acupuncture.[110] However, in a recent, large, randomized, and well-controlled study, acupuncture was not seen to be any more effective than sham controls.[111]

■ PHARMACOECONOMIC CONSIDERATIONS

There are substantial economic ramifications with OA, as the disease is extremely common, and OA ranks second in causes of disability in the United States.[1,40]

One of the highest costs associated with the pharmacotherapy of OA is hospitalization for treatment of NSAID-related complications, particularly serious GI adverse events. Several cost analysis have been performed to determine the cost-effectiveness of gastroprotective therapy in NSAID users. The cost-effectiveness of using NSAIDS or COX-2–selective inhibitors with or without concomitant PPI therapy in both high-risk and low-risk patients was reported, based on estimates of the risk of GI complications in these settings.[112] The cost of avoiding one serious GI complication would be $61,933 if all NSAID patients were given a PPI, but only $4,355 if PPIs were limited to high-risk patients. In the same analysis, the cost of avoiding one serious GI complication would be $62,467 if all NSAID patients were given a COX-2–selective inhibitor. The cost-effectiveness of an NSAID plus a PPI for high-risk patients has been demonstrated by others as well.[113] Historically, gastroprotective therapy or the use of COX-2–selective inhibitors for low-risk patients has not been cost-effective because of the large number needed to treat to prevent serious events, but current data suggest that concomitant PPI therapy in low-risk patients is cost-effective if the agent selected is a generic, multisource product.[114] The use of COX-2–selective inhibitors to protect gastric mucosa in aspirin users is not cost-effective, because aspirin negates most, if not all, of the gastroprotective effects of these agents.[112,113]

Pharmacoeconomic considerations for OA involve the selection of therapy for the initial treatment of patients with OA. Use of the nonprescription analgesic acetaminophen as initial therapy has greatly reduced medication costs in comparison with the use of NSAIDs, many of which are by prescription only. NSAID costs range from $20 to $150 per month, depending on the medication, daily dose, and regimen selected. As NSAIDs as a class are therapeutically similar, use of less-expensive NSAIDs, such as nonprescription ibuprofen or naproxen or a multisource generic product, may minimize the cost of medicine to the patient. More-expensive NSAIDs can be prescribed if neither of these offers benefit after a 2-week trial at sufficient doses.

Nearly all elderly patients are eligible for prescription drug coverage through Medicare Part D insurance programs or other private insurance to assist with the costs of prescription medications for the treatment of OA. The use of nonformulary or noncovered medications can significantly increase patient drug costs. Careful attention to selection of appropriately covered medications will increase the affordability of medication for patients receiving drug therapy for OA.

EVALUATION OF THERAPEUTIC OUTCOMES

Pharmacotherapy monitoring in OA is patient specific. It should be guided by aspects of disease that are most troubling to the patient, such as pain or decreased function, as well as the patient's risk of adverse effects. To monitor efficacy, the patient's baseline pain can be assessed with a visual analog scale, and range of motion for affected joints can be assessed, providing baseline measures to monitor the success of therapy. Baseline radiographs are helpful to document the extent of joint involvement and to follow progression of disease with therapy. Additional tests of OA severity may include measurement of grip strength, 50 ft (15.2 m) walking time, patient and physician global assessment of OA severity, and the Western Ontario and McMaster Universities Arthrosis Index or Stanford Health Assessment Questionnaire to monitor ability to perform activities of daily living. A decrease in the use of analgesics or NSAIDs would suggest a beneficial effect of nonpharmacologic interventions. Lastly, disease-specific quality of life is valuable in assessing clinical response to interventions.

Adverse events with acetaminophen are uncommon. NSAID toxicity is more problematic and requires continued individual attention to minimize serious consequences from this drug therapy option. Each patient's gastrointestinal, cardiovascular, renal, and other risks, as well as age and comorbidities, should be assessed. When assessing toxicity of therapy, patients should be asked first if they are having any "problems" with their medications. This open-ended question can be followed with direct questions relating to the most common adverse effects associated with the respective medication. Symptoms of abdominal pain, heartburn, nausea, or change in stool color provide valuable clues to the presence of GI complications, although serious GI complications can occur without warning. Patients also should be monitored for the

development of hypertension, weight gain, edema, skin rash, and CNS adverse effects such as headaches and drowsiness. Baseline serum creatinine, complete blood count, and serum transaminases are repeated at 6- to 12-month intervals to identify GI, renal, and hepatic toxicities.

For patients receiving intraarticular corticosteroids, improvement should begin with 2 to 3 days and last 4 to 8 weeks. Patients should be advised about possible injection site reactions, as well as possible systemic effects, especially for those with hypertension or diabetes, as there is a potential for increased blood pressure or blood glucose. Modest improvement with the use of intraarticular HA can begin within 3 to 4 weeks and can last several months, and patients should be advised about possible injection-site reactions and allergic reactions.

For patients receiving opioids or tramadol, relief from pain is expected to occur rapidly. Patients, especially if frail or elderly, should be monitored carefully and cautioned about sedation, dysphoria, nausea, risk of falls, and constipation. Additional monitoring should include strategies to assess development of opioid tolerance and addiction.

CONCLUSIONS

OA is a very common, slowly progressive disorder that affects diarthrodial joints and is characterized by progressive deterioration of articular cartilage, subchondral sclerosis, and osteophyte production. Clinical manifestations include gradual onset of joint pain, stiffness, and limitation of motion. The primary treatment goals are to reduce pain, maintain function, and prevent further destruction. An individualized approach based on education, rest, exercise, weight loss as needed, and analgesic medication can succeed in meeting these goals. Recommended drug treatment starts with acetaminophen ≤4 g/day and topical analgesics as needed. If acetaminophen is ineffective, NSAIDs may be used, often providing satisfactory relief of pain and stiffness. Individuals at increased risk for toxicity from NSAIDs, especially for GI, cardiovascular, or renal events, deserve special attention. Coxibs may have advantages in some OA patients, but their safety relative to other NSAIDS and their role in OA remain in a state of flux. Glucosamine–chondroitin may be useful in moderate to severe arthritis and is safe. Experimental therapy aimed at preventing the progression of OA requires further clinical investigation before entering widespread clinical use.

ABBREVIATIONS

ADAPT: Alzheimer's Disease Antiinflammatory Prevention Trial

APC: Adenoma Prevention with Celecoxib

APPROVe: Adenomatous Polyp Prevention on VIOXX

ASUs: avocado/soy unsaponifiables

CLASS: Celecoxib Long-Term Arthritis Safety Study

COX: cyclooxygenase

CINOD: cyclooxygenase-inhibiting nitric oxide–donor compound

ECM: extracellular matrix

FDA: Food and Drug Administration

GI: gastrointestinal

GWAS: genome-wide linkage studies

HA: hyaluronic acid

IDEA: Intensive Diet and Exercise for Arthritis

IR: immediate release

LOX: lipoxygenase

MEDAL: Multinational Etoricoxib and Diclofenac Arthritis Long-Term Program

MMP: matrix metalloproteinase

NSAID: nonsteroidal antiinflammatory drug

OA: osteoarthritis

OARSI: Osteoarthritis Research International

PPI: proton pump inhibitor

QALE: quality-adjusted life expectancy

SR: sustained release

TARGET: Therapeutic Arthritis Research and Gastrointestinal Event Trial

TIMP: tissue inhibitors of metalloproteinase

TNF: tumor necrosis factor

VIGOR: Vioxx Gastrointestinal Outcomes Research Study

REFERENCES

1. Hunter DJ. Insights from imaging on the epidemiology and pathophysiology of osteoarthritis. Radiol Clin North Am 2009;47:539–551.
2. Rosenberg AE. Bones, Joints and Soft Tissue Tumors. In: Kumar V, Abbas AK, Fausto N, Aster J, eds. Robbins and Cotran Pathologic Basis of Disease, Professional Edition, 8th ed. Philadelphia, PA: W.B. Saunders; 2009:1235–1236.
3. Lane NE. Clinical practice. osteoarthritis of the hip. N Engl J Med 2007;357:1413–1421.
4. Hunter DJ. In the clinic. osteoarthritis. Ann Intern Med 2007;147: ITC 8–16.
5. Roach HI. The complex pathology of osteoarthritis: Even mitochondria are involved. Arthritis Rheum 2008;58:2217–2218.
6. Dagenais S, Garbedian S, Wai EK. Systematic review of the prevalence of radiographic primary hip osteoarthritis. Clin Orthop Relat Res 2009;467:623–637.
7. Feydy A, Pluot E, Guerini H, Drape JL. Osteoarthritis of the wrist and hand, and spine. Radiol Clin North Am 2009;47:723–759.
8. Kopec JA, Rahman MM, Sayre EC, et al. Trends in physician-diagnosed osteoarthritis incidence in an administrative database in British Columbia, Canada, 1996–1997 through 2003–2004. Arthritis Rheum 2008;59:929–934.
9. Garstang SV, Stitik TP. Osteoarthritis: Epidemiology, risk factors, and pathophysiology. Am J Phys Med Rehabil 2006;85(11 suppl):S2,S11, quiz S12–S14.
10. Gelber AC, Hochberg MC, Mead LA, Wang NY, Wigley FM, Klag MJ. Body mass index in young men and the risk of subsequent knee and hip osteoarthritis. Am J Med 1999;107:542–548.
11. Felson DT, Niu J, Clancy M, Sack B, Aliabadi P, Zhang Y. Effect of recreational physical activities on the development of knee osteoarthritis in older adults of different weights: The Framingham study. Arthritis Rheum 2007;57:6–12.
12. Vincent TL, Saklatvala J. Is the response of cartilage to injury relevant to osteoarthritis? Arthritis Rheum 2008;58:1207–1210.
13. Tanamas S, Hanna FS, Cicuttini FM, Wluka AE, Berry P, Urquhart DM. Does knee malalignment increase the risk of development and progression of knee osteoarthritis? A systematic review. Arthritis Rheum 2009;61:459–467.
14. Hunter DJ, Niu J, Felson DT, et al. Knee alignment does not predict incident osteoarthritis: The Framingham osteoarthritis study. Arthritis Rheum 2007;56:1212–1218.
15. Gelber AC, Hochberg MC, Mead LA, Wang NY, Wigley FM, Klag MJ. Joint injury in young adults and risk for subsequent knee and hip osteoarthritis. Ann Intern Med 2000;133:321–328.
16. Sun BH, Wu CW, Kalunian KC. New developments in osteoarthritis. Rheum Dis Clin North Am 2007;33:135–148.
17. Valdes AM, Spector TD. The contribution of genes to osteoarthritis. Med Clin North Am 2009;93:45,66.
18. Botha-Scheepers SA, Watt I, Slagboom E, et al. Influence of familial factors on radiologic disease progression over two years in siblings with osteoarthritis at multiple sites: A prospective longitudinal cohort study. Arthritis Rheum 2007;57:626–632.
19. Valdes AM, Doherty M, Spector TD. The additive effect of individual genes in predicting risk of knee osteoarthritis. Ann Rheum Dis 2008;67:124–127.
20. Rego-Perez I, Fernandez-Moreno M, Fernandez-Lopez C, Arenas J, Blanco FJ. Mitochondrial DNA haplogroups: Role in the prevalence and severity of knee osteoarthritis. Arthritis Rheum 2008;58: 2387–2396.
21. Sandell LJ, Heinegard D, Hering TH. Cell biology, biochemistry, and molecular biology of articular cartilage in osteoarthritis. In: Moscowitz RW, Altman RD, Hochberg MC, Buckwalter JA, Goldberg VM, eds. Osteoarthritis: Diagnosis and Medical/Surgical Management, 4th ed. Philadelphia: Lippincott, Williams, & Wilkins; 2007:73–106.
22. Felson DT. Osteoarthritis. In: Fauci AS, Braunwald E, Kaspar DL, Hauser DL, Longo DLJ, Loscalzo J, eds. Harrison's Principles of Internal Medicine. New York, NY: McGraw-Hill; 2009:2158–2165.
23. Goldring MB, Marcu KB. Cartilage homeostasis in health and rheumatic diseases. Arthritis Res Ther 2009;11:224.
24. Xu L, Peng H, Glasson S, et al. Increased expression of the collagen receptor discoidin domain receptor 2 in articular cartilage as a key event in the pathogenesis of osteoarthritis. Arthritis Rheum 2007;56:2663–2673.
25. Dell'accio F, De Bari C, Eltawil NM, Vanhummelen P, Pitzalis C. Identification of the molecular response of articular cartilage to injury, by microarray screening: Wnt-16 expression and signaling after injury and in osteoarthritis. Arthritis Rheum 2008;58:1410–1421.
26. Fukui N, Ikeda Y, Ohnuki T, et al. Regional differences in chondrocyte metabolism in osteoarthritis: A detailed analysis by laser capture microdissection. Arthritis Rheum 2008;58:154–163.
27. Wu J, Liu W, Bemis A, et al. Comparative proteomic characterization of articular cartilage tissue from normal donors and patients with osteoarthritis. Arthritis Rheum 2007;56:3675–684.
28. Karsdal MA, Leeming DJ, Dam EB, et al. Should subchondral bone turnover be targeted when treating osteoarthritis? Osteoarthritis Cartilage 2008;16:638–646.
29. Altman RD. Laboratory diagnosis of osteoarthritis. In: Moscowitz RW, Altman RD, Hochberg MC, Buckwalter JA, Goldberg VM, eds. Osteoarthritis: Diagnosis and Medical/Surgical Management, 4th ed. Philadelphia: Lippincott, Williams, & Wilkins; 2007:201–214.
30. Hough AB. Pathology of Osteoarthritis. In: Moscowitz RW, Altman RD, Hochberg MC, Buckwalter JA, Goldberg VM, eds. Osteoarthritis: Diagnosis and Medical/Surgical Management, 4th ed. Philadelphia, PA: Lippincott Williams & Wilkins; 2007:51–72.
31. *http://www.rheumatology.org/publications/*.
32. Zhang W, Doherty M, Leeb BF, et al. EULAR evidence based recommendations for the management of hand osteoarthritis: Report of a task force of the EULAR standing committee for international clinical studies including therapeutics (ESCISIT). Ann Rheum Dis 2007;66:377–388.
33. Felson DT. Clinical practice. osteoarthritis of the knee. N Engl J Med 2006;354:841–848.
34. Roddy E, Zhang W, Doherty M, et al. Evidence-based recommendations for the role of exercise in the management of osteoarthritis of the hip or knee—The MOVE consensus. Rheumatol (Oxford) 2005;44:67–73.
35. Hunter DJ, Felson DT. Osteoarthritis. BMJ 2006;332:639–642.
36. Zhang W, Moskowitz RW, Nuki G, et al. OARSI recommendations for the management of hip and knee osteoarthritis, part II: OARSI evidence-based, expert consensus guidelines. Osteoarthritis Cartilage 2008;16:137–162.
37. Juni P, Reichenbach S, Dieppe P. Osteoarthritis: Rational approach to treating the individual. Best Pract Res Clin Rheumatol 2006;20: 721–740.
38. Tannenbaum H, Bombardier C, Davis P, Russell AS, Third Canadian Consensus Conference Group. An evidence-based approach to prescribing nonsteroidal antiinflammatory drugs. Third Canadian Consensus Conference. J Rheumatol 2006;33:140–157.

39. American Academy of Orthopedic Surgeons Multi-Disciplinary Workgroup. Treatment of Osteoarthritis of the Knee (Non-Arthroplasty). Rosemont, IL: American Academy of Orthopedic Surgeons; 2008. 1–247.

40. American College of Rheumatology Subcommittee on Osteoarthritis Guidelines. Recommendations for the medical management of osteoarthritis of the hip and knee: 2000 update. Arthritis Rheum 2000;43:1905–1915.

41. http://www.arthritis.org/disease-center.php?disease_id=32&df= treatments.

42. Christensen R, Bartels EM, Astrup A, Bliddal H. Effect of weight reduction in obese patients diagnosed with knee osteoarthritis: A systematic review and meta-analysis. Ann Rheum Dis 2007;66: 433–439.

43. Felson DT, Lawrence RC, Dieppe PA, et al. Osteoarthritis: New insights. part 1: The disease and its risk factors. Ann Intern Med 2000;133: 635–646.

44. Reijman M, Pols HA, Bergink AP, et al. Body mass index associated with onset and progression of osteoarthritis of the knee but not of the hip: The rotterdam study. Ann Rheum Dis 2007;66:158–162.

45. Christensen R, Bartels EM, Astrup A, Bliddal H. Symptomatic efficacy of avocado-soybean unsaponifiables (ASU) in osteoarthritis (OA) patients: A meta-analysis of randomized controlled trials. Osteoarthritis Cartilage 2008;16:399–408.

46. Messier SP, Loeser RF, Miller GD, et al. Exercise and dietary weight loss in overweight and obese older adults with knee osteoarthritis: The arthritis, diet, and activity promotion trial. Arthritis Rheum 2004;50:1501–1510.

47. Messier SP, Legault C, Mihalko S, et al. The intensive diet and exercise for arthritis (IDEA) trial: Design and rationale. BMC Musculoskelet Disord 2009;10:93.

48. Jenkinson CM, Doherty M, Avery AJ, et al.. Effects of dietary intervention and quadriceps strengthening exercises on pain and function in overweight people with knee pain: Randomised controlled trial. BMJ 2009;339:b3170.

49. National Institutes of Health (NIH) Consensus Development Panel on Total Knee Replacement. National institutes of health consensus statement on total knee replacement. U.S. Department of Health and Human Services; 2004

50. Fitzpatrick R, Shortall E, Sculpher M, et al. Primary total hip replacement surgery: A systematic review of outcomes and modelling of cost-effectiveness associated with different prostheses. Health Technol Assess 1998;2:1–64.

51. Losina E, Walensky RP, Kessler CL, et al. Cost-effectiveness of total knee arthroplasty in the united states: Patient risk and hospital volume. Arch Intern Med 2009;169:1113,1121; discussion 1121–1122.

52. Kuo CK, Li WJ, Mauck RL, Tuan RS. Cartilage tissue engineering: Its potential and uses. Curr Opin Rheumatol 2006;18:64–73.

53. Towheed TE, Maxwell L, Judd MG, Catton M, Hochberg MC, Wells G. Acetaminophen for osteoarthritis. Cochrane Database Syst Rev 2006; CD004257.

54. Pepper GA. Nonsteroidal anti-inflammatory drugs: New perspectives on a familiar drug class. Nurs Clin North Am 2000;35:223–244.

55. Fraenkel L, Bogardus ST, Jr, Concato J, Wittink DR. Treatment options in knee osteoarthritis: The patient's perspective. Arch Intern Med 2004;164:1299–1304.

56. Henrich WL, Agodoa LE, Barrett B, et al. Analgesics and the kidney: Summary and recommendations to the scientific advisory board of the national kidney foundation from an ad hoc committee of the national kidney foundation. Am J Kidney Dis 1996;27:162–165.

57. Federal Register. Rockville, MD: Department of Health and Human Services Vol. 74, No. 81; 2009.

58. Watkins PB, Kaplowitz N, Slattery JT, et al. Aminotransferase elevations in healthy adults receiving 4 grams of acetaminophen daily: A randomized controlled trial. JAMA 2006;296:87–93.

59. Larson AM, Polson J, Fontana RJ, et al. Acute Liver Failure Study Group. Acetaminophen-induced acute liver failure: Results of a United States multicenter, prospective study. Hepatology 2005;42:1364–1372.

60. Laine L, White WB, Rostom A, Hochberg M. COX-2 selective inhibitors in the treatment of osteoarthritis. Semin Arthritis Rheum 2008;38:165–187.

61. Chou R, Hefland M, Peterson K, Dana T, Roberts C. Comparative effectiveness and safety of analgesics for osteoarthritis. Comparative Effectiveness Review No. 4; 2006

62. Frampton JE, Keating GM. Celecoxib: A review of its use in the management of arthritis and acute pain. Drugs 2007;67:2433–2472.

63. Wolfe MM, Lichtenstein DR, Singh G. Gastrointestinal toxicity of nonsteroidal antiinflammatory drugs. N Engl J Med 1999;340: 1888–1899.

64. Crofford LJ, Lipsky PE, Brooks P, Abramson SB, Simon LS, van de Putte LB. Basic biology and clinical application of specific cyclooxygenase-2 inhibitors. Arthritis Rheum 2000;43:4–13.

65. Grosser T. The pharmacology of selective inhibition of COX-2. Thromb Haemost 2006;96:393–400.

66. Grosser T, Fries S, FitzGerald GA. Biological basis for the cardiovascular consequences of COX-2 inhibition: Therapeutic challenges and opportunities. J Clin Invest 2006;116:4–1115.

67. Angst F, Ewert T, Lehmann S, Aeschlimann A, Stucki G. The factor subdimensions of the western ontario and McMaster universities osteoarthritis index (WOMAC) help to specify hip and knee osteoarthritis. a prospective evaluation and validation study. J Rheumatol 2005;32:1324–1330.

68. Lanas A. Nonsteroidal antiinflammatory drugs and cyclooxygenase inhibition in the gastrointestinal tract: A trip from peptic ulcer to colon cancer. Am J Med Sci 2009;338:96–106.

69. Lazzaroni M, Porro GB. Management of NSAID-induced gastrointestinal toxicity: Focus on proton pump inhibitors. Drugs 2009;69: 51–69.

70. Rostom A, Moayyedi P, Hunt R, Canadian Association of Gastroenterology Consensus Group. Canadian consensus guidelines on long-term nonsteroidal anti-inflammatory drug therapy and the need for gastroprotection: Benefits versus risks. Aliment Pharmacol Ther 2009;29:481–496.

71. Laine L, Smith R, Min K, Chen C, Dubois RW. Systematic review: The lower gastrointestinal adverse effects of non-steroidal anti-inflammatory drugs. Aliment Pharmacol Ther 2006;24:751–767.

72. Zhang W, Moskowitz RW, Nuki G, et al. OARSI recommendations for the management of hip and knee osteoarthritis, part I: Critical appraisal of existing treatment guidelines and systematic review of current research evidence. Osteoarthritis Cartilage 2007;15:981–1000.

73. Singh G, Fort JG, Goldstein JL, et al. Celecoxib versus naproxen and diclofenac in osteoarthritis patients: SUCCESS-I study. Am J Med 2006;119:255–266.

74. Chan FK, Hung LC, Suen BY, et al. Celecoxib versus diclofenac and omeprazole in reducing the risk of recurrent ulcer bleeding in patients with arthritis. N Engl J Med 2002;347:2104–2110.

75. Bombardier C, Laine L, Reicin A, et al. Comparison of upper gastrointestinal toxicity of rofecoxib and naproxen in patients with rheumatoid arthritis. VIGOR study group. N Engl J Med 2000;343:1520–1528.

76. Bresalier RS, Sandler RS, Quan H, et al. Cardiovascular events associated with rofecoxib in a colorectal adenoma chemoprevention trial. N Engl J Med 2005;352:1092–1102.

77. Farkouh ME, Kirshner H, Harrington RA, et al. Comparison of lumiracoxib with naproxen and ibuprofen in the therapeutic arthritis research and gastrointestinal event trial (TARGET), cardiovascular outcomes: Randomised controlled trial. Lancet 2004;364:675–684.

78. Laine L, Curtis SP, Cryer B, Kaur A, Cannon CP, MEDAL Steering Committee. Assessment of upper gastrointestinal safety of etoricoxib and diclofenac in patients with osteoarthritis and rheumatoid arthritis in the multinational etoricoxib and diclofenac arthritis long-term (MEDAL) programme: A randomised comparison. Lancet 2007;369:465–473.

79. Solomon SD, McMurray JJ, Pfeffer MA, et al. Cardiovascular risk associated with celecoxib in a clinical trial for colorectal adenoma prevention. N Engl J Med 2005;352:1071–1080.

80. Cannon CP, Curtis SP, FitzGerald GA, et al. Cardiovascular outcomes with etoricoxib and diclofenac in patients with osteoarthritis and rheumatoid arthritis in the multinational etoricoxib and diclofenac arthritis long-term (MEDAL) programme: A randomised comparison. Lancet 2006;368(9549):1771–1781.

81. Kearney PM, Baigent C, Godwin J, Halls H, Emberson JR, Patrono C. Do selective cyclo-oxygenase-2 inhibitors and traditional non-steroi-

dal anti-inflammatory drugs increase the risk of atherothrombosis? Meta-analysis of randomised trials. BMJ 2006;332:1302–1308.

82. Solomon SD, Wittes J, Finn PV, et al. Cardiovascular risk of celecoxib in 6 randomized placebo-controlled trials: The cross trial safety analysis. Circulation 2008;117:2104–2113.

83. McGettigan P, Henry D. Cardiovascular risk and inhibition of cyclooxygenase: A systematic review of the observational studies of selective and nonselective inhibitors of cyclooxygenase 2. JAMA 2006;296:1633–1644.

84. Barkin RL, Buvanendran A. Focus on the COX-1 and COX-2 agents: Renal events of nonsteroidal and anti-inflammatory drugs-NSAIDs. Am J Ther 2004;11:124–129.

85. Epstein M. Non-steroidal anti-inflammatory drugs and the continuum of renal dysfunction. J Hypertens Suppl 2002;20:S17–S23.

86. Zhang J, Ding EL, Song Y. Adverse effects of cyclooxygenase 2 inhibitors on renal and arrhythmia events: Meta-analysis of randomized trials. JAMA 2006;296:1619–1632.

87. Soni P, Shell B, Cawkwell G, Li C, Ma H. The hepatic safety and tolerability of the cyclooxygenase-2 selective NSAID celecoxib: Pooled analysis of 41 randomized controlled trials. Curr Med Res Opin 2009;25:1841–1851.

88. Martin-Garcia C, Hinojosa M, Berges P, Camacho E, Garcia-Rodriguez R, Alfaya T, Iscar A. Safety of a cyclooxygenase-2 inhibitor in patients with aspirin-sensitive asthma. Chest 2002;121:1812–1817.

89. Garnett WR. Clinical implications of drug interactions with coxibs. Pharmacotherapy 2001;21:1223–1232.

90. http://www.fda.gov/medwatch/safety/2006/safety06.htm#aspirin.

91. Eccles M, Freemantle N, Mason J. North of England evidence based guideline development project: Summary guideline for non-steroidal anti-inflammatory drugs versus basic analgesia in treating the pain of degenerative arthritis. the north of England non-steroidal anti-inflammatory drug guideline development group. BMJ 1998;317:526–530.

92. Mason L, Moore RA, Derry S, Edwards JE, McQuay HJ. Systematic review of topical capsaicin for the treatment of chronic pain. BMJ 2004;328:991.

93. Zacher J, Altman R, Bellamy N, et al. Topical diclofenac and its role in pain and inflammation: An evidence-based review. Curr Med Res Opin 2008;24:925–950.

94. Stanos SP. Topical agents for the management of musculoskeletal pain. J Pain Symptom Manage 2007;33:342–355.

95. Mason L, Moore RA, Edwards JE, McQuay HJ, Derry S, Wiffen PJ. Systematic review of efficacy of topical rubefacients containing salicylates for the treatment of acute and chronic pain. BMJ 2004;328:995.

96. Samson DJ, Grant MD, Ratko TA, Bonnell CJ, Ziegler KM, Aronson N. Treatment of Primary and Secondary Osteoarthritis of the Knee. Rockville, MD: Agency for Healthcare Research and Quality; 2007, http://ahrq.gov/clinic/tp/oakneetp.htm

97. Clegg DO, Reda DJ, Harris CL, et al. Glucosamine, chondroitin sulfate, and the two in combination for painful knee osteoarthritis. N Engl J Med 2006;354:795–808.

98. Bellamy N, Campbell J, Robinson V, Gee T, Bourne R, Wells G. Intraarticular corticosteroid for treatment of osteoarthritis of the knee. Cochrane Database Syst Rev 2006;CD005328.

99. Pyne D, Ioannou Y, Mootoo R, Bhanji A. Intra-articular steroids in knee osteoarthritis: A comparative study of triamcinolone hexacetonide and methylprednisolone acetate. Clin Rheumatol 2004;23:116–120.

100. Bellamy N, Campbell J, Robinson V, Gee T, Bourne R, Wells G. Viscosupplementation for the treatment of osteoarthritis of the knee. Cochrane Database Syst Rev 2006;CD005321.

101. Hunter DJ. Osteoarthritis: Hyaluronic acid is not effective in symptomatic hip OA. Nat Rev Rheumatol 2009;5:359–3560.

102. Pergolizzi J, Boger RH, Budd K, et al. Opioids and the management of chronic severe pain in the elderly: Consensus statement of an international expert panel with focus on the six clinically most often used world health organization step III opioids (buprenorphine, fentanyl, hydromorphone, methadone, morphine, oxycodone). Pain Pract 2008;8:287–313.

103. Cepeda MS, Camargo F, Zea C, Valencia L. Tramadol for osteoarthritis: A systematic review and metaanalysis. J Rheumatol 2007;34:543–555.

104. Silverfield JC, Kamin M, Wu SC, Rosenthal N, CAPSS-105 Study Group. Tramadol/acetaminophen combination tablets for the treatment of osteoarthritis flare pain: A multicenter, outpatient, randomized, double-blind, placebo-controlled, parallel-group, add-on study. Clin Ther 2002;24:282–297.

105. Pelletier JP, Martel-Pelletier J. DMOAD developments: Present and future. Bull NYU Hosp Jt Dis 2007;65:242–248.

106. Brandt KD, Mazzuca SA, Katz BP, et al. Effects of doxycycline on progression of osteoarthritis: Results of a randomized, placebo-controlled, double-blind trial. Arthritis Rheum 2005;52:2015–2025.

107. Cicero AF, Laghi L. Activity and potential role of licofelone in the management of osteoarthritis. Clin Interv Aging 2007;2:73–79.

108. Fidelix TS, Soares BG, Trevisani VF. Diacerein for osteoarthritis. Cochrane Database Syst Rev 2006;CD005117.

109. Wallace JL, Viappiani S, Bolla M. Cyclooxygenase-inhibiting nitric oxide donors for osteoarthritis. Trends Pharmacol Sci 2009;30:112–117.

110. Kwon YD, Pittler MH, Ernst E. Acupuncture for peripheral joint osteoarthritis: A systematic review and meta-analysis. Rheumatology (Oxford) 2006;45:1331–1337.

111. Scharf HP, Mansmann U, Streitberger K, et al. Acupuncture and knee osteoarthritis: A three-armed randomized trial. Ann Intern Med 2006;145:12–20.

112. Spiegel BM, Chiou CF, Ofman JJ. Minimizing complications from nonsteroidal antiinflammatory drugs: Cost-effectiveness of competing strategies in varying risk groups. Arthritis Rheum 2005;53:185–197.

113. Hur C, Chan AT, Tramontano AC, Gazelle GS. Coxibs versus combination NSAID and PPI therapy for chronic pain: An exploration of the risks, benefits, and costs. Ann Pharmacother 2006;40:1052–1063.

114. Latimer N, Lord J, Grant RL, et al. Cost effectiveness of COX 2 selective inhibitors and traditional NSAIDs alone or in combination with a proton pump inhibitor for people with osteoarthritis. BMJ 2009;339:b2538.

MICHAEL E. ERNST AND ELIZABETH C. CLARK

CHAPTER 102

Gout and Hyperuricemia

KEY CONCEPTS

❶ In the absence of a history of gout, asymptomatic hyperuricemia does not require treatment.

❷ Acute gouty arthritis may be treated effectively with short courses of high-dose nonacetylated nonsteroidal antiinflammatory drugs (NSAIDs), corticosteroids, or colchicine.

❸ Colchicine is highly effective at relieving acute attacks of gout but has the lowest benefit-to-toxicity ratio of the available pharmacotherapy for gout.

❹ Uric acid nephrolithiasis should be treated with adequate hydration (2 to 3 L/day), a daytime urine-alkalinizing agent, and 60 to 80 mEq/day (60 to 80 mmol/L) of potassium bicarbonate or potassium citrate.

❺ Treatment with urate-lowering drugs to reduce risk of recurrent attacks of gouty arthritis is considered cost-effective for patients having two or more attacks of gout per year.

❻ Xanthine oxidase inhibitors are efficacious for the prophylaxis of recurrent gout attacks in both underexcreters and overproducers of uric acid. Allopurinol should be started with a low dose (100 mg/day) after the acute attack has resolved and increased by 100 mg/day at 1-week intervals until the goal serum urate concentration of <6 mg/dL (<357 µmol/L) is achieved. Febuxostat 40 to 80 mg/day can be used for patients intolerant to allopurinol or who have mild to moderate renal insufficiency. Colchicine (0.6 mg once daily) or an NSAID should be administered for at least the first 8 weeks of therapy to minimize the risk of acute attacks that may occur during initiation of uric acid–lowering therapy.

❼ Uricosuric agents should be avoided for patients with renal impairment [a creatinine clearance below 50 mL/min (0.84 mL/s)], a history of renal calculi, or overproduction of uric acid.

❽ Patients with hyperuricemia or gout should undergo comprehensive evaluation for signs and symptoms of cardiovascular disease, and aggressive management of cardiovascular risk factors (i.e., weight loss, reduction of alcohol intake, control of blood pressure, glucose, and lipids) should be undertaken as indicated.

Learning objectives, review questions, and other resources can be found at
www.pharmacotherapyonline.com.

The term *gout* describes a heterogeneous clinical spectrum of diseases including elevated serum urate concentration (hyperuricemia), recurrent attacks of acute arthritis associated with monosodium urate crystals in synovial fluid leukocytes, deposits of monosodium urate crystals (tophi) in tissues in and around joints, interstitial renal disease, and uric acid nephrolithiasis.[1]

The underlying metabolic disorder of gout is hyperuricemia, defined physiochemically as serum that is supersaturated with monosodium urate. At 37°C (98.6°F), serum urate concentrations above (or around) 7 mg/dL (416 µmol/L) begin to exceed the limit of solubility for monosodium urate.[1] For determination of the risk of gout, hyperuricemia is defined statistically as serum urate concentrations greater than 2 standard deviations above the population means for age- and sex-matched healthy populations, usually 7.0 mg/dL (416 µmol/L) for men and 6.0 mg/dL (357 µmol/L) for women.[1,2] Although hyperuricemia is fundamental to the development of gout, the mere presence of hyperuricemia itself is often an asymptomatic condition.

EPIDEMIOLOGY

Historically, gout has been referred to as the "disease of kings" since it was often associated with affluent societies and lifestyles of overindulgence, gluttony, and intemperance.[1] The incidence and prevalence of gout are increasing in Western industrialized countries, but contrary to history, the disease is no longer limited strictly to populations with a high standard of living.[3,4] Epidemiologic data indicate that the prevalence of gout is also increasing in less industrialized Eastern countries.[5-7] Numerous factors may explain this finding, including increased longevity, dietary habits, and increasing prevalence of obesity and the metabolic syndrome.

There is a direct correlation between serum uric acid concentration and both the incidence and prevalence of gout. Population studies have shown that serum urate concentration correlates with increasing age, serum creatinine, blood urea nitrogen, male gender, blood pressure, body weight, and alcohol intake. The incidence of gout is consistently higher for individuals who are obese or who consume large amounts of alcohol or higher amounts of meat or fish.[8-10]

Elevated serum urate levels are the single most important risk factor for the development of gout, and the relationship between the risk of an attack of acute gouty arthritis and serum urate levels is linearly correlated. The 5-year cumulative risk of gout for patients with serum urate concentrations <7 mg/dL (<416 µmol/L) is 0.6%, compared with a risk of 30.5% for those with urate levels >10 mg/dL (>595 µmol/L).[11] Sustained elevation of serum urate is virtually essential for the development of gout; however, hyperuricemia does not always lead to gout, and many patients with hyperuricemia remain asymptomatic.[2] Although unusual, acute gouty arthritis has been reported to occur in the presence of normal serum uric acid concentrations.[12]

Gout affects men about seven to nine times more often than women.[13] The incidence of gout increases with age, peaking at 30 to 50 years of age, with an annual incidence ranging from 1 in 1,000 for men ages 40 to 44 years and 1.8 in 1,000 for those ages 55 to 64 years.[10] The lowest rates of gout are observed in young women, approximately 0.8 cases per 10,000 patient-years.[14] Serum uric acid levels in women approach those of men once menopause has occurred; thus, in older age groups the gender gap narrows, and approximately half of newly diagnosed cases of gout are found in women.[2,4] Gout in men younger than 30 years of age or in premenopausal women may indicate an inherited enzyme defect or the presence of renal disease. Although no genetic marker has been isolated for gout, the familial nature of gout strongly suggests an interaction between genetic and environmental factors.

ETIOLOGY AND PATHOPHYSIOLOGY

In humans, the production of uric acid is the terminal step in the degradation of purines. Uric acid serves no known physiologic purpose and is regarded as a waste product. Normal uric acid levels are near the limits of urate solubility, because of the delicate balance that exists between the amount of urate produced and excreted.[15] Humans have higher uric acid levels than other mammals because they do not express the enzyme uricase, which converts uric acid to the more soluble allantoin.[16]

Gout occurs exclusively in humans in whom a miscible pool of uric acid exists. Under normal conditions, the amount of accumulated uric acid is about 1,200 mg in men and about 600 mg in women. The size of the urate pool is increased severalfold in individuals with gout. This excess accumulation may result from either overproduction or underexcretion of uric acid. Several conditions are associated with either decreased renal clearance or an overproduction of uric acid, leading to hyperuricemia. Table 102–1 lists some of these conditions.

OVERPRODUCTION OF URIC ACID

The purines from which uric acid is produced originate from three sources: dietary purine, conversion of tissue nucleic acid to purine nucleotides, and de novo synthesis of purine bases. The purines derived from these three sources enter a common metabolic pathway leading to the production of either nucleic acid or uric acid. Under normal circumstances, uric acid may accumulate excessively if production exceeds excretion. The average human produces about 600 to 800 mg of uric acid each day. Dietary purines play an unimportant role in the generation of hyperuricemia in the absence of some derangement in purine metabolism or elimination.

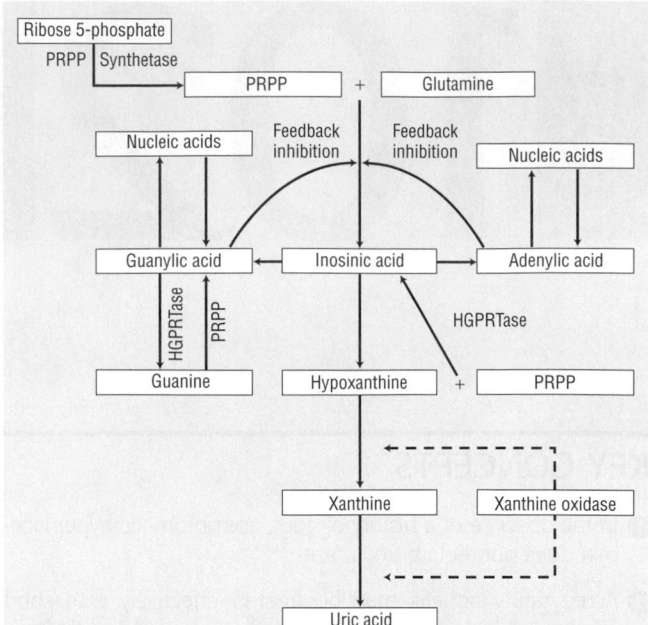

FIGURE 102-1. Purine metabolism (HGPRT, hypoxanthine-guanine phosphoribosyltransferase; PRPP, phosphoribosyl pyrophosphate).

However, diet modifications are important for patients with such problems who develop symptomatic hyperuricemia.

Several enzyme systems regulate purine metabolism. Abnormalities in these regulatory systems can result in overproduction of uric acid. Uric acid may also be overproduced as a consequence of increased breakdown of tissue nucleic acids and excessive rates of cell turnover, as observed with myeloproliferative and lymphoproliferative disorders, polycythemia vera, psoriasis, and some types of anemias. Cytotoxic medications used to treat these disorders can result in overproduction of uric acid secondary to lysis and breakdown of cellular matter.

Two enzyme abnormalities resulting in an overproduction of uric acid have been well described (Fig. 102–1). The first is an increase in the activity of phosphoribosyl pyrophosphate (PRPP) synthetase, which leads to an increased concentration of PRPP. PRPP is a key determinant of purine synthesis and uric acid production. The second is a deficiency of hypoxanthine-guanine phosphoribosyltransferase (HGPRT). HGPRT is responsible for the conversion of guanine to guanylic acid and hypoxanthine to inosinic acid. These two conversions require PRPP as the cosubstrate and are important reactions involved in the synthesis of nucleic acids. A deficiency in the HGPRT enzyme leads to increased metabolism of guanine and hypoxanthine to uric acid and to more PRPP to interact with glutamine in the first step of the purine pathway.[17] Complete absence of HGPRT results in the childhood Lesch-Nyhan syndrome, characterized by choreoathetosis, spasticity, mental retardation, and markedly excessive production of uric acid. A partial deficiency of the enzyme may be responsible for marked hyperuricemia in otherwise normal, healthy individuals.

UNDEREXCRETION OF URIC ACID

Normally, uric acid does not accumulate as long as production is balanced with elimination. About two thirds of the daily uric acid production is excreted in the urine and the remainder is eliminated through the gastrointestinal tract after enzymatic degradation by colonic bacteria. The vast majority of patients (80% to 90%) with gout have a relative decrease in the renal excretion of uric acid for an unknown reason (primary idiopathic hyperuricemia).[2]

TABLE 102-1	Conditions Associated with Hyperuricemia
Primary gout	Obesity
Diabetic ketoacidosis	Sarcoidosis
Myeloproliferative disorders	Congestive heart failure
Lactic acidosis	Renal dysfunction
Lymphoproliferative disorders	Down syndrome
Starvation	Lead toxicity
Chronic hemolytic anemia	Hyperparathyroidism
Toxemia of pregnancy	Acute alcoholism
Pernicious anemia	Hypoparathyroidism
Glycogen storage disease type 1	Acromegaly
Psoriasis	Hypothyroidism
Hypoxanthine-guanine phosphoribosyl-transferase deficiency	Phosphoribosylpyrophosphate synthetase overactivity
Polycythemia vera	Berylliosis
Renal transplantation	

TABLE 102-2	Drugs Capable of Inducing Hyperuricemia and Gout

Diuretics	Ethanol	Ethambutol
Nicotinic acid	Pyrazinamide	Cytotoxic drugs
Salicylates (<2 g/day)	Levodopa	Cyclosporine

A decline in the urinary excretion of uric acid to a level below the rate of production leads to hyperuricemia and an increased miscible pool of sodium urate. Almost all the urate in plasma is freely filtered across the glomerulus. The concentration of uric acid appearing in the urine is determined by multiple renal tubular transport processes in addition to the filtered load. Evidence favors a four-component model including glomerular filtration, tubular reabsorption, tubular secretion, and postsecretory reabsorption.

Approximately 90% of filtered uric acid is reabsorbed in the proximal tubule, probably by both active and passive transport mechanisms. There is a close linkage between proximal tubular sodium reabsorption and uric acid reabsorption; so conditions that enhance sodium reabsorption (e.g., dehydration) also lead to increased uric acid reabsorption. The exact site of tubular secretion of uric acid has not been determined; this too appears to involve an active transport process. Postsecretory reabsorption occurs somewhere distal to the secretory site. Table 102–2 lists the drugs that decrease renal clearance of uric acid through modification of filtered load or one of the tubular transport processes. By enhancing renal urate reabsorption, insulin resistance is also associated with gout.

The pathophysiologic approach to the evaluation of hyperuricemia requires determining whether the patient is overproducing or underexcreting uric acid. This can be accomplished by placing the patient on a purine-free diet for 3 to 5 days and then measuring the amount of uric acid excreted in the urine in 24 hours. As it is very difficult to maintain a purine-free diet for several days, this test is done infrequently in clinical practice. Nevertheless, when it is performed, individuals who excrete more than 600 mg on a purine-free diet may be considered overproducers. Hyperuricemic individuals who excrete less than 600 mg of uric acid per 24 hours on a purine-free diet may be classified as underexcreters of uric acid. On a regular diet, excretion of more than 1,000 mg per 24 hours reflects overproduction; less than this is probably normal.

CLINICAL PRESENTATION

❶ Gout is diagnosed clinically by symptoms rather than laboratory tests of uric acid. In fact, asymptomatic hyperuricemia discovered incidentally generally requires no therapy because many individuals with hyperuricemia will never experience an attack of gout. These patients should still be encouraged to implement lifestyle measures to reduce serum urate concentrations.

PRESENTATION OF ACUTE GOUTY ARTHRITIS

General

- Gout classically presents as an acute inflammatory monoarthritis. The first metatarsophalangeal joint is often involved ("podagra"), but any joint of the lower extremity can be affected and occasionally gout will present as a monoarthritis of the wrist or finger. The spectrum of gout also includes nephrolithiasis, gouty nephropathy, and aggregated deposits of sodium urate (tophi) in cartilage, tendons, synovial membranes, and elsewhere.

Signs and Symptoms

- Fever, intense pain, erythema, warmth, swelling, and inflammation of involved joints

Laboratory Tests

- Elevated serum uric acid levels; leukocytosis

Other Diagnostic Tests

- Observation of monosodium urate crystals in synovial fluid or a tophus

- For patients with long-standing gout, radiographs may show asymmetric swelling within a joint on or subcortical cysts without erosions

ACUTE GOUTY ARTHRITIS

A classic acute attack of gouty arthritis is characterized by rapid and localized onset of excruciating pain, swelling, and inflammation. The attack is typically monarticular at first, most often affecting the first metatarsophalangeal joint (great toe) and then, in order of frequency, the insteps, ankles, heels, knees, wrists, fingers, and elbows. In one half of initial attacks, the first metatarsophalangeal joint is affected, a condition commonly referred to as *podagra* (see Fig. 102–2). Up to 90% of patients with gout will experience podagra at some point in the course of their disease.[15]

Atypical presentations of gout also occur. For elderly patients, gout can present as a chronic polyarticular arthritis that can be confused with rheumatoid arthritis or osteoarthritis. Additionally, the onset of gout may be less dramatic than the typical acute attack and have fewer clinical findings. Multiple small joints in the hands may be involved, especially in elderly women.[2] Table 102–3 summarizes the different clinical manifestations of gout.

The predilection of acute gout for peripheral joints of the lower extremity is probably related to the low temperature of these joints combined with high intraarticular urate concentration. Synovial effusions are likely to occur transiently in weight-bearing joints during the course of a day with routine activity. At night, water is reabsorbed from the joint space, leaving behind a supersaturated solution of monosodium urate, which can precipitate attacks of acute arthritis. Attacks generally begin at night with the patient awakened from sleep by excruciating pain.

The development of crystal-induced inflammation involves a number of chemical mediators causing vasodilation, increased vascular permeability, complement activation, and chemotactic activity for polymorphonuclear leukocytes.[18] Phagocytosis of urate crystals by the leukocytes results in rapid lysis of cells and a discharge of lysosomal and proteolytic enzymes into the cytoplasm.

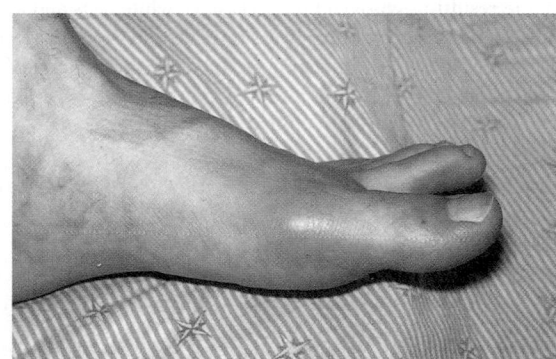

FIGURE 102-2. Acute gout attack of the first metatarsophalangeal joint. (From Imboden J, Hellmann DB, Stone JH. Current Rheumatology Diagnosis and Treatment, 2d ed. New York: McGraw-Hill, 2004:316.)

TABLE 102-3	Clinical Manifestations of Gout
Classic acute gout ("podagra")	Monoarticular arthritis
	Frequently attacks the first metatarsophalangeal joint, although other joints of the lower extremities are also frequently involved.
	Affected joint is swollen, erythematous, and tender.
Interval gout	Asymptomatic period between attacks.
Tophaceous gout	Deposits of monosodium urate crystals in soft tissues.
	Complications include soft tissue damage, deformity, joint destruction, and nerve compression syndromes such as carpal tunnel syndrome.
Atypical gout	Polyarthritis affecting any joint, upper or lower extremity.
	May be confused with rheumatoid arthritis or osteoarthritis.
Renal effects	Nephrolithiasis
	Acute and chronic gouty nephropathy

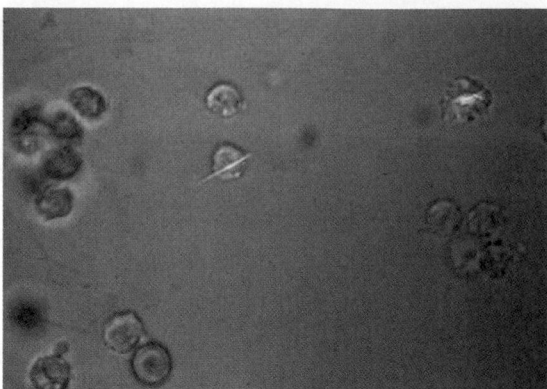

FIGURE 102-3. Urate crystal ingested by a polymorphonuclear leukocyte in synovial fluid. *(From Imboden J, Hellmann DB, Stone JH. Current Rheumatology Diagnosis and Treatment, 2d ed. New York: McGraw-Hill, 2004:317.)*

The ensuing inflammatory reaction is associated with intense joint pain, erythema, warmth, and swelling. Fever is common, as is leukocytosis. Untreated attacks may last from 3 to 14 days before spontaneous recovery.

Although acute attacks of gouty arthritis may occur without apparent provocation, a number of conditions may precipitate an attack. These include stress, trauma, alcohol ingestion, infection, surgery, rapid lowering of serum uric acid by ingestion of uric acid-lowering agents, and ingestion of certain drugs known to elevate serum uric acid concentrations (see Table 102–2). Other crystal-induced arthropathies that may resemble gout on clinical presentation are caused by calcium pyrophosphate dihydrate crystals (pseudogout) and calcium hydroxyapatite crystals, which are associated with calcific periarthritis, tendinitis, and arthritis.[19,20]

Acute flares of gouty arthritis may occur infrequently, but over time the interval between attacks may shorten if appropriate measures to correct hyperuricemia are not undertaken. Later in the disease, tophaceous deposits of monosodium urate crystals in the skin or subcutaneous tissues may be found. These tophi can be anywhere but are often found on the hands, wrists, elbows, or knees. It is estimated to take 10 or more years for tophi to develop.

Diagnostic Evaluation

Table 102–4 lists the differential diagnosis of an acute monoarthritis.[21] A definitive diagnosis of gout requires aspiration of synovial fluid from the affected joint and identification of intracellular crystals of monosodium urate monohydrate in synovial fluid leukocytes.[2] Identification of monosodium urate crystals is highly dependent on the experience of the observer. Crystals are needle shaped, and when examined under polarizing light microscopy, they are strongly negatively birefringent (see Fig. 102–3). Crystals can be observed in synovial fluid during asymptomatic periods.[22] If an affected joint is tapped, the resulting synovial fluid may have white cells and appear purulent. Such findings should always raise the question of infection. If any clinical features of infection are present, such as high fever, elevated white blood cell count, multiple joints affected, or an identi-

fied source of infection, proper diagnosis and treatment are critical. Patients with gout can have septic arthritis. Diabetes, alcohol abuse, and advanced age increase the likelihood of septic arthritis.

In lieu of obtaining a synovial fluid sample from an affected joint to inspect for urate crystals, the clinical triad of inflammatory monoarthritis, elevated serum uric acid level, and response to colchicine can be used to diagnose gout. However, this approach has limitations, including a failure to recognize atypical gout presentations and the fact that serum uric acid levels can be normal or even low during an acute gout attack.[11,23] In addition, use of colchicine as a diagnostic tool for gout is limited by lack of sensitivity and specificity for the disease. Other conditions such as psoriatic arthritis, sarcoidosis, and Mediterranean fever can respond to colchicine therapy. Table 102–5 shows the American College of Rheumatology classification criteria for an acute gouty arthritis attack.[24]

For patients with long-standing gout, radiographs may show punched-out marginal erosions and secondary osteoarthritic changes; however, in an acute first attack radiographs will be unremarkable.[21,25] The presence of chondrocalcinosis on radiographs may indicate pseudogout. Some studies have recently examined the use of magnetic resonance imaging and computed tomography to obtain images for patients with gout; however, this is not currently considered part of normal practice.

URIC ACID NEPHROLITHIASIS

Clinicians should be suspicious of hyperuricemic states for patients who present with kidney stones, as nephrolithiasis occurs in 10% to

TABLE 102-4	Differential Diagnosis of Acute Monoarthritis

1. Pseudogout (pyrophosphate crystal related arthritis)
2. Palindromic rheumatism
3. Seronegative inflammatory arthritis
4. Trauma or hemarthrosis
5. Septic arthritis
6. Cellulitis
7. Type II dyslipidemia
8. Unrelated hyperuricemia (as in psoriasis, hypertension) when joint pain is not caused by gout.

TABLE 102-5	American College of Rheumatology Criteria for the Clinical Diagnosis of Gout[a]

1. More than one attack of acute arthritis
2. Maximum inflammation developed within 1 day
3. Monoarthritis attack
4. Redness observed over joints
5. First metatarsophalangeal joint painful or swollen
6. Unilateral first metatarsophalangeal joint attack
7. Unilateral tarsal joint attack
8. Tophus (proven or suspected)
9. Hyperuricemia
10. Asymmetric swelling within a joint on x-ray images
11. Subcortical cysts without erosions on x-ray images
12. Monosodium urate monohydrate microcrystals in joint fluid during attack
13. Joint fluid culture negative for organisms during attack

[a]The combination of crystals, tophi, and/or six or more criteria is highly suggestive of gout.
Source: Reference 24.

25% of patients with gout.[26] The frequency of urolithiasis depends on serum uric acid concentrations, acidity of the urine, and urinary uric acid concentration. Typically, patients with uric acid nephrolithiasis have a urinary pH of less than 6.0. Uric acid has a negative logarithm of the acid ionization constant of 5.5. Therefore, when the urine is acidic, uric acid exists primarily in the unionized, less soluble form. At a urine pH of 5.0, urine is saturated at a uric acid level of 15 mg/dL (0.89 mmol/L). When the urine pH is 7.0, the solubility of uric acid in urine is increased to 200 mg/dL (11.9 mmol/L).[1] For patients with uric acid nephrolithiasis, urinary pH typically is less than 6.0 and frequently less than 5.5. When acidic urine is saturated with uric acid, spontaneous precipitation of stones may occur.

Other factors that predispose individuals to uric acid nephrolithiasis include excessive urinary excretion of uric acid and highly concentrated urine. The risk of renal calculi approaches 50% in individuals whose renal excretion of uric acid exceeds 1,100 mg/day (6.5 mmol/day). In addition to pure uric acid stones, hyperuricosuric individuals are at increased risk for mixed uric acid–calcium oxalate stones and pure calcium oxalate stones. Uric acid stones are usually small, round, and radiolucent. Uric acid stones containing calcium are radiopaque.[26]

GOUTY NEPHROPATHY

There are two types of gouty nephropathy: acute uric acid nephropathy and chronic urate nephropathy.[27] In acute uric acid nephropathy, acute renal failure occurs as a result of blockage of urine flow secondary to massive precipitation of uric acid crystals in the collecting ducts and ureters. This syndrome is a well-recognized complication for patients with myeloproliferative or lymphoproliferative disorders and is a result of massive malignant cell turnover, particularly after initiation of chemotherapy.

Chronic urate nephropathy is caused by the long-term deposition of urate crystals in the renal parenchyma. Microtophi may form, with a surrounding giant-cell inflammatory reaction. A decrease in the kidneys' ability to concentrate urine and the presence of proteinuria may be the earliest pathophysiologic disturbances. Hypertension and nephrosclerosis are common associated findings. Although renal failure occurs in a higher percentage of gouty patients than expected, it is not clear if hyperuricemia per se has a harmful effect on the kidneys. The chronic renal impairment seen in individuals with gout may result largely from the coexistence of hypertension, diabetes mellitus, and atherosclerosis.

TOPHACEOUS GOUT

Tophi (urate deposits) are uncommon in the general population of gouty subjects and are a late complication of hyperuricemia. The most common sites of tophaceous deposits for patients with recurrent acute gouty arthritis are the base of the great toe, helix of the ear, olecranon bursae, Achilles tendon, knees, wrists, and hands (Fig. 102–4).[2] Eventually, even the hips, shoulders, and spine may be affected. In addition to causing obvious deformities, tophi may damage surrounding soft tissue, cause joint destruction and pain, and even lead to nerve compression syndromes including carpal tunnel syndrome.

TREATMENT

Gout and Hyperuricemia

The goals in the treatment of gout are to terminate the acute attack, prevent recurrent attacks of gouty arthritis, prevent complications associated with chronic deposition of urate crystals in tissues, and

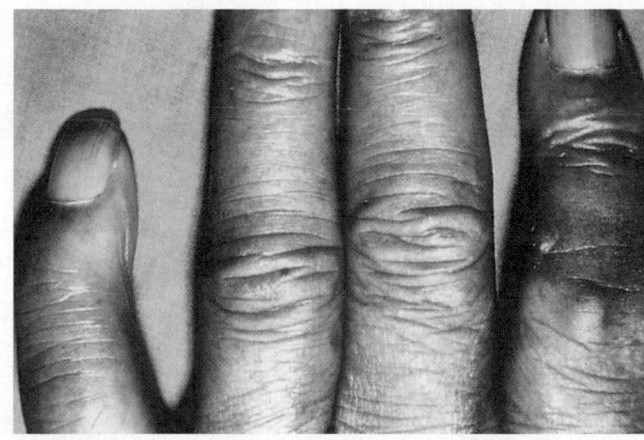

FIGURE 102-4. Tophaceous gout with subcutaneous nodule almost breaking through the skin. *(From South-Paul JE, Matheny SC, Lewis EL. Current Diagnosis and Treatment in Family Medicine. New York: McGraw-Hill, 2004:275.)*

prevent or reverse features commonly associated with the illness including obesity, elevated triglycerides, and hypertension.[1] This can be accomplished through a combination of nonpharmacologic and pharmacologic methods. Table 102–6 summarizes the available pharmacotherapy for gout.

■ ACUTE GOUTY ARTHRITIS

❷ For most patients without contraindications, acute attacks of gouty arthritis may be treated successfully with short courses of high-dose nonsteroidal antiinflammatory drugs (NSAIDs), corticosteroids, or colchicine (Fig. 102–5).[28,29]

Nonsteroidal Antiinflammatory Drugs

NSAIDs are the mainstay of therapy for acute attacks of gouty arthritis because of their excellent efficacy and minimal toxicity with short-term use. Indomethacin has been historically favored as the NSAID of choice for acute gout flares, but there is little evidence to support one NSAID as being more efficacious than another. Three agents (indomethacin, naproxen, and sulindac) have actual U.S. Food and Drug Administration (FDA)-approved labeling for the treatment of gout, although several have been studied (see Table 102–6).[2] The most important determinant of therapeutic success with NSAIDs appears not to be which one is chosen but rather how soon it is initiated. Therapy should be initiated with maximum dosages at the onset of symptoms and continued for 24 hours after complete resolution of an acute attack, then tapered quickly over 2 to 3 days. Resolution of an acute attack for most patients generally occurs within 5 to 8 days after initiating therapy.

All NSAIDs have the potential to cause similar adverse effects. The most common areas affected include the gastrointestinal system (gastritis, bleeding, perforation), kidneys (renal papillary necrosis, reduced creatinine clearance), cardiovascular system (sodium and fluid retention, increased blood pressure), and central nervous system (impaired cognitive function, headache, dizziness). Caution should be exercised when using NSAIDs for individuals with a history of peptic ulcer disease, congestive heart failure, uncontrolled hypertension, renal insufficiency, coronary artery disease or who are concurrently receiving anticoagulants or antiplatelets. Patients with active peptic ulcer disease, uncompensated congestive heart failure, severe renal impairment, or a history of hypersensitivity to aspirin or other NSAIDs should not be prescribed an NSAID.

TABLE 102-6 Pharmacotherapy of Acute and Chronic Gout

Therapeutic Agent	Typical Regimen	Considerations
Acute gout		
Nonsteroidal antiinflammatory drugs		
Etodolac	300 mg twice daily	Avoid for patients with peptic ulcer disease, active bleeding. May cause renal dysfunction, gastritis (worse with concurrent aspirin), fluid retention, and hypertension. Use caution in congestive heart failure. Consider coadministration with a proton-pump inhibitor for patients at risk for gastrointestinal bleeding.
Fenoprofen	300–600 mg three to four times daily	
Ibuprofen	800 mg four times daily	
Indomethacin[a]	25–50 mg four times daily initially for 3 days, then taper to twice daily for 4–7 days	
Ketoprofen	75 mg four times daily	
Naproxen[a]	500 mg twice daily initially for 3 days, then 250–500 mg once daily for 4–7 days	
Piroxicam	20 mg once daily or divided twice daily	
Sulindac[a]	200 mg twice daily for 7–10 days	
Oral colchicine	1.2 mg initially, followed by 0.6 mg 1 hour later	In the presence of renal impairment, dosing should be repeated no more than once every 2 weeks. Dose-dependent gastrointestinal side effects (diarrhea, nausea, vomiting). Avoid coadministration with p-glycoprotein or strong CYP3A4 inhibitors (e.g., clarithromycin).
Corticosteroids		
Oral	30–60 mg prednisone equivalent once daily for 3–5 days, then taper in 5 mg decrements spread over 10–14 days until discontinuation	Use with caution in diabetics. Avoid long-term use. May cause fluid retention and impaired wound healing. Intraarticular administration is preferred for monoarticular involvement; avoid use if joint sepsis is not excluded.
Intramuscular	Triamcinolone acetonide 60 mg IM once, or methylprednisolone 100–150 mg/day for 1–2 days	
Intraarticular	Triamcinolone acetonide 10–40 mg (large joints), 5–20 mg (small joints)	
Corticotropin	25 USP units subcutaneously for acute small-joint monoarticular gout; 40 USP units IM or IV for larger joints or polyarticular involvement	Repeat injections (every 6–8 hours for 2–3 days) may be needed. Requires intact pituitary-adrenal axis. Less effective for patients receiving long-term oral corticosteroid therapy.
Intercritical gout		
NSAIDs	Lowest effective dosage	NSAID gastropathy (See above.)
Oral colchicine	0.6 once daily or every other day	Reversible axonal neuromyopathy and rhabdomyolysis.
Xanthine oxidase inhibitors		
Allopurinol	50–300 mg daily [can be titrated up to 800 mg/day to achieve serum urate concentration <6.0 mg/dL (<357 μmol/L)]	Can be used in both urate overproduction and urate underexcretion. Side effects include rash, gastrointestinal symptoms, and potential for fatal hypersensitivity syndrome. Dose reduction necessary for patients with renal insufficiency.
Febuxostat	40–80 mg/daily	Can be used for allopurinol-intolerant patients. No dosage adjustment necessary for patients with mild-moderate renal dysfunction [creatinine clearance 30–59 mL/min (0.50–0.99 mL/s)]. Side effects include liver enzyme elevations, nausea, arthralgias, and rash.
Uricosurics		
Probenecid	250 mg twice daily, titrated up to 500–2000 mg/day [target serum urate concentration <6 mg/dL (<357 μmol/L)]	Useful in urate underexcretion. Avoid for patients with history of urolithiasis.
Sulfinpyrazone	50 mg twice daily, titrated to 100–400 mg/day [target serum urate concentration <6 mg/dL (<357 μmol/L)]	

[a]FDA-approved for treatment of acute gouty arthritis.

Although the risk for gastric ulceration and bleeding is relatively small with short-term therapy normally employed when treating acute gout flares, consideration should be given to administering a proton pump inhibitor to protect from NSAID-induced gastric problems for elderly patients and for others who are at risk for these complications (e.g., presence of multiple comorbidities, alcoholism, previous history of ulcer, or concurrent anticoagulant use).[30,31] The efficacy and safety of selective cyclooxygenase-2 inhibitors have not been assessed for patients with gouty arthritis, but they are more costly than older NSAIDs and unlikely to result in fewer gastrointestinal complications because of the short courses of therapy routinely used to treat acute attacks.

Corticosteroids

Corticosteroids have typically been reserved for treatment of acute gout flares when contraindications to NSAIDs exist, largely due to lack of evidence from controlled clinical trials. However, evidence that is more recent indicates that corticosteroids are equivalent to NSAIDs in the treatment of acute gout flares.[29] They can be used either systemically or by intraarticular injection. Oral corticosteroids are usually administered in doses of 30 to 60 mg of prednisone equivalent for 3 to 5 days.[2] Patients with multiple joint involvement may be good candidates to consider for this regimen.

A hypothetical risk for a rebound attack upon steroid withdrawal exists; therefore, the dose of corticosteroid should be tapered gradually in 5 mg decrements spread over 10 to 14 days and then discontinued. Intraarticular administration of triamcinolone acetonide in a dose of 20 to 40 mg may be useful in treating acute gout limited to one or two joints. Injection should be done under aseptic technique in a joint determined not to be infected. A single intramuscular injection of a long-acting corticosteroid, such as methylprednisolone, can be used as an alternative to the oral route if patients are unable to take oral therapy.[2] If not contraindicated,

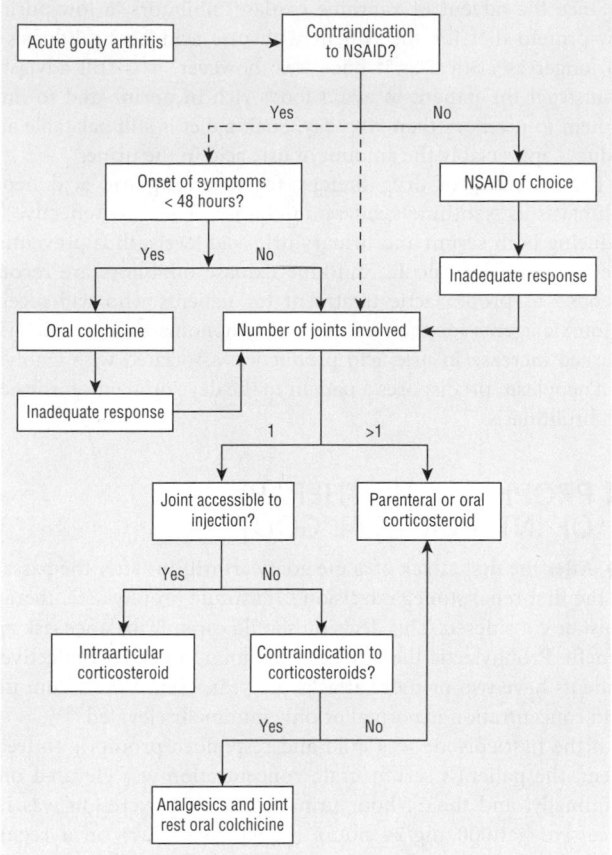

FIGURE 102-5. Treatment algorithm for acute gouty arthritis (NSAID, nonsteroidal antiinflammatory drug).

low-dose colchicine can be used as adjunctive therapy to injectable corticosteroids to prevent rebound flare-ups.

The adverse effects of corticosteroids are generally dose and duration dependent. Short-term use for treatment of acute attacks is generally well tolerated. Corticosteroids should be used with caution for patients with diabetes as they can increase blood sugar. In addition, patients with a history of gastrointestinal problems, bleeding disorders, cardiovascular disease, and psychiatric disorders should be monitored closely. Long-term corticosteroid use should be avoided because of the risk for osteoporosis, hypothalamic–pituitary axis suppression, cataracts, and muscle deconditioning that can occur with their use.

CLINICAL CONTROVERSY

NSAIDs have historically been used as the first-line therapy for treatment of acute attacks of gout. Some clinicians prefer to start therapy instead with a corticosteroid, believing them to be tolerated better and equally effective. Presently, there is no compelling evidence for superiority of either class of agents. The choice of therapy should be individualized based on the characteristics of the patient and the profile of the drug(s). Regardless of the selection, therapy should be initiated quickly, and side effects carefully monitored.

Corticotropin, or adrenocorticotropic hormone (ACTH), which stimulates the adrenal cortex to produce cortisol and corticosterone, can be administered in acute gout. Doses of 40 to 80 United States Pharmacopeia (USP) units are given intramuscularly every 6 to 8 hours for 2 to 3 days, and then discontinued. Studies with

ACTH are limited, but it appears to provide similar efficacy to systemic antiinflammatory doses of corticosteroids.[32] When administered alone or in combination with colchicine, ACTH may provide earlier efficacy compared with indomethacin but with fewer adverse effects.[33] Unfortunately, ACTH is often difficult to obtain in the United States as a result of manufacturing problems. Because the studies have several limitations, the regimen should be considered only as an alternative, one that is especially for patients with comorbidities where other regimens are contraindicated.[34] Examples of patients where ACTH has been used safely when other first-line gout therapies were contraindicated include those with congestive heart failure, chronic renal failure, and history of gastrointestinal bleeding.[35]

Colchicine

❸ Colchicine is an antimitotic drug that is highly effective at relieving acute attacks of gout but has the lowest benefit-to-toxicity ratio of the available pharmacotherapy for gout.[36] When begun within the first 24 hours of an acute attack, colchicine produces a response in two thirds of patients within hours of administration.[37] If the initiation of colchicine is delayed longer than 48 hours after the onset of acute symptoms, the probability of success with the drug diminishes substantially. Although it is a highly effective therapy, oral colchicine can cause dose-dependent gastrointestinal adverse effects, including nausea, vomiting, and diarrhea, in 50% to 80% of patients.[2] Other important nongastrointestinal adverse effects include neutropenia and axonal neuromyopathy, which may be worsened for patients taking other myopathic drugs such as β-hydroxy-β-methylglutaryl-coenzyme A reductase inhibitors (statins) or for those with renal insufficiency.

Colchicine has been used for many years as an unapproved drug with no FDA-approved prescribing information, dosage recommendations, or drug interaction warnings. Recently, the FDA approved a 0.6 mg tablet of colchicine (Colcrys) for oral use. Data submitted in support of the safety and efficacy of colchicine in acute gout flares demonstrated that a substantially lower dose of colchicine (1.2 mg initially, followed by 0.6 mg 1 hour later) was as effective as higher doses traditionally used (continued hourly dosing until symptoms subside or gastrointestinal symptoms become intolerable).[38] These findings suggest that prior use of high-dose colchicine regimens, as traditionally recommended, may unnecessarily expose patients to increased toxicity with no additional efficacy. Additionally, comprehensive review of post-marketing safety data revealed an increased risk of adverse events for patients receiving colchicine administered concurrently with P-glycoprotein or cytochrome P450 3A4 inhibitors (e.g., clarithromycin).[39-42] This interaction is thought to result from decreased biliary excretion of colchicine leading to increased plasma levels of colchicine.

Colchicine should be used carefully for patients with renal insufficiency, with dosing repeated no more than once every 2 weeks. Patients undergoing dialysis should receive a reduced dose of 0.6 mg, administered as a one-time dose only. As a consequence of the high incidence of adverse effects and the low benefit-to-toxicity ratio, colchicine is used less often than NSAIDs in the United States, and it should be reserved as a second-line therapy when NSAIDs or corticosteroids are contraindicated or ineffective.

Intravenous colchicine has resulted in fatalities and is no longer available.[43]

Nonpharmacologic Therapies

Gout is influenced by several dietary factors, including obesity, alcohol intake, hyperlipidemia, and the insulin resistance syndrome.[44] Because of the elevated risk for development of gout that exists with hyperuricemia, even the asymptomatic patient should receive interventions directed toward modifying or correcting some of these underlying contributors.

Patients suffering from acute gouty arthritis should be advised to reduce their dietary intake of saturated fats and meats high in purines (e.g., organ meats). Some consideration may be given to a rigid purine-free diet, although they may only be moderately effective in lowering serum uric acid levels and they can rarely be sustained for long periods of time.[44] Because of the increased risk of developing nephrolithiasis, clinicians should counsel patients with gout to increase fluid intake and decrease salt consumption.[45] In addition, joint rest for 1 to 2 days should be encouraged, and local application of ice may be beneficial.[44,46] Joint exercise and application of heat to the affected area should be avoided, as they can worsen the condition.

Weight loss through caloric restriction and exercise should be promoted in all patients with gout or asymptomatic hyperuricemia, and this may enhance renal excretion of urate.[47] Restriction of alcohol intake is of great importance, as alcohol consumption is closely correlated with gout symptoms.[8] Acute ingestions of alcohol cause lactic acidemia, which reduces renal urate excretion, whereas long-term alcohol intake promotes production of purines as a by-product of the conversion of acetate to acetyl coenzyme A in the metabolism of alcohol.[44]

The presence of gout should not be a contraindication to the use of thiazide diuretics in hypertensive patients, although clinicians should be aware that diuretics are independent risk factors for gout and can increase serum uric acid levels.[9] It may be important to avoid using diuretics if other agents can be used to control blood pressure, particularly if the patient has had frequent gout attacks or continues to have an elevated serum uric acid level despite appropriate therapy for gout.

■ NEPHROLITHIASIS

❹ The medical management of uric acid nephrolithiasis includes hydration sufficient to maintain a urine volume of 2 to 3 L/day, alkalinization of urine, avoidance of purine-rich foods, moderation of protein intake, and reduction of urinary uric acid excretion.

Maintenance of a 24-hour urine volume of 2 to 3 L with an adequate intake of fluids is desirable for all gout patients, but especially for those with excessive [>1 g/day (>6 mmol/day)] uric acid excretion. Alkalinizing agents should be used with the objective of making the urine less acidic. Urine pH should be maintained at 6 to 6.5. In this pH range, up to 85% of uric acid will be in the form of the soluble urate ion.

Reduction of urine acidity is usually accomplished by the administration of potassium bicarbonate or potassium citrate 60 to 80 mEq/day.[48,49] Administration of alkali via sodium salts is a less desirable option for two reasons. First, the sodium-induced volume expansion will increase sodium excretion and can secondarily cause hypercalcemia because calcium passively follows the reabsorption of sodium in the proximal tubule and loop of Henle. In the presence of uric acid, the resultant hypercalcemia can lead to calcium oxalate stone formation. Second, older patients with uric acid kidney stones may also have hypertension, congestive heart failure, or renal insufficiency. Because of these conditions, they should not be overloaded with alkalinizing sodium salts or unlimited fluid intake, as these agents can worsen these conditions. Acetazolamide, a carbonic anhydrase inhibitor, produces rapid and effective urinary alkalinization and sometimes is used in conjunction with alkali therapy. When a 250 mg dose of acetazolamide is given at bedtime, the excretion of acidic urine in the early morning hours is avoided. The usual tachyphylaxis (rapid tolerance) to this drug is obviated by a daily repletion dose of bicarbonate.

Since the advent of xanthine oxidase inhibitors, a low-purine, low-protein diet for the patient with uric acid nephrolithiasis is no longer as critical as it once was; however, it is still advisable to instruct the patient to avoid foods rich in purine and to limit protein to no more than 90 g/day. Such a diet is still palatable and reduces appreciably the amount of uric acid in the urine.

The mainstay of drug therapy for recurrent uric acid nephrolithiasis is xanthine oxidase inhibitors. They are effective in reducing both serum and urinary uric acid levels, thus preventing the formation of calculi. Xanthine oxidase inhibitors are recommended as prophylactic treatment for patients who will receive cytotoxic agents for the treatment of lymphoma or leukemia. The marked increase in uric acid production associated with cytolysis of a neoplasm predisposes a patient to the development of uric acid nephrolithiasis.

■ PROPHYLACTIC THERAPY OF INTERCRITICAL GOUT

❺ After the first attack of acute gouty arthritis or after the passage of the first renal stone, a decision to institute prophylactic therapy must be considered. This decision should carefully balance risk and benefit. Prophylactic therapy has been found to be cost-effective if patients have two or more attacks per year, even if the serum uric acid concentration is normal or only minimally elevated.[50,51]

If the first episode was mild and responded promptly to treatment, the patient's serum urate concentration was elevated only minimally, and the 24-hour urinary uric acid excretion was not excessive [<1,000 mg/24 hours (<5.95 mmol/day) on a regular diet], then prophylactic treatment can be withheld. Some patients never have a second attack or a second stone. Others may not experience a second gouty episode for 5 to 10 years. Consequently, a wait-and-see approach seems justified for patients who meet these conditions.[52]

On the other hand, if the patient had a severe attack of gouty arthritis, a complicated course of uric acid nephrolithiasis, a substantially elevated serum uric acid level [>10 mg/dL (>595 μmol/L)], or a 24-hour urinary excretion of uric acid of more than 1,000 mg (5.95 mmol), then prophylactic treatment should be instituted immediately after resolution of the acute episode. Patients with tophi should also be administered prophylactic therapy. When implemented, urate-lowering therapy should not commence during an acute attack but 6 to 8 weeks after resolution.

Prophylactic therapy with low-dose oral colchicine, 0.6 mg once daily, may be effective in preventing recurrent arthritis for patients with no evidence of visible tophi and a normal or slightly elevated serum urate concentration. Patients do not become resistant to or tolerant of daily colchicine, and if they sense the beginning of an acute attack, they should increase the dose to 1.2 mg, followed by one repeat dose of 0.6 mg in 1 hour. If the serum urate concentration is within the normal range and the patient has been symptom free for 1 year, maintenance colchicine may be discontinued. The patient should be advised, however, that discontinuation of the treatment program may be followed by an exacerbation of acute gouty arthritis.

Patients with a history of recurrent acute gouty arthritis and a significantly elevated serum uric acid concentration probably are best managed with uric acid–lowering therapy. The goal of initiating urate-lowering therapies is to achieve and maintain a serum uric acid concentration of less than 6 mg/dL (357 μmol/L), and preferably below 5 mg/dL (297 μmol/L).[52] Reduction of the serum urate concentration can be accomplished pharmacologically by decreasing the synthesis of uric acid (xanthine oxidase inhibitors) or by increasing the renal excretion of uric acid (uricosurics). Colchicine at a dose of 0.6 mg once daily should be administered for at least the first 8 weeks of antihyperuricemic therapy to minimize the risk of acute attacks that may occur during initiation of uric acid–lowering therapy.

Xanthine Oxidase Inhibitors

6 Xanthine oxidase inhibitors reduce uric acid by impairing the ability of xanthine oxidase to convert hypoxanthine to xanthine and xanthine to uric acid. Because they are efficacious for prophylaxis in both underexcreters and overproducers of uric acid, xanthine oxidase inhibitors are the most widely prescribed agents for the long-term prevention of recurrent attacks of gout. For nearly 40 years, allopurinol was the only agent available in the United States; however, a second xanthine oxidase inhibitor (febuxostat; Uloric) was recently made available.

Allopurinol lowers uric acid levels in a dose-dependent manner. Because of the long half-life of its metabolite (oxypurinol), it can be given once daily. It is typically initiated at a dose of 100 mg/day and then titrated by 100 mg/day at 1-week intervals to achieve a serum uric acid level of 6 mg/dL (357 μmol/L) or less, which will promote shrinkage of tophi.[53] Serum uric acid levels can be checked approximately 1 week after initiating or modifying the dose of allopurinol. Typical doses of 100 to 300 mg/day are used, although tophaceous gout may require doses of 400 to 600 mg/day and the maximum recommended dose of allopurinol is 800 mg/day. Allopurinol should be considered for long-term use when prescribed, as intermittent administration has been found to be less effective in controlling gouty attacks.[54]

Allopurinol is an effective urate-lowering agent, but up to 5% of patients are unable to tolerate it because of adverse effects, and long-term adherence with allopurinol is low.[55] Mild adverse effects such as skin rash, leukopenia, gastrointestinal problems, headache, and urticaria can occur with allopurinol administration. More severe adverse reactions including severe rash (toxic epidermal necrolysis, erythema multiforme, or exfoliative dermatitis), hepatitis, interstitial nephritis, and eosinophilia reportedly occur in approximately 2% of patients and are associated with a 20% mortality.[56] Although direct evidence is lacking, the presence of renal insufficiency is believed to predispose patients to this "allopurinol hypersensitivity syndrome."[56] It is traditionally recommended that the dose of allopurinol be reduced for patients with renal insufficiency [200 mg/day for creatinine clearance of 60 mL/min (1.00 mL/s), and 100 mg/day for creatinine clearance of 30 mL/min (0.50 mL/s)].

Similar to allopurinol, febuxostat lowers serum urate concentrations in a dose-dependent manner.[57,58] In clinical trials, 40 mg/day of febuxostat was noninferior to conventionally dosed allopurinol (300 mg/day) in achieving the primary endpoint of serum urate concentration <6.0 mg/dL (<357 μmol/L), while 80 mg/day of febuxostat was more effective. The incidence of gout flares occurring during the initial months of administration was similar for both drugs. Febuxostat is well tolerated, with adverse events mostly limited to nausea, arthralgias, and minor liver transaminase elevations.

One criticism of the studies comparing allopurinol and febuxostat is that a fixed dose of allopurinol was used, rather than titrating the dose to achieve the targeted serum urate level. However, the 300 mg/day dosing of allopurinol reflects what is typically used in the majority of clinical practice.[59]

An advantage of febuxostat is that it does not require dose adjustment for patients with mild to moderate hepatic or renal impairment [creatinine clearances of 30 to 89 mL/min (0.50 to 1.49 mL/s)]. Due to the rapid mobilization of urate deposits occurring with initiation of febuxostat, concomitant therapy with colchicine or a NSAID to prevent acute gout flares should be overlapped for at least the first 8 weeks after initiation of therapy.

CLINICAL CONTROVERSY

Which xanthine oxidase inhibitor is preferred for use? Although allopurinol is approved for treatment of hyperuricemia in doses up to 800 mg/day, the majority of prescriptions for allopurinol are for doses ≤300 mg/day, a dose that is inadequate to achieve serum urate concentration <6.0 mg/dL (<357 μmol/L) for many patients. The underdosing of allopurinol is likely due to the belief that dose should be calibrated to renal function in order to avoid the rare allopurinol hypersensitivity syndrome. Unfortunately, little evidence examines the risk-to-benefit ratio of uptitrating doses of allopurinol to optimize urate lowering, and severe allopurinol hypersensitivity reactions are not necessarily dose dependent. Febuxostat is more potent on a milligram-per-milligram basis in lowering serum urate than allopurinol, but there is no evidence to suggest superiority of effect in reducing recurrent gout attacks when equipotent doses are used.

Uricosuric Drugs

Uricosuric drugs increase the renal clearance of uric acid by inhibiting postsecretory renal proximal tubular reabsorption of uric acid. The drugs used most widely to increase uric acid excretion are probenecid and sulfinpyrazone. Several other uricosuric drugs are available in Europe, but they have not been approved for use in the United States.

Therapy with uricosuric drugs should be started at a low dose to avoid marked uricosuria and possible stone formation. They should be used only for patients with documented underexcretion of urate (less than 800 mg in 24 hours on a regular diet or 600 mg on a purine-restricted diet). The maintenance of adequate urine flow and alkalinization of the urine during the first several days of uricosuric therapy further diminish the possibility of uric acid stone formation. Probenecid is given initially at a dose of 250 mg twice a day for 1 to 2 weeks and then 500 mg twice a day for 2 weeks. Thereafter the daily dose is increased by 500 mg increments every 1 to 2 weeks until satisfactory control is achieved or a maximum dose of 2 g is reached. The initial dose of sulfinpyrazone is 50 mg twice a day for 3 to 4 days and then 100 mg twice a day, increasing the daily dose by 100 mg increments each week up to 800 mg/day.

The major adverse effects associated with uricosuric therapy are gastrointestinal irritation, rash and hypersensitivity, precipitation of acute gouty arthritis, and stone formation. Of the two agents, probenecid is the most frequently used uricosuric, as sulfinpyrazone is associated with more severe adverse effects. A disadvantage of uricosurics is that salicylates may interfere with this mechanism and result in treatment failure; however, low doses (325 mg/day or less) of enteric-coated aspirin may be used cautiously. In addition, probenecid can inhibit the tubular secretion of other organic acids; thus, increased plasma concentrations of penicillins, cephalosporins, sulfonamides, and indomethacin can occur. Because it is chemically related to phenylbutazone, sulfinpyrazone can act as an antiplatelet agent and should be used with great caution for anticoagulated patients or for those with peptic ulcer disease.

7 Uricosuric drugs are contraindicated for patients who are allergic to them and for patients with impaired renal function [a creatinine clearance <50 mL/min (<0.84 mL/s)] and a history of renal calculi and for patients who are overproducers of uric acid; for such patients, a xanthine oxidase inhibitor should be used.

Miscellaneous Agents

Several other medications have been effective in gout. Benzbromarone is a uricosuric that is efficacious for patients with renal insufficiency, but it is not available in the United States.[2] Oxypurinol, a metabolite of allopurinol, is not commercially available in the United States but can be obtained through the manufacturer on a compassionate basis.[44] Several newer medications, including uric acid oxidase (uricase), are currently under investigation and may offer additional options in the future.[44] A recombinant form of uricase (rasburicase) is currently available and indicated for use in the management of hyperuricemia in children with leukemia, lymphoma, or solid-tumor malignancies who are likely to experience tumor lysis syndrome. The efficacy of rasburicase has not been assessed outside of the oncology setting in adults with acute gouty arthritis.

Lipid-lowering agents, in particular fenofibrate, can also be prescribed for patients with gout. Although dyslipidemia is common in gout patients, the fibrates are believed to exert their effects as an ancillary benefit by increasing the clearance of hypoxanthine and xanthine, leading to a sustained reduction in serum urate concentrations. Reductions of 20% to 30% in urate levels are observed with fenofibrate use.[60,61] Importantly, fenofibrate does not appear to not cause an acute gout flare when initiated and is well tolerated overall.[62,63]

Losartan, an angiotensin II receptor antagonist, has also demonstrated benefit in reducing serum urate concentrations independently of angiotensin receptor antagonism.[64] Losartan inhibits renal tubular reabsorption of uric acid and increases urinary excretion, and this effect seems to be a unique property of losartan that is not shared with other angiotensin II receptor antagonists.[65] In addition, it alkalinizes the urine, which helps reduce the risk for stone formation.

ASYMPTOMATIC HYPERURICEMIA

Questions are often raised regarding the indications for drug therapy for asymptomatic hyperuricemia. The purported benefits include prevention of acute gouty arthritis, tophi formation, nephrolithiasis, and chronic urate nephropathy. The first three complications are easily controlled should they develop; therefore, antihyperuricemic therapy is not warranted to prevent these conditions. The prevention of urate nephropathy might be a stronger indication because it is irreversible even with proper treatment. Available data indicate, however, that gouty nephropathy is extremely rare in the absence of clinical gout, and evidence that elevation of uric acid by itself may cause renal disease is weak and inconclusive. As discussed previously, renal impairment is very rare in the absence of concurrent hypertension and atherosclerosis. In addition, it is unclear whether uric acid–lowering therapy protects renal function in such individuals. Thus, the routine treatment of asymptomatic hyperuricemia on the grounds of reducing renal complications is presently not recommended.

The relationship between elevated serum urate concentrations and cardiovascular disease is controversial. In observational studies, hyperuricemia has been shown to be a risk factor for ischemic heart disease.[66–69] However, hyperuricemia is also associated with other known risk factors for cardiovascular disease, such as diabetes mellitus, dyslipidemia, and hypertension, and the individual contribution of hyperuricemia on the risk for cardiovascular disease is difficult to separate from these associated factors. Recently, a 12-year follow-up of the Health Professionals Study revealed a 28% higher risk of death from all causes, 38% higher risk of cardiovascular disease death, 55% higher risk of death from coronary heart disease, and a 59% higher risk of nonfatal myocardial infarction for men with a self-reported history of gout compared with those who do not have these conditions.[70] These associations remained significant even after adjusting for age, body mass index, smoking, family history of myocardial infarction, and comorbidities such as diabetes

and hypertension. To date, this study is the only one providing prospective data that implicate gout as an independent risk for coronary heart disease. No studies have examined whether drug treatment of asymptomatic hyperuricemia or gout is protective against coronary artery disease. At this time, it is premature to implement therapy for patients with asymptomatic hyperuricemia in the absence of a history of gout. Instead, efforts should be directed toward aggressive management of cardiovascular risk factors.

CLINICAL CONTROVERSY

While asymptomatic hyperuricemia is not generally treated, some clinicians have begun recommending treatment to reduce the risk of coronary artery disease. Hyperuricemia is associated with both hypertension and coronary artery disease, and patients with elevated uric acid levels and hypertension may have an increased risk of cardiovascular morbidity and mortality.

PHARMACOECONOMIC CONSIDERATIONS

Assuming patients with asymptomatic hyperuricemia are not treated with pharmacologic therapy, pharmacoeconomic considerations apply only to the management of the acute and chronic clinical manifestations of gout.

In a cost-effectiveness analysis for patients with nontophaceous recurrent gouty arthritis, urate-lowering therapy was found to reduce costs if patients experienced two or more recurrent attacks per year.[50] Generic allopurinol was associated with a lower incremental cost-effectiveness ratio than were either probenecid or sulfinpyrazone. No studies have examined the cost-effectiveness of febuxostat.

In the case of chronic tophaceous gout, the need to continue long-term therapy with a urate-lowering drug clearly exists. Allopurinol is less expensive than uricosuric therapy and may be more effective. Comparative trials are lacking. For severe cases, combination therapy may be indicated. Many clinicians will add colchicine to the regimen to reduce the likelihood of precipitating acute gouty arthritis, but this does not appear to be a cost-effective measure.

EVALUATION OF THERAPEUTIC OUTCOMES

Follow-up of the gout sufferer depends on the frequency of attacks and on the medications used to treat symptoms. For a patient who is experiencing a first attack of gout, long-term therapy is generally not indicated. As previously mentioned, most experts agree that treatment should be started only after two or three attacks of gout, because the treatment is long term and relatively expensive, the drugs used are potentially toxic, and adherence for patients without symptoms is generally poor.[51,55] Patients having a first attack should be educated about the likelihood of recurrence and what to do if another attack occurs. Approximately 60% of patients have a second attack within the first year, and 78% have a second attack within 2 years. Only 7% of patients do not have a recurrence within a 10-year period.[71]

Baseline blood work for patients receiving hypouricemic medications chronically should include renal function (serum creatinine, blood urea nitrogen), liver enzymes (aspartate aminotransferase, alanine aminotransferase), complete blood count, and electrolytes. There is generally no need to recheck these laboratory parameters for patients undergoing acute therapy with an NSAID or colchicine of limited duration. However, for patients requiring long-term therapy or prophylaxis, they should be rechecked every 6 to 12 months or as clinically indicated. For patients without evident tophi, consideration can be given to discontinuing long-term therapy 6 to 12 months after normal scrum urate levels are obtained.

For patients suspected of having an acute attack of gouty arthritis, it is reasonable to check a serum uric acid level, particularly if it is not the first attack and a decision is to be made regarding initiation of prophylactic therapy. However, clinicians should be mindful that acute gouty arthritis can occur in the presence of normal serum uric acid concentrations.[12] Repeat serum uric acid levels do not need to be routinely monitored in patients, with the exception of during the titration phase of allopurinol or febuxostat to achieve a goal serum urate concentration of <6 mg/dL (<357 μmol/L).[72]

❽ Because of comorbidity with diabetes mellitus, lipid abnormalities, hypertension, and stroke, elevated uric acid levels or gout should prompt evaluations for signs of cardiovascular disease and the need for appropriate risk reduction measures.[28] Additionally, clinicians should look for a possible correctable cause of hyperuricemia, such as medications (e.g., thiazide diuretics, niacin, cyclosporine), obesity, malignancy, and alcohol abuse. Patients should be encouraged to exercise, lose weight, reduce alcohol intake, and control blood pressure and to have periodic follow-up to address these conditions.

CONCLUSIONS

Hyperuricemia may lead to acute arthritis, chronic gout, or kidney stones or to no sequelae at all. Asymptomatic hyperuricemia need not be treated, although lifestyle modifications (e.g., weight loss, reduction of alcohol intake, control of blood pressure) should be encouraged to help reduce serum urate and overall cardiovascular health.

Acute gouty arthritis responds well to short courses of NSAIDs to treat the underlying inflammatory condition. Colchicine is also highly effective, but has the lowest benefit-to-toxicity ratio of the available pharmacotherapy for acute gouty arthritis. Oral or intraarticular corticosteroids can be used, particularly if contraindications to NSAIDs or colchicine are present, there is lack of response to these agents, or polyarticular involvement is noted. The management of uric acid nephrolithiasis includes hydration and alkalinization of the urine. Prevention of recurrent gouty arthritis or recurrent nephrolithiasis and treatment of chronic gout require hypouricemic therapy with either a uricosuric drug or xanthine oxidase inhibitor. Xanthine oxidase inhibitors are effective in both underexcreters and overproducers of uric acid, making them the hypouricemic drugs of choice for most patients with gout.

ABBREVIATIONS

ACTH: adrenocorticotropic hormone

HGPRT: hypoxanthine guanine phosphoribosyl transferase

NSAID: nonsteroidal antiinflammatory drug

PRPP: phosphoribosyl pyrophosphate (synthetase)

REFERENCES

1. Wortmann RL. Chapter 87: Gout and hyperuricemia. In: Firestein GS, Budd RC, Harris ED Jr, et al, eds. Kelley's Textbook of Rheumatology. 8th ed. Philadelphia, PA: WB Saunders; 2008.
2. Rott KT, Agudelo CA. Gout. JAMA 2003;289:2857–2860.
3. Johnson RJ, Rideout BA. Uric acid and diet—Insights into the epidemic of cardiovascular disease. N Engl J Med 2004;350:1071–1073.
4. Wallace KL, Riedel AA, Joseph-Ridge N, Wortmann R. Increasing prevalence of gout and hyperuricemia over 10 years among older adults in a managed care population. J Rheumatol 2004;31:1582–1587.
5. Annemans L, Spaepen E, Gaskin M, et al. Gout in the UK and Germany: prevalence, comorbidities and management in general practice 2000–2005. Ann Rheum Dis 2008;67:960–966.
6. Chen SY, Chen CL, Shen ML, Kamatani N. Trends in the manifestations of gout in Taiwan. Rheumatol 2003;42:1529–1533.
7. Miao Z, Li C, Chen Y, et al. Dietary and lifestyle changes associated with high prevalence of hyperuricemia and gout in the Shandong coastal cities of Eastern China. J Rheumatol 2008;35:1859–1864.
8. Choi HK, Atkinson K, Karlson EW, et al. Alcohol intake and risk of incident gout in men: A prospective study. Lancet 2004;363:1277–1281.
9. Choi HK, Atkinson K, Karlson EW, Curhan G. Obesity, weight change, hypertension, diuretic use, and risk of gout in men: The health professionals follow-up study. Arch Intern Med 2005;165:742–748.
10. Choi HK, Atkinson K, Karlson EW, et al. Purine-rich foods, dairy and protein intake, and the risk of gout in men. N Engl J Med 2004;350:1093–1103.
11. Campion EW, Glynn RJ, DeLabry LO. Asymptomatic hyperuricemia. Risks and consequences in the Normative Aging Study. Am J Med 1987;82:421–426.
12. McCarty DJ. Gout without hyperuricemia. JAMA 1994;271:302–303.
13. Kramer HM, Curhan G. The association between gout and nephrolithiasis: The National Health and Nutrition Examination Survey III, 1988–1994. Am J Kidney Dis 2002;40:37–42.
14. Mikuls TR, Farrar JT, Bilker WB, et al. Gout epidemiology: Results from the UK General Practice Research Database, 1990-1999. Ann Rheum Dis 2005;64:267–272.
15. Terkeltaub RA. Gout. N Engl J Med 2003;349:1647–1655.
16. Choi HK, Mount DB, Reginato AM. Pathogenesis of gout. Ann Intern Med 2005;143:499–516.
17. Wilson JM, Young AB, Kelley WN. Hypoxanthine-guanine phosphoribosyltransferase deficiency. N Engl J Med 1983;309:900–910.
18. Beutler A, Schumacher HR. Gout and "pseudogout": When are arthritis symptoms caused by crystal deposition? Postgrad Med 1994;95:103–116.
19. McGill NW. Gout and other crystal arthropathies. Med J Aust 1997;166:33–38.
20. Schumacher HR. Crystal-reduced arthritis: An overview. Am J Med 1996;100(suppl 2A):46S–52S.
21. Pal B, Foxall M, Dysart T, et al. How is gout managed in primary care? A review of current practice and proposed guidelines. Clin Rheumatol 2000;19:21–25.
22. Agudelo CA, Weinberger A, Schumacher HR, et al. Definitive diagnosis of gout by identification of urate crystals in asymptomatic metatarsophalangeal joints. Arthritis Rheum 1979;22:559–560.
23. Logan JA, Morrison E, McGill PE. Serum uric acid in acute gout. Ann Rheum Dis 1997;56:696–697.
24. Wallace SL, Robinson H, Masi AT, et al. Preliminary criteria for the classification of the acute arthritis of primary gout. Arthritis Rheum 1977;20:895–900.
25. Zhang W, Doherty M, Pascual E, et al. EULAR evidence based recommendations for gout. Part I. Diagnosis. Report of a task force of the Standing Committee for International Clinical Studies Including Therapeutics (ESCISIT). Ann Rheum Dis 2006;65:1301–1311.
26. Yu T. Nephrolithiasis in patients with gout. Postgrad Med 1978;63:164–170.
27. Klineberg JR. Role of the kidneys in the pathogenesis of gout. Postgrad Med 1978;63:145–150.
28. Zhang W, Doherty M, Bardin T, et al. EULAR evidence based recommendations for gout. Part II. Management. Report of a task force of the EULAR Standing Committee for International Clinical Studies Including Therapeutics (ESCISIT). Ann Rheum Dis 2006;65:1312–1324.
29. Janssens HJ, Janssen M, van de Lisdonk EH, et al. Use of oral prednisolone or naproxen for the treatment of gout arthritis: a double-blind, randomised equivalence trial. Lancet 2008;371:1854–1860.

30. Hawkey CJ, Karrasch JA, Szczepanski L, et al. Omeprazole compared with misoprostol for ulcers associated with nonsteroidal anti-inflammatory drugs. Omeprazole versus Misoprostol for NSAID-induced Ulcer Management (OMNIUM) Study Group. N Engl J Med 1998;338:727–734.

31. Yeomans ND, Tulassay Z, Juhasz L, et al. A comparison of omeprazole with ranitidine for ulcers associated with nonsteroidal anti-inflammatory drugs. Acid Suppression Trial: Ranitidine versus Omeprazole for NSAID-associated Ulcer Treatment (ASTRONAUT) Study Group. N Engl J Med 1998;338:719–726.

32. Siegel LB, Alloway JA, Nashel DJ. Comparison of adrenocorticotropic hormone and triamcinolone acetonide in the treatment of acute gouty arthritis. J Rheumatol 1994;21:1325–1327.

33. Axelrod D, Preston S. Comparison of parenteral adrenocorticotropic hormone with oral indomethacin in the treatment of acute gout. Arthritis Rheum 1988;31:803–805.

34. Taylor CT, Brooks NC, Kelley KW. Corticotropin for acute management of gout. Ann Pharmacother 2001;35:365–368.

35. Ritter J, Kerr LD, Valeriano-Marcet J, Spiera H. ACTH revisited: Effective treatment for acute crystal induced synovitis in patients with multiple medical problems. J Rheumatol 1994;21:696–699.

36. Schlesinger N, Schumacher R, Catton M, Maxwell L. Colchicine for acute gout. Cochrane Database Syst Rev 2006;4:CD006190.

37. Ahern MJ, Reid C, Gordon TP, et al. Does colchicine work? The results of the first controlled study in acute gout. Aust N Z J Med 1987;17:301–304.

38. Terkeltaub RA, Furst DE, Bennett K, et al. High versus low dosing of oral colchicine for early acute gout flare: Twenty-four-hour outcome of the first multicenter, randomized, double-blind, placebo-controlled, parallel-group, dose-comparison colchicine study. Arthritis Rheum 2010;62:1060–1068.

39. Dogukan A, Oymak FS, Taskapan H, et al. Acute fatal colchicine intoxication in a patient on continuous ambulatory peritoneal dialysis (CAPD). Possible role of clarithromycin administration. Clin Nephrol 2001;55:181–182.

40. Rollot F, Pajot O, Chauvelot-Moachon L, et al. Acute colchicine intoxication during clarithromycin administration. Ann Pharmacother 2004;38:2074–2077.

41. Hung IF, Wu AK, Cheng VC, et al. Fatal interaction between clarithromycin and colchicine in patients with renal insufficiency: A retrospective study. Clin Infect Dis 2005;41:291–300.

42. Cheng VC, Ho PL, Yuen KY. Two probable cases of serious drug interaction between clarithromycin and colchicine. South Med J 2005;98:811–813.

43. Bonnel RA, Villalba ML, Karwoski CB, Beitz J. Deaths associated with inappropriate intravenous colchicine administration. J Emerg Med 2002;22:385–387.

44. Schlesinger N. Management of acute and chronic gouty arthritis: Present state-of-the-art. Drugs 2004;64:2399–2416.

45. Kramer HJ, Choi HK, Atkinson K, et al. The association between gout and nephrolithiasis in men: The Health Professionals' Follow-Up Study. Kidney Int 2003;64:1022–1026.

46. Schlesinger N, Detry MA, Holland BK, et al. Local ice therapy during bouts of acute gouty arthritis. J Rheumatol 2002;29:331–334.

47. Dessein PH, Shipton EA, Stanwix AE, et al. Beneficial effects of weight loss associated with moderate calorie/carbohydrate restriction, and increased proportional intake of protein and unsaturated fat on serum urate and lipoprotein levels in gout: A pilot study. Ann Rheum Dis 2000;59:539–543.

48. Riese RJ, Sakhaee K. Uric acid nephrolithiasis: Pathogenesis and treatment. J Urol 1992;148:765–771.

49. Pak CY, Sakhaee K, Fuller C. Successful management of uric acid nephrolithiasis with potassium citrate. Kidney Int 1986;30:422–428.

50. Ferraz MB, O'Brien B. A cost effectiveness analysis of urate lowering drugs in nontophaceous recurrent gouty arthritis. J Rheumatol 1995;22:908–914.

51. Dincer HE, Dincer AP, Levinson DJ. Asymptomatic hyperuricemia: To treat or not to treat. Cleve Clin J Med 2002;69:594–602.

52. Shoji A, Yamanaka H, Kamatani N. A retrospective study of the relationship between serum urate level and recurrent attacks of gouty arthritis: Evidence for reduction of recurrent gouty arthritis with anti-hyperuricemic therapy. Arthritis Rheum 2004;51:321–325.

53. Li-Yu J, Clayburne G, Sieck M, et al. Treatment of chronic gout. Can we determine when urate stores are depleted enough to prevent attacks of gout? J Rheumatol 2001;28:577–580.

54. Bull PW, Scott JT. Intermittent control of hyperuricemia in the treatment of gout. J Rheumatol 1989;16:1246–1248.

55. Riedel AA, Nelson M, Joseph-Ridge N, et al. Compliance with allopurinol therapy among managed care enrollees with gout: A retrospective analysis of administrative claims. J Rheumatol 2004;31:1575–1581.

56. Hande KR, Noone RM, Stone WJ. Severe allopurinol toxicity. Description and guidelines for prevention in patients with renal insufficiency. Am J Med 1984;76:47–56.

57. Ernst ME, Fravel MA. Febuxostat: a selective xanthine-oxidase/xanthine-dehydrogenase inhibitor for the management of hyperuricemia in adults with gout. Clin Ther 2009;31:2503-2518.

58. Becker MA, Schumacher HR, Wortmann RL, et al. Febuxostat compared with allopurinol in patients with hyperuricemia and gout. N Engl J Med 2005;353:2450–2461.

59. Chao J, Terkeltaub R. A critical reappraisal of allopurinol dosing, safety, and efficacy for hyperuricemia in gout. Curr Rheumatol Rep 2009;11:135–140.

60. de la Serna G, Cadarso C. Fenofibrate decreases plasma fibrinogen, improves lipid profile, and reduces uricemia. Clin Pharmacol Ther 1999;66:166–172.

61. Feher MD, Hepburn AL, Hogarth MB, et al. Fenofibrate enhances urate reduction in men treated with allopurinol for hyperuricaemia and gout. Rheumatol 2003;42:321–325.

62. Hepburn AL, Kaye SA, Feher MD. Long-term remission from gout associated with fenofibrate therapy. Clin Rheumatol 2003;22:73–76.

63. Hepburn AL, Kaye SA, Feher MD. Fenofibrate: A new treatment for hyperuricaemia and gout? Ann Rheum Dis 2001;60:984–986.

64. Wurzner G, Gerster JC, Chiolero A, et al. Comparative effects of losartan and irbesartan on serum uric acid in hypertensive patients with hyperuricaemia and gout. J Hypertens 2001;19:1855–1860.

65. Shahinfar S, Simpson RL, Carides AD, et al. Safety of losartan in hypertensive patients with thiazide-induced hyperuricemia. Kidney Int 1999;56:1879–1885.

66. Abbott RD, Brand FN, Kannel WB, et al. Gout and coronary heart disease: The Framingham Study. J Clin Epidemiol 1988;41:237–242.

67. Freedman DS, Williamson DF, Gunter EW, et al. Relation of serum uric acid to mortality and ischemic heart disease. The NHANES I Epidemiologic Follow-up Study. Am J Epidemiol 1995;141:637–644.

68. Langford HG, Blaufox MD, Borhani NO, et al. Is thiazide-produced uric acid elevation harmful? Analysis of data from the Hypertension Detection and Follow-up Program. Arch Intern Med 1987;147:645–649.

69. Bengtsson C, Lapidus L, Stendahl C, Waldenstrom J. Hyperuricaemia and risk of cardiovascular disease and overall death. A 12-year follow-up of participants in the population study of women in Gothenburg, Sweden. Acta Med Scand 1988;224:549–555.

70. Choi HK, Curhan G. Independent impact of gout on mortality and risk for coronary heart disease. Circ 2007;116:894–900.

71. Gutman AB. The past four decades of progress in the knowledge of gout, with an assessment of the present status. Arthritis Rheum 1973;16:431–445.

72. Mikuls TR, MacLean CH, Olivieri J, et al. Quality of care indicators for gout management. Arthritis Rheum 2004;50:937–943.

OPHTHALMIC AND OTOLARYNGOLOGICAL DISORDERS

CHAPTER

103

Glaucoma

RICHARD G. FISCELLA, TIMOTHY S. LESAR, AND DEEPAK P. EDWARD

KEY CONCEPTS

❶ Primary open-angle glaucoma (POAG) or ocular hypertension is more prevalent than closed- or narrow-angle glaucoma.

❷ In any form of glaucoma, reduction of intraocular pressure (IOP) is essential.

❸ IOP is a very important risk factor for glaucoma, but the most important considerations are progression of glaucomatous changes in the back of the eye (optic disk and nerve fiber layer) and visual field changes when diagnosing and monitoring for POAG or ocular hypertension.

❹ Optic nerve changes often occur before visual field changes are exhibited.

❺ Recent studies demonstrate that reduction in IOP prevents progression or even onset of glaucoma.

❻ Newer medications simplify treatment regimens for patients. Prostaglandin analogs are considered the most potent topical medications for reducing IOP and flattening diurnal variations in intraocular pressure.

❼ Local adverse events are common with topical glaucoma medications, but patient education and reinforcing adherence are essential to prevent glaucoma progression.

The glaucomas are a group of ocular disorders that lead to an optic neuropathy characterized by changes in the optic nerve head (optic disk) that is associated with loss of visual sensitivity and field. Increased intraocular pressure (IOP), a traditional diagnostic criterion for glaucoma, is thought to play an important role in the pathogenesis of glaucoma, but it is no longer a diagnostic criterion for glaucoma.[1-10] Two major types of glaucoma

Learning objectives, review questions, and other resources can be found at **www.pharmacotherapyonline.com**.

have been identified: open angle and closed angle. Open-angle glaucoma accounts for the great majority of cases. Either type can be a primary inherited disorder, congenital, or secondary to disease, trauma, or drugs and can lead to serious complications.[11-16] Both primary and secondary glaucomas may be caused by a combination of open-angle and closed-angle mechanisms (Table 103–1).

BASIC CONCEPTS

AQUEOUS HUMOR DYNAMICS AND INTRAOCULAR PRESSURE

An understanding of IOP and aqueous humor dynamics will assist the reader in understanding the drug therapy of glaucoma.[1,2,17-19]

Aqueous humor is formed in the ciliary body and its epithelium (Figs. 103–1 and 103–2) through both filtration and secretion. Because ultrafiltration depends on pressure gradients, blood pressure and IOP changes influence aqueous humor formation. Osmotic gradients produced by active secretion of sodium and bicarbonate and possibly by other solutes such as ascorbate from the ciliary body epithelial cells into the aqueous humor result in movement of water from the pool of ciliary stromal ultrafiltrate into the posterior

TABLE 103-1	General Classification of Glaucoma
I. Primary glaucoma	
A. Open angle	
B. Angle closure	
1. With pupillary block	
2. Without pupillary block	
II. Secondary glaucoma	
A. Open angle	
1. Pretrabecular	
2. Trabecular	
3. Posttrabecular	
B. Angle closure	
1. Without pupillary block	
2. With pupillary block	
III. Congenital glaucoma	

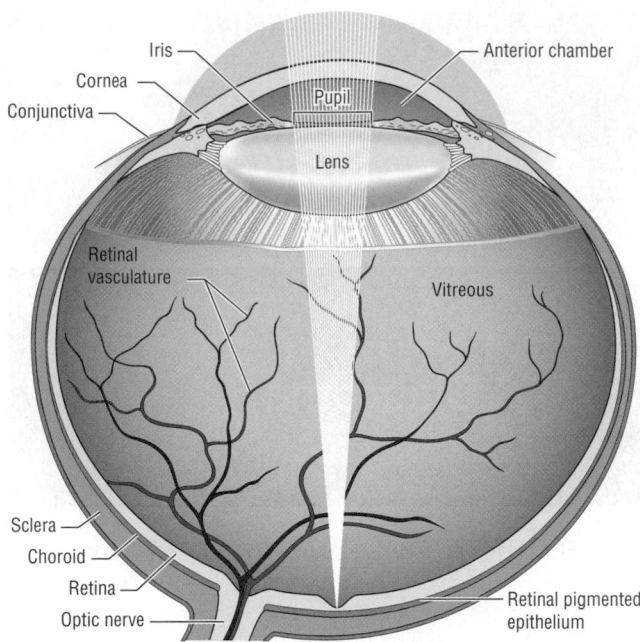

FIGURE 103-1. Anatomy of the eye.

chamber, forming aqueous humor. Carbonic anhydrase (primarily isoenzyme type II), α- and β-adrenergic receptors, and sodium- and potassium-activated adenosine triphosphatases are found on the ciliary epithelium and appear to be involved in this secretion of the solutes sodium and bicarbonate.

Receptor systems controlling aqueous inflow have not been elucidated fully. Pharmacologic studies suggest that β-adrenergic agents increase inflow, whereas α_2-adrenergic blocking, β-adrenergic blocking dopamine-blocking, carbonic anhydrase-inhibiting, and adenylate cyclase-stimulating agents decrease aqueous inflow. Aqueous humor produced by the ciliary body is secreted into the posterior chamber at a rate of approximately 2 to 3 μL/min. The pressure in the posterior chamber produced by the constant inflow pushes the aqueous humor between the iris and lens and through the pupil into the anterior chamber of the eye (see Fig. 103–2).[1,2,17–22]

Aqueous humor in the anterior chamber leaves the eye by two routes: (1) filtration through the trabecular meshwork (conventional outflow) to the Schlemm canal (80% to 85%) and (2) through the ciliary body and the suprachoroidal space (uveoscleral outflow or unconventional outflow). Cholinergic agents such as pilocarpine increase outflow by physically opening the meshwork pores secondary to ciliary muscle contraction. The uveoscleral outflow of aqueous humor is also increased by prostaglandin analogs and β- and α_2-adrenergic agonists. Constant inflow of aqueous humor from the ciliary body and resistance to outflow result in an IOP great enough to produce an outflow rate equal to the inflow rate (see Fig. 103–2).

The median IOP measured in large populations is 15.5 $\pm$ 2.5 mm Hg (2.1 $\pm$ 0.3 kPa); however, the distribution of pressures around the mean is skewed to the right (toward higher readings). IOP is not constant and changes with pulse, blood pressure, forced expiration or coughing, neck compression, and posture. IOP is measured by tonometry: indentation tonometry, applanation tonometry, or a noncontact method using an air pulse. These methods may result in slightly different pressure readings. IOPs consistently greater than 21 mm Hg (2.8 kPa) are found in 5% to 8% of the general population. The incidence increases with age, such that "abnormal" (i.e., >22 mm Hg [>2.9 kPa]) IOP is found in 15% of those 70 to 75 years of age. Intermittently high IOP (>40 mm Hg [>5.3 kPa]) is found in patients with closed-angle glaucoma (CAG). The increased IOP in all types of glaucoma results from the decreased facility for aqueous humor outflow through the trabecular meshwork. Aqueous humor production in primary open-angle glaucoma (POAG) is normal.[1,2,17–19]

IOP demonstrates considerable circadian variation (often referred to as *diurnal* IOP or the IOP during the daily 24-hour cycle) primarily because of changes in the rate of aqueous humor formation. This circadian variation results in a minimum IOP at approximately 6 PM and a maximum IOP at awakening, although some studies suggest that both healthy and glaucoma patients may have their highest IOP at night after falling asleep.[20] Low systemic blood pressure in conjunction with high IOPs (decreased ocular perfusion pressure) at night can result in optic nerve head damage.[20] Generally, the circadian IOP variation is usually less than 3 to 4 mm Hg (0.4 to 0.5 kPa); however, it may be greater for patients with glaucoma. This circadian variation and the poor rela-

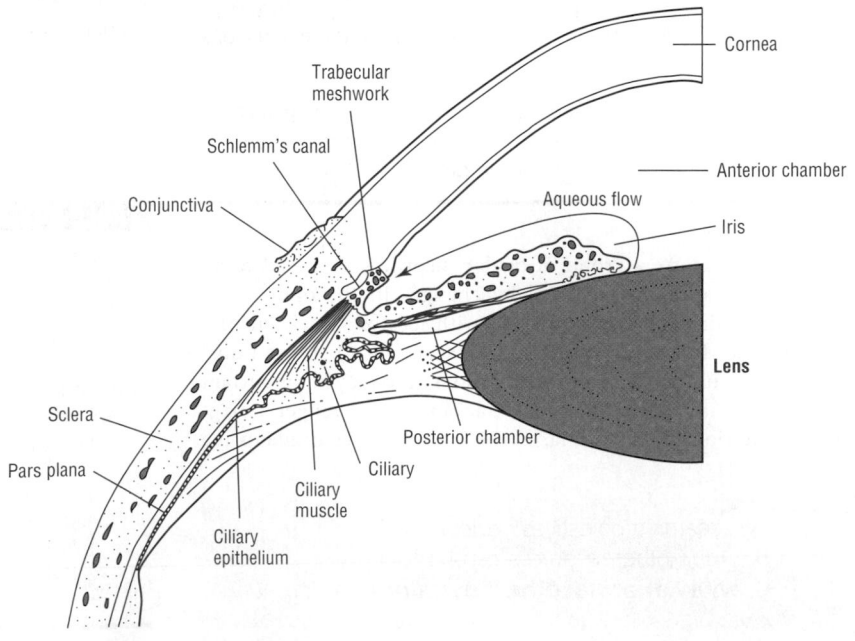

FIGURE 103-2. Anterior chamber of the eye and aqueous humor flow.

tionship of IOP with visual loss make measurement of IOP a poor screening test for glaucoma.

Although increased IOP within any range is associated with a higher risk of glaucomatous damage, it is both an insensitive and nonspecific diagnostic and monitoring tool. Of individuals with IOP between 21 and 30 mm Hg (2.8 and 4.0 kPa), only 0.5% to 1% per year will develop optic disk changes and visual field loss (i.e., glaucoma) over 5 to 15 years. However, more subtle retinal damage, such as alteration of color vision or decreased contrast sensitivity, occurs in a higher percentage of patients with IOPs greater than 21 mm Hg (2.8 kPa), and the incidence of visual field defects increases to as high as 28% in individuals with IOPs above 30 mm Hg (4.0 kPa). For a given abnormal IOP, the incidence of glaucoma increases with age. For patients with preexisting optic nerve damage, the worse the existing damage, the more sensitive the eye is to a given IOP. As many as 20% to 30% of patients with glaucomatous visual field loss have an IOP of less than 21 mm Hg (2.8 kPa) (called *normal-tension glaucoma*, referring to the normal IOP). Thus the absolute IOP is a less-precise predictor of optic nerve damage. More direct measurements of therapeutic outcome, such as optic disk examination and visual field evaluation, also must be used as monitors of disease progression.[1-7,17-24] Taking the above factors into consideration, glaucoma medications that provide maximal reduction of IOP over 24 hours and have minimal influence on blood pressure may be advantageous in treating glaucoma patients.

OPTIC DISK AND VISUAL FIELDS

The optic disk is the portion of the optic nerve ophthalmoscopically visible as it leaves the eye. It consists of approximately 1 million retinal ganglion nerve cell axons, blood vessels, and supporting connective tissue structures (lamina cribrosa). The small depression within the disk is termed the *cup* (Fig. 103–3). A normal physiologic cup does not extend beyond the optic nerve rim and has a varying diameter of less than one third to one half that of the disk (cup-to-disk ratio: 0.33 to 0.5). Table 103–2 lists the common alterations of the optic disk found in glaucoma. These disk changes result from optic nerve axonal degeneration and remodeling of the supporting structures. As the nerve axons die, the cup becomes larger in relation to the whole disk. A loss of retinal nerve fiber layer visibility might be visualized in glaucoma patients with detectable visual field loss. This pattern of changes is consistent with visual field losses and loss of visual sensitivity seen in glaucoma.[1,2,17-24] Damage to the optic nerve can be documented by optic disk photographs, and disease stability or progression

TABLE 103-2 Optic Disk and Visual Field Findings

Optic disk
Cup-to-disk ratio >0.5
Progressive increase in cup size
Cup-to-disk ratio asymmetry >0.2
Vertical elongation of the cup
Excavation of the cup
Increased exposure of lamina cribrosa
Pallor of the cup
Splinter hemorrhages
Cupping to edge of disk
Notching of the cup (usually superior or inferior)
Nerve fiber defects
Visual field findings
General peripheral field constriction
Isolated scotomas (blind spots)
Nasal visual field depression ("nasal step")
Enlargement of blind spot
Large arc-like scotomas
Reduced contrast sensitivity
Reduced peripheral acuity
Altered color vision

may be monitored by examining sequential photographs. Newer methods of assessing damage to the retinal nerve fiber layer and optic disk have been described. These include scanning laser polarimetry (GDX), confocal laser ophthalmoscopy (Heidelberg retinal tomography, or HRT), and optical coherence tomography (OCT). These methods offer the ability to assess the damage to the optic nerve quantitatively.

Determination of the visual field allows assessment of optic nerve damage and is an important monitoring parameter in treatment. However, visual field changes lag behind optic disk changes, and a loss of 25% to 35% of retinal ganglion cells is usually required before detectable visual field defects are noted. The peripheral visual field is measured using a visual field instrument called a *perimeter*. Characteristic visual field loss occurs in glaucoma (Fig. 103–4; see also Table 103–2), but loss of central visual acuity usually does not occur until late in the disease. Other indicators, such as color vision changes and contrast sensitivity, may allow earlier and more sensitive detection of glaucomatous changes.[1,2]

GENETICS

Glaucoma is often inherited as a complex multifactorial disease, but it can also be inherited as a Mendelian autosomal-dominant or autosomal-recessive trait form. The common age-related adult-onset glaucoma, like POAG, although containing heritability of some significance, is more complex and is influenced by environmental factors. Genetic studies have more clearly defined the underlying molecular events responsible for the Mendelian forms of the disease. However, the chromosome locations identified may play some factor in the more complex forms. A number of major gene loci associated with POAG have been identified. The molecular mechanism of how mutations in any of these genes result in increased IOP with loss of visual field has not been elucidated. The future of genetic studies in glaucoma will include discovery of new glaucoma genes, determination of clinical phenotypes associated with these genes and mutations, understanding how environmental factors interact, and developing a database that can be used for further testing. It is hoped that improved understanding of the genetic origins of POAG will lead to new diagnostic tools and therapies that target the underlying causes of the disease.[1,2,25,26]

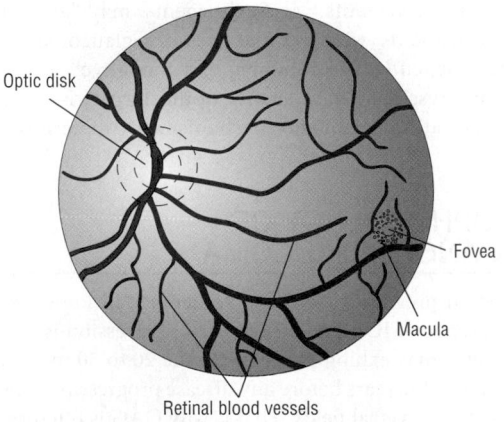

FIGURE 103-3. Normal fundus of the eye and optic disk and cup.

Optic disk
Fovea
Macula
Retinal blood vessels

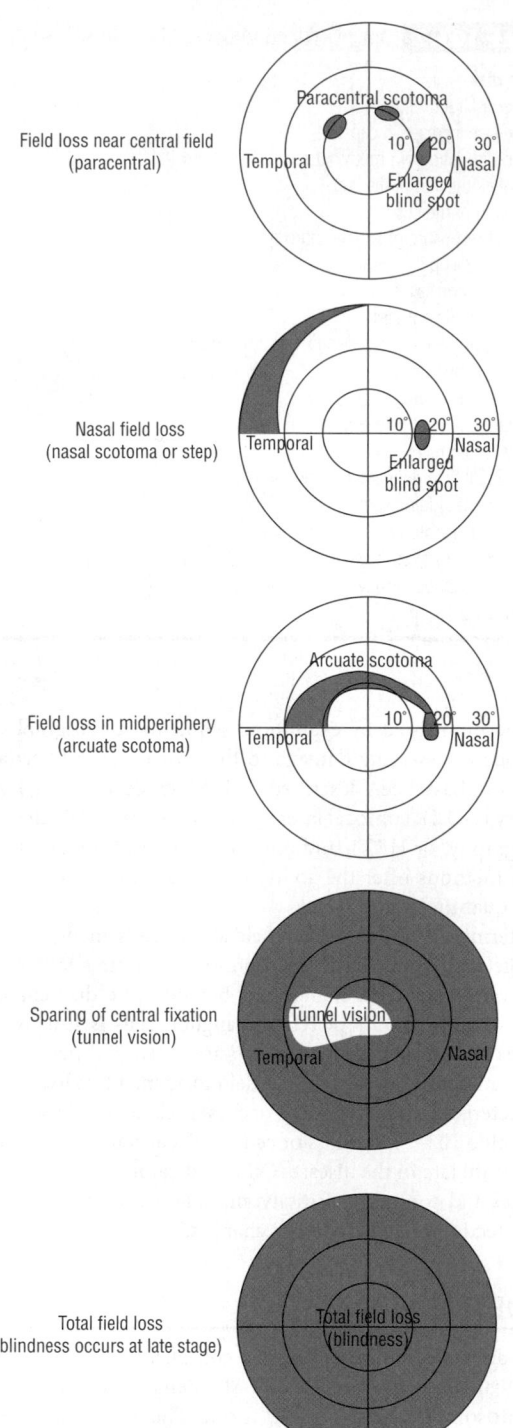

FIGURE 103-4. Schematic of the progression of visual field loss in glaucoma.

approximately 4.74% and 3.56% of people affected, respectively.[27] The incidence of OAG increases with increasing age. The incidence of the disease for patients 80 years of age is 3% in whites and 5% to 8% in blacks.

ETIOLOGY OF OPEN-ANGLE GLAUCOMA

❷ The specific cause of glaucomatous optic neuropathy is presently unknown. Previously, increased IOP was considered to be the sole cause of the damage; however, it is now recognized that IOP is only one of many factors associated with the development and progression of glaucoma.[1–10] Increased susceptibility of the optic nerve to ischemia (a reduced or dysregulated blood flow), excitotoxicity, autoimmune reactions, and other abnormal physiologic processes are likely additional contributory factors. The final outcome of these processes is believed to be apoptosis of the retinal ganglion cells, which results in axonal degeneration and finally permanent loss of vision.[11–16] Interestingly enough, there appears to be a fair amount of similarity between neuronal cell death by apoptosis in Alzheimer disease and glaucoma.[13] Indeed, OAG may represent a number of distinct diseases or conditions that simply manifest the same symptoms. Susceptibility to visual loss at a given IOP varies considerably; some patients do not demonstrate damage at high IOPs, whereas other patients have progressive visual field loss despite an IOP in the normal range (normal-tension glaucoma).

Although IOP poorly predicts which patients will have visual field loss, the risk of visual field loss clearly increases with increasing IOP within any range. In fact, recent studies demonstrate that lowering IOP, no matter what the pretreatment IOP, reduces the risk of glaucomatous progression or may even prevent the onset to early glaucoma in patients with ocular hypertension.[3–7]

The mechanism by which a certain level of IOP increases the susceptibility of a given eye to nerve damage remains controversial. Multiple mechanisms are likely to be operative in a spectrum of combinations to produce the death of retinal ganglion cells and their axons in glaucoma. Pressure-sensitive astrocytes and other cells in the optic disk supportive matrix may produce changes and remodeling of the disk, resulting in axonal death. Vasogenic theories suggest that optic nerve damage results from insufficient blood flow to the retina secondary to the increased perfusion pressure required in the eye, dysregulated perfusion, or vessel wall abnormalities, and results in degeneration of axonal fibers of the retina. Another theory suggests that the IOP may disrupt axoplasmal flow at the optic disk.

Recently, focus on the mechanisms of the retinal ganglion cell apoptosis and the role of excessive glutamate and nitric oxide found in glaucoma patients has broadened the focus of drug therapy research to include evaluation of agents that act as neuroprotectants.[12–15] Such agents may be particularly useful for patients with normal-pressure glaucoma, in whom pressure-independent factors may play a relatively larger role in disease progression. These agents would target risk factors and underlying pathophysiologic mechanisms of disease other than IOP.[11–16]

PATHOPHYSIOLOGY OF OPEN-ANGLE GLAUCOMA

❸ As stated previously, optic nerve damage in POAG can occur at a wide range of IOPs, and the rate of progression is highly variable. Patients may exhibit pressures in the 20 to 30 mm Hg (2.7 to 4.0 kPa) range for years before any disease progression is noticed in the optic disk or visual fields. That is why OAG is often referred to as the "sneak thief of sight."

EPIDEMIOLOGY OF OPEN-ANGLE GLAUCOMA

❶ Open-angle glaucoma (OAG) is the second leading cause of blindness, affecting up to 3 million individuals in the United States and up to 60.5 million individuals worldwide by 2010. It is estimated that by 2010, 135,000 persons in the United States and about 4.5 million in the world will have bilateral blindness. The prevalence rate varies with age, race, diagnostic criteria, and other factors. In the United States, OAG occurs in 1.5% of the population older than 30 years of age, 1.3% of whites and 3.5% of blacks. Recent study data have also suggested that the prevalence of OAG and ocular hypertension is also high among Latinos of Mexican ancestry, with

CLINICAL PRESENTATION OF GLAUCOMA

General

- Glaucoma can be detected in otherwise asymptomatic patients, or patients can present with characteristic symptoms, especially vision loss. POAG is a chronic, slowly progressive disease found primarily in patients older than 50 years of age, whereas CAG is more typically associated with symptomatic acute episodes.

Symptoms

- POAG: None until substantial visual field loss occurs.
- CAG: Nonsymptomatic or prodromal symptoms (blurred or hazy vision with halos around lights that is caused by a hazy, edematous cornea, and occasionally headache) may be present. Acute episodes produce symptoms associated with a cloudy, edematous cornea, ocular pain, or discomfort, nausea, vomiting, abdominal pain, and diaphoresis.

Signs

- POAG: Disk changes and visual field loss (see Table 103–2); IOP can be normal or elevated (>21 mm Hg [>2.8 kPa]).
- CAG: Hyperemic conjunctiva, cloudy cornea, shallow anterior chamber, and occasionally an edematous and hyperemic optic disk; IOP is generally elevated markedly (40 to 90 mm Hg [5.3 to 12.0 kPa]) when symptoms are present.

Laboratory Tests

- None

Other Diagnostic Tests

- Emerging tests include OCT, retinal nerve fiber analyzers, and confocal scanning laser tomography of the optic nerve.

CLINICAL PRESENTATION OF OPEN-ANGLE GLAUCOMA

POAG is a bilateral, genetically determined disorder constituting 60% to 70% of all glaucomas and 90% to 95% of primary glaucomas (see Clinical Presentation of Glaucoma above). An increased IOP is not required for diagnosis of POAG. Symptoms do not present until substantial visual field constriction occurs. Central visual acuity typically is maintained, even in the late stages of the disease. Even though POAG is a bilateral disease, it may have greater progression and severity in one eye.

❹ Detection and diagnosis involve evaluation of the optic disk and retinal nerve fiber layer, assessment of the visual fields, and measurement of IOP. The presence of characteristic disk changes and visual field loss with or without increased IOP confirms the diagnosis of glaucoma. Typical disk changes and field loss occurring at an IOP of less than 21 mm Hg (2.8 kPa) account for 20% to 30% of patients and are referred to as *normal-tension glaucoma*. Elevated IOP (>21 mm Hg [>2.8 kPa]) without disk changes or visual field loss is observed in 5% to 7% of individuals (known as *glaucoma suspects*) and is referred to as *ocular hypertension*. New technologies such as OCT, retinal nerve fiber analyzers, or confocal scanning laser tomography of the optic nerve head may allow early identification of signs of glaucomatous retinal changes in ocular hypertensives, thus allowing for earlier initiation of therapy.[1–3,17]

Secondary OAG has many causes, including exfoliation syndrome, pigmentary glaucoma, systemic diseases, trauma, surgery, ocular inflammatory diseases, and medications. A system for classifying secondary glaucomas into pretrabecular, trabecular, and posttrabecular forms has been proposed. This classification allows drug therapy to be chosen on the basis of the pathogenic mechanism involved. In pretrabecular forms, a normal meshwork is covered and does not permit aqueous humor outflow. Trabecular forms of secondary glaucoma result from either an alteration of meshwork or an accumulation of material in the intertrabecular spaces. The posttrabecular forms result primarily from disorders causing increased episcleral venous blood pressure.[1,2,15–17]

PROGNOSIS OF OPEN ANGLE GLAUCOMA

❺ In most cases of POAG, the overall prognosis is excellent when it is discovered early and treated adequately. Even patients with advanced visual field loss can have continued visual field loss reduced if the IOP is maintained at low enough pressures (often <10 to 12 mm Hg [<1.3 to 1.6 kPa]). Progression of visual field loss still occurs in 8% to 20% of patients despite reaching standard therapy IOP goals. However, for untreated patients and for those who fail to achieve target IOP reduction, up to 80% have continued visual field loss. Estimates of progression to bilateral blindness in treated patients range from 4% to 22%. Thus, the keys to medical treatment of POAG are an effective, well-tolerated drug regimen, close monitoring of therapy, and adherence. Medications will control IOP successfully in 60% to 80% of patients over a 5-year period. Availability of newer, highly effective, well-tolerated agents may improve the prognosis further.[1,2,5,17–19,23–28]

EPIDEMIOLOGY OF CLOSED-ANGLE GLAUCOMA

The incidence of CAG varies by ethnic group, with a higher incidence in individuals of Inuit, Chinese, and Asian-Indian descent. Incidence rates of 1% to 4% have been reported in these populations.[1,2]

ETIOLOGY OF CLOSED-ANGLE GLAUCOMA (ANGLE-CLOSURE GLAUCOMA)

Primary CAG accounts for 5% or less of primary glaucomas; however, when CAG occurs, it may need to be treated as an emergency to avoid visual loss. CAG results from mechanical blockage of the (usually normal) trabecular meshwork by the peripheral iris. Partial or complete blockage of the meshwork occurs intermittently, resulting in extreme fluctuations between normal IOP with no symptoms and very high IOP with symptoms of acute CAG. Between attacks of CAG, the IOP is usually normal unless the patient has concomitant OAG or nonreversible blockage of the meshwork with synechiae ("creeping" angle closure) that develops over time in the narrow-angle eye. Primary CAG occurs for patients with inherited shallow anterior chambers, which produce a narrow angle between the cornea and iris or tight contact between the iris and lens (pupillary block). The presence of a narrow angle is determined mainly by visualization of the angle by gonioscopy. Other tests for CAG involve provocation of an angle-closure–induced IOP increase. These tests, which attempt to produce angle closure through mydriasis (darkroom test or mydriasis test) or gravity (prone test), are rarely performed in the clinical setting.

Two major types of classic, reversible primary CAG have been described: CAG with pupillary block and CAG without pupillary block. CAG with pupillary block results when the iris is in firm contact with the lens. This produces a relative block of aqueous flow through the pupil to the anterior chamber (pupillary block), resulting in a bowing forward of the iris, which blocks the trabecular meshwork. CAG with pupillary block occurs most commonly when the pupil is in middilation. In this position, the combination of pupillary block and relaxed iris allows the greatest bowing of the iris; however, angle closure may occur during miosis or mydriasis.

CAG can occur without significant pupillary block for patients with an abnormality called a *plateau iris*. The ciliary processes in these cases are situated anteriorly, which indent the iris forward and cause closure of the trabecular meshwork, especially during mydriasis. The mydriasis produced by anticholinergic drugs or any other drug results in precipitation of both types of CAG glaucoma, whereas drug-induced miosis may produce pupillary block.

PATHOPHYSIOLOGY OF CLOSED-ANGLE GLAUCOMA

The mechanism of IOP elevation in CAG is clearer than that of POAG. In CAG, a physical blockage of trabecular meshwork is present. In many cases, single or multiple episodes of excessively high IOP (>40 mm Hg [>5.3 kPa]) result in optic nerve damage. Very high IOP (>60 mm Hg [>8.0 kPa]) may result in permanent loss of visual field within a matter of hours to days.

One type of CAG, known as "creeping" angle closure, occurs in patients with narrow angles in which the iris adheres to the trabecular meshwork and may result in continuously increased IOP in ranges more similar to those of POAG, and the clinical behavior is similar to POAG, with individuals differing in the degree and rapidity of visual loss from any given elevated IOP.[1]

CLINICAL PRESENTATION OF CLOSED-ANGLE GLAUCOMA

Patients with untreated CAG typically experience intermittent nonsymptomatic or prodromal symptoms brought on by precipitating events (see Clinical Presentation of Glaucoma above). Increased IOP during such prodromal episodes is not great enough or long enough to produce the other symptoms of a full-blown attack. Such prodromal attacks last 1 to 2 hours, at which time pupillary block is broken by further mydriasis or miosis, or when miosis or mydriasis occurs in patients with plateau iris. The rate at which IOP increases may be a determinant of when full-blown symptoms occur. Visual fields demonstrate generalized constriction or typical glaucomatous defects. In prolonged attacks, total loss of vision may occur if the IOP is high enough. Tonometry reveals IOPs as high as 40 to 90 mm Hg (5.3 to 12.0 kPa). Patients who have developed adhesions between the iris and meshwork (anterior synechiae) may have chronic IOP elevation with intermittent spikes of high IOP when angle closure occurs.

DRUG-INDUCED GLAUCOMA

A number of medications are associated with increased IOP or carry labeling that cautions against use of the medication in glaucoma patients. The potential for a medication to produce or worsen glaucoma depends on the type of glaucoma and whether the patient is treated adequately.[25]

Patients with treated, controlled POAG are at minimal risk of induction of an increase in IOP by systemic medications with anticholinergic properties or vasodilators; however, for patients with untreated glaucoma or uncontrolled POAG, the potential of these medications to increase IOP should be considered. Topical anticholinergic agents used to produce mydriasis may result in an increase in IOP. Potent anticholinergic agents such as atropine or homatropine are most likely to increase IOP. Weaker anticholinergics, such as tropicamide, that produce less cycloplegia are less likely to increase IOP and are favored, along with phenylephrine, when mydriasis is desired for POAG patients. Inhaled, nasal, topical, or systemic glucocorticoids may increase IOP for both normal individuals and patients with POAG.

Patients with POAG appear to be particularly susceptible to glucocorticoid-induced increases in IOP. Glucocorticoids reduce

TABLE 103-3	Drugs that may Induce or Potentiate Increased Intraocular Pressure

Open-angle glaucoma
Ophthalmic corticosteroids (high risk)
Systemic corticosteroids
Nasal/inhaled corticosteroids
Fenoldopam
Ophthalmic anticholinergics
Succinylcholine
Vasodilators (low risk)
Cimetidine (low risk)

Closed-angle glaucoma
Topical anticholinergics
Topical sympathomimetics
Systemic anticholinergics
Heterocyclic antidepressants
Low-potency phenothiazines
Antihistamines
Ipratropium
Benzodiazepines (low risk)
Theophylline (low risk)
Vasodilators (low risk)
Systemic sympathomimetics (low risk)
Central nervous system stimulants (low risk)
Serotonin selective reuptake inhibitors
Imipramine
Venlafaxine
Topiramate
Tetracyclines (low risk)
Carbonic anhydrase inhibitors (low risk)
Monoamine oxidase inhibitors (low risk)
Topical cholinergics (low risk)

the facility of aqueous humor outflow through the trabecular meshwork. The decreased facility of outflow appears to result from the accumulation of extracellular material blocking the trabecular channels. The potential of a glucocorticoid to increase IOP is related to its antiinflammatory potency and intraocular penetration. Thus, patients should be treated with the lowest potency and dose and for the shortest time possible when steroids are indicated.

For patients predisposed to CAG (i.e., narrow anterior chambers), angle closure may be produced by any drug that causes mydriasis (e.g., anticholinergics). A wide range of sulfa compounds causes idiosyncratic reactions that result in anterior choroidal effusions with anterior movement of the iris and lens, resulting in angle closure. The topical use of anticholinergics or sympathomimetic agents most likely will result in angle closure. Systemic and inhaled anticholinergic and sympathomimetic agents also must be used with caution in such patients. As discussed previously, potent miotic agents such as echothiophate may produce angle closure by increasing pupillary block. Table 103–3 lists the drugs associated with potentiation of glaucoma.

TREATMENT

Ocular Hypertension

Treatment of the patient with possible glaucoma (ocular hypertension; i.e., patients with IOP >22 mm Hg [>2.9 kPa]) is less controversial with the recent results of the Ocular Hypertensive Treatment Study (OHTS) than it was in the past,.[3] The OHTS helped to identify risk factors for treatment. Patients with IOPs higher than 25 mm Hg (3.3 kPa), vertical cup-to-disk ratio of more than 0.5, and central corneal thickness of less than 555 μm are at greater risk for developing glaucoma. Risk factors such as family history of glaucoma, black ethnicity, severe myopia, and patients with only one eye must also be taken into consideration when deciding which individuals need treatment.

Patients without risk factors typically are not treated and are monitored for the development of glaucomatous changes. Patients with significant risk factors usually are treated with a well-tolerated topical agent such as a β-blocking agent, an α_2-agonist (brimonidine), a topical carbonic anhydrase inhibitor (CAI), or a prostaglandin analog, depending on individual patient characteristics. Optimally, therapy is initiated in one eye to assess efficacy and tolerance. Use of second- or third-line agents (e.g., pilocarpine or dipivefrin) when first-line agents fail to reduce IOP depends on the risk-to-benefit assessment of each patient. The cost, inconvenience, and frequent adverse effects of combination therapies, anticholinesterase inhibitors, and oral CAIs result in an unfavorable risk-to-benefit ratio for patients with possible glaucoma.[29]

The goal of therapy is to lower the IOP to a level associated with a decreased risk of optic nerve damage, usually at least a 20%, if not a 25% to 30% decrease from the baseline IOP. Greater decreases may be required in high-risk patients or those with higher initial IOPs. Drug therapy should be monitored by measurement of IOP, examination of the optic disk, assessment of the visual fields, and evaluation of the patient for drug adverse effects and compliance with therapy. Patients who are unresponsive to or intolerant of a drug should be switched to an alternative agent rather than given an additional drug. Many clinicians prefer to discontinue all medications for patients who fail to respond adequately to simple topical therapy, closely monitor for development of disk changes or visual field loss, and treat again when such changes occur.[1,2,17–19,29]

More recently, risk calculators have been suggested as a means of determining who are at greatest risk in developing glaucoma. It is hoped that with future improvement in such calculators, one would be able to tailor treatment to those at greatest risk for developing glaucoma.

TREATMENT

Open-Angle Glaucoma

All patients with elevated IOP and characteristic optic disk changes and/or visual field defects not caused by other factors (i.e., glaucoma by definition) should be treated. Recent findings that 1 in 5 patients with "normal" IOP and glaucomatous retinal nerve findings (i.e., normal-tension glaucoma) do not have progression of visual field loss if left untreated have prompted recommendations to monitor normal-tension glaucoma patients without immediate threat of loss of central vision and to treat only when progression is documented. Some controversy exists as to whether the initial therapy of glaucoma should be surgical trabeculectomy (filtering procedure), argon or selective laser trabeculectomy, or medical therapy.[1,2,17,18] Presently, drug therapy remains the most common initial treatment modality. Drug therapy of patients with documented glaucomatous change with either elevated or normal IOP is initiated in a stepwise manner (Fig. 103–5), starting with lower concentrations of a single, well-tolerated topical agent. The goal of therapy is to prevent further visual loss. A "target" IOP is chosen based on a patient baseline IOP and the amount of existing visual field loss. Typically, an initial target IOP reduction of 30% is desired. Greater reductions may be desired for patients with very high baseline IOPs or advanced visual field loss. Patients with normal baseline IOPs (normal-tension glaucoma) may have target IOPs of less than 10 to 12 mm Hg (1.3 to 1.6 kPa).

■ PHARMACOTHERAPEUTIC APPROACH

❻ Medications most commonly used to treat glaucoma are the nonselective β-blockers, the prostaglandin analogs (latanoprost, travoprost, and bimatoprost), brimonidine (an α_2-agonist), and the fixed combination products of timolol/dorzolamide or timolol/brimonidine.[21–22]

Before 1996, a β-blocker was used provided no contraindications existed, because this class of drugs has a long history of successful use, providing a combination of clinical efficacy and tolerability. The newer agents, in particular the prostaglandin analogs, brimonidine, and topical CAIs, are also considered suitable first-line therapy or alternative initial therapy for patients with contraindications to or other concerns with β-blockers (see Fig. 103–5). Pilocarpine and dipivefrin are used as third-line therapies because of their increased frequency of adverse effects or reduced efficacy.

Therapy optimally is started as a single agent in one eye (except for patients with very high IOP or advanced visual field loss) to evaluate drug efficacy and tolerance. Monitoring of therapy should be individualized: Initial response to therapy is typically done 4 to 6 weeks after the medication is started. A monocular trial of medication is recommended when possible. Once IOPs reach acceptable levels, the IOP is monitored every 3 to 4 months (more frequently after any change in drug therapy).

Visual fields and disk changes are typically monitored annually or earlier if the glaucoma is unstable or there is suspicion of disease worsening. Patients should always be questioned regarding adherence to and tolerance of prescribed therapy. Initial IOP response does not predict long-term IOP control. Using more than one drop per dose does not improve response, but increases the likelihood of adverse effects and the cost of therapy. When using more than one medication, separation of drop instillation of each agent by at least 5 to 10 minutes is suggested to provide optimal ocular contact for each agent.

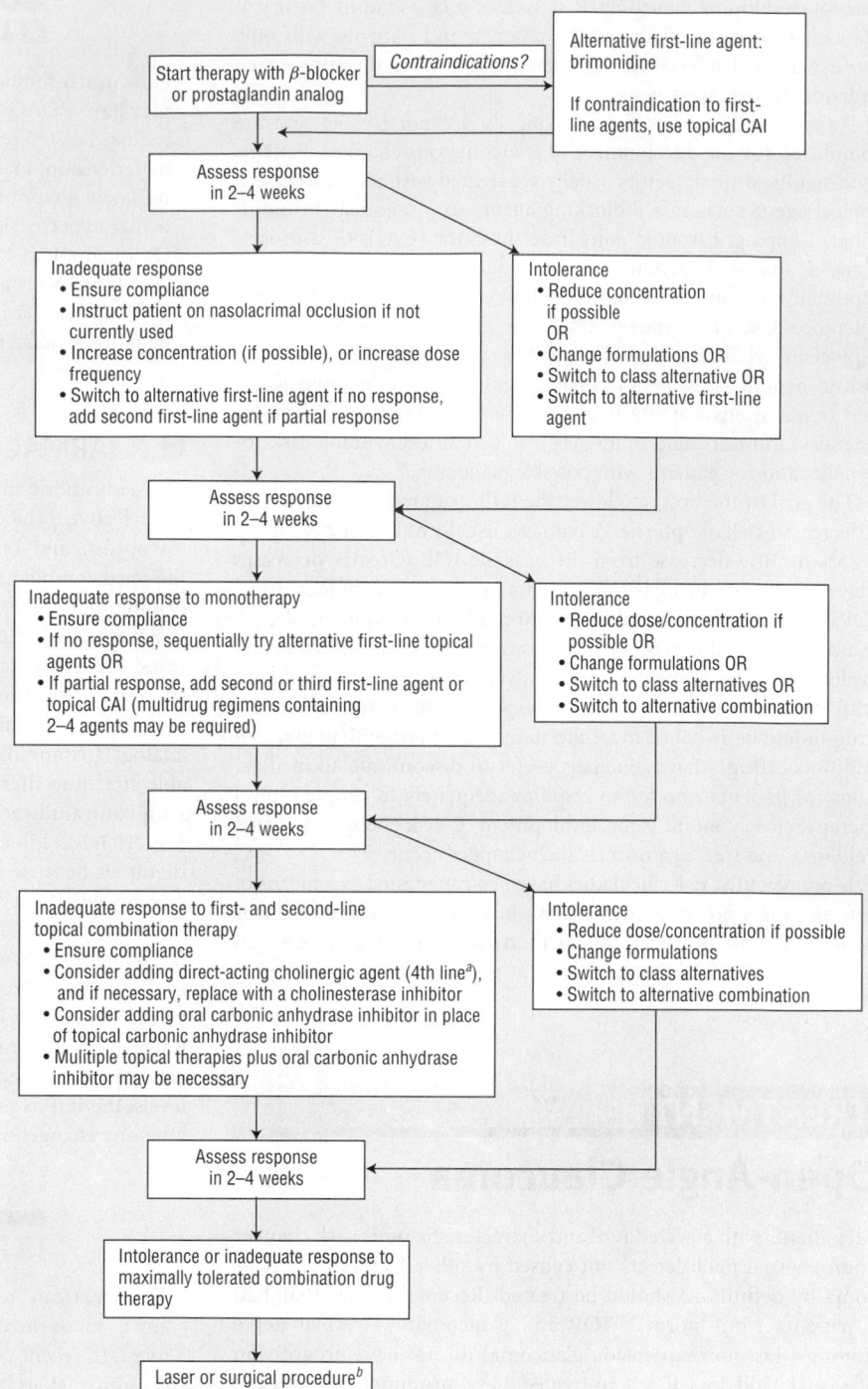

FIGURE 103-5. Algorithm for the pharmacotherapy of open-angle glaucoma. [a]Fourth-line agents not commonly used any longer. [b]Most clinicians believe laser procedure should be performed earlier (e.g., after three-drug maximum, poorly adherent patient). (CAI, carbonic anhydrase inhibitor.)

The value of an agent with which the patient has shown a drop in IOP following an initial response can be measured by discontinuing the medication completely and determining if an increase in IOP occurs. Patients responding to but intolerant of initial therapy may be switched to another drug or to an alternative dosage form of the same medication. For patients failing to respond to the highest tolerated concentrations of an initial drug, a switch to an alternative agent after 1 day of concurrent therapy should be considered. Alternatively, if only a partial response occurs, addition of another topical drug to be used in combination is a possibility. A number of drugs or drug combinations may need to be tried before an effective and well-tolerated regimen is identified. Because of the frequency of adverse effects, carbachol, topical cholinesterase inhibitors, and oral CAIs are considered last-line agents to be used for patients who fail less-toxic combination topical therapy.

■ NONPHARMACOLOGIC THERAPY: LASER AND SURGICAL PROCEDURES

When drug therapy fails, is not tolerated, or is excessively complicated, surgical procedures such as laser trabeculoplasty (argon or selective) or a surgical trabeculectomy (filtering procedure) may be performed to improve outflow. Laser trabeculoplasty is usually an intermediate step between drug therapy and trabeculectomy. Procedures with higher complication rates, such as those involving placement of draining tubes or destruction of the ciliary body (cyclodestruction), may be required when other methods fail (see Fig. 103–2).[1,2,25]

Surgical methods for reduction of IOP involve the creation of a channel through which aqueous humor can flow from the anterior chamber to the subconjunctival space (filtering bleb), where it is reabsorbed by the vasculature. A major reason for failure of the procedure is healing and scarring of the site.

Modification of the healing process to maintain patency is possible with the use of antiproliferative agents. The antiproliferative agents 5-fluorouracil and mitomycin C are used for patients undergoing glaucoma-filtering surgery to improve success rates by reducing fibroblast proliferation and consequent scarring. Although used most commonly for patients with increased risk for suboptimal surgical outcome (after cataract surgery and a previous failed filtering procedure), use of these agents also improves success in low-risk patients.[30-33]

TREATMENT

Closed-Angle Glaucoma

The goal of initial therapy for acute CAG with high IOP is rapid reduction of the IOP to preserve vision and to avoid surgical or laser iridectomy on a hypertensive, congested eye. Iridectomy (laser or surgical) is the definitive treatment of CAG; it produces a hole in the iris that permits aqueous humor flow to move directly from the posterior chamber to the anterior chamber, opening up the block at the trabecular meshwork. Drug therapy of an acute attack typically involves administration of pilocarpine, hyperosmotic agents, and a secretory inhibitor (a β-blocker, α_2-agonist, prostaglandin $F_2\alpha$ analog, or a topical or systemic CAI). With miosis produced by pilocarpine, the peripheral iris is pulled away from the meshwork. Although traditionally the drug of choice, pilocarpine used as initial therapy is controversial. Miotics may worsen angle closure by increasing pupillary block and producing anterior movement of the lens because of drug-induced accommodation.

At IOPs greater than 60 mm Hg (8.0 kPa), the iris may be ischemic and unresponsive to miotics; as the pressure drops and the iris responds, miosis occurs. During this time, the urge to use excessive amounts of pilocarpine must be resisted. The dose of pilocarpine commonly used is a 1% or 2% solution instilled every 5 minutes for two or three doses and then every 4 to 6 hours. However, many practitioners withhold application of pilocarpine until the IOP has been reduced by other agents, and then apply a single drop of 1% to 2% pilocarpine to produce miosis. In either case, the unaffected contralateral eye should be treated with the miotic every 6 hours to prevent development of angle closure. An osmotic agent also is commonly administered because these drugs produce the most rapid decrease in IOP. Oral glycerin 1 to 2 g/kg can be used if an oral agent is tolerated; if not, intravenous mannitol 1 to 2 g/kg should be used. Osmotic agents reduce IOP by withdrawing water from the eye secondary to the osmotic gradient between the blood and the eyes. These drugs are among the first-line agents in the short-term treatment of CAG or other forms of acute very high IOP elevations. Topical corticosteroids often are used to reduce the ocular inflammation and reduce the development of synechiae in CAG eyes. In classic CAG, once the IOP is controlled, pilocarpine may be given every 6 hours until iridectomy is performed. Patients failing therapy altogether will require an emergency iridectomy.

Peripheral iridectomy essentially "cures" primary CAG without significant synechiae. Long-term drug therapy is not used unless IOP remains high because of the presence of synechiae blocking the trabecular meshwork or concurrent POAG. In such cases, the pharmacotherapeutic approach is essentially identical to that for the POAG patient, or laser or surgical procedures are performed.[1,2]

PHARMACOLOGIC AGENTS USED IN GLAUCOMA

β-BLOCKING DRUGS

The topical β-blocking agents are one of the most commonly used antiglaucoma medications (Table 103–4). β-Blockers lower IOP by 20% to 30% with a minimum of local ocular adverse effects. These are commonly one of the agents of first choice in treating POAG if no contraindications exist.[1,2,17–19,34–36]

The β-blocking agents produce ocular hypotensive effects by decreasing the production of aqueous humor by the ciliary body without producing substantial effects on aqueous humor outflow facility. The mechanism by which β-blockers decrease aqueous humor inflow remains controversial, but it is most frequently attributed to β_2-adrenergic receptor blockade in the ciliary body.

Five ophthalmic β-blockers are presently available: timolol, levobunolol, metipranolol, carteolol, and betaxolol. Timolol, levobunolol, and metipranolol are nonspecific β-blocking agents, whereas betaxolol is a relatively β_1-selective agent. Carteolol is a nonspecific blocker with intrinsic sympathomimetic activity. Despite differences in potency, selectivity, lipophilicity, and intrinsic sympathomimetic activity, the five agents reduce IOP to a similar degree, although betaxolol has been reported to produce somewhat less lowering of IOP than timolol and levobunolol. Levobunolol may be more effective than timolol and betaxolol in reducing postcataract surgery IOP increases. Levobunolol solution is more effective in controlling IOP than other agents when given as aqueous solutions on a once-daily schedule (up to 70% of patients). Timolol in the form of a gel-forming solution (Timoptic-XE) provides equivalent IOP control with once-daily administration when compared with the same concentration of the aqueous solution administered twice daily. The choice of a specific β-blocking agent generally is based on differences in adverse effect potential, individual patient response, and cost. Long-term treatment with topical β-blockers results in tachyphylaxis in 20% to 25% of patients. The mean IOP reduction from baseline may be smaller for patients receiving topical β-blockers with concurrent systemic β-blockers.[29]

Local adverse effects with β-blockers usually are tolerable, although stinging on application occurs commonly, particularly with betaxolol solution (less with betaxolol suspension) and metipranolol. Other local effects include dry eyes, corneal anesthesia, blepharitis, blurred vision, and, rarely, conjunctivitis, uveitis, and keratitis. Some local reactions may be a result of preservatives used in the commercially available products. Switching from one agent to another or switching the type of formulation may improve tolerance in patients experiencing local adverse effects.

Systemic effects are the most important adverse effects of β-blockers. Drug absorbed systematically may produce decreased heart rate, reduced blood pressure, negative inotropic effects, conduction defects, bronchospasm, central nervous system effects, and alteration of serum lipids and may block the symptoms of hypoglycemia. The β_1-specific agents betaxolol and possibly carteolol (as a consequence of intrinsic sympathomimetic activity) are less likely to produce the systemic adverse effects caused by β-adrenergic blockade, such as the cardiac effects and bronchospasm, but a real risk still exists. The use of timolol as a gel-forming liquid or betaxolol as a suspension allows for administration of less drug per day and, therefore, reduces the chance for systemic adverse effects compared with the aqueous solutions.

TABLE 103-4 Topical Drugs Used in the Treatment of Open-Angle Glaucoma

Drug	Pharmacologic Properties	Common Brand Names	Dose Form	Strength (%)	Usual Dose[a]	Mechanism of Action
β-Adrenergic blocking agents						
Betaxolol	Relative β_1-selective	Generic	Solution	0.5	1 drop twice a day	All reduce aqueous production of ciliary body
		Betoptic-S	Suspension	0.25	1 drop twice a day	
Carteolol	Nonselective, intrinsic sympathomimetic activity	Generic	Solution	1	1 drop twice a day	
Levobunolol	Nonselective	Betagan	Solution	0.25, 0.5	1 drop twice a day	
Metipranolol	Nonselective	OptiPranolol	Solution	0.3	1 drop twice a day	
Timolol	Nonselective	Timoptic, Betimol, Istalol	Solution	0.25, 0.5	1 drop every day–one to two times a day	
		Timoptic-XE	Gelling solution	0.25, 0.5	1 drop every day[a]	
Nonspecific adrenergic agonists						
Dipivefrin	Prodrug	Propine	Solution	0.1	1 drop twice a day	Increased aqueous humor outflow
α_2-Adrenergic agonists						
Apraclonidine	Specific α_2-agonists	Iopidine	Solution	0.5, 1	1 drop two to three times a day	Both reduce aqueous humor production; brimonidine known to also increase uveoscleral outflow; only brimonidine has primary indication
Brimonidine		Alphagan P	Solution	0.15, 0.1	1 drop two to three times a day	
Cholinergic agonists direct acting						
Carbachol	Irreversible	Carboptic, Isopto Carbachol	Solution	1.5, 3	1 drop two to three times a day	All increase aqueous humor outflow through trabecular meshwork
Pilocarpine	Irreversible	Isopto Carpine, Pilocar	Solution	0.25, 0.5, 1, 2, 4, 6, 8, 10	1 drop two to three times a day 1 drop four times a day	
		Pilopine HS	Gel	4	Every 24 h at bedtime	
Cholinesterase inhibitors						
Echothiophate		Phospholine Iodide	Solution	0.125	Once or twice a day	
Carbonic anhydrase inhibitors						
Topical						
Brinzolamide	Carbonic anhydrase type II inhibition	Azopt	Suspension	1	Two to three times a day	All reduce aqueous humor production of ciliary body
Dorzolamide		Trusopt	Solution	2	Two to three times a day	
Systemic						
Acetazolamide		Generic	Tablet	125 mg, 250 mg	125–250 mg two to four times a day	
		Injection	500 mg/vial	250–500 mg		
		Diamox Sequels	Capsule	500 mg	500 mg twice a day	
Methazolamide		Generic	Tablet	25 mg, 50 mg	25–50 mg two to three times a day	
Prostaglandin analogs						
Latanoprost	Prostaglandin $F_{2\alpha}$ analog	Xalatan	Solution	0.005	1 drop every night	Increases aqueous uveoscleral outflow and to a lesser extent trabecular outflow
Bimatoprost	Prostamide analog	Lumigan	Solution	0.03	1 drop every night	
Travoprost		Travatan Z	Solution	0.004	1 drop every night	
Combinations						
Timolol-dorzolamide		Cosopt	Solution	Timolol 0.5% dorzolamide 2%	1 drop twice daily	
Timolol-brimonidine		Combigan	Solution	Timolol 0.5% brimonide 0.2%	1 drop twice daily	

[a]Use of nasolacrimal occlusion will increase the number of patients successfully treated with longer dosage intervals.

Because of their systemic adverse effects, all ophthalmic β-blockers should be used with caution for patients with pulmonary diseases, sinus bradycardia, second- or third-degree heart block, congestive heart failure, atherosclerosis, diabetes, and myasthenia gravis, as well as for patients receiving oral β-blocker therapy. Use of nasolacrimal occlusion (NLO; see Patient Education below for description) technique during administration reduces the risk or severity of systemic adverse effects, as well as optimizes response. Overall, β-adrenergic blocking agents are well tolerated by most patients, and most potential problems can be avoided by appropriate patient evaluation, drug choice, and monitoring of drug therapy. For patients failing or having an inadequate response to single-drug therapy with a β-blocking agent, the addition of a CAI, parasympathomimetic agent, prostaglandin analog, or an α_2-adrenergic receptor agonist usually will result in additional IOP reduction. Dipivefrin added to a β-blocking agent (particularly nonspecific β-blockers) usually results in only minimal additional IOP reduction.[1–3,17–19,29]

α_2-ADRENERGIC AGONISTS

Brimonidine and the less lipid-soluble and less receptor-selective apraclonidine are α_2-adrenergic agonists structurally similar to clonidine. Apraclonidine is indicated and brimonidine is effective for prevention or control of postoperative or postlaser treatment increases in IOP. Brimonidine is considered a first-line or adjunctive agent in the therapy of POAG, and apraclonidine is seen as a second-line or adjunctive therapy. Use of apraclonidine has fallen dramatically because of a high incidence of loss of control of IOP (tachyphylaxis) and a more severe and prevalent ocular allergy rate.

α_2-Agonists reduce IOP by decreasing the rate of aqueous humor production (some increase in uveoscleral outflow also occurs with brimonidine). The drugs reduce IOP by 18% to 27% at peak (2 to 5 hours) and by 10% at 8 to 12 hours. Comparative trials demonstrate a reduction in IOP similar to that obtained with 0.5% timolol. Use of brimonidine 0.2% every 8 to 12 hours appears to provide maximum IOP-lowering effects in long-term use. Use of NLO (see Patient Education below) may improve response and allow the longer dosing frequency (i.e., every 12 hours). Combinations of α_2-agonists with β-blockers, prostaglandin analogs, or CAIs produce additional IOP reduction.

An allergic-type reaction characterized by lid edema, eye discomfort, foreign-object sensation, itching, and hyperemia occurs in approximately 30% of patients with apraclonidine. Brimonidine produces this adverse effect in up to 8% of patients. This reaction commonly necessitates drug discontinuation. Systemic adverse effects with brimonidine include dizziness, fatigue, somnolence, dry mouth, and possibly a slight reduction in blood pressure and pulse. α_2-Agonists should be used with caution for patients with cardiovascular diseases, renal compromise, cerebrovascular disease, and diabetes, as well as in those taking antihypertensives and other cardiovascular drugs, monoamine oxidase inhibitors, and tricyclic antidepressants.

Brimonidine is also contraindicated in infants because of apneic spells and hypotensive reactions. In terms of overall efficacy and tolerability, brimonidine approximates that achieved with β-blockers.[1,2,17–19,29]

Brimonidine purite 0.15% or 0.1% is a formulation of brimonidine in a lower concentration than the original product that contains a less-toxic preservative than the most commonly employed benzalkonium chloride. The newer formulations are as effective as the original because the more neutral pH of brimonidine purite (0.15% pH 7.2; 0.1% pH 7.7) allows for higher concentrations of brimonidine in the aqueous humor with a similar reduction in IOP and a reduced incidence of ocular allergy.[29]

The combination product timolol 0.5% and brimonidine 0.2% (Combigan) may provide additional IOP lowering than either agent alone. A new treatment option, this product is marketed in solution that is dosed twice daily.

CLINICAL CONTROVERSY

Many animal trials demonstrate that brimonidine has excellent neuroprotective properties.[12–15] Some clinicians believe that one of the major advantages of using brimonidine lies in its potential neuroprotective properties. However, neuroprotection has not been demonstrated in human trials.

PROSTAGLANDIN ANALOGS

The prostaglandin analogs, including latanoprost, travoprost, and bimatoprost, reduce IOP by increasing the uveoscleral and, to a lesser extent, trabecular outflow of aqueous humor. Some differences in receptor sites and mechanisms of action may exist between the two prostaglandins (latanoprost and travoprost), the prostamide (bimatoprost). Bimatoprost may be slightly more effective in lowering IOP, getting a larger percentage of patients to lower IOPs, and for patients unresponsive to latanoprost.[29,37–39] If the patient does not respond to trovaprost or latanoprost, a switch to bimatoprost may be beneficial.[39]

Reduction in IOP with once-daily doses of prostaglandin $F_2\alpha$ analogs (a 25% to 35% reduction) is often greater than that seen with timolol 0.5% twice daily. In addition, nocturnal control of IOP is improved compared with timolol. Interestingly, administration of prostaglandin $F_2\alpha$ analogs twice daily may reduce the IOP similarly to once-daily dosing. The drugs are administered at nighttime, although they are probably as effective if given in the morning.

Prostaglandin analogs are well tolerated and produce fewer systemic adverse effects than timolol. Local ocular tolerance generally is good, but ocular reactions such as punctate corneal erosions and conjunctival hyperemia do occur. Local intolerance occurs in 10% to 25% of patients with these agents.

With prostaglandin analogs, altered iris pigmentation occurs in 15% to 30% of patients, particularly those with mixed-color irises (blue-brown, green-brown, blue-gray-brown, or yellow-brown eyes), which become browner in color over 3 to 12 months. The change in iris pigmentation will often appear within 2 years, and long-term consequences of this pigment change appear to be mostly cosmetic but irreversible upon discontinuation. Hypertrichosis is common and reverses upon discontinuation of the drug. Hyperpigmentation around the lids and lashes has also been reported and appears to reverse upon discontinuation.

These agents are associated with uveitis, and caution is recommended for patients with ocular inflammatory conditions. Cystoid macular edema also has been reported. Cases of worsening of herpetic keratitis have been reported.

Prostaglandin analogs can be used in combination with other antiglaucoma agents for additional IOP control because of their unique mechanism of action. Given their excellent efficacy and side-effect profile, prostaglandin analogs provide effective monotherapy or adjunctive therapy for patients who are not responding to or tolerating other agents. The use of prostaglandin analogs as first-line therapy in POAG is approved for latanoprost and bimatoprost. Long-term studies demonstrate these agents are safe, efficacious, and well tolerated in glaucoma therapy.[17–19,29,37,38]

CARBONIC ANHYDRASE INHIBITORS

Topical Agents

CAIs reduce IOP by decreasing ciliary body aqueous humor secretion. CAIs appear to inhibit aqueous production by blocking active secretion of sodium and bicarbonate ions from the ciliary body to the aqueous humor.[1,2,29] Topical CAIs such as dorzolamide and brinzolamide are well tolerated and are indicated for monotherapy or adjunctive therapy of OAG and ocular hypertension. Relatively specific inhibitors of carbonic anhydrase enzyme II such as dorzolamide and brinzolamide reduce IOP by 15% to 26%.

Topical CAIs generally are well tolerated. Local adverse effects include transient burning and stinging, ocular discomfort and transient blurred vision, tearing, and, rarely, conjunctivitis, lid reactions, and photophobia. A superficial punctate keratitis occurs in 10% to 15% of patients. Brinzolamide produces more blurry vision but is less stinging than dorzolamide. Systemic adverse effects are unusual despite the accumulation of drug in red blood cells. Because of their favorable adverse-effect profile, topical CAIs provide a useful alternative agent for monotherapy or adjunctive therapy for patients with inadequate response to or who are unable to use other agents. The drugs may add additional IOP reduction for patients using other single or multiple topical agents. The usual dose of a topical CAI is 1 drop every 8 to 12 hours. Administration every 12 hours produces somewhat less IOP reduction than administration every 8 hours. Use of NLO should optimize response to CAI given at any interval.[1,2,17–19,29,34,36] The combination product timolol 0.5% and dorzolamide 2% (Cosopt) is dosed twice daily and produces equivalent IOP lowering to each product dosed separately.

Systemic Agents

Systemic CAIs are indicated for patients failing to respond to or tolerate maximum topical therapy. Systemic and topical CAIs should not be used in combination because no data exist concerning improved IOP reduction, and the risk for systemic adverse effects is increased. Oral CAIs reduce aqueous humor inflow by 40% to 60% and IOP by 25% to 40%. The available systemic CAIs (see Table 103–4) produce equivalent IOP reduction but differ for potency, adverse effects, dosage forms, and duration of action. Despite their excellent effects on elevated IOP of any etiology, the systemic CAIs frequently produce intolerable adverse effects. As a result, CAIs are considered third-line agents in the treatment of POAG and often used for short-term administration to lower IOP.

On average, only 30% to 60% of patients are able to tolerate oral CAI therapy for prolonged periods. Intolerance to CAI therapy results most commonly from a symptom complex attributable to systemic acidosis and including malaise, fatigue, anorexia, nausea, weight loss, altered taste, depression, and decreased libido. Other adverse effects include renal calculi, increased uric acid, blood dyscrasias, diuresis, and myopia. Elderly patients do not tolerate CAIs as well as younger patients. The available CAIs produce the same spectrum of adverse effects; however, the drugs differ in the frequency and severity of the adverse effects listed.

CAIs should be used with caution for patients with sulfa allergies (all CAIs, topical or systemic, contain sulfonamide moieties), sickle cell disease, respiratory acidosis, pulmonary disorders, renal calculi, electrolyte imbalance, hepatic disease, renal disease, diabetes mellitus, or Addison disease. Concurrent use of a CAI and a diuretic may rapidly produce hypokalemia. High-dose salicylate therapy may increase the acidosis produced by CAIs, whereas the acidosis produced by CAIs may increase the toxicity of salicylates.[1,2,17–19,21,29,34,35]

PARASYMPATHOMIMETIC AGENTS

The parasympathomimetic (cholinergic) agents reduce IOP by increasing aqueous humor trabecular outflow. The increase in outflow is a result of physically pulling open the trabecular meshwork secondary to ciliary muscle contraction, thereby reducing resistance to outflow. These agents may reduce uveoscleral outflow. Cholinergic agents work well to decrease IOP, but their use as primary or even adjunctive agents in the treatment of glaucoma has decreased significantly because of local ocular adverse effects and/or frequent dosing requirements.

Pilocarpine, the parasympathomimetic agent of choice in POAG, is available as an ophthalmic solution, an ocular insert, and a hydrophilic polymer gel (see Table 103–4). Pilocarpine produces similar (20% to 30%) reductions in IOP as those seen with β-blocking agents. Pilocarpine in POAG or "glaucoma suspects" is initiated as 0.5% or 1% solution, 1 drop three to four times daily. The use of NLO improves response and reduces the need for an every-6-hour

dosing frequency. The use of 1 drop of 2% pilocarpine every 6 to 12 hours and NLO provides optimal response in many patients. Both drug concentration and frequency may be increased if IOP reduction is inadequate. Patients with darkly pigmented eyes frequently require higher concentrations of pilocarpine than do patients with lightly pigmented eyes. Concentrations of pilocarpine above 4% rarely improve IOP control in patients, other than those patients with darkly pigmented eyes.

Pilocarpine 4% gel (Pilopine HS) once daily is equivalent to treatment with pilocarpine solution 4% four times daily or timolol 0.5% twice daily. When using every-24-hour dosing of pilocarpine gel, the adequacy of IOP control late in the dosing interval should be confirmed. Ocular adverse effects of pilocarpine include miosis, which decreases night vision and vision in patients with central cataracts. Visual field constriction may be seen secondary to miosis and should be considered when evaluating visual field changes in a glaucoma patient. Pilocarpine ciliary muscle contraction produces accommodative spasm, particularly in young patients still able to accommodate (prepresbyopic). Pilocarpine may also produce frontal headache, brow ache, periorbital pain, eyelid twitching, and conjunctival irritation or injection early in therapy, which tends to decrease in severity over 3 to 5 weeks of continued therapy.

Cholinergics produce a breakdown of the blood–aqueous humor barrier and may result in a worsening of an ocular inflammatory reaction or condition. Systemic cholinergic adverse effects of pilocarpine—such as diaphoresis, nausea, vomiting, diarrhea, cramping, urinary frequency, bronchospasm, and heart block—are rare but may be seen in patients who are using products with high pilocarpine concentrations (6% to 8%) or in those patients who are using such products overzealously in treatment of acute-angle closure. Other adverse effects associated with direct-acting miotics include retinal tears or detachment, allergic reaction, permanent miosis, cataracts, precipitation of CAG, and, rarely, miotic cysts of the pupillary margin.

Carbachol is a potent direct-acting miotic agent; its duration of action is longer than that of pilocarpine (8 to 10 hours) because of resistance to hydrolysis by cholinesterases. This drug also may act as a weak inhibitor of cholinesterase. Patients with an inadequate response to or intolerance of pilocarpine as a result of ocular irritation or allergy frequently do well on carbachol. The ocular and systemic adverse effects of carbachol are similar to but more frequent, constant, and severe than those of pilocarpine.[1,2,17–19,29,34,35] Clinical use of carbachol is limited and may not be commercially available in the near future.

The cholinesterase inhibitors used most commonly in the treatment of POAG are the long-acting, relatively irreversible agents demecarium and echothiophate (limited commercial availability; see Table 103–4). These agents are potent inhibitors of pseudocholinesterase, but they also inhibit true cholinesterase. Because of the serious ocular and systemic toxic effects of these agents, the cholinesterase inhibitors are reserved primarily for patients who are either not responding to or are intolerant of other therapy. Because of their cataractogenic properties, most ophthalmologists use these agents only for patients without lenses (aphakia) and for patients with artificial lenses (pseudophakia). The ocular and periocular parasympathomimetic adverse effects are more common and more severe than with pilocarpine or carbachol.

In addition to the parasympathomimetic effects, the cholinesterase inhibitors may produce severe fibrinous iritis (particularly with the irreversible inhibitors), synechiae, iris cysts, conjunctival thickening, occlusion of the nasolacrimal ducts, and cataracts. The inhibition of systemic pseudocholinesterase by these agents decreases the rate of succinylcholine hydrolysis, resulting in prolonged muscle paralysis. Cholinesterase inhibitors should be discontinued at least 2 weeks before procedures in which succinylcholine is used.

The role of cholinesterase inhibitors in glaucoma is limited by the frequency and potential toxicity of these agents. For phakic patients, cholinesterase inhibitors should be administered only if intolerance or failure results with other antiglaucoma medications. Cholinesterase inhibitors have been shown to provide additional IOP-lowering effects when used with β-blockers, CAIs, and sympathomimetic (adrenergic) agents. As with all agents for glaucoma, therapy should be initiated with lower concentrations of these agents. A once-daily administration frequency should be used for most patients unless very high IOP is present.

Use of NLO likely improves response, reduces systemic adverse effects, and should be performed by all patients administering cholinesterase inhibitors. These agents should be used with caution for patients with asthma, retinal detachments, narrow angles, bradycardia, hypotension, heart failure, Down syndrome, epilepsy, parkinsonism, peptic ulcer, and ocular inflammation, as well as in those receiving cholinesterase inhibitor therapy for myasthenia gravis or exposure to carbamate or organophosphate insecticides and pesticides.[1,2,17–19,29,34,35]

EPINEPHRINE AND DIPIVEFRIN

The mechanism of action by which epinephrine lowers IOP has not been fully elucidated; however, a β_2-receptor–mediated increase in outflow facility through the trabecular meshwork and the uveoscleral route appears to be the primary mechanism. Compared with β-blockers or miotics, epinephrine is less effective for reducing IOP. With the advent of the better-tolerated and more-efficacious agents to treat glaucoma, the clinical use of epinephrines has decreased dramatically.

Epinephrine is not commercially available in the United States anymore. Use of the prodrug of epinephrine, dipivefrin, allows use of lower concentrations secondary to improved intraocular absorption (10- to 15-fold higher). The 0.1% dipivefrin produces equivalent IOP reduction to 1% to 2% epinephrine. Consequently, dipivefrin may be tolerated by patients who are unable to tolerate epinephrine solutions.

A factor limiting the usefulness of dipivefrin is the high frequency of local ocular adverse effects. Tearing, burning, ocular discomfort, brow ache, conjunctival hyperemia, punctate keratopathy, allergic blepharoconjunctivitis, rare loss of eyelashes, stenosis of the nasolacrimal duct, and blurred vision may occur. Prolonged use (>1 year) may result in deposition of pigment (adrenochrome) in the conjunctiva and cornea. Pigment also may deposit in soft contact lenses, turning them black. These adverse effects occur less frequently with dipivefrin than with epinephrine. Dipivefrin may produce mydriasis (particularly when combined with a β-blocker) and may precipitate acute CAG in patients with narrow anterior chambers. A transient increase in IOP may occur with initial therapy, particularly for patients not using other antiglaucoma medications. A relative contraindication to the use of dipivefrin is aphakia (i.e., after cataract removal) or lens dislocation because of the development of swelling of the macular portion of the retina. The edema is dose dependent and disappears with drug discontinuation.

Systemic adverse effects of epinephrine and dipivefrin include headache, faintness, increased blood pressure, tachycardia, arrhythmias, tremor, pallor, anxiety, and increased perspiration. Epinephrine and dipivefrin should be used with caution for patients with cardiovascular diseases, cerebrovascular diseases, aphakia, CAG, hyperthyroidism, and diabetes mellitus, as well as for patients undergoing anesthesia with halogenated hydrocarbon anesthetics. Using NLO with epinephrine and dipivefrin will improve therapeutic response and reduce the risk of systemic adverse effects.[1,2,17–19,29,34,35]

FUTURE DRUG THERAPIES

It is hoped that new agents, improved formulations, and novel approaches to the reduction of IOP and other methods of prevention of glaucomatous visual field loss will provide more effective and better-tolerated therapies. Agents that are neuroprotective and act through mechanisms other than IOP reduction are likely to be part of glaucoma therapy in the future.[13–15,40]

EVALUATION OF THERAPEUTIC OUTCOMES

The ultimate goal of drug therapy for the patient with glaucoma is to preserve visual function through reduction of IOP to a level at which no further optic nerve damage occurs. Because of the poor relationship between IOP and optic nerve damage, no specific target IOP exists. Indeed, drugs used to treat glaucoma may act in part to halt visual field loss through mechanisms separate from or in addition to IOP reduction, such as improvements in retinal or choroidal blood flow. Often a 25% to 30% reduction is desired, but greater reductions (40% to 50%) may be desired for patients with initially high IOPs. For patients with glaucoma, an IOP of less than 21 mm Hg (2.8 kPa) generally is desired, with progressively lower target pressures needed for greater levels of glaucomatous damage. Even lower IOPs (possibly even below 10 mm Hg [1.3 kPa]) are required for patients with very advanced disease, those showing continued damage at higher IOPs, and those with normal-tension glaucoma and pretreatment pressures in the low to middle teens. The IOP considered acceptable for a patient is often a balance of desired IOP and acceptable treatment-related toxicity and of patient quality of life.

PATIENT EDUCATION

❼ An important consideration for patients failing to respond to drug therapy is adherence. Poor adherence or nonadherence occurs in 25% to 60% of glaucoma patients.

A large percentage of patients also fail to use topical ophthalmic drugs correctly. Patients should be taught the following procedure:

1. Wash and dry the hands; shake the bottle if it contains a suspension.

2. With a forefinger, pull down the outer portion of the lower eyelid to form a "pocket" to receive the drop.

3. Grasp the dropper bottle between the thumb and fingers with the hand braced against the cheek or nose and the head held upward.

4. Place the dropper over the eye while looking at the tip of the bottle; then look up and place a single drop in the eye.

5. The lids should be closed (but not squeezed or rubbed) for 1 to 3 minutes after instillation. This increases the ocular availability of the drug.

6. Recap bottle and store as instructed.

Note that many patients are physically unable to administer their own eyedrops without assistance. NLO also should be used to improve ocular bioavailability and reduce systemic absorption.[1,2,17–19,29,34,35] The patient induces NLO for 1 to 3 minutes by closing the eyes and placing the index finger over the nasolacrimal drainage system in the inner corner of the eye. This maneuver, as well as eyelid closure itself, decreases nasolacrimal drainage of drug, thereby decreasing the amount of drug available for systemic absorption by the nasopharyngeal mucosa. The use of NLO may improve drug response significantly, reduce adverse effects, and allow less-frequent dosing intervals and the use of lower drug concentrations.

Use of more than 1 drop per dose increases costs, does not improve response significantly, and may increase adverse effects. When two drugs are to be administered, instillations should be separated by at least 3 to 5 minutes (preferably 10 minutes) to prevent the drug administered first from being washed out. The patient should be taught not to touch the dropper bottle tip with eye, hands, or any surface.

Adherence to glaucoma therapy usually is inadequate, and it always should be considered as a possible cause of drug therapy failure. Assessment of adherence by healthcare providers generally is poor; so all patients should be encouraged continually to administer prescribed therapy diligently as instructed. To improve adherence, the patient, family, and care providers should be fully informed of the expectations of therapy and the need to continue therapy despite a lack of symptoms. Possible adverse effects of the medication and ways to reduce them should be discussed. Adherence will be improved by good communication, simplified and well tolerated dosing regimens, reminder devices, education, close monitoring, and individualized care planning.[1,2,17–19,29,41]

CONCLUSIONS

The glaucomas are a group of primary and secondary diseases whose management presents a considerable challenge to the clinician. Successful therapy requires rational use of antiglaucoma medications and patient adherence to the selected regimen, combined with conscientious monitoring for adverse effects and disease progression. The reward for successful therapy is considerable—the maintenance of vision. The overview of the clinical findings, pathology, and drug therapy presented in this chapter provides the clinician with the fundamentals necessary to understand and treat glaucoma.

ABBREVIATIONS

CAG: closed-angle glaucoma

CAI: carbonic anhydrase inhibitor

IOP: intraocular pressure

NLO: nasolacrimal occlusion

OHTS: Ocular Hypertensive Treatment Study

POAG: primary open-angle glaucoma

REFERENCES

1. Coleman AL. Glaucoma. Lancet 1999;354:1803–1810.
2. Kwon YH, Fingert JH, Kuehn MH, and Alward WLM. Primary open-angle glaucoma. N Engl J Med 2009;360:1113–1124.
3. Kass MA, Heuer DK, Higginbotham EJ, et al. The ocular hypertension treatment study: A randomized trial determines that topical ocular hypotensive medication delays or prevents the onset of primary open-angle glaucoma. Arch Ophthalmol 2002;120:701–713, discussion 829, 830.
4. Leske MC, Heijl A, Hussein M, et al. Factors for glaucoma progression and the effect of treatment: The early manifest glaucoma trial. Arch Ophthalmol 2003;121:48–56.
5. Van Veldhuisen PC, Schwartz AL, Gaasterland DE, et al. The advanced glaucoma intervention study (AGIS): 7. The relationship between control of intraocular pressure and visual field deterioration. Am J Ophthalmol 2000;130:429–440.
6. Janz NK, Wren PA, Lichter PR, et al. Quality of life in newly diagnosed glaucoma patients: The collaborative initial glaucoma treatment study. Ophthalmology 2001;108:887–897.
7. Collaborative Normal-Tension Glaucoma Study Group. Comparison of glaucomatous progression between untreated patients with normal-tension glaucoma and patients with therapeutically reduced intraocular pressures. Am J Ophthalmol 1998;126:487–497.
8. Khaw PT, Cordiero MF. Towards better treatment of glaucoma. BMJ 2000;320:1619–1620.
9. Weinreb RN, Khaw PT. Primary open-angle glaucoma. Lancet 2004;363:1711–1720.
10. Tsai JC, Kanner EM. Current and emerging medical therapies for glaucoma. Expert Opin Emerg Drugs, 2005;10:109–118.
11. Chung HS, Harris A, Evans DW, et al. Vascular aspects in the pathophysiology of glaucomatous optic neuropathy. Surv Ophthalmol 1999;43(suppl 1):S43–S50.
12. Galanopoulos A, Goldberg I. Clinical efficacy and neuroprotective effects of brimonidine in the management of glaucoma and ocular hypertension. Clin Ophthalmol. 2009;3:117–122.
13. Tatton W, Chen D, Chalmers-Redman R, et al. Hypothesis for a common basis for neuroprotection in glaucoma and Alzheimer's disease: Anti-apoptosis by α-2-adrenergic receptor activation. Surv Ophthalmol 2003;48(Suppl 1):S25–S37.
14. Levin LA. Extrapolation of animal models of optic nerve injury to clinical trial design. J Glaucoma 2004;13:1–5.
15. Nickells, RW. From ocular hypertension to ganglion cell death: A theoretical sequence of events leading to glaucoma. Can J Ophthalmol 2007;42:278–284.
16. Yu DY, Su EN, Cringle SJ, et al. Systemic and ocular vascular roles of the antiglaucoma agents β-adrenergic antagonists and Ca^{2+} entry blockers. Surv Ophthalmol 1999;43(suppl 1):S214–S222.
17. Marquis RE, Whitson JT. Management of glaucoma: focus on pharmacological therapy. Drugs Aging. 2005;22:1–21.
18. King A, Migdal C. Clinical management of glaucoma. J R Soc Med 2000;93:175–177.
19. Hoyng PF, van Beek LM. Pharmacological therapy for glaucoma: A review. Drugs 2000;59:411–434.
20. Wax MB, Camras CB, Fiscella RG, et al. Emerging perspectives in glaucoma: Optimizing 24-hour control of intraocular pressure. Am J Ophthalmol 2002;133:S1–S10.
21. Law SK. Switching within glaucoma medication class. Curr Opin Ophthalmol 2009;20:10–115.
22. Kaufman PL, Gabelt B, Tian B, Liu X. Advances in glaucoma diagnosis and therapy for the next millennium: New drugs for trabecular and uveoscleral outflow. Semin Ophthalmol 1999;14:130–143.
23. Ocular Hypertension Treatment Study Group; European Glaucoma Prevention Study Group; Gordon MO, Torri V, Miglior S, Beiser JA, Floriani I, Miller JP, Gao F, Adamsons I, Poli D, D'Agostino RB, Kass MA. Validated prediction model for the development of primary open-angle glaucoma in individuals with ocular hypertension. Ophthalmology 2007;114:10–19.
24. Kamal D, Hitchings R. Normal-tension glaucoma: A practical approach. Br J Ophthalmol 1998;82:835–840.
25. Triptahi RC, Tripathi BJ, Haggerty C. Drug-induced glaucomas. Drug Saf 2003;26:749–767.
26. Wiggs JL. Genetic etiologies of glaucoma. Arch Ophthalmol, 2007;125:30–37.
27. Varma R, Ying-Lai M, Francis BA, et al. Prevalence of open-angle glaucoma and ocular hypertension in Latinos. Ophthalmology 2004;111:1439–1448.
28. Quigley HA, Broman AT. The number of people with glaucoma worldwide in 2010 and 2020. Br J Ophthalmol 2006;90:262–267.
29. Cantor L. Achieving low target pressures with today's glaucoma medications. Surv Ophthalmol 2003;48(suppl 1):S8–S16.
30. Cooper R. Surgical management of the glaucomas. Aust N Z J Ophthalmol 1999;27:352.
31. Mearza AA, Aslanides IM. Uses and complications of mitomycin C in ophthalmology. Expert Opin Drug Saf 2007;6:27–32.
32. Donohue EK, Cioffi GA. Glaucoma surgery: Are there new perspectives in perioperative pharmacology? Curr Opin Ophthalmol 1999;10:93–98.

33. Loon SC, Chew PT. A major review of antimetabolites in glaucoma therapy. Ophthalmologica 1999;213:234–245.

34. Schuman JS. Antiglaucoma medications: A review of safety and tolerability issues related to their use. Clin Ther 2000;22:167–208.

35. Kanner E, Tsai JC. Glaucoma medications. Use and safety in the elderly population. Drugs Aging 2006;23:321–332.

36. Han JA, Frishman WH, Sun SW, et al. Cardiovascular and respiratory considerations with pharmacotherapy of glaucoma and ocular hypertension. Cardiol Rev 2008;16:95–108.

37. Noecker R, Dirks M, Choplin N. A six-month randomized clinical trial comparing the IOP lowering efficacy of bimatoprost and latanoprost in patients with ocular hypertension or glaucoma. Am J Ophthalmol 2003;135:55–63.

38. van der Valk R, Webers CA, Schouten JSAG, et al. Intraocular pressure-lowering effects of all commonly used glaucoma drugs. A meta-analysis of randomized clinical trials. Ophthalmology 2005;112:1177–1185.

39. Gandolfi SA, Cimino L. Effect of bimatoprost on patients with primary open-angle glaucoma or ocular hypertension who are nonresponders to latanoprost. Ophthalmology 2003;110:609–614.

40. Naskar R, Vorwerk CK, Dreyer EB. Saving the nerve from glaucoma: Memantine to caspases. Semin Ophthalmol 1999;14:152–158.

41. Gray TA, Orton LC, Henson D, et al. Interventions for improving adherence to ocular hypotensive therapy. Cochrane Database of Systematic Reviews 2009, issue 2. Art. No.:CD006132. DOI:10.1002/14651858. CD006132.pub2.

104

Allergic Rhinitis

J. RUSSELL MAY AND PHILIP H. SMITH

KEY CONCEPTS

❶ Allergic rhinitis is a common disease. Treatment is justified in most cases because of the potential for complications.

❷ Because an immediate immune response to allergens results in release of inflammatory mediators that cause allergic rhinitis symptoms, patients must understand the rationale for the proper timing and administration of prophylactic regimens.

❸ Proven therapies include avoidance of allergens and pharmacologic management with antihistamines, topical and systemic decongestants, topical steroids, cromolyn sodium, leukotriene receptor antagonists, and immunotherapy.

❹ Immunotherapy can be highly successful, offering long-term benefits, but expense, potential risks, and a major time commitment makes proper patient selection critical.

Allergic rhinitis involves inflammation of the nasal mucous membrane. In a sensitized individual, allergic rhinitis occurs when inhaled allergenic materials contact mucous membranes and elicit a specific response mediated by immunoglobulin E (IgE). This acute response involves the release of inflammatory mediators and is characterized by sneezing, nasal itching, and watery rhinorrhea, often associated with nasal congestion. Itching of the throat, eyes, and ears frequently accompanies allergic rhinitis.

Allergic rhinitis may be regarded as seasonal allergic rhinitis, commonly known as *hay fever*, or perennial allergic rhinitis (increasingly called *intermittent* and *persistent*). Seasonal rhinitis occurs in response to specific allergens usually present at predictable times of the year, during plants' blooming seasons (typically the spring or fall). Seasonal allergens include pollen from trees, grasses, and weeds. Perennial allergic rhinitis is a year-round disease caused by nonseasonal allergens, such as house-dust mites, animal dander, and molds, or multiple allergic sensitivities. It typically results in subtler, chronic symptoms. Many patients have a combination of these two types of allergic rhinitis, with symptoms year-round and seasonal exacerbations. About one third to one half of sufferers have recognizable seasonal disease with the remainder having perennial or a combination of both.[1]

EPIDEMIOLOGY AND ETIOLOGY

❶ Allergic rhinitis is one of the most common medical disorders found in humans. Using questionnaires, investigators have found the prevalence of seasonal and perennial allergic rhinitis, respectively, to range between 1% and 40% and from 1% to 13% with some believing the percentage to be higher.[2,3] It ranks as the sixth most prevalent chronic illness in the United States.[1] In the populations of Europe, United States, Australia, and New Zealand, the prevalence of an IgE sensitization to aeroallergens measured by allergen-specific IgE in serum or skin tests is more than 40% to 50%.[3] Most but not all of these patients have allergic rhinitis and/or asthma. Patients are limited in their ability to carry out normal daily functions; higher levels of general fatigue, mental fatigue, anxiety, depressive disorders, and learning disabilities (secondary to sleep loss and fatigue) are seen.[3,4]

In addition, the impact of allergic rhinitis goes well beyond these central-nervous-system issues. Allergic rhinitis is associated with several other serious medical conditions, including asthma, chronic rhinosinusitis, otitis media, nasal polyposis, respiratory infections, and orthodontic malocclusions.

PREDISPOSING FACTORS

The development of allergic rhinitis is determined by genetics, allergen exposure, and the presence of other risk factors. A family history of allergic rhinitis, atopic dermatitis, or asthma suggests that rhinitis is allergic. The risk of developing allergic disease appears to increase if one parent is atopic and further increases if two are allergic; however, small sample sizes and the lack of reproducibility prevent generalization.[3]

Allergen exposure is another necessary factor. For allergic rhinitis to occur, an individual must be exposed over time to a protein that elicits the allergic response in that individual. Many potential sufferers never develop symptoms because they do not come into contact with the allergen that would produce symptoms in them.

Evidence suggests microbial exposure in the first years of life could help prevent allergic disease by stimulating a nonatopic immune response.[5] Farm children are exposed to higher concentrations of endotoxin, derived from cell walls of gram-negative bacteria, in stables and in dust around the farmhouse. Consumption of nonpasteurized farm milk may cause further exposure. This concept has led to the idea that allergic disease could be prevented by proactively increasing exposure to harmless bacteria early in life (see Alternative Treatment Options below). This could explain why positive skin tests indicating allergen sensitization have been observed more frequently for people in higher socioeconomic classes and for people who live in suburban areas.

Other predisposing factors include an elevated serum IgE (>100 international units/mL [>100 kIU/L]) before the age of 6 years, eczema, and heavy exposure to secondhand cigarette smoke.[6]

ALLERGENS

Allergens that produce seasonal rhinitis include protein components of airborne pollen grains, often enzymes, from a variety of trees, grasses, and weeds. Ragweed and grass pollen are the most common offenders in the United States; however, this varies with the geographic region. In general, tree pollens cause symptoms in the spring, grass pollens cause symptoms in the late spring and summer, and weed pollens are the culprits from late summer through fall. Patients who are hypersensitive to all three may have overlapping problem periods and may be described as having perennial rhinitis when they are actually experiencing prolonged seasonal rhinitis. For this reason and the fact that most patients with seasonal problems are sensitive to at least some of the perennial allergens, there is little practical difference between the two types of allergic rhinitis. To complicate matters further, the antigenic components of many grasses—including fescue, Kentucky bluegrass, orchard, redtop, and timothy—cross-react extensively. By contrast, tree allergens are antigenically distinct. These trees include ash, beech, birch, cedar, hickory, maple, oak, poplar, and sycamore. Flowering plants that depend on insect pollination do not cause allergic rhinitis because their pollen is too heavy and sticky and is not carried in the air.

Mold spores are also important but cause allergy much less frequently. Various spores are present year-round; however, mold growth on decaying vegetation increases seasonally. Just walking through uncut fields or raking leaves can increase exposure. Thus, mold spores can be responsible for both perennial and seasonal allergies.

Indoor allergens are always present. Most important among these are house-dust mite fecal proteins, animal dander, cockroaches, and certain mold species. Dust mite levels are on the rise, possibly because of the construction of energy-efficient homes and offices with reduced ventilation and increased humidity, use of wall-to-wall carpeting, and the popularity of cool-water detergents and cold-water washing.[3]

PATHOPHYSIOLOGY

Knowledge of nasal physiology aids in the understanding of allergic rhinitis. The nose performs three "air conditioning" functions to prepare incoming gases for the lungs. During the fraction of a second that air is in the nose, it is heated, humidified, and cleaned. The cleaning process plays a role in the development of allergic rhinitis. As the air passes through the nose, the turbulence throws particulate matter against a mucous blanket. The rhythmic movements of the nasal cilia cause the mucous blanket to move posteriorly at approximately 9 mm/min, where it is eventually swallowed; thus, trapped foreign particles are removed via the gastrointestinal tract and do not reach the lungs. It also concentrates foreign protein material into the posterior throat, where lymph tissues identify them and produce most of the allergic antibody that drives allergic rhinitis.

The vascular tissue in the nose is erectile. Stimulation of sympathetic fibers causes vasoconstriction, reduction in erectile tissue size and the size of the membranes and turbinates, and airway widening. Parasympathetic stimulation causes opposite effects.

Located in the nasal mucosa are the mast cells, which participate in the regulation of nasal patency by releasing such mediators as histamine. These are described below.

IMMUNE RESPONSE TO ALLERGENS

❷ Allergic reactions in the nose are mediated by antigen–antibody responses, during which allergens interact with specific IgE molecules bound to nasal mast cells and basophils. In allergic people, these cells are increased in both number and reactivity. During inhalation, airborne allergens enter the nose and are processed by lymphocytes, which produce antigen-specific IgE, thereby sensitizing genetically predisposed hosts to those agents. Upon nasal reexposure, IgE bound to mast cells interacts with airborne allergen, triggering release of inflammatory mediators (Fig. 104–1).[7]

Both immediate and late-phase reactions are observed after allergen exposure. The immediate reaction occurs within seconds to minutes, resulting in the rapid release of preformed mediators and newly generated mediators from the arachidonic acid cascade as the mast cell membrane is disturbed (Table 104–1). These mediators of immediate hypersensitivity include histamine; leukotrienes C_4, D_4, and E_4; prostaglandin D_2; tryptase; and kinins.[7] In addition, the mast cell has been found to be a source of several cytokines that probably are relevant to the chronicity of the mucosal inflammation that characterizes allergic rhinitis.[8] Sensory nerve stimulation produces itching, and sneezing occurs via reflex stimulation of efferent vagal

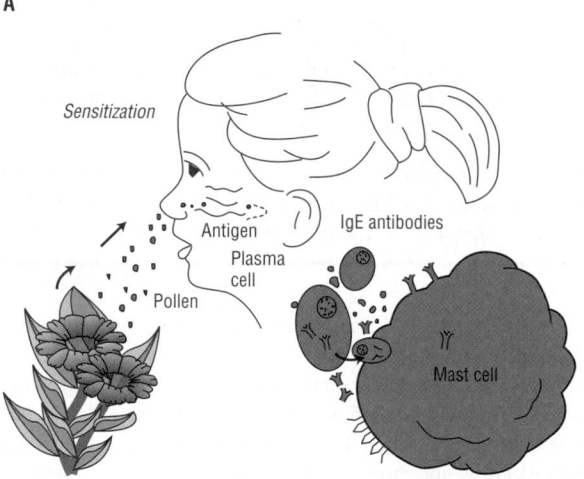

A

Sensitization

Antigen
Plasma cell
Pollen
IgE antibodies
Mast cell

B

Reexposure to antigen

Antigen
Histamine
Antigen–antibody complex
Degranulation
Leukotrienes
Platelet-activating factor

FIGURE 104-1. Allergen sensitization and the allergic response. (A) Exposure to antigen stimulates IgE production and sensitization of mast cells with antigen-specific IgE antibodies. (B) Subsequent exposure to the same antigen produces an allergic reaction when mast cell mediators are released.

TABLE 104-1 Mast Cell Mediators

Mediator	Effect
Preformed and rapidly released	
Histamine	Stimulates irritant receptors
	Pruritus
	Vascular permeability
	Mucosal permeability
	Smooth muscle contraction
Neutrophil chemotactic factor	Influx of inflammatory cells
Eosinophil chemotactic factor	Influx of inflammatory cells
Kinins	Vascular permeability
N-α-tosyl L-arginine methyl esterase	Vascular permeability
Newly generated	
Leukotrienes	Smooth muscle contraction
	Vascular permeability
	Mucus secretion
	Chemotaxis
	Neutrophil chemotaxis
Thromboxanes	Smooth muscle spasm
Platelet-activating factor	Mucus secretion
	Airway permeability
	Chemotaxis
	Vascular permeability
Granule matrix contents	
Heparin	Antiinflammatory
Tryptase	Protein hydrolysis
Kallikrein	Protein hydrolysis

pathways. Neuropeptides substance P and calcitonin gene-related peptide from nonadrenergic, noncholinergic nerves affect vascular engorgement directly and via modulation of sympathetic tone. Histamine produces rhinorrhea, itching, sneezing, and obstruction, with the obstruction only partially blocked by H_1- or H_2-blocking agents.[9] Nasal obstruction is also caused by kinins, prostaglandin D_2, and leukotrienes C_4/D_4. Kinins, when directly administered, produce pain rather than itching.[10] These inflammatory mediators also produce vasodilation, increased vascular permeability, and production of increased nasal secretions.[11]

Four to 8 hours after the initial exposure to an allergen, a late-phase reaction occurs symptomatically in 50% of allergic rhinitis patients.[12] This response, thought to be caused by cytokines released primarily by mast cells and thymus-derived helper lymphocytes, is characterized by profound infiltration and activation of migrating cells. This inflammatory response likely is responsible for the persistent, chronic symptoms of allergic rhinitis, including nasal congestion. The inflamed mucosa becomes hyperresponsive, a state characterized by exacerbation of nasal reactions to nonspecific or irritant triggers. In this state, the patient also reacts to increasingly lower amounts of the same allergen.[13] The process also causes significant increases in nonspecific irritability (as seen in asthma) and the notion among patients that they have become "allergic to everything."

CLINICAL PRESENTATION

SYMPTOMS AND DIAGNOSIS

The patient with allergic rhinitis typically complains of clear rhinorrhea, paroxysms of sneezing, nasal congestion, postnasal drip, and pruritic eyes, ears, nose, or palate. Symptoms of allergic conjunctivitis are associated more frequently with seasonal than perennial allergic rhinitis, because a majority of the perennial allergens, such as dust mites and molds, are indoors, where air velocity is too low

for substantial deposition of allergenic particles on the conjunctivae. However, with heavy exposure from animal or mold allergens, allergic conjunctivitis can be pronounced.

Symptoms secondary to the late-phase reaction, predominantly nasal congestion, begin 3 to 5 hours after antigen exposure and peak at 12 to 24 hours. Subsequent symptoms, both allergic and irritant, are elicited more easily because of the priming effect. For instance, a ragweed-sensitive patient, when exposed to ragweed pollen out of season, responds with modest symptoms and may be very tolerant of irritants such as air pollution or tobacco smoke. During the ragweed season, however, when the nasal mucosa is already inflamed, exposure to small doses of pollen or to irritants to which the patient is usually tolerant elicits a response clinically indistinguishable from the patient's allergy.

Allergic rhinitis is distinguished from other causes of rhinitis by a thorough history, physical examination, and certain diagnostic tests. The medical history consists of a careful description of symptoms, environmental factors and exposures, results of previous therapy, use of other medications, previous nasal injuries, previous nasal or sinus surgery, family history, and the presence of other medical problems and medications. Historical identification of specific causative allergens may be difficult. For example, a reaction induced by mowing the lawn may not be caused by grass pollens but may be caused by the disturbance of various weeds, molds, or other plants in the lawn. With perennial allergic rhinitis, the cause–effect and temporal relationships are less clear, making the diagnosis of specific causes more difficult, especially with such covert allergens as house-dust mites and molds.

In children, physical examination may reveal allergic shiners—a transverse nasal crease caused by repeated rubbing of the nose—and adenoidal breathing. Pale, bluish, edematous nasal turbinates coated with thin, clear secretions are characteristic of a purely allergic reaction. Tearing, conjunctival injection and edema, and periorbital swelling may be present. Physical findings are generally less clear-cut for adults.

Nasal scrapings will provide a representative sample of cells infiltrating the nasal mucosa and can be helpful in supporting the diagnosis.[14] Microscopic examination of the nasal smear from an allergic individual typically will show numerous eosinophils. The blood eosinophil count may be elevated in allergic rhinitis, but it is nonspecific and has limited usefulness.[15]

Allergy testing can help determine whether a patient's rhinitis is caused by an allergen. Immediate-type hypersensitivity skin tests are used for the diagnosis of allergic rhinitis. These include skin tests performed by the percutaneous route, where the diluted allergen is pricked or scratched into the skin surface, or by the intradermal route, where a small volume (0.01 to 0.05 mL) of diluted allergen is injected between the layers of skin. Percutaneous tests are more commonly performed and are safer and more generally accepted, with intradermal tests reserved for patients requiring confirmation in special circumstances.

In all allergy testing, a positive control (histamine) and a negative control are essential for correct interpretation. After 15 minutes of the application of the allergen, the site is examined for a positive reaction (defined as a wheal-and-flare reaction). Because correct testing is done with extremely minute doses, undetectable by nonsensitized individuals, this reaction is evidence of the presence of mast cell-bound IgE specific to the allergen tested. Many, but not all, common allergens are available as standardized allergenic extracts.

Antihistamines and a few other medications interfere with the wheal-and-flare reaction. First-generation antihistamines should be stopped 3 to 5 days before testing, and second-generation, nonsedating antihistamines should be stopped for 10 days before testing.[16] Medications with antihistamine properties (e.g., sympathomimetic agents, phenothiazines, and tricyclic antidepressants) should be discontinued before skin testing.

The radioallergosorbent test (RAST) was the first commonly used method for detecting IgE antibodies in the blood that are specific for a given allergen. Several other quantitative assays that include a reference curve calculated against standardized IgE are available. These tests are highly specific but may be slightly less sensitive than percutaneous tests.

CLINICAL PRESENTATION

General

- Allergic rhinitis occurs with exposure to allergens specific to a given patient. Intermittent symptoms occur with seasonal allergens such as pollens, and persistent symptoms occur with perennial allergens such as dust mites.

Symptoms

- The patient typically complains of clear rhinorrhea, paroxysms of sneezing, nasal congestion, postnasal drip, and pruritic eyes, ears, nose, or palate. Late-phase reaction consists of primarily nasal congestion.

Signs

- For children, physical exam may reveal allergic shiners, a transverse nasal crease caused by repeated rubbing of the nose, and adenoidal breathing. Nasal turbinates are coated with thin, clear secretions. Tearing and periorbital swelling may be present.

Laboratory

- Microscopic examination of the nasal smear will show numerous eosinophils. Blood eosinophil count may be elevated in allergic rhinitis, but it is nonspecific.

Other Diagnostic Tests

- Percutaneous skin tests with diluted allergen, positive control (histamine), and negative control are used to identify to what the patient has sensitivities. Also, a radioallergosorbent test can detect IgE antibodies in the blood that are specific for a given allergen.

COMPLICATIONS

Not only is allergic rhinitis aggravating, it also frequently leads to further complications, particularly if the patient does not receive adequate treatment. Symptoms of untreated rhinitis may lead to disturbed sleep, chronic malaise, fatigue, and poor work or school performance. Patients often are plagued by loss of smell or taste, with sinusitis or polyps underlying many cases of allergy-related hyposmia. Postnasal drip with cough, hoarseness, and even vocal polyps also can be bothersome.

The role of allergic rhinitis in the development of acute otitis media or chronic middle ear effusion is often less clear. Children with allergic rhinitis appear to be at greater risk of these conditions because of nasal obstruction and negative middle ear pressure. Hearing problems in children related to middle ear effusion may lead to delayed development of language in young children or to school problems in older children.

Structural facial and dental problems can result from chronic allergic rhinitis.[17,18] The chronic edema and venous stasis may contribute to the development of a high-arched, V-shaped palate. Mouth breathing caused by nasal obstruction can be responsible for dental malocclusion and orthodontic problems. Constant upward rubbing of the nose (allergic salute) can cause a transverse crease across the lower nose; nasal congestion often leads to venous pooling and dark circles under the eyes known as *allergic shiners*.

Allergic rhinitis is clearly a risk factor for asthma. The majority of asthma patients have nasal symptoms, whereas approximately 10% to 40% of rhinitis patients have asthma.[3] It is not known if allergic rhinitis is an early clinical manifestation of asthma or if the nasal disease itself is causative for asthma.

Recurrent sinusitis and chronic sinusitis are relatively common complications of allergic rhinitis. The structure of the mucus blanket breaks down, with decreased water production by serous glands, leaving hair cells trapped in the thicker mucus layer. This greatly reduces the clearance of trapped bacteria and offers ideal breeding grounds for the bacteria. Nasal polyps are less common but nonetheless bothersome; they require specific therapy but may improve with management of the underlying allergic state. Epistaxis also can be a problem; it is related to mucosal hyperemia and inflammation.

TREATMENT

Allergic Rhinitis

■ DESIRED OUTCOME

The therapeutic goal for patients with allergic rhinitis is to minimize or prevent symptoms and prevent long-term complications. This goal should be accomplished with no or minimal adverse medication effects and reasonable medication expenses. The patient should be able to maintain a normal lifestyle, including participating in outdoor activities, yard work, and playing with pets as desired.

■ GENERAL APPROACH TO TREATMENT

❸ Once the causative allergens and the specific symptoms are identified, management consists of three possible approaches: (1) allergen avoidance, (2) pharmacotherapy for prevention or treatment of symptoms, and (3) specific immunotherapy. The pharmacotherapy for symptoms approach includes several options that are based on patient-specific information (Table 104–2). Figure 104–2 depicts an algorithm for treatment options.

■ AVOIDANCE

Avoidance of offending allergens is the most direct method of preventing allergic rhinitis, but it is often the most difficult to accomplish, especially for perennial allergens. Mold growth can be reduced by maintaining household humidity below 50% and removing obvious growth with bleach or disinfectant. Patients sensitive to animals will benefit most by removing pets from the home; however, most animal lovers are reluctant to comply with this approach. Dog and cat allergens may produce symptoms in sensitized individuals.[8] After removing a cat from the home, it may take as long as 20 weeks for the home to reach allergen levels of a pet-free home. Washing cats weekly may reduce allergens but studies are inconclusive.[8] Some dogs display antigens more profusely than do others; clinically, a sensitized person may tolerate one animal better than another.

Evidence to support avoidance measures for house dust mites suggests that accepted notions for reducing exposure have little practical effect.[19] While some evidence shows allergen levels can be reduced by washing bedding on a hot cycle, replacing carpets with hard flooring and using vacuum cleaners with HEPA filters, there is no documented evidence for a clinical benefit. Only encasing bedding in impermeable covers has some clinical benefit in children

TABLE 104-2 Pharmacotherapeutic Options for Allergic Rhinitis

Medication Class	Symptoms Controlled	Comments
Antihistamines		
Systemic	Sneezing, rhinorrhea, itching, conjunctivitis	For seasonal allergic rhinitis, begin treatment before allergen exposure. Nonsedating agents should be tried first. If ineffective or too expensive for the patient, the older agents may be used. For perennial allergic rhinitis, use an intranasal steroid as an alternative to or in combination with systemic antihistamines.
Ophthalmic	Conjunctivitis	Logical addition to nasal steroids if ocular symptoms are present.
Intranasal	Sneezing, rhinorrhea, nasal pruritus	Option for seasonal allergic rhinitis. Warn patients of potential drowsiness.
Decongestants		
Systemic	Nasal congestion	Only needed when nasal congestion is present.
Topical	Nasal congestion	Only needed when nasal congestion is present. Do not exceed 3–5 days.
Intranasal corticosteroids	Sneezing, rhinorrhea, itching, nasal congestion	For seasonal allergic rhinitis, an option when congestion is present. Must begin therapy before allergen exposure. Excellent choice for perennial rhinitis.
Mast cell stabilizers	See comments.	Prevents symptoms; therefore, for seasonal allergic rhinitis, use before offending allergen's season starts. For perennial rhinitis, improvement may not be seen for up to 1 month.
Intranasal anticholinergics	Rhinorrhea	Reserve for use when above therapies fail or cannot be tolerated.
Leukotriene receptor antagonists	See comments.	When combined with antihistamines, more effective than antihistamines alone. May be used as monotherapy in children with asthma and coexisting allergic rhinitis.

but not adults. Future studies are needed to determine if environmental control of allergens may be helpful in forestalling further rhinitis and preventing later asthma.

General recommendations have been made to prevent poor air quality in homes.[20] Steps include avoiding wall-to-wall carpeting, using moisture control to prevent the accumulation of molds, and controlling sources of pollution such as cigarette smoke. Patients with seasonal allergic rhinitis should keep windows closed and minimize time spent outdoors during pollen seasons. Immediate hair washing and change of clothes are recommended upon returning indoors. Use of fans that direct outside air into the house should be avoided. Filter masks can be worn while gardening or mowing the lawn. Avoidance of upholstery and stuffed toys in the bedroom are easy steps to accomplish. Table 104–3 summarizes recommendations for environmental control. While these steps are logical, there is little existing evidence that environmental control measures provide clinical benefit. These measures are intended to be a part of a comprehensive treatment strategy that will likely include pharmacotherapy and, in selected cases, immunotherapy.

■ PHARMACOLOGIC THERAPY

First-line therapeutic modalities for treating allergic rhinitis are directed at relief of symptoms (see Table 104–2). Antihistamines and decongestants (both oral and topical) generally are used first in treating allergic rhinitis with medications. Several options in these two categories are available without a prescription, but patients will need sound advice to make appropriate choices. Knowledge of pathophysiology and the inflammatory state has led to prophylactic therapy for those with more severe disease using agents such as cromolyn and topical steroids. However, in attempting to assess the evidence supporting any particular therapy, clinicians have difficulty interpreting the medical literature for a variety of reasons, including lack of uniformity in the research methodologies, inappropriate drug controls, and failure to identify types of rhinitis in study subjects (perennial versus seasonal and allergic versus nonallergic).

Antihistamines

Histamine (H_1)-receptor antagonists are competitive antagonists to histamine. They bind to H_1 receptors without activating them, preventing histamine binding and action. Second-generation antihistamines may also affect components of the inflammatory response

such as histamine release, generation of adhesion molecules, and influx of inflammatory cells. Although it was once thought that the older antihistamines had no antiinflammatory action, some were shown to have these effects as early as the 1950s.[21] Antihistamines are available in oral, ophthalmic, and intranasal dosage forms.

The oral antihistamines are the most commonly used and can be divided into two major categories: nonselective (first generation) and peripherally selective (second generation). Nonselective agents are commonly referred to as *sedating antihistamines*, and peripherally selective agents are referred to as *nonsedating antihistamines*. These generalizing terms can be misleading. Individual agents should be judged on their specific characteristics because variation within these broad categories exists. Also, the nonsedating claim is only valid when the agents are used at recommended doses.[22] This is of particular concern as some of these antihistamines are available without a prescription. The mechanism for sedation is not well understood, but its central effect depends on the drugs' ability to cross the blood–brain barrier. Most older antihistamines are lipid soluble and cross this barrier easily. The peripherally selective agents have little or no central or autonomic nervous system effects. Table 104–4 lists common antihistamines, their chemical classifications, their relative potential for causing sedation, and their relative anticholinergic effects.

Antihistamines are much more effective in preventing the actions of histamines than in reversing these actions once they have taken place. Reversal of symptoms is largely caused by the anticholinergic properties of these drugs. This activity is responsible for the drying effect of antihistamines, which reduces the problem of nasal, salivary, and lacrimal gland hypersecretion. Antihistamines antagonize increased capillary permeability, wheal-and-flare formation, and itching.

In general, the antihistamines are well absorbed, have large volumes of distribution, and are metabolized by the liver. Serum half-lives vary considerably between patients. In addition, the therapeutic effects of these agents are more prolonged than might be predicted by their half-lives.

Drowsiness is usually the chief complaint of patients who take antihistamines. It can interfere with a patient's ability to drive a car or operate machinery and may interfere with the patient's ability to function adequately at the workplace. Remember that these problems can also be a reflection of the disease itself. For this reason, many recommend the use of peripherally selective agents as first-line treatment for any patient who is at high risk

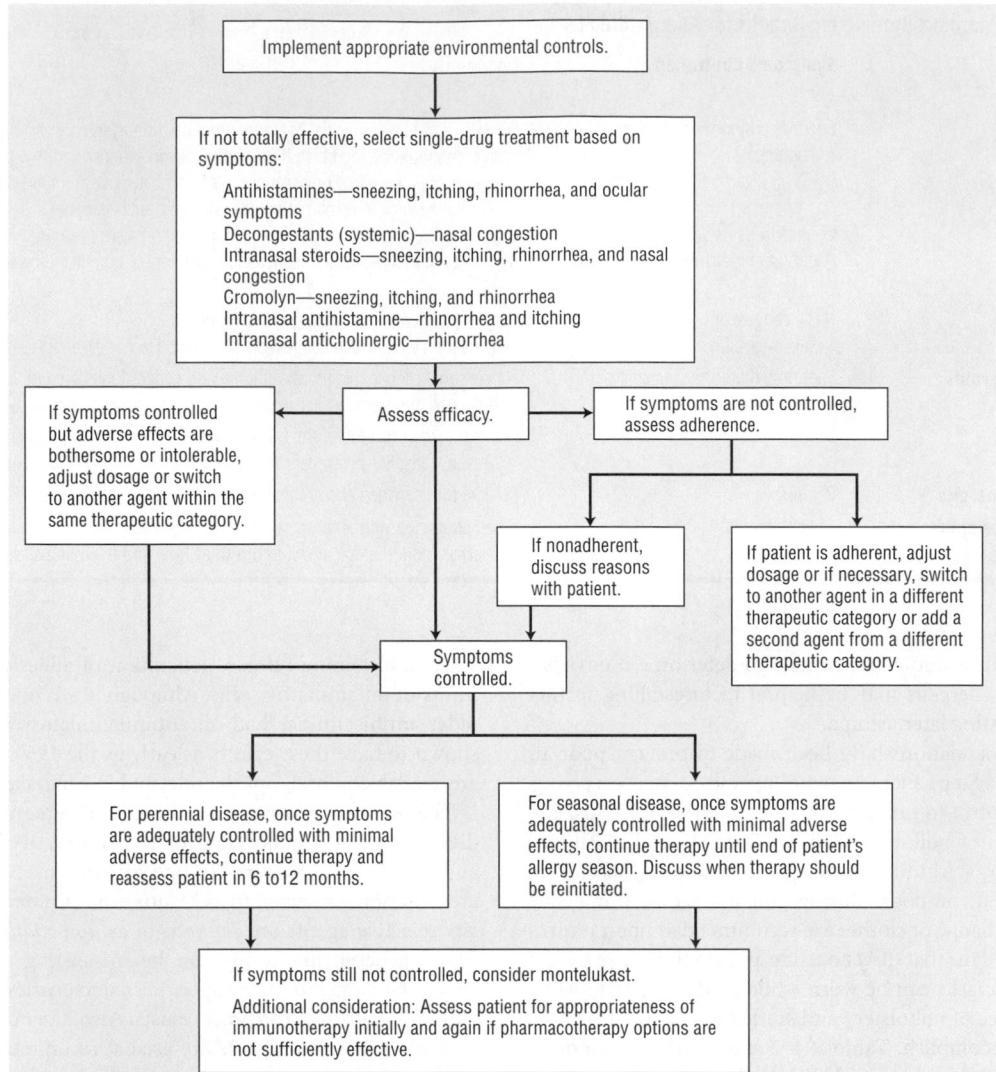

FIGURE 104-2. Treatment algorithm for allergic rhinitis.

for the development of adverse events. This includes patients with renal or hepatic impairment, those with small weights (for whom adult doses may provide larger-than-recommended doses on a milligram-per-kilogram basis), patients with preexisting central-nervous-system or cardiac disorders, patients who require higher doses, and patients who have shown a tendency to overuse nonprescription or prescription medications.[21]

The sedative effects of antihistamines can be useful for patients who suffer from sleeplessness caused by the symptoms of allergic rhinitis. In these patients, a bedtime dose may prove beneficial. However, they may cause residual daytime sedation, decreased alertness, and performance impairment.

The logic of preferentially using the second-generation agents is not clear-cut. A metaanalysis of performance-impairment trials did not show a clear and consistent distinction between diphenhydramine and the peripherally selective agents.[23] Another study showed that tolerance to sedation secondary to diphenhydramine developed by day 4 of treatment, becoming indistinguishable from placebo,[24] but sedation must be distinguished from impairment since the two are not equivalent.

Anticholinergic (drying) effects contribute to the agents' therapeutic efficacy, but they also cause most adverse effects. Dry mouth, difficulty in voiding urine, constipation, and potential cardiovascular effects may be troublesome. Keep in mind that the differences may be small. Patients with a predisposition to urinary retention

(e.g., older men and those on concurrent anticholinergic therapy) should use antihistamines with caution. Caution also should be used for patients with increased intraocular pressure, hyperthyroidism, and cardiovascular disease.

Other adverse effects of oral antihistamines include loss of appetite (and paradoxically, weight gain with increased appetite), nausea, vomiting, and epigastric distress.

Antihistamines are only fully effective when taken approximately 1 to 2 hours before anticipated exposure to the offending allergen. This must be discussed with patients who face exposure daily during a pollen season and with those who have indoor perennial allergens where daily scheduled use is necessary. If tolerance develops to the therapeutic effect, a change to an agent in a different chemical class is usually effective.

Patients should be counseled about the proper use of antihistamines. Adverse effects, especially drowsiness, should be emphasized. Patients should be warned against taking other central-nervous-system depressants, including the use of alcohol. Patients should be told not to take a double dose when a dose is missed. Taking the antihistamine with meals or at least a full glass of water will help prevent gastrointestinal adverse effects such as nausea, vomiting, and epigastric distress. Patients should check with their healthcare professional and read labels before taking nonprescription medications. Many cold products and sleep aids contain antihistamines. Patients should be instructed not to use

TABLE 104-3 Environmental Controls to Prevent Allergic Rhinitis

Pollens
- Keep windows and doors closed during pollen season
- Avoid fans that draw in outside air
- Use air conditioning
- If possible, eliminate outside activities during times of high pollen counts
- Shower, shampoo, and change clothes following outdoor activity
- Use a vented dryer rather than an outside clothesline

Molds
- Use similar controls as above
- Avoid walking through uncut fields, working with compost or dry soil, and raking leaves
- Clean indoor moldy surfaces
- Fix all water leaks in home
- Reduce indoor humidity to <50% if possible

House-dust mites
- Encase mattress, pillow, and box springs in an allergen-impermeable cover
- Wash bedding in hot water weekly
- Remove stuffed toys from bedroom
- Minimize carpet use and upholstered furniture
- Reduce indoor humidity to <50% if possible

Animal allergens (if removal of pet is not acceptable)
- Keep pet out of patient's bedroom
- Isolate pet from carpet and upholstered furniture
- Wash pet weekly

Cockroaches
- Keep food and garbage in tightly closed containers
- Take out garbage regularly
- Clean up dirty dishes promptly
- Use roach traps

Other recommendations
- Do not allow smoking around the patient, in the patient's house, or in the family car
- Minimize the use of wood-burning stoves and fireplaces

Adapted from reference 3.

TABLE 104-4 Relative Adverse-Effect Profiles of Antihistamines

Medication	Relative Sedative Effect	Relative Anticholinergic Effect
Alkylamine class, nonselective		
Brompheniramine maleate	Low	Moderate
Chlorpheniramine maleate	Low	Moderate
Dexchlorpheniramine maleate	Low	Moderate
Ethanolamine class, nonselective		
Carbinoxamine maleate	High	High
Clemastine fumarate	Moderate	High
Diphenhydramine hydrochloride	High	High
Ethylenediamine class, nonselective		
Pyrilamine maleate	Low	Low to none
Tripelennamine hydrochloride	Moderate	Low to none
Phenothiazine class, nonselective		
Promethazine hydrochloride	High	High
Piperidine class, nonselective		
Cyproheptadine hydrochloride	Low	Moderate
Phenindamine tartrate	Low to none	Moderate
Phthalazinone class, peripherally selective		
Azelastine (nasal only)	Low to none	Low to none
Piperazine class, peripherally selective		
Cetirizine	Low to moderate	Low to none
Levocetirizine	Low to moderate	Low to none
Piperidine class, peripherally selective		
Desloratadine	Low to none	Low to none
Fexofenadine	Low to none	Low to none
Loratadine	Low to none	Low to none

more than one antihistamine at a time. Table 104–5 lists the recommended dosages of the commonly used agents with their prescription status.

Many patients respond to and tolerate the older agents quite well. Because many of the older agents are available generically, they are much less expensive. Patient cost for many of the older nonprescription agents is less than $5 for a 30-day supply, compared with more than $20 for some of the nonprescription selective agents and more than $70 dollars for the selective prescription-only products. Although cost is a concern, patient safety should be the first consideration. Interestingly, the most frequently recommended nonprescription antihistamine to adults by pharmacists was diphenhydramine.[25] This may be because the use of diphenhydramine as a sleep aid. With the heavy promotion of competing brands of nonprescription loratadine, this ranking may change. Loratadine in combination with pseudoephedrine did show up in the same survey as the top pharmacists' pick in the "adult multisymptom allergy" category. The over-the-counter availability of cetirizine further broadens the range of suggestions.

For seasonal and perennial allergic rhinitis, an intranasal antihistamine, azelastine, is available. The 0.1% product can be used in children and is effective in seasonal allergies, while the 0.15% product is used in adults only and may be used for either type of allergic rhinitis. Azelastine has been used successfully for patients who did not respond to loratadine.[26] Using the nasal route offers an alternative to switching to another oral antihistamine. Patient satisfaction has been varied because while the product produces rapid symptom relief, patients complain of drying effects, headache, and diminished effectiveness over time. Patients should be warned

of the medication's potential to produce drowsiness, as its systemic availability is approximately 40%.[27,28]

Allergic conjunctivitis, often associated with allergic rhinitis, can be treated with an ophthalmic antihistamine such as levocabastine. Because systemic antihistamines usually are also effective for allergic conjunctivitis, levocabastine is a logical addition to nasal steroids when ocular symptoms occur, and it is an acceptable approach for patients whose only symptoms involve the eyes or to add for those whose symptoms persist on oral treatment.

CLINICAL CONTROVERSY

Although many clinicians strongly prefer a peripherally selective agent as the first antihistamine choice, economic considerations still result in the first-line choice of the less expensive and more sedating products by some prescription plans and clinicians.

Decongestants

Topical and systemic decongestants are sympathomimetic agents that act on adrenergic receptors in the nasal mucosa, producing vasoconstriction. Decongestants shrink swollen mucosa and improve ventilation. When nasal congestion is part of the clinical picture, decongestants work well in combination with antihistamines.

■ TOPICAL DECONGESTANTS

Topical decongestants are applied directly to swollen nasal mucosa via drops or sprays. Table 104–6 lists the common topical decongestants and their durations of action. The use of these agents results in little or no systemic absorption.

TABLE 104-5 Oral Dosages of Commonly Used Oral Antihistamines and Decongestants

| Medication | Availability | Dosage and interval[a] | |
		Adults	*Children*
Nonselective (first-generation) antihistamines			
Chlorpheniramine maleate, plain[b]	OTC	4 mg every 6 h	6–12 y: 2 mg every 6 h 2–5 y: 1 mg every 6 h
Chlorpheniramine maleate, sustained-release	OTC	8–12 mg daily at bedtime or 8–12 mg every 8 h	6–12 y: 8 mg at bedtime <6 y: Not recommended
Clemastine fumarate[b]	OTC	1.34 mg every 8 h	6–12 y: 0.67 mg every 12 h
Diphenhydramine hydrochloride[b]	OTC	25–50 mg every 8 h	5 mg/kg per day divided every 8 h (up to 25 mg per dose)
Peripherally selective (second-generation) antihistamines			
Loratadine[b]	OTC	10 mg once daily	6–12 y: 10 mg once daily 2–5 y: 5 mg once daily
Fexofenadine	Rx	60 mg twice daily or 180 mg once daily	6–11 y: 30 mg twice daily
Cetirizine[b]	OTC	5–10 mg once daily	>6 y: 5 mg once daily Infants 6–11 month[c]
Levocetirizine	Rx	5 mg every evening	6–11 y: 2.5 mg every evening
Oral decongestants			
Pseudoephedrine, plain[b]	OTC[e]	60 mg every 4–6 h	6–12 y: 30 mg every 4–6 h 2–5 y: 15 mg every 4–6 h
Pseudoephedrine, sustained-release[d]	OTC[e]	120 mg every 12 h	Not recommended
Phenylephrine[f]	OTC	10–20 mg every 4 h	6–12 y: 10 mg every 4 h 2–6 y: 0.25% drops, 1 mL every 4 h

OTC, nonprescription; Rx, prescription.

[a]Dosage adjustment may be needed in renal/hepatic dysfunction. Refer to manufacturers' prescribing information.

[b]Available in liquid form.

[c]0.25 mg/kg orally demonstrated to be safe.[31]

[d]Controlled-release product available: 240 mg once daily (60-mg immediate-release with 180-mg controlled-release).

[e]See text regarding nonprescription requirements.

[f]Phenylephrine has replaced pseudoephrine in many nonprescription antihistamine–decongestant combination products. Read product labels carefully.

Because these agents are extremely effective and are available to patients without a prescription, they are widely used. However, prolonged use of these agents (for more than 3 to 5 days) can result in a condition known as *rhinitis medicamentosa*, or *rebound vasodilation*, with even more severe congestion. Patients who develop this condition use increasingly more spray more often with less response. Although the methods used to treat this "addiction" have not been studied formally, several are used commonly. Abrupt cessation works, but it is difficult because of rebound congestion that may leave the patient congested for several days or weeks. Sleeping may become difficult. Nasal steroids have been used successfully, but they take several days to work. Weaning the patient off topical decongestants can be accomplished by decreasing the dosing frequency or the concentration over several weeks. Combining the weaning process with nasal steroids may prove useful. Ultimately, the success of any plan depends on the patient's resolve and clear understanding of the importance of stopping the drug to end the problem.

Other adverse effects of topical decongestants include burning, stinging, sneezing, and dryness of the nasal mucosa.

TABLE 104-6 Duration of Action of Topical Decongestants

Medication	Duration (h)
Short acting	
Phenylephrine hydrochloride	Up to 4
Intermediate acting	
Naphazoline hydrochloride	4–6
Tetrahydrozoline hydrochloride	
Long acting	
Oxymetazoline hydrochloride	Up to 12
Xylometazoline hydrochloride	

Patients should be counseled on the use of topical decongestants to prevent rhinitis medicamentosa. Patients should be instructed to use as small a dose as possible as infrequently as possible and only when absolutely necessary (e.g., at bedtime to aid in falling asleep). Duration of therapy always should be limited to 3 to 5 days.

Systemic Decongestants

Oral decongestants are not as effective on an immediate basis as the topical agents, but their effects sometimes last longer and they cause less local irritation. In addition, rhinitis medicamentosa is not a problem with oral agents. The most commonly used agent is pseudoephedrine. Table 104–5 lists the usual doses for the regular and sustained-release versions. The use of phenylephrine is increasing because of new regulations related to pseudoephedrine described below.

Concerns of safety have greatly limited the systemic decongestant options. Legal requirements for the sale of pseudoephedrine were put into place to combat the misuse of the drug as a component in making methamphetamine. Pseudoephedrine must now be sold behind the counter, and the monthly amount a patient can purchase is limited. Until this requirement, pseudoephedrine was the most frequently used systemic decongestant, and it was considered the safest. Doses of 180 mg have been shown to produce no measurable change in blood pressure or heart rate.[29] In higher doses (210 to 240 mg), pseudoephedrine has raised both blood pressure and heart rate.[30] Pseudoephedrine can cause mild central-nervous-system stimulation, even at therapeutic doses. Stroke, related to use of oral decongestants such as pseudoephedrine, can occur in patients with hypertension and/or vasospasm.[31] Although stroke complications seem to be associated with higher-than-recommended doses, there is also a stroke risk when these agents are taken properly. Severe hypertensive reactions can occur when pseudoephedrine is given concomitantly with monoamine

TABLE 104-7	Dosage of Nasal Steroids
Medication	**Dosage and Interval**
Beclomethasone dipropionate, monohydrate	>12 y: 1–2 inhalations (42–84 mcg) twice daily in each nostril
	6–12 y: 1 inhalation per nostril (42 mcg) twice daily to start
Budesonide	>6 y: 2 sprays (64 mcg) per nostril in am and pm or 4 sprays per nostril in am (maximum: 256 mcg)
Flunisolide	Adults: 2 sprays (50 mcg) per nostril twice daily (maximum: 400 mcg)
	Children: 1 spray per nostril three times a day
Fluticasone	Adults: 2 sprays (100 mcg) per nostril once daily; after a few days decrease to 1 spray per nostril
	Children >4 y and adolescents: 1 spray per nostril once daily (maximum: 200 mcg/day)
Mometasone furoate	>12 y: 2 sprays (100 mcg) per nostril once daily
Triamcinolone acetonide	>12 y: 2 sprays (110 mcg) per nostril once daily (maximum: 440 mcg/day)

oxidase inhibitors.[32] Hypertensive patients should, unless necessary, avoid systemic decongestants.

Combination Products

Numerous products combine an antihistamine with a decongestant. While the combination may be rational because of the different mechanisms of action, remember that antihistamines must be taken on a regular schedule, but decongestants should only be used when needed. Both nonselective and peripherally selective antihistamines are available in such combinations. As mentioned previously, patients should read labels to avoid therapeutic duplication. Consideration should be given to how often the patient is congested before recommending these combinations.

■ NASAL STEROIDS

Nasal steroids are an excellent choice for treating perennial rhinitis, and can be useful in seasonal rhinitis, especially if begun in advance of symptoms. Nasal steroids appear to be effective with minimal adverse effects. Some believe that nasal steroids should be recommended as initial therapy over antihistamines because of their high level of efficacy when used properly and along with avoidance of allergens.[8] Multiple mechanisms are involved with the effects of nasal steroids on the nasal mucosa: reducing inflammation by reducing mediator release, suppressing neutrophil chemotaxis, reducing intracellular edema, causing mild vasoconstriction, and inhibiting mast cell-mediated late-phase reactions. Table 104–7 lists the available nasal steroids and their usual doses.

Topical steroids produce only minor adverse effects, most commonly sneezing, stinging, headache, and epistaxis. Despite concerns about safety of systemic steroids, nasal steroids have been found to have no significant association with hypothalamic–pituitary axis suppression, cataract formation, glaucoma, or bone mineral density changes in the doses used for allergic rhinitis. Growth suppression remains a question with some evidence showing that nasal steroids with higher bioavailability (e.g., beclomethasone) may have a greater growth-suppression effect than less bioavailable agents.[33] These findings require more study. Most likely, all currently available nasal steroids are safe in the majority of patients, and their clinical benefits outweigh any small growth suppressive effect. Other concerns include local infections with *Candida albicans*, which occur rarely.

The therapeutic benefits of topical steroids are not immediate, and they are not decongestants. Patients need to understand this to ensure cooperation and continuation of therapy. Some patients notice improvement in a few days, but peak responses may not be observed for 2 to 3 weeks. Once a response is achieved, the dosage may be reduced. Blocked nasal passages should be cleared with a decongestant or saline irrigation before administration to ensure adequate penetration of the spray. Patients should be advised to avoid sneezing or blowing their noses for at least 10 minutes after administration. Topical steroids should not be used for patients with nasal septum ulcers or recent nasal surgery or trauma.

One additional benefit of nasal steroids in treating allergic rhinitis in individuals with asthma and upper airway conditions is that they may confer some protection against exacerbations of asthma, leading to fewer emergency room visits. The overall relative risk for an emergency visit among asthma patients who received intranasal steroids was 0.7.[34] No effect was seen for patients receiving antihistamines.

■ OTHER INHALANT MEDICATIONS

Cromolyn sodium and ipratropium bromide offer two additional approaches for treating allergic rhinitis. Cromolyn sodium is a mast cell stabilizer. Increased interest in this product has resulted from it becoming available without a prescription. Ipratropium bromide is an anticholinergic agent useful in perennial allergic rhinitis.

Cromolyn sodium nasal spray is used for the symptomatic prevention and treatment of allergic rhinitis. It curtails antigen-triggered mast cell degranulation and release of the mediators of allergic reactions, including histamine. Cromolyn sodium has no direct antihistaminic, anticholinergic, or antiinflammatory properties. Similarly to topical steroids, the most common adverse effects—sneezing and nasal stinging—result from local irritation. The dose in adults and children at least 2 years of age is one spray in each nostril three to four times per day at regular intervals every 4 to 6 hours. Cromolyn sodium must cover the entire nasal lining; therefore, patients should be instructed to clear nasal passages before administration. Inhaling gently through the nose during administration aids in this process. Dosing must be repeated at 6-hour intervals to maintain the effect.

For seasonal rhinitis, treatment with cromolyn sodium should be initiated just before the usual start of the offending allergen's season and continued throughout the season. In perennial rhinitis, the effects may not be seen for 2 to 4 weeks; therefore, antihistamines or decongestants may be needed during this initial phase of therapy. As cromolyn sodium begins to work, the need for these medications should decrease.

Ipratropium nasal spray is an anticholinergic agent that exhibits antisecretory properties when applied locally. It provides symptomatic relief of rhinorrhea associated with allergic and other forms of chronic rhinitis. The 0.03% solution is given as two sprays (42 mcg) two to three times daily. The optimal dose should be determined based on the specific patient's symptoms and response. Adverse effects are mild, with the most common being headache, nosebleeds, and nasal dryness.

■ IMMUNOTHERAPY

❹ The first report of the successful use of grass pollen extract injections to treat allergic rhinitis was published in 1911 by Noon.[35] The therapy was first called *desensitization*; however, this did not seem appropriate because skin reactivity sometimes remained. The name was later changed to *hyposensitization*. Although this term is still used today, *immunotherapy* is used more commonly and is less confusing.

Immunotherapy is the slow, gradual process of injecting increasing doses of antigens responsible for eliciting allergic symptoms into a patient with the hope of inducing tolerance to the allergen when natural exposure occurs. Several mechanisms have been proposed to explain the beneficial effects of immunotherapy, including induction of IgG-blocking antibodies, reduction in specific IgE (long-term), reduced recruitment of effector cells, altered T-cell cytokine balance (a shift from T-helper type 1 to T-helper type 2), T-cell anergy, and induction of regulatory T cells.[36]

Immunotherapy is moderately expensive, has significant potential risks, and requires a major time commitment from the patient. However, the cost of immunotherapy is usually covered by insurance, including Medicaid. Long-term savings can be realized since decades of treatment with medication can be averted through successful immunotherapy. Candidates for immunotherapy should have significant symptoms unsuccessfully controlled by avoidance and pharmacotherapy or should stand to benefit in other significant ways, such as with asthma. Immunotherapy may postpone the onset of asthma or possibly even prevent it.[37] Patients who are unable to tolerate the adverse effects of properly managed drug therapy also should be considered. Patients must be committed to the necessary regular office visits required to complete this course of therapy over several years.

The effectiveness of immunotherapy for seasonal allergic rhinitis appears to be better than that seen with perennial rhinitis, in part because it is more difficult to determine which allergen is responsible for perennial symptoms, and it is more often due to multiple sensitizations. Effectiveness has been shown in a number of clinical studies using a variety of pollen extracts, even for patients with severe disease resistant to pharmacotherapy.[36] Specific immunotherapy for house-dust mites has had good results in appropriately selected patients, while several studies have described marked improvement for patients with allergy to cats. Data indicate that for some patients 3 years of immunotherapy may be sufficient to give lasting benefit;[38] however, many require longer treatment.

The selection of antigens should be based on patient history and skin test results. Numerous regimens for administration of selected allergens have been suggested. In the beginning, very dilute solutions are given initially one to two times per week. The concentration is increased until the maximum tolerated or highest planned or effective dose is achieved. This maintenance dose is continued in slowly increasing intervals over several years, depending on clinical response. In light of the present understanding of the immunologic results of immunotherapy, it should be given year-round rather than seasonally.

Adverse reactions can occur with immunotherapy and range from mild to life threatening. Among the most common are mild local reactions, consisting of induration and swelling at the site of the injection. These may be immediate or delayed. Other more serious reactions (e.g., generalized urticaria, bronchospasm, laryngospasm, and vascular collapse) occur rarely; deaths can result from anaphylactic reactions. Severe reactions are treated with epinephrine as well as other modalities recommended for anaphylaxis. Because of this potential risk, immunotherapy must not be given without adequate direct observation in a medical facility.

Several patient types have been identified as poor candidates for immunotherapy, including patients with any medical condition that would compromise the ability to tolerate an anaphylactic-type reaction, patients with impaired immune systems, and patients with a history of nonadherence to therapy.[39]

■ LEUKOTRIENE RECEPTOR ANTAGONISTS

Leukotriene receptor antagonists inhibit the cysteinyl leukotriene receptor. The cysteinyl leukotrienes are one type of inflammatory mediators released from mast cells in allergy. Montelukast is approved for the treatment of perennial allergic rhinitis in children as young as 6 months and for seasonal allergic rhinitis in children as

TABLE 104-8	Dosage Regimens for Montelukast in Treatment of Allergic Rhinitis
Age	**Dosage**
Adults and adolescents >14 years	10 mg tablet daily
Children 6–14 years	5 mg chewable tablet daily
Children 6 months to 5 years	4 mg chewable tablet or oral granule packet daily

young as 2 years. Montelukast is effective alone or in combination with an antihistamine.[8]

Studies published to date show leukotriene receptor antagonists to be no more effective than peripherally selective antihistamines and less effective than intranasal steroids. However, when combined with antihistamines, they are more effective than the antihistamine alone.[40] In children with mild persistent asthma and coexisting allergic rhinitis, montelukast as monotherapy has been recommended.[41] Table 104–8 lists dosage regimens.

CLINICAL CONTROVERSY

The exact role of montelukast in treating allergic rhinitis remains to be defined. Although expensive, it may be advantageous in men with significant prostatic hypertrophy who cannot tolerate antihistamines and for patients who have difficulty stopping antihistamines a week before skin testing.

■ ALTERNATIVE TREATMENT OPTIONS

The development of monoclonal antibodies directed against the binding site of IgE provides an additional way to treat allergic respiratory diseases. Omalizumab, a recombinant humanized anti-IgE monoclonal antibody, is the first to show efficacy in allergic rhinitis.[42] The actual mechanism of how this agent is thought to work is quite complex.[43] Anti-IgE antibodies bind to the site on the IgE molecule that recognizes the IgE receptor, thereby preventing the IgE molecule from binding to mast cells or basophils. The half-life of IgE antibodies on the mast cell surface is about 6 weeks, and as the antibodies turn over, they become available for binding to anti-IgE antibodies. Thus by giving repeated doses of omalizumab, the number of IgE antibodies on the mast cell surface can be significantly reduced over time. These new IgE molecules are not eliminated but remain in circulation as small immune complexes. IgE receptor numbers on basophils and mast cells may be decreased as a result of downregulation. Because of the extremely expensive nature of this therapy, omalizumab's role strictly limited to allergic asthma.

CLINICAL CONTROVERSY

Omalizumab may offer significant long-term benefits to allergic rhinitis patients, but it may prove to be too expensive to gain widespread acceptance.

As mentioned earlier in this chapter, microbial exposure in the early years of life could help prevent allergic disease by favoring a nonatopic immune response.[5] This concept was further studied by administering *Lactobacillus rhamnosus* prenatally to mothers who had at least one first-degree relative or partner with atopic disease (eczema, allergic rhinitis, or asthma) and postnatally for 6 months to their infants.[44] However, their use may be limited to treatment or prevention of childhood eczema as available evidence shows little benefit in allergic airway diseases.[45]

Other avenues for treating allergic rhinitis include Chinese herbal medicine and acupuncture. Although study designs and the small number of patients included have been questioned, these treatments deserve further study.[46]

PHARMACOECONOMIC CONSIDERATIONS

The economic impact of allergic rhinitis is enormous. The direct costs have grown significantly over the past few years because of the increasing use of peripherally selective antihistamines and nasal steroids. The most recent review of the annual costs of allergic rhinitis in the United States has been estimated at $2 billion and $5 billion.[47] In an older study detailing drug use in allergic rhinitis, 51% of prescribed agents were peripherally selective antihistamines, 25% intranasal steroids, and 5% older antihistamines.[48] A total of 58% of patients received one or more agents. The mean prescription medication expenditure was $103 per patient for those on Medicaid, $155 for patients with private insurance, and $69 for patients with no insurance. Estimates of work productivity losses ranged from $2.4 billion to $4.6 billion.[49] Direct-to-consumer advertising for prescription-only allergic rhinitis treatment options has also increased significantly. How this will affect the prescription market is unknown.

The most cost-effective choice of treatment for allergic rhinitis is an individualized decision. Seasonal allergic rhinitis patients who see improvement and can tolerate nonprescription and/or generic antihistamines will experience the least impact on out-of-pocket medical and drug expenses. If these are ineffective, the economic picture becomes more complicated. Choices should follow the logical path based on symptoms, tolerance, and efficacy, as described earlier in this chapter. Knowledge of an individual patient's drug coverage or lack of drug coverage may drive drug choices.

EVALUATION OF THERAPEUTIC OUTCOMES

With allergic rhinitis, major outcomes include the effect of the disease on a patient's life, the efficacy and tolerability of treatment, and patient satisfaction. Consideration must be given to how the condition is affecting the patient's job or school performance, family and social interactions, and other aspects of quality of life. The drug therapy should prevent or minimize symptoms with minimal or no adverse effects. The patient should not have difficulty obtaining needed medication for financial or other reasons. Patients should be questioned about their satisfaction with the management of their allergic rhinitis. The management should result in minimal disruption to their lives.

Both the Medical Outcomes Study 36-Item Short Form Health Survey and the Rhinoconjunctivitis Quality of Life Questionnaire have been used to evaluate outcomes of treatment for seasonal and perennial allergic rhinitis.[47–49] These tools go beyond measuring improvement in symptoms and include such items as sleep quality, nonallergic symptoms (e.g., fatigue, poor concentration, and others), emotions, and participation in a variety of activities. How well each of the current treatment modalities performs and how they compare in improving patient outcomes remain to be determined.

Clinicians caring for allergic rhinitis patients should develop a comprehensive pharmaceutical care plan that addresses several areas. Discuss and agree on therapeutic end points for allergic rhinitis, including the patient's acceptable level of symptom relief, onset of symptom relief expectations, and seasonal starts and stops. Discuss adverse drug reaction self-monitoring and prevention based on treatment selection. Assess patient attitude toward adherence to and persistence with oral, ocular, intranasal, or immunologic therapies. Ensure proper matching of treatment to symptoms and intervene with the prescriber if necessary. Conduct seasonal or annual review with patient.

The therapeutic goal for all patients with allergic rhinitis is to minimize or prevent symptoms. Evaluation of success is accomplished primarily through the discussions with the patient, in whom both relief of symptoms and tolerance of drug therapy must be discussed.

CONCLUSIONS

Allergic rhinitis is a common disease with symptoms ranging from mild to severe. If avoidance measures are unsuccessful, it should be treated to improve quality of life and prevent long-term complications. Timing of treating is essential. Treatment regimens should be individualized based on patient symptoms and response. Care should be taken to correctly identify allergy as the cause of the patient's rhinitis before committing them to chromic treatment.

ABBREVIATION

IgE: immunoglobulin E

REFERENCES

1. McCrory DC, Williams JW, Dolor RJ, et al. Management of Allergic Rhinitis in the Working-Age Population. Evidence Report/Technology Assessment No. 67. Prepared by Duke Evidence-based Practice Center under Contract No. 290-97-0014. Washington, DC: Agency for Healthcare Research and Quality; 2003.
2. Plaut M, Valentine MD. Allergic rhinitis. N Engl J Med 2005;353:1934–1944.
3. Bousquet J, Khaltaev N, Cruz AA, et al. Allergic rhinitis and its impact on asthma (ARIA) 2008. Allergy 2008;63(suppl 86):8–160.
4. Sauder A, Kovacs M. Anxiety symptoms in allergic patients: Identification and risk factors. Psychosom Med 2003;65:816–823.
5. von Mutius E, Radon K, Living on a farm: Impact on asthma induction and clinical course. Immunol Allergy Clin North Am. 2008;28:631–647.
6. Wallace DV, Dykewicz MS, Bernstein DI, et al. The diagnosis and management of rhinitis: An updated practice parameter. J Allergy Clin Immunol 2008;122:S1–S83.
7. Wilson SJ, Shute JK, Holgate ST, et al. Localization of interleukin (IL)-4 but not 5 to human mast cell secretory granules by immuno-electron microscopy. Clin Exp Allergy 2000;30:493–500.
8. Riccio AAM, Tosco MA, Cosentino C, et al. Cytokine pattern in allergic and non-allergic chronic rhinosinusitis in asthmatic children. Clin Exp Allergy 2002;32:422–426.
9. Wood-Baker R, Lau L, Howarth PH. Histamine and the nasal vasculature: The influence of H1 and H2-histamine receptor antagonism. Clin Otolaryngol 1996;21:348–352.
10. Howarth PH. Mediators of nasal blockage in allergic rhinitis. Allergy 1997;52(40 suppl):12–18.
11. Howarth PH. Leukotrienes in rhinitis. Am J Respir Crit Care Med 2000;161:S133–S136.
12. Clark RR, Baroody FM. What drives the symptoms of allergic rhinitis? J Respir Dis 1998;19:S6–S15.
13. Gerth van Wijk R. Perennial allergic rhinitis and nasal hyperreactivity. Am J Rhinol 1998;12:33–35.
14. Klaewsongkram J, Ruxrungtham K, Wannakrairot P, et al. Eosinophil count in nasal mucosa is more suitable than the number of ICAM-1-positive nasal epithelial cells to evaluate the severity of house dust mite-sensitive allergic rhinitis: A clinical correlation study. Int Arch Allergy Immunol 2003;132:68–75.

15. Braunstahl GJ, Fokkens WJ, Overbeek SE, et al. Mucosal and systemic inflammatory changes in allergic rhinitis and asthma: A comparison between upper and lower airways. Clin Exp Allergy 2003;33:579–587.

16. Hill SL, Krouse JH. The effects of montelukast on intradermal wheal and flare. Otolarygol Head Neck Surg 2003;129:199–203.

17. Trask G, Shapiro G, Shapiro P. The effects of perennial allergic rhinitis on dental and skeletal development: A comparison of sibling pairs. Am J Orthod Dentofacial Orthop 1987;92:286–293.

18. Shapiro G, Shapiro P. Nasal airway obstruction and facial development. Clin Rev Allergy 1984;2:225–236.

19. Custovic A, Wuk RC. The effectiveness of measures to change the indoor environment in the treatment of allergic rhinitis and asthma: ARIA update. Allergy 2005;60:1112–1115.

20. Franchi M, Carrier P, Kotzias D, et al. Working toward healthy air in dwellings in Europe. Allergy 2006;61:864–868.

21. Casale TB, Blaiss MS, Gelfand E, et al. First do no harm: Managing antihistamine impairment in patients with allergic rhinitis. J Allergy Clin Immunol 2003;111:S835–S842.

22. Sansgiry SS, Shringarpure GS. Springtime confusion: Are consumers getting the right information on how to treat seasonal allergies? J Allergy Clin Immunol 2003;112:627–628.

23. Bender BG, Berning S, Dudden R, et al. Sedation and performance impairment of diphenhydramine and second-generation antihistamines: A meta-analysis. J Allergy Clin Immunol 2003;111:770–776.

24. Richardson GS, Roehrs TA, Rosenthal L, et al. Tolerance to daytime sedative effects of H1 antihistamines. J Clin Psychopharmacol 2002;22:511–515.

25. 2003 Survey Pharmacist Survey of OTC Products. Pharm Today 2003;(October suppl):22–26.

26. Berger WE, White MV. Efficacy of azelastine nasal spray in patients with an unsatisfactory response to loratadine. Ann Allergy Asthma Immunol 2003;91:205–211.

27. Astelin. Product Information. Somerset, NJ: Meda Pharmaceuticals; April 2007.

28. Astepro. Product Information, Somerset, NJ: Meda Pharmaceuticals; September 2009.

29. Empey DE, Young GA, Letley E, et al. Dose response study of the nasal decongestant and cardiovascular effects of pseudoephedrine. Br J Clin Pharmacol 1980;9:351–358.

30. Drew CDM, Knight GT, Hughes DTD, et al. Comparison of the effects of D-()-ephedrine and L-(+)-pseudoephedrine on the cardiovascular and respiratory systems in man. Br J Clin Pharmacol 1978;6:221–225.

31. Cantu C, Arauz A, Murilla-Bonilla LM, et al. Stroke associated with sympathomimetics contained in over-the-counter cough and cold drugs. Stroke 2003;34:1667–1673.

32. Facts and Comparisons 4.0 Online Version. St. Louis: Wolters Kluwer; 2006.

33. Mehle ME. Are nasal steroids safe? Curr Opin Otolaryngol Head Neck Surg 2003;11:201–205.

34. Adams RJ, Fuhlbrigge AL, Finkelstein JA, Weiss ST. Intranasal steroids and the risk of emergency department visits for asthma. J Allergy Clin Immunol 2002;109:636–642.

35. Noon L. Prophylactic inoculation against hay fever. Lancet 1911;1:1572–1573.

36. Frew AJ. Immunotherapy of allergic disease. J Allergy Clin Immunol 2003;111:S712–S719.

37. Moller C, Dreborg S, Ferdousi HA, et al. Pollen immunotherapy reduces the development of asthma in children with seasonal rhinoconjunctivitis (the PAT-study). J Allergy Clin Immunol 2002;109:251–256.

38. Durham SR, Walker SM, Varga EM, et al. Long-term clinical efficacy of grass pollen immunotherapy. N Engl J Med 1999;341:468–475.

39. Li JT, Lockey RF, Bernstein IL, et al. Allergen immunotherapy: A practice parameter. Ann Allergy Asthma Immunol 2003;90:1–40.

40. Rodrigo GT, Yanez A. The role of antileukotriene therapy in seasonal allergic rhinitis: A systematic review randomized trials. Ann Allergy Asthma Immunol 2006;96:779–786.

41. Polos PG, Montelukast is an effective monotherapy for mild asthma and for asthma with co-morbid allergic rhinitis. Prim Care Respir J 2006;15:310,311.

42. Casale TB, Condemi J, LaForce C, et al. Effect of omalizumab on symptoms of seasonal allergic rhinitis. JAMA 2001;286:2956–2967.

43. Frew AJ. Anti-IgE and asthma. Ann Allergy Asthma Immunol 2003;91:117–118.

44. Kalliomaki M, Salminen S, Arvilommi H, et al. Probiotics in primary prevention of atopic disease: A randomized placebo-controlled trial. Lancet 2001;357:1076–1079.

45. Boyle RJ, Tang ML. The role of probiotics in the management of allergic disease. Clin Exp Allergy 2006;36:568–576.

46. Xue CC, Li CG, Hugel HM, et al. Does acupuncture or Chinese herbal medicine have a role in the treatment of allergic rhinitis. Curr Opin Allergy Clin Immunol 2006;6:175–179.

47. Reed SD, Lee TA, McCrory DC. The economic burden of allergic rhinitis: A critical evaluation of the literature. Pharmacoeconomics 2004;22:345–361.

48. Law AW, Reed SD, Sundy JS, Schulman KA. Direct costs of allergic rhinitis in the United States: Estimates from the 1996 medical expenditure survey. J Allergy Clin Immunol 2003;111:296–300.

49. Crystal-Peters J, Crown WH, Goetzel RZ, Schutt DC. The cost of productivity losses associated with allergic rhinitis. Am J Manag Care 2000;6:373–378.

CHAPTER

105

Dermatologic Drug Reactions and Common Skin Conditions

REBECCA M. LAW AND DAVID T.S. LAW

KEY CONCEPTS

① The skin is the largest organ of the human body. It performs many vital functions such as (a) protecting the body against injury, physical agents, and UV radiation; (b) regulating body temperature; (c) preventing dehydration, thus helping to maintain fluid balance; (d) acting as a sense organ; and (e) acting as an outpost for immune surveillance. Skin also has a role in vitamin D production and absorption.

② There are age-related factors affecting the epidermis and dermis. Pediatric skin is thinner and better hydrated, which enhances topical drug absorption and potential drug toxicities. Elderly skin is drier, thinner, and more friable, which may predispose to external insults.

③ Patients presenting with a skin condition should be interviewed thoroughly regarding signs and symptoms, urgency, medication history, etc. The skin eruption should be carefully assessed to help distinguish between a disease condition and a drug-induced skin reaction.

④ Drug-induced skin reactions can be irritant or allergic in nature.

⑤ Allergic drug reactions can be classified into exanthematous, urticarial, blistering, and pustular eruptions. Exanthematous reactions include maculopapular rashes and drug hypersensitivity syndrome. Urticarial reactions include urticaria, angioedema, and serum sickness-like reactions. Blistering reactions include fixed drug eruptions, Stevens-Johnson syndrome, and toxic epidermal necrolysis. Pustular eruptions include acneiform drug reactions and acute generalized exanthematous pustulosis. There are other drug-induced skin reactions including hyperpigmentation and photosensitivity.

⑥ Not all skin reactions are drug-induced.

Learning objectives, review questions, and other resources can be found at **www.pharmacotherapyonline.com**.

⑦ Contact dermatitis is a common skin disorder caused either by an irritant or an allergic sensitizer.

⑧ The first goal of therapy in the management of contact dermatitis involves identification, withdrawal, and avoidance of the offending agent. A thorough history, including work history, must be carefully reviewed for potential contactants.

⑨ Other goals of therapy for contact dermatitis include providing symptomatic relief, implementing preventative measures, and providing coping strategies and other information for patients and caregivers.

⑩ Diaper dermatitis is most often seen in infants although the condition may also be seen in older adults who wear diapers for incontinence. Management includes frequent diaper changes, air drying, gentle cleansing, and the use of barriers.

⑪ Skin cancers include squamous cell carcinoma, basal cell carcinoma, and malignant melanoma.

---

① Skin is an essential part of our body. Although it is not commonly thought of as such, skin is an organ. In fact, it is the human body's largest organ, with an average surface area of about 1.8 m².[1] The organ system that includes our skin is known as *the integumentary system*.

The human skin consists of an outer epidermis and an inner dermis. The epidermis primarily provides protection from the environment and performs a critical barrier function—keeping water and other vital substances in and foreign elements out. The dermis is a connective tissue layer that primarily provides resiliency and support for various skin structures or appendages such as sweat glands, sebaceous glands, hair, and nails.

Since the skin surface is such a visible part of our body, changes that are slow or subtle often go unnoticed. Slowly enlarging and evolving moles or dry skin conditions can go undetected, even though such changes can be life threatening in some cases (e.g., malignancy). Health professionals who have direct contact with patients should be able to distinguish between common self-treatable skin lesions and common skin lesions that must be seen and treated professionally, such as melanoma or squamous cell carcinoma.

Skin infections and infestations are not covered in this chapter but are discussed in Chap. 119. Acne, psoriasis, and atopic dermatitis are discussed in Chaps. 106–108.

STRUCTURE AND FUNCTIONS OF THE SKIN

The integumentary system comprises the epidermis and dermis. The epidermis, which is derived from ectoderm, is further divided into four layers: *stratum basale* (basal layer), *stratum spinosum* (prickle cell layer), *stratum granulosum* (granular layer), and *stratum corneum* (horny layer). The *stratum corneum* is the outermost layer of skin and primarily is responsible for the barrier function. The epidermis is thick on the palms and soles and thin on other parts of the body, with some variations. For example, palms and soles contain sweat glands but lack sebaceous glands, which are found almost everywhere else in the skin, with the highest concentration on the face and trunk areas. Sebaceous glands and small hair follicles together form pilosebaceous units, which originate in the dermis and have follicular ducts extending through the epidermis to the skin surface. Sebaceous glands produce sebum, a lipid-like substance.[1] (Increased production by sebaceous glands is partially responsible for acne.[2])

Skin cells are called keratinocytes. They produce keratin, a protein network that gives epithelial cells resilience to mechanical stress. Keratinocytes begin at the *stratum basale* as box-shaped basal cells. As the cells mature, they migrate toward the skin surface, elongating and flattening as they divide and differentiate, ending as corneocytes in the *stratum corneum*. Corneocytes are flattened keratinocytes containing keratin tonofibrils (filaments composed of keratin and keratohyalin granules). They are often termed *dead* since they do not contain nuclei and are not capable of mitosis. Each cell covers a much larger surface area as a corneocyte compared with its basal origin. Overlapping corneocytes provide for the skin barrier.[1] (Note that abnormal keratinocyte activity accounts for some skin diseases. For example, psoriasis is associated with increased keratinocyte cell turnover, and acne is partially caused by increased keratin production.[2])

Melanocytes are pigment-producing cells in the *stratum basale*. They produce melanin, a yellow–brown/black pigment. Melanin granules are spread out into a protective layer in the *stratum corneum*, reducing UV penetration into the skin. UV radiation causes human skin to increase both melanin production and keratinocyte proliferation as a protective effort.[1]

The skin surface is normally covered with a hydrolipid film composed of sweat, oils (sebaceous lipids and free fatty acids), corneocytes, protein decomposition products, and transepidermal water. Some of these are natural moisturizing factors that help the skin retain water. Thus, the hydrolipid film is a permeability barrier that keeps the skin supple.[1]

Due to the presence of lactic acid and various amino acids from sweat, free fatty acids from sebum, and amino acids from shedding corneocytes, our skin is normally acidic, generally with a pH of 5.5 to 6. Bacteria thrive in an alkaline environment. As a result, our skin also functions as a protective acid mantle against invasion by pathogenic bacteria and fungi.[1]

The dermis, which is derived from mesoderm, is a much thicker layer that contains nerve endings and blood vessels. It is made up of collagen and elastin, which provides support for various skin structures and appendages. Eccrine (sweat) glands, hair follicles, sebaceous glands, and arrector pili muscles originate in the dermis. Subcutaneous tissue (adipose tissue with nerves and blood vessels) lies beneath the dermis.[1]

Skin is also involved in regulating body temperature, preventing dehydration, acting as a sense organ, and playing a role in vitamin D production and absorption.

AGE-RELATED CHANGES AND OTHER SKIN-RELATED CONSIDERATIONS

❷ Age-related changes in the structure and functions of the epidermis and dermis are important.

In general, pediatric skin contains more water and is thinner, allowing for enhanced topical drug absorption in both the rate and amount of drug absorbed. This increases the potential for drug toxicities. Increased topical absorption and toxicity has been reported with the use of rubbing alcohol, boric acid powders, and hexachlorophene emulsions and soaps in infants and young children. Even drugs that are not normally used topically may be systemically absorbed. For example, a theophylline gel (17 mg spread over an area 2 cm in diameter) applied to the abdomen of premature infants produced therapeutic serum theophylline concentrations.[3]

Well-hydrated, unbroken skin provides maximal protection against microbial invaders. Aged skin tends to be drier, thinner, and more friable, which increases susceptibility to external insults. In addition, the healing time after skin injury may be prolonged in aged skin. For a video presentation of skin changes due to aging, see *http://www.eucerin.com/en/skin-expertise/journey-through-the-skin*.

UV radiation is associated with accelerated skin aging and skin cancers (e.g., malignant melanoma, basal cell carcinoma). Skin should be constantly protected from UV damage by the use of sunscreens that block both UVA and UVB, with a sun protection factor (SPF) of at least 15, preferably 30 or higher. Sunscreens should be applied 20 minutes before sun exposure and reapplied after sweating or swimming.

It should not be surprising that skin health is related to overall health. Exercise and adequate sleep along with maintaining a healthy, well-balanced diet are key factors. Ample daily fluid intake and regular use of moisturizers are important for skin hydration. Malnourishment can cause a patient to become immunocompromised, which may adversely affect the ability of the skin to act as a barrier. Nutritional deficiencies can cause skin problems including dry skin. Specific food allergies can cause skin reactions (e.g., rashes, hives). Patients with atopic dermatitis often have multiple food sensitivities and allergies resulting in hives and skin rashes, and/or systemic manifestations. For skin cleansing, soapless cleansers may be preferable to soap since they may cause less skin irritation. Repeated and frequent exposure to soap or other cleansers that cause cumulative irritation (e.g., with surfactants and emulsifiers) can result in irritant contact dermatitis.

PATIENT ASSESSMENT

When patients present with dermatologic disorders, a standard approach to assessment should be used. This is especially important for pharmacists who must decide whether to recommend nonprescription therapies or refer patients to medical practitioners, and to nurse practitioners and physician assistants, who must evaluate symptoms and decide whether a supervising physician or dermatologist should be involved.

PATIENT HISTORY: QUESTIONS TO ASK

❸ With all skin conditions, including possible drug-induced reactions, a comprehensive patient history is important. These include questioning and physically assessing the patient to obtain the following information:

- Signs and symptoms
  - *Onset.* When did the lesions first appear? It is important to distinguish between an acute versus a chronic condition.

- *Progression.* Are the lesions improving or worsening/spreading? If lesions are worsening, how quickly are the lesions becoming more severe or widespread?

- *Timeframe.* Did the occurrence of skin lesions correlate temporally with the use of any medications? This may help to distinguish between a drug-induced condition versus a disease-related condition.

- *Location(s) and description of the lesions.* Specific details about where the lesions occur and what they look like will help to identify the type of skin condition. For example, plaque psoriasis is usually diagnosed in this manner and not through laboratory means. However, for conditions such as skin cancers,[4] a skin biopsy may be needed to establish a definitive histopathologic diagnosis.

- *Presenting symptoms.* Is there pruritus? Are the lesions painful? Pruritus is a common symptom for various skin conditions (e.g., atopic dermatitis, allergic and irritant contact dermatitis, psoriasis, bullous pemphigoid, lichen planus, pityriasis rosea) as well as systemic conditions (e.g., chronic renal failure, hepatobiliary diseases, malignancy, parasitosis) and drug reactions.[5]

- *Previous occurrence.* Has the patient presented with similar lesions before? If so, that may be extremely helpful in establishing a diagnosis and deciding on a course of treatment.

- Urgency

  - *Severity, area, and extent of skin involvement.* If a large area of the body is involved, or if signs of severe disease such as skin sloughing or hives (and in some cases if the face is involved) are present, more urgent treatment may be required; and an immediate referral to a physician would be appropriate if the patient were first seen by another health professional such as a pharmacist. In some cases a dermatology consult or an emergency hospital admission would be needed.

  - *Signs of a systemic/generalized reaction or disease condition.* Is there a fever? If there is any indication that the patient has a systemic disease condition, whether drug-induced or disease-related, and particularly if the patient is febrile, this generally indicates a more urgent situation requiring immediate medical attention. For example, erythrodermic psoriasis is distinguishable from plaque psoriasis and would require immediate referral to a physician. (See Chap. 107 for details about psoriasis.)

- Medication history

  - Is the patient using any medication that could potentially cause the observed skin condition? Temporal correlation with medication use is important in evaluating for a potential drug-induced skin reaction. Although possible, drug-induced skin reactions do not generally begin after the offending agent has already been discontinued. However, it is possible for the patient to have used the offending drug for months to years before a skin reaction occurs.

  - If the patient had presented with similar skin lesions previously, was the patient on the same or similar medication(s) at that time? If so, did the skin lesions improve after drug discontinuation?

- Differential diagnosis

  - What other possible diseases or conditions might present in this manner? Is this a disease-related problem, a drug-induced problem, or a food allergy? It is not possible to provide a thorough discussion about differential diagnoses of skin lesions in this chapter. The reader should be aware

that there are differential diagnoses for each type of skin lesion. For example, besides drugs (e.g., antimalarials, cyclophosphamide, clofazimine, busulfan), other causes of hyperpigmentation include Wilson disease, malabsorption syndromes, lymphomas, porphyria cutanea tarda, physical trauma, and others.[6] Besides drugs (e.g., aspirin, nonsteroidal antiinflammatory drugs [NSAIDs], penicillins, sulfonamides, opiates), other causes of urticaria include infection (viral, bacterial, fungal, parasitic), insect stings, foods and food additives, cold, pressure, dermatographism, cholinergic stimulation (exercise, hot shower, emotional stress), hereditary C1 inhibitor deficiency, and others.[7]

LESION ASSESSMENT

As discussed briefly in the following section, the appearance of skin lesions can give some clues as to their causes. Lesions may be categorized as macules (Fig 105-1A and B), papules (Fig 105-2A, B, and C), nodules (Fig 105-3A, B, and C), blisters (Fig 105-4A, B, and C), or plaque and lichenification (Fig 105-5A, B, and C).

However, some skin conditions may cause more than one type of lesion. For example, patients with acne vulgaris may present with macules, papules, nodules, or a combination of these. Another example is psoriasis—the most common type is plaque psoriasis noted by discrete, well-defined plaques; however, there are other types of psoriasis such as guttate or erythrodermic with varying lesions. Wheals developing as a result of a drug reaction may present as papules or plaques. In contrast, some skin conditions present with a characteristic lesion. For example, lichenification is a thickening of the skin usually caused by chronic rubbing or scratching and can be seen in patients with chronic pruritus or atopic dermatitis.

Drug-Induced Skin Reactions

4 Drug-induced skin reactions can be irritant or allergic in origin.

Irritant reactions are localized. Examples include chemical vaginitis, such as those resulting from vaginal douches, spermicides, and imidazoles; and vesication, produced by drug extravasation, as with agents such as anthracyclines.

Allergic reactions depend on inducing an immune response from the host; thus, the reaction may be systemic rather than limited to skin manifestations.

5 Allergic drug reactions can be classified as exanthematous, urticarial, blistering, and pustular eruptions (Fig. 105-6).[8] Skin reactions accompanied by fever are generally more serious systemic disorders. These may be life threatening in some cases, although afebrile skin reactions are not always minor (e.g., urticaria, angioedema).

Maculopapular skin reaction is an afebrile exanthematous eruption that is considered the most commonly encountered allergic skin reaction. Signs and symptoms of a maculopapular skin rash include erythematous macules and papules that may be pruritic. There is no fever, blisters, or pustules. The lesions usually begin within 7–10 days after starting the offending medication, and generally resolve within 7–14 days after drug discontinuation. However, in a previously sensitized patient the onset may be earlier (within 2–3 days). The lesions may spread and become confluent. Usual drug culprits include penicillins, cephalosporins, sulfonamides, and some anticonvulsant medications.

Drug Hypersensitivity Syndrome is an exanthematous eruption accompanied by fever, lymphadenopathy, and multiorgan involvement (including kidneys, liver, lung, bone marrow, heart, and brain). Signs and symptoms begin 1–4 weeks after starting

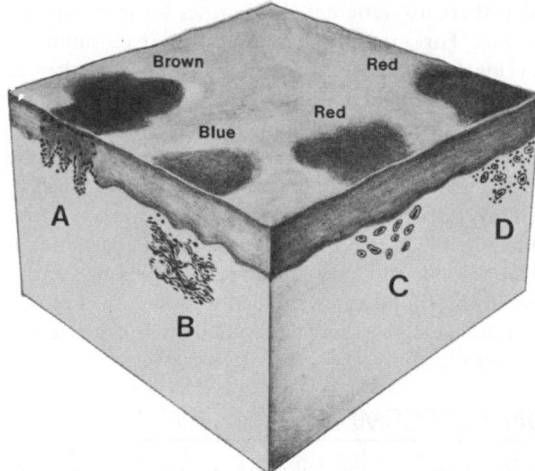

A.

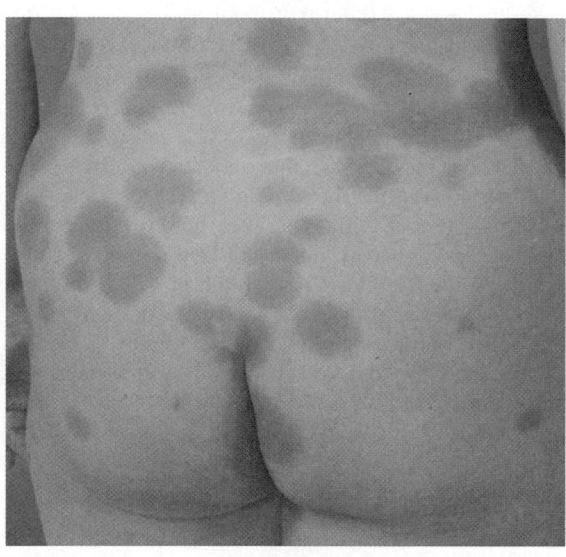

B.

FIGURE 105-1. Macules are circumscribed, flat lesions of any shape or size that differ from surrounding skin because of their color. A. Macules may be the result of hyperpigmentation (*a*), hypopigmentation, dermal pigmentation (*b*), vascular abnormalities, capillary dilation (erythema) (*c*), or purpura (*d*). B. The clinical appearance of a drug reaction that has produced an eruption consisting of multiple, well-defined red macules of varying size that blanch upon pressure (diascopy) and are thus a result of inflammatory vasodilation. (*Reprinted with permission from Stewart MI, Bernhard JD, Cropley TG, Fitzpatrick TB. The structure of skin lesions and fundamentals of diagnosis. In: Freedberg IM, Eisen AZ, Wolff K, et al., eds. Fitzpatrick's Dermatology in General Medicine, 6th ed. New York, NY:McGraw-Hill, 2003:18.*)

the offending drug, and the reaction may be fatal if not promptly treated.

This condition is also known as drug reaction with eosinophilia and systemic symptoms. It is commonly referred to by the acronym DRESS.

Usual drug culprits include allopurinol, sulfonamides, some anticonvulsants (barbiturates, phenytoin, carbamazepine, lamotrigine), and dapsone. For patients taking allopurinol, several factors increase the risk of serious skin reactions: renal impairment, hypertension, and use of thiazide diuretics or excessive allopurinol doses (i.e., not dose-adjusted for renal impairment).[9,10]

Urticaria and angioedema are simple eruptions that are caused by drugs in about 5% to 10% of cases. Other causes include foods (likely the most significant offenders) and physical factors such as

cold or pressure, infections, and exposure to latex. The condition may also be idiopathic.

Urticaria has been called the cutaneous manifestation of anaphylaxis. It is an IgE-related (Type 1) allergic reaction that may be the first symptom of an emerging anaphylactic reaction. It is characterized by hives, extremely pruritic red raised wheals, angioedema, and mucous membrane swelling that typically occurs within minutes to hours (anaphylactoid) (Fig. 105–7). Individual lesions typically last less than 24 hours, but new lesions may continually develop. Offending drugs include penicillins and related antibiotics, aspirin, sulfonamides, X-ray contrast media, opiates, and others. Latex allergy is linked to the natural rubber latex (NRL) proteins, which bind with human IgE and result in contact urticaria, asthma, and anaphylaxis.[11] Aside from latex gloves and medical products, other sources of NRL proteins include rubber insoles of shoes, balloons, inflatable mattresses, and poinsettia plants.

Serum sickness-like reactions are complex urticarial eruptions presenting with fever, rash (usually urticarial), and arthralgias, usually within 1–3 weeks after starting the offending drug. This is not a true serum sickness and there is no immune complex formation, vasculitis, or renal lesions.[8]

Fixed drug eruptions are simple eruptions presenting as pruritic, red, raised lesions that may blister. Symptoms can include burning or stinging. Lesions may evolve into plaques.[8] These so called "fixed" drug eruptions recur in the same area each time the offending drug is given. Lesions appear within minutes to days and also disappear within days, leaving hyperpigmented skin for months (Fig. 105–8). Usual drug culprits include tetracyclines, barbiturates, sulfonamides, codeine, phenolphthalein, acetaminophen, and NSAIDs.

Stevens-Johnson syndrome (SJS) and *toxic epidermal necrolysis* (TEN) are complex blistering eruptions that, together with erythema multiforme (EM), are known as acute bullous disorders. They are histologically similar and have been considered part of an "EM spectrum of diseases."[12] EM may be considered a dermatologic disorder not associated with a drug reaction, whereas SJS and TEN are immune complex or cell-mediated allergic responses to offending agents, including drugs.[12] Because of their histologic similarity, SJS and TEN have been considered either distinct disorders or progressions of the same disorder based on the percentage of skin area involved, and these two entities are often discussed together.[12]

SJS/TEN are rare, severe, and life-threatening conditions with an acute onset (within 7–14 days of drug exposure). Patients present with generalized tender/painful bullous formation with accompanying systemic signs and symptoms, including fever, headache, and respiratory symptoms, that rapidly deteriorate. Lesions show rapid confluence and spread, resulting in extensive epidermal detachment and sloughing.[12] This may result in marked loss of fluids, drop in blood pressure, electrolyte imbalances, and secondary infections, including *Staphylococcus epidermidis* and methicillin-resistant *Staphylococcus aureus* (MRSA). Usual drug culprits include sulfonamides, penicillins, some anticonvulsants (hydantoins, carbamazepine, barbiturates, lamotrigine), NSAIDs, and allopurinol.

Acneiform drug reactions are simple pustular eruptions caused by medications that induce acne (whiteheads or blackheads). The onset is usually about one to three weeks. Common drug culprits include corticosteroids, androgenic hormones, some anticonvulsants, isoniazid, and lithium. Topical acne treatments can be used to manage symptoms if the offending drug cannot be discontinued or replaced.

Acute generalized exanthematous pustulosis (AGEP) is a complex pustular eruption characterized by acute onset (within days after starting the offending drug), fever, diffuse erythema, and many pustules. About one half of patients have other cutaneous lesions, and one quarter have mucosal erosions. Generalized desquamation occurs two weeks later.[8] Usual drug culprits include beta-lactam antibiotics, macrolides, and calcium channel blockers.

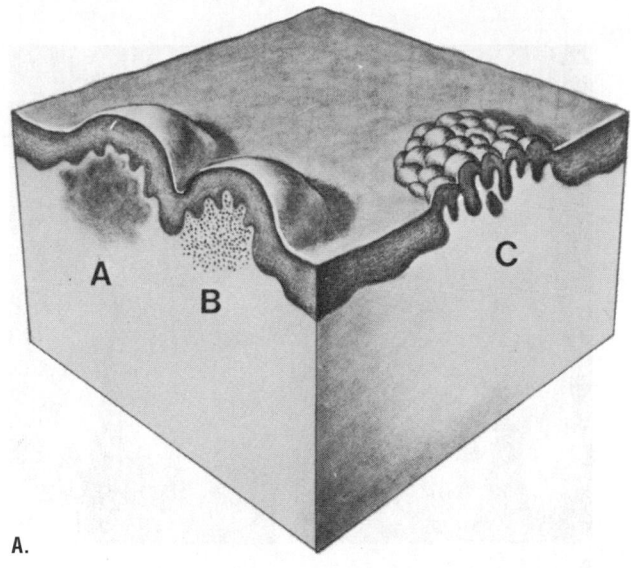

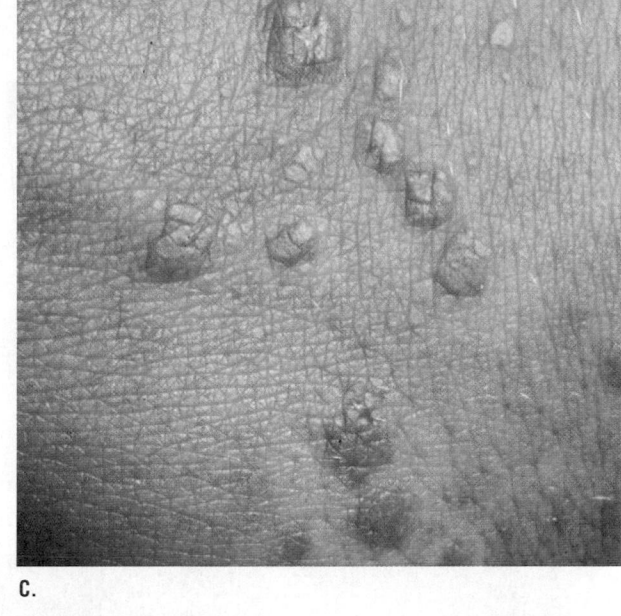

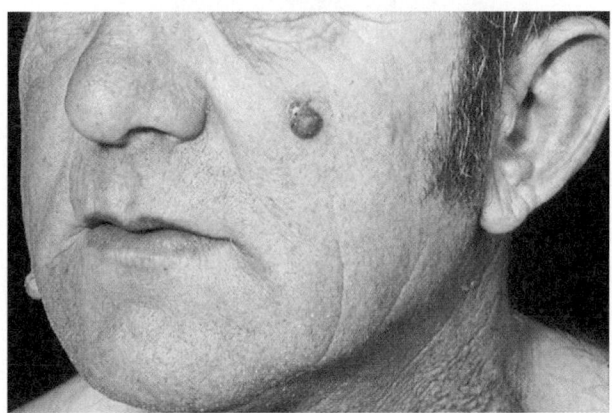

FIGURE 105-2. Papules are small, solid, elevated lesions that are usually less than 1 cm in diameter. The major portion of a papule projects above the plane of the surrounding skin. *A.* Papules may result, for example, from metabolic deposits in the dermis (*a*), from localized dermal cellular infiltrates (*b*), and from localized hyperplasia of cellular elements in the dermis and epidermis (*c*). Papules with scaling are referred to as papulosquamous lesions, as in psoriasis (see Chap. 107). *B.* Clinical examples of papules. The examples are two well-defined and dome-shaped papules of firm consistency and brownish color, which are dermal melanocytic nevi. *C.* Multiple, well-defined, and coalescing papules of varying size are seen. Their violaceous color, glistening surface, and flat tops are characteristic of lichen planus. (*Reprinted with permission from Stewart MI, Bernhard JD, Cropley TG, Fitzpatrick TB. The structure of skin lesions and fundamentals of diagnosis. In: Freedberg IM, Eisen AZ, Wolff K, et al., eds. Fitzpatrick's Dermatology in General Medicine, 6th ed. New York, NY: McGraw-Hill, 2003:18.*)

Other Drug-Induced Skin Reactions *Hyperpigmentation* of the skin (Fig. 105–8) may be related to increased melanin (e.g., hydantoins), direct deposition (e.g., silver, mercury, tetracyclines, antimalarials), or other mechanisms (some cytotoxic drugs, such as 5-fluorouracil, may cause banding on nails or tracking along veins).

Photosensitivity reactions (Fig. 105–9) may be phototoxic or photoallergic. Drugs that induce phototoxic reactions absorb ultraviolet A (UVA) light, resulting in skin damage. Severity tends to be proportional to the drug dose. Usual drug culprits include amiodarone, tetracyclines, sulfonamides, psoralens, and coal tar.

Drug-induced photoallergic reactions result from UVA transformation of medications into allergens. In this syndrome, skin damage may occasionally spread beyond sun-exposed skin. These reactions require sensitization to the offending drug and are not dose-related. Usual drug culprits include sulfonamides, sulfonylureas, thiazides, NSAIDs, chloroquine, and carbamazepine.

Management and Prevention of a Drug-Induced Skin Reaction ❻ The first rule of thumb in managing skin reactions is to remember that not all are drug-induced. In clinical practice, a diagnosis of drug-induced skin reaction is often a diagnosis of

exclusion (i.e., the diagnosis is reached after other possible diagnoses have been ruled out). Potential foods and other causes have to be thoroughly investigated, and a detailed patient interview is important, as discussed earlier. Consistent with the assessment for any adverse drug reaction, the likelihood of a drug-induced skin reaction should be categorized as probable, possible, or not probable (unlikely). It may not be possible to categorize a drug-induced skin reaction as definite, as this requires rechallenge with the potentially offending agent, and this should not be done with most reactions. Reactions are often unpredictable adverse drug reactions unrelated to the normal pharmacologic effects of the drug. Fortunately, unpredictable adverse drug reactions (e.g. allergic, idiosyncratic, carcinogenic) usually affect only a small percentage of patients.

If a drug-induced skin reaction is suspected, the most important treatment in nearly all cases is discontinuing the suspected drug as quickly as possible and avoiding the use of potential cross-sensitizers. In most instances, that is the only specific treatment required. In severe cases a short course of systemic corticosteroids may be needed. In a few instances it may be possible to continue the offending drug and "treat through" the reaction[8] (e.g., ampicillin-associated maculopapular skin rash).

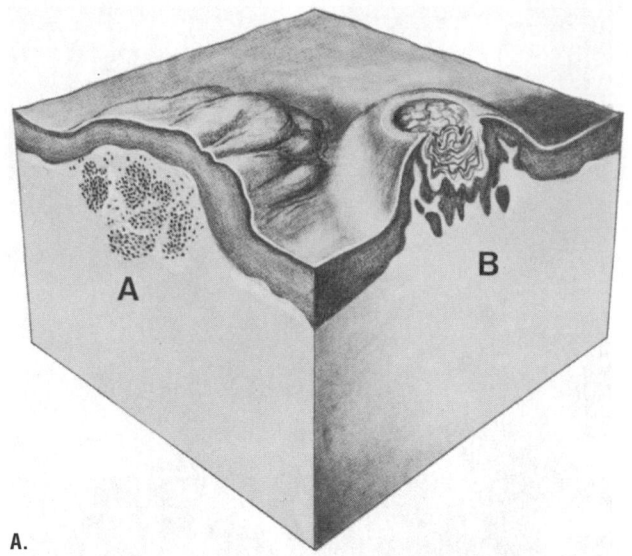

A.

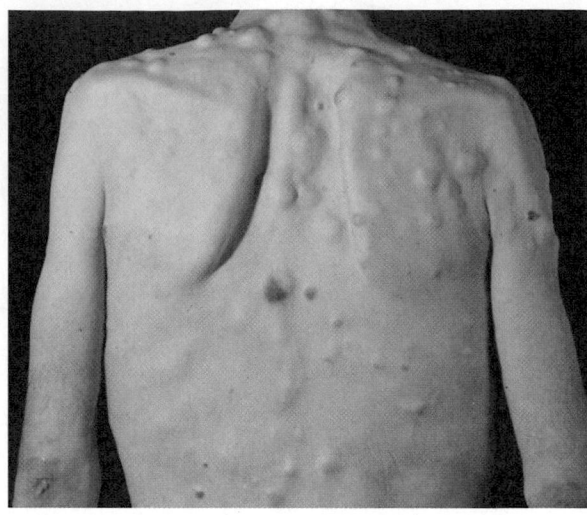

C.

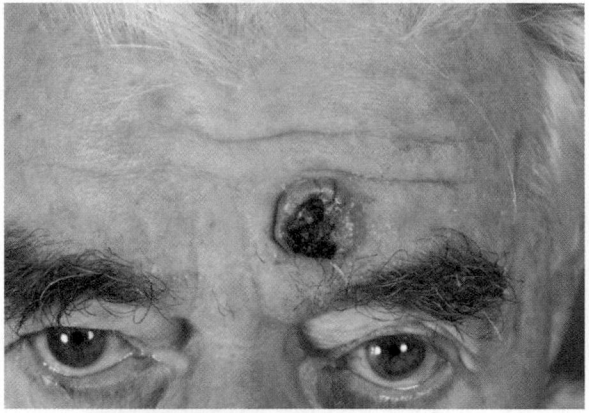

B.

FIGURE 105-3. Nodules are palpable, solid, round or ellipsoidal lesions. Depth of involvement and/or substantive palpability, rather than diameter, differentiates a nodule from a papule. *A.* Nodules may extend into the dermis or subcutaneous tissue (*a*) or be located in the epidermis (*b*). *B.* This photograph shows a well-defined, firm nodule with a smooth and glistening surface through which telangiectasia (dilated capillaries) can be seen; there is central crusting indicating tissue breakdown and thus incipient ulceration (nodular basal cell carcinoma). *C.* Multiple nodules of varying size can be seen (melanoma metastases). (*Reprinted with permission from Stewart MI, Bernhard JD, Cropley TG, Fitzpatrick TB. The structure of skin lesions and fundamentals of diagnosis. In: Freedberg IM, Eisen AZ, Wolff K, et al., eds. Fitzpatrick's Dermatology in General Medicine, 6th ed. New York, NY: McGraw-Hill, 2003:18.*)

The next step is to control symptoms associated with the drug reaction (e.g., pruritus). Furthermore, any signs or symptoms of a systemic or generalized reaction may require additional supportive therapies specific to the severity and type of signs and symptoms seen. For high fevers, an antipyretic such as acetaminophen is more appropriate than aspirin or an NSAID, as these may exacerbate skin lesions for some reactions. Depending on the type of skin reaction, the affected skin condition may take days to weeks or months to resolve.

For patients with life-threatening SJS/TEN, supportive measures such as maintenance of adequate blood pressure, fluid and electrolyte balance, use of broad-spectrum antibiotics and vancomycin for secondary infections, and intravenous immunoglobulin (IVIG) may all be appropriate. IVIG has been shown to halt disease progression and enhance recovery for SJS/TEN.[12] The use of corticosteroids for SJS/TEN is somewhat controversial; although they may curb disease progression they may also increase the risk of infection and thus contribute to increased mortality.[12] If used, relatively high initial doses followed by rapid tapering as soon as disease progression halts is indicated.[12] Refer to the Drug-Induced Skin Reactions case in the *Pharmacotherapy Casebook* to further explore management.

Patient education should be provided. Advice to the patient should include information about the suspected drug and potential drugs to avoid in the future, and which drugs may be used. Potential cross-sensitizers should be identified. For patients with photosensitivity reactions, provide information about preventive measures such as the use of sunscreens and sun avoidance (Fig. 105–9). For patients with severe reactions (e.g., anaphylaxis), information about MedicAlert programs may be appropriate. Genetic predisposition has not been established for most drug-induced reactions, but for severe reactions such as SJS/TEN or hypersensitivity syndromes, the risk may be higher in first-degree relatives of affected patients.

COMMON SKIN DISORDERS

Contact Dermatitis

❼ Contact dermatitis is defined as an inflammation of the skin caused by irritants or allergic sensitizers.[13] It describes and includes all skin reactions resulting from direct contact of the skin or mucous membranes with an exogenous agent, which may be a "foreign" molecule such as a drug or chemical, UV light, or temperature.[13]

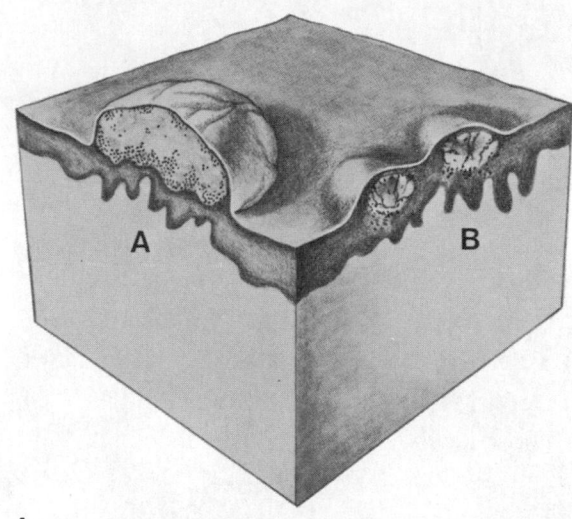

A.

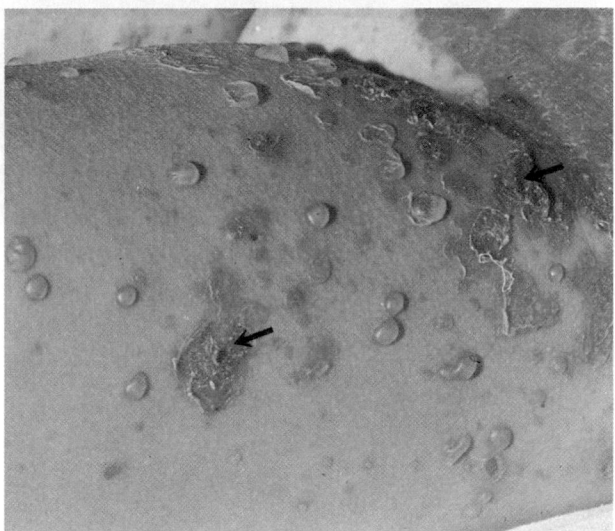

B.

FIGURES 105-4. Vesicles and bullae are the technical terms for blisters. Vesicles are circumscribed lesions that contain fluids, while bullae are vesicles that are larger than 0.5 cm in diameter. *A.* Subcorneal vesicles (*a*) result from fluid accumulation just below the stratum corneum, whereas spongiotic vesicles (*b*) result from intercellular edema. *B.* Multiple translucent subcorneal vesicles are extremely fragile, collapse easily, and thus lead to crusting (arrows). These lesions are staphylococcal impetigo. (*Reprinted with permission from Stewart MI, Bernhard JD, Cropley TG, Fitzpatrick TB. The structure of skin lesions and fundamentals of diagnosis. In: Freedberg IM, Eisen AZ, Wolff K, et al., eds. Fitzpatrick's Dermatology in General Medicine, 6th ed. New York: McGraw-Hill, 2003:18.*)

The skin or mucous membranes may react nonimmunologically and/or immunologically to an exogenous agent, resulting in either an irritant or allergic skin reaction as described earlier. However, the distinction between an allergic contact dermatitis (ACD) and irritant contact dermatitis (ICD) has become increasingly blurred[13]; ICD is often a diagnosis of exclusion, as in cases where patch test results for ACD are negative.[13]

In addition, an exogenous dermatitis can be superimposed on an endogenous skin eruption such as acne.[13] Irritant effects may be considerably enhanced by occlusion. Contact dermatitis must also be distinguished from atopic dermatitis and other dermatologic conditions such as dyshidrotic dermatitis, Lichen simplex

dermatitis, acne rosacea, and other conditions. (See Chap. 108 for a discussion on atopic dermatitis).

Contact dermatitis is a common skin problem for which 5.7 million physician visits are made per year.[13] Almost any of the more than 85,000 chemicals in the world environment may be a skin irritant, and more than 3,700 substances have been identified as contact allergens.[13] Although all age groups may be affected, ACD is rare in the first years of life (<10 years), but the rate of occurrence in older children may exceed that in adults.[13]

The prevalences of ACD to individual allergens is similar in children and adults; allergens include nickel, fragrances, *Toxicodendron* (formerly known as *Rhus*), and rubber chemicals.[13] There may be a slight female preponderance, presumably due to exposure to specific contactants in jewelry and cosmetics.[13]

The clinical presentation of contact dermatitis is that of an eczematous inflammation, with erythema, vesicles, papules, crusting, fissuring, or scaling (see Figs. 105–10 and 105–11A and B). The area may itch, burn, or sting and may be extremely pruritic. The severity may range from a mild, short-lived condition to a severe and persistent condition but is rarely life-threatening.[13] The gross and histologic appearances of ICD and ACD are often similar and may be difficult to distinguish.[13] However, the rash/lesion for ICD is frequently localized whereas for ACD it may extend beyond the borders of the exposed area of contact, and the reaction may rarely become systemic (e.g., latex allergy).

ICD is generally a multifactorial response involving contact with a substance that chemically abrades, irritates, or otherwise damages the skin; cellular damage in ICD occurs via T-cells (activated by irritant or innate mechanisms) releasing proinflammatory cytokines.[13] ACD is the clinical manifestation of contact hypersensitivity;[14] skin allergens tend to be low-molecular weight molecules (haptens) that become immunogenic after conjugation with skin proteins, resulting in a complex series of interactions that involve antigen-presenting Langerhans and/or other dendritic cells, or CD4+ and CD8+ T cells,[13] including IL-17–producing T_H17 cells.[14]

Since ACD is immunologically-mediated the patient may have tolerated exposure to the offending agent for some time, making it more difficult to pinpoint the culprit. Furthermore, the reaction may continue to develop for some time after the offending agent is removed.

❽ The first goal of therapy in the management of contact dermatitis involves identifying, withdrawal, and avoidance of the offending agent. A thorough history including work history must be carefully reviewed for potential contactants. Nonwork activities such as hobbies (e.g., painting, gardening, camping, fishing) may be additional potential sources of exposure. Patch testing is the gold standard for identifying a contact allergen[13] but it is impractical to test an unlimited number of allergens.

Standard panels of allergens have been designed and validated by collaborative research dermatologic societies; however, these may account for only 25% to 30% of the most relevant contact allergens.[13] Many patients need additional testing, Customized patch tests may be needed, depending on the patient's exposure history.[13]

The most common causes of occupational contact dermatitis are chromium (leather exposure), rubber and rubber additives (gloves), nickel (work tools and metal working), food ingredients including intact proteins (for food processing workers), fertilizers and pesticides (for farmers), and handwashing (disinfectants, irritants in soaps).[13]

The most common cause of plant dermatitis is *Toxicodendron* (*Rhus*) dermatitis. This genus includes poison ivy, poison oak, and poison sumac. These plants contain the offender urushiol oil, one of several oleoresins that are sensitizers and irritants. Urushiol oil is also found in mango skin, cashew nut oil, ginkgo (female) leaves, Japanese lacquer, and Indian marking ink.[13]

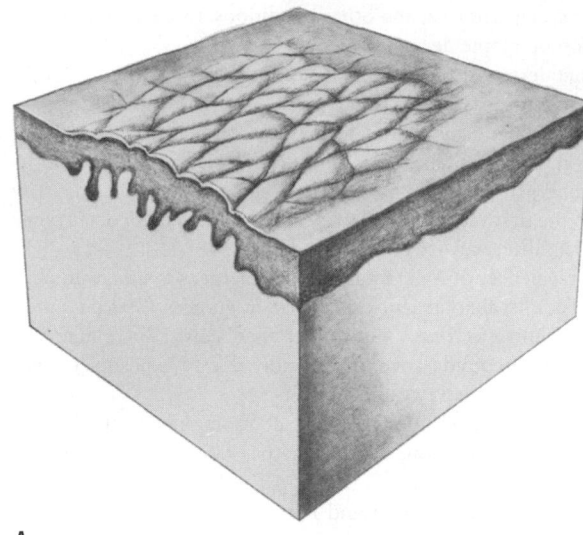

A.

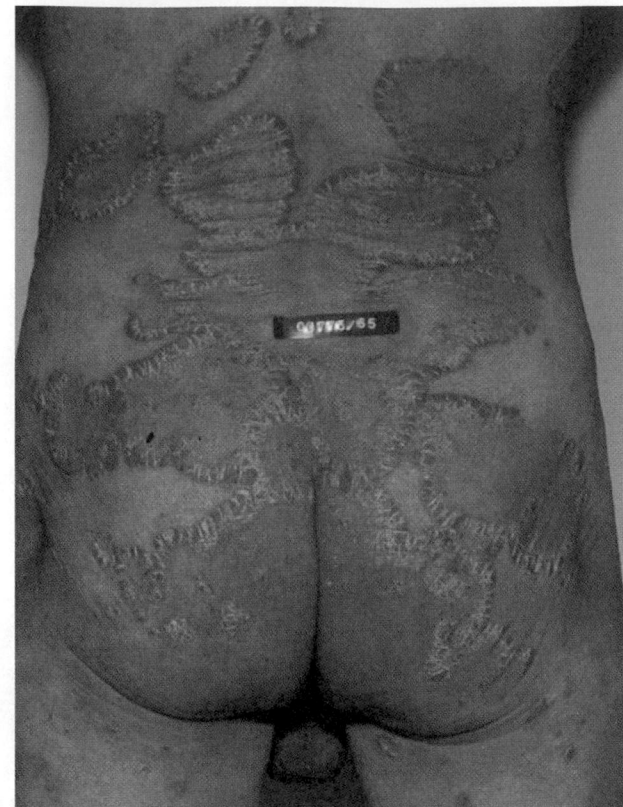

B.

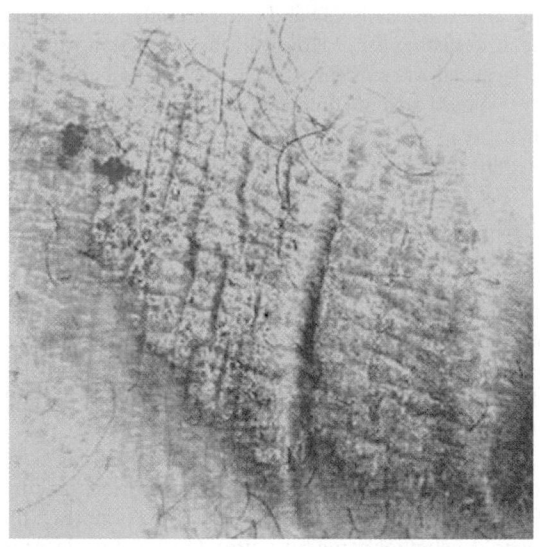

C.

FIGURE 105-5. *A.* Plaque is a mesa-like elevation that occupies a relatively large surface area relative to its height above the skin surface. *B.* Well-defined, reddish, scaling plaques can coalesce to cover large areas of the back and buttocks, with some regression in the center as is common in psoriasis (see Chap. 107). *C.* Lichenification, a thickening of the skin and accentuation of skin, can result from repeated rubbing. It develops frequently in patients with atopy, and also occurs in eczematous dermatitis or other conditions associated with pruritus. Lesions of lichenification are not as well defined as most plaques and often show signs of scratching, such as in excoriations and crusts. (*Reprinted with permission from Stewart MI, Bernhard JD, Cropley TG, Fitzpatrick TB. The structure of skin lesions and fundamentals of diagnosis. In: Freedberg IM, Eisen AZ, Wolff K, et al., eds. Fitzpatrick's Dermatology in General Medicine, 6th ed. New York: McGraw-Hill, 2003:18, and Garg Amit, Levin Nikki A, Bernhard Jeffrey D. Structure of Skin Lesions and Fundamentals of Clinical Diagnosis. In: Wolff K, Goldsmith LA, Katz SI, Gilchrest B, Paller AS, Leffell DJ, eds. Fitzpatrick's Dermatology in General Medicine, 7th ed. http://www.accessmedicine.com/content.aspx?aID=2965385*).

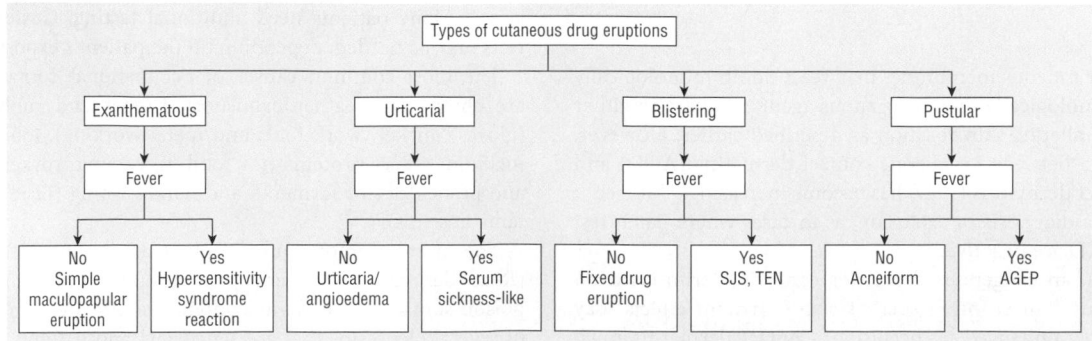

FIGURE 105-6. Types of cutaneous drug eruptions. Adapted from Knowles S. Drug-induced Skin Reactions, Figure 46–1. In: Patient Self-Care (PSC). Ontario, Canada: Canadian Pharmacists Association, 2002.[8]

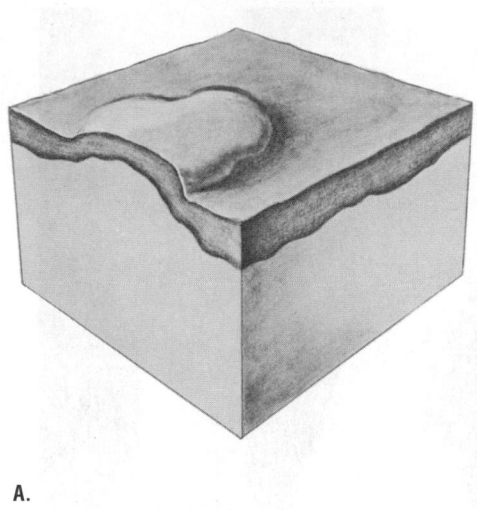
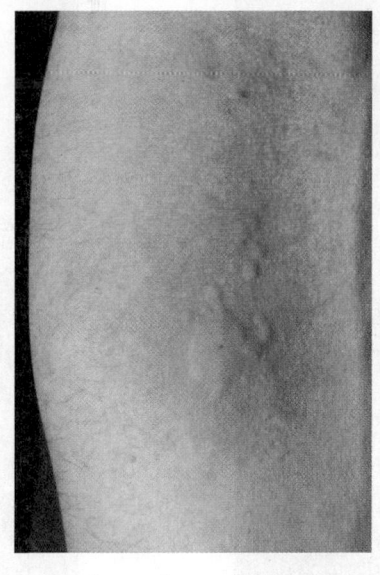
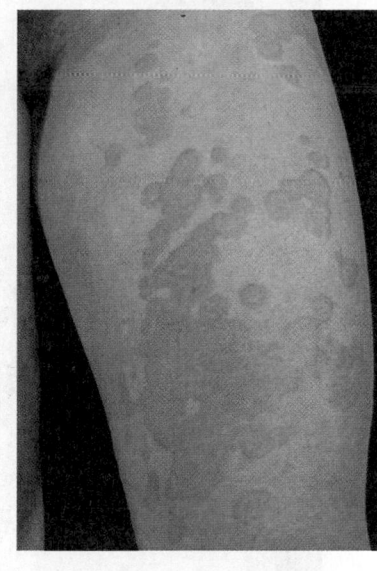

FIGURE 105-7. *A.* Wheals are rounded or flat-topped papules or plaques that are characteristically evanescent, disappearing within hours. An eruption consisting of wheals is termed urticaria and usually itches. *B.* Wheals may be tiny papules 3 to 4 mm in diameter, as in cholinergic urticaria. *C.* Alternatively, wheals may present as large, coalescing plaques, as in allergic reactions to penicillin, other drug, or alimentary allergens. (*Reprinted with permission from Stewart MI, Bernhard JD, Cropley TG, Fitzpatrick TB. The structure of skin lesions and fundamentals of diagnosis. In: Freedberg IM, Eisen AZ, Wolff K, et al., eds. Fitzpatrick's Dermatology in General Medicine, 6th ed. New York: McGraw-Hill, 2003:18.*)

Cosmetics and personal hygiene products, such as hair conditioners and shampoos, nail polishes and hardeners, mascara, foundations, antiperspirants and deodorants, and toothpastes, may all contain potential causes of contact dermatitis. The most important classes are fragrances, preservatives, formulation excipients, glues, and sunblocks;[13] fragrances are among the most common causes of contact dermatitis in the United States.[13]

❾ The second goal of therapy in contact dermatitis is to provide symptomatic relief while decreasing skin lesions. The affected skin may require supportive treatment such as the use of cold compresses to sooth and cleanse the skin, or topical corticosteroids to help resolve the inflammatory process. Compresses are applied to wet or oozing lesions, removed, remoistened, and reapplied every few minutes for a 20–30 minute period. Calamine lotion or Burow solution (aluminum acetate) may be soothing.

Topical corticosteroids are considered the mainstay of treatment, and ACD responds better than ICD. Generally, higher potency corticosteroids are used initially, switching to medium or lower potency corticosteroids as the condition improves.[13] Refer to the

FIGURE 105-8. Hyperpigmentation. This patient exhibits a striking amiodarone-induced, slate-gray pigmentation of the face. The blue color (ceruloderma) is caused by deposition of a brown pigment in the dermis, contained in macrophages, and endothelial cells. (*Reprinted with permission from Ortonne J-P, Bahadoran P, Fitzpatrick TB, et al. Hypomelanoses and hypermelanoses. In: Freedberg IM, Eisen AZ, Wolff K, et al., eds. Fitzpatrick's Dermatology in General Medicine, 6th ed. New York: McGraw-Hill, 2003:876.*)

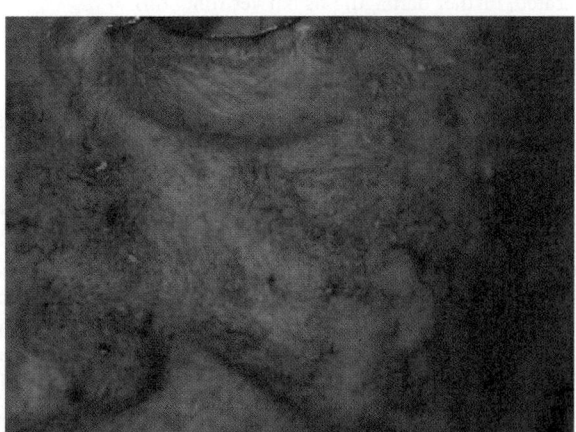

FIGURE 105-9. Photosensitivity. Severe solar damage of the face revealing both telangiectasias and actinic keratoses at different stages in development, including the flat, pink macules and hyperkeratotic papules. (*Reprinted with permission from Duncan KO, Leffell DJ. Epithelial precancerous lesions. In: Freedberg IM, Eisen AZ, Wolff K, et al., eds. Fitzpatrick's Dermatology in General Medicine, 6th ed. New York: McGraw-Hill, 2003:722.*)

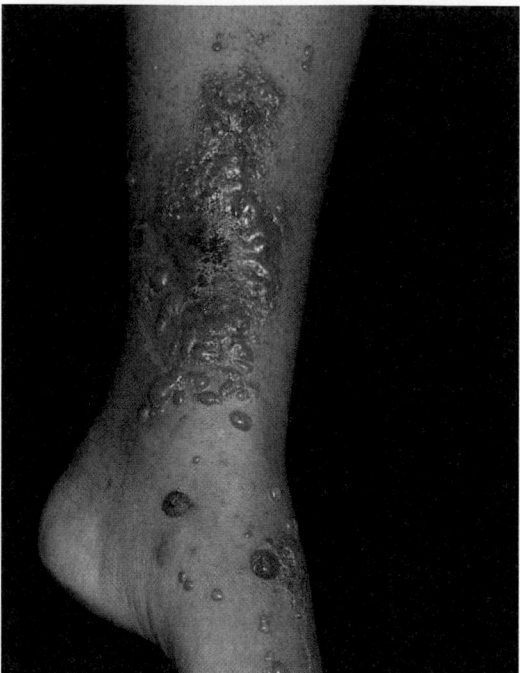

FIGURE 105-10. Acute dermatitis caused by poison ivy. Note the linear arrangement of lesions typical of phytodermatitis acquired by inadvertent contact with the plant. The severe vesiculobullous reaction is typical for urushiol, an oily poisonous irritant found in Toxicodendron spp. (*Reprinted with permission from Belsito DV. Allergic contact dermatitis. In: Freedberg IM et al., eds. Fitzpatrick's Dermatology in General Medicine, 6th ed. New York: McGraw-Hill, 2003:1167.*)

Topical Corticosteroid Potency Chart in Chap. 107 (Table 107–2) for specific examples.

Other treatments may be effective. Tacrolimus ointment has been shown to be effective for nickel-induced ACD in a small randomized placebo-controlled clinical trial.[15] Oatmeal baths or oral first-generation antihistamines may provide relief for excessive itching. If the affected areas are already dry or hardened (e.g., lichenification), wet dressings applied as soaks (without removal for up to 20–30 minutes) will soften and hydrate the skin (these should not be used for acute exudating lesions, as the skin area may become macerated, further damaging its barrier function).

The third goal of contact dermatitis therapy is to implement preventive measures. Prevention involves both primary and secondary measures.

Primary prevention may be done in the workplace, by initiating surveillance programs and educating workers about proper skin care and chemical exposure.

Secondary prevention involves the use of moisturizers to prevent dryness and fissuring of the skin. The efficacy of barrier creams is controversial.[13] The damaged skin may need to be protected against secondary infections, at least until the acute stage subsides. Debris, produced by oozing, scaling, or crusting, should not be allowed to accumulate. Rarely, some workers may have persistent dermatitis despite removal of offenders, and a small number of workers change jobs because of severe recalcitrant OCD.[13]

A final goal of therapy is to provide patient and caregiver information and support, helping them to develop coping strategies for contact dermatitis, as required.

Diaper Dermatitis

❿ Diaper dermatitis, more commonly known as diaper rash, is most often seen in infants, although the condition may also be

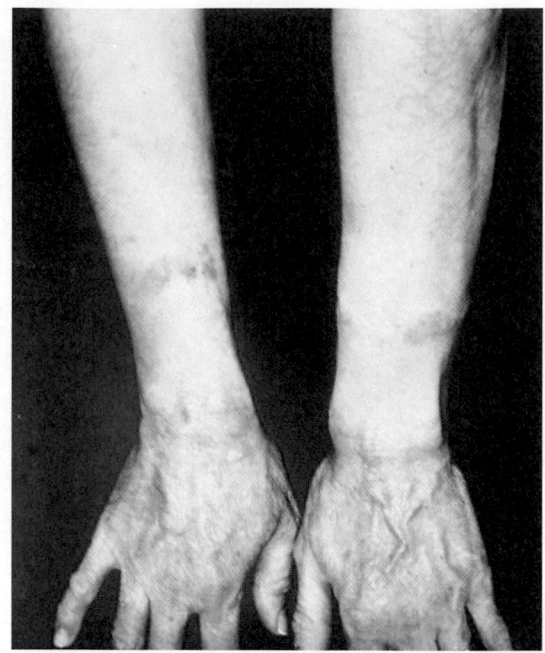

A.

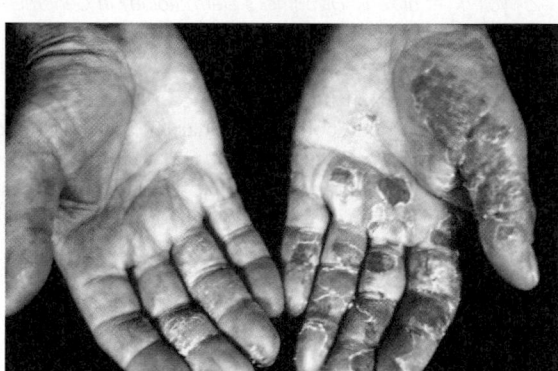

B.

FIGURE 105-11A AND 105-11B. 105–11A This patient has allergic chronic dermatitis involving the dorsal aspects of the hands and the distal forearms, but with minimal involvement of the palms. In this case, contact dermatitis is secondary to use of thiuram present in rubber gloves, prescribed for treatment of an irritant hand dermatitis. 105–11B. This patient, a florist, has allergic contact dermatitis as a consequence of exposure to tuliposide A, the allergen in Peruvian lilies (Alstroemeria spp.). Note the more prominent involvement of the palms of the dominant hand. (*Reprinted with permission from Belsito DV. Allergic contact dermatitis. In: Freedberg IM et al., eds. Fitzpatrick's Dermatology in General Medicine, 6th ed. New York: McGraw-Hill, 2003:1167.*)

seen in older adults who wear diapers for incontinence. It is an acute inflammatory dermatitis affecting the buttocks, genital, and perineum regions that are covered by the diaper. The rash is erythematous, and severe rashes may have vesicles or oozing erosions. The rash may be infected by *Candida* species and present with confluent red plaques, papules, and pustules.

Management of diaper dermatitis includes frequent diaper changes, air drying (removing the diaper as long as practical), gentle cleansing (preferably with nonsoap cleansers and lukewarm water), and the use of barriers. Commercial diaper wipes containing fragrance or alcohol should be avoided. Zinc oxide has astringent and absorbent properties, and provides an effective barrier. Petrolatum also provides a water-impermeable barrier but has no absorbent ability and may trap moisture.

Patients with candidal (yeast) diaper rash should be treated with a topical antifungal agent then covered by a barrier product. Imidazoles are the treatment of choice for this type of diaper rash. Once the rash subsides, the antifungal agent should be stopped and the barrier product continued.

In severe inflammatory diaper rashes a very low potency topical corticosteroid (hydrocortisone 0.5% to 1%) may be used for short periods of one to two weeks.

Skin Cancers

Actinic keratoses are precursors to the development of skin cancers. UV radiation (with UVA a greater risk than UVB) may induce abnormal keratinocyte changes. These present as actinic keratoses. These lesions can develop into squamous cell or basal cell carcinomas.

Actinic keratoses are most often found in elderly fair-skinned patients and on chronically sun-exposed areas, such as hands, forearms, head, and neck.

Squamous Cell Carcinoma (SCC) is a skin cancer most commonly seen in older patients (Fig. 105–12). Risk factors include fair complexion, prolonged sun exposure, UV radiation (including PUVA used for treatment of psoriasis), long-term immunosuppression (including the use of biologic response modifiers for treatment of conditions such as psoriasis). Most SCCs present as firm, flesh-colored, or erythematous papules or plaques. Treatment is primarily via surgical excision.

Basal Cell Carcinoma (BCC) is a very common skin disorder (Fig. 105–13). BCC most commonly presents as a pigmented nodule on the head and neck. Treatment may vary based on histology and may involve surgical excision as well as the use of topical agents such as imiquimod or antineoplastic agents, such as 5-fluorouracil.

Malignant melanoma, unless detected early and excised, often produces systemic metastases. Its incidence has increased over the past few decades, with an estimated 1 in 65 Americans developing melanoma during their lifetimes.[16]

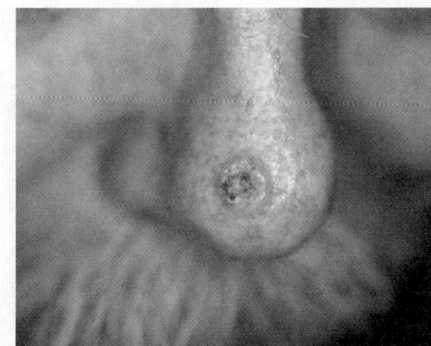

A.

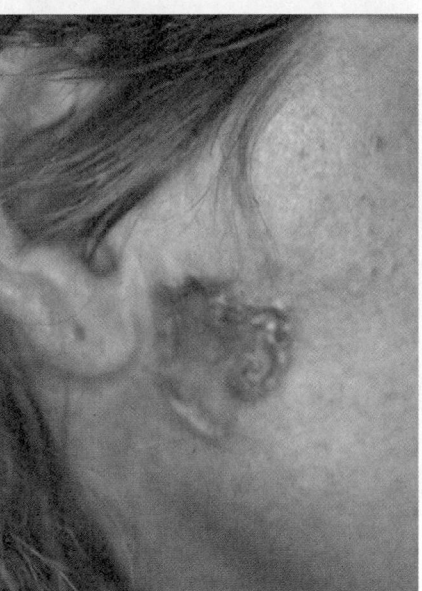

B.

FIGURE 105-13A AND 105-13B. Basal Cell Carcinoma. 105-13A. Basal cell carcinoma, nodular type. 105-13B. An ulcerated nodular basal cell carcinoma. (*Reprinted with permission from Carucci JA, Leffell DJ. Basal cell carcinoma. In: Freedberg IM, Eisen AZ, Wolff K, et al., eds. Fitzpatrick's Dermatology in General Medicine, 6th ed. New York: McGraw-Hill, 2003:749.*)

A changing mole is often a harbinger of melanoma. These are detected by skin examination; dermatologists often have melanoma clinics for this purpose. Moles are examined for asymmetry, irregular borders, variegated colors, and size. (See Fig. 105–14A and B). Full-body skin exams are important in screening for melanoma, as it can occur anywhere on the skin.[16]

Other risk factors include prolonged sun exposure and ability to tan, family history, and drug treatments such as PUVA or biologic response modifiers used for psoriasis.

Suspicious pigmented lesions should be fully excised as soon as possible rather than biopsied; malignant melanomas are best diagnosed and microstaged with an excisional biopsy of the entire lesion.[17] Delayed diagnosis of malignant melanoma directly affects patient survival adversely.[16] Treatment may also include systemic antineoplastic therapy, such as temozolomide or dacarbazine for metastatic melanoma.

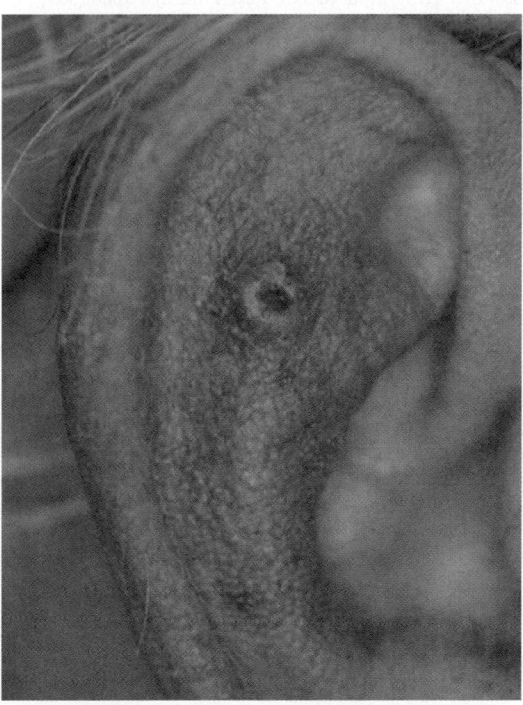

FIGURE 105-12. Squamous Cell Carcinoma. This case of squamous cell carcinoma must be differentiated in diagnosis from chondrodermatitis nodularis helicis, which, unlike the carcinoma, is painful. (*Reprinted with permission from Grossman D, Leffell DJ. Squamous cell carcinoma. In: Freedberg IM, Eisen AZ, Wolff K, et al., eds. Fitzpatrick's Dermatology in General Medicine, 6th ed. New York: McGraw-Hill, 2003:738.*)

CONCLUSIONS

This chapter provided coverage about the skin and associated age-related changes, lesion assessment and recognition, drug-induced skin reactions, contact dermatitis, diaper dermatitis, and briefly discussed common skin cancers. Other common skin disorders

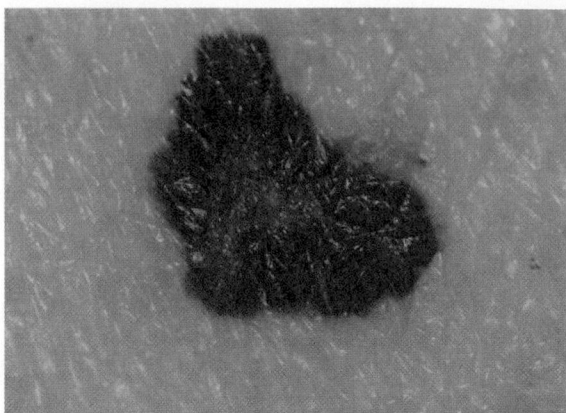

A.

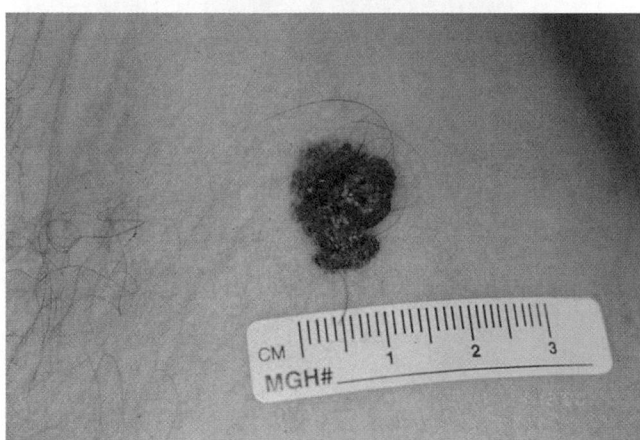

B.

FIGURE 105-14A AND 105-14B. Melanomas. These two superficial spreading melanomas illustrate the ABCDs of melanoma. *A*, asymmetry. The lesions are not symmetrical and often have irregular borders. *B*, border. Note the highly irregular, uneven, and notched border. *C*, color. The color is variegated with different shades of brown, black, and tan. *D*, diameter. The diameter is usually (but not always) more than 6 mm in melanomas. (*Reprinted with permission from Langley RGB, Barnhill RL, Mihm MC Jr, et al. Neoplasms: Cutaneous melanoma. In: Freedberg IM, Eisen AZ, Wolff K, et al., eds. Fitzpatrick's Dermatology in General Medicine, 6th ed. New York: McGraw-Hill, 2003:925.*)

are covered in the following three chapters, including acne (see Chap. 106), psoriasis (see Chap. 107), and atopic dermatitis (see Chap. 108). Skin and soft tissue infections (Chap. 119) and parasitic diseases (Chap. 124) are detailed later in this text.

ABBREVIATIONS

ACD: allergic contact dermatitis

BCC: basal cell carcinoma

EM: erythema multiforme

ICD: irritant contact dermatitis

IVIG: intravenous immunoglobulin

NRL: natural rubber latex

NSAID: nonsteroidal antiinflammatory agent

SCC: squamous cell carcinoma

SJS: Stevens-Johnson syndrome

TEN: toxic epidermal necrolysis

UV: ultraviolet

UVA: ultraviolet A

REFERENCES

1. Franz TJ, Lehman PA. The skin as a barrier: Structure and function. In: Kydonieus AF, Wille JJ, eds. Biochemical modulation of skin reactions: Transdermals, topicals, cosmetics. New York, NY: CRC Press, 2000.
2. Law RM. The pharmacist's role in the treatment of acne. Am Pharm 2003;125(6):35–42.
3. Evans NJ, Rutter N, Hadgraft J et al. Percutaneous administration of theophylline in the preterm infant. Journal Pediatr 1985:107(2): 307–311.
4. Sober AJ. 177. Screening for Skin Cancers In: Goroll AH, Mulley AG, eds. Primary Care Medicine: Office Evaluation and Management of the Adult Patient, 4th ed. Philadelphia, PA: Lippincott Williams & Wilkins, 2000:995–1001.
5. Shellow WVR. 178. Evaluation of Pruritus. In: Goroll AH, Mulley AG, eds. Primary Care Medicine: Office Evaluation and Management of the Adult Patient, 4th ed. Philadelphia, PA: Lippincott Williams & Wilkins, 2000:1001–1004.
6. Shellow WVR. 180. Evaluation of Disturbances in Pigmentation. In: Goroll AH, Mulley AG, eds. Primary Care Medicine: Office Evaluation and Management of the Adult Patient, 4th ed. Philadelphia, PA: Lippincott Williams & Wilkins, 2000:1008–1010.
7. Shellow WVR. 181. Evaluation of Urticaria and Angioedema. In: Goroll AH, Mulley AG, eds. Primary Care Medicine: Office Evaluation and Management of the Adult Patient, 4th ed. Philadelphia, PA: Lippincott Williams & Wilkins, 2000:1011–1015.
8. Knowles S. Drug-induced Skin Reactions. In: Patient Self-Care (PSC). Ontario, Canada: Canadian Pharmacists Association, 2002:584–591.
9. Arellano F, Sacristan JA. Allopurinol hypersensitivity syndrome: A review. Ann Pharmacother 1993:27(3):337–343.
10. Lee HY, Ariyasinghe JTN, Thirumoorthy T. Allopurinol hypersensitivity syndrome: A preventable severe cutaneous adverse reaction? Singapore Med J 2008;49(5):384–387.
11. Bernstein J. Allergic Occupational Disease Among Healthcare Workers: Latex Allergy and Beyond. American Academy of Allergy, Asthma & Immunology 62nd Annual Meeting, 2006.
12. Fritsch PO, Sidoroff A. Drug-induced Stevens-Johnson Syndrome/ Toxic Epidermal Necrolysis. Am J Clin Dermatol 2000;1(6):349–360.
13. Beltrani VS, Bernstein IL, Cohen DE, Fonacier L. Contact dermatitis: A practice parameter. Ann Allergy Asthma Immunol 2006;97(9) Suppl:S1–S38.
14. Larsen JM, Bonefeld CM, Poulsen SS et al. Il-23 and T_H17-mediated inflammation in human allergic contact dermatitis. J Allergy Clin Immunol 2009;123:486–492.
15. Saripalli YV, Gadzia JE, Belsito DV. Tacrolimus ointment 0.1% in the treatment of nickel-induced allergic contact dermatitis. J Am Acad Dermatol 2003;49:477–482.
16. Matzke TJ, Bean AK, Ackerman T. Avoiding delayed diagnosis of malignant melanoma. J Nurse Pract 2009;5(1):42–46.
17. Ng JC, Swain S, Dowling JP, Wolfe R, Simpson P, Kelly JW. The impact of Partial Biopsy on Histopathologic Diagnosis of Cutaneous Melanoma. *Arch Dermatol.* 2010;146:234–239.

106

Acne Vulgaris

DEBRA SIBBALD

KEY CONCEPTS

1 Acne is a highly prevalent disorder affecting many adolescents and adults.

2 It is an extremely complex disease with an etiology originating from multiple causative and contributory factors.

3 Elements of pathogenesis involve defects in epidermal keratinization, androgen secretion, sebaceous function, bacterial growth, inflammation, and immunity.

4 Acne vulgaris cannot be "cured." Goals of treatment of this chronic disorder include control and alleviation of symptoms by reducing the number and severity of lesions, slowing progression, and limiting disease duration and recurrence. Key elements for patient adherence to therapy include prevention of long-term disfigurement associated with scarring and hyperpigmentation and avoidance of psychologic suffering.

5 The most critical target for treatment is the microcomedone, as the entire pathogenic cascade of acne is arrested if follicular occlusion is minimized or reversed. This involves a combination of treatment measures, integrating pharmacologic protocols targeting all four mechanisms involved in acne pathogenesis: increased follicular keratinization, increased sebum production, bacterial lipolysis of sebum triglycerides to free fatty acids, and inflammation.

6 Nondrug measures are aimed at both long-term prevention and treatment. Patients should eliminate aggravating factors, maintain a balanced, low-glycemic load diet, and control stress. They should wash twice daily with a mild soap or soapless cleanser, and restrict cosmetic use to oil-free products. Comedone extraction results in immediate cosmetic improvement in about 10% of patients. Shaving should be done as lightly and infrequently as possible, using a sharp blade or electric razor.

7 First-, second-, and third-line therapies should be selected and altered as appropriate for the severity and staging of the clinical presentation.

8 Treatment is directed at controlling the disorder, not curing it. Regimens should be tapered over time, adjusting to response. The smallest number of agents should be used at the lowest

possible dosages to ensure efficacy, safety, avoidance of resistance, and patient adherence.

9 Once control is achieved, simplify the regimen but continue with some suppressive therapy. It takes 8 weeks for a microcomedone to mature; thus, any therapy must be continued beyond this duration to assess efficacy in terms of comedonal and inflammatory lesion count, control or progression of severity, and management of associated anxiety or depression. Safety endpoints include monitoring for adverse effects of treatment.

10 Through empathic and informative counseling, the health professional can motivate the patient to continue long-term therapy.

In this chapter, we review the latest developments in understanding acne vulgaris and its treatment. The contents provide an analysis of the physiology of the pilosebaceous unit; the epidemiology, etiology and pathophysiology of acne; relevant treatment with nondrug measures; and comparisons of pharmacologic agents, including drugs of choice recommended in best-practice guidelines. Options include a variety of alternatives such as retinoids, antimicrobial agents, hormones, and light therapy. Formulation principles are discussed in relation to drug delivery. Patient assessment, general approaches to individualized therapy plans, and monitoring evaluation strategies are presented.

EPIDEMIOLOGY

1 Acne vulgaris is a chronic disease and the most common one treated by dermatologists. The lifetime prevalence of acne approaches 90%, with the highest incidence in adolescents. Prevalence data available from the European Union, United States, Australia, and New Zealand shows that acne affects 80% of individuals between puberty and 30 years of age.[1] Other studies have reported acne in 28% to 61% of school children aged 10–12 years; 79% to 95% of those 16–18 years of age; and even in children aged 4–7 years.[2-4]

The onset of acne vulgaris during puberty occurs at a younger chronologic age in girls than boys. Most patients continue to have symptoms into their mid-20s, and there is evidence that the duration of acne may last into middle age for most women, recorded in 54% of women and 40% of men older than 25 years of age.[5] In puberty, acne is often more severe in boys in about 15% of cases, which is tenfold greater than in girls. Women often have more severe forms during adulthood. When untreated, acne usually lasts for several years until it spontaneously remits.

There are believed to be no gender differences in acne prevalence, although such differences are often reported and may represent social biases. In urban clinics, there is a clear preponderance of girls seeking treatment. There is also a perception that acne is less prevalent in rural populations. This is supported by the data from Varanasi where 21.35% of boys (13–18 years) from rural areas had acne versus 37.5% of those from the urban areas.[6]

An international group of epidemiologists, community medicine specialists, and anthropologists have questioned whether acne might be predominantly a disease of Western civilization.[7] They assert that since acne vulgaris is nearly universal in westernized societies (afflicting 79% to 95% of the adolescent population), one causative factor might be the Western glycemic diet. While this hypothesis is based on the observation that primitive societies subsisting on traditional (low glycemic) diets have no acne, the theory awaits validation and acceptance by the dermatologic community.

ETIOLOGY

❷ Acne is a multifactorial disease. Genetic, racial, hormonal, dietary, and environmental factors have been implicated in its development. Its psychologic impact can be severe.

Four major etiologic factors are involved in the development of acne: increased sebum production, due to hormonal influences; hyperproliferation of ductal epidermis; bacterial colonization of the duct with *Propionibacterium acnes;* and production of inflammation in acne sites. These are reviewed in the Pathophysiology section later in this chapter.

The role of heredity in acne has not been clearly defined; however, there is a significant tendency toward more serious involvement if one or both parents had severe acne during their youth.

Environmental factors play a major role in determining the severity and extent of acne and may influence the choice of topical treatments. Heat and humidity may induce comedones; pressure or friction caused by protective devices such as helmets, shoulder pads, or pillows, and excessive scrubbing or washing can exacerbate existing acne by causing microcomedones to rupture. Hair styles that are low on the forehead or neck may cause excessive sweating and occlusion, exacerbating acne. In most cases acne is worse in winter and improves during the summer, suggesting a salutary effect of sunlight. However, in some cases exposure to sunlight worsens the disease.[8]

The importance of psychologic factors in this prolonged and capricious condition has been repeatedly stressed. Emotions such as intense anger and stress can exacerbate acne, causing flares or increasing mechanical manipulation. This is probably the result of increased glucocorticoid secretion by the adrenal glands, which appears to potentiate the effects of androgens.[9]

Dietary influences are the focus of current investigations. In the past, acne was not felt to be influenced by diet, but patients could restrict certain foods they perceive exacerbate acne (chocolate, cola drinks, milk and milk products).[10,11] These recommendations, which still persist in some guidelines, are based on one or two poorly designed studies conducted more than 40 years ago. They have largely been discounted by well-designed current studies. A discussion of the issues surrounding dietary influences is elaborated as a Current Controversy later in this chapter.

PATHOPHYSIOLOGY

❸ The pathogenesis of acne progresses through the following four major stages:

1. Increased follicular keratinization
2. Increased sebum production
3. Bacterial lipolysis of sebum triglycerides to free fatty acids
4. Inflammation

Acne usually begins in the prepubertal period, when the adrenal glands mature, and progresses as androgen production and sebaceous gland activity increase with gonad development.

As shown in Figure 106–1, acne results from the development of an obstructed sebaceous follicle, called a *microcomedone.* Sebaceous glands increase their size and activity in response to circulating androgens. Most patients with acne do not overproduce androgens (with some exceptions); instead, they have sebaceous glands that are hyperresponsive to androgens.[12] The composition of sebum is changed, with a reduction in linoleic acid. The growth of keratinocytes changes. The infrainfundibulum increases its keratinization of cells with hypercornification and development of the microcomedone, the primary lesion of both noninflammatory and inflammatory acne.[13] Cells adhere to each other in an expanding mass, which forms a dense keratinous plug. In particular androgens, hormones could be a stimulus to pilosebaceous duct hypercornification. Sebum, produced in increasing amounts by the active gland, becomes trapped behind the keratin plug and solidifies, contributing to open or closed comedone formation.

The pooling of sebum in the follicle provides ideal substrate conditions for proliferation of the anaerobic bacterium *Propionibacterium acnes,* generating a T cell response, which results in inflammation.[13] *P. acnes* produces a lipase that hydrolyzes sebum triglycerides into free fatty acids. These free fatty acids may trigger the changes that lead to an increase in keratinization and microcomedone formation.[14,15] This closed comedone, or whitehead, is the first clinically visible lesion of acne. It takes approximately 5 months to develop. The closed comedone is almost completely obstructed to drainage and has a tendency to rupture.[16–18]

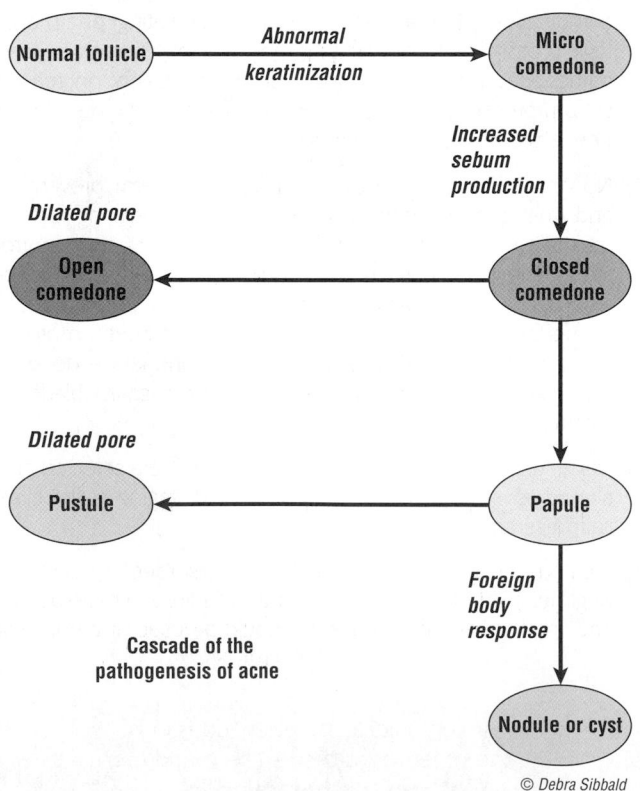

Cascade of the
pathogenesis of acne

© Debra Sibbald

FIGURE 106–1. Cascade of the Pathogenesis of Acne

As the plug extends to the upper canal and dilates its opening, an open comedone, or blackhead, is formed. Its dark color is not due to dirt but to either oxidized lipid and melanin or to the impacted mass of horny cells. The cylindrically shaped, open comedone is very stable and may persist for a long time as soluble substances and liquid sebum escape more easily. Acne that is characterized by open and closed comedones is termed *noninflammatory acne*.

Both recruitment of polymorphs into the follicle during the inflammatory process and release of *P. acnes*-generated chemokines lead to pus formation. The pus eventually bursts on the surface with resolution of the inflammation or into the dermis. *P. acnes* also produces enzymes which increase the permeability of the follicular wall, causing it to rupture, releasing keratin, hair, and lipids and irritating free fatty acids into the dermis. Several different types of inflammatory lesions may form, including pustules, nodules, and cysts and may lead to scarring.

Hyperpigmentation and scarring are two sequelae of acne. A time delay of up to 3 years between acne onset and adequate treatment correlates to degree of scarring and emphasizes the need for early therapy.[10,11]

ACNE VULGARIS CAN BE NONINFLAMMATORY OR INFLAMMATORY.

- Noninflammatory acne is characterized by open and closed comedones.
  - The closed comedo is visible as a 1 to 2 mm whitehead most easily seen when the skin is stretched.
    - Is the first clinical sign of acne
    - Has a tendency to rupture
  - The open comedo, or blackhead, is larger, approximately 2 to 5 mm and is dark-topped with contents extruding
    - Is relatively stable
- Inflammatory acne is traditionally characterized as having papulopustular and/or nodular lesions
  - A pustule is formed from a superficial aggregation of neutrophils
    - Appears as a raised white lesion filled with pus, usually less than 5 mm in diameter
    - Superficial pustules usually resolve within a few days without scarring
  - A nodule is produced through deeper, dermal, inflammatory infiltration.
    - Is the most severe variant of acne
    - Appears as warm, tender, firm lesions, with a diameter of 5 mm or greater
    - May be suppurative or hemorrhagic within the dermis, may involve adjacent follicles and sometimes extend down to fat
  - Cysts are suppurative nodules named because they resemble inflamed epidermal cysts.
    - Cystic acne may show double comedones, resulting from prior inflammation and fistulous links between neighboring sebaceous units.
  - Progression of inflammatory lesions:
    - Pustules and cysts often rupture spontaneously and drain a purulent or bloody but odorless discharge.[19]
    - Inflammatory lesions may itch as they erupt and can be tender or painful.

- Often resolution of these lesions leaves erythematous or pigmented macules that can persist for months or longer, especially in dark-skinned individuals.
- Nodules and deep lesions may result in scarring.
- Acne lesions can occur anywhere on the body apart from the palms and soles.
  - Are usually located on the face, back, neck, shoulders, and chest
  - May extend to buttocks or extremities
  - One or more anatomic areas may be involved in any given patient
  - The pattern of involvement, once present, tends to remain constant.
- Skin, scalp, and hair are frequently oily.

CLINICAL PRESENTATION AND DIAGNOSTIC CONSIDERATIONS

To correctly diagnose acne vulgaris, the clinician considers patient assessment which includes distinguishing all the presenting signs and symptoms of the clinical presentation (see box), as well as considering a differential diagnosis and the possibility of drug-induced acne.

PATIENT ASSESSMENT

Patient assessment begins with establishing a therapeutic relationship with the patient, in which their understanding, expectations, concerns, and behaviors are considered. All relevant information must be elicited from the patient to determine if their drug-related needs are being met and to identify drug therapy problems. Rational drug therapy decisions and a plan for delivering patient goals, along with follow-up evaluation, are made.

CONDUCTING A PATIENT ASSESSMENT

When acne is the chief complaint, the clinician begins by eliciting all details of presenting signs and symptoms.

Determine Signs and Symptoms

Palliating factors (e.g., sunlight) and provoking factors (e.g., premenstrual flares, humid environments, excessive sweating; exposure to chemicals; occlusive clothing; friction; oily cosmetics; manual manipulation; stress) should be determined.

Next, the quality and quantity of lesions should be considered (comedonal or inflammatory).

Then, determine the regions of involvement (e.g., face, back, chest) and areas of radiation (e.g., localized, generalized, symmetric or nonsymmetric).

To assess severity grading, several taxonomies are used but none are accepted universally. The following system includes factors such as lesion type, location of lesions, and number and status of irreversible sequelae:[20,21]

Type 1: Comedones only, fewer than 10 lesions on the face, no lesions on the trunk, and no scarring

Type 2: Papules, 10–25 lesions on the face and trunk, mild scarring

Type 3: Pustules, more than 25 lesions, moderate scarring

Type 4: Nodules or cysts, extensive scarring

Inflammatory acne can also be graded using a mild, moderate, and severe hierarchy that addresses the kind of inflammatory lesion. Severity grading under this scheme is as follows:

Mild: few to several papules or pustules and no nodules

Moderate: several to many papules or pustules and few to several nodules

Severe: numerous and/or extensive papules or pustules and many nodules[22]

In addition to determining severity, the patient should be asked about associated symptoms (e.g., itch, pain, fever). Finally, the time of onset of lesions and time patterns (e.g., intermittent, constant, progressive) must be established.

Medical Conditions

Once the full picture of signs and symptoms is clarified, ascertain if the patient has medical conditions which either contribute to or co-exist with acne and confuse the clinical presentation, if endocrine factors are significant in the patient (e.g. irregular menses, hirsutism, alopecia), and if the patient is pregnant or atopic.

Medication History

A full medication history should be established. Determine if the patient is taking or using a product that could cause or interact with acne signs and symptoms, based on literature evidence. Has the patient tried any nondrug measures, and what was the effect on acne signs and symptoms? Has the patient used any product successfully or unsuccessfully to treat acne lesions recently or during past episodes? Has a health care practitioner or another individual (friend, relative, media) made a treatment recommendation for the acne signs and symptoms? If so, was this attempted and what was the result?

Allergies

Determine if specific allergies affect drug therapy. Could an allergy be causing the acne symptoms, or could an allergy present a contraindication to acne therapy? Social habits, such as diet, smoking, or alcohol use, should be discussed.

Family History

Family history should be elicited. Is there a genetic predisposition to acne? If so, determine the nature of the acne presentation in these individuals.

Psychosocial Issues

Are there significant psychosocial issues affecting control of acne? Have global and disease specific quality of life (QOL) indicators or health-state utilities been assessed? QOL indicators represent patients' perceptions and reactions to their health. Assessing QOL impairment in patients with acne may aid in management by evaluating psychologic impacts, which may not correlate with clinical severity; aid in detection of depression or need for psychologic care; and improve therapeutic outcomes.

Examples of global scales that have been used to evaluate acne include Skindex[23] and Dermatology QOL Index;[24] examples of acne specific scales include the Acne-specific QOL questionnaire[25] and the Acne QOL Scale.[26] Health-state utilities (such as time trade-off [TTO]) are quantitative measures of patient preferences of health outcomes ranging from 0 (death) to 1 (perfect health) and can be used in clinical trials as outcome measures of treatment effects. TTO utilities for acne in the range of 0.94 to 0.96 can be compared with those of other diseases (e.g., 0.92 for epilepsy, 0.94 for myopia),

and help to identify the impact of acne on self-perception and psychologic functioning.[27]

DIFFERENTIAL DIAGNOSIS

Acne vulgaris is rarely misdiagnosed. The conditions most commonly mistaken for acne vulgaris include rosacea, perioral dermatitis, gram-negative folliculitis, and drug-induced acne.[28]

Acne rosacea (adult acne) is a chronic relapsing condition, occurring after age 30 in fair-complexioned persons and involving blood vessels. The first sign is easy flushing followed by development of inflammatory lesions, with edema, papules, and pustules appearing on the nose, cheeks, chin, and forehead, and telangiectasia (spider veins) developing as the condition progresses. The affected area may be sensitive to the touch.

Rosacea differs from acne vulgaris in several ways. Its onset is not linked to increased androgens or endocrine changes; comedones are not usually present; aggravating factors are different and include ingestion of alcohol, spicy foods, or hot drinks (especially those containing caffeine); smoking; overexposure to sunlight; and exposure to temperature extremes, friction, irritating cosmetics, and steroids. Rosacea is not curable, progressively worsens, and may ultimately result in rhinophyma (enlarged nose). Refer patients to a physician for treatment, as antibiotics, particularly topical metronidazole, may be required.[29]

Perioral dermatitis occurs primarily in young women and adolescents and is characterized by erythema, scaling, and papulopustular lesions commonly clustered around the nasolabial folds, mouth, and chin. The cause is unknown.[29]

Gram-negative folliculitis (*Proteus, Pseudomonas, Klebsiella*) may complicate acne, with a sudden change to pustules or large inflammatory cysts occurring after long-term treatment of acne with oral antibiotics. Folliculitis may be caused by staphylococci. There is a sudden onset of superficial pustules around the nose, chin, and cheeks. Patients with suspected folliculitis should be referred to a physician.[29]

Several conditions include acne vulgaris as a characteristic component, and understanding the mechanisms involved in these syndromes provides insight into the pathogenesis of acne. These include polycystic ovary syndrome (elevated androgen levels); PAPA syndrome (pyogenic arthritis, pyoderma gangrenosum, acne; early onset arthritis with increased inflammatory activity), and SAPHO syndrome (synovitis, acne, pustulosis, hyperostosis, osteitis syndrome; sterile inflammatory arthro-osteitis, with *P. acnes* as a possible trigger).[13]

DRUG-INDUCED ACNE

In addition to the conditions induced by drugs that were presented in Chap. 105, acneiform eruptions can also be caused by medications. Systemic corticosteroids can cause a pustular inflammatory form of acne, especially on the trunk. Onset is abrupt at 2 to 6 weeks after initiation of therapy. Acne has also been associated with most of the potent topical steroids, but not with hydrocortisone, which lacks the ability to inhibit protein synthesis. Discontinuation of the steroid results in an initial worsening of appearance due to removal of the antiinflammatory action of the steroid itself. Caution patients about this reaction, which can be subdued through judicious use of topical hydrocortisone.[30–32]

Antiepileptics and tuberculostatics are the most commonly implicated in drug-induced acne, followed by lithium. Other heavy metals inducing acne include cobalt in vitamin B_{12}.[33] Halogens, especially an excess of iodide in seafood, salt, and health foods, can exacerbate acne.

In addition, certain minor ingredients in cosmetics have been implicated in cosmetic acne, including isopropyl myristate, cocoa butter, and fatty acids.

TREATMENT

The first step in determining a safe and efficacious treatment regimen for acne vulgaris is to establish desired outcomes for the patient, regarding both short- and long-term goals.

■ DESIRED OUTCOME (GOALS OF TREATMENT)

4 Acne vulgaris requires long-term control, as it cannot be cured. This basic principle needs to be stressed with the patient to establish motivation to adhere to lengthy treatment regimens, which involve both addressing current symptoms and signs and taking preventive measures. Basic goals of treatment include alleviation of symptoms by reducing the number and severity of lesions, slowing the progression of signs and symptoms, limiting the disease duration and recurrence, prevention of long-term disfigurement associated with scarring and hyperpigmentation, and avoidance of psychologic suffering.

■ GENERAL APPROACH TO TREATMENT

5 The most critical target for treatment is the microcomedone, because by eliminating the follicular occlusion the whole cascade of acne is arrested. This will involve a combination of preventive measures to reduce or eliminate risk and aggravating factors and treatment measures. These should integrate nondrug and pharmacologic protocols aimed at cleansing as well as targeting all four mechanisms involved in acne pathogenesis. First-line, second-line, and third-line therapies should be selected and altered as appropriate for the severity and staging of the clinical presentation. Treatment is directed at controlling the disorder, not curing it. Regimens should be tapered over time, adjusting to response. The smallest number of agents should be used at the lowest possible dosages to ensure efficacy, safety, avoidance of resistance, and patient adherence. Once control is achieved, simplify the regimen but continue with some suppressive therapy. It takes 8 weeks for a microcomedone to mature, thus any therapy must be continued beyond this duration in order to assess efficacy.[32]

■ NONPHARMACOLOGIC THERAPY

6 Encourage patients with acne to discontinue or avoid any aggravating factors, maintain a balanced, low-glycemic-load diet and control stress. Evidence shows that by being empathic and informative during counseling, the health professional may motivate the patient to continue long-term therapy.[8,9,28] One of the first approaches to nondrug management of acne is attention to cleansing techniques. Shaving recommendations, comedone extraction, dietary considerations, issues relating to ultraviolet light, and prevention of cosmetic acne should be reviewed with patients.

Cleansing

Cleansers often contain surfactant systems to remove fat from the skin surface. The oil is dispersed from the skin into the surfactant system; however, the active ingredient is sometimes trapped and removed upon rinsing, Also, the balance between cleanliness and drying or irritation should be taken into account. Most patients prefer products with foaming action, and these must contain additional secondary surfactants to enhance the foam and condition the skin.

Soaps are the most widely used cleansing products, but do not lend themselves to efficient delivery of active drug. Two main disadvantages exist. As soaps are rinsed off, the deposit of active agent will be small; and the high pH required in soaps may degrade some active ingredients and be less tolerable on sensitive skin. Soapless cleansers are an alternatives to soaps.[34]

Patients should wash no more than twice daily with a mild, nonfragranced opaque or glycerin soap or a soapless cleanser. Acne patients often wash too frequently, attempting to remove surface oils. There is no evidence indicating that this is helpful, as surface lipids do not affect acne.[35] Contributory lipids are deep in the follicle and are not removed through washing. Antiseptic cleansers, while producing a clean, refreshed feeling, remove only surface dirt, oil, and aerobic bacteria. They do not affect *P. acnes*. There is no evidence that any particular washing regimen is superior. Scrubbing should be minimized to prevent follicular rupture. Soaps produce a drying effect on the skin due to detergent action. As medicated cleansers require increased contact time, this drying action is pronounced, especially with peeling agents. Avoid cream-based cleansers.

Polyester cleansing sponges (e.g., Buf-Puf) are synthetics that abrade the skin surface, removing superficial debris. They are unlikely to unseat comedones, considering the structure of these lesions. The sponges are available in soft or coarse textures, with or without soap. Caution patients against using a circular or rubbing motion that will increase irritation, and instruct them to use single, gentle, continuous strokes on each side of the face, from the midline out toward the ears.

Cationic-bond strips that become activated by water are available. The dirt and oil in the pores is anionic. As the strip dries, the cationic-bond binds the anionic dirt and removes it when the strip is peeled off.

Shaving

Males should try both electric and safety razors to determine which is more comfortable for shaving. When using a safety razor, the beard should be softened with soap and warm water or shaving gel. Shaving should be done as lightly and infrequently as possible, using a sharp blade and being careful to avoid nicking lesions. Strokes should be in the direction of hair growth, shaving each area only once.

Comedone Extraction

Comedone extraction is useful and painless and results in immediate cosmetic improvement although it has not been widely tested in clinical trials. Pretreatment with a peeler for 4 to 6 weeks often facilitates the procedure.[32] Following cleansing with hot water, a comedone extractor is placed over the lesion and gentle pressure applied until the contents are expressed. This removes unsightly lesions, preventing progression to inflammation. A correctly sized extractor allows the central keratin plug to extrude through the opening. The small end of a plastic eye dropper, with bulb removed, may also be used. These instruments should be cleaned with alcohol after each use. Some initial reddening may be apparent. If the contents are not expressed with modest pressure, patients should not continue since improper extraction may further irritate the skin. A physician should be consulted if this technique is too difficult for the patient to manage. Since the follicle is difficult to remove completely, comedones may recur between 25 and 50 days following expression. Fewer than 10% of comedone extractions are a complete success, but the process is useful when done properly.[19]

Comedo removal may be helpful in the management of comedones resistant to other therapies, but it has not been well studied despite long-standing clinical use. Also, while the procedure cannot affect the clinical course of the disease, it can improve the patient's appearance, which may positively affect adherence with the treatment program.

Ultraviolet Light

Although ultraviolet light was recommended in the past for desquamation, the practice is no longer advisable because of the well-established carcinogenic and photoaging effects of ultraviolet exposure. Moreover, inflamed skin is more susceptible to the damaging effects of ultraviolet light. Patients taking tretinoin may show heightened sensitivity.[36]

Before exposure to sunlight, patients with acne should apply sunscreens (SPF 15) in alcohol or oil-free bases and avoid using the acnegenic benzophenones. Sunscreen should be applied as the first product.

CLINICAL CONTROVERSY: LIGHT THERAPY

Recently some authors proposed "diverse" light therapies (using various wavelengths) as a new acne treatment. The outcomes of existing trials are contradictory. Light therapies for acne are believed to work by killing *P. acnes* and by damaging and shrinking sebaceous glands, reducing sebum output. Studies report few adverse effects,[117] and any adverse effects are temporary.[119] Light therapies may be given once or twice weekly as a course of 6 to 10 treatments, with each irradiation lasting 10 to 20 minutes.[119] Treatment is not available universally; it is accessed privately via dermatologists or clinics, and can be expensive. *P. acnes* produce endogenous porphyrins that absorb light to form highly reactive singlet oxygen, which destroys the bacteria.[119] Since porphyrins have peak absorption at blue light wavelengths, blue light is often used to treat acne. Red light is also absorbed by porphyrins and can penetrate deeper into the skin,[120] where it may directly affect inflammatory mediators. Other light therapies attempt to selectively target and damage sebaceous glands directly, reducing their size and thus sebum output.[121] These include infrared lasers, low-energy pulsed dye lasers, and radiofrequency devices.[119]

Photodynamic therapy (PDT) uses specific light-activating creams, which are absorbed into the skin and amplify the response to light therapy but tend to produce more severe adverse effects. There are concerns that PDT may interfere with the skin's natural immune mechanisms[122] and cause long-term skin damage.

An increase in transforming growth factor (TGF)-β1 mRNA 24 hours after treatment with lasers has been observed. TGF-β1, an immunosuppressive cytokine, stimulates the formation of collagen. Its increase following laser treatment may promote resolution of inflammation.[123]

Light therapies are increasingly popular among consumers. Medical science is needed to establish whether light of different wavelengths is effective.[119] A Cochrane review protocol will investigate the current state of evidence for use of light therapy in acne.[124]

Prevention of Cosmetic Acne

Persistent low-grade acne in women after their mid-20s is frequently caused by heavy cosmetic use. Adolescent acne in younger women may be exacerbated with makeup overuse. The problem is perpetuated when the resultant blemishes are concealed with more cosmetics.

Advise patients to stop using oil-containing cosmetics and avoid cosmetic programs that advocate applying multiple layers of cream-based cleansers and cover-ups. These are advertised through the media and often available through Internet shopping with promotional bonuses. Three-step basic systems usually combine medicated and nonmedicated ingredients, although it may not be apparent by their cosmetic names that therapeutic agents are included. They often start with cleansers, in lotions or creams, which may contain a multitude of unnecessary ingredients, including medicated peelers, oils, fragrances, and preservatives. Often drugs are included in subtherapeutic or low doses, including salicylic acid, sulfur, or benzoyl peroxide. The second step is generally a "toner" or "refresher" which is usually water- or alcohol-based and might contain medicated ingredients such as alpha-hydroxy acids (e.g., glycolic acid), which are mild comedolytic agents, or even glycerin as a humectant. The final product, often called intensive or repairing solutions, usually contains the lowest strength of peelers such as benzoyl peroxide, sulfur, or salicylic acid; plus potentially sensitizing fragrances and preservatives; or oil-soluble sunscreens that are not identified on the label. Bases may have significant oil content. There may be additional products to supplement as necessary to the base routine of 3 steps, such as masks or spot treatments. Multiple-step cosmetic programs are often costly, and should be avoided in favor of simple cleansers and more effective single-ingredient peelers at optimal concentrations.

The term *noncomedogenic* may refer to either water-based vehicles or products that are free of substances known to induce comedones. They are not necessarily oil-free. Water-based cosmetics may contain significant amounts of oil in the form of undiluted vegetable oils, lanolin, fatty acid esters (butyl stearate, isopropyl myristate), fatty acids (stearic acid), fatty acid alcohols, cocoa butter, coconut oil, red veterinary petrolatum, and sunscreens containing benzophenones. Water-based products are more likely to contribute to pore blockage than oil-free products.

Oil-free makeups are well-tolerated and lipstick, eye shadow, eyeliner, eyebrow pencils, and loose face powders are relatively innocuous. Heavier, oil-based preparations, particularly moisturizers and hairsprays, clog pores and accelerate comedone formation.[37]

The patient should restrict cosmetic use to products labeled oil-free rather than water-based, including makeup, moisturizers, or sunscreens. Coverup cosmetics for acne are available in several skin tones and in lotion and cream forms. They often contain peeling agents, antibacterial agents, or hydroquinone. Most contain sulfur. They may be applied as cosmetics 2 or 3 times daily, over the entire face or to individual lesions. However, since the spread time of oil-free makeup is decreased, best results are achieved if applied to one-quarter of the face at a time. Topical medication should be applied after gentle cleansing and a foundation lotion may be used sparingly as a concealer.[38,39,40]

Since the action of most therapeutic acne agents is to dry the skin, the use of moisturizers is counterproductive. Active agents such as alpha-hydroxy acids (glycolic, lactic, pyruvic, and citric acids) may be present in the cosmetic formulation, since they reduce corneocyte adhesion.[41] Patients with acne should be restricted to oil-free alpha-hydroxy acid products unless absolutely necessary because of treatment with strong drying agents or isotretinoin.

Vehicles

The formulation of an acne vehicle must consider the technical characteristics of maintaining and delivering the drug in an active state together with the need for an elegant product that the patient will enjoy using, so that it is more likely to be applied as required and deliver the full benefit. Physically and chemically, the vehicle will be used with one or more of the following goals: reduce excess oil, control bacteria associated with acne, reduce the effects of hyperkeratinization, and unclog pores. Performance, safety, and stability should be maximized while addressing technical and commercial factors.

Immiscible liquids might be delivered in oil-in-water or water-in-oil emulsions. In addition to having undesirable oil content, these vehicles also contain humectants, thickeners, preservatives, and fragrance, all of which may be problematic.

Solutions are simpler formulations, and there is a trend to use them as the soaking liquid for wipe products made with fibrous cloths. The viability of these kinds of products must take into consideration whether packages are resealable if they contain multiple wipes, and whether the volatility of the solvent will affect storage and availability of the active agent or cause crystallization. Solutions are used mainly with topical antibiotics, which are often dissolved in specific types of alcohol. While some antibiotics are only soluble in ethyl alcohol, isopropyl alcohol is generally better able to remove oil from the skin surface and is preferred for nonmedicated vehicles. An 8% glycolic acid solution is available for use alone or for incorporation in topical antibiotic preparations. Solutions and washes can be more easily applied to large areas such as the back.[42]

Nongreasy solutions, gels, lotions and creams should be selected as bases for topical acne preparations. Gels are very useful as they are totally oil-free along with mixtures of water or alcohol. Lotions and creams will contain some oil-phase ingredients. Discourage moisturizers and oil-based products. Lotions are slightly less drying than gels, and creams are more emollient. Many gels contain ethanol or isopropyl alcohol. Propylene glycol is sometimes present in small amounts to add viscosity and lessen the drying effects of strong peeling agents. Gels are drying but may cause a burning irritation in some patients and may prevent certain kinds of cosmetics from adhering to the skin.[43] Propylene glycol gels are easy to apply and dry without a visible or sticky film. Nonalcoholic gels may be as effective and less drying than alcoholic solutions. Alcoholic or acetone gels are usually more drying and provide better penetration of the active ingredient.

Consider the patient's skin type and preferences in the choice of vehicle for topical agents. Patients with oily skin often prefer vehicles with higher proportions of alcohol (solutions and gels), while those with dry or sensitive skin prefer nonirritating lotions and creams. Lotions can be used with any skin type and can be easily spread over hair-bearing skin, but will cause burning or dryness if they contain propylene glycol. Compatibility of vehicles and agents with cosmetics should also be considered.

How to Use Topical Preparations

Topical preparations should not be applied to individual lesions but to the whole area affected by acne to prevent new lesions from developing, using care around the eyelid, mouth, and neck to avoid chafing. Lotions should be applied with a cotton swab once or twice a day after washing or at bedtime if they leave a visible residue.

Psychologic Approaches/ Hypnosis/Biofeedback

The psychologic effects of acne may be profound and the American Academy of Dermatology expert workgroup unanimously concluded that effective acne treatment can improve the emotional outlook of patients.[44] There is weak evidence of the possible benefit of biofeedback-assisted relaxation and cognitive imagery.[45,46]

Dressings

A pilot double-blind, randomized study of 20 patients has shown some benefit of treatment with a hydrocolloid acne dressing when compared with tape dressings for improving mild to moderate inflammatory acne vulgaris. Results showed greater reduction over 3 to 7 days in the overall severity of acne and inflammation, along with greater improvement in redness, oiliness, dark pigmentation, and sebum casual level. Less ultraviolet B light reaches the skin surface with the hydrocolloid dressing in place.[47]

■ PHARMACOLOGIC THERAPY

Successful pharmacologic therapy must address one of the four mechanisms involved in the pathogenesis of acne. There are numerous agents available that prove one or more of these actions and are therefore effective. However The choice of active pharmacologic therapy depends on severity.

Mechanisms of drug action relating to acne pathogenesis are illustrated in Figure 106–2.

Drug Treatments of First Choice

For mild to moderate acne with predominantly noninflammatory lesions (comedones), few inflammatory lesions, and no scars, active agents of first choice include those that correct the defect in keratinization by producing exfoliation most efficaciously. Such agents include topical retinoids, salicylic acid, and benzoyl peroxide. Sulfur

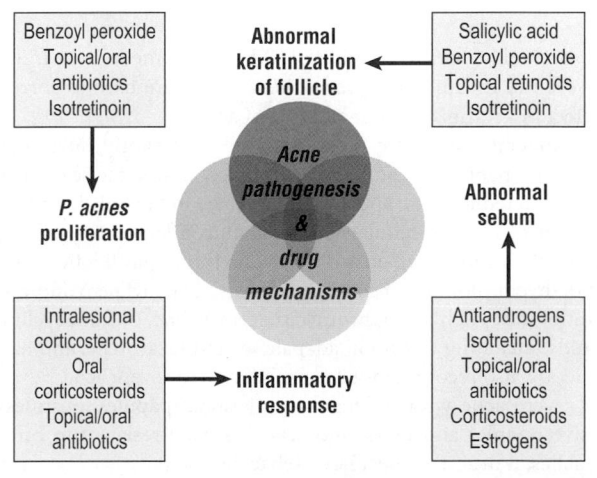

© Debra Sibbald

FIGURE 106-2. Acne Pathogenesis and Drug Mechanisms

CLINICAL CONTROVERSY

The role of dietary influences in acne has always been controversial. Guidelines asserting little or no psychologic influences are largely based upon results of a 1969 single-blind crossover study, which had a number of methodologic flaws, showing no significant differences in lesion count or sebum characteristics following ingestion of enriched chocolate bar versus a control bar without cocoa butter and chocolate liquor. A subsequent small study also showed no differences in count or grade of acne in medical students who were asked to consume the food they thought most likely to worsen acne for 7 days.[131] It is now suggested that this information has been widely overinterpreted, resulting in an inappropriate dismissal of potential effects of dietary ingestions on acne.[132]

More recent studies have reported association between various dietary influences and presentation of acne, including an association between acne and intake of milk, perhaps due to natural hormonal components and/or other bioactive molecules in milk.[133,134] Other studies suggest that insulin-like growth factor (IGF), increased by ingestion of high glycemic loads, may play a role in acne.[135,136]

Patients who consumed a low-glycemic-load diet, compared with a conventional high-glycemic-load diet, had improvements of facial acne after 12 weeks. Accompanying changes in physical and endocrinologic parameters suggest that decreases in total energy intake, body weight, and indices of androgenicity and insulin resistance may also be associated with observed improvements in acne.[137] Further studies that examined the effect of a low-glycemic-load diet versus controls on acne and fatty acid composition of skin surface triglycerides showed increases in the ratio of saturated to monounsaturated fatty acids which correlated with acne lesion counts and increased sebum outflow. This suggests a possible role of desaturase enzymes in sebaceous lipogenesis and the clinical manifestation of acne; these require further investigation.[138] Another study that reported an improvement in acne and insulin sensitivity in low-glycemic-load diets compared with controls, suggests nutrition-related lifestyle factors play a role in the etiology of acne. Independent effects of weight loss versus dietary intervention need to be isolated.[139]

While still controversial, diet is thought to play a role in the development or progression of acne vulgaris and further studies are ongoing.

and resorcinol are weaker exfoliators. Since the comedo is the initial lesion even in inflammatory acne, these agents are used to correct the defect in keratinization in all cases of acne.

For moderate to severe acne, with predominantly inflammatory lesions (papules, pustules, few nodules) and some scars, it is important to reduce the population of *P. acnes* in the follicle and the generation of its extracellular products and inflammatory effects. Drugs of choice include benzoyl peroxide; topical antibiotics, such as clindamycin, alone or in combination with benzoyl peroxide; and oral antibiotics, such as erythromycin, tetracycline, or minocycline. Retinoids, including tretinoin, adapalene, and tazarotene, and azaleic acid are also recommended for moderate to severe acne.

For severe acne with inflammatory lesions (papules, pustules), extensive nodules and cysts, and scars, or acne resistant to other approaches, a drug that decreases sebaceous activity, such as antiandrogens, isotretinoin, or topical and oral antibiotics, should be added to the regimen.[48]

Published Guidelines

There is considerable heterogeneity in the acne literature. Various evidence-based guidelines available from multiple American, Canadian, European, Scandinavian, and South African sources do not provide concordance or clarity on all issues. Recommendations should be based on critical appraisal and interpretation of the literature combined with clinical experience.

An expert committee of the American Academy of Dermatology convened in 2007 to define guidelines for acne therapy and identify nine clinical questions to structure the primary issues in diagnosis and management (Table 106–1).[44] These guidelines address the management of adolescent and adult patients presenting with acne but not the consequences of disease, including the scarring, postinflammatory erythema, or postinflammatory hyperpigmentation. The use of light and laser therapy was not addressed in the guidelines.

General Information Regarding Efficacy and Safety

The guidelines and recommendations of the American Academy of Dermatology considered the efficacy and safety of various treatments, such as topical agents, systemic antibacterial agents, hormonal agents, isotretinoin, miscellaneous therapies, complementary and alternative therapies, and dietary restriction, based on levels of evidence and best clinical practice.[44] More specific information about the efficacy and safety of each of these specific modalities is outlined below in sections on each individual agent.

Alternative Drug Treatments

Herbal and alternative therapies have been used to treat acne. Although these products appear to be well tolerated, very limited data exist regarding their safety and efficacy.

Tea Tree Oil This contains terpinen-4-ol which appears responsible for some antimicrobial activity. One clinical trial has demonstrated that topical tea tree oil is effective for the treatment of acne, although the onset of action is slower than with other topical treatments.[49] In a study comparing 5% tea tree oil gel with 5% benzoyl peroxide lotion, both reduced the number of inflamed and noninflamed lesions. A randomized double-blind clinical trial performed in 60 patients with mild to moderate acne vulgaris reported 5% tea tree oil gel was more effective than placebo in terms of total acne lesions counting (TLC, 3.55 times) and acne severity index (ASI, 5.75 times) after a period of 45 days.[50] A systematic review of randomized clinical trials concludes there is no compelling evidence showing that tea tree oil is effective in any dermatologic condition.[51]

Tea Lotion Tea lotion is another natural plant extract that has been tested in acne vulgaris. A single-blind randomized controlled study of 60 patients compared a freshly prepared 2% tea lotion with placebo twice daily for 2 months in the treatment of acne vulgaris.[52] The authors reported significantly reduced mean lesion count of papules and pustules after 8 weeks for the tea lotion, and the difference between the 2 study groups was statistically significant.

Other Herbal Agents Topical and oral ayurvedic compounds have been reported to have value in the treatment of acne.[53,54] Notwithstanding, the use of botanical preparations, which are nonstandardized, should be discouraged in favor of traditional quality-controlled preparations that have evidence of efficacy.[55]

Glycolic Acid Another agent considered as an alternative therapy for acne vulgaris is glycolic acid. The efficacy and tolerability of a 0.1% retinaldehyde/6% glycolic acid combination (Diacneal) has been evaluated for mild to moderate acne vulgaris.[56] Physician and

TABLE 106-1 Guidelines for Managing Acne Vulgaris

Clinical Question Issues	Recommendation	Strength of Recommendation[a]	Level of Evidence[a]
I			
Systems for the grading and classification of acne	Use a grading/classification system	B	II
IIa			
Role of microbiologic testing	Do microbiologic testing	B	II
IIb			
Role of endocrinologic testing	Do endocrinologic testing	A	I
III			
Use of specific agents for topical therapy	Retinoids	A	I
	Benzoyl peroxide	A	I
	Antibiotics	A	I
	Other agents	A	I
IV			
Efficacy and safety of systemic antibiotics	Tetracyclines	A	I
	Macrolides	A	I
	Trimethoprim–sulfamethoxaxole	A	I
V			
Efficacy and safety of hormonal agents	Contraceptive agents	A	I
	Spironolactone	B	II
	Antiandrogens	B	II
	Oral corticosteroids	B	II
VI			
Efficacy and safety of isotretinoin	Isotretinoin	A	I
VII			
Efficacy and safety of miscellaneous therapy	Intralesional steroids	C	III
	Chemical peels	C	III
	Comedo removal	C	III
VIII			
Efficacy and safety of complementary therapy	Herbal agents	B	I
	Psychologic approaches	C	III
	Hypnosis/biofeedback	B	II
IX			
Efficacy and safety of dietary restrictions[b]	Effect of diet	B	II

[a]An expert panel of the American Academy of Dermatology developed these clinical recommendations using the best available evidence. The panel rated evidence using the Strength of Recommendation
   Taxonomy (SORT), which uses this three-point scale:
I. Good quality patient-oriented evidence.
II. Limited quality patient-oriented evidence.
III. Other evidence including consensus guidelines, extrapolations from bench research, opinion, or case studies.
Similarly, recommendations were ranked as follows:
A. Recommendation based on consistent and good quality patient-oriented evidence.
B. Recommendation based on inconsistent or limited quality patient-oriented evidence.
C. Recommendation based on consensus, opinion, or case studies.
[b]See Current Controversies: Dietary Influences
Reprinted from Am Acad Dermatol, Vol. 56, Strauss JS, Kowchk DP, Leyden JJ et al, Guidelines of care for acne vulgaris management, 651–63, Copyright © 2007, with permission from Elsevier.

patient ratings of acne symptom severity and tolerance performed at baseline and months 1, 2, and 3 showed mean numbers of papules, pustules, and comedones were significantly reduced from month 1 on, demonstrating that glycolic acid is effective and well tolerated in mild-to-moderate acne vulgaris.

Both glycolic acid–based and salicylic acid–based peeling preparations have been used in the treatment of acne. There is very little evidence from clinical trials published in peer-reviewed literature supporting the efficacy of peeling regimens.[44] Further research on the use of peeling in the treatment of acne needs to be conducted to establish best practices for this modality.

Hydroquinone To control pigmentation, hydroquinone, which reversibly damages melanocytes, has been used as a hypopigmenting agent in concentrations of 2% to 4%, in preparations of clear or tinted gels, which are more drying, and as vanishing or opaque, flesh-tinted creams, with or without alpha-hydroxy acids or sunscreens. Hydroquinone causes fading of epidermal but not dermal pigmentation. Onset of response is usually 3 to 4 weeks, and the depigmentation lasts for 2 to 6 months but is reversible. While effective in the removal of melanin, hydroquinone has been

clinically found to be a possible carcinogen and causes a blue-black discoloration known as ochronosis.[57]

After considering new data and information on the safety of hydroquinone, the U.S. Food and Drug Administration (FDA) issued a proposed ruling in 2006 about hydroquinone products. The FDA proposed reversing earlier rules that hydroquinone is generally recognized as safe and effective; however, the FDA has also allowed the products to stay on the U.S. market until a final rule is issued. The FDA is also considering all prescription hydroquinone products to be new drugs requiring an approved new drug application for continued marketing.

Hydroquinone has already been banned in Japan, much of the European Union, and Africa.

Treatment of Scarring Drug and non measures for scar resolution are important in acne vulgaris since many patients are scarred despite adequate treatment. For patients with mild scarring, nonprescription alpha-hydroxy acids may be used, while severe scarring may be corrected with other treatment modalities that require consultation with a dermatologist. Dermabrasion, local excision, collagen implants, chemical peels (e.g., 70% glycolic acid) and laser therapy have been used to improve scarring. Atrophic scars can be treated with laser resurfacing. Usually the scar is not completely removed, but a more cosmetically acceptable result is achieved. Keloids and hypertrophic scars can be treated with intralesional triamcinolone, cryotherapy, topical steroids and silicone sheeting. Surgical options for scars include excision, augmentation with collagen or fat, chemical peels, subcision, and injection of autologous fibroblasts.[58]

Special Populations

About 20% of young infants (2 to 3 months of age) develop papules, pustules, and less commonly closed or open comedones, primarily on the cheeks, due to placental transfer of maternal androgens (neonatal acne). The acne subsides within a few months with regular maturation. Boys are affected more often than girls because of a transient increase in testosterone secretion during the third and fourth month of intrauterine life. *Malassezia* spp. may be involved in pathogenesis.[19] Resolution occurs without therapy.[59] Infants with neonatal acne may have more severe teenage acne.[19]

Drug Class Information

This section reviews the pharmacology and mechanisms as related to pathophysiology for pharmacologic options recommended in the guidelines for mild, moderate, and severe acne. It will also review evidence of efficacy and safety as well as kinetics, interactions, dosing, and administration when relevant.

Exfoliants (Peeling Agents) Exfoliants induce continuous mild drying and peeling by primary irritation, damaging the superficial layers of the skin, and inciting inflammation. This stimulates mitosis, thickening the epidermis, and increasing horny cells, scaling, and erythema. A decrease in sweating results in a dry, less oily surface and may superficially resolve pustular lesions.

In the past, a rabbit model was used to study the efficacy of topical exfoliants in retarding tar-induced comedone formation and accelerating their loss (comedolysis). In this animal model, retinoic acid (tretinoin) was most active, compared with benzoyl peroxide and salicylic acid, which were respectively less active. Data from peer-reviewed literature regarding the efficacy of sulfur, resorcinol, sodium sulfacetamide, aluminum chloride, and zinc are limited. Traditional nonprescription exfoliants, including phenol, resorcinol, betanaphthol, sulfur, Vleminckx's solution, and sodium thiosulfate, are weak or ineffective. These agents are not comedolytic given that they affect the superficial epidermis rather than the hair canal. They have been supplanted by superior effective agents.[60,61]

Resorcinol. This phenol derivative is less keratolytic than salicylic acid. It is said to be both bactericidal and fungicidal. Products containing resorcinol 1% to 2% have been used for acne, often in combination with other peeling agents, such as sulfur or salicylic acid. The FDA considers resorcinol 2% and resorcinol monoacetate 3%, in combination with sulfur 3% to 8%, to be safe and effective and that the combination may enhance the activity of sulfur. However, the FDA is not convinced that resorcinol and resorcinol acetate are safe and effective when used as single ingredients, and has placed such products in Category II (not generally recognized as safe and effective, or misbranded).[61]

Resorcinol is an irritant and sensitizer and should not be applied to large areas of the skin or on broken skin. It produces a reversible, dark brown scale on some dark-skinned individuals.

Protective packaging is important as resorcinol is reactive to light and oxygen. It has good solubility in both water and alcohol and is heat stabile Thus, it is incorporated into a variety of products, including emulsions.[62]

Salicylic Acid. Salicylic acid has been used for many years for the treatment of acne, although few well-designed trials of its safety and efficacy exist. It is a natural ingredient in many plants, such as willow tree or willow bark, is a beta-hydroxy acid, and penetrates the pilosebaceous unit. It has comedolytic activity, although the concentrations in commercial preparations (less than 2% to 3%) are generally low. While concentrations less than 2% may actually increase keratinization, concentrations between 3% and 6% are keratolytic, softening the horny layer and producing shedding of scales. Its mechanism remains unresolved, attributed to either reduced cohesion of corneocytes or shedding of epidermal cells, rather than breakdown of keratin.

Salicylic acid has no effect on the mitotic activity of normal epidermis and does not influence disordered cornification.[63] It may also provide mild antibacterial value, as it is active against *P. acnes*. It also offers slight antiinflammatory activity at concentrations ranging from 0.5% to 5%. Its efficacy against comedones helps to prevent development of inflamed lesions, thus providing a delayed efficacy.[64]

Salicylic acid is an effective agent. As a peeling agent, its relative strength compared with others in this class varies according to the model used in measurement. It is slightly *less* potent than equal-strength benzoyl peroxide when measured with the rabbit ear animal model, and slightly *more* potent when measured with a biologic microcomedone model.[64] It may have antiinflammatory properties that help dry inflammatory lesions.[62] Its comedolytic properties are considered less potent than topical retinoids. It is often used when patients cannot tolerate a topical retinoid because of skin irritation.[65]

Its keratolytic effect may enhance the absorption of other agents. Salicylic acid may cause some degree of local skin peeling and discomfort (burning or reddening) as it is a mild irritant. It is not a sensitizer. Although the FDA recognizes salicylic acid as safe and effective, the compound offers no advantages over more modern topical agents such as benzoyl peroxide.[61,63,65]

Salicylic acid products are often used as first-line therapy for mild acne because of their widespread availability without a prescription. They are often available in alcohol–detergent impregnated pads as well as washes, bars, and semisolid vehicles. Lower concentrations are sometimes combined with sulfur to produce an additive keratolytic effect. Concentrations of up to 5% to 10% can be used for acne, beginning with a low concentration and increasing as tolerance to the irritation develops. However, the maximum strength allowed in nonprescription acne products is 2%. In high concentrations of 20% to 30% in hydroethanolic vehicles, salicylic acid, either alone or in combination, can be used as a peeling agent for comedonal acne and hyperpigmentation. It has been shown to extrude closed and open comedones several days after peel, but it must be applied under strict control to offer this adjunctive benefit when treating acne vulgaris.[66]

Sulfur. Sulfur medications often lessen the severity of acne, presumably because of keratolytic and antibacterial action. Sulfur helps resolve comedones by its exfoliant action. Its popularity is due to its ability to quickly resolve pustules and papules, mask and conceal lesions (similar to a thick foundation lotion), and produce irritation leading to skin peeling and mild antibacterial action. Sulfur is used in the precipitated or colloidal form in concentrations of 2% to 10%, since it is practically insoluble in water and must be well-dispersed. Its stability depends on effective maintenance of the dispersion.[62] Sulfur compounds (e.g., sulfides, thioglycolates, sulfites, thiols, cysteines, and thioacetates) are also available and somewhat weaker. Sulfur can cause slight ophthalmic and dermatologic irritation, and patients should be cautioned to avoid eye contact. Use should be discontinued if excessive irritation results. Although it is often combined with salicylic acid or resorcinol to increase its effect, its use is limited by its offensive odor and the availability of more effective agents.[67]

Sulfur has met the criteria of the FDA Advisory Review Panel for nonprescription topical acne products and is considered safe and effective when used alone, although its antibacterial effects were not recognized by this panel. Sodium thiosulfate, zinc sulfate, and zinc sulfide were not considered safe and effective.

Topical Retinoids.
Normal epithelial cell differentiation is a vitamin A–dependent process, and the most powerful peeling agents identified to date are related retinoid compounds. The effectiveness of topical retinoids in the treatment of acne is well documented. There is no consensus about the relative efficacy of currently available topical retinoids (tretinoin, adapalene, tazarotene) and oral isotretinoin.

These agents act to reduce obstruction within the follicle and therefore are useful in the management of both comedonal and inflammatory acne. As a group, the retinoids reverse abnormal keratinocyte desquamation.[68] Thus, the retinoid family are highly active peelers. They improve acne vulgaris by inhibiting microcomedone formation, diminishing the number of mature comedones and subsequently, inflammatory lesions. In addition, they normalize follicular epithelium maturation and desquamation. The third-generation retinoids (i.e., adapalene and tazarotene) are receptor specific. Topical retinoids, unlike isotretinoin, do not decrease production of sebum, but primarily decrease inflammation, normalize keratinocyte differentiation, and increase keratinocyte proliferation and migration.[68]

Retinoids have a secondary effect that facilitates acne clearance. By loosening and decreasing corneocytes, they increase skin permeability, facilitate absorption of other agents, such as antimicrobials or benzoyl peroxide, and increase penetration of oral antibiotics into the follicular canal. This decreases the overall duration of antibiotic treatment and lessens the possibility of resistance. Therefore, combination products with oral or topical antimicrobials are available for increased efficacy, faster onset of effects, decreased total antibiotic use and risk of resistance, and shorter duration of treatment.[68] Retinoids may also improve and prevent postinflammatory hyperpigmentation often seen in people with darker complexions who have acne.

Retinoic acid (vitamin A acid or tretinoin) slows the desquamation process, reducing numbers of both microcomedones and comedones.[14] It is a powerful exfoliant and is not to be used in pregnant women because of risk to the fetus. Gels and creams are less irritating than solutions.

Adapalene is a stable, fast-acting, antiacne treatment that has significant antiinflammatory and comedolytic properties.[68–72] It causes epidermal and follicular epithelium hyperplasia, increased desquamation, keratinocyte differentiation, and loosening of corneocyte connections. Its antiinflammatory effect is due to the inhibition of oxidative metabolism of arachidonic acid and inhibition of chemotactic reponses.[72] It is better at reducing inflammatory lesions and total lesion count[72] and causes less local irritation due to its mechanisms and receptor specificity than tretinoin or tazarotene.[68–75] Release from lotions and hydroalcoholic gels is more effective than from creams and aqueous gels.[68,74] It is a good first-line therapy for colder climates or in patients with sensitive skin.[57]

Tazarotene is also a specific agent with superior efficacy to parent retinoids, reducing both noninflammatory and inflammatory lesions.[68] Its exact mechanism is unknown, but it is thought to activate retinoid receptors and thereby affect keratinocyte differentiation, as well as inhibit proinflammatory transcription factors to decrease cell proliferation and inflammation.[68] It penetrates skin but accumulates in the upper dermis. It is as effective as adapalene in reducing noninflammatory and inflammatory lesion counts when applied half as frequently. Compared with tretinoin, it is as effective for comedonal and more effective for inflammatory lesions when applied once daily.[76–78] Short contact therapy, 1–5 minutes every other night, gradually increasing to overnight, is frequently advocated for dosing in patients with sensitive skin, while oily complexions may tolerate twice daily short contact time. Tazarotene is not degraded by sunlight.[14]

Retinoids include the systemic agent isotretinoin, which has effects on comedogenesis and sebum control, and is reviewed below under Antisebum Agents.

Retinoids tend to produce remissions that are maintained for extended periods of time, provided the accompanying irritation does not impede patient adherence. However, such adverse effects including erythema, xerosis, burning, and desquamation, are issues for many patients. The concentration and/or vehicle of any particular retinoid may decrease tolerability.[69,70] Most retinoids are unstable and insoluble in water.

Topical retinoids are not teratogenic; however, tretinoin should be used cautiously in pregnancy and tazarotene is contraindicated. Tretinoin and adapalene are in FDA category C, while tazarotene, based on large surface area use in psoriasis (see Chap. 107), is in FDA category X.[19]

Application of retinoids should be at night, a half hour after cleansing, starting with every other night for 1 to 2 weeks to adjust to irritation. Short contact time starting with 2 minutes and adding 30 seconds per dose can be advised for patients with sensitive skin or in the winter, discontinuing and resuming after a 3-day rest if undue irritation results. Doses can be increased only after beginning with 4 to 6 weeks of the lowest concentration and least irritating vehicle. Adapalene and tazarotene are photoirritants (not photosensitizers), and sun avoidance and sunscreen use are imperative.[68]

Overall, topical retinoids are the cornerstone of acne treatment and provide safe, effective, and economical means of treating all but the most severe cases of acne vulgaris. They should be the first step in moderate acne, alone or in combination with antibiotics and benzoyl peroxide, reverting to retinoids alone for maintenance once adequate results are achieved.

Antibacterial Agents
Choices for antibacterial therapy include benzoyl peroxide, prescription topical and systemic antibiotics, and combination products. These drugs kill *P. acnes* and inhibit the production of proinflammatory mediators by organisms that are not killed.[14]

Benzoyl Peroxide.
Benzoyl peroxide is a bactericidal agent that has proven effective in the treatment of acne. Because of concerns of resistance, it is often used in the management of patients treated with oral or topical antibiotics. It is available in a variety of concentrations and vehicles; however, there is insufficient evidence to evaluate and compare the efficacy of these different formulations. It has the ability to prevent or eliminate the development of *P. acnes* resistance.

Benzoyl peroxide is a derivative of coal tar and was first used for acne vulgaris in the mid-1960s, becoming popular once stable formulations aimed at its heat-lability were developed in the mid-1970s.[79] These preparations are the single most useful group of topical nonprescription drugs and agents of first choice for most patients with mild to moderate acne vulgaris. Benzoyl peroxide is well absorbed through the stratum corneum and concentrates in the pilosebaceous unit.[80] It has three principle actions useful in both noninflammatory and inflammatory acne. It produces powerful anaerobic antibacterial activity due to slow release of oxygen, thereby acting against gram-positive and -negative bacteria, yeasts, and fungi. This nonspecific antibacterial mechanism does not induce resistance with long-term use.[79] It has a rapid (within 2 hours) cidal effect that lasts at least 48 hours. As a result, it may decrease the number of inflamed lesions within 5 days. As an indirect effect, it induces suppression of sebum production; it does not reduce skin surface lipids, but is effective in reducing free fatty acids, which are comedogenic agents and triggers of inflammation.[80] Topical benzoyl peroxide 5% lowers free fatty acids 50% to 60% after daily application for 14 days, and decreases aerobic bacteria by 84% and anaerobic bacteria (primarily *P. acnes*) by 98%. It also produces comedolysis.

While earlier rabbit model studies showed a benzoyl peroxide effect greater than that of salicylic acid, these animal comedones were not physiologic but induced by tar. More recent studies using native microcomedones show an anticomedogenic effect that is only comparatively slight, compared with tretinoin or salicylic acid.[81,82] Finally, a supplementary benefit of benzoyl peroxide is an indirect antiinflammatory action, which is due either to its antibacterial or oxidizing effects. This has been reported in several studies and thus can be used to support treatment of predominantly inflamed lesions.[79] The drug's antiacne effect is augmented by increased blood flow, dermal irritation, local anesthetic properties, and promotion of healing.[83–86] Since the primary effect of benzoyl peroxide is antibacterial, it is most effective for inflammatory acne. Many patients with noninflammatory comedonal acne will respond to its peeling action.

Cleansers containing benzoyl peroxide are available as nonprescription liquid washes and solid bars of various strengths. The desquamative and antibacterial effectiveness in a soap or wash is minimized by limited contact time and removal with proper rinsing. Stable lotions are available in 2.5%, 5%, and 10%. Alcohol and acetone gels facilitate bioavailability and may be more effective, while water-based vehicles are less irritating and better tolerated. A 4% hydrophase gel is available that suspends crystals of benzoyl peroxide in a dimethylisosorbide solvent as the water in the base evaporates. The resulting solution is absorbed by the skin, leaving no film. The manufacturer claims the resulting efficacy is equal to 10% benzoyl peroxide with the minimal irritation of a 2.5% aqueous base gel. This may be an alternative for the patient with easily irritated skin who requires additional potency. This vehicle is easily combined with prepackaged clindamycin or erythromycin powders. Paste vehicles are stiffer and more drying than ointments or creams, which facilitate absorption and allow the active ingredients to stay localized.

Concentrations of 2.5%, 5%, and 10% in a water-based gel have been compared with the vehicle alone. The 2.5% formulation is equivalent to the 5% and 10% formulation in reducing the number of inflammatory lesions. The lower strength may not be as effective a peeler compared to higher strengths, which is due to an irritancy reaction. Thus, irritant side effects with the 2.5% gel are less frequent than with the 10% gel but are equivalent to the 5% gel. The lowest concentration of benzoyl peroxide should be used for treating patients with easily irritated skin and may lessen irritation when used in combination topical therapy with comedolytic agents.

Benzoyl peroxide may bleach hair and clothing. It produces a mild primary irritant dermatitis that subsides with continued use and is more likely to occur in those with fair complexions, a tendency to irritancy, or propensity to sunburn. This irritation is dependent on the concentration and the vehicle, being higher with alcoholic gels compared with emulsion bases.[80] There are rare reports of contact allergic dermatitis. Cross-reactions with other sensitizers, notably Peruvian balsam and cinnamon, are well established. It may cross-sensitize to other benzoic acid derivatives such as topical anesthetics. Concomitant use of an abrasive cleanser may initiate or enhance sensitization.[87]

Another side effect is body odor from breakdown of the benzoyl peroxide that remains on clothing and bed sheets.

There is no indication that the normal use of benzoyl peroxide in the treatment of acne is associated with an increased risk of facial skin cancer. Although links have been made in experiments with mice, human relevance has not been established. The weak in vitro genotoxic potential is not manifested in vivo based on a lack of initiating or complete carcinogenic activity.[80] Overall, the cutaneous use of benzoyl peroxide is relatively safe, and is recognized by the FDA as category 3, which means that more information is required to make a final determination of safety and efficacy for nonprescription use.[88–91] Safety is also confirmed by the American Academy of Dermatology and the German BGA-Monograph.[79]

Benzoyl peroxide has been used in combination with other antiacne medications, such as sulfur and chlorhydroxyquinoline, or in formulations with urea to facilitate drug delivery. No significant improvement has been demonstrated.

Benzoyl peroxide has also been combined with prescription agents to improve efficacy, reduce dosing strengths, decrease irritation, and reduce resistance of antibiotics.[92–94]

A combination of benzoyl peroxide with butenafine, an allylamine, was compared with benzoyl peroxide alone in an open-label, patient-satisfaction, 8-week comparative study of 23 patients with mild to moderate facial acne.[95] The allylamine-benzoyl peroxide combination therapy outperformed benzoyl peroxide action alone during 2-week evaluations in reduction of comedones, inflammatory lesions, and degree of oiliness. There was a marked preference for the allylamine-benzoyl peroxide combination in terms of patient satisfaction, although the patient sample is too small to reach significant conclusions.

The adjunctive use of clindamycin/benzoyl peroxide gel with tazarotene cream promotes greater efficacy and may also enhance tolerability. Increased tolerability might be attributed to emollients in the clindamycin/benzoyl peroxide gel formulation.[96] A patented gel formulation of benzoyl peroxide 5%/clindamycin phosphate 1% (clindamycin) containing dimethicone and glycerin was studied both as a monotherapy and in combination with topical retinoid use. Certain additives, such as silicates and specific humectants, reduced irritation by maintaining barrier integrity.[97]

Preparations of benzoyl peroxide are available without prescription in concentrations up to 5%. Recommend the weakest concentration (2.5%) in a water-based formulation or the 4% hydrophase, for anyone with a history of skin irritation, or who must use combination therapy.[98] There are many suggested routines to initiate therapy. One is to gently cleanse the skin and apply the preparation for 15 minutes the first evening, avoiding the eyes and mucous membranes. A mild stinging and reddening will appear. Each evening the time should be doubled until the product is left on for 4 hours and subsequently all night. Dryness and peeling will appear after a few days. Once tolerance is achieved, the strength may be increased to 5% or the base changed to the acetone or alcohol gels, or to paste. Alternatively, benzoyl peroxide can be applied for 2 hours for 4 nights, 4 hours for 4 nights, and then left on all night. It is important to wash the product off in the morning. Other drying agents should be discontinued. Patients with very sensitive skin or demonstrated sensitivity to benzoyl peroxide should not use the product, and it should be discontinued if irritation becomes severe upon use. Contact with eyes, lips, or mouth should be avoided.

A sunscreen is recommended if benzoyl peroxide is used. To avoid interactions, apply the sunscreen during the day and the benzoyl peroxide at night.

Comparison of Salicylic Acid and Benzoyl Peroxide.
While both salicylic acid and benzoyl peroxide are used for mild to moderate acne, their mechanisms differ and therefore different types

of acne respond to each. Benzoyl peroxide is a strong antibacterial agent, while salicylic acid acts primarily through keratolysis.

Studies have shown salicylic acid to be equal or slightly superior to benzoyl peroxide in reducing number of comedones and subsequently number of inflammatory lesions. Any superiority salicylic acid demonstrates is likely because it interferes with an earlier step in pathogenesis—formation of the primary lesion of acne, the microcomedone.[63,65] However, studies of the compound did not use identical formulations. Instead, they compared salicylic acid cleansers to benzoyl peroxide washes and salicylic acid solutions to benzoyl peroxide creams. The effect of different bases is critical in determining differences in efficacy and therefore comparability of action since the base itself has an effect and influences penetration and duration of action.

In summary, the two products have similar efficacy, with salicylic acid noted as stronger in terms of retarding comedone formation. Benzoyl peroxide, as an antibacterial with some peeling effects, is considered the nonprescription and cosmetic gold standard for milder versions of the condition, used alone or in combination to increase efficacy and improve tolerability; however, salicylic acid is included in many of these products because of the perception of efficacy and safety for comedonal acne of type 1 or milder presentation.[64]

Topical Antibacterials. The value of topical antibiotics in the treatment of acne has been investigated in many clinical trials. In addition to reduction of *P. acnes* as the primary mechanism for efficacy in acne, certain antibiotic drugs are also potent antiinflammatory agents via other mechanisms.

Macrolides, including topical erythromycin and topical clindamycin, have been demonstrated to be effective and are well tolerated, well established acne treatments. However, they have become less effective since the early 1990s due to resistance by *P. acnes*.[99] Decreased sensitivity of *P. acnes* to these antibiotics can limit the use of either drug as a single therapeutic agent. Resistant strains are usually resistant to all of the macrolides.

Addition of benzoyl peroxide or topical retinoids to the macrolide antibiotic regimen is more effective than monotherapy and mitigates against survival of resistant *P. acnes* populations. Clindamycin is preferred because of potent action, lack of absorption, and its limited systemic use because it can cause pseudomembranous colitis when given orally or by injection. It is available as a single ingredient topical preparation and can also be combined with benzoyl peroxide.

Erythromycin is available alone and in combination with retinoic acid or benzoyl peroxide.

Some topical antibiotic–benzoyl peroxide combinations require refrigeration.[44]

Oral Antibacterials. Systemic antibiotics are a standard of care in the management of moderate and severe acne and treatment-resistant forms of inflammatory acne. There is evidence to support the use of tetracycline, doxycycline, minocycline, erythromycin, trimethoprim–sulfamethoxazole, trimethoprim, and azithromycin. Studies do not exist for the use of ampicillin, amoxicillin, or cephalexin. However, any antibiotic that can reduce the *P. acnes* population in vivo and interfere with the organism's ability to generate inflammatory agents should be effective.[44] Although erythromycin is effective, use should be limited to those who cannot use one of the tetracyclines (i.e., pregnant women or children under 8 years of age because of the potential for damage to the skeleton or teeth). Ciprofloxacin, trimethoprim–sulfamethoxazole, and trimethoprim alone are also effective in instances where other antibiotics cannot be used or for patients who do not respond to conventional treatment.[61,100]

The tetracycline antibiotic family has multiple modes of action, well understood antibacterial effects, and antiinflammatory effects

that target an additional aspect of pathogenesis.[99–101] Agents such as tetracycline, minocycline, and doxycycline are used only as systemic agents. Through calcium chelation, they inhibit neutrophil and monocyte chemotaxis. Doxycycline and minocycline are tenfold more effective than tetracycline, and there is evidence that minocycline is superior to doxycycline in reducing *P. acnes*. Concentrations below the antibiotic threshold still inhibit inflammation, and improve both acne vulgaris and acne rosacea.

Tetracycline is no longer the drug of choice in this family; its disadvantages include diet-related effects on absorption and the drug's lower antiinflammatory and antibacterial activity. Clinically, minocycline appears stronger than doxycycline and will produce a response in patients who do not respond to doxycycline.[99] This may be due to greater lipophilicity; there is a tenfold greater reduction of *P. acnes* by minocycline compared with doxycycline.[102]

Bacterial resistance to antibiotics is an increasing problem particularly because therapy is directed at control over a long period of time.[99] Patients with less severe forms of acne should not be treated with oral antibiotics, and where possible the duration of such therapy should be limited. Resistance has been seen with all antibiotics, but is most common with erythromycin. Resistance is less with tetracyclines than with macrolides, with cross-resistance occurring between tetracycline and doxycycline but not minocycline.[99]

The incidence of significant adverse effects with oral antibiotic use is low. However, adverse effect profiles may be helpful for each systemic antibiotic used in the treatment of acne. Vaginal candidiasis may complicate the use of all oral antibiotics.[44] Doxycycline is very commonly a photosensitizer especially at higher doses. Minocycline has been associated with pigment deposition in the skin, mucous membranes, and teeth, particularly among patients receiving long-term therapy and/or higher doses of the medication. Pigmentation occurs most often in acne scars, anterior shins, and mucous membranes.

Minocycline may cause dose-related dizziness, which resolves with dose titration. Urticaria; autoimmune hepatitis, a systemic lupus erythematosus-like syndrome; and serum sickness-like reactions occur rarely with minocycline.[44,99]

Often, when oral antibiotics are combined with topical agents, the antibiotic may be discontinued after 6 months of therapy.[103] Prolonged oral administration may cause overgrowth of gram-negative organisms, producing a refractory folliculitis and necessitating discontinuation. Regimens should be optimized to minimize antibiotic exposure and reduce resistance. Methods to consider include early use of combination therapy with retinoids. Nearly 70% of patients with acne require antibiotics for 12 weeks or less if aggressive retinoid therapy is used during that time.[99] In addition, initiating use of isotretinoin earlier in indicated patients, rather than prolonging antibiotic courses, and using benzoyl peroxide as part of the regimen when long-term antibiotic therapy is required are two additional strategies to reduce long-term antibiotic use and resistance in acne patients.[99]

Azelaic Acid. Azelaic acid has been shown effective in clinical trials studied with topical 2% erythromycin, topical 5% benzoyl peroxide gel, and topical 0.05% tretinoin cream in the treatment of mild to moderate inflammatory acne. However, the agent has limited efficacy, compared with other antiacne therapies.[44]

Azelaic acid possesses activity against all four pathogenic factors that produce acne. It has antiinflammatory and antibacterial activities. Azelaic acid also normalizes keratinization, which accounts for its anticomedogenic effect. It is a competitive inhibitor of mitochondrial oxidoreductases and of 5-α reductase, inhibiting the conversion of testosterone to 5-dehydrotestosterone. It also possesses bacteriostatic activity to both aerobic and anaerobic bacteria including *P. acnes*. Azelaic acid is an antikeratinizing agent, displaying antiproliferative cytostatic effects on keratinocytes and modulating the early and terminal phases of epidermal differentiation.[104] It may produce hypopigmentation. Inhibition of thioredoxin reductase by azelaic acid provides a rationale for its depigmenting property.

Azelaic acid 20% cream is used in the treatment of mild to moderate inflammatory acne, has an excellent safety profile with minimal adverse effects, and is well-tolerated in comparison with other acne treatments. The most common adverse effects, occurring in approximately 1% to 5% of patients, are pruritus, burning, stinging, and tingling. Adverse reactions are generally transient and mild in nature. Other adverse reactions, such as erythema, dryness, rash, peeling, irritation, dermatitis, and contact dermatitis, have been reported in less than 1% of patients.[104]

Azelaic acid should be applied twice a day, in the morning and evening. A majority of patients with inflammatory lesions may experience an improvement in their acne within 4 weeks of beginning treatment. However, treatment may be continued over several months, if necessary.

Azelaic acid is in a Pregnancy Category B and should only be used in pregnant women if medically necessary. Patients with dark complexions should be monitored for early signs of hypopigmentation.

Intralesional Steroids. Intralesional corticosteroid injections are effective in the treatment of individual inflammatory acne nodules. The effect of intralesional injection with corticosteroids is a well-established and recognized treatment for large inflammatory lesions. Cystic acne improved in patients receiving intralesional steroids.[44]

Systemic absorption of steroids may occur with intralesional injections. Adrenal suppression was observed in one study. The injection of intralesional steroids may be associated with local atrophy. Lowering the concentration and/or volume of steroid may minimize these complications.

Antisebum Agents No topical agents directly influence the production of sebum. Systemic drugs that influence sebum production include high-dose estrogens, antiandrogens (cyproterone acetate), spironolactone, and the retinoid isotretinoin.

Estrogen-containing oral contraceptives can be useful in the treatment of acne in some women. Oral antiandrogens, such as spironolactone and cyproterone acetate, can also be useful in the treatment of acne. While flutamide can be effective, hepatotoxicity limits its use. There is no evidence to support the use of finasteride. There are limited data to support the effectiveness of oral corticosteroids in the treatment of acne. Oral corticosteroid therapy is of temporary benefit in patients who have severe inflammatory acne. In patients who have well-documented adrenal hyperandrogenism, low-dose oral corticosteroids may be useful in treatment of acne.[44]

Oral Contraceptives. Estrogen-containing contraceptive agents have been studied for the treatment of acne. Those currently approved by the US Food and Drug Administration (FDA) for the management of acne contain norgestimate with ethinyl estradiol and norethindrone acetate with ethinyl estradiol. There is good evidence and consensus opinion that other estrogen-containing oral contraceptives are also equally effective.[44] The effect on acne of other estrogen-containing contraceptives (e.g., transdermal patches, vaginal rings) has not been studied.

Spironolactone. At higher doses, spironolactone is an antiandrogenic compound. Dosages of 50 mg to 200 mg have been shown to be effective in acne. Spironolactone may cause hyperkalemia, particularly when higher doses are prescribed or when there is cardiac or renal compromise. It occasionally causes menstrual irregularity.[105–107]

Cyproterone Acetate. Cyproterone combined with ethinyl estradiol (in the form of an oral contraceptive) has been found effective in the treatment of acne in females. Higher doses have been found more effective than lower doses. No cyproterone/estrogen-containing oral contraceptives are approved for use in the United States.[108]

Oral Corticosteroids. Oral corticosteroids have two potential modes of activity in the treatment of acne. One study demonstrated that low-dose corticosteroids suppress adrenal activity in patients who have proven adrenal hyperactivity.[109] Expert opinion is that short courses of higher dose oral corticosteroids may be beneficial in patients with highly inflammatory disease.

Oral Isotretinoin. Oral isotretinoin is a natural metabolite of vitamin A. Its mechanism is elusive, as it does not bind to retinoid receptors. It has been shown to reduce sebogenesis and may also inhibit sebaceous gland activity, growth of *P. acnes*, inflammation, and improve follicular epithelial differentiation.[110] Systemic isotretinoin exerts a primary effect on comedogenesis, causing a decrease in size and reduction in formation of new comedones.[14] Isotretinoin is the only drug treatment for acne that produces prolonged remission.

Oral isotretinoin is approved for the treatment of severe recalcitrant nodular acne. Oral isotretinoin is also useful for the management of less severe acne that is treatment-resistant (unresponsive to adequate treatment, reasonable courses of antibiotic, or combination peelers and antibiotics administered for 6 weeks to 3 months) or that is producing either physical or psychologic scarring.[44]

The teratogenic effects of oral retinoid therapy are well documented. Because of its teratogenicity and the potential for many other adverse effects, this drug should be prescribed only by those physicians knowledgeable in its appropriate administration and monitoring. Female patients of child-bearing potential must only be treated with oral isotretinoin if they are participating in the approved pregnancy prevention and management program (iPLEDGE). Two different forms of contraception must be started 1 month before and continue at least 1 month (but normally 4 months) after therapy.

The approved dosage of isotretinoin is 0.5 to 2.0 mg/kg/day. The drug is usually given over a 20-week course. Drug absorption is greater when the drug is taken with food. Initial flaring can be minimized with a beginning dose of 0.5 mg/kg/day or less. Alternatively, lower doses can be used for longer time periods, with a total cumulative dose of 120 to 150 mg/kg. In patients with severely inflamed acne, an even greater initial dose reduction may be required. In the most severe cases of acne, consideration of pretreatment with oral corticosteroids may also be appropriate. When used, drying agents must be discontinued, and replaced with moisturizers.

Isotretinoin, a vitamin A derivative, interacts with many of the biologic systems of the body, and consequently has a significant pattern of adverse effects. The pattern is similar to that seen in hypervitaminosis A. Side effects include those of the mucocutaneous, musculoskeletal, and ophthalmic systems, as well as headaches and central nervous system effects. Most of the adverse effects are temporary and resolve after the drug is discontinued. Laboratory monitoring during therapy should include triglycerides, cholesterol, transaminases, and complete blood counts.

Mood disorders, depression, suicidal ideation, and suicides have been reported sporadically in patients taking this drug. However, a causal relationship has not been established. Nonetheless, there are instances in which withdrawal of isotretinoin has resulted in improved mood and reintroduction of isotretinoin has resulted in the return of mood changes. The symptoms mentioned are quite common in adolescents and young adults, the age range of patients who are likely to receive isotretinoin. Treatment of severe acne with isotretinoin is often associated with mood improvement. There is epidemiologic evidence that the incidence of these events is less in patients treated with isotretinoin than in an age-matched general population. There is also evidence that the risk of depressed mood is no greater during isotretinoin therapy than during therapy of an age-matched acne group treated with conservative therapy. Nonetheless, patients must be made aware of this possibility and treating physicians should monitor patients for psychiatric adverse effects.[44]

Some patients experience a relapse of acne after the first course of treatment with isotretinoin. Relapses are more common in younger adults or when lower doses are used.

Pharmacologic Cleansing Options

Medicated Soaps and Washes. Medicated soaps, washes, and foams may contain topical antiseptics, or peeling agents such as salicylic acid, sulfur, benzoyl peroxide, or clindamycin, alone or in combination in low concentrations, and may be nonprescription or prescription status. Most washes should remain on the skin from 15 seconds to 5 minutes followed by thorough rinsing. This limits the amount of time the active ingredient is in contact with the skin. Other cleansers are applied after washing and left on the skin without rinsing.

Quaternary ammonium compounds are cationic detergents that are inactivated quickly in the presence of organic material, such as sebum. The duration of action of these products is short.

Bacteriostatic soaps, such as hexachlorophene, carbanilides, and salicylanilides (halogenated hydroxyphenols), are acnegenic.[111] Few ordinary soaps induce acne. However, acne patients are particularly susceptible to comedogenic contactants, and if these soaps are applied several times daily for long periods, they may become troublesome.

Soaps containing coal tar, which can induce folliculitis, are not indicated for acne.

Chlorhexidine inhibits in vitro growth of *P. acnes.*[112] A 4% chlorhexidine gluconate preparation in a detergent base has been shown to be as effective as benzoyl peroxide washes in patients with mild acne, and both preparations reduced the number of inflammatory and noninflammatory lesions after 8 and 12 weeks, compared with vehicle alone.[113]

Alcohol-detergent medicated pads, impregnated with salicylic acid 0.5%, have reduced inflammatory lesions and open comedones in mild to moderate acne. This type of medication is less abrasive, not rinsed off, and convenient.[114]

Alcohol-detergent wipes, swabs, or "pledgets" impregnated with antibiotics, such as clindamycin or lincomycin, are available. The antibiotic is deposited in low concentrations on the surface of the skin, and may not penetrate to the depths of the pilosebaceous duct. Although patients may like the convenience and perception of using an active agent, they should not be recommended over simple cleansing.

Abrasives consist of finely divided particles of fused aluminum or plastic together with cleansing and wetting agents. Abrasives peel and remove surface debris and may assist resorption of papules and pustules. Despite vigorous rubbing, removal of comedones is not accomplished. Particles containing active agents, such as sodium tetraborate decahydrate, dissolve on use, and their abrasiveness is therefore limited.[115] The effectiveness of an abrasive cleanser with and without polyethylene granules showed no difference in results in patients with mild to moderate acne. These products are not indicated in most cases but may be used in a patient who responds empirically.[116]

EVALUATION OF THERAPEUTIC OUTCOMES

9 Provide a monitoring framework for patients with acne. Parameters should be monitored by the patient and recorded in a diary. Therapy should be appropriately tapered in response to improvement or resolution. The health care professional should be responsible for ensuring that the treatment plan remains on schedule and is effective with no adverse effects. The patient should be contacted within 2–3 weeks to determine progress.

Acne is poorly understood by adolescents. These patients often lack knowledge of the cause of the disorder and aggravating factors, indications for self-care versus prescription treatment, and concerns regarding safety and duration of treatment and appropriate application of topical agents. Clinicians should review patient understanding of each of these important factors to ensure patient adherence. There is often a need to supplement counseling sessions with written materials to which the patient can refer at home.

MONITORING OF THE PHARMACEUTICAL CARE PLAN

Tables 106–2 and 106–3 provide a guide for monitoring patients with acne. Table 106–2 outlines general effectiveness and safety

---

TABLE 106-2 Monitoring Therapy for Acne: Parameters and Frequency

Person Responsible and Frequencies for Monitoring:
Patient: daily while on drug therapy; Pharmacist: every 4–8 weeks of therapy or next pharmacy visit

Short-Term
Effectiveness Endpoints (Acne Resolution/Control)

Parameter	Time Frame/Degree of Change	Actions
Lesion count	Decrease by 10–25% within 4–8 wks, with control, or more than a 50% decrease within 2–4 months	If endpoints not achieved, refer to a physician for further therapy.
Comedones	Resolve by 3–4 months	
Inflammatory lesions	Resolve within a few weeks	
Anxiety, depression	Achieve control or improvement within 2–4 months	

Long Term

Parameter	Time Frame/Degree of Change	Actions
Progression of severity	No progression of severity	If endpoints not achieved, refer to a physician for further therapy.
Recurrent episodes	Lengthening of acne-free periods throughout therapy	
Scarring or pigmentation	No further scarring or pigmentation throughout therapy	

Safety Endpoints (Treatment Side Effects)

Dermatitis, increased dryness, gastrointestinal upset, photosensitivity	No adverse effects	Refer to a physician for alternate therapy, dose reduction, discontinuation or additive palliative treatment or preventative measures for adverse effects.

TABLE 106-3 Monitoring Care Plans for Acne Types I Through IV

Acne Type	Description	Suggested Options	Follow-up Action if Patient Responds	Follow-up Action If Patient Does Not Respond in 3 Months	Adjustment in Therapy If Patient Does Not Respond Adequately to Previous Action
Type I	Mainly comedones with an occasional small inflamed papule or pustule; no scarring present	Topical retinoid is the drug of choice; can also consider benzoyl peroxide or salicylic acid	Continue until lesions are completely cleared and then stop or taper therapy	Treat as Type II acne	
Type II	Comedones and more numerous papules and pustules (mainly facial); mild scarring	Topical retinoid plus benzoyl peroxide, topical or antibiotic	Continue until lesions are completely cleared and then stop or taper therapy	Treat as Type III acne	
Type III	Numerous comedones, papules and pustules, spreading to the back, chest and shoulders, with an occasional cyst or nodule; moderate scarring	Systemic antibiotic plus topical retinoid, or benzoyl peroxide *Or* Topical retinoid plus benzoyl peroxide plus antibiotic	Oral antibiotics typically are prescribed for daily use over 4–6 months, with subsequent tapering and discontinuation as acne improves. Other agents can also be stopped or tapered at this time	Add oral contraceptive or antiandrogen (women only)	Oral isotretinoin (except in women who are or who may become pregnant; consider safety endpoints (potential adverse effects) before initiating therapy
Type IV	Numerous large cyst on the face, neck and upper trunk; sever scarring	Systemic antibiotic plus topical retinoid, and benzoyl peroxide +/- oral contraceptive or anti-androgen (females only)	Oral antibiotics typically are prescribed for daily use over 4–6 months, with subsequent tapering and discontinuation as acne improves Other agents can also be stopped or tapered at this time	If no response after 3–6 months, oral isotretinoin (except in women who are or who may become pregnant) Consider safety endpoints (potential adverse effects) before initiating therapy	

endpoints, monitoring parameters, and degree of change and timeframes for short- and long-term outcomes. Table 106–3 is a guide for monitoring acne patients with consideration to the severity grading of acne types I through IV.

TGF: transforming growth factor

TLC: total lesion count

TTO: health state utilities

UV: ultraviolet

CONCLUSIONS

Considerable gaps remain in the understanding of acne, despite all that is known about the pathogenesis of acne and the mechanisms of effective drugs for controlling its symptoms, progression, and complications at structural, biochemical, and physiologic levels. It is still not possible to precisely define the cause of one of the most common skin diseases, nor is it possible to identify a cure for a condition that affects a very large proportion of the global population.

ABBREVIATIONS

AAD: American Academy of Dermatology

ACI: acne severity index

BGA: best guidelines acne

FDA: U.S. Food and Drug Administration

IGF insulin growth factor

LGL: low glycemic load

P. acnes: Propionibacterium acnes

PAPA: pyogenic arthritis, pyoderma gangrenosum, acne

PDT: photodynamic therapy

QOL: quality of life

SAPHO: synovitis, acne, pustulosis, hyperostosis, osteitis syndrome

SPF: sun protection factor

REFERENCES

1. Cunliffe WJ, Gould DJ. Prevalence of facial acne vulgaris in late adolescence and in adults. Br Med J 1979;1:1109–1110.
2. Rademaker M, Garioch JJ, Simpson NB. Acne in schoolchildren: No longer a concern for dermatologists. BMJ 1989;298:1217–1219.
3. Kilkenny M, Merlin K, Plunkett A, Marks R. The prevalence of common skin conditions in Australian school children, III: Acne vulgaris. Br J Dermatol 1998;139:840–845.
4. Lello J, Pearl A, Arroll B, Yallop J, Birchall NM. Prevalence of acne vulgaris in Auckland senior high school students. N Z Med J 1995;108:287–289.
5. Goulden V, Stables GI, Cunliffe WJ. Prevalence of facial acne in adults. J Am Acad Dermatol 1999;41:577–580.
6. Pandey SS. Epidemiology of acne vulgaris (Thesis abstract VII). Indian J Dermatol 1983;28:109–110.
7. Kubba R, Bajaj AK, Thappa DM, et al. Acne in India: Guidelines for management—IAA Consensus Document: Epidemiology of acne. Indian J Dermatol Venereol Leprol 2009;75(Suppl 1):S3.
8. Shalita AR. Acne vulgaris: Pathogenesis and treatment. Cosmet Toiletries 1983;98:57–60.
9. Malus M, LaChance PA, Lamy L, Macaulay A, Vanasse M. Priorities in adolescent health care: the teenagers' viewpoint. J Fam Pract 1987;25:159–162.
10. Rosenberg EW. Acne diet reconsidered. Arch Dermatol 1981;117(4):193–195.
11. Fulton JE, Plewig G, Kligman AM. Effect of chocolate on acne vulgaris. JAMA 1969;210:2071.
12. Leyden JJ. Therapy for acne vulgaris. N Engl J Med 1997; 336(16): 1156–1162.

13. Chu A. Acne Vulgaris. In Lebwohl MG, Heyman WR, Berth-Jones J and Couslon I, eds. Treatment of Skin Diseases 2nd ed., Philadelphia, PA: Mosby Elsevier 2006:6–12.

14. Shalita AR. Genesis of free fatty acids. J Invest Dermatol 1974;62: 332–335.

15. Tucker SB, Rogers S, Winkleman RK. Inflammation in acne vulgaris: Leukocyte attraction and cytotoxicity by comedonal material. J Invest Dermatol 1985;74:21–25.

16. Winston MH, Shalita AR. Acne vulgaris. Pediatr Clin North Am 1991;38(4):889–903.

17. Plewig G, Kligman AM. The dynamics of primary comedo formation. In: Plewig G, Kligman AM, eds. Acne: Morphogenesis and Treatment. New York, NY: Springer-Verlag, 1975:58–107.

18. Puissegur-Lupo M. Acne vulgaris, treatments and their rationale. Postgrad Med 1985;78(7):76–88.

19. Batra RS. Acne. In: Arndt KA and Tsu JTS eds. Manual of Dermatologic Therapeutics 7th ed. Philadelphia, PA: Lippincott, Williams and Wilkins 2007;3–18.

20. Nguyen QH, Kim YA, Schwartz RA. Management of acne vulgaris. Am Fam Physician 1994;50:89.

21. Harrison-Atlas R, Bernhard JD, O'Connor RC, Weinraub LF. What to do when typical teenage acne strikes. JCOM 1996;3:9.

22. Pochi PE, Shalita AR, Straus JC, et al. Report of the consensus conference on acne classification. J Am Acad Dermatol 1991;24(3):495–500.

23. Chren MM, Lasek RJ, Quinn LM et al. Skindex, a quality-of-life measure for patients with skin disease. Reliability, validity and responsiveness. J Invest Dermatol 1996;107(5):707–713

24. Finlay AY, Khan GK Dermatology Quality of Life Index (DLQI): A simple practical measure for routine clinical use. Clin Exp Dermatol 1994;19(3):210–106.

25. Girman CJ, Hartmaier S,Thiboutot D, et al Evaluating health-related quality of life in patients with facial acne: Development of a self-administered questionnaire for clinical trials. Qual Lif Res 1996;5(5): 481–490

26. Gupta MA, Johnson AM, Gupta AK. The development of an acne quality of life scale: Reliability, validity and relationship to subjective acne severity in mild to moderate acne vulgaris. Acta Derm Venereol 1998;78(6):451–456.

27. Wang KC and Zane LT. Recent advances in acne vulgaris research: Insights and clinical implications. In: James, WD, ed. Advances in Dermatology. Philadelphia, PA: Elsevier, 2008:197–209.

28. Johnson BA, Nunley JR. Topical therapy for acne vulgaris: How do you choose the best drug for each patient? Postgrad Med J 2000;107(3):69–80.

29. Habif TP. Acne, rosacea, and related disorders. In: Klein EA, Menczer BS, eds. Clin Dermatol. Toronto: Mosby:1990:756.

30. Kelly AP. Acne and related disorders. In: Sams WM, Lynch PJ, eds: Principles and Practice of Dermatology. New York, NY: Churchill Livingstone, 1990:1014.

31. MacDonald Hull S, Sunliffe WJ. The use of a corticosteroid cream for immediate reduction in the clinical signs of acne vulgaris. Acta Derm Venereol 1989;69(5):452–453.

32. Brodell RT, O'Brien MR. Topical corticosteroid-induced acne: three treatment strategies to break the 'addiction cycle'. Postgrad Med 1999;106(6):225–229.

33. Hitch JM. Acneform eruption induced by drugs and chemicals. JAMA 1969;200:879.

34. Boothroyd, S. Topical Therapy and Formulation Principles. In: Webster G F & Rawlings AV, eds. Acne and its therapy. New York, NY: Informa Healthcare USA, 2007:253–274.

35. Plewig G, Kligman AM. Acne detergicans. In: Plewig G, Kligman AM, eds. Acne: Morphogenesis and Treatment. New York, NY: Springer-Verlag, 1975:270–325.

36. Food and Drug Administration. Non-prescription drugs. 2009, http://www.fda.gov/OHRMS/DOCKETS/98fr/78n-0065-npr0003.pdf.

37. Walzer RA. Acne: some answers to a complexion problem In: Walzer RA, ed. Skintelligence: How to be Smart About Your Skin. New York, NY: ACC, 1981:53–69.

38. Epinette WW, Gresit MC, Osols II. The role of cosmetics in postadolescent acne. Cutis 1982;29(5):500–514.

39. Plewig G, Kligman AM. Acne cosmetica. In: Plewig G, Kligman AM, eds. Acne: Morphogenesis and Treatment. New York, NY: Springer-Verlag, 1975:226–229

40. Mills OH, Kligman AM. Comedogenicity of sunscreens. experimental observations in rabbits. Arch Dermatol 1982;18(6):417–419.

41. Cappel M Mauger D, Thiboutet D. Correlation between serum levels of insulin-like growth factor 1, dehydroepiandrosterone sulfate, an dihydrotestosterone and acne lesion counts in adult women. Arch Dermatol 2005;141:333.

42. Thiboutot DM. New treatments and therapeutic strategies for acne. Arch Fam Med 2000;9(2):179–187.

43. Russell JJ. Topical therapy for acne. Am Fam Physician 2000; 61(2):357–365.

44. Strauss JS, Kowchk DP, Leyden JJ et al. Guidelines of care for acne vulgaris management. J Am Acad Dermatol 2007;56:651–663.

45. Ellerbroek WC. Hypotheses toward a unified field theory of human behavior with clinical application to acne vulgaris. Perspect Biol Med 1973;16:240–262.

46. Hughes H, Brown BW, Lawlis GF, Fulton JE Jr. Treatment of acne vulgaris by biofeedback relaxation and cognitive imagery. J Psychosom Res 1983;27:185–191.

47. Chao CM, Lai WY, Wu BY, Chang HC, Huang WS and Chen YF. A pilot study on efficacy treatment of acne vulgaris using a new method: Results of a randomized double-blind trial with Acne Dressing. J Cosmet Sci. 2006;57(2):95–105.

48. Rhei LD, Zatz JL, Motwani MR. Targeted delivery of actives from topical treatment products to the pilosebaceous unit. In: Webster G F & Rawlings AV, eds. Acne and its therapy. New York, NY: Informa Healthcare USA, 2007:223–252.

49. Bassett IB, Pannowitz DL, Barnetson RS. A comparative study of tea-tree oil versus benzoyl peroxide in the treatment of acne. Med J Aust 1990;153:455–458.

50. Enshaieh S. Jooya A. Siadat AH. Iraji F. The efficacy of 5% topical tea tree oil gel in mild to moderate acne vulgaris: a randomized, double-blind placebo-controlled study. Indian J Dermatol Venereol Leprol 2007;73(1):22–25.

51. Ernst E, Huntley A. Tea tree oil: A systematic review of randomized clinical trials. Forsh-Komplementarmed 2000;7(1):17–20.

52. Sharquie KE. Al-Turfi IA. Al-Shimary WM. Treatment of acne vulgaris with 2% topical tea lotion. Saudi Medical Journal. 2006;27(1): 83–85.

53. Paranjpe P, Kulkarni PH. Comparative efficacy of four Ayurvedic formulations in the treatment of acne vulgaris: a double-blind randomised placebo-controlled clinical evaluation. J Ethnopharmacol 1995;49:127–132.

54. Lalla JK, Nandedkar SY, Paranjape MH, Talreja NB. Clinical trials of ayurvedic formulations in the treatment of acne vulgaris. J Ethnopharmacol 2001;78:99–102.

55. Combest, W. Tea tree oil. US Pharm 1999(April):35–38.

56. Poli F, Ribet V, Lauze C, Adhoute H, and Morinet P. Efficacy and safety of 0.1% retinaldehyde/6% glycolic acid (Diacneal) for mild to moderate acne vulgaris. A multicentre, double-blind, randomized, vehicle-controlled trial. Dermatol 2005; 210(Suppl 1):14–21.

57. Food and Drug Administration. Non-prescription drugs. 2009, http://www.fda.gov/OHRMS/DOCKETS/98fr/78n-0065-npr0003.pdf.

58. Strasburger VC. Acne: what every pediatrician should know about treatment. Pediatr Clin North Am 1997;44(6):1505–1523.

59. Katsambas AD, Katoulis AC, Stavropoulos P. Acne neonatorum: a study of 22 cases. Int J Dermatol 1999;38(2)128–30.

60. Brown S. Therapeutic potpourri. Dermatol Clin 1989;7(1):71–74.

61. Sykes NL, Webster GF. Acne: a review of optimum treatment. Drugs 1994;48(1):59–70.

62. Zouboulis CC. Moderne aknetherapie. Akt Dermatol 2003;29:49–57.

63. Zander E, Weisman S. Treatment of acne vulgaris with salicylic acid pads. Clin Ther 1992;14:247–253.

64. Gross, G. Benzoyl peroxide and salicylic acid therapy. In: Webster G F & Rawlings AV eds Acne and its therapy. New York, NY: Informa Healthcare USA;2007:117–136.

65. Shalita AR. Treatment of mild and moderate acne vulgaris with salicylic acid in an alcohol-detergent vehicle. Cutis 1981;28:556–561.

66. Kligman D, Kligman AM. Salicylic acid as a peeling agent for the treatment of acne. Cosmetic Dermatol 1997;10:44–47.

67. Lin AN, Reimer RJ, Carter DM. Sulfur revisited. J Am Acad Dermatol 1988;18:553–558.

68. Kroshinsky D and Shalita AR, Topical Retinoids. In Webster, G F & Rawlings AV eds Acne and its therapy. New York, NY: Informa Healthcare USA, 2007:103–112.

69. Galvin SA, Gilbert R, Baker M, Guibal F, Tuley MR. Comparative tolerance of adapalene 0.1% gel and six different tretinoin formulations. Br J Dermatol 1998;139(suppl 52):34–40.

70. Mills OH Jr, Berger RS. Irritation potential of a new topical tretinoin formulation and a commercially-available tretinoin formulation as measured by patch testing in human subjects. J Am Acad Dermatol 1998;38:S11–S16.

71. Jeremy AHT, Holland DB, Roberts SG, et al. Inflammatory events are involved in acne lesion initiation. J Invest Dermatol 2003;139: 897–900.

72. Shroot B, Michel S. Pharmacology and chemistry of adapalene. J Am Acad Dermatol 1997;36(6):S96–S103.

73. Weiss JS, Shavin JS. Adapalene for the treatment of acne vulgaris. J Am Acad Dermatol 1998;39(2):50–54.

74. Brogden R, Goa K. Adapalene: A review of its pharmacological properties and clinical potential in the management of mild to moderate acne. Drugs 1997;53(3):511–519.

75. Verschoore M, Langner A, Wolska M, Jablonska S, Czernielewski J, Schaefer H. Vehicle controlled study of CD 271 lotion in the topical treatment of acne vulgaris. J Invest Dermatol 1993;100:221.

76. Russell JJ. Topical therapy for acne. Am Fam Physician 2000; 61(2):357–365.

77. Gibson JR. Rationale for the development of new topical treatments for acne vulgaris. Cutis 1996;57:13–19.

78. Kakita L. Tazarotene versus tretinoin or adapalene in the treatment of acne vulgaris. J Am Acad Dermatol 2000;43 (2pt3):851–854.

79. Gross, G. Benzoyl peroxide and salicylic acid therapy, In: Webster G F & Rawlings AV, eds. Acne and its therapy. New York, NY: Informa Healthcare USA, 2007:117–136.

80. Zander E, Weisman S. Treatment of acne vulgaris with salicylic acid pads. Clin Ther 1992;14:247–253.

81. Zouboulis CC. Moderne aknetherapie. Akt Dermatol 2003;29:49–57.

82. Gollnick H, Schramm M. Topical Drug Treatments in Acne. Dermatol 1998;196:119–125.

83. Cotterill JA. Benzoyl peroxide. Acta Derm Venereol (Stock) 1980;89(suppl):57–63.

84. Cunliffe WJ, Holland KT. The effect of benzoyl peroxide on acne. Acta Derm Venereol (Stock) 1981;61(3):267–269.

85. Lassus A. Local treatment of acne. A clinical study and evaluation of the effect of different concentrations of benzoyl peroxide gel. Curr Med Res Opin 1981;7(6):370–373.

86. Cunliffe WJ, Dodman B, Eady R. Benzoyl peroxide in acne. Practitioner 1978;220(3):470–482.

87. Maddin S. Benzoyl peroxide. Can J Dermatol 1989;1(4):92.

88. Report of the Expert Advisory Committee on Dermatology. The carcinogenic activity of benzoyl peroxide. Information Letter Ottawa: Health Protection Branch (Canada) 1987;711:1–9.

89. Cunliffe WJ, Burke B. Benzoyl peroxide: Lack of sensitization. Acta Derm Venereol (Stock) 1982;62(5):458–459.

90. Tkach JR. Allergic contact urticaria to benzoyl peroxide. Cutis 1982;29(2)187–188.

91. Rietschel RL, Duncan SH. Benzoyl peroxide reactions in an acne study group. Contact Dermatitis 1982;8:323–326.

92. Bowman S, Gold M, Nasir A, Vamvakias G. Comparison of clindamycin/benzoyl peroxide, tretinoin plus clindamycin, and the combination of clindamycin/benzoyl peroxide and tretinoin plus clindamycin in the treatment of acne vulgaris: A randomized, blinded study. J Drug Dermatol 2005; 4(5):611–618.

93. Korkut C and Piskin S. Benzoyl peroxide, adapalene, and their combination in the treatment of acne vulgaris. J Dermatol 2005;2(3):169–173.

94. Bikowski JB. Clinical experience results with clindamycin 1% benzoyl peroxide 5% gel (Duac) as monotherapy and in combination. J Drug Dermatol 2005; 4(2):164–171.

95. Burkhart CG, Burkhart CN. Treatment of acne vulgaris without antibiotics: Tertiary amine-benzoyl peroxide combination vs. benzoyl peroxide alone (Proactiv Solution). Int J Dermatol 2007;46(1):89–93.

96. Tanghetti E, Abramovits W, Solomon B, Loven K, Shalita A. Tazarotene versus tazarotene plus clindamycin/benzoyl peroxide in the treatment of acne vulgaris: A multicenter, double-blind, randomized parallel-group trial. J Drugs Dermatol. 2006;5(3):256–261.

97. Del Rosso JQ and Tanghetti E. The clinical impact of vehicle technology using a patented formulation of 5%/clindamycin 1% gel: Comparative assessments of skin tolerability and evaluation of combination use with a topical retinoid. J Drug Dermatol 2006;5(2):160–164.

98. Mills OH, Kligman AM, Pochi P, Comite H. Comparing 2.5% 5% and 10% benzoyl peroxide on inflammatory acne vulgaris. Int J Dermatol 1986;25(12):664–667.

99. Webster, G. Antimicrobial therapy in acne. In: Webster G F & Rawlings AV, eds. Acne and its therapy. New York, NY: Informa Healthcare USA, 2007:97–102.

100. Bottomly WW, Cunliffe WJ. Oral trimethoprim as a third line antibiotic in the management of acne vulgaris. Dermatol 1993;187:193–196.

101. Dalzeil K, Dykes PJ, Marks R. The effect of tetracycline and erythromycin in a model of acne-type inflammation. Br J Exp Pathol 1987;68:67–70.

102. Leyden, JJ. The antimicrobial effects in vivo of minocycline doxycycline and tetracycline in humans. J Dermatol Treat 1996;7:223–225.

103. Hughes BR, Murphy CE, Barnett J, Cunliffe WJ. Strategy of acne therapy with long-term antibiotics. Br J Dermatol 1989;121:623–628.

104. Passi S, Picardo M, De Luca C, Nazzaro-Porro M. Mechanism of azelaic acid action in acne. G Ital Dermatol Venereol 1989;10:455–463.

105. Goodfellow A, Alaghband-Zadeh J, Carter G, Cream JJ, Holland S, Scully J, et al. Oral spironolactone improves acne vulgaris and reduces sebum excretion. Br J Dermatol 1984;111:209–214.

106. Muhlemann MF, Carter GD, Cream JJ, Wise P. Oral spironolactone: an effective treatment for acne vulgaris in women. Br J Dermatol 1986;115:227–2232.

107. Hatwal A, Bhatt RP, Agrawal JK, Singh G, Bajpai HS. Spironolactone and cimetidine in treatment of acne. Acta Derm Venereol 1988;68:84–87.

108. Fugere P, Percival-Smith RK, Lussier-Cacan S, Davignon J, Farquhar D. Cyproterone acetate/ethinyl estradiol in the treatment of acne. A comparative dose-response study of the estrogen component. Contraception 1990;42:225–234.

109. Nader S, Rodriguez-Rigau LJ, Smith KD, Steinberger E. Acne and hyperandrogenism: Impact of lowering androgen levels with glucocorticoid treatment. J Am Acad Dermatol 1984;11:256–259.

110. Rawlings, AV. The molecular biology of retinoids and their receptors. In: Webster G F & Rawlings AV, eds. Acne and its therapy. New York, NY: Informa Healthcare USA, 2007:45–53.

111. Plewig G, Kligman AM. Acne detergicans. In: Plewig G, Kligman AM, eds. Acne: Morphogenesis and Treatment. New York, NY: Springer-Verlag, 1975:270–325.

112. Stoughton RB. Comparative in vitro bioassay of skin penetration and activity of chlorhexidine preparations and other topical agents against P. acnes: An assessment of their potential use in the treatment of acne vulgaris. ICI: American Inc. Research report on file, CLR-120, Mar 1979.

113. Stoughton RB, Leyden JJ. Efficacy of 4 percent chlorhexidine gluconate skin cleanser in the treatment of acne vulgaris. Cutis 1987;39(6):551–553.

114. Shalita AR. Treatment of mild and moderate acne vulgaris with salicylic acid in an alcohol-detergent vehicle. Cutis 1982; 28(11):556–568.

115. Arndt KA. Acne. In: Arndt KA, ed. Manual of Dermatologic Therapeutics, 4th ed. Toronto: Little Brown, 1989:3–13.

116. Fulgha CC, Caltalano PM, Childers RC et al. Abrasive cleansing in the management of acne vulgaris. Arch Dermatol 1982;118(9):658–659.

117. Elman M. The effective treatment of acne vulgaris by a high-intensity, narrow band 405–420 nm light source. J Cosmet Laser Ther 2003;5:111.

118. Friedman PM. Treatment of inflammatory facial acne vulgaris with the 1450-nm diode laser: A pilot study. Dermatol Surg 2004;30:147.

119. Mariwalla K. Use of lasers and light-based therapies for treatment of acne vulgaris. Laser Surg Med 2005;37:33.

120. Ross EV. Optical treatments for acne. Dermatol Ther 2005;18:253.

121. Lloyd JR. Selective photothermolysis of the sebaceous glands for acne treatment. Laser Surg Med 2002;31:115.

122. Böhm M, Luger TA. The Pilosebaceous Unit Is Part of the Skin Immune System. Dermatol 1998;196(1):75–79.

123. Seaton E. Investigation of the mechanism of action of nonablative pulsed-dye laser therapy in photorejuvenation and inflammatory acne vulgaris. Brit J Dermatol 2006;155:748.

124. Car J, Car M, Hamilton F, et al. Light therapies for acne (Protocol). The Cochrane Library 2009. Issue 4, The Cochrane Collaboration. New York NY: John Wiley & Sons. *http://www.thecochranelibrary.com.*

125. Mills CM, Peters TJ, Finlay AY. Does smoking influence acne? Clin Exper Dermatol 1993;18(2):100–101.

126. Chuh AAT, Zawar V, Wong WCW, Lee A. The association of smoking and acne in men in Hong Kong and in India: A retrospective case-control study in primary care settings. Clin Exper Dermatol 2004;29:597–599.

127. Schafer T, Nienhaus A, Vieluf D, Berger J, Ring J. Epidemiology of acne in the general population: The risk of smoking. British Journal of Dermatology 2001;145(1):100–104.

128. Firooz A, Sarhangnejad R, Davoudi SM, Nassiri-Kashani M. Acne and smoking: Is there a relationship? BMC Dermatol 2005;5(1):2

129. Jemec GB, Linneberg A, Nielsen NH, Frolund L, Madsen F, Jorgensen T. Have oral contraceptives reduced the prevalence of acne? a population-based study of acne vulgaris, tobacco smoking and oral contraceptives. Dermatol 2002;204(3):179–184.

130. Heilig L, Cerahill C, Freeman S, et al. Tobacco smoking cessation for treating acne (Protocol). The Cochrane Library 2009. Issue 4, The Cochrane Collaboration. New York, NY: John Wiley & Sons. *http://www.thecochranelibrary.com.*

131. Anderson, PC. Foods as the cause of acne. Am Fam Physician 1971;3(3):n102–n103.

132. Fulton, JE, Plewig G, Kligman AM. Effect of chocolate on acne vulgaris. JAMA 1969;210(11):2071–2074.

133. Adebamowo CA, Spiegelman D, Danby FW et al. High school dietary dairy intake and teenage acne. J Am Acad Dermatol 2005;52:360.

134. Danby FW. Acne and milk, the diet myth, and beyond. J Am Acad Dermatol 2005;52:360.

135. Thiboutot D. Acne: hormonal concepts and therapy. Clin Dermatol 2004;22:419.

136. Cappel M, Mauger D, Thiboutet D. Correlation between serum levels of insulin-like growth factor 1, dehydroepiandrosterone sulfate, an dihydrotestosterone and acne lesion counts in adult women. Arch Dermatol 2005;141:333.

137. Smith RN, Mann NJ, Braue A, et al The effect of a high protein, low-glycemic load diet versus a conventional high-glycemic load diet on biochemical parameters associated with acne vulgaris: a randomized, investigator-masked controlled trial. Am J Acad Dermatol. 2007;57(2);247–256.

138. Smith RN, Braue A, Varigos GA, Mann NJ. The effect of a low-glycen-load diet on acne vulgaris and the fatty acid composition of skin surface triglycerides. J Dermatol Sci. 2008;50(1):41–52.

139. Smith RN, Mann NJ, Braue A., Makelainen H, and Varigos GA. A low-glycemic-load diet improves symptoms in acne vulgaris patients: a randomized controlled trial. Am J Clin Nutr. 2007;86(1): 107–115.

CHAPTER

107

Psoriasis

REBECCA M. LAW AND WAYNE P. GULLIVER

KEY CONCEPTS[1]

❶ Patients with psoriasis have a lifelong illness that may be very visible and emotionally distressing. There is a strong need for empathy and a caring attitude in interactions with these patients.

❷ Psoriasis is a T-lymphocyte–mediated inflammatory disease that results from a complex interplay between multiple genetic factors and environmental influences. Genetic predisposition coupled with some precipitating factor triggers an abnormal immune response, resulting in the initial psoriatic skin lesions. Keratinocyte proliferation is central to the clinical presentation of psoriasis.

❸ Diagnosis of psoriasis is usually based on recognition of the characteristic psoriatic lesion and not based on laboratory tests.

❹ Treatment goals for patients with psoriasis are to minimize signs such as plaques and scales, alleviate symptoms such as pruritus, reduce the frequency of flare-ups, ensure appropriate treatment of associated conditions such as psoriatic arthritis or clinical depression, and minimize treatment-related morbidity.

❺ Management of patients with psoriasis generally involves both nonpharmacologic and pharmacologic therapies.

❻ Nonpharmacologic alternatives such as stress reduction and the liberal use of moisturizers may be very beneficial and should always be considered and initiated when appropriate.

❼ Pharmacologic alternatives for psoriasis include topical agents, phototherapy, and systemic agents (both traditional agents and newer biologic response modifiers).

❽ In initiating pharmacologic treatment, the choice of therapy is generally guided by the severity of disease. Topical agents are appropriate for mild to moderate disease, while systemic agents are better choices for moderate to severe disease. Phototherapy or photochemotherapy are used for patients with moderate to severe psoriasis, generally when topical therapies alone are inadequate. Patient-specific concerns such as existing comorbid conditions (e.g., diabetes mellitus, hypertension, renal impairment, or hepatic disease) must also be taken into consideration in the choice of therapy. Once the

disease is under control, therapy should be stepped down to the least potent, least toxic agent(s) that maintain control.

❾ Rotational therapy (i.e., rotating systemic drug interventions) is a means to minimize drug-associated toxicities. However, continuous treatment has replaced rotational or sequential therapy and is now the standard of care for many dermatologists.

❿ Some biologic response modifiers have proven efficacy for psoriasis; however, there are differences among these agents, including mechanism of action, duration of remission, and adverse-effect profile. In general, due to their immunomodulatory effects, risk of infection is increased with most of these agents. The use of live or live-attenuated vaccines during therapy is generally contraindicated. Currently, biologic response modifiers are often considered for patients with moderate to severe psoriasis when other systemic agents are inadequate or relatively contraindicated. It has also been recommended that biologic response modifiers be considered as first-line therapy, alongside conventional systemic agents, for patients with moderate to severe psoriasis; however, in practice, drug access due to cost considerations may be a limiting factor. They may be appropriate if comorbidities exist.

Psoriasis is a chronic disease that waxes and wanes. It is never cured, and it is now known to be associated with multiple comorbidities including heart disease, diabetes, and the metabolic syndrome. The signs and symptoms of psoriasis may subside totally (go into remission) and then flare-up again (exacerbation). Triggers include stress, seasonal changes, and some drugs. Disease severity may vary from mild to disabling. Psoriasis imposes a burden of disease that extends beyond the physical dermatologic manifestations.

❶ Patients with psoriasis have a lifelong illness that may be very visible and emotionally distressing. There is a strong need for empathy and a caring attitude in interactions with these patients. Thus, management of this condition is necessarily long-term and multifaceted, and management modalities may change according to the severity of illness at the time.

EPIDEMIOLOGY

Psoriasis is likely the most common immune modulated inflammatory disease in North America and Europe, as it is thought to affect 17 million people, or about 2% of the population.[2,3] Worldwide prevalences vary between 0.1% and 3%, with reasons for variation ranging from racial to geographic and environmental.[3] Higher prevalences than 3% have been reported occasionally in Canada and the United States. Lower frequencies of between 0.4% and 0.7% are seen for people of African and Asian descent.[4,5] Of interest is the fact that

Learning objectives, review questions, and other resources can be found at **www.pharmacotherapyonline.com**.

psoriasis is seldom seen in North and South American Aboriginal Indians. It affects males and females equally.[3,6] The majority of patients (approximately 75%) have onset before the age of 40,[3] but psoriasis has been observed at birth and as late as the ninth decade of life.[3] Many studies report two peak ages of onset: at 20 to 30 and 50 to 60 years of age.[3,5]

ETIOLOGY

❷ Psoriasis is a T-lymphocyte–mediated inflammatory disease that results from a complex interplay between multiple genetic factors and environmental influences. Genetic predisposition coupled with some precipitating factor triggers an abnormal immune response, resulting in the initial psoriatic skin lesions. Keratinocyte proliferation is central to the clinical presentation of psoriasis.

GENETICS

Dermatologists have recognized the familial tendencies of psoriasis for many years. Monozygotic twins have a concordance rate in the 80% range. Rates of family history in a psoriasis family range between 36% and 91%.[6–9] A study utilizing the founder population of Newfoundland and Labrador noted that more than 80% of the patients had a positive family history.

Genetic studies suggested at least seven loci are involved in psoriasis.[3] In 2009, studies of the Newfoundland and Labrador population confirmed that major histocompatibility complex antigen HLA-Cw6 and tumor necrosis factor (TNF)-α as major psoriasis susceptibility genes, along with IL-23 loci that had previously been reported.[3,10] The findings have recently been confirmed in multiple populations from North America, Europe, and China.[11,12]

PREDISPOSING FACTORS AND PRECIPITATING FACTORS

Injury to the skin, infection, drugs, smoking, alcohol consumption, obesity, and psychogenic stress have been implicated in development of psoriasis. Examples of these precipitating factors include a horse-fly bite causing skin trauma (known as the *Koebner phenomenon*),[13] a viral or streptococcal infection, or the use of β-adrenergic blockers.[14] Factors exacerbating preexisting psoriasis include drugs [e.g., lithium, nonsteroidal antiinflammatory drugs (NSAIDS), antimalarials, β-adrenergic blockers, and withdrawal of corticosteroids], and psoriatic patients commonly have exacerbations during times of stress.[1,14] Stressful situations occur for many patients, and it is thought that patients with a genetic predisposition to psoriasis and a precipitating event or trigger factor plays a role.

PATHOPHYSIOLOGY

Psoriasis is a common chronic inflammatory disease of the skin that most likely involves both acquired and innate immunity. The interaction between dermal dendritic cells activated T cells of the TH-1, TH-17 lineage in concert with a multitude of cytokines and growth factors are responsible for the epidermal hyperplasia and dermal inflammation that is seen in psoriasis. These inflammatory cells form lymphoid structures in psoriatic dermis, allowing the unimpeded inflammatory process to continue.[15] When therapeutic intervention is initiated and positive the psoriatic phenotype is completely reversible without residual damage. This is in contrast to significant damage often seen in psoriatic arthritis that, if not treated early, is irreversible.

COMORBIDITIES

It is now well documented that psoriasis patients have significant associated comorbidities. Psoriatic arthritis is one of the most common and well-known extracutaneous manifestations of disease. Other associated comorbidities include metabolic syndrome, other immune-mediated disorders such as Crohn's disease, multiple sclerosis, and some psychological illnesses (anxiety, depression, and alcoholism).[16] Also, malignancies such as cutaneous T-cell lymphoma are associated with psoriasis and melanoma and nonmelanoma skin cancer are associated with psoriasis treatments.

The National Psoriasis Foundation published a clinical consensus on psoriasis comorbidities with recommendations for screening and addressing issues such as cardiovascular risk, metabolic syndrome, and obesity.[17] The importance of screening for comorbidities in psoriasis patients cannot be overemphasized: Nearly half of the psoriatic patients over age 65 have at least three comorbidities, (with two thirds of this patient population having two or more comorbidities).[18] The presence of a specific comorbidity in a patient with psoriasis may influence the choice of pharmacotherapy.

Psoriatic arthritis (PsA) usually develops after the onset of psoriasis,[3] typically 10 years later.[16] However, 10% to 15% of patients report that the PsA appeared first.[3] The prevalence of PsA in psoriatic patients is about 30% but varies by disease severity.[16] In one U.S. study, the prevalences were 14% for patients with mild psoriasis, 18% for those with moderate psoriasis, and 56% for patients with severe psoriasis.[19] TNF-α and HLA-Cw6 are linked to both PsA and psoriasis.[20] Although immunomodulating treatments for psoriasis (such as methotrexate or TNF-α inhibitors) are useful for PsA, NSAIDs effective for joint symptoms of PsA may exacerbate psoriasis.

Metabolic syndrome is a cluster of risk factors including abdominal obesity, atherogenic dyslipidemia, hypertension, insulin resistance or glucose intolerance, prothrombotic state, and proinflammatory state.[17] Patients with psoriasis are at increased risk of developing metabolic syndrome.[17] The syndrome is a strong predictor of cardiovascular diseases, stroke, and diabetes.[17,21,22] Patients with this syndrome are three times as likely to have a myocardial infarction (MI) or stroke, twice as likely to die from the MI or stroke, and five times as likely to develop type 2 diabetes.[17]

Patients with psoriasis also have a decreased life expectancy and increased rates of mortality. Psoriasis is an independent risk factor for atherosclerosis, especially for younger patients with severe disease.[17] A 2006 study found that a relative risk (RR) of death for a 30-year-old person with severe psoriasis was 3.10, after controlling for traditional cardiovascular risk factors[e.g. age, gender, hypertension, dyslipidemia, diabetes mellitus, smoking, body mass index (BMI), C-reactive protein (CRP), and family history of cardiovascular disease].[17,22]

TYPES OF PSORIASIS

Plaque psoriasis, also known as *psoriasis vulgaris*, is the most common type of psoriasis (Table 107–1) and is seen in about 90% of

TABLE 107-1	Phenotypic Classifications of Psoriasis
Plaque	
Flexural and/or intertriginous	
Seborrheic	
Scalp	
Acrodermatitis of Hallopeau	
Palm and/or soles	
Erythrodermic	
Guttate	
Generalized pustular psoriasis	

psoriasis patients. Plaque psoriasis presents as shown in the Clinical Presentations box.

CLINICAL PRESENTATION

Signs and Symptoms of Plaque Psoriasis	Description (From Reference 23)
Lesions (plaques)	Erythematous Red-violet in color At least 0.5 cm in diameter Well demarcated—clearly distinguished from normal skin Typically covered by silver, flaking scales
Skin involvement	Either as single lesions at predisposed areas (e.g., knees, elbows) or Generalized over a wide body surface area (BSA) Mild psoriasis: ≤5% BSA involvement Moderate psoriasis: PASI ≥8 (higher in trials of biologics) Severe psoriasis: The rule of tens: PASI ≥10 or DLQI ≥10 or BSA ≥10% (in some phototherapy trials, BSA ≥20% used as lower limit)
Pruritus	More than 50% of patients with psoriasis have associated pruritus May be severe in some patients and may require treatment to minimize excoriations from constant scratching
Other associated concerns	Lesions may also be physically debilitating or socially isolating. Potential comorbidities: PsA, depression, hypertension, obesity, diabetes mellitus, Crohn's disease, anxiety, alcoholism

DIAGNOSTIC CONSIDERATIONS

❸ The diagnosis of psoriasis is a diagnosis based upon recognition of the characteristic psoriatic lesion and not on laboratory tests. Diagnostic testing is rarely performed as a biopsy may be suggested but is not diagnostic of psoriasis.

Psoriasis is classified into mild, moderate, or severe. In clinical practice, assessment of the severity of disease includes both an objective evaluation of the extent and symptoms as well as a subjective evaluation of the impact of disease on the patient's quality of life.[23] Assessment typically includes measures of symptom and involvement such as body surface area (BSA), Psoriasis Area and Severity Index (PASI), or Physician's Global Assessment (static PGA), as well as quality-of-life measures such as the Dermatology Life Quality Index (DLQI) or the Short Form (SF-36) Health Survey.[23]

Classification of psoriasis as mild, moderate, or severe disease is generally based on BSA or PASI measurements (see Clinical Presentations box). Practically, to give a rough estimate of BSA involvement, palm size is approximately 1% BSA, head and neck involvement is about 10% BSA, both upper limbs about 20% BSA, trunk involvement (front and back) about 30% BSA, and both lower limbs about 40% BSA.

TREATMENT

Treatment of psoriasis is based on managing the underlying pathophysiology. Agents that modulate the abnormal immune response, such as corticosteroids and biologic response modifiers, are important treatment strategies for psoriasis. Topical therapies that affect cell turnover are also effective for psoriasis. In addition, nonpharmacologic therapies are effective adjuncts and should be considered for all patients with psoriasis. A treatment regimen should always be individualized, taking into consideration severity of disease, patient responses, and tolerability to various interventions. Furthermore, if they exist, comorbidities must be taken into treatment considerations. Optimal psoriasis care needs to maintain a focus on the patient's overall health-related quality of life.

■ DESIRED OUTCOMES

❹ Goals of treatment[1]:

- Minimizing or eliminating the signs of psoriasis such as plaques and scales
- Alleviating pruritus and minimizing excoriations
- Reducing the frequency of flare-ups
- Ensuring appropriate treatment of associated conditions such as PsA, hypertension, dyslipidemia, diabetes, clinical depression, or itching
- Avoiding or minimizing adverse effects from topical or systemic treatments used
- Providing cost-effective therapy
- Providing guidance or counseling as needed (e.g., stress-reduction techniques)
- Maintaining or improving the patient's quality of life

■ GENERAL APPROACH TO TREATMENT

❺ Management of patients with psoriasis generally involves both nonpharmacologic and pharmacologic therapies. Nonpharmacologic therapies are important and should be used for all patients with psoriasis, regardless of the severity of disease. Pharmacologic therapies are always tailored to the individual patient with psoriasis and different treatment strategies would be used depending on psoriatic disease severity, presence or absence of comorbid illnesses, and any special considerations such as hepatic or renal dysfunction.

■ NONPHARMACOLOGIC THERAPY

❻ Nonpharmacologic alternatives may be very beneficial and should always be considered and initiated when appropriate.[1] These include stress-reduction strategies, moisturizers, oatmeal baths, and skin protection using sunscreens.[24]

In particular, stress reduction has been shown to improve both the extent and severity of psoriasis and to include methods such as guided imagery and stress-management clinics. Liberal use of nonmedicated moisturizers, applied ad lib, helps to maintain skin moisture, reduces skin shedding, controls associated scaling, and may reduce pruritus. Oatmeal baths further reduce pruritus and with regular use may minimize the need for systemic antipruritic drugs.

Sunscreens, preferably with a sun protection factor (SPF) of 30 or more, should be regularly used since sunburns can trigger an exacerbation of psoriasis. Irritation to the skin should be minimized—harsh soaps or detergents should not be used. Cleansing should be done with tepid water and preferably with lipid-free and fragrance-free cleansers.[1,24]

■ PHARMACOLOGIC THERAPY

❼ Pharmacologic alternatives for psoriasis are topical agents, phototherapy, and systemic agents, including biologic response modifiers.

Drug Treatments of First Choice

❽ For limited or mild to moderately severe disease, topical treatments are the usual standard of care, with phototherapy and photochemotherapy used in moderate to severe cases. For patients presenting with extensive or moderate to severe disease, systemic therapies with or without the use of topical treatments are the usual standard of care. Newer systemic treatments such as biologic response modifiers (BRMs) may be the treatments of choice, especially for patients with comorbidities such as PsA or if traditional systemic treatments (such as methotrexate or cyclosporine) are contraindicated. Once the disease is under control, it would be important to step down to the least potent, least toxic agent(s) that maintain control. **❾** Sequential therapy and rotational therapy may minimize drug-associated toxicities; however, continuous treatment is now the standard of care for many dermatologists. Different treatment algorithms are used, depending on the severity of the plaque psoriasis (Figs. 107–1 and 107–2).[1]

Published Guidelines or Treatment Protocols Treatment guidelines have recently been updated in both the United States and Canada.[23,25-32] All U.S. guidelines are endorsed by the American Academy of Dermatology or the National Psoriasis Foundation, and Canadian guidelines are endorsed by the Canadian Dermatology Association. These guidelines represent the current standards of care.

Topical Therapies

Approximately 80% of patients with psoriasis have mild to moderate disease,[27] and the majority of these patients can be treated with topical therapies alone.[27] Individualized approaches are essential because of the wide variation in patients' presentations, their psychosocial health, and their personal opinions as to what would be acceptable treatment.[23] Topical therapies include corticosteroids, vitamin D3 analogues, retinoids, anthralin, and coal tar. These are generally efficacious and safe for this patient population. Topical agents are also used as adjunctive therapy for patients with more extensive disease who are being treated concurrently with phototherapy or systemic agents.

To determine the quantity of topical agents required, the fingertip unit[33] can be used. One fingertip unit is approximately 500 mg,[27,33] which is sufficient to cover one hand (front and back) or about 2% BSA.[34] The trunk (front and back) is about 30% BSA;

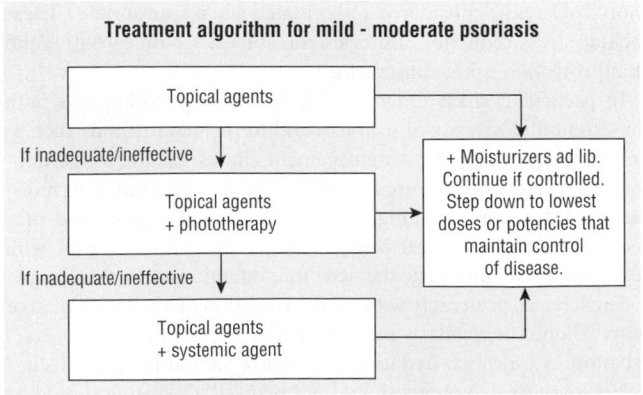

FIGURE 107-1. Treatment algorithm for mild to moderate psoriasis. *(Reprinted from reference 1 with permission from the publisher.)*

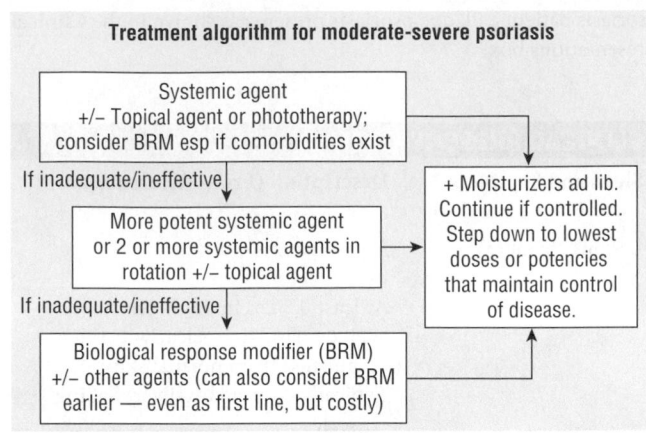

FIGURE 107-2. Treatment algorithm for moderate to severe psoriasis. *(Reprinted from reference 1 with permission from the publisher.)*

to cover the entire trunk once, about 15 fingertip units, or 7500 mg (7.5 g), would be required.

Corticosteroids Topical corticosteroids have been the mainstay of therapy for the majority of patients with psoriasis for over half a century. They are generally well tolerated, although adverse effects can occur, including systemic ones. Table 107–2 provides a summary of topical corticosteroid formulations—including ointments, creams, gels, foams, lotions, sprays, shampoos, tape, and solutions[27]—and potencies.

The choice of vehicle affects corticosteroid potency: Ointments, being the most occlusive, enhance drug penetration and provide the most potent formulations. However, patients may prefer a less greasy formulation, such as a cream or lotion for daytime use, although they may be willing to apply the more effective ointment-based corticosteroid during the night.[27] Providing additional occlusion will increase drug penetration of a topical preparation, resulting in enhanced potency. For example, flurandrenolide cream and lotion are potency class 5, but flurandrenolide tape was found to have higher efficacy than diflorasone diacetate ointment (potency class 1).[27,35]

Despite their widespread use, there have been few large-scale, randomized placebo-controlled corticosteroid trials and even fewer head-to-head comparisons with other therapies. The most comprehensive review to date is the analysis of topical psoriasis therapies done in 2002.[23,36] This systemic review found that all topical corticosteroid treatments considered were efficacious and significantly better than placebo and that the highest potency corticosteroids were the most efficacious, followed by vitamin D3 analogues.[23]

Corticosteroids have antiinflammatory, antiproliferative, immunosuppressive, and vasoconstrictive effects.[27] These are mediated through a variety of mechanisms. Mechanisms of action include binding to intracellular corticosteroid receptors and regulation of gene transcription (in particular those which code for proinflammatory cytokines).[27]

Appropriate use of topical corticosteroids should include an assessment of disease severity and disease location as well as knowledge of the patient's preference and age. Lower potency corticosteroids should be used for infants and for lesions on the face, intertriginous areas, and areas with thin skin. For other areas of the body in adults, mid- to high-potency agents are generally recommended as initial therapy.[27] The highest potency corticosteroids are generally reserved for patients with very thick plaques or recalcitrant disease, such as plaques on palms and soles. The use of potency class 1 corticosteroids should be limited to a duration of 2 to 4 weeks,[27] recognizing that the risk of cutaneous and systemic side effects increases with continued use.

TABLE 107-2 Topical Corticosteroid Potency Chart

Potency Rating	Corticosteroid–Topical Preparations
Class 1: Superpotent	Betamethasone dipropionate 0.05% ointment (Diprolene and Diprosone ointment)
	Clobetasone propionate 0.05% lotion/spray/shampoo (Clobex lotion/spray/shampoo, OLUX foam)
	Clobetasone propionate 0.05% cream and ointment (Cormax, Temovate)
	Diflorasone diacetate 0.05% ointment (Florone, Psorcon)
	Halobetasol propionate 0.05% cream and ointment (Ultravate)
	Flurandrenolide tape 4 mcg/cm² (Cordran)
Class 2: Potent	Amcinonide 0.1% ointment (Cyclocort ointment)
	Betamethasone dipropionate 0.05% cream/gel (Diprolene cream, gel, and Diprosone cream)
	Desoximetasone 0.25% cream (Topicort)
	Fluocinonide 0.05% cream, gel, ointment (Lidex)
	Halcinonide 0.1% cream (Halog)
Class 3: Upper mid-strength	Amcinonide 0.1% cream (Cyclocort cream)
	Betamethasone valerate 0.1% ointment (Betnovate/Valisone ointment)
	Diflorasone diacetate 0.05% cream (Psorcon cream)
	Fluticasone propionate 0.005% ointment (Cutivate ointment)
	Mometasone furoate 0.1% ointment (Elocon ointment)
	Triamcinolone acetonide 0.5% cream and ointment (Aristocort)
Class 4: Mid-strength	Betamethasone valerate 0.12% foam (Luxiq)
	Clocortolone pivolate 0.1% cream (Cloderm)
	Desoximetasone 0.05% cream and gel (Topicort LP)
	Fluocinolone acetonide 0.025% ointment (Synalar ointment)
	Fluocinolone acetonide 0.2% cream (Synalar-HP)
	Hydrocortisone valerate 0.2% ointment (Westcort ointment)
	Mometasone furoate 0.1% cream (Elocon cream)
	Triamcinolone acetonide 0.1% ointment (Kenalog)
Class 5: Lower mid-strength	Betamethasone dipropionate 0.05% lotion (Diprosone lotion)
	Betamethasone valerate 0.1% cream and lotion (Betnovate/Valisone cream & lotion)
	Desonide 0.05% lotion (DesOwen)
	Fluocinolone acetonide 0.01% shampoo (Capex shampoo)
	Fluocinolone acetonide 0.01%, 0.025%, 0.03% cream (Synalar cream)
	Flurandrenolide 0.05% cream and lotion (Cordran)
	Fluticasone propionate 0.05% cream and lotion (Cutivate cream and lotion)
	Hydrocortisone butyrate 0.1% cream (Locoid)
	Hydrocortisone valerate 0.2% cream (Westcort cream)
	Prednicarbate 0.1% cream (Dermatop)
	Triamcinolone acetonide 0.1% cream and lotion (Kenalog cream and lotion)
Class 6: Mild	Alclometasone dipropionate 0.05% cream and ointment (Aclovate)
	Betamethasone valerate 0.05% cream and ointment
	Desonide 0.05% cream, ointment, gel (DesOwen, Desonate, Tridesilon)
	Desonide 0.05% foam (Verdeso)
	Fluocinonide acetonide 0.01% cream and solution (Synalar)
	Fluocinonide acetonide 0.01% FS oil (Derma-Smoothe)
Class 7: Least Potent	Hydrocortisone 0.5%, 1%, 2%, 2.5% cream, lotion, spray, and ointment (various brands)

Adapted from The National Psoriasis Foundation—Mild Psoriasis: Steroid potency chart, http://www.psoriasis.org/netcommunity/sublearn03_mild_potency. Rosso JD, Friedlander SF. Corticosteroids: Options in the era of steroid-sparing therapy. J Am Acad Dermatol 2005;53:S50–S58; Leung DYM, Nicklas RA, Li JT, et al. Disease management of atopic dermatitis: An updated practice parameter. Ann Allergy Asthma Immunol 2004;93:S1–S17.

Cutaneous adverse effects include skin atrophy, acne, contact dermatitis, hypertrichosis, folliculitis, hypopigmentation, perioral dermatitis, striae, telangiectases, and traumatic purpura.[23,27] Systemic adverse effects have been reported not only with superpotent corticosteroids but also with extended or widespread use of mid-potency agents.[27] Systemic adverse effects include hypothalamic–pituitary–adrenal (HPA) axis suppression and less commonly Cushing syndrome, osteonecrosis of the femoral head, cataracts, and glaucoma.[27]

All topical corticosteroids are pregnancy category C.[27]

Tachyphylaxis can occur with prolonged use, although its clinical significance is difficult to verify.[23] It is recommended that the frequency of use be gradually reduced once clinical response is seen, although there are no established tapering regimens.[27] Other approaches include transitioning to weaker potency agents or combination with other nonsteroidal topical therapies.[27] Pulse dosing has also been used to minimize tachyphylaxis and adverse effects.[37]

Vitamin D3 Analogues Topical vitamin D3 analogues include calcipotriol (calcipotriene), calcitriol (the active metabolite of vitamin D), and tacalcitol. Only calcipotriol is currently available in the United States[27] and Canada.[23] Other analogues currently under study include maxacalcitol and becocalcidiol.[27] Their mechanisms of action include binding to vitamin D receptors, which results in inhibition of keratinocyte proliferation and enhancement of keratinocyte differentiation.[23,27] They also inhibit T-lymphocyte activity.[23]

The efficacy of calcipotriol for patients with mild psoriasis is well established in randomized double-blind placebo-controlled trials. In head-to-head comparison studies with other topical agents, calcipotriol was found to be more effective than anthralin (dithranol)[38] and comparable or slightly more effective than potency class 3 (upper mid-strength) topical corticosteroid ointments such as betamethasone valerate 0.1% ointment.[23,39,40] In an analysis of topical psoriasis therapies done in 2002,[37] calcipotriol was found to be as effective as all but the most potent topical corticosteroids.[23]

Vitamin D3 analogues are generally well tolerated and have a good safety profile in comparison with other topical therapies.[41] Cutaneous adverse effects most commonly include a mild irritant contact dermatitis; others include burning, pruritus, edema, peeling, dryness, and erythema.[23,27] These adverse effects may be mitigated with continued use.[27] Systemic adverse effects, including hypercalcemia and parathyroid hormone suppression, are rare unless patients are using more than the recommended maximum of 5 mg calcipotriol (100 g of calcipotriol 50 mcg/g cream or ointment) per week[23,27] or if there is underlying renal disease or impaired calcium metabolism.[27]

Calcipotriol is pregnancy category C. It is inactivated by ultraviolet A (UVA) light thus it should be applied after rather than before UVA exposure.[27]

Retinoids Tazarotene is a topical retinoid that acts through the following mechanisms: normalizing abnormal keratinocyte differentiation, diminishing keratinocyte hyperproliferation, and clearing the inflammatory infiltrate in the psoriatic plaque.[23,27] It is effective in clearing psoriatic plaque lesions and achieving remission.

In a placebo-controlled trial of tazarotene 0.1% and 0.05% gels for patients with plaque psoriasis, tazarotene provided a 50% or greater improvement in 63% (0.1% gel) and 50% (0.05% gel) of patients, respectively, after 12 weeks of use.[42] The therapeutic benefit appears to be maintained for 12 weeks after cessation of therapy.[42] Later clinical trials with tazarotene 0.1% and 0.05% creams versus a placebo vehicle provided similar findings.[43]

Adverse effects of tazarotene include a high incidence of irritation at the site of application, a dose-dependent effect.[23] This results in burning, itching, and erythema, which can occur in lesional and perilesional skin.[27] Irritation may be reduced by using the cream formulation, lower concentration, alternate-day application, or short-contact (30 to 60 minutes) treatment.[27] Ad lib use of moisturizers is also beneficial. Tazarotene is also potentially photosensitizing, due to thinning of the epidermis that can occur with continued use.[27]

Tazarotene is pregnancy category X and should not be used in women of childbearing age unless effective contraception is being used.

Anthralin Anthralin is not as commonly used as other topical therapies currently available for psoriasis; however, there are situations where its use is appropriate and efficacious. It has a direct antiproliferative effect on epidermal keratinocytes,[1,14] normalizing keratinocyte differentiation.[27] Although the exact mechanism of action is unknown, it may have a direct effect on mitochondria[27,44] and reduce the mitotic activity. It also prevents T-lymphocyte activation.[27] Small placebo-controlled studies demonstrated efficacy for anthralin used continuously or as very short contact (1 minute of treatment).[27]

Currently, short-contact anthralin therapy (SCAT) is usually the preferred regimen, where the anthralin ointment is applied only to the thick plaque lesions for 2 hours or less and then wiped off.[1,27] Since lesions are generally well demarcated, zinc oxide ointment or a nonmedicated stiff paste should be applied to the surrounding normal skin to protect it from irritation and burning. Anthralin should be used with caution, if at all, on the face and intertriginous areas due to the risk of severe skin irritation.[27]

Concentrations for SCAT range from 1% to 4% or as tolerated; concentrations for continuous anthralin therapy vary from 0.05% to 0.4%. Aside from significant and often severe skin irritation, other adverse effects include folliculitis and allergic contact dermatitis, but these are uncommon.

Anthralin is Pregnancy Category C. People who handle the dry anthralin powder should avoid skin contact (e.g., by wearing gloves while compounding).[1]

Coal Tar Coal tar was one of the earliest agents used to treat psoriasis. It is keratolytic and may have antiproliferative and antiinflammatory effects.[1] Coal tar formulations include crude coal tar and tar distillates (liquor carbonis detergens) in ointments, creams, and shampoos. Due to limited efficacy coupled with patient acceptance/compliance issues, coal tar preparations are less commonly used today, especially in North American countries.

A 2007 comparative study in Thailand reported that betamethasone valerate was significantly more effective than coal tar.[23,45] Although coal tar may have similar efficacy as calcipotriol, it has a slower onset of action.[22] In addition, coal tar has an unpleasant odor and will stain clothing; thus, it may be cosmetically unappealing to patients.

Adverse effects include folliculitis, acne, local irritation, and phototoxicity.[23] It is carcinogenic in animals, but for humans no convincing data have emerged regarding carcinogenicity with topical use.[27]

Coal tar concentrations as used in psoriasis treatments (0.5% to 5%) are considered safe by the FDA.[30] However, occupational exposure to coal tar, especially in very high concentrations such as coal tar used in industrial paving,[30] was reported to increase the risk of lung cancer, scrotal cancer, and skin cancer.[27,30] The risk of teratogenicity when used in pregnancy is likely to be small, if it exists.[27]

Salicylic Acid Salicylic acid has keratolytic properties and has been used in various formulations including shampoos or bath oils for patients with scalp psoriasis. In combination with topical corticosteroids, it enhances steroid penetration thus increasing efficacy. It should not be used in combination with ultraviolet B (UVB) phototherapy due to a filtering effect that may reduce efficacy. Systemic absorption and toxicity can occur, especially when applied to more than 20% BSA or when used for patients with renal impairment.

Avoid the use of salicylic acid in children. However, it may be used for limited and localized plaque psoriasis in pregnancy.[27]

Calcineurin Inhibitors Topical calcineurin inhibitors such as pimecrolimus 1% cream (Elidel) are used for the treatment of inflammatory skin diseases such as atopic dermatitis.[46–48] Pimecrolimus was found to be effective for plaque psoriasis when used under occlusion[47] and also effective for patients with moderate to severe inverse psoriasis (intertriginous areas are affected).[48] Since this cream is less irritating than calcipotriol and also avoids steroid adverse effects such as skin atrophy, it may be a useful alternative for patients with lesions in intertriginous areas.

Phototherapies and Photochemotherapy

Phototherapy has been used for treating psoriasis for years and is still an important treatment modality today. It has been known for centuries that some skin diseases improve with sun exposure, and clinical studies with phototherapies have been reported since the late 19th century.[25] Phototherapy consists of using nonionizing electromagnetic radiation, either UVA or UVB, as light therapy to treat psoriatic lesions.[49]

UVB is given alone as either broadband or narrowband UVB (NB-UVB), currently with NB-UVB being the preferred method. Broadband UVB is also given as photochemotherapy with topical agents such as crude coal tar (Goeckerman regimen)[49] or anthralin (Ingram regimen) for enhanced efficacy.[25]

UVA is generally given with a photosensitizer, such as an oral psoralens, to enhance efficacy—this regimen is known as PUVA.[49]

With respect to comparative efficacy, NB-UVB is more efficacious than broadband UVB, but may be slightly less effective than PUVA.[25,28] PUVA is very effective in the majority of patients, with the potential for long remissions.[28] However, due to greater availability of UVB treatment centers, more evidence of the efficacy of UVB treatments for psoriasis (in particular, NB-UVB), and especially the increasing concerns about PUVA toxicities (including skin cancers), phototherapy for psoriasis currently uses UVB or NB-UVB where available. Failure of NB-UVB may justify PUVA therapy.[49]

UVB interferes with protein and nucleic acid synthesis, leading to decreased proliferation of epidermal keratinocytes.[25] UVA has similar effects on epidermal keratinocytes. However, because of deeper penetration into the dermis, it also has effects on dermal dendritic cells, fibroblasts, endothelial cells, mast cells, and skin-infiltrating inflammatory cells including granulocytes and T lymphocytes.[25]

Adverse effects of phototherapy include erythema, pruritus, xerosis, hyperpigmentation, and blistering, especially with higher dosages. It should be used with caution for patients with photosensitivity concerns, and drug interactions include photosensitizing medications such as tetracyclines. Patients must be provided with eye protection during UVB, NB-UVB, or PUVA treatments, and for 24 hours[49] or the remainder of the day[25] after PUVA treatments. In addition, patients receiving PUVA therapy may experience gastrointestinal symptoms such as nausea or vomiting, which may be minimized by taking the oral psoralens with food or milk.[25] For patients also receiving oral retinoids (RE-PUVA), the UVA dose should be reduced by one third.[25]

Long-term PUVA use can lead to photoaging and the development of PUVA lentigines. Psoralens bind to proteins in the lens of the eye; thus, there is a potential for increased cataract formation. Furthermore, although UVB has a theoretical risk of photocarcinogenesis, the risk is significantly higher with PUVA and is dose related.[25,49] A metaanalysis reported a 14-fold increase in the incidence of squamous cell carcinoma (SCC) in patients receiving high-dose PUVA when compared with low-dose PUVA, with SCC of the male genitalia particularly elevated.[25,50] PUVA may also increase the risk of basal cell carcinoma and possibly melanoma,[25] which may occur 15 years after the first treatment.[49]

Systemic Therapies

Systemic therapies are the mainstay of treatment for patients with moderate to severe psoriasis, with topical therapies remaining as useful adjuncts. However, as discussed below under combination therapies, topical calcipotriol and betamethasone dipropionate ointment may provide sufficient disease control for some patients.[23,51] Conversely, a subset of patients with limited disease may have debilitating symptoms, and the use of systemic therapies would be warranted.[26] Systemic therapies include the following traditional agents acitretin, cyclosporine, methotrexate, mycophenolate mofetil (MMF), and hydroxyurea; as well as the newer BRMs, specifically adalimumab, alefacept, etanercept, infliximab, and ustekinumab.

Acitretin In the 1980s, etretinate became the first oral retinoid, or vitamin A acid derivative, available for the treatment of psoriasis. It has since been replaced by acitretin, its active metabolite.

Retinoids may be less effective than methotrexate or cyclosporine when used as monotherapy. Currently, acitretin is more commonly used in combination with topical calcipotriol or phototherapy.[23,26] Its efficacy appears to be dose dependent,[26] but low-dose acitretin (25 mg/day) is safer and better tolerated than higher-dose (50 mg/day) therapy.[23]

Common adverse effects of acitretin include hypertriglyceridemia and mucocutaneous adverse effects such as dryness of the eyes, nasal and oral mucosa, chapped lips, cheilitis, epistaxis, xerosis, brittle nails, and burning or sticky skin.[23,26] Less commonly,

"retinoid dermatitis" may occur. Periungual pyogenic granulomas are sometimes seen after long-term use of acitretin.[26] Rarely, skeletal abnormalities—such as disseminated idiopathic skeletal hyperostosis (DISH) syndrome—may occur.[23]

All retinoids are teratogenic and are pregnancy category X, including topical retinoids. Acitretin should not be used for women of childbearing age unless they are able and willing to use effective birth control not only for the duration of acitretin therapy but also for 3 years after discontinuing the agent.[23,26] Men receiving acitretin should not donate blood for a similar time period.

Ethanol should be avoided during therapy and for 2 months after drug discontinuation since it causes the transesterification of acitretin to etretinate, which has a much longer elimination half-life.

Cyclosporine Cyclosporine is a systemic calcineurin inhibitor. The original formulation, marketed as Sandimmune, was first approved as a posttransplant immunosuppressant to prevent organ rejection. The more bioavailable microemulsion formulation, Neoral, was approved by the FDA in 1997 for the treatment of psoriasis and rheumatoid arthritis.[29]

Cyclosporine is efficacious for both inducing remission and maintenance therapy for patients with moderate to severe plaque psoriasis. It is also effective in treating pustular, erythrodermic, and nail psoriasis.[29]

In comparative randomized controlled trials, cyclosporine was significantly more effective than etretinate[52] and similar or slightly better in efficacy than methotrexate.[23,29,53] After inducing remission, maintenance therapy using low doses (1.25 mg/kg/day to 3.0 mg/kg/day) may prevent relapse.[29] The dose should always be titrated to the lowest effective dose for maintenance. In one placebo-controlled study, the relapse rate was 42% for patients on 3.0 mg/kg/d versus 84% for patients on placebo.[54]

For patients discontinuing cyclosporine, a gradual taper of 1 mg/kg/day each week may prolong the time before relapse, as compared with abrupt discontinuation.[26,29] Abrupt discontinuation resulted in a dramatic rebound of psoriasis in a few cases.[23] Because more than half of patients discontinuing cyclosporine will relapse within 4 months, patients should be provided with appropriate alternative treatments shortly before or after discontinuing cyclosporine therapy.[29]

Adverse effects of cyclosporine include cumulative renal toxicity, hypertension, and hypertriglyceridemia. The latter two are particularly significant for patients with prior elevation of diastolic blood pressure or triglycerides.[23] Hypertriglyceridemia can occur in up to 15% of patients with psoriasis who are treated with cyclosporine, although this effect is generally reversible upon cessation of therapy.[26]

The risk of SCC and other nonmelanoma skin cancers increases with duration of treatment[23] and with prior PUVA treatments.[26] Thus, although continuous therapy for up to 2 years may be efficacious,[29] it should be used only in a subset of patients[23] in whom renal function is monitored with annual determinations of glomerular filtration rate (GFR) and monthly measurements of blood pressure and creatinine clearance, with more frequent measurements during the initial 6 weeks of treatment.[23]

Baseline blood pressure, serum creatinine, serum urea nitrogen, triglycerides, complete blood count, uric acid, potassium and magnesium should be obtained before initiating therapy, every 2 weeks for the first 12 weeks of therapy, and monitored monthly thereafter during therapy.[23,29] Age-appropriate malignancy screens should also be done, and patients should be seen for dental examinations at least yearly because of the risk of gingival hyperplasia.[29]

The 2009 Canadian Guidelines recommended that cyclosporine be normally reserved for intermittent use in periods up to 12 weeks for most patients with psoriasis,[23] although other recommendations are for periods of 1 year or up to 2 years.[29] Risk of toxicity increases with treatment duration.

As a CYP3A4 substrate, cyclosporine has significant drug interactions. Serum concentration monitoring is not routinely needed for patients with psoriasis because doses used are lower than in transplant recipients, although monitoring may be advisable for patients taking interacting drugs.

Drugs that can increase cyclosporine concentrations include calcium channel blockers (verapamil, diltiazem, and nicardipine), amiodarone, thiazide diuretics, macrolide antibiotics, allopurinol, oral contraceptives, ezetimibe, selective serotonin reuptake inhibitors (fluoxetine, sertraline), fluoroquinolones (ciprofloxacin, norfloxacin), antifungals (ketoconazole, itraconazole, fluconazole, voriconazole), and cimetidine.[29] Grapefruit juice will also increase cyclosporine concentrations.

Drugs that can reduce cyclosporine concentrations include anticonvulsants (carbamazepine, oxcarbazepine, phenobarbital, phenytoin, valproic acid), efavirenz, and St. John's wort.[29]

Conversely, cyclosporine may also affect the drug levels of some drugs. Concurrent use of potentially interacting drugs should be avoided when possible.

Methotrexate For decades, methotrexate has been the mainstay of systemic therapy for patients with moderate to severe psoriasis. It has direct antiinflammatory benefits due to its effects on T-cell gene expression and also has cytostatic effects.[23] It is more efficacious than acitretin and similar or slightly less efficacious than cyclosporine.[23,31]

Although it also has a significant adverse effects profile, methotrexate is generally considered a safer alternative than cyclosporine unless there are preexisting contraindications such as liver disease. In some head-to-head clinical studies more patients dropped out of the cyclosporine treatment arms due to adverse effects.[26,31] While BRMs are undoubtedly more efficacious, they are much more costly, and some insurance companies require an inadequate response or intolerance to methotrexate (the gold standard) as a prerequisite for approving their use.[31] In a recent placebo-controlled comparative study with adalimumab, the efficacy of methotrexate was 36% versus 80% for adalimumab and 19% for placebo.[55] Adalimumab also provided a more rapid response; however, the duration of remission is unclear. Methotrexate can be used continuously for years or decades with sustained benefits.[23]

Methotrexate inhibits folate biosynthesis; and the use of folate supplementation during prolonged methotrexate therapy as seen in dermatology remains controversial (see Clinical Controversy box).

CLINICAL CONTROVERSY: FOLATE SUPPLEMENTATION FOR METHOTREXATE THERAPY

Although some experts recommend folate supplementation for all patients receiving methotrexate for psoriasis, others add folate only when patient issues occur, such as gastrointestinal adverse effects or early bone marrow toxicity (as manifested by an increased mean corpuscular volume) that can be caused by megaloblastic anemia.[26,31] Lack of folate supplementation has also been listed as a risk factor for hepatotoxicity from methotrexate use.[31] One small placebo-controlled study suggested that folate supplementation may result in a slight decrease in efficacy of treatment;[92] but the study methodology has been questioned.[26,31]

The most significant adverse effect is cumulative liver toxicity; and total lifetime dose of methotrexate must be monitored. Traditionally, patients received a pretreatment liver biopsy and subsequent biopsies when a cumulative dose of 1.5 g is reached. Currently, it is recognized that pretreatment liver biopsies may not be practical or appropriate in all cases[23,31] and that baseline liver biopsies only be considered for patients with a history of significant liver disease.[31] It has also been recommended that a baseline liver biopsy be delayed for 2 to 6 months so that medication efficacy and tolerability can first be established[31] (i.e., intention to continue with methotrexate use). Risk factors for hepatotoxicity from methotrexate include the following: a history of or current alcohol consumption, persistent abnormal liver chemistry studies, history of liver disease including chronic hepatitis B or C, family history of inheritable liver disease, history of significant exposure to hepatotoxic drugs or chemicals, diabetes mellitus, obesity, and hyperlipidemia.[26,31] For patients without preexisting risk factors for hepatotoxicity, it is recognized that they would likely have a low risk of fibrosis and would not require a baseline liver biopsy; furthermore, consideration can be made to continue methotrexate treatment for these patients without biopsies at all, to perform a liver biopsy after 3.5 to 4.0 g total cumulative dose, or to switch therapy to an alternate drug at that point.[26,31]

Other adverse effects include significant nausea, pulmonary toxicity, pancytopenia, acute myelosuppression, megaloblastic anemia, and a small but significant increase in lymphoma.[23] Although rare, pancytopenia can occur anytime with the use of low-dose weekly methotrexate and even after single doses of methotrexate.[26] Methotrexate is an abortifacient and is teratogenic (pregnancy category X) and should not be used in pregnancy. After methotrexate therapy is discontinued, it is recommended that men continue an effective birth control for 3 months (since one cycle of spermatogenesis is 74 days), and women should be on effective birth control for at least one ovulatory cycle.[23,26]

Significant drug interactions include serum albumin binding interactions with salicylates, phenytoin, sulfonamides/trimethoprim, ciprofloxacin, and thiazide diuretics, potentially increasing toxicity. Drugs that can reduce methotrexate renal elimination (such as acidic drugs, including salicylates or vitamin C) will also increase serum methotrexate levels and hence increase toxicity. In addition, drugs with hepatotoxic potential may pose an additive risk with methotrexate use.[26]

Systemic Therapy with Biologic Response Modifiers

❿ Some BRMs have proven efficacy for psoriasis; however, there are differences among these agents, including mechanism of action, duration of remission, and adverse-effect profile. In general, due to their immunomodulatory effects, there is an increased risk of infection with most of these agents. The use of live or live-attenuated vaccines during therapy is generally contraindicated. Currently, BRMs are often considered for patients with moderate to severe psoriasis when other systemic agents are inadequate or relatively contraindicated. BRMs are sometimes recommended for first-line therapy, alongside conventional systemic agents, for patients with moderate to severe psoriasis; however, in practice, drug access due to cost considerations may be a limiting factor. BRMs may be appropriate if comorbidities exist. For example, BRMs such as etanercept would be an appropriate treatment option for patients with both plaque psoriasis and active PsA. BRMs currently available for treatment of psoriasis include adalimumab, alefacept, etanercept, infliximab, and ustekinumab.[56]

Tumor Necrosis Factor-α Inhibitors. Dysregulation of TNF-α production has been associated with various inflammatory conditions, including rheumatoid arthritis, inflammatory bowel disease, ankylosing spondylitis, PsA, and psoriasis.[57] Elevated TNF-α levels are seen in both the affected skin and serum of patients with psoriasis; and these elevated levels have a significant correlation with psoriasis severity.[28] The biologic agents etanercept, adalimumab, and infliximab are TNF-α inhibitors. They offer the prospect of more rapid disease control than is commonly seen with the other BRMs.[23] After successful control of psoriasis, TNF-α levels are reduced to normal.[28]

There are safety concerns common to TNF-α inhibitors, mainly from observations made through their use in rheumatoid arthritis and inflammatory bowel disease. One concern is an increased risk of infections, most commonly upper respiratory tract infections, and less commonly serious infections including sepsis, new-onset or reactivation tuberculosis, and opportunistic infections such as histoplasmosis, cryptococcosis, aspergillosis, candidiasis, and pneumocystis.[23,28] There have been reports of serious pulmonary and disseminated histoplasmosis, coccidioidomycosis, and blastomycosis infections,[60,61] sometimes with fatal outcomes when these infections were not consistently recognized and promptly treated in the patients taking TNF-α inhibitors.[60]

A second concern is the development or worsening of autoimmune diseases such as peripheral and central demyelinating disorders including multiple sclerosis and drug-induced lupus-like syndromes.[23,28,61] A third concern is the potential increased risk of malignancies such as lymphoma,[23,28,61] melanoma, and non-melanoma skin cancer.[28] A fourth concern is the potential for other cutaneous adverse effects including vasculitis, granulomatous reactions, cutaneous infections, psoriasiform eruptions, and infusion or injection site reactions.[57] Flares of pustular psoriasis have been reported primarily for patients undergoing treatment for nondermatologic conditions such as rheumatoid arthritis.[23] There is also a concern about congestive heart failure (CHF), although this has now become controversial due to conflicting studies demonstrating both worsening and improvement.[28]

The current recommendation from the American Academy of Dermatology is that TNF-α inhibitors be avoided in patients with severe CHF (New York Heart Association class III or IV), and those with milder CHF should have their TNF-α inhibitors withdrawn at the onset of new symptoms or worsening of preexisting CHF.[28]

Although the above are safety concerns common to etanercept, adalimumab, and infliximab, their safety profiles are not identical. For example, the risk for tuberculosis (TB) is lowest with etanercept and highest with infliximab.[23] They are pregnancy category B and safe to use in pregnancy.[28]

Adalimumab is a human monoclonal antibody that provides rapid and efficacious control of psoriasis.[28] In a double-blind, randomized controlled and open-label extension study of patients with moderate to severe psoriasis, significant improvement was often seen within 1 week of therapy, complete or nearly complete clearance was seen forn some patients, and clinical benefits were maintained for at least 1 year with continuous therapy for most patients.[23,59] As discussed in the methotrexate section, in a recent head-to-head study adalimumab was significantly more efficacious than methotrexate.[55] Adalimumab is given as 80 mg subcutaneously in the first week, then 40 mg the following week, and thereafter 40 mg every other week continuously.[23,28] More frequent dosing has been explored.[23]

Etanercept was one of the earliest BRMs available on the market for use in inflammatory diseases. It has demonstrated efficacy for rheumatoid arthritis. It was approved for use in PsA in the United States in June 2002 and approved in 2004 for use in moderate to severe psoriasis.[61] It is also approved for treatment of juvenile rheumatoid arthritis and ankylosing spondylitis. Thus, as opposed to some of the other BRMs approved for psoriasis, etanercept has been extensively used in rheumatology both for adults and children.

The dosing of etanercept in psoriasis differs from its other indications, reflective of the dosing regimens found to be effective for psoriasis in clinical trials. Etanercept is used continuously, given as 50 mg subcutaneously twice weekly for the first 12 weeks, followed by 25 mg twice weekly[23] or 50 mg once weekly.[28,61] Significant improvement was seen in about 50% of patients in clinical trials by week 12 and more than 50% of participants by week 24; with continuing therapy, weaker responders continued to improve for up to 1 year.[23,26,62] Continuing therapy using 50 mg twice weekly regimens are being explored and may provide greater benefit.[23] Etanercept was efficacious in children and adolescents (aged 4 to 17 years) with plaque psoriasis dosed at 0.8 mg/kg (maximum 50 mg) once weekly.[63]

Infliximab also received approval for rheumatologic diseases before psoriasis and was on the market before adalimumab. Unlike etanercept or adalimumab, infliximab is a chimeric antibody with both murine and human components; thus, antibodies to the drug can develop, resulting in infusion reactions.[28] Regular therapy rather than intermittent dosing on an as-needed basis may minimize this occurrence.[28] The standard dosing regimen is three intravenous infusions of 5 mg/kg given over a 6-week induction period, followed by regular infusions every 8 weeks.[23]

Clinical response is seen rapidly. In a randomized controlled phase III trial, 80% of patients responded by week 10 (after 3 doses of infliximab); however, the response dropped to about 50% by week 50.[64,65] Rare reports of serious adverse events, including fatal cases of hepatosplenic T-cell lymphomas, have been associated with infliximab use.[28] Other rare instances of cholecystitis and autoimmune hepatitis, which may be a class effect for TNF-α inhibitors, have also been reported.[23]

Alefacept Alefacept was the first BRM to receive approval for the treatment of psoriasis, in January 2003 in the United States and in October 2004 in Canada. Over the years, it has accumulated an extensive and reassuring safety record, with no evidence of increased incidence of infections, cancers, or any other serious adverse events beyond background levels. The exception is that CD4 T lymphocytes can be depleted, and CD4 cell counts must be monitored.[23,66]

In comparison with other BRMs, alefacept monotherapy provides only limited control of psoriasis, and as discussed later, it is often explored in combination regimens to enhance response.[23] However, even with monotherapy, long periods of near complete remission can be seen occasionally.[23]

Dosing is intended to be intermittent. Alefacept is given for a 12-week course, then repeated only when the loss of control becomes unacceptable (up to two more courses per year).[23] Maximal response was generally seen by 6 to 8 weeks in responders, and currently there is no measure to predict which patients will respond.[28]

Ustekinumab Ustekinumab is an IL-12/23 monoclonal antibody and the newest BRM, having been approved for the treatment of psoriasis in adults 18 years or older with moderate to severe plaque psoriasis in Canada in December 2008 and in the United States in September 2009.[67] It selectively targets IL-12 and IL-23, two cytokines that play a role in the pathogenesis of psoriasis.

Two large randomized placebo-controlled trials demonstrated clinical efficacy of ustekinumab, with approximately 70% of patients achieving 75% skin clearance after two doses and maintaining the response for 1 year with continued treatment.[67]

Dosing is 45 mg for patients weighing 100 kg (220 lb) or less, and 90 mg for those of higher weights. Ustekinumab is administered subcutaneously at weeks 0 and 4, then every 12 weeks as maintenance therapy.

Common adverse effects include upper respiratory infections, headache, and tiredness. Serious adverse effects include those seen with other BRMs, including serious tubercular, fungal, viral infections, and cancers. In addition, a reversible posterior leukoencephalopathy syndrome (RPLS) has been reported.[67]

Combination Therapies

Combination therapies may be beneficial in the management of plaque psoriasis: generally to either enhance efficacy or minimize toxicity. As shown in Figures 107–1 and 107–2, combinations can include two topical agents, a topical agents plus phototherapy, a systemic agent plus topical therapy, a systemic agent plus phototherapy, two systemic agents used in rotation, or a systemic agent and a BRM. Rotational therapy is not commonly used in practice, and the use of a BRM added to a systemic agent is still under investigation.

The combination of a topical corticosteroid and a topical vitamin D3 analogue is particularly useful. This was shown in several studies to be efficacious and safe, with less skin irritation than monotherapy with either agent, and the combination product containing calcipotriol and betamethasone dipropionate ointment has demonstrated efficacy in randomized controlled trials for patients with relatively severe psoriasis.[23,27] The combination may also be steroid sparing.[27]

The combination of retinoids with phototherapy has also been shown to increase efficacy. Since retinoids may be photosensitizing and increase the risk of burning after UV exposure, doses of phototherapy should be reduced to minimize adverse effects. A randomized controlled trial with tazarotene and broadband UVB not only showed significant enhancement of UVB efficacy but also reduced the number of UVB treatment sessions needed for response.[25,27,68] The combination of acitretin and broadband UVB reduced the number of needed treatments, compared with UVB alone.[23,69] Acitretin with NB-UVB (RE-UVB) was highly effective for patients with difficult-to-control psoriasis.[26,70] The combination of acitretin and PUVA (RE-PUVA) also showed greater efficacy than monotherapy with either agent.[25,71] RE-PUVA can be used to achieve clearance with up to a twofold reduction in total UV exposure.[23] Phototherapy has also been used with other topical agents, such as UVB with coal tar (Goeckerman regimen)[49] to increase treatment response, since coal tar is also photosensitizing.

BRMs used in combination with other therapies are being explored. Some beneficial combinations have been found. Alefacept and NB-UVB in combination significantly reduced the number of UVB treatments needed with clearance seen in 43% of patients within 12 weeks.[23,72] Infliximab given concurrently with immunosuppressive agents such as methotrexate or azathioprine may result in a lower incidence of infusion reactions to infliximab.[28]

Alternative Drug Treatments

Mycophenolate Mofetil MMF is a systemic agent occasionally used for patients with resistant cases of moderate to severe psoriasis.[23] This is currently not an approved indication in either Canada or the United States.

A few reports and small studies are available describing the efficacy of MMF when used as monotherapy or adjuvant therapy.[73] In addition, one small study evaluated the switch for eight patients with severe psoriasis from cyclosporine to MMF after a washout period of 2 to 4 weeks. On cyclosporine, seven of these patients had deteriorating renal function and hypertension, and one experienced loss of efficacy.[74] After the switch to MMF, there was significant loss of psoriasis control in five of the eight patients but also significant improvement in renal function for six patients.[73,74]

Conversely, another small study evaluated the sequential use of MMF followed by cyclosporine in eight patients with moderate to severe psoriasis.[75] There was significant improvement with MMF in all patients, and all patients further improved when switched to cyclosporine.[75]

MMF has some uncommon but significant adverse effects, including increased incidence of opportunistic infections such as cytomegalovirus, cryptococcosis, candidiasis, and *Pneumocystis jirovecii*.[73] Cases of progressive multifocal leukoencephalopathy have also been reported.[73] There may be an associated risk of malignancy.[76]

Hydroxyurea Hydroxyurea is an antimetabolite usually used for cancer treatments, but it has also been used in the systemic treatment of psoriasis for more than 30 years.[23,26] It is still occasionally tried for patients with recalcitrant severe psoriasis, although BRMs may be a better option for these patients.

Hydroxyurea has been compared with methotrexate for patients with moderate to severe psoriasis.[77] Weekly regimens showed greater efficacy for methotrexate with a faster clearance rate, although hydroxyurea was also efficacious. The authors concluded that weekly doses of hydroxyurea may be an alternative to methotrexate for patients experiencing intolerable methotrexate side effects or have reached the recommended cumulative dose.[77]

Adverse effects of hydroxyurea include significant bone marrow suppression, lesional erythema, localized tenderness, and reversible hyperpigmentation.[23,77]

Complementary and Alternative Medicines. The use of complementary and alternative medicines (CAM) among patients with psoriasis is common, with a prevalence of 43% to 69% in various studies.[78] Most of these patients use herbs, special diets, or dietary supplements in conjunction with their usual antipsoriatic medications and not as replacements. Most patients do not discuss CAM use with their physicians.[78]

A 2009 systematic review of randomized controlled trials found that, although there is a large body of literature on CAM use in psoriasis, the quality of most studies was relatively low.[78] CAM agents and interventions with documented clinical efficacy in psoriasis include *Mahonia aquifolium*, fish oil, climatotherapy (Dead Sea salts), and stress reduction techniques.

Mahonia aquafolium (Oregon grape, Mountain grape, or barberry but *not* European barberry) is an evergreen native to southern British Columbia, western Oregon, and northern Idaho. The rhizome and root contain berberine as the primary active constituent. Berberine is an alkaloid that inhibits keratinocyte growth and reduces keratinocyte proliferation, and it also has antibacterial and antifungal activities. In at least two clinical trials *Mahonia aquifolium* was efficacious in reducing disease severity: In one randomized placebo-controlled study a *Mahonia aquifolium* 10% preparation applied topically twice daily resulted in a significant improvement in the PASI score and the Quality of Life Index (QLI), compared with placebo.[79] Adverse effects in clinical trials included rash, burning sensation, redness, and itching.

Fish oil contains two important long-chain polyunsaturated fatty acids eicosapentaenoic acid (EPA) and docosahexaenoic acid (DHA). EPA and DHA are omega-3 fatty acids. They act as substrates competing with arachidonic acid for cyclooxygenase and lipoxygenase, thus reducing the production of proinflammatory molecules in psoriatic plaques.[78] Several randomized, placebo-controlled, and/or comparative trials for patients with psoriasis have demonstrated efficacy of fish oils. One study comparing EPA plus etretinate to etretinate monotherapy found significantly greater efficacy with the combination of EPA plus etretinate.[80]

Climatotherapy refers to the practice of traveling to the Dead Sea and sunbathing and/or bathing in the sea—the beneficial effects are likely from the high salinity of the sea and UV rays.[78] Several studies have demonstrated efficacy, including two studies using saline spa baths. One study used highly concentrated (25% to 27%) saline spa baths plus UVB compared with UVB alone, and the other used low concentrated (4.5% to 12%) saline spa bath plus UVB again compared with UVB alone. In both studies the clinical response was significantly better with the saline spa bath plus UVB combination.[78,81,82]

Stress-reduction techniques have inconsistently shown some benefit. One randomized study demonstrated that both meditation or meditation and imagery were efficacious as adjunctive treatments for patients with scalp psoriasis.[83] A second randomized study for patients with psoriasis receiving either UVB or PUVA therapy showed that the addition of a mindfulness-based stress-reduction audiotape played during light treatments reduced response times for patients receiving UVB but not PUVA therapy.[84] This confirmed the belief that psychological stress plays a role in psoriasis. More recently, in a case-control study of risk factors during the year before the onset of psoriasis, stressful life events were found to be significant.[85,86]

Special Populations

Psoriasis in Children Pediatric psoriasis is more often attributable to direct precipitating factors such as skin trauma, infections, drugs, or stress.[23,87] Compared with adults, plaque lesions in children are often smaller, thinner, and less scaly, which can make diagnosis more difficult. Face and flexures are more commonly involved than for adults. Psoriatic diaper rash can occur up to age 2. PsA is rare.[23]

Topical treatment is the standard of care for children with psoriasis, with topical corticosteroids often the treatment of first choice.[23] Other useful pharmacologic therapies include calcipotriol and anthralin; calcipotriol with or without topical corticosteroids has also been recommended as treatment of first choice[88] because it produces minimal adverse effects.[23] Since children's skin is thinner and better hydrated than that of adults, they are at higher risk of drug absorption leading to systemic adverse effects. The lowest potency corticosteroid that provides control should be used, and it should be tapered as the lesions improve. If long-term calcipotriol is used, monitoring of ionized calcium is recommended because of the risk of hypercalcemia.[23]

Systemic therapies are reserved for children with severe and recalcitrant psoriasis.[23,88] Methotrexate can provide near to complete clearance[88] and has been safely used to control severe childhood psoriatic episodes and then withdrawn as lesions improve.[23] Regular monitoring for liver and blood toxicity is required.[23] The BRM etanercept was recently studied in a randomized, placebo-controlled trial of 211 children and adolescents (4 to 17 years) with moderate to severe plaque psoriasis. It significantly reduced disease severity; however, four serious adverse events occurred (ovarian cyst requiring removal, gastroenteritis, gastroenteritis-associated dehydration, and left basilar pneumonia).[89] Etanercept has been studied in children with polyarticular juvenile rheumatoid arthritis without new safety concerns emerging.[23]

Phototherapy should be used with caution, especially for younger children, because of long-term carcinogenic risks and phototoxicities. For older children and adolescents with severe, extensive, or treatment-resistant disease, UVB may be a treatment option.[23]

Psoriasis in Pregnancy Hormonal changes in pregnancy can improve symptoms for patients with plaque psoriasis. In one study, 55% of patients showed improvements during pregnancy.[23,90] For patients with more than 10% BSA involvement who reported improvement, lesions decreased by more than 80% during pregnancy.[90] This appeared to correlate with high estrogen but not progesterone levels.[90] Thus, some pregnant women may require minimal treatment for their psoriasis.

Some antipsoriatic drugs have significant teratogenic risks, placing them in pregnancy category X. Thus, women of childbearing potential must use effective birth control during therapy, and

may need to continue effective contraception after discontinuing therapy for a period of time, as discussed in detail throughout this chapter. In addition, drugs listed as pregnancy category C may carry known teratogenic risks in animal studies or have limited available data for use in pregnancy.

UVB has been considered the safest treatment for extensive psoriasis during pregnancy. It is recommended for patients with widespread disease not controlled by topical agents. One problem with this therapy is an increased potential for reactivation of herpes simplex, which may be transmitted to the infant at delivery.[23]

For more detailed information about antipsoriatic drugs in pregnancy, a systematic, drug-by-drug review of case reports and case-control studies is available.[91] The 2009 Canadian Guidelines for the Management of Plaque Psoriasis provides a drug-by-drug summary of recommendations for topical agents, phototherapy, and systemic agents in pregnancy.[23]

Psoriasis in the Elderly. Age-related changes in organ function/drug clearance and greater drug sensitivity increase the risk of adverse drug events for elderly patients with psoriasis.

Methotrexate is hepatotoxic and should be used with caution in the elderly. Cyclosporine has nephrotoxic potential and may also increase blood pressure. Both drugs have significant drug interactions, and polypharmacy, common in older patients, makes management of interactions challenging.

In addition, older patients may have preexisting comorbidities, such as hyperlipidemia and metabolic syndrome, and this may further limit drug use. Topical psoriasis treatments are often prescribed for elderly patients as first-line therapy[23]; however, even with topicals, adverse effects—including systemic ones—can occur with greater frequency in these patients.[23]

Psoriasis in Patients with a History of Solid Tumors. As discussed throughout this chapter, many antipsoriatic therapies carry significant cancer risks. PUVA, systemic therapies such as cyclosporine, and some BRMs are associated with increased risks of oncologic disorders.

A systematic review of the risk of malignancy associated with therapies for moderate to severe psoriasis confirmed the following[76]: PUVA is associated with an increased risk of cutaneous SCC and malignant melanoma; UVB is a much safer therapeutic modality than PUVA; cyclosporine increases risks of lymphoma, internal malignancies, and skin cancers; methotrexate may be associated with increased melanoma and Epstein–Barr virus–associated lymphomas; MMF may be associated with lymphoproliferative disorders; and the malignancy risk may be increased for biologic agents, especially the TNF-α inhibitors.[76]

The 2009 Canadian guidelines recommend that TNF-α inhibitors be used with caution for patients with a history of malignancy or existing malignancies, and the T-cell modulator alefacept is contraindicated for these patients.[23]

PHARMACOECONOMIC CONSIDERATIONS

❿ The wide gap in costs of agents for psoriasis makes economics and availability of insurance or other coverage important considerations in formulating a therapeutic plan.

Currently, the expensive BRMs are often considered for patients with moderate to severe psoriasis when less expensive systemic agents are inadequate or relatively contraindicated. BRMs have also been recommended as first-line therapy, alongside conventional systemic agents, for patients with moderate to severe psoriasis; however, in practice, drug access secondary to cost considerations can limit use. These agents may be needed early, though, for some patients with comorbidities.

A recent pharmacoeconomic analysis of BRMs in the treatment of psoriasis suggests that the cost-to-benefit ratio for BRMs may be favorable.[58]

CONCLUSIONS

Psoriasis is a life-long illness with no known cure. Significant comorbidities may coexist. Treatment should be patient specific, with consideration given to disease severity, patient risk factors, age, and comorbidities. Newer treatment modalities, including numerous BRMs, are now part of the armamentarium available in the management of this disease.

ABBREVIATIONS

BRM: biologic response modifier

BSA: body surface area

CYP3A4: cytochrome P450 isoenzyme 3A4

DISH: disseminated (or diffuse) idiopathic skeletal hyperostosis

DLQI: Dermatology Life Quality Index

HLA: major histocompatibility complex antigen

HPA: hypothalamic–pituitary–adrenal

IL: Interleukin

MMF: mycophenolate mofetil

NSAIDS: nonsteroidal antiinflammatory drugs

NB-UVB: narrowband ultraviolet B (311 nm ultraviolet B light)

PASI: Psoriasis Area and Severity Index

PGA: Physician's Global Assessment

PML: progressive multifocal leukoencephalopathy

PUVA: psoralens plus ultraviolet A

QLI: Quality of Life Index

RE-PUVA: retinoid plus PUVA (as combination therapy)

RE-UVB: retinoid plus NB-UVB (as combination therapy)

RPLS: reversible posterior leukoencephalopathy syndrome

SCAT: short-contact anthralin therapy

SCC: squamous cell carcinoma

SF-36: Short Form Health Survey

SPF: sun protection factor

TNF-α: Tumor necrosis factor-α

UVA: ultraviolet A (315 to 400 nm ultraviolet A light)

UVB: ultraviolet B, or broadband UVB (28 to 315 nm ultraviolet B light)

REFERENCES

1. Law RM. Chapter 64: Psoriasis. In: Chisholm-Burns M, ed. Pharmacotherapy Principles and Practice, 2nd ed. New York: McGraw-Hill; 2010.
2. de Rie MA, Goedkoop AY, Bos JD. Overview of psoriasis. Dermatol Ther 2004;17:341–349.
3. Gulliver WP, Pirzada SM. Psoriasis; More than skin deep. In: Saeland S, ed. Recent Advances in Skin Immunology. Kevala, India: Research Signpost; 2008:167–179.
4. Christopher E. Psoriasis-Epidemiology and Clinical spectrum. Clinical and Experimental Dermatol 2001;26:314–320.
5. Lowes, MA, Bowcock AM, Krueger JG. Pathogenesis and Therapy of Psoriasis. Nature 2007;445(7130):866–873.
6. Farber EM, Nall ML. The Natural History of Psoriasis in 5600 pts, Dermatol 1974;148:118.
7. Farber E, Bright R, Nall M. Psoriasis: A questionnaire survey of 2144 pts. Arch Derm 1974;98:248–259.
8. Lomboldt G. Psoriasis: Prevalence, spontaneous course and genetics, GEC. Gad, Copenhagen; 1963.
9. Farber EM, Nall ML, Watson W. Natural history of psoriasis in 61 twin pairs. Arch of Dermatol 1974;109:207–211.
10. Nall L, Gulliver WP, Charmley P, et al. Search for the psoriasis susceptibility gene: The Newfoundland Study. Cutis 1999;64:323–329.
11. Nair RP, Duffin KC, Helms C, et al. Genome-wide scan reveals association of psoriasis with IL-23 and NF-kB pathways. Nature Genetics 2009;41:199–204.
12. Zhang XJ, Huang W, Yang S, et al. Psoriasis genome-wide association study identified susceptibility variants within LCE gene cluster at 1q21. Nature Genetics; 2009;41:205–210.
13. Raychaudhuri SP, Jiang W-Y, Raychaudhuri SK. Revisiting the Koebner Phenomenon. Am J Pathol 2008;172:961–971.
14. Clarke C. Psoriasis—first-line treatments. Pharm J 2005;274:623–626.
15. Nickoloff BJ, Nestle FO. Recent insight into the immunopathogenesis of psoriasis provide new therapeutic opportunities. J Clin Invest 2004;113:1664–1675.
16. Guenther L, Gulliver W. Psoriasis comorbidities. Journal of Cutaneous Medicine and Surgery 2009;13(suppl. 2):S77–S87.
17. Kimball AB, Gladman D, Gelfand JM, et al. National Psoriasis Foundation clinical consensus on psoriasis comorbidities and recommendations for screening. J Am Acad Dermatol 2008;58: 1031–1042.
18. Gulliver WP. Importance of screening for comorbidities in psoriasis patients. Expert Rev Dermatol 2008;3:133–135.
19. Gelfand JM, Gladman Dd, Mease PJ, et al. Epidemiology of psoriatic arthritis in the population of the United States. J Am Acad Dermatol 2005;53:573–577.
20. Rahman P, O'Reilly DD. Psoriatic arthritis genetic susceptibility and pharmacogenetics. Pharmacogenomics 2008;9:195–205.
21. Wilson PW, D'Agostino RB, Parise H, et al. Metabolic syndrome as a precursor of cardiovascular disease and type 2 diabetes mellitus. Circulation 2005;112:3066–3072.
22. Gelfand JM, Neimann AL, Shin DB, et al. Risk of myocardial infarction in patients with psoriasis. JAMA 2006;296:1735–1741.
23. Papp KA, Gulliver W, Lynde CW, Poulin Y (Steering Committee). 2009 Canadian Guidelines for the Management of Plaque Psoriasis— Canadian Guidelines for the Management of Plaque Psoriasis. 1st ed. Endorsed by the Canadian Dermatology Association; 2009, *http://www.dermatology.ca/guidelines/cdnpsoriasisguidelines.pdfwww.dermatology.ca/psoriasisguidelines.html.*
24. Law RMT, Gulliver WP. Psoriasis: The harried school teacher. Section 14: Dermatological Disorders, Chapter 103. In: Schwinghammer TL, Koehler JM, eds. Pharmacotherapy Casebook: A Patient-Focused Approach. 7th ed. and In: Instructor's Guide [to accompany] Pharmacotherapy Casebook: A Patient-Focused Approach. 7th ed., Chapter 103. New York: McGraw-Hill; 2008.:256–258.
25. Menter A, Korman NJ, Elmets CA, et al. 2009 guidelines of care for the management of psoriasis and psoriatic arthritis—Section 5. Guidelines of care for the treatment of psoriasis with phototherapy and photochemotherapy. J Am Acad Dermatol 2010;62:114–135.
26. Menter A, Korman NJ, Elmets CA, et al. 2009 Guidelines of care for the management of psoriasis and psoriatic arthritis—Section 4. Guidelines of care for the management and treatment of psoriasis with traditional systemic agents. J Am Acad Dermatol 2009;61: 451–485.
27. Menter A, Korman NJ, Elmets CA, et al. 2009 Guidelines of care for the management of psoriasis and psoriatic arthritis—Section 3. Guidelines of care for the management and treatment of psoriasis with topical therapies. J Am Acad Dermatol 2009;60:643–659.
28. Menter A. Gottlieb A, Feldman SR, et al. Guidelines of care for the management of psoriasis and psoriatic arthritis. Section 1. Overview of psoriasis and guidelines of care for the treatment of psoriasis with biologics. J Am Acad Dermatol 2008;58:826–850.

29. Rosmarin DM, Lebwohl M, Elewski BE, et al. Cyclosporine and psoriasis: 2008 National psoriasis Foundation Consensus Conference. J Am Acad Dermatol 2010;62:838–853.

30. National Psoriasis foundation—Topical treatments for psoriasis including steroids; 2009, *http://www.psoriasis.org/NetCommunity/Document.Doc?id=164.*

31. Kalb RE, Strober B, Weinstein G, Lebwohl M. Methotrexate and psoriasis: 2009 National Psoriasis Foundation Consensus Conference. J Am Acad Dermatol 2009;60:824–837.

32. Guenther L, Langley RG, Shear NH, et al. Integrating biologic agents into management of moderate-to-severe psoriasis: a consensus of the Canadian Psoriasis Expert Panel. J Cutan Med Surg 2004;8:321–337.

33. Long CC, Finlay AY. The finger-tip unit—a new practical measure. Clin Exp Dermatol 1991;16:444–447.

34. Menter Kamili. Topical treatment of psoriasis. In: Yawalkar N, ed. Current Problems in Dermatology. Basel, Switzerland: S. Karger AG; 2009.

35. Krueger GG, O'Reilly MA, Weidner M, et al. Comparative efficacy of once-daily flurandrenolide tape versus twice-daily diflorasone diacetate ointment in the treatment of psoriasis. J Am Acad Dermatol 1998;38:186–190.

36. Mason J, Mason AR, Cork MJ. Topical preparations for the treatment of psoriasis: a systemic review. Br J Dermatol 2002;146:351–364.

37. Katz HI, Prawer SE, Medansky RS, et al. Intermittent corticosteroid maintenance treatment of psoriasis: A double-blind multicenter trial of augmented betamethasone dipropionate ointment in a pulse dose treatment regimen. Dermatol 1991;183:269–274.

38. Wall ARJ, Poyner TF, Menday AP. A comparison of treatment with dithranol and calcipotriol on the clinical severity and quality of life in patients with psoriasis. Br J Dermatol 1998;139:1005–1011.

39. Cunliffe WJ, Berth-Jones J, Claudy A, et al. Comparative study of calcipotriol (MC 903) ointment and betamethasone 17-valerate ointment in patients with psoriasis vulgaris. J Am Acad Dermatol 1992;26:736–743.

40. Kragballe K, Gjertsen BT, De Hoop D, et al. Double-blind, right/left comparison of calcipotriol and betamethasone valerate in treatment of psoriasis vulgaris. Lancet 1991;337:193–196.

41. Bruner CR, Feldman SR, Wentrapragada M, et al. A systemic review of adverse effects associated with topical treatments for psoriasis. Dermatol Online J 2003;9:2.

42. Weinstein GD, Krueger GG, Lowe NJ, et al. Tazarotene gel, a new retinoid, for topical therapy of psoriasis: vehicle-controlled study of safety, efficacy, and duration of therapeutic effect. J Am Acad Dermatol 1997;37:85–92.

43. Weinstein GD, Koo JY, Krueger GG, et al. Tazarotene cream in the treatment of psoriasis: two multicenter, double-blind, randomized, vehicle-controlled studies of the safety and efficacy of tazarotene cream 0.05% and 0.1% applied once daily for 12 weeks. J Am Acad Dermatol 2003;48:760–767.

44. McGill A, Frank A, Emmett N, et al. The anti-psoriatic drug anthralin accumulates in keratinocyte mitochondria, dissipates mitochondrial membrane potential, and induces apoptosis through a pathway dependent on respiratory competent mitochondria. FASEB J 2005;19:1012–1014.

45. Thawornchaisit P, Harncharoen K. A comparative study of tar and betamethasone valerate in chronic plaque psoriasis: a study in Thailand. J Med Assoc Thai 2007;90:1997–2002.

46. Stuetz A, Grassberger M, Meingassner JG. Pimecrolimus (Elidel, SDZ ASM 981)—Preclinical pharmacologic profile and skin selectivity. Semin Cutan Med Surg 2001;20:233–241.

47. Mrowietz U, Graeber M, Brautigam M, et al. The novel ascomycin derivative SDZ ASM 981 is effective for psoriasis when used topically under occlusion. Br J Dermatol 1998;139:992–996.

48. Gribetz C, Ling M, Lebwohl M, et al. Pimecrolimus cream 1% in the treatment of intertriginous psoriasis: A double-blind, randomized study. J Am Acad Dermatol 2004;51:731–738.

49. Matz H. Phototherapy for psoriasis: what to choose and how to use: facts and controversies. Clini Dermatol 2010;28:73–80.

50. Stern RS. Genital tumors among men with psoriasis exposed to psoralens and ultraviolet A radiation (PUVA) and ultraviolet B radiation: the photochemotherapy follow-up study. N Engl J Med 1990;322:1093–1097.

51. Anstey AV, Kragballe K. Retrospective assessment of PASI 50 and PASI 75 attainment with a calcipotriol/betamethasone dipropionate ointment. Int J Dermatol 2006;45:970–975.

52. Mahrie G, Schulze HJ, Farber L, et al. Low-dose short-term cyclosporine versus etretinate in psoriasis: improvement of skin, nail, and joint involvement. J Am Acad Dermatol 1995;32:78–88.

53. Heydendael VM, Spuls POL, Opmeer BC, et al. Methotrexate versus cyclosporine in moderate-to-severe chronic plaque psoriasis. N Engl J Med 2003;349:658–665.

54. Shupack J, Abel E, Bauer E, et al. Cyclosporine as maintenance therapy in patients with severe psoriasis. J Am Acad Dermatol 1997;36:423–432.

55. Saurat JH, Stingl G, Dubertret L, et al. Efficacy and safety results from the randomized controlled comparative study of adalimumab vs. methotrexate vs. placebo in patients with psoriasis (CHAMPION). Br J Dermatol 2008;158:558–566.

56. Ferrandiz C, Carrascosa JM, Boada A. A new era in the management of psoriasis? The biologics: facts and controversies. Clinics in Dermatol 2010;28:81–87.

57. Moustou A-E, Matekovits A, Dessinioti C, et al. Cutaneous side effects of anti-tumor necrosis factor biologic therapy: A clinical review. J Am Acad Dermatol 2009;61:486–504.

58. Poulin Y, Langley R, Teiseira HD, et al. Biologics in the treatment of psoriasis: Clinical and economic overview. J Cutan Med Surg 2009;13(suppl. 2):S49–S57.

59. Gordon KB, Langley RG, Leonard C, et al. Clinical response to adalimumab treatment in patients with moderate to severe psoriasis: double-blind, randomized controlled trial and open-label extension study. J Am Acad Dermatol 2006;55:598–606.

60. Health Canada. Association of Enbrel (etanercept) with Histoplasmosis and Other Invasive Fungal Infections—For Health Professionals; 2009, *http://www.hc-sc.gc.ca/dhp-mps/medeff/advisories-avis/prof/_2009/enbrel_hpc-cps-eng.php.*

61. Bissonnette R. Etanercept for the treatment of psoriasis. Skin Ther Lett 2006;11:1–4, *http://www.skintherapyletter.com/2006/11.1/1.html.*

62. Leonardi CL, Powers JL, Matheson RT, et al. Etanercept as monotherapy in patients with psoriasis. N Engl J Med 2003;349:2014–2022.

63. Paller AS, Siegfried EC, Langley RG, et al. Etanercept treatment for children and adolescents with plaque psoriasis. N Engl J Med 2008;358:241–251.

64. Reich K, Nestle FO, Papp K, et al. Infliximab induction and maintenance therapy for moderate-to-severe psoriasis: A phase III, multi-center, double-blind trial. Lancet 2005;366:1367–1374.

65. Menter A, Feldman SR, Weinstein GD, et al. A randomized comparison of continuous vs intermittent infliximab maintenance regimens over 1 year in the treatment of moderate-to-severe plaque psoriasis. J Am Acad Dermatol 2007;56:e1–e15.

66. Goffe B, Papp K, Gratton D, et al. An integrated analysis of thirteen trials summarizing the long-term safety of alefacept in psoriasis patients who have received up to nine courses of therapy. Clin Ther 2005;27:1912–1921.

67. Stelara (ustekinumab) anti IL-12/23—receives FDA approval for treatment of moderate to severe plaques psoriasis with four-times-a-year maintenance dosing. Johnson & Johnson; 2009, *http://www.jnj.com/connect/news/all/20090925_150000.*

68. Koo JY, Lowe NJ, Lew-Kaya DA, et al. Tazarotene plus UVB phototherapy in the treatment of psoriasis. J Am Acad Dermatol 2000;43:821–828.

69. Lowe NJ, Prystowsky JH, Bourget T, et al. Acitretin plus UVB therapy for psoriasis: comparisons with placebo plus UVB and acitretin alone. J Am Acad Dermatol 1991;24:591–594.

70. Spuls PI, Rozenblit M, Lebwohl M. Retrospective study of the efficacy of narrowband UVB and acitretin. J Dermatolog Treat 2003;14(suppl):17–20.

71. Tanew A, Guggenbichler A, Honigsmann H, et al. Photochemotherapy for severe psoriasis without or in combination with acitretin: a randomized, double-blind comparison study. J Am Acad Dermatol 1991;25:682–684.

72. Legat FJ, Hofer A, Wackernagel A, et al. Narrowband UV-B phototherapy, alefacept, and clearance of psoriasis. Arch Dermatol 2007;143:1016–1022.

73. Orvis AK, Wesson SK, Breza TS, et al. Mycophenolate mofetil in dermatology. J Am Acad Dermatol 2009;60:183–199.

74. Davidson SC, Morris-Jones R, Powles AV, et al. Change of treatment from cyclosporin to mycophenolate mofetil in severe psoriasis. Br J Dermatol 2000;143:405–407.

75. Pedraz J, Dauden E, Delgado-Jimenez Y, et al. Sequential study on the treatment of moderate-to-severe chronic plaque psoriasis with mycophenolate mofetil and cyclosporin. J Eur Acad Dermatol Venereol 2006;20:702–706.

76. Patel RV, Clark LN, Lebwohl M, et al. Treatments for psoriasis and the risk of malignancy. J Am Acad Dermatol 2009;60:1001–1017.

77. Ranjan N, Sharma NL, Shanker V, et al. Methotrexate versus hydroxy-carbamide (hydroxyurea) as a weekly dose to treat moderate-to-severe chronic plaque psoriasis: A comparative study. J Dermatol Treatment 2007;18:295–300.

78. Smith N, Weymann A, Tausk FA, et al. Complementary and alternative medicine for psoriasis: A qualitative review of the clinical trial literature. J Am Acad Dermatol 2009;61:841–856.

79. Bernstein S, donsky H, Gulliver W, et al. Treatment of mild to moderate psoriasis with Relieva, a Mahonia aquifolium extract—A double-blind, placebo-controlled study. Am J Ther 2006;13:121–126.

80. Danno K, Sugie N. Combination therapy with low-dose etretinate and eicosapentaenoic acid for psoriasis vulgaris. J Dermatol 1998;25:703–705.

81. Brochow T, Schiener R, Franke A, et al. A pragmatic randomized controlled trial on the effectiveness of highly concentrated saline spa water baths followed by UVB compared to UVB only in moderate to severe psoriasis. J Altern Complement Med 2007;13:725–732.

82. Brochow T, Schiener R, Franke A, et al. A pragmatic randomized controlled trial on the effectiveness of low concentrated saline spa water baths followed by ultraviolet B (UVB) compared to UVB only in moderate to severe psoriasis. J Eur Acad Dermatol Venereol 2007;21:1027–1037.

83. Gaston L, Crombez J, Lassonde M, et al. Psychological stress and psoriasis: experimental and prospective correlational studies. Acta Derm Venereol 1991;156:37–43.

84. Kabat-Zinn J, Wheeler E, Light T, et al. Influence of a mindfulness meditation-based stress reduction intervention on rates of skin clearing in patients with moderate to severe psoriasis undergoing phototherapy (UVB) and photochemotherapy (PUVA). Psychosom Med 1998;60:625–632.

85. Treloar V. Integrative dermatology for psoriasis: facts and controversies. Clin Dermatol 2010;28:93–99.

86. Naldi L, Chatenoud L, Linder D, et al. Cigarette smoking, body mass index, and stressful life events as risk factors for psoriasis: results from an Italian case-control study. J Invest Dermatol 2005;125:61–67.

87. Benoit S, Hamm H. Childhood psoriasis. Clin Dermatol 2007;25:555–562.

88. De Jager MEA, de Jong EMG, van de Kerkhof PCM, et al. Efficacy and safety of treatments for childhood psoriasis: A systemic literature review. J Am Acad Dermatol 10.1016/j.jaad.2009.06.048 [corrected proof, November 2009].

89. Paller AS, Siegfried EC, Langley RG, et al. Etanercept treatment for children and adolescents with plaque psoriasis. N Engl J Med 2008;358:241–251.

90. Murase JE, Chan KK, Garite TJ, et al. Hormonal effect on psoriasis in pregnancy and post partum. Arch Dermatol 2005;141:601–606.

91. Lam J, Polifka JE, and Dohil MA. Safety of dermatologic drugs used in pregnant patients with psoriasis and other inflammatory skin diseases. J Am Acad Dermatol 2008;59:295–315.

92. Salim A, Tan E, Ilchyshyn A, et al. Folic acid supplementation during treatment of psoriasis with methotrexate: a randomized, double-blind, placebo-controlled trial. Br J Dermatol 2006;154:1169–1174.

108

Atopic Dermatitis

REBECCA M. LAW AND PO GIN KWA

KEY CONCEPTS

❶ Atopic dermatitis is a chronic skin disorder involving inflammation associated with intense pruritus, a hallmark symptom. Management of atopic dermatitis must always include appropriate management of the associated pruritus.

❷ Atopic dermatitis is associated with other atopic diseases such as asthma and allergic rhinitis in the same patient or family. The three conditions are known as the *atopic triad*.

❸ The prevalence of atopic dermatitis appears to have increased two- to threefold in many developed and developing countries during the past three decades. Recent data indicate age and country or regional differences, with some countries showing no change or even a decrease. Rural areas appear to have lower prevalence rates.

❹ There are genetic and environmental factors in the pathogenesis and pathophysiologic manifestations of atopic dermatitis. The inheritance pattern is not straightforward. More than one gene may be involved in the disease, with the filaggrin gene (*FLG*) being a key player.

❺ Atopic dermatitis often presents in infants and young children. The clinical presentation differs somewhat depending on the age of the patient.

❻ Secondary bacterial skin infections are common in patients with atopic dermatitis and must be promptly treated.

❼ Management of atopic dermatitis must always include appropriate nonpharmacologic management of any controllable environmental factors, such as avoidance of identified triggers. These may include aeroallergens (e.g., mold, grass, pollen), foods (e.g., peanuts, eggs, tomatoes), chemicals (e.g., detergents, soaps), clothing material (e.g., wool, polyester), temperature (e.g., excessive heat), and humidity (e.g., low humidity).

❽ Nonpharmacologic management of atopic dermatitis entails managing the symptoms associated with pruritus and encouraging appropriate skin care habits such as proper bathing techniques and the copious use of moisturizers, which is a standard of care.

Learning objectives, review questions, and other resources can be found at **www.pharmacotherapyonline.com**.

❾ Topical corticosteroids are the drugs of first choice for atopic dermatitis.

❿ Topical calcineurin inhibitors (tacrolimus and pimecrolimus) are alternate treatment options for adults and children over the age of 2 years.

⓫ This chronic illness has substantial socioeconomic impact. The cost may be magnified by undertreatment.

❶ Atopic dermatitis (AD) is a common skin disease. It is often referred to as *eczema*, which is a general term for several types of skin inflammation. Atopic dermatitis is the most common type of eczema (Table 108–1).[1] It is a chronic skin disorder involving inflammation with pruritus as the hallmark symptom/presentation. This disorder is often the prelude to atopic diathesis, which includes asthma and other allergic diseases.

❷ This form of dermatitis is commonly associated with other atopic disorders, such as allergic rhinitis and asthma. Atopic dermatitis, allergic rhinoconjunctivitis, and asthma are known collectively as the *atopic triad*.[2] Atopic dermatitis has also been defined as the cutaneous manifestation of atopy.[2]

The disease can have periods of exacerbation, or flare ups, followed by periods of remission. These flare ups may be disruptive to the patient's quality of life and may affect the entire family. Disease flare-ups are difficult to manage and may be complicated by

TABLE 108-1 Types of Eczema (Dermatitis)[1]

- **Allergic contact eczema (allergic contact dermatitis):** A red, itchy, weepy reaction where the skin has come into contact with a substance that the immune system recognizes as foreign, such as poison ivy or certain preservatives in creams and lotions.
- **Atopic dermatitis (or irritant contact dermatitis):** A chronic skin disease characterized by itchy, inflamed skin.
- **Contact eczema:** A localized reaction that includes redness, itching, and burning where the skin has come into contact with an allergen (an allergy-causing substance) or with an irritant such as an acid, cleaning agent, or other chemical.
- **Dyshidrotic eczema:** Irritation of the skin on the palms of hands and soles of the feet characterized by clear, deep blisters that itch and burn.
- **Neurodermatitis:** Scaly patches of the skin on the head, lower legs, wrists, or forearms caused by a localized itch (such as an insect bite) that become intensely irritated when scratched.
- **Nummular eczema:** Coin-shaped patches of irritated skin—most common on the arms, back, buttocks, and lower legs—that may be crusted, scaling, and extremely itchy.
- **Seborrheic eczema:** Yellowish, oily, scaly patches of skin on the scalp, face, and occasionally other parts of the body.
- **Stasis dermatitis:** A skin irritation on the lower legs, generally related to circulatory problems.

secondary infections. About one half (estimate up to 65%) of cases in children first manifest before age 1 year [1-4]; these cases are termed *early-onset atopic dermatitis*.[5] About 85% of patients develop symptoms before age 5.[1]

Of the children with atopic dermatitis diagnosed before age 1 year, approximately 40% to 60% will have the same skin condition continuing into their adulthood.[1,3]

Onset after age 30 is much less common and is often caused by exposure to harsh or wet conditions[1] such as repeated skin trauma or exposure to harsh chemicals. In adults, the prevalence is believed to be 1% to 3%, with an overall lifetime prevalence of about 7%.[1]

EPIDEMIOLOGY

❸ The prevalence of atopic dermatitis is generally said to have increased two- to threefold in developed and developing countries during the past three decades.[5] Currently in developed countries, an estimated 15% to 30% of children and 2% to 10% of adults are affected.[5,6] The prevalence appears to be increasing worldwide, since earlier prevalence rates were estimated at 10% to 15% in children.[4]

❸ A 2008 study has found both age and country differences in prevalence rates.[7] This international study included 187,943 children aged 6 to 7 years from 64 centers in 35 countries and 302,159 adolescents aged 13 to 14 years from 105 centers in 55 countries. For children aged 6 to 7 years, most countries showed an increase of 2 standard deviations (SDs) in mean annual prevalence over a 5- to 10-year period. In contrast, for adolescents aged 13 to 14 years, the trends differ from country to country. Large increases in prevalence were seen in developing countries (e.g., Mexico, Chile, Kenya, and Algeria, and seven countries in Southeast Asia). But in other countries with formerly very high prevalences, the mean annual prevalence in eczema symptoms has either leveled off or decreased. Most of the largest decreases (SD ≥2) in prevalence were reported from developed countries in northwest Europe, (e.g., the United Kingdom, Ireland, Sweden, Germany) and New Zealand.[7]

There were no differences according to the sex of the study participant, or with gross national income at a country level.[7] This is consistent with other reports that atopic dermatitis affects males and females at about the same rate.[1] This international study demonstrating different trends according to age group is partly corroborated by a study from the United Kingdom suggesting that the prevalence of allergic disorders (eczema and hay fever) might have leveled off or decreased over the past 10 years in those aged 12 years or older, but increased among younger children.[8]

There appears to be a lower prevalence of atopic dermatitis in rural areas when compared with urban areas, suggesting a link to the *hygiene hypothesis*, which postulates that the absence of early childhood exposure to infectious agents increases susceptibility to allergic diseases.[9-11] In contrast, children attending day care centers before 3 months of age have less atopy and asthma in later childhood,[11,12] and areas with diffuse and chronic helminth infestations have a low prevalence of allergic diseases.[11] In addition, a recent European birth cohort study involving 1,133 newborns showed that children born to farm families had a lower prevalence of sensitization to seasonal inhaled allergens such as grass pollen.[13] Maternal exposure during pregnancy (i.e., prenatal exposure) to animal sheds correlated with the lower prevalence rate in the farm children.[12] However, there were no differences in prevalence related to inhaled perennial allergens.

ETIOLOGY

❹ Atopic dermatitis is a complex genetic disease that arises from gene–gene and gene–environment interactions. There are two major groups of genes involved. First, there are the genes encoding for epidermal or other epithelial structural proteins. Second, there are genes encoding for the major elements of the immune system.[5]

The inheritance pattern is not straightforward. More than one gene is likely involved in the disease. There is an increased risk for a child to have atopic dermatitis if there is a family history of other atopic diseases, such as hay fever or asthma. The risk is significantly higher if both parents have an atopic disease.[1] Studies of identical twins show that a person whose identical twin has atopic dermatitis is seven times more likely to have atopic dermatitis than someone in the general population.[1] And a person whose fraternal twin has atopic dermatitis is three times more likely to have atopic dermatitis than someone in the general population.[1]

Thus, genetic predispositions to developing atopic dermatitis exist. Specifically, there are several possible genes on the chromosomes 3q21, 1q21, 16q, 17q25, 20p, and 3p26. Of these chromosomes, 1q21 has the highest linkage region. This region has a family of epithelium-related genes called the epidermal differentiation complex.[5] One of these genes, the filaggrin gene (*FLG*), on chromosome 1q21.3, was initially identified as the gene involved in ichthyosis vulgaris, and several mutations of this gene were subsequently identified in European and Japanese patients with atopic dermatitis.[14] *FLG* encodes for a key protein in epidermal differentiation. Mutations or deficiency of *FLG* results in an abnormality in permeability barrier function.[15]

Epidermal barrier dysfunction is a prerequisite for the penetration of high-molecular-weight allergens in pollens, house dust mite products, microbes, and food.[5] In mice studies, this barrier abnormality alters thresholds for irritant and acute allergic contact dermatitis, and *FLG* deficiency predisposes to the development of an atopic dermatitis-like dermatosis.[15] In humans, two common *FLG* variants (*R501X* and *2282del4*) with an estimated combined allele frequency of about 6% have been identified in individuals of European descent.[16] Eighteen other less common variants have also been identified in Europeans, with an additional 17 mutations restricted to individuals of Asian descent.[16] Each of these variants leads to nonsense mutations which either prevent or severely diminish the production of filaggrin in the epidermis.[16] Mutations of *FLG* seem to occur mainly in early-onset atopic dermatitis patients and may be associated with the development of asthma in patients with atopic dermatitis.[5,16] However, *FLG* mutations are identified in only 30% of European patients with atopic dermatitis; implying that other genetic mutations affecting other epidermal structures may be important (e.g., changes in the cornified envelope proteins involucrin and loricrin, or lipid composition).[5]

There are other genes encoding for the immune system that may be associated with atopic dermatitis, especially those found on chromosome 5q31-33.[5] These genes code for cytokines that regulate IgE synthesis. Cytokines are produced mainly by type 1 and type 2 helper T cells. Type 1 helper T cells (Th1) produce cytokines which suppress IgE production (e.g., interferon-γ and interleukin 12 [IL-12]).[5] Type 2 helper T cells (Th2) produce cytokines which increase IgE production (e.g., IL-5 and IL-13).[5,17] In patients with atopic dermatitis, there is an imbalance between Th1 and Th2 immune responses. These patients are genetically predisposed to Th2 predominance, seen as increased Th2 cell activity.[2,5,17] Increased Th2 activity causes the release of IL-3, IL-4, IL-5, IL-10, and IL-13, resulting in blood eosinophilia, increased serum IgE, and increased growth and development of mast cells.[2,5,17,18] In addition, these cytokines affect the maturation of B cells and cause a genomic rearrangement in these cells that favors isotype class switching from IgM to IgE.[5]

In summary, recent data suggests that *FLG* deficiency alone can provoke a barrier abnormality in the epidermis and predispose to the development of dermatitis by enhancing allergen absorption through the skin.[19] Furthermore, there appears to be complex relationships, including genetic and nongenetic risk factors, that modify an individual's susceptibility to allergic disease.[20] Complex genetic factors contribute to the increased susceptibility to atopic dermatitis (*FLG* mutations and gene–gene interactions). These, along with environmental factors (gene–environment interactions), result in the pathophysiologic changes and clinical presentations associated with atopic dermatitis.

PATHOPHYSIOLOGY

The initial mechanisms that trigger inflammatory changes in the skin in patients with atopic dermatitis are unknown. Neuropeptides, irritation, or pruritus-induced scratching may be causing the release of proinflammatory cytokines from keratinocytes. Alternatively, allergens in the epidermal barrier or in food may cause T-cell mediated but IgE-independent reactions. Allergen-specific IgE is not a prerequisite.[5]

Skin barrier dysfunction plays a critical role in the development of atopic dermatitis,[21,22] and loss of function mutations in the skin structural protein *filaggrin* is a major risk factor.[22] Other factors may include a deficiency of skin barrier proteins, increased peptidase activity, lack of certain protease inhibitors, and lipid abnormalities.[22] There must be epidermal barrier dysfunction for high-molecular-weight allergens in pollens, house dust mite particles, microbes, and foods to penetrate the skin barrier. Atopic skin has reduced antimicrobial peptides (AMPs). AMPs are normally produced by keratinocytes, sebocytes, and mast cells and they form a chemical shield on the surface of the skin. Reduced AMPs result in a diminished antimicrobial barrier, which correlates with increased susceptibility to infections and superinfections seen in these patients.[23]

Upon penetration of the epidermal barrier, allergens are met by dendritic cells (DCs). DCs are antigen-presenting cells populating the skin, respiratory tract, and mucosa of the GI tract (i.e., at the front line of pathogen entry).[24] DCs then enhance Th2 polarization, resulting in increased production of IgE. Keratinocytes in the skin of patients with atopic dermatitis also produce high levels of an interleukin-7–like protein, which again drives dendritic cells to enhance Th2 polarization. Epidermal dendritic cells in patients with atopic dermatitis bear IgE and express its high-affinity receptor (FcεRI).[25-27] Serum IgE is often elevated in patients with atopic dermatitis,[1,18] especially during an exacerbation.

However, upon initial presentation, patients with early-onset atopic dermatitis generally do not have increased IgE levels (i.e., there is no detectable IgE-mediated allergic sensitization). IgE-mediated allergic sensitization may occur several weeks or months after the initial atopic dermatitis lesions appear. Although in some children—mostly girls—this sensitization never occurs.[5]

PREDISPOSING FACTORS

Several factors can predispose patients to development of atopic dermatitis. These include climate, infection, genetics, environmental aeroallergens, and food.

Hot and extremely cold climates are both poorly tolerated by patients with this condition. Dry weather, common in the winter, causes increased skin dryness. Hot weather causes increased sweating, resulting in pruritus.

Patients with atopic dermatitis are commonly colonized by *Staphylococcus aureus* bacteria. Clinical infections with *S aureus* frequently cause flare-ups of atopic dermatitis.

As discussed previously, genetics plays a role in atopic dermatitis. Family history of atopic dermatitis is common.

Exposure to environmental aeroallergens is another risk factor. Dust mites, pollens, molds, cigarette smoke, and dander from animal hair or skin may worsen the symptoms of atopic dermatitis.[1,18]

The role of food as antigens in the pathogenesis of atopic dermatitis is controversial. Small amounts of environmental foods (low-dose exposure from foods on tabletops, hands, dust) may penetrate the skin barrier and be taken up by Langerhans cells, leading to Th2 responses and IgE production.[28] However, early high-dose oral food consumption induces oral tolerance. The timing and balance of cutaneous and oral exposure determines whether a child will have allergy or tolerance.[28] Increased serum IgE antibodies to a particular food is consistent with a food allergy.[1] Eczema may frequently be a manifestation of food allergy,[28] and patients with atopic dermatitis have a higher prevalence of food allergy than those in the general population.[1]

This is consistent with the known epidermal barrier dysfunction in atopic dermatitis, allowing for increased low-level skin permeability to allergenic foods. Certain foods may trigger acute reactions, including urticaria and anaphylaxis. The most commonly reported allergenic foods are eggs, milk, peanuts, wheat, soy, tree nuts, shellfish, and fish.[1] Individual food allergies, such as peanut allergy, have increased in prevalence in the past decade;[28,29] new food allergies may also be increasing in prevalence, particularly kiwi allergy[28,30] and sesame seed allergy.[28,31] Consistent with the oral tolerance concept, early results from recent studies using sublingual and oral immunotherapy to specific food allergens (e.g., milk or peanut) appear to indicate that it may be possible to induce oral tolerance, and that it may be possible to desensitize children to some allergenic foods. Currently, these treatment protocols have only been done in highly supervised research settings and with small numbers of patients.[32]

CLINICAL PRESENTATION

Diagnosis of atopic dermatitis is generally based on clinical presentation (Table 108–2)[1] There is no objective diagnostic test for the clinical confirmation of atopic dermatitis.[1,33] Filaggrin gene mutations may be associated with persistent and more severe atopic dermatitis as well as early-onset cases.[22]

TABLE 108-2 Skin Features Associated with Atopic Dermatitis[1]

- **Atopic pleat (Dennie–Morgan fold)**: An extra fold of skin that develops under the eye.
- **Cheilitis**: Inflammation of the skin on and around the lips.
- **Hyperlinear palms**: Increased number of skin creases on the palms.
- **Hyperpigmented eyelids**: Eyelids that have become darker in color from inflammation or hay fever.
- **Ichthyosis**: Dry, rectangular scales on the skin.
- **Keratosis pilaris**: Small, rough bumps, generally on the face, upper arms, and thighs.
- **Lichenification**: Thick, leathery skin resulting from constant scratching and rubbing.
- **Papules**: Small raised bumps that may open when scratched and become crusty and infected.
- **Urticaria**: Hives (red, raised bumps) that may occur after exposure to an allergen, at the beginning of flares, or after exercise or a hot bath.

❺ The clinical presentation of atopic dermatitis differs somewhat depending on the age of the patient. In infancy, the earliest onset of atopic dermatitis usually occurs between 2 and 6 months of age, and especially between the sixth and twelfth weeks of life.[1,2] It has been reported that 75% of cases have their onset within the first six months.[2] A more conservative estimate is that at least 65% of patients develop symptoms within the first year of life, and at least 85% will have developed symptoms before the age of 5.[1] The initial presentation in infancy is an erythematous, papular skin rash that may first appear on the cheeks and chin as a patchy facial rash[1,2] and that can progress to red, scaling, oozing skin.[1] The rash shows a centrifugal distribution affecting the malar region of the cheeks, forehead, scalp, chin, and behind the ears while sparing the central areas (i.e., the nose and paranasal creases).[2] Lesions occur in the flexor surfaces, such as antecubital and popliteal fossae. Over the next few weeks and as the infant becomes more mobile and begins crawling, the lesions spread to the extensors of the lower legs, and eventually the entire body may be involved, with sparing of the diaper area and the nose.[1] These lesions are associated with uncontrollable itchiness, and the infant will become irritable and may try to rub his or her face to relieve the itch. Scratching may occur quite early, and infants with atopic dermatitis may scratch themselves continuously, mainly when they are undressed or during sleep.[2] Excessive rubbing or scratching may result in excoriation and development of secondary infections.

In childhood, the skin often appears dry, flaky, rough, cracked, and may bleed due to scratching. With repeated scratching and rubbing the skin becomes lichenified. Lichenification, usually localized to the flexural folds of the extremities,[33] is very characteristic of childhood atopic dermatitis in older children and adults.[33,34] Lichenification signifies repeated rubbing of the skin and is seen mostly over the folds, bony protuberances, and forehead.[34] Excoriations and crusting are also commonly seen, along with secondary infections. Sometimes increased folds are seen underneath the eyes (so called Dennie–Morgan folds).[34] Lesions are still most commonly seen in the flexor surfaces of the body, particularly the flexural creases of the antecubital and popliteal fossae.[34]

Sleep disturbances also occur. One study reported that there are both brief and longer awakenings associated with scratching episodes that affect sleep efficiency in school-age children with atopic dermatitis.[35]

In adulthood, lesions are more diffuse with underlying erythema. The face is commonly involved and may be dry and scaly. Lichenification may again be seen. A brown macular ring around the neck, representing a localized deposit of amyloid, is typical but not always present.[34]

Although no objective diagnostic test confirms presence of atopic dermatitis,[1] some signs, symptoms, and other factors are commonly used in its diagnosis. These include pruritus, early age of onset, eczematous skin lesions that vary with age, chronic and relapsing courses, dry and flaky skin, IgE reactivity, family or personal history of asthma or hay fever, or other atopic diseases (Table 108-3).[18] In addition, allergy skin testing may be helpful in identifying factors that trigger flares of atopic dermatitis.[1] Negative results may help rule out certain substances as triggers; however, positive results may be unrelated to disease activity, and false positives are common.[1]

❶ Pruritus is a quintessential feature of atopic dermatitis, and a diagnosis cannot be made if there is no history of itching.[1–4] Atopic dermatitis has been called the itch that, when scratched, erupts.[2] Scratching or rubbing itchy, atopic skin characterizes this type of eczema.[2] Scratching and rubbing further irritates the skin, increases inflammation, and exacerbates itchiness.[3] Atopic skin can itch dur-

TABLE 108-3 Major and Minor Signs and Symptoms of Atopic Dermatitis[1]

Major indicators
- Pruritus (intense itching)
- Characteristic rash in locations typical of the disease
- Chronic or repeatedly occurring symptoms
- Personal or family history of atopic disorders (eczema, hay fever, asthma)

Selected minor indicators
- Early age of onset
- Dry skin that may also have patchy scales or rough bumps
- Increased serum IgE
- Numerous skin creases on the palms
- Hand or foot involvement
- Inflammation around the lips
- Nipple eczema
- Susceptibility to skin infection
- Positive allergy skin tests

ing sleep. This nighttime itching is a problem for many children with the disease, since there is no conscious control of scratching during sleep.[1,18,35]

Pruritus can be triggered by a variety of factors. The most common triggers of itch have been reported as heat and perspiration (96%), wool (91%), emotional stress (81%), certain foods (49%), alcohol (44%), upper respiratory infections (36%), and house dust mites (>35%).[36]

Once pruritus occurs, the surrounding normally nonpruritic skin area (whether inflamed or noninflamed) may be very sensitive and react to light stimuli and begin itching (allokinesis). Allokinesis is typical of atopic dermatitis.[18,36] As a result of allokinesis, patients with atopic dermatitis may experience pruritic attacks when their skin is touched accidentally by mechanical factors such as clothing,[18] especially wool products.[36]

Elevated serum IgE may be seen, consistent with the genetically predetermined dominance of Th2 cytokines causing increased IgE. In addition, increased serum IgE antibodies to a particular food, consistent with a food allergy,[3] is common in patients with atopic dermatitis. The radioallergosorbent test (RAST) is an allergen-specific IgE antibody test used to screen for allergy to a specific substance or substances. In some cases the RAST test may be used to monitor immunotherapy or to see if a child has outgrown a specific allergy. Positive (elevated) RAST usually indicates an allergy to a suspected or known allergen. However, the level of IgE may not correlate with the severity of an allergic reaction, and the IgE level may remain elevated for years after an allergy has been outgrown.[18]

A clinically useful set of criteria for the diagnosis of atopic dermatitis is as follows: atopy, pruritus, eczema, and altered vascular reactivity.[18,36]

COMPLICATIONS

❻ Patients with atopic dermatitis are prone to skin infections. Atopic skin is drier and the stratum corneum has weakened protective abilities; combined with the abnormal skin barrier function and immune defense, there is an increased risk of secondary bacterial skin infections with staphylococci or streptococci, and viral infections such as herpes simplex or even fungal infections.[1] Constant scratching to relieve pruritus may cause excoriations, further compromising the integrity of the skin barrier. S aureus is a common cause of secondary bacterial infections in atopic dermatitis. Binding of S aureus is enhanced by skin inflammation as seen in atopic dermatitis.[21] Many patients with atopic dermatitis are colonized with S aureus and may have exacerbations after skin infections of this organism.[21] Secondary bacterial infections may present as yellowish crusty lesions and should be promptly treated. Oral (systemic) antibiotics are generally more effective than topical treatment.[1,21]

Patients with atopic dermatitis are also more prone to disseminated infections with herpes simplex or vaccinia virus.[21] Severe viral infections such as eczema herpeticum or eczema vaccinatum might be linked to the severity of atopy.[21] Smallpox vaccination is contraindicated in patients with atopic dermatitis.[21]

TREATMENT

In treating patients with atopic dermatitis, clinicians generally have the following clinical goals in mind:

1. Provide symptomatic relief—control the itching
2. Control the atopic dermatitis
3. Identify and, when possible, eliminate triggers and environmental aeroallergens
4. Identify and minimize predisposing factors for exacerbations including any stressors
5. Prevent future exacerbations
6. Provide any social and psychological support needed for the patient, family, and caregivers
7. Minimize or prevent adverse events from medications and other treatment modalities
8. Treat to cure any secondary skin infections, if present

❼ Both nonpharmacologic and pharmacologic therapies are important in managing the signs and symptoms of atopic dermatitis. Nonpharmacologic strategies include identifying and minimizing or eliminating preventable risk factors such as known triggers and allergens, as well as appropriate skin care.

Treatment guidelines and protocols for atopic dermatitis are available. These are listed in Table 108–4.

■ NONPHARMACOLOGIC THERAPY

❽ Nonpharmacologic approaches to the treatment of infants and children with atopic dermatitis include the following[1]:

- Give lukewarm baths.
- Apply lubricant immediately after bathing (moisturizers are a standard of care).[10]
- Keep child's fingernails filed short.
- Select clothing made of soft cotton fabrics.
- Consider using sedating antihistamines to reduce scratching at night.
- Keep the child cool; avoid situations in which overheating occurs.
- Learn to recognize skin infections and seek treatment promptly.
- Attempt to distract the child with activities to keep him or her from scratching.
- Identify and remove irritants and allergens.

Hydration is crucial, and adequate skin hydration is a fundamental part of managing atopic dermatitis.[3] Transepidermal water loss is greater in atopic skin than in normal skin. Thus, any measures to improve skin moisturization, such as liberal use of moisturizers, would be beneficial. Moisturizers are a standard of care and may be steroid-sparing.[10] They are useful for both prevention and

TABLE 108–4	Useful Sources of Information About Treatment of Atopic Dermatitis

Published Guidelines or Treatment Protocols

- National Guideline Clearinghouse. Guidelines of care for atopic dermatitis – current release updated Nov. 16, 2009. www.guideline.gov/summary/summary.aspx?ss=15&doc_id=4361&nbr=3286. Accessed Nov. 21, 2009.
- National Institute of Arthritis and Musculoskeletal and Skin Diseases. Handout on Health: Atopic Dermatitis. US Department of Health and Human Services, May 2009. NIH Publication No. 09-4272. www.niams.nih.gov/Health_Info/Atopic_Dermatitis/default.asp. Accessed Nov. 19, 2009.
- Lynde C, Barber K, Claveau J, Gratton D, et al. Canadian Practical Guide for the Treatment and Management of Atopic Dermatitis. Journal of Cutaneous Medicine and Surgery (incorporating Medical and Surgical Dermatology), published online June 30, 2005. (Online First) http://www.springerlink.com/content/r5432000056r2748/fulltext.html. Accessed Nov. 19, 2009.
- Eichenfield LF, Hanifin JM, Luger TA, et al. Consensus conference on pediatric atopic dermatitis. J Am Acad Dermatol. 2003;49:1088–1095.
- Leung DYM, Nicklas RA, Li JT, et al. Disease management of atopic dermatis: an updated practice parameter. Ann Allergy Asthma Immunol. 2004;93(9):S1–S21.
- Abramovits W. A clinician's paradigm in the treatment of atopic dermatitis. J Am Acad Dermatol. 2005;53:S70–S77.

Useful Web Sites

- National Institute of Arthritis and Musculoskeletal and Skin Diseases (NIAMS), U.S. National Institutes of Health. http://www.niams.nih.gov/Health_Info/Atopic_Dermatitis/default.asp
- American Academy of Allergy Asthma & Immunology (AAAAI). http://www.aaaai.org/patients/allergic_conditions/atopic_dermatitis.stm
- American Academy of Dermatology. http://www.aad.org/public/publications/pamphlets/skin_eczema.html
- DermNet NZ. http://dermnetnz.org/dermatitis/atopic.html
- FDA Public Health Advisory: Elidel (pimecrolimus) Cream and Protopic (tacrolimus) Ointment http://www.fda.gov/Drugs/DrugSafety/PublicHealthAdvisories/ucm051760.htm
- EczemaNet: http://www.skincarephysicians.com/eczemanet/phototherapy.html

maintenance therapy.[10] They can be categorized based on their specific effects on the skin:

- *Occlusives:* These agents provide an oily layer on the skin surface to slow transepidermal water loss, increasing the moisture content of the stratum corneum. These are the best moisturizers for patients with atopic dermatitis.[3]
- *Humectants:* In the stratum corneum, these agents increase the water-holding capacity. However, they are not useful in patients with atopic dermatitis because they have a stinging effect on open skin.[3]
- *Emollients:* These agents smooth out the surface of the skin by filling the spaces with droplets of oil. These are the least effective moisturizers.[3]

The humidity in the home should be kept at or above 50% and the room temperature kept on the cool side.[18]

Appropriate skin care is crucial in preventing flare-ups.[1] A daily skin care routine should include the following[18]:

- Using scent-free moisturizers liberally as needed each day.
- Bathing in lukewarm water (never hot) for about 5 minutes once[3,37] or twice[3] daily. Adding a capful of emulsifying oil may help the body retain moisture; baths are better than showers. If showering, mild liquid cleansers are preferred over soaps.[3]
- The skin should be air dried or lightly towel dried (pat to dry, avoid rubbing or brisk drying).[1,37,38]
- Scent-free moisturizer should then be applied while the skin is still moist or slightly damp (within 3 minutes of towel drying).[3,38] Some fragrance-free moisturizers include Aveeno

Baby Soothing Relief Moisture Cream, Cetaphil, Neutrogena Hand Cream, and Vanicream products. Lotions may be used on the scalp and other hairy areas and for mild dryness on the face, trunk, and limbs; creams are more occlusive than lotions; ointments are the most occlusive and can be used for drier, thicker, or more scaly areas.[3] Occlusive moisturizers are best.[3]

- Using nonsoap skin cleansers[1] may cause less skin irritation. Lipid- and fragrance-free skin cleansers may be particularly advantageous (e.g., Cetaphil Gentle Skin Cleanser, Free and Clear Liquid Cleanser, Spectro Derm Cleanser). Aquanil, Dove, Neutrogena, and pHisoderm sensitive skin products have also been recommended as low-irritant products, and some are lipid free.

- Avoiding alcohol-containing topical products including lotions, swabs, and wipes, as they may be drying.

- Clothing should be double-rinsed. Mild detergents should be used to wash clothing, with no bleach or fabric softener.[3]

■ PHARMACOLOGIC THERAPY

Topical Corticosteroids

❽ *Topical corticosteroids* are the standard of care to which other treatments are compared.[10] They remain the drug treatment of choice for atopic dermatitis. However, despite their extensive use, supporting data are limited regarding optimal corticosteroid concentrations, duration and frequency of therapy, and quantity of application.[10] The use of long-term intermittent application of topical corticosteroids was beneficial and safe in two randomized controlled studies;[10] however, independent studies of other formulations are needed.[10]

To maximize the antiinflammatory benefit and minimize adverse effects, the choice of corticosteroid should be matched with the severity and site of disease.[3] Low-potency corticosteroids, such as hydrocortisone 1%, are suitable for the face, and medium-potency corticosteroids, such as betamethasone valerate 0.1%, may be used for the body.[3] For longer-duration maintenance therapy, low-potency corticosteroids are recommended.[33] Mid-strength and high-potency corticosteroids should be used for short-term management of exacerbations.[33] Ultra-high and high-potency corticosteroids, such as betamethasone dipropionate 0.05% or clobetasone propionate 0.05%, are typically reserved for short-term treatment of lichenified areas in adults.[39] After the lesions have cleared or significantly improved, a lower-potency steroid should be used for maintenance when necessary.[39] Potent fluorinated corticosteroids should be avoided not only on the face, but also the genitalia and the intertriginous areas, and in young infants.[33] (For a corticosteroid potency comparison chart, see Table 107–2 or the National Psoriasis Foundation Website at *http://www.psoriasis.org/ netcommunity/sublearn03_mild_potency.*)

It is also important to remember that altering the local environment through hydration and/or occlusion as well as changing the vehicle[39] may alter the absorption and effectiveness of the topical corticosteroid.[10] Some vehicles are better suited for certain body areas,[39] such as a lotion for the scalp and hairy areas. Foams may be more cosmetically pleasing to some patients, as they easily disappear into the skin. The surface area of the skin involved and the skin thickness also play a role.[33] In addition, tachyphylaxis is a clinical concern, but there is no experimental documentation.[10]

Adverse effects of topical corticosteroids may be systemic in nature, and they are directly related to the steroid potency, duration of use, and other factors as discussed above. Local adverse effects include striae and skin atrophy, perioral dermatitis, acne,

rosacea, telangiectasias, and allergic contact dermatitis (often related to the vehicle).[33,40] The potential for systemic adverse effects is related to the potency of the topical corticosteroid, the site of application, the occlusiveness of the preparation, the percentage of body surface area covered, and the duration of use.[33] Potential systemic effects include hypothalamic–pituitary–adrenal (HPA) axis suppression, infections, hyperglycemia, cataracts, glaucoma, and growth retardation (in children).[1,3,9,18,40] However, growth retardation may also be related to the chronicity of the illness rather than to corticosteroid use or dietary factors.[3] Although less likely, systemic adverse effects can occur with low-potency topical corticosteroids. For example, a recent phase II study of a mild-potency corticosteroid (desonide 0.05% foam) in children and adolescents 3 months to 17 years showed that 4% (3 of 75) of patients experienced mild reversible HPA-axis suppression after a 4-week treatment period.[41]

When topical steroid therapy has failed for efficacy or safety reasons, numerous agents and interventions can be used as alternative or add-on therapy in patients with atopic dermatitis.

Topical Calcineurin Inhibitors

❾ Topical immunomodulators such as the calcineurin inhibitors tacrolimus ointment (Protopic) and pimecrolimus cream (Elidel) have been shown to reduce the extent, severity, and symptoms of atopic dermatitis in adults and children.[10] Tacrolimus has been reported to inhibit the activation of key cells involved in atopic dermatitis, including T cells, dendritic cells, mast cells, and keratinocytes.[33] Pimecrolimus acts similarly to tacrolimus, inhibiting T-cell proliferation, preventing gene transcription of Th1 and Th2 cytokines, and reducing mediator release from mast cells and basophils.[33] However, pimecrolimus has more favorable lipophilic characteristics and, in animal studies, appears to preferentially distribute to the skin as opposed to the systemic circulation.[33,42] Both tacrolimus ointment and pimecrolimus cream are approved for atopic dermatitis in adults and children older than age 2.[3,10,42] Although clinical trials conducted in younger infants (e.g., 2–23 months old) also showed significant efficacy without appreciable adverse effects, use in children younger than age 2 is not FDA approved.[43] Tacrolimus 0.03% ointment is approved for moderate to severe atopic dermatitis for ages 2 and above, with the 0.1% ointment limited to ages 16 and above; pimecrolimus 1% cream is approved for mild to moderate atopic dermatitis for ages 2 and above.[43]

Due to continuing concerns regarding a possible risk of cancer with tacrolimus and pimecrolimus,[43] both drugs are recommended for use as second-line treatments in atopic dermatitis.[9,10,37] They may be appropriate in patients with corticosteroid-related adverse effects, patients with large body-surface areas of disease, patients unresponsive to corticosteroids, or when treatment with corticosteroids is inadvisable.[3] Children and adults with a weakened or compromised immune system should not be treated with these agents. Unlike topical corticosteroids, calcineurin inhibitors can be used on all body locations for prolonged periods,[3] although episodic use is recommended.[37] Skin atrophy does not occur.[33]

The most common adverse effect of topical calcineurin inhibitors is transient discomfort (burning sensation) at the application site.[3] There is a potential for local skin carcinogenesis as seen in animal studies, or for systemic effects if high blood levels are reached (for example, increased susceptibility to infections due to immunosuppressive effects).[43] Since there is a possible risk of cutaneous malignancy,[3,37] sun protection is recommended.[3,18,37,43] Patients should be encouraged to apply a high sun protection factor broad-spectrum sunblock daily to all exposed skin (e.g., SPF 30 or higher); and this counseling should especially be emphasized for those patients with the highest risk of developing skin cancer, including patients with red hair and/or Fitzpatrick skin types I and II, and patients receiving phototherapy or using tanning beds.[43]

Topical calcineurin inhibitors are very effective in relieving the associated pruritus. Pimecrolimus therapy has been shown in a controlled long-term (6-month) study in adults with atopic dermatitis to significantly reduce pruritus within 48 hours (48.3% reduction versus 15.9% reduction in the placebo group; P <0.001).[3,44]

Phototherapy

Phototherapy is effective for atopic dermatitis and is recommended[10] especially when the disease is not controlled by tacrolimus or pimecrolimus ointment. Phototherapy may be steroid sparing, allowing for the use of lower-potency topical corticosteroids, or even eliminating the need for maintenance corticosteroids in some cases. Phototherapy may also help prevent secondary bacterial skin infections, commonly seen in patients with atopic dermatitis. However, in a few patients, phototherapy may worsen the atopic dermatitis; it is not recommended in patients whose disease flares up when exposed to sunlight. Relapse following cessation of therapy frequently occurs.[10]

Phototherapy may consist of either ultraviolet light therapy alone, or ultraviolet light therapy alongside drug or topical ointment (commonly called photochemotherapy). Psoralens plus ultraviolet A light (PUVA) is one type of photochemotherapy. The photosensitizer (psoralens) is administered either orally or in a bath immediately prior to UVA therapy. Topical ointments (such as crude coal tar) may also be used concomitantly with ultraviolet light therapy (e.g., Crude coal tar + UVB).

Ultraviolet lamps include UVA (315–400 nm), UVA1 (340–400 nm), broadband UVB (280–315 nm), and narrowband UVB (311 nm). Phototherapies used for atopic dermatitis have included PUVA, high- or medium-dose UVA1, wideband UVB, and narrowband UVB.[10,45] There is weaker evidence supporting the use of PUVA in atopic dermatitis.[45] Narrowband UVB is more effective than broadband UVB therapy. Broadband UVB may not effectively treat the scalp and skin fold areas. Medium-dose UVA1 is very effective for patients with an acute exacerbation of severe atopic dermatitis; however, the effect may be relatively short-lived and symptoms recurred within 3 months of stopping therapy in one adult study.[45,46] A recent adult study comparing medium-dose UVA1 and narrowband UVB found no difference in efficacy; however, the sample size was quite small (N = 13), and the follow-up period was confounded by the use of topical corticosteroids.[47] On-going clinical trials are comparing UVA1 and UVB light therapy for atopic dermatitis and other inflammatory skin conditions.

Patients need to wear eye protection during UV therapy to prevent damage to the retina. Short-term adverse effects include erythema, skin pain, skin burning or sunburn, pruritus, and pigmentation.[33] Long-term adverse effects include premature aging of the skin (photoaging) and skin cancer.[33,45] For example, PUVA has been associated with squamous cell carcinoma and possibly melanoma, which may occur years after PUVA therapy has ceased.[45]

Coal Tar

Although tar preparations had been widely used for atopic dermatitis and are recommended as alternative topical therapy,[10] few randomized controlled studies support their efficacy.[33] Their anti-inflammatory properties are not well characterized, and part of the improvement with the agent may be the result of a placebo effect, which can be significant in atopic dermatitis.[33]

Coal tar products are also staining and malodorous, although newer products may be more cosmetically acceptable. They are not recommended on acutely inflamed skin, since this may result in additional skin irritation.[33]

The use of coal tar in pregnancy has not been studied. Few data are available about tar excretion into breast milk; in addition, safety in children has not been established.[48] Adverse effects include tar folliculitis, acneiform eruptions, irritant dermatitis, burning, stinging, photosensitivity, and a risk of tar intoxication if used extensively in a young child.[48] Although animal studies showed that tar components can be converted to carcinogenic/mutagenic entities, there is inconclusive epidemiologic evidence supporting the claim that human use of topical tar preparations in dermatology leads to skin cancer.[48]

■ SYSTEMIC THERAPIES

Systemic therapies for the treatment of atopic dermatitis are generally not well studied or approved by FDA. Small case series or open studies are available for some agents, but few well-conducted randomized controlled trials exist. Agents described in published papers have included systemic corticosteroids, cyclosporine, interferon-γ, azathioprine, methotrexate, mycophenolate mofetil, intravenous immunoglobulin (IVIG), and more recently biologic response modifiers.

Systemic corticosteroids, such as oral prednisone, rarely may be required as a short term treatment for severe, recalcitrant, chronic atopic dermatitis.[33] While not routinely recommended,[37] systemic corticosteroids can provide rapid relief of severe refractory disease during transition to other therapies.[45] The dosage of the drug must be tapered during discontinuance to minimize a rebound flare-up. Intensified skin care, particularly with topical corticosteroids and moisturizers, is also important during the taper to minimize a rebound flare-up.[33]

Cyclosporine is considered effective for severe atopic dermatitis,[10] but its usefulness is limited by significant side effects, including hypertension and nephrotoxicity. There is also the potential for significant drug–drug and drug–food (e.g., grapefruit juice) interactions. It should be reserved for short-term use in adults or children with severe refractory disease.[45] Maximal benefit is usually seen after about 2 weeks of use and relapse may occur quickly after cessation of therapy.[45]

Recombinant interferon-γ may be effective in a subset of patients with atopic dermatitis.[10] Two randomized placebo-controlled trials in patients with severe atopic dermatitis demonstrated significant improvement in symptoms.[49,50] Short-term adverse effects, such as headache, myalgias, and chills, occurred in substantial proportions of study patients. Transient liver transaminase elevations and granulocytopenia have also occurred.[51] Long-term therapy (up to 24 months) did not appear to be associated with significant adverse events.[33] Some recommend that a higher dose of this agent be used initially followed by a lower dosage during maintenance therapy.[45]

Azathioprine,[33,52] *methotrexate,*[53] *mycophenolate mofetil,*[33] and *IVIG* have shown efficacy in small case series or open-label studies primarily in adults with recalcitrant atopic dermatitis. They are rarely used. Oral methotrexate, with a long history of pediatric use for various inflammatory conditions, appeared to be effective in a case series of children (aged 2–16 years) with severe atopic dermatitis.[53]

Biologic response modifiers, unlike for psoriasis, are currently not approved for atopic dermatitis. The safety and efficacy of various biologic response modifiers in patients with atopic dermatitis have been studied,[51] mostly in case reports, small case series, or open-label studies with a limited number of patients. Theoretically, using protein-based therapies is inherently risky in a patient population more prone to developing IgE sensitization to protein antigens than the general population. Type 1 immediate hypersensitivity reactions such as anaphylaxis could result, and patients with severe disease are potentially the patients at greatest risk of anaphylaxis. None has been reported in the published literature, which detail 261 patients with atopic dermatitis treated with various biologics,[51] but these numbers are too small to generalize their findings to larger numbers of people or specific populations.

More specifically, the TNF-α inhibitors infliximab and etanercept appeared effective in a few patients but not others, and adverse events have included infusion reactions with flushing and dyspnea, urticaria, and recurrent skin infections of methicillin-resistant *S aureus*. Similarly, omalizumab, rituximab, and alefacept have been shown in a few case reports and small case series to be somewhat effective.

Additional research is needed to determine the therapeutic potential and safety of biologics in patients with atopic dermatitis.[51]

Complementary and Alternative Therapies

Traditional Chinese herbal therapy has been studied in placebo-controlled trials and appeared to provide temporary benefit for patients with severe atopic dermatitis. However, the effectiveness may wear off despite continued treatment, and long-term toxicity is unknown.[10,33,54,55]

Mycobacterium vaccae (killed) injected intradermally was found to be effective in reducing the severity of skin disease in a placebo-controlled trial in children with moderate to severe atopic dermatitis.[56] This suggests that down-regulation of the Th2 response in atopic dermatitis may potentially be beneficial.[33]

Probiotics of various types have been studied in placebo-controlled trials with mixed results. One study group reported that prenatal and postnatal exposure for 6 months to *Lactobacillus rhamnosus GG* halved the frequency of atopic dermatitis at 2, 4 and 7 years but had no effect on atopic sensitization. Other study groups also administered lactobacilli, including *L rhamnosus GG*, but with mixed results. One study showed that *L acidophilus* supplementation actually increased the risk of atopic sensitization.

A recent placebo-controlled study comparing *Bifidobacterium lactis* and *L rhamnosus HN001* found that *L rhamnosus HN001* may be effective in preventing the development of atopic dermatitis in high-risk infants.[57]

More research is needed about the role of probiotics in treating patients with atopic dermatitis.

Immunotherapy using allergen-specific desensitization techniques in controlled settings for patients with atopic dermatitis may also be beneficial, and much research is ongoing. Double-blind controlled studies have not shown consistent efficacy.

More research is also needed to adequately assess the role of homeopathy, hypnotherapy, acupuncture, massage therapy, and biofeedback therapy in the treatment of atopic dermatitis.[10]

PHARMACOECONOMICS AND OTHER CONSIDERATIONS

⑪ Atopic dermatitis may have significant implications not only for the patients themselves, but also their families and caregivers.

In 2006, an international study of 2,002 patients and caregivers from 8 countries addressed the effect of atopic dermatitis on the lives of patients and society.[58] This European study found that, on average, patients experienced 9 flares per year, with those having severe disease experiencing more flares and taking significantly longer to clear. The flares were associated with disturbed sleep, and 86% of patients avoided at least one type of everyday activity. Schoolwork performance and productivity were negatively

affected. Patients missed an average of 2.5 days of school or work per year, and an analysis of adult patient performance at work and occupational absence showed that the social cost of lost productivity could amount to more than 2 billion euros per year across the European Union. There were also emotional consequences; half of the patients experienced depression or unhappiness about their condition, and one third reported that atopic dermatitis had eroded their self-confidence. In addition, concern about adverse effects from topical corticosteroid treatments resulted in poor adherence to therapy. On average, patients endured the symptoms of atopic dermatitis without initiating specific treatment 47% of the time they had an exacerbation. About one half of the respondents were concerned about using topical corticosteroids, and 58% restricted them to particular sites, 39% used them less frequently or for shorter time periods than prescribed, and 66% used them as a last resort. The study concluded that atopic dermatitis is "an undertreated disease that has a significant, yet mostly avoidable, negative effect on patients, their caregivers, and society."[58]

Thus, health care professionals play an integral role in providing patient and caregiver education about this disease and specific treatment plans. The importance of adequate and appropriate education for the patient, family, and caregivers about atopic dermatitis and its management cannot be overemphasized. Patients should be involved in their own care.

CLINICAL CONTROVERSY

Animal studies showed that coal tar components can be converted to carcinogenic/mutagenic entities, and tar keratoses (small nodules that develop from cutaneous tar exposure) have the potential to regress, fall off, or develop into a squamous cell carcinoma. However, there is inconclusive epidemiologic evidence supporting the claim that human use of topical tar preparations in dermatology leads to skin or internal cancers such as bladder cancer or lymphoma.[48]

CLINICAL CONTROVERSY

With topical calcineurin inhibitors, there is a potential for local skin carcinogenesis as seen in animal and in vitro studies. In addition, pigmented melanocytic lesions have been seen in treated areas, raising concern about melanoma.[43] FDA has a black-box warning for both tacrolimus ointment and pimecrolimus cream about their potential cancer risk, but no causal relationship has been proven between use of a topical calcineurin inhibitor and the development of lymphoma or nonmelanoma skin cancer.[43]

EVALUATION OF THERAPEUTIC OUTCOMES

Successful management of atopic dermatitis should include not only clearance of skin lesions, which may take days to weeks depending on the severity of disease, but also control of the itch, minimizing or eliminating triggers, monitoring the patient to minimize or prevent adverse events from medications or other treatment modalities, and providing adequate social and psychological support for the patient, family, and caregivers. The ultimate goal is to provide enough control of this chronic disease that future exacerbations are prevented, thus ensuring that the patient's quality of life is minimally affected by atopic dermatitis.

CONCLUSIONS

Atopic dermatitis is a chronic skin condition that generally presents at an early age, It affects the patient, family, and caregivers. Nonpharmacologic management strategies are important in treatment; these include appropriate skin care, hydration, avoidance of triggers, and psychosocial support. Pharmacologic treatment emphasizes topical corticosteroids as the standard of care. Patient and caregiver education about atopic dermatitis and treatment strategies is critical to minimize nonadherence. Successful outcomes result when patients and caregivers are partners with health care professionals in the management of this chronic disease.

ACKNOWLEDGMENT

Portions of this chapter have been adapted with permission from Law RM, Kwa PG. Atopic dermatitis: The Itch that Erupts when Scratched. Chapter 104, Instructor's Guide. Schwinghammer T, Koehler J, eds. Pharmacotherapy Casebook: A Patient Focused Approach, 7th ed. New York, NY: McGraw-Hill, 2008.

ABBREVIATIONS

AMPs: antimicrobial peptides

DCs: dendritic cells

FLG: filaggrin gene

IL: interleukin

RAST: radioallergosorbent test

Th1: Type 1 helper T cells

Th2: Type 2 helper T cells

UVA: ultraviolet A

UVB: ultraviolet B

REFERENCES

1. National Institute of Arthritis and Musculoskeletal and Skin Diseases. Handout on Health: Atopic Dermatitis. US Department of Health and Human Services. 2009, *http://www.niams.nih.gov/Health_Info/ Atopic_Dermatitis/default.asp*.
2. Gimenez JCM. Atopic Dermatitis. Alergol Immunol Clin 2000;15: 279–295.
3. Lynde C, Barber K, Claveau J, Gratton D, et al. Canadian Practical Guide for the Treatment and Management of Atopic Dermatitis. Journal of Cutaneous Medicine and Surgery (incorporating Medical and Surgical Dermatology). 2005, *http://www.springerlink.com/ content/r5432000056r2748/fulltext.html*.
4. Hanifin JM. Epidemiology of Atopic Dermatitis. Immunology Clinics of North America. 2002;22:1–24.
5. Bieber T. Mechanisms of Disease: Atopic Dermatitis. N Engl J Med 2008;358:1483–494.
6. Williams H, Flohr C. How epidemiology has challenged 3 prevailing concepts about atopic dermatitis. J Allergy Clin Immunol 2006;118:209–213.
7. Williams H, Stewart A, von Mutius E, Cookson W et al. Is eczema really on the increase worldwide? J Allergy Clin Immunol 2008;121: 947–954.
8. Gupta R, Sheikh A, Strachan DP, Anderson HR. Time trends in allergic disorders in the UK. Thorax 2007;62:91–96.
9. Hanifin JM, Cooper KD, Ho VC, et al. Guidelines of care for atopic dermatitis. J Am Acad Dermatol 2004;50:391–404.
10. National Guideline Clearinghouse. Guidelines of care for atopic dermatitis. 2009, *http://www.guideline.gov/summary/summary.aspx?ss= 15&doc_id=4361&nbr=3286*.
11. Akdis CA. New insights into mechanisms of immunoregulation in 2007. J Allergy Clin Immunol 2008;122:700–709.
12. Rothers J, Stern DA, Spangenberg A, Lohman IC, et al. Influence of early day-care exposure on total IgE levels through age 3 years. J Allergy Clin Immunol 2007;120:1201–1207.
13. Ege MJ, Herzum I, Buchele G, Krauss-Etschmann S, et al. Prenatal exposure to a farm environment modifies atopic sensitization at birth. J Allergy Clin Immunol 2008;122:407–412.
14. O'Regan GM, Sandilands A, McLean WHI, Irvine AD. Filaggrin in atopic dermatitis. J Allergy Clin Immunol 2008;122:689–693.
15. Scharschmidt TC, Man MQ, Hatano Y, Crumrine D, et al. Filaggrin deficiency confers a paracellular barrier abnormality that reduces inflammatory thresholds to irritants and haptens. J Allergy Clin Immunol 2009;124:496–506.
16. Rodriguez E, Baurecht H, Herberich E, Wagenpfeil S, et al. Meta-analysis of filaggrin polymorphisms in eczema and asthma: robust rick factors in atopic disease. J Allergy Clin Immunol 2009;123:1361–1370.
17. Honey B, Steinhoff M, Ruzicka T, Leung DYM. Cytokines and chemokines orchestrate atopic skin inflammation. J Allergy Clin Immunol 2006;118:178–189.
18. Law RM, Kwa PG. Atopic Dermatitis: The Itch that Erupts when Scratched. Instructor's Guide. In Schwinghammer TL, Koehler JM. Pharmacotherapy Casebook: A Patient-Focused Approach, 7th ed. New York, NY: McGraw-Hill, 2009:104–1 to 104–5.
19. Leung DYM. Our evolving understanding of the functional role of filaggrin in atopic dermatitis. J Allergy Clinical Immunol 2009;124: 494–495.
20. Steinke JW, Rich SS, Borish L. Genetics of allergic disease. J Allergy Clin Immunol 2008;121(Supplement):S384–S387.
21. Akdis CA, Akdis M, Bieber T, et al. Diagnosis and treatment of atopic dermatitis in children and adults: European Academy of Allergology and Clinical Immunology / American Academy of Allergy, Asthma and Immunology / PRACTALL Consensus Report. J Allergy Clin Immunol 2006;118:152–169.
22. Sicherer SC, Leung DYM. Advances in allergic skin disease, anaphylaxis and hypersensitivity reactions to foods, drugs, and insects in 2008. J Allergy Clin Immunol 2009;123:319–327.
23. Schauber J, Gallo RL. Antimicrobial peptides and the skin immune defense system. J Allergy Clin Immunol 2008;122:261–266.
24. Novak N, Bieber T. Dendritic cells as regulators of immunity and tolerance. J Allergy Clin Immunol 2008;121(Suppl):S370–S374.
25. Biebe T, de la Salle H, Wollenberg A, et al. Human epidermal Langerhans cells express the high affinity receptor for immunoglobulin E (Fc epsilon RI). J Exp Med 1992;175:1285–1290.
26. Wang B, Rieger A, Kilgus O, et al. Epidermal Langerhans cells from normal human skin bind monomeric IgE via Fc epsilon RI. J Exp Med 1992;175:1353–1365.
27. Novak N, Bieber T. The role of dendritic cell subtypes in the pathophysiology of atopic dermatitis. J Am Acad Dermatol 2005;53:Suppl 2:S171–S176.
28. Lack G. Epidemiologic risks for food allergy. J Allergy Clin Immunol 2008;121:1331–1336.
29. Grundy J, Matthews S, Bateman B, et al. Rising prevalence of allergy to peanut in children: Data from 2 sequential cohorts. J Allergy Clin Immunol 2002;110:784–789.
30. Lucas JSA, Lewis SA, Jourihane JO'B. Kiwi fruit allergy: A review. Pediatr Allergy Immunol 2003;14:420–428.
31. Cohen A, Goldberg M, Levy B et al. Sesame food allergy and sensitization in children: The natural history and long-term follow-up. Pediatr Allergy Immunol 2007;18:217–223.
32. Burks AW, Laubach S, Jones SM. Oral tolerance, food allergy, and immunotherapy: Implications for future treatment. J Allergy Clin Immunol 2008;121:1344–350.
33. Leung DYM, Nicklas RA, Li JT, Bernstein L, et al. Disease management of atopic dermatitis: an updated practice parameter. change to: Ann Allergy Asthma Immunol 2004;93(9):S1–S17.
34. Krafchik BR. Atopic Dermatitis. 2008, *http://emedicine.medscape.com* (eMedicine Specialties > Dermatology > Allergy & Immunology).

35. Stores G, Burrows A, Crawford C. Physiological sleep disturbance in children with atopic dermatitis: A case control study. Pediatr Dermatol 1998;15(4):264–268.

36. Beltrani VS, Boguneiwicz M. Atopic Dermatitis. Dermatology Online Journal. 2003, *http://dermatology.cdlib.org/92/reviews/atopy/beltrani.html.*

37. Eichenfield LF, Hanifin JM, Luger TA, et al. Consensus conference on pediatric atopic dermatitis. J Am Acad Dermatol 2003;49:1088–1095.

38. Lewis E. Atopic dermatitis: Disease overview and the development of topical immunomodulators. Formulary 2002;37(Suppl 2):3–15.

39. Rosso JD, Friedlander SF. Corticosteroids: Options in the era of steroid-sparing therapy. J Am Acad Dermatol 2005;53:S50–S58.

40. Hengge UR, Ruzicka T, Schwartz RA, et al. Adverse effects of topical glucocorticosteroids. J Am Acad Dermatol 2006;54:1–15.

41. Hebert AA and the Desonide Foam Phase III Clinical Study Group. Desonide foam 0.05%: Safety in children as young as 3 months. J Am Acad Dermatol 2008;59:334–340.

42. Stuetz A, Grassberger M, Meingassner JG. Pimecrolimus (Elidel,SDZ ASM 981)—Preclinical pharmacologic profile and skin selectivity. Semin Cutan Med Surg 2001;20:233–241.

43. Berger TG, Duvic M, Van Voorhees AS, Frieden IJ. The use of topical calcineurin inhibitors in dermatology: Safety concerns. J Am Acad Dermatol 2006;54:818–823.

44. Meurer M, Folster-Holst R, Wozel G, et al. Pimecrolimus cream in the long-term management of atopic dermatitis in adults: A six-month study. Dermatology 2002;205(3):271–277.

45. Abramovits W. A clinician's paradigm in the treatment of atopic dermatitis. J Am Acad Dermatol 2005;53:S70–S77.

46. Abeck D, Schnidt T, Fesq H et al. Long-term efficacy of medium-dose UVA1 phototherapy in atopic dermatitis. J Am Acad Dermatol 2000;42:254–257.

47. Majoie IML, Oldhoff JM, van Weelden H, et al. Narrowband ultraviolet B and medium-dose ultraviolet A1 are equally effective in the treatment of moderate to severe atopic dermatitis. J Am Acad Dermatol 2009;60:77–84.

48. Pughdal KV, Schwartz RA. Topical tar: Back to the future. J Am Acad Dermatol 2009;61:294–302.

49. Hanifin JM, Schneider LC, Leung DY, et al. Recombinant interferon gamma therapy for atopic dermatitis. J Am Acad Dermatol 1993;28:189–197.

50. Jang IG, Yang JK, Lee HJ, et al. Clinical improvement and immunohistochemical findings in severe atopic dermatitis treated with interferon gamma. J Am Acad Dermatol 2000;42:1033–1040.

51. Bremmer MS, Bremmer SF, Baig-Lewis S, et al. Are biologics safe in the treatment of atopic dermatitis? A review with a focus on immediate hypersensitivity reactions. J Am Acad Dermatol 2009;61:666–676.

52. Langan S, Rogers S. A retrospective review of the use of azathioprine in the therapy of severe atopic eczema. J Am Acad Dermatol 2005;52(3)Suppl:P84, Abstract P1001.

53. Rouse C, Siegfried E. Methotrexate for atopic dermatitis in children. J Am Acad Dermatol 2008;58(2)Suppl2:AB7, Abstract P608.

54. Koo J, Arain S. Traditional Chinese medicine for the treatment of dermatologic disorders. Arch Dermatol 1998;134:1388–1393.

55. Harper J. Traditional Chinese medicine for eczema. BMJ 1994;308:489–490.

56. Arkwright PD, David TJ. Intradermal administration of a killed *Mycobacterium vaccae* suspension (SRL 172) is associated with improvement in atopic dermatitis in children with moderate-to-severe disease. J Allergy Clin Immunol 2001;107:531–534.

57. Wickens K, Black PN, Stanley TV, et al. A differential effect of 2 probiotics in the prevention of eczema and atopy: A double-blind, randomized, placebo-controlled trial. J Allergy Clin Immunol 2008;122:788–794.

58. Zuberbier T, Orlow SJ, Paller AS, et al. Patient perspectives on the management of atopic dermatitis. J Allergy Clin Immunol 2006;118:226–232.

SECTION 15
HEMATOLOGIC DISORDERS

109

Anemias

KRISTEN COOK, BEATA A. INECK, AND WILLIAM L. LYONS

KEY CONCEPTS

❶ Anemia is a group of diseases characterized by a decrease in either hemoglobin (Hb) or the volume of red blood cells (RBCs), which results in decreased oxygen-carrying capacity of the blood. Anemia is defined by the World Health Organization as Hb <13g/dL (<130 g/L; <8.07 mmol/L) in men and <12g/dL (<120 g/L; <7.45 mmol/L) in women.

❷ Acute onset anemias are most likely to present with tachycardia, lightheadedness, and dyspnea. Chronic anemia often presents with weakness, fatigue, headache, vertigo, and pallor.

❸ Iron-deficiency anemia (IDA) is characterized by decreased levels of ferritin (most sensitive marker) and serum iron, as well as decreased transferrin saturation. Hb and hematocrit decrease later. RBC morphology includes hypochromia and microcytosis. Most patients are adequately treated with oral ferrous sulfate therapy, although parenteral iron therapy is necessary in selected patient populations.

❹ Vitamin B_{12} deficiency, a macrocytic anemia, can be due to inadequate intake, malabsorption syndromes, and inadequate utilization. Anemia caused by lack of intrinsic factor, resulting in decreased vitamin B_{12} absorption, is called *pernicious anemia*. Neurologic symptoms can be present and can become irreversible if the vitamin B_{12} deficiency is not treated promptly. Oral or parenteral therapy can be used for replacement.

❺ Folic acid deficiency, a macrocytic anemia, results from inadequate intake, decreased absorption, and increased folate requirements. Treatment consists of oral administration of folic acid, even for patients with absorption problems. Adequate folic acid intake is essential in women of childbearing age to decrease the risk of neural tube defects in their children.

❻ Anemia of chronic disease is a diagnosis of exclusion. It results from chronic inflammation, infection, or malignancy and can occur as early as 1 to 2 months after the onset of the disease. The serum iron level usually is decreased, but in contrast to IDA, the serum ferritin concentration is normal or increased. Treatment is aimed at correcting the underlying pathology.

❼ Anemia is a common complication in critically ill patients. Contributing factors include sepsis, frequent blood samples, surgical blood loss, immune mediated functional iron deficiency, decreased erythropoietin (EPO) production, reduced RBC life span, and active bleeding. Whether exogenous EPO improves clinical outcomes for critically ill patients is not clear.

❽ Anemia is one of the most prevalent clinical problems in the elderly, although not an inevitable complication of aging. Anemia is associated with an increased risk of hospitalization and mortality, reduced quality of life, and decreased physical functioning in the elderly.

❾ IDA is a leading cause of infant morbidity and mortality. Age- and sex-adjusted norms must be used in the interpretation of laboratory results for pediatric patients. Primary prevention of IDA is the goal. A therapeutic trial of oral iron is the standard of care.

❿ Hemolytic anemia results in decreased survival of RBCs secondary to destruction in the spleen or circulation. Treatment is directed toward correcting or controlling the underlying pathology.

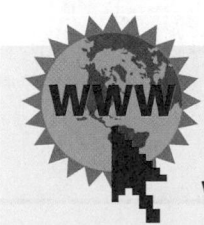

The complete chapter, learning objectives, and other resources can be found at **www.pharmacotherapyonline.com**.

Anemia affects a large part of the world's population. According to the World Health Organization, almost 1.6 billion people (25% of the world's population) are anemic. Anemia is defined by the World Health Organization as hemoglobin (Hb) <13 g/dL (<130 g/L; <8.07 mmol/L) in men or <12 g/dL (<120 g/L; <7.45 mmol/L) in women. In the United States approximately 3.5 million Americans have anemia based on self-reported data from the National Center for Health Statistics. It is estimated that millions of people are unaware they have anemia, making it one of the most underdiagnosed conditions in the United States. Iron deficiency is considered to be the leading cause of anemia worldwide, accounting for as many as 50% of cases.[1] Recent data have shown that overall anemia has declined in the United States in preschool-aged children and women of childbearing age over the past 20 years. However, the prevalence of iron-deficiency anemia did not change significantly in these groups and the difference remains unclear.[2] Although nutritional deficiencies are less common in the United States, obesity surgery, which can cause deficiencies, is becoming increasingly common. Gastric bypass may result in folate, vitamin B_{12}, and iron deficiencies. Prevalence data are confounded by the lack of a standardized definition of anemia and lack of screening guidelines for several populations. The U.S. Preventive Services Task Force (USPSTF) guidelines for pregnant women recommend routine screening for iron-deficiency anemia (IDA).

Anemia is not an innocent bystander; it may affect both length and quality of life. Retrospective observational studies of hemodialysis patients and heart failure patients suggest that anemia is an independent risk factor for mortality.[3] In addition, anemia significantly influences morbidity, as shown for patients with end-stage renal disease, chronic kidney disease, and heart failure.[4] Anemia is associated with psychomotor and cognitive abnormalities in

children. Similarly, among adults, anemia is associated with cognitive dysfunction in patients with renal failure, with those having cancer, and with community-dwelling elders.[5] Anemia during pregnancy is associated with increased risk for low birth weights, preterm delivery, and perinatal mortality.[6] Maternal IDA may be associated with postpartum depression and poor performance by offspring on mental and psychomotor tests. The effect of treatment on patient outcomes must be the focus of research on each specific type of anemia. Global goals of treatment in anemic patients are to alleviate signs and symptoms, correct the underlying etiology, and prevent recurrence of anemia.

❶ Anemia is a group of diseases characterized by a decrease in either Hb or circulating red blood cells (RBCs), resulting in reduced oxygen-carrying capacity of the blood. Anemia can result from inadequate RBC production, increased RBC destruction, or blood loss. It can be a manifestation of a host of systemic disorders, such as infection, chronic renal disease, or malignancy. Because anemia is often a sign of underlying pathology, rapid diagnosis of the cause is essential.

Anemia can be classified on the basis of the morphology of the RBCs, etiology, or pathophysiology (see Table 109–1 for examples). This chapter focuses on IDA, anemia associated with vitamin B_{12} or folic acid deficiency, and anemia of chronic disease (ACD). Characteristic changes in the size of RBCs seen in erythrocyte indices can be the first step in the morphologic classification and understanding of the anemia.

TABLE 109-1	Classification Systems for Anemias
I. Morphology	Gastritis
Macrocytic anemias	Hemorrhoids
Megaloblastic anemias	Chronic hemorrhage
Vitamin B_{12} deficiency	Vaginal bleeding
Folic acid deficiency anemia	Peptic ulcer
Microcytic hypochromic anemias	Intestinal parasites
Iron-deficiency anemia	Aspirin and other nonsteroidal antiinflammatory agents
Genetic anomaly	Excessive RBC destruction
Sickle cell anemia	Extracorpuscular (outside the cell) factors
Thalassemia	RBC antibodies
Other hemoglobinopathies (abnormal hemoglobins)	Drugs
Normocytic anemias	Physical trauma to RBC (artificial valves)
Recent blood loss	Excessive sequestration in the spleen
Hemolysis	Intracorpuscular factors
Bone marrow failure	Heredity
Anemia of chronic disease	Disorders of hemoglobin synthesis
Renal failure	Inadequate production of mature RBCs
Endocrine disorders	Deficiency of nutrients (B_{12}, folic acid, iron, protein)
Myelodysplastic anemias	Deficiency of erythroblasts
II. Etiology	Aplastic anemia
Deficiency	Isolated (often transient) erythroblastopenia
Iron	Folic acid antagonists
Vitamin B_{12}	Antibodies
Folic acid	Conditions with infiltration of bone marrow
Pyridoxine	Lymphoma
Central, caused by impaired bone marrow function	Leukemia
Anemia of chronic disease	Myelofibrosis
Anemia of the elderly	Carcinoma
Malignant bone marrow disorders	Endocrine abnormalities
Peripheral	Hypothyroidism
Bleeding (hemorrhage)	Adrenal insufficiency
Hemolysis (hemolytic anemias)	Pituitary insufficiency
III. Pathophysiology	Chronic renal disease
Excessive blood loss	Chronic inflammatory disease
Recent hemorrhage	Granulomatous diseases
Trauma	Collagen vascular diseases
Peptic ulcer	Hepatic disease

RBC, red blood cell.

Anemia is classified by RBC size as macrocytic, normocytic, or microcytic. Vitamin B$_{12}$ deficiency and folic acid deficiency both are macrocytic anemias. An example of a microcytic anemia is iron deficiency, whereas a normocytic anemia may be associated with recent blood loss or chronic disease. More than one anemia and etiology can occur concurrently. Inclusion of the underlying cause of the anemia makes diagnostic terminology easier to understand (e.g., microcytic anemia secondary to iron deficiency).

Microcytic anemias are pathogenically a result of a quantitative deficiency in Hb synthesis, usually due to iron deficiency or impaired iron utilization. As a result, erythrocytes containing insufficient Hb are formed. Microcytosis and hypochromia are the morphologic abnormalities that provide evidence of impaired Hb synthesis.

Macrocytic anemias can be divided into megaloblastic and nonmegaloblastic anemias. The type of macrocytic anemia can be distinguished microscopically by peripheral blood smear examination. Megaloblasts are distinctive cells that express a biochemical abnormality of retarded DNA synthesis, resulting in unbalanced cell growth. Megaloblastic anemias may affect all hematopoietic cell lines. The most common cause of megaloblastic anemia is vitamin B$_{12}$ and/or folate deficiency. Nonmegaloblastic macrocytic anemias may arise from liver disease, hypothyroidism, hemolytic processes, and alcoholism. Hemolytic anemias often are macrocytic, reflecting the increased numbers of circulating reticulocytes, which are larger on average than mature red cells.

MATURATION AND DEVELOPMENT OF RED BLOOD CELLS

In adults, RBCs are formed in the marrow of the vertebrae, ribs, sternum, clavicle, pelvic (iliac) crest, and proximal epiphyses of the long bones. In children, most bone marrow space is hematopoietically active to meet increased RBC requirements.

In normal RBC formation, a pluripotent stem cell yields an erythroid burst-forming unit. Erythropoietin (EPO) and cytokines such as interleukin-3 and granulocyte–macrophage colony-stimulating factor stimulate this cell to form an erythroid colony-forming unit in the marrow. The erythroid colony-forming unit is sensitive to EPO and produces proerythroblasts. Subsequent divisions yield basophilic erythroblasts, polychromatic erythroblasts, pyknotic erythroblasts, reticulocytes, and finally erythrocytes. During this process, the nucleus becomes smaller with each division, finally disappearing in the normal erythrocyte (Fig. 109–1). Hb and iron are incorporated into the gradually maturing RBC, which eventually is released from the marrow into the circulating blood as a reticulocyte. The maturation process usually takes approximately 1 week. The reticulocyte loses its nucleus and becomes an erythrocyte within several days. The circulating erythrocyte is a nonnucleated, nondividing cell. More than 90% of the protein content of the erythrocyte consists of the oxygen-carrying molecule Hb. Erythrocytes have a normal survival time of 120 days.[7]

STIMULATION OF ERYTHROPOIESIS

The hormone EPO, 90% of which is produced by the kidneys, initiates and stimulates the production of RBCs. Erythropoiesis is regulated by a feedback loop. The main mechanism of action of EPO is preventing apoptosis, or programmed cell death, of erythroid precursor cells and allowing their proliferation and subsequent maturation. A decrease in tissue oxygen concentration signals the kidneys to increase the production and release of EPO into the plasma, which increases production and maturation of RBCs.

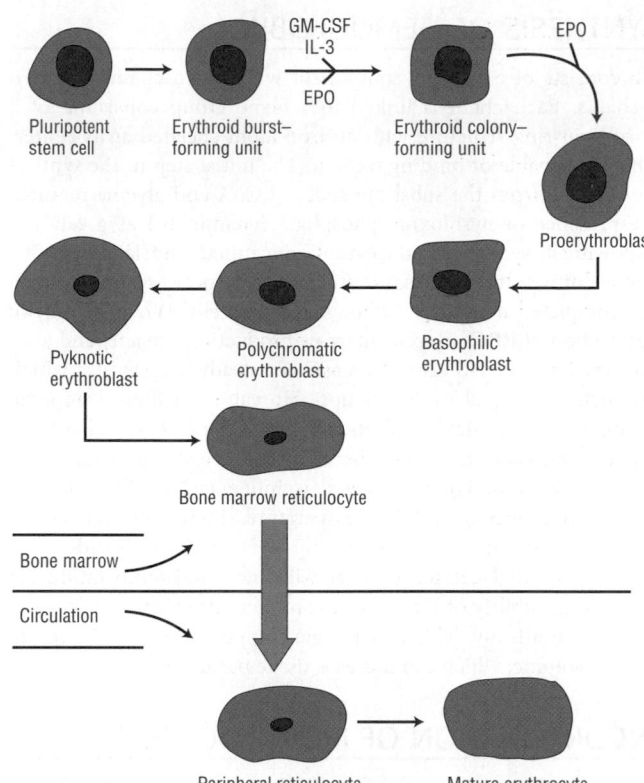

FIGURE 109-1. Erythrocyte maturation sequence (EPO, erythropoietin; GM-CSF, granulocyte-macrophage colony-stimulating factor; IL-3, interleukin-3).

Under normal circumstances, the RBC mass is kept at an almost constant level by EPO matching new erythrocyte production to the natural rate of loss of RBCs. A feedback mechanism stops further RBC nucleic acid synthesis, causing an earlier release of reticulocytes. This feedback loop and summary of erythropoiesis are shown in Figure 109–2. Early appearance of large quantities of reticulocytes in the peripheral circulation (reticulocytosis) is an indication of increased RBC production.[7]

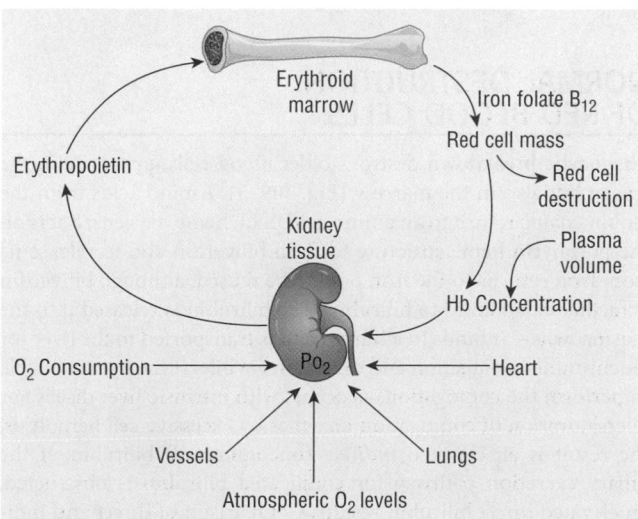

FIGURE 109-2. Physiologic regulation of red cell production by tissue oxygen tension. (*Reproduced with permission from Adamson JW., Longo DL. Anemia and polycythemia. In: Fauci AS, Braunwald E, Kasper DL, et al, eds. Harrison's Principles of Internal Medicine. 17th ed. New York: Copyright © McGraw-Hill; 2008:355.*)

SYNTHESIS OF HEMOGLOBIN

Hb consists of a protein component with two α-chains and two β-chains. Each chain is linked to a heme group consisting of a porphyrin ring structure with an iron atom chelated at its center, which is capable of binding oxygen. The initial step in the synthesis of heme from the substrate succinyl CoA and glycine requires the presence of pyridoxine phosphate (vitamin B_6) as a catalyst. Following its synthesis in the cytoplasmic mitochondria of the RBC, heme diffuses into the extramitochondrial space, combines with the completed α- and β-chains, and forms Hb. When hemolytic destruction of RBCs exceeds marrow production capacity and anemia develops, the Hb value decreases to a steady-state level at which production is equal to destruction. Hb values in these hemolytic anemias, such as sickle cell anemia (see Chap. 111), will remain stable unless other factors further shorten the RBC life span.

The affinity of Hb for oxygen is influenced by three intracellular components and by temperature. Increasing concentrations of hydrogen ion (decreasing pH), carbon dioxide, and 2,3-bisphosphoglycerate, together with increased temperature, all enhance the ability of Hb to release oxygen into tissue by decreasing oxygen affinity. This physiologic compensation also increases plasma volume, which can increase tissue perfusion.[8]

INCORPORATION OF IRON INTO HEME

Iron is an essential part of hemoglobin. The specific plasma transport protein transferrin delivers iron to the bone marrow for incorporation into the Hb molecule. Transferrin enters cells by binding to transferrin receptors, which circulate and then attach to cells needing iron. Conversely, there are fewer transferrin receptors on the surface of cells that do not need iron, thus preventing iron-replete cells from receiving excess iron.[9]

Circulating transferrin normally is approximately 30% saturated with iron. Transferrin delivers extra iron to other body storage sites, such as the liver, marrow, and spleen, for later use. This iron is stored within macrophages as ferritin or hemosiderin. Ferritin consists of a Fe^{3+} hydroxyphosphate core surrounded by a protein shell called *apoferritin*. Hemosiderin can be described as compacted ferritin molecules with an even greater iron-to-protein shell ratio. Physiologically it is a more stable, but less available, form of storage iron. Total body iron storage is generally reflected by ferritin levels.[10]

NORMAL DESTRUCTION OF RED BLOOD CELLS

Phagocytic breakdown destroys older blood cells, primarily in the spleen but also in the marrow (Fig. 109–3). Amino acids from the globin chains return to an amino acid pool; heme oxygenase acts on the porphyrin heme structure to form biliverdin and to release its iron. Iron returns to the iron pool to be reused, although biliverdin is further catabolized to bilirubin. The bilirubin is released into the plasma, where it binds to albumin and is transported to the liver for glucuronide conjugation and excretion via bile. If the liver is unable to perform the conjugation, as occurs with intrinsic liver disease or oversaturation of conjugation enzymes by excessive cell hemolysis, the result is an elevated *indirect* (unconjugated) bilirubin. If the biliary excretion pathway for conjugated bilirubin is obstructed, an elevated *direct* bilirubin results. Comparison of direct and indirect bilirubin values helps to determine if the defect in bilirubin clearance occurs before or after bilirubin enters the liver. The Hb in RBCs, which is destroyed by intravascular hemolysis, becomes attached to haptoglobin and is carried back to the marrow for processing in the normal manner.[11]

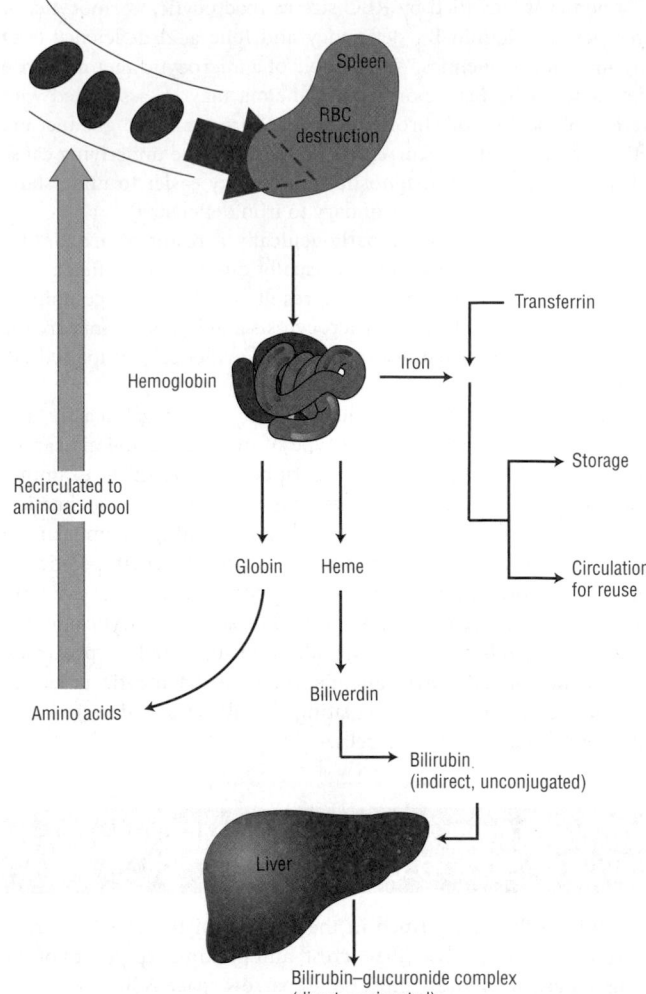

FIGURE 109-3. Destruction of red blood cells (RBCs).

DIAGNOSIS OF ANEMIA

GENERAL PRESENTATION

History, physical examination, and laboratory testing are used in the evaluation of the patient with anemia. The workup determines if the patient is bleeding and investigates potential causes of the anemia, such as increased RBC destruction, bone marrow suppression, or iron deficiency. Diet can also be important in identifying causes of anemia. Additionally, information about concurrent non-hematologic disease states and a drug ingestion history are essential when evaluating the cause of the anemia (see Chap. 112). History of blood transfusions and exposure to toxic chemicals also should be obtained.

Presenting signs and symptoms of anemia depend on the rate of development and the age of the patient, as well as the cardiovascular status of the patient. Severity of symptoms does not always correlate with the degree of anemia. Healthy patients may acclimate to very low Hb concentrations if the anemia develops slowly. Mild anemia often is associated with no clinical symptoms and may be found incidentally upon obtaining a complete blood count (CBC) for other reasons. The signs and symptoms in elderly patients with anemia may be attributed to their age or concomitant disease states. The elderly may not tolerate levels of Hb tolerated by younger persons. Patients with cardiac or pulmonary disease may be less tolerant of mild anemia. Premature infants with anemia may be asymptomatic or have tachycardia, poor weight gain, increased supplemental oxygen needs, or increased episodes of apnea or bradycardia.

CLINICAL PRESENTATION OF ANEMIA

General

- Patients may be asymptomatic or have vague complaints
- Patients with vitamin B_{12} deficiency may develop neurologic consequences
- In ACD, signs and symptoms of the underlying disorder often overshadow those of the anemia

Symptoms

- Decreased exercise tolerance
- Fatigue
- Dizziness
- Irritability
- Weakness
- Palpitations
- Vertigo
- Shortness of breath
- Chest pain
- Neurologic symptoms in vitamin B_{12} deficiency

Signs

- Tachycardia
- Pale appearance (most prominent in conjunctivae)
- Decreased mental acuity
- Increased intensity of some cardiac valvular murmurs
- Diminished vibratory sense or gait abnormality in vitamin B_{12} deficiency

Laboratory Tests

- Hb, hematocrit (Hct), and RBC indices may remain normal early in the disease and then decrease as the anemia progresses
- Serum iron is low in IDA and ACD
- Ferritin levels are low in IDA and normal to increased in ACD
- TIBC is high in IDA and is low or normal in ACD
- Mean cell volume is elevated in vitamin B_{12} deficiency and folate deficiency
- Vitamin B_{12} and folate levels are low in their respective types of anemia
- Homocysteine is elevated in vitamin B_{12} deficiency and folate deficiency
- Methylmalonic acid is elevated in vitamin B_{12} deficiency

Other Diagnostic Tests

- Schilling test may help uncover intrinsic factor deficiency
- Bone marrow testing with iron staining can indicate low iron levels in IDA and adequate stores in ACD

❷ Anemia of rapid onset is most likely to present with cardiorespiratory symptoms such as tachycardia, palpitations, angina, hypotension, lightheadedness, and breathlessness due to decreased oxygen delivery to tissues or hypovolemia in those with acute bleeding.

If onset is more chronic, presenting symptoms may include fatigue, weakness, headache, symptoms of heart failure, vertigo, faintness, sensitivity to cold, pallor, and loss of skin tone. Traditional signs of anemia, such as pallor, have limited sensitivity, and specificity and may be misinterpreted. With chronic bleeding, there is time for equilibration within the extravascular space.

Possible manifestations of IDA include glossal pain, smooth tongue, reduced salivary flow, pica (compulsive eating of nonfood items), and pagophagia (compulsive eating of ice). These symptoms are not likely to appear until the Hb concentration falls to a level of 9 g/dL (90 g/L; 5.59 mmol/L) or below.

Neurologic findings in vitamin B_{12} deficiency, which often precede hematologic findings, may be partly due to impairment of conversion of homocysteine to methionine, as methionine is necessary for production of choline and choline-containing phospholipids. Neurologic effects of vitamin B_{12} deficiency may occur even in the absence of anemia. Early neurologic findings include numbness and paraesthesias, then peripheral neuropathy, ataxia, diminished vibratory sense, decreased proprioception, and imbalance, as demyelination of the dorsal columns and corticospinal tract develop. Vision changes may result from optic nerve involvement. Psychiatric findings include irritability, personality changes, memory impairment, depression, and, infrequently, psychosis. Pernicious anemia is associated with increased risk of gastric cancer.

Anemia associated with folate deficiency is typically macrocytic but, unlike B_{12} deficiency, occurs without neurological symptoms. Although the symptoms of anemia will improve with folate replacement and a partial hematologic response will occur, the neurologic manifestations of vitamin B_{12} deficiency will not be reversed with folic acid replacement therapy and consequently may progress or become irreversible if not treated.

LABORATORY EVALUATION

The initial evaluation of anemia involves a CBC (including RBC indices), reticulocyte index, and examination of a stool sample for occult blood. The results of the preliminary evaluation determine the need for other studies, such as examination of a peripheral blood smear. Based on laboratory test results, anemia can be categorized into three functional defects: RBC production failure (hypoproliferative), cell maturation ineffectiveness, or increased RBC destruction or loss.

Table 109–2 lists normal hematologic values, although these values may differ in certain populations such as individuals living at high altitudes and endurance athletes.

Figure 109–4 shows a broad, general algorithm for the diagnosis of anemia based on laboratory data. There are many exceptions and additions to this algorithm, but it can serve as a guide to the typical presentation of common types and causes of anemia. The algorithm is less useful in the presence of more than one cause of anemia.

Hemoglobin

Values given for Hb represent the amount of Hb per volume of whole blood. The higher values seen in males are due to stimulation of RBC production by androgenic steroids, whereas the lower values in females are due to decrease in Hb as a result of blood loss during menstruation. The Hb level can be used as a very rough estimate of the oxygen-carrying capacity of blood. Hb levels may be diminished because of a decreased quantity of Hb per RBC or because of a decrease in the actual number of RBCs. In pregnancy, Hb may not reflect red cell mass changes.

Hematocrit

Expressed as a percentage, hematocrit (Hct) is the actual volume of RBCs in a unit volume of whole blood. In general, it is

TABLE 109-2	Normal Hematologic Values			
	Reference Range			
Test	**2–6**	**6–12**	**12–18**	**18–49**
Hemoglobin (g/dL)	11.5–15.5	11.5–15.5	M 13.0–16.0 F 12.0–16.0	M 13.5–17.5 F 12.0–16.0
Hematocrit (%)	34–40	35–45	M 37–49 F 36–46	M 41–53 F 36–46
MCV (fL)	75–87	77–95	M 78–98 F 78–102	80–100
MCHC (%)	–	31–37	31–37	31–37
MCH (pg)	24–30	25–33	25–35	26–34
RBC (million/mm³)	3.9–5.3	4.0–5.2	M 4.5–5.3	M 4.5–5.9
Reticulocyte count, absolute (%)				0.5–1.5
Serum iron (mcg/dL)		50–120	50–120	M 50–160 F 40–150
TIBC (mcg/dL)	250–400	250–400	250–400	250–400
RDW (%)				11–16
Ferritin (ng/mL)	7–140	7–140	7–140	M 15–200 F 12–150
Folate (ng/mL)				1.8–16.0[a]
Vitamin B₁₂ (pg/mL)				100–900[a]
Erythropoietin (mU/mL)				0–19

F, female; M, male; MCH, mean corpuscular hemoglobin; MCHC, mean corpuscular hemoglobin concentration; MCV, mean corpuscular volume; RBC, red blood cell; RDW, red blood cell distribution; TIBC, total iron-binding capacity.
[a]Varies by assay method.

approximately three times the Hb value. An alteration in this ratio may occur with abnormal cell size or shape and often indicates the pathology. A low Hct indicates a reduction in either the number or the size of RBCs or an increase in plasma volume.

Red Blood Cell Count

The RBC count is an indirect estimate of the Hb content of the blood; it is an actual count of RBCs per unit of blood.

Red Blood Cell Indices

Wintrobe indices describe the size and Hb content of the RBCs and are calculated from the Hb, Hct, and RBC count. RBC indices, such as mean corpuscular volume (MCV) and mean corpuscular Hb (MCH), are single mean values that do not express the variation that can occur in cells.

Mean Cell Volume (Hct/RBC Count) MCV represents the average volume of RBCs. It may reflect changes in MCH. Cells are considered macrocytic if they are larger than normal, microcytic if they are smaller than normal, and normocytic if their size falls within normal limits. Folic acid and vitamin B₁₂ deficiency anemias yield macrocytic cells, whereas iron deficiency and thalassemia are examples of microcytic anemias. MCV is falsely elevated in the presence of cold agglutinins and hyperglycemia. When IDA (decreased MCV) is accompanied by folate deficiency (increased MCV), the overall MCV may be normal. Failure to understand that the MCV represents an average RBC size creates the potential for overlooking some causes of the anemia.

Mean Cell Hemoglobin (Hb/RBC Count) MCH is the amount of Hb in a RBC. It reflects the adequacy of iron supply. Two morphologic changes, microcytosis and hypochromia, can reduce MCH. A microcytic cell contains less Hb because it is a smaller cell, while a hypochromic cell has a low MCH because of the decreased amount of Hb present in the cell. Cells can be both microcytic and hypochromic, as seen with IDA. The MCH alone can not distinguish between

microcytosis and hypochromia. The most common cause of an elevated MCH is macrocytosis (e.g., vitamin B₁₂ or folate deficiency).

Mean Cell Hemoglobin Concentration (Hb/Hct) The concentration of Hb per volume of cells is the mean corpuscular Hb concentration (MCHC). Because MCHC is independent of cell size, it is more useful than MCH in distinguishing between microcytosis and hypochromia. A low MCHC indicates hypochromia; a microcyte with a normal Hb concentration will have a low MCH but a normal MCHC. A decreased MCHC is seen most often in IDA.

Total Reticulocyte Count

The total reticulocyte count is an indirect assessment of new RBC production. It reflects how quickly immature RBCs (reticulocytes) are produced by bone marrow and released into the blood. Reticulocytes circulate in the blood approximately 2 days before maturing into RBCs. About 1% of RBCs are normally replaced daily, representing a reticulocyte count of 1%. The reticulocyte count in normocytic anemia can differentiate hypoproliferative marrow from a compensatory marrow response to an anemia. A lack of reticulocytosis in anemia indicates impaired RBC production. Examples include iron deficiency, B₁₂ deficiency, ACD, malnutrition, renal insufficiency, and malignancy. A high reticulocyte count may be seen in acute blood loss or hemolysis. A patient's Hct occasionally decreases while the absolute number of reticulocytes remains the same, resulting in a falsely elevated reticulocyte percentage. Multiplying the reticulocyte percentage by the patient's Hct and then dividing the product by an average normal Hct (for men or women) produces a corrected percentage of reticulocytes. When the reticulocyte count is >2.5%, hemolysis may be present.

Red Blood Cell Distribution Width

The higher the RBC distribution width (RDW) is, the more variable is the size of the RBCs. The RDW increases in early IDA because of the release of large, immature, nucleated RBCs to compensate for the anemia, but this change is not specific for IDA. The RDW also can be helpful in the diagnosis of a mixed anemia. A patient can have a normal MCV yet have a wide RDW. This finding indicates the presence of microcytes and macrocytes, which would yield a "normal" average RBC size. Use of RDW to distinguish IDA from ACD is not recommended.

Peripheral Blood Smear

The peripheral blood smear can supplement other clinical data and help establish a diagnosis. Peripheral blood smears provide information on the functional status of the bone marrow and defects in RBC production. Additionally, it provides information on variations in cell size (anisocytosis) and shape (poikilocytosis). Automated blood counters, used for the CBC, can flag specific RBC changes that can be confirmed by a peripheral blood smear. Blood smears are placed on a microscope slide and stained as appropriate. Morphologic examination includes assessment of size, shape, and color. The extent of anisocytosis correlates with increased range of cell sizes. Poikilocytosis suggests a defect in the maturation of RBC precursors in the bone marrow.

Serum Iron

The level of serum iron is the concentration of iron bound to transferrin. Transferrin is normally approximately one-third bound (saturated) to iron. The serum iron level of many patients with IDA may remain within the lower limits of normal because a considerable amount of time is required to deplete iron stores. Serum iron levels show diurnal variation (higher in the morning, lower in the afternoon), but this variation is probably not clinically significant in

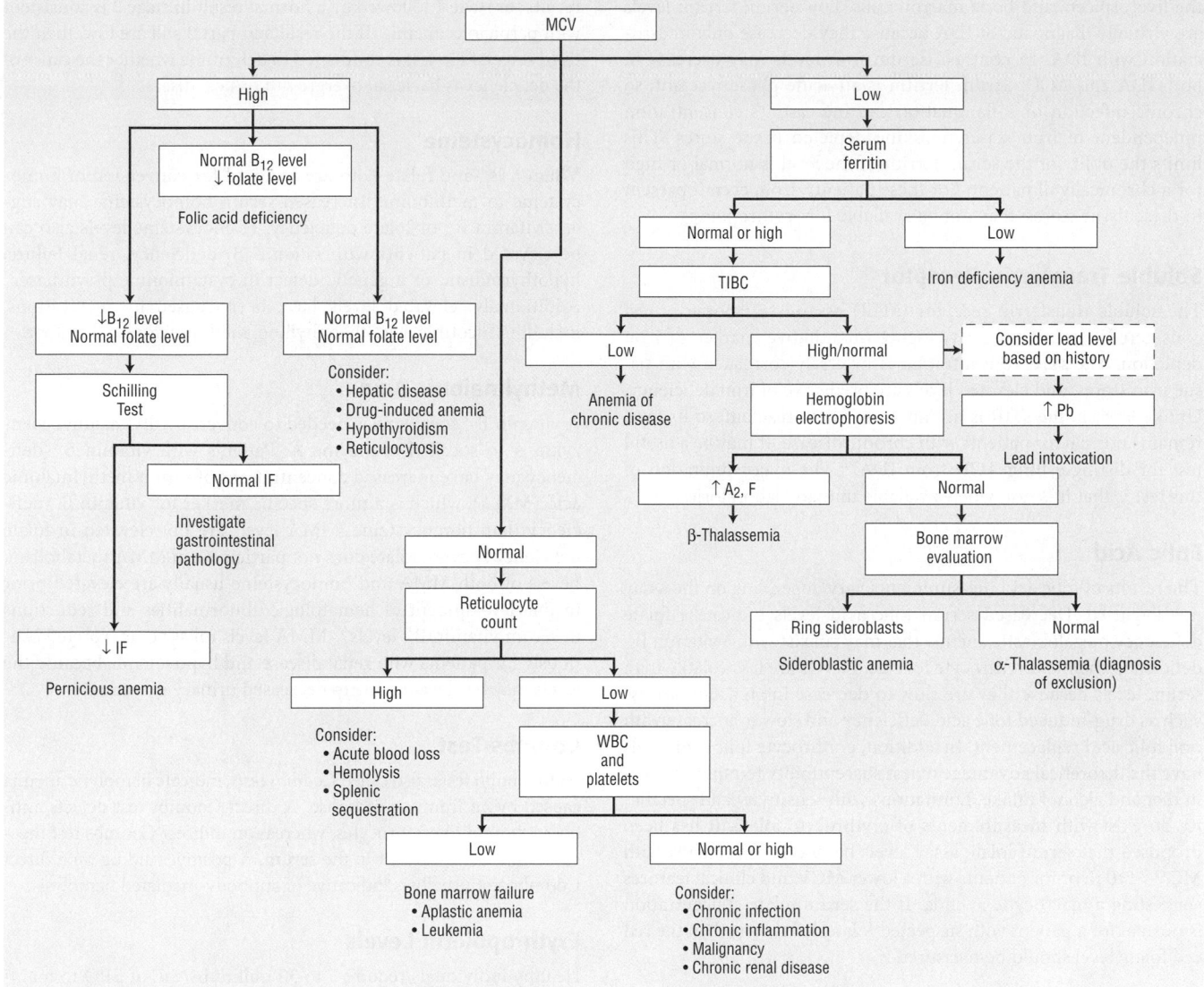

FIGURE 109-4. General algorithm for diagnosis of anemias (↑, increased; ↓, decreased; A$_2$, hemoglobin A$_2$; F, hemoglobin F; IF, intrinsic factor; MCV, mean corpuscular volume; Pb, lead; TIBC, total iron-binding capacity; WBC, white blood cells).

timing of levels.[10] Since serum iron levels are decreased by infection and inflammation, serum iron levels are best interpreted in conjunction with the TIBC. The serum iron level decreases with IDA and ACD and increases with hemolytic anemias and iron overload.

Total Iron-Binding Capacity

An indirect measurement of the iron-binding capacity of serum transferrin, total iron-binding capacity (TIBC) evaluation is performed by adding an excess of iron to plasma to saturate all transferrin with iron. Each transferrin molecule can carry two iron atoms. Normally, approximately 30% of available iron-binding sites are filled. With this laboratory test, all binding sites are filled to measure TIBC. The excess (unbound) iron is then removed and the serum iron concentration determined. Unlike the serum iron level, the TIBC does not fluctuate over hours or days. TIBC usually is higher than normal when body iron stores are low. The finding of a low serum iron level and a high TIBC suggests IDA. The TIBC is actually a measurement of protein serum transferrin, which can be affected by a variety of factors. Patients with infection, malignancy, inflammation, liver disease, and uremia may have a decreased TIBC and a decreased serum iron level, which are consistent with the diagnosis of ACD. Oral contraceptive use and pregnancy can

increase TIBC because serum transferrin production is increased with a variety of other proteins.

Percentage Transferrin Saturation

The ratio of serum iron level to TIBC indicates transferrin saturation. It reflects the extent to which iron-binding sites are occupied on transferrin and indicates the amount of iron readily available for erythropoiesis. It is expressed as a percentage, as described in the following formula:

$$\text{Transferrin saturation} = \frac{\text{serum iron}}{\text{TIBC}} \times 100$$

Transferrin normally is 20% to 50% saturated with iron. In IDA, transferrin saturation of 15% or lower is commonly seen.[10] Transferrin saturation is a less sensitive and specific marker of iron deficiency than are ferritin levels.

Serum Ferritin

The concentration of ferritin (storage iron) is proportional to total iron stores and therefore is the best indicator of iron deficiency or iron overload. Ferritin levels indicate the amount of iron stored in the liver, spleen, and bone marrow cells. Low serum ferritin levels are virtually diagnostic of IDA because they decrease only in association with IDA. In contrast, serum iron levels may decrease in both IDA and ACD. Serum ferritin is an acute phase reactant; so chronic infection or inflammation can increase its concentration independent of iron status, masking depleted tissue stores. This limits the utility of the serum ferritin if the level is normal or high for a chronically ill patient. For these patients, iron, even if present in these tissue stores, may not be available for erythropoiesis.

Soluble Transferrin Receptor

The soluble transferrin receptor (sTfR) assay is a laboratory test considered a sensitive, early, highly quantitative marker of iron depletion. The sTfR concentration is inversely correlated with tissue iron stores, and elevated levels are predictive of iron deficiency. Unlike ferritin, the sTfR is not an acute phase reactant; so its level remains normal for patients with chronic disease. It may be a useful test for distinguishing ACD from IDA.[10] The major limitation of this test is that it is not available in many laboratories.

Folic Acid

The results of folic acid measurements vary depending on the assay method used. Decreased serum folic acid levels indicate a folate deficiency megaloblastic anemia that may coexist with a vitamin B_{12} deficiency anemia. Erythrocyte folic acid levels are less volatile than serum levels because they are slow to decrease in an acute process such as drug-induced folic acid deficiency and slow to increase with oral folic acid replacement. In addition, erythrocyte folic acid levels have the theoretical advantage of less susceptibility to rapid changes in diet and alcohol intake. Limitations with sensitivity and specificity do exist with measurements of erythrocyte folate. It has been proposed that serum folate assay levels be drawn for patients with MCV >110 fL or for patients with a lower MCV and clinical features suggesting a macrocytic anemia. If the serum folate concentration is normal for a patient with suspected folate deficiency, then the red cell folate level should be measured.[12]

Vitamin B_{12}

Low levels of vitamin B_{12} (cyanocobalamin) indicate deficiency. However, a deficiency may exist prior to the recognition of low serum levels. Serum values are maintained at the expense of vitamin B_{12} tissue stores. Vitamin B_{12} and folate deficiency may overlap, thus serum levels of both vitamins should be determined. Vitamin B_{12} levels may be falsely low with folate deficiency, pregnancy, and use of oral contraceptives.[13]

Schilling Test

The purpose of the rarely used Schilling urinary excretion test is to diagnose vitamin B_{12} deficiency anemia caused by a B_{12} absorption defect resulting from a lack of intrinsic factor (pernicious anemia). The patient initially receives an oral dose of radiolabeled vitamin B_{12}. Two hours later, the patient receives a large intramuscular dose of nonlabeled vitamin B_{12} to saturate plasma transport proteins. Any excess vitamin B_{12} that is not taken up by the transport proteins or stored in the liver is excreted in the urine. A 24-hour urine collection then is measured for radioactivity. If production of gastrointestinal intrinsic factor is sufficient, the radiolabeled B_{12} will be absorbed initially, displaced by the injected B_{12}, and excreted in the urine.

If oral absorption is impaired, stage 2 of the test is conducted 5 to 7 days later. The second stage of the Schilling test differentiates inadequate secretion of intrinsic factor by the stomach from an abnormality in absorption by the ileum. Generally, the finding of abnormal results for stage 1 followed by a normal result in stage 2 is consistent with pernicious anemia. If the results in part 2 still are low, then the third stage of the test is conducted to determine whether the cause of the deficiency is bacterial overgrowth or ileal disease.[14]

Homocysteine

Vitamin B_{12} and folate both are required for conversion of homocysteine to methionine. Increased serum homocysteine may suggest vitamin B_{12} or folate deficiency. Homocysteine levels also can be elevated in patients with vitamin B_6 deficiency, renal failure, hypothyroidism, or a genetic defect in cystathionine β-synthase.[15] Additionally, elevated levels have been caused by medications, including nicotinic acid, theophylline, methotrexate, and L-dopa.

Methylmalonic Acid

A vitamin B_{12} coenzyme is needed to convert methylmalonyl coenzyme A to succinyl coenzyme A. Patients with vitamin B_{12} deficiency may have increased concentrations of serum methylmalonic acid (MMA), which is a more specific marker for vitamin B_{12} deficiency than homocysteine. MMA levels are not elevated in folate deficiency because folate does not participate in MMA metabolism. Levels of both MMA and homocysteine usually are elevated prior to the development of hematologic abnormalities and reductions in serum vitamin B_{12} levels.[13] MMA levels must be interpreted cautiously for patients with renal disease and hypovolemia because the levels may be elevated due to decreased urinary excretion.

Coombs Test

Antiglobulin tests, also called *Coombs tests*, indicate hemolytic anemia caused by an immune response. A direct Coombs test detects antibodies bound to erythrocytes, whereas an indirect Coombs test measures antibodies present in the serum. A positive finding on a direct Coombs test usually is indicative of antibody-mediated hemolysis.

Erythropoietin Levels

Healthy individuals require 5 to 30 milliunits/mL of EPO to maintain normal Hb and Hct concentrations. Endogenous EPO levels can increase during hypoxia or anemia, but this marked increase does not occur for patients with significant renal disease, for patients receiving chemotherapy, and for patients with acquired immunodeficiency syndrome (AIDS), especially those taking zidovudine. These patients will have an EPO response that is insufficient to correct their anemia.

SPECIFIC ANEMIAS

IRON-DEFICIENCY ANEMIA

Epidemiology

Iron deficiency is the most common nutritional deficiency in developing and developed countries. Data from the National Health and Nutrition Examination Survey (NHANES) indicates the prevalence of IDA in young children and women of childbearing age is 1.2% and 4.5%, respectively.[2] The normal ranges for Hb and Hct are so wide that a patient may lose up to 15% of RBC mass and still have a Hct within the normal range. Therefore, iron deficiency may precede the appearance of anemia.

Iron Balance

The normal iron content of the body is approximately 3 to 4 g. Iron is a component of Hb, myoglobin, and cytochromes. Approximately

2 g of the iron exists in the form of Hb, and approximately 140 mg exists as iron-containing proteins such as myoglobin. Approximately 3 mg of iron is bound to transferrin in plasma, and 1,000 mg of iron exists as storage iron in the form of ferritin or hemosiderin. The rest of the iron is stored in other tissues such as cytochromes.[10] Due to the toxicity of inorganic iron, the body has an intricate system for iron absorption, transport, storage, assimilation, and elimination. Hepcidin is a regulator of intestinal iron absorption, iron recycling, and iron mobilization from hepatic stores. It is a peptide made in the liver, distributed in plasma, and excreted in urine. Hepcidin inhibits efflux of iron through ferroportin. Hepcidin synthesis is increased by iron loading and decreased by anemia and hypoxia. Hepcidin is induced during infections and inflammation, which allows iron to sequester in macrophages, hepatocytes, and enterocytes.[16] As a result, hepcidin is likely an important mediator of ACD.

Most people lose approximately 1 mg of iron daily. Menstruating women can lose up to 0.6% to 2.5% more per day. Pregnancy requires an additional 700 mg of iron and a blood donation can result in as much as 250 mg of iron loss;[17] these populations are at higher risk for deficiency.

Iron is best absorbed in its ferrous (Fe^{2+}) form. The normal daily Western diet contains approximately 12 to 15 mg of iron, mainly in the ferric (Fe^{3+}) nonabsorbed form. After iron is ionized by stomach acid and then reduced to the Fe^{2+} state, it is absorbed primarily in the duodenum, and to a smaller extent in the jejunum, via intestinal mucosal cell uptake. Subsequently, it is transferred across the cell into the plasma. Iron absorption is not directly correlated to iron intake. As physiologic iron levels decrease, gastrointestinal absorption of iron increases.

The daily recommended dietary allowance for iron is 8 mg in adult males and postmenopausal females and 18 mg in menstruating females. Children require more iron because of growth-related increases in blood volume, and pregnant women have an increased iron demand brought about by fetal development. In the absence of hemachromatosis, iron overload does not occur, because only the amount of iron lost per day is absorbed. The amount of iron absorbed from food depends on the body stores, the rate of RBC production, the type of iron provided in the diet, and the presence of any substances that may enhance or inhibit iron absorption.

Heme iron, which is found in meat, fish, and poultry, is approximately three times more absorbable than the nonheme iron found in vegetables, fruits, dried beans, nuts, grain products, and dietary supplements. Gastric acid and other dietary components such as ascorbic acid increase the absorption of nonheme iron. Dietary components that form insoluble complexes with iron (phytates, tannates, and phosphates) decrease absorption. Phytates, a natural component of grains, brans, and some vegetables, can form poorly absorbed complexes and partially explain the increased prevalence of IDA in poorer countries, where grains and vegetables compose a disproportionate amount of the normal diet. Polyphenols bind the iron and decrease nonheme iron absorption when large amounts of tea or coffee are consumed with a meal. Although the mechanism is unknown, calcium inhibits absorption of both heme and nonheme iron. Finally, because gastric acid improves iron absorption, patients who have undergone a gastrectomy or have achlorhydria have decreased iron absorption.[18]

Etiology

Iron deficiency results from prolonged negative iron balance. This can occur due to increased iron demand or hematopoiesis, increased loss, or decreased intake/absorption. The onset of iron deficiency depends on an individual's initial iron stores and balance between iron absorption and loss. Multiple etiologic factors usually are involved. Certain groups at higher risk for iron deficiency include children younger than 2 years, adolescent girls, pregnant/lactating females, and those older than 65 years. Patients older than 65 years of age with IDA should be considered for screening for occult gastrointestinal cancer.[17] Blood loss must initially be considered a cause of IDA in adults. Blood loss may occur as a result of many disorders, including trauma, hemorrhoids, peptic ulcers, gastritis, gastrointestinal malignancies, arteriovenous malformations, diverticular disease, copious menstrual flow, nosebleeds, and postpartum bleeding. In less industrialized nations, the risks for developing IDA are largely related to dietary factors.

The USPSTF recommends routine screening for IDA in all pregnant women.[19] The USPSTF has concluded that evidence is insufficient to recommend for or against routine iron supplementation for nonanemic pregnant women.[19] However, iron deficiency in pregnant women is so common that the Centers for Disease Control and Prevention (CDC) guidelines recommend initiation of low-dose iron supplements or prenatal vitamins with 30 mg/day of iron at the woman's first prenatal visit.

Medication history, specifically regarding recent or past use of iron or hematinics, alcohol, corticosteroids, aspirin, and nonsteroidal antiinflammatory drugs, is a vital part of the history. Other possible causes of hypochromic microcytic anemia include ACD, thalassemia, sideroblastic anemia, and heavy metal (mostly lead) poisoning (Fig. 109–4).

Pathophysiology

Iron is vital to the function of all cells. It is a critical element in iron-containing enzymes such as the mitochondrial cytochrome system. Without iron, cells lose their capacity for electron transport and energy metabolism. Because iron is a cofactor for oxidative metabolism, dopamine and DNA synthesis, and free radical function in neutrophils, IDA can be associated with abnormal neurotransmitter function and altered immunologic and inflammatory defenses. Iron deficiency usually is the result of a long period of negative iron balance. Manifestations of iron deficiency occur in three stages. In the initial stage, iron stores are reduced without reduced serum iron levels and can be assessed with serum ferritin measurement. In this first stage, iron stores can be depleted without causing anemia. The stores allow iron to be utilized when there is an increased need for Hb synthesis. Once stores are depleted, there still is adequate iron from daily RBC turnover for Hb synthesis. Further iron losses would make the patient vulnerable to anemia development. In the second stage, iron deficiency occurs when iron stores are depleted, and Hb is above the lower limit of normal for the population but may be reduced for a given patient. This can be determined by serial CBC measurements. Findings include reduced transferrin saturation and increased TIBC. The third stage is IDA and occurs when the Hb falls to less than normal values.

Laboratory Findings

❸ Abnormal laboratory findings for patients with IDA generally include low serum iron and ferritin levels and high TIBC. The first apparent sign of iron deficiency is the increased RDW, although the finding is not specific to IDA. In the early stages of IDA, RBC size is not changed. Low ferritin concentration is the earliest and most sensitive indicator of iron deficiency. However, ferritin may not correlate with iron stores in the bone marrow because renal or hepatic disease, malignancies, infection, or inflammatory processes may increase ferritin values.[10] Hb, Hct, and RBC indices usually remain normal.

In the later stages of IDA, Hb and Hct fall below normal values, and a microcytic hypochromic anemia develops. Microcytosis may precede hypochromia, as erythropoiesis is programmed to maintain normal Hb concentration in preference to cell size. As a result, even slightly abnormal Hb and Hct levels may indicate significant depletion of iron stores and should not be ignored. In terms of RBC indices, MCV is reduced earlier in IDA than Hb concentration.

Transferrin saturation (i.e., serum iron level divided by the TIBC) is useful for assessing IDA. Low values may indicate IDA, although low serum transferrin saturation values also may be present in inflammatory disorders. The TIBC may help to differentiate the diagnosis in these patients: TIBC >400 mcg/dL (71.6 mol/L) suggests IDA, whereas values <200 mcg/dL (35.8 mol/L) usually represent inflammatory disease. With continued progression of IDA, anisocytosis occurs and poikilocytosis develops, as seen on peripheral blood smear and indicated by increased RDW. In microcytic anemias due to all other causes, iron stores are detectable. Serum transferrin receptor can be used to diagnose iron-store depletion and defects in iron delivery to the marrow. An elevated serum transferrin receptor level would be expected in IDA and a normal level in ACD.

TREATMENT

Iron-Deficiency Anemia

The severity and cause of IDA determines the approach to treatment. Treatment is focused on replenishing iron stores. Because iron deficiency can be an early sign of other illnesses, treatment of the underlying disease may aid in the correction of iron deficiency.

■ DIETARY SUPPLEMENTATION AND ORAL IRON PREPARATIONS

Treatment of IDA usually consists of dietary supplementation and administration of oral iron preparations. Food high in iron are listed in Table 109–3. Iron is best absorbed from meat, fish, and poultry. These foods, as well as certain iron-fortified cereals can help with IDA. Orange juice and other ascorbic acid–rich foods can be included with meals to increase absorption. Milk and tea reduce absorption and should be consumed in moderation. In most cases of IDA, oral administration of iron therapy with soluble Fe^{2+} iron salts is appropriate.

CLINICAL CONTROVERSY

Daily ferrous sulfate is not tolerated by all patients and can be difficult to administer in populations of developing countries. Weekly rather than daily supplements have been used, with conflicting efficacy results. The weekly approach follows the natural pattern of mucosal cell turnover.

TABLE 109-3	Good Sources of Iron	
Food	**Serving Size**	**Amount (mg)**
Total cereal	1 cup	18
Grape-Nuts cereal	1 cup	18
Instant Cream of Wheat	1 cup	8.2
Instant plain oatmeal	1 cup	6.7
Wheat germ	1 oz	2.6
Broccoli	1 medium stalk	2.1
Baked potato	1 medium	2.7
Raw tofu	½ cup	4
Lentils	½ cup	3.3
Beef chuck	3 oz	3.2

TABLE 109-4	Oral Iron Products	
Salt	**Elemental Iron Percentage**	**Elemental Iron Provided**
Ferrous sulfate	20%	60–65 mg/324–325 mg tablet
		18 mg iron/5 mL syrup
		44 mg iron/5 mL elixir
		15 mg iron/0.6 mL drop
Ferrous sulfate (exsiccated)	30%	65 mg/200 mg tablet
		60 mg/187 mg tablet
		50 mg/160 mg tablet
Ferrous gluconate	12%	36 mg/325 mg tablet
		27 mg/240 mg tablet
Ferrous fumarate	33%	33 mg/100 mg tablet
		63–66 mg/200 mg tablet
		106 mg/324–325 mg tablet
		15 mg/0.6 mL drop
		33 mg/5 mL suspension
Polysaccharide iron complex	100%	150 mg capsule 50 mg tablet
		100 mg/5 mL elixir
Carbonyl iron	100%	50 mg caplet

Fe^{2+} sulfate, succinate, lactate, fumarate, glycine sulfate, glutamate, and gluconate are absorbed similarly. The addition of copper, cobalt, molybdenum, or other minerals or hematinics provides no advantage but adds expense. The carbonyl iron may be advantageous because of lower risk for death in cases of accidental overdose. Iron is best absorbed in the reduced Fe^{2+} form, with maximal absorption occurring in the duodenum, primarily due to the acidic medium of the stomach. Slow-release or sustained-release iron preparations do not undergo sufficient dissolution until they reach the small intestine. In the alkaline environment of the small intestine, iron tends to form insoluble complexes, which significantly reduces absorption. The dose of iron replacement therapy depends on the patient's ability to tolerate the administered iron. Tolerance of iron salts improves with a small initial dose and gradual escalation to the full dose. For patients with IDA, the general recommendation is administration of approximately 200 mg of elemental iron daily, usually in two or three divided doses to maximize tolerability. If patients cannot tolerate this daily dose of elemental iron, smaller amounts of elemental iron (e.g., single 325 mg tablet of Fe^{2+} sulfate) usually is sufficient to replace iron stores, although at a slower rate. Table 109–4 lists the percentage of elemental iron of commonly available iron salts. The percentage of iron absorbed decreases progressively as the dose increases, although the absolute amount absorbed increases. Iron preferably is administered at least 1 hour before meals because food interferes with iron absorption. Many patients must take iron with food because they experience gastrointestinal upset when iron is administered on an empty stomach.

Adverse reactions to therapeutic doses of iron are primarily gastrointestinal in nature and consist of dark discoloration of feces, constipation or diarrhea, nausea, and vomiting. Gastrointestinal side effects usually are dose related and are similar among iron salts when equivalent amounts of elemental iron are administered. Administration of smaller amounts of iron with each dose may minimize these adverse effects. Histamine-2 blockers or proton pump inhibitors reduce gastric acidity and may impair iron absorption. Table 109–5 lists drug interactions with iron. Failure to develop at least some mild gastrointestinal symptoms may suggest nonadherence. If these side effects become intolerable, the total daily dose can be decreased or the dose can be taken with meals.

Failure to respond to appropriate treatment regimens necessitates reevaluation of the patient's condition. Occasionally a "therapeutic trial of iron" approach will be used to confirm a presumptive

TABLE 109-5 Iron Salt–Drug Interactions

Drugs That Decrease Iron Absorption	Object Drugs Affected by Iron
Al-, Mg-, and Ca^{+2}-containing antacids	Levodopa ↓ (chelates with iron)
Tetracycline and doxycycline	Methyldopa ↓ (decreases efficacy of methyldopa)
Histamine$_2$ antagonists	Levothyroxine ↓ (decreased efficacy of levothyroxine)
Proton pump inhibitors	
Cholestyramine	Penicillamine ↓ (chelates with iron)
	Fluoroquinolones ↓ (forms ferric ionquinolone complex)
	Tetracycline and doxycycline ↓ (when administered within 2 hours of iron salt)
	Mycophenolate ↓ (decreases absorption)

diagnosis of IDA. Common causes of treatment failure include poor patient adherence, inability to absorb iron, incorrect diagnosis, continued bleeding, or a concurrent condition that impairs full reticulocyte response. Even when iron deficiency is present, response may be impaired when a coexisting cause for anemia exists. Rarely a patient has diminished ability to absorb iron, most often due to previous gastrectomy, such as gastric bypass surgery, or celiac disease. Malabsorption can be ruled out by the iron test, in which plasma iron levels are determined at half-hour intervals for 2 hours following the administration of 50 mg of elemental iron as liquid Fe^{2+} sulfate. If plasma iron levels increase by >50 mcg/dL (>9.0 mol/L) during this time, absorption is satisfactory. Regardless of the form of oral therapy used, treatment should continue for 3 to 6 months after the anemia is resolved to allow for repletion of iron stores and to prevent relapse. Patients should be instructed to store oral iron out of reach of children and pets as small amounts

can result in a fatal overdose. Products containing more than 30 mg of elemental iron are required to be packaged as individual dosage units to prevent toxicity. Treatment for acute iron poisoning is discussed in Chapter 14.

■ PARENTERAL IRON THERAPY

Indications for parenteral iron therapy include intolerance to oral, malabsorption, and long-term nonadherence. Patients with significant blood loss who refuse transfusions and can not take oral iron therapy also may require parenteral iron therapy. Parenteral iron therapy is also used for patients with chronic kidney disease (see Chap. 53), especially those undergoing hemodialysis, and for some cancer patients receiving chemotherapy on erythropoiesis stimulating agents (see Chap. 135). Four different parenteral iron preparations currently available in the United States are iron dextran, sodium ferric gluconate, iron sucrose, and ferumoxytol (Table 109–6). They differ in their molecular size, degradation kinetics, bioavailability, and side-effect profiles. Although toxicity profiles of these agents differ, clinical studies indicate that each is efficacious. Most of the recent research on intravenous iron has been performed in hemodialysis patients. Iron dextran parenteral preparations have been associated with death due to anaphylactic reactions. These reactions may be related to immune reactions to the iron–carbohydrate or iron–dextran complex. Another theory for the anaphylaxis is the high-molecular-weight dextran component, which may be antigenic even when not complexed to iron. The safety profile of parenteral iron is largely assessed by spontaneous reports to the Food and Drug Administration (FDA) and observational studies. All parenteral iron preparations carry a risk for anaphylactic reactions but likely to a lesser extent than iron dextran.[20,21] A concern with parenteral iron is that iron may be released

TABLE 109-6 Comparison of Parenteral Iron Preparations

	Ferumoxytol	Sodium Ferric Gluconate	Iron Dextran	Iron Sucrose
Amount of elemental iron	30mg/mL	62.5 mg iron/5 mL	50 mg iron/mL	20 mg iron/mL
Molecular weight	Feraheme: 75,000 Da	Ferrlecit: 289,000–444,000 Da	InFeD: 165,000 Da DexFerrum: 267,000 Da	Venofer: 34,000–60,000 Da
Composition	Superparamagnetic iron oxide that is coated with a carbohydrate shell	Ferric oxide hydrate bonded to sucrose chelates with gluconate in a molar rate of 2 iron molecules to 1 gluconate molecule	Complex of ferric hydroxide and dextran	Complex of polynuclear iron hydroxide in sucrose
Preservative	None	Benzyl alcohol 9 mg/5 mL 20% (975 mg in 62.5 mg iron)	None	None
Indication	Treatment of iron deficiency anemia for adult patients with chronic kidney disease (CKD)	Treatment of iron-deficiency anemia for patients undergoing chronic hemodialysis who are receiving supplemental erythropoietin therapy	Treatment of patients with documented iron deficiency in whom oral therapy is unsatisfactory or impossible	Treatment of iron-deficiency anemia for patients undergoing chronic hemodialysis who are receiving supplemental epoetin alfa therapy
Warning	No black-box warning: hypersensitivity reactions	No black-box warning: hypersensitivity reactions	Black-box warning: anaphylactic-type reactions	Black-box warning: anaphylactic-type reactions
IM injection	No	No	Yes	No
Usual dose	Initial 510 mg intravenous injection followed by a second 510 mg intravenous injection 3 to 8 days later (rate 30 mg/s)	125 mg (10 mL) diluted in 100 mL normal saline, infused over 60 minutes; also can be administered as a slow IV injection (rate of 12.5 mg/min).	100 mg undiluted at a rate not to exceed 50 mg (1 mL) per minute	100 mg into the dialysis line at a rate of 1 mL (20 mg of iron) undiluted solution per minute
Treatment	2 doses × 510 mg = 1,020 mg	8 doses × 125 mg = 1,000 mg	10 doses × 100 mg = 1,000 mg	Up to 10 doses × 100 mg = 1,000 mg
Common adverse effects	Diarrhea, constipation, nausea, dizziness, hypotension, peripheral edema,	Cramps, nausea and vomiting, flushing, hypotension, rash, pruritus	Pain and brown staining at injection site, flushing, hypotension, fever, chills, myalgia, anaphylaxis	Leg cramps, hypotension

too quickly and overload the ability of transferrin to bind it, leading to free iron reactions that can interfere with neutrophil function. In regards to general estimation of total dose of parenteral iron needed to correct anemia, the following formula can be used:

Dose of iron (mg) =
whole blood hemoglobin deficit (g/dl) × body weight (lb)

An additional quantity of iron to replenish stores should be added. This is approximately 600 mg for women and 1,000 mg for men.[10]

Iron dextran, a complex of Fe^{3+} hydroxide and the carbohydrate dextran, contains 50 mg of iron per milliliter and can be given via the intramuscular or intravenous route. Different brands of iron dextran are available and differ in their molecular weight. They are not interchangeable. Iron dextran must be processed by macrophages for the iron to be biologically available. The absorption and metabolism vary with the route and amount of drug given. The intramuscular route is no longer used routinely.[22] The intramuscular administration of iron dextran requires Z-tract injection technique to minimize staining of the skin and pain. This technique is used for delivering intramuscular injections of irritating substances to minimize tracking of the medication through surrounding tissues. If intramuscular doses are given, they should not exceed 25 mg for patients weighing less than 5 kg, 50 mg for patients weighing less than 10 kg, and 100 mg for all other patients. Problems with intramuscular administration include patient discomfort, unpredictable delivery, sterile abscesses, tissue necrosis, and atrophy.[23]

The iron dextran package insert carries a black-box warning regarding the risk of anaphylaxis. A test dose is required prior to administration of any dose. Fatal reactions have also occurred in patients who tolerated the test dose. Patients with a history of multiple drug allergies and those who are concomitantly taking angiotensin-converting enzyme inhibitors may be at higher risk. Patients should also be monitored throughout the complete administration of iron dextran and resuscitative equipment should be readily available. Methods of intravenous administration include multiple slow injections of undiluted iron dextran solution or an infusion of a diluted preparation. This latter method often is referred to as total dose infusion.

Equations for calculating the appropriate doses of parenteral iron dextran for patients with IDA or anemia secondary to blood loss are listed in Table 109–7. Doses given by intravenous administration should not exceed 50 mg of iron per minute (1 mL/min). It is suggested that all patients considered for an iron dextran injection receive a test dose of 25 mg intramuscularly or intravenously or a 5- to 10-minute infusion of the diluted solution. Patients then should be observed for more than 1 hour for untoward reactions. An anaphylaxis-like reaction generally responds to intravenous

TABLE 109-7	Equations for Calculating Doses of Parenteral Iron Dextran

For patients with iron deficiency anemia:
Adults + children >15 kg
    Dose (mL) = 0.0442 (Desired Hb − Observed Hb) × LBW + (0.26 × LBW)
LBW males = 50 kg + 2.3 × (inches over 5 ft)
LBW females = 45.5 kg + 2.3 × (inches over 5 ft)
Children 5–15 kg
    Dose (mL) = 0.0442(Desired Hb − Observed Hb) × W + (0.26 × W)
For patients with anemia secondary to blood loss (hemorrhagic diathesis or long-term dialysis):
    mg of iron = blood loss × hematocrit,
where blood loss is in milliliters and hematocrit is expressed as a decimal fraction.

Hb, hemoglobin; LBW, lean body weight; mL, milliliter; W, weight.

epinephrine, diphenhydramine, and corticosteroids. If the test dose is tolerated, patients receiving total dose infusions can undergo infusion of the remaining solution during the next 2 to 6 hours.[23]

Total replacement doses of intravenous iron dextran have been given as a single dose. A test dose still is required. The ability to give a total dose infusion is a benefit of iron dextran over the other parenteral iron products.[17] Iron dextran is best utilized when smaller frequent doses of sodium ferric gluconate or iron sucrose are impractical. Patients who receive total dose infusions are at higher risk for adverse reactions, such as arthralgias, myalgias, flushing, malaise, and fever. Other adverse reactions of iron dextran include staining of the skin, pain at the injection site, allergic reactions, and rarely anaphylaxis. Patients with preexisting immune-mediated diseases, such as active rheumatoid arthritis or systemic lupus erythematosus, are considered at high risk for adverse reactions because of their hyperreactive immune response capabilities.

Sodium ferric gluconate is a complex of iron bound to one gluconate and four sucrose molecules in a repeating pattern. Its molecular weight is 289 kDa to 440 kDa. Sodium ferric gluconate is available in an aqueous solution. No direct transfer of iron from the Fe^{3+} gluconate to transferrin occurs. The complex is taken up quickly by the mononuclear phagocytic system and has a half-life of approximately 1 hour in the bloodstream. Sodium ferric gluconate appears to produce fewer anaphylactic reactions than iron dextran does. Side effects of sodium ferric gluconate include cramps, nausea, vomiting, flushing, hypotension, intense upper gastric pain, rash, and pruritus.[24]

Iron sucrose is a polynuclear iron (III) hydroxide in sucrose complex with a molecular weight of approximately 34 kDa to 60 kDa. It is available in 5 mL single-dose vials. Each vial contains 100 mg (20 mg/mL) of iron sucrose. Following intravenous administration of iron sucrose, the iron is released directly from the circulating iron sucrose to transferrin and is taken up by the mononuclear phagocytic system and metabolized. The half-life is approximately 6 hours, with a volume of distribution similar to that of iron dextran. Iron sucrose injection should not be administered concomitantly with oral iron preparations because it will reduce the absorption of oral iron.[25] Adverse effects include leg cramps and hypotension. Overall, iron sucrose has been shown to be safe and efficacious.

A fourth parenteral iron product, ferumoxytol, was approved in the United States in June 2009. Ferumoxytol is FDA approved to treat iron deficiency in adults with chronic kidney disease who are on or off diaylsis. The drug enters the macrophages in the liver, spleen, and bone marrow. The iron is then released and enters the storage pool as ferritin or is transported by transferrin for incorporation into Hb. Ferumoxytol can be administered at a quicker rate than other parenteral iron products with a rate up to 30 mg/s. Typical dosing is 510 mg intravenous dose followed by a second 510 mg dose 3 to 8 days later. The dose can be readministered after 1 month if anemia persists. No test dose is required but anaphylaxis can occur and patients should be observed for at least 30 minutes after each dose. Compared with oral iron replacement therapy, ferumoxytol has a higher incidence of hypotension and dizziness but less diarrhea, nausea, constipation, and peripheral edema. The clinical significance of this new preparation is yet to be determined as it just started being marketed.[26]

■ TRANSFUSIONS

Another treatment for IDA is blood transfusion. The decision to manage anemia with blood transfusions is based on the evaluation of risks and benefits. Transfusion of allogeneic blood is indicated in acute situations of blood loss when hemodynamic support is needed. Transfusions may also be necessary for patients with cardiac instability or when blood loss cannot be immediately alleviated.

Blood transfusion in chronic anemia can elevate Hb concentration in the short term but does not address the underlying disorder.

Evaluation of Therapeutic Outcomes

A positive response to a trial of oral iron therapy results in a modest reticulocytosis in a few days, with an increase in Hb around 2 weeks with continued rapid rise in Hb. As the Hb level approaches normal, the rate of increase slows progressively. A Hb response of <2 g/dL (<20 g/L; <1.24 mmol/L) over a 3-week period warrants further evaluation. Hb should reach a normal level after 2 months of therapy and often sooner.[10] If the patient does not develop reticulocytosis, reevaluation of the diagnosis or iron replacement therapy is necessary.

Iron therapy should continue for a period sufficient for complete restoration of iron stores. Serum ferritin concentrations should return to the normal range prior to discontinuation of iron. The time interval required to accomplish this goal varies, although at least 6 to 12 months of therapy usually is warranted. Patients with negative iron balances caused by bleeding may require iron replacement therapy for only 1 month after correction of the underlying lesion, whereas patients with recurrent negative balances may require long-term treatment with as little as 30 to 60 mg of elemental iron daily.

When large amounts of parenteral iron are administered, by either total dose infusion or multiple intramuscular or intravenous doses, the patient's iron status should be closely monitored. Patients receiving regular intravenous iron should be monitored for clinical or laboratory evidence of iron toxicity or overload. Iron overload may be indicated by abnormal hepatic function tests, serum ferritin >800 ng/mL (>800 g/L), or transferrin saturation >50%. Serum ferritin and transferrin saturation should be measured in the first week after doses of 100 to 200 mg and 2 weeks after larger intravenous iron doses. Hb and Hct should be measured weekly, and serum iron and ferritin levels should be measured at least monthly. Serum iron values can be obtained reliably 48 hours after intravenous dosing.

MEGALOBLASTIC ANEMIAS

Macrocytic anemias are divided into megaloblastic and nonmegaloblastic anemias. Macrocytosis, as seen in megaloblastic anemias, is caused by abnormal DNA metabolism resulting from vitamin B_{12} or folate deficiency. It also can be caused by administration of various drugs, such as hydroxyurea, zidovudine, cytarabine, methotrexate, azathioprine, 6-mercaptopurine, and cladribine. In vitamin B_{12}– or folate-deficiency anemia, megaloblastosis results from interference with folic acid– and vitamin B_{12}–interdependent nucleic acid synthesis in the immature erythrocyte. The rate of RNA and cytoplasm production exceeds the rate of DNA production. The maturation process is retarded, resulting in immature large RBCs (macrocytosis). RNA and DNA synthesis depend on a series of reactions catalyzed by vitamin B_{12} and folic acid because of their role in the conversion of uridine to thymidine. As shown in Fig. 109–5, dietary folates are absorbed in this process and converted to 5-methyltetrahydrofolate (A), which then is converted via a B_{12}-dependent reaction (B) to tetrahydrofolate (C). After gaining a carbon, tetrahydrofolate is converted to 5,10-methyl-tetrahydrofolate (D), a folate cofactor used by thymidylate synthetase (E) in the biosynthesis of nucleic acids. The 5,10-methyl-tetrahydrofolate cofactor is converted to dihydrofolate (F) during biosynthesis. Dihydrofolate reductase normally reduces dihydrofolate back to tetrahydrofolate (C), which can again pick up a carbon and be recycled to produce more 5,10-methyl-tetrahydrofolate (D).

Although vitamin B_{12} and folate deficiency are common causes of macrocytosis, other possible causes must be considered if these deficiencies are not found. Other causes of macrocytosis include

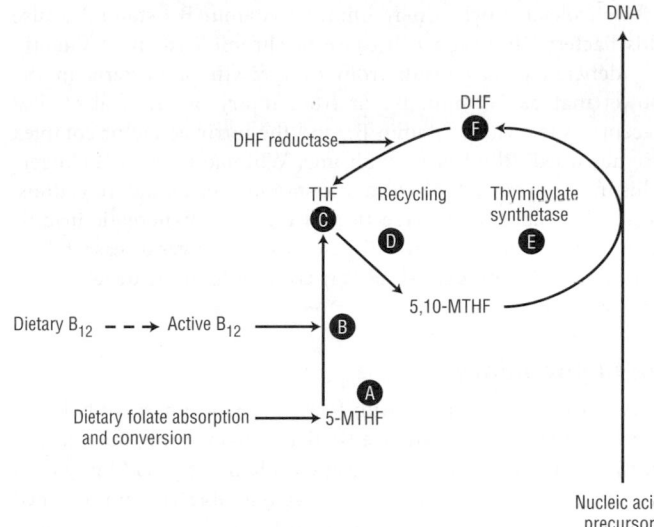

FIGURE 109-5. Drug-induced megaloblastosis (DHF, dihydrofolate; 5-MTHF, 5-methyl-tetrahydrofolate; 5,10-MTHF, 5,10-methyl-tetrahydrofolate THF; THF, tetrahydrofolate).

(1) a shift to immature or stressed RBCs as seen in reticulocytosis, aplastic anemia, and pure RBC aplasia; (2) a primary bone marrow disorder such as myelodysplastic syndromes, congenital dyserythropoietic anemias, and large granular lymphocyte leukemia; (3) lipid abnormalities as seen with liver disease, hypothyroidism, or hyperlipidemia; and (4) unknown mechanisms resulting from alcohol abuse and multiple myeloma. Macrocytosis is the most typical morphologic abnormality associated with excessive alcohol consumption. Even with adequate folate and vitamin B_{12} levels and the absence of liver disease, patients with high alcohol intake may present with an alcohol-induced macrocytosis. Cessation of alcohol ingestion results in resolution of the macrocytosis within a couple of months.

VITAMIN B_{12} DEFICIENCY ANEMIA

The prevalence of vitamin B_{12} deficiency causing anemia in the United States is unknown. Risk increases with age.[27] Increased use of gastric acid–suppressing agents, which may inhibit the release of cobalamin from food, is also associated with an increased risk. Older adults in the United States have a high prevalence (up to 15%) of elevated MMA levels and associated low or low–normal vitamin B_{12} levels, likely due to atrophic gastritis and malabsorption of food-bound vitamin B_{12}.[27]

Etiology

❹ The three major causes of vitamin B_{12} deficiency are inadequate intake, malabsorption syndromes, and inadequate utilization. Inadequate dietary consumption of vitamin B_{12} is rare. It usually occurs only in patients who are strict vegans and their breast-fed infants, chronic alcoholics, and elderly patients who consume a "tea and toast" diet because of financial limitations or poor dentition. Decreased vitamin B_{12} absorption is seen in patients with pernicious anemia, which is caused by the absence of intrinsic factor due to autoimmune destruction of the gastric parietal cells, atrophy of the gastric mucosa, or stomach surgery. One of the most frequent causes of low serum B_{12} levels is malabsorption, which results from the inability of vitamin B_{12} to be cleaved and released from proteins in food because of inadequate gastric acid production. In these individuals, supplemental cobalamin is well absorbed because it is not protein bound. Treatment of Helicobacter pylori may improve vitamin B$_{12}$ status because this bacterial infection is a cause of chronic gastritis.[28] Vitamin B$_{12}$ deficiency may result from overgrowth of bacteria in the bowel that use vitamin B$_{12}$ or from injury or removal of ileal receptor sites where vitamin B$_{12}$ and the intrinsic factor complex are absorbed. Blind loop syndrome, Whipple disease, Zollinger-Ellison syndrome, tapeworm infestations, intestinal resections, tropical sprue, surgical resection of the ileus, pancreatic insufficiency, inflammatory bowel disease, advanced liver disease, tuberculosis, and Crohn disease all may contribute to the development of vitamin B$_{12}$ deficiency.[27]

Pathophysiology

Vitamin B$_{12}$ works closely with folate in the synthesis of building blocks for DNA and RNA, is essential in maintaining the integrity of the neurologic system, and plays a role in fatty acid biosynthesis and energy production. It is a water-soluble vitamin obtained exogenously by ingestion of meat, fish, poultry, dairy products, and fortified cereals. The body stores several years of vitamin B$_{12}$, of which approximately one half is in the liver. The recommended daily allowance is 2 mcg in adults and 2.6 mcg in pregnant or breast-feeding women. The average western diet provides 5 to 15 mcg of vitamin B$_{12}$ daily, of which 1 to 5 mcg is absorbed.[27] Vitamin B$_{12}$ deficiency takes several years to develop following vitamin deprivation because of efficient enterohepatic circulation and stores of the vitamin.

Once dietary cobalamin enters the stomach, pepsin and hydrochloric acid release the cobalamin from animal proteins. The free cobalamin then binds to R-protein, which is released from parietal and salivary cells. In the duodenum, the cobalamin–R-protein is degraded, releasing free cobalamin. The cobalamin then binds with intrinsic factor that serves as a cell-directed carrier protein similar to transferrin for iron. This complex attaches to mucosal cell receptors in the distal ileum, the intrinsic factor is discarded, and the cobalamin is bound to transport proteins (transcobalamin I, II, and III). The cobalamin bound to transcobalamin II is secreted into the circulation and is taken up by the liver, bone marrow, and other cells. Most circulating cobalamin is bound to transcobalamin I and transcobalamin III. An alternate pathway for vitamin B$_{12}$ absorption independent of intrinsic factor or an intact terminal ileum accounts for a small amount of vitamin B$_{12}$ absorption.[27] This alternate pathway involves passive diffusion and accounts for approximately 1% absorption of the ingested vitamin B$_{12}$.

Vitamin B$_{12}$ deficiency can also cause neurologic complications. These usually start with bilateral paraesthesia in extremities; deficits in proprioception and vibration can also be present. If not treated, this can progress to ataxia, dementia-like symptoms, and psychotic symptoms. In children prolonged deficiency can lead to poor brain development.[14,29] Patients with unexplained neuropathies should be evaluated for vitamin B$_{12}$ deficiency.

Laboratory Findings

In macrocytic anemias, MCV usually is elevated >100 fL, but some patients deficient in vitamin B$_{12}$ may have a normal MCV. If there is a coexisting cause of microcytosis, the MCV may not be elevated.[29] Mild leukopenia and thrombocytopenia are often present because abnormal DNA synthesis can affect all blood cells. A peripheral blood smear demonstrates macrocytosis accompanied by hypersegmented polymorphonuclear leukocytes (one of the earliest and most specific indications of this disease), oval macrocytes, anisocytosis, and poikilocytosis. Serum lactate dehydrogenase and indirect bilirubin levels may be elevated as a result of hemolysis or ineffective erythropoiesis.[14] Other laboratory findings include a

low reticulocyte count, low serum vitamin B$_{12}$ level [<150 pg/mL <111 pmol/L], and low Hct.

In the early stages of vitamin B$_{12}$ deficiency, classic signs and symptoms of megaloblastic anemia may not be evident, and serum levels of vitamin B$_{12}$ may be within normal limits. Therefore, measurement of MMA and homocysteine may be useful because these parameters are often the first to change. Because MMA and homocysteine are involved in enzymatic reactions that depend on vitamin B$_{12}$, a deficiency in vitamin B$_{12}$ leads to accumulation of serum MMA and homocysteine. Elevations in MMA are more specific for vitamin B$_{12}$ deficiency. Homocysteine is also elevated in several other situations including: folate deficiency, chronic renal disease, alcoholism, smoking, use of steroid or cyclosporine therapy, and smoking.[29] Low levels of vitamin B$_{12}$ result in hyperhomocysteinemia, which some studies have reported to be an independent risk factor for cerebrovascular, peripheral vascular, coronary, and venous thromboembolic disease.[30]

Blood levels of vitamin B$_{12}$ should be drawn for all patients with suspected vitamin B$_{12}$ deficiency. Vitamin B$_{12}$ values <150 pg/mL (<111 pmol/L) for patients with macrocytosis, hypersegmented polymorphonuclear leukocytes, peripheral neuropathy, or dementia are suggestive of B$_{12}$ deficiency. Approximately one third of patients with pernicious anemia do not demonstrate macrocytosis if their condition is complicated by iron deficiency, thalassemia. Some patients with a clinical B$_{12}$ deficiency with neurological involvement may have normal hematological parameters.

A Schilling test may be performed to diagnose pernicious anemia, but the usefulness of this test is questionable and rarely alters the clinical management of the vitamin B$_{12}$ deficiency. The Schilling test was once performed to determine whether replacement of vitamin B$_{12}$ should occur via an oral or parenteral route, but evidence now shows that oral replacement is as efficacious as parenteral supplementation because of the vitamin B$_{12}$ absorption pathway independent of intrinsic factor.[27,31]

Other potentially useful tests include antibody testing and serum gastrin levels. Positive antiintrinsic factor antibodies may be present in approximately half of patients with pernicious anemia but is highly specific for the disease.[13] In addition, an estimated 85% of patients have antiparietal cell antibodies, but this test is not specific because 3% to 10% of healthy patients have these antibodies.[13] When evaluating low serum vitamin B$_{12}$ levels, other causes besides dietary deprivation and malabsorption should be ruled out. For example, levels may be falsely low for patients receiving antibiotics, anticonvulsants, cytotoxic agents, oral contraceptives, and high-dose vitamin C.

TREATMENT

Vitamin B$_{12}$ Deficiency Anemia

The goals of treatment for vitamin B$_{12}$ deficiency include reversal of hematologic manifestations, replacement of body stores, and prevention or resolution of neurologic manifestations. Early treatment is of paramount importance because neurologic damage may be irreversible if the deficiency is not detected and corrected within months. In addition to replacement therapy, any underlying etiology that is treatable, such as bacterial overgrowth, should be remedied. Indications for starting oral or parenteral therapy include megaloblastic anemia or other hematologic abnormalities and neurologic disease from deficiency.[29] Those with borderline low levels of B$_{12}$ but no hematologic abnormalities should be followed at yearly intervals.[29] Patients should be counseled on

TABLE 109-8	Good Sources of Vitamin B_{12}	
Food	**Serving Size**	**Amount (mcg)**
Beef liver, cooked	3 oz	60
Breakfast cereal, fortified (100%)	¾ cup	6
Rainbow trout, cooked	3 oz	5.3
Sockeye salmon, cooked	3 oz	4.9
Beef, cooked	3 oz	2.1
Breakfast cereal, fortified (25%)	¾ cup	1.5
Haddock, cooked	3 oz	1.2
Clams, breaded and fried	¾ cup	1.1
Oysters, breaded and fried	6 pieces	1
Tuna, canned in water	3 oz	0.9
Milk	1 cup	0.9
Yogurt	8 oz	0.9

the types of foods high in vitamin B_{12} content such as fortified cereals as seen in Table 109–8. Orally administered vitamin B_{12} can be used effectively to treat pernicious anemia because of the aforementioned alternate pathway of passive absorption, independent of intrinsic factor.[14] Daily oral doses (1–2 mg) of vitamin B_{12} is as effective as intramuscular administration in achieving hematologic and neurologic responses.[27,31] If vitamin B_{12} levels are marginally low and either MMA or both MMA and homocysteine levels are elevated, administration of 1 mg of oral vitamin B_{12} daily should be strongly considered.[32] Timed-release preparations of oral cobalamin should be avoided.[33] Nonprescription 1 mg cobalamin tablets are available, among several other strengths. A commonly used initial parenteral vitamin B_{12} regimen consists of daily injections of 1,000 mcg of cyanocobalamin for 1 week to saturate vitamin B_{12} stores in the body and resolve clinical manifestations of the deficiency. Thereafter, it can be given weekly for 1 month and monthly thereafter for maintenance. Hydroxocobalamin is a less popular formulation of parenteral vitamin B_{12}. Its low utilization rate may be due to the occasional development of antibodies to the hydroxocobalamin–transcobalamin II complex. Parenteral therapy is preferred for patients exhibiting neurologic symptoms until resolution of symptoms and hematologic indices because the most rapid-acting therapy is necessary.[34] When patients are converted from the parenteral to the oral form of cobalamin, 1 mg of oral cobalamin daily can be initiated on the due date of the next injection.

In addition to the oral and parenteral forms, vitamin B_{12} is available as a nasal spray for patients in remission following intramuscular vitamin B_{12} therapy who have no nervous system involvement. The nasal spray is administered once weekly. Intranasal administration should be avoided for patients with nasal diseases or those receiving medications intranasally in the same nostril. Patients should not administer the spray 1 hour before or after ingestion of hot foods or beverages, which can impair cobalamin absorption. The efficacy of the nasal spray formulation has not been well studied, and it should be used for maintenance therapy only after hematologic parameters have normalized.

Potential adverse effects with vitamin B_{12} replacement therapy are rare. Uncommon side effects include hyperuricemia and hypokalemia due to marked increase in potassium utilization during production of new hematopoietic cells. Rebound thrombocytosis may precipitate thrombotic events. Another side effect of vitamin B_{12} therapy is fluid retention, which is more likely to occur for patients with compromised cardiovascular status because of an expansion in intravascular volume secondary to the sudden increase in production of RBCs. Rare cases of anaphylaxis with parenteral administration of cobalamin have been reported.

Evaluation of Therapeutic Outcomes

Most patients respond rapidly to vitamin B_{12} therapy. The typical patient will experience an improvement in strength and well-being within a few days. Bone marrow begins to become normoblastic in 2 to 3 days. Reticulocytosis is evident in 3 to 5 days. Hb begins to rise after the first week and should normalize in 1 to 2 months. CBC count and serum cobalamin levels usually are drawn 1 to 2 months after initiation of therapy and 3 to 6 months thereafter for surveillance monitoring. Homocysteine and MMA levels should be repeated 2 to 3 months after initiation of replacement therapy to evaluate for normalization of levels, although levels begin to decrease in 1 to 2 weeks. Neuropsychiatric signs and symptoms can be reversible if treated early. If permanent neurologic damage has resulted, progression should cease with replacement therapy. Slow response to therapy or failure to observe normalization of laboratory results may suggest the presence of an additional abnormality such as iron deficiency, thalassemia trait, infection, malignancy, nonadherence, or misdiagnosis.

FOLIC ACID DEFICIENCY ANEMIA

Epidemiology

Folic acid deficiency is one of the most common vitamin deficiencies occurring in the United States, largely because of its association with excessive alcohol intake and pregnancy.

Etiology

❺ Major causes of folic acid deficiency include inadequate intake, decreased absorption, and increased folate requirements. Poor eating habits make this deficiency more common for elderly patients, teenagers whose diets consist of "junk food," alcoholics, food faddists, the impoverished, and those who are chronically ill or demented. Folic acid absorption may decrease for patients who have malabsorption syndromes or those who have received certain drugs. In alcoholics with poor dietary habits, alcohol interferes with folic acid absorption, interferes with folic acid utilization at the cellular level, and decreases hepatic stores of folic acid.

Increased folate requirements may occur when the rate of cellular division is increased, as seen in pregnant women; patients with hemolytic anemia, myelofibrosis, malignancy, chronic inflammatory disorders such as Crohn disease, rheumatoid arthritis, or psoriasis; patients undergoing long-term dialysis; burn patients; and for adolescents and infants during their growth spurts. This hyperutilization eventually can lead to anemia, particularly when the daily intake of folate is borderline, resulting in inadequate replacement of folate stores.

Several drugs have been reported to cause a folic acid deficiency megaloblastic anemia. Some drugs (e.g., azathioprine, 6-mercaptopurine, 5-fluorouracil, hydroxyurea, and zidovudine) directly inhibit DNA synthesis. Other drugs are folate antagonists; the most toxic is methotrexate (other examples include pentamidine, trimethoprim, and triamterene). A number of drugs (e.g., phenytoin, phenobarbital, and primidone) antagonize folate via poorly understood mechanisms but are thought to reduce vitamin absorption by the intestine (see Chap. 112). Since folic acid doses as low as 1 mg/day may affect serum phenytoin levels, routine folic acid supplementation is not generally recommended. The decline in phenytoin concentration usually occurs within the first 10 days and may decrease phenytoin levels by 15% to 50%.[35]

Pathophysiology

Folic acid is a water-soluble vitamin readily destroyed by cooking or processing. It is necessary for the production of nucleic acids, proteins, amino acids, purines, and thymine and hence DNA and RNA. It acts as a methyl donor to form methylcobalamin, which is used in the remethylation of homocysteine to methionine. Because humans are unable to synthesize sufficient folate to meet total daily requirements, they depend on dietary sources. Major dietary sources of folate include fresh, green leafy vegetables, citrus fruits, yeast, mushrooms, dairy products, and animal organs such as liver and kidney. Most folate in food is present in the polyglutamate form, which must be broken down into the monoglutamate form prior to absorption in the small intestine. Once absorbed, dietary folate must be converted to the active form tetrahydrofolate through a cobalamin-dependent reaction. In 1997, the U.S. government mandated the fortification of grain products with folic acid in an attempt to increase the dietary intake of folate by 100 mcg of folate daily per person. This amount of supplementation was chosen to decrease the incidence of neural tube defects without masking occult vitamin B_{12} deficiency.

As a result of grain product fortification, neural tube defect frequency has decreased by 25% to 30%.[36] Although body demands for folate are high because of high rates of RBC synthesis and turnover, the minimum daily requirement is 50 to 100 mcg. In the general population, the recommended daily allowance for folate is 400 mcg in nonpregnant females, 600 mcg for pregnant females, and 500 mcg for lactating females.[36] Because the body stores approximately 5 to 10 mg of folate, primarily in the liver, cessation of dietary folate intake can result in megaloblastosis within 3 to 4 months. Folate is distributed to the other tissues primarily via enterohepatic recirculation. The methylated form of folate is reabsorbed from the bile into the serum. As folate enters the tissues, including erythrocytes, it endures for the remaining life span of the cell.

Laboratory Findings

It is of paramount importance to rule out vitamin B_{12} deficiency when folate deficiency is suspected. Laboratory changes associated with folate deficiency are similar to those seen in vitamin B_{12} deficiency, except vitamin B_{12} levels are normal. Serum folate levels decrease to less than 3 ng/mL (7 nmol/L) within a few days of reduced dietary folate intake. The RBC folate level (<150 ng/mL [<340 nmol/L]) also declines, and levels remain constant throughout the life span of the erythrocyte. An estimated 60% of patients with pernicious anemia have low RBC folate levels, probably because of the cobalamin requirement for normal transfer of methyl-tetrahydrofolate from plasma to cells.[13] If serum or erythrocyte folate levels are borderline, serum homocysteine usually is increased with a folic acid deficiency. If serum MMA levels also are elevated, vitamin B_{12} deficiency must be ruled out given that folate does not participate in MMA metabolism.

TREATMENT

Folic Acid Deficiency Anemia

Therapy for folic acid deficiency consists of administration of exogenous folic acid to induce hematologic remission, replace body stores, and resolve signs and symptoms. In most cases, 1 mg daily is sufficient to replace stores, except in cases of deficiency due to malabsorption, in which case doses of 1 to 5 mg daily may be necessary. Parenteral folic acid is available but rarely necessary. Synthetic folic acid is almost completely absorbed by the gastrointestinal tract and is converted to tetrahydrofolate without cobalamin. Therapy should continue for approximately 4 months if the underlying cause of the deficiency can be identified and corrected to allow for clearance of all folate-deficient RBCs from the circulation. Foods high in folic

TABLE 109-9	Good Sources of Folate	
Food	**Serving**	**Amount (mcg)**
Chicken liver	3.5 oz	770
Cereal	½ to 1½ cups	100–400
Lentils, cooked	½ cup	180
Chickpeas	½ cup	141
Asparagus	½ cup	132
Spinach, cooked	½ cup	131
Black beans	½ cup	128
Pasta	2 oz	100–120
Kidney beans	½ cup	115
Lima beans	½ cup	78
White rice, cooked	¾ cup	60
Tomato juice	1 cup	48
Brussels sprouts	½ cup	47
Orange	1 medium	47

acid should also be encouraged in the diet as seen in Table 109–9. Long-term folate administration may be necessary in chronic conditions associated with increased folate requirements. Low-dose folate therapy (500 mcg daily) can be administered when anticonvulsant drugs produce a megaloblastic anemia so that discontinuation of anticonvulsant therapy may not be necessary. Adverse effects have not been reported with folic acid doses used for replacement therapy. It is considered nontoxic at high doses and is rapidly excreted in the urine.

Although megaloblastic anemia during pregnancy is rare, the most common cause is folate deficiency. The condition usually manifests as an underweight premature infant and suboptimal health of the mother. Periconceptional folic acid supplementation is recommended to decrease the occurrence and recurrence of neural tube defects, specifically anencephaly and spinal bifida. Folic acid supplementation at a dose of 400 mcg daily is recommended for all women. Women who have previously given birth to offspring with neural tube defects or those with a family history of neural tube defects should ingest 4 mg daily of folic acid.[35,36,37] Higher levels of folic acid supplementation should not be attained via ingestion of excess multivitamins because of the risk for vitamin A toxicity.[37] Prenatal vitamins usually have a higher amount of folic acid as compared with general multivitamins to ensure adequate supplementation is attained. It is essential that women in their childbearing years maintain adequate folic acid intake.

Evaluation of Therapeutic Outcomes

Symptomatic improvement, as evidenced by increased alertness and appetite, often occur early during the course of treatment. Reticulocytosis begins in the first week. Hct begins to rise within 2 weeks and should reach normal levels within 2 months. MCV initially increases because of an increase in reticulocytes but gradually decreases to normal.

ANEMIA OF CHRONIC DISEASE

Epidemiology

6 ACD is one of the most common forms of anemia seen clinically, particularly among the elderly. It is especially important in the differential diagnosis of iron deficiency. ACD is associated with common disease states that may mimic the symptoms of anemia, which causes the diagnosis of ACD to sometimes be overlooked.

Etiology

The diagnosis of ACD usually is one of exclusion. It is important to exclude IDA as the true or competing etiology. Various

| TABLE 109-10 | Diseases Causing Anemia of Chronic Disease |

Common causes
Chronic infections
  Tuberculosis
  Other chronic lung infections (e.g., lung abscess, bronchiectasis)
  Human immunodeficiency virus
  Subacute bacterial endocarditis
  Osteomyelitis
  Chronic urinary tract infections
Chronic inflammation
  Rheumatoid arthritis
  Systemic lupus erythematosus
  Inflammatory bowel disease
  Inflammatory osteoarthritis
  Gout
  Other (collagen vascular) diseases
  Chronic inflammatory liver diseases
Malignancies
  Carcinoma
  Lymphoma
  Leukemia
  Multiple myeloma
Less common causes
Alcoholic liver disease
Congestive heart failure
Thrombophlebitis
Chronic obstructive pulmonary disease
Ischemic heart disease

| TABLE 109-11 | Laboratory Value Differences Between Anemia of Chronic Disease and Iron-Deficiency Anemia |

	Anemia of Chronic Disease	Iron-Deficiency Anemia	Both
Iron	↓	↓	↓
Transferrin	↓ or nl	↓	↓
Transferrin saturation	↓	↓	↓
Ferritin	↑ or nl	↓	↓ or nl
Soluble transferrin receptor	nl	↑	↑ or nl

nl, normal limits.

conditions associated with ACD may predispose patients to blood loss [malignancy, gastrointestinal blood loss from treatments with aspirin, nonsteroidal antiinflammatory drugs (NSAIDs), or corticosteroids]. ACD is often observed for patients with diseases that last longer than one to two months, although it can occur in conditions with a more rapid onset of several weeks, such as pneumonia. ACD tends to be a mild (Hb >9.5 g/dL [>95 g/L; >5.90 mmol/L]) or moderate (Hb >8 g/dL [80 g/L; >4.97 mmol/L]) anemia.[38] Anemia associated with human immunodeficiency virus (HIV), autoimmune conditions, cancer, and heart failure are common forms of ACD. A 1 g/dL (10 g/L; 0.62 mmol/L) decrease in Hb was independently associated with significantly increased mortality risk in several studies of the heart failure population.[39] The degree of anemia in ACD is generally associated with the severity of underlying disease. Table 109–10 lists common diseases associated with ACD.

ACD commonly develops in AIDS patients, especially those with opportunistic infections or malnutrition, and is associated with increased morbidity and mortality. For patients with HIV, anemia is a predictor of progression to AIDS and is independently associated with an increased risk of death.[40] The etiology of anemia for patients with HIV is complex. HIV infects hematopoietic cells, which can lead to abnormal hematopoiesis and bone marrow suppression. In addition, the drugs used to treat AIDS and associated illness can cause bone marrow suppression.

Pathophysiology

ACD is a response to stimulation of the cellular immune system by various underlying disease processes. ACD is a hypoproliferative anemia that traditionally has been associated with infectious or inflammatory processes, tissue injury, and conditions associated with release of proinflammatory cytokines. Alternative names include anemia of inflammation and cytokine-mediated anemia. The pathogenesis of ACD is multifactorial and is characterized by a blunted EPO response to anemia, an impaired proliferation of erythroid progenitor cells, and a disturbance of iron homeostasis.

Increased iron uptake and retention occur within cells of the mononuclear phagocytic system. The RBCs have a shortened life span, and the bone marrow's capacity to respond to EPO is inadequate to maintain normal Hb concentration. The cause of this defect is uncertain but appears to involve blocked release of iron from cells in the bone marrow. Iron availability to erythroid progenitor cells then is limited. Various cytokines, such as interleukin-1, interferon-γ, and tumor necrosis factor released during illness may inhibit the production or action of EPO or the production of RBCs.[38] Hepcidin may decrease duodenal absorption of iron and block release of iron from macrophages.[38]

Laboratory Findings

No definitive test can confirm the diagnosis of ACD. The practitioner should maintain a high index of suspicion for any patient with a chronic inflammatory or neoplastic disease. ACD may coexist with IDA and folic acid deficiency because many patients with these conditions have poor dietary intake or gastrointestinal blood loss. Examination of the bone marrow reveals an abundance of iron, suggesting that the release mechanism for iron is the central defect. Patients with ACD usually have a decreased serum iron level, but unlike patients with IDA, their serum ferritin level is normal or increased and their TIBC is decreased. Transferrin saturation is typically decreased. ACD usually is normocytic and normochromic with mildly depressed Hb. With ACD, hypochromia usually precedes microcytosis, with the opposite finding in IDA. Patients with concurrent ACD and IDA usually have microcytes and a more severe anemia. Table 109–11 shows lab values seen in ACD and IDA. Erythrocyte survival may be reduced for patients with ACD, but a compensatory erythropoietic response usually does not occur. A low reticulocyte count indicates underproduction of red cells.[38]

TREATMENT

Anemia of Chronic Disease

Treatment of ACD depends on the underlying etiology. Guidelines exist for management of anemia for patients with cancer or chronic kidney disease (see Chaps. 53 and 135). Although the goals of therapy should include treating the underlying disorder and correcting reversible causes of anemia, accomplishment of these goals may not totally reverse hematologic and physiologic abnormalities. Iron is effective only if iron deficiency is present. During inflammation, oral or parenteral iron therapy is not as effective. Absorption is impaired because of downregulation of ferroportin and iron diversion mediated by cytokines.[38] Because iron is a required nutrient for proliferating microorganisms, supplementation may theoretically increase the risk of infections. Iron therapy should be reserved for those patients with an absolute iron deficiency.[38]

RBC transfusions are effective but should be limited to situations in which oxygen transport is inadequate due to concomitant medical problems. Transfusions are typically considered for those with severe anemia (Hb <8 g/dL [<80 g/L; <4.97 mmol/L]) but can be considered for those between 8 to 10 g/dL (80 to 100 g/L; 4.97 to 6.21 g/L) based on factors such as cost, convenience, and risk of complications. Risks may include transmission of bloodborne infections, development of autoantibodies, transfusion reactions, and iron overload. Transfusion is of doubtful benefit for patients with Hb >8 g/dL (>80 g/L; >4.97 mmol/L) if they are not symptomatic with anemia.

Erythropoiesis-stimulating agents (ESAs) have been used to stimulate erythropoiesis for patients with ACD since a relative EPO deficiency exists for the degree of anemia. Two agents are available: recombinant epoetin alfa and recombinant darbepoetin alfa. Although both agents share the same mechanism of action, darbepoetin alfa has a longer half-life and can be administered less frequently. Although these agents are sometimes used to treat ACD, this is currently not an FDA-approved indication. Patients with chronic disease may have a relatively impaired response to ESAs. The initial dosage of epoetin alfa and darbepoetin alfa are typically 50 to 100 units per kilogram three times per week and 0.45 mcg per kilogram once weekly, respectively. These doses are typical starting doses for those with chronic kidney disease. Response to ESAs varies depending on dose and cause of the anemia. ESA treatment is effective when the marrow has an adequate supply of iron, cobalamin, and folic acid. Whether EPO levels are a useful predictor of response is controversial.

Iron deficiency can occur in patients treated with ESAs; so close monitoring of iron levels is necessary. Some patients develop "functional" iron deficiency, in which the iron stores are normal but the supply of iron to the erythroid marrow is less than necessary to support the demand for RBC production. Therefore, many practitioners routinely supplement ESA therapy with oral iron therapy. Potential toxicities of exogenous ESA administration include increases in blood pressure, nausea, headache, fever, bone pain, and fatigue. Less common adverse effects include seizures, thrombotic events, and allergic reactions such as rashes and local reactions at the injection site. If ESAs are used the practitioner must monitor to ensure the patient's Hb does not exceed 12 g/dL (120 g/L; 7.45 mmol/L) with treatment or that Hb does not rise >1 g/dL (>10 g/L; >0.62 mmol/L) every 2 weeks since both of these events have been associated with increased mortality and cardiovascular events.[41] Tumor progression with these agents can also occur and is discussed in Chap. 135. Further discussion of dosing guidelines and potential adverse outcomes of ESA treatment in populations for which treatment is FDA approved are discussed in Chaps. 53 and 135.

Evaluation of Therapeutic Outcomes

One of the earliest responses to increased endogenous or exogenous EPO is an increase in blood reticulocyte count, which usually occurs in the first few days. Baseline iron status should be checked before and during treatment, as many patients receiving ESAs require supplemental iron therapy. The optimal form and schedule of iron supplementation are not known. Hb levels should be monitored twice a week until stabilized. Hb should also be monitored twice weekly for 2 to 6 weeks after a dose adjustment.[41] A fall in Hb during ESA therapy may indicate a need for iron supplementation or signal occult blood loss. Baseline and periodic monitoring of iron, TIBC, transferrin saturation, or ferritin levels may be useful in optimizing iron repletion and limiting the need for ESAs. Patients who do not respond to 8 weeks of optimal dosage should not continue taking ESAs. Target Hb levels should be 11 to 12 g/dL (110 to 120 g/L; 6.83 to 7.45 mmol/L). Cost is an issue with ESA therapy; therefore, drug expense must be weighed against the effects on transfusions and hospitalizations.

ANEMIA OF CRITICAL ILLNESS

Epidemiology

❼ Anemia is a common complication in critically ill patients and is found almost universally in this patient population.[42] Approximately 95% of patients have less than normal Hb levels by their third day in the intensive care unit (ICU).[43]

Etiology

Factors that may contribute to anemia in critically ill patients include sepsis, taking of frequent blood samples, hemodilution, surgical blood loss, immune-mediated functional iron deficiency, decreased production of endogenous EPO, reduced RBC life span, and active bleeding, especially in the gastrointestinal tract. More commonly, a combination of these factors exists. Additional comorbid factors include coagulopathies and nutritional deficits such as malnourishment and altered absorption of vitamins and minerals, including iron, vitamin B$_{12}$, and folate.[44] Deleterious effects of anemia include an increased risk of cardiac-related morbidity and mortality, especially for patients with known cardiovascular disease. Persistent tissue hypoxia can result in cerebral ischemia, myocardial ischemia, multiple organ deterioration, lactic acidosis, and death. Consequences of anemia in critically ill patients may be enhanced because of the increased metabolic demands of critical illness. Weaning anemic patients from mechanical ventilation may be more difficult.[45]

Pathophysiology

In anemia of critical illness, the mechanism for RBC replenishment and homeostasis is altered. The effect of various inflammatory cytokines on EPO may partly explain anemia of critical illness because inflammatory cytokines are associated with a blunted erythropoietic response.[46] Inflammatory cytokines appear to directly inhibit RBC production and stimulate synthesis of iron-binding proteins that sequester iron and limit RBC production.[46]

Laboratory Findings

The pattern of laboratory findings in anemia of critical illness is similar to that of ACD. Laboratory findings frequently seen in anemia of critical illness are low serum iron, TIBC, and iron/TIBC ratio. Transferrin saturation usually is less than 20% in anemia of critical illness due to functional iron deficiency. Serum ferritin is normal to high, as seen with ACD, and EPO levels usually are slightly decreased despite the presence of anemia, with minimal reticulocyte response.[42,46] These findings differ from those for patients with IDA, who generally have elevated EPO concentrations in response to a low Hct.

TREATMENT

Anemia of Critical Illness

Patients with anemia of critical illness require the necessary substrates of iron, folic acid, and vitamin B$_{12}$ for RBC production. Parenteral iron is generally preferred in this population because patients often are undergoing enteral therapy or because of concerns regarding inadequate iron absorption. The disadvantage of parenteral therapy is the theoretical risk of infection.

Pharmacologic doses of ESAs have been used to treat the anemia of critical illness. Few randomized controlled trials have evaluated the role of ESAs in critically ill patients, and the results of these trials have not consistently shown a decrease in transfusion requirements in ESA-treated patients.[46] Further investigation is necessary to determine the effectiveness and the cost effectiveness of ESAs in critically ill patients.[43]

Many critically ill patients receive RBC transfusions despite the inherent risks associated with transfusions. Stored RBCs may not function as well as endogenous blood. Although RBC transfusions may increase oxygen delivery to tissues, cellular oxygen may not increase.[47] Transfusion practices in ICUs vary, and clinicians use different Hb concentrations as thresholds for administering transfusions. Study results suggest that RBC transfusions may decrease the likelihood of survival in some subgroups of critically ill patients.[48] Decisions to use transfusions must consider the risks, including transmission of infections; volume overload, especially for patients with renal or heart failure; iron overload; and immune-mediated reactions such as febrile reactions, hemolysis, and anaphylaxis. The clinician also must consider administrative, logistic, and economic factors, including the shortage of blood supplies.

Evaluation of Therapeutic Outcomes

Goals of therapy include maintenance of adequate tissue oxygenation and perfusion and immediate correction of severe anemia. The role of monitoring RBCs, Hb, Hct, EPO levels, and reticulocyte counts remains to be determined. Outcomes used in ESA studies are transfusion requirements and transfusion independence. Morbidity, mortality, and length of stay also should be assessed. Iron lab studies should be monitored to ensure that adequate amounts of iron are present to support an optimal erythropoietic response to ESAs.

ANEMIA IN THE ELDERLY

Epidemiology

❽ One of the most common clinical problems observed in the elderly is anemia. Anemia is a prevalent and increasing problem in the elderly, with approximately 20% of people 85 years and older affected.[49] Elderly patients with the highest incidence of anemia are those who are hospitalized, followed by residents of nursing homes and institutions, with an estimated rate of 31% to 40%.[50] The lowest incidence is seen in elderly patients who are community dwellers. Although the incidence of anemia is high in the elderly, anemia should not be regarded as an inevitable outcome of aging. The body's set point of hemoglobin does not fall with age. An underlying cause can be identified in approximately two thirds of older patients. Undiagnosed and untreated anemia has been associated with adverse outcomes, including all-cause hospitalization, hospitalization secondary to cardiovascular disease, and all-cause mortality.[51] Anemia is an independent predictor of death and major clinical adverse events in elderly patients with stable symptomatic coronary artery disease.[52] Anemia can exacerbate neurologic and cognitive conditions and can adversely influence quality of life and physical performance in the elderly.[53] Anemia may be an indication of serious diseases such as gastrointestinal cancer.

Pathophysiology

Aging is associated with a progressive reduction in hematopoietic reserve, which makes individuals more susceptible to developing anemia in times of hematopoietic stress.[54] Dysregulation of proinflammatory cytokines, most notably interleukin-6, may inhibit EPO production or interact with EPO receptors.[55] Although Hb levels may remain normal, the diminished marrow reserve leaves the elderly patient more susceptible to other causes of anemia. Renal insufficiency, which also is common in elderly patients, may reduce the ability of the kidneys to produce EPO. Older patients often have a normal creatinine level but a diminished glomerular filtration rate. Myelodysplastic syndromes are another common cause of anemia in the elderly, but most anemia cases in the elderly are multifactorial.

Etiology

In the acute care setting, the top three causes of anemia in the elderly are chronic disease (35%), unexplained cause (17%), and iron deficiency (15%), whereas in community-based outpatient clinics, the most common causes are unexplained (36%), infection (23%), and chronic disease (17%).[56] Risk factors for the development of anemia in the elderly include race and ethnicity. The highest prevalence is seen for elderly blacks, those with serum albumin and serum creatinine abnormalities, and patients with recent hospitalization or placement in an institution.[50]

Anemia in the elderly usually is typically hypoproliferative and reflects an inability of the aging hematopoietic system to replace the peripheral blood loss or respond to marrow insults. Unexplained causes may be due to inadequate diagnostic evaluation or absolute or relative EPO deficiency. Absolute EPO deficiency may be associated with renal insufficiency, whereas relative deficiency may be due to the body's inability to provide adequate response to declining Hb levels.[56]

Another common problem in the elderly is vitamin B_{12} deficiency. The most common causes of clinically overt vitamin B_{12} deficiency are food/cobalamin malabsorption (more than 60% of cases) and pernicious anemia (15% to 20% of cases).[57]

One often-overlooked major factor that may contribute to anemia in the older population is nutritional status. Cognitive and functional impairments in the older population may create barriers for patients to obtain and prepare a nutritious diet. Nutritional deficiencies that are not severe enough to affect the hematopoietic system in the younger population may contribute to anemia in the elderly. Edentulous or infirm elderly who may be too ill to prepare their meals are at risk for nutritional folate deficiency. Risk factors for inadequate folate intake in the elderly include low energy intake, inadequate consumption of fortified cereals, and failure to take a vitamin/mineral supplement.[58] However, unlike cobalamin levels, folate levels often increase rather than decline with age. High folic acid intake can occur if the elderly patient regularly uses a supplement and consumes fortified cereals.[58,59]

Other common anemias in the elderly include IDA and ACD. Bleeding with resultant iron deficiency in the elderly may be due to carcinoma, ulcer, atrophic gastritis, drug-induced gastritis, postmenopausal vaginal bleeding, or bleeding hemorrhoids. Elderly women have a much lower incidence of IDA compared with younger, menstruating women. Until proven otherwise, iron deficiency in the elderly should be considered a sign of chronic blood loss. Steps should be taken to rule out bleeding, especially from the gastrointestinal or female reproductive tract. ACD is more common in the elderly, as diseases that contribute to ACD such as cancer, infection, and rheumatoid arthritis are more prevalent in this population.

Laboratory Findings

For practical purposes, it is best to use usual adult reference values and WHO criteria for laboratory tests in the elderly. Anemia in elderly persons usually is normocytic and mild, with Hb values ranging between 10 and 12 g/dL (100 to 120 g/L; 6.21 to 7.45 mmol/L) in most anemic patients.[49] Evaluation of an elderly patient should be similar to strategies described previously for younger adults, perhaps with more emphasis on identifying occult blood loss and vitamin B_{12} deficiency. Vitamin B_{12} deficiency may be present even when plasma levels of vitamin B_{12} are within the normal range, but elevated MMA levels will detect the deficiency. A refractory macrocytic anemia in the elderly should raise suspicion of a myelodysplastic syndrome.

TREATMENT

Anemia in the Elderly

Treatment of anemia in the elderly is the same as that described for each type of anemia discussed in this chapter. With IDA it is essential to treat the underlying cause, if known (i.e., bleeding), and administer iron supplementation. Lower doses of iron supplementation are often recommended in the elderly (e.g., 325 mg of ferrous sulfate once daily) to decrease the incidence of gastrointestinal adverse effects, which can lead to additional morbidity and poor adherence. The goal of treatment of ACD is resolution of the underlying cause, although curing the underlying chronic illness for elderly patients can be difficult. Routine treatment with ESAs is not currently standard of care for ACD in the elderly. The medical and economic implications of anemia correction remain to be defined for ACD or undefined anemia.

Evaluation of Therapeutic Outcomes

Responses and monitoring of treatment are similar in the elderly as described for the general adult population described earlier in the chapter. If the reticulocyte count rises but the anemia does not improve, inadequate absorption of iron or continued blood loss should be suspected. As with any form of anemia, symptomatic improvement should be evident shortly after starting therapy, and Hb/Hct should begin to rise within a few weeks of initiating therapy. A key component of symptom assessment among older adults is the functional domain. Patients should be asked about changes in self-care abilities, mobility, and stamina.

ANEMIA IN PEDIATRIC POPULATIONS

Epidemiology

❾ IDA is a leading cause of infant morbidity and mortality around the world.[60] Data from NHANES III indicated that 9% of children ages 12 to 36 months in the United States had iron deficiency and 3% had IDA.[61,62] Lack of a normal Hb at birth directly affects nonstorage iron and increases the risk of IDA in the first 3 to 6 months of life. African- or Hispanic-American children have a higher incidence of anemia.[63] Requirements for iron absorption peak during puberty. An anemia of prematurity can occur 3 to 12 weeks after birth in infants younger than 32 weeks' gestation and spontaneously resolves by 3 to 6 months. The prevalence of vitamin B_{12} deficiency has been identified as 1 in 1,255 for levels <100 pg/mL (<74 pmol/L)

and 1 in 200 for levels of <200 pg/mL (<148 pmol/L), with the lowest levels in non-Hispanic whites.[64]

Pathophysiology

In contrast to anemias in adults, which tend to be manifestations of a broader underlying pathology, anemias in the pediatric population are more often due to a primary hematologic abnormality. The amount of iron present at birth depends on gestational length and weight. Erythropoiesis normally decreases after birth. A concurrent decrease in EPO production results in a physiologic anemia at peaking at 2 months.[65] Iron stores are mostly depleted by age 6 months.

Etiology

The age of the child can yield some clues regarding the etiology of the anemia. The optimal amount of nutritional iron and folate required varies among individuals based on life-cycle stages. Two peak periods place children at risk of developing IDA. The first peak period occurs during late infancy and early childhood, when children undergo rapid body growth, have low levels of dietary iron, and exhaust stores accumulated during gestation. The second peak period occurs during adolescence, which is associated with rapid growth, poor diets, and onset of menses in girls. Some studies suggest that overweight children are at significantly higher risk for IDA. Proposed factors include genetic influences; physical inactivity, leading to decreased myoglobin breakdown and lower amounts of released iron into the blood; and inadequate diet with limited intake of iron-rich foods.[66]

Conditions in the newborn period that can lead to IDA include prematurity and insufficient dietary intake. Premature infants are at increased risk for IDA because of their smaller total blood volume, increased blood loss through phlebotomy, and poor gastrointestinal absorption. Blood loss and hemolysis are other common causes of anemia in neonates. Factors leading to unbalanced iron metabolism in infants include insufficient iron intake, decreased absorption, early introduction of cow's milk, intolerance of cow's milk, medications, and malabsorption. Dietary deficiency of iron in the first 6 to 12 months of life is less common today because of the increased use of iron supplementation during breast-feeding and use of iron-fortified formulas. Iron deficiency becomes more common when children change to regular diets.

When screening for iron deficiency in young children, a careful dietary history can help identify children at risk. High iron needs and the tendency to eat fewer iron-containing foods contribute to the etiology of iron deficiency during adolescence.

Other causes of microcytic anemia include thalassemia, lead poisoning, and sideroblastic anemia. Use of homeopathic or herbal medications and exposure to paint or certain cooking materials may place children at risk for lead exposure. Normocytic anemias in children include infection with human parvovirus B19 and glucose-6-phosphate dehydrogenase (G6PD) deficiency. Macrocytic anemias are caused by deficiencies in vitamin B_{12} and folate, chronic liver disease, hypothyroidism, and myelodysplastic disorders. Folic acid deficiency usually is due to inadequate dietary intake, but human milk and cow's milk provide adequate sources. Folic acid deficiency may be seen in infants and children who primarily consume goat's milk or health food milk alternatives, or in children with insufficient intake of green leafy vegetables. Vitamin B_{12} deficiency due to nutritional reasons is rare but may occur due to a congenital pernicious anemia.

Laboratory Findings

When evaluating laboratory values for pediatric patients, the clinician must use age- and sex-adjusted norms. It is important to know that many blood samples are capillary samples, such as heel or finger sticks, which may have slightly different results than venous samples. The USPSTF has concluded that evidence is insufficient to recommend for or against routine screening for IDA in asymptomatic, low risk, children aged 6 to 12 months. The Hb is a sensitive test for iron deficiency, but it has low specificity in childhood anemias. If an abnormality is found, a CBC should be ordered to evaluate MCV and determine whether the anemia is microcytic, normocytic, or macrocytic. A peripheral blood smear and reticulocyte count also may be helpful. The peripheral blood smear can indicate the etiology based on RBC morphology, and the reticulocyte count helps differentiate between decreased RBC production and increased RBC destruction or loss. Other laboratory tests include serum iron, ferritin, TIBC, and transferrin saturation. Mild hereditary anemias may produce a mild hypochromic microcytic anemia that can be confused with IDAs. The RDW may be high with iron deficiency and is more likely to be normal with thalassemia. Laboratory features of anemia of prematurity include normocytic normochromic cells, low reticulocyte count, low serum EPO concentrations, and decreased RBC precursors in bone marrow. Laboratory diagnosis of vitamin B_{12} and folate deficiency in children is similar to that of adults.

TREATMENT

Anemia in Pediatric Populations

Primary prevention of IDA in infants, children, and adolescents is the most appropriate goal because delays in mental and motor development are potentially irreversible. In 2006, the USPSTF published revised recommendations to screen and supplement iron deficiency in the United States, focusing on children and pregnant women.[19] The USPSTF recommends routine iron supplementation for asymptomatic children aged 6 to 12 months who are at increased risk for IDA. Fair evidence was found that iron supplementation (e.g., iron-fortified formula or iron supplements) might improve neurodevelopmental outcomes in children at risk for IDA. Evidence of benefit for children 6 to 12 months of age not at risk for IDA was poor.

Interventions likely to prevent anemia include diverse foods with bioavailable forms of iron, food fortification for infants and children, and individual supplementation. Routine screening for iron deficiency in nonpregnant adolescents is recommended only for those with risk factors, which include vegetarian diets, malnutrition, low body weight, chronic illness, or history of heavy menstrual blood loss.

Anemia of prematurity is frequently treated with RBC transfusions, with wide variations in transfusion practices among neonatal ICUs. Reasons for transfusions include improved oxygen delivery, intravascular volume, reduced fatigue during feeding, and improved growth. ESAs have been used to treat anemia of prematurity, but it is important to note that ESA pharmacokinetics differ depending on the developmental age of the infant. ESA use is controversial because it has not been shown to clearly reduce transfusion requirements. Other questions regarding safety and proper use of ESAs in anemia of prematurity remain unanswered.

For infants aged 9 to 12 months with a mild microcytic anemia, the most cost-effective treatment is a therapeutic trial of iron. Fe^{2+} sulfate at a dose of 3 mg/kg of elemental iron once or twice daily between meals for 4 weeks is recommended. In children who respond, iron should be continued for 2 more months to replace storage iron pools, along with dietary intervention and patient education.[67] Parenteral iron therapy has a limited role and is rarely necessary.

For the macrocytic anemias in children, folate can be administered in a dose of 1 to 3 mg daily. However, vitamin B_{12} deficiency due to congenital pernicious anemia requires lifelong vitamin B_{12}

supplementation. Dose and frequency should be titrated according to clinical response and laboratory values. No data regarding the use of oral vitamin B_{12} supplementation in children are available.

Evaluation of Therapeutic Outcomes

Therapeutic outcomes are assessed in children by monitoring Hb, Hct, and RBC indices 6 to 8 weeks after initiation of iron therapy. For premature infants, Hb or Hct should be monitored weekly.

HEMOLYTIC ANEMIA

Pathophysiology

10 Hemolytic anemia results from decreased survival time of RBCs secondary to destruction in the spleen or circulation. The severity of hemolytic anemia varies with the mechanism. Hemolysis may be mild, chronic, and compensated or acute, severe, and life threatening.

The normal 120-day life span of a RBC depends upon its inherent flexibility in passing through the microvasculature and spleen without disruption of the cell membrane or sequestration and phagocytosis by the mononuclear phagocytic system. Hemolysis, as defined by an RBC life span of less than 120 days, results from one of three primary defects that are intrinsic or extrinsic in origin: membrane defects, alterations in Hb solubility or stability, and changes in intracellular metabolic processes. Intrinsic defects are intracorpuscular changes and often are genetically determined. Extrinsic defects, or extracorpuscular changes, usually are the cause of acquired hemolytic anemia. Acquired disorders result mainly from a direct effect on the membrane and less often from alterations in Hb or metabolism. Table 109–12 lists examples of the different classes of hemolytic anemias.

Causes of hemolytic anemia in younger patients differ from causes in elderly patients. Most younger patients exhibit congenital disease, while older patients most often experience autoimmune hemolytic anemia. A positive Coombs test is diagnostic in the latter group.

Alterations in Hb solubility or stability, as seen with sickle cell anemia and the thalassemias, cause cell deformations leading to hemolysis (see Chap. 111).

Finally, alterations in cell metabolism (enzymopathies) lead to hemolytic disease by changing cell dimensions and Hb solubility.

The most common metabolic abnormality resulting in a hemolytic syndrome is G6PD deficiency in the hexose monophosphate shunt pathway described in Chap. 112. The disease more typically occurs in those of Mediterranean descent upon exposure to oxidant drugs (e.g., sulfamethoxazole and dapsone) and chemicals or with infection. Some drugs and ingested toxins (e.g., nitrofurantoin, cancer chemotherapy agents, phenazopyridine, sulfones, amyl nitrate, mothballs, paraquat, and hydrogen peroxide) can cause direct oxidative damage to erythrocytes (see Chap. 112).

TABLE 109-12 Common Classes of Hemolytic Anemias

Intrinsic (intracorpuscular; usually genetically inherited)
Membrane defect
Spherocytosis and elliptocytosis
Hemoglobin defect
Sickle cell anemia
Thalassemia syndrome
Metabolic defect
Glucose-6-phosphate dehydrogenase (G6PD) deficiency
Many other enzyme deficiencies
Extrinsic
Membrane defect
Autoimmune hemolytic anemias
Oxidants; may cause unstable hemoglobin to clump

Laboratory Findings

The appearance of RBCs varies greatly depending on the cause of the hemolytic anemia. An increased reticulocyte count is evidence of an attempt to maintain RBC mass. Depending on the disease, a peripheral blood smear may reveal sickle cells, target cells, spherocytes, elliptocytes, or fragmented RBCs. Decreased haptoglobin is seen, caused by increased Hb–haptoglobin complex formation. Lactate dehydrogenase level often is elevated secondary to release from RBCs, but this enzyme is very nonspecific. Hemoglobinuria may result, and an increase in indirect bilirubin often occurs.

TREATMENT

Hemolytic Anemia

Therapy for hemolytic anemia consists of managing the underlying cause of the anemia. Patients with G6PD deficiency should avoid use of precipitating oxidant medications and chemicals. No specific therapy compensates for this enzyme deficiency. Steroids and other immunosuppressive agents have been used for management of autoimmune hemolytic anemias. A splenectomy is sometimes indicated in an attempt to reduce RBC destruction.

PHARMACOECONOMIC CONSIDERATIONS

Anemia has an independent impact on many clinical, functional, and economic indicators, and evidence suggests that treatment can improve patient outcomes. The implications of treating anemia are becoming increasingly recognized, especially for the elderly. The cost of the complications associated with anemia in the elderly is considerable because anemia has been associated with an increased risk of falls, dementia, depression, and general functional disability that increases the demand for long-term care services.[68] However, the causal link between anemia and the costs of these conditions is not well established. Studies show that treatment of anemia in elderly patients with renal failure and heart failure is beneficial.[69] More research is needed to assess the costs and benefits of anemia therapies in other conditions, especially when treatment of mild anemia is considered.[69]

Although the direct medical costs of anemia are unknown, the direct costs of drug treatment must be weighed against the indirect costs associated with anemia.[70] The costs of laboratory tests used to diagnose anemia, the role of screening for anemia, and the prevention of anemia are components that must be considered in the pharmacoeconomic analysis. Additionally, the frequency of blood transfusions must be considered because it impacts cost and therapeutic decision making for patients. Blood products are a scarce resource that also must be factored into decision making.

For IDA, intravenous iron is costly but may have superior bioavailability compared with oral preparations. In some individuals, the bioavailability advantage of parenteral iron over oral iron can be the difference in achieving a successful outcome. The benefits of using combination oral iron products designed to enhance absorption probably are not warranted.

With regard to vitamin B_{12} deficiency, the cost of oral cyanocobalamin tablets and intramuscular injections is inexpensive. However, the parenteral route has significant additional costs, including the cost of a physician or nurse's visit for the injection or the cost of a home health visit. Additionally, many elderly patients may have difficulties attending extra clinic appointments because of transportation difficulties. A 90-day supply of nonprescription 1 mg oral tablets can be purchased for a few dollars. The disadvantage of the nasal spray is its higher cost compared with the oral or parenteral route.

For ACD, ESA cost needs to be taken into consideration along with safety as it is expensive. The cost of intravenous iron is low compared with the cost of ESAs. Because most patients with ACD are not symptomatic, they may feel no improvement with therapy. Symptom severity should be considered in the decision to use ESAs. Transfusion use for treatment of ACD as an alternative to ESAs must consider cost, convenience, and risk of complications.

Formal economic evaluation of treatment approaches for anemia of critical illness is generally lacking. Future studies may need to assess the cost per unit of RBC saved, which differs among institutions. Other pharmacoeconomic factors for consideration include morbidity and mortality of transfusion reactions, related infections, potential for medical errors, and availability of RBCs as a resource. Length of ICU stay, total hospital stay, length of time on mechanical ventilation, and mortality are other key factors.

ABBREVIATIONS

ACD: anemia of chronic disease

AIDS: acquired immunodeficiency syndrome

AIP: acute intermittent porphyria

CBC: complete blood count

CDC: Centers for Disease Control and Prevention

EPO: erythropoietin

ESA: erythropoiesis-stimulating agent

FDA: Food and Drug Administration

Fe^{2+}: ferrous iron

Fe^{3+}: ferric iron

G6PD: glucose-6-phosphate dehydrogenase

Hb: hemoglobin

Hct: hematocrit

HIV: human immunodeficiency virus

ICU: intensive care unit

IDA: iron-deficiency anemia

MCH: mean corpuscular hemoglobin

MCHC: mean corpuscular hemoglobin concentration

MCV: mean corpuscular volume

MMA: methylmalonic acid

NHANES: National Health and Nutrition Examination Survey

RBC: red blood cell

RDW: red blood cell distribution width

TIBC: total iron-binding capacity

USPSTF: U.S. Preventive Services Task Force

WHO: World Health Organization

REFERENCES

1. Benoist B, McLean E, Egli M, et al. Worldwide prevalence of anaemia 1993–2005: WHO global database on anaemia. World Health Organization; 2008.
2. Cusick SE, Mei Z, Freedman DS, et al. Unexplained decline in the prevalence of anemia among US children and women between 1988–1994 and 1999–2002. Am J Clin Nutr 2008;88:1611–1617.

3. Nissenson A. Anemia not just an innocent bystander. Arch Intern Med 2003;163:1400–1404.

4. Mozaffarian D. Anemia predicts mortality in severe heart failure: The prospective randomized amlodipine survival evaluation (PRAISE). J Am Coll Cardiol 2003;41:1933–1939.

5. Chaves PHM, Carlson MC, et al. Association between mild anemia and executive function impairment in community-dwelling older women: The Women's Health and Aging Study II. J Am Geriatr Soc 2006;54:1429–1435.

6. Anemia in pregnancy. ACOG Practice Bulletin No.95. American College of Obst and Gynecologists. Obstet Gynecol 2008;112:201–207.

7. Prchal JT. Production of erythrocytes. In: Lichtman MA, Beutler E, Kipps TJ, et al, eds. Williams Hematology, 7th ed. New York: McGraw-Hill; 2006:393–403.

8. Benz EJ. Disorders of hemoglobin. In: Fauci AS, Braunwald E, Kasper DL, et al, eds. Harrison's Principles of Internal Medicine, 17th ed. New York:. McGraw-Hill;2008:635–643.

9. Wians FH, Urban JE, Keffer JH, Kroft SH. Discriminating between iron deficiency anemia and anemia of chronic disease using traditional indices of iron status vs. transferrin receptor concentration. Am J Clin Pathol 2001;115:112–118.

10. Beutler E. Disorders of iron metabolism. In: Lichtman MA, Beutler E, Kipps TJ, et al, eds. Williams Hematology, 7th ed. New York: McGraw-Hill; 2006:511–553.

11. Beutler E. Destruction of erythrocytes. In: Lichtman MA, Beutler E, Kipps TJ, et al, eds. Williams Hematology, 7th ed. New York: McGraw-Hill; 2006:405–410.

12. Galloway M, Rushworth L. Red cell or serum folate? Results from the National Pathology Alliance benchmarking review. J Clin Pathol 2003;56:924–926.

13. Snow CF. Laboratory diagnosis of vitamin B_{12} and folate deficiency. Arch Intern Med 1999;159:1289–1298.

14. Babior B. Folate, cobalamin, and megaloblastic anemias. In: Lichtman MA, Beutler E, Kipps TJ, et al, eds. Williams Hematology, 7th ed. New York: McGraw-Hill; 2006:477–509.

15. Dharmarajan TS, Norkus EP. Approaches to vitamin B_{12} deficiency. Early treatment may prevent devastating complications. Postgrad Med 2001;110:99–105.

16. Ganz T. Hepcidin—A regulator of intestinal iron absorption and iron recycling by macrophages. Best Pract Res Clin Haematol 2005;18:171–182.

17. Killip S, Bennett J, Chambers M. Iron deficiency anemia. Am Fam Physician 2007;75:671–678.

18. Hershko C, Ianculovich M, Souroujon M. A hematologist's view of unexplained iron deficiency anemia in males: Impact of Helicobacter pylori eradication. Blood Cells Mol Dis 2007;38:45–53.

19. U.S. Preventive Services Task Force (USPSTF). Screening for Iron Deficiency Anemia—Including Iron Supplementation for Children and Pregnant Women. Rockville, MD: Agency for Healthcare Research and Quality (AHRQ); 2006.

20. Faich G, Strobos J. Sodium Fe^{3+} gluconate complex in sucrose: Safer IV iron therapy than iron dextrans. Am J Kidney Dis 1999;33:464–470.

21. Chandler G, Harchowal J, Macdougall IC. Intravenous iron sucrose: Establishing a safe dose. Am J Kidney Dis 2001;38:988–991.

22. Silverstein SB, Gilreath JA, Rodgers GM. Intravenous iron therapy: a summary of treatment options and review of guidelines. J Pharm Practice 2008;21:431–443.

23. InFeD [package insert]. Morristown, NJ: Watson Pharma;2009.

24. Ferrlecit [package insert] Morristown, NJ: Watson Pharma;2006.

25. Venofer [package insert] Shirley, NY: American Regent;2008.

26. Feraheme [package insert] Lexington, MA: AMAG Pharmaceuticals; 2009.

27. Oh RC, Brown DL. Vitamin B_{12} deficiency. Am Fam Physician 2003; 67:979–986, 993–994.

28. Kaptan K, Beyan C, Ural AU, et al. Helicobacter pylori—Is it a novel causative agent in vitamin B_{12} deficiency? Arch Intern Med 2000;160:1349–1353.

29. Hoffbrand AV. Megaloblastic anemias. In: Fauci AS, Braunwald E, Kasper DL, et al, eds. Harrison's Principles of Internal Medicine, 17th ed. New York: McGraw-Hill;2008:643–651.

30. Aronow WS. Homocysteine. The association with atherosclerotic vascular disease in older persons. Geriatrics 2003;58:22–28.

31. Vidal-Alaball J, Butler CC, Cannings-John R, et al. Oral vitamin B_{12} versus intramuscular vitamin B_{12} for vitamin B_{12} deficiency. Cochrane Database Syst Rev 2005;3:CD004655.

32. Cravens DD, Nashelsky J, Oh RC. How do we evaluate a marginally low B_{12} level? J Fam Pract 2007;56:62–63.

33. Solomon LR. Oral vitamin B_{12} therapy: A cautionary note. Blood 2004;103:2863.

34. Lane LA, Rojas-Fernandez. Treatment of vitamin B_{12}-deficiency anemia: Oral versus parenteral therapy. Ann Pharmacother 2002;36:1268–1272.

35. Yerby MS. Clinical care of pregnant women with epilepsy: Neural tube defects and folic acid supplementation. Epilepsia 2003;44(suppl 3):33–40.

36. Pitkin RM. Folate and neural tube defects. Am J Clin Nutr 2007;85:285S–288S.

37. American College of Obstetricians and Gynecologists (ACOG). Neural Tube Defects. ACOG Practice Bulletin No. 44. Washington, DC: American College of Obstetricians and Gynecologists; 2003.

38. Weiss GW, Goodnough LT. Anemia of chronic disease. N Engl J Med 2005;352:1011–1023.

39. Tang Y, Katz S. Anemia in Chronic Heart Failure. Circulation 2006;113:2454–2461.

40. Belperio PS, Rhew DC. Prevalence and outcomes of anemia in individuals with human immunodeficiency virus: A systemic review of the literature. Am J Med 2004;116:27S–43S.

41. Procrit [package insert]. Thousand Oaks, CA: Amgen;2009.

42. Corwin HL, Gettinger A, Pearl RG, et al. The CRIT Study: Anemia and blood transfusion in the critically ill—Current clinical practice in the United States. Crit Care Med 2004;32:39–52.

43. Stubbs JR. Alternatives to blood product transfusion in the critically ill: Erythropoietin. Crit Care Med 2006;34(suppl.):S160–S169.

44. Rodriguez RM, Corwin HL, Gettinger A, et al. Nutritional deficiencies and blunted erythropoietin response as cause of anemia of critical illness. J Crit Care 2001;16:36.

45. Silver MR. Anemia in the long-term ventilator-dependent patient with respiratory failure. Chest 2005;128(suppl):568S–575S.

46. Rudis M, Jacobi J, Hassan E, et al. Managing anemia in the critically ill patient. Pharmacotherapy 2004;24:229–247.

47. Hébert PC, Wells G, Martin C, et al. Do blood transfusions improve outcomes related to mechanical ventilation? Chest 2001;119:1850–1857.

48. Vincent JL, Piagnerelli M. Transfusion in the intensive care unit. Cit Care Med 2006;34(suppl.):S96–S101.

49. Guralnik JM, Eisenstaedt RS, Ferrucci L, et al. Prevalence of anemia in person 65 years and older in the United States: Evidence for a high rate of unexplained anemia. Blood 2004;104:2263–2268.

50. Carmel R. Anemia and aging: An overview of clinical, diagnostic, and biological issues. Blood Rev 2001;15:9–18.

51. Culleton BF, Manns BJ, Zhang J, et al. Impact of anemia on hospitalization and mortality in older adults. Blood 2006;107:3841–3846.

52. Muzzarelli S, Pfisterer M, TIME Investigators. Anemia as independent predictor of major events in elderly patients with chronic angina. Am Heart J 2006;152:991–996.

53. Woodman R, Ferrucci L, Guralnik J. Anemia in older adults. Curr Opin Hematol 2005;12:123–128.

54. Balducci L, Hardy CL, Lyman GH. Hematopoietic growth factors in the older cancer patient. Curr Opin Hematol 2001;8:170–187.

55. Eisenstaedt R, Penninx BW, Woodman RC. Anemia in the elderly: Current understanding and emerging concepts. Blood Rev 2006;20:213–226.

56. Balducci L. Epidemiology of anemia in the elderly: Information on diagnostic evaluation. J Am Geriatr Soc 2003;51(suppl):S2–S9.

57. Andres E, Loukili N, Noel E, et al. Vitamin B_{12} (cobalamin) deficiency in elderly patients. CMAJ 2004;171:251–259.

58. Mulligan JE, Greene GW, Caldwell M. Sources of folate and serum folate levels in older adults. J Am Diet Assoc 2007;107:495–499.

59. Ford ES, Bowman BA. Serum and red blood cell folate concentrations, race, and education: Findings from the third National Health and Nutrition Examination Survey. Am J Clin Nutr 1999;69:476–481.

60. Milman N. Iron prophylaxis in pregnancy—General or individual and in which dose? Ann Hematol 2006;85:821–828.

61. Recommendations to prevent and control iron deficiency in the United States. Morb Mortal Wkly Rep 1998;47:1–36.

62. Moy RJ. Prevalence, consequences and prevention of childhood nutritional iron. Clin Lab Haematol 2006;28:291–298.

63. Coyer S. Anemia: Diagnosis and management. J Pediatr Health Care 2005;19:380–385.

64. Wright JD, Bialostosky K, Gunter EW, et al. Blood folate and vitamin B_{12}: United States, 1988–94. Vital Health Stat 1998;11:1–78.

65. Segel GB, Palis J. Hematology of the newborn. In: Lichtman MA, Beutler E, Kipps TJ, et al, eds. Williams Hematology, 7th ed. New York: McGraw-Hill; 2006: 81–99.

66. Nead KG, Halterman JS, Kaczorowski JM, et al. Overweight children and adolescents: A risk group for iron deficiency. Pediatrics 2004;114:104–108.

67. Kazal LA. Prevention of iron deficiency in infants and toddlers. Am Fam Physician 2002;66:1217–1224.

68. Robinson B. Cost of anemia in the elderly. J Am Geriatr Soc 2003;51(suppl):S14–S17.

69. Cogswell M, Kettel-Khan L, Ramakrishnan V. Iron supplement use among women in the United States: Science, policy and practice. J Nutr 2003;133(suppl):1974S–1977S.

70. Tice JA, Ross E, Coxson PG, et al. Cost-effectiveness of vitamin therapy to lower plasma homocysteine levels for the prevention of coronary heart disease. JAMA 2001;286:936–943.

110

Coagulation Disorders

BETSY BICKERT POON, CHAR WITMER, AND JANE PRUEMER

KEY CONCEPTS

❶ Hemophilia is an inherited bleeding disorder resulting from a congenital deficiency in factor VIII or IX.

❷ The goal of therapy for hemophilia is to prevent bleeding episodes and their long-term complications and to arrest bleeding when it occurs.

❸ Recombinant factor concentrates are usually first-line treatment of hemophilia because they have the lowest risk of infection.

❹ The goal of therapy for von Willebrand disease is to increase von Willebrand factor and factor VIII levels to prevent bleeding during surgery or arrest bleeding when it occurs.

❺ Factor VIII concentrates that contain von Willebrand factor are the agents of choice for treatment of type 3 von Willebrand disease and some type 2 von Willebrand disease, and for serious bleeding in type 1 von Willebrand disease.

❻ Desmopressin acetate is often effective for treatment of type 1 von Willebrand disease. It may also be effective for treatment of some forms of type 2 von Willebrand disease.

❼ The optimal approach for patients with disseminated intravascular coagulation remains to be determined. The goal of treatment is to diagnose and treat the underlying cause.

❽ Prophylactic use of phytonadione can effectively prevent vitamin K–dependent bleeding in newborns.

A series of complex procoagulant and anticoagulant actions and reactions regulate hemostasis. Maintenance of hemostasis involves the interplay of four major components: (a) the vessel wall, (b) platelets, (c) the coagulation system, and (d) the fibrinolytic system. Coagulation disorders result from an imbalance in the regulation of these components. Bleeding disorders are the result of a decreased number of platelets, decreased function of platelets, coagulation factor deficiency, or enhanced fibrinolytic activity.

The traditional view of the coagulation cascade consists of intrinsic (propagation), extrinsic, and common pathways where coagulation proteins directed and controlled coagulation. This consisted of a sequential activation of clotting factors as shown in Figure 110–1. Although the historical model in Figure 110–1 shows the basic dependency of the various coagulation factors, it does not reflect the interactions with platelets and the endothelium. Thus it has been replaced by the cell-based model that more accurately describes these interactions (Fig. 110–2). This is known as the *tissue factor pathway* because it recognizes the central role of tissue factor in coagulation.

REGULATION OF HEMOSTASIS

COAGULATION FACTORS

Twelve plasma proteins are considered coagulation factors (Table 110–1). The coagulation factors can be divided into three groups on the basis of biochemical properties: vitamin K–dependent factors (II, VII, IX, and X), contact activation factors (XI and XII, prekallikrein, high-molecular-weight kininogen), and thrombin-sensitive factors (V, VIII, XIII, and fibrinogen).

Coagulation factors circulate as inactive precursors (zymogens). Coagulation of blood entails a cascading series of proteolytic reactions. At each step, a clotting factor undergoes limited proteolysis and becomes an active protease (designated by a lowercase "a," as in Xa). These coagulation factors play key roles in the coagulation pathway.

VESSEL WALL AND PLATELETS

Two distinct pathways are involved in platelet activation: the collagen pathway and the tissue factor pathway. Activated platelets play a central role in primary hemostasis. Damage to a vessel wall initiates vasoconstriction and the exposure of collagen and tissue factor to blood. Exposed collagen triggers platelet recruitment and activation.[1] Tissue factor initiates coagulation via the tissue factor pathway, which leads to the generation of thrombin and activates platelets.

Primary hemostasis occurs in response to vascular injury and includes local vascular smooth muscle contraction, platelet activation, platelet adhesion and aggregation, and elaboration of procoagulant activity.[2] Platelet glycoprotein VI interacts with collagen from exposed vessels, and platelet glycoprotein Ib-V-IX interacts with collagen-bound von Willebrand factor to cause adhesion of platelets at the site.[1] Glycoprotein VI stimulates platelets to release granular contents, such as adenosine diphosphate and thromboxane A_2, which lead to platelet aggregation.[1] A platelet plug is formed that occludes the blood vessel lesion. Activated coagulation factors are generated at the site of bleeding on the activated platelets to form fibrin and stabilize the platelet plug. Factor XIIIa cross-links the fibrin and stabilizes the fibrin clot.[1]

INTRINSIC PATHWAY

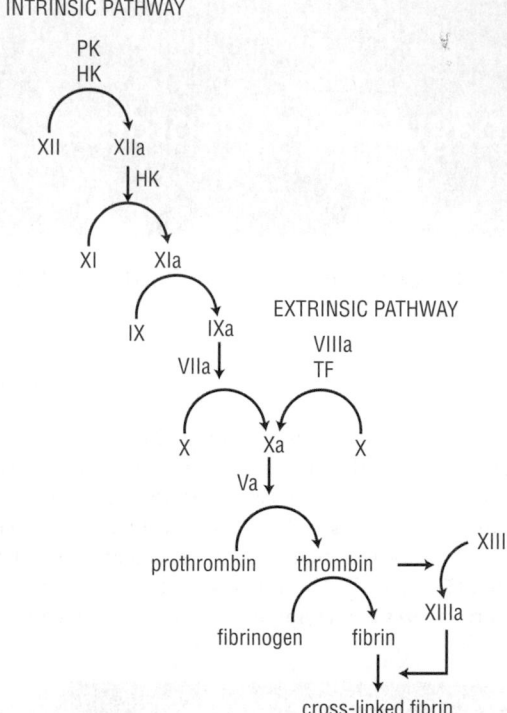

FIGURE 110-1. Cascade model of coagulation demonstrates activation via the intrinsic or extrinsic pathway. This model shows successive activation of coagulation factors proceeding from the top to the bottom where thrombin and fibrin are generated. (PK, prekallikrein; HK, high-molecular, weight kininogen; TF, tissue factor.) *(Reproduced from Roberts HR, Monroe DM, Hoffman M. Molecular biology and biochemistry of the coagulation factors and pathways of hemostasis. In: Lichtman MA, Beutler E, Coller BS, et al., eds. Williams Hematology. 7th edition. New York: McGraw-Hill; 2006:1665–1694.*

Simultaneously, the body works to localize clotting to the site of injury and prevent clotting in the intact vascular system. Unbound factors IIa, IXa, Xa, XIa, and XIIa are inactivated by antithrombin when they migrate to the endothelial cell surface. Heparin and heparin-like substances present on the surface of endothelial cells

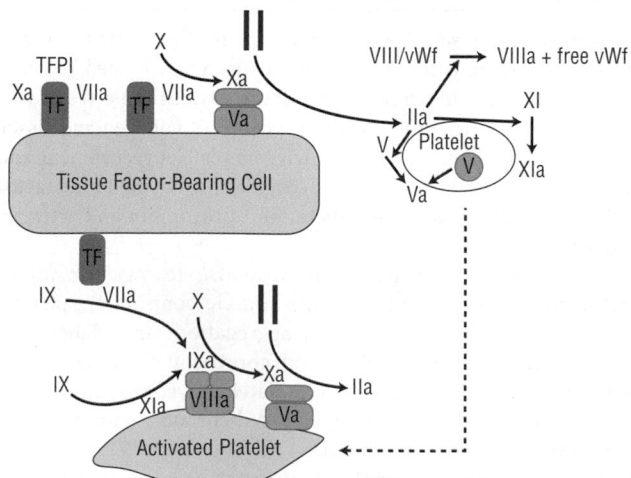

FIGURE 110-2. Cell-based model of hemostasis. (TF, tissue factor; TFPI, tissue factor pathway inhibitor; vWf, von Willebrand factor.) *(Reproduced from Roberts HR, Monroe DM, Hoffman M. Molecular biology and biochemistry of the coagulation factors and pathways of hemostasis. In: Lichtman MA, Beutler E, Coller BS, et al., eds. Williams Hematology. 7th ed. New York: McGraw-Hill; 2006:1665–1694.*

TABLE 110-1	Blood Coagulation Factors		
Factor[a]	Synonym	Biologic Half-life (h)	Blood Product Source
I	Fibrinogen	100–150	Cryoprecipitate (200–300 mg/bag)
II	Prothrombin	50–80	FFP, PCC
V	Proaccelerin	12–36	FFP
VII	Proconvertin	4–6	Recombinant VIIa, FFP, PCC
VIII	Antihemophilic factor	12–15	FFP, factor concentrates, cryoprecipitate
IX	Christmas factor	18–30	FFP, PCC, factor concentrates
X	Stuart-Power factor	25–60	FFP, PCC
XI	Plasma thromboplastin antecedent	40–80	FFP
XII	Hageman factor	50–70	Not associated with bleeding diathesis
XIII	Fibrin-stabilizing factor	150	FFP, cryoprecipitate, factor concentrate
VWF	von Willebrand factor	8–12	FFP, cryoprecipitate, factor concentrate

[a]Coagulation factors are numbered with Roman numerals in order of their discovery. The most common synonyms are listed. Factor III (tissue factor) and factor IV (calcium ions) have been omitted. There is no factor VI.

FFP, fresh-frozen plasma; PCC, prothrombin complex concentrate.

enhance the inhibitory capacity of antithrombin.[1] Thrombomodulin binds thrombin and activates protein C. Activated protein C and its cofactor, protein S, are vitamin K–dependent proteins that inactivate factor Va and VIIIa on the endothelial cell surface.

TISSUE FACTOR PATHWAY

Tissue factor is a membrane protein found in organs, circulating blood, and smooth muscle cells of vessel walls. Tissue factor is activated as a consequence of vessel wall damage or inflammatory cytokine release from endothelial cells or monocytes.[1,3] Coagulation is initiated when factor VIIa binds to activated tissue factor (Fig. 110–2).[1] The factor VIIa–tissue factor complex activates factors IX and X.[1,3] Activated platelets form complexes with factor IXa–factor VIIIa (tenase) and factor Xa-factor Va (prothrombinase).[1] Tenase activates factor X, and prothrombinase converts prothrombin to thrombin.[1] Thrombin activates platelets and catalyzes the conversion of fibrinogen to fibrin. Thrombin also amplifies coagulation by activating factors V, VIII, and XI, which leads to amplification of thrombin production by activated tenase and prothrombinase without the need to replenish active tissue factor.[1]

FIBRINOLYSIS

The coagulation system regulates fibrin clot formation, whereas the fibrinolytic system dissolves the polymerized clot and restores blood flow. As a regulatory mechanism for maintaining blood flow, the fibrinolytic system removes fibrin deposits and prevents formation of unnecessary fibrin clots. It also contributes to localized repair of damaged endothelium.

Plasminogen is the primary compound of the fibrinolytic enzyme system. Plasminogen activators include tissue-type plasminogen activator and urokinase-type plasminogen activator.[4] Activators convert plasminogen to plasmin in the presence of fibrin. Plasmin enzymatically digests fibrin, dissolves the clot, and releases a number of fibrin degradation products (FDPs). The interaction among plasminogen activators, plasminogen, and fibrin restricts the fibrinolytic activity to the site of the clot. Plasminogen activator inhibitor type 1 (PAI-1) blocks the plasminogen activators, whereas antiplasmin directly inhibits circulating plasmin to prevent systemic fibrinolysis.[4]

SIMPLE LABORATORY TESTS

The diagnosis of coagulation disorders can be established from a detailed clinical history, physical examination, and laboratory test results. The most common screening tests are prothrombin time (PT), activated partial thromboplastin time (aPTT), thrombin time, platelet count, and bleeding time. The results of these standard laboratory procedures can distinguish bleeding disorders caused by defects in the intrinsic, extrinsic, and common coagulation pathways (see Fig. 110–1) or alterations in the number of functioning platelets. Specific assays of individual coagulation factors and platelet function tests can be performed after abnormalities are identified by initial screening tests. The following is a brief review of widely available tests (summarized in Table 110–2).

Bleeding Time and Platelet Function Analyzer

Bleeding time assesses platelet and capillary function. Bleeding time reflects the time to cessation of bleeding following a standardized skin cut. This technique is patient and operator dependent and has fallen out of favor.[2] The bleeding time is insensitive to mild platelet defects and does not consistently predict a bleeding tendency.[5] The platelet function analyzer (PFA-100) is an in vitro screen for platelet function.[5] This test measures the time to occlude an aperture in a cartridge containing a membrane coated with either collagen/epinephrine or collagen/adenosine phosphate.[2] Platelet function analyzers are becoming a common screening test for primary hemostasis. The test is more sensitive than bleeding time for evaluating von Willebrand disease but still has limitations.[2] The PFA-100 has not been validated in patients with liver dysfunction.[4]

A prolonged bleeding time can be caused by incorrect performance of the test, thrombocytopenia, platelet dysfunction, von Willebrand disease, use of antiplatelet drugs (i.e., aspirin), renal failure (uremia), fibrinogen disorders, abnormal blood vessels, or collagen disorders.

Prothrombin Time

PT assesses the activity of fibrinogen and factors II, V, VII, and X.[6] PT reflects the time required for fibrin strands to appear after the addition of tissue thromboplastin (tissue factor) and calcium chloride to the platelet-poor plasma. Thus PT provides information about the current synthetic capacity of the liver, the adequacy of vitamin K absorption, and the inhibition of clotting factor synthesis by warfarin. PT is expressed as an international normalized ratio that normalizes values based on the international sensitivity index of the test reagents for patients on vitamin K antagonists.[6]

Activated Partial Thromboplastin Time

aPTT measures the activity of the intrinsic system and common pathway (factors II, V, VIII, IX, X, XI, and XII, high-molecular-weight kininogen, prekallikrein, and fibrinogen). aPTT reflects the time required for a fibrin clot to form after a partial thromboplastin (tissue factor) and a foreign material (usually silica) are added to platelet-poor plasma. aPTT is widely used for monitoring heparin therapy.

Thrombin Time

The thrombin time measures the conversion of fibrinogen to fibrin and is affected by quantitative or qualitative abnormalities of fibrinogen, the presence of thrombin inhibitors, and fibrinogen degradation products. The thrombin time measures the time required for the formation and appearance of the fibrin clot after thrombin is added to plasma.

TABLE 110-2 Laboratory Procedures			
Procedure	**Identifies**	**Cause of Prolonged Value**	**Clinical Manifestations**
Bleeding time	Platelet number and function	Acquired platelet disorders (uremia)	Bleeding from the gums
		Vasculitis	Easy bruising
		Connective tissue disorder	Bleeding following surgery or tooth extraction
		Thrombocytopenia	Epistaxis
		Inherited qualitative platelet defects	Menorrhagia
		Antiplatelet drugs	
		von Willebrand disease	
		Factor V or XI deficiency	
		Afibrinogenemia, dysfibrinogenemia	
Prothrombin time (PT)	Factors I, II, V, VII, X	Newborn	Bleeding following surgery, trauma, etc.
		Vitamin K deficiency	Easy bruising
		Inherited factor deficiencies[a]	
		Warfarin	
		Liver disease	
		Lupus anticoagulant	
		Afibrinogenemia	
Activated partial thromboplastin time (aPTT)	Factors I, II, V, VIII, IX, X	Inherited factor deficiencies[a]	Joint and muscle bleeding
		Lupus anticoagulant	Bleeding after surgery, trauma, etc.
		Heparin therapy	
		Liver disease	
		Afibrinogenemia	
	HMWK, prekallikrein		No bleeding manifestations
	Factor XII		Increased incidence of thrombotic disease possible with factor XII deficiency
	Factor XI		Variable bleeding tendency
			Bleeding following surgery, trauma, etc.
Thrombin time (TT)	Fibrinogen	Afibrinogenemia, dysfibrinogenemia	Lifelong hemorrhagic disease
	Inhibitors of fibrin aggregation	Heparin therapy	

[a]Bleeding manifestations dependent on factor levels.
HMWK, high-molecular-weight kininogen.

CONGENITAL COAGULATION DISORDERS

HEMOPHILIA

❶ Hemophilia is a bleeding disorder that results from a congenital deficiency in a plasma coagulation protein. Hemophilia A (classic hemophilia) is caused by a deficiency of factor VIII, while hemophilia B (Christmas disease) is caused by a deficiency of factor IX. The incidence of hemophilia is approximately 1 in 5,000 male births, 80% to 85% hemophilia A and 15% to 20% hemophilia B.[7,8] There are no significant racial differences in the incidence of hemophilia.

Approximately one third of patients with hemophilia have a negative family history, presumably representing a spontaneous mutation. Both hemophilia A and hemophilia B are recessive X-linked diseases; that is, the defective gene is located on the X chromosome. The disease usually affects only males; females are carriers. Affected males have the abnormal allele on their X chromosome and no matching allele on their Y chromosome, their sons would be normal (assuming the mother is not a carrier), and their daughters would be obligatory carriers. Female carriers have one normal allele and therefore do not usually have a bleeding tendency. Sons of a female carrier and a normal male have a 50% chance of having hemophilia, whereas daughters have a 50% chance of being carriers. Thus there is a "skipped generation" mode of inheritance in which the female carriers, who are the children of patients with hemophilia, do not express the disease but can pass it on to the next male generation.

Hemophilia has been observed in a small number of females. It can occur if both factor VIII and IX genes are defective,[9,10] if a female patient has only one X chromosome, as in Turner syndrome, or if the normal X chromosome is excessively inactivated through a process called *lyonization* or highly skewed X inactivation.[11–13]

In 1984, researchers isolated and cloned the human factor VIII gene.[14] It is a large gene, consisting of 186 kilobases (kb).[14,15] More than 900 unique mutations in the factor VIII gene, including point mutations, deletions, and insertions, have been reported (*http://hadb.org.uk/*). Deletions and nonsense mutations are often associated with the more severe forms of factor VIII deficiency because no functional factor VIII is produced. In 1993, researchers identified an inversion in the factor VIII gene at intron 22 that accounts for approximately 45% of severe hemophilia A gene abnormalities.[16] That discovery has greatly simplified carrier detection and prenatal diagnosis in families with this gene mutation. A more recently discovered inversion mutation involving intron 1 of the factor VIII gene accounts for an additional 5% of severe hemophilia mutations.[17]

The factor IX gene, cloned and sequenced in 1982, consists of only 34 kb and thus is significantly smaller than the factor VIII gene.[15,18] Unlike the factor VIII gene in patients with severe hemophilia A, the factor IX gene in patients with hemophilia B has no predominant mutation. Direct gene mutation analysis is simpler in hemophilia B because of the smaller gene size, and to date more than 900 different mutations have been reported (*http://kcl. ac.uk/ip/petergreen/haemBdatabase.html*). Most of these mutations are single base pair substitutions. Approximately 3% of factor IX gene mutations are deletions or complex rearrangements, and the presence of these mutations is associated with a severe phenotype.[14]

Hemophilia B Leyden is a rare variant in which factor IX levels are initially low but rise at puberty. The mechanism underlying the pathogenesis of this disorder has been controversial. Some propose that the binding of androgen receptor and other transcription factors is responsible.[19,20] Recently, other molecular mechanisms for

TABLE 110-3 Laboratory and Clinical Manifestations of Hemophilia

	Severe (<0.01 units/mL)	Moderate (0.01–0.05 units/mL)	Mild (>0.05 units/mL)
Age at diagnosis	1 year	1–2 years	2 years–adult
Neonatal symptoms			
PCB	Usually	Usually	Rarely
ICH	Occasionally	Uncommonly	Rarely
Muscle/joint hemorrhage	Spontaneous	Minor trauma	Minor trauma
CNS hemorrhage	High risk	Moderate risk	Rare
Postsurgical hemorrhage (without prophylaxis)	Frank bleeding, severe	Wound bleeding, common	Wound bleeding
Oral hemorrhage following trauma, tooth extraction	Usually	Common	Common

Normal range of factor VIII/IX activity level is 0.5–1.5 units/mL (50%–150%). 1 unit/mL corresponds to 100% of the factor found in 1 mL of normal plasma.
CNS, central nervous system; ICH, intracranial hemorrhage; PCB, postcircumcisional bleeding.

age-related gene regulation have been discovered and implicated in factor IX Leyden.[21] Identification of this genotype is clinically important because it confers a better prognosis.

Clinical Presentation

The characteristic bleeding manifestations of hemophilia include palpable ecchymoses, bleeding into joint spaces (hemarthroses), muscle hemorrhages, and excessive bleeding after surgery or trauma. The severity of clinical bleeding generally correlates with the degree of deficiency of factor VIII or factor IX. Factor VIII and factor IX activity levels are usually measured in units per milliliter, with 1 unit/mL representing 100% of the factor found in 1 mL of normal plasma.[22] Normal plasma levels range from 0.5 to 1.5 units/mL (50 to 150%). Patients with less than 0.01 units/mL (1%) of either factor are classified as having severe hemophilia, those with 0.01 to 0.05 units/mL (1%–5%) are moderate, and those with greater than 0.05 units/mL (5%) have mild hemophilia (Table 110–3).

Patients with severe disease experience frequent spontaneous hemorrhages and joint space bleeding, whereas those with moderate disease have excessive bleeding following mild trauma and rarely experience spontaneous hemarthroses. Patients with mild hemophilia may have so few symptoms that their condition can be undiagnosed for many years, and they usually have excessive bleeding only after significant trauma or surgery. Occasionally those with severe disease (less than 1% factor activity) may not display a severe phenotype; conversely, some with milder forms of the disease may have more severe bleeding. Patients with hemophilia usually present with clinical manifestations after age 1 year, when they begin to walk and increase their risk of bleeding.

Diagnosis

The diagnosis of hemophilia should be considered in any male with unusual bleeding. A family history of bleeding is helpful in the diagnosis but is absent in up to one third of patients.[23] Brothers of patients with hemophilia should be screened; sisters should undergo carrier testing.

Advances in molecular genetic analysis have greatly improved the accuracy of carrier status evaluation. Thus female relatives of patients with hemophilia who are at risk of being carriers should be tested. Additionally, the appropriate factor level should be measured in female carriers to identify those with levels less than 0.3 units/mL (30%) who themselves might be at risk for bleeding.

CLINICAL PRESENTATION OF HEMOPHILIA

Signs and Symptoms

- Ecchymoses (palpable)
- Hemarthrosis (especially knee, ankle, and elbow)
- Joint pain
- Joint swelling and erythema
- Decreased range of motion
- Muscle hemorrhage
- Swelling
- Pain with motion of affected muscle
- Signs of nerve compression
- Potential life-threatening blood loss, especially with thigh bleeding
- Oral bleeding with dental extractions or trauma
- Hematuria
- Intracranial hemorrhage (spontaneous or following trauma)
- Excessive bleeding with surgery

Laboratory Testing

- Prolonged aPTT
- Decreased factor VIII or factor IX level
- Normal PT
- Normal platelet count
- Normal von Willebrand factor antigen and activity
- Normal bleeding time

Patients with severe hemophilia A should be tested for the common factor VIII gene inversions. If the patient has this mutation, female family members should undergo testing to determine whether they also have the mutation and thus are carriers. In patients with hemophilia A who lack the inversion mutation, the gene can be sequenced to determine the exact mutation.[24,25] Techniques for determining carrier status in families with hemophilia B are similar, although no predominant mutation like the factor VIII inversion has been found. The smaller size of the factor IX gene facilitates direct DNA mutational analysis.[25]

Hemophilia can be diagnosed prenatally by chorionic villus sampling in gestational weeks 10 to 11 or by amniocentesis after 15 weeks' gestation.[15,24] Fetal blood can be sampled and assayed directly for factor VIII levels by 18 to 20 weeks' gestation.[15,24] This procedure is less useful for diagnosing factor IX deficiency because factor IX levels are physiologically low in fetuses and infants.

TREATMENT

Hemophilia

The comprehensive care of hemophilia requires a multidisciplinary approach. The patient is best managed in specialized centers with trained personnel and appropriate laboratory, radiologic, and pharmaceutical services. The healthcare team includes hematologists, orthopedic surgeons, nurses, physical therapists, dentists, genetic counselors, psychologists, pharmacists, case managers, and social workers.

Patients with hemophilia should receive routine immunizations, including immunization against hepatitis B. Hepatitis A vaccine is also recommended for patients with hemophilia because of the risk

(albeit small) of transmitting the causative agent through factor concentrates.[26] Use of a small-gauge needle can prevent excessive bleeding. Many healthcare providers advocate subcutaneous rather than intramuscular immunizations to decrease the risk of intramuscular bleeding or hematoma formation.

A few special considerations apply to the perinatal care of male infants of hemophilia carriers. Intracranial or extracranial hemorrhage has been estimated to occur in 1% to 4% of newborns with hemophilia.[27] Vacuum extraction and forceps delivery increase the risk of cranial bleeding. Elective cesarean section has not been shown to prevent intracranial bleeding. There is no clear consensus on the optimal mode of delivery or the use of prophylactic factor replacement in male infants of hemophilia carriers.[27] Circumcision should be postponed until a diagnosis of hemophilia is excluded. Factor levels can be assayed from cord blood samples or from peripheral venipuncture. Arterial puncture should be avoided because of the risk of hematoma formation. If an infant has hemophilia, many clinicians recommend a screening head ultrasound to rule out an intracranial hemorrhage prior to discharge from the nursery.

❷ Intravenous factor replacement therapy for the treatment or prevention of bleeding is the mainstay of treatment of hemophilia. Parents usually learn how to infuse with factor concentrate to facilitate home treatment. Older children and adult patients learn self-administration. Home healthcare nursing support may be helpful, particularly for the youngest patients in whom venous access may be difficult. In the setting of poor venous access a central line may be indicated. Administration of factor at home is more convenient for families and allows for earlier treatment of acute bleeding episodes. However, serious bleeding episodes always require medical evaluation.

■ HISTORY OF HEMOPHILIA TREATMENT

Therapy for hemophilia has undergone dramatic advances over the past few decades. Fifty years ago, administration of fresh-frozen plasma was the only available treatment. The introduction of cryoprecipitate in the early 1960s allowed more specific therapy for hemophilia A.[14] Intermediate-purity factor VIII and IX concentrates became available in the 1970s.[14] Plasma-derived factor concentrates are made from the donations of thousands of people. Contamination of plasma pools with hepatitis B, hepatitis C, and the human immunodeficiency virus (HIV) during the late 1970s and early 1980s resulted in transmission to most patients with severe hemophilia. Since the mid-1980s, plasma-derived concentrates have been manufactured with a variety of virus-inactivating techniques, including dry heat, pasteurization, and treatment with chemicals (e.g., solvent detergent mixtures).[14] Since 1986, no transmission of HIV through factor concentrates to patients with hemophilia in the United States has been reported.[14] Protein purification, introduced in the 1990s, produced high-purity concentrates with increased amounts of factor VIII or factor IX relative to the product's total protein content. Recombinant factor VIII and then factor IX also became available.[14] The first-generation recombinant factor VIII products utilize human and animal proteins in culture and add human albumin as a protein stabilizer.[14] Second-generation recombinant factor VIII concentrates removed albumin as a protein stabilizer, and third-generation products lack human and animal proteins in the culture media.[28] Gene therapy for treatment of hemophilia is now in the early stages of clinical trials.

■ HEMOPHILIA A

Table 110–4 summarizes the factor VIII products currently available in the United States. Most patients are treated with high-purity products. In general, products that have the lowest risk of transmitting

TABLE 110-4 Factor Concentrates

Brand Name	Product Type	Viral Inactivation or Exclusion Method	Other Contents
Factor VIII concentrates			
Alphanate	Plasma	Solvent detergent, dry heat	Albumin, heparin, vWF
Hemophil M	Plasma	Solvent detergent, monoclonal antibody	Albumin
Humate-P	Plasma	Pasteurization	Albumin, vWF
Koate-DVI	Plasma	Solvent detergent, dry heat	Albumin, heparin, vWF
Monarc-M	Plasma	Solvent detergent, monoclonal antibody	Albumin
Monoclate P	Plasma	Pasteurization, monoclonal antibody	Albumin
Advate	Recombinant	None	
Bioclate	Recombinant	None	Albumin
Helixate FS	Recombinant	Solvent detergent	Albumin (fermentation only); sucrose
Kogenate FS	Recombinant	Solvent detergent, monoclonal antibody	Albumin (fermentation only); sucrose
Recombinate	Recombinant	Monoclonal antibody	Albumin
ReFacto B domain deleted	Recombinant	None	Albumin (fermentation only); sucrose
Factor IX Concentrates			
AlphaNine SD	Plasma	Solvent detergent, filtered	Heparin
Mononine	Plasma	Monoclonal antibody, ultrafiltration	Heparin
BeneFix	Recombinant	None	
aPCC			
Autoplex T	Plasma	Dry heat	Heparin, IIa, VIIa, trace VIIIa, IXa, Xa
Feiba VH Immuno	Plasma	Vapor heat	IIa, VIIa, VIIIa, IXa, Xa
PCC			
Bebulin VH	Plasma	Vapor heat	Heparin, II, IX, X
Profilnine SD	Plasma	Solvent detergent	II, VII, IX, X
Proplex T	Plasma	Dry heat	Heparin, II, VII, IX, X
Other			
NovoSeven	Recombinant VII	None	
Hyate:C[a]	Porcine VIII	Freeze-dried	Citrate

aPCC, activated prothrombin complex concentrate; PCC, prothrombin complex concentrate; vWF, von Willebrand factor.
[a]No longer available in the United States.

infectious disease should be used. Thus recombinant products, when available, are generally used rather than plasma-derived products.

Recombinant Factor VIII

❸ Derived from cultured Chinese hamster ovary cells or baby hamster kidney cells transfected with the human factor VIII gene, recombinant factor VIII is produced with recombinant DNA technology.[14] Because it is not derived from blood donations, the risk of transmitting infections through administration of recombinant factor VIII is low. For this reason, recombinant products are generally favored over plasma-derived products. There is still a small risk of viral infection of the cell lines used to produce the clotting factor.[29] Furthermore, human and/or animal proteins are utilized in the production process of some recombinant products.[28] Therefore, these products have a theoretical risk of transmitting infection, although hepatitis and HIV infection have never been reported with their use.[14] The presence of parvovirus B19 DNA has been reported in recombinant factor VIII products.[30] First-generation recombinant factor VIII products contain human albumin as a stabilizing protein.[14] Second-generation recombinant factor VIII products add sucrose instead of human albumin as a stabilizer, but human albumin is utilized in the culture process. One second-generation product (ReFacto) has deletion of the B domain of the factor VIII gene, yielding a smaller protein product.[14] This B domain does not appear to be necessary for coagulation function. Third-generation recombinant factor VIII products contain no human protein in either the culture or the stabilization processes.[28]

Clinical trials have demonstrated that recombinant factor VIII products are comparable in effectiveness to plasma-derived products.[14] The risk of patients with severe hemophilia A developing an inhibitory antibody to factor VIII with use of recombinant factor VIII is 25% to 32%.[31] There is concern that this risk is higher than

what was previously reported with plasma-derived products. The difference may be partly attributable to more frequent screening for inhibitors in the recombinant product trials, with detection of transient inhibitors that might have been missed in the trials with plasma-derived products.[32] A recent multicenter retrospective cohort study of 316 patients with severe hemophilia did not find a difference in inhibitor development in patients who received recombinant products versus plasma-derived products.[33] A prospective international clinical trial comparing inhibitor development in patients receiving recombinant products versus plasma-derived products has been initiated.

Plasma-Derived Factor VIII Products

Several different plasma-derived factor VIII products are available (see Table 110–4). These products are derived from the plasma of thousands of donors and therefore can potentially transmit infection. Donor screening, testing plasma pools for evidence of infection, viral reduction through purification steps, and viral inactivation procedures (e.g., dry heat, pasteurization, and solvent detergent treatment) have all resulted in a safer product.[28] No cases of HIV transmission from factor concentrates have been reported since 1986.[14] However, isolated cases of hepatitis C infection with use of plasma-derived products have been reported.[14] Additionally, outbreaks of hepatitis A viral infections associated with plasma-derived products, likely because solvent detergent treatment does not inactivate this nonenveloped virus, have been reported. Parvovirus has been reported to be present in both plasma-derived and recombinant factor VIII products.[29,30] Finally, possible infection with as yet unidentified viruses that currently used methods would not inactivate remains a concern. There is a new concern that prion disease may be present in plasma derived factor VIII products.[29,34]

Factor VIII concentrates can be classified according to their level of purity, which refers to the specific activity of factor VIII in the product. Cryoprecipitate is a low-purity product. Cryoprecipitate also contains von Willebrand factor, fibrinogen, and factor XIII. Current American Association of Blood Banks standards call for a minimum of 80 international units of factor VIII per pack.[14] This product is no longer considered a primary treatment of factor VIII deficiency in countries where factor VIII concentrates are available because cryoprecipitate does not undergo a viral inactivation process. Intermediate-purity products have a specific activity of factor VIII of 5 units/mg of protein, whereas high-purity products have up to 2,000 units/mg of protein.[14] Ultrahigh-purity plasma-derived products are prepared with monoclonal antibody purification steps and have a specific activity of 3,000 units/mg of protein prior to addition of albumin as a stabilizer.

Factor VIII Concentrate Replacement

Appropriate dosing of factor VIII concentrate depends on the half-life of the infused factor, the patient's body weight, and the volume of distribution. The presence or absence of an inhibitory antibody to factor VIII and the titer of this antibody also influence treatment. Recovery studies, which measure the immediate postinfusion factor level, and survival studies, which assess the half-life of the factor, can establish patient-specific pharmacokinetics. The location and magnitude of the bleeding episode determine the percent correction to target as well as the duration of treatment. Serious or life-threatening bleeding requires peak factor levels of greater than 0.75 to 1 units/mL (75%–100%); less severe bleeding may be treated with a goal of 0.3 to 0.5 units/mL (30%–50% peak plasma levels. Table 110–5 provides general guidelines for the management of bleeding in different locations.

Factor VIII is a large molecule that remains in the intravascular space. Therefore, the plasma volume (approximately 50 mL/kg) can be used to estimate the volume of distribution. In general, each unit of factor VIII concentrate infused per kilogram of actual body weight yields a 2% rise in plasma factor VIII levels. The following equation can be used to calculate an initial dose of factor VIII:

Factor VIII (units) = (Desired level [in units/mL] – Baseline level [in units/mL]) × 0.5 × (Weight [in kilograms]).

The baseline level is usually omitted from the equation because it is negligible compared with the desired level. The half-life of

factor VIII ranges from 8 to 15 hours. It is generally necessary to administer half of the initial dose approximately every 12 hours to sustain the desired level of factor VIII. A single treatment may be adequate for minor bleeding, such as oral bleeding or slight muscle hemorrhages. However, because of the potential for long-term joint damage with hemarthroses, 2 or 3 days of treatment is often recommended for these bleeds. Serious bleeding episodes may require maintenance of 70% to 100% factor activity for 1 week or longer. As previously mentioned, factor VIII dosing depends on several variables, and each case must be considered individually. Individual pharmacokinetics may help guide treatment, particularly for serious bleeding episodes.

Alternatively, factor VIII can be administered as a continuous infusion when prolonged treatment is required (e.g., in the perioperative period or for serious bleeding episodes). Infusion rates ranging from 2 to 4 units/kg per hour are usually given in fixed-dose continuous infusion protocols, with the aim of maintaining a steady-state level of 60% to 100%.[35,36] Administration of factor concentrate via continuous infusion may reduce factor requirements by 20% to 50% because unnecessarily high peaks of factor VIII that occur with bolus injections are avoided.[36] A gradual decrease in factor VIII clearance during the first 5 to 6 days of treatment contributes to the lower factor concentrate requirements.[36] Daily monitoring of factor level can help determine the appropriate rate of infusion.

Administration of factor VIII concentrate via continuous infusion has been shown to be safe and effective, and it may be more convenient than bolus therapy for hospitalized patients.[35,36] The advantages of continuous infusion include maintenance of a steady-state plasma level with avoidance of potentially subtherapeutic trough levels and a reduction in cost associated with decreased factor requirements. A potential side effect with continuous infusion is thrombophlebitis at the delivery site. Concomitant infusion of saline or the addition of heparin (2–5 units/mL) to the infusion bag can minimize this risk.[36] Bacterial contamination of the concentrate is another theoretical concern, and preparation of the infusion bag should occur under sterile conditions (i.e., under laminar flow).[36] Finally, concerns about the stability of the formulations appear to be unwarranted, as most high-purity factor VIII concentrates have been shown to remain stable for at least 7 days after reconstitution.[36] Exposure of factor VIII to light for 10 hours postreconstitution can cause a 30% decrease in the activity.[36] It would be prudent to shield the container with foil wrap or an appropriate bag.

TABLE 110-5	Guidelines for Factor Replacement Therapy for Hemorrhage in Hemophilia A and B	
Site of Hemorrhage	**Desired Hemostatic Factor Level (% of normal)**	**Comments**
Joint	50%–70%	Rest/immobilization/physical therapy rehabilitation following bleed; several doses may be necessary to prevent or treat target joint
Muscle	30%–50% for most sites 70%–100% for thigh, iliopsoas, or nerve compression	Risk of significant blood loss with femoral/retroperitoneal bleed; bed rest for iliopsoas or other retroperitoneal bleeding
Oral mucosa	30%–50%	May try antifibrinolytic or topical thrombin prior to factor replacement for minor bleeding; higher factor levels may be needed for tongue swelling or risk of airway compromise; antifibrinolytic therapy should be used following factor replacement; do not use with aPCCs or PCCs
Gastrointestinal	Initially 100%, then 30% until healing occurs	Endoscopy is highly recommended; antifibrinolytic therapy may be useful
Hematuria	30% if no trauma 70%–100% if traumatic	If no pain or trauma, consider bed rest and fluids for 24 hours; factor should be given if hematuria persists; evaluate if hematuria persists; if trauma to abdomen or back, perform imaging and give aggressive factor replacement
Central nervous system	Initially 100%, then 50%–100% for 10–14 days	Lumbar puncture requires prophylactic factor coverage
Trauma or surgery	Initially 100%, then 50% until wound healing complete	Perioperative and postoperative management plan must be in place preoperatively; evaluation for inhibitors is crucial prior to elective surgery

aPCC, activated prothrombin complex concentrate; PCC, prothrombin complex concentrate.

Other Pharmacologic Therapy

Treatment with desmopressin acetate is often adequate for minor bleeding episodes in patients with mild hemophilia A. A synthetic analogue of the antidiuretic hormone vasopressin, desmopressin causes release of von Willebrand factor and factor VIII from endogenous endothelial storage sites. It appears to be most effective in patients with higher baseline factor VIII levels (0.1–0.15 units/mL or 10–15%).[37] The recommended dose of desmopressin is 0.3 mcg/kg diluted in 50 mL of normal saline and infused IV over 15 to 30 minutes.[15,37] Patients with mild or moderate hemophilia A should undergo a desmopressin trial to determine their response to this medication. At least a twofold rise in factor VIII to a minimal level of 0.3 units/mL (30%) within 60 minutes is considered an adequate response.[38] In adults with mild hemophilia A, the response rate to desmopressin has been reported to be 80% to 90%.[38] Pediatric studies have reported a lower rate of response ranging from 40% to 47%.[38] Furthermore, the pediatric response rate was related to age; some nonresponding children became responders at an older age.[38]

Infusion of desmopressin can be repeated daily for up to 2 to 3 days. Tachyphylaxis, an attenuated response with repeated dosing, may develop after that time. The factor increase after the second dose of desmopressin is approximately 30% lower than after the initial dose.[37] Factor concentrate therapy may be necessary if the patient requires additional treatment. Factor levels should be measured to ensure that an adequate response has been achieved. Treatment with desmopressin will not result in hemostasis in patients who have severe hemophilia and those who are only marginally responsive. Desmopressin should not be used as primary therapy for life-threatening bleeding episodes such as intracranial hemorrhage or for major surgical procedures when a minimum factor VIII concentration of 0.7 to 1 units/mL (70%–100% [0.70–1.00]) is required.[37]

Desmopressin can be administered intranasally via a concentrated nasal spray.[37,38] It elicits a slower and less marked response, with a peak effect in 60 to 90 minutes after administration, somewhat longer than with desmopressin administered intravenously.[37,38] The dosage is one spray (150 mcg) for patients who weigh less than 50 kg (110 lbs) and two sprays (300 mcg) for those who weigh more than 50 kg (110 lbs).[15] The nasal spray may serve as an alternative to the intravenous formulation, especially in patients with mild bleeding episodes.

Few adverse effects are associated with desmopressin. The most commonly observed side effect is facial flushing.[37] Less frequently reported side effects include mild headaches, increased heart rate, and decreased blood pressure. Thrombosis is a rare complication associated with desmopressin.[38] Because of its antidiuretic effects, desmopressin has the potential to cause water retention, which may lead to severe hyponatremia. This may be a particular problem in children younger than 2 years, in whom hyponatremic seizures have been reported.[36] Therefore, desmopressin should be used with caution in this age group.[37,38] Patients with congestive heart failure may be at increased risk for developing hyponatremia with use of desmopressin.[37] Fluid restriction for 24 hours after the desmopressin dose and monitoring of urine output are recommended with desmopressin administration.[38]

Antifibrinolytic therapy inhibits clot lysis and is therefore a useful adjunctive therapy for the treatment of hemophilia. Antifibrinolytic agents are particularly beneficial for treatment of oral bleeding because of the high concentration of fibrinolytic enzymes present in saliva. Two antifibrinolytics are aminocaproic acid and tranexamic acid. Aminocaproic acid is given at a dosage of 100 mg/kg (maximum 6 g) every 6 hours and can be administered orally or intravenously.[15] The dosage of tranexamic acid is 25 mg/kg (maximum 1.5 g) orally every 8 hours or 10 mg/kg (maximum 1 g) intravenously every 8 hours.[15]

■ HEMOPHILIA B

Therapeutic options for hemophilia B have improved greatly over the past several years, first with the development of monoclonal antibody–purified plasma-derived products and then with the licensure of recombinant factor IX. Products currently available in the United States for treatment of hemophilia B are listed in Table 110–4.

Recombinant Factor IX

First marketed in the United States in 1999, recombinant factor IX is produced in Chinese hamster ovary cells transfected with the factor IX gene.[14] Blood and plasma products are not used to produce recombinant factor IX or to stabilize the final product; thus recombinant factor IX has an excellent viral safety profile.[14] Clinical trials have shown the product to be safe and efficacious in the treatment of acute bleeding episodes and in the management of bleeding associated with surgical procedures.[14,39] Although the half-life of recombinant factor IX is similar to that of the plasma-derived products, recovery is approximately 30% lower.[40] As a result, doses of recombinant factor IX concentrate must be higher than those of plasma-derived products to achieve equivalent plasma levels. Because individual pharmacokinetics may vary, recovery and survival studies should be performed to determine optimal treatment.[14,39,40] Recombinant factor IX is considered the treatment of choice for hemophilia B.

Plasma-Derived Factor IX Products

High-purity factor IX plasma concentrates have been available in the United States since the early 1990s.[14,39,40] These products are derived from plasma through biochemical purification and monoclonal immunoaffinity techniques. Other viral inactivation measures, such as solvent detergent or chemical treatment, are also used.

Before the high-purity products were approved for use, hemophilia B patients were treated with factor IX concentrates that also contained other vitamin K–dependent proteins (factors II, VII, and X), known as prothrombin complex concentrates (PCCs). These products contain small amounts of activated factors generated during processing, and their use has been associated with thrombotic complications, including deep-vein thrombosis, pulmonary embolism, myocardial infarction, and disseminated intravascular coagulation (DIC).[14,41] The risk of such complications is highest in patients who are receiving high or repeated doses of PCCs, in those who have hepatic disease (the liver removes the activated factors from circulation), in neonates, and in patients who have experienced crush injuries or who are undergoing major surgery.[14,41] Concomitant use of PCCs and antifibrinolytics should be avoided because of the risk for thrombosis.

Because of the lower purity of PCCs and their thrombogenic potential, these products are not first-line treatment of hemophilia B, although they are still used for treatment of patients with hemophilia A or B who have developed inhibitory antibodies against factor VIII or factor IX, respectively. High-purity factor IX concentrates have excellent efficacy in the treatment of bleeding episodes and in the control of bleeding associated with surgical procedures.[42] Their viral safety profile has been reported to be excellent, and the risk of thromboembolic complications is low.[42]

Factor IX Concentrate Replacement

Factor IX is a relatively small protein. Unlike factor VIII, it is not limited to the intravascular space; it also passes into the extravascular compartment.[40] This results in a volume of distribution that is about twice that of factor VIII. In general, for plasma-derived factor IX concentrates, each unit of factor IX infused per kilogram of actual body weight yields a 1% rise in the plasma level of factor IX (range 0.67%–1.28%).[14] The following equation can be used to calculate the initial dose:

Plasma-derived factor IX (units) = (Desired level – Baseline level) × (Weight [in kilograms]).

As with the similar calculation for factor VIII dosing, the baseline level term can be omitted from the formula. Because recovery of recombinant factor IX is lower than that of the plasma-derived products, the following adjustment is made:

Pediatric dosing:

Recombinant factor IX (units) = (Desired level[in units/mL] – Baseline level [in units/mL]) × 1.4 × (Weight [in kilograms]).

Adult dosing:

Recombinant factor IX (units) = (Desired level [in units/mL] – Baseline level [in units/mL]) × 1.2 × (Weight [in kilograms]).

A recovery study to determine optimal dosing is recommended for patients who receive recombinant factor IX because of the wide interpatient variability in pharmacokinetics.

Because the half-life of factor IX is approximately 24 hours, dosing can be less frequent than with factor VIII. Table 110–5 provides general guidelines for dosing factor IX, based on the site and severity of the bleeding episode. As with factor VIII replacement therapy, individual pharmacokinetics may vary, and monitoring the patient's factor IX levels helps optimize therapy.

■ PROPHYLACTIC REPLACEMENT THERAPY

Traditionally, factor concentrates for hemophilia patients have been given on demand, as the bleeding episode occurs. However, recurrent joint bleeding can damage the joint and lead to development of severe physical disability. Thus it would be preferable to prevent bleeding episodes and avoid the resultant damage. Known as *prophylactic factor replacement therapy*, this approach entails regular infusion of concentrate to maintain the deficient factor at a minimum of 0.01 units/mL (1%).

In effect, prophylactic replacement therapy converts severe hemophilia into a milder form of the disease. The rationale for this approach is that patients with moderate hemophilia rarely experience spontaneous hemarthroses, and they have a much lower incidence of chronic arthropathy. Patients with hemophilia A usually require 25 to 40 units of factor VIII per kilogram of body weight, given every other day or three times per week.[15] For hemophilia B, the usual dosage is 40 to 100 units/kg of factor IX given twice weekly instead of three times weekly because of the longer half-life of factor IX.[43]

Primary prophylaxis is regular replacement therapy started at a young age (usually before age 2 years), prior to the onset of joint bleeding.[44,45] In the Swedish experience, children who began prophylaxis at age 1 to 2 years experienced almost no bleeding episodes and had normal joint examinations and radiographs over a 5-year period.[14,46] Secondary prophylaxis begins after significant joint bleeding has already occurred. It is associated with a significant reduction in the number of joint bleeding episodes and a better clinical and orthopedic outcome.[47,48] However, radiographic evidence of joint disease rarely improves and often progresses despite the institution of secondary prophylaxis.[14,46] Therefore, it may not be possible to avoid chronic arthropathy when prophylaxis is initiated after significant joint bleeding has already occurred; this supports a need for earlier intervention. Manco-Johnson et al. completed the first pediatric randomized clinical trial comparing prophylaxis to enhanced episodic treatment to prevent joint disease in boys (age <30 months) with severe hemophilia.[49] They demonstrated that prophylaxis prevented joint damage and decreased the frequency of joint and other hemorrhages in boys with hemophilia.[49]

In 2001 the Medical and Scientific Advisory Council of the National Hemophilia Foundation of the United States recommended primary prophylaxis (prior to onset of frequent bleeding) beginning at age 1 to 2 years for children with severe hemophilia. The use of primary prophylaxis has many challenges and has not been widely accepted in the United States. Many institutions continue to use some form of secondary prophylaxis, in which prophylaxis is started after a pattern of bleeding has been established.

Several disadvantages are associated with primary prophylaxis. Perhaps most important is the high cost of prophylactic replacement therapy. Factor requirements are estimated to be twofold to threefold higher with prophylactic regimens than with treatment on demand.[46,50] Use of individual pharmacokinetics to titrate dosage may help to lessen costs.[50] Other issues to consider are the inconvenience to families and possible difficulties with compliance. Central venous lines may be necessary for frequent administration of factor concentrates, particularly in children younger than 5 years, who are at the age targeted for initiation of primary prophylaxis regimens. Potential complications of central venous access include surgical risks, infection, and catheter-related deep-vein thrombosis.[51] Catheter-related infections are common in patients with hemophilia and have been reported to occur in up to 0.2-2 per 1,000 catheter days.[52] Catheter-related infectious complications appear to be more common in hemophilia patients who have developed inhibitory antibodies.[52] Finally, routine use of primary prophylaxis may overtreat some patients with severe hemophilia who do not have a severe clinical phenotype.

CLINICAL CONTROVERSY

Hemophilia patients may receive prophylactic factor concentrate therapy to prevent or decrease bleeding episodes, or they may receive on-demand factor concentrate therapy in response to a bleeding episode. In addition, prophylaxis may be primary or secondary. Controversy exists over whether the benefits of prophylaxis justify the cost, appropriate time to initiate prophylaxis, and appropriate dosing for prophylaxis.

■ TREATMENT OF INHIBITORS IN HEMOPHILIA

Neutralizing antibodies to factor VIII and IX, known as *inhibitors*, develop in a subset of patients with hemophilia, challenging the management of these patients. The development of an inhibitor is the most serious complication of factor replacement therapy. The reported prevalence of inhibitor development varies considerably, depending on the population studied, the study design, the method of detection, and the frequency and duration of testing. In one systematic review, the overall prevalence of inhibitors in unselected patients with hemophilia was 5% to 7%.[32] The prevalence among patients with severe hemophilia was approximately 12% to 13%, which is higher than for unselected patients.[32] The reported cumulative incidence of inhibitors in hemophilia B is much lower, occurring in only 1% to 4% of patients.[31]

Most inhibitors develop in childhood, often after relatively few exposure days (median 9–12 days).[31] Patients with severe hemophilia are much more likely to develop inhibitors than those with milder forms of the disease.[32] It is possible that the low levels of factor produced in patients with mild and moderate hemophilia induce immune tolerance in these individuals. In contrast, factor levels are undetectable in patients with severe hemophilia, and infused factor VIII, regarded as a foreign protein, may provoke an antibody response. The rate of inhibitor formation varies even among patients with identical mutations, which suggests that host factors modify the risk. One possibility is that human leukocyte antigen (HLA) genotype may influence the risk of inhibitor formation, but studies have been inconclusive.[53]

Inhibitors are usually immunoglobulins of the immunoglobulin G subclass that are directed against the factor coagulant portion of the complex. The presence of an inhibitor is suspected when a decreased clinical response to factor replacement is observed. It may be discovered incidentally on routine laboratory screening. Inhibitors are measured with the Bethesda assay, and titers are reported in Bethesda units (BU). One BU is the amount of inhibitor needed to inactivate half of the factor VIII or factor IX in a mixture of inhibitor-containing plasma and pooled normal plasma.[14] Patients with inhibitors to factor VIII or factor IX are divided into two groups: low responders, who have low levels of inhibitors (<5 BU/mL) and generally have little or no rise in antibody titers after exposure to the factor; and high responders (>5 BU/mL), who have higher inhibitor levels and develop an increase in antibody titer after exposure (anamnestic response).[14]

Therapy for patients with inhibitors involves treatment of acute bleeding episodes and treatment directed at eradicating the inhibitor. The inhibitor titer, the site and magnitude of bleeding, and the patient's past response to therapy determine the approach to treatment. For patients with a low inhibitor titer, administration of high doses of the specific factor can often control bleeding episodes. Two to three times the usual replacement dose and more frequent dosing intervals are often necessary to overcome the antibody. Factor level monitoring and clinical assessments help to evaluate the adequacy of treatment. Additional supportive measures, such as immobilization and administration of antifibrinolytic agents, should be used, where appropriate.

In the presence of a high-titer inhibitor, it may be impossible to administer enough factor VIII or factor IX to neutralize the antibody and achieve a hemostatic plasma level. Therefore, in these patients treatment of bleeding episodes consists of use of agents that bypass the factor to which the antibody is directed. These include PCCs, activated PCCs, and recombinant activated factor VII.

PCCs contain the vitamin K–dependent factors II, VII, IX, and X. Small quantities of activated factors VII and IX are present in these products. Activated PCCs (aPCCs) contain greater quantities of the activated factors.[54] The usual dosage is 50 to 100 units/kg administered every 12 to 24 hours, depending on the severity of the bleeding episode.[32] The maximum dose should not exceed 200 units/kg/day. Use of PCCs and aPCCs, when not restricted to one or two doses, is effective in obtaining hemostasis in approximately 80% of bleeding episodes in patients with inhibitors, and aPCCs appear to be more effective than PCCs. As previously mentioned, there is a risk of serious thrombotic complications, including pulmonary emboli, deep-vein thrombosis, and myocardial infarction associated with use of PCCs and aPCCs.[54] Additionally, because these products contain trace amounts of factor VIII and larger amounts of factor IX, they can stimulate an anamnestic response in patients with hemophilia A and, more commonly, in those with hemophilia B.[54] Other minor side effects include dizziness, nausea, hives, flushing, and headaches.[54] Patients with factor IX inhibitors occasionally develop severe allergic reactions in response to infusion of factor IX–containing products, so these patients should be monitored closely.[55]

Recombinant factor VIIa, a newer bypassing agent, is thought to be hemostatically active only at the site of tissue injury where tissue factor is present; thus the risk of systemic thrombotic events associated with this agent is minimal.[56] Additionally, because recombinant VIIa is not a plasma-derived product, both viral transmission and anamnestic responses to factor VIII or factor IX are unlikely.[54] The initial dose for bleeding episodes ranges from 35 to 120 mcg/kg.[54] Doses of 70 mcg/kg or higher are more effective, and often a dose of 90 to 120 mcg/kg is used for treatment of patients with hemophilia and inhibitors.[54,57] A drawback is the product's short half-life, which necessitates dosing every 2 hours. Continuous infusion of recombinant factor VIIa, which may be more convenient and cost effective, has been successful, although studies are limited. Recombinant factor VIIa appears to be efficacious in controlling bleeding episodes and managing hemophilia during surgical procedures.[54] Patients treated with bypassing agents must be monitored clinically because no laboratory test directly measures the effectiveness of treatment.

Porcine factor VIII is an alternative therapeutic option for patients who have hemophilia A and inhibitors. The rationale is that porcine factor VIII is enough like human factor VIII to participate in the coagulation cascade, yet most factor VIII inhibitors have absent or only weak neutralizing activity against nonhuman factor VIII. However, cross-reactivity with porcine factor VIII does occur, and a high titer of antibody against porcine factor VIII can develop. Although the rise in antibody titer with porcine factor VIII is generally lower than that seen with administration of human factor VIII, anamnestic rises in inhibitor titers to both porcine and human factor VIII may occur and can limit future use.[54] Other potential side effects include severe allergic reactions and thrombocytopenia.[54] Porcine factor VIII is no longer commercially available but can be obtained for use in specific patients. Because of these limitations, porcine factor VIII is usually indicated only after the patient has not responded to recombinant factor VIIa and PCC or when the patient has severe hemorrhages.[54] An advantage to porcine factor VIII is that treatment response can be monitored with factor VIII levels.

The ideal therapy for patients with hemophilia and inhibitors eradicates the inhibitor so that future treatment with factor VIII or factor IX concentrates is possible. Immune tolerance therapy, which involves the regular infusion of high doses of the factor to which the antibody is directed, may accomplish this eradication. A variety of different dosing regimens, ranging from 25 units/kg every other day to more than 200 units/kg every day, have been used. Some treatment protocols include adjunctive immunomodulatory therapy, such as administration of cyclophosphamide, prednisone, and intravenous immune globulin.[58] The overall success rate is 50% to 70% and is higher in patients with low inhibitor titers and in those with recent development of inhibitor.[53] Weeks to years of therapy may be required to eradicate the antibody. Unfortunately, immune tolerance therapy is costly, time consuming, and often requires placement of a central venous catheter.[59] Once achieved, however, immune tolerance facilitates the management of bleeding episodes with specific factor replacement therapy. Rituximab, an anti-CD20 monoclonal antibody, has been used with some success in a few patients with acquired factor VIII inhibitors.[60] The mechanism of action involves the rapid depletion of circulating B cells, which produce antibodies, including the anti–factor VIII antibody. An ongoing clinical trial is assessing the use of rituximab in patients with hemophilia and inhibitors who have previously failed immune tolerance.

Figure 110–3 summarizes the therapeutic options in the management of hemophilia A patients with inhibitors. The same algorithm can be applied to the management of hemophilia B patients, except that factor IX should be substituted for factor VIII. Use of porcine factor VIII is not indicated for inhibitors in hemophilia B.

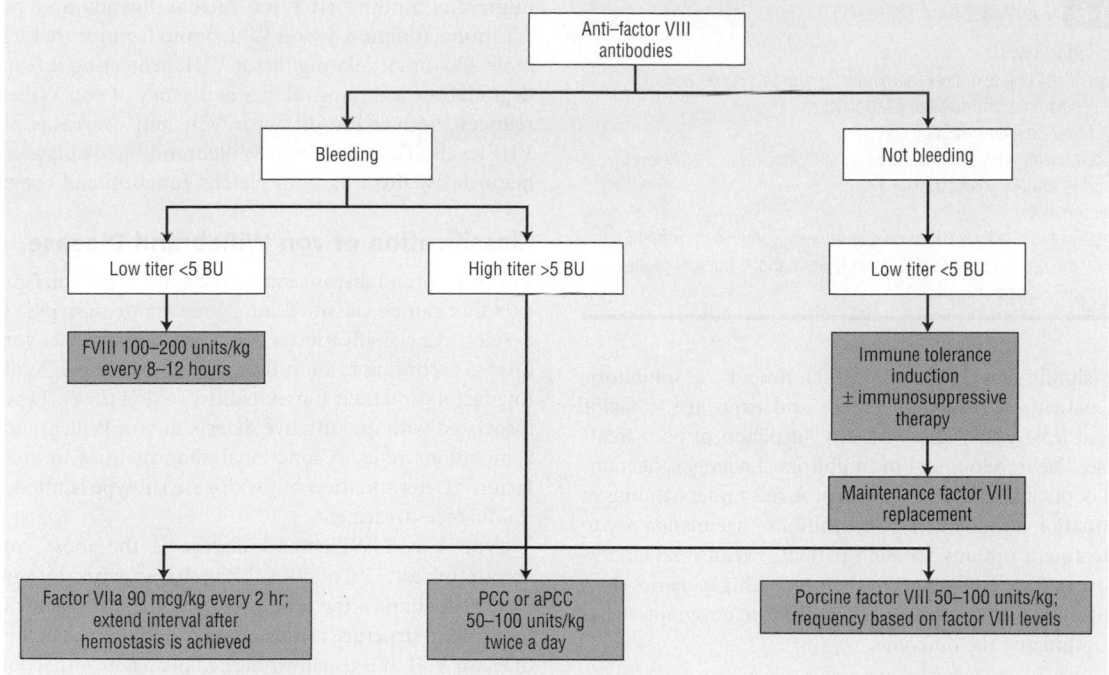

FIGURE 110-3. Treatment algorithm for the management of patients with hemophilia A and factor VIII antibodies. (aPCC, activated prothrombin complex concentrate; BU, Bethesda unit; PCC, prothrombin complex concentrate.)

GENE THERAPY IN HEMOPHILIA

Use of gene therapy for hemophilia A and B is currently under investigation and continues to face significant challenges. A number of different viral and nonviral vectors have been used to transfer the recombinant factor gene to human cells, such as liver and muscle cells.[61] Even low levels of factor expression through gene therapy should reduce bleeding episodes in patients with severe hemophilia, a rationale for gene therapy similar to that for prophylactic factor replacement. Furthermore, given the broad range of physiologically normal factor levels, very tight regulation of gene expression is not necessary. The safety and efficacy of this approach to treatment remain to be determined. A total of five clinical trials have been completed but none have had significant enough results to progress to phase III clinical studies.[61] Potential benefits to gene therapy include patient convenience, viral safety, and decreased cost. Possible drawbacks to gene therapy include a risk of inhibitor formation, tumorigenesis related to integration of the viral vector, possible germ-line transmission, and concerns about long-term gene expression.[62]

PAIN MANAGEMENT IN HEMOPHILIA

Pain, both acute and chronic, can be a common occurrence in patients with hemophilia. The likely cause of acute pain is bleeding, and control of the bleeding episode should ease the pain. Chronic pain may be the result of permanent joint changes. Surgical intervention may help to alleviate the pain, as may an intensive physical therapy program.[63] Intraarticular administration of dexamethasone may also be useful.[64] Acetaminophen can be used, although narcotic analgesia may be required for more severe pain. Nonsteroidal antiinflammatory drugs impair platelet function and may increase the risk of bleeding in patients with hemophilia, although these drugs have been used for the management of chronic arthropathy. Cyclooxygenase-2 inhibitors have less antiplatelet activity and may be an option for pain management.

SURGERY IN HEMOPHILIA

In the patient with hemophilia undergoing a surgical procedure, the goal of treatment is maintaining factor levels of at least 0.5 to 0.7 units/mL (50%–70%) during surgery and in the postoperative period in order to prevent excessive bleeding. Intermittent dosing or continuous infusion factor replacement may accomplish this goal. Before surgery, factor concentrate is usually infused to obtain a plasma level of 1 unit/mL (100%). Replacement therapy is continued to maintain plasma levels greater than 0.5 units/mL (50%) for 5 to 7 days or longer, depending on the type of surgery. Preoperative evaluation for elective procedures should include measurement of an inhibitor titer and assessment of the recovery and half-life of infused factor in the patient. Elective surgery should not proceed unless therapeutic plasma levels can be obtained.

Evaluation of Therapeutic Outcomes

The main goal in the treatment of hemophilia is controlling and preventing bleeding episodes and their long-term sequelae, such as chronic arthropathies. Pharmacologic and nonpharmacologic interventions should be aimed at achieving this goal. Treatment response can be monitored through clinical parameters, such as cessation of bleeding and resolution of symptoms. Determination of plasma factor levels may also be helpful, particularly for severe bleeding episodes. Home therapy for administration of factor concentrates is common among these patients because this approach can lead to earlier treatment and more independence for the patient. Diaries in which the patient documents symptoms, the dose of factor replacement, adjuvant therapies used, and treatment response can help the caregiver evaluate the success of home therapy. Monitoring the number and type of bleeding episodes and measuring trough plasma factor levels make it possible to evaluate the adequacy of prophylactic regimens. Physical examination with evaluation of joint range of motion and radiographs of target joints indicates the long-term success of preventing and treating arthropathies.

TABLE 110-6 Von Willebrand Disease

von Willebrand factor (vWF)
  Large multimeric glycoprotein that is necessary for normal platelet adhesion, normal bleeding time, and stabilizing factor VIII.
von Willebrand factor antigen (vWF:Ag)
  Antigenic determinant(s) on vWF measured by immunoassays; usually low in types 1 and 2; virtually absent in type 3.
Ristocetin cofactor activity
  Functional assay of vWF activity based on platelet aggregation with ristocetin. Reduced by the same degree as vWF:Ag in types 1 and 3, but to a greater extent in type 2 disease (except 2B).

Clinicians should check for the development of inhibitors, especially in patients with severe disease and exposure to factor concentrates, at least yearly and with any suspicion of poor treatment response. The development of inhibitors challenges the management and control of bleeding episodes. A full understanding of the clinical situation and the titer of the inhibitor are mandatory to address all treatment options for each patient. Because no laboratory test measures the effectiveness of therapy in this scenario, close clinical monitoring for worsening or resolution of symptoms is essential for optimizing the outcome.

VON WILLEBRAND DISEASE

The most common congenital bleeding disorder in the United States and in the world, von Willebrand disease, has a prevalence of 1% to 2%.[65] Von Willebrand disease refers to a family of disorders caused by a quantitative and/or qualitative defect of von Willebrand factor, a glycoprotein that plays a role in both platelet aggregation and coagulation (Table 110–6). Unlike hemophilia, von Willebrand disease has an autosomal inheritance pattern, resulting in an equal frequency of disease in males and females.

The gene for von Willebrand factor is located on chromosome 12 and is 178 kb in length.[66,67] Transcription and translation produce a large primary product that subsequently undergoes complex modifications, resulting in von Willebrand factor multimers of various sizes with molecular weights ranging from 500 to 20,000 kDa. Von Willebrand factor is synthesized in endothelial cells, where it is either stored in Weibel-Palade bodies or secreted constitutively.[68] It is also synthesized in megakaryocytes and stored in α-granules, from which it is released following platelet activation.

Von Willebrand factor is important for both primary and secondary hemostasis. In response to vascular injury, it promotes platelet adhesion by interacting with the glycoprotein Ib receptor on platelets.[66,68] It can facilitate platelet aggregation by binding to the platelet glycoprotein IIb/IIIa receptor, although fibrinogen is the main ligand for this receptor.[66] The highest-molecular-weight von Willebrand factor multimers appear to be the most important in platelet adhesion because their large surface area contains numerous binding sites for various ligands and receptors. An additional function of von Willebrand factor is that it is the carrier molecule for circulating factor VIII, protecting it from premature degradation and removal.[69] A deficiency of von Willebrand factor reduces the half-life of factor VIII and decreases plasma factor VIII levels. Therefore, von Willebrand factor plays a dual role in hemostasis, affecting both platelet function and coagulation.

Classification of von Willebrand Disease

Von Willebrand disease consists of a heterogeneous group of disorders that can be classified into three major subtypes. The NIH has developed a classification scheme that characterizes von Willebrand disease according to both the quantity of the von Willebrand clotting factors and their functionality (Table 110–7). Types 1 and 3 are associated with quantitative defects in von Willebrand factor; type 2 mutations refer to functional abnormalities in von Willebrand factor.[70] Determination of the disease subtype is important because it influences treatment.

Type 1 von Willebrand disease is the most common type, accounting for 75% of cases.[65] It is characterized by a mild-to-moderate reduction in the level of von Willebrand factor (although its multimeric structure is normal) and a similar reduction in the level of factor VIII. It is usually inherited in an autosomal dominant fashion with variable penetrance and expression.[71] Bleeding symptoms are often very mild to moderate.[69] Patients with von Willebrand disease can experience easy bruising, nosebleeds, or other mucosal bleeding such as gastrointestinal or heavy menstrual bleeding. Subjects may be at risk of bleeding following surgery, traumatic injury, or childbirth.[65]

Type 2 von Willebrand disease, diagnosed in 9% to 30% of affected patients, is characterized by a qualitative abnormality of von Willebrand factor.[69] Bleeding manifestations may be more severe than with type 1 disease. Inheritance is most often autosomal dominant but may be recessive.[71] Type 2 von Willebrand disease can be subdivided into four variants. Type 2A is the most frequent subtype and is characterized by a reduced von Willebrand factor–platelet interaction and an absence of high- and intermediate-molecular-weight factor multimers. Type 2B is a less common variant characterized by an abnormal von Willebrand factor that has an increased affinity for the platelet glycoprotein Ib receptor. This is associated with thrombocytopenia, which is usually mild. In addition, there is usually an absence of high-molecular-weight forms of von Willebrand factor. Type 2M arises from a qualitative defect in von Willebrand factor that impairs its binding to platelets; it is similar to type 2A, except that there is no measurable reduction in the high-molecular-weight multimers.[71] Finally, type 2N von Willebrand disease (Normandy) is a rare form of the disease in which von Willebrand factor has a markedly reduced affinity for factor VIII. This leads to a moderate-to-severe reduction of factor VIII plasma levels with normal von Willebrand factor levels.[71]

TABLE 110-7 VWD Classification and Laboratory Values

Condition	Description	VWF-RCo (IU/dL)	VWF-Ag (IU/DL)	FVIII	VWF-RCo/VWF-Ag Ratio
Type 1	Partial quantitative VWF deficiency	<30	<30	↓ or Normal	>0.5–0.7
Type 2A	↓ VWF-dependent platelet adhesion with selective deficiency of high-MW VWF multimer	<30	<30–200	↓ or Normal	<0.5–0.7
Type 2B	↑ VWF affinity for platelet GP Ib; ± ↓ platelet numbers	<30	<30–200	↓ or Normal	Usually <0.5–0.7
Type 2M	↑ VWF-dependent platelet adhesion without selective deficiency of high-MW VWF multimers	<30	<30–200	↓ or Normal	<0.5–0.7
Type 2N	Markedly ↓ VWF binding affinity for FVIII	30–200	30–200	↓↓	>0.5–0.7
Type 3	Virtually complete deficiency of VWF	<3	<3	↓↓↓ (<10 IU/dL)	Not applicable
"Low VWF"		30–50	30–50	Normal	>0.5–0.7
Normal		50–200	50–200	Normal	>0.5–0.7

(Modified from Reference A.)

TABLE 110-8 Questions to Ask Patient

1. Have you or a blood relative ever needed medical attention for a bleeding problem or been told you have a bleeding disorder or problem?
   - During or after surgery?
   - With dental procedures or extractions?
   - During childbirth or for heavy menses?
   - Ever had bruises with lungs?
2. Do you have or have you ever had:
   - Liver or kidney disease?
   - A blood or bone marrow disorder?
   - A high or low platelet count?
3. Do you take aspirin, NSAID, clopidogrel, warfarin, or heparin?

If yes to any of the above questions, ask additional questions:

1. Do you have a blood relative who has a bleeding disorder, such as von Willebrand disease or hemophilia?
2. Have you ever had prolong bleeding from trivial wounds, lasting more than 15 minutes or recurring spontaneously during the 7 days after the wound?
3. Have you ever had heavy, prolonged, or recurrent bleeding after surgical procedures, such as tonsillectomy?
4. Have you ever had bruising, with minimal or no apparent trauma, especially if you could feel a lump under the bruise?
5. Have you ever had a spontaneous nosebleed that required more than 10 minutes to stop or needed medical attention?
6. Have you ever had heavy, prolonged, or recurrent bleeding after dental extractions that required medical attention?
7. Have you ever had blood in your stool, unexplained by a specific anatomic lesion (such as an ulcer in the stomach or polyp in the colon), that required medical attention?
8. Have you ever had anemia requiring treatment or received a blood transfusion?
9. For women, have you ever had heavy menses, characterized by the presence of clots greater than an inch in diameter and/or changing a pad or tampon more than hourly or resulting in anemia or low iron level?

(Adapted from the National Heart, Lung, and Blood Institute Expert Panel for Assessment of VWD. Reference 65.)
NSAID, non-steroidal antiinflammatory drug.

Type 3 von Willebrand disease refers to a severe quantitative variant of the disease in which von Willebrand factor is nearly undetectable and factor VIII levels are very low. It is often inherited in an autosomal recessive fashion.[69] Type 3 von Willebrand disease is rare, affecting only about 1 person in 1,000,000.[65] The clinical phenotype is severe, reflecting major deficits in primary hemostasis and coagulation.

There is a platelet-type pseudo–von Willebrand disease in which von Willebrand factor is normal but a defect in the platelet glycoprotein Ib receptor causes an increased affinity for normal von Willebrand factor.[69] As a result, platelet-type pseudo–von Willebrand disease is phenotypically similar to type 2B disease but should be distinguished from it because the treatment is different.

Acquired von Willebrand disease is a rare bleeding disorder that is similar to the congenital form of the disease. It has been reported primarily in association with autoimmune disorders, such as systemic lupus erythematosus, lymphoproliferative disorders, myeloproliferative disorders, hypothyroidism, and certain neoplastic diseases such as Wilms tumor and lymphoma.[69,72] It has been reported in situations of high shear stress, such as aortic stenosis. Certain medications have been associated with acquired von Willebrand disease, including valproic acid, griseofulvin, hydroxyethyl starch, and ciprofloxacin.[72] Bleeding manifestations vary from mild to severe, and the condition often resolves with treatment of the underlying disease. Various mechanisms have been proposed, including autoantibodies to von Willebrand factor resulting in rapid removal from the plasma, adsorption to tumor cells or activated platelets, increased proteolysis, or mechanical destruction.[72]

CLINICAL PRESENTATION OF VON WILLEBRAND DISEASE

- Clinical manifestations are variable; some patients are asymptomatic.
- Mucocutaneous bleeding: epistaxis, gingival bleeding with minor manipulation, menorrhagia
- Easy bruising
- Postoperative bleeding

Diagnosis

When a patient has a lifelong history of mucocutaneous bleeding and a family history of abnormal bleeding, the clinician should suspect von Willebrand disease. For a review of clinical questions to ask the patient, refer to the National Heart, Lung, and Blood Institute (NHLBI) guidelines (Table 110–8).[65] Several different laboratory tests are helpful in the diagnosis of this hemostatic abnormality. Initial screening tests include determinations of PT, aPTT, and platelet count. PT is normal, whereas aPTT may be normal or prolonged in relation to the reduction in plasma factor VIII levels. A normal aPTT does not rule out von Willebrand disease; specific laboratory assessment of the von Willebrand factor is required. The platelet count is usually is normal, although thrombocytopenia is common in type 2B and platelet-type pseudo–von Willebrand disease. The bleeding time or PFA-100 may be prolonged but can be normal in patients with milder forms of the disease.

Specific laboratory tests for determining the presence of von Willebrand disease include measurement of von Willebrand factor antigen (vWF:Ag) level, factor VIII assay, determination of von Willebrand factor (ristocetin cofactor) activity, and von Willebrand factor multimer analysis (see Table 110–6). Plasma concentrations of von Willebrand factor increase with age, cigarette smoking, exercise, pregnancy starting in the second trimester, and infection, as well as with use of certain medications, such as corticosteroids, high-dose estrogen birth control pills, and desmopressin.[73] Repeated test measurements may be necessary to make the diagnosis because of physiologic variations in plasma levels.

Electroimmunoassay, immunoradiometric assay, or enzyme-linked immunosorbent assay can be used to quantify vWF:Ag.[69] vWF:Ag levels are known to vary with different ABO blood types.[74] The vWF:Ag level is usually low in types 1 and 2 von Willebrand disease and virtually absent in type 3 disease. Factor VIII levels are normal or mildly decreased in patients with type 1 or 2 disease and very low (<10%) in those with type 3 disease.[69] Ristocetin, an antibiotic that causes platelet aggregation in the presence of functional von Willebrand factor, is used to measure von Willebrand factor activity. The assay is performed by mixing platelet-free patient plasma, normal formalin-fixed platelets, and ristocetin and then quantitating the extent of platelet agglutination. Ristocetin cofactor activity is usually reduced in parallel to vWF:Ag levels in types

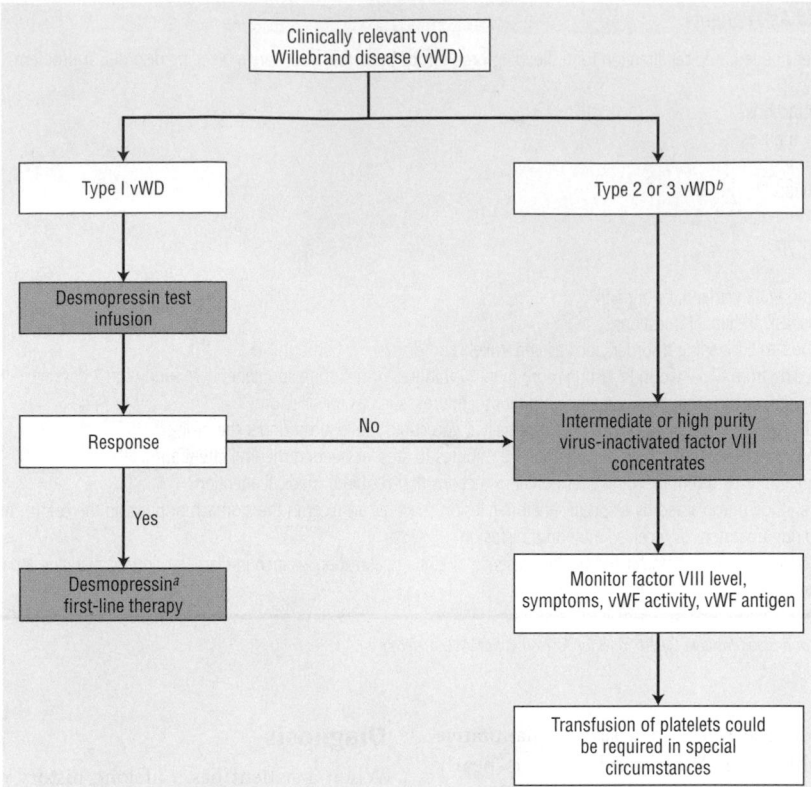

aUse factor VIII concentrate for life-threatening bleeding.
bSome patients with type 2 or 3 von Willebrand disease may respond to desmopressin.

FIGURE 110-4. Guidelines for treatment of von Willebrand disease.

1 and 3 disease and decreased to a greater extent than vWF:Ag in type 2 disease (except type 2B).[71] Ristocetin-induced platelet agglutination is useful for further distinguishing type 2B disease, as a low concentration of ristocetin induces excessive aggregation in type 2B disease. The reader is referred to Table 110–7 for a summary of the various types of von Willebrand disease.

Von Willebrand factor multimers can be analyzed by separating them by size on an agarose gel. All multimer sizes are present in type 1 disease, whereas reduced levels of intermediate- and high-molecular-weight multimers are characteristic of type 2 disease. Type 3 patients lack all types of von Willebrand factor multimers.

The von Willebrand factor gene was cloned in the mid-1980s, and now the role of molecular genetics is coming into play in the diagnosing of von Willebrand disease. Molecular genetic testing for von Willebrand disease is now a feasible option in some instances.[75] Genetic testing may be used to clarify diagnostic uncertainty that may remain after coagulation testing and clinical evaluation.

TREATMENT

von Willebrand Disease

❹ The specific type of von Willebrand disease, as well as the location and severity of bleeding, determines the approach to treatment. Local measures, including pressure, ice, and topical thrombin, can often control superficial bleeding. Systemic treatment is used for bleeding that cannot be controlled in this manner and for prevention of bleeding with surgery. The goal of systemic therapy is correction of platelet adhesion and coagulation defects by stimulating the release of endogenous von Willebrand factor or

by administering products that contain von Willebrand factor and factor VIII.[68] General guidelines for treatment of von Willebrand disease are shown in Figure 110–4. The von Willebrand disease guidelines are available at the NHLBI Web site (http://www.nhlbi.nih.gov/guidelines/vwd/index.htm). In addition, a consensus guideline for the treatment of von Willebrand disease and other bleeding disorders in women was published in 2009.[76]

■ REPLACEMENT THERAPY

❺ The treatment of choice for patients with types 2B, 2M, and 3 von Willebrand disease and for patients with type 1 or 2A von Willebrand disease who are unresponsive to desmopressin (which is discussed in the next section) is replacement therapy with plasma-derived von Willebrand factor–containing products.[77] Several virus-inactivated, intermediate- or high-purity factor VIII concentrates contain sufficient amounts of functional von Willebrand factor.[77] Humate-P is a lyophilized, pasteurized, VWF/FVIII complex (human) that contains the high-molecular-weight multimers of von Willebrand factor.[78] Ultrahigh-purity (monoclonal antibody-derived) plasma-derived products and recombinant factor VIII products contain only negligible amounts of von Willebrand factor and are inadequate for treatment of von Willebrand disease. A very high purity plasma-derived von Willebrand factor concentrate and a recombinant von Willebrand factor product are currently in clinical trials.[79] Because these von Willebrand factor concentrates do not contain appreciable factor VIII, concomitant administration of a factor VIII–containing product may be necessary for patients with severe disease and low levels of factor VIII.[80] Cryoprecipitate contains approximately 80 to 100 units of von Willebrand factor per unit (5–10 times more von Willebrand factor and factor VIII than fresh-frozen plasma), and in the past it was the mainstay of therapy

TABLE 110-9	Replacement Therapy in von Willebrand Disease[a]
Condition	**Therapy**
Major surgery	Maintain factor VIII level ≥50% for 1 week
	Prolonged treatment in type 3 patients (>7 days)
Minor surgery	Maintain factor VIII level ≥50% for 1–3 days
	Maintain factor VIII level >20%–30% for an additional 4–7 days
Dental extraction	Single infusion to achieve factor VIII level >50%
	Desmopressin prior to procedure for type I
Spontaneous or posttraumatic bleeding	Usually single infusion of 20–40 units/kg

[a]The yield of factor VIII after first infusion is similar to that observed in hemophilia A (about 2% increment over baseline amount for every 1 unit/kg of factor VIII infused).

for von Willebrand disease.[69] However, because cryoprecipitate is not virally inactivated, it should not be used as first-line treatment. General guidelines for the dosing of replacement therapy in patients with von Willebrand disease unresponsive to desmopressin are provided in Table 110–9.

■ OTHER PHARMACOLOGIC THERAPY

6 Desmopressin stimulates the endothelial cell release of von Willebrand factor and factor VIII. It is effective for patients with von Willebrand disease who have adequate endogenous stores of functional von Willebrand factor. This group includes most patients with type 1 disease and some patients with type 2A disease. Conversely, desmopressin is not appropriate for patients with type 3 disease, who lack stores of von Willebrand factor.

CLINICAL CONTROVERSY

Some hematologists find desmopressin beneficial in treating patients with type 2B von Willebrand disease, whereas others believe it may exacerbate thrombocytopenia.

Desmopressin is not usually recommended for treatment of type 2B disease because the release of additional abnormal von Willebrand factor may exacerbate thrombocytopenia.[69] However, desmopressin has been reported to be beneficial in some patients with type 2B disease.[69] If desmopressin is used for treatment of type 2B disease, close monitoring is necessary.

The dose of desmopressin used for treatment of von Willebrand disease is identical to that used for treatment of mild factor VIII deficiency, 0.3 mcg/kg diluted in 30 to 50 mL of normal saline and given intravenously over 15 to 30 minutes. In general, patients with von Willebrand disease have a better response to desmopressin than those with hemophilia, with an average threefold to fivefold rise in von Willebrand factor and factor VIII levels.[69] These levels remain elevated for approximately 6 to 8 hours. The response to desmopressin in a given patient is usually consistent, and a trial of desmopressin should establish if the medication will likely be effective for the individual. Desmopressin is preferable to use of plasma-derived products for patients who have an adequate response because desmopressin does not carry a risk of viral transmission. An added benefit is the substantially lower cost of desmopressin compared with the plasma-derived products. (For a discussion of the side effects of desmopressin, see earlier Treatment of Hemophilia A.)

Desmopressin can be administered every 12 to 24 hours, but the response diminishes with repeated treatment. After three to four doses, desmopressin is often no longer effective, and alternative replacement therapy may be necessary if prolonged treatment is required. Laboratory monitoring, including vWF:Ag measurements, factor VIII assays, vWF:activity assessments, and clinical examinations, will determine the adequacy of treatment.

Intranasal administration of desmopressin at the same dosage as that used for mild factor VIII deficiency can be useful for treatment of mild bleeding episodes. One or two doses administered at the start of menses may be helpful in controlling menorrhagia.[81] Oral contraceptives may also be very effective in controlling this symptom. Antifibrinolytic agents, such as aminocaproic acid and tranexamic acid, may be of special value in tissues rich in plasminogen activators, such as the mouth, especially with tooth extractions.[69] They can also be used in the management of epistaxis, gastrointestinal bleeding, and menorrhagia. However, these agents should be avoided in urinary tract bleeding because of the risk of thrombosis and obstruction.

In acquired von Willebrand disease, low levels of plasma von Willebrand factor are the result of accelerated removal of protein from plasma through the action of different pathogenic mechanisms. Acquired von Willebrand disease may be associated with monoclonal gammopathy, lymphoproliferative or myeloproliferative syndromes, or cardiovascular disease. The treatment of the underlying lymphoproliferative disease with rituximab, a monoclonal antibody against CD-20 on lymphocytes, has been reported to be relatively ineffective in the management of the acquired von Willebrand disease.[82] Therefore, intravenous gammaglobulin remains an additional therapy in acquired von Willebrand disease, along with von Willebrand factor concentrate and/or desmopressin.

■ GENE THERAPY

Patients with the most severe bleeding phenotypes of von Willebrand disease (type 3 and some severe cases of types 1 and 2) may be the most likely candidates for gene therapy, which may offer the potential of a long-term, if not lifelong, correction of von Willebrand factor deficiency. Studies placing von Willebrand factor cDNA into a lentiviral vector are currently ongoing.[67] Preclinical trials are being conducted to test the feasibility of gene transfer to be utilized in the management of von Willebrand disease.

OTHER CONGENITAL FACTOR DEFICIENCIES

In addition to deficiencies in factors VIII and IX, congenital deficiencies in fibrinogen, in factors II, V, VII, X, XI, and XIII, and in combinations of factor deficiencies have been reported.[83] Contact factor abnormalities, including deficiencies in factor XII, high-molecular-weight kininogen, and prekallikrein, prolong the aPTT but do not lead to any bleeding diathesis. Identification of these disorders is important so that inappropriate treatment is not given. The only contact factor deficiency associated with bleeding symptoms is factor XI deficiency. Also known as hemophilia C, this deficiency is particularly common in people of Ashkenazi Jewish descent.[83] Bleeding manifestations are variable. Bleeding does not usually occur spontaneously, but excessive bleeding may occur after trauma or surgery. Most other deficiencies are inherited as autosomal recessive disorders and are rare. Some patients with abnormal molecules, such as a dysfibrinogenemia, may have an increased tendency to develop thromboembolic disease. Most of these deficiencies are treated with fresh-frozen plasma. Newer specific concentrates are becoming available. For example, a factor XIII plasma-derived concentrate is available, and recombinant factor VIIa is approved for use in patients with congenital VII deficiency. Cryoprecipitate, which is rich in fibrinogen, can be used to treat patients with fibrinogen deficiency or dysfunctional fibrinogen (dysfibrinogenemia).

COMPLICATIONS OF REPLACEMENT THERAPY

Transmission of bloodborne infectious diseases is always a concern when blood and blood-derived products are used. Most patients with hemophilia who received plasma-derived products were infected with hepatitis viruses and HIV during the 1980s prompting the development of viral inactivation methods for use during the manufacturing of factor concentrates.[29] All currently available plasma-derived factor concentrates come from screened donors and undergo viral inactivation procedures in an effort to reduce the risk of viral transmission. Heat treatment, which includes dry and wet heat, is one method of viral inactivation. Wet heat is applied while the concentrate is in suspension or in solution (pasteurization) and appears to be more effective than dry heat. Other methods of viral inactivation include chemical (solvent detergent) and affinity chromatography with monoclonal antibodies. Solvent detergent treatment inactivates lipid-coated viruses such as HIV and hepatitis B and C, but it is not effective against parvovirus B19, transfusion transmitted virus, hepatitis A, or prions.[29] Parvovirus B19 has been found in both plasma-derived and recombinant factor VIII concentrates (due to the use of albumin as a stabilizer in some recombinant products).[29,30] Parvovirus B19, may be particularly important for patients with hemophilia and HIV infection because it can cause chronic anemia in patients with immune deficiency.[23] Concern has arisen as prions are not inactivated by either solvent detergent treatment or heat, so there is a risk of transmission.[29]

Other complications associated with factor administration include allergic reactions, fever, chills, urticaria, and nausea. PCCs and aPCCs also have the potential to cause thromboembolic complications, including deep-vein thrombosis, pulmonary embolism, myocardial infarction, and DIC, likely related to the presence of activated factors.[14] Antifibrinolytic agents should not be given to patients receiving PCCs or aPCCs to avoid thrombotic complications.

Porcine factor VIII, used in the treatment of patients with inhibitors to factor VIII, is not known to transmit human viruses. However, allergic-type reactions (e.g., fever, chills, skin rashes, nausea, and headaches) have been reported.[54] Patients who experience these reactions can be treated with steroids and/or diphenhydramine. Thrombocytopenia is another potential complication of porcine factor VIII use.[54]

Recombinant factor VIII or IX has a low risk of viral transmission. Adverse effects of these products include metallic taste, mild dizziness, mild rash, burning at the infusion site, and a small drop in blood pressure.

PHARMACOECONOMIC CONSIDERATIONS

Treatment of severe hemophilia is often expensive, with a substantial portion of the cost related to the expense of factor concentrates. The highly purified plasma-derived products and recombinant factor concentrates are considerably more expensive than the low- and intermediate-purity products. However, the viral safety of recombinant products must be weighed against the added cost. Recombinant products are often used, particularly for children with hemophilia. With the widespread use of prophylactic factor replacement regimens to prevent chronic arthropathy, factor usage and cost of treatment have increased over those for on-demand therapy.[14] The positive impact on patient lifestyle must be weighed against the drawbacks of cost, the potential need for permanent venous access, and patient compliance. Finally, the use of immune tolerance therapy is associated with extremely high factor usage and cost, but with the potential benefit of eradicating an inhibitor, a life-threatening complication of hemophilia.

Optimal management of von Willebrand disease starts with adequate identification of the patient's disease type. Desmopressin is considerably less expensive than plasma-derived factor VIII concentrates.[69] It should be the treatment of choice for all patients responsive to the test dose because of its viral safety, reduced cost, and ease of administration.

ACQUIRED COAGULATION DISORDERS

DISSEMINATED INTRAVASCULAR COAGULATION

Systemic inflammation is associated with systemic activation of coagulation. The most severe variant of this is disseminated intravascular coagulation (DIC). Systemic activation of coagulation may be the result of cytokine release as part of an inflammatory response or due to the release of, or exposure to, procoagulant substances. DIC leads to fibrin clot formation in the microvasculature, often with compensatory bleeding owing to consumption of coagulation factors and platelets. Although the causes for DIC can be diverse (see Table 110–10), the pathophysiology leading to DIC is the same once the triggering event occurs (Fig. 110–5). An overwhelming insult leads to the formation of thrombin and plasmin beyond the control of the regulatory systems. Once formed, thrombin leads to the cleavage of fibrinopeptide A and B from fibrinogen, leaving a fibrin monomer. The monomer polymerizes into a clot, leading to microvascular and macrovascular thrombosis while consuming platelets by trapping them in the clots. Thrombosis ultimately decreases blood flow to multiple organs, leading to organ damage. Plasmin cleaves fibrinogen into fibrin(ogen) degradation products (FDPs), which can combine with the fibrin monomer before polymerization. This forms a soluble fibrin monomer that impairs hemostasis and leads to hemorrhage. Some of the FDPs may adhere to platelets, causing platelet dysfunction that may contribute to clinically significant hemorrhage. In addition, plasmin is a proteolytic enzyme that can degrade factors V, VIII, IX, and XI and other plasma proteins. Circulation of plasmin can activate the complement system, leading to red blood cell and platelet lysis. The activated complement system also increases vascular permeability that can cause hypotension and shock.

Complicating this process is an intricate web of feedback systems. Thrombin induces activation of factors V and XI, while it also activates protein C that inhibits the activation of the same. Antithrombin is a serine protease that mediates the antithrombotic effect of heparin. It also inhibits the activation of thrombin, plasmin, and factors IXa, Xa, XIa, and XIIa.[80] Acute DIC is characterized by rapid and extensive depletion of coagulation factors and inhibitors and excessive fibrinolysis in an attempt to compensate for microvascular clotting. Normally, a balanced dynamic process of clotting and fibrinolysis operates to prevent organ dysfunction, bleeding, or clotting. In acute DIC, excessive intravascular coagulation overcomes the normal inhibitory processes. In subacute or chronic DIC, the balance between depletion and synthesis of coagulation factors in the circulation may make the diagnosis difficult, because patients may be asymptomatic. Thrombosis predominates over bleeding in chronic DIC.[1]

In summary, bleeding problems observed during DIC can be the result of consumption of coagulation factors during clotting, depletion or dysfunction of platelets, interference in fibrin formation by FDPs, and lysis of clots by plasmin. Thrombosis occurs in parallel with the bleeding process, and the extent of microvascular obstruction will determine the degree of organ damage.

TABLE 110-10 Conditions Associated with Disseminated Intravascular Coagulation

Cardiovascular

Acute myocardial infarction

Angiopathy

Aortic aneurysm
Aortic balloon assist devices
Giant hemangiomas
Peripheral vascular disease
Postcardiac arrest
Prosthetic devices
Raynaud syndrome

Infectious

Arbovirus
Aspergillus
Candida albicans
Cytomegalovirus
Ebola virus
Gram-negative bacteria
Gram-positive bacteria
Herpesvirus
Histoplasma
Human immunodeficiency virus
Influenza
Kala-azar
Malaria
Mycobacteria
Mycoplasma
Paramyxoviruses
Rocky Mountain spotted fever
Rubella
Typhoid
Varicella
Variola

Intravascular hemolysis

Hemolytic transfusion reaction
Hemolytic uremic syndrome
Minor hemolysis
Massive transfusion

Newborn

Birth asphyxia
Hypothermia
Meconium or amniotic fluid aspiration
Necrotizing enterocolitis
Respiratory distress syndrome
Shock

Obstetrics

Abortion
Amniotic fluid embolism
Fatty liver of pregnancy
Placental abruption
Preeclampsia/eclampsia
Retained fetus syndrome

Pulmonary

Acute respiratory distress syndrome
Empyema
Hyaline membrane disease
Pulmonary embolism
Pulmonary infarction

Tissue injury

Burns
Crush injuries
Extensive surgery
Head trauma
Multiple trauma

Miscellaneous

Acid–base imbalance
Acute liver failure
Amphetamines
Anaphylaxis
Autoimmune diseases
Cholestasis
Chronic inflammatory diseases
Collagen vascular disease
Craniotomy
Extracorporeal circulation
Extracorporeal membrane oxygenation
Fat embolism
Heat stroke
Hemorrhagic telangiectasia
Hepatitis
Leukemia
Lightning strikes
Near drowning
Organic solvent poisoning
Paroxysmal nocturnal hemoglobinuria
Peritoneovenous or pleurovenous shunts
Polycythemia rubra vera
Renal vascular disorders
Severe anoxia
Snake bite
Solid tumors
Transplant rejection

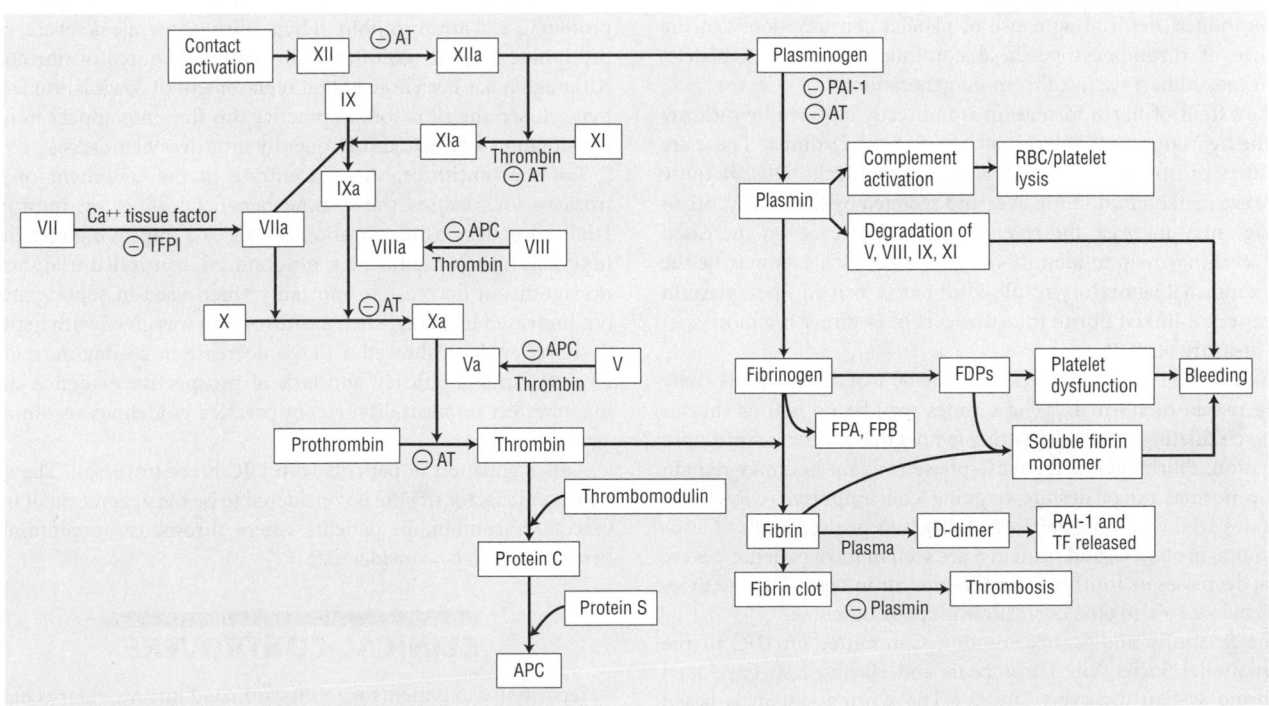

FIGURE 110-5. Pathophysiology of disseminated intravascular coagulation. (APC, activated protein C; AT, antithrombin; FDP, fibrin degradation product; FPA, fibrinopeptide A; FPB, fibrinopeptide B; PAI-1, plasminogen activator inhibitor type 1; RBC, red blood cell; TFPI, tissue factor pathway inhibitor.)

CLINICAL PRESENTATION OF DISSEMINATED INTRAVASCULAR COAGULATION

General

☐ Underlying illness (Table 110–10)

Signs and Symptoms

☐ Bleeding, thrombosis, or both

☐ Petechiae and purpura

☐ Peripheral cyanosis

☐ Hemorrhagic bullae

Laboratory Tests

☐ Elevated D-dimer

☐ Decreased antithrombin

☐ Decreased fibrinogen

☐ Thrombocytopenia

☐ Decreased proteins C and S

☐ Increased fibrinopeptides A and B

☐ Elevated prothrombin fragments 1 and 2

☐ Evidence of end-organ dysfunction or failure

Laboratory Diagnosis

No single laboratory test has adequate sensitivity and specificity to confirm or exclude a diagnosis of DIC. PT, aPTT, and platelet count are used to screen for hemostatic function and indirectly evaluate the degree of coagulation factor consumption and activation. The most common laboratory abnormalities in decreasing order of frequency are: thrombocytopenia, elevated FDP, prolonged PT, prolonged aPTT, and low fibrinogen.[84]

Thrombocytopenia is a sensitive, but not specific, sign of DIC.[84] It is present in up to 98% of DIC cases. Thrombin-induced platelet aggregation is the leading cause of platelet consumption.[84] In the absence of thrombocytopenia, a continuous decline in platelet count may indicate active thrombin generation.

The extent of fibrin formation is indirectly assessed by measuring the byproducts of its lysis, such as FDP or D-dimer. These are measures of fibrinolytic activity and not specific to DIC. Because FDPs are metabolized in the liver and secreted by the kidney, organ damage may increase the level of FDPs. However, an increased FDP level may help to identify compensated DIC, as it may be the only abnormal laboratory result. D-dimer is formed when plasmin digests cross-linked fibrin; thus the level of D-dimer is a more specific measure of FDPs.

PT and aPTT are prolonged in 50% to 60% of cases, but they may be decreased or normal.[84] These times may be normal or shorter due to circulating activated clotting factors that accelerate thrombin formation. Fibrinogen is an acute-phase reactant and may remain in the normal range despite ongoing consumption. A low level indicates DIC with only 28% sensitivity.[84] Depressed levels of antithrombin, protein C, and protein S are seen in most patients. Severe initial decreases in antithrombin levels occur in septic DIC. Activity levels below 50% to 60% correlate with poor outcome.[80]

The Scientific and Standardisation Committee on DIC of the International Society on Thrombosis and Haemostasis developed a scoring system for overt DIC.[84,85] The scoring system is based on routine coagulation tests. The scoring system is only valid if the patient has an underlying condition associated with DIC. The committee has suggested that the score not be used in patients with liver failure or within the first 24 hours in trauma patients. One drawback to this score is that it is static and does not account for the dynamic coagulation changes in DIC. This score has been validated

in children and adults and is sensitive for infectious and noninfectious etiologies. A strong correlation has been established between increasing score and mortality.[84,85]

The most commonly used fibrin-related markers for the DIC score are FDP and D-dimer. D-dimer assays are not standardized and the definition of elevated levels varies among the validation studies for the DIC score. In general, moderate increase has been defined as 2 to 5 times the upper limit of normal and a strong increase is greater than 5 to 10 times the upper limit of normal.

TREATMENT

Disseminated Intravascular Coagulation

❼ If unrecognized and left untreated, DIC may lead to death as a result of hemorrhage or thrombosis. However, there is some controversy regarding optimal treatment because of the different mechanisms and clinical manifestations that can occur with DIC. Even so, there is a consensus that the most important step in therapy for DIC is treatment of the underlying disease.[84] In a pregnant woman with placental abruption or retained placenta in whom the disease is self-limited, delivery of the fetus with the products of conception usually returns hemostasis to normal. In patients who have overwhelming sepsis or shock, antibiotics and treatment of hypotension are the mainstays of therapy. In patients who are receiving maximum treatment for the underlying condition but in whom the process is worsening or in whom bleeding develops, additional treatments may be necessary.

The efficacy of fresh-frozen plasma or platelet transfusions has not been proven in randomized clinical trials but is rational for patients who are bleeding or require invasive procedures.[84] Fresh-frozen plasma replaces clotting factors, fibrinogen, protein S, protein C, and antithrombin. If hypofibrinogenemia is severe, cryoprecipitate may be useful as a concentrated source of fibrinogen. Although it has been argued that replacement of coagulation factors may worsen the situation, in practice this does not appear to make the situation worse, and it frequently improves hemostasis.

Trials of antithrombin concentrate in the treatment of DIC from various causes show some beneficial effect on improving DIC score, decreasing duration of DIC, or improving end-organ function. A large multicenter, randomized, controlled trial showed no significant decrease in mortality when used in septic patients but increased bleeding when antithrombin was given with heparin. A subset analysis showed a 14.6% decrease in 28-day mortality.[86] Due to variable efficacy and lack of prospective evidence showing an effect on mortality, recent practice guidelines recommend against its use.[84]

Anticoagulation in patients with DIC is controversial. The main pathogenic factor of DIC is considered to be the generation of intravascular thrombin. In patients where thrombosis predominates, heparin should be considered.[84]

CLINICAL CONTROVERSY

Heparin use in patients with disseminated intravascular coagulation may prevent the formation of new blood clots. The most common complication of heparin therapy is bleeding, so some clinicians find the risk too high to justify heparin use.

The main advantage of heparin is that it can prevent further thrombosis and consumption of hemostatic factors, but it has no effect on an already established microthrombus within the vasculature. Because the major complication of heparin therapy is bleeding, some experts argue against heparin use in patients with an existing bleeding disorder. Although case reports have shown improvement in individual patients, heparin has not been shown to reduce morbidity or mortality in controlled clinical trials. Heparin rarely restores the coagulopathy to normal, although both the deficiency of coagulation factors and the thrombocytopenia may improve. If the patient does not respond to the replacement of coagulation factors, the addition of heparin may improve the coagulopathy by forming the heparin–antithrombin complex to inhibit thrombin.

Heparin may be given subcutaneously or as a continuous IV infusion. The dosage of heparin for DIC is controversial, ranging anywhere from full-dose to low-dose heparin. Full-dose heparin in adults requires administration of 5,000 units as an IV bolus, followed by a continuous infusion at 1,000 units per hour or according to a weight-based heparin dosing regimen. Some experts advocate low-dose heparin for patients at high risk of bleeding, such as an infusion of 10 units per kilogram per hour in adults.[84] Monitoring of heparin therapy is difficult because the aPTT is often elevated before initiation of heparin therapy, so following D-dimer and fibrinogen levels may be necessary.

Anticoagulation is contraindicated in patients with life-threatening or serious bleeding (e.g., intracranial, retroperitoneal, or pericardial). Patients with symptomatic thromboemboli, extensive fibrin deposition, and persistent coagulation abnormalities despite replacement of hemostatic factors, solid tumors, or chronic DIC may benefit from heparin therapy. Venous thromboembolism prophylaxis is recommended for critically ill, nonbleeding patients with DIC.[84]

Use of antifibrinolytics in patients with DIC is not recommended.[84] Since antifibrinolytics increase fibrin deposition, many experts believe that they are usually contraindicated. In patients with chronic liver disease who manifest dominant fibrinolysis, attempts to inhibit the fibrinolytic system have generally been unsuccessful. Although patients with acute promyelocytic leukemia have hyperfibrinolysis as the dominant clinical feature of their condition, there is no clear role for the routine use of heparin or antifibrinolytic therapy.[87]

Activated protein C modulates coagulation (Fig. 110–5). Activation of protein C may be impaired during sepsis. Drotrecogin alfa (recombinant human activated protein C) administration resulted in an absolute reduction in mortality of 6.1% from severe sepsis without undue bleeding in the Recombinant Human Activated Protein C Worldwide Evaluation in Severe Sepsis (PROWESS) trial.[84] In a post hoc analysis, adults with DIC scores ≥5 have a more favorable response to drotecogin resulting in a 20% relative risk reduction in mortality over those with lower scores.[88] The pediatric trials closed prematurely due to lack of benefit. Patients must be carefully chosen to minimize bleeding complications. A recent retrospective review compared patients treated with bleeding precautions listed in the drotrecogin package insert that were not allowed in the PROWESS trial with those who did not.[89] Examples of these bleeding precautions include concurrent heparin use, platelet inhibitor use within 7 days, platelet count less than 30,000 cells/mm³ (30 × 10⁹/L), and recent surgery. This review found serious bleeding events in 35% of patients with any baseline bleeding precaution versus only 3.8% in patients without.[89]

Evaluation of Therapeutic Outcomes

The management of DIC is surrounded by controversy, and the optimal approach to these patients is still to be determined. Diagnosis and treatment of the underlying disease should be the goal in all cases. Determination of the dominant process

(i.e., hemorrhage vs. thrombosis) can help focus the treatment approach but is often impossible.

Risk versus benefit, as well as any contraindications, should be considered at the start of any given therapy for each patient. Monitoring therapy for DIC with laboratory tests can be difficult because the underlying process can cause a variety of laboratory abnormalities. Trending of the DIC score over time may offer some benefit. In addition, it is important to combine laboratory parameters with clinical assessment to make rational treatment adjustments. Aggressive hemodynamic stabilization and other supportive measures to prevent organ failure are also important in the overall management and prognosis of patients with DIC.

VITAMIN K DEFICIENCY

Vitamin K is a fat-soluble vitamin. Vitamin K_1, phytonadione, is found in green vegetables. Bacteria in the large intestine produce vitamin K_2, the menaquinones, which require bile salts to be solubilized and absorbed.[90] Vitamin K_3, manadion, is a synthetic, water-soluble product associated with hemolytic anemia, indirect hyperbilirubinemia, and kernicterus when given in high doses.[90]

Vitamin K is a cofactor for activation of factors II, VII, IX, and X.[90] Vitamin K is required for γ-carboxylation of these clotting factors. Without vitamin K, these factors cannot bind calcium or bind to negatively charged phospholipid membranes and thus remain inactive precursors. Vitamin K is also necessary for the active forms of proteins C and S, which inhibit factors Va and VIIIa.[90] In most clinical situations, vitamin K deficiency causes a bleeding diathesis as a result of marked deficiency of factors II, VII, IX, and X referred to as vitamin K deficiency bleeding (VKDB). A diagnosis of VKDB is considered if the INR is ≥4 or PT ≥4 seconds above normal in the presence of a normal platelet count and fibrinogen level and the absence of a known etiology.[90] VKDB can be confirmed if coagulation tests normalize within 2 hours of parenteral vitamin K administration.[90]

Hemorrhagic Disease of the Newborn

Newborns have limited vitamin K stores at birth since transplacental passage is limited.[90] The level may continue to fall during the neonatal period because the infant's gut has not had sufficient time to undergo bacterial colonization, so the infant lacks hepatic stores. Normal menaquinone stores are not present in the liver until 2 to 3 months of age.[90] Breast milk contains a low content of vitamin K in comparison with infant formulas; therefore, breast-fed infants are more vulnerable to developing VKDB.[90] Premature infants are at increased risk for VKDB.[90]

Bleeding within 24 hours of birth, early VKDB, is almost exclusively the result of maternal ingestion of drugs that inhibit vitamin K, such as carbamazepine, phenytoin, barbiturates, warfarin, rifampin, or isoniazid. The incidence of drug-induced early VKDB without maternal vitamin K supplementation is 6% to 12%.[90] Clinical presentation is severe bleeding, usually intracranial or intraabdominal.

Classic VKDB usually appears during the first week of life and results from the lack of prophylactic vitamin K administration at birth. The incidence of classic VKDB is less than 2% without supplementation. Clinical presentation is often mild consisting of bruising, umbilical bleeding, or gastrointestinal bleeding.

Risk factors for late VKDB, which occurs at 2 to 12 weeks, include cholestatic liver disease, cystic fibrosis, α_1-antitrypsin deficiency, exclusive breast-feeding, and failure to give adequate vitamin K at birth.[90] The incidence of late VKDB is approximately 1 in 20,000 births without supplementation.[90] Clinical presentation is severe bleeding, most commonly intracranial (50%) with a mortality rate of 20%.[90] Use of oral vitamin K at birth is associated with a higher incidence of late VKDB most likely due to a lack of compliance with the long treatment course required. It is presumed that the intramuscular route of administration allows the vitamin K to act as a depot preparation and may explain the virtual eradication of late VKDB with this route.

The levels of vitamin K–dependent coagulation factors are low at birth. Without adequate vitamin K, these levels may fall even further. In this situation, PT and aPTT are prolonged, but the thrombin time, fibrinogen level, and platelet count are normal. Most infants achieve adult levels by 6 months of age if intramuscular phytonadione was given at birth.

❽ In the United States, infants usually receive 1 mg of phytonadione intramuscularly at birth for VKDB prophylaxis. Reduced doses are recommended for preterm infants: 0.3 mg for birth weight less than 1,000 g and 0.5 mg for those 1,000 to 1,500 g at birth.[90] The speed of repletion depends on the amount of milk or formula received. Controversy has arisen over whether the high plasma vitamin K levels achieved with intramuscular injection lead to an increased incidence of childhood cancer. This risk has not been substantiated, and the benefits of widespread use outweigh the minimal risk.[91] Fresh-frozen plasma is used to treat life-threatening hemorrhages.

Malabsorption

Patients may become deficient in vitamin K as a result of poor nutrition or malabsorption. A careful dietary history is important in this regard. Broad-spectrum antibiotics may sterilize the large intestine and prevent vitamin K_2 production.

Vitamin K absorption depends on both bile acids and pancreatic enzymes to create micelles.[90] Malabsorption resulting from diseases of the intestines or pancreas, such as cystic fibrosis, Crohn disease, ulcerative colitis, cholestatic liver disease, celiac disease, amyloidosis, Whipple disease, and short-bowel syndrome, may cause abnormal development in children, weight loss, muscle wasting, steatorrhea, vitamin deficiencies, and anemia. Significant malabsorption can occur even without the symptoms of diarrhea or steatorrhea. VKDB may be the first sign of malabsorption.

TREATMENT

Vitamin K Deficiency

Phytonadione is used to treat vitamin K deficiency. The dose, frequency, and duration of vitamin K administration depend on the severity of the deficiency and the patient's response. Vitamin K can be administered orally, intramuscularly, subcutaneously, or intravenously. After an oral dose of vitamin K_1, blood coagulation factors increase within 6 to 12 hours. When vitamin K_1 is administered parenterally, PT may take 12 to 24 hours to normalize, although improvement usually occurs within 1 to 2 hours. Failure of vitamin K_1 to correct PT after 48 hours should raise suspicion about the etiology of the coagulation abnormality (e.g., liver disease).

The appropriate route of administration depends on the severity and the cause of the vitamin K deficiency. For instance, in patients with severe hypoprothrombinemia, it is best to avoid the intramuscular route because of the risk of hematoma formation. Due to polyethoxylated castor oil use as an emulsifier causing rare anaphylactic reactions when phytonadione is given intravenously, this route often is restricted to patients who are thrombocytopenic or unable to absorb the drug via the gastrointestinal tract.[90] Vitamin K can be administered subcutaneously to patients without intravenous access. Patients with life-threatening bleeding should receive

fresh-frozen plasma as a source of vitamin K–dependent factors to ensure immediate correction.

Patients with malabsorption, cholestasis, or obstructive jaundice may require parenteral administration of vitamin K. Phytonadione 10 mg weekly usually is sufficient in adults. Children with chronic cholestasis receiving 2.5 to 5 mg orally 2 to 7 times per week continue to have low vitamin K levels, but normal PT.[90] Doses sufficient to maintain normal PT may not be enough for osteocalcin carboxylation and may not prevent osteopenia.[90] Patients on long-term total parenteral nutrition should receive daily supplementation.

COAGULOPATHY AND LIVER DISEASE

Bleeding disorders can be associated with acute or chronic liver disease. The degree of coagulopathy correlates with the degree of hepatocellular disease. The liver synthesizes the blood coagulation factors and inhibitors of coagulation (e.g., antithrombin and proteins C and S), so patients are at risk for bleeding and clotting. All clotting factors except factor VIII and von Willebrand factor are decreased in liver failure.[6] Vitamin K–dependent clotting factors may be defective due to decreased gamma-carboxylation secondary to vitamin K deficiency.[92] The ability of the liver to clear activated clotting factors and their degradation products is reduced with liver failure. Primary fibrinolysis occurs due to decreased levels of the inhibitors of plasmin activation.[6,93]

Dysfibrinogenemia, portal hypertension, endothelial dysfunction, and renal failure may also confound the situation in patients with advanced disease.[92] Platelet count and function are decreased in patients with liver disease. Hypersplenism is the main cause of thrombocytopenia. Decreased platelet function may result from increased production of endothelial-derived platelet inhibitors. The development of DIC may worsen the coagulopathy.

PT, aPTT, and thrombin time are useful in screening for a deficiency of liver-dependent factors. PT is sensitive to deficiencies in the vitamin K–dependent factors. International Normalized Ratio should not be used in these patients unless the relevant international sensitivity index for this category of patients is used.[6] aPTT helps to determine deficiencies in factor IX and other factors. The accuracy of PT/aPTT in patients with cirrhosis is dependent on many factors, and these are often poor predictors of bleeding.[6,92] Thrombin time can help to detect hypofibrinogenemia, dysfibrinogenemia, and the presence of FDPs that interfere with fibrin polymerization. Defects in polymerization may occur before severe hypofibrinogenemia and may be an indication of the degree of liver dysfunction. Relatively stable platelet count, normal or high factor VIII, and normal D-dimer should distinguish from DIC.

Factor V is synthesized by hepatic cells but is not dependent on vitamin K. Therefore, it may be useful in distinguishing vitamin K deficiency from liver disease. Deficiency of antithrombin occurs with severe hepatocellular disease and may contribute to the development of DIC. In acute hepatic failure, the level of plasminogen may be low, reflecting decreased synthesis or increased catabolism associated with DIC.

TREATMENT

Coagulopathy and Liver Disease

The inherent problem with treating patients with liver dysfunction prophylactically or in response to coagulopathy is the inadequacy of conventional laboratory tests to measure the bleeding risk. Despite this, correction of coagulation parameters (e.g., PT and aPTT) prior to an invasive procedure is common practice.[92] Major bleeding may occur with normal coagulation parameters secondary to esophageal varices or peptic ulcer disease. To ensure that vitamin K deficiency is not contributing to the abnormalities, adults may receive 10 mg of vitamin K for 3 days. Treatment of the coagulopathy associated with liver disease is recommended for overt bleeding.

When a patient bleeds in association with a coagulopathy, replacement therapy with platelets and fresh-frozen plasma may decrease bleeding. Fresh-frozen plasma supplies all of the missing coagulation factors, but fluid overload may exacerbate portal hypertension. If fluid overload becomes an issue, plasma exchange may be considered. If the patient has ascites, the half-life of many of these factors is decreased, and correcting the coagulopathy is difficult. PCCs can be given, but they may increase the risk of intravascular coagulation and cause DIC if not already present. In general, use of these concentrates is not recommended. Only when administration of fresh-frozen plasma does not correct the coagulopathy and the patient continues to have serious bleeding should PCCs be considered.

The use of antifibrinolytic drugs is controversial. Aminocaproic acid is effective in decreasing soft tissue and subcutaneous bleeding.[93] Aprotinin has variable effect on decreasing blood transfusions during liver transplantation surgery.[93] Antithrombin concentrates have been evaluated in fulminant liver failure with no benefit on mortality, clinical complications, or coagulation laboratory findings. Desmopressin may decrease the bleeding time in patients with liver failure, but clinical trials in cirrhosis have been disappointing.[92]

Recombinant human factor VIIa augments thrombin burst at the site of bleeding, enhances platelet action despite thrombocytopenia or renal failure, and has the advantage of not causing fluid overload. Administration of recombinant factor VIIa has been successful for liver biopsies but not effective in treating variceal bleeding.[93] Recombinant human factor VIIa improves PT and INR, but that has not resulted in a clear reduction in bleeding for these patients.[93] The greatest risk is the risk of thrombosis. The duration of effect is generally 2 to 4 hours.[92,93]

ABBREVIATIONS

aPCC: activated prothrombin complex concentrate

aPTT: activated partial thromboplastin time

BU: Bethesda unit

DIC: disseminated intravascular coagulation

FDP: fibrin degradation product

HIV: human immunodeficiency virus

NHLBI: National Heart, Lung, and Blood Institute

PAI-1: plasminogen activator inhibitor type 1

PCC: prothrombin complex concentrate

PT: prothrombin time

VKDB: vitamin K deficiency bleeding

vWF:Ag: von Willebrand factor antigen

REFERENCES

1. Furie B, Furie BC. Mechanisms of Thrombus Formation. N Engl J Med 2008;359(9):938–49.
2. Lippi G, Favaloro EJ, Franchini M, Guidi GC. Milestones and perspectives in coagulation and hemostasis. Semin Thromb Hemost 2009;35(1):9–22.
3. Tilley R, Mackman N. Tissue factor in hemostasis and thrombosis. Semin Thromb Hemost 2006;32:5–10.
4. Wiman B. The fibrinolytic enzyme system: Basic principles and links to venous and arterial thrombosis. Hematol Oncol Clin North Am 2000;14:325–38.
5. Harrison P. The role of PFA-100 testing in the investigation and management of haemostatic defects in children and adults. Br J Haematol 2005;130:3–10.
6. Tripodi A. Tests of coagulation in liver disease. Clin Liver Dis 2009;13:55–61.
7. Rosendaal FR, Briet E. The increasing prevalence of haemophilia. Thromb Haemost 1990 Feb 19;63(1):145.
8. Soucie JM, Evatt B, Jackson D. Occurrence of hemophilia in the United States. The Hemophilia Surveillance System Project Investigators. Am J Hematol 1998 Dec;59(4):288–294.
9. David D, Morais S, Ventura C, Campos M. Female haemophiliac homozygous for the factor VIII intron 22 inversion mutation, with transcriptional inactivation of one of the factor VIII alleles. Haemophilia 2003 Jan;9(1):125–130.
10. Shetty S, Ghosh K, Mohanty D. Hemophilia B in a female. Acta Haematol 2001;106(3):115–117.
11. Espinos C, Lorenzo JI, Casana P, Martinez F, Aznar JA. Haemophilia B in a female caused by skewed inactivation of the normal X-chromosome. Haematologica 2000 Oct;85(10):1092–1095.
12. Favier R, Lavergne JM, Costa JM, Caron C, Mazurier C, Viemont M, Delpech M, Valleix S. Unbalanced X-chromosome inactivation with a novel FVIII gene mutation resulting in severe hemophilia A in a female. Blood 2000;96(13):4373–4375.
13. Weinspach S, Siepermann M, Schaper J, Sarikaya-Seiwert S, Rieder H, Gerigk M, Hohn T, Laws HJ. Intracranial hemorrhage in a female leading to the diagnosis of severe hemophilia A and Turner syndrome. Klin Padiatr 2009;221(3):167–171.
14. Lee C, Berntorp E, Hoots W, eds. Textbook of Hemophilia. Malden, MA: Blackwell Publishing Ltd; 2005.
15. Dunn AL, Abshire TC. Recent advances in the management of the child who has hemophilia. Hematol Oncol Clin North Am 2004;18(6):1249–1276, viii.
16. Lakich D, Kazazian HH, Jr., Antonarakis SE, Gitschier J. Inversions disrupting the factor VIII gene are a common cause of severe haemophilia A. Nat Genet 1993;5(3):236–241.
17. Bagnall RD, Waseem N, Green PM, Giannelli F. Recurrent inversion breaking intron 1 of the factor VIII gene is a frequent cause of severe hemophilia A. Blood 2002;99(1):168–174.
18. Kurachi K, Davie EW. Isolation and characterization of a cDNA coding for human factor IX. Proc Natl Acad Sci U S A 1982;79(21):6461–6464.
19. Crossley M, Ludwig M, Stowell KM, De Vos P, Olek K, Brownlee GG. Recovery from hemophilia B Leyden: An androgen-responsive element in the factor IX promoter. Science 1992;257(5068):377–379.
20. Picketts DJ, Lillicrap DP, Mueller CR. Synergy between transcription factors DBP and C/EBP compensates for a haemophilia B Leyden factor IX mutation. Nat Genet 1993;3(2):175–179.
21. Kurachi S, Huo JS, Ameri A, Zhang K, Yoshizawa AC, Kurachi K. An age-related homeostasis mechanism is essential for spontaneous amelioration of hemophilia B Leyden. Proc Natl Acad Sci U S A 2009;106(19):7921–7926.
22. Orkin S, Nathan D, Ginsburg D, Look A, Fisher D, Lux S, eds. Nathan and Oski's Hematology of Infancy and Childhood. 7th ed. Philadelphia, PA: Saunders Elsevier; 2009.
23. Bolton-Maggs PH, Pasi KJ. Haemophilias A and B. Lancet 2003 May 24;361(9371):1801–9.
24. Ljung R, Tedgard U. Genetic counseling of hemophilia carriers. Semin Thromb Hemost 2003 Feb;29(1):31–6.
25. Peyvandi F, Jayandharan G, Chandy M, Srivastava A, Nakaya SM, Johnson MJ, Thompson AR, Goodeve A, Garagiola I, Lavoretano S, Menegatti M, Palla R, Spreafico M, Tagliabue L, Asselta R, Duga S, Mannucci PM. Genetic diagnosis of haemophilia and other inherited bleeding disorders. Haemophilia 2006;12(suppl 3):82–89.
26. Steele M, Cochrane A, Wakefield C, Stain AM, Ling S, Blanchette V, Gold R, Ford-Jones L. Hepatitis A and B immunization for individuals with inherited bleeding disorders. Haemophilia 2009;15(2):437–447.
27. Ljung RC. Intracranial haemorrhage in haemophilia A and B. Br J Haematol 2008;140(4):378–384.

28. Guidelines on the selection and use of therapeutic products to treat haemophilia and other hereditary bleeding disorders. Haemophilia 2003;9(1):1–23.

29. Valentino LA, Oza VM. Blood safety and the choice of anti-hemophilic factor concentrate. Pediatr Blood Cancer 2006;47(3):245–254.

30. Soucie JM, Siwak EB, Hooper WC, Evatt BL, Hollinger FB. Human parvovirus B19 in young male patients with hemophilia A: Associations with treatment product exposure and joint range-of-motion limitation. Transfusion 2004;44(8):1179–1185.

31. Key NS. Inhibitors in congenital coagulation disorders. Br J Haematol 2004;127(4):379–391.

32. Wight J, Paisley S. The epidemiology of inhibitors in haemophilia A: A systematic review. Haemophilia 2003;9(4):418–435.

33. Gouw SC, van der Bom JG, Auerswald G, Ettinghausen CE, Tedgard U, van den Berg HM. Recombinant versus plasma-derived factor VIII products and the development of inhibitors in previously untreated patients with severe hemophilia A: The CANAL cohort study. Blood 2007;109(11):4693–4697.

34. Ward HJ, MacKenzie JM, Llewelyn CA, Knight RS, Hewitt PE, Connor N, Molesworth A, Will RG. Variant Creutzfeldt-Jakob disease and exposure to fractionated plasma products. Vox Sang 2009;97(3):207–210.

35. Batorova A, Martinowitz U. Continuous infusion of coagulation factors: Current opinion. Curr Opin Hematol 2006;13(5):308–315.

36. Schulman S. Continuous infusion. Haemophilia 2003;9(4):368–375.

37. Lethagen S. Desmopressin in mild hemophilia A: Indications, limitations, efficacy, and safety. Semin Thromb Hemost 2003;29(1):101–106.

38. Castaman G. Desmopressin for the treatment of haemophilia. Haemophilia 2008;14(suppl 1):15–20.

39. Shapiro AD, Di Paola J, Cohen A, Pasi KJ, Heisel MA, Blanchette VS, Abshire TC, Hoots WK, Lusher JM, Negrier C, Rothschild C, Roth DA. The safety and efficacy of recombinant human blood coagulation factor IX in previously untreated patients with severe or moderately severe hemophilia B. Blood 2005;105(2):518–525.

40. Berntorp E, Bjorkman S. The pharmacokinetics of clotting factor therapy. Haemophilia 2003;9(4):353–359.

41. Luu H, Ewenstein B. FEIBA safety profile in multiple modes of clinical and home-therapy application. Haemophilia 2004;10(suppl 2):10–16.

42. Shapiro AD, Ragni MV, Lusher JM, Culbert S, Koerper MA, Bergman GE, Hannan MM. Safety and efficacy of monoclonal antibody purified factor IX concentrate in previously untreated patients with hemophilia B. Thromb Haemost 1996;75(1):30–35.

43. Bjorkman S. Prophylactic dosing of factor VIII and factor IX from a clinical pharmacokinetic perspective. Haemophilia 2003;9(suppl 1):101–108; discussion 109–110.

44. Berntorp E, Astermark J, Bjorkman S, Blanchette VS, Fischer K, Giangrande PL, Gringeri A, Ljung RC, Manco-Johnson MJ, Morfini M, Kilcoyne RF, Petrini P, Rodriguez-Merchan EC, Schramm W, Shapiro A, van den Berg HM, Hart C. Consensus perspectives on prophylactic therapy for haemophilia: summary statement. Haemophilia 2003;9(suppl 1):1–4.

45. Petrini P. How to start prophylaxis. Haemophilia 2003;9(suppl 1):83–85; discussion 86–87.

46. van den Berg HM, Fischer K. Prophylaxis for severe hemophilia: Experience from Europe and the United States. Semin Thromb Hemost 2003;29(1):49–54.

47. Astermark J. When to start and when to stop primary prophylaxis in patients with severe haemophilia. Haemophilia 2003;9(suppl 1):32–36; discussion 37.

48. Panicker J, Warrier I, Thomas R, Lusher JM. The overall effectiveness of prophylaxis in severe haemophilia. Haemophilia 2003;9(3):272–278.

49. Manco-Johnson MJ, Abshire TC, Shapiro AD, Riske B, Hacker MR, Kilcoyne R, Ingram JD, Manco-Johnson ML, Funk S, Jacobson L, Valentino LA, Hoots WK, Buchanan GR, DiMichele D, Recht M, Brown D, Leissinger C, Bleak S, Cohen A, Mathew P, Matsunaga A, Medeiros D, Nugent D, Thomas GA, Thompson AA, McRedmond K, Soucie JM, Austin H, Evatt BL. Prophylaxis versus episodic treatment to prevent joint disease in boys with severe hemophilia. N Engl J Med 2007;357(6):535–544.

50. Fischer K, Van Den Berg M. Prophylaxis for severe haemophilia: Clinical and economical issues. Haemophilia 2003;9(4):376–381.

51. Ljung R. Central venous lines in haemophilia. Haemophilia 2003;9(suppl 1):88–92; discussion 93.

52. Ljung R. The risk associated with indwelling catheters in children with haemophilia. Br J Haematol 2007;138(5):580–586.

53. Wight J, Paisley S, Knight C. Immune tolerance induction in patients with haemophilia A with inhibitors: a systematic review. Haemophilia 2003;9(4):436–463.

54. Lloyd Jones M, Wight J, Paisley S, Knight C. Control of bleeding in patients with haemophilia A with inhibitors: a systematic review. Haemophilia 2003;9(4):464–520.

55. Shibata M, Shima M, Misu H, Okimoto Y, Giddings JC, Yoshioka A. Management of haemophilia B inhibitor patients with anaphylactic reactions to FIX concentrates. Haemophilia 2003;9(3):269–271.

56. Hedner U. Mechanism of action of factor VIIa in the treatment of coagulopathies. Semin Thromb Hemost 2006;32(suppl 1):77–85.

57. von Depka M. Managing acute bleeds in the patient with haemophilia and inhibitors: options, efficacy and safety. Haemophilia 2005;11 (suppl 1):18–23.

58. Paisley S, Wight J, Currie E, Knight C. The management of inhibitors in haemophilia A: Introduction and systematic review of current practice. Haemophilia 2003;9(4):405–417.

59. Gringeri A, Mantovani LG, Scalone L, Mannucci PM. Cost of care and quality of life for patients with hemophilia complicated by inhibitors: The COCIS Study Group. Blood 2003;102(7):2358–2363.

60. Collins PW. Novel therapies for immune tolerance in haemophilia A. Haemophilia 2006;12(suppl 6):94–100; discussion 101.

61. Viiala NO, Larsen SR, Rasko JE. Gene therapy for hemophilia: Clinical trials and technical tribulations. Semin Thromb Hemost 2009;35(1):81–92.

62. Walsh CE. Gene therapy progress and prospects: Gene therapy for the hemophilias. Gene Ther 2003;10(12):999–1003.

63. Dunn AL. Management and prevention of recurrent hemarthrosis in patients with hemophilia. Curr Opin Hematol 2005;12(5):390–394.

64. Fernandez-Palazzi F, Caviglia HA, Salazar JR, Lopez J, Aoun R. Intraarticular dexamethasone in advanced chronic synovitis in hemophilia. Clin Orthop Relat Res 1997(343):25–29.

65. Nichols WL, Rick ME, Ortel TL. Clinical and laboratory diagnosis of von Willebrand disease: A synopsis of the 2008 NHLBI/NIH guidelines. Am J Hematol 2009;84:366–370.

66. Kreutz W. Von Willebrand's disease: From discovery to therapy—milestones in the last 25 years. Haemophilia 2008;14(suppl 5):1–2.

67. DeMeyer SF, Deckmyn H, Vanhoorelbeke K. Von Willebrand factor to the rescue. Blood 2009;113:5049–5057.

68. Reininger AJ. Function of von Willebrand factor in haemostasis and thrombosis. Haemophilia2008;14(suppl 5):11–26.

69. Federici AB, Castaman G, Mannucci PM. Guidelines for the diagnosis and management of von Willebrand disease in Italy. Haemophilia 2002; 8:607–621.

70. Budde U. Diagnosis of von Willebrand disease subtypes: Implications for treatment. Haemophilia 2008;14(suppl 5):27–38.

71. Federici AB, Mannucci PM. Advances in the genetics and treatment of von Willebrand disease. Curr Opin Pediatr 2002;14:23–33.

72. Mohri H. Acquired von Willebrand syndrome: Features and management. Am J Hematol 2006;81:616–623.

73. Kouides PA. Aspects of the laboratory identification of von Willebrand disease in women. Semin Thromb Hemost 2006;32:480–484.

74. Gill JC, Endres-Brooks J, Bauer PJ, Marks WJJ, Montgomery RR. The effect of ABO blood group on the diagnosis of von Willebrand disease. Blood 1987;69:1691–1695.

75. James P, Lillicrap DP. The role of molecular genetics in diagnosing von Willebrand disease. Semin Thromb Hemost 2008;34:502–508.

76. James AH, Kouides PA, Abdul-Kadir R. Von Willebrand disease and other bleeding disorders in women: Consensus on diagnosis and management from an international expert panel. Am J Obstet Gynecol 2009;201(1):12e1–18.

77. Schramm W. Haemate P. Von Willebrand factor/factor VIII concentrate: 25 years of clinical experience. Haemophilia 2008;14(suppl 5):3–10.

78. Auerswald G, Kreutz W. Haemate P/Humate P for the treatment of von Willebrand disease: Considerations for use and clinical experience. Haemophilia 2008;14(suppl 5):39–46.

79. Berntorp E. Prophylaxis in von Willebrand disease. Haemophilia 2008;14(suppl 5):47–53.

80. Bolton-Maggs PH, Lillicrap DP, Goudemand J, Berntorp E. Von Willebrand disease update: Diagnostic and treatment dilemmas. Haemophilia 2008;14(suppl 5):56–61.

81. Mannucci PM. Treatment of von Willebrand's disease. N Engl J Med 2004;351:683–694.

82. Mazoyer E, Fain O, Dhote R, Laurian Y. Is rituximab effective in acquired von Willebrand syndrome? (Letter). Br J Haematol 2008;144:967–968.

83. Peyvandi F, Duga S, Akhavan S, Mannucci PM. Rare coagulation deficiencies. Haemophilia 2002;8:308–321.

84. Levi M, Toh CH, Thachil J, Watson HG. Guidelines for the diagnosis and managment of disseminated intravascular coagulation. Br J Haematol 2009;145:24–33.

85. Toh CH, Hoots WK. The scoring system of the Scientific and Standardisation Committee on Disseminated Intravascular Coagulation of the International Society on Thrombosis and Haemostasis: A 5-year overview. J Thromb Haemost 2006;5:604–606.

86. Kienast J, Juers M, Wiedermann CJ, Hoffmann JN, Ostermann H. Treatment effects of high-dose antithrombin without concomitant heparin in patients with severe sepsis with or without disseminated intravascular coagulation. J Thromb Haemost 2006;4:90–97.

87. Stein E, McMahon B, Kwaan H, Altman JK, Frankfurt O, Tallman MS. The coagulopathy of acute promyelocytic leukaemia revisited. Best Prac Res Clin Haematol 2009;22:153–163.

88. Dhainaut JF, Yan SB, Joyce DE, Pettila V, Basson B. Treatment effects of drotecogin alfa (activated) in patients with severe sepsis with or without overt disseminated intravascular coagulation. J Thromb Haemost 2004;2:1924–1933.

89. Gentry CA, Gross KB, Sud B, Drevets DA. Adverse outcomes associated with the use of drotrecogin alfa (activated) in patients with severe sepsis and baseline bleeding precautions. Crit Care Med 2009;37:19–25.

90. VanWinckel M, De Bruyne R, Van De Velde S, Van Biervliet S. Vitamin K, an update for the paediatrician. Eur J Pediatr 2009;168:127–134.

91. Ross JA, Davies SM. Vitamin K prophylaxis and childhood cancer. Med Pediatr Oncol 2000;34:434–437.

92. Caldwell SH, Hoffman M, Lisman T, Macik BG. Coagulation disorders and hemostasis in liver disease: Pathophysiology and critical assessment of current management. Hepatology 2006;44:1039–1046.

93. Shah NL, Caldwell SH. The role of anti-fibrinolytics, rFVIIa and other pro-coagulants: Prophylactic versus rescue. Clin Liver Dis 2009;13:87–93.

111

Sickle Cell Disease

C. Y. JENNIFER CHAN AND REGINALD MOORE

KEY CONCEPTS

❶ Sickle cell disease is an inherited disorder caused by a defect in the gene for hemoglobin. Patients can have one defective gene (sickle cell trait) or two defective genes (sickle cell disease).

❷ Although sickle cell disease usually occurs in persons of African ancestry, other ethnic groups can be affected. Different mutation variants can result in variation in clinical manifestations.

❸ Sickle cell disease involves multiple organ systems. Usual clinical signs and symptoms include anemia, pain crisis, hepatosplenomegaly, and pulmonary diseases. Sickle cell disease can be identified by routine neonatal screening programs. Early diagnosis allows early comprehensive care.

❹ Patients with sickle cell disease are at risk for infection. Prophylaxis against pneumococcal infection reduces death during childhood.

❺ Hydroxyurea has been shown to decrease the incidence of painful crises, but patients treated with hydroxyurea should be carefully monitored.

❻ Neurologic complications caused by vasoocclusion can lead to stroke. Chronic transfusion therapy programs have been shown to be beneficial in decreasing the occurrence of stroke in children with sickle cell disease.

❼ Patients with fever greater than 38.5°C (101.3°F) should be evaluated, and appropriate antibiotics should include coverage for encapsulated organisms, especially pneumococcal organisms.

❽ Pain episodes can usually be managed at home. Hospitalized patients usually require parenteral analgesics. Analgesic options include opioids, nonsteroidal antiinflammatory agents, and acetaminophen. The patient characteristics and the severity of the crisis should determine the choice of agent and regimen.

❾ Patients with sickle disease should be followed regularly for healthcare maintenance issues and monitored for changes in organ functions

Learning objectives, review questions, and other resources can be found at **www.pharmacotherapyonline.com**.

❶ Sickle cell syndromes, which can be divided into sickle cell disease (SCD) and sickle cell trait (SCT), are a group of hereditary disorders characterized by the presence of sickle cell hemoglobin (HbS) in red blood cells. SCT is the heterozygous inheritance of one normal cell and one sickle cell hemoglobin (HbAS) gene. Individuals with SCT are usually asymptomatic. SCD can be of homozygous or compounded heterozygous inheritance. Homozygous HbS (HbSS) is called sickle cell anemia (SCA); heterozygous inheritance of HbS compounded with another mutation results in sickle cell hemoglobin C (HbSC), sickle cell β-thalassemia (HbSβ^+-thal and HbSβ^0-thal), and some other rare phenotypes.[1,2]

Over the years, much progress has been made in identifying the molecular and functional defects and understanding the relationship between genotypes and clinical severity of the disease. Ongoing research involves investigation of pharmacotherapy with various effects on the pathogenesis of the disease.[1–5]

SCD is a chronic illness with significant burden for family and society.[2,6,7] Frequent crisis episodes can interrupt schooling and result in employment difficulties. Acute complications of the disease can be unpredictable, rapidly progressive, and life threatening. Later in life, chronic organ damage can develop. Because of the complexity and seriousness of the illness, it is essential that comprehensive care is available and that all providers involved have a good understanding of the disease and its management options.[1–3]

EPIDEMIOLOGY

❷ SCD affects millions of people worldwide and is most common in people with African heritage. In particular, the disease is common among those with ancestors from sub-Saharan Africa, India, Saudi Arabia, and Mediterranean countries. In the United States, about 70,000 Americans have SCD occurring in 1 in 500 African American births. Approximately 2 million Americans have SCT with a prevalence rate of 1 in 12 African Americans. The most common SCD genotype is HbSS (~65%), followed by HbSC (~25%), HbSβ^+-thal (~8%), and HbSβ^0-thal (~2%). Other variants account for less than 1% of patients.[2,5,8–10]

In Africa, more than 200,000 infants are born with the disease each year. In some areas of sub-Saharan Africa, SCD occurred in up to 2% of all children. The prevalence rate of SCT in Africa varies across regions, ranging from 15 to 45% in West Africa, 1 to 2% on the North African coast, and less than 1% in South Africa. The frequencies of SCT directly determine the prevalence of SCD at birth. For example, 24% of the Nigerian population are carriers, and the prevalence of SCD is about 20 per 1,000 births, resulting in more than 100,000 infants born with SCD each year.[8–11]

The distribution of SCT reflects the survival advantage in regions (tropical areas) where malaria is endemic as the gene mutation offers partial protection against serious malarial infection.

Abnormal red blood cells (RBCs) are less easily parasitized by *Plasmodium falciparum* than normal RBCs. The incidence of the sickle cell gene in a population correlates with the historical incidence of malaria.[2,8,11]

Other areas with sickle cell mutation are the Arabian Peninsula, the Indian subcontinent, and the Mediterranean region. HbS has been reported in up to 25% in certain Middle Eastern populations and greater than 30% in Greece and Cyprus. Genetic analysis shows that the mutation found in Arabic patients is different from the mutation in those of African descent. Sickle cell gene mutation variants have been associated with different geographic locations and may be responsible for variations in clinical manifestations. In Africa, the variants are Senegal (Atlantic West Africa), Benin (Central West Africa), Bantu (Central African Republic), and Cameroon. Arab-Indian haplotype is seen in certain areas of Saudi Arabia and India. Genetic studies performed through newborn screening programs in the United States showed that Benin haplotype was the most frequent (63%), followed by the Bantu (14%), Senegal (9%), Cameroon (4%), and Saudi Arabia (2%).[2,8,11]

ETIOLOGY

Normal hemoglobin (hemoglobin A [HbA]) is composed of two α chains and two β chains ($\alpha_2\beta_2$). The biochemical defect that leads to the development of HbS involves the substitution of valine for glutamic acid as the sixth amino acid in the β-polypeptide chain. Another type of abnormal hemoglobin, hemoglobin C (HbC), is produced by the substitution of lysine for glutamic acid as the sixth amino acid in the β-chain. Structurally, the α-chains of HbS, HbA, and HbC are identical. Therefore, it is the chemical differences in the β-chain that account for sickling and its related sequelae.[1,2,5,11]

SCA is a form of SCD in which the patient has inherited both genes that code for formation of HbS, one from each parent (HbSS). Figures 111–1, 111–2, 111–3, and 111–4 show the probability of inheritance with each pregnancy for the offspring of parents with HbA, SCT, and SCA. If both parents are carriers, the offspring will have a 25% risk of having SCD and a 50% risk of being a carrier (see Fig. 111–1). β-Thalassemia can be found in conjunction with HbS. Because patients with HbSS and HbSβ^0-thal do not have normal β-globin production, they usually have a more severe course than those with HbSC and HbSβ^+-thal. As discussed earlier, several haplotypes characterize the sickle cell gene, resulting in different clinical and hematologic courses. Included among these types are the three most commonly found

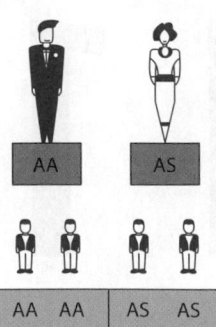

FIGURE 111-2. Sickle cell gene inheritance scheme for one parent with sickle cell trait (SCT) and one parent with no sickle cell gene. Possibilities with each pregnancy: 50% normal (AA); 50% SCT (AS). (A, normal hemoglobin; S, sickle cell hemoglobin.)

in the United States: the Bantu haplotype, characterized by severe disease; the Senegal haplotype, characterized by mild disease; and the Benin haplotype, characterized by a course intermediate to that of the other two haplotypes. Although there are a number of other haplotypes seen around the world, the major types include Saudi Arabian and Cameroon. Both of these types usually follow milder courses of illness.[2,5,11]

PATHOPHYSIOLOGY

Normal adult RBCs contain predominantly HbA (96%). Other forms of hemoglobin are HbA$_2$ (2% to 3%) and fetal hemoglobin (less than 2%). Fetal hemoglobin (HbF) is present predominantly in fetal RBCs. Instead of β chains in HbA or HbS, HbF contains two γ chains ($\alpha_2\gamma_2$). The switch from production of γ chains to β chains occurs shortly before birth. A few red cell clones remain to produce HbF postnatally. Increased production of HbF is seen under severe erythroid stress, such as anemia, hematopoietic stem cell transplantation, or chemotherapy. Both water and hemoglobin content in the RBCs determine the mean corpuscular hemoglobin concentration (MCHC). Passive diffusion and active transport regulate intracellular cation and volume contents, which determine the intracellular viscosity of RBC. Normal RBCs are biconcave shape and able to deform to squeeze through capillaries. As RBCs age, MCHC increases, deformability decreases, and the cells are removed by the mononuclear phagocytic system.[5,11,12,13]

In the pathogenesis of SCD, three known problems are primarily responsible for various clinical manifestations: impaired circulation, destruction of RBCs, and stasis of blood flow. These three problems

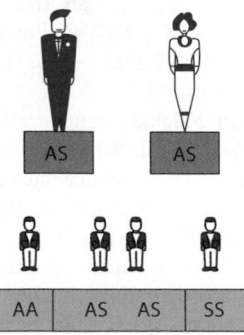

FIGURE 111-1. Sickle cell gene inheritance scheme for both parents with sickle cell trait (SCT). Possibilities with each pregnancy: 25% normal (AA); 50% SCT (AS); 25% sickle cell anemia (SS). (A, normal hemoglobin; S, sickle cell hemoglobin.)

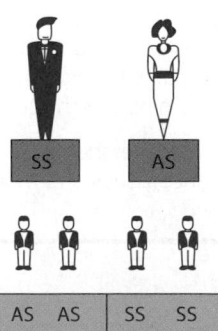

FIGURE 111-3. Sickle cell gene inheritance scheme for one parent with sickle cell trait (SCT) and one parent with sickle cell anemia (SCA). Possibilities with each pregnancy: 50% SCA (SS); 50% SCT (AS). (A, normal hemoglobin; S, sickle cell hemoglobin.)

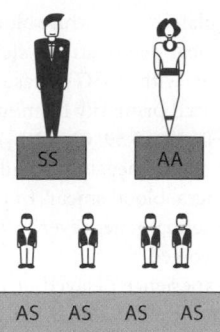

FIGURE 111-4. Sickle cell inheritance scheme for one parent without sickle cell gene and one parent with sickle cell anemia (SCA). Possibilities with each pregnancy: 100% SCT (AS). (A, normal hemoglobin; S, sickle cell hemoglobin.)

probably relate directly to two major disturbances involving RBCs: polymerization and membrane damage (Fig. 111–5).

The solubilities of HbS and HbA are the same when oxygenated. Because of increased hydrophobicity as a result of valine-substituting glutamic acid, solubility of deoxygenated HbS is reduced to 17 g/dL (170 g/L; 10.55 mmol/L). Saturation of deoxy-HbS leads to intermolecular binding and formation of thin bundles of fibers, which initially are unstable, but increased binding of deoxy-HbS eventually results in cross-linking fibers and stable polymers. This process is influenced by MCHC, temperature, intracellular pH, and the amount of HbS. Polymerization allows deoxygenated hemoglobin molecules to exist as a semisolid gel that protrudes into the cell membrane, leading to distortion of RBCs (sickle shaped) and loss of deformability. The presence of sickled RBCs increases blood viscosity and encourages sludging in the capillaries and small venous vessels. Such obstructive events lead to local tissue hypoxia, which tends to accentuate the pathologic process.[12–14]

When reoxygenated, polymers within the RBCs are lost, and the RBCs eventually return to normal shape. This process contributes to the vasoocclusive manifestation in that HbS is able to squeeze into microvasculature when oxygenated, but becomes sickled when deoxygenated. This cycle of sickling and unsickling results in damage to the cell membrane, loss of membrane flexibility, and rearrangement of surface phospholipids. Membrane damage also alters ion transport, resulting in potassium and water loss, which can lead to a dehydrated state that enhances the formation of sickled forms. After continual repetitions of the process, the RBC membrane develops into a more rigid form, irreversibly sickled cell (ISC). Unlike the reversible sickle cells, which have normal morphology when oxygenated, ISCs are elongated cells and remain sickled when oxygenated. More rigid membranes of HbS-containing RBC retard their flow, particularly through the microcirculation. In addition, sickled RBCs tend to adhere to vascular endothelial cells, which further increase polymerization and obstruction.

Intermolecular binding and polymer formation are reduced by HbF and to a lesser degree by HbA_2. RBCs that contain HbF sickle less readily than cells without. ISCs, not surprisingly, have a low HbF level. Increased levels of HbF, as in the case of the Saudi Arabian genotype, result in more benign forms of SCD. The amount of HbF and HbA_2 in relation to HbS influences clinical manifestations and accounts for the variability in severity among different SCD genotypes.

Intravascular destruction of sickle cells can occur at an accelerated rate. The stresses of circulation, and repetitive sickle–unsickle cycles are likely to lead to cell fragmentation. Damage to the cell membrane promotes cell recognition by macrophages. Rigid ISCs are easily trapped, resulting in short circulatory survival and chronic hemolysis. The typical sickled cell survives for about 10 to 20 days, whereas the life span of a normal RBC is 100 to 120 days.

In addition to sickling, other factors are also responsible for the clinical manifestations associated with SCD. Obstruction of blood flow to the spleen by sickle cells can result in functional asplenia, defined as the loss of splenic function with an intact spleen. These patients can also have deficient opsonization. Impaired splenic function increases susceptibility to infection by encapsulated organisms, particularly pneumococcal disease. Coagulation abnormalities in SCD can be the result of continuous activation of the hemostatic system or disorganization of the membrane layer.[1,11–14]

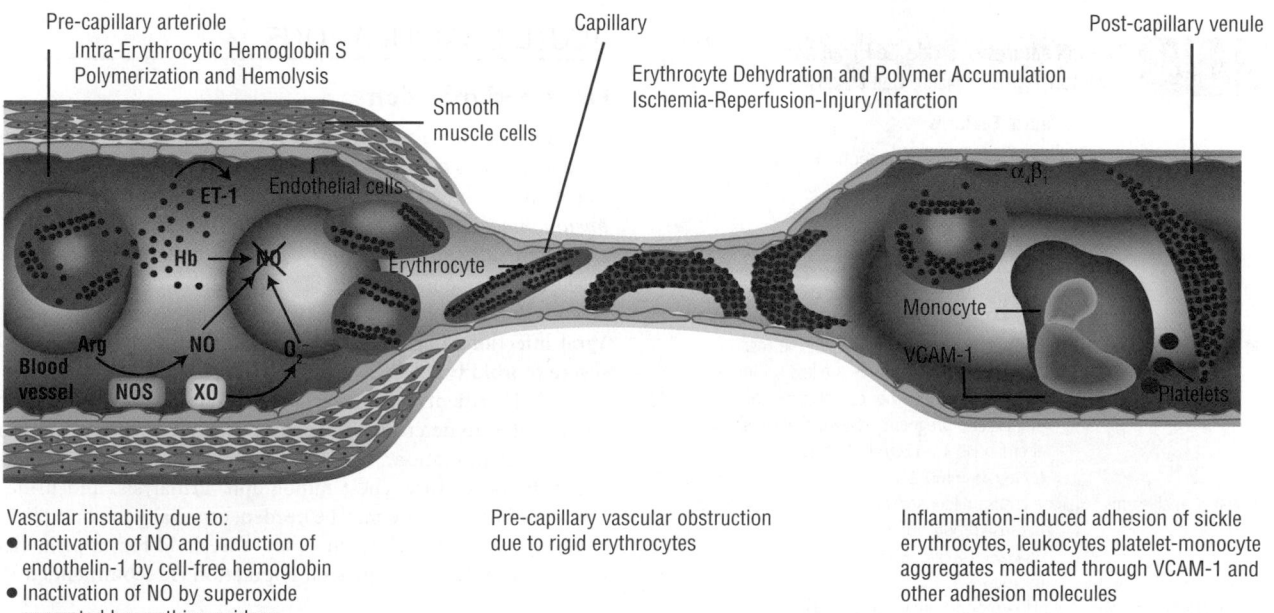

FIGURE 111-5. Pathophysiology of sickle cell disease. (Arg, arginine; ET-1, endothelin-1; Hb, hemoglobin; NO, nitric oxide; NOS, nitrous oxide synthase; VCAM-1, vascular cell adhesion molecule 1; XO, xanthine oxidase.) *(From Kato GJ, Gladwin MT. Sickle cell disease. In: Hall JB, Schmidt GA, Wood LDH. Principles of Critical Care, 3rd ed. New York: McGraw-Hill, 2005:1658.)*

CLINICAL PRESENTATION

❸ SCD is usually identified by routine neonatal screening programs. The sensitivity and specificity of screening methods (isoelectric focusing, high-performance liquid chromatography, or electrophoresis) are 93.1 to 100% and 99.9 to 100%, respectively. For infants with a positive screening result, a second test should be performed by 2 months of age to confirm the diagnosis. More than 98% newborns in the United States are screened for SCD to identify the disease. Even with universal screening, infants with SCD are sometimes not identified at birth because of extreme prematurity, prior blood transfusion, inability to contact family, or clerical errors.[2,5,9]

SCD involves multiple organ systems, and its clinical manifestations vary greatly between and among genotypes (Table 111-1). Persons with SCT are usually asymptomatic and are not considered to have clinical disease. However, some clinical signs and symptoms can occur, and patients should be cautious when participating in exercise under extreme conditions, such as high altitude or military training. Sickling of RBCs in the renal medulla can result in loss of ability to maximally concentrate urine. Patients with such impairment can be at risk of dehydration during periods in which the body normally conserves water. Microscopic hematuria has been observed, and gross hematuria can occur after heavy exercise. An increased incidence of urinary tract infection in women, especially during pregnancy, has been reported.[9,11,15]

The feature presentations of SCD are hemolytic anemia and vasoocclusion. In patients who are homozygous for HbS, anemia usually appears from 4 to 6 months after birth. The delay in presentation is because, during those months, HbF in the infant's RBC is gradually replaced by HbS, which typically leads to attacks of pain frequently accompanied by fever. Pneumonia and splenomegaly are also common findings. Infants can also present with pain and swelling of the hands and feet, commonly referred to as *hand-and-foot syndrome* or *dactylitis*.[1,2,5,7,9]

The usual clinical signs and symptoms associated with SCA include chronic anemia; fever and pallor; arthralgia; scleral icterus; abdominal pain; weakness; anorexia; fatigue; enlargement of the liver, spleen, and heart; and hematuria. Laboratory findings include low hemoglobin level around 8 g/dL (80 g/L; 4.97 mmol/L) and increased reticulocyte, platelet, and white blood cell (WBC) counts. The peripheral blood smear demonstrates sickle cell forms.[1,2,5,8,9]

Presentation of patients with HbSC disease is less severe than that of SCA and is characterized primarily by mild anemia (hemoglobin levels above 9 g/dL [90 g/L; 5.59 mmol/L]), infrequent episodes of pain, persistence of splenomegaly into adult life, and excessive target cells in the peripheral blood smear. In patients with heterozygous HbS and β-thalassemia gene, severity of disease depends on the thalassemia gene involved.[1,2,5,9,11]

Patients with SCD experience delayed growth and sexual maturation. Both height and weight are usually below average, and the poor growth cannot be explained by nutritional factors alone. Fertility problems tend to occur more often, and some menstrual abnormalities are more common in female SCD patients than in normal women. Other typical physical characteristics include a protuberant abdomen with exaggerated lumbar lordosis, usually an asthenic appearance with rather long extremities and tapered fingers, and frequently a barrel-shaped chest.[1,2,5,9,11,16]

The previously high mortality rate of early childhood has been reduced for patients with SCD with availability of public health programs and comprehensive care.[1,9,17] The median survival rate is estimated to be 42 years for males and 48 years for females for HbA, and 60 years for males and 68 years for females for HbSC.[9] Predictors for severe disease in children who are less than 10 years of age include dactylitis before 1 year of age, an average hemoglobin level less than 7 g/dL (70 g/L; 4.34 mmol/L) in the second year of life, and WBC count greater than 13,700 cells/mm³ (13.7 × 10⁹/L) in the absence of infection. Early acute chest syndrome during the first 3 years of life is a predictor for recurrent episodes throughout childhood. Children with concomitant SCD and asthma have increased episodes of acute chest syndrome and stroke and increased mortality. Risk factors for early death in adults with SCD include acute complications such as pain crisis, anemic events, acute chest syndrome, renal failure, and pulmonary disease.[3,5,17–22] Today, with longer survival for SCD, chronic manifestations of the disease contribute to the morbidity later in life.

COMPLICATIONS

ACUTE COMPLICATIONS

Fever and Infection

Functional asplenia and failure to make antibodies against encapsulated organisms contribute to the high risk of overwhelming sepsis in patients with SCD. The most common pathogen is *Streptococcus pneumoniae*. Other encapsulated organisms are *Haemophilus influenzae* and *Salmonella*, and the latter has been known to cause osteomyelitis and pneumonia in SCD. *Mycoplasma pneumoniae* should be considered in older children with infiltrates on chest radiograph. Viral infections (e.g., influenza and parvovirus B19) can result in severe morbidity.[1,5,23,24]

All SCD patients with fever greater than 38.5°C (101.3°F) must be evaluated to determine the extent of sepsis; workup can include physical examination, complete blood count with reticulocyte count, blood culture, chest radiograph, urinalysis, and urine culture. Lumbar puncture may be needed, especially in young children and toxic-appearing children. A low threshold for empiric therapy compared to that in the general population is recommended.[1,5,9,11,24]

Neurologic

Neurologic abnormalities can occur in both adults and children. Vasoocclusive processes occasionally lead to cerebrovascular

TABLE 111-1	Clinical Features of Sickle Cell Trait and Common Types of Sickle Cell Disease
Type	**Clinical Features**
Sickle cell trait (SCT)	Rare painless hematuria; normal Hb level; heavy exercise under extreme conditions can provoke gross hematuria and complications
Sickle cell anemia (SCA)	Pain crises, microvascular disruption of organs (spleen, liver, bone marrow, kidney, brain, and lung), gallstone, priapism, leg ulcers; anemia (Hb 7–10 g/dL [70–100 g/L; 4.34–6.21 mmol/L])
Sickle cell hemoglobin C	Painless hematuria and rare aseptic necrosis of bone; vasoocclusive crises are less common and occur later in life; other complications are ocular disease and pregnancy-related problems; mild anemia (Hb 10–12 g/dL [100–120 g/L; 6.21–7.45 mmol/L])
Sickle cell β^+-thalassemia	Rare crises; milder severity than sickle cell disease because production of HbA; Hb 10–14 g/dL (100–140 g/L; 6.21 –8.69 mmol/L) with microcytosis
Sickle cell β^0-thalassemia	No HbA production; severity similar to SCA; Hb 7–10 g/dL (70–100 g/L; 4.34–6.21 mmol/L) with microcytosis

HbA, hemoglobin A; Hb, hemoglobin.

occlusion that manifests itself as the signs and symptoms of stroke, such as drowsiness, paralysis, transitory or permanent blindness, aphasia, visual disturbances, spinal cord infarction, and convulsions. Behavioral and performance changes can occur in patients with asymptomatic infarction. The risk of cerebral infarct in HbSS is 11% by age 20 years and 24% by age 45 years with a recurrence rate as high as 70% in 3 years. Some patients recover rapidly and completely, although others are left with permanent neurologic deficits. Evaluation of acute events include computed tomography (CT) scan and magnetic resonance imaging (MRI), magnetic resonance angiography (MRA) for asymptomatic infarction, and transcranial Doppler (TCD) ultrasound to detect abnormal velocity and identify high-risk patients. In addition, electroencephalography (EEG) can be used if there is a history of seizure. Some patients who have SCA with no prior history of stroke have been found to have changes on MRI of the brain consistent with infarction or ischemia. These "silent infarcts" have been reported to occur in up to 22% of HbSS patients and can be associated with increased risk of stroke and decreased neurocognitive functions.[1,5,25–28]

Acute Chest Syndrome

Acute chest syndrome is the leading cause of death among patients with SCD. It is characterized by a new pulmonary infiltrate associated with one or more other symptoms (such as cough, dyspnea, tachypnea, chest pain, fever, wheezing, and new-onset hypoxia), and an equivocal response to antibiotic therapy. As many as one-half of patients with SCD experience at least one episode of acute chest syndrome. Pulmonary infarcts often involve the lower lobes of the lungs and are a frequent cause of pleural effusions. Pneumonia occurs most often in the middle and upper lobes. These pulmonary manifestations must be recognized early and managed aggressively because the patient can rapidly progress to pulmonary failure and death.[29–32]

Priapism

Sickling in the sinusoids of the penis can cause priapism, a sustained painful erection that can last several hours or days; 30 to 45% of patients with SCD will present at least one episode of priapism during their lifetime. Impotence has been reported after repeated episodes. Recurrent and severe priapism is a predictor for other end-organ damage. ASPEN (association of sickle cell disease, priapism, exchange transfusion, and neurologic events) syndrome has occurred in some patients with priapism 1 to 11 days after partial exchange transfusion. This syndrome can range from headaches and seizures to obtundation requiring ventilation.[1,9,11,33]

Sickle Cell Crisis

Chronic hemolytic anemia in the SCD patient is periodically interrupted by crises, particularly in childhood (see Table 111–2). Patients with HbSS disease experience crises more often than do patients with HbSC disease or some other variants. Although fever, infections, dehydration, hypoxia, acidosis, and sudden temperature alterations can precipitate crises, multiple factors often contribute to development of a crisis.

Vasoocclusive Pain Crisis The most common type of crisis is the vasoocclusive crisis, which is usually characterized by pain affecting the involved areas, without changes in hemoglobin. Laboratory changes that can be seen include leukocytosis, increased fibrinogen levels, and decreased serum pH and bicarbonate level. Dactylitis (hand-and-foot syndrome) occurs in infancy and early childhood and is characterized by redness and swelling of the dorsal aspects of the hands, feet, fingers, and toes. The episodes are painful but usually do not result in permanent damage.[1,5,8,9,11,34]

TABLE 111-2 Sickle Cell Crisis

Vasoocclusive pain crisis[a]

Clinical features: Acute painful infarction without changes in Hb; almost all patients with SCA will have episodes of acute pain. Recurrent acute crises result in bone, joint, and organ damage and chronic pain. Vasoocclusive crisis most commonly involves the bones, liver, spleen, brain, lungs, and penis. Acute long bone pains can be accompanied by signs of inflammation, making it difficult to differentiate from osteomyelitis. Abdominal involvement can resemble a surgical abdomen. Precipitating factors include infection, extreme weather conditions, dehydration, and stresses.

Signs and symptoms: Deep throbbing pain; local tenderness, erythema, and swelling can be seen. Fever and leukocytosis are common. Dactylitis usually occurs in young infants. Jaundice and increased transaminases present if liver is involved.

Evaluation: Frequent physical examination, CBC, reticulocyte count, and urinalysis; based on symptomatology. The following can be needed: needle aspiration to rule out osteomyelitis, abdominal studies (radiograph, computed tomography scan, etc.), liver function tests, bilirubin, culture, and chest radiograph.

Aplastic crisis[b]

Clinical features: Acute decrease in Hb with decreased reticulocyte count (usually less than 1%); transient suppression of RBC production in response to bacterial or viral infection, most common being parvovirus B19

Signs and symptoms: Headache, fatigue, dyspnea, pallor, and tachycardia; can also present with fever, upper respiratory or gastrointestinal infection symptoms

Evaluation: CBC, reticulocyte count, radiograph, cultures (blood, urine, and throat), evaluation of viral infection (e.g., parvovirus titers)

Acute splenic sequestration crisis[c]

Clinical features: Acute exacerbation of anemia due to sequestration of large blood volume by the spleen. More commonly seen in patients with functioning spleens (e.g., infants and adults with HbSC disease); onset often is associated with viral or bacterial infections; recurrences are common and can be fatal.

Signs and symptoms: Sudden onset of fatigue, dyspnea, and distended abdomen; rapid decrease in Hb and Hct with elevated reticulocyte count, abdominal pain, splenomegaly, vomiting, hypotension, and shock

Evaluation: Close monitoring of vital signs, spleen size, and oxygen saturation, CBC, reticulocyte count, and cultures

CBC, complete blood count; HbSC, sickle cell hemoglobin C; Hb, hemoglobin; Hct, hematocrit; RBC, red blood cell; SCA, sickle cell anemia.

[a]From Montalembert,[1] Driscoll,[5] National Institutes of Health,[9] Stuart and Nagel,[11] and Fellison and Shaw.[34]

[b]From Creary and Williamson et al.,[2] Driscoll,[5] and National Institutes of Health.[9]

[c]From Montalembert,[1] Driscoll,[5] National Institutes of Health,[9] and Stuart and Nagel.[11]

Aplastic Crisis Aplastic crisis is characterized by a decrease in the reticulocyte count and a rapidly developing severe anemia. The bone marrow is hypoplastic. There can be associated pain. The crisis is typically caused by a viral infection, particularly parvovirus B19.[2,5,9,23,24]

Splenic Sequestration Crisis This is a sudden massive enlargement of the spleen resulting from the sequestration of blood from the mononuclear phagocytic system. Hematocrit and hemoglobin concentrations dramatically fall, with reticulocytosis and no evidence of marrow failure or accelerated hemolysis. The trapping of the sickled RBCs by the spleen also leads to a decrease in circulating blood volume, which can result in hypotension and shock. The condition is most often seen in infants and children because their spleens are intact, and can cause sudden death in young children. Repeated infarctions lead to autosplenectomy as the disease progresses; the incidence therefore declines as adolescence approaches.[1,5,9,11]

CHRONIC COMPLICATIONS

SCD manifests in a variety of chronic problems involving multiple organs. Pulmonary hypertension has been reported to be a risk factor for death in adult patients with SCD.[19,35] Pulmonary hypertension is frequently reported in children and adolescents, although its significance has not been established.[36,37] Headache and weakness of one leg or arm is a symptom associated with acute neurologic events, and pseudotumor cerebri presenting with severe headache and blurred vision has also been reported.[25,38]

Bone diseases are common in SCD. Osteonecrosis, particularly of the femoral or humeral heads, causes permanent damage and disability.[39,40] Osteopenia associated with low bone formation has been reported in both boys and girls.[41] Patients with SCD also have an increased incidence of osteomyelitis; the organism most often responsible is *Salmonella*.[5,9,24] In addition to necrosis of joints, chronic leg ulcers can become a difficult skeletal problem. Ulcers are often seen after trauma or infection and are usually slow to heal.[5,9]

Ocular problems seen in patients with SCD include transient monocular blindness, visual field defects from retinal hemorrhage, retinal detachment, vitreous hemorrhage, venous microaneurysms, and neovascularization. The incidence of proliferative retinopathy in SCD patients varies from 5% to 10%. Vasoocclusion in the eye can occur as early as 20 months of age, and clinically detectable retinal diseases usually occur during adolescence and early adulthood. Despite the less systemic manifestations, patients with HbSC develop serious retinal complications more often and earlier. Annual examination with retinal evaluation is recommended for patients with SCD to prevent blindness from retinopathy and other complications.[9,42]

Cholelithiasis is a common occurrence in the SCD patient. It is the result of the chronic hemolysis that results in increased bilirubin production, leading to biliary sludge and/or stone formation. The risk of gallstones increases with age, with 14% younger than age 10 years and 50% by age 22 years. Cholecystitis, exemplified by pain in the right iliac fossa, can be confused with abdominal pain crisis.[5,9,43]

As with any anemia, cardiovascular abnormalities, including cardiac enlargement and various murmurs, can occur in patients with SCD. Patients complain of various degrees of exertional dyspnea, tachycardia, and palpitation because of the decreased oxygen-carrying capacity of the blood. Left ventricular diastolic dysfunction has been reported in 18% of adult patients and is associated with increased mortality, especially in patients with pulmonary hypertension. In children, left ventricular stiffness and left ventricular hypertrophy have been reported, and the progression is speculated to lead to diastolic dysfunction later in life. Acute myocardial infarction in young adults with SCD may not be recognized.[9,44–46]

Renal complications include hematuria, tubular acidosis, proteinuria, and hyposthenuria (inability to concentrate urine maximally). Enuresis, as a result of increased urine production, is a common complaint. Nephrotic syndrome and end-stage renal disease have also been reported in 5% to 10% of patients.[5,9]

Depression and anxiety are more common in children and adults with SCD than in the general population and have a significant impact on quality of life.[47–49] Reduced cognitive function has been reported, even in children with no evidence of cerebral infarction.[2] Delays in growth and sexual development are seen in patients with SCD.[49] Adults with SCD have decreased fertility. Finally, pregnancy introduces an increased risk for the mother with SCD and for the fetus. Some patients can experience increased frequency of pain crisis during pregnancy. The anemia of SCD can lead to intrauterine growth retardation. Preterm labor and premature delivery are common occurrences in mothers with SCD, and the risk of spontaneous abortion is increased. The incidences of cesarean delivery and pregnancy-related complications are higher when compared with mothers who do not have SCD.[9,11,50]

TREATMENT

Sickle Cell Disease

Patients with SCD require lifelong multidisciplinary care. All patients with SCD should receive regularly scheduled comprehensive medical evaluations. The goal of comprehensive care is to reduce hospitalizations, complications, and mortality. Because of the complexity of the disease, a multidisciplinary team is needed to provide medical care, education, counseling, and psychosocial support. Appropriate comprehensive care can have a positive impact on both longevity and general quality of life. This care includes the use of traditional prophylactic and general symptomatic supportive care and the use of newer, more specific therapies aimed at altering hematologic capacity and function.[1,2,5,9,11]

Treatment for patients with SCD involves the use of general measures to meet the unique demands for increased erythropoiesis. Additional interventions can be aimed at preventing or treating complications of the disease. When a crisis occurs, the type and severity of the crisis determine the appropriate therapeutic plan.

■ HEALTH MAINTENANCE

Immunizations

Administration of routine immunizations as recommended by the American Academy of Pediatrics is crucial. In addition to the routine immunizations, SCD patients 6 months and older should receive influenza vaccine annually. Meningococcal vaccine is also recommended for patients older than 2 years of age who are undergoing splenectomy or are functionally asplenic.[9,24,51]

Patients with SCD have impaired splenic function, which increases their susceptibility to infection by encapsulated organisms, particularly pneumococci. Prior to the routine use of penicillin prophylaxis and the development of pneumococcal vaccines, invasive pneumococcal disease was 20- to 100-fold more common in children with SCD than in healthy children. Reduced mortality rate has been associated with the introduction of the pneumococcal vaccines.[17,24,52,53]

Two different pneumococcal vaccines are available. The 13-valent pneumococcal conjugate vaccine (PCV13; Prevnar) induces good antibody responses in infants. Immunization with the PCV13 is recommended for all children younger than 24 months of age. Infants should receive the first dose after 6 weeks of age. Two additional doses should be given at 2-month intervals, followed by a fourth dose at age 12 to 15 months. The 23-valent pneumococcal polysaccharide vaccine (PPV 23; Pneumovax 23) is not recommended for use in children younger than 2 years of age because of poor antibody response. To cover for different serotypes, PPV 23 should be given at 2 years of age, administered about 2 months after the last dose of the PCV7/PCV13 and a booster dose at age 5. The recommended immunization schedule and catch-up schedule for PCV13 and PPV 23 are presented in Table 111–3.[5,9,24,54]

In addition to pneumococcal disease, the risk of meningococcal disease can be higher in SCD. Revaccination with meningococcal conjugate vaccine (MCV4) is recommended for persons with anatomic or functional asplenia due to prolonged increased risk for meningococcal disease. Those patients should be revaccinated 5 years after the previous vaccine if given at age 7 or older or 3 years after the previous vaccine if given between ages 2 and 6.[51]

TABLE 111-3	Pneumococcal Immunization for Children with Sickle Cell Disease
Recommended Schedule	
Previously unvaccinated	
Age 2–6 months	**PCV13 (Prevnar):** 3 doses 6–8 wk apart; then 1 dose at 12–15 months
Age 7–11 months	**PCV13 (Prevnar):** 2 doses 6–8 wk apart; then 1 dose at 12–15 months
Age ≥12–23 months	**PCV13 (Prevnar):** 2 doses 6–8 wk apart
Age 24–59 months	**PCV13 (Prevnar):** 2 doses 6–8 wk apart
	PPV 23 (Pneumovax): 2 doses; first dose at least 6–8 wk after last PCV7/PCV13 dose; second dose 3–5 years after the first PPV 23 dose
Age 5 years or older	**PCV13 (Prevnar):** 1 dose
	PPV 23 (Pneumovax): 2 doses; first dose at least 6–8 wk after last PCV7/PCV13 dose; second dose 3–5 years (for those age 10 years or younger) or more than 5 years (for those older than 10 years) after the first PPV 23 dose
Previously vaccinated	
Age 12–23 months, incomplete PCV7/PCV13 series	**PCV13 (Prevnar):** 2 doses 6–8 wk apart
Age 24–59 months, received four doses of PCV7/PCV13	**PPV 23 (Pneumovax):** 2 doses; first dose at least 6–8 wk after last PCV7 dose; second dose 3–5 years after the first PPV 23 dose
Age 24–59 months, three doses PCV7/PCV13 given before 24 months of age	**PCV13 (Prevnar):** 1 dose
	PPV 23 (Pneumovax): 2 doses; first dose at least 6–8 wk after last PCV7/PCV13 dose; second dose 3–5 y after the first PPV 23 dose
Age 24–59 months, 1 dose PPV 23 given	**PCV13 (Prevnar):** 2 doses 6–8 wk apart; first dose at least 8 wk after PPV 23 dose
	PPV 23 (Pneumovax): second dose 3–5 years after first PPV 23
Age 5 years or older, received PPV 23	**PCV13 (Prevnar):** 1 dose 6–8 wk after PPV 23
	If only received 1 dose of PPV 23 (Pneumovax): Second dose 6–8 wk after PCV7/PCV13 *and* 3–5 years (for those age 10 years or less) or more than 5 years (for those age older than 10 years) after the first PPV 23 dose

PCV7, 7-valent pneumococcal conjugated vaccine; PCV13, 13-valent pneumococcal conjugated vaccine; PPV 23, 23-valent pneumococcal polysaccharide vaccine.
From MMWR.[54]

Penicillin

④ Penicillin prophylaxis until at least 5 years of age is recommended in children with SCD, even if they have been immunized with PCV7 as prophylaxis against pneumococcal infections. Prophylactic treatment should begin at 2 months of age or earlier. An effective regimen that reduces the risk of pneumococcal infections by 84% is penicillin V potassium at a dosage of 125 mg orally twice daily until the age of 3 years, followed by 250 mg twice daily until the age of 5 years. An alternate regimen is benzathine penicillin, 600,000 units given intramuscularly every 4 weeks for children age 6 months to 6 years, and 1.2 million units every 4 weeks for those over 6 years of age for whom continued therapy is warranted. Patients who are allergic to penicillin can be given erythromycin 20 mg/kg per day twice daily. Penicillin prophylaxis is not routinely given in older children, based on a study demonstrating no benefit over placebo beyond the age of 5 years. However, continuation of oral pneumococcal prophylaxis should be evaluated on a case-by-case basis, especially in patients with a history of invasive pneumococcal infection or surgical splenectomy.[5,9,24,54]

CURRENT CONTROVERSY

The need for routine penicillin prophylaxis is controversial in HbSβ⁺-thal patients because these patients have less severe disease.

Folic Acid

Patients with SCD have an increased demand for folic acid because of accelerated erythropoiesis. Conversion of homocysteine (Hcy) to methionine depends on folate, and vitamins B_6 and B_{12}. Plasma homocysteine level has been used as a marker for folate and vitamins B_6 and B_{12} status, and increased homocysteine levels have been associated with endothelial damage in pediatric SCD patients. In general, folic acid supplementation at a dose of 1 mg/day is recommended in adult patients, women who are contemplating pregnancy, and patients of all ages with chronic hemolysis.[5,9]

CURRENT CONTROVERSY

Daily supplementation with folic acid, vitamin B_{12}, and vitamin B_6 has been suggested for SCD patients to reduce risk of endothelial damage.

■ FETAL HEMOGLOBIN INDUCERS

HbF reduces polymer formation of HbS due to its high oxygen affinity. Increases in HbF levels significantly correlate with decreased RBC sickling and RBC adhesion. Epidemiologic studies show a relationship between HbF concentration and severity of the disease. Patients with low HbF levels have more frequent crises and higher mortality. It has been suggested that HbF level of 20% is the threshold for reduction of acute symptoms. Based on these observations, HbF induction has become a treatment modality for patients with SCD.[4,14,55]

Hydroxyurea

Hydroxyurea, a chemotherapeutic agent, increases HbF levels by stimulating the production of HbF. It also increases in the number of HbF-containing reticulocytes and intracellular HbF. Its antineoplastic activity is related to inhibition of DNA synthesis by blocking the conversion of ribonucleoside to deoxyribonucleotides. The exact mechanism of HbF production is unknown, but its cytotoxic effect in the bone marrow triggers rapid erythroid regeneration and increases erythrocyte precursors becoming HbF. In addition, hydroxyurea increases nitric oxide (NO) levels, reduces neutrophils and monocytes, has antioxidant properties, alters RBC membrane properties, increases RBC deformability by increasing intracellular water content, and decreases RBC adhesion to endothelium.[4,9,55–57]

Hydroxyurea can prevent painful crises and is FDA approved for adult patients based on a double-blind, placebo-controlled study called the Multicenter Study of Hydroxyurea in Sickle Cell Anemia (MSH). In that study of 299 adults with moderate-to-severe SCD, hydroxyurea significantly reduced the frequency of painful episodes, incidence of acute chest syndrome, need for blood transfusions, and number of hospitalizations.[56] The average number of crises was 44% lower in those who received hydroxyurea, declining from 4.5 to 2.5 crises per year. The incidence of severe crises, defined as those requiring hospitalization, was also lower, with a median rate of 2.4 severe crises per year in the placebo group versus one severe crisis per year in the hydroxyurea group. The risk of acute chest syndrome was also significantly reduced in patients receiving hydroxyurea. Of the 152 patients in the hydroxyurea group, 25 (16%) developed acute chest syndrome, as compared with 51 (35%) of the 147 patients in the placebo group. Blood transfusion requirements were decreased by 34% in the hydroxyurea group. The study was terminated early after interim analyses revealed the significant benefits. The incidence of death, stroke, and hepatic sequestration in the hydroxyurea and placebo groups was not significantly different during the 29-month evaluation period. However, the follow-up study showed a 40% reduction in mortality with hydroxyurea over a 9-year period.[56]

Although hydroxyurea is not FDA approved for children and adolescents with SCD, its use in this patient population is supported by the National Institutes of Health (NIH).[9,57] Studies in pediatric patients (Pediatric Hydroxyurea in Sickle Cell Anemia) showed similar benefits as in adults with no adverse effects on growth and development. In addition, patients treated with hydroxyurea therapy had possible recovery or preservation of splenic and brain functions, including cognitive performances. When given with a transfusion program, hydroxyurea can play an important role in preventing recurrent strokes and reducing iron overload from transfusion.[56-63] Two NIH studies are under way in children with SCD. The Pediatric Hydroxyurea Phase III Clinical Trial (BABY HUG) evaluates whether hydroxyurea therapy prevents chronic end-organ damage in young children ages 9 to 17 months. The SCA and Stroke with Transfusions Changing to Hydroxyurea (SWiTCH) trial compares hydroxyurea and phlebotomy to standard therapy for prevention of secondary stroke and management of iron overload.[62,64]

The most common side effect of hydroxyurea is bone marrow suppression, including neutropenia, thrombocytopenia, anemia, and/or decreased reticulocyte count. These hematologic side effects usually recover within 2 weeks with discontinuation of therapy. Other side effects include dry skin and hyperpigmentation of skin or nails.[56] Long-term side effects of hydroxyurea therapy in patients with SCD are not fully known. Studies in children have not demonstrated delays in growth or puberty. Myelodysplasia, acute leukemia, and chronic opportunistic infection associated with T-lymphocyte abnormalities have been reported. Longer follow-up is needed to determine its carcinogenic or leukemogenic effects. Reproductive toxicity is another concern. High-dose hydroxyurea has been shown to be teratogenic in animals, but normal pregnancies have been reported in women who received hydroxyurea during pregnancy.[5,9,55-58-61]

Clinical indications for hydroxyurea use include frequent painful episodes, severe symptomatic anemia, a history of acute chest syndrome, or other severe vasoocclusive complications. The starting dose for hydroxyurea is 10 to 15 mg/kg per day as a single daily dose (Fig. 111–6). The dosage can be increased after 8 to 12 weeks if the patient can tolerate the adverse effects and blood counts are stable. Hydroxyurea dosage should be individualized based on response and toxicity. In general, 3 to 6 months of daily administration are required before improvement is observed. Medication adherence can be an issue. Since the mean corpuscular volume (MCV) generally increases as the level of HbF increases, monitoring the MCV is an inexpensive and convenient method of monitoring response. With close monitoring, hydroxyurea can be increased by 5 mg/kg per day up to 35 mg/kg per day.[9,56]

❺ Patients receiving hydroxyurea should be closely monitored for toxicity. Blood counts should be checked every 2 weeks during dose titration and every 4 to 6 weeks thereafter. Treatment should be interrupted if hematologic indices fall below the following values: absolute neutrophil count, 2,000 cells/mm³ (2×10^9/L); platelet count, 80,000 cells/mm³ (80×10^9/L); hemoglobin, 5 g/dL (50 g/L; 3.1 mmol/L); or reticulocytes, 80,000 cells/mm³ if the hemoglobin concentration is less than 9 g/dL (90 g/L; 5.59 mmol/L). Other laboratory abnormalities warranting temporary discontinuation of therapy are a 50% increase in serum creatinine and a 100% increase in transaminase. After recovery has occurred, treatment should be resumed at a dose that is 2.5 to 5 mg/kg per day lower than the dose associated with toxicity. If no toxicity occurs after 12 weeks with the lower dose, the dose can be increased by 2.5 to 5 mg/kg per day. A given dose that twice produces a toxic hematologic response should not be tried again. Failure to see an increase in the MCV with hydroxyurea therapy can indicate that the marrow is unable to respond, the hydroxyurea dose is inadequate, or the patient is nonadherent.[5,9,56]

Butyrate

Butyrate, a naturally occurring fatty acid, increases HbF by altering gene expression, which leads to increased γ-globin chain production. Unlike hydroxyurea, butyrate does not appear to be cytotoxic.

Butyrate has been studied in a small number of adult patients. Initial trials with continuous-infusion butyrate showed an increase not only in HbF but also in total hemoglobin and in the number of cells containing HbF. However, a sustained effect or an associated clinical benefit has not been observed. A later study with arginine butyrate in a pulse regimen reported a sustained increase in HbF and reduction of hospitalized days in a small number of adult patients. In that study, adult patients received a 4-day course of arginine butyrate, followed by a 10- to 24-day drug-free period before the administration of the next dose. Arginine butyrate was given at a daily dose of 250 to 500 mg/kg over 6 to 12 hours. Although the results are encouraging, the need for intravenous administration can limit widespread use of the regimen.[4,9,55]

HbF production by butyrate appears to depend on pretreatment HbF. Young children may be better candidates for this therapy because they have a higher level of HbF. Oral sodium phenylbutyrate has been used for years in young children with urea cycle disorders. At high doses, side effects include transient fluid retention, rashes, and unusual body odor. Increased HbF levels were seen in patients with SCA who received both high-dose (15 to 20 g/day) and low-dose (1 to 11 g/day) regimens. In the study of low-dose sodium phenylbutyrate, increased HbF was seen within 5 weeks but may not be sustained.[4,9,55] Butyrate has been shown to heal intractable leg ulcers, and the use of arginine butyrate in patients with SCD and refractory leg ulcers is being evaluated.[65]

5-Aza-2′-Deoxycytidine (Decitabine)

5-Azacytidine and 5-aza-2′-deoxycytidine (decitabine) induce HbF by inhibiting DNA methylation, thus preventing the switch from γ- to β-globin production. Compared with 5-azacytidine, decitabine has a more favorable safety profile and is a more potent DNA methylation inhibitor. Virtually abandoned in the past because of concerns regarding the cytotoxicity of 5-azacytidine, decitabine has been studied in a small number of patients with SCD who did not respond to hydroxyurea. In one study, an increase in HbF was seen in adult patients who were resistant or intolerant to hydroxyurea with 5-aza-2′-deoxycytidine was given at a dose of 0.2 mg/kg one to three times a week subcutaneously. Reduction of vasoocclusive crisis and improved performance status were reported in four adult patients with severe SCD. The only significant toxicities observed were neutropenia and increased platelet count. Long-term clinical effects and side effects of this agent have not been fully evaluated. This agent may have a role in treating patients who fail to respond to hydroxyurea.[4,9,55,66]

Combinations of Hemoglobin F Inducers

Erythropoietin therapy has been used in some patients with SCD, and the clinical results have been inconsistent; therefore its routine

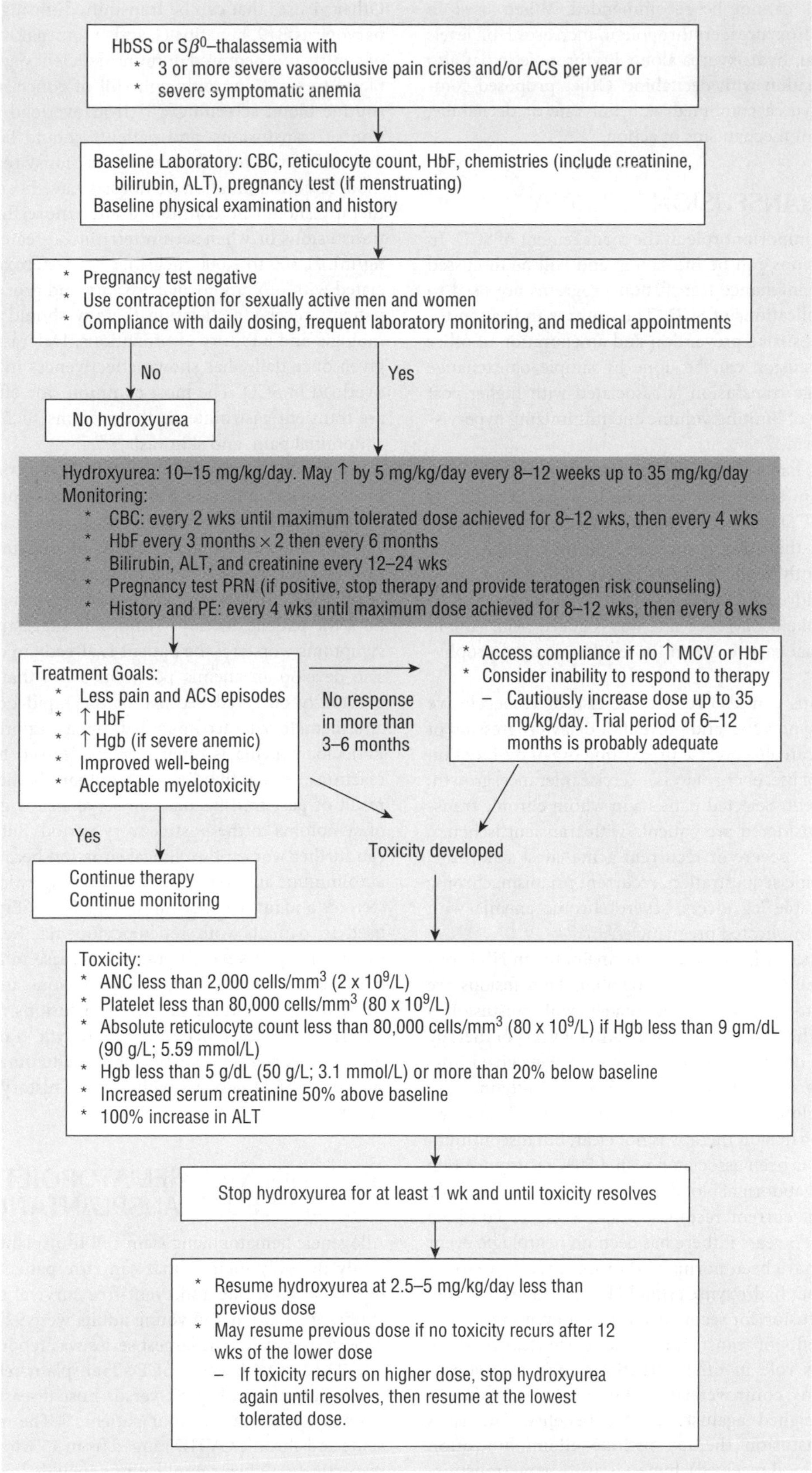

HbSS or Sβ⁰–thalassemia with
* 3 or more severe vasoocclusive pain crises and/or ACS per year or
* severe symptomatic anemia

↓

Baseline Laboratory: CBC, reticulocyte count, HbF, chemistries (include creatinine, bilirubin, ALT), pregnancy test (If menstruating)
Baseline physical examination and history

↓

* Pregnancy test negative
* Use contraception for sexually active men and women
* Compliance with daily dosing, frequent laboratory monitoring, and medical appointments

No → Yes ↓

No hydroxyurea

Hydroxyurea: 10–15 mg/kg/day. May ↑ by 5 mg/kg/day every 8–12 weeks up to 35 mg/kg/day
Monitoring:
* CBC: every 2 wks until maximum tolerated dose achieved for 8–12 wks, then every 4 wks
* HbF every 3 months × 2 then every 6 months
* Bilirubin, ALT, and creatinine every 12–24 wks
* Pregnancy test PRN (if positive, stop therapy and provide teratogen risk counseling)
* History and PE: every 4 wks until maximum dose achieved for 8–12 wks, then every 8 wks

Treatment Goals:
* Less pain and ACS episodes
* ↑ HbF
* ↑ Hgb (if severe anemic)
* Improved well-being
* Acceptable myelotoxicity

No response in more than 3–6 months →

* Access compliance if no ↑ MCV or HbF
* Consider inability to respond to therapy
  – Cautiously increase dose up to 35 mg/kg/day. Trial period of 6–12 months is probably adequate

Yes ↓

Continue therapy
Continue monitoring

Toxicity developed

↓

Toxicity:
* ANC less than 2,000 cells/mm³ (2 x 10⁹/L)
* Platelet less than 80,000 cells/mm³ (80 x 10⁹/L)
* Absolute reticulocyte count less than 80,000 cells/mm³ (80 x 10⁹/L) if Hgb less than 9 gm/dL (90 g/L; 5.59 mmol/L)
* Hgb less than 5 g/dL (50 g/L; 3.1 mmol/L) or more than 20% below baseline
* Increased serum creatinine 50% above baseline
* 100% increase in ALT

↓

Stop hydroxyurea for at least 1 wk and until toxicity resolves

↓

* Resume hydroxyurea at 2.5–5 mg/kg/day less than previous dose
* May resume previous dose if no toxicity recurs after 12 wks of the lower dose
  – If toxicity recurs on higher dose, stop hydroxyurea again until resolves, then resume at the lowest tolerated dose.

FIGURE 111-6. Hydroxyurea use in sickle cell disease. (ACS, acute chest syndrome; ALT, alanine aminotransferase; ANC, absolute neutrophil count; CBC, complete blood cell count; HbF, fetal hemoglobin; Hb, hemoglobin; HbSS, homozygous sickle cell hemoglobin; HBSSβ⁰, sickle cell β⁰-thalassemia; MCV, mean corpuscular volume; PE, physical examination; PRN, as needed; RBC, red blood cell.) *(From Stuart et al.,[7] Sickle Cell Disease Care Consortium,[46] and Halsey and Roberts.[51])*

use in these patients cannot be recommended. When used in combination with hydroxyurea, erythropoietin increases HbF levels to a greater extent than hydroxyurea alone. Erythropoietin has also been used in combination with decitabine. Other proposed combinations are hydroxyurea combined with butyrate or decitabine, based on their different mechanisms of action.[4,11,63,66]

■ CHRONIC TRANSFUSION THERAPY

Transfusions play an important role in the management of SCD. In acute illness, transfusions can be life saving and will be discussed in a later section. Maintenance transfusion programs are used to prevent serious complications of SCD. The primary indication for chronic transfusion is stroke prevention and amelioration of other organ damage. Transfusion can be done by simple or exchange transfusions. Exchange transfusion is associated with higher cost but has the advantage of limiting volume and minimizing hyperviscosity and iron overload.[4,5,67]

❻ In children who had a stroke, chronic transfusions can reduce stroke recurrence from about 50% to about 10% over 3 years. As the initial stroke in SCD can be devastating, transfusions are usually given to prevent the initial stroke. In one trial, prophylactic transfusions significantly reduced the incidence of first stroke over a 2-year period in children 2 to 16 years of age with abnormal TCD ultrasonography. Stroke occurrence rate was reduced from 16% in patients receiving usual care to 2% in those who received prophylactic transfusions.[67-69]

Chronic transfusions can also reduce the risk of vasoocclusive pain and acute chest syndrome, and prevent or delay progression of organ damage. They can also reverse preexisting organ dysfunction and improve quality of life, energy levels, exercise tolerance, growth, and sexual development. Selected patients in whom chronic transfusions should be considered are patients with transient ischemic attack, abnormal TCD, severe or recurrent acute chest syndrome, debilitating pain, splenic sequestration, recurrent priapism, chronic organ failure, intractable leg ulcers, severe chronic anemia with cardiac failure, and complicated pregnancies.[5,9,68,70]

The goal of transfusions is to achieve and maintain an HbS concentration of less than 30% of total hemoglobin. Transfusions are usually given every 3 to 4 weeks, but the frequency of transfusion is adjusted to maintain the desired HbS levels. After 4 years of therapy without development of complications, many clinicians give transfusions less frequently and allow the HbS concentration to increase to 50% of total hemoglobin.[9,67] The optimal duration of chronic primary prophylactic transfusion therapy is not clear, but discontinuation of transfusions has been associated with a 50% recurrence rate within 12 months and abnormal blood flow velocity in children. For secondary prevention, current recommendations are to continue transfusion for at least 5 years if there has been no neurologic event and imaging studies have been normalized or until age 18 years. A pilot study suggests that hydroxyurea should be started prior to discontinuation of transfusion for secondary stroke prevention.[9,67-72]

Although the benefits of transfusion therapy are clear in some clinical situations, its role in other situations such as priapism and leg ulcer remains controversial.[67] The risks of transfusion therapy must be weighed against possible benefits. The risks associated with transfusion therapy include alloimmunization (sensitization to the blood received), hyperviscosity, viral transmission, volume overload, iron overload, and transfusion reactions. Alloimmunization occurs in 18% to 36% of SCD patients who receive blood transfusions. The use of leukocyte-reduced RBC transfusions or human leukocyte antigen (HLA)-matched units in chronically transfused patients can reduce the risk of alloimmunization. Transfusion-related infections also remain a concern. All patients should be immunized with hepatitis A and B vaccines.

Other viruses that can be transmitted through blood products are parvovirus B19, hepatitis C, and cytomegalovirus (CMV). The risk of contracting acquired immune deficiency syndrome (AIDS) from blood transfusions, although still of concern, has decreased with routine blood screening.[5,24,67] Iron overload is another complication of transfusions, and patients should be counseled to avoid excess dietary iron. Abnormal liver biopsy results showing mild to moderate inflammation or fibrosis have been reported. Chelation therapy should be considered after more than 1 year of chronic transfusions or when serum ferritin is greater than 1,500 to 2,000 ng/mL (1,500 to 2,000 mcg/L).[5,9,11,67] Deferoxamine has been associated with oto- and ocular toxicity and growth failure. Therefore, patients receiving chelation therapy should have yearly ophthalmologic and auditory examinations. Deferasirox, an oral chelator given once daily, has shown effectiveness in management of iron overload in SCD. The most common side effects with deferasirox are transient gastrointestinal symptoms such as nausea, vomiting, abdominal pain, and skin rash.[5,9,73-75]

Unique to the population with SCD is a constellation of features that can occur in response to blood transfusion; this is often referred to as the sickle cell hemolytic transfusion reaction syndrome. This syndrome includes manifestations of an acute or delayed transfusion reaction caused by alloimmunization. Delayed reactions can occur 2 to 20 days after transfusion. During the hemolytic reaction, the patient develops symptoms suggestive of a pain crisis, or symptoms worsen if the patient is already in crisis. The patient can also develop an anemia posttransfusion that is more severe than previously observed because of the rapid decline in hemoglobin and hematocrit, accompanied by a suppressed erythropoiesis. Reticulocytopenia is often seen in delayed hemolytic transfusion reactions. Alloantibodies and autoantibodies that formed as a result of past transfusions can serve as a trigger, causing a return of symptoms in the postrecovery period. Subsequent transfusions can further worsen the clinical situation because of the presence of autoimmune antibodies. Life-threatening events can be treated with steroids and intravenous immunoglobulin. Erythropoietin has been used in patients with reticulocytopenia. Recovery, as evidenced by reticulocytosis with a gradual increase in the hemoglobin level, may occur only after further transfusions are withheld. Although some patients tolerate further transfusions after recovery, others experience a recurrence of the hemolytic transfusion reaction. To prevent recurrent hemolytic anemia, rituximab has been used with success in SCD patients with a prior history of a life-threatening event.[9,14,67,76]

■ ALLOGENEIC HEMATOPOIETIC STEM CELL TRANSPLANTATION

Allogeneic hematopoietic stem cell transplantation (HSCT) is currently the only therapy that can cure patients with SCD.[77-79] The overall survival rate and event-free survival rate reported in three studies in children and young adults were 92% to 94% and 83% to 86%, respectively. The largest series was reported in 87 patients age 2 to 22 years with severe SCD. Transplant-related deaths occurred in six patients, with graft-versus-host disease (GVHD) being the main cause of death in four patients.[78] The reported incidences of acute and chronic GVHD ranged from 15% to 20% and 12% to 20%, respectively. Other complications included seizure, marrow rejection, and sepsis. Improved growth, stabilization or improvement of CNS abnormalities, and recovery of splenic dysfunction were observed in post-transplant SCD patients, but gonadal failure and delayed sexual development in females requiring hormonal replacements have been reported.[77,79,80]

The best candidates for allogeneic HSCT are SCD patients who are younger than 16 years of age; have severe complications such as refractory pain, stroke, or recurrent acute chest syndrome; and have an HLA-matched donor. Although allogeneic HSCT in young children before organ damage and alloimmunization occur can be associated with an increased success rate, disease progression is unpredictable, making it difficult to determine the optimal time for transplantation. The risks associated with allogeneic HSCT must be carefully considered, as the transplant-related mortality rate is about 5% to 10%, and graft rejection is about 10%. Other risks associated with allogeneic HSCT include secondary malignancies. Neurologic events, such as intracranial hemorrhage and seizures during transplant, were seen more frequently in patients with a history of stroke.[9,77,79]

Experience with unrelated HLA-matched or related HLA-mismatched donor transplants is very limited. Studies in thalassemia patients do not support the use of these alternate donors at this time. Umbilical cord blood is another donor source. Its advantages include a lower incidence of severe GVHD and the potential of using umbilical cord blood from unrelated donors, but such advantages are balanced by longer duration for engraftment and a higher rate of graft rejection.[5,77,79,81] Finally, a recent study reports the use of nonmyeloablative allogeneic stem-cell transplantation in 10 adult patients to achieve mixed donor-recipient chimerism and reversal of SCD.[82]

TREATMENT OF COMPLICATIONS

■ GENERAL MANAGEMENT

Parents and older children should be educated on the signs and symptoms of complications and conditions that require urgent evaluation. During acute illness, patients should be evaluated promptly, as deterioration can occur rapidly. It is essential to maintain a balanced fluid status because dehydration and fluid overload can worsen complications associated with SCD. Oxygen saturation by pulse oximetry should be maintained at least 92% or at baseline. New or increasing supplemental oxygen requirements should be investigated.[5,8,9,11]

■ EPISODIC TRANSFUSIONS FOR ACUTE COMPLICATIONS

Indications for RBC transfusions include (a) acute exacerbation of baseline anemia, such as aplastic crisis if the anemia is severe, hepatic or splenic sequestration, or severe hemolysis; (b) severe vasoocclusive episodes, such as acute chest syndrome, stroke, or acute multiorgan failure; and (c) preparation for procedures that require the use of general anesthesia or ionic contrast. Other patients in whom transfusions can be useful include patients with complicated obstetric problems, refractory leg ulcers, or refractory and protracted painful episodes or severe priapism. Simple transfusion or partial exchange transfusion can be used. If simple transfusion is used, volume overload leading to congestive heart failure can occur if anemia is corrected too rapidly in patients with severe anemia. In addition, increases in hemoglobin levels to greater than 10 to 11 g/dL (100 to 110 g/L; 6.21 to 6.83 mmol/L) can cause hyperviscosity and should be avoided.[5,9,67]

■ INFECTION AND FEVER

Patients with SCD should be evaluated as soon as possible for any fever greater than 38.5°C (101.3°F). Criteria for hospitalization include an infant younger than 1 year old, history of previous bacteremia or sepsis, temperature greater than 40°C (104°F), WBC greater than 30,000 cells/mm³ (30 × 10⁹/L) or less than 5,000 cells/mm³ (5 × 10⁹/L) and/or platelets less than 100,000 cells/mm³ (100 × 10⁹/L), and evidence of other acute complications or toxic appearance. Outpatient management can be considered in older nontoxic children with reliable family caregivers. Antibiotic choice should provide adequate coverage for encapsulated organisms.

❼ Ceftriaxone should be used for outpatient management because it provides coverage for 24 hours. If admitted, cefotaxime can also be used. For patients with cephalosporin allergy, clindamycin can be used. Vancomycin should be considered for acutely ill children or if *Staphylococcus* is suspected. A macrolide antibiotic should be added if *Mycoplasma pneumoniae* is suspected. Penicillin prophylaxis should be discontinued while the patient is receiving broad-spectrum antibiotics. Acetaminophen or ibuprofen can be used for fever control. Increased fluid requirements can be needed because of dehydration and/or increased insensible loss.[1,5,9,11,24]

■ CEREBROVASCULAR ACCIDENTS

Patients with acute neurologic events must be hospitalized and monitored closely. Physical and neurologic examination should be performed every 2 hours. Acute treatment for children should include exchange transfusion or simple transfusion to maintain hemoglobin at about 10 g/dL (100 g/L; 6.21 mmol/L) and HbS less than 30%, anticonvulsants for patients with a seizure history, and therapy for increased intracranial pressure if needed. Chronic transfusion therapy should be initiated for children with ischemic stroke as discussed earlier. In adults presenting with ischemic stroke, thrombolytic therapy should be considered if it is less than 3 hours since the onset of symptoms.[9,11,25,27,68]

■ ACUTE CHEST SYNDROME

Patients with acute chest syndrome should use incentive spirometry frequently (e.g., at least every 2 hours while awake) to reduce atelectasis development. In addition, proper management of pain is important. The goal is to provide relief while avoiding analgesic-induced hypoventilation. Appropriate fluid therapy is important as overhydration can cause pulmonary edema and exacerbate respiratory distress. Early use of broad-spectrum antibiotics, including a macrolide or quinolone, is also recommended. Studies indicate that infection is common with acute chest syndrome and can involve gram-positive, gram-negative, or atypical bacteria. Oxygen therapy is indicated for all patients who are hypoxic or in acute distress. In a patient with a history of reactive airway disease or wheezing on examination, a trial of bronchodilators is appropriate. Transfusions are often used in the treatment of acute lung disease.[1,5,9,11,31]

Steroids can decrease inflammation and endothelial cell adhesion. Glucocorticoids can decrease the duration of hospitalization, transfusions, and need for other supportive care but can increase the readmission rate for SCA-related complications.[83] Another promising therapy is the use of NO, which relaxes and dilates blood vessels. Its hematologic effects include inhibition of platelet aggregation and reduction in the polymerization tendency of HbS. Marked improvement of pulmonary status and cardiac output has been reported in a patient with acute chest syndrome. Both inhaled NO and oral L-arginine, the precursor of NO, are being evaluated for management of acute chest syndrome.[3,4,31]

■ PRIAPISM

Stuttering priapism, episodes that last a few minutes to 2 hours, resolve spontaneously. Prolonged episodes lasting more than 2 to

3 hours require prompt medical attention. The initial goals of treatment are to provide appropriate analgesic therapy, reduce anxiety, produce detumescence, and preserve testicular function and fertility. Treatment given within 4 to 6 hours can usually reduce erection. Aggressive hydration and adequate pain control should be initiated. Use of ice packs is not recommended. Heat (hot water bottles, hot packs, or sitz baths) can provide comfort without precipitating pain crisis. Although transfusions have been given to these patients, the efficacy of this therapeutic intervention has not been established.[1,9,33,84]

Clinicians have used both vasoconstrictors and vasodilators in the treatment of priapism. Vasoconstrictors, such as diluted phenylephrine (10 mcg/mL) or epinephrine (1:1,000,000), are thought to work by forcing blood out of the corpus cavernosum into the venous return. In one uncontrolled open-label study, aspiration followed by intrapenile irrigation with epinephrine was effective and well tolerated. In that study, blood was first aspirated from the corpus cavernosum, and then the area was irrigated with a 1:1,000,000 solution of epinephrine. The priapism resolved in 37 of the 39 occasions. A follow-up study reported that 3 out of 20 patients required a repeat procedure within 24 hours. The therapy was well tolerated with no serious immediate or long-term side effects, but on two occasions, a small intrapenile hematoma formed after treatment.[33,84]

Vasodilators, such as terbutaline and hydralazine, relax the smooth muscle of the vasculature. This relaxation allows oxygenated arterial blood to enter the corpus cavernosum, which displaces or washes out the damaged sickle cells that are stagnant in the corpus cavernosum. Terbutaline has been used to treat priapism, but it has not been formally studied in patients with SCA. In one case report, a single oral sildenafil dose at onset of priapism aborted episodes. Surgical interventions used in severe refractory priapism have included a variety of shunt procedures. These surgical procedures have been successful in some cases, but they have a high failure rate and potential serious complications, which include impotence, skin sloughing, cellulitis, and urethral fistulas.[9,11,33,84]

Modalities to prevent priapism are limited and not well studied. Pseudoephedrine (30 or 60 mg/day given orally at bedtime) and leuprolide, a gonadotropin-releasing hormone, have been used to decrease the number of recurrent episodes of priapism. Hydroxyurea therapy can also be useful. Finally, antiandrogens (bicalutamide, and finasteride) and sildenafil have been used in SCD for treatment of recurrent or refractory priapism without major side effects. The role of RBC transfusion in preventing priapism remains unclear.[4,9,11,33,67,84,85]

CURRENT CONTROVERSY

Some clinicians transfuse patients to maintain an HbS level less than 30% to prevent recurrent priapism. Duration of such regimens should be limited to 6 to 12 months.

■ MANAGEMENT OF CRISIS

Aplastic Crisis

Treatment of aplastic crisis is primarily supportive, and most patients recover spontaneously. The patient can need blood transfusions if the anemia is severe or symptomatic. The reticulocyte count can determine if there is red cell production and the need for transfusions. The most common cause for aplastic crisis is acute infection with human parvovirus B19. As parvovirus is contagious, infected patients should be placed in isolation. In addition, contact with pregnant healthcare providers should be avoided because parvovirus infection during the midtrimester of pregnancy can result in hydrops fetalis and stillbirth.[5,9,11]

Sequestration Crisis

Splenic sequestration crisis is a major cause of mortality in young patients with SCD. The sequestration of RBCs in the spleen can result in a rapid drop of hematocrit, leading to hypovolemia, shock, and death. Immediate treatment is RBC transfusion to correct hypovolemia. Broad-spectrum antibiotic therapy, which includes coverage for pneumococci and *H. influenzae*, can also be beneficial because infection can precipitate crises.[5,9,11]

Recurrent episodes occur in about half of patients and are associated with increased mortality. Options for management of recurrence include observation, chronic transfusion, and splenectomy. Adults are often observed because they tend to have milder episodes. Increased risk of invasive infection after splenectomy is a concern in young children. Chronic transfusions delay splenectomy and temporarily restore splenic function, but it is associated with its own risks. Splenectomy is probably indicated, even after a single sequestration crisis, if that event is life threatening. Splenectomy should be considered after repetitive episodes, even if they are less serious. For children younger than 2 years of age, chronic blood transfusions are recommended to prevent sequestration and delay splenectomy until the age of 2 years, when there is less risk of postsplenectomy septicemia. Finally, splenectomy should also be considered for patients with chronic hypersplenism.[5,9,11,86]

Vasoocclusive Pain Crisis

Hydration and analgesia are the mainstays of treatment for vasoocclusive (painful) crises (Table 111–4). Patients with mild pain crisis can be treated as outpatients with rest, increased fluid intake, warm compresses, and oral analgesics. Hospitalization is necessary for moderate to severe crisis. As infection can precipitate crises, an infectious etiology should be ruled out, and appropriate empiric therapy should be initiated in patients who have fever or are critically ill. In anemic patients, transfusion to maintain the hemoglobin level at baseline can be needed. Fluid replacement given intravenously or orally at 1.5 times the maintenance requirement is recommended. Close monitoring of fluid status is essential as aggressive hydration, particularly with sodium-containing fluids, can lead to volume overload, acute chest syndrome, and heart failure.[1,3,5,9,11]

The frequency and severity of acute pain episodes associated with SCD are variable, and pain should be assessed, and analgesic therapy should be tailored for each patient. Several pain assessment tools are available and should be used to measure the intensity of pain. Unfortunately, they have not been validated for sickle cell pain. The healthcare provider should choose one tool appropriate for age and use it routinely to assess pain. Other useful information to guide choice of analgesics should include previous effective agents and their dosages, response to therapy and previous clinical course, and duration of pain crisis.[5,9,11,87,88]

❽ Aggressive therapy that relieves pain and enables the patient to attain maximum functional ability should be initiated in patients with pain crisis. Treatment of mild to moderate pain should include the use of nonsteroidal antiinflammatory drugs (NSAIDs) or acetaminophen, unless there are contraindications to their use. Ketorolac is useful for patients requiring intravenous therapy. Because of concerns about gastrointestinal bleeding, it is recommended to limit the duration of therapy to 5 days or less. When acetaminophen is used, it is important to review the total dose of acetaminophen administered in patients who may also be receiving

TABLE 111-4	Management of Acute Pain of Sickle Cell Disease

Principles

- Treat underlying precipitating factors
- Avoid delays in analgesia administration
- Use pain scale to assess severity
- Choice of initial analgesic should be based on previous pain crisis pattern, history of response, current status, and other medical conditions
- Schedule pain medication; avoid as-needed dosing
- Provide rescue dose for breakthrough pain
- If adequate pain relief can be achieved with one or two doses of morphine, consider outpatient management with a weak opioid; otherwise hospitalization is needed for parenteral analgesics
- Frequently assess to evaluate pain severity and side effects; titrate dose as needed
- Treating adverse effects of opioids is part of pain management
- Consider nonpharmacologic intervention (e.g., relaxation techniques, guided imagery, deep breathing)
- Transition to oral analgesics as the patient improves; choose an oral agent based on previous history, anticipated duration, and ability to swallow tablets; if sustained-release products are used, a product with a rapid onset is also needed for breakthrough pain

Analgesic regimens

Mild-to-moderate pain: nonopioid ± weak opioid
Moderate-to-severe pain: weak opioid or low dose of a strong opioid ± nonopioid
Severe pain: strong opioid + nonopioid

Weak opioid

Acetaminophen with codeine

Dose based on codeine–children: 1 mg/kg per dose every 6 hours; adult: 30 to 60 mg/dose

Hydrocodone + acetaminophen

Dose based on hydrocodone–children: 0.2 mg/kg per dose every 6 hours; adults: 5 to 10 mg/dose

Nonopioid

Oral antiinflammatory agents

Use with caution in patients with renal failure (dehydration) and bleeding
Ibuprofen–children: 10 mg/kg every 6 to 8 hours; adult: 200 to 400 mg/dose
Naproxen: 5 mg/kg every 12 hours; adult 250 to 500 mg/dose

Intravenous antiinflammatory agents:

Ketorolac: 0.5 mg/kg up to 30 mg/dose every 6 hours

Strong opioid

Morphine: 0.1 to 0.15 mg/kg per dose every 3 to 4 hours for children; 5 to 10 mg/ dose for adults

Continuous infusion: 0.04 to 0.05 mg/kg per hour; titrate to effect

Hydromorphone: 0.015 mg/kg per dose every 3 to 4 hours for children; 1.5 to 2 mg/dose for adults

Continuous infusion: 0.004 mg/kg per hour; titrate to effect

Patient-controlled analgesics:

Morphine: 0.01 to 0.03 mg/kg per hours basal; demand 0.01 to 0.03 mg/kg every 6 to 10 min; 4-hour lock out 0.4 to 0.6 mg/kg

Hydromorphone: 0.003 to 0.005 mg/kg per hour basal; demand 0.03 to 0.05 mg/kg every 6–10 minutes; 4 hour lock out 0.06 to 0.08 mg/kg

Rescue therapy:

For breakthrough, give 1/4 to 1/2 of the scheduled dose as bolus every 1 to 2 hour; assess amount of rescue dose used in 8 to 12 hours and readjust scheduled dose or infusion rate as needed

Other adjunct therapy:

Hydration, heating pads, relaxation, and distraction
Stool softener and/or stimulants for constipation
Antihistamine for itching
Antiemetics for nausea or vomiting

From Montalembert,[1] Driscoll,[5] National Institutes of Health,[9] Stuart and Nagel,[11] Richard,[87] Dumaplin.[88]

the agent for fever or another acetaminophen-containing product for pain. If mild to moderate pain persists, an opioid should be added. Effective combination therapy, such as an NSAID combined with an opioid, can enhance analgesic efficacy while decreasing side effects.[5,9,11,87,88]

Severe pain should be treated aggressively until the pain is tolerable. Commonly used opioids include morphine, hydromorphone, fentanyl, and methadone. The weak opioids, codeine and hydrocodone, are used to manage mild to moderate pain. Meperidine has no advantages as an analgesic. Its duration of action is short compared with the half-life of the metabolite normeperidine. The accumulation of normepcridine can cause central nervous system side effects, ranging from dysphoria to seizures. Therefore, meperidine should be avoided if possible and used only for a very brief duration in patients who are allergic or intolerant to other opioids.[9,11,87,88]

Both prior history and current assessment should be considered in the management of pain crisis. For patients whose typical crisis improves in a short time, preparations with a short duration of action are appropriate. For patients whose crises require many days to resolve, sustained-release preparations combined with a short-acting product for breakthrough pain are more appropriate. If the patient has been on long-term opioid therapy at home, tolerance can develop. In these cases, the pain of acute crises can be treated with a different potent opioid or a larger dose of the same medication. Intravenous administration provides a rapid onset of action and therefore is preferred for severe pain. Intramuscular injections should be avoided. Children might actually deny pain because of fear of injections. Analgesics should be titrated to pain relief. In patients with continuous pain, the analgesic should be given as a scheduled dose or continuous infusion. Continuous infusion has the advantage of less fluctuation of blood levels between dosing intervals. As-needed dosing is only appropriate for breakthrough pain. Patient-controlled analgesia (PCA) is commonly used. When used properly, PCA allows patients to have control over pain therapy and minimizes the lag time between perception of pain and administration of analgesics. The transdermal fentanyl patch has also been used successfully, but its role in sickle cell pain crisis is unclear because of its long time of onset of pain relief (12 to 16 hours) and fixed dosage form, which makes it difficult to titrate the dose. Other alternative pain management techniques such as physical therapy and relaxation therapy can be helpful as adjunct therapy.[9,11,87–89]

Suboptimal pain relief has been reported in both emergency room and hospitalized patients. The most common cause of suboptimal pain control in children with SCA is the suspicion of addiction. This obstacle is especially common in adolescents. In one study, 53% of emergency physicians believed that 20% of SCD patients are addicted to analgesics. Another barrier for effective pain control is the difference in perception between patients, family, and healthcare providers. Patients with SCD often suffer from chronic pain, and they may cope with the pain by being inactive. Patients who have inadequate pain control can exhibit anxiety and drug-seeking behavior for fear of pain. Tolerance to narcotics can also be misinterpreted as drug addiction by healthcare providers and families. Aggressive pain control, frequent monitoring of pain during crises, and tapering medication according to response are factors that minimize physical dependence. The use of a protocol has been shown to result in optimal management of pain control in SCD.[87,88,90,91]

Intracellular adhesion of RBCs contributes to vasoocclusion in SCD. Agents that can alter adhesion molecules on RBCs can potentially reduce or ameliorate clinical manifestation of SCD. Omega-3 fatty acids are important components of cell membranes and organelles and may be important for erythrocyte integrity and play a role in reducing hemolysis. In addition, omega-3 fatty acids have antiadhesion activity by modulating adhesive molecules in the membrane. Reduction of disease severity has been reported in clinical trials.[92]

PHARMACOECONOMIC CONSIDERATIONS

Patients with SCD incur considerable healthcare costs. Pharmacoeconomic considerations should include newborn screening, cost of managing acute and chronic complications, and the economic impact of new treatment modalities. Early penicillin prophylaxis prevents pneumococcal sepsis in infants. Newborn screening targeted at African Americans has been shown to be cost-effective. Whether it is cost-effective to screen all infants depends on the prevalence of high-risk infants in the area. In general, universal screening identifies more infants with disease, prevents more deaths, and can provide for a certain degree of cost-effectiveness because targeted screening might not detect all infants with the disease.[2,93]

Hospitalization is an important societal financial burden. Studies conducted in various regions have shown that a small number of patients consume a disproportionate amount of care as a result of severe illness, and most of the total cost is related to hospitalizations. In 2004, an estimated 113,098 patients with SCD were hospitalized, of whom, about three-quarters were adult patients. The average cost for each hospitalization was $6,223, and the total estimated cost was $488 million.[94] Patients who are not being followed in settings that provide comprehensive medical care tend to acquire higher costs for emergency room and hospital visits. A study examining relationships between socioeconomic factors and geographic distribution in Alabama reported that use of comprehensive care was lower for those living in rural areas.[95-97]

Newer therapies, diagnostic methods such as TCD, and chronic transfusions further increase cost. The estimated mean cost in SCD patients receiving iron chelation was $69,259 per year.[98] Using the data from the MSH trial, researchers estimated the average annual cost for medical care to be lower in the hydroxyurea group as compared with the placebo group ($12,160 vs. $22,020). Hospitalization for pain crisis accounted for the highest cost in both groups, and savings of more than $5,000 per patient per year of medical costs could be achieved if every eligible patient received the agent. However, this cost-saving was not demonstrated in one analysis performed in Maryland.[98,99] Allogeneic HSCT can potentially cure the disease and if successful can reduce long-term costs, but it requires a high up-front cost. New therapies, although expensive, might reduce visits to emergency departments and inpatient hospitalizations, improving the cost-effectiveness of those therapies over a patient's lifetime.[9]

EVALUATION OF THERAPEUTIC OUTCOMES

❾ SCD is a complex disorder that requires multidisciplinary comprehensive care. All patients should be medically evaluated regularly to establish baseline, monitor changes, and provide education appropriate for age. For infants younger than 1 year old, medical evaluations every 2 to 4 months are needed. Beyond 1 year of age, evaluation can be extended to every 6 to 12 months with modifications depending on severity of the illness.[5,9]

It is important to establish baseline laboratory values and imaging studies. Routine laboratory evaluation includes complete blood cell counts and reticulocyte counts every 3 months up to 2 years of age, then every 6 months; HbF level should be taken every 6 months until 2 years of age, then annually. Evaluation of renal, hepatobiliary, and pulmonary function should be done annually. TCD screening is recommended to start at age 2 years, then annually. Ophthalmologic examination to screen for retinopathy is recommended at around age 10 years. In patients with recurrent acute chest syndrome, pulmonary function tests should be done to establish baseline values and identify declines in lung function.

It is essential that immunizations and prophylactic antibiotics are given. When infections do occur, appropriate antibiotic therapy should be initiated, and the patient should be monitored for laboratory and clinical improvement. The efficacy of hydroxyurea can best be assessed in terms of the decrease in number, severity, and duration of sickle cell pain crises. HbF concentrations or MCV values can also provide some indication of the patient's response to therapy. When painful crises do occur, the effectiveness of analgesics can be measured by subjective assessments made by the patient, family, and healthcare practitioners. The success of post-stroke blood transfusions can be measured by clinical progression or the occurrence of subsequent strokes.

CONCLUSIONS

The goals of the general management of SCA are to decrease the number of sickle cell crises, decrease the complications arising from the disease, and improve the overall quality of the patient's life. The general care of SCA patients still includes early penicillin prophylaxis and appropriate immunization. HbF inducers such as hydroxyurea can decrease the frequency and severity of painful episodes. Continued studies of other possible agents and treatment modalities that can reduce crises or reverse organ damage are warranted.

ABBREVIATIONS

ASPEN syndrome: association of sickle cell disease, priapism, exchange transfusion, and neurologic events

HbA: hemoglobin A

HbAS: one normal (hemoglobin A) and one sickle cell hemoglobin (hemoglobin S) gene

HbC: hemoglobin C

HbF: fetal hemoglobin

HbSβ^+-thal, HbSβ^0-thal: hemoglobin sickle cell β^+-thalassemia and hemoglobin sickle cell β^0-thalassemia

HbSC: sickle cell hemoglobin C

HbSS: homozygous sickle cell hemoglobin (hemoglobin S)

HbS: sickle cell hemoglobin

HLA: human leukocyte antigen

HSCT: hematopoietic stem cell transplantation

ISC: irreversibly sickled cell

MCHC: mean corpuscular hemoglobin concentration

MCV: mean corpuscular volume

MSH: Multicenter Study of Hydroxyurea in Sickle Cell Anemia

NO: nitric oxide

NSAID: nonsteroidal antiinflammatory drug

PCA: patient-controlled analgesia

PCV7: 7-valent pneumococcal conjugate vaccine

PPV 23: 23-valent pneumococcal polysaccharide vaccine

RBC: red blood cell

SCA: sickle cell anemia

SCD: sickle cell disease

SCT: sickle cell trait

TCD: transcranial Doppler

WBC: white blood cell

REFERENCES

1. Montalembert M. Management of sickle cell disease. BMJ 2008;337:626–630.

2. Creary M, Williamson D, and Kulkarni R. Sickle cell disease: Current activities, public health implications, and future directions (report from the CDC). J Womens Health 2007;16:575–582.

3. Hagar W, Vichinsky E. Advances in clinical research in sickle cell disease. Br J Haematol 2008;141:346–356.

4. Hankins J, Aygun B. Pharmacotherapy in sickle cell disease—state of the art and future prospects. Br J Haematol 2009;145:296–308.

5. Driscoll CM. Sickle cell disease. Pediatr Rev 2007;28:259–267.

6. van den Tweel XW, Hatzmann J, Ensink E, et al. Quality of life of female caregivers of children with sickle cell disease: A survey. Haematologica 2008;93:588–593.

7. Mann-Jiles V, Morris DL. Quality of life of adult patients with sickle cell disease. J Am Acad Nurse Pract 2009;21:340–349.

8. Sickle-cell anemia. Report by the Secretariat. World Health Organization. D Executive Board 117th Session provisional agenda item 4.8 December 2005;EB117/34:1–5.

9. National Institutes of Health, Division of Blood Diseases and Resources, Public Health Service. The Management of Sickle Cell Disease. Bethesda, MD: U.S. Department of Health and Human Services, June 2002:1–88. NIH publication 02–2117.

10. National Heart, Lung and Blood Institute, National Institute of Health. Sickle cell anemia: Who is at risk? 2008, *http://www.nhlbi.nih.gov/health/dci/Diseases/Sca/SCA_WhoIsAtRisk.html.*

11. Stuart MJ, Nagel RL. Sickle-cell disease. Lancet 2004;364:1343–1360.

12. Hebbel RP, Osarogiagbon R, Kaul D. The endothelial biology of sickle cell disease: inflammation and a chronic vasculopathy. Microcirculation 2004;11:129–151.

13. Kutlar A. Sickle cell disease: A multigenic perspective of a single gene disorder. Hemoglobin 2007;31:209–224.

14. Ballas SK, Mohandas N. Sickle red cell microheology and sickle blood rheology. Microcirculation 2004;11:209–225.

15. Mitchell BL. Sickle cell trait and sudden death—bring it home. J Natl Med Assoc 2008;99:300–305.

16. Al-Saqladi AW, Cipolotti R, Fijnvandraat K, Brabin B. Growth and nutritional status of children with homozygous sickle cell disease. Ann Trop Paediatr 2008;29:165–189.

17. Yanni E, Grosse SD, Yang Q eta al. Trends in sickle cell disease-related mortality in the United States, 1983–2002. J Pediatr 2009;154:541–545.

18. Quinn CT, Rogers ZR, Buchanan GR. Survival of children with sickle cell disease. Blood 2004;103:4023–4027.

19. Darbari DS, Kple-Faget P, Kwagyan J, et al. Circumstances of death in adult sickle cell disease patients. Am J Hematol 2006;81:858–863.

20. Quinn CT, Shull EP, Ahmad N, et al. Prognostic significance of early vaso-occlusive complications in children with sickle cell anemia. Blood 2006;109:40–45.

21. Nordness ME, Lynn J, Zacharisen MC, et al. Asthma is a risk factor for acute chest syndrome and cerebral vascular accidents in children with sickle cell disease. Clin Molecular Allergy 2005;3:2–6.

22. Boyd JH, Macklin EA, Strunk RC, Debaun MR. Asthma is associated with increased mortality in individuals with sickle cell anemia. Haematological 2007;92:1115–1118.

23. Smithy-Whitley K, Zhao H, Hodinka RL, et al. The epidemiology of human parvovirus B 19 in children with sickle cell disease. Blood 2004;103:422–427.

24. Booth C, Inusa B, Obaro S. Infection in sickle cell disease: A review. Int J Infect Dis 2010;14:e2–e12.

25. Wong W, Powars DR. Overt and incomplete (silent) cerebral infarction in sickle cell anemia: Diagnosis and management. Hematol Oncol Clin North Am 2005;19:839–855.

26. Prengler M, Pavlakis SG, Boyd S, et al. Sickle cell disease: Ischemia and seizures. Ann Neurology 2005;58:290–302.

27. Wang WC. The pathophysiology, prevention and treatment of stroke in sickle cell disease. Curr Opin Hematol 2007;14:191–197.

28. Adams RJ. Big strokes in small persons. Arch Neurol 2007;64:1567–1574.

29. Caboot JB, Allen JL. Pulmonary complications of sickle cell disease in children. Curr Opin Pediatr 2008;20:279–287.

30. Sylvester KP, Patey RA, Milligan P, et al. Impact of acute chest syndrome on lung function of children with sickle cell disease. J Pediatr 2006.149:17–22.

31. Johnson CS. The acute chest syndrome. Hematol Oncol Clin North Am 2005;198:857–879.

32. Gladwin MT, Vichinsky E. Pulmonary complications of sickle cell disease NEJM 2008;359:2254–2265.

33. Rogers ZR. Priapism in sickle cell disease. Hematol Oncol Clin North Am 2005;19:917–928.

34. Fellison AM, Shaw, KS. Management of vasoocclusive pain events in sickle cell disease. Pediatr Emergency Care 2007;23:832–838.

35. Dessap AM, Leon R, Habibi A, et al. Pulmonary hypertension and cor pulmonale during severe acute chest syndrome in sickle cell disease. Am J Respir Crit Care Med 2008;177:646–653.

36. Sedrak A, Rao SP, Miller ST, et al. A prospective appraisal of pulmonary hypertension in children with sickle cell disease. J Pediatr Hematol Oncol 2009;31:97–100.

37. Nelson SC, Adade BB, McDonough EA, et al. High prevalence of pulmonary hypertension in children with sickle cell disease. J Pediatr Hematol Oncol 2007;29:334–337.

38. Henry M, Driscoll CM, Miller M, et al. Pseudotumor cerebri in children with sickle cell disease: A case series. Pediatrics 2004;113:e265–e269.

39. Al-Mousawi FR, Malki AA. Managing femoral head osteonecrosis in patients with sickle cell disease. Surgeon 2007;5:282–289.

40. Akinyoola AL, Adediran IA, Asaleye CM, Bolarinwa AR. Risk factors for osteonecrosis of the femoral head in patients with sickle cell disease. Int Orthop 2009;33:923–926.

41. Chapelon E, Garabedian M, Brousse V, et al. Osteopenia and vitamin D deficiency in children with sickle cell disease. Eur J Haematol 2009;83:572–578.

42. Emerson GG, Lutty GA. Effects of sickle cell disease on the eye: Clinical features and treatment. Hematol Oncol Clin North Am 2005;957–973.

43. Suell MN, Horton TM, Dishop MK, et al. Outcomes for children with gallbladder abnormalities and sickle cell disease. J Pediatr 2004;145:617–621.

44. Sachdev V, Machado RF, Shizukuda Y, et al. Diastolic dysfunction is an independent risk factor for death in patients with sickle cell disease. J Am Coll Cardiol 2007;49;472–479.

45. Zilberman MV, Du W, Das S, Sarnaik SA. Evaluation of left ventricular diastolic function in pediatric sickle cell disease patients. Am J Hematol 2007;82:433–438.

46. Pannu R, Zhang J, Andraws R, Armani A, et al. Acute myocardial infarction in sickle disease: A systematic review. Crit Pathways in Cardiol 2008;7:133–138.

47. Levenson JL, McClish DK, Dahman BA, Bovbjerg VE, et al. Depression and anxiety in adults with sickle cell disease: The PiSES project. Psychosom Med 2008;70:192–196.

48. Simon K, Barakat LP, Ptterson A, Dampier C. Symptoms of depression and anxiety in adolescents with sickle cell disease: The role of intrapersonal characteristics and stress processing variables. Child Psychiatry Hum Dev 2009;40:317–330.

49. Benton TD, Ifeagwu JA, Smith-Whitley K. Anxiety and depression in children and adolescents with sickle cell disease. Curr Psychiatry Rep 2007;9:114–121.

50. Villers MS, Jamison MG, DeCastro LM, James AH. Morbidity associated with sickle cell disease in pregnancy. Am J Obstet Gynecol 2008;199:125.e1–125.e5.

51. Update recommendation from the advisory committee on immunization practices (ACIP) for revaccination of persons at prolonged increased risk for meningococcal disease. MMWR Morb Mortal Wkly Rep 2009;58:1042–1043.

52. Halasa NB, Shankar SM, Talbot TR, et al. Incidence of invasive pneumococcal disease among individuals with sickle cell disease before and after the introduction of the pneumococcal conjugate vaccine. Clin Infect Dis 2007;44:1428–1433.

53. Adamkiewicz TV, Silk BJ, Howgate J, et al. Effectiveness of the 7-valent pneumococcal conjugate vaccine in children with sickle cell disease in the first decade of life. Pediatrics 2008;121:562–569.

54. Licensure of a 13-valent pneumococcal conjugate vaccine (PCV13) and recommendations for use among children—Advisory Committee on Immunization Practice (ACIP). MMWR Morb Mortal Wkly Rep 2010;59:258–261.

55. Coleman E, Inusa B. Sickle cell anemia: Targeting the role of fetal hemoglobin in therapy. Clin Pediatr 2007;46:386–391.

56. Heeney MM, Ware RE. Hydroxyurea for children with sickle cell disease. Pediatr Clin N Am 2008;5;483–501.

57. Brawley OW, Comelius LJ, Edwards LR. National Institutes of Health consensus development conference statement: Hydroxyurea treatment for sickle cell disease. Ann Intern Med 2008;148:932–938.

58. Strouse JJ, Lanzkron S, Beach MC, et al. Hydroxyurea for sickle cell disease: A systematic review for efficacy and toxicity in children. Pediatrix 2008;122:1332–1342.

59. Thornburg CD, Dixon N, Burgett S, et al. A pilot study of hydroxyurea to prevent chronic organ damage in young children with sickle cell anemia. Pediatr Blood Cancer 2009;52:609–615.

60. Hankins JS, Helton KJ, McCarville MB, et al. Preservation of spleen and brain function in children with sickle cell anemia treated with hydroxyurea. Pediatr Blood Cancer 2008;50:293–297.

61. Hankins JS, Ware RE, Rogers ZR, et al. Long-term hydroxyurea therapy for infants with sickle cell anemia: The HUSOFT extension study. Blood 2005;106:2269–2275.

62. Thompson BW, Miller ST, Rogers ZR, et al. The pediatric hydroxyurea phase III clinical trial (BABY HUG): Challenges of study design. Pediat Blood Cancer 2010;54:250–255.

63. Little JA, McGowan VR, Kato GJ, et al. Combination erythropoietin hydroxyurea therapy in sickle cell disease: Experience from National Institute of Health and a literature review. Haematologica 2006;91:1076–1083.

64. National Heart, Lung, and Blood Institute (NHLBI). Stroke with Transfusions Changing to Hydroxyurea (SWiTCH). NCT00122980 Study Details. 2009, *http://www.clinicaltrials.gov*.

65. National Heart, Lung, and Blood Institute (NHLBI). Phase II randomized trial of arginine butyrate plus standard local therapy in patients with refractory sickle cell ulcers. NCT00004412 Study Details. 2009, *http://www.clinicaltrials.gov*.

66. Saunthararajah Y, Molokie R, Saraf S, et al. Clinical effectiveness of decitabine in severe sickle cell disease. Br J Haematol 2008;141:120–131.

67. Wanko SO, Telen MJ. Transfusion management in sickle cell disease. Hematol Oncol Clin North Am 2005;19:803–826.

68. Switzer J, Hess DC, Nichols FT, et al. Pathophysiology and treatment of stroke in sickle cell disease: Present and future. Lancet Neurol 2006;5:501–512.

69. Bader-Meunier B, Verthac S, Elmaleh-Berges M, et al. Effect of transfusion therapy on cerebral vasculopathy in children with sickle-cell anemia. Haematologica 2008;93:123–126.

70. Adams RJ, Brambilla D. Discontinuing prophylactic transfusions used to prevent stroke in sickle cell disease. N Engl J Med 2005;29:2769–2778.

71. Ware RE, Zimmerman SA, Sylvestre PB, et al. Prevention of secondary stroke and resolution of transfusional iron overload in children with sickle cell anemia using hydroxyurea and phlebotomy. J Pediatr 2004;145:346–352.

72. Lee MT, Piomelli S, Granger S, et al. Stroke prevention trial in sickle cell anemia (STOP) extended follow-up and final results. Blood 2006:108:847–852.

73. Vichinsky E, Onyekwere O, Porter J, et al. A randomized comparison of deferasirox versus deferoxamine for the treatment of transfusion iron overload in sickle cell disease. Br J Haematol 2007;136:501–508.

74. Porter JB. Concepts and goals in the management of transfusional iron overload. Am J Hematol 2007;82:1136–1139.

75. Raphael J, Bernhardt MB, Mahoney DH, Mueller U. Oral iron chelation and the treatment of iron overload in a pediatric hematology center. Pediatr Blood Cancer 2009:52:616–620.

76. Naizat-Pirenne F, Bachir D, Chadebech P, et al. Rituximab for prevention of delayed hemolytic transfusion reaction in sickle cell disease. Haematol 2007;92:e132–e135.

77. Bhatia M, Walters MC. Hematopoietic cell transplantation for thalassemia and sickle cell disease: Past, present and future. Bone Marrow Transplant 2008;41:109–117.

78. Bemaudin F, Socie G, Kuentz M, et al. Long-term results of related myelooblative stem-cell transplantation to cure sickle cell disease. Blood 2007;110:2749–2756.

79. Shenoy S. Has stem cell transplantation come of age in the treatment of sickle cell disease? Bone Marrow Transplant 2007;40:813–821.

80. Brachet C, Heinrichs C, Tenoutasse S, et al. Children with sickle cell disease: Growth and gonadal function after hematopoietic stem cell transplantation. J Pediatr Hematol Oncol 2007;29:445–450.

81. Adamkiewicz TV, Szabolcs P, Haight A, et al. Unrelated cord blood transplantation in children with sickle cell disease: Review of four-center experience. Pediatr Transplant 2007;11:641–644.

82. Hsieh MM, Kang, EM, Fitzhugh CD, et al. Allogeneic hematopoietic stem-cell transplantation for sickle cell disease. NEJM 2009;361:2309–2317.

83. Strouse JJ, Takemoto CM, Keefer JR, et al. Corticosteroids and increased risk of readmission after acute chest syndrome in children with sickle cell disease. Pediatr Blood Cancer 2008;50:1006–1012.

84. Muneer A, Minhas S, Arya M, Ralph DJ. Stuttering priapism—a review of the therapeutic options. Int J Clin Pract 2008;62:1265–1270.

85. Rachid-Filho D, Cavalcanti AG, Favorito LA, et al. Treatment of recurrent priapism in sickle cell anemia with finasteride: A new approach. Urology 2009;74:1054–1057.

86. Al-salem AH. Indications and complications of splenectomy for children with sickle cell disease. J Pediatr Surg 2006;41:1909–1915.

87. Richard RE. The management of sickle cell pain. Curr Pain Headache Rep 2009;12:295–297.

88. Dumaplin CA. Avoiding admission for afebrile pediatric sickle cell pain: Pain management methods. J Pediatr Health Care 2006;20:115–122.

89. van Beers EJ, van Tuijn CF, Nieuwkerk PT, et al. Patient-controlled analgesia versus continuous infusion of morphine during vaso-occlusive crisis in sickle cell disease: A randomized controlled trial. Am J Hematol 2007;82:955–960.

90. Labbe E, Herbert D, Haynes J. Physicians' attitude and practices in sickle cell disease pain management. J Palliat Care 2005;21:246–251.

91. Morrissey LK, O'Brien Shea J, Kalish L, et al. Clinical practice guideline improves the treatment of sickle cell disease vasoocclusive pain. Pediatr Blood Cancer 2009;52:369–372.

92. Okpala IE. New therapies for sickle cell disease. Hematol Oncol Clin North Am 2005;19:975–987.

93. Grosse S, Olney R, Baily M. The cost effectiveness of universal versus selective newborn screening for sickle cell disease in the US and the UK: A critique. Appl Health Econ Health Policy 2005;4:239–244.

94. Steiner CA, Miller JL. Sickle cell disease patients in U.S. Hospitals, 2004. Healthcare Cost and Utilization Project (HCUP) Statistical Brief No.21. December 2006. Rockville, MD: Agency for Health Care Research Quality, *http://www.hcup-us.ahrq.gov/reports/statbriefs/sb21.jsp*.

95. Telfair J, Haque A, Etienne M, et al. Rural/urban difference in access to and utilization of services among people in Alabama with sickle cell disease. Public Health Rep 2003;118:27–36.

96. Ballas SK. The cost of health care for patients with sickle cell disease. Am J Hematol 2009;84:320–322.

97. Raphael JL, Dietrich CL, Whitmire D, et al. Healthcare utilization and expenditures for low income children with sickle cell disease. Pediatr Blood Cancer 2009;52:263–267.

98. Delea TE, Hagiwara M, Thomas SK. Outcomes, utilization and costs among thalassemia and sickle cell disease patients receiving deferoxamine therapy in the United States. Am J Hematol 2008;83:263–270.

99. Lanzkron S, Haywood C, Segal JB, et al. Hospitalization rates and costs of care of patients with sickle-cell anemia in the state of Maryland in the era of hydroxyurea. Am J Hematol 2006;81:927–932.

CHAPTER 112

Drug-Induced Hematologic Disorders

CHRISTINE N. HANSEN AND AMY F. ROSENBERG

KEY CONCEPTS

❶ The most common drug-induced hematologic disorders include aplastic anemia, agranulocytosis, megaloblastic anemia, hemolytic anemia, and thrombocytopenia.

❷ Drug-induced hematologic disorders are generally rare adverse effects associated with drug therapy.

❸ Reporting during postmarketing surveillance of a drug is usually the method by which the incidence of rare adverse drug reactions is established.

❹ Because drug-induced blood disorders are potentially dangerous, rechallenging a patient with a suspected agent in an attempt to confirm a diagnosis may not be ethical.

❺ The mechanisms of drug-induced hematologic disorders are the result of direct toxicity or an immune reaction.

❻ The primary treatment of drug-induced hematologic disorders is removal of the drug in question and symptomatic support of the patient.

❼ Frequent laboratory monitoring may be warranted for agents commonly demonstrating severe hematologic reactions.

---

❶ Hematologic disorders have long been a potential risk of modern pharmacotherapy. Granulocytopenia (agranulocytosis) was reported in association with one of medicine's early therapeutic agents, sulfanilamide, in 1938.[1] Some agents cause predictable hematologic disease (e.g., antineoplastics), but others induce idiosyncratic reactions not directly related to the drugs' pharmacology. The most common drug-induced hematologic disorders include aplastic anemia, agranulocytosis, megaloblastic anemia, hemolytic anemia, and thrombocytopenia.

❷ The incidence of idiosyncratic drug-induced hematologic disorders varies depending on the condition and the associated drug. Few epidemiologic studies have evaluated the actual incidence of these adverse reactions, but these reactions appear to be rare. A multinational study in Latin American countries estimated the incidence of agranulocytosis was 0.38 cases per 1 million inhabitant-years and reported a rate of 1.6 cases of aplastic anemia per million per year.[2,3] Similar results were reported in epidemiologic

studies conducted in Thailand and Barcelona.[4,5] The incidence of drug-induced thrombocytopenia is more frequent, with some reports suggesting that as many as 5% of patients who receive heparin develop heparin-induced thrombocytopenia.[6]

Although drug-induced hematologic disorders are less common than other types of adverse reactions, they are important because they are associated with significant morbidity and mortality. An epidemiologic study conducted in the United States estimated that 4,490 deaths in 1984 were attributable to blood dyscrasias from all causes. Aplastic anemia was the leading cause of death, followed by thrombocytopenia, agranulocytosis, and hemolytic anemia.[7] Like most other adverse drug reactions, drug-induced hematologic disorders are more common in the elderly than in the young; the risk of death also appears to be greater with increasing age. The risk of agranulocytosis has been reported to be higher in women than in men, with some studies suggesting a biphasic distribution, with peaks in patients <10 years of age and those >60 years of age.[3]

❸ Because of the seriousness of drug-induced hematologic disorders, it is necessary to track the development of these disorders to predict their occurrence and to estimate their incidence. Reporting during postmarketing surveillance of a drug is the most common method of establishing the incidence of adverse drug reactions. The MedWatch program supported by the Food and Drug Administration is one such program.[8] Many facilities have similar drug-reporting programs to follow adverse drug reaction trends and to determine whether an association between a drug and an adverse drug reaction is causal or coincidental. In the case of drug-induced hematologic disorders, these programs can enable practitioners to confirm that an adverse event is indeed the result of drug therapy rather than one of many other potential causes; general guidelines are readily available.[9,10]

❹ Because drug-induced blood disorders are potentially dangerous, rechallenging a patient with a suspected agent in an attempt to confirm a diagnosis may not be ethical. In vitro studies with the offending agent and cells or plasma from the patient's blood can be performed to determine causality.[11] These methods are often expensive, however, and require facilities and expertise that are not generally available. Therefore, it is extremely important that practitioners be able to clinically evaluate suspect drugs quickly and to interrupt therapy when necessary.

Throughout the past decades, lists of drugs that have been associated with adverse events have been developed to help clinicians identify possible causes. Unfortunately, these lists are comprehensive and include commonly used drugs, making it difficult to determine the cause of any abnormality. Furthermore, the absence of a drug from such a list should not discourage the investigation and reporting of an agent associated with an adverse event. It is imperative that clinicians use a rational approach to determine causality and identify the agents associated with a reaction. The clinician should focus on the issue, perform a rigorous investigation, develop

---

Learning objectives, review questions, and other resources can be found at **www.pharmacotherapyonline.com**.

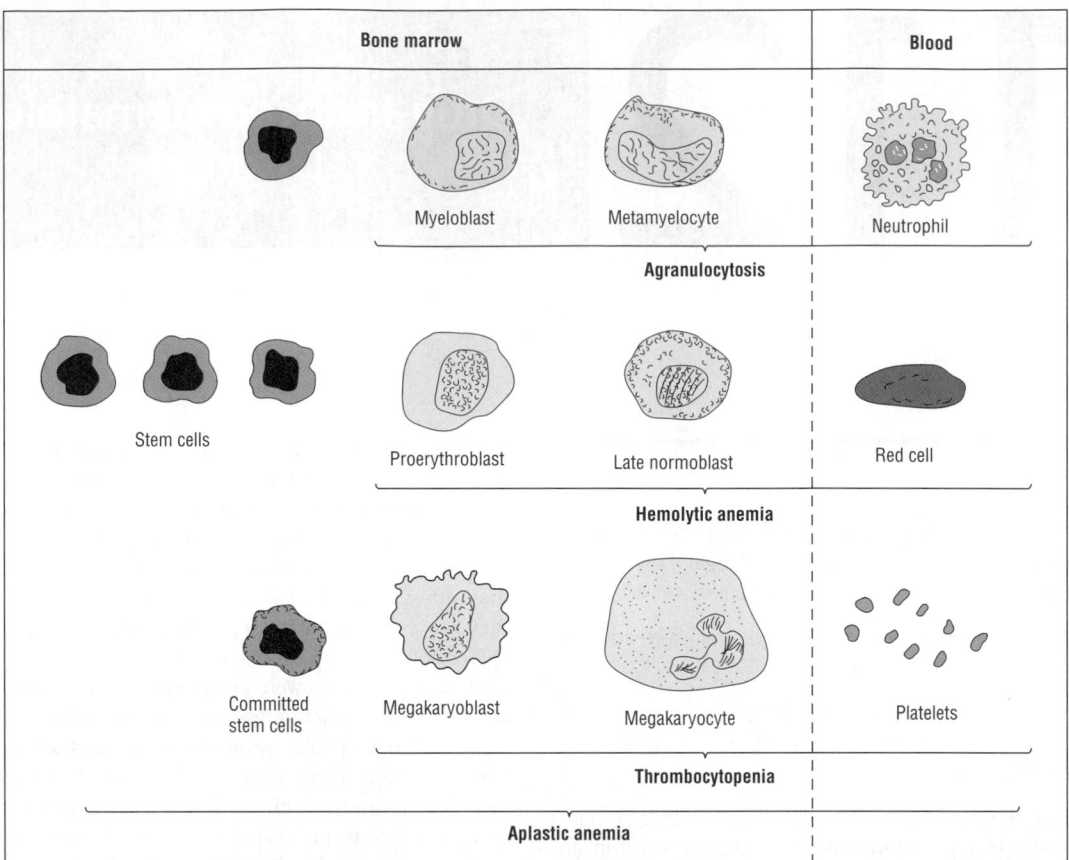

FIGURE 112-1. Differentiation of the stem cell into committed cell lines, illustrating the origins of various drug-induced hematologic disorders.

appropriate criteria, use objective criteria to grade the response, and complete a quantitative summary. A systematic approach to evaluate the information available in the literature also helps the clinician to focus and intervene in the cause of the disorder.

A common tool employed by clinicians to rate the likelihood of causality in adverse drug reaction (ADR) investigations is an ADR probability scale (algorithm). One such scale was developed and tested by Naranjo and colleagues.[12] This tool provides a series of scored questions that leads an investigator to the likelihood that an ADR was caused by the suspected medication. Depending on the aggregate score, the causality is rated as *doubtful, possible, probable, or definite*. The scale gives the most weight to the temporal relationship of the reaction with relation to administration of the drug, observations following a rechallenge of the suspected medication, and alternate explanations for the ADR. As mentioned earlier, it is often unethical to rechallenge patients who experience severe hematologic toxicities. Thus, without a rechallenge it is difficult to achieve a causality rating of *definite* with such an algorithm.

In determining the likelihood that an observed reaction is caused by a particular medication, clinicians should review the medical literature for past reports supporting the observation. Using an evidence-based approach such as that proposed by Sackett,[13] the investigator assigns greater weight to prospective study designs such as clinical trials or cohort studies than to case reports or expert opinion. This will provide a framework for the investigator's confidence in published literature describing ADRs.

In this chapter, we use both methods described to review and present published information on hematologic drug toxicities. When only case reports were available, the Naranjo algorithm was applied to the cases (if not already used). *Definite* and those rated as *probable* when only a lack of rechallenge prevented a rating of *definite* were included in the lists. An evidence-based approach was

incorporated through a review of the medical literature for prospective and retrospective studies of the adverse reactions and medications of interest. Drugs significantly associated with an adverse reaction of interest through studies were also deemed to have a causal relationship to the reaction.

The understanding of drug-induced hematologic disorders requires a basic understanding of hematopoiesis. The pluripotential hematopoietic stem cells in the bone marrow, which have the ability to self-reproduce, maintain the blood. These pluripotential hematopoietic stem cells further differentiate to intermediate precursor cells, which are also called *progenitor cells or colony-forming cells*. Committed to a particular cell line, these intermediate stem cells differentiate into colonies of each type of blood cell in response to specific colony-stimulating factors (Fig. 112–1).

Drug-induced hematologic disorders can affect any cell line, including white blood cells (WBCs), red blood cells (RBCs), and platelets. When a drug causes decreases in all three cell lines accompanied by a hypoplastic bone marrow, the result is drug-induced aplastic anemia. The decrease in WBC count alone by a medication is drug-induced agranulocytosis. Drugs can affect RBCs by causing a number of different anemias, including drug-induced immune hemolytic anemia, drug-induced oxidative hemolytic anemia, or drug-induced megaloblastic anemia. A drug-induced decrease in platelet count is drug-induced thrombocytopenia.

DRUG-INDUCED APLASTIC ANEMIA

Aplastic anemia is a rare, serious disease of unclear etiology. It was first described by Ehrlich in 1888 following an episode of failed hematopoiesis identified during the autopsy of a pregnant woman.[14] Since that first report, numerous cases of aplastic anemia have been described, but the true incidence of the disease remains uncertain. Best estimates report an incidence of two to seven cases per million inhabitants.[15,16,17] Interestingly, the incidence of aplastic anemia is different in different regions, which suggests an environmental component to the etiology of this condition.[4,15,16] There is also debate regarding the peak age at which aplastic anemia is most common. Some authors have reported a peak incidence in patients younger than age 30 years while others report the highest incidence in those older than age 60 years.[4,15–18,19] When the results of all studies are considered, the young and elderly appear to be at increased risk for the development of aplastic anemia.

Aplastic anemia can be broken down into two very broad categories—inherited and acquired. Although this chapter will focus on one specific type of acquired aplastic anemia, it is important to be aware of inherited disorders of bone marrow failure because they can be misdiagnosed as acquired.[18] Inherited types of bone marrow failure typically present in the first decade of life, are often associated with physical anomalies (e.g., short stature and café-au-lait spots), and rarely respond to immunosuppressive therapies.[18] Acquired aplastic anemia accounts for the large majority of cases, and as with many other autoimmune disorders, genetic factors may predispose some patients to acquire aplastic anemia.[20,21] A number of variables can incite immune destruction of the bone marrow; the most common are drugs, insecticides, benzene and other chemical exposure, viruses, and radiation. It has been estimated that 25% to 40% of aplastic anemia cases are related to one of these external factors.[22] However, in the large majority of modern cases, a definitive causative agent cannot be identified.[18,23]

Aplastic anemia is characterized by pancytopenia (presence of anemia, neutropenia, and thrombocytopenia) with a hypocellular bone marrow and no gross evidence of increased peripheral blood cell destruction.[24] A diagnosis of aplastic anemia can be made by the presence of two of the following criteria: a WBC count of 3,500 cells/mm³ (3.5×10^9/L) or less, a platelet count of 55,000 cells/mm³ (55×10^9/L) or less, or a hemoglobin value of 10 g/dL (100 g/L; 6.21 mmol/L) or less with a reticulocyte count of 30,000 cells/mm³ (30×10^9/L) or less.[25] However, all of these blood counts do not decrease at the same rate.

Once diagnosed, acquired aplastic anemia can be classified as nonsevere, severe, or very severe based on the degree of bone marrow cellularity and peripheral neutrophil, platelet, and reticulocyte counts. Severe aplastic anemia is defined by at least two of the following three peripheral blood findings: neutrophil count of less than 500 cells/mm³ (500×10^6/L), platelet count of less than 20,000 cells/mm³ (20×10^9/L), and anemia with a corrected reticulocyte index of less than 1%.[26,27] The prognosis is poor if the neutrophil count declines to less than 200 cells/mm³ (200×10^6/L), which is the definition of very severe.[28,29] A bone marrow aspirate and biopsy are required to exclude other causes of pancytopenia.[30] There must also be no history of iatrogenic exposure to cytotoxic chemotherapy that is known to cause transient bone marrow suppression or to intensive radiation.

Aplastic anemia is considered the most serious drug-induced blood dyscrasia because of the associated high mortality rate as compared with other blood dyscrasias.[26,31] The onset of drug-induced aplastic anemia is variable and insidious. Symptoms have been reported to appear from days to months after initiation of the offending drug, with the average being approximately 6.5 weeks.[29] In some instances, symptoms appear after the drug has been discontinued. Neutropenia typically presents first, followed by thrombocytopenia, and finally, because of the longer life span of the RBCs, anemia evolves slowly.[32] Clinical features of drug-induced aplastic anemia depend on the degree to which each cell line is suppressed, similar to idiopathic disease. Symptoms of anemia include pallor, fatigue, and weakness, whereas fever, chills, pharyngitis, or other signs of infection can characterize neutropenia. Thrombocytopenia, often the initial clue to diagnosis, is manifest by easy bruisability, petechiae, and bleeding.

5 The cause of drug-induced aplastic anemia is damage to the pluripotential hematopoietic stem cells before their differentiation to committed stem cells. This damage effectively reduces the normal levels of circulating erythrocytes, neutrophils, and platelets. Three mechanisms have been proposed as causes of damage to the pluripotent hematopoietic stem cells.[28] The first is direct, dose-dependent drug toxicity. This type of injury leads to transient marrow failure secondary to direct suppression of proliferating cell lines, and hematopoietic suppression continues with dose escalation. Most often caused by chemotherapy or radiotherapy, this injury is frequently iatrogenic. The second mechanism is idiosyncratic and may operate through toxic metabolites of the parent drug. Furthermore, individual variations in the pharmacokinetics of the suspected drug, genetic polymorphisms altering metabolism, or a hypersensitivity of the stem cells to the destructive effects of the implicated drug may increase the potential for toxicity. The third mechanism is a drug- or metabolite-induced immune reaction specific to the stem-cell population, and it is this mechanism that has received much attention over the past few decades. Currently, it is believed that most cases of aplastic anemia are immune mediated.[17] It is proposed that exposure to an inciting antigen (drug) activates cells and cytokines of the immune system, leading to the death of stem cells.[28] Table 112–1 lists drugs that have been associated with drug-induced aplastic anemia.

The antineoplastic agents exemplify the dose-dependent mechanism for the development of aplastic anemia. Many of these agents have the ability to suppress one or more cell lines in a reversible manner. The degree of suppression and the cell line involved depend on the nature of the particular drug and its potential for inhibiting marrow proliferation. Chloramphenicol, an antimicrobial agent, also causes a bone marrow depression that is dose dependent and reversible.[33]

Idiosyncratic drug-induced aplastic anemia secondary to direct toxicity can be characterized by dose independence, a latent period prior to the onset of anemia, and continued marrow injury following drug discontinuation.[34] Chloramphenicol, already known to cause a dose-dependent reaction, is the prototype drug for the idiosyncratic mechanism. The estimated incidence of chloramphenicol-induced aplastic anemia is 1 case per 20,000 patients treated,[29] but the overall prevalence has fallen with decreased use of this agent.[34] The idiosyncratic mechanism is believed to result from abnormal metabolism of chloramphenicol. The nitrobenzene ring on chloramphenicol is thought to be reduced to form a nitroso group on the chloramphenicol molecule.[33] The nitroso group may then interact with DNA in the stem cell, causing damage to the chromosomes, and eventually cell death. Other investigators have hypothesized that bacteria from the gastrointestinal tract may metabolize chloramphenicol to marrow-toxic metabolites.[35] The dose-dependent and idiosyncratic reactions seen with chloramphenicol do not appear to be related.

Other drugs thought to induce aplastic anemia through toxic metabolites include phenytoin and carbamazepine. Investigators have theorized that metabolites of phenytoin and carbamazepine bind covalently to macromolecules in the cell and then cause cell death either by exerting a direct toxic effect on the stem cell or by causing the death of lymphocytes involved in regulating hematopoiesis.[36]

Of the three potential mechanisms, the most common cause of drug-induced aplastic anemia is the development of an immune reaction. Early laboratory studies showed that removal of T lymphocytes from patients with aplastic anemia improved in vitro colony formation.[37] Furthermore, overproduction of cytokines

TABLE 112-1 Drugs Associated with Aplastic Anemias

Observational study evidence
Carbamazepine
Furosemide
Gold salts
Mebendazole
Methimazole
NSAIDs
Oxyphenbutazone
Penicillamine
Phenobarbital
Phenothiazines
Phenytoin
Propylthiouracil
Sulfonamides
Thiazides
Tocainide

Case report evidence (*probable* or *definite* causality rating)
Acetazolamide
Aspirin
Captopril
Chloramphenicol
Chloroquine
Chlorothiazide
Chlorpromazine
Dapsone
Felbamate
Interferon alfa
Lisinopril
Lithium
Nizatidine
Pentoxifylline
Quinidine
Sulindac
Ticlopidine

NSAID, nonsteroidal antiinflammatory drug.

(e.g., tumor necrosis factor and interferon-γ) from activated T lymphocytes appears to be responsible for hematopoietic failure, as well as for the initiation of apoptosis.[17,38] The observation of improved hematopoiesis in aplastic anemia patients who receive a conditioning regimen with antithymocyte globulin and cyclophosphamide prior to allogeneic hematopoietic stem cell transplantation (HSCT) supports this hypothesis.[39] After the initiation of immunosuppressive therapy, bone marrow concentrations of interferon-γ decreased, whereas all cell lines improved.[40]

Additional support for an immunologic basis as a mechanism of aplastic anemia comes from a prospective, randomized, placebo-controlled trial evaluating the efficacy of antilymphocyte globulin and methylprednisolone, with or without cyclosporine, in patients with severe aplastic anemia.[41] The primary response variable was an improvement in blood counts (i.e., platelets, erythrocytes, and leukocytes) at 3 months. Patients receiving therapy with antilymphocyte globulin, methylprednisolone, and cyclosporine had a response rate of 65% versus a response rate of 39% in the group not receiving cyclosporine. The favorable response rate with immunosuppressant drugs supports the overall hypothesis of an immune-based mechanism for aplastic anemia. One can also conclude that the degree of immunosuppression is related to a better response rate.

Genetic predisposition can also influence the development of drug-induced aplastic anemia. Studies in animals and a case report of chloramphenicol-induced aplastic anemia in identical twins suggest a genetic predisposition to the development of drug-induced aplastic anemia.[29,33] Furthermore, pharmacogenetic research that focuses on patients who may be slow or

normal metabolizers of drugs can increase the clinician's ability to predict the development of aplastic anemia. Initial case-control studies have not had the statistical power necessary to identify a significant difference between controls and cases, but continued research may establish the role of altered metabolism in patients with aplastic anemia.[42]

TREATMENT

Drug-Induced Aplastic Anemia

Because of the high mortality rate associated with severe and very severe aplastic anemia, it is imperative that drug-induced aplastic anemia be diagnosed quickly and therapy initiated immediately. Treatment should be based on the degree of cytopenia, and the goals of therapy are to improve peripheral blood counts, which limits the requirement for transfusions and minimizes the risk for opportunistic infections.

6 As with all cases of drug-induced hematologic disorders, the first step is to remove the suspected offending agent. Early withdrawal of the drug can allow for reversal of the aplastic anemia.[29] The next step is to provide adequate supportive care, including appropriate antimicrobial therapy for the treatment of infection and transfusion support with erythrocytes and platelets. The routine use of recombinant human erythropoietin has been shown to be ineffective and is not recommended for the management of aplastic anemia. Appropriate supportive care is essential because the major causes of mortality in patients with aplastic anemia are bacterial or fungal infections and bleeding. Current treatment guidelines for aplastic anemia recommend the use of prophylactic antibiotic and antifungal agents when neutrophil counts are below 200 cells/mm³ (200 × 10⁶/L), but do not recommend prophylaxis for *Pneumocystis jirovecii* or use of antivirals unless the patient has undergone an HSCT. Therefore, fever of unknown origin should be initially managed with broad-spectrum antibiotics and not with agents that were used for prophylaxis. The use of granulocyte colony-stimulating factor (G-CSF) may be considered in patients not responding to antimicrobial therapy, but these agents should be discontinued after 1 week if there is no increase in neutrophil count.[30]

The clinical course of aplastic anemia is variable. The condition can progress to severe or very severe disease in some patients, although it can remain relatively stable or even resolve in others.[17] The treatment of moderate disease ranges from no clinical intervention to immunosuppressive regimens, and treatment should be based on the degree of cytopenias.[17,18]

For patients with disease requiring treatment, the two major treatment options for patients with drug-induced aplastic anemia are allogeneic HSCT and immunosuppressive therapy. Most experts consider allogeneic HSCT the treatment of choice for young patients who have human leukocyte antigen (HLA)-matched sibling donors.[30] Most patients are cured after HSCT, and the 5-year survival of patients following a matched sibling donor transplant has been reported to be 77% for adults and up to 80% to 90% in children.[17,43] Despite these promising results, relatively few patients are eligible for HSCT because less than 30% of patients have a matched sibling donor.[44] For those patients who do not have a matched sibling donor, mismatched related and matched unrelated donor transplants may be an option, but the prognosis is less optimistic. A recent published review of unrelated donor stem cell transplantation in severe aplastic anemia reported a 5-year overall survival rate ranging between 28% and 94% from eight studies.[44] The highest mortality rate was seen in older patients and those with poorer clinical status at the time of transplantation. Complications for HSCT, such as graft-versus-host disease (GVHD) and graft rejection, require all patients to be closely monitored for an extended period of time.

An alternative to allogeneic HSCT is immunosuppressive therapy, which tends to be first-line therapy for older patients and those who are not candidates for HSCT. The current standard regimen against which new therapies are measured is combination therapy with antithymocyte globulin (ATG) and cyclosporine.[45] This combination has been reported to achieve 5-year survival rates between 75% and 85%, but the response rates in older patients are lower.[44] ATG is composed of polyclonal immunoglobulin G (IgG) against human T-lymphocytes derived from either horses or rabbits, and it has been a standard component of immunosuppressive therapy for aplastic anemia for many years. Most of the studies used horse-derived ATG, and one recent trial reported a lower response rate in patients whose regimen contained rabbit-derived ATG versus those who received horse-derived ATG.[47] However, rabbit-derived ATG can produce satisfactory responses in patients who had failed previous treatment with horse-derived ATG.[46] More data are needed to determine the role of rabbit-derived ATG in the treatment of aplastic anemia. Since response to immunosuppressive therapy is often delayed (3–4 months), patients will need to continue supportive care until recovery. Patients will require monitoring for adverse effects, including serum sickness, which can occur approximately 1 week after ATG begins.[44]

Cyclosporine plays a key role in immunosuppressant therapy for aplastic anemia. Although cyclosporine monotherapy has been used in moderate cases of aplastic anemia, it is more often used in combination with ATG. The addition of cyclosporine to ATG therapy has been shown to increase response rate, improve failure-free survival, and reduce the number of immunosuppressive courses needed.[45,47] Cyclosporine inhibits interleukin-2 production and release and subsequent activation of resting T cells. Cyclosporine dosing has varied from 4 to 6 mg/kg per day to 10 to 12 mg/kg per day, with the most frequently reported initial dose of 5 mg/kg per day in two divided doses. Cyclosporine doses are titrated to a target blood concentration that can be patient and institution specific but is usually in the range of 150 to 250 mcg/L (125 to 208 nmol/L) for adult patients. Increased rates of relapse have been seen when tapering cyclosporine rapidly, and it is recommended that cyclosporine be continued for at least 12 months after response and then tapered slowly.[44] Corticosteroids are added to ATG-based immunosuppression due to their ability to reduce adverse reactions associated with ATG administration. In an effort to improve outcomes, several other agents have also been investigated in the treatment of aplastic anemia. The additive benefits of other immunosuppressive agents such as mycophenolate, cyclophosphamide, and sirolimus have been evaluated.[17] However, they have not been shown to be superior to the combination of ATG and cyclosporine, and their place in therapy is not defined.[48]

CLINICAL CONTROVERSY

Allogeneic HSCT has long been the established treatment of drug-induced aplastic anemia. More recently, immunosuppressive regimens combining antithymocyte globulin, glucocorticoids, and cyclosporine are gaining favor. The usefulness of each treatment modality is limited by various factors. Clinical data suggest that there is no difference in survival achieved with the two treatments among patients followed for 6 years. Parity between the treatments will necessitate that clinicians individualize treatment decisions, while considering risk factors, economics, and quality of life.

DRUG-INDUCED AGRANULOCYTOSIS

Agranulocytosis is defined as a reduction in the number of mature myeloid cells in the blood (granulocytes and immature granulocytes [bands]) to a total count of 500 cells/mm^3 (500 × 10^6/L) or less. It occurs most commonly in females and the elderly (i.e., >60 years of age),[49] with an estimated annual incidence of 1.1 to 12 cases per million population.[16,50] However, a multinational case-control study in Latin American countries demonstrated a much lower rate of 0.38 cases per million inhabitant-years.[3] The overall mortality rate of agranulocytosis is estimated to be 3.5% to 16%, and that rate is highest among the elderly and patients with renal failure, bacteremia, or shock at the time of diagnosis.[16,50] Of those cases reported since 1990, approximately 5% to 6% have resulted in fatal outcomes.[51] Symptoms of agranulocytosis include sore throat, fever, malaise, weakness, chills, and other signs and symptoms of infection. These symptoms can appear rapidly, within days to weeks after the initiation of the offending drug. The median duration of exposure prior to the development of agranulocytosis ranges from 19 to 60 days for most drugs associated with this adverse event, but the time to onset is greater than 1 month for most of these agents.[51] Drug-induced agranulocytosis will usually resolve over time with supportive care and management of infection. Time to neutrophil recovery has typically been reported to range from 4 to 24 days.[51] Table 112–2 provides a list of medications that have been associated with drug-induced agranulocytosis.

The cause of drug-induced agranulocytosis is not fully understood, and several mechanisms have been proposed. Initially, it was thought that drugs affected only the mature granulocytes, causing a *maturation arrest*. However, more recent studies have demonstrated that drugs may have either a direct toxic effect or an antibody-mediated effect on the bone marrow, neutrophils, or stem cells. Several immune-mediated mechanisms have been proposed.[49]

The first type of immune-mediated mechanism involves the drug or drug metabolite, antibodies, and neutrophils. This mechanism involves drug adsorption on the membrane of the neutrophil. The drug-membrane complex then acts as a hapten to stimulate antibody formation. The antibodies produced bind to the drug–membrane complex, causing WBC destruction through complement activation and removal by the phagocytic system (Fig. 112–2). This hapten-type reaction is often seen when drugs, such as the penicillin derivatives, are given in large doses. Continuous presence of the drug is required for the destruction of neutrophils in this type of reaction.

The second mechanism of immune-mediated agranulocytosis is called the *innocent bystander phenomenon*. In this reaction, the drug combines with a drug-specific antibody. The complex is nonspecifically adsorbed to the neutrophil membrane, resulting in complement activation. The activated complement then destroys the cell (Fig. 112–3). Quinidine has been associated with this type of reaction. Functioning in a manner somewhat similar to that of the second mechanism, the third mechanism of immune response involves a protein carrier that combines with the drug and then attaches to the cell membrane. This in turn causes antibody formation. The antibodies bind to the drug protein carrier–membrane complex and activate complement. The cells are then cleared by the phagocytic system (Fig. 112–4).

In addition, there are several other immune-mediated mechanisms that have been identified. The production of autoantibodies to a *spoiled membrane* is a mechanism in which the offending drug alters the neutrophil membrane. This alteration induces the formation of autoantibodies (antibodies that attach directly to the neutrophil), which causes cellular destruction by the phagocytic system. High concentrations of β-lactam antibiotics, carbamazepine, and valproic acid have been associated with inhibition of colony-forming units of granulocytes and macrophages.

TABLE 112-2 Drugs Associated with Agranulocytosis

Observational Study Evidence	Case Report Evidence (*Probable* or *Definite* Causality Rating)	
β-Lactam antibiotics	Acetaminophen	Levodopa
Carbamazepine	Acetazolamide	Meprobamate
Carbimazole	Ampicillin	Methazolamide
Clomipramine	Captopril	Methyldopa
Digoxin	Carbenicillin	Metronidazole
Dipyridamole	Cefotaxime	Nafcillin
Ganciclovir	Cefuroxime	NSAIDs
Glyburide	Chloramphenicol	Olanzapine
Gold salts	Chlorpromazine	Oxacillin
Imipenem-cilastatin	Chlorpropamide	Penicillamine
Indomethacin	Chlorpheniramine	Penicillin G
Macrolide antibiotics	Clindamycin	Pentazocine
Methimazole	Clozapine	Phenytoin
Mirtazapine	Colchicine	Primidone
Phenobarbital	Doxepin	Procainamide
Phenothiazines	Dapsone	Propylthiouracil
Prednisone	Desipramine	Pyrimethamine
Propranolol	Ethacrynic acid	Quinidine
Spironolactone	Ethosuximide	Quinine
Sulfonamides	Flucytosine	Rifampin
Sulfonylureas	Gentamicin	Streptomycin
Ticlopidine	Griseofulvin	Terbinafine
Valproic acid	Hydralazine	Ticarcillin
Zidovudine	Hydroxychloroquine	Tocainide
	Imipenem-cilastatin	Tolbutamide
	Imipramine	Vancomycin
	Lamotrigine	

NSAID, nonsteroidal antiinflammatory drug.

Finally, drug-induced apoptosis and direct toxicity for pluripotent or bipotent hematopoietic progenitor stem cells have also been associated with clozapine and ticlopidine, respectively.[49]

In the case of penicillin-induced agranulocytosis, the patient can often begin taking penicillin again, at a lower dosage, after the neutropenia has resolved without any relapse of drug-induced agranulocytosis.[52] Because of the rapid onset of symptoms and the dose-related phenomenon, a second mechanism could possibly be involved with penicillin-induced agranulocytosis. That mechanism involves an accumulation of drug to toxic concentrations in hypersensitive individuals. Researchers have shown with in vitro cell cultures that penicillin derivatives in high concentrations inhibit the growth of myeloid colony-forming units in patients recovering from drug-induced agranulocytosis.[53] Penicillin derivatives, therefore, may suppress WBCs by several mechanisms.

Antithyroid medications, such as propylthiouracil and methimazole, have been reported to cause agranulocytosis. The current incidence of this adverse effect is unknown, but early publications report agranulocytosis in approximately 0.3% to 0.6% of patients.[54] In two more recent reports, antithyroid medications accounted for 7% to 23% of drug-induced agranulocytosis cases investigated.[55,56] The mechanism by which antithyroid agents cause agranulocytosis is unknown, but antineutrophil cytoplasmic antibodies have been identified.[57] In a study by Cooper and coworkers, agranulocytosis occurred more frequently in older patients (>40 years old) and appeared within 2 months after the initiation of therapy; a possible dose-response relationship was also observed.[54] More recently Takata and colleagues found the prevalence of neutropenia to be significantly greater in patients receiving methimazole 30 mg daily compared with those receiving 15 mg per day.[58] No dose-response

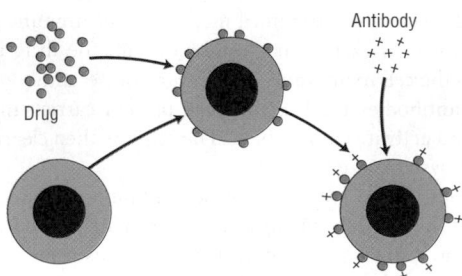

FIGURE 112-2. Drug adsorption mechanism. The drug binds to the membrane of the blood cell. Antibodies are formed to the drug–membrane complex (hapten). The antibodies then attach to the complex, and cell toxicity occurs. *(This article was published in Transfus Med Rev, Vol 7(Oct), Petz LD, Drug-induced autoimmune hemolytic anaemia, pages 242–254, Copyright © Elsevier 1993.)*

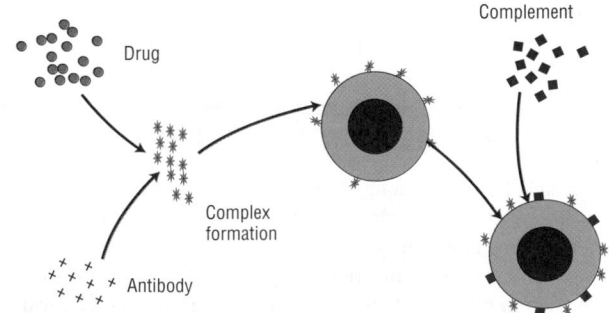

FIGURE 112-3. Innocent bystander mechanism. The drug induces antibody formation. The antibodies and drug form a complex in the serum, and the complex nonspecifically binds to the cell membrane. Complement is activated, and the cell is lysed. *(This article was published in Ballieres Clin Haematol, Vol 91, Petz LD, Drug-induced haemolytic anaemia, pages 455–482, Copyright © Elsevier 1980.)*

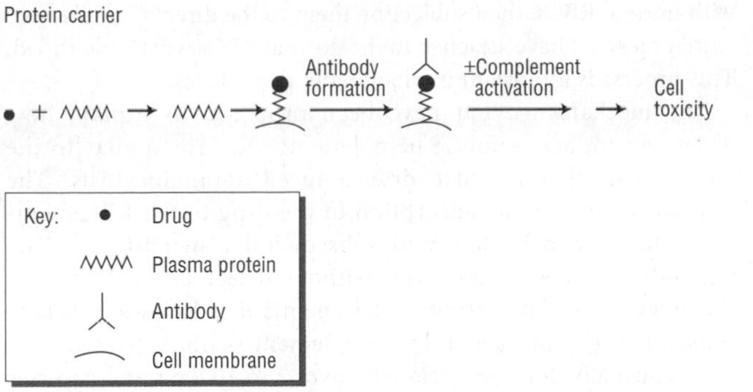

Protein carrier

FIGURE 112-4. Protein carrier mechanism. The drug combines with a plasma protein. The complex then attaches to the cell membrane, and antibody formation is stimulated. Antibodies later attach to the complex and activate complement. The cell is then lysed by the complement. (*This article was published in Clin Haematol, Vol 9(Oct), Young GA, Vincent PC, Drug-induced agranulocytosis, pages 483–504, Copyright © Elsevier 1980.*)

relationship has been observed with conventional doses of propylthiouracil. However, another study demonstrated no relationship between age or dose and the incidence of thionamide-induced agranulocytosis.[59]

Ticlopidine is an antiplatelet agent indicated for the treatment of cerebrovascular disease and the prevention of reocclusion associated with stent placement. It produces neutropenia in approximately 2.4% of patients and agranulocytosis in 0.8%,[60] possibly by inhibiting hematopoietic progenitor stem cells.[49] Patient factors that can be associated with the development of agranulocytosis include poor bone marrow reserve and age. Agranulocytosis most commonly occurs within 1 to 3 months from the initiation of ticlopidine. Removal of the drug is the best treatment option, with counts usually returning to normal within 2 to 4 weeks. The phenothiazine class of drugs is known to cause drug-induced agranulocytosis by the innocent bystander mechanism. The onset of phenothiazine-induced agranulocytosis is approximately 2 to 15 weeks after the initiation of therapy, with a peak onset between 3 and 4 weeks.[61,62] The mechanism by which phenothiazines cause drug-induced agranulocytosis has been studied primarily with chlorpromazine,[63] which is thought to affect cells in the cell cycle phase that manufactures enzymes needed for DNA synthesis (G_1 phase), or the phase in which cells are resting and not committed to cell division (G_0 phase).[63] The antipsychotic agents are known to precipitate proteins and may co-precipitate polynucleotides so they can no longer participate in nucleic acid synthesis. Chlorpromazine also increases the loss of macromolecules from the intracellular pools that are essential for cellular replication.[63] When the bone marrow from a patient with phenothiazine-induced agranulocytosis is examined, it initially appears to have no cellularity (aplastic), but over time it becomes hyperplastic. It is believed that toxic effects of the phenothiazines are not seen in all patients taking the medications because most patients have enough bone marrow reserve to overcome the toxic effects.[63]

Clozapine, an antipsychotic agent, is associated with a significantly higher risk of agranulocytosis as compared with other antipsychotic medications and has received much attention over recent years.[64] The annual incidence of clozapine-induced agranulocytosis in the United States is reported to be 1.3% and can occur at any time during treatment, although the risk is highest at around 3 months after initiation.[65] Because of the frequency and seriousness of clozapine-induced agranulocytosis and because of its reversible nature if detected early in therapy, clozapine is currently only available through a limited distribution program that requires strict WBC count monitoring.[65] In vitro studies have suggested that the formation of a nitrenium ion unstable metabolite may be responsible for clozapine-induced agranulocytosis.[49] The resulting oxidative stress caused by this metabolite may cause cytotoxicity or an immune reaction.[66]

TREATMENT

Drug-Induced Agranulocytosis

The primary treatment of drug-induced agranulocytosis is the removal of the offending drug. Following discontinuation of the drug, most cases of neutropenia resolve over time, and only symptomatic treatment (e.g., antimicrobials for infections) and appropriate vigilant hygiene practices are necessary. Sargramostim (GM-CSF) and filgrastim (G-CSF) have been shown to shorten the duration of neutropenia, length of antibiotic therapy, and hospital length of stay.[50] Although the use of both agents has been reported in the literature, a commonly reported regimen is G-CSF 300 mcg/day via subcutaneous injection. The only prospective, randomized trial to date did not confirm the benefit of these growth factors.[67] However, some experts have questioned the validity of these results based on the small sample size ($n = 24$) and the lower than standard dose of filgrastim used (i.e., 100–200 mcg/day). One systematic review found that patients with a neutrophil nadir less than 100 cells/mm³ (100×10^6/L) had a higher rate of infections and fatal complications as compared to those with a higher nadir.[51] Therefore, some clinicians recommend the use of growth factors in patients with a neutrophil nadir less than 100 cells/mm³ (100×10^6/L), regardless of the presence of infection.

DRUG-INDUCED HEMOLYTIC ANEMIA

Following their release from the bone marrow, normal RBCs survive for approximately 120 days before they are removed by phagocytic cells of the spleen and liver. The process of premature RBC destruction is referred to as hemolysis, which can occur because of either defective RBCs or abnormal changes in the intravascular environment. Drugs can promote hemolysis by both processes.

The causes of drug-induced hemolytic anemia can be divided into two categories: immune or metabolic. Those in the first category may operate much like the process that leads to immune-mediated agranulocytosis, or they can suppress regulator cells, which can lead to the production of autoantibodies. The second category involves the induction of hemolysis by metabolic abnormalities in the RBCs. Patients with drug-induced hemolytic anemia can present with signs of intravascular or extravascular hemolysis. Intravascular hemolysis, the lysis of RBCs in the circulation, can result from trauma, complement fixation to the RBC, or exogenous toxic factors. Extravascular hemolysis refers to the ingestion of RBCs by macrophages in the spleen and liver, a process that requires the presence of surface abnormalities on RBCs, such as bound immunoglobulin.[68]

The onset of drug-induced hemolytic anemia is variable and depends on the drug and mechanism of the hemolysis. Symptoms of hemolytic anemia can include fatigue, malaise, pallor, and shortness of breath. Table 112–3 provides a list of drugs that have been associated with drug-induced immune hemolytic anemia.

DRUG-INDUCED IMMUNE HEMOLYTIC ANEMIA

In immune hemolytic anemia, IgG and/or immunoglobulin M (IgM) bind to antigens on the surface of RBCs and initiate their destruction through the complement and mononuclear phagocytic systems.[69]

TABLE 112-3 Drugs Associated with Hemolytic Anemia

Observational study evidence
Phenobarbital
Phenytoin
Ribavirin

Case report evidence (*probable* or *definite* causality rating)
Acetaminophen
Angiotensin-converting enzyme inhibitors
β-Lactam antibiotics
Cephalosporins
Ciprofloxacin
Clavulanate
Erythromycin
Hydrochlorothiazide
Indinavir
Interferon alfa
Ketoconazole
Lansoprazole
Levodopa
Levofloxacin
Methyldopa
Minocycline
NSAIDs
Omeprazole
p-Aminosalicylic acid
Phenazopyridine
Probenecid
Procainamide
Quinidine
Rifabutin
Rifampin
Streptomycin
Sulbactam
Sulfonamides
Sulfonylureas
Tacrolimus
Tazobactam
Teicoplanin
Tolbutamide
Tolmetin
Triamterene

NSAID, nonsteroidal antiinflammatory drug.

Depending on the antigenic stimulus, immune hemolytic anemia is either classified as autoimmune, alloimmune, or drug-induced.[69] Drug-induced antibodies may recognize the host's intrinsic RBC antigens or RBCs bound to drug. If the antibodies react against RBC-bound drug, then the drug must be present to induce hemolysis.[69]

A laboratory test called the direct Coombs test (or direct antiglobulin test [DAT]), which identifies foreign immunoglobulins either in the patient's serum or on the RBCs themselves, is the best means to diagnose drug-induced immune hemolytic anemia. The Coombs test begins with the antiglobulin serum, which is produced by injecting rabbits with preparations of human complement, crystallizable fragment (of immunoglobulin) (Fc), or immunoglobulins. The rabbits produce antibodies against human immunoglobulins and complement. The direct Coombs test involves combining the patient's RBCs with the antiglobulin serum. If the patient's RBCs are coated with antibody or complement (as a result of a drug-induced process), the antibodies in the serum (produced by the rabbit) will attach to the Fc regions of the autoimmune globulins on separate RBCs, creating a lattice formation called agglutination.[70] This agglutination is considered positive for the presence of IgG or complement on the cell surfaces.

An indirect Coombs test can identify antibodies in a patient's serum. This test is performed by combining the patient's serum with normal RBCs, then subjecting them to the direct Coombs test. Antibodies that have attached to the normal RBCs will be identified. This process is important in blood bank procedures.

The mechanisms that have been proposed to explain how drugs can induce immune hemolytic anemia are similar to the mechanisms that produce drug-induced agranulocytosis. The first mechanism is the adsorption of the drug to the RBC membrane to form a hapten, and subsequently, an antibody. The antibody attaches to the drug without direct interaction with the erythrocyte. The extravascular anemia that follows is usually caused by IgG, and generally complement is not activated. The anemia usually develops gradually over 7 to 10 days and reverses over a couple of weeks after the offending drug is discontinued. The direct Coombs test may remain positive for several weeks. The penicillin and cephalosporin derivatives given in high doses are primarily associated with this type of immune reaction.[71] Other drugs that have been reported to cause drug-induced immune hemolytic anemia by this process include minocycline, tolbutamide, and semisynthetic penicillins.[71] Streptomycin is also associated with this type of reaction and is associated with activation of the complement system.[72]

Like drug-induced agranulocytosis, immune hemolytic anemia has been associated with the formation of immune complexes in a reaction formally known as the *innocent bystander phenomenon*. Quinidine and phenacetin are the prototype drugs of this reaction, but many other drugs have been implicated, including quinine and several sulfonamides. Drugs that induce this reaction bind weakly to a normal RBC component. The immune system identifies this complex as foreign, a *neoantigen*, and initiates lysis of the RBC via the complement system.[69] As soon as complement is activated, the complex can detach and move on to other RBCs, and to WBCs or platelets. Because of this low affinity, only a small amount of drug is needed to cause the reaction, and the direct Coombs test is positive for complement only. RBCs are essentially victims, or "innocent bystanders," of the immunologic reaction. This type of mechanism is associated with acute intravascular hemolysis that can be severe, sometimes leading to hemoglobinuria and renal failure. Following discontinuation and clearance of the drug from the circulation, the direct Coombs test will become negative.

The third mechanism is drug-induced autoimmune hemolytic anemia. The first drug implicated in this type of hemolytic anemia was methyldopa.[73] Like some other drugs, methyldopa is known to induce true autoantibodies to RBCs; the antibodies can be identified without the presence of the offending drug or its metabolites. Approximately 10% to 20% of patients receiving methyldopa will develop a positive Coombs test, usually within 6 to 12 months of initiating therapy.[74] However, less than 1% of these patients experience hemolysis, and hemolysis can develop from 4 to 6 months to more than 2 years after the start of therapy. After the withdrawal of the drug, results of the Coombs test can remain positive for many months.[72] The mechanism by which methyldopa induces antibody production is not completely known, but there are two main hypotheses.[73] The first suggests that methyldopa or its metabolites acts on the immune system and impairs immune tolerance. An alternative hypothesis suggests that the offending drug may bind to immature RBCs, altering the membrane antigens and inducing autoantibodies.

The fourth and newest mechanism that has been suggested is that of nonimmune protein adsorption (NIPA). With this mechanism, the drug alters the RBC membrane such that normal plasma proteins, including IgG, become adsorbed to the RBC membrane. RBCs coated with IgG then interact with macrophages, thereby resulting in hemolysis.[75,76]

It is not known why only some patients develop autoantibodies, and why only some of the patients who have autoantibodies develop hemolytic disease. In an effort to explain why patients have a positive result from a Coombs test and no hemolysis, Kelton demonstrated that methyldopa impairs the ability of these patients to remove antibody-sensitized cells.[77] In Coombs-positive patients receiving methyldopa, patients with impairment of the mononuclear phagocytic system could not clear the RBCs coated with autoantibodies from their bloodstream, and therefore hemolysis did not occur. Patients with hemolysis had no impairment of the mononuclear phagocytic system. Procainamide has also been reported to cause a positive result on the indirect Coombs test and hemolytic anemia.[78] Other drugs that have been reported to cause autoimmune hemolytic anemia include levodopa, mefenamic acid, and diclofenac.[79]

DRUG-INDUCED OXIDATIVE HEMOLYTIC ANEMIA

A hereditary condition, drug-induced oxidative hemolytic anemia, most often accompanies a glucose-6-phosphate dehydrogenase (G6PD) enzyme deficiency, but it can occur because of other enzyme defects (reduced nicotinamide adenine dinucleotide phosphate [NADPH] methemoglobin reductase or reduced glutathione peroxidase). A G6PD deficiency is a disorder of the hexose monophosphate shunt, which is responsible for producing NADPH in RBCs, which in turn keeps glutathione in a reduced state. Reduced glutathione is a substrate for glutathione peroxidase, an enzyme that removes peroxide from RBCs, thus protecting them from oxidative stress.[80] Without reduced glutathione, oxidative drugs can oxidize the sulfhydryl groups of hemoglobin, removing them prematurely from the circulation (i.e., causing hemolysis).

A G6PD deficiency is the most common of all enzyme defects, affecting millions of people. Because the G6PD gene is located on the X chromosome, the disorder is therefore inherited through a sex-linked mode. Both homozygotes and heterozygotes can be symptomatic, but homozygotes tend to have the most severe cases.[81] There are many G6PD variants, but the most common types occur in American and African blacks (approximately 10%), people from Mediterranean areas (e.g., Greeks, Sardinians, and Khurdic and Sephardic Jews), and Asians.[81]

The degree of hemolysis depends on the severity of the enzyme deficiency and the amount of oxidative stress. However, the dose required for hemolysis to occur is often less than prescribed quantities of the suspected drug.[72,80] Although severe hemolysis is rare, any drug that places oxidative stress on RBCs can cause drug-induced oxidative hemolytic anemia. One case of drug-induced oxidative hemolytic anemia has been reported in a child when dapsone (an oxidizing agent) was transferred through the breast milk of the mother, who was taking the drug.[82] For a list of agents associated with drug-induced oxidative hemolytic anemia, refer to Table 112–4.

TABLE 112-4 Drugs Associated with Oxidative Hemolytic Anemia

Observational study evidence
Dapsone
Case report evidence (*probable* or *definite* causality rating)
Ascorbic acid
Metformin
Methylene blue
Nalidixic acid
Nitrofurantoin
Phenazopyridine
Primaquine
Sulfacetamide
Sulfamethoxazole
Sulfanilamide

TREATMENT

Drug-Induced Hemolytic Anemia

■ DRUG-INDUCED IMMUNE HEMOLYTIC ANEMIA

The severity of drug-induced immune hemolytic anemia depends on the rate of hemolysis. Hemolytic anemia caused by drugs through the hapten/adsorption and autoimmune mechanisms tends to be slower in onset and mild to moderate in severity. Conversely, hemolysis prompted through the neoantigen mechanism (innocent bystander) phenomenon can have a sudden onset, lead to severe hemolysis, and result in renal failure. The treatment of drug-induced immune hemolytic anemia includes the removal of the offending agent and supportive care. In severe cases, glucocorticoids can be helpful,[69] but some practitioners have questioned their efficacy.[79] Other agents such as the chimeric anti-CD20 monoclonal antibody rituximab and immunoglobulin treatments have been used, but their role is yet to be clearly defined.[83,84]

■ DRUG-INDUCED OXIDATIVE HEMOLYTIC ANEMIA

Removal of the offending drug is the primary treatment for drug-induced oxidative hemolytic anemia. No other therapy is usually necessary, as most cases of drug-induced oxidative hemolytic anemia are mild in severity. Patients with these enzyme deficiencies should be advised to avoid medications capable of inducing the hemolysis.

DRUG-INDUCED MEGALOBLASTIC ANEMIA

In drug-induced megaloblastic anemia, the development of RBC precursors called megaloblasts in the bone marrow is abnormal.

Deficiencies in either vitamin B_{12} or folate are responsible for the impaired proliferation and maturation of hematopoietic cells, resulting in cell arrest and subsequent sequestration. Examination of peripheral blood shows an increase in the mean corpuscular hemoglobin concentration. These megaloblastic changes are caused by the direct or indirect effects of the drug on DNA synthesis. Some patients can have a normal-appearing cell line, and the diagnosis must be made by measurement of vitamin B_{12} and folate concentrations. The abnormality can be seen in any portion of the replication process, including DNA assembly, base precursor metabolism, or RNA synthesis.[85]

Because of their pharmacologic action on DNA replication, the antimetabolite class of chemotherapeutic agents is most frequently associated with drug-induced megaloblastic anemia. Methotrexate, an irreversible inhibitor of dihydrofolate reductase, causes megaloblastic anemia in 3% to 9% of patients.[86] Dihydrofolate reductase is an enzyme responsible for generating tetrahydrofolate, an essential factor in making deoxythymidine triphosphate, which is necessary for DNA synthesis. Other drugs such as cotrimoxazole, phenytoin, or the barbiturates have also been implicated in megaloblastic anemia. Cotrimoxazole, for example, has been reported to cause drug-induced megaloblastic anemia with both low and high doses,[87,88] particularly in patients with a partial vitamin B_{12} or folate deficiency.[85] Because the drug's affinity for human dihydrofolate reductase is low, patients with adequate stores of these vitamins are at low risk of developing drug-induced megaloblastic anemia. It has been postulated that phenytoin, primidone, and phenobarbital cause drug-induced megaloblastic anemia by either inhibiting folate absorption or by increasing folate catabolism. In both instances,

TABLE 112-5 Drugs Associated with Megaloblastic Anemia

Case Report Evidence (*Probable* or *Definite* Causality Rating)

Azathioprine
Chloramphenicol
Colchicine
Cotrimoxazole
Cyclophosphamide
Cytarabine
5-Fluorodeoxyuridine
5-Fluorouracil
Hydroxyurea
6-Mercaptopurine
Methotrexate
Oral contraceptives
p-Aminosalicylate
Phenobarbital
Phenytoin
Primidone
Pyrimethamine
Sulfasalazine
Tetracycline
Vinblastine

the patient develops a relative deficiency of folate. Table 112–5 provides a list of drugs that have been suggested as causative factors in drug-induced megaloblastic anemia.

TREATMENT

Drug-Induced Megaloblastic Anemia

When drug-induced megaloblastic anemia is related to chemotherapy, no real therapeutic option is available, and the anemia becomes an accepted side effect of therapy. If drug-induced megaloblastic anemia results from cotrimoxazole, a trial course of folinic acid, 5 to 10 mg up to four times a day, can correct the anemia.[87,88] Folic acid supplementation of 1 mg every day often corrects the drug-induced megaloblastic anemia produced by either phenytoin or phenobarbital, but some clinicians suggest that folic acid supplementation can decrease the effectiveness of the antiepileptic medications.[89]

DRUG-INDUCED THROMBOCYTOPENIA

Thrombocytopenia is usually defined as a platelet count below 100,000 cells/mm³ (100×10^9/L) or >50% reduction from baseline values. Thrombocytopenia can be caused by numerous conditions such as blood loss, infection, diffuse intravascular coagulation, and the use of some medications. The annual incidence of drug-induced thrombocytopenia is approximately 10 cases per 1,000,000 population (excluding those cases associated with heparin).[90] Although numerous epidemiologic studies have been reported, none of them have identified patient-specific risk factors that are associated with an increased risk for the development of drug-induced thrombocytopenia.[90]

Drug-induced thrombocytopenia can result from immune-mediated mechanisms or through a nonimmune-mediated mechanism. Nonimmune-mediated mechanisms, such as direct-toxicity-type reactions, are associated with medications that cause bone marrow suppression. This results in suppressed thrombopoiesis and a decreased number of megakaryocytes. This type of reaction is commonly associated with chemotherapeutic agents. Several mechanisms have been proposed for the development of immune-mediated

drug-induced thrombocytopenia: hapten-type immune reactions, drug-dependent antibodies, fiban-induced thrombocytopenia, drug-specific antibodies, autoantibody induction, and immune complex thrombocytopenia (heparin-induced thrombocytopenia).[91] While direct toxicity reactions result in decreased megakaryocytes, in contrast, immune reactions result in an increased peripheral destruction of platelets and an increased number of megakaryocytes. The clinical consequences of thrombocytopenia associated with each one of these mechanisms except the immune complex mechanism is hemorrhage. In contrast, immune complex thrombocytopenia or HIT is associated with thrombosis. Early symptoms of drug-induced thrombocytopenia include increased bruising, petechiae, ecchymoses, and epistaxis. Bleeding from mucous membranes and severe purpura can appear later in the disorder. A list of medications (excluding cancer chemotherapeutic agents) associated with drug-induced thrombocytopenia can be found in Table 112–6.

Most of the drugs that induce thrombocytopenia by their toxic effects are cancer chemotherapy agents, but organic solvents, pesticides, drugs that influence folic acid metabolism, and inamrinone (formally named amrinone) have also been implicated. Although orally administered inamrinone has been reported to cause thrombocytopenia in up to 18.6% of patients,[92] only the intravenous formulation is currently commercially available in the United States. Some studies suggest that this toxic effect might be caused by the metabolite of inamrinone, instead of the parent drug.[93] Regardless of the cause, inamrinone use has been largely replaced by other phosphodiesterase-3 inhibitors that are not associated with the same high risk of side effects.

The agents most commonly implicated in immune-mediated thrombocytopenia are quinine, quinidine, gold salts, sulfonamide antibiotics, rifampin, glycoprotein IIb/IIIa (GPIIb/IIIa) receptor antagonists, and heparin.[91] Studies of these agents have helped to elucidate the mechanisms of drug-induced immune thrombocytopenia. In hapten-type reactions, the offending drug binds covalently to certain platelet glycoproteins. Antibodies are generated that bind to these drug-bound glycoprotein epitopes. After the binding of antibodies to the platelet surface, lysis occurs through complement activation or through clearance from the circulation by macrophages.[94] Hapten-mediated immune thrombocytopenia usually occurs at least 7 days after the initiation of the drug, although it can occur much sooner if the exposure is actually a reexposure to a previously administered drug. The recovery period, once the suspected drug is discontinued, is often short in duration with a median recovery time within 1 week.[95] Although relatively rare, penicillins and cephalosporins can cause thrombocytopenia through this mechanism.[90]

Quinine, anticonvulsants, and nonsteroidal anti-inflammatory medications are thought to induce thrombocytopenia through the drug-dependent antibody mechanism.[91] This mechanism is slightly different from the hapten-type mechanism. In this type of reaction it is thought that antibodies exist within the patient's circulation that recognize an epitope on the platelet glycoprotein, but this recognition is too weak to result in antibody binding to the platelet surface. However, the drug contains structural elements that are noncovalently complementary to regions of the antibody and the glycoproteins on the platelet surface. This causes an improved fit or increased K_A between the antibody and the platelet surface, with the drug "trapped" in between, resulting in antibody binding of platelet.[91] A recently published study suggests that vancomycin-induced thrombocytopenia is related to drug-dependent antibodies.[96,97]

Eptifibatide and tirofiban are platelet glycoprotein IIb/IIIa receptor antagonists that prevent platelet activation and binding of fibrinogen, thereby inhibiting platelet thrombus formation. In clinical trials and postmarketing studies it was found that approximately 0.1% to 2% of patients treated with these medications experienced acute profound thrombocytopenia within several hours of their first exposure to the drug.[91,97] This acute drop in platelets without prior drug exposure

TABLE 112-6 Drugs Associated with Thrombocytopenia

Observational study evidence	Diazoxide	Morphine
Carbamazepine	Diclofenac	Nalidixic acid
Phenobarbital	Diethylstilbestrol	Naphazoline
Phenytoin	Digoxin	Naproxen
Valproic acid	Ethambutol	Nitroglycerin
Case report evidence (*probable* or *definite* causality rating)	Felbamate	Octreotide
Abciximab	Fluconazole	Oxacillin
Acetaminophen	Gold salts	p-Aminosalicylic acid
Acyclovir	Haloperidol	Penicillamine
Albendazole	Heparin	Pentoxifylline
Aminoglutethimide	Hydrochlorothiazide	Piperacillin
Aminosalicylic acid	Ibuprofen	Primidone
Amiodarone	Inamrinone	Procainamide
Amphotericin B	Indinavir	Pyrazinamide
Ampicillin	Indomethacin	Quinidine
Aspirin	Interferonalfa	Quinine
Atorvastatin	Isoniazid	Ranitidine
Captopril	Isotretinoin	Recombinant hepatitis B vaccine
Chlorothiazide	Itraconazole	Rifampin
Chlorpromazine	Levamisole	Simvastatin
Chlorpropamide	Linezolid	Sirolimus
Cimetidine	Lithium	Sulfasalazine
Ciprofloxacin	Low-molecular-weight heparins	Sulfonamides
Clarithromycin	Measles, mumps, and rubella vaccine	Sulindac
Clopidogrel	Meclofenamate	Tamoxifen
Danazol	Mesalamine	Tolmetin
Deferoxamine	Methyldopa	Trimethoprim
Diazepam	Minoxidil	Vancomycin

suggested initially that this reaction was mediated by a nonimmune mechanism. However, a plausible immune-mediated mechanism has since been proposed. After binding to the GPIIb/IIIa receptor, these medications cause a conformational change in the receptor that allows it to be recognized by naturally occurring antibodies already in the patient's blood (i.e., a ligand-induced binding site). In contrast to the two previously discussed immune-mediated mechanisms (hapten-type and drug dependent), the drug is not present within the binding between the antibody and the platelet surface. The drug has been removed from the platelet surface before the antibody binds, but the conformational change in the GPIIb/IIIa receptor remains.[91]

Abciximab, a GPIIb/IIIa receptor antagonist like tirofiban and eptifibatide is also associated with thrombocytopenia. Abciximab-induced thrombocytopenia appears to occur through a different drug-specific antibody mechanism as opposed to a ligand-induced binding site mechanism with eptifibatide and tirofiban. Unlike tirofiban and eptifibatide, abciximab is a chimeric (human–mouse) monoclonal antibody. As such, it is not surprising that this molecule may exhibit some immunogenic properties. It has been demonstrated that patients who experience thrombocytopenia after the administration of abciximab have circulating antibodies that directly recognize the drug. Because the drug is bound to platelets, thrombocytopenia results. Approximately 2% of patients experience thrombocytopenia with the first administration, and 10% to 12% with subsequent administrations.[98,99] Further, in those patients who experience the reaction with the first administration, some experience immediate thrombocytopenia, while in a small subset of patients, this does not occur until approximately a week after drug administration. In patients who experience immediate thrombocytopenia, drug-specific antibodies are naturally occurring and present at the time of drug administration. For those with a delayed response (6 to 8 days later), drug-specific antibodies are produced during this time, and because abciximab remains bound to platelets for up to 2 weeks, the reaction can still occur.[100] Because all three GPIIb/IIIa receptor antagonists are coadministered with heparin, it is impor-

tant to distinguish between GPIIb/IIIa receptor antagonist-induced and heparin-induced thrombocytopenia. A heparin-induced platelet aggregation study can help to determine the offending agent. Pseudothrombocytopenia, defined as in vitro platelet aggregation in blood anticoagulated with ethylenediamine tetraacetic acid (EDTA), is clinically insignificant, but it must also be differentiated from thrombocytopenia induced by GPIIb/IIIa receptor antagonists. In this case, microscopic examination of a peripheral blood smear, along with repeated platelet counts in citrate-anticoagulated blood samples, makes the distinction possible.[101]

CLINICAL CONTROVERSY

Profound thrombocytopenia (i.e., platelet count less than 20,000 cells/mm³ [20 × 10⁹/L]) has been reported with the GPIIb/IIIa receptor antagonists. Before this effect was fully appreciated, many clinicians attributed this event to heparin. The current challenge for clinicians is to distinguish between GPIIb/IIIa receptor antagonist-induced and heparin-induced thrombocytopenia, so that the patient's adverse event is documented properly. Thrombocytopenia associated with GPIIb/IIIa receptor antagonists can present with a nadir of platelet counts of 1,000 to 4,000 cells/mm³ (1 to 4 × 10⁹/L) occurring from 2 to 31 hours following bolus infusion, which is much sooner than the 5 to 10 days observed with initial heparin exposure. However, reexposure to heparin can produce profound thrombocytopenia within hours. The ubiquity of heparin use for flushing catheters makes it difficult to determine previous exposure in many cases. Clinicians can choose from several types of assays to aid in the diagnosis of heparin-induced thrombocytopenia, including platelet activation assays, platelet aggregation studies, and enzyme-linked immunosorbent assay methods, each with varying sensitivity, specificity, and availability.

Gold compounds and procainamide appear to induce thrombocytopenia through the platelet-specific autoantibody-type reaction.[90] In this type of reaction, a drug induces the production of autoantibodies that bind to platelet membranes and cause destruction, but the causative drug does not have to be present for the reaction to occur. In contrast, the drug-dependent antibody reaction requires the presence of the drug to allow antibody binding. Although several mechanisms of drug-induced thrombocytopenia have been proposed, it is often not possible to determine the mechanism for an individual drug or patient, and more than one mechanism can be responsible for the condition.

The final type of immune-mediated thrombocytopenia has been categorized as immune complex–induced thrombocytopenia.[91] This describes the mechanism of the most serious type of heparin-induced thrombocytopenia, HIT type II.

At least two types of heparin-induced thrombocytopenia (HIT) have been identified. The most common, type I, occurs in approximately 10% to 20% of patients treated with heparin.[102] It is a mild, reversible, nonimmune-mediated reaction that usually occurs within the first 2 days of therapy.[6] The platelet count slowly returns to baseline following an initial decline, despite continued heparin therapy. HIT type I is usually an asymptomatic condition and is thought to be related to platelet aggregation.[6]

HIT type II is less common but more severe and can be associated with more complications. Approximately 1% to 5% of patients receiving unfractionated heparin and up to 0.8% of patients receiving low-molecular-weight heparin (LMWH) can develop HIT.[6,102] Patients typically present with a low platelet count (e.g., below 150,000 cells/ mm³ [150 × 10⁹/L]) or a 50% or more decrease in platelet count from baseline, and thrombosis can occur.[103] The platelet count generally begins to decline 5 to 10 days after the start of heparin therapy. However, this decline can occur within hours of receiving heparin if the patient has recently received heparin (i.e., within 100 days).[103] Thrombocytopenia and thrombosis can develop with low-dose heparin,[104] heparin-coated catheters,[105] or even heparin flushes. Certain patient populations have a higher risk for developing HIT than others; patients who have had recent, major surgery are one of the highest-risk groups.[102] The next highest risk groups include patients receiving heparin for thrombosis prophylaxis following peripheral vascular surgery, cardiac surgery, and orthopedic surgery.[106] A lower incidence is seen in medical, obstetric, and pediatric patients, especially those receiving LMWH instead of unfractionated heparin.[102] The most recent practice guidelines by the American College of Chest Physicians recommend varying degrees of platelet monitoring based on the relative risk of developing HIT.[107]

HIT is caused by the development of antibodies against platelet factor-4 (PF-4) and heparin complexes[103] (Fig. 112–5). Low-molecular-weight heparins bind less well to PF-4 than unfractionated heparin, and therefore antibody formation is less common. However, there is cross-reactivity between antibodies developed by patients receiving unfractionated heparin and LMWH; thus LMWH should not be used in patients with HIT.[102] Once the antibodies bind to the complexes, platelet activation and aggregation occur, with subsequent release of more circulating PF-4 to interact with heparin. In addition, procoagulant microparticles are also released that increase the risk of thrombosis.[102] Thrombosis is one of the major complications of HIT and can occur in up to 20% to 50% of patients with HIT.[103] In fact, thrombosis is the precipitating factor that leads the clinician to diagnose HIT in many patients. This high risk of thrombosis continues for days to weeks after heparin discontinuation and platelet recovery, and continued anticoagulation with an alternative agent is essential during this time period.[103] Other less frequent manifestations of HIT include heparin-induced

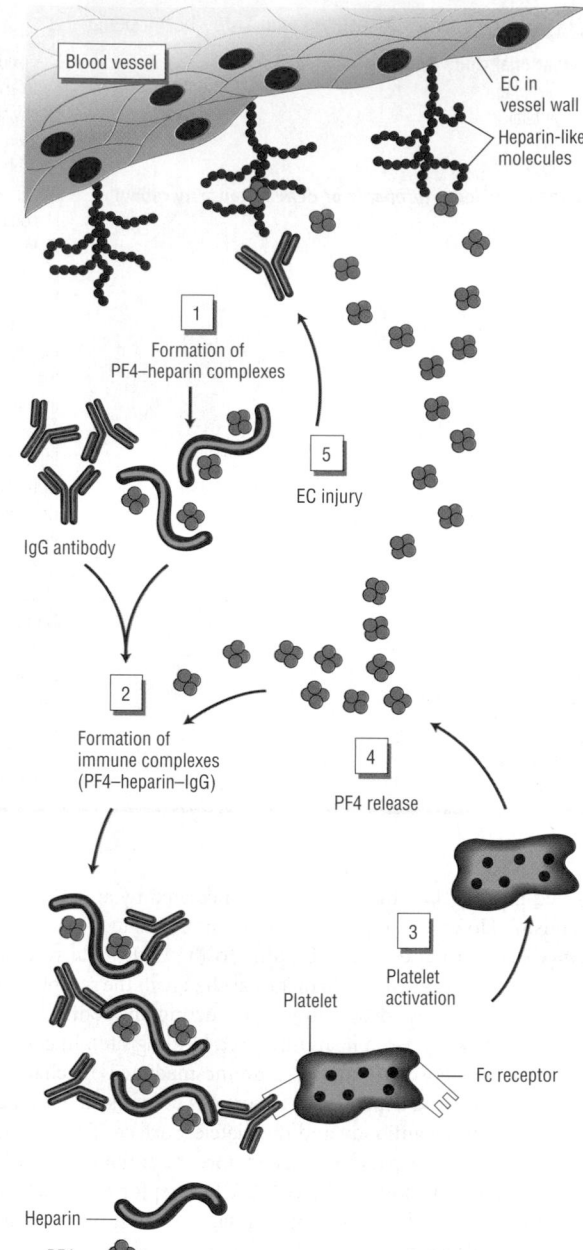

FIGURE 112-5. Proposed explanation for the presence of both thrombocytopenia and thrombosis in heparin-sensitive patients who are treated with heparin. Injected heparin reacts with platelet factor-4 (PF-4), which is normally present on the surface of endothelial cells (ECs) or released in small quantities from circulating platelets, to form PF-4–heparin complexes *(1)*. Specific immunoglobulin G (IgG) antibodies react with these conjugates to form immune complexes *(2)* that bind to crystallizable fragment (Fc) receptors on circulating platelets. Fc-mediated platelet activation *(3)* releases PF-4 from α-granules in platelets *(4)*. Newly released PF-4 binds to additional heparin, and the antibody forms more immune complexes, establishing a cycle of platelet activation. PF-4 released in excess of the amount that can be neutralized by available heparin binds to heparin-like molecules (glycosaminoglycans) on the surface of ECs to provide targets for antibody binding. This process leads to immune-mediated EC injury *(5)* and heightens the risk of thrombosis and disseminated intravascular coagulation. *(Aster RH. Heparin-induced thrombocytopenia and thrombosis. N Engl J Med 1995;332:1374–1376. Copyright © 1995 Massachusetts Medical Society. All rights reserved.)*

skin necrosis and venous gangrene of the limbs.[102,103] The diagnosis of HIT is frequently a clinical one, supported by laboratory testing. Several types of assays are available to aid in the diagnosis of HIT, including platelet activation assays, platelet aggregation studies, and enzyme-linked immunosorbent assay methods, each with varying sensitivities and specificities.[6]

TREATMENT

Drug-Induced Thrombocytopenia

The primary treatment of drug-induced thrombocytopenia is removal of the offending drug and symptomatic treatment of the patient. The use of corticosteroid therapy in the treatment of drug-induced thrombocytopenia is controversial, although some authors recommend it in severe symptomatic cases.[108]

In the case of HIT, the main goal of management is to reduce the risk of thrombosis or reduce thrombosis-associated complications in patients who have already developed a clot. All forms of heparin must be discontinued, including heparin flushes, and alternative anticoagulation must begin immediately.[109] The direct thrombin inhibitors are the alternative anticoagulants most commonly used in current practice. Three direct thrombin inhibitors are currently available: lepirudin, argatroban, and bivalirudin. Lepirudin, the first drug that was approved for the treatment of HIT, is a recombinant analogue of hirudin, a natural anticoagulant found in leeches. Lepirudin is renally eliminated and requires dosage adjustment in those patients with kidney dysfunction. It is also important to note that antibodies to lepirudin develop in approximately 30% of patients who receive this agent for the first time, and it is therefore recommended that patients receive only one treatment course of lepirudin.[103] Argatroban is another intravenous thrombin inhibitor indicated for the management of HIT. But unlike lepirudin, argatroban is metabolized in the liver and can be used in patients with end-stage renal disease. However, dosage adjustment is needed for patients with significant hepatic impairment. The most recently approved direct thrombin inhibitor is bivalirudin. It is similar to lepirudin in that is a parenteral bivalent analogue of hirudin. It requires dosage adjustment only in severe renal failure. Fondaparinux, an anticoagulant pentasaccharide that inhibits factor Xa, has been proposed by some as a potential treatment for HIT because it does not appear to cause in vitro cross-reactivity with HIT antibodies.[110,111] Clinical data, however, to support the use of fondaparinux in the treatment of HIT-induced thrombosis are lacking. The most recent guidelines by the American College of Chest Physicians suggest that fondaparinux is most appropriately used in patients at relatively low risk of having HIT but for whom the use of either UFH or LMWH is not desired.[107] These agents should also be considered for the treatment of patients who have acute HIT without thrombosis because of the increased risk of thrombosis occurring in these patients. Because of the increased risk of venous limb gangrene, warfarin should not be used alone to treat acute HIT complicated by deep vein thrombosis.[107]

SUMMARY

❼ Drug-induced hematologic disorders are rare but potentially life-threatening conditions. Clinicians should be cognizant of medications with the potential of causing hematologic disorders and educate patients to recognize the symptoms associated with such events. Frequent laboratory monitoring of patients taking medications associated with severe hematologic events can facilitate diagnosis and treatment. Identifying the etiology of the event and documenting the causative agents can serve to prevent a recurrence secondary to the use of a related medication. Reporting these events to national adverse event reporting services and in the peer-reviewed medical literature can serve to improve the understanding of the prevalence and risk factors for this disorder.

ABBREVIATIONS

ADR: adverse drug reaction

ATG: antithymocyte globulin

DAT: direct antiglobulin test

EDTA: ethylenediamine tetraacetic acid

Fc: crystallizable fragment (of immunoglobulin)

G6PD: glucose-6-phosphate dehydrogenase

G-CSF: granulocyte colony-stimulating factor

GM-CSF: granulocyte-macrophage colony-stimulating factor

GPIIb/IIIa: glycoprotein IIb/IIIa

GVHD: graft-versus-host disease

HIT: heparin-induced thrombocytopenia

HLA: human leukocyte antigen

HSCT: hematopoietic stem cell transplantation

IgG: immunoglobulin G

IgM: immunoglobulin M

LMWH: low-molecular-weight heparin

NADPH: reduced nicotinamide adenine dinucleotide phosphate

PF-4: platelet factor-4

RBC: red blood cell

WBC: white blood cell

REFERENCES

1. Johnston FD. Granulocytopenia following the administration of sulfanilamide compounds. Lancet 1938;2:1004–1047.
2. Maluf E, Hamerschlak N, Cavalcanti A, et al. Incidence and risk factors of aplastic anemia in Latin American countries: the LATIN case-control study. Haematologica 2009;94:1220–1226.
3. Hamerschlak N, Maluf E, Cabalcanti A, et al. Incidence and risk factors for agranulocytosis in Latin American countries—the Latin study. Eur J Clin Pharmacol 2008;64:921–929.
4. Montane E, Ibanez L, Vidal X, et al. Epidemiology of aplastic anemia: A prospective multicenter study. Haematologica 2008;93:518–523.
5. Kaufman DW, Kelly JP, Issaragrisil S, et al. Relative incidence of agranulocytosis and aplastic anemia. Am J Hematol 2006;81:65–67.
6. Franchini M. Heparin-induced thrombocytopenia: An update. Thromb J 2005;3:1–5, http://www.thrombosisjournal.com/content/3/1/14.
7. Hine LK, Gerstman BB, Wise RP, et al. Mortality resulting from blood dyscrasias in the United States, 1984. Am J Med 1990;88:151–153.
8. Kessler DA. Introducing MEDWatch: A new approach to reporting medication and device adverse effects and product problems. JAMA 1993;269:2765–2768.
9. ASHP guidelines on adverse drug reaction monitoring and reporting. American Society of Hospital Pharmacy. Am J Health Syst Pharm 1995;52:417–419.
10. Rieder MJ. In vivo and in vitro testing for adverse drug reactions. Pediatr Clin North Am 1997;44:93–111.
11. Parent-Massin DM, Sensebe L, Leglise MC, et al. Relevance of in vitro studies of drug-induced agranulocytosis. Report of 14 cases. Drug Saf 1993;9:463–469.
12. Naranjo CA, Busto U, Sellers EM, et al. A method for estimating the probability of adverse drug reactions. Clin Pharmacol Ther 1981;30:239–245.

13. Sackett D. Clinical Epidemiology: A Basic Science for Clinical Medicine, 2nd ed. Boston: Little, Brown; 1991:xiii, 370, plates 1.

14. Ehrlich P. Ueber einem Fall von Anamie mit Berner-kungen uber regenerative Veranderungen des Knochenmarks. Charite-Annalen 1888;13:301–309.

15. Issaragrisil S, Kaufman DW, Anderson T, et al. The epidemiology of aplastic anemia in Thailand. Blood 2006;107:1299–1307.

16. Kaufman DW, Kelly JP, Issaragrisil S, et al. Relative incidence of agranulocytosis and aplastic anemia. Am J Hematol 2006;81:65–67.

17. Young NS, Calado RT, Scheinberg P. Current concepts in the patho-physiology and treatment of aplastic anemia. Blood 2006;108: 2509–2519.

18. Brodsky RA, Jones RJ. Aplastic anaemia. Lancet 2005;365:1647–1656.

19. Gale RP, Champlin RE, Feig SA, et al. Aplastic anemia: Biology and treatment. Ann Intern Med 1981;95:477–494.

20. Nimer SD, Ireland P, Meshkinpour A, et al. An increased HLA DR2 frequency is seen in aplastic anemia patients. Blood 1994;84:923–927.

21. Poonkuzhali B, Shaji RV, Salamun DE, et al. Cytochrome P4501A1 and glutathione S transferase gene polymorphisms in patients with aplastic anemia in India. Acta Haematol 2005;114:127–132.

22. Kaufman DW, Kelly JP, Levy M, et al. The Drug Etiology of Agranulocytosis and Aplastic Anemia, 1st ed. New York: Oxford University Press; 1991.

23. Gewirtz AM, Hoffman R. Current considerations of the etiology of aplastic anemia. Crit Rev Oncol Hematol 1985;4:1–30.

24. Council for International Organizations of Medical Sciences. Standardization of definitions and criteria of assessment of adverse drug reactions: Drug-induced cytopenia. Int J Clin Pharmacol Ther Toxicol 1991;29:75–81.

25. Heimpel H. Epidemiology and etiology of aplastic anemia. In: Schrezenmeier H, ed. Aplastic Anemia: Pathophysiology and Treatment. Cambridge, UK: Cambridge University Press; 2000:97–116.

26. The International Agranulocytosis and Aplastic Anemia Study Group. Risks of agranulocytosis and aplastic anemia: A first report of their relation to drug use with special reference to analgesics. JAMA 1986;256:1749–1757.

27. Camitta BM, Thomas ED, Nathan DG, et al. A prospective study of androgens and bone marrow transplantation for treatment of severe aplastic anemia. Blood 1979;53:504–514.

28. Young NS, Maciejewski J. The pathophysiology of acquired aplastic anemia. N Engl J Med 1997;336:1365–1372.

29. Shadduck R. Aplastic anemia. In: Beutler E, Lichtman MA, Coller BS, Kipps TJ, eds. Williams Hematology. New York: McGraw-Hill, 1995:238–251.

30. Marsh J, Ball S, Cavenagh J, et al. Guidelines for the diagnosis and management of aplastic anemia. Br J Haematol 2009;147:43–70.

31. Howard SC, Naidu PE, Hu XJ, et al. Natural history of moderate aplastic anemia in children. Pediatr Blood Cancer 2004;43:545–551.

32. Vandendries ER, Drews RE. Drug-associated disease: Hematologic dysfunction. Crit Care Clin 2006;22:347–355, viii.

33. Yunis AA, Miller AM, Salem Z, et al. Chloramphenicol toxicity: Pathogenetic mechanisms and the role of the p-NO$_2$ in aplastic anemia. Clin Toxicol 1980;17:359–373.

34. Malkin D, Koren G, Saunders EF. Drug-induced aplastic anemia: Pathogenesis and clinical aspects. Am J Pediatr Hematol Oncol 1990;12:402–410.

35. Jimenez JJ, Arimura GK, Abou-Khalil WH, et al. Chloramphenicol-induced bone marrow injury: Possible role of bacterial metabolites of chloramphenicol. Blood 1987;70:1180–1185.

36. Gerson WT, Fine DG, Spielberg SP, et al. Anticonvulsant-induced aplastic anemia: increased susceptibility to toxic drug metabolites in vitro. Blood 1983;61:889–893.

37. Kagan WA, Ascensao JA, Pahwa RN, et al. Aplastic anemia: Presence in human bone marrow of cells that suppress myelopoiesis. Proc Natl Acad Sci USA 1976;73:2890–2894.

38. Selleri C, Sato T, Anderson S, et al. Interferon-gamma and tumor necrosis factor-alpha suppress both early and late stages of hematopoiesis and induce programmed cell death. J Cell Physiol 1995;165:538–546.

39. Mathe G, Amiel JL, Schwarzenberg L, et al. Bone marrow graft in man after conditioning by antilymphocytic serum. Br Med J 1970;2: 131–136.

40. Platanias L, Gascon P, Bielory L, et al. Lymphocyte phenotype and lymphokines following anti-thymocyte globulin therapy in patients with aplastic anaemia. Br J Haematol 1987;66:437–443.

41. Frickhofen N, Kaltwasser JP, Schrezenmeier H, et al. Treatment of aplastic anemia with antilymphocyte globulin and methylprednisolone with or without cyclosporine. The German Aplastic Anemia Study Group. N Engl J Med 1991;324:1297–1304.

42. Marsh JC, Chowdry J, Parry-Jones N, et al. Study of the association between cytochromes P450 2D6 and 2E1 genotypes and the risk of drug and chemical induced idiosyncratic aplastic anaemia. Br J Haematol 1999;104:266–270.

43. Horowitz MM. Current status of allogeneic bone marrow transplantation in acquired aplastic anemia. Semin Hematol 2000;37:30–42.

44. Peinemann F, Grouven U, Kroger N, et al. Unrelated donor stem cell transplantation in acquired severe aplastic anemia: A systemic review. Haematologica 2009;94:1–11.

45. Frickhofen N, Heimpel H, Kaltwasser JP, et al. Antithymocyte globulin with or without cyclosporin A: 11-year follow-up of a randomized trial comparing treatments of aplastic anemia. Blood 2003;101: 1236–1242.

46. Miura K, Hatta Y, Kobayashi S, et al. Feasibility and eligibility of retreatment with rabbit anti-T lymphocyte globulin for aplastic anemia previously treated with horse anti-thymocyte globulin. Int J Hematol. 2009; 90:426–428.

47. Zheng Y, Liu Y, Chu Y. Immunosuppressive therapy for acquired severe aplastic anemia (SAA): A prospective comparison of four different regimens. Exp Hematol 2006;34:826–831.

48. Scheinberg P, Wu C, Nunez O, et al. Treatment of severe aplastic anemia with combination of horse antithymocyte globulin and cyclosporine, with or without sirolimus: A prospective randomized study. Haematologica 2009;94:348–354.

49. Bhatt V, Saleem A. Review: Drug-induced neutropenia—pathophysiology, clinical features, and management. Ann Clin Lab Sci 2004;34: 131–137.

50. Andres E, Noel E, Kurtz JE, et al. Life-threatening idiosyncratic drug-induced agranulocytosis in elderly patients. Drugs Aging 2004;21: 427–435.

51. Andersohn F, Konzen C, Garbe E. Systematic review: Agranulocytosis induced by nonchemotherapy drugs. Ann Intern Med 2007;146: 657–665.

52. Neftel K, Muller M, Hauser S, et al. More on penicillin-induced leukopenia. N Engl J Med 1983;308:901–902.

53. Neftel KA, Hauser SP, Muller MR. Inhibition of granulopoiesis in vivo and in vitro by beta-lactam antibiotics. J Infect Dis 1985;152:90–98.

54. Cooper DS, Goldminz D, Levin AA, et al. Agranulocytosis associated with antithyroid drugs: Effects of patient age and drug dose. Ann Intern Med 1983;98:26–29.

55. Andres E, Maloisel F, Kurtz JE, et al. Modern management of nonchemotherapy drug-induced agranulocytosis: A monocentric cohort study of 90 cases and review of the literature. Eur J Intern Med 2002;13:1–4, http://www.ispub.com/journals/ijim.htm.

56. Ibanez L, Vidal X, Ballarin E, et al. Population-based drug-induced agranulocytosis. Arch Intern Med 2005;165:869–874.

57. Akamizu T, Ozaki S, Hiratani H, et al. Drug-induced neutropenia associated with anti-neutrophil cytoplasmic antibodies (ANCA): Possible involvement of complement in granulocyte cytotoxicity. Clin Exp Immunol 2002;127:92–98.

58. Takata K, Kubota S, Fukata S, et al. Methimazole-induced agranulocytosis in patients with Graves' disease is more frequent with an initial dose of 30 mg daily than with 15 mg daily. Thyroid 2009;19:559–563.

59. Werner MC, Romaldini JH, Bromberg N, et al. Adverse effects related to thionamide drugs and their dose regimen. Am J Med Sci 1989;297:216–219.

60. Ticlid (ticlopidine). Prescribing information. 2001, http://www.roche usa.com/products/ticlid/pi.pdf.

61. Young GA, Vincent PC. Drug-induced agranulocytosis. Clin Haematol 1980;9:483–504.

62. Stubner S, Grohmann R, Engel R, et al. Blood dyscrasias induced by psychotropic drugs. Pharmacopsychiatry 2004;37(suppl 1): S70–S78.

63. Pisciotta V. Drug-induced agranulocytosis. Drugs 1978;15:132–143.

64. Schulte PF. Risk of clozapine-associated agranulocytosis and mandatory white blood cell monitoring. Ann Pharmacother 2006;40:683–688.

65. Bosco A, Kidson-Gerber G, Dunkley S. Delayed tirofiban-induced thrombocytopenia: Two case reports. J Thromb Haemost 2005;3:1109–1110.

66. Fischer V, Haar JA, Greiner L, et al. Possible role of free radical formation in clozapine (Clozaril)-induced agranulocytosis. Mol Pharmacol 1991;40:846–853.

67. Fukata S, Kuma K, Sugawara M. Granulocyte colony-stimulating factor (G-CSF) does not improve recovery from antithyroid drug-induced agranulocytosis: A prospective study. Thyroid 1999;9:29–31.

68. Tabbara IA. Hemolytic anemias: Diagnosis and management. Med Clin North Am 1992;76:649–668.

69. Gehrs BC, Friedberg RC. Autoimmune hemolytic anemia. Am J Hematol 2002;69:258–271.

70. McKenzie SB. Hemolytic anemias due to extrinsic factors. In: McKenzie SB. Textbook of Hematology. Baltimore: Williams & Wilkins; 1996;245–274.

71. Thomas A. Autoimmune hemolytic anaemias. In: Lee R, Foerster J, Lukens J, et al., eds. Wintrobe's Clinical Hematology. Baltimore: Williams & Wilkins; 1999:1233–1263.

72. Jandl J. Immunohemolytic anemias. In: Strangis J, ed. Textbook of Hematology. Boston: Little, Brown; 1996:421–518.

73. Dacie SJ. The immune haemolytic anaemias: A century of exciting progress in understanding. Br J Haematol 2001;114:770–785.

74. Aldomet (methyldopa). Prescribing information. 1998, http:// www.merck.com/product/usa/pi_circulars/a/aldomet/aldomet_pi.pdf.

75. Garraty G, Arndt P. Positive direct antiglobulin tests and haemolytic anemia following therapy with beta lactamase inhibitor containing drugs may be associated with non-immune protein adsorption onto red blood cells. Br J Haemotol 1998;100:777–783.

76. Garraty, G. Drug induced hemolytic anemia. In: Hematology 2009. American Society of Hematology Education Program Book: 73–79.

77. Kelton JG. Impaired reticuloendothelial function in patients treated with methyldopa. N Engl J Med 1985;313:596–600.

78. Kleinman S, Nelson R, Smith L, et al. Positive direct antiglobulin tests and immune hemolytic anemia in patients receiving procainamide. N Engl J Med 1984;311:809–812.

79. Packman C, Leddy J. Drug-related immune hemolytic anemia. In: Beutler E, Lichtman MA, Coller BS, Kipps TJ, eds. Williams. Hematology. New York: McGraw-Hill; 1995:691–697.

80. Beutler E. G6PD deficiency. Blood 1994;84:3613–3636.

81. Frank JE. Diagnosis and management of G6PD deficiency. Am Fam Physician 2005;72:1277–1282.

82. Sanders SW, Zone JJ, Foltz RL, et al. Hemolytic anemia induced by dapsone transmitted through breast milk. Ann Intern Med 1982;96:465–466.

83. Ahrens N, Kingreen D, Seltsam A, et al. Treatment of refractory autoimmune haemolytic anaemia with anti-CD20 (rituximab). Br J Haematol 2001;114:244–245.

84. Flores G, Cunningham-Rundles C, Newland AC, et al. Efficacy of intravenous immunoglobulin in the treatment of autoimmune hemolytic anemia: Results in 73 patients. Am J Hematol 1993;44:237–242.

85. Scott JM, Weir DG. Drug-induced megaloblastic change. Clin Haematol 1980;9:587–606.

86. Weinblatt ME. Toxicity of low dose methotrexate in rheumatoid arthritis. J Rheumatol 1985;12(suppl 12):35–39.

87. Kobrinsky NL, Ramsay NK. Acute megaloblastic anemia induced by high-dose trimethoprim-sulfamethoxazole. Ann Intern Med 1981;94:780–781.

88. Magee F, O'Sullivan H, McCann SR. Megaloblastosis and low-dose trimethoprim-sulfamethoxazole. Ann Intern Med 1981;95:657.

89. Rivey MP, Schottelius DD, Berg MJ. Phenytoin-folic acid: A review. Drug Intell Clin Pharm 1984;18:292–301.

90. Van den Bemt PM, Meyboom RH, Egberts AC. Drug-induced immune thrombocytopenia. Drug Saf 2004;27:1243–1252.

91. Aster RH, Curtis BR, McFarland JG, Bougie DW. Drug-induced immune thrombocytopenia: Pathogenesis, diagnosis, and management. J Thromb Haemost 2009;7:911–918.

92. Ansell J, Tiarks C, McCue J, et al. Amrinone-induced thrombocytopenia. Arch Intern Med 1984;144:949–952.

93. Sadiq A, Tamura N, Yoshida M, et al. Possible contribution of acetylamrinone and its enhancing effects on platelet aggregation under shear stress conditions in the onset of thrombocytopenia in patients treated with amrinone. Thromb Res 2003;111:357–361.

94. Aster RH. Drug-induced immune thrombocytopenia: an overview of pathogenesis. Semin Hematol 1999;36(suppl 1):2–6.

95. George JN, Raskob GE, Shah SR, et al. Drug-induced thrombocytopenia: A systematic review of published case reports. Ann Intern Med 1998;129:886–890.

96. Von Drygalski A, Curtis BR, Bougie DW, et al. Vancomycin-induced immune thrombocytopenia. N Engl J Med 2007;356:904–910.

97. Ortel T. Heparin-induced thrombocytopenia: When a low platelet count is a mandate for anticoagulation. In: Hematology 2009. American Society of Hematology Education Program Book: 225–232.

98. Jubelirer SJ, Koenig BA, Bates MC. Acute profound thrombocytopenia following C7E3 Fab(Abciximab) therapy: Case reports, review of the literature and implications for therapy. Am J Hematol 1999;61:205–208.

99. Dery JP, Braden GA, Lincoff AM, et al. Final results of the ReoPro readministration registry. Am J Cardiol 2004;93:979–984.

100. Mascelli MA, Lance ET, Damaraju L, Wagner CL, Weisman HF, Jordan RE. Pharmacodynamic profile of short-term abciximab treatment demonstrates prolonged platelet inhibition with gradual recovery from GP IIb/IIIa receptor blockade. Circulation 1998;97:1680–1688.

101. Aster RH. Immune thrombocytopenia caused by glycoprotein IIb/IIIa inhibitors. Chest 2005;127(suppl):53S–59S.

102. Menajovsky LB. Heparin-induced thrombocytopenia: Clinical manifestations and management strategies. Am J Med 2005;118(suppl 8A):21S–30S.

103. Arepally GM, Ortel TL. Clinical practice: Heparin-induced thrombocytopenia. N Engl J Med 2006;355:809–817.

104. Girolami B, Prandoni P, Stefani PM, et al. The incidence of heparin-induced thrombocytopenia in hospitalized medical patients treated with subcutaneous unfractionated heparin: A prospective cohort study. Blood 2003;101:2955–2959.

105. Laster JL, Nichols WK, Silver D. Thrombocytopenia associated with heparin-coated catheters in patients with heparin-associated antiplatelet antibodies. Arch Intern Med 1989;149:2285–2287.

106. Lindhoff-Last E, Wenning B, Stein M, et al. Risk factors and long-term follow-up of patients with the immune type of heparin-induced thrombocytopenia. Clin Appl Thromb Hemost 2002;8:347–352.

107. Warkentin T, Greinacher A, Koster A, Lincoff M. Treatment and prevention of heparin-induced thrombocytopenia. American College of Chest Physicians Evidence-Based Clinical Practice Guidelines (8th edition). Chest 2008;133(6):340S–380S.

108. Pedersen-Bjergaard U, Andersen M, Hansen PB. Drug-induced thrombocytopenia: Clinical data on 309 cases and the effect of corticosteroid therapy. Eur J Clin Pharmacol 1997;52:183–189.

109. Dager WE, Dougherty JA, Nguyen PH, et al. Heparin-induced thrombocytopenia: Treatment options and special considerations. Pharmacotherapy 2007;27:564–587.

110. Warkentin TE, Cook RJ, Marder VJ, et al. Anti-platelet factor 4/heparin antibodies in orthopedic surgery patients receiving antithrombotic prophylaxis with fondaparinux or enoxaparin. Blood 2005;106:3791–3796.

111. Elalamy I, Lecrubier C, Potevin C, et al. Absence of in vitro cross-reaction of pentasaccharide with the plasma heparin-dependent factor of twenty-five patients with heparin-associated thrombocytopenia. Thromb Haemost 1995;74:1384–1385.

CHAPTER

113

Laboratory Tests to Direct Antimicrobial Pharmacotherapy

MICHAEL J. RYBAK, JEFFREY R. AESCHLIMANN, AND KERRY L. LAPLANTE

KEY CONCEPTS

❶ Familiarity with normal host flora and typical pathogens will help to determine whether a patient is truly infected or merely colonized.

❷ Direct examination of tissue and body fluids by Gram stain provides simple and rapid information about the causative pathogen.

❸ Isolation of the offending organism by culture assists in the diagnosis of infection and allows for more definitive directed treatment.

❹ The development of molecular testing systems has improved our ability to diagnose infection and determine the antimicrobial susceptibilities for numerous fastidious or slow growing pathogens, such as mycobacteria and viruses.

❺ Although highly standardized, in vitro antimicrobial susceptibility testing has limitations and often cannot truly mimic the conditions found at the site of an infection. This can cause discordance between in vitro susceptibility results and in vivo response to therapy.

❻ The laboratory evaluation of antimicrobial activity is an important component of the pharmacotherapeutic management of infectious diseases.

❼ Antimicrobial pharmacodynamics have become a crucial consideration the selection of both empirical and pathogen-directed therapy in the current era of antimicrobial resistance.

❽ When used appropriately, rapid automated susceptibility test systems appear to improve therapeutic outcomes of patients with infection, especially when they are linked with other clinical information systems.

❾ Laboratory tests such as minimal bactericidal concentration tests, time-kill tests, post-antibiotic effect tests, and antimicrobial combination testing are important for the clinician to understand because they help to determine antimicrobial pharmacodynamic properties.

❿ Routine monitoring of serum concentrations is currently used for a select few antimicrobials (e.g., aminoglycosides, chloramphenicol, and vancomycin) in an attempt to minimize toxicity and maximize efficacy.

⓫ Appropriate timing for the collection of serum samples when measuring antimicrobial serum concentrations is crucial to ensure that proper data are generated on the pharmacokinetics of antimicrobials.

⓬ The monitoring of aminoglycoside serum concentrations and the use of extended-interval doses can help to maximize the probability of therapeutic success and minimize the probability of aminoglycoside-related toxicity.

⓭ Vancomycin and aminoglycoside serum concentration monitoring should be routinely done to ensure adequate serum concentrations, minimize toxicity, and avoid the potential for resistance.

⓮ Optimization of antimicrobial pharmacodynamic parameters such as the ratio of the peak serum concentration to minimum inhibitory concentration or the time that the serum concentration remains above the minimum inhibitory concentration and area above the curve over minimum inhibitory concentration can improve infection treatment outcomes.

Learning objectives, review questions, and other resources can be found at
www.pharmacotherapyonline.com.

Selection of an appropriate antimicrobial therapeutic regimen for a given infectious disease requires knowledge of the infecting pathogen, host characteristics, and the drug's expected activity against the pathogen. The most fundamental aspect of therapy starts with an appropriate diagnosis. A vast array of laboratory tests is available to assist in verifying the presence of infection and for monitoring the response to therapy. Although useful, these tests are subject to interpretation and cannot be substituted for sound clinical judgment. Organism susceptibility to the administered antimicrobials is key to determining the outcome from therapy. Host characteristics, however, such as immune status, infection site location, and body organ function, play a significant role in selecting the most appropriate antimicrobial for a given individual.[1] This chapter reviews the routine laboratory tests that are used to assist in the diagnosis and treatment of infection.

LABORATORY TESTS CONFIRMING THE PRESENCE OF INFECTION

NONSPECIFIC TESTS

Many tests are used to determine whether a patient has an infection. Although no single test can prove that a patient is infected, when used in combination with clinical findings, tests are helpful to establish the diagnosis of infection. Because many tests are nonspecific, there are factors other than infection that can cause a test to be reported as positive when no infection exists. Therefore, the importance of careful interpretation and sound clinical judgment cannot be overemphasized.

White Blood Cell Count and Differential

Understanding the role of the white blood cell (WBC) in fighting infection is important in the diagnosis of infection, the selection of drug therapy, and the monitoring of patient progress. The major role of the WBC is to defend the body against invading organisms such as bacteria, viruses, and fungi. The typical normal range of the WBC is 4,500 to 11,000 cells/mm³ and depends on many factors such as patient age, gender, sample population and test method. White blood cells usually are elevated in response to infection. The WBC count can also become elevated in response to noninfectious causes, including stress, inflammatory conditions such as rheumatoid arthritis, and leukemia or in response to certain drugs (e.g., corticosteroids).

White blood cells are divided into two groups: the granulocytes, which have prominent cytoplasmic granules, and the agranulocytes, which lack granules. Polymorphonuclear (PMN) granulocytes are made up of neutrophils, basophils, and eosinophils. The two other classes of WBCs are the monocytes and lymphocytes. Neutrophils are the most common type of WBCs in the blood, comprising approximately 70% of the total WBC count. In response to infection, they leave the bloodstream and enter the tissue to interact with and phagocytize offending pathogens. Mature neutrophils sometimes are referred to as *segs* because of their segmented nucleus, which usually consists of two to five lobes. Immature neutrophils lack this segmented feature and are referred to as *bands*. During an acute infection, immature neutrophils, such as bands (single-lobed nucleus), are released from the bone marrow into the bloodstream

at an increased rate, and the percentage of bands (usually 5%) can increase in relationship to mature cells. The change in the ratio of mature to immature cells is often referred to as a "shift to the left" because of the way the cells were counted by hand with a microscope and charted from immature to mature cells.

Leukocytosis, an increase in WBCs, is a normal host defense to infection. Unfortunately, bacterial infection is a common complication of neutropenia from cancer chemotherapy. Neutropenia occurs when the bone marrow does not produce enough WBCs to fight infection. Patients who are neutropenic are incapable of increasing their WBCs in response to infection. In fact, susceptibility to infection in these patients is highly dependent on their WBC status. Patients with neutrophil counts of less than 500 cells/mm³ are at high risk for the development of bacterial or fungal infections. The absence of leukocytosis also occurs in the elderly and in severe cases of sepsis.[2,3]

Lymphocytes comprise 15% to 40% of all WBCs and are of central importance to the immune system. Two functional types of lymphocytes are the T cell, which is involved in cell-mediated immunity, and the B cell, which produces antibodies involved in humoral immunity. Lymphocytosis is frequently associated with acute viral infections such as Epstein-Barr virus infection (mononucleosis) and Cytomegalovirus (CMV) infection and rarely with unusual bacterial infections (i.e., *Brucella* species infections).

T lymphocytes are characterized on the basis of function (i.e. T-helper cells, Th_1 and Th_2) and on the basis of surface protein. Most type 1 and type 2 T cells carry a T4 (CD4) marker that recognizes class II major histocompatibility complex (MHC) antigens, and most cytoxic T cells carry a T8 (CD8) marker that recognizes class I MHC antigens. A severe deficiency of CD4 cells is associated with human immunodeficiency virus (HIV) infection and opportunistic infections.[4] Malignancies also can adversely affect cellular immunity. Patients with Hodgkin's disease and other types of lymphoma exhibit defective cell-mediated immunity that predisposes them to a variety of infections, notably fungal diseases and infections by the *Listeria* species. Drug treatment with cytotoxic chemotherapy and corticosteroids also can have profound deleterious effects on cell-mediated immunity.[5] Defects in cell-mediated immune function can be demonstrated by a variety of simple laboratory tests, including quantification of lymphocytes on a routine complete blood cell count and skin testing for anergy. A more detailed investigation includes quantitative measurements of CD4+ and CD8+ cells. Monocytosis is correlated less frequently with acute bacterial infection, although its presence has been associated with the response of certain infections (e.g., tuberculosis) to chemotherapy. Eosinophilia can result from parasitic infection.[6] Figure 113–1 describes a number of cell types and their biologic function.

Cell type	Cellular function	
Macrophage/monocyte	Antigen presenting cell Surveillance of foreign antigens	
Neurophils	Defense against bacteria and fungus	
Eosinophils	Defense against parasites Response against allergic reactions	
Basophil	Allergic response	
B lymphocyte	Antibody production Antigen presenting cell	
T lymphocytes	Cellular immunity against virus and tumors Regulation of the immune system	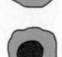

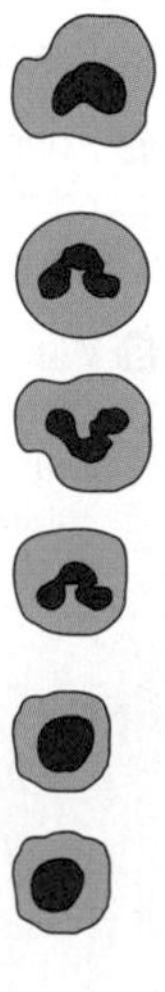

FIGURE 113-1. Various cell types and their biologic functions.

TABLE 113-1 Examples of Normal Bacterial Flora

| | Gram-Positive | | Gram-Negative | | |
	Cocci	Rods	Cocci	Rods	Other
Skin	*Staphylococcus* spp (e.g., S. epidermidis), *Streptococcus* spp	*Corynebacterium* spp, *Propionibacterium* spp		Enteric bacilli (some sites), *Acinetobacter* spp (Coccobacilli)	
Oropharynx	Streptococci–viridans group Micrococcus	*Corynebacterium* spp	Neisseria	*Haemophilus* spp	Spirochetes
Gastrointenstinal tract	*Enterococcus* spp, *Peptostreptococcus* spp	*Lactobacillus, Clostridium*		*Bacteroides* spp, Enteric bacilli (*E coli, Klebsiella* spp)	
Genital tract	*Streptococcus* spp, *Staphylococcus* spp	*Lactobacillus, Corynebacterium* spp		Enterobacteriacea, *Prevotella* spp	*Mycoplasma*

Other Tests

Some nonspecific laboratory tests are useful to support the diagnosis of infection. The inflammatory process initiated by an infection sets up a complex host response. Activation of the nuclear factor-κ_B (NF-κ_B) transcription factors plays an important role in the regulation of the immune system. NF-κ_B is activated by bacterial and viral antigens, which lead to the production of proinflammatory cytokines and chemokines. The rapid detection of activated NF-κ_B can be measured by transcription factor enzyme-linked immunoassay (TF-ELISA) during a systemic inflammatory response syndrome (SIRS) and is considered to be crucial for the treatment of patients with septicemia. Acute-phase reactants, such as the erythrocyte sedimentation rate (ESR) and the C-reactive protein concentration, are elevated in the presence of an inflammatory process but do not confirm the presence of infection because they are often elevated in noninfectious conditions, such as collagen-vascular diseases and arthritis. Large elevations in ESR are associated with infections such as endocarditis, osteomyelitis, and intraabdominal infections.[8,9]

Changes in endothelial membranes and the presence of a foreign pathogen and its endotoxins cause inflammatory cytokines, such as interleukin 1 (IL-1), IL-6, and IL-8 and tumor necrosis factor-α (TNF-α), to be produced by macrophages or lymphocytes. Fluctuations in cytokine levels occur during the course of an infection, which can be useful in staging and monitoring the response to therapy. Although abnormally high levels of TNF have been associated with a variety of noninfectious causes, spiked elevations in TNF are found in patients with serious infections, such as sepsis. Studies of the relationship of circulating mediators to patient outcome have determined the value of endotoxin and cytokine measurements in patients with sepsis. Although the combination of elevations in endotoxin and individual cytokines has correlated well with the mortality rate, measurement of IL-6 was by far the best individual cytokine that predicted patient outcome.[9] Understanding the balance between these proinflammatory and antiinflammatory processes likely will lead to interventions that can have a direct impact on the outcome of patients with sepsis.[11]

LABORATORY IDENTIFICATION OF PATHOGENS

COLONIZATION VERSUS INFECTION

❶ Pathogens are organisms that are capable of damaging host tissues and that elicit specific host responses and symptoms that are consistent with an infectious process. These organisms are transferred from patient to patient, vector to patient (animals, insects, and so on), environment to patient (e.g., hospital settings) or are derived from the patient's own flora. Conversely, the human body contains a vast variety of microorganisms that colonize body systems and make up the so-called normal flora. These organisms occur naturally in

the tissues of the host and provide some benefits, including defense by occupying space, competing for essential nutrients, stimulating cross-protective antibodies, and suppressing the growth of potentially pathogenic bacteria and fungi (Table 113–1).

Organisms that comprise the normal flora can become pathogenic when host defenses become impaired or if they are translocated to other body sites during trauma. The identification of an organism that is considered to be normal flora in a wound or otherwise sterile body cavity or fluid often becomes a dilemma for the clinician in deciding whether or not a patient is infected and whether or not the patient requires treatment. Such is the case with *Staphylococcus epidermidis* when it is identified in the blood of a hospitalized patient. *S epidermidis* is considered normal skin flora and commonly colonizes intravenous catheters. In these conditions, identification of the organism must be taken in light of the patient circumstances (signs and symptoms, laboratory indices supporting infection) and the probability of the organism being responsible for the infection. Often the simple removal of the catheter can eliminate the organism from the bloodstream, thereby preventing misdiagnosis and unnecessary application of antimicrobials.[12]

DIRECT EXAMINATION

❷ Direct examination of tissue or body fluids believed to be infected can provide simple, rapid information to the clinician. Microscopic examination of wet-mount specimen preparations can provide valuable information regarding potential pathogens. Applications of this procedure with or without staining preparations include direct examination of sputum, bronchial aspirates, scrapings of mucosal lesions, and urinary sediment. The Gram stain is one of the first identification tests run on a specimen brought to the laboratory. For this procedure, crystal violet is applied as the primary stain, with iodine added to enhance the staining process and to form a crystal violet–iodine complex. Alcohol decolorization is the next step in the procedure. Gram-negative cells are decolorized by the addition of alcohol, and they take in a red color when counterstained by safranin. Gram-positive cells are not decolorized by alcohol and retain the crystal violet color and appear purple. Gram staining in conjunction with microscopic examination can provide a presumptive diagnosis and some indication of the organism's morphologic characteristics (gram-positive, gram-negative, gram-variable, bacillus, or cocci). This is extremely useful information for the selection of empirical antibiotic therapy.

Gram stains are performed routinely on cerebrospinal fluid (CSF) in cases of suspected meningitis, on urethral smears for venereal diseases, and on abscess or effusion specimens. They are helpful in identifying organisms that may not grow on culture and which otherwise would be missed. Although Gram stains of sputum are performed routinely when respiratory tract infections are suspected, there is controversy regarding the usefulness of this test because the sputum is often contaminated with mixed or normal flora. The predominance of one particular organism, the overall

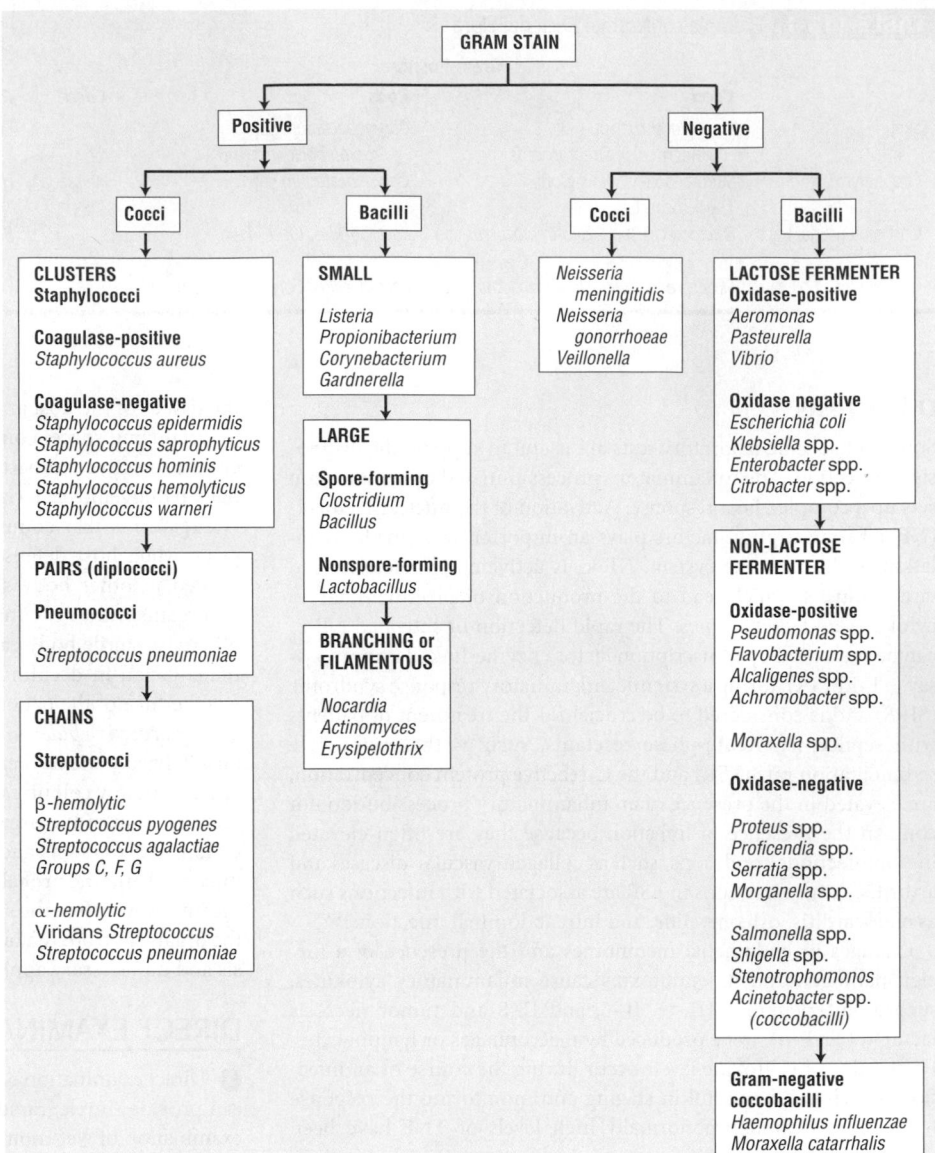

FIGURE 113-2. Important bacterial pathogens classified according to Gram stain and morphologic characteristic.

number of organisms present, the amount of PMN granulocyte present, and the presence or absence of a significant amount of squamous epithelial cells (<10 per low-power field) can improve the significance of the sputum Gram stain specimen. Figure 113–2 lists some common infecting pathogens grouped according to Gram stain and other characteristics.

Other staining techniques are used to identify pathogens such as those that are best identified microscopically because of their poor growth characteristics in the laboratory setting. The best examples of these are the Ziehl-Neelsen stain for acid-fast bacilli, which is used for the identification of mycobacteria species, and the India ink, potassium hydroxide (KOH), and Giemsa stains, which are useful for detecting certain fungi.[13]

CULTURES

❸ Isolation of the etiologic agent by culture is the most definitive method available for the diagnosis and eventual treatment of infection. Although suspicion of a specific pathogen or group of pathogens is helpful to the laboratory for the selection of a specific cultivating medium, the more common procedure for the laboratory is to screen for the presence of any potential pathogen. After receipt of a clinical specimen, the laboratory will inoculate the

specimen in a variety of artificial media. Some culture media are designed to differentiate various organisms on the basis of biochemical characteristics or to select specific organisms on the basis of resistance to certain antimicrobials. Other media are employed commonly for the isolation of more fastidious organisms, such as *Listeria, Legionella, Mycobacterium,* or *Chlamydia.* Cultures for viruses are more difficult to perform and are undertaken primarily by larger institutions or outside laboratories because of the technical expense and time involved in processing samples.

When a culture is obtained, careful attention must be paid to ensuring that specimens are collected and transported appropriately to the laboratory. Every effort should be made to avoid contamination with normal flora and to ensure that the specimen is placed in the appropriate transport medium. Culture specimens should be transported to the laboratory as soon as possible because organisms can perish from prolonged exposure to air or drying. This is especially important for swab specimen preparations. Transport media may not be ideal for all organisms. Specimens that contain fastidious organisms or anaerobes require special transport media and should be forwarded immediately to the laboratory for processing. Finally, the source of the specimen should be clearly recorded and forwarded along with the culture to the laboratory. This process will aid the laboratory in differentiating true pathogens from the expected normal flora, and it will help in the selection of the appropriate culture media. Detection of microorganisms in the bloodstream by standard culturing techniques is difficult because of the inherently low yield of organisms diluted by blood, humoral factors with bactericidal activity, and the potential of antimicrobial pretreatment affecting organism growth. Most blood collection bottles dilute the blood specimen 1:10 with growth medium to neutralize the bactericidal properties of blood and antimicrobials. The addition of a polyanionic anticoagulant abolishes the effect of complement and antiphagocytic activity in the specimen. Some laboratories also add β-lactamase to their blood collection bottles.

Rapid detection of bacteria or fungi within a few hours of specimen collection is now possible by the use of automated culturing systems, such as BACTEC (Becton Dickinson Diagnostic Instruments, Sparks, MD), that use bottles of growth medium containing a fluorescent sensor to monitor culture bottles every 10 minutes for the presence of carbon dioxide (CO_2) as a by-product of microorganism growth. Computers monitoring the system alert laboratory personnel of positive culture results by both audible and visual alarms. Once detected, a battery of testing can be performed rapidly that shortens the reporting time and that enables clinicians to obtain preliminary information about the organism.[13,14] The initial identity of the organism can be determined by a variety of testing procedures. General schemes differentiate organisms into primary groups, such as Gram-positive and Gram-negative bacteria. This can be accomplished by simple Gram staining, as described previously, by evaluating organism growth patterns on selective media, and by testing for the presence or absence of specific enzymes and chemical characteristics, such as hemolytic and fermentation properties. For example, non–lactose-fermenting gram-negative bacilli that are oxidase-positive can suggest *Pseudomonas aeruginosa* as opposed to a variety of other potential gram-negative organisms. This preliminary information, which is readily obtainable from the laboratory, can greatly assist the clinician in choosing the appropriate empirical therapy. Definitive identification of organisms requires more complex testing procedures and devices that can further differentiate the organism on the basis of specific fermentation and biochemical reactive properties. Commercially available automated systems can inoculate the test organism into a series of panels containing a variety of test media, sugars, and other reagents. The system can then photo-metrically determine the results and compare the findings to a library of organism characteristics to produce a definitive identification.[14]

Viral agents can be detected by direct observation of inoculated culture cells for cytopathic effects or by detection of antigens after incubation by immunofluorescent methods. The culture method is most useful for organisms such as CMV or herpes simplex virus because these viral agents are rapidly propagated in culture cells, making them easily detected.[15]

DIAGNOSIS OF INFECTION USING IMMUNOLOGIC AND MOLECULAR METHODS

ANTIBODY AND ANTIGEN DETECTION

❹ The use of immunologic methods for the diagnosis and monitoring of human host immune response to infection has become an indispensable laboratory tool. This is especially important in the detection of microorganisms, such as bacteria, fungi, and viruses, that otherwise would elude detection or severely delay results from conventional culturing techniques. The primary immunologic methods involve the detection and quantification of antibodies directed against a specific pathogen or its components. These

methods have the advantage of a rapid turnaround time and an acceptable level of sensitivity and specificity. Some tests (e.g., identification of group A streptococci and the Rapid Influenza diagnostic test) are simple to use, can be performed conveniently in the physician's office, and often can be used to decide whether antimicrobials should be administered for a suspected infection. Limitations with these tests exist as antigens will still exist even if the pathogen is not longer alive, hence allowing for a false positive test. In addition, the positive test result indicating the presence of the pathogen does not assist in determining if the patient was infected or simply colonized with the pathogen.

Antibody or antigen detection can be accomplished by a variety of techniques, including immunofluorescence, which has been used routinely for the detection of CMV, respiratory syncytial virus, varicella-zoster virus, *Treponema pallidum* (syphilis), *Borrelia burgdorferi* (Lyme disease), and *Chlamydia trachomatis*. Latex agglutination is useful for detecting meningococcal capsular antigens in CSF of patients suspected of having bacterial meningitis and as an aid in the diagnosis of *Legionella pneumophila*. Enzyme-linked immunosorbent assay (ELISA) is a commonly employed method for detecting HIV, herpes simplex virus, respiratory syncytial virus, pneumococcal serum antibody, *Neisseria gonorrhoeae*, and *Haemophilus pylori*.[15]

MOLECULAR TECHNIQUES FOR THE DETECTION OF MICROORGANISMS

Hybridization DNA Probes

❹ Highly sensitive and specific molecular methods are now available for the rapid detection and identification of a variety of pathogens. The two primary molecular techniques used commonly are nucleic acid hybridization, which involves the binding of a specific DNA or RNA probe to its target, and DNA amplification schemes. Probe-based methods require the extraction of DNA or RNA from a clinical specimen (i.e., body fluid, tissue, or WBC) or directly from a microorganism culture. The extract is then tested for the presence of pathogen DNA or RNA using a probe that contains a specific oligonucleic acid–based sequence for the organism. For example, a probe with a sequence of ACTGTT would bind to the complementary organism nucleic acid sequence of TGACAA. Because the probe is labeled with a signal-emitting molecule (i.e., radiolabeled, colorimetric, or chemoluminescent), a match would be detected.

The primary means for detection involves the use of separation of the organism DNA into specific fragments (gel electrophoresis), transfer and fixation of the mixture to specialized paper or nylon membranes (Southern or Northern blotting), the mixing of the DNA fragments with the labeled probe (hybridization), and transfer to radiographic or photographic film for processing. These techniques have been used for many years and are fairly standardized methods for the detection of a variety of organisms. Hybridization probes are useful for a variety of diagnostic and clinical applications, including the direct examination of organisms in tissue, which enables the evaluation and documentation of organism infestation, location, distribution, and host response. The use of hybridization probes is particularly helpful for the detection of slow-growing organisms such as *Mycobacterium tuberculosis*, *N gonorrhoeae*, and certain species of fungi. This technique is also used to document the presence or absence of antimicrobial-resistant genes in a cell culture and to track the spread of resistant microorganisms in hospital and outpatient settings. Although employed widely, the use of hybridization probes is often limited by their lack of sensitivity. Probe amplification methods are available that improve the sensitivity of these assays. The principle of these probe-amplification schemes is to boost the probe's signal-emitting molecule to make it more easily detected. A more advanced signal-amplification system available is the branched DNA (bDNA) probe system (Chiron Corp., Emeryville, CA) which is often used to identify retroviruses such as HIV. This system uses multiple probes and multiple signal-emitting molecules (reporters). The target-binding probe contains two hybridization regions. One region is complementary to the target, and the other region is capable of binding with the bDNA amplification multimer. The amplification multimer binds multiple reporter molecules (as many as 3,000), which provides a significant boost in the probe's signal. Branched DNA probe systems are being developed for rapid detection of hepatitis B and C, HIV-1, and CMV. Because of the system's high specificity and quantitative ability, bDNA probe assays can be useful for therapeutic monitoring, such as in the case of monitoring the response to antiretroviral therapy in acquired immunodeficiency syndrome (AIDS).[16,17]

Nucleic Acid Amplification Methods

Nucleic acid amplification methods are now considered a standard laboratory tool. They have had a tremendous impact on the diagnosis and treatment of infectious diseases. These highly sensitive methods have the capability to detect and quantitate minute amounts of target nucleic acid in a rapid manner. The polymerase chain reaction (PCR) is based on the capability of a DNA polymerase to copy and elongate a targeted strand of DNA. This is accomplished by the use of short oligonucleotide primers (20 to 25 nucleotides long) that correspond to the DNA targeted to be expanded. After an excess of primers and heat-stable DNA polymerases are added to the targeted DNA mixture, the targeted DNA is denatured and separated by a process of cycling hot and cool temperatures. Each cycle doubles the amount of DNA originally present at the start of the cycle, thereby exponentially increasing the overall number of DNA copies. In theory, more than 1 million copies of the original DNA can be generated from as few as 20 cycles. Although this amplification technique is very sensitive and has tremendous application potential, it is not without problems. The powerful amplification procedure can yield false-positive results when samples are contaminated by nucleic acid left over from previously amplified DNA or by dead pathogens that exist in the sample. Other problems include primer artifact formation and nonspecific hybridization of primers to DNA samples. Several modifications to the original PCR technology have been made over the years to improve the sensitivity and application potential for PCR, including the use of multiple sets of amplification primers, multiplex PCR, PCR amplification of RNA by converting targeted RNA with reverse transcriptase to complementary DNA templates and real-time quantitative PCR. The cost-benefit ratio of PCR as compared with traditional microbiologic methods must be evaluated. Molecular amplification schemes such as PCR have become routine in situations in which rapid turnaround time is essential to improve patient diagnosis and outcome, for example, real-time universal screening for acute HIV infection and routine testing and monitoring of patients receiving treatment for HIV infection, and the isolation and detection of fastidious or slow-growing organisms such as *M tuberculosis*, *B burgdorferi*, and *Helicobacter pylori*. Another potential application for this technology is the early detection of multidrug-resistant organisms. Amplification of resistant gene markers would aid in rapid selection of the most appropriate therapy in the treatment of organisms in which days or weeks traditionally are required for culturing and determining basic susceptibility. Examples fitting this description include the rapid detection of isoniazid and rifampin gene markers for *M tuberculosis*, early detection of the *mecA* gene responsible for

methicillin-resistance in *Staphylococcus aureus*, and identification of resistant genes responsible for production of β-lactamase capable of destroying specific cephalosporins and multidrug-resistant *H pylori*.[17–20]

EVALUATION OF ANTIMICROBIAL ACTIVITY AND DETERMINATION OF ANTIMICROBIAL PHARMACODYNAMICS

⑤ The laboratory evaluation of antimicrobial activity is an important component of the pharmacotherapeutic management of infectious diseases. The integration of this activity **⑥** with various pharmacokinetic properties of the antimicrobial agent determines the drug's pharmacodynamic characteristics. Antimicrobial pharmacodynamics have become a crucial consideration for the clinician for selecting both empirical and pathogen-directed therapy, formulary decision making, developing antimicrobial streamlining programs, and for intravenous-to-oral antimicrobial switch protocols.

⑤ Most antimicrobial susceptibility testing methods that are used in the clinical laboratory are well characterized and have been standardized by the Clinical and Laboratory Standards Institute (CLSI). However, controversies exist about which test methods provide the most useful information, how to report these results, and how to apply them to the treatment of patients.[21] Nevertheless, there are many investigations that show that the general antimicrobial susceptibility or resistance profile of an infecting organism correlates with clinical and/or microbiologic responses to therapy.

Most of the standardized and well-accepted test methods evaluate the susceptibility of aerobic, nonfastidious bacteria. However, substantial progress has been made to develop sensitive, specific, reproducible, and clinically useful susceptibility tests for anaerobic bacteria, yeasts, mycobacteria, and viruses. Continued advances in technology should further improve test methods and the rapidity with which the results can be applied to the management of patients. Although these newer systems are often expensive, the increased quality and decreased overall costs of patient care can determine their cost-effectiveness.

QUANTITATIVE ANTIMICROBIAL SUSCEPTIBILITY TESTING

MINIMAL INHIBITORY CONCENTRATIONS

⑤ The *minimal inhibitory concentration* (MIC) is defined as the lowest antimicrobial concentration that prevents visible growth of an organism after approximately 24 hours of incubation in a specified growth medium. The MIC quantitatively determines in vitro antibacterial activity. Classically, MICs were determined through the macrotube dilution method, which uses liquid growth medium (broth), doubling serial dilutions of antimicrobials in test tubes, and a standard inoculum of bacteria (approximately 10^5 colony-forming units [CFU]/mL). The tubes (up to 10 mL) were incubated at approximately 35°C (95°F) for 18 to 24 hours and then examined for visible bacterial growth (Fig. 113–3). Because macrodilution MIC testing is laborious and supply intensive, it is not used often in the contemporary clinical microbiology laboratory. However, one advantage of this method is that it tests a large inoculum of bacteria—a factor that can improve the detection of small numbers of resistant subpopulations or document the presence of inducible resistance.

1803

CHAPTER 113

Laboratory Tests to Direct Antimicrobial Pharmacotherapy

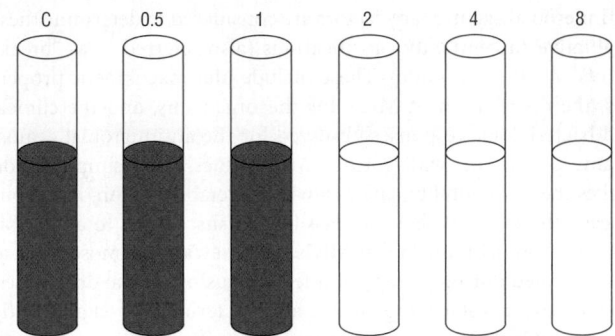

FIGURE 113-3. Macrotube minimal inhibitory concentration (MIC) determination. The growth control *(C)*, 0.5 mg/L, and 1 mg/L tubes are visibly turbid, indicating bacterial growth. The MIC is read as the first clear test tube (2 mg/L).

The use of 96-well microtiter plates substantially reduces the amount of growth medium and preparation time needed for broth-dilution MIC testing in the clinical laboratory. Volumes of 100 to 200 microliters (mcL) or less of medium are used, and multichannel pipets and/or automated systems allow efficient preparation of numerous tests (Fig. 113–4). The microdilution MIC test method is currently the most commonly used susceptibility test method in the clinical microbiology laboratory. Although microdilution MIC testing is a vast improvement over macrodilution MIC testing, it still has important shortcomings. These include both limitations in the numbers and various types of antimicrobials to use in the test (especially with premade or premanufactured trays) and a limited ability to detect some forms of antimicrobial resistance (e.g., β-lactamases in gram-negative bacteria).[22]

The MIC also can be determined using solid agar growth medium. For the agar dilution MICs, the test antimicrobial is added to the molten agar at the desired concentration just prior to its solidification. After the agar has hardened, suspensions of test bacteria are applied to the agar. As with broth MICs, the agar dilution MIC is defined as the lowest concentration that prevents the visible growth of the organism after an overnight incubation period. The primary advantages of the agar dilution MICs are the ability to test many bacteria on the same agar plate and the flexibility to choose specific antimicrobials. These advantages often are outweighed by the need to prepare agar plates manually and the instability of the antimicrobial in the agar as compared with commercially prepared microtiter MIC trays. Although agar dilution MIC once was considered the standard susceptibility test for many bacteria

and for certain slow-growing organisms such as *M tuberculosis*, its use has declined in most clinical laboratories with the advent of more rapidly performed and less cumbersome susceptibility testing methods (e.g., microtiter MICs, PCR, radiometric, and/or fluorometric tests).

LIMITATIONS AND PROBLEMS WITH MIC TESTING

❺ Some of the limitations and problems of MIC testing are academic in nature, whereas others can have important implications for the management of patients with serious infections. For example, because the MIC only represents the concentration of antimicrobial that is needed to inhibit visual growth of the most resistant cells within the tested bacterial population, there can be a small percentage of bacteria present within the large numbers at the site of infection that are more antimicrobial-resistant than the MIC would indicate. Use of the antimicrobial then could select these more resistant subpopulations, resulting in poor clinical response. This phenomenon can be observed with intermediate vancomycin resistance in *S aureus*, as well as in strains of gram-negative bacteria such as the *Enterobacteriaceae* species that produce both plasmid-borne and chromosomal β-lactamases.[22,23]

Many other factors also can influence the in vitro MIC value obtained and its subsequent application to the in vivo situation. The bacterial growth medium used and cation content can affect the activity of many drugs significantly. For example, aminoglycosides are more active against *P aeruginosa* in a medium supplemented with physiologic concentrations of magnesium and calcium (CLSI standardized method) than in a medium without these cations. MIC values of antibiotics that are highly bound to plasma proteins are significantly higher when the test medium contains human serum. As testing of these drugs in a serum-supplemented medium has not gained widespread acceptance, their in vivo activity can be overestimated by in vitro MIC test results. Fortunately, the standardized guidelines for testing and quality assurance procedures proposed by the CLSI attempt to minimize the impact of these problems and are followed by most clinical and research laboratories.[24] However, when a patient infected with an apparently susceptible organism fails therapy, it is important for the clinician to consider these potential confounding factors as possibly being related to the observed failure. In such situations, consideration of antimicrobial pharmacokinetics and pharmacodynamics also often can help to better predict therapeutic response as compared with organism susceptibility alone.

	128	64	32	16	8	4	2	1	0.5	0.25	0.125	GC
Aztreonam	○	○	○	○	○	○	●	●	●	●	●	●
Cefepime	○	○	○	○	○	○	○	●	●	●	●	●
Ceftazidime	○	○	○	○	○	○	●	●	●	●	●	●
Ciprofloxacin	○	○	○	○	○	○	○	○	●	●	●	●
Gentamicin	○	○	○	○	○	○	○	○	●	●	●	●
Meropenem	○	○	○	○	○	○	○	●	●	●	●	●
Piperacillin	○	○	○	●	●	●	●	●	●	●	●	●
Tobramycin	○	○	○	○	○	○	○	○	○	●	●	●

FIGURE 113-4. Depiction of a 96-well microtiter plate with minimal inhibitory concentration (MIC) assays for antibiotics used commonly against gram-negative pathogens. The shaded wells indicate visible bacterial growth. The MICs (milligrams per liter) for this organism would be 16 for piperacillin, 4 for aztreonam, 2 for ceftazidime and cefepime, 1 for meropenem, 0.5 for ciprofloxacin and gentamicin, and 0.25 for tobramycin. GC is the growth control (no antibiotic added).

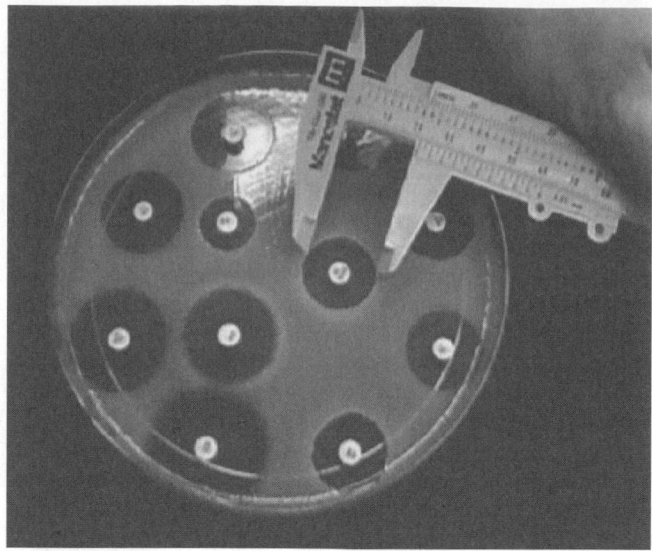

FIGURE 113-5. Disk diffusion susceptibility test. Antibiotic-impregnated disks are placed on the surface of a plate previously inoculated with the test organism. The plate is incubated for 18 hours, and the subsequent zones of inhibition are measured. The zone size correlates with the sensitivity of the organism. The larger the zone, the more sensitive is the organism to the specific antibiotic. On the basis of predetermined zone breakpoints, organisms can be classified as susceptible, resistant, or intermediately susceptible to the antibiotic. *(Photograph courtesy of the Anti-Infective Research Laboratory, Wayne State University, Detroit, MI.)*

QUALITATIVE ANTIMICROBIAL SUSCEPTIBILITY TEST METHODS

DISK DIFFUSION ASSAY

The disk diffusion assay method for susceptibility testing (Kirby-Bauer method) was developed in the 1960s by Bauer and coworkers as a way to reduce the labor needed for tube dilution susceptibility testing.[25] It still remains one of the more common susceptibility test methods used in the clinical microbiology laboratory owing to its high degree of standardization, reliability, flexibility, low cost, and simplicity of test interpretation. Up to 12 user-selected antibiotic-impregnated paper disks are placed on an agar plate previously streaked with a standard suspension of bacteria (1–2 × 10⁸ CFU/ mL). The drug contained in the disk diffuses in a concentration gradient out into the agar. The plate is incubated (18 to 24 hours at 35°C), and visual bacterial growth occurs only in areas in which the drug concentrations are below those required for growth inhibition. The diameters of the zones of inhibition are measured via calipers or automated scanners and are compared with standard zone size ranges that determine susceptibility, intermediate susceptibility, or resistance to the antimicrobials that were tested (Fig. 113–5). Although factors such as agar composition, incubation temperature, bacterial inoculum, and antibiotic paper disk composition can influence results, the standards for testing conditions and interpretive zone sizes are well defined by the CLSI.

QUALITATIVE VERSUS QUANTITATIVE SUSCEPTIBILITY TESTING OF MICROORGANISMS

Quantitative MIC data often are reported to the clinician qualitatively by deeming an organism "susceptible," "intermediate or indeterminate" or "moderately susceptible," or "resistant" to a given

antimicrobial agent. Many factors are considered to determine these qualitative susceptibility classifications (also referred to as "breakpoints" for the antibiotic). These include pharmacokinetic properties, the distribution of MICs for the organisms, and the clinical and bacteriologic responses observed for the antimicrobial against strains of bacteria with various MIC values. This simplification makes the susceptibility data easily interpretable by non–infectious disease clinicians. Pathogens classified as susceptible to an antibiotic are those with the lowest MICs, and they are the most likely to be eradicated during therapy of infections using typical drug doses. Conversely, resistant organisms are bacteria with significantly higher MICs that, when treated with the antimicrobial, will result in a less-than-optimal clinical response, even at the highest doses. The indeterminate classification exists when the number of strains with MICs in the given range is too small to derive robust conclusions on susceptibility or resistance to the antimicrobial. Responses to therapy for organisms that are moderately susceptible/intermediately susceptible/indeterminate can be variable. These organisms can respond to treatment with maximal doses of the antimicrobial or can respond when the drug is known to be concentrated at the site of infection (e.g., urinary tract infections treated by drugs excreted by the kidneys).

There are concerns that the "user friendly" susceptible/resistant classification system can oversimplify the decision-making process for treating infections. For example, a critically ill patient may not respond to the antimicrobial therapy of a susceptible organism at the usual doses. If serum concentrations or concentrations at the site of infection could be assayed (not practically done), one might discover suboptimal concentrations as a result of inadequate tissue perfusion. Likewise, a patient with severe vascular insufficiency and a diabetic foot infection may fail a course of therapy with normal doses of an antimicrobial and a susceptible organism because of inadequate drug delivery. Additionally, some investigators have shown that different outcomes can be achieved for "susceptible" organisms with different MIC values[26] and also that substantial (although not clinically acceptable) clinical and/ or microbiologic cure rates can occur for infections that are caused by resistant organisms.[27] These reports emphasize that in vitro susceptibility does not correlate unequivocally with clinical success and that resistant organisms do not always equate with impending clinical failure.

CLINICAL CONTROVERSY

Some clinicians believe that the MICs for all antimicrobials for which susceptibility testing was performed should be reported to allow for the most appropriate antimicrobial selection for the patient. However, others believe that only selective antimicrobial susceptibility should be reported to avoid overprescribing of more costly broad spectrum antimicrobials.

Similarities in the spectrum of activity for classes of antibiotics have led to the concept of *class testing*. Thus cephalothin susceptibility results are extrapolated to other first-generation cephalosporins, such as cephalexin or cefazolin. Likewise, susceptibility to an antibiotic that typically has minimal activity usually ensures that other more potent agents in its class will have activity as well. However, many gram-negative organisms have now developed extended-spectrum β-lactamases (ESBLs) that often have different activity against members of the same drug class. These developments significantly limit the utility of class testing to reduce susceptibility testing workload.

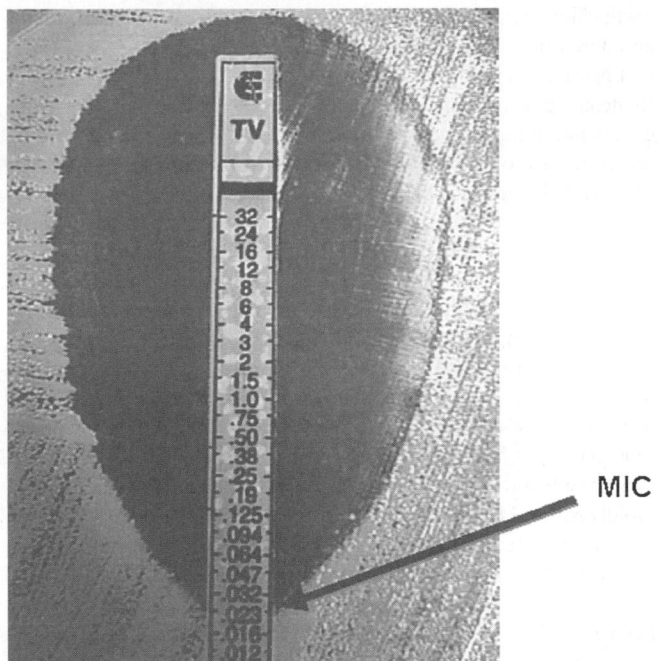

FIGURE 113-6. Photograph of E test susceptibility strip. The minimal inhibitory concentration (MIC) is determined from the point where the zone of inhibition intersects with the numerical scale. *(Photograph courtesy of the Anti-Infective Research Laboratory, Wayne State University, Detroit, MI.)*

OTHER SUSCEPTIBILITY TESTS

EPSILOMETER TEST

❽ The Epsilometer test (Etest; AB bioMérieux, Nouvelle, France) combines the benefits of quantitative MIC test methods with the ease of agar diffusion testing. The Etest is a plastic strip impregnated with a known, prefixed concentration gradient of antibiotic that is placed on an agar plate streaked with a suspension of known bacterial inoculum. The drug instantly diffuses from the plastic strip to form an effective concentration gradient within the agar. After overnight incubation, elliptical zones of inhibition are formed; the point where the bottom of the ellipse crosses the plastic strip is correlated with an MIC value printed on the strip (Fig. 113–6). A similar product (M.I.C. Evaluator; Oxoid Limited, Hampshire, United Kingdom) is also available. Many investigators have analyzed the Etest's correlation with standard susceptibility methods and assessed its potential clinical use. In general, values obtained with Etest methods are comparable with or even more consistent and accurate than standard methods. In fact, the Etest method is the recommended method for susceptibility testing of *Streptococcus pneumoniae*. However, the widespread clinical use of the Etest has been limited primarily by the excessive costs of the test strips (nearly 10 times more costly than antibiotic-impregnated disks) in relation to the benefits that may be gained from their use.

AUTOMATED ANTIMICROBIAL SUSCEPTIBILITY TESTING

❽ Various degrees of automation have been applied to susceptibility testing. Early advances included automated preparation of microtiter trays, instrument-assisted readers, and computer-assisted result databases. Rapid automated susceptibility tests became available in the 1980s, and their use has increased substantially in the two subsequent decades. These systems often incorporate microprocessors, robotics, and microcomputers to rapidly identify organisms and produce susceptibility test results in as few as 3 hours.

There are three rapid automated susceptibility test systems in common use in clinical microbiology laboratories. The Vitek system (bioMerieux, Durham, NC) uses small plastic reagent "cards" that contain 64 microwells for the testing of various antimicrobials or indicator chemicals. Bacterial test suspensions enter the wells by capillary diffusion, and growth is monitored automatically via photometric assessment of turbidity every hour for up to 15 hours. When the growth control reaches a specified turbidity level, growth curves for all wells are calculated and compared with the growth control curve for slope normalization. Computerized linear regression and the use of best-fit line coefficients produce an algorithm-derived MIC. The clinical laboratory can control the result output that is generated (qualitative susceptibility, quantitative susceptibility, or both).

The Microscan Walkaway system (Siemens Healthcare Diagnostics, Deerfield, IL) is a rapid test system that uses fluorogenic substrate hydrolysis as an indicator of bacterial growth. This system uses standard microdilution test trays and a computer-controlled incubator and reader unit that can perform robotic manipulations, such as reagent addition and tray rotation, to allow for spectrophotometric or fluorometric growth assessments. As with the Vitek system, growth curves are generated, and algorithms applied for the determination of MICs; output is via computer or video display.

The final system is the BD Phoenix Automated Microbiology System (BD Diagnostics, Sparks, MD). This system utilizes an oxidation-reduction detector and a turbidometric growth detection system to determine antibiotic resistance/susceptibility. Output of data is similar to the other two automated systems previously described.

❽ The results obtained from all of these three systems generally are comparable. However, there have been documented differences in the ability of these systems to accurately detect emerging resistance mechanisms such as vancomycin resistance in Staphylococci and carbapenem resistance in gram-negative pathogens.[28,29] Importantly, all of the systems contain information management software that allow for the storage and rapid retrieval of historical susceptibility data. They can produce chartable patient data reports, antibiograms (summaries of overall resistance for organisms causing infections in a given hospital), and epidemiologic reports. These systems also can be interfaced with other clinical information systems, such as the pharmacy, infection control, or other laboratory data systems, which can help to improve clinical outcomes.[30]

ADVANCES IN SUSCEPTIBILITY TESTING FOR MYCOBACTERIA, FUNGI, AND VIRUSES

Impressive advances have been made in the past decade in the areas of mycobacterial, fungal, and viral susceptibility testing. The use of radio-metric techniques, such as the BACTEC TB460 system (Becton Dickinson Biosciences, Sparks, MD), has revolutionized the analysis of antimicrobial susceptibility for *M tuberculosis* and other slow-growing mycobacteria.[31] Radiometric susceptibility testing involves the incubation of *M tuberculosis* in liquid medium containing carbon-14 (^{14}C)-labeled growth substrate. As organisms grow, respiration causes the release of ^{14}C, which is then detected. The growth indices for antimicrobial-containing bottles are compared with those of a control bottle with the calculation of an MIC. Use of this method, when coupled with the rapid processing of samples, can reduce the time to susceptibility result generation to approximately 1 week. A newer mycobacterial susceptibility testing method (the BACTEC Mycobacteria Growth Indicator Tube [MGIT 960]; Becton Dickinson Diagnostic Instruments, Sparks, MD) that is fully automated and that employs detection of fluorescence related to growth also has been developed. It produces results in a similar time frame and with similar reliability as the radiometric method.[32] Primary advantages of this system are its automation, the elimination of radioactivity, and the elimination of needle use. Although the slower agar proportion susceptibility method (generating results in approximately 1 month) is still considered the reference standard for mycobacterial susceptibility testing by the CLSI, the group now recommends the use of a rapid susceptibility testing method to ensure that the Centers for Disease Control and Prevention (CDC) guidelines for reporting susceptibility results for *M tuberculosis* infections within 28 days of specimen receipt in the laboratory can be met.[33] In the future, the use of molecular probes for mycobacterial resistance genes most likely will become a more important component of mycobacterial susceptibility determinations, especially in light of the increasing problems with antimicrobial resistance.[34]

There has been a substantial increase in the prevalence of fungal infections in the past two decades and an increase in the development and use of antifungal agents has followed. Historically, antifungal susceptibility testing was imprecise and fraught with many inconsistencies. However, pioneering research in the past decade has resulted in the development of CLSI guidelines for the antifungal susceptibility testing methods of both yeasts and filamentous fungi (molds).[35,36] Use of these techniques can result in greater than 90% inter- and intralaboratory reproducibility. Although routine antifungal testing of every isolate is not generally necessary for most clinical microbiology laboratories, periodic batch testing for the development of antibiograms and for the surveillance of resistance and/or antifungal testing of patients with such infections as cryptococcal meningitis or oropharyngeal candidiasis refractory to therapy are warranted.

DETECTION OF RESISTANCE FACTORS

There are a number of methods in use that directly detect the production of antimicrobial resistance in pathogens. β-Lactamase production can be detected rapidly and easily in the clinical laboratory with the use of nitrocephin disks. Nitrocephin is a chromogenic cephalosporin derivative that changes color on hydrolysis by β-lactamase. Colonies from a growing bacterial culture can be touched to a disk, with β-lactamase production noted within a few minutes. Although rapid and reliable, this method is limited to the assessment of strains of staphylococci, enterococci, *H influenzae*, *Moraxella catarrhalis*, and *N gonorrhoeae*. The nitrocephin disk also cannot detect β-lactam resistance caused by altered penicillin-binding proteins or by some of the newer ESBLs. The use of PCR or DNA probes for detection of β-lactamases improves sensitivity/specificity but is still limited to the research setting. In the years to come, these molecular biologic techniques should become more refined and more prominent in the clinical microbiology laboratory.

PCR has now become a standard method to quantify the replication of the HIV and hepatitis viruses in infected patients (the *viral load*, described as copies per milliliter).[37] Similar methods are used to determine the presence of genetic mutations in the HIV that are associated with increased resistance to one or more of the many antiretroviral medications available for clinical use. The use of these genotyping methods as an aid to select an optimized antiretroviral regimen has been correlated with an improved clinical response to therapy, as well as with a more potent reduction in the viral load.[37]

The detection of methicillin resistance in *Staphylococcus* (methicillin-resistant *S aureus* [MRSA]) is crucial to ensure appropriate therapy.

Methicillin resistance is the result of the *mecA* gene, which encodes for an altered penicillin-binding protein (penicillin-binding protein 2a) that has a low binding affinity for β-lactams. It is particularly difficult to detect this resistance, although, because of the heterogeneous expression of the phenotype—it is common for only 1 in 10^{4-6} tested bacterial cells to express methicillin resistance (even though all cells may have the genetic ability to do so). Screening via oxacillin disks or by oxacillin-containing agar (6 mcg/mL) was once considered the gold standard for resistance detection prior to the development of PCR and DNA probes that were specific for *mecA*. The *mecA* PCR test is available for clinical use, is 99% sensitive and specific, and allows for the rapid (within 6 hours) determination of the presence of methicillin resistance. Although the *mecA* PCR test has been available for many years, many laboratories do not use it commonly because of its high cost relative to other screening methods with acceptable sensitivity/specificity. For example, the presence of MRSA in a nasal swab or a blood culture sample can now be determined directly and rapidly within 24 hours using chromogenic technology (CHROMagar MRSA). This technology uses chromogenic substrates and a cephalosporin; MRSA strains will grow in the presence of cephalosporins such as cefoxitin and will produce mauve-colored colonies resulting from hydrolysis of the chromogenic substrates. The sensitivity and specificity for this test is as high as 97% and 99%, respectively.[38,39] In addition, fluorescence in situ hybridization (FISH) is a novel technique that uses peptide nucleic acid probes to target ribosomal RNA (rRNA) to rapidly identify both bacteria and yeasts in culture. Peptide nucleic acid probes that specifically target 16S rRNA of *S aureus* have now been developed for rapid and specific identification of *S aureus* directly from blood cultures that are gram-stain positive for gram-positive cocci. The assay has 100% sensitivity and 96% specificity.[40]

The detection of decreased vancomycin susceptibility in gram-positive organisms has become more important with the increased prevalence of both vancomycin-resistant Enterococcus (VRE) and vancomycin-intermediate-resistant and vancomycin-resistant *S aureus* (VISA and VRSA). The vancomycin agar screening method (Brain-Heart Infusion agar containing 6 mg/L of vancomycin) is an inexpensive and reliable way to detect vancomycin resistance. With this test, the growth of any colonies from a sample of the test organism (10^5–10^6 CFU) after 24 hours of incubation would indicate the presence of decreased vancomycin susceptibility (VISA) or vancomycin resistance (VRE, VRSA) within the test strain. This screening method appears to work well for VRE, but it appears to be less reliable for detecting VISA or VRSA strains when compared to the CLSI broth microdilution reference method.[28] It is important to note that most of the MIC testing methods currently used in the clinical microbiology laboratory do appear to reliably detect these VISA and VRSA strains.[28]

SPECIAL IN VITRO TESTS OF ANTIMICROBIAL ACTIVITY

MINIMAL BACTERICIDAL CONCENTRATION

❾ In certain infections (e.g., Gram-positive bacterial meningitis and endocarditis), the bactericidal (killing) activity may be more predictive of a favorable infection outcome than the MIC.[41] The minimal bactericidal concentration (MBC) can be performed in conjunction with the broth microtiter MIC test by taking aliquots of broth from microtiter wells that demonstrate no visible growth and plating the samples onto antibiotic-free agar plates for subsequent incubation. The MBC is defined as the lowest concentration of drug that kills 99.9% of the total initially viable cells (representing a 3 $\log_{10}$ CFU/mL or greater reduction in the starting inoculum).

For certain antibiotic classes such as the aminoglycosides and the quinolones, the MIC often approximates the MBC. However, for β-lactam antibiotics and glycopeptides, the MBC can exceed the MIC substantially, resulting in an overestimation of in vivo bactericidal activity. When the MBC exceeds the MIC by 32-fold or more, an organism is said to be *tolerant* to the antimicrobial's killing activity. Although the phenomenon of tolerance has been documented for β-lactams and glycopeptides against certain staphylococci, streptococci, and enterococci, its impact on the outcome of infections caused by organisms other than those just mentioned appears to be limited.

TIMED-KILL CURVE TESTS

Timed-kill curve tests are not performed routinely in the clinical laboratory but can provide important additional data on the effects of an antimicrobial on bacteria. For timed-kill curve tests, a standard inoculum of bacteria (10^6 CFU/mL) is placed in a test tube containing liquid growth medium with or without desired test concentrations of antimicrobial. Samples are removed periodically to determine the number of living cells at the given time points. The viable cell counts are plotted versus time to construct the timed-kill profile of the antimicrobial. The tested concentration of antimicrobial is considered to be bactericidal if it causes at least a 3 $\log_{10}$ CFU/mL reduction in viable inoculum. Comparisons of the relative rates of bacterial killing also can be performed in timed-kill curve experiments. Additionally, the presence of concentration-dependent killing activity (where killing increases with increasing drug concentrations above the MIC) versus concentration-independent killing activity can be determined from a timed-kill curve experiment. An example of results from a timed-kill curve experiment is depicted in Figure 113–7. These data can help to predict the best way to administer an antimicrobial to maximize activity. For example, lower-dose, more frequent (or continuous) infusions would be preferable for concentration-independent antibiotics, while higher-dose intermittent administrations would maximize activity for concentration-dependent antibiotics.

POSTANTIBIOTIC EFFECT

The *postantibiotic effect* (PAE) is defined as the persistent suppression of an organism's growth after a brief exposure to an antibiotic.[42] A PAE experiment is performed by exposing a fixed

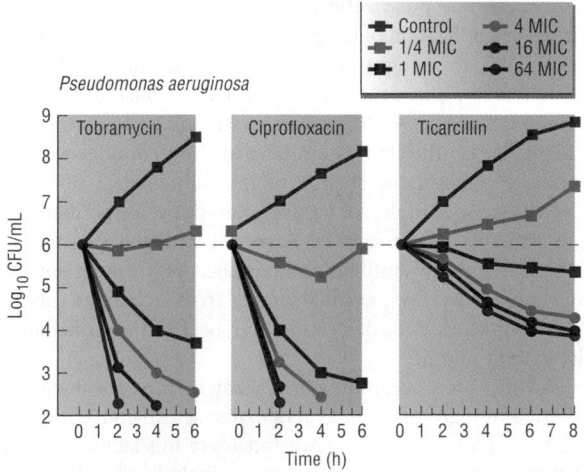

FIGURE 113-7. Killing curve depicting the effect of concentration on antibiotic bactericidal activity. (CFU, colony-forming unit; MIC, minimal inhibitory concentration [0.25-64 times the MIC; the organism tested was *P aeruginosa* ATCC 27853]) *(From Craig WA, Ebert SC. Killing and regrowth of bacteria in vitro: a review. Scand J Infect Dis Suppl 1991;74:63–70).*

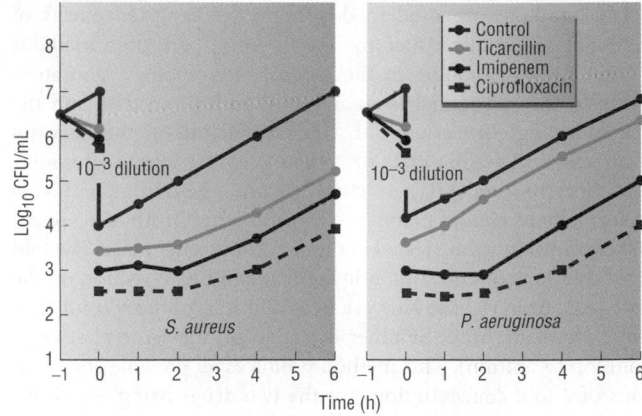

FIGURE 113-8. Postantibiotic effect. In this experiment, fixed inocula of *Staphylococcus aureus* and *Pseudomonas aeruginosa* are exposed to ticarcillin, imipenem, and ciprofloxacin at a set concentration of four times the MIC. The organism and the antibiotic are then diluted 1,000-fold to a point where the antibiotic concentration is far below the MIC of the organism. Growth suppression of *S aureus* following exposure to the three drugs (postantibiotic effect [PAE]) occurs for approximately 2 hours. Growth suppression of *P aeruginosa*, however, is only demonstrated for imipenem and ciprofloxacin. The ß-lactam ticarcillin has no effect on the growth of *P aeruginosa*. (CFU, colony-forming unit; MIC, minimal inhibitory concentration.) *(From Craig WA, Ebert SC. Killing and regrowth of bacteria in vitro: a review. Scand J Infect Dis Suppl 1991;74:63–70)*

inoculum of organism to a set concentration of antibiotic (typically some multiple of the MIC) (Fig. 113–8). The antibiotic is then removed either by inactivation (e.g., inactivation by a β-lactamase or binding the antibiotic to a resin) or by filtration/centrifugation of the mixture. The cells are resuspended in antibiotic-free growth medium, and samples are removed frequently (every 0.5 to 2 hours) to determine resumption of normal growth. The PAE is quantified as the difference in time that it takes the organism exposed to the antibiotic to demonstrate a 10-fold increase in viable cells per milliliter as compared with a separate culture of organism not subjected to the antibiotic. A PAE equal to or greater than 1 hour has been demonstrated for most antibiotics against gram-positive bacteria (β-lactams, vancomycin, daptomycin, linezolid, telavancin). As a general rule, antibiotics that inhibit DNA or protein synthesis (e.g., quinolones and aminoglycosides) demonstrate significant PAEs against gram-negative organisms. An exception to this rule are the carbapenem cell wall synthesis inhibitors (e.g., ertapenem, imipenem, and meropenem), which demonstrate PAEs against selected strains of gram-negative organisms. The primary clinical application of the PAE is to allow for less frequent administration of antimicrobials while still maintaining adequate antibacterial activity (e.g., extended-interval aminoglycoside administration).[43]

ANTIMICROBIAL COMBINATION EFFECT TEST

Antimicrobial combination therapy is used frequently to treat serious infections. Combination therapy can be used prior to knowing the pathogen or antibiotic susceptibility for the treatment of infections in neutropenic patients and in patients with enterococcal endocarditis or bacteremia, sepsis, or pneumonia caused by *P aeruginosa*. In these cases, it is important to know whether the combination will have beneficial (or detrimental) effects on the overall antibacterial activity of the regimen. For example, the combination can result in activity that is significantly greater than the sum of activity of either agent alone (i.e., synergy). Conversely, the combination can result in activity that is worse than either agent alone (i.e., antagonism). Combination activity that is neither synergistic nor antagonistic is said to be *indifferent* or *additive*.[44]

Two methods are used to determine the expected effects of combination antibiotic therapy. For the most part, both methods are not used commonly in the clinical microbiology laboratory owing to the substantial labor involved with these tests and the lack of strong correlation with clinical outcome in the majority of infections. The first method is the microtiter fractional inhibitory concentration (FIC, or "checkerboard" method). The FIC is performed in a similar manner to the microtiter broth MIC except that two antibiotics are tested in the same microtiter plate. Twofold serial dilutions of one antibiotic are made in one direction on the plate (e.g., from right to left), whereas dilutions of the second antibiotic are made from the other direction on the same plate (e.g., from top to bottom). This method produces all possible combinations of 2-fold concentrations for the two drugs being tested. An inoculum of test bacteria is added to all wells, and the results are read in a similar manner as the MIC test. The FIC is expressed mathematically by calculation of the FIC index. The FIC index is calculated as

$$ \text{FIC index} = \frac{A}{\text{MIC}_A} + \frac{B}{\text{MIC}_B} $$

where A or B is the lowest concentration of the drug that is inhibitory in the presence of the second drug, and the MIC is the minimal inhibitory concentration of each drug tested alone. Synergism is defined as an FIC index of 0.5 or less, indifference is defined as an FIC index of between 0.6 and 4.0, and antagonism is defined as an FIC index of greater than 4.0.[44] The microtiter FIC methods have been adapted to allow the use of Etest antibiotic-susceptibility test strips.[45] In this method, two antibiotic Etest strips are crossed at the individual MIC of each antibiotic; an extension of the zone of inhibition beyond that from either antibiotic alone is considered additive or synergistic activity, and an FIC index can be calculated in a similar manner as the microtiter method.

The second most common method to determine the effects of antibiotic combinations is an adaptation of timed-kill curve tests. Two antibiotics are added to the same test tube at fixed concentration fractions of the MIC for each drug, and killing is quantified. With this method, synergism is defined as a 100-fold decrease in viable organisms at 24 hours for the combination as compared with the most potent antibiotic tested alone. Antagonism is defined as a 100-fold or greater increase in viable organism count[44] (Fig. 113–9). It is important to note that although antagonism has been demonstrated for several combinations in vitro (e.g., penicillin plus tetracycline, chloramphenicol and an aminoglycoside, fluoroquinolones and rifampin), antagonism in vivo has been demonstrated only infrequently.

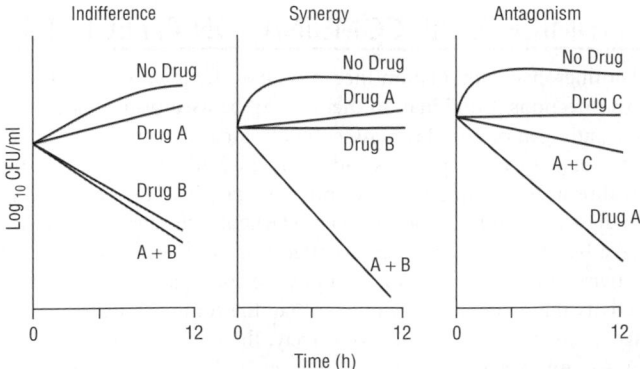

FIGURE 113-9. Timed-kill curve illustrating indifference, synergy, and antagonism. (CFU, colony-forming unit.)

Although the methods for testing the effects of antimicrobial combinations are well described, the results from these tests have not been adequately studied in the context of many infection outcomes. There is little debate that the combination of a β-lactam antibiotic and an aminoglycoside is required for successful treatment of enterococcal endocarditis. For enterococci, susceptibility to high concentrations of aminoglycosides (e.g., gentamicin, 500 mg/mL) is evaluated in the clinical laboratory because it correlates closely with synergy when the drug is combined with β-lactam antibiotics.

The concept of combination therapy is not universally accepted for the treatment of other infections. There is ongoing debate as to whether the combination of a broad-spectrum β-lactam and an aminoglycoside is needed (versus the β-lactam alone) for the therapy of such infections as gram-negative bloodstream infections or infections in neutropenic patients. In individual studies, combination therapy has resulted in improved outcomes in patients with severe illness and in patients with *P aeruginosa* bloodstream infections, but pooled meta-analyses have disputed these results.[46]

LABORATORY MONITORING OF ANTIMICROBIAL THERAPY

🔟 The clinician should have an understanding of in vivo antimicrobial agent disposition to select the most appropriate therapy for a given infection and to help monitor for clinical or bacteriologic efficacy. Serum concentration monitoring is the most common method used to attempt to maximize efficacy and minimize toxicity of antimicrobials. Because most antimicrobials are well tolerated at their usual doses, only a select few agents (e.g., aminoglycosides, chloramphenicol, and vancomycin) are monitored routinely in the current clinical environment. There are a number of direct and indirect methods that are used to quantify the concentration of antimicrobial in an experimental sample.

METHODS OF ANTIMICROBIAL CONCENTRATION DETERMINATION IN CLINICAL SAMPLES

Fluorescence-Polarization Immunoassay

The fluorescence-polarization immunoassay (FPIA) technique involves the application of the principles of fluorescence when molecules are exposed to light. A fluorescein-labeled drug and antibody that is directed against the drug are added in constant amounts to samples with unknown drug concentrations and to concentration standards. When the fluorescein-labeled drug complexes with the antibody, a quantifiable change in the fluorescence polarization occurs. When a sample containing non–fluorescein-labeled drug (i.e., a patient's serum sample) is mixed with the standard mixture, competition for antibody binding occurs. Comparison of the change caused by the patient's sample to the changes caused by standard concentrations determines the specific drug concentration in the patient sample.

FPIA is the most commonly used assay method for the determination of aminoglycoside and vancomycin serum concentrations in the clinical laboratory setting. Advantages of this technique include its automation, and the disadvantages include the expenses for reagents and the cost for the purchase of the automated system.

Radioimmunoassay

Radioimmunoassay (RIA) uses a radiolabeled drug and an antibody directed against the specific drug to determine the concentration contained in an unknown sample. The theory behind the assay is similar to FPIA because radiolabeled antibiotic and unlabeled antibiotic (in the patient's serum sample) are equilibrated with the antibody. The amount of free radiolabeled drug is measured and compared with the values obtained with standard concentrations of the radiolabeled drug alone to determine the concentration in the patient sample. Although RIA has good sensitivity and specificity, its main disadvantage compared with FPIA is the expense and hassle of handling and disposal of the radioactive waste generated during the test.

High-Pressure Liquid Chromatography

High-performance liquid chromatography (HPLC) permits the separation of different molecular species by passing a mobile solvent phase over a stationary phase. Drugs with a polarity similar to that of the stationary phase are retained for a time on the chromatographic column and then released after various retention times. Detection can be accomplished via fluorescence, electrochemical, or radiometric methods. The detector signal is proportional to the amount of molecules present. Standard curves are generated from known concentrations of the drug (usually recorded as peak area or peak height). Advantages of HPLC include a rapid turnaround time, precision, and an ability to detect the test drug in the presence of its metabolites and/or other drugs. Disadvantages include the high cost of HPLC instruments and the expertise required to perform the assays. These disadvantages usually relegate HPLC drug assay to the experimental and/or research settings.

Microbiologic Assay

Microbioassay of antimicrobial agents can be performed by several methods. The most common method is a modification of the disk diffusion antimicrobial-susceptibility technique. Typically, paper disks are placed on agar that contains an inoculum of a bacterium known to be highly susceptible to the antimicrobial agent to be assayed. Fixed volumes (usually 10 mcL) of a range of prepared concentration standards of the test drug are placed on the disks. The zones of growth inhibition are measured and plotted versus the drug concentration to generate a standard curve. Zone sizes from samples containing the unknown concentrations of the test drug are measured, and the concentrations are determined from the plotted

curve; the drug concentration in unknown samples is determined from the standard curve generated from the known concentrations of the drug. The advantages of this method include its relative ease of performance and the minimal cost for equipment. The disadvantages of this method include interference from other antibiotics that can be present in the unknown sample, a lack of sensitivity/specificity for certain antimicrobials, and a slow turnaround time (usually 24 to 48 hours) for generation of results.

TIMING OF COLLECTION OF SERUM SAMPLES

❿ Peak and/or trough concentrations are monitored routinely for only a select few antimicrobials (e.g., aminoglycosides and vancomycin) during the contemporary management of infections. It is crucial for the healthcare team to ensure that the antimicrobial's administration time and serum sample time(s) are meticulously recorded because even small errors in recording these (e.g., 1 hour) can have a substantial impact on the calculation of pharmacokinetics for antibiotics such as the aminoglycosides, which have relatively short elimination half-lives.

⓫ Samples ideally should be obtained after steady state is achieved (usually defined as the passage of at least 3 to 4 anticipated half-lives), but in certain situations, this may not be possible (e.g., critically ill patients with fluctuations in drug elimination owing to fluctuating hemodynamics, kidney function, and/or liver function). Generally, the timing of the peak serum sample collection is usually more critical than the trough concentration because adequate time must elapse to allow for completion of the distribution phase and to avoid underestimating the drug's volume of distribution.

SPECIFIC AGENTS

The aminoglycosides (i.e., amikacin, gentamicin, and tobramycin) and vancomycin remain the most common agents for which serum concentrations are monitored. A summary of the recommendations for serum concentration monitoring of these agents is shown in Table 113–2.

Aminoglycosides

⓬ There are many studies that have linked serum aminoglycoside concentrations with clinical response and with the occurrence of nephrotoxicity. One of the classic investigations into the

---

TABLE 113-2 Suggested Therapeutic Serum Concentrations for Selected Antimicrobial Agents

Drug	Sample	Target Concentrations (mg/L)	Comments
Gentamicin, Tobramycin (traditional dosage regimens)	Peak (1 h after start of 15- to 45-min infusion)	<5	Urinary tract infections
		>5	Bacteremia
		>6	Bacterial pneumonia
		>12	Endocarditis caused by *Pseudomonas aeruginosa*
	Trough	<2–3	High trough concentrations are most likely a result of and not a cause of nephrotoxicity
Amikacin	Peak	>15	Urinary tract infections
		>20	Bacteremia
		>24	Bacterial pneumonia, other serious infections
	Trough	>9–10	See comments regarding trough gentamicin/tobramycin concentrations
Single daily dosage regimens[49]			
Gentamicin Netilmicin Tobramycin	8-h postdose (*mid-dose*)	1.5–6	Concentrations above this range associated with nephrotoxicity in one study with netilmicin
Vancomycin	Trough	15–20	Recent data suggest this higher trough range due to low lung penetration, potential for resistance and increasing vancomycin MICs/MBCs[50]

MIC, minimal inhibitory concentration; MBC, minimal bactericidal concentration.
Data from Nicolau et al.,[49] and Rybak et al.[51]

relationship between serum aminoglycoside activity and clinical outcome revealed that peak serum concentrations of at least 5 mcg/mL for gentamicin and tobramycin and at least 20 mcg/mL for amikacin were associated with a lower prevalence of clinical failure rates during the treatment of gram-negative bacteremia.[47] Although earlier studies suggested that trough concentrations exceeding 2 to 4 mcg/mL for gentamicin and tobramycin and 10 mcg/mL for amikacin predisposed patients to nephrotoxicity, other investigations indicated that the development of aminoglycoside-related ototoxicity and nephrotoxicity is more complex and also is associated with the total exposure to the aminoglycoside (as measured by the AUC) and/or the total duration of aminoglycoside therapy.[48] The specific recommended serum peak and trough concentrations for the various aminoglycosides are described in Table 113–2.

Newer regimens of high dose once-daily or extended-interval aminoglycoside administration have gained widespread acceptance for use in the clinical setting. These regimens exploit the pharmacodynamic properties of these agents (i.e., concentration-dependent bacterial killing and a substantial PAE) to maximize activity while also attempting to minimize drug nephrotoxicity by reducing the total aminoglycoside exposure time for the patient's kidneys. The doses employed for extended-interval treatment typically range from 5 to 7 mg/kg of lean body weight (administered every 24 to 48 hours), with the dose and/or interval adjusted based on renal function or observed mid-dose serum concentrations.[49] Many prospective studies have been performed to evaluate the safety and efficacy of once-daily aminoglycoside dosing, and most have revealed similar rates of efficacy and toxicity, or trends toward improved efficacy and reduced toxicity for once-daily dosage regimens as compared with traditional (thrice daily) regimens.

Traditional methods of aminoglycoside serum concentration monitoring (evaluating peak and trough serum concentrations) cannot be applied to extended-interval dosing because the serum concentrations 24 hours after a dose ideally should be undetectable. A mid-interval serum sample can be taken approximately 6 to 12 hours after the dose to allow for use of first-order pharmacokinetic equations.

CLINICAL CONTROVERSY

Some clinicians believe that there is sufficient clinical data to support widespread use of once-daily aminoglycoside dosing without determination of individual patient pharmacokinetics. However, there are some clinicians that believe that the data is incomplete and that patients should receive individualized pharmacokinetic assessments and dosage adjustments.

Vancomycin

13 The area under the concentration-time curve to MIC ratio (AUC/MIC) is the most likely parameter predicting efficacy as demonstrated by animal and limited human data.[50] Although intravenous vancomycin has been associated with oto- and nephrotoxicity in humans, most of these reports occurred with older, impure formulations of the drug, with extremely high concentrations uncommon with contemporary dosing regimens, or when vancomycin was combined with known nephrotoxic agents. Although serum peak and trough concentrations were previously recommended for monitoring vancomycin therapy, now, only the trough concentration is routinely monitored since vancomycin is not a concentration-dependent killing antibiotic.

Weight-based dosage regimens and/or nomogram-based dosage methods were developed to help minimize monitoring of serum concentrations for the vast majority of patients. Most of these methods of empirical vancomycin dosing resulted in trough concentrations between 5 and 10 mcg/mL. However, higher vancomycin trough concentrations are now believed to be needed because of its poor penetration into tissue such as the lung, the association of the emergence of vancomycin nonsusceptible strains for those patients for which trough serum concentrations were maintained below 10 mg/L and the trend toward an increased prevalence of strains of staphylococci with higher vancomycin MICs and/or MBCs. There is some animal data and limited clinical data that suggest that targeting an AUC/MIC of ≥400 may improve patient outcome in patients with Staphylococcus aureus infections. Consensus-review guidelines for the dosing and monitoring of vancomycin suggest that vancomycin trough concentrations should be considered as the most accurate and practical means for monitoring efficacy.[51] Trough serum concentrations should be maintained above 10 mg/L to avoid the emergence of resistance. A serum trough concentration of 15 to 20 mg/L is recommended for patients with serious infections such as complicated bacteremia endocarditis, meningitis, and hospital-acquired pneumonia caused by S aureus.[52] A target trough concentration of 15 to 20 mg/L should achieve an AUC/MIC of ≥400 when the S aureus vancomycin MIC is ≤1 mg/L. Although more data are needed, targeting these higher troughs may result in an increased risk of renal dysfunction in some patients.[51]

CLINICAL CONTROVERSY

Some clinicians believe that vancomycin should no longer be considered as the drug of first-choice for treatment of serious staphylococcal infections—even when it is administered to target the new, higher trough range of 15 to 20 mg/L. The desired target attainment of an AUC/MIC of ≥400 may not be achieved with conventional doses of vancomycin with S aureus exhibiting a vancomycin MIC of ≥2 mg/L.

INTEGRATING ORGANISM SUSCEPTIBILITY WITH SERUM CONCENTRATION DATA TO IMPROVE ANTIMICROBIAL THERAPY

7 **14** We have advanced our understanding substantially of the importance of considering both antimicrobial pharmacokinetics and organism susceptibility when selecting therapy for the treatment of infections. Antimicrobial regimens should be selected and/or designed to maximize the probability that bacterial killing is optimized and that the probability of resistance is minimized. For example, the activity of antimicrobials such as the fluoroquinolones and the aminoglycosides can be maximized if the ratio of the peak serum concentration to the organism MIC (peak-to-MIC ratio) is greater than or equal to 10.[52] Similarly, the probability of clinical and/or microbiologic infection cure can be maximized if a fluoroquinolone is chosen that achieves an area under the curve (AUC)-to-MIC ratio of 100 to 125 or greater for gram-negative bacteria (e.g., P aeruginosa) and 30 to 40 or greater for gram-positive bacteria (e.g., S pneumoniae). The clinical application of these principles to aminoglycoside dosage regimen optimization is depicted in Figure 113–10. Although the maintenance of concentrations above the infecting organism's MIC (the time above the MIC) best predicts the clinical efficacy of the β-lactam antimicrobials, the AUC-to-MIC ratio also appears to be a strong predictor for treatment outcome for certain organisms and in certain clinical situations (e.g., vancomycin for staphylococcal infections).[51]

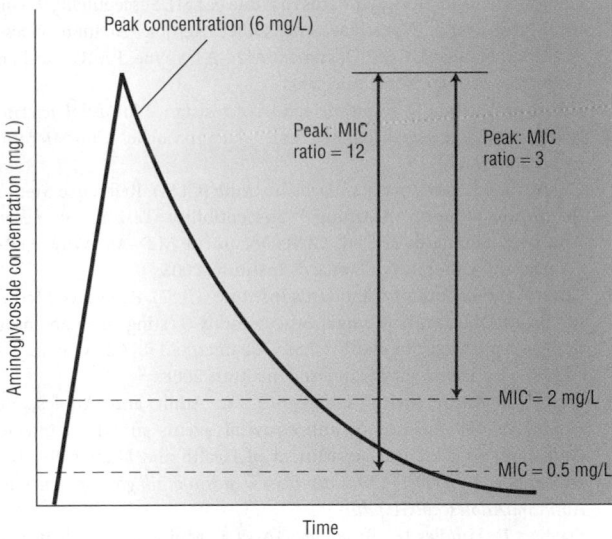

FIGURE 113-10. Illustration of the concept of peak concentration to the minimal inhibitory concentration (MIC) ratio for aminoglycosides. The MIC for the given organism to gentamicin is 2 mg/L, whereas the tobramycin MIC is 0.5 mg/L. Administration of gentamicin would result in a suboptimal peak:MIC ratio (<10), which could increase the chances for development of resistance or an inadequate response. Administration of tobramycin would result in a peak:MIC ratio of 12, which should improve efficacy. Note that modification of the gentamicin regimen to produce peak serum concentrations of 20 mg/L or more (as commonly done with once-daily administration) also would result in a peak:MIC ratio of ≥10.

Most of the data on optimization of antimicrobial pharmacodynamics have been generated in in vitro models of infection, in animal models of infection, within the context of controlled clinical trials, or through mathematical modeling of small data sets. However, research continues to emerge on the best ways to apply these valuable data to the everyday management of patients in the clinical setting. The recognition of the importance of antimicrobial pharmacodynamics already has resulted in such therapeutic innovations such as (1) the expansion of serum concentration monitoring for select antimicrobials (e.g., antiretroviral agents, antifungal agents), (2) suggested revisions of breakpoint values that define antimicrobial susceptibility and/or resistance, (3) development of nomograms or computer programs that can suggest optimal drugs and doses for a given infection, (4) novel administration methods such as prolonged infusion times for antibiotics such as β-lactams with time-dependent activity, and (5) the development of newer antimicrobial agents with minimized risks of suboptimal pharmacodynamics. These developments present exciting opportunities for healthcare providers to improve the outcomes of patients with infections in a variety of different healthcare settings.

ABBREVIATIONS

AIDS: acquired immunodeficiency syndrome

AUC: area under the curve

bDNA: branched DNA

CDC: Centers for Disease Control and Prevention

CLSI: Clinical and Laboratory Standards Institute

CFU: colony-forming unit

CMV: cytomegalovirus

CSF: cerebrospinal fluid

ELISA: enzyme-linked immunosorbent assay

ESBL: extended-spectrum β-lactamase

ESR: erythrocyte sedimentation rate

FIC: fractional inhibitory concentration

FISH: fluorescence in situ hybridization

FPIA: fluorescence-polarization immunoassay

HIV: human immunodeficiency virus

HPLC: high-performance liquid chromatography

KOH: potassium hydroxide

MBC: minimum bactericidal concentration

MHC: major histocompatibility complex

MIC: minimum inhibitory concentration

MRSA: methicillin-resistant *Staphylococcus aureus*

PAE: postantibiotic effect

PCR: polymerase chain reaction

PMN: polymorphonuclear leukocyte

RIA: radioimmunoassay

SBT: serum bactericidal titer

SIRS: systemic inflammatory response syndrome

SIT: serum inhibitory titer

TNF: tumor necrosis factor

VISA: vancomycin-intermediate *Staphylococcus aureus*

VRE: vancomycin-resistant enterococci

VRSA: vancomycin-resistant *Staphylococcus aureus*

REFERENCES

1. Reese RE, Betts RF. Principles of Antibiotic Use. In: Betts RF, Chapman SW, Penn RL, eds. A Practical Approach to Infectious Diseases, 5th ed. Philadelphia, PA: Lippincott Williams & Wilkins, 2003:969–988.
2. Andro V, Cainelli F. Infections in patients with cancer undergoing chemotherapy: Aetiology, prevention, and treatment. Lancet Oncol 2003;595–604.
3. Crawford J, Dale DC, Lyman GH. Chemotherapy-induced neutropenia: Risks, consequences, and new directions for its management. Cancer 2003;100:228–237.
4. Day CL, Walker BD. Progress in defining CD4 helper cell responses in chronic viral infections. J Exp Med 2003;198:1773–1777.
5. Smith JM, Nemeth TL, McDonald RA. Current immunosuppressive agents: Efficacy, side effects and utilization. Pediatr Clin North Am 2003;6:1283–1300.
6. Penn RL, Betts RF. Lower respiratory tract infections (including tuberculosis). In: Betts RF, Chapman SW, Penn RL, eds. A Practical Approach to Infectious Diseases, 5th ed. Philadelphia, PA: Lippincott Williams & Wilkins, 2003:295–371.
7. Lannergard A, Larsson A, Kragsbjerg P, Friman G. Correlation between serum amyloid A protein and C-reactive protein in infectious diseases. Scand J Clin Lab Invest 2003;4:267–272.
8. Priest DH, Peacock JE Jr. Hematogenous vertebral osteomyelitis due to Staphylococcus aureus in the adult: Clinical features and therapeutic outcomes. South Med J 2005;98:854–862.
9. Cavaillon JM, Adib-Conquy M, Fitting C, et al. Cytokine cascade in sepsis. Scand J Infect Dis 2003;35:535–544.
10. Lekkou A, Karakantza M, Mouzaki A, et al. Cytokine production and monocyte HLH-DR expression as predictors of outcome for patients with community-acquired severe infections. Clin Diagn Lab Immunol 2004;11:161–167.
11. Dorman NJ. Sepsis. In: Betts RF, Chapman SW, and Penn RL, eds. A Practical Approach to Infectious Diseases, 5th ed. Philadelphia, PA: Lippincott Williams & Wilkins, 2003:19–66.

12. Safdar N, Kluger DM, Maki DG. A review of risk factors for catheter-related bloodstream infection caused by percutaneously inserted, non-cuffed central venous catheters: Implications for preventive strategies. Medicine 2002;86:466–479.

13. Graman PS, Menegus MA. Microbiology laboratory tests In: Betts RF, Chapman SW, Penn RL, eds. A Practical Approach to Infectious Diseases, 5th ed. Philadelphia, PA: Lippincott Williams & Wilkins, 2003:929–956.

14. O'Hara CM, Weinstein MP, Miller JM. Manual and automated systems for detection and identification of microorganisms. In: Murry PR, Baron EJ, Jorgensen JH, et al., eds. Manual of Clinical Microbiology, 8th ed. Washington, DC: ASM Press, 2003:185–207.

15. Constantine NT, Lana DP. Immunoassays for the diagnosis of infectious diseases. In: Murray PR, Baron EJ, Jorgensen JH, et al., eds. Manual of Clinical Microbiology, 8th ed. Washington, DC: ASM Press, 2003:218–256.

16. Gill VJ, Fedorko DP, Witebsky FG. The clinician and the microbiology laboratory. In: Mandell GL, Bennet JE, Dolin R, eds. Principles and Practice of Infectious Diseases, 6th ed. New York: Churchill-Livingstone, 2005:203–241.

17. Nolte FS, Caliendo AM. Molecular detection and identification of microorganisms. In: Murry PR, Baron EJ, Jorgensen JH, et al., eds. Manual of Clinical Microbiology, 8th ed. Washington, DC: ASM Press, 2003:234–256.

18. Pilcher CD, McPherson JD, Leone PA, et al. Real-time, universal screening for acute HIV infection in a routine HIV counseling and testing population. JAMA 2002;288:216–221.

19. Bryant P, Venter D, Robins-Browne R, Curtis N. Chips with everything: DNA microarrays in infectious diseases. Lancet Infect Dis 2004;4:100–111.

20. Owen RJ. Molecular testing for antibiotic resistance in *Helicobacter pylori*. Gut 2002;50:285–289.

21. Varaldo PE. Antimicrobial resistance and susceptibility testing: An evergreen topic. J Antimicrob Chemother 2002;50:1–4.

22. Pfaller MA, Segreti J. Overview of the epidemiological profile and laboratory detection of extended-spectrum beta-lactamases. Clin Infect Dis 2006;42(Suppl 4):S153–S163.

23. Appelbaum PC. The emergence of vancomycin-intermediate and vancomycin-resistant Staphylococcus aureus. Clin Microbiol Infect 2006;12(Suppl 1):16–23.

24. Clinical and Laboratory Standards Institute (CLSI). Methods for Antimicrobial Susceptibility Tests for Bacteria that Grow Aerobically; Approved Standard, 7th ed. CLSI document M7-A7. Wayne, PA: Clinical and Laboratory Standards Institute.

25. Bauer AW, Kirby MM, Sherris JC, et al. Antibiotic susceptibility testing by a standardized, single-disk method. Am J Clin Pathol 1966;45:493–496.

26. Hidayat LK, Hsu DI, Quist R, Shriner KA, Wong-Beringer A. High-dose vancomycin therapy for methicillin-resistant Staphylococcus aureus infections: Efficacy and toxicity. Arch Intern Med 2006;166:2138–2144.

27. Craig WA. Does the dose matter? Clin Infect Dis 2001;33(Suppl 3):S233–S237.

28. Swenson JM, Anderson KF, Lonsway DR, et al. Accuracy of commercial and reference susceptibility testing methods for detecting vancomycin-intermediate Staphylococcus aureus. J Clin Microbiol 2009;47:2013–2017.

29. Kulah C, Aktas E, Comert F, et al. Detecting imipenem resistance in *Acinetobacter baumannii* by automated systems (BD Phoenix, Microscan WalkAway, Vitek 2); high error rates with Microscan WalkAway. BMC Infect Dis 2009;9:30.

30. Pestotnik SL. Expert clinical decision support systems to enhance antimicrobial stewardship programs: Insights from the Society of Infectious Diseases Pharmacists. Pharmacotherapy 2005;25:1116–1125.

31. Woods GL. Susceptibility testing for mycobacteria. Clin Infect Dis 2000;31:1209–1215.

32. Ardito F, Posteraro B, Sanguinetti M, et al. Evaluation of BACTEC Mycobacteria Growth Indicator Tube (MGIT 960) automated system for drug susceptibility testing of *Mycobacterium tuberculosis*. J Clin Microbiol 2001;38:4440–4444.

33. Clinical and Laboratory Standards Institute (CLSI). Susceptibility Testing for Mycobacteria, Nocardiae, and Other Aerobic Actinomycetes—Approved Standard. CLSI Document M24-A. Wayne, PA: Clinical and Laboratory Standards Institute, 2003.

34. Garcie de Viedma D. Rapid detection of resistance in *Mycobacterium tuberculosis*: A review discussing molecular approaches. Clin Microbiol Infect 2003;9:349–359.

35. Clinical and Laboratory Standards Institute (CLSI). Reference Method for Broth Dilution Antifungal Susceptibility Testing of Yeasts; Approved Standard, 3rd ed. CLSI Document M27-A3. Wayne, PA: Clinical and Laboratory Standards Institute, 2008.

36. Clinical and Laboratory Standards Institute (CLSI). Reference Method for Broth Dilution Antifungal Susceptibility Testing of Filamentous Fungi—Approved Standard. CLSI Document M38-A2. Wayne, PA: Clinical and Laboratory Standards Institute, 2008.

37. Panel on Antiretroviral Guidelines for Adult and Adolescents. Guidelines for the use of antiretroviral agents in HIV-1-infected adults and adolescents. Department of Health and Human Services. November 3, 2008:1–139. *http://www.aidsinfo.nih.gov/ContentFiles/AdultandAdolescentGL.pdf.*

38. Flayhart D, Hindler JF., Bruckner DA, et al. Multicenter evaluation of BBL CHROMagar MRSA medium for direct detection of methicillin-resistant *Staphylococcus aureus* from surveillance cultures of the anterior nares. J Clin Microbiol 2005;43:5336–5340.

39. Pape J, Waldlin J, Nackamkin I. Use of BBL CHROMagar MRSA medium for identification of methicillin-resistant *Staphylococcus aureus* directly from blood cultures. J Clin Microbiol 2006;44:2575–2576.

40. Oliveira K, Procop GW, Wilson D, et al. Rapid identification of *Staphylococcus aureus* directly from blood cultures by fluorescence in situ hybridization with peptide nucleic acid probes. J Clin Microbiol 2002;40:247–251.

41. Rodriguez CA, Atkinson R, Bitar W, et al. Tolerance to vancomycin in pneumococci: detection with a molecular marker and assessment of clinical impact. J Infect Dis 2004;190:1481–1487.

42. Craig WA, Ebert SC. Killing and regrowth of bacteria in vitro: a review. Scand J Infect Dis Suppl 1991;74:63–70.

43. Craig WA, Gudmundsson S. Postantibiotic effect. In: Lorian V, ed. Antibiotics in Laboratory Medicine, 5th ed. Baltimore, MD: Williams & Wilkins, 2005:296–329.

44. Elipoulos G, Moellering RC Jr. Antimicrobial combinations. In: Lorian V, ed. Antibiotics in Laboratory Medicine, 5th ed. Baltimore, MD: Williams & Wilkins, 2005:330–397.

45. White RL, Burgess DS, Manduru M, Bosso JA. Comparison of three different in vitro methods of detecting synergy: Time-kill, checkerboard, and E test. Antimicrob Agents Chemother 1996;40:1914–1918.

46. Paul M, Silbiger I, Grozinsky S, Soares-Weiser K, Leibovici L. Beta lactam antibiotic monotherapy versus beta lactam-aminoglycoside antibiotic combination therapy for sepsis. Cochrane Database Syst Rev 2006(1):CD003344.

47. Moore RD, Smith CR, Lietman PS. The association of aminoglycoside plasma levels with mortality in patients with gram-negative bacteremia. J Infect Dis 1984;149:443–448.

48. Rybak MJ, Abate BJ, Kang SL, Ruffing MJ, Lerner SA, Drusano GL. Prospective evaluation of the effect of an aminoglycoside dosing regimen on rates of observed nephrotoxicity and ototoxicity. Antimicrob Agents Chemother 1999;43:1549–1555.

49. Nicolau DP, Freeman CD, Belliveau PP, et al. Experience with a once-daily aminoglycoside program administered to 2,184 adult patients. Antimicrob Agents Chemother 1995;39:650–655.

50. Rybak MJ. The pharmacokinetic and pharmacodynamic properties of vancomycin. Clin Infect Dis 2006;42(Suppl 1):S35–S39.

51. Rybak MJ, Lomaestro BM, Rotschafer JC, et al. Therapeutic monitoring of vancomycin in adults summary of consensus recommendations from the American Society of health-system pharmacists, the infectious diseases society of America, and the society of infectious diseases pharmacists. Pharmacotherapy 2009;29:1275–1279.

52. DeRyke CA, Lee SY, Kuti JL, Nicolau DP. Optimising dosing strategies of antibacterials utilising pharmacodynamic principles: impact on the development of resistance. Drugs 2006;66:1–14.

DAVID S. BURGESS

CHAPTER

114

Antimicrobial Regimen Selection

KEY CONCEPTS

❶ Every attempt should be made to obtain specimens for culture and sensitivity testing prior to initiating antibiotics.

❷ Empirical antibiotic therapy should be based on knowledge of likely pathogens for the site of infection, information from patient history (e.g., recent hospitalizations, work-related exposure, travel, and pets), and local susceptibility.

❸ Patients with delayed dermatologic reactions (i.e., rash) to penicillin generally can receive cephalosporins. Patients with type I hypersensitivity reactions (i.e., anaphylaxis) to penicillins should not receive cephalosporins. Alternatives to the cephalosporins include aztreonam, quinolones, sulfonamide antibiotics, or vancomycin based on type of coverage indicated.

❹ Estimated creatinine clearance should be calculated for every patient who is to receive antibiotics and the antibiotic dose interval adjusted accordingly. Hepatic function should be considered for drugs eliminated through the hepatobiliary system, such as clindamycin, erythromycin, and metronidazole.

❺ All concomitant drugs and nutritional supplements should be reviewed when an antibiotic is added to a patient's therapy to ensure drug–drug interactions will be avoided.

❻ Combination antibiotic therapy may be indicated for polymicrobial infections (intra-abdominal, gynecologic infections), to produce synergistic killing (such as β-lactam plus aminoglycoside versus *Pseudomonas aeruginosa*), or to prevent the emergence of resistance.

❼ All patients receiving antibiotics should be monitored for resolution of infectious signs and symptoms (e.g., decreasing temperature and white blood cell count) and adverse drug events.

❽ Antibiotics with the narrowest effective spectrum of activity are preferred. Antibiotic route of administration should be evaluated daily, and conversion from intravenous to oral therapy should be attempted as signs of infection improve for patients with functioning gastrointestinal tracts (general exceptions are endocarditis and central nervous system infections).

❾ Patients not responding to an appropriate antibiotic treatment in 2 to 3 days should be reevaluated to ensure (a) the correct diagnosis, (b) that therapeutic drug concentrations are being achieved, (c) that the patient is not immunosuppressed, (d) that the patient does not have isolated infection (i.e., abscess, foreign body), or (e) that resistance has not developed.

Choosing an antimicrobial agent to treat an infection is far more complicated than matching a drug to a known or suspected pathogen.[1,2] Most clinicians generally follow a systematic approach to select an antimicrobial regimen (Table 114–1). Problems arise when this systematic approach is replaced by prescribing broad-spectrum therapy to cover as many organisms as possible. Consequences of not using the systematic approach include the use of more expensive and potentially more toxic agents, which can, in turn, lead to widespread resistance and difficult-to-treat superinfections. Another abuse of antimicrobial agents is administration when they are not needed such as when they are prescribed for self-limited clinical conditions that are most likely viral in origin (i.e., the common cold).

Initial selection of antimicrobial therapy is nearly always empirical, which is prior to documentation and identification of the offending organism. Infectious diseases generally are acute, and a delay in antimicrobial therapy can result in serious morbidity or even mortality. Thus empirical antimicrobial therapy selection should be based on information gathered from the patient's history and physical examination and results of Gram stains or of rapidly performed tests on specimens from the infected site. This information, combined with knowledge of the most likely offending organism(s) and an institution's local susceptibility patterns, should result in a rational selection of antibiotics to treat the patient. This chapter introduces a systematic approach to the selection of antimicrobial therapeutic regimens.

TABLE 114-1 Systematic Approach for Selection of Antimicrobials
Confirm the presence of infection
Careful history and physical
Signs and symptoms
Predisposing factors
Identification of the pathogen (see Chap. 113)
Collection of infected material
Stains
Serologies
Culture and sensitivity
Selection of presumptive therapy considering every infected site
Host factors
Drug factors
Monitor therapeutic response
Clinical assessment
Laboratory tests
Assessment of therapeutic failure

Learning objectives, review questions, and other resources can be found at **www.pharmacotherapyonline.com**.

CONFIRMING THE PRESENCE OF INFECTION

FEVER

The presence of a temperature greater than the expected 37°C (98.6°F) "normal" body temperature is considered a hallmark of infectious diseases. Body temperature is controlled by the hypothalamus. In addition, the circadian rhythm, a built-in temperature cycle, is also operational. The daily temperature rhythm can vary for each individual. In a healthy person, the internal thermostat is set between the morning low temperature and the afternoon peak as controlled by the circadian rhythm. During fever, the hypothalamus is reset at a higher temperature level.

Fever is defined as a controlled elevation of body temperature above the normal range. The average normal body temperature range taken orally is 36.7 to 37°C (98.0–98.6°F). Body temperatures obtained rectally generally are 0.6°C (1°F) higher and axillary temperatures are 0.6°C (1°F) lower than oral temperatures, respectively. Skin temperatures are also less than the oral temperature but can vary depending on the specific measurement method.

Fever can be a manifestation of disease states other than infection. Collagen-vascular (autoimmune) disorders and several malignancies can have fever as a manifestation. Fever of unknown or undetermined origin is a diagnostic dilemma and is reviewed extensively elsewhere.[3]

Many drugs have been identified as causes of fever.[4] *Drug-induced fever* is defined as persistent fever in the absence of infection or other underlying condition. The fever must coincide temporally with the administration of the offending agent and disappear promptly on its withdrawal, after which the temperature remains normal. Possible mechanisms of drug-induced fever are either a hypersensitivity reaction or development of antigen-antibody complexes that result in the stimulation of macrophages and the release of interleukin 1 (IL-1). Although this is not a common drug effect (accounting for no more than 5% of all drug reactions), it should be suspected when obvious reasons for fever are not present. Almost any medication can produce fever, but β-lactam antibiotics, anticonvulsants, allopurinol, hydralazine, nitrofurantoin, sulfonamides, phenothiazines, and methyldopa appear to be responsible more often than others.

Noninfectious etiologies of fever can be referred to as "false-positives." Although these certainly can confuse the clinician, even more troublesome are false-negatives: the absence of fever in a patient with signs and symptoms consistent with an infectious disease. Careful questioning of the patient or family is vital to assess the ingestion of any medication that can mask fever (e.g., aspirin, acetaminophen, nonsteroidal antiinflammatory agents, and corticosteroids). The use of antipyretics should be discouraged during the treatment of infection unless absolutely necessary because they can mask a poor therapeutic response. Moreover, elevated body temperature, unless very high (>40.5°C [105°F]), is not harmful and may be beneficial.

SIGNS AND SYMPTOMS

White Blood Cell Count

Most infections result in elevated white blood cell (WBC) counts (leukocytosis) because of the increased production and mobilization of granulocytes (neutrophils, basophils, and eosinophils), lymphocytes, or both to ingest and destroy invading microbes. The generally accepted range of normal values for WBC counts is between 4,000 and 10,000 cells/mm³. Values above or below this range hold important prognostic and diagnostic value.

Bacterial infections are associated with elevated granulocyte counts, often with immature forms (band neutrophils) seen in peripheral blood smears. Mature neutrophils are also referred to as *segmented neutrophils* or *polymorphonuclear* (PMN) *leukocytes*. The presence of immature forms (left shift) is an indication of an increased bone marrow response to the infection. With infection, peripheral WBC counts can be very high, but they are rarely higher than 30,000 to 40,000 cells/mm³. Because leukocytosis indicates the normal host response to infection, low leukocyte counts after the onset of infection indicate an abnormal response and generally are associated with a poor prognosis.

The most common granulocyte defect is neutropenia, a decrease in absolute numbers of circulating neutrophils. A thorough description of the consequences of neutropenia is given in Chapter 131. Lymphocytosis, even with normal or slightly elevated total WBC counts, generally is associated with tuberculosis and viral or fungal infections. Increases in monocytes can be associated with tuberculosis or lymphoma, and increases in eosinophils can be associated with allergic reactions to drugs or infections caused by metazoa. Many types of infections can be accompanied by a completely normal WBC count and differential.

Local Signs

The classic signs of pain and inflammation can manifest as swelling, erythema, tenderness, and purulent drainage. Unfortunately, these are only visible if the infection is superficial or in a bone or joint. The manifestations of inflammation in deep-seated infections (e.g., meningitis, pneumonia, endocarditis, and urinary tract infection) must be ascertained by examining tissues or fluids. For example, the presence of neutrophils in spinal fluid, lung secretions (sputum), or urine is highly suggestive of a bacterial infection.

Symptoms referable to an organ system must be sought out carefully because not only do they help in establishing the presence of infection, but they also aid in narrowing the list of potential pathogens. For example, a febrile patient with complaints of flank pain and dysuria can well have pyelonephritis. In this situation, enteric gram-negative bacilli, especially *Escherichia coli*, are the predominant pathogens. If a febrile patient has no symptoms suggestive of an organ system but only constitutional complaints, the list of possible infectious diseases is lengthy.[3] A febrile individual with cough and sputum production probably has a pulmonary infection. What is not so evident, however, is the etiologic organism in this situation, because it can be caused by bacteria, mycobacteria, viruses, chlamydia, or mycoplasmas.[5] In this situation, attention to the patient's history and background disease states is important. Even more important is a careful examination of the infected material (in this case sputum) to ascertain the identity of the pathogen.

IDENTIFICATION OF THE PATHOGEN

MICROBIOLOGY ISSUES

❶ Infected body materials must be sampled, if at all possible or practical, before institution of any antimicrobial therapy for two reasons. First, a Gram stain of the material might reveal bacteria, or an acid-fast stain might detect mycobacteria or actinomycetes. Second, a delay in obtaining infected fluids or tissues until after antimicrobial therapy is started might result in false-negative culture results or alterations in the cellular and chemical composition of infected fluids. This is particularly true in patients with urinary tract infections, meningitis, and septic arthritis.[6]

Blood cultures usually should be performed in the acutely ill febrile patient. Blood culture collection should coincide with sharp elevations in temperature, suggesting the possibility of microorganisms or microbial antigens in the bloodstream. Ideally, blood should be obtained from peripheral sites as two sets (one set consists of an aerobic bottle and one set an anaerobic bottle) from two different sites approximately 1 hour apart. In selected infections, bacteremia is qualitatively continuous (e.g., endocarditis), so cultures can be obtained at any time.[7]

In addition to the infected materials produced by the patient (e.g., blood, sputum, urine, stool, and wound or sinus drainage), other less accessible fluids or tissues must be obtained if they are suspected to be the infected site (e.g., spinal fluid in meningitis and joint fluid in arthritis). Abscesses and cellulitic areas also should be aspirated.

INTERPRETING RESULTS

After a positive Gram stain, culture results, or both are obtained, the clinician must be cautious in determining whether the organism recovered is a true pathogen, a contaminant, or a part of the normal flora (see Chap. 113). This latter consideration is especially problematic with cultures obtained from the skin, oropharynx, nose, ears, eyes, throat, and perineum. These surfaces are heavily colonized with a wide variety of bacteria, some of which can be pathogenic in certain settings. For example, coagulase-negative staphylococci are found in cultures of all the aforementioned sites yet are seldom regarded as pathogens unless recovered from blood, venous access catheters, or prosthetic devices.

Importantly, cultures of specimens from purportedly infected sites that are obtained by sampling from or through one of these contaminated areas might contain significant numbers of the normal flora. In the case of urine cultures, the urinalysis should be used in combination with culture results to assess the presence of WBCs, nitrite, and leukocyte esterase to help confirm infection and rule out colonization.

Particularly problematic are expectorated sputum specimens that must be evaluated carefully by determination of the presence of squamous epithelial cells and leukocytes.[5] A predominance of epithelial cells in sputum specimens reduces the likelihood that recovered bacteria are pathogenic, especially when multiple types of organisms are seen on Gram stain. In contrast, the discovery of leukocytes in large numbers with one predominant type of organism is a more reliable indicator of a valid collection. In general, however, sputum evaluation has poor sensitivity and specificity as a diagnostic test.[5]

Caution also must be used in the evaluation of positive culture results from normally sterile sites (e.g., blood, cerebrospinal fluid, or joint fluid). The recovery of bacteria normally found on the skin in large quantities (e.g., coagulase-negative staphylococci or diphtheroids) from one of these sites can be a result of contamination of the specimen rather than a true infection. However, these organisms can be pathogenic in certain settings.

Gram-staining techniques, culture methods, and serologic identification, as well as susceptibility testing, are discussed in detail in Chapter 113. Emphasis must be placed on the proper collection and handling of specimens and careful assessment of Gram stain or other test results in guiding the clinician toward appropriate selection of initial antimicrobial therapy.[8]

SELECTION OF PRESUMPTIVE THERAPY

❷ To select rational antimicrobial therapy for a given clinical situation, a variety of factors must be considered. These include the severity and acuity of the disease, host factors, factors related to the drugs used, and the necessity for using multiple agents. In addition, there are generally accepted drugs of choice for the treatment of most pathogens (see Appendix 114–1).

Drugs of choice are compiled from a variety of sources and are intended as guidelines rather than as specific rules for antimicrobial use. These choices are influenced by local antimicrobial susceptibility data rather than information published by other institutions or national compilations. Each institution should publish an annual summary of antibiotic susceptibilities (antibiogram) for organisms cultured from patients. Antibiograms contain both the number of nonduplicate isolates for common species and the percentage susceptible to the antibiotics tested. To further guide empirical antibiotic therapy, some hospitals publish unit-specific antibiograms in unique patient care areas, such as intensive care units or burn units.

Susceptibility of bacteria can differ substantially among hospitals within a community. For example, the prevalence of hospital-acquired methicillin-resistant *Staphylococcus aureus* (HA-MRSA) in some centers is quite high, whereas in other centers the problem might be nonexistent. This particular situation will influence the selection of therapy for possible *S aureus* infection, where the clinician must choose either a β-lactam or vancomycin. The problem of differing susceptibilities is not limited only to gram-positive bacteria but also is evident gram-negative organisms, and all drug classes are affected.

Empirical therapy is directed at organisms that are known to cause the infection in question. These organisms are discussed for different sites of infection in Chapters 115 to 132. To define the most likely infecting organisms, a careful history and physical examination must be performed. The place where the infection was acquired should be determined, for example, the home (community acquired), nursing home environment, or hospital acquired (nosocomial). Nursing home patients can be exposed to potentially more resistant organisms because they are often surrounded by ill patients who are receiving antibiotics. Other important questions to ask infected patients regarding the history of present illness include the following:

1. Are any other people sick at home, especially children?

2. Are any unusual pets kept in the home such as pigeons?

3. Where are you employed (i.e., are you exposed to contaminated meat or infectious biohazards)?

4. Has there been any recent travel (i.e., to endemic areas of fungal infections or developing countries)?

HOST FACTORS

Several host factors should be considered when evaluating a patient for antimicrobial therapy. The most important factors are drug allergies, age, pregnancy, genetic or metabolic abnormalities, renal and hepatic function, site of infection, concomitant drug therapy, and underlying disease states.

Allergy

❸ Allergy to an antimicrobial agent generally precludes its use. Careful assessment of allergy histories must be performed because many patients confuse common adverse drug effects (i.e., gastrointestinal disturbance) with true allergic reactions.[9] Among the most commonly cited antimicrobial allergies are those to penicillin, penicillin-related compounds, or both. In the absence of complete penicillin skin testing capabilities, a rule of thumb for giving cephalosporins to patients allergic to penicillin is to avoid giving them to patients who give a good history for immediate or accelerated reactions (e.g., anaphylaxis, laryngospasm) and to give them under close supervision in patients with a history of delayed reactions, such as a rash.[10] If a gram-negative infection is suspected or documented, therapy with a monobactam may be appropriate because cross-reactivity with other β-lactams is nonexistent.

Age

The patient's age is an important factor both in trying to identify the likely etiologic agent and in assessing the patient's ability to eliminate the drug(s) to be used. The best example of an age determinant of organisms is in bacterial meningitis, where the pathogens differ as the patient grows from the neonatal period through infancy and childhood into adulthood.[6]

In the case of the neonate, hepatic and liver functions are not well developed. Therefore, bilirubin excretion is decreased resulting in increased concentration of unconjugated bilirubin that can cause kernicterus. Neonates (especially when premature) can develop kernicterus when given sulfonamides. This results from displacement of bilirubin from serum albumin. In addition, neonates have more body water content that results in a larger volume of distribution leading to adjustments in antibiotic dosing regimens. Additional special drug considerations for pediatric patients include low frequency of adverse effects and compliance-enhancing features (e.g., absorption not affected by food, once- to twice-daily dosing, and good taste).[11]

The major physiologic change in persons older than 65 years of age is a decline in the number of functioning nephrons that, in turn, results in decreased renal function.[12] This is usually manifested by an increased incidence of side effects caused by antimicrobials that are eliminated renally. For example, renal toxicity caused by aminoglycosides may be apparent much sooner during therapy than in younger patients.

Pregnancy

During pregnancy, not only is the fetus at risk for drug teratogenicity, but also the pharmacokinetic disposition of certain drugs can be altered.[13] Penicillins, cephalosporins, and aminoglycosides are cleared from the peripheral circulation more rapidly during pregnancy. This is probably a result of marked increases in intravascular volume, glomerular filtration rate, and hepatic and metabolic activities. The net result is that maternal serum antimicrobial concentrations can be as much as 50% lower during this period than in the nonpregnant state. Increased dosages of certain compounds might be necessary to achieve therapeutic levels during late pregnancy.

Metabolic Abnormalities

Inherited or acquired metabolic abnormalities will influence the therapy of infectious diseases in a variety of ways. For example, patients with impaired peripheral vascular flow may not absorb drugs given by intramuscular injection. In addition, certain metabolic states can predispose patients to enhanced drug toxicity. For instance, patients who are phenotypically slow acetylators of isoniazid are at greater risk for peripheral neuropathy.[14] Patients with severe deficiency of glucose-6-phosphate dehydrogenase can develop significant hemolysis when exposed to such drugs as sulfonamides, nitrofurantoin, nalidixic acid, antimalarials, and dapsone. Although mild deficiencies are found in African Americans, the more severe forms of the disease generally are confined to persons of eastern Mediterranean origin.

Organ Dysfunction

❹ Patients with diminished renal or hepatic function or both will accumulate certain drugs unless the dosage is adjusted.[15,16] Recommendations for dosing antibiotics in patients with liver dysfunction are not as formalized as guidelines for patients with renal dysfunction. Antibiotics that should be adjusted in severe liver disease include clindamycin, erythromycin, metronidazole, and rifampin. Significant accumulation can occur when both liver dysfunction and renal dysfunction are present for the following drugs: cefotaxime, nafcillin, piperacillin, and sulfamethoxazole.

Concomitant Drugs

❺ Any concomitant therapy that the patient is receiving can influence the drug selection, dose, and monitoring. For instance, administration of isoniazid to a patient who is also receiving phenytoin can result in phenytoin toxicity secondary to inhibition of phenytoin metabolism by isoniazid. Furthermore, drugs that possess similar adverse-effect profiles can increase the risk for effects, (i.e., two drugs that cause nephrotoxicity or neutropenia). A detailed review of drug interactions is beyond the scope of this chapter, but an excellent textbook on this subject is available.[17] Lists of potentially severe drug-drug interactions are provided in Table 114–2.

Concomitant Disease States

Concomitant disease states can influence the selection of therapy. Certain diseases will predispose patients to a particular infectious disease or will alter the type of infecting organism. For example, patients with diabetes mellitus and the resulting peripheral vascular disease often develop infections of the lower extremity soft tissue. Moreover, the alterations in peripheral blood flow associated with the disease and perhaps altered immunity make such infections more difficult to treat than in nondiabetics. Patients with chronic lung disease or cystic fibrosis develop frequent pulmonary infections that can be caused by somewhat different microorganisms than are found in otherwise normal hosts.

Patients with immunosuppressive diseases, such as malignancies or acquired immunologic deficiencies, are highly predisposed to infections, and the types of causative or pathogenic organisms can be vastly different from what would be expected (see Chap. 131). For instance, patients undergoing chemotherapy for acute forms of leukemia often are profoundly granulocytopenic and are predisposed to infections caused by bacteria and fungi.[18] Patients with the acquired immunodeficiency syndrome (AIDS) often become infected with an enormous variety of organisms (see Chap. 134).

Many factors predisposing to infection are related to disruption of the host's integumentary barriers. For example, trauma, burns, and iatrogenic wounds induced in surgery can lead to a substantial risk of infection depending on the severity and location of the injury or disruption. For a complete discussion of the various risks involved in surgical procedures, see Chapter 132.

DRUG FACTORS

Pharmacokinetic and Pharmacodynamic Considerations

Integration of both pharmacokinetic and pharmacodynamic properties of an agent is important when choosing antimicrobial therapy to ensure efficacy and to prevent resistance.[19] Early researchers relied solely on pharmacokinetic properties such as the area under the (drug concentration) curve (AUC), maximum observed concentration (peak), and drug half-life to optimize therapy. Pharmacodynamics is the study of the relationship between drug concentration and the effects on the microorganism. There is an important relationship between both pharmacokinetic and microbiologic parameters that has resulted in measurements such as AUC:minimal inhibitory concentration (MIC) ratio, peak: MIC ratio, and time (T) the concentration is above MIC ($T > \text{MIC}$).[19-23]

Aminoglycosides exhibit concentration-dependent bactericidal effects. An example of the integration of pharmacokinetics and microbiological activity is the use of high-dose, once-daily aminoglycosides. For these regimens, the drug is given as a single large daily dose to maximize the peak:MIC ratio. Aminoglycosides also

TABLE 114-2 Major Drug Interactions with Antimicrobials

Antimicrobial	Other Agent(s)	Mechanism of Action/Effect	Clinical Management
Aminoglycosides	Neuromuscular blocking agents	Additive adverse effects	Avoid
	Nephrotoxins (N) or ototoxins (O) (e.g., amphotericin B (N) cisplatin (N/O), cyclosporine (N), furosemide (O), NSAIDs (N), radio contrast (N), vancomycin (N)	Additive adverse effects	Monitor aminoglycoside SDC and renal function
Amphotericin B	Nephrotoxins (e.g., aminoglycosides, cidofovir, cyclosporine, foscarnet, pentamidine)	Additive adverse effects	Monitor renal function
Azoles	See Chap. 130		
Chloramphenicol	Phenytoin, tolbutamide, ethanol	Decreased metabolism of other agents	Monitor phenytoin SDC, blood glucose
Foscarnet	Pentamidine IV	Increased risk of severe nephrotoxicity/hypocalcemia	Monitor renal function/serum calcium
Isoniazid	Carbamazepine, phenytoin	Decreased metabolism of other agents (nausea, vomiting, nystagmus, ataxia)	Monitor drug SDC
Macrolides/azalides	Digoxin	Decreased digoxin bioavailability and metabolism	Monitor digoxin SDC; avoid if possible
	Theophylline	Decreased metabolism of theophylline	Monitor theophylline SDC
Metronidazole	Ethanol (drugs containing ethanol)	Disulfiram-like reaction	Avoid
Penicillins and cephalosporins	Probenecid, aspirin	Blocked excretion of β-lactams	Use if prolonged high concentration of β-lactam desirable
Ciprofloxacin/norfloxacin	Theophylline	Decreased metabolism of theophylline	Monitor theophylline
Quinolones	Classes Ia and III Antiarrhythmics	Increased Q-T interval	Avoid
	Multivalent cations (antacids, iron, sucralfate, zinc, vitamins, dairy, citric acid) didanosine	Decreased absorption of quinolone	Separate by 2 hours
Rifampin	Azoles, cyclosporine, methadone propranolol, PIs, oral contraceptives, tacrolimus, warfarin	Increased metabolism of other agent	Avoid if possible
Sulfonamides	Sulfonylureas, phenytoin, warfarin	Decreased metabolism of other agent	Monitor blood glucose, SDC, PT
Tetracyclines	Antacids, iron, calcium, sucralfate	Decreased absorption of tetracycline	Separate by 2 hours
	Digoxin	Decreased digoxin bioavailability and metabolism	Monitor digoxin SDC; avoid if possible

PI, protease inhibitor; PT, prothrombin time; SDC, serum drug concentrations.

Azalides: azithromycin; azoles: fluconazole, itraconazole, ketoconazole, and voriconazole; macrolides: erythromycin, clarithromycin; protease inhibitors: amprenavir, indinavir, lopinavir/ritonavir, nelfinavir, ritonavir, and saquinavir; quinolones: ciprofloxacin, gemifloxacin, levofloxacin, moxifloxacin.

possess a postantibiotic effect (persistent suppression of organism growth after concentrations decrease below the MIC) that appears to contribute to the success of high-dose, once-daily administration. Fluoroquinolones exhibit concentration-dependent killing activity, but optimal killing appears to be characterized by the AUC:MIC ratio.

β-Lactams display time-dependent bactericidal effects. Killing activity is enhanced only marginally if drug concentration exceeds the MIC. Therefore, the important pharmacodynamic relationship for these antimicrobials is the duration that drug concentrations exceed the MIC ($T > MIC$). Effective dosing regimens require serum drug concentrations to exceed the MIC for at least 40% to 50% of the dosing interval. Frequent small doses, continuous infusion, or prolonged infusion of β-lactams appears to be correlated with positive outcomes.

A detailed discussion on antimicrobial pharmacokinetics-pharmacodynamics is beyond the scope of this chapter. However, excellent sources of information on this topic are available.[19–23]

Tissue Penetration

The importance of tissue penetration varies with site of infection. Some of the difficulties in interpreting data include a lack of correlation with clinical outcomes and poor understanding of whether the antimicrobial agents are present in a biologically active form. An example of the former problem is the recognized efficacy of drugs with low biliary fluid concentrations in the treatment of cholecystitis, cholangitis, or both and the absence of the enhanced efficacy of drugs whose primary route of elimination is biliary excretion of active drug. An example of the latter difficulty is with penetration to deep infections, such as abscesses, where various factors such as acid pH, WBC products, and various enzymes can inactivate even high concentrations of certain drugs.

The central nervous system (CNS) is one body site where antimicrobial penetration is relatively well defined, and correlations with clinical outcomes are established.[6,24] Cerebrospinal fluid (CSF) concentrations of antimicrobial agents necessary to cure bacterial meningitis have been defined, and drugs that do not reach significant concentrations in the CSF should either be avoided or instilled directly, if feasible.

Caution must be exercised when selecting an antimicrobial agent for clinical use on the basis of tissue or fluid penetration. Body fluids where drug concentration data are clinically relevant include CSF, urine, synovial fluid, and peritoneal fluid. Apart from these areas, more attention should be paid to clinical efficacy, antimicrobial spectrum, toxicity, and cost than to comparative data on penetration into a given body site.

The proper route of administration for an antimicrobial depends on the site of infection. Parenteral therapy is warranted when patients are being treated for febrile neutropenia or deep-seated infections such as meningitis, endocarditis, and osteomyelitis. Severe pneumonia often is treated initially with intravenous antibiotics and switched to oral therapy as clinical improvement is evident.[5,25] Patients treated in the ambulatory setting for upper respiratory tract infections (e.g., pharyngitis, bronchitis, sinusitis, and otitis media), lower respiratory tract infections, skin and soft tissue infections, uncomplicated urinary tract infections, and selected sexually transmitted diseases can usually receive oral therapy.

Drug Toxicity

It is incumbent on health professionals to avoid toxic drugs whenever possible. Antibiotics associated with CNS toxicities, usually when not dose-adjusted for renal function, include penicillins, cephalosporins, quinolones, and imipenem. Hematologic toxicities generally are manifested with prolonged use of nafcillin (neutropenia), piperacillin (platelet dysfunction), cefotetan (hypoprothrombinemia), chloramphenicol (bone marrow suppression, both idiosyncratic and dose-related toxicity), and trimethoprim (megaloblastic anemia). Reversible nephrotoxicity classically is associated with aminoglycosides and vancomycin. Reversible ototoxicity can occur with aminoglycosides or erythromycin. In the outpatient setting, patients must be counseled regarding photosensitivity with azithromycin, quinolones, tetracyclines, pyrazinamide, sulfamethoxazole, and trimethoprim. Lastly, all antibiotics have been implicated in causing diarrhea and colitis secondary to *Clostridium difficile*[26] (see Chap. 122).

Aside from consideration of drug toxicity, some antimicrobial use requires more intensive risk-benefit analysis. An example of this is the decision to use isoniazid prophylactically to prevent tuberculosis. Because the hepatotoxicity of isoniazid increases in frequency with age, older persons (>45 years of age) who are candidates for isoniazid prophylaxis (positive skin test) must have additional risk factors for tuberculosis to balance the potential toxic effects. These include evidence of recent skin-test conversion, immunosuppression, or previous gastrectomy. Older patients without additional risk factors are more likely to suffer toxicity from isoniazid than derive benefit from its use.[27]

Cost

The costs of drug therapy are increasing dramatically, especially as new products, derived from biotechnology, are introduced. Greater attention is being paid to the pharmacoeconomics of drug therapy, where patient outcomes are valued, and the costs to arrive at those outcomes are estimated. Understanding the true cost of antimicrobial therapy is more important than ever. The total cost of antimicrobial therapy includes much more than just the acquisition cost of the drugs.[28]

Many ancillary costs and factors affect the true cost of therapy. These include factors such as storage, preparation, distribution, and administration, as well as all the costs incurred from monitoring for adverse effects and factors such as length of hospitalization, readmissions, and all directly provided healthcare goods and services. More difficult to value but equally as important are indirect costs such as patient quality-of-life issues. Pharmacoeconomic and outcomes analyses are becoming more widely applied and used in order to derive values such as cost-benefit ratios and the cost-effectiveness of various products as compared with other products. A great deal more research in this area is needed, and multidisciplinary, collaborative efforts with the involvement of pharmacy, medicine, nursing, and microbiology are essential.

Many oral antimicrobials have been approved, including cephalosporins, linezolid, and fluoroquinolones, which can be used in place of more expensive parenteral therapy. These agents offer extended-spectrum killing activity, increased tissue penetration, and excellent safety and pharmacokinetic profiles. When oral therapy is being considered, the choice between convenient once-a-day expensive agents versus multiple-dose inexpensive agents arises. It is easy to calculate the difference in acquisition cost; however, the overall cost between agents is more difficult to determine. Factors to weigh include safety, effectiveness, tolerability, patient compliance, and potential drug–drug interactions. In some instances, more expensive agents can be warranted to avoid adverse outcomes.

COMBINATION ANTIMICROBIAL THERAPY

❻ In selecting a drug regimen for a given patient, consideration must be given to the necessity of using more than one drug. Combinations of antimicrobials generally are used to broaden the spectrum of coverage for empirical therapy, achieve synergistic activity against the infecting organism, and prevent the emergence of resistance.

Broadening the Spectrum of Coverage

Increasing the coverage of antimicrobial therapy generally is necessary in mixed infections where multiple organisms are likely to be present. This is the case in intraabdominal and female pelvic infections, in which a variety of aerobic and anaerobic bacteria can produce disease.[29] Traditionally, a combination of a drug active against aerobic gram-negative bacilli, such as an aminoglycoside, and a drug active against anaerobic bacteria, such as metronidazole or clindamycin, is selected. Newer compounds, which possess good activity against both of these types of organisms, such as the β-lactam/β-lactamase inhibitor combinations, carbapenems or glycylcyclines, might be adequate to replace the combination and thereby reduce the cost of therapy. The other clinical situation in which an increased spectrum of activity is desirable is with nosocomial infections.[25]

Synergism

The achievement of synergistic antimicrobial activity is advantageous for infections caused by enteric gram-negative bacilli in immunosuppressed patients. Laboratory tests to identify synergy between antibiotic combinations are described in Chapter 113. Traditionally, combinations of aminoglycosides and β-lactams have been used because these drugs together generally act synergistically against a wide variety of bacteria. However, the data supporting superior efficacy of synergistic over nonsynergistic combinations are weak. At best, it would appear that synergistic combinations produce better results in certain infections caused by *P aeruginosa* and *Enterococcus* species.[30-32]

The most obvious example of the use of synergy is the treatment of enterococcal endocarditis. The causative organism is usually only inhibited by penicillins, but it is killed rapidly by the addition of streptomycin or gentamicin to a penicillin.[7] The need for bactericidal activity in the treatment of endocarditis underscores the need for these synergistic combinations.

Preventing Resistance

The use of combinations to prevent the emergence of resistance is applied widely but not often realized. The only circumstance where this has been clearly effective is in the treatment of tuberculosis. The prevalence of resistance to a first-line drug such as isoniazid or rifampin in a population of organisms may be as high as 1 in 10^6 to 10^8. Because the bacterial load in a patient with active tuberculosis often exceeds this, two drugs are given to reduce the likelihood of encountering resistance to less than 1 in 10^{13}.[27] There is ample evidence from in vitro data and experimental bacterial infections that combinations of drugs with different mechanisms are effective in the prevention of the emergence of resistance. Data from clinical trials, however, are either conflicting or do not convincingly support this concept.[32]

Disadvantages of Combination Therapy

Although there are potentially beneficial effects from combining drugs, there also are potential disadvantages, including increased cost, greater risk of drug toxicity such as nephrotoxicity with aminoglycosides, amphotericin, and possibly vancomycin, and superinfection with even more resistant bacteria.[30-32]

The combination of two or more antibiotics can result in antagonistic effects. Clinically, the effect of antagonism may be evident when one drug induces β-lactamase production and another drug is β-lactamase unstable. Cefoxitin and imipenem are examples of drugs capable of inducing β-lactamases and may result in more rapid inactivation of penicillins when used together.

MONITORING THERAPEUTIC RESPONSE

❼ After antimicrobial therapy has been instituted, the patient must be monitored carefully for a therapeutic response. Culture and sensitivity reports from specimens sent to the microbiology laboratory must be reviewed and the therapy changed accordingly. Use of agents with the narrowest spectrum of activity against identified pathogens is recommended. If anaerobes are suspected, even if they are not identified, anaerobic therapy should be continued.

Patient monitoring should include many of the same parameters used to diagnose the infection. The WBC count and temperature should start to normalize. Physical complaints from the patient also should diminish (i.e., decreased pain, shortness of breath, cough, or sputum production). Appetite should improve. However, radiologic improvement can lag behind clinical improvement.

Determinations of serum (or other fluid) levels of antimicrobials can be useful in ensuring outcome, preventing toxicity, or both. There are only a few antimicrobials that require serum concentration monitoring and then only in selected situations. These include the aminoglycosides, flucytosine, and chloramphenicol. Achievement of adequate aminoglycoside concentrations within the first few days of therapy of gram-negative infection has been correlated with better therapeutic outcome.[33]

Changes in the volume of distribution can have a significant impact on the efficacy, safety, or both of therapy. An unexpectedly low volume of distribution (such as in the dehydrated patient) will result in higher, potentially toxic drug concentrations, whereas a larger-than-expected volume of distribution (such as in patients with edema or ascites) will result in low, potentially subtherapeutic concentrations. The most effective methods use measured serum concentrations of the drugs rather than estimations from renal function tests to assess true drug clearance from the body.

❽ As patients improve clinically, the route of administration should be reevaluated. Streamlining therapy from parenteral to oral (switch therapy) has become an accepted practice for many infections.[5] Criteria that should be present to justify a switch to oral therapy include (1) overall clinical improvement, (2) lack of fever for 8 to 24 hours, (3) decreased WBC count, and (4) a functioning gastrointestinal tract. Drugs that exhibit excellent oral bioavailability when compared with intravenous formulations include ciprofloxacin, clindamycin, doxycycline, levofloxacin, metronidazole, moxifloxacin, linezolid, and trimethoprim-sulfamethoxazole.

FAILURE OF ANTIMICROBIAL THERAPY

❾ A variety of factors may be responsible for an apparent lack of response to therapy. Patients who fail to respond over 2 to 3 days require a thorough reevaluation. It is possible that the disease is not infectious or is nonbacterial in origin, or there is an undetected pathogen in a polymicrobial infection. Other factors include those directly related to drug selection, the host, or the pathogen. Laboratory error in identification, susceptibility testing, or both (presence of inoculum effect or resistant subpopulations) is a rare cause of antimicrobial failure.

Failures Caused by Drug Selection

Factors related directly to the drug selection include an inappropriate drug selection, dosage, or route of administration. Malabsorption of a drug product because of gastrointestinal disease, such as a short-bowel syndrome, or a drug interaction, such as complexation of fluoroquinolones with multivalent cations resulting in reduced absorption, can lead to potentially subtherapeutic serum concentrations. Accelerated drug elimination is also possible. This can occur in patients with cystic fibrosis or during pregnancy, when more rapid clearance or larger volumes of distribution can result in low serum concentrations, particularly for aminoglycosides. A common cause of failure of therapy is poor penetration into the site of infection. This is especially true for sites such as the CNS, eye, and prostate gland. Drug failure also can result from drugs that are highly protein bound or that are chemically inactivated at the site of infection.

Failures Caused by Host Factors

Host defenses must be considered when evaluating a patient who is not responding to antimicrobial therapy. Patients who are immunosuppressed (e.g., granulocytopenia from chemotherapy or AIDS) may respond poorly to therapy because their defenses are inadequate to eradicate the infection despite seemingly adequate drug regimens. A good example is the poor response of infection in granulocytopenic patients that is seen when their WBC counts remain low during therapy. This contrasts with a much better response when granulocyte counts increase during therapy.

Other host factors are related to the need for surgical drainage of abscesses or removal of foreign bodies, necrotic tissue, or both. If these situations are not corrected, they result in persistent infection and, occasionally, bacteremia despite adequate antimicrobial therapy.

Failures Caused by Microorganisms

There are two types of resistance, intrinsic and acquired resistance. Intrinsic resistance is when the antimicrobial agent never had activity against the bacterial species. For example, gram-negative bacteria are naturally resistant to vancomycin because the drug cannot penetrate the outer membrane of gram-negative bacteria. Acquired resistance is when the antimicrobial agent was originally active against the bacterial species but the genetic makeup of the bacteria has changed so the drug can no longer be effective.[34]

The strategies used by bacteria to develop acquired resistance are primarily classified into four general mechanisms of resistance: (1) alteration in the target site, (2) change in membrane permeability, (3) efflux pump, and (4) drug inactivation. Bacteria can use one or more of these mechanisms against a specific antibiotic class. Furthermore, a single mechanism of resistance can result in resistance to multiple related or unrelated classes of antibiotics.

Drug inactivation either through β-lactamases or aminoglycoside modifying enzymes is the predominant mechanism of resistance. For example, β-lactamases can either be plasmid or chromosomally mediated. In addition, the expression of β-lactamases can be induced or constitutive. There are now multiple types and classes of β-lactamases identified which is beyond the scope of this chapter. However, there are several outstanding papers discussing all of the different types of β-lactamases.[35-37]

The increase in resistance among bacteria is believed to be a result of continued overuse of antimicrobials in the community, as well as in hospitals, and the increasing prevalence of immunosuppressed patients receiving long-term suppressive antimicrobials for the prevention of infections. These resistance patterns are regionally variable, and susceptibility patterns in the community (or hospital) should be monitored closely to promote rational antimicrobial selection.[34]

Enterococci have been isolated with multiple resistance patterns. They may be resistant to β-lactams (by virtue of β-lactamase production, altered penicillin-binding proteins [PBPs], or both), vancomycin (via alterations in peptidoglycan synthesis), and high levels of aminoglycosides (via enzymatic degradation). Pneumococci resistant to penicillins, certain cephalosporins, and macrolides are increasingly common. These organisms generally are susceptible to vancomycin, the new fluoroquinolones, and cefotaxime or ceftriaxone. However, antimicrobial agents such as linezolid, daptomycin, telavancin, and tigecycline have been targeted at resistant gram-positive bacteria.

Treatment of an infection caused by *Enterobacter, Citrobacter, Serratia,* or *P aeruginosa* with a third-generation cephalosporin or aztreonam may produce an initial clinical response by eradicating all the susceptible bacteria in the population. Within a few days, however, the highly resistant subpopulations have a selective advantage and can overgrow the infection site to produce a relapse.[37] These bacteria usually retain susceptibility to aminoglycosides, carbapenems, and fluoroquinolones but are resistant to all other β-lactams. Host defenses are extremely important in this scenario. Debilitated patients with pulmonary infections, abscesses, or osteomyelitis are at high risk for drug failure. In these situations, a combination regimen to prevent the emergence of resistance or the use of carbapenem or a fluoroquinolone may be warranted for empirical therapy.

ANTIMICROBIAL USE MANAGEMENT

ANTIBIOTIC FORMULARY

Institutions must decide which antibiotics to include on their formularies. The actual decision to have a formulary remains controversial; however, restricting choices does encourage familiarity with a core of antibiotics for residents and attending physicians. Open formularies allow the empirical use of any commercially available antibiotics, with recommended guidelines for changes when culture and sensitivity results are finalized. Many institutions have developed an antibiotic stewardship team.[38,39] The team is generally a multidisciplinary group including representation from microbiology, infection control, administration, information technology, pharmacy including an infectious disease trained clinical pharmacists, and physicians from several disciplines, including infectious disease. The actual implementation of the guidelines and restrictions recommended by such groups requires the cooperation of the entire medical staff. Education is vital to the success of the antibiotic formulary.[38,39]

ANTIMICROBIAL CYCLING

An interesting topic in formulary management that gained interest and scientific research is *antimicrobial cycling*. Antimicrobial cycling is a predetermined change in an antimicrobial recommendation for empirical therapy of a specific infection at a predetermined time. It also has been called *rotation of antimicrobials*. This strategy should not be confused with *antimicrobial switch therapy*, which involves changes in the route of administration of antimicrobial therapy (i.e., intravenous to oral).

Antimicrobial cycling is employed as a mechanism to reduce or prevent antimicrobial resistance. *Proactive cycling* is a planned switch to preempt resistance at a predetermined point or series of points with a predetermined schedule. *Reactive cycling* is a response to high or unacceptable resistance and is often a one-time switch. Most programs incorporate aspects of both types of cycling. Cycling implies returning to the original drug after other choices have been used. Rotation implies several planned changes.

Antimicrobial cycling is based on the assumptions that the resistance problem is (1) caused by the overuse of a particular agent or class of agents and (2) that discontinuation of the particular agent

or class of agents will restore susceptibility. These assumptions correlate best with nosocomial gram-negative organisms that can rapidly develop resistance. Theoretically, antimicrobial agents should be sequenced in such an order that mechanisms of resistance do not overlap (i.e., changing drug classes).[39,40] However, data have provided insufficient evidence to clearly demonstrate the usefulness of antibiotic cycling.

KEEPING CURRENT

Attention must be paid to the literature on antimicrobials to assist in the selection of therapy. The results from prospective, controlled, randomized clinical trials should be evaluated whenever possible when considering appropriate antimicrobial therapy. Results from prelicensing open trials offer only limited information that can be useful in this regard because patients in these trials generally are not seriously ill and are not infected with multiple resistant bacteria. Other confounding factors found in most clinical situations are excluded by virtue of the study design. Therefore, comparative data in more seriously ill patients are essential for the appropriate application of new agents.

Postmarketing trials are also important because results can demonstrate superiority of one regimen over another, either in efficacy, safety, or cost-effectiveness. Appropriate antimicrobial therapy can change as new organisms are discovered, susceptibility patterns change, new drugs become available, and new clinical trial results are published. Classical thinking in the treatment of infectious diseases will continue to change and evolve to maintain antimicrobial efficacy. Optimal use of modern antimicrobials is just beginning to be defined.

ABBREVIATIONS

AUC: area under the curve

IL: interleukin

MIC: minimal inhibitory concentration

PBP: penicillin-binding protein

PMN: polymorphonuclear leukocytes

WBC: white blood cell

REFERENCES

1. Hessen MT, Kaye D. Principles of selection and use of antibacterial agents: In vitro activity and pharmacology. Infect Dis Clin North Am 2004;18:435–450.
2. Slama TG, Amin A, Brunton SA, et al. A clinician's guide to the appropriate and accurate use of antibiotics: The Council for Appropriate and Rational Antibiotic Therapy (CARAT) criteria. Am J Med 2005;118(7A):1S–6S.
3. Mackowiak PA, Durach DT. Fever of unknown origin. In: Mandell GL, Bennett JE, Dolin R, eds. Mandell, Douglas and Bennett's Principles and Practice of Infectious Diseases, 6th ed. New York: Churchill Livingstone, 2005:718–729.
4. Cunha BA. Antibiotic selection in the penicillin-allergic patient. Med Clin North Am 2006;90:1257–1264.
5. Mandell LA, Wunderink RG, Anzueto A, et al. Infectious Diseases Society of America/American Thoracic Society Consensus Guidelines on the management of community-acquired pneumonia in adults. Clin Infect Dis 2007;44:S27–S72.
6. Tunkel AR, Hartman BJ, Kaplan SL, et al. Practice guidelines for the management of bacterial meningitis. Clin Infect Dis 2004;39:1267–1284.
7. Baddour LM, Wilson WR, Bayer AS, et al. Infective Endocarditis. Diagnosis, Antimicrobial Therapy, and Management of Complications: A Statement for Healthcare Professionals from the Committee on

Rheumatic Fever, Endocarditis, and Kawasaki Disease, Council on Cardiovascular Disease in the Young, and the Councils on Clinical Cardiology, Stroke, and Cardiovascular Surgery and Anesthesia, American Heart Association. Circulation 2005;111:e394–e434.

8. Thomson RB Jr, Miller JM. Specimen collection, transport, and processing: Bacteriology. In: Murray PR, Baroon EJ, Jorgensen JH, et al. eds. Manual of Clinical Microbiology, 8th ed. Washington, DC: ASM Press, 2003:286–330.

9. Park MA, Li JTC. Diagnosis and management of penicillin allergy. Mayo Clin Proc 2005;80:405–410.

10. Gruchalla RS, Pirmohamed M. Antibioitic allcrgy. N Engl J Med 2006;354:601–609.

11. Bowlware KL, Stull T. Antibacterial agents in pediatrics. Infect Dis Clin North Am 2004;18:513–531.

12. Stalam M, Kaye D. Antibiotic agents in the elderly. Infect Dis Clin North Am 2004;18:533–549.

13. Anderson GD. Pregnancy-induced changes in pharmacokinetics. Clin Pharmacokinetic 2005;44:989–1008.

14. Weinshilboum R. Inheritance and drug response. N Engl J Med 2003;348:529–537.

15. Livornese LL, Slavin D, Benz RL, et al. Use of antibacterial agents in renal failure. Infect Dis Clin North Am 2004;18:551–579.

16. Tschida SJ, Vance-Bryan K, Zaske DE. Anti-infective agents in hepatic disease. Med Clin North Am 1995;79:895–917.

17. Piscitelli SC, Rodvold KA. Drug Interactions in Infectious Diseases, 2nd ed. Totowa, NJ: Humana Press, 2005.

18. Hughes WT, Armstrong D, Bodey GP, et al. 2002 Guidelines for the use of antimicrobial agents in neutropenic patients with cancer. Clin Infect Dis 2002;34:730–751.

19. Drusano GL. Pharmacokinetics and pharmacodynamics of antimicrobials. Clin Infect Dis 2007;45:s89–s95.

20. Ambrose PG, Bhavnani SM, Rubino CM, et al. Pharmacokinetics-pharmacodynamics of antimicrobial therapy: it's not just for mice anymore. Clin Infect Dis 2007;44:79–86.

21. Nightingale Ch, Ambrose PG, Drusano GL, et al. Antimicrobial Pharmacodynamics in Theory and Clinical Practice, 2nd ed. New York: Marcel Dekker, 2007.

22. DeRyke CA, Lee SY, Kuti JL, et al. Optimising dosing strategies of antibacterials utilizing pharmacodynamic principles. Drugs 2006;66:1–14.

23. Lodise TP, Lomaestro, Drusano GL. Applications of antimicrobial pharmacodynamic concepts into clinical practice: focus on β-lactam antibiotics. Pharmacotherapy 2006;26:1320–1332.

24. Sinner SW, Tunkel AR. Antimicrobial agents in the treatment of bacterial meningitis. Infect Dis Clin North Am 2004;18:581–602.

25. American Thoracic Society (ATS), Infectious Diseases Society of America (IDSA). Official ATS and IDSA statement: Guidelines for the management of adults with hospital-acquired, ventilator-associated, and healthcare-associated pneumonia Am J Respir Crit Care Med 2005;171:388–416.

26. Starr J. *Clostridium difficile* associated diarrhoea: Diagnosis and treatment. BMJ 2005;331:498–501.

27. Recommendations from the American Thoracic Society, Centers for Disease Control and Prevention, and Infectious Diseases Society of America. Controlling tuberculosis in the United States. MMWR Recomm Rep 2005;54(RR-12):1–81.

28. Goldman MP, Nair R. Antibacterial treatment strategies in hospitalized patients: What role for pharmacoeconomics? Cleve Clin J Med 2007;74;s38–s47.

29. Solomkin JS, Mazuski JE, Bradley JS, et al. Diagnosis and management of complicated intra-abdominal infection in adults and children: Guidelines by the Surgical Infection Society and the Infectious Diseases Society of America. Clin Infect Dis 2010;50:133–164.

30. Paul M, Leibovici L. Combination antimicrobial treatment versus monotherapy: the contribution of meta-analyses. Infect Dis Clin N Am 2009;23:277–293.

31. Bliziotis IA, Samonis G, Vardakas KZ, et al. Effect of aminoglycoside and β-lactam combination therapy versus β-lactam monotherapy on the emergence of antimicrobial resistance: A meta-analysis of randomized, controlled trials. Antimicrob Agents Chemother 2005;41:149–158.

32. Safdar N, Handelsman J, Maki DG. Does combination antimicrobial therapy reduce mortality in gram-negative bacteraemia? A meta-analysis. Lancet Infect Dis 2004;4:519–527.

33. Turnidge J. Pharmacodynamics and dosing of aminoglycosides. Infect Dis Clin N Am 2003;17:503–528.

34. Kaye KS, Engemann JJ, Fraimiw HS, et al. Pathogens resistant to antimicrobial agents: epidemiology, molecular mechanisms, and clinical management. Infect Dis Clin North Am 2004;18:467–511.

35. Queenan AM, Bush K. Carbapenemases: the versatile β-lactamases. Clin Microbiol Rev 2007;20:440–458.

36. Paterson DL, Bonomo RA. Extended-spectrum β-lactamases: a clinical update. Clin Microbiol Rev 2005;18:657–686.

37. Jacoby GA. AmpC β-lactamases. Clin Microbiol Rev 2009;22:161–182.

38. MacDougall C, Polk RE. Antimicrobial stewardship programs in health care systems. Clin Microbiol Rev 2005;18:638–656.

39. Dellit TH, Owens RC, McGowan JE, et al. Infectious Diseases Society of America and the Society for Healthcare Epidemiology of America guidelines for developing an institutional program to enhance antimicrobial stewardship. Clin Infect Dis 2007;44:159–177.

40. Brown EM, Nathwani D. Antibiotic cycling or rotation: a systematic review of the evidence of efficacy. J Antimicrob Chemother 2005;55:6–9.

Appendix 114-1
Drugs of Choice, First Choice, *Alternative(s)*

GRAM-POSITIVE COCCI

Enterococcus faecalis (generally not as resistant to antibiotics as *Enterococcus faecium*)

- Serious infection (endocarditis, meningitis, pyelonephritis with bacteremia)
  - Ampicillin (or penicillin G) + (gentamicin or streptomycin)
  - *Vancomycin + (gentamicin or streptomycin), daptomycin, linezolid, telavancin, tigecycline[a]*
- Urinary tract infection (UTI)
  - Ampicillin, amoxicillin
  - *Fosfomycin or nitrofurantoin*

E faecium (generally more resistant to antibiotics than *E faecalis*)

- Recommend consultation with infectious disease specialist
  - *Linezolid, quinupristin/dalfopristin, daptomycin, tigecycline[a]*

Staphylococcus aureus/Staphylococcus epidermidis

- Methicillin (oxacillin)-sensitive
  - Nafcillin or oxacillin
  - *FGC,[b,c] trimethoprim-sulfamethoxazole, clindamycin, BL/BLI[j]*
- Hospital-acquired methicillin (oxacillin)–resistant
  - Vancomycin ± (gentamicin or rifampin)
  - *Daptomycin, linezolid, telavancin, tigecycline,[a] trimethoprim-sulfamethoxazole, or quinupristin-dalfopristin*
- Community-acquired methicillin (oxacillin)-resistant
  - Clindamycin, trimethoprim-sulfamethoxazole, doxycylcine[a]
  - *Daptomycin, linezolid, telavancin, tigecycline,[a] or vancomycin*

Streptococcus (groups A, B, C, G, and *Streptococcus bovis*)

- Penicillin G or V or ampicillin
- *FGC,[b,c] erythromycin, azithromycin, clarithromycin*

Streptococcus pneumoniae

- Penicillin-sensitive (MIC <0.1 mcg/mL)
  - Penicillin G or V or ampicillin
  - *FGC,[b,c] doxycycline,[a] azithromycin, clarithromycin, erythromycin*
- Penicillin intermediate (MIC 0.1–1.0 mcg/mL)
  - High-dose penicillin (12 million units/day for adults) or ceftriaxone[c] or cefotaxime[c]
  - *Levofloxacin,[a] moxifloxacin,[a] gemifloxacin,[a] or vancomycin*
- Penicillin-resistant (MIC ≥1.0 mcg/mL)
  - Recommend consultation with infectious disease specialist.
    - *Vancomycin ± rifampin*
    - *Per sensitivities: cefotaxime,[c] ceftriaxone,[c] levofloxacin,[a] moxifloxacin,[a] or gemifloxacin[a]*

Streptococcus, viridans group

- Penicillin G ± gentamicin[d]
- *Cefotaxime,[c] ceftriaxone,[c] erythromycin, azithromycin, clarithromycin, or vancomycin ± gentamicin*

GRAM-NEGATIVE COCCI

Moraxella (Branhamella) catarrhalis

- Amoxicillin-clavulanate, ampicillin-sulbactam
- *Trimethoprim-sulfamethoxazole, erythromycin, azithromycin, clarithromycin, doxycycline,[a] SGC,[c,e] cefotaxime,[c] ceftriaxone,[c] or TGC PO[c,f]*

Neisseria gonorrhoeae (also give concomitant treatment for *Chlamydia trachomatis*)

- Disseminated gonococcal infection
  - Ceftriaxone[c] or cefotaxime[c]
  - *Oral follow-up: cefpodoxime,[c] ciprofloxacin,[a] or levofloxacin[a]*
- Uncomplicated infection
  - Ceftriaxone,[c] cefotaxime,[c] or cefpodoxime[c]
  - *Ciprofloxacin[a] or levofloxacin[a]*

Neisseria meningitides

- Penicillin G
- *Cefotaxime[c] or ceftriaxone[c]*

GRAM-POSITIVE BACILLI

Clostridium perfringens

- Penicillin G ± clindamycin
- *Metronidazole,[a] clindamycin, doxycycline,[a] cefazolin,[c] carbapenem[g,h]*

Clostridium difficile

- Oral metronidazole[a]
- *Oral vancomycin*

GRAM-NEGATIVE BACILLI

Acinetobacter spp

- Doripenem, imipenem or meropenem ± aminoglycoside[i] (amikacin usually most effective)
- *Ampicillin-sulbactam, colistin,[h] or tigecycline[a]*

Bacteroides fragilis (and others)

- Metronidazole[a]
- *BL/BLI,[j] clindamycin, cefoxitin,[c] cefotetan,[c] or carbapenem[g,h]*

Enterobacter spp

- Carbapenem,[g] or cefepime ± aminoglycoside[i]
- *Ciprofloxacin,[a] levofloxacin,[a] piperacillin-tazobactam, ticarcillin-clavulanate*

Escherichia coli

- Meningitis
  - Cefotaxime,[c] ceftriaxone,[c] meropenem
- Systemic infection
  - Cefotaxime[c] or ceftriaxone[c]
  - *BL/BLI,[j] fluoroquinolone,[a,k] carbapenem[g,h]*
- Urinary tract infection
  - Most oral agents: check sensitivities
  - Ampicillin, amoxicillin-clavulanate, doxycyline,[a] or cephalexin[c]
  - *Aminoglycoside,[i] FGC,[b,c] nitrofurantoin, fluoroquinolone[a,k]*

Gardnerella vaginalis

- Metronidazole[a]
- *Clindamycin*

Haemophilus influenzae

- Meningitis
  - Cefotaxime[c] or ceftriaxone[c]
  - *Meropenem[h]*

- Other infections
  - BL/BLI,[j] or if β-lactamase-negative, ampicillin or amoxicillin
  - *Trimethoprim-sulfamethoxazole, cefuroxime,[c] azithromycin, clarithromycin, or fluoroquinolone[a,k]*

Klebsiella pneumoniae

- BL/BLI,[j] cefotaxime,[c] ceftriaxone,[c] cefepime[c]
- *Carbapenem,[g,h] fluoroquinolone[a,k]*

Legionella spp

- Azithromycin, erythromycin ± rifampin, or fluoroquinolone[a,k]
- *Trimethoprim-sulfamethoxazole, clarithromycin, or doxycycline[a]*

Pasteurella multocida

- Penicillin G, ampicillin, amoxicillin
- *Doxycycline,[a] BL/BLI,[j] trimethoprim-sulfamethoxazole or ceftriaxone[c]*

Proteus mirabilis

- Ampicillin
- *Trimethoprim-sulfamethoxazole*

Proteus (indole-positive) (including *Providencia rettgeri, Morganella morganii,* and *Proteus vulgaris*)

- Cefotaxime,[c] ceftriaxone,[c] or fluoroquinolone[a,k]
- *BL/BLI,[j] aztreonam,[l] aminoglycosides,[i] carbapenem[g,h]*

Providencia stuartii

- Amikacin, cefotaxime,[c] ceftriaxone,[c] fluoroquinolone[a,k]
- *Trimethoprim-sulfamethoxazole, aztreonam,[l] carbapenem[g,h]*

Pseudomonas aeruginosa

- UTI only
  - Aminoglycoside[i]
  - *Ciprofloxacin,[a] levofloxacin[a]*
- Systemic infection
  - Cefepime,[c] ceftazidime,[c] doripenem,[h] imipenem,[h] meropenem,[h] piperacillin-tazobactam, or ticarcillin-clavulanate + aminoglycoside[i]
  - *Aztreonam,[l] ciprofloxacin,[a] levofloxacin,[a] colistin[h]*

Salmonella typhi

- Ciprofloxacin,[a] levofloxacin,[a] ceftriaxone,[c] cefotaxime[c]
- *Trimethoprim-sulfamethoxazole*

Serratia marcescens

- Ceftriaxone,[c] cefotaxime,[c] cefepime,[c] ciprofloxacin,[a] levofloxacin[a]
- *Aztreonam,[l] carbapenem,[g,h] piperacillin-tazobactam, ticarcillin-clavulanate*

Stenotrophomonas (Xanthomonas) maltophilia (generally very resistant to all antimicrobials)

- Trimethoprim-sulfamethoxazole
- *Check sensitivities to ceftazidime,[c] doxycycline,[a] minocycline,[a] and ticarcillin-clavulanate*

MISCELLANEOUS MICROORGANISMS

Chlamydia pneumoniae

- Doxycycline[a]
- *Azithromycin, clarithromycin, erythromycin, or fluoroquinolone[a,k]*

Chlamydia trachomatis

- Azithromycin or doxycycline[a]
- *Levofloxacin,[a] erythomycin*

Mycoplasma pneumoniae

- Azithromycin, clarithromycin, erythromycin, fluoroquinolone[a,k]
- *Doxycycline[a]*

SPIROCHETES

Treponema pallidum

- Neurosyphilis
  - Penicillin G
  - *Ceftriaxone[c]*
- Primary or secondary
  - Benzathine penicillin G
  - *Ceftriaxone[c] or doxycycline[a]*

Borrelia burgdorferi (choice depends on stage of disease)

- Ceftriaxone[c] or cefuroxime axetil,[c] doxycycline,[a] amoxicillin
- *High-dose penicillin, cefotaxime[c]*

MIC, minimal inhibitory concentration; PO, orally

[a]Not for use in pregnant patients or children.

[b]First-generation cephalosporins—IV: cefazolin; PO: cephalexin, cephradine, or cefadroxil.

[c]Some penicillin-allergic patients may react to cephalosporins.

[d]Gentamicin should be added if tolerance or moderately susceptible (MIC >0.1 g/mL) organisms are encountered; streptomycin is used but can be more toxic.

[e]Second-generation cephalosporins—IV: cefuroxime; PO: cefaclor, cefditoren, cefprozil, cefuroxime axetil, and loracarbef.

[f]Third-generation cephalosporins—PO: cefdinir, cefixime, cefetamet, cefpodoxime proxetil, and ceftibuten.

[g]Carbapenem: doripenem, ertapenem, imipenem/cilastatin, meropenem.

[h]Reserve for serious infection.

[i]Aminoglycosides: gentamicin, tobramycin, and amikacin; use per sensitivities.

[j]β-lactam/β-lactamase inhibitor combination—IV: ampicillin-sulbactam, piperacillin-tazobactam, ticarcillin-clavulanate; PO: amoxicillin-clavulanate.

[k]Fluoroquinolones - IV/PO: ciprofloxacin, levofloxacin, and moxifloxacin.

[l]Generally reserved for patients with hypersensitivity reactions to penicillin.

ISAAC F. MITROPOULOS, ELIZABETH D. HERMSEN,
AND JOHN C. ROTSCHAFER

CHAPTER

115

Central Nervous System Infections

KEY CONCEPTS

❶ The three most likely pathogens of bacterial meningitis in the United States are *Streptococcus pneumoniae*, *Neisseria meningitidis*, and *Hemophilus influenzae*, although routine vaccination is having a dramatic effect on the incidence of these pathogens causing infection.

❷ In cases of meningitis, initial findings can include (a) *presenting signs and symptoms*: fever, headache, nuchal rigidity (the classic triad), Brudzinski's or Kernig's sign, and altered mental status; and (b) *abnormal cerebrospinal fluid (CSF) chemistries*: elevated white blood cell (WBC) count (>100 cells/mm³), elevated protein (>50 mg/dL), and decreased glucose levels (<40 mg/dL).

❸ Two main microbiologic tests that should be obtained include a Gram stain and culture of the CSF.

❹ Three primary goals of treatment in meningitis include (a) *eradication* of infection, (b) *amelioration* of signs and symptoms, and (c) *prevention* of the development of neurologic sequelae, such as seizures, deafness, coma, and death.

❺ When selecting antibiotics, the clinician must consider the antibiotic concentration at the site of infection, as well as the spectrum of antibacterial activity. Empirical choices should be based on age, predisposing conditions, and comorbidities. (a) *Ceftriaxone* or *cefotaxime* and *vancomycin* are reasonable initial choices for empirical coverage of community-acquired meningitis in adult patients. (b) *Listeria monocytogenes* is a common pathogen in infants and elderly; therefore, *ampicillin* should be added empirically to antimicrobial coverage.

❻ Empirical coverage with an appropriate antibiotic should be started as soon as possible when clinical suspicion of meningitis exists. If there is a delay in doing a lumbar puncture (even 30–60 minutes), or if the patient is to undergo neuroimaging, the first dose of an antibiotic *should not* be withheld. Changes in the CSF after initiation of antibiotics usually take 12 to 24 hours.

❼ In contrast to the treatment of other infectious diseases, antibiotic dosages in the treatment of meningitis should be maximized to optimize CNS penetration.

Learning objectives, review questions, and other resources can be found at **www.pharmacotherapyonline.com**.

❽ The duration of antibiotic treatment for meningitis has not been standardized; however, the duration generally is based on the causative organism and the individual case and may range from 7 to 21 days.

❾ Close contacts and relatives of the index case should be assessed for appropriate prophylaxis, particularly with *N. meningitidis* and *H. influenzae* meningitis.

❿ Steroid treatment includes dexamethasone 0.15 mg/kg per dose to be given 4 times daily for 4 days in infants and children older than 2 months of age with proven or strongly suspected bacterial meningitis. Steroids should be given *prior* to antibiotics.

Central nervous system (CNS) infections are caused by a variety of pathogens, including bacteria, viruses, fungi, and parasites. Infections are the result of hematogenous spread from a primary infection site, seeding from a parameningeal focus, reactivation from a latent site, trauma, or congenital defects within the CNS. Newer diagnostic techniques have enabled more rapid and definitive diagnoses, thus diminishing the number of unknown "aseptic meningitis" diagnoses and improving targeted therapy. Bacteria resistant to multiple antibiotics present new challenges in the management of meningitis. This chapter presents the etiologies, pathophysiology, therapy, and prophylaxis of these infections but will concentrate predominantly on bacterial meningitis.

EPIDEMIOLOGY

Approximately 1.2 million cases of acute bacterial meningitis, excluding epidemics, occur every year around the globe, resulting in 135,000 deaths.[1] Overall mortality rates for patients with meningitis range from 2% to 30% depending on the causative microorganism, approaching 20% in most cases of bacterial meningitis.[2] Neurologic sequelae frequently associated with meningitis include seizures, sensorineural hearing loss, and hydrocephalus. Risk for the development of neurologic sequelae depends on the infecting organism, with pneumococcal meningitis being associated with the highest risk.[3] Generally, 30% to 50% of patients who survive meningitis may develop neurologic disabilities.[4,5] Despite the availability of antimicrobial therapy against the most common CNS pathogens, CNS infections continue to have significant morbidity and mortality.

Two findings that have the potential for great epidemiologic impact on bacterial meningitis are (a) passive and active exposures to cigarette smoke are risk factors for bacterial meningitis, especially meningococcal disease[6] and (b) children with cochlear implants that include a positioner are at increased risk of bacterial meningitis, specifically pneumococcal meningitis. The incidence of meningitis due to *Streptococcus pneumoniae* in children with cochlear implants was more than 30 times the incidence in a similar cohort of the U.S. population without implants.[7]

ETIOLOGY

❶ CNS infections are caused by a variety of microorganisms. Historically, CNS infections were primarily community acquired; however, an increasing number are now nosocomial.[8] *Hemophilus influenzae* was the most commonly identified cause of bacterial meningitis (45%), followed by *S. pneumoniae* (18%) and *Neisseria meningitidis* (14%). However, in 1995, approximately 5 years after introduction of the *H. influenzae* type b conjugate (Hib) vaccine, *S. pneumoniae* became the most commonly identified cause of bacterial meningitis (47%), followed by *N. meningitidis* (25%), group B streptococcus (13%), *Listeria monocytogenes* (8%), and *H. influenzae* (7%).

The incidence of invasive *H. influenzae* infections has decreased by more than 90% since the introduction of the Hib vaccine.[9] Mass immunization with the Hib vaccine also has resulted in alterations in the age distribution of bacterial meningitis. While the median age was 15 months in 1986, by 1995 that age increased to 25 years. Accordingly, the proportion of cases in those 18 years of age and older increased from 20.8% to 51.5%.[9] However, many developing countries have not adopted the Hib vaccine as part of the standard vaccines offered to children because of cost. Thus approximately 350,000 to 700,000 children die each year worldwide due to invasive *H. influenzae* infections.[1]

Following the release of the heptavalent protein-polysaccharide conjugate vaccine, the rate of invasive pneumococcal disease dropped from 24.3 cases per 100,000 people in 1999 to 17.3 per 100,000 in 2001. The largest impact was in children younger than 2 years of age where a nearly 70% decline in infection rate was reported as a result of implementation in the routine childhood vaccination schedule. Among children younger than 5 years of age, the rates of pneumococcal meningitis were reduced nearly 60% from 10.3 cases per 100,000 to 4.2 cases during the same time period. Interestingly, the effect carried into the adult population as well with significant reduction in invasive pneumococcal disease across all age groups.[10] Both the Hib and pneumococcal vaccines are of limited availability in developing countries where cost is often prohibitive.

ANATOMY AND PHYSIOLOGY OF THE CENTRAL NERVOUS SYSTEM

MENINGES

The skull and vertebrae protect the CNS from blunt or penetrating trauma (Fig. 115–1). The brain is suspended in these structures by cerebrospinal fluid (CSF) and is surrounded by the meninges. The meninges are made up of three separate membranes: dura mater, arachnoid, and pia mater.[11] Dura mater, or pachymeninges, lies directly beneath and is adherent to the skull. The other two membranes are referred to collectively as *leptomeninges*. Pia mater lies directly over brain tissue. Arachnoid, the middle layer, lies between the dura mater and the pia mater. The subarachnoid space, located between the arachnoid and the pia mater, is the conduit for CSF. By definition, meningitis refers to inflammation of the subarachnoid space or spinal fluid, whereas encephalitis is

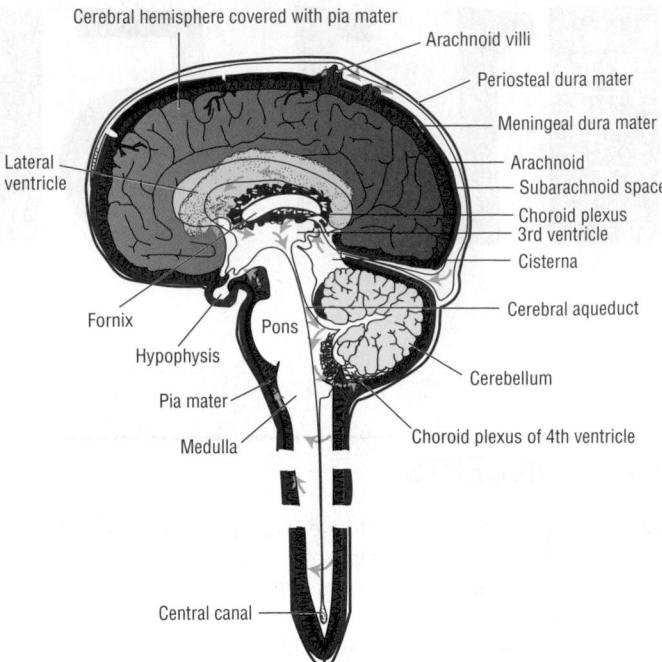

FIGURE 115-1. Diagram of the central nervous system.

an inflammation of the brain itself. Since infectious microorganisms frequently are an underlying cause of these inflammatory processes, the terms *meningitis* and *encephalitis* frequently are used to denote an infectious process. The decision regarding the diagnosis of meningoencephalitis depends on radiographic, laboratory, and clinical information but would refer to inflammation of both tissue and fluid.

CEREBROSPINAL FLUID

Approximately 85% of the CSF is produced within the third, fourth, and lateral ventricles by the choroid plexus (see Fig. 115–1). CSF volume in the CNS is related to patient age: Infants have approximately 40 to 60 mL of CSF, older children have 60 to 100 mL, and adults have 115 to 160 mL. Normally, CSF is produced at the rate of approximately 500 mL/day and flows unidirectionally downward through the spinal cord. The CSF is removed by the arachnoid villi and vertebral venous plexus located in the spinal cord and does not recommunicate with the point of production.[11]

The CSF normally is clear, with a protein content of less than 50 mg/dL, a glucose concentration of approximately 50% to 66% of the simultaneous peripheral serum glucose concentration, and a pH of approximately 7.4; also, it typically contains fewer than five white blood cells (WBCs) per cubic millimeter, all of which should be lymphocytes (Table 115–1). As meninges become inflamed, the constituency of the CSF will change, and these changes can be used diagnostically as markers of infection.

BLOOD–BRAIN BARRIER/ BLOOD–CSF BARRIER

Natural barriers to the exchange of drugs and endogenous compounds among the blood, brain, and CSF are the blood–brain barrier (BBB) and the blood–CSF barrier (BCSFB) (Fig. 115–2). The BBB consists of tightly joined capillary endothelial cells. Drug entry into brain tissue is accomplished by direct passage through the capillary endothelial cells and further penetration of the glial cells that envelop the capillary structure.[11]

TABLE 115-1 Mean Values of the Components of Normal and Abnormal Cerebrospinal Fluid[9,92]

Type	Normal	Bacterial	Viral	Fungal	Tuberculosis
WBC (cells/mm³)	<5	1,000–5,000	100–1,000	40–400	100–500
Differential (%)	>90[a]	≥80 PMNs	50[b,c]	>50[b]	>80[b,c]
Protein (mg/dL)	<50	100–500	30–150	40–150	≤40–150
Glucose (mg/dL)	50%–66% simultaneous serum value	<40 (<60% simultaneous serum value)	<30–70	<30–70	<30–70

[a]Monocytes.
[b]Lymphocytes.
[c]Initial cerebrospinal fluid (CSF), while blood cell (WBC) count may reveal a predominance of polymorphonuclear neutrophils (PMNs).

Passage of drugs into the CSF is controlled by the BCSFB. This barrier is created by ependymal cells of the choroid plexus, which function as an active transport system similar to the renal tubular epithelial cells. The inflammatory process associated with meningitis inhibits the active transport system of the choroid plexus.[12] As in the active transport system in the kidney, the secretion of substances out of the choroid plexus also can be inhibited by the administration of probenecid.[11]

PATHOPHYSIOLOGY OF THE CNS INFECTION

The development of bacterial meningitis occurs following bacterial invasion of the host and CNS, bacterial multiplication with subsequent inflammation of the CNS, specifically the subarachnoid space and the ventricular space, pathophysiologic alterations owing to progressive inflammation, and the resulting neuronal damage.[13] The critical first step in the acquisition of acute bacterial meningitis is nasopharyngeal colonization of the host. Immunoglobulins (Igs) such as secretory IgA are found in high concentrations within nasopharyngeal secretions and work to inhibit bacterial colonization. However, the mucus barrier is deteriorated by IgA proteases secreted by the bacteria, which then extend pili that allow adherence to the host cell surface receptors.[14] Bacterial pathogens attach themselves to nasopharyngeal epithelial cells and are phagocytized into the host's bloodstream. After accessing the patient's bloodstream, bacteria must overcome the host's defense mechanisms.[1] Commonly, CNS bacterial pathogens will produce an extensive polysaccharide capsule resistant to neutrophil phagocytosis and complement opsonization. *H. influenzae, E. coli,* and *N. meningitidis* strains lacking polysaccharide capsules are unable to cause meningitis. Capsular polysaccharides activate the alternate complement pathway, which promotes phagocytosis and clearance of infecting pathogens. Patients unable to activate the alternative complement pathway, such as asplenic and sickle cell patients, are predisposed to bacterial infections caused by encapsulated microorganisms and therefore are at increased risk for meningitis.

Although the exact site and mechanism of bacterial invasion into the CNS is unknown, studies suggest that invasion into the subarachnoid space occurs by continuous exposure of the CNS to large bacterial inocula. Bacteremia with inoculum densities of at least 10³ colony-forming units (CFU)/mL appears to be essential for subarachnoid space invasion.[5] Although several sites of bacterial invasion have been theorized; the most plausible sites are the choroid plexus and/or the cerebral microvasculature. Successful translocation of *E. coli* across the BBB requires a high bacterial inoculum, *E. coli* binding to and invading the brain microvascular endothelial cells through specific ligand-receptor interactions, host cytoskeletal reorganization, and activation of various signaling pathways.[5] Host defense mechanisms within the subarachnoid space are inadequate to combat bacterial pathogens; bacteria, therefore, replicate freely within the CSF until either overgrowth occurs or an effective antibiotic regimen is administered that terminates the process.

The effects of meningitis, namely, inflammation within the subarachnoid space and the ensuing neurologic damage, are not necessarily a direct result of the pathogens themselves. The neurologic sequelae occur due to the activation of the host's inflammatory pathways, which is induced by the pathogens or their products.[2] Bacterial cell lysis and subsequent death can result in the release of cell wall components, such as lipopolysaccharide (LPS), lipid A (endotoxin), lipoteichoic acid, teichoic acid, and peptidoglycan, depending on whether the pathogen is gram-positive or gram-negative (Fig. 115–3). These cell wall components cause capillary endothelial cells and CNS macrophages to release cytokines (interleukin 1 [IL-1] and tumor necrosis factor [TNF]) and other inflammatory mediators (IL-6, IL-8, platelet-activating factor [PAF], nitric oxide, arachadonic acid metabolites [e.g., prostaglandin and prostacycline], and macrophage-derived proteins). Proteolytic products and toxic oxygen radicals are released from the capillary endothelium, causing an alteration in the permeability of the BBB. PAF activates the coagulation cascade, and arachidonic acid metabolites stimulate vasodilation. These events propagate other sequential events that lead to cerebral edema, elevated intracranial pressure (ICP), CSF pleocytosis, decreased cerebral blood flow, cerebral ischemia, and death.[2]

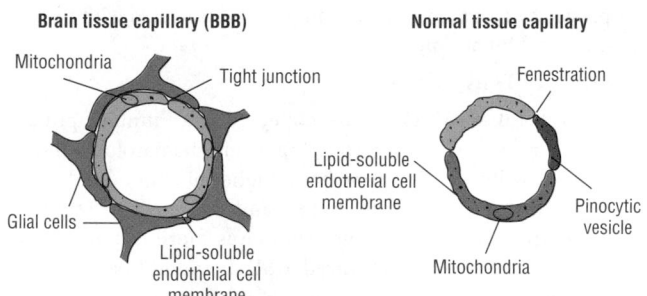

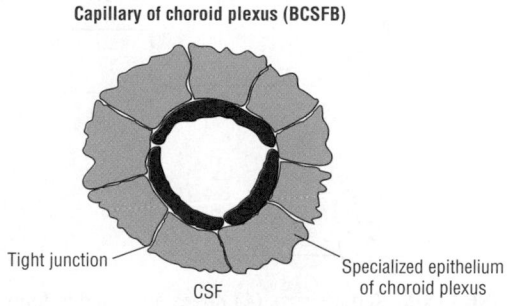

FIGURE 115-2. Schematic representation of a blood–cerebrospinal fluid barrier capillary, brain tissue capillary, and normal tissue capillary (*below*).

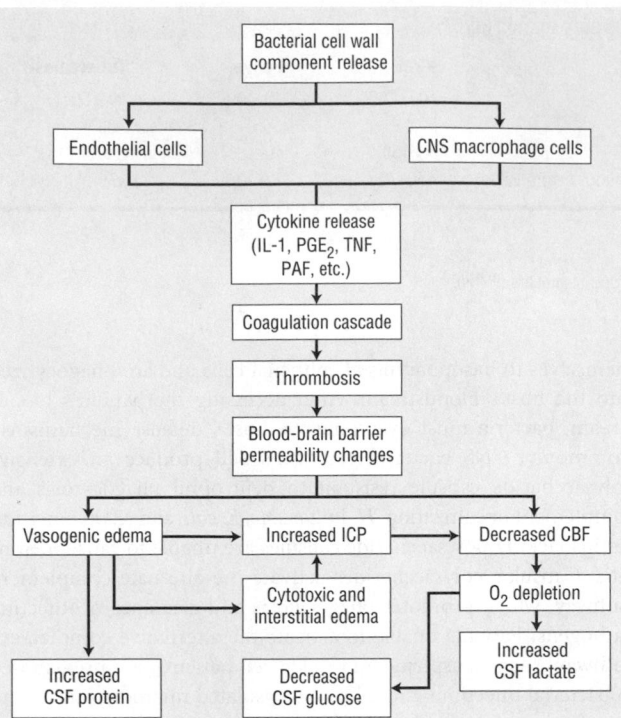

FIGURE 115-3. Hypothetical schema of pathophysiologic events that occur during bacterial meningitis. (IL-1, interleukin 1; TNF, tumor necrosis factor; PAF, platelet-activating factor; CBF, cerebral blood flow; CSF, cerebrospinal fluid; PGE$_2$, prostaglandin E$_2$; ICP, intracranial pressure.)

CLINCAL PRESENTATION AND DIAGNOSIS

CLINICAL PRESENTATION OF ACUTE MENINGITIS

General

- Clinical presentation varies with age, and generally, the younger the patient, the more atypical and the less pronounced is the clinical picture.

- Up to 50% of patients may receive antibiotics before a diagnosis of meningitis is made, delaying presentation to the hospital. Prior antibiotic therapy may cause the Gram stain and CSF culture to be negative, but the antibiotic therapy rarely affects CSF protein or glucose.[15]

Signs And Symptoms

- ❷ Classic signs and symptoms include fever, nuchal rigidity, altered mental status (the classic triad), chills, vomiting, photophobia, and severe headache; Kernig's and Brudzinski's signs may also be present but are poorly sensitive and frequently are absent in children.[15,16] (Figs. 115–4 and 115–5).

- Other signs and symptoms include irritability, delirium, drowsiness, lethargy, and coma.

- Clinical signs and symptoms in young children may include bulging fontanelle, apneas, purpuric rash, and convulsions in addition to those just mentioned.[15]

- Seizures occur more commonly in children (20%–30%) than in adults (0%–12%).[17]

Differential Signs And Symptoms[2]

- Purpuric and petechial skin lesions typically indicate meningococcal involvement, although the lesions may be present

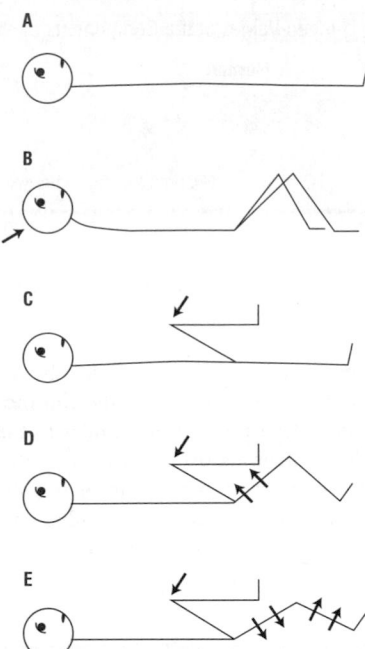

FIGURE 115-4. (A,B) Brudzinski's neck signs. Hip and knee flexion occurs as a result of flexion of the neck (B). (C–E) Brudzinski's leg signs. (C) Patient's leg is flexed by examiner (arrow). (D) The contralateral leg begins to flex—identical contralateral sign (arrows). (E) The contralateral leg now begins to extend spontaneously, resembling a little kick (arrows).

with *H. influenzae* meningitis. Rashes rarely occur with pneumococcal meningitis.

- Waterhouse-Friderichsen syndrome, a rapid eruption of multiple hemorrhagic lesions associated with a shock-like state, is associated with meningococcal meningitis.

- *H. influenzae* meningitis and meningococcal meningitis both can cause involvement of the joints during the illness.

- A history of head trauma with or without skull fracture or presence of a chronically draining ear is associated with pneumococcal involvement.

Laboratory Tests

- Several tubes of CSF are collected via lumbar puncture for chemistry, microbiology, and hematology tests. Theoretically, the first tube has a higher likelihood of being contaminated with both blood and bacteria during the puncture, although the total volume is more important in practice than the tube cultured. CSF should not be refrigerated or stored on ice.[18]

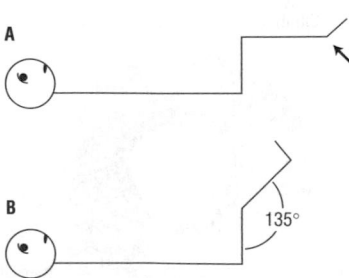

FIGURE 115-5. Kernig's sign. (A) Knees are raised to form a 90-degree angle relative to the trunk, and the examiner attempts to extend the knees. (B) Once the knee angle reaches approximately 135 degrees, contracture or extensor spasm occurs.

- Analysis of CSF chemistries typically includes measurement of glucose and total protein concentrations. An elevated CSF protein of ≥100 mg/dL and a CSF glucose concentration of less than 50% of the simultaneously obtained peripheral value suggest bacterial meningitis (see Table 115–1).

- The values for CSF glucose, protein, and WBC concentrations found with bacterial meningitis overlap significantly with those for viral, tuberculous, and fungal meningitis (see Table 115–1). Therefore, CSF WBC counts and CSF glucose and protein concentrations cannot always distinguish the different etiologies of meningitis.

Other Diagnostic Tests[18]

- In patients presenting with new-onset seizures, signs of space-occupying lesions or moderate to severe impairment of consciousness, cranial imaging via magnetic resonance imaging (MRI) or cranial computed tomography (CT) should precede a lumbar puncture. MRI is generally preferred as it more clearly identifies areas of cerebral edemas. In these instances, the withdrawal of CSF fluid from a lumbar puncture reduces counterpressure that may result in compression of the brain from above with risk of brain herniation complicating the clinical course.[19,20] Neuroimaging should not however delay initiation of antibiotic therapy as doing so can result in a poor outcome in this disease.[21]

- Blood and other specimens should be cultured according to clinical judgment because meningitis frequently can arise via hematogenous dissemination or can be associated with infections at other sites. A minimum of 20 mL of blood in each of two to three separate cultures per each 24-hour period is necessary for the detection of most bacteremias.

- ❸ Gram stain and culture of the CSF are the most important laboratory tests performed for bacterial meningitis. The Gram stain continues to be the most rapid and accurate method of presumptively diagnosing acute bacterial meningitis. When performed before antibiotic therapy is initiated, Gram stain is both rapid and sensitive and can confirm the diagnosis of bacterial meningitis in 75% to 90% of cases. The sensitivity of the Gram stain decreases to 40% to 60% in patients who received prior antibiotic therapy. Culture is required to differentiate the various bacterial etiologies.

- Polymerase chain reaction (PCR) techniques can be used to diagnose meningitis caused by *N. meningitidis*, *S. pneumoniae*, and Hib. PCR is considered to be highly sensitive and specific, but use of this powerful diagnostic approach is limited due to expense and availability.

- Latex fixation, latex coagglutination, and enzyme immunoassay (EIA) tests provide for the rapid identification of several bacterial causes of meningitis, including *S. pneumoniae*, *N. meningitidis*, and Hib.[13] Rapid-identification latex tests work by bringing potential capsular antigens of the pathogen causing meningitis in contact with a specific antibody, causing an antigen-antibody reaction. This capsular antigen-antibody reaction can be observed visually and quickly without waiting for culture results. The rapid antigen tests should be used in situations in which the Gram stain is negative.[17] The sensitivity and specificity of latex fixation and coagglutination tests can vary with the manufacturer of the antibody, density of the antigen present in the CSF, and pathogen being tested.

- Diagnosis of tuberculosis meningitis employs acid-fast staining, culture, and PCR of the CSF.

- PCR testing of the CSF is the preferred method of diagnosing most viral meningitis infections.

- The standard diagnostic tests for fungal meningitis include culture, direct microscopic examination of stained and unstained specimens of CSF, antigen detection of cryptococcal or histoplasmal antigens, and antibody assay of serum and/or CSF.

TREATMENT

CNS Infections

■ DESIRED OUTCOME

Supportive care, particularly early in the course of treatment, is critically important. Administration of fluids, electrolytes, antipyretics, analgesics, and other supportive measures is indicated for patients presenting with acute bacterial meningitis. Although supportive care is important initially, appropriate antibiotic therapy (empirical or definitive) should be started as soon as possible. ❹ Understanding antibiotic selection and the issues surrounding antibiotic penetration will assist in meeting the goals of treatment, which include eradication of infection with amelioration of signs and symptoms and prevention of neurologic sequelae, such as seizures, deafness, coma, and death.

■ APPROACH TO TREATMENT

This section discusses issues surrounding the approach to treatment, such as antibiotic penetration within the CNS, duration of antibiotic therapy, and the use of adjunctive corticosteroids. Until a pathogen is identified, prompt empirical antibiotic coverage is often needed. ❺ Based on the patient's profile (i.e., allergies, age, and concurrent medical conditions), extent of antibiotic CNS penetration, and spectrum of activity, appropriate recommendations can be made, and therapy should last at least 48 to 72 hours or until the diagnosis of bacterial meningitis can be ruled out (Tables 115–2 and 115–3). ❻ The first dose of antibiotics should not be withheld, even when lumbar puncture is delayed or neuroimaging is being performed. Changes in the CSF after antibiotic administration usually take 12 to 24 hours. Continued therapy should be based on the assessment of clinical improvement, cultures, and susceptibility testing results. Once a pathogen is identified, antibiotic therapy should be tailored to the specific pathogen (Tables 115–4 and 115–5). Throughout the course of treatment, efficacy parameters, such as signs and symptoms, microbiologic findings, and CSF examination, should be followed to evaluate the success of meeting the desired outcomes.

Several factors influence the transfer of antibiotic from capillary blood into the CNS, including inflammation of the meninges, which increases antibiotic penetration through damage to tight junctions between capillary endothelial cells and decreases the activity of an energy-dependent efflux pump in the choroid plexus responsible for movement of penicillins and, to a much lesser extent, fluoroquinolones and aminoglycosides (see Table 115–3). Antibiotics having low molecular weights are passed more easily through biologic barriers than compounds of higher molecular weight. Only antibiotics that are nonionized at physiologic or pathologic pH are capable of diffusion. Highly lipid-soluble compounds penetrate more readily than water-soluble compounds. Antibiotics not extensively protein bound in the serum provide a larger free fraction of drug capable of passing into the CSF. Passage

TABLE 115-2 Bacterial Meningitis: Most Likely and Empirical Therapy by Age Group

Age Commonly Affected	Most Likely Organisms	Empirical Therapy	Risk Factors for All Age Groups
Newborn–1 mo	Group B *Streptococcus* Gram-negative enterics[a] *Listeria monocytogenes*	Ampicillin + cefotaxime or ceftriaxone or aminoglycoside	Respiratory tract infection Otitis media Mastoiditis Head trauma Alcoholism High-dose steroids
1 mo–4 y	*S. pneumoniae* *N. meningitidis* *H. influenzae*	Vancomycin[b] and cefotaxime or ceftriaxone	Splenectomy Sickle cell disease Immunoglobulin deficiency
5–29 y	*N. meningitidis* *S. pneumoniae* *H. influenzae*	Vancomycin[b] and cefotaxime or ceftriaxone	Immunosuppression
30–60 y	*S. pneumoniae* *N. meningitidis*	Vancomycin[b] and cefotaxime or ceftriaxone	
>60 y	*S. pneumoniae* Gram-negative enterics *L. monocytogenes*	Vancomycin[b] plus ampicillin plus cefotaxime or ceftriaxone	

[a]*E. coli*, *Klebsiella* spp, *Enterobacter* spp common.
[b]Vancomycin use should be based on local incidence of penicillin-resistant *S. pneumoniae* and until cefotaxime or ceftriaxone minimum inhibitory concentration results are available.

TABLE 115-3 Penetration of Antimicrobial Agents into the Cerebrospinal Fluid

Therapeutic levels in CSF with or without inflammation

Choramphenicol	Pyrazinamide
Cycloserine	Rifampin
Ethionamide	Sulfonamides
Isoniazid	Trimethoprim
Metronidazole	

Therapeutic levels in CSF with inflammation of meninges

Acyclovir	Ganciclovir
Ampicillin ± sulbactam	Imipenem
Aztreonam	Levofloxacin
Carbenicillin	Linezolid
Cefotaxime	Meropenem
Ceftazidime	Mezlocillin
Ceftizoxime	Moxifloxacin
Ceftriaxone	Nafcillin
Cefuroxime	Ofloxacin
Ciprofloxacin	Penicillin G
Colistin	Piperacillin
Daptomycin	Pyrimethamine
Ethambutol	Quinupristin/dalfopristin
Fluconazole	Ticarcillin ± clavulanic acid
Flucytosine	Vancomycin
Foscarnet	Vidarabine

Non-therapeutic levels in CSF with or without inflammation

Aminoglycosides	Cephalosporins (Second Generation)[a]
Amphotericin B	Clindamycin[b]
Cefoperazone	Itraconazole[c]
Cephalosporins (first generation)	Ketoconazole

[a]Cefuroxime is an exception.
[b]Achieves therapeutic brain tissue concentrations.
[c]Achieves therapeutic concentrations for *Cryptococcus neoformans* therapy.
CSF, cerebrospinal fluid.

of large, polar antibiotics into the CSF may be assisted, however, by a carrier transport system. ❼ Unlike the treatment of many other infections, antibiotic dosages in the treatment of CNS infections must be maximized to optimize penetration to the site of infection.

Problems of CSF penetration may be overcome by direct instillation of antibiotics intrathecally, intracisternally, or intraventricularly (Table 115–6). Advantages of direct instillation, however, must be weighed against the risks of invasive CNS procedures. Intrathecal administration of antibiotics is unlikely to produce therapeutic concentrations in the ventricles possibly owing to the unidirectional flow of CSF.[22] Although intraventricular administration from a therapeutic standpoint may be preferred over intrathecal administration, the former requires neurosurgical placement of a subcutaneous reservoir. Intraventricular delivery may be necessary when bacteria that require treatment with aminoglycosides, such as *L. monocytogenes, Pseudomonas aeruginosa* or enterococci, are isolated. Children who received both parenteral antibiotics and intrathecal gentamicin had higher CSF endotoxin levels, higher CSF IL-1β levels, and higher mortality than children receiving only parenteral antibiotics. Interestingly, the differences were attributed to direct CSF administration of gentamicin, which generally is thought to blunt the endotoxin release caused by β-lactam antibiotics.[23]

❽ Although the length of treatment for bacterial meningitis generally is based on the causative organism, there is no universally accepted standard (Table 115–4). Meningitis caused by *S. pneumoniae* has been treated successfully with 10 to 14 days of antibiotic therapy. Meningitis caused by *N. meningitidis* usually can be treated with a 7-day course of antibiotics. In contrast, a longer duration (≥21 days) has been recommended for patients infected with *L. monocytogenes* (A-III). Therapy should be individualized, and some patients may require enduring courses.

■ CAUSATIVE AGENTS

N. Meningitidis (Meningococcus)

N. meningitidis is the leading cause of bacterial meningitis in children and young adults in the United States.[24] The source of infection usually is an asymptomatic carrier. Most cases occur in the winter or spring, a time when viral meningitis is relatively uncommon. Five serogroups of *N. meningitidis* (A, B, C, Y, and W-135) are primarily responsible. Clusters of meningococcal disease, defined as two or more cases of the same serogroup that are closer in time and space than expected for the population or group under observation, generally are associated with schools.[25] Although some of these clusters have been due to serogroup B, the majority have been due to serogroup C. Serogroup A, although associated with meningococcal outbreaks in Africa and Asia, is a rare cause of disease in the United States.[26] Serogroup Y, although frequently associated with pneumonia, is emerging as an important cause of invasive meningococcal disease in select areas.[27,28] Overall, *N. meningitidis* accounts for 25% of all meningitis cases, 60% of cases in persons aged 2 to 18 years, and carries a case-fatality rate of approximately 10%.[9,27]

Initially, patients are colonized and, at some point, develop a bacteremia, which most likely occurs prior to hospital admission. Meningitis occurs after the bacteria seeds into the meninges, which can occur in 50% of the cases of meningococcal disease.[29] After the acute phase of meningitis has resolved, there is a unique immune reaction that distinguishes meningococcal meningitis from other bacterial causes. The patient develops a characteristic immunologic reaction of fever, arthritis (usually involving large joints), and pericarditis approximately 10 to 14 days after the onset of disease

TABLE 115-4 Antimicrobial Agents of First Choice and Alternative Choice in the Treatment of Meningitis Caused by Gram-Positive and Gram-Negative Microorganisms

Organism	Antibiotic of First Choice	Alternative Antibiotics	Recommended Duration of Therapy
Gram-positive			
Streptococcus pneumoniae			10–14 days
Penicillin susceptible	Penicillin G or Ampicillin (A-III)	Cefotaxime (A-III), Ceftriaxone (A-III), Chloramphenicol (A-III)	
Penicillin intermediate	Cefotaxime or Ceftriaxone (A-III)	Cefepime (B-II), Meropenem (B-II), Moxifloxacin (B-II), Linezolid (C-III)	
Penicillin resistant	Vancomycin^a plus Cefotaxime or Ceftriaxone (A-III)	Cefepime (B-II), Meropenem (B-II), Moxifloxacin (B-II), Linezolid (C-III)	
Group B Streptococcus	Penicillin G or Ampicillin ± Gentamicin^a (A-III)	Cefotaxime (B-III), Ceftriaxone (B-III), Chloramphenicol (B-III)	14–21 days
Staphylococcus aureus			14–21 days^e
Methicillin susceptible	Nafcillin or Oxacillin (A-III)	Vancomycin^a (A-III), Meropenem (B-III)	
Methicillin resistant	Vancomycin^a (A-III)	Trimethoprim-sulfamethoxazole (A-III), Linezolid (B-III)	
Staphylococcus epidermidis	Vancomycin^a (A-III)	Linezolid (B-III)	14–21 days^e
Listeria monocytogenes	Penicillin G or Ampicillin ± Gentamicin^a (A-III)	Trimethoprim-sulfamethoxazole (A-III), Meropenem (B-III)	≥21 days
Gram-negative			
Neisseria meningitis			7 days
Penicillin susceptible	Penicillin G or Ampicillin (A-III)	Cefotaxime (A-III), Ceftriaxone (A-III), Chloramphenicol (A-III)	
Penicillin resistant	Cefotaxime or Ceftriaxone (A-III)	Chloramphenicol (A-III), Meropenem (A-III), Fluoroquinolone (A-III)	
Haemophilus influenzae			7 days
β-Lactamase negative	Ampicillin (A-III)	Cefotaxime (A-III), Ceftriaxone (A-III), Chloramphenicol (A-III), Cefepime (A-III), Fluoroquinolone (A-III)	
β-Lactamase positive	Cefotaxime or Ceftriaxone (A-I)	Cefepime (A-I), Fluoroquinolone (A-III), Chloramphenicol (A-III)	
Enterobacteriaceae^d	Cefotaxime or Ceftriaxone (A-II)	Cefepime (A-III), Fluoroquinolone (A-III), Meropenem (A-III), Aztreonam (A-III)	21 days
Pseudomonas aeruginosa	Cefepime or Ceftazidime (A-II) ± Tobramycin^{a,b} (A-III)	Ciprofloxacin (A-III), Meropenem (A-III), Piperacillin plus Tobramycin^{a,b} (A-III), Colistin sulfomethate^{a,c} (B-III), Aztreonam (A-III)	21 days

Strength of recommendation: (A) Good evidence to support a recommendation for use; should always be offered. (B) Moderate evidence to support a recommendation for use; should generally be offered.

Quality of evidence: (I) Evidence from ≥1 properly randomized, controlled trial. (II) Evidence from ≥1 well-designed clinical trial, without randomization; from cohort or case-controlled analytic studies (preferably from >1 center) or from multiple time-series. (III) Evidence from opinions of respected authorities, based on clinical experience, descriptive studies, or reports of expert committees.

^{a}Monitor drug levels in serum.
^{b}Direct central nervous system administration may be added; see Table 115–6 for dosage.
^{c}Should be reserved for multidrug-resistant pseudomonal or *Actinetobacter* infections for which all other therapeutic options have been exhausted.
^{d}Includes *E. coli* and *Klebsiella* spp.
^{e}Based on clinical experience; no clear recommendations.

and despite successful treatment.[30] At this time, examination of the synovial fluid reveals a large number of polymorphonuclear cells, elevated protein concentrations, normal glucose concentrations, and sterile cultures. The reaction may last a week or longer, and no additional antibiotic therapy is required. Patients, however, may benefit from nonsteroidal antiinflammatory agents and supportive care.[30]

Seizures and coma are uncommon with meningococcal meningitis. Patients may behave aggressively, however, and often are maniacal. Patients may develop deafness and transiently impaired ocular movements. Deafness unilaterally or, more commonly, bilaterally may develop early or late in the disease course.[30] Hearing loss secondary to sensory nerve damage (sensorineural hearing) is usually permanent, whereas conductive hearing impairment, such as damage to the tympanic membrane, is often reversible.

The presence of petechiae may be the primary clue that the underlying pathogen is *N. meningitidis*. Approximately 50% of patients with meningococcal meningitis have purpuric lesions, petechiae, or both. Patients may have an obvious or subclinical picture of disseminated intravascular coagulation (DIC), which may progress to infarction of the adrenal glands and renal cortex and cause widespread thrombosis.

Aggressive, early intervention with high-dose intravenous crystalline penicillin G, 50,000 units/kg every 4 hours, is usually recommended for the treatment of *N. meningitidis* meningitis. Chloramphenicol is bactericidal for *N. meningitidis* and may be used in place of penicillin G. However, chloramphenicol has unpredictable metabolism in young infants and several drug–drug

interactions which largely preclude its use in developed countries.[2] Several third-generation cephalosporins (i.e., cefotaxime, ceftriaxone, ceftazidime and ceftizoxime) have indications for the treatment of meningitis and are acceptable alternatives to penicillin G (see Table 115–5). Meropenem and fluoroquinolones are also suitable alternatives for the treatment of penicillin nonsusceptible meningiococci (A-III).

Cases of meningitis caused by relatively penicillin-resistant meningococci (minimun inhibitory concentration [MIC] 0.1–1 mg/L) and highly (MIC ≥ 256 mg/L) have been reported. Prevalence varies geographically, ranging from 0.4% to 42.6%.[31] Isolated reports of treatment failure with penicillin have surfaced in recent years.[32,33] Completely resistant strains produce β-lactamase, whereas relatively resistant strains have an alteration of penicillin-binding proteins. The emergence of β-lactamase producing strains of meningococci are causing more practitioners to utilize third-generation cephalosporins (cefotaxime or ceftriaxone) instead of penicillin, which has long been considered the drug of choice for meningococcal meningitis.[34]

N. meningitidis is spread by direct person-to-person close contact, including respiratory droplets and pharyngeal secretions.[29] Close contacts of patients contracting *N. meningitidis* meningitis are at an increased risk of developing meningitis. Close contacts include day-care center contacts, members of the household, or anyone who has been exposed to respiratory or oral secretions through activities such as coughing, sneezing, or kissing. Household contacts of people who have sporadic disease are estimated to have an incidence of meningococcal meningitis that is 500 to 800 times

TABLE 115-5 Dosing of Antimicrobial Agents by Age Group

Antimicrobial Agent	Infants and Children	Adults
Antibacterials		
Ampicillin	75 mg/kg every 6 h	2 g every 4 h
Aztreonam		2 g every 6–8 h
Cefepime	50 mg/kg every 8 h	2 g every 8 h
Cefotaxime	75 mg/kg every 6–8 h	2 g every 4–6 h
Ceftazidime	50 mg/kg every 8 h	2 g every 8 h
Ceftriaxone	100 mg/kg once daily	2 g every 12–24 h
Chloramphenicol	25 mg/kg every 6 h	1–1.5 g every 6 h
Ciprofloxacin	10 mg/kg every 8 h	400 mg every 8–12 h
Colistin[a,c]	5 mg/kg once daily	5 mg/kg once daily
Gentamicin[a,b]	2.5 mg/kg every 8 h	2 mg/kg every 8 h
Levofloxacin	10 mg/kg once daily	750 mg once daily
Linezolid	10 mg/kg every 8 h	600 mg every 12 h
Meropenem	40 mg/kg every 8 h	2 g every 8 h
Moxifloxacin		400 mg once daily
Oxacillin/Nafcillin	50 mg/kg every 6 h	2 g every 4 h
Penicillin G	0.05 mUnits/kg every 4–6 h	4 mUnits every 4 h
Piperacillin	50 mg/kg every 4–6 h	3 g every 4–6 h
Tobramycin[a,b]	2.5 mg/kg every 8 h	2 mg/kg every 8 h
TMP-SMZ[d]	5 mg/kg every 6–12 h	5 mg/kg every 6–12 h
Vancomycin[a]	15 mg/kg every 6 h	15 mg/kg every 8–12 h
Antimycobacterials		
Isoniazid[e]	10–15 mg/kg once daily	5 mg/kg once daily
Rifampin	10–20 mg/kg once daily	600 mg once daily
Pyrazinamide	15–30 mg/kg once daily	15–30 mg/kg once daily
Ethambutol	15–25 mg/kg once daily	15–2 5mg/kg once daily
Antifungals		
Amphotericin B		0.7–1 mg/kg once daily
Lipid amphotericin B		4 mg/kg once daily
Flucytosine		25 mg/kg every 6 h
Fluconazole		400–800 mg once daily
Voriconazole		6 mg/kg every 12 h × 2 doses then 4 mg/kg every 12 h
Antivirals		
Acyclovir	20 mg/kg every 8 h	10 mg/kg every 8 h
Foscarnet		60 mg/kg every 8–12 h

[a]Monitor drug levels in serum.
[b]Direct central nervous system administration may be added; see Table 115-6 for dosage.
[c]Should be reserved for multidrug-resistant pseudomonal or *Actinetobacter* infections for which all other therapeutic options have been exhausted.
[d]Dosing based on trimethoprim component.
[e]Supplemental pyridoxine hydrochloride (vitamin B₆) 50 mg/day is recommended.

TABLE 115-6 Intraventricular and Intrathecal Antibiotic Dosage Recommendation

Antibiotic	Dose (mg)	Expected CSF Concentration[a] (mg/L)	Reference
Ampicillin	10–50	60–300	114–116
Methicillin	25–100	160–600	114–116
Nafcillin	75	500	115
Cephalothin	25–100	160–600	114–116
Chloramphenicol	25–100	160–600	114, 116, 117
Gentamicin	1–10	6–60	114–118
Quinupristin/ dalfopristin	1–2	7–13	119
Tobramycin	1–10	6–60	118
Vancomycin	5	30	120–122
Amphotericin B	0.05–0.25 mg/day or 0.05–1 mg 1–3 times weekly	–	123

[a]Assumes adult CSF volume = 150 mL.
CSF, cerebrospinal fluid.

S. Pneumoniae (Pneumococcus or Diplococcus)

S. pneumoniae is the leading cause of meningitis in adults. Moreover, *S. pneumoniae* is the most common cause of bacterial meningitis in children younger than 2 years of age, accounting for 4 to 6 cases per 100,000 of this population, and the second most common cause in children older than 2 years of age.[37] Case-fatality rates in children are highest with this organism and approach 20%. Approximately 50% of cases are secondary infections resulting from primary infections of parameningeal foci, such as the ear or paranasal sinuses. Pneumonia, endocarditis, CSF leak secondary to head trauma, splenectomy, alcoholism, sickle cell disease, and bone marrow transplantation may predispose the patient to the development of pneumococcal meningitis.

Neurologic complications, such as coma and seizures, are common with pneumococcal meningitis. Children with pneumococcal meningitis have lower mortality rates (4%–17%) compared with the mortality rates in adults (20%–30%), but children who survive suffer from a high rate of neurologic sequelae (29%–56%).[38,39] Risk factors for recurrent pneumococcal meningitis include traumatic tears of the dura, fracture of the cribriform plate or paranasal sinuses, nasal meningoceles, repeated episodes of otitis media, basilar skull fractures, and CSF leaks. The prognosis of pneumococcal meningitis depends on a variety of factors, including the number of WBCs in the CSF, the number of WBCs in the periphery, the CSF glucose concentration, the CSF protein concentration, the serum sodium concentration, and the presence of a comatose state and/or shock.[40]

Based on resistance patterns and the fact that sufficient CSF concentrations of penicillin are difficult to achieve with standard intravenous doses, penicillin should not be used as empirical therapy if *S. pneumoniae* is a suspected pathogen. Furthermore, appropriate Clinical Laboratory Standards Institute (CLSI)-approved testing of all CSF isolates for penicillin resistance is recommended. Ceftriaxone and cefotaxime have served as alternatives to penicillin in the treatment of penicillin intermediate- and high-resistant pneumococci. Of note, treatment failures with third-generation cephalosporins in the management of penicillin-resistant pneumococci have been reported.[34] Therapeutic approaches to cephalosporin-resistant pneumococcus include the addition of vancomycin and rifampin, which have demonstrated synergistic activity with ceftriaxone. However, no data from controlled clinical

greater than that of the overall population.[29] Secondary cases of meningitis usually develop within the first week following exposure, but they may take up to 60 days after contact with the index case.[35] Young children are at the greatest risk of contracting *N. meningitidis;* however, all ages are at risk, especially close contacts exposed via household, daycare, or military contact.

❾ Prophylaxis of close contacts should be started only after consultation with the local health department. In general, rifampin is given as prophylaxis for 2 days.[26] The adult dose is 600 mg every 12 hours, whereas children aged 1 month and older should receive 10 mg/kg every 12 hours, and children younger than 1 month should receive 5 mg/kg every 12 hours (A-III). Intramuscular ceftriaxone (250 mg in adults, 125 mg in children younger than 12 years of age) and oral ciprofloxacin (500 mg in adults and children older than 12 years) are alternatives to rifampin (A-III).[15] Further discussion of who should receive prophylaxis is beyond the scope of this chapter; interested readers can refer to the recommendations of the U.S. Centers for Disease Control and Prevention for that information.[36]

trials supporting the use of rifampin are available. Therefore, the combination of vancomycin and ceftriaxone has been suggested as empirical treatment until the results of antimicrobial susceptibility testing are available.[2,34] Some investigators have suggested that the addition of vancomycin to the initial empirical regimen may not be necessary because the prevalence of β-lactam–resistant pneumococci has been reduced greatly as a result of the pneumococcal vaccines.[2]

Ceftriaxone and vancomycin are the agents of choice to treat presumed pneumococcal meningitis empirically until the susceptibility is known. Penicillin may be used for drug-susceptible isolates with MICs of 0.06 mg/L or less, but for intermediate isolates, ceftriaxone is used, and for highly drug resistant isolates, a combination of ceftriaxone and vancomycin should be used. Vancomycin should not be used as monotherapy.[34] In severe cases, therapeutic drug monitoring of the CSF and possibly even direct antibiotic instillation may be necessary.

Some pneumococcal strains exhibit tolerance to vancomycin and are of great concern, but the clinical significance is unknown.[41,42] Based on concern about the limited therapeutic options for penicillin- and cephalosporin-resistant pneumococcal meningitis, newer agents have been evaluated. Meropenem is approved by the U.S. Food and Drug Administration (FDA) for the treatment of bacterial meningitis in children aged 3 months and older and has shown similar clinical and microbiologic efficacy to cefotaxime or ceftriaxone. Meropenem is currently recommended as an alternative to a third generation cephalosporin in penicillin nonsusceptible isolates (B-II). Some caution is warranted with the use of imipenem for CNS infections because of the possibility of drug-induced seizures, especially when not properly dose adjusted for declining renal function. Of note, seizures may be caused by meningitis itself or by imipenem, and the cause is difficult to differentiate. The newer fluoroquinolones represent another therapeutic option owing to favorable activity against multidrug-resistant pneumococci and good penetration into the CSF.[43] However, clinical data to date regarding fluoroquinolone treatment of pneumococcal meningitis are limited mainly to animal models. Comparative, controlled clinical efficacy trials in patients with meningitis will be necessary before routine use of the fluoroquinolones is viable.

Linezolid, and daptomycin have emerged as therapeutic options for treating multidrug-resistant gram-positive infections. Linezolid in combination with ceftriaxone has been used to treat a limited number of cases of pneumococcal meningitis with outcomes similar to standard treatment.[44] The penetration of daptomycin in the CSF was approximately 6% following a 15mg/kg bolus achieving maximum concentration approximately four hours after the dose in a rabbit meningitis model. The 15 mg/kg dose produces similar serum concentrations in rabbits as the 6 mg/kg dose in humans. In this study, daptomycin was able to clear both the penicillin-resistant and the quinilone-resistant pneumococci from the CSF more rapidly than the standard regimen of vancomycin and ceftriaxone.[45] Additionally, daptomycin may reduce the inflammatory response caused by cell wall components in pneumococcal meningitis compared with ceftriaxone.[46] However, limited data are available, and these agents cannot be recommended for use in the treatment of pneumococcal meningitis.

CLINICAL CONTROVERSY

Some investigators believe that the use of vancomycin in the empirical treatment of pneumococcal meningitis is no longer necessary because the widespread use of pneumococcal vaccines has greatly reduced the prevalence of β-lactam–resistant pneumococci. However, because the infecting organism is rarely known initially, most clinicians still use the combination of a third-generation cephalosporin and vancomycin for empirical treatment.

Pneumococcal vaccines help in reducing the risk of invasive pneumococcal disease. Virtually all serotypes of *S. pneumoniae* exhibiting intermediate or complete resistance to penicillin are found in the 23-serotype pneumococcal polysaccharide vaccine. However, in 1997, only 30% of people 65 years of age and older had been immunized against pneumococcal disease.[47] Therefore, the CDC issued stronger recommendations for the use of the pneumococcal polysaccharide vaccine, calling for vaccination of the following high-risk groups: persons over the age of 65 years; persons aged 2 to 64 years who have a chronic illness, who live in high-risk environments (e.g., Alaskan Natives and residents of long-term care facilities), and who lack a functioning spleen (e.g., sickle cell disease and splenectomy); and immunocompromised persons over the age of 2 years, including those with HIV infection. Additionally, the question of whether or not college students living in dormitories, a possible high-risk environment, should be vaccinated remains debatable. Unfortunately, variability in the host's ability to mount an immune response to the vaccine limits its usefulness for penicillin-resistant pneumococci in children younger than 2 years of age and in immunocompromised adults.

In 2000, a heptavalent pneumococcal conjugate vaccine (Prevnar) was approved for use in children 2 months of age and older. Use of the vaccine has reduced invasive pneumococcal infections, including sepsis and meningitis more than 90%.[48] Moreover, the vaccine is safe and effective in low-birth-weight and preterm infants.[49,50] Widespread vaccination is expected to have a significant impact on the prevalence of pneumococcal meningitis, including infection caused by antibiotic-resistant strains. A cohort study of 3.8 million healthy infants projected that vaccination would prevent more than 12,000 cases of invasive disease for each U.S. birth cohort, resulting in substantial decreases in morbidity and mortality, as well as possible cost savings.[51] Current recommendations are for all healthy infants younger than 2 years of age to be immunized with the heptavalent vaccine at 2, 4, 6, and 12 to 15 months. The recommendations are extended to include Alaskan Native, Native American, and African American children between the ages of 2 and 5 years. The CDC has issued a recommendation that all persons with cochlear implants receive age-appropriate vaccination with the pneumococcal conjugate vaccine, pneumococcal polysaccharide vaccine, or both.[52]

H. Influenzae

Historically, *H. influenzae* was the most common cause of meningitis in children 6 months to 3 years of age. Since the introduction of effective vaccines, however, the incidence of *H. influenzae* type B disease in the United States has declined dramatically. Widespread vaccination of infants and children has decreased the incidence of bacterial meningitis due to *H. influenzae* in children between the ages of 1 month and 5 years by 87%, resulting in a 55% decline in all cases of bacterial meningitis.[14] Worldwide, in countries that have adopted universal immunization, the incidence of bacterial meningitis caused by *H. influenzae* type b has decreased more than 99%.[2] In children older than 3 years and adults, meningitis caused by *H. influenzae* may indicate a parameningeal focus of infection such as middle ear infection, paranasal sinus infection, or CSF leakage. Spread of the organism occurs either through direct spread from infected sinuses, draining of these areas via the veins, or bacteremia originating from the local focus of infection.[53]

Since approximately 30% to 40% of *H. influenzae* are now ampicillin-resistant, a third-generation cephalosporin is recommended empirically until sensitivities are available. If the organism is then sensitive to ampicillin, the patient can be switched to ampicillin and the the the cephalosporin discontinued (A-1). Third-generation cephalosporins (cefotaxime and ceftriaxone) are active against β-lactamase–producing and non–β-lactamase–producing strains of *H. influenzae.* In addition, they are relatively free of toxicity, and do not require serum concentration monitoring. Cefepime (A-I) and fluoroquinolones (A-III) are suitable alternatives regardless of β-lactamase activity.

Secondary cases resulting from close contact with an index case occur within 30 days of the onset of disease. Close contacts, which include household members, individuals sharing sleeping quarters, daycare attendees, nursing home residents, and crowded, confined populations, may be at 200 to 1,000 times the risk of the general population for acquiring *H. influenzae* meningitis. The risk of acquiring *H. influenzae* meningitis is low without intimate contact with the index patient's respiratory secretions.[54]

❾ Prophylaxis is to protect close contacts from the index case by eliminating nasopharyngeal and oropharyngeal carriage of *H. influenzae.* Invasive disease should be reported to the local public health department and the CDC. Prophylaxis of close contacts should be started only after consultation with the local health department. In general, children should receive rifampin 20 mg/kg per day (maximum 600 mg) and adults 600 mg/day in one dose for 4 days. Any unvaccinated children between the ages of 12 and 48 months should receive one dose of the vaccine, whereas those between the ages of 2 and 11 months should be given three doses of the vaccine.[15] Individuals fully vaccinated are not recommended to receive prophylaxis.[26] Further discussion of who should receive prophylaxis is beyond the scope of this chapter; interested readers can refer to the recommendations of the American Academy of Pediatrics for that information.[55]

Vaccination includes a series of doses and usually is begun in children at 2 months of age. The DTaP/Hib combination vaccine (diphtheria, tetanus, acellular pertusis, *H. influenzae* type B) is also available as a booster following the Hib series. In addition to pediatric immunization, the vaccine also should be considered in patients older than 5 years of age with the following underlying conditions: sickle cell disease, asplenia, and immunocompromising diseases. Refer to Chapter 133 for further information on dosing and administration.

L. Monocytogenes

L. monocytogenes is a gram-positive diphtheroid-like organism responsible for 8% of all reported cases of meningitis. This disease primarily affects neonates, alcoholics, immunocompromised adults, and the elderly. Infections caused by *Listeria* in healthy individuals are extremely rare. *L. monocytogenes* is implicated in 20% of meningitis cases in those older than 60 years of age and carries a case-fatality rate of approximately 15%.[9]

Transmission usually involves colonization of the patient's gastrointestinal (GI) tract with the organisms, which then penetrate the gut lumen. Coleslaw, unpasteurized milk, Mexican-style soft cheese, ready-to-eat foods, and raw beef and poultry all have been identified as sources of this food-borne pathogen.[26] If a sufficient cell-mediated immune response (T-lymphocytes, macrophages) is not produced, bacteremia, meningitis, meningoencephalitis, or cerebritis may develop. Infection of the CNS may be diffuse or localized, possibly involving the cerebral hemispheres, thalamus, and brain stem. In immunocompromised hosts, approximately 75% of *L. monocytogenes* infections result in transmission into the CNS.[56]

Incidence of *L. monocytogenes* meningitis tends to peak in the summer and early fall. As with gram-negative meningitis, presentation may be subtle and insidious, and clinical suspicion should prompt lumbar puncture. *L. monocytogenes* produces primarily a mononuclear CSF response.[56] One common laboratory error seen with *L. monocytogenes* is a tendency to misidentify the organism on Gram stain as a diphtheroid, streptococcus, or a poorly staining gram-negative rod.

Treatment of *L. monocytogenes* meningitis with penicillin G or ampicillin may result in only a bacteriostatic effect and possible persistence of infection. Usually the combination of penicillin G or ampicillin with an aminoglycoside results in a bactericidal effect. Patients should be treated for 2 to 3 weeks after defervescence (A-III).[15] Combination therapy is usually employed for a minimum of 10 days, with the remaining course of therapy completed with penicillin G or ampicillin alone. Trimethoprim-sulfamethoxazole may be an effective alternative because adequate CSF penetration is achieved (A-III). Chloramphenicol and vancomycin both possess in vitro activity against *Listeria*, but they are not be recommended for use in meningitis caused by *L. monocytogenes* owing to unacceptably high failure rates.[34]

Gram-Negative Meningitis

During the last several years, the incidence of gram-negative bacillary meningitis, excluding *H. influenzae,* has been increasing in both children and adults. Enteric gram-negative organisms are the fourth leading cause of meningitis, with only *S. pneumoniae, H. influenzae,* and *N. meningitidis* having a higher incidence.

Several factors predispose patients to the development of gram-negative meningitis: congenital defects involving the CNS, accidental cranial trauma, neurosurgery, the use of antimicrobial agents with exclusive gram-positive activity preoperatively in neurosurgery, any form of communication between the skin and subarachnoid space (such as a dermal sinus), diabetes, malignancy, urinary tract infection in neonates, cirrhosis, parameningeal infection, spinal anesthesia, advanced age, immunosuppression, and hospitalization in general.

Elderly debilitated patients are at an increased risk of gram-negative meningitis but typically lack the classic signs and symptoms of the disease. Nuchal rigidity may be difficult to detect secondary to cervical arthritis. Presence of a low-grade fever and changes in mental status without other obvious cause should prompt consideration of meningitis and a lumbar puncture. Neonates are also at risk for gram-negative meningitis with *E. coli* and *Klebsiella pneumoniae,* which are responsible for 60% to 70% of cases.

Optimal antimicrobial therapies for gram-negative bacillary meningitis have not been fully defined. The therapy of gram-negative meningitis is complex because of the variety of organisms that can infect the CNS. The treatment of meningitis due to *P. aeruginosa* remains a unique problem because antibiotics showing good antibacterial activity against *P. aeruginosa,* such as antipseudomonal penicillins and aminoglycosides, penetrate the CSF poorly. Furthermore, many isolates of *P. aeruginosa* are resistant to multiple, if not all, commonly used agents, and this trend in resistance is increasing. Initially, cases of *P. aeruginosa* meningitis should be treated with an extended-spectrum β-lactam such as ceftazidime or cefepime (A-II), or alternativly piperacillin ± tazobactam, or meropenem plus an aminoglycoside, usually tobramycin.[2] Since aminoglycosides penetrate the CSF poorly, their inclusion is predominantly to aid in the treatment of extracerebral infections. If multidrug-resistant *Pseudomonas* is suspected initially, intraventricular administration of aminoglycoside should be considered along with intravenous administration. Preservative-free forms of gentamicin and tobramycin are available and should be used for direct administration into the CSF. Intraventricular aminoglycoside dosages should be adjusted to the estimated CSF volume (0.03 mg tobramycin or gentamicin per milliliter of CSF and 0.1 mg amikacin per milliliter of CSF every 24 hours). Since CSF flows unidirectionally with gravity, intraventricular aminoglycoside administration is more likely to produce therapeutic concentrations throughout the CSF than intrathecal administration. While intraventricular administration of aminoglycosides is considered for treatment of *P. aeruginosa* meningitis, this method produced higher mortality in a sample of infants treated for gram-negative bacillary meningitis.[22] Thus intraventricular administration of aminoglycosides to infants is not recommended routinely. Ventricular levels of aminoglycoside should be monitored every 2 or 3 days, just prior to the next intraventricular dose, and should approximate 2 to 10 mg/L. Interpretation of drug levels may be difficult because determinations often are contaminated with residual aminoglycoside from the preceding dose.

Multidrug-resistant *Pseudomonas* and *Acinetobacter* infections are of concern to clinicians because of the limited therapeutic options available for the treatment. This concern has led to the reemergence of the use of older antibiotics, such as colistin. Colistin can be used, both intravenously and intrathecally, in the treatment of multidrug-resistant *Pseudomonas* or *Acinetobacter* CNS infections.[57–59] Furthermore, there is synergistic activity with the combination of colistin and ceftazidime against multidrug-resistant *P. aeruginosa*.[60] The use of colistin should be reserved for only the most severe cases.

Other gram-negative organisms causing meningitis, excluding *P. aeruginosa* and *Acinetobacter* spp, most likely can be treated with a third or fourth-generation cephalosporin, such as cefotaxime, ceftriaxone, ceftazidime or cefepime. Ceftazidime, however, may not be the best choice of empirical antibiotic for situations where the offending organism is not known initially because CSF antibiotic concentrations greater than 10 times the minimal bactericidal concentration (MBC) may not be produced reliably for gram-positive organisms. In adults, daily doses of 8 to 12 g/day of third-generation cephalosporins (2 g twice a day of ceftriaxone) should produce CSF concentrations of 5 to 20 mg/L. Ceftriaxone is not recommended for use in the neonatal period because of the potential for the displacement of bilirubin from albumin-binding sites.[2] Cefotaxime should be used in place of ceftriaxone in this situation.

Trimethoprim-sulfamethoxazole is useful in the management of the Enterobacteriaceae family and also may be useful in the management of *L. monocytogenes*.[2,8] One advantage of trimethoprim-sulfamethoxazole is that its penetration into the CSF does not depend on meningeal inflammation. Trimethoprim-sulfamethoxazole is not, however, bactericidal. Trimethoprim-sulfamethoxazole produces CSF levels of 1.9 to 5.7 mg/L for the former and 20 to 63 mg/L for the latter when given parenterally in doses of 10 mg/kg per day (trimethoprim) and 50 mg/kg per day (sulfamethoxazole).

Fluoroquinolones have good penetration into the CSF and are effective in animal models of both gram-negative and gram-positive meningitis. However, there are limited data on the efficacy of fluoroquinolones in clinical practice. Ciprofloxacin is recommended as an alternative for the treatment of *E. coli* and other *Enterobacterianeae* as well as *Pseudomonas aeruginosa* (A-III). Cefepime and meropenem represent other therapeutic options for the treatment of gram-negative bacterial meningitis, as does aztreonam (A-III).[2,34]

CSF cultures may remain positive for several days or more with a regimen that eventually will be curative. Therapeutic efficacy can be monitored through bacterial colony counts every 2 or 3 days, which should decrease progressively over the period of therapy. Therapy for gram-negative meningitis should be continued for a minimum of 21 days from the start of treatment.[15]

Bacillus Anthracis

B. anthracis is a large, endospore-forming, aerobic, gram-positive bacteria capable of producing infection via the cutaneous, pulmonary, or GI routes. Cases of meningitis have been reported following both cutaneous and inhalational infection. Prior to the bioterrorism-related outbreak of 11 inhalational and 12 suspected or confirmed cases of cutaneous anthrax in 2001, only 18 sporadic cases had occurred in the United States in the 20th century, with the last occurrence in 1976.[61] However, since the terrorist attack on the United States on September 11, 2001, heightened awareness of biologic warfare agents, which include *B. anthracis*, has percolated throughout the United States.

The major neurologic complication of anthrax infection is fulminant, rapidly fatal hemorrhagic meningoencephalitis. The inhalational form of anthrax seems to be a potent inducer of neurologic symptoms, and death usually occurs within a week for those with neurologic complications.[61] Neurologic manifestations may be the initial symptoms leading to the diagnosis of anthrax. An index case of fatal inhalational anthrax from bioterrorism developed acute fever, emesis, disorientation, and confusion. A computed tomographic (CT) scan of the head showed no abnormalities, but spinal tap revealed cloudy CSF, low CSF glucose concentration, high CSF protein concentration, increased leukocytes in the CSF, and large gram-positive bacilli in chains. Shortly thereafter, the patient developed a generalized seizure and died on the third hospital day.[62]

Consistent findings in the CSF of anthrax meningitis cases include a low CSF glucose level, marked infiltration of WBCs into the CSF, and the presence of gram-positive bacilli in chains. High suspicion of anthrax meningitis is warranted in the additional presence of grossly visible blood or elevated red blood cell counts in the CSF with hemorrhagic changes on a CT scan. Recent molecular advances can aid in the rapid diagnosis of *B. anthracis* infections. Rapid PCR techniques, such as the Light Cycler (Roche Applied Science, Indianapolis, IN), can produce molecular confirmation for the presence of anthrax within 1 hour.[61] Extreme caution is warranted for diagnosis without the use of molecular techniques because *B. anthracis* can be confused easily with *B. cereus*, which is found commonly in soil and often considered a contaminant if identified.

B. anthracis typically is susceptible to penicillin, amoxicillin, erythromycin, doxycycline, ciprofloxacin, and chloramphenicol. The bioterrorism-related strain was susceptible to the fluoroquinolones, rifampin, tetracycline, vancomycin, imipenem, meropenem, chloramphenicol, clindamycin, and the aminoglycosides. However, the strain was resistant to third-generation cephalosporins and trimethoprim-sulfamethoxazole. Ciprofloxacin or doxycycline plus one or two of the aforementioned antibiotics is the currently recommended regimen for the treatment of inhalational anthrax, but doxycycline is not recommended for the treatment of anthrax meningitis owing to poor CNS penetration and recent in vitro resistance.[61]

Dexamethasone as an Adjunctive Treatment for Meningitis In addition to antibiotics, dexamethasone has become a commonly used therapy in the treatment of meningitis. Corticosteroids inhibit the production of TNF and IL-1, both potent proinflammatory cytokines. A series of clinical studies assessing the efficacy of corticosteroid therapy for the initial treatment of bacterial meningitis indicates conflicting results.[63–67] A fundamental problem with corticosteroid investigations to date is that the majority of patients in the trials had *H. influenzae* meningitis. While *H. influenzae* was the most commonly identified causative pathogen responsible for bacterial meningitis in the United States in 1986, the incidence of *H. influenzae* meningitis has decreased dramatically because of the introduction of polysaccharide conjugate vaccines. Additionally, the majority of studies examining dexamethasone use for pneumococcal meningitis were conducted before the widespread problem of penicillin-resistant pneumococcus had emerged, or in parts of the world where penicillin resistance is minimal. Whether or not steroids are beneficial in meningitis caused by penicillin-resistant *S. pneumoniae*, *N. meningitidis*, and group B streptococci is unclear at this time.

Significant improvement in markers of active infection, such as CSF levels of proinflammatory cytokines, as well as CSF protein, glucose, and lactate concentrations, have been shown after corticosteroid administration as adjunctive treatment.[14] Trials consistently detected a significantly lower incidence of neurologic sequelae commonly associated with bacterial meningitis with corticosteroid use. In trials that measured inflammatory mediators, lower levels of TNF, PAF, or IL-1 were detected in patients treated with dexamethasone.[63,64,67]

Most clinical trials on the use of adjunctive dexamethasone in bacterial meningitis have involved children. A retrospective analysis of pediatric patients with pneumococcal meningitis and one unblinded, noncontrolled trial suggested that adjunctive steroids may decrease the neurologic sequelae and mortality associated with *S. pneumoniae* meningitis.[63,68] A meta-analysis suggests that with the possible exception of hearing loss, dexamethasone does not protect against neurologic sequelae.[69] The protective effect of dexamethasone was observed to be strongest in those with meningitis due to *H. influenzae*.

❿ The American Academy of Pediatrics suggests that dexamethasone be considered for infants and children 2 months of age or older with pneumococcal meningitis (C-II) and be given to those with *H. influenzae* meningitis.[55,70] The recommended intravenous dose is 0.15 mg/kg every 6 hours for 4 days. Alternatively, prospective, randomized, double-blind studies have found dexamethasone 0.15 mg/kg every 6 hours for 2 days or dexamethasone 0.4 mg/kg every 12 hours for 2 days to be equally effective and potentially less toxic.[67,71] Dexamethasone should be administered prior to or with the first antibiotic dose and not after antibiotics already have been started (A-I).[14] Additionally, serum hemoglobin and stool guaiac should be monitored for evidence of GI bleeding.[64,66,68,71] Dexamethasone should not be used in neonates or any infant younger than 6 weeks of age.[14,22] The use of dexamethasone interferes with the interpretation of clinical response to treatment. For example, corticosteroid use interferes with the resolution of fever. Thus all infants and children are recommended to undergo a repeat lumbar puncture after 24 to 48 hours of treatment to verify CSF sterilization.[14]

Data supporting the use of corticosteroids in adults with meningitis is scarce. A prospective, randomized, double-blind multicenter study evaluated the use of adjuvant therapy plus dexamethasone compared with adjuvant therapy plus placebo in adults with acute bacterial meningitis.[72] Early treatment with dexamethasone improved clinical outcome in adults with bacterial meningitis, reducing the risk of both unfavorable outcome and death. However, the study did not show a beneficial effect of dexamethasone on neurologic sequelae, including hearing loss. Furthermore, a meta-analysis of five trials involving 623 adults with actue bacterial meningitis described a significant reduction in mortality in patiens treated with steroids and antibiotics compared to those treated with antibiotics alone. There was not however a significant reduction in neurologic sequelae, but this could have been limited by the sample size considering two of the five trials did not investigate neurologic complications. The safety and adverse events were similar between those who received steroids and those who did not.[73]

If pneumococcal meningitis is suspected or proven, it is recommended that adults receive dexamethasone 0.15 mg/kg every 6 hours for 2 to 4 days with the first dose administered 10 to 20 minutes prior to first dose of antibiotics. Patient outcome is unlikely to improve if dexamethasone is given after first dose of antibiotic and should therefore be avoided (A-I). It is often difficult to ascertain the responsible pathogen on presentation therefore some clinicians recommend initiating dexamethasone in all adult patients presenting with meningitis (B-III).

Routine use of dexamethasone in meningitis is not without controversy. A potential concern is that adjunctive dexamethasone therapy might reduce the penetration of antibiotics into the CSF by inhibiting meningeal inflammation. In experimental models of meningitis, steroids decreased the CSF concentrations of ampicillin, rifampin, vancomycin, and gentamicin.[67,74] Ceftriaxone and vancomycin penetration into CSF was unaffected by concurrent dexamethasone administration in pediatric patients.[75,76]

CLINICAL CONTROVERSY

Some clinicians believe that dexamethasone should be initiated in all patients over the age of 2 months with bacterial meningitis and continued for the recommended 2 to 4 days regardless of bacterial etiology. Others, however, believe corticosteroids have limited proven benefit in the treatment of non-pneumococcal meningitis and recommend stopping dexamethasone if another bacterial pathogen is identified.

Mycobacterium Tuberculosis

M. tuberculosis is the primary cause of tuberculous meningitis. Tuberculous meningitis is associated with significant morbidity and mortality and is difficult to diagnose in a timely manner. The most life-threatening form of extrapulmonary tuberculosis is tuberculous meningitis.[77] The epidemiology of tuberculous meningitis as a cause of extrapulmonary tuberculosis has changed. Between the years 1997 and 1990, an average of 193 cases of tuberculous meningitis were reported to the CDC, representing 4.7% of extrapulmonary cases. The number of cases reported in 1990 was 284, or 6.2% of extrapulmonary cases. This change is most likely secondary to HIV/AIDS and rising rates among minority adults leading to increased tuberculosis in their children.[78] The incidence of tuberculosis in general has increased 15% since 1985, and the increase is more substantial in children than in adults.[77]

The most useful clue to diagnose tuberculous meningitis is the presence of inflammation of the CSF in an individual who is at epidemiologic risk for tuberculosis. Although up to 40% of patients may present with evidence of pulmonary involvement with hilar adenopathy, tuberculous meningitis still may exist in the absence of disease in the lung or extrapulmonary sites. The tuberculin skin test (purified protein derivative [PPD]) is also negative in 5% to 50% of cases.[79]

On initial examination, CSF usually contains from 100 to 1,000 WBCs/mm³, which may be 75% to 80% polymorphonuclear cells. Over time, the pattern of WBCs in the CSF will shift to lymphocytes and monocytes (see Table 115–1). CSF glucose concentration may be normal initially but gradually decreases as the disease progresses.[79,80] Protein concentration within the CSF may be normal or elevated, with high protein levels shown to correlate with advanced disease.[79–81] CSF cultures often are positive for *M. tuberculosis* even if the patient is asymptomatic.

One potentially useful diagnostic sign unique to tuberculous meningitis is paralysis of the VI cranial nerve, which initially is unilateral and then progresses to bilateral.[30] Initial acid-fast bacilli (AFB) smears are approximately 37% sensitive and as high as 87% sensitive following subsequent smears. Sensitivity of the AFB smear is enhanced by the examination of multiple CSF specimens collected on consecutive days. Cultures of CSF are positive in 45% to 90% of cases depending on the quantity of CSF used in the culture, pathogen density, and experience of the laboratory in culturing *M. tuberculosis*. Some clinicians will obtain fluid from the base of the brain or the ventricles in an attempt to increase the yield. Positive culture results may take up to 8 weeks, providing little help with the initial diagnosis.[79,80] Several systems employing rapid broth culture (Organon Teknika MB/BacT, Organon Teknika, Durham, NC; ESP system, Trek Diagnostic Systems, Inc., Westlake, OH; and Bactec 9000 TB series or Bactec 460, Becton Dickinson Diagnostic Instruments, Sparks, MD) have considerably shortened the time to detection and are able to detect organisms in less than 3 weeks.[18] Nucleic acid amplification products, such as Amplicor (Roche) and MTD (Genprobe), allow for the direct identification of *M. tuberculosis* within 48 hours and yield higher sensitivity than a smear.

Unfortunately, the incidence of multidrug-resistant strains of *M. tuberculosis* has increased, necessitating the use of at least three antitubercular agents to treat active pulmonary disease. The CDC recommends an initial regimen of four drugs for empirical treatment of *M. tuberculosis*.[82] This regimen consists of isoniazid, rifampin, pyrazinamide, and ethambutol 15 to 20 mg/kg per day (maximum 1.6 g/day) for the first 2 months, generally followed by isoniazid plus rifampin for the remaining duration of therapy. The recommended therapy for HIV-positive individuals is the same as for immunocompetent patients, although rifabutin may be considered in place of other rifamycins in an effort to minimize drug interactions with protease inhibitors and nonnucleoside reverse-transcriptase inhibitors. Therapy in HIV-negative and HIV-positive patients should be individualized based on susceptibility patterns and guidelines from the CDC and the American Thoracic Society, which are updated frequently and available on the Internet (*www.cdc.gov/nchstp/tb/pubs/mmwrhtml/maj_guide.htm*). Patients with *M. tuberculosis* meningitis should be treated for 9 months or longer with multiple-drug therapy, and patients with rifampin-resistant strains should receive 18 to 24 months of therapy.

Isoniazid, the mainstay in virtually any regimen to treat *M. tuberculosis*, penetrates the CSF with or without meningeal inflammation and achieves concentrations of more than 30 times the MIC of *M. tuberculosis* (MICs of 0.05–0.2 mg/L).[56,79,80] Rifampin's penetration of CSF approximates only 20% of serum concentrations in the presence of meningeal inflammation. *M. tuberculosis* typically is so exquisitely sensitive to rifampin, however, that the low penetration ratio is of little clinical significance.[79,80,83] However, the incidence of *M. tuberculosis* resistance to rifampin has increased, necessitating empirical multiple-antibiotic regimens.

Pyrazinamide is a small molecule that penetrates the CSF well in the presence or absence of meningeal inflammation. Streptomycin, an aminoglycoside, penetrates the CSF poorly, even in the presence of meningeal inflammation. The incidence of resistance to streptomycin is increasing, and this drug should not be recommended unless susceptibility is known. Ethambutol is a weak antitubercular agent that reaches the CSF in moderate concentrations. Ethambutol's use is also limited by a high incidence of dose-related optic neuritis. Ethionamide and cycloserine are two other agents that sometimes are used to treat tuberculous meningitis. These agents both penetrate the CSF well in the absence of meningeal inflammation.[79,80]

The usual dose of isoniazid in children is 10 to 15 mg/kg per day (maximum 300 mg/day), and adults usually receive 5 mg/kg per day or a daily dose of 300 mg.[82] Supplemental doses of pyridoxine hydrochloride (vitamin B_6) 50 mg/day are recommended to prevent the peripheral neuropathy associated with isoniazid administration.[79,80] Concurrent administration of rifampin is recommended at doses of 10 to 20 mg/kg per day (maximum 600 mg/day) for children and 600 mg/day for adults. The addition of pyrazinamide (children and adults 15–30 mg/kg per day; maximum in both 2 g/day) to the regimen of isoniazid and rifampin is recommended.[82] Duration of concomitant pyrazinamide therapy generally should be limited to 2 months to avoid hepatotoxicity.

The role of steroids in the management of tuberculous meningitis remains unclear. The administration of oral prednisone 60 to 80 mg/day or 0.2 mg/kg per day of intravenous dexamethasone for adults and prednisone 1 to 2 mg/kg per day for children, tapered over 4 to 8 weeks, has been used in clinical practice. Corticosteroids improve neurologic sequelae and survival in adults and decrease mortality, long-term neurologic complications, and permanent sequelae in children. Concerns regarding the use of steroids include a possible interference with CSF chemistry studies and decreased penetration of antitubercular agents because of a decrease in inflammation. Despite the controversy, the trend toward an improved outcome generally supports their use for tuberculous meningitis.[84,85]

Tuberculous meningitis has a mortality rate of 10% to 50% despite early diagnosis and treatment.[79,80,86] The level of patient consciousness at the start of therapy is the most useful prognostic indicator. Patients who are comatose at the beginning of therapy have a mortality rate of approximately 75%.[80] Other negative prognostic factors include old age, poor nutrition, evidence of miliary disease, high initial CSF protein concentrations, presence of hydrocephalus, and evidence of elevated ICP.[80] Bewteen 10% and 30% of patients surviving the disease have physical or mental sequelae, including deafness, vertigo, and short-term memory loss.[79,80]

Cryptococcus Neoformans

Cryptococcal meningitis is the most common form of fungal CNS infection in the United States and is a major cause of morbidity and mortality in immunosuppressed patients. In the United States, 85% of cases occur in HIV-infected patients. *C. neoformans* is a soil fungus acquired by inhalation of spores from the environment leading to pneumonia, which is usually asymptomatic. Most patients present initially with disseminated disease, especially meningoencephalitis. The incubation period in AIDS patients may be very short, as opposed to a relatively normal host, in whom it may be very long.

Symptoms of cryptococcal meningitis are insidious and may be present for varying periods, depending on the host involved, before the definitive diagnosis is made. Fever and a history of headaches are the most common symptoms, although altered mentation and evidence of focal neurologic deficits may be present. Examination of the CSF usually reveals small numbers of WBCs (<150/mm^3), which are primarily lymphocytes (see Table 115–1). Diagnosis is based on the presence of a positive CSF, blood, sputum, or urine culture for *C. neoformans*. The CSF cultures are positive in more than 90% of cases. Organisms may be seen by microscope when stained with india ink and are more likely to be seen in AIDS patients compared with other hosts. An additional rapid test helpful in diagnosis is latex agglutination, which detects the presence of cryptococcal antigens.[89] Latex agglutination is positive in more than 90% of culture-positive cases. A cryptococcal antigen test can be used to follow the prognosis of non-AIDS patients, but cryptococcal antigen titers do not correlate well with treatment efficacy in AIDS patients.[88] A cryptococcal antigen detection test needs to be considered in any patient presenting initially with meningitis. Risk factors predictive of a poor outcome include lethargy at presentation, high CSF cryptococcal antigen titer, and low CSF WBC count.[89]

Despite poor penetration into the CSF, amphotericin B has long been the drug of choice for the treatment of acute *C. neoformans* meningitis. Amphotericin B 0.5 to 1 mg/kg per day combined with flucytosine 100 mg/kg per day is more effective than amphotericin alone, with successful outcomes in 75% of non-AIDS patients and

50% in AIDS patients.[90] Unfortunately, in the AIDS population, flucytosine is often poorly tolerated, causing bone marrow suppression and GI distress. Amphotericin B alone, although less effective, has been used in AIDS patients with preexisting granulocytopenia.[90,91] Because of the high acute mortality rate of up to 40% and a relapse rate of 50% in AIDS patients receiving therapy, many new agents and regimens are being investigated in this population.[89] A small, noncomparative open study evaluating the safety and efficacy of liposomal amphotericin B (AmBisome) found the product to be well tolerated and moderately effective.[92] A second study found high-dose liposomal amphotericin B (4 mg/kg) to clear CSF cultures more rapidly relative to standard amphotericin B, although clinical efficacy was not significantly different.[93]

Azole therapy is the most studied alternative regimen for the treatment of *C. neoformans* meningitis in AIDS patients. Fluconazole at doses of 200 mg/day was compared with amphotericin B alone (0.4 mg/kg/day) with no significant difference in overall mortality between groups. However, patients receiving fluconazole had a higher 2-week mortality rate and time to CSF conversion.[94] High-dose fluconazole therapy (800 mg/day) was tried as salvage therapy in eight AIDS patients who failed previous antifungal therapy, but success was limited.[95] A randomized trial in Thailand compared amphotericin B (0.7mg/kg daily), amphotericin B plus flucytosine (100mg/kg daily), amphotericin B plus fluconazole (400mg daily) and triple therapy with amphotericin B, flucytosine and fluconazole daily for the treatment of HIV-associated cryptococcal meningitis. The addition of fluconazole to the standard therapy of amphotericin B plus flucytosine resulted in less fungicidal activity against *C. neoformans* than the current standard of amphotericin B plus flucytosine.[96] Itraconazole 200 mg orally twice daily was less effective than amphotericin B plus flucytosine in a small nonblinded study.[97] Voriconazole has demonstrated good in vitro activity against *C. neoformans*, however there are currently no comparative data to suggest an improvement over fluconazole.[98] Posaconazole has demonstrated clinical activity against cryptococcal and other fungal infections of the CNS in patients with refractory disease or otherwise intolerant to standard antifungal agents. Posaconazole appeared well tolerated at oral doses of 800 mg/day divided.[99] More data is needed to determine what role the new azole antifungal agents will play in future treatment of cryptococcal meningitis.

Patients with AIDS often require lifelong maintenance or suppressive therapy because of high relapse rates following acute therapy for *C. neoformans*. A large multicenter, controlled trial compared fluconazole (200 mg/day) and amphotericin B (1 mg/kg/wk) in the prevention of relapse.[100] Two percent of patients receiving fluconazole versus 18% of patients on amphotericin B relapsed. In addition, the amphotericin B group had significantly more frequent bacterial infections, bacteremias, and drug-related toxicity.[100] Fluconazole is superior to itraconazole in the prevention of relapse.[101] Current guidelines for patients with AIDS-associated cryptococcal meningitis recommend 2 weeks of therapy with a combination of amphotericin B 0.7 to 1 mg/kg/day and flucytosine 100 mg/kg/day. This is often referred to as the induction phase and is followed by 8 weeks of fluconazole 400 mg/day as part of the consolidation phase. Therapy should then be continued thereafter with fluconazole 200 mg/day until immune reconstitution takes place. Guidelines for the prevention of opportunistic infections in HIV-infected persons are updated frequently and can be found at *www.aidsinfo.nih.gov*.

Viral Encephalitis

The epidemiology of viral encephalitis in the United States has changed dramatically since the mid-1960s because of the introduction of large-scale polio and mumps immunization programs.

In the United States, the incidence of mumps has decreased 98% between 1967 and 1985. Worldwide, mumps remains a causative agent of viral encephalitis in countries with low vaccination rates. Poliomyelitis, once a significant cause of encephalitis, is now confined to only a few less developed countries and likely soon will be eradicated as an infectious agent.

Nonpolio enteroviruses such as coxsackieviruses A and B, echoviruses, and enteroviruses 70 and 71 cause approximately 85% of all viral encephalitis cases.[102,103] The remaining 10% to 15% of viral encephalitis cases are caused by a variety of pathogens, such as arboviruses, adenoviruses, influenzae virus A and B, rotavirus, corona virus, cytomegalovirus, varicella-zoster, herpes simplex virus, Epstein-Barr virus, and lymphocytic choriomeningitis.[18,102] In the past, the St. Louis and LaCrosse viruses have been the most common cause of arbovirus encephalitis.[18] However, in 2002, the largest arboviral meningoencephalitis epidemic in the western hemisphere was caused by the West Nile Virus, accounting for 4,156 human cases of West Nile disease in 44 states and the District of Columbia.[104] To date, nearly 20,000 cases of West Nile disease and almost 800 deaths have been reported in the United States since surveillance began in 1999.[105]

Viral encephalitis is acquired primarily by hematogenous spread or, alternatively, by neuronal spread of the causative pathogen. After entry into the host, viral replication occurs, resulting in dissemination through the reticuloendothelial system or vasculature. Infection of the capillary endothelial cells and choroid plexus may provide a conduit for CNS infections. Viruses such as polio, herpes, and varicella-zoster virus also may gain access to the CNS by axonal retrograde transmission from peripheral nerve endings.[106] Once a virus gains access to the CNS, the course of infection depends on the virulence of the particular virus and the host immune response. Host response to aseptic CNS infections is mediated by a complex cascade of inflammatory cytokines in a manner similar to purulent meningitis. In contrast with purulent meningitis, host response to viral encephalitis is mediated primarily through cytotoxic T-lymphocytes. Although TNF is a prominent mediator in purulent bacterial meningitis, TNF concentrations are not increased in viral encephalitis, whereas increases in concentrations of IL-1 and interferon (INF)-α and -γ occur. TNF concentrations have been suggested as a diagnostic tool for differentiating between bacterial meningitis and viral encephalitis.[107] While cytokine assays are available for investigational use, they are not used routinely in the clinical diagnosis of viral encephalitis.

The clinical syndrome associated with viral encephalitis generally is independent of viral etiology and may vary depending on the patient's age. Common signs in adults include headache, mild fever (<40°C [<104°F]), nuchal rigidity, malaise, drowsiness, nausea, vomiting, and photophobia. Only fever and irritability may be evident in the infant, and meningitis must be ruled out as a cause of fever when no other localized findings are observed in a child. Duration of symptoms generally is 1 to 2 weeks, and specific manifestations outside the meninges also can occur depending on the viral etiology.

Laboratory examination of the CSF usually reveals a pleocytosis with 100 to 1,000 WBCs/mm³, which are primarily lymphocytic; however, 20% to 75% of patients with viral encephalitis may have a predominance of polymorphonuclear cells on initial examination of the CSF, especially in enteroviral meningitis.[90] On repeat lumbar puncture, 90% of patients presenting initially with a predominance of neutrophils experience a shift to a predominance of mononuclear cells. Other laboratory findings include normal to mildly elevated protein concentrations and normal or mildly reduced glucose concentrations (see Table 115–1).[102]

Historically, pathogens responsible for viral encephalitis were not identified.[108] Poor laboratory recovery of viral pathogens and limited treatment options for viral encephalitis made the need for specific identification of pathogens of questionable value. Advances in diagnostic laboratory techniques and the potential for decreased costs associated with longer duration of hospitalization for patients with unconfirmed viral encephalitis have led to a reevaluation of the need for confirmatory pathogen diagnosis.[109] When clinical signs warrant pathogen identification, appropriate laboratory diagnostic techniques, including PCR, should be undertaken. Molecular methods are preferred to conventional laboratory tests in the diagnosis of viral encephalitis owing to the ability to detect a specific virus in 30% to 70% of cases as compared with the 14% to 24% sensitivity of viral culture.[18]

Although there are numerous pathogenic causes of viral encephalitis, much of the clinical presentation, diagnosis, and treatment are similar. The most commonly isolated viral etiologies are described here.

Commonly, the incidence of enteroviral encephalitis peaks in late summer and continues into early fall. Enteroviruses are transmitted in the host via the fecal-oral route. Clinical presentation of enteroviral infection frequently is nonspecific and characterized by fever, nausea, vomiting, and malaise; however, GI symptoms may not be present. Following a prodrome of 1 to 2 days, headache, photophobia, and neck stiffness develop. Diagnosis can be confirmed by cell culture from the CSF, where the incidence of successful isolation has ranged from 40% to 80%.[107] In addition, enterovirus can be isolated from throat swabs (60%) and stool cultures (80%), but they are not necessarily diagnostic because the virus is shed in the stool for 1 to 2 weeks following infection.[108] Conversely, an enterovirus-specific reverse-transcriptase polymerase chain reaction (EV-PCR) test can provide prompt results within 24 hours with a sensitivity and a specificity of 100%.[110] Treatment for enteroviral encephalitis consists of supportive care, fluids, antipyretics, and analgesics. Generally, disease progression is self-limiting, and the patient recovers fully without long-term neurologic complications.

Both herpes simplex virus types 1 and 2 have been associated with infections of the CNS. Herpes simplex type 1 (HSV1) is associated with encephalitis in adults, whereas herpes simplex type 2 (HSV2) is associated predominantly with encephalitis in newborns.[103] An HSV infection of the CNS most likely is spread via retrograde movement from the dorsal root ganglion. Sexually active adults acquire herpes simplex meningitis during or after an attack of genital or rectal herpes. Although HSV2 frequently can be cultured from CSF, HSV1 cannot. As such, PCR may be more useful than culture in detecting infection with HSV; diagnosis is usually made by PCR, culture, or a 4-fold rise in complement-fixing antibody to the virus. Establishing the correct diagnosis as early as possible is paramount because mortality rates are between 50% and 85% without treatment, and unlike other viral encephalitides, specific and effective therapy is available. As a result, empirical therapy of suspected HSV encephalitis while laboratory results are pending is necessary. Additionally, a clinical decision to treat may need to be made regardless of test results.

Acyclovir is the drug of choice for herpes simplex encephalitis. In patients with normal renal function, acyclovir is usually administered as 10 mg/kg intravenously every 8 hours for 2 to 3 weeks.[103] Herpes virus resistance to acyclovir has been reported with increasing incidence, particularly from immunocompromised patients with prior or chronic exposures to acyclovir.[111] The alternative treatment for acyclovir-resistant herpes simplex virus is foscarnet.[103] The dose for patients with normal renal function is 40 mg/kg infused over 1 hour every 8 to 12 hours for 2 to 3 weeks. Ensuring adequate hydration is imperative. In addition, patients receiving foscarnet should be monitored for seizures related to alterations in plasma electrolyte levels.

Historically, the four most important arboviral pathogens in the United States were the St. Louis virus, the La Crosse virus, and the eastern and western equine viruses. However, the West Nile virus has been recognized as an emerging pathogen and has been implicated in an epidemic occurring in the United States since 1999. Transmission occurs through the bites of mosquitoes. Typically, an incubation period of 2 to 14 days precedes the onset of clinical symptoms. Infection of the brain tissue results in fever, headache, paralysis, and coma. While many patients have a benign presentation, symptomatic cases are associated with a higher degree of mortality. Mortality rates of 50% to 75% have been reported for eastern equine virus, whereas mortality rates for western equine and St. Louis viruses are 3% to 4% and 10% to 20%, respectively.[103,106] Treatment is supportive, including treatment for seizures and increased ICP, and in the majority of cases, the disease is self-limiting.[106]

Because of the recent epidemic in the United States, a separate discussion of the West Nile virus is warranted. Although West Nile virus is transmitted primarily by mosquitoes, transmission of the virus via blood products, organ transplantation, transplacental transfer, and breast milk has been documented.[104] Similar to the other arboviruses, the incubation period for West Nile virus ranges from 3 days to 2 weeks. West Nile virus infection is asymptomatic in most adults or causes a mild flulike syndrome characterized by fever, malaise, myalgia, and lymphadenopathy. Typically, less than 1% of patients develop neurologic disease, and approximately two-thirds have encephalitis, with the remainder having meningitis without encephalitis.[14] Many patients develop a maculopapular, erythematous rash, which is more common in children than in adults and is uncommon in other forms of viral encephalitis. The other neurologic manifestations include fever, nausea, vomiting, headache, altered mental status, movement disorders, and/or a syndrome much like poliomyelitis.[14,112,113] The primary risk factor for this manifestation seems to be advanced age. The poliomyelitis syndrome is characterized by an early prodromic phase of fevers and weakness followed by the sudden onset of flaccid paralysis. Among patients hospitalized with West Nile virus, the mortality rate is approximately 10% to 15%, whereas patients with encephalitis and weakness have a mortality rate of 30%. CSF examination of West Nile virus encephalitis typically shows pleocytosis and a slightly elevated CSF protein concentration.[14] Several diagnostic methods have been developed for West Nile virus, including a PCR assay and enzyme-linked immunosorbent assay (ELISA) tests. However, serologic tests (ELISA) can cross-react with other flaviviruses causing a false-positive result. Moreover, the IgM antibodies for West Nile virus can persist for up to 1 year, leading to confusion regarding whether the infection is an acute or previous infection.[14] Ribavirin has shown inhibitory effects on the West Nile virus in neural tissue cultures, but this has not been studied in controlled trials.

HIV encephalitis is the most common CNS complication associated with AIDS. Frequently, patients may complain of headache, photophobia, or stiff neck at the time of presumed seroconversion. As the disease progresses, however, neurologic symptoms are reported frequently secondary to other opportunistic infections. Diagnosis of viral encephalitis is difficult because mental status and neurologic examinations are not sensitive enough to detect early changes. Direct evidence of HIV encephalitis can be obtained through CSF culture, p24 antigen testing, or qualitative or quantitative PCR for HIV RNA. Diagnostic workup of other potential copathogens, such as herpes simplex virus (HSV), *Toxoplasma gondii*, *M. tuberculosis*, *Aspergillus* spp, and *Cryptococcus* also should be performed. Refer to Chapter 134 for a complete discussion of infectious complications in HIV-positive individuals.

EVALUATION OF THERAPEUTIC OUTCOMES

SIGNS AND SYMPTOMS

Because of the potential for rapid deterioration associated with meningitis, signs and symptoms of fever, headache, meningismus (e.g., nuchal rigidity, Brudzinski's or Kernig's sign), vital signs, and signs of cerebral dysfunction should be evaluated every 4 hours for the initial 3 days and then daily thereafter. The Glasgow Coma Scale should be used in severely ill patients. Trends in improvement and resolution rather than single evaluations in time are more important in monitoring the signs and symptoms of meningitis.

MICROBIOLOGIC FINDINGS

CSF and blood samples for Gram stain, cultures, and sensitivity testing should be taken prior to starting antibiotic therapy. If lumbar puncture is delayed, however, antibiotics should be started. Although the CSF cultures may be negative, antibiotic therapy rarely interferes with the protein and/or glucose concentrations in the CSF.[15] Furthermore, if the laboratory is made aware of the antibiotic therapy, steps can be taken to diminish the effects of the antibiotic during the detection process.[18] Gram stain results can be obtained immediately and can guide empirical antibiotic treatment. Identification of the organism can be made within 24 hours, and sensitivities should be available within 48 hours. Repeat cultures should be performed to help determine if sterilization is achieved. A second tube of blood should be taken to allow for latex agglutination tests of antigens to common meningeal pathogens (*H. influenzae, S. pneumoniae, N. meningitidis, E. coli,* and group B streptococcus) if the Gram stain has not been helpful.

CSF EXAMINATION

In bacterial meningitis, the CSF WBC count usually is greater than 1,000 cells/mm^3, the CSF protein concentration is elevated, and the CSF glucose concentration (hypoglycorachia) is often low (<50 mg/dL or 50%–60% of a simultaneous blood glucose value). Viral encephalitis, in contrast, results in relatively normal CSF protein and glucose levels and typically does not result in greater than 90% polymorphonuclear neutrophils (PMNs) in the CSF (see Table 115–1).

ABBREVIATIONS

AFB: acid-fast bacilli

AIDS: acquired immunodeficiency syndrome

BBB: blood–brain barrier

BCSFB: blood–cerebrospinal fluid barrier

CBF: cerebral blood flow

CDC: U.S. Centers for Disease Control and Prevention

CFU: colony forming unit

CNS: central nervous system

CSF: cerebrospinal fluid

CT: computed tomography

DIC: disseminated intravascular coagulation

EV-PCR: enterovirus-specific reverse-transcriptase polymerase chain reaction

FDA: U.S. Food and Drug Administration

GI: gastrointestinal

Hib: *H. influenzae* type b

HIV: human immunodeficiency virus

ICP: intracranial pressure

IL-1: interleukin 1

INF: interferon

LPS: lipopolysaccharide

MBC: minimum bactericidal concentration

MIC: minimum inhibitory concentration

NCCLS: National Committee for Clinical Laboratory Standards

PAF: platelet-activating factor

PCR: polymerase chain reaction

PGE$_2$: prostaglandin E$_2$

PPD: purified protein derivative

TNF: tumor necrosis factor

WBC: white blood cell

REFERENCES

1. Scheld WM, Koedel U, Nathan B et al. Pathophysiology of bacterial meningitis: Mechanism(s) of neuronal injury. J Infect Dis 2002;186(Suppl 2):S225–S233.
2. Saez-Llorens X, McCracken Jr GH. Bacterial meningitis in children. Lancet 2003;361:2139–2148.
3. van de Beek D, de Gans J, Spanjaard L, et al. Clinical features and prognostic factors in adults with bacterial meningitis. N Engl J Med 2004;351:1849–1859.
4. Meli DN, Christen S, Leib SL, et al. Current concepts in the pathogenesis of meningitis caused by *Streptococcus pneumoniae.* Curr Opin Infect Dis 2002;15:253–257.
5. Kim KS. Pathogenesis of bacterial meningitis: from bacteraemia to neuronal injury. Nature Rev Neurosci 2003;4:376–385.
6. Gold R. Epidemiology of bacterial meningitis. Infect Dis Clin North Am 1999;13:515–525, v.
7. Reefhuis J, Honein MA, Whitney CG, et al. Risk of bacterial meningitis in children with cochlear implants. N Engl J Med 2003;349:435–445.
8. Parodi S, Lechner A, Osih R et al. Nosocomial enterobacter meningitis: risk factors, management, and treatment outcomes. Clin Infect Dis 2003;37:159–166.
9. Schuchat A, Robinson K, Wenger JD, et al. Bacterial meningitis in the United States in 1995. Active Surveillance Team. N Engl J Med 1997;337:970–976.
10. Whitney CG, Farley MM, Hadler J et al. Decline in invasive pneumococcal disease after the introduction of protein-polysaccharide conjugate vaccine. N Engl J Med 2003;348:1737–1746.
11. Bleck TP, Greenlee JE. Anatomic considerations in central nervous system infections. In: Mandell GL, Bennett JE, Dolin R, eds. Principles and Practice of Infectious Diseases, 5th ed. New York: Churchill Livingstone, 2000:950–959.
12. Spector R, Lorenzo AV. Inhibition of penicillin transport from the cerebrospinal fluid after intracisternal inoculation of bacteria. J Clin Invest 1974;54:316–325.
13. Leib SL, Tauber MG. Pathogenesis of bacterial meningitis. Infect Dis Clin North Am 1999;13:527–548.
14. Bonthius DJ, Karacay B. Meningitis and encephalitis in children: an update. Neurol Clin North Am 2002;20:1013–1038.
15. Bashir HE, Laundy M, Booy R. Diagnosis and treatment of bacterial meningitis. Arch Dis Child 2003;88:615–620.
16. Thomas KE, Hasbun R, Jekel J, et al. The diagnostic accuracy of Kernig's sign, Brudzinski's sign, and nuchal rigidity in adults with suspected meningitis. Clin Infect Dis 2002;35:46–52.
17. Kaplan SL. Clinical presentations, diagnosis, and prognostic factors of bacterial meningitis. Infect Dis Clin North Am 1999;13:579–593.
18. Thomson RB, Bertram H. Laboratory diagnosis of central nervous system infections. Infect Dis Clin North Am 2001;15:1047–1071.

19. van Crevel H, Hijdra A, de Gans J. Lumbar puncture and the risk of herniation: when should we first perform CT? J Neurol 2002;249: 129–137.

20. Hasbun R, Abrahams J, Jekel J, et al. Computed tomography of the head before lumbar puncture in adults with suspected meningitis. N Engl J Med 2001;345:1727–1733.

21. Proulx N, Frechette D, Toye B, et al. Delays in the administration of antibiotics are associated with mortality from adult acute bacterial meningitis. QJM 2005;98:291–298.

22. Heath PT, Yusoff NK, Baker CJ. Neonatal meningitis. Arch Dis Child Fetal Neonatal Ed 2003;88:F173–F178.

23. Prins JM, van Deventer SJ, Kuijper EJ, et al. Clinical relevance of antibiotic-induced endotoxin release. Antimicrob Agents Chemother 1994;38:1211–1218.

24. Shepard CW, Rosenstein NE, Fischer M. Neonatal meningococcal disease in the United States, 1990 to 1999. Pediatr Infect Dis J 2003;22:418–422.

25. Gold R. Epidemiology of bacterial meningitis. Infect Dis Clin North Am 1999;13:515–525, v.

26. Spach DH, Jackson LA. Bacterial meningitis. Neurologic Clin 1999;17:711–735.

27. Moura AS, Mendez AP, Layton M, et al. Epidemiology of meningococcal disease, New York City, 1989–2000. Emerg Infect Dis 2003;9: 355–361.

28. Rosenstein NE, Perkins BA, Stephens DS, et al. The changing epidemiology of meningococcal disease in the United States. J Infect Dis 1999;180:1894–1901.

29. Kelleher JA, Raebel MA. Meningococcal vaccine use in college students. Ann Pharmacother 2002;36:1776–1784.

30. Weinstein L. Bacterial meningitis. Specific etiologic diagnosis on the basis of distinctive epidemiologic, pathogenetic, and clinical features. Med Clin North Am 1985;69:219–229.

31. Klugman KP, Madhi SA. Emergence of drug resistance. Impact on bacterial meningitis. Infect Dis Clin North Am 1999;13:637–646, vii.

32. Glodani LZ. Inducement of Neisseria meningitidis resistance to ampicillin and penicillin in a patient with meningococcemia treated with high doses of ampicillin. Clin Infect Dis 1998;26:772.

33. Casado-Flores J, Osona B, Domingo P, et al. Meningococcal meningitis during penicillin therapy for meningococcemia. Clin Infect Dis 1997;25:1479.

34. Chowdhury MH, Tunkel AR. Antibacterial agents in infections of the central nervous system. Infect Dis Clin North Am 2000;14:391–407.

35. Schwartz B. Chemoprophylaxis for bacterial infections: principles of and application to meningococcal infections. Rev Infect Dis 1991;13(Suppl 2):S170–S173.

36. Bilukha OO, Rosenstein N. Prevention and control of meningococcal disease. Recommendations of the Advisory Committee on Immunization Practices (ACIP). MMWR Morb Mortal Wkly Rep 2005;54(RR-07):1–21.

37. Kaplan SL. Management of pneumococcal meningitis. Pediatr Infect Dis J 2002;21:589–591.

38. Aronin SI. Current pharmacotherapy of pneumococcal meningitis. Expert Opin Pharmacother 2002;3:121–129.

39. Kastanbauer S, Pfister HW. Pneumococcal meningitis in adults. Brain 2003;126:1015–1025.

40. Kaplan SL. Clinical presentations, diagnosis, and prognostic factors of bacterial meningitis. Infect Dis Clin North Am 1999;13:579–593.

41. Mitchell L, Tuomanen E. Vancomycin-tolerant Streptococcus pneumoniae and its clinical significance. Pediatr Infect Dis J 2001;20:531–533.

42. Novak R, Henriques B, Charpentier E, et al. Emergence of vancomycin tolerante in Streptococcus pneumoniae. Nature 1999;399:590–593.

43. Ross GH, Wright DH, Ibrahim KH, et al. Use of fluoroquinolones in central nervous system infections. J Infect Dis Pharmacother 2001;4:47–72.

44. Faella F, Pagliano P, Fusco U, et al. Combined treatment with ceftriaxone and linezolid of pneumococcal meningitis: a case series including penicillin-resistant strains. Clin Microbiol Infect 2006;12:391–394.

45. Cottagnoud P, Pfister M, Acosta F, et al. Daptomycin is highly efficacious against penicillin-resistant and penicillin- and quinolone-resistant pneumococci in experimental meningitis. Antimicrob Agents Chemother 2004;48:3928–3933.

46. Stucki A, Cottagnoud M, Winkelmann V, et al. Daptomycin produces an enhanced bactericidal activity compared to ceftriaxone, measured by [³H]choline release in the cerebrospinal fluid, in experimental meningitis due to a penicillin-resistant pneumococcal strain without lysing its cell wall. Antimicrob Agents Chemother 2007;51(6):2249–2252.

47. Centers for Disease Control and Prevention. Prevention of pneumococcal disease: recommendations of the advisory committee on immunization practices. MMWR 1997;46(RR-08):1–24.

48. Black S, Shinefield H, Fireman B, et al. Efficacy, safety and immunogenicity of heptavalent pneumococcal conjugate vaccine in children. Northern California Kaiser Permanente Vaccine Study Center Group [see comments]. Pediatr Infect Dis J 2000;19:187–195.

49. Shinefield H, Black S, Ray P, et al. Efficacy, immunogenicity and safety of heptavalent pneumococcal conjugate vaccine in low birth weight and preterm infants. Pediatr Infect Dis J 2002;21:182–186.

50. Black S, Shinefield H. Safety and efficacy of the seven-valent pneumococcal conjugate vaccine: evidence from Northern California. Eur J Pediatr 2002;161(Suppl 2):S127–S131.

51. Lieu TA, Ray GT, Black SB, et al. Projected cost-effectiveness of pneumococcal conjugate vaccination of healthy infants and young children. JAMA 2000;283:1460–1468.

52. Centers for Disease Control and Prevention. Pneumococcal vaccination for cochlear implant candidates and recipients: updated recommendations of the Advisory Committee on Immunization Practices. MMWR 2003;52(31):739–740.

53. Tang LM, Chen ST, Wu YR. Haemophilus influenzae meningitis in adults. Diagn Microbiol Infect Dis 1998;32:27–32.

54. Lieberman JM, Greenberg DP, Ward JI. Prevention of bacterial meningitis. Vaccines and chemoprophylaxis. Infect Dis Clin North Am 1990;4:703–729.

55. Pediatrics AA. Haemophilus influenzae infections. In: 2000 Red Book: Report of the Committee on Infectious Diseases, 25th ed. Pickering LK, ed. Elk Grove Village, IL: American Academy of Pediatrics, 2000: 262–272.

56. Rubin RH, Hooper DC. Central nervous system infection in the compromised host. Med Clin North Am 1985;69:281–296.

57. Levin AS, Barone AA, Penco J, et al. Intravenous colistin therapy for nosocomial infections caused by multidrug-resistant Pseudomonas aeruginosa and Acinetobacter baumannii. Clin Infect Dis 1999;28: 1008–1011.

58. Jimenez-Mejias ME, Pichardo-Guerrero C, Marquez-Rivas FJ, et al. Cerebrospinal fluid penetration and pharmacokinetic/pharmacodynamic parameters of intravenously administered colistin in a case of multidrug-resistant Acinetobacter baumannii meningitis. Eur J Clin Microbiol Infect Dis 2002;21:212–214.

59. Vasen W, Desmery P, Ilutovich S, et al. Intrathecal use of colistin. J Clin Microbiol 2000;38:3523.

60. Gunderson BW, Ibrahim KH, Hovde LB, et al. Synergistic activity of colistin and ceftazidime against multiantibiotic-resistant Pseudomonas aeruginosa in an in vitro pharmacodynamic model. Antimicrob Agents Chemother 2003;47:905–909.

61. Meyer MA. Neurologic complications of anthrax. Arch Neurol 2003;60:483–488.

62. Bush LM, Abrams BH, Beall A, et al. Index case of fatal inhalational anthrax due to bioterrorism in the United States. N Engl J Med 2001;345:1607–1610.

63. Girgis NI, Farid Z, Mikhail IA, et al. Dexamethasone treatment for bacterial meningitis in children and adults. Pediatr Infect Dis J 1989;8:848–851.

64. Lebel MH, Freij BJ, Syrogiannopoulos GA, et al. Dexamethasone therapy for bacterial meningitis. Results of two double-blind, placebo-controlled trials. N Engl J Med 1988;319:964–971.

65. Lebel MH, Hoyt MJ, Waagner DC, et al. Magnetic resonance imaging and dexamethasone therapy for bacterial meningitis. Am J Dis Child 1989;143:301–306.

66. Odio CM, Faingezicht I, Paris M, et al. The beneficial effects of early dexamethasone administration in infants and children with bacterial meningitis [see comments]. N Engl J Med 1991;324:1525–1531.

67. Schaad UB, Lips U, Gnehm HE, et al. Dexamethasone therapy for bacterial meningitis in children. Swiss Meningitis Study Group. Lancet 1993;342(8869):457–461.

68. Kennedy WA, Hoyt MJ, McCracken GH Jr. The role of corticosteroid therapy in children with pneumococcal meningitis. Am J Dis Child 1991;145:1374–1378.

69. McIntyre PB, Berkey CS, King SM, et al. Dexamethasone as adjunctive therapy in bacterial meningitis. A meta-analysis of randomized clinical trials since 1988. JAMA 1997;278:925–931.

70. Pediatrics AAP. Pneumococcal infections. In: 2000 Red Book: Report of the Committee on Infectious Diseases, 25th ed. Pickering LK, ed. Elk Grove Village, IL: American Academy of Pediatrics, 2000:452–460.

71. Syrogiannopoulos GA, Lourida AN, Theodoridou MC, et al. Dexamethasone therapy for bacterial meningitis in children: 2- versus 4-day regimen. J Infect Dis 1994;169:853–858.

72. De Gans J, Van De Beek D. Dexamethaxone in adults with bacterial meningitis. N Engl J Med 2002;347:1549–1556.

73. van de Beek D, de Gans J, McIntyre P, et al. Steroids in adults with acute bacterial meningitis: a systematic review. Lancet Infect Dis 2004;4:139–143.

74. Paris MM, Hickey SM, Uscher MI, et al. Effect of dexamethasone on therapy of experimental penicillin- and cephalosporin-resistant pneumococcal meningitis. Antimicrob Agents Chemother 1994;38:1320–1324.

75. Klugman KP, Friedland IR, Bradley JS. Bactericidal activity against cephalosporin-resistant Streptococcus pneumoniae in cerebrospinal fluid of children with acute bacterial meningitis. Antimicrob Agents Chemother 1995;39:1988–1992.

76. Gaillard JL, Abadie V, Cheron G, et al. Concentrations of ceftriaxone in cerebrospinal fluid of children with meningitis receiving dexamethasone therapy. Antimicrob Agents Chemother 1994;38:1209–1210.

77. Tung YR, Lai MC, Lui CC, et al. Tuberculous meningitis in infancy. Pediatr Neurol 2002;27:262–266.

78. Iseman MD. Extrapulmonary tuberculosis in adults. In: A Clinician's Guide to Tuberculosis. Iseman MD, ed. Philadelphia, PA: Lippincott Williams & Wilkins, 2000:145–197.

79. Leonard JM, Des Prez RM. Tuberculous meningitis. Infect Dis Clin North Am 1990;4:769–787.

80. Holdiness MR. Management of tuberculosis meningitis. Drugs 1990;39:224–233.

81. Kent SJ, Crowe SM, Yung A, et al. Tuberculous meningitis: a 30-year review [see comments]. Clin Infect Dis 1993;17:987–994.

82. Centers for Disease Control and Prevention. Treatment of tuberculosis. MMWR 2003;52(RR11):1–77.

83. Ellard GA, Humphries MJ, Allen BW. Cerebrospinal fluid drug concentrations and the treatment of tuberculous meningitis. Amn Rev Resp Dis 1993;148:650–655.

84. Byrd T, Zinser P. Tuberculosis meningitis. Curr Treat Options Neurol 2001;3:427–432.

85. Waecker NJ. Tuberculosis meningitis in children. Curr Treat Options Neurol 2002;4:249–257.

86. Alzeer AH, FitzGerald JM. Corticosteroids and tuberculosis: risks and use as adjunct therapy [see comments]. Tuber Lung Dis 1993;74:6–11.

87. Sugar AM, Stern JJ, Dupont B. Overview: treatment of cryptococcal meningitis. Rev Infect Dis 1990;12(Suppl 3):S338–S348.

88. Powderly WG, Cloud GA, Dismukes WE, et al. Measurement of cryptococcal antigen in serum and cerebrospinal fluid: value in the management of AIDS-associated cryptococcal meningitis. Clin Infect Dis 1994;18:789–792.

89. Powderly WG, Saag MS, Cloud GA, et al. A controlled trial of fluconazole or amphotericin B to prevent relapse of cryptococcal meningitis in patients with the acquired immunodeficiency syndrome. The NIAID AIDS Clinical Trials Group and Mycoses Study Group [see comments]. N Engl J Med 1992;326:793–798.

90. Bennett JE, Dismukes WE, Duma RJ, et al. A comparison of amphotericin B alone and combined with flucytosine in the treatment of cryptoccal meningitis. N Engl J Med 1979;301:126–131.

91. Chuck SL, Sande MA. Infections with Cryptococcus neoformans in the acquired immunodeficiency syndrome [see comments]. N Engl J Med 1989;321:794–799.

92. Coker RJ, Viviani M, Gazzard BG, et al. Treatment of cryptococcosis with liposomal amphotericin B (AmBisome) in 23 patients with AIDS. Aids 1993;7:829–835.

93. Leenders AC, Reiss P, Portegies P, et al. Liposomal amphotericin B (AmBisome) compared with amphotericin B both followed by oral fluconazole in the treatment of AIDS-associated cryptococcal meningitis. AIDS 1997;11:1463–1471.

94. Saag MS, Powderly WG, Cloud GA, et al. Comparison of amphotericin B with fluconazole in the treatment of acute AIDS-associated cryptococcal meningitis. The NIAID Mycoses Study Group and the AIDS Clinical Trials Group [see comments]. N Engl J Med 1992;326:83–89.

95. Berry AJ, Rinaldi MG, Graybill JR. Use of high-dose fluconazole as salvage therapy for cryptococcal meningitis in patients with AIDS. Antimicrob Agents Chemother 1992;36:690–692.

96. Brouwer AE, Rajanuwong A, Chierakul W, et al. Combination antifungal therapies for HIV-associated cryptococcal meningitis: a randomised trial. Lancet 2004;363(9423):1764–1767.

97. de Gans J, Portegies P, Tiessens G, et al. Itraconazole compared with amphotericin B plus flucytosine in AIDS patients with cryptococcal meningitis. AIDS 1992;6:185–190.

98. Pfaller MA, Messer SA, Boyken L, et al. Global trends in the antifungal susceptibility of Cryptococcus neoformans (1990 to 2004). J Clin Microbiol 2005;43:2163–2167.

99. Pitisuttithum P, Negroni R, Graybill JR, et al. Activity of posaconazole in the treatment of central nervous system fungal infections. J Antimicrob Chemother 2005;56(4):745–755.

100. Powderly WG. Therapy for cryptococcal meningitis in patients with AIDS. Clin Infect Dis 1992;14(Suppl 1):S54–S59.

101. Saag MS, Cloud GA, Graybill JR, et al. A comparison of itraconazole versus fluconazole as maintenance therapy of AIDS-associated cryptococcal meningitis. Clin Infect Dis 1999;28:291–296.

102. Maxson S, Jacobs RF. Viral meningitis. Tips to rapidly diagnose treatable causes. Postgrad Med 1993;93:153–156, 159–160, 163–166.

103. Roos KL. Encephalitis. Neurol Clin 1999;17:813–833.

104. Centers for Disease Control and Prevention. Epidemic/epizootic West Nile Virus in the United States: Guidelines for surveillance, prevention, and control. National Center for Infectious Diseases, Division of Vector-Borne Infectious Diseases; 2003. http://www.cdc.gov/ncidod/dvbid/arbor/wn_surv_guide_mar_2000.pdf.

105. Centers for Disease Control and Prevention. Summary of West Nile Virus Activity, United States 2005. National Center for Infectious Diseases, Division of Vector-Borne Infectious Diseases; 2006. http://www.cdc.gov/ncidod/dvbid/westnile/conf/2006pdf/2006wnvsumm_ecf_final.pdf.

106. Rubeiz H, Roos RP. Viral meningitis and encephalitis. Sem Neurol 1992;12(3):165–177.

107. Glimaker M. Enteroviral meningitis. Diagnostic methods and aspects on the distinction from bacterial meningitis. Scand J Infect Dis Suppl 1992;85:1–64.

108. Overall JC Jr. Is it bacterial or viral? Laboratory differentiation. Pediatr Rev 1993;14:251–261.

109. Dalton M, Newton RW. Aseptic meningitis. Dev Med Child Neurol 1991;33:446–451.

110. Sawyer MH, Holland D, Aintablian N, et al. Diagnosis of enteroviral central nervous system infection by polymerase chain reaction during a large community outbreak. Pediatr Infect Dis J 1994;13:177–182.

111. Gateley A, Gander RM, Johnson PC, et al. Herpes simplex virus type 2 meningoencephalitis resistant to acyclovir in a patient with AIDS. J Infect Dis 1990;161:711–715.

112. Kelley TW, Prayson RA, Ruiz AI, et al. The neuropathology of West Nile virus meningoencephalitis. Am J Clin Pathol 2003;119:749–753.

113. Sejvar JJ, Haddad MB, Tierney BC, et al. Neurologic manifestations and outcome of West Nile virus infection. JAMA 2003;290:511–515.

114. Salmon JH. Ventriculitis complicating meningitis. Am J Dis Child 1972;124:35–40.

115. Wald SL, McLaurin RL. Cerebrospinal fluid antibiotic levels during treatment of shunt infections. J Neurosurg 1980;52:41–46.

116. McLaurin RL. Infected cerebrospinal fluid shunts. Surg Neurol 1973;1:191–195.

117. Sells CJ, Shurtleff DB, Loeser JD. Gram-negative cerebrospinal fluid shunt-associated infections. Pediatrics 1977;59:614–618.

118. Kaiser AB, McGee ZA. Aminoglycoside therapy of gram-negative bacillary meningitis. N Engl J Med 1975;293:1215–1220.

119. Williamson JC, Glazier SS, Peacock JE. Successful treatment of ventriculostomy-related meningitis caused by vancomycin-resistant Enterococcus with intravenous and intraventricular quinupristin/dalfopristin. Clin Neurol Neurosurg 2002;104:54–56.

120. Congeni B, Tan J, Salstrom S. Kinetics of vancomycin after intraventricular and intravenous administration. Pediatr Res 1979;13:459–463.

121. Pau AK, Smego RA Jr, Fisher MA. Intraventricular vancomycin: Observations of tolerance and pharmacokinetics in two infants with ventricular shunt infections. Pediatr Infect Dis 1986;5:93–96.

122. Visconti EB, Peter G. Vancomycin treatment of cerebrospinal fluid shunt infections: Report of two cases. J Neurosurg 1979;51:245–246.

123. Wen DY, Bottini AG, Hall WA, et al. Infections in neurologic surgery: The intraventricular use of antibiotics. Neurosurg Clin North Am 1992;3:343–354.

CHAPTER

116

Lower Respiratory Tract Infections

MARTHA G. BLACKFORD, MARK L. GLOVER, AND MICHAEL D. REED

KEY CONCEPTS

❶ Respiratory infections remain the major cause of morbidity from acute illness in the United States and likely represent the most common reasons why patients seek medical attention.

❷ The majority of pulmonary infections follow colonization of the upper respiratory tract with potential pathogens, whereas microbes less commonly gain access to the lungs via the blood from an extrapulmonary source or by inhalation of infected aerosol particles. The competency of a patient's immune status is an important factor influencing the susceptibility to infection, etiologic cause, and disease severity.

❸ An appropriate treatment regimen for the patient with uncomplicated lower respiratory tract infection can be established by following the patient history, physical examination, chest radiograph, and properly collected sputum for culture and interpreted in light of current knowledge of the most common lung pathogens and their antibiotic susceptibility patterns within the community.

❹ Acute bronchitis is caused most commonly by respiratory viruses and almost always is self-limiting. Therapy targets associated symptoms, such as lethargy, malaise, or fever (ibuprofen or acetaminophen), and fluids for rehydration. Routine use of antibiotics should be avoided and medication to suppress cough is rarely indicated.

❺ Chronic bronchitis is caused by several interacting factors, including inhalation of noxious agents (most prominent are cigarette smoke and exposure to occupational dusts, fumes, and environmental pollution) and host factors including genetic factors and bacterial (and possibly viral) infections. The hallmark of this disease is a chronic cough, excessive sputum production, and expectoration with persistent presence of microorganisms in the patient's sputum.

❻ Treatment of acute exacerbations of chronic bronchitis includes attempts to mobilize and enhance sputum expectoration (chest physiotherapy, humidification of inspired air), oxygen if needed, aerosolized bronchodilators (albuterol) in select patients with demonstrated benefit, and antibiotics.

❼ Respiratory syncytial virus is the most common cause of acute bronchiolitis, an infection that mostly affects infants during

their first year of life. In the well infant, bronchiolitis usually is a self-limiting viral illness, whereas in the child with underlying respiratory disease, cardiac disease, or both, the child may develop severe respiratory compromise (failure) necessitating in-hospital treatment, such as rehydration, oxygen, and, in select patients, bronchodilators, ribavirin aerosol, or both.

❽ The most prominent pathogen causing community-acquired pneumonia in otherwise healthy adults is *S. pneumoniae*, whereas the most common pathogens causing hospital-acquired pneumonia (including nursing home residents) are *S. aureus* and gram-negative aerobic bacilli. Anaerobic bacteria are the most common etiologic agents in pneumonia that follows aspiration of gastric or oropharyngeal contents.

❾ Treatment of community-acquired pneumonia may consist of humidified oxygen for hypoxemia, bronchodilators (albuterol) when bronchospasm is present, rehydration fluids, and chest physiotherapy for marked accumulation of retained respiratory secretions. Antibiotic regimens should be selected based on presumed causative pathogens and pulmonary distribution characteristics and should be adjusted to provide optimal activity against pathogens identified by culture (sputum or blood).

❿ Treatment of nosocomial pneumonia requires aggressive therapy with careful consideration of the dominance and susceptibility patterns of the pathogens present within the institution. The epidemiology of these common pathogens should be evaluated on a regular basis in order to identify changing resistance patterns and subsequent alternation of treatment guidelines.

---

❶ Respiratory tract infections remain the major cause of morbidity from acute illness in the United States and most likely represent the single most common reason patients seek medical attention. This chapter focuses on bacterial and viral infections involving the lower respiratory tract, which includes the tracheobronchial tree and lung parenchyma.

❷ The respiratory tract has an elaborate system of host defenses, including humoral immunity, cellular immunity, and anatomic mechanisms.[1] When functioning properly, the host defenses of the respiratory tract are markedly effective in protecting against pathogen invasion and removing potentially infectious agents from the lungs. For the most part, infections in the lower respiratory tract occur only when these defense mechanisms are impaired, as in cases of dysgammaglobulinemia or compromised ciliary function, such as that caused by the chronic inflammation accompanying cigarette smoking. In addition, local defenses may be overwhelmed when a particularly virulent microorganism or excessive inoculum invades lung parenchyma. The majority of pulmonary infections follow colonization of the upper respiratory tract with potential pathogens, which, after achieving sufficiently high concentrations, gain access to the lung via aspiration of oropharyngeal secretions. Less commonly, microbes enter the lung via the blood from an extrapulmonary source or by inhalation of infected aerosolized particles. The specific type of pulmonary infection caused by an invading microorganism is determined by a variety of host factors, including age, anatomic features of the airway, and specific characteristics of the infecting agent.

The most common infections involving the lower respiratory tract are bronchitis, bronchiolitis, and pneumonia. Lower respiratory tract infections in children and adults most commonly result from either viral or bacterial invasion of lung parenchyma. The diagnosis of viral infections rests primarily on the recognition of a characteristic constellation of clinical signs and symptoms. Because treatment is largely supportive, only occasionally does the diagnosis require laboratory confirmation; this is achieved through serologic tests or identification of the organism by culture or antigen detection in respiratory secretions.[2] Laboratory techniques using polymerase chain reaction (PCR) and genetic "fingerprinting" technology have emerged as a means to identify specific pathogens rapidly and accurately.[3]

In contrast, because bacterial pneumonia usually necessitates expedient, effective, and specific antibiotic therapy, its management depends, in large part, on an understanding of the risk factors for acquiring pneumonia, predominate pathogens within the community and, if necessary, isolation of the etiologic agent by culture from lung tissue or secretions.[4-7] The pharynx is colonized with many organisms that can cause pneumonia; therefore, culture of expectorated sputum can be misleading unless the specimen is examined to ensure that it has originated from the lower respiratory tract. The Gram stain provides the easiest method for distinguishing lower from upper respiratory tract secretions; moreover, through determination of the shape and color of the bacteria, the Gram stain frequently narrows the microbiologic differential diagnosis sufficiently to allow accurate initial therapy. Scanned under low-power microscopy, Gram-stained expectorated upper respiratory tract secretions contain many irregularly shaped epithelial cells with little evidence of inflammation and may not reflect the pathogen. In contrast, a lower-tract specimen from a patient with bacterial pneumonia usually contains multiple neutrophils per high-powered field and a single or predominant bacterial species. Culture of specimens confirmed to originate from the lower tract by Gram stain provides valuable diagnostic information for the majority of patients with bacterial pneumonia. In addition, pneumonia promotes the release of inflammatory mediators and acute phase proteins such as C-reactive protein, which is significantly elevated in serum in the presence of respiratory tract infections.[8]

❸ An appropriate treatment regimen for the patient with an uncomplicated lower respiratory tract infection usually can be established by history, physical examination, chest radiograph, and properly collected sputum cultures interpreted in light of the most common lung pathogens and their antibiotic susceptibility patterns within the community.[2,4,5,9,10] More sophisticated or invasive diagnostic methods (e.g., computed tomography, bronchoscopy, and lung biopsy)[11,12] should be reserved for very ill patients who are unable to expectorate sputum or who are not responding to empirical therapy or for pulmonary infections occurring in immunocompromised patients.

BRONCHITIS

Bronchitis and bronchiolitis are inflammatory conditions of the large and small elements, respectively, of the tracheobronchial tree. The inflammatory process does not extend to the alveoli. Bronchitis

frequently is classified as acute or chronic. Acute bronchitis occurs in individuals of all ages, whereas chronic bronchitis primarily affects adults. Bronchiolitis is a disease of infancy.

ACUTE BRONCHITIS

Epidemiology and Etiology

Acute bronchitis occurs most commonly during the winter months, following a pattern similar to those of other acute respiratory tract infections. Cold, damp climates and the presence of high concentrations of irritating substances (e.g., air pollution, cigarette smoke) may precipitate attacks.

❹ Respiratory viruses are by far the most common infectious agents associated with acute bronchitis.[13] The common cold viruses (rhinovirus and coronavirus) and lower respiratory tract pathogens (influenza virus and adenovirus) account for the majority of cases. Wider use of reverse transcriptase PCR diagnostic evaluations has identified respiratory viral pathogens previously undescribed as etiologic agents in acute bronchitis and bronchiolitis including the human metapneumovirus and bocavirus.[14] In children, similar pathogens are observed, with the addition of the parainfluenza viruses. Although the true incidence remains to be defined, *M. pneumoniae* appears to be a frequent cause of acute bronchitis. Additionally, *C. pneumoniae* (also referred to as *Chlamydophila*)[15,16] and *B. pertussis*[17] (agent responsible for whooping cough) have been associated with acute respiratory tract infections. Although a variety of bacteria, including *S. pneumoniae*, *Streptococcus* species, *Staphylococcus* species, and *Haemophilus* species, may be isolated from throat or sputum culture, these organisms probably represent contamination by normal flora of the upper respiratory tract rather than true pathogens. Although a primary bacterial etiology for acute bronchitis appears rare, secondary bacterial infection may be involved.

Pathogenesis

❹ Because acute bronchitis is primarily a self-limiting illness and rarely a cause of death, few data describing the pathology are available. In general, infection of the trachea and bronchi yields hyperemic and edematous mucous membranes with an increase in bronchial secretions. Destruction of respiratory epithelium can range from mild to extensive and may affect bronchial mucociliary function. In addition, the increase in desquamated epithelial cells and bronchial secretions, which can become thick and tenacious, further impairs mucociliary activity. The probability of permanent damage to the airways as a result of acute bronchitis remains unclear but appears very unlikely. However, epidemiologic evaluations support the belief that recurrent acute respiratory infections may be associated with increased airway hyperreactivity and possibly the pathogenesis of asthma or chronic obstructive pulmonary disease (COPD).

Clinical Presentation

Acute bronchitis usually begins as an upper respiratory infection with nonspecific complaints.[13,18] Cough is the hallmark of acute bronchitis and occurs early. The onset of cough may be insidious or abrupt, and the symptoms persist despite resolution of nasal or nasopharyngeal complaints; cough may persist for up to 3 or more weeks. Frequently, the cough initially is nonproductive but then progresses, yielding mucopurulent sputum. In older children and adults, the sputum is raised and expectorated; in the young child, sputum often is swallowed and can result in gagging and vomiting. Substantial discomfort may result from the coughing. Dyspnea, cyanosis, or signs of airway obstruction are observed rarely unless the patient has underlying pulmonary disease, such as emphysema or COPD. Fever, when present, rarely exceeds 39°C (102.2°F) and appears most commonly with adenovirus, influenza virus, and *M. pneumoniae* infections. The diagnosis typically is made on the basis of a characteristic history and physical examination. Bacterial cultures of expectorated sputum generally are of limited use because of the inability to avoid normal nasopharyngeal flora by the sampling technique. In routine cases, viral cultures are unnecessary and frequently unavailable. Viral antigen detection tests, developed to identify respiratory viral antigens from nasal secretions rapidly, can be obtained in many hospital laboratories and in some practice settings when a specific diagnosis is necessary for clinical or epidemiologic reasons. Cultures, serologic or PCR diagnosis of *M. pneumoniae,* and culture direct fluorescent antibody detection or PCR for *B. pertussis* should be obtained in prolonged or severe cases when epidemiologic considerations would suggest their involvement.

TREATMENT

Acute Bronchitis

■ DESIRED OUTCOME

In the absence of a complicating bacterial superinfection, acute bronchitis almost always is self-limiting. The goals of therapy are to provide comfort to the patient and, in the unusually severe case, to treat associated dehydration and respiratory compromise.[13]

■ GENERAL APPROACH TO TREATMENT

❹ Treatment of acute bronchitis is symptomatic and supportive in nature. Reassurance and antipyretics frequently are all that are needed. Bed rest for comfort may be instituted as desired. Patients should be encouraged to drink fluids to prevent dehydration and possibly to decrease the viscosity of respiratory secretions. Mist therapy (use of a vaporizer) may promote the thinning and loosening of respiratory secretions.

■ PHARMACOLOGIC THERAPY

Mild analgesic–antipyretic therapy often is helpful in relieving the associated lethargy, malaise, and fever. Aspirin or acetaminophen (650 mg in adults or 10 to 15 mg/kg per dose in children; maximum daily pediatric dose 60 mg/kg; maximum daily adult dose 4 g) or ibuprofen (200 to 800 mg in adults or 10 mg/kg per dose in children; maximum daily pediatric dose 40 mg/kg; maximum daily adult dose 3.2 g) should be administered every 4 to 6 hours. In children, aspirin should be avoided and acetaminophen used as the preferred agent because of the possible association between aspirin use and the development of Reye syndrome.[19]

Use of ibuprofen as an antipyretic has increased. The drug's antipyretic efficacy appears identical to that of aspirin or acetaminophen, although its duration of antipyretic effect may be slightly longer (e.g., 3 to 4 hours for aspirin and acetaminophen versus 5 to 6 hours for ibuprofen). Caution should be exercised in the administration of ibuprofen for patients younger than 3 months, elderly patients, and individuals with poor renal function. Aspirin and ibuprofen inhibit prostaglandin synthesis and may adversely influence renal function in these predisposed patient populations.

Patients may present with mild to moderate wheezing. In otherwise healthy patients, no meaningful benefits have been described with the use of oral or aerosolized β_2-receptor agonists and/or oral or aerosolized corticosteroids. A Cochrane Review showed limited benefit of β_2-receptor agonists even for patients with airflow obstruction. Nevertheless and despite no data, some clinicians may initiate a brief trial (e.g., ~5 to 7 days) of oral or inhaled corticosteroid for patients with persistent (>14 to 20 days), troublesome cough. Despite several studies, none support the use of mucolytic agents.

Patients suffering from acute bronchitis frequently medicate themselves with nonprescription cough and cold remedies containing various combinations of antihistamines, sympathomimetics, and antitussives despite the lack of definitive evidence supporting their effectiveness. In fact, the tendency of these agents to dehydrate bronchial secretions could aggravate and prolong the recovery process. Although not recommended for routine use, persistent, mild cough, which may be bothersome, can be treated with dextromethorphan; more severe coughs may require intermittent codeine or other similar agents.[13,18] In severe cases, the cough may be persistent enough to disrupt sleep, and use of a mild sedative–hypnotic, concomitantly with a cough suppressant (e.g. codeine), may be desirable. However, antitussives should be used cautiously when the cough is productive. The primary or supplemental use of expectorants is questionable because their clinical effectiveness has not been well established.

Routine use of antibiotics for treatment of acute bronchitis should be discouraged.[13] In previously healthy patients who exhibit persistent fever or respiratory symptoms for more than 4 to 6 days or for predisposed patients (e.g., elderly, immunocompromised), the possibility of a concurrent bacterial infection should be suspected. When possible, antibiotic therapy should be directed toward anticipated respiratory pathogen(s) (i.e., *S. pneumoniae). M. pneumoniae,* if suspected by history or if confirmed by culture serology or PCR, can be treated with azithromycin. Alternatively and empirically, a fluoroquinolone antibiotic with activity against these suspected pathogens (e.g., levofloxacin) can be used. During known epidemics involving the influenza A virus, amantadine or rimantadine may be effective in minimizing associated symptoms if administered early in the course of the disease though treatment with adamantanes is no longer CDC recommended due to increasing influenza resistance to these two agents.[20] The neuraminidase inhibitors (e.g., zanamivir and oseltamivir) are active against both influenza A and B viral infections and may reduce the severity and duration of the influenza episode if administered promptly during the onset of the viral infection and are the preferred treatment (see Chap. 118).[21,22] Unfortunately, the incidence of influenzae virus resistance to available antiviral drugs is increasing.[20,23]

CHRONIC BRONCHITIS

Epidemiology and Etiology

Chronic bronchitis, a component of the COPD is a clinical diagnosis for a nonspecific disease that primarily affects adults. An indepth presentation of the spectrum and management of the COPDs is in Chap. 34. This section will focus solely on chronic bronchitis, a disease that affects most patients with COPD. In developed countries the prevalence of chronic bronchitis is nearly equal in men and woman and possibly more common in whites.[24,25]

❺ Chronic bronchitis is defined clinically as the presence of a chronic cough productive of sputum lasting more than 3 consecutive months of the year for 2 consecutive years without an underlying etiology of bronchiectasis or tuberculosis. The disease is a result of several contributing factors; the most prominent include cigarette smoking, exposure to occupational dusts, fumes, and environmental pollution; and host factors [e.g., genetic factors and bacterial (and possibly viral) infections]. The contribution of each of these factors and of others (either alone or in combination) to chronic bronchitis is unknown. Cigarette smoke is a well-known airway irritant and is believed to be the predominant factor in the etiology of chronic bronchitis. Although previously assumed the most common etiologic cause of chronic bronchitis, more strict prohibition of public smoking and the resultant decrease in chronic tobacco smokers, particularly in developed countries, underscores the importance of other factors as causes of this chronic disease. Additional airway irritants including occupational dust, chemicals, or air pollution, either alone or more probably in combination, are also responsible for the pathogenesis of chronic bronchitis. Furthermore, it appears from candidate gene association studies that a genetic basis for some COPD phenotypes will be identified in the near future.[25] Lastly, the influence of recurrent respiratory tract infections during childhood or young adult life on the later development of chronic bronchitis remains obscure, but recurrent respiratory infections may predispose individuals to the development of chronic bronchitis.[26] Whether these recurrent respiratory tract infections are a result of unrecognized anatomic abnormalities of the airways or impaired pulmonary defense mechanisms is unclear.

Chronic bronchitis is a disease of the bronchi and as noted above is manifested by cough and excessive sputum expectoration that occurs on most days of the week for a minimum of 3 consecutive months per year for at least 2 consecutive years that is unrelated to other pulmonary or cardiac disease. Numerous consensus statements and published authoritative guidelines define chronic bronchitis and emphysema as the two main components of COPD/chronic obstructive lung disease (COLD).[18,24,27] The Global Initiative for Chronic Obstruction Lung Disease (GOLD)[24] guidelines document does not distinguish these two diagnoses (e.g., emphysema or chronic bronchitis) in the definition of COPD, but it does define COPD as a disease characterized by airflow obstruction that is not fully reversible and progressive.[28] The GOLD guidelines provide a COPD classification scoring system according to severity that can be very helpful in staging patients for intensity of therapy and prognosis.[24] Unfortunately, differences in definitions between authoritative organizations[18,24,27] may cause confusion in the assignment of patients in clinical trials and thus to assessment and applications of study results to clinical care.

Pathogenesis

Chronic inhalation of an irritating noxious substance compromises the normal secretory and mucociliary function of bronchial mucosa. Bronchial biopsy specimens in bronchitic patients underscore the importance of proinflammatory cytokines [e.g., interleukins 1β, 6, and 8, transforming growth factor-β, leukotriene B4 and tumor necrosis factor-α] in the pathogenesis and propagation of the observed inflammatory changes. In chronic bronchitis, the bronchial wall is thickened, and the number of mucus-secreting goblet cells on the surface epithelium of both larger and smaller bronchi is increased markedly. In contrast, goblet cells generally are absent from the smaller bronchi of normal individuals. In addition to the increased number of goblet cells, hypertrophy of the mucous glands and dilation of the mucous gland ducts are observed. As a result of these changes, chronic bronchitics have substantially more mucus in their peripheral airways, further impairing normal lung defenses. This increased quantity of tenacious secretions within the bronchial tree frequently causes mucous plugging of the smaller airways. Accompanying these changes are squamous cell metaplasia of the surface epithelium, edema, and increased vascularity of the basement membrane of larger airways and variable chronic inflammatory cell infiltration. In addition, the amounts of several proteases derived from inflammatory cells are increased and due to COPD-induced defective antiproteases leads to continued destruction of connective tissue. Continued progression of this pathology can result in residual scarring of small bronchi and peribronchial fibrosis augmenting airway obstruction and weakening of bronchial walls.

Clinical Presentation

⑤ The hallmark of chronic bronchitis is a cough that may range from a mild to a severe, incessant coughing productive of purulent sputum. Coughing may be precipitated by multiple stimuli, including simple, normal conversation. Expectoration of the largest quantity of sputum usually occurs on arising in the morning, although many patients expectorate sputum throughout the day. The expectorated sputum usually is tenacious and can vary in color from white to yellow-green. Patients with chronic bronchitis often expectorate as much as 100 mL/day more than normal. As a result, many patients complain of a frequent bad taste in their mouth and of halitosis.

The diagnosis of chronic bronchitis is based primarily on clinical assessment and history. Any patient who reports coughing sputum on most days for at least 3 consecutive months each year for 2 consecutive years presumptively has chronic bronchitis.[28] The diagnosis of chronic bronchitis is made only when the possibilities of bronchiectasis, cardiac failure, cystic fibrosis, and lung carcinoma have been effectively excluded. In an attempt to be more specific in the diagnosis, some investigators have added the criteria of lost wages for 3 or more weeks. In addition, many clinicians attempt to subdivide their patients based on severity of disease to guide therapeutic interventions. A useful diagnostic/clinical severity-based classification system is often used to categorize patients to assist in defining an acute therapeutic strategy. The classification system used most often utilizes three descriptive categories: I. *Simple chronic bronchitis* best describes patients with no major risk factors and sputum flora reflects the common associated pathogens where the patient usually responds well to first-line oral antibiotic therapy; II. *Complicated chronic bronchitis* are those patients with what would be considered a "simple chronic bronchitis" exacerbation, but the patients have two or more disease-associated risk factors such as FEV$_1$ <50% predicted, age >64 years, >4 exacerbations per year, home oxygen use, underlying cardiac disease, use of immunosuppressants, or use of antibiotics for an exacerbation within the past 3 months. These group II patients may also harbor drug-resistant pathogens; III. *Severe complicated chronic bronchitis* are those patients with group II symptoms but clinically are much worse, for example, FEV$_1$ <35% predicted, >4 acute exacerbations per year, increased risk for infection with *P. aeruginosa* and presence of pathogens that are multidrug resistant (MDR). These later patients often require hospitalization and aggressive parenteral antibiotics including combination therapy. A clinical algorithm for the diagnosis and treatment of chronic bronchitic patients with an acute exacerbation incorporating the principles of the clinical classification system is shown in Figure 116–1. The importance of accurate classification for grouping patients of similar disease involvement cannot be overemphasized with respect to assessing publications outlining treatment strategies for these patients.[29] Although gross, these classifications attempt to capture specific subphenotypes of chronic bronchitis patients. It is hoped that within the next 2 to 4 years, pharmacogenomic advances will provide a more sophisticated tool for defining specific phenotypes linked to specific, optimal therapies.[30] The typical clinical presentation of chronic bronchitis is listed in Table 116–1. Comparison of the trends in changes in patient physical activity, symptoms and clinical/physical findings from the patient's "routine" is extremely helpful in determining the presence and severity of an acute exacerbation. In general, a good clinical relationship exists between the purulence of the sputum and the bacterial load (>90% of cases) and for sputum color, for example,

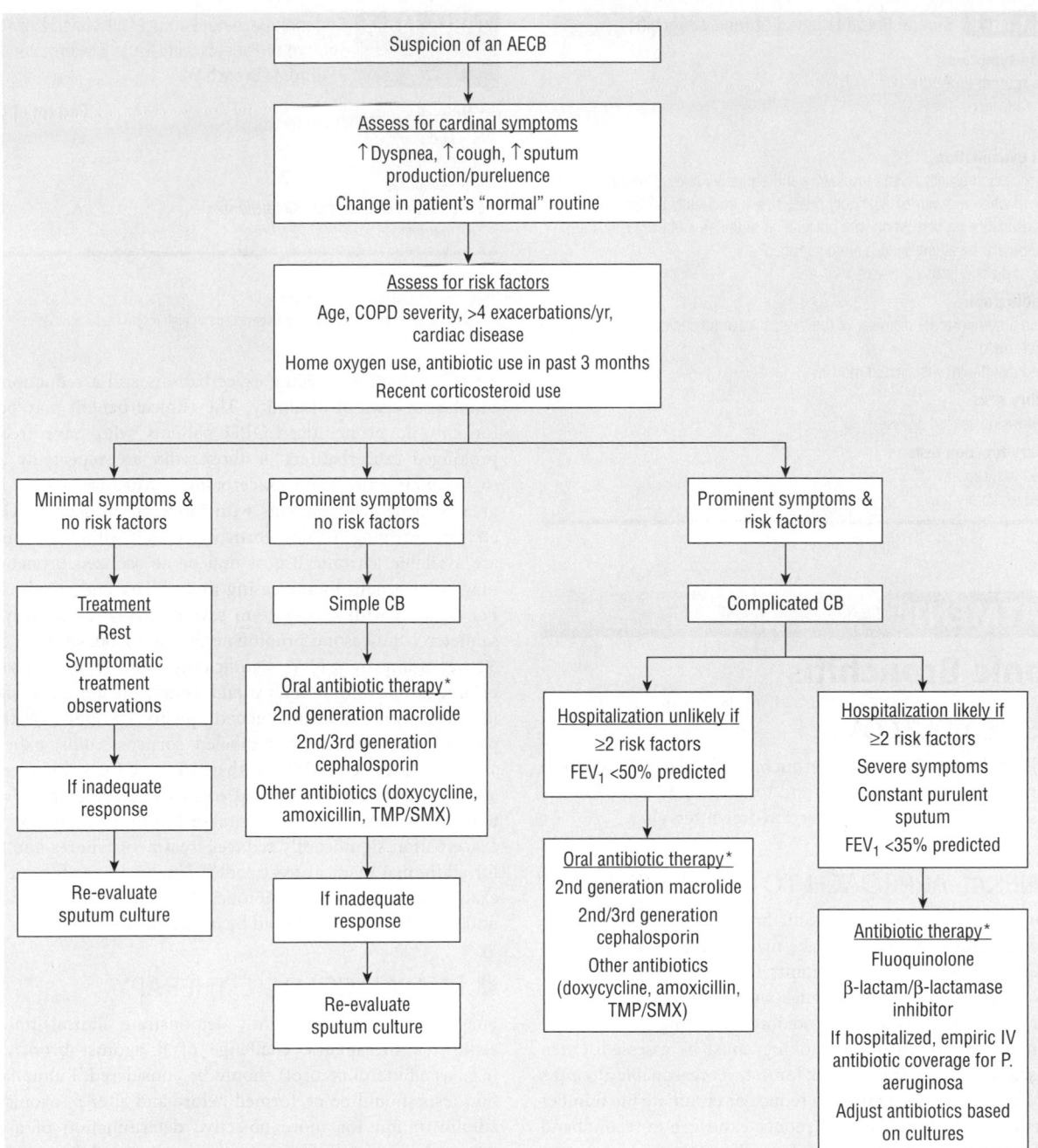

FIGURE 116-1. Clinical algorithm for the diagnosis and treatment of chronic bronchitic patients with an acute exacerbation incorporating the principles of the clinical classification system (AECB, acute exacerbation of chronic bronchitis; COPD, chronic obstructive pulmonary disease; CB, chronic bronchitis; TMP/SMX, trimethoprim/sulfamethoxazole). *See Table 116–4 for commonly used antibiotics and doses. *(Adapted from reference 36.)*

the greener the color the greater the amount of leukocyte myeloperoxidase (indicating that more inflammatory cells are present).

In more advanced stages of chronic bronchitis, physical findings associated with cor pulmonale, including cardiac enlargement, hepatomegaly, and edema of the lower extremities, are observed. In general, chronic bronchitics tend to maintain at least normal body weight and commonly are obese. Radiographic studies are of limited value in either the diagnosis or follow-up of a patient. The microscopic and laboratory assessments of sputum are considered important components in the overall evaluation of patients with chronic bronchitis. A fresh sputum specimen obtained as an early-morning sample is preferred. Comparison of the cellular constituents of chronic bronchitic sputum with those of normal sputum can provide insight into the degree of activity of the disease processes. An increased number of polymorphonuclear granulocytes often suggests continual bronchial irritation, whereas an increased number of eosinophils suggests an allergic component that should be further investigated. Gram staining of the sputum often reveals a mixture of both gram-positive and gram-negative bacteria, reflecting normal oropharyngeal flora and chronic tracheal colonization (in order of frequency) by nontypeable *H. influenzae, S. pneumoniae,* and *M. catarrhalis.* Table 116–2 lists the most common bacterial isolates identified from sputum culture for patients experiencing an acute exacerbation of chronic bronchitis. For patients with more severe airflow disease [e.g., forced expiratory volume in the first second of expiration (FEV_1) <40%], enteric gram-negative bacilli, *E. coli, Klebsiella* species, *Enterobacter* species, and *P. aeruginosa* may be significant pathogens during acute exacerbations.[31]

TABLE 116-1	Clinical Presentation of Chronic Bronchitis

Signs and symptoms
Excessive sputum expectoration
Cyanosis (advanced disease)
Obesity

Physical examination
Chest auscultation usually reveals inspiratory and expiratory rales, rhonchi,
    and mild wheezing with an expiratory phase that is frequently prolonged;
    hyperresonance on percussion with obliteration of the area of cardiac dullness
Normal vesicular breathing sounds are diminished
Clubbing of digits (advanced disease)

Chest radiograph
Increase in anteroposterior diameter of the thoracic cage (observed as
    a barrel chest)
Depressed diaphragm with limited mobility

Laboratory tests
Erythrocytosis (advanced disease)

Pulmonary function tests
Decreased vital capacity
Prolonged expiratory flow

TABLE 116-2	Common Bacterial Pathogens Isolated from Sputum of Patients with Acute Exacerbation of Chronic Bronchitis

Pathogen	Percent of Cultures
H. influenzae[a,b]	45
M. catarrhalis[a]	30
S. pneumoniae[c]	20
E.coli, Enterobacter species, Klebsiella species, P. aeruginosa	5

[a]Often β-lactamase positive.
[b]Vast majority are nontypeable strains.
[c]As many as 25% of strains may have intermediate or high resistance to penicillin.

TREATMENT

Chronic Bronchitis

■ DESIRED OUTCOME

The goals of therapy for chronic bronchitis are twofold: to reduce the severity of chronic symptoms and to ameliorate acute exacerbations and achieve prolonged infection-free intervals.

■ GENERAL APPROACH TO TREATMENT

The approach to treatment of chronic bronchitis is multifactorial. First and foremost, attempts must be made to reduce the patient's exposure to known bronchial irritants (e.g., smoking, workplace pollution). A complete occupational and environmental history for determination of exposure to noxious, irritating gases, as well as preference toward cigarette smoking, must be assessed. Often easier discussed than accomplished, honest, yet reasonable attempts should be made with the patient to reduce or eliminate the number of cigarettes smoked daily and to reduce exposure to secondhand smoke. In an organized, coordinated, smoking cessation program, including counseling and hypnotherapy, the adjunctive use of nicotine substitutes (e.g., nicotine gum or patch) or other pharmacotherapy (e.g. bupropion) may promote the reduction or complete withdrawal from cigarette smoking. Often just as difficult is modification of exposure to irritating substances within the home and workplace.

❻ Measures to provide pulmonary toilet can be instituted. During acute pulmonary exacerbations of the disease, the patient's ability to mobilize and expectorate sputum may be reduced dramatically. In these instances, attempts at postural drainage techniques, with instruction, active participation, or both from a respiratory therapist, may assist in promoting clearance of pulmonary secretions. In addition, humidification of inspired air may promote the hydration (liquefaction) of tenacious secretions, allowing for removal that is more productive. Use of mucolytic aerosols, such as N-acetylcysteine and DNAse, is of questionable therapeutic value, particularly considering their propensity to induce bronchospasm (N-acetylcysteine) and their excessive cost. A Cochrane metaanalysis of mucolytic therapy in subjects with chronic bronchitis or COPD found that treatment with mucolytics was associated with

a small reduction in acute exacerbations and a reduction in total number of days of disability. The clinical benefit may be greater for chronic bronchitics/COPD patients who have frequent or prolonged exacerbations or those who are repeatedly admitted to hospitals with acute exacerbations. Mucolytics may have the greatest benefit for patients with moderate or severe COPD who are not receiving inhaled corticosteroids.[32] Although limited data are available, chronic use of oral or aerosolized bronchodilators may be of benefit by increasing mucociliary and cough clearance. For patients with moderate to severe COPD, twice-daily inhaled salmeterol/fluticasone propionate 50:250 or 50:500 mcg for 24 to 52 weeks improves FEV_1 significantly more than does salmeterol or fluticasone monotherapy and results in clinically significant improvements in health-related quality of life.[33] Furthermore, patients may benefit from inhaled corticosteroids; patients with severe disease (FEV_1 <50%) with a history of frequent exacerbations should receive chronic inhaled corticosteroid therapy. Use of systemic corticosteroid therapy (oral or IV) for patients with an acute exacerbation significantly reduces treatment failures and the need for additional medical treatment.[34] Finally, in the face of an acute exacerbation, a trial of antibiotics directed against the most likely underlying pathogens should be initiated.

■ PHARMACOLOGIC THERAPY

For patients who consistently demonstrate clinical limitation in airflow, a therapeutic challenge of β_2-agonist bronchodilators (e.g., as albuterol aerosol) should be considered. Pulmonary function tests should be performed before and after β_2-agonist aerosol administration for more objective determination of a patient's propensity to benefit from supplemental aerosol therapy. Sufficient published experience supports the use of inhalation therapy with a β_2-agonist for patients with chronic bronchitis (COPD) to improve pulmonary function and exercise tolerance and to reduce the sense of breathlessness.[28] Regular use of a long-acting β-receptor agonist aerosol (e.g., salmeterol, formoterol) in responsive patients may be more effective and probably more convenient than short-acting β_2-receptor agonists. The aerosol route for β_2-receptor agonist and/or corticosteroid administration is favored over systemic formulations for improved patient acceptance, compliance and to minimize the number and magnitude of associated adverse effects.[24] Chronic inhalation of the salmeterol/fluticasone combination has been associated with improved pulmonary function and quality of life.

Published experience with inhaled anticholinergic drugs, including ipratropium and tiotropium, is limited. In stable patients, long-term inhalation of ipratropium has been associated with a decreased frequency of cough, less severe coughing, and a decrease in the volume of expectorated sputum. Once-daily tiotropium inhalation was associated with significant bronchodilation and dyspnea relief compared with placebo but had no significant effect on the incidence or severity of cough.[24,28] Although chronic theophylline administration has been used extensively in the past, this therapy is used with decreasing frequency in favor of aerosolized β_2-receptor agonists. A salmeterol/fluticasone combination markedly reduced the number of chronic bronchitis-associated emergency room visits and hospitalizations compared to an ipratropium-based regimen.[35]

Use of antimicrobials for treatment of chronic bronchitis has been controversial but is becoming more accepted. Numerous comparative evaluations, including placebo-controlled studies of antibiotic administration with acute and chronic treatment of chronic bronchitics, have suggested definite clinical benefit, whereas other similar studies have not.[24,27,29,31,36] The antibiotics selected most frequently possess variable in vitro activity against the common sputum isolates *H. influenzae*, *S. pneumoniae*, *M. catarrhalis*, and *M. pneumoniae*. In general, conflicting published results appear independent of the antibiotic used or the regimen compared. The wide disparity that exists in the results from these studies, combined with the difficulties in recognition and lack of standardized diagnostic criteria for acute exacerbations of chronic bronchitis, serves as the basis for the enormous controversy surrounding the use of antibiotics in this condition.[37] A review of 14 double-blinded randomized clinical trials compared fluoroquinolones with more standard antibiotic regimens (e.g., macrolides, azalides, oral cephalosporins, and the combination drug amoxicillin/clavulanate).[31] As expected, no significant differences were observed between treatment arms. However, in a small subset of studies ($n = 4$), the sputum culture became negative in a significantly higher number of fluoroquinolone-treated patients. Other studies showed an increase in the interval between acute exacerbations for patients who received fluoroquinolone therapy. An additional advantage of fluoroquinolone therapy is the short course (e.g., 5 days) and once-daily dosing compared to other antibiotic regimens. A useful paradigm for the assessment and treatment of acute exacerbations of chronic bronchitis and antibiotic decision making is shown in Figure 116–1. Furthermore, many clinicians will use the so-called Anthonisen criteria to determine if antibiotic therapy is indicated. The Anthonisen criteria are as follows:[38] If a patient exhibits two of the following three criteria during an acute exacerbation of chronic bronchitis, the patient will most likely benefit from antibiotic therapy and thus, should receive a treatment course: (1) increase in shortness of breath; (2) increase in sputum volume; (3) production of purulent sputum. There are greater healthcare costs for patients who are noncompliant with their antibiotic regimen for their acute exacerbation of chronic bronchitis.[39]

The increasing resistance of the common bacterial pathogens to first-line agents further complicates antibiotic selection. As many as 30% to 40% of *H. influenzae* and 95% to 100% of *M. catarrhalis* isolates produce β-lactamases. Moreover, up to 40% of *S. pneumoniae* isolates demonstrate resistance to penicillin [minimum inhibitory concentration (MIC) = 0.1 to 2 mg/L], with approximately 20% of isolates being highly resistant (MIC>2 mg/L). Concern regarding *S. pneumoniae* resistance is increasing, now ≥30% for macrolides. Despite these changes in bacterial susceptibility, the current recommendation is to initiate therapy with first-line agents in less severely affected patients (see Fig. 116–1). Trimethoprim/sulfamethoxazole has been extremely useful for patients with less severe disease.[40] However, the public campaign in the United Kingdom by the Committee of Safety of Medicines to discourage the use of trimethoprim/sulfamethoxazole based on rare but possibly life-threatening cases of Stevens-Johnson syndrome has markedly reduced the use of this agent worldwide. For patients with more moderate to severe disease, many clinicians will begin antibiotic therapy with the second line agents, amoxicillin/clavulanate, a macrolide (such as azithromycin or clarithromycin) (they are being used less frequently) and more frequently with a fluoroquinolone, such as levofloxacin (see Fig. 116–1).[24,31,36,41]

TABLE 116-3 Oral Antibiotics Commonly Used for the Treatment of Acute Respiratory Exacerbations in Chronic Bronchitis

Antibiotic	Usual Adult Dose (mg)	Dose Schedule (Doses/Day)
Preferred drugs		
Ampicillin	250–500	4
Amoxicillin	500–875	3–2
Amoxicillin/clavulanate	500–875	3–2
Ciprofloxacin	500–750	2
Levofloxacin	500–750	1
Moxifloxacin	400	1
Doxycycline	100	2
Minocycline	100	2
Tetracycline HCl	500	4
Trimethoprim/sulfamethoxazole[a]	1 DS	2
Supplemental drugs		
Azithromycin	250–500	1
Erythromycin	500	4
Clarithromycin	250–500	2
Cephalexin	500	4

[a]DS, double-strength tablet (160-mg trimethoprim/800-mg sulfamethoxazole).

Regardless of the antibiotic selected, careful attention to predetermined outcome measures should be monitored closely for each patient to determine the success or failure of the therapeutic intervention. Oral antibiotics with broader antibacterial spectra (e.g., amoxicillin/clavulanate, fluoroquinolones, or azalides) that possess potent in vitro activity against sputum isolates are increasingly becoming first-line antibiotics as initial therapy for treatment of acute exacerbations of chronic bronchitis.[24,31,35,36,40]

An important clinical outcome variable directing drug selection and criteria for beginning antibiotics in individual patients is the infection-free period when chronic bronchitics are off antibiotics. The actual length of the infection-free time period and the change in the number of physician office visits and hospital admissions with a particular antibiotic regimen are extremely important to identify, whenever possible, for each patient. The antibiotic regimen that results in the longest infection-free period defines the "regimen of choice" for specific patients for future acute exacerbations of their disease.

Antibiotics should be selected that are effective against responsible pathogens, demonstrate the least risk of drug interactions, and can be administered in a manner that promotes compliance. Antibiotics commonly used for treatment of these patients and their respective adult starting doses are listed in Table 116–3. Doses of antibiotics should be adjusted as needed to the desired clinical effect and the lowest incidence of acceptable side effects. A frequently used clinical strategy to enhance the duration of symptom-free periods incorporates higher-dose antibiotic regimens using the upper limit of the recommended daily antibiotic dose for a period of 5 to 7 days. More clinicians are electing to limit their antibiotic treatment regimen to 5 days as compelling data continue to support equal efficacy and possibly less side effects with short duration antibiotic therapy versus longer treatment regimens (>7 days).[42]

For the patient whose history suggests recurrent exacerbations of disease that might be attributable to specific events (e.g., seasonal or related to the winter months), a trial of prophylactic antibiotics might be beneficial. If no clinical improvement is noted over an appropriate period (2 to 3 months per year for 2 to 3 years), further attempts at prophylactic therapy can be discontinued. Similarly, patient-specific antibiotic trials can be performed in individuals experiencing acute exacerbations, focusing on attaining the maximum infection-free period. Although less than desirable, this method of clinical assessment may distinguish patients who will benefit from prophylactic antibiotic therapy from those who will not.

BRONCHIOLITIS

EPIDEMIOLOGY AND ETIOLOGY

7 Bronchiolitis is an acute viral infection of the lower respiratory tract that affects approximately 50% of children during the first year of life and 100% by age 3 years. The occurrence of bronchiolitis peaks during the winter months and persists through early spring. Bronchiolitis remains the major reason for hospital admission during the first year of life. The incidence of bronchiolitis appears to be more common in males than in females.[43,44]

Respiratory syncytial virus (RSV) is the most common cause of bronchiolitis, accounting for up to 75% of all cases. During epidemic periods, the incidence of RSV-induced bronchiolitis may approach 90% of cases. Other detectable viruses include parainfluenza, adenovirus, and influenza. Bacteria serve as secondary pathogens in a minority of cases.[43,45]

CLINICAL PRESENTATION

A prodrome suggesting an upper respiratory tract infection, usually lasting from 2 to 8 days, precedes the onset of clinical symptoms (Table 116–4). Due to limited oral intake because of coughing combined with fever, vomiting, and diarrhea, infants frequently are dehydrated. The increased work of breathing and tachypnea most likely further increases fluid loss. In most cases, this clinical picture persists between 3 and 7 days. Although the hospital course of bronchiolitic children often is variable, substantial clinical improvement usually is observed within the first 2 days, with gradual improvement and complete resolution sometimes requiring 4 to 8 weeks.

The diagnosis of bronchiolitis is based primarily on history and clinical findings. It is important for the clinician to attempt to differentiate between bronchiolitis and a host of other clinical entities affecting infants, which may produce a similar picture of dyspnea and wheezing. Asthma, congestive heart failure, anatomic airway abnormalities, cystic fibrosis, foreign bodies, and gastroesophageal reflux are the primary disease entities that may present with wheezing in children. Isolation of a viral pathogen in the respiratory secretions of a wheezing child establishes a presumptive diagnosis of infectious bronchiolitis. However, the ability to identify specific viral pathogens often is hindered by the limited availability of special virology laboratories. In addition, in the elderly and in immunocompromised patients, antigen detection lacks adequate sensitivity, and patients frequently seek medical care after the acute stage of the infection, thus compromising the ability of the available tests to diagnose RSV. However, the proliferation of commercial enzyme-linked immunosorbent assays and fluorescent antibody staining techniques of nasopharyngeal secretions has increased the ability to identify viral antigens within several hours.[43] Identification of RSV by PCR should be available routinely from most clinical laboratories, but its relevance to the clinical management of bronchiolitis remains obscure.

Multiple clinical laboratory determinations have been used to assist in the management of cases of bronchiolitis. Radiographic evaluation of the chest in children with bronchiolitis yields variable findings but may help to distinguish this illness from other entities characterized by wheezing. In children requiring hospitalization, abnormalities in blood gas tensions are frequent and appear to relate to disease severity. Hypoxemia is common and increases the respiratory drive, whereas hypercarbia is seen in only the most severe cases. Despite the presence of moderate degrees of hypoxemia, clinical cyanosis is unusual.

TREATMENT

Bronchiolitis

■ DESIRED OUTCOME

7 In the well infant, bronchiolitis usually is a self-limiting illness, and reassurance, antipyretics, and adequate fluid intake usually are all that are necessary while waiting for resolution of the underlying viral infection. In-hospital support is necessary for the child suffering from respiratory failure or marked dehydration; underlying cardiac and pulmonary diseases potentiate these conditions.

■ GENERAL APPROACH TO TREATMENT

7 Almost all otherwise healthy babies with bronchiolitis can be followed as outpatients. Such infants are treated for fever, provided generous amounts of oral fluids, and observed closely for evidence of respiratory deterioration.[46] In severely affected children, the mainstays of therapy for bronchiolitis are oxygen therapy and intravenous fluids. In a subset of patients, aerosolized bronchodilators may have a role. For selected infants, particularly those with underlying pulmonary disease, cardiac disease, or both, therapy with the antiviral agent ribavirin can be considered.[47]

■ PHARMACOLOGIC THERAPY

7 Aerosolized β_2-adrenergic therapy appears to offer little benefit for the majority of patients and may even be detrimental.[43,45] However, this therapy may offer some benefit to the child with a predisposition toward bronchospasm. In addition, although clinical trials have demonstrated varied results, nebulized epinephrine seems to be more efficacious than salbutamol in hospitalized patients with bronchiolitis.[43,48] For such patients, bronchodilator therapy may be offered initially but should not be pursued in the absence of a clearcut clinical benefit. Similarly, controlled trials of corticosteroids in bronchiolitic infants have not shown therapeutic effects or significant harmful effects.[45,47] As a result, the routine use of systemically administered corticosteroids is discouraged. Conversely, the combined use of oral dexamethasone with nebulized epinephrine may act synergistically to reduce hospital admissions and shorten the time to discharge and the duration of symptoms; however, more trials are needed to confirm these findings.[49] Although placing

---

TABLE 116-4 Clinical Presentation of Bronchiolitis

Signs and symptoms
Prodrome with irritability, restlessness, and mild fever
Cough and coryza
Vomiting, diarrhea, noisy breathing, and increased respiratory rate as symptoms progress
Labored breathing with retractions of the chest wall, nasal flaring, and grunting

Physical examination
Tachycardia and respiratory rate of 40–80 per minute in hospitalized infants
Wheezing and inspiratory rales
Mild conjunctivitis in one third of patients
Otitis media in 5–10% of patients

Laboratory tests
Peripheral white blood cell count normal or slightly elevated
Abnormal arterial blood gases (hypoxemia and, rarely, hypercarbia)

children with bronchiolitis in mist tents has been common practice, no data have documented the effectiveness of this practice.

Ribavirin may offer benefit to a subset of infants with bronchiolitis. Although ribavirin, a synthetic nucleoside, possesses in vitro antiviral properties against a variety of RNA and DNA viruses, including influenza A, influenza B, parainfluenza, and adenovirus,[45] it is approved only in aerosolized form against RSV. Use of the drug requires special equipment (small-particle aerosol generator) and specially trained personnel for administration via oxygen hood or mist tent. Special care must be taken to avoid drug particle deposition and the resulting clogging of respiratory tubing and valves in mechanical ventilators. Among hospital admissions for RSV infection, ribavirin therapy failed to decrease length of hospital stay, number of days in the intensive care unit, or number of days receiving mechanical ventilation. Consequently, the American Academy of Pediatrics has modified its recommendation for the use of ribavirin from "should be used" to "may be considered."[45] In light of this and because of the requirement for special aerosolization equipment and the cost of the drug itself, most experts recommend reserving use of ribavirin for severely ill patients, especially those with chronic lung disease (particularly bronchopulmonary dysplasia), congenital heart disease, prematurity, and immunodeficiency [especially severe combined immunodeficiency and human immunodeficiency virus (HIV) infection].

CLINICAL CONTROVERSY

Because bacteria are not primary pathogens in the etiology of bronchiolitis, antibiotics should not be administered routinely. Despite this, many clinicians frequently administer antibiotics while awaiting culture results because the clinical and radiographic findings in bronchiolitis often are suggestive of possible bacterial pneumonia.

For infants with underlying pulmonary or cardiovascular disease, prophylaxis against RSV may be warranted. When administered monthly during the RSV season, both RSV immune globulin[50] and palivizumab[51,52] (a monoclonal antibody for RSV) may decrease the number of RSV episodes and the need for hospitalization. Between the two, palivizumab appears to be preferred, given its ease of administration, lack of administration-related adverse effects, and noninterference with select immunizations.

There is no vaccine marketed for RSV. Of note, in the 1960s, a formalin-inactivated vaccine induced a promising IgG response; however, the severity of subsequent infections was increased in immunized patients. In addition, aside from the need to induce immunity to multiple strains of the virus, a series of boosters would be required as natural infection with RSV does not prevent subsequent infections.[47]

PNEUMONIA

EPIDEMIOLOGY

Pneumonia is the most common infectious cause of death in the United States, where approximately three million cases are diagnosed annually at a cost of more than $20 billion to the healthcare system.[53,54] Pneumonia occurs throughout the year, with the relative prevalence of disease resulting from different etiologic agents varying with the seasons. It occurs in persons of all ages, although the clinical manifestations are most severe in the very young, the elderly, and the chronically ill.

PATHOGENESIS

Microorganisms gain access to the lower respiratory tract by three routes. They may be inhaled as aerosolized particles, or they may enter the lung via the bloodstream from an extrapulmonary site of infection; however, aspiration of oropharyngeal contents, a common occurrence in both healthy and ill persons during sleep, is the major mechanism by which pulmonary pathogens gain access to the normally sterile lower airways and alveoli. When pulmonary defense mechanisms are functioning optimally, aspirated microorganisms are cleared from the region before infection can become established; however, aspiration of potential pathogens from the oropharynx can result in pneumonia if lung defenses are impaired.[1] Factors that promote aspiration, such as altered sensorium and neuromuscular disease, may result in an increase in the size of the inoculum delivered to the lower respiratory tract, thereby overwhelming local defense mechanisms. Lung infections with viruses suppress the antibacterial activity of the lung by impairing alveolar macrophage function and mucociliary clearance, thus setting the stage for secondary bacterial pneumonia. Mucociliary transport is also depressed by ethanol and narcotics and by obstruction of a bronchus by mucus, tumor, or extrinsic compression. All these factors can severely impair pulmonary clearance of aspirated bacteria.

❽ The most prominent pathogen causing community-acquired pneumonia (CAP) in otherwise healthy adults is *S. pneumoniae* and accounts for up to 75% of all acute cases. Other common pathogens include *M. pneumoniae*, *Legionella species*, *C. pneumoniae*, *H. influenzae*, and a variety of viruses including influenza.[6,53,54] Healthcare-associated pneumonia (HCAP) has been a recently accepted classification used to distinguish nonhospitalized patients at risk for MDR pathogens [e.g., *P. aeruginosa*, *Acinetobacter species*, and methicillin-resistant *S. aureus* (MRSA)] from those with CAP.[6,55] The term *atypical* may be applied to pneumonia to indicate that the pneumonia may be caused by an atypical pathogen (e.g., bilateral lobar pneumonia with a negative Gram stain of sputum) caused by *M. pneumoniae*, *C. pneumoniae*, or *Legionella species*.[56]

Gram-negative aerobic bacilli, *S. aureus*, and MDR pathogens are the leading causative agents in hospital-acquired pneumonia (HAP).[7] Anaerobic bacteria are the most common etiologic agents in pneumonia that follows the gross aspiration of gastric or oropharyngeal contents. Ventilator-associated pneumonia (VAP) is also associated with MDR pathogens.

Pneumonia in infants and children is caused by a wider range of microorganisms, and, unlike adults, nonbacterial pathogens predominate. Most pneumonias occurring in the pediatric age group are caused by viruses, especially RSV, parainfluenza, and adenovirus.[45] *M. pneumoniae* is an important pathogen in older children. Beyond the neonatal period, *S. pneumoniae* is the major bacterial pathogen in childhood pneumonia, followed by group A *Streptococcus* and *S. aureus*. *H. influenzae* type b, once a major childhood pathogen, has become an infrequent cause of pneumonia since the introduction of active vaccination against this organism in the late 1980s.

Based on the differences in severity and outcome for patients with CAP, genetic factors likely play a role.[57] Multiple variations in genes affecting inflammation, cough and airway protection, pattern recognition molecules, and organ function along with environmental factors may alter a patient's response to CAP. In the future, as specific genetic polymorphisms are better associated with disease response, therapy should become better targeted.

TABLE 116-5	Clinical Presentation of Pneumonia

Signs and symptoms
Abrupt onset of fever, chills, dyspnea, and productive cough
Rust-colored sputum or hemoptysis
Pleuritic chest pain

Physical examination
Tachypnea and tachycardia
Dullness to percussion
Increased tactile fremitus, whisper pectoriloquy, and egophony
Chest wall retractions and grunting respirations
Diminished breath sounds over affected area
Inspiratory crackles during lung expansion

Chest radiograph
Dense lobar or segmental infiltrate

Laboratory tests
Leukocytosis with predominance of polymorphonuclear cells
Low oxygen saturation on arterial blood gas or pulse oximetry

CLINICAL PRESENTATION

Bacterial pneumonia is caused most commonly by gram-positive streptococci and staphylococci and gram-negative organisms that normally inhabit the gastrointestinal tract (enterics) and soil and water (nonenterics). In addition, *Legionella,* itself a weakly staining gram-negative nonenteric organism, accounts for a small percentage of community- and hospital-acquired bacterial pneumonia, although the true incidence may be underreported.[58] Finally, *M. tuberculosis,* an acid-fast staining bacillus, has reemerged as an important cause of pneumonia in urban centers throughout the United States.

A wide array of gram-positive and gram-negative organisms can cause pneumonia, but they usually present a similar clinical appearance (Table 116–5). *S. pneumoniae, S. aureus,* the enteric gram-negative rods, and occasionally other organisms may produce local irritation or destruction of blood vessels leading to rust-colored sputum or hemoptysis. Pleural effusions, both sterile and empyematous, may be associated with many of these entities, as evidenced by distant breath sounds and a wide area of dulled percussion. The chest radiograph and sputum examination and culture are the most useful diagnostic tests for gram-positive and gram-negative bacterial pneumonia. Typically, the chest radiograph reveals a dense lobar or segmental infiltrate. However, patchy consolidation may be seen occasionally with virtually all these pathogens. Occasionally, pneumonia resulting from hematogenous spread of the organisms results in a diffuse, alveolar pattern on chest radiograph. Gram stain of the expectorated sputum demonstrates many polymorphonuclear cells per high-powered field in the presence of a predominant organism, which is reflected as heavy growth of a single species on culture. Other laboratory tests are less sensitive or specific. Blood cultures may be helpful in identifying the offending organism but are positive in only a minority of patients. The complete blood count usually reflects a leukocytosis with a predominance of polymorphonuclear cells; in some instances, particularly with *S. pneumoniae,* elevation of the white blood cell (WBC) count may be pronounced. Normal or mildly elevated WBC counts, however, do not exclude bacterial pneumonic disease. The patient also may be hypoxic, as reflected by low oxygen saturation on arterial blood gas or pulse oximetry.

Although the clinical appearance of gram-positive and gram-negative pneumonias is similar, epidemiologic and clinical clues render one more likely than the other.

Community-Acquired Pneumonia

❽ *S. pneumoniae* is the most common community-acquired bacterial pneumonia, accounting for up to 76% of cases.[54] It is particularly prevalent and severe for patients with splenic dysfunction, diabetes mellitus, chronic cardiopulmonary or renal disease, or HIV infection. Community-acquired disease with *S. aureus* is identified most frequently in young infants, patients with early cystic fibrosis, and those recovering from an antecedent respiratory viral infection. Group A *Streptococcus* is an uncommon cause of CAP and frequently occurs after a viral respiratory tract infection. Only occasionally is it associated with streptococcal pharyngitis. The organism is pyogenic, and the presentation can be severe. Community-acquired enteric gram-negative pneumonia is identified most frequently among patients with chronic illness, especially alcoholism and diabetes mellitus.

Severity scores, with varying strengths and weaknesses, have been utilized to assist healthcare professionals in predicting outcomes for patients with CAP.[59] Definitions of severe CAP may vary depending on the institution; however, patients with severe CAP are more likely to require intensive care, mechanical ventilation, or complications with sepsis, bacteremia, or multiorgan failure.[55] Severe CAP may be difficult to distinguish from HCAP or HAP; however, the pathogens, *S. pneumoniae, H. influenzae,* and anaerobic bacteria are not usually MDR. Patients at greater risk for severe CAP are those with underlying medical conditions or at risk for aspiration, animal exposure, or exposure to other infected patients or seasonal epidemics.[55]

Healthcare-Associated Pneumonia

Over the past several decades, the types of facilities where patients can receive healthcare has changed with infusion therapies, wound care, and dialysis available in an outpatient environment.[60] This, along with patients residing in a nursing home or long-term care facility or patients recently discharged from a hospital, has blurred the distinction between the pneumonia acquired as an inpatient versus an outpatient. See Table 116–6 for HCAP criteria. Patients diagnosed with HCAP are more similar to hospitalized patients based on comorbid conditions (e.g., heart disease, chronic kidney disease, immunocompromised, or dementia) than patients with CAP and are at a greater risk for multidrug-resistant pathogens.[7,55] The more common pathogens isolated from residents of long-term care facilities/nursing homes have MRSA, enteric gram-negative rods, and *Pseudomonas* species.[7] Compared with patients with CAP, patients with HCAP are more likely to receive inappropriate antibiotics initially and have a higher risk of mortality.[61] Thus, it is important to recognize the difference between HCAP and CAP for appropriate empiric antibiotics.

Pneumonia in the HIV-Infected Patient

HIV infects and destroys helper T lymphocytes bearing the CD4 surface molecule; these cells are critical for orchestrating a wide variety of immunologic responses. Their depletion consequently results in dysfunction of both cell-mediated and humoral immunity. As a result, a broad range of pathogens can cause pneumonia in HIV infection (Table 116–7).[62] The HIV-infected patient may be afflicted with pneumonia multiple times in his or her lifetime, particularly in the advanced stages of the disease, and a given episode may be caused by more than one species.

The clinical presentation of pneumonia in HIV-infected persons frequently is not helpful in distinguishing one pathogen from another. The pneumonia usually is subacute in onset and consists of fever, nonproductive cough, and dyspnea. Radiographically, most of these entities produce a multilobular or diffuse pattern. Some practitioners initially treat the HIV-infected patient with pneumonia empirically, covering the most common entities (bacteria and *P. jiroveci*). However, given the wide array of possible pathogens, more frequently a specific microbiologic diagnosis is aggressively

TABLE 116-6	Pneumonia Classifications and Risk Factors	
Type of Pneumonia	**Definition**	**Risk Factors**
Community acquired (CAP)	Pneumonia developing in patients with no contact to a medical facility	• Age >65 years • Diabetes Mellitus • Asplenia • Chronic cardiovascular, pulmonary, renal and/or liver disease • Smoking and/or alcohol abuse
Healthcare associated (HCAP)	Pneumonia developing in patients not in medical facility but two or more risk factors for MDR pathogens	• Recent hospitalization ≥2 days within past 90 days • Nursing home or long-term care facility resident • Recent (past 30 days) antibiotic use, chemotherapy, wound care or infusion therapy either at a healthcare facility or home • Hemodialysis patients • Contact with a family member with infection caused by MDR pathogen
Hospital-acquired (HAP)	Pneumonia developing >48 hours after hospital admission	• Witnessed aspiration • COPD, ARDS, or coma • Administration of antacids or H2-antagonists • Supine position • Enteral nutrition, nasogastric tube • Reintubation, tracheostomy, or patient transport • Prior antibiotic exposure • Head trauma, ICP monitoring • Age >60 years • See healthcare associated for MDR risk factors
Ventilator associated (VAP)	Pneumonia developing >48 hours after intubation and mechanical ventilation	• Same as hospital acquired

TABLE 116-7	Pulmonary Complications of Human Immunodeficiency Virus Infection

Infections
  Viruses
    Cytomegalovirus
    Herpes simplex virus
    Varicella-zoster virus
    Respiratory syncytial virus and other common respiratory pathogens (parainfluenza virus, adenovirus)
    Measles virus
  Bacteria
    Pyogenic organisms (especially *S. pneumoniae, H. influenzae*; in late disease, *S. aureus* and gram-negative organisms)
    M. tuberculosis
    M. avium complex and other nontuberculous mycobacteria
  Fungi
    Histoplasma capsulatum
    Coccidioides immitis
    Cryptococcus neoformans
    Candida species
    Aspergillus species
  Parasites
    Pneumocystis carinii
    Toxoplasma gondii
    Cryptosporidia
    Strongyloides stercoralis
Malignancies
  Kaposi's sarcoma
  Non-Hodgkin's lymphoma
  Smooth muscle tumors
Lymphocytic interstitial pneumonitis
Nonspecific interstitial pneumonitis
Drug-induced pneumonitis

From reference 63.

radiation or chemotherapy or infiltration of the lung parenchyma by the tumor itself.

Hospital-Acquired Pneumonia

After the urinary tract and the bloodstream, the lungs are the most frequent site of infection acquired in the hospital. HAP is seen most commonly in critically ill patients and usually caused by bacteria.[7,65] Factors predisposing patients to the development of HAP include the severity of illness, duration of hospitalization, supine positioning, witnessed aspiration, coma, acute respiratory distress syndrome, patient transport, and prior antibiotic exposure (see Table 116–6).[66] The strongest predisposing factor, however, is mechanical ventilation (intubation). The length of stay for hospital admissions is increased, on average, by 7 to 9 days for patients who develop HAP.[7]

The organisms most commonly associated with HAP are *S. aureus* and enteric (e.g., *K. pneumoniae* or *E. coli*) and nonenteric (e.g., *P. aeruginosa*) gram-negative bacilli, organisms that colonize the pharynx of the hospitalized, critically ill patient. Patients with longer lengths of hospital admission prior to the development of HAP are more likely to have MDR organisms.[7] The diagnosis of HAP usually is established by the presence of a new infiltrate on chest radiograph, fever, worsening respiratory status, and the appearance of thick, neutrophil-laden respiratory secretions. In actuality, the diagnosis often is difficult to make in the intensively ill patient with underlying lung pathology that itself can be associated with an abnormal changing radiograph, as occurs with congestive heart failure or chronic lung disease. If patients develop fever, leukocytosis, purulent sputum, and have positive sputum/tracheal cultures but radiographic imaging does not indicate new infiltrates, the patient may have

pursued early in the patient's course through sputum induction or bronchoalveolar lavage to allow a rational choice of an antimicrobial regimen. The diagnosis and treatment of HIV-infected patients with pulmonary disease is discussed in detail in Chap. 134.

Pneumonia in the Neutropenic Host

Neutropenia in the cancer patient is a common complication of aggressive chemotherapy but occasionally results from the cancer itself. The risk of infection for the cytopenic patient is increased significantly when the absolute neutrophil count falls below 500 cells/mm³ and the neutropenia persists for more than 7 days.[63] For many patients, the duration of chemotherapy-induced cytopenia can be reduced by judicious application of colony-stimulating factors.[64]

The organisms that cause pneumonia in the cytopenic cancer patient include a broad range of bacteria and fungi. The most prominent among these are gram-positive bacteria (staphylococci and streptococci); others include enteric and nonenteric (particularly *P. aeruginosa*) gram-negative rods as well as the fungi (*Candida, Aspergillus*). The chest radiograph may reveal the lobar pattern typical of bacterial infection in the normal host, or it may exhibit a diffuse pattern. Sometimes the pneumonia remains invisible by chest radiograph until the neutropenia resolves. Noninfectious entities that may cause pulmonary symptoms include toxicity from tracheobronchitis as opposed to HAP.[7] Broad-spectrum antibiotics frequently are started empirically even in equivocal circumstances, with bronchoscopy reserved for poorly responsive patients.[7]

Gram-Positive Bacteria

S. aureus is a prominent cause of HAP and may result from hematogenous spread from a distant source. In both settings, it is characteristically severe and accompanied by the formation of pneumatoceles (air-containing cavities within the lung). Infections caused by MDR organisms such as MRSA and more recently vancomycin-intermediate and vancomycin-resistant *S. aureus* are increasing among patients with HAP. Group B *Streptococcus,* although rare in adults, is the most common cause of bacterial pneumonia among neonates, in whom it typically causes a clinical and radiographic picture nearly indistinguishable from hyaline membrane disease.[67]

Enteric Gram-Negative Bacteria

The enteric gram-negative bacteria are leading causes of HAP because the upper respiratory tract becomes rapidly colonized with gram-negative organisms after hospitalization, particularly among critically ill patients and those receiving antibiotics.[68] *K. pneumoniae* is the most frequently encountered pathogen among the gram-negative enteric bacteria, although the relative prominence of these organisms varies among hospitals. The gram-negative bacilli are associated with high mortality, sometimes exceeding 50%; their potential to produce significant morbidity and mortality has been enhanced by the emergence of highly MDR organisms in some hospital settings.[7]

Nonenteric Gram-Negative Bacteria

The most prominent nonenteric gram-negative rods associated with pneumonia include *P. aeruginosa, H. influenzae,* and *M. catarrhalis.* Like the enteric gram-negative organisms, *P. aeruginosa* is a frequent cause of HAP and is particularly prominent among neutropenic and burn patients.[7] In addition, cystic fibrosis patients suffer from chronic, multilobar infections with *P. aeruginosa* as well as other *Pseudomonas* species; these infections are punctuated with acute exacerbations.[69] *H. influenzae* type b historically has been a prominent pathogen in childhood pneumonia. However, the incidence of all invasive disease due to this organism in the pediatric age group has dropped dramatically since the introduction of the conjugated *Haemophilus* vaccines in the late 1980s. However, two different clinical presentations of *H. influenzae* pneumonia still are seen in adults. The most common by far is the bronchopneumonia form, which develops most frequently for patients with underlying chronic lung disease and is believed to represent, in most patients, an exacerbation of chronic bronchitis. In the second form of *H. influenzae* pneumonia, segmental or lobar involvement predominates. The course of this illness is more acute, with sudden onset of cough, fever, and pleuritic chest pain. Finally, *M. catarrhalis,* an important cause of otitis media and sinusitis, is an increasingly important cause of lower respiratory tract infections in immunoincompetent and hospitalized patients.

Anaerobic Bacteria

8 Anaerobic pneumonitis is most likely to occur in individuals predisposed to aspiration by impaired consciousness and may be more prevalent in those with periodontal disease or dysphagia. Bronchogenic carcinoma is an associated underlying condition. A variety of gram-positive and gram-negative anaerobic bacteria indigenous to the upper airway may cause pneumonitis when large quantities of oropharyngeal secretions are aspirated into the lower airways. The organisms most frequently implicated are *Peptostreptococcus* species, *Fusobacteria, B. melaninogenicus, B. fragilis,* and *Peptococcus* species; polymicrobial infections with anaerobes and aerobes, such as *S. aureus, S. pneumoniae,* and gramnegative bacilli, are common.[70]

The course of illness typically is indolent, with cough, low-grade fever, and weight loss, although an acute presentation may occur. Rigors are notably absent, and bacteremia is rare. Putrid sputum, when present, is highly suggestive of the diagnosis. Chest radiographs reveal infiltrates typically located in dependent lung segments, and lung abscesses develop in 20% of patients 1 to 2 weeks into the course of the illness.

Ventilator-Associated Pneumonia

VAP is defined as pneumonia occurring >48 hours post endotracheal intubation. The risk for developing pneumonia in the hospital increases by 6 to 21 times after a patient is intubated[7] because it bypasses the natural airway defenses against the migration of upper respiratory tract organisms into the lower tract. This situation is exacerbated by the wide use of H2-receptor blocking agents in the intensive care unit, which increases the pH of gastric secretions and may promote the proliferation of microorganisms in the upper gastrointestinal tract. Subclinical microaspirations are events that occur routinely in intubated patients and result in the inoculation of bacteria-contaminated gastric contents into the lung and a higher incidence of nosocomial pneumonia. VAP can be diagnosed accurately by any one of multiple standard criteria, including histopathologic examination of lung tissue obtained by open-lung biopsy, rapid cavitation of a pulmonary infiltrate in the absence of cancer or tuberculosis, positive pleural fluid culture, and same species with an identical antibiogram for a pathogen(s) isolated from blood and respiratory secretions without another identifiable source of bacteremia.[10] *P. aeruginosa* is the most common organism associated with VAP. Outbreaks of HAP may be caused occasionally by contaminated respiratory therapy equipment.

Atypical Pneumonia

Viruses, *Mycoplasma* species, *Chlamydia* species, and fungi are recognized causes of pneumonia syndromes in all age groups. The designation *atypical pneumonia,* distinct from the typical bacterial pneumonia seen most commonly in adults, has been used to describe the illness caused by many of these agents.[71]

Legionella Pneumophila

Of the several *Legionella* species known to cause pneumonia in humans, *L. pneumophila* is by far the most important, accounting for 2% to 15% of all CAPs in North America and Europe.[58] *Legionella* is a water and soil organism and most probably is transmitted by inhalation of aerosols containing the organism or by microaspiration of contaminated water. Outbreaks of illness caused by *L. pneumophila* have been linked to excavation sites and to contaminated water from air conditioners and showers. Person-to-person transmission has not been demonstrated. In addition to epidemics, *L. pneumophila* causes sporadic illness that peaks in summer and fall. Individuals who are male, middle aged or older, immunocompromised, chronic bronchitics, or cigarette smokers are at increased risk.

Infection with *L. pneumophila* is characterized by multisystem involvement, including rapidly progressive pneumonia.[71] It has a gradual onset, with prominent constitutional symptoms (e.g., malaise, lethargy, weakness, anorexia) occurring early in the course of the illness. A dry, nonproductive cough is present initially and becomes productive of mucoid or purulent sputum over several days. Fevers exceeding 40°C (104°F) develop in more than half of patients, typically are unremitting, and are associated with a relative bradycardia. Pleuritic chest pain and progressive dyspnea may be seen. Extrapulmonary symptoms, particularly diarrhea, nausea, and vomiting, remain evident throughout the course of the illness. Myalgias and arthralgias also occur. Substantial changes in the patient's mental status, often out of proportion to the degree of fever, are seen in approximately one fourth of patients. Obtundation, hallucinations, grand mal seizures, and focal neurologic findings are also associated with this illness. Chest roentgenograms initially reveal patchy alveolar infiltrates that may be bilateral and asymmetric. Pulmonary infiltrates may worsen even when the patient is receiving appropriate antibiotics. Progression to lobar or multilobar consolidation is frequent, as are small pleural effusions.

Laboratory findings include leukocytosis with a predominance of mature and immature granulocytes in 50% to 75% of patients. Urinalysis may reveal proteinuria, hematuria, and casts; liver function tests may be abnormal. Hyponatremia and hypophosphatemia have been reported frequently. Because *L. pneumophila* stains poorly with commonly used stains, routine microscopic examination of sputum is of little diagnostic value. Although it exhibits slow growth and has highly selective growth requirements, *L. pneumophila* has been isolated successfully from tissue using a specialized medium. Direct fluorescent antibody examination of respiratory tract secretions, lung tissue, or pleural fluid is the most rapid means of establishing the diagnosis. The sensitivity of this method approaches 70% for sputum and 90% for lung tissue, and diagnostic specificity is high for both. Commercially available urine antigen tests have been developed for *L. pneumophila*. These tests are 70% sensitive and remain positive for weeks, even after effective antibiotics have been started. Because these diagnostic tests are unavailable in many clinical laboratories, the diagnosis of Legionnaires' disease often is presumptive and based on a suggestive clinical presentation.

Mycoplasma Pneumonia

Taxonomically, the mycoplasmas are included in their own class labeled *Mollicutes*. Although their small size and filterability are similar to viruses, the structure of their ribosomal RNA indicates that they have evolved from bacteria, and, unlike any virus, they contain cytoplasm and can replicate in an extracellular environment. They are distinguished from eubacteria by their low genetic content. In addition, the mycoplasmas lack a cell wall and are surrounded instead by a lipid membrane. This latter characteristic explains the resistance of these pathogens to cell-wall active antibiotics.

M. pneumoniae causes human disease throughout the year, with a slightly increased incidence in fall and early winter. During the summer months when other causes of pneumonia are less common, *M. pneumoniae* is responsible for a greater proportion of cases. Both infection and disease from *M. pneumoniae* are common, with two thirds of children ages 2 to 5 years and 97% of persons older than 17 years having detectable serum antibody to the organism. Overall, *M. pneumoniae* is responsible for approximately 20% of pneumonia cases, although in enclosed populations, such as military recruits and college dormitory residents, it may cause more than 50%. Infection is spread by close person-to-person contact, and the incubation period is 2 to 3 weeks. *M. pneumoniae* infections are unusual in children younger than 5 years and show a peak incidence in older children and young adults. Only 3% to 10% of persons infected with *M. pneumoniae* develop pneumonia, with the majority of respiratory tract involvement manifested as pharyngitis and tracheobronchitis. Asymptomatic infection is common.

M. pneumoniae usually presents with a gradual onset of fever, headache, and malaise, with the appearance 3 to 5 days after the onset of illness of a persistent, hacking cough that initially is nonproductive. Sore throat, ear pain, and rhinorrhea often are present. Chills are seen only occasionally, and pleuritic pain is uncommon. Lung findings generally are limited to rales and rhonchi; findings of consolidation are rare. Nonpulmonary manifestations are extremely common and include nausea, vomiting, diarrhea, myalgias, arthralgias, polyarticular arthritis, skin rashes, myocarditis and pericarditis, hemolytic anemia, meningoencephalitis, cranial neuropathies, and Guillain-Barré syndrome. Systemic symptoms generally clear in 1 to 2 weeks, whereas respiratory symptoms may persist for up to 4 weeks. Although the course of mycoplasmal pneumonia usually is benign and self-limited, severe respiratory disease may develop in patients with sickle cell disease, agammaglobulinemia, and COPD.[71]

Radiographic findings generally are more impressive than the patient's physical findings and include patchy or interstitial infiltrates, which are seen most commonly in the lower lobes. Small unilateral, transient pleural effusions are common, but large effusions and empyema are rare. Roentgenographic abnormalities resolve slowly, and 4 to 6 weeks may be required for complete resolution.

Sputum Gram stain may reveal mononuclear or polymorphonuclear leukocytes, with no predominant organism. Although *M. pneumoniae* can be cultured from respiratory secretions using specialized medium, its growth is slow, and 2 to 3 weeks may be necessary for culture identification. Indirect evidence of infection by *M. pneumoniae* is the presence of elevated levels of serum cold hemagglutinins. These immunoglobulin M antibodies develop in approximately half of patients with mycoplasmal pneumonia and can be elevated in other illnesses, especially viral infection. A definitive diagnosis also can be made by demonstrating a fourfold or greater rise in serum antibodies to *M. pneumoniae*. However, because this test also requires 2 to 4 weeks for results, the diagnosis of mycoplasmal pneumonia during the acute phase of the illness must be based on the characteristic history, appropriate clinical setting, and typical physical findings.

Chlamydophila Pneumonia

C. pneumoniae has received the new taxonomic classification of *Chlamydophila*; however, it may still be referred to as *Chlamydia pneumoniae* in some references.[16] *C. pneumoniae*, formally designated the *TWAR* agent after the laboratory designations for the first two isolates, is antigenically similar to *C. psittaci*. *C. pneumoniae* infection is ubiquitous worldwide, but only a small percentage of infections result in clinically apparent pneumonia. Conversely, approximately 5% to 15% of pneumonia is associated with this pathogen.[16] Primary infection with *Chlamydia* pneumonia typically occurs in young adults and is characterized by mild respiratory symptoms with a gradual onset. Constitutional manifestations, particularly fever and headache, are common. The radiographic findings are nonspecific and usually consist of multilobular interstitial infiltrates. Immunity is incomplete, and reinfection with *C. pneumoniae* is common, particularly among the elderly. Definitive diagnosis of *C. pneumoniae*–associated pneumonia depends on identification of the organism in sputum. Culture of this organism is difficult, and commercially available antigen detection systems are insensitive.

Viral Pneumonia

Viruses are an uncommon cause of pneumonia in adults, except in the immunosuppressed.[3] Influenza virus, usually type A, is the most common cause of pneumonia in the adult civilian population causing CAP;[6] adenoviruses cause most cases in military trainees. In contrast, viruses are by far the most common agents producing pneumonia in infants and young children, with RSV, parainfluenza, and adenovirus producing most cases.[7,43]

All viral respiratory tract infections occur more commonly in the winter, and rapid person-to-person spread through susceptible populations is typical. Underlying cardiac or pulmonary disease predisposes to an increased incidence and severity of viral lower respiratory tract infection, especially with influenza virus in adults and RSV in children. Radiographic findings are nonspecific and include bronchial wall thickening and perihilar and diffuse interstitial infiltrates. Pleural effusions may be seen, especially in adenovirus and parainfluenza pneumonia.

The clinical pictures produced by respiratory viruses are sufficiently variable and overlap to such a degree that an etiologic diagnosis can not be made confidently based on clinical grounds alone. Although virus isolation in tissue culture is possible, a period of 7 or more days often is required for virus identification; thus, this method usually cannot be used for definitive diagnosis during the acute phase of illness. Serologic tests for virus-specific antibodies are used often in the diagnosis of viral infections. The diagnostic fourfold rise in titer between acute and convalescent phase sera may require 2 to 3 weeks to develop. Same-day diagnosis of viral infections now is possible using indirect immunofluorescence tests on exfoliated cells from the respiratory tract. The immunofluorescence technique frequently uses a battery of monoclonal antibodies, including those against influenza A and B, RSV, parainfluenza, and adenovirus, to provide rapid diagnosis of a range of viral infections.[3]

Tuberculosis

The acid-fast bacillus *M. tuberculosis* causes tuberculosis. After years of steady decline, the number of cases of pneumonia caused by *M. tuberculosis* in the United States began to increase in the middle to late 1980s. The new epidemic was a consequence of an increased incidence among prison inmates, intravenous drug abusers, immigrants, and, most prominently, HIV-infected patients.[72] It is most prominent in urban neighborhoods afflicted with crowded conditions and poor access to healthcare. Unlike previous eras in which tuberculosis was seen most frequently in elderly men, infection currently is identified in increasing numbers of young minority adults. As mentioned, the resurgence of tuberculosis is at least partially related to coinfection with HIV; HIV-infected patients are more likely to develop symptomatic disease with its associated fits of coughing than are their immunocompetent counterparts, and this enables further spread of infection. Other groups prone to tuberculosis include the homeless and patients in chronic care facilities and homes for the elderly. Fortunately, since 1992, the incidence of tuberculosis in the United States has declined, reaching a record low. However, the incidence of tuberculosis worldwide continues to increase. Both the sustained worldwide increase in tuberculosis and the reemergence of tuberculosis in the United States are important reasons for the development of multiple-drug resistance, that is, mycobacteria that are resistant to two or more of the first-line antituberculosis drugs. Infection caused by these organisms is poorly responsive to alternative therapy and is associated with mortality rates exceeding 50% (see Chap. 121).

Tuberculosis is spread from person to person by inhalation of droplet nuclei generated by vigorous coughing. Adult disease (from adolescence onward) begins with constitutional complaints, followed by a prominent chronic, troublesome cough productive of mucopurulent material. The infection initially appears in the lung apices with little or no hilar adenopathy and, in advanced disease, results in lung necrosis, producing a cavity containing enormous numbers of organisms. In contrast, pediatric tuberculosis commonly is associated with little cough even in the presence of extensive pulmonary infection. Instead, the child presents with a subacute course of poor appetite, weight loss, lethargy, fever, and sweats.

Severe Acute Respiratory Syndrome

In November 2002, an extremely contagious atypical pneumonia manifested in China that since has been termed *severe acute respiratory syndrome* (SARS).[73] The etiology of SARS is an enveloped RNA virus, a coronavirus, referred to as SARS-CoV. The virus is transmitted primarily via large-droplet spread; however, surface contamination and airborne and fecal spread are possible. Signs and symptoms associated with SARS include high fever, myalgias, headache, diarrhea, and a dry nonproductive cough. Respiratory symptoms may progress to shortness of breath and hypoxemia, necessitating the need for intubation and mechanical ventilation. Diagnostic tests for patients suspected of contracting SARS should include chest x-ray film, blood cultures, sputum cultures and Gram stain, pulse oximetry, and identification of other potential pathogens, including influenza A and B, *Legionella,* and RSV. For unclear reasons, SARS appears to be less severe for pediatric patients.

Avian Influenza (Bird Flu)

All influenza viruses may be present in aquatic birds, with the H5N1 subtype being extremely pathogenic and fatal to fowl.[74,75] The first known cases of humans infected with this subtype occurred in Hong Kong in 1997, with 6 deaths among 18 infected patients. Signs and symptoms typical of the H5N1 virus are those common to other subtypes and include conjunctivitis, fever, rhinitis, and pharyngitis. However, pneumonia, respiratory distress syndrome, lymphopenia, and clotting abnormalities tend to occur rapidly in patients infected with this highly virulent subtype. Laboratory tests used to detect the H5N1 virus include immunoassays and reverse-transcription PCR.

H1N1 Influenza (Swine Flu)

In April 2009, a novel influenza A virus of swine origin, H1N1, was identified as the causative pathogen in a recent outbreak of respiratory illness and influenza-like illness in Mexico.[76] Due to a report of atypical pneumonia and an increase in the number of respiratory illnesses in North America, surveillance increased that resulted in the WHO raising alert status to phase 6, global pandemic, in June 2009. Signs and symptoms of the H1N1 virus are similar to other subtypes and include fever, cough, sore throat, body and headaches, chills, and fatigue; however, more serious infections have resulted in hospitalization and death. It has also affected normally healthy young adults as opposed to other flu viruses, which tend to be more severe in the young and the elderly. Transmission of the virus is thought to be similar to seasonal flu and spread via coughing, sneezing, and touching infected objects. PCR diagnostic kits have been developed to facilitate the detection of the virus.

TREATMENT

Pneumonia

■ DESIRED OUTCOME

Eradication of the offending organism through selection of the appropriate antibiotic and complete clinical cure are the goals of therapy for bacterial pneumonia. Therapy should minimize associated morbidity, including one or both of the following: reversible or irreversible disease and drug-induced organ toxicity (e.g., renal, lung, or hepatic dysfunction). Most cases of viral pneumonia are self-limiting, although therapy of influenza pneumonia with specific antiviral agents (oseltamivir and zanamivir) may hasten recovery. All efforts should focus on the design of the most cost-effective approach to therapy. Whenever possible, the oral (vs parenteral) route for drug administration should be selected, encouraging outpatient management rather than hospitalization.

■ GENERAL APPROACH TO TREATMENT

⑨ The first priority in assessing the patient with pneumonia is to evaluate the adequacy of respiratory function and to determine the presence of signs of systemic illness, specifically dehydration or sepsis with resulting circulatory collapse. Oxygen or, in severe cases, mechanical ventilation and fluid resuscitation should be provided as necessary. Further supportive care of the patient with pneumonia includes humidified oxygen for hypoxemia, administration of bronchodilators (albuterol) when bronchospasm is present, and chest physiotherapy with postural drainage if evidence of retained secretions is present. Additional therapeutic adjuncts include adequate hydration (intravenously if necessary), optimal nutritional support, and control of fever. Appropriate sputum samples may be obtained to determine the microbiologic etiology. Rehydration should be provided to replace losses that may have occurred as a result of fever, poor intake, and/or associated vomiting. Selection of an appropriate antimicrobial must be made based on the patient's probable or documented microbiology, distribution in the respiratory tract, side effects, and cost. Respiratory track infection diagnosis and treatment guideline reports have been published by authoritative professional organizations that focus on proper treatment regimens and should be consulted for evidence-based treatment recommendations across the spectrum of community- and/or hospital-associated pneumonias.[77,78]

■ PHARMACOLOGIC THERAPY

Antibiotic Concentrations

Antibiotic concentrations in respiratory secretions in excess of the pathogen MIC are necessary for successful treatment of pulmonary infections.[78,79] The concept of a blood–bronchus barrier, analogous but dissimilar to the blood–brain barrier, has been used to assess the characteristics of drug penetration into pulmonary secretions. The ability of a drug to penetrate respiratory secretions depends on multiple physicochemical factors, including molecular size, lipid solubility, and degree of ionization at serum and biologic fluid pH and extent of protein binding. Studies performed in animals and cystic fibrosis patients suggest that larger molecular size favors the accumulation of drugs in bronchial secretions. This finding contrasts with data on drug penetration of other physiologic compartments, such as the cerebrospinal fluid, and may be a result of the trapping of lower-molecular-weight compounds in mucin pores. Nevertheless, the rate at which a drug may accumulate in certain respiratory secretions appears to remain an important factor relative to the drug's clinical efficacy in treating pulmonary infections. The un-ionized form of drug and lipid solubility also appears to favor drug penetration. Of note, the pH of the infected bronchi often is more acidic than that of normal tissue and blood. These factors combined underscore the importance of considering the inhaled route of antimicrobial drugs for the treatment of patients with moderate to severe pneumonia, particularly in high-risk patient groups.[79-81]

Limited data are available for assessing the influence of drug protein binding on the rate and amount of respiratory secretion penetration. Clearly, it is the free antibiotic fraction reaching the infected site capable of binding to the bacterial cell target that is responsible for antibacterial activity. Given that the degree of protein binding influences a drug's ability to traverse membranes, a similar relationship would be expected within the lung. However,

focusing on the absolute amount of an antibiotic bound to plasma/tissue proteins without accounting for the drug's overall antibacterial potency is errant. To completely assess an antibiotic's therapeutic potential in the treatment of pneumonia or any infectious process, it is prudent to assess the antibiotic's integrated pharmacokinetic–pharmacodynamic (PK-PD) characteristics (e.g., bacterial killing may be concentration dependent or time dependent) that account for the drug's degree of binding to serum proteins, tissue distribution, and in vitro potency. Thus, simply focusing on a drug's degree of protein binding is an errant, overly simplistic approach that does not account for the drug's inherent antibacterial activity or distribution characteristics.

These concepts relating to antibiotic activity and overall drug penetration of respiratory secretions underscore the importance of applying the advances realized in our knowledge of antimicrobial PK and PD to the design of optimal antibiotic dosing regimens. Integration of an individual antimicrobial drug's PK-PD has afforded the development of just such optimal antibiotic dosing regimens (improved efficacy and safety) based upon drug- and patient-specific factors.[77,78] A primary example of antibiotic PK-PD designed optimal dosing is reflected in the clinical practice of administering certain antibiotics (aminoglycosides) to achieve high peak serum concentrations on the assumption that higher (and possibly more effective) biologic fluid concentrations of the drug will be achieved. The aminoglycosides are large polar molecules that diffuse poorly into tissue and respiratory secretions; however, with increasing concentrations obtained with once-daily dosing, increased target-tissue concentrations would be expected with increasing individual doses. Further, recognizing that the peak drug concentration-to-pathogen MIC ratio (Cmax:MIC) is the primary PK-PD correlate for aminoglycosides and that the target Cmax:MIC ratio for aminoglycosides is ~10, the single daily dose strategy is most likely to achieve the desired PK-PD target at the desired anatomic site. Similarly for the so-called respiratory fluoroquinolones (e.g., levofloxacin, moxifloxacin, gemifloxacin) higher individual dose therapy targeting a greater Cmax:MIC ratio or the more commonly targeted area under the concentration time curve (AUC) to pathogen MIC ratio, i.e.,AUC:MIC, for fluoroquinolones. The target 24 hour AUC:MIC ratio for fluoroquinolones is 35+ (possible minimum of 25) for gram-positive and 125+ (possible minimum of 100) for gram-negative pathogens. For greatest probability of success, the antibiotic concentrations projected in these PK-PD correlates should include the expected free (not protein bound) antibiotic concentration. Conversely, concentration-dependent killing characteristics best correlate with successful therapy with the β-lactam/carbapenem and macrolide classes of antimicrobials.[77,78]

Sputum is frequently assessed as possibly representing the PD interface for pulmonary infections. Sputum is only one of many pulmonary fluids and secretions, and it may serve as a reservoir for pathogen growth. These beliefs have led many investigators to assess antibiotic concentrations in sputum, frequently describing sputum drug concentrations as a ratio of serum to sputum drug concentration. Although sputum drug concentrations provide some insight into the characteristics of drug penetration of respiratory secretions, caution should be exercised in the interpretation of these data. Data describing sputum drug concentrations often are difficult to interpret because of differences in analytic techniques, method of sputum sampling, and random nature of sampling times relative to drug dose. Moreover, representation of sputum drug concentrations as a ratio of serum drug concentration can be misleading and most probably should be described relative to absolute drug concentration or apparent area under the drug concentration versus time curve in sputum. To more accurately describe the distribution characteristics of antimicrobial agents in sputum, research studies should be designed to allow sequential repeated sputum sampling over a specified dosage interval under both first-dose and steady-state conditions. Thus, until greater sophistication is achieved in our understanding of the relationships between antibiotic concentrations in specific anatomic sites, plasma (blood)-based integrated PK-PD correlates should be used for antibiotic and dose selection.

Selection of Antimicrobial Agents

Treatment of bacterial pneumonia, like the treatment of most infectious diseases, initially involves the empirical use of a relatively broad-spectrum antibiotic that is effective against probable pathogens after appropriate cultures and specimens for laboratory evaluation have been obtained.[6,7,82] Therapy should be narrowed to cover specific pathogens after the results of cultures are known. Multiple factors that help to define the potential pathogens involved include patient age, previous and current medication history, underlying disease(s), major organ function, and present clinical status. These factors must be evaluated to select an appropriate and effective empirical antibiotic regimen as well as the most appropriate route for drug administration (oral or parenteral). For a more detailed discussion on the principles of antibiotic selection, see Chap. 114.

Numerous antibiotics are available, and many are effective in the treatment of bacterial pneumonia. Superiority of one antibiotic over another when both demonstrate similar dose-normalized in vitro activity and tissue distribution characteristics is difficult to define. Our opinions on appropriate empirical choices for the treatment of bacterial pneumonias relative to a patient's underlying disease are listed in Table 116–8 for adults and Table 116–9 for children. A complete listing of antimicrobial agents for specific pathogens is beyond the scope of this chapter and is presented in Chap. 114.

A patient's previous medical history of responding/not responding to one of these antibiotics in the recent past will assist greatly in the decision to continue their use. In contrast and for patients with risk factors, regardless of the patient's setting at the time of infection, i.e., community, long-term care facility, acute care hospital, etc., the fluoroquinolone antibiotics represent important treatment tools based on their highly favorable PK (tissue and intracellular distribution) and PD (potency, broad spectrum) characteristics combined with ease of administration (IV, oral) and patient tolerability. Furthermore, optimal dosing directed by the projected 24 hour free fluoroquinolone AUC-to-pathogen MIC ratio (see above) has markedly decreased the emergence of pathogen resistance, fostered maximal bacteriologic kill and enhanced patient safety.

Table 116–10 lists dosages for selected antibiotics used for the treatment of bacterial pneumonia. The list of commercially available antimicrobial agents with documented bacterial and clinical effectiveness in the treatment of pneumonia can appear endless.

TABLE 116–8 Evidence-Based Empiric Antimicrobial Therapy for Pneumonia in Adults[a]

Clinical Setting	Usual Pathogens	Empiric Therapy
Outpatient/community acquired		
• Previously healthy	S. pneumoniae, M. pneumoniae, H influenza, C. pneumoniae, M. catarrhalis	Macrolide/azalide[b], or tetracycline[c]
• Comorbidities (diabetes, heart/lung/liver/ renal disease, alcoholism		Fluoroqinolone[d] or β-lactam + macrolide[b]
• Elderly	S. pneumoniae, Gram-negative bacilli	Piperacillin/tazobactam or cephalosporin[e] or carbapenem[f]
Inpatient/community acquired		
• Non-ICU	S. pneumoniae, H. influenza, M. pneumoniae, C. pneumoniae, Legionella sp.	Fluoroquinolone[d] or β-lactam + macrolide[b]
• ICU	S. pneumoniae, S.aureus, Legionella sp, gram-negative bacilli, H. influenza	β-lactam + macrolide[b] or fluoroquinolone[d]; piperacillin/taxobactam or meropenem or cefepime + fluoroquinolone[d], or β-lactam + AMG + azithromycin or β-lactam + AMG + respiratory fluoroquinolone[d]
	If MRSA suspected	Above + vancomycin or linezolid
Hospital acquired, ventilator associated, or healthcare associated		
• No risk factors for MDR pathogens	S. pneumoniae, H. influenzae, MSSA enteric Gram-negative bacilli	Ceftriaxone or fluoroquinolone[d] or ampicillin/sulbactam or ertapenem or doripenem
• Risk factors for MDR pathogen	P. aeruginosa, K. pneumoniae (ESBL), Acinetobacter sp.,	Antipseudomonal cephalosporin[e] or antipseudomonal carbapenem or β-lactam/β-lactamase + antipseudomonal fluoroquinolone[d] or AMG[g]
	If MRSA or Legionella sp. suspected	Above + vancomycin or linezolid
• Aspiration	Mouth anaerobes, S. aereus, enteric Gram-negative bacilli	Penicillin or clindamycin or piperacillin/tazobactum + AMG[g]
Atypical pneumonia[h]		
• Legionella pneumophilia		Fluoroquinolone[d] or doxycycline
• Mycoplasma pneumonia		Fluoroquinolone[d] or doxycycline
• Chlamydophila pneumonia		Fluoroquinolone[d] or doxycycline
• SARS		Fluoroquinolone[d] or macrolides[b]
• Avian Influenza		Oseltamivir
• H1N1 Influenza		Oseltamivir

MRSA, methicillin resistance staphylococcus aureus; AMG, aminoglycoside; SARS, severe acute respiratory syndrome; ESBL, extended-spectrum β-lactamases.

[a]See section on treatment of bacterial pneumonia
[b]Macrolide/azalide: erythromycin, clarithromycin, azithromycin
[c]Tetracycline: tetracycline, HC1, doxycycline
[d]Fluoroquinolone: ciprofloxacin, levofloxacin, moxifloxacin
[e]Antipseudomonal cephalosporin: cefepime, ceftazidime
[f]Antipseudomonal carbapenem: imipenem, meropenem
[g]Aminoglycoside: amikacin, gentamicin, tobramycin
[h]For tuberculosis, see Chap. 121.
Data from references 6 and 7.

TABLE 116-9 Empirical Antimicrobial Therapy for Pneumonia in Pediatric Patients[a]

Age	Usual Pathogen(s)	Empirical Therapy
1 month	Group B streptococcus, H. influenzae (nontypeable), E. coli, S. aureus, Listeria, CMV, RSV, adenovirus	Ampicillin/sulbactam, cephalosporin,[b] carbapenem[c] Ribavirin for RSV[g]
1–3 months	C. pneumoniae, possibly Ureaplasma, CMV, Pneumocystis carinii (afebrile pneumonia syndrome)	Macrolide/azalide,[d] trimethoprim-sulfamethoxazole
	RSV	Ribavirin
	S. pneumoniae, S. aureus	Semisynthetic penicillin[e] or cephalosporin[f]
3 months to 6 years	S. pneumoniae, H. influenzae, RSV, adenovirus, parainfluenza	Amoxicillin or cephalosporin[f] Ampicillin/sulbactam, amoxicillin–clavulanate Ribavirin for RSV
>6 years	S. pneumoniae, M. pneumoniae, adenovirus	Macrolide/azalide[d] cephalosporin,[f] amoxicillin–clavulanate

CMV, cytomegalovirus; RSV, respiratory syncytial virus.
[a]See section on treatment of bacterial pneumonia.
[b]Third-generation cephalosporin: ceftriaxone, cefotaxime, cefepime. Note that cephalosporins are not active against Listeria.
[c]Carbapenem: imipenem–cilastatin, meropenem.
[d]Macrolide/azalide: erythromycin, clarithromycin/azithromycin.
[e]Semisynthetic penicillin: nafcillin, oxacillin.
[f]Second-generation cephalosporin: cefuroxime, cefprozil.
[g]See text for details regarding ribavirin treatment for RSV infection.

TABLE 116-10 Antibiotic Doses for Treatment of Bacterial Pneumonia

Antibiotic Class	Antibiotic	Daily antibiotic dose[a] Pediatric (mg/kg/day)	Adult (Total Dose/Day)
Macrolide	Clarithromycin	15	0.5–1 g
	Erythromycin	30–50	1–2 g
Azalide	Azithromycin	10 mg/kg × 1 day, then 5 mg/kg/day 4 days	500 mg day 1, then 250 mg/day × 4 days
Tetracycline[b]	Doxycycline	2–5	100–200 mg
	Tetracycline HCl	25–50	1–2 g
Penicillin	Ampicillin	100–200	2–6 g
	Amoxicillin ± clavulanate[c]	40–90	0.75–1 g
	Piperacillin/ tazobactam	200–300	12–18 g
	Ampicillin/ sulbactam	100–200	4–8 g
Extended-spectrum cephalosporins	Ceftriaxone	50–75	1–2 g
	Ceftazidime	150	4–6 g
	Cefepime	100–150	2–6 g
Fluoroquinolones[d]	Moxifloxacin		400 mg
	Gemifloxacin	–	320 mg
	Levofloxacin	10–15	0.75 g
	Ciprofloxacin	20–30	1.2 g
Aminoglycosides	Gentamicin	7.5–10	7.5 mg/kg
	Tobramycin	7.5–10	7.5 mg/kg
Carbapenems	Imipenem	60–100 g	2–4 g
	Meropenem	30–60	1–3 g
Other	Vancomycin	45–60	2–3 g
	Linezolid	20–30	1.2 g

[a]Doses can be increased for more severe disease and may require modification for patients with organ dysfunction.
[b]Tetracyclines are rarely used in pediatric patients, particularly in those younger than 8 years because of tetracycline-induced permanent tooth discoloration.
[c]Higher-dose amoxicillin, amoxicillin/clavulanate (e.g., 90 mg/kg/day) is used for penicillin-resistant S. pneumoniae.
[d]Fluoroquinolones have been avoided for pediatric patients because of the potential for cartilage damage; however, they have been used for MDR bacterial infection safely and effectively in infants and children (see text).

The large number of expensive drugs mandates critical evaluation for formulary selection and clinical use. Similarities of in vitro activity, resistance to bacterial-inactivating enzymes, and overall effectiveness often make rational therapeutic decisions difficult and even appear random. However, some general principles can be applied to guide rational antibiotic choice, including direct comparison of the antibiotic's likely attainment of the defined PK-PD target correlate for specific bacterial species within the infected site. These PK-PD principals are outlined above. An understanding and application of inherent drug characteristics appears to be of the utmost importance for the selection of an optimal therapeutic regimen. Thus, whenever possible, identification of the causative pathogen and expected/defined antibiotic activity (e.g., MIC) is of paramount importance to the selection/design of the optimal antibiotic regimen.

Community-Acquired Pneumonia

Table 116–8 provides evidence-based guidelines for the treatment of CAP.[6] The bacterial causes are relatively constant, even across geographic areas and patient populations. Unfortunately, pathogen resistance to standard antimicrobials is increasing (e.g., penicillin-resistant pneumococci), necessitating careful attention by the clinician to local and regional bacterial susceptibility patterns.[53] Thus, whenever possible, initial therapy should be based on presumed antibacterial susceptibility and consist of older, less-expensive agents, with newer and more expensive antibiotics reserved for unresponsive illness or special circumstances. Indiscriminate use of recently introduced agents increases healthcare costs and, in some instances (e.g., widespread use of fluoroquinolones), induces resistance among a significant percentage of community-acquired organisms.[6] It must be emphasized, however, that the rapidly evolving epidemiology of bacterial resistance, including the increasing emergence of penicillin-resistant S. pneumoniae in many areas of the United States and Europe, forces the clinician to be vigilant and knowledgeable about antibiotic sensitivity patterns in each community. Indiscriminate use of antimicrobials for treatment of pneumonia has contributed to the problem of antimicrobial resistance, underscoring the need for defining the optimal antibiotic regimen for each patient.

❾ Evidence-based empirical therapy differs among outpatients, hospitalized patients, and hospitalized patients admitted to an intensive care unit (Table 116–8).[6,83,84] Antimicrobial therapy should be initiated for hospitalized patients with acute pneumonia within 8 hours of admission because an increase in mortality has been demonstrated when therapy was delayed beyond 8 hours of admission.

Healthcare-Associated Pneumonia

It is important to identify patients at risk for HCAP and initiate appropriate empiric antibiotic therapy since these patients are at risk for MDR organisms. Delaying treatment of appropriate antibiotics in these patients increases mortality.[55] Antibiotic selection will be similar to those used in HAP and VAP. Broad spectrum antibiotics should be used empirically for pneumonia developing ≥5 days after hospital admission or if the patient has risk factors for MDR pathogens.[7] See Table 116–8 for recommended empiric antimicrobial therapy.

Hospital-Acquired Pneumonia

❿ Antibiotic selection within the hospital environment demands greater care because of constant changes in antibiotic resistance patterns in vitro and in vivo. Ironically, some β-lactam antibiotics, which were developed to treat MDR hospital-acquired organisms, can themselves induce broad-spectrum bacterial β-lactamases and thereby lead to even greater problems with resistance.[85] These facts underscore the importance of regularly documenting the epidemiology of pathogens and infectious diseases within a specific practice or institution. As a result, an antimicrobial agent for a specific infectious disease favored in one practice site may not be the most desirable selection in another site despite similarities in size and patient profile. Strict and careful control and, possibly, rotation of empirical antibiotics in the hospital environment may help to limit the emergence of resistant organisms. Newer antibiotics developed for treatment of resistant, hospital-acquired pathogens are costly; therefore, their use must be moderated to some extent in an era where capitated hospital costs and mandated budget cuts will not tolerate careless antibiotic use. Broad spectrum antibiotics are more appropriate choices for patients with risk factors for MDR pathogens or if HAP develops after at least 5 days of hospitalization.[7] See Table 116–8 for recommended antimicrobial therapy.

Ventilator-Associated Pneumonia

The approach to treating VAP is similar to antibiotic selection in HAP and HCAP (see Table 116–8). Patients should be carefully evaluated to determine whether they are at risk for MDR pathogens as this is essential in selecting appropriate empiric antibiotic therapy.[7] It is also important to identify patients with VAP early since delays in initiating appropriate antibiotic therapy are associated with increased mortality. Aerosolized antibiotic delivery has been considered for more targeted therapy; however, there are limited studies at this time supporting the safety and efficacy in pneumonia.[86]

CLINICAL CONTROVERSY

Prior to the availability of newer β-lactam and fluoroquinolone antibiotics possessing consistently potent activity against multiple gram-negative pathogens, some investigators promoted the administration of antibiotics by direct endotracheal instillation. This method of drug administration attempts to provide increased topical concentrations of antibiotics that do not appear to penetrate respiratory secretions effectively while reducing the likelihood of systemic toxicity. In addition, greater local concentrations of antibiotics, particularly of the polymyxins and aminoglycosides, are believed to overcome partially the substantial decrease in antibiotic bioactivity observed when these agents interact with the purulent material present in infectious foci. Despite these potential theoretical advantages, the role of antibiotic aerosols or direct endotracheal instillation in clinical practice remains controversial.[78–82]

Atypical Pneumonia

Pneumonia caused by atypical pathogens may be more difficult to treat with antibiotics than "typical" pathogens. It is debatable whether empiric treatment for hospitalized patients with CAP should include antibiotic coverage of atypical pathogens. Currently there does not appear to be any benefit in terms of survival or clinical efficacy to providing atypical coverage for all patients.[87]

For *Legionella* pneumonia, fluoroquinolones are superior to macrolides, the previous drug of choice.[88] *Mycoplasma* pneumonia is difficult to treat due to the organism's lack of a cell wall, limiting certain antibiotics, and is found on epithelial cells in the respiratory tract instead of inside the cells.[71] Macrolides and tetracyclines are generally effective against *Mycoplasma*. *Chlamydophila* organisms are sensitive to macrolides, doxycycline, and fluoroquinolones. For viral causes of pneumonia, antivirals such as amantadine and oseltamivir can be used, depending on viral susceptibility. Management of TB is discussed in Chap. 121. See Table 116–8 for a summary of the evidence-based guidelines on management.

Severe Acute Respiratory Syndrome

Treatment of SARS involves primarily supportive care and procedures to prevent transmission to others.[73] Owing to the uncertainty associated with the diagnosis of SARS, empirical therapy with broad-spectrum antibiotics should be used. To date, fluoroquinolones (e.g., moxifloxacin, levofloxacin) or macrolides/azalides (e.g., erythromycin, clarithromycin, azithromycin) typically have been used. Although its efficacy is unproven, ribavirin also has been used to treat patients. Owing to the potential benefit of corticosteroids in the presence of progressive pulmonary disease, methylprednisolone has been used in doses ranging from 80 to 500 mg/day.

Avian Influenza

Treatment of avian influenza is primarily supportive, with the majority of patients requiring aggressive oxygen therapy and intensive care monitoring.[74,75] Due to observed resistance with amantadine, the neuraminidase inhibitors are the recommended treatment of avian influenza, with oseltamivir being the preferred agent. For optimal efficacy, treatment should be initiated within 48 hours of the first sign of infection. Of note, there is concern regarding oseltamivir, with a resistant A/H5N1 isolate identified in Vietnam.[75]

H1N1 Influenza (Swine Flu)

Treatment of H1N1 influenza is primarily supportive, with the majority of patients being treated as outpatients. The H1N1 virus is currently susceptible to oseltamivir and zanamivir and resistant to amantadine and rimantadine. Therefore, antivirals should only be administered to patients at high risk for influenza complications (i.e., hospitalized patients and those at high risk for seasonal flu complications). Vaccinations are being developed for H1N1 virus.

PREVENTION

Prevention of some cases of pneumonia is possible through the use of vaccines and medications against selected infectious agents. Polyvalent polysaccharide vaccines are available for two of the leading causes of bacterial pneumonia, *S. pneumoniae* and *H. influenzae* type b. In addition, evidence-based guidelines for preventing HCAP have been published (Table 116–11).[89] (See Chap. 118 for a full discussion of prevention of influenza and Chap. 133.)

EVALUATION OF THERAPEUTIC OUTCOMES

After therapy has been instituted, appropriate clinical parameters should be monitored to ensure the efficacy and safety of the therapeutic regimen. For patients with bacterial infections of the upper or lower respiratory tract, the time to resolution of initial presenting symptoms and the lack of appearance of new associated symptomatology are important to determine. For patients with CAP or pneumonia from any source of mild to moderate clinical severity, the time to resolution of cough, decreasing sputum production, and

TABLE 116-11 Evidenced-Based Guidelines for Preventing Healthcare-Associated Pneumonia

Recommendation	Recommendation Grade[a]
For nebulizers, use aerosolized medications in single-dose vials. If multidose medication vials are used, follow manufacturers' instructions for handling, storing, and dispensing the medications.	1B
Pneumococcal vaccination is recommended for patients at high risk for severe pneumococcal infections.	1A
Unless contraindicated, administer a macrolide to any person who has had close contact with persons having pertussis.	1B
In acute-care settings, offer vaccine to inpatients and outpatients at high risk for complications from influenza beginning in September and throughout the influenza season.	1A
Unless contraindicated, provide prophylactic treatment to all patients without influenza illness in the involved unit with amantadine, rimantadine, or oseltamivir for a minimum of 2 weeks or until approximately 1 week after the end of the outbreak.	1A
Unless contraindicated, patients with influenza should receive amantadine, rimantadine, oseltamivir, or zanamivir within 48 hours of the onset of symptoms.	1A

[a]Grade IA, strongly recommended for implementation and strongly supported by well-designed experimental, clinical, or epidemiologic studies; grade IB, strongly recommended for implementation and supported by certain clinical or epidemiologic studies and by strong theoretical rationale.

fever, as well as other constitutional symptoms of malaise, nausea, vomiting, and lethargy, should be noted. If the patient requires supplemental oxygen therapy, the amount and need should be assessed regularly. A gradual and persistent improvement in the resolution of these symptoms and therapies should be observed. Initial resolution should be observed within the first 2 days and progression to complete resolution within 5 to 7 days but usually no more than 10 days. For patients with HAP/HCAP, substantial underlying diseases, or both, additional parameters can be followed, including the magnitude and character of the peripheral blood WBC count, chest radiograph, and blood gas determinations. Similar to patients with less severe disease, some resolution of symptoms should be observed within 2 days of instituting antibiotic therapy. If no resolution of symptoms is observed within 2 days of starting seemingly appropriate antibiotic therapy or if the patient's clinical status is deteriorating, the appropriateness of initial antibiotic therapy should be critically reassessed. The patient should be evaluated carefully for deterioration of underlying concurrent disease(s). Additionally, the caregiver should consider the possibility of changing the initial antibiotic therapy to expand antimicrobial coverage not included in the original regimen (e.g., *Mycoplasma, Legionella,* and anaerobes). Furthermore, the need for antifungal therapy (lipid-based amphotericin B) should be considered. Some resolution of symptoms should be observed within 2 days of starting proper antibiotic therapy, with complete resolution expected within 10 to 14 days.

ABBREVIATIONS

CAP: community-acquired pneumonia

COPD: chronic obstructive pulmonary disease

HAP: hospital-acquired pneumonia

HCAP: healthcare-associated pneumonia

MDR: multidrug resistant

MIC: minimum inhibitory concentration

MRSA: methicillin-resistant *S. aureus*

PCR: polymerase chain reaction

PK-PD: pharmacokinetic–pharmacodynamic

RSV: respiratory syncytial virus

SARS: severe acute respiratory syndrome

VAP: ventilator-associated pneumonia

WBC: white blood cell

REFERENCES

1. Mason CM, Nelson S. Pulmonary host defenses and factors predisposing to lung infection. Clin Chest Med 2005;26:11–17.
2. Zaas AK, Alexander BD. New developments in the diagnosis and treatment of infections in lung transplant recipients. Respir Care Clin N Am 2004;10:531–547.
3. Yip TT, Chan JW, Cho WC, et al. Protein chip array profiling analysis in patients with severe acute respiratory syndrome identified serum amyloid a protein as a biomarker potentially useful in monitoring the extent of pneumonia. Clin Chem 2005;51:47–55.
4. Don M, Fasoli L, Paldanius M, Vainionpää R, et al. Aetiology of community-acquired pneumonia: serological results of a paediatric survey. Scand J Infect Dis 2005;37:806–812.
5. Koulenti D, Rello J. Hospital-acquired pneumonia in the 21st century: a review of existing treatment options and their impact on patient care. Expert Opin Pharmacother 2006;7:1555–1569.
6. Mandell LA, Wunderink RG, Anzueto A, et al. Infectious Diseases Society of America/American Thoracic Society consensus guidelines on the management of community-acquired pneumonia in adults. Clin Infect Dis 2007;44 (suppl 2):S27–S72.
7. Guidelines for the management of adults with hospital-acquired, ventilator-associated, and healthcare-associated pneumonia. Am J Respir Crit Care Med 2005;171:388–416.
8. Almirall J, Bolíbar I, Toran P, et al. Contribution of C-reactive protein to the diagnosis and assessment of severity of community-acquired pneumonia. Chest 2004;125:1335–1342.
9. Howard LS, Sillis M, Pasteur MC, Kamath AV, Harrison BD. Microbiological profile of community-acquired pneumonia in adults over the last 20 years. J Infect 2005;50:107–113.
10. Porzecanski I, Bowton DL. Diagnosis and treatment of ventilator-associated pneumonia. Chest 2006;130:597–604.
11. Trotman-Dickenson B. Radiology in the intensive care unit (Part I). J Intensive Care Med 2003;18:198–210.
12. Donnelly LF. Imaging in immunocompetent children who have pneumonia. Radiol Clin North Am 2005;43:253–265.
13. Wenzel RP, Fowler AA, 3rd. Clinical practice. Acute bronchitis. N Engl J Med 2006;355:2125–2130.
14. Brodzinski H, Ruddy RM. Review of new and newly discovered respiratory tract viruses in children. Pediatr Emerg Care 2009;25:352–360.
15. Tsai MH, Huang YC, Chen CJ, et al. Chlamydial pneumonia in children requiring hospitalization: effect of mixed infection on clinical outcome. J Microbiol Immunol Infect 2005;38:117–122.
16. Blasi F, Tarsia P, Aliberti S. Chlamydophila pneumoniae. Clin Microbiol Infect 2009;15:29–35.
17. Crowcroft NS, Pebody RG. Recent developments in pertussis. Lancet 2006;367:1926–1936.
18. Braman S. Chronic cough due to acute bronchitis: ACCP evidence-based clinical practice guidelines. Chest 2006;129(1 suppl): 95S–103S.
19. Glasgow JF. Reye's syndrome: the case for a causal link with aspirin. Drug Saf 2006;29:1111–1121.
20. Hersh A, Maselli J, Cabana M. Changes in prescribing of antiviral medications for influenza associated with new treatment guidelines. Am J Public Health 2009;99(suppl 2):S362–S364.
21. Jefferson TO, Demicheli V, Di Pietrantonj C, Jones M, Rivetti D. Neuraminidase inhibitors for preventing and treating influenza in healthy adults. Cochrane Database Syst Rev 2006;3:CD001265.

22. Jefferson T, Jones M, Doshi P, Del Mar C. Neuraminidase inhibitors for preventing and treating influenza in healthy adults: Systematic review and meta-analysis. BMJ 2009;339:b5106.

23. Regoes RR, Bonhoeffer S. Emergence of drug-resistant influenza virus: population dynamical considerations. Science 2006;312:389–391.

24. Rodriguez-Roisin R, Anzueto A, Bourbeau J, et al. Global Strategy for the Diagnosis, Management, and Prevention of Chronic Obstructive Pulmonary Disease, Medical Communications Resources, Inc., www.goldcopd.org; 2009.

25. Molfino NA. Genetics of COPD. Chest 2004;125:1929–1940.

26. Holtzman MJ, Tyner JW, Kim EY, et al. Acute and chronic airway responses to viral infection: implications for asthma and chronic obstructive pulmonary disease. Proc Am Thorac Soc 2005;2:132–140.

27. Pierson DJ. Clinical practice guidelines for chronic obstructive pulmonary disease: A review and comparison of current resources. Respir Care 2006;51:277–288.

28. Braman S. Chronic cough due to chronic bronchitis: ACCP evidence-based clinical practice guidelines. Chest 2006;129(1 suppl):104S–115S.

29. Wilson R, Jones P, Schaberg T, Arvis P, Duprat-Lomon I, Sagnier PP. Antibiotic treatment and factors influencing short and long term outcomes of acute exacerbations of chronic bronchitis. Thorax 2006;61:337–342.

30. Wood A, Tan S, Stockley R. Chronic obstructive pulmonary disease: towards pharmacogenetics. Genome Med 2009;1:112.

31. Mensa J, Trilla A. Should patients with acute exacerbation of chronic bronchitis be treated with antibiotics? Advantages of the use of fluoroquinolones. Clin Microbiol Infect 2006;12(suppl 3):42–54.

32. Poole PJ, Black PN. Mucolytic agents for chronic bronchitis or chronic obstructive pulmonary disease. Cochrane Database Syst Rev 2006;3:CD001287.

33. Fenton C, Keating GM. Inhaled salmeterol/fluticasone propionate: A review of its use in chronic obstructive pulmonary disease. Drugs 2004;64:1975–1996.

34. Wood-Baker RR, Gibson PG, Hannay M, Walters EH, Walters JA. Systemic corticosteroids for acute exacerbations of chronic obstructive pulmonary disease. Cochrane Database Syst Rev 2005:CD001288.

35. Delea TE, Hagiwara M, Dalal AA, Stanford RH, Blanchette CM. Healthcare use and costs in patients with chronic bronchitis initiating maintenance therapy with fluticasone/salmeterol vs other inhaled maintenance therapies. Curr Med Res Opin 2009;25:1–13.

36. Hayes D, Jr., Meyer KC. Acute exacerbations of chronic bronchitis in elderly patients: pathogenesis, diagnosis and management. Drugs Aging 2007;24:555–572.

37. Miravitlles M, Torres A. No more equivalence trials for antibiotics in exacerbations of COPD, please. Chest 2004;125:811–813.

38. Anthonisen NR, Manfreda J, Warren CP, Hershfield ES, Harding GK, Nelson NA. Antibiotic therapy in exacerbations of chronic obstructive pulmonary disease. Ann Intern Med 1987;106:196–204.

39. Sorensen SV, Baker T, Fleurence R, et al. Cost and clinical consequence of antibiotic non-adherence in acute exacerbations of chronic bronchitis. Int J Tuberc Lung Dis 2009;13:945–954.

40. Korbila IP, Manta KG, Siempos, II, Dimopoulos G, Falagas ME. Penicillins vs trimethoprim-based regimens for acute bacterial exacerbations of chronic bronchitis: meta-analysis of randomized controlled trials. Can Fam Physician 2009;55:60–67.

41. Dimopoulos G, Siempos, II, Korbila IP, Manta KG, Falagas ME. Comparison of first-line with second-line antibiotics for acute exacerbations of chronic bronchitis: a metaanalysis of randomized controlled trials. Chest 2007;132:447–455.

42. Falagas ME, Avgeri SG, Matthaiou DK, Dimopoulos G, Siempos, II. Short- versus long-duration antimicrobial treatment for exacerbations of chronic bronchitis: a meta-analysis. J Antimicrob Chemother 2008;62:442–450.

43. Stempel HE, Martin ET, Kuypers J, Englund JA, Zerr DM. Multiple viral respiratory pathogens in children with bronchiolitis. Acta Paediatr 2009;98:123–126.

44. Mejías A, Chávez-Bueno S, Jafri HS, Ramilo O. Respiratory syncytial virus infections: old challenges and new opportunities. Pediatr Infect Dis J 2005;24(11 suppl):S189–S196, discussion S96–S97.

45. King VJ, Viswanathan M, Bordley WC, et al. Pharmacologic treatment of bronchiolitis in infants and children: a systematic review. Arch Pediatr Adolesc Med 2004;158:127–137.

46. Panitch HB. Respiratory syncytial virus bronchiolitis: supportive care and therapies designed to overcome airway obstruction. Pediatr Infect Dis J 2003;22(2 suppl):S83–S87; discussion S7–S8.

47. Yanney M, Vyas H. The treatment of bronchiolitis. Arch Dis Child 2008;93:793–798.

48. Langley JM, Smith MB, LeBlanc JC, Joudrey H, Ojah CR, Pianosi P. Racemic epinephrine compared to salbutamol in hospitalized young children with bronchiolitis; a randomized controlled clinical trial [ISRCTN46561076]. BMC Pediatr 2005;5:7.

49. Plint AC, Johnson DW, Patel H, et al. Epinephrine and dexamethasone in children with bronchiolitis. N Engl J Med 2009;360:2079–2089.

50. Prais D, Danino D, Schonfeld T, Amir J. Impact of palivizumab on admission to the ICU for respiratory syncytial virus bronchiolitis: A national survey. Chest 2005;128:2765–71.

51. Feltes TF, Cabalka AK, Meissner HC, Piazza FM, Carlin DA, Top FH, Jr., Connor EM, Sondheimer HM. Palivizumab prophylaxis reduces hospitalization due to respiratory syncytial virus in young children with hemodynamically significant congenital heart disease. J Pediatr 2003;143:532–540.

52. Pedraz C, Carbonell-Estrany X, Figueras-Aloy J, Quero J. Effect of palivizumab prophylaxis in decreasing respiratory syncytial virus hospitalizations in premature infants. Pediatr Infect Dis J 2003;22:823–827.

53. File TM, Jr., Garau J, Blasi F, et al. Guidelines for empiric antimicrobial prescribing in community-acquired pneumonia. Chest 2004;125:1888–1901.

54. Bjerre LM, Verheij TJ, Kochen MM. Antibiotics for community acquired pneumonia in adult outpatients. Cochrane Database Syst Rev 2004;CD002109.

55. Anand N, Kollef MH. The alphabet soup of pneumonia: CAP, HAP, HCAP, NHAP, and VAP. Semin Respir Crit Care Med 2009;30:3–9.

56. Shefet D, Robenshtok E, Paul M, Leibovici L. Empirical atypical coverage for inpatients with community-acquired pneumonia: systematic review of randomized controlled trials. Arch Intern Med 2005;165:1992–2000.

57. Wunderink RG, Waterer GW. Genetics of community-acquired pneumonia. Semin Respir Crit Care Med 2005;26:553–562.

58. Roig J, Sabria M, Pedro-Botet ML. Legionella spp.: Community acquired and nosocomial infections. Curr Opin Infect Dis 2003;16:145–151.

59. Buising KL, Thursky KA, Black JF, et al. A prospective comparison of severity scores for identifying patients with severe community acquired pneumonia: reconsidering what is meant by severe pneumonia. Thorax 2006;61:419–424.

60. Zilberberg MD, Shorr AF. Epidemiology of healthcare-associated pneumonia (HCAP). Semin Respir Crit Care Med 2009;30:10–15.

61. Micek ST, Kollef KE, Reichley RM, Roubinian N, Kollef MH. Health care-associated pneumonia and community-acquired pneumonia: a single-center experience. Antimicrob Agents Chemother 2007;51:3568–3573.

62. Feldman C. Pneumonia associated with HIV infection. Curr Opin Infect Dis 2005;18:165–170.

63. Viscoli C, Varnier O, Machetti M. Infections in patients with febrile neutropenia: epidemiology, microbiology, and risk stratification. Clin Infect Dis 2005;40(suppl 4):S240–S245.

64. Smith TJ, Khatcheressian J, Lyman GH, et al. 2006 update of recommendations for the use of white blood cell growth factors: an evidence-based clinical practice guideline. J Clin Oncol 2006;24:3187–3205.

65. Rello J, Diaz E. Pneumonia in the intensive care unit. Crit Care Med 2003;31:2544–2551.

66. Kollef MH. Prevention of hospital-associated pneumonia and ventilator-associated pneumonia. Crit Care Med 2004;32:1396–1405.

67. Gibbs RS, Schrag S, Schuchat A. Perinatal infections due to group B streptococci. Obstet Gynecol 2004;104(5 Pt 1):1062–1076.

68. Lim W, Macfarlane J. Hospital acquired pneumonia. Clin Med 2001;1:180–184.

69. Starner TD, McCray PB, Jr. Pathogenesis of early lung disease in cystic fibrosis: a window of opportunity to eradicate bacteria. Ann Intern Med 2005;143:816–822.

70. Brook I. Anaerobic pulmonary infections in children. Pediatr Emerg Care 2004;20:636–640.

71. Cunha BA. Atypical pneumonias: current clinical concepts focusing on Legionnaires' disease. Curr Opin Pulm Med 2008;14:183–194.

72. Nahid P, Daley CL. Prevention of tuberculosis in HIV-infected patients. Curr Opin Infect Dis 2006;19:189–193.

73. Sampathkumar P, Temesgen Z, Smith TF, Thompson RL. SARS: Epidemiology, clinical presentation, management, and infection control measures. Mayo Clin Proc 2003;78:882–890.

74. Liu JP. Avian influenza—A pandemic waiting to happen? J Microbiol Immunol Infect 2006;39:4–10.

75. Wong SS, Yuen KY. Avian influenza virus infections in humans. Chest 2006;129:156–168.

76. Update: novel influenza A (H1N1) virus infections—Worldwide, May 6, 2009. MMWR Morb Mortal Wkly Rep 2009;58:453–458.

77. Sharpe B. Guideline-recommended antibiotics in community-acquired pneumonia: not perfect, but good. Arch Intern Med 2009; 169: 1462–1464.

78. Owens RJ, Shorr A. Rational dosing of antimicrobial agents: pharmacokinetic and pharmacodynamic strategies. Am J Health Syst Pharm 2009;66(12 suppl 4):S23–S30.

79. Calbo E, Garau J. Application of pharmacokinetics and pharmacodynamics to antimicrobial therapy of community-acquired respiratory tract infections. Respiration 2005;72:561–571.

80. Safdar A, Shelburne S, Evans S, Dickey B. Inhaled therapeutics for prevention and treatment of pneumonia. Expert Opin Drug Saf 2009;8:435–449.

81. Palmer L. Aerosolized antibiotics in critically ill ventilated patients. Curr Opin Crit Care 2009;15:413–418.

82. Muscedere J, Dodek P, Keenan S, Fowler R, Cook D, Heyland D. Comprehensive evidence-based clinical practice guidelines for ventilator-associated pneumonia: diagnosis and treatment. J Crit Care 2008;23:138–147.

83. Mandell LA, Bartlett JG, Dowell SF, File TM, Jr., Musher DM, Whitney C. Update of practice guidelines for the management of community-acquired pneumonia in immunocompetent adults. Clin Infect Dis 2003;37:1405–1433.

84. Cunha BA. Empiric therapy of community-acquired pneumonia: guidelines for the perplexed? Chest 2004;125:1913–1919.

85. Owens RC, Jr., Rice L. Hospital-based strategies for combating resistance. Clin Infect Dis 2006;42(suppl 4):S173–S181.

86. Luyt CE, Combes A, Nieszkowska A, Trouillet JL, Chastre J. Aerosolized antibiotics to treat ventilator-associated pneumonia. Curr Opin Infect Dis 2009;22:154–158.

87. Robenshtok E, Shefet D, Gafter-Gvili A, Paul M, Vidal L, Leibovici L. Empiric antibiotic coverage of atypical pathogens for community acquired pneumonia in hospitalized adults. Cochrane Database Syst Rev 2008;CD004418.

88. Forgie S, Marrie TJ. Healthcare-associated atypical pneumonia. Semin Respir Crit Care Med 2009;30:67–85.

89. Tablan OC, Anderson LJ, Besser R, Bridges C, Hajjeh R. Guidelines for preventing health-care—Associated pneumonia, 2003: Recommendations of CDC and the Healthcare Infection Control Practices Advisory Committee. MMWR Recomm Rep 2004;53(RR-3):1–36.

Upper Respiratory Tract Infections

CHRISTOPHER FREI, BRADI FREI, AND GEORGE ZHANEL

KEY CONCEPTS

❶ Most upper respiratory tract infections have a viral etiology and tend to resolve spontaneously without pharmacologic therapy.

❷ The most common bacterial causes are *Streptococcus pneumoniae* (acute otitis media and acute sinusitis) and group A β-hemolytic *Streptococcus* (acute pharyngitis).

❸ Vaccination against influenza and pneumococcus may decrease the risk of acute otitis media.

❹ Because upper respiratory tract infections are so common, antibiotics used to treat them serve as catalysts for the emergence and spread of antibiotic resistance, thereby making prudent antibiotic use critically important.

❺ When antibiotics are prescribed, the empiric medications of choice are amoxicillin for acute otitis media and acute sinusitis and penicillin for acute pharyngitis.

❻ For otitis media, high-dose amoxicillin (80–90 mg/kg/day) is recommended if the patient is at high risk for a penicillin-resistant pneumococcal infection.

Patients visit medical clinics and emergency rooms more for upper respiratory tract infections than any other reason.[1,2] Otitis media, sinusitis, and pharyngitis are the three most common upper respiratory tract infections. Other, less common infections are laryngitis, rhinitis, and epiglottitis. Because they are so common, community and emergency healthcare workers must be familiar with the diagnosis, assessment, and management of these infections. Furthermore, antibiotics used for the treatment of upper respiratory tract infections serve as catalysts for the emergence and spread of antibiotic resistance, thereby making prudent antibiotic use critically important.

ACUTE OTITIS MEDIA

The term *otitis media* comes from the Latin *oto-* for "ear," *-itis* for "inflammation," and *medi-* for "middle;" otitis media, then, is an inflammation of the middle ear. There are three subtypes of otitis

Learning objectives, review questions, and other resources can be found at **www.pharmacotherapyonline.com**.

media: acute otitis media, otitis media with effusion, and chronic otitis media. The three are differentiated by onset, signs and symptoms of infection, and the presence of fluid in the middle ear.[3,4] Acute otitis media is the subtype with the greatest role for antibiotics and will be discussed in detail.

EPIDEMIOLOGY

Otitis media is the 11th most common reason for an emergency room visit and the 15th most common reason for an office visit in the United States, accounting for more than 15 million emergency room and clinic visits annually.[1,2] It is common in infants and children, 75% of whom will have at least one episode in the first 12 months of life.[5] More than 80% of patients seen for acute otitis media receive a prescription, and the direct and indirect costs associated with managing otitis media add up to almost $3 billion annually in the United States.[3]

ETIOLOGY

❶ Approximately 40% to 75% of acute otitis media cases are caused by viral pathogens.[3] ❷ Common bacterial pathogens include *Streptococcus pneumoniae* (25–50%), nontypeable *Haemophilus influenzae* (15–30%), and *Moraxella catarrhalis* (3–20%).[3] The microbial etiology may be changing as a result of the introduction and widespread use of the pneumococcal conjugate vaccine. Specifically, the proportion of *S. pneumoniae* cases may be declining, and the proportion of *H. influenzae* cases may be on the rise.[6,7]

S. pneumoniae, *H. influenzae*, and *M. catarrhalis* can all possess resistance to β-lactams. *S. pneumoniae* develops resistance through alteration of penicillin-binding proteins, whereas *H. influenzae* and *M. catarrhalis* produce β-lactamases.[3] Between 15% and 50% of *S. pneumoniae* isolates from the upper respiratory tract are not susceptible to penicillin, and up to half of these have high-level penicillin resistance.[8] Half of the *H. influenzae* and 100% of *M. catarrhalis* isolates from the upper respiratory tract produce β-lactamases.[9]

The risk factors for amoxicillin-resistant bacteria in acute otitis media are attendance at child care centers, recent receipt of antibiotic treatment (within the past 30 days), and age younger than 2 years.[3]

PATHOPHYSIOLOGY

Acute bacterial otitis media usually follows a viral upper respiratory tract infection that causes eustachian tube dysfunction and mucosal swelling in the middle ear.[10] The middle ear is the space behind the tympanic membrane, or eardrum. A noninfected ear has a thin, clear tympanic membrane. In otitis media, this space becomes blocked with fluid, resulting in a bulging and erythematous tympanic membrane. Bacteria that colonize the nasopharynx enter the middle ear and are not cleared properly by the mucociliary system.[11]

The bacteria proliferate and cause infection.[10,11] Children tend to be more susceptible to otitis media than adults because the anatomy of their eustachian tube is shorter and more horizontal, facilitating bacterial entry into the middle ear.[10]

CLINICAL PRESENTATION

Patients or caregivers frequently characterize acute otitis media as having an acute onset of ear pain. For parents of young children, irritability and tugging on the ear are often the first clues that a child has acute otitis media. The diagnosis of acute otitis media and otitis media with effusion are easily confused, and careful attention to history, signs, and symptoms is important. Otitis media with effusion is characterized by fluid in the middle ear without signs and symptoms of acute ear infection, such as pain and a bulging eardrum.[4]

A diagnosis of acute otitis media requires that three criteria be satisfied: acute onset of signs and symptoms, middle ear effusion, and middle ear inflammation.[3] Middle ear effusion is indicated by any of the following: bulging of the tympanic membrane, limited or absent mobility of the tympanic membrane, air-fluid level behind the tympanic membrane, or otorrhea.[3] Signs and symptoms of middle ear inflammation include either distinct erythema of the tympanic membrane or distinct ear otalgia (or ear pain).[3] A diagnosis is considered to be "uncertain" if the patient does not have all three of these diagnostic criteria.

CLINICAL PRESENTATION OF ACUTE BACTERIAL OTITIS MEDIA

General

- Acute onset of signs and symptoms of middle ear infection following cold symptoms of runny nose, nasal congestion, or cough

Signs and Symptoms

- Ear pain that can be severe (>75% of patients)
- Children may be irritable, tug on the involved ear, and have difficulty sleeping
- Fever is present in less than 25% of patients and, when present, occurs more often in younger children
- Examination shows a discolored (gray), thickened, bulging eardrum
- Pneumatic otoscopy or tympanometry demonstrates an immobile eardrum; 50% of cases are bilateral
- Draining middle ear fluid occurs in less than 3% of patients and usually has a bacterial etiology

Laboratory Tests

- Gram stain, culture, and sensitivities of draining fluid or aspirated fluid if tympanocentesis is performed

---

Adapted from Hendley JO. Clinical practice: Otitis media. N Engl J Med 2002;347(15):1169–1174.

TREATMENT

■ DESIRED OUTCOME

❻ Treatment goals include pain management, prudent antibiotic use, and secondary disease prevention. These will be discussed in detail, but first, it is important to consider primary prevention of acute otitis media through the use of bacterial and viral vaccines.

❸ A systematic review demonstrated that the seven-valent pneumococcal conjugate vaccine Prevnar (with CRM197 carrier protein) reduced the occurrence of acute otitis media episodes by 6% to 7% when the vaccine was administered during infancy.[12] Other, currently nonlicensed pneumococcal conjugate vaccines had mixed results. Children with a history of acute otitis media did not benefit when the seven-valent vaccine was administered at an older age.[12] An *H. influenzae* type b (Hib) vaccine is now available and reduces invasive Hib disease;[13] however, it is the nontypeable *H. influenzae* that is of greatest concern in acute otitis media. Other vaccines, including nontypeable *H. influenzae* and *M. catarrhalis* vaccines, are in development. Finally, because acute otitis media cases often follow influenza cases, influenza vaccination should be considered as a possible means to prevent acute otitis media. Refer to the U.S. Centers for Disease Control and Prevention website (*www.cdc.gov*) and statements from the Advisory Committee on Immunization Practices (ACIP) for the most up-to-date information regarding recommended pneumococcal and influenza immunization practices.[14,15]

■ GENERAL APPROACH TO TREATMENT

The first step in the treatment of otitis media is to differentiate acute otitis media from otitis media with effusion or chronic otitis media, as the latter two types do not benefit substantially from antibiotic therapy. The second step is to address pain with oral analgesics. The third step is to consider if a brief observation period is warranted or if the disease severity or patient characteristics require immediate antibiotic therapy. If a bacterial infection is suspected, consider if the patient has risk factors for penicillin resistance. Recognize that amoxicillin is the mainstay of therapy and that penicillin resistance can be overcome, in many cases, with high-dose amoxicillin therapy. The therapeutic strategy should be changed if complications develop or if symptoms fail to resolve within 3 days.

■ NONPHARMACOLOGIC THERAPY

Regardless of the decision to administer antibiotics, acetaminophen or a nonsteroidal antiinflammatory drug (NSAID), such as ibuprofen, should be offered early to relieve pain in acute otitis media.[3] In addition, eardrops with a local anesthetic, such as ametocaine, benzocaine, or lidocaine, provide pain relief when administered with oral pain medication to children ages 3 to 18 years.[16] Because of minimal benefit and increased side effects, neither decongestants nor antihistamines should be routinely recommended in cases of acute otitis media or otitis media with effusion.[3,4,17,18]

■ PHARMACOLOGIC THERAPY

National clinical practice guidelines for appropriate diagnosis and treatment of acute otitis media were first published in 2004 by the American Academy of Pediatrics (AAP) and the American Academy of Family Physicians (AAFP).[3] Three pertinent systematic reviews have also been released.[19–21] The AAP/AAFP guidelines for acute otitis media are focused on children 2 months through 12 years of age with uncomplicated cases. These guidelines do not pertain to children with systemic illness or with underlying conditions that may alter the course of acute otitis media (e.g., anatomic abnormalities, genetic conditions such as Down syndrome, immunodeficiencies, and cochlear implants).[3]

❸ Antibiotic therapy for upper respiratory diseases must be balanced with possible increases in adverse drug events and increased antibiotic pressure. One strategy to reduce antibiotic use in this setting is "delayed therapy."[22] Delayed therapy most often means that a healthcare worker provides the patient with a prescription but encourages the patient to wait to use the medication for 48 to 72 hours to see if the symptoms will resolve on their own. Candidates for delayed therapy include (a) children 6 months to 2 years of age without severe symptoms plus uncertain diagnosis, (b) children 2 years and older without severe symptoms, and (c) children 2 years and older with an uncertain diagnosis.[3] Delayed therapy decreases antibiotic use but also decreases patient satisfaction. Ultimately, this strategy is no better than avoiding antibiotics altogether.[22]

❹ ❺ If antibiotics are to be administered, then amoxicillin should be given to most children, at a dose of 80 to 90 mg/kg/day.[3] S. pneumoniae resistance to penicillin can be overcome with this high amoxicillin dose. If pathogens that produce β-lactamase are known or suspected, then amoxicillin should be given in combination with a β-lactamase inhibitor: amoxicillin-clavulanate at a dose of 90 mg/kg/day of amoxicillin with 6.4 mg/kg/day of clavulanate in two divided doses.[23]

Clinical trials have not provided a clear answer as to which antibiotics are most efficacious;[24] therefore, the choice of amoxicillin is largely based on microbiology and pharmacokinetic-pharmacodynamic studies. Amoxicillin has the best pharmacodynamic profile against drug-resistant S. pneumoniae of all available oral antibiotics. In addition, amoxicillin has a long record of safety, possesses a narrow spectrum, and is inexpensive. Higher middle ear fluid concentrations of amoxicillin as a result of higher dosing overcome most drug-resistant S. pneumoniae even with its increased minimum inhibitory concentration (MIC).[25] Its excellent efficacy against S. pneumoniae outweighs the issue of β-lactamase-producing H. influenzae and M. catarrhalis, against which amoxicillin may not be effective. This is because H. influenzae and M. catarrhalis are both more likely than S. pneumoniae to lead to a spontaneous resolution of the infection. In patients with moderate to severe illness (temperature >39°C [102°F] and/or severe otalgia), amoxicillin-clavulanate is recommended. Table 117-1 lists antibiotic recommendations for acute otitis media.

If treatment failure occurs with amoxicillin, an antibiotic should be chosen with activity against β-lactamase-producing H. influenzae and M. catarrhalis, as well as drug-resistant S. pneumoniae.[10] High-dose amoxicillin-clavulanate is recommended. Other choices are cefuroxime, cefdinir, cefpodoxime, and intramuscular ceftriaxone.[3] Second-generation cephalosporins, though β-lactamase stable, are expensive, have an increased incidence of side effects, and may increase selective pressure for resistant bacteria. Furthermore, most cephalosporins do not achieve adequate middle ear fluid concentrations against drug-resistant S. pneumoniae for the desired duration of the dosing interval. Use of trimethoprim-sulfamethoxazole and erythromycin-sulfisoxazole is discouraged because of high rates of resistance.[3] Intramuscular ceftriaxone is the only antibiotic other than amoxicillin that achieves middle ear fluid concentrations above the MIC for >40% of the dosing interval.[26] Although single doses of ceftriaxone have been used, daily doses for 3 days are recommended to optimize clinical outcomes.[3,10] Ceftriaxone should be reserved for severe and unresponsive infections or for patients for whom oral medication is inappropriate because of vomiting, diarrhea, or possible nonadherence. Ceftriaxone is an expensive antibiotic, and the intramuscular injections are painful. The drug can be given intravenously, but the risk-to-benefit ratio of starting an IV line must also be examined. Tympanocentesis can also be considered for treatment failure or persistent acute otitis media. It has a therapeutic effect of relieving pain and pressure and can be used to collect fluid to identify the causative agent. Clindamycin may also be considered at this point for coverage of documented penicillin-resistant S. pneumoniae.[3] Patients with a penicillin allergy can be treated with several alternative antibiotics. If the reaction is not type I hypersensitivity, cefdinir, cefpodoxime, or cefuroxime can be used.[3] If the reaction is type I, a macrolide such as azithromycin or clarithromycin may be used. If S. pneumoniae is documented, clindamycin is an alternative. However, the incidence of resistance is much higher with these antibiotics,[10] and of these antibiotics, only clindamycin is recommended by the AAP guidelines.[3]

There is debate regarding the optimal duration of therapy for acute otitis media. Traditional recommendations were for 10 to 14 days of antibiotic therapy; however, 5 days of therapy may be as effective as 10 days.[27] The advantages of short-term therapy are an increased likelihood the patient will adhere to the full course of treatment, decreased side effects and cost, and decreased bacterial-selective pressure for both the individual and the community. Short treatment courses in children younger than 2 years are not recommended.[25] In children at least 6 years old who have mild to moderate acute otitis media, a 5- to 7-day course may be used.

Recurrent acute otitis media is defined as at least three episodes in 6 months or at least four episodes in 12 months. Recurrent infections are of concern because patients younger than 3 years are at high risk for hearing loss and language and learning disabilities.[28] Data from studies generally do not favor prophylaxis. A meta-analysis demonstrated that prophylaxis prevents one infection each time one child is treated for 9 months.[29] Of further concern is antibiotic resistance. Treatment can be delayed until the onset of symptoms of an upper respiratory tract infection (viral symptoms), or antibiotic prophylaxis can be limited to 6 months' duration during the winter months. Surgical insertion of tympanostomy tubes (T-tubes) is an effective method for the prevention of recurrent

---

TABLE 117-1 Acute Otitis Media Antibiotic Recommendations

| | Initial Diagnosis | | Failure at 48–72 Hours | |
	Nonsevere	Severe[a]	Nonsevere	Severe[a]
First line	Amoxicillin, high-dose; 80–90 mg/kg/day divided twice daily	Amoxicillin-clavulanate, high-dose;[b] 90 mg/kg/day of amoxicillin plus 6.4 mg/kg/day of clavulnate divided twice daily	Amoxicillin-clavulanate, high-dose;[b] 90 mg/kg/day of amoxicillin plus 6.4 mg/kg/day of clavulanate divided twice daily	Ceftriaxone (1–3 days)
Non–type 1 allergy	Cefdinir, cefuroxime, cefpodoxime	Ceftriaxone (1–3 days)	Ceftriaxone (1–3 days)	Clindamycin
Type 1 allergy	Azithromycin, clarithromycin		Clindamycin	Clindamycin

[a]Severe = temperature ≥39°C (102°F) and/or severe otalgia.
[b]Amoxicillin-clavulanate 90:6.4 or 14:1 ratio is available in the United States; 7:1 ratio is available in Canada (use amoxicillin 45 mg/kg for one dose, amoxicillin 45 mg/kg with clavulanate 6.4 mg/kg for second dose).
Adapted from McCaig LF, Nawar EW. National Hospital Ambulatory Medical Care Survey: 2004 emergency department summary. Adv Data 2006(372):1–29.

otitis media. These small tubes are placed through the inferior portion of the tympanic membrane under general anesthesia and aerate the middle ear. Children with recurrent acute otitis media should be considered for T-tube placement. Finally, there may be an emerging role for oral fluoroquinolones when acute otitis media does recur or persist.

CLINICAL CONTROVERSY

Fluoroquinolones have not been used extensively in acute otitis media because of concerns regarding the safety of these antibiotics when used in children. This is primarily due to animal studies in which juvenile laboratory animals experienced cartilage lesions in weight-bearing joints.[80] However, the concern for β-lactam resistance has prompted some to investigate the safety and efficacy profile of oral fluoroquinolones in children with acute otitis media. Three studies by a single group of investigators with oral fluoroquinolone used in children with recurrent or persistent acute otitis media demonstrated similar efficacy compared with amoxicillin-clavulanate.[81-83] None demonstrated more frequent adverse drug effects with fluoroquinolones compared with amoxicillin-clavulanate, although these studies were underpowered to evaluate uncommon adverse effects, such as cartilage lesions. On July 8, 2008, the United States Food and Drug Administration (FDA) strengthened the fluoroquinolone labeling by adding a boxed warning concerning the "increased risk of developing tendinitis and tendon rupture in patients taking fluoroquinolones for systemic use."

PHARMACOECONOMIC CONSIDERATIONS

Pharmacoeconomic considerations are minimal in the treatment of acute otitis media, as the medications of choice are widely available from several generic manufacturers. There is some debate regarding the cost-effectiveness of routine recommendations for childhood influenza and pneumococcal immunization as a means to reduce acute otitis media.

EVALUATION OF THERAPEUTIC OUTCOMES

Patients with acute otitis media should be reassessed after 3 days. Pain and fever tend to resolve after 2 or 3 days, with most children becoming asymptomatic at 7 days. Treatment failure is a lack of clinical improvement in the signs and symptoms of infection, including pain, fever, and erythema/bulging of the tympanic membrane, after 3 days. If antibiotics were withheld initially, they should be instituted now. If the patient initially received an antibiotic, then the antibiotic should be changed (Table 117–1).

Early reevaluation of the eardrum when signs and symptoms are improving can be misleading because effusions persist. Over a period of 1 week, changes in the eardrum normalize, and the pus becomes serous fluid. Air-fluid levels are apparent behind the eardrum, at which point the stage is now referred to as *otitis media with effusion*. This does not represent ongoing infection, nor are additional antibiotics required. Two weeks after an acute otitis media episode, 60% to 70% of children still have a middle ear effusion; 40% at 1 month, and 10% to 25% at 3 months.[3] Younger children and those with a history of recurrent infections have a further delay in resolution.[11] Immediate reevaluation is appropriate if hearing loss results from persistent middle ear effusions following infection.[4] Complications of otitis media are infrequent but include mastoiditis, bacteremia, meningitis, and auditory sequelae with the potential for speech and language impairment.[3,4]

ACUTE BACTERIAL SINUSITIS

Sinusitis is an inflammation and/or infection of the paranasal sinuses, or membrane-lined air spaces, around the nose.[30,31] The term *rhinosinusitis* is used by some specialists because sinusitis typically also involves the nasal mucosa.[30] Even though the majority of these infections are viral in origin, antibiotics are prescribed frequently. It is thus important to differentiate between viral and bacterial sinusitis to aid in optimizing treatment decisions. This chapter will focus on acute bacterial sinusitis.

EPIDEMIOLOGY

More than 31 million cases of sinusitis are diagnosed annually in the United States.[32] ❶ Most sinusitis infections have a viral etiology; nevertheless, sinusitis accounts for 9% and 21% of all adult and pediatric antibiotic prescriptions, respectively.[33] Acute bacterial sinusitis is overdiagnosed by family physicians; thus, antibiotics are overprescribed.[30,34] Children have six to eight viral upper respiratory tract infections per year, yet only 5% to 13% of these are complicated by a secondary bacterial sinusitis infection.[35] Only 0.5% to 2% of viral upper respiratory tract infections in adults are complicated by sinusitis.[30,31,35] Ultimately, sinusitis results in 5.8 billion expenditures annually in the United States.[36]

ETIOLOGY

Viruses are responsible for most cases of acute sinusitis; however, when symptoms persist for 7 days or more or become severe, bacteria may be a primary or secondary cause of infection.[30] ❷ Acute bacterial sinusitis is caused most often by the same bacteria implicated in acute otitis media: *S. pneumoniae* and *H. influenzae*. These organisms are responsible for ~70% of bacterial causes of acute sinusitis in both adults and children.[33] *M. catarrhalis* is also frequently implicated in children (~25%).[33,35] *Streptococcus pyogenes*, *Staphylococcus aureus*, fungi, and anaerobes are associated less frequently with acute sinusitis.[30,33] Issues of bacterial resistance are similar to those found with otitis media.

PATHOPHYSIOLOGY

Similar to acute otitis media, acute bacterial sinusitis usually is preceded by a viral respiratory tract infection that causes mucosal inflammation.[30,31,35] This can lead to obstruction of the sinus ostia—the pathways that drain the sinuses. Mucosal secretions become trapped, local defenses are impaired, and bacteria from adjacent surfaces begin to proliferate. The maxillary and ethmoid sinuses are the ones most frequently involved. The pathogenesis of chronic sinusitis has not been well studied. Whether it is caused by more persistent pathogens or there is a subtle defect in the host's immune function, some patients develop chronic symptoms after their acute infection.

CLINICAL PRESENTATION

The greatest barrier to efficient use of antibiotics in acute bacterial sinusitis is the lack of a simple and accurate diagnostic test. The gold standard for the diagnosis of acute bacterial sinusitis is sinus puncture with recovery of bacteria in high density ($\geq 10^4$ colony-forming units/mL);[30,35] however, sinus puncture is an invasive procedure, so it is not routinely done. Sinus radiography can help, but it is not routinely recommended for uncomplicated sinusitis.

Because there is no simple and accurate office-based test for acute bacterial sinusitis, clinicians rely on clinical findings to make the diagnosis.

In general, patients with acute bacterial sinusitis present with nonspecific upper respiratory symptoms that persist for 7 to 14 days. Children may have nasal discharge, cough, fever (>39°C [>102°F]), and facial or sinus swelling and/or pain. Likewise, adults may have nasal congestion or discharge, maxillary tooth pain, facial or sinus swelling and/or pain, and fever. For chronic sinusitis, symptoms are similar, but they may be even more nonspecific. Chronic sinusitis patients may also have chronic unproductive cough, laryngitis, or headache.

CLINICAL PRESENTATION AND DIAGNOSIS OF BACTERIAL SINUSITIS

General

- A nonspecific upper respiratory tract infection that persists beyond 7 to 14 days

Signs and Symptoms

- Acute
  - *Adults*
    - Nasal discharge/congestion
    - Maxillary tooth pain, facial or sinus pain that may radiate (unilateral in particular), as well as deterioration after initial improvement
    - Severe or persistent (>7 days) signs and symptoms are most likely bacterial and should be treated with antibiotics
  - *Children*
    - Nasal discharge and cough for longer than 10 to 14 days or severe signs and symptoms such as temperature above 39°C (102°F) or facial swelling or pain are indications for antibiotic therapy
- Chronic
  - Symptoms are similar to acute sinusitis but more nonspecific
  - Rhinorrhea is associated with acute exacerbations
  - Chronic unproductive cough, laryngitis, and headache may occur
  - Chronic/recurrent infections occur three or four times per year and are unresponsive to steam and decongestants

Laboratory Tests

- Gram stain, culture, and sensitivities of draining fluid or aspirated fluid if sinus puncture is performed

---

From Hickner JM, Bartlett JG, Besser RE, et al. Principles of appropriate antibiotic use for acute rhinosinusitis in adults: Background. Ann Intern Med 2001;134(6):498–505; Piccirillo JF. Clinical practice: Acute bacterial sinusitis. N Engl J Med 2004;351(9):902–910; Anon JB, Jacobs MR, Poole MD, et al. Antimicrobial treatment guidelines for acute bacterial rhinosinusitis. Otolaryngol Head Neck Surg 2004;130(1 Suppl):1–45; Scheid DC, Hamm RM. Acute bacterial rhinosinusitis in adults: 2. Treatment. Am Fam Physician 2004;70(9):1697–1704; Subcommittee on Management of Sinusitis and Committee on Quality Improvement. Clinical practice guideline: Management of sinusitis. Pediatrics 2001;108(3):798–808; and Ip S, Fu L, Balk E, et al. Update on Acute Bacterial Rhinosinusitis: Evidence Report/Technology Assessment No. 124 (Prepared by Tufts-New England Medical Center Evidence-based Practice Center under Contract No. 290-02-0022). AHRQ Pub. No. 05-E020-2. Rockville, MD: Agency for Healthcare Research and Quality; 2005.

TREATMENT

■ DESIRED OUTCOME

The goals of treatment for acute sinusitis are to reduce signs and symptoms, achieve and maintain patency of the ostia, limit antibiotic treatment to those who may benefit, eradicate the bacterial infection with appropriate antibiotic therapy, minimize the duration of illness, prevent complications, and prevent progression from acute disease to chronic disease.[33,35]

■ GENERAL APPROACH TO TREATMENT

A clinical practice guideline outlined 17 action statements for the management of sinusitis, 7 of which pertain to acute bacterial sinusitis.[37,38] The cumulative evidence behind all seven recommendations was assigned a grade of B, indicating that the evidence came from "randomized controlled trials or diagnostic studies with minor limitations or overwhelmingly consistent evidence from observational studies." See Table 117–2 for abbreviated definitions of the terms used to describe this evidence and Table 117–3 for the actual evidence-based statements.

The first step in the assessment and treatment of sinusitis is to delineate viral and bacterial sinusitis. This is based on disease duration, rather than symptomatology, as signs and symptoms are generally similar for viral and bacterial sinusitis. Viral sinusitis typically improves in 7 to 10 days; therefore, a diagnosis of acute bacterial sinusitis requires persistent symptoms (≥10 days) or a worsening of symptoms after 5 to 7 days. Bacterial sinusitis may also be suspected if symptoms do not respond to nonprescription nasal decongestants and acetaminophen.

If a bacterial infection is suspected, the next step is to decide whether the infection is complicated or uncomplicated. Acute bacterial sinusitis is considered to be complicated if the patient has mental status changes, immunosuppressive illness, unilateral findings, significant coexisting illnesses, risk factors for β-lactam-resistant strains, history of antibiotic failure, isolated frontal or sphenoid sinusitis, or intense periorbital swelling, erythema, and facial pain. When a complicated infection is suspected, the patient should be referred to a specialist for computed tomography to assess the severity and extent of disease and identify the underlying causes. The remainder of this chapter focuses on the management of uncomplicated acute bacterial sinusitis. Antibiotics, such as amoxicillin, are recommended to reduce disease duration for patients with acute bacterial sinusitis. Adjuvant, nonantibiotic therapies have a limited role.

■ NONPHARMACOLOGIC THERAPY

Many symptoms of sinusitis will resolve within 48 hours without medical therapy. When they persist, pharmacotherapy should be

TABLE 117-2 Abbreviated Definitions for Evidence-Based Statements

Statement	Definition
Strong recommendation	The benefits of the recommended approach clearly exceed the risks
Recommendation	The benefits exceed the risks
Option	Either the quality of evidence that exists is suspect, or well-done studies show little clear advantage of one approach over another
No recommendation	Both a lack of pertinent evidence and an unclear balance between benefits and harms

From Rosenfeld RM, Andes D, Bhattacharyya N, et al. Clinical practice guideline: Adult sinusitis. Otolaryngol Head Neck Surg 2007;137(3 Suppl):S1–S31.

TABLE 117-3 Abbreviated Guideline Statements for Acute Bacterial Sinusitis

Practice	Evidence-Based Statement
Consider a sinusitis infection to be of bacterial origin if symptoms persist 10 days or more or if symptoms worsen within 10 days after initial improvement	Strong recommendation
Do not obtain radiographic imaging for patients who meet diagnostic criteria for acute bacterial sinusitis unless a complication or alternative diagnosis is suspected	Recommendation against
Management of acute bacterial sinusitis should include pain assessment and severity-based treatment	Strong recommendation
Clinicians may prescribe therapies for symptomatic relief in acute bacterial sinusitis	Option
Delayed therapy is an option in selected patients with uncomplicated acute bacterial sinusitis who have mild pain, temperature <31°C (101°F), and assurance of follow-up	Option
Amoxicillin should be used as first-line therapy for most adults	Recommendation
If the patient fails therapy, or if the disease worsens with the initial management option by 7 days after diagnosis, then reassess, detect complications, and initiate alternative antibiotic therapy	Recommendation

Adapted from Rosenfeld RM, Andes D, Bhattacharyya N, et al. Clinical practice guideline: Adult sinusitis. Otolaryngol Head Neck Surg 2007;137(3 Suppl):S1–S31.

directed toward symptomatic relief, restoring and improving sinus function, and eradicating the causative pathogen.

Data regarding supportive therapy are limited, but such therapy may be useful in reducing symptoms in some patients.[34] Nasal decongestant sprays that reduce inflammation by vasoconstriction, such as phenylephrine and oxymetazoline, are used often in sinusitis.[30] Use should be limited to no more than 3 days to prevent the development of tolerance and/or rebound congestion. Oral decongestants also may aid in nasal/sinus patency. Irrigation of the nasal cavity with saline and steam inhalation may be used to increase mucosal moisture, and mucolytics (e.g., guaifenesin) may be used to decrease the viscosity of nasal secretions.[30]

Antihistamines should not be used for acute bacterial sinusitis due to of their anticholinergic effects that can dry mucosa and disturb clearance of mucosal secretions.[35] Second-generation antihistamines may play a role in chronic sinusitis, which is frequently accompanied by concomitant allergic rhinitis. Glucocorticoids intranasally may decrease inflammation causing headache, nasal congestion, and facial pain;[39] however, there are limited data to support their use in acute sinusitis.[40]

CLINICAL CONTROVERSY

Proponents of intranasal corticosteroids have suggested that they may alleviate symptoms and hasten recovery due to their local antiinflammatory properties. A systematic review of four studies with 1,943 participants found that patients receiving intranasal corticosteroids were more likely to have symptom resolution or improvement in symptoms than those patients receiving placebo.[40] Furthermore, there appeared to be a dose–response relationship with higher doses of intranasal corticosteroids resulting in a stronger effect. There were no significant differences in adverse effects, drop-outs, or recurrence rates between participants who received intranasal corticosteroids and those who received placebo. This systematic review supports the use of intranasal corticosteroids as monotherapy or adjuvant therapy to antibiotics for the treatment of acute bacterial sinusitis.[40]

■ PHARMACOLOGIC THERAPY

Several sets of clinical practice guidelines and thought papers have been published in the last few years, and more are in development by professional societies, including the Infectious Diseases Society of America. These include statements from the AAP;[35] the Sinus and Allergy Health Partnership,[33] the American Academy of Otolaryngology–Head and Neck Surgery (AAO-HNS);[37,38] the Agency for Healthcare Research and Quality (AHRQ);[41] and the Joint Task Force on Practice Parameters, representing the American Academy of Allergy, Asthma, and Immunology, the American College of Allergy, Asthma, and Immunology, and the Joint Council of Allergy, Asthma, and Immunology.[42] In addition, there have been several high-quality reviews.[30,31,43,44]

❹ Amoxicillin is first-line treatment for acute bacterial sinusitis (Table 117–4). The advantages of amoxicillin include proven efficacy and safety, a relatively narrow antibacterial spectrum, and good tolerability. It is cost-effective in acute uncomplicated disease, and systematic reviews have failed to demonstrate the superiority of alternative antibiotic therapies as compared with amoxicillin.[41,45] High-dose amoxicillin is recommended in situations with a high risk of penicillin-resistant S. pneumoniae. See Table 117–5 for dosing guidelines.

If the patient has a penicillin allergy, but it is not a type I, immunoglobulin (Ig) E–mediated reaction (e.g., hives or anaphylaxis), a second-generation cephalosporin is initially recommended

TABLE 117-4 Acute Bacterial Sinusitis Antibiotic Recommendations[a,b]

	Uncomplicated	Treatment Failure or Prior Antibiotic Therapy in Past 4 to 6 Weeks	High Suspicion of Penicillin-resistant Streptococcus pneumoniae
First line	Amoxicillin	Amoxicillin-clavulanate (high-dose) or cephalosporin	Amoxicillin (high-dose) or clindamycin
Second line	–	Respiratory fluoroquinolone	Respiratory fluoroquinolone
Non–type 1 allergy	Cephalosporin	Cephalosporin	Clindamycin or respiratory fluoroquinolone
Type 1 allergy	Clarithromycin, azithromycin, trimethoprim-sulfamethoxazole, doxycycline, or a respiratory fluoroquinolone	Respiratory fluoroquinolone	Clindamycin or respiratory fluoroquinolone

[a]See Table 117–5 for dosing guidelines in children and adults.
[b]From Anon JB, Jacobs MR, Poole MD, et al. Antimicrobial treatment guidelines for acute bacterial rhinosinusitis. Otolaryngol Head Neck Surg 2004;130(1 Suppl):1–45; Subcommittee on Management of Sinusitis and Committee on Quality Improvement. Clinical practice guideline: Management of sinusitis. Pediatrics 2001;108(3):798–808; and Ip S, Fu L, Balk E, et al. Update on Acute Bacterial Rhinosinusitis: Evidence Report/Technology Assessment No. 124 (Prepared by Tufts-New England Medical Center Evidence-based Practice Center under Contract No. 290-02-0022). AHRQ Pub. No. 05-E020-2. Rockville, MD: Agency for Healthcare Research and Quality; 2005.

TABLE 117-5 Oral Dosing Guidelines for Acute Bacterial Sinusitis

Medication	Adult Dosage	Pediatric Dosage
Amoxicillin	Low dose: 500 mg three times daily High dose: 2 g twice daily	Low dose: 45 mg/kg/day divided in three doses High dose: 90 mg/kg/day divided in two doses
Amoxicillin-clavulanate	Low dose: 500/125 mg three times daily High dose: 2 g/125 mg twice daily	Low dose: 45 mg/kg/day of amoxicillin and 3.2 mg/kg/day of clavulanate divided in three doses High dose: 90 mg/kg/day of amoxicillin and 6.4 mg/kg/day of clavulanate divided in two doses
Cefuroxime	250–500 mg twice daily	15 mg/kg/day divided in two doses
Cefaclor	250–500 mg three times daily	20 mg/kg/day divided in three doses
Cefixime	200–400 mg twice daily	8 mg/kg/day in one dose or divided in two doses
Cefdinir	600 mg daily or divided in two doses	14 mg/kg/day in one dose or divided in two doses
Cefpodoxime	200 mg twice daily	10 mg/kg/day in two divided doses (maximum 400 mg daily)
Cefprozil	250–500 mg twice daily	15–30 mg/kg/day divided in two doses
Doxycycline	100 mg every 12 hours	–
Trimethoprim- sulfamethoxazole	160/800 mg every 12 hours	6–8 mg/kg/day trimethoprim, 30–40 mg/kg/day sulfamethoxazole divided in two doses
Clindamycin	150–450 mg every 6 hours	30–40 mg/kg/day divided in three doses
Clarithromycin	250–500 mg twice daily	15 mg/kg/day divided in two doses
Azithromycin	500 mg day 1, then 250 mg/day × days 2–5	10 mg/kg day 1, then 5 mg/kg/day × days 2–5
Levofloxacin	500 mg daily	–

From Piccirillo JF. Clinical practice: Acute bacterial sinusitis. N Engl J Med 2004;351(9):902–910; Scheid DC, Hamm RM. Acute bacterial rhinosinusitis in adults: 2. Treatment. Am Fam Physician 2004;70(9):1697–1704; and Subcommittee on Management of Sinusitis and Committee on Quality Improvement. Clinical practice guideline: Management of sinusitis. Pediatrics 2001;108(3):798–808.

(e.g., cefprozil, cefuroxime, or cefpodoxime).[35,46] Patients with type I IgE-mediated reactions to penicillin may be treated with trimethoprim-sulfamethoxazole, doxycycline, azithromycin, or clarithromycin. There is concern, however, regarding increasing resistance to trimethoprim-sulfamethoxazole and macrolides,[33] as well as the high failure rate of all these antibiotics. Respiratory fluoroquinolones may also be suitable alternatives in penicillin-allergic patients.

In the case of treatment failure with amoxicillin (i.e., no improvement in symptoms 72 hours after starting therapy) or in patients who have received antibiotic therapy in the prior 4 to 6 weeks, limitations of initial treatment coverage must be considered.[33] Improved coverage of *H. influenzae* and *M. catarrhalis* with either high-dose amoxicillin plus clavulanate or a β-lactamase-stable cephalosporin that covers *S. pneumoniae* (e.g., cefprozil, cefuroxime, or cefpodoxime) is an option.[33,35] Other alternatives are cefdinir, azithromycin, clarithromycin, and trimethoprim-sulfamethoxazole.[34,35] Clinical cure rates are similar among antibiotics,[47] although local-area resistance rates also must be considered, as well as increasing resistance of *S. pneumoniae*, *H. influenzae*, and *M. catarrhalis* to trimethoprim-sulfamethoxazole, and of *S. pneumoniae* to macrolides. Respiratory fluoroquinolones and ceftriaxone have also been recommended.

If drug-resistant *S. pneumoniae* is suspected (daycare attendance, recent antibiotic use, age younger than 2 years), then high-dose amoxicillin should be given. Some recommend clindamycin, but it is important to note that this drug is not active against *H. influenzae* and *M. catarrhalis*.[35] In adults, respiratory fluoroquinolones are considered to be second line in patients who have failed other therapies, have recently received other antibiotics, or in whom there is a high suspicion for drug-resistant *S. pneumoniae*.[33]

The duration of therapy for treatment of sinusitis is not well established. Most trials have used 10- to 14-day antibiotic courses for uncomplicated sinusitis.[45] A 3-day course of azithromycin was approved for use in sinusitis in both Canada and the United States. A randomized, double-blind study demonstrated that azithromycin 500 mg daily for 3 or 5 days was as effective as amoxicillin-clavulanate over 10 days.[46] Furthermore, an extended-release single-dose preparation of azithromycin approved in the United States. However, data supporting these short regimens are limited, and new guidelines express concern over macrolide-resistant *S. pneumoniae*.[33] The current recommendations are 10 to 14 days of antibiotic therapy or at least 7 days after signs and symptoms are under control.[30,33,43]

PHARMACOECONOMIC CONSIDERATIONS

Similar to acute otitis media, pharmacoeconomic considerations in acute bacterial sinusitis are minimal, as the empiric antibiotic of choice is generically available, and meta-analyses have failed to demonstrate superior efficacy with more costly therapies.[41,45] More expensive therapies may be justified if drug-resistant pathogens are suspected or documented.

EVALUATION OF THERAPEUTIC OUTCOMES

Persistent or worsening symptoms 72 hours after initiating antibiotic therapy should be considered treatment failure.[30,33,43] Referral to a specialist should be considered for patients who have not responded to first- or second-line therapy; for those with severe, recurrent, and chronic disease; and for patients who are at risk for complications. Patients who experience changes in visual acuity or mental status should be referred immediately. Surgery may be considered in more complicated patients. Acute bacterial sinusitis lasts less than 30 days with complete resolution of symptoms, whereas chronic sinusitis is defined as episodes of inflammation lasting more than 3 months with persistence of respiratory symptoms.[30,35]

ACUTE PHARYNGITIS

1 **2** Pharyngitis is an acute infection of the oropharynx or nasopharynx.[48] It is responsible for 1% to 2% of all outpatient visits.[49] Although viral causes are most common, group A β-hemolytic streptococci (GABHS; also known as *S. pyogenes*), is the primary bacterial cause.[48,50] GABHS is commonly known as "strep throat."

EPIDEMIOLOGY

Acute pharyngitis accounts for ~2 million emergency department and outpatient department visits per year,[51] at a cost of approximately $1.2 billion total and up to $539 million for children alone.[52] Although viral causes are most common, GABHS is the primary bacterial cause and is associated with rare but severe sequelae if not treated appropriately.[48,50] Nonsuppurative complications such as acute rheumatic fever, acute glomerulo-nephritis, and reactive arthritis may occur, as well as suppurative complications, such as peritonsillar abscess, retropharyngeal abscess, cervical lymphadenitis, mastoiditis, otitis media, sinusitis, and necrotizing fasciitis.

Although all age groups are susceptible, epidemiologic data demonstrate certain groups are at higher risk. Children ages 5 to 15 years are most susceptible; parents of school-age children and those who work with children are also at increased risk. Pharyngitis in a child younger than 3 years of age is rarely caused by GABHS.[48,50]

Seasonal outbreaks occur, and the incidence of GABHS is highest in winter and early spring.[48,53] The incubation period is 2 to 5 days, and the illness often occurs in clusters.[53,54] Spread occurs via direct contact (usually from hands) with droplets of saliva or nasal secretions, and transmission is thus worse in institutions, schools, families, and areas of crowding.[54,55] Untreated, patients with streptococcal pharyngitis are infectious during the acute illness and for another week thereafter.[56] Effective antibiotic therapy reduces the infectious period to about 24 hours.

Acute rheumatic fever is rarely seen in developed countries. In the United States, acute rheumatic fever secondary to GABHS infection was a cause of concern in the 1950s and was the major reason for penicillin therapy, but the annual incidence of this disease today is extremely rare (≤1 case per 1 million population). However, some risk does remain; outbreaks have been reported in the United States as recently as the late 1980s and early 1990s. Furthermore, acute rheumatic fever is widespread in developing countries.[57] South Central Asia's median incidence of acute rheumatic fever is 54 cases per 100,000 compared with 10 cases per 100,000 in established markets.[57]

ETIOLOGY

Viruses cause the majority of acute pharyngitis cases. Specific etiologies include rhinovirus (20%), coronavirus (<5%), adenovirus (5%), herpes simplex virus (4%), influenza virus (2%), parainfluenza virus (2%), and Epstein-Barr virus (<1%).[48,50] A bacterial etiology is far less likely. Of all the bacterial causes, GABHS is the most common (10–30% of persons of all ages with pharyngitis) and is the only commonly occurring form of acute pharyngitis for which antibiotic therapy is indicated.[48] In the pediatric population, GABHS causes 15% to 30% of pharyngitis cases. In adults, GABHS is responsible for 5% to 15% of all symptomatic episodes of pharyngitis.[48–50,54]

Other, less-common causes of acute pharyngitis are groups C and G *Streptococcus, Corynebacterium diphtheriae, Neisseria gonorrhoeae, Mycoplasma pneumoniae, Arcanobacterium haemolyticum, Yersinia enterocolitica,* and *Chlamydia pneumoniae.* Treatment options for these organisms are not addressed in this chapter.[48,50]

PATHOPHYSIOLOGY

The mechanism by which GABHS causes pharyngitis is not well defined. Asymptomatic pharyngeal carriers of the organism may have an alteration in host immunity (e.g., a breach in the pharyngeal mucosa) and the bacteria of the oropharynx, allowing colonization to become an infection. Pathogenic factors associated with the organism itself may also play a role. These include pyrogenic toxins, hemolysins, streptokinase, and proteinase.

CLINICAL PRESENTATION

The most common symptom of pharyngitis is sore throat. Accurate differentiation of GABHS from pharyngitis caused by other agents is key for treatment decisions; however, this can be difficult even for

TABLE 117–6 Modified Centor Criteria for Clinical Prediction of Group A β-Hemolytic Streptococcal Pharyngitis[a]

Criteria	Points
Temperature >38°C (101°F)	1
Absence of cough	1
Swollen, tender anterior cervical nodes	1
Tonsillar swelling or exudate	1
Age	
3–14 years	1
15–44 years	0
45 years or older	−1

Score	Risk of streptococcal infection
≤0	1%–2.5%
1	5%–10%
2	11%–17%
3	28%–35%
≥4	51%–53%

[a]The original Centor score applies to adults only. This modified version allows for age.
From McIsaac WJ, Kellner JD, Aufricht P, et al. Empirical validation of guidelines for the management of pharyngitis in children and adults. JAMA 2004;291(13):1587–1595.

experienced clinicians. Therefore, incorporation of microbiologic testing is recommended if the patient meets the appropriate clinical criteria.

Clinical scoring systems such as the Centor criteria,[58] or modifications of the Centor criteria,[59] have been advocated for clinical diagnosis in adults as a way to overcome the lack of sensitivity and specificity of clinician judgment and to avoid laboratory testing of all patients.[49,54] Table 117–6 lists the modified Centor criteria. The modified Centor criteria include age as a factor for scoring. Concern exists that use of these criteria alone leads to overprescribing.[48,50,60] Guidelines from the American Heart Association (AHA), which are endorsed by the AAP, suggest that testing be done in all patients with signs and symptoms of streptococcal pharyngitis. Only those with a positive test for GABHS require antibiotic treatment.[48,53,60] Limiting testing to patients who meet two or more Centor criteria will minimize overtesting.[59,60] The simplest approach is likely point-of-care testing with culture confirmation in cases of negative results. This ensures those with the condition are not undertreated. Table 117–7 compares recommendations for diagnostic testing and antibiotic treatment among recent GABHS pharyngitis guidelines.

Laboratory testing should not be used without consideration of clinical criteria. This is because a positive test does not necessarily indicate disease. A positive test may indicate the patient is a carrier for GABHS (not active infection), and the cause of pharyngitis could be viral. Approximately 5% to 20% of children are carriers; the prevalence is lower among adults.[53] Table 117–8 lists the evidence-based principles for diagnosis of GABHS. There are several options to test for GABHS. A throat swab can be sent for culture or used for the rapid antigen-detection test (RADT). Cultures are the gold standard, but they require 24 to 48 hours for results.[50] The RADT is more practical in that it provides results quickly, it can be performed at the bedside, and it is less expensive than culture. If RADT yields negative test results, it is generally recommended to follow up with a throat culture to confirm results. Cultures are recommended for children and adolescents who have a negative RADT.[48] However, the AHA, which is the most recent position statement, recommends follow-up throat cultures for all patients after a negative RADT.[61] Delaying therapy while awaiting culture results does not affect the risk of complications (although some argue that symptomatic benefit is postponed, and contagion remains), and patients must be educated as to the value of waiting, given the low false-negative rate of RADT.[62]

TABLE 117-7 Recommendations for Diagnostic Testing and Indications for Antibiotic Treatment in Suspected Group A β-hemolytic Streptococcal Pharyngitis[a]

Guideline	Population	Tests		Antibiotic Treatment
ACP-ASIM, AAFP, CDC[54]	Suspected pharyngitis evaluated using Centor criteria	0 or 1 criteria	None	No treatment
		2 or 3 criteria	RADT	Yes, if test positive
		3 or 4 criteria	None	Yes (empiric)
				Negative RADT with sensitivity > 80% does not need follow-up throat culture
IDSA[48]	Suspected pharyngitis with clinical and epidemiologic factors suggestive of GABHS pharyngitis[b]	RADT or throat culture		Yes, if test positive
				Negative RADT results must be confirmed with throat culture for children and adolescents only
AHA[a61]	Suspected pharyngitis with clinical and epidemiologic factors suggestive of GABHS pharyngitis[b]	RADT or throat culture		Yes, if test positive
				Negative RADT results must be confirmed with throat culture for all patients tested

[a]The American Academy of Pediatrics endorses the American Heart Association statement.[61]
[b]Epidemiologic factors suggestive of GABHS pharyngitis include history of exposure, presentation in winter or early spring, and patient age 5 to 15 years.
AAFP = American Academy of Family Physicians, ACP-ASIM = American College of Physicians–American Society of Internal Medicine, AHA = American Heart Association, CDC = Centers for Disease Control and Prevention, GABHS = group A β-hemolytic streptococci, IDSA = Infectious Disease Society of America, RADT = rapid antigen detection test.
From Bisno AL, Gerber MA, Gwaltney JM, Jr., et al. Practice guidelines for the diagnosis and management of group A streptococcal pharyngitis: Infectious Diseases Society of America. Clin Infect Dis 2002;35(2):113–125; Cooper RJ, Hoffman JR, Bartlett JG, et al. Principles of appropriate antibiotic use for acute pharyngitis in adults: Background. Ann Intern Med 2001;134(6):509–517; and Gerber MA, Baltimore RS, Eaton CB, et al. Prevention of rheumatic fever and diagnosis and treatment of acute streptococcal pharyngitis: A scientific statement from the American Heart Association Rheumatic Fever, Endocarditis, and Kawasaki Disease Committee of the Council on Cardiovascular Disease in the Young, the Interdisciplinary Council on Functional Genomics and Translational Biology, and the Interdisciplinary Council on Quality of Care and Outcomes Research: endorsed by the American Academy of Pediatrics. Circulation 2009;119(11):1541–1551.

CLINICAL PRESENTATION AND DIAGNOSIS OF GROUP A STREPTOCOCCAL PHARYNGITIS

General

- A sore throat of sudden onset that is mostly self-limited
- Fever and constitutional symptoms resolving in about 3 to 5 days
- Clinical signs and symptoms are similar for viral causes and nonstreptococcal bacterial causes

Signs and Symptoms

- Sore throat
- Pain on swallowing
- Fever
- Headache, nausea, vomiting, and abdominal pain (especially children)
- Erythema/inflammation of the tonsils and pharynx with or without patchy exudates
- Enlarged, tender lymph nodes
- Red swollen uvula, petechiae on the soft palate, and a scarlatiniform rash
- Several symptoms that are not suggestive of group A streptococci are cough, conjunctivitis, coryza, and diarrhea

Signs Suggestive of Viral Origin for Pharyngitis

- Conjunctivitis
- Coryza
- Cough
- Diarrhea

Laboratory Tests

- Throat swab and culture
- Rapid antigen detection testing (RADT)

From Bisno AL, Gerber MA, Gwaltney JM, Jr., et al. Practice guidelines for the diagnosis and management of group A streptococcal pharyngitis: Infectious Diseases Society of America. Clin Infect Dis 2002;35(2):113–125; Snow V, Mottur-Pilson C, Cooper RJ, Hoffman JR.

Principles of appropriate antibiotic use for acute pharyngitis in adults. Ann Intern Med 2001;134(6):506–508; Cooper RJ, Hoffman JR, Bartlett JG, et al. Principles of appropriate antibiotic use for acute pharyngitis in adults: Background. Ann Intern Med 2001;134(6):509–517; and Gerber MA, Baltimore RS, Eaton CB, et al. Prevention of rheumatic fever and diagnosis and treatment of acute streptococcal pharyngitis: A scientific statement from the American Heart Association Rheumatic Fever, Endocarditis, and Kawasaki Disease Committee of the Council on Cardiovascular Disease in the Young, the Interdisciplinary Council on Functional Genomics and Translational Biology, and the Interdisciplinary Council on Quality of Care and Outcomes Research: endorsed by the American Academy of Pediatrics. Circulation 2009;119(11):1541–1551.

TREATMENT

■ DESIRED OUTCOME

The goals of treatment for pharyngitis are to improve clinical signs and symptoms, minimize adverse drug reactions, prevent transmission to close contacts, and prevent acute rheumatic fever and suppurative complications, such as peritonsillar abscess, cervical lymphadenitis, and mastoiditis.[48,49]

■ GENERAL APPROACH TO TREATMENT

Once the diagnosis of GABHS pharyngitis has been made, the clinician must decide appropriate supportive care, when to initiate antibiotic therapy, the appropriate antibiotic, and the duration of therapy. The selection of appropriate antibiotic therapy will involve careful consideration of cost, safety, efficacy, potential for regimen adherence, and bacterial resistance rates. Clinicians should be aware of the local resistance patterns, which may differ from the national patterns.

Antibiotic overuse has been well documented.[48,60] Antibiotic therapy should be reserved for those patients with clinical and epidemiologic features of GABHS pharyngitis, preferably with a positive laboratory test. Empiric therapy is not recommended unless there is a high index of suspicion based on clinical or epidemiologic data and laboratory results are pending. However, it is very important to discontinue empiric antibiotics if laboratory results are negative.

TABLE 117-8 Evidence-Based Principles for Diagnosis of Group A *Streptococcus*

Recommendations	Level
Selective use of diagnostic testing only in those with clinical features suggestive of group A *Streptococcus* will increase the proportion of positive tests as well as results of those truly infected, not carriers.	A-II
Clinical diagnosis cannot be made with certainty even by the most experienced clinician; bacteriologic confirmation is required.	A-II
Throat culture remains the diagnostic standard, with a sensitivity of 90% to 95% for detection of group A *Streptococcus* if done correctly.	A-II
Rapid identification and treatment of patients with disease can reduce transmission, allow patients to return to work or school earlier, and reduce the acute morbidity of the disease.	A-II
The majority of rapid antigen detection tests available have a specificity >95% (minimizes overprescribing to those without disease) and a sensitivity of 80% to 90% compared with culture.	A-II
Early initiation of antibiotic therapy results in faster resolution of signs and symptoms. Delays in therapy (if awaiting cultures) can be made safely for up to 9 days after symptom onset and still prevent major complications such as rheumatic fever.	A-I

Rating:

   Strength of recommendation: A to E

   Evidence to support use: A, good; B, moderate; C, poor

   Evidence against use: D, moderate; E, good

   Quality of evidence: I, II, or III

      I: At least one randomized controlled trial

      II: At least one well-designed clinical trial, not randomized, or a cohort or case-controlled analytical study, or from multiple time series, or from dramatic results of an uncontrolled trial

      III: Opinions of respected authorities

From Bisno AL, Gerber MA, Gwaltney JM, Jr., et al. Practice guidelines for the diagnosis and management of group A streptococcal pharyngitis: Infectious Diseases Society of America. Clin Infect Dis 2002;35(2):113–125.

■ NONPHARMACOLOGIC THERAPY

Supportive care should be offered for all patients with acute pharyngitis. In a prospective study of the care of patients with "sore throat," patient satisfaction with their care was strongly associated with whether the physician addressed the patient's concerns rather than antibiotic prescribing.[63] Pharmacologic interventions include antipyretic medications and nonprescription lozenges and sprays containing menthol and topical anesthetics for temporary relief of pain.[50] Because pain is often the primary reason for visiting a physician, emphasis on analgesics such as acetaminophen and NSAIDs to aid in pain relief is strongly recommended.[64] However, acetaminophen is a better option because there is some concern that NSAIDs may increase the risk for necrotizing fasciitis/toxic shock syndrome. Toxic shock syndrome has been linked to GABHS pharyngitis. Symptoms may resolve 1 or 2 days sooner with such interventions.[48,50,54]

■ PHARMACOLOGIC THERAPY

❹ For over 30 years, GABHS isolated in the United States has shown susceptibility to penicillin. Because penicillin has a narrow spectrum of activity and is readily available, safe, and inexpensive, it is considered the treatment of choice.[48,49] The only controlled studies that have demonstrated that antibiotic therapy prevents rheumatic fever following GABHS pharyngitis were done with procaine penicillin, which was later replaced with benzathine penicillin.[65,66] Penicillin given by other routes is assumed to be equally efficacious. The ability of other antibiotics to eradicate GABHS has led to extrapolation that these antibiotics will also prevent rheumatic fever.[54] Amoxicillin can be used in children because the suspension is more palatable than penicillin.[48,55] Gastrointestinal (GI) adverse effects and rash, however, are more common. A once-daily, extended-release formulation of amoxicillin has been approved

for treatment of GABHS pharyngitis in adults and children ages 12 years and older; however, use of once-daily dosing in GABHS pharyngitis is controversial.

CLINICAL CONTROVERSY

Once-daily amoxicillin given at a dose of 750 mg is as effective as penicillin 250 mg given three times daily (duration 10 days each) in children ages 4 to 18 years with GABHS pharyngitis.[84] This dosing regimen has not yet been endorsed by expert panels but may gain support in the future if the results are reproducible.[48,49,54]

In penicillin-allergic patients, erythromycin or a first-generation cephalosporin such as cephalexin can be used if the reaction is non-IgE-mediated.[50] Newer macrolides such as azithromycin and clarithromycin are equally effective as erythromycin and cause fewer GI adverse effects. Second-generation cephalosporins, such as cefuroxime and cefprozil, or third-generation cephalosporins, such as cefpodoxime and cefdinir, which are β-lactamase-stable, have been advocated for clinical failures with penicillin. In cases of documented macrolide resistance (owing to low-level macrolide resistance—erythromycin MIC 1 to 8 mcg/mL—because of expression of the *mefA/E* gene leading to efflux of macrolide out of the bacterial cell), clindamycin is an alternative. If patients are unable to take oral medications, intramuscular benzathine penicillin can be given, although it is painful.[48]

There are no definitive trial data to support a particular antibiotic regimen preferentially over another to treat multiple recurring episodes of culture-positive GABHS pharyngitis. Amoxicillin-clavulanate or clindamycin may be considered for recurrent episodes of pharyngitis to maximize bacterial eradication in potential carriers and to counter co-pathogens that produce β-lactamases.[48,53] Surgical removal of tonsils may be indicated in patients whose frequency of episodes does not diminish over time, and there is no other explanation for recurrence.[48] Tables 117–9 and 117–10 outline dosing for acute and recurrent episodes of GABHS pharyngitis.

To date, no resistance of GABHS to penicillin has been reported in clinical isolates.[48,49,53,67,68] Macrolide resistance is low (<5%) and is not widespread.[67–73] There has been a report of an outbreak of macrolide-resistant GABHS pharyngitis in the United States and increasing rates in New York City.[68] Internationally, higher rates have also been reported,[73] and as usage of macrolides increases, these rates will continue to rise. Consequently, use of newer macrolides as first-line therapy is discouraged in febrile patients with upper respiratory tract infections. GABHS resistance rates to tetracyclines and sulfonamides are high; therefore, use of these antibiotics is no longer recommended.[48]

The ideal time to start antibiotic therapy has not been established. The immediate start of antibiotic therapy does not affect the risk of developing rheumatic fever, and no evidence suggests it reduces recurrent infection.[74,75] Clinical guidelines recommend withholding antibiotics unless the patient has a positive laboratory test or three or four of the Centor criteria. Nevertheless, a survey of clinicians treating children and adolescents with acute pharyngitis revealed that 42% of clinicians would start antibiotic therapy before diagnostic results were received and continue antibiotics despite a negative test result.[76]

The impact of appropriate antibiotic therapy is limited to decreasing the duration of signs and symptoms by 1 or 2 days.[49,77] It can decrease the severity of pharyngitis symptoms when initiated within 2 or 3 days of onset in patients with proven GABHS.

TABLE 117-9 Dosing Guidelines for Pharyngitis

Medication	Adult Dosage	Pediatric Dosage	Duration	Rating
Preferred antibiotics				
Penicillin V	250 mg three or four times daily or 500 mg twice daily	50 mg/kg/day divided in three doses	10 days	IB
Penicillin benzathine	1.2 million units intramuscularly	0.6 million units for weight ≤27 kg (50,000 units/kg)	One dose	IB
Penicillin G procaine and benzathine mixture	Not recommended in adolescents and adults	1.2 million units (benzathine 0.9 million units, procaine 0.3 million units)	One dose	
Additional effective antibiotics				
Amoxicillin	500 mg three times daily	40–50 mg/kg/day divided in three doses	10 days	IB
Amoxicillin, extended release	775 mg daily	775 mg daily[b]	10 days	IIaB
Cephalexin[a]	250–500 mg orally four times daily	25–50 mg/kg/day divided in four doses	10 days	IB
Clindamycin[a]	20 mg/kg per day divided into 3 doses (maximum 1.8 g/day)		10 days	IIaB
Azithromycin[a]	12 mg/kg once daily (maximum 500 mg)		5 days	IIaB
Clarithromycin[a]	15 mg/kg per day divided in two doses (maximum 250 mg twice daily)		10 days	IIaB
Erythromycin[a]	Variable depending on formulation	Variable depending on formulation	10 days	IIaB

[a]To be prescribed as an alternative to penicillin in penicillin-allergic patients.
[b]Children ages 12 years and older.
Classification of recommendations:

Class I: Conditions for which there is evidence and/or general agreement that a given procedure or treatment is beneficial, useful, and effective.

Class II: Conditions for which there is conflicting evidence and/or a divergence of opinion about the usefulness/efficacy of a procedure or treatment.

Class IIa: Weight of evidence/opinion is in favor of usefulness/efficacy.

Class IIb: Usefulness/efficacy is less well established by evidence/opinion.

Class III: Conditions for which there is evidence and/or general agreement that a procedure/treatment is not useful/effective and in some cases may be harmful.

Level of evidence:

Level of evidence A: Data derived from multiple randomized clinical trials or meta-analyses.

Level of evidence B: Data derived from a single randomized trial or nonrandomized studies.

Level of evidence C: Only consensus opinion of experts, cases studies, or standard of care.

From Bisno AL, Gerber MA, Gwaltney JM, Jr., et al. Practice guidelines for the diagnosis and management of group A streptococcal pharyngitis: Infectious Diseases Society of America. Clin Infect Dis 2002;35(2):113–125; Bisno AL. Acute pharyngitis. N Engl J Med 2001;344(3):205–211; American Academy of Pediatrics. Group A streptococcal infections. In: Pickering LK, ed. Red Book 2003: Report of the Committee on Infectious Diseases. 26th ed. Elk Grove Village, IL: American Academy of Pediatrics, 2003:526–536; and Gerber MA, Baltimore RS, Eaton CB, et al. Prevention of rheumatic fever and diagnosis and treatment of acute streptococcal pharyngitis: A scientific statement from the American Heart Association Rheumatic Fever, Endocarditis, and Kawasaki Disease Committee of the Council on Cardiovascular Disease in the Young, the Interdisciplinary Council on Functional Genomics and Translational Biology, and the Interdisciplinary Council on Quality of Care and Outcomes Research: endorsed by the American Academy of Pediatrics. Circulation 2009;119(11):1541–1551.

Microbiologic eradication will occur in 48 to 72 hours, which aids in decreasing transmission.[49] However, antibiotics may be delayed up to 9 days after diagnosis without affecting the incidence of acute rheumatic fever.[62]

The duration of therapy for GABHS pharyngitis is 10 days to maximize bacterial eradication.[48] Although some clinicians have proposed shorter courses of treatment for pharyngitis, confounding factors from these studies, such as the lack of strict entry criteria or differentiation between new or failed infections, limit the widespread application of short antibiotic courses at this time.[48]

CLINICAL CONTROVERSY

Short-course therapy has been advocated to help overcome compliance issues that lead to bacteriologic failure.[85] A 6-day course of amoxicillin demonstrated promising results;[86] in addition, studies with newer broad-spectrum antibiotics (e.g., azithromycin, cefuroxime, cefprozil, cefdinir, cefixime, and cefpodoxime) have demonstrated durations of 5 days or less to be effective.[87,88] A Cochrane review examining short-course (3–6 days) versus standard-duration (10-day course of penicillin) antibiotic therapy for acute GABHS pharyngitis in children reported no significant difference in early bacteriologic treatment failure or late clinical recurrence.[89] Unfortunately, the overall risk of late bacteriologic treatment failure was worse for short-duration treatment. When low-dose azithromycin (10 mg/kg) regimens were eliminated from the analysis, the overall risk of late bacteriologic treatment failure was not different between short-course and standard-duration therapy. The review noted that shorter-duration treatment resulted in better compliance.

Additionally, newer antibiotics that have been studied in this fashion are more expensive and may be more likely to lead to resistance in light of their broad-spectrum of activity.[50]

Overprescribing is common in acute pharyngitis. Antibiotics are prescribed for 73% of patients who visit their provider with a complaint of "sore throat."[78] This is well above the incidence of GABHS pharyngitis. For those who receive antibiotics, 68% of prescriptions are described as being nonrecommended treatments, for example, extended-spectrum macrolides (e.g., azithromycin or clarithromycin) or fluoroquinolones (e.g., ciprofloxacin, levofloxacin, or moxifloxacin). Factors including cost and resistance should discourage this practice.

Approximately 25% of household contacts of a person with acute GABHS pharyngitis harbor GABHS in their upper respiratory tracts.[48] Routine testing of asymptomatic household contacts of an index patient is not recommended. If tested, it is not necessary to treat these asymptomatic carriers. However, it is difficult to ascertain the cause of symptomatic pharyngitis in carriers of GABHS if they do develop symptoms. In cases of acute pharyngitis in GABHS carriers, a treatment course of appropriate antibiotics is recommended.[61]

Patients with documented histories of rheumatic fever (including cases manifested solely by Sydenham chorea) and those with definite evidence of rheumatic heart disease should receive continuous prophylaxis initiated as soon as the patient is diagnosed and the initial infection has been treated. The duration of secondary prophylaxis is individualized based on patient risk of recurrence of rheumatic fever and/or rheumatic heart disease. Intramuscular benzathine penicillin G every 4 weeks is the recommended regimen for secondary prevention in the United States in most circumstances.[61] Additional options for secondary prophylaxis include oral penicillin V and sulfadiazine. Medication adherence is key to successful secondary prevention with oral antibiotics. Sulfadiazine is an effective antibiotic for the

TABLE 117-10 Antibiotics and Dosing for Recurrent Episodes of Pharyngitis

Drug	Adult Dosage	Pediatric Dosage
Clindamycin	600 mg orally divided in two to four doses	20 mg/kg/day orally in three divided doses (maximum 1.8 g/day)
Amoxicillin-clavulanate	500 mg orally twice daily	40 mg/kg/day orally in three divided doses
Penicillin benzathine	1.2 million units intramuscularly for one dose	0.6 million units intramuscularly for weight <27 kg (50,000 units/kg)
Penicillin benzathine with rifampin	As above	As above
	Rifampin 20 mg/kg/day orally in two divided doses during last 4 days of treatment with penicillin (maximum daily dose 600 mg)	Rifampin dose same as adults

From Bisno AL, Gerber MA, Gwaltney JM, Jr., et al. Practice guidelines for the diagnosis and management of group A streptococcal pharyngitis: Infectious Diseases Society of America. Clin Infect Dis 2002;35(2):113–125.

prevention of infection and is appropriate if the patient is penicillin-allergic. Sulfonamides are not appropriate for treatment of GABHS pharyngitis because they are not effective for eradication of GABHS. If individuals are allergic to penicillin and sulfadiazine, a macrolide is recommended; however, this recommendation is based on expert opinion rather than clinical trial data.[61]

PHARMACOECONOMIC CONSIDERATIONS

Adherence to acute pharyngitis guidelines is difficult for many clinicians.[79] A retrospective analysis of visits to a primary care clinic for acute pharyngitis demonstrated that 66% of providers did not adhere to any of the recommended pharyngitis guidelines.[79]

Pharmacoeconomic studies support the use of guideline-concordant therapies for the reduction of healthcare costs and antibiotic resistance in acute pharyngitis. In one pharmacoeconomic study, the annual expenditures for acute pharyngitis were determined to be $1.2 billion, with antibiotic resistance contributing 36% of these costs in a cost of illness analysis.[52] These figures were based on common prescribing practices, including inappropriate antibiotic prescribing for viral pharyngitis. The authors suggested that adherence to guideline recommendations would decrease costs by ~53%.

EVALUATION OF THERAPEUTIC OUTCOMES

Most pharyngitis cases are self-limited; however, antibiotics hasten resolution when given early for proven cases of GABHS pharyngitis.[48] Generally, fever and other symptoms resolve within 3 or 4 days of onset without antibiotics; however, symptoms will improve 16 hours to 2½ days earlier with antibiotic therapy.[48] Follow-up testing is generally not necessary for index cases or in asymptomatic contacts of the index patient.[48,50,53] However, for patients who remain symptomatic or when symptoms recur despite completion of treatment, posttreatment throat cultures 2 to 7 days after completion of antibiotics should be done.[61]

ABBREVIATIONS

MIC: Minimum inhibitory concentration

MIC_{90}: Minimum inhibitory concentration for 90% of isolates

NSAID: Nonsteroidal antiinflammatory drug

GABHS: Group A β-hemolytic streptococci

RADT: Rapid antigen detection testing

REFERENCES

1. Hing E, Cherry DK, Woodwell DA. National Ambulatory Medical Care Survey: 2004 summary. Adv Data 2006(374):1–33.
2. McCaig LF, Nawar EW. National Hospital Ambulatory Medical Care Survey: 2004 emergency department summary. Adv Data 2006(372):1–29.
3. Subcommittee on Management of Acute Otitis Media. Diagnosis and management of acute otitis media. Pediatrics 2004;113(5):1451–1465.
4. American Academy of Family Physicians, American Academy of Otolaryngology–Head and Neck Surgery and American Academy of Pediatrics Subcommittee on Otitis Media With Effusion. Otitis media with effusion. Pediatrics 2004;113(5):1412–1429.
5. Faden H, Duffy L, Boeve M. Otitis media: Back to basics. Pediatr Infect Dis J 1998;17(12):1105–1112.
6. Block SL, Hedrick J, Harrison CJ, et al. Community-wide vaccination with the heptavalent pneumococcal conjugate significantly alters the microbiology of acute otitis media. Pediatr Infect Dis J 2004;23(9):829–833.
7. Arguedas A, Dagan R, Pichichero M, et al. An open-label, double tympanocentesis study of levofloxacin therapy in children with, or at high risk for, recurrent or persistent acute otitis media. Pediatr Infect Dis J 2006;25(12):1102–1109.
8. Jacobs MR, Felmingham D, Appelbaum PC, Gruneberg RN. The Alexander Project 1998–2000: Susceptibility of pathogens isolated from community-acquired respiratory tract infection to commonly used antimicrobial agents. J Antimicrob Chemother 2003;52(2):229–246.
9. Doern GV, Jones RN, Pfaller MA, Kugler K. *Haemophilus influenzae* and *Moraxella catarrhalis* from patients with community-acquired respiratory tract infections: Antimicrobial susceptibility patterns from the SENTRY antimicrobial Surveillance Program (United States and Canada, 1997). Antimicrob Agents Chemother 1999;43(2):385–389.
10. Hoberman A, Marchant CD, Kaplan SL, Feldman S. Treatment of acute otitis media consensus recommendations. Clin Pediatr (Phila) 2002;41(6):373–390.
11. Hendley JO. Clinical practice: Otitis media. N Engl J Med 2002;347(15):1169–1174.
12. Jansen AG, Hak E, Veenhoven RH, et al. Pneumococcal conjugate vaccines for preventing otitis media. Cochrane Database Syst Rev 2009(2):CD001480.
13. Swingler GH. Chickenpox. Clin Evid (Online) 2007.
14. Fiore AE, Bridges CB, Cox NJ. Seasonal influenza vaccines. Curr Top Microbiol Immunol 2009;333:43–82.
15. Fiore AE, Shay DK, Broder K, et al. Prevention and control of seasonal influenza with vaccines: recommendations of the Advisory Committee on Immunization Practices (ACIP), 2009. MMWR Recomm Rep 2009;58(RR-8):1–52.
16. Foxlee R, Johansson A, Wejfalk J, et al. Topical analgesia for acute otitis media. Cochrane Database Syst Rev 2006;3:CD005657.
17. Coleman C, Moore M. Decongestants and antihistamines for acute otitis media in children. Cochrane Database Syst Rev 2008(3):CD001727.
18. Griffin GH, Flynn C, Bailey RE, Schultz JK. Antihistamines and/or decongestants for otitis media with effusion (OME) in children. Cochrane Database Syst Rev 2006(4):CD003423.
19. Glasziou PP, Del Mar CB, Sanders SL, Hayem M. Antibiotics for acute otitis media in children. Cochrane Database Syst Rev 2004(1):CD000219.
20. Rovers MM, Glasziou P, Appelman CL, et al. Antibiotics for acute otitis media: A meta-analysis with individual patient data. Lancet 2006;368(9545):1429–1435.
21. Thanaviratananich S, Laopaiboon M, Vatanasapt P. Once or twice daily versus three times daily amoxicillin with or without clavulanate for the treatment of acute otitis media. Cochrane Database Syst Rev 2008(4):CD004975.

22. Spurling GK, Del Mar CB, Dooley L, Foxlee R. Delayed antibiotics for respiratory infections. Cochrane Database Syst Rev 2007;(3):CD004417.

23. Dagan R, Hoberman A, Johnson C, et al. Bacteriologic and clinical efficacy of high dose amoxicillin/clavulanate in children with acute otitis media. Pediatr Infect Dis J 2001;20(9):829–837.

24. Dagan R, McCracken GH, Jr. Flaws in design and conduct of clinical trials in acute otitis media. Pediatr Infect Dis J 2002;21(10):894–902.

25. Cohen R, Levy C, Boucherat M, et al. A multicenter, randomized, double-blind trial of 5 versus 10 days of antibiotic therapy for acute otitis media in young children. J Pediatr 1998;133(5):634–669.

26. McCracken GH, Jr. Prescribing antimicrobial agents for treatment of acute otitis media. Pediatr Infect Dis J 1999;18(12):1141–1146.

27. Kozyrskyj A, Hildes-Ripstein GE, Longstaffe SE, et al. Short course antibiotics for acute otitis media. Cochrane Database Syst Rev 2000;(2):CD001095.

28. Luotonen M, Uhari M, Aitola L, et al. Recurrent otitis media during infancy and linguistic skills at the age of nine years. Pediatr Infect Dis J 1996;15(10):854–858.

29. Williams RL, Chalmers TC, Stange KC, et al. Use of antibiotics in preventing recurrent acute otitis media and in treating otitis media with effusion: A meta-analytic attempt to resolve the brouhaha. JAMA 1993;270(11):1344–1351.

30. Hickner JM, Bartlett JG, Besser RE, et al. Principles of appropriate antibiotic use for acute rhinosinusitis in adults: Background. Ann Intern Med 2001;134(6):498–505.

31. Piccirillo JF. Clinical practice: Acute bacterial sinusitis. N Engl J Med 2004;351(9):902–910.

32. Pleis JR, Lethbridge-Cejku M. Summary health statistics for U.S. adults: National Health Interview Survey, 2005. Vital Health Stat 2006;10(232):1–153.

33. Anon JB, Jacobs MR, Poole MD, et al. Antimicrobial treatment guidelines for acute bacterial rhinosinusitis. Otolaryngol Head Neck Surg 2004;130(1 Suppl):1–45.

34. Scheid DC, Hamm RM. Acute bacterial rhinosinusitis in adults: 2. Treatment. Am Fam Physician 2004;70(9):1697–1704.

35. Subcommittee on Management of Sinusitis and Committee on Quality Improvement. Clinical practice guideline: Management of sinusitis. Pediatrics 2001;108(3):798–808.

36. Anand VK. Epidemiology and economic impact of rhinosinusitis. Ann Otol Rhinol Laryngol Suppl 2004;193:3–5.

37. Rosenfeld RM. Clinical practice guideline on adult sinusitis. Otolaryngol Head Neck Surg 2007;137(3):365–377.

38. Rosenfeld RM, Andes D, Bhattacharyya N, et al. Clinical practice guideline: Adult sinusitis. Otolaryngol Head Neck Surg 2007;137(3 Suppl):S1–S31.

39. Meltzer EO, Bachert C, Staudinger H. Treating acute rhinosinusitis: Comparing efficacy and safety of mometasone furoate nasal spray, amoxicillin, and placebo. J Allergy Clin Immunol 2005;116(6):1289–1295.

40. Zalmanovici A, Yaphe J. Steroids for acute sinusitis. Cochrane Database Syst Rev 2007;(2):CD005149.

41. Ip S, Fu L, Balk E, et al. Update on Acute Bacterial Rhinosinusitis: Evidence Report/Technology Assessment No. 124 (Prepared by Tufts-New England Medical Center Evidence-based Practice Center under Contract No. 290-02-0022). AHRQ Pub. No. 05-E020-2. Rockville, MD: Agency for Healthcare Research and Quality; 2005.

42. Slavin RG, Spector SL, Bernstein IL, et al. The diagnosis and management of sinusitis: A practice parameter update. J Allergy Clin Immunol 2005;116(6 Suppl):S13–S47.

43. Snow V, Mottur-Pilson C, Hickner JM. Principles of appropriate antibiotic use for acute sinusitis in adults. Ann Intern Med 2001;134(6):495–497.

44. Rosenfeld RM, Singer M, Jones S. Systematic review of antimicrobial therapy in patients with acute rhinosinusitis. Otolaryngol Head Neck Surg 2007;137(3 Suppl):S32–S45.

45. Ahovuo-Saloranta A, Borisenko OV, Kovanen N, et al. Antibiotics for acute maxillary sinusitis. Cochrane Database Syst Rev 2008;(2):CD000243.

46. Henry DC, Riffer E, Sokol WN, et al. Randomized double-blind study comparing 3- and 6-day regimens of azithromycin with a 10-day amoxicillin-clavulanate regimen for treatment of acute bacterial sinusitis. Antimicrob Agents Chemother 2003;47(9):2770–2774.

47. Piccirillo JF, Mager DE, Frisse ME, et al. Impact of first-line vs second-line antibiotics for the treatment of acute uncomplicated sinusitis. JAMA 2001;286(15):1849–1856.

48. Bisno AL, Gerber MA, Gwaltney JM, Jr., et al. Practice guidelines for the diagnosis and management of group A streptococcal pharyngitis: Infectious Diseases Society of America. Clin Infect Dis 2002;35(2):113–125.

49. Snow V, Mottur-Pilson C, Cooper RJ, Hoffman JR. Principles of appropriate antibiotic use for acute pharyngitis in adults. Ann Intern Med 2001;134(6):506–508.

50. Bisno AL. Acute pharyngitis. N Engl J Med 2001;344(3):205–211.

51. Hing E, Hall MJ, Xu J. National Hospital Ambulatory Medical Care Survey: 2006 outpatient department summary. Natl Health Stat Report 2008;(4):1–31.

52. Salkind AR, Wright JM. Economic burden of adult pharyngitis: The payer's perspective. Value Health 2008;11(4):621–627.

53. American Academy of Pediatrics. Group A streptococcal infections. In: Pickering LK, ed. Red Book 2003: Report of the Committee on Infectious Diseases. 26th ed. Elk Grove Village, IL: American Academy of Pediatrics, 2003:526–536.

54. Cooper RJ, Hoffman JR, Bartlett JG, et al. Principles of appropriate antibiotic use for acute pharyngitis in adults: Background. Ann Intern Med 2001;134(6):509–517.

55. Hayes CS, Williamson H, Jr. Management of group A beta-hemolytic streptococcal pharyngitis. Am Fam Physician 2001;63(8):1557–1564.

56. Vincent MT, Celestin N, Hussain AN. Pharyngitis. Am Fam Physician 2004;69(6):1465–1470.

57. Carapetis JR, Steer AC, Mulholland EK, Weber M. The global burden of group A streptococcal diseases. Lancet Infect Dis 2005;5(11):685–694.

58. Centor RM, Witherspoon JM, Dalton HP, et al. The diagnosis of strep throat in adults in the emergency room. Med Decis Making 1981;1(3):239–246.

59. McIsaac WJ, Kellner JD, Aufricht P, et al. Empirical validation of guidelines for the management of pharyngitis in children and adults. JAMA 2004;291(13):1587–1595.

60. Humair JP, Revaz SA, Bovier P, Stalder H. Management of acute pharyngitis in adults: Reliability of rapid streptococcal tests and clinical findings. Arch Intern Med 2006;166(6):640–644.

61. Gerber MA, Baltimore RS, Eaton CB, et al. Prevention of rheumatic fever and diagnosis and treatment of acute streptococcal pharyngitis: A scientific statement from the American Heart Association Rheumatic Fever, Endocarditis, and Kawasaki Disease Committee of the Council on Cardiovascular Disease in the Young, the Interdisciplinary Council on Functional Genomics and Translational Biology, and the Interdisciplinary Council on Quality of Care and Outcomes Research: endorsed by the American Academy of Pediatrics. Circulation 2009;119(11):1541–1551.

62. Catanzaro FJ, Stetson CA, Morris AJ, et al. The role of the streptococcus in the pathogenesis of rheumatic fever. Am J Med 1954;17(6):749–756.

63. Little P, Gould C, Williamson I, et al. Clinical and psychosocial predictors of illness duration from randomised controlled trial of prescribing strategies for sore throat. BMJ 1999;319(7212):736–737.

64. Dickinson JA. Acute pharyngitis. N Engl J Med 2001;344(19):1479–1480.

65. Chamovitz R, Catanzaro FJ, Stetson CA, Rammelkamp CH, Jr. Prevention of rheumatic fever by treatment of previous streptococcal infections: 1. Evaluation of benzathine penicillin G. N Engl J Med 1954;251(12):466–471.

66. Denny FW, Wannamaker LW, Brink WR, et al. Prevention of rheumatic fever; treatment of the preceding streptococcic infection. JAMA 1950;143(2):151–153.

67. Kaplan EL, Johnson DR, Del Rosario MC, Horn DL. Susceptibility of group A beta-hemolytic streptococci to thirteen antibiotics: Examination of 301 strains isolated in the United States between 1994 and 1997. Pediatr Infect Dis J 1999;18(12):1069–1072.

68. Lin K, Tierno PM, Jr., Komisar A. Increasing antibiotic resistance of streptococcus species in New York City. Laryngoscope 2004;114(7):1147–1150.

69. De Azavedo JC, Yeung RH, Bast DJ, et al. Prevalence and mechanisms of macrolide resistance in clinical isolates of group A streptococci from Ontario, Canada. Antimicrob Agents Chemother 1999;43(9):2144–2147.

70. Martin JM, Green M, Barbadora KA, Wald ER. Erythromycin-resistant group A streptococci in schoolchildren in Pittsburgh. N Engl J Med 2002;346(16):1200–1206.

71. Seppala H, Klaukka T, Vuopio-Varkila J, et al. The effect of changes in the consumption of macrolide antibiotics on erythromycin resistance in group A streptococci in Finland: Finnish Study Group for Antimicrobial Resistance. N Engl J Med 1997;337(7):441–446.

72. Littauer P, Caugant DA, Sangvik M, et al. Macrolide-resistant *Streptococcus pyogenes* in Norway: Population structure and resistance determinants. Antimicrob Agents Chemother 2006;50(5):1896–1899.

73. Grivea IN, Al-Lahham A, Katopodis GD, et al. Resistance to erythromycin and telithromycin in *Streptococcus pyogenes* isolates obtained between 1999 and 2002 from Greek children with tonsillopharyngitis: Phenotypic and genotypic analysis. Antimicrob Agents Chemother 2006;50(1):256–261.

74. Rammelkamp CH, Jr. Rheumatic heart disease: A challenge. Circulation 1958;17(5):842–851.

75. Gerber MA, Randolph MF, DeMeo KK, Kaplan EL. Lack of impact of early antibiotic therapy for streptococcal pharyngitis on recurrence rates. J Pediatr 1990;117(6):853–858.

76. Park SY, Gerber MA, Tanz RR, et al. Clinicians' management of children and adolescents with acute pharyngitis. Pediatrics 2006;117(6):1871–1878.

77. Del Mar CB, Glasziou PP, Spinks AB. Antibiotics for sore throat. Cochrane Database Syst Rev 2000(4):CD000023.

78. Linder JA, Stafford RS. Antibiotic treatment of adults with sore throat by community primary care physicians: A national survey, 1989–1999. JAMA 2001;286(10):1181–1186.

79. Linder JA, Chan JC, Bates DW. Evaluation and treatment of pharyngitis in primary care practice: The difference between guidelines is largely academic. Arch Intern Med 2006;166(13):1374–1379.

80. Burkhardt JE, Walterspiel JN, Schaad UB. Quinolone arthropathy in animals versus children. Clin Infect Dis 1997;25(5):1196–1204.

81. Noel GJ, Blumer JL, Pichichero ME, et al. A randomized comparative study of levofloxacin versus amoxicillin/clavulanate for treatment of infants and young children with recurrent or persistent acute otitis media. Pediatr Infect Dis J 2008;27(6):483–489.

82. Saez-Llorens X, Rodriguez A, Arguedas A, et al. Randomized, investigator-blinded, multicenter study of gatifloxacin versus amoxicillin/clavulanate treatment of recurrent and nonresponsive otitis media in children. Pediatr Infect Dis J 2005;24(4):293–300.

83. Sher L, Arguedas A, Husseman M, et al. Randomized, investigator-blinded, multicenter, comparative study of gatifloxacin versus amoxicillin/clavulanate in recurrent otitis media and acute otitis media treatment failure in children. Pediatr Infect Dis J 2005;24(4):301–308.

84. Feder HM, Jr., Gerber MA, Randolph MF, et al. Once-daily therapy for streptococcal pharyngitis with amoxicillin. Pediatrics 1999;103(1):47–51.

85. Guay D. Short-course antimicrobial therapy of respiratory tract infections. Drugs 2003;63(20):2169–2184.

86. Cohen R, Levy C, Doit C, et al. Six-day amoxicillin vs. ten-day penicillin V therapy for group A streptococcal tonsillopharyngitis. Pediatr Infect Dis J 1996;15(8):678–682.

87. Cohen R, Reinert P, De La Rocque F, et al. Comparison of two dosages of azithromycin for three days versus penicillin V for ten days in acute group A streptococcal tonsillopharyngitis. Pediatr Infect Dis J 2002;21(4):297–303.

88. Scholz H. Streptococcal-A tonsillopharyngitis: A 5-day course of cefuroxime axetil versus a 10-day course of penicillin V. results depending on the children's age. Chemotherapy 2004;50(1):51–54.

89. Altamimi S, Khalil A, Khalaiwi KA, et al. Short versus standard duration antibiotic therapy for acute streptococcal pharyngitis in children. Cochrane Database Syst Rev 2009(1):CD004872.

118

Influenza

JESSICA C. NJOKU AND ELIZABETH D. HERMSEN

KEY CONCEPTS

❶ Influenza is a viral illness associated with high mortality and high hospitalization rates among persons younger than age 65 years. The aging of the population is contributing to an increased disease burden in the United States.

❷ Seasonal influenza epidemics are the result of viral antigenic drift, which is why the influenza vaccine is changed on a yearly basis. Antigenic drift forms the foundation of the recommendation for annual influenza vaccination.

❸ The acquisition of a new hemagglutinin and/or neuraminidase by the influenza virus is called *antigenic shift*, which results in a novel influenza virus that has the potential to cause a pandemic.

❹ The primary route of influenza transmission is person-to-person via inhalation of respiratory droplets, and transmission can occur for as long as the infected person is shedding virus from the respiratory tract.

❺ Clinical diagnosis of influenza is difficult. Classic signs and symptoms include abrupt onset of fever, muscle pain, headache, malaise, nonproductive cough, sore throat, and rhinitis. These signs and symptoms usually resolve within 1 week of presentation.

❻ In the United States, the primary mechanism of influenza prevention is annual vaccination. Vaccination not only prevents influenza illness and influenza-related hospitalizations and deaths, but also may decrease healthcare resource use and the overall cost to society.

❼ The trivalent influenza vaccine (TIV) and the live-attenuated influenza vaccine (LAIV) are the two commercially available vaccines for prevention of seasonal influenza. Both vaccines contain influenza A subtypes H3N2 and H1N1 and influenza B virus, which are initially grown in hens' eggs. Monovalent live attenuated and inactivated vaccine formulations against novel influenza A H1N1 were distributed during the 2009–2010 season to combat the pandemic. For

the 2010–2011 influenza season, the novel H1N1 virus is incorporated within the usual seasonal influenza vaccine.

❽ Antiviral drugs for prophylaxis of influenza should be considered adjuncts to vaccine and are not replacements for annual vaccination.

❾ The sooner the antivirals are started after the onset of illness, the more effective they are.

❿ Oseltamivir and zanamivir are neuraminidase inhibitors that have activity against both influenza A and influenza B viruses, while the adamantanes have activity against only some influenza A H1N1 viruses. Anti-influenza agents are most effective if started within 48 hours of the onset of illness.

Influenza causes significant morbidity and mortality, particularly among young children and the elderly. Seasonal influenza epidemics result in 25 to 50 million influenza cases, approximately 200,000 hospitalizations, and more than 30,000 deaths each year in the United States. Globally, influenza causes nearly 500,000 deaths each year. Overall, more people die of influenza than of any other vaccine-preventable illness. Significant societal consequences associated with influenza include visits to physicians' offices and emergency departments and days lost from school and/or work. The societal costs associated with influenza are more than $37 billion in the United States alone.[1]

Vaccination is the primary mechanism of prevention of influenza in the United States. The antiviral armamentarium for treatment and prophylaxis of influenza is limited, which further emphasizes the importance of prevention with vaccination and appropriate use of infection control measures during outbreaks. Research toward the development of novel antivirals and vaccines is needed for effective control of seasonal epidemics and for pandemic preparedness.

ETIOLOGY AND EPIDEMIOLOGY

Influenza infection can occur at any time during the year with the highest rates of influenza-associated illness during the winter months. The highest rate of infection occurs in children, but the highest rates of severe illness, hospitalization, and death occur among those older than age 65 years, young children (<2 years old), and those who have underlying medical conditions, including pregnancy and cardiopulmonary disorders, that increase their risk of complications from influenza. ❶ The seasonal influenza epidemics from 1979 through 2000 resulted in an average of 226,000 hospitalizations per year with more than 63% of the hospitalizations occurring in those older than age 65 years.[2] More than 90% of seasonal influenza-related deaths occur in those older than age 65 years.[3] Thus the aging of the population is contributing to an

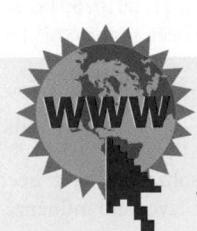

The complete chapter, learning objectives, and other resources can be found at **www.pharmacotherapyonline.com**.

increased disease burden. Deaths associated with influenza often result from secondary bacterial pneumonia, primary viral pneumonia, and/or exacerbation of underlying comorbidities.

INFLUENZA VIRUSES A, B, AND C

Influenza virus types A, B, and C are members of the Orthomyxoviridae family and affect many species, including humans, pigs, horses, and birds. Influenza A and B viruses are the two types that cause disease in humans. Influenza A viruses are responsible for the regular, seasonal epidemics of the flu, whereas influenza B viruses are typically associated with sporadic outbreaks, particularly among residents of long-term care facilities. Influenza A viruses are further categorized into different subtypes based on changes in two surface antigens—hemagglutinin and neuraminidase. Influenza B viruses are not categorized into subtypes.

Hemagglutinin allows the influenza virus to enter host cells by attaching to sialic acid receptors and is the major antigen to which antibodies are directed upon exposure.[5] Neuraminidase allows the release of new viral particles from host cells by catalyzing the cleavage of linkages to sialic acid.[4]

Sixteen hemagglutinin subtypes (H1–H16) and nine neuraminidase subtypes (N1–N9) of influenza A have been isolated from birds. However, the only influenza A subtypes that have circulated among humans since the 1918 pandemic (see Pandemics and Antigenic Shift below) are H1 to H3 and N1 and N2.[4] The primary subtypes of influenza A that have been circulating among humans for the last three decades are H3N2 and H1N1.

ANTIGENIC DRIFT AND ANTIGENIC SHIFT

❷ Immunity to influenza virus occurs as a result of the development of antibody directed at the surface antigens, particularly hemagglutinin. However, immunity to one influenza subtype does not offer protection against other subtypes or types of influenza. Moreover, immunity to one antigenic variant of a subtype of influenza may not confer protection against other antigenic variants. Antigenic variants are created by point mutations in the surface antigens of a particular subtype, resulting in small changes in the hemagglutinin and/or neuraminidase molecules, which is called *antigenic drift*. Antigenic drift is the basis for seasonal epidemics of influenza, the reason for changes in the annual influenza vaccine, and the rationale behind the recommendation for annual vaccination.

Immunity to one subtype of influenza does not confer protection against other subtypes or types. **❸** Antigenic shift occurs when the influenza virus acquires a new hemagglutinin and/or neuraminidase via genetic reassortment rather than point mutations.[4] Most likely, the genetic reassortment occurs when an animal that supports the growth of multiple subtypes of influenza, such as a pig, is concurrently infected with two subtypes of the influenza virus. Conversely, antigenic shift may occur directly from avian strains that have gained competency in the human host. Antigenic shift results in the emergence of a novel influenza virus and carries the potential of causing a pandemic. However, novelty alone is insufficient to cause an influenza pandemic; the virus must be able to replicate in humans, spread person-to-person, and affect a susceptible population.[4]

Spanish Influenza of 1918

The influenza pandemic of 1918 was the most significant infectious disease outbreak known to man, causing approximately 40 to 50 million deaths in a year, with more than 500,000 deaths occurring in the United States.[4–6] Although the reports of the first illnesses associated with this pandemic occurred in Spain, there is no evidence that the virus associated with this pandemic actually originated

there, indicating a misnomer. The pandemic occurred almost concurrently in Europe, Asia, and North America.[5]

The 1918 pandemic was caused by a particularly virulent influenza A H1N1 virus, which was entirely of avian origin.[7] In contrast to the other pandemics of the 20th century, the 1918 pandemic resulted in an unusual mortality pattern. The mortality peaked for those younger than age 4 years, those between the ages of 25 and 35 years, and those older than 65 years of age, which resulted in a W-shaped mortality curve, as opposed to the U- or J-shaped curve typically associated with influenza.[6] Over half of the deaths occurred in persons ages 20 to 40 years. The death toll associated with this pandemic culminated in an almost 10-year drop in the life expectancy of the population at the time.[6]

Asian Influenza of 1957

The Asian flu pandemic began when a new H2 subtype of influenza A surfaced in Hunan province in China in 1957.[8] The virus appears to have formed from coinfection with an avian H2N2 virus and a human H1N1 virus in a common host, possibly a pig or a human.[9] The H2N2 virus quickly spread to Japan, South America, the United States, New Zealand, and Europe, resulting in approximately 4 million deaths worldwide, with 70,000 deaths occurring in the United States.[5,6,8] Unlike the Spanish flu of 1918, the mortality curve for the Asian flu pandemic was U- or J-shaped, with infants and elderly being most affected.[5]

Hong Kong Influenza of 1968

The H2N2 virus of the Asian flu circulated in the human population until 1968, when a new H3 subtype emerged in China and Hong Kong[8] following genetic reassortment with the H2N2 virus.[5,8] The H3N2 virus quickly spread to the United States and later to Europe. This pandemic caused more than 30,000 deaths in the United States and approximately 2 million deaths worldwide.[5,6,8] The lower morbidity and mortality associated with the Hong Kong flu may be explained by previous exposure of the population to the N2 subtype.[10] Similar to the Asian flu of 1957, the mortality curve for the Hong Kong flu pandemic was U- or J-shaped, primarily affecting infants and elderly.

Avian Influenza

Influenza viruses are in circulation in southern China during all months of the year.[4] Given this fact and the close proximity of dense populations of people, pigs, and wild and domestic birds, this area proves ideal for the development of new influenza viruses via genetic reassortment (antigenic shift), as demonstrated by the pandemics of 1957 and 1968 and, most recently, the emergence of what is known as avian influenza.[4]

The first report of human infection with the avian H5N1 virus occurred in 1997 in Hong Kong in a 3-year-old who had a direct link with chickens and later died.[11] This was followed by 18 confirmed cases and 6 deaths.[12] The virus reemerged in 2003 as an antigenically and genetically different virus that has spread widely through wild and domestic bird populations in Asia, Africa, and Europe as well as infecting humans in 15 countries: Azerbaijan, Bangladesh, Cambodia, China, Djibouti, Egypt, Indonesia, Iraq, Lao People's Democratic Republic, Myanmar, Nigeria, Pakistan, Thailand, Turkey, and Vietnam.[5,13] As of August 21, 2010, 504 cases and 229 deaths caused by H5N1 infection have been reported.[13] The current overall case fatality is 45.4%.

In contrast to the animal-to-human transmission of the 1997 epidemic, occasional human-to-human transmission has been suggested during the outbreaks associated with the H5N1 virus,[14,15] although no cases of transmission via aerosolization have been identified.[16] Clinical presentation includes high fever and influenza-like illness, and watery diarrhea without blood may occur up to

1 week prior to respiratory symptoms.[16] Almost all patients have clinically apparent pneumonia. Progression to death, most commonly as a consequence of respiratory failure, occurs a mean of 9 to 10 days after the onset of illness.[16] The neuraminidase inhibitors, oseltamivir and zanamivir, have activity against the H5N1 virus, although higher doses may be needed. Oseltamivir resistance has been detected in several patients infected with the H5N1 virus who were treated with oseltamivir.[16] Amantadine and rimantadine are ineffective against H5N1. An inactivated monovalent influenza virus vaccine against H5N1 is currently available for vaccination of persons 18 through 64 years of age at increased risk of exposure to the H5N1 influenza virus. Two 1-mL doses given intramuscularly at least 28 days apart (range, 21–35 days) are recommended. The vaccine is supplied in a 5-mL multidose vial, with ~50 mcg thimerosal per dose added as a preservative.[17]

The potential for H5N1 to cause a pandemic is of concern as it could spread more quickly than pandemics of the past because of the mobility of people in today's world. International travel has increased 73% since 1990, with 763 million people crossing international borders in 2004.[18] A severe pandemic, like that of 1918, could cause more than 9 million hospitalizations and more than 1.9 million deaths, whereas a moderate pandemic, like those of 1957 and 1968, could result in more than 800,000 hospitalizations and more than 200,000 deaths in the United States alone.[5]

Swine Influenza of 2009

An outbreak of a novel influenza A H1N1 (formerly swine origin influenza virus [SOIV]) was initially detected in Mexico in March 2009 and subsequently in the United States in April 2009 in California and Texas.[19-21] Since that time, the virus has extended throughout North America, Europe, Asia and subsequently worldwide, prompting the World Health Organization (WHO) on June 11, 2009 to declare phase 6, indicating widespread human infection, for the influenza pandemic.[20] Since 1998, triple reassortant swine influenza A (H1) viruses, containing genes from swine, avian, and human lineages, have circulated among swine in the United States.[21] However, the novel influenza A H1N1 virus is unique in that although much of the genome is similar to the triple reassortant swine viruses previously seen in the United States, the genes encoding for neuraminidase (NA) and matrix proteins (M) are most similar to those circulating in the Eurasian swine population. This particular genetic combination has not been seen before.[21]

Several characteristics of the novel influenza A H1N1 outbreak differs compared with a typical seasonal influenza outbreak. Symptomatology associated with the novel influenza include fever (94%), cough (92%), sore throat (66%), diarrhea (25%), and vomiting (25%).[21,22] The majority of novel influenza A H1N1 cases have occurred in otherwise healthy children and young adults including pregnant women, with the highest incidence reported among those aged 5 to 24 years. Among those who were deceased due to novel H1N1 infection, the median age was 37 years and only ~8% of these were among patients aged ≥65 years.[23] As of August 28, 2009, there were 43,771 confirmed cases, 8,843 hospitalizations, and 556 deaths (15 deaths in individuals 0–4 years, 86 deaths in individuals 5–24 years, 235 deaths in adults 25–49 years, 158 deaths in adults 50–64 years, 50 deaths in adults age ≥65, and 12 deaths for which age was not reported).[24]

Pandemic Preparedness

This chapter is not meant to provide an exhaustive review of the biology of influenza or pandemic preparedness. This topic is rapidly changing and interested readers are referred to the following Websites: www.pandemicflu.gov, www.who.int/csr/disease/avian_influenza/en/, and www.cdc.gov/h1n1flu.

A vital component of pandemic preparedness is forethought—plans must be established for how to effectively triage large numbers of ill patients, prioritize and/or ration vaccine and antivirals, and communicate with the public through mass media during a period of severe labor shortage (a result of stress and illness amongst healthcare workers) and supply shortfall (a result of societal and economic disruption).

PATHOGENESIS

4 The route of influenza transmission is person-to-person via inhalation of respiratory droplets, which can occur when an infected person coughs or sneezes.[25] Transmission may also occur if a person touches an object contaminated with respiratory secretions and then touches their mucus membranes. The incubation period for influenza ranges between 1 and 7 days, with an average incubation of 2 days.[22] Transmission can occur for as long as the infected person is shedding virus from the respiratory tract. Adults are considered infectious within one day before until 7 days after onset of illness. Children, especially younger children, might potentially be infectious for longer periods (>10 days).[22,26,27] Viral shedding can persist for weeks to months in severely immunocompromised people.[27]

The pathogenesis of influenza in humans is not well understood. The severity of the infection is determined by the balance between viral replication and the host immune response.[4] Severe illness is likely a result of both a lack of ability of host defense mechanisms to inhibit viral replication and an overproduction of cytokines leading to tissue damage in the host.[28]

CLINICAL PRESENTATION AND DIAGNOSIS OF INFLUENZA

General

☐ The clinical diagnosis of influenza can be difficult because the presentation is similar to a number of other respiratory illnesses. The sensitivity of clinical diagnosis ranges from 38% for children to 77% for adults and largely depends on the relative prevalence of influenza and other respiratory viruses circulating in a community.[30]

☐ The clinical course and outcome are affected by age, immunocompetence, viral characteristics, smoking, comorbidities, pregnancy, and the degree of preexisting immunity.

☐ Complications of influenza may include exacerbation of underlying comorbidities, primary viral pneumonia, secondary bacterial pneumonia or other respiratory illnesses (e.g., sinusitis, bronchitis, otitis), encephalopathy, transverse myelitis, myositis, myocarditis, pericarditis, and Reye syndrome.

Signs and Symptoms

5 Classic signs and symptoms of influenza include rapid onset of fever, myalgia, headache, malaise, nonproductive cough, sore throat, and rhinitis.

☐ Nausea, vomiting, and otitis media are also commonly reported in children.[31]

☐ Signs and symptoms typically resolve in approximately 3 to 7 days, although cough and malaise may persist for more than 2 weeks.

☐ Primary viral pneumonia, occurring predominantly in pregnant women and in those with underlying cardiovascular disease, usually begins with fever and dry cough, which changes to a productive cough of bloody sputum. This rapidly progresses to dyspnea, hypoxemia, and cyanosis with radiologic evidence of bilateral interstitial infiltrates.[32]

Secondary bacterial pneumonia is usually seen in individuals with underlying pulmonary disorders and presents during the early stages of defervescence from the influenza infection. These patients usually present with fever, productive cough, and radiologic evidence of consolidation.[32]

Laboratory Tests

Complete blood count and chemistry panels should be obtained to assess the overall status of the patient.

The gold standard for diagnosis of influenza is viral culture, which can provide information on the specific strain and subtype. Viral culture has a high sensitivity but can take as long as a week to develop, limiting the clinical relevance of the results.

Tests such as the rapid antigen and point-of-care (POC) tests, direct fluorescence antibody (DFA) test, and the reverse-transcription polymerase chain reaction (RT-PCR) assay may be used for rapid detection of virus.

Other Diagnostic Tests

Cultures of potential sites of infection should be obtained if co-infection, superinfection, or secondary infection is suspected.

Chest radiograph should be obtained if pneumonia is suspected.

Rapid Tests

Rapid tests have allowed for prompt diagnosis and initiation of antiviral therapy and decreased inappropriate use of antibiotics. Rapid antigen or POC tests use enzyme immunoassay (EIA) technology to provide results within 1 hour of specimen collection. Appropriate specimens for collection, in decreasing order of sensitivity, are nasopharyngeal aspirates, nasopharyngeal swabs/washes, and oropharyngeal swabs.[30] POC tests allow for differentiation of influenza viruses A and B, with sensitivity and specificity ranging from 57% to 90% and 65% to 99%, respectively.[30] In general, use of POC tests is contraindicated in those who have had symptoms for longer than 3 days, and results may be confounded following recent immunization with live-attenuated influenza vaccine.[30]

DFA testing requires more technical expertise and infrastructure than POC tests. The advantages of DFA are increased sensitivity over POC tests and simultaneous detection of other respiratory viruses, such as respiratory syncytial virus and adenovirus.[30] DFA provides results between 1 and 4 hours after specimen collection and may serve as a confirmatory assay for a POC test.

RT-PCR assay is a nucleic acid amplification test and is the most sensitive, specific, and versatile diagnostic test for influenza.[30] RT-PCR is replacing viral isolation as the reference standard and can determine the type, subtype, and strain of influenza. Results are provided within 4 to 6 hours of specimen collection. A new RT-PCR for detection of novel influenza A H1N1 is available through the CDC.[22]

PREVENTION

The best means to decrease the morbidity and mortality associated with influenza is to prevent infection through vaccination.[23,26] Appropriate infection control measures, such as hand hygiene, basic respiratory etiquette (e.g., cover your cough, throw tissues

away), and contact avoidance, are also important in preventing the spread of influenza. Additionally, chemoprophylaxis is useful in certain situations.

VACCINATION

6 The primary means of influenza prevention employed in the United States is annual vaccination. Vaccination can help prevent hospitalization and death among those at high risk, decrease influenza-like illness, decrease visits to physicians' offices and emergency rooms, decrease otitis media in children, and prevent school and/or work absenteeism. Annual vaccination is now recommended for all peasons aged 6 months or older.

Vaccination is also recommended for those who live with and/or care for people who are at high risk, including household contacts and healthcare workers.

The ideal time for all influenza vaccination is during October or November to allow for the development and maintenance of immunity during the peak of the influenza season.[23,26] Table 118–1 lists the vaccination coverage rates and goals for various patient populations.

Seasonal influenza vaccine will not likely provide protection against the novel influenza A (H1N1) due to absence of or low levels of cross reacting antibodies.[23,26] As a result, new monovalent live-attenuated (mLAIV) and inactivated monovalent influenza vaccine (MIV) formulations against the novel H1N1 virus are available (Table 118–2).[29] Simultaneous administration of inactivated vaccines against seasonal and novel influenza A H1N1 is permissible if given at different sites. However, administration of live attenuated vaccine formulations against seasonal and novel H1N1 simultaneously is not recommended.[23] Based on evolving burden of illness, the age distribution and risk groups most affected, and anticipated vaccine supply, novel H1N1 vaccination efforts were targeted toward certain patient groups[23] with more widespread vaccination possible only after vaccine supply was adequate for demand.[22,23]

7 The two vaccines currently available for prevention of seasonal influenza are the trivalent influenza vaccine (TIV) and the live-attenuated influenza vaccine (LAIV). Both vaccines contain two influenza A subtypes (H3N2 and H1N1) and influenza B virus; the specific strains included in the vaccine each year change based on antigenic drift. The viruses used for both vaccines are initially grown in embryonated hens' eggs, which explains the contraindication for vaccination of persons with a severe allergic reaction to eggs.[26] Afluria is contraindicated in patients with hypersensitivity to

TABLE 118-1	Influenza Vaccination Rates and Goals by Patient Population	
Patient Population	**Vaccination Coverage**	**Vaccination Coverage National Goal (2000/2010)**
Children age 6–23 mo	18%[a]	N/A
Persons age 18–49 y with high-risk conditions	26%[b]	60%/60%
Persons age 50–64 y	36%[b]	60%/60%
Persons age 50–64 y with high-risk conditions	46%[b]	60%/60%
Persons age >65 y	66%[a]	60%/90%
Nursing home residents	83%[c]	80%/90%
Pregnant women without other high-risk conditions	13%[b]	N/A
Healthcare workers	42%[a]	N/A

N/A, not applicable; no goals established.
[a]2004 data.
[b]2006–2007 data.
[c]1998 data.
From Fiore et al.[26]

TABLE 118-2 Approved Monovalent Novel Influenza H1N1 Vaccines for Different Age Groups—United States, 2009–2010

Vaccine	Trade Name	Manufacturer	How Supplied	Thimerosal Mercury Content (mcg/0.5 mL)	Age Group	Number of Doses
MIV	No trade name	Sanofi Pasteur	0.25-mL prefilled syringe	0	6–35 mo	2[a]
			0.5-mL prefilled syringe	0	36 mo–9 y	2[a]
			0.5-mL prefilled syringe	0	≥10 y	1
			5-mL multidose vial	25	≥6 mo	1 or 2[a]
MIV	No trade name	Novartis Vaccines	0.5-mL prefilled syringe	≤1	4–9 y	2[a]
			5-mL multidose vial	25	≥10 y	1
mLAIV	No trade name	MedImmune LLC	0.2-mL sprayer	0	2–49 y	1 or 2[b]
MIV	No trade name	CSL Limited	0.5-mL prefilled syringe	0	≥18 y	1
			5-mL multidose vial	24.5		

[a]Two doses administered at least 1 month apart are recommended for children age 6 months to less than 9 years who are receiving vaccine for the first time.
[b]Two doses administered 4 weeks apart are recommended for children age 2 to 9 years who are receiving influenza vaccine for the first time.
MIV, monovalent influenza vaccine; mLAIV, monovalent live-attenuated influenza vaccine.
From FDA Approved Vaccines.[29]

neomycin or polymyxin.[29] Novel influenza A H1N1vaccines from 2009 were manufactured via a similar process as the seasonal influenza vaccines but are monovalent. Likewise, novel influenza vaccine is contraindicated if known hypersensitivity to eggs or chicken protein exists.[29] As with every new vaccine, the CDC encourages individuals to use the Vaccine Adverse Event Reporting System to aide in collecting and analyzing adverse events following vaccination with the novel influenza H1N1 monovalent vaccine.[23]

Trivalent Influenza Vaccine

❼ TIV is FDA approved for use in people older than 6 months of age, regardless of their immune status. Of note, several commercial products are available and are approved for different age groups (Table 118–3). TIV is administered intramuscularly and is made with killed viruses, meaning it cannot cause signs and symptoms of influenza-like illness (Table 118–4). Age and immune status can affect the efficacy of TIV as can the similarity of the vaccine to the viruses in circulation.

In children between 6 and 24 months of age, a 2-year randomized study of TIV exhibited 89% seroconversion and efficacy of 66% in year 1 and 7% in year 2 versus culture-confirmed influenza.[33] In children between 1 and 15 years of age, the efficacy of TIV was

91.4% and 77.3% against culture-confirmed influenza A H1N1 and H3N2, respectively. Two doses of TIV are important for children under the age of 9 years, supporting the rationale for the recommendation of a booster dose of TIV at least 1 month after the initial dose in children between 6 months and less than 9 years of age (see Table 118–3).[26]

TIV is also effective in adult populations under and older than the age of 65 years. A double-blind, randomized, controlled trial evaluating TIV in healthy adults younger than the age of 65 years demonstrated an efficacy of 50% against serologically confirmed influenza during a season in which the vaccine and the circulating viruses were not well matched and an efficacy of 86% during a season in which the vaccine and the circulating viruses were well matched.[34] These findings were corroborated by a large Cochrane Database System review, which found that TIV had an efficacy of 70% in healthy adults younger than 65 years of age, regardless of virus and vaccine concordance.[35] Vaccination of those younger than 65 years old during seasons when the virus and vaccine are well-matched results in decreased work absenteeism and healthcare resource use.[34,35]

Adults older than the age of 65 years benefit from influenza vaccination, including prevention of complications and decreased risk of influenza-related hospitalization and death. However, people in

TABLE 118-3 Approved Influenza Vaccines for Different Age Groups—United States, 2010–2011 Season

Vaccine	Trade Name	Manufacturer	Dose/Presentation	Thimerosal Mercury Content (mcg Hg/0.5 mL dose)	Age Group	Number of Doses
TIV	Fluzone	Sanofi Pasteur	0.25-mL prefilled syringe	0	6–35 mo	1 or 2[a]
			0.5-mL prefilled syringe	0	≥36 mo	1 or 2[a]
			0.5-mL vial	0	≥36 mo	1 or 2[a]
			5-mL multidose vial	25	≥6 mo	1 or 2[a]
TIV	Fluvirin	Novartis Vaccine	0.5-mL prefilled syringe	<1	≥4 y	1 or 2[a]
			5-mL multidose vial	25	≥4 y	1 or 2[a]
TIV	Fluarix	GlaxoSmithKline ID Biomedical	0.5-mL prefilled syringe 5-mL mutlidose vial	0	≥3 y	1
TIV	FluLaval	Corp of Quebec	0.5-mL prefilled syringe	25	≥18 y	1
TIV	Afluria	CSL limited	5-mL multidose vial	0 24.5	≥6 mo	1
TIV High Dose	Fluzone HD	Sanofi Pasteur	0.5 mL prefilled syringe	0.0	≥65	1
LAIV	FluMist	MedImmune	0.2-mL sprayer	0	2–49 y	1 or 2[b]

[a]Two doses administered at least 1 month apart are recommended for children age 6 months to less than 9 years who are receiving influenza vaccine for the first time or received 1 dose in first year of vaccination during the previous influenza season.
[b]Two doses administered 4 weeks apart are recommended for children age 2 to less than 9 years who are receiving influenza vaccine for the first time.
LAIV, live-attenuated influenza vaccine; TIV, trivalent influenza vaccine.
From Fiore et al.[26]

TABLE 118-4 Comparison of Trivalent (TIV) and Live-Attenuated Influenza Vaccine (LAIV)

Characteristic	TIV	LAIV
Age groups approved for use	>6 mo	2–49 y
Immune status requirements	Immunocompetent or immunocompromised	Immunocompetent
Viral properties	Inactivated (killed) influenza A (H3N2), A (H1N1), and B viruses	Live-attenuated influenza A (H3N2), A (H1N1), and B viruses
Route of administration	Intramuscular	Intranasal
Immune system response	High serum IgG antibody response	Lower IgG response and high serum IgA mucosal response

this population may not generate a strong antibody response to the vaccine and may remain susceptible to infection. In patients older than the age of 60 years who do not reside in a long-term care facility, TIV efficacy was 58% against influenza illness.[26] Although the efficacy against influenza illness for those living in long-term care facilities is between 30% and 40%, the vaccine is 50% to 60% effective in preventing influenza-related hospitalization or pneumonia and 80% effective in preventing influenza-related death.[26]

The most frequent adverse effect associated with TIV is soreness at the injection site that lasts for less than 48 hours. TIV may cause fever and malaise in those who have not previously been exposed to the viral antigens in the vaccine.[26] Allergic-type reactions (hives, systemic anaphylaxis) rarely occur after influenza vaccination and are likely a result of a reaction to residual egg protein in the vaccine.

The 1976 swine influenza vaccine was linked to a rise in the incidence of Guillain-Barré syndrome (GBS), and this has propagated the belief that TIV may cause GBS.[26] However, there is insufficient evidence to establish causality. Although several studies have failed to establish a relationship between influenza vaccination and increased frequency of GBS, two studies have demonstrated a small but significant increase in GBS following influenza vaccination.[36,37] Therefore, vaccination should be avoided in persons who are not at high risk for influenza complications and who have experienced GBS within 6 weeks of receiving a previous influenza vaccine.[26] The potential benefits of influenza vaccination in terms of prevention of severe illness, hospitalization, and mortality significantly outweigh the risks of GBS, and vaccination is recommended for all groups previously discussed.

The multidose vials and a few of the single-dose preparations of TIV contain trace to small amounts of a preservative, thimerosal, which is a mercury-containing compound (see Table 118-3). Some individuals are concerned about thimerosal exposure, particularly among children, because of the unfounded belief that thimerosal exposure is linked to the development of autism. No scientifically persuasive evidence exists to suggest harm from thimerosal exposure from a vaccine. Conversely, accumulating evidence reports the lack of harm from such exposure.[38-40] Thus, similar to GBS, the potential benefits of influenza vaccination in terms of prevention of severe illness, hospitalization, and mortality significantly outweigh the theoretical risk associated with thimerosal exposure, and vaccination is recommended for all groups previously discussed. However, to maximize the public health benefit and placate concerned individuals, thimerosal-free vaccine is available (see Table 118-3).

Live-Attenuated Influenza Vaccine

❼ LAIV is made with live, attenuated viruses and is approved for intranasal administration in healthy people between 2 and 49 years

of age (see Table 118-4). Advantages of LAIV include its ease of administration, intranasal rather than intramuscular administration, and the potential induction of broad mucosal and systemic immune response.[26] The mucosal response occurs at the site of viral entry and may prevent infection before viral replication occurs.[41] LAIV is more expensive than TIV and is approved for use in a more limited population.

Controlled studies support the use of LAIV in healthy people between the ages of 2 and 49 years. Although LAIV was previously FDA approved for children who were at least 5 years old, three pivotal trials led the FDA to approve LAIV for children who were at least 2 years old.[42] LAIV recipients aged 2 to 5 years had 52.5% and 54.4% fewer cases of influenza illness against matched and mismatched strains, respectively, as compared with TIV recipients.

Although LAIV is FDA approved for adults younger than the age of 49 years, LAIV is effective in healthy adults between 18 and 64 years old.[43] Vaccination reduced the number of severe febrile illnesses by 18.8% and febrile upper respiratory tract illnesses by 23.6%.[43] Additionally, vaccination led to fewer days of illness, fewer days lost from work, fewer visits to healthcare providers, and decreased use of prescription antibiotics and nonprescription medications.[43]

The adverse effects typically associated with LAIV administration include runny nose, congestion, sore throat, and headache. Because LAIV contains live, attenuated viruses, viral shedding may occur for several days following vaccination with LAIV, although this should not be equated with person-to-person transmission.[26] Additionally, because LAIV contains live-attenuated viruses, which carry a theoretical infection risk, LAIV should not be given to immunosuppressed patients or given by healthcare workers who are severely immunocompromised. Moreover, for the reasons discussed in the TIV section, LAIV should not be administered to persons with a history of GBS or hypersensitivity to eggs.

CLINICAL CONTROVERSY

LAIV is not recommended in several populations, including people older than 50 years and pregnant women, largely because the vaccine has not been studied extensively in these populations. However, many clinicians believe the use of LAIV in these populations is acceptable.

POSTEXPOSURE PROPHYLAXIS

❽ Antiviral drugs available for prophylaxis of influenza should be considered adjuncts but are not replacements for annual vaccination. The two classes of antiviral drugs available for influenza prophylaxis are the adamantanes and the neuraminidase inhibitors. Adamantane monotherapy is currently not recommended for prophylaxis or treatment in the United States because of the rapid emergence of resistance.[26,27,49] Both of the neuraminidase inhibitors, oseltamivir and zanamivir, are effective prophylactic agents against influenza in terms of preventing laboratory-confirmed influenza when used for seasonal prophylaxis (67% and 85% effective for zanamivir and oseltamivir, respectively) and preventing influenza illness among persons exposed to a household contact who was diagnosed with influenza (79%–81% and 68%–89% effective for zanamivir and oseltamivir, respectively).[37,44-46] Additionally, oseltamivir was 92% effective against influenza and also reduced associated complications when used as seasonal prophylaxis among immunized, institutionalized, elderly patients.[47] However, recent surveillance data and susceptibility testing have identified strains of influenza A, mainly H1N1, with reduced susceptibility to oseltamivir, resulting in alterations to the recommendations for oseltamivir

TABLE 118-5 Antiviral Susceptibilities of Circulating Viruses

	Oseltamivir	Zanamivir	Adamantanes
Novel influenza A (H1N1) 2009	Susceptible[a]	Susceptible	Resistant
Seasonal A (H1N1)	Mostly resistant	Susceptible	Mostly susceptible
Seasonal A (H3N2)	Susceptible	Susceptible	Resistant
Influenza B	Susceptible	Susceptible	Resistant
Avian influenza (H5N1)	Susceptible	Susceptible	Variable

[a]Small number of isolates shown to be resistant to oseltamivir.
From WHO.[49]

use for influenza treatment and chemoprophylaxis (Tables 118–5 and 118–6).[48,49] Due to the emergence of novel H1N1 influenza, in 2009 dosing recommendations for oseltamivir were expanded by the FDA to include children older than 3 months of age, and zanamivir is approved for prophylaxis in those older than the age of 5 years.[50] Table 118–7 gives dosing recommendations.

In those patients who did not receive the influenza vaccination and are receiving an antiviral drug for prevention of disease during the influenza season, the medication should optimally be taken for the entire duration of influenza activity in the community. The use of prophylaxis requires clinical judgment and depends on a variety of factors, but prophylaxis for seasonal influenza should be considered during influenza season for the following groups of patients:

- Persons at high risk of serious illness and/or complications who cannot be vaccinated
- Persons at high risk of serious illness and/or complications who are vaccinated after influenza activity has begun in their community since the development of sufficient antibody titers after vaccination takes approximately 2 weeks

TABLE 118-6 Interim Recommendations for the Selection of Antiviral Treatment Based on Confirmed Influenza Subtypes

Laboratory Test	Predominant Circulating Virus	Preferred	Alternative
Not performed or negative, but influenza suspected clinically	H1N1 (seasonal or novel) or unknown	Zanamivir	Oseltamivir + rimantadine[a,b]
Not performed or negative, but influenza suspected clinically	H3N2 or B	Oseltamivir or zanamivir	None
Positive novel H1N1	NA	Oseltamivir	Zanamivir
Positive A	H1N1 (seasonal or novel) or unknown	Zanamivir	Oseltamivir + rimantadine[a,b]
Positive A	H3N2 or B	Oseltamivir or Zanamivir	None
Positive B	Any	Oseltamivir or Zanamivir	None
Positive A + B	H1N1 (seasonal or novel) or unknown	Zanamivir	Oseltamivir + rimantadine[a,b]
Positive A + B	H3N2 or B	Oseltamivir or zanamivir	None

[a]Preferred if severely ill.
[b]Amantadine can be substituted for rimantadine but has increased risk of adverse events.
Modified from CDC on olsetamivir resistance[48] and Harper et al.[27]

- Unvaccinated persons who have frequent contact with those at high risk
- Persons who may have an inadequate response to vaccination (e.g., advanced HIV disease)
- Long-term care facility residents, regardless of vaccination status, when an outbreak has occurred in the institution
- Unvaccinated household contacts of someone who was diagnosed with influenza

Prophylaxis for novel H1N1 influenza should be considered in the following groups:

- Persons at high risk of serious illness and/or complications who have had close contact with persons with laboratory- or clinically confirmed novel H1N1 infection during that person's infectious period
- Healthcare/public health personnel who have had recognized, unprotected close contact with persons with laboratory- or clinically confirmed novel H1N1 infection during that person's infectious period

LAIV should not be administered until 48 hours after influenza antiviral therapy has stopped, and influenza antiviral drugs should not be administered for 2 weeks after the administration of LAIV because the antiviral drugs inhibit influenza virus replication.[38] No contraindication exists for concomitant use of TIV and influenza antiviral drugs.

SPECIAL POPULATIONS

Pregnant women and immunocompromised hosts are special populations at increased risk of influenza complications and are also populations in whom careful consideration must be given in regard to prevention strategies.

Pregnant Women

Pregnant women, regardless of trimester, should receive annual influenza vaccination with TIV but not with LAIV.[23,26] No studies have demonstrated an increased incidence of adverse effects in mothers or their infants related or potentially related to TIV, but no such data exist for LAIV.[51] TIV is also safe for breastfeeding mothers. No data exist for LAIV and breast-feeding, but caution is warranted because of the potential for viral shedding.[26] The effects of the monovalent vaccines against the novel H1N1 virus on fetal development or reproductive capacity is unknown due to lack of data (pregnancy category C).[23]

Immunocompromised Hosts

Immunocompromised hosts should receive annual influenza vaccination with TIV but not LAIV. TIV was 100% effective against laboratory-confirmed influenza in HIV-positive patients with no significant effect on viral load or CD4 cell count.[52] However, antibody titers may not be as high as in immunocompetent individuals and are not improved with a second dose of vaccine.[53] Similarly, antibody titers may not be as high in solid-organ transplant patients as in immunocompetent persons, but conversely, antibody titers were increased significantly after a second dose of TIV in adult liver transplant patients.[54] Although this suggests a potential benefit from a two-dose regimen, such a regimen is not currently recommended for solid-organ transplant recipients. Data is currently limited in this arena for the novel H1N1 vaccines. However, no contraindication has been noted to date based on preliminary data from clinical trials. Additionally, immune response to vaccine may be less than desired in immunocompromised patients.[23,29]

Large clinical trials evaluating the use of influenza antivirals for prophylaxis are lacking in immunocompromised hosts. Viral

TABLE 118-7 Recommended Daily Dosage of Influenza Antiviral Medications for Treatment and Prophylaxis—United States

Drug	Adult Treatment	Adult Prophylaxis[a]	Pediatric Treatment	Pediatric Prophylaxis

Oseltamivir	75-mg capsule twice daily for 5 days	75-mg capsule daily	≤3 mo[b]: 12 mg twice daily
			3–5 mo[b]: 20 mg twice daily
			6–11 mo[b]: 25 mg twice daily
			≥1 year
			  <15 kg: 30 mg twice daily
			  16–23 kg: 45 mg twice daily
			  23–40 kg: 60 mg twice daily
			  >40 kg: 75 mg twice daily
			All for 5 days
				≤3 mo. Not recommended situation judged critical due to limited data in this group
				3–5 mo[b]: 20 mg daily
				6–11 mo[b]: 25 mg daily
				≥1 year
				  ≤15 kg: 30 mg daily
				  16–23 kg: 45 mg daily
				  23–40 kg: 60 mg daily
				  >40 kg: 75 mg daily

Zanamivir	2 inhalations twice daily × 5 days	2 inhalations daily	2 inhalations twice daily × 5 days for ≥7 years old	2 inhalations daily for ≥5 years old
Rimantadine[c]	200 mg/day in 1–2 doses × 7 days	200 mg/day in 1–2 doses	1–9 years old or <40 kg: 6.6 mg/kg/day divided twice daily (max 150 mg/day) ≥10 years old: 200 mg/day in 1–2 doses Treat 5–7 days	1–9 years old: 5 mg/kg daily (max 150 mg/day) ≥10 years old: 200 mg/day in 1–2 doses
Amantadine[c]	200 mg/day in 1–2 doses until 24–48 h after symptom resolution	Same as treatment doses	>12 years old: same as adult 1–9 years old: 5 mg/kg/day in 1–2 doses; max 150 mg/day ≥10–12 years old: 100 mg orally twice daily	Same as treatment doses

[a]If influenza vaccine is administered, prophylaxis can generally be stopped 14 days after vaccination for non-institutionalized persons. When prophylaxis is being administered following an exposure, prophylaxis should be continued for 10 days after the last exposure. In persons at high risk for complications from influenza for whom vaccination is contraindicated or expected to be ineffective, chemoprophylaxis should be continued for the duration that influenza viruses are circulating in the community during influenza season.
[b]Emergency use authorization for pandemic H1N1 virus from the CDC.
[c]Monotherapy not recommended due to rapid emergence of resistance when used alone.
Modified from Fiore et al.[26]

shedding occurs for prolonged periods in this population and may promote the development of antiviral resistance, which has already been documented with oseltamivir in HIV-positive patients.[55,56]

TREATMENT

Influenza

When prevention efforts fail or are not used, clinicians must turn to the agents available for treatment of influenza. Currently, the antiviral treatment options are limited, particularly in the face of resistance to the adamantanes and oseltamivir.

CLINICAL CONTROVERSY

Some clinicians debate the cost-benefit of the use of diagnostic tests for influenza as well as treatment of influenza in otherwise healthy individuals who are likely to experience resolution without treatment. This controversy is compounded by the fact that the diagnostic tests and the benefits associated with treatment of influenza are highest early in the disease process, and many patients present after this time period.

■ GOALS OF THERAPY

The four primary goals of therapy of influenza are as follows:

1. Control symptoms
2. Prevent complications
3. Decrease work and/or school absenteeism
4. Prevent the spread of infection

■ GENERAL APPROACH TO TREATMENT

In the era of pandemic preparedness and increasing resistance, early and definitive diagnosis of influenza is crucial. ❾ The currently available antiviral drugs are most effective if started within 48 hours of the onset of illness. Moreover, the sooner the antiviral drugs are started after the onset of illness, the more effective they are. Antiviral drugs shorten the duration of illness and provide symptom control. Adjunct agents, such as acetaminophen for fever or an antihistamine for rhinitis, may be used concomitantly with the antiviral drugs.

■ NONPHARMACOLOGIC THERAPY

Patients suffering from influenza should get adequate sleep and maintain a low level of activity. They should stay home from work and/or school in order to rest and prevent the spread of infection. Appropriate fluid intake should be maintained. Cough/throat lozenges, warm tea, or soup may help with symptom control (cough, sore throat).

■ PHARMACOLOGIC THERAPY

The two classes of antiviral drugs available for treatment of influenza are the same as those available for prophylaxis and include the adamantanes, amantadine and rimantadine, and the neuraminidase inhibitors, oseltamivir and zanamivir. Although adamantanes maintain activity against most seasonal influenza A H1N1 viruses, they are not currently recommended as monotherapy due to rapid emergence of resistance. A limited discussion of these two agents can be found below, but the focus will be on oseltamivir and zanamivir.

Amantadine and Rimantadine

Amantadine and rimantadine are adamantanes that have activity against seasonal influenza A H1N1 only. The adamantanes block the M2 ion channel, which is specific to influenza A viruses, and inhibit viral uncoating. Rapid emergence of resistance is a problem with these agents because cross-resistance is conferred by a single point mutation, which is why adamanatane monotherapy is not recommended.[26,27,49] Because oseltamivir resistance among seasonal influenza A H1N1 is increasing, the addition of an adamantine to oseltamivir is recommended when this specific subtype is suspected (Table 118–6). However, adamantanes do not have activity against influenza A H3N2 or influenza B viruses, and thus should not be used for infections due to these viruses.

Oseltamivir and Zanamivir

❿ Oseltamivir and zanamivir are neuraminidase inhibitors that have activity against both influenza A and influenza B viruses, although resistance to oseltamivir among seasonal influenza A H1N1 is on the rise.[26,27] Without neuraminidase, release of the virus from infected cells is impaired, and thus, viral replication is decreased. When administered within 48 hours of the onset of illness, oseltamivir and zanamivir may reduce the duration of illness by approximately 1 day versus placebo.[26,27] In a pivotal trial, oseltamivir reduced the time to return to normal health in adults by 1.9 days and the time to return to normal activity by 2.8 days.[57] These reductions have a significant effect on not only the quality of life for the patient but also the societal costs associated with influenza. ❾ Of note, the benefits of treatment are highly dependent on the timing of the initiation of treatment, with the ideal initiation period being within 12 hours of illness onset.[58]

Oseltamivir treatment in adults and adolescents with documented influenza illness resulted in a 26.7% reduction in overall antibiotic use, a 55% reduction in lower respiratory tract complications (bronchitis, pneumonia), and a 59% reduction in hospitalizations.[59] Zanamivir treatment in adults and adolescents with influenza-like illness resulted in a 28% reduction in antibiotic use and a 40% reduction in lower respiratory tract complications.[60] The data in these studies largely come from healthy individuals rather than those at highest risk for complications associated with influenza. The impact of appropriate treatment in high-risk populations may be even greater than that which has been documented to date.

Oseltamivir is approved for treatment in those older than the age of 1 year, while zanamivir is approved for treatment in those older than the age of 7 years. Given the recent pandemic of novel H1N1 in 2009, the FDA issued an emergency use authorization (EUA) for oseltamivir that expanded its use to children younger than 1 year of age.[50] The recommended doses vary by agent and age (see Table 118–7), and the recommended duration of treatment for both agents is 5 days. As of June 23, 2010, the expanded use of oseltamivir under the EUA expired. Therefore, oseltamivir and zanamivir can only be used for approved indications and populations.

Neuropsychiatric complications consisting of delirium, seizures, hallucinations, and self-injury in pediatric patients (mostly from Japan) have been reported following treatment with oseltamivir.[61] Since influenza itself can be associated with neuropsychiatric manifestations, a causal relationship between oseltamivir and neuropsychiatric effects has not been delineated.[62–64] However, the label for oseltamivir has been updated to include neuropsychiatric events as a precaution,[62] and their occurrence with use of oseltamivir should not be ignored.

Influenza resistance to the neuraminidase inhibitors has been documented but cross-resistance between the neuraminidase inhibitors has not been reported.[26] Surveillance during the 2008 to 2009 influenza season identified oseltamivir resistance among most influenza A H1N1 virus isolates.[24] Antiviral susceptibility testing of circulating viruses confirmed that seasonal influenza A H3N2 maintains susceptibility to oseltamivir and zanamivir, but the seasonal H1N1 strain is generally oseltamivir resistant. This prompted the CDC and Infectious Diseases Society of America to issue an

interim recommendation summarized in Table 118–6, regarding the use of antiviral agents for the management of persons with suspected seasonal influenza A virus infection.[48] The burden of surveillance rests on clinicians to identify local patterns of influenza circulation to guide antiviral therapy.

CLINICAL CONTROVERSY

Some debate exists regarding the benefit of antiviral administration >48 hours after onset. While clinicians agree that the most benefit is achieved the earlier the medications are started, some data suggest benefit even beyond 48 hours after onset, albeit more limited.

■ SPECIAL POPULATIONS

Inadequate data exist regarding the use of antiinfluenza medications in special populations, such as immunocompromised hosts. Furthermore, limited data exist regarding use of influenza antivirals during pregnancy. The adamantanes are embryotoxic and teratogenic in rats, and limited case reports of adverse fetal outcomes following amantadine use in humans have been published. Oseltamivir and zanamivir have been used but lack solid safety clinical data in pregnant women. Pregnancy should not be considered a contraindication to oseltamivir or zanamivir use. Oseltamivir is preferred for treatment of pregnant women because of its systemic activity; however, the drug of choice for chemoprophylaxis is not yet defined. Zanamivir may be preferred because of its limited systemic absorption, but respiratory complications need to be considered, especially in women with underlying respiratory diseases. Both the adamantanes and the neuraminidase inhibitors are excreted in breast milk and should be avoided by mothers who are breastfeeding their infants. More studies are needed in these populations who are at high risk for serious disease and complications from influenza.

EVALUATION OF THERAPEUTIC OUTCOMES

Patients should be monitored daily for resolution of signs and symptoms associated with influenza, such as fever, myalgia, headache, malaise, nonproductive cough, sore throat, and rhinitis. These signs and symptoms will typically resolve within approximately 1 week. If the patient continues to exhibit signs and symptoms of illness beyond 10 days or a worsening of symptoms after 7 days, a physician visit is warranted as this may be an indication of a secondary bacterial infection. Ideally, antiviral therapy should not be started until influenza is confirmed via the laboratory. However, therapy should be initiated within 48 hours of illness onset, emphasizing the need for rapid diagnosis. Repeat diagnostic tests to demonstrate clearance of the virus are not necessary.

CONCLUSIONS

Influenza is associated with significant morbidity and mortality and substantial burden to society in terms of both direct and indirect costs. Prevention of influenza by vaccination may yield significant benefit to society in terms of reductions in influenza-related complications, decreased work/school absenteeism, reductions in hospitalizations and deaths, and general cost savings. Two highly effective seasonal influenza vaccines are currently available in the United States, yet influenza remains the leading cause of vaccine-preventable mortality. This underscores the need for targeted efforts toward populations at high risk for serious disease and complications as well as the need for more vaccines, particularly for certain populations (e.g., those younger than 6 months old, those with hypersensitivity to eggs).

Four antiviral drugs are available for treatment and prophylaxis of influenza. Thus, the antiinfluenza antiviral armamentarium is limited and has been further reduced by significant resistance to the adamantanes and oseltamivir in recent years. Importantly, these agents are not a replacement for vaccination but rather an adjunct. Although the neuraminidase inhibitors remain useful as agents for treatment and prophylaxis of influenza, information on the use of these agents in special populations, such as immunocompromised hosts, pregnant women, and very young children, is limited. The best mechanism to decrease the morbidity, mortality, and societal burden associated with influenza remains prevention of the disease through annual vaccination.

ABBREVIATIONS

CDC: U.S. Centers for Disease Control and Prevention

FDA: U.S. Food and Drug Administration

GBS: Guillain-Barré syndrome

HIV: human immunodeficiency virus

LAIV: live-attenuated influenza vaccine

MIV: monovalent inactivated vaccine

mLAIV: monovalent live-attenuated influenza vaccine

TIV: trivalent influenza vaccine

WHO: World Health Organization

REFERENCE

1. American Lung Association. Trends in Pneumonia and Influenza Morbidity and Mortality. American Lung Association. New York: Research and Scientific Affairs Epidemiology and Statistics Unit, 2004.

2. Thompson WW, Shay DK, Weintraub E, et al. Influenza-associated hospitalizations in the United States. JAMA 2004;292(11): 1333–1340.

3. Thompson WW, Shay DK, Weintraub E, et al. Mortality associated with influenza and respiratory syncytial virus in the United States. JAMA 2003;289(2):179–186.

4. Nicholson KG, Wood JM, Zambon M. Influenza. Lancet 2003; 362(9397):1733–1745.

5. Monto AS, Comanor L, Shay DK, Thompson WW. Epidemiology of pandemic influenza: Use of surveillance and modeling for pandemic preparedness. J Infect Dis 2006;194(Suppl 2):S92–S97.

6. Palese P. Influenza: Old and new threats. Nat Med 2004;10 (12 Suppl):S82–S87.

7. Taubenberger JK, Morens DM. 1918 influenza: The mother of all pandemics. Emerg Infect Dis 2006;12(1):15–22.

8. Oxford JS. Influenza a pandemics of the 20th century with special reference to 1918: Virology, pathology and epidemiology. Rev Med Virol 2000;10(2):119–133.

9. Belshe RB. The origins of pandemic influenza—lessons from the 1918 virus. N Engl J Med 2005;353(21):2209–2211.

10. Lipatov AS, Govorkova EA, Webby RJ, et al. Influenza: Emergence and control. J Virol 2004;78(17):8951–8959.

11. Yuen KY, Chan PK, Peiris M, et al. Clinical features and rapid viral diagnosis of human disease associated with avian influenza A H5N1 virus. Lancet 1998;351(9101):467–471.

12. Mounts AW, Kwong H, Izurieta HS, et al. Case-control study of risk factors for avian influenza A (H5N1) disease, Hong Kong, 1997. J Infect Dis 1999;180(2):505–508.

13. Anonymous. Epidemic and Pandemic Alert and Response: Avian Influenza. http://www.who.int/csr/disease/avian_influenza/en/index.html.

14. Tran TH, Nguyen TL, Nguyen TD, et al. Avian influenza A (H5N1) in 10 patients in Vietnam. N Engl J Med 2004;350(12):1179–1188.

15. Ungchusak K, Auewarakul P, Dowell SF, et al. Probable person-to-person transmission of avian influenza A (H5N1). N Engl J Med 2005;352(4):333–340.

16. Beigel JH, Farrar J, Han AM, et al. Avian influenza A (H5N1) infection in humans. N Engl J Med 2005;353(13):1374–1385.

17. Avian Influenza H5N1Vaccine. http://www.fda.gov/downloads/ BiologicsBloodVaccines/Vaccines/ApprovedProducts/UCM112836.pdf.

18. Hill DR. The burden of illness in international travelers. N Engl J Med 2006;354(2):115–117.

19. Centers for Disease Control and Prevention. Update: novel influenza A (H1N1) virus infections – worldwide, May 6, 2009. MMWR Morb Mortal Wkly Rep 2009;58:453–458.

20. Influenza A (H1N1) – update 14. Geneva: World Health Organization, 2009. http://www.who.int/csr/don/2009_05_04a/en/index.html.

21. Dawood FS, Jain S, Finelli L, Shaw MW, Lindstrom S, Garten RJ, et al. Novel swine-origin influenza A (H1N1) virus investigation team. Emergence of a novel swine-origin influenza A (H1N1) virus in humans. N Engl J Med 2009;360:2605–2615.

22. Centers for Disease Control and Prevention. Interim guidance on antiviral recommendations for patients with novel influenza A (H1N1) virus infection and their close contacts. Atlanta, GA: CDC; 2009. www. cdc.gov/h1n1flu/recommendations.htm.

23. Schuchat A. Use of influenza A (H1N1) 2009 monovalent vaccine: recommendations of the Advisory Committee on Immunization Practices (ACIP), 2009. MMWR 2009;58(ER):1-8. http://www.cdc.gov/ mmwr/preview/mmwrhtml/rr58e0821a1.htm.

24. CDC. Flu Activity & Surveillance [updated in weekly CDC surveillance reports]. http://www.cdc.gov/flu/weekly/fluactivity.htm.

25. Bridges CB, Kuehnert MJ, Hall CB. Transmission of influenza: Implications for control in health care settings. Clin Infect Dis 2003; 37(8):1094–1101.

26. Fiore AE, Shay DK, Broder K, Iskander JK, Uyeki TM, Mootrey G, et al. Prevention and control of influenza: recommendations of the Advisory Committee on Immunization Practices (ACIP), 2009. MMWR 2009;58(RR-8):1–52.

27. Harper SA, Bradley JS, Englund JA, et al. Expert Panel of the Infectious Diseases Society of America. Seasonal influenza in adults and children — diagnosis, treatment, chemoprophylaxis, and institutional outbreak management: clinical practice guidelines of the Infectious Diseases Society of America. Clin Infect Dis 2009;48(8):1003–1032.

28. Cheung CY, Poon LL, Lau AS, et al. Induction of proinflammatory cytokines in human macrophages by influenza A (H5N1) viruses: A mechanism for the unusual severity of human disease? Lancet 2002;360(9348):1831–1837.

29. FDA Approved Vaccines. http://www.fda.gov/BiologicsBloodVaccines/ Vaccines/ApprovedProducts/ucm093833.htm.

30. Petric M, Comanor L, Petti CA. Role of the laboratory in diagnosis of influenza during seasonal epidemics and potential pandemics. J Infect Dis 2006;194(Suppl 2):S98–S110.

31. Neuzil KM, Zhu Y, Griffin MR, et al. Burden of interpandemic influenza in children younger than 5 years: A 25-year prospective study. J Infect Dis 2002;185(2):147–152.

32. Newton DW, Treanor JJ, Menegus MA. Clinical and laboratory diagnosis of influenza virus infections. Am J Manag Care 2000;6(5 Suppl):S265–S275.

33. Hoberman A, Greenberg DP, Paradise JL, et al. Effectiveness of inactivated influenza vaccine in preventing acute otitis media in young children: A randomized controlled trial. JAMA 2003;290(12):1608–1616.

34. Bridges CB, Thompson WW, Meltzer MI, et al. Effectiveness and cost-benefit of influenza vaccination of healthy working adults: A randomized controlled trial. JAMA 2000;284(13):1655–1663.

35. Demicheli V, Rivetti D, Deeks JJ, Jefferson TO. Vaccines for preventing influenza in healthy adults. Cochrane Database Syst Rev 2004;(3):CD001269.

36. Juurlink DN, Stukel TA, Kwong J, et al. Guillain-Barré syndrome after influenza vaccination in adults: A population-based study. Arch Intern Med 2006;166(20):2217–2221.

37. Lasky T, Terracciano GJ, Magder L, et al. The Guillain-Barré syndrome and the 1992–1993 and 1993–1994 influenza vaccines. N Engl J Med 1998;339(25):1797–1802.

38. Summary of the joint statement on thimerosal in vaccines. American Academy of Family Physicians, American Academy of Pediatrics, Advisory Committee on Immunization Practices, Public Health Service. MMWR Morb Mortal Wkly Rep 2000;49(27):622, 631.

39. McCormick MC. The autism "epidemic": Impressions from the perspective of immunization safety review. Ambul Pediatr 2003;3(3): 119–120.

40. Verstraeten T, Davis RL, DeStefano F, et al. Safety of thimerosal-containing vaccines: A two-phased study of computerized health maintenance organization databases. Pediatrics 2003;112(5):1039–1048.

41. Boyce TG, Poland GA. Promises and challenges of live-attenuated intranasal influenza vaccines across the age spectrum: A review. Biomed Pharmacother 2000;54(4):210–218.

42. Belshe RB, Ambrose CS, Yi T. Safety and efficacy of live attenuated influenza vaccine in children 2-7 years of age. Vaccine 2008;26 (Suppl 4):D10-D16.

43. Nichol KL, Mendelman PM, Mallon KP, et al. Effectiveness of live, attenuated intranasal influenza virus vaccine in healthy, working adults: A randomized controlled trial. JAMA 1999;282(2): 137–144.

44. Hayden FG, Atmar RL, Schilling M, et al. Use of the selective oral neuraminidase inhibitor oseltamivir to prevent influenza. N Engl J Med 1999;341(18):1336–1343.

45. Hayden FG, Pavia AT. Antiviral management of seasonal and pandemic influenza. J Infect Dis 2006;194(Suppl 2):S119–S126.

46. Monto AS, Pichichero ME, Blanckenberg SJ, et al. Zanamivir prophylaxis: An effective strategy for the prevention of influenza types A and B within households. J Infect Dis 2002;186(11): 1582–1588.

47. Peters PH Jr, Gravenstein S, Norwood P, et al. Long-term use of oseltamivir for the prophylaxis of influenza in a vaccinated frail older population. J Am Geriatr Soc 2001;49(8):1025–1031.

48. Centers for Disease Control and Prevention. CDC Issues Interim Recommendations for the Use of Influenza Antiviral Medications in the Setting of Oseltamivir Resistance among Circulating Influenza A (H1N1) Viruses, 2008-09 Influenza Season. *http://www2a.cdc.gov/HAN/ArchiveSys/ViewMsgV.asp?AlertNum=00279.*

49. WHO Guidelines for Pharmacological Management of Pandemic (H1N1) 2009 Influenza and other Influenza Viruses. *http://www.who.int/csr/resources/publications/swineflu/h1n1_guidelines_pharmaceutical_mngt.pdf.*

50. Centers for Disease Control and Prevention. Emergency Use Authorization of Tamiflu (oseltamivir). *http://www.cdc.gov/h1n1flu/eua/tamiflu.htm.*

51. Englund JA. Maternal immunization with inactivated influenza vaccine: Rationale and experience. Vaccine 2003;21(24):3460–3464.

52. Tasker SA, Treanor JJ, Paxton WB, Wallace MR. Efficacy of influenza vaccination in HIV-infected persons. A randomized, double-blind, placebo-controlled trial. Ann Intern Med 1999;131(6):430–433.

53. Kroon FP, van Dissel JT, de Jong JC, et al. Antibody response after influenza vaccination in HIV-infected individuals: A consecutive 3-year study. Vaccine 2000;18(26):3040–3049.

54. Soesman NM, Rimmelzwaan GF, Nieuwkoop NJ, et al. Efficacy of influenza vaccination in adult liver transplant recipients. J Med Virol 2000;61(1):85–93.

55. Ison MG, Gubareva LV, Atmar RL, et al. Recovery of drug-resistant influenza virus from immunocompromised patients: A case series. J Infect Dis 2006;193(6):760–764.

56. Whitley RJ, Monto AS. Prevention and treatment of influenza in high-risk groups: Children, pregnant women, immunocompromised hosts, and nursing home residents. J Infect Dis 2006;194(Suppl 2):S133–S138.

57. Treanor JJ, Hayden FG, Vrooman PS, et al. Efficacy and safety of the oral neuraminidase inhibitor oseltamivir in treating acute influenza: A randomized controlled trial. US Oral Neuraminidase Study Group. JAMA 2000;283(8):1016–1024.

58. Aoki FY, Macleod MD, Paggiaro P, et al. Early administration of oral oseltamivir increases the benefits of influenza treatment. J Antimicrob Chemother 2003;51(1):123–129.

59. Kaiser L, Wat C, Mills T, et al. Impact of oseltamivir treatment on influenza-related lower respiratory tract complications and hospitalizations. Arch Intern Med 2003;163(14):1667–1672.

60. Kaiser L, Keene ON, Hammond JM, et al. Impact of zanamivir on antibiotic use for respiratory events following acute influenza in adolescents and adults. Arch Intern Med 2000;160(21):3234–3240.

61. Bridges A. FDA. Tamiflu patients need monitoring. Washington, DC: Associated Press, November 14, 2006.

62. Tamiflu [prescribing information]. Genentech USA, Inc/Roche Group; April 2010. *http:/www.rocheusa.com/products/tamiflu/pi.pdf.*

63. Newland JG, Laurich VM, Rosenquist AW, et al. Neurologic complications in children hospitalized with influenza: characteristics, incidence, and risk factors. J Pediatr 2007;150:306–310.

64. Chung BH, Tsang AM, Wong VC. Neurologic complications in children hospitalized with influenza: comparison between USA and Hong Kong. J Pediatr 2007;151:e17–e8.

119

Skin and Soft-Tissue Infections

DOUGLAS N. FISH, SUSAN L. PENDLAND AND LARRY H. DANZIGER

KEY CONCEPTS

❶ Folliculitis, furuncles (boils), and carbuncles begin around hair follicles and are caused most often by *Staphylococcus aureus*. Folliculitis and small furuncles are generally treated with warm, moist heat to promote drainage; large furuncles and carbuncles require incision and drainage. A penicillinase-resistant penicillin such as dicloxacillin is commonly used for extensive or serious infections (e.g., fever).

❷ Erysipelas, a superficial skin infection with extensive lymphatic involvement, is caused by *Streptococcus pyogenes*. The treatment of choice is penicillin, administered orally or parenterally, depending on the severity of the infection.

❸ Impetigo is a superficial skin infection that occurs most commonly in children. It is characterized by fluid-filled vesicles that develop rapidly into pus-filled blisters that rupture to form golden-yellow crusts. Effective therapy includes penicillinase-resistant penicillins (dicloxacillin), first-generation cephalosporins (cephalexin), and topical mupirocin. *S. aureus* is the primary cause of impetigo, with infections caused by community-associated methicillin-resistant *S. aureus* (CA-MRSA) emerging in recent years.

❹ Lymphangitis, an infection of the subcutaneous lymphatic channels, is generally caused by *S. pyogenes*. Acute lymphangitis is characterized by the rapid development of fine, red, linear streaks extending from the initial infection site toward the regional lymph nodes, which are usually enlarged and tender. Penicillin is the drug of choice.

❺ Cellulitis is an infection of the epidermis, dermis, and superficial fascia most commonly caused by *S. pyogenes* and *S. aureus*. Lesions generally are hot, painful, and erythematous, with nonelevated, poorly defined margins. Treatment generally consists of a penicillinase-resistant penicillin (dicloxacillin) or first-generation cephalosporin (cephalexin) for 5 to 10 days. Trimethoprim-sulfamethoxazole, with or without a β-lactam agent, or doxycycline should be considered for treatment of suspected staphylococcal infections in areas with a high prevalence of CA-MRSA.

❻ Necrotizing fasciitis is a rare but life-threatening infection of subcutaneous tissue that results in progressive destruction of superficial fascia and subcutaneous fat. Early and aggressive surgical debridement is an essential part of therapy for treatment of necrotizing fasciitis. Infections caused by *S. pyogenes* or *Clostridium* species should be treated with the combination of penicillin and clindamycin.

❼ Diabetic foot infections are managed with a comprehensive treatment approach that includes both proper wound care and antimicrobial therapy. Antimicrobial regimens for diabetic foot infections should include broad-spectrum coverage of staphylococci, streptococci, enteric gram-negative bacilli, and anaerobes. Outpatient therapy with oral antimicrobials should be used whenever possible for less severe infections.

❽ Prevention is the single most important aspect in the management of pressure sores. After a sore develops, successful local care includes a comprehensive approach consisting of relief of pressure, proper cleaning (debridement), disinfection, and appropriate antimicrobial therapy if an infection is present. Good wound care is crucial to successful management.

❾ All bite wounds (either animal or human) should be irrigated thoroughly with large volumes of sterile normal saline, and the injured area should be immobilized and elevated. Depending on the severity of the bite wound, amoxicillin-clavulanic acid or ampicillin-sulbactam are often used for treatment of animal bites because of their coverage of *Pasteurella multocida*, *S. aureus*, and anaerobes typically present in the oral flora of dogs and cats.

❿ Although antimicrobial prophylaxis of dog or cat bites is not recommended routinely, patients with human bite injuries should be given prophylactic antimicrobial therapy for 3 to 5 days. Infected wounds, particularly clenched-fist injuries, should be treated for 7 to 14 days with ampicillin-sulbactam, cefoxitin, or other combination that has activity against *Eikenella corrodens*, *S. aureus*, and β-lactamase–producing anaerobes.

Learning objectives, review questions, and other resources can be found at **www.pharmacotherapyonline.com**.

The skin serves as a barrier between humans and their environment, therefore functioning as a primary defense mechanism against infections. The skin consists of the epidermis, the dermis, and subcutaneous fat. The epidermis is the outermost, nonvascular layer of the skin. It varies in thickness from approximately 0.1 mm on most areas of the body to a maximum of 1.5 mm on the soles of the feet. Although extremely thin, the epidermis is composed of several layers. The innermost layer consists of continuously dividing cells. The outer layers are renewed as cells are gradually pushed outward. As the cells approach the surface, they become flattened, lose their nuclei, and are filled with keratin. The outermost layer, the stratum corneum, is composed of flattened, cornified, nonnucleated cells. The dermis is the layer of skin directly beneath the epidermis. It consists of connective tissue and contains blood vessels and lymphatics, sensory nerve endings, sweat and sebaceous glands, hair follicles, and smooth muscle fibers. Beneath the dermis is a layer of loose connective tissue containing primarily fat cells. This subcutaneous fat layer is of variable thickness over the body. Beneath the subcutaneous fat lies the fascia, which separates the skin from underlying muscle. It is generally divided into superficial fascia, which is located immediately beneath the skin, and deep fascia, which forms sheaths for muscles.

Skin and soft-tissue infections (SSTIs) may involve any or all layers of the skin, fascia, and muscle. They also may spread far from the initial site of infection and lead to more severe complications, such as endocarditis, gram-negative sepsis, or streptococcal glomerulonephritis. Sometimes the treatment of SSTIs may necessitate both medical and surgical management. This chapter presents details of the pathogenesis and management of some of the most common infections involving the skin and soft tissues. The first part of the chapter discusses a variety of SSTIs that range in severity from superficial to life threatening. The remainder of the chapter discusses diabetic foot infections, pressure sores, and human and animal bites.

EPIDEMIOLOGY

Classification schemes have been developed to describe SSTIs. Bacterial infections of the skin can be classified as primary or secondary (Table 119–1). Primary bacterial infections usually involve areas of previously healthy skin and are caused by a single pathogen. In contrast, secondary infections occur in areas of previously damaged skin and are frequently polymicrobic. SSTIs are also classified as complicated or uncomplicated. Complicated infections are those that involve deeper skin structures (e.g., fascia, muscle layers), require significant surgical intervention, or occur in patients with

compromised immune function [e.g., diabetes mellitus, human immunodeficiency virus (HIV) infection].[1]

A newer classification system also divides SSTIs into four classes based on severity of signs and symptoms, as well as the presence and stability of any comorbidities.[2] The classification was used to develop an algorithm to help with admission and treatment decisions. Class 1 includes patients who are afebrile and otherwise healthy. These infections are generally managed on an outpatient basis with topical or oral antimicrobials. Class 2 includes patients who are febrile and ill appearing but who have no unstable comorbid conditions. Some class 2 patients may be treated with oral antimicrobials, but most are likely to require some parenteral therapy, either as an outpatient or with short-term hospitalization. Class 3 includes patients having a toxic appearance, unstable comorbidity, or a limb-threatening infection. Class 4 includes patients with sepsis syndrome or another life-threatening infection, such as necrotizing fasciitis. Patients in classes 3 and 4 require hospitalization and parenteral antimicrobial therapy initially but may be candidates for oral or outpatient parenteral therapy once their condition has stabilized. Patients in class 4 also usually require some type of surgical intervention.

SSTIs are among the most common infections seen in both community and hospital settings.[3–5] However, most infections are believed to be mild and are treated in an outpatient setting, making it difficult to accurately quantify community-acquired SSTIs. SSTIs were diagnosed in 0.8% of physician office visits between 1993 and 2005; this corresponded to approximately 82 million diagnoses of SSTI, being more common among elderly patients (70 years of age and older).[3] Another description of office visits among health plan members listed cellulitis and impetigo as the primary diagnoses for 2.2% and 0.3% of patients, respectively.[4] According to an Agency for Healthcare Research and Quality (AHRQ) report, in 2007 SSTIs were responsible for over 600,000 hospitalizations and represented 2.0% of all admissions in males and 1.2% in females.[5]

While the exact incidence of SSTIs is unknown, the frequency of infections caused by invasive group A streptococci and drug-resistant gram-positive cocci has been increasing.[1] Group A streptococci (*Streptococcus pyogenes*) are among the most common etiologic agents of SSTIs. Although they may be found in many mild, superficial skin infections, they are also responsible for life-threatening cases of necrotizing fasciitis.[1] A documented increase in necrotizing fasciitis caused by *S. pyogenes* is a major concern because of the high morbidity and mortality associated with these infections.

Another concerning trend is the increased in vitro resistance reported among other gram-positive bacteria.[1] While the high incidence of nosocomial methicillin-resistant *Staphylococcus aureus* (MRSA) has been a major concern for many years,[6–8] the emergence of community-associated MRSA (CA-MRSA) is even more problematic.[9–15] CA-MRSA strains are characteristically isolated from patients lacking typical risk factors (e.g., prior hospitalization, long-term care facility) and are often susceptible to non-β-lactam antibiotics (trimethoprim-sulfamethoxazole, doxycycline, clindamycin).[9,11,13] They also differ genetically from nosocomial strains of MRSA with methicillin resistance carried on the type IV staphylococcal chromosomal cassette *mec* (SCC*mec*) element of the *mecA* gene. CA-MRSA strains often harbor genes for Panton-Valentine leukocidin, a cytotoxin responsible for leukocyte destruction and tissue necrosis. In contrast, nosocomial strains usually lack genes for Panton-Valentine leukocidin and are associated with SCC*mec* alleles I to III.[10,11,15] Clinicians should suspect CA-MRSA in geographic areas with a high prevalence of these strains or in recurrent or persistent infections that are not responding to appropriate β-lactam therapy. In addition to the emergence of CA-MRSA,

TABLE 119-1	Bacterial Classification of Important Skin and Soft-Tissue Infections
Primary infections	
Erysipelas	Group A streptococci
Impetigo	*Staphylococcus aureus*, group A streptococci
Lymphangitis	Group A streptococci; occasionally *S. aureus*
Cellulitis	Group A streptococci, *S. aureus* (potentially including methicillin-resistant strains); occasionally other gram-positive cocci, gram-negative bacilli, and/or anaerobes
Necrotizing fasciitis	
Type I	Anaerobes (*Bacteroides* spp., *Peptostreptococcus* spp.) and facultative bacteria (streptococci, Enterobacteriaceae)
Type II	Group A streptococci
Secondary infections	
Diabetic foot infections	*S. aureus*, streptococci, Enterobacteriaceae, *Bacteroides* spp., *Peptostreptococcus* spp., *Pseudomonas aeruginosa*
Pressure sores	*S. aureus*, streptococci, Enterobacteriaceae, *Bacteroides* spp., *Peptostreptococcus* spp., *P. aeruginosa*
Bite wounds	
Animal	*Pasteurella multocida*, *S. aureus*, streptococci, *Bacteroides* spp.
Human	*Eikenella corrodens*, *S. aureus*, streptococci, *Corynebacterium* spp., *Bacteroides* spp., *Peptostreptococcus* spp.
Burn wounds	*P. aeruginosa*, Enterobacteriaceae, *S. aureus*, streptococci

TABLE 119-2	Predominant Microorganisms of Normal Skin

Bacteria
Gram-positive
    Coagulase-negative staphylococci
    Micrococci (*Micrococcus luteus*)
    Corynebacterium species (diphtheroids)
    Propionibacterium species
Gram-negative
    Acinetobacter species
Fungi
Malassezia species
Candida species

treatment choices for SSTIs have been further complicated by the increased incidence of macrolide-resistant strains of *S. aureus* and *S. pyogenes*.[1,8,11]

ETIOLOGY

The majority of SSTIs are caused by gram-positive organisms present on the skin surface.[1] Gram-positive bacteria (coagulase-negative staphylococci, diphtheroids) are the predominant flora of the skin, with gram-negative organisms (*Escherichia coli* and other Enterobacteriaceae) being relatively uncommon[16] (Table 119–2). *S. aureus*, as well as a variety of gram-negative bacteria, including *Acinetobacter* species, can be found in moist intertriginous areas (e.g., axilla, groin, and toe webs) of the body.[17] *S. aureus* also inhabits the anterior nares of approximately 30% of healthy individuals.[16] Colonization, whether transient or permanent, provides a nidus for infection should the integrity of the epidermis be compromised.

S. aureus and *S. pyogenes* account for the majority of community-acquired SSTIs.[1] Data from large surveillance studies showed *S. aureus* to be the most common cause (45%) of SSTIs in hospitalized patients.[6,7] Also of note in these studies was the 36% incidence of methicillin resistance among strains of *S. aureus*. Other common nosocomial pathogens included *Pseudomonas aeruginosa* (11%), enterococci (9%), and *E. coli* (7%).[6,7]

PATHOPHYSIOLOGY

The skin and subcutaneous tissues normally are extremely resistant to infection but may become susceptible under certain conditions. Even when high concentrations of bacteria are applied topically or injected into the soft tissue, resulting infections are rare.[16] Several host factors act together to confer protection against skin infections. Because the surface of the skin is relatively dry and has a pH of approximately 5.6, it is not conducive to bacterial growth.[16] Continuous renewal of the epidermal layer results in the shedding of keratocytes, as well as skin bacteria. In addition, sebaceous secretions are hydrolyzed to form free fatty acids that strongly inhibit the growth of many bacteria and fungi.[4] Conditions that may predispose a patient to the development of skin infections include (a) high concentrations of bacteria ($>10^5$ microorganisms), (b) excessive moisture of the skin, (c) inadequate blood supply, (d) availability of bacterial nutrients, and (e) damage to the corneal layer allowing for bacterial penetration.[4,16]

The majority of SSTIs result from the disruption of normal host defenses by processes such as skin puncture, abrasion, or underlying diseases (e.g., diabetes). The nature and severity of the infection depend on both the type of microorganism present and the site of innoculation.

FOLLICULITIS, FURUNCLES, AND CARBUNCLES

❶ Folliculitis is inflammation of the hair follicle and is caused by physical injury, chemical irritation, or infection.[4] Infection occurring at the base of the eyelid is referred to as a stye. While folliculitis is a superficial infection with pus present only in the dermis, furuncles and carbuncles occur when a follicular infection extends from around the hair shaft to involve deeper areas of the skin. A furuncle, commonly known as an *abscess* or *boil*, is a walled-off mass of purulent material arising from a hair follicle.[4] The lesions are called *carbuncles* when they coalesce and extend to the subcutaneous tissue. This aggregate of infected hair follicles forms deep masses that generally open and drain through multiple sinus tracts.[4] *S. aureus* is the most common cause of folliculitis, furuncles, and carbuncles. Inadequate chlorine levels in whirlpools, hot tubs, and swimming pools have been responsible for outbreaks of folliculitis caused by *P. aeruginosa*.[17] Outbreaks of furunculosis caused by *S. aureus* and CA-MRSA have been reported in settings involving close contact (such as with families, prisons), especially when skin injury was common (such as with sports). In addition, some individuals experience repeated attacks of furunculosis. The major predisposing factor in this population is the presence of *S. aureus* in the anterior nares.[11]

CLINICAL PRESENTATION

Folliculitis

- Pruritic, erythematous papules typically appear within 48 hours (range: 6 to 72 hours) of exposure to large numbers of organisms.
- Papules evolve into pustules that generally heal in several days.
- Systemic signs such as fever and malaise are uncommon, although they have been reported in cases caused by *P. aeruginosa*.

Furuncles

- Furuncles can occur anywhere on hairy skin but generally develop in areas subject to friction and perspiration.
- Furuncles are discrete lesions, whether occurring as singular or multiple nodules.
- The lesion starts as a firm, tender, red nodule that becomes painful and fluctuant.
- Lesions often drain spontaneously.
- Lesions caused by CA-MRSA often have necrotic centers characteristic of "spider bites."

Carbuncles

- Carbuncles are broad, swollen, erythematous, deep, and painful follicular masses.
- Carbuncles commonly develop on the back of the neck and are more likely to occur in patients with diabetes.
- Unlike folliculitis and furuncles, carbuncles are commonly associated with fever, chills, and malaise.
- Bacteremia with secondary spread to other tissues is common.

TREATMENT

Folliculitis, Furuncles, and Carbuncles

Table 119–3 summarizes evidence-based treatment recommendations from clinical guidelines for SSTIs.[11,18] Treatment of folliculitis generally requires only local measures, such as warm moist compresses or topical therapy (e.g., clindamycin, erythromycin, mupirocin, or benzoyl peroxide).[19] Topical agents generally are applied two to four times daily for 7 days. Small furuncles generally can be treated with moist heat, which promotes localization and drainage of pus.[19] Large and/or multiple furuncles and carbuncles require incision and drainage.[19] Systemic antibiotics are usually not necessary unless accompanied by fever or extensive cellulitis.[11] Treatment of more severe infections generally consists of a penicillinase-resistant penicillin (such as dicloxacillin) or a first-generation cephalosporin (such as cephalexin) for 5 to 10 days (refer to Table 119–4 for adult and pediatric doses). An alternative agent for penicillin-allergic patients is clindamycin. For individuals with nasal colonization, application of mupirocin ointment twice daily in the anterior nares for the first 5 days of each month decreases recurrent furunculosis by almost half.[11] In addition, a single oral daily dose of clindamycin 150 mg for 3 months reduced recurrent infections caused by susceptible strains of *S. aureus* by approximately 80%.[11]

EVALUATION OF THERAPEUTIC OUTCOMES

Many follicular infections resolve spontaneously without medical or surgical intervention. Lesions should be incised if they do not respond to a few days of moist heat and nonprescription topical agents. Following drainage, most lesions begin to heal within several days without antimicrobial therapy. Any patient who is unresponsive to several days of therapy with a penicillinase-resistant penicillin or first-generation cephalosporin should have a culture and sensitivity performed because of the increasing frequency of CA-MRSA.

ERYSIPELAS

❷ Erysipelas is an infection of the more superficial layers of the skin and cutaneous lymphatics.[20] The intense red color and burning pain associated with this skin infection led to the common name of "St. Anthony's fire." The infection is almost always caused by β-hemolytic streptococci, with the organisms gaining access via small breaks in the skin. Group A streptococci (*S. pyogenes*) are responsible for most infections.[11,19,20] Infections are more common

---

TABLE 119-3 Evidence-Based Recommendations for Treatment of Skin and Soft-Tissue Infections[11,19]

Recommendations	Recommendation Grade
Folliculitis, furuncles, carbuncles	
Folliculitis and small furuncles can be treated with moist heat; large furuncles and carbuncles require incision and drainage. Antimicrobial therapy is unnecessary unless extensive lesions or fever are present.	EIII
Erysipelas	
Most infections are caused by *Streptococcus pyogenes*. Penicillin (oral or intravenous depending on clinical severity) is the drug of choice.	AI
If *Staphylococcus aureus* is suspected, a penicillinase-resistant penicillin or first-generation cephalosporin should be used.	AI
Impetigo	
S. aureus accounts for the majority of infections; consequently, a penicillin-resistant penicillin or first-generation cephalosporin is recommended.	AI
Topical therapy with mupirocin is equivalent to oral therapy.	AI
Cellulitis	
Mild-moderate infections can generally be treated with oral agents (dicloxacillin, cephalexin, clindamycin) unless resistance is high in the community.	AI
Serious infections should be treated intravenously with a penicillinase-resistant penicillin (nafcillin) or first-generation cephalosporin (cefazolin). Patients with penicillin allergies should be treated with vancomycin or clindamycin.	AI
Vancomycin, linezolid, and daptomycin should be used to treat serious infections caused by methicillin-resistant *S. aureus*.	AI
Necrotizing fasciitis	
Early and aggressive surgical debridement of all necrotic tissue is essential.	AIII
Necrotizing fasciitis caused by *S. pyogenes* should be treated with the combination of clindamycin and penicillin.	AII
Clostridial gas gangrene (myonecrosis) should be treated with clindamycin and penicillin.	BIII
Diabetic foot infections	
Many mild to moderate infections can be treated with oral agents that possess high bioavailability.	AII
All severe infections should be treated with intravenous therapy. After initial response, step-down therapy to oral agents can be used.	CIII
Broad-spectrum antimicrobial therapy is not generally required, except for some severe cases.	BIII
Definitive therapy should be based on results of appropriately collected cultures and sensitivities, as well as clinical response to empiric antimicrobial agents.	CIII
Optimal wound care, in additional to appropriate antimicrobial therapy, is essential for wound healing.	AI
Animal bites	
Many bite wounds can be treated on an outpatient basis with amoxicillin-clavulanic acid.	BII
Serious infections requiring intravenous antimicrobial therapy can be treated with a β-lactam/β-lactamase inhibitor combination or second-generation cephalosporin with activity against anaerobes (cefoxitin).	BII
Penicillinase-resistant penicillins, first-generation cephalosporins, macrolides, and clindamycin should not be used for treatment because of their poor activity against *Pasteurella multocida*.	DIII
Human bites	
Antimicrobial therapy should provide coverage against *Eikenella corrodens*, *S. aureus*, and β-lactamase–producing anaerobes.	BIII

Strength of recommendation: A, good evidence for use; B, moderate evidence for use; C, poor evidence for use, optional; D, moderate evidence to support not using; E, good evidence to support not using.
Quality of evidence: I, evidence from ≥1 properly randomized, controlled trials; II, evidence from ≥1 well-designed clinical trials without randomization, case-controlled analytic studies, multiple time series, or dramatic results from uncontrolled experiments; III, evidence from expert opinion, clinical experience, descriptive studies, or reports of expert committees.

TABLE 119-4 Recommended Drugs and Dosing Regimens for Outpatient Treatment of Mild–Moderate Skin and Soft-Tissue Infections

Infection	Oral Adult Dose	Oral Pediatric Dose
Folliculitis	None; warm saline compresses usually sufficient	
Furuncles and carbuncles	Dicloxacillin 250–500 mg every 6 h Cephalexin 250–500 mg every 6 h Clindamycin 300–600 mg every 6–8 h[a]	Dicloxacillin 25–50 mg/kg in four divided doses Cephalexin 25–50 mg/kg in four divided doses Clindamycin 10–30 mg/kg/day in three to four divided doses[a]
Erysipelas	Procaine penicillin G 600,000 units intramuscularly every 12 h Penicillin VK 250–500 mg every 6 h Clindamycin 150–300 mg every 6–8 h[a] Erythromycin 250–500 mg every 6 h[a]	Penicillin VK 25,000–90,000 units/kg in four divided doses Clindamycin 10–30 mg/kg in three to four doses[a] Erythromycin 30–50 mg/kg in four divided doses[a]
Impetigo	Dicloxacillin 250–500 mg every 6 h Cephalexin 250–500 mg every 6 h Cefadroxil 500 mg every 12 h Clindamycin 150–300 mg every 6–8 h[a] Mupirocin ointment every 8 h[a] Retapamulin ointment every 12 h[a]	Dicloxacillin 25–50 mg/kg in four divided doses Cephalexin 25–50 mg/kg in two to four divided doses Cefadroxil 30 mg/kg in two divided doses Clindamycin 10–30 mg/kg/day in three to four divided doses[a] Mupirocin ointment every 8 h[a] Retapamulin ointment every 12 h[a]
Lymphangitis	Initial intravenous therapy, followed by penicillin VK 250–500 mg every 6 h Clindamycin 150–300 mg every 6–8 h[a]	Initial intravenous therapy, followed by penicillin VK 25,000–90,000 units/kg in four divided doses Clindamycin 10–30 mg/kg/day in three to four divided doses[a]
Diabetic foot infections	Amoxicillin-clavulanic acid 875 mg/125 mg every 12 h Fluoroquinolone (levofloxacin 750 mg every 24 h or moxifloxacin 400 mg every 24 h) + metronidazole 250–500 mg every 8 h or clindamycin 300–600 mg every 6–8 h[a]	
Animal bite	Amoxicillin-clavulanic acid 875 mg/125 mg every 12 h Doxycycline 100–200 mg every 12 h[a] Dicloxacillin 250–500 mg every 6 h + penicillin VK 250–500 mg every 6 h Cefuroxime axetil 500 mg every 12 h + metronidazole 250–500 mg every 8 h or clindamycin 300–600 mg every 6–8 h Fluoroquinolone (levofloxacin 500–750 mg every 24 h or moxifloxacin 400 mg every 24 h) or clindamycin 300-600 mg every 6–8 h[a] Erythromycin 500 mg every 6 h + metronidazole 250–500 mg every 8 h or clindamycin 300–600 mg every 6–8 h[a]	Amoxicillin-clavulanic acid 40 mg/kg (of the amoxicillin component) in two divided doses Dicloxacillin 25–50 mg/kg in four divided doses + penicillin VK 40,000–90,000 units/kg in four divided doses Cefuroxime axetil 20–30 mg/kg in two divided doses + metronidazole 30 mg/kg in three to four divided doses or clindamycin 10–30 mg/kg/day in three to four divided doses Trimethoprim-sulfamethoxazole 4–6 mg/kg (of the trimethoprim component) every 12 h + metronidazole 30 mg/kg in three to four divided doses or clindamycin 10–30 mg/kg/day in three to four divided doses[a] Erythromycin 30–50 mg/kg in four divided doses + every 12 h + metronidazole 30 mg/kg in three to four divided doses or clindamycin 10–30 mg/kg/day in three to four divided doses[a]
Human bite	Amoxicillin-clavulanic acid 875 mg/125 mg every 12 h Doxycycline 100–200 mg every 12 h[a] Dicloxacillin 250–500 mg every 6 h + penicillin VK 250–500 mg every 6 h Cefuroxime axetil 500 mg every 12 h metronidazole 250–500 mg every 8 h or clindamycin 300–600 mg every 6–8 h Fluoroquinolone (levofloxacin 500–750 mg every 24 h or moxifloxacin 400 mg every 24 h) + metronidazole 250–500 mg every 8 h or clindamycin 300–600 mg every 6–8 h[a]	Amoxicillin-clavulanic acid 40 mg/kg (of the amoxicillin component) in two divided doses Dicloxacillin 25–50 mg/kg in four divided doses + penicillin VK 40,000–90,000 units/kg in four divided doses Cefuroxime axetil 20–30 mg/kg in two divided doses + metronidazole 30 mg/kg in three to four divided doses or clindamycin 10–30 mg/kg/day in three to four divided doses Trimethoprim-sulfamethoxazole 4–6 mg/kg (of the trimethoprim component) every 12 h + metronidazole 30 mg/kg in three to four divided doses or clindamycin 10–30 mg/kg/day in 3–4 divided doses[a]

[a]Recommended for patients with penicillin allergy.

in infants, young children, the elderly, and patients with nephrotic syndrome.[19] Erysipelas also commonly occurs in areas of preexisting lymphatic obstruction or edema.[19] Diagnosis is made on the basis of the characteristic lesion.

CLINICAL PRESENTATION

General

- The lower extremities are the most common sites for erysipelas.

Symptoms

- Patients often experience flu-like symptoms (fever, malaise) prior to the appearance of the lesion.
- The infected area is described as painful or as a burning pain.

Signs

- The lesion is bright red and edematous, often with lymphatic streaking.
- Temperature is often mildly elevated.

Laboratory Tests

- The causative organism usually cannot be cultured from the surface skin but sometimes may be aspirated from the edge of the advancing lesion.
- Cultures may be considered in more severe cases or those with atypical clinical findings such as fluid-filled blisters.

Other Diagnostic Tests

- A complete blood count is often performed because leukocytosis is common.
- C-reactive protein is also generally elevated.

TREATMENT

Erysipelas

The goal of treatment of erysipelas is rapid eradication of the infection. Mild to moderate cases of erysipelas are treated with intramuscular procaine penicillin G or penicillin VK for 7 to 10 days (see Table 119–4)[19,20] Penicillin-allergic patients can be treated with clindamycin or erythromycin. For more serious infections, the patient should be hospitalized and aqueous penicillin G 2 to 8 million units daily administered intravenously.[19,20] Marked improvement usually is seen within 48 hours, and the patient often may be switched to oral penicillin to complete the course of therapy. Although one study has shown that the median time for cure, intravenous antibiotics, and hospital stay was reduced in patients receiving prednisolone in addition to antibiotics, further studies are needed before corticosteroids can be recommended for routine use.[11,19]

EVALUATION OF THERAPEUTIC OUTCOMES

Erysipelas generally responds quickly to appropriate antimicrobial therapy. Temperature and white blood cell count should return to normal within 48 to 72 hours. Erythema, edema, and pain also should resolve gradually.

IMPETIGO

❸ Impetigo is a superficial skin infection that is seen most commonly in children.[21] The infection is generally classified as bullous or nonbullous based on clinical presentation.[4] Impetigo is most common during hot, humid weather, which facilitates microbial colonization of the skin.[19] Minor trauma, such as scratches or insect bites, allows entry of organisms into the superficial layers of skin, and infection ensues.[19] Impetigo is highly communicable and readily spreads through close contact, especially among siblings and children in daycare centers and schools.[19,20]

Although historically caused by *S. pyogenes*, *S. aureus* has also emerged as a principle cause of impetigo (either alone or in combination with *S. pyogenes*).[21] The bullous form is caused by strains of *S. aureus* capable of producing exfoliative toxins.[21] The bullous form most frequently affects neonates and accounts for approximately 10% of all cases of impetigo.[19,21]

CLINICAL PRESENTATION

General

- Exposed skin, especially the face, is the most common site for impetigo.

Symptoms

- Pruritus is common, and scratching of the lesions may further spread infection through excoriation of the skin.
- Other systemic signs of infection are minimal.
- Weakness, fever, and diarrhea sometimes are seen with bullous impetigo.

Signs

- Nonbullous impetigo manifests initially as small, fluid-filled vesicles.
- These lesions rapidly develop into pus-filled blisters that rupture readily.
- Purulent discharge from the lesions dries to form golden-yellow crusts that are characteristic of impetigo.

- In the bullous form of impetigo, the lesions begin as vesicles and turn into bullae containing clear yellow fluid.
- Bullae soon rupture, forming thin, light brown crusts.
- Regional lymph nodes may be enlarged.

Laboratory Tests

- Cultures should be collected.
- Crusted tops of lesions should be raised so that purulent material at the base of the lesion can be cultured.
- Cultures should not be collected from open, draining skin pustules because they may be colonized with staphylococci and other normal skin flora.

Other Diagnostic Tests

- A complete blood count is often performed because leukocytosis is common.

TREATMENT

Impetigo

Although impetigo may resolve spontaneously, antimicrobial treatment is indicated to relieve symptoms, prevent formation of new lesions, and prevent complications such as cellulitis. Penicillinase-resistant penicillins (such as dicloxacillin) are preferred for treatment because of the increased incidence of infections caused by *S. aureus*.[11] First-generation cephalosporins (such as cephalexin) are also commonly used. Penicillin, administered as a single intramuscular dose of benzathine penicillin G (300,000 to 600,000 units in children, 1.2 million units in adults) or as oral penicillin VK, is effective for infections known to be caused by *S. pyogenes*. Penicillin-allergic patients can be treated with clindamycin. The duration of therapy is 7 to 10 days. Topical therapy with mupirocin ointment or retapamulin ointment (applied three times daily or twice daily, respectively, for 7 days) is also effective for mild cases.[11] With proper treatment, healing of skin lesions generally is rapid and occurs without residual scarring. Removal of crusts by soaking in soap and warm water also may be helpful in providing symptomatic relief.[19,20]

EVALUATION OF THERAPEUTIC OUTCOMES

Clinical response should be seen within 7 days of initiating antimicrobial therapy for impetigo. Treatment failures could be a result of noncompliance or antimicrobial resistance. A followup culture of exudates should be collected for culture and sensitivity, with treatment modified accordingly.[21]

LYMPHANGITIS

❹ Acute lymphangitis is an inflammation involving the subcutaneous lymphatic channels. Lymphangitis usually occurs secondary to puncture wounds, infected blisters, or other skin lesions. Most infections are caused by *S. pyogenes*.[22]

CLINICAL PRESENTATION

General

- Lymphadenitis (acute or chronic inflammation of the lymph nodes) also may occur when microorganisms reach the lymph nodes and elicit an inflammatory response.

Symptoms

- Systemic manifestations of infection (i.e., fever, chills, malaise, and headache) often develop rapidly before any sign of infection is evident at the initial site of inoculation or even after the initial lesion has subsided.
- Systemic symptoms often are more profound than would be expected based on examination of the cutaneous lesion.

Signs

- Identification of a peripheral lesion associated with proximal red linear streaks directed toward the regional lymph nodes is diagnostic of acute lymphangitis.
- Lymph nodes usually are enlarged and tender.
- Peripheral edema of the involved extremity often is present.
- Thrombophlebitis and acute lymphangitis in the lower extremities may be confused because both are associated with red linear streaking and tender areas; however, in thrombophlebitis, no portal of entry is identifiable.

Laboratory Tests

- Cultures of the affected lesions often yield negative results because the infection resides within the lymphatic channels.
- Offending pathogens often can be identified by Gram stain of the initial lesion if done early in the course of the disease.

Other Diagnostic Tests

- A complete blood count frequently is performed because leukocytosis is common.

TREATMENT

Lymphangitis

The goal of therapy for lymphangitis is rapid eradication of infection and prevention of further systemic complications. Penicillin is the antibiotic of choice. Because these infections are potentially serious and rapidly progressive, initial treatment should be with intravenous penicillin G 1 to 2 million units every 4 to 6 hours. Parenteral treatment should be continued for 48 to 72 hours, followed by oral penicillin VK for a total of 10 days.[22] Nondrug therapy includes immobilization and elevation of the affected extremity and warm-water soaks every 2 to 4 hours.[22] For penicillin-allergic patients, clindamycin may be used.

EVALUATION OF THERAPEUTIC OUTCOMES

Lymphangitis usually responds rapidly to appropriate therapy; signs and symptoms often are decreased markedly or absent within 24 hours of starting antibiotics.

CELLULITIS

❺ Cellulitis is an acute infectious process that represents a serious type of SSTI. Cellulitis initially affects the epidermis and dermis and may spread subsequently within the superficial fascia. Cellulitis is considered a serious disease because of the propensity of the infection to spread through lymphatic tissue and to the bloodstream. *S. pyogenes* and *S. aureus* are the most frequent bacterial causes. However, many bacteria have been implicated in various types of cellulitis (see Table 119–1). Approximately 4 million patients were hospitalized for cellulitis between 1998 and 2006, representing 10% of all infection-related admissions.[23] The rising incidence of

infections caused by MRSA is a major concern in both the community and hospital settings.[6,7,9–15]

Injection-drug users are predisposed to a number of infectious complications, including abscess formation and cellulitis at the site of injection.[24] These SSTIs are located most frequently on the upper extremities and often are polymicrobic in nature.[25] Infecting organisms are believed to originate from the skin and/or oropharynx, as well as from contaminated needles, syringes, and diluents.[25] *S. aureus* is the most common pathogen isolated from these infections. The incidence of MRSA is also rising in SSTIs for injection-drug users.[26,27] Anaerobic bacteria, especially oropharyngeal anaerobes, are also found commonly, particularly in polymicrobic infections.[25] Outbreaks caused by *Clostridium* species have also been reported in injection-drug users, particularly as a consequence of injection of contaminated black-tar heroin.[28,29]

Acute cellulitis with mixed aerobic and anaerobic pathogens may occur in diabetics, following traumatic injuries, at sites of surgical incisions to the abdomen or perineum, or where host defenses have been otherwise compromised (vascular insufficiency). In older patients, cellulitis of the lower extremities also may be complicated by thrombophlebitis. Other complications of cellulitis include local abscess, osteomyelitis, and septic arthritis.[11,30]

CLINICAL PRESENTATION

General

- There is usually a history of an antecedent wound from a minor trauma, abrasion, ulcer, or surgery.
- Because these infections occur often for patients with alterations in host defense mechanisms, poor nutrition, or both, systemic findings such as hypotension, dehydration, and altered mental status are common.

Symptoms

- Patients often experience fever, chills, or malaise and complain that the affected area feels hot and painful.

Signs

- Cellulitis is characterized by erythema and edema of the skin.
- Lesions, which may be extensive, are nonelevated and have poorly defined margins.
- Affected areas generally are warm to touch.
- Inflammation generally is present with little or no necrosis or suppuration of soft tissue.
- Tender lymphadenopathy associated with lymphatic involvement is common.

Laboratory Tests

- Cultures should be collected when possible.
- A Gram stain of fluid obtained by injection and aspiration of 0.5 mL of saline (using a small 22-gauge needle) into the advancing edge of the lesion may aid the microbiologic diagnosis but often yields negative results.
- Diagnosis usually is made on clinical grounds, that is, the appearance of the lesion.

Other Diagnostic Tests

- A complete blood count frequently is performed because leukocytosis is common.
- Because bacteremia may be present in as many as 30% of cases of cellulitis, blood cultures may be useful for diagnosis of some patients.

TREATMENT

Cellulitis

The goal of therapy of acute bacterial cellulitis is rapid eradication of the infection and prevention of further complications. Antimicrobial therapy is directed against the type of bacteria either documented or suspected to be present based on the clinical presentation. Local care of cellulitis includes elevation and immobilization of the involved area to decrease swelling. Cool sterile saline dressings may decrease pain and can be followed later with moist heat to aid in localization of the cellulitis. Surgical intervention (incision and drainage) as a mode of therapy is rarely indicated in the treatment of uncomplicated cellulitis. The use of inappropriate antibiotic therapy for cellulitis is associated with significantly higher risk of clinical treatment failures.[30] Therefore, in the selection of antibiotics for treatment of cellulitis, particular attention must be paid to patients with risk factors for more atypical or resistant bacterial pathogens (e.g., gram-negative bacteria, anaerobes, MRSA).

Because staphylococcal and streptococcal cellulitis are indistinguishable clinically,[1,20] administration of a penicillinase-resistant penicillin (nafcillin or oxacillin) or first-generation cephalosporin (cefazolin) is recommended until a definitive diagnosis, by skin or blood cultures, can be made (Table 119–5).[2,11,19,20,30] Mild to moderate infections not associated with systemic symptoms may

TABLE 119-5	Initial Treatment Regimens for Cellulitis Caused by Various Pathogens	
Antibiotic	**Adult Dose and Route**	**Pediatric Dose and Route**
Staphylococcal or unknown gram-positive infection		
Mild infection	Dicloxacillin 0.25–0.5 g orally every 6 h[a,b]	Dicloxacillin 25–50 mg/kg/day orally in four divided doses[a,b]
Mild infection· suspected CA-MRSA	Trimethoprim-sulfamethoxazole 80 mg/160 mg orally every 8–12 h Doxycycline 100 mg orally every 12 h	Trimethoprim-sulfamethoxazole 4 mg/kg (trimethoprim component) orally every 8–12 h
Moderate to severe infection	Nafcillin or oxacillin 1–2 g IV every 4–6 h[a,b]	Nafcillin or oxacillin 150–200 mg/kg/day (not to exceed 12 g/24 h) IV in four to six equally divided doses[a,b]
Streptococcal (documented)		
Mild infection	Penicillin VK 0.5 g orally every 6 h[a] or procaine penicillin G 600,000 units IM every 8–12 h[a]	Penicillin VK 125–250 mg orally every 6–8 h, or procaine penicillin G 25,000–50,000 units/kg (not to exceed 600,000 units) IM every 8–12 h[a]
Moderate to severe infection	Aqueous penicillin G 1–2 million units IV every 4–6 h[a,c]	Aqueous penicillin G 100,000–200,000 units/kg/day IV in four divided doses[a]
Gram-negative bacilli		
Mild infection	Cefaclor 0.5 g orally every 8 h[d] or cefuroxime axetil 0.5 g orally every 12 h[d]	Cefaclor 20–40 mg/kg/day (not to exceed 1 g) orally in three divided doses or cefuroxime axetil 0.125–0.25 g (tablets) orally every 12 h
Moderate to severe infection	Aminoglycoside[e] or IV cephalosporin (first-or second-generation depending on severity of infection or susceptibility pattern)[d]	Aminoglycoside[e] or intravenous cephalosporin (first- or second-generation depending on severity of infection or susceptibility pattern)
Polymicrobic infection without anaerobes		
	Aminoglycoside[e] + penicillin G 1–2 million units every 4–6 h or a semisynthetic penicillin (nafcillin 1–2 g every 4–6 h) depending on isolation of staphylococci or streptococci[b]	Aminoglycoside[e] + penicillin G 100,000–200,000 units/kg/day IV in four divided doses or a semisynthetic penicillin [nafcillin 150–200 mg/kg/day (not to exceed 12 g/24 h)] IV in four to six equally divided doses] depending on isolation of staphylococci or streptococci[b]
Polymicrobic infection with anaerobes		
Mild infection	Amoxicillin/clavulanate 0.875 g orally every 12 h or a fluoroquinolone (ciprofloxacin 0.4 g orally every 12 h or levofloxacin 0.5–0.75 g orally every 24 h) plus clindamycin 0.3–0.6 g orally every 8 h or metronidazole 0.5 g orally every 8 h	Amoxicillin/clavulanic acid 20 mg/kg/day orally in three divided doses
Moderate to severe infection	Aminoglycoside[e,f] + clindamycin 0.6–0.9 g IV every 8 h or metronidazole 0.5 g IV every 8 h	Aminoglycoside[e] plus clindamycin 15 mg/kg/day IV in three divided doses or metronidazole 30–50 mg/kg/day IV in three divided doses
	Or Monotherapy with second- or third-generation cephalosporin (cefoxitin 1–2 g IV every 6 h or ceftizoxime 1–2 g IV every 8 h) Or Monotherapy with imipenem 0.5 g IV every 6–8 h, meropenem 1 g IV every 8 h, ertapenem 1 g IV every 24 h, doripenem 0.5 g every 8 h, extended-spectrum penicillins with a β-lactamase inhibitor (piperacillin/tazobactam 4.5 g IV every 6 h), or tigecycline 100 mg IV as loading dose, then 50 mg IV every 12 h	

IM, intramuscularly; IV, intravenous; CA-MRSA, community-associated methicillin-resistant *Staphylococcus aureus*.
[a]For penicillin-allergic patients, use clindamycin 150–300 mg orally every 6–8 h (pediatric dosing: 10–30 mg/kg/day in three to four divided doses).
[b]For methicillin-resistant staphylococci, use vancomycin 0.5–1 g orally every 6–12 h (pediatric dosing 40 mg/kg/day in divided doses) with dosage adjustments made for renal dysfunction.
[c]For type II necrotizing fasciitis, use clindamycin 0.6–0.9 g IV every 8 h (in children, clindamycin 15 mg/kg/day IV in 3 divided doses).
[d]For penicillin-allergic adults, use a fluoroquinolone (ciprofloxacin 0.5–0.75 g orally every 12 h or 0.4 g IV every 12 h; levofloxacin 0.5–0.75 g orally or IV every 24 h; or moxifloxacin 0.4 g orally or IV every 24 h).
[e]Gentamicin or tobramycin, 2 mg/kg loading dose, then maintenance dose as determined by serum concentrations.
[f]A fluoroquinolone or aztreonam 1 g IV every 6 h may be used in place of the aminoglycoside in patients with severe renal dysfunction or other relative contraindications to aminoglycoside use.

be treated orally with dicloxacillin or cephalexin. Other oral cephalosporins, such as cefadroxil, cefaclor, cefprozil, cefpodoxime proxetil, and cefdinir, are also effective in the treatment of cellulitis but are more expensive.[11,20,30] If documented to be a mild cellulitis secondary to streptococci, oral penicillin VK or intramuscular procaine penicillin may be administered. More severe infections, either staphylococcal or streptococcal, should be treated initially with intravenous antibiotic regimens. Ceftriaxone 50 to 100 mg/kg as a single daily dose is efficacious in the treatment of cellulitis in pediatric patients.[31] The usual duration of therapy for cellulitis is 5 to 10 days.[11,19,30]

In penicillin-allergic patients, oral or parenteral clindamycin may be used.[1,2] Alternatively, a first-generation cephalosporin may be used cautiously for patients without a history of immediate or anaphylactic reactions to penicillin. In severe cases in which cephalosporins can not be used because of suspected and/or documented MRSA or severe β-lactam allergies, vancomycin should be administered.[2,11]

Infection with CA-MRSA should be considered for patients with skin abscesses, subjective history of insect bites, or more severe infections.[30,32] Appropriate clinical specimens for culture and susceptibility testing should be collected whenever possible for such patients.[30,32] Incision and drainage is the primary therapy for CA-MRSA infections such as furuncles and small abscesses in otherwise uncomplicated patients with mild infections, and systemic antibiotic therapy is often unnecessary in such cases. Antibiotic therapy should be added to incision and drainage for patients with more complicated cases such as rapidly progressive infection; abscesses in association with more severe cellulitis; signs and symptoms of systemic illness; complicating factors such as extreme age, comorbidities, or immunosuppression; or lack of response to previous drainage alone.[30,32-35]

Although the most optimal treatment for CA-MRSA infections is not known, initial therapy with trimethoprim-sulfamethoxazole, doxycycline, or clindamycin appears to be effective in most cases and should be considered in geographic areas in which CA-MRSA infections are commonly encountered.[9,13,14,32-35] Hospital-acquired strains of MRSA tend to be more antibiotic resistant and vancomycin is a more appropriate choice for initial treatment of patients in whom hospital-acquired MRSA is a suspected or documented pathogen. Alternative agents for infections with resistant gram-positive bacteria such as MRSA and vancomycin-resistant enterococci include linezolid, quinupristin-dalfopristin, daptomycin, tigecycline, and telavancin.[1,2,32-39] The excellent activity of these drugs against resistant gram-positive pathogens but significantly higher cost make them most appropriate for treatment of complicated or refractory infections, or those documented as caused by multidrug-resistant pathogens, rather than as initial therapy. The availability of orally administered linezolid may provide a cost-effective "step-down" option for many patients with more complicated infections and/or those patients who require initial hospitalization as an alternative to prolonged treatment with parenteral agents.[40] Tigecycline may be considered in complicated infections, particularly those in which the presence of mixed gram-negative and/or anaerobic pathogens is suspected or documented alongside resistant gram-positive bacteria.[38,39]

CLINICAL CONTROVERSY

Because numerous studies have documented the increasing prevalence of CA-MRSA, there is considerable debate regarding the optimal treatment recommendations for empiric antimicrobial therapy of SSTIs.[9,13,14,32-35]

Trimethoprim-sulfamethoxazole has excellent in vitro activity against CA-MRSA, but few clinical trials have been published that correlate susceptibility data with clinical outcomes. Another concern is the lack of activity of trimethoprim-sulfamethoxazole against *S. pyogenes*, another organism commonly found in SSTIs. The combination of trimethoprim-sulfamethoxazole plus a β-lactam antibiotic has been suggested when empiric therapy is needed for coverage of both organisms, but there are no data confirming that combination therapy improves outcomes.[9,13,14,32-35] Doxycycline has activity against both *S. aureus* and *S. pyogenes,* but only limited data suggests efficacy for SSTIs caused by CA-MRSA.[41,42] The optimal role of doxycycline relative to trimethoprim-sulfamethoxazole remains unclear. Clindamycin is often active against CA-MRSA, but there is concern of inducible clindamycin resistance during therapy, and the role of this agent is still not well-defined.[9,13,14,32-35]

The carbapenems (i.e., imipenem, meropenem, ertapenem, and doripenem) and the β-lactam–β-lactamase inhibitor combination antibiotics (ampicillin-sulbactam, ticarcillin-clavulanic acid, and piperacillin-tazobactam) appear to be equivalent to standard therapies for adults.[1,2,11,43] However, the greater cost of these newer agents without increased efficacy compared with other reliable regimens, particularly given the increasing problem of MRSA, makes them less desirable for empiric therapy.[1,2,11]

For cellulitis caused by gram-negative bacilli or a mixture of microorganisms, immediate antimicrobial chemotherapy, as determined by Gram stain, is essential (see Table 119-5). Surgical debridement of necrotic tissue and drainage also may be appropriate. Gram-negative cellulitis may be treated appropriately with an aminoglycoside (such as gentamicin or tobramycin), or first- or second-generation cephalosporin (such as cephalexin or cefaclor/cefuroxime, respectively). If gram-positive aerobic bacteria are also present, penicillin G or a penicillinase-resistant penicillin should be added to the regimen. Ceftazidime and the fluoroquinolones are effective in the treatment of cellulitis caused by both gram-negative and gram-positive bacteria.[1,2,11,43]

CLINICAL CONTROVERSY

Fluoroquinolones are attractive options for SSTIs due to a broad spectrum of activity and availability of highly bioavailable oral agents. They also have demonstrated efficacy similar to parenteral β-lactam antibiotics in the treatment of SSTIs, including diabetic foot infections.[1,11,18,43] Lower eradication rates for streptococci have been reported with fluoroquinolones when compared with cephalexin and other agents in the treatment of uncomplicated SSTIs.[1,11,44] Levofloxacin and moxifloxacin are approved by the Food and Drug Administration for both uncomplicated and complicated SSTIs. However, the use of fluoroquinolones is of concern because of increasing resistance among both gram-positive and gram-negative bacteria.[1,11,45,46] Despite potential in vitro susceptibility, the optimal role of the fluoroquinolones for treatment of MRSA infections is not well-defined and they are not routinely recommended due to inconsistent efficacy and concerns regarding resistance.[9,11,13,14,32-35] Also, fluoroquinolones are not approved for use in children because of toxicity concerns.

Because some infections may be polymicrobic, antibiotic therapy may need to be broadened to include agents with good activity against anaerobic bacteria. Many different treatment regimens are possible depending on the bacteriology of the lesion (see Table 119–5). Usually an aminoglycoside combined with an antianaerobic cephalosporin (such as cefoxitin or ceftizoxime), extended-spectrum penicillin (such as piperacillin), or clindamycin is used. Second- or third-generation cephalosporins (such as cefaclor/cefuroxime or ceftizoxime, respectively) have been suggested as single-agent therapy in certain instances.[1,2,11] Monotherapy with a β-lactam plus β-lactamase inhibitor combination antibiotic (such as piperacillin-tazobactam) or a carbapenem (such as imipenem or ertapenem) also may be appropriate for seriously ill patients.[1,2,11] Therapy should be 10 to 14 days in duration.

Because gram-negative and mixed aerobic–anaerobic cellulitis can progress quickly to serious tissue invasion, therapeutic intervention should be immediate. If treated early, a rapid response can be seen. Unfortunately, because these infections often occur for patients with compromised immune defenses, they may still progress, even with therapeutic intervention. If the infectious process is secondary to a systemic cause (e.g., diabetes), the treatment course often is prolonged and may be associated with high morbidity and mortality.

Infections in injection-drug users generally are treated similarly to those in other types of patients.[11,12,25] It is important that blood cultures be obtained in these cases because 25% to 35% of patients may be bacteremic.[1,11,25] Also, patients should be assessed for the presence of abscesses; incision, drainage, and culture of these lesions are of extreme importance.[11] Initial antimicrobial therapy while awaiting culture results of abscesses should include broad coverage for gram-negative and anaerobic organisms, in addition to *S. aureus* (including MRSA in areas with high prevalence) and streptococci.[1,2,11,25]

EVALUATION OF THERAPEUTIC OUTCOMES

If treated promptly with appropriate antibiotics, the majority of patients with cellulitis are cured rapidly. Culture and sensitivity results should be evaluated carefully both for the adequacy of culture material and the presence of resistant organisms. Additional high-quality samples for culture may be needed for microbiologic analysis. Failure to respond to therapy also may be indicative of an underlying local or systemic problem or a misdiagnosis.

NECROTIZING SOFT-TISSUE INFECTIONS

Necrotizing soft-tissue infections consist of a group of highly lethal infections that require early and aggressive surgical debridement in addition to appropriate antibiotics and intensive supportive care.[47–49] A number of different terms have been used to classify necrotizing infections based on factors such as predisposing conditions, onset of symptoms, pain, skin appearance, etiologic agent, gas production, muscle involvement, and systemic toxicity. While many types of necrotizing soft-tissue infections have been designated as unique infectious processes, they all share similar pathophysiologies, clinical features, and treatment approaches.[47–49] The major clinical entities of necrotizing infections are *necrotizing fasciitis* and *clostridial myonecrosis* (gas gangrene).[47,48]

❻ Necrotizing fasciitis is a rare but very severe infection of the subcutaneous tissue that may be caused by aerobic and/or anaerobic bacteria and results in progressive destruction of the superficial fascia and subcutaneous fat. It is generally characterized as one of two different types based on bacterial etiology. Type I necrotizing fasciitis generally occurs after trauma

and surgery and involves a mixture of anaerobes (*Bacteroides, Peptostreptococcus*) and facultative bacteria (streptococci and members of Enterobacteriaceae) that act synergistically to cause destruction of fat and fascia. Type I necrotizing fasciitis is also being reported more commonly among injection-drug users.[47–49] In type I infections, the skin may be spared, and the speed at which the infection spreads is somewhat slower than type II. Necrotizing fasciitis affecting the male genitalia is termed *Fournier gangrene*. Type II necrotizing fasciitis is caused by virulent strains of *S. pyogenes* and is more commonly referred to as *streptococcal gangrene*. This type of infection has often been called *flesh-eating bacteria* by the lay press. Unlike previous reports of streptococcal gangrene that affected older individuals with underlying diseases, recent reports have occurred primarily in young, previously healthy adults following some type of minor trauma. It differs from the polymicrobial type I infections in its clinical presentation. Type II infections have rapidly extending necrosis of subcutaneous tissues and skin, gangrene, severe local pain, and systemic toxicity.[20,47,48] Type II infections are also highly associated with an early onset of shock and organ failure and are present in approximately half the cases of streptococcal toxic shock-like syndrome.[20]

Clostridial myonecrosis is a necrotizing infection that involves the skeletal muscle. Gas production and muscle necrosis are prominent features of this infection, which readily explains why this infection is commonly referred to as *gas gangrene*.[47,48] The infection advances rapidly, often over a matter of a few hours.[47,48] Most infections occur after surgery or trauma, with *Clostridium perfringens* identified as the most common etiologic agent.

CLINICAL PRESENTATION

General

☐ These infections may occur in almost any anatomic location but most frequently involve the abdomen, the perineum, and the lower extremities.

☐ Patients often have predisposing factors such as diabetes mellitus, local trauma or infection, or recent surgery.

Symptoms

☐ Systemic symptoms generally are marked (e.g., fever, chills, and leukocytosis) and may include shock and organ failure, especially for patients with type II infections.

☐ In general, pain in the affected area and systemic toxicity are more pronounced than would be expected with cellulitis.

Signs

☐ At the beginning of an infection, it may be difficult to differentiate between necrotizing fasciitis and cellulitis.

☐ Like cellulitis, the affected area is initially hot, swollen, and erythematous without sharp margins.

☐ The affected area is often shiny, exquisitely tender, and painful.

☐ Diffuse swelling of the area is followed by the appearance of bullae filled with clear fluid.

☐ The infectious process progresses rapidly, with the skin taking on a maroon or violaceous color after several days.

☐ Without appropriate intervention, the infection will evolve rapidly into a frank cutaneous gangrene, sometimes with myonecrosis (involvement of skin and muscle).

☐ Because of the aggressive nature and high mortality (20% to 50%) associated with these infections, a rapid diagnosis is critical.

Laboratory Tests

▪ Although computed tomography and magnetic resonance imaging studies can distinguish these infections, the best and most rapid diagnosis of necrotizing infections is obtained via surgical exploration.

▪ Intraoperative samples should be collected for culture and sensitivity, as well as for histologic examination.

▪ Unlike necrotizing fasciitis, clostridial myonecrosis shows little inflammation on histologic examination.

Other Diagnostic Tests

▪ Because marked systemic symptoms are seen commonly in necrotizing infections, blood samples should be collected for complete blood count and chemistry profile, as well as for bacterial culture.

TREATMENT

Necrotizing Soft-Tissue Infections

After the diagnosis is made, immediate and aggressive surgical debridement of all necrotic tissue is essential.[47-49] Initial surgical debridement performed greater than 14 hours after the diagnosis of necrotizing infection was independently associated with increased patient mortality, including a 34-fold increased risk of death for patients with septic shock.[50] Patients often require further surgical intervention following initial debridement to ensure that all necrotic tissue has been removed.[2,11,47-50] Broad-spectrum antibiotics must include coverage against streptococci, Enterobacteriaceae, and anaerobes. A number of antibiotic regimens have been used to successfully treat necrotizing soft-tissue infections; these are generally similar to those used for severe polymicrobic cellulitis involving anaerobes (see Table 119-5). Other combination antibiotic regimens that may be used empirically include ampicillin with gentamicin and clindamycin (or metronidazole), ampicillin-sulbactam with gentamicin, and imipenem with metronidazole.[19,47-49]

Antibiotic therapy can be modified after Gram stain and culture reports are available. If a diagnosis of type II necrotizing fasciitis is established, broad-spectrum empirical therapy should be replaced with the combination of penicillin and clindamycin.[20] Although *S. pyogenes* remains susceptible to penicillin, clindamycin is more effective.[20] A number of factors have been postulated to explain the greater efficacy of clindamycin, including the mechanism of action (inhibition of protein synthesis), which may cause decreased production of bacterial exotoxins.[20,47-49] In addition, clindamycin has immunomodulatory properties that may account for the higher efficacy.[20] The combination of penicillin and clindamycin is also recommended for treatment of clostridial myonecrosis.[11,47,48] Hyperbaric oxygen also may be of some benefit for clostridial myonecrosis.[47,48,51]

EVALUATION OF THERAPEUTIC OUTCOMES

Because of the high mortality associated with necrotizing infections, rapid and complete debridement of all devitalized and necrotic tissue is essential. Surgical debridement, coupled with appropriate antimicrobial therapy and supportive measures for management of shock and organ failure, should stabilize the patient. Vital signs and laboratory tests should be monitored carefully for signs of resolution of the infection. Change in antimicrobial therapy or additional surgical debridement may be needed for patients who do not show signs of improvement.

DIABETIC FOOT INFECTIONS

Three major types of foot infections are seen in diabetic patients: deep abscesses, cellulitis of the dorsum, and mal perforans ulcers.[52-55] Most deep abscesses involve the central plantar space (arch) and are caused by minor penetrating trauma or by an extension of infection of a nail or web space of the toes. Infections of the dorsal area generally arise from infections in the toes that are related to routine care of the nails, nail beds, and calluses of the toes. Mal perforans ulcer is a chronic ulcer of the sole of the foot. The ulcer develops on thickened, hardened calluses over the first or fifth metatarsal. Mal perforans ulcers are associated with neuropathy, which is responsible for the misalignment of the weight-bearing bones of the foot.[52-55] Osteomyelitis is one of the most serious complications of foot problems in diabetic patients and may occur in 30% to 40% of infections.[18,52-55]

EPIDEMIOLOGY

Infections of the foot are among the most common complications of diabetes, accounting for as many as 20% of all hospitalizations of diabetic patients at an annual cost of $200 to $350 million.[18,52-55] Approximately 25% of diabetic patients experience significant soft-tissue infection at some time during their lifetime. Approximately 55,000 lower-extremity amputations, often sequelae of uncontrolled infection, are performed each year on diabetic patients; this represents 50% of all nontraumatic amputations in the United States.[52-54] Between 10% and 20% of diabetics will undergo additional surgery or amputation of a second limb within 12 months of the initial amputation.[52-54] By 5 years, this increases to 25% to 50%, with death reported in as much as two thirds of patients.[52-54]

ETIOLOGY

Diabetic foot infections begin with local bacterial invasion and are typically polymicrobic in nature, with an average of 2.3 to 5.8 isolates per culture (Table 119-6).[18,52-59] Staphylococci (especially *S. aureus*) and streptococci are the most common pathogens, although gram-negative bacilli and/or anaerobes occur in approximately 50% of cases.[18,54-59] Common gram-negative isolates include *E. coli*,

TABLE 119-6 Bacterial Isolates from Foot Infections in Diabetic Patients

Organisms	Percentage of Isolates
Aerobes	63–75%
Gram-positive	42–64%
Staphylococcus aureus	15–20%
Streptococcus spp.	6–12%
Enterococcus spp.	7–20%
Coagulase-negative staphylococci	6–10%
Other gram-positive aerobes	0–12%
Gram-negative	16–18%
Proteus spp.	5–6%
Enterobacter spp.	1–2%
Escherichia coli	3–5%
Klebsiella spp.	1–2%
Pseudomonas aeruginosa	1–3%
Other gram-negative bacilli	3–8%
Anaerobes	25–40%
Peptostreptococcus spp.	8–12%
Bacteroides fragilis group	4–7%
Other *Bacteroides* spp.	3–6%
Clostridium spp.	0–2%
Other anaerobes	7–10%

Compiled from references 18, 62, 65.

Klebsiella spp., *Proteus* spp., and *P. aeruginosa. Bacteroides fragilis* and *Peptostreptococcus* spp. are among the most common anaerobes isolated. Methicillin-resistant *S. aureus* has been reported in up to 30% of diabetic foot wounds.[60] However, whether MRSA is associated with worse patient outcomes is still somewhat controversial, and the clinical relevance of MRSA in this setting is not clear.[57]

The optimum technique for obtaining culture material from ulcerated lesions is still debated.[52–56] Routine swab cultures of ulcerative lesions or sinus tracts are difficult to interpret because of organisms that colonize the wounds. The correlation between superficial cultures and true deep cultures (via biopsy or needle aspiration of drainage or abscess fluid) is often poor, particularly in chronic lesions.[18,54–56] Therefore, cultures and sensitivity tests should be done with specimens obtained from a deep culture whenever possible. Before the wound is cultured, it should be scrubbed vigorously with saline-moistened sterile gauze to remove any overlying necrotic debris.[18,54–56] Cultures then can be obtained from the wound base, preferably from expressed pus.[54–56] Specimens obtained from curettage of the base of the ulcer correlate best with results from deep-tissue or bone biopsies.[61–63]

PATHOPHYSIOLOGY

Three key factors are involved in the development of diabetic foot problems:

1. Neuropathy
2. Angiopathy and ischemia
3. Immunologic defects

Any of these disorders can occur in isolation; however, they frequently occur together.

Neuropathic changes to the autonomic nervous system as a consequence of diabetes may affect the motor nerve supply of small intrinsic muscles of the foot, resulting in muscular imbalance, abnormal stresses on tissues and bone, and repetitive injuries.[52–54] Diminished sensory perception causes an absence of pain and unawareness of minor injuries and ulceration. The sympathetic nerve supply may be damaged, resulting in an absence of sweating, which may lead to dry cracked skin and secondary infection.[18,52–54]

Atherosclerosis is more common, appears at a younger age, and progresses more rapidly in the diabetic than in the nondiabetic. Diabetics may have problems with both small vessels (microangiopathy) and large vessels (macroangiopathy) that can result in varying degrees of ischemia, ultimately leading to skin breakdown and infection.

Diabetic patients typically have normal humoral immunity, normal levels of immunoglobulins, and normal antibody responses. Patients with diabetes, however, have impaired phagocytosis and intracellular microbicidal function as compared with nondiabetics; this may be related to angiopathy and low tissue levels of oxygen.[18,52,53] These defects in cell-mediated immunity make patients with diabetes more susceptible to certain types of infection and impair the patients' ability to heal wounds adequately.[52–54,57]

CLINICAL PRESENTATION

General

- Infections are often much more extensive than they appear initially.

Symptoms

- Patients with peripheral neuropathy often do not experience pain but seek medical care for swelling or erythema in the foot.

Signs

- Clinical signs of infection in the diabetic foot may not be present secondary to the angiopathy and neuropathy.
- When present, lesions vary in size and clinical features (e.g., erythema, edema, warmth, presence of pus, draining sinuses, pain, and tenderness).
- A foul-smelling odor suggests the presence of anaerobic organisms.
- Temperature may be mildly elevated or normal.

Laboratory Tests

- Specimens for culture and sensitivities should be collected.
- If possible, deep intraoperative samples should be obtained during surgical debridement.
- Because of the complex microbiology of these infections, wounds must be cultured for both aerobic and anaerobic organisms.

Other Diagnostic Tests

- The presence of osteomyelitis also must be assessed via radiograph, bone scan, or both, as appropriate.

TREATMENT

Diabetic Foot Infections

❼ The goal of therapy of diabetic foot infections is preservation of as much normal limb function as possible while preventing additional infectious complications. Up to 90% of infections can be treated successfully with a comprehensive treatment approach that includes both wound care and antimicrobial therapy.[18,57–59] After carefully assessing the extent of the lesion and obtaining necessary cultures, necrotic tissue must be thoroughly debrided, with wound drainage and amputation as required. Wounds must be kept clean and dressings changed frequently (two to three times daily). Because of the relationship between hyperglycemia and immune system defects, glycemic control must be maximized to ensure optimal wound healing. In addition, the patient's activities should be restricted initially to bedrest for leg elevation and control of edema, if present. Adequate pressure relief from a foot wound (i.e., off-loading) is crucial to the healing process.[18,64] Finally, appropriate antimicrobials must be initiated.[18,54–59] However, the optimal antimicrobial therapy for diabetic foot infections has yet to be defined. Empirical therapy that is totally comprehensive in its coverage of all possible pathogens does not seem to be necessary unless the infection is life or limb threatening.[18,57–59] This is particularly true regarding MRSA and *P. aeruginosa*, the perceived need for coverage of these organisms often leading to use of broad-spectrum drug regimens. One comparative study showed good efficacy rates despite that fact that neither agent (ertapenem and piperacillin-tazobactam) had consistently good activity against these organisms.[65]

The majority of mild, uncomplicated infections can be managed successfully on an outpatient basis with oral antimicrobials and good wound care. Many different agents have been studied, including cephalosporins, fluoroquinolones, clindamycin, and amoxicillin-clavulanic acid, and provide clinical cure rates of 60% to 85%.[18,54–59] However, significant failure and/or relapse rates have been reported with the use of oral agents. In addition, the development of resistance was problematic in some infections involving *P. aeruginosa* and staphylococci.[18,57] Many clinicians consider amoxicillin-clavulanic acid to be the preferred agent because of its broad spectrum of activity, which includes staphylococci, streptococci, enterococci, and many Enterobacteriaceae and anaerobes.[18,57-59] However, this agent does not have activity against *P. aeruginosa*. Fluoroquinolones, which provide coverage against *P. aeruginosa*, have been studied extensively as monotherapy but are perhaps most appropriately used in combination with metronidazole or clindamycin to provide anaerobic activity.[2,18,57] Oral antimicrobials should be used cautiously in serious infections, especially those complicated by osteomyelitis, extensive ulceration, areas of necrosis, or a combination of these. The use of topical antimicrobials, including medical-grade honey, has been advocated for the treatment of diabetic foot infections in an attempt to minimize the cost of therapy and systemic antibiotic exposure leading to adverse effects and resistance. However, use of topical agents is quite controversial and not routinely recommended outside of the treatment of infected burn wounds.[66,67]

Initial therapy for patients requiring hospitalization for moderate to severe infections is similar to that for polymicrobic cellulitis with anaerobes (see Table 119–5). Monotherapy with broad-spectrum parenteral antimicrobials, along with appropriate medical or surgical management, or both, is often effective in treating these infections, including those in which osteomyelitis is present.[18,57-59,63] Monotherapy is particularly attractive because of the potential advantages of convenience, cost, and avoidance of toxicities. Microbiological and clinical cure rates ranging from 60% to 90% may be expected from any of these agents; selection of a specific regimen is determined primarily by cost. In penicillin-allergic patients, metronidazole or clindamycin plus either a fluoroquinolone, aztreonam or possibly a third-generation cephalosporin is appropriate.[2,18,57-59] Vancomycin also is used frequently in severe infections because of its excellent activity against gram-positive pathogens. With the increased incidence of MRSA, linezolid, quinupristin-dalfopristin, daptomycin, and tigecycline are alternatives for treatment of this pathogen.[1,2,18,57-59] Tigecycline may be particularly useful in this setting because of its activity against gram-negative aerobes and anaerobic bacteria, thus allowing it to be used as monotherapy for the treatment of mixed infections. Because many patients already have some degree of diabetic nephropathy that may place them at higher risk of nephrotoxicity, strong recommendations have been made against the use of aminoglycoside antibiotics unless no alternative agents are available.[18,57] When an aminoglycoside is used, care must be taken to avoid further compromising renal function. All antibiotic regimens should be adjusted as necessary for renal dysfunction.

Mild to moderate infections can be treated with highly bioavailable oral agents. Duration of therapy is usually 7 to 14 days, although some infections may require an additional 1 to 2 weeks of therapy. More severe infections require initial parenteral therapy. Duration of therapy for most moderate to severe infections ranges from 2 to 4 weeks.[18,57] In cases of underlying osteomyelitis, treatment should continue for 6 to 12 weeks.[18,57-59,63] After healing of the infection has occurred, a well-designed program for prevention of further infections should be instituted. The use of adjunctive agents such as colony stimulating factors and hyperbaric oxygen for either prevention or treatment of diabetic foot infections are controversial and not widely recommended.[68,69]

EVALUATION OF THERAPEUTIC OUTCOMES

Therapy should be reevaluated carefully after 48 to 72 hours to assess favorable response. Change in therapy (or route of administration, if oral) should be considered if clinical improvement is not observed at this time. For optimal results, drug therapy should be appropriately modified according to information from deep-tissue culture and the clinical condition of the patient. Infections in diabetic patients often require extended courses of therapy because of impaired host immunity and poor wound healing.

TABLE 119-7	Pressure Sore Classification
Suspected deep tissue injury	Area of discolored intact skin or blood-filled blister due to damage of underlying soft tissue from pressure and/or shear. Area may be preceded by tissue that is painful, firm, mushy, boggy, warmer, or cooler as compared with adjacent tissue.
Stage 1	Pressure sore is generally reversible, is limited to the epidermis, and resembles an abrasion. Intact skin with nonblanchable redness of a localized area, usually over a bony prominence. The area may be painful, firm, soft, warmer, or cooler as compared with adjacent tissue.
Stage 2	A stage 2 sore also may be reversible; partial thickness loss of dermis presenting as a shallow open ulcer with a red pink wound bed. May also present as an intact or open/ruptured serum-filled blister or as a shiny or dry shallow ulcer.
Stage 3[a]	Full thickness tissue loss. Subcutaneous fat may be visible, but bone, tendon, or muscles are not exposed. May include undermining and tunneling. Depth of the ulcer varies by anatomical location; may range from shallow to extremely deep over areas of significant adiposity.
Stage 4[a]	Full thickness tissue loss with exposed bone, tendon, or muscle; can extend into muscle and/or supporting structures (e.g., fascia, tendon, or joint capsule) making osteomyelitis possible. Often include undermining and tunneling; depth of the ulcer varies by anatomical location.
Unstageable[a]	Full thickness tissue loss in which the base of the ulcer is covered by slough (yellow, tan, gray, green, or brown) and/or eschar (tan, brown, or black) in the wound bed. True depth, and therefore stage, cannot be determined.

[a]Stage 3, Stage 4, and unstageable lesions are unlikely to resolve on their own and often require surgical intervention.
From reference 70.

PRESSURE SORES

The terms *decubitus ulcer, bed sore,* and *pressure sore* are used interchangeably. The decubitus ulcer and the bed sore are types of pressure sores. The term *decubitus ulcer* is derived from the Latin word *decumbere,* meaning "lying down." Pressure sores, however, can develop regardless of a patient's position.

Numerous systems for classification of pressure sores have been described. The 2007 recommendations of the National Pressure Ulcer Advisory Panel are shown in Table 119–7 and illustrate the various stages of progression through which a pressure sore may pass.[70]

Complications of pressure sores are not uncommon and may be life threatening. Infection is one of the most serious and most frequently encountered complications of pressure ulcers. Bacterial colonization must be differentiated from true bacterial infection. Although most pressure sore wounds are colonized, the majority of these eventually heal.[71-75] When the tissue is infected, there is bacterial invasion of previously healthy tissue. Without treatment, an initial small, localized area of ulceration can rapidly progress to large ulcers within days. The visible ulcer is just a small portion of the actual wound; up to 70% of the total wound is below the skin. A pressure-gradient phenomenon is created by which the wound takes on a conical nature; the smallest point is at the skin surface, and the largest portion of the defect is at the base of the ulcer (Fig. 119–1).

EPIDEMIOLOGY

Pressure sores are most common among chronically debilitated persons, the elderly, and persons with serious spinal cord injury.

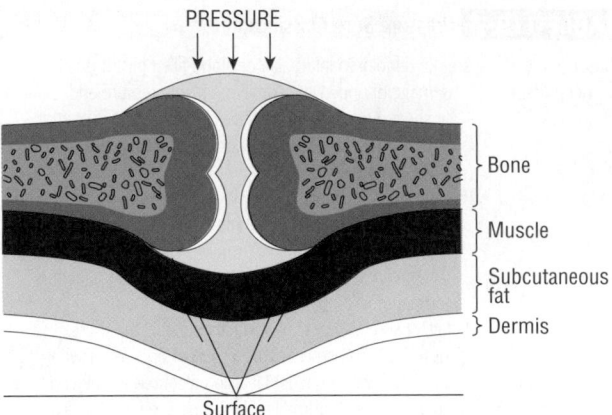

FIGURE 119-1. Distribution of forces involved with sore formation in a conical fashion.

Generally, patients who are at risk for pressure sores are elderly or chronically ill young patients who are immobilized, either in bed or a wheelchair, and who may have altered mental status and/or incontinence.

ETIOLOGY

Similar to diabetic foot infections, a large variety of aerobic gram-positive and gram-negative organisms, as well as anaerobes, frequently are isolated from wound cultures.[73] Curettage of the ulcer base after debridement provides more reliable culture information than does needle aspiration.[71-75] Biopsy specimens give the most reliable data but may not be practical to obtain. Deep-tissue cultures from different sites may give different results. Cultures collected from pressure ulcers reveal polymicrobial growth. A culture collected by swab is likely to identify surface bacteria colonizing the wound rather than to diagnose the infection.[71-75]

PATHOPHYSIOLOGY

Many factors apparently predispose patients to the formation of pressure sores: paralysis, paresis, immobilization, malnutrition, anemia, infection, and advanced age. Factors thought to be most critical to their formation are pressure, shearing forces, friction, and moisture; however, there is still debate as to the exact pathophysiology of pressure sore formation.

Pressure is the essential element in the formation of pressure sores. The areas of highest pressure are generated most often over the bony prominences. When the pressure is relieved intermittently within a 2-hour period, only minimal changes occur in soft-tissue and skin structures.[71,72] Therefore, both the degree of pressure and the length of time that the pressure is applied are important.

Shearing forces are caused by the sliding of adjacent parallel surfaces of soft tissues in an unequal fashion. This situation can occur when the head of a bed is raised, causing the upper torso to slide downward, transmitting pressure to the sacrum and other areas. This effect results in occlusion or distortion of vessels, leading to compromise of the dermis. At the same time, sitting and gravity create shearing forces; the posterior sacral skin area can become fixed secondary to friction with the bed. The effects of friction and shearing forces combine, resulting in transmission of force to the deep portion of the superficial fascia and leading to further damage of soft-tissue structures.[71-75]

Compounding the problems of shearing and friction forces are the macerating effects of excessive moisture in the local environment, resulting from incontinence and perspiration. This factor is of critical importance because when combined with the other forces, it increases the risk of pressure sore formation fivefold.[71,72]

General

- Pressure sores can occur anywhere on the body.

- However, more than 95% of all pressure sores are located on the lower part of the body (65% in the region of the pelvis and 3.4% on the lower extremities; see Fig. 119–2).

- The most common sites on the lower portion of the body are the sacral and coccygeal areas, ischial tuberosities, and greater trochanter.

Symptoms

- Patients with pressure sores commonly have other medical problems that may mask the typical signs and symptoms of infection.

Signs

- Clinical infection is recognized by the presence of surrounding redness, heat, and pain.

- Purulent discharge, foul odor, and systemic signs (e.g., fever and leukocytosis) of infection may be present.

Laboratory Tests

- Cultures should be collected from either a biopsy or fluid obtained by needle aspiration.

Other Diagnostic Tests

- Because clinicians also must be aware of the possibility of underlying osteomyelitis, magnetic resonance imaging or other radiographic procedures should be considered.

TREATMENT

Pressure Sores

❽ Prevention is the single most important aspect in the management of pressure sores. Prevention is far easier and less costly than the intensive care necessary for the healing and eventual closure of pressure sores. Of primary importance, then, is the ability to identify patients who are at high risk so that preventive measures may be instituted.

The medical approach to the treatment of pressure sores depends on the stage of the disease. Medical management generally is indicated for lesions that are of moderate size and relatively shallow depth (stage 1 or 2 lesions) and are not located over a bony prominence. Depending on their location and severity, from 30% to 80% of these ulcers will heal without an operation. Surgical intervention is almost always necessary for ulcers that extend through superficial layers or into bone (stage 3, stage 4 and unstageable lesions).[70,71]

The goal of therapy is to clean and decontaminate the ulcer to promote wound healing by permitting the formation of healthy granulation tissue or to prepare the wound for an operative procedure. The main factors to be considered for successful topical therapy (local care) are (a) relief of pressure, (b) debridement of necrotic tissue as needed, (c) wound cleansing, (d) dressing selection, and (e) prevention, diagnosis, and treatment of infection.[71-75]

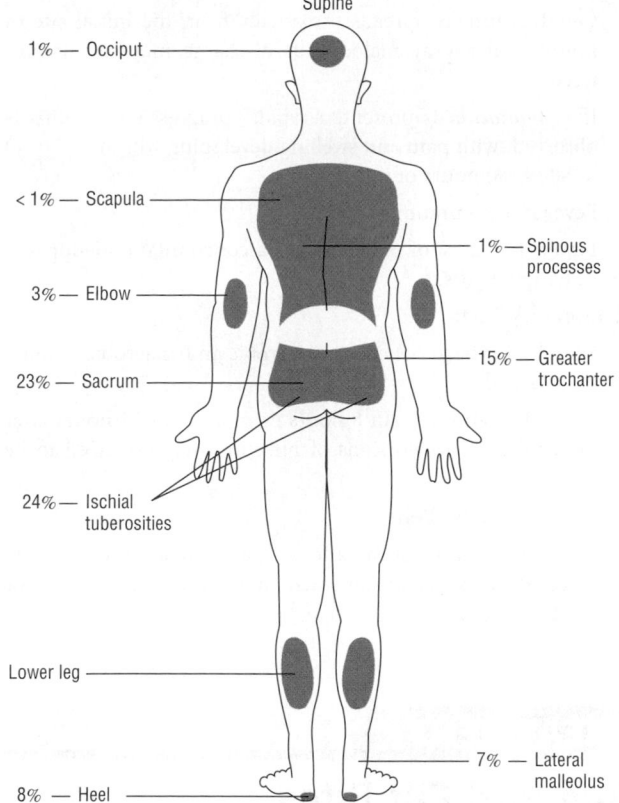

FIGURE 119-2. Supine view of areas where pressure sore formation tends to occur.

1% — Occiput
< 1% — Scapula
1% — Spinous processes
3% — Elbow
15% — Greater trochanter
23% — Sacrum
24% — Ischial tuberosities
Lower leg
7% — Lateral malleolus
8% — Heel

Friction and shearing forces can be minimized with proper positioning. Skin care and prevention of soilage are important, with the intent being to keep the surface relatively free of moisture. Patients with problems of incontinence should be cleaned frequently, and efforts should be made to keep the involved areas dry. Natural sheepskin is believed to be useful in minimizing the effects of moisture, shearing forces, and friction. Relief of pressure is probably the single most important factor in preventing pressure sore formation. Relief for a period of only 5 minutes once every 2 hours is believed to give protection against pressure sore formation.[71-75]

The goals of debridement and cleansing measures are removal of devitalized tissue and reduction of bacterial contamination, which can slow granulation time and, therefore, impede healing. Debridement can be accomplished by surgical, mechanical, or chemical means. Surgical debridement rapidly removes necrotic material from the wound and is recommended for urgent situations (e.g., cellulitis and sepsis).[71-75] Mechanical debridement generally involves wet-to-dry dressing changes. Saline-soaked gauze is applied to the wound; after drying, the gauze is removed and with it any adherent necrotic tissue. Other effective mechanical therapies include hydro-therapy (use of the whirlpool [Hubbard tank] to remove necrotic tissue and debris), wound irrigation, and dextranomers (beads placed in the wound to absorb exudate and bacteria). Chemical debridement includes enzymatic and autolytic agents. Enzymatic debridement involves application of topical debriding agents to remove devitalized tissue. This method is recommended for patients who cannot tolerate surgery or are in a long-term care or home setting. Autolytic debridement involves the use of synthetic dressings that allow devitalized tissue to self-digest via enzymes present in wound fluids. Autolytic debridement is contraindicated in the treatment of infected pressure sores.

Pressure sore wounds should be cleaned with normal saline. Cleansing agents that are cytotoxic, such as povidone-iodine, iodophor, sodium hypochlorite solution, hydrogen peroxide, and acetic acid, should be avoided.[71-75] Many of these agents impair healing. Many different types of dressings are available for pressure sores. Wound dressing materials should keep the wound moist, allow free exchange of air, act as a physical barrier to bacteria, and prevent physical damage. Controlled studies of the various types of wound dressings have shown no significant differences in healing outcomes.[71] Occlusive dressings should be avoided if infection is present.[71-75] If occlusive dressings are used, any infection should be controlled or the dressing frequency increased.

Systemic treatment (see Table 119–5) of an infected pressure ulcer should be guided by results from appropriately collected cultures. Systemic antibiotics generally are reserved for treatment of bacteremia, sepsis, cellulitis, or osteomyelitis.[71-75] However, a 2-week trial of topical antibiotics (silver sulfadiazine or triple antibiotic) may be considered for a clean ulcer that is not healing or is producing a moderate amount of exudate despite appropriate care.[71]

Other nonpharmacologic approaches to shortening the healing time have included the use of hyperbaric oxygenation, hydrotherapy, high-frequency/high-intensity sound waves, and electrotherapy.[71-75] Electrical stimulation is the only adjunctive therapy that is proven effective.[71-75]

EVALUATION OF THERAPEUTIC OUTCOMES

With appropriate wound care and antimicrobial therapy, infected pressure sores can heal. A reduction in erythema, warmth, pain, and other signs and symptoms should be seen in 48 to 72 hours.

BITE WOUNDS

Approximately half the population in the United States will be bitten by either an animal or another human sometime during their lifetimes.[76] Bite wounds have a substantial potential for infectious complications. If left untreated, complications such as soft-tissue infection and osteomyelitis may occur, possibly requiring extensive débridement or amputation.

ANIMAL BITES

Animal bites (typically from dogs or cats) are common causes of injury, particularly to children, and are associated with significant risk of infection without prompt attention to appropriate management.

Epidemiology

Dog bites account for approximately 80% of all animal bite wounds requiring medical attention. Data from U.S. emergency departments reported 368,245 visits for new dog bite-related injuries in 2001.[76] Based on this study, approximately 1,000 new dog bite injuries are seen in emergency departments every day. Approximately one half of dog bites occur in individuals younger than 20 years of age, usually males (55%). More than 70% of bites are to the extremities. Facial bites are also seen, particularly in children younger than 5 years of age. Up to 65% of bite wounds in young children involve the head and neck, and can be a lethal event because of blood loss. From 1979 through 1994, 279 deaths were the result of attacks by dogs.[77]

Patients at greatest risk of acquiring a bite-related infection have had a puncture wound (usually the hand), have not sought medical attention within 12 hours of the injury, and are older than 50 years of age.[78,79]

Cat bites, with an estimated incidence of 5% to 15% of all animal bites, are the second most common cause of animal bite wounds in the United States.[78] Bites and scratches occur most commonly on the upper extremities, with most injuries reported in women.[78] Infection rates, estimated at 30% to 50%, are more than double those seen with dog bites.[78,79]

Etiology

Infections from dog bite wounds are caused predominantly by mouth flora from the animal.[80–82] Most infections are polymicrobial, with approximately five bacterial isolates per culture.[80–82] *Pasteurella multocida* is the most frequent isolate. Other common aerobes include streptococci, staphylococci, *Moraxella,* and *Neisseria.* The most common anaerobes are *Fusobacterium, Bacteroides, Porphyromonas,* and *Prevotella.*[80–82] Wound-site cultures in both infected and noninfected patients have similar bacteria present, with aerobic organisms isolated from 74% to 90% and anaerobic organisms isolated from 41% to 49% of patients.[78,80]

Infections arising from cat bites or scratches are frequently (75%) caused by *P. multocida,* which has been isolated in the oropharynx of 50% to 70% of healthy cats.[78,82] Mixed aerobic and anaerobic infections have been reported in 63% of cat bite wounds, whereas approximately one third of cultures grow aerobes only.[78,82] Both tularemia (*Pasteurella tularensis*) and rabies also have been transmitted by cat bites.[78,82]

Pathophysiology

The potential for infection from an animal bite is great owing to the pressure that can be exerted during the bite and the vast number of potential pathogens that make up the normal oral flora.[81] Cats' teeth are slender and extremely sharp. Their teeth easily penetrate into bones and joints, resulting in a higher incidence of septic arthritis and osteomyelitis.[78] Although a dog's teeth may not be as sharp, they can exert a pressure of 200 to 450 lb/in² and therefore result in a serious crush injury with much devitalized tissue.[81] Known human pathogens such as *S. aureus, P. multocida,* and anaerobes are among the more than 64 species of bacteria that are harbored in the average dog mouth.[81] In addition, the polymicrobic (aerobic and anaerobic) nature of animal bites provides a synergistic relationship, thus making an infection harder to eradicate.[81]

CLINICAL PRESENTATION

General

- Healthcare providers see two distinct groups of patients seeking medical attention for dog bites.
- The first group presents within 12 hours of the injury; these patients require general wound care, repair of tear wounds, or rabies and/or tetanus treatment. The second group of patients presents more than 12 hours after the injury has occurred; these patients usually have clinical signs of infection and seek medical attention for infection-related complaints.

Symptoms

- Patients seek medical care for infection-related complaints (i.e., pain, purulent discharge, and swelling).

Signs

- Patients with infected dog bite wounds generally present with a localized cellulitis and pain at the site of injury.

- Cellulitis usually spreads proximally from the initial site of injury, and a gray malodorous discharge may be encountered.
- If *P. multocida* is present, a rapidly progressing cellulitis is observed, with pain and swelling developing within 24 (70%) to 48 (90%) hours of initial injury.
- Fever is uncommon.
- Fewer than 20% of patients have a concomitant adenopathy or lymphangitis.

Laboratory Tests

- Samples for bacterial cultures (aerobic and anaerobic) should be obtained.
- Wounds seen less than 8 hours or more than 24 hours after injury that show no signs of infection may not need to be cultured.

Other Diagnostic Tests

- A roentgenogram of the affected part should be considered when infection is documented in proximity to a bone or joint.

TREATMENT

Dog and Cat Bites

Table 119–4 lists the recommended drugs and dosing regimens for animal bite wounds.

Cultures obtained from early, noninfected bite wounds are not of great value in predicting the subsequent development of infection. Documentation of the mechanism of injury is important; if possible, an immunization history of the animal should be obtained. It is also important for the patient's tetanus immune status to be determined.

Wounds should be irrigated thoroughly with a copious volume (>150 mL) of sterile normal saline. Proper irrigation reduces the bacterial count in the wound. Antibiotic or iodine solutions do not offer any advantage over saline and actually may increase tissue irritation. Several management techniques used in the treatment of bite wounds remain controversial, including the extent and type of debridement,[78,83,84] suturing wounds within 8 hours of the injury,[11] and indications for the use of antibiotics.

The role of prophylactic antimicrobial therapy for the early, noninfected bite wound remains controversial.[78,82,85,86] Unfortunately, suggestions concerning the use of prophylactic antibiotics are based on minimal data because few clinical trials have been performed. Most reports are of retrospective studies or observations of complicated cases. A systematic review of eight randomized trials of bite wounds (caused by both animals and humans) evaluated the use of antibiotics for the prevention of infectious complications and concluded that antibiotics did not significantly reduce the risk of infection for patients with dog or cat bites but that wounds involving the hands may benefit from antimicrobial prophylaxis.[86] However, this review also concluded that additional studies are required to support these conclusions.[86]

Controlled studies have not shown benefits definitively with prophylactic antibiotics for noninfected bites. Because up to 20% of bite wounds may become infected, a 3- to 5-day course of antimicrobial therapy generally is recommended.[11,78,82] This is especially important for patients at greater risk for infection (patients older than 50 years of age and those with puncture wounds and wounds to the hands, and those who are immunocompromised).[82,85]

Treatment should be directed at the typical aerobic and anaerobic oral flora of dogs, as well as at potential pathogens from the skin flora of the bite victim. The length of antimicrobial therapy depends on the severity of the injury/infection.[11,78] Amoxicillin-clavulanic acid is commonly recommended for oral outpatient therapy.[11,78,82] Alternative oral agents include doxycycline or the combination of penicillin VK and dicloxacillin. Trimethoprim-sulfamethoxazole and fluoroquinolones have activity against *P. multocida* and are recommended as alternatives for patients who are allergic to penicillins.[11,78] However, these agents should not be used in children and/or pregnant women; trimethoprim-sulfamethoxazole also should be avoided during pregnancy. Macrolides or azalides may be considered as alternatives for growing children or pregnant women.[11,78,83] If erythromycin or similar-class agent is selected, bacterial sensitivities should be obtained and clinical response monitored carefully because most strains of *P. multocida* are resistant. Cefuroxime is another viable alternative for patients with mild penicillin allergies. Many of these alternative agents will likely require an additional agent (metronidazole, clindamycin) with activity against anaerobes. Failure to provide adequate initial treatment of bite wounds results in treatment failures and increased need for hospitalization for administration of parenteral antibiotics.[87]

Treatment options for patients requiring intravenous therapy include β-lactam–β-lactamase inhibitor combinations (ampicillinsulbactam, piperacillin-tazobactam), second-generation cephalosporins with antianaerobic activity (cefoxitin), and carbapenems.[11,78,82]

In addition to irrigation and antibiotics, when indicated, the injured area should be immobilized and elevated. Clinical failures due to edema have occurred despite appropriate antibiotic therapy.[78] Therefore, it is important to stress to patients that the affected area should be elevated for several days or until edema has resolved.

Tetanus does not occur commonly after dog bites; however, it is possible. If the immunization history of a patient with anything other than a clean, minor wound is unknown, tetanus-diphtheria (TD) toxoids should be administered (0.5 mL intramuscularly).[88] Both TD toxoids and tetanus immune globulin (250 units intramuscularly) should be administered to patients who have never been immunized.[82,89]

Because the rabies virus can be transmitted via saliva, rabies may be a potential complication of a bite. When the symptoms of rabies develop after a bite, the prognosis for survival is poor. Roughly 3% of rabies cases documented in animals were in dogs (the most frequent vectors are skunks, raccoons, and bats).[90]

After a patient has been exposed to rabies, the treatment objectives consist of thorough irrigation of the wound, tetanus prophylaxis, antibiotic prophylaxis, if indicated, and immunization. Prompt, thorough irrigation of the wound with soap or iodine solution may reduce the development of rabies.[90] Postexposure prophylaxis immunization against rabies consists of the administration of both passive antibody and vaccine.[89,90] The vaccine is administered as a series of five 1 mL intramuscular injections given on days 0, 3, 7, 14, and 28, beginning on the day of exposure or as soon as possible afterward. Rabies hyperimmune globulin is administered at a dose of 40 international units/kg; as much of the total dose as possible should be infiltrated into and around the wound, with the remainder being injected intramuscularly at a site different from that of the vaccine.[89] The only exceptions to administration of hyperimmune globulin are patients who were immunized previously and who have the appropriate degree of documented rabies antibody titers. However, even individuals who have been fully vaccinated should receive two doses of vaccine on days 0 and 3 after actual rabies exposure.[89,90]

The management of cat bites is similar to that discussed for dog bites. Cat scratches typically involve the same organisms as bites and should be treated accordingly.

Evaluation of therapeutic outcomes

Bite victims treated on an outpatient basis with oral antimicrobials should be followed up within 24 hours either by phone or office visit.[11] Hospitalization or change to intravenous therapy should be considered if the infection has progressed. For hospitalized patients with no improvement in signs and symptoms following 24 hours of appropriate therapy, then surgical debridement may be needed.

HUMAN BITES

Human bite wounds are often deceptively severe and frequently require aggressive management to reduce the risk of infectious complications.

Epidemiology

Human bites are the third most frequent type of bite. Infected human bites can occur as bites from the teeth or from blows to the mouth (clenched-fist injuries). Human bites generally are more serious than animal bites and carry a higher likelihood of infection than do most animal bites. Infectious complications occur in 10% to 50% of patients with human bites.[78,91]

Self-inflicted bites most commonly occur on the lips or around the fingernails (from sucking or biting the nails). Bites by others can occur to any part of the body but most often involve the hands. Bites to the hand are most serious and become infected more frequently. The clenched-fist injury is a traumatic laceration caused by one person hitting another in the mouth and is a very serious bite wound. The areas most commonly affected by this injury are the third and fourth metacarpophalangeal joints.[92]

Etiology

Infections caused by these injuries are similar and are caused most often by the normal oral flora, which include both aerobic and anaerobic microorganisms. *Streptococcus* spp. (especially *Streptococcus anginosus*) are the most common isolates, followed by *Staphylococcus* spp. (predominately *S. aureus*).[93] *Eikenella corrodens* is isolated from human bite wounds approximately 30% of the time.[78,93] Anaerobic microorganisms have been isolated in approximately 40% of human bites and 55% of clenched-fist injuries. Common anaerobes recovered from human bite infections include *Fusobacterium, Prevotella, Porphyromonas,* and *Peptostreptococcus* species.[93]

Pathophysiology

Human bites generally are more serious and more prone to infection than animal bites, particularly clenched-fist injuries.[81] While the force of a punch may sever a tendon or nerve or break a bone, it most often causes a breach in the capsule of the metacarpophalangeal joint, leading to direct inoculation of bacteria into the joint or bone.[78] When the hand is relaxed, the tendons carry bacteria into deeper spaces of the hand, resulting in more extensive infection.[78]

CLINICAL PRESENTATION

General

- Most clenched-fist injuries are already infected by the time patients seek medical care, and most require hospitalization.

Symptoms

- Patients with infected bites to the hand may develop a painful, throbbing, swollen extremity.

- Wounds often have a purulent discharge, and the patient complains of a decreased range of motion.

Signs

- Signs of infection include erythema, swelling, and clear or pussy discharge.
- Adjacent lymph nodes may be enlarged.
- In clenched-fist injuries, edema may limit the ability of tendons to glide in their sheaths, thereby limiting a joint's range of motion.

Laboratory Tests

- Samples for bacterial cultures (aerobic and anaerobic) should be collected as per animal bites.
- In severe infections, a peripheral leukocytosis of 15,000 to 30,000 cells/mm³ may be seen; therefore, the white blood count should be monitored for resolution of infection.

Other Diagnostic Tests

- If damage to a bone or joint is suspected, radiographic evaluation should be undertaken.

TREATMENT

Human Bites

Table 119–4 lists the recommended drugs and dosing regimens for human bite wounds.

❾ Management of bite wounds consists of aggressive irrigation and topical wound cleansing. Surgical debridement and immobilization of the affected area is often required. Prophylactic antimicrobial agents should be given as soon as possible to all patients, regardless of the appearance of the wound, unless it can be documented that the wound does not involve hands, feet, or joints and penetrates no deeper than the epidermis.[11,79,82] Patients with clenched-fist injuries should be seen by a specialist in hand care to evaluate for penetration into the synovium, joint capsule, and bone.[11,78] Primary closure for human bites generally is not recommended. Tetanus toxoid and antitoxin may be indicated. Because transmission of viruses (HIV, herpes, hepatitides B and C) is a possibility with human bites, information about the biter is important. Although the possibility of acquiring HIV through bites is believed to be unlikely, the presence of the virus in the saliva makes disease transmission possible.[94] If the biter is HIV positive, the victim should have a baseline blood specimen drawn to determine preexposure HIV status and then be retested in 3 months and 6 months.[82,91,94] The bite wound should be irrigated thoroughly and vigorously with a virucidal agent such as povidone-iodine.[78] Bite victims exposed to blood-tainted saliva may be offered antiretroviral chemoprophylaxis, but each case should be individually assessed based on the potential for significant exposure and potential risks and benefits of antiretroviral therapy.[94]

❿ Patients with human bite injuries should receive prophylactic antibiotic therapy for 3 to 5 days.[82,91,95] First-generation cephalosporins, macrolides, clindamycin, and aminoglycosides are not recommended because the sensitivity of these agents to E. corrodens is variable.[78,85,95]

Hospitalization for minor wounds is unnecessary if surgical repair of vital structures has not been performed. Patients suffering serious injuries or clenched-fist injuries should be started on intravenous antibiotics. Recommended agents include cefoxitin (1 g IV every 6 to 8 hours), ampicillin-sulbactam (1.5 to 3 g IV every 6 hours), or ertapenem (1 g IV every 24 hours).[11] Therapeutic failures have been documented when either first-generation cephalosporins or penicillinase-resistant penicillins have been used alone, most

likely because of their poor and variable activity against E. corrodens. Therapy should be continued from 7 to 14 days.[11,91]

Evaluation of Therapeutic Outcomes

Evaluation of treatment should follow the same general guidelines as discussed for animal bite wounds. Complications with clenched-fist injuries are common and may result in residual joint stiffness and loss of function. Physical therapy can be needed to improve these complications.

ABBREVIATIONS

HIV: human immunodeficiency virus

MRSA: methicillin-resistant *Staphylococcus aureus*

CA-MRSA: community-associated methicillin-resistant *S. aureus*

SSTI: skin and soft-tissue infection

TD: tetanus-diphtheria

REFERENCES

1. Fung HB, Chang JY, Kuczynski S. A practical guide to the treatment of complicated skin and soft tissue infections. Drugs 2003;63: 1459–1480.
2. Eron LJ, Lipsky BA, Low DE, et al. Managing skin and soft tissue infections: Expert panel recommendations on key decision points. J Antimicrob Chemother 2003;59;52(suppl S1):i3–i17.
3. Pallin DJ, Espinola JA, Leung DY, et al. Epidemiology of dermatitis and skin infections in United States physicians offices, 1993–2005. Clin Infect Dis 2009;49:901–907.
4. Stulberg DL, Penrod MA, Blatny RA. Common bacterial skin infections. Am Fam Physician 2002;66:119–124.
5. Levit K, Wier L, Stranges E, Ryan K, Elixhauser A. HCUP Facts and Figures: Statistics on Hospital-based Care in the United States; 2007. Rockville, MD: Agency for Healthcare Research and Quality; 2009 *http://www.hcup-us.ahrq.gov/reports.jsp*.
6. Rennie RP, Jones RN, Mutnick AH, and the SENTRY Program Study Group (North America). Occurrence and antimicrobial susceptibility patterns of pathogens isolated from skin and soft tissue infections: Report from the SENTRY Antimicrobial Surveillance Program (United States and Canada, 2000). Diagn Microbiol Infect Dis 2003;45:287–293.
7. Moet GJ, Jones RN, Biedenbach DJ, Stilwell MG, Fritsche TR. Contemporary causes of skin and soft tissue infections in North America, Latin America, and Europe: Report from the SENTRY Antimicrobial Surveillance Program (1998–2004). Diagn Microbiol Infect Dis 2007;57:7–13.
8. Wilson MA. Skin and soft-tissue infections: Impact of resistant gram-positive bacteria. Am J Surg 2003;186(suppl 5A):35S–41S.
9. Stryjewski ME, Chambers HF. Skin and soft tissue infections caused by community-acquired methicillin-resistant Staphylococcus aureus. Clin Infect Dis 2008;46(suppl 5):S368–377.
10. Tenover FC, Goering RV. Methicillin-resistant Staphylococcus aureus strain USA300: origin and epidemiology. J Antimicrob Chemother 2009;64:441–446.
11. Stevens DL, Bisno AL, Chambers HF, et al. Practice guidelines for the diagnosis and management of skin and soft-tissue infections. Clin Infect Dis 2005;41:1373–1406.
12. Frazee BW, Lynn J, Charlebois ED, Lambert L, Lowery D, Perdreau-Remington F. High prevalence of methicillin-resistant Staphylococcus aureus in emergency department skin and soft tissue infections. Ann Emerg Med 2005;45:311–320.
13. Daum RS. Skin and soft tissue infections caused by methicillin-resistant Staphylococcus aureus. N Engl J Med 2007;357:380–390.
14. Moran GJ, Krishnadasan A, Gorwitz RJ, et al. Methicillin-resistant S. aureus infections among patients in the emergency department. N Eng J Med 2006;355:666–674.

15. King MD, Humphrey BJ, Wang YF, et al. Emergence of community-acquired methicillin-resistant Staphylococcus aureus USA 300 clone as the predominant cause of skin and soft-tissue infections. Ann Intern Med 2006;144:309–317.

16. Granato PA. Pathogenic and indigenous microorganisms of humans. In: Murray PR, Baron EJ, Jorgensen JH, et al., eds. Manual of Clinical Microbiology, 8th ed. Washington, DC: ASM Press; 2003:44–54.

17. Yu Y, Cheng AS, Wang L, et al. Hot tub folliculitis or hand-foot syndrome caused by Pseudomonas aeruginosa. J Am Acad Dermatol 2007;57:596–600.

18. Lipsky BA, Berendt AR, Deery HG, et al. Diagnosis and treatment of diabetic foot infections. Clin Infect Dis 2004;39:885–910.

19. Swartz MN, Pasternak MS. Cellulitis and subcutaneous tissue infections. In: Mandell GL, Bennett JE, Dolin R, eds. Principles and Practice of Infectious Diseases, 6th ed. New York: Churchill-Livingstone; 2005:1172–1193.

20. Bhumbra NA, McCullough SG. Skin and subcutaneous infections. Prim Care Clin Office Pract 2003;30:1–24.

21. Brown J, Shriner DL, Schwartz RA, Janniger CK. Impetigo: An update. Int J Dermatol 2003;42:251–255.

22. Pasternak MS, Swartz MN. Lymphadenitis and lymphangitis. In: Mandell GL, Bennett JE, Dolin R, eds. Principles and Practice of Infectious Diseases, 6th ed. New York: Churchill-Livingstone; 2005:1204–1214.

23. Christensen KLY, Holman RC, Steiner CA, et al. Infectious diseases hospitalizations in the United States. Clin Infect Dis 2009;49: 1025–1035.

24. Lloyd-Smith E, Kerr T, Hogg RS, et al. Prevalence and correlates of abscesses among a cohort of injection drug users. Harm Reduct J 2005;2:24–28.

25. Takahashi TA, Merrill JO, Boyko EJ, Bradley KA. Type and location of injection drug use-related soft tissue infections predict hospitalization. J Urban Health 2003;80:127–136.

26. Bassetti S, Battegav M. Staphylococcus aureus infections in injection drug users: Risk factors and prevention strategies. Infection 2004;32:163–169.

27. Young DM, Harris HW, Charlebois ED, et al. An epidemic of methicillin-resistant Staphylococcus aureus soft tissue infections among medically underserved patients. Arch Surg 2004;139:947–953.

28. Kimura AC, Higa JI, Levin RM, Simpson G, Vargas Y, Vugla DJ. Outbreak of necrotizing fasciitis due to Clostridium sordellii among black-tar heroin users. Clin Infect Dis 2004;38:e87–e91.

29. Brett MM, Hood J, Brazier JS, Duerden BI, Hahne SJ. Soft tissue infections caused by spore-forming bacteria in injecting drug users in the United Kingdom. Epidemiol Infect 2005;133:575–582.

30. Stevens DL, Eron LL. Cellulitis and soft tissue infections. Ann Intern Med 2009;150:ITC1–11.

31. Ladhani S, Garbash M. Staphylococcal skin infections in children: Rational drug therapy recommendations. Paediatr Drugs 2005;7: 77–102.

32. Gorwitz RJ, Jernigan DB, Powers JH, et al. Strategies for clinical management of MRSA in the community: Summary of an experts' meeting convened by the Centers for Disease Control and Prevention; 2006. http://www.cdc.gov/ncidod/dhqp/ar_mrsa_ca.html.

33. Herman RA, Kee VR, Moores KG, et al. Etiology and treatment of community-acquired methicillin-resistant Staphylococcus aureus. Am J Health-Syst Pharm 2008;65:219–225.

34. Moellering RC Jr. Current treatment options for community-acquired methicillin-resistant Staphylococcus aureus infection. Clin Infect Dis 2008;46:1032–1037.

35. Nathwani D, Morgan M, Masterton RG, et al. Guidelines for UK practice for the diagnosis and management of methicillin-resistant Staphylococcus aureus (MRSA) infections presenting in the community. J Antimicrob Chemother 2008;61:976–994.

36. Arbeit RD, Maki D, Tally FP, et al. The safety and efficacy of daptomycin for the treatment of complicated skin and skin-structure infections. Clin Infect Dis 2004;38:1673–1681.

37. Leonard SN, Rybak MJ. Telavancin: an antimicrobial with a multifunctional mechanism of action for the treatment of serious gram-positive infections. Pharmacother 2008;28:458–468.

38. Breedt J, Teras J, Gardovskis J, et al. Safety and efficacy of tigecycline in treatment of skin and skin structure infections: Results of a double-blind phase 3 comparison study with vancomycin-aztreonam. Antimicrob Agents Chemother 2005;49:4658–4666.

39. Micek ST. Alternatives to vancomycin for the treatment of methicillin-resistant Staphylococcus aureus infections. Clin Infect Dis 2007;45(suppl 3):S184-S190.

40. McKinnon PS, Sorensen SV, Liu LZ, Itani KM. Impact of linezolid on economic outcomes and determinants of cost in a clinical trial evaluating patients with MRSA complicated skin and soft-tissue infections. Ann Pharmacother 2006;40:1017–1023.

41. Ruhe JJ, Menon A. Tetracyclines as an oral treatment option for patients with community onset skin and soft tissue infections caused by methicillin-resistant Staphylococcus aureus. Antimicrob Agents Chemother 2007;51:3298–3303.

42. Cenizal MJ, Skiest D, Luber S, et al. Prospective randomized trial of empiric therapy with trimethoprim-sulfamethoxazole or doxycycline for outpatient skin and soft tissue infections in an area of high prevalence of methicillin-resistant Staphylococcus aureus. Antimicrob Agents Chemother 2007;51:2628–2630.

43. Giordano P, Song J, Pertel P, et al. Sequential intravenous/oral moxifloxacin versus intravenous piperacillin-tazobactam followed by oral amoxicillin-clavulanate for the treatment of complicated skin and skin structure infection. Int J Antimicrob Agents 2005;26:357–365.

44. Parish LC, Routh HB, Miskin B, et al. Moxifloxacin versus cephalexin in the treatment of uncomplicated skin infections. Int J Clin Pract 2000;54:497–503.

45. Zervos MJ, Hershberger E, Nicolau DP, et al. Relationship between fluoroquinolone use and changes in susceptibility to fluoroquinolones of selected pathogens in 10 United States teaching hospitals, 1991–2000. Clin Infect Dis 2003;37:1643–1648.

46. Neuhauser MM, Weinstein RA, Rydman R, et al. Antibiotic resistance among gram-negative bacilli in US intensive care units. Implications for fluoroquinolone use. JAMA 2003;289:885–888.

47. Cainzos M, Gonzales-Rodriguez FJ. Necrotizing soft tissue infections. Curr Opin Infect Dis 2007;13:433–439.

48. Vinh DC, Embil JM. Rapidly progressive soft tissue infections. Lancet Infect Dis 2005;5:501–513.

49. Bellapianta JM, Ljungquist K, Tobin E, et al. Necrotizing fasciitis. J Am Acad Orthop Surg 2009;17:174–182.

50. Boyer A, Vargas F, Coste F, et al. Influence of surgical treatment timing on mortality from necrotizing soft tissue infections requiring intensive care management. Intensive Care Med 2009;35:847–853.

51. Jallali N, Withey S, Butler PE. Hyperbaric oxygen as adjuvant therapy in the management of necrotizing fasciitis. Am J Med 2005;189: 462–466.

52. Laverly LA, Armstrong DG, Wunderlich RP, et al. Risk factors for foot infections in persons with diabetes mellitus. Diabetes Care 2006;29:1288–1293.

53. Boulton AJ, Kirsner RS, Vileikyte L. Clinical practice: neuropathic diabetic foot ulcers. N Engl J Med 2004;351:48–55.

54. Wieman TJ. Principles of management: the diabetic foot. Am J Surg 2005;190:295–299.

55. Lipsky BA. A report from the international consensus on diagnosing and treating the infected diabetic foot. Diabetes Metab Res Rev 2004;20(S1):S68–77.

56. Zgonis T, Roukis TS. A systematic approach to diabetic foot infections. Adv Ther 2005; 22:244–262.

57. Rao N, Lipsky BA. Optimising antimicrobial therapy in diabetic foot infections. Drugs 2007;67:195–214.

58. Nelson EA, O'Meara S, Craig D, et al. Systematic review of antimicrobial treatments for diabetic foot ulcers. Diabetic Med 2006;23:348–359.

59. Senneville E. Antimicrobial interventions for the management of diabetic foot infections. Expert Opin Pharmacother 2005;6:263–273.

60. Tentolouris N, Petrikkos G, Vallianou N, et al. Prevalence of methicillin-resistant Staphylococcus aureus in infected and uninfected diabetic foot ulcers. Clin Microbiol Infect 2006;12:186–189.

61. Senneville E, Melliez H, Beltrand E, et al. Culture of percutaneous bone biopsy specimens for diagnosis of diabetic foot osteomyelitis. Clin Infect Dis 2006;42:57–62.

62. Kessler L, Piemont Y, Ortega F, et al. Comparison of microbiological results of needle puncture vs. superficial swab in infected diabetic foot ulcer with osteomyelitis. Diabetic Med 2006;23:99–102.

63. Jeffcoate WJ, Lipsky BA. Controversies in diagnosing and managing osteomyelitis of the foot in diabetes. Clin Infect Dis 2004;39(suppl 2):S115–122.

64. Armstrong DG, Lavery LA, Nixon BP, Boulton AJ. It's not what you put on, but what you take off; techniques for debriding and off-loading the diabetic foot wound. Clin Infect Dis 2004;39(suppl 2):S92–S99.

65. Lipsky BA, Armstrong DG, Citron DM, et al. Ertapenem versus piperacillin/tazobactam for diabetic foot infections (SIDESTEP): Prospective, randomized, controlled, double-blinded, multicentre trial. Lancet 2005;366:1695–1703.

66. Lipsky BA, Hoey C. Topical antimicrobial therapy for treating chronic wounds. Clin Infect Dis 2009;49:1541–1549.

67. Kwakman PHS, Van den Akker JPC, Guciu A, et al. Medical-grade honey kills antibiotic-resistant bacteria in vitro and eradicates skin colonization. Clin Infect Dis 2008;46:1677–1682.

68. Cruciani M, Lipsky BA, Mengoli C, et al. Are granulocyte colony-stimulating factors beneficial in treating diabetic foot infections? A meta-analysis. Diabetes Care 2005;28:454–460.

69. Kranke P, Bennette M, Roeckl-Wiedmann I, et al. Hyperbaric oxygen therapy for chronic wounds. Cochrane Database Syst Rev 2004;2:CD004123.

70. Black J, Baharestani M, Cuddigan J, et al. National Pressure Ulcer Advisory Panel's updated pressure ulcer staging system. Derm Nursing 2007;19:343–349.

71. Reddy M, Gill SS, Kalkar SR, et al. Treatment of pressure ulcers. A systematic review. JAMA 2008;300:2647–2662.

72. Levi B, Rees R. Diagnosis and management of pressure ulcers. Clin Plastic Surg 2007;34:735–748.

73. Garcia AD, Thomas DR. Assessment and management of chronic pressure ulcers in the elderly. Med Clin North Am 2006;90:925–944.

74. Keast DH, Parslow N, Houghton PE, et al. Best practice recommendations for the prevention and treatment of pressure ulcers: update 2006. Advances Skin Wound Care 2007;20:447–460.

75. Ho CH, Bogie K. The prevention and treatment of pressure ulcers. Phys Med Rehab Clin North Am 2007;18:235–253.

76. Centers for Disease Control and Prevention. Nonfatal dog bite-related injuries treated in hospital emergency departments—United States, 2001. MMWR 2003;52:605–610.

77. Anonymous. Dog bite related fatalities—United States, 1995–1996. MMWR 1997;46:463–467.

78. Brook, I. Management of human and animal bite wounds: An overview. Adv Skin Wound Care 2005;18:197–203.

79. Broder J, Jerrard D, Olshaker J, Witting M. Low risk of infection in selected human bites treated without antibiotics. Am J Emerg Med 2004;22:10–13.

80. Oehler RL, Velez AP, Mizrachi M, et al. Bite-related and septic syndromes caused by cats and dogs. Lancet Infect 2009;9:439–447.

81. Brook I. Microbiology and management of human and animal bite wound infections. Prim Care 2003;30:25–39.

82. Goldstein EJC. Bites. In: Mandell GL, Bennett JE, Dolin R, eds. Principles and Practice of Infectious Diseases, 6th ed. New York: Churchill-Livingstone; 2005:3552–3556.

83. Benson LS, Edwards SL, Schiff AP, et al. Dog and cat bites to the hand: Treatment and cost assessment. J Hand Surg 2006;31:468–473.

84. Stefanopoulos PK, Tarantzopoulou AD. Facial bite wounds: Management update. Int J Oral Maxillofac Surg 2005;34:464–472.

85. Taplitz RA. Managing bite wounds. Currently recommended antibiotics for treatment and prophylaxis. Postgrad Med 2004;116:49–52, 55–56.

86. Medeiros I, Saconato H. Antibiotic prophylaxis for mammalian bites. Cochrane Database Syst Rev 2001;2:CD001738.

87. Holm M, Tarnvik A. Hospitalization due to Pasteurella multocida-infected animal bite wounds: Correlation with inadequate primary antibiotic medication. Scand J Infect Dis 2000;32:181–183.

88. Centers for Disease Control and Prevention. Preventing Tetanus, Diphtheria, and Pertussis Among Adults: Use of Tetanus Toxoid, Reduced Diphtheria Toxoid and Acellular Pertussis Vaccine. Recommendations of the Advisory Committee on Immunization Practices (ACIP). MMWR 2006;55(RR17):1–33.

89. Orenstein WA, Wharton M, Bart KJ, Hinman AR. Immunization. In: Mandell GL, Bennett JE, Dolin R, eds. Principles and Practice of Infectious Diseases, 6th ed. New York: Churchill-Livingstone; 2005:3557–3588.

90. Human rabies prevention—United States, 2008. Recommendations of the Advisory Committee on Immunization Practices (ACIP). MMWR 2008;57(RR03):1–26,28.

91. Stierman KL, Lloyd KM, De Luca-Pytell DM, et al. Treatment and outcome of human bites in the head and neck. Otolaryngol Head Neck Surg 2003;128:795–801.

92. Henry FP, Purcell EM, Eadie PA. The human bite injury: A clinical audit and discussion regarding the management of this alcohol fuelled phenomenon. Emerg Med 2007;24:455–458.

93. Talan DA, Abrahamian FM, Moran PM, et al. Clinical presentation and bacteriologic analysis of infected human bites in patients presenting to emergency departments. Clin Infect Dis 2003;37:1481–1489.

94. Antiretroviral Postexposure Prophylaxis After Sexual, Injection-Drug Use, or Other Nonoccupational Exposure to HIV in the United States. Recommendations from the U.S. Department of Health and Human Services. MMWR 2005;54(RR2):1–20.

95. Rittner AV, Fitzpatrick K, Corfield A. Best evidence topic report. Are antibiotics indicated following human bites? Emerg Med J 2005;22:654.

120

Infective Endocarditis

ANGIE VEVERKA AND MICHAEL A. CROUCH

KEY CONCEPTS

❶ Infective endocarditis is an uncommon infection usually occurring in persons with preexisting cardiac valvular abnormalities (e.g., prosthetic heart valves) or with other specific risk factors (e.g., intravenous drug abuse).

❷ Three groups of organisms cause a majority of infective endocarditis cases: streptococci, staphylococci, and enterococci.

❸ The clinical presentation of infective endocarditis is highly variable and nonspecific, although a fever and murmur usually are present. Classic peripheral manifestations (e.g., Osler nodes) may or may not occur.

❹ The diagnosis of infective endocarditis requires the integration of clinical, laboratory, and echocardiographic findings. The two major diagnostic criteria are bacteremia and echocardiographic changes (e.g., valvular vegetation).

❺ Treatment of infective endocarditis involves isolation of the infecting pathogen and determination of antimicrobial susceptibilities, followed by high-dose, parenteral, bactericidal antibiotics for an extended period.

❻ Surgical replacement of the infected heart valve is an important adjunct to endocarditis treatment in certain situations (e.g., patients with acute heart failure).

❼ β-Lactam antibiotics, such as penicillin G (or ceftriaxone), nafcillin, and ampicillin, remain the drugs of choice for streptococcal, staphylococcal, and enterococcal endocarditis, respectively.

❽ Aminoglycoside antibiotics are essential to obtain a synergistic bactericidal effect in the treatment of enterococcal endocarditis. Adjunctive aminoglycosides also may decrease the emergence of resistant organisms (e.g., prosthetic valve endocarditis caused by coagulase-negative staphylococci) and hasten the pace of clinical and microbiologic response (e.g., some streptococcal and staphylococcal infections).

❾ Vancomycin is reserved for patients with immediate β-lactam allergies and the treatment of resistant organisms.

❿ Antimicrobial prophylaxis is used as an attempt to prevent infective endocarditis for patients who are at the highest risk (such as persons with prosthetic heart valves) before a bacteremia-causing procedure (e.g., dental extraction).

Learning objectives, review questions, and other resources can be found at **www.pharmacotherapyonline.com**.

Endocarditis is an inflammation of the endocardium, the membrane lining the chambers of the heart and covering the cusps of the heart valves.[1,2] More commonly, *endocarditis* refers to infection of the heart valves by various microorganisms. Although it typically affects native valves, it also may involve nonvalvular areas or implanted mechanical devices (e.g., mechanical heart valves). Bacteria primarily cause endocarditis, but fungi and other atypical microorganisms can lead to the disease; hence, the more encompassing term *infective endocarditis* is preferred.[2,3]

Endocarditis is often referred to as *acute* or *subacute* depending on the pace and severity of the clinical presentation. The acute, fulminating form is associated with high fevers and systemic toxicity. Virulent bacteria, such as *Staphylococcus aureus*, frequently cause this syndrome, and if untreated, death may occur within days to weeks. On the other hand, subacute infective endocarditis is more indolent, and it is caused by less-invasive organisms, such as viridans streptococci, usually occurring in preexisting valvular heart disease. Although infective endocarditis is often referred to as acute or subacute, it is best classified based on the etiologic organism, the anatomic site of infection, and pathogenic risk factors.[1,4,5] Infection also may follow surgical insertion of a prosthetic heart valve, resulting in prosthetic-valve endocarditis (PVE).[6]

EPIDEMIOLOGY AND ETIOLOGY

Infective endocarditis is an uncommon, but not rare, infection. Population-based studies have reported incidence rates of 2 to 15 cases per 100,000 person-years.[2,7,8] In the United States, the infection is listed as the primary or secondary diagnosis of 30,000 hospital discharges.[9] Yet, the incidence of infective endocarditis may be increasing, and it is now the fourth leading cause of infectious disease syndromes that are life threatening, after urosepsis, pneumonia, and intraabdominal sepsis.[10] The mean male-to-female ratio is 1.7:1. As the population ages and as valve replacement surgery becomes more common, the mean age of patients with infective endocarditis increases. Overall, most cases occur in individuals older than 50 years of age, and it is uncommon in children.[11,12] PVE accounts for 20% to 25 % of cases of infective endocarditis.[3,12] Those with a history of intravenous drug abuse (IVDA) are also at high risk. Of note, the incidence of healthcare-associated infective endocarditis is rising, especially in the elderly population.[11,12] Other conditions associated with a higher incidence of infective endocarditis include diabetes, long-term hemodialysis, and poor dental hygiene.[2,5]

❶ Most persons with infective endocarditis have risk factors, such as preexisting cardiac valvular abnormalities. Many types of structural heart disease result in turbulent blood flow that increases the risk for infective endocarditis. A predisposing risk factor, however, may be absent in up to 25% of cases. Some of the more important risk factors include:[2,5,12,13]

- Presence of a prosthetic valve (highest risk)
- Previous endocarditis (highest risk)
- Congenital heart disease
- Chronic intravenous access
- Diabetes mellitus
- Healthcare-related exposure
- Acquired valvular dysfunction (e.g., rheumatic heart disease)
- Hypertrophic cardiomyopathy
- Mitral valve prolapse with regurgitation
- IVDA

In the past, rheumatic heart disease was a prevalent risk factor for infective endocarditis, but the incidence of this disease continues to decline. The risk of infective endocarditis in persons with mitral valve prolapse and regurgitation is small; however, because the condition is prevalent, it is an important contributor to the overall number of infective endocarditis cases.[2,5] Prosthetic valve endocarditis occurs in 1% to 3% of patients undergoing valve replacement surgery in the first postoperative year.[3,14]

❷ Nearly every organism causing human disease has been reported to cause infective endocarditis, but three groups of organisms result in a majority of cases: streptococci, staphylococci, and enterococci (Table 120–1).[1,3,4,14] The incidence of staphylococci, particularly *S. aureus*, continues to increase, and recent case series document staphylococci have surpassed viridans streptococci as the leading cause of infective endocarditis.[12,13] In general, streptococci cause infective endocarditis in patients with underlying cardiac abnormalities, such as mitral valve prolapse or rheumatic heart disease. Staphylococci (*S. aureus* and coagulase-negative staphylococci) are the most common cause of PVE within the first year after valve surgery, and *S. aureus* is common in those with a history of IVDA. Although polymicrobial infective endocarditis is uncommon, it is encountered most often in association with IVDA.[2,3,5] Enterococcal endocarditis tends to follow genitourinary manipulations (older men) or obstetric procedures (younger women).[3] There are many exceptions to the preceding generalizations; thus, isolation of the causative pathogen and determination of its antimicrobial susceptibilities offer the best chance for successful therapy.

The mitral and aortic valves are affected most commonly in cases involving a single valve. Subacute endocarditis tends to involve the mitral valve, whereas acute disease often involves the aortic valve. Up to 35% of cases involve concomitant infections of both the aortic and the mitral valves. Infection of the tricuspid valve is less common, with a majority of these cases occurring for patients with a history of IVDA. It is rare for the pulmonary valve to be infected.[1,3,12,13]

PATHOPHYSIOLOGY

The development of infective endocarditis via hematogenous spread, the most common route, requires the sequential occurrence of several factors. These components are complex and not fully elucidated.[2,3,15]

- *The endothelial surface of the heart is damaged.* This injury occurs with turbulent blood flow associated with the valvular lesions previously described.
- *Platelet and fibrin deposition occurs on the abnormal epithelial surface.* These platelet-fibrin deposits are referred to as *nonbacterial thrombotic endocarditis.*
- *Bacteremia gives organisms access to and results in colonization of the endocardial surface.* Bacteremia is the result of trauma to a mucosal surface with a high concentration of resident bacteria, such as the oral cavity and gastrointestinal tract. Transient bacteremia commonly follow certain dental, gastrointestinal, urologic, and gynecologic procedures. Staphylococci, viridans streptococci, and enterococci are most likely to adhere to nonbacterial thrombotic endocarditis, probably because of production of specific adherence factors, such as dextran by some oral streptococci and glycocalyx for staphylococci. Gram-negative bacteria rarely adhere to heart valves and are uncommon causes of infective endocarditis.
- *After colonization of the endothelial surface, a "vegetation" of fibrin, platelets, and bacteria forms.* The protective cover of fibrin and platelets allows unimpeded bacterial growth to concentrations as high as 10^9 to 10^{10} organisms per gram of tissue.

The pathogenesis of early PVE differs from the infective endocarditis acquired by the hematogenous route because surgery may directly inoculate the valve with bacteria from the patient's skin or operating room personnel. A recently placed nonendothelialized valve is more susceptible to bacterial colonization than are native valves. Bacteria also may colonize the new valve from contaminated bypass pumps, cannulas, and pacemakers or from a nosocomial bacteremia subsequent to an intravascular catheter.[1,13] The mechanism of bacterial colonization and pathogenesis in late PVE is similar to native-valve endocarditis.[1]

The vegetations seen in infective endocarditis may be single or multiple and vary in size from a few millimeters to centimeters. Bacteria within the vegetation grow slowly and are protected from antibiotics and host defenses. The adverse effects of infective endocarditis and the resulting lesions can be far-reaching and include (a) local perivalvular damage, (b) embolization of septic fragments with potential hematogenous seeding of remote sites, and (c) formation of antibody complexes.[1–3]

Formation of vegetations may destroy valvular tissue, and continued destruction can lead to acute heart failure via perforation of the valve leaflet, rupture of the chordae tendineae or papillary muscle, or for patients with PVE, valve dehiscence. Occasionally, valvular stenosis may occur. Abscesses can develop in the valve ring or in myocardial tissue itself. Even with resolution of the process, fibrosis of tissue with some residual dysfunction is possible.

Vegetations may be friable, and fragments may be released downstream. These infected particles, termed *septic emboli*, can result in organ abscess or infarction. Septic emboli from right-sided endocarditis commonly lodge in the lungs, causing pulmonary

TABLE 120-1 Etiologic Organisms in Infective Endocarditis	
Agent	**Percentage of Cases (%)**
Streptococci	25–35
Viridans streptococci	10–20
Other streptococci	5–10
Staphylococci	45–70
Coagulase positive	30–60
Coagulase negative	3–25
Enterococci	5–18
Gram-negative aerobic bacilli	1.5–13
Fungi	1–4
Miscellaneous bacteria	<5
Mixed infections	1–2
"Culture negative"	<5–24

Adapted from references 2 and 12.

abscesses. Emboli from left-sided vegetations commonly affect organs with high blood flow, such as the kidneys, spleen, and brain.[1-3]

Circulating immune complexes consisting of antigen, antibody, and complement may deposit in organs, producing local inflammation and damage (e.g., glomerulonephritis in the kidneys). Other potential pathologic changes that result from immune-complex deposition or septic emboli include the development of "mycotic" aneurysms (although the aneurysm is usually bacterial in origin, not fungal), cerebral infarction, splenic infarction and abscess, and skin manifestations such as petechiae, Osler nodes, and Janeway lesions.[1,3]

CLINICAL PRESENTATION

❸ The clinical presentation of infective endocarditis is highly variable and nonspecific. Fever is the most common finding and is often accompanied by other vague symptoms (Table 120–2). Fever may be relatively low grade, particularly in subacute cases. Heart murmurs are found in a majority of patients, most often preexisting, with some documented as new or changing. Infective endocarditis usually begins insidiously and worsens gradually. Patients may present with nonspecific findings, such as fever, chills, weakness, dyspnea, night sweats, weight loss, or malaise. In contrast, patients with acute disease, such as those with a history of IVDA and *S. aureus* infective endocarditis, may appear with classic signs of sepsis.

Splenomegaly is a frequent finding for patients with prolonged endocarditis. Other important clinical signs especially prevalent in subacute illness may include the following peripheral manifestations ("stigmata") of endocarditis[5,11-13]:

- Osler nodes: Purplish or erythematous subcutaneous papules or nodules on the pads of the fingers and toes. These lesions are 2 to 15 mm in size and are painful and tender. These nodes are not specific for infective endocarditis and may be the result of embolism, immunologic phenomena, or both.
- Janeway lesions: Hemorrhagic, painless plaques on the palms of the hands or soles of the feet. These lesions are believed to be embolic in origin.

- Splinter hemorrhages: Thin, linear hemorrhages found under the nail beds of the fingers or toes. These lesions are not specific for infective endocarditis and more commonly are the result of traumatic injuries. Distal lesions are more likely the result of trauma, whereas proximal lesions tend to be associated with infective endocarditis.
- Petechiae: Small (usually 1 to 2 mm in diameter), erythematous, painless, hemorrhagic lesions. These lesions appear anywhere on the skin but more frequently on the anterior trunk, buccal mucosa and palate, and conjunctivae. Petechiae are nonblanching and resolve after a few days.
- Clubbing of the fingers: Proliferative changes in the soft tissues about the terminal phalanges observed in long-standing endocarditis.
- Roth spots: Retinal infarct with central pallor and surrounding hemorrhage.
- Emboli: Embolic phenomena occur in up to one-third of cases and may result in significant complications. Left-sided endocarditis can result in renal artery emboli causing flank pain with hematuria, splenic artery emboli causing abdominal pain, and cerebral emboli, which may result in hemiplegia or alteration in mental status. Right-sided endocarditis may result in pulmonary emboli, causing pleuritic pain with hemoptysis.

Patients with infective endocarditis typically have laboratory abnormalities; however, none of these changes is specific for the disease. Anemia (normocytic, normochromic), leukocytosis, and thrombocytopenia may be present. The white blood cell count is often normal or only slightly elevated, sometimes with a mild left shift. Acute bacterial endocarditis, however, may present with an elevated white blood cell count, consistent with a fulminant infection. The erythrocyte sedimentation rate and C-reactive protein may be elevated in approximately 60% of patients. Often the urinary analysis is abnormal, with proteinuria and microscopic hematuria occurring in approximately 25% of individuals.[5,12]

The hallmark of infective endocarditis is a continuous bacteremia caused by bacteria shedding from the vegetation into the bloodstream; 90% to 95% of patients with infective endocarditis have positive blood cultures.[2,3,12] Three sets of blood cultures, each from separate venipuncture sites, should be collected over 24 hours, and antibiotics should be withheld until adequate blood cultures are obtained. On the other hand, if a patient has a toxic appearance, several blood cultures should be collected promptly, followed by immediate empirical antimicrobial treatment. The blood cultures for patients who have received previous antibiotics should be monitored more closely because pathogen growth may be suppressed.[2,14] "Culture negative" endocarditis describes a patient in whom a clinical diagnosis of infective endocarditis is likely but blood cultures do not yield a pathogen. This condition is often the consequence of previous antibiotic therapy, improperly collected blood cultures, or unusual organisms.[4] When blood cultures from patients suspected of having infective endocarditis show no growth after 48 to 72 hours, the laboratory should be advised and cultures held for up to a month to detect growth of fastidious organisms.[2-4,14]

An electrocardiogram, chest radiograph, and echocardiogram are performed for patients suspected of endocarditis. The electrocardiogram rarely shows important diagnostic findings but may reveal heart block, suggesting extension of the infection. The chest radiograph may provide more diagnostic information, especially in a patient with right-sided endocarditis. Septic pulmonary emboli may occur, leading to multiple lung foci. The echocardiogram is the most important test and should be performed for all patients suspected of this infection.

TABLE 120-2	Clinical Presentation of Infective Endocarditis

General
The clinical presentation of infective endocarditis is highly variable and nonspecific.

Symptoms
The patient may complain of fever, chills, weakness, dyspnea, night sweats, weight loss, and/or malaise.

Signs
Fever is common, as is a heart murmur (sometimes new or changing). The patient may have embolic phenomenon, splenomegaly, or skin manifestations (e.g., Osler nodes, Janeway lesions).

Laboratory tests
The patient's white blood cell count may be normal or only slightly elevated. Nonspecific findings include anemia (normocytic, normochromic), thrombocytopenia, an elevated erythrocyte sedimentation rate or C-reactive protein, and altered urinary analysis (proteinuria/microscopic hematuria). The hallmark laboratory finding is continuous bacteremia; three sets of blood cultures should be collected over 24 hours.

Other diagnostic tests
An electrocardiogram, chest radiograph, and echocardiogram are commonly performed. Echocardiography to determine the presence of valvular vegetations plays a key role in the diagnosis of infective endocarditis; it should be performed in all suspected cases.

Echocardiography plays an important role in the diagnosis and management of infective endocarditis.[4] The chosen approach, transthoracic echocardiography (TTE) or transesophageal echocardiography (TEE), depends on the clinical setting. The TEE technique is more sensitive for detecting vegetations (90% to 100%) as compared with TTE (58% to 63%), and TEE maintains good specificity (85% to 95%).[3,4] TTE appears reasonable in the evaluation of children or adults in whom the clinical suspicion of infective endocarditis is relatively low.[4,16] TEE is preferred in high-risk patients such as those with prosthetic heart valves, many congenital heart diseases, previous endocarditis, new murmur, heart failure, or other stigmata of endocarditis.[4,17] The lack of vegetation on echocardiogram does not exclude infection even if the transesophageal approach is used. Conversely, the test may reveal an unsuspected large vegetation, extension of the disease into surrounding tissue, valvular defects, abscess formation, cordial rupture, or an intracardiac fistula. Thus, in addition to helping in the diagnosis of infective endocarditis, the echocardiogram allows the physician to evaluate hemodynamic stability and the need for urgent surgical intervention; it also provides a rough estimate of the likelihood of embolism.[4,18]

DIAGNOSIS

❹ The signs and symptoms of infective endocarditis are not specific, and the diagnosis is often unclear. The identification of infective endocarditis requires the integration of clinical, laboratory, and echocardiographic findings. The Duke diagnostic criteria include major and minor variables (Table 120–3).[19,20] Based on the number of major and minor criteria that are fulfilled, patients suspected of infective endocarditis are categorized into three separate groups: definite infective endocarditis, possible infective endocarditis, or infective endocarditis rejected.[20]

PROGNOSIS

The outcome for endocarditis is improved with rapid diagnosis, appropriate treatment (i.e., antimicrobial therapy, surgery, or both), and prompt recognition of complications should they arise. Factors associated with increased mortality include (a) heart failure, (b) increasing age, (c) endocarditis caused by resistant organisms such as fungi or gram-negative bacteria, (d) left-sided endocarditis caused by *S. aureus*, (e) paravalvular complications, (f) healthcare-acquired infection, and (g) PVE.[4,5,12,13] The presence of heart failure has the greatest negative impact on the short-term prognosis.[4] For native-valve infective endocarditis, mortality rates range from 20% to 25%; lower rates occur with viridans streptococci (4% to 16%), and higher rates occur with left-sided infective endocarditis caused by enterococci (15% to 25%) and staphylococci (25% to 47%). Even higher rates of mortality are seen with unusually encountered organisms (e.g., mortality greater than 50% for *Pseudomonas aeruginosa*).[4] The mortality rate for right-side infective endocarditis associated with IVDA is generally low (e.g., 10%).[4,5] For those who relapse after treatment for infective endocarditis, most will do so within the first 2 months after discontinuation of antimicrobials. Relapse rates for viridans streptococcus are generally low (2%), whereas relapse is more likely in those with enterococcal infection (8% to 20%) and PVE (10% to 15%).[1,5] After appropriate treatment and recovery, the risk of morbidity and mortality following infective endocarditis persist for years, although it gradually declines annually. Morbidity remains elevated because of a greater likelihood of recurrent infective endocarditis, heart failure, and embolism or, if a valve is replaced, the risk of anticoagulation, valve thrombosis, or additional valve surgery.[21]

TABLE 120-3 Diagnosis of Infective Endocarditis According to the Modified Duke Criteria

Major Criteria
Blood culture positive for infective endocarditis
Typical microorganisms consistent with infective endocarditis from two separate blood cultures:
  Viridans streptococci, *Streptococcus bovis*, HACEK group, *Staphylococcus aureus*; or
  Community-acquired enterococci, in the absence of a primary focus; or
Microorganisms consistent with infective endocarditis from persistently positive blood cultures, defined as follows:
  At least two positive cultures of blood samples drawn greater than 12 hours apart; or
  All of three or a majority of four or more separate cultures of blood (with first and last sample drawn at least 1 hour apart)
Single positive blood culture for *Coxiella burnetii* or antiphase I immunoglobulin G antibody titer >1:800.
Evidence of endocardial involvement
Echocardiogram positive for infective endocarditis (transesophageal echocardiography recommended for patients with prosthetic valves, rated at least "possible infective endocarditis" by clinical criteria, or complicated infective endocarditis [paravalvular abscess]; transthoracic echocardiography as first test for other patients), defined as follows:
  Oscillating intracardiac mass on valve or supporting structures, in the path of regurgitant jets or on implanted material in the absence of an alternative anatomic explanation; or
  Abscess; or
  New partial dehiscence of prosthetic valve
New valvular regurgitation (worsening or changing of preexisting murmur not sufficient)
Minor Criteria
Predisposition, predisposing heart condition, or injection drug use
Fever, temperature >38°C (100.4°F)
Vascular phenomena, major arterial emboli, septic pulmonary infarcts, mycotic aneurysm, intracranial hemorrhage, conjunctival hemorrhages, and Janeway lesions
Immunologic phenomena: glomerulonephritis, Osler nodes, Roth spots, and rheumatoid factor
Microbiologic evidence: Positive blood culture but does not meet a major criterion as noted above or serologic evidence of active infection with organism consistent with infective endocarditis
Echocardiographic minor criteria eliminated

HACEK, *Haemophilus* species (*H. parainfluenzae, H. aphrophilus, H. paraphrophilus*), *Actinobacillus actinomycetemcomitans, Cardiobacterium hominis, Eikenella corrodens*, and *Kingella kingae*.
Note: Cases are defined clinically as *definite* if they fulfill two major criteria, one major criterion plus three minor criteria, or five minor criteria; cases are defined as *possible* if they fulfill one major and one minor criterion or three minor criteria. Cases are rejected if there is a firm alternate diagnosis explaining evidence of infective endocarditis; resolution of infective endocarditis syndrome with antibiotic therapy for <4 days; no pathologic evidence of infective endocarditis at surgery or autopsy, with antibiotic therapy for <4 days; or does not meet criteria for possible infective endocarditis, as above.
Adapted from references 19 and 20.

TREATMENT

Infective Endocarditis

■ DESIRED OUTCOMES

The desired outcomes for treatment and prophylaxis of infective endocarditis are to:

- Relieve the signs and symptoms of the disease.
- Decrease morbidity and mortality associated with the infection.
- Eradicate the causative organism with minimal drug exposure.
- Provide cost-effective antimicrobial therapy determined by the likely or identified pathogen, drug susceptibilities,

hepatic and renal function, drug allergies, and anticipated drug toxicities.

- Prevent infective endocarditis from occurring or recurring in high-risk patients with appropriate prophylactic antimicrobials.

■ GENERAL APPROACH TO TREATMENT

❺ The most important approach in the treatment of infective endocarditis is isolation of the infecting pathogen and determination of antimicrobial susceptibilities, followed by high-dose, parenteral, bactericidal antibiotics for an extended period.[1,2,5] Identification of susceptibilities is crucial given the escalating level of antibiotic resistance to commonly encountered pathogens. Treatment usually is started in the hospital, but for select patients it is often completed in the outpatient setting so long as defervescence has occurred and followup blood cultures show no growth.[5,22] Large doses of parenteral antimicrobials usually are necessary to achieve bactericidal concentrations within vegetations. An extended duration of therapy is required, even for susceptible pathogens, because microorganisms are enclosed within valvular vegetations and fibrin deposits. These barriers impair host defenses and protect microbes from phagocytic cells. In addition, high bacterial concentrations within vegetations may result in an inoculum effect that further resists killing (see Chap. 113 for additional discussion). Many bacteria are not actively dividing, further limiting the rate of bacterial death. For most patients, 4 to 6 weeks of therapy is required.[2,3]

■ NONPHARMACOLOGIC THERAPY

❻ Surgery is an important adjunct in the management of endocarditis. In most surgical cases, valvectomy and valve replacement are performed to remove infected tissue and to restore hemodynamic function. Echocardiographic features that suggest the need for surgery include persistent vegetation or an increase in vegetation size after prolonged antibiotic treatment, valve dysfunction, or paravalvular extension (e.g., abscess).[4,23] Surgery also may be considered in cases of PVE endocarditis caused by resistant organisms (e.g., fungi or gram-negative bacteria), or if there is persistent bacteremia or other evidence of failure despite appropriate antimicrobial therapy.[1,3,23,24] Surgical intervention is also appropriate if heart failure is present in left-sided infective endocarditis and when there is persistent infection in right-sided infective endocarditis.[1,5,23]

■ PHARMACOLOGIC THERAPY

Specific treatment recommendations from the American Heart Association (AHA) provide guidance for the management of infective endocarditis and these were updated in 2005.[4] Guidelines, published in 2009 by the European Society of Cardiology, are consistent with the AHA.[25] Both guidelines use an evidence-based scoring system where recommendations are given a classification as well as level of evidence. Class I recommendations are conditions for which there is evidence, general agreement, or both that a given procedure or treatment is useful and effective. Class II recommendations are conditions for which there is conflicting evidence, a divergence of opinion, or both about the usefulness/efficacy of a procedure or treatment (IIa implies the weight of evidence/opinion is in favor of usefulness/efficacy whereas IIb implies usefulness/efficacy is less well established by evidence/opinion). Class III recommendations are conditions for which there is evidence, general agreement, or both that the procedure/treatment is not useful/effective and in some cases may be harmful. Level of evidence is listed as A (data derived from multiple randomized clinical trials), B (data derived from a single randomized trial or nonrandomized studies), and C (consensus opinion of experts).

❼ β-Lactam antibiotics, such as penicillin G (or ceftriaxone), nafcillin, and ampicillin, remain the drugs of choice for streptococcal, staphylococcal, and enterococcal endocarditis, respectively. Tables 120–4 through 120–11 summarize these recommendations, which are discussed in more detail in the following sections. Because these guidelines focus on common causes of endocarditis, readers are referred to other references for more in-depth discussion of unusually encountered organisms.[4,10,26]

❽ For some pathogens, such as enterococci, the use of synergistic antimicrobial combinations (including an aminoglycoside) is essential to obtain a bactericidal effect. Combination antibiotics also may decrease the emergence of resistant organisms during treatment (e.g., PVE caused by coagulase-negative staphylococci) and hasten the pace of clinical and microbiologic response (e.g., some streptococcal and staphylococcal infections). Occasionally, combination treatment will result in a shorter treatment course.

■ STREPTOCOCCAL ENDOCARDITIS

Streptococci are a common cause of infective endocarditis, with most isolates being viridans streptococci. *Viridans streptococci* refer to a large number of different species, such as *Streptococcus sanguinis, Streptococcus oralis, Streptococcus salivarius, Streptococcus mutans,* and *Gemella morbillorum.*[4] These bacteria are common inhabitants of the human mouth and gingiva, and they are especially common causes of endocarditis involving native valves.[4,13,27] During dental surgery, and even when brushing the teeth, these organisms can cause a transient bacteremia. In susceptible individuals, this may result in infective endocarditis. Streptococcal endocarditis is usually subacute, and the response to medical treatment is very good. *Streptococcus bovis* is not a viridans streptococcus, but it is included in this treatment group because it is penicillin sensitive and requires the same treatment as viridans streptococci. *S. bovis* is a nonenterococcal group D *Streptococcus* that resides in the gastrointestinal tract. Infective endocarditis caused by this organism is often associated with a gastrointestinal pathology, especially colon carcinoma. Endocarditis caused by *Streptococcus pneumoniae, Streptococcus pyogenes,* and groups B, C, and G streptococci are uncommon, and their treatment is not well defined.[4,27]

Antimicrobial regimens for viridans streptococci are well studied, and in uncomplicated cases, response rates as high as 98% can be expected. Viridans streptococci are penicillin susceptible, although some are more susceptible than others. Most are exquisitely sensitive to penicillin G and have minimal inhibitory concentrations (MICs) of less than 0.12 mcg/mL.[4,27] Approximately 10% to 20% are moderately susceptible (MIC 0.12 to 0.5 mcg/mL). This difference in in vitro susceptibility led to recommendations that the MIC be determined for all viridans streptococci and that the results be used to guide therapy. Some streptococci are deemed tolerant to the killing effects of penicillin, where the minimal bactericidal concentration (MBC) exceeds the MIC by 32 times. A tolerant organism is inhibited but not killed by an antibiotic normally considered bactericidal.[4] Bactericidal activity is required for successful treatment of infective endocarditis; therefore, infections with a tolerant organism may relapse after treatment. Despite some animal studies of endocarditis suggesting that tolerant strains do not respond as readily to β-lactam therapy as nontolerant ones, this phenomenon is primarily a laboratory finding with little clinical significance.[3,4] Treatment for tolerant strains is identical to that for nontolerant organisms, and measurement of the MBC is not recommended.[4]

An assortment of regimens can be used to treat uncomplicated, native-valve endocarditis caused by fully susceptible viridans streptococci (Table 120–4). Two single-drug regimens consist of high-dose parenteral penicillin G or ceftriaxone for 4 weeks. If a shorter course of therapy is desired, the guidelines suggest high-dose

TABLE 120-4 Therapy of Native Valve Endocarditis Caused by Highly Penicillin-Susceptible Viridans Group Streptococci and *Streptococcus bovis*

Regimen	Dosage[a] and Route	Duration (week)	Strength of Recommendation	Comments
Aqueous crystalline penicillin G sodium	12–18 million units/24 hours IV either continuously or in four or six equally divided doses	4	I A	Preferred for most patients older than age 65 years or patients with impairment of 8th cranial nerve function or renal function
or				
Ceftriaxone sodium	2 g/24 hours IV/IM in one dose Pediatric dose[b]: penicillin 200,000 units/kg per 24-hour IV in four to six equally divided doses; ceftriaxone 100 mg/kg per 24 hours IV/IM in 1 dose	4	I A	
Aqueous crystalline penicillin G sodium	12–18 million units/24 hours IV either continuously or in six equally divided doses	2	I B	2-week regimen not intended for patients with known cardiac or extracardiac abscess or for those with creatinine clearance of <20 mL/min, impaired 8th cranial nerve function, or *Abiotrophia, Granulicatella,* or *Gemella* spp. infection; gentamicin dosage should be adjusted to achieve peak serum concentration of 3–4 mcg/ mL and trough serum concentration of <1 mcg/mL when three divided doses are used (second option to single daily dose)
or				
Ceftriaxone sodium	2 g/24 hours IV/IM in 1 dose	2	I B	
plus				
Gentamicin sulfate[c]	3 mg/kg per 24 hours IV/IM in 1 dose Pediatric dose: penicillin 200,000 units/kg per 24 hours IV in four to six equally divided doses; ceftriaxone 100 mg/kg per 24 hours IV/IM in 1 dose; gentamicin 3 mg/kg per 24 hours IV/IM in one dose or three equally divided doses[d]	2		
Vancomycin hydrochloride[e]	30 mg/kg per 24 hours IV in two equally divided doses not to exceed 2 g/24 hours unless concentrations are inappropriately low Pediatric dose: 40 mg/kg per 24 hours IV in two to three equally divided doses	4	I B	Vancomycin therapy recommended only for patients unable to tolerate penicillin or ceftriaxone; vancomycin dosage should be adjusted to obtain peak (1 hour after infusion completed) serum concentration of 30–45 mcg/mL and a trough concentration range of 15–20 mcg/mL

Minimum inhibitory concentration <0.12 mcg/mL.
[a]Dosages recommended are for patients with normal renal function.
[b]Pediatric dose should not exceed that of a normal adult.
[c]Other potentially nephrotoxic drugs (e.g., nonsteroidal antiinflammatory drugs) should be used with caution for patients receiving gentamicin therapy.
[d]Data for once-daily dosing of aminoglycosides for children exist, but no data for treatment of infective endocarditis exist.
[e]Vancomycin dosages should be infused during course of at least 1 hour to reduce risk of histamine-release "red man" syndrome.
From reference 4, with permission. Copyright 2005, American Medical Association.

TABLE 120-5 Therapy of Native Valve Endocarditis Caused by Strains of Viridans Group Streptococci and *Streptococcus bovis* Relatively Resistant to Penicillin

Regimen	Dosage[a] and Route	Duration (week)	Strength of Recommendation	Comments
Aqueous crystalline penicillin G sodium	24 million units/24 hours IV either continuously or in four to six equally divided doses	4	I B	Patients with endocarditis caused by penicillin-resistant (MIC >0.5 mcg/mL) strains should be treated with regimen recommended for enterococcal endocarditis (see Table 120–9)
or				
Ceftriaxone sodium	2 g/24 hours IV/IM in one dose	4	I B	
plus				
Gentamicin sulfate[b]	3 mg/kg per 24 hours IM/IV in one dose Pediatric dose[c]: penicillin 300,000 units/24 hours IV in four to six equally divided doses; ceftriaxone 100 mg/kg per 24 hours IV/IM in one dose; gentamicin 3 mg/kg per 24 hours IV/IM in one dose or three equally divided doses	2		Although it is preferred that gentamicin (3 mg/kg) be given as a single daily dose to adult patients, as a second option, gentamicin can be administered daily in three equally divided doses
Vancomycin hydrochloride[c]	30 mg/kg per 24 hours IV in two equally divided doses not to exceed 2 g/24 hours unless serum concentrations are inappropriately low Pediatric dose: 40 mg/kg per 24 hours in two or three equally divided doses	4	I B	Vancomycin[d] therapy recommended only for patients unable to tolerate penicillin or ceftriaxone therapy

Minimum inhibitory concentration (MIC) >0.12 mcg/mL to ≥0.5 mcg/mL.
[a]Dosages recommended are for patients with normal renal function.
[b]See Table 120–4 for appropriate dosage of gentamicin.
[c]Pediatric dose should not exceed that of a normal adult.
[d]See Table 120–4 for appropriate dosage of vancomycin.
From reference 4, with permission. Copyright 2005, American Medical Association.

TABLE 120-6 Therapy for Endocarditis of Prosthetic Valves or Other Prosthetic Material Caused by Viridans Group Streptococci and *Streptococcus bovis*

Regimen	Dosage[a] and Route	Duration (week)	Strength of Recommendation	Comments
Penicillin-susceptible strain (minimum inhibitory concentration ≤0.12 mcg/mL)				
Aqueous crystalline penicillin G sodium	24 million units/24 hours IV either continuously or in four to six equally divided doses	6	I B	Penicillin or ceftriaxone together with gentamicin has not demonstrated superior cure rates compared with monotherapy with penicillin or ceftriaxone for patients with highly susceptible strain; gentamicin therapy should not be administered to patients with creatinine clearance of <30 mL/min
or				
Ceftriaxone sodium	2 g/24 hours IV/IM in one dose	6	I B	
with or without				
Gentamicin sulfate[b]	3 mg/kg per 24 hours IM/IV in one dose	2		
	Pediatric dose[c]: penicillin 300,000 units/24 hours IV in four to six equally divided doses; ceftriaxone 100 mg/kg per 24 hours IV/IM in one dose; gentamicin 3 mg/kg per 24 hours IV/IM in one dose or three equally divided doses			
Vancomycin hydrochloride[d]	30 mg/kg per 24 hours IV in two equally divided doses	2	I B	Vancomycin therapy recommended only for patients unable to tolerate penicillin or ceftriaxone therapy
	Pediatric dose: 40 mg/kg per 24 hours in two or three equally divided doses			
Penicillin relatively or fully resistant strain (minimum inhibitory concentration >0.12 mcg/mL)				
Aqueous crystalline penicillin sodium	24 million units per 24 hours IV either continuously or in four to six equally divided doses	6	I B	
or				
Ceftriaxone	2 g/24 hours IV/IM in one dose	6	I B	
plus				
Gentamicin sulfate	3 mg/kg per 24 hours IV/IM in one dose	6		
	Pediatric dose: penicillin 300,000 units/kg per 24 hours IV in four to six equally divided doses			
Vancomycin hydrochloride	30 mg/kg per 24 hours IV in two equally divided doses	6	I B	Vancomycin therapy recommended only for patients unable to tolerate penicillin or ceftriaxone therapy
	Pediatric dose: 40 mg/kg per 24 hours IV in two or three equally divided doses			

[a]Dosages recommended are for patients with normal renal function.
[b]See Table 120–4 for appropriate dosage of gentamicin.
[c]Pediatric dose should not exceed that of a normal adult.
[d]See text and Table 120–4 for appropriate dosage of vancomycin.
From reference 4, with permission. Copyright 2005, American Medical Association.

parenteral penicillin G plus an aminoglycoside.[4] When used in select patients, this combination is as effective as 4 weeks of penicillin alone. Although streptomycin was listed in previous guidelines, gentamicin is the preferred aminoglycoside because serum drug concentrations are obtained easily, clinicians are more familiar with its use, and the few strains of streptococci resistant to the effects of streptomycin-penicillin remain susceptible to gentamicin-penicillin. Other aminoglycosides are not recommended.

The decision of which regimen to use depends on the perceived risk versus benefit. For example, a 2-week course of gentamicin in an elderly patient with renal impairment may be associated with ototoxicity, worsening renal function, or both. Furthermore, the 2-week regimen is not recommended for patients with known extracardiac infection. On the other hand, a 4-week course of penicillin alone generally entails greater expense, especially if the patient remains in the hospital. Monotherapy with once-daily ceftriaxone offers ease of administration, facilitates home healthcare treatment, and may be cost-effective.[4,28]

The British Society for Antimicrobial Chemotherapy guidelines suggest that all of the following conditions be present to consider a 2-week treatment regimen for penicillin-sensitive streptococcal endocarditis:[26,29]

- Penicillin-sensitive viridans streptococcus or *S. bovis* (penicillin MIC <0.1 mcg/mL)
- No cardiovascular risk factors such as heart failure, aortic insufficiency, or conduction abnormalities
- No evidence of thromboembolic disease

- Native-valve infection
- No vegetation of greater than 5 mm diameter on echocardiogram
- Clinical response within 7 days (the temperature should return to normal, the patient should feel well, and the patient's appetite should return to normal)

⑨ When a patient has a history of an immediate-type hypersensitivity to penicillin, vancomycin should be chosen for infective endocarditis caused by viridans streptococci. When vancomycin is used, the addition of gentamicin is not recommended.[4] Most patients who report a penicillin allergy have a negative penicillin skin test and consequently are at low risk of anaphylaxis.[30] The published experience with penicillin is more extensive than with alternative regimens; consequently, a thorough allergy history must be obtained before a second-line therapy is administered.

For patients with complicated infections (e.g., extracardiac foci) or when the streptococcus has an MIC of 0.12 to less than or equal to 0.5 mcg/mL, combination therapy with an aminoglycoside for the first 2 weeks and penicillin (higher dose) or ceftriaxone is recommended, followed by penicillin or ceftriaxone alone for an additional 2 weeks (Table 120–5).[4] Some viridans streptococci have biologic characteristics that complicate diagnosis and treatment, previously referred to as nutritionally variant streptococci. *Abiotrophia defectiva* and *Granulicatella* species have nutritional deficiencies that hinder growth in routine culture media.[3,4,27] These organisms require special broth supplemented with pyridoxal hydrochloride or cysteine. For patients infected with nutritionally

TABLE 120-7 Therapy for Endocarditis Caused by Staphylococci in the Absence of Prosthetic Materials

Regimen	Dosage[a] and Route	Duration	Strength of Recommendation	Comments
Oxacillin-susceptible strains				
Nafcillin or oxacillin[b] **with**	12 g/24 hours IV in four to six equally divided doses	6 weeks	I A	For complicated right-sided infective endocarditis and for left-sided infective endocarditis; for uncomplicated right-sided infective endocarditis, 2 weeks (see text)
Optional addition of gentamicin sulfate[c]	3 mg/kg per 24 hours IV/IM in two or three equally divided doses	3–5 days		Clinical benefit of aminoglycosides has not been established
For penicillin-allergic (nonanaphylactoid type) patients:				Consider skin testing for oxacillin-susceptible staphylococci and questionable history of immediate-type hypersensitivity to penicillin
Cefazolin **with**	6 g/24 hours IV in three equally divided doses	6 weeks	I B	Cephalosporins should be avoided in patients with anaphylactoid-type hypersensitivity to β-lactams; vancomycin should be used in these cases[d]
Optional addition of gentamicin sulfate	3 mg/kg per 24 hours IV/IM in two or three equally divided doses Pediatric dose: cefazolin 100 mg/kg per 24 hours IV in three equally divided doses; gentamicin 3 mg/kg per 24 hours IV/IM in three equally divided doses	3–5 days		Clinical benefit of aminoglycosides has not been established
Oxacillin-resistant strains				
Vancomycin[e]	30 mg/kg per 24 IV in two equally divided doses Pediatric dose: 40 mg/kg per 24 hours IV in two or three equally divided doses	6 weeks	I B	Adjust vancomycin dosage to achieve 1-hour serum concentration of 30–45 mcg/mL and trough concentration of 15–20 mcg/mL

[a]Dosages recommended are for patients with normal renal function.
[b]Penicillin G 24 million units/24 hours IV in four to six equally divided doses may be used in place of nafcillin or oxacillin if strain is penicillin susceptible (minimum inhibitory concentration ≤0.1 mcg/mL) and does not produce β-lactamase.
[c]Gentamicin should be administered in close temporal proximity to vancomycin, nafcillin, or oxacillin dosing. See Table 120–4 for appropriate dosage of gentamicin.
[d]Pediatric dose should not exceed that of a normal adult.
[e]For specific dosing adjustment and issues concerning vancomycin, see Table 120–4 footnotes.
From reference 4, with permission. Copyright 2005, American Medical Association.

variant streptococci or when the *Streptococcus* has an MIC of more than 0.5 mcg/mL, treatment should follow the enterococcal endocarditis treatment guidelines.[4]

The rationale for combination therapy of penicillin-susceptible viridans streptococci is that enhanced activity against these organisms usually is observed when cell-wall active agents are combined with aminoglycosides in vitro.[31] Combined treatment results in quicker sterilization of vegetations in animal models of endocarditis and probably explains the high response rates observed for patients treated for a total of 2 weeks.[4,32] The combined treatment, however, is not superior to penicillin alone. Some authors question the need for combination therapy in relatively resistant streptococci, emphasizing that few human data suggest that patients with endocarditis caused by these organisms respond less well to penicillin alone.[31,33]

For patients with endocarditis of prosthetic valves or other prosthetic material caused by viridans streptococci and *S. bovis*, choices of treatment are similar to those without prosthetic material (e.g., penicillin or ceftriaxone); however, treatment courses are extended to 6 weeks (Table 120–6). In fact, if the organism is relatively resistant, gentamicin is recommended for 6 weeks.

Whether extended-interval aminoglycoside dosing has a role in infective endocarditis continues to be debated. At this time, data support extended-interval dosing for the treatment of streptococcal infective endocarditis, and as compared with three-times-daily dosing this approach may have greater efficacy.[34–37] One study specifically evaluated the combination of ceftriaxone (2 g daily) with gentamicin (3 mg/kg daily) for 2 weeks compared with ceftriaxone (2 g daily) alone for 4 weeks for penicillin-sensitive streptococci. Both regimens were safe and effective with similar clinical cure rates at 3 months following treatment.[32]

CLINICAL CONTROVERSY

In the past, the AHA guidelines recommended traditional aminoglycoside dosing (three times daily) whenever clinicians use these antibiotics. Extended-interval dosing (once-daily administration) is an intriguing dosing strategy, but data only support this approach for the treatment of streptococcal infective endocarditis.

■ STAPHYLOCOCCAL ENDOCARDITIS

Endocarditis caused by staphylococci has become more prevalent, mainly because of increased IVDA, more frequent use of peripheral and central venous catheters, and increased frequency of valve-replacement surgery.[38,39] *S. aureus* is the most common organism causing infective endocarditis among those with IVDA and persons with venous catheters. Coagulase-negative staphylococci (usually *Staphylococcus epidermidis*) are prominent causes of PVE.

Staphylococcal endocarditis is not a homogeneous disease; appropriate management requires consideration of several questions: Is the organism methicillin resistant? Should combination therapy be used? Is the infection on a native or prosthetic valve? Does the patient have a history of IVDA? Is the infection on the left or right side of the heart? Another consideration in staphylococcal endocarditis is that some organisms may exhibit tolerance to antibiotics. Similar to streptococci, however, the concern for tolerance among staphylococci should not affect antibiotic selection.[4]

TABLE 120-8 Therapy for Prosthetic Valve Endocarditis Caused by Staphylococci

Regimen	Dosage*a* and Route	Duration (week)	Strength of Recommendation	Comments
Oxacillin-susceptible strains				
Nafcillin or oxacillin **plus**	12 g/24 hours IV in four to six equally divided doses	≥6	I B	Penicillin G 24 million units per 24 hours IV in four to six equally divided doses may
Rifampin **plus**	900 mg per 24 hours IV/orally in three equally divided doses	≥6		be used in place of nafcillin or oxacillin if strain is penicillin susceptible (minimum inhibitory concentration ≤0.1 mcg/ mL) and
Gentamicin*b*	3 mg/kg per 24 hours IV/IM in two or three equally divided doses	2		does not produce β-lactamase; vancomycin should be used in patients with immediate-
	Pediatric dose*c*: nafcillin or oxacillin 200 mg/kg per 24 hours IV in four to six equally divided doses; rifampin 20 mg/kg per 24 hours IV/orally in three equally divided doses; gentamicin 3 mg/kg per 24 hours IV/IM in three equally divided doses			type hypersensitivity reactions to β-lactam antibiotics (see Table 120–4 for dosing guidelines); cefazolin may be substituted for nafcillin or oxacillin for patients with nonimmediate-type hypersensitivity reactions to penicillins
Oxacillin-resistant strains				
Vancomycin **plus**	30 mg/kg per 24 hours in two equally divided doses	≥6	I B	Adjust vancomycin to achieve 1-hour serum concentration of 30–45 mcg/mL and trough concentration of 15–20 mcg/mL
Rifampin **plus**	900 mg/24 hours IV/orally in three equally divided doses	≥6		
Gentamicin	3 mg/kg per 24 hours IV/IM in two or three equally divided doses	2		
	Pediatric dose: vancomycin 40 mg/kg per 24 hours IV in two or three equally divided doses; rifampin 20 mg/kg per 24 hours IV/orally in three equally divided doses (up to adult dose); gentamicin 3 mg/kg per 24 hours IV or IM in three equally divided doses			

*a*Dosages recommended are for patients with normal renal function.
*b*Gentamicin should be administered in close proximity to vancomycin, nafcillin, or oxacillin dosing. See Table 120–4 for appropriate dosage of gentamicin.
*c*Pediatric dose should not exceed that of a normal adult.
From reference 4, with permission. Copyright 2005, American Medical Association.

TABLE 120-9 Therapy for Native Valve or Prosthetic Valve Enterococcal Endocarditis Caused by Strains Susceptible to Penicillin, Gentamicin, and Vancomycin

Regimen	Dosage*a* and Route	Duration (week)	Strength of Recommendation	Comments
Ampicillin sodium **or**	12 g/24 hours IV in six equally divided doses	4–6	I A	Native valve: 4-week therapy recommended for patients with symptoms of illness less than 3 months; 6-week therapy recommended for patients with symptoms greater than 3 months
Aqueous crystalline penicillin G sodium **plus**	18–30 million units per 24 hours IV either continuously or in six equally divided doses	4–6	I A	
Gentamicin sulfate*b*	3 mg/kg per 24 hours IV/IM in three equally divided doses	4–6		Prosthetic valve or other prosthetic cardiac material: minimum of 6 weeks of therapy recommended
Vancomycin hydrochloride*d* **plus**	30 mg/kg per 24 hours IV in 2 equally divided doses	6	I B	Vancomycin therapy recommended only for patients unable to tolerate penicillin or ampicillin
Gentamicin sulfate	3 mg/kg per 24 hours IV/IM in three equally divided doses	6		6 weeks of vancomycin therapy recommended because of decreased activity against enterococci
	Pediatric dose*c*: vancomycin 40 mg/kg per 24 hours IV in two or three equally divided doses; gentamicin 3 mg/kg per 24 hours IV/IM in three equally divided doses			

*a*Dosages recommended are for patients with normal renal function.
*b*Dosage of gentamicin should be adjusted to achieve peak serum concentration of 3–4 mcg/mL and a trough concentration of less than 1 mcg/mL. See Table 120–4 for appropriate dosage of gentamicin.
*c*Pediatric dose should not exceed that of a normal adult.
*d*See text and Table 120–4 for appropriate dosing of vancomycin.
From reference 4, with permission. Copyright 2005, American Medical Association.

TABLE 120-10 Therapy for Both Native and Prosthetic Valve Endocarditis Caused by HACEK[a] Microorganisms

Regimen	Dosage and Route	Duration (week)	Strength of Recommendation	Comments
Ceftriaxone[b] sodium	2 g/24 hours IV/IM in one dose	4	I B	Cefotaxime or another third- or fourth-generation cephalosporin may be substituted
or				
Ampicillin-sulbactam[c]	12 g/24 hours IV in four equally divided doses	4	IIa B	
or				
Ciprofloxacin[c,d]	1,000 mg/24 hours orally or 800 mg/24 hours IV in two equally divided doses Pediatric dose[e]: Ceftriaxone 100 mg/kg per 24 hours IV/IM once daily; ampicillin-sulbactam 300 mg/kg per 24 hours IV divided into four or six equally divided doses; ciprofloxacin 20–30 mg/kg per 24 hours IV/orally in two equally divided doses	4	IIb C	Fluoroquinolone therapy recommended only for patients unable to tolerate cephalosporin and ampicillin therapy; levofloxacin, gatifloxacin, or moxifloxacin may be substituted; fluoroquinolones generally not recommended for patients younger than 18 years old Prosthetic valve: Patients with endocarditis involving prosthetic cardiac valve or other prosthetic cardiac material should be treated for 6 weeks.

[a]*Haemophilus parainfluenzae, H. aphrophilus, Actinobacillus actinomycetemcomitans, Cardiobacterium hominis, Eikenella corrodens,* and *Kingella kingae.*
[b]Patients should be informed that IM injection of ceftriaxone is painful.
[c]Dosage recommended for patients with normal renal function.
[d]Fluoroquinolones are highly active in vitro against HACEK microorganisms. Published data on use of fluoroquinolone therapy for endocarditis caused by HACEK are minimal.
[e]Pediatric dose should not exceed that of a normal adult.
From reference 4, with permission. Copyright 2005, American Medical Association.

Any patient who develops staphylococcal bacteremia is at risk for endocarditis. Many investigators have attempted to develop criteria that identify the bacteremic patient likely to have infective endocarditis.[38,39] In the past, patients were considered to be at high risk for infective endocarditis if *S. aureus* bacteremia was community acquired versus hospital acquired.[19] However, nosocomial *S. aureus* bacteremia is now considered as a major criterion for development of infective endocarditis.[20] In hospitalized patients with *S. aureus* bacteremia and an identified focus of infection, such as a vascular catheter, the risk of concomitant infective endocarditis is low, and treatment of the bacteremia can be reduced to 2 weeks. This approach applies only if the patient does not have a prosthetic valve or additional clinical evidence for endocarditis.[39,40] Additionally, the following parameters predict higher risk of infective endocarditis for patients with *S. aureus* bacteremia: (a) the absence of a primary site of infection, (b) metastatic signs of infection, and (c) valvular vegetations detected by echocardiography.[10,20]

The recommended therapy for patients with left-sided, native-valve infective endocarditis caused by methicillin-sensitive *S. aureus* (MSSA) is 6 weeks of nafcillin or oxacillin, often combined with a short course of gentamicin (Table 120–7). Four weeks of mono-therapy with nafcillin or oxacillin may be sufficient for uncomplicated infections (no perivalvular abscess or septic metastatic complications). From in vitro studies, the combination of an aminoglycoside and penicillinase-resistant penicillin or vancomycin enhances the activity of these drugs for MSSA. In animal models of endocarditis, combinations of penicillin with an aminoglycoside eradicate organisms from vegetations more rapidly than penicillins alone.[31,41] In human studies, the addition of an aminoglycoside to nafcillin hastens the resolution of fever and bacteremia, but it does not affect survival or relapse rates and can increase renal toxicity.[31,42,43] Traditional twice- or three-times-daily dosing of aminoglycosides is recommended when administered for staphylococcal infective endocarditis, however there is a report with gentamicin given once a day.[44]

If a patient has a mild, delayed allergy to penicillin, first-generation cephalosporins (such as cefazolin) are effective alternatives, but they should be avoided for patients with a history of immediate-type hypersensitivity reactions to penicillins (see Table 120–7). The potential for

a true immediate-type allergy should be assessed carefully. A penicillin skin test should be conducted before giving antibiotic treatment to any patient with infective endocarditis caused by MSSA if there is a questionable penicillin allergy.[45] ❾ For a patient with a positive skin test or a history of immediate hypersensitivity to penicillin, vancomycin is chosen. Vancomycin, however, kills *S. aureus* slowly and is regarded as inferior to penicillinase-resistant penicillins for MSSA.[39] Alternatively, patients with immediate-type hypersensitivity reactions to penicillin who fail to respond to vancomycin therapy should be considered for penicillin desensitization.[4] Generally, antibiotic therapy should be continued for 6 weeks. Unfortunately, left-sided infective endocarditis caused by *S. aureus* continues to have a poor prognosis, with a mortality rate of 25% to 47%.[5] For reasons discussed in the following section, those with infective endocarditis associated with IVDA have a more favorable response to therapy.

During the past decade, staphylococci more commonly are resistant to penicillinase-resistant penicillins (e.g., methicillin). ❾ Vancomycin is used in this situation because most methicillin-resistant *S. aureus* (MRSA) and coagulase-negative staphylococci are susceptible to it (see Table 120–7). Reports of *S. aureus* strains resistant to vancomycin are emerging.[46] This is concerning as there are currently no standard treatment regimens to treat *S. aureus* infective endocarditis if the strain is resistant to both methicillin and vancomycin. There is literature documenting success with daptomycin or linezolid for these patients.[46–53] Based on available data, daptomycin (at a dose of 6 mg/kg per day) was approved by the Food and Drug Administration (FDA) in 2006 for the treatment of *S. aureus* bacteremia associated with right-sided infective endocarditis.[46,50,54] To date, linezolid has not been approved by the FDA for use in endocarditis as most available data are based on case reports, and there is concern regarding use of a bacteriostatic agent for this condition.[46,47,54] Furthermore, the FDA issued a warning for linezolid in 2007 following reports from one study that patients with catheter-related bacteremia treated with linezolid had an increased incidence of death due to gram-negative bacillary infections.[55] The presence or lack of a prosthetic heart valve in patients with a methicillin-resistant organism guides therapy and determines whether vancomycin should be used alone or, if a prosthetic valve is present, whether combination therapy is necessary (Table 120–8).[4,56]

TABLE 120-11 Therapy for Culture-Negative Endocarditis Including *Bartonella* Endocarditis

Regimen	Dosage[a] and Route	Duration (week)	Strength of Recommendation	Comments
Native valve				
Ampicillin-sulbactam	12 g/24 hours IV in four equally divided doses	4–6	IIb C	Patients with culture-negative endocarditis should be treated with consultation with an infectious diseases specialist
plus				
Gentamicin sulfate[b]	3 mg/kg per 24 hours IV/IM in three equally divided doses	4–6		
Vancomycin[c]	30 mg/kg per 24 hours IV in 2 equally divided doses	4–6	IIb C	Vancomycin recommended only for patients unable to tolerate penicillins
plus				
Gentamicin sulfate	3 mg/kg per 24 hours IV/IM in three equally divided doses	4–6		
plus				
Ciprofloxacin	1,000 mg/24 hours orally or 800 mg/24 hours IV in two equally divided doses	4–6		
	Pediatric dose[d]: ampicillin-sulbactam 300 mg/kg per 24 hours IV in four to six equally divided doses; gentamicin 3 mg/kg per 24 hours IV/IM in three equally divided doses; vancomycin 40 mg/kg per 24 hours in two or three equally divided doses; ciprofloxacin 20–30 mg/kg per 24 hours IV/orally in two equally divided doses			
Prosthetic valve (early, <1 year)				
Vancomycin	30 mg/kg per 24 hours IV in two equally divided doses	6	IIb C	
plus				
Gentamicin sulfate	3 mg/kg per 24 hours IV/IM in three equally divided doses	2		
plus				
Cefepime	6 g/24 hours IV in three equally divided doses	6		
plus				
Rifampin	900 mg/24 hours orally/IV in three equally divided doses	6		
	Pediatric dose: vancomycin 40 mg/kg per 24 hours IV in two or three equally divided doses; gentamicin 3 mg/kg per 24 hours IV/IM in three equally divided doses; cefepime 150 mg/kg per 24 hours IV in three equally divided doses; rifampin 20 mg/kg per 24 hours orally/IV in three equally divided doses			
Prosthetic valve (late, >1 year)		6	IIb C	Same regimens as listed above for native valve endocarditis with the addition of rifampin
Suspected *Bartonella*, culture negative				
Ceftriaxone sodium	2 g/24 hours IV/IM in one dose	6	IIa B	Patients with *Bartonella* endocarditis should be treated in consultation with an infectious diseases specialist
plus				
Gentamicin sulfate	3 mg/kg per 24 hours IV/IM in three equally divided doses	2		
with/without				
Doxycycline	200 mg per 24 hours IV/orally in two equally divided doses	6		
Documented *Bartonella*, culture positive				
Doxycycline	200 mg/24 hours IV or orally in two equally divided doses	6	IIa B	If gentamicin cannot be given, then replace with rifampin, 600 mg/24 hours orally/IV in two equally divided doses
plus				
Gentamicin sulfate	3 mg/kg per 24 hours IV/IM in three equally divided doses	2		
	Pediatric dose: ceftriaxone 100 mg/kg per 24 hours IV/IM once daily; gentamicin 3 mg/kg per 24 hours IV/IM in three equally divided doses; doxycycline 2–4 mg/kg per 24 hours IV/orally in two equally divided doses; rifampin 20 mg/kg per 24 hours orally/IV in two equally divided doses			

[a]Dosages recommended are for patients with normal renal function.
[b]See text and Table 120–4 for appropriate dosing of gentamicin.
[c]See Table 120–4 for appropriate dosing of vancomycin.
[d]Pediatric dose should not exceed that of a normal adult.
From reference 4, with permission. Copyright 2005, American Medical Association.

Staphylococcus Endocarditis: Intravenous Drug Abuser

Infective endocarditis in those with IVDA is frequently (60% to 70%) caused by *S. aureus*, although other organisms may be common in certain geographic locations.[57] In this setting, the tricuspid valve is frequently infected, resulting in right-sided infective endocarditis. Most patients have no history of valve abnormalities, are usually otherwise healthy, and have a good response to medical treatment. Nonetheless, surgery may be required.

An uncomplicated, left-sided MSSA endocarditis may be treated sufficiently with 4 weeks of monotherapy with penicillinase-resistant penicillin.[4] For the intravenous drug abuser, however, the clinical response with right-sided MSSA endocarditis is usually excellent. These patients may be treated effectively (clinical and microbiologic cure exceeding 85%) with a 2-week course of nafcillin or oxacillin plus an aminoglycoside.[57–64] Short-course vancomycin, in place of nafcillin or oxacillin, appears ineffective.[59] Another trial suggested that a 2-week regimen of a penicillinase-resistant penicillin alone, without the addition of an aminoglycoside, is as effective as combined therapy in MSSA tricuspid valve endocarditis.[65] Although these data suggest that an aminoglycoside is unnecessary for short-course treatment in the intravenous drug abuser with right-sided infective endocarditis, most clinicians are uncomfortable with monotherapy and choose combination treatment so long as there are no reasons to avoid an aminoglycoside. Short-course therapy should not be used in left-sided endocarditis, and it is inappropriate for patients with underlying acquired immunodeficiency syndrome, renal failure, meningitis, or substantial pulmonary complications, such as lung abscess from right-sided infective endocarditis.[4]

An intriguing therapeutic approach for staphylococcal endocarditis in those with IVDA is oral treatment. Preliminary data suggest that short-course intravenous treatment (primarily nafcillin; mean: 16 days) followed by oral treatment (dicloxacillin or oxacillin; mean: 26 days) might be effective for tricuspid valve MSSA endocarditis.[66] The positive results of this trial can be explained by the duration of intravenous antibiotics (>2 weeks), which may be a sufficient treatment course. Yet, two other studies that predominantly used oral therapy (ciprofloxacin and rifampin) found this approach to be effective (cure rates exceeding 90%) in addicts with uncomplicated right-sided endocarditis caused by MSSA.[67,68] At this time, concerns with resistance (e.g., ciprofloxacin) and limited published data preclude routine use of oral antibacterial regimens for the treatment of infective endocarditis in the intravenous drug abuser.[4]

Staphylococcal Endocarditis: Prosthetic Valves

PVE accounts for approximately 15% of all infective endocarditis cases.[7] An episode of PVE occurring within 2 months of surgery strongly suggests that the cause is staphylococci implanted during the procedure.[1] Yet the risk of staphylococcal endocarditis remains elevated for up to 12 months after valve replacement. Because this type of infective endocarditis is typically a nosocomial infection, methicillin-resistant organisms are common, and vancomycin is the cornerstone of therapy. Combination antimicrobials are recommended because of the high morbidity and mortality associated with PVE and its refractoriness to therapy.[4,12] Although the addition of rifampin to a penicillinase-resistant penicillin or vancomycin does not result in predictable bacterial synergism, rifampin may have unique activity against staphylococcal infection that involves prosthetic material, where its addition results in a higher microbiologic cure rate.[54] Combination therapy also decreases the emergence of resistance to rifampin, which frequently occurs when it is used alone. For methicillin-resistant staphylococci (both MRSA and coagulase-negative staphylococci), vancomycin is recommended with rifampin for 6 weeks or more (see Table 120–8). An aminoglycoside is added for the first 2 weeks if the organism is aminoglycoside susceptible. For MSSA, penicillinase-resistant penicillin is administered in place of vancomycin. PVE responds poorly to medical treatment and has a higher mortality compared with native-valve endocarditis. Valve dehiscence and incompetence can result in acute heart failure, and surgery is often a component of treatment.[4,38]

Twelve months or more after valve replacement, the likely organism for PVE parallels that of native-valve endocarditis. As with native-valve endocarditis, antimicrobial therapy should be based on the identified organism and in vitro susceptibility. If an organism is identified other than staphylococci, the treatment regimen should be guided by susceptibilities and should be at least 6 weeks in duration.[4] Additionally, a concomitant aminoglycoside is recommended if streptococci or enterococci are identified. Once-daily aminoglycoside regimens have not been adequately evaluated in PVE and are not recommended.[4]

The use of anticoagulation is controversial in PVE. In general, those who require anticoagulation for a prosthetic valve should continue the anticoagulant cautiously during endocarditis therapy, unless a contraindication to therapy exists. It is recommended to hold all anticoagulation for at least 2 weeks for patients with *S. aureus* PVE if a recent central-nervous-system (CNS) embolic event has occurred.[4]

CLINICAL CONTROVERSY

Oral antibiotics for the treatment of infective endocarditis have been assessed primarily in those with IVDA. Although treating infective endocarditis with oral antibiotics would decrease adverse events associated with prolonged use of intravenous catheters, the paucity of data preclude this being a routine treatment. Oral rifampin is used as part of combination therapy in PVE caused by staphylococci. The AHA guidelines recently added ciprofloxacin orally as an option for treatment of infective endocarditis caused by the HACEK group of organisms.

■ ENTEROCOCCAL ENDOCARDITIS

Enterococci are normal inhabitants of the human gastrointestinal tract and, occasionally, of the anterior urethra. These organisms are usually of low virulence but can become pathogens in predisposed patients following genitourinary manipulations (older men) or obstetric procedures (younger women).[3] Historically, enterococci were considered group D streptococci, but they have been reclassified into the genus *Enterococcus* (*E. faecalis* and *E. faecium*). *E. faecalis* is the most common clinical isolate (approximately 90%) of the two species. Enterococci cause 5% to 18% of endocarditis cases, but they are more resistant to therapy than staphylococci and streptococci. Enterococci are noteworthy for these reasons: (a) no single antibiotic is bactericidal, (b) MICs to penicillin are relatively high (1 to 25 mcg/mL), (c) intrinsic resistance occurs to all cephalosporins and relative resistance occurs to aminoglycosides (e.g., "low-level" aminoglycoside resistance), (d) combinations of a cell-wall active agent such as a penicillin or vancomycin and an aminoglycoside are necessary for killing, and (e) resistance to all available drugs is increasing.[4,69,70]

Monotherapy with penicillin for infective endocarditis caused by enterococci results in relapse rates of 50% to 80%. When used alone, penicillins are only bacteriostatic against enterococci, and combination therapy is always recommended for susceptible strains.[4] The relapse rate following penicillin-gentamicin therapy for susceptible strains is less than 15%.[5] The killing of enterococci by the bactericidal combination of an aminoglycoside antibiotic and a penicillin is the best clinical example of antibiotic synergy. Because the aminoglycoside cannot penetrate the bacterial cell in the absence of the penicillin, enterococci usually will appear to be resistant to aminoglycosides by routine susceptibility testing (low-level resistance). However, in the presence of an agent that disrupts the cell wall such as penicillin, the aminoglycoside can gain entry, attach to bacterial ribosomes, and cause rapid cell death. An aminoglycoside-vancomycin combination is also synergistic against enterococci and is appropriate therapy for the penicillin-allergic patient.[3,4]

Enterococcal endocarditis ordinarily requires 4 to 6 weeks of ampicillin or high-dose penicillin G plus an aminoglycoside for cure (Table 120–9). Ampicillin has greater in vitro activity than penicillin G, although there are no clinical data to document differences in efficacy. A 6-week course is recommended for patients with symptoms lasting longer than 3 months and those with PVE. Streptomycin has been the most extensively studied aminoglycoside, but gentamicin is presently favored. Because of resistance, other aminoglycosides, such as tobramycin and amikacin, cannot be substituted routinely. In the treatment of enterococcal endocarditis, relatively low serum concentrations of aminoglycosides appear adequate for successful therapy, such as a gentamicin peak concentration of approximately 3 to 4 mcg/mL.[4,71] Treatment of enterococcal endocarditis does not have the high success rate seen with infective endocarditis caused by viridans streptococci, presumably because the organism is more resistant to killing.

Although some data support the use of extended-interval aminoglycoside dosing for other types of endocarditis (i.e., streptococci), the data are more vague regarding this strategy in enterococcal infective endocarditis.[72] Even though some studies suggest that extended-interval aminoglycoside dosing and short-interval (traditional) dosing are clinically equivalent,[73–75] discordant studies imply otherwise.[76,77] The paucity of human data precludes routine use of extended-interval aminoglycoside dosing in this setting and the guidelines recommend three-times-daily dosing.[4]

Resistance among enterococci to penicillins and aminoglycosides is increasing.[4] Enterococci that exhibit high-level resistance to streptomycin (MIC >2000 mcg/mL) are not synergistically killed by penicillin and streptomycin because the aminoglycoside either no longer binds to the ribosome or is inactivated by an aminoglycoside-modifying enzyme, streptomycin adenylase. Because enterococci will appear resistant to aminoglycosides on routine susceptibility testing, the only way to distinguish high-level from low-level resistance is by performing special susceptibility tests using 500 to 2,000 mcg/mL of the aminoglycoside. High-level streptomycin-resistant enterococci occur with a frequency approaching 60%, and high-level resistance to gentamicin is now found in 10% to 50% of isolates. Although most gentamicin-resistant enterococci are resistant to all aminoglycosides (including amikacin), 30% to 50% remain susceptible to streptomycin.[3,69] High-level gentamicin resistance is mediated by a bifunctional aminoglycoside-modifying enzyme, 6-acetyltransferase/2-phosphotransferase, and most strains also possess streptomycin adenylase. These organisms do not commonly cause infective endocarditis; data on appropriate therapy are sparse, and therapeutic options are few.[69,70,78]

In addition to isolates with high-level aminoglycoside resistance, β-lactamase–producing enterococci (especially E. faecium) have been reported.[79] If these organisms are discovered, use of vancomycin or ampicillin-sulbactam in combination with gentamicin should be considered. Vancomycin-resistant enterococci are reported increasingly, primarily with E. faecium. Vancomycin resistance occurs when the bacterium replaces the normal vancomycin target with a peptidoglycan precursor that does not bind vancomycin.[70]

Treating multidrug-resistant enterococci is difficult, and data on appropriate therapy are sparse. Current guidelines suggest either linezolid or quinupristin-daltopristin for resistant strains of E. faecium and combination β-lactam therapy (ampicillin with either imipenem-cilastatin or ceftriaxone) for E. faecalis.[4] Daptomycin has produced conflicting results.[80–83] Surgery and replacement of the infected cardiac valve may be the only cure.

HACEK Group

Fastidious gram-negative bacteria from the HACEK group account for 5% to 10% of native-valve, community-acquired infective endocarditis.[4] Frequently, these types of infective endocarditis present as subacute illnesses with large vegetations and emboli.[3] These oropharyngeal organisms typically are slow growing and should be considered as possible causes of "culture negative" endocarditis. In the past, high-dose ampicillin with gentamicin for 4 weeks was an acceptable treatment regimen for HACEK endocarditis, but β-lactamase–producing organisms are occurring more often; hence, HACEK organisms should be considered resistant to ampicillin alone. Numerous treatments are reasonable for the treatment of HACEK infective endocarditis, including ceftriaxone and ampicillin-sulbactam; the newest addition to the guidelines is oral ciprofloxacin for select patients (Table 120–10).[4] Treatment is usually for 4 weeks, but it should be extended to 6 weeks in PVE caused by one of these organisms.

■ LESS-COMMON TYPES OF INFECTIVE ENDOCARDITIS

Atypical Microorganisms

Endocarditis caused by organisms such as Bartonella; Coxiella burnetii; Brucella, Candida, and Aspergillus spp.; Legionella; and gram-negative bacilli (e.g., Pseudomonas) is relatively uncommon. Medical therapy for infective endocarditis caused by these organisms is usually unsuccessful.[4,5] Consultation with an infectious disease expert is warranted when these microorganisms are identified.

In addition to Pseudomonas spp., other gram-negative bacilli that have been implicated include Salmonella spp., Escherichia coli, Citrobacter spp., Klebsiella-Enterobacter spp., Serratia marcescens, Proteus spp., and Providencia spp.[84] Generally, these infections have a poor prognosis, with mortality rates as high as 60% to 80%.[84] Cardiac surgery in concert with extended course antibacterial therapy is the recommended course (class IIa; level of evidence: B) for most patients with gram-negative bacillary infective endocarditis. Readers are referred to the AHA guidelines for more extensive review of Pseudomonas spp. infective endocarditis and unusual gram-negative bacteria treatment regimens.[4]

Fungi cause between 2% and 4% of endocarditis cases; most patients with fungal endocarditis have undergone recent cardiovascular surgery, are intravenous drug abusers, have received prolonged treatment with intravenous catheters or antibiotics, or are immunocompromised.[3,85] Candida spp. and Aspergillus spp. are the most commonly involved, and the mortality rate is high (greater than 80%) for these reasons: (a) large, bulky vegetations that often form, (b) systemic septic embolization that may occur, (c) the tendency for fungi to invade the myocardium, (d) poor penetration of vegetations by antifungals, (e) the low toxic-to-therapeutic ratio of agents such as amphotericin B, and (f) the lack of consistent fungicidal activity of available antifungal agents.[3,86] When fungal infective endocarditis is identified, the combined medical–surgical approach is recommended. Because these infections occur infrequently, scant clinical data are available to make solid treatment recommendations; however, the use of antifungal agents alone has been globally unsuccessful. Amphotericin B has been the mainstay pharmacologic approach. The availability of newer antifungal agents challenges this historical approach, although clinical trial data are lacking.[4]

C. burnetii (Q fever) may be recovered from blood cultures, but infection is more likely to be identified via serologic tests. It is a common cause of infective endocarditis in certain areas of the world where goat, cattle, and sheep farming are widespread.

The most favorable therapy for Q fever is unknown but may include doxycycline with trimethoprim-sulfamethoxazole, rifampin, or fluoroquinolones.[3,10] *Brucella* are facultative intracellular gram-negative bacilli. Humans are infected by this organism after ingesting infected unpasteurized milk or undercooked meat, inhalation of infectious aerosols, or contact with infected tissues. This type of infective endocarditis is more common in veterinarians and livestock handlers. Cure requires valve replacement and antimicrobial agents including doxycycline with streptomycin or gentamicin or doxycycline with trimethoprim-sulfamethoxazole or rifampin for an extended period (8 weeks to months).[10]

Culture-Negative Endocarditis

Sterile blood cultures are reported in 5% to 20% of patients with infective endocarditis if strict diagnostic criteria are used.[5,12] This type of infective endocarditis may occur as a result of unidentified subacute right-sided infective endocarditis, previous antibiotic therapy, slow-growing fastidious organisms, nonbacterial etiologies (e.g., fungi), and improperly collected blood cultures. When blood cultures from patients suspected of infective endocarditis show no growth after 48 to 72 hours, the laboratory should be advised, and cultures should be held for up to a month to detect growth of fastidious organisms.[4]

The AHA guidelines provide general recommendations for culture-negative infective endocarditis (Table 120–11), although clinicians should individualize therapy, as necessary. Selection of treatment can be difficult, balancing the need to cover all likely organisms against potential toxic drug effects (e.g., aminoglycosides). Antimicrobial selection should be in consultation with an infectious diseases specialist. Irrespective of the chosen treatment, extended antimicrobial therapy is required. The preceding empirical approaches for culture-negative infective endocarditis highlight the need for proper collection and monitoring of blood cultures and an extensive medication history.

PHARMACOECONOMIC CONSIDERATIONS

Infective endocarditis remains an uncommon disease, but the cost of treatment can be substantial. In the past, the long duration of hospitalization required to administer intravenous antimicrobials was the major expense. In select cases, abbreviated and/or outpatient, oral antimicrobial therapy may appreciably reduce the cost of care.

Shorter-course antimicrobial regimens are advocated when possible. For instance, in exquisitely sensitive streptococcal endocarditis (MICs less than 0.12 mcg/mL), a 2-week regimen of high-dose parenteral penicillin G or ceftriaxone in combination with an aminoglycoside is as effective as 4 weeks of penicillin alone.[4] Uncomplicated right-sided MSSA endocarditis in the intravenous drug abuser may be treated with a 2-week course. Treatment with nafcillin or oxacillin in combination with an aminoglycoside appears to be cost-effective.

The initiation of outpatient parenteral antibiotics should be considered early in the treatment of infective endocarditis, after the patient is stable clinically and responds favorably to initial antibiotics. Outpatient treatment is safe and cost-effective in select situations.[22,87] Patients considered for home therapy must be hemodynamically stable, compliant with therapy, have careful medical monitoring, understand the potential complications of the disease, and have immediate access to medical care. Advances in technology allow for the outpatient administration of complex antibiotic regimens that significantly reduce the cost of therapy. Simple regimens, such as single daily doses of ceftriaxone for streptococcal infective

endocarditis, are particularly attractive. Although endocarditis is common in those with a history of IVDA and home healthcare would substantially reduce the cost of treatment, many clinicians are uncomfortable with outpatient intravenous therapy because central venous access is required. Sudden cardiac decompensation in an outpatient setting is also of concern.[4,88]

EVALUATION OF THERAPEUTIC OUTCOMES

The evaluation of patients treated for infective endocarditis includes assessment of disease signs and symptoms, blood cultures, microbiologic tests, serum drug concentrations, and other tests that evaluate organ function.

SIGNS AND SYMPTOMS

Fever usually subsides within 1 week of initiating therapy.[1,5,88] Persistence of fever may indicate ineffective antimicrobial therapy, emboli, infections of intravascular catheters, or drug reactions. For some patients, low-grade fever may persist even with appropriate antimicrobial therapy. With defervescence, the patient should begin to feel better, and other symptoms, such as lethargy or weakness, should subside. Echocardiography should be performed when antibiotic therapy has been completed to determine new baseline cardiac function (i.e., ventricular size and function). A TTE is usually sufficient.

BLOOD CULTURES

Blood cultures should be negative within a few days, although microbiologic response to vancomycin may be slower. If bacteria continue to be isolated from blood beyond the first few days of therapy, it may indicate that the antimicrobials are inactive against the pathogen or that the doses are not producing adequate concentrations at the site of infection. After the initiation of therapy, blood cultures should be rechecked until negative. During the remainder of therapy, frequent blood culturing is not necessary. Additional blood cultures should be rechecked after successful treatment (e.g., once or twice within the 8 weeks after treatment) to ensure cure.[4]

MICROBIOLOGIC TESTS

For all isolates from blood cultures, MICs should be determined; MBCs are no longer recommended.[4] The agent currently being used should be tested, as well as alternatives that may be required if intolerance, allergy, or resistance occurs. Occasionally, it is useful to determine whether synergy exists for antimicrobial combinations, although synergistic regimens usually can be predicted from the literature. Chapter 113 summarizes the methods for in vitro determinations of synergy.

Serum bactericidal titers (SBTs; also called *Schlichter tests*) have been used in the past in association with a number of infectious diseases. The SBT is the greatest dilution of a patient's serum sample that is obtained while receiving antimicrobial treatment that kills greater than 99.9% of an inoculum of the infecting pathogen in vitro over 18 to 24 hours.

Although specific SBTs have been evaluated in endocarditis, at present, SBTs have little value in monitoring treatment of common types of infective endocarditis and should not be recommended routinely.[4,89] This test may be useful when the causative organisms are only moderately susceptible to antimicrobials, when less-well-established regimens are used, or when response to therapy is suboptimal and dosage escalation is being considered.

SERUM DRUG CONCENTRATIONS

Of the agents used commonly for infective endocarditis, measurement of serum drug concentrations is routinely available for aminoglycosides (except streptomycin) and vancomycin. Few data, however, support attaining any specific serum concentrations for patients with infective endocarditis. In general, serum concentrations of the antimicrobial should exceed the MBC of the organisms. Aminoglycoside concentrations rarely exceed the MBC for certain organisms, such as streptococci and enterococci, and concentrations of aminoglycosides and vancomycin for staphylococci have not been correlated with response.[89,90]

When aminoglycosides are administered for infective endocarditis caused by gram-positive cocci with a traditional three-times-daily regimen, peak serum concentrations are recommended to be on the low side of the traditional ranges (3 to 4 mcg/mL for gentamicin). If extended-interval dosing is used, which is only recommended in streptococcal infective endocarditis, the most appropriate method of monitoring has not been determined. When vancomycin is administered, the most recent treatment guidelines for infective endocarditis recommend serum drug monitoring of peak and trough concentrations.[4] However, it is now generally accepted that peak concentrations of vancomycin have limited clinical applicability and the primary goal of serum vancomycin monitoring is to ensure adequate trough concentrations, in this case 15 to 20 mcg/mL, are achieved.[4,91]

PREVENTION

🔟 Antimicrobial prophylaxis is used as an attempt to prevent infective endocarditis for patients who are at the highest risk.[6,15] The use of antimicrobials for this purpose requires consideration of (a) cardiac conditions associated with endocarditis, (b) procedures causing bacteremia, (c) organisms likely to cause endocarditis, and (d) pharmacokinetics, spectrum, cost, adverse effects, and ease of administration of available antimicrobial agents. The objective of prophylaxis is to diminish the likelihood of infective endocarditis in high-risk individuals from procedures that result in bacteremia. Although there are no prospective, controlled human trials demonstrating that prophylaxis in high-risk individuals protects against the development of endocarditis during bacteremia-induced procedures, animal studies suggest possible benefit.[15] Many causes of infective endocarditis, however, appear not to be secondary to an invasive procedure. Bacteremia as a consequence of daily activities may, in fact, be the major culprit, and the value of antibiotic prophylaxis before bacteremia-causing procedures has been questioned.[92] Retrospective human studies, though, support that a reduction of endocarditis occurs for select patients following dental surgery where prophylaxis is employed.[15] The common practice of using antimicrobial therapy in this setting remains controversial. The mechanism of a beneficial effect in humans is unclear, but antibiotics may decrease the number of bacteria at the surgical site, kill bacteria after they are introduced into the blood, and prevent adhesion of bacteria to the valve. Prophylaxis does not reduce the frequency of bacteremia immediately following tooth extraction as compared with a control group, suggesting that a reduction in adhesion or effects after the bacteria adhere to the endocardium are more likely mechanisms.[93,94] Other studies have further questioned the benefit of antibiotic prophylaxis.[95]

Regardless of the controversy about whether prophylactic antibiotics should be used, infective endocarditis prophylaxis is recommended in select situations, specifically dental procedures, in those with underlying high-risk cardiac conditions. Recently the AHA released new guidelines that better define who should and should

TABLE 120-12	Cardiac Conditions Associated with the Highest Risk of Adverse Outcome from Endocarditis for Which Prophylaxis with Dental Procedures is Recommended

Prosthetic cardiac valves
Previous infective endocarditis
Congenital heart disease (CHD)[a]
  Unrepaired cyanotic CHD, including palliative shunts and conduits
  Completely repaired congenital heart defect with prosthetic material or device, whether placed by surgery or by catheter intervention, during the first 6 months after the procedure[b]
  Repaired CHD with residual defects at the site or adjacent to the site of a prosthetic patch or prosthetic device (that inhibit endothelialization)
Cardiac transplantation recipients who develop cardiac valvulopathy

[a]Except for the conditions listed above, antibiotic prophylaxis is no longer recommended for any other form of CHD.
[b]Prophylaxis is recommended because endothelialization of prosthetic material occurs within 6 months after the procedure.
From reference 4, with permission. Copyright 2005, American Medical Association.

not receive infective endocarditis prophylaxis.[15] This update is timely as data show overuse of infective endocarditis prophylaxis occurs in low-risk patients and underuse occurs in those at greater risk.[96]

CLINICAL CONTROVERSY

The common practice of administering antibiotics to high-risk individuals before a bacteremia-causing procedure is controversial. Despite limited data supporting this approach and the fact that 100% compliance with AHA preventative guidelines would have only a modest benefit, the use of single-dose antibiotics for the prevention of endocarditis remains a standard of care.

Key points of this report are that (a) only a small number of cases of infective endocarditis might be prevented with antibiotic prophylaxis for dental procedures, even if 100% effective; (b) infective endocarditis prophylaxis for dental procedures should be recommended only for patients with underlying cardiac conditions associated with the highest risk; (c) for those with high-risk underlying cardiac conditions, prophylaxis is recommended for all dental procedures involving manipulation of gingival tissue or the periapical region of teeth or perforation of the oral mucosa; (d) prophylaxis is not recommended based solely on an increased lifetime risk of acquisition of infective endocarditis; and (e) administration of antibiotics solely to prevent endocarditis is not recommended for patients who undergo a genitourinary or gastrointestinal tract procedure.

To determine whether a patient should receive prophylactic antibiotics, one needs to assess the patient's risk (Table 120–12) and whether they are undergoing a procedure resulting in bacteremia (Table 120–13). When antibiotic prophylaxis is appropriate,

TABLE 120-13	Dental Procedures for Which Endocarditis Prophylaxis Is Recommended for Patients Described in Table 120–12

All dental procedures that involve manipulation of gingival tissue or the periapical region of teeth or perforation of the oral mucosa[a]

[a]The following procedures and events do not need prophylaxis: routine anesthetic injections through noninfected tissue, taking dental radiographs, placement of removable prosthodontic or orthodontic appliances, adjustment of orthodontic appliances, placement of orthodontic brackets, shedding of deciduous teeth, and bleeding from trauma to the lips or oral mucosa.
From reference 4, with permission. Copyright 2005, American Medical Association.

TABLE 120-14 Antibiotic Regimens for a Dental Procedure

| Situation | Agent | Regimen: Single Dose 30 to 60 Minutes Before Procedure | |
		Adults	Children
Oral	Amoxicillin	2 g	50 mg/kg
Unable to take oral medication	Ampicillin	2 g IM or IV	50 mg/kg IM or IV
	or		
	Cefazolin or ceftriazone	1 g IM or IV	50 mg/kg IM or IV
Allergic to penicillins or ampicillin (oral)	Cephalexin[a,b]	2 g	50 mg/kg
	or		
	Clindamycin	600 mg	20 mg/kg
	or		
	Azithromycin or clarithromycin	500 mg	15 mg/kg
Allergic to penicillins or ampicillin and unable to take oral medication	Cefazolin or ceftriaxone[b]	1 g IM or IV	50 mg/kg IM or IV
	or		
	Clindamycin	600 mg IM or IV	20 mg/kg IM or IV

[a]Or other first- or second-generation oral cephalosporin in equivalent adult or pediatric dosage.
[b]Cephalosporins should not be used for an individual with a history of anaphylaxis, angioedema, or urticaria with penicillins or ampicillin.
From reference 4, with permission. Copyright 2005, American Medical Association.

a single 2 g dose of amoxicillin is recommended for adult patients at risk, given 30 to 60 minutes before undergoing procedures associated with bacteremia (Table 120–14). Because the duration of antimicrobial prophylaxis appears to be relatively short, these guidelines do not advocate a second oral dose of amoxicillin, which was recommended previously. Alternative prophylaxis regimens for patients allergic to penicillins or those unable to take oral medications are also provided.

ABBREVIATIONS

AHA: American Heart Association

HACEK: The group of bacteria including *Haemophilus parainfluenzae, Haemophilus aphrophilus, Actinobacillus actinomycetemcomitans, Cardiobacterium hominis, Eikenella corrodens*, and *Kingella kingae*

IVDA: intravenous drug abuse

MBC: minimal bactericidal concentration

MIC: minimal inhibitor concentration

MRSA: methicillin-resistant *Staphylococcus aureus*

MSSA: methicillin-sensitive *Staphylococcus aureus*

PVE: prosthetic valve endocarditis

SBT: serum bactericidal titer

TEE: transesophageal echocardiogram

TTE: transthoracic echocardiogram

REFERENCES

1. Hill EE, Herijgers P, Herregods MC, Peetermans WE. Evolving trends in infective endocarditis. Clin Microbiol Infect 2006;12:5–12.
2. Moreillon P, Que YA. Infective endocarditis. Lancet 2004;363:139–149.
3. Bashore TM, Cabell C, Fowler V Jr. Update on infective endocarditis. Curr Probl Cardiol 2006;31:274–352.
4. Baddour LM, Wilson WR, Bayer AS, et al. Infective endocarditis: diagnosis, antimicrobial therapy, and management of complications: A statement for healthcare professionals from the Committee on Rheumatic Fever, Endocarditis, and Kawasaki Disease, Council on Cardiovascular Disease in the Young, and the Councils on Clinical Cardiology, Stroke, and Cardiovascular Surgery and Anesthesia, American Heart Association: Endorsed by the Infectious Diseases Society of America. Circulation 2005;111:e394–e434.
5. Mylonakis E, Calderwood SB. Infective endocarditis in adults. N Engl J Med 2001;345:1318–1330.
6. Nishimura RA, Carabello BA, Faxon DP, et al. ACC/AHA 2008 guideline update on valvular heart disease: Focused update on infective endocarditis: A report of the American College of Cardiology/American Heart Association Task Force on Practice Guidelines: Endorsed by the Society of Cardiovascular Anesthesiologists, Society for Cardiovascular Angiography and Interventions, and Society of Thoracic Surgeons. Circulation 2008;118:887–896.
7. Berlin JA, Abrutyn E, Strom BL, et al. Incidence of infective endocarditis in the Delaware Valley, 1988–1990. Am J Cardiol 1995;76:933–936.
8. Hogevik H, Olaison L, Andersson R, Lindberg J, Alestig K. Epidemiologic aspects of infective endocarditis in an urban population. A 5-year prospective study. Medicine (Baltimore) 1995;74:324–339.
9. Lloyd-Jones D, Adams R, Carnethon M, et al. Heart disease and stroke statistics—2009 update: A report from the American Heart Association Statistics Committee and Stroke Statistics Subcommittee. Circulation 2009;119:480–486.
10. Bayer AS, Bolger AF, Taubert KA, et al. Diagnosis and management of infective endocarditis and its complications. Circulation 1998;98:2936–2948.
11. Durante-Mangoni E, Bradley S, Selton-Suty C, et al. Current features of infective endocarditis in elderly patients: Results of the International Collaboration on Endocarditis Prospective Cohort Study. Arch Intern Med 2008;168:2095–2103.
12. Murdoch DR, Corey GR, Hoen B, et al. Clinical presentation, etiology, and outcome of infective endocarditis in the 21st century: The International Collaboration on Endocarditis-Prospective Cohort Study. Arch Intern Med 2009;169:463–473.
13. Benito N, Miro JM, de Lazzari E, et al. Health care-associated native valve endocarditis: Importance of non-nosocomial acquisition. Ann Intern Med 2009;150:586–594.
14. Winston LG, Bolger AF. Modern epidemiology, prophylaxis, and diagnosis and therapy for infective endocarditis. Curr Cardiol Rep 2006;8:102–108.
15. Wilson W, Taubert KA, Gewitz M, et al. Prevention of infective endocarditis: Guidelines from the American Heart Association: A guideline from the American Heart Association Rheumatic Fever, Endocarditis, and Kawasaki Disease Committee, Council on Cardiovascular Disease in the Young, and the Council on Clinical Cardiology, Council on Cardiovascular Surgery and Anesthesia, and the Quality of Care and Outcomes Research Interdisciplinary Working Group. Circulation 2007;116:1736–1754.
16. Cheitlin MD, Armstrong WF, Aurigemma GP, et al. ACC/AHA/ASE 2003 guideline update for the clinical application of echocardiography—Summary article: A report of the American College of Cardiology/American Heart Association Task Force on Practice Guidelines (ACC/AHA/ASE Committee to Update the 1997 Guidelines for the Clinical Application of Echocardiography). J Am Coll Cardiol 2003;42:954–970.
17. Sachdev M, Peterson GE, Jollis JG. Imaging techniques for diagnosis of infective endocarditis. Cardiol Clin 2003;21:185–195.
18. Flachskampf FA, Daniel WG. Role of transoesophageal echocardiography in infective endocarditis. Heart 2000;84:3–4.
19. Durack DT, Lukes AS, Bright DK. New criteria for diagnosis of infective endocarditis: Utilization of specific echocardiographic findings. Duke Endocarditis Service. Am J Med 1994;96:200–209.
20. Li JS, Sexton DJ, Mick N, et al. Proposed modifications to the Duke criteria for the diagnosis of infective endocarditis. Clin Infect Dis 2000;30:633–638.

21. Pokorski RJ. Long-term survival of patients with infective endocarditis. J Insur Med 1998;30:76–87.

22. Rehm SJ. Outpatient intravenous antibiotic therapy for endocarditis. Infect Dis Clin North Am 1998;12:879–901, vi.

23. Bonow RO, Carabello BA, Chatterjee K, et al. 2008 Focused update incorporated into the ACC/AHA 2006 guidelines for the management of patients with valvular heart disease: A report of the American College of Cardiology/American Heart Association Task Force on Practice Guidelines (Writing Committee to Revise the 1998 Guidelines for the Management of Patients With Valvular Heart Disease): Endorsed by the Society of Cardiovascular Anesthesiologists, Society for Cardiovascular Angiography and Interventions, and Society of Thoracic Surgeons. Circulation 2008;118:e523–e661.

24. Ferguson E, Reardon MJ, Letsou GV. The surgical management of bacterial valvular endocarditis. Curr Opin Cardiol 2000;15:82–85.

25. Habib G, Hoen B, Tornos P, et al. Guidelines on the prevention, diagnosis, and treatment of infective endocarditis (new version 2009): The Task Force on the Prevention, Diagnosis, and Treatment of Infective Endocarditis of the European Society of Cardiology (ESC). Eur Heart J 2009.

26. Elliott TS, Foweraker J, Gould FK, et al. Guidelines for the antibiotic treatment of endocarditis in adults: Report of the Working Party of the British Society for Antimicrobial Chemotherapy. J Antimicrob Chemother 2004;54:971–981.

27. Hoen B. Special issues in the management of infective endocarditis caused by gram-positive cocci. Infect Dis Clin North Am 2002;16:437–452, xi.

28. Francioli PB. Ceftriaxone and outpatient treatment of infective endocarditis. Infect Dis Clin North Am 1993;7:97–115.

29. Shanson DC. New guidelines for the antibiotic treatment of streptococcal, enterococcal and staphylococcal endocarditis. J Antimicrob Chemother 1998;42:292–296.

30. Gruchalla RS, Pirmohamed M. Clinical practice. Antibiotic allergy. N Engl J Med 2006;354:601–609.

31. Falagas ME, Matthaiou DK, Bliziotis IA. The role of aminoglycosides in combination with a beta-lactam for the treatment of bacterial endocarditis: A meta-analysis of comparative trials. J Antimicrob Chemother 2006;57:639–647.

32. Sexton DJ, Tenenbaum MJ, Wilson WR, et al. Ceftriaxone once daily for four weeks compared with ceftriaxone plus gentamicin once daily for two weeks for treatment of endocarditis due to penicillin-susceptible streptococci. Endocarditis Treatment Consortium Group. Clin Infect Dis 1998;27:1470–1474.

33. Paul M, Leibovici L. Combination antimicrobial treatment versus monotherapy: The contribution of meta-analyses. Infect Dis Clin North Am 2009;23:277–293.

34. Blatter M, Fluckiger U, Entenza J, et al. Simulated human serum profiles of one daily dose of ceftriaxone plus netilmicin in treatment of experimental streptococcal endocarditis. Antimicrob Agents Chemother 1993;37:1971–1976.

35. Francioli P, Ruch W, Stamboulian D. Treatment of streptococcal endocarditis with a single daily dose of ceftriaxone and netilmicin for 14 days: A prospective multicenter study. Clin Infect Dis 1995;21:1406–1410.

36. Francioli PB, Glauser MP. Synergistic activity of ceftriaxone combined with netilmicin administered once daily for treatment of experimental streptococcal endocarditis. Antimicrob Agents Chemother 1993;37:207–212.

37. Gavalda J, Pahissa A, Almirante B, et al. Effect of gentamicin dosing interval on therapy of viridans streptococcal experimental endocarditis with gentamicin plus penicillin. Antimicrob Agents Chemother 1995;39:2098–2103.

38. Fernandez Guerrero ML, Gonzalez Lopez JJ, Goyenechea A, et al. Endocarditis caused by *Staphylococcus aureus*: A reappraisal of the epidemiologic, clinical, and pathologic manifestations with analysis of factors determining outcome. Medicine (Baltimore) 2009;88:1–22.

39. Petti CA, Fowler VG, Jr. *Staphylococcus aureus* bacteremia and endocarditis. Cardiol Clin 2003;21:219–233, vii.

40. Mermel LA, Allon M, Bouza E, et al. Clinical practice guidelines for the diagnosis and management of intravascular catheter-related infection: 2009 Update by the Infectious Diseases Society of America. Clin Infect Dis 2009;49:1–45.

41. Graham JC, Gould FK. Role of aminoglycosides in the treatment of bacterial endocarditis. J Antimicrob Chemother 2002;49:437–444.

42. Cosgrove SE, Vigliani GA, Fowler VG Jr., et al. Initial low-dose gentamicin for *Staphylococcus aureus* bacteremia and endocarditis is nephrotoxic. Clin Infect Dis 2009;48:713–721.

43. Korzeniowski O, Sande MA. Combination antimicrobial therapy for *Staphylococcus aureus* endocarditis in patients addicted to parenteral drugs and in nonaddicts: A prospective study. Ann Intern Med 1982;97:496–503.

44. Gavalda J, Lopez P, Martin T, et al. Efficacy of ceftriaxone and gentamicin given once a day by using human-like pharmacokinetics in treatment of experimental staphylococcal endocarditis. Antimicrob Agents Chemother 2002;46:378–384.

45. Dodek P, Phillips P. Questionable history of immediate-type hypersensitivity to penicillin in Staphylococcal endocarditis: Treatment based on skin-test results versus empirical alternative treatment—A decision analysis. Clin Infect Dis 1999;29:1251–1256.

46. Garau J, Bouza E, Chastre J, et al. Management of methicillin-resistant *Staphylococcus aureus* infections. Clin Microbiol Infect 2009;15:125–136.

47. Falagas ME, Manta KG, Ntziora F, et al. Linezolid for the treatment of patients with endocarditis: A systematic review of the published evidence. J Antimicrob Chemother 2006;58:273–280.

48. Fowler VG, Jr., Boucher HW, Corey GR, et al. Daptomycin versus standard therapy for bacteremia and endocarditis caused by *Staphylococcus aureus*. N Engl J Med 2006;355:653–665.

49. Howden BP, Ward PB, Charles PG, et al. Treatment outcomes for serious infections caused by methicillin-resistant *Staphylococcus aureus* with reduced vancomycin susceptibility. Clin Infect Dis 2004;38:521–528.

50. Levine DP, Lamp KC. Daptomycin in the treatment of patients with infective endocarditis: Experience from a registry. Am J Med 2007;120(10 suppl 1):S28–33.

51. Rehm SJ, Boucher H, Levine D, et al. Daptomycin versus vancomycin plus gentamicin for treatment of bacteraemia and endocarditis due to *Staphylococcus aureus*: Subset analysis of patients infected with methicillin-resistant isolates. J Antimicrob Chemother 2008;62:1413–1421.

52. Segreti JA, Crank CW, Finney MS. Daptomycin for the treatment of gram-positive bacteremia and infective endocarditis: A retrospective case series of 31 patients. Pharmacotherapy 2006;26:347–352.

53. Woods CW, Cheng AC, Fowler VG, Jr., et al. Endocarditis caused by *Staphylococcus aureus* with reduced susceptibility to vancomycin. Clin Infect Dis 2004;38:1188–1191.

54. Gold HS, Pillai SK. Antistaphylococcal agents. Infect Dis Clin North Am 2009;23:99–131.

55. Linezolid (marketed as Zyvox)—Healthcare Professional Sheet text version; 2009, *http://www.fda.gov/Drugs/DrugSafety/PostmarketDrugSafetyInformationforPatientsandProviders/ucm126262.htm*.

56. Drinkovic D, Morris AJ, Pottumarthy S, et al. Bacteriological outcome of combination versus single-agent treatment for staphylococcal endocarditis. J Antimicrob Chemother 2003;52:820–825.

57. Miro JM, del Rio A, Mestres CA. Infective endocarditis and cardiac surgery in intravenous drug abusers and HIV-1 infected patients. Cardiol Clin 2003;21:167–184, v–vi.

58. Chambers HF. Short-course combination and oral therapies of Staphylococcus aureus endocarditis. Infect Dis Clin North Am 1993;7:69–80.

59. Chambers HF, Miller RT, Newman MD. Right-sided *Staphylococcus aureus* endocarditis in intravenous drug abusers: Two-week combination therapy. Ann Intern Med 1988;109:619–624.

60. DiNubile MJ. Abbreviated therapy for right-sided *Staphylococcus aureus* endocarditis in injecting drug users: The time has come? Eur J Clin Microbiol Infect Dis 1994;13:533–534.

61. DiNubile MJ. Short-course antibiotic therapy for right-sided endocarditis caused by *Staphylococcus aureus* in injection drug users. Ann Intern Med 1994;121:873–876.

62. Espinosa FJ, Valdes M, Martin-Luengo F, et al. Right endocarditis caused by *Staphylococcus aureus* in parenteral drug addicts: Evaluation of a combined therapeutic scheme for 2 weeks versus conventional treatment. Enferm Infecc Microbiol Clin 1993;11:235–240.

63. Torres-Tortosa M, de Cueto M, Vergara A, et al. Prospective evaluation of a two-week course of intravenous antibiotics in intravenous drug addicts with infective endocarditis. Grupo de Estudio

de Enfermedades Infecciosas de la Provincia de Cadiz. Eur J Clin Microbiol Infect Dis 1994;13:559–564.

64. Yung D, Kottachchi D, Neupane B, et al. Antimicrobials for right-sided endocarditis in intravenous drug users: A systematic review. J Antimicrob Chemother 2007;60:921–928.

65. Ribera E, Gomez-Jimenez J, Cortes E, et al. Effectiveness of cloxacillin with and without gentamicin in short-term therapy for right-sided *Staphylococcus aureus* endocarditis. A randomized, controlled trial. Ann Intern Med 1996;125:969–974.

66. Parker RH, Fossieck BE, Jr. Intravenous followed by oral antimicrobial therapy for staphylococcal endocarditis. Ann Intern Med 1980;93: 832–834.

67. Dworkin RJ, Lee BL, Sande MA, et al. Treatment of right-sided *Staphylococcus aureus* endocarditis in intravenous drug users with ciprofloxacin and rifampicin. Lancet 1989;2:1071–1073.

68. Heldman AW, Hartert TV, Ray SC, et al. Oral antibiotic treatment of right-sided staphylococcal endocarditis in injection drug users: Prospective randomized comparison with parenteral therapy. Am J Med 1996;101:68–76.

69. Fernandez Guerrero ML, Goyenechea A, Verdejo C, et al. Enterococcal endocarditis on native and prosthetic valves: A review of clinical and prognostic factors with emphasis on hospital-acquired infections as a major determinant of outcome. Medicine (Baltimore) 2007;86:363–377.

70. Sood S, Malhotra M, Das BK, et al. Enterococcal infections & antimicrobial resistance. Indian J Med Res 2008;128:111–121.

71. Wilson WR, Wilkowske CJ, Wright AJ, et al. Treatment of streptomycin-susceptible and streptomycin-resistant enterococcal endocarditis. Ann Intern Med 1984;100:816–823.

72. Tam VH, Preston SL, Briceland LL. Once-daily aminoglycosides in the treatment of gram-positive endocarditis. Ann Pharmacother 1999;33:600–606.

73. Gavalda J, Cardona PJ, Almirante B, et al. Treatment of experimental endocarditis due to *Enterococcus faecalis* using once-daily dosing regimen of gentamicin plus simulated profiles of ampicillin in human serum. Antimicrob Agents Chemother 1996;40:173–178.

74. Houlihan HH, Stokes DP, Rybak MJ. Pharmacodynamics of vancomycin and ampicillin alone and in combination with gentamicin once daily or thrice daily against *Enterococcus faecalis* in an in vitro infection model. J Antimicrob Chemother 2000;46:79–86.

75. Schwank S, Blaser J. Once-versus thrice-daily netilmicin combined with amoxicillin, penicillin, or vancomycin against *Enterococcus faecalis* in a pharmacodynamic in vitro model. Antimicrob Agents Chemother 1996;40:2258–2261.

76. Fantin B, Carbon C. Importance of the aminoglycoside dosing regimen in the penicillin-netilmicin combination for treatment of *Enterococcus faecalis*-induced experimental endocarditis. Antimicrob Agents Chemother 1990;34:2387–2391.

77. Marangos MN, Nicolau DP, Quintiliani R, et al. Influence of gentamicin dosing interval on the efficacy of penicillin-containing regimens in experimental *Enterococcus faecalis* endocarditis. J Antimicrob Chemother 1997;39:519–522.

78. Lipman ML, Silva J, Jr. Endocarditis due to *Streptococcus faecalis* with high-level resistance to gentamicin. Rev Infect Dis 1989;11:325–328.

79. Wells VD, Wong ES, Murray BE, et al. Infections due to beta-lactamase-producing, high-level gentamicin-resistant *Enterococcus faecalis*. Ann Intern Med 1992;116:285–292.

80. Arias CA, Torres HA, Singh KV, et al. Failure of daptomycin monotherapy for endocarditis caused by an *Enterococcus faecium* strain with vancomycin-resistant and vancomycin-susceptible subpopulations and evidence of in vivo loss of the vanA gene cluster. Clin Infect Dis 2007;45:1343–1346.

81. Cunha BA, Mickail N, Eisenstein L. *E. faecalis* vancomycin-sensitive enterococcal bacteremia unresponsive to a vancomycin tolerant strain successfully treated with high-dose daptomycin. Heart Lung 2007;36:456–461.

82. Hidron AI, Schuetz AN, Nolte FS, et al. Daptomycin resistance in *Enterococcus faecalis* prosthetic valve endocarditis. J Antimicrob Chemother 2008;61:1394–1396.

83. Jenkins I. Linezolid- and vancomycin-resistant *Enterococcus faecium* endocarditis: Successful treatment with tigecycline and daptomycin. J Hosp Med 2007;2:343–344.

84. Morpeth S, Murdoch D, Cabell CH, et al. Non-HACEK gram-negative bacillus endocarditis. Ann Intern Med 2007;147:829–835.

85. Falcone M, Barzaghi N, Carosi G, et al. Candida infective endocarditis: Report of 15 cases from a prospective multicenter study. Medicine (Baltimore) 2009;88:160–168.

86. Pierrotti LC, Baddour LM. Fungal endocarditis, 1995–2000. Chest 2002;122:302–310.

87. Rehm S, Campion M, Katz DE, et al. Community-based outpatient parenteral antimicrobial therapy (CoPAT) for *Staphylococcus aureus* bacteraemia with or without infective endocarditis: Analysis of the randomized trial comparing daptomycin with standard therapy. J Antimicrob Chemother 2009;63:1034–1042.

88. Andrews MM, von Reyn CF. Patient selection criteria and management guidelines for outpatient parenteral antibiotic therapy for native valve infective endocarditis. Clin Infect Dis 2001;33:203–209.

89. Weinstein MP, Stratton CW, Ackley A, et al. Multicenter collaborative evaluation of a standardized serum bactericidal test as a prognostic indicator in infective endocarditis. Am J Med 1985;78:262–269.

90. McCormack JP, Jewesson PJ. A critical reevaluation of the "therapeutic range" of aminoglycosides. Clin Infect Dis 1992;14:320–339.

91. Rybak M, Lomaestro B, Rotschafer JC, et al. Therapeutic monitoring of vancomycin in adult patients: A consensus review of the American Society of Health-System Pharmacists, the Infectious Diseases Society of America, and the Society of Infectious Diseases Pharmacists. Am J Health Syst Pharm 2009;66:82–98.

92. Roberts GJ. Dentists are innocent! "Everyday" bacteremia is the real culprit: A review and assessment of the evidence that dental surgical procedures are a principal cause of bacterial endocarditis in children. Pediatr Cardiol 1999;20:317–325.

93. Hall G, Hedstrom SA, Heimdahl A, et al. Prophylactic administration of penicillins for endocarditis does not reduce the incidence of postextraction bacteremia. Clin Infect Dis 1993;17:188–194.

94. Van der Meer JT, Van Wijk W, Thompson J, et al. Efficacy of antibiotic prophylaxis for prevention of native-valve endocarditis. Lancet 1992;339(8786):135–139.

95. Strom BL, Abrutyn E, Berlin JA, et al. Risk factors for infective endocarditis: Oral hygiene and nondental exposures. Circulation 2000;102:2842–2848.

96. Seto TB, Kwiat D, Taira DA, et al. Physicians' recommendations to patients for use of antibiotic prophylaxis to prevent endocarditis. JAMA 2000;284:68–71.

CHARLES A. PELOQUIN AND ROCSANNA NAMDAR

KEY CONCEPTS

❶ Tuberculosis (TB) is the most prevalent communicable infectious disease on earth; it remains out of control in many developing nations. These nations require medical and financial assistance from developed nations in order to control the spread of TB globally.

❷ In the United States, TB disproportionately affects ethnic minorities as compared with whites, reflecting greater ongoing transmission in ethnic minority communities. Additional TB surveillance and preventive treatment are required within these communities.

❸ Coinfection with human immunodeficiency virus (HIV) and TB accelerates the progression of both diseases, thus requiring rapid diagnosis and treatment of both diseases.

❹ Mycobacteria are slow-growing organisms; in the laboratory, they require special stains, special growth media, and long periods of incubation to isolate and identify.

❺ TB can produce atypical signs and symptoms in infants, the elderly, and immunocompromised hosts, and it can progress rapidly in these patients.

❻ Latent TB infection (LTBI) can lead to reactivation disease years after the primary infection occurred.

❼ The patient suspected of having active TB disease must be isolated until the diagnosis is confirmed and the patient is no longer contagious. Often, isolation takes place in specialized "negative-pressure" hospital rooms to prevent the spread of TB.

❽ Isoniazid and rifampin are the two most important TB drugs; organisms resistant to both these drugs [multidrug-resistant TB (MDR-TB)] are much more difficult to treat.

❾ Never add a single drug to a failing TB treatment regimen!

❿ Directly observed treatment should be used whenever possible to reduce treatment failures and the selection of drug-resistant isolates.

> Learning objectives, review questions, and other resources can be found at **www.pharmacotherapyonline.com**.

❶ Tuberculosis (TB) remains a leading infectious killer globally. TB is caused by *Mycobacterium tuberculosis*, which can produce either a silent, latent infection or a progressive, active disease.[1] Left untreated or improperly treated, TB causes progressive tissue destruction and, eventually, death. Because of renewed public health efforts, TB rates in the United States continue to decline. In contrast, TB remains out of control in many developing countries—to the point that one-third of the world's population currently is infected.[1] Given increasing drug resistance, it is critical that a major effort be made to control TB before the most effective drugs are lost permanently.

M. tuberculosis preferentially infects humans, and the closely related *Mycobacterium bovis* causes a similar disease in cattle and other livestock. Although uncommon today, humans frequently developed TB by drinking milk contaminated with *M. bovis*— a threat that spurred the development of pasteurization. Today, airborne *M. tuberculosis* is the main threat to humans.

Evidence of TB has been found in ancient human remains, and ancient texts describe it.[1–3] TB commonly was known as "consumption" because of the pronounced weight loss that it caused.[1] Other common names included "wasting disease" and the "white plague." As the term *plague* implies, TB had a profound impact on human history, most notably in Europe. (Note: The "black plague," or bubonic plague, is a separate disease caused by *Yersinia pestis*.)

TB rates generally have risen with increasing urbanization and overcrowding because it is easier for an airborne disease to spread when people are packed closely together.[3] Hence TB became a significant pathogen in Europe during the Middle Ages and peaked during the Industrial Revolution, when it caused approximately 25% of all deaths in Europe and in the United States.[1–3] This dire threat led to the rise of public health departments and to procedures such as the isolation of infected patients. Thus, TB was directly responsible for many of the healthcare practices that we take for granted today. Unfortunately, in developing nations, some of these practices are not widely available, and TB continues to rage unabated.

EPIDEMIOLOGY

Globally, roughly 2 billion people are infected by *M. tuberculosis*, and roughly 2 million people die from active TB each year despite the fact that it is curable.[1,2,4] In the United States, about 13 million people are latently infected with *M. tuberculosis*, meaning that they are not currently sick but that they could fall ill with TB at any time. The United States had 12,904 new cases of active TB in 2008 and about 644 deaths in 2006.[5] [For detailed data analysis, visit the Centers for Disease Control and Prevention (CDC) website at *www.cdc.gov/nchstp/tb*.)] The annual incidence of TB in the United States declined by approximately 5% per year from 1953 to 1983[6]

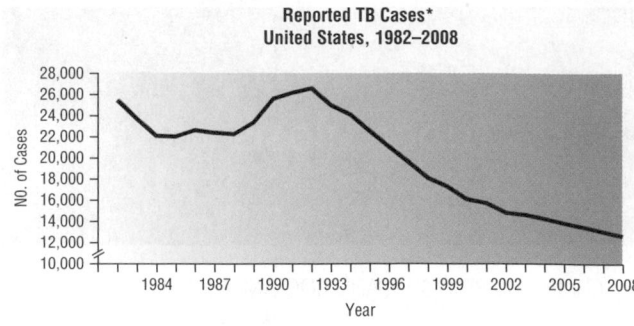

FIGURE 121-1. Reported tuberculosis cases in the United States, 1982 to 2008. *(From the Centers for Disease Control and Prevention. www.cdc.gov.)*

(Fig. 121–1). In 1984, this decline slowed, and then the incidence of TB rose from 1988 to 1992, reaching 10.5 cases per 100,000 population. Since 1992, more effective infection control practices and treatment protocols have reduced TB rates to 4.2 per 100,000 population as of 2008.[5] Despite this good news, the eradication of TB from the United States remains very difficult. One reason is that we continue to import new cases from countries where TB remains out of control.[4,5]

RISK FACTORS FOR INFECTION

Location and Place of Birth

TB can infect anyone, but the risk is not evenly distributed across the U.S. population. The major points of entry into the United States have the most TB cases. Four states (California, Florida, New York, and Texas) reported more than 500 cases each for 2008; combined, these four states accounted for 49% (6,350 cases) of the national total.[5] Within these states, TB is most prevalent in large urban areas.[4]

The TB rate among foreign-born persons was 10 times that of U.S.-born persons in 2008.[5] The percentage of foreign-born TB patients in the United States has increased annually since 1986, reaching 59% in 2008.[5] More than half (59.0%) of the foreign-born cases in 2008 were reported in persons from Mexico (1,752), the Philippines (855), Vietnam (582), India (596), and China (398).[5] Therefore, healthcare workers must "think TB" when caring for patients from these countries who experience symptoms such as cough, fever, and weight loss.

Close contacts of pulmonary TB patients are most likely to become infected.[2-4] These include family members, coworkers, or coresidents in places such as prisons, shelters, or nursing homes. The more prolonged the contact, the greater is the risk, with infection rates as high as 30%.[5,6] Although many circumstances exist, TB patients frequently have limited access to healthcare, live in crowded conditions, or are homeless.[2,4] Many patients have histories of alcohol abuse or illicit drug use, and many are coinfected with hepatitis B or human immunodeficiency virus (HIV). These concurrent social and health problems make treating some TB patients particularly difficult.

Race, Ethnicity, Age, and Gender

❷ In the United States, TB disproportionately affects ethnic minorities. Hispanics, blacks, and Asians had TB rates 7.4, 8.0, and 23.2 times, respectively, higher than whites in 2008.[5] Hispanics accounted for 29% of all TB cases, followed by Asians at 26%[5] and blacks accounted for 25%, whereas non-Hispanic whites accounted for only 17% of the new TB cases.[5]

TB is most common among people 25 to 44 years of age (33% of all U.S. cases in 2008), followed by those 45 to 64 years of age (30%) and 65 years of age and older (19%).[5] TB is more common in older whites and Asians compared with younger people from these groups. This reflects reactivation of latent infection acquired many years earlier when TB was very common. Older blacks and Hispanics also have more TB than younger individuals, but the differences by age are not as pronounced.[5] This reflects a greater recent transmission among younger blacks and Hispanics compared with younger whites and Asians. Until the age of 15 years, TB rates are similar for males and females, but after that, the male predominance increases with each decade of life.[5]

Coinfection with Human Immunodeficiency Virus

❸ HIV is the most important risk factor for active TB, especially among people 25 to 44 years of age.[2,4,5,7] TB and HIV seem to act synergistically within patients and across populations, making each disease worse than it might otherwise be. *Approximately 6% of U.S. TB patients are coinfected with HIV, and 10% of TB patients ages 25 to 44 years are coinfected.*[5] These numbers are estimates because laws and regulations in some states prohibit sharing HIV status of TB patients with the TB program. HIV coinfection may not increase the risk of acquiring *M. tuberculosis* infection, but it does increase the likelihood of progression to active disease.[1,7] There is evidence for higher mortality rates in HIV coinfected with MDR and XDR-TB.[8] Furthermore, TB and HIV patients share a number of behavioral risk factors that contribute to the high rates of coinfection.[2,9,10]

RISK FACTORS FOR DISEASE

Once infected with *M. tuberculosis*, a person's lifetime risk of active TB is approximately 10%.[2,4,7] The greatest risk for active disease occurs during the first 2 years after infection. Children younger than 2 years of age and adults older than 65 years of age have two to five times greater risk for active disease compared with other age groups. Patients with underlying immune suppression (e.g., renal failure, cancer, and immunosuppressive drug treatment) have 4 to 16 times greater risk than other patients. Finally, HIV-infected patients with *M. tuberculosis* infection are 100 times more likely to develop active TB than normal hosts.[4,11] HIV-infected patients have an annual risk of active TB of approximately 10%, rather than a lifetime risk at that rate. Therefore, all patients with HIV infection should be screened for tuberculous infection, and those known to be infected with *M. tuberculosis* should be tested for HIV infection.

ETIOLOGY

M. tuberculosis is a slender bacillus with a waxy outer layer.[2,7] It is 1 to 4 μm in length, and under the microscope, it is either straight or slightly curved in shape.[1,12,13] It does not stain well with Gram stain, so the Ziehl-Neelsen stain or the fluorochrome stain must be used instead.[1,2,7] After Ziehl-Neelsen staining with carbol-fuchsin, mycobacteria retain the red color despite acid–alcohol washes. Hence, they are called *acid-fast bacilli*.[12] After staining, microscopic examination ("smear") detects about 8,000 to 10,000 organisms per milliliter of specimen, so a patient can be "smear negative" but still grow *M. tuberculosis* on culture. Microscopic examination also cannot determine which of the more than 100 mycobacterial species is present or whether the organisms in the original samples were alive or dead.[1,12,13] On smear, they are all dead. On culture, *M. tuberculosis* grows slowly, doubling about every 20 hours. This is slow compared with gram-positive and gram-negative bacteria, which double about every 30 minutes.

Among the mycobacteria, only *M. tuberculosis* is a frequent human pathogen. Some nontuberculous mycobacteria such as *Mycobacterium kansasii*, *Mycobacterium fortuitum*, and *Mycobacterium avium* complex (MAC) cause infections in patients with other medical problems, especially the acquired immunodeficiency syndrome (AIDS). The treatment of these infections is discussed in Chap. 134.

CULTURE AND SUSCEPTIBILITY TESTING

❹ Direct susceptibility testing involves inoculating specialized media with organisms taken directly from a concentrated, smear-positive specimen.[1,12,13] This approach produces susceptibility results in 2 to 3 weeks. Indirect susceptibility testing involves inoculating the test media with organisms obtained from a pure culture of the organisms, which can take several more weeks. The most common agar method, known as the *proportion method*, uses the ratio of colony counts on drug-containing agar to that on drug-free agar.[1,13] In the United States, the critical proportion for resistance is 1%. That means that if a drug-containing plate shows only 2% of the growth seen on a drug-free plate, some of the organisms from the specimen were resistant to that drug. Therefore, it is likely that many of the organisms in the patient also are resistant to that drug, and it should not be used to treat that patient.

The proportion method's limitations include many weeks to obtain results, drug degradation during the incubation, and a qualitative result (susceptible or resistant). The BACTEC system (Becton-Dickinson, Sparks, MD) uses liquid medium (7H12 broth) and detects live mycobacteria based on the release of radiolabeled CO_2.[12] Advantages of the BACTEC system include reduced incubation time (as few as 9 to 14 days), reduced drug loss in the medium, and when multiple concentrations are tested, a truly quantitative end point [minimal inhibitory concentration (MIC)].[1,12,13] Newer, nonradiometric rapid methods such as the MGIT system are now being used by many laboratories.[14]

Rapid-identification tests are now available.[14] Nucleic acid probes such as the AccuProbe (Gen-Probe, San Diego, CA) use DNA probes to identify the presence of complementary ribosomal ribonucleic acid (rRNA) for several mycobacterial species.[7,12,15] DNA fingerprinting using restriction-fragment-length polymorphism analysis has been used to identify clusters of cases.[1,12,15] Amplification of the genetic material can be achieved through polymerase chain reaction (Roche Molecular Systems, Branchburg, NJ), the amplified *M. tuberculosis* direct (MTD) test (Gen-Probe, San Diego, CA), and strand-displacement amplification (SDA; Becton-Dickinson, Sparks, MD).[12,16] Thin-layer chromatography, high-performance liquid chromatography for mycolic acid identification, and gas chromatography for short-chain fatty acids (methyl esters) have been used to speciate mycobacterial isolates.[1,12,15] Other tests are designed to detect common genetic changes associated with drug resistance, such as changes in the *katG* gene associated with isoniazid resistance and the *rpoB* gene associated with rifampin resistance.[7,17–19] One such test, the Hain test, is being evaluated by the FDA and has entered into limited clinical use in the United States. These tests offer clinicians a chance to know rapidly what organism they are treating and what drugs might be good initial choices.

TRANSMISSION

M. tuberculosis is transmitted from person to person by coughing or sneezing.[2,7,14] This produces "droplet nuclei" that are dispersed in the air. Each droplet nuclei contains one to three organisms. Riley and colleagues showed that air circulated from a hospital TB ward could cause disease in guinea pigs.[20] When this air was filtered or treated with ultraviolet radiation, the animals were not infected. Approximately 30% of individuals who experience prolonged contact with an infectious TB patient will become infected.

A person with cavitary, pulmonary TB and a cough may infect roughly one person per month until that person is treated effectively, although this number can vary significantly. A person with the uncommon laryngeal form of TB can spread organisms even when talking, so the transmission rates can be very high. HIV-infected patients acquire the organisms through the lungs just like normal hosts, but their weakened immune system puts them at very high risk for active disease.[2,4,7,14]

PATHOPHYSIOLOGY

IMMUNE RESPONSE

Good T-lymphocyte responses are essential to controlling *M. tuberculosis* infections.[2,7,21,22] In the mouse model, two different T-cell responses—the T-helper type 1 (TH_1) response and the T-helper type 2 (TH_2) response—have been described. The TH_1 response is the preferred response to TB, and the TH_2 response, including the potentially subversive influence of interleukin (IL) 4, is undesirable.[2,21,22] Some workers have argued that this dichotomy is clearer in the mouse model, and in many humans, the T-cell response may be classified as TH_0 (elements of both TH_1 and TH_2).[21] In either case, T lymphocytes activate macrophages that, in turn, engulf and kill mycobacteria. T lymphocytes also destroy immature macrophages that harbor *M. tuberculosis* but are unable to kill the invaders.[21,22] CD4+ cells are the primary T cells involved, with contributions by γδ T cells and CD8+ T cells.[20] CD4+ T cells produce interferon-γ (INF-γ) and other cytokines, including IL-2 and IL-10, that coordinate the immune response to TB.[21] Because CD4+ cells are depleted in HIV-infected patients, these patients are unable to mount an adequate defense to TB.[21,22]

Although B-cell responses and antibody production can be demonstrated in TB-infected mammals, these humoral responses do not appear to contribute much to the control of TB within the host.[2,7,21] T cells are responding to certain mycobacterial antigens, but the key antigen(s) invoking the immune response have not been identified.[21] Tumor necrosis factor-α (TNF-α) and INF-γ are important cytokines involved in coordinating the host's cell-mediated response. Rheumatoid arthritis patients treated with TNF-α inhibitors (such as infliximab) have high rates of reactivation TB.[23] Therefore, patients known to be deficient in the activity of TNF-α or INF-γ should be screened for TB infection and offered appropriate treatment.

M. tuberculosis has several ways of evading or resisting the host immune response.[21,22] In particular, *M. tuberculosis* can inhibit the fusion of lysosomes to phagosomes inside macrophages. This prevents the destructive enzymes found in the lysosomes from getting to the bacilli captured in the phagosomes. This inhibition of destructive mechanisms allows time for *M. tuberculosis* to escape into the cytoplasm. Virulent *M. tuberculosis* is able to multiply in the macrophage cytoplasm, thus perpetuating their spread. Finally, lipoarabinomannan (LAM), the principal structural polysaccharide of the mycobacterial cell wall, inhibits the host immune response.[21,22] Lipoarabinomannan induces immunosuppressive cytokines, thus blocking macrophage activation; additionally, lipoarabinomannan scavenges O_2, thus preventing attack by superoxide anions, hydrogen peroxide, singlet oxygen, and hydroxyl radicals.[21,22] These survival mechanisms make *M. tuberculosis* a particularly difficult organism to control. Any defects in the host immune system make it likely that *M. tuberculosis* will not be controlled and that active disease will ensue.

PRIMARY INFECTION

Primary infection usually results from inhaling airborne particles that contain *M. tuberculosis*.[2,7,22] These particles, called *droplet nuclei,* contain one to three bacilli and are small enough (1 to 5 mm) to reach the alveolar surface. Ingestion (swallowing) and inoculation (puncture wound) are other rare pathways to acquire *M. tuberculosis* infection.[22]

The progression to clinical disease depends on three factors: (a) the number of *M. tuberculosis* organisms inhaled (infecting dose), (b) the virulence of these organisms, and (c) the host's cell-mediated immune response.[2,5,7,14,22,24] At the alveolar surface, the bacilli that were delivered by the droplet nuclei are ingested by pulmonary macrophages.[22] If these macrophages inhibit or kill the bacilli, infection is aborted.[22] If the macrophages cannot do this, the organisms continue to multiply. The macrophages eventually rupture, releasing many bacilli, and these mycobacteria are then phagocytized by other macrophages. This cycle continues over several weeks until the host is able to mount a more coordinated response.[22] During this early phase of infection, *M. tuberculosis* multiplies logarithmically.[22]

Some of the intracellular organisms are transported by the macrophages to regional lymph nodes in the hilar, mediastinal, and retroperitoneal areas. The cycle of phagocytosis and cell rupture continues. During lymph node involvement, the mycobacteria may be held in check. More frequently, *M. tuberculosis* spreads throughout the body through the bloodstream.[2,7,22] When this intravascular dissemination occurs, *M. tuberculosis* can infect any tissue or organ in the body. Most commonly, *M. tuberculosis* infects the posterior apical region of the lungs. This may be so because of the high oxygen content, and it may be because of a less vigorous immune response in this area.

After about 3 weeks of infection, T lymphocytes are presented with *M. tuberculosis* antigens. These T cells become activated and begin to secrete INF-γ and the other cytokines noted earlier. The processes described in the immune response section earlier then begin to occur. First, T-lymphocytes stimulate macrophages to become bactericidal.[22] Large numbers of activated microbicidal macrophages surround the solid caseous (cheese-like) tuberculous foci (the necrotic area of infection).[22] This process of creating activated microbicidal macrophages is known as *cell-mediated immunity* (CMI).[22]

At the same time that cell-mediated immunity occurs, delayed-type hypersensitivity also develops through the activation and multiplication of T lymphocytes. Delayed-type hypersensitivity (DTH) refers to the cytotoxic immune process that kills nonactivated immature macrophages that are permitting intracellular bacillary replication.[22] These immature macrophages are killed when the T lymphocytes initiate Fas-mediated apoptosis (programmed cell death).[22] The bacilli released from the immature macrophages then are killed by the activated macrophages.[22]

By this time (>3 weeks), macrophages have begun to form granulomas to contain the organisms. In a typical tuberculous granuloma, activated macrophages accumulate around a caseous lesion and prevent its further extension.[22] At this point, the infection is largely under control, and bacillary replication falls off dramatically. Depending on the inflammatory response, tissue necrosis and calcification of the infection site plus the regional lymph nodes may occur.

Over 1 to 3 months, activated lymphocytes reach an adequate number, and tissue hypersensitivity results. This is shown by a positive tuberculin skin test. Any remaining mycobacteria are believed to reside primarily within granulomas or within macrophages that have avoided detection and lysis, although some residual bacilli have been found in various types of cells.[2,7,21]

Approximately 90% of infected patients have no further clinical manifestations. Most patients only show a positive skin test (70%), whereas some also have radiographic evidence of stable granulomas (approximately 20%). This radiodense area on chest radiograph is called a *Ghon complex*. Approximately 5% of patients (usually children, the elderly, and the immunocompromised) experience "progressive primary" disease that occurs before skin test conversion.[25,26] This presents as a progressive pneumonia, usually in the lower lobes. Disease frequently spreads, leading to meningitis and other severe forms of TB.[25,26] Because of this risk of severe disease, very young, elderly, and immunocompromised patients, including those with HIV, should be evaluated and treated for latent or active TB.

REACTIVATION DISEASE

6 Roughly 10% of infected patients develop reactivation disease at some point in their lives. Nearly half of these cases occur within 2 years of infection.[2,7,14] In the United States, most cases of TB are believed to result from reactivation. Reinfection is uncommon in the United States because of the low rate of exposure and because previously sensitized individuals possess some degree of immunity to reinfection.[2,22] Exceptions include patients coinfected with HIV who live in areas of higher exposure to *M. tuberculosis.*

The apices of the lungs are the most common sites for reactivation (85% of cases).[2] This reflects the fact that *M. tuberculosis* prefers areas with high oxygen content and possibly because the immune response may not be as effective in this region.[2,22] For reasons that are not entirely known (waning cellular immunity, loss of specific T-cell clones, blocking antibody), organisms within granulomas emerge and begin multiplying extracellularly.[22] The inflammatory response produces caseating granulomas, which eventually will liquefy and spread locally, leading to the formation of a hole (cavity) in the lungs.

The immune response contributes to the severity of the lung damage. There is targeted killing of immature macrophages that are allowing mycobacterial multiplication (DTH).[21,22] In addition, there is "innocent bystander" killing of host cells and locally thrombosed blood vessels.[22] The killing of mycobacteria, macrophages, and neutrophils that have entered the battle releases cytokines and lysozymes into the infectious foci. This toxic mixture can be too much for the surrounding alveoli and airway cells, causing regional necrosis and structural collapse.[2,22] These unstable foci liquefy, spreading the infection to neighboring areas of the lung, creating a cavity. Some of this necrotic material is coughed out, producing droplet nuclei. Bacterial counts in the cavities can be as high as 10^8 per milliliter of cavitary fluid. Partial healing may result from fibrosis, but these lesions remain unstable and may continue to expand.[2,22] If left untreated, pulmonary TB continues to destroy the lungs, resulting in hypoxia, respiratory acidosis, and eventually death.

EXTRAPULMONARY AND MILIARY TUBERCULOSIS

Caseating granulomas at extrapulmonary sites can undergo liquefaction, releasing tubercle bacilli and causing symptomatic disease.[2,7] Extrapulmonary TB without concurrent pulmonary disease is uncommon in normal hosts but more common in HIV-infected patients. Because of these unusual presentations, the diagnosis of TB is difficult and often delayed in immunocompromised hosts.[2,4,7] Lymphatic and pleural diseases are the most common forms of extrapulmonary TB, followed by bone, joint, genitourinary, meningeal, and other forms.[2,7] Left untreated, these forms will spread to other organs and may result in death.

Occasionally, a massive inoculum of organisms enters the bloodstream, causing a widely disseminated form of the disease known as *miliary TB*. It is named for the millet seed appearance of the small granulomas seen on chest radiographs, and it can be rapidly fatal.[21] Miliary TB is a medical emergency requiring immediate treatment.

INFLUENCE OF HIV INFECTION ON PATHOGENESIS

❸ HIV infection is the largest risk factor for active TB.[2,7,21] As CD4+ lymphocytes multiply in response to the mycobacterial infection, HIV multiplies within these cells and selectively destroys them. In turn, the TB-fighting lymphocytes are depleted.[21] This vicious cycle puts HIV-infected patients at 100 times the risk of active TB compared with HIV-negative people.[27] In addition, the combination of HIV infection and certain social behaviors increases the risk of newly acquired TB. In select areas of the United States, up to 50% of new TB cases are the result of recent infection, particularly among HIV-infected individuals.[27–29]

As mycobacteria spread throughout the body, HIV replication accelerates in lymphocytes and macrophages. This leads to progression of HIV disease.[21,30] HIV-infected patients who are infected with TB deteriorate more rapidly unless they receive antimycobacterial chemotherapy.[31,32] Most clinicians now recommend beginning TB treatment first, and 2 weeks later, begin HIV treatment. Some patients will experience paradoxical worsening of the TB.[14,33] This appears to result from a reinvigorated inflammatory response to TB. Because TB can be very dangerous in HIV-positive patients, they should be screened for tuberculous infection or disease soon after they are shown to be HIV-positive.[2,4,7,21]

CLINICAL PRESENTATION

The classical presentation of TB is shown below. The onset of TB may be gradual, and the diagnosis may not be considered until a chest radiograph is performed. Unfortunately, many patients do not seek medical attention until more dramatic symptoms, such as hemoptysis, occur. At this point, patients typically have large cavitary lesions in the lungs. These cavities are loaded with *M. tuberculosis.*

CLINICAL PRESENTATION OF TUBERCULOSIS

Signs and Symptoms

  Patients typically present with weight loss, fatigue, a productive cough, fever, and night sweats.[1,2,7,24]

  Frank hemoptysis.

Physical Examination

  Dullness to chest percussion, rales, and increased vocal fremitus are observed frequently on auscultation.

Laboratory Tests

  Moderate elevations in the white blood cell (WBC) count with a lymphocyte predominance.

Chest Radiograph

  Patchy or nodular infiltrates in the apical areas of the upper lobes or the superior segment of the lower lobes.[2,7,24]

  Cavitation that may show air-fluid levels as the infection progresses.

Expectoration or swallowing of infected sputum may spread the disease to other areas of the body.[1,2,7,24] Physical examination is nonspecific but suggestive of progressive pulmonary disease.

❺ Patients coinfected with HIV may have atypical presentations.[1,2,7,24,34] As their CD4+ counts decline, HIV-positive patients are less likely to have positive skin tests, cavitary lesions, or fever. Pulmonary radiographic findings may be minimal or absent. HIV-positive patients have a higher incidence of extrapulmonary TB and are more likely to present with progressive primary disease. Because their symptoms are not specific to TB, a thorough workup for TB is essential.[2,7,21,24]

Extrapulmonary TB typically presents as a slowly progressive decline in organ function.[2,7,24] Patients may have low-grade fever and other constitutional symptoms. Patients with genitourinary TB may present with sterile pyuria and hematuria. Lymphadenitis often involves the cervical and supraclavicular nodes and may appear as a neck mass with spontaneous drainage. Tuberculous arthritis and osteomyelitis occur most commonly in the elderly and usually affect the lower spine and weight-bearing joints. TB of the spine is known as *Pott disease.*[2] Abnormal behavior, headaches, or convulsions suggest tuberculous meningitis. Involvement of the peritoneum, pericardium, larynx, and adrenal glands also occurs.[2,7,24]

THE ELDERLY

❺ TB in the elderly is easily confused with other respiratory diseases. Many clinical findings are muted or absent altogether. Compared with younger patients, TB in the elderly is far less likely to present with positive skin tests, fevers, night sweats, sputum production, or hemoptysis.[2,24,35,36] Weight loss may occur but is nonspecific. In contrast, mental status changes are twice as common in the elderly, and mortality is six times higher.[2,24,35] TB is a preventable cause of death in the elderly that should not be overlooked.

CHILDREN

❺ TB in children, especially those younger than 12 years of age, may present as a typical bacterial pneumonia and is called *progressive primary TB.*[24–26] Clinical disease often begins 1 to 2 months after exposure and precedes skin-test positivity. Unlike adults, pulmonary TB in children often involves the lower and middle lobes.[24–26] Dissemination to the lymph nodes, gastrointestinal and genitourinary tracts, bone marrow, and meninges is common. Because of delays in recruitment of cellular immunity, cavitary disease is infrequent, and the number of organisms present typically is smaller than in an adult. Because cavitary lesions are uncommon, children do not spread TB readily. However, TB can be rapidly fatal in a child, and it requires prompt chemotherapy.

DIAGNOSIS

DIAGNOSTIC TESTING

The key to stopping the spread of TB is early identification of infected individuals.[1,2,7,24] Table 121–1 lists the populations most likely to benefit from testing (column 1 patients are at highest risk for TB, followed by those in column 2). Members of these high-risk groups should be tested for TB infection and educated about the disease.

The Mantoux test is a TB skin test. It uses tuberculin purified protein derivative (PPD), and unlike the Heaf or tine test, the Mantoux test is quantitative. The standard 5-tuberculin-unit PPD dose is placed intracutaneously on the volar aspect of the forearm with a 26- or 27-gauge needle.[2,24,31] This injection should produce a small, raised, blanched wheal. An experienced professional should read

TABLE 121-1 Criteria for Tuberculin Positivity by Risk Group

Reaction 5 mm of Induration	Reaction ≥10 mm of Induration	Reaction ≥15 mm of Induration
Human immunodeficiency virus (HIV)-positive persons	Recent immigrants (i.e., within the last 5 years) from high-prevalence countries	Persons with no risk factors for TB
Recent contacts of tuberculosis (TB) case patients	Injection-drug users	
Fibrotic changes on chest radiograph consistent with prior TB	Residents and employees[a] of the following high-risk congregate settings: prisons and jails; nursing homes and other long-term care facilities for the elderly; hospitals and other healthcare facilities; residential facilities for patients with acquired immunodeficiency syndrome (AIDS); homeless shelters	
Patients with organ transplants and other immuno-suppressed patients (receiving the equivalent of ≥15 mg/day of prednisone for 1 month or more)[b]	Mycobacteriology laboratory personnel	
	Persons with the following clinical conditions that place them at high risk: silicosis; diabetes mellitus; chronic renal failure; some hematologic disorders (e.g., leukemias and lymphomas); other specific malignancies (e.g., carcinoma of the head or neck and lung); weight loss of ≥10% of ideal body weight; gastrectomy; jejunoileal bypass	
	Children younger than 4 years of age or infants, children, and adolescents exposed to adults at high risk	

[a]For persons who are otherwise at low risk and who are tested at the start of employment, a reaction of ≥15 mm induration is considered positive.
[b]Risk of TB for patients treated with corticosteroids increases with higher dose and longer duration.
Adapted from Centers for Disease Control and Prevention. Screening for tuberculosis and tuberculosis infection in high-risk populations: Recommendations of the Advisory Council for the Elimination of Tuberculosis. MMWR 1995;44(RR-11):19–34.

the test in 48 to 72 hours. The area of induration (the "bump") is the important end point, not the area of redness. Table 121-1 lists the criteria for interpretation.[1,2,7,24,31] The CDC does not recommend the routine use of anergy panels.[31,37] Aplisol and Tubersol 5-tuberculin-unit products are available commercially, but because of more predictable results, Tubersol appears to be the preferred product.

The "booster effect" occurs for patients who do not respond to an initial skin test but show a positive reaction if retested about a week later.[24,37] Patients with past *M. tuberculosis* infection and some patients with past immunization with bacillus Calmetté-Guerin (BCG) vaccine or past infection with other mycobacteria may "boost" with a second skin test. Individuals who require periodic skin testing, such as healthcare workers, should receive a two-stage test initially.[24,37,38] Once they are shown to be skin-test negative, any positive skin test later shows recent infection, and this requires treatment.

The PPD skin test is an imperfect diagnostic tool. Up to 20% of patients with active TB are falsely skin-test negative, presumably because their immune systems are overwhelmed.[21,37] False-positive results are more common in low-risk patients and those recently vaccinated with BCG. Despite BCG vaccination, one should not ignore a positive PPD result. These patients require careful evaluation for active disease, and they may be offered preventive treatment because many come from areas where TB infection is common.

Interferon gamma release assays (IGRA) measure the release of INF-γ in blood in response to the TB antigens.[39] They may provide quick and specific results for identifying *M. tuberculosis*. IGRAs do not trigger a booster effect and are more specific for testing M. tuberculosis than the PPD. The QuantiFERON-TB Gold test (QFT-G) is an enzyme-linked immunosorbent assay (ELISA) and was approved by the U.S. Food and Drug Administration in 2005.[40] The T-SPOT.TB, an enzyme linked immunospot (ELISPOT) assay, was approved by the U.S. Food and Drug Administration in 2008.[41] Both tests can be used for diagnosing latent tuberculosis infection and tuberculosis disease caused by *M. tuberculosis*. The antigenic proteins are absent from BCG vaccine strains and from most nontuberculosis mycobacteria. Therefore, QFT-G does not trigger a booster effect and is more specific for testing of *M. tuberculosis* than the PPD. Although these tests can provide results to diagnose both latent infection and disease, they can not differentiate between the two. Results are available within <24 hours, instead of the 2 to 3 days required for the traditional PPD skin test. Therefore, the patient does not have to return to the clinic as required by the PPD skin test, making it more convenient. The CDC recognizes the use of these tests in all circumstances in which the PPD is currently used; however, the sensitivity for young children, immunocompromised patients has not been determined.[42–45]

ADDITIONAL TESTS

When active TB is suspected, attempts should be made to isolate *M. tuberculosis* from the site of infection.[2,7,24,37] Sputum collected in the morning usually has the highest yield.[2,12,24] Daily sputum collection over 3 consecutive days is recommended.

For patients unable to expectorate, sputum induction with aerosolized hypertonic saline may produce a diagnostic sample. Bronchoscopy, or aspiration of gastric fluid via a nasogastric tube, may be attempted for select patients.[24] For patients with suspected extrapulmonary TB, samples of draining fluid, biopsies of the infected site, or both may be attempted. Blood cultures are positive occasionally, especially in AIDS patients.[24,34,46]

TREATMENT

Tuberculosis

■ DESIRED OUTCOMES

The desired outcomes for the treatment of tuberculosis are

1. Rapid identification of a new TB case

2. Initiation of specific antituberculosis treatment

3. Prompt resolution of the signs and symptoms of disease

4. Achievement of a noninfectious state in the patient, thus ending isolation

5. Adherence to the treatment regimen by the patient

6. Cure of the patient as quickly as possible (generally at least 6 months of treatment)

It is also important that patients with active disease are isolated to prevent spread of the disease and that appropriate samples for smears and cultures are collected. Secondary goals are identification of the index case that infected the patient, identification of all persons infected by both the index case and the new case of TB ("contact investigation"), and completion of appropriate treatments for those individuals.

GENERAL APPROACHES TO TREATMENT

Drug treatment is the cornerstone of TB management.[2,7,14,47] Monotherapy can be used only for infected patients who do not have active TB (latent infection, as shown by a positive skin test). Once active disease is present, a minimum of two drugs, and generally three or four drugs, must be used simultaneously.[2,7,14,47] The duration of treatment depends on the condition of the host, extent of disease, presence of drug resistance, and tolerance of medications. The shortest duration of treatment generally is 6 months, and 2 to 3 years of treatment may be necessary for cases of multidrug-resistant TB (MDR-TB).[2,7,14,47] Because the duration of treatment is so long and because many patients feel better after a few weeks of treatment, careful follow-up is required. Directly observed therapy by a healthcare worker is a cost-effective way to ensure completion of treatment.[2,7,14,47–49]

PRINCIPLES FOR TREATING LATENT INFECTION AND FOR TREATING DISEASE

Asymptomatic patients with tuberculous infection have a bacillary load of about 10^3 organisms, compared with 10^{11} organisms in a patient with cavitary pulmonary TB.[2,7,50] As the number of organisms increases, the likelihood of naturally occurring drug-resistant mutants also increases. Naturally occurring resistant mutants are found at rates of 1 in 10^6 to 1 in 10^8 organisms for the antituberculosis drugs.[2,47,50] When treating asymptomatic latent infection with isoniazid monotherapy, the risk of selecting out isoniazid-resistant organisms is low. The isoniazid mutation rate is about 1 in 10^6, but only about 10^3 organisms are present in the body. In contrast, the risk of selecting out isoniazid-resistant organisms is unacceptably high for patients with cavitary TB. One can prevent selection of these resistant mutants by adding more drugs because the rates for resistance mutations to multiple drugs are additive functions of the individual rates. For example, only 1 in 10^{13} organisms would be naturally resistant to both isoniazid (1 in 10^6) and rifampin (1 in 10^7).[2,47,50] It is unlikely that such rare organisms are present in a previously untreated patient.

Combination chemotherapy is required for treating active TB disease. The patient should receive at least two drugs to which the isolate is susceptible, and generally, four drugs are given at the outset of treatment. Rifampin and isoniazid are the best drugs for preventing drug resistance, followed by ethambutol, streptomycin, and pyrazinamide.[2,7,47,50,51]

Three subpopulations of mycobacteria are proposed to exist within the body, and each appears to respond to certain drugs.[2,47,50] Most numerous are the extracellular, rapidly dividing bacteria, often found within cavities (about 10^7 to 10^9 organisms). These are killed most readily by isoniazid, followed by rifampin, streptomycin, and the other drugs. A second group resides within caseating granulomas (possibly 10^5 to 10^7 organisms). These organisms appear to be in a semidormant state, with occasional bursts of metabolic activity. Pyrazinamide, through its conversion within *M. tuberculosis* to pyrazinoic acid, appears most active against these organisms. Rifampin and isoniazid also may be active against this subpopulation. The third subset is the intracellular mycobacteria present within macrophages (10^4 to 10^6). Rifampin, isoniazid, and the quinolones appear to be most active against intracellular *M. tuberculosis*. While this appears to explain what happens during the treatment of TB, there is no practical way to quantitate these populations within a given patient.

NONPHARMACOLOGIC THERAPY

❼ Nonpharmacologic interventions aim to (a) prevent the spread of TB, (b) find where TB has already spread using contact investigation, and (c) replenish the weakened (consumptive) patient to a state of normal weight and well-being. The first two items are performed by public health departments. Clinicians involved in the treatment of TB should verify that the local health department has been notified of all new cases of TB.

Workers in hospitals and other institutions must prevent the spread of TB within their facilities.[2,4,14,31] All such workers should learn and follow each institution's infection control guidelines. This includes using personal protective equipment, including properly fitted respirators, and closing doors to "negative pressure" rooms. These hospital isolation rooms draw air in from surrounding areas rather than blowing air (and *M. tuberculosis*) into these surrounding areas. The air from the isolation room may be treated with ultraviolet lights and then vented safely outside. However, these isolation rooms work properly only if the door is closed.

Debilitated TB patients may require therapy for other medical problems, including substance abuse and HIV infection, and some may need nutritional support. Therefore, clinicians involved in substance abuse rehabilitation and nutritional support services should be familiar with the needs of TB patients.

Surgery may be needed to remove destroyed lung tissue, space-occupying infected lesions (*tuberculomas*), and certain extrapulmonary lesions.[2,14,47] Vaccines against TB include BCG and *M. vaccae*.[47] However, these vaccines are of limited value, and neither can prevent infection by *M. tuberculosis*. BCG (discussed below) may prevent extreme forms of TB in infants, whereas *Mycobacterium vaccae* can not be recommended.[47,52]

PHARMACOLOGIC THERAPY

Treating Latent Infection

Isoniazid is the preferred drug for treating latent TB infection.[2,7,14,47] Generally, isoniazid alone is given for 9 months. The treatment of latent TB infection (LTBI) reduces a person's lifetime risk of active TB from approximately 10% to approximately 1%. Because TB is spread easily through the air, each case prevented also prevents a second wave of cases that each prevented case would have produced. Historically, the treatment of LTBI has been called *prophylaxis, chemoprophylaxis,* or *preventive treatment*. By any name, it is one of the primary mechanisms for reducing TB in the United States. Table 121–2 lists the LTBI treatment options.

Because young children, the elderly, and HIV-positive patients are at greater risk of active disease once infected with *M. tuberculosis*, they require careful evaluation. Once active TB is ruled out, they should receive treatment for latent infection.[2,23,24,47]

The keys to successful treatment of LTBI are (a) infection by an isoniazid-susceptible isolate, (b) adherence to the 9-month regimen, and (c) no exogenous reinfection.[2] Isoniazid adult doses are usually 300 mg daily (5 to 10 mg/kg of body weight)[47] (see Table 121–2). Lower doses are less effective.[2,53,54] Isoniazid should be given on an empty stomach, and antacids should be avoided within 2 hours of dosing. When adherence is an issue, twice-weekly isoniazid (900 mg in an adult) can be given using directly observed treatment. Nine months of treatment is recommended, but 6 months still provides considerable benefit.

Rifampin 600 mg daily for 4 months can be used when isoniazid resistance is suspected or when the patient cannot tolerate isoniazid.[2,26,47] Rifabutin 300 mg daily might be substituted for rifampin for patients at high risk of drug interactions. The combination of pyrazinamide plus rifampin is no longer recommended because of higher than expected rates of hepatotoxicity. When resistance to isoniazid and rifampin is suspected in the isolate causing infection, there is no regimen proved to be effective.[2,47] Regimens that *might* be effective include ethambutol plus levofloxacin, but data regarding efficacy are lacking.

TABLE 121-2 Recommended Drug Regimens for Treatment of Latent Tuberculosis (TB) Infection in Adults

Drug	Interval and Duration	Comments	Rating[a] (Evidence)[b] HIV−	Rating[a] (Evidence)[b] HIV+
Isoniazid	Daily for 9 months[b,c]	In human immunodeficiency virus (HIV)-infected patients, isoniazid may be administered concurrently with nucleoside reverse transcriptase inhibitors (NRTIs), protease inhibitors, or nonnucleoside reverse transcriptase inhibitors (NNRTIs)	A (II)	A (II)
	Twice weekly for 9 months[b,c]	Directly observed therapy (DOT) must be used with twice-weekly dosing.	B (II)	B (II)
Isoniazid	Daily for 6 months[c]	Not indicated for HIV-infected persons, those with fibrotic lesions on chest radiographs, or children	B (I)	C (I)
	Twice weekly for 6 months[c]	DOT must be used with twice-weekly dosing	B (II)	B (III)
Rifampin	Daily for 4 months	For persons who are contacts of patients with isoniazid-resistant, rifampin-susceptible TB who can not tolerate pyrazinamide	B (II)	C (I)

[a]Strength of recommendation: A, preferred; B, acceptable alternative; C, offer when A and B can not be given.
[b]Quality of evidence: I, randomized clinical trial data; II, data from clinical trials that are not randomized or were conducted in other populations; III, expert opinion.
[c]Recommended regimen for children younger than 18 years of age.
[d]Recommended regimen for pregnant women. Some experts would use rifampin and pyrazinamide for 2 months as an alternative regimen in HIV-infected pregnant women, although pyrazinamide should be avoided during the first trimester.
Adapted from Centers for Disease Control and Prevention. Targeted tuberculin testing and treatment of latent tuberculosis infection. MMWR 2000;49(RR-6):31.

For recent skin-test converters of all ages, the risk of active TB outweighs the risk for drug toxicity.[31,47] Pregnant women, alcoholics, and patients with poor diets who are treated with isoniazid should receive pyridoxine (vitamin B6) 10 to 50 mg daily to reduce the incidence of central nervous system (CNS) effects or peripheral neuropathies. All patients who receive treatment of LTBI should be monitored monthly for adverse drug reactions and for possible progression to active TB.

Treating Active Disease

❽ The treatment of active TB requires the use of multiple drugs. There are two primary antituberculosis drugs, isoniazid and rifampin, with the rest of the drugs having specific roles.[47,50,51] Isoniazid and rifampin should be used together whenever possible. Typically, *M. tuberculosis* is either very susceptible or very resistant to a given drug. This contrasts with *M. avium*, where moderately resistant organisms are a frequent occurrence. Theoretically, MIC results could be used to guide dosing in the treatment of moderately resistant *M. tuberculosis*, but this remains to be studied prospectively.[2,14,47]

Drug-susceptibility testing should be done on the initial isolate for all patients with active TB. These data should guide the selection of drugs over the course of treatment.[2,7,14,47] However, some patients are unable to provide a suitable specimen for laboratory testing. If susceptibility data are not available for a given patient, the drug-susceptibility data for the suspected source case or regional susceptibility data should be used.[2,47]

Drug resistance should be expected for patients presenting for the retreatment of TB. These patients require retesting of drug susceptibility using freshly collected specimens. It is imperative to learn what drugs the patient received and for how long the patient received them.[2,14,47] A treatment history, often called a *drug-o-gram*, shows the start and stop dates of all antimycobacterial drugs on a horizontal bar graph.[2,47] A drug-o-gram should be constructed for all retreatment patients.

❿ The standard TB treatment regimen is isoniazid, rifampin, pyrazinamide, and ethambutol for 2 months, followed by isoniazid and rifampin for 4 months, a total of 6 months of treatment.[2,14,47] If susceptibility to isoniazid, rifampin, and pyrazinamide is shown, ethambutol can be stopped at any time. Without pyrazinamide, a total of 9 months of isoniazid and rifampin treatment is required. Table 121–3 shows the recommended treatment regimens. When intermittent therapy is used, directly observed treatment is essential. Doses missed during an intermittent TB regimen decrease its efficacy and increase the relapse rate. Note that Table 121–3 shows recommendations that differ for HIV-negative and HIV-positive

patients. HIV-positive patients should not receive highly intermittent regimens. In general, regimens given daily five times each week or three times weekly can be used for HIV-positive patients. Less-frequent dosing is associated with higher failure and relapse rates and the selection of rifampin-resistant organisms.[47]

When a patient's sputum smears convert to a negative, the risk of the patient infecting others is greatly reduced, but it is not zero.[2,22,47] Such patients can be removed from respiratory isolation, but they must be careful not to cough on others and should meet with others only in well-ventilated places. Smear-negative patients still may be culture positive, so they still can transmit TB to others.

Patients who are slow to respond clinically, those who remain culture positive at 2 months of treatment, those with cavitary lesions on chest radiograph, and perhaps HIV-positive patients should be treated for a total of 9 months and for at least 6 months from the time that they convert to smear and culture negativity.[2,7,14,47] Some authors recommend therapeutic drug monitoring for such patients.[2,47,51,53] When isoniazid and rifampin can not be used, treatment durations become 2 years or more regardless of immune status.[2,14,47,51]

Adjustments to the regimen should be made once the susceptibility data are available.[2,14,47] If the organism is drug-resistant, careful consideration of the remaining therapeutic options must be made. Two or more drugs with in vitro activity against the patient's isolate and that the patient has not received previously should be added to the regimen, as needed.[2,14,47] TB specialists should be consulted regarding cases of drug-resistant TB.[2,14,47]

❾ There is no standard regimen for MDR-TB.[2,14,47] Each patient's exposure history, previous treatment history (including toxicity and adherence issues), and current susceptibility data must be considered simultaneously. *It is critical to avoid monotherapy, and it is critical to avoid adding a single drug to a failing regimen.*[2,14,47] Adding one drug at a time leads to the sequential selection of drug resistance until there are no drugs left. The treatment of MDR-TB should be managed by TB specialists. It may take several months for a patient with MDR-TB to become culture negative because the drugs used lack the potency of isoniazid and rifampin.[2,50,51] Consequently, prolonged respiratory isolation may be required.

Drug resistance should be suspected in the following situations:

- Patients who have received prior therapy for TB
- Patients from areas with a high prevalence of resistance (South Africa, Mexico, Southeast Asia, the Baltic countries, and the former Soviet states)
- Patients who are homeless, institutionalized, intravenous drug abusers, or infected with HIV

TABLE 121-3 Drug Regimens for Culture-Positive Pulmonary Tuberculosis Caused by Drug-Susceptible Organisms

		Initial phase			Continuation Phase			Rating[a] (Evidence)[b]	
Regimen	Drugs	Interval and Doses[c] (Minimal Duration)	Regimen	Drugs	Interval and Doses[c,d] (Minimal Duration)	Range of Total Doses (Minimal Duration)		HIV-	HIV+
1	Isoniazid, rifampin, pyrazinamide, ethambutol	Seven days per week for 56 doses (8 weeks) or 5 days/week for 40 doses (8 weeks)[c]	1a	Isoniazid/ rifampin	Seven days per week for 126 doses (18 weeks) or 5 days/week for 90 doses (18 weeks)[c]	182–130 (26 weeks)		A (I)	A (II)
			1b	Isoniazid/ rifampin	Twice weekly for 36 doses (18 weeks)	92–76 (26 weeks)		A (I)	A (II)[f]
			1c[g]	Isoniazid/ rifapentine	Once weekly for 18 doses (18 weeks)	74–58 (26 weeks)		B (I)	E (I)
2	Isoniazid, rifampin, pyrazinamide, ethambutol	Seven days per week for 14 doses (2 weeks), then twice weekly for 12 doses (6 weeks) or 5 days/week for 10 doses (2 weeks)| then twice weekly for 12 doses (6 weeks)	2a	Isoniazid/ rifampin	Twice weekly for 36 doses (18 weeks)	62–58 (26 weeks)		A (II)	B (II)[f]
			2b[g]	Isoniazid/ rifapentine	Once weekly for 18 doses (18 weeks)	44–40 (26 weeks)		B (I)	E (I)
3	Isoniazid, rifampin, pyrazinamide, ethambutol	Three times weekly for 24 doses (8 weeks)	3a	Isoniazid/ rifampin	Three times weekly for 54 doses (18 weeks)	78 (26 weeks)		B (I)	B (II)
4	Isoniazid, rifampin, ethambutol	Seven days per week for 56 doses (8 weeks) or 5 days/week for 40 doses (8 weeks)[c]	4a	Isoniazid/ rifampin	Seven days per week for 217 doses (31 weeks) or 5 days/week for 155 doses (31 weeks)|	273–195 (39 weeks)		C (I)	C (II)
			4b	Isoniazid/ rifampin	Twice weekly for 62 doses (31 weeks)	118–102 (39 weeks)		C (I)	C (II)

[a]Ratings: A, preferred; B, acceptable alternative; C, offer when A and B can not be given; E, should never be given.

[b]Evidence ratings: I, randomized clinical trial; II, data from clinical trials that were not randomized or were conducted in other populations; III, expert opinion.

[c]When directly observed therapy is used, drugs may be given 5 days per week, and the necessary number of doses adjusted accordingly. Although there are no studies that compare five with seven daily doses, extensive experience indicates this would be an effective practice.

[d]Patients with cavitation on initial chest radiograph and positive cultures at completion of 2 months of therapy should receive a 7-month [31-week; either 217 doses (daily) or 62 doses (twice weekly)] continuation phase.

[e]Five-day-a-week administration is always given by directly observed therapy. Rating for 5-day-per-week regimens is A (III).

[f]Not recommended for HIV-infected patients with CD4+ cell counts <100 cells/µL.

[g]Options 1c and 2b should be used only in HIV-negative patients who have negative sputum smears at the time of completion of 2 months of therapy and who do not have cavitation on initial chest radiograph (see text). For patients started on this regimen and found to have a positive culture from the 2-month specimen, treatment should be extended an extra 3 months.

From Centers for Disease Control and Prevention. Treatment of tuberculosis. MMWR 2003;52 (RR-11).

- Patients who still have acid-fast bacilli-positive sputum smears after 1 to 2 months of therapy
- Patients who still have positive cultures after 2 to 4 months of therapy
- Patients who fail treatment or relapse after treatment
- Patients known to be exposed to MDR-TB cases

The patients just listed should be considered infected with drug-resistant TB until proved otherwise. Empirical therapy with four or more drugs may be needed for acutely ill patients.[2,14,47] These regimens may be altered when the susceptibility pattern becomes known. If the index case is known, then the same effective regimen should be employed for the new case. Again, MDR-TB cases should be referred to specialists. A new term in use, *XDR-TB*, refers to "extensively drug-resistant TB." Such organisms are resistant to at least isoniazid, rifampin, a fluoroquinolone and one second-line injectable drug (amikacin, capreomycin, or kanamycin).[55]

Special Populations

Tuberculous Meningitis and Extrapulmonary Disease

Patients with CNS tuberculosis usually are treated for longer periods (9 to 12 months instead of 6 months) (Table 121–4).[2,14,47]

In general, isoniazid, pyrazinamide, ethionamide, and cycloserine penetrate the cerebrospinal fluid readily, but rifampin, ethambutol, and streptomycin have variable CNS penetration.[54] Of the quinolones, levofloxacin may be preferred based on current data. Extrapulmonary TB of the soft tissues can be treated with conventional regimens.[2,14,47] TB of the bone typically is treated for 9 months, occasionally with surgical debridement.[2,14,47]

Children TB in children may be treated with regimens similar to those used in adults, although some physicians still prefer to extend treatment to 9 months.[2,14,24,25,47,56,57] Pediatric doses of isoniazid and rifampin on a milligram-per-kilogram basis are higher than those used in adults (Table 121–5).[47]

Pregnancy Women with TB should be cautioned against becoming pregnant because the disease poses a risk to the fetus and to the mother. If already pregnant, the usual treatment is isoniazid, rifampin, and ethambutol for 9 months.[47] Isoniazid or ethambutol are relatively safe for use in pregnant women.[2,47,54,56,57] B vitamins are particularly important during pregnancy and should be provided to women being treated for TB. Rifampin is associated rarely with birth defects, including limb reduction and CNS lesions.[54] In general, rifampin is used in pregnant women with TB. Pyrazinamide has not been studied in large numbers

TABLE 121-4 Evidence-Based[a] Guidelines for the Treatment of Extrapulmonary Tuberculosis and Adjunctive Use of Corticosteriods[b]

Site	Length of Therapy (month)	Rating (Duration)	Corticosteroids[c]	Rating (Corticosteroids)
Lymph node	6	A (I)	Not recommended	D (III)
Bone and joint	6–9	A (I)	Not recommended	D (III)
Pleural disease	6	A (II)	Not recommended	D (I)
Pericarditis	6	A (II)	Strongly recommended	A (I)
CNS tuberculosis including meningitis	9–12	B (II)	Strongly recommended	A (I)
Disseminated disease	6	A (II)	Not recommended	D (III)
Genitourinary	6	A (II)	Not recommended	D (III)
Peritoneal	6	A (II)	Not recommended	D (III)

[a]For rating system, see Table 121–3.
[b]Duration of therapy for extrapulmonary tuberculosis caused by drug-resistant organisms is not known.
[c]Corticosteroid preparations vary among studies.

of pregnant women, but anecdotal data suggest that it may be safe.[47]

Streptomycin use during pregnancy may lead to hearing loss in the newborn, including complete deafness. Streptomycin and the other aminoglycosides must be reserved for critical situations where alternatives do not exist.[2,47] Although the polypeptide capreomycin has not been studied, it probably carries the same risks.

Ethionamide may cause premature delivery and congenital deformities when used during pregnancy.[47,54] Mongolism also has been reported with ethionamide, so it cannot be recommended in this setting. p-Aminosalicylic acid has been used safely in pregnancy, but specific data are lacking.[47,54] Cycloserine is known to cross the placenta, but the effects on the developing fetus are not known. Therefore, cycloserine generally cannot be recommended during pregnancy.[54]

Ciprofloxacin, levofloxacin, moxifloxacin, and the other quinolones are associated with permanent damage to cartilage in the weight-bearing joints of immature animals, especially dogs and rabbits.[47,54] Although these drugs do not frequently cause joint problems in humans, other antituberculosis agents should be used during pregnancy.

Pregnant women with LTBI are not at the same level of risk compared with those with active disease. Therapy with isoniazid for LTBI may be delayed until after pregnancy or, if recent skin-test conversion has occurred, started during the second trimester of pregnancy.[47,54–57] Although most antituberculosis drugs are excreted in breast milk, the amount of drug received by the infant through nursing is insufficient to cause toxicity. Quinolones should be avoided in nursing mothers, if possible.

HIV Infection Patients with AIDS and other immunocompromised hosts may be managed with chemotherapeutic regimens similar to those used in immunocompetent individuals, although treatment is often extended to 9 months (see Table 121–3).[2,14,47] The precise duration to recommend remains a matter of debate. Highly intermittent regimens (twice or once weekly) are not recommended for HIV-positive TB patients. Prognosis has been particularly poor for HIV-infected patients infected with MDR-TB, so all efforts should be made to reduce the time between clinical presentation, diagnosis of TB, and start of appropriate treatment. Recommendations for management of HIV and TB published by the World Health Organization and others have provided guidance on monitoring of treatment, side effects, and drug interactions of HIV and TB. MDR, XDR-TB. [8,58] Differentiation must be made between infection with *M. tuberculosis* and nontuberculous mycobacteria, such as MAC, because the drugs used are different. While awaiting laboratory results, the patient can be treated empirically for TB if there is any doubt about the causative organism. Some patients with AIDS malabsorb their oral medications; this is

discussed under Therapeutic Drug Monitoring below.[2,47,51,53] The major issue of drug interactions is discussed further below under Rifampin.

CLINICAL CONTROVERSY

The recommended duration of treatment often is the same for HIV-negative and HIV-positive patients. However, some clinicians believe that therapy should be extended for patients with weakened immune systems. These clinicians treat HIV-positive patients with drug-susceptible TB for 9 months rather than the usual 6 months.

Renal Failure For nearly all patients, isoniazid and rifampin do not require dose modification in renal failure. They are eliminated primarily by the liver.[51,54,59] In the unlikely event that peripheral neuropathies develop, the frequency of isoniazid dosing may be reduced. Pyrazinamide and ethambutol typically require a reduction in dosing frequency from daily to three times weekly (Table 121–6).[47,59]

Renally cleared TB drugs include the aminoglycosides (amikacin, kanamycin, and streptomycin), capreomycin, ethambutol, cycloserine, and levofloxacin.[47,54,50,60] Dosing intervals need to be extended for these drugs (see Table 121–6). Ciprofloxacin and moxifloxacin are approximately 50% cleared by the kidneys but may not require a change in dose from once daily, as used for TB. The metabolites of isoniazid, pyrazinamide, and p-aminosalicylic acid are cleared primarily by the kidneys. The role of these metabolites in causing toxicity is unknown, so their accumulation in renal failure may carry some risk.

Ethionamide and its sulfoxide metabolite are hepatically cleared, so dosing is unchanged.[47,60] p-Aminosalicylic acid is converted largely to metabolites prior to renal elimination; these metabolites may accumulate in renal failure.[60] For patients on hemodialysis, the usual 12-hour dosing interval for p-aminosalicylic acid granules seems to be safe. Dialysis will remove the metabolites. Serum concentration monitoring must be performed for cycloserine to avoid dose-related toxicities in renal failure patients.[51,53,60]

Hepatic Failure Antituberculosis drugs that rely on hepatic clearance for most of their elimination include isoniazid, rifampin, pyrazinamide, ethionamide, and p-aminosalicylic acid.[54] Ciprofloxacin and moxifloxacin are approximately 50% cleared by the liver. Elevations of serum transaminase concentrations generally are not correlated with the residual capacity of the liver to metabolize drugs, so these markers cannot be used as guides for drug dosing. Furthermore, isoniazid, rifampin, pyrazinamide, and, to a lesser degree, ethionamide,

TABLE 121-5 Doses[a] of Antituberculosis Drugs for Adults and Children[b]

Drug	Preparation	Adults/Children	Daily	1 × per week	2 × per week	3 × per week
			Doses			
First-line drugs						
Isoniazid	Tablets (50 mg, 100 mg, 300 mg); elixir (50 mg/5 mL); aqueous solution (100 mg/mL) for intravenous or intramuscular injection	Adults (max)	5 mg/kg (300 mg)	15 mg/kg (900 mg)	15 mg/kg (900 mg)	15 mg/kg (900 mg)
		Children (max)	10–15 mg/kg (300 mg)	–	20–30 mg/kg (300 mg)	–
Rifampin	Capsule (150 mg, 300 mg); powder may be suspended for oral administration; aqueous solution for intravenous injection	Adults[c] (max)	10 mg/kg (600 mg)	–	10 mg/kg (600 mg)	10 mg/kg (600 mg)
		Children (max)	10–20 mg/kg (600 mg)	–	10–20 mg/kg (600 mg)	–
Rifabutin	Capsule (150 mg)	Adults[c] (max)	5 mg/kg (300 mg)	–	5 mg/kg (300 mg)	5 mg/kg (300 mg)
		Children	Appropriate dosing for children is unknown	Appropriate dosing for children is unknown	Appropriate dosing for children is unknown	Appropriate dosing for children is unknown
Rifapentine	Tablet (150 mg, film coated)	Adults	–	10 mg/kg (continuation phase) (600 mg usual adult dose)	–	–
		Children	The drug is not approved for use in children	The drug is not approved for use in children	The drug is not approved for use in children	The drug is not approved for use in children
Pyrazinamide	Tablet (500 mg, scored)	Adults	1,000 mg (40–55 kg)	–	2,000 mg (40–55 kg)	1,500 mg (40–55 kg)
			1,500 mg (56–75 kg)	–	3,000 mg (56–75 kg)	2,500 mg (56–75 kg)
			2,000 mg (76–90 kg)[y]	–	4,000 mg (76–90 kg)[y]	3,000 mg (76–90 kg)[y]
		Children (max)	15–30 mg/kg (2 g)	–	50 mg/kg (2 g)	–
Ethambutol	Tablet (100 mg, 400 mg)	Adults	800 mg (40–55 kg)	–	2,000 mg (40–55 kg)	1,200 mg (40–55 kg)
			1,200 mg (56–75 kg)	–	2,800 mg (56–75 kg)	2,000 mg (56–75 kg)
			1,600 mg (76–90 kg)[y]	—	4,000 mg (76–90 kg)[y]	2,400 mg (76–90 kg)[y]
		Children[d] (max)	15–20 mg/kg daily (1 g)	–	50 mg/kg (2.5 g)	–
Second-line drugs						
Cycloserine	Capsule (250 mg)	Adults (max)	10–15 mg/kg/day (1 g in two doses), usually 500–750 mg/day in two doses[e]	There are no data to support intermittent administration	There are no data to support intermittent administration	There are no data to support intermittent administration
		Children (max)	10–15 mg/kg/day (1 g/day)	–	–	–
Ethionamide	Tablet (250 mg)	Adults[f] (max)	15–20 mg/kg/day (1 g/day), usually 500–750 mg/day in a single daily dose or two divided doses[f]	There are no data to support intermittent administration	There are no data to support intermittent administration	There are no data to support intermittent administration
		Children (max)	15–20 mg/kg/day (1 g/day)	There are no data to support intermittent administration	There are no data to support intermittent administration	There are no data to support intermittent administration
Streptomycin	Aqueous solution (1-g vials) for intravenous or intramuscular administration	Adults (max)	g	g	g	g
		Children (max)	20–40 mg/kg/day (1 g)	–	20 mg/kg	–
Amikacin/kanamycin	Aqueous solution (500 mg and 1 g vials) for intravenous or intramuscular administration	Adults (max)	g	g	g	g
		Children (max)	15–30 mg/kg/day (1 g) intravenous or intramuscular as a single daily dose	–	15–30 mg/kg	–
Capreomycin	Aqueous solution (1 g vials) for intravenous or intramuscular administration	Adults (max)	g	g	15–30 mg/kg	g
		Children (max)	15–30 mg/kg/day (1 g) as a single daily dose	–	–	–
p-Amino-salicylic acid (PAS)	Granules (4 g packets) can be mixed with food; tablets (500 mg) are still available in some countries, but not in the United States; a solution for intravenous administration is available in Europe	Adults	8–12 g/day in two or three doses	There are no data to support intermittent administration	There are no data to support intermittent administration	There are no data to support intermittent administration
		Children (max)	200–300 mg/kg/day in two to four divided doses (10 g)	There are no data to support intermittent administration	There are no data to support intermittent administration	There are no data to support intermittent administration

(continued)

TABLE 121-5 Doses[a] of Antituberculosis Drugs for Adults and Children[b] (continued)

Drug	Preparation	Adults/Children	Daily	Doses		
				1× per week	2× per week	3×per week
Moxifloxacin[h]	Tablets (400 mg); aqueous solution (400 mg/250 mL) for intravenous injection	Adults	400 mg daily	There are no data to support intermittent administration	There are no data to support intermittent administration	There are no data to support intermittent administration

[a]Dose per weight is based on ideal body weight. Children weighing more than 40 kg should be dosed as adults.

[b]For purposes of this document, adult dosing begins at age 15 years.

[c]Dose may need to be adjusted when there is concomitant use of protease inhibitors or nonnucleoside reverse transcriptase inhibitors.

[d]The drug can likely be used safely in older children but should be used with caution in children less than 5 years of age, in whom visual acuity can not be monitored. In younger children, ethambutol at the dose of 15 mg/kg per day can be used if there is suspected or proven resistance to isoniazid or rifampin.

[e]It should be noted that although this is the dose recommended generally, most clinicians with experience using cycloserine indicate that it is unusual for patients to be able to tolerate this amount. Serum concentration measurements are often useful in determining the optimal dose for a given patient.

[f]The single daily dose can be given at bedtime or with the main meal.

[g]Dose: 15 mg/kg per day (1 g) but 10 mg/kg in persons older than 59 years of age (750 mg). Usual dose: 750–1,000 mg administered intramuscularly or intravenously, given as a single dose 5–7 days/ week and reduced to two or three times per week after the first 2–4 months or after culture conversion, depending on the efficacy of the other drugs in the regimen.

[h]The long-term (more than several weeks) use of moxifloxacin in children and adolescents has not been approved because of concerns about effects on bone and cartilage growth. The optimal dose is not known.

p-aminosalicylic acid, and, rarely, ethambutol may cause hepatotoxicity.[47,51,54] For some patients with drug-susceptible TB, a "liver-sparing" regimen of streptomycin, levofloxacin, and ethambutol may be used, at least temporarily.[47,51,54] Because this regimen requires 18 or more months of treatment to be successful, patients usually are switched to isoniazid- and rifampin-containing regimens as soon as they are able.

TABLE 121-6 Dosing Recommendations for Adult Patients with Reduced Renal Function and for Adult Patients Receiving Hemodialysis

Drug	Change in Frequency?	Recommended Dose and Frequency for Patients with Creatinine Clearance <30 mL/min or for Patients Receiving Hemodialysis
Isoniazid	No change	300 mg once daily or 900 mg three times per week
Rifampin	No change	600 mg once daily or 600 mg three times per week
Pyrazinamide	Yes	25–35 mg/kg per dose three times per week (not daily)
Ethambutol	Yes	15–25 mg/kg per dose three times per week (not daily)
Levofloxacin	Yes	750–1,000 mg per dose three times per week (not daily)
Cycloserine	Yes	250 mg once daily or 500 mg/dose three times per week[a]
Ethionamide	No change	250–500 mg/dose daily
p-Aminosalicylic acid	No change	4 g/dose, twice daily
Streptomycin	Yes	12–15 mg/kg per dose two or three times per week (not daily)
Capreomycin	Yes	12–15 mg/kg per dose two or three times per week (not daily)
Kanamycin	Yes	12–15 mg/kg per dose two or three times per week (not daily)
Amikacin	Yes	12–15 mg/kg per dose two or three times per week (not daily)

Standard doses are given unless there is intolerance.

The medications should be given after hemodialysis on the day of hemodialysis.

Monitoring of serum drug concentrations should be considered to ensure adequate drug absorption, without excessive accumulation, and to assist in avoiding toxicity.

Data currently are not available for patients receiving peritoneal dialysis. Until data become available, begin with doses recommended for patients receiving hemodialysis, and verify adequacy of dosing, using serum concentration monitoring.

[a]The appropriateness of 250 mg daily doses has not been established. There should be careful monitoring for evidence of neurotoxicity.

Morbid Obesity Data are not available for dosing the TB drugs for patients with morbid obesity.[54] Relatively hydrophilic drugs (isoniazid, pyrazinamide, the aminoglycosides, capreomycin, ethambutol, *p*-aminosalicylic acid, and cycloserine) can be dosed initially based on ideal body weight. Very low or very high serum concentrations can be avoided by checking the serum concentrations.

The TB Drugs

The interested reader is referred to several other publications for more detailed information regarding these drugs.[2,13,47,50,51,53,54,61–63] Note that although the American Thoracic Society (ATS)/CDC guidelines recommend "maximum" doses. (see Table 121–5).[47] In the author's view, the "maximum" dose for a given patient is the dose that produces the desired response with an acceptable level of toxicity.[51,53] This can only be determined on a case-by-case basis. Artificially capping doses may deprive patients of needed drug.

Primary Antituberculosis Drugs *Isoniazid* Isoniazid is one of the two most important TB drugs. It is highly specific for mycobacteria, with a MIC against *M. tuberculosis* of 0.01 to 0.25 mcg/mL. Most nontuberculous mycobacteria such as *M. avium* are resistant to isoniazid, although *M. kansasii* and *Mycobacterium xenopi* are susceptible. The most common mechanisms of resistance result from mutations in the *katG* or *inhA* genes.

Isoniazid is readily absorbed from the gastrointestinal tract and from intramuscular injection sites. It also can be given as a short intravenous infusion over 5 minutes if diluted in about 20 mL of normal saline.[64] Isoniazid should be given on an empty stomach whenever possible.[65] *N*-Acetyltransferase 2 forms the principal metabolite acetylisoniazid, which lacks antimycobacterial activity. The rate at which humans acetylate isoniazid is determined genetically; slow acetylation is an autosomal recessive trait and reflects a relative lack of *N*-acetyltransferase 2. Fast acetylators have isoniazid half-lives of less than 2 hours. Approximately 50% of whites and blacks and 80% to 90% of Asians and Eskimos are rapid acetylators. Slow acetylators have isoniazid half-lives of 3 to 4 hours and may be at an increased risk of neurotoxicity. The association of acetylator status and risk of hepatotoxicity, however, appears to be weak.[66] Poor absorption and rapid clearance of isoniazid for patients receiving highly intermittent therapy are associated with poor clinical outcomes.[67,68]

Transient elevations of the serum transaminases occur in 12% to 15% of patients receiving isoniazid and usually occur within the first 8 to 12 weeks of therapy.[47] Overt hepatotoxicity, however, occurs in only 1% of cases. Risk factors for hepatotoxicity include patient age, preexisting liver disease, excessive alcohol intake, pregnancy, and the postpartum state. Isoniazid also may result in neurotoxicity, most frequently presenting as peripheral neuropathy or, in overdose, as seizures and coma. Patients with pyridoxine deficiency, such as pregnant women, alcoholics, children, and the malnourished, are at increased risk. Isoniazid may inhibit the metabolism of phenytoin, carbamazepine, primidone, and warfarin.[51] Patients who are being treated with these agents should be monitored closely, and appropriate dose adjustments should be made when necessary.

Rifampin The introduction of rifampin into routine use during the 1970s allowed for true short-course treatment of TB (6 to 9 months).[2,14,47] Without rifampin, treatment is generally 18 months or longer. Drug resistance to rifampin is an ominous prognostic factor because it is frequently associated with isoniazid resistance and leaves the patient with few good therapeutic options. Clinicians *must* take care to protect susceptibility to rifampin by carefully treating their patients. Rifampin shows bactericidal activity against *M. tuberculosis* and several other mycobacterial species, including *M. bovis* and *M. kansasii*.[69] Other nontuberculous mycobacteria, including MAC, show variable susceptibility to rifampin. Rifampin also is active against a broad array of other bacteria. Alteration of the target site on RNA polymerase, primarily through changes in the *rpoB* gene, leads to most forms of rifampin resistance.[47,69]

Rifampin usually is given orally, but it also can be given as a 30-minute intravenous infusion.[61,69] Oral doses are best given on an empty stomach.[70] Patients with AIDS, diabetes, and other gastrointestinal problems appear to have difficulty absorbing rifampin after oral doses, and this has been associated with therapeutic failures in some cases.[51,53,68,71] Rifampin is metabolized to 25-desacetylrifampin, which retains some of rifampin's activity; most of rifampin and its metabolite are cleared in the bile. Rifampin generally is given at 600 mg daily or intermittently, although this dose does not take full advantage of rifampin's concentration-dependent killing.[51,53] Higher doses should be tested in humans within the context of clinical trials.

Elevations in hepatic enzymes have been attributed to rifampin in 10% to 15% of patients, with overt hepatotoxicity occurring in less than 1%.[47,69] More frequent adverse effects of rifampin include rash, fever, and gastrointestinal distress. Allergic reactions to rifampin have been reported and occur more frequently with intermittent rifampin doses 900 mg or more twice weekly. These reactions may take the form of a flu-like syndrome with development of fever, chills, headache, arthralgias, and, rarely, hypotension and shock.[47,62] Alternatively, hemolytic anemia or acute renal failure may occur, requiring permanent discontinuation.

Rifampin's potent induction of hepatic enzymes, especially cytochrome P450 3A4, may enhance the elimination of many other drugs, most notably the protease inhibitors used to treat HIV (Table 121–7). HIV-positive patients may benefit from the use of rifabutin instead of rifampin (see below).[47,72–75] Furthermore, women who use oral contraceptives must use another form of contraception during therapy because increased clearance of the hormones may lead to unexpected pregnancies. Patient records should be reviewed for potential drug interactions before dispensing rifampin.[61] Rifampin may turn urine and other secretions orange-red and may permanently stain some types of contact lenses.

Other Rifamycins Rifabutin is used for disseminated *M. avium* infection in AIDS patients and is quite active against *M. tuberculosis*. Most rifampin-resistant organisms are resistant to rifabutin.

Because rifabutin is a less potent enzyme inducer than rifampin, it may be used for patients who are receiving protease inhibitors.[47,72–75] For HIV-positive patients, the ATS/CDC recommends regimens with three or more doses of the TB drugs per week (see Table 121–3). Rifapentine is a long-acting rifamycin that can be used once weekly in the continuation phase of treatment (after the first 2 months) in carefully selected HIV-negative patients. Rifapentine is approximately 85% as potent an enzyme inducer as rifampin, so similar drug interactions are likely.[47,72–75]

Pyrazinamide Adding pyrazinamide to the first 2 months of treatment with isoniazid and rifampin shortens the duration to 6 months for most patients.[2,47] It is usually well absorbed and displays a fairly long half-life.[76,77] The most common toxicities of pyrazinamide are gastrointestinal distress, arthralgias, and elevations in the serum uric acid concentrations.[47,62] Most patients do not experience true gout. Hepatotoxicity is the major limiting adverse effect and is dose-related when pyrazinamide is given daily.

A fixed-combination product (Rifater, Aventis) of rifampin 120 mg, isoniazid 50 mg, and pyrazinamide 300 mg is designed to prevent drug resistance by keeping the self-medicating patient from using only one drug at a time. If the patient is receiving directly observed treatment, there is no particular advantage to this product. The typical dose of Rifater will be five to six tablets daily. When pyrazinamide is discontinued after 2 months of treatment, the combination product Rifamate (isoniazid 150 mg and rifampin 300 mg) can be substituted.

Ethambutol Ethambutol replaced *p*-aminosalicylic acid as a first-line agent in the 1960s because it was better tolerated by patients.[2,47] Ethambutol is used as a fourth drug for TB while awaiting susceptibility data.[47] If the organism is susceptible to isoniazid, rifampin, and pyrazinamide, ethambutol can be stopped. Ethambutol is active against most mycobacteria, including *M. tuberculosis* and *M. avium*, but it is generally bacteriostatic.

Ethambutol should not be given with antacids.[78] For patients with renal failure, the ethambutol dose should be reduced to three times per week.[59,79] Retrobulbar neuritis is the major adverse effect. Patients may complain of a change in visual acuity, the inability to see the color green, or both. They should be monitored monthly while on the drug using Snellen wall charts for visual acuity and Ishihara red-green color discrimination cards.[47,61,62]

Second-Line Antituberculosis Drugs **Streptomycin** Streptomycin is one of three aminoglycoside antibiotics (along with amikacin and kanamycin) that are active against mycobacteria. Streptomycin is quite active against MAC and several other mycobacteria, enterococci, *Brucella*, *Yersinia*, and various other bacteria. Although labeled only for intramuscular dosing, streptomycin can be given safely as intravenous infusions (100 mL of dextrose 5% water or normal saline) over 30 minutes, similar to the other aminoglycosides.[80] Streptomycin, like other aminoglycosides, is renally cleared by glomerular filtration and must be given less often to patients with renal dysfunction.[47,51,61]

TABLE 121-7 Clinically Significant Drug–Drug Interactions Involving the Rifamycins

Drug Class	Drugs Whose Concentrations Are Substantially Decreased by Rifamycins (References)	Comments
Antiinfectives	HIV-1 protease inhibitors	Can be used with rifabutin. Ritonavir, 400–600 mg twice daily, probably can be used with rifampin. The combination of saquinavir and ritonavir can also be used with rifampin.
	Nonnucleoside reverse transcriptase inhibitors	Delavirdine should not be used with any rifamycin. Doses of nevirapine and efavirenz need to be increased if given with rifampin; no dose increase needed if given with rifabutin.
	Macrolide antibiotics (not azithromycin)	Azithromycin has no significant interaction with rifamycins.
	Doxycycline	May require use of a drug other than doxycycline.
	Azole antifungal agents	Itraconazole, ketoconazole, and voriconazole concentrations may be subtherapeutic with any of the rifamycins. Fluconazole can be used with rifamycins, but the dose of fluconazole may have to be increased.
	Atovaquone	Consider alternate form of **Pneumocystis carinii** treatment or prophylaxis.
	Chloramphenicol	Consider an alternative antibiotic.
	Mefloquine	Consider alternate form of malaria prophylaxis.
Hormone therapy	Ethinylestradiol, norethindrone	Women of reproductive potential on oral contraceptives should be advised to add a barrier method of contraception when taking a rifamycin.
	Tamoxifen	May require alternate therapy or use of a nonrifamycin-containing regimen.
	Levothyroxine	Monitoring of serum thyroid-stimulating hormone recommended; may require increased dose of levothyroxine.
Narcotics	Methadone	Rifampin and rifapentine use may require methadone dose increase; rifabutin infrequently causes methadone withdrawal.
Anticoagulants	Warfarin	Monitor prothrombin time; may require two- to threefold dose increase.
Immunosuppressive agents	Cyclosporine, tacrolimus	Rifabutin may allow concomitant use of cyclosporine and a rifamycin; monitoring of cyclosporine serum concentrations may assist with dosing.
	Corticosteroids	Monitor clinically; may require two- to threefold increase in corticosteroid dose.
Anticonvulsants	Phenytoin, lamotrigine	Therapeutic drug monitoring recommended; may require anticonvulsant dose increase.
Cardiovascular agents	Verapamil, nifedipine, diltiazem (a similar interaction is also predicted for felodipine and nisoldipine)	Clinical monitoring recommended; may require change to an alternate cardiovascular agent.
	Propranolol, metoprolol	Clinical monitoring recommended; may require dose increase or change to an alternate cardiovascular drug.
	Enalapril, losartan	Monitor clinically; may require a dose increase or use of an alternate cardiovascular drug.
	Digoxin (among patients with renal insufficiency), digitoxin	Therapeutic drug monitoring recommended; may require digoxin or digitoxin dose increase.
	Quinidine	Therapeutic drug monitoring recommended; may require quinidine dose increase.
	Mexiletine, tocainide, propafenone	Clinical monitoring recommended; may require change to an alternate cardiovascular drug.
Bronchodilators	Theophylline	Therapeutic drug monitoring recommended; may require theophylline dose increase.
Sulfonylurea hypoglycemics	Tolbutamide, chlorpropamide, glyburide, glimepiride, repaglinide	Monitor blood glucose; may require dose increase or change to an alternate hypoglycemic drug.
Hypolipidemics	Simvastatin, fluvastatin	Monitor hypolipidemic effect; may require use of an alternate hypolipidemic drug.
Psychotropic drugs	Nortriptyline	Therapeutic drug monitoring recommended; may require dose increase or change to alternate psychotropic drug.
	Haloperidol, quetiapine	Monitor clinically; may require a dose increase or use of an alternate psychotropic drug.
	Benzodiazepines, zolpidem, buspirone	Monitor clinically; may require a dose increase or use of an alternate psychotropic drug.

Streptomycin occasionally causes nephrotoxicity, although it tends to be mild and reversible. It also is capable of causing ototoxicity (vestibular and cochlear), which may become permanent with continued use.[47,62] Older patients and those receiving long durations of treatment are most likely to experience hearing loss, whereas vestibular toxicity is highly unpredictable.

Resistance to amikacin and kanamycin is frequently linked but independent of resistance to streptomycin and independent of resistance to capreomycin. Therefore, susceptibility tests should guide the selection of these injectable drugs.

p-Aminosalicylic Acid In the United States, only the enteric-coated, sustained-release granule form (Paser) is available.[81–83] Gastrointestinal disturbances are the most common adverse effects from p-aminosalicylic acid. Diarrhea is usually self-limited, with symptoms improving after the first 1 to 2 weeks of therapy. Occasionally, a few doses of an opioid will resolve the problem. It also is important to tell the patient that the empty granules will appear in the stool. Although FDA approved for three daily doses, pharmacokinetic data support twice-daily dosing.[82]

Various types of malabsorption, including steatorrhea, were reported with previous dosage forms of p-aminosalicylic acid. Hypersensitivity and, rarely, severe hepatitis may occur. p-Aminosalicylic acid is known to produce goiter, with or without myxedema, that seems to occur more frequently with concomitant ethionamide therapy.

Cycloserine Cycloserine is only used to treat MDR-TB. It is well absorbed orally and is best taken on an empty stomach.[84] It is cleared primarily through the kidneys by glomerular filtration and requires dosage reduction in renal failure. Cycloserine can produce dose-related CNS toxicity, including lethargy, confusion, or unusual behavior. Seizures, although reported, are exceedingly rare in U.S. patients.[2,47,61] Therapy is improved by maintaining 2-hour postdose serum concentrations between 20 and 35 mcg/mL.[51,53] Most patients reach a maximum dose of 750 mg daily, divided unevenly into two doses. This can be achieved by starting with 250 mg daily for 2 days, followed by 250 mg increments over 2-day intervals. This dose of cycloserine can be maintained if the patient complains of only occasional mild CNS effects, such as difficulty concentrating. Serum concentrations can be checked 1 to 2 weeks into therapy. The addition of pyridoxine 50 mg daily may improve patient tolerance of cycloserine.

Ethionamide Ethionamide shares structural features with two other antimycobacterial agents, isoniazid and, more distantly, thiacetazone, a drug not used in the United States. Prothionamide, the n-propyl derivative of ethionamide, is used in Europe. Ethionamide is only active against organisms of the genus *Mycobacterium*, and it should be considered primarily bacteriostatic because it is difficult to achieve serum concentrations that would be bactericidal.[47,51,53]

Gastrointestinal toxicity is the dose-limiting adverse effect. The drug should be introduced gradually in 250 mg increments, as described earlier for cycloserine. Rarely will a patient tolerate more than 1,000 mg daily in divided oral doses. Ethionamide may be administered with a light snack or prior to bedtime to minimize gastrointestinal intolerance. Food does not affect absorption significantly.[85] Little ethionamide is recovered in the urine, so doses remain the same in renal failure. Ethionamide may cause goiter with or without hypothyroidism (especially when given with p-aminosalicylic acid), gynecomastia, alopecia, impotence, menorrhagia, photodermatitis, and acne. The management of diabetes also may be more difficult for patients receiving ethionamide. Because of these problems, ethionamide only is used when necessary.

Clofazimine Clofazimine is a drug with good activity against *Mycobacterium leprae* and weak activity against *M. tuberculosis* and *M. avium*. It is used in doses of 100 mg daily in advanced cases of MDR-TB or MAC, especially when therapeutic options are limited.[47,51] The drug has a terminal elimination half-life that is weeks long. Gastrointestinal distress and skin discoloration are the most important adverse reactions. Although uncommon, severe gastrointestinal pain may occur because of deposition of clofazimine crystals within the intestines; this may require surgical correction.

Thiacetazone Thiacetazone is a weak agent used rarely in parts of the developing world because of its low cost. Skin reactions, including rash and Stevens-Johnson syndrome, may occur. Thiacetazone must be discontinued permanently as soon as a rash appears. Similar to trimethoprim-sulfamethoxazole, the incidence of skin reactions is much higher for AIDS patients.[86]

Quinolones Levofloxacin, gatifloxacin (outside of the United States), and moxifloxacin are sometimes used to treat MDR-TB because of their excellent activity against *M. tuberculosis*. Several studies have suggested a potential role for moxifloxacin as a possible replacement for certain first-line agents.[2,14,47,51,87-89] Moxifloxacin has been compared with isoniazid and ethambutol during the first 8 weeks of therapy for pulmonary TB. Moxifloxacin did not demonstrate a significant increase in 8-week culture negativity when compared to isoniazid. However, shorter time to culture conversion was seen when compared with ethambutol. Quinolones are useful because most are available in oral and intravenous dosage forms, so they can be used in critically ill patients.

β-Lactam and β-Lactamase Inhibitor Combinations The β-lactams have limited activity against mycobacteria because of β-lactamases and because β-lactams fail to enter macrophages.[47,51,90] Cefoxitin, a β-lactamase–stable cephalosporin, has useful activity against rapidly growing mycobacteria, such as *M. fortuitum* and *Mycobacterium chelonae*. Combinations of β-lactam with β-lactamase inhibitors have been used in salvage regimens for TB patients with no other options, but they are not used routinely to treat TB.

Macrolides/Azalides The macrolide clarithromycin and azalide azithromycin represent substantial advances in the treatment of MAC but demonstrate limited activity against *M. tuberculosis* and are not used frequently for TB.[2,14,47,51]

New Drugs and Delivery Systems The nitroimidazole derivatives PA824 and OPC67683, which are chemically related to metronidazole and tinidazole, have activity against *M. tuberculosis* in vitro and in animal models.[91,92] Early clinical data appear to be promising. Aerosol dry powder formulation is a promising delivery system for PA824.[93] This class, along with the oxazolidinones, may produce useful agents for TB. The diarylquinoline TMC207 has potent in vitro and in vivo activity against both TB and MDR-TB. TMC207 works through targeting the ATP synthase pump. Phase I studies in humans have shown the drug to be well tolerated.[94] Linezolid has been used in some patients with MDR-TB.[95] Long-term use of linezolid requires careful monitoring of hematologic indices for potential anemia and thrombocytopenia. It may be possible to reduce the incidences of these toxicities by giving linezolid 600 mg daily or 300 mg twice daily for the slow-growing *M. tuberculosis* rather than the usual 600 mg twice-daily dose used for gram-positive organisms, and clinical investigations are under way. Chemical modification of existing compounds, such as pyrazinamide, may produce new TB drugs. Finally, continuing research on the construction of the mycobacterial cell wall and intracellular pathways may lead to agents with unique activity against this genus.

Liposomes have been investigated as delivery systems for various agents against mycobacteria, including isoniazid, rifampin, and the aminoglycosides. Liposomes also could be used to deliver β-lactams or other agents that generally are excluded from macrophages. By changing the pharmacokinetic profile of such agents, their use in the treatment of mycobacterial infections could be enhanced greatly. Currently, no such product is licensed for use against TB.

Corticosteroids Adjunctive therapy with corticosteroids may be of benefit for some patients with tuberculous meningitis or pericarditis to relieve inflammation and pressure (see Table 121–4).[2,47] They should be avoided in most other circumstances because they detract from the immune response to TB.

Bacille Calmette-Guérin Vaccine The BCG vaccine is an attenuated, hybridized strain of *M. bovis*. It was developed in 1921 and is used as a prophylactic vaccine against TB. Administration of BCG vaccine is compulsory in many developing countries and is officially recommended in many others. Vaccination with BCG produces a subclinical infection resulting in sensitization of T lymphocytes and cross-immunity to *M. tuberculosis*, as well as cutaneous hypersensitivity and, in many cases, a positive tuberculin skin test.

In the published clinical trials, several different BCG preparations were used, and the efficacy of these vaccinations ranged from negative 56% (some patients did worse with the vaccine) to positive 80%.[2,47] Trials within the United States and Puerto Rico have shown efficacy rates of 6% to 29%. The primary benefit of BCG vaccination appears to be the prevention of severe forms of TB in children. Data from the BCG trials show that the incidence of tuberculous meningitis and miliary TB is 52% to 100% lower and that the incidence of pulmonary TB is 2% to 80% lower in vaccinated children younger than 15 years of age than it was in unvaccinated controls.

Unfortunately, BCG does not appear to be very reliable in preventing disease by *M. tuberculosis* in other segments of the population. Side effects occur in 1% to 10% of vaccinated persons and usually include severe or prolonged ulceration at the vaccination site, lymphadenitis, and lupus vulgaris. It is recommended that pregnant women and patients with impaired immune systems, including those with HIV infection, avoid vaccination. The World Health Organization had recommended, however, that in populations where the risk of TB is high, HIV-infected infants who are asymptomatic should receive BCG vaccine at birth or as soon as possible thereafter. Because BCG infection has occurred in AIDS patients given the vaccine, individuals with symptomatic HIV infection should not be vaccinated.[2,47]

In the United States, BCG vaccination is recommended only for uninfected children who are at unavoidable risk of exposure to TB and for whom other methods of prevention and control have failed or are not feasible.[2,47] Its use is very limited.

PHARMACOECONOMIC CONSIDERATIONS

The World Health Organization and the World Bank agree that the control of TB is one of the most cost-effective health interventions any nation can pursue. Early identification of TB cases and the effective use of isoniazid, rifampin, and pyrazinamide (plus ethambutol) while the isolate is still drug susceptible always should be the primary goals of public health departments. Contact investigation and treatment of those infected but without disease are important secondary goals to reduce the number of future cases.

Patients who complete all their treatment for drug-susceptible TB have cure rates over 95%. Noncompliance (nonadherence), drug resistance, extrapulmonary disease, and concomitant disease states reduce the overall effectiveness of chemotherapy of TB to approximately 75%.

The treatment of TB is not particularly expensive, especially if hospitalization is not required.[96] Furthermore, TB is quite curable. Because the various TB drugs each have a role to play in the treatment of TB or MDR-TB, all the antituberculosis drugs approved by the Food and Drug Administration should be on institutional formularies. Centers that see little MDR-TB need not keep stocks of the second-line drugs, provided that they are readily available should the need arise. Because the treatment of MDR-TB is difficult and because missteps are potentially disastrous, such patients should be referred to centers experienced in the management of MDR-TB.[2,47,97-99]

EVALUATION OF THERAPEUTIC OUTCOMES

MONITORING OF THE PHARMACEUTICAL CARE PLAN

The most serious problem with TB therapy is patient nonadherence to the prescribed regimens.[99,100] Unfortunately, there is no reliable way to identify such patients a priori. In the study by Brudney and Dobkin,[99] 89% of the patients were noncompliant with therapy. It is critical to the control of TB that such adherence rates be improved dramatically. The most effective way to achieve this end is with directly observed treatment.[2,14,47] Despite criticisms that it will cost more money, it is far cheaper in the long run to prevent the further spread of disease with directly observed treatment than to track down and treat additional cases of TB continuously.

The homeless and other underprivileged individuals are assumed to constitute the group of patients considered "unreliable," and directly observed treatment should be reserved for them; it is also assumed that "responsible" patients cared for by private physicians may be treated with daily, unsupervised therapy. A study conducted in Baltimore, however, compared outcomes (sputum culture conversion to negative at 3 months) for patients with pulmonary TB who were treated by private physicians with outcomes for patients treated via directly observed treatment in a city-run clinic. Surprisingly, 3-month culture conversion occurred in only 40% of the private-care patients, compared with 90% in the city clinic-care patients.[101] Clearly, expansion of the use of directly observed treatment to nearly all patients with TB may be of benefit.

For patients who are acid-fast bacilli smear positive, they should have sputum samples sent for acid-fast bacilli stains every 1 to 2 weeks until two consecutive smears are negative. This provides early evidence of a response to treatment.[47] Once on maintenance therapy, sputum cultures can be performed monthly until two consecutive cultures are negative, which generally occurs over 2 to 3 months. If sputum cultures continue to be positive after 2 months, drug susceptibility testing should be repeated, and serum concentrations of the drugs should be checked.

Serum chemistries, including blood urea nitrogen, creatinine, aspartate transaminase, and alanine transaminase, and a complete blood count with platelets should be performed at baseline and periodically thereafter, depending on the presence of other factors that may increase the likelihood of toxicity (e.g., advanced age, alcohol abuse, pregnancy).[2,47] Hepatotoxicity should be suspected for patients whose transaminases exceed five times the upper limit of normal or whose total bilirubin concentration exceeds 3 mg/dL and for patients with symptoms such as nausea, vomiting, or jaundice. At this point, the offending agent(s) should be discontinued. Sequential reintroduction of the drugs with frequent testing of liver enzymes is often successful in identifying the offending agent; other agents may be continued. Alternative agents should be selected as needed. Audiometric testing should be performed at baseline and monthly for patients who must receive aminoglycosides for more than 1 to 2 months. Vision testing (Snellen visual acuity charts and Ishihara color discrimination plates) should be performed on all patients who receive ethambutol. All patients diagnosed with TB should be tested for HIV infection.

THERAPEUTIC DRUG MONITORING

Therapeutic drug monitoring (TDM), or applied pharmacokinetics, is the use of serum drug concentrations to optimize therapy.[47,51,53,101] Non-AIDS patients with drug-susceptible TB generally do well, and TDM generally should be used if they are failing appropriate directly observed treatment (no clinical improvement after 2 to 4 weeks or smear positive after 4 to 6 weeks). On the other hand, patients with AIDS, diabetes, cystic fibrosis, and various gastrointestinal disorders often fail to absorb these drugs properly and are candidates for TDM. Furthermore, patients with hepatic or renal disease should be monitored, given their potential for overdoses.

CLINICAL CONTROVERSY

Some TB centers employ TDM for many of their patients at the outset of treatment in order to identify drug-delivery problems early. Other centers wait to see how the patient responds and perform TDM only if problems arise. An argument can be made for either approach. The latter can save money, but delays in effective treatment can affect the patient's outcome adversely. Most otherwise healthy TB patients will absorb their drugs adequately. Patients who are critically ill or who have MDR-TB can benefit from early TDM.

In the treatment of MDR-TB, the differences between the maximum serum concentration (C_{max}) and the MIC for the second-line agents are much smaller that with isoniazid and rifampin. Therefore, alterations in the absorption of these drugs can have significant impact on the outcome of therapy.[51,53] Although the optimal serum concentrations for TB are not known, target serum peak concentrations have been proposed.[51,53] Blood samples collected at 2 and 6 hours after a dose have been used with some success, although they may not be the optimal sampling times for all the drugs. Long–half-life drugs (e.g., pyrazinamide and cycloserine) can be sampled at 2 and 10 hours if an estimate of the half-life is desired. Finally, TDM of the TB and HIV drugs is perhaps the most logical way to untangle the complex drug interactions that take place (see Table 121–7).[103,104]

CONCLUSIONS

Good patient adherence to treatment regimens is the cornerstone to effective antimycobacterial chemotherapy. Pharmacists should monitor TB therapy with particular interest in drug–drug interactions, drug malabsorption, and avoiding the error of adding a single drug to a failing regimen. They should educate patients on the importance of continuing their chemotherapy despite symptomatic improvement. Pharmacists should become part of a multidisciplinary team (with nurses, physicians, and social workers) devoted to successful chemotherapy of TB patients and their families.

ABBREVIATIONS

ATS: American Thoracic Society

BCG: bacillus Calmette-Guérin

CDC: Centers for Disease Control and Prevention

CMI: cell-mediated Immunity

DTH: delayed-type hypersensitivity

IGRA: interferon gamma release assay

INF: interferon

IL: interleukin

LTBI: latent tuberculosis infection

MAC: *Mycobacterium avium* complex

MDR: multidrug resistance

MIC: minimal inhibitory concentration

PPD: purified protein derivative

TB: tuberculosis

TDM: therapeutic drug monitoring

TH: T-helper cell

TNF: tumor necrosis factor

XDR: extensively drug resistant

REFERENCES

1. World Health Organization Report on the Global Tuberculosis Epidemic. Geneva: WHO; 1998.
2. Iseman MD. A Clinician's Guide to Tuberculosis. Philadelphia, PA: Lippincott Williams & Wilkins; 2000.
3. Stead WW. The origin and erratic global spread of tuberculosis. Clin Chest Med 1997;18:65–77.
4. McCray E, Weinbaum CM, Braden CR, Onorato IM. The epidemiology of tuberculosis in the United States. Clin Chest Med 1997;18:99–113.
5. Centers for Disease Control and Prevention. Reported Tuberculosis in the United States, 2008. Department of Health and Human Services, Atlanta: CDC; 2009.
6. Centers for Disease Control and Prevention. Tuberculosis in the United States, 2002. Atlanta, GA: CDC; 2005.
7. Haas DW. Mycobacterium tuberculosis. In: Mandell GL, Bennett JE, Dolin R, eds. Principles and Practice of Infectious Diseases, 5th ed. New York: Churchill-Livingstone; 2000:2576–2607.
8. Scano F, Vitoria M, Burman W, et al. Management of HIV-infected patients with MDR and XDR-TB in resource limited settings. Int J Tuberc Lung Dis 2008; 12:1370–1375.
9. Small PM, Shafer RW, Hopewell PC, et al. Exogenous reinfection with multidrug-resistant Mycobacterium tuberculosis in patients with advanced HIV infection. N Engl J Med 1993;328:1137–1144.
10. Beck-Sague C, Dooley SW, Hutton MD, et al. Hospital outbreak of multidrug-resistant Mycobacterium tuberculosis infections: Factors in transmission to staff and HIV-infected patients. JAMA 1992;268:1280–1286.
11. Centers for Disease Control and Prevention. Meeting the challenge of multidrug-resistant tuberculosis: Summary of a conference. MMWR 1992;41:51–71.
12. Heifets L. Mycobacteriology laboratory. Clin Chest Med 1997;18:35–53.
13. Heifets LB. Drug susceptibility tests in the management of chemotherapy of tuberculosis. In: Heifets LB, ed. Drug Susceptibility in the Chemotherapy of Mycobacterial Infections. Boca Raton, FL: CRC Press; 1991:89–122.
14. Daley CL, Chambers HF. *Mycobacterium tuberculosis* complex. In: Yu VL, Weber R, Raoult D, eds. Antimicrobial Therapy and Vaccines, Vol I. Microbes, 2d ed. New York: Apple Trees Productions; 2002:841–865.
15. Roberts GD, Böttger EC, Stockman L. Methods for the rapid identification of mycobacterial species. Clin Lab Med 1996;16:603–615.
16. Sandin RL. Polymerase chain reaction and other amplification techniques in mycobacteriology. Clin Lab Med 1996;16:617–639.
17. Blanchard JS. Molecular mechanisms of drug resistance in Mycobacterium tuberculosis. Annu Rev Biochem 1996;65:215–239.
18. Somoskovi A, Parsons LM, Salfinger M. The molecular basis of resistance to isoniazid, rifampin, and pyrazinamide in Mycobacterium tuberculosis. Respir Res 2001;2:164–168.
19. Marin M, Garcia de Viedma D, Ruiz-Serrano MJ, Bouza E. Rapid direct detection of multiple rifampin and isoniazid resistance mutations in Mycobacterium tuberculosis in respiratory samples by real-time PCR. Antimicrob Agents Chemother 2004;48:4293–4300.
20. Riley RL, Mills CC, Nyka W, et al. Aerial dissemination of pulmonary tuberculosis: A two-year study of contagion in a tuberculosis ward. Am J Hygiene 1959;70:185–196.
21. Daniel TM, Boom WH, Ellner JJ. Immunology of tuberculosis. In: Reichman LB, Hershfield ES, eds. Tuberculosis: A Comprehensive International Approach, 2d ed. New York: Marcel Dekker; 2000:157–185.
22. Piessens WF, Nardell EA. Pathogenesis of tuberculosis. In: Reichman LB, Hershfield ES, eds. Tuberculosis: A Comprehensive International Approach, 2d ed. New York: Marcel Dekker; 2000:241–260.
23. Long, R, Gardam, M. Tumour necrosis factor-α inhibitors and the reactivation of latent tuberculosis infection. CMAJ 2003;168:1153–1156.
24. American Thoracic Society/Centers for Disease Control and Prevention. Diagnostic standards and classification of tuberculosis in adults and children. Am J Respir Crit Care Med 2000;161:1376–1395.
25. Peloquin CA, Berning SE. Tuberculosis and multi-drug resistant tuberculosis in children. Pediatr Nurs 1995;21:566–572.
26. Correa AG. Unique aspects of tuberculosis in the pediatric population. Clin Chest Med 1997;18:89–98.
27. Alland D, Kalkut GE, Moss AR, et al. Transmission of tuberculosis in New York City: An analysis of DNA fingerprinting and conventional epidemiologic methods. N Engl J Med 1994;330:1710–1716.
28. Small PM, Hopewell PC, Singh SP, et al. The epidemiology of tuberculosis in San Francisco: A population-based study using conventional and molecular methods. N Engl J Med 1994;330:1703–1709.
29. Daley CL, Small PM, Schecter GF, et al. An outbreak of tuberculosis with accelerated progression among persons infected with the human immunodeficiency virus: An analysis using restricted-fragment-length polymorphisms. N Engl J Med 1992;326:231–235.
30. Wallis RS, Vjecha M, Amir-Tahmasseb M, et al. Influence of tuberculosis on human immunodeficiency virus (HIV-1): Enhanced cytokine expression and elevated β_2-microglobulin in HIV-1–associated tuberculosis. J Infect Dis 1993;167:43–48.

31. American Thoracic Society/Centers for Disease Control and Prevention. Targeted tuberculin skin testing and treatment of latent tuberculosis infection. Am J Respir Crit Care Med 2000;161:S221-S247.

32. Pape JW, Jean SS, Ho JL, et al. Effect of isoniazid prophylaxis on incidence of active tuberculosis and progression of HIV infection. Lancet 1993;342:268-272.

33. Narita M, Ashkin D, Hollender ES, Pitchenik AE. Paradoxical worsening of tuberculosis following antiretroviral therapy in patients with AIDS. Am J Respir Crit Care Med 1998;158:157-161.

34. Barnes PF, Bloch AB, Davidson PT, Snider DE. Tuberculosis in patients with human immunodeficiency virus infection. N Engl J Med 1991;324:1644-1650.

35. Alvarez S, Shell C, Berk SL. Pulmonary tuberculosis in elderly men. Am J Med 1987;82:602-606.

36. Umeki S. Comparison of younger and elderly patients with pulmonary tuberculosis. Respiration 1989;55:75-83.

37. Centers for Disease Control and Prevention. Anergy skin testing and preventive therapy for HIV-infected persons: Revised recommendations. MMWR 1997;46:1-10.

38. Rosenberg T, Manfreda J, Hershfield ES. Two-step tuberculin testing in staff and residents of a nursing home. Am Rev Resp Dis 1993;148:1537-1540.

39. Centers for Disease Control and Prevention. Guidelines for using the QuantiFERON-TB test for detecting Mycobacterium tuberculosis infection, United States. MMWR 2005;54:49-55.

40. Mazurek GH, Villarino ME. Guidelines for using the quantiferon-TB test for diagnosing latent Mycobacterium tuberculosis infection. United States. MMWR 2003; 52:15-18.

41. Barnes PF. Weighing gold or counting spots. Am J Respir Crit Care Med 2006;174:731-735.

42. Nicol MP, Davies MA, Wood K, Hatherill M, et al. Comparison of T-SPOT. TB assay and tuberculosis skin test for the evaluation of young children at high risk for tuberculosis in community setting. Pediatrics 2009; 123:38-43.

43. Bergamini BM, Losi M, Vaienti F, et al. Performance of commercial blood tests for the diagnosis of latent tuberculosis infection in children and adolescents. Pediatrics 2009; 123:e419-e424.

44. Lighter J, Rigaud M, Eduardo R, Peng CH, et al. Latent tuberculosis diagnosis in children by using the quantiferon-TB gold in tube test. Pediatrics 2009;123: 30-37.

45. Richeldi L, Losi M, D'Amico R, et al. Performance of tests for latent tuberculosis in different groups of immunocompromised patients. Chest 2009;136:198-204.

46. Bouza E, Diaz-Lopez MD, Moreno S, et al. Mycobacterium tuberculosis bacteremia in patients with and without human immunodeficiency virus infection. Arch Intern Med 1993;153:496-500.

47. American Thoracic Society/Centers for Disease Control/Infectious Disease Society of America. Treatment of tuberculosis. Am J Respir Crit Care Med 2003;167:603-662.

48. Fujiwara PI, Larkin C, Frieden TR. Directly observed therapy in New York City. Clin Chest Med 1997;18:135-148.

49. Weis SE. Universal directly observed therapy. Clin Chest Med 1997;18:155-163.

50. Mitchison DA. Basic mechanisms of chemotherapy. Chest 1979;1994; 76(suppl):771-781.

51. Peloquin CA. Pharmacological issues in the treatment of tuberculosis. Ann N Y Acad Sci 2001;953:157-164.

52. Fourie PB, Ellner JJ, Johnson JL. Whither Mycobacterium vaccae—Encore. Lancet 2002;360:1032-1033.

53. Peloquin CA. Therapeutic drug monitoring in the treatment of tuberculosis. Drugs 2002;62:2169-2183.

54. Peloquin CA. Antituberculosis drugs: Pharmacokinetics. In: Heifets LB, ed. Drug Susceptibility in the Chemotherapy of Mycobacterial Infections. Boca Raton, FL: CRC Press; 1991:59-88.

55. Lawn SD, Wilkinson R. Extensively drug resistant tuberculosis. BMJ 2006;333;559-560.

56. Hamadeh MA, Glassroth J. Tuberculosis and pregnancy. Chest 1992;101:1114-1120.

57. Vallejo JG, Starke JR. Tuberculosis and pregnancy. Clin Chest Med 1992;13:693-707.

58. World Health Organization Report on antiretroviral therapy for HIV infection in adults and adolescents: towards universal access. Geneva: WHO; 2006.

59. Malone RS, Fish DN, Spiegel DM, et al. The effect of hemodialysis on isoniazid, rifampin, pyrazinamide, and ethambutol. Am J Respir Crit Care Med 1999;159:1580-1584.

60. Malone RS, Fish DN, Spiegel DM, et al. The effect of hemodialysis on cycloserine, ethionamide, para-aminosalicylate, and clofazimine. Chest 1999;116:984-990.

61. McEvoy GK, ed. AHFS Drug Information. Bethesda, MD: American Society of Health-Systems Pharmacists; 2003.

62. Girling DJ. Adverse effects of antituberculous drugs. Drugs 1982;23: 56-74.

63. Holdiness MR. Clinical pharmacokinetics of the antituberculosis drugs. Clin Pharmacokinet 1984;9:511-544.

64. Crabbe SJ. Drug infosearch—Intravenous isoniazid. P&T 1990;15: 1483-1484.

65. Peloquin CA, Namdar R, Dodge AA, Nix DE. Pharmacokinetics of isoniazid under fasting conditions, with food, and with antacids. Intl J Tuberc Lung Dis 1999;3:703-710.

66. Berning SE, Peloquin CA. Antimycobacterial agents: Isoniazid. In: Yu VL, Merigan TC, Barriere S, White NJ, eds. Antimicrobial Chemotherapy and Vaccines. Baltimore: Williams & Wilkins; 1998:654-663.

67. Weiner M, Burman W, Vernon A, et al. Low isoniazid concentration associated with outcome of tuberculosis treatment with once-weekly isoniazid and rifapentine. Am J Respir Crit Care Med 2003;167: 1341-1347.

68. Weiner M, Benator D, Burman W, et al. Association between acquired rifamycin resistance and the pharmacokinetics of rifabutin and isoniazid among patients with HIV and tuberculosis. Clin Infect Dis 2005;40:1481-1491.

69. Morris AB, Kanyok TP, Scott J, et al. Rifamycins. In: Yu VL, Merigan TC, Barriere S, White NJ, eds. Antimicrobial Chemotherapy and Vaccines. Baltimore: Williams & Wilkins; 1998:901-963.

70. Peloquin CA, Namdar R, Singleton MD, Nix DE. Pharmacokinetics of rifampin under fasting conditions, with food, and with antacids. Chest 1999;115:12-18.

71. Barroso EC, Pinheiro VG, Facanha MC, et al. Serum concentrations of rifampin, isoniazid, and intestinal absorption, permeability in patients with multidrug resistant tuberculosis. Am J Trop Med Hyg 2009;81:322-329.

72. Centers for Disease Control and Prevention. Prevention and treatment of tuberculosis among patients infected with human immunodeficiency virus: Principles of therapy and revised recommendations. MMWR 1998;47:1-58.

73. Centers for Disease Control and Prevention. Updated guidelines for the use of rifabutin or rifampin for the treatment and prevention of tuberculosis among HIV-infected patients taking protease inhibitors on nonnucleoside reverse transcriptase inhibitors. MMWR 2000;49:185-189.

74. Burman WJ, Gallicano K, Peloquin CA. Therapeutic implications of drug interactions in the treatment of HIV-related tuberculosis. Clin Infect Dis 1999;28:419-430.

75. Burman WJ, Gallicano K, Peloquin CA. Comparative pharmacokinetics and pharmacodynamics of the rifamycin antibiotics. Clin Pharmacokinet 2001:40:327-341.

76. Peloquin CA, Jaresko GS, Yong CL, et al. Population pharmacokinetic modeling of isoniazid, rifampin, and pyrazinamide. Antimicrob Agents Chemother 1997;41:2670-2679.

77. Peloquin CA, Bulpitt AE, Jaresko GS, et al. Pharmacokinetics of pyrazinamide under fasting conditions, with food, and with antacids. Pharmacotherapy 1998;18:1205-1211.

78. Peloquin CA, Bulpitt AE, Jaresko GS, et al. Pharmacokinetics of ethambutol under fasting conditions, with food, and with antacids. Antimicrob Agents Chemother 1999;43:568-572.

79. Summers KK, Hardin TC. Treatment of tuberculosis in hemodialysis patients. J Infect Dis Pharmacother 1996;2:37-55.

80. Peloquin CA, Berning SE. Comment: Intravenous streptomycin. Ann Pharmacother 1993;27:1546-1547.

81. Peloquin CA, Henshaw TL, Huitt GA, et al. Pharmacokinetic evaluation of p-aminosalicylic acid granules. Pharmacotherapy 1994;14:40–46 (and correction: Pharmacotherapy 1994;14:2).

82. Peloquin CA, Berning SE, Huitt GA, et al. Once-daily and twice-daily dosing of p-aminosalicylic acid (PAS) granules. Am J Respir Crit Care Med 1999;159:932–934.

83. Peloquin CA, Zhu M, Adam RD, et al. Pharmacokinetics of p-aminosalicylate under fasting conditions, with orange juice, food, and antacids. Ann Pharmacother 2001;35:1332–1338.

84. Zhu M, Nix DE, Adam RD, et al. Pharmacokinetics of cycloserine under fasting conditions, with orange juice, food, and antacids. Pharmacotherapy 2001;21:891–897.

85. Zhu M, Namdar R, Stambaugh JJ, et al. Population pharmacokinetics of ethionamide in patients with tuberculosis. Tuberculosis 2002;82:91–96.

86. Elliott AM, Foster SD. Thiacetazone: Time to call a halt? Tuber Lung Dis 1996;77:27–29.

87. Burman WJ, Goldberg S, Johnson JL, et al. Moxifloxacin versus ethambutol in the first 2 months of treatment for pulmonary tuberculosis. Am J Respir Crit Care Med 2006;174:331–338.

88. Conde MB, Efron A, Loredo C, et al. Moxifloxacin versus ethambutol in the initial treatment of tuberculosis: A double blind, randomized, controlled phase II trial. Lancet 2009; 373:1183–1189.

89. Dorman SE, Johnson JL, Goldberg S, et al. Substitution of moxifloxadin for isoniazid during intensive phase treatment of pulmonary tuberculosis. Am J Respir Crit Care Med; 2009; 180:273–280.

90. Zhang Y, Steingrube VA, Wallace RJ. Beta-lactamase inhibitors and the inducibility of the beta-lactamase of Mycobacterium tuberculosis. Am Rev Respir Dis 1992;145:657–660.

91. Stover CK, Warrener P, VanDevanter DR, et al. A small-molecule nitroimidazopyran drug candidate for the treatment of tuberculosis. Nature 2000;405:962–966.

92. Nuermberger E, Rosenthal I, Tyagi S, et al. Combination chemotherapy with the nitroimidazopyran PA-824 and first-line drugs in the murine model of tuberculosis. Antimicrob Agents Chemother 2006;50:2621–2625.

93. Sung JC, Garcia-Contreras Lucila, VerBerkmoes JL et al. Dry Powder nitroimidazopyran antibiotic PA-824 aerosol for inhalation. Antimicrob Agents Chemother 2009; 53:1338–1343.

94. Andries K, Verhasselt P, Guillemont J, et al. A diarylquinolone drug active on the ATP synthase of Mycobacterium tuberculosis. Science 2005; 307:223–227.

95. Forun J, Martin-Davila P, Navas E, et al. Linezolid for the treatment of multidrug resistant tuberculosis. J Antimicrob Chemother 2005; 56:180–185.

96. Reves R, Burman W, Dalton C, et al. A cost-effectiveness analysis of directly-observed therapy versus self-administered therapy for treatment of tuberculosis. Am J Respir Crit Care Med 1997;155(Suppl): A33.

97. Goble M, Iseman MD, Madsen LA, et al. Treatment of 171 patients with pulmonary tuberculosis resistant to isoniazid and rifampin. N Engl J Med 1993;328:527–532.

98. Iseman MD. Treatment of multidrug-resistant tuberculosis. N Engl J Med 1993;329:784–791.

99. Brudney K, Dobkin J. Resurgent tuberculosis in New York City: Human immunodeficiency virus, homelessness, and the decline of tuberculosis control programs. Am Rev Respir Dis 1991;144:745–749.

100. Mahmoudi A, Iseman MD. Pitfalls in the care of patients with tuberculosis: Common errors and their association with the acquisition of drug resistance. JAMA 1993;270:65–68.

101. Chaulk CP, Friedman M, Dunning R. Modeling the epidemiology and economics of directly observed therapy in Baltimore. Int J Tuberc Lung Dis 2000;4:201–207.

102. Tappero JW, Bradford WZ, Agerton TB, et al. Serum concentrations of antimycobacterial drugs in patients with pulmonary tuberculosis in Botswana. Clin Infect Dis 2005;41:461–469.

103. Perlman DC, Segal Y, Rosenkranz S, et al. The clinical pharmacokinetics of rifampin and ethambutol in HIV-infected persons with tuberculosis. Clin Infect Dis 2005;41:1638–1647.

104. Peloquin CA. Agents for tuberculosis. In: Piscitelli SC, Rodvold KA, eds. Drug Interactions in Infectious Diseases. Totowa, NJ: Humana Press; 2001:109–120.

CHAPTER

122

Gastrointestinal Infections and Enterotoxigenic Poisonings

STEVEN MARTIN AND ROSE JUNG

KEY CONCEPTS

❶ The etiology of infectious diarrhea includes bacteria, viruses, and protozoans. Viral infections are the leading cause of diarrhea in the world.

❷ Fluid and electrolyte replacement is the cornerstone of therapy. Oral rehydration therapy is preferred in most cases of mild and moderate diarrhea. The necessary components of oral replacement therapy are glucose, sodium, potassium, chloride, and water.

❸ Antimicrobial therapy often is not indicated for enteritis because many cases are mild and self-limited or are viral in nature.

❹ Diarrheal illness can be prevented by following simple rules of personal hygiene and safe food preparation.

❺ The most common pathogens for traveler's diarrhea include enterotoxigenic *Escherichia coli*, *Shigella*, *Campylobacter*, *Salmonella*, and viruses.

❻ Patient education in prevention strategies and self-treatment of traveler's diarrhea is recommended. Prophylaxis with antibiotics is not recommended in most situations.

❼ Common pathogens responsible for food poisoning include *Staphylococcus*, *Salmonella*, *Shigella*, and *Clostridium*.

Gastrointestinal (GI) infections encompass a wide variety of syndromes from mild gastroenteritis to life-threatening systemic disease. Dehydration from GI infections is the second leading cause of morbidity and mortality worldwide, and infants and children younger than age 5 years are at the highest risk. From 1992 to 2000, the median incidence of diarrhea for all children younger than age 5 years was 3.2 episodes per child per year. The incidence of diarrhea was higher in younger children, with 4.8 episodes per child per year among children ages 6 to 11 months, compared with 1.4 episodes per child per year for children age 4 years. Younger children also had a higher risk of death from acute dehydrating diarrhea. For children younger than age 1 year and those age 1 to 4 years, the median mortality rates were 8.5 and 3.8 per 1,000 children per year, respectively.[1] Although this was a decrease from

13.6 per 1,000 children per year during 1955–1979 and 5.6 per 1,000 children per year during 1980 to 1989, diarrhea remains a major health problem in children, especially in those younger than age 1 year.[2,3]

Although outbreaks of infectious diarrhea and deaths in the United States are not as common as in other parts of the world, the economic burden of GI infections still remains high. The estimates by the Centers for Disease Control and Prevention (CDC) suggest that 211 million episodes of acute gastroenteritis occur each year in the United States, resulting in more than 900,000 hospitalizations and more than 6,000 deaths. In contrast to the developing world, where the risk of death is highest among young children, in the United States, most of those who die of diarrheal illness are elderly. According to the National Center for Health Statistics, during 1979 to 1987, 51% of deaths caused by diarrheal illness were among patients older than age 74 years, and 27% were among the ages of 55 to 74 years; only 11% of deaths were in those younger than age 5 years.[2] Similarly, a study of the McDonnell-Douglas Health Information System database revealed that 25% of all hospitalizations and 85% of all mortality associated with diarrhea involved the elderly (≥age 60 years).[3] In addition to children and elderly, other groups at risk for GI infections include travelers and campers, patients in chronic care facilities, military personnel assigned overseas, and immunocompromised patients such as those with acquired immunodeficiency syndrome (AIDS).

Fortunately, diarrheal mortality has declined substantially in the past two decades, especially among children younger than age 1 year. Interventions for diarrheal disease such as breast-feeding, better weaning practices, improved sanitation, and increased use of oral rehydration therapy are responsible for the decrease in case-fatality rates. Although this reduction in mortality is reassuring, diarrhea still remains among the top 10 leading causes of death world wide.[4] To achieve further declines in mortality, a more complex approach needs to be adopted that includes distinguishing acute watery diarrhea from dysentery and persistent diarrhea, and providing appropriate case management for each syndrome.

❶ A variety of pathogens are responsible for acute infectious diarrhea. Viruses are suspected to be the most common cause of gastroenteritis worldwide, especially in children. However, in the United States, bacterial species are the most commonly identified cause of infectious diarrhea. This chapter focuses on the bacterial and viral etiologies of GI infections such as *Vibrio cholerae*, *Escherichia coli*, *Salmonella*, *Shigella*, *Campylobacter jejuni*, rotaviruses, noroviruses, astrovirus, and enteric adenovirus. Clinical presentation, diagnosis, treatment, and prevention strategies are discussed in general terms initially for all GI infections, and further elaborated in regards to specific etiologies in subsequent sections.

CLINICAL PRESENTATION AND DIAGNOSIS

Gastroenteritis is an illness characterized by diarrhea which may be accompanied by nausea, vomiting, fever, and abdominal pain.[5] Diarrhea is usually defined as a decrease in consistency of bowel movements (i.e., unformed stool) and an increase of stools to ≥3 per day. For best diagnosis and management, it is important to distinguish secretory diarrhea that produces watery diarrhea from inflammatory diarrhea. Caused by invasive pathogens, inflammatory diarrhea often presents as fever, tenesmus, or bloody stool. Symptoms of and enteric pathogens that cause watery and inflammatory diarrhea are listed in Table 122–1.

A careful history and physical examination that includes information about symptoms, the length of time the patient has been sick, the number of individuals affected, and recent history of travel, diet, and medications are important factors in making a diagnosis. Stool cultures are also an invaluable tool in making an organism-specific diagnosis and determining sensitivity to antimicrobial agents. The stool culture will identify the presence of *Campylobacter, Salmonella,* and *Shigella* species. Other pathogens such as *Yersinia* and *Vibrio* species may also be detected using selective media. Unfortunately, the yield of positive stool cultures is very low. In order to improve the usefulness of stool cultures, fecal testing is recommended in patients with inflammatory diarrhea.[5] For community-acquired or traveler's diarrhea, stool samples should be sent for culture of *Salmonella, Shigella,* and *Campylobacter,* and toxin testing of *E. coli* O157:H7 and *C. difficile* toxins A and B. In hospitalized patients who develop diarrhea 3 days after hospitalization, stool specimen should be tested for *C. difficile* toxins A and B, especially in those who are exposed to antimicrobial therapy or chemotherapy. Stool culture is also recommended in patients with persistent diarrhea, especially if they are immunocompromised (i.e., persons age 65 years and older with comorbid diseases, neutropenia, or human immunodeficiency virus [HIV] infection). In immunocompromised hosts, a wide range of viral, bacterial, and parasitic organisms should be sought. In addition to stool cultures, microscopic examination for fecal polymorphonuclear cells, or a simple immunoassay for the neutrophil marker lactoferrin can further provide evidence of an inflammatory process and increase the yield of cultures for invasive pathogens in patients presenting with fever or bloody stool.

TREATMENT

Diarrhea

■ GENERAL APPROACHES TO MANAGEMENT

Rehydration Therapy

Initial assessment of fluid loss is essential for rehydration and should include acute weight loss, as it is the most reliable means of determining the extent of water loss. However, if accurate baseline weight is not available, clinical signs are helpful in determining approximate deficits (Table 122–2).[6,7] Physical assessment generally is more reliable in young children and infants than in adults.

❷ Fluid replacement is the cornerstone of therapy for dehydration due to diarrhea regardless of etiology. For the treatment of mild to moderate dehydration, oral rehydration therapy (ORT) is superior to administration of intravenous (IV) fluids. ORT reverses dehydration in nearly all patients with mild to moderate diarrhea with 94% to 97% efficacy.[6] ORT offers the advantages of being inexpensive, noninvasive, and does not require hospitalization for administration. Moreover, thirst drives use of ORT and provides a safeguard against overhydration.

The necessary components of oral rehydration solutions (ORS) include carbohydrates (typically glucose), sodium, potassium, chloride, and water. Glucose-based ORS takes advantage of glucose-coupled sodium transport in the small bowel that enhances sodium and subsequently water transport across intestinal walls. In 2002, the World Health Organization/United Nations Children's Fund (WHO/UNICEF) recommended a reduced osmolarity solution (Osm = 245 mmol/L) for ORT in response to reports that this reduced osmolarity solution reduced stool output, vomiting, and the need for intravenous therapy.[7] The composition of commercial ORS and commonly consumed beverages are listed in Table 122–3.[8] Clear fluids, such as soft drinks, sweetened fruit drinks, broth, and sports drinks should be avoided in the treatment of dehydration. Those solutions may cause an osmotic diarrhea and hypernatremia.

In the treatment of severe dehydration, IV therapy remains the therapy of choice. Severely dehydrated patients should be resuscitated initially with Lactated Ringer's solution or normal saline intravenously to restore hemodynamic stability. Lactated Ringer's solution is preferred over normal saline because normal saline does not correct metabolic acidosis. Rapid IV rehydration is preferred over more prolonged replacement regimens for restoring extracellular fluids and electrolytes because it more effectively reestablishes gastrointestinal and renal perfusion. ORT should be instituted as soon as it can be tolerated.

Treatment of dehydration consists of rehydration, replacement of ongoing losses, and continuation of normal feeding. Guidelines on rehydration therapy based on degree of dehydration and replacement of ongoing losses are outlined in Table 122–2. ORS should be given in small and frequent volumes (5 mL every 2 to 3 minutes in a teaspoon or oral syringe). Nasogastric administration of ORT is

TABLE 122-1	Acute Infectious Diarrhea Clinical Syndromes: Watery vs. Inflammatory	
	Watery	**Inflammatory**
Percentage of patients	90	5–10
Stools		
Appearance	Watery	Bloody
Volume	Increased: ++/+++	Increased: +/++
Number per day	<10	>10
Reducing substances	0 to +++	0
pH	5.0–7.5	6.0–7.5
Occult blood	Negative	Positive
Fecal polymorpho-nuclear cells	Absent or few	Many
Mechanisms	Toxins Reduced absorption	Mucosal invasion
Complications		
Dehydration	Could be severe	Mild
Others	Acidosis, shock, electrolyte imbalance	Tenesmus, rectal pro-lapse, seizures
Etiology	*Vibrio cholerae* Enterotoxigenic *Escherichia coli* (ETEC) Enteropathogenic *E. coli* (EPEC) Rotaviruses Noroviruses	*Shigella* *Salmonella* *Campylobacter* *Yersinia* Enterohemorrhagic *E. coli* (EHEC) Enteroinvasive *E. coli* (EIEC) Enteroaggregative *E. coli* (EAEC) Cytotoxigenic *C. difficile*

From Guerrant et al.[5] and Holtz et al.[25]

TABLE 122-2 Clinical Assessment of Degree of Dehydration in Children Based on Percentage of Body Weight Loss[a]

Variable	Minimal or No Dehydration (<3% Loss of Body Weight)	Mild to Moderate (3–9% Loss of Body Weight)	Severe (≥10% Loss of Body Weight
Blood pressure	Normal	Normal	Normal to reduced
Quality of pulses	Normal	Normal or slightly decreased	Weak, thready, or not palpable
Heart rate	Normal	Normal to increased	Increased (bradycardia in severe cases)
Breathing	Normal	Normal to fast	Deep
Mental status	Normal	Normal to listless	Apathetic, lethargic, or comatose
Eyes	Normal	Sunken orbits/decreased tears	Deeply sunken orbits/absent tears
Mouth and tongue	Moist	Dry	Parched
Thirst	Normal	Eager to drink	Drinks poorly; too lethargic to drink
Skin fold	Normal	Recoil in <2 seconds	Recoil in >2 seconds
Extremities	Warm, normal capillary refill	Cool, prolonged capillary refill	Cold, mottled, cyanotic, prolonged capillary refill
Urine output	Normal to decreased	Decreased	Minimal
Hydration therapy	None	ORS 50–100 mL/kg over 3–4 hours	Lactated Ringer's solution or normal saline 20 mL/kg in 15–30 minutes intravenously until mental status or perfusion improve; Followed by 5% dextrose ½ normal saline intravenously at twice maintenance rates or ORS 100 mL/kg over 4 hours.
Replacement of ongoing losses	<10kg body weight: 60–120 mL ORS per >10kg body weight: 120–240 mL ORS per diarrheal stool or emesis	Same	If unable to tolerate ORS, administer through nasogastric tube or administer 5% dextrose ½ normal saline with 20 mEq/L potassium chloride intravenously

ORS, oral rehydration solution.

[a]Percentages vary among authors for each dehydration category; hemodynamic and perfusion status is most important; when unsure of category, therapy for more severe category is recommended.

Data from King et al. (6) and World Health Organization (7)

an alternative method of administration in a child with persistent vomiting. For breastfed infants, nursing should be continued.

Early refeeding as tolerated is recommended.[6,7] Age-appropriate unrestricted diet is recommended as soon as dehydration is corrected. Early initiation of feeding can shorten the course of diarrhea. In a study of severely malnourished children with diarrhea younger than age 5 years, the use of a standardized protocol of slow oral rehydration, immediate feeding, and intensive management of complications resulted in a significant reduction of mortality as compared with standard therapy. Initially, easily digested foods such as bananas, applesauce, and cereal may be added. Foods high in fiber, sodium, and sugar should be avoided. Lactase deficiency may be exacerbated among known lactase-deficient patients and may persist up to 10 days.

Antimicrobial Therapy

The indiscriminate use of antimicrobial therapy in GI infections produces increases in antimicrobial resistance, side effects of antimicrobial agents, and the threat of superinfections owing to eradication of normal flora. Increasing fluoroquinolone resistance in *Campylobacter* and multidrug resistance in *Salmonella* species worldwide reinforce the importance of judicious use of antibiotics and prudent infection control measures.[9,10] Furthermore,

it is important to take local susceptibility patterns into consideration in the selection of initial therapy with an antimicrobial regimen.

❸ Antibiotics are not essential in the treatment of most mild diarrheas, and empirical therapy for acute GI infections may result in courses of unnecessary antibiotics. However, appropriate antibiotic therapy shortens the duration of illness and reduces morbidity in some bacterial (cholera, enterotoxigenic *E. coli*, shigellosis, campylobacteriosis, yersiniosis) infections and can be lifesaving in invasive infections (*C. difficile*, salmonellosis). Antibiotic treatment also reduces the duration and shedding of organisms in infections with susceptible *Shigella* species and possibly in infection with susceptible *Campylobacter* species. Table 122-4 summarizes antibiotic recommendations. Further details regarding treatment of specific infections are discussed in appropriate sections.

It is also important to note that outcomes of some bacterial diarrheal illnesses may be worsened by the use of antibiotics. Antibiotic treatment may prolong asymptomatic carriage of *Salmonella*.[11] In patients infected with *E. coli* O157, use of an antimicrobial agent may worsen the risk of hemolytic uremic syndrome (HUS), which is defined by the triad of acute renal failure, thrombocytopenia, and microangiopathic hemolytic anemia, by increasing the production of shiga-like toxin.[12]

TABLE 122-3 Comparison of Common Solutions Used in Oral Rehydration and Maintenance

Product	Na (mEq/L)	K (mEq/L)	Base (mEq/L)	Carbohydrate (mmol/L)	Osmolality (mOsm/L)
WHO/UNICEF (2002)	75	20	30	75	245
Naturalyte	45	20	48	140	265
Pedialyte	45	20	30	140	250
Infalyte	50	25	30	70	200
Rehydralyte	75	20	30	140	250
Cola[a]	2	0	13	700	750
Apple juice[a]	5	32	0	690	730
Chicken broth[a]	250	8	0	0	500
Sports beverage[a]	20	3	3	255	330

[a]These solutions should be avoided in dehydration.

From Stone et al (8) and World Health Organization (7)

TABLE 122-4 Recommendations for Antibiotic Therapy

Pathogen	First-Line Agents	Alternative Agents
Enterotoxigenic (cholera-like) diarrhea		
Vibrio cholerae O1 or O139	Doxycycline 300 mg orally × 1	Tetracycline 500 mg orally four times daily × 3 days; ciprofloxacin 500 mg orally every 12 hours × 3 days or 1 g orally single dose; norfloxacin 400 mg orally every 12 hours × 3 days; levofloxacin 500 mg orally once daily × 3 days; trimethoprim-sulfamethoxazole DS tablet twice daily × 3 days; erythromycin 250–500 mg orally every 6–8 hours; azithromycin 1,000 mg orally × 1
Enterotoxigenic *Escherichia coli*	Ciprofloxacin 500 mg orally every 12 hours, norfloxacin 400 mg orally every 12 hours, levofloxacin 500 mg orally once daily × 3 days	Rifaximin 200 mg 3 times daily × 3 days; azithromycin 1,000 mg orally × 1 or 500 mg orally daily × 3 days
Invasive (dysentery-like) diarrhea		
Shigella species[a]	Ciprofloxacin 500 mg orally every 12 hours, norfloxacin 400 mg orally every 12 hours, levofloxacin 500 mg orally 1 daily × 5 days	Azithromycin 500 mg orally × 1, then 250 mg orally daily × 4 days
Salmonella Nontyphoidal[a]	Gastroenteritis: Ciprofloxacin 500 mg every 12 hours × 5–7 days Bacteremia: Ceftriaxone 2 g IV daily × 7–14 days Chronic carriers: Ciprofloxacin 750 mg orally every 12 hours × 1 month	Gastroenteritis: Azithromycin 1,000 mg orally × 1 day, followed by 500 mg orally once daily × 6 days; trimethoprim-sulfamethoxazole DS orally every 12 hours × 5–7 days Chronic carriers: amoxicillin 1,000 mg orally every 8 hours × 3 months; trimethoprim-sulfamethoxazole DS orally every 12 hours × 3 months
Campylobacter[a]	Erythromycin 500 mg orally twice daily, azithromycin 1,000 mg orally × 1 day followed by 500 mg daily or clarithromycin 500 mg orally twice daily × 5 days	Ciprofloxacin 500 mg or norfloxacin 400 mg orally twice daily × 5 days
Yersinia species[a]	A combination therapy with doxycycline, aminoglycosides, trimethoprim-sulfamethoxazole, or fluoroquinolones	
Clostridium difficile	Mild to moderate disease: Metronidazole 250 mg every 6 hours to 500 mg every 8 hours orally or intravenously daily × 10–14 days Severe disease: Vancomycin 125 mg every 6 hours orally × 10–14 days First relapse: same as above Subsequent relapses: Tapered pulse dose of oral vancomycin (125 mg every 6 hours × 2 weeks, every 12 hours × 1 week, every 24 hours × 1 week, every 48 hours × 8 days (4 doses), every 72 hours × 15 days (5 doses)	Subsequent relapses: Oral vancomycin 125 mg every 6 hours × 10–14 days followed by rifaximin 400 mg every 12 hours orally × 2 weeks; Nitazoxanide 500 mg every 12 hours × 10 days
Traveler's diarrhea		
Prophylaxis[a]	Norfloxacin 400 mg or ciprofloxacin 750 mg orally daily	Rifaximin 200 mg one to three times daily up to 2 weeks
Treatment	Norfloxacin 800 mg orally × 1 or 400 mg orally every 12 hours × 3 days, or Ciprofloxacin 750 mg orally ×1 or 500 mg orally every 12 hours × 3 days, or Levofloxacin 1,000 mg orally × 1 or 500 mg orally daily × 3 days Azithromycin 1,000 mg orally × 1 or 500 mg orally daily × 3 days	Rifaximin 200 mg 3 times daily × 3 days

[a]For high-risk patients only. See the preceding text for the high-risk patients in each infection.

Antimotility Agents

Antiperistaltic drugs such as diphenoxylate and loperamide offer symptomatic relief in patients with mild diarrhea. However, these agents are contraindicated in most toxin-mediated diarrheal illnesses (enterohemorrhagic *E. coli*, pseudomembranous colitis, shigellosis) and thus should be avoided in patients with high fever and bloody diarrhea. Slowing of fecal transit time is thought to result in extended toxin-associated damage, worsening diseases such as HUS.

CLINICAL CONTROVERSY

Loperamide should not be used in patients with fever or bloody stool. There is evidence that the use of such agents can increase the risk for development of HUS, possibly by delaying intestinal clearance of the organism and thereby increasing toxin absorption.

PREVENTION OF GASTROINTESTINAL INFECTIONS

❹ Public health measures of improved water supply and sanitation facilities and the quality control of commercial products are important for the control of the majority of enteric infections. In addition, many diarrheal diseases can be prevented by following simple rules of personal hygiene and safe food preparation. Handwashing with soap and running water is instrumental in preventing the spread of illness and should be emphasized for caregivers and persons with diarrheal illnesses. Safe food handling and preparation practices can significantly decrease the incidence of certain types of enteric infections.

Reporting suspected outbreaks and cases of notifiable illness to local health authorities is vital in investigation of threats of enteric infection arising from increasingly global and industrialized food supplies. The reporting of specific infectious diseases to the appropriate public health authorities is the cornerstone of public health surveillance, outbreak detection, and prevention and control efforts.

Vaccines are used to boost specific immune processes directed against the bacteria themselves or against adherence appendages, cytotoxins, or enterotoxins. Unfortunately, there are only a few vaccines available for prevention of gastroenteritis. Currently available vaccines for typhoid fever are the parenteral Vi capsular polysaccharide vaccine and the oral live-attenuated Ty21a vaccine.[13] Efficacy rates for both vaccines range from 50% to 80%. There are 2 vaccines (RotaTeq and Rotarix) available for reducing rotaviral gastroenteritis.[14]

PATIENT ASSESSMENT

Appropriate follow-up care of patients with acute diarrhea is based on successful restoration of fluid losses. The clinical signs and symptoms (see Table 122–1) that lead to the diagnosis also can assess adequate rehydration, and should be monitored frequently. Since oral rehydration therapy is now preferred, routine laboratory testing often is unnecessary. Electrolytes should be measured in those receiving IV fluids, when oral replacement fails, or when signs of hypernatremia or hypokalemia are present. Follow-up stool samples to ensure complete evacuation of the infecting pathogen may be necessary only in patients who are at high risk to initiate or contribute to a community outbreak. All patients should be monitored for complications associated with the infecting pathogen, resolution of the diarrhea, and adverse reactions to the pharmacologic agents used. Prompt discharge of hospitalized patients is recommended when rehydration is achieved, intravenous fluids have not been required, oral intake equals or exceeds losses, or adequate education and medical follow-up are ensured. For most patients, discharge can occur in 16 to 24 hours.

SPECIFIC BACTERIAL INFECTIONS

Bacterial agents are important causes of GI infections, and syndromes caused by these pathogens are better understood than viral gastroenteritis. For a simple generalization, the bacterial pathogens presented in this section are divided into either those that cause watery (enterotoxigenic) diarrhea or those that cause dysentery (invasive diarrhea). Watery diarrhea is usually self-limiting, whereas those who present with dysenteric symptoms, such as fever, tenesmus, and blood and/or pus in the stool, require close monitoring and intensive follow-up. Table 122–1 lists the clinical signs and symptoms of these two broad categories.

WATERY (CHOLERA-LIKE) DIARRHEA

Cholera (*Vibrio Cholerae*)

Epidemiology Cholera has been endemic in the Ganges delta, West Bengal, Bangladesh, and southern Asia (including Southeast Asia) since at least 1817. A 1994 outbreak of a multidrug-resistant strain of cholera among Rwandan refugees resulted in more than 20,000 deaths. Cholera epidemics in 1991 and 1998 caused more than 1 million deaths in Latin America. As international travel has increased, cholera has also been reported in all major regions of the United States. However, the incidence, 1 case per 1 million persons, is extremely low.[15]

V. cholerae O1 is the most common serogroup associated with epidemics and pandemics. Within this serogroup, there are two biotypes, classic and El Tor.[16] In 1992, a new serogroup, *V. cholerae* O139 Bengal, appeared in India and spread rapidly through Southeast Asia. Four mechanisms for transmission have been proposed, including animal reservoirs, chronic carriers, asymptomatic or mild disease victims, and water reservoirs.

A relatively large inoculum of 10^3 to 10^6 organisms is required for infection if water is the vehicle, and 10^2 to 10^4 if the vehicle is food. Approximately half of the people infected with *V. cholerae* O1 are symptomatic, whereas only 1% to 5% of those infected with *V. cholerae* O139 manifest symptoms. The hallmark of cholera is the production of profuse, watery diarrhea, and severe dehydration may develop within a few hours, causing death within 24 hours. An estimated 25% to 50% of cases are fatal if left untreated. The prevention of cholera transmission depends on the provision of clean drinking water and public sanitation, which is difficult in impoverished and developing countries.[17]

Pathogenesis *V. cholerae* is a gram-negative bacillus sharing similar characteristics with the family Enterobacteriaceae. Most pathology of cholera results from an enterotoxin (cholera toxin) produced by the bacteria.[17] Conditions that reduce gastric acidity, such as the use of antacids, histamine receptor blockers, or proton pump inhibitors, or infections with *Helicobacter pylori,* increase the risk for clinical disease. Cholera toxin stimulates adenylate cyclase, which increases intracellular cyclic adenosine monophosphate (cAMP) and results in inhibition of sodium and chloride absorption by microvilli and promotes the secretion of chloride and water by crypt cells. The toxin likely acts along the entire intestinal tract, but most fluid loss occurs in the duodenum. The net effect of the cholera toxin is isotonic fluid secretion (primarily in the small intestine) that exceeds the absorptive capacity of the intestinal tract (primarily the colon). This results in the production of watery diarrhea with electrolyte concentrations similar to that of plasma.

Clinical Presentation The average incubation period for *V. cholerae* infection is 1 to 3 days.[17] The clinical presentation can vary from asymptomatic to life-threatening dehydration owing to watery diarrhea. Patients may lose up to 1 L of isotonic fluid every hour. The onset of diarrhea is abrupt and is followed rapidly or sometimes preceded by vomiting. Fever occurs in less than 5% of patients, and the physical examination correlates well with the severity of dehydration. In some cases, fluid accumulates within the intestinal lumen causing abdominal distension and ileus and may cause intravascular depletion without diarrhea. In the most severe state, this disease can progress to death in 2 to 4 hours if not treated.

Laboratory abnormalities, such as increased packed red blood cell volume and total protein, magnesium, and calcium levels, are a result of hemoconcentration. Hypoglycemia, seizures, fever, and mental alterations are seen more often in children, perhaps as a reflection of the greater degree of dehydration and electrolyte losses observed with diarrhea in children. Other complications include metabolic acidosis, prerenal azotemia, iatrogenic water intoxication from overhydration, and aspiration pneumonia. Children, the elderly, and pregnant women are at an increased risk of complications caused by cholera.

TREATMENT

Regardless of the serotypes, the primary goal of therapy is rapid restoration of fluid losses, correction of metabolic acidosis, and replacement of potassium deficiency. In restoring fluid and electrolyte balance in cholera infections, rice-based ORT may be more efficacious than glucose-based ORT, reducing fluid requirements by 32% to 35% when rice-based instead of glucose-based ORT solutions are used (50 to 80 grams rice instead of 20 grams glucose/L).[18] In patients who cannot tolerate ORT, lactated Ringer's solution IV is preferred. After rehydration, maintenance fluid is given based on accurate recording of intake and output volumes.

Antibiotics are not necessary in most cholera cases. However, in severe cases, antibiotics shorten the duration of diarrhea, decrease fluid loss, and shorten the duration of the carrier state.[17] There appears to be substantial mobility in genetic elements encoding antibiotic resistance in *V. cholerae*, and the drug resistance patterns may change between outbreaks. For example, O139 strains isolated during 1992 and 1993 showed a trend toward increased resistance to trimethoprim-sulfamethoxazole, but those isolated in India during 1996 and 1997 showed susceptibility to the same agent. A single dose of doxycycline is the preferred agent, especially in endemic areas, although it has been associated with prolonged fecal excretion of bacteria.[11] In areas of high tetracycline resistance, fluoroquinolones such as ciprofloxacin are effective, and in areas of high fluoroquinolone resistance, azithromycin has been shown to be effective.[19] In children and pregnant women, erythromycin and azithromycin can be used.[20]

The manufacture of the only licensed whole-cell cholera vaccine in the United States has been discontinued. Two oral vaccines are available in other countries.[17] Dukoral consists of killed *V. cholerae* organisms and the cholera B subunit, and Orochol is an avirulent mutant of *V. cholerae* strain CVD103HgR. Both vaccines are effective in field trials and volunteer studies, but their cost-effectiveness in endemic settings is uncertain. The World Health Organization (WHO) does not require vaccination for international travel to or from endemic areas because the series of two injections is effective in only 50% of people and immunity wanes in 6 months or less.

Escherichia Coli

Diarrheagenic *E. coli* is differentiated into several distinct categories based on pathogenic features of diarrheal disease: enterotoxigenic *E. coli* (ETEC), enteroinvasive *E. coli* (EIEC), enteropathogenic *E. coli* (EPEC), enteroaggregative *E. coli* (EAEC), and enterohemorrhagic *E. coli* (EHEC). The most common diarrheagenic *E. coli* infection is caused by ETEC manifested by watery (enterotoxigenic) diarrhea. Dysentery is caused by EHEC. In this section, commonly known categories of diarrheagenic *E. coli* that cause watery diarrhea are discussed separately from EHEC that cause bloody diarrhea.

Epidemiology ETEC occurs most commonly, and accounts for about half of all cases of *E. coli* diarrhea. There are an estimated 79,420 cases in the United States each year.[21] TEC is the most common cause of traveler's diarrhea and a common cause of food- and water-associated outbreaks. Infections with EIEC and EPEC are primarily a disease of children in developing countries.[22,23] EAEC strains are implicated in persistent diarrhea (≥14 days) in HIV-infected patients.[24]

Recognized as a common and potentially deadly cause of infectious diarrhea, EHEC is believed to be the major etiologic factor responsible for the development of hemorrhagic colitis and HUS. The CDC estimates the annual disease burden of *E. coli* O157:H7 in the United States to be more than 20,000 infections and as many as 250 deaths, but the failure of many clinical laboratories to screen for this organism greatly complicates any estimates.[25] In the United States, serotype O157:H7 causes 50% to 80% of all EHEC infections, but in the southern hemisphere, such as in Argentina, Australia, Chile, and South Africa, non-O157:H7 serotypes are often more important. Transmission usually occurs via food and water, and outbreaks have been associated with undercooked ground beef and feces-contaminated vegetables.

Pathogenesis *E. coli* is a gram-negative bacillus commonly found in the human GI tract as well as in intestines of healthy cattle, deer, goats, and sheep. Enterotoxigenic *E. coli* are capable of producing either or both plasmid-mediated enterotoxins: heat-labile toxin and heat-stable toxin.[21] A cholera-like toxin, heat-labile toxin has two subunits (A and B) that have similar antigenic properties and action on the gut mucosa. The net effect is luminal accumulation of electrolytes that draws water into the intestine, and production of

a cholera-like secretory diarrhea. Heat-stable toxin is nonantigenic and produces watery diarrhea by acting on the small intestine.

The mode of pathogenesis of the non-ETEC varieties is less well understood. The hallmark histopathologic lesions of EPEC infections is the effacing of microvilli and intimate adherence between the bacterium and the epithelial cell membrane throughout the intestine.[23] The attaching and effacing lesions disrupt the integrity of the intestinal epithelium, leading to diarrhea. EAEC adheres to intestinal mucosal cells by mucus production and deposition of bacteria in a bacterium–mucus biofilm.[24] This persistent colonization of EAEC potentially leads to cytotoxic damage of intestinal cells, resulting in persistent diarrhea. EIEC closely resembles *Shigella* species and penetrates the intestinal mucosa, predominantly the lining of the large intestine. The resulting histological damage is inflammation and mucosal ulceration which are characteristic of bacillary dystentery.[22]

The pathogenicity of EHEC is related to the production of shiga-like toxins, so named because of their resemblance to the shiga toxin of *Shigella dysenteriae*.[25] The cytotoxic effect of shiga-like toxins disrupts the mucosal integrity of the large intestine, causing diarrhea. In addition, the toxin is able to pass through the intestinal epithelium to reach the endothelial cells lining small blood vessels that supply the gut, kidney, and other viscera, causing the myriad metabolic events that eventually lead to HUS.

Clinical Presentation Nausea and watery stools, with or without abdominal cramping, are characteristic of the disease caused by ETEC. Usually there is no blood or pus in the stool. Signs and symptoms depend directly on the extent of fluid loss, which in most cases is subclinical. Most ETEC diarrhea is typically abrupt in onset and resolves within 24 to 48 hours without complication. Common symptoms of EPEC infection include acute onset of profuse watery diarrhea, vomiting, and low-grade fever. The clinical features of EAEC diarrhea are characterized as persistent, watery, mucoid, secretory diarrhea with low-grade fever and little or no vomiting. EIEC infection presents most commonly as watery diarrhea, which can be indistinguishable from the secretory diarrhea seen with ETEC. However, in a minority of cases, patients experience the dysentery syndrome, manifested as blood, mucus, and leukocytes in the stool with tenesmus and fever.

Symptoms from EHEC infection can be severe, with as many as 12 bloody stools per day.[22] Initially, EHEC infections typically manifest as cramping abdominal pain, abdominal distension, and watery diarrhea. Nausea occurs in about two-thirds of patients, and vomiting occurs in less than half. The white blood cell count is elevated and accompanied by a left shift, but patients often remain afebrile. Within 1 to 2 days the diarrhea becomes bloody with increased abdominal pain. The illness typically resolves in 1 week; however in approximately 2% to 7% of cases, particularly in children younger than age 5 years and the elderly, the disease is complicated by development of HUS. Death may occur rarely, usually as a result of HUS.[25]

TREATMENT

The cornerstone of management of all diarrheagenic *E. coli* infection is to prevent dehydration by correcting fluid and electrolyte imbalances. ORT is often lifesaving in infants and children.[21] Although antimicrobial prophylaxis is effective in preventing ETEC diarrhea, the growing problem of antibiotic resistance and the possibility of adverse effects from antimicrobial agents deter recommendations of prophylaxis. Instead, recommendations involve avoiding risk factors while traveling. In addition, loperamide and to a lesser extent, bismuth subsalicylate, are effective in decreasing the severity of ETEC diarrhea; empirical antibiotics shorten the duration of the disease. Fluoroquinolones (e.g., ciprofloxacin, norfloxacin, and levofloxacin) are the most commonly recommended agents owing to increasing antimicrobial resistance among other drug classes.[21]

The use of antibiotics remains controversial in EHEC infection.[25] Their use may be harmful because of lysis of bacteria leading to increased release of toxin and alteration of normal intracolonic bacterial flora, thereby increasing the systemic absorption of the toxin. Treatment of EHEC infection is primarily limited to supportive care, which may include dialysis, hemofiltration, transfusion of packed erythrocytes, platelet infusions, and other interventions as indicated clinically.[25] Severe disease may cause chronic kidney failure and require renal transplant.

INFLAMMATORY (DYSENTERY-LIKE) DIARRHEA

Bacillary Dysentery (Shigellosis)

Epidemiology Approximately 450,000 cases of shigellosis occur in the United States and 165 million cases occur in the world annually, resulting in more than 1 million global deaths each year.[26] Shigellosis is primarily a disease of children, with the highest incidence in children between the ages of 6 months and 5 years. Only a third of all cases occur in adults. Most cases result from fecal–oral transmission. A few well-documented food- and water-associated outbreaks have been reported. The peak incidence in the United States is in late summer.

The shigellae have worldwide distribution, with regional differences in prevalence of subgroups responsible for disease. Four species most often associated with disease are *S. dysenteriae* type I, *Shigella flexneri*, *Shigella boydii*, and *Shigella sonnei*.[26] In the United States, the common causes of shigellosis are *S. sonnei* and *S. flexneri*. Cases caused by other shigellae are commonly acquired during travel to developing countries. Because of overuse of antibiotics in human and animal feed, Southeast Asia and India have higher levels of resistance. Poor sanitation, poor personal hygiene, inadequate water supply, malnutrition, and increased population density are associated with an increased risk of *Shigella* gastroenteritis epidemics, even in developed countries.

Pathogenesis The shigellae are gram-negative bacilli belonging to the family Enterobacteriaceae. Ingestion of as few as 10 to 200 viable organisms of the *Shigella* species causes disease in healthy adults, explaining the ease with which the disease is transmitted from person to person.[26] The bacteria multiply and spread within the submucosa of the small bowel, but they rarely extend beyond the mucosa. Penetration of the mucosa is conferred genetically by large "invasion plasmids" and results in distortion of the crypts, death to intestinal epithelium, causing focal ulceration, sloughing of mucosal cells, bloody mucoid exudate into the gut lumen, and submucosal accumulation of inflammatory cells with microabscess formation.[27] Microabscesses eventually may coalesce, forming larger abscesses. Infection frequently involves the entire colon. In addition to the virulence characteristics of invasiveness, *S. dysenteriae* type 1 and, to a lesser degree, *S. flexneri* and *S. sonnei,* produce a cytotoxin, or shiga toxin, the pathogenic role of which is unclear, although it is thought to damage endothelial cells of the lamina propria, resulting in microangiopathic changes that can progress to HUS.[21]

Clinical Presentation Initial signs and symptoms include abdominal pain, cramping, and fever followed by frequent watery stools.[26] Within a few days, patients experience a decrease in fever, severe abdominal pain, and tenderness prior to the development of bloody diarrhea and other signs of dysentery (see Table 122–4). Stools are often greenish in color and contain leukocytes. Fluid and electrolyte losses may be significant, particularly in infants and elderly patients. In the early stages of the disease, stool cultures are positive. A rapid diagnostic test kit that uses DNA amplification by polymerase chain reaction is also available.

If left untreated, bacillary dysentery usually lasts about 1 week (range: 1 to 30 days). Complications are unusual but may include severe dehydration, generalized seizures, septicemia, toxic megacolon, perforated colon, arthritis, protein-losing enteropathy, and HUS. Mortality is rare, but it may be more likely with *S. dysenteriae* type I. Less than 3% of persons who are infected with *S. flexneri* will later develop Reiter syndrome, characterized by pains in the joints, irritation of the eyes, and painful urination. This can lead to chronic arthritis.[28]

TREATMENT

Shigellosis is usually a self-limiting disease. Most patients recover in 4 to 7 days, although 10% may experience a recurrence. ORT is the foundation of treatment (dysentery is not generally associated with significant fluid loss). However, intravenous fluid replacement therapy may be necessary, especially in children and the elderly.

Owing to the self-limiting nature of the illness and rapid development of antimicrobial resistance, antibiotic treatment is reserved for the elderly, those who are immunocompromised, children in daycare centers, malnourished children, and healthcare workers. Antibiotics shorten the period of fecal shedding and attenuate the clinical illness. Due to multidrug resistance, the preferred agents of choice are fluoroquinolones (ciprofloxacin, levofloxacin, or norfloxacin). A single dose is reasonable for mild to moderate illness, but for complicated bacillary dysentery or proven *S. dysenteriae* type 1 infection 5 days of therapy is recommended.[26] In children and pregnant women, azithromycin can be used.[29] Antimotility agents such as loperamide are contraindicated because they can worsen bacillary dysentery and could be involved in the development of toxic dilatation of the colon.

Salmonellosis

Epidemiology *Salmonella enterica* are gram-negative bacilli belonging to the family Enterobacteriaceae. The most prevalent *Salmonella enterica* serotypes are Typhi or Paratyphi, which cause enteric fever. Gastroenteritis (enterocolitis) is caused by *S. enterica* serotypes Typhimurium or Enteritidis. Other clinical manifestations produced by nontyphoidal salmonellosis include bacteremia, and extraintestinal localized infection.

In the United States, the largest burden of *Salmonella* infection is due to nontyphoidal serotypes, causing approximately 1.4 million cases of salmonellosis, 16,000 hospitalizations, and 600 deaths, occurring annually.[30] The incidence of salmonellosis in the United States is decreasing, which is believed to be a result of improved food-handling practices and water treatment. Salmonellosis is a disease primarily of infants, children, and adolescents. Children younger than age 5 years account for approximately 25% of all diagnosed cases. Conditions that may predispose to infection include those which decrease gastric acidity, antibiotic use, malnutrition, and immunodeficiency states. Contaminated food or water has been implicated in the majority of cases. Direct fecal–oral transmission occurs less frequently but is particularly important in children. Foods most often implicated in human salmonellosis are poultry, poultry products, beef, pork, and dairy products.[31] Pets, particularly reptiles, are a common source of infection.

Pathogenesis The incubation period, symptoms, and disease severity depend on the amount of organism ingested. The inoculum necessary for clinical illness is estimated to be 10^6 organisms, and this infectious dose is lowered in patients with achlorhydria (gastric pH >4.0). Once ingested and successfully beyond host defense mechanisms such as low gastric pH and bile salts, organisms can attach and invade the distal ileum and proximal colon. Gastroenteritis often is characterized by massive neutrophil infiltration followed by lymphocytes and macrophages.[31] The serotypes that are responsible for human illness cause intestinal epithelial cells to secrete interleukin 8, a potent neutrophil chemo-tactic factor. Degranulation and release of toxic substances by neutrophils may contribute to inflammation and result in tissue damage, fluid secretion, or leakage across the intestinal mucosa.

Clinical Presentation Most patients experience symptoms within 72 hours of ingestion of contaminated food or water.[31] Patients often complain of nausea and vomiting followed by abdominal cramps, headache, fever, and diarrhea, although the actual presentation is quite variable. Some patients do not have increased stool frequency, whereas others have more than 1 stool per hour. Stools generally are loose and may be mucoid or bloody (dysentery-like) or both. Febrile episodes usually range between 37.7°C and 38.8°C (100°F and 102°F) but may be higher. Some evidence suggests that fever of 40°C (104°F) or higher is associated with shorter bacterial excretion. Diarrhea and fever usually resolve spontaneously within 1 to 5 days but may last 2 weeks.[31]

Stool cultures inevitably yield the causative organism if obtained early (i.e., in patients hospitalized less than 3 days). Recovery of organisms continues to decrease with time such that by 3 to 4 weeks, only 5% to 15% of adult patients are passing *Salmonella*. Infants and children tend to pass bacteria for longer periods than adults (up to 7 weeks). Chronic fecal shedding of *Salmonella* has been associated with chronic biliary infection and cholelithiasis.

Bacteremia is the most common complication of gastroenteritis. This clinical syndrome is most frequent with serovars Choleraesuis and Dublin. In addition, high-risk patients include infants, elderly, and patients with severe underlying illness or immunosuppression, including those with AIDS. The clinical syndrome is characterized by persistent bacteremia and prolonged intermittent fever with chills. Stool cultures frequently are negative. Leukocyte counts are often within the normal range. Vascular complications such as seeding of athrerosclerotic plaques or aneurysms in arterial vessels occur in 10% to 25% of adults with bacteremia.

Localized infections develop in 5% to 10% of patients with bacteremia. Extraluminal infection or abscess formation or both can occur at any site. They may follow any of the other syndromes, or they may be the primary presentation. Metastatic infections may involve bone, cysts, heart, kidney, liver, lungs, pericardium, spleen, and tumors. The clinical presentation usually is determined by the organ systems involved. Polymorphonuclear leukocyte counts often are elevated.

TREATMENT

Gastroenteritis is usually self-limiting, and fluid and electrolyte replacement is the primary mode of treatment. Most patients respond well to ORT.[31] Antimotility drugs should be avoided because they increase the risk of mucosal invasion and complications. Antibiotic therapy is not indicated in otherwise healthy adults. Antibiotics have no effect on the duration of fever or diarrhea, and their frequent use increases the likelihood of resistance and the duration of fecal shedding.[32] Antibiotics should be used in high-risk patients: (a) neonates or infants younger than age 1 year, because young children have an increased risk of complicated infection; (b) persons older than age 50 years; (c) patients with primary or secondary immunodeficiency such as AIDS, or chemotherapy

patients; and (d) patients with vascular abnormalities (valvular heart disease, severe atherosclerosis), or those with prosthetic joints. Susceptibility testing is recommended because many drug-resistant strains of *Salmonella* have emerged.[10] For high-risk patients, ciprofloxacin for 5–7 days is recommended.[32] Depending on susceptibility results, azithromycin, trimethoprim-sulfamethoxazole, and amoxicillin can also be used.[32] In chronic carrier states, the choice of antibiotic should be based upon sensitivity testing of the colonizing isolate. The chronic carriage state has been reduced with long-term use of ciprofloxacin, trimethoprim-sulfamethoxazole, or amoxicillin.

Increased resistance concerns dictate that empiric therapy for life-threatening bacteremia or focal infections following nontyphoidal *Salmonella* infection should include a combination of a third-generation cephalosporin (such as ceftriaxone 2 g IV daily) and a fluoroquinolone (ciprofloxacin 500 mg orally twice daily) until the susceptibilities are known.[33] The duration of antibiotic therapy is dictated by the site of infection. Bacteremia without endovascular infection should be treated for 7 to 14 days. In documented or suspected endovascular infection, 6 weeks of intravenous therapy with ampicillin or ceftriaxone is recommended. Chloramphenicol is no longer recommended in patients with endovascular infection because of high failure rates.

Campylobacteriosis

Epidemiology The *Campylobacter* species are flagellated, curved, gram-negative rods that are thought to be one of the most common bacterial causes of diarrheal illnesses worldwide. Although there are 14 different species, *C. jejuni* is the species responsible for more than 99% of *Campylobacter*-associated gastroenteritis. In the United States, the incidence of *Campylobacter* infection decreased 26% from 1996 to 1999.[34] However, surveillance studies indicate that *Campylobacter* species remain the most commonly isolated enteric pathogen, detected two to seven times more frequently than *Salmonella* or *Shigella*. The CDC estimates that 2.4 million persons are affected each year in the United States, involving almost 1% of the entire population.

In developed countries, the peak incidence of *Campylobacter* infections occurs in children younger than age1 year and in young adults ages 15 to 44 years. The incidence is also higher in males than in females, although the reason for this is unknown. Patients with AIDS are particularly susceptible; the incidence in AIDS patients is 40 times that of the general population.[34] Most reported cases occur during the summer months, beginning in May and peaking in August. In tropical developing countries, *Campylobacter* infections are common among children younger than age 2 years, and asymptomatic infections of children and adults are more common than those seen in industrialized nations. This decrease in the case-to-infection ratio suggests that previous exposure confers immunity to the infecting strain.

The transmission of infection occurs primarily by ingestion of contaminated food or water. Although *Campylobacter* species have varied reservoirs, such as livestock, dogs, cats, and birds, the consumption of chicken is the major vector of infections in industrialized nations. Poultry products are nearly always contaminated with *Campylobacter* species during the slaughtering process, and it is estimated that 1 drop of chicken juice may contain 500 infectious organisms.[35] Although public education emphasizes safe handling and cooking of chicken, it is easy to see how simple errors may result in human illness.

Pathogenesis *Campylobacter* species are labile in acidic environments, much like *Salmonella*. Therefore, an inoculum of approximately 800 organisms is required to initiate infection. Conditions in the upper small intestine are favorable for multiplication.

Flagella-mediated adherence and tissue invasion by bacteria have been demonstrated in the jejunum, ileum, and colon. Infection results in an acute inflammatory enteritis. *C. jejuni* can produce an enterotoxin or cytotoxin.[36] Both cytotoxins and enterotoxins may be produced in many strains. Symptom manifestation depends on immunity. Patients infected with *Campylobacter* develop specific immunoglobulin (Ig) G, IgM, and IgA antibodies in serum and IgA antibodies in intestinal secretions. Volunteer studies indicate that immunity does protect against illness.

Clinical Presentation The average incubation period of *Campylobacter* is 2 to 4 days.[34] The most common presenting symptoms include diarrhea, abdominal pain, and fever. Nausea, vomiting, headache, myalgia, and malaise also may occur. Bowel movements may be numerous, bloody (dysentery-like), and foul smelling, and range from loose to watery. Cramping and abdominal pain usually are relieved by defecation. In 75% of cases, leukocytes and red blood cells are detected in the stool samples. Peripheral leukocytosis also may be present. The disease usually is self-limited to about 1 week, but it may persist for several weeks in 10% to 20% of patients. The case-fatality rate is 0.05 per 1,000 infections.

Complications, including pseudoappendicitis, pancreatitis, gastrointestinal hemorrhage, thrombophlebitis, abscess, septicemia, peritonitis, empyema, urinary tract infection, and cholecystitis, are uncommon, but occur more frequently in those who are immunocompromised. *C. jejuni* has been associated with Guillain-Barré syndrome (GBS), but the relationship is not well understood.[34] *C. jejuni* infections are a common trigger of GBS, accounting for approximately 30% of GBS cases, but the risk of developing GBS after *C. jejuni* infection appears to be low (<1 case of GBS per 1,000 *C. jejuni* infections). A reactive arthritis may develop several weeks after infection in persons with the HLA-B27 histocompatibility antigens.[28] Diagnosis is made by stool culture, but the bacteria sometimes are identifiable with Gram's stain or carbol-fuchsin stain.

TREATMENT

The primary treatment of campylobacteriosis is oral fluid and electrolyte replacement.[34] Most people recover from this self-limiting disease in 4 to 7 days. Antibiotics are not useful unless started within 4 days of the start of the illness because they do not shorten the duration or severity of diarrhea but only shorten the duration of bacterial excretion. However, antibiotics are warranted in patients with high fevers, severe bloody diarrhea, prolonged illnesses (>1 week), pregnancy, and immunocompromised states, including HIV infection (see Table 122–4).

C. jejuni is susceptible to a wide variety of antimicrobial agents. Fluoroquinolone resistance has increased, and is now 10% to 13% in the United States (41% to 88% in Europe and Asia). Resistance may be the result of the use of fluoroquinolone antibiotics in poultry feed, and the frequent use of these agents internationally in treating enteric infections. Erythromycin is considered the drug of choice due to its low cost, high efficacy, safety profile, and ease of administration. Macrolides such as clarithromycin and azithromycin are equally effective. Tetracycline, chloramphenicol, clindamycin, and aminoglycosides may be effective. Antimotility agents such as loperamide are contraindicated because slowing fecal transit time may extend the duration of infection and increase toxin mucosal invasion.

Yersiniosis

Yersinia species are non-lactose-fermenting gram-negative coccobacilli that are widely distributed in nature. The genus *Yersinia* includes six species known to cause disease in humans. *Y. enterocolitica* and, to a lesser extent, *Yersinia pseudotuberculosis,* are most likely associated with intestinal infection, but overall both are a relatively infrequent cause of diarrhea and abdominal pain. More than 50 serotypes of *Y. enterocolitica* exist; of these, serotypes 0:3, 0:8, and 0:9 are associated most frequently with enterocolitis.[37] Infections are reported commonly from northern Europe, and the peak incidence occurs during the winter months.

Children are the most likely to experience illness with *Y. enterocolitica* infection.[38] Transmission of infection occurs frequently by ingestion of contaminated food or water. The organisms have been isolated from a variety of food sources, including pigs, raw goat milk, and cow milk. Refrigeration does not deter the development of adherence and invasive virulence factors.

Y. enterocolitica invade the intestinal epithelium and penetrate the intestinal mucosa.[39] An inoculum of 10^9 organisms may be required for infection. Most strains produce an enterotoxin, but the role of toxin production in causing diarrhea is not well established. However, this infection causes mucosal ulcerations in the terminal ileum, necrotic lesions in Peyer patches, and enlargement of mesenteric lymph nodes.

Clinical Presentation These bacteria cause a wide spectrum of clinical syndromes.[38] Most patients with *Y. enterocolitica* infection present with enterocolitis that is mild and self-limiting. Symptoms include vomiting, abdominal pain, diarrhea, and fever; up to 60% of patients will have blood-streaked stools. Diarrhea resolves after 1 to 3 weeks, but bacteria excretion may continue for up to 3 months after diarrhea subsides. Most patients with this type of infection are younger than age 5 years. In older children and adolescents, mesenteric adenitis and/or terminal ileitis with fever, right lower quadrant pain, and leukocytosis are common. Mesenteric adenitis, which is difficult to distinguish from acute appendicitis, is also seen in patients infected with *Y. pseudotuberculosis.*

Approximately 10% to 30% of adult patients develop a reactive arthritis 1 to 2 weeks after recovery from enteritis. This arthritis, involving the knees, ankles, toes, fingers, and wrists, usually resolves in 1 to 4 months but may persist in approximately 10% of patients.[28] This complication is more common in persons with the HLA-B27 antigen. Other postinfection complications include erythema nodosum, exudative pharyngitis, pneumonia, empyema, and lung abscess. Although rare, *Y. enterocolitica* bacteremia has been reported in patients with diabetes mellitus, severe anemia, hemochromatosis, cirrhosis, and malignancy. Other groups at risk include the elderly and those who received frequent red blood cell transfusions (iron overload).[40] These patients are at increased risk for hepatic or splenic abscesses, peritonitis, septic arthritis, osteomyelitis, wound infections, meningitis, and endocarditis.

TREATMENT

Oral fluid and electrolyte replacement is an important initial approach. Owing to the self-limiting nature of the illness, antibiotics may not alter the time to resolution of the diarrhea or the rate of bacteriologic cure. Antibiotics should be used in high risk patients who develop bacteremia (i.e., infants younger than age 3 months and patients with cirrhosis or iron overload) or in patients with bone and joint infections.[38] The drugs of choice remains unclear. Fluoroquinolones alone or in combination with third-generation cephalosporins or aminoglycosides may be effective for *Yersinia* bacteremia or for those with bone and joint infections.[38] Other antibiotics effective in vitro are chloramphenicol, tetracyclines, and trimethoprim-sulfamethoxazole. Agents frequently resistant to *Yersinia* are penicillin G, ampicillin, and first-generation cephalosporins.

CLOSTRIDIUM DIFFICILE

Epidemiology

C. difficile is the most commonly known cause of infectious diarrhea in hospitalized patients in North America and Europe. *C. difficile* infection (CDI) is associated with use of broad-spectrum antimicrobials, including clindamycin, ampicillin, cephalosporins, and fluoroquinolones. Other agents that have been implicated, albeit at a lower incidence rate, include aminoglycosides, erythromycin, trimethoprim-sulfamethoxazole, vancomycin, and metronidazole. Although in most cases CDI occurs during or shortly after the completion of antimicrobial therapy, disease onset can be delayed for 2 or 3 months.[41] CDI occurs most often in high-risk groups, such as the elderly, debilitated patients, cancer patients, surgical patients, patients receiving antibiotics, patients with nasogastric tubes, and patients who frequently use laxatives.

Unfortunately, the incidence and severity of disease have increased dramatically since 2000. These changes are assumed to be due to the emergence of a single-strain type (North American pulsed-field type [NAP-1]) in outbreaks.[42] NAP-1 strain is highly resistant to fluororquinolones and carries deletion mutations in a regulatory gene (tcdC) believed to inhibit toxin production, causing higher levels of toxin production responsible for more serious diseases. The NAP-1 strain is also refractory to standard therapy.

Pathogenesis

C. difficile is a gram-positive spore-forming anaerobic bacillus and causes a toxin-mediated disease. Once antibiotics disrupt normal colonic flora and colonization of *C. difficile* occurs, two toxins (A and B) are released to mediate diarrhea and colitis. This toxin production is essential in disease manifestation. Toxin A is the major pathogenic factor and has been characterized as an enterotoxin that causes intestinal fluid secretion, mucosal injury, and inflammation through actin disaggregation, intracellular calcium release, and damage to neurons. Toxin B is a nonenterotoxic cytotoxin that causes depolymerization of filamentous actin and mediates more potent damage to human colonic mucosa than toxin A. Initially, raised white and yellowish plaques form, and the surrounding mucosa may be inflamed. With progression of disease, these pseudomembranous plaques become enlarged and scatted over the colorectal mucosa.[41]

Clinical Presentation

Clinical diagnosis is based on the onset of diarrhea during or after antimicrobial use and often is associated with abdominal discomfort, fever, and polymorphonuclear leukocytosis. A spectrum of disease ranges from mild diarrhea to life-threatening toxic megacolon and pseudomembranous entercolitis.[41] In colitis without pseudomembrane formation, patients present with malaise, abdominal pain, nausea, anorexia, watery diarrhea, low-grade fever, and leukocytosis. Fulminant disease is characterized by severe abdominal pain, perfuse diarrhea, high fever, marked leukocytosis, and classic pseudomembrane formation evident with sigmoidoscopic examination.

CDI should be suspected in patients experiencing diarrhea with a recent history of antibiotic use (within the previous 3 months) or in those whose diarrhea began 72 hours after hospitalization. Diagnosis can be established by detection of toxin A or B, stool culture for *C. difficile,* or endoscopy. If the stool sample is negative, a second analysis is recommended because the testing sensitivity may be increased with repeat testing. Endoscopy should be reserved for situations where rapid diagnosis is needed, ileus is present, stool is not available, or other colonic diseases are in the differential diagnosis.

TREATMENT

Initial therapy should include discontinuation of the offending agent.[41] Fluid and electrolyte replacement therapy is necessary. Although diarrhea will resolve in up to 25% of patients within 48 hours of discontinuing the offending agent without therapy, most patients require antibiotics. Both vancomycin and metronidazole are similar in time to resolution of diarrhea, incidence of side effects, and relapse rates. Metronidazole is the drug of choice for mild to moderate CDI because its oral formation is less expensive and there are concerns for vancomycin resistant-enterococci with oral vancomycin use. In patients with severe disease, contraindication or intolerance to metronidazole, and inadequate response to metronidazole, oral vancomycin is recommended. Vancomycin must be administered orally because intravenous vancomycin does not achieve gut lumen concentrations high enough for effective bacterial elimination. In patients with an ileus (where oral vancomycin reaching site of infection is questioned) vancomycin may be delivered by retention enema or add intravenous metronidazole.

Relapse after metronidazole or vancomycin therapy occurs in approximately 20% of patients and increases in frequency with subsequent recurrences. Patients with 1 prior episode of relapse have a greater than 40% risk of additional recurrences, whereas those with 2 or more previous episodes have a greater than 60% risk.[43] Relapse typically develops in 1 to 2 weeks after stopping metronidazole or vancomycin but can be delayed for up to 12 weeks. Risk factors for recurrent CDI include a history of recurrence, advancing age, use of additional antimicrobials, and an inadequate protective immune response to *C. difficile* toxins. Management of the first relapse is identical to a primary episode because relapse is rarely due to resistance to metronidaole or to vancomycin. Instead, relapse occurs because treatment fails to eradicate the spore forms of pathogen or treatment makes patients vulnerable to another infection by impairing normal flora.

The optimal management of patients with multiple relapses is not clear. The most effective regimen is a prolonged tapered pulse-dosing of oral vancomycin and should be considered for second relapse.[43,44] Alternative regimens that have shown efficacy include drugs in rifamycin class: vancomycin + rifampin[45] or vancomycin followed by rifaximin.[46] Concern with these regimens includes drug interactions with rifampin and development of resistance, especially if either rifampin or rifaximin is used as monotherapy. Nitazoxanide is another alternative agent in patients with relapse following metronidazole therapy.[47] There are two other modalities that have been shown to have efficacy against CDI: IVIG and fecal transplantation. Individuals with low concentration of circulating IgG antitoxin are susceptible to more severe disease and frequent relapses. In those with multiple relapses due to impaired antigenic response to toxins, IVIG 400 mg/kg may be a worthwhile intervention.[48] It is, however, expensive and its efficacy is reported in case series and anecdotal reports. Fecal transplantation uses a small amount of fresh feces from a healthy donor, suspended in saline, filtered and administered through a nasogastric tube or by retention enema.[49] Although it was efficacious in a case series, it is a difficult option to offer to patients.

Agents that have lost favor due to poor efficacy or resistance include bacitracin, cholestyramine, colestipol, and fusidic acid. Probiotics using *Saccharomycin boulardii* or *Lactobacilli* species to augment colonization resistance and prevent recurrent CDI have been studied but data are too limited for recommendation.[50] Their use in conjunction with antibiotics for the treatment of relapses and their risk of bacteremia and fungemia, especially in immunocompromised hosts, require further study. Agents that are in clinical trials include Ramoplanin (a new lipoglycodepsipeptide), difimicin (an 18-membered macrocyclic antibiotic) and tolevamer (a large anionic polymer that binds *C. difficile* toxins A and B). Tolevamer is inferior to metronidazole and vancomycin in the treatment of the first episode of CDI but the relapse rate was lower.[51] An active vaccine has been studied in 1 small case series.

Drugs that inhibit peristalsis, such as diphenoxylate, are contraindicated in CDI.[41] Slowing of fecal transit time is thought to result in extended toxin-associated damage. Strict hand washing and contact precautions are imperative measures in preventing the spread of the organism. *C. difficile* can be cultured in rooms of infected individuals up to 40 days after discharge.

CLINICAL CONTROVERSY

Some investigators have found prophylaxis with competing, nonpathogenic organisms such as *Lactobacillus* spp. or *Saccharomyces* spp. to be helpful in preventing relapses in small numbers of patients with *C. difficile* infection. It is thought that these organisms help to restore the natural flora in the gut and make patients more resistant to colonization by *C. difficile* when used in conjunction with appropriate antibiotics.

ACUTE VIRAL GASTROENTERITIS

Acute viral gastroenteritis was unknown until the 1970s. Viruses are now recognized as the leading cause of diarrhea in the world, although in many cases an exact pathogen cannot be determined. In Asia, Africa, and Latin America, viral gastroenteritis accounts for an estimated 3 to 5 billion cases and is associated with 5 to 10 million deaths.[52] Viruses that cause gastroenteritis include rotavirus, norovirus (belonging to calicivirus), enteric adenovirus, and astrovirus. Other viruses, such as toroviruses, coronaviruses, picobirnaviruses, and pestiviruses, are being identified increasingly as causative agents of diarrhea. Characteristics of common viral pathogens causing gastroenteritis are outlined in Table 122–5.

ROTAVIRUSES

Epidemiology

Rotavirus is the most common cause of diarrhea in infants and children worldwide, and 1 million people die annually from the infection. In the United States, approximately 3.5 million cases of diarrhea, 500,000 physician visits, 50,000 hospitalizations, and 20 deaths occur each year in children younger than age 5 years.[52] Serologic surveys show that nearly all children are infected by age 5 years, but dehydrating diarrhea occurs primarily among young children ages 3 to 35 months during their initial infection.[53] Thereafter, young children are shielded from the severity of subsequent infection. In fact, after the initial infection with rotavirus, 40% of children are protected against subsequent infection, 75% are protected against subsequent gastroenteritis, and up to 88% are protected against severe gastroenteritis. Unfortunately, both immunocompromised children and adults are at increased risk for severe, prolonged, and even fatal rotavirus gastroenteritis.

Pathogenesis

Rotaviruses are double-stranded, wheel-shaped, RNA viruses. The outermost layer contains two structural viral proteins. The protease-cleaved protein (P protein) VP4 and the glycoprotein (G protein) VP7 define the serotype of the virus and are the basis for vaccine development. Once ingested, these strains cause diarrhea by inducing changes in transepithelial fluid balance, malabsorption as a consequence of destruction of epithelial lining of intestine, and vascular damage and ischemia of villi. Changes to the villi include shortening of villus height, crypt hyperplasia, and mononuclear cell infiltration of the lamina propria.[53]

Clinical Presentation

The incubation period of rotavirus infection is typically 1 to 3 days. Clinical manifestations vary from asymptomatic (which is common in adults) to severe nausea, vomiting, and diarrhea with dehydration. Because the first infection tends to be the most severe, dehydration and electrolyte disturbances occur more frequently in children. The symptoms begin abruptly, with vomiting often preceding the onset of diarrhea. Fever is present in a third of patients. Other signs and symptoms include respiratory symptoms, irritability, lethargy, pharyngeal erythema, rhinitis, red tympanic membranes, and palpable cervical lymph nodes. These gastrointestinal symptoms resolve in 3 to 7 days.[53]

Laboratory findings reflect the degree of vomiting, diarrhea, or both. Transient rises in liver enzymes may be seen in 60% of children hospitalized for rotavirus diarrhea. The white blood cell count is usually normal. Stools rarely contain blood or leukocytes. Rotavirus detection in stool samples is possible with an enzyme

TABLE 122-5	Characteristics of Agents Responsible for Acute Viral Gastroenteritis and Diarrhea				
Virus	**Peak Age of Onset**	**Time of Year**	**Duration**	**Mode of Transmission**	**Symptoms**
Rotavirus	6 months–2 years	October to April	3–8 days	Fecal–oral, water, food	Vomiting, diarrhea, fever, abdominal pain, lactose intolerance
Norovirus	3 months–6 years	Peak in winter	4 days	Fecal–oral, water, shellfish	Vomiting, diarrhea
Astrovirus	<7 years	Winter	1–4 days	Fecal–oral, water, shellfish	Diarrhea, headache, malaise, nausea,
Enteric adenovirus	<2 years	Year-round	7–9 days	Fecal–oral	Diarrhea, respiratory symptoms, vomiting, fever
Pestivirus	<2 years	NR	3 days	NR	Mild
Coronavirus-like particles	<2 years	Fall and early winter	7 days	NR	Respiratory disease
Enterovirus	NR	NR	NR	NR	Mild diarrhea, secondary organ damage
Norwalk	>5 y	Variable	12–24 hours	Fecal–oral, food, aerosol	Nausea, vomiting, diarrhea, abdominal cramps, headache, fever, chills, myalgia

NR, not reported.

immunoassay and a latex agglutination assay, both of which are available commercially.

TREATMENT

Oral fluid and electrolyte replacement is the cornerstone of treatment.[53] Probiotic therapy with *Lactobacillus* may reduce the duration of diarrhea and of viral excretion. There is no role for antibiotics in acute infection. Bismuth subsalicylate, although shown to decrease the duration of diarrhea and stool output, is not recommended for routine use because of the self-limiting nature of the disease and the risk of bismuth subsalicylate overdose. Antimotility agents are not recommended because they do not decrease the duration or volume of diarrhea.

The first vaccine (RotaShield) to prevent rotavirus infection was licensed for use in the United States in 1998, but it was withdrawn after 1 year because of an increased rate of idiopathic intussusception. Post-licensure surveillance found that the risk for intussusception was the highest within 3 to 14 days after receipt of the first dose, which was estimated to be 1 case per 10,000 vaccine recipients.[54] There was also a suggestion that the risk was age-dependent, and possibly infants younger than 3 months were in less danger than older ones.

There are currently 2 vaccines that are licensed for use in the United States.[14] RotaTeq is a live, oral vaccine that contains five human/bovine reassortant rotaviruses. Because these viral strains are derived by inserting the gene encoding capsid protein from G1, G2, G3, or G4 human rotavirus strain into a bovine rotavirus backbone, they contain segmented genome from different parents and are referred to as *reassortant rotaviruses*. Four reassortant rotaviruses express one of the outer capsid proteins, G types (G1 to G4), and the fifth expresses the attachment protein, P1A. Therefore, this vaccine provides protection against the serotypes G1, G2, G3, and G4 when administered. In clinical trials, the vaccine offered 74% efficacy against gastroenteritis of any severity and 98% efficacy against severe disease.[55] This oral vaccine decreased office visits by 86%, emergency department visits by 94%, and hospitalizations by 96%. Moreover, the vaccinated children showed similar cases of intussusception as nonvaccinated children (six cases versus five cases; adjusted relative risk of 1.6; confidence interval [CI] = 0.4 to 6.4). Other serious side effects, including deaths, were similar among vaccine and placebo recipients. There were small but significantly greater rates of vomiting, diarrhea, nasopharyngitis, otitis media, and bronchospasm among vaccine recipients. Three doses at age 2, 4, and 6 months are recommended.[14]

Another rotavirus vaccine, RotaRix, is a live-attenuated human rotavirus vaccine prepared from a single human strain of P1A G1. A trial of this vaccine has shown a clinical efficacy of 79% against gastroenteritis of any severity and 96% efficacy against severe rotavirus disease. Rotarix reduced hospitalizations by 100%, medically attended visits by 92% in the first rotavirus season, and reduced hospitalizations by 96% through 2 seasons. There were no increases in intussusception among vaccine recipients.[56] Two doses, administered at 2 and 4 months are recommended.[14]

CALICIVIRUSES

The human caliciviruses are assigned to two genera, Norovirus and Sapovirus, responsible for gastroenteritis. The Norovirus causes illness in all age groups, whereas Sapovirus causes illness mainly in children. Although the relative importance of these viruses as causes of GI infections is unknown, Noroviruses are important

causes of outbreaks.[57] The Norwalk virus was the first norovirus to be described in 1972 in Norwalk, Ohio.

As with most viruses, the epidemiology of the norovirus is not well understood. The disease commonly affects children and adults, but it is not often associated with disease in neonates and preschool children.[57] Outbreaks occur throughout the year and have been documented in families, healthcare systems, cruise ships, and college dormitories.

The pathophysiology of this disease is similar to that caused by the rotavirus. Human volunteer studies show histopathologic changes in the jejunum within 24 hours of viral challenge, and clinical manifestations appear within 48 hours.[57] The exact mechanisms of virus-induced vomiting or diarrhea are unknown. Brush-border enzyme activity may be decreased, resulting in lactose intolerance, but it generally returns to preinfection levels within 2 weeks. Virus shedding in the stool can occur over the first 24 to 48 hours after illness.

Gastroenteritis caused by norovirus is characterized by sudden onset of abdominal cramps with nausea, vomiting, or both. Adults frequently experience non-bloody diarrhea; children experience vomiting more often than diarrhea. Other complaints are myalgia, headache, and malaise, which are accompanied by fever in approximately 50% of patients. Signs and symptoms generally last 12 to 48 hours.

The disease is generally self-limiting. Oral fluid and electrolyte replacement should be used, if necessary. A norovirus vaccine produced via expression of viral antigens in a baculovirus or transgenic plants is under investigation.[58]

OTHER POTENTIAL VIRAL PATHOGENS

Astroviruses increasingly are being recognized as important causes of gastroenteritis. Astroviral illness is often reported in children younger than age 3 years, but it has also been described in adults and the elderly.[59] Astroviruses have been detected in the stools of children, as well as in patients with immunodeficiency conditions such as HIV infection or bone marrow transplantation. Outbreaks have been reported in schools, daycare settings, and pediatric wards. The pathogenesis of astroviral infection is believed to be similar to that noted for rotavirus. The clinical presentation consists of diarrhea, headache, malaise, nausea, and to lesser extent, vomiting. These symptoms appear to be similar to those observed with rotavirus but milder. Maintenance of adequate hydration and electrolyte balance is the only therapeutic issue. The duration of viral shedding may be as long as 35 days.

Adenovirus is an icosahedral virus previously associated with respiratory, ocular, and genitourinary infections; however, serotypes 40 and 41 are GI pathogens. Low-grade fever and respiratory symptoms are also common. The diagnosis can be made by enzyme immunoassay that identifies serotypes.

Although less commonly associated with severe GI disease, pestivirus, torovirus, and coronavirus-like particles have been recovered from diarrheal stools. In HIV-infected patients, the presence of diarrhea is associated with virus in 35% of stool specimens.[60] Astrovirus, picobirnavirus, calicivirus, and adenovirus appear to be the most commonly isolated viral pathogens. Table 122–5 presents specific characteristics of these agents.

TRAVELER'S DIARRHEA

Traveler's diarrhea describes the clinical syndrome manifested by malaise, anorexia, and abdominal cramps followed by the sudden onset of diarrhea that incapacitates many travelers. Traveler's diarrhea interferes with planned activities or work in 30% of those affected.[61] In particular, an increased risk lies with North Americans and northern Europeans traveling to Latin America, southern Europe, Africa, and Asia. The highest risk is observed with patients with immuno-compromised conditions, achlorhydria, inflammatory bowel disease, and people with chronic debilitating medical conditions. Overall, an estimated 20% to 50% of people traveling to high-risk areas will develop the illness.

⑤ The onset of symptoms usually occurs during the first week of travel but can occur anytime during the visit or after returning home. Traveler's diarrhea is caused by contaminated food or water. The most common pathogens are bacterial in nature and include ETEC (20% to 72%), *Shigella* (3% to 25%), *Campylobacter* (3% to 17%), and *Salmonella* (3% to 7%).[61] Viruses (0% to 30%) are also potential causes, as are parasites, although they are rare during short-term travels, accounting for less than 5% of cases. The severity of the syndrome is determined by the number of stools per day and the presence or absence of cramping, nausea, and vomiting. Mild diarrhea is defined as 1 to 3 loose stools per day that are associated with abdominal cramps lasting less than 14 days. Moderate diarrhea indicates more than 4 loose stools daily associated with dehydration, and severe diarrhea is defined as presence of fever or blood in stools. Traveler's diarrhea is rarely life-threatening and in most cases, symptoms resolve in several days without treatment. Travelers to high-risk areas should pack a kit that includes a thermometer, loperamide, 3 days of antibiotics (see Prevention below), oral rehydration solution salts, and a water purification method.[61]

PREVENTION

⑥ Patient education in avoiding high-risk food and beverages should be the best method for minimizing the risk. High-risk foods and beverages include raw or undercooked meat and seafood, moist foods served at room temperature, fruits that cannot be peeled, vegetables, milk from a questionable source, hot sauces on the table, tap water, unsealed bottled water, iced drinks, and food from a street vendor. Slogans such as "Peel it, boil it, cook it, or forget it" remind travelers to avoid contaminated food and to use water purification or reliable bottled beverages. Unfortunately, a recent meta-analysis concluded that the incidence of diarrhea was similar in travelers who followed the old adage and those that engaged in riskier eating habits.[62] A potential reason for a lack of difference may be due to the fact that cooking foods does not always kill pathogens and food should not be considered safe unless it is cooked until steaming hot. Nonetheless, advisement of avoidance measures regarding safe foods, beverages, and eating establishments is recommended to heighten awareness.

Bismuth subsalicylate 524 mg (2 tablets, tablespoonfuls) orally four times daily for up to 3 weeks is a commonly recommended prophylactic regimen.[63] Bismuth subsalicylate may inhibit enterotoxin activity and prevent diarrhea. Persons taking this regimen should be informed of adverse events, including temporary black discoloration of tongue and stools, and, rarely, tinnitus.

Although efficacy of prophylactic antibiotics have been documented, their uses are not recommended for most travelers owing to potential side effects of antibiotics (e.g., photosensitivity), predisposition to other infections such as CDI or vaginal candidiasis, the increased risk of selection of drug-resistant organisms, cost, lack of data on the safety and efficacy of antibiotics given for more than 2 or 3 weeks, and availability of rapidly effective antibiotics for treatment. Prophylactic antibiotics (see Table 122–4) are recommended only in high-risk individuals or in situations in which short-term illness could ruin the purpose of the trip, such as a military mission.[64] A fluoroquinolone is a drug of choice when traveling to most areas of the world.[61,64] Due to fluoroquinolone-resistance among

Campylobacter spp., azithromycin can be considered when traveling to South Asia and Southeast Asia.

A nonabsorbed oral rifamycin, rifaximin, has activity against enteric pathogens and may have a role in prevention of traveler's diarrhea in select populations. A randomized, double-blind trial of rifaximin 200 mg once, twice, or three times daily with meals for 2 weeks resulted in equal protection of 72% with each of the three dosing regimens compared to placebo.[65] Since rifaximin is effective against traveler's diarrhea due to noninvasive strains of *E. coli*, this agent should be reserved for travel regions where *E. coli* predominates, such as Latin America and Africa. Rifaximin has a tolerability and safety profile comparable to that of placebo. The concern with this class of agents is emergence of resistance when used as monotherapy.

TREATMENT

Traveler's Diarrhea

The goals of treatment are to avoid dehydration, reduce the severity and duration of symptoms, and prevent interruption to planned activities. Fluid and electrolyte replacement should be initiated at the onset of diarrhea. ORT is generally not required in otherwise healthy individuals; flavored mineral water ad libitum offers a good source of sodium and glucose.[64] In infants and young children, elderly, and those with chronic debilitating medical conditions, ORT is recommended. For symptom relief, loperamide (preferred because of its quicker onset and longer duration of relief relative to bismuth) may be taken (4 mg orally initially and then 2 mg with each subsequent loose stool to a maximum of 16 mg/day in patients without bloody diarrhea and discontinued if symptoms persist for more than 48 hours). Other symptomatic therapy in mild diarrhea includes bismuth subsalicylate 525 mg every 30 minutes up to 8 doses. There is insufficient evidence to warrant the recommendation of probiotics.

Since behavioral modification has limited efficacy and chemoprophylaxis is not recommended in most travelers, the current recommendation relies on self treatment. Most trials indicate that a single dose or up to three days will improve the condition within 24 to 36 hours, shortening the duration of diarrhea by 1–2 days.[66,67] A single dose of fluoroquinolone is recommended initially and if diarrhea is improved within 12–24 hours, antibiotic should be discontinued. Otherwise, it can be continued for up to three days. A fluoroquinolone is recommended when traveling to most areas of the world. When fluoroquinolone-resistant *Campylobacter* is common, such as in south Asia and Southeast Asia, azithromycin can be used.[68] Azithromycin can also be used in pregnant women and children younger than age 16 years. Empiric treatment of young children should be cautioned.

Rifaximin was as effective as a 3-day course of ciprofloxacin in shortening the duration of diarrhea in noninvasive traveler's diarrhea.[69] However, rifaximin was not as effective in patients with fever and bloody diarrhea and in those with invasive pathogens. Therefore, a 3-day course of rifaximin has been approved for the treatment of traveler's diarrhea caused by noninvasive strains of *E. coli* in people ≥ 12 years of age and can be considered when traveling to areas where E. coli-associated traveler's diarrhea is common, such as Mexico and Jamaica.

For rapid improvement in symptoms, antibiotic therapy with adjustive treatment with loperamide has shown benefit.[70] All clinical trials concluded that the combination therapy was safe and worsening of disease with the use of antimotility treatment has not been encountered.

CLINICAL CONTROVERSY

Most trials have shown that a short course of antibiotic therapy reduces the duration of traveler's diarrhea by 1–2 days with mild side effects. Some clinicians advocate a self-treatment with antibiotics for moderate to severe traveler's diarrhea, while others urge a more cautious approach. The final decision on self-treatment should rely on discussions with individual travelers, taking into consideration their ability and willingness to adhere to prevention strategies and to tolerate diarrheal illness during the trip.

FOOD POISONING

❼ Food poisoning results from the ingestion of food containing pathogenic microorganisms, preformed toxins that were produced by microorganisms, or other toxic compounds. In the United States, food-borne disease causes approximately 76 million illnesses, 325,000 hospitalizations, and 5,200 deaths each year.[3] Food-borne transmission may account for up to 35% of acute gastroenteritis cases caused by unknown agents. A number of bacteria can cause food poisoning (Table 122–6). Common bacterial (*Campylobacter, Salmonella, Shigella, E. coli, Yersinia, Vibrio*) and viral (Norovirus) causes of GI infections were discussed in the preceding sections. Other common food-borne pathogens that cause gastroenteritis include *S. aureus, Bacillus cereus, C. perfringens,* and *Clostridium botulinum.* Unfortunately, sporadic illnesses caused by these agents are not reportable through passive or active systems, and thus it is difficult to determine their disease burden.

Because food-borne disease can appear as sporadic cases or outbreaks, the diagnosis should be suspected whenever two or more people present with acute gastrointestinal or neurologic manifestations after sharing a meal within the previous 72 hours. Important clues about etiologic agents can be gathered from demographic information (age, gender, etc.), the clinical syndrome, incubation period, medical history, type of foods consumed, seasonality, and geographic location of the outbreak.

Staphylococcal food poisoning results from the ingestion of food contaminated by an enterotoxin produced by certain strains of *S. aureus* growing within the food.[71] Enterotoxin production generally results from leaving foods at room temperature, allowing the staphylococci to grow. Symptoms are rapid in onset, generally occurring within 1 to 6 hours of ingestion of preformed toxin-containing foods. The condition is characterized by nausea and vomiting (75%), although abdominal cramps and diarrhea also may be present. Symptoms resolve in less than 12 hours. ORT should be provided in severe cases, but antibiotics are not indicated.

B. cereus causes two different types of clinical syndromes.[72] The first one is characterized by a short incubation period with vomiting, abdominal cramps, and to a lesser extent, diarrhea, within 1 to 6 hours of ingestion of contaminated food. This syndrome is caused by a preformed heat-stable toxin. Similar to staphylococcal food poisoning, illnesses caused by *B. cereus* usually last less than 12 hours. The second syndrome has a longer incubation period (8 to 16 hours) and is caused by toxins produced in vivo after the ingestion of contaminated food. In this syndrome, patients experience diarrhea, abdominal cramps, and less frequently, vomiting. The heat-labile enterotoxin produced in this syndrome activates intestinal adenylate cyclase and causes intestinal fluid secretion. This illness usually resolves within 24 hours, but symptom durations of several days to weeks also have been observed.

Food-borne *C. perfringens* infection may present as two distinct syndromes.[73] Type A organisms are seen in Western nations and result in a 24-hour illness characterized by watery diarrhea and epigastric pain. Symptoms generally resolve within 24 hours. This enterotoxin-related syndrome damages the brush borders of

TABLE 122–6	Food Poisonings					
Organism	Time to Symptoms (Hours)	Principal Foods	Peak Incidence (U.S.)	Principal Mechanism of Pathophysiology	Duration	Treatment
Staphylococcus aureus	1–6	Salad, pastries, ham, poultry	Summer	Preformed toxins A–E (heat stable)	12 hours	Supportive
Bacillus cereus	1–6	Meats, vegetables, fried rice	None	Preformed toxin	12 hours	Supportive
	8–16			Toxin production (in vivo)	24 hours	Supportive
Clostridium perfringens (type A)	6–24	Meats, poultry	Fall, winter, spring	Toxin production (in vivo)	24 hours	Supportive
Vibrio parahaemolyticus	16–72	Shellfish	Spring, summer, fall	Toxin production and tissue invasion	2–7 days	Supportive
Salmonella spp.	16–48	Beef, poultry, water, eggs, dairy products	Summer	Tissue invasion	2–7 days	Supportive
Shigella spp.	16–48	Salad, water	Summer	Tissue invasion	2–7 days	Supportive
EPEC	16–48	Water	None	Tissue invasion	2–7 days	Supportive
Campylobacter	16–48	Poultry, dairy products, clams, water	Spring, summer	Tissue invasion	2–7 days	Supportive
ETEC	16–72	Water	None	Toxin production (in vivo)	1–7 days	Supportive
Vibrio cholerae	16–72	Water		Toxin production (in vivo)	2–12 days	Supportive, antibiotics
Yersinia enterocolitica	16–48	Dairy products		Toxin production and/or tissue invasion	1–30 days	Supportive
Clostridium botulinum	12–72	Canned fruits, vegetables, meats, honey	None	Preformed toxins A, B, and E (children and adults)		
				Toxin production (in vivo) (infants)		Supportive (including mechanically assisted ventilation), trivalent antitoxin

EPEC, enteropathogenic *E. coli*; ETEC, enterotoxigenic *E. coli*.

epithelial cells at the villus tips to cause a noninflammatory diarrhea. Type C organisms can be found in undercooked pork and occur in underdeveloped tropical regions. Type C organisms can produce a toxin-related syndrome called *enteritis necroticans,* which is a coagulative transmural necrosis of the intestinal wall. This syndrome can result in intestinal perforation leading to sepsis and mortality in approximately 40% of victims.

Food-borne botulism results from the ingestion of food contaminated with preformed toxins or toxin-producing spores from *C. botulinum. C. botulinum* poisoning is relatively rare; only 110 cases are reported per year in the United States.[74,75] Botulism is almost always associated with improper preparation or storage of food. Seven distinct toxins (A to G) have been described. The toxins, which are produced by the bacteria and released on lysis, are the most potent biologic or chemical toxins known to humans. The toxin prevents the release of acetylcholine at the peripheral cholinergic nerve terminal. Toxin activity has prompted the use of minute locally injected doses to treat select spastic disorders, such as blepharospasm, hemifacial spasm, and certain dystonias.

Food-borne botulism is suspected when patients present with acute GI symptoms concurrently or just prior to the onset of a symmetric descending paralysis without sensory or central nervous system involvement. Symptoms usually begin 18 to 24 hours after ingestion and progress over days to weeks. Other symptoms can include blurred vision, photophobia (90%), dysphagia (76%), generalized weakness (58%), nausea and vomiting (56%), and dysphonia (55%). Diagnosis is made by culturing *C. botulinum* from the stool. Guillain-Barré syndrome associated with *C. jejuni* infection has been a common differential diagnosis in patients who present with these symptoms.[76] The difference lies in the onset of neurologic symptoms, which typically occur 1 to 3 weeks after the onset of *C. jejuni* infection, and the condition usually is manifested by an ascending paralysis in *C. jejuni*-associated Guillain-Barré syndrome.[77]

Treatment consists primarily of respiratory support and use of botulinum antitoxin.[75] Respiratory failure may occur prior to involvement of other upper muscle groups. If evaluation is performed within several hours of ingestion, gastric lavage or induction of vomiting is suggested. Cathartics and enemas also can be used to remove residual toxin from the bowel, but they are contraindicated in cases of ileus. Although the effectiveness of antitoxins is unknown, patients diagnosed with botulism should receive botulinum antitoxin. Botulinum antitoxin is a concentrated preparation of equine globulins obtained from horses immunized with toxins A, B, and E. Because trivalent antitoxin is equine in origin, patients should be tested for hypersensitivity before receiving the product intravenously. Other agents used experimentally as adjunctive therapy are guanidine, which antagonizes the effect of botulinum toxin at the neuromuscular junction, and 4-aminopyridine, which increases acetylcholine release. Newer and more effective methods of treatment and prevention are under development, including a botulinum toxin vaccine consisting of nontoxic botulinum fragments. Prevention always should be stressed. Botulinum toxins are heat labile and readily destroyed by 10 minutes of boiling. All home-canned foods should be processed according to directions and boiled, not just warmed, prior to consumption.

In food-borne illnesses, the cornerstone of therapy remains supportive care. ORT is preferred in replenishing and maintaining fluid and electrolyte balance, and intravenous fluid therapy should be reserved for those who are severely ill and cannot tolerate oral therapy. Antiemetics and antiperistaltic agents offer symptomatic relief, but the latter should not be given in patients who present with high fever, bloody diarrhea, or fecal leukocytes. Antimicrobial therapy is not effective in the management of *S. aureus, C. perfringens,* or *B. cereus* food poisonings. In developed countries, many of the food-borne illnesses can be prevented with proper food selection, preparation, and storage. However, in developing countries, sanitation and clean water supply are larger concerns.

ABBREVIATIONS

AIDS: acquired immunodeficiency syndrome

CDC: Centers for Disease Control and Prevention

CDI: *Clostridium difficile* infection

EAEC: enteroaggregative *Escherichia coli*

EHEC: enterohemorrhagic *Escherichia coli*

EIEC: enteroinvasive *Escherichia coli*

EPEC: enteropathogenic *Escherichia coli*

ETEC: enterotoxigenic *Escherichia coli*

GBS: Guillain-Barré syndrome

HUS: hemolytic uremic syndrome

ORT: oral rehydration solution

REFERENCES

1. Kosek M, Bern C, Guerrant RL. The global burden of diarrhoeal disease, as estimated from studies published between 1992 and 2000. Bull World Health Organ.2003;81(3):197–204.

2. Gangarosa RE, Glass RI, Lew JF, Boring JR. Hospitalizations involving gastroenteritis in the United States, 1985: the special burden of the disease among the elderly. Am J Epidemiol.1992;135(3):281–290.

3. Mead PS, Slutsker L, Dietz V, et al. Food-related illness and death in the United States. Emerg Infect Dis.1999;5(5):607–625.

4. Lopez AD, Mathers CD, Ezzati M, et al. Global and regional burden of disease and risk factors, 2001: systematic analysis of population health data. Lancet. 2006;367(9524):1747–1757.

5. Guerrant RL, Van Gilder T, Steiner TS, et al. Practice guidelines for the management of infectious diarrhea. Clin Infect Dis. 2001;32(3):331–351.

6. King CK, Glass R, Bresee JS, Duggan C. Managing acute gastroenteritis among children: oral rehydration, maintenance, and nutritional therapy. MMWR Recomm Rep. 2003;52(RR-16):1–16.

7. World Health Organization. The treatment of diarrhoea: a manual for physicians and other senior health workers *http://whqlibdoc.who.int/publications/2005/9241593180.pdf*>. Geneva, Switzerland: World Health Organization; 2005.

8. Stone B. Fluid and electrolytes. In: Robertson J, Shikofski N. The Johns Hopkins Hospital: The Harriet Lane Handbook, 17th ed. St. Louis, MO: Mosby; 2005. AU: Missing page numbers.

9. Payot S, Bolla JM, Corcoran D, et al. Mechanisms of fluoroquinolone and macrolide resistance in *Campylobacter* spp. Microbes Infect. 2006;8(7):1967–71.

10. Parry CM, Threlfall EJ. Antimicrobial resistance in typhoidal and nontyphoidal salmonellae. Curr Opin Infect Dis.2008;21(5):531–538.

11. Graham SM. Salmonellosis in children in developing and developed countries and populations. Curr Opin Infect Dis. 2002;15(5):507–512.

12. Panos GZ, Betsi GI, Falagas ME. Systematic review: are antibiotics detrimental or beneficial for the treatment of patients with *Escherichia coli* O157:H7 infection? Aliment Pharmacol Ther. 2006;24(5):731–742.

13. Typhoid immunization. Recommendations of the Immunization Practices Advisory Committee (ACIP). MMWR Recomm Rep. 1990;39(RR-10):1–5.

14. Cortese MM, Parashar UD. Prevention of rotavirus gastroenteritis among infants and children: recommendations of the Advisory Committee on Immunization Practices (ACIP). MMWR Recomm Rep. 2009;58(RR-2):1–25.

15. Chang MH, Glynn MK, Groseclose SL. Endemic, notifiable bioterrorism-related diseases, United States, 1992–1999. Emerg Infect Dis. 2003;9(5):556–564.

16. Bhuiyan NA, Nusrin S, Alam M, et al. Changing genotypes of cholera toxin (CT) of Vibrio cholerae O139 in Bangladesh and description of three new CT genotypes. FEMS Immunol Med Microbiol. 2009;57(2):136–141.

17. Sack DA, Sack RB, Nair GB, Siddique AK. Cholera. Lancet. 2004;363(9404):223–233.

18. Gregorio GV, Gonzales ML, Dans LF, Martinez EG. Polymer-based oral rehydration solution for treating acute watery diarrhoea. Cochrane Database Syst Rev. 2009(2):CD006519.

19. Khan WA, Bennish ML, Seas C, et al. Randomised controlled comparison of single-dose ciprofloxacin and doxycycline for cholera caused by Vibrio cholerae O1 or O139. Lancet.1996;348(9023):296–300.

20. Khan WA, Saha D, Rahman A, et al. Comparison of single-dose azithromycin and 12-dose, 3-day erythromycin for childhood cholera: a randomised, double-blind trial. Lancet. 2002;360(9347):1722–1727.

21. Flores J, Okhuysen PC. Enteroaggregative Escherichia coli infection. Curr Opin Gastroenterol. 2009;25(1):8–11.

22. Holtz LR, Neill MA, Tarr PI. Acute bloody diarrhea: a medical emergency for patients of all ages. Gastroenterology. 2009;136(6): 1887–98.

23. Robins-Browne RM, Hartland EL. Escherichia coli as a cause of diarrhea. J Gastroenterol Hepatol. 2002;17(4):467–475.

24. Ochoa TJ, Barletta F, Contreras C, Mercado E. New insights into the epidemiology of enteropathogenic Escherichia coli infection. Trans R Soc Trop Med Hyg. 2008;102(9):852–856.

25. Nataro JP, Kaper JB. Diarrheagenic Escherichia coli. Clin Microbiol Rev. 1998;11(1):142–201.

26. Niyogi SK. Shigellosis. J Microbiol. 2005;43(2):133–143.

27. Fernandez MI, Sansonetti PJ. Shigella interaction with intestinal epithelial cells determines the innate immune response in shigellosis. Int J Med Microbiol. 2003;293(1):55–67.

28. Garg AX, Pope JE, Thiessen-Philbrook H, et al. Arthritis risk after acute bacterial gastroenteritis. Rheumatology (Oxford). 2008;47(2):200–204.

29. Basualdo W, Arbo A. Randomized comparison of azithromycin versus cefixime for treatment of shigellosis in children. Pediatr Infect Dis J. 2003;22(4):374–377.

30. Voetsch AC, Van Gilder TJ, Angulo FJ, et al. FoodNet estimate of the burden of illness caused by nontyphoidal Salmonella infections in the United States. Clin Infect Dis. 2004;38 Suppl 3:S127–134.

31. Crum-Cianflone NF. Salmonellosis and the gastrointestinal tract: more than just peanut butter. Curr Gastroenterol Rep. 2008;10(4): 424–431.

32. Sirinavin S, Garner P. Antibiotics for treating salmonella gut infections. Cochrane Database Syst Rev. 2000(2):CD001167.

33. Thaver D, Zaidi AK, Critchley JA, et al. Fluoroquinolones for treating typhoid and paratyphoid fever (enteric fever). Cochrane Database Syst Rev. 2008(4):CD004530.

34. Allos BM. Campylobacter jejuni Infections: update on emerging issues and trends. Clin Infect Dis. 2001;32(8):1201–1206.

35. DuPont HL. The growing threat of foodborne bacterial enteropathogens of animal origin. Clin Infect Dis. 2007;45(10):1353–1361.

36. Janssen R, Krogfelt KA, Cawthraw SA, et al. Host-pathogen interactions in Campylobacter infections: the host perspective. Clin Microbiol Rev. 2008;21(3):505–518.

37. Hoogkamp-Korstanje JA, de Koning J, Samsom JP. Incidence of human infection with Yersinia enterocolitica serotypes O3, O8, and O9 and the use of indirect immunofluorescence in diagnosis. J Infect Dis. 1986;153(1):138–141.

38. Marks MI, Pai CH, Lafleur L, et al. Yersinia enterocolitica gastroenteritis: a prospective study of clinical, bacteriologic, and epidemiologic features. J Pediatr. 1980;96(1):26–31.

39. San Joaquin VH. Aeromonas, Yersinia, and miscellaneous bacterial enteropathogens. Pediatr Ann. 1994;23(10):544–548.

40. Haverly RM, Harrison CR, Dougherty TH. Yersinia enterocolitica bacteremia associated with red blood cell transfusion. Arch Pathol Lab Med. 1996;120(5):499–500.

41. Leffler DA, Lamont JT. Treatment of Clostridium difficile-associated disease. Gastroenterology. 2009;136(6):1899–1912.

42. Loo VG, Poirier L, Miller MA, et al. A predominantly clonal multi-institutional outbreak of Clostridium difficile-associated diarrhea with high morbidity and mortality. N Engl J Med. 2005;353(23):2442–2449.

43. McFarland LV, Elmer G, Surawicz CM. Breaking the cycle: Treatment strategies for 163 cases of recurrent Clostridium difficile disease. Am J Gastroenterol. 2002;97(7):1769–1775.

44. Kelly C. A 76-year-old man with recurrent Clostridium difficile-associated diarrhea. JAMA. 2009;301(9):954–962.

45. Buggy BP, Fekety R, Silva J Jr. Therapy of relapsing Clostridium difficile-associated diarrhea and colitis with the combination of vancomycin and rifampin. J Clin Gastroenterol. 1987;9:155–159.

46. Johnson S, Schriever C, Galang M, et al. Interruption of recurrent Clostridium difficile-associated diarrhea episodes by serial therapy with vanocmycin and rifaximin. Clin Infect Dis. 2007;44: 846–848.

47. Musher DM, Logan N, Mehendiratta V, et al. Clostridium difficile colitis that fails conventional metronidazole therapy: response to nitazoxanide. J Antimicrob Chemother. 2007;59:705–710.

48. Wilcox W. Descriptive study of intravenous immunoglobulin for the treatment of recurrent Clostridium difficile diarrhea. J Antimicrobial Chemother. 2004;53:882–884.

49. Aas J, Gessert CE, Bakken JS. Recurrent Clostridium difficile colitis: case series involving 18 patients treated with donor stool administered via a nasogastric tube. Clin Infect Dis. 2003;36:580–585.

50. Pillai A, Nelson R. Probiotics for treatment of Clostridium difficile-associated colitis in adults. Cochrane Database Syst Rev. 2008;1:CD004611.

51. Louie TJ, Peppe J, Watt CK, et al. Tolevamer, a novel nonantibiotic polmer, compared wtih vancomycin in the treatmetn of mild to moderately severe Clostridium difficile-associated diarrhea. Clin Infect Dis. 2006;43:411–20.

52. Charles MD, Holman RC, Curns AT, et al. Hospitalizations associated with rotavirus gastroenteritis in the United States, 1993–2002. Pediatr Infect Dis J. 2006;25(6):489–493.

53. Greenberg HB, Estes MK. Rotaviruses: from pathogenesis to vaccination. Gastroenterology. 2009 May;136(6):1939–1951.

54. Intussusception among recipients of rotavirus vaccine–United States, 1998–1999. MMWR Morb Mortal Wkly Rep. 1999;48(27): 577–581.

55. Vesikari T, Matson DO, Dennehy P, et al. Safety and efficacy of a pentavalent human-bovine (WC3) reassortant rotavirus vaccine. N Engl J Med. 2006;354(1):23–33.

56. Ruiz-Palacios GM, Perez-Schael I, Velazquez FR, et al. Safety and efficacy of an attenuated vaccine against severe rotavirus gastroenteritis. N Engl J Med. 2006;354(1):11–22.

57. Patel MM, Widdowson MA, Glass RI, et al. Systematic literature review of role of noroviruses in sporadic gastroenteritis. Emerg Infect Dis. 2008;14(8):1224–1231.

58. Ball JM, Graham DY, Opekun AR, et al. Recombinant Norwalk virus-like particles given orally to volunteers: phase I study. Gastroenterology.1999;117(1):40–48.

59. Walter JE, Mitchell DK. Astrovirus infection in children. Curr Opin Infect Dis. 2003;16(3):247–253.

60. Cello JP, Day LW. Idiopathic AIDS enteropathy and treatment of gastrointestinal opportunistic pathogens. Gastroenterology. 2009;136(6):1952–1965.

61. Hill DR. Occurrence and self-treatment of diarrhea in a large cohort of Americans traveling to developing countries. Am J Trop Med Hyg. 2000;62(5):585–589.

62. Shlim D. Looking for evidence that personal hygiene precautions prevent traveler's diarrhea. Clin Infect Dis. 2005;41(Suppl 8): S531–S535.

63. DuPont HL, Ericsson CD, Johnson PC, et al. Prevention of travelers' diarrhea by the tablet formulation of bismuth subsalicylate. JAMA. 1987;257(10):1347–1350.

64. Hill DR, Ericson CD, Pearson RD, et al. The practice of travel medicine: guidelines by the Infectious Diseases Society of America. Clin Infect Dis. 2006;43(12):1499–1539.

65. DuPont HL, Jiang ZD, Okhuysen PC, et al. A randomized, double-blind, placebo-controlled trial of rifaximin to prevent travelers' diarrhea. Ann Intern Med. 2005;142(10):805–812.

66. DuPont HL, Ericsson CD, Farthing MJ, et al. Expert review of the evidence base for self-therapy of travelers' diarrhea. J Travel Med. 2009;16(3):161–171.

67. De Bruyn G, Hahn S, Borwick A. Antibiotic treatment for travelers' diarrhea. Cochrane Database Syst Rev. 2000;3:CD0002242.

68. Tribble DR, Sanders JW, Pang LW, et al. Traveler's diarrhea in Thailand: randomized, double-blind trial comparing single-dose and 3-day azithromycin-based regimens with a 3-day levofloxacin regimen. Clin Infect Dis. 2007;44(3):338–346.

69. Taylor DN, Bourgeois AL, Ericsson CD, et al. A randomized, double-blind, multicenter study of rifaximin compared with placebo and with ciprofloxacin in the treatment of travelers' diarrhea. Am J Trop Med Hyg. 2006;74(6):1060–1066.

70. Riddle MS, Arnold S, Tribble DR. Effect of adjunctive loperamide in combination with antibiotics on treatment outcomes in traveler's diarrhea: a systematic review and meta-analysis. Clin Infect Dis. 2008;47(8):1007–1014.

71. Le Loir Y, Baron F, Gautier M. *Staphylococcus aureus* and food poisoning. Genet Mol Res. 2003;2(1):63–76.

72. Schoeni JL, Wong AC. *Bacillus cereus* food poisoning and its toxins. J Food Prot. 2005;68(3):636–648.

73. Brynestad S, Granum PE. *Clostridium perfringens* and foodborne infections. Int J Food Microbiol. 2002;74(3):195–202.

74. Sobel J. Botulism. Clin Infect Dis. 2005;41(8):1167–1173.

75. Sobel J, Tucker N, Sulka A, et al. Foodborne botulism in the United States, 1990–2000. Emerg Infect Dis. 2004;10(9):1606–1611.

76. Lindstrom M, Korkeala H. Laboratory diagnostics of botulism. Clin Microbiol Rev. 2006;19(2):298–314.

77. van Belkum A, Jacobs B, van Beek E, et al. Can *Campylobacter coli* induce Guillain-Barre syndrome? Eur J Clin Microbiol Infect Dis. 2009;28(5):557–560.

123

Intraabdominal Infections

JOSEPH T. DIPIRO AND THOMAS R. HOWDIESHELL

KEY CONCEPTS

❶ Most intraabdominal infections are "secondary" infections that are polymicrobic and are caused by a defect in the gastrointestinal tract that must be treated by surgical drainage, resection, and/or repair.

❷ Primary peritonitis is generally caused by a single organism (*Staphylococcus aureus* in patients undergoing chronic ambulatory peritoneal dialysis [CAPD] or *Escherichia coli* in patients with cirrhosis).

❸ Secondary intraabdominal infections are usually caused by a mixture of bacteria, including enteric gram-negative bacilli and anaerobes, which enhances the pathogenic potential of the bacteria.

❹ For peritonitis, early and aggressive intravenous fluid resuscitation and electrolyte replacement therapy are essential. A common cause of early death is hypovolemic shock caused by inadequate intravascular volume and tissue perfusion.

❺ Cultures of secondary intraabdominal infection sites are generally not useful for directing antimicrobial therapy. Treatment is generally initiated on a "presumptive" or empirical basis.

❻ Antimicrobial regimens for secondary intraabdominal infections should include coverage for enteric gram-negative bacilli and anaerobes. Antimicrobials that may be used for the treatment of secondary intraabdominal infections include (a) a β-lactam–β-lactamase inhibitor combination (such as piperacillin-tazobactam), (b) a carbapenem (imipenem or meropenem), (c) quinolone (ciprofloxacin) plus metronidazole, or an aminoglycoside (gentamicin) plus clindamycin (or metronidazole).

❼ Treatment of primary peritonitis for CAPD patients should include an antistaphylococcal antimicrobial such as a first-generation cephalosporin (cefazolin) or vancomycin (usually given by the intraperitoneal route).

❽ The duration of antimicrobial treatment should be for a total of 5 to 7 days for most secondary intraabdominal infections.

❾ Patients treated for intraabdominal infections should be assessed for the occurrence of drug-related adverse effects,

particularly hypersensitivity reactions (β-lactam antimicrobials), diarrhea (most agents), fungal infections (most agents), and nephrotoxicity (aminoglycosides).

Intraabdominal infections are those contained within the peritoneal cavity or retroperitoneal space. The peritoneal cavity extends from the undersurface of the diaphragm to the floor of the pelvis and contains the stomach, small bowel, large bowel, liver, gallbladder, and spleen. The duodenum, pancreas, kidneys, adrenal glands, great vessels (aorta and vena cava), and most mesenteric vascular structures reside in the retroperitoneum. Intraabdominal infections may be generalized or localized. They may be contained within visceral structures, such as the liver, gallbladder, spleen, pancreas, kidney, or female reproductive organs. Two general types of intraabdominal infections are discussed throughout this chapter: peritonitis and abscess. *Peritonitis* is defined as the acute inflammatory response of the peritoneal lining to microorganisms, chemicals, irradiation, or foreign-body injury. This chapter deals only with peritonitis of infectious origin.

An *abscess* is a purulent collection of fluid separated from surrounding tissue by a wall consisting of inflammatory cells and adjacent organs. It usually contains necrotic debris, bacteria, and inflammatory cells. These processes differ considerably in presentation and approach to treatment.

EPIDEMIOLOGY

Peritonitis may be classified as primary, secondary, or tertiary.[1–3] Primary peritonitis, also called *spontaneous bacterial peritonitis*, is an infection of the peritoneal cavity without an evident source in the abdomen. Bacteria may be transported from the bloodstream to the peritoneal cavity, where the inflammatory process begins. In secondary peritonitis, a focal disease process is evident within the abdomen. Secondary peritonitis may involve perforation of the gastrointestinal (GI) tract (possibly because of ulceration, ischemia, or obstruction), postoperative peritonitis, or posttraumatic peritonitis (blunt or penetrating trauma). Tertiary peritonitis occurs in critically ill patients and is infection that persists or recurs at least 48 hours after apparently adequate management of primary or secondary peritonitis.

❶ Primary peritonitis develops in up to 10% to 30% of patients with alcoholic cirrhosis.[4] Patients undergoing chronic ambulatory peritoneal dialysis (CAPD) average one episode of peritonitis every 33 months.[5] Epidemiologic data for secondary and tertiary intraabdominal infections are limited. Secondary peritonitis may be caused by perforation of a peptic ulcer; traumatic perforation of the stomach, small or large bowel, uterus, or urinary bladder; appendicitis; pancreatitis; diverticulitis; bowel infarction; inflammatory

TABLE 123-1	Causes of Bacterial Peritonitis

Primary bacterial peritonitis

Peritoneal dialysis
Cirrhosis with ascites
Nephrotic syndrome

Secondary bacterial peritonitis

Miscellaneous causes
  Diverticulitis
  Appendicitis
  Inflammatory bowel diseases
  Salpingitis
  Biliary tract infections
  Necrotizing pancreatitis
Neoplasms
  Intestinal obstruction
  Perforation
Mechanical gastrointestinal problems
  Any cause of small bowel obstruction (adhesions, hernia)
Vascular causes
  Mesenteric arterial or venous occlusion (atrial fibrillation)
  Mesenteric ischemia without occlusion
Trauma
  Blunt abdominal trauma with rupture of intestine
  Penetrating abdominal trauma
Iatrogenic intestinal perforation (endoscopy)
Intraoperative events
Peritoneal contamination during abdominal operation
Leakage from gastrointestinal anastomosis

bowel disease, cholecystitis; operative contamination of the peritoneum; or diseases of the female genital tract, such as septic abortion, postoperative uterine infection, endometritis, and salpingitis. Appendicitis is one of the most common causes of intraabdominal infection. In 1998, 278,000 appendectomies were performed in the United States for suspected appendicitis.[6]

ETIOLOGY

Primary peritonitis in adults occurs most commonly in association with alcoholic cirrhosis, especially in its end stage, or with ascites caused by postnecrotic cirrhosis, chronic active hepatitis, acute viral hepatitis, congestive heart failure, malignancy, systemic lupus erythematosus, or nephritic syndrome. It may also result from the use of a peritoneal catheter for dialysis or central nervous system ventriculoperitoneal shunting for hydrocephalus. Rarely, primary peritonitis occurs without apparent underlying disease.

Table 123–1 summarizes many of the potential causes of bacterial peritonitis. Causes include inflammatory processes of the GI tract or abdominal organs, bowel obstruction, vascular occlusions that may lead to gangrene of the intestines, and neoplasia that may cause

intestinal perforation or obstruction. Other possible causes include those resulting from traumatic injuries or postoperative infections.

Abscesses are the result of chronic inflammation and may occur without preceding generalized peritonitis. They may be located within one of the spaces of the peritoneal cavity or within one of the visceral organs, and may range from a few milliliters to a liter or more in volume. These collections often have a fibrinous capsule and may take from a few weeks to years to form.

The causes of intraabdominal abscess overlap those of peritonitis and, in fact, may occur sequentially or simultaneously. Appendicitis is the most frequent cause of abscess. Other potential causes of intraabdominal abscess include pancreatitis, diverticulitis, lesions of the biliary tract, genitourinary tract infections, perforating tumors in the abdomen, trauma, and leaking intestinal anastomoses. In addition, pelvic inflammatory disease in women may lead to tuboovarian abscess. For some diseases, such as appendicitis and diverticulitis, abscesses occur more frequently than generalized peritonitis.

MICROFLORA OF THE GASTROINTESTINAL TRACT AND FEMALE GENITAL TRACT

A full appreciation of intraabdominal infection requires an understanding of the normal microflora within the GI tract. There are striking differences in bacterial species and concentrations of flora within the various segments of the GI tract (Table 123–2), and this bacterial environment usually determines the severity of infectious processes in the abdomen. Generally, the low gastric pH eradicates bacteria that enter the stomach. With achlorhydria, bacterial counts may rise to 10^5 to 10^7 organisms/mL. The normally low bacterial count may also increase by 1,000- or 10,000-fold with gastric outlet obstruction, hemorrhage, gastric cancer, and in patients receiving histamine 2 (H_2)-receptor antagonists, proton pump inhibitors, or antacids.

The biliary tract (gallbladder and bile ducts) is sterile in most healthy individuals, but in people older than 70 years of age, those with acute cholecystitis, jaundice, or common bile duct stones, it is likely to be colonized by aerobic gram-negative bacilli (particularly *Escherichia coli* and *Klebsiella* spp.) and enterococci.[7] Patients with biliary tract bacterial colonization are at greater risk of intraabdominal infection.

In the distal ileum, bacterial counts of aerobes and anaerobes are quite high. In the colon, there may be 500 to 600 different types of bacteria in stool, with concentrations often reaching 10^{11} organisms/mL and anaerobic bacteria outnumbering aerobic bacteria by more than 1,000 to 1.[2,8] In fact, up to 50% of the dry mass of stool is bacteria. Fortunately, most colonic bacteria are not pathogens because they cannot survive in environments outside the colon. Perforation of the colon results in the release of large numbers of anaerobic and aerobic bacteria into the peritoneum. The colonic flora are generally consistent unless broad-spectrum antimicrobials have been used, in which case there are increases in *Candida* or gram-negative bacteria.

TABLE 123-2	Usual Microflora of the Gastrointestinal Tract			

Site	Commonly Found Bacteria	Approximate Concentration (Log No. Organisms/mL)	
		Aerobes	*Anaerobes*
Stomach[a]	*Streptococcus, Lactobacillus*	10–100	Rare
Biliary tract	Normally sterile (*Escherichia coli, Klebsiella*, or enterococci in some patients)	0	0
Proximal small bowel	*Streptococcus* (including enterococci), *E. coli, Klebsiella, Lactobacillus*, diphtheroids	100	Few
Distal ileum	*E. coli, Klebsiella, Enterobacter*, enterococci, *Bacteroides fragilis, Clostridium*, peptostreptococci	10^4–10^6	10^5–10^7
Colon	*Bacteroides* spp., peptostreptococci, *Clostridium, E. coli, Klebsiella*, enterococci, *Enterobacter*, and many others	10^5–10^8	10^9–10^{11}

[a]With achlorhydria, H_2-antagonist therapy, gastric cancer, or gastric outlet obstruction, bacterial counts may rise to 10^5/mL.

The lower female genital tract is generally colonized by a large number of aerobic and anaerobic bacteria. Anaerobes may number 10^9 organisms per milliliter and often include lactobacilli, eubacteria, clostridia, anaerobic streptococci, and, less frequently, *Bacteroides fragilis.* Aerobic bacteria most often are streptococci and *Staphylococcus epidermidis,* and these may number 10^8 organisms per milliliter.

PATHOPHYSIOLOGY

Intraabdominal infection results from bacterial entry into the peritoneal or retroperitoneal spaces or from bacterial collections within intraabdominal organs. In primary peritonitis, bacteria may enter the abdomen via the bloodstream or the lymphatic system by transmigration through the bowel wall, through an indwelling peritoneal dialysis catheter, or via the fallopian tubes in females. Hematogenous bacterial spread (through the bloodstream) occurs more frequently with tuberculosis peritonitis or peritonitis associated with cirrhotic ascites. When peritonitis results from peritoneal dialysis, skin surface flora are introduced via the peritoneal catheter. In secondary peritonitis, bacteria most often enter the peritoneum or retroperitoneum as a result of perforation of the GI or female genital tracts caused by diseases or traumatic injuries. Also, peritonitis or abscess may result from contamination of the peritoneum during a surgical procedure or following anastomotic leak.

The physiologic characteristics of the peritoneal cavity determine the nature of the response to infection or inflammation within it.[1] The peritoneum is lined by a highly permeable serous membrane with a surface area approximately that of skin. The peritoneal cavity is lubricated with less than 100 mL of sterile, clear yellow fluid, normally with fewer than 300 cells/mm^3, a specific gravity below 1.016, and protein content below 3 g/dL. These conditions change drastically with peritoneal infection or inflammation, as described below.

After bacteria are introduced into the peritoneal cavity, there is an immediate response to contain the insult. Humoral and cellular defenses respond first; then the omentum adheres to the affected area. A limited bacterial inoculum is handled rapidly by defense mechanisms, including complement activation and a leukocyte response. Under certain conditions, the bacterial insult is not contained, and bacteria disseminate throughout the peritoneal cavity, resulting in peritonitis. This is more likely to occur in the presence of a foreign body, hematoma, dead tissue, a large bacterial inoculum, continuing bacterial contamination, and contamination involving a mixture of synergistic organisms. Protein-calorie malnutrition, antecedent steroid therapy, and diabetes mellitus may also contribute to the formation of an intraabdominal abscess.

When bacteria become dispersed throughout the peritoneum, the inflammatory process involves most of the peritoneal lining. There is an outpouring into the peritoneum of fluid containing leukocytes, fibrin, and other proteins that form exudates on the inflamed peritoneal surfaces and begin to form adhesions between peritoneal structures. This process, combined with a paralysis of the intestines (ileus), may result in confinement of the contamination to one or more locations within the peritoneum. Fluid also begins to collect in the bowel lumen and wall, and distension may result.

The fluid and protein shift into the abdomen (called *third-spacing*) may be so dramatic that circulating blood volume is decreased, which causes decreased cardiac output and hypovolemic shock. Accompanying fever, vomiting, or diarrhea may worsen the fluid imbalance. A reflex sympathetic response, manifested by sweating, tachycardia, and vasoconstriction, may be evident. With an inflamed peritoneum, bacteria and endotoxins are absorbed easily into the bloodstream (translocation), and this may result in septic shock.[1] Other foreign substances present in the peritoneal cavity

potentiate peritonitis. These adjuvants, notably feces, dead tissues, barium, mucus, bile, and blood, have detrimental effects on host defense mechanisms, particularly on bacterial phagocytosis.

Many of the manifestations of intraabdominal infections, particularly peritonitis, result from cytokine activity. Inflammatory cytokines, such as tumor necrosis factor-α (TNF-α), interleukin (IL) 1, IL-6, IL-8, and interferon γ (INF-γ), are produced by macrophages and neutrophils in response to bacteria and bacterial products or in response to tissue injury resulting from the surgical incision.[1,9] These cytokines produce wide-ranging effects on the vascular endothelium of organs, particularly the liver, lungs, kidneys, and heart. With uncontrolled activation of these mediators, sepsis may result (see Chap. 128).[10]

Peritonitis may result in death because of the effects on major organ systems. Fluid shifts and endotoxin may result in hypovolemic and septic shock. Hypoalbuminemia may result from protein loss into the peritoneum exacerbating intravascular volume loss. Pulmonary function may be compromised by the inflamed peritoneum, producing splinting (muscle rigidity caused by pain) that inhibits adequate diaphragmatic movement leading to atelectasis and pneumonia. Increased lung vascular permeability and resulting shunting of blood may induce onset of the respiratory distress syndrome and associated hypoxemia and hypercarbia. With fluid loss, hypotension, endotoxemia, and renal and hepatic perfusion may be compromised, and acute renal and hepatic failure are potential threats.

If peritoneal contamination is localized but bacterial elimination is incomplete, an abscess results. This collection of necrotic tissue, bacteria, and white blood cells may be at single or multiple sites and may be within one of the spaces of the peritoneal cavity or in one of the visceral organs. The location of the abscess is often related to the site of primary disease. For example, abscesses resulting from appendicitis tend to appear in the right lower quadrant or the pelvis; those resulting from diverticulitis tend to appear in the left lower quadrant or pelvis.

An abscess begins by the combined action of inflammatory cells (such as neutrophils), bacteria, fibrin, and other inflammatory mediators. Bacteria may release heparinases that cause local thrombosis and tissue necrosis or fibrinolysins, collagenases, or other enzymes that allow extension of the process into surrounding tissues. Neutrophils gathered in the abscess cavity die in 3 to 5 days, releasing lysosomal enzymes that liquefy the core of the abscess. A mature abscess may have a fibrinous capsule that isolates bacteria and the liquid core from antimicrobials and immunologic defenses.

Within the abscess, the oxygen tension is low and anaerobic bacteria thrive; thus the size of the abscess may increase because it is hypertonic, resulting in an additional influx of fluid. Hypertonicity promotes the formation of bacterial L forms, which are resistant to antimicrobial agents that disrupt cell walls. Abscess formation may continue and mature for long periods of time and may not be readily evident to either patient or physician. In some instances, the abscess may resolve spontaneously, and, infrequently, it may erode into adjacent organs or rupture and cause diffuse peritonitis. If the abscess erodes through the skin, it may result in an enterocutaneous fistula, connecting bowel to skin, or in a draining sinus tract.

The overall outcome from an intraabdominal infection depends on five key factors: inoculum size, virulence of the contaminating organisms, the presence of adjuvants within the peritoneal cavity that facilitate infection, the adequacy of host defenses, and the adequacy of initial treatment.[11]

MICROBIOLOGY OF INTRAABDOMINAL INFECTION

❷ Primary bacterial peritonitis is often caused by a single organism. In children, the pathogen is usually group A *Streptococcus, E. coli,*

Streptococcus pneumoniae, or *Bacteroides* species.[12] When peritonitis occurs in association with cirrhotic ascites, *E. coli* is isolated most frequently. Other potential pathogens are: *Haemophilus pneumoniae*, *Klebsiella*, *Pseudomonas*, anaerobes, and *S. pneumoniae*.[13] Occasionally, primary peritonitis may be caused by *Mycobacterium tuberculosis*. Peritonitis in patients undergoing peritoneal dialysis is caused most often by common skin organisms, such as coagulase-negative staphylococci, *Staphylococcus aureus*, streptococci, and enterococci. Gram-negative bacteria associated with peritoneal dialysis infections include *E. Coli*, *Klebsiella*, and *Pseudomonas*.[5] Mortality from primary peritonitis caused by gram-negative bacteria is much greater than that from gram-positive bacteria.[14]

❸ Because of the diverse bacteria present in the GI tract, secondary intraabdominal infections are often polymicrobial.[2] The mean number of different bacterial species isolated from infected intraabdominal sites ranged from 2.9 to 3.7, including an average of 1.3 to 1.6 aerobes and 1.7 to 2.1 anaerobes.[15,16] With proper anaerobic specimen collection, anaerobic organisms are isolated in most patients. In one report of patients with gangrenous and perforated appendicitis, an average of 10.2 different organisms was isolated from each patient, including 2.7 aerobes and 7.5 anaerobes.[17] Purely aerobic or anaerobic infections are uncommon, as are infections caused by fungi. Table 123–3 gives the frequencies with which specific bacteria were isolated from patients with peritonitis and other intraabdominal infections.[3,18] Nosocomial infections tend to have a more diverse array of pathogens and higher likelihood of multidrug resistance compared with isolates from community-acquired infections.[18] *E. coli*, *Streptococcus* spp., and *Bacteroides* spp. were isolated most often from the infection site, as well as from blood cultures. In patients diagnosed with severe infections, the pattern of bacterial isolates may change and commonly includes *Candida*, enterococci, Enterobacteriaceae, and *S. epidermidis*.

Visceral organ abscesses differ in character from the typical intraabdominal abscess. Hepatic abscesses may be polymicrobial (involving *E. coli*, *Klebsiella*, and anaerobes) or occasionally may be caused by amoeba.[8] Pancreatic abscesses are often polymicrobial, involving enteric bacteria that ascend through the biliary system. Splenic abscesses usually result from hematogenous dissemination of bacteria, such as *E. coli*, *S. aureus*, *Proteus mirabilis*, *Enterococcus*, and *K. pneumoniae*, as well as anaerobes.[8] Pelvic inflammatory disease is associated initially with *Neisseria gonorrhoeae* or *Chlamydia trachomatis*. However, tuboovarian abscesses are usually polymicrobial, having a mix of gram-positive and gram-negative aerobes and anaerobes.

BACTERIAL SYNERGISM

The size of the bacterial inoculum and the number and types of bacterial species present in intraabdominal infections influence patient outcome. The combination of aerobic and anaerobic organisms appears to increase the severity of infection greatly. In animal studies, combinations of aerobic and anaerobic bacteria were much more lethal than infections caused by aerobes or anaerobes alone.

Facultative bacteria may provide an environment conducive to the growth of anaerobic bacteria.[2] Although many bacteria isolated in mixed infections are nonpathogenic by themselves, their presence may be essential for the pathogenicity of the bacterial mixture.[4] The role of facultative bacteria in mixed infections can include (a) promotion of an appropriate environment for anaerobic bacterial growth through oxygen consumption, (b) production of nutrients necessary for anaerobes, and (c) production of extracellular enzymes that promote tissue invasion by anaerobes.

Rat models of intraabdominal infection demonstrate that uncontrolled infection with an implanted mix of aerobes and anaerobes leads to a two-stage (biphasic) infectious process. There is an early peritonitis phase with a high mortality rate and isolation of *E. coli* from blood and a late abscess formation phase in all survivors with isolation of anaerobes such as *B. fragilis* and *Fusobacterium varium*. These experiments and others support the concept that aerobic enteric organisms and anaerobes are pathogens in intraabdominal infection. Aerobic bacteria, particularly *E. coli*, appear responsible for the early mortality from peritonitis, whereas anaerobic bacteria are major pathogens in abscesses, with *B. fragilis* predominating.[19]

Enterococcus can be isolated from many intraabdominal infections in humans, but its role as a pathogen is not clear. Enterococcal infection occurs more commonly in postoperative peritonitis, in the presence of specific risk factors indicating failure of the host's defenses (immunocompromised patients), or with the use of broad-spectrum antibiotics.[20,21]

CLINICAL PRESENTATION

Intraabdominal infections have a wide spectrum of clinical features often depending on the specific disease process, the location and magnitude of bacterial contamination, and concurrent host factors. Peritonitis is usually recognized easily, but intraabdominal abscess may often continue for considerable periods of time, either going unrecognized or being attributed to an unrelated disease process. Patients with primary and secondary peritonitis present quite differently (Table 123–4).[1]

Primary peritonitis can develop over a period of days to weeks and is usually a more indolent process than secondary peritonitis. The first sign of peritonitis may be a cloudy dialysate in patients undergoing peritoneal dialysis or worsening encephalopathy in a cirrhotic patient.

The patient with generalized bacterial peritonitis presents most often in acute distress. The patient lies still, usually on his or her back, possibly with the hips slightly flexed. Any movement of the patient, including rocking the bed or breathing, worsens the generalized abdominal pain.

If peritonitis continues untreated, the patient may experience hypovolemic shock from third-space fluid loss into the peritoneum, bowel wall, and lumen. This may be accompanied by sepsis because the inflamed peritoneum absorbs bacteria and toxins into mesenteric blood vessels and lymph nodes, initiating production of inflammatory cytokines. Hypovolemic shock is the major factor contributing to mortality in the early stage of peritonitis.

Intraabdominal abscess may pose a difficult diagnostic challenge because the symptoms are neither specific nor dramatic. The patient may complain of abdominal pain or discomfort, but these

TABLE 123-3	Pathogens Isolated from Patients with Intraabdominal Infection		
	Secondary Peritonitis[3]	**Community-Acquired Infection**[18]	**Nosocomial Infection**[18]
Gram-negative bacteria			
Escherichia coli	32–61%	29%	22.5%
Enterobacter	8–26%	5.2%	8.0%
Klebsiella	6–26%	2.8%	4.5%
Proteus	4–23%	1.7%	2.4%
Gram-positive bacteria			
Enterococci	18–24%	10.6%	18%
Streptococci	6–55%	13.7%	10%
Staphylococci	6–16%	3.1%	4.8%
Anaerobic bacteria			
Bacteroides	25–80%	13.7%	10.3%
Clostridium	5–18%	3.5%	3.4%
Fungi	2–5%	3%	4%

TABLE 123-4 Clinical Presentation of Peritonitis

Primary Peritonitis

General
The patient may not be in acute distress, particularly with peritoneal dialysis.

Signs and symptoms
The patient may complain of nausea, vomiting (sometimes with diarrhea), and abdominal tenderness.
  Temperature may be only mildly elevated or not elevated in patients undergoing peritoneal dialysis.
  Bowel sounds are hypoactive.
  The cirrhotic patient may have worsening encephalopathy.
  Cloudy dialysate fluid with peritoneal dialysis.

Laboratory tests
The patient's white blood cell (WBC) count may be only mildly elevated.
  Ascitic fluid usually contains greater than 300 leukocytes/mm³, and bacteria may be evident on Gram stain of a centrifuged specimen.
  In 60–80% of patients with cirrhotic ascites, the Gram stain is negative.

Other diagnostic tests
Culture of peritoneal dialysate or ascitic fluid should be positive.

Secondary Peritonitis

Signs and symptoms
Generalized abdominal pain
  Tachypnea
  Tachycardia
  Nausea and vomiting
  Temperature is normal initially then increases to 37.7°C to 38.8°C (100°F to 102°F) within the first few hours and may continue to rise for the next several hours
  Hypotension and shock if volume is not restored
  Decreased urine output due to dehydration

Physical examination
Voluntary abdominal guarding changing to involuntary guarding and a "board-like abdomen"
  Abdominal tenderness and distension
  Faint bowel sounds that cease over time

Laboratory tests
Leukocytosis (15,000–20,000 WBC/mm³, with neutrophils predominating and an elevated percentage of immature neutrophils (bands)
  Elevated hematocrit and blood urea nitrogen because of dehydration
  Patient progresses from early alkalosis because of hyperventilation and vomiting to acidosis and lactic acidemia

Other diagnostic tests
Abdominal radiographs may be useful because free air in the abdomen (indicating intestinal perforation) or distension of the small or large bowel is often evident.

symptoms are not reliable. Fever is usually present; often it is low grade, but it may be high, with a spiking pattern. The patient may have a paralytic ileus and abdominal distension. The abdominal examination is unreliable; tenderness and pain may be present, and a mass may be palpated.

Peritonitis may result from an abscess that ruptures, spreading bacteria and toxins throughout the peritoneum. In other patients, the entry of bacterial toxins into the systemic circulation from the abscess may lead to sepsis and progressive multisystem organ failure (e.g., renal, hepatic, pulmonary, or cardiovascular).

Laboratory studies are not generally helpful in the diagnosis of intraabdominal abscess, although most patients will have leukocytosis. Some patients may have positive blood cultures, whereas others, particularly diabetics, may have hyperglycemia. The finding of *Bacteroides* or any two enteric bacteria in the bloodstream is often indicative of an intraabdominal infectious process.

Radiographic methods are used to make the diagnosis of an intraabdominal abscess. Plain radiographs may show air–fluid levels or a shift of normal intraabdominal contents by the abscess mass. GI contrast studies may also demonstrate this displacement of abdominal structures. Both of these modalities provide indirect

evidence of abscess presence but are not generally helpful in precisely locating the abscess.

Ultrasound is a frequent first diagnostic method used when an intraabdominal abscess is suspected. The procedure may be done at the bedside, which is particularly helpful when the patient is in the intensive care unit.

Computed tomographic (CT) scanning is frequently used to evaluate the abdomen for the presence of an abscess and is the imaging modality of greatest value. An oral radiocontrast agent should be given to allow differentiation of the abscess from the bowel. Intravenous radiocontrast material will be taken up preferentially in the wall of the abscess, creating a unique radiographic appearance, so-called rim enhancement.

Magnetic resonance imaging is used infrequently to locate an intraabdominal abscess, particularly in the retroperitoneum, but this modality offers no significant advantage when compared with CT scanning.

Radioactive isotope imaging with ^{67}Ga citrate-, ^{99m}Tc-, or ^{111}In-labeled leukocytes may also be used.[22] These studies require long preparation and image acquisition and are not used routinely unless CT scanning fails to demonstrate a suspected abscess.

Intraabdominal infection caused by disease processes at specific sites often produces characteristic manifestations that are helpful in diagnosis. For example, a patient with diverticulitis may exhibit stabbing left-lower-quadrant abdominal pain and constipation. Fever and leukocytosis are frequently present, and a tender mass is sometimes palpable. With appendicitis, the findings may be inconsistent, but many patients have a sudden onset of periumbilical or epigastric pain that is usually colicky and later shifts to the right lower quadrant. The location of pain may vary because the appendix can be in many locations (e.g., retrocecal or pelvic) in the abdomen. A mass may be palpable on abdominal, pelvic, or rectal examination. The patient's temperature is generally mildly elevated early and then increases. If perforation and peritonitis occur, findings would include diffuse abdominal pain, rigidity, and sustained fever. More often, however, appendiceal perforation results in a local abscess.

TREATMENT

Intraabdominal Infections

■ DESIRED OUTCOME

The primary goals of treatment are correction of the intraabdominal disease processes or injuries that have caused infection and the drainage of purulent collections (abscesses). A secondary objective is to achieve a resolution of infection without major organ system complications (pulmonary, hepatic, cardiovascular, or renal failure) or adverse drug effects. Ideally, the patient should be discharged from the hospital after treatment with full function for self-care and routine daily activities.

■ GENERAL APPROACH TO TREATMENT

The treatment of intraabdominal infection most often requires hospitalization and the coordinated use of three major modalities: (a) prompt drainage of the infected site, (b) hemodynamic resuscitation and support of vital functions, and (c) early administration of appropriate antimicrobial therapy to treat infection not eradicated by surgery.[2]

Antimicrobials are an important adjunct to drainage procedures in the treatment of secondary intraabdominal infections; however, the use of antimicrobial agents without surgical intervention is usually inadequate. For most cases of primary peritonitis, drainage procedures may not be required, and antimicrobial agents become the mainstay of therapy.

❹ In the early phase of serious intraabdominal infections, attention should be given to the maintenance of organ system functions. With generalized peritonitis, large volumes of intravenous (IV) fluids are required to restore vascular volume, to improve cardiovascular function, and to maintain adequate tissue perfusion and oxygenation. Adequate urine output should be maintained to ensure adequate resuscitation and proper renal function. Respiratory function can be assisted by a variety of methods, including oxygen therapy, pulmonary physiotherapy, and ventilatory support in severely ill patients. Often the critically ill patient with intraabdominal infection will require intensive care management, particularly if there is cardiovascular or respiratory instability. Also, isolation procedures may be required if the infectious process poses a threat to other hospitalized patients.

An additional important component of therapy is nutrition. Intraabdominal infections often directly involve the GI tract or disrupt its function (paralytic ileus). The return of GI motility may take days, weeks, and, occasionally, months. In the interim, enteral or parenteral nutrition as indicated facilitates improved immune function and wound healing to ensure recovery.

■ NONPHARMACOLOGIC TREATMENT

Drainage Procedures

Primary peritonitis is treated with antimicrobials and rarely requires drainage. Secondary peritonitis requires surgical correction of the underlying pathology. The drainage of the purulent material is the critical component of management of an intraabdominal abscess. Without adequate drainage of the abscess, antimicrobial therapy and fluid resuscitation can be expected to fail.

Secondary peritonitis is treated surgically; this is often called *source control*, which refers to all the physical measures undertaken to eradicate the focus of infection.[2,23] At the time of laparotomy (surgical opening and exploration of the abdomen) attempts are made to correct the cause of the peritonitis. This may include patching a perforated ulcer with omentum, removal of a segment of perforated colon, or excision of a portion of gangrenous small intestine. Also, the surgeon may elect to leave the abdomen open after the laparotomy, plan a re-laparotomy at a later time regardless of the patient's condition, or, perform re-laparotomy if the patient develops reinfection.[23] The goal of all these procedures is to repair or remove the inflamed or gangrenous viscus and to prevent further bacterial contamination. The presence of active inflammation increases the difficulty of the surgical procedure, which results in a higher morbidity and mortality rate than if the same procedures were performed in an elective setting without inflammation.

The presence of active inflammation may make it technically impossible to perform the definitive surgical procedure. In this situation, attempts are made to provide drainage of the infected or gangrenous structures. If an intraabdominal abscess, separate from any intraabdominal organ, is discovered during an exploratory laparotomy, it may be debrided, excised, or drained. If the intraabdominal abscess involves an abdominal structure, then a resection of part or all of that organ may be required. An example of this situation is an abscess associated with diverticular disease of the colon. Management may include drainage of the abscess and resection of the involved part of the colon. All foreign material, necrotic tissue, feces, blood, or pus should be removed from the operative field, and the peritoneum should be copiously irrigated with 0.9% sodium chloride to decrease the concentrations of bacteria or other noxious substances.

After an abscess is located, it must be drained. This may be performed surgically or with percutaneous, image-guided techniques.[24]

Typically, image-guided techniques employ ultrasonography or CT scanning. The management of an intraabdominal abscess with percutaneous catheter drainage may be sufficient to resolve the infection. Some patients may require a subsequent procedure to treat the underlying gastrointestinal conditions; however, a significant advantage is obtained by first draining the abscess percutaneously. This allows the surgical procedure to be performed on a patient who is no longer suffering the systemic manifestations of uncontrolled infection. Drainage techniques may be performed using endoscopy or laparoscopy. These minimal-access techniques may offer advantages when compared with traditional surgery but will probably be used less often than radiologically assisted percutaneous drainage techniques.

The most valuable microbiologic information may be obtained at the time of percutaneous or operative abscess drainage. If pus or fluid is found that is believed to be infected, it is best to aspirate 2 to 3 mL into a syringe, remove any air, and tightly cap the syringe. The specimen should be taken promptly to the microbiology laboratory, where a Gram stain should be performed immediately and cultures prepared for identification of aerobic and anaerobic bacteria. If no fluid is available for collection, culture swab devices may be applied to the infected area; however, anaerobic organisms often are not isolated from swabs.

Fluid Therapy

❹ Aggressive fluid repletion and management are required for successful treatment of intraabdominal infections. Fluid therapy is instituted for the purposes of achieving or maintaining proper intravascular volume to ensure adequate cardiac output, tissue perfusion, and correction of acidosis. Loss of fluid through vomiting, diarrhea, or nasogastric suction contributes to dehydration. Intravascular volume can be assessed by blood pressure and heart rate but more accurately by measurement of central venous pressure, pulmonary capillary wedge pressure, or urinary output. When a contracted vascular volume is accompanied by hemorrhage, the initial hematocrit may be normal, but if there is no associated hemorrhage, the hematocrit is usually elevated as an indication of hemoconcentration. Urine output should be monitored continuously in severely ill patients by use of a urinary bladder catheter, quantitated hourly, and should equal or exceed 0.5 mL/kg of body weight per hour.

In patients with peritonitis, hypovolemia is often accompanied by acidosis, so a reasonable IV fluid would be lactated Ringer's solution, which contains the bicarbonate precursor lactate, as well as sodium, chloride, potassium, and calcium. In the initial hour of treatment, large volumes of solution may be required to restore intravascular volume. Thereafter, fluids may be required at a rate of 1 L/h. Maintenance fluids should be instituted (after intravascular volume is restored) with 0.9% sodium chloride and potassium chloride (20 mEq/L) or 5% dextrose and 0.45% sodium chloride with potassium chloride (20 mEq/L). The administration rate should be based on estimated daily fluid loss through urine and nasogastric suction, including 0.5 to 1.0 L for insensible fluid loss. Potassium would not be included routinely if the patient is hyperkalemic or has renal insufficiency.

In patients with significant blood loss, blood transfusion may be indicated. This is generally in the form of packed red blood cells. The criteria for blood transfusion are controversial, but a hematocrit of 25% is generally accepted. In the individual patient, the decision is often determined by the overall clinical status and the ability of the patient to compensate for the reduction in oxygen-carrying capacity associated with an acute anemia. Additional blood component therapy with fresh-frozen plasma or platelets is also based on the needs of the individual patient. Aggressive fluid therapy must often be continued in the postoperative period because fluid will continue to sequester in the peritoneal cavity, bowel wall, and lumen.

■ PHARMACOLOGIC TREATMENT

Antimicrobial Therapy

The goals of antimicrobial therapy are (a) to control bacteremia and prevent the establishment of metastatic foci of infection, (b) to reduce suppurative complications after bacterial contamination, and (c) to prevent local spread of existing infection. After suppuration has occurred (e.g., an abscess has formed), a cure by antibiotic therapy alone is very difficult to achieve; antimicrobials may serve to improve the results obtained with surgery.

⑤ An empirical antimicrobial regimen should be started as soon as the presence of intraabdominal infection is suspected. Therefore, antibiotics are usually initiated after culture specimens are collected but before identification of the infecting organisms is complete. Therapy must be initiated based on the likely pathogens. Predominant pathogens, as discussed in the preceding section, vary depending on the site of intraabdominal infection and the underlying disease process. Table 123–5 lists the likely pathogens against which antimicrobial agents should be directed.

Antimicrobial Experience Many studies have been conducted evaluating or comparing the effectiveness of antimicrobials for the treatment of intraabdominal infections. Substantial differences in patient outcomes from treatment with a variety of agents have not generally been demonstrated.[25]

Important findings from over 20 years of clinical trials regarding selection of antimicrobials for intraabdominal infections are the following:

- Antimicrobial regimens used for secondary infections should cover a broad spectrum of aerobic and anaerobic bacteria from the gastrointestinal tract. Treatment of healthcare-associated infections should consider the high prevalence of resistant bacterial and fungal pathogens.

- Single-agent regimens (such as antianaerobic cephalosporins, extended-spectrum penicillins with β-lactamase inhibitors,

and carbapenems) are as effective as combinations of aminoglycosides with antianaerobic agents. This is also true for antimicrobial treatment of acute bacterial contamination from penetrating abdominal trauma.[26,27]

- Clindamycin and metronidazole appear to be equivalent in efficacy when combined with agents effective against aerobic gram-negative bacilli (gentamicin or aztreonam).

- For most patients, antimicrobial treatment can be completed orally with amoxicillin-clavulanate or the combination of ciprofloxacin and metronidazole.

- Five to seven days of antimicrobial treatment is sufficient for most uncomplicated intraabdominal infections of mild to moderate severity.

Intraabdominal infection presents in many different ways and with a wide spectrum of severity. The regimen employed and duration of treatment depend on the specific clinical circumstances (i.e., the nature of the underlying disease process and the condition of the patient). Compromised patients require more aggressive therapies than do otherwise healthy patients who experience the same intraabdominal infection.

Recommendations ⑥ For most intraabdominal infections, the antimicrobial regimen should be effective against both aerobic and anaerobic bacteria.[28] When initial antimicrobial therapy is inappropriate, morbidity and mortality rates are higher than when appropriate agents are used.[29] Although it is impossible to provide antimicrobial activity against every possible pathogen, agents with activity against enteric gram-negative bacilli such as *E. coli* and *Klebsiella*, and anaerobes such as *B. fragilis* and *Clostridium* spp. should be administered. If most of the organisms can be eliminated through drainage or antimicrobials, the synergistic effect may be removed, and the patient's defenses may be able to resolve the remaining infection.

Table 123–6 presents the recommended agents for treatment of community-acquired and complicated intraabdominal infections from the Infectious Diseases Society of America and the Surgical Infection Society.[28,30,31] These recommendations were formulated using an evidence-based approach. Table 123–7 lists additional evidence-based recommendations. Most community-acquired infections are "mild to moderate," whereas healthcare-associated infections tend to be more severe, more difficult to treat, and more commonly resistant with bacteria or fungi. Table 123–8 presents guidelines for treatment and alternative regimens for specific situations. These are general guidelines; there are many factors that cannot be incorporated into such a table.

Most patients with severe intraabdominal infection, generalized peritonitis, or sepsis should be placed on a β-lactam–β-lactamase inhibitor combination or carbapenem such as imipenem, ertapenem, or meropenem. Combinations of an aminoglycoside with an antianaerobic agent, such as clindamycin or metronidazole, may be used, but such combinations are considered to be obsolete.[25] Gentamicin is the aminoglycoside of choice based on its lower cost. Other aminoglycosides, such as tobramycin or amikacin have no advantage in intraabdominal infection and generally are not drugs of first choice. Aztreonam may be used as an alternative to an aminoglycoside to avoid potential nephrotoxicity.

The dosage for aminoglycosides should be determined initially based on the patient's weight and renal function. Dosage adjustment should be performed by applying pharmacokinetic principles and by using peak and trough serum drug levels. Unless relatively resistant bacteria are suspected, a gentamicin or tobramycin peak concentration of 5 to 6 mcg/mL is usually effective. To achieve these serum concentrations, gentamicin or tobramycin dosage may range from 1 to 3 mg/kg per dose given as often as every 6 hours or as infrequently as every 48 hours if the patient has renal failure.

TABLE 123–5	Likely Intraabdominal Pathogens	
Type of Infection	**Aerobes**	**Anaerobes**
Primary bacterial peritonitis		
Children (spontaneous)	Group A *Streptococcus, E. coli*, pneumococci	–
Cirrhosis	*E. coli, Klebsiella,* pneumococci (many others)	–
Peritoneal dialysis	*Staphylococcus, Streptococcus, E. coli, Klebsiella, Pseudomonas*	–
Secondary bacterial peritonitis		
Gastroduodenal	*Streptococcus, E. coli*	–
Biliary tract	*E. coli, Klebsiella,* enterococci	*Clostridium* or *Bacteroides* (infrequent)
Small or large bowel	*E. coli, Klebsiella* spp., *Proteus* spp.	*Bacteroides fragilis* and other *Bacteroides, Clostridium*
Appendicitis	*E. coli, Pseudomonas*	*Bacteroides* spp.
Abscesses	*E. coli, Klebsiella,* enterococci	*B. fragilis* and other *Bacteroides, Clostridium,* anaerobic cocci
Liver	*E. coli, Klebsiella,* enterococci staphylococci, amoeba	*Bacteroides* (infrequent)
Spleen	*Staphylococcus, Streptococcus*	

TABLE 123-6 Recommended Agents for the Treatment of Community-Acquired Complicated Intraabdominal Infections

Agents Recommended for Mild to Moderate Infections	Agents Recommended for High-Severity Infections
β-Lactamase inhibitor combinations	
Ampicillin-sulbactam[a]	Piperacillin-tazobactam
Ticarcillin-clavulanate	
Carbapenems	
Ertapenem	Imipenem/cilastatin
	Meropenem, doripenem
Combination regimens	
Cefazolin or cefuroxime plus metronidazole	Third- or fourth-generation cephalosporins (cefotaxime, ceftriaxone, ceftizoxime, ceftazidime, cefepime) plus metronidazole
Ciprofloxacin, levofloxacin, moxifloxacin, or gatifloxacin in combination with metronidazole	Ciprofloxacin in combination with metronidazole
	Aztreonam plus metronidazole

[a]Use of ampicillin-sulbactam may be associated with treatment failure due to increasing resistance of E. coli.
From Solomkin et al.,[28] and Mazuski et al.[30,32]

Because aminoglycosides have concentration-dependent killing and a relatively long postantibiotic effect for aerobic gram-negative bacilli, once-daily administration (5 to 7 mg/kg) is a reasonable alternative and appears to be equivalent to multiple daily dosing.

When used for intraabdominal infection, aminoglycosides should be combined with agents that are effective against the majority of *B. fragilis*. Clindamycin or metronidazole is the agent of first choice, but others, such as antianaerobic cephalosporins (e.g., cefoxitin, cefotetan, or ceftizoxime), piperacillin, mezlocillin, and combinations of extended-spectrum penicillins with β-lactamase inhibitors, would be suitable alternatives. Clindamycin should be administered intravenously in a dosage of 600 or 900 mg every 8 hours. Patients receiving multiple broad-spectrum antimicrobial agents who are immunocompromised should receive an oral antifungal agent (nystatin) for prevention of fungal overgrowth in the mouth and GI tract. The benefits of systemic antifungal prophylaxis (with fluconazole) have not been established for intraabdominal infection and should not be used routinely.

With intraabdominal contamination from the upper GI tract (perforation of a peptic ulcer or biliary tract disease), *B. fragilis* is an uncommon pathogen, and other agents therefore may be substituted for clindamycin or metronidazole. Alternatives include ampicillin, penicillin, or first-generation cephalosporins.

CLINICAL CONTROVERSY

Enterococci are often isolated from intraabdominal infections, and many antimicrobials are ineffective against enterococci (such as cephalosporins and fluoroquinolones). Regimens without activity against enterococci (gentamicin with clindamycin or cephalosporins) are generally effective in treating intraabdominal infections; however, there are numerous reports of enterococcal superinfection in immunocompromised patients, particularly after broad-spectrum antimicrobial use. The Infectious Disease Society of America guidelines state that "Routine coverage against enterococcus is not necessary for patients with community-acquired intraabdominal infections. Antimicrobial therapy for enterococci (e.g., ampicillin, penicillin, or vancomycin) should be given when enterococci are recovered from patients with "healthcare-associated infections."

TABLE 123-7 Evidence-Based Recommendations for Treatment of Complicated Intraabdominal Infections

	Grade of recommendation[a]
Acute contamination as a result of trauma	
Bowel injuries caused by penetrating, blunt, or iatrogenic trauma that are repaired within 12 hours and intraoperative contamination of the operative field by enteric contents under other circumstances should be treated with antibiotics ≤24 hours.	A-1
Acute appendicitis	
Acute appendicitis without evidence of gangrene, perforation, abscess, or peritonitis requires only prophylactic administration of inexpensive regimens active against facultative and obligate anaerobes.	A-1
Community-acquired infections	
Antibiotics used for empirical treatment of community-acquired intraabdominal infections should be active against empiric gram-negative aerobic and facultative bacilli and β-lactam–susceptible gram-positive cocci.	A-1
For patients with mild-to-moderate community-acquired infections, agents that have a narrower spectrum of activity, such as ampicillin-sulbactam, cefazolin, or cefuroxime-metronidazole, ticarcillin-clavulanate, and ertapenem are preferable to more costly agents that have broader coverage against gram-negative organisms and/or greater risk of toxicity.	A-1
Anaerobic coverage	
Coverage against obligate anaerobic bacilli should be provided for distal small-bowel and colon-derived infections and for more proximal gastrointestinal perforations when obstruction is present.	A-1
Nosocomial infections	
Agents used to treat nosocomial infections in the intensive care unit (e.g., expanded gram-negative bacterial spectrum) should not be routinely used to treat community-acquired infections.	B-2
If a patient with diagnosed infection has previously been treated with an antibiotic, that patient should be treated as if he or she has had a healthcare-associated (nosocomial) infection.	B-3
Aminoglycosides	
Aminoglycosides are not recommended for routine use in community-acquired intraabdominal infections.	A-1
Oral completion therapy	
Completion of the antimicrobial course with oral forms of a quinolone plus metronidazole,	A-1
or with amoxicillin-clavulanic acid is acceptable for patients who are able to tolerate an oral diet.	B-3
Suspected fungal infection	
Antiinfective therapy for *Candida* should be withheld until the infecting species is identified.	C-3
Enterococcal infection	
Routine coverage against *Enterococcus* is not necessary for patients with community-acquired intraabdominal infections.	A-1

[a]Strength of recommendations: A, B, C = good, moderate, and poor evidence to support recommendation, respectively. Quality of evidence: 1 = Evidence from >1 properly randomized, controlled trial. 2 = Evidence from >1 well-designed clinical trial with randomization, from cohort or case-controlled analytic studies; from multiple time series, or from dramatic results from uncontrolled experiments. 3 = Evidence from opinions of respected authorities, based on clinical experience, descriptive studies, or reports of expert communities.
From Solomkin et al.,[28] and Mazuski et al.[30,31]

Coverage for enterococci for most community-acquired intraabdominal infections is not recommended.[23] The failure of host defenses may be a critical factor in the pathogenicity of enterococci. In immunocompromised patients, patients with valvular heart disease or a prosthetic heart valve, those who have had prior cephalosporin or carbapenem therapy, or those who have severe sepsis or septic shock, there is justification to provide specific antimicrobial activity against enterococci. In patients with healthcare-associated intraabdominal infections it is reasonable to include coverage of enterococcus in the initial regimen.[32] Ampicillin or other penicillins that are active against enterococci (e.g., penicillin, piperacillin, and mezlocillin) should be used in patients at high risk, patients with persistent or recurrent intraabdominal infection, or patients who are immunosuppressed, such as after organ transplantation. Ampicillin remains the drug of choice for this indication because it is most active in vitro against enterococcus and is relatively inexpensive. Vancomycin is active against most enterococci; however, resistance is increasing, and this agent should be reserved for established infections when first-line therapies cannot be used.

❼ Intraperitoneal administration of antibiotics is preferred over IV therapy in the treatment of peritonitis that occurs in patients undergoing CAPD.[33] The International Society of Peritoneal Dialysis guidelines for the diagnosis and pharmacotherapy of peritoneal dialysis–associated infections provide dosing recommendations for intermittent and continuous therapy based on the modality of dialysis (CAPD or automated peritoneal dialysis) and the extent of the patient's residual renal function.[34] Third-generation cephalosporins, such as cefotaxime, remain the treatments of choice for primary peritonitis associated with cirrhosis.[35]

Antimicrobial agents effective against both gram-positive and gram-negative organisms should be used for initial intraperitoneal empiric therapy for peritonitis in peritoneal dialysis patients. The most important factors to take into consideration for initial antimicrobial selection are the dialysis center's and the patient's history of infecting organisms and their sensitivities. The use of cefazolin (loading dose [LD] 500 mg/L; maintenance dose [MD] 125 mg/L) plus ceftazidime (LD 500 mg/L; MD 125 mg/L) or cefepime (LD 500 mg/L; MD 125 mg/L) or an aminoglycoside (gentamicin-tobramycin LD 8 mg/L; MD 4 mg/L) is suitable for initial empiric therapy; if patients are allergic to cephalosporin antibiotics, vancomycin (LD 1,000 mg/L; MD 25 mg/L) or an aminoglycoside should be substituted. Another option is monotherapy with imipenem-cilastin (LD 500 mg/L; MD 200 mg/L) or cefepime. Antimicrobial doses should empirically be increased by 25% in patients with residual renal function (more than 100 mL/day urine output).[34] Antimicrobial therapy should be continued for at least 1 week after the dialysate fluid is clear and for a total of at least 14 days. The reader is referred to these guidelines for additional information.[34]

After acute bacterial contamination, such as with abdominal trauma where GI contents spill into the peritoneum, combination antimicrobial regimens are not required. If the patient is seen soon after injury (within 2 hours) and surgical measures are instituted promptly, antianaerobic cephalosporins (such as cefoxitin or cefotetan) or extended-spectrum penicillins are effective in preventing most infectious complications. Antimicrobials should be administered as soon as possible after injury.

For appendicitis, the antimicrobial regimen used should depend on the appearance of the appendix at the time of operation, which may be normal, inflamed, gangrenous, or perforated. Because the condition of the appendix is unknown preoperatively, it is advisable to begin antimicrobial agents before the appendectomy is performed. Reasonable regimens would be antianaerobic cephalosporins or, if the patient is seriously ill, a carbapenem or β-lactam–β-lactamase inhibitor combination. If, at operation, the appendix is normal or inflamed, postoperative antimicrobials are not required. If the appendix is gangrenous or perforated, a treatment course of 5 to 7 days with the agents listed in Table 123–8 is appropriate.

❽ The necessary duration of treatment for intraabdominal infections is not clearly defined. Acute intraabdominal contamination, such as after a traumatic injury, may be treated with a very short course (24 hours).[36] For established infections (i.e., peritonitis or intraabdominal abscess), an antimicrobial course limited to 5 to 7 days is justified. This allows eradication of bacteria remaining in the peritoneum after a surgical procedure that may enter the peritoneum through healing suture lines. Under certain conditions, therapy for longer than 7 days would be justified (e.g., if the patient remains febrile or is in poor general condition, when relatively resistant bacteria are isolated, or when a focus of infection in the abdomen may still be present). For some abscesses, such as pyogenic liver abscess, antimicrobials may be required for a month or longer.

Intraperitoneal irrigation of antimicrobial agents for treatment of intraabdominal infection has been studied, often with conflicting results.[37] Intraoperative antimicrobial irrigation does not improve patient outcomes in comparison with copious intraoperative irrigation with normal saline. Possibly the most important aspect of peritoneal irrigation is the dilutional effect on bacteria and adjuvants that promotes infection (intestinal contents and hemoglobin). Most systemically administered antimicrobials easily cross the peritoneal membrane so that peritoneal fluid concentrations are similar to serum. Confined areas, such as an abscess, can be expected to attain much lower antimicrobial concentrations.

EVALUATION OF THERAPEUTIC OUTCOMES

Whichever antimicrobial regimen is chosen, the patient should be reassessed continually to determine the success or failure of therapies. The clinician should recognize that there are many reasons for poor patient outcome with intraabdominal infection; improper antimicrobial administration is only one. The patient may be immunocompromised, which decreases the likelihood of successful outcome with any regimen. It is impossible for antimicrobials to compensate for a nonfunctioning immune system. There may be surgical reasons for poor patient outcome. Failure to identify all intraabdominal foci of infection or leaks from a GI anastomosis may cause continued intraabdominal infection. Even when intraabdominal infection is controlled, accompanying organ system failure, most often renal or respiratory, may lead to patient demise. Finally, antimicrobial resistance may relate to treatment failure as isolates from intraabdominal infections are increasingly drug resistant.[38]

The outcome from intraabdominal infection is not determined solely by what transpires in the abdomen. Unsatisfactory outcomes in patients with intraabdominal infections may result from complications that arise in other organ systems. Infectious complications commonly associated with mortality after intraabdominal infection are urinary tract infections and pneumonia.[39] A high APACHE (Acute Physiology and Chronic Health Evaluation) II score, low serum albumin concentration, and high New York Heart Association cardiac function status were significantly and independently associated with increased mortality from intraabdominal infection.[40]

❾ Once antimicrobials are initiated and the other important therapies described earlier are used, most patients should show improvement within 2 to 3 days. Usually, temperature will return to near normal, vital signs should stabilize, and the patient should not appear in distress, with the exception of recognized discomfort and pain from incisions, drains, and the nasogastric tube. At 24 to 48 hours, aerobic bacterial culture results should return. If a suspected pathogen is not sensitive to the antimicrobial agents being given, the regimen should be changed if the patient has not shown sufficient improvement. If the isolated pathogen is extremely sensitive to one antimicrobial and the patient is progressing well, concurrent antimicrobial therapy may often be discontinued.

TABLE 123-8 Guidelines for Initial Antimicrobial Agents for Intraabdominal Infections

	Primary Agents	Alternatives
Primary bacterial peritonitis		
Cirrhosis	Cefotaxime	1. Add clindamycin or metronidazole if anaerobes are suspected
		2. Other third-generation cephalosporins, extended-spectrum penicillins, aztreonam, and imipenem as alternatives
		3. Piperacillin–tazobactam
Peritoneal dialysis	Initial empiric regimens	1. An aminoglycoside may be used in place of ceftazidime or cefepime
	Cefazolin or cephalothin plus ceftazidime or cefepime	2. Imipenem/cilastatin or cefepime may be used alone
		3. Quinolones may be used in place of ceftazidime or cefepime if local susceptibilities allow
	1. *Staphylococcus*: penicillinase-resistant penicillin or first-generation cephalosporin	1. Alternative for methicillin resistant staphylococci is vancomycin
		2. For vancomycin-resistant *Staphylococcus aureus*, linezolid, daptomycin, or quinupristin-dalfopristin must be used
	2. *Streptococcus or Enterococcus:* ampicillin	1. An aminoglycoside may be added for enterococcal peritonitis
		2. Linezolid or quinupristin-dalfopristin should be used to treat vancomycin-resistant enterococcus not susceptible to ampicillin
	3. Aerobic gram-negative bacilli: ceftazidime or cefepime	1. The regimen should be based on in vitro sensitivity tests
	4. *Pseudomonas aeruginosa*: two agents with differing mechanisms of action, such as an oral quinolone plus ceftazidime, cefepime, tobramycin, or piperacillin	
Secondary bacterial peritonitis		
Perforated peptic ulcer	First-generation cephalosporins	1. Antianaerobic cephalosporins[a]
		2. Possibly add aminoglycoside if patient condition is poor
		3. Aminoglycoside with clindamycin or metronidazole; add ampicillin if patient is immunocompromised or if biliary tract origin of infection
Other	Imipenem-cilastatin, meropenem, ertapenem, or extended-spectrum penicillins with β-lactamase inhibitor	1. Ciprofloxacin with metronidazole
		2. Aztreonam with clindamycin or metronidazole
		3. Antianaerobic cephalosporins[a]
Abscess		
General	Imipenem-cilastatin, meropenem, ertapenem, or extended-spectrum penicillins with β-lactamase inhibitor	1. Aztreonam with clindamycin or metronidazole
		2. Ciprofloxacin with metronidazole
		3. Aminoglycoside with clindamycin or metronidazole;
Liver	As above but add a first-generation cephalosporin	Use metronidazole if amoebic liver abscess is suspected
Spleen	Aminoglycoside plus penicillinase-resistant penicillin	Alternatives for penicillinase-resistant penicillin are first-generation cephalosporins or vancomycin
Appendicitis		
Normal or inflamed	Antianaerobic cephalosporins[a] (discontinued immediately postoperation)	1. Ampicillin-sulbactam
Gangrenous or perforated	Imipenem-cilastatin, meropenem, ertapenem, antianaerobic cephalosporins, or extended-spectrum penicillins with β-lactamase inhibitor	1. Aztreonam with clindamycin or metronidazole
		2. Ciprofloxacin with metronidazole
		3. Aminoglycoside with clindamycin or metronidazole
Acute cholecystitis	First-generation cephalosporin	Aminoglycoside plus ampicillin if severe infection
Cholangitis	Aminoglycoside with ampicillin with or without clindamycin or metronidazole	Use vancomycin instead of ampicillin if patient is allergic to penicillin
Acute contamination from abdominal trauma	Antianaerobic cephalosporins[a] or ampicillin-sulbactam	1. A carbapenem
		2. Ciprofloxacin plus metronidazole
Pelvic inflammatory disease	Cefotetan or cefoxitin with doxycycline	1. Clindamycin with gentamicin
		2. Ciprofloxacin with doxycycline and metronidazole

[a]Cefoxitin, cefotetan, and ceftizoxime.

CLINICAL CONTROVERSY

Although some investigators suggest that routine culturing of patients with community-acquired intraabdominal infections contributes little to their management,[33] other investigators suggest that antimicrobial therapy should be based on susceptibility of the bacteria collected from the operative site because this correlates with clinical outcome.[34]

With anaerobic culturing techniques and the slow growth of these organisms, anaerobes are often not identified until 4 to 7 days after culture, and sensitivity information is difficult to obtain. For this reason, there are usually few data with which to alter the antianaerobic component of the antimicrobial regimen. A report indicating that anaerobes were not isolated should not be the sole justification for discontinuing antianaerobic drugs because anaerobic bacteria that were present in the infectious process may not have been transported properly to the microbiology laboratory, or other problems may have led to cell death in vitro.

Reasons for antimicrobial failure may not always be apparent. Even when antimicrobial susceptibility tests indicate that an organism is susceptible in vitro to the antimicrobial agent, therapeutic failures may occur. Possibly there is poor penetration of the antimicrobial agent into the focus of infection, or bacterial resistance may develop after initiation of antimicrobial therapy. Also, it is possible that an antimicrobial regimen may encourage the development of infection by organisms not susceptible to the regimen being used. Superinfection in patients being treated for intraabdominal infection can be caused by *Candida;* however, enterococci or opportunistic gram-negative bacilli such as *Pseudomonas* or *Serratia* may be involved.

Treatment regimens for intraabdominal infection can be judged as successful if the patient recovers from the infection without recurrent peritonitis or intraabdominal abscess and without the need for additional antimicrobials. A regimen can be considered unsuccessful if a significant adverse drug reaction occurs, reoperation or percutaneous drainage is necessary, or patient improvement is delayed beyond 1 or 2 weeks. The costs of treatment can be significantly reduced if parenteral antimicrobials can be switched to oral agents for completion of therapy.[41]

ABBREVIATIONS

CAPD: chronic ambulatory peritoneal dialysis

CT: computed tomography

IL: interleukin

LD: loading dose

MD: maintenance dose

REFERENCES

1. Ordonez CA, Puyana JC. Management of peritonitis in the critically ill patient. Surg Clin North Am 2006;86:1323–1349.
2. Marshall JC. Intra-abdominal infections. Microbes Infect 2004;6:1015–1025.
3. Marshall JC, Innes M. Intensive care unit management of intraabdominal infection. Crit Care Med 2003;31:2228–2237.
4. Mowat C, Stanley AJ. Spontaneous bacterial peritonitis—diagnosis, treatment, and prevention. Aliment Pharmacol Ther 2001;15:1851–1859.
5. Mujais S. Microbiology and outcomes of peritonitis in North America. Kidney International. 2006;70:555–562.
6. DeFrances CJ, Lucas CA, Buie VC, Golosinskiy A. 2006 National Hospital Discharge Survey, #5. National Center for Health Statistics; July 30, 2008.
7. Toloza EM, Wilson SE. Cholecystitis and cholangitis. In: Fry DE, ed. Surgical Infections. Boston: Little, Brown; 1995:254–263.
8. Brook I. Microbiology and management of abdominal infections. Dig Dis Sci 2008;53:2585–2591.
9. Schein M, Wittman DH, Holzheimer R, et al. Hypothesis: Compartmentalization of cytokines in intraabdominal infection. Surgery 1996;119:694–700.
10. Riche FC, Cholley BP, Panis YH, et al. Inflammatory cytokine response in patients with septic shock secondary to generalized peritonitis. Crit Care Med 2000;28:433–437.
11. Malangoni MA. Contributions to the management of intraabdominal infection. Am J Surg 2005;190:255–259.
12. Thompson AE, Marshall JC, Opal SM. Intraabdominal infections in infants and children: Descriptions and definitions. Pediatr Crit Care Med 2005;6:S30–S35.
13. Johnson DH, Cuhna BA. Infections in cirrhosis. Infect Dis Clin North Am 2001;15:363–371.
14. Troidle L, Gordon-Brennan N, Kliger A, Finkelstein F. Differing outcomes of gram-positive and gram-negative peritonitis. Am J Kidney Dis 1998;32:623–628.
15. Brook I, Frazier EH. Aerobic and anaerobic microbiology of retroperitoneal abscesses. Clin Infect Dis 1998;26:938–941.
16. Bennion RS, Baron EJ, Thompson JE, et al. The bacteriology of gangrenous and perforated appendicitis—Revisited. Ann Surg 1990;211:165–171.
17. Sawyer RG, Rosenlof LK, Adams RB, et al. Peritonitis into the 1990s: Changing pathogens and changing strategies in the critically ill. Am Surg 1992;58:82–87.
18. Montravers P, Lepape A, Dubreuil L, et al. Clinical and microbiological profiles of community-acquired and nosocomial infections: Results of

19. the French prospective, observational EBIIA study. J Antimicrob Chemother. 2009;63:785–794.
19. Onderdonk AB, Bartlett JG, Louie T, et al. Microbial synergy in experimental intraabdominal abscess. Infect Immun 1997;13:22–26.
20. Donskey CJ, Chowdhry TK, Hecker MT, et al. Effect of antibiotic therapy on the density of vancomycin-resistant enterococci in the stool of colonized patients. Ann Surg 2000;343:1925–1932.
21. Sitges-Serra A, Lopez MJ, Girvent M, et al. Postoperative enterococcal infection after treatment of complicated intraabdominal sepsis. Br J Surg 2002;89:361–367.
22. Youssef IM, Milardovic R, Perone RWM, Heiba SI, Abdel-Dayem HM. Importance of 99mTc-sulfur colloid liver-spleen scans performed before 111indium labeled leukocyte imaging for localization of abdominal infection. Clin Nucl Med 2005;30:87–90.
23. Pieracci FM, Barie PS. Intra-abdominal infections. Curr Opin Crit Care 2007;13:440–449.
24. Jaffe TA, Nelson RC, Delong DM, Paulson EK. Practice patterns in percutaneous image-guided intraabdominal abscess drainage: Survey of academic and private practice centers. Radiology 2004;233:750–756.
25. Wong PF, Gilliam AD, Kumar S, et al. Antibiotic regimens for secondary peritonitis of gastrointestinal origin in adults. Cochrane Database Syst Rev 2007;2;CD 004539.
26. Hooker KD, DiPiro JT, Wynn JJ. Aminoglycoside combinations versus single β-lactams for penetrating abdominal trauma: A meta analysis. J Trauma 1991;31:1155–1160.
27. Solomkin JS, Dellinger EP, Christou NV, et al. Results of a multicenter trial comparing imipenem/cilastatin to tobramycin/clindamycin for intraabdominal infections. Ann Surg 1990;212:581–591.
28. Solomkin JS, Mazuski JE, Baron EJ, et al. Guidelines for the selection of anti-infective agents for complicated intraabdominal infections. Clin Infect Dis 2003;37:997–1005.
29. Gauzit R, Pean Y, Mistretta F, Lalaude O. Epidemiology, management, and prognosis of secondary non-postoperative peritonitis: A French prospective observational multicenter study. Surg Infect 2009;10;119–127.
30. Mazuski JE, Sawyer RG, Nathens AB, et al. The Surgical Infection Society guidelines on antimicrobial therapy for intraabdominal infections: An executive summary. Surg Infect (Larchmt) 2002;3:161–174.
31. Mazuski JE, Sawyer RG, Nathens AB, et al. The Surgical Infection Society guidelines on antimicrobial therapy for intraabdominal infections: Evidence for recommendations. Surg Infect (Larchmt) 2002;3:175–234.
32. Solomkin JS, Mazuski J. Intra-abdominal sepsis: Newer interventional and antimicrobial therapies. Infect Dis Clin N Am 23:209:593–608.
33. Wiggins KJ, Craig JC, Johnson DW, Strippoli GF. Treatment for peritoneal dialysis-associated peritonitis. Cochrane Database of Systematic Reviews. 2008 (1):CD005284.
34. Piraino B, Bailie GR, Bernardini J, et al. Peritoneal dialysis related infections: 2005, update. Perit Dial Int 2005;25:107–131.
35. Runyon BA. Management of adult patients with ascites due to cirrhosis: An update. Hepatology 2009;49:2087–2107.
36. Bozorgzadeh A, Pizzi WF, Barie PS, et al. The duration of antibiotic administration in predicting abdominal trauma. Am J Surg 1999;172:125–135.
37. Schein M, Gecelter G, Freinkel W, et al. Peritoneal lavage in abdominal sepsis: A controlled clinical study. Arch Surg 1990;125:1132–1135.
38. Baquero F, Hsueh P, Paterson DL, et al. In vitro susceptibilities of aerobic and facultatively anaerobic gram-negative bacilli isolated from patients with intra-abdominal infections worldwide: 2005 results from study for monitoring antimicrobial resistance trends. Surg Infect 2009;10:99–104.
39. Merlino JI, Yowler CJ, Malangoni MA. Nosocomial infections adversely affect the outcomes of patients with serious intraabdominal infections. Surg Infect (Larchmt) 2004;5:21–27.
40. Christou NV, Barie PS, Dellinger EP, et al. Surgical infection society intraabdominal infection study. Arch Surg 1993;128:193–199.
41. Paladino JA, Gilliland-Johnson KK, Adelman MH, Coohn SM. Pharmacoeconomics of ciprofloxacin plus metromidazole vs. piperacillin-tazobactam for complicated intra-abdominal infections. Surg Infect 2008;9:325

CHAPTER 124

Parasitic Diseases

J. V. ANANDAN

KEY CONCEPTS

❶ All symptomatic adults and children older than 8 years of age with giardiasis can be treated with metronidazole 250 mg 3 times daily for 5 to 10 days, or tinidazole 2 g once, or nitazoxanide 500 mg twice daily for 3 days.

❷ Amebic liver abscesses can spread to the lungs and pleura. Pericardial infections, although rare, may be associated with extension of the amebic abscess from the left lobe of the liver. Erosion of liver abscesses also present as peritonitis.

❸ Asymptomatic cyst passers and patients with mild intestinal amebiasis should receive one of the following luminal agents: paromomycin 25 to 35 mg/kg/day 3 times daily for 7 days, iodoquinol 650 mg 3 times daily for 20 days, or diloxanide furoate 500 mg 3 times daily for 10 days.

❹ Mebendazole (Vermox), an oral synthetic benzimidazole, is the agent of first choice for hookworm. It is also effective against ascariasis, enterobiasis, and trichuriasis.

❺ Administration of corticosteroids or other immunosuppressive drugs to an infected individual with strongyloidiasis can result in hyperinfections and disseminated strongyloidiasis.

❻ The most serious complication of cysticercosis is invasion of the central nervous system which results in neurocysticercosis. Neurocysticercosis can cause obstructive hydrocephalus, strokes, and seizures; antihelminthic treatment for these conditions remains controversial.

❼ When intravenous quinidine is not readily available, intravenous artesunate (available under an investigational new drug (IND) from the CDC at *www.cdc.gov/malaria/features/artesunate_now_available.htm*), a water-soluble artemisinin derivative, administered at 2.4 mg/kg/dose for 3 days at 0, 12, 24, 48, and 72 hours is the recommended drug if severe *Plasmodium falciparum* is suspected.

❽ Because *falciparum* malaria is associated with serious complications, including pulmonary edema, hypoglycemia, jaundice, renal failure, confusion, delirium, seizures, coma, and death, careful monitoring of fluid status and hemodynamic parameters is mandatory. Either hemofiltration or hemodiafiltration is indicated in renal failure.

Learning objectives, review questions, and other resources can be found at **www.pharmacotherapyonline.com**.

❾ The drugs that have been used to treat *Trypanosoma cruzi* infections include nifurtimox (Lampit, Bayer 2502) and benznidazole (Rochagan).

❿ Permethrin (1% and 5%) for pediculosis and scabies, respectively, is the preferred agent and remains the safest agent, especially in infants and children.

Parasitic diseases continue to receive increasing attention from clinicians in the United States because of the high frequency of travel, deployment of personnel for humanitarian and military missions (e.g., Peace Corps volunteers), inflow of immigrants from a wider geographic distribution, and the presence of immunosuppressed populations (e.g., acquired immunodeficiency syndrome [AIDS] and transplant patients). Migrant farm workers who work and live in substandard hygienic conditions, the large and growing Central and South American immigrant population, and other inadequately screened immigrants from Asia represent significant sources of parasitic infections in the United States.[1-9] Clinicians need to have a heightened awareness of parasitic diseases and how to treat them. Clinical signs and symptoms, together with the patient's travel history, should be used with other diagnostic aids in the identification of parasitic diseases. Parasitic infections caused by pathogenic protozoa or helminths affect more than 3 billion people worldwide and impose tremendous health and economic burdens on developing countries.[9]

This chapter discusses the major parasitic diseases, including protozoan diseases (giardiasis, amebiasis, malaria, and Chagas disease), helminthic infections (ascariasis, enterobiasis, hookworm, strongyloidiasis, and cestodiasis), and ectoparasitic infestations (head and body lice). Emphasis is placed on diseases seen more frequently in the United States. World distribution of parasites depends on the presence of suitable hosts, habitats, and environmental conditions.[9] A human parasite that does not use an intermediate host is likely to be found in any inhabited region of the world as long as the environmental conditions are suitable. *Ascaris* (roundworm) and *Trichuris* (whipworm) require carelessness of habits for transfer and require time outside the human body, where they are exposed to heat and dryness, to reach the infective stage. The distribution of the hookworm is more limited because the free-living forms are unprotected by resistant shells or cysts. African trypanosomiasis never occurs outside the range of the tsetse fly; malaria normally never occurs beyond the range of the infective *Anopheles* mosquito; and schistosomiasis never occurs in the absence of a specific water snail. The prevalence of clonorchiasis (Chinese liver fluke) is an example of the impact of both environmental and geographic factors. Clonorchiasis requires the simultaneous presence of not only humans, specific snail species, and certain fish, but also unsanitary conditions that make the eggs accessible to the snails, an association of the snail and fish, and the established local habit of eating raw fish. The ability of some parasites to infect hosts other than humans may perpetuate an infection even when human habits preclude the possibility of more than occasional access to the human body. In North America, the broad tapeworm (*Diphyllobothrium latum*) would perish if it were not that dogs and other carnivores, such as the brown bear, serve as reservoir hosts.

HOST–PARASITE RELATIONSHIP

Symbiosis is the association of two species for the purpose of obtaining food for either one or the other. *Parasitism* is a symbiotic relationship in which one species, the host, is injured through the activities of the other. Through evolution, parasites have made specific morphologic adaptations. Adaptation to the host has taken a number of forms: loss of locomotor organelles in the protozoan *Sporozoa*; partial and complete lack of digestive systems in the trematodes and cestodes, respectively; elaboration of proteolytic enzymes to penetrate the host intestinal mucosa by *Entamoeba histolytica*; the cercariae of the blood fluke that penetrate the skin of the host by elaborate enzymes; and, finally, the ability to infect an intermediate host to increase reproductive capacity, as seen among the cestodes and trematodes.[9]

Parasites normally inflict some degree of injury to the host, the extent of which depends on such factors as parasite load, nutritional status, and immunologic competence of the host. *Entamoeba coli* is considered commensal because it subsists on the bacterial flora of the gut and does not cause any harm to the host. Unlike *Entamoeba coli*, *Fasciolopsis buski*, the giant intestinal fluke, can produce severe local damage to the intestinal wall. *Ascaris*, the roundworm, can perforate the bowel wall, cause intestinal obstruction, and invade the appendix and bile duct. Malarial parasites destroy red blood cells by multiplying inside them. *Diphyllobothrium latum*, or the broad fish tapeworm, removes vitamin B_{12} from the gastrointestinal tract (GI) tract, resulting in megaloblastic anemia.[9]

PROTOZOAN DISEASES

GIARDIASIS

Epidemiology and Etiology

Giardia lamblia (also known as *Giardia intestinalis* or *Giardia duodenalis*), an enteric protozoan, is the most common intestinal parasite responsible for diarrheal syndromes throughout the world.[10–13] *Giardia* is the most frequently identified intestinal parasite in the United States, with a prevalence rate of 15% in some areas. *G lamblia* is the first enteric pathogen seen in children in developing countries, with prevalence rates between 15% and 30%.[12]

There are two stages in the life cycle of *G lamblia*: the trophozoite and the cyst. *G lamblia*, which is found in the small intestine, the gallbladder, and biliary drainage, is a pear-shaped trophozoite with four pairs of flagella. Two nuclei lie in the area of the sucking disk, giving the protozoan a characteristic face-like image.

The distribution of giardiasis is worldwide. Children seem to be affected more frequently than adults. Children in day care centers may infect parents and other family members.[12] In less developed countries, fecal contamination of the environment and lack of potable water, education, and housing continue to be risk factors for giardiasis among children.

Pathology

Giardiasis results from ingestion of *G lamblia* cysts in fecally contaminated water or food. The protozoan excysts under the stimulus

TABLE 124-1	Clinical Presentation of Giardiasis

Acute onset
Diarrhea, cramp-like abdominal pain, bloating, and flatulence[10–12]
Malaise, anorexia, nausea, and belching[12]

Chronic
Diarrhea: foul-smelling, copious, light-colored, fatty stools; weight loss
Periods of diarrhea alternating with constipation
Steatorrhea, lactose intolerance, vitamin B_{12}, and fat-soluble vitamin deficiencies[10–14]

of low gastric pH to release the trophozoite.[12] Colonization and multiplication of the trophozoite lead to mucosal invasion, localized edema, and flattening of the villi, resulting in malabsorption states in the host.[10–13]

Lactose intolerance precipitated by giardiasis can persist even after eradication of the protozoan. Achlorhydria, hypogammaglobulinemia, or deficiency in secretory immunoglobulin A (IgA) are predispositions for giardiasis.[10,12,13] Table 124-1 describes the clinical presentation of giardiasis.

Diagnosis of giardiasis is made by examination of fresh stool or a preserved specimen during the acute diarrheal phase. Fresh stool specimens may show the trophozoites, whereas preserved specimens usually yield the cysts. If both the stool examination and string test prove unsuccessful, it may be necessary to attempt duodenal aspiration and biopsy to confirm the diagnosis; this may be more important in AIDS patients and in patients with hypogammaglobulinemia.[10,12] Most clinicians advocate a clinical trial of the standard therapy before undertaking invasive diagnostic tests. Detection of the trophozoites or cysts in fecal samples by enzymelinked immunosorbent assay (ELISA) or immunofluorescence or identification of the *Giardia* antigen by counterimmunoelectrophoresis are alternative ways for diagnosis of giardiasis.[9,10,12,15]

TREATMENT

Giardiasis

■ DESIRED OUTCOME

To reduce morbidity and to avoid complications in patients identified with prolonged diarrhea and malabsorption and who have a recent history of travel to an endemic area, rapid identification by ova and parasite examination or by antigen detection test should be used to institute appropriate therapy.[13]

■ PHARMACOLOGIC THERAPY

❶ All symptomatic adults and children older than 8 years of age with giardiasis can be treated with metronidazole 250 mg 3 times daily for 5 to 10 days, or tinidazole 2 g once, or nitazoxanide 500 mg twice daily for 3 days.[16] The alternative drugs include furazolidone 100 mg 4 times daily or paromomycin 25 to 35 mg/kg/day in divided doses daily for 1 week.[11–14,16,17] Paromomycin 25 to 35 mg/kg/day in three doses for 7 to 10 days is a safe agent in pregnancy.[10,12,16] The pediatric dose for metronidazole is 15 mg/kg/day 3 times daily for 5 to 7 days.[16] The pediatric dose of tinidazole is 50 mg/kg (maximum 2 g) once while nitazoxanide (Alinia) suspension is dosed at 100 mg every 12 hours (1–3 years), 200 mg every 12 hours (4–11 years) and the adult dose is recommended for children older than 12 years; all are administered for 3 days.[12,16] Quinacrine, which was the drug of choice in giardiasis, has been discontinued by the manufacturer but is obtained in the United States from a specialized pharmacy (see Appendix 124–1). Albendazole 400 mg daily for 5 days has been cited to produce cure rates of 97% and as being equivalent to metronidazole in children. However, other investigators have disputed the efficacy of this agent.[17]

Evaluation of Therapeutic Outcomes

Patients with symptomatic giardiasis, positive stool samples, or the detection of *Giardia* antigen by counterimmunoelectrophoresis or ELISA should be treated with metronidazole for 5 to 7 days. Metronidazole produces cure rates of between 85% and 95%.[10,17] Diarrhea will stop within a few days, although in some patients it may take 1 to 2 weeks. Cyst excretion will cease within days; however, intestinal dysfunction (manifested as increased transit time) and radiologic changes (irregular thickening of the folds in the upper small intestine) may take a few months to resolve.[10] Patients who fail initial therapy with metronidazole should receive a second course of therapy. Nitazoxanide (500 mg twice daily for 3 days) is effective in patients who are not responding to metronidazole.[12] Pregnant patients can receive paromomycin 25 to 35 mg/kg/day in divided doses for 7 days. Metronidazole has been used in the second and third trimesters of pregnancy.[12] Giardiasis can be prevented by good personal hygiene and by caution in food and drink consumption.

AMEBIASIS

Epidemiology and Etiology

Because of its worldwide distribution and serious gastrointestinal manifestations, amebiasis is one of the most important parasitic diseases of humans.[9,18–21] The major causative organism in amebiasis is *E histolytica*, which inhabits the colon and must be differentiated from the *Entamoeba dispar* and a recently identified species, *E moshkovskii* which are associated with an asymptomatic carrier state. *E dispar* is considered nonpathogenic, while the status of *E moshkovskii* remains to be defined.[19] Although *E histolytica* and *E dispar* are indistinguishable morphologically, monoclonal antibodies have been used to separate the two.[20,21] The *Entamoeba histolytica* II kit (TechLab, Blacksburg, VA) remains the most specific test for *E histolytica*.[19] Invasive amebiasis is almost exclusively the result of *E histolytica* infection. Approximately 50 million cases of invasive disease result each year worldwide, leading to an excess of 100,000 deaths.[19,21] The incidence of amebiasis is estimated at approximately 4% in the general U.S. population.[21] The highest incidence is found in institutionalized mentally retarded patients, sexually active homosexuals, patients with AIDS, and new immigrants from endemic areas (e.g., Mexico, India, West and South Africa, and portions of Central and South America).[19,21]

Pathology

E histolytica invades mucosal cells of colonic epithelium, producing the classic flask-shaped ulcer in the submucosa.[19–23] The trophozoite has a cytolethal effect on cells through a toxin. If the trophozoite gets into the portal circulation, it will be carried to the liver, where it produces abscess and periportal fibrosis.[19–24] Amebic ulcerations can affect the colon, perineum, and genitalia, and abscesses may occur in the lung and brain.[20–24]

Clinical Presentation

The most frequent clinical manifestations of the disease are gastrointestinal (Table 124–2).
❷ Amebic liver abscesses can spread to the lungs and pleura.[20,21] Pericardial infections, although rare, may be associated with extension of the amebic abscess from the left lobe of the liver. Erosion of liver abscesses also present as peritonitis.[19–22]

TABLE 124–2 Most Common Manifestations of Amebiasis

Intestinal disease
Vague abdominal discomfort, malaise to severe abdominal cramps, flatulence, bloody diarrhea (heme-positive in 100% of cases) with mucus[19–21]
Eosinophilia is usually absent, although moderate leukocytosis is not unusual[20,21]

Amebic liver abscess
High fever, rigors and profuse sweating, significant leukocytosis with left shift, elevated alkaline phosphatase, and liver tenderness on palpation[21,22,24]
Right-upper-quadrant pain, hepatomegaly, and liver tenderness, with referred pain to the left or right shoulder
Erosion of liver abscesses may also present as peritonitis[19–21]

Review of the patient's history and recent travel should be strongly emphasized. Intestinal amebiasis is diagnosed by demonstrating *E histolytica* cysts or trophozoites (may contain ingested erythrocytes) in fresh stool or from a specimen obtained by sigmoidoscopy. Three stool samples obtained 24 to 36 hours apart will produce a 60% to 90% yield for *E histolytica*. Microscopy may not differentiate between the pathogenic *E histolytica* and the nonpathogenic *E dispar* in stools. Sensitive techniques are available to detect *E histolytica* in stool, including ELISA and antigen detection.[19–21,23] Endoscopy with scraping or biopsy may provide more definitive diagnosis where stool examinations do not provide adequate evidence.[19,21]

When amebic liver abscess is suspected from initial physical examination and history, confirmatory diagnostic procedures will include serology and liver scans (using isotopes by ultrasound or computed tomography) or magnetic resonance imaging.[20,21] Leukocytosis (>10,000/mm³) and an elevated alkaline phosphatase concentration (>75%) are common findings. In rare instances, needle aspiration of the hepatic abscess may be attempted using ultrasound guidance.[20–22,24]

TREATMENT

Amebiasis

■ DESIRED OUTCOME

In amebiasis, the goals of therapy are initially to eradicate the parasite by use of specific amebicides and then to render supportive therapy.

■ TREATMENT REGIMENS

A number of different regimens have been suggested depending on the category of amebiasis: asymptomatic cyst passers, intestinal amebiasis, and amebic liver abscess.[13,19–22] Electrolyte replacement, antibiotic therapy, and nutritional support are essential adjunctive treatment modalities. Large hepatic abscess or amebic pericarditis may require needle aspiration, percutaneous catheter drainage, or, rarely, surgery before drug therapy.[20–22] Most regimens require a combination of drugs administered concurrently or sequentially.[19,21,24]

A careful history should be taken when one of the differential diagnoses is ulcerative colitis because corticosteroid administration has the potential to unmask amebiasis and produce toxic megacolon.[22]

■ PHARMACOLOGIC THERAPY

Metronidazole (Flagyl), dehydroemetine, and chloroquine (Aralen) are tissue-acting agents, whereas iodoquinol (Yodoxin), diloxanide furoate (Furamide), and paromomycin (Humatin) are luminal amebicides. A systemic agent may be so well absorbed that only small amounts of the drug stay in the bowel, which might prove ineffective as a luminal agent.[20-23] A luminal-acting agent, on the other hand, may be too poorly absorbed to be effective in the tissue. In the asymptomatic cyst passer, it is necessary to eradicate the causative agent from the lumen to prevent intestinal amebiasis or the development of amebic liver abscess. Drug effectiveness must be monitored by stool examination, that is, from one to three negative specimens from 1 to 3 months after treatment.

❸ Asymptomatic cyst passers and patients with mild intestinal amebiasis should receive one of the following luminal agents: paromomycin 25 to 35 mg/kg/day 3 times daily for 7 days, iodoquinol 650 mg 3 times daily for 20 days, or diloxanide furoate 500 mg 3 times daily for 10 days.[16] These regimens have cure rates of between 84% and 96%.[21] Diloxanide furoate is available only from Ponorama Compounding Pharmacy (6744 Balboa Blvd., Van Nuys, CA 91406, (800) 247–9767; or Medical Center Pharmacy, New Haven, CT, (203) 688–6816].[16] The pediatric dose for paromomycin is the same as in adults, whereas the dose of iodoquinol is 30 to 40 mg/kg/day (maximum:2 g) in three doses for 20 days, and the dose of diloxanide furoate is 20 mg/kg/day in three doses for 10 days.[16] Paromomycin is the preferred luminal agent in pregnant patients.[13,21]

Patients with severe intestinal disease or liver abscess should receive metronidazole 750 mg 3 times daily for 10 days, followed by a course of one of the luminal agents indicated earlier.[13,20-21] Tinidazole 2 g mg once daily for 5 days has been suggested for amebic liver abscess.[16,22] In the pediatric patient, the dose of oral metronidazole is 50 mg/kg/day in divided doses to be followed by a luminal agent.[16] Patients who are too ill to take oral metronidazole should receive the drug in equivalent doses by the intravenous route.[21]

Evaluation of Therapeutic Outcomes

Followup in patients with amebiasis should include repeat stool examination, serology, colonoscopy (for colitis), or computed tomography (CT) (for liver abscess) between days 5 and 7, at the end of the course of therapy, and a month after the end of therapy. Most patients with either intestinal amebiasis or colitis will respond in 3 to 5 days with amelioration of symptoms. Patients with liver abscesses may take from 7 to 10 days to respond; patients not responding during this period may require aspiration of abscesses or exploratory laparotomy. Serial liver scans have demonstrated healing of liver abscesses over 4 to 8 months after adequate therapy.[22]

Sanitation and Preventive Measures

Travelers and tourists visiting an epidemic area should avoid local tap water, ice, salads, and unpeeled fruits. Water can be disinfected by the use of iodine (tincture of iodine or commercial sources: Potable Aqua tablet (Wisconsin Pharmacal) or 5% to 10% acetic acid, but boiled water is probably the safest. An alternative or additional measure may be to carry a portable water purifier (such as Safewater, Durango, CO, www.outgear.com). Because food handlers in Asia and Latin America may be a source of amebiasis, travelers should avoid eating at food stalls and open markets.

HELMINTHIC DISEASES

Most intestinal helminthic infections may not be associated with clearly defined manifestation of disease, but they can cause significant pathology.[9,25-33] One factor that determines the pathogenicity of helminths is their population density. Light infections may be fairly well tolerated, whereas high populations of intestinal helminths can result in predictable disease presentations. In the United States,

TABLE 124-3	Clinical Presentations of Nematode Infections and Cysticercosis

Hookworm[27]
Mild epigastric pain and tenderness, headache, fatigue, anemia, hypoproteinemia, and cutaneous larva migrans

Ascariasis[26]
Abdominal pain, right-upper-quadrant pain, biliary coli, cholangitis, pancreatitis, and abdominal obstruction

Enterobiasis[25]
Mild abdominal discomfort and perianal itch

Strongyloidiasis[35,37]
Gastrointestinal: abdominal pain, bloating, nausea, constipation, and small bowel obstruction
Cardiopulmonary: cough, wheezing, pleural effusion, chest pain, and dyspnea
Dermatologic/hematologic: pruritic linear streaks of lower thighs and buttocks and eosinophilia
Central nervous system: headache, altered mental status, and meningitis

Cysticercosis[41,42,45]
Abdominal pain, nausea, diarrhea, painless nodules on arms, chest, and legs, and myalgia
Neurocysticercosis: headache, intracranial hypertension, hydrocephalus, and seizures

these infections are seen most frequently in recent immigrants from Southeast Asia, the Caribbean, Mexico, and Central America.[1,8,26,27] Other populations that have a high risk of infestation include institutionalized patients (both young and elderly), preschool children in daycare centers, residents of Indian reservations, and homosexual individuals. Certain conditions and drugs (fever, corticosteroids, and anesthesia) can cause atypical localization of worms.[34-38] Immunocompromised hosts can be overwhelmed by some helminthic infections, such as strongyloidiasis.[34]

NEMATODES

Hookworm Disease

This is an infection of the small intestine caused by either *Ancylostoma duodenale* or *Necator americanus*. *N americanus* is found in the southeastern United States, where the temperature and humidity provide the proper environment. *Ancylostoma* is seen rarely in the United States.[25,27]

The life cycles of both species of hookworm are similar. The adult worms live in the small intestine attached to the mucosa. The females liberate eggs, which are eliminated in the feces and develop into larvae. Infective larva enter the host in contaminated food or water or penetrate the skin, where a papular eruption with localized edema and erythema can result.

In the small intestine, where the adult worm lives attached to the mucosa, injury is usually caused by mechanical and lytic destruction of tissue. The loss of blood can lead to anemia and hypoproteinemia (Table 124–3).[26-29]

Stool should be examined for eggs and the rhabditiform larvae. Eosinophilia (30%–60%) may be present in patients during early infection.

TREATMENT

Hookworm Disease

❹ Mebendazole (Vermox), an oral synthetic benzimidazole, is the agent of first choice in hookworm. It is also effective against ascariasis, enterobiasis, trichuriasis.[16,25,26] The adult dose for treatment of hookworm infestation is 100 mg twice daily for 3 days. Pediatric patients older than 2 years of age should receive the same dose as adults.[13] Albendazole is an alternative agent.[13]

Ascariasis

Ascariasis is caused by the giant roundworm *Ascaris lumbricoides.* Female worms range from 20 to 35 cm in length. The worm is found worldwide but more commonly in areas where sanitation is poor. In the United States, endemic areas include southeastern parts of the Appalachian range and the Gulf Coast states.

Clinical Manifestations During migration of the larvae through the lungs, patients can present with pneumonitis, fever, cough, eosinophilia, and pulmonary infiltrates.[9,25,26] Other symptoms of ascariasis include abdominal discomfort, abdominal obstruction, vomiting, and appendicitis (see Table 124–3).[9,25,31,32] Diagnosis is made by demonstrating the characteristic egg in the stool.

TREATMENT

Ascariasis

In both adults and pediatric patients older than 2 years of age, the treatment for ascariasis is mebendazole (Vermox) 100 mg twice daily for 3 days.[16] An alternative drug for ascariasis is albendazole 400 mg as a single dose.[16]

Enterobiasis

Enterobiasis, or pinworm infection, is caused by *Enterobius vermicularis.* The pinworm is a small, thread-like, spindle-shaped worm about 1 cm in length. It is the most widely distributed helminthic infection in the world. There are estimated to be 42 million cases in the United States.[25] The majority of those infected are children.

The most common problem with enterobiasis is cutaneous irritation in the perianal region, made by the migrating females or the presence of eggs. However, there are reports of other complications, including appendicitis and intestinal perforation.[33] The intense pruritus and scratching can cause dermatitis and secondary bacterial infections. In children, the itching can cause loss of sleep and restlessness (see Table 124–3).

The most effective method of diagnosing pinworm infections is by the use of perianal swab using adhesive Scotch tape. The Scotch tape, which is applied to the perianal region with a tongue depressor, is examined microscopically for eggs.[9,25]

TREATMENT

Enterobiasis

The common agents for treatment include pyrantel pamoate, mebendazole, or albendazole (Albenza). The dose of pyrantel pamoate is 11 mg/kg (maximum 1 g) as a single dose that can be repeated in 2 weeks. The dose of mebendazole for adults and children older than 2 years of age is 100 mg as a single dose; this may be repeated in 2 weeks.[16,25] The dose of albendazole for adults and children older than 2 years of age is 400 mg, and should be repeated in 2 weeks.[25] Following treatment, all bedding and underclothes should be sterilized by steaming or washing in the hot water cycle of a regular washing machine; this will eradicate the eggs. Bathroom rugs and toilet accessories also should be cleaned in a similar way.

Strongyloidiasis

Strongyloidiasis is caused by *Strongyloides stercoralis*, which has a worldwide distribution and is predominantly prevalent in South America (Brazil and Columbia) and in Southeast Asia. Strongyloidiasis is primarily seen among institutionalized populations (mental homes, mentally disabled children's homes) and immunocompromised individuals (patients with human immunodeficiency virus [HIV], AIDS, and hematologic malignancies).[8,34-38] The worm is usually found in the upper intestine where the eggs are deposited and hatch to form the rhabditiform larvae. The rhabditiform larvae (male and female) migrate to the bowel where they may be excreted in the feces. If excreted in the feces, the larvae can evolve into either one of two forms after copulation: (a) free-living noninfectious rhabditiform larvae or (b) infectious filariform larvae. The filariform larvae can penetrate host skin, travel to the lungs via the bronchi and glottis and make their way to the small intestine. At times, the filariform larvae may not pass out in the feces but instead migrate to the lungs and produce progeny, a process called autoinfection. This can result in hyperinfection (i.e., increased number of larvae in intestine, lungs, and other internal organs), especially in immunocompromised hosts.[34-36]

Symptoms with acute infection may appear with localized pruritic rash but heavy infestations can produce eosinophilia (10%–15%), diarrhea, abdominal pain, and intestinal obstruction (see Table 124–3).[37-39]

⑤ Administration of corticosteroids or other immunosuppressive drugs to an infected individual can result in hyperinfections and disseminated strongyloidiasis.[34,36,38] Diagnosis of strongyloidiasis is made by identification of the rhabditiform larvae in stool, sputum, duodenal fluid, and cerebrospinal fluid, by small bowel biopsy specimens, or by antigen testing (ELISA assay).[37]

TREATMENT

Strongyloidiasis

The drug of choice for strongyloidiasis is oral ivermectin 200 mcg/kg/day for 2 days and the alternative is albendazole 400 mg twice daily for 7 days.[16,34,39,40] In a patient with hyperinfection or disseminated strongyloidiasis, immunosuppressive drugs should be discontinued and treatment initiated with ivermectin 200 mcg/kg/day until all symptoms are resolved (duration, 5 to 14 days). Patients should be tested periodically to ensure the elimination of the larvae.[39] Individuals from endemic areas, who are candidates for organ transplantation, must be screened for *S stercoralis.*

Taenia solium: Cysticercosis and Neurocysticercosis

Tapeworm infection caused by *Taenia solium* is a result of ingestion of poorly cooked pork that contains the larvae or cysticercus.[41,42] Cysticercus, when released from the contaminated meat by host digestive juices, matures into the adult tapeworm and attaches to the host jejunum. Cysticercosis is a systemic disease caused by the larva of *T solium* (oncosphere) and is usually acquired by ingestion of eggs in contaminated food or by autoinfection.[41-43] The larvae can penetrate the bowel and migrate through the bloodstream to infect different organs including the central nervous system (neurocysticercosis).[43,44,46] The larvae matures in about 8 weeks and remain as a semitransparent, oval-shaped, fluid-filled bladder in tissues. In the United States, the highest incidence of cysticercosis has been reported in immigrants from Mexico.[41-43] Cysticercosis in most tissues may not produce major symptoms and usually manifest as subcutaneous nodules, primarily in the arms, legs, and chest. However, penetration of the larval stage (cysticercus) into the central nervous system can produce hydrocephalus, intracranial hypertension, stroke, and seizure activity.[42] Epileptic seizures (50% to 80%) may be the presenting symptoms in patients with neurocysticercosis (see Table 124–3).[42,45] Clinical presentation, primarily seizure history, together with radiographic demonstration (CT and magnetic resonance imaging) of the cysticercus within the bladder or calcified cysts in the central nervous system, is diagnostic for neurocysticercosis.[41,42] Serologic diagnosis is made by the use of an enzyme-linked immunoelectrotransfer blot assay, which is considered highly sensitive and specific for cysticercosis.[41,42,45,46]

CLINICAL CONTROVERSY

❹ Cysticercosis (excluding neurocysticercosis) is normally not treated. The management for neurocysticercosis remains controversial but may include surgery, anticonvulsants (neurocysticercosis-induced seizures), and antihelminthic therapy.[41,42,45,47] Antihelminthic therapy, if one decides this is an option, is albendazole 400 mg twice daily for 8 to 30 days.[16] However, the dose and duration of therapy with albendazole is not clearly defined.[42,47] The pediatric dose of albendazole is 15 mg/kg (maximum 800 mg) in two divided doses for 8 to 30 days. The doses for both adults and pediatric subjects may be repeated if necessary. Praziquantel is an alternative therapy.[16]

TREATMENT

Helminthic Diseases

Evaluation of Therapeutic Outcome

Morbidity and disease with intestinal nematodes are related to the intensity of infection or worm burden; subjects with transient exposure have less severe disease. The major adverse effects of intestinal nematodes are malnutrition, fatigue, and diminished work capacity. Treatment with antihelminthic agents results in complete eradication and significant change in the well-being of patients. Unlike other nematode infections, strongyloidiasis can perpetuate itself by autoinfection, and in the immunosuppressed host, the filariform larvae can invade various organs (e.g., lungs, central nervous system, and the like) to produce disseminated infection that can be fatal.[9,43–47]

❻ The most serious complication of cysticercosis is invasion of the central nervous system which results in neurocysticercosis. Neurocysticercosis can cause obstructive hydrocephalus, strokes and seizures; antihelminthic treatment for these conditions remains controversial.[42,45,46]

MALARIA

Malaria represents the most devastating disease in terms of human suffering and economics. It affects the largest number of people (between 300 and 500 million new infections are reported annually) in the world, and between 1 to 2 million deaths worldwide.[3,5,48–50] In the United States, deaths from malaria are preventable. The primary reasons for deaths are failure to take chemoprophylaxis,

inappropriate chemoprophylaxis, delay in seeking medical care, and misdiagnosis.[3,4,7,50]

EPIDEMIOLOGY

The exact geographic distribution of the various species is not well documented; it is reported that *Plasmodium vivax* is more prevalent in India, Pakistan, Bangladesh, Sri Lanka, and Central America; whereas *P falciparum* is predominant in Africa, Haiti, Dominican Republic, the Amazon region of South America, and New Guinea. Most of the infections with *Plasmodium ovale* occur in Africa, and the distribution of *Plasmodium malariae* is considered worldwide.[7,49,60]

In the United States, most cases of malaria are reported in immigrants from endemic areas and in American travelers. Blood transfusion also has been cited as a cause of malarial infection.[48,51]

ETIOLOGY

Malaria is transmitted by the bite of an infected *Anopheles* mosquito that introduces the sporozoites (tissue parasites) of the plasmodia (*P falciparum, P vivax, P malariae,* and *P ovale*) into the bloodstream. The asexual reproduction stage develops in humans, whereas the sexual stage occurs in the mosquito.[9,48,49] The sporozoites invade parenchymal hepatocytes, multiply in stages referred to as *exoerythrocytic stages*, and become hepatic vegetative forms or schizonts. Schizonts rupture to release daughter cells, or merozoites, that then infect erythrocytes.

P falciparum and *P malariae* remain in the primary exoerythrocytic stage in the liver for about 4 weeks before invading erythrocytes, whereas *P vivax* and *P ovale* can exist in the liver in the latent exoerythrocytic form for extended periods, and, therefore, infected subjects can experience relapses. The merozoites that invade the erythrocytes develop sequentially into ring forms, trophozoites, schizonts, and finally, merozoites, which can invade other erythrocytes or can develop into gametocytes, which undergo the sexual stage in the *Anopheles* vector. Because erythrocytic forms never reinvade the liver without developing into sporozoites in the vector, malaria infections from transfusion never result in the exoerythrocytic, or "liver," form.[9,49] *P falciparum* can result in high levels of parasitemia because of its ability to invade erythrocytes of all ages, unlike *P vivax* and *P ovale*, which only invade young cells.[48,49]

PATHOLOGY

The erythrocytic phase causes extensive hemolysis, which results in anemia and splenomegaly. The most serious complications usually are associated with *P falciparum* infections.[48–50,52–60] Infants and children younger than 5 years of age and nonimmune pregnant women are at high risk for severe complications from falciparum malaria.[52–55] The complications associated with falciparum malaria are primarily a result of the high parasitemia and the ability of the parasites to sequester in capillaries and postcapillary vessels of organs such as the brain and the kidney. It has been postulated that tissue hypoxia from anemia, together with *P falciparum*–parasitized red blood cell adherence to endothelial cells in capillaries, contribute to extensive vascular disease and severe metabolic effects.[52,53] *P malariae* is implicated in immune-mediated glomerulonephritis and nephrotic syndrome (Table 124–4).[49,52]

To ensure a positive diagnosis, blood smears should be obtained every 12 to 24 hours for 3 consecutive days.[9,49,52] The presence of parasites in the blood 3 to 5 days after initiation of therapy suggests drug resistance. Recent advances for detecting malaria parasite

TABLE 124-4 Clinical Presentation of Malaria

Initial presentation

Nonspecific fever, chills, rigors, diaphoresis, malaise, vomiting[48,49,52]

Orthostatic hypotension

Electrolyte abnormalities

Erythrocytic phase

Prodrome: headache, anorexia, malaise, fatigue, myalgia

Nonspecific complaints such as abdominal pain, diarrhea, chest pain, and arthralgia

Paroxysm: high fever, chills, and rigor[9,49,52,59]

Cold phase: severe pallor and cyanosis of the lips[9,49,52]

Hot phase: fever between 40.5°C (104.9°F) and 41°C (105.8°F)

Sweating phase:

    Follows hot phase by 2–6 hours

    Fever resolves

    Marked fatigue and drowsiness, warm, dry skin, tachycardia, cough, severe headache, nausea, vomiting, abdominal pain, diarrhea, and delirium

    Lactic acidosis and hypoglycemia (with falciparum malaria)[48,49,52,59]

Anemia

Splenomegaly

P falciparum infections

Hypoglycemia, acute renal failure, pulmonary edema, severe anemia, thrombocytopenia, high-output heart failure, cerebral congestion, seizures and coma, and adult respiratory syndrome[49,52,59]

have included DNA or RNA probes by polymerase chain reaction (PCR) and rapid dipstick tests (_Para_ Sight F, Becton-Dickinson, Cockeysville, MD) and OptiMAL.[48,49,52] The dipstick is reported to have a sensitivity of 88% and a specificity of 97%; however, microscopy is still considered the optimal test.

TREATMENT

Malaria

■ DESIRED OUTCOME

The primary goal in the management of malaria is the rapid diagnosis of the _Plasmodia_ spp by blood smears (repeated every 12 hours for 3 days) so as to initiate timely antimalarial therapy to eradicate the infection within 48 to 72 hours and to avoid complications such as hypoglycemia, pulmonary edema, and renal failure that are responsible for increased mortality in malaria.[49]

■ PHARMACOLOGIC THERAPY

In adults (including pregnant women), the chemoprophylaxis for all species of _Plasmodium_ is chloroquine phosphate 300 mg (base) once weekly beginning 1 to 2 weeks prior to departure and continued for 4 weeks after leaving an endemic area.[16,48,49,52,61–63] The pediatric dose of chloroquine phosphate is 5 mg (base) per kilogram of body weight (maximum 300 mg). When departing an area endemic for _P vivax_ or _P ovale_, primaquine phosphate 30 mg (base) daily for 14 days beginning the last 2 weeks of chloroquine prophylaxis should be added to the regimen. The pediatric dose of primaquine is 0.6 mg (base) per kilogram of body weight per day for 14 days. The pediatric doses of chloroquine can be calculated based on body weight, and the tablets can be pulverized and placed in gelatin capsules. Parents can be instructed to suspend the dose in food, simple syrup, chocolate milk, or in a drink.[61]

In areas where chloroquine-resistant _P falciparum_ strains exist, travelers should receive mefloquine (Lariam) for prophylaxis. The adult dose of mefloquine is 250 mg once weekly beginning

1 week prior to departure and continuing for the full period of exposure, followed by 250 mg for 4 weeks after last exposure.[16,48,49] The pediatric dose of mefloquine for prophylaxis is based on body weight.[16]

Body Weight (kg)	Dose
5 to 10 kg	one-eighth tablet/week
11 to 20 kg	one-quarter tablet/week
21 to 30 kg	one-half tablet/week
31 to 45 kg	three-quarters tablet/week
>45 kg	1 tablet/week

For travelers who are at immediate risk for drug-resistant _falciparum_ malaria, a loading dose of mefloquine may be considered (except for travel to Thailand, Myanmar, Vietnam, Laos, and Cambodia, where atovaquone-proguanil combination, one tablet daily 2 days prior to departure and through the stay and 1 week after leaving area, may be an alternative).[49] Mefloquine is administered at 250 mg daily for 3 days before travel, followed by 250 mg once weekly while in the endemic area and continued for 4 weeks after last exposure.[48,49] Patients may experience neuropsychiatric reactions from mefloquine and may need to be monitored closely.[16,62–64]

An alternative regimen for prophylaxis in chloroquine-resistant areas for those who cannot tolerate mefloquine or Malarone, is to take oral doxycycline 100 mg daily starting 1 to 2 days prior to departure, during the exposure period, and continuing for 4 weeks after leaving the endemic area.[16] Children older than 8 years of age should receive 2 mg/kg/day (up to 100 mg) of doxycycline. Doxycycline is contraindicated in children younger than 8 years of age, in pregnant women, and during breastfeeding.[16,49,63,65]

In an uncomplicated attack of malaria (for all plasmodia except chloroquine-resistant _P falciparum_), the recommended regimen is chloroquine 600 mg (base) initially, followed by 300 mg (base) 6 hours later, and then 300 mg (base) daily for 2 days. In severe illness or when oral therapy is not tolerated or parenteral quinine is not available, quinidine gluconate 10 mg/kg as a loading dose (maximum 600 mg) in 250 mL normal saline should be administered slowly over 1 to 2 hours, followed by continuous infusion of 0.02 mg/kg/minute until oral therapy can be started.[16,48,49] In patients who have received either quinine or mefloquine, the loading dose of quinidine should be omitted. Oral quinine (650 mg every 8 hours) together with doxycycline 100 mg twice daily should follow the intravenous dose of quinidine to complete a total of 7 days of therapy.[16,48,60] The pediatric dose of intravenous quinidine gluconate is the same as the dose for adults.[16] The pediatric dose of quinine is 30 mg/kg/day in three divided doses for 7 days. Children younger than age 8 years and pregnant women should get clindamycin 20 mg/kg/day in divided doses for 7 days instead of doxycycline.[16,49,60]

❼ When intravenous quinidine is not readily available, intravenous artesunate (available under an IND from the CDC at _www.cdc.gov/malaria/features/artesunate_now_available.htm_), a water-soluble artemisinin derivative, administered at 2.4 mg/kg/dose for 3 days at 0, 12, 24, 48, and 72 hours is the recommended drug if severe _P falciparum_ is suspected.[16,58]

In _P falciparum_ (chloroquine-resistant) infections, a dose of 750 mg mefloquine followed by 500 mg 12 hours later is recommended. The pediatric dose of mefloquine is 15 mg/kg (<45 kg body weight) followed by 10 mg/kg 8 to 12 hours later.[16] Intravenous quinidine gluconate (or intravenous artesunate) followed by oral quinine plus doxycycline to complete a total of 7 days of therapy should follow in a severe illness, as already indicated.[16,49] An alternative oral treatment for chloroquine-resistant _P falciparum_ infection in adults, especially in those with a history of seizures or psychiatric disorders, is the combination of atovaquone 250 mg and proguanil 100 mg (Malarone) (4 tablets daily for 3 days).[16,48,49] An alternative to Malarone is the combination product of artemether 20 mg and lumefantrine 120 mg (Coartem) recently approved by the FDA in the United States (for regimen, see *http://www.cdc.gov/malaria/pdf/treatmenttable.pdf*). The intravenous quinidine regimen requires close monitoring of the electrocardiogram and other vital signs (e.g., hypotension, QT interval prolongation, and hypoglycemia).[16,49,55,60]

8 Because *falciparum* malaria is associated with serious complications, including pulmonary edema, hypoglycemia, jaundice, renal failure, confusion, delirium, seizures, coma, and death, careful monitoring of fluid status and hemodynamic parameters is mandatory.[48,49,55,60] Either hemofiltration or hemodiafiltration is indicated in renal failure.[55]

Malarial infection does not produce immunity in patients, and active research has been initiated to develop a malaria vaccine.[66-68] A vaccine that blocks the entry of sporozoites into the liver cells will prevent malaria at this stage. However, immunity to sporozoites does not protect the host against parasites in the erythrocytic cycle. Infective sporozoites of *P falciparum* are covered by a polypeptide, circumsporozoite protein. Isolation and identification of the gene encoding for this circumsporozoite protein have led to the development of a monoclonal antibody by recombinant DNA technology; *P falciparum* sporozoite vaccine is now under investigation.[68]

CLINICAL CONTROVERSY

Because there remains public concern with mefloquine therapy, primarily about its neuropsychiatric effects,[16,63] an alternative regimen for chemoprophylaxis is the combination of atovaquone and proguanil (Malarone): 1 tablet daily beginning 1 to 2 days prior to travel and continuing for the duration of stay and 1 week after leaving the area.[16,62] Daily primaquine 30 mg (base) also has been recommended for prophylaxis for both *P vivax* and *P falciparum* malaria.[16]

EVALUATION OF THERAPEUTIC OUTCOMES

When advising potential travelers on prophylaxis for malaria, be aware of the incidence of chloroquine-resistant *P falciparum* malaria and the countries where this is prevalent.[16,62,63] Detailed recommendations for prevention of malaria may be obtained by checking the websites *www.cdc.gov/travel/* or *www2.cdc.gov/mmwr/*[63,69] or calling the U.S. Centers for Disease Control and Prevention (CDC) (see Appendix 124–1). In view of the increasing incidence of *P falciparum* resistance to antimalarials, newer drugs are under active study and include the water-soluble artesunate and the oil-soluble artemether and combinations with other agents.[7,16,49,63,70-75]

Acute *P falciparum* malaria resistant to chloroquine should be treated with intravenous quinidine or artesunate.[16,58] Patients receiving intravenous quinidine should have a central venous catheter to follow fluid status, and the electrocardiogram should be monitored closely. Hypoglycemia that is associated with *P falciparum* should be checked and corrected with dextrose infusions.[48,49,55] Quinidine infusion should be slowed temporarily or stopped if electrocardiogram shows a QT interval of greater than 0.6 seconds, an increase in the QRS complex to greater than 50%, or hypotension unresponsive to fluid challenge results. The suggested quinidine levels should be maintained at 3 to 7 mg/L.[49] Blood smears should be checked every 12 hours until parasitemia is less than 1%. Resolution of fever should take place between 36 and 48 hours after initiation of the intravenous quinidine therapy and the blood should be clear of parasites in 5 days.[48,49,52] If parenteral

therapy is required for more than 48 hours, the dose of quinidine should be lowered by half.[16]

Travelers to endemic areas for malaria should be advised to remain in well-screened areas, to wear clothes that cover most of the body, and to sleep in mosquito nets.[4,7,49,71] It is prudent to carry the insect repellent DEET (N,N,diethyl-metatol) or Picaridin (Cutter Advanced) insect spray for use in mosquito-infested areas. Readers are urged to check publications from the CDC for the list of countries where chloroquine-resistant *P falciparum* exist.[16,69]

AMERICAN TRYPANOSOMIASIS

ETIOLOGY

Two distinct forms of the genus *Trypanosoma* occur in humans. One is associated with African trypanosomiasis (sleeping sickness) and the other with American trypanosomiasis (Chagas disease).[76-79] *Trypanosoma brucei gambiense* and *Trypanosoma brucei rhodesiense* are the causative organisms for the East African and West African trypanosomiasis, respectively. *T brucei rhodesiense* causes the acute disease and is the more virulent of the two species. Both East and West African trypanosomiasis are transmitted by various species of tsetse fly belonging to the genus *Glossina*. Further discussion of this subject will focus on American trypanosomiasis.

Trypanosoma cruzi is the agent that causes American trypanosomiasis. American trypanosomiasis is transmitted by a number of species of a reduviid bug (*Triatoma infestans*, *Rhodnius prolixus*) that live in wall cracks of houses in rural areas of North, Central, and South America. The reduviid bug is infected by sucking blood from animals (e.g., opossums, dogs, and cats) or humans infected with circulating trypomastigotes (Table 124–5).

In chronic trypanosomiasis, patients present with cardiomyopathy and heart failure. Electrocardiograms are usually abnormal, demonstrating extrasystoles, first-degree heart block, right bundle-branch block, and other serious conduction disturbances.[77-79] Degeneration of the autonomic ganglia in the smooth muscle of the esophagus and colon leads to uncoordinated peristalsis. The end result has been reported to be "megasyndromes" of affected organs.[78-79] Penetration of the central nervous system results in meningoencephalitis, strokes, seizures, and focal paralysis.[78-80]

A history to verify the possible exposure to *T cruzi* should be an important initial diagnostic workup. Recovery of *T cruzi* is definitive, but this is not always possible, especially in chronic disease. Positive serologic tests using indirect immunofluorescent antibody test and ELISA (Chagas' EIA, Abbott Laboratories, Abbott Park, IL) may be diagnostic for the disease. The only serologic test available in the United States is Chagas' Kit (Hemagen Diagnostics, Inc., Columbia, MD).[78] A PCR test has also been used for diagnosis of *T cruzi*.[81] Specimens may be sent to the CDC for testing. All candidates from an endemic area for Chagas disease who are candidates for transplantation should be tested for *T cruzi*.[82]

TABLE 124-5 Clinical Presentation of South American Trypanosomiasis

Acute
Unilateral orbital edema ("Romana sign")[78,79]
Granuloma or "chagoma"
Fever, hepatosplenomegaly, and lymphadenopathy

Chronic
Cardiac: cardiomyopathy and heart failure
ECG: first-degree heart block, right bundle-branch block, and arrhythmias[76-78]
Gastrointestinal: enlargement of esophagus and colon ("mega" syndrome)[76,78]
Central nervous system: meningoencephalitis, strokes, seizures, and focal paralysis[78-80]

TREATMENT

American Trypanosomiasis

■ DESIRED OUTCOME

The primary goal of drug therapy in trypanosomiasis is to reduce the duration and severity of the illness and to decrease mortality.

■ PHARMACOLOGIC THERAPY

9 The drugs that have been used to treat *T cruzi* infections include nifurtimox (Lampit, Bayer 2502) and benznidazole (Rochagan).[16,78,79,83] Oral nifurtimox is available from the CDC, whereas benznidazole is only available in Brazil. Neither of these agents are optimal therapy and there is ongoing search for newer agents.[76,78] The adult dose of nifurtimox is 8 to 10 mg/kg/day in divided doses for 120 days. Because pediatric patients tolerate the drug better than adults, the dose for children age 1 to 10 years is 15 to 20 mg/kg/day, and for children age 11 to 16 years it is 12.5 to 15 mg/kg/day in divided doses.[16] Symptomatic treatment for heart failure includes digitalis and diuretics; the gastrointestinal complications, however, may require surgical revisions and reconstruction.[78,79]

EVALUATION OF THERAPEUTIC OUTCOMES

American trypanosomiasis (Chagas disease), which is endemic in all Latin American countries, can be transmitted congenitally, by blood transfusion, and by organ transplantation.[78,79] Treatment with nifurtimox of the acute phase (i.e., fever, malaise, edema of face, generalized lymphadenopathy, and hepatosplenomegaly) produces between 10% and 30% cure rates.[78] Treatment of chronic infection with nifurtimox is not recommended. It is essential to identify *T cruzi*–infected patients by serology and to monitor the cardiovascular status of these patients by electrocardiogram periodically. The congestive failure of cardiomyopathic Chagas disease is treated the same way as cardiomyopathies from other causes.[76,78]

ECTOPARASITES

A parasite that lives on the outside of the body of the host is called an *ectoparasite*. Approximately 6 to 12 million people become infested with pediculosis yearly in the United States.[84] Pediculosis usually is associated with poor personal hygiene, and infections are passed from person to person through social and sexual contact. The three types of human lice belong to two genera: *Pediculus*, including the head and body lice, and *Phthirus*, with only one species, the crab louse.[9,84,85] The human louse is detectable to the human naked eye and measures approximately 2 to 3 mm in length.

LICE

The two species that belong to this group include *Pediculus humanus capitis* (head louse) and *Pediculus humanus corporis* (body louse). Female lice deposit eggs on the hair. The eggs (or nits) remain firmly attached to the hair, and in about 10 days, the lice hatch to form nymphs, which mature in 2 weeks. Using both their piercing mouth parts and a pumping device, the larva and adults feed on the blood of the host. The body louse and head louse are essentially identical, although they live on different parts of the body. Unlike the head louse, which lives on the hair, the body louse is more frequently found on clothing of the infected host.

Pubic or crab lice are found on the hairs around the genitals, although they can occur in other areas of the body (e.g., eyelashes, beards, and axillae). Patients usually complain of severe pruritus from papular lesions produced by the bite of the louse. Hypersensitivity to foreign material injected by the lice can produce macular swellings and occasionally can lead to secondary bacterial infections.[84]

TREATMENT

Lice

The goal of therapy is to eradicate the causative organisms and provide symptomatic relief to patients. The agent of choice for all three infections (body, head, and crab lice) is 1% permethrin (Nix).[84-88] Permethrin is a derivative of the flowers of the plant *Chrysanthemum cinerariifolium*. The term *pyrethrin* is usually applied to several esters of chrysanthemic acid and pyrethric acid. Permethrin has both pediculicidal and ovicidal activity against *P humanus* var *capitis*. The cure rate is reported to be in the range of 85% to 95%.[84] Individuals who have a history of ragweed or chrysanthemum allergy should use this compound with caution. The side effects reported with permethrin products include itching, burning, stinging, and tingling. Permethrin 1% is applied to the scalp after the hair has been dried following a shampooing. The scalp should be saturated with permethrin liquid, and a towel should be wrapped around the scalp to allow the application to stay on for 10 minutes. The hair then should be rinsed thoroughly. A cream rinse of permethrin 1% (Nix-Creme Rinse) is also available. To ensure complete eradication, especially of newly hatched lice, it may be necessary to repeat the application. Recently the FDA-approved benzyl alcohol 5% (Ulesfia; Sciele Pharma Inc, Atlanta, GA) as an alternative therapy for head lice.[86]

There is increasing lice resistance to permethrin 1%.[85,88,89] An alternative preparation for lice is 0.5% malathion (Ovide), which is very effective.[16,87] To ensure complete eradication of lice infestation, the malathion application should be left on the scalp for about 90 minutes.[87] For the relief of pruritus, a soothing lotion of calamine liniment or lotion with 0.1% menthol may be used. Other members of the family or sexual partners also should be treated. All bedding and clothes should be sterilized by boiling or washing in the hot water cycle of the washing machine to avoid reinfections. Seams of clothes should be examined to verify that all organisms are eradicated. An ocular lubricant (e.g., Lacri-Lube S.O.P.) applied twice daily may be used to remove crab louse infection of the eyelids.

SCABIES

Scabies is caused by the itch mite *Sarcoptes scabiei*, which affects both humans and animals. Mange in domestic animals is caused by the same organism. Infection usually affects the interdigital and popliteal folds, axillary folds, the umbilicus, and the scrotum.[89-92]

Clinical Presentation

Patients will complain of severe itching and an inability to sleep and may have excoriations in the interdigital web spaces, wrists, elbows, buttocks, groin, and scalp. Excoriations may lead to secondary bacterial infections. The diagnosis is made by looking for burrows formed by the mite and taking skin scrapings, which will demonstrate the mite on a wet mount.

TREATMENT

Scabies

Because these infections cause a great deal of discomfort and distress to patients and families, the goals of therapy are to eradicate the infestations rapidly, to institute symptomatic treatment, and to provide counseling and reassurance. The treatment of choice is permethrin 5% (Elimite) cream.[16,90–92] To initiate the treatment, the skin should be scrubbed thoroughly in a warm soapy bath using a soft brush to remove all scabs. The lotion is then applied to the whole body, avoiding the face, mucous membranes, and eyes. The application should be left on for 8 to 14 hours before bathing. A single application eradicates 97% of scabies in subjects.[90] All close contacts should be checked and treated appropriately.

Other agents used to treat scabies include topical crotamiton 10% (Eurax) and oral ivermectin (Stromectol) 200 mcg/kg as a single dose which may be repeated in 2 weeks.[16,92] Crotamiton and oral ivermectin may be used in patients who have hypersensitivity to permethrin preparations. Topical corticosteroids and antihistamines may be used to decrease pruritus.

❿ Permethrin (1% and 5%) for pediculosis and scabies, respectively, is the preferred agent and remains the safest agent, especially in infants and children.[84,92] One application of permethrin is consistently effective in eradicating more than 90% of all infections. However, pruritus may persist for 2 to 4 weeks because of the remnants of mite parts in the skin. Ivermectin is an alternative therapy for scabies.

ABBREVIATIONS

AIDS: acquired immunodeficiency syndrome

ELISA: enzyme-linked immunosorbent assay

PCR: polymerase chain reaction

REFERENCES

1. Garg PK, Perry S, Dorn M, Hardcastle L, Parsonnet J. Risk of intestinal helminth and protozoan infection in a refugee population. Am J Trop Med Hyg 2005;73:386–391.
2. Nair P, Mohamed JA, DuPont HL, et al. Epidemiology of Crytosporidiosis in North American Travelers to Mexico. Am J Trop Med Hyg 2008;79:210–214.
3. Breman JG, Alilo MS, White NJ. Defining and defeating the intolerable burden of malaria. III. Progress and Perspectives. Am J Trop Med Hyg 2007;77(Suppl 6): vi–xi.
4. Murray CK, Horvath LL. An approach to prevention of infectious diseases during military deployments. Clin Infect Dis 2007;44:424–430.
5. Malaria Surveillance—United States, 2007. MMWR 2009;58(SS-02): 1–16.
6. Castro E. Chagas' disease: lessons from routine donation testing. Transfusion Med 2009;19:16–23.
7. Franco-Paredes C, Santos-Preciado JI. Problem pathogens: Prevention of malaria in travelers. Lancet Infect Dis 2006;6:139–149.
8. Nuesch R, Zimmerli L, Stockli R, Gyr N, Hatz CFR. Imported strongyloidosis: A longitudinal analysis of 31 cases. J Travel Med 2005;29:80–84.
9. John DT, Petri WA Jr. Markell and Voge's Medical Parasitology, 9th ed. Philadelphia, PA: WB Saunders, 2006.
10. Farthing MJG, Cevellos AM, Kelly P. Intestinal protozoa. The Mastigophora (flagellates): Giardia intestinalis. In: Cook GC, Zumla A, eds. Manson's Topical Diseases, 22nd ed. London: Saunders Elsevier; 2009:1387–1395.
11. Farthing MJG. Treatment options for the eradication of intestinal protozoa. Nat Clin Pract Gastroenterol Hepatol 2006;3:436–445.
12. Hill DR, Nash TE. Giardia lamblia. In: Mandell GL, Bennett JE, Dolin R, eds. Principles and Practice of Infectious Diseases, 7th ed. New York: Elsevier Churchill Livingstone; 2010;3527–3534.
13. Hill DR, Nash TE. Intestinal flagellate and ciliate infections. In: Guerrant RL, Walker DH, Weller PF, eds. Topical Infectious Diseases. Principles, Pathogens & Practice, 2nd ed. Philadelphia, PA: Elsevier Churchill Livingstone; 2006:984–1002.
14. Fuglestad AJ, Lehmann A, Kroupina MG, et al. Iron deficiency in international adoptees from Eastern Europe. J Pediatr 2008;153: 272–277.
15. Weitzel T, Dittrich S, Mohl I, Adursu E, Jelinek T. Evaluation of seven commercial antigen detection tests for Giardia and Cryptosporidium in stool samples. Clin Microbiol Infect 2006;12:656–659.
16. Abramowicz M, ed. Drugs for parasitic infections. In: Handbook of Antimicrobial Therapy, 18th ed. New Rochelle, NY: Medical Letter; 2008:225–280.
17. Escobedo AA, Cimerman S. Giardiasis: A pharmacotherapy review. Expert Opin Pharmacother 2007;8:1885–1902.
18. Hung C-C, Deng H-Y, Hsiao W-H, et al. Invasive amebiasis as an emerging parasite disease in patients with human immunodeficiency virus type 1 infection in Taiwan. JAMA 2005;165:409–415.
19. Farthing MJG. Intestinal protozoa. Entamoeba histolytica. In: Cook GC, Zumla A, eds. Mansons Tropical Diseases, 22nd ed. London: Saunders Elsevier; 2009:1375–1386.
20. Haque R, Huston CD, Hughes M, et al. Amebiasis. N Engl J Med 2003;348:1565–1573.
21. Petri Jr WA, Haque R. Entamoeba species, including Amebiasis. In: Mandell GL, Bennett JA, Dolin R, eds. Principles and Practice of Infectious Diseases, 7th ed. New York: Elsevier Churchill Livingstone; 2010;3411–3425.
22. Salles JM, Moraes LA, Salles MC. Hepatic Amebiasis. Brazilian J Infect Dis 2003;7:96–110.
23. Bercu TE, Petri Jr WA, Behm BW. Amebic colitis: new insights into pathogenesis and treatment. Curr Gastroenterol Rep 2007;9:429–433.
24. Rao S, Solaymani-Mohammadi S, Petri Jr WA, Parker SK. Hepatic amebiasis: a reminder of the complications. Curr Opin Pediatr 2009;21:145–149.
25. Maguire JH. Intestinal nematodes (Roundworms). In: Mandell GL, Bennett JE, Dolin R, eds. Principles and Practice of Infectious Diseases, 7th ed. New York: Elsevier Churchill-Livingstone;2010; 3577–3586.
26. Bethony J, Brooker S, Albonico M, et al. Soil-transmitted helminth infection: Ascariasis, trichuriasis, and hookworm. Lancet 2006;367: 1521–1532.
27. Hotez PJ, Brooker S, Bethony JM, et al. Hookworm Infection. N Engl J Med 2004;357:799–807.
28. Pasricha S-R, Caruana SR, Phu TQ, et al. Anemia, iron deficiency, meat consumption, and hookworm in women of reproductive age in Northwest Vietnam. Am J Trop Med Hyg 2008;78:375–381.
29. Jarim-Botelho A, Raff S, Gazzinelli MF, et al. Hookworm, Ascaris lumbricoides infection and polyparasitism associated with poor cognitive performance in Brazilian schoolchildren. Trop Med Int Health 2008;13:994–1004.
30. Keiser J, Utzinger J. Efficacy of current drugs against soil-transmitted helminth infections: Systematic review and meta-analysis. JAMA 2008;299:1937–1948.
31. Malik AH, Saima BD, Wani MY. Management of hepatobiliary and pancreatic ascariasis in children of endemic area. Pediatr Surg Int 2006;22:164–168.
32. Huratado RM, Sahani DV, Kradin RL. Case records of the Massachusetts General Hospital. Case 9–2006. A 35-year-old woman with recurrent upper-quadrant pain. N Engl J Med 2006;354:1295–1303.
33. Jardine M, Kokai GK, Dalzell AM. Enterobius vermicularis and colitis in children. J Pediatr Gastroenterol 2006;43:610–612.
34. Balagopal A, Mills L, Shah A, Subramaniam A. Detection and treatment of Strongyloides syndrome following lung transplantation. Transplant Infect Dis 2009;11:149–154.
35. Bush LM, de Almeida KNF, Perez MT. Severe strongyloidiasis associated with subclinical human T-cell leukemia/lymphoma virus-1 infection. An illustrative case and review. Infect Dis Clin Pract 2009;17:84–89.

36. Lichtenberger P, Rosa-Cunha I, Morris M, et al. Hyperinfection strongyloidiasis in a liver transplant recipient treated with parenteral ivermectin. Transplant Infect Dis 2009;11:137–142.

37. Concho R, Harrington W, Rogers AI. Intestinal strongyloidiasis: Recognition, management, and determinants of outcome. Clin Gastroenterol 2005;39:203–211.

38. Lichentenberger P, Rosa-Cunha I, Morris M, et al. Hyperinfection Strongyloidiasis in liver transplantation recipient treated with parenteral ivermectin. Transplant Infect Dis 2009;11:137–142.

39. Aregawi D, Lopez D, Wick M, Schell WM, Schiff D. Disseminated strongloidiasis complicating glioblastoma therapy: A case report. J Neurooncol 2009;94:439–443.

40. Segarra-Newnham M. Manifestations, diagnosis, and treatment of *Strongyloides stercoralis* infection. Ann Pharmacother 2007;41:1992–2001.

41. King CH, Farley JK. Cestodes (Tapeworms). In: Mandell GL, Dolin R, Bennett JE, eds. Principles and Practice of Infectious Diseases, 6th ed. New York: Elsevier Churchill Livingstone; 2010;3607–3616.

42. Garcia HH, Wittner M, Coyle CM, Tanowitz HB, White Jr AC. Cysticercosis. In: Guerrant RL, Walker DH, Weller PF, eds. Tropical Infectious Diseases. Principles, Pathogens, & Practice, 2nd ed. Philadelphia, PA: Elsevier Churchill Livingstone; 2006:1289–1303.

43. Del La Garza Y, Graviss EA, Daver NG, et al. Epidemiology of neurocysticercosis in Houston, Texas. Am J Trop Med Hyg 2005;73:766–770.

44. Buneo JG, Plener I, Garcia HH. Neurocysticercosis in a patient in Canada. CMAJ 2009;180:639–642.

45. Carpio A, Kelvin EA, Bagiella E, et al. Effects of albendazole treatment on neurocysticercosis: a randomized controlled trial. J Neurol Neurosurg Psychiatry 2008;79:1050–1055.

46. White Jr AC. New developments in the management of neurocysticercosis. J Infect Dis 2009;199:1261–1262.

47. Singh G, Prabhakar S. The effects of antimicrobial and antiepiletic treatment on the outcome of epilepsy associated with central nervous system (CNS) infections. Epilepsia 2008;49(Suppl 6):42–46.

48. Fairhurst RM, Wellems TE. Plasmodium species (Malaria). In: Mandell GL, Dolin R, Bennett JE, eds. Principles and Practice of Infectious Diseases, 7th ed. New York: Elsevier Churchill Livingstone; 2010:3437–3462.

49. White NJ, Breman JG. Malaria. In: Fauci AS, Kasper DL, Longo DL, et al. eds. Harrison's Principles of Internal Medicine, 18th ed. New York: McGraw-Hill; 2008:1280–1294.

50. Krause G, Schoneberg I, Altmann D, Stark K. Chemoprophylaxis and malaria death rates. Emerging Infect Dis 2006;12:447–451.

51. Kitchen AD, Chiodini PL. Malaria and blood transfusion. Vox Sang 2006;90:77–84.

52. White NJ. Malaria. In: Cook GC, Zumla A, eds. Manson's Tropical Diseases, 22nd ed. London: Saunders Elsevier; 2009:1201–1300.

53. John CC, Bangirana P, Byarugaba J, et al. Cerebral malaria in children is associated with long-term cognitive impairment. Pediatrics 2008;122:e92–e99.

54. Idro R, Jenkins NE, Newton CR. Pathogenesis, clinical features, and neurological outcome of cerebral malaria. Lancet Neurol 2005;4:827–840.

55. Pasvol G. Management of severe malaria: Interventions and controversies. Infect Dis Clin North Am 2005;19:211–240.

56. Phillips A, Bassett P, Zeki S, Newman S, Pasvol G. Risk factors for severe disease in adults with Falciparum malaria. Clin Infect Dis 2009;48:871–878.

57. Idro R, Ndiritu M, Ogatu B, et al. Burden, features, and outcome of neurological involvement in acute Falciparum malaria in Kenyan children. JAMA 2007;297:2232–2240.

58. Rosenthal PJ. Artesunate for the treatment of severe Falciparum malaria. N Engl J Med 2008;358:1829–1836.

59. Day N, Dondorp AM. The management of patients with severe malaria. Am J Trop Med Hyg 2007;77(Suppl 6):29–35.

60. Griffith KS, Lewis LS, Mali S, Parise ME. Treatment of malaria in the United States. A systematic review. JAMA 2007;297:2264–2277.

61. Freedman DO. Malaria prevention in short-term travelers. N Engl J Med 2008;359:603–612.

62. Chen LH, Wilson ME, Schlagenhauf P. Controversies and misconceptions in malaria chemoprophylaxis for travelers. JAMA 2007;290:2251–2263.

63. Shanks GD, Edstein MD. Modern malaria chemoprophylaxis. Drugs 2005;65:2091–2110.

64. Taylor WRJ, White NJ. Antimalarial drug toxicity. Drug Saf 2004;27:25–61.

65. Rogerson SJ, Mwapasa V, Meshnick SR. Malaria in pregnancy: linking immunity and pathogenesis to prevention. Am J Trop Med Hyg 2007;77(Suppl 6):14–22.

66. Winzeler EA. Malaria research in the post-genomic era. Nature 2008;455:751–756.

67. Abdulla S, Oberholzer R, Juma O, et al. Safety and immunogenicity of RTS, S/ASO2D malaria vaccine in infants. N Engl J Med 2008;359:2533–2544.

68. Roestenberg M, McCall M, Hopman J, et al. Protection against a malaria challenge by sporozoite inoculation. N Engl J Med 2009;361:468–477.

69. Keystone JS, Steffen R, Kozarsky P. Health advice for International Travel. In: Guerrant RL, Walker DH, Weller PF, eds. Tropical Infectious Diseases. Principles, Pathogens, & Practice, 2nd ed. Philadelphia, PA: Elsevier Churchill Livingstone; 2006:1400–1424.

70. Rathore D, McCutchan TF, Sullivan M, Kumar S. Antimalarial drugs: Current status and new developments. Expert Opin Investig Drugs 2006;14:871–883.

71. Chen LH, Keystone JS. New strategies for the prevention of malaria in travelers. Infect Dis Clin North Am 2005;19:185–210.

72. Wongsrichanalai C, Meshnick SR. Declining artesunate-mefloquine efficacy against Falciparum malaria on the Cambodia-Thailand border. Emerg Infect Dis 2008;14:716–719.

73. Nosten F, White NJ. Artemisinin-based combination treatment of Falciparum malaria. Am J Trop Med Hyg 2007;77(Suppl 6):181–192.

74. Dondorp AM, Nosten F, Yi P, et al. Artemisinin resistance in *Plasmodium falciparum* malaria. N Engl J Med 2009;361:455–467.

75. Rosenthal PJ. Antiprotozoal drugs. In: Katzung BG, Masters SB, Trevor AJ, eds. Basic and Clinical Pharmacology, 11th ed. New York: Lange Medical Books/McGraw-Hill; 2009:899–921.

76. Bern C, Montgomery SP, Herwaldt BL, et al. Evaluation and treatment of Chagas disease in the United States. A systematic review. JAMA 2007;298:2171–2181.

77. Gascont J, Albajar P, Canas E, et al. Diagnosis, management, and treatment of chronic Chagas' heart disease in areas Trypansoma cruzi infection is not endemic. Rev Esp Cardiol 2007;60:285–293.

78. Kirchhoff LV. Trypanosoma species (American trypanosomiasis, Chagas' disease): Biology of trypanosomes. In: Mandell GL, Bennett JE, Dolin R, eds. Principles and Practice of Infectious Diseases, 6th ed. New York: Elsevier Churchill Livingstone; 2010:3481–3488.

79. Miles MA. American trypanosomiasis (Chagas' disease). In: Cook GC, Zumla A, eds. Manson's Tropical Diseases, 22nd ed. London: Saunders Elsevier; 2009:1327–1340.

80. Nunes MCP, Barbosa MM, Ribeiro ALP. Ischemic cerebrovascular events in patients with Chagas cardiomyopathy. A prospective follow-up study. J Neurol Sci 2009;278:96–101.

81. Bern C, Montgomery SP, Katz L, Caglioti S, Stramer SL. Chagas disease and US blood supply. Curr Opin Infect Dis 2008;21:476–482.

82. Kun H, Moore A, Mascola L, et al. Transmission of *Trypanosoma cruzi* by heart transplantation. Clin Infect Dis 2009;48:1534–1540.

83. Viotti R, Vigliano C, Lococo B, et al. Long-term cardiac outcomes of treating chronic Chagas' disease with benznidazole versus no treatment. A nonrandomized trial. Ann Intern Med 2006;144:724–734.

84. Diaz JH. Lice (pediculosis). In: Mandell GL, Bennett JR, Dolin R, eds. Principles and Practice of Infectious Diseases, 6th ed. New York: Elsevier Churchill Livingstone; 2010:3629–3632.

85. Diamantis SA, Morrell DS, Burkhart CN. Treatment of head lice. Dermatol Ther 2009;22:273–278.

86. [No author]. Benzyl alcohol for head lice. Med Lett 2009;51:57–58.

87. Idriss S, Levitt J. Malathion for head lice and scabies: Treatment and safety considerations. J Drugs Dermatol 2009;8:715–720.

88. Lebwohl M, Clark L, Levitt J. Therapy for head lice based on life cycle, resistance, and safety considerations. Pediatr 2007;119:965–974.

89. Leone PA. Scabies and Pediculosis pubis: An update of treatment regimens and general review. Clin Infect Dis 2007;44:S153–S159.

90. Heukelbach J, Feldmeier H. Scabies. Lancet 2006;1767–1774.

91. Hicks MI, Elston DM. Scabies. Dermatol Ther 2009;22:279–292.

92. Chosidow O. Scabies. N Engl J Med 2006;354:1718–1727.

Appendix 124-1 Antiparasitic Drugs

Drug	Indications	Side Effects	Comments	References
Albendazole 200 mg tablet (Albenza)	Giardiasis, Ascariasis, Neurocysticercosis	GI: abdominal pain, nausea, diarrhea, increase in liver function enzymes	Not recommended in children <2 years old	9, 16, 42, 45, 46
Artemether 20 mg/Lumefantrine 120 mg tablet (Coartem	Acute uncomplicated Falciparum malaria	Headache, dizziness, asthenia, fatigue, and arthralgia	Approved for patients >5 kg body weight	52, 75
Artesunate[a]	Severe *falciparum* malaria	Rash, dizziness, and pruritus	Obtained by IND from CDC (when IV Quinidine is not readily available)	16, 58
Atovaquone 250 mg *plus* proguanil 100 mg (Malarone)[b]	Prevention and treatment of *Plasmodium falciparum* malaria	Abdominal pain, nausea, vomiting, and headache		9, 16, 48, 49, 52, 61, 62, 75
Chloroquine phosphate (Aralen, Nivaquine) 250- and 500-mg tablets; 50 mg/mL (as HCl); 5-mL ampule	Malaria	GI: nausea, vomiting, diarrhea CNS: dizziness, headache, blurring of vision, confusion, fatigue Derm: pruritus	Administer oral dose after meals IV route: recommend ECG monitoring *Contraindication*: patients with psoriasis or porphyria	9, 16, 48, 49, 52, 61, 62, 75
Diloxanide furoateb (Furamide) 500-mg tablet[c]	Amebiasis	GI: nausea, flatulence Derm: pruritus		9, 16, 19, 20, 21, 23, 75
Furazolidone (Furoxone) 100-mg tablet Suspension: 50 mg/5 mL	Giardiasis Alternative to metronidazole	GI: nausea, vomiting Hypersensitivity: hypotension, fever, arthralgia, urticaria Other: headache	Disulfiram-like reaction with alcohol; avoid in G6PD deficiency; may cause hemolysis; changes color of urine to brown	9,16
Iodoquinol (Yodoxin) 210-mg tablet	Amebiasis	GI: abdominal pain, diarrhea Derm: rash	May interfere with thyroid function test *Contraindication*: patients with iodine intolerance	9, 16, 19–23, 75
Ivermectin (Stromectol) 6-mg tablet	Strongyloidiasis Pediculosis Scabies	Dizziness, somnolence, tremor, vertigo, pruritus, abdominal pain	Should be taken with a full glass of water	9, 16, 34, 37, 39, 92
Mebendazole (Vermox) 100-mg chewable tablet	Ascariasis, trichuriasis, hookworm, pinworm	GI: abdominal pain, diarrhea CNS: headache, dizziness Other: pyrexia, neutropenia	Drug should be taken with meals *Contraindication*: pregnancy *Drug interaction*: can increase serum levels of theophylline	9, 16, 25, 26
Mefloquine (Lariam) 250-mg tablet	*P falciparum* malaria	Incidence 17% GI: nausea, vomiting, abdominal pain, diarrhea Card: sinus bradycardia CNS: vertigo, dizziness, confusion, hallucinations, psychosis, convulsions Derm: itching, skin rash	Patients given doses in excess of 12 mg/kg should be monitored carefully because the side effects are dose related	9, 16, 48–50, 52, 55, 61, 62, 75
Metronidazole (Flagyl) Oral: 250-mg, 500-mg tablets	Amebiasis Giardiasis	GI: nausea, anorexia, vomiting, diarrhea, abdominal cramping, glossitis, metallic taste CNS: dizziness, vertigo, headache, paresthesia	Avoid alcohol; alcohol ingestion will cause the disulfiram reaction: abdominal distress, vomiting, hypotension *Contraindication*: First trimester of pregnancy	9, 11–13, 16,19–21
Nifurtimox[c] (Lampit, Bayer 2502)	South American trypanosomiasis	GI: anorexia, nausea CNS: peripheral neuritis, psychosis Hemat: hemolysis in G6PD deficiency patients	Monitor pulmonary function and hematologic parameters	9, 16, 75, 76, 78, 79
Nitazoxanide (Alinia) 100-mg/5-mL suspension	Cryptosporidiosis Giardiasis	Abdominal pain, diarrhea, vomiting, and headache	Rarely may produce yellow sclerae	12, 16, 17
Primaquine phosphate 26.3-mg tablet	Malaria *(P vivax) (P ovale)*	GI: nausea, abdominal pain CNS: mental depression	In G6PD deficiency can cause hemolysis	9, 16, 48, 49, 52, 55, 62

(continued)

Appendix 124-1 Antiparasitic Drugs (continued)

Drug	Indications	Side Effects	Comments	References
Pyrimethamine 25 mg *plus* sulfadoxine 500 mg (Fansidar)	*P falciparum*-resistant malaria	GI: nausea, abdominal pain, stomatitis, headache, and glossitis Hemat: agranulocytosis, aplastic anemia, leukopenia, megaloblastic anemia, hemolytic anemia, hemolysis in patients with G6PD deficiency	Combination was recently reported to cause the Stevens-Johnson syndrome; patients should be advised to call their physician/pharmacist if a skin rash or other reaction is seen	9, 16, 48, 49, 75
Quinacrine 100 mg[c]	Giardiasis	GI: nausea, anorexia, vomiting Headache, toxic psychosis, hepatitis, and aplastic anemia	Avoid in pregnancy, psychosis, and psoriasis	9, 12, 16
Quinidine gluconate 500 mg base/mL; 10 mL	Acute malaria	GI: nausea, vomiting, diarrhea Card: hypotension, widening of QRS and QT on ECG, heart block	Administration of IV quinidine requires close monitoring; should normally monitor ECG and all vital signs	9, 16, 48, 49, 52
Quinine sulfate 325-mg and 650-mg tablets	Acute malaria	Cinchonism: flushing, dizziness, nausea, vomiting, diarrhea (levels over 10 mcg/mL) Card: hypotension, widening of QRS complex Hemat: hemolysis, leukopenia, thrombocytopenia	When drug is administered IV, it should be administered by slow infusion (600 mg over 8 hours); close monitoring of vitals and ECG *Avoid use:* IM administration	9, 16, 48, 49, 52, 55

Card, cardiologic; Derm, dermatologic; ECG, elecetrocardiogram; G6PD, glucose-6-phosphate dehydrogenase; Hemat, hematologic; IND, investigational new drug.

[a]Investigational new drug from Centers for Disease Control and Prevention, Atlanta, GA 30333(404–639–3670).

[b]Atovaquone 62.5 mg/proguanil 25 mg (Malarone), pediatric strength.

[c]Investigational drugs obtained from Ponorama Compounding Pharmacy, 6744 Balboa Blvd, Van Nuys, CA 91406 (800–247–9767).

Available from CDC drug service, Centers for Disease Control and Prevention, Atlanta, GA 30333 (404–639–3670).

125

Urinary Tract Infections and Prostatitis

ELIZABETH A. COYLE AND RANDALL A. PRINCE

KEY CONCEPTS

❶ Urinary tract infections (UTIs) are classified as uncomplicated and complicated. *Uncomplicated* refers to an infection in an otherwise healthy female who lacks structural or functional abnormalities of the urinary tract. Most often complicated infections are associated with a predisposing lesion of the urinary tract; however, the term may be used to refer to all other infections, except for those in the otherwise healthy adult female.

❷ Recurrent UTIs are considered either reinfections or relapses. Reinfection usually happens more than 2 weeks after the last UTI, and is treated as a new uncomplicated UTI. Relapse usually happens within 2 weeks of the original infection and is a relapse of the original infection either because of unsuccessful treatment of the original infection, a resistant organism, or anatomical abnormalities.

❸ Eighty-five percent of uncomplicated urinary tract infections are caused by *Escherichia coli*, and the remainder are caused primarily by *Staphylococcus saprophyticus, Proteus* spp., and *Klebsiella* spp. Complicated infections are more frequently associated with gram-negative organisms and *Enterococcus faecalis*.

❹ Symptoms of lower urinary tract infections include dysuria, urgency, frequency, nocturia, and suprapubic heaviness, whereas upper urinary tract infections involve more systemic symptoms such as fever, nausea, vomiting, and flank pain.

❺ Significant bacteriuria traditionally has been defined as bacterial counts of greater than 100,000 (10^5)/mL of urine. Many clinicians, however, have challenged this as too general a statement. Indeed, significant bacteriuria in patients with symptoms of a urinary tract infection may be defined as greater than 10^2 organisms per milliliter.

❻ The goals of treatment of urinary tract infections are to eradicate the invading organism(s), prevent or treat systemic consequences of infections, and prevent the recurrence of infection.

❼ Uncomplicated urinary tract infections can be managed most effectively with short-course (3 days) therapy with either trimethoprim-sulfamethoxazole or a fluoroquinolone. Complicated infections require longer treatment periods (2 weeks) usually with one of these agents.

❽ In choosing appropriate antibiotic therapy, practitioners need to be cognizant of antibiotic resistance patterns, particularly to *E. coli*. Trimethoprim-sulfamethoxazole has demonstrated diminished activity against *E. coli* in some areas of the country, with reported resistance in some areas almost 30%.

❾ Acute bacterial prostatitis can be managed with many agents that have activity against the causative organism. Chronic prostatitis requires an agent that is not only active against the causative organism but also concentrates in the prostatic secretions. Therapy with trimethoprim-sulfamethoxazole or a fluoroquinolone is preferred for 4 to 6 weeks.

Infections of the urinary tract represent a wide variety of syndromes, including urethritis, cystitis, prostatitis, and pyelonephritis. Urinary tract infections (UTIs) are the most commonly occurring bacterial infections, especially in females of child-bearing age.[1-3] Approximately 60% of females will develop a UTI during their lifetime, with about one fourth having a recurrence within a year.[2] Infections in men occur much less frequently until the age of 65 years, at which point the incidence rates in men and women are similar.

A UTI is defined as the presence of microorganisms in the urinary tract that cannot be accounted for by contamination. The organisms present have the potential to invade the tissues of the urinary tract and adjacent structures. Infection may be limited to the growth of bacteria in the urine, which frequently may not produce symptoms. A UTI can present as several syndromes associated with an inflammatory response to microbial invasion and can range from asymptomatic bacteriuria to pyelonephritis with bacteremia or sepsis.

UTIs are classified by lower and upper urinary tract infections. Typically, they have been described by anatomic site of involvement. Lower tract infections correspond to cystitis (bladder), and pyelonephritis (an infection involving the kidneys) represents upper tract infection.

❶ Also, UTIs are designated as uncomplicated or complicated. Uncomplicated infections occur in individuals who lack structural or functional abnormalities of the urinary tract that interfere with the normal flow of urine or voiding mechanism. These infections occur in females of child-bearing age (15 to 45 years) who are otherwise normal, healthy individuals. Infections in males generally are not classified as uncomplicated because these infections are rare and most often represent a structural or neurologic abnormality.

Complicated UTIs are the result of a predisposing lesion of the urinary tract, such as a congenital abnormality or distortion of the urinary tract, a stone, indwelling catheter, prostatic hypertrophy, obstruction, or neurologic deficit that interferes with the normal

Learning objectives, review questions, and other resources can be found at **www.pharmacotherapyonline.com**.

TABLE 125-1	Diagnostic Criteria for Significant Abacteriuria

$\geq 10^2$ CFU coliforms/mL or $\geq 10^5$ CFU noncoliforms/mL in a symptomatic female
$\geq 10^3$ CFU bacteria/mL in a symptomatic male
$\geq 10^5$ CFU bacteria/mL in asymptomatic individuals on two consecutive specimens
Any growth of bacteria on suprapubic catheterization in a symptomatic patient
$\geq 10^2$ CFU bacteria/mL in a catheterized patient

CFU, colony-forming unit.

flow of urine and urinary tract defenses. Complicated infections occur in both genders and frequently involve the upper and lower urinary tract.

❷ Recurrent UTIs in healthy nonpregnant women—three or more UTIs occurring within 1 year—are a common problem. They are characterized by multiple symptomatic infections with asymptomatic periods occurring between each episode and may be either reinfections or relapses. Reinfections are caused by a different organism than originally isolated and account for the majority of recurrent UTIs. Relapses are the development of repeated infections with the same initial organism and usually indicate a persistent infectious source.[2]

Asymptomatic bacteriuria is a common finding, particularly among those 65 years of age and older, when there is significant bacteriuria ($>10^5$ bacteria/mL of urine) in the absence of symptoms. Symptomatic abacteriuria or acute urethral syndrome consists of symptoms of frequency and dysuria in the absence of significant bacteriuria. This syndrome is commonly associated with *Chlamydia* infections.

Significant abacteriuria is a term used to distinguish the presence of microorganisms that represent true infection versus contamination of the urine as it passes through the distal urethra prior to collection. Historically, bacterial counts equal to or greater than 100,000 organisms/mL of urine in a "clean-catch" specimen were judged to indicate true infection.[4-6] Counts less than 100,000 organisms/mL of urine, however, may represent true infection in certain situations. For example, with concurrent antibacterial drug administration, rapid urine flow, low urinary pH, or upper tract obstruction.[6] Table 125–1 lists the clinical definitions of significant bacteriuria, which are dependent on the clinical setting and the method of specimen collection.[6] These criteria allow for more appropriate specificity and sensitivity in documenting infection under differing clinical circumstances.

EPIDEMIOLOGY

The prevalence of UTIs varies with age and gender. In newborns and infants up to 6 months of age, the prevalence of abacteriuria is approximately 1% and is more common in boys. Most of these infections are associated with structural or functional abnormalities of the urinary tract and also have been correlated with noncircumcision.[7] Between the ages of 1 and 6 years, UTIs occur more frequently in females. The prevalence of abacteriuria in females and males of this age group is 7% and 2%, respectively.[7,8] Infections occurring in preschool boys usually are associated with congenital abnormalities of the urinary tract. These infections are difficult to recognize because of the age of the patient, but they often are symptomatic. In addition, the majority of renal damage associated with UTI develops at this age.[7,8]

Through grade school and before puberty, the prevalence of UTI is approximately 1%, with 5% of females reported to have significant bacteriuria prior to leaving high school. This percentage increases dramatically to 1% to 4% after puberty in nonpregnant females primarily as a result of sexual activity. Approximately 1 in 5 women will suffer a symptomatic UTI at some point in their lives. Many women have recurrent infections, with a significant proportion of these women having a history of childhood infections. In contrast, the prevalence of bacteriuria in adult men is very low (<0.1%).[9]

In the elderly, the ratio of bacteriuria in women and men is dramatically altered and is approximately equal in persons older than age 65 years.[10] The overall incidence of UTI increases substantially in this population, with the majority of infections being asymptomatic. The rate of infection increases further for elderly persons who are residing in nursing homes, particularly those who are hospitalized frequently. The increase is probably the result of factors such as obstruction from prostatic hypertrophy in males, poor bladder emptying as a result of prolapse in females, fecal incontinence in demented patients, neuromuscular disease including strokes, and increased urinary instrumentation (catheterization).

ETIOLOGY

❸ The bacteria causing UTIs usually originate from bowel flora of the host. Although virtually every organism is associated with UTIs, certain organisms predominate as a result of specific virulence factors. The most common cause of uncomplicated UTIs is *Escherichia coli*, which accounts for 80% to 90% of community-acquired infections. Additional causative organisms in uncomplicated infections include *Staphylococcus saprophyticus*, *Klebsiella pneumoniae*, *Proteus* spp., *Pseudomonas aeruginosa*, and *Enterococcus* spp.[11] Because *Staphylococcus epidermidis* is frequently isolated from the urinary tract, it should be considered initially a contaminant. Repeat cultures should be performed to help confirm the organism as a real pathogen.

Organisms isolated from individuals with complicated infections are more varied and generally are more resistant than those found in uncomplicated infections. *E. coli* is a frequently isolated pathogen, but it accounts for less than 50% of infections. Other frequently isolated organisms include *Proteus* spp., *K. pneumoniae*, *Enterobacter* spp., *P. aeruginosa*, staphylococci, and enterococci. Enterococci represent the second most frequently isolated organisms in hospitalized patients.[11,12] In part, this finding may be related to the extensive use of third-generation cephalosporin antibiotics, which are not active against the enterococci. Vancomycin-resistant *Enterococcus faecalis* and *Enterococcus faecium* (vancomycin-resistant enterococci) have become more widespread, especially in patients with long-term hospitalizations or underlying malignancies. Vancomycin-resistant enterococci are major therapeutic and infection control issues because the organisms are susceptible to few antimicrobials.[12]

Staphylococcus aureus infections may arise from the urinary tract, but they are more commonly a result of bacteremia producing metastatic abscesses in the kidney. *Candida* spp. are common causes of UTI in the critically ill and chronically catheterized patient.

Most UTIs are caused by a single organism; however, in patients with stones, indwelling urinary catheters, or chronic renal abscesses, multiple organisms may be isolated. Depending on the clinical situation, the recovery of multiple organisms may represent contamination, and a repeat evaluation should be done.

PATHOPHYSIOLOGY

ROUTE OF INFECTION

Organisms typically gain entry into the urinary tract via three routes: the ascending, hematogenous (descending), and lymphatic pathways. The female urethra usually is colonized by bacteria believed to originate from the fecal flora. The short length of the female urethra and its proximity to the perirectal area make colonization of the urethra likely. Other factors that promote urethral colonization include the use of spermicides and diaphragms as methods of contraception.[2,3] Although there is evidence in females that bladder infections follow colonization of the urethra, the mode of ascent of the microorganisms is incompletely understood. Massage of the female urethra and sexual intercourse allow bacteria to reach the bladder.[13] Once bacteria have reached the bladder, the organisms quickly multiply and can ascend the ureters to the kidneys. This sequence of events is more likely to occur if vesicoureteral reflux (reflux of urine into the ureters and kidneys while voiding) is present. UTIs are more common in females than in males because the anatomic differences in location and length of the urethra tend to support the ascending route of infections as the primary acquisition route.

Infection of the kidney by hematogenous spread of microorganisms usually occurs as the result of dissemination of organisms from a distant primary infection in the body. Infections via the descending route are uncommon and involve a relatively small number of invasive pathogens. Bacteremia caused by *S. aureus* may produce renal abscesses. Additional organisms include *Candida* spp., *Mycobacterium tuberculosis*, *Salmonella* spp., and enterococci. Of particular interest, it is difficult to produce experimental pyelonephritis by intravenously administering common gram-negative organisms such as *E. coli* and *P. aeruginosa*. Overall, less than 5% of documented UTIs result from hematogenous spread of microorganisms.

There appears to be little evidence supporting a significant role for renal lymphatics in the pathogenesis of UTIs. There are lymphatic communications between the bowel and kidney, as well as between the bladder and kidney. There is no evidence, however, that microorganisms are transferred to the kidney via this route.

After bacteria reach the urinary tract, three factors determine the development of infection: the size of the inoculum, the virulence of the microorganism, and the competency of the natural host defense mechanisms. Most UTIs reflect a failure in host defense mechanisms.

HOST DEFENSE MECHANISMS

The normal urinary tract generally is resistant to invasion by bacteria and is efficient in rapidly eliminating microorganisms that reach the bladder. The urine under normal circumstances is capable of inhibiting and killing microorganisms. The factors thought to be responsible include a low pH, extremes in osmolality, high urea concentration, and high organic acid concentration. Bacterial growth is further inhibited in males by the addition of prostatic secretions.[14,15]

The introduction of bacteria into the bladder stimulates micturition, with increased diuresis and efficient emptying of the bladder. These factors are critical in preventing the initiation and maintenance of bladder infections. Patients who are unable to void urine completely are at greater risk of developing UTIs and frequently have recurrent infections. Also, patients with even small residual amounts of urine in their bladder respond less favorably to treatment than patients who are able to empty their bladders completely.[16]

An important virulence factor of bacteria is their ability to adhere to urinary epithelial cells, resulting in colonization of the urinary tract, bladder infections, and pyelonephritis. Various factors that act as antiadherence mechanisms are present in the bladder, preventing bacterial colonization and infection. The epithelial cells of the bladder are coated with a urinary mucus or slime called *glycosaminoglycan*. This thin layer of surface mucopolysaccharide is hydrophilic and strongly negatively charged. When bound to the uroepithelium, it attracts water molecules and forms a layer between the bladder and urine. The antiadherence characteristics of the glycosaminoglycan layer are nonspecific, and when the layer is removed by dilute acid solutions, rapid bacterial adherence results.[17]

In addition, the Tamm-Horsfall protein is a glycoprotein produced by the ascending limb of Henle and distal tubule that is secreted into the urine and contains mannose residues. These mannose residues bind *E. coli* that contain small surface-projecting organellae on their surfaces called *pili* or *fimbriae*. Type 1 fimbriae are mannose sensitive, and this interaction prevents the bacteria from binding to similar receptors present on the mucosal surface of the bladder. Other factors that possibly prevent adherence of bacteria include immunoglobulins (Ig) G and A. Investigators have documented both systemic and local kidney immunoglobulin synthesis in upper tract infections. The role of immunoglobulins in preventing bladder infection is less clear. Patients with reduced urinary levels of secretory IgA are, however, at increased risk of infections of the urinary tract.

After bacteria actually have invaded the bladder mucosa, an inflammatory response is stimulated with the mobilization of polymorphonuclear leukocytes (PMNs) and resulting phagocytosis. PMNs are primarily responsible for limiting the tissue invasion and controlling the spread of infection in the bladder and kidney. They do not play a role in preventing bladder colonization or infections and actually contribute to renal tissue damage.

Other host factors that may play a role in the prevention of UTIs are the presence of *Lactobacillus* in the vaginal flora and circulating estrogen levels. In premenopausal women, circulating estrogen supports the vaginal tract growth of lactobacilli, which produce lactic acid to help maintain a low vaginal pH, thereby preventing *E. coli* vaginal colonization.[18] Topical estrogens are used for the prevention of UTI in postmenopausal women who have more than 3 recurrent UTI episodes per year and are not on oral estrogens.[19]

BACTERIAL VIRULENCE FACTORS

Pathogenic organisms have differing degrees of pathogenicity (virulence), which play a role in the development and severity of infection. Bacteria that adhere to the epithelium of the urinary tract are associated with colonization and infection. The mechanism of adhesion of gram-negative bacteria, particularly *E. coli*, is related to bacterial fimbriae that are rigid, hair-like appendages of the cell wall.[9] These fimbriae adhere to specific glycolipid components on epithelial cells. The most common type of fimbriae is type 1, which binds to mannose residues present in glycoproteins. Glycosaminoglycan and Tamm-Horsfall protein are rich in mannose residues that readily trap those organisms that contain type 1 fimbriae, which are then washed out of the bladder.[20] Other fimbriae are mannose resistant and are associated more frequently with pyelonephritis, such as P fimbriae, which bind avidly to specific glycolipid receptors on uroepithelial cells. These bacteria are resistant to washout or removal by glycosaminoglycan and are able to multiply and invade tissue, especially the kidney. In addition, PMNs, as well as secretory IgA antibodies, contain receptors for type 1 fimbriae, which facilitate phagocytosis, but they lack receptors for P fimbriae.

Other virulence factors include the production of hemolysin and aerobactin.[21] Hemolysin is a cytotoxic protein produced by bacteria that lyses a wide range of cells, including erythrocytes, PMNs, and monocytes. *E. coli* and other gram-negative bacteria require iron for aerobic metabolism and multiplication. Aerobactin facilitates the binding and uptake of iron by *E. coli*; however, the significance of this property in the pathogenesis of UTIs remains unknown.

PREDISPOSING FACTORS TO INFECTION

The normal urinary tract typically is resistant to infection and colonization by pathogenic bacteria. In patients with underlying structural abnormalities of the urinary tract, the typical host defenses previously discussed usually are lacking. There are several known abnormalities of the urinary tract system that interfere with its natural defense mechanisms, the most important of which is obstruction. Obstruction can inhibit the normal flow of urine, disrupting the natural flushing and voiding effect in removing bacteria from the bladder and resulting in incomplete emptying. Common conditions that result in residual urine volumes include prostatic hypertrophy, urethral strictures, calculi, tumors, bladder diverticula, and drugs such as anticholinergic agents. Additional causes of incomplete bladder emptying include neurologic malfunctions associated with stroke, diabetes, spinal cord injuries, tabes dorsalis, and other neuropathies. Vesicoureteral reflux represents a condition in which urine is forced up the ureters to the kidneys. Urinary reflux is associated not only with an increased incidence of UTIs and pyelonephritis, but also with renal damage.[8,16] Reflux may be the result of a congenital abnormality or, more commonly, bladder overdistension from obstruction.

Other risk factors include urinary catheterization, mechanical instrumentation, pregnancy, and the use of spermicides and diaphragms.

CLINICAL PRESENTATION

❹ The presenting signs and symptoms of UTIs in adults are recognized easily (Table 125–2). Women frequently will report gross hematuria. Systemic symptoms, including fever, typically are absent in this setting. Unfortunately, large numbers of patients with significant bacteriuria are asymptomatic. These patients may be normal, healthy patients, elderly patients, children, pregnant patients, and patients with indwelling catheters. It is important to note that attempts at differentiating upper tract from lower tract infections on the basis of symptoms alone are not reliable.

Elderly patients frequently do not experience specific urinary symptoms, but they will present with altered mental status, change in eating habits, or gastrointestinal symptoms. In addition, patients with indwelling catheters or neurologic disorders commonly will not have lower tract symptoms, whereas flank pain and fever may be recognized. Many of the aforementioned patients, however, frequently will develop upper tract infections with bacteremia and no or minimal urinary tract symptoms.

Symptoms alone are unreliable for the diagnosis of bacterial UTIs. The key to the diagnosis of UTI is the ability to demonstrate significant numbers of microorganisms in an appropriate urine specimen to distinguish contamination from infection. The type and extent of laboratory examination required depends on the clinical situation.

TABLE 125-2	Clinical Presentation of Urinary Tract Infections in Adults

Signs and symptoms
  Lower UTI: dysuria, urgency, frequency, nocturia, suprapubic heaviness
  Gross hematuria
  Upper UTI: flank pain, fever, nausea, vomiting, malaise
Physical examination
  Upper UTI: costovertebral tenderness
Laboratory tests
  Bacteriuria
  Pyuria (white blood cell count >10/mm³)
  Nitrite-positive urine (with nitrite reducers)
  Leukocyte esterase-positive urine
  Antibody-coated bacteria (upper UTI)

UTI, urinary tract infection.

URINE COLLECTION

Examination of the urine is the cornerstone of laboratory evaluation for UTIs. There are three acceptable methods of urine collection. The first is the *midstream clean-catch method*. After cleaning the urethral opening area in both men and women, 20 to 30 mL of urine is voided and discarded. The next part of the urine flow is collected and should be processed immediately (refrigerated as soon as possible). Specimens that are allowed to sit at room temperature for several hours may result in falsely elevated bacterial counts. The midstream clean-catch is the preferred method for the routine collection of urine for culture. When a routine urine specimen cannot be collected or contamination occurs, alternative collection techniques must be used.

The two acceptable alternative methods include catheterization and suprapubic bladder aspiration. Catheterization may be necessary for patients who are uncooperative or who are unable to void urine. If catheterization is performed carefully with aseptic technique, the method yields reliable results. Note, however, that introduction of bacteria into the bladder may result, and the procedure is associated with infection in 1% to 2% of patients. Suprapubic bladder aspiration involves inserting a needle directly into the bladder and aspirating the urine. This procedure bypasses the contaminating organisms present in the urethra, and any bacteria found using this technique generally are considered to represent significant bacteriuria.[24,25] Suprapubic aspiration is a safe and painless procedure that is most useful in newborns, infants, paraplegics, seriously ill patients, and others in whom infection is suspected and routine procedures have provided confusing or equivocal results.

BACTERIAL COUNT

❺ The diagnosis of UTI is based on the isolation of significant numbers of bacteria from a urine specimen. Microscopic examination of a urine sample is an easy-to-perform and reliable method for the presumptive diagnosis of bacteriuria. The examination may be performed by preparing a Gram stain of unspun or centrifuged urine. The presence of at least one organism per oil-immersion field in a properly collected uncentrifuged specimen correlates well with more than 100,000 colony-forming units (CFU)/mL (10^5 CFU/mL) of urine. For detecting smaller numbers of organisms, a centrifuged specimen is more sensitive. Such examinations detect more than 10^5 bacteria/mL with a sensitivity of greater than 90% and a specificity of greater than 70%.[22,23] A quantitative count of greater than or equal to 10^5 CFU/mL is considered indicative of a UTI; however, up to 50% of women will present with clinical symptoms of a UTI with lower counts (10^3 CFU/mL).[4]

PYURIA, HEMATURIA, AND PROTEINURIA

Microscopic examination of the urine for leukocytes is also used to determine the presence of pyuria. The presence of pyuria in a symptomatic patient correlates with significant bacteriuria.[24] Pyuria is defined as a white blood cell (WBC) count of greater than 10 WBC/mm³ of urine. A count of 5 to 10 WBC/mm³ is accepted as the upper limit of normal. It should be emphasized that pyuria is nonspecific and signifies only the presence of inflammation and not necessarily infection. Thus patients with pyuria may or may not have infection. Sterile pyuria has long been associated with urinary tuberculosis, as well as chlamydial and fungal urinary infections.

Hematuria, microscopic or gross, is frequently present in patients with UTI but is nonspecific. Hematuria may indicate the presence of other disorders, such as renal calculi, tumors, or glomerulonephritis. Proteinuria is found commonly in the presence of infection.

CHEMISTRY

Several biochemical tests have been developed for screening urine for the presence of bacteria. A common dipstick test detects the presence of nitrite in the urine, which is formed by bacteria that reduce nitrate normally present in the urine. False-positive tests are uncommon. False negative tests are more common and frequently are caused by the presence of gram-positive organisms or *P. aeruginosa* that do not reduce nitrate.[25] Other causes of false tests include low urinary pH, frequent voiding, and dilute urine.

The leukocyte esterase dipstick test is a rapid screening test for detecting the presence of pyuria. Leukocytes esterase is found in primary neutrophil granules and indicates the presence of WBCs. The leukocyte esterase test is a sensitive and highly specific test for detecting more than 10 WBC/mm^3 of urine. When the leukocyte esterase test is used with the nitrite test, the reported positive predictive value and specificity is 79% and 82%, respectively, for the detection of bacteriuria.[27] These tests can be useful in the outpatient evaluation of uncomplicated UTIs. However, urine culture is still the "gold standard" test in determining the presence of UTIs.

CULTURE

The most reliable method of diagnosing UTI is by quantitative urine culture. Urine in the bladder is normally sterile, making it statistically possible to differentiate contamination of the urine from infection by quantifying the number of bacteria present in a urine sample. This criterion is based on a properly collected midstream clean-catch urine specimen. Patients with infection usually have greater than 10^5 bacteria/mL of urine. It should be emphasized that as many as one third of women with symptomatic infection have less than 10^5 bacteria/mL. A significant portion of patients with UTIs, either symptomatic or asymptomatic, also have less than 10^5 bacteria/mL of urine.

Several laboratory methods are used to quantify bacteria present in the urine. The most accurate method is the pour-plate technique. This method is unsuitable for a high-volume laboratory because it is expensive and time-consuming. The streak-plate method is an alternative that involves using a calibrated-loop technique to streak a fixed amount of urine on an agar plate. This method is used most commonly in diagnostic laboratories because it is simple to perform and less costly.

After identification and quantification are complete, the next step is to determine the susceptibility of the organism. There are several methods by which bacterial susceptibility testing may be performed. Knowledge of bacterial susceptibility and achievable urine concentration of the antibiotics puts the clinician in a better position to select an appropriate agent for treatment.

Infection Site

Several methods have been evaluated to determine the location of infection within the urinary system and differentiate upper tract from lower tract involvement. The most direct method is a ureteral catheterization procedure as described by Stamey and colleagues.[28] The method involves the passage of a catheter into the bladder and then into each ureter, where quantitative cultures are obtained. History and physical examination were of little value in predicting the site of infection. Although this method provides direct quantitative evidence for UTI, it is invasive, technically difficult, and expensive. The Fairley bladder washout technique is a modification of the Stamey procedure that involves Foley catheterization only.[29] After the catheter is passed into the bladder, bladder samples are obtained, and the bladder is washed out, with culture samples taken at 10, 20, and 30 minutes. The procedure shows that up to 50% of patients have renal involvement regardless of signs and symptoms. Other investigators found 10% to 20% of tests to be equivocal.[29]

Noninvasive methods of localization may be more acceptable for routine use; however, they have limited clinical value. Patients with pyelonephritis can have abnormalities in urinary concentrating ability. The use of concentrating ability for localization of UTIs, however, is associated with high false-positive and false-negative responses and is not useful clinically.[25] The antibody-coated bacteria test is an immunofluorescent method that detects bacteria coated with Ig in freshly voided urine, indicating upper urinary tract infection. The sensitivity and specificity of this test to localize the site of infection are reported to average 88% and 76%, respectively.[30] Because of the high incidence of false-positive and false-negative results, antibody-coated bacteria testing is not used routinely in the management of UTIs.

Virtually all patients with uncomplicated lower tract infections can be cured with a short course of antibiotic therapy, and this assumption sometimes can be used to distinguish between patients with lower and upper tract infections. Patients who do not respond or who relapse do so because of upper tract involvement. It is rarely necessary to localize the site of infection to direct the clinical management of such patients.

TREATMENT

■ DESIRED OUTCOME

6 The goals of UTI treatments are (a) to eradicate the invading organism(s), (b) to prevent or to treat systemic consequences of infection, and (c) to prevent the recurrence of infection.

■ MANAGEMENT

The management of a patient with a UTI includes initial evaluation, selection of an antibacterial agent and duration of therapy, and followup evaluation. The initial selection of an antimicrobial agent for the treatment of UTI is based primarily on the severity of the presenting signs and symptoms, the site of infection, and whether the infection is determined to be uncomplicated or complicated. Other considerations include antibiotic susceptibility, side-effect potential, cost, and the comparative inconvenience of different therapies.

Various pharmacologic factors may affect the action of antibacterial agents. Certainly, the ability of the agent to achieve appropriate concentrations in the urine is of utmost importance. Factors that affect the rate and extent of excretion through the kidney include the patient's glomerular filtration rate and whether or not the agent is actively secreted. Filtration depends on the molecular size and degree of protein binding of the agent. Agents such as sulfonamides, tetracyclines, and aminoglycosides enter the urine via filtration. As the glomerular filtration rate is reduced, the amount of drug that enters the urine is reduced. Most β-lactam agents and quinolones are filtered and are actively secreted into the urine. For this reason, these agents achieve high urinary concentrations despite unfavorable protein-binding characteristics or the presence of renal dysfunction.

The ability to eradicate bacteria from the urine is related directly to the sensitivity of the microorganism and the achievable concentrations of the antimicrobial agent in the urine. Unfortunately, most susceptibility testing is directed at achievable concentrations in the blood. There is a poor correlation between achievable blood levels of antimicrobial agents and the eradication of bacteria from the urine.[31] In the treatment of lower tract infections, plasma concentrations of antibacterial agents may not be important, but achieving appropriate plasma concentrations appears critical in patients with bacteremia and renal abscesses.

Nonspecific therapies have been advocated in the treatment and prevention of UTIs. Fluid hydration has been used to produce rapid dilution of bacteria and removal of infected urine by increased voiding. A critical factor appears to be the amount of residual volume remaining after voiding. As little as 10 mL of residual urine can alter the eradication of infection significantly.[16] Paradoxically, increased diuresis also may promote susceptibility to infection by diluting the normal antibacterial properties of the urine. Often in clinical practice the concentrations of antimicrobial agents in the urine are so high that dilution has little effect on efficacy.

The antibacterial activity of the urine is related to the low pH, which is the result of high concentrations of various organic acids. Large volumes of cranberry juice increase the antibacterial activity of the urine and prevent the development of UTIs.[3,32–34] Apparently, the fructose and other unknown substances (condensed tannins) in cranberry juice act to interfere with adherence mechanisms of some pathogens, thereby preventing infection. Acidification of the urine by cranberry juice does not appear to play a significant role. The use of other agents (ascorbic acid) to acidify the urine to hinder bacterial growth does not achieve significant acidification. Consequently, attempts to acidify urine with systemic agents are not recommended. *Lactobacillus* probiotics also may aid in the prevention of female UTIs by decreasing the vaginal pH, thereby decreasing *E. coli* colonization.[19,33] In postmenopausal women, estrogen replacement may be of help in the prevention of recurrent UTIs. After 1 month of topical estrogen replacement, decreases in vaginal *Lactobacillus*, as well as decreases in vaginal pH and *E. coli* colonization, have been found.[18,33]

Urinary analgesics such as phenazopyridine hydrochloride are used frequently by many clinicians.[3] If the pain or dysuria present in a UTI is a consequence of infection, then urinary analgesics have little clinical role because most patients' symptoms respond quite rapidly to appropriate antibacterial therapy. Urinary analgesics also may mask signs and symptoms of UTIs not responding to antimicrobial therapy.

CLINICAL CONTROVERSY

The role of nonantibiotic alternatives such as cranberry juice, estrogens, and lactobacilli in the prevention of urinary tract infections has long been discussed. Lactobaccillus potentially helps keep the vaginal pH in the normal range (pH 4–4.5), regulating genitourinary bacteria assisting in the prevention of UTIs.[33] Possible clinical benefits with cranberry juice in sexually active adult women with recurrent UTI have been suggested. However, the consistency of study results has varied, as have the types of cranberry products tested, leading to inconclusive evidence.[32,34] In a randomized, double-blind, placebo-controlled study, postmenopausal women receiving topical estriol vaginal cream had significantly fewer UTIs than did those receiving placebo.[18,19] Estrogens are only recommended in topical formulation in postmenapausal females having ≥ 3 recurrent UTIs/year and are not taking oral estrogens.[19] More thorough studies on the overall effectiveness of cranberry juice, lactobacilli, and/or estrogen replacement needs to be performed before a uniform opinion of the role of these agents in UTIs can be formulated.

■ PHARMACOLOGIC THERAPY

Ideally, the antimicrobial agent chosen should be well tolerated, well absorbed, achieve high urinary concentrations, and have a spectrum of activity limited to the known or suspected pathogen(s).

Table 125–3 lists the most common agents used in the treatment of UTIs along with comments concerning their general use. Table 125–4 presents an overview of various therapeutic options for outpatient therapy of UTI. Table 125–5 describes empirical treatment regimens for selected clinical situations.

❽ The therapeutic management of UTIs is best accomplished by first categorizing the type of infection: acute uncomplicated cystitis, symptomatic abacteriuria, asymptomatic bacteriuria, complicated UTIs, recurrent infections, or prostatitis. In choosing the appropriate antibiotic therapy, it is important to be aware of the increasing resistance of *E. coli* and other pathogens to many frequently prescribed antimicrobials. Resistance to *E. coli* is as high as 37% for ampicillin.[35] Overall, most *E. coli* remain susceptible to trimethoprim-sulfamethoxazole, although resistance is continuing to increase and has been reported as high as 27%.[35] Although resistance to the fluoroquinolones remains low, these agents are being utilized more frequently and the incidence of fluoroquinolone-resistant *E. coli* is increasingly being reported and is of great concern.[35–40] Current or recent antibiotic exposure is the most significant risk factor associated with *E. coli* resistance, and with the extensive use of the fluoroquinolones and trimethoprim-sulfamethoxazole for various infections, including UTIs, resistance will continue to increase.[35–39] In light of rising resistance and in order to decrease the overuse of broad-spectrum antimicrobials, agents such as nitrofurantoin and fosfomycin may be reliable options in the treatment of acute uncomplicated cystitis. In addition, *E. coli* remains highly susceptible to both nitrofurantoin and fosfomycin.[3,41–45] Antibiotic therapy should be determined based on the geographic resistance patterns, as well as the patient's recent history of antibiotic exposure.

CLINICAL CONTROVERSY

The problem of antibiotic resistance is increasing in the treatment of uncomplicated urinary tract infections. The majority of infections are treated with trimethoprim-sulfamethoxazole or a fluoroquinolone; however, resistance to these agents is continuing to rise with rates as high as 29.6% and 9%, respectively.[40] These agents have very broad antimicrobial coverage, are used for various types of infections, and have a high impact on gastrointestinal flora, increasing the risk for resistant *E. coli* pathogens.[35–37,40,41] Although these agents remain highly effective in the empiric treatment of the majority of uncomplicated UTIs, the need for more selective agents for management of such infections may be warranted. Therefore, the utilization of more selective antimicrobials as first line agents, such as nitrofurantoin and fosfomycin, may become common in the coming years.[42,43]

■ ACUTE UNCOMPLICATED CYSTITIS

Acute uncomplicated cystitis is the most common form of UTI. These infections typically occur in women of childbearing age and often are related to sexual activity. Although the presence of dysuria, frequency, urgency, and suprapubic discomfort frequently is associated with lower tract infection, a significant number of patients have upper tract involvement as well.[3] Because these infections are predominantly caused by *E. coli*, antimicrobial therapy initially should be directed against this organism. Other common causes include *S. saprophyticus* and occasionally, *K. pneumoniae* and *Proteus mirabilis*. Because the causative organisms and their susceptibility generally are known, many clinicians advocate a cost-effective approach to management. This approach includes

TABLE 125-3 Commonly Used Antimicrobial Agents in the Treatment of Urinary Tract Infections

Agent	Comments
Oral therapy	
Trimethoprim-sulfamethoxazole	This combination is highly effective against most aerobic enteric bacteria except *Pseudomonas aeruginosa*. High urinary tract tissue levels and urine levels are achieved, which may be important in complicated infection treatment. Also effective as prophylaxis for recurrent infections.
Penicillins	Ampicillin is the standard penicillin that has broad-spectrum activity. Increasing *Escherichia coli*
Ampicillin	resistance has limited amoxicillin use in acute cystitis. Drug of choice for enterococci sensitive
Amoxicillin-clavulanic acid	to penicillin. Amoxicillin-clavulanate is preferred for resistance problems.
Cephalosporins	There are no major advantages of these agents over other agents in the treatment of UTIs, and they
Cephalexin	are more expensive. They may be useful in cases of resistance to amoxicillin and trimethoprim–
Cefaclor	sulfamethoxazole. These agents are not active against enterococci.
Cefadroxil	
Cefuroxime	
Cefixime	
Cefprozil	
Cefpodoxime	
Tetracyclines	These agents have been effective for initial episodes of urinary tract infections; however, resistance
Tetracycline	develops rapidly, and their use is limited. These agents also lead to candidal overgrowth. They are
Doxycycline	useful primarily for chlamydial infections.
Minocycline	
Fluoroquinolones	The newer quinolones have a greater spectrum of activity, including *P. aeruginosa*. These agents
Ciprofloxacin	are effective for pyelonephritis and prostatitis. Avoid in pregnancy and children. Moxifloxacin
Levofloxacin	should not be used owing to inadequate urinary concentrations.
Nitrofurantoin	This agent is effective as both a therapeutic and prophylactic agent in patients with recurrent UTIs. Main advantage is the lack of resistance even after long courses of therapy. Adverse effects may limit use (GI intolerance, neuropathies, pulmonary reactions).
Azithromycin	Single-dose therapy for chlamydial infections.
Fosfomycin	Single-dose therapy for uncomplicated infections.
Parenteral therapy	
Aminoglycosides	Gentamicin and tobramycin are equally effective; gentamicin is less expensive. Tobramycin has
Gentamicin	better pseudomonal activity, which may be important in serious systemic infections. Amikacin
Tobramycin	generally is reserved for multiresistant bacteria.
Amikacin	
Penicillins	These agents generally are equally effective for susceptible bacteria. The extended-spectrum
Ampicillin	penicillins are more active against *P. aeruginosa* and enterococci and often are preferred over
Ampicillin-sulbactam	cephalosporins. They are very useful in renally impaired patients or when an aminoglycoside
Ticarcillin-clavulanate	is to be avoided.
Piperacillin-tazobactam	
Cephalosporins, first-, second-, and third-generation	Second- and third-generation cephalosporins have a broad spectrum of activity against gram-negative bacteria but are not active against enterococci and have limited activity against *P. aeruginosa*. Ceftazidime and cefepime are active against *P. aeruginosa*. They are useful for nosocomial infections and urosepsis due to susceptible pathogens.
Carbapenems/Monobactams	These agents have a broad spectrum of activity, including gram-positive, gram-negative, and
Imipenem-cilastatin	anaerobic bacteria.
Meropenem	Imipenem, meropenem, and doripenem are active against *P. aeruginosa* and enterococci,
Ertapenem	but ertapenem is not. All may be associated with candidal superinfections.
Doripenem	
Aztreonam	A monobactam that is only active against gram-negative bacteria, including some strains of *P. aeruginosa*. Generally useful for nosocomial infections when aminoglycosides are to be avoided and in penicillin-sensitive patients.
Fluoroquinolones	These agents have broad-spectrum activity against both gram-negative and gram-positive bacteria.
Ciprofloxacin	They provide urine and high-tissue concentrations and are actively secreted in reduced renal
Levofloxacin	function.

a urinalysis and initiation of empirical therapy without a urine culture (Fig. 125–1).[1] Therefore, the susceptibility patterns of the geographic area drive the choice of empiric therapy, not necessarily the specific organism causing the infection.

The goal of treatment for uncomplicated cystitis is to eradicate the causative organism and to reduce the incidence of recurrence caused by relapse or reinfection. The ability to reduce the chance of recurrence depends on the agent's efficacy in eradicating the uropathogenic bacteria from the vaginal and gastrointestinal reservoir. In the past, conventional therapy consisted of an effective oral antibiotic administered for 7 to 14 days. However, acute cystitis is a superficial mucosal infection that can be eradicated

with much shorter courses of therapy (3 days). Advantages of short-course therapy include increased compliance, fewer side effects, decreased cost, and less potential for the development of resistance.

❼ Three-day courses of trimethoprim-sulfamethoxazole or a fluoroquinolone (e.g., ciprofloxacin or levofloxacin) are superior to single-dose therapies.[44,46–48] The fluoroquinolone moxifloxacin is not recommended for use in UTIs owing to the inadequate urinary concentrations.[49] A 5-day course of nitrofurantoin is as effective as a 3-day course of trimethoprim-sulfamethoxazole, and can be considered an alternative therapy.[50] The use of amoxicillin or amoxicillin/clavulanate is not recommended because of the high

TABLE 125-4 Overview of Outpatient Antimicrobial Therapy for Lower Tract Infections in Adults

Indications	Antibiotic	Dose[a]	Interval	Duration
Lower tract infections Uncomplicated	Trimethoprim-sulfamethoxazole	1 DS tablet	Twice a day	3 days
	Ciprofloxacin	250 mg	Twice a day	3 days
	Levofloxacin	250 mg	Once a day	3 days
	Amoxicillin	500 mg	Twice a day	5–7 days
	Amoxicillin-clavulanate	500 mg	Every 8 hours	5–7 days
	Trimethoprim	100 mg	Twice a day	3–5 days
	Nitrofurantoin macrocrystal	100 mg	Every 6 hours	7 days
	Nitrofurantoin monohydrate	100 mg	Twice a day	5 days
	Fosfomycin	3 g	Single dose	1 day
Complicated	Trimethoprim-sulfamethoxazole	1 DS tablet	Twice a day	7–10 days
	Ciprofloxacin	250–500 mg	Twice a day	7–10 days
	Levofloxacin	250 mg	Once a day	10 days
		750 mg	Once a day	5 days
	Amoxicillin-clavulanate	500 mg	Every 8 hours	7–10 days
Recurrent infections	Nitrofurantoin	50 mg	Once a day	6 months
	Trimethoprim-sulfamethoxazole	1/2 SS tablet	Once a day	6 months
Acute urethral syndrome	Trimethoprim-sulfamethoxazole	1 DS tablet	Twice a day	3 days
Failure of trimethoprim-sulfamethoxazole	Azithromycin	1 g	Single dose	
	Doxycycline	100 mg	Twice a day	7 days
Acute pyelonephritis	Trimethoprim-sulfamethoxazole	1 DS tablet	Twice a day	14 days
	Ciprofloxacin	500 mg	Twice a day	14 days
	Levofloxacin	250 mg	Once a day	10 days
		750 mg	Once a day	5 days
	Amoxicillin-clavulanate	500 mg	Every 8 hours	14 days

DS, double strength; SS, single strength.
[a]Dosing intervals for normal renal function.

incidence of resistant *E. coli*. For most adult females, short-course therapy is the treatment of choice for uncomplicated lower UTIs. Short-course therapy is inappropriate for patients who have had previous infections caused by resistant bacteria, for male patients, and for patients with complicated UTIs. If symptoms recur or do not respond to therapy, a urine culture should be obtained and conventional therapy with a suitable agent instituted.[1]

■ SYMPTOMATIC ABACTERIURIA

Symptomatic abacteriuria or acute urethral syndrome represents a clinical syndrome in which females present with dysuria and pyuria, but the urine culture reveals less than 10^5 bacteria/mL of urine. Acute urethral syndrome accounts for more than half the complaints of dysuria seen in the community today. These women

TABLE 125-5 Evidence-Based Empirical Treatment of Urinary Tract Infections and Prostatitis

Diagnosis	Pathogens	Treatment Recommendation	Comments
Acute uncomplicated cystitis	*Escherichia coli* *Staphylococcus saprophyticus*	1. Trimethoprim-sulfamethoxazole × 3 days (A, I)[a] 2. Fluoroquinolone × 3 days (A, II)[a] 3. Nitrofurantion × 5 days (B, I)[a] 4. β-lactams × 3 days (E, III)[a]	Short-course therapy more effective than single dose β-Lactams as a group are not as effective in acute cystitis then trimethoprim-sulfamethoxazole or the fluoroquinolones[a]
Pregnancy	As above	1. Amoxicillin-clavulanate × 7 days 2. Cephalosporin × 7 days 3. Trimethoprim-sulfamethoxazole × 7 days	Avoid trimethoprim-sulfamethoxazole during third trimester
Acute pyelonephritis Uncomplicated	*E. coli*	1. Quinolone × 14 days (A, II)[a] 2. Trimethoprim-sulfamethoxazole (if susceptible) × 14 days (B, II)[a]	Can be managed as outpatient
	Gram-positive bacteria	1. Amoxicillin or amoxicillin-clavulanic acid × 14 days (B, III)[a]	
Complicated	*E. coli* *Proteus mirabilis* *Klebisella pneumoniae* *Pseudomonas aeruginosa* *Enterococcus faecalis*	1. Quinolone × 14 days (B, III)[a] 2. Extended-spectrum penicillin plus aminoglycoside (B, III)[a]	Severity of illness will determine duration of IV therapy; culture results should direct therapy Oral therapy may complete 14 days of therapy
Prostatitis	*E. coli* *K. pneumoniae* *Proteus* spp. *P. aeruginosa*	1. Trimethoprim-sulfamethoxazole × 4–6 weeks 2. Quinolone × 4–6 weeks	Acute prostatitis may require IV therapy initially Chronic prostatitis may require longer treatment periods or surgery

[a]Strength of recommendations: A, good evidence for; B, moderate evidence for; C, poor evidence for and against; D, moderate against; E, good evidence against. Quality of evidence: I, at least one proper randomized, controlled study; II, one well-designed clinical trial; III, evidence from opinions, clinical experience, and expert committees.
Data from Warren JW, Abrutyn E, Hebel JR, et al. Guidelines for antimicrobial treatment of uncomplicated acute bacterial cystitis and acute pyelonephritis. Clin Infect Dis 1999;29:745–758.

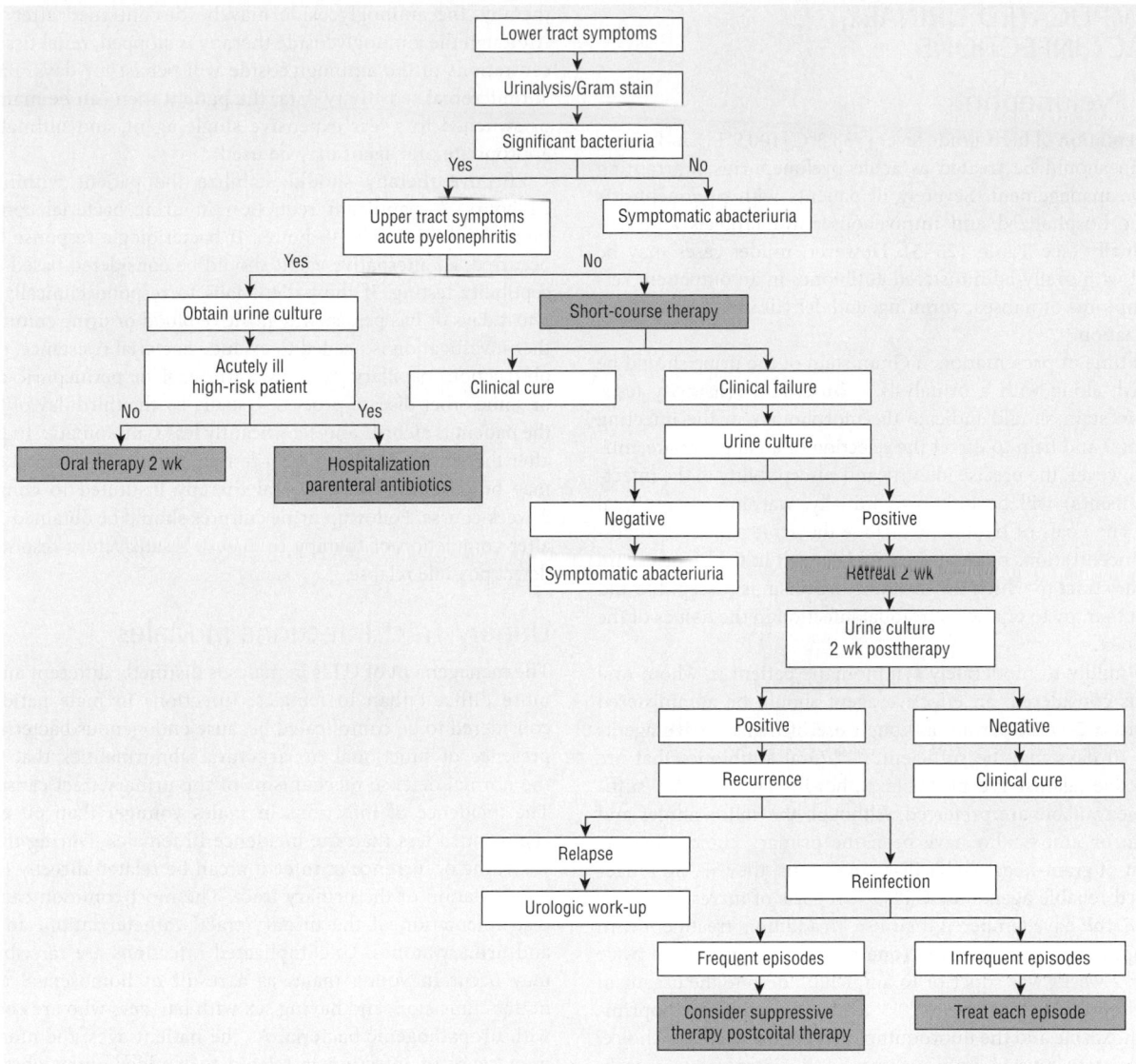

FIGURE 125-1. Management of UTIs in females.

most likely are infected with small numbers of coliform bacteria, including *E. coli*, *Staphylococcus* spp., or *Chlamydia trachomatis*. Additional causes include *Neisseria gonorrhoeae*, *Gardnerella vaginalis*, and *Ureaplasma urealyticum*.

Most patients presenting with pyuria will, in fact, have infection that requires treatment. Single-dose or short-course therapy with trimethoprim-sulfamethoxazole has been used effectively, and prolonged courses of therapy are not necessary for most patients. If single-dose or short-course therapy is ineffective, a culture should be obtained. If the patient reports recent sexual activity, therapy for *C. trachomatis* should be considered. Chlamydial treatment should consist of 1 g azithromycin or doxycycline 100 mg twice daily for 7 days. Often, concomitant treatment of all sexual partners is required to cure chlamydial infections and prevent reacquisition (see Chap. 126).

■ ASYMPTOMATIC BACTERIURIA

Asymptomatic bacteriuria is the finding of two consecutive urine cultures with $>10^5$ organisms/mL of the same organism in the absence of urinary symptoms. Most patients with asymptomatic bacteriuria are elderly and female. Pregnant women frequently present with asymptomatic bacteriuria. Although this group of

patients typically responds to treatment, relapse and reinfection are very common, and chronic asymptomatic bacteriuria is difficult to eradicate.

The management of asymptomatic bacteriuria depends on the age of the patient and whether or not the patient is pregnant. In children, because of a greater risk of developing renal scarring and long-standing renal damage, treatment should consist of the same conventional courses of therapy as that used for symptomatic infection. The greatest risk of renal damage occurs during the first 5 years of life.[51] In nonpregnant females, therapy is controversial; however, treatment has little effect on the natural course of infections. Two groups characterize asymptomatic bacteriuria in the elderly: those with persistent bacteriuria and those with intermittent bacteriuria.

Several studies in hospitalized elderly subjects, however, have not found antimicrobial therapy to be efficacious for abacteriuria.[52–55] A number of questions remains unanswered, for example: What is the effect of eradication of bacteriuria on life expectancy? What are the cost-effectiveness and risk-to-benefit ratio of therapy? What is the effect on morbidity? Certainly, with the information available and the high adverse reaction rate in the elderly, vigorous treatment and screening programs cannot be advocated.

■ COMPLICATED URINARY TRACT INFECTIONS

Acute Pyelonephritis

The presentation of high-grade fever (>38.3°C [100.9°F]) and severe flank pain should be treated as acute pyelonephritis, warranting aggressive management. Severely ill patients with pyelonephritis should be hospitalized and intravenous antimicrobials administered initially (see Table 125–5). However, milder cases may be managed with orally-administered antibiotics in an outpatient setting. Symptoms of nausea, vomiting, and dehydration may require hospitalization.

At the time of presentation, a Gram stain of the urine should be performed, along with a urinalysis, culture, and sensitivity tests. The Gram stain should indicate the morphology of the infecting organism(s) and help to direct the selection of an appropriate antibiotic. However, the precise identity and susceptibility of the infecting organism(s) will be unknown initially, warranting empirical therapy. The goals of treatment include the achievement of therapeutic concentrations of an antimicrobial agent in the bloodstream and urinary tract to which the invading organism is susceptible and sufficient therapy to eradicate residual infection in the tissues of the urinary tract.

In the mildly to moderately symptomatic patient in whom oral therapy is considered, an effective agent should be administered for at least a 2-week period, although use of highly active agents for 7 to 10 days may be sufficient.[1,56-60] Oral antibiotics that are highly active against the probable pathogens and that are sufficiently bioavailable are preferred. Although the sulfonamides and ampicillin or amoxicillin have been the primary choices for the treatment of gram-negative bacillary infections, they are no longer considered reliable agents for UTIs;[40,61] reports of increasing resistance to *E. coli* have tempered their use. In addition, treatment with trimethoprim-sulfamethoxazole (one double-strength tablet twice daily) for 2 weeks was superior to ampicillin, despite the organism being susceptible to both agents.[1,59,61] Agents such as trimethoprim-sulfamethoxazole and the fluoroquinolones are the agents of choice. If a Gram stain reveals gram-positive cocci, *Enterococcus faecalis* should be considered and treatment directed against this potential pathogen (ampicillin). Close followup of outpatient treatment is mandatory to ensure success.

In the seriously ill patient, parenteral therapy should be administered initially. Therapy should provide a broad spectrum of coverage and should be directed toward bacteremia or sepsis, if present. A number of antibiotic regimens have been used as empirical therapy, including an intravenous fluoroquinolone, an aminoglycoside with or without ampicillin, and extended-spectrum cephalosporins with or without an aminoglycoside.[1,62] Other options include aztreonam, the β-lactamase inhibitor combinations (e.g., ampicillin-sulbactam, ticarcillin-clavulanate, and piperacillin-tazobactam), carbapenems (e.g., imipenem, meropenem, doripenem or ertapenem), or intravenous trimethoprim-sulfamethoxazole.[63] If the patient has been hospitalized within the past 6 months, has a urinary catheter, or is a nursing home resident, the possibility of *P. aeruginosa* and enterococci, as well as multiple resistant organisms, should be considered. In this setting, ceftazidime, ticarcillin-clavulanate, piperacillin, aztreonam, meropenem, or imipenem in combination with an aminoglycoside is recommended. Ertapenem should not be used in this case owing to its inactivity against enterococci and *P. aeruginosa*.[62] The rationale for combination therapy is that in experimental animals, 3 days of aminoglycoside combination therapy followed by nonaminoglycoside single-agent therapy for 7 days resulted in a 100% cure rate.[56,61] If the patient responds to initial combination therapy, the aminoglycoside may be discontinued after 3 days. Although the aminoglycoside therapy is stopped, renal tissue concentrations of the aminoglycoside will persist for days. Based on antimicrobial sensitivity data, the patient then can be maintained or switched to a less expensive single agent, and ultimately, an appropriate oral agent may be used.

Effective therapy should stabilize the patient within 12 to 24 hours. A significant reduction in urine bacterial concentrations should occur in 48 hours. If bacteriologic response has not occurred, an alternative agent should be considered based on susceptibility testing. If the patient fails to respond clinically within 3 to 4 days or has persistently positive blood or urine cultures, further investigation is needed to exclude bacterial resistance, possible obstruction, papillary necrosis, intrarenal or perinephric abscess, or some other disease process. Usually by the third day of therapy the patient is afebrile and significantly less symptomatic. In general, after the patient has been afebrile for 24 hours, parenteral therapy may be discontinued, and oral therapy instituted to complete a 2-week course. Followup urine cultures should be obtained 2 weeks after completion of therapy to ensure a satisfactory response and detect possible relapse.

Urinary Tract Infections in Males

The management of UTIs in males is distinctly different and often more difficult than in females. Infections in male patients are considered to be complicated because endogenous bacteria in the presence of functional or structural abnormalities that disrupt the normal defense mechanisms of the urinary tract cause them. The incidence of infections in males younger than 60 years of age is much less than the incidence in females. During the adult years, the occurrence of infection can be related directly to some manipulation of the urinary tract. The most common causes are instrumentation of the urinary tract, catheterization, and renal and urinary stones. Uncomplicated infections are rare, but they may occur in young males as a result of homosexual activity, noncircumcision, and having sex with partners who are colonized with uropathogenic bacteria. As the patient ages, the most common cause of infection is related to bladder outlet obstruction because of prostatic hypertrophy. In addition, the prostate gland may become infected and provide a nidus for recurrent infection in males.

The conventional view is that therapy in males requires prolonged treatment (Fig. 125–2). A urine culture should be obtained before treatment because the cause of infection in men is not as predictable as in women. Single-dose or short-course therapy is not recommended in males. Considerably fewer data are available comparing various antimicrobial agents in males as compared with females. If gram-negative bacteria are presumed, trimethoprim-sulfamethoxazole or the quinolone antimicrobials should be considered because these agents achieve high renal tissue, urine, and prostatic concentrations.[15]

Initial therapy should be for 10 to 14 days. Factors associated with treatment success are isolation of a single organism, the absence of significant obstruction or anatomic abnormalities, a normally functioning urinary tract, and the absence of prostatic involvement. Parenteral therapy may be required in certain situations, such as in severely ill patients, in the presence of acute prostatitis or epididymitis, and in patients who cannot tolerate oral medications. A comparison of 2-week vs. 6-week therapy in males with recurrent infections who were given trimethoprim-sulfamethoxazole had cure rates of 29% and 62%, respectively.[64] Other investigators advocate longer treatment periods in males as well.[65] Followup cultures at 4 to 6 weeks after treatment are important in males to ensure bacteriologic cure. Many patients

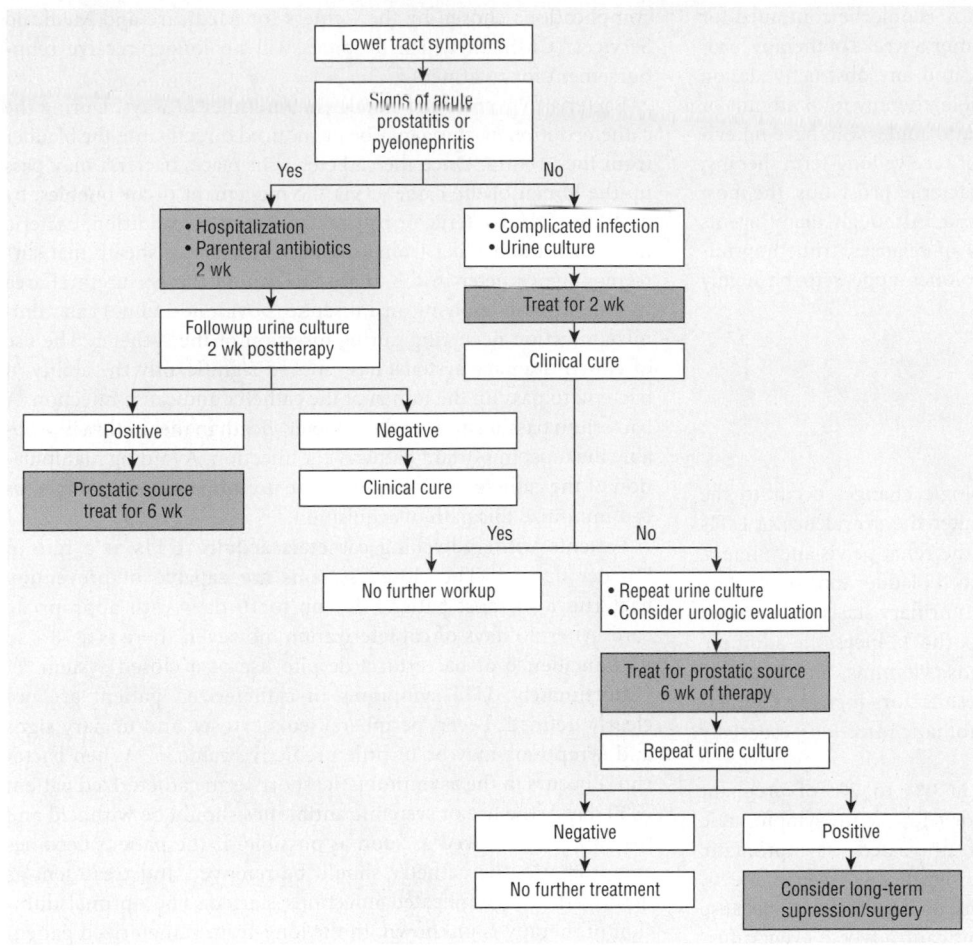

FIGURE 125-2. Management of UTIs in male.

require longer periods of treatment and possible alterations in antibiotics, depending on culture and sensitivity results and clinical response.

Recurrent Infections

Recurrent episodes of UTI account for a significant portion of all UTIs. Of the patients suffering from recurrent infections, 80% can be considered reinfections, that is, the recurrence of infection by an organism different from the organism isolated from the preceding infection. These patients most commonly are female, and recurrence develops in approximately 20% of females with cystitis. Reinfections can be divided into two groups: those with less than three episodes per year and those who develop more frequent infections.

Management strategies depend on predisposing factors, number of episodes per year, and the patient's preference. Factors commonly associated with recurrent infections include sexual intercourse and diaphragm or spermicide use for birth control. Therapeutic options include self-administered therapy, postcoital therapy, and continuous low-dose prophylaxis. In patients with infrequent infections (less than 3 infections per year), each episode may be treated as a separately occurring infection. Short-course therapy is appropriate in this setting. Many women have been treated successfully with self-administered short-course therapy at the onset of symptoms.[66]

In patients with more frequent symptomatic infections and no apparent precipitating event, long-term prophylactic antimicrobial therapy may be instituted. Prophylactic therapy reduces the frequency of symptomatic infections in elderly men, women, and children. In women, most studies show a reinfection rate of 2 to 3 per patient-year reduced to 0.1 to 0.2 per patient-year with

treatment.[67] Before prophylaxis is initiated, patients should be treated conventionally with an appropriate agent. Trimethoprim-sulfa-methoxazole (one-half of a single-strength tablet), trimethoprim (100 mg daily), a fluoroquinolone (levofloxacin 500 mg daily) and nitrofurantoin (50 or 100 mg daily) all reduce the rate of reinfection as single-agent therapy.[67] Full-dose therapy with these agents is unnecessary, and single daily doses can be used. Therapy generally is prescribed for a period of 6 months, during which time urine cultures are followed monthly. If symptomatic episodes develop, the patient should receive a full course of therapy with an effective agent and should be restarted on prophylactic therapy.

In women who experience symptomatic reinfections in association with sexual activity, voiding after intercourse may help to prevent infection. Also, single-dose prophylactic therapy with trimethoprim-sulfamethoxazole taken after intercourse reduces the incidence of recurrent infection significantly.[68]

In postmenopausal women with recurrent infections, the lack of estrogen results in changes in the bacterial flora of the vagina, resulting in increased colonization with uropathogenic *E. coli*. Topically administered estrogen cream reduces the incidence of infections in this population.[18,19]

The remaining 20% of recurrent UTIs are relapses, that is, persistence of infection with the same organism after therapy for an isolated UTI. The recurrence of symptomatic or asymptomatic bacteriuria after therapy usually indicates that the patient has renal involvement, a structural abnormality of the urinary tract, or chronic bacterial prostatitis. In the absence of structural abnormalities, relapse often is related to renal infection and requires a long duration of treatment. Women who relapse after short-course therapy should receive a 2-week course of therapy. In patients who relapse after 2 weeks of therapy, therapy should be continued for another 2 to 4 weeks. If relapse occurs after 6 weeks of therapy, urologic evaluation should be performed, and any obstructive lesion should be corrected. If this is not possible, therapy for 6 months or longer may be considered. Asymptomatic adults who have no evidence of urinary obstruction should not receive long-term therapy.

In males, relapse usually indicates bacterial prostatitis, the most common cause of persistent bacteriuria. Although many agents have been used for long-term therapy of relapses, trimethoprim-sulfamethoxazole and the fluoroquinolones appear to be highly effective.

■ SPECIAL CONDITIONS

UTIs in Pregnancy

During pregnancy, significant physiologic changes occur to the entire urinary tract that dramatically alter the prevalence of UTIs and pyelonephritis. Severe dilation of the renal pelvis and ureters, decreased ureteral peristalsis, and reduced bladder tone occur during pregnancy.[69] These changes result in urinary stasis and reduced defenses against reflux of bacteria to the kidneys. In addition, increased urine content of amino acids, vitamins, and nutrients encourages bacterial growth. All of these factors increase the incidence of bacteriuria, resulting in symptomatic infections, especially during the third trimester.

Asymptomatic bacteriuria occurs in 4% to 7% of pregnant patients. Of these, 20% to 40% will develop acute symptomatic pyelonephritis during pregnancy. If untreated, asymptomatic bacteriuria has the potential to cause significant adverse effects, including prematurity, low birth weight, and stillbirth.[70,71] Because pyelonephritis is associated with significant adverse events during pregnancy, routine screening tests for bacteriuria should be performed at the initial prenatal visit and again at 28 weeks' gestation. In patients with significant bacteriuria, symptomatic or asymptomatic, treatment is recommended so as to avoid possible complications. Organisms associated with bacteriuria are the same as those seen in uncomplicated UTIs, with *E. coli* isolated most frequently.

Therapy should consist of an agent administered for 7 days that has a relatively low adverse-effect potential and is safe for the mother and baby. The administration of amoxicillin, amoxicillin-clavulanate, or cephalexin, is effective in 70% to 80% of patients. Nitrofurantoin has been utilized in pregnancy, however must be used with caution as occurrences of birth defects have been reported. Tetracyclines should be avoided because of teratogenic effects, and sulfonamides should not be administered during the third trimester because of the possible development of kernicterus and hyperbilirubinemia. In addition, the available fluoroquinolones should not be given because of their potential to inhibit cartilage and bone development in the newborn. A follow-up urine culture 1 to 2 weeks after completing therapy and then monthly until gestation is complete is recommended.

Catheterized Patients

The use of an indwelling catheter frequently is associated with infection of the urinary tract and represents the most common cause of hospital-acquired infection. The incidence of catheter-associated infection is related to a variety of factors, including method and duration of catheterization, the catheter system (open or closed), the care of the system, the susceptibility of the patient, and the technique of the healthcare personnel inserting the catheter. Catheter-related infections are reasonably preventable infections, and are now considered one of the hospital-acquired

complications chosen by the Centers for Medicare and Medicaid Services (CMS) in which hospitals will no longer receive reimbursement for treatment.[72,73]

Bacteria may enter the bladder in a number of ways. During the catheterization, bacteria may be introduced directly into the bladder from the urethra. Once the catheter is in place, bacteria may pass up the lumen of the catheter via the movement of air bubbles, by motility of the bacteria, or by capillary action. In addition, bacteria may reach the bladder from around the exudative sheath that surrounds the catheter in the urethra. Cleaning the periurethral area thoroughly and applying an antiseptic (povidone-iodine) can minimize infection occurring during insertion of the catheter. The use of closed drainage systems has reduced significantly the ability of bacteria to pass up the lumen of the catheter and cause infection. A bacterium passing around the catheter sheath in the urethra is probably the most important pathway for infection. Avoiding manipulation of the catheter and trauma to the urethra and urethral meatus can minimize this path of acquisition.

Patients with indwelling catheters acquire UTIs at a rate of 5% per day.[72-74] The closed systems are capable of preventing bacteriuria in most patients for up to 10 days with appropriate care. After 30 days of catheterization, however, there is a 78% to 95% incidence of bacteriuria despite use of a closed system.[73,75] Unfortunately, UTI symptoms in catheterized patient are not clearly defined. Fever, peripheral leukocytosis, and urinary signs and symptoms may be of little predictive value.[72,73] When bacteriuria occurs in the asymptomatic, short-term catheterized patient (<30 days), the use of systemic antibiotics should be withheld and the catheter removed as soon as possible. If the patient becomes symptomatic, the catheter should be removed and treatment as described for complicated infections started. The optimal duration of therapy is unknown. In the long-term catheterized patient (>30 days), bacteriuria is inevitable.[72,73] The administration of systemic antibiotics active against the infecting organism will sterilize the urine; however, reinfection occurs rapidly in more than 50% of patients. In addition, resistant organisms recolonize the urine. Symptomatic patients must be treated because they are at risk of developing pyelonephritis and bacteremia. Bacteria adhere to the catheter and produce a biofilm consisting of bacterial glycocalyces, Tamm-Horsfall protein, as well as apatite and struvite salts, that act to protect the bacteria from antibiotics.[74] Recatheterization with a new, sterile unit should be performed in those symptomatic patients if the existing catheter has been in place for more than 2 weeks.

Various methods have been proposed to prevent the development of bacteriuria and infection in the patient with an indwelling catheter (see Table 125–5). The success of these methods depends on the type of catheter and the length of time it is in place. The use of constant bladder irrigation with antiseptic or antibacterial solutions reduces the incidence of infection in those with open drainage systems, but this approach has no advantage in those with closed systems. The use of prophylactic systemic antibiotics in patients with short-term catheterization reduces the incidence of infection over the first 4 to 7 days.[73,75] In long-term catheterized patients, however, antibiotics only postpone the development of bacteriuria and lead to the emergence of resistant organisms.

PROSTATITIS

Bacterial prostatitis is an inflammation of the prostate gland and surrounding tissue as a result of infection. It is classified as either acute or chronic. By definition, pathogenic bacteria and significant inflammatory cells must be present in prostatic secretions and urine to make the diagnosis of bacterial prostatitis. Prostatitis occurs rarely in young males, but it is commonly associated with recurrent infections in persons older than 30 years of age. As many as 50% of all males develop some form of prostatitis at some period in their life.[76][78] The acute form typically is an acute infectious disease characterized by a sudden onset of fever, tenderness, and urinary and constitutional symptoms. Chronic prostatitis presents with few symptoms related to the prostate but rather symptoms of urinating difficulty, low back pain, perineal pressure, or a combination of these. It represents a recurring infection with the same organism that results from incomplete eradication of bacteria from the prostate gland.

PATHOGENESIS AND ETIOLOGY

The exact mechanism of bacterial infection of the prostate is not well understood. The possible routes of infection are the same as those for UTIs. Reflux of infected urine into the prostate gland is thought to play an important role in causing infection. Intraprostatic reflux of urine occurs commonly and results in direct inoculation of infected urine into the prostate.[76-78] In addition, intraprostatic reflux of sterile urine can result in a chemical prostatitis and may be the cause of nonbacterial prostatitis. Sexual intercourse may contribute to infection of the prostate gland because prostatic secretions from men with chronic prostatitis and vaginal cultures from their sexual partners grow identical organisms. Other known causes of bacterial prostatitis include indwelling urethral and condom catheterization, urethral instrumentation, and transurethral prostatectomy in patients with infected urine.

A number of physiologic factors are believed to contribute to the development of prostatitis. Functional abnormalities found in bacterial prostatitis include altered prostate secretory functions. Prostatic fluid obtained from normal males contains prostatic antibacterial factor. This heat-stable, low-molecular-weight cation is a zinc-complexed polypeptide that is bactericidal to most urinary tract pathogens.[79] The antibacterial activity of prostatic antibacterial factor is related directly to the zinc content of prostatic fluid. Prostate fluid zinc levels and prostatic antibacterial factor activity also appear diminished in patients with prostatitis, as well as in the elderly.[79] Whether these changes are a cause or effect of prostatitis remains to be determined.

The pH of prostatic secretions in patients with prostatitis is altered.[80] Normal prostatic secretions have a pH in the range of 6.6 to 7.6. With increasing age, the pH tends to become more alkaline. In patients with inflammation of the prostate, prostatic secretions may have an alkaline pH in the range of 7 to 9. These changes suggest a generalized secretory dysfunction of the prostate that not only can affect the pathogenesis of prostatitis but also can influence the mode of therapy.

Gram-negative enteric organisms are the most frequent pathogens in acute bacterial prostatitis.[76-78] E. coli is the predominant organism, occurring in 75% of cases. Other gram-negative organisms frequently isolated include K. pneumoniae, P. mirabilis, and less frequently, P. aeruginosa, Enterobacter spp., and Serratia spp. Occasionally, cases of gonococcal and staphylococcal prostatitis occur, but they are infrequent.

E. coli most commonly causes chronic bacterial prostatitis, with other gram-negative organisms isolated less frequently. The importance of gram-positive organisms in chronic bacterial prostatitis remains controversial. S. epidermidis, S. aureus, and diphtheroids have been isolated in some studies.

CLINICAL PRESENTATION

Acute bacterial prostatitis presents as other acute infections (Table 125–6). Massage of the prostate will express a purulent

TABLE 125-6	Clinical Presentation of Bacterial Prostatitis

Signs and symptoms

Acute bacterial prostatitis: high fever, chills, malaise, myalgia, localized pain (perineal, rectal, sacrococcygeal), frequency, urgency, dysuria, nocturia, and retention

Chronic bacterial prostatitis: voiding difficulties (frequency, urgency, dysuria), low back pain, and perineal and suprapubic discomfort

Physical examination

Acute bacterial prostatitis: swollen, tender, tense, or indurated gland

Chronic bacterial prostatitis: boggy, indurated (enlarged) prostate in most patients

Laboratory tests

Bacteriuria

Bacteria in expressed prostatic secretions

discharge that will readily grow the pathogenic organism. Prostatic massage is contraindicated in acute bacterial prostatitis, however, because of the risk of inducing bacteremia and associated local pain. The diagnosis of acute bacterial prostatitis can be made from the patient's clinical presentation and the presence of significant bacteriuria. As with other UTIs, the infecting organism can be isolated from a midstream specimen.

In contrast, chronic bacterial prostatitis is more difficult to diagnose and treat. Chronic bacterial prostatitis typically is characterized by recurrent UTIs with the same pathogen and is the most common cause of recurrent UTI in males. The patient's clinical presentation can vary widely (see Table 125–6). Many adults, however, are asymptomatic.

Because physical examination of the prostate is often normal, urinary tract localization studies are critical to the diagnosis of chronic bacterial prostatitis. The method of quantitative localization culture, as described by Meares and Stamey,[81] remains the diagnostic standard (Fig. 125–3). The method compares the bacterial growth in sequential urine and prostatic fluid cultures obtained during micturition. The first 10 mL of voided urine is collected (voiding bladder 1, or VB_1) and constitutes urethral urine. After approximately 200 mL of urine has been voided, a 10-mL midstream sample is collected (VB_2). This specimen represents bladder urine. After the patient voids, the prostate is massaged, and expressed prostatic secretions (EPS) are collected. After prostatic massage, the patient voids again, and 10 mL of urine is collected (VB_3).

The diagnosis of bacterial prostatitis is made when the number of bacteria in EPS is 10 times that of the urethral sample (VB_1) and midstream sample (VB_2). If no EPS is available, the urine sample following massage (VB_3) should contain a bacterial count 10-fold greater than that of VB_1 or VB_2. If significant bacteriuria is present, ampicillin,

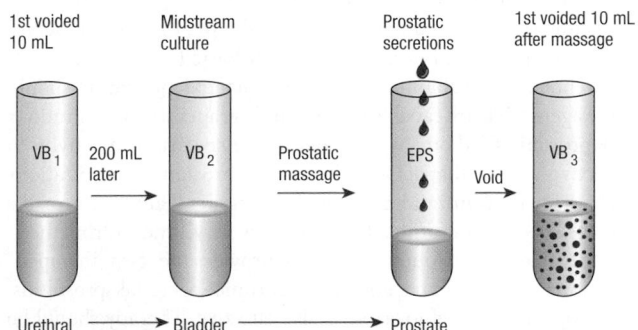

FIGURE 125-3. Segmented cultures of the lower tract in men. (EPS, expressed prostatic secretions; VB_1, voiding bladder 1; VB_2, voiding bladder 2; VB_3, voiding bladder 3.)

cephalexin, or nitrofurantoin should be given for 2 to 3 days to steril-ize the urine prior to performing the localization study.

TREATMENT

❾ The goals in the management of bacterial prostatitis are, in general, the same as those for UTIs. Acute bacterial prostatitis responds well to appropriate antimicrobial therapy that is directed at the most commonly isolated organisms. Prostatic penetration of antimicrobials occurs because the acute inflammatory reaction alters the cellular membrane barrier between the bloodstream and the prostate. Most patients can be managed with oral antimicrobial agents, such as trimethoprim-sulfamethoxazole and the fluoro-quinolones (e.g., ciprofloxacin, levofloxacin) (see Table 125–5). Other effective agents in this setting include cephalosporins, and β-lactam–β-lactamase combinations. Although intravenous therapy is rarely necessary for total treatment, intravenous to oral sequential therapy with trimethoprim-sulfamethoxazole or the fluoroquinolo-nes is appropriate. The conversion to an oral antibiotic can be con-sidered after the patient is afebrile for 48 hours or after 3 to 5 days of intravenous therapy. The total course of antibiotic therapy should be 4 weeks in order to reduce the risk of development of chronic prostatitis. Therapy may be prolonged with chronic prostatitis (6 to 12 weeks). Long-term suppressive therapy also may be initiated for recurrent infections, such as three times weekly ciprofloxacin, trimethoprim-sulfamethoxazole regular-strength tablet daily, or nitrofurantoin 100 mg daily.[81]

Chronic bacterial prostatitis often presents a more vexing situation because cures are obtained rarely. Despite high serum concentrations of antibacterial drugs in excess of the minimal inhibitory concentrations of the infecting organisms, bacteria persist in prostatic fluid. Most likely the failure to eradicate sensi-tive bacteria is caused by the inability of antibiotics to reach suf-ficient concentrations in the prostatic fluid and cross the prostatic epithelium.

Several factors that determine antibiotic diffusion into prostatic secretions were delineated from the canine model. Lipid solubility is a major determinant in the ability of drugs to diffuse from plasma across epithelial membranes. The degree of ionization in plasma also affects the diffusion of drugs. Only unionized molecules can cross the lipid barrier of prostatic cells, and the drug's pK_a (negative logarithm of acid ionization constant) directly determines the frac-tion of unchanged drug.

The pH gradient across the membrane has an influence on tissue penetration as well. A pH gradient of at least 1 pH unit between separate compartments allows for ion trapping. As the unionized drug crosses the epithelial barrier into prostatic fluid, it becomes ionized, allowing less drug to diffuse back across the lipid barrier. In early studies with the canine model, the prostatic pH was reported to be acidic (6.4).[80] In humans, however, the pH of prostatic secre-tions from an inflamed prostate is actually basic (8.1 to 8.3).[80]

The choice of antibiotics in chronic bacterial prostatitis should include agents that are capable of reaching therapeutic concentrations in the prostatic fluid and which possess the spectrum of activity to be effective. Agents that achieve therapeutic prostatic concentrations include trimethoprim and the fluoroquinolones. Sulfamethoxazole penetrates poorly and probably contributes very little to trimethop-rim. The fluoroquinolones appear to provide the best therapeu-tic options in the management of chronic bacterial prostatitis. Trimethoprim-sulfamethoxazole is also effective. Therapy should be continued for 4 to 6 weeks initially. Longer treatment periods may be necessary in some cases. If therapy fails with these regimens, chronic suppressive therapy may be used or surgery considered.

PHARMACOECONOMIC CONSIDERATIONS

The cost-effective management of UTIs requires knowledge of its pathogenesis and causative organisms associated with the various clinical syndromes described in this chapter. The costs associated with managing a UTI include direct costs, such as laboratory tests, medication, and healthcare visits. The indirect costs include lost work time and general quality-of-life issues such as disease or therapy adverse effects.

Direct costs are those associated with diagnosis, treatment, and followup. The cost of pharmaceuticals varies according to the agents used and the duration of therapy. Trimethoprim-sulfamethoxazole and ampicillin are rather inexpensive; however with rates of resis-tance, the risk of therapy failure is high, leading to increased costs. The fluoroquinolones also are highly effective agents but generally are more expensive, and a rise in their utilization is now being associated with increasing resistance.[61,82] In general, the outcome and total cost depend on whether therapy is empirical or definitive (based on a culture diagnosis for acute infection), and if the indi-vidual patient is compliant with the regimen.

ABBREVIATIONS

CFU: colony forming unit

EPS: expressed prostatic secretions

PMN: polymorphonuclear leukocyte

UTI: urinary tract infection

WBC: white blood cell

REFERENCES

1. Warren JW, Abrutyn E, Hebel JR, et al. Guidelines for antimicrobial treatment of uncomplicated acute bacterial cystitis and acute pyelone-phritis. Clin Infect Dis 1999;29:745–758.
2. Naber KG, Cho YH, Matsumoto T, et al. Immunoactive prophylaxis of recurrent urinary tract infections: a meta-analysis. Int J Antimicrob Agents 2009;33:111–119.
3. Fihn SD. Acute uncomplicated urinary tract infection in women. N Engl J Med 2003;349:259–266.
4. Nicolle LE. Uncomplicated Urinary Tract Infection in Adults Including Uncomplicated Pyelonephritis. Urol Clin N Am 2008;35:1–12.
5. Little P, Turner S, Rumsby K, et al. Developing clinical rules to predict urinary tract infection in primary care settings: sensitivity and specific-ity of near patient tests (dipsticks) and clinical scores. Br J Gen Prac 2006;56:606–612.3
6. Platt R. Quantitative definition of bacteriuria. Am J Med 1983;75:44–52.
7. Alper BS, Curry SH. Urinary tract infection in children. Am Fam Physician 2005;72(12):2483–2488.
8. Bauer R, Kogan BA. New Developments in the Diagnosis and Management of Pediatric UTIs. Urol Clin N Am 2008;35:47–58.
9. Sobel JD, Kaye D. Urinary tract infections. In: Mandell GL, Bennett JE, Dolin R, eds. Principles and Practice of Infectious Diseases, 6th ed. New York: Churchill-Livingstone, 2005:906–926.
10. Shortliffe LM, McCue JD. Urinary tract infections at the age extremes: Pediatrics and geriatrics. Am J Med 2002;113(Suppl 1A):55S–66S.
11. Nicolle L, Anderson PAM, Conly J, et al. Uncomplicated Urinary Tract Infection in Women, Current Practice and the Effect of Antibiotic Resistance on Empiric Treatment. Can Fam Phys 2006;52:612–618.
12. Shigemura K, Arakawa S, Tanaka K, et al. Clinical investigation of isolated bacteria from urinary tracts of hospitalized patients and their susceptibilities to antibiotics. J Infect Chemother 2009;15:18–22.
13. Stamatiou C, Bovis C, Panaguopoulos P, Petrakos G, Economou A, Lycoudt A. Sex-induced cystitis—Patient burden and other epidemio-logical features. Clin Exp Obstet Gynecol 2005;32(13):180–182.

14. Stamey TA, Fair WR, Timothy MM, et al. Antibacterial nature of prostatic fluid. Nature 1968;218:444–447.

15. Naber KG. Management of bacterial prostatitis: what's new? BJU International 2008;101(Suppl 3):7–10.

16. Shand DG, Nimmon CC, O'Grady F, et al. Relation between residual urine volume and response to treatment of urinary infection. Lancet 1970;1:1305–1306.

17. Parsons CL, Schrom SH, Hanno P, et al. Bladder surface mucin: Examination of possible mechanisms for its antibacterial effect. Invest Urol 1978;6:196–200.

18. Raz R, Stamm WE. A controlled trial of intravaginal estriol in postmenopausal women with recurrent urinary tract infections. N Engl J Med 1993;329:753–756.

19. Stamm WE. Estrogens and Urinary Tract Infection. J Infect Dis 2007; 195:623–624.

20. Orskov I, Ferencz A, Orskov F. Tamm-Horsfall protein or uromucoid is the normal urinary slime that traps type-1 fimbriated Escherichia coli. Lancet 1980;1:887.

21. Measley RE, Levison ME. Host defense mechanisms in the pathogenesis of urinary tract infection. Med Clin North Am 1991;75:275–286.

22. Jenkins RD, Fenn JP, Matsen JM. Review of urine microscopy for bacteriuria. JAMA 1986;255:3397–3403.

23. Pezzlo M. Detection of urinary tract infections by rapid methods. Clin Microbiol Rev 1988;2:268–280.

24. Stamm WE. Measurement of pyuria and its relation to bacteriuria. Am J Med 1983;75(Suppl 1):53–58.

25. Pappas PG. Laboratory in the diagnosis and management of urinary tract infections. Med Clin North Am 1991;75:313–325.

26. St John A, Boyd JC, Lowes AJ, Price CP. The use of urinary dipstick tests to exclude urinary tract infection: A systematic review of the literature. Am J Clin Pathol 2006;126(3):428–436.

27. Nys S, van Merode T, Bartelds AIM, et al. Urinary tract infections in general practice patients: diagnostic tests versus bacteriological culture. J Antimicrob Chemother 2006;57:955–958.

28. Stamey TA, Govan DE, Palmer JM. The localization and treatment of urinary tract infections: The role of bactericidal urine levels as opposed to serum levels. Medicine (Baltimore) 1965;44:1–36.

29. Fairley KF, Bond AG, Brown RB, et al. Simple test to determine the site of urinary tract infection. Lancet 1967;2:427–428.

30. Thomas VC, Forland M. Antibody-coated bacteria in urinary tract infection. Kidney Int 1982;21:1–7.

31. Stamey TA, Fair WR, Timothy MM, et al. Serum versus urinary antimicrobial concentrations in cure of urinary tract infections. N Engl J Med 1974;291:1159–1163.

32. Cimolai N, Cimolai T. The cranberry and urinary tract. Eur J Clin Microbiol Infect Dis 2007;26:767–776.

33. Barrons R, Tassone D. Use of Lactobacillus Probiotics for bacterial genitourinary infections in women: A Review. Clin Ther 2008;30(3):453–468.

34. Masson P, Matheson S, Webster AC. Meta-analyses in prevention and treatment of urinary tract infections. Infect Dis Clin N Am 2009;23:355–385.

35. Olson RP, Harrell LJ, Kaye KS. Antibiotic resistance in urinary isolates of escherichia coli from college women with urinary tract infections. Antimicrob Agents Chemother 2009;53(3):1285–1286.

36. Bergman M, Nyberg ST, Huovinen P, et al. Association between antimicrobial consumption and resistance in Escherichia coli. Antimicrob Agents Chemother 2009; 53(3):912–917.

37. Talan DA, Krishnadasan A, Abrahamian FM, et al. Prevalence and risk factor analysis of trimethoprim-sulfamethoxazole and fluoroquinolone-resistant Escherichia coli infection among emergency department patients with pyelonephritis. Clin Infect Dis 2008;47: 1150–1158.

38. Goettsch W, VanPelt W, Naglekerke N, et al. Increasing resistance to fluoroquinolones in Escherichia coli from urinary tract infections in the Netherlands. J Antimicrob Chemother 2000;46:223–228.

39. Karlowsky JA, Hoban DJ, DeCarby MR, Laing NM, Zhanel GG. Fluoroquinolone-resistant urinary isolates of Escherichia coli from outpatients are frequently multi-drug resistant: Results from the North American urinary tract infection collaborative. Antimicrob Agents Chemother 2006;50:2251–2254.

40. Johnson L, Sabel A, Burman WJ, et al. Emergence of Fluoroquinolone Resistance in Outpatient Urinary Escherichia coli isolates. Am J Med 2008;121(10):876–884.

41. Wagenlehner FME, Weidner W, Naber KG. An update on uncomplicated urinary tract infections in women. Curr Opin Urol 2009;19:368–374.

42. Kashanian J, Hakimian P, Blute M, et al. Nitrofurantoin: the return of an old friend in the wake of growing resistance. Br J Urol Intern 2008; 102:1634–1637.

43. Knottnerus BJ, Nys S, ter Riet G, et al. Fosfomycin tromethamine as a second agent for the treatment of acute, uncomplicated urinary tract infections in adult female patients in the Netherlands? J Antimicrob Chemother 2008;62:356–359.

44. Tice AD. Short course therapy of acute cystitis: A brief review of therapeutic strategies. J Antimicrob Chemother 1999;43(Suppl A):85–93.

45. Stein GE. Comparison of single-dose fosfomycin and a 7-day course of nitrofurantoin in female patients with uncomplicated urinary tract infections. Clin Ther 1999;21:1864–1872.

46. Cox CE, Marbury TC, Pittman WG, et al. A randomized, double-blind, multicenter comparison of gatifloxacin versus ciprofloxacin in the treatment of complicated urinary tract infection and pyelonephritis. Clin Ther 2002;24:223–236.

47. Irvani A, Klimberg I, Briefer C, et al. A trial comparing low-dose, short-course ciprofloxacin and standard 7-day therapy with cotrimoxazole or nitrofurantoin in the treatment of uncomplicated urinary tract infections. J Antimicrob Chemother 1999;43(Suppl A):67–75.

48. McCarty JM, Richard G, Huck W, et al. A randomized trial of short-course ciprofloxacin, ofloxacin, or trimethoprim-sulfamethoxazole for treatment of acute urinary tract infections in women. Am J Med 1999;106:292–299.

49. Stass H, Kubitza D. Pharmacokinetics and elimination of moxifloxacin after oral and intravenous administration in man. J Antimicrob Chemother 1999;43(Suppl B):83–90.

50. Gupta K, Hooton TM, Roberts PL, et al. Short-Course Nitrofurantoin for the Treatment of Acute Uncomplicated Cystitis in Women. Arch Intern Med. 2007; 167(20): 2207–2212.

51. Chang SL, Shortliffe LD. Pediatric urinary tract infections. Pediatr Clin North Am 2006;53(3):379–400.

52. Nicolle LE, Bradley S, Colgan R, et al. Infectious Disease Society of America guidelines for diagnosis and treatment of asymptomatic bacteriuria in adults. Clin Infect Dis 2005;40:643–654.

53. U.S. Preventive Services Task Force. Screening for Asymptomatic Bacteriuria in Adults: U.S. Preventive Services Task Force Reaffirmation Recommendation Statement. Ann Intern Med 2008;149:43–47.

54. Juthani-Mehta M, Quagliarello V, Perrelli E, et al. Clinical Features to Identify Urinary Tract Infection in Nursing Home Residents: A Cohort Study. J Am Geriatr Soc 2009;57:963–970.

55. Nicolle LE, Bjornson J, Harding GKM, et al. Bacteriuria in elderly institutionalized men. N Engl J Med 1983;309:1420–1425.

56. Neal DE. Complicated Urinary Tract Infections. Urol Clin N Am 2008;35:13–22.

57. Talan DA, Stamm WE, Hooton TM, et al. Comparison of ciprofloxacin (7 days) and trimethoprim-sulfamethoxazole (14 days) for acute uncomplicated pyelonephritis in women: a randomized trial. JAMA 2000;283(12):1583–1590.

58. van Nieuwkoop C, van't Wout JW, Assendelft WJJ, et al. Treatment duration of febrile urinary tract infection (FUTIRST trial): a randomized placebo-controlled multicenter trial comparing short (7 days) antibiotic treatment with conventional treatment (14 days). BMC Infect Dis 2009;9:131–140.

59. Katchman EA, Milo G, Paul M, Christiaens T, Baerheim A, Leibovici L. Three days vs. longer duration of antibiotic treatment for cystitis in women: A systemic review and meta-analysis. Am J Med 2005;118(11):1196–1207.

60. Peterson J, Kaul S, Khashab M, et al. A double-blind, randomized comparison of levofloxacin 750 mg once-daily for five days with ciprofloxacin 400/500 mg twice-daily for 10 days for the treatment of complicated urinary tract infections and acute pyelonephritis. Urol 2008;71(1):17–22.

61. Brown P, Moran K, Foxman B. Acute pyelonephritis among adults, cost of illness and considerations for the economic evaluation of therapy. Pharmacoeconomics 2005;23(11):1123–1142.

62. Curran MP, Simpson D, Perry CM. Ertapenem, a review of its use in the management of bacterial infections. Drugs 2003;63:1855–1878.

63. Wagenlehner FME, Wagenlehner C, Redman R, et al. Urinary bactericidal activity of doripenem versus that of levofloxacin in patients with complicated urinary tract infections or pyelonephritis. Antimicrob Agents Chemother 2009;53(4):1567–1573.

64. Gleckman R, Crowley M, Natsios GA. Therapy of recurrent invasive urinary tract infection in men. N Engl J Med 1979;301: 878–880.

65. Lipsky GA. Urinary tract infections in men: Epidemiology, pathophysiology, diagnosis, and treatment. Ann Intern Med 1989;110: 138–150.

66. Wong ES, McKevitt M, Running K, et al. Management of recurrent urinary tract infections with patient-administered single-dose therapy. Ann Intern Med 1985;102:302–307.

67. Hooton TM. Recurrent urinary tract infection in women. Int J Antimicrob Agents 2001;17:259–268.

68. Stapleton A, Latham RH, Johnson C, et al. Post-coital antimicrobial prophylaxis for recurrent urinary tract infection. JAMA 1990;264:703–706.

69. Macejko AM, Shaeffer AJ. Asymptomatic bacteruria and symptomatic urinary tract infections during pregnancy. Urol Clin North Am 2007;34(1):35–42.

70. Christensen B. Which antibiotics are appropriate for treating bacteriuria in pregnancy? J Antimicrob Chemother 2000;46(Suppl S1): 29–34.

71. McDermott S, Daguise V, Mann H, Szwejbka L, Callaghan W. Perinatal risk for mortality and mental retardation associated with maternal urinary tract infections. J Fam Pract 2001;50:433–437.

72. Saint S, Meddings JA, Calfee D, et al. Catheter-associated urinary tract infection and the medicare rule changes. Ann Intern Med 2009;150(12):877–884.

73. Nicolle LE. Catheter-related urinary tract infection. Drugs Aging 2005;22(8):627–639.

74. Ohkawa M, Sugata T, Sawaki M, et al. Bacterial and crystal adherence to the surfaces of indwelling urethral catheters. J Urol 1990;143:717–721.

75. Johnson JR, Duskowski MA, Wilt TJ. Systemic review: Antimicrobial urinary catheters prevent catheter-associated urinary tract infections in hospital patients. Arch Intern Med 2006;144(2):116–126.

76. Murphy AB, Macejko A, Taylor A, et al. Chronic prostatitis management strategies. Drugs 2009;69(1):71–84.

77. Lipsky BA. Prostatitis and urinary tract infection in men: what's new; what's true? The Amer J Med 1999;106:327–334.

78. Drieger JN, Nyberg L, Nickel JC. NIH consensus definition and classification of prostatitis. JAMA 1999;282:236–237.

79. Fair WR, Couch J, Wehner M. Prostatic antibacterial factor: Identity and significance. Urology 1976;7:169–177.

80. Pfau A, Perlberg S, Shapiro A. The pH of prostatic fluid in health and disease: Implications of treatment in chronic bacterial prostatitis. J Urol 1978;119:384–387.

81. Wagenlehner FM, Naber KG. Current challenges in the treatment of complicated urinary tract infections and prostatitis. Clin Microbiol Infect 2006;12(Suppl 3):67–80.

82. Alam MF, Cohen D, Butler C, et al. The additional costs of antibiotics and re-consultations for antibiotic-resistant Escherichia coli urinary tract infections managed in general practice. Int J Antimicrob Agents 2009;33:255–257.

CHAPTER 126

Sexually Transmitted Diseases

LEROY C. KNODEL

KEY CONCEPTS

❶ All recommended treatment regimens for gonorrhea include antibiotic therapy directed against *Chlamydia* species because of the high prevalence of coexisting infections, unless chlamydia has been ruled out.

❷ Parenteral penicillin is the treatment of choice for all syphilis infections. For patients who are penicillin allergic, few well-studied alternative agents are available, and all are oral medications that require 2 to 4 weeks of therapy to be effective. Patient compliance and thus efficacy are a concern when alternative regimens must be used.

❸ Chlamydia genital tract infections represent the most frequently reported communicable disease in the United States. In females, these infections are frequently asymptomatic or minimally symptomatic and, if left untreated, are associated with the development of pelvic inflammatory disease and attendant complications such as ectopic pregnancy and infertility. As a result, all sexually active females aged 20 to 25 years and sexually active women with multiple sexual partners should be screened annually for this infection.

❹ Oral acyclovir, famciclovir, and valacyclovir are effective in reducing viral shedding, duration of symptoms, and time to healing of first-episode genital herpes infections, with maximal benefits seen when therapy is initiated at the earliest stages of infection. The benefit of these agents for recurrent infections has not been demonstrated. Patient-initiated, single-day antiviral therapy started within 6 to 12 hours of prodromal symptom onset offers an alternative to continuous suppressive therapy of recurrent infection in some individuals.

❺ Metronidazole and tinidazole are the only agents currently approved in the United States to treat trichomoniasis. Although a single 2-g dose of either agent is widely used for compliance and other reasons, the alternative 7-day metronidazole regimen may be a better choice if sexual partners of treated individuals cannot be treated concurrently.

The spectrum of sexually transmitted diseases (STDs) has broadened from the classic venereal diseases—gonorrhea, syphilis, chancroid, lymphogranuloma venereum, and granuloma inguinale—to include

Learning objectives, review questions, and other resources can be found at **www.pharmacotherapyonline.com**.

a variety of pathogens known to be spread by sexual contact (Table 126–1). Because of the large number of infected individuals, the diversity of clinical manifestations, the changing drug-susceptibility patterns of some pathogens, and the high frequency of multiple STDs occurring simultaneously in infected individuals, the diagnosis and management of patients with STDs are much more complex today than they were even a decade ago.[1–4]

Despite a higher reported incidence of most major STDs in men, the complications of STDs generally are more frequent and severe in women. In particular, serious effects on maternal and infant health during pregnancy are well documented.[1,4] Damage to reproductive organs, increased risk of cancer, complications associated with pregnancy, and transmission of disease to the fetus or newborn are associated with several STDs. As a result of the physiologic, psychosocial, and economic consequences of STDs, and because of the increasing prevalence of some viral STDs, such as human immunodeficiency virus (HIV) and genital herpes, for which curative therapy is not available, there is continuing research into STDs and the primary prevention of these diseases.[2–5]

With the exception of HIV infection, which is reviewed in detail in Chapter 134, the most frequently occurring STDs in the United States are discussed in this chapter. For other less common STDs, only recommended treatment regimens are presented. The most current information on the epidemiology, diagnosis, and treatment of STDs provided by the U.S. Centers for Disease Control and Prevention (CDC) can be obtained at the CDC Website (*www.cdc.gov*).

Numerous interrelated factors contribute to the epidemic nature of STDs. Sociocultural, demographic, and economic factors, together with patterns of sexual behavior, host susceptibility to infection, changing properties of the causative pathogens, disease transmission by asymptomatic individuals, and environmental factors, are important determinants of the frequency and distribution of STDs in the United States and worldwide.

Age is one of the most important demographic determinants of STD incidence. Two thirds of STD cases each year occur in persons in their teens and twenties, the peak years of sexual activity. With increasing age, the incidence of most STDs decreases exponentially. In sexually active teenagers, STD rates are highest in the youngest, suggesting that physiologic differences may contribute to increased susceptibility.[2–5]

Age-specific rates of STDs are higher in men than in women; however, reported rates may not represent true gender differences but rather may reflect greater ease of detection in men. In recent years, the ratio of male-to-female cases for most STDs has declined, possibly reflecting improvements in the diagnosis of STDs in asymptomatic women or changes in female sexual behavior following the availability of improved methods of contraception. Although some racial disparity exists for rates of STD infection, it is possible that this is a reflection of socioeconomic differences.[1–5]

TABLE 126-1 Sexually Transmitted Diseases

Disease	Associated Pathogens
Bacterial	
Gonorrhea	*Neisseria gonorrhoeae*
Syphilis	*Treponema pallidum*
Chancroid	*Haemophilus ducreyi*
Granuloma inguinale	*Calymmatobacterium granulomatis*
Enteric disease	*Salmonella* spp, *Shigella* spp, *Campylobacter* fetus
Campylobacter infection	*Campylobacter jejuni*
Bacterial vaginosis	*Gardnerella vaginalis, Mycoplasma hominis, Bacteroides* spp, *Mobiluncus* spp
Group B streptococcal infections	Group B *Streptococcus*
Chlamydial	
Nongonococcal urethritis	*Chlamydia trachomatis*
Lymphogranuloma venereum	*Chlamydia trachomatis*, type L
Viral	
Acquired immunodeficiency syndrome	Human immunodeficiency virus
Herpes genitalis	Herpes simplex virus, types I and II
Viral hepatitis	Hepatitis A, B, C, and D viruses
Condylomata acuminata	Human papillomavirus
Molluscum contagiosum	Poxvirus
Cytomegalovirus infection	Cytomegalovirus
Mycoplasmal	
Nongonococcal urethritis	*Ureaplasma urealyticum*
Protozoal	
Trichomoniasis	*Trichomonas vaginalis*
Amebiasis	*Entamoeba histolytica*
Giardiasis	*Giardia lamblia*
Fungal	
Vaginal candidiasis	*Candida albicans*
Parasitic	
Scabies	*Sarcoptes scabiei*
Pediculosis pubis	*Phthirus pubis*
Enterobiasis	*Enterobius vermicularis*

The single greatest risk factor for contracting STDs is the number of sexual partners. As the number of sexual partners increases, the risk of being exposed to someone infected with an STD increases. Sexual preference also plays a major role in the transmission of STDs. For all major STDs, rates are disproportionately greater in men who have sex with men (MSM) than in heterosexuals. Also, a number of less common STDs, including several caused by enteric protozoans and bacterial pathogens, occur primarily in MSM. The major risk factors for MSM appear to be related to the greater number of sexual partners and the practice of unprotected anal-genital, oral-genital, and oral-anal intercourse. In addition, prostitution and illicit drug use are associated with a higher incidence of most STDs.[1-5]

Some of the most serious sequelae of STDs are associated with congenital or perinatal infections. Most neonatal infections are acquired at birth, after infant passage through an infected cervix or vagina. Neonatal *Chlamydia trachomatis, Neisseria gonorrhoeae,* and herpes simplex virus (HSV) infections are associated with this type of spread. For pregnant women with syphilis, infection is usually transmitted transplacentally, producing a congenital infection. Depending on the organism, neonatal infections can manifest in a variety of ways, produce significant morbidity, and in some cases result in infant death.[1-4]

Other than complete abstinence, the most effective way to prevent STD transmission is by maintaining a mutually monogamous sexual relationship between uninfected partners. Short of this, use of barrier contraceptive methods, such as the male and female condoms, diaphragm, cervical cap, vaginal sponges, and vaginal spermicides alone

or in combination, provides varying degrees of protection from a number of STDs. When used correctly and consistently, male latex condoms with or without spermicide are more effective than natural skin condoms in protecting against STD transmission, including HIV, gonorrhea, chlamydia, trichomoniasis, HSV, and human papillomavirus (HPV). When lubrication is desired with latex condoms, water-based products, such as K-Y jelly, are recommended because oil-based agents (e.g., petroleum jelly) can weaken latex condoms and reduce their effectiveness. For latex-allergic individuals, other synthetic condoms (e.g., polyurethane) appear to possess efficacy against STD transmission similar to latex condoms. The female condom is a lubricated polyurethane sheath with a diaphragm-like ring on each end that can be used as a protective device for women with male sexual partners who do not desire to use a condom. Limited data suggest that the female condom blocks penetration of viruses, including HIV; for nonviral STDs, the female condom provides STD protection similar to the male condom.[1,3,5,6] At one time, use of nonoxynol-9, a vaginal spermicide with cytolytic activity, was advocated to reduce the transmissibility of several STDs. This was based in large part on in vitro and animal data. However, nonoxynol-9 does not reduce the risk of transmission of common STDs and actually can increase the risk of HIV transmission. Frequent use of nonoxynol-9 damages vaginal, cervical, and rectal epithelium, leading to increased transmissibility of HIV and possibly other STDs. Diaphragms may protect against cervical gonorrheal, chlamydial, and trichomonal infections.[1,5-8]

The varied spectrum of clinical syndromes produced by common STDs is determined not only by the etiologic pathogen(s) but also by differences in male and female anatomy and reproductive physiology. For a number of STDs, the signs and symptoms overlap sufficiently to prevent accurate diagnosis without microbiologic confirmation. Frequently, symptoms are minimal or absent despite the presence of infection. Table 126–2 lists common clinical syndromes associated with STDs.[1-4]

GONORRHEA

EPIDEMIOLOGY AND ETIOLOGY

The gram-negative diplococcus *N. gonorrhoeae* is the causative organism of gonorrhea. Although the rate of reported cases in the United States has remained relatively stable over the last decade, over 300,000 cases were reported in 2008.[1,9] Of concern, however, are the substantial number of infections that remain undiagnosed and unreported.[1,9] Humans are the only known natural host of this intracellular parasite. Because of its rapid incubation period and the large number of infected individuals with asymptomatic disease, gonorrhea is difficult to control.[1,10-15]

Although the risk of a female acquiring a cervical infection after a single episode of vaginal intercourse with an infected male partner is high and increases with multiple exposures, the risk of transmission from an infected female to an uninfected male is not as great following a single act of coitus. No data are available on the risk of transmission after other types of sexual contact.[10-14]

PATHOPHYSIOLOGY

On contact with a mucosal surface lined by columnar, cuboidal, or noncornified squamous epithelial cells, the gonococci attach to cell membranes by means of surface pili and are then pinocytosed. The virulence of the organism is mediated primarily by the presence of pili and other outer membrane proteins. After mucosal damage is established, polymorphonuclear (PMN) leukocytes invade the tissue, submucosal abscesses form, and purulent exudates are secreted.[10-15]

TABLE 126-2 Selected Syndromes Associated with Common Sexually Transmitted Pathogens

Syndrome	Commonly Implicated Pathogens	Common Clinical Manifestations[a]
Urethritis	Chlamydia trachomatis, herpes simplex virus, Neisseria gonorrhoeae, Trichomonas vaginalis, Ureaplasma urealyticum	Urethral discharge, dysuria
Epididymitis	C. trachomatis, N. gonorrhoeae	Scrotal pain, inguinal pain, flank pain, urethral discharge
Cervicitis/vulvovaginitis	C. trachomatis, Gardnerella vaginalis, herpes simplex virus, human papillomavirus, N. gonorrhoeae, T. vaginalis	Abnormal vaginal discharge, vulvar itching/irritation, dysuria, dyspareunia
Genital ulcers (painful)	Haemophilus ducreyi, herpes simplex virus	Usually multiple vesicular/pustular (herpes) or papular/pustular (H ducreyi) lesions that can coalesce; painful, tender lymphadenopathy[b]
Genital ulcers (painless)	Treponema pallidum	Usually single papular lesion
Genital/anal warts	Human papillomavirus	Multiple lesions ranging in size from small papular warts to large exophytic condylomas
Pharyngitis	C. trachomatis (?), herpes simplex virus, N. gonorrhoeae	Symptoms of acute pharyngitis, cervical lymphadenopathy, fever[c]
Proctitis	C. trachomatis, herpes simplex virus, N. gonorrhoeae, T. pallidum	Constipation, anorectal discomfort, tenesmus, mucopurulent rectal discharge
Salpingitis	C. trachomatis, N. gonorrhoeae	Lower abdominal pain, purulent cervical or vaginal discharge, adnexal swelling, fever[d]

[a]For some syndromes, clinical manifestations can be minimal or absent.
[b]Recurrent herpes infection can manifest as a single lesion.
[c]Most cases of pharyngeal gonococcal infection are asymptomatic.
[d]Salpingitis increases the risk of subsequent ectopic pregnancy and infertility.

CLINICAL PRESENTATION

Individuals infected with gonorrhea can be symptomatic or asymptomatic, have complicated or uncomplicated infections, and have infections involving several anatomic sites. Interestingly, most of the symptomatic patients who are not treated become asymptomatic within 6 months, with only a few becoming asymptomatic carriers of the disease.[10–13] The most common clinical features of gonococcal infections are presented in Table 126–3.

Complications associated with untreated gonorrhea appear more pronounced in women, likely a result of a high percentage who experience signs and symptoms that are nonspecific and minimally symptomatic. As a result, many women do not seek treatment until after the development of serious complications, such as pelvic inflammatory disease (PID). Approximately 15% of women with gonorrhea develop PID. Left untreated, PID can be an indirect cause of infertility and ectopic pregnancies. In 0.5% to 3.0% of patients with gonorrhea, the gonococci invade the bloodstream and produce disseminated disease. Disseminated gonococcal infection (DGI) is 3 times more common in women than in men. The usual clinical manifestations of DGI are tender necrotic skin lesions, tenosynovitis, and monarticular arthritis.[1,10–14]

DIAGNOSIS

Diagnosis of gonococcal infections can be made by gram-stained smears, culture, or methods based on the detection of cellular components of the gonococcus (e.g., enzymes, antigens, DNA, or lipopolysaccharide) in clinical specimens. Various stains have been used to identify gonococci microscopically, with the Gram stain the most widely used in clinical practice. Gram-stained smears are positive for gonococci when gram-negative diplococci of typical kidney bean morphology are identified within PMN leukocytes.[1,10–14] In the presence of equivocal smears (extracellular gonococcal forms that can be nonpathogenic, commensal Neisseria, or gram-negative diplococci of atypical morphology), culture is mandatory. In urethral smears from men with symptomatic urethritis, the smear is highly sensitive and specific, and is considered diagnostic for infection. Because of their low sensitivity, gram-stained smears are not recommended in the diagnosis of endocervical, rectal, cutaneous, and asymptomatic male urethral infections. Because of the presence of nonpathogenic Neisseria in the pharynx, the Gram stain is not useful in the diagnosis of pharyngeal infection.[1,10,12–14]

Although no longer considered the most sensitive of diagnostic tests for gonorrhea, culture is considered the test of choice because

TABLE 126-3 Presentation of Gonorrhea Infections

	Males	Females
General	Incubation period 1–14 days	Incubation period 1–14 days
	Symptom onset in 2–8 days	Symptom onset in 10 days
Site of infection	Most common: urethra	Most common: endocervical canal
	Others: rectum (usually caused by rectal intercourse in MSM), oropharynx, eye	Others: urethra, rectum (usually caused by perineal contamination), oropharynx, eye
Symptoms	Can be asymptomatic or minimally symptomatic	Can be asymptomatic or minimally symptomatic
	Urethral infection: dysuria and urinary frequency	Endocervical infection: usually asymptomatic or mildly symptomatic
	Anorectal infection: asymptomatic to severe rectal pain	Urethral infection: dysuria, urinary frequency
	Pharyngeal infection: asymptomatic to mild pharyngitis	Anorectal and pharyngeal infection: symptoms same as for men
Signs	Purulent urethral or rectal discharge can be scant to profuse	Abnormal vaginal discharge or uterine bleeding; purulent urethral or rectal discharge can be scant to profuse
	Anorectal: pruritus, mucopurulent discharge, bleeding	
Complications	Rare (epididymitis, prostatitis, inguinal lymphadenopathy, urethral stricture)	Pelvic inflammatory disease and associated complications (i.e., ectopic pregnancy, infertility)
	Disseminated gonorrhea	Disseminated gonorrhea (3 times more common than in men)

MSM, men who have sex with men.

of its high specificity in medicolegal situations (e.g., suspected abuse, rape); in diagnosing anorectal, pharyngeal, and conjunctival infections; and in screening populations with a low prevalence. Anatomic sites to be cultured depend on the individual's sexual preferences and body areas exposed. In women, because the urethra and other sites are rarely the sole locus of infection, cervical cultures produce the highest yield and frequently are performed in conjunction with rectal cultures. Urethral cultures are recommended in women who have had hysterectomies and heterosexual men.[1,10–14]

Because technical constraints and cost preclude the use of culture techniques in many office settings and clinics, alternative methods of diagnosis have been developed, including enzyme immunoassay, DNA probe techniques, and nucleic acid amplification techniques (NAATs). With the exception of Gram stain for symptomatic gonococcal urethritis, these tests offer increased sensitivity and/ or specificity over both Gram stain and culture.[10,13,14] Additionally, many of these tests can provide a more rapid means of diagnosis than culture. Of particular clinical importance is the high sensitivity of NAATs for detecting *N. gonorrhoeae* using noninvasive specimens (e.g., self-collected urine specimens, vaginal swabs). This technology is also being used to concurrently test for *C. trachomatis*

using a single specimen. However, a major drawback of NAATs is their inability to provide resistance data on isolated gonococcal strains.[1,14,15]

TREATMENT

Gonorrhea

❶ With the CDC recommendation in 2007 that fluoroquinolones no longer be considered a preferred treatment of gonorrhea because of the increasing rate of resistance, ceftriaxone and cefixime are now the only agents included in the recommended regimens for gonorrhea treatment.[16] (Table 126–4). These regimens have documented efficacy in the treatment of urethral, cervical, rectal, and pharyngeal infections. Coexisting chlamydial infection, which is documented in up to 50% of women and 20% of men with gonorrhea, constitutes the major cause of postgonococcal urethritis, cervicitis, and salpingitis in patients treated for gonorrhea for whom concurrent chlamydial infection has not been ruled out.[1,14] As a result, concomitant treatment with doxycycline or azithromycin is recommended in all patients treated for gonorrhea. Although none

---

TABLE 126-4 Treatment of Gonorrhea

Type of Infection	Recommended Regimens[a]	Alternative Regimens[b]
Uncomplicated infections of the cervix, urethra, and rectum in adults[c,d]	Ceftriaxone 125 mg IM once,[e] or cefixime 400 mg PO once (tablet or suspension) *plus* A treatment regimen for presumptive *C. trachomatis* coinfection if chlamydial infection has not been ruled out (see Table 126–8)	Spectinomycin 2 g IM once,[f] or ceftizoxime 500 mg IM once, or cefotaxime 500 mg IM once, or cefoxitin 2 g IM once with probenecid 1 g PO once *plus* A treatment regimen for presumptive *C. trachomatis* coinfection if chlamydial infection has not been ruled out (see Table 126–8)
Gonococcal infections in pregnancy	Ceftriaxone 125 mg IM once,[g,h] or cefixime 400 mg PO once (tablet or suspension) *plus* A recommended treatment regimen for presumptive *C. trachomatis* infection during pregnancy,[h] if chlamydial infection has not been ruled out (see Table 126–8)	Spectinomycin 2 g IM once,[f] or ceftizoxime 500 mg IM once, or cefotaxime 500 mg IM once, or cefoxitin 2 g IM once with probenecid 1 g PO once *plus* A recommended treatment regimen for presumptive *C. trachomatis* infection during pregnancy,[h] if chlamydial infection has not been ruled out (see Table 126–8)
Disseminated gonococcal infection in adults (>45 kg)[h,i,j,k]	Ceftriaxone 1 g IM or IV every 24 hours[k]	Cefotaxime 1 g IV every 8 hours[k] or ceftizoxime 1 g IV every 8 hours,[k] or spectinomycin 2 g IM every 12 hours[f,k]
Uncomplicated infections of the cervix, urethra, and rectum in children (<45 kg)	Ceftriaxone 125 mg IM once[l]	Spectinomycin 40 mg/kg IM once (not to exceed 2 g)[f]
Gonococcal conjunctivitis in adults	Ceftriaxone 1 g IM once[m]	
Ophthalmia neonatorum	Ceftriaxone 25–50 mg/kg IV or IM once (not to exceed 125 mg)	
Infants born to mothers with gonococcal infection (prophylaxis)	Erythromycin (0.5%) ophthalmic ointment in a single application[n]; or Tetracycline (1%) ophthalmic ointment in a single application[n,o]	

CDC, Centers for Disease Control and Prevention; *C. trachomatis*, *Chlamydia trachomatis*; PO, orally.
[a]Recommendations are those of the CDC.
[b]A number of other antimicrobials have demonstrated efficacy in treating uncomplicated gonorrhea but are not included in the CDC guidelines.
[c]Treatment failures are usually caused by reinfection and necessitate patient education and sex-partner referral; additional treatment regimens for gonorrhea and chlamydia infections should be administered. Epididymitis should be treated for 10 days (see Table 126–8).
[d]Patients allergic to β-lactams should receive a quinolone. Persons unable to tolerate a β-lactam (penicillin or cephalosporin) or a quinolone should receive spectinomycin.
[e]Also recommended for the treatment of uncomplicated infections of the pharynx in combination with a treatment regimen for presumptive *C. trachomatis* infection, if chlamydial infection has not been ruled out.
[f]Spectinomycin is currently not available in the United States (January 9, 2010).
[g]Another recommended IM or PO cephalosporin also can be used.
[h]Tetracyclines are contraindicated during pregnancy.
[i]Patients treated with one of the recommended regimens should be treated with doxycycline or azithromycin for possible coexistent chlamydial infection.
[j]Patients with gonococcal meningitis should be treated for 10 to 14 days and those with endocarditis for at least 4 weeks with ceftriaxone 1–2 g IV every 12 hours.
[k]All treatment regimens should be continued for 24–48 hours after improvement begins; at this time therapy can be switched to one of the following oral regimens to complete a 7-day course of treatment: cefixime 400 mg PO twice daily (tablet or suspension) or spectinomycin 2 g IM every 12 hours; fluoroquinolones may be an acceptable alternative if susceptibility can be documented by culture.
[l]Patients with bacteremia or arthritis should receive ceftriaxone 50 mg/kg (max. 1 g) IM or IV once daily for 7 days.
[m]A single lavage of the infected eye should be considered.
[n]Efficacy in preventing chlamydial ophthalmia is unclear.
[o]Tetracycline ophthalmic ointment (1%) is currently not available in the United States (January 9, 2010).

of the single-dose regimens recommended for gonorrhea in the CDC guidelines is effective against chlamydia, azithromycin (2 g) as a single dose is highly effective in eradicating both gonorrhea and chlamydia.[1,17,18]

Although oral therapy with cefixime offers a more patient acceptable alternative to intramuscular ceftriaxone, it may not be preferred for all cases of gonorrhea. Of the regimens of choice, only ceftriaxone is effective in eradicating both gonorrhea and incubating syphilis. Because the overall incidence of concomitant infection with both gonorrhea and syphilis appears low in most areas, selection of ceftriaxone based on this criterion should be considered only in areas in which the incidence of syphilis infection is high. Resistance to the broad-spectrum cephalosporins included in the recommended and alternativeregimens for gonorrhea treatmenthas not been reported. Spectinomycin is the preferred alternative for patients unable to tolerate one of the recommended cephalosporins; however, it is currently not available in the United States. Although some resistance to spectinomycin is reported, its limited use appears to have prevented widespread resistance from developing. Unlike ceftriaxone, spectinomycin has only limited efficacy in treating pharyngeal infections.[1,10,12–15]

CLINICAL CONTROVERSY

Some clinicians advocate that a single 2-g dose of azithromycin should be the treatment of choice for gonorrhea because it is also effective in eradicating concomitant chlamydial infection. However, because of concerns regarding the development of resistance and the relatively high incidence of gastrointestinal side effects, azithromycin is not a recommended first-line therapy.

Pregnant women infected with *N. gonorrhoeae* should be treated with either a cephalosporin or spectinomycin. For presumed or diagnosed concurrent *C. trachomatis* infection, either azithromycin or amoxicillin is the preferred treatment.[1,10,11]

Ceftriaxone is the recommended therapy for DGI, gonococcal meningitis, endocarditis, and any type of gonococcal infection in children. In cases of DGI, patients should be hospitalized and treated initially with one of the recommended parenteral antibiotics (see Table 126–4). Although marked improvement is usually noted within 48 hours of initiating therapy, treatment should be continued as an outpatient with one of the recommended oral antibiotics to complete at least 7 days of antibiotic therapy.[1,13,14] Gonococcal ophthalmia is highly contagious in adults and neonates and requires IM ceftriaxone therapy. Single-dose therapy is adequate for gonococcal conjunctivitis, although some physicians recommend continuing therapy until cultures are negative at 48 to 72 hours. Topical antibiotics are not sufficiently effective when used alone for ocular infections and are not necessary with appropriate systemic therapy. Infants with either type of ophthalmologic infection should be evaluated for signs of DGI.[1,10,13–14,19]

Treatment of gonorrhea during pregnancy is essential to prevent ophthalmia neonatorum. Gonococcal infection in newborns results primarily from passage through an infected birth canal, but it also can be transmitted in utero. Ophthalmia neonatorum is the most common ophthalmic infection in newborns (1.6%–12%), although membranes of the vagina, pharynx, or rectum also can become colonized. Conjunctival involvement usually develops within 7 days of delivery and is characterized by intense, bilateral conjunctival inflammation with chemosis. If not treated promptly, corneal ulceration and blindness can develop. Because the law in most states

requires neonatal prophylaxis with topical ocular antimicrobials, gonococcal ophthalmia neonatorum is rare in the United States. The CDC recommends that either erythromycin (0.5%) ophthalmic ointment or tetracycline (1%) ophthalmic ointment be instilled in each conjunctival sac immediately postpartum. At present, tetracycline ophthalmic ointment is not commercially available in the United States.[1,10–14,19]

EVALUATION OF THERAPEUTIC OUTCOMES

Although some clinicians recommend obtaining follow-up cultures at least 3 days after treatment, combination gonorrhea and chlamydial therapy rarely results in treatment failures, and routine follow-up of patients treated with a regimen included in the CDC guidelines is not recommended. Persistence of symptoms following any treatment requires culture of the site(s) of gonorrheal infection, as well as susceptibility testing if gonococci are isolated. In most cases, the presence of gonococci indicates reinfection rather than treatment failure and reflects the need for improved patient education and sex partner referral. Persistence of symptoms also can be caused by other infectious causes, such as *C. trachomatis*.[1,10–15]

SYPHILIS

EPIDEMIOLOGY AND ETIOLOGY

Although the 13,500 cases of primary and secondary syphilis reported in the United States in 2008 is still relatively low, this number represents the highest number of cases reported in over a decade.[9] In addition to being highly contagious, syphilis is of major concern because, if left untreated, it can progress to a chronic systemic disease that can be fatal or seriously disabling.[21–29]

Syphilis usually is acquired by sexual contact with infected mucous membranes or cutaneous lesions, although on rare occasions it can be acquired by nonsexual personal contact, accidental inoculation, or blood transfusion. The causative organism of syphilis is *Treponema pallidum*, a spirochete. The risk of acquiring syphilis from an infected individual after a single sexual encounter is approximately 50% to 60%. After sexual contact, the organism penetrates the intact mucous membrane or a break in the cornified epithelium, and spirochetemia occurs.[21,24,25–29]

There is strong evidence of an association between syphilis and HIV infection. Syphilis, similar to other sexually transmitted genital ulcer diseases, can increase the risk of acquiring HIV in exposed individuals. Also, immunologic defects in HIV-infected individuals can produce an atypical serologic response to syphilis. In particular, the possibility of delayed seroreactivity, markedly elevated serologic titers, and increased false-positive results could complicate the diagnosis, as well as assessment of treatment efficacy, in HIV-positive individuals infected with syphilis. Furthermore, anecdotal evidence suggests that compromised immune function can result in an accelerated progression of syphilis, particularly to neurosyphilis, requiring more aggressive antibiotic therapy in comparison with an immunocompetent host. As a result of this association, the CDC recommends that all patients diagnosed with syphilis be tested for HIV infection.[1,22–24,26,27]

CLINICAL PRESENTATION

The clinical presentation of syphilis is varied with progression through multiple stages possible in untreated or inadequately treated patients (Table 126–5).

TABLE 126-5 Presentation of Syphilis Infections

General

Primary	Incubation period 10–90 days (mean, 21 days)
Secondary	Develops 2–8 weeks after initial infection in untreated or inadequately treated individuals
Latent	Develops 4–10 weeks after secondary stage in untreated or inadequately treated individuals
Tertiary	Develops in approximately 30% of untreated or inadequately treated individuals 10–30 years after initial infection

Site of infection

Primary	External genitalia, perianal region, mouth, and throat
Secondary	Multisystem involvement secondary to hematogenous and lymphatic spread
Latent	Potentially multisystem involvement (dormant)
Tertiary	CNS, heart, eyes, bones, and joints

Signs and symptoms

Primary	Single, painless, indurated lesion (chancre) that erodes, ulcerates, and eventually heals (typical); regional lymphadenopathy is common; multiple, painful, purulent lesions possible but uncommon
Secondary	Pruritic or nonpruritic rash, mucocutaneous lesions, flulike symptoms, lymphadenopathy
Latent	Asymptomatic
Tertiary	Cardiovascular syphilis (aortitis or aortic insufficiency), neurosyphilis (meningitis, general paresis, dementia, tabes dorsalis, eighth cranial nerve deafness, blindness), gummatous lesions involving any organ or tissue

Primary Syphilis

The primary stage, characterized by the appearance of a chancre on cutaneous or mucocutaneous tissue exposed to the organism, is highly infectious. Even without treatment, chancres persist only for 1 to 8 weeks before healing spontaneously. Because syphilitic chancres can be confused with other infectious etiologies, appropriate diagnostic testing is important.[21–24,26,28]

Secondary Syphilis

The secondary stage of syphilis is characterized by a variety of mucocutaneous eruptions resulting from widespread hematogenous and lymphatic spread of *T. pallidum*. Skin lesions can be either generalized or localized to a small portion of the body and, with the exception of follicular lesions, are nonpruritic. Generalized lymphadenopathy also is seen in the majority of patients, as are nonspecific symptoms such as mild and transitory malaise, fever, pharyngitis, headache, anorexia, and arthralgia. If untreated, secondary syphilis disappears in 4 to 10 weeks; however, lesions can recur at any time within 4 years.[21–28]

Latent Syphilis

By definition, persons with a positive serologic test for syphilis but with no other evidence of disease have latent syphilis. Latent syphilis is further divided into early and late latency. During early latency, the patient is considered potentially infectious because of the 25% risk of spontaneous mucocutaneous relapse. The U.S. Public Health Service defines early latency as 1 year from the onset of infection, although other investigators propose a longer interval, such as 2 to 4 years. With the exception of pregnancy in which the mother can pass the disease to the fetus, late latency is considered noninfectious, although the patient remains a host.[1,21–28]

Most untreated patients with late latent syphilis have no further sequelae; however, approximately 25% to 30% progress either to neurosyphilis or to late syphilis with clinical manifestations other than neurosyphilis. Treatment of all patients with latent syphilis is essential because there is no way to predict which patients will have progression of their disease.[21–28]

Tertiary Syphilis and Neurosyphilis

If left untreated, syphilis can slowly produce an inflammatory reaction in virtually any organ in the body. Manifestations of this disease progression were referred to previously as *tertiary syphilis*. These clinical manifestations now are differentiated into two subgroups based on the presence or absence of central nervous system (CNS) involvement: neurosyphilis or tertiary syphilis (i.e., gumma and cardiovascular syphilis).[1,21–27]

Currently, the term *neurosyphilis* encompasses any patient with cerebrospinal fluid (CSF) abnormalities consistent with CNS infection. Approximately 40% of patients with primary or secondary syphilis exhibit such abnormalities, although most remain asymptomatic. Persistence of CSF abnormalities into late latency is associated with a greater risk of progression to symptomatic neurosyphilis. Although data are conflicting, some investigators suggest that HIV-infected patients are at greater risk of developing symptomatic neurosyphilis than patients with intact immune systems.[1,21–25]

Rarely seen, the most common manifestations of disease progression from late latency are benign gumma formation and cardiovascular syphilis. The gumma, a nonspecific granulomatous lesion, is the classic lesion of late syphilis and develops in 50% of patients with disease progression. These chronic, destructive lesions characteristically infiltrate the skin, bone, soft tissue, and liver but can be found in any organ or tissue. Gummas of critical organs, such as the heart or brain, can be fatal.[1,21–24,27]

Congenital Syphilis

In pregnant women with syphilis, *T. pallidum* can cross the placenta at any time during pregnancy. The risk of fetal infection is greatest in pregnant women with primary and secondary syphilis and declines in pregnant women with late disease. Transmission of syphilis during pregnancy occurs primarily transplacentally and can result in fetal death, prematurity, or congenital syphilis. Symptoms can be seen during the first months of life (early congenital syphilis) or later in childhood or adolescence (late congenital syphilis). Manifestations of early congenital syphilis resemble those of secondary syphilis, whereas those of late congenital syphilis correspond to the tertiary stage in adults.[22–24]

DIAGNOSIS

Because *T. pallidum* is difficult to culture in vitro, diagnosis is based primarily on microscopic examination of serous material from a suspected syphilitic lesion or on results from serologic testing. In primary syphilis, diagnosis is established by the presence of *T. pallidum* on dark-field microscopic examination of material from cutaneous lesions and enlarged lymph nodes in patients with secondary syphilis. In incubating syphilis, confirmation frequently is by dark-field microscopic examination because serologic tests can be unreactive early in the disease. Another method of direct microscopic examination, the direct fluorescent antibody (test) for *T. pallidum* (DFA-TP), which uses monoclonal or polyclonal antibodies specific for *T. pallidum*, has greater specificity and sensitivity than dark-field examination, and does not require the immediate examination of fresh specimens.[24–29]

Serologic tests are the mainstay in the diagnosis of syphilis and traditionally are categorized as nontreponemal or treponemal. Common nontreponemal tests include the Venereal Disease Research Laboratory (VDRL) slide test, rapid plasma reagin (RPR) card test, unheated serum reagin (USR) test, and the toluidine red unheated serum test (TRUST). Nontreponemal tests, which are inexpensive and easily performed, rely on the detection of treponemal antibodies directed against an alcoholic solution of cardiolipin, lecithin, and cholesterol contained in these tests. A positive nontreponemal test can indicate the presence of any stage of syphilis or congenital syphilis, although incubating syphilis and very early primary syphilis produce a negative reaction; however, because they are nonspecific tests, false-positive reactions occur, making them inappropriate to confirm the diagnosis alone. Transiently false-positive results can be seen in patients with acute febrile illnesses, after immunizations, and during pregnancy. Chronic false-positive results are commonly associated with heroin addiction, aging, chronic infections, autoimmune diseases, and malignant disease. In some cases, false-positive reactions are familial and are related to abnormal serum globulin levels.[23–29]

Nontreponemal tests are used primarily as screening tests; however, because T. pallidum antibody titers also can be quantitated by testing serial dilutions of the patient's serum for reactivity, they are useful in following the progression of the disease, recovery after therapy, and possible reinfection. Because antibody titers vary to some extent between tests, it is important that sequential serologic testing be performed using the same method each time. In patients treated successfully for primary and secondary syphilis, nontreponemal tests almost always will return to seronegativity. If these tests are going to return to negative in patients with early latent syphilis, they will do so within the first 4 years after adequate therapy; patients with disease of longer duration usually remain seropositive for life. In addition to their use in serologic testing, nontreponemal tests often are used on CSF to diagnose neurosyphilis.[23–29]

In some patients with secondary syphilis, a prozone phenomenon occurs that produces a negative VDRL test despite the presence of high reaginic antibody titers. This is corrected by diluting the patient's serum prior to testing.[26,27] For HIV-positive individuals with syphilis, the reactivity of nontreponemal tests can vary depending on the stage of the HIV infection. In the early stages, reaginic titers higher than in non–HIV-infected patients have been seen, resulting in the prozone phenomenon. During the later stages of HIV infection, however, when immune function deteriorates to a greater extent, serologic responses can be reduced or delayed. As a result, the diagnosis of syphilis in HIV-infected individuals can be more difficult.[1,24–29]

In diagnosing all stages of syphilis, treponemal tests are more sensitive than nontreponemal tests. Because these tests are technically more demanding and are more expensive, they are used primarily as confirmatory rather than as screening tests. For many years, the fluorescent treponemal antibody absorption (FTA-ABS) test was the most frequently used treponemal test. The FTA-ABS test uses the T. pallidum antigen to detect specific antibodies to treponemal organisms. However, the FTA-ABS test has largely been replaced by card assays such as the T. pallidum hemagglutination assay (TPHA), the micro-hemagglutination assay for antibodies to T. pallidum (MHA-TP), and the T. pallidum particle agglutination assay (TPPA) which can be automated and are less expensive to perform. Despite adequate antibiotic therapy for any stage of syphilis, the antibody tests, usually remain reactive for life and therefore are not useful in assessing serologic response to therapy, relapse, or reinfection.[1,24–29]

Several enzyme immunoassays for T. pallidum have become available and are gaining wide use as confirmatory tests. Polymerase chain reaction (PCR)-based tests also are being investigated, particularly in situations in which serologic testing has poor sensitivity and specificity (e.g., congenital syphilis, early primary syphilis, and neurosyphilis). Additionally, multiplex PCR tests that can identify the presence of T. pallidum, herpes simplex virus type 1 (HSV-1) and herpes simplex virus type 1 (HSV-2), and Haemophilus ducreyi from genital ulcer specimens are under study.[22–24,29]

TREATMENT

Syphilis

Table 126–6 presents the CDC's treatment recommendations.[1] Parenteral penicillin G is the treatment of choice for all stages of syphilis. Because T. pallidum multiplies slowly, single doses of short- or intermediate-acting penicillins do not provide the prolonged, low-level exposure to penicillin required for eradication of the treponeme. As a result, benzathine penicillin G is the only penicillin effective for single-dose therapy.[1,22–28]

The recommended treatment for syphilis of less than 1 year's duration is benzathine penicillin G 2.4 million units as a single dose. Although the relapse rate for this regimen is less than 3%, some investigators advocate that 2.4 million units be administered once a week for 2 consecutive weeks. In patients with syphilis of longer than 1 year's duration and normal CSF examination, benzathine penicillin G is administered weekly for three successive doses. Although not specifically recommended by the CDC, this three-dose regimen is used by some experts to treat HIV-infected patients with syphilis of less than 1 year's duration based on data suggesting a greater risk of treatment failure with single-dose therapy.[1,24–28]

CLINICAL CONTROVERSY

Some experts even prefer to treat all patients with syphilis of less than 1 year's duration with the three-dose regimen because single-dose therapy is not consistently effective in eradicating treponemes from the CSF; this is of primary concern in patients with undiagnosed CSF involvement, such as HIV-infected individuals.

Patients with abnormal CSF findings should be treated as having neurosyphilis. Preferred regimens for neurosyphilis provide treatment over 10 to 14 days with parenteral penicillin G administered every 4 hours. Benzathine penicillin G alone in standard weekly doses and procaine penicillin G in doses under 2.4 million units do not consistently provide treponemicidal levels in the CSF and have resulted in treatment failures. Because T. pallidum resistance to penicillin has not emerged, the primary need for alternative drugs in treating syphilis is for penicillin-allergic patients.[1,24–28]

❷ Alternative regimens recommended for penicillin-allergic patients are doxycycline 100 mg orally twice daily or tetracycline 500 mg orally 4 times daily for 2 to 4 weeks depending on the duration of syphilis infection. These regimens should be used only in cases of documented penicillin allergy, and given concerns regarding patient compliance with these regimens, follow-up serologic testing is of particular importance.[1,24–28]

Other antibiotics used successfully in treating syphilis include various β-lactam antibiotics; however, none offers significant advantages over benzathine penicillin G. Even though ceftriaxone is considered effective in eradicating incubating syphilis when given as a single 125-mg dose, higher doses and more frequent administration (e.g., 1,000 mg daily for 8 to 10 days) appear necessary for more advanced syphilis, and treatment failures are reported in HIV-infected patients. Although azithromycin 2 g as a single dose produces good results in patients with early syphilis, treatment failures and resistance to azithromycin are reported.[1,21,24–28]

TABLE 126-6 Drug Therapy and Follow-up of Syphilis

Stage/Type of Syphilis	Recommended Regimens[a,b]	Follow-up Serology
Primary, secondary, or early latent syphilis (<1 year's duration)	Benzathine penicillin G 2.4 million units IM in a single dose[c]	Quantitative nontreponemal tests at 6 and 12 months for primary and secondary syphilis; at 6, 12, and 24 months for early latent syphilis[d]
Late latent syphilis (>1 year's duration) or latent syphilis of unknown duration	Benzathine penicillin G 2.4 million units IM once a week for 3 successive weeks (7.2 million units total)	Quantitative nontreponemal tests at 6, 12, and 24 months[e]
Neurosyphilis	Aqueous crystalline penicillin G 18–24 million units IV (3–4 million units every 4 hours or by continuous infusion) for 10–14 days[f] *or* Aqueous procaine penicillin G 2.4 million units IM daily plus probenecid 500 mg PO four times daily, both for 10–14 days[f]	CSF examination every 6 months until the cell count is normal; if it has not decreased at 6 months or is not normal by 2 years, retreatment should be considered
Congenital syphilis (infants with proven or highly probable disease)	Aqueous crystalline penicillin G 50,000 units/kg IV every 12 hours during the first 7 days of life and every 8 hours thereafter for a total of 10 days *or* Procaine penicillin G 50,000 units/kg IM daily for 10 days	Serologic follow-up only recommended if antimicrobials other than penicillin are used
Penicillin-allergic patients[g]		
Primary, secondary, or early latent syphilis	Doxycycline 100 mg PO 2 times daily for 14 days[g,h] *or* Tetracycline 500 mg PO 4 times daily for 14 days[h] Ceftriaxone 1 g IM or IV daily for 8–10 days	Same as for non–penicillin-allergic patients
Late latent syphilis (>1 year's duration) or syphilis of unknown duration	Doxycycline 100 mg PO twice a day for 28 days[h,i] *or* Tetracycline 500 mg PO 4 times daily for 28 days[h,i]	Same as for non–penicillin-allergic patients

CDC, Centers for Disease Control and Prevention; CSF, cerebrospinal fluid; PO, orally.
[a]Recommendations are those of the CDC.
[b]The CDC recommends that all patients diagnosed with syphilis be tested for HIV infection.
[c]Some experts recommend multiple doses of benzathine penicillin G or other supplemental antibiotics in addition to benzathine penicillin G in HIV-infected patients with primary or secondary syphilis; HIV-infected patients with early latent syphilis should be treated with the recommended regimen for latent syphilis of more than 1 year's duration.
[d]More frequent follow-up (i.e., 3, 6, 9, 12, and 24 months) recommended for HIV-infected patients.
[e]More frequent follow-up (i.e., 6, 12, 18, and 24 months) recommended for HIV-infected patients.
[f]Some experts administer benzathine penicillin G 2.4 million units IM once per week for up to 3 weeks after completion of the neurosyphilis regimens to provide a total duration of therapy comparable to that used for late syphilis in the absence of neurosyphilis.
[g]For nonpregnant patients; pregnant patients should be treated with penicillin after desensitization.
[h]Pregnant patients allergic to penicillin should be desensitized and treated with penicillin.
[i]Limited data suggest that ceftriaxone my be effective, although the optimal dosage and treatment duration are unclear.

For pregnant patients, penicillin is the treatment of choice at the dosage recommended for that particular stage of syphilis. To ensure treatment success and prevent transmission to the fetus, some experts advocate an additional IM dose of benzathine penicillin G 2.4 million units 1 week after completion of the recommended regimen. In women allergic to penicillin, safe and effective alternatives are not available; therefore, skin testing should be performed to confirm a penicillin allergy. It is recommended that women with positive skin tests undergo penicillin desensitization and receive the appropriate treatment regimen for their stage of disease.[1,22–24]

Most patients treated for primary and secondary syphilis experience the Jarisch-Herxheimer reaction after treatment. This benign, self-limiting reaction is characterized by flulike symptoms, such as transient headache, fever, chills, malaise, arthralgia, myalgia, tachypnea, peripheral vasodilation, and aggravation of syphilitic lesions. The exact mechanism of the reaction is unknown, although proposed etiologies, including immunologic mechanisms and release of endotoxin or other toxic treponemal products, are not substantiated. The Jarisch-Herxheimer reaction is independent of the drug and dose used and should not be confused with penicillin allergy. It usually begins within 2 to 4 hours of initiating therapy, peaks at 8 hours, and is complete within 12 to 24 hours. Most reactions can be managed symptomatically with analgesics, antipyretics, and rest. Steroids and antihistamines have been administered prior to initiation of syphilitic therapy but are of limited value.[1,22–24]

EVALUATION OF THERAPEUTIC OUTCOMES

Table 126–6 lists the CDC recommendations for serologic follow-up of patients treated for syphilis.[1] Quantitative nontreponemal tests should be performed at 6 and 12 months in all patients treated for primary and secondary syphilis and at 6, 12, and 24 months for early and late latent disease. The CDC recommends more frequent monitoring of HIV-infected individuals (i.e., 3, 6, 9, 12, and 24 months after therapy). In general, the time to reach seronegativity is proportional to the duration of the disease. Table 126–6 also includes specific testing recommendations for other stages of syphilis. Despite adequate therapy, some patients can remain seropositive based on nontreponemal test results. In these cases, stabilization of low antibody titers is indicative of adequate therapy. For women treated during pregnancy, monthly quantitative nontreponemal tests are recommended in those at high risk of reinfection.[22–24]

CHLAMYDIA TRACHOMATIS

EPIDEMIOLOGY AND ETIOLOGY

Based on CDC data, the number of reported cases of chlamydia infection, the most frequently reported infectious disease in the United States, has almost doubled in the past 10 years.[1,9] Although this most likely is a result of improved screening and detection, it can also represent a true increase in the infection rate. Chlamydial infections represent the most common cause of nongonococcal urethritis (NGU), accounting for as much as 50% of such infections.[1,30–34]

PATHOPHYSIOLOGY

C. trachomatis is an obligate intracellular parasite that shares properties of both viruses and bacteria. Like viruses, chlamydiae require cellular material from host cells for replication; however, unlike viruses, chlamydiae maintain their cellular identity throughout development. Although *C. trachomatis* lacks a cell-wall peptidoglycan, its major outer membrane is similar to gram-negative bacteria. At least 18 serovars (subspecies) of *C. trachomatis* exist, of which only the lymphogranuloma venereum strains produce potentially invasive infections. The remaining serovars are involved primarily with superficial infection of epithelial cells.[30–34]

The risk of transmissibility of chlamydia after exposure is unknown but is believed to be less than that following exposure to *N. gonorrhoeae*. Coinfection with chlamydia occurs in a substantial number of individuals with gonorrhea and all individuals diagnosed with *N. gonorrhoeae* should be assumed also to have *C. trachomatis* present, if chlamydial infection has not been ruled out.[1] Of major concern is that chlamydial infections are associated with a significantly increased risk of acquiring HIV infection. In addition to genital infections, ocular infections in adults owing to autoinoculation and infants owing to vaginal delivery through an infected birth canal are reported. Pharyngeal and rectal infections can develop secondary to orogenital or receptive anal intercourse, respectively, with an infected individual.[1,30–37]

CLINICAL PRESENTATION

In comparison with gonorrhea, chlamydial genital tract infections are more frequently asymptomatic, and when present, symptoms tend to be less noticeable. Urethral discharge usually is less profuse and more mucoid or watery than the urethral discharge associated with gonorrhea.[31–34] Table 126–7 summarizes the usual clinical presentation of chlamydial infections.

Similar to gonorrhea, chlamydia can be transmitted to an infant during contact with infected cervicovaginal secretions. Nearly two-thirds of infants acquire chlamydial infection after endocervical exposure, with the primary morbidity associated with seeding of the infant's eyes, nasopharynx, rectum, or vagina. In exposed infants, neonatal conjunctivitis develops in as many as 50%, and pneumonia develops in up to 16%. Inclusion conjunctivitis in newborns is usually self-limited, but it can result in scarring and micropannus of the cornea. Interstitial pneumonitis occurring secondary to carriage in the nasopharynx typically is mild, but it can be severe and require hospitalization.[1,31–34,36]

DIAGNOSIS

❸ Because of the high rate of asymptomatic disease and the high prevalence of chlamydial infection in sexually active females 25 years of age or younger and sexually active women with new sex partners or multiple sex partners, the CDC recommends routine annual screening in these individuals. Laboratory confirmation of chlamydial infection is important because of the relative lack of specificity of symptoms when present.[1]

Cell culture is the reference standard against which all other diagnostic tests are measured. Because chlamydiae are obligate intracellular parasites, specimens for culture must be obtained from endocervical (women) or urethral (men) epithelial cell scrapings rather than from urine or urethral discharges. Although tissue culture techniques have close to 100% specificity, the sensitivity is reported to be as low as 70% in part because of problems of improper specimen collection, transport, or processing. Because of the technical demands, expense, and length of time until results are available (3–7 days), culture is not used widely for diagnostic purposes today. However, culture remains the diagnostic standard in medicolegal cases such as sexual assault and child abuse because of its high specificity and ability to detect only viable organisms.[31–34,37–40]

Tests that detect chlamydial antigens and nucleic acid provide more rapid results, are technically less demanding to perform, are less costly, and in some situations have greater sensitivity than culture. Commonly used nonculture tests for detection of *C. trachomatis* are the enzyme immunosorbent assay (EIA), DNA hybridization probe, and NAATs.[32,34,37,39]

Although still widely used both as rapid office tests and as laboratory-based tests, EIA methods for diagnosis of *C. trachomatis* are no longer recommended because of their poor sensitivity in comparison to NAATs. NAATs, which can detect small amounts of chlamydial DNA, are highly sensitive and specific for detecting infection in urogenital and anal specimens, as well as in urine. Use of self-collected vaginal or anal specimens or first-void urine samples offers greater patient acceptability, particularly when used to screen asymptomatic individuals. A further advantage of tests that can screen urine for the presence of infection is that up to 30% of women are reported to have urethral infection only, which would be missed using a test on endocervical samples. Because of their ability to detect as little as a single gene copy in a specimen, nucleic acid residues that persist following successful antibiotic therapy of a chlamydial infection can result in a false-positive test for several weeks following eradication of the organism.[33,34]

TREATMENT

Chlamydia

A number of antimicrobials, including tetracyclines, macrolides, azithromycin, and some fluoroquinolones, display good in vitro and in vivo activity against *C. trachomatis*. In most clinical

TABLE 126–7	Presentation of *Chlamydia* Infections	
	Males	**Females**
General	Incubation period: 35 days	Incubation period: 7–35 days
	Symptom onset: 7–21 days	Usual symptom onset: 7–21 days
Site of infection	Most common: urethra	Most common: endocervical canal
	Others: rectum (receptive anal intercourse), oropharynx, eye	Others: urethra, rectum (usually caused by perineal contamination), oropharynx, eye
Symptoms	More than 50% of urethral and rectal infections are asymptomatic	More than 66% of cervical infections are asymptomatic
	Urethral infection: mild dysuria, discharge	Urethral infection: usually sub-clinical; dysuria and frequency uncommon
	Pharyngeal infection: asymptomatic to mild pharyngitis	Rectal and pharyngeal infection: symptoms same as for men
Signs	Scant to profuse, mucoid to purulent urethral or rectal discharge	Abnormal vaginal discharge or uterine bleeding, purulent urethral or rectal discharge can be scant to profuse
	Rectal infection: pain, discharge, bleeding	
Complications	Epididymitis, Reiter syndrome (rare)	Pelvic inflammatory disease and associated complications (i.e., ectopic pregnancy, infertility) Reiter syndrome (rare)

	Recommended Regimens[a]	Alternative Regimen
urethral, endocervical, ...fection in adults	Azithromycin 1 g PO once, or doxycycline 100 mg PO twice daily for 7 days	Ofloxacin 300 mg PO twice daily for 7 days, or levofloxacin 500 mg PO once daily for 7 days, or erythromycin base 500 mg PO 4 times daily for 7 days, or erythromycin ethyl succinate 800 mg PO 4 times daily for 7 days
infections during pregnancy	Azithromycin 1 g PO as a single dose or amoxicillin 500 mg PO 3 times daily for 7 days	Erythromycin base 500 mg PO 4 times daily for 7 days, or erythromycin base 250 mg PO 4 times daily for 14 days, or erythromycin ethyl succinate 800 mg PO 4 times daily for 7 days (or 400 mg PO 4 times daily for 14 days)
...nctivitis of the newborn or ...neumonia in infants	Erythromycin base 50 mg/kg/day PO in four divided doses for 14 days[b]	

...C, Centers for Disease Control and Prevention; PO, orally.
...Recommendations are those of the CDC.
[b]Topical therapy alone is inadequate and is unnecessary when systemic therapy is administered.

trials, cure rates exceeding 90% are reported for these agents. All these antimicrobials also appear to have good efficacy against *Ureaplasma urealyticum*, the second most common cause of NGU.[31-34]

Azithromycin 1 g orally as a single dose and doxycycline 100 mg orally twice daily for 7 days are the regimens of choice for the treatment of uncomplicated chlamydial infections[1] (Table 126-8). Because of its prolonged serum and tissue half-life, azithromycin is the only single-dose therapy that is effective in treating *C. trachomatis*. Of the fluoroquinolones, ofloxacin and levofloxacin are included in the CDC recommendations, but neither appears to offer an advantage over other first-line or alternative therapies. Although ciprofloxacin and some other fluoroquinolones have activity against *C. trachomatis* and *U. urealyticum*, high dosages have not consistently eradicated chlamydial infections.[1,31-37]

For pregnant women with chlamydial urogenital infections, treatment can reduce the risk of pregnancy complications and transmission to the newborn significantly. Because the use of tetracyclines and fluoroquinolones is contraindicated during pregnancy, azithromycin and amoxicillin are the recommended drug treatments (see Table 126-8). When compliance with a multiday regimen is a concern, azithromycin is the preferred treatment in women, regardless of pregnancy status. It is recommended that post-treatment cultures be obtained for pregnant patients treated for chlamydial infections to ensure eradication of the infection. Persons treated for chlamydia should abstain from sexual intercourse for 7 days following the initiation of treatment.[1,34-37,41,42]

C. trachomatis transmission during perinatal exposure can result in infections of the eye, oropharynx, lungs, urogenital tract, and rectum of the neonate or infant. Despite their efficacy in preventing gonococcal ophthalmia, topical erythromycin ointment (0.5%), and tetracycline ointment (1%) appear less effective in preventing chlamydial ophthalmia. Additionally, topical therapy has no effect on nasal carriage or colonization of other parts of the infant's body, so the potential for other infections, including pneumonia, remains. Because of the high percentage of treatment failures, topical therapy is not recommended to treat ophthalmia caused by *C. trachomatis*. Instead, an oral erythromycin regimen is recommended.[1,31-34]

EVALUATION OF THERAPEUTIC OUTCOMES

Treatment of chlamydial infections with the recommended regimens is highly effective; therefore, post-treatment laboratory testing is not recommended routinely unless symptoms persist or there are other specific concerns (e.g., pregnancy). Post-treatment tests should not be performed for at least 3 weeks following completion of therapy.[1] When post-treatment tests are positive, they usually

represent noncompliance, failure to treat sexual partners, or laboratory error rather than inadequate therapy or resistance to therapy. Infants with pneumonitis should receive follow-up testing because erythromycin is only 80% effective, and a second course of therapy can be necessary.[1,31-34]

GENITAL HERPES

EPIDEMIOLOGY AND ETIOLOGY

Genital herpes infections represent the most common cause of genital ulceration seen in the United States. More than 50 million Americans have genital herpes, and this number is increasing by at least 500,000 each year.[1,43-48] Because of its morbidity, recurrent nature, and potential for complications, as well as its ability to be transmitted asymptomatically, genital herpes is of major public health importance.[45-54] Similar to syphilis and other STDs, the presence of genital herpes lesions is associated with an increased risk of acquiring HIV following exposure.[1,43-49]

PATHOPHYSIOLOGY

Herpes comes from the Greek word meaning "to creep" and is used to describe two distinct but antigenically related serotypes of herpes simplex virus. HSV-1 is associated most commonly with oropharyngeal disease, and HSV-2 is associated most closely with genital disease; however, each virus is capable of causing clinically indistinguishable infections in both anatomic areas.[43-45,48]

Humans are the sole known reservoir for HSV. Infection is transmitted via inoculation of virus from infected secretions onto mucosal surfaces (e.g., urethra, oropharynx, cervix, and conjunctivae) or through abraded skin. Evidence that the virus survives for a limited time on environmental surfaces suggests the possibility of fomitic transfer as a nonvenereal route of transmission.[43-45,48]

The cycle of HSV infection occurs in five stages: primary muco-cutaneous infection, infection of the ganglia, establishment of latency, reactivation, and recurrent infection. After viral inoculation, HSV infection is associated with cytoplasmic granulation, ballooning degeneration of cells, and production of mononucleated giant cells. Initially, the cellular response is predominantly polymorphonuclear, followed by a lymphocytic response. Replication occurs with viral spread to contiguous cells and peripheral sensory nerves. Latency then is established in sensory or autonomic nerve root ganglia. Latency appears to be lifelong, interrupted only by reactivation of the viral infection. It is unclear what factors are important in maintaining latency, but

TABLE 126-9 Presentation of Genital Herpes Infections

General	Incubation period 2–14 days (mean, 4 days)
	Can be caused by either HSV-1 or HSV-2
Classification of infection	
First-episode primary	Initial genital infection in individuals lacking antibody to either HSV-1 or HSV-2
First-episode nonprimary	Initial genital infection in individuals with clinical or serologic evidence of prior HSV (usually HSV-1) infection
Recurrent	Appearance of genital lesions at some time following healing of first-episode infection
Signs and symptoms	
First-episode infections	Most primary infections are asymptomatic or minimally symptomatic
	Multiple painful pustular or ulcerative lesions on external genitalia developing over a period of 7–10 days; lesions heal in 2–4 weeks (mean, 21 days)
	Flulike symptoms (e.g., fever, headache, malaise) during first few days after appearance of lesions
	Others–local itching, pain or discomfort; vaginal or urethral discharge, tender inguinal adenopathy, paresthesias, urinary retention
	Severity of symptoms greater in females than in males
	Symptoms are less severe (e.g., fewer lesions, more rapid lesion healing, fewer or milder systemic symptoms) with nonprimary infections
	Symptoms more severe and prolonged in the immunocompromised
	On average viral shedding lasts approximately 11–12 days for primary infections and 7 days for nonprimary infections
Recurrent	Prodrome seen in approximately 50% of patients prior to appearance of recurrent lesions; mild burning, itching, or tingling are typical prodromal symptoms
	Compared to primary infections, recurrent infections associated with (1) fewer lesions that are more localized, (2) shorter duration of active infection (lesions heal within 7 days), and (3) milder symptoms
	Severity of symptoms greater in females than in males
	Symptoms more severe and prolonged in the immunocompromised
	On average viral shedding lasts approximately 4 days
	Asymptomatic viral shedding is more frequent during the first year after infection with HSV
Therapeutic implications of HSV-1 vs HSV-2 genital infection	Primary infections caused by HSV-1 and HSV-2 virtually indistinguishable
	Recurrent infections and subclinical viral shedding are less frequent with HSV-1
	Recurrent infections with HSV-2 tend to be more severe
Complications	Secondary infection of lesions; extragenital infection because of autoinoculation; disseminated infection (primarily in immunocompromised patients); meningitis or encephalitis; neonatal transmission

HSV-1, herpes simplex virus type 1; HSV-2, herpes simplex virus type 2.

immune responses and emotional and physical stresses appear important in reactivating latent virus.[43–45,48]

CLINICAL PRESENTATION

The signs and symptoms of genital herpes infection are influenced by many factors, including previous exposure to HSV, viral type, and host factors such as age and site of infection. Because a high percentage of initial and recurrent infections are asymptomatic, and because viral shedding can occur in the absence of apparent lesions or symptoms, identification and education of individuals with genital herpes are essential in controlling its transmission.[43–52] A summary of the clinical presentation of genital herpes is provided in Table 126–9.

Complications

Complications from genital herpes infections result from both genital spread and autoinoculation of the virus and occur most commonly with primary first episodes. Lesions at extragenital sites, such as the eye, rectum, pharynx, and fingers, are not uncommon. CNS involvement is seen occasionally and can take several forms, including an aseptic meningitis, transverse myelitis, or sacral radiculopathy syndrome.[43–52]

A major concern is the effect of genital herpes on neonates exposed during pregnancy. Neonatal herpes is associated with a high mortality and significant morbidity. It is transmitted to the newborn primarily through exposure to HSV in the birth canal but, in rare cases, also is transmitted transplacentally. The risk of transmission during birth appears much greater for first-episode primary infections than for recurrent infections. Neonatal herpes infection has a case-fatality rate of approximately 50%, with a large proportion of surviving infants experiencing significant morbidity, including permanent neurologic damage.[43,44,48]

DIAGNOSIS

Confirmation of a genital herpes infection can be made only with laboratory testing. Tissue culture is the most specific (100%) and sensitive method (80%–90%) of confirming the diagnosis of first-episode genital herpes; however, culture is relatively insensitive in detecting HSV in ulcers in the latter stages of healing and in recurrent infections, as a result, in part, of reduced viral load. Viral culture is expensive and time consuming, and improper collection or transport of specimens can result in false-negative results. In most situations, HSV isolation on tissue culture takes 48 to 96 hours. Following isolation, it is recommended that typing of the virus be performed because of prognostic implications (HSV-1 is associated with a lower rate of asymptomatic and symptomatic recurrence). In instances in which rapid detection is necessary, such as an impending birth, other detection methods can be more useful. Amplified culture techniques that combine cell culture for 24 hours and subsequent staining for HSV antigen have sensitivities and specificities only slightly less than those of culture.[43–48,53–55]

Several serologic tests capable of distinguishing HSV-1 and HSV-2 antibodies are available. These tests detect antibodies to type-specific HSV-1 and HSV-2 proteins gG-1 and gG-2, respectively. Whereas antibody formation begins immediately following a primary herpes infection, complete seroconversion (i.e., complete antibody development) can take several months. Until the full expression of all antigenic determinants of HSV-1 and HSV-2 occurs, these tests are not useful in differentiating HSV-1 and HSV-2 infection. Older antibody detection tests, some of which are still marketed, are unable to distinguish between HSV-1 and HSV-2 owing to the considerable cross-reactivity between the two serotypes. Given the high prevalence of HSV-1 antibody in the adult population, accurate interpretation of positive results is not possible.[43–48,53–55]

PCR assays that detect HSV DNA and differentiate HSV-1 and HSV-2 infections are more sensitive than culture and are considered the diagnostic test of choice for suspected CNS infections (i.e., HSV encephalitis and HSV meningitis). PCR assays are highly sensitive in detecting asymptomatic viral shedding.[43–48,53–55]

Although the diagnosis of genital herpes can be confirmed only by laboratory tests, less stringent diagnostic criteria (e.g., characteristic physical findings or clinical history) frequently are used in clinical practice. A presumptive diagnosis of genital herpes commonly is made based on the presence of dark-field-negative, vesicular, or ulcerative genital lesions. A prior history of similar lesions or recent sexual contact with an individual with similar lesions also is useful in making the diagnosis. Other STDs, including chancroid, lymphogranuloma venereum, and granuloma inguinale, and causes such as trauma, allergic reactions, and bacterial or fungal infections are considered in the differential diagnosis.[43–48,53–55]

TREATMENT

Genital Herpes

The most achievable goals in the management of genital herpes are to relieve symptoms and to shorten the clinical course, to prevent complications and recurrences, and to decrease disease transmission. Although research has focused primarily on the treatment of active infection and suppression of recurrences, increasing emphasis is being placed on various approaches, including immunotherapy that might provide protection from disease transmission or possibly eliminate established latency.[47–48]

Palliative and supportive measures are the cornerstone of therapy for patients with genital herpes. Pain and discomfort usually respond to warm saline baths or the use of analgesics, antipyretics, or antipruritics; good genital hygiene can prevent the development of bacterial superinfection.

❹ Specific chemotherapeutic approaches to treating genital herpes include antiviral compounds, topical surfactants, photodynamic dyes, immune modulators, vaccines, and interferons. Few of these have undergone extensive evaluation, however, and only the antiviral agents have demonstrated any consistent clinical efficacy. The most recent CDC recommendations for the treatment of genital herpes include the antiviral agents acyclovir, valacyclovir, and famciclovir[1] (Table 126–10). The overall efficacy of these agents in treating genital HSV infection appears comparable, although patient compliance can be improved with regimens requiring less frequent dosing.[1,43,44]

■ FIRST-EPISODE INFECTIONS

Oral formulations of acyclovir, famciclovir, and valacyclovir have demonstrated efficacy in reducing viral shedding, duration of symptoms, and time to healing of first-episode genital herpes infections, with maximal benefits seen when therapy is initiated at the earliest stages of infection. Table 126–10 lists the recommended acyclovir, famciclovir, and valacyclovir oral regimens for first-episode infections. In immunocompromised patients or those with severe symptoms or complications necessitating hospitalization, parenteral acyclovir can be beneficial; however, the IV regimen has been associated with renal, gastrointestinal, bone marrow, and CNS toxicity, particularly in patients with renal dysfunction receiving high doses. No antiviral regimen is known to prevent latency or alter the subsequent frequency and severity of recurrences in humans.[1,43–48,51,52,56–59]

TABLE 126-10	Treatment of Genital Herpes	
Type of Infection	**Recommended Regimens[a,b]**	**Alternative Regimen**
First clinical episode of genital herpes[c]	Acyclovir 400 mg PO 3 times daily for 7–10 days,[d] or Acyclovir 200 mg PO 5 times daily for 7–10 days,[d] or Famciclovir 250 mg PO 3 times daily for 7–10 days,[d] or Valacyclovir 1 g PO twice daily for 7–10 days[d]	Acyclovir 5–10 mg/kg IV every 8 hours for 2–7 days or until clinical improvement occurs, followed by oral therapy to complete at least 10 days of total therapy[e]
Recurrent infection Episodic therapy	Acyclovir 400 mg PO 3 times daily for 5 days,[g] or Acyclovir 800 mg PO twice daily for 5 days,[g] or Acyclovir 800 mg PO 3 times daily for 2 days,[g] or Famciclovir 125 mg PO twice daily for 5 days,[g] or Famciclovir 1,000 mg PO twice daily for 1 day,[g] or Valacyclovir 500 mg PO twice daily for 3 days,[g] or Valacyclovir 1 g PO once daily for 5 days[g]	
Suppressive therapy	Acyclovir 400 mg PO twice daily, or Famciclovir 250 mg PO twice daily, or Valacyclovir 500 mg or 1,000 mg PO once daily[h]	

CDC, Centers for Disease Control and Prevention; HIV, human immunodeficiency virus; PO, orally.
[a]Recommendations are those of the CDC.
[b]HIV-infected patients can require more aggressive therapy.
[c]Primary or nonprimary first episode.
[d]Treatment duration can be extended if healing is incomplete after 10 days.
[e]Only for patients with severe symptoms or complications that necessitate hospitalization.
[f]Recommendations based on studies using this dosage regimen rather than the lower dosage regimens recommended for first clinical episodes of genital herpes. It is not clear whether lower dosage regimens would have comparable efficacy. Famciclovir and valacyclovir are probably also effective for proctitis and oral infection, but clinical experience is limited.
[g]Requires initiation of therapy within 24 hours of lesion onset or during the prodrome that precedes some outbreaks.
[h]Valacyclovir 500 mg appears less effective than valacyclovir 1,000 mg in patients with approximately 10 recurrences per year.

■ RECURRENT INFECTIONS

There are two approaches to management of recurrent episodes: episodic or chronic suppressive therapy. Episodic therapy is initiated early during the course of the recurrence, preferably within 6 to 12 hours of the onset of prodromal symptoms but no more than 24 hours after the appearance of lesions. In most patients, appreciable effects on symptomatology are not seen. Patients with prolonged episodes of recurrent infection or severe symptomatology are most likely to benefit from episodic therapy. Table 126–10 lists the recommended acyclovir, famciclovir, and valacyclovir suppressive regimens. One concern with episodic therapy is that some patients continue to shed virus despite the absence of lesions or presence of prodromal symptoms. Because of the relative mildness and brevity of recurrent infections, parenteral administration of acyclovir usually is not justifiable.[1,43–48,51,52,56–59]

Suppressive therapy with recommended antivirals reduces the frequency and severity of recurrences in 70% to 80% of patients experiencing frequent recurrences. Asymptomatic viral shedding is markedly reduced in patients receiving suppressive therapy; however, the extent to which this decreases disease transmission to sexual partners remains to be determined. Despite antiviral suppressive therapy, low-level virus shedding still occurs. However, this virus shedding may be less than that seen in patients treated episodically for recurrences, and thus may be associated with a lower risk of disease transmission. Because the frequency of recurrences tends to diminish over time, periodic "drug holidays" are advocated to assess changes in the underlying recurrence rate and determine if continued suppressive therapy is warranted.[1,43–48,51,52,56–59]

CLINICAL CONTROVERSY

The role of antiviral agents in the treatment of most recurrent genital herpes episodes is controversial. Because signs and symptoms of recurrent infections generally are milder and of shorter duration than those of first-episode infections in immunocompetent hosts, demonstration of clinically important therapeutic benefits is difficult. However, as episodic, asymptomatic viral shedding is common in HSV-2 infection, suppressive therapy in combination with use of condoms provides some protection to uninfected sexual partners.

Resistant HSV isolates have been identified in some patients experiencing breakthrough recurrences while taking acyclovir. Although there is concern about the development of resistant strains with suppressive therapy, clinical trials have found no evidence of cumulative toxicity or significant resistance in patients treated continuously with the recommended antivirals.[43–48]

■ SELECTED POPULATIONS

Immunocompromised patients are at greatest risk for severe and recurrent HSV infections. Acyclovir, valacyclovir, and famciclovir have been used to prevent reactivation of infection in patients seropositive for HSV who undergo transplantation procedures or induction chemotherapy for acute leukemia. Immunocompromised individuals, such as patients with acquired immunodeficiency syndrome (AIDS), who fail treatment or prophylaxis with recommended antiviral doses frequently demonstrate improved response with higher doses. If resistance is suspected or confirmed with recommended first-line antivirals, foscarnet is usually effective. However, its use is associated with a greater risk of serious adverse effects. Lesional application of an extemporaneous compounded cidofovir (1%) gel or trifluridine ophthalmic solution appears to offer some benefits also.[1,43–48]

The safety of acyclovir, famciclovir, and valacyclovir during pregnancy is not established, although considerable experience with acyclovir in pregnant patients has produced no evidence of teratogenic effects. Because of the high maternal and infant morbidity associated with first-episode primary genital infections or severe recurrent infections at or near term, many clinicians advocate the use of systemic acyclovir as the standard of care in such cases; however, the effectiveness of such therapy is unknown. The use of acyclovir to suppress recurrent episodes near term is more controversial primarily because of the lack of data demonstrating significant benefits in this situation.[1,43–48,60–63]

With the increasing prevalence of genital herpes worldwide, the potential exists for widespread use and misuse of acyclovir, valacyclovir, and famciclovir, resulting in development of resistant HSV isolates. In vitro resistance to these three agents usually is mediated by alterations in viral thymidine kinase; most resistant isolates are either thymidine kinase–deficient or have altered thymidine kinase. The incidence and clinical implications of HSV resistance require further study particularly with respect to immunocompromised hosts, in whom resistance can develop with greater frequency and be of greater clinical importance. Unlike acyclovir, valacyclovir, and famciclovir, foscarnet does not require the presence of thymidine kinase to be effective.[43–48]

Numerous agents for the prophylaxis and treatment of genital herpes infections are being studied. Neither topical nor systemic interferons have demonstrated consistent beneficial effects in genital HSV infections; however, a reduction in pain and time of healing of lesions has been reported with an interferon preparation incorporated into a gel containing nonoxynol-9. Other treatments under investigation include cidofovir and immune modulators such as imiquimod and resiquimod.[43–48] Agents that can eliminate ganglionic latency and prevent recurrent HSV infections are not expected to be available in the near future. Development of vaccines capable of protecting against HSV infection has proved challenging given the relative lack of protection offered by humoral and cell-mediated immunity in preventing naturally occurring recurrent infections. Safety concerns with live attenuated virus vaccines resulted in research focused primarily on recombinant protein vaccines that have exhibited relatively poor immunogenicity. Use of heterologous vaccines (bacillus Calmette-Guérin and influenza vaccines) to stimulate the immune system in patients with recurrent genital herpes has proved of no significant benefit.[43–48,64]

EVALUATION OF THERAPEUTIC OUTCOMES

Available antiviral compounds are of greatest benefit in patients experiencing first-episode primary infections, immunocompromised patients, and patients with frequent or severe recurrent infections. Antivirals, however, are palliative and not curative, and patients receiving these agents should be monitored closely for adverse drug effects. CDC guidelines suggest that discontinuation of suppressive therapy after 1 year should be considered to assess for possible changes in the patient's intrinsic pattern of recurrence. In many patients, decreases in recurrence rates and the severity of symptoms occur over time. However, some clinicians prefer to continue suppressive therapy indefinitely because it significantly reduces asymptomatic viral shedding, a potential benefit in reducing the risk of disease transmission to uninfected sexual partners.[1,43–48]

TRICHOMONIASIS

EPIDEMIOLOGY AND ETIOLOGY

Trichomonas vaginalis, a flagellated, motile protozoan is responsible for 3 to 5 million cases of trichomoniasis annually in the United States. Humans are host to two other *Trichomonas* species, *Trichomonas tenax* and *Trichomonas hominis*, but *T. vaginalis* is the only species thought to be pathogenic. Although infection by nonsexual contact is reported, it is rare. Contamination of inanimate objects and spread of infection via communal bathing or contact with infected bath or toilet articles is possible because *T. vaginalis* can survive for up to 45 minutes on moist surfaces. Neonatal infections also represent another possible nonvenereal route of disease transmission.[65–69]

Coinfection with other STDs is not unusual in patients diagnosed with trichomoniasis. Women infected with *T. vaginalis* are three times more likely to have gonorrhea than those who do not have trichomoniasis; approximately 20% of men with gonococcal urethritis also have trichomoniasis.[65–69] In patients treated appropriately for genital *C. trachomatis* or *U. urealyticum* infection, persistent urethritis can result from coexisting trichomonal infection. Although not well documented, the inflammatory response produced by trichomoniasis may increase the risk of acquiring HIV.[1,65–70]

PATHOPHYSIOLOGY

Trichomonads typically can be isolated from the vagina, urethra, and paraurethral ducts and glands in the majority of infected women. Infrequently, they are recovered from the endocervix. Extragenital sites are epidemiologically important because infection can persist and result in reinfection of the vagina if local therapy alone is used. This may account for the higher relapse rates reported for local versus systemic therapy. After attachment to the vaginal or urethral mucosa, trichomonads usually elicit an inflammatory response that manifests as a discharge containing large numbers of PMN leukocytes.[65-74]

CLINICAL PRESENTATION

Trichomonal infections are reported more commonly in women than in men. In part this might be because of the smaller number of organisms found in the male urethra making detection more difficult, greater disease transmission rates from males to females, and the nature of male infections, which have a high spontaneous cure rate even in the absence of treatment.[66,67,70-72,75] The typical clinical presentation of trichomoniasis in males and females is presented in Table 126–11.

DIAGNOSIS

T. vaginalis produces nonspecific symptoms also consistent with bacterial vaginosis; as a result, laboratory diagnosis is required.

TABLE 126-11	Presentation of *Trichomonas* Infections	
	Males	**Females**
General	Incubation period 3–28 days Organism can be detectable within 48 hours after exposure to infected partner	Incubation period 3–28 days
Site of infection	Most common: urethra Others: rectum (usually caused by rectal intercourse in MSM), oropharynx, eye	Most common: endocervical canal Others: urethra, rectum (usually caused by perineal contamination), oropharynx, eye
Symptoms	Can be asymptomatic (more common in males than females) or minimally symptomatic Urethral discharge (clear to mucopurulent) Dysuria, pruritus	Can be asymptomatic or minimally symptomatic Scant to copious, typically malodorous vaginal discharge (50%–75%) and pruritus (worse during menses) Dysuria, dyspareunia
Signs	Urethral discharge	Vaginal discharge Vaginal pH 4.5–6 Inflammation/erythema of vulva, vagina, and/or cervix Urethritis
Complications	Epididymitis and chronic prostatitis (uncommon) Male infertility (decreased sperm motility and viability)	Pelvic inflammatory disease and associated complications (i.e., ectopic pregnancy, infertility) Premature labor, premature rupture of membranes, and low–birth-weight infants (risk of neonatal infections is low) Cervical neoplasia

MSM, men who have sex with men.

Because *T. vaginalis* requires a pH range of 4.9 to 7.5 for survival, a vaginal discharge pH of greater than 5.0 usually indicates the presence of either *T. vaginalis* or *Gardnerella vaginalis*, a common cause of bacterial vaginosis. The simplest and most reliable means of diagnosis is a wet-mount examination of the vaginal discharge.[67,70-72,75] Trichomoniasis is confirmed if characteristic pear-shaped, flagellating organisms are observed. The wet mount is only about 60% to 80% sensitive in detecting the presence of trichomonads, with lower sensitivities reported in men and in women with low-grade, subacute, or chronic infections.[68-70,72,74]

Although the presence of trichomonads may be reported on a Papanicolaou (Pap) smear, the sensitivity of this cytologic technique is less than for wet mount and also is associated with a high number of false-positive and false-negative results. Stained smears of cervical specimens have been used in diagnosis, but they are less sensitive and more time consuming than the wet mount and therefore are not recommended. Culture techniques for trichomonads are highly specific and more sensitive than the wet mount, but they are not useful in rapid diagnosis because up to 48 hours or longer is necessary for growth. Cultures can be necessary, however, to confirm the diagnosis in the absence of a positive wet mount or to determine antimicrobial susceptibility in intractable cases.[1,65-72,74,75]

Newer diagnostic tests such as monoclonal antibody or DNA probe techniques, as well as PCR tests that can detect small amounts of trichomonal DNA, have been developed. These office-based tests are highly sensitive and specific for detecting infection in both vaginal specimens and urine. However, these tests are still not widely used.[65-69]

In males, demonstration of trichomonads in urethral specimens or urine sediment by wet mount is difficult, and diagnosis depends largely on culture. Specimens from males should be taken prior to first voiding because the small number of trichomonads in males may be reduced by micturition.[65-71]

TREATMENT

Trichomoniasis

Recommended and alternative treatment regimens for *T. vaginalis* include either metronidazole or tinidazole, both of which produce high cure rates in these infections. In only a few cases have *T. vaginalis* isolates been resistant to standard metronidazole or tinidazole doses. In these instances, longer courses of therapy or doses higher than those recommended routinely as initial therapy usually produce a cure.[1,65-69,72,75,76]

Table 126–12 provides treatment recommendations for trichomonas infections.[1] The standard therapy for trichomoniasis is either metronidazole or tinidazole 2 g orally as a single dose; cure rates are comparable with the recommended alternative regimen of metronidazole 500 mg twice daily for 7 days. When sexual partners are treated simultaneously, cure rates greater than 95% are reported. If sexual partners are not treated concurrently, cure rates are somewhat lower. In limited clinical testing, single metronidazole doses of less than 1.5 g are associated with high failure rates.[1,65-69,72,75,76]

Advantages of single-dose therapy over the multidose alternative regimen include better patient compliance, lower total dose, lower cost, and shorter exposure of the patient's gastrointestinal and urogenital anaerobic bacterial flora to the drug. As a result of the latter, the likelihood of developing pseudomembranous colitis or symptomatic candidal vulvovaginitis is decreased.[65-69,72] Because high doses of metronidazole have mutagenic effects in bacteria and oncogenic effects in mice, a reduced time of exposure in humans can be beneficial. There is no conclusive evidence for either of these

TABLE 126-12 Treatment of Trichomoniasis

Type	Recommended Regimen[a]	Alternative Regimen
Symptomatic and asymptomatic infections	Metronidazole 2 g PO in a single dose[b] *or* Tinidazole 2 g PO in a single dose	Metronidazole 500 mg PO 2 times daily for 7 days[c] *or* Tinidazole 2 g PO in a single dose[d]
Treatment in pregnancy	Metronidazole 2 g PO in a single dose[e]	

CDC, Centers for Disease Control and Prevention; PO, orally.

[a]Recommendations are those of the CDC.

[b]Treatment failures should be treated with metronidazole 500 mg PO twice daily for 7 days. Persistent failures should be managed in consultation with an expert. Metronidazole or tinidazole 2 g PO daily for 5 days has been effective in patients infected with *Trichomonas vaginalis* strains mildly resistant to metronidazole, but experience is limited; higher doses also have been used.

[c]Metronidazole labeling approved by the FDA does not include this regimen. Dosage regimens for treatment of trichomoniasis included in the product labeling are the single 2 g dose; 250 mg 3 times daily for 7 days; and 375 mg twice daily for 7 days. The 250 mg and 375 mg dosage regimens are currently not included in the CDC recommendations.

[d]For treatment failures with metronidazole 2 g as a single dose.

[e]Metronidazole is pregnancy category B and tinidazole is pregnancy category C; both drugs are contraindicated in the first trimester of pregnancy. Some clinicians recommend deferring metronidazole treatment in asymptomatic pregnant women until after 37 weeks gestation.

effects in humans after short-term therapy with recommended doses. Gastrointestinal complaints (e.g., anorexia, nausea, vomiting, and diarrhea) are more common with the single 2-g dose of either metronidazole or tinidazole, occurring in 5% to 10% of treated patients. Some patients also complain of a bitter metallic taste in the mouth with metronidazole. Patients intolerant of the single 2-g dose because of gastrointestinal adverse effects usually tolerate the alternative metronidazole multidose regimen.[65–69,72,75,76]

⑤ To achieve maximal cure rates and prevent relapse with either metronidazole or tinidazole as a single 2-g dose, simultaneous treatment of infected sexual partners is necessary. In women treated with the alternative 7-day course, however, relapse rates are not appreciably different regardless of whether or not sexual partners are treated. It is speculated that in men, spontaneous resolution of trichomonal infection or a reduction in the number of trichomonads below the inoculum necessary to transmit disease may occur during the 7 days of a female's therapy. In patients who fail to respond to an initial course of metronidazole therapy, a second course of therapy with metronidazole 500 mg twice daily for 7 days or a single 2-g dose of tinidazole is recommended. Patients refractory to a second course of treatment usually respond to a regimen using higher dosages of either agent (i.e., 2–4 g daily for 5–14 days). Good response rates also are reported for metronidazole 2 to 3 g orally plus either a single 500-mg tablet administered intravaginally or intravaginal metronidazole gel (0.75%) for 7 to 14 days.[61,65–69,71,76,77] Topical vaginal therapy alone is associated with low cure rates because infections involving the urethra or periurethral glands are unaffected and can serve as the source of reinfection.[67] Use of intravenous metronidazole can be warranted for rare cases of intolerance to oral medication or infections resistant to high-dose oral metronidazole. Sexual partners of all patients who require retreatment also should be treated or retreated because the majority of apparent treatment failures appear to be caused by reinfection or noncompliance.[65–69]

Concerns regarding the use of metronidazole in women who are pregnant or breast-feeding have been raised. Because metronidazole is secreted in breast milk, it is recommended that breastfeeding be interrupted for 12 to 24 hours after maternal ingestion of a single 2-g dose. Metronidazole (pregnancy category B) and tinidazole (pregnancy category C) are contraindicated during the first trimester of pregnancy based on Food and Drug Administration (FDA)–approved labeling. Although some experts recommend avoiding use of either agent throughout pregnancy, others advocate the use of metronidazole during any stage of pregnancy because of the potential adverse pregnancy outcomes associated with trichomoniasis. Currently no consensus exists on whether or how to treat trichomonas infections in pregnant women.[1,65–69]

Various local therapies for trichomoniasis have been proposed, particularly for pregnant patients. Clotrimazole vaginal suppositories, 100 mg at bedtime for 1 to 2 weeks, relieve symptoms in many women and produce cure rates of 50% or greater. An alternative therapy is gentle douching with either a diluted solution of vinegar or a 1% zinc sulfate solution until symptoms improve and then less frequently thereafter. This therapy generally provides some symptomatic improvement but few cures. Although once recommended, povidone-iodine douches should be avoided during pregnancy because of the risk of fetal thyroid suppression.[65–69]

Several other nitroimidazole antibiotics related to metronidazole and tinidazole (e.g., nimorazole, ornidazole, and carnidazole) are being investigated worldwide for the treatment of trichomoniasis. Unfortunately, none of these agents differs significantly from metronidazole or tinidazole in terms of efficacy (i.e., cross-resistance is high) or toxicity against metronidazole-susceptible strains of *T. vaginalis*.[65–69]

EVALUATION OF THERAPEUTIC OUTCOMES

Follow-up is considered unnecessary in patients who become asymptomatic after treatment with recommended therapy. When patients remain symptomatic, it is important to determine if reinfection has occurred. In these cases, a repeat course of therapy, as well as identification and treatment or retreatment of infected sexual partners, is recommended. In situations in which reinfection can be excluded, a relative resistance to metronidazole or tinidazole should be assumed, and an alternative regimen should be prescribed. Culture and sensitivity are warranted for infections unresponsive to alternative regimens.

HUMAN PAPILLOMAVIRUS AND OTHER STDS

Several STDs other than those just discussed occur with varying frequency in the United States and throughout the world. Although an in-depth discussion of these diseases is beyond the scope of this chapter, Table 126–13 lists recommended treatment regimens.[1] Of notable importance among these other STDs, however, is genital HPV infection, the most common viral STD in the United States. More than 100 HPV types have been characterized by genomic makeup, with approximately 30 types associated with genital tract lesions.[79–81] Of these, types 6 and 11 are associated most commonly with the development of low-grade dysplasia manifested as exophytic genital warts. In most individuals, genital infection with HPV is subclinical, and patients with visible acuminate warts represent less than 1% of all infected individuals. When present, genital warts can be large and multifocal, producing variable degrees of discomfort. Based on HPV DNA detection methods, most warts will regress spontaneously within 1 to 2 years of their initial appearance. However, reinfection is common in young, sexually active populations.[1,78,79]

Infection with several HPV types, particularly HPV-16 and HPV-18, is considered the major risk factor for the development

TABLE 126-13 Treatment Regimens for Miscellaneous Sexually Transmitted Diseases

Infection	Recommended Regimen[a]	Alternative Regimen
Chancroid (*Haemophilus ducreyi*)	Azithromycin 1 g PO in a single dose, *or* Ceftriaxone 250 mg IM in a single dose, *or* Ciprofloxacin 500 mg PO twice daily for 3 days,[b] *or* Erythromycin base 500 mg PO 4 times daily for 7 days	
Lymphogranuloma venereum	Doxycycline 100 mg PO twice daily for 21 days[c]	Erythromycin base 500 mg PO 4 times daily for 21 days
Human papillomavirus (HPV) infection		
External genital warts	*Provider-Administered Therapies:* Cryotherapy (e.g., liquid nitrogen or cryoprobe), *or* Podophyllin resin 10%–25% in compound tincture of benzoin applied to lesions; repeat weekly if necessary,[d,e] *or* Trichloroacetic acid 80%–90% *or* Bichloracetic acid 80%–90% applied to warts; repeat weekly if necessary, *or* Surgical removal (tangential scissor excision, tangential shave excision, curettage, or electrosurgery) *Patient-Applied Therapies:* Podofilox 0.5% solution or gel applied twice daily for 3 days, followed by 4 days of no therapy; cycle is repeated as necessary for up to four cycles,[e] *or* Imiquimod 5% cream applied at bedtime 3 times weekly for up to 16 weeks[e]	Intralesional interferon or laser surgery
Vaginal and anal warts	Cryotherapy with liquid nitrogen, or TCA or BCA 80%–90% as for external HPV warts; repeat weekly as necessary[f] Surgical removal (not for vaginal or urethral meatus warts)	
Urethral meatus warts	Cryotherapy with liquid nitrogen, or podophyllin resin 10%–25% in compound tincture of benzoin applied at weekly intervals[e,g]	

[a]Recommendations are those of the Centers for Disease Control and Prevention (CDC).
[b]Ciprofloxacin is contraindicated for pregnant and lactating women and for persons aged <18 years.
[c]Azithromycin 1 g PO once weekly for 3 weeks can be effective.
[d]Some experts recommended washing podophyllin off after 1–4 hours to minimize local irritation.
[e]Safety during pregnancy is not established.
[f]Surgical removal of anal warts is also a recommended treatment.
[g]Some specialists recommend the use of podofilox and imiquimod for treating distal meatal warts.

of cervical neoplasia, the second most common cancer in women worldwide. Although epidemiologic, virologic, and clinical data strongly support this association, HPV infection alone is insufficient to cause cervical cancer development because only a small percentage of infected women develop the disease. It appears that the interplay of host immune defenses, genetic factors, and infection with HPV types containing a more aggressive variant all contribute to the risk of developing cervical neoplasia.[78,79]

The Pap smear is the most cost-effective and frequently used diagnostic test for HPV. It can detect abnormal cytology in patients with clinical manifestations and those with subclinical disease (i.e., no overt condylomata) but not latent HPV infection. Visual inspection of genital surfaces under magnification can assist in making the diagnosis. Various tests for detecting HPV DNA also are available, and unlike the Pap smear do not require subjective interpretation of the results. Currently HPV DNA testing is only approved in women with abnormal Pap smears or women older than 30 years of age. However, use of HPV DNA testing as a routine screening test in lieu of Pap smears is expected in the near future. In women identified to have high-risk HPV infections by these tests, follow-up cytology would be performed.[78,79]

No consensus exists on the best approach to treating patients with genital HPV infection, particularly because most cases appear to be transient with spontaneous regression of lesions. A number of treatments are recommended (see Table 126–13), but none is clearly superior to the others. Treatment generally is directed toward patients with manifestations of genital warts, with the goal of removing or destroying these lesions and grossly infected surrounding tissue. Because such treatment neither stops viral expression in surrounding tissue nor eliminates viral latency, recurrence of lesions is not uncommon.[78,79]

Two HPV vaccines are marketed in the United States. Cervarix, a bivalent vaccine for HPV-16 and -18, and Gardasil, a quadrivalent vaccine for HPV-6, -11, -16, and -18. Both vaccines are indicated for preventing cervical precancers and cervical cancer in females 9 to 26 years of age. In addition, Gardasil is indicated for the prevention of genital warts caused by HPV-16 and -18 in males between the ages of 9 and 25 years. Clinically important differences in the magnitude and duration of the immune response, as well as prevention of HPV infections and cervical cancer remain to be determined.[80-83]

ABBREVIATIONS

AIDS: acquired immunodeficiency syndrome

CDC: Centers for Disease Control and Prevention

CSF: cerebrospinal fluid

DFA-TP: direct fluorescent-antibody test

DGI: disseminated gonorrhea infection

EIA: enzyme immunoassay

FDA: Food and Drug Administration

FTA-ABS: fluorescent treponemal antibody absorption

HIV: human immunodeficiency virus

HPV: human papillomavirus

HSV: herpes simplex virus

HSV-1: herpes simplex virus type 1

LPS: lipopolysaccharide

MHA-TP: microhemagglutination assay for antibodies to *T. pallidum*

MSM: men who have sex with men

NAATs: nucleic acid amplification tests

NGU: nongonococcal urethritis

Pap: Papanicolaou smear

PCR: polymerase chain reaction

PID: pelvic inflammatory disease

PMN: polymorphonuclear

QRNG: quinolone-resistant *N. gonorrhoeae*

RPR: rapid plasma reagin

STD: sexually transmitted disease

TPHA: *T. pallidum* hemagglutination assay

TPPA: *T. pallidum* particle agglutination assay

TRUST: toluidine red unheated serum test

USR: unheated serum reagin

VDRL: Venereal Disease Research Laboratory

REFERENCES

1. Centers for Disease Control and Prevention. Workowski KA, Berman SM. Sexually transmitted diseases treatment guidelines 2006. MMWR Recomm Rep 2006;21;55(RR 11):1–94.
2. Holmes KK. Sexually transmitted diseases: Overview and clinical approach. In: Fauci AS, Kasper DL, Longo DL, et al., eds. Harrison's Principles of Internal Medicine, 17th ed [electronic version]; 2008. *http://online.statref.com.libproxy.uthscsa.edu/TOC/TOC.aspx?SessionId=1143C56YWJTAOWJY.*
3. Aral SO, Holmes KK. The epidemiology of STIs and their social and behavioral determinants: Industrialized and developing countries. In: Holmes KK, Sparling PF, Stamm WE, et al., eds. Sexually Transmitted Diseases, 4th ed. New York: McGraw-Hill; 2008:53–92.
4. Sulak PJ. Sexually transmitted diseases. Semin Reprod Med 2003;21:399–413.
5. Rietmeijer CA, McMillan A. Some aspects of the prevention of sexually transmissible infections. In: McMillan A, Young H, Ogilvie MM, Scott GR, eds. Clinical Practice in Sexually Transmissible Infections. London: WB Saunders, 2002:11–28.
6. Steiner MJ, Warner L, Stone KM, Cates W Jr. Condoms and other barrier methods for prevention of STD/HIV infection and pregnancy. In: Holmes KK, Sparling PF, Stamm WE, et al., eds. Sexually Transmitted Diseases, 4th ed. New York: McGraw-Hill; 2008:1821–1829.
7. Roddy RE, Zekeng L, Ryan KA, et al. Effect of nonoxynol-9 gel on urogenital gonorrhea and chlamydial infection: A randomized, controlled trial. JAMA 2002;287:1117–1122.
8. Food and Drug Administration, HHS. Over-the-counter vaginal contraceptive and spermicide drug products containing nonoxynol 9; required labeling. Final rule. Fed Regist 2007;72:71769–71785.
9. Centers for Disease Control and Prevention. Sexually Transmitted Disease Surveillance, 2008. Atlanta, GA: U.S. Department of Health and Human Services; November 2009. *http://www.cdc.gov/std/stats08/surv2008-Complete.pdf.*
10. Ram S, Rice PA. Gonococcal infections. In: Fauci AS, Kasper DL, Longo DL, et al., eds. Harrison's Principles of Internal Medicine, 17th ed [electronic version]; 2008. *http://online.statref.com.libproxy.uthscsa.edu/TOC/TOC.aspx?SessionId=1143C56YWJTAOWJY.*
11. Marrazzo JM, Handsfield HH, Sparling PF. *Neisseria gonorrhoeae.* In: Mandell GL, Bennett JE, Dolin R, eds. Mandell, Douglas, and Bennett's Principles and Practice of Infectious Diseases, 7th ed [electronic version]; MD Consult, 2010. *http://www.mdconsult.com.libproxy.uthscsa.edu/book/player/book.do?method=display&type=aboutPage&decorator=header&eid=4-u1.0-B978-0-443-06839-3..X0001-X--TOP&isbn=978-0-443-06839-3&uniq=177288689.*
12. Newman LM, Moran JS, Workowski KA. Update on the management of gonorrhea in adults in the United States. Clin Infect Dis 2007;44:S84–101.
13. Marrazzo JM, Hofmann J. Infections due to *Neisseria.* In: Nabel EG (editor in chief), Federman DD (founding editor). ACP Medicine [electronic version]; 2009. *http://online.statref.com.libproxy.uthscsa.edu/Document/Document.aspx?docAddress=SaoWxNG8S1byvtPckclkVw%3d%3d&offset=7&SessionId=11469E6MHHSOSKLN.*
14. Hook EW III, Handsfield HH. Gonococcal infections in the adult. In: Holmes KK, Sparling PF, Stamm WE, et al., eds. Sexually Transmitted Diseases, 4th ed. New York: McGraw-Hill; 2008:627–645.
15. Centers for Disease Control and Prevention. Updated recommended treatment regimens for Gonococcal infections and associated conditions – United States, April 2007. *http://www.cdc.gov/std/treatment/2006/updated-regimens.htm.*
16. Gaydos CA. Nucleic acid amplification tests for gonorrhea and chlamydia: Practice and applications. Infect Dis Clin North Am 2005;19:367–386.
17. Lyss SB, Kamb ML, Peterman TA, et al. *Chlamydia trachomatis* among patients infected with and treated for *Neisseria gonorrhoeae* in sexually transmitted disease clinics in the United States. Ann Intern Med 2003;139:178–185.
18. Workowski KA, Berman SM, Douglas JM Jr. Emerging antimicrobial resistance in *Neisseria gonorrhoeae*: Urgent need to strengthen prevention strategies. Ann Intern Med 2008;148:606–613.
19. Woods CR. Gonococcal infections in neonates and young children. Semin Pediatr Infect Dis 2005;16:258–270.
20. LaFond RE, Lukehart SA. Biological basis for syphilis. Clin Microbiol Rev 2006;19:29–49.
21. Golden MR, Marra CM, Holmes KK. Update on syphilis: Resurgence of an old problem. JAMA 2003;290:1510–1514.
22. Lukehart SA. Syphilis. In: Fauci AS, Kasper DL, Longo DL, et al., eds. Harrison's Principles of Internal Medicine, 17th ed [electronic version]; 2008. *http://online.statref.com.libproxy.uthscsa.edu/Document/Document.aspx?docAddress=41ATb9F8ccLkXnJpdO9gbw%3d%3d&offset=71&SessionId=11465DDAHROTSXMQ.*
23. Augenbraun M. Syphilis. In: Klausner JD, Hook EW III, eds. Current Diagnosis & Treatment of Sexually Transmitted Diseases [electronic version]; AccessMedicine, 2007. *http://www.accessmedicine.com.libproxy.uthscsa.edu/content.aspx?aID=3025480.*
24. Sparling PF, Swartz MN, Musher DM, Healy BP. Clinical manifestations of syphilis. In: Holmes KK, Sparling PF, Stamm WE, et al., eds. Sexually Transmitted Diseases, 4th ed. New York: McGraw-Hill; 2008:661–688.
25. Zeltser R, Kurban AK. Syphilis. Clin Dermatol 2004;22:461–468.
26. Goh BT. Syphilis in adults. Sex Transm Infect 2005;81:448–452.
27. Kent ME, Romanelli F. Reexamining syphilis: An update on epidemiology, clinical manifestations, and management. Ann Pharmacother 2008;42:226–236.
28. Eccleston K, Collins L, Higgins SP. Primary syphilis. Int J STD AIDS 2008;19:145–151.
29. Hall CS, Klausner JD. Diagnostic tests for common STDs and HSV-2. MLO Med Lab Obs 2004;36:10–16.
30. Hafner L, Beagley K, Timms P. *Chlamydia trachomatis* infection: Host immune responses and potential vaccines. Mucosal Immunol 2008;1:116–130.
31. Stamm WE, Batteiger BE. *Chlamydia trachomatis* (trachoma, perinatal infections, lymphogranuloma venereum, and other genital infections). In: Mandell GL, Bennett JE, Dolin R, eds. Mandell, Douglas, and Bennett's Principles and Practice of Infectious Diseases, 7th ed [electronic version]; MD Consult, 2010. *http://www.mdconsult.com.libproxy.uthscsa.edu/book/player/book.do?method=display&type=aboutPage&decorator=header&eid=4-u1.0-B978-0-443-06839-3..X0001-X--TOP&isbn=978-0-443-06839-3&uniq=177288689.*
32. Stamm WE. Chlamydial infections. In: Fauci AS, Kasper DL, Longo DL, et al., eds. Harrison's Principles of Internal Medicine, 17th ed [electronic version]; 2008. *http://online.statref.com.libproxy.uthscsa.edu/Document/Document.aspx?docAddress=41ATb9F8ccLkXnJpdO9gbw%3d%3d&offset=71&SessionId=11465DDAHROTSXMQ.*
33. Stamm WE. *Chlamydia trachomatis* infections of the adult. In: Holmes KK, Sparling PF, Stamm WE, et al., eds. Sexually Transmitted Diseases, 4th ed. New York: McGraw-Hill; 2008:575–593.
34. Geisler WM, Stamm WE. Genital chlamydial infections. In: Klausner JD, Hook EW III, eds. Current Diagnosis & Treatment of Sexually

Transmitted Diseases [electronic version]; AccessMedicine, 2007. *http://www.accessmedicine.com.libproxy.uthscsa.edu/content.aspx?aID=3025480.*

35. Geisler WM. Approaches to the management of uncomplicated genital *Chlamydia trachomatis* infections. Expert Rev Anti Infect Ther 2004;2:771–785.

36. Zar HJ. Neonatal chlamydial infections: Prevention and treatment. Paediatr Drugs 2005;7:103–110.

37. Peipert JF. Genital chlamydial infections. N Engl J Med 2003;349: 2424–2430.

38. Hollblad-Fadiman K, Goldman SM. American College of Preventive Medicine practice policy statement: Screening for *Chlamydia trachomatis*. Am J Prev Med 2003;24:287–292.

39. Ostergaard L. Microbiological aspects of the diagnosis of *Chlamydia trachomatis*. Best Pract Res Clin Obstet Gynaecol 2002;16:789–799.

40. Watson EJ, Templeton A, Russell I, et al. The accuracy and efficacy of screening tests for *Chlamydia trachomatis*: A systematic review. J Med Microbiol 2002:51:1021–1031.

41. Guaschino S, Ricci G. How, and how efficiently, can we treat *Chlamydia trachomatis* infections in women? Best Pract Res Clin Obstet Gynaecol 2002:16:875–888.

42. Anonymous. Drugs for sexually transmitted infections. Treat Guidelines Med Lett 2007;5:81–88.

43. Leone P. Genital Herpes. In: Klausner JD, Hook EW III, eds. Current Diagnosis & Treatment of Sexually Transmitted Diseases [electronic version]; AccessMedicine, 2007. *http://www.accessmedicine.com.libproxy.uthscsa.edu/content.aspx?aID=3025480.*

44. Schiffer, JT, Corey L. Herpes simplex virus. In: Mandell GL, Bennett JE, Dolin R, eds. Mandell, Douglas, and Bennett's Principles and Practice of Infectious Diseases, 7th ed [electronic version]; MD Consult, 2010. *http://www.mdconsult.com.libproxy.uthscsa.edu/book/player/book.do?method=display&type=aboutPage&decorator=header&eid=4-u1.0-B978-0-443-06839-3..X0001-X--TOP&isbn=978-0-443-06839-3&uniq=177288689.*

45. Gupta R, Warren T, Wald A. Genital herpes. Lancet 2007; 370-2127–2137.

46. Kimberlin DW, Rouse DJ. Genital herpes. N Engl J Med 2004;350: 1970–1977.

47. Corey L, Wald A. Genital herpes. In: Holmes KK, Sparling PF, Stamm WE, et al., eds. Sexually Transmitted Diseases, 4th ed. New York: McGraw-Hill; 2008:399–437.

48. Corey L. Herpes simplex viruses. In: Fauci AS, Kasper DL, Longo DL, et al., eds. Harrison's Principles of Internal Medicine, 17th ed [electronic version]; 2008. *http://online.statref.com.libproxy.uthscsa.edu/Document/Document.aspx?docAddress=41ATb9F8ccLkXnJpdO9gbw%3d%3d&offset=71&SessionId=11465DDAHROTSXMQ.*

49. Dwyer DE, Cunningham AL. Herpes simplex and varicella-zoster virus infections. Med J Aust 2002;177:267–273.

50. Chayavichitslip P, Buckwalter J V, Krakowski AC, Friedlander SF. Herpes simplex. Pediatr Rev 2009;30:119–130.

51. Simmons A. Clinical manifestations and treatment considerations of herpes simplex virus infection. J Infect Dis 2002;186(Suppl 1): S71–S77.

52. Beauman JG. Genital herpes: A review. Am Fam Physician 2005;72:1527–1534.

53. Wald A, Ashley-Morrow R. Serological testing for herpes simplex virus (HSV)-1 and HSV-2 infection. Clin Infect Dis 2002;35(Suppl 2): S173–S182.

54. Wald A. Testing for genital herpes: How, who, and why. Curr Clin Top Infect Dis 2002;22:166–180.

55. Scoular A. Using the evidence base on genital herpes: Optimising the use of diagnostic tests and information provision. Sex Transm Infect 2002;78:160–165.

56. Cernik C, Gallina K, Brodell RT. The treatment of herpes simplex infections: An evidence-based review. Arch Intern Med 2008;168: 1137–1144.

57. Martinez V, Caumes E, Chosidow O. Treatment to prevent recurrent genital herpes. Curr Opin Infect Dis 2008;21:42–48.

58. Mell HK. Management of oral and genital herpes in the emergency department. Emerg Med Clin North Am 2008;26:457–473.

59. Patel R, Stanberry L, Whitley RJ. Review of recent HSV recurrent-infection treatment studies. Herpes 2007;14:23–26.

60. Hill J, Roberts S. Herpes simplex virus in pregnancy: New concepts in prevention and management. Clin Perinatol 2005;32:657–670.

61. Mills J, Mindel A. Genital herpes simplex infections: Some therapeutic dilemmas. Sex Transm Dis 2003;30:232–233.

62. Jones CA. Vertical transmission of genital herpes: Prevention and treatment options. Drugs 2009;69:421–434.

63. Hollier LM, Wendell GD. Third trimester antiviral prophylaxis for preventing maternal genital herpes simplex virus (HSV) recurrences and neonatal infection. Cochrane Database Syst Rev 2009;4:1–19.

64. Stanberry LR. Clinical trials of prophylactic and therapeutic herpes simplex virus vaccines. Herpes 2004;11(Suppl 3):161A–169A.

65. Weller PF. Protozoal intestinal infections and trichomoniasis. In: Fauci AS, Kasper DL, Longo DL, et al., eds. Harrison's Principles of Internal Medicine, 17th ed [electronic version]; 2008. *http://online.statref.com.libproxy.uthscsa.edu/Document/Document.aspx?docAddress=41ATb9F8ccLkXnJpdO9gbw%3d%3d&offset=71&SessionId=11465DDAHROTSXMQ.*

66. Soper D. Trichomoniasis: Under control or undercontrolled? Am J Obstet Gynecol 2004;190:281–290.

67. Hobbs MM, Sena AC, Swygard H, Schwebke JR. *Trichomonas vaginalis* and trichomoniasis. In: Holmes KK, Sparling PF, Stamm WE, et al., eds. Sexually Transmitted Diseases, 4th ed. New York: McGraw-Hill; 2008:771–793.

68. Schwebke J. Trichomoniasis. In: Klausner JD, Hook EW III, eds. Current Diagnosis & Treatment of Sexually Transmitted Diseases [electronic version]; AccessMedicine, 2007. *http://www.accessmedicine.com.libproxy.uthscsa.edu/content.aspx?aID=3025480.*

69. Schwebke JR. *Trichomonas vaginalis*. In: Mandell GL, Bennett JE, Dolin R, eds. Mandell, Douglas, and Bennett's Principles and Practice of Infectious Diseases, 7th ed [electronic version]; MD Consult, 2010. *http://www.mdconsult.com.libproxy.uthscsa.edu/book/player/book.do?method=display&type=aboutPage&decorator=header&eid=4-u1.0-B978-0-443-06839-3..X0001-X--TOP&isbn=978-0-443-06839-3&uniq=177288689.*

70. Schwebke JR, Burgess D. Trichomoniasis. Clin Microbiol Rev 2004;17:794–803.

71. Wendel KA, Workowski KA. Trichomoniasis: Challenges to appropriate management. Clin Infect Dis 207;44(Suppl 3):S123–S129.

72. Say PJ, Jacyntho C. Difficult-to-manage vaginitis. Clin Obstet Gynecol 2005;48:753–768.

73. Faro S. Vaginitis: Differential Diagnosis and Management. Boca Raton, FL: Parthenon Publishing, 2004:67–92.

74. Eckert LO. Acute vulvovaginitis. N Engl J Med 2006;355:1244–1252.

75. Sobel JD. What's new in bacterial vaginosis and trichomoniasis. Infect Dis Clin North Am 2005;19:387–406.

76. Forna F, Gülmezoglu AM. Interventions for treating trichomoniasis in women. Cochrane Database Syst Rev 2009;4:1–93.

77. Cudmore SL, Delgaty KL, Hayward-McClelland SF, et al. Treatment of infections caused by metronidazole-resistant *Trichomonas vaginalis*. Clin Microbiol Rev 2004;17:783–793.

78. Huh WK. Human papillomavirus infection: A concise review of natural history. Obstet Gynecol 2009;114:139–143.

79. Winer RL, Koutsky LA. Genital human papillomavirus infection. In: Holmes KK, Sparling PF, Stamm WE, et al., eds. Sexually Transmitted Diseases, 4th ed. New York: McGraw-Hill; 2008:489–508.

80. Hutchinson DJ, Klein KC. Human papillomavirus disease and vaccines. Am J Health Syst Pharm 2008;65:2105–2112.

81. Hershey JH, Velez LF. Public health issues related to HPV vaccination. J Public Health Manag Pract 2009;15:384–392.

82. Hager WD. Human papilloma virus infection and prevention in the adolescent population. J Pediatr Adolesc Gynecol 2009;22:197–204.

83. Medeiros LR, Rosa DD, da Rosa MI, et al. Efficacy of human papillomavirus vaccines: A systematic quantitative review. Int J Gynecol Cancer 2009;19:1166–1176.

EDWARD P. ARMSTRONG AND ALLAN D. FRIEDMAN

KEY CONCEPTS

❶ The most common cause of osteomyelitis (particularly that acquired by hematogenous spread) and infectious arthritis is *Staphylococcus aureus*.

❷ Culture and susceptibility information are essential as a guide for antimicrobial treatment of osteomyelitis and infectious arthritis.

❸ Joint aspiration and examination of synovial fluid are extremely important to evaluate the possibility of infectious arthritis.

❹ The most important treatment modality of acute osteomyelitis is the administration of appropriate antibiotics in adequate doses for a sufficient length of time.

❺ Antibiotics generally are given in high doses so that adequate antimicrobial concentrations are reached within infected bone and joints.

❻ The standard duration of antimicrobial treatment for acute osteomyelitis is 4 to 6 weeks.

❼ Oral antimicrobial therapy can be used for osteomyelitis to complete a parenteral regimen in children who have had a good clinical response to intravenous (IV) antibiotics and in adults without diabetes mellitus or peripheral vascular disease when the organism is susceptible to the oral antimicrobial, a suitable oral agent is available, and compliance is ensured.

❽ The three most important therapeutic maneuvers in the management of infectious arthritis are appropriate antibiotics, joint drainage, and joint rest.

❾ Monitoring of antibiotic therapy is important and typically involves noting clinical signs of inflammation, periodic white blood cell counts, C-reactive protein (or erythrocyte sedimentation rate) determinations, and radiographic findings.

Bone and joint infections are composed of two disease processes known, respectively, as *osteomyelitis* and *septic* or *infectious arthritis*. They are unique and separate infectious entities with different signs and symptoms and infecting organisms. Despite advances in therapy, these infections continue to cause significant morbidity

Learning objectives, review questions, and other resources can be found at **www.pharmacotherapyonline.com**.

from residual damage and chronic recurring infections. Emphasis on initiating antibiotic therapy as soon as possible is important in reducing long-term complications.

EPIDEMIOLOGY

Osteomyelitis generally is an uncommon disease. One classic publication reported that 247 patients had osteomyelitis in a prominent American teaching hospital during a 4-year period.[1] Acute osteomyelitis has an estimated annual incidence of 0.4 per 1,000 children.[2] Osteomyelitis caused by contiguous spread, including postoperative, direct puncture, and that associated with adjacent soft tissue infections, comprises 47% of infections. Hematogenous osteomyelitis comprises 19% of infections, and osteomyelitis occurring in patients with significant peripheral vascular disease comprises 34% of infections. A review of osteomyelitis cases based on duration of disease shows that acute disease constitutes 56% of patients and that chronic osteomyelitis, defined as having a previous hospitalization for the same infection, constitutes 44% of patients.

Infectious or septic arthritis is an inflammatory reaction within the joint space. Distinct from osteomyelitis, septic arthritis is a more common disease and is one of the most common causes of new cases of arthritis. One study identified 22 patients with culture-proven septic arthritis at a tertiary teaching hospital over 10 years.[3] Another hospital reported 15 cases of neonatal septic arthritis of the hip in a 3-year period.[4] Overall, the yearly incidence of bacterial arthritis varies from 2 to 10 per 100,000 inhabitants.[5]

ETIOLOGY

OSTEOMYELITIS

The most common method of classifying osteomyelitis is based on the route in which the infecting organism reaches the bone. Infection that results from spread through the bloodstream is termed *hematogenous osteomyelitis*. When the organism reaches the bone from an adjoining soft tissue infection, it is termed *contiguous osteomyelitis*. Osteomyelitis that results from direct inoculation, such as from trauma, puncture wounds, or surgery, generally is also classified under the contiguous osteomyelitis category. Patients with peripheral vascular disease are at risk for the development of osteomyelitis, and these patients often are separated into a third distinct category because of their unique management features. Osteomyelitis also can be classified based on the duration of the disease. Acute osteomyelitis describes infections of recent onset, usually several days to 1 week, whereas chronic infections are those of a longer duration. Some authors describe chronic infections as those with symptoms for more than 1 month before therapy, whereas

TABLE 127-1	Types of Osteomyelitis, Age Distribution, Common Sites, and Risk Factors		
Type of Osteomyelitis	**Typical Age (years)**	**Site(s) Involved**	**Risk Factors**
Hematogenous	Younger than 1	Long bones and joints	Prematurity, umbilical catheter or venous cutdown, respiratory distress syndrome, perinatal asphyxia
	1–20	Long bones (femur, tibia, humerus)	Infection (pharyngitis, cellulitis, respiratory infections), trauma, sickle cell disease, puncture wounds to feet
	Older than 50	Vertebrae	Diabetes mellitus, blunt trauma to spine, urinary tract infection
Contiguous	Older than 50	Femur, tibia, mandible	Hip fractures, open fractures
Vascular insufficiency	Older than 50	Feet, toes	Diabetes mellitus, peripheral vascular disease, pressure sores

other authors define chronic infections as relapse of an initial infection. Yet a third system sometimes used to classify osteomyelitis is based on the anatomic location of the infection (medullary or superficial) and the physiologic status of the patient (otherwise healthy, systemic immunologic compromise, or local immunologic compromise).[6,7] This classification system can be useful when comparing patients among different studies and attempting to categorize the severity of infection.

INFECTIOUS ARTHRITIS

Infectious arthritis can occur from many different types of microorganisms.[8] Most infecting organisms are known to produce an infection in a single joint, termed *monarthritic infections*; however, infections also can involve two or more joints.[9] As with osteomyelitis, joint infections can be classified according to the mechanisms by which the infecting organism reaches the joint. Infectious arthritis can result from the spread of an adjacent bone infection, direct contamination of the joint space, or hematogenous dissemination. Hematogenous spread of the disease comprises the majority of infections; spread from osteomyelitis and direct inoculation are much less frequent.[10] Infectious arthritis occurs most commonly in patients older than age 16 years; however, approximately one-fourth of cases occur in children 15 years or younger.[11]

PATHOPHYSIOLOGY

HEMATOGENOUS OSTEOMYELITIS

Hematogenous osteomyelitis is described classically as a disease of children because most cases occur in patients younger than 16 years of age.[7] Table 127–1 summarizes the primary characteristics of osteomyelitis. Less commonly, these infections occur in adults. One exception, vertebral osteomyelitis, involves the vertebrae and occurs most frequently in patients older than 50 years.

Unique features of the anatomy and physiology of some bones appear to predispose them to become infected.[12] The vascular structure within the long bones appears to predispose the bone for hematogenous infections to begin within the metaphyses (Fig. 127–1). The nutrient arteries of the long bones divide within the medullary canal of the bone into small arterioles. These end in hairpin turns near the growth plate and flow into veins, of much wider diameter, that drain the medullary cavity.[1] An infection in hematogenous disease is initiated within the bend of the arterioles. There is considerable slowing of blood flow passing through the hairpin turns within the arterioles and then into the wider venous structures. This sludging of blood flow allows bacteria present within the bloodstream to settle and initiate an inflammatory response. In addition to these structural features, there appears to be less active phagocytosis within the metaphysis. After the bacteria settle in the bone, avascular necrosis can occur from occlusion of the nutrient vessels and release of bacterial enzymes.

In addition to these anatomic and functional features, there is some evidence that trauma is associated with developing an infection in specific bones. Children who develop hematogenous osteomyelitis may report some type of trauma as an etiologic event. Animal data also indicate that traumatized bone is more likely to become infected than normal bone.

Once the infection is initiated, exudate begins to form within the bone, which produces increased pressure. The age of the patient largely determines the next stage in the pathophysiology. In children older than 12 to 18 months, the infection that started in the metaphysis of a long bone is prevented from spreading into the joint because of the growth plate; however, the exudate often expands laterally through the thin outer cortex of the bone and raises the loose periosteum. The periosteum is thick and not easily broken, and the resulting pus usually remains subperiosteal. If there is significant periosteal damage, a soft tissue abscess can develop. Impairment of blood flow to the outer portion of the cortical bone can occur, producing dead bone that separates from healthy bone, termed *sequestra*. The elevated periosteum remains viable because its blood supply, derived from the overlying muscle, is unaffected. The raised periosteum will continue to produce bone; however, this new bone is now separated from the cortex because the periosteum has been raised from the infection. This new bone is termed *involucrum*.

In adults, the periosteum is tightly bound, and the cortex is thick. These anatomic features generally cause the infections to remain intramedullary. As expected, subperiosteal abscess formations are less common in this population. The infection can spread to adjacent bone structures through the haversian and Volkmann canals.

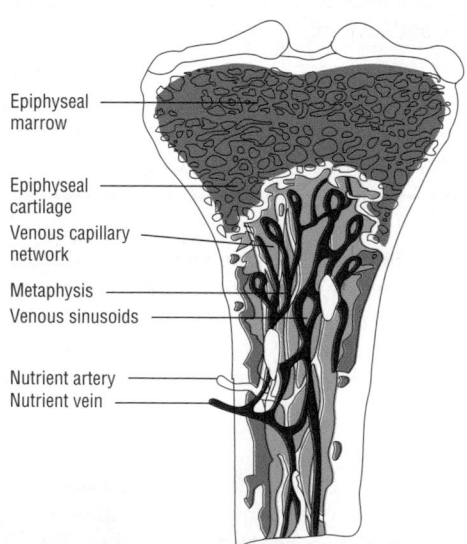

Epiphyseal marrow

Epiphyseal cartilage

Venous capillary network

Metaphysis

Venous sinusoids

Nutrient artery
Nutrient vein

FIGURE 127-1. Cross section of normal bone.

Chronic osteomyelitis is more likely to occur if large segments of bone become avascular and necrotic.

Neonatal patients also have unique characteristics, blood vessels that spread through the cortex of the metaphyses and up into the epiphyses. This enables an infection that started within the metaphyseal area to spread easily to involve the epiphyses and then into the joint.[13] Therefore, in infants, not only can the infection spread to involve the periosteum and the shaft as in children, but the infection also can spread to involve the joint.[14]

Hematogenous osteomyelitis also is known to have a predilection for certain bones, depending on the age of the patient. Children most commonly develop infections within the femur, tibia, humerus, and fibula.[14] Vertebral infections are more common in patients older than 50 years.[15] Neonatal infections commonly involve multiple bones.

❶ The bacteriology of hematogenous osteomyelitis is unique compared with osteomyelitis caused by other routes of infection. A single organism is responsible for the vast majority of hematogenous infections. *Staphylococcus aureus* is isolated most frequently with hematogenous infections in children. In immunocompetent children who have been fully vaccinated with the *Haemophilus influenzae* type B vaccine, this is now an uncommon pathogen causing bone and joint infections.[16] However, neonatal osteomyelitis has a wider spectrum of infecting organisms. The three most common etiologic agents are *S. aureus,* group B streptococcus, and *Escherichia coli.* The infections from *S. aureus* and *E. coli* have been linked to complications occurring during pregnancy or delivery, and they are involved most frequently in multiple-bone infections.

Vertebral osteomyelitis has several unique features and occurs most commonly in adults 50 to 60 years of age. The lumbar and thoracic regions are the locations of most infections. Hematogenous infections are most likely to develop in the vascular areas near the subchondral plate region of the vertebral body. Staphylococci cause ~60% of these infections; however, gram-negative organisms now play a significant role. These gram-negative organisms, particularly *E. coli,* most likely originate within the urinary tract. *E. coli* vertebral infections have been associated with urinary tract infections, positive urine cultures, and bacteremias. *Mycobacterium tuberculosis* also is known to cause infections in the spine. Skin and respiratory tract infections are other foci of infections known to lead to vertebral infections.

A unique category of osteomyelitis patients consists of individuals with a history of IV drug abuse. More than 50% of the osteomyelitis infections in this group of patients are found in the vertebral column. Less than 20% of infections are located in either the sternoarticular or pelvic girdle. Infections are much less frequent within the extremities. An unusual feature of osteomyelitis in the IV drug-abusing population is the spectrum of organisms. Gram-negative organisms are responsible for 88% of infections. *Pseudomonas aeruginosa,* either singly or in combination with other organisms, is cultured in 78% of all infections. *Klebsiella, Enterobacter,* and *Serratia* species also can be found but less commonly. In addition, staphylococcal and streptococcal organisms are sometimes cultured.

Patients with sickle cell anemia and related hemoglobinopathies have a much higher rate of infection with *Salmonella* species as compared with other populations.[17] *Salmonella* species are responsible for two-thirds of the infections in these patients. Bowel infarctions from the sickle cell disease can facilitate salmonellae entry into the bloodstream from the colon and spread hematogenously to the bone. Osteomyelitis in patients with sickle cell disease may occur in any bone, but it is observed to be most common in the medullary cavity of long or tubular bones. Because of the difficulty in separating bone pain during a sickle cell crisis from that of an infection, osteomyelitis can be relatively advanced in these patients when the diagnosis is made. Although salmonellae are cultured most frequently, staphylococci and other gram-negative organisms also can be isolated.

CONTIGUOUS-SPREAD OSTEOMYELITIS

This category of osteomyelitis includes infections caused by direct entrance of organisms from a source outside the body or progressive spread of an infection from tissue adjacent to the bone. Penetrating wounds (e.g., trauma), open fractures, and various invasive orthopedic procedures can result in direct inoculation of organisms into the bone. Infections also can occur secondary to pressure ulcers. More than 80% of cases of postoperative osteomyelitis are known to occur following open reductions of fractures. Specifically, these infections occur most commonly after internal fixation of a hip fracture or femoral or tibial shaft fracture.

Osteomyelitis secondary to an adjoining soft tissue infection comprises another very important group of contiguous infections and most often involves the fingers and toes. Less commonly, infections can spread from infected teeth to involve the mandible or occur secondary to sinus infections by spreading through the mucosal lining of the sinuses into the vascular system surrounding the bone.[18,19]

In contrast to hematogenous osteomyelitis, which occurs most commonly in children, contiguous-spread osteomyelitis occurs most commonly in patients older than age 50. Most likely this is so because important predisposing factors, such as hip fractures, are more common in this age group.

Contiguous-spread disease has several important differences compared with hematogenous osteomyelitis. Although *S. aureus* is still the most common organism isolated, infections with multiple organisms, including gram-negative bacilli, occur frequently. *P. aeruginosa,* streptococcus, *E. coli, Staphylococcus epidermidis,* and anaerobes all can be isolated. One important exception to this wide range of organisms is puncture wounds of the feet. There is a correlation between puncture wounds of the feet and gram-negative osteomyelitis (sometimes classified as osteochondritis), especially infections caused by *P. aeruginosa.*

Patients with osteomyelitis in association with severe vascular insufficiency are extremely difficult to manage.[20,21] As anticipated, most of these patients have diabetes mellitus or severe atherosclerosis, and they develop their infections from contiguous-spread mechanisms. Generally, these patients are between the ages of 50 and 70 years when they develop osteomyelitis. Frequently, patients with vascular disease develop osteomyelitis in their toes and fingers, and there is usually an adjacent area of infection, such as cellulitis or dermal ulcers.

Another important characteristic of osteomyelitis in association with vascular insufficiency is the spectrum of infecting organisms. Infections in these patients almost always include multiple organisms. The mixed-flora infections often include staphylococcus and streptococcus or the combination of staphylococcus, streptococcus, and Enterobacteriaceae. Enterococci and anaerobic organisms also can be involved.

Anaerobic organisms also play a role in osteomyelitis. When anaerobes are grown from cultures, they usually are found in association with other organisms, including aerobic bacteria. Predisposing factors in patients who have anaerobic osteomyelitis include vascular disease, bites, contiguous infections, peripheral neuropathy, hematogenous spread, and trauma.[22] The anaerobic infections in association with diabetes mellitus almost always occur within the feet. *Bacteroides fragilis* and *Bacteroides melaninogenicus* comprise the majority of anaerobic isolates.

INFECTIOUS ARTHRITIS

Distinct from osteomyelitis, infectious arthritis usually is acquired by hematogenous spread.[9] The synovial tissue is highly vascular and does not have a basement membrane, so organisms in the blood

TABLE 127-2 Characteristics of Acute Infectious Arthritis

Feature	Finding
Peak incidence	Children younger than 16 years
	Adults older than 50 years
Clinical findings	Fever of 38–40°C (100.4–104°F) in children; painful swollen joint in the absence of trauma
	Physical examination: effusion, restriction of joint motion, tenderness, and warmth of joint
Most commonly affected joints	Knee, hip, ankle, elbow, wrist, and shoulder
Laboratory findings:	
Erythrocyte sedimentation rate	Elevated in 90% of cases
White blood cell count	Elevated in 30–60% of cases
Left shift	Seen in two-thirds of patients
Blood culture	Positive in 40% of cases
Needle aspiration of joint	Gram stain diagnostic in 30–50% of cases. Synovial fluid cultures are positive in 60–80% of cases. Synovial fluid differential reveals 90% polymorphonuclear leukocytes. Synovial fluid glucose decreased relative to serum glucose. Lactic acid levels elevated in nongonococcal infectious arthritis but not in gonococcal infectious arthritis

TABLE 127-3 Clinical Presentation of Hematogenous Osteomyelitis

Signs and symptoms
Significant tenderness of the affected area, pain, swelling, fever, chills, decreased motion, and malaise

Laboratory tests
Elevated erythrocyte sedimentation rate, C-reactive protein, and white blood cell count. Fifty percent of patients will have positive blood cultures.

Diagnostic studies
Bone changes observed on radiographs 10–14 days after the onset of infection. Technetium and gallium scans are positive as early as 1 day after the onset of infection.

can easily reach the synovial fluid. Table 127–2 summarizes the characteristics of acute infectious arthritis. Some organisms, such as *Neisseria gonorrhoeae*, are especially likely to infect a joint during bacteremia. In addition, organisms can gain access to the joint from a deep-penetrating wound, an intraarticular steroid injection, arthroscopy, prosthetic joint surgery, and contiguous osteomyelitis expansion into the joint.[3]

The risk factors associated with adult infectious arthritis (more than one factor may be present) are systemic corticosteroid use, preexisting arthritis, arthrocentesis, distant infection, diabetes mellitus, trauma, and other diseases.[23]

Trauma also appears to be a risk factor in facilitating microorganism entry into the synovial space. One study found that 35% of patients with infectious arthritis had preexisting joint disease.[11] Unlike children, adults often have significant systemic diseases that predispose them to infectious arthritis, such as diabetes mellitus, immunosuppressive states (e.g., cancer and liver disease), and preexisting arthritis. IV drug abusers also are prone to develop septic arthritis.

Arthritis, joint trauma, and surgery are other important risk factors because chronic inflammation or trauma makes the joint more susceptible to infection. In addition, patients with rheumatoid arthritis can be prone to bacterial infection because of an inherent phagocytic defect, as well as concomitant corticosteroid therapy. Hormonal factors appear to play a role in *N. gonorrhoeae* infectious arthritis. Women are more prone to develop disseminated gonococcal infections than men. The second and third trimesters of pregnancy and during menstruation appear to be the times of greatest risk for developing gonococcal bacteremia.

After bacteria gain access to the joint, the organisms begin to multiply and produce a persistent purulent effusion within the joint. If this joint effusion is present beyond 7 days, chronic, and sometimes irreversible, damage can occur. Purulent effusions can promote cartilage destruction by increasing leukocyte enzyme activity. In conjunction with the development of the effusion, almost all patients will develop a hot, swollen, painful joint. The proteolytic enzymes within the effusion and pressure necrosis can lead to cartilage and bone damage.

❶ *S. aureus*, the single most common infecting organism, is found in 48% of cases of nongonococcal bacterial arthritis. Streptococcal infections account for 18% of cases, and gram-

negative organisms are less common.[11] Overall, *E. coli* is the most common of the gram-negative organisms; however, *P. aeruginosa* is the most frequent organism in IV drug abusers. Neonates may have infectious arthritis because of a broad range of organisms, with *S. aureus*, streptococcus, and gram-negative organisms being most common. *S. aureus* and streptococcus are the most common pathogens in children younger than 5 years. If the child has not been fully vaccinated or is immunocompromised, *H. influenzae* type B may be a cause. Within the adult population, *S. aureus* is responsible for the vast majority of nongonococcal infections. The most common cause of bacterial arthritis in adults 18 to 30 years of age is *N. gonorrhoeae*, which are the most common infections in women.[24] Patients with a terminal complement deficiency (C5–C9) are at increased risk of disseminated infections with *Neisseria* species. Although less common, nonbacterial causes of osteomyelitis and septic arthritis include fungi and viruses.[25]

CLINICAL PRESENTATION

The clinical presentation of acute hematogenous osteomyelitis is summarized in Table 127–3. Although neonatal hematogenous osteomyelitis can spread rapidly to involve the joint, often there are few systemic symptoms present. A joint effusion is present in 60% to 70% of neonatal infections. Decreased limb motion and edema over the affected area may be the only signs from which to make a diagnosis. Pyogenic vertebral osteomyelitis produces nonspecific symptoms, such as severe back pain, fever or night sweats, and weight loss. The pain typically is present at rest and increases in severity with movement. Neurologic symptoms can occur if the infection extends and compresses the spinal cord. With contiguous-spread osteomyelitis, there is often an area of localized tenderness, warmth, edema, and erythema over the infected site. Patients with significant vascular insufficiency usually have local symptoms, such as pain, swelling, and redness. Less commonly, patients with vascular disease also can have a fever and elevated white blood cell (WBC) count. The presentation of osteomyelitis from surgery or trauma depends on the precipitating cause. If the infection follows surgery or bone trauma, the symptoms usually are noted within 1 month. The most frequent symptom is simply pain in the area of infection. Less commonly, patients also can develop a fever and elevated WBC count.

Patients with nongonococcal bacterial arthritis almost always present with a fever, and 50% of patients have an elevated WBC count (see Table 127–2). The average initial synovial WBC count is $10 \times 10^3/mm^3$ or greater in nongonococcal bacterial disease. The most frequent initial sign of disseminated gonococcal infections is a migratory polyarthralgia. In addition, two-thirds of patients complain of fever, dermatitis, and tenosynovitis (inflammation of the tendon sheath).

Nongonococcal bacterial arthritis almost always involves only a single joint. The knee is the most commonly involved joint, but infections also can occur in the shoulder, wrist, hip, ankle, interphalangeal joints, and elbow joints. Usually, the initial focus of infection that acted as the source for bacterial or microbial entrance can be identified. Common routes for bacterial entrance are infections of the respiratory tract, skin, and urinary tract. Blood cultures are important in these patients because they can be positive in 50% of patients.

Another type of infectious arthritis occurs following prosthetic joint surgery. With these infections, the erythrocyte sedimentation rate (ESR) usually is elevated, although a leukocytosis often is absent. Infections that result from postoperative contamination usually become apparent within 1 year of surgery.

RADIOLOGIC AND LABORATORY TESTS

The evaluation of a patient who may have osteomyelitis has several unusual aspects. Radiographs of the involved area should be obtained; however, bone changes characteristic of osteomyelitis are not seen for at least 10 to 14 days after the onset of the infection. Radiologists may note soft tissue swelling before any bone changes become obvious. Bone lesions do not appear on roentgenogram films until 10 days after infection because >50% of the bone matrix must be removed before the lesions can be detected. To aid in improving the diagnosis, magnetic resonance imaging (MRI) and bone scanning are commonly used.[26,27]

Despite the seriousness of osteomyelitis, often there are few laboratory abnormalities. The ESR, C-reactive protein, and WBC count may be the only laboratory abnormalities.[14] The degree of abnormality of these laboratory findings does not correlate with the disease outcome; however, they are useful for monitoring therapy. C-reactive protein can be elevated because of the presence of inflammation, and it can be substituted for the ESR. It is generally the more sensitive and specific marker of response to therapy and often increases and decreases before the ESR.

When a clinical assessment of osteomyelitis is suspected, it is important to establish a bacteriologic diagnosis by culture of the infected bone. Accurate culture information is especially important as a guide for treatment of osteomyelitis. Bone aspiration is valuable in determining an accurate bacteriologic diagnosis. In addition, performing a bone aspiration determines whether or not there is an abscess present. If an abscess is located, the pus is cultured, and a Gram stain is performed. If an abscess is found, the fluid needs to be drained and cultured. Aspirates of subperiosteal pus or metaphyseal fluid yield a pathogen in 70% of cases. Cultures should be done for both aerobic and anaerobic bacteria. A Gram stain of the aspirate can be useful in initiating empirical antibiotic therapy. This allows a more appropriate choice of antibiotics from the first day of therapy rather than waiting several days while culture results are pending.

If a specimen is obtained from a previously undrained or unopened wound abscess, the pathogen usually can be identified. In chronic osteomyelitis, however, identification can be more difficult.[28] Open wounds and draining sinuses frequently are contaminated with other organisms and thus provide inaccurate culture information. Therefore, because of the inaccuracies with sinus tract cultures, they cannot be relied on to reflect the pathogen. Cultures of loculated pus aspirates in the area of orthopedic devices removed from infected bone can be trusted, however, to identify the infecting organism. The preferable time to obtain culture material in a patient with a chronic draining sinus is at the time of open surgical débridement.

❷ In addition to performing cultures from the involved bone, it is important to obtain blood cultures from any site believed to be the source of a bacteremia. Approximately 50% of patients with hematogenous osteomyelitis will have positive blood cultures.

❸ When evaluating the possibility of a patient having infectious arthritis, immediate joint aspiration with subsequent analysis of the synovial fluid is extremely important. The presence of purulent fluid usually indicates the presence of a septic joint. The synovial fluid WBC count is usually 50 to 200 × 10³/mm³ when an infection is present. Approximately half the patients with an infected joint have a low synovial glucose level, usually <40 mg/dL. Gram stains of joint fluid demonstrate bacteria in 50% of patients with septic arthritis; however, such stains can be positive in only 25% of patients with gonococcal arthritis infections. Synovial fluid cultures usually are positive in patients with nongonococcal infections. Both blood and joint fluid should be cultured aerobically and anaerobically in a patient suspected of having an infected joint. Blood cultures are positive in half of patients with nongonococcal infections but in only 20% of those with gonococcal infections. Pharyngeal, rectal, cervical, or urethral smears and cultures, as well as cultures of cutaneous lesions, should be performed if a disseminated gonococcal infection is considered. As with osteomyelitis, most patients will have an elevated C-reactive protein concentration and ESR. Radiographs of infected joints often reveal distention of the joint capsule with soft tissue swelling in the adjacent space. MRI can be helpful in identifying an infected hip. In patients who have developed an infected prosthetic joint, loosening of the prosthesis can be seen radiographically.

TREATMENT

■ DESIRED OUTCOME

The goals of treatment are resolution of the infection and prevention of long-term sequelae. The ultimate outcome of osteomyelitis depends on the acute or chronic nature of the disease and how rapidly appropriate therapy is initiated. Patients with acute osteomyelitis have the best prognosis. Cure rates exceeding 80% can be expected for patients with acute osteomyelitis who have surgery as indicated and receive appropriate injectable antibiotics for 4 to 6 weeks. In contrast, patients with chronic osteomyelitis have a much poorer prognosis. Dead bone and other necrotic material from the infection act as a bacterial reservoir and make the infection very difficult to eliminate. Adequate surgical debridement to remove all the dead bone and necrotic material, combined with prolonged administration of antibiotics, provides the best chance to obtain a cure. The inability to remove all the dead bone can allow residual infection and require suppressive antibiotics to control the infection.

In comparison, many patients who develop infectious arthritis recover with no long-term sequelae. Gonococcal arthritis usually resolves rapidly with antibiotics; however, patients with staphylococcal arthritis have a higher incidence of joint damage. Individuals at greatest risk for long-term sequelae are those who have symptoms present for more than 7 days before starting therapy and those with infections occurring within the hip joint and infections caused by gram-negative organisms. Common long-term residual effects following infectious arthritis are limited joint motion and persistent pain. Shortening of the affected extremity is another well-known complication. More than half the children in one hospital who subsequently developed residual joint damage were believed normal at the time of hospital discharge.

■ GENERAL APPROACH TO TREATMENT

❹ Following completion of the steps needed to determine the infecting organism, the most important treatment modality of acute osteomyelitis is the administration of appropriate antibiotics in adequate doses for a sufficient length of time. It is important to stress that early antibiotic therapy can mitigate the need for surgery.[29] A delay in treatment can allow bone necrosis to occur and make eradication of the infection much more difficult. In these patients, recurrent exacerbations of the infection can result if all necrotic tissue is not removed surgically and all microorganisms eliminated. Adjunctive treatment with hyperbaric oxygen or antibiotic-impregnated implants during surgery also has been used.[30,31]

If a patient with hematogenous osteomyelitis does not respond by having a decrease in fever, local swelling, redness, and pain following the initiation of adequate antibiotic therapy, the patient should undergo surgical debridement of the infected area. It is important to emphasize the priority of starting antibiotics immediately after the cultures have been obtained. No treatment failures have been reported when injectable antibiotics were started within 48 hours of the onset of symptoms in children with osteomyelitis.

▇ PHARMACOLOGIC THERAPY

Antibiotic Bone Concentration

❺ Antibiotics used in the management of acute osteomyelitis generally are given in high doses (adjusted for weight and renal and/or hepatic function) so that adequate antimicrobial concentrations are reached within the infected bone and joint.[32] Between 8 and 12 g/day of a penicillinase-resistant penicillin (nafcillin or oxacillin), ampicillin, or cephalosporin or a similar large dose of another parenteral antibiotic is used in the initial management of adults with osteomyelitis. These dosing recommendations, however, are empirical; the relationship between a specific dose of a given antibiotic and its resulting concentration within the infected bone is largely unknown. Semisynthetic penicillins, cephalosporins, clindamycin, and the aminoglycosides can be detected in bone homogenates soon after their administration.

Daptomycin may also be an effective empiric therapy for the treatment of osteomyelitis in adults.[33] It is effective against most methicillin-sensitive and -resistant *S. aureus*. Although a retrospective study, these results support the use of daptomycin, especially when other standard therapies have failed. Further prospective studies are needed to define the situations in which daptomycin might be best used and its optimal dosing.

▇▇▇▇▇▇
CLINICAL CONTROVERSY

Some clinicians recommend coverage empirically for methicillin-resistant *Staphylococcus aureus* (MRSA) when staphylococcal infection is suspected. Others believe that culture results and sensitivity testing or lack of response to routine staphylococcal antibiotics should trigger use of antibiotics directed against MRSA. The frequency of MRSA in a community may help govern which approach is used.

Duration of Antibiotic Therapy

❻ The specific duration of antibiotic therapy needed in the management of osteomyelitis is usually 4 to 6 weeks.[34] Failure rates approaching 20% have been observed in children treated with injectable antibiotics for 3 weeks or less. Thus, with the data indicating a minimum of 3 weeks of antibiotic therapy, the standard treatment for osteomyelitis has been parenteral antibiotics for 4 to 6 weeks.[35] Although these data were largely evaluated in children, this duration-of-therapy recommendation is also used in adults.[36] Treatment failures may be due to the presence of infected necrotic

bone or infected hardware (wires, plates, screws, and rods) that could not be removed.

A modification of this recommendation has been used in some patients. Children receiving an appropriate oral antibiotic regimen and adults receiving an oral fluoroquinolone antibiotic, such as ciprofloxacin, for a duration of 6 weeks have been treated successfully. Monitoring the patient's clinical signs and symptoms and the C-reactive protein level or ESR is an important parameter to assess therapy. If signs or symptoms are still present at 6 weeks, therapy should be extended. In contrast, children who have had a puncture wound of the foot resulting in *P. aeruginosa* osteochondritis and who have had surgical debridement of infected material can be treated with parenteral antibiotics for 10 days.

Oral Antibiotic Therapy

❼ One of the most significant changes in the management of osteomyelitis is the use of oral antibiotics to complete therapy.[37] Criteria for the use of oral outpatient antibiotic therapy for osteomyelitis include the following:

- Confirmed osteomyelitis
- Initial clinical response to parenteral antibiotics
- Suitable oral agent available
- Compliance ensured

Suitable candidates are children with good clinical response to IV therapy and adults without diabetes mellitus or peripheral vascular disease.

Two primary populations have benefited from oral treatment. Children responding to initial parenteral therapy may be excellent candidates to receive follow-up oral therapy with an agent such as dicloxacillin, cephalexin, or amoxicillin, depending on their culture and sensitivity results.[38] Although more controversial, the other population to benefit from oral therapy is adults with an infecting organism sensitive to a fluoroquinolone.[39] These two populations now no longer routinely require expensive and complicated courses of long-term parenteral antibiotics.

The use of oral antibiotics is well studied in children.[40] Several studies documenting the effectiveness of oral therapy used injectable antibiotics initially, then switched to oral antibiotics when there was a decrease in the signs of inflammation and the ESR or when the patient was afebrile for 3 days.[38] If pus was obtained on the initial needle aspirate, or if a reduction in fever, local swelling, and tenderness did not occur despite adequate rest, immobilization, and intensive antibiotic therapy, the patients underwent surgical drainage.

The patients enrolled in oral antibiotic trials generally had disease of recent onset, identification of a specific infecting organism, enforced compliance, and surgery as indicated. In patients who meet these criteria, oral antibiotics appear to offer a great advantage in the treatment of osteomyelitis.[41] Patients not meeting these criteria are more likely to develop chronic osteomyelitis with resulting recurrent exacerbations of the infection if oral therapy is attempted. Limited retrospective data in adults indicated that parenteral therapy for less than 4 weeks followed by oral therapy may be effective.[42]

Ciprofloxacin is effective in the treatment of osteomyelitis caused by gram-negative strains, such as *Enterobacter cloacae* and *Serratia marcescens*;[43] however, many strains of streptococci are relatively resistant. Activity of ciprofloxacin against gram-negative bacilli allows patients to be treated orally and avoids the potential toxic complications of 4 to 6 weeks of aminoglycoside therapy. Ciprofloxacin and other fluoroquinolones also have demonstrated effectiveness in the treatment of chronic osteomyelitis along with adequate surgical debridement.[44,45] Another benefit with this agent is that it can be administered on an every-12-hour schedule. An important limitation of this antibiotic class, however, is that fluoroquinolones should not be used in children younger than 16 to 18 years of age or in pregnant women because of the potential to cause cartilage damage. Other limitations of ciprofloxacin are that it has poor coverage against anaerobic organisms and staphylococci and that *P. aeruginosa* can develop resistance. Newer fluoroquinolones have additional gram-positive activity; however, additional well-controlled clinical trials are needed to determine most appropriately their role in the treatment of osteomyelitis.[46]

Concern has been raised about staphylococci resistance to fluoroquinolones. Methicillin-resistant *S. aureus* infections do not respond well to ciprofloxacin; however, resistance also can be troublesome for methicillin-sensitive strains. It is now recommended that when ciprofloxacin is to be used to treat osteomyelitis with mixed etiologies that include *S. aureus,* it should be combined with an antistaphylococcal drug such as dicloxacillin, cephalexin, or clindamycin.

CLINICAL CONTROVERSY

Some clinicians believe that oral fluoroquinolones should be preferred treatments for osteomyelitis, whereas others believe that there have been inadequate studies to date to determine their comparative clinical effectiveness.

Antibiotic Selection

A critical component in the management of osteomyelitis is the selection of appropriate antibiotics. Empirical therapy must be selected on the basis of the most likely infecting organism while the results of culture and sensitivity data are pending. Table 127–4 summarizes empirical therapy recommendations. It is difficult to make evidence-based recommendations on the treatment of these infections, as little high-quality clinical evidence exists. Experimental evidence, case series, and published expert opinion are used to suggest preferred treatment options.[29] Dosages expressed in terms of milligrams per kilograms per day generally are given in divided doses every 6 to 8 hours (three or four times a day).

Because *S. aureus,* streptococci, and *E. coli* are the most common infecting organisms in newborns, an IV dosage of 150 mg/kg/day (given in four divided doses) of oxacillin or nafcillin plus cefotaxime 150 mg/kg/day (given in three or four divided doses) is appropriate. For children 5 years of age or younger, *S. aureus* and streptococci are the most common infecting organisms. Appropriate therapy in this age group is an IV dosage of nafcillin or oxacillin 150 mg/kg/day or cefazolin 100 mg/kg/day. If the patient is immunocompromised or has not been fully vaccinated, empirical therapy is needed to also cover *H. influenzae* type B. In this setting, IV dosage of cefuroxime 150 mg/kg/day is appropriate empirical therapy. For children older than 5 years, *S. aureus* is the most likely infecting organism, and either nafcillin 150 to 200 mg/kg/day IV or cefazolin 100 mg/kg/day IV is recommended. If patients are allergic to penicillins or cephalosporins or are infected with MRSA, vancomycin, clindamycin, or linezolid can be used.[47–49] Children with culture-negative osteomyelitis can be managed as presumed staphylococcal disease with excellent long-term results.[50] Empiric therapy may need to be modified if community-acquired methicillin-resistant *S. aureus* is prevalent.[51] Children with osteomyelitis usually can be treated successfully with 4 weeks of parenteral therapy or parenteral followed by oral therapy.

An oral regimen can be an alternative to the previous recommendation in many cases of osteomyelitis in children. Children who have undergone surgery, if needed, and have had a good clinical response to IV therapy may be candidates for the alternate oral antibiotic regimen. Parenteral antibiotic therapy should be initiated and continued until there has been a resolution in the erythema, swelling, and tenderness and until the patient is afebrile. Dicloxacillin, cloxacillin, and cephalexin (100 mg/kg/day) are effective oral agents. Patients should be monitored with periodic WBC counts, C-reactive protein (or ESR) determinations, and radiographic findings. When oral antibiotics are used, the total duration of oral and injectable therapy is usually at least 4 to 6 weeks. As stated previously, because of the risk of cartilage damage, fluoroquinolones should not be used in children. Hematogenous osteomyelitis in adults is caused most frequently by *S. aureus* and thus is treated appropriately with 8 to 12 g/day of a penicillinase-resistant penicillin, such as nafcillin. A similar dose of a first-generation cephalosporin (e.g., cefazolin), clindamycin 2.4 g/day, or vancomycin 2 g/day (with normal renal function) can be used in adults allergic to penicillin. If the infection

TABLE 127–4 Empirical Treatment of Osteomyelitis

Patient Subtype	Likely Infecting Organism	Antibiotic[a]	Recommendation Grades[b]
Newborn	*Staphylococcus aureus,* streptococci, *Escherichia coli*	Nafcillin or oxacillin 50–150 mg/kg/day IV plus cefotaxime 100–200 mg/kg/day IV	B–3
Children 5 years of age or younger	If vaccinated for *Haemophilus influenzae* type B: *S. aureus* or streptococci	Nafcillin 150 mg/kg/day IV or cefazolin 100 mg/kg/day IV	B–3
	If not vaccinated against *H. influenzae* type B	Cefuroxime 150 mg/kg/day IV	B–3
Children older than 5 years of age	*S. aureus*	Nafcillin 150 mg/kg/day IV or cefazolin 100 mg/kg/day IV	A–3
Adults	*S. aureus*	Nafcillin 2 g IV every 4 hours or cefazolin 2 g IV every 8 hours	A–3
IV drug abusers	Pseudomonas	Ciprofloxacin 750 mg PO twice daily or ceftazidime 2 g IV every 8 hours plus tobramycin 5 mg/kg/day IV	B–3
Postoperative or posttrauma patients	Gram-positive and gram-negative organisms	Nafcillin 2 g IV every 4 hours plus ceftazidime 2 g IV every 8 hours or ticarcillin-clavulanate 3.1 g IV every 4 hours	B–3
Patients with vascular insufficiency	Gram-positive and gram-negative organisms	Nafcillin 2 g IV every 4 hours or cefazolin 2 g IV every 8 hours plus ceftazidime 2 g IV every 8 hours	B–3
	If anaerobes suspected	Cefotetan 2 g IV every 12 hours or clindamycin 900 mg IV every 8 hours plus ceftazidime 2 g IV every 8 hours	C–3

[a]Dosage should be adjusted for some agents in patients with renal and/or hepatic dysfunction.
[b]Strength of recommendations: A, B, C = good, moderate, and poor evidence to support recommendation, respectively. Quality of evidence: 1 = Evidence from more than one properly randomized, controlled trial. 2 = Evidence from more than one well-designed clinical trial with randomization, from cohort or case-controlled analytic studies or multiple time series; or dramatic results from uncontrolled experiments. 3 = Evidence from opinions of respected authorities, based on clinical experience, descriptive studies, or reports of expert communities. PO = orally.

is located within the vertebrae, *E. coli* must be considered; thus, depending on the culture and sensitivity data, a switch to a cephalosporin may be needed.[52] After institution of appropriate antibiotic therapy, the antimicrobial agent should be continued for at least 4 to 6 weeks total (parenteral plus oral).

CLINICAL CONTROVERSY

Some clinicians believe that empirical therapy of osteomyelitis and septic arthritis in a child younger than 5 years of age no longer requires *H. influenzae* type B coverage, whereas others are concerned about children not being fully vaccinated and desire to use an antibiotic with activity against this organism.

Special Populations Osteomyelitis in a patient with a hemoglobinopathy, such as sickle cell anemia, is commonly caused by either *Salmonella* or *S. aureus*.[17] Thus, empirical antibiotics of first choice are ceftriaxone and cefotaxime. Alternatives are chloramphenicol and ciprofloxacin (in adults). Bone infections in adults with a history of IV drug abuse require coverage for gram-negative organisms; therefore, empirical treatment with ceftazidime 2 g IV every 8 hours plus an aminoglycoside is indicated. If compliance can be ensured, these patients are excellent candidates to receive oral ciprofloxacin 750 mg twice daily. Antibiotic therapy in these patients should be continued for at least 4 to 6 weeks.

As discussed previously, several microorganisms can cause bone infections that occur after surgery or from contiguous spread of an adjacent soft tissue infection. *S. aureus* is the single most common organism, but multiple organisms can be involved. To provide the required broad-spectrum coverage, nafcillin 2 g IV every 4 hours plus ceftazidime 2 g intravenously every 8 hours should be used as initial therapy. An alternative single agent is ticarcillin–clavulanate potassium 3.1 g IV every 4 hours in adults; however, there is less experience with this agent. Other broad-spectrum alternatives can be cefepime and imipenem. The antibiotic regimen can require modification after culture and sensitivity information is evaluated. Based on the culture and sensitivity data, ciprofloxacin can be an appropriate oral alternative for these patients. Frequently, the antibiotics must be continued for 6 weeks to obtain a cure, and surgery often is required to remove any infected or devitalized tissue.

Patients with established vascular insufficiency who subsequently develop osteomyelitis are extremely difficult to manage.[6] Impaired blood flow to the extremities impedes the healing process, possibly requiring vascular bypass surgery.[53] Infections in these patients involve a wide range of organisms, including *S. aureus, Streptococcus,* anaerobes, and gram-negative organisms. Bone culture–based antibiotic therapy has been associated with cure in diabetics with osteomyelitis of the foot.[54] Broad-spectrum therapy with a penicillinase-resistant penicillin in combination with ceftazidime is the preferred initial therapy. If anaerobes are suspected, an antianaerobic cephalosporin (e.g., cefoxitin) or clindamycin plus ceftazidime can be substituted. Ampicillin may need to be added to the regimen to provide coverage against enterococci. Despite aggressive antibiotic therapy along with surgical debridement, these patients continue to have low cure rates.[55,56] Amputation of the involved area may be required to obtain a cure of the infection.[57,58]

Home Antibiotic Therapy Because the management of bone and joint infections frequently requires prolonged parenteral antibiotics,

newer antibiotic regimens have been used. Administration of antibiotics in the home environment and use of antibiotics with extended elimination half-lives are possible. Although acute osteomyelitis is one of the more common infectious diseases that can be treated with home IV antibiotics, not all patients are acceptable candidates for home administration.[59] Patients must be screened to include only those who are receiving a stable treatment program, those who are interested and are motivated in participating, and those who have good venous access, as well as those who have support from family members or neighbors and have home facilities for storage and refrigeration. Patients with adequate vascular access may be able to use a peripheral IV catheter; however, a central IV catheter may be required if venous access difficulties occur. Certain exclusion criteria also must be considered. Complications of other preexisting diseases, such as diabetic retinopathy, intention tremor, disabling inflammation or degenerative joint disease, coagulopathies, or various neurologic disorders can prevent individuals from receiving home antibiotics. A history of alcoholism or of IV drug abuse also is an important exclusion criterion. Patients who are fluent only in a foreign language and those who are illiterate or hard of hearing may have to be excluded if a qualified guardian is unavailable. In addition to meeting these initial screening criteria, patients must complete a thorough training program successfully before hospital discharge. Aseptic technique, proper catheter care, and correct administration techniques must be documented. Once a patient is receiving therapy in the home environment, continued monitoring of his or her antimicrobial therapy is important. It is vital to ensure compliance with the antimicrobial regimen. Catheter-related complications are common in patients receiving prolonged courses of parenteral antibiotics.[60]

In addition, the specific antibiotic regimen characteristics must be considered when evaluating a patient for home antibiotics.[61] Some important features are microbiologic culture and sensitivity data, the number of required daily antimicrobial doses, antibiotic stability data, and requirements for unique monitoring for the specific antimicrobial regimen, such as serum creatinine and peak and trough concentration measurements with aminoglycosides. Although an organism can be sensitive to several antimicrobial agents, one antibiotic can provide practical benefits over other agents. Patients who have an infecting organism that is sensitive to one of the longer-acting (less frequently dosed) cephalosporins and is resistant to less expensive agents (cefazolin) may benefit from the newer antibiotics. It is important, however, to monitor for the development of resistant strains and superinfections.

Infectious Arthritis ❽ The three most important therapeutic maneuvers in the management of infectious arthritis are appropriate antibiotics, joint drainage, and joint rest. Smears of the synovial fluid can be useful to select appropriate antibiotic therapy initially.[62] If bacteria are not observed on the Gram stain in a patient who has a purulent joint effusion, antibiotics still should be initiated because of the high risk of an infection being present.[63] A delay in initiating antibiotics significantly increases the likelihood for long-term complications.[64,65]

The specific antibiotic selected depends on the most likely infecting organism.[66] In infants younger than 1 month, the infecting organisms vary widely, and empirical therapy thus must provide broad-spectrum coverage. A penicillinase-resistant penicillin such as nafcillin or oxacillin plus an aminoglycoside is appropriate. Children younger than 5 years who have been immunized for *H. influenzae* type B should receive nafcillin, oxacillin, or cefazolin.

In children older than 5 years and in adults, initial therapy with a penicillinase-resistant penicillin is appropriate to provide the necessary coverage against *S. aureus*. Therapy should be changed to clindamycin, vancomycin, or linezolid if the *S. aureus* is resistant to methicillin.[67,68] Preliminary data indicate that children with infectious arthritis can be converted to oral therapy after initial IV therapy.[69] As with osteomyelitis, IV drug abusers require coverage for *P. aeruginosa*; therefore, combination therapy with an aminoglycoside is needed. The antibiotics selected usually are administered parenterally. Antibiotics administered by this route achieve sufficient concentrations within the synovial fluid; thus, intraarticular antibiotic injections are unnecessary. Although studies to define clearly the appropriate length of therapy have not been conducted, 2 to 3 weeks of antibiotic therapy generally is adequate in nongonococcal infections. Less than 2 weeks of therapy combined with one joint aspiration was effective in closely monitored children with infectious arthritis.[70,71] Joint fluid cultures usually are no longer positive after 7 days of antibiotics.

Disseminated gonococcal infections often respond quickly to antibiotics.[72] Ceftriaxone 1 g/day for 7 to 10 days is the treatment of choice for adults. After culture and sensitivity results are available, and the organism is determined to be sensitive, therapy can be switched on the fourth day to oral amoxicillin or to doxycycline or tetracycline to complete the 7- to 10-day course. Clinical resolution of signs and symptoms usually is rapid.

Closed-needle aspiration is recommended for all infected joints except the hip.[72,73] Joint drainage can be repeated daily for 5 to 7 days until effusions no longer reaccumulate. Open drainage is required in hip infections because closed-needle aspiration is difficult and inadequate. During the initial phase of the infection, weight bearing, such as walking, on the joint should be avoided. Passive range-of-motion exercises should be initiated when the pain begins to subside to maintain joint mobility.[74] Approximately one-third of patients with bacterial arthritis have a poor joint outcome, such as severe functional deterioration. Poor joint outcomes are associated with older patients, those with preexisting joint disease, and patients with an infected joint containing synthetic material. Treatment guidelines are useful with septic arthritis of the hip.[75,76]

PHARMACOECONOMIC CONSIDERATIONS

Cost and outcome issues are important in osteomyelitis and infectious arthritis. If long-term sequelae develop, such as impaired joint motion or draining sinus tracts, or if amputation is required, patient quality of life can be significantly diminished. Cost and quality-of-life issues have clearly played a major role in evaluating other treatment alternatives (oral therapy or home antibiotic treatment) rather than requiring patients to remain hospitalized to receive 4 to 6 weeks of parenteral antibiotics. In addition, adverse events commonly occur with prolonged outpatient parenteral antibiotic therapy. One study in 45 children noted that 85.7% of patients receiving vancomycin had adverse drug events, and 42.9% of patients required the drug be discontinued.[77] This analysis also noted that cefazolin had the lowest rate of adverse drug events in this population.

EVALUATION OF THERAPEUTIC OUTCOMES

❾ Patients with bone and joint infections must be monitored closely. Table 127–5 summarizes a pharmaceutical care monitoring protocol. An assessment of a therapy's success or failure is based on the patient's clinical findings and laboratory values. The clinical signs of inflammation, such as swelling, tenderness, pain, redness, and fever, should resolve with appropriate therapy. Initially, the

TABLE 127–5 Monitoring Protocol

Parameter	Frequency	Notes
Culture and sensitivity	At initiation of treatment	
White blood cell count	One time per week until within normal range	
C-reactive protein or ESR	Weekly	May not decrease to normal range until several weeks of therapy
Clinical signs of inflammation (redness, pain, swelling, tenderness, fever)	Daily during initiation of therapy	
Compliance of outpatient therapy	Reinforce before starting oral therapy and with each healthcare visit	Compliance is critical if treatment is to be successful

ESR = erythrocyte sedimentation rate.

clinical signs are assessed daily until improvement, then periodically thereafter. Elevations in WBC count also should decline gradually. The ESR usually is determined weekly. Elevations in the C-reactive protein or ESR may not return to normal for several weeks of therapy. The WBC count usually is obtained once or twice per week until it returns to the normal range. If by the end of the 4- to 6-week antibiotic course the clinical findings of osteomyelitis are no longer present, and the C-reactive protein or ESR is within normal limits, the patient can be considered a clinical cure. Patients can relapse, however, after initially appearing to be cured. No relapse for 1 year generally is considered a complete cure.

If a patient fails to resolve the clinical signs and symptoms of inflammation after appropriate empirical antibiotics, surgical debridement may be needed. In addition, the patient might have a resistant infecting organism or an atypical infecting organism that can require a modification of the antibiotic therapy. It is especially important to note the infecting organism and its sensitivity pattern. Follow-up cultures at subsequent debridements can be useful to assess the antibiotic therapy.

Despite apparently adequate surgery and antibiotics, some patients can fail therapy and have recurrent relapses in their infection. This scenario is more common in the population with chronic osteomyelitis. These patients can require long-term oral antibiotics to keep the infection under control.

ABBREVIATIONS

ESR: Erythrocyte sedimentation rate

MRSA: Methicillin-resistant *Staphylococcus aureus*

WBC: White blood cell

REFERENCES

1. Waldvogel FA, Medoff G, Swartz MN. Osteomyelitis: A review of clinical features, therapeutic considerations and unusual aspects. N Engl J Med 1970;282:198–206, 260-266, 316–322.
2. Van den Bruel A, Bartholomeeusen S, Aertgeerts B, Truyers C, Buntinx F. Serious infections in children: An incidence study in family practice. BMC Family Practice 2006;7–23.
3. Uthman I, Bizri AR. Clinical features of septic arthritis at a tertiary teaching hospital in Lebanon. Clin Rheumatol 2003;22:359–360.
4. Deshpande SS, Taral N, Modi N, Singrakhia M. Changing epidemiology of neonatal septic arthritis. J Orthop Surg (Hong Kong) 2004;12:10–13.

5. Garcia-De La Torre I. Advances in the management of septic arthritis. Rheum Dis Clin North Am 2003;29:61–75.

6. Gutierrez K. Bone and joint infections in children. Pediatr Clin North Am 2005;52:779–794.

7. Berendt T, Byren I. Bone and joint infection. Clin Med 2004;4:510–518.

8. Lavy CBD, Thyoka M. For how long should antibiotics be given in acute paediatric septic arthritis? A prospective audit of 96 cases. Trop Doct 2007;37:195–197.

9. Smith JW, Chalupa P, Shabaz HM. Infectious arthritis: Clinical features, laboratory findings and treatment. Clin Microbial Infect 2006;12:309–314.

10. Shetty AK, Avinash K, Gedalia A. Management of septic arthritis. Indian J Pediatr 2004;71:819–824.

11. Levine M, Siegel LB. A swollen joint: Why all the fuss? Am J Ther 2003;10:219–224.

12. McCarthy JJ, Dormans JP, Kozin SH, Pizzutillo PD. Musculoskeletal infections in children: Basic treatment principles and recent advancements. Instr Course Lect 2005;54:515528.

13. Dessi A, Crisafulli M, Accossu S, et al. Osteo-articular infections in newborns: Diagnosis and treatment. J Chemother 2008;20:542–550.

14. Offiah AC. Acute osteomyelitis, septic arthritis and discitis: Differences between neonates and older children. Eur J Radiol 2006;60:221–232.

15. Livorsi DJ, Daver NG, Atmar RL, et al. Outcomes of treatment for hematogenous Staphylococcus aureus vertebral osteomyelitis in the MRSA era. J Infect 2008;57:128–131.

16. Goergens ED, McEvoy A, Watson M, Barrett IR. Acute osteomyelitis and septic arthritis in children. J Paediatr Child Health 2005;41:59–62.

17. Marti-Carvajal AJ, Agreda-Perez LH, Cortes-Jofre M. Antibiotics for treating osteomyelitis in people with sickle cell disease. Cochrane Database of Systematic Reviews 2009;2:cd007175.

18. Prasad KC, Prasad SC, Mouli N, Agarwal S. Osteomyelitis in the head and neck. Acta Oto-Laryngologica 2007;127:194–205.

19. Ducic Y. Osteomyelitis of the mandible. South Med J 2008;101:465.

20. Ansari MA, Shukla VK. Foot infections. Int J Low Extrem Wounds 2005;4:74–87.

21. Brem H, Sheehan P, Boulton AJ. Protocol for treatment of diabetic foot ulcers. Am J Surg 2004;187:1S–10S.

22. Brook I. Microbiology and management of joint and bone infections due to anaerobic bacteria. J Orthop Sci 2008;13:160–169.

23. Smith JW, Chalupa P, Hasan MS. Infectious arthritis: clinical features, laboratory findings and treatment. Clin Microbiol Infect 2006;12:309–314.

24. Rice PA. Gonococcal arthritis (disseminated gonococcal infection). Infect Dis Clin North Am 2005;19:853–861.

25. Kohli R, Hadley S. Fungal arthritis and osteomyelitis. Infect Dis Clin North Am 2005;19:831–851.

26. Delcourt A, Huglo D, Prangere T, et al. Comparison between Leukoscan (Sulesomab) and gallium-67 for the diagnosis of osteomyelitis in the diabetic foot. Diabetes Metab 2005;31:125–133.

27. Kan JH, Hilmes MA, Martus JE, et al. Value of MRI after recent diagnostic or surgical intervention in children with suspected osteomyelitis. Am J Roentgenol 2008;191:1595–1600.

28. Coviello V, Stevens MR. Contemporary concepts in the treatment of chronic osteomyelitis. Oral Maxillofacial Surg Clin N Am 2007;19:523–534.

29. Davis JS. Management of bone and joint infections due to Staphylococcus aureus. Internal Med J 2005;35:S79–S96.

30. Sancineto CF, Barla JD. Treatment of long bone osteomyelitis with a mechanically stable intramedullar antibiotic dispenser: Nineteen consecutive cases with a minimum of 12 months' follow-up. J Trauma 2008;65:1416–1420.

31. Wright BA, Roberts CS, Seligson CS, et al. Cost of antibiotic beads is justified: A study of open fracture wounds and chronic osteomyelitis. J Long Term Eff Med Implants 2007;17:181–185.

32. Pea F. Penetration of antibacterials into bone: What do we really need to know for optimal prophylaxis and treatment of bone and joint infections? Clin Pharmacokinet 2009;48:125–127.

33. Lamp KC, Friedrich LV, Mendez-Vigo L, et al. Clinical experience with daptomycin for the treatment of patients with ostmyelitis. Am J Med 2007;120:S13–S20.

34. Lazzarini L, Lipsky BA, Mader JT. Antibiotic treatment of osteomyelitis: What have we learned from 30 years of clinical trials? Int J Infect Dis 2005;9:127–138.

35. Weichert S, Sharland M, Clarke NMP, Faust SN. Acute haematogenous osteomyelitis in children: Is there any evidence for how long we should treat? Curr Opin Infect Dis 2008;21:258–262.

36. Roblot F, Besnier JM, Juhel L, et al. Optimal duration of antibiotic therapy in vertebral osteomyelitis. Semin Arthritis Rheum 2007;36:269–277.

37. Steer AC, Carapetis JR. Acute hematogenous osteomyelitis in children: Recognition and management. Paediatr Drugs 2004;6:333–346.

38. Darville T, Jacobs RF. Management of acute hematogenous osteomyelitis in children. Pediatr Infect Dis J 2004;23:255–257.

39. Karamanis EM, Matthaiou DK, Moraitis LI, Falagas ME. Fluoroquinolones versus β-lactam based regimens for the treatment of osteomyelitis: A meta-analysis of randomized controlled trials. Spine 2008;33:E297–E304.

40. Zaoutis T, Localio AR, Leckerman K, et al. Prolonged intravenous therapy versus early transition to oral antimicrobial therapy for acute osteomyelitis in children. Pediatrics 2009;123:636–642.

41. Bachur R, Pagon Z. Success of short-course parenteral antibiotic therapy for acute osteomyelitis of childhood. Clin Pediatr 2007;46:30–35.

42. Daver NG, Shelburne SA, Atmar RL, et al. Oral step-down therapy is comparable to intravenous therapy for Staphylococcus aureus osteomyelitis. J Infect 2007;54:539–544.

43. Shuford JA, Steckelberg JM. Role of oral antimicrobial therapy in the management of osteomyelitis. Curr Opin Infect Diseas 2003;16:515–519.

44. Grady RW. Systemic quinolone antibiotics in children: A review of the use and safety. Expert Opin Drug Saf 2005;4:623–630.

45. Senneville E, Poissy J, Legout L, et al. Safety of prolonged high-dose levofloxacin therapy for bone infections. J Chemother 2007;19:688–693.

46. Andriole VT. The quinolones: Past, present, and future. Clin Infect Dis 2005;41(Suppl 2):S113–S119.

47. Chen CJ, Chiu CH, Lin TY, et al. Experience with linezolid therapy in children with osteoarticular infections. Pediatr Infect Dis J 2007;26:985–988.

48. Joshi AY, Huskins WC, Henry NK, Boyce TG. Empiric antibiotic therapy for acute osteoarticular infections with suspected methicillin-resistant Staphylococcus aureus or Kingella. Pediatr Infect Dis J 2008;27:765–767.

49. Kaplan SL. Challenges in the evaluation and management of bone and joint infections and the role of new antibiotics for gram-positive infections. Adv Exp Med Biol 2009;634:111–120.

50. Floyed RL, Steele RW. Culture-negative osteomyelitis. Pediatr Infect Dis J 2003;22:731–735.

51. Afghani B, Kong V, Wu FL. What would pediatric infectious disease consultants recommend for management of culture-negative acute hematogenous osteomyelitis? J Pediatr Orthop 2007;27:805–809.

52. Jones ME, Karlowsky JA, Draghi DC, et al. Antibiotic susceptibility of bacteria most commonly isolated from bone related infections: The role of cephalosporins in antimicrobial therapy. Int J Antimicrob Agents 2004;23:240–246.

53. Brem H, Sheehan P, Boulton AJ. Protocol for treatment of diabetic foot ulcers. Am J Surg 2004;187:1S–10S.

54. Senneville E, Lombart A, Beltrand E, et al. Outcome of diabetic foot osteomyelitis treated nonsurgically. Diabetes Care 2008;31:637–642.

55. Berendt AR, Peters EJG, Bakker K, et al. Specific guidelines for treatment of diabetic foot osteomyelitis. Diabetes Metab Res Rev 2008;24(Suppl 1):S190–S191.

56. Berendt AR, Peters EJG, Bakker K, et al. Diabetic foot osteomyelitis: A progress report on diagnosis and a systematic review of treatment. Diabetes Metab Res Rev 2008;24(Suppl 1):S145–S161.

57. Aksoy DY, Gurlek A, Cetinkaya Y, et al. Change in the amputation profile in diabetic foot in a tertiary reference center: Efficacy of team working. Exp Clin Endocrinol Diabetes 2004;112:526–530.

58. Game FL, Jeffcoate WJ. Primarily non-surgical management of osteomyelitis of the foot in diabetes. Diabetologia 2008;51:962–967.

59. Tice AD, Hoaglund PA, Shoultz DA. Outcomes of osteomyelitis among patients treated with outpatient parenteral antimicrobial therapy. Am J Med 2003;114:723–728.

60. Pulcini C, Couadau T, Bernard E, et al. Adverse effects of parenteral antimicrobial therapy for chronic bone infections. Eur J Clin Microbiol Infect Dis 2008;27:1227–1232.

61. Tice AD, Hoaglund PA, Shoultz DA. Outcomes of osteomyelitis among patients treated with outpatient parenteral antimicrobial therapy. Am J Med 2003;114:723–728.

62. Ross JJ. Septic arthritis. Infect Dis Clin North Am 2005;19:799–817.

63. De Boeck H. Osteomyelitis and septic arthritis in children. Acta Orthop Belg 2005;71:505–515.

64. Balabaud L, Gaudias J, Boeri C, et al. Results of treatment of septic knee arthritis: A retrospective series of 40 cases. Knee Surg Sports Traumatol Arthrosc 2007;15:387–392.

65. Nunn TR, Cheung WY, Rollinson PD. A prospective study of pyogenic sepsis of the hip in childhood. J Bone Joint Surg Br 2007;89:100–106.

66. Mathews CJ, Kingsley G, Field M, et al. Management of septic arthritis: a systematic review. Postgrad Med J 2008;84:265–270.

67. Rao N, Hamilton CW. Efficacy and safety of linezolid for gram-positive orthopedic infections: A prospective case series. Diagn Microbiol Infect Dis 2007;59:173–179.

68. Falagas ME, Siempos II, Papagelopoulos PJ, Vardakas KZ. Linezolid for the treatment of adults with bone and joint infections. Int J Antimicrob Agents 2007;29:233–239.

69. Nade S. Septic arthritis. Best Pract Res Clin Rheumatol 2003;17:183–200.

70. Peltola H, Paakkonen M, Kallio P, et al. Prospective, randomized trial of 10 days versus 30 days of antimicrobial treatment, including a short-term course of parenteral therapy, for childhood septic arthritis. Clin Infect Dis 2009;48:1201–1210.

71. Bradley JS. What is the appropriate treatment course for bacterial arthritis in children? Clin Infect Dis 2009;48:1211–1212.

72. Bardin T. Gonococcal arthritis. Best Pract Res Clin Rheumatol 2003;17:201–208.

73. Mathews CJ, Coakley G. Septic arthritis: Current diagnostic and therapeutic algorithm. Curr Opin Rheumatol 2008;20:457–462.

74. Mathews CJ, Coakley G. Acute hot joint. Br J Hosp Med 2006;67:232–234.

75. Kocher MS, Mandiga R, Murphy JM, et al. A clinical practice guideline for treatment of septic arthritis in children: Efficacy in improving process of care and effect on outcome of septic arthritis of the hip. J Bone Joint Surg Am 2003;85A:994–999.

76. Ravindran V, Logan I, Bourke BE. Septic arthritis: clinical audits would help optimize the management. Clin Rheumatol 2008;27:1565–1567.

77. Faden D, Faden HS. The high rate of adverse drug events in children receiving prolonged outpatient parenteral antibiotic therapy for osteomyelitis. Pediatr Infect Dis J 2009;28:539–541.

128

Severe Sepsis and Septic Shock

S. LENA KANG-BIRKEN AND KARLA KILLGORE-SMITH

KEY CONCEPTS

❶ The spectrum of microorganisms associated with sepsis has changed from predominantly gram-negative bacteria in the late 1970s and 1980s to gram-positive bacteria as the major pathogens since the 1990s.

❷ Candidemia is a major cause of morbidity and mortality. *Candida albicans* remains the most common pathogen (45.6%); however, non–*C. albicans Candida* species collectively is more frequently isolated (54.4%).

❸ Sepsis presents a complex pathophysiology, characterized by the activation of multiple overlapping and interacting cascades leading to systemic inflammation, a procoagulant state, and decreased fibrinolysis.

❹ Mortality rates with sepsis are higher for patients with preexisting disease, intensive care unit care, and multiple organ failure.

❺ Prompt initiation of broad-spectrum, parenteral antibiotic therapy is required due to the high incidence of complications and mortality with sepsis.

❻ A significant volume of fluid leaks from the vasculature occurs with sepsis, and initial fluid resuscitation with large volumes of fluid is required. There is no clinical outcome difference between colloid and crystalloid fluid resuscitation.

❼ Norepinephrine is generally preferred over dopamine as the vasopressor to correct hypotension in septic shock. Low-dose dopamine does not maintain or improve renal function.

❽ Early goal-directed therapy of sepsis, consisting of hemodynamic monitoring with a central venous catheter, volume resuscitation, inotropic therapy, and red blood cell transfusions, demonstrated a significant clinical outcome benefit with a 16% absolute reduction in 28-day mortality.

❾ A blood glucose level less than 150 mg/dL is recommended for the majority of critically ill patients to reduce morbidity and mortality without the detrimental effects associated with hypoglycemia.

❿ IV hydrocortisone is recommended for adult patients with septic shock whose blood pressure is unresponsive to fluids and vasopressors.

Learning objectives, review questions, and other resources can be found at **www.pharmacotherapyonline.com**.

⓫ Drotrecogin (recombinant human activated protein C), which has both antiinflammatory and anticoagulant properties, was associated with a 6.1% reduction in 28-day all-cause mortality in comparison to placebo and should be used in patients at high risk of death.

Severe sepsis and septic shock continue to pose major healthcare problems. More than 750,000 cases of sepsis occur each year in the United States, and slightly more than half of the patients are admitted to the intensive care unit (ICU) with a mean length of stay of 15.7 days.[1] Despite aggressive medial care and advances, overall mortality from severe sepsis or septic shock ranges from 30% to 60%.[1] Septic shock is the 10th leading cause of death.[2] With the annual cost of approximately $16.7 billion, there is a vital need for clinicians to comprehend the pathophysiology and to appreciate the management options available for acutely ill patients with severe sepsis or septic shock.[1]

DEFINITIONS

In 1992, a joint committee of the American College of Chest Physicians and the Society of Critical Care Medicine standardized the terminology related to sepsis for several reasons: (a) widespread confusion with the use of these terms, (b) the need to provide a flexible classification scheme for patient identification, (c) identification of an earlier therapeutic intervention, and (d) standardization of research protocols.[3]

The criteria for the new terms provide specific physiologic variables that can be used to categorize a patient as having bacteremia, systemic inflammatory response syndrome (SIRS), sepsis, severe sepsis, septic shock, or multiple-organ dysfunction syndrome (MODS), suggesting an important continuum of progressive physiologic decline (Table 128–1). Introduction of the term *SIRS* reflects the knowledge that a physiologically similar systemic inflammatory response can be seen even in the absence of identifiable infection (Fig. 128–1).[4] More recently, the classification of sepsis was modified to include severe sepsis, septic shock, and refractory septic shock.[5] *Severe sepsis* refers to patients with an acute organ dysfunction, such as acute renal failure or respiratory failure. *Septic shock* refers to sepsis patients with arterial hypotension that is refractory to adequate fluid resuscitation, thus requiring vasopressor administration. It is important to note that progression from sepsis to MODS can occur in the absence of an intervening period of septic shock. Finally, *refractory septic shock* exists if dopamine IV infusion greater than 15 mcg/kg/min or norepinephrine greater than 0.25 mcg/kg/min is required to maintain a mean blood pressure greater than 60 mm Hg.[5]

TABLE 128-1 Definitions Related to Sepsis

Condition	Definition
Bacteremia (fungemia)	Presence of viable bacteria (fungi) in the bloodstream
Infection	Inflammatory response to invasion of normally sterile host tissue by the microorganisms
Systemic inflammatory response syndrome (SIRS)	Systemic inflammatory response to a variety of clinical insults, which can be infectious or noninfectious. The response is manifested by two or more of the following conditions: temperature >38°C or <36°C; HR >90 beats/min; RR >20 breaths/min or PaCO₂ <32 torr; WBC >12,000 cells/mm³, <4,000 cells/mm³, or >10% immature (band) forms; positive fluid balance (>20 mL/kg over 24 h); hyperglycemia; plasma C-reactive protein/procalcitonin >2 SD above normal value; arterial hypotension; CI >3.5 L/min; arterial hypoxemia; acute oliguria; creatinine increase >0.5 mg/dL; coagulation abnormalities; ileus, platelets <100,000 mcL; bilirubin >4 mg/dL; hyperlactatemia; decreased capillary refill
Sepsis	SIRS secondary to infection
Severe sepsis	Sepsis associated with one or more organ dysfunctions, hypoperfusion, or hypotension. Hypoperfusion and perfusion abnormalities may include, but are not limited to, lactic acidosis, oliguria, and acute alteration in mental status
Septic shock	Sepsis with persistent hypotension despite fluid resuscitation, along with the presence of perfusion abnormalities. Patients who are on inotropic or vasopressor agents may not be hypotensive at the time perfusion abnormalities are measured
Refractory septic shock	Persistent septic shock, requiring dopamine >15 mcg/kg/min or norephinephrine >0.25 mcg/kg/min to maintain mean arterial blood pressure
Multiple organ dysfunction syndrome (MODS)	Presence of altered organ function requiring intervention to maintain homeostasis

CI = cardiac index, HR = heart rate, RR = respiratory rate, SD = standard deviation, T = temperature, WBC = white blood cell (count).

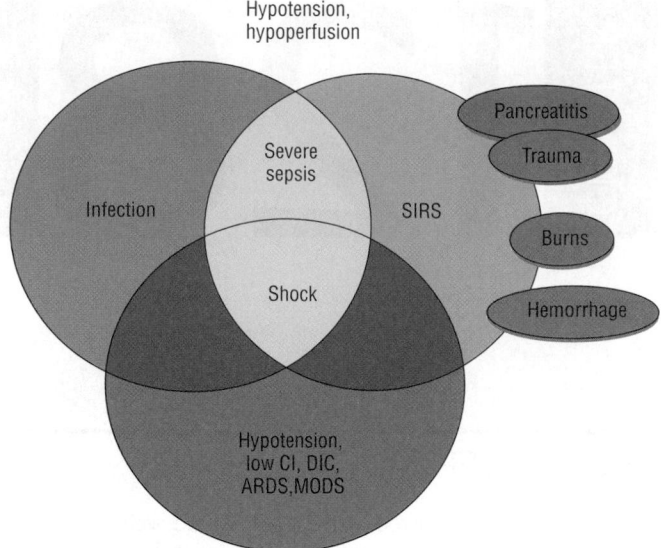

FIGURE 128-1. Relationship of infection, systemic inflammatory response syndrome (SIRS), sepsis, severe sepsis, and septic shock. ARDS, acute respiratory distress syndrome; CI, cardiac index; DIC, disseminated intravascular coagulation; MODS, multiple-organ dysfunction syndrome.

INFECTION SITES AND PATHOGENS

Predisposing factors of septic shock include age, male gender, nonwhite ethnic origin in North Americans, comorbid diseases, malignancy, immunodeficiency or immunocompromised state, chronic organ failure, alcohol dependence, and genetic factors.[1,6]

The leading primary sites of microbiologically documented infections that led to sepsis were the respiratory tract (21%–68%), intraabdominal space (14%–22%), and urinary tract (14%–18%).[5,7–9] Although almost any microorganism can be associated with sepsis and septic shock, the most common etiologic pathogens are gram-positive bacteria (40% of patients), followed by gram-negative bacteria (38%) and fungi (17%).[5] Certain viruses and rickettsiae can produce a similar syndrome.

GRAM-POSITIVE BACTERIAL SEPSIS

❶ Since 1987, gram-positive organisms have been the predominant pathogens in sepsis and septic shock, accounting for approximately 40% to 50% of all cases.[1] They are commonly caused by *Staphylococcus aureus*, *Streptococcus pneumoniae*, coagulase-negative staphylococci, and *Enterococcus* species. *Streptococcus pyogenes* and viridans streptococci are less commonly involved.[5,8–11]

S. pneumoniae sepsis is associated with an overall mortality rate of >25%. Factors related to a higher mortality include shock, respiratory insufficiency, preexisting renal failure, and the presence of a rapidly fatal underlying disease. *Staphylococcus epidermidis* is most often related to infected intravascular devices, such as artificial heart valves and stents and the use of IV and intraarterial catheters. The rates of nosocomial enterococcal bacteremia and associated sepsis are also increasing. Enterococci are isolated most commonly in blood cultures following a prolonged hospitalization and treatment with broad-spectrum cephalosporins.

GRAM-NEGATIVE BACTERIAL SEPSIS

A greater proportion of patients with gram-negative bacteremia develop clinical sepsis, and gram-negative bacteria are also more likely to produce septic shock in comparison to gram-positive organisms, 50% versus 25%, respectively.[8,11,12] Gram-negative sepsis also results in a higher mortality rate compared with sepsis from any other group of organisms.[12] The major factor associated with the outcome of gram-negative sepsis appears to be the severity of any underlying condition. Patients with rapidly fatal conditions, such as acute leukemia, aplastic anemia, and burn injury to >70% of the body's surface, have a significantly worse prognosis than do those patients with nonfatal underlying conditions, such as diabetes mellitus and chronic renal insufficiency.[1,2,12]

Escherichia coli and *Pseudomonas aeruginosa* are the most commonly isolated gram-negative microorganisms in sepsis.[5,7–12] Other common gram-negative pathogens are *Klebsiella* species, *Serratia* species, *Enterobacter* species, and *Proteus* species. *P. aeruginosa*, although not considered predominant in human endogenous flora, is found widely in the environment and is the most frequent cause of sepsis fatality. In a European study evaluating sepsis occurring in acutely ill patients, *P. aeruginosa* was isolated from 14% of all cultures.[5]

ANAEROBIC AND MISCELLANEOUS BACTERIAL SEPSIS

Anaerobic bacteria are usually considered low-risk organisms for the development of sepsis. If present, anaerobes are often found together with other pathogenic bacteria that are commonly found in sepsis. Polymicrobial infections accounted for 5% to 39% of sepsis.[1,5,7–9,12] Mortality rates associated with polymicrobial infections are similar to sepsis caused by a single organism. Although some clinicians believe the particular combination of organisms present in polymicrobial sepsis can provide clues to the source of infection, no clear source for the infection can be identified in up to 25% of cases. Other less common pathogens are meningococcus, gonococcus, rickettsia, chlamydia, and spirochetes.

FUNGAL SEPSIS

❷ Candidemia is among the most common etiologic agents of bloodstream infections. Although *C. albicans* was the most commonly isolated fungus from blood cultures (45.6%), collectively, non–*C. albicans Candida* species were more frequently isolated (54.4%).[13] Non-*Candida* species include *C. glabrata* (26%), *C. parapsilosis* (15.7%), *C. tropicalis* (8.1%), and *C. krusei* (2.5%). Other fungi identified as causes of sepsis are Cryptococcus, Coccidioides, Fusarium, and Aspergillus. Risk factors for fungal infection include abdominal surgery, poorly controlled diabetes mellitus, prolonged granulocytopenia, broad-spectrum antibiotic treatment, corticosteroid treatment, prolonged hospitalization, central venous catheter, total parenteral nutrition, hematologic malignancy, and chronic, indwelling bladder (Foley) catheter.

In a prospective analysis of the Antifungal Therapy Alliance database, the overall crude 12-week mortality rate for sepsis due to candidemia was 35.2%.[13] The highest mortality rate of 52.9% was observed in patients with *C. krusei* candidemia; *C. parapsilosis* candidemia was associated with the lowest 12-week mortality rate (23.7%). Hematologic diseases, neutropenia, and a higher number of positive blood cultures were associated with poor outcome irrespective of the patient's gender, age, or days of antifungal drug treatment.

PATHOPHYSIOLOGY

Sepsis is the result of complex interactions among the invading pathogen, the host immune system, and the inflammatory responses. Proinflammatory mediators that contribute to eradication of invading microorganisms are produced, and antiinflammatory mediators control this response. The inflammatory response leads to damage to host tissue, and the antiinflammatory response causes leukocytes to activate. Once the balance to control the local inflammatory process to eradicate the invading pathogens is lost, systemic inflammatory response occurs, converting the infection to sepsis, severe sepsis, or septic shock.[14]

CELLULAR COMPONENTS FOR INITIATING THE INFLAMMATORY PROCESS

The pathophysiologic focus of gram-negative sepsis has been on the lipopolysaccharide component of the gram-negative bacterial cell wall. Commonly referred to as endotoxin, this substance is unique to the outer membrane of the gram-negative cell wall and is generally released with bacterial lysis. Lipid A, the innermost region of the lipopolysaccharide, is highly immunoreactive and is considered responsible for most of the toxic effects observed with gram-negative sepsis. Although lipid A can affect tissues directly, its predominant effect is to activate macrophages and trigger inflammatory cascades critical in the progression to sepsis and septic shock.[14] Endotoxin forms a complex with an endogenous protein called a lipopolysaccharide-binding protein, which then engages the CD14 receptor on the surface of a macrophage. Subsequently, cytokine mediators are activated and released by the macrophage.

In gram-positive sepsis, the exotoxin peptidoglycan appears to exhibit proinflammatory activity. Peptidoglycan comprises up to 40% of a gram-positive cell mass and is exposed on the cell wall surface. Although it competes with lipid A for similar binding sites on CD14, the potency of peptidoglycan is less than that of endotoxin.[14] However, an important feature of gram-positive bacteria such as *S. aureus* and *S. pyogenes* is the production of potent exotoxins, some of which have been associated with septic shock.

PRO- AND ANTIINFLAMMATORY MEDIATORS

Sepsis involves activation of inflammatory pathways, and a complex interaction between proinflammatory and antiinflammatory mediators plays a major role in the pathogenesis of sepsis. The key proinflammatory mediators are tumor necrosis factor-α (TNF-α), interleukin-1 (IL-1), and interleukin-6 (IL-6), which are released by activated macrophages.[14–16] Other mediators that may be important for the pathogenesis of sepsis are interleukin-8 (IL-8), platelet-activating factor (PAF), leukotrienes, and thromboxane A$_2$.

The TNF-α is considered the primary mediator of sepsis.[15,16] Although the TNF-α levels in plasma can be increased in patients with a variety of diseases and in many healthy people, there is a correlation of plasma TNF-α levels with the severity of sepsis. The plasma TNF-α level is highly elevated early in the inflammatory response in most patients with sepsis.[17] In meningococcemia, increased morbidity and mortality are associated with high plasma concentrations of TNF-α. The TNF-α release leads to activation of other cytokines (IL-1 and IL-6) associated with cellular damage. In addition, TNF-α stimulates the release of cyclooxygenase-derived arachidonic acid metabolites (thromboxane A$_2$ and prostaglandins) that contribute to vascular endothelial damage.

Although IL-1 serum levels have been inconsistently associated with sepsis, IL-6 is a more consistent predictor of sepsis, as it remains elevated for a longer period of time than TNF-α.[15] The highest circulating levels of IL-6 in addition to IL-8 have been associated with severity and mortality.[15,18,19]

The significant antiinflammatory mediators include interleukin-1 receptor antagonist (IL-1RA), interleukin-4 (IL-4), and interleukin-10 (IL-10).[14–16] These antiinflammatory cytokines inhibit the production of the proinflammatory cytokines and downregulate some inflammatory cells. Levels of IL-10 and IL-1RA are higher in septic shock than in sepsis, and higher levels are found among nonsurviving patients than in survivors.[15]

The net effect of a given mediator can vary depending on the state of activation of the target cell, the presence of other mediators near the target cell, and the ability of the target cell to release mediators that can augment or inhibit the primary mediator. As Fig. 128–2 illustrates, when there is a systemic spillover of excessive proinflammatory mediators, the patient presents with SIRS and possibly MODS. Shortly after this initial phase, counterregulatory pathways become activated, and there is a systemic spillover of excessive antiinflammatory mediators, representing a compensatory antiinflammatory response syndrome (CARS). The balance between pro- and antiinflammatory mechanisms determines the degree of inflammation, ranging from local antibacterial activity to systemic tissue toxicity or organ failure.[14]

CASCADE OF SEPSIS

❸ The cascade leading to development of sepsis is complex and multifactorial, involving various mediators and cell lines.[14–16] Endothelial cells produce a variety of cytokines that mediate a primary mechanism of injury in sepsis. When injured, endothelial cells allow circulating cells such as granulocytes and plasma constituents to enter inflamed tissues, which can result in organ damage.

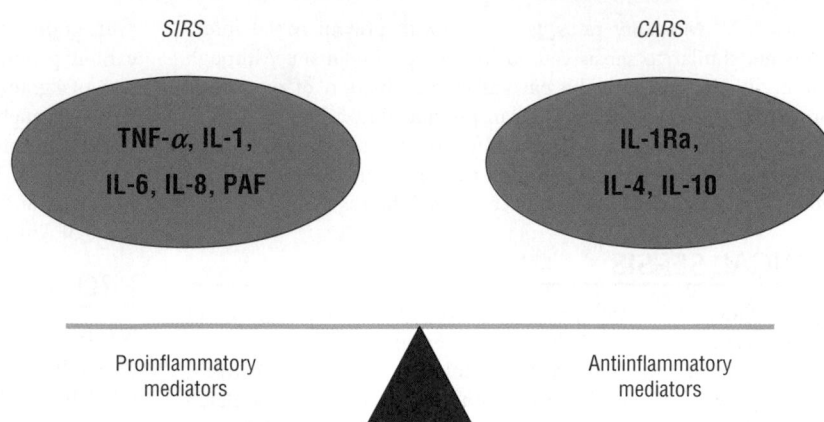

FIGURE 128-2. The balance between pro- and antiinflammatory mediators. CARS, compensatory antiinflammatory response syndrome; IL, interleukin; IL-1RA, interleukin-1 receptor antagonist; SIRS, systemic inflammatory response syndrome; TNF, tumor necrosis factor.

The microcirculation is affected by sepsis-induced inflammation.[20] The arterioles become less responsive to either vasoconstrictors or vasodilators. The capillaries are less perfused, and there is neutrophil infiltration and protein leakage into the venules. Pulmonary dysfunction can result from the destructive mechanisms of neutrophils that are attracted to lung tissue through the action of mainly IL-8.

Activation of complement in sepsis leads to pathophysiologic consequences, including generation of anaphylactic toxins and other substances that augment or exaggerate the inflammatory response. Stimulation of leukocyte chemotaxis, phagocytosis with lysosomal enzyme release, increased aggregation and adhesion of platelets and neutrophils, and the production of toxic superoxide radicals are attributed, in part, to complement activation. Among these responses are the release of histamine from mast cells and the resultant increase in capillary permeability and the "third-spacing" of fluid in interstitial spaces.

The inflammatory process in sepsis is also directly linked to the coagulation system. Proinflammatory mechanisms that promote sepsis are also procoagulant and antifibrinolytic, whereas fibrinolytic mechanisms can be antiinflammatory.[21] A key endogenous substance involved in inflammation of sepsis is activated protein C, which enhances fibrinolysis and inhibits inflammation. Levels of protein C are reduced in patients with sepsis.[22]

COMPLICATIONS

The majority of patients with severe sepsis have dysfunction of two organs, and the three most frequent organ dysfunctions are respiratory, circulatory, and renal.[9] Shock is the most ominous complication associated with sepsis, and mortality occurs in approximately half of the patients with septic shock. Severe hypotension appears to be caused, in part, by the release of vasoactive peptides, such as bradykinin and serotonin, and by endothelial cell damage leading to the extravasation of fluids into interstitial spaces. Septic shock is associated with several complications, including disseminated intravascular coagulation, acute respiratory distress syndrome, and multiple organ failure.

DISSEMINATED INTRAVASCULAR COAGULATION

Disseminated intravascular coagulation (DIC) is the inappropriate activation of the clotting cascade that causes formation of microthrombi, resulting in consumption of coagulation factors, organ dysfunction, and bleeding. Sepsis remains the most common cause of DIC. The incidence of DIC increases as the severity of sepsis increases. In sepsis alone, the incidence was 16% in comparison to 38% in septic shock.[23] DIC occurs in up to 50% of patients with

gram-negative sepsis, but it is also common in patients with gram-positive sepsis.

DIC begins with the activation and production of the proinflammatory cytokines, such as TNF, IL-1, and IL-6, which appear to be the principal mediators, along with endotoxin, of endothelial injury, activation of the coagulation cascade, and inhibition of fibrinolysis. The combination of excessive fibrin formation, inhibited fibrin removal from a depressed fibrinolytic system, and endothelial injury results in microvascular thrombosis and DIC.[23]

Complications of DIC vary and depend on the target organ affected and the severity of the coagulopathy. DIC can produce acute renal failure, hemorrhagic necrosis of the GI mucosa, liver failure, acute pancreatitis, acute respiratory distress syndrome, and pulmonary failure. Furthermore, as the procoagulant state appears to be the key in the pathogenesis of MODS, coagulation dysfunction and MODS often coexist in sepsis.

ACUTE RESPIRATORY DISTRESS SYNDROME

Pulmonary dysfunction usually precedes dysfunction in other organs, and it can even initiate the development of SIRS with resultant MODS. Activated neutrophils and platelets adhere to the pulmonary capillary endothelium, initiating multiple inflammatory cascades with a release of a variety of toxic substances. There is diffuse pulmonary endothelial cell injury, increased capillary permeability, and alveolar epithelial cell injury.[24] Consequently, interstitial pulmonary edema occurs that gradually progresses to alveolar flooding and collapse. The end result is loss of functional alveolar volume, impaired pulmonary compliance, and profound hypoxemia.

Abnormalities of pathways of fibrin turnover after the pathogenesis of acute inflammation responses and fibrotic repair.[25] Coagulation is locally upregulated in the injured lung, whereas fibrinolytic activity is depressed. These abnormalities occur concurrently and favor alveolar fibrin deposition. Anticoagulant interventions that block the extrinsic coagulation pathway can protect against the development of pulmonary fibrin deposition as well as lung dysfunction and acute inflammation.[26] Overall, fibrin deposition in the injured lung and abnormalities of coagulation and fibrinolysis are integral to the pathogenesis of acute respiratory distress syndrome (ARDS).

HEMODYNAMIC EFFECTS

The hallmark of the hemodynamic effect of sepsis is the hyperdynamic state characterized by high cardiac output and an abnormally low systemic vascular resistance (SVR).[27] TNF-α and endotoxin directly depress cardiovascular function. Endotoxin depresses left ventricular function independent of changes in left ventricular volume or vascular resistance.

Persistent hypotension raises concern for the balance of oxygen delivery (DO_2) to the tissues and oxygen consumption (VO_2) by the tissues.[24,27] Sepsis results in a distributive shock characterized by inappropriately increased blood flow to particular tissues at the expense of other tissues, which is independent of specific tissue oxygen needs. This perfusion defect is accentuated by an increased precapillary atrioventricular shunt. If perfusion decreases, oxygen extraction increases, and the arteriovenous oxygen gradient widens. Cellular DO_2 is decreased, but VO_2 remains unaffected. When increased oxygen demand occurs without increased blood flow, the increased VO_2 is compensated by increased oxygen extraction. If perfusion decreases sufficiently in the face of high metabolic demands, then the reserve DO_2 can be exceeded, and tissue ischemia results. Significant tissue ischemia leads to organ dysfunction and failure. Therefore, systemic DO_2 relative to VO_2 should be optimized by increasing oxygen delivery or decreasing oxygen consumption in a hypermetabolic patient.

ACUTE RENAL FAILURE

Early acute kidney injury occurs in 42% to 64% of adult patients with sepsis and septic shock.[28,29] Without normal urine output, fluid overload in extravascular space including the lungs develops, leading to impairment of pulmonary gas exchange and severe hypoxemia. Consequently, compromised oxygen delivery exacerbates peripheral ischemia and organ damage. Adequate renal perfusion and a trial of loop diuretics should be initiated promptly in oliguric or anuric patients with MODS. In addition, renal replacement therapy such as continuous hemofiltration or intermittent hemodialysis should be used to facilitate volume and electrolytes.[30]

CLINICAL PRESENTATION

Table 128–2 lists some of the common clinical features of sepsis, although several of these findings are not limited to infectious processes. The initial clinical presentation can be referred to as signs and symptoms of early sepsis, defined as the first 6 hours. They are typically fever, chills, and change in mental status. Hypothermia can occur with a systemic infection, and this is often associated with a poor prognosis.[3,6] In patients with sepsis caused by gram-negative bacilli, hyperventilation can occur even before fever and chills, and it can lead to respiratory alkalosis as the earliest metabolic change.

Progression of uncontrolled sepsis leads to clinical evidence of organ system dysfunction as represented by the signs and symptoms attributed to late sepsis. With the exception of rapidly progressing cases as in meningococcemia, *P. aeruginosa,* or *Aeromonas* infection, the onset of shock is slow and usually follows a period of

TABLE 128-2	Signs and Symptoms Associated with Sepsis
Early Sepsis	**Late Sepsis**
Fever or hypothermia	Lactic acidosis
Rigors, chills	Oliguria
Tachycardia	Leukopenia
Tachypnea	DIC
Nausea, vomiting	Myocardial depression
Hyperglycemia	Pulmonary edema
Myalgias	Hypotension (shock)
Lethargy, malaise	Hypoglycemia
Proteinuria	Azotemia
Hypoxia	Thrombocytopenia
Leukocytosis	ARDS
Hyperbilirubinemia	GI hemorrhage
	Coma

ARDS = acute respiratory distress syndrome; DIC = disseminated intravascular coagulation; GI = gastrointestinal.

several hours of hemodynamic instability. Oliguria often follows hypotension. Increased glycolysis with impaired clearance of the resulting lactate by the liver and kidneys and tissue hypoxia because of hypoperfusion result in elevated lactate levels, contributing to metabolic acidosis. Altered glucose metabolism, including impaired gluconeogenesis and excessive insulin release, is evidenced by either hyperglycemia or hypoglycemia.

PROGNOSIS

❹ As the patient progresses from SIRS to sepsis to severe sepsis to septic shock, mortality increases in a stepwise fashion. Mortality rates are higher for patients with advanced age; preexisting disease, including chronic obstructive pulmonary disease, neoplasm, and human immunodeficiency virus (HIV) disease; ICU care; more failed organs; positive blood cultures; and *Pseudomonas* species infection.[5,9] In one analysis of cases, mortality increased with age from 10% in children to 38.4% in those 85 years or older.[1] ICU admission was required in 51.1% of patients with severe sepsis; of those patients, mortality was reported in 34.1%.[1] Mortality from severe sepsis and MODS is most closely related to the number of dysfunctioning organs. As the number of failing organs increased from two to five, mortality increased from 54% to 100% (Fig. 128–3).[24] Duration of organ dysfunction can also affect the overall mortality rate.

An elevated lactate concentration of >4 mmol/L in the presence of SIRS significantly increases ICU admission rates, and persistent

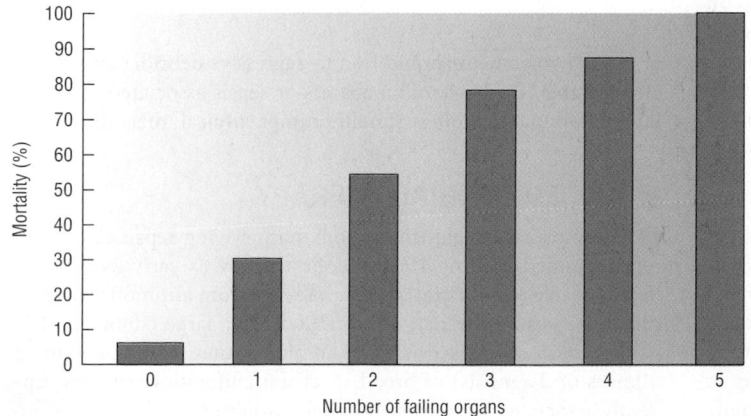

FIGURE 128-3. Mortality related to the number of failing organs.

elevations in lactate for more than 24 hours are associated with a mortality rate as high as 89%.[31] Inversely, patients with higher lactate clearance after 6 hours of emergency department intervention have improved outcome compared with those with lower lactate clearance. There was an ~11% decrease in the likelihood of mortality for each 10% increase in lactate clearance.[31]

TREATMENT

In 2008, a "surviving sepsis" campaign guideline for management of severe sepsis and septic shock was published as an international effort to increase awareness and improve outcome in severe sepsis.[32] The primary goals of therapy for patients with sepsis are (a) timely diagnosis and identification of the pathogen, (b) rapid elimination of the source of infection medically and/or surgically, (c) early initiation of aggressive antimicrobial therapy, (d) interruption of pathogenic sequence leading to septic shock, and (e) avoidance of organ failure. Supportive care such as stress ulcer prophylaxis and nutritional support is important to prevent complications during the stay in the ICU. Table 128–3 describes the summary of the surviving sepsis campaign treatment recommendations.

■ IDENTIFICATION OF THE PATHOGEN

The presence of clinical features suggesting sepsis should prompt further evaluation of the patient. In addition to obtaining a careful history of any underlying conditions and recent travel, injury, animal exposure, infection, or use of antibiotics, a complete physical examination should be performed to determine the source of the infection.

A collection of specimens should be sent for culture prior to initiating any antimicrobial therapy. Generally, at least two sets of blood samples from a peripheral vein and through a vascular access device should be obtained for aerobic and anaerobic culture. In critically ill septic patients, two or three sets of blood cultures should be collected without temporal separation between the sets.[33] With suspected catheter-related infection, a pair of blood cultures obtained through the catheter hub and a peripheral site should be obtained simultaneously.[33] In severe community-acquired pneumonia, blood cultures and respiratory secretions must be obtained. Urinary antigen detection of *Legionella* serogroup 1 is recommended during outbreaks. To document a soft tissue infection, a Gram stain and bacterial culture of any obvious wound exudates should be performed. A needle aspiration of a closed infection such as cellulitis or abscess may be needed for stain and bacterial culture. In abdominal infections, fluid collections identified by imaging studies should be aspirated for Gram stains and aerobic and anaerobic cultures.[33] A lumbar puncture is indicated in case of mental alteration, severe headache, or a seizure, assuming there are no focal cranial lesions identified by computed tomography scan. Further tests can be indicated to assess any systemic organ dysfunction caused by severe sepsis. The laboratory tests should include hemoglobin, white blood cell count with differential, platelet count, complete chemistry profile, coagulation parameters, serum lactate, procalcitonin, and arterial blood gases.

■ ELIMINATION OF THE SOURCE OF INFECTION

After the source of infection is identified, prompt efforts to eradicate that source should be initiated.[34] With an infected intravascular catheter, the catheter should be removed and cultured. Urinary tract catheters should be removed if association with sepsis is suspected. Suspicion of soft tissue (cellulitis or wound infection)

TABLE 128-3 Evidence-based Treatment Recommendations for Sepsis and Septic Shock

Recommendations	Recommendation Grades[a]
Initial resuscitation (first 6 hours)	
Early goal-directed goals, including CVP 8–12 mm Hg, MAP ≥65 mm Hg, central venous oxygen saturation ≥70%	1C
Antibiotic therapy	
IV broad-spectrum antibiotic within 1 hour of diagnosis of septic shock and severe sepsis against likely bacterial/fungal pathogens	1B
Reassess antibiotic therapy daily with microbiology and clinical data to narrow coverage	1C
Fluid therapy	
No clinical outcome difference between colloids and crystalloids	1B
Fluid challenges of 1000 mL of crystalloids or 300–500 mL of colloids over 30 minutes	1D
Vasopressors	
Norepinephrine and dopamine are the initial choices	1C
Maintain MAP ≥65 mm Hg	1C
Inotropic therapy	
Use dobutamine when cardiac output remains low despite fluid resuscitation and combined inotropic/vasopressor therapy	1C
Glucose control	
Use IV insulin to keep blood glucose ≤150 mg/dL	2C
Steroids	
IV hydrocortisone for septic shock when hypotension remains poorly responsive to adequate fluid resuscitation and vasopressors	2C
Hydrocortisone dose should be <300 mg/day	1A
Recombinant human activated protein C (drotrecogin)	
Consider in sepsis-induced organ dysfunction with high risk of death (typically APACHE II ≥25 or multiple organ failure) in the absence of contraindications	2B
Deep vein thrombosis prophylaxis	
Use either low-molecular-weight heparin or low-dose unfractionated heparin in preventing deep vein thrombosis	1A
Stress ulcer prophylaxis	
H2 receptor blocker or proton pump inhibitor is effective	1A, 1B

[a]Grades of Recommendation, Assessment, Development, and Evaluation (GRADE) system: a structured system for rating quality of evidence and grading strength of recommendation in clinical practice. Quality of evidence: high (grade A), moderate (grade B), low (grade C), or very low (grade D). Strength of recommendation: strong (grade 1) or weak (grade 2).
CVP = central venous pressure, MAP = mean arterial pressure.
Adapted from Dellinger RP, Levy MM, Carlet JM, et al. Surviving sepsis campaign: International guidelines for management of severe sepsis and septic shock: 2008. Crit Care Med 2008;36: 296–327.

or bone involvement should lead to aggressive debridement of the affected area. Evidence of an abscess or sepsis associated with any intraabdominal pathology should prompt surgical intervention.

■ ANTIMICROBIAL THERAPY

❺ The most recent guidelines from the Surviving Sepsis Campaign recommended starting IV antibiotic therapy as early as possible because early administration of broad-spectrum antibiotics is critical in decreasing the risk of mortality.[32] In a large cohort of ICU patients with severe sepsis, early administration (within 1 hour vs 6 hours of diagnosis) of broad-spectrum antibiotics was independently associated with lower hospital mortality.[35]

In a study evaluating 904 patients with microbiologically confirmed severe sepsis or septic shock, appropriate initial antimicrobial therapy was an important determinant of survival.[7] The 28-day mortality was 24% in patients who received appropriate initial antimicrobial treatment versus 39% in those who received inappropriate initial treatment. Furthermore, in patients who had septic shock, delays in the initiation of effective antimicrobial therapy after the onset of hypotension were significant predictors of mortality.[36,37] Therefore, early administration of appropriate antimicrobial therapy is critical in the treatment of severe sepsis.

Selection of Antimicrobial Agents

The selection of an empiric regimen should be based on the suspected site of infection, the most likely pathogens, acquisition of the organism from the community or hospital, the patient's immune status, and the antibiotic susceptibility and resistance profile for the institution. All patients should be treated initially with parenteral antibiotics for optimal drug concentrations within the first hour of recognition of severe sepsis after appropriate cultures have been taken.[32] Empiric therapy for an immunocompromised patient should be broad enough to cover likely pathogens and penetrate adequately into the presumed infection site. Once the pathogen and its susceptibility pattern are known, the antimicrobial regimen should be modified accordingly.

Table 128–4 lists antimicrobial regimens that can be used empirically based on the possible source of infection. In the nonneutropenic patient with a urinary tract infection, ceftriaxone and fluoroquinolones are generally recommended. When there is increased risk of *P. aeruginosa* in sepsis or hospital-acquired infections, an antipseudomonal antibiotic, such as ceftazidime, is recommended.[38]

S. pneumoniae is the most common cause of community-acquired pneumonia, and it accounts for ~60% of all deaths. The rising incidence of penicillin-resistant *S. pneumoniae* requires empiric use of newer "respiratory" fluoroquinolones. Newer fluoroquinolones, such as levofloxacin and moxifloxacin, can be used as monotherapy, as they offer excellent coverage against penicillin-resistant pneumococci and aerobic gram-negative bacteria, as well as atypical pathogens, including *Legionella pneumophila, Mycoplasma pneumoniae,* and *Chlamydia pneumoniae.*[39] Clarithromycin and azithromycin are effective against atypical pathogens and better tolerated than erythromycin.

In nosocomial pneumonia, enteric gram-negative bacteria such as *Enterobacter* and *Klebsiella* species and *P. aeruginosa* are the major pathogens, in addition to *S. aureus.* If *P. aeruginosa* infection is suspected, β-lactam antipseudomonal agents (ceftazidime or cefepime), antipseudomonal fluoroquinolone (ciprofloxacin or levofloxacin), or an aminoglycoside should be included in the regimen[40] When *S. aureus* is likely to be methicillin-resistant, linezolid may be preferred to vancomycin because of the poor penetration of vancomycin into the lungs, as well as the worldwide emergence of glycopeptide intermediately resistant *S. aureus.*[41,42]

Secondary peritonitis as a consequence of perforation of the GI tract is usually polymicrobial involving enteric aerobes and anaerobes, and as many as five organisms are isolated per patient. In general, if resistance for a given antibiotic is greater than 10% to 20% for a common intraabdominal pathogen in the community, that agent should be avoided. Because of widespread resistance of *Escherichia coli* to ampicillin/sulbactam, it is no longer recommended.[43] Emerging fluoroquinolone-resistant *E. coli,* as well as areas of high prevalence of extended-spectrum β-lactamase-producing strains of *Klebsiella* species and *E coli,* should be considered in choosing empiric therapy.[43] *Bacteroides fragilis,* the major pathogen, has shown uniform susceptibility to metronidazole, carbapenems, and β-lactam/β-lactamase inhibitors.[44] Although moxifloxacin demonstrates activity against *B. fragilis,* it should be avoided in patients who recently received quinolone therapy.

In addition to surgical intervention, broad-spectrum antibiotics, such as β-lactamase inhibitor combination agent (piperacillin/tazobactam), are appropriate in treating intraabdominal infections.[45] Carbapenems such as imipenem, meropenem, and doripenem are indicated in the treatment of resistant pathogens, including Enterobacteriaceae and *P. aeruginosa,* in critically ill patients.[45,46]

Skin and soft tissue infections (SSTIs) range from cellulitis to rapidly progressive necrotizing fasciitis, which may be associated with septic shock and toxic shock syndrome. Staphylococci and streptococci long have been the leading causes of SSTIs, but severe SSTIs can be caused also by indigenous aerobes and anaerobes such as *Clostridium* species.[47] Early initiation of appropriate empiric broad-spectrum antimicrobial therapy is essential and should include coverage against methicillin-resistant *S. aureus* (MRSA) due to the high prevalence of community-associated MRSA strains.[47,48] Vancomycin, daptomycin, and linezolid have comparable clinical efficacy and safety data for complicated skin and skin-structure infections caused by MRSA.[49,50]

The antimicrobial regimen should be reassessed after 48 to 72 hours based on the microbiological and clinical data. Once the culture results and antimicrobial susceptibility data return, therapy should be directed toward the isolated pathogen as part of good antibiotic stewardship to prevent drug toxicities and the development of nosocomial superinfections with *Candida* species, *Clostridium difficile,* or vancomycin-resistant enterococcus.[51] Furthermore, improved patient care outcomes have been demonstrated with such deescalation of antibiotic therapy.[52]

Pathophysiologic changes have been reported in sepsis that can affect drug distribution, and adjusted dosing regimens are required

TABLE 128-4 Empiric Antimicrobial Regimens in Sepsis

Infection (Site or Type)	Antimicrobial Regimen	
	Community-acquired	Hospital-acquired
Urinary tract	ceftriaxone or ciprofloxacin/levofloxacin	ciprofloxacin/levofloxacin or ceftriaxone or ceftazidime
Respiratory tract	levofloxacin[a]/moxifloxacin or ceftriaxone + clarithromycin/azithromycin	piperacillin/tazobactam or ceftazidime or cefepime + levofloxacin/ciprofloxacin or aminoglycoside
Intraabdominal	piperacillin/tazobactam or ciprofloxacin + metronidazole	piperacillin/tazobactam or carbapenem[b]
Skin/soft tissue	vancomycin or linezolid or daptomycin	vancomycin + ampicillin/sulbactam or piperacillin/tazobactam
Catheter-related		vancomycin
Unknown		piperacillin/tazobactam or ceftazidime/cefepime or imipenem/meropenem } +/- vancomycin not gentamicin.

[a]750 mg orally once daily.
[b]Imipenem, meropenem, doripenem.

in critically ill patients with sepsis.[53] Initially high creatinine clearance can be seen in patients with normal serum creatinine because of increased renal preload. Volume of distribution can increase because of fluid accumulation from leaky capillaries and/or altered protein binding. Consequently, some antimicrobial agents, including aminoglycosides, β-lactams, carbapenems, and vancomycin, can result in lower peak serum concentrations with usual doses. However, as sepsis progresses, organ perfusion decreases because of significant myocardial depression and leads to multiple organ dysfunction. Consequently, clearance of antimicrobial agents is decreased, prolonging the elimination half-life and accumulation of metabolites. Hence, in addition to selecting the most appropriate antimicrobial agents, a clinician must ensure effective antibiotic usage, such as proper dosing, interval of administration, optimal duration of treatment, monitoring of drug levels when appropriate, and avoidance of unwanted drug interactions. The lack of adherence to these requirements can lead to suboptimal or excessive tissue concentrations that can promote antibiotic resistance, toxicity, and inadequate efficacy despite appropriate antibiotic selection.

Monotherapy with a broad-spectrum β-lactam antibiotic is as efficacious as and less toxic than a combination of β-lactam and an aminoglycoside as empirical therapy for critically ill patients with severe sepsis or septic shock.[54,55] There is no evidence that combination therapy is more effective than monotherapy. However, some experts prefer combination therapy for patients with *Pseudomonas* infections and for neutropenic patients with severe sepsis or septic shock.[32,56]

CLINICAL CONTROVERSIES

The rationale of antibiotic combination therapy for severe infections includes broadening the antibacterial spectrum, exertion of additive or synergistic effects, and possible reduction of emergence of resistant bacteria or superinfection. Combinations such as a β-lactam and an aminoglycoside have been evaluated[54,55] However, superiority of the combination therapy over single-agent therapy was not demonstrated with the exception of those patients with rapidly declining diseases such severe sepsis. With the introduction of highly bactericidal, broad-spectrum antibiotics such as piperacillin/tazobactam, ceftazidime, cefepime and the carbapenems, more studies have compared the efficacy and toxicities of monotherapy against a β-lactam and an aminoglycoside combination regimen during the last two decades.

Monotherapy with a broad-spectrum β-lactam antibiotic is as efficacious and less toxic than a combination of β-lactam and an aminoglycoside as empirical therapy for critically ill patients with severe sepsis or septic shock.[32,54] However, it would be premature to initiate monotherapy for all patients with severe sepsis as standard of care due to limitations in the clinical trials such as small sample sizes (less than 200 patients) and the variability in antimicrobials used.[55,56]

Antifungal Therapy

Candida species are most frequently associated with fungal infections, and the resulting candidemia is frequently associated with sepsis syndrome and a high mortality rate.[13,57] Septic shock caused by *C. albicans* demonstrated 24.6% survival with initial appropriate therapy but only 4.6% survival without (ninefold decrease).[11] Empirical fluconazole therapy for suspected nosocomial bloodstream infections can be appropriate for hospitalized patients at high risk for fungal infections, including those receiving total parenteral nutrition, with bowel perforation, or with persistent or new signs and symptoms of infections despite receiving broad-spectrum antibacterial therapy. Of the patients with candidemia, mortality rates were lowest for those who began empirical fluconazole therapy on day 0 (15%) and highest for those who began on day 3 or later (41%).[58] Although prompt empirical fluconazole therapy significantly affects mortality rates of hospitalized patients with candidemia, it can increase overprescribing of antifungal agents for patients without candidemia. Rapid diagnostic tests or identification of unique risk factors for bloodstream infections caused by *Candida* species are needed.

Treatment of invasive candidiasis involves amphotericin B–based preparations, azole antifungal agents, and echinocandin antifungal agents, or combinations. The choice depends on the clinical status of the patient, the fungal species and its susceptibility, the relative drug toxicity, the presence of organ dysfunction that would affect drug clearance, and the patient's prior exposure to antifungal agents.

Fluconazole is less toxic and easier to administer than amphotericin B. However, fluconazole resistance in *C. albicans* has been well described among HIV-infected individuals and is increasing in immunocompetent adults.[59] *C. glabrata* often has reduced susceptibility to fluconazole. Itraconazole exhibits a similar activity profile as fluconazole and is well known to be active against mucosal forms of candidiasis. However, the parenteral form of itraconazole is no longer available. Voriconazole appears to be active against *Candida* species, including fluconazole-resistant isolates. A worldwide study will aid in analyzing voriconazole for the indication of treatment of serious invasive, fluconazole-resistant *Candida* infections, including *C. krusei*.[59,60]

Caspofungin, the first echinocandin antifungal agent, appears to be potent against all *Candida* species, including *C. glabrata*, *C. krusei*, and *Candida lusitaniae,* as well as *Aspergillus* species. IV caspofungin was equally effective but better tolerated than amphotericin B deoxycholate for invasive candidiasis.[61] In an international, randomized, double-blind trial, the micafungin 100 mg group was noninferior to caspofungin for the treatment of candidemia and other forms of invasive candidiasis demonstrated (76.4% vs 72.3%).[62] Anidulafungin, the latest echinocandin to be approved, achieved a success rate of 73.2% against invasive candidiasis in comparison to the 61.1% treatment success rate of fluconazole.[63] The difference was not statistically significant.

In general, suspected systemic mycotic infection leading to sepsis in nonneutropenic patients should be treated empirically with parenteral fluconazole, caspofungin, anidulafungin, or micafungin.[59] An echinocandin is preferred for a patient with recent azole exposure or if the patient is clinically unstable because of its greater activity against fluconazole-resistant *Candida* species and non-*Albicans* species, including *C. glabrata* and *C. krusei*.[59,64] In neutropenic patients, a lipid formulation of amphotericin, caspofungin, or voriconazole is recommended. Azoles should be avoided for empiric therapy in patients who have received an azole for prophylaxis.[59]

Duration of Therapy

The average duration of antimicrobial therapy in the normal host with sepsis is 7 to 10 days, and fungal infections can require 10 to 14 days.[7,32,40,59] However, the duration can be longer in patients with a slow clinical response, undrainable focus of infection, or neutropenia. After the patient is hemodynamically stable, has been afebrile for 48 to 72 hours, has a normalizing white blood cell (WBC) count, and is able to take oral medications, then a "step-down" from parenteral to oral antibiotics can be considered for the remaining duration of therapy. Treatment can continue considerably longer if the infection is persistent. In a neutropenic patient, therapy is usually continued until the patient is no longer neutropenic and has been afebrile for at least 72 hours.

Procalcitonin may also be used to guide the length of antibiotic therapy. Procalcitonin is a biomarker that increases in response to endotoxins and inflammatory cytokines released during systemic bacterial infections.[65,66] A reduction in antibiotic exposure has been reported in patients with lower respiratory tract infections using procalcitonin levels as a guide for discontinuing antibiotics. Results from a limited number of studies using procalcitonin as a marker to discontinue antibiotics in patients with severe sepsis or septic shock and surgical intensive care patients are promising, and more trials are expected in the near future.[65,66]

■ HEMODYNAMIC SUPPORT

A high cardiac output and a low systemic vascular resistance characterize septic shock. Patients can have hypotension as a result of low systemic vascular resistance and abnormal distribution of blood flow in the microcirculation, resulting in compromised tissue perfusion. Because approximately half of patients with septic shock die of multiple organ system failure, they should be monitored carefully, and aggressive hemodynamic support should be initiated.

Hemodynamics change rapidly in sepsis, and noninvasive evaluation can give inaccurate assessment of filling pressures and cardiac output, requiring a right-sided heart catheter in the ICU setting.[67] Hemodynamic support can be divided into three main categories: fluid therapy, vasopressor therapy, and inotropic therapy.

Fluid Therapy

6 Septic patients have enormous fluid requirements as a result of peripheral vasodilation and capillary leakage.[67] In ~50% of septic patients who initially present with hypotension, fluids alone will reverse hypotension and restore hemodynamic stability. Rapid fluid resuscitation improves the 28-day survival rate in patients with sepsis-induced hypoperfusion.[32] The goal of fluid therapy is to maximize cardiac output by increasing the left ventricular preload, which will ultimately restore tissue perfusion.[67] Fluid administration should be titrated to clinical end points such as heart rate, urine output, blood pressure, and mental status. Increased serum lactate, a by-product of cellular anaerobic metabolism, should normalize as tissue perfusion improves.

Isotonic crystalloids, such as 0.9% sodium chloride (normal saline), and lactated Ringer solution are commonly used for fluid resuscitation. A patient in septic shock typically requires up to 10 L of crystalloid solution during the first 24-hour period. These solutions distribute into the extracellular compartment. Approximately 25% of the infused volume of crystalloid remains in the intravascular space, whereas the balance distributes to extravascular spaces. Although this could impair diffusion of oxygen to tissues, clinical impact is unproven.

The most commonly used colloids are 5% albumin, a naturally occurring plasma protein, and 6% hetastarch, a synthetic colloid formulation. These solutions offer more rapid restoration of intravascular volume because they produce greater intravascular volume expansion per quantity of volume infused. Colloids produce less peripheral edema than crystalloid, but there is no significant clinical impact. The use of colloid solutions and blood products can be particularly important if there is significant blood loss associated with sepsis or if the patient had severe preexisting anemia.

Meta-analysis of clinical studies comparing crystalloid and colloid resuscitation indicated no clinical outcome differences.[68] The Saline versus Albumin Fluid Evaluation (SAFE) trial found no difference in the 28-day mortality rate in critically ill patients (21.1% with saline vs 20.9% with albumin).[69] Although crystalloid solutions require two to four times more volume than colloids, they are generally recommended for fluid resuscitation because of the lower cost. However, colloids can be preferred, especially when the serum albumin is less than 2.0 g/dL.

Central venous pressure (CVP) is used to monitor fluid status in patients with septic shock. Initial fluid resuscitation should target a CVP between 8 and 12 mm Hg within the first 6 hours of presentation.[32] Fluid challenges should continue until hemodynamic stability is reached as long as CVP is at goal. The rate of fluid administration should be reduced if hemodynamic measures do not improve despite adequate or increasing cardiac filling pressures. Resuscitation typically includes IV normal saline 500 mL every 15 minutes until the target CVP is reached.

Patients receiving fluid challenges require close monitoring of volume status to avoid pulmonary and systemic edema. Aggressive volume expansion can cause an increase in pulmonary capillary pressure, leading to an increase in lung water and associated hypoxemia.[70] There is no significant difference in the incidence of pulmonary edema between the crystalloid and colloid solutions.

Vasopressor and Inotropic Therapy

When fluid resuscitation alone provides inadequate arterial pressure and organ perfusion, vasopressors and inotropic agents should be initiated. Inotropic agents such as dopamine and dobutamine have been effective in improving cardiac output by increasing cardiac contractility. Vasopressors such as norepinephrine should be considered when a systolic blood pressure is less than 90 mm Hg or mean arterial pressure (MAP) is <65 mm Hg after adequate left ventricular preload and inotrope therapy. Although inotropes and vasopressors are effective in life-threatening hypotension and in improving cardiac index, there are significant complications such as tachycardia and myocardial ischemia and infarction as a result of the change in myocardial oxygen consumption in patients with coexisting coronary disease. Thus, a catecholamine infusion should be titrated gradually to restore MAP without impairing stroke volume.

7 Agents commonly considered for vasopressor or inotropic support include dopamine, dobutamine, norepinephrine, phenylephrine, and epinephrine (Table 128–5).[71] Norepinephrine should generally be considered to be the first-choice vasopressor in septic shock after failure to restore adequate blood pressure and organ perfusion with appropriate fluid resuscitation. Norepinephrine is a potent α-adrenergic agent with less pronounced β-adrenergic activity. It increases MAP and systemic vascular resistance because of its vasoconstrictive effects on peripheral

TABLE 128–5	Receptor Activity of Cardiovascular Agents Commonly used in Septic Shock				
Agent	α_1	α_2	β_1	β_2	**Dopaminergic**
Dopamine	++/+++	?	++++	++	++++
Dobutamine	+	+	++++	++	0
Norepinephrine	+++	+++	+++	+/++	0
Phenylephrine	++/+++	+	?	0	0
Epinephrine	++++	++++	++++	+++	0

$\alpha_1 = \alpha_1$-adrenergic receptor, $\alpha_2 = \alpha_2$-adrenergic receptor, $\beta_1 = \beta_1$-adrenergic receptor, $\beta_2 = \beta_2$-adrenergic receptor, 0 = no activity, ++++ = maximal activity, ? = unknown activity.

vascular beds. Doses of 0.01 to 3 mcg/kg/min can reliably increase blood pressure with little changes in heart rate or cardiac index (CI). Despite the earlier concern of decreased renal blood flow associated with norepinephrine, data in humans and animals demonstrate a norepinephrine-induced renal blood flow as well as urine and cardiac output.[71] Norepinephrine is a more potent agent than dopamine in refractory septic shock. Norepinephrine resulted in greater increases in arterial blood pressure in comparison to patients with septic shock who were treated with dopamine (93% with norepinephrine vs 31% with dopamine).[72] Norepinephrine was also associated with a higher rate of survival compared with dopamine and epinephrine.[73]

Dopamine is a natural precursor of norepinephrine and epinephrine, and it exhibits dose-dependent pharmacologic effects. It is an α- and β-adrenergic agent with dopaminergic activity. Doses of >5 mcg/kg/min increase MAP and cardiac output, primarily because of the increase in heart rate and cardiac contractility through stimulation of β-adrenergic receptors. At higher doses, α-adrenergic effects predominate, resulting in arterial vasoconstriction. Because of combined vasopressor and inotropic effects, dopamine is more useful in patients with hypotension and compromised systolic function. However, it is also more arrhythmogenic and can cause more tachycardia.[32,73,74] It should be used with caution in patients who have underlying heart disease.

Phenylephrine, a selective $α_1$-agonist, has rapid onset, short duration, and primary vascular effects, and it is least likely to produce tachycardia. Limited data suggest it can increase blood pressure modestly in fluid-resuscitated patients, and it does not appear to impair cardiac or renal function. Phenylephrine appears useful when tachycardia limits the usage of other vasopressors.[67,71]

Epinephrine is a nonspecific α- and β-adrenergic agonist. Ranging from 0.1 to 0.5 mcg/kg/min, cardiac output is increased at lower doses, and vasoconstriction occurs predominantly at higher doses. Epinephrine should be reserved for patients who fail to respond to traditional therapies for increasing or maintaining blood pressure, as it impairs blood flow to the splanchnic system, increases the lactate level, and causes dysrhythmia more frequently than other vasoactive agents.[67,73]

During hypotension, endogenous vasopressin levels increase and maintain arterial blood pressure, as vasopressin is a direct vasoconstrictor without inotropic or chronotropic effects. However, there is a vasopressin deficiency in septic shock most likely caused by inadequate production. Low doses of vasopressin (0.01–0.04 units/min) produce a significant increase in MAP in septic shock, and it may be beneficial to add vasopressin in severe sepsis and septic shock that is refractory to other vasopressors.[71] Vasopressin should not be used as a single agent for refractory hypotension. Although it can be used to reduce norepinephrine requirements, this has not been shown to improve mortality rates.[75]

Dobutamine is a β-adrenergic inotropic agent that many clinicians consider to be the preferred drug for improvement of cardiac output and oxygen delivery, particularly in early sepsis before significant peripheral vasodilation has occurred. Doses of 2 to 20 mcg/kg/min increases the CI, ranging from 20% to 66%. However, heart rate often increases significantly.[67] Dobutamine should be considered in severely septic patients with low CI but adequate filling pressures and blood pressure. A vasopressor such as norepinephrine and an inotrope such as dobutamine can be used to maintain both MAP and cardiac output.

In summary, for the septic patient with clinical signs of shock and significant hypotension unresponsive to aggressive fluid therapy, norepinephrine is the preferred agent for increasing MAP. Epinephrine should be considered for refractory hypotension. Dopamine and epinephrine are more likely to induce or exacerbate tachycardia than norepinephrine and phenylephrine.

In a septic patient with low CI after adequate fluid therapy and adequate MAP, dobutamine is the first-line agent. Alternatively, dopamine in moderate doses (5–10 mcg/kg/min) can also be used as an initial agent because of its selective effect on increasing cardiac output with its minimal effect on systemic vascular resistance.

■ EARLY GOAL-DIRECTED THERAPY

8 Initial resuscitation of a patient in severe sepsis or sepsis-induced tissue hypoperfusion should begin as soon as the syndrome is recognized. A randomized, controlled trial evaluated the timing of the goal-directed therapy involving adjustments of cardiac preload, afterload, and contractility to balance oxygen delivery with demand prior to admission to the ICU.[76] The goals during the first 6 hours included CVP of 8 to 12 mm Hg, MAP ≥65 mm Hg, urine output ≥0.5 mL/kg/h, and a central venous or mixed venous oxygen saturation ≥70%. During the first 6 hours of resuscitation, the early goal-directed therapy group had a central venous catheter placed and received more fluid than with traditional therapy (5 vs 3.5 L), dobutamine therapy to a maximum of 20 mcg/kg/min, and red blood cell transfusions. The 28-day mortality rate was 30% in the early goal-directed therapy group, in comparison to 46.5% in the traditional therapy group consisting of fluid resuscitation, followed by vasopressor therapy if required. Increased oxygen delivery from the red blood cell transfusions to achieve a hematocrit of ≥30% in the early goal-directed therapy group appeared to be the primary difference between the two groups. One institution evaluated the impact of 6-hour sepsis care bundle and found the compliance rate to be 52%.[77] The noncompliant group had a more than twofold increase in hospital mortality in comparison to the compliant group (49% vs 23%).

■ ADJUNCTIVE THERAPIES

ARDS and hypoxia are common in septic patients, even in those without pulmonary infection. Oxygen therapy is indicated to maintain oxygen saturation greater than 90%, and with progressive pulmonary insufficiency, the patient can require assisted ventilation.

9 Hyperglycemia is frequently associated with sepsis regardless of the presence of diabetes prior to sepsis, and it is usually quite refractory to exogenous insulin. Intensive insulin therapy is no longer the standard of care in critically ill patients. Results from a parallel, randomized control trial showed that more patients receiving intensive insulin therapy (target serum glucose of 81–108 mg/dL) at 90 days died compared with patients receiving conventional insulin therapy (target ≤180 mg/dL).[78,79] Hypoglycemia is the most common adverse effect of intensive insulin therapy. Even though there was no difference in mortality in the subgroup of patients with severe sepsis, a glucose range of 140 to 180 mg/dL or less than 150 mg/dL is recommended for the majority of critically ill patients to improve the outcome while reducing the risk of hypoglycemia.[32,80]

10 The role of corticosteroids has been the subject of much controversy in the management of septic patients.[81,82] Inflammatory cytokines contribute to adrenal insufficiency during sepsis. Corticosteroids have been advocated as adjunctive therapy in patients with severe sepsis and septic shock, as they prevent the release of proinflammatory cytokines.

A multicenter, randomized, controlled trial demonstrated significant shock reversal and decrease in mortality (absolute reduction 10%) in patients with severe septic shock who were given low-dose corticosteroids.[83] Fludrocortisone 50 mcg orally and hydrocortisone 200 to 300 mg/day for 7 days in three or four divided doses or by continuous infusion were used in patients with adrenal insufficiency, requiring high-dose or increasing vasopressor therapy within the first 8 hours of septic shock.[83] There was no benefit for those patients without adrenal insufficiency. An adrenocorticotropic hormone (ACTH) stimulation test has been used to identify those patients who have a relative adrenal insufficiency who should then receive supplemental steroid. However, in the large multicenter trial, the Corticosteroid Therapy of Septic Shock (CORTICUS), the patients benefited regardless of ACTH stimulation test outcome.[82]

The Surviving Sepsis Campaign recommends IV hydrocortisone for adult patients with septic shock whose blood pressure is unresponsive to fluids and vasopressors.[32,84] Corticosteroids should be weaned once a patient is off vasopressors, although comparative clinical trials comparing whether steroids should be abruptly discontinued or tapered are lacking.

CLINICAL CONTROVERY

A systematic review reported a significant reduction in 28-day all cause mortality and hospital mortality in patients receiving prolonged courses (>5 days) of low-dose corticosteroid therapy (≤300 mg hydrocortisone or equivalent/day).[81] The Corticosteroid Therapy of Septic Shock (CORTICUS) trial found no survival benefit among patients who received prolonged courses of hydrocortisone, but reported a trend in shock reversal for patients who received hydrocortisone.[82] Based on the current Surviving Sepsis guidelines, corticosteroids should be reserved for patients who continue to be hypotensive despite adequate fluids and vasopressor therapy, are maintained on an outpatient corticosteroid regimen, or may be initiated at physician discretion.

Deep vein thrombosis prophylaxis with either low-dose unfractionated heparin or low-molecular-weight heparin should be initiated in general ICU patients, including those with severe sepsis and septic shock.[32] Similarly, stress ulcer prophylaxis should be initiated in all patients with severe sepsis and septic shock.[32] Proton pump inhibitors and H_2 receptor antagonists are equivalent in their ability to increase gastric pH.

■ IMMUNOTHERAPY

Despite the initial enthusiasm for immunotherapeutic interventions for sepsis, overall results have been generally disappointing, with the exception of drotrecogin alfa (recombinant human activated protein C, rhAPC), an endogenous anticoagulant with antiinflammatory properties. During severe sepsis, the activation of protein C is inhibited by inflammatory cytokines.

⑪ Drotrecogin, the first antiinflammatory agent to be approved for sepsis, promotes fibrinolysis and the inhibition of coagulation and inflammation. The Recombinant Human Activated Protein C Worldwide Evaluation in Severe Sepsis (PROWESS) trial studied the effects of 96 hours of continuous infusion (24 mcg/kg/h) of rhAPC.[22] All-cause mortality at 28 days was significantly reduced from 30.8% with placebo to 24.7% in those receiving drotrecogin. However, a major risk associated with drotrecogin is hemorrhage. Serious bleeding, including intracranial hemorrhage and a life-threatening bleeding episode, occurred in 3.5% of patients who received drotrecogin in comparison to 2% of patients in the placebo group. Regardless, drotrecogin appears to have a significant role in the treatment of septic shock. Currently, drotrecogin is recommended in patients at high risk of death, including Acute Physiology and Chronic Health Evaluation (APACHE) II score ≥25, sepsis-induced multiple organ failure, septic shock, and sepsis-

induced ARDS and with no absolute contraindication related to bleeding risk.[85] Cost–benefit analysis studies support the use of drotrecogin for patients at high risk of death, especially for those with APACHE II scores greater than 25.[22,86]

Subanalysis of the PROWESS trial demonstrated significant absolute risk reductions in 28-day and in-hospital mortality among patients 75 years or older (15.5% and 15.6%, respectively) in comparison to the placebo group.[87,88] There was no significant difference between the drotrecogin-treated group and the placebo group with respect to the incidences of serious bleeding (3.9% vs 2.2%). A randomized, placebo-controlled multicenter trial evaluating the efficacy of drotrecogin for adults who had severe sepsis and a low risk of death defined by an APACHE score <25 or single organ failure showed no significant difference between the placebo and the treatment groups in terms of the 28-day mortality rate (17% vs 18.5%, respectively).[89] The incidence of serious bleeding was higher in the treatment group than in the placebo group (3.9% vs 2.2%). Consequently, drotrecogin should not be used in patients with severe sepsis and low risk of death.

CONCLUSION

The diagnosis and management of severe sepsis and septic shock are challenging. The updated Surviving Sepsis Campaign international guidelines for management of severe sepsis and septic shock incorporate newer evidence-based interventions with the purpose of improving morbidity and mortality. Many institutions are following sepsis protocols, including initiation of early appropriate empiric antibiotics, restoration of tissue perfusion, initiation of vasopressor support, and other supportive measures to improve overall patient outcomes. The use of standardized treatment protocols in addition to newer treatment modalities in patients with severe sepsis and septic shock can continue to have an impact on the overall morbidity and mortality rate.

ABBREVIATIONS

ACTH: Adrenocorticotropic hormone

APACHE: Acute Physiology and Chronic Health Evaluation

ARDS: Acute respiratory distress syndrome

CARS: Compensatory antiinflammatory response syndrome

CI: Cardiac index

CORTICUS: Corticosteroid Therapy of Septic Shock (trial)

CVP: Cardiac venous pressure

DIC: Disseminated intravascular coagulation

DO_2: Oxygen delivery to tissues

HIV: Human immunodeficiency virus

ICU: Intensive care unit

IL: Interleukin

IL-1RA: Interleukin-1 receptor antagonist

MAP: Mean arterial pressure

MODS: Multiple-organ dysfunction syndrome

MRSA: Methicillin-resistant *Staphylococcus aureus*

PAF: Platelet-activating factor

PROWESS: Recombinant Human Activated Protein C Worldwide Evaluation in Severe Sepsis (trial)

rhAPC: Recombinant human activated protein C

SAFE: Saline versus Albumin Fluid Evaluation (trial)

SIRS: Systemic inflammatory response syndrome

SSTIs: Skin and soft tissue infections

SVR: Systemic vascular resistance

TNF: Tumor necrosis factor

VO$_2$: Oxygen consumption

WBC: White blood cell

REFERENCES

1. Angus DC, Linde-Zwirble WT, Lidicker J, et al. Epidemiology of severe sepsis in the United States: Analysis of incidence, outcome, and associated costs of care. Crit Care Med 2001;29:1303–1310.

2. Kung HC, Hoyert DL, Xu, et al. Deaths: Final data for 2005. Natl Vital Stat Rep 2008;56:1–120.

3. American College of Chest Physicians/Society of Critical Care Medicine Consensus Conference. Definitions for sepsis and organ failure and guidelines for the use of innovative therapies in sepsis. Crit Care Med 1992;20:864–874.

4. Robertson CM, Coopersmith CM. The systemic inflammatory response syndrome. Microbes Infect 2006;8:1382–1389.

5. Vincent JL, Sakr Y, Sprung CL, et al. Sepsis in European intensive care units: Results of the SOAP study. Crit Care Med 2006;34:344–353.

6. Levy MM, Fink MP, Marshall JC, et al. 2001 SCCM/ESICM/ACCP/ATS/SIS International Sepsis Definitions Conference. Crit Care Med 2003;31:1250–1256.

7. Harbarth S, Garbino J, Pugin J, et al. Inappropriate initial therapy and its effect on survival in a clinical trial of immunomodulating therapy for severe sepsis. Am J Med 2003;115:529–535.

8. Valles J, Rello J, Ochagavia A, et al. Community-acquired bloodstream infection in critically ill adult patients. Chest 2003;123:1615–1624.

9. Guidet B, Aegerter P, Gauzit R, et al. Incidence and impact of organ dysfunctions associated with sepsis. Chest 2005;127:942–951.

10. Garnacho-Montero J, Garcia-Garmendia JL, Barrero-Almodovar A, et al. Impact of adequate empirical antibiotic therapy on the outcome of patients admitted to the intensive care unit with sepsis. Crit Care Med 2003;31:2742–2751.

11. Kumar A, Ellis P, Arabi Y, et al. Initiation of inappropriate antimicrobial therapy results in a fivefold reduction of survival in human septic shock. Chest 2009;136:1237–1248.

12. Laupland KB, Kirkpatrick AW, Church DL, et al. Intensive-care-unit-acquired bloodstream infections in a regional critically ill population. J Hosp Infect 2004;58:137–145.

13. Horn DL, Neofytos D, Anaissie EJ, et al. Epidemiology and outcomes of candidemia in 2019 patients: Data from the prospective antifungal therapy alliance registry. Clin Infect Dis 2009;48:1695–1703.

14. Annane D, Bellissant E, Cavaillon JM. Septic shock. Lancet 2005;365:63–78.

15. Cavaillon JM, Adib-Conquy M, Fitting C, et al. Cytokine cascade in sepsis. Scand J Infect Dis 2003;35:535–544.

16. Kim PK, Deutschman CS. Inflammatory responses and mediators. Surg Clin North Am 2000;80:885–894.

17. Heper Y, Akalin EH, Mistik R, et al. Evaluation of serum C-reactive protein, procalcitonin, tumor necrosis factor alpha, and interleukin-10 levels as diagnostic and prognostic parameters in patients with community-acquired sepsis, severe sepsis, and septic shock. Eur J Clin Microbiol Infect Dis 2006;25:481–491.

18. O'Malley K, Moldawer LL. Interleukin-6: Still crazy after all these years. Crit Care Med 2006;34:2690–2691.

19. Lin KJ, Lin J, Hanasawa K, et al. Interleukin-8 as a predictor of the severity of bacteremia and infectious disease. Shock 2000;14:95–100.

20. Ellis CG, Jagger J, Sharpe M. The microcirculation as a functional system. Crit Care 2005;9(Suppl 4):S3–S8.

21. Esmon CT. The interactions between inflammation and coagulation. Br J Haematol 2005;131:416–430.

22. Bernard GR, Vincent JL, Laterre PF, et al. Efficacy and safety of recombinant human activated protein C for severe sepsis. N Engl J Med 2001;344:699–709.

23. Nimah M, Brill RJ. Coagulation dysfunction in sepsis and multiple organ failure. Crit Care Clin 2003;19:441–458.

24. Awad SS. State-of-the-art therapy for severe sepsis and multisystem organ failure. Am J Surg 2003;186:23S–30S.

25. Bastarache JA, Ware LB, Bernard GR. The role of the coagulation cascade in the continuum of sepsis and acute lung injury and acute respiratory distress syndrome. Semin Respir Crit Care Med 2006;27:365–376.

26. Guidelines for the diagnosis and management of disseminated intravascular coagulation. Br J Haematol 2009;145:24–33.

27. Young JD. The heart and circulation in severe sepsis. Br J Anaesth 2004;93:114–120.

28. Bagshaw SM, George C, Bellomo R. Early acute kidney injury and sepsis: A multicentre evaluation. Crit Care 2008;12:R47.

29. Bagshaw SM, Lapinsky S, Dial S, et al. Acute kidney injury in septic shock: Clinical outcomes and impact of duration of hypotension prior to initiation of antimicrobial therapy. Intensive Care Med 2009;35:871–881.

30. Bagshaw SM, Berthiaume LR, Delaney A, et al. Continuous versus intermittent renal replacement therapy for critically ill patients with acute kidney injury: A meta-analysis. 2008;36:610–617.

31. Nguyen HB, Rivers EP, Knoblich BP, et al. Early lactate clearance is associated with improved outcome in severe sepsis and septic shock. Crit Care Med 2004;32:1637–1642.

32. Dellinger RP, Levy MM, Carlet JM, et al. Surviving sepsis campaign: International guidelines for management of severe sepsis and septic shock: 2008. Crit Care Med 2008;36:296–327.

33. Cohen J, Brun-Buisson C, Torres A, Jorgensen J. Diagnosis of infection in sepsis: An evidence-based review. Crit Care Med 2004:32:S466–S494.

34. Marshall JC, Maier RV, Jimenez M, et al. Source control in the management of severe sepsis and septic shock: An evidence-based review. Crit Care Med 2004;32(11 Suppl):S513–526.

35. Ferrer R, Artigas A, Suarez D, et al. Effectiveness of treatments for severe sepsis: A prospective, multicenter, observational study. Am J Respir Crit Care Med 2009;180:861–866.

36. Morrell M, Franser VJ, Kollef MH. Delaying the empiric treatment of candida bloodstream infection until positive blood culture results are obtained: A potential risk factor for hospital mortality. Antimicrob Agents Chemother 2005;49:3640–3645.

37. Kumar A, Roberts D, Wood KE, et al. Duration of hypotension before initiation of effective antimicrobial therapy is the critical determinant of survival in human septic shock. Crit Care Med 2006;34:1589–1596.

38. Liu H, Mulholland G. Appropriate antibiotic treatment of genitourinary infections in hospitalized patients. Am J Med 2005;118:14S–20S.

39. Mandell LA, Wunderinnk RG, Anzueto A, et al. Infectious Disease Society of America/American Thoracic Society consensus guidelines on management of community-acquired pneumonia in adults. Clin Infect Dis 2007;44:S27–S72

40. American Thoracic Society Documents. Guidelines for the management of adults with hospital-acquired, ventilator-associated, and healthcare-associated pneumonia. Am J Respir Crit Care Med 2005;171:388–416.

41. Wunderink RG, Rello J, Cammarata SK, et al. Linezolid vs vancomycin: Analysis of two double-blind studies of patients with methicillin-resistant Staphylococcus aureus nosocomial pneumonia. Chest 2003;124:1789–1797.

42. Mullins CD, Kuznik A, Shaya FT, et al. Cost-effectiveness analysis of linezolid compared with vancomycin for the treatment of nosocomial pneumonia caused by methicillin-resistant Staphylococcus aureus. Clin Ther 2006;28:1184–1198.

43. Paterson DL, Rossi F, Basquero F, et al. In vitro susceptibilities of aerobic and facultative gram-negative bacilli isolated from patients with intra-abdominal infections worldwide: The 2003 Study for Monitoring Antimicrobial Resistance Trends (SMART). J Antimicrob Chemother 2005;55:965–973.

44. Snydman DR, Jacobus NV, McDermott LA, et al. National survey on the susceptibility of Bacteroides fragilis group: Report and analysis of trends in the United States from 1997 to 2004. Antimicrob Agents Chemother 2007;51:1649–1655.

45. Solomkin JS, Mazuski JE, Baron EJ, et al. Guidelines for the selection of anti-infective agents for complicated intra-abdominal infections. Clin Infect Dis 2003;37:997–1005.

46. Lucasti C, Jasovich A, Umeh O, et al. Efficacy and tolerability of IV doripenem versus meropenem in adults with complicated intra-abdominal infection: A phase III, prospective, multicenter, randomized, double-blind, noninferiority study. Clin Ther 2008;30:868–883.

47. Stevens BL, Bisno AL, Chambers HF, et al. Practice guidelines for the diagnosis and management of skin and soft-tissue infections. Clin Infect Dis 2005;41:1373–1406.

48. Ruhe JJ, Smith N, Bradsher RW, et al. Community-onset methicillin-resistant *Staphylococcus aureus* skin and soft tissue infections: Impact of antimicrobial therapy on outcome. Clin Infect Dis 2007;44:777–784.

49. Arbeit RD, Maki D, Tally FP, et al. The safety and efficacy of daptomycin for the treatment of complicated skin and skin-structure infections. Clin Infect Dis 2004;38:1673–1681.

50. Sharpe JN, Shively EH, Polk HC. Clinical and economic outcomes of oral linezolid versus intravenous vancomycin in the treatment of MRSA-complicated, lower-extremity skin and soft-tissue infections caused by methicillin-resistant *Staphylococcus aureus*. Am J Surg 2005;189:425–428.

51. Dellit TH, Owens RC, McGowan JE Jr, et al. Infectious Disease Society of America and the Society for Healthcare Epidemiology of America guidelines for developing an institutional program to enhance antimicrobial stewardship. Clin Infect Dis 2007;44:159–177.

52. Micek ST, Roubinian N, Heuring T, et al. Before-after study of a standardized hospital order set for the management of septic shock. Crit Care Med 2006;34:2707–2713.

53. Roberts JA, Lipman J. Pharmacokinetic issues for antibiotics in the critically ill patients. Crit Care Med 2009;37:840–851.

54. Paul M, Benuri-Silbiger I, Soares-Weiser K, et al. β-lactam monotherapy versus β-lactam-aminoglycoside combination therapy for sepsis in immunocompetent patients: Systematic review and meta-analysis of randomized trials. BMJ 2004;328:668–681.

55. Safdar N, Handelsman, Maki D. Does combination antimicrobial therapy reduce mortality in gram-negative bacteraemia? A meta-analysis. Lancet Infect Dis 2004;4:519–527.

56. Paul M, Leibovici L. Combination antibiotic therapy for *Pseudomonas aeruginosa* bacteraemia. Lancet Infect Dis 2005;5:192–194.

57. Shorr AF, Gupta V, Sun X, et al. Burden of early-onset candidemia: Analysis of culture-positive bloodstream infections from a large U.S. database. Crit Med Med 2009;37:2519–2526.

58. Garey KW, Rege M, Pai MP, et al. Time to initiation of fluconazole therapy impacts mortality in patients with candidemia: A multiinstitutional study. Clin Infect Dis 2006;43:25–31.

59. Pappas PG, Kauffman CA, Andes D, et al. Clinical practice guidelines for management of candidiasis: 2009 update by the Infectious Diseases Society of America. Clin Infect Dis 2009;48:503–535.

60. Kullberg BJ, Sobel JD, Ruhnke M, et al. Voriconazole versus a regimen of amphotericin B followed by fluconazole for candidemia in nonneutropenic patients: A randomized non-inferiority trial. Lancet 2005;366:1435–1442.

61. Mora-Duarte J, Betts R, Rotstein R, et al. Comparison of caspofungin and amphotericin B for invasive candidiasis. N Engl J Med 2002;347:2020–2029.

62. Pappas PG, Rotstein CMF, Betts RF, et al. Micafungin versus caspofungin for treatment of candidemia and other forms of invasive candidiasis. Clin Infect Dis 2007;45:883–893.

63. Reboli AC, Rotstein C, Pappas PG, et al. Anidulafungin versus fluconazole for invasive candidiasis. N Engl J Med 2007;356:2472–2482.

64. Mohr J, Johnson M, Cooper T, et al. Current options in antifungal pharmacotherapy. Pharmacother 2008;28:614–645.

65. Schroeder S, Hochreiter M, Koehler T, et al. Procalcitonin-guided algorithm reduces length of antibiotic treatment in surgical intensive care patients with severe sepsis: Results of a prospective randomized study. Langenbecks Arch Surg 2009;394:221–226.

66. Vandack N, Harbarth S, Graf JD, et al. Use of procalcitonin to shorten antibiotic treatment duration in septic patients. Am J Respir Crit Care Med 2008;177:498–505.

67. Hollenberg SM, Ahrens TS, Annane D, et al. Practice parameters for hemodynamic support of sepsis in adult patients: 2004 Update. Crit Care Med 2004;32:1928–1948.

68. Choi PTL, Yip G, Quinonez LG, et al. Crystalloids versus colloids in fluid resuscitation: Systemic review. Crit Care Med 1999;27:200–210.

69. Finfer S, Bellomo R, Boyce N, et al. A comparison of albumin and saline for fluid resuscitation in the intensive care unit. N Engl J Med 2004;350:2247–2256.

70. Durairaj L, Schmidt GA. Fluid therapy in resuscitated sepsis: Less is more. Chest 2008;133:252–263.

71. Hollenberg SM. Vasopressor support in septic shock. Chest 2007;132:1678–1687.

72. Levy MM, Macias WL, Vincent JL, et al. Early changes in organ function predict eventual survival in severe sepsis. Crit Care Med 2005;33:2194–2201.

73. De Backer D, Creteur J, Silva E, et al. Effects of dopamine, norepinephrine, and epinephrine on the splanchnic circulation in septic shock: Which is best? Crit Care Med 2003;31:1659–1667.

74. Sakr Y, Reinhart K, Vincent JL, et al. Dose dopamine administration in shock influence outcome? Results of the sepsis occurrence in acutely ill patients (SOAP) study. Crit Care Med 2006;34:589–597.

75. Russell JA, Walley KR, Singer J, et al. Vasopressin versus norepinephrine infusion in patients with septic shock. N Engl J Med 2008;358:877–887.

76. Rivers E, Nguyen B, Havstad S, et al. Early goal-directed therapy in the treatment of severe sepsis and septic shock. N Engl J Med 2001;345:1368–1377.

77. Gao F, Melody T, Daniels D, et al. The impact of compliance with 6-hour and 24-hour sepsis bundles on hospital mortality in patients with severe sepsis: A prospective observational study. Crit Care 2005;9:R764–R770.

78. Brunkhorst FM, Engel C, Bloos F, et al. Intensive insulin therapy and pentastarch resuscitation in severe sepsis. N Engl J Med 2008;358:125–139.

79. The NICE-SUGAR Investigators. Intensive versus conventional glucose control in critically ill patients. N Engl J Med 2009;360:1283–1297.

80. Moghissi ES, Korytkowski MT, DiNardo M, et al. American Association of Clinical Endocrinologists and American Diabetes Association consensus statement on inpatient glycemic control. Endocr Pract 2009;15:1–17.

81. Annane D, Bellissant E, Bollaert PE, et al. Corticosteroids in the treatment of severe sepsis and septic shock in adults: A systematic review. JAMA 2009;301:2362–2375.

82. Sprung CL, Annane D, Keh D, et al. Hydrocortisone therapy for patients with septic shock. N Engl J Med 2008;358:111–124.

83. Annane D, Sebille V, Charpentier C, et al. Effects of treatment with low-dose hydrocortisone and fludrocortisone on mortality in patients with septic shock. JAMA 2002;288:862–871.

84. Russell JA, Walley KR, Gordon AC, et al. Interaction of vasopressin infusion, corticosteroid treatment and mortality of septic shock. Crit Care Med 2009;37:811–818.

85. Vincent JL, Bernard GR, Beasle R, et al. Drotrecogin alfa (activated) treatment in severe sepsis from the global open-label trial ENHANCE: Further evidence for survival and safety and implications for early treatment. Crit Care Med 2005;33:2266–2277.

86. Angus DC, Linde-Zwirble WT, Clermont G, et al. Cost-effectiveness of drotrecogin alfa (activated) in the treatment of severe sepsis. Crit Care Med 2003;31:1–11.

87. Alexander SL, Ernst FR. Use of drotrecogin alfa (activated) in older patients with severe sepsis. Pharmacotherapy 2006;26:533–538.

88. Ely EW, Angus DC, Williams MD, et al. Drotrecogin alfa (activated) treatment of older patients with severe sepsis. Clin Infect Dis 2003;37:187–195.

89. Abraham E, Laterre PF, Garg R, et al. Drotrecogin alfa (activated) for adults with severe sepsis and a low risk of death. N Engl J Med 2005;353:1332–1341.

CHAPTER 129

Superficial Fungal Infections

THOMAS E. R. BROWN, LINDA D. DRESSER AND THOMAS W. F. CHIN

KEY CONCEPTS

❶ Vulvovaginal candidiasis (VVC) can be classified as uncomplicated or complicated. This classification is useful in determining appropriate pharmacotherapy.

❷ *Candida albicans* is the major pathogen responsible for VVC. The number of cases of non–*C. albicans* species appears to be increasing.

❸ Signs and symptoms of VVC are not pathognomonic, and reliable diagnosis must be made with laboratory tests.

❹ *C. albicans* is the predominant species causing all forms of mucosal candidiasis. Important host and exogenous risk factors have been identified that predispose an individual to the development of mucosal candidiasis. In oropharyngeal and esophageal candidiasis, the key risk factor is impaired host immune system.

❺ A topical agent is the first choice for treating oropharyngeal candidiasis. Systemic therapy can be used in patients who are not responding to an adequate trial of topical treatment or are unable to tolerate topical agents and in those at high risk for systemic candidiasis. Fluconazole and itraconazole solution are the most effective azole agents.

❻ In esophageal candidiasis, topical agents are not of proven benefit; fluconazole or itraconazole solution is the first choice.

❼ Patients with human immunodeficiency virus (HIV) infection must be on concurrent optimal antiretroviral therapy, which is important for the prevention of recurrent and refractory candidiasis.

❽ Primary or secondary prophylaxis of fungal infection is not recommended routinely for HIV-infected patients; use of secondary prophylaxis should be individualized for each patient.

❾ Topical agents are first-line treatment for fungal skin infections. Oral therapy is preferred for the treatment of extensive or severe infection or those of tinea capitis or onychomycosis.

❿ Oral agents, in particular terbinafine and itraconazole, are first-line treatment for toenail and fingernail onychomycosis.

Learning objectives, review questions, and other resources can be found at **www.pharmacotherapyonline.com**.

Superficial mycoses are among the most common infections in the world and the second most common vaginal infections in North America. Mucocutaneous candidiasis can occur in three forms—oropharyngeal, esophageal, and vulvovaginal disease—with oropharyngeal and vulvovaginal disease being the most common. These infections were reported in humans as far back as 1839. Over the past 15 to 20 years, the occurrence rates of some fungal infections have increased dramatically. The prevalence of fungal skin infections varies throughout different parts of the world, from the most common causes of skin infections in the tropics to relatively rare disorders in the United States. This chapter reviews the pharmacotherapy of vulvovaginal candidiasis, oropharyngeal and esophageal candidiasis, and common dermatophyte infections.

VULVOVAGINAL CANDIDIASIS

❶ *Vulvovaginal candidiasis* (VVC) refers to infections in individuals with or without symptoms who have positive vaginal cultures for *Candida* species. Depending on episodic frequency, VVC can be classified as either sporadic or recurrent.[1] This classification is essential to understanding the pathophysiology, as well as the pharmacotherapy, of VVC. Furthermore, VVC may be defined as uncomplicated, which refers to sporadic infections that are susceptible to all forms of antifungal therapy regardless of the duration of treatment, or complicated, in which consideration of factors affecting the host, microorganism, and pharmacotherapy all have an essential role in successful treatment.[1] Complicated VVC includes recurrent VVC, severe disease, non–*Candida albicans* candidiasis, and host factors, including diabetes mellitus, immunosuppression, and pregnancy.[1]

EPIDEMIOLOGY

Minimal information on the incidence and prevalence of VVC exists. Healthcare workers are not required to report cases of VVC; therefore, estimates are derived from self-reported histories. Epidemiologic data are limited because VVC usually is diagnosed without microscopy and/or cultures, and antifungal nonprescription preparations are available for self-treatment.[1] By 25 years of age, ~50% of college women will have had at least one episode of VVC.[1] It is rare before menarche and increases dramatically at about 20 years of age, with the peak incidence between age 30 and 40. It is associated with the initial act of sexual intercourse. As many as 75% of women experience one bout of symptomatic VVC in their lifetime. Between 40% and 50% of women who experience one episode of VVC experience a second episode, and 5% experience recurrent VVC.[2,3] Black women appear to be at higher risk than white women of developing VVC (62.8% vs 55%, respectively).[4] The incidence after menopause remains unknown.

Costs from VVC can be direct (medical visits and self-treatment) and indirect (nonmedical expenses, e.g., time losses from work, costs of travel, and time required in obtaining treatment). There are an estimated 6 million visits to healthcare providers each year, resulting in more than $1 billion spent annually on these medical visits and self-treatment.[5]

PATHOPHYSIOLOGY

❷ *Candida albicans* is the major pathogen responsible for VVC, accounting for 80% to 92% of symptomatic episodes. The remainder are caused by non–*C. albicans* species, with *Candida glabrata* dominating.[6] The number of cases of non–*C. albicans* candidiasis appears to be increasing, possibly related to the use of nonprescription vaginal antifungal preparations and short-course therapy and/or the increased use of long-term maintenance therapy in preventing recurrent infections.[1]

Candida species can act as commensal members of the vaginal flora. Asymptomatic colonization with *Candida* species has been found in 10% to 20% of women of reproductive age.[6,7] *Candida* organisms are dimorphic; blastospores are believed to be responsible for colonization (transmission and spread), whereas germinated *Candida* forms are associated with tissue invasion and symptomatic infections.[8] To colonize the vagina, *Candida* species must be able to attach to the mucosa. The attachment process is complex. Not only are candidal surface structures important for attachment, but appropriate receptors for attachment must be present in the epithelial tissue. Not all women have the same range of receptors, which may explain variation in colonization.[7] Changes in the host's vaginal environment or response are necessary to induce a symptomatic infection. Unfortunately, in most cases of symptomatic VVC, no precipitating factor can be identified.[8]

RISK FACTORS

Several factors predispose a woman to VVC. VVC is not considered to be a sexually transmitted disease, although sexual factors can be important. There is a dramatic increase in the frequency of VVC when women become sexually active. In addition, oral-genital contact can increase the risk.[1] However, current guidelines do not recommend the treatment of asymptomatic partners.[6] Contraceptive agents, including the diaphragm with spermicide, the contraceptive sponge, and the intrauterine device, increase the risk of VVC. Oral contraceptive users demonstrated increased risk of candidiasis; however, these reports were with the higher-dose oral contraceptive pills, and the risk may not be as great with the lower-estrogen-dose oral contraceptives.[9]

Antibiotic use can increase the risk of VVC, but it is significant in only a small number of women. The mechanism by which antibiotics can increase the risk of VVC is unknown; colonization, however, is a prerequisite.[1] Diet (excess refined carbohydrates), douching, and tight-fitting clothing often are listed as important risk factors; however, no association has been established between these factors and increased risk of VVC.[1]

CLINICAL PRESENTATION

❸ The clinical presentation of VVC is given in Table 129–1.[1,6] These signs and symptoms are not pathognomonic, and a reliable diagnosis cannot be made without laboratory tests. Self-diagnosis has a sensitivity of 35%, a specificity of 89%, and a positive predictive value of 62%.[4] More than 50% of women who had self-diagnosed VVC did not have yeast as the causative agent.[10] This limits the value of self-diagnosis and the success of self-treatment. The American College of Obstetricians and Gynecologists (ACOG) recommend that whenever possible women requesting treatment

TABLE 129-1	Clinical Presentation of Vulvovaginal Candidiasis
General Symptoms	Often involves both the vulva and the vagina Intense vulvar itching, soreness, irritation, burning on urination, and dyspareunia
Signs	Erythema, fissuring, curdy "cheese"-like discharge, satellite lesions, edema
Laboratory tests	Vaginal pH–normal, saline and 10% KOH microscopy–blastospores or pseudohyphae
Other diagnostic tests	*Candida* cultures not recommended unless classic signs and symptoms with normal vaginal pH and microscopy are inconclusive or recurrence is suspected

KOH = potassium hydroxide.

for VVC should be examined and evaluated. They only recommend self-diagnosis in compliant women with multiple confirmed prior cases of VVC who report the same symptoms. They further recommend that if these individuals fail to improve on a short course of therapy, they be evaluated for a further diagnosis.[11] Therefore, in most instances the diagnosis should be based on both clinical presentation and investigations, including vaginal pH, saline microscopy, and 10% potassium hydroxide (KOH) microscopy. The vaginal pH remains normal in VVC, and microscopic investigations should detect blastospores or pseudohyphae. *Candida* cultures usually are not required in the diagnosis of uncomplicated VVC; however, they are recommended when an individual presents with classic signs and symptoms of VVC, has a normal vaginal pH, but microscopy is inconclusive or recurrence is suspected.[6]

TREATMENT

■ GOALS OF THERAPY

The goal of therapy is complete resolution of symptoms in patients who have symptomatic VVC. A test of the cure is not necessary if symptoms resolve.[6] Antimycotic agents used in the treatment of VVC do not meet the definition of being fungicidal agents because of their slower killing rate. At the end of therapy, the number of viable organisms drops below the detectable range. However, by 6 weeks after a course of therapy, 25% to 40% of women will have positive yeast cultures and remain asymptomatic.[1] Asymptomatic colonization with *Candida* species does not require therapy.

■ GENERAL APPROACHES TO TREATMENT

The approach to therapy is to remove or improve any predisposing factors if they can be identified. A pharmacologic agent should have limited local and systemic side effects, a high cure rate, and easy administration. Additionally, it would be advantageous to use a therapy that is able to resolve symptoms within 24 hours, that has broad antimycotic activity (to cover increasing rates on non–*C. albicans* species), that prevents recurrence, and that can be used over a shortened period of time, such as 1 to 3 days. Many topical azoles are available without a prescription, and although this may increase public access to these medications, there is concern that having them available without a prescription may lead to inappropriate use. A study conducted using 10 actors as simulated paients who visited 60 pharmacies found that vaginal antifungals were more likely to be supplied to appropriate individuals as more information was exchanged, if interactions involved a pharmacist, and if questions regarding specific symptoms were used.[12]

Patients should be advised to avoid harsh soaps and perfumes that can cause or worsen vulvar irritation. The genital area must be kept clean and dry by avoiding constrictive clothing and frequent or prolonged exposure to hot tub use.[3] Douching is not recommended for either prevention or treatment.[11] Cool baths can soothe the skin.[3] Daily ingestion of 240 mL yogurt containing *Lactobacillus acidophilus* has been shown to decrease colonization and symptomatic infections of VVC in women with recurrent infections.[13]

Treatment of VVC will be considered to have positive outcomes if the symptoms of VVC are resolved within 24 to 48 hours and no adverse medication events are experienced. Self-assessment of symptom relief is appropriate for most cases of VVC. If symptoms remain unresolved or recur, then further testing and treatment can be required.

■ PHARMACOLOGIC TREATMENTS

Uncomplicated Vulvovaginal Candidiasis

Cure rates for uncomplicated VVC are between 80% and 95% with topical or oral azoles and between 70% and 90% with nystatin preparations. Table 129–2 lists available topical and oral preparations for the treatment of uncomplicated VVC. There are many topical nonprescription preparations for the treatment of VVC. No significant differences in in vitro activity or clinical efficacy exist between the topical azole agents.[1,3,6,11] The selection of a topical azole should be based primarily on an individual patient's preference as to product formulation. Some topical products can cause vaginal burning, stinging, or irritation; conversely, the vehicle used in topical creams or gels can provide initial symptomatic relief.[1] Of note, most topical preparations can decrease the efficacy of latex condoms and diaphragms.

Oral azoles have been used in the treatment of VVC. Patients may prefer oral therapy because of its convenience.[14] Oral and topical therapy are therapeutically equivalent.[1] A Cochrane review of 19 trials analyzing 22 oral versus topical antifungal comparisons concluded that there were no differences between the routes in short-term mycologic cure rates. There was a significant difference between long-term cure rates in favor of long-term follow-up; however, the authors stated that the clinical significance of this finding is uncertain.[15]

In the treatment of uncomplicated VVC, the duration of therapy is not critical. Cure rates with different lengths of treatment have not demonstrated that one therapy is significantly better.[14,15,16] Shorter-duration therapies (e.g., clotrimazole 1-day therapy) consist of higher concentrations of azoles that maintain the local therapeutic effect for up to 72 hours and allow for resolution of signs and symptoms.[17] A review of 14 trials that examined 1-day treatments showed less than 7% difference in short-term cure rates or improvement between any two treatments in any two studies and no significant differences in short- or long-term clinical cure rates among 1-day regimens.[16] Table 129–2 lists the therapeutic options for the treatment of uncomplicated VVC.

Complicated Vulvovaginal Candidiasis

Complicated VVC occurs in patients who are immunocompromised or have uncontrolled diabetes mellitus.[1] These individuals need a more aggressive treatment plan.[11] Current recommendations are to lengthen therapy to 10 to 14 days regardless of the route of administration.[11] Therapeutic options include those listed in Table 129–2; however, regimens should be continued for 10 to 14 days. A study of oral fluconazole therapy in women with complicated VVC demonstrated that cure rates increased from 67% with single-dose therapy to 80% when the 150 mg dose of fluconazole was repeated 72 hours after the initial dose.[18]

VVC during pregnancy can be considered complicated because consideration of host factors such as hormonal changes that can affect normal flora are essential in selecting therapeutic regimens. Topical agents are considered to be safe throughout pregnancy. A systematic review of 10 trials demonstrated that imidazole topical agents were more effective than nystatin. Two of the trials showed that treatment for 7 days was more effective than treatments of 4 days or less.[19] Oral agents are contraindicated in pregnancy because of the concern for fetal complications. A prospective assessment of pregnancy outcomes in 226 women exposed to fluconazole in the first trimester did not indicate increased risk of congenital abnormalities or other adverse outcomes.[20] The median dose of fluconazole was 200 mg, with 46.5% of the cohort receiving a single dose of fluconazole 150 mg.[21] However, the ACOG recommends avoiding oral therapy, as larger doses of fluconazole have been linked to birth defects.[21] Instead, the ACOG recommends a topical imidazole therapy for 7 days.[11]

Recurrent Vulvovaginal Candidiasis

Recurrent vulvovaginal candidiasis (RVVC) is defined as having more than four episodes of VVC within a 12-month period.[1,6] Fewer than 5% of women develop RVVC, and its pathogenesis is poorly understood. A proper diagnosis should be obtained to rule out other infections or nonmycotic contact dermatitis. RVVC is best treated in two stages: an initial intensive stage followed by prolonged antifungal therapy to achieve mycologic remission. This was demonstrated in a randomized controlled trial in which women were assigned to receive 150 mg fluconazole daily for 10 days followed by 6 months of either fluconazole 150 mg weekly or placebo. Ninety percent of women receiving both active treatments were symptom free for the 6 months following initial treatment (during the weekly fluconazole therapy), and there were 50% fewer symptomatic episodes in the 6 months following weekly suppressive therapy.[22] The Infectious Diseases Society of America stated that there is good evidence from more than one properly randomized controlled trial to recommend 10 to 14 days of induction therapy with a topical or oral azole, followed by 150 mg of fluconazole once weekly for 6 months for recurring *Candida* VVC.[23]

TABLE 129-2	Treatment for Uncomplicated Vulvovaginal Candidiasis	
Active Ingredient	**Preparation**	**Regimen**
Over-the-counter/topical vaginal products		
Butoconazole	2% cream	One applicator × 3 days
Clotrimazole	1% cream	One applicator × 1 day
	100 mg tablet	One 100 mg tablet × 7 days
	2% cream	One applicator × 1 day
	200 mg tablet	One 200 mg tablet × 3 days
	10% cream	One applicator × 1 day
	500 mg tablet	One 500 mg tablet × 1 day
Miconazole[a]	2% cream	One applicator × 1 day
	100 mg suppository	One 100 mg suppository × 7 days
	200 mg suppository	One 200 mg suppository × 3 days
	1200-mg ovule	One ovule × 1 day
Ticonazole	2% cream	One applicator × 3 days
	6.5% cream	One applicator × 1 day
Prescription/topical		
Nystatin	100,000-unit tablet	One tablet × 14 days
Terconazole	0.4% cream	One applicator × 7 days
	0.8% cream	One applicator × 3 days
Oral products		
Fluconazole	150 mg	One tablet × 1 day

[a]The FDA warns of the possible increase in the anticoagulant effects of warfarin with concomitant use.

Antifungal-Resistant Vulvovaginal Candidiasis

Resistance to azole antifungals should be considered in individuals who have persistently positive yeast cultures and fail to respond to therapy despite adherence to prescribed regimens.[1] These infections can be treated with boric acid or 5-flucytosine.[24,25] Boric acid is administered as a 600 mg intravaginal capsule daily for 14 days of induction therapy, followed by a maintenance regimen of one capsule intravaginally twice weekly. Boric acid should not be administered orally, as it is toxic. 5-Flucytosine cream is administered vaginally, 1,000 mg inserted nightly for 7 days. The prevalence of *C. glabrata* is higher in those with diabetes. In a study of 111 consecutive diabetic patients with VVC, 68% had isolates for *C. glabrata* compared with 28.8% for *C. albicans*. Those with *C. glabrata* had significantly higher mycological cure rates with 600 mg of boric acid suppositories for 14 days compared with a single dose of fluconazole 150 mg.[26]

OROPHARYNGEAL AND ESOPHAGEAL CANDIDIASIS

Oropharyngeal candidiasis (OPC), or *thrush,* refers to an infection of the oral mucosa. *Candida* is responsible for the majority of oral fungal infections, and *C. albicans* is the principal species causing the infection, commonly referred to as *candidiasis* (the proper but less commonly used term being *candidosis*). The infection may extend into the esophagus, causing esophageal candidiasis.

MICROBIOLOGY AND EPIDEMIOLOGY

Candida species are normal inhabitants of the human GI tract. They can be isolated from the oral cavity in up to 65% of healthy adults without producing any signs or symptoms.[27] This is referred to as *asymptomatic colonization*. The incidence of candidal carriage is increased under immunocompromised conditions, and the organism is capable of rapid conversion to a pathogen causing symptomatic mucosal infections. In HIV-infected individuals, asymptomatic colonization may be as high as 88%.[28] *C. albicans* is the predominant colonizing *Candida* species (70% to 80%), but any of the non–*C. albicans* species can be colonizers. Colonization rates are influenced by the severity and nature of the underlying medical illness and the duration of hospitalization, as well as age (highest in infants younger than 18 months of age and in adults older than 60 years of age). A variety of host and exogenous factors (Table 129–3) can lead to the transformation of asymptomatic colonization to symptomatic disease, such as oropharyngeal and esophageal candidiasis. *C. albicans* is the most common species causing all forms of mucosal candidiasis in humans. Less frequently, non–*C. albicans* species can be pathogenic and cause disease. These include *C. glabrata, Candida tropicalis, Candida krusei, Candida guilliermondii,* and *Candida parapsilosis*.[29,30] *C. krusei,* although relatively uncommon, generally is recovered from mucosal surfaces of neutropenic patients with hematologic malignancies.[29] Another species, *Candida dubliniesis,* has been identified in both HIV-infected and -noninfected patients, and may cause ~15% of infections previously ascribed to *C. albicans*.[29] In patients with cancer, non–*C. albicans* species account for almost half of all *Candida* infections.

Oropharyngeal candidiasis is the most common opportunistic infection in patients with HIV disease, and it may be the first clinical manifestation of the HIV infection in the majority of untreated patients. OPC occurs in 50% to 90% of HIV-infected patients at some point during the progressive course of the disease to acquired immunodeficiency syndrome (AIDS),[27,28,30] although significant reductions in the incidence have been observed after the introduction of highly active antiretroviral therapy (HAART). The incidence of OPC increases as the level of immunity decreases, especially when the CD4 T-cell counts are between 500 and 200 cells/mm[3] and is further increased when the CD4 T-cell counts drop below 200 cells/mm[3].[27] OPC is considered one of the earliest indicators of HIV infection and is a relatively reliable indirect marker of disease progression. Regardless of the CD4 T-cell count, OPC is predictive for the development of AIDS-related illnesses if left untreated.[27,30] In non-HIV diseases, such as cancer, the incidence of OPC varies depending on the type of malignant neoplastic disease, level of immune suppression, and type and duration of treatment, but it is less common than in HIV-infected patients. OPC was initially reported in ~25% of patients with solid tumors and up to 60% in those with hematologic malignancies or bone marrow transplant recipients.[31] Current rates of OPC have decreased significantly in these patients because of widespread use of antifungal prophylaxis.

OPC can predispose patients to develop more invasive disease, including esophageal candidiasis.[30] The esophagus is the second most common site of GI candidiasis. The prevalence of esophageal candidiasis has increased mainly because of the number of individuals with AIDS, as well as the increased numbers of other severely immunocompromised patients, especially those with hematologic malignancies.[29] Esophageal candidiasis is the first opportunistic infection in 3% to 10% of HIV-infected patients and is the second most common AIDS-defining disease after *Pneumocystis jiroveci* pneumonia.[30] The mean incidence of esophageal candidiasis among HIV-infected patients is less than OPC and ranges from 15% to 20%.[30] The risk of esophageal candidiasis is increased in HIV-infected patients when the CD4 T-cell count has dropped below 100 to 200 cells/mm[3], as well as in those with OPC.[32,33] However, the absence of OPC does not necessarily exclude the possibility of esophageal disease. Like OPC, the presence of esophageal candidiasis can help predict HIV disease progression and prognosis.[30] The incidence of esophageal candidiasis in non-HIV-infected immunocompromised patients is not well established. *C. albicans* is the most common cause of esophageal candidiasis, accounting for ~80% of cases, with the rest being caused by non–*C. albicans* species.[29,30]

The epidemiology of mucosal candidiasis has been affected by two factors. The introduction of HAART appears to have resulted in a significant decline in the incidence of OPC and esophageal candidiasis.[27,28] This is postulated to be caused both by enhanced immune responsiveness and by direct action on the organism by HAART.[28] The widespread use of the azole agents has led to a decline in the prevalence of mucosal candidiasis while leading to the emergence of refractory infections that have become difficult to treat.

PATHOGENESIS AND HOST DEFENSES

The pathogenesis of OPC is most clearly elucidated in the setting of HIV infection. There appear to be several levels of immune defense against the development of OPC in HIV-infected persons, and they involve both systemic and local immunity. The primary line of host defense against *C. albicans* is cell-mediated immunity (CMI) at the mucosal surfaces, which is mediated by CD4 T cells.[27] The efficacy of the CD4 T cells is reduced when the number of cells drops below

TABLE 129-3 Risk Factors for the Development of Oropharyngeal and/or Esophageal Candidiasis

Local factors	Potential mechanisms
Use of steroids and antibiotics	Suppression of cellular immunity and inhibition of phagocytosis by steroids, including chronic use of inhaled and topical steroids
	Alteration of endogenous oral flora by broad-spectrum antibiotics, especially when used with steroids, creates a milieu for proliferation of *Candida* species because of reduced environmental and nutritional competition
Dentures	Enhanced adherence of *Candida* species to the acrylic material of dentures, reduced saliva flow under surfaces of denture fittings, improperly fitted dentures, and poor oral hygiene provide a milieu conducive to the survival of microorganisms
Xerostomia caused by drugs (e.g., tricyclic antidepressants and phenothiazine), chemotherapy, radiotherapy to the head/neck, and various diseases (e.g., Sjögren syndrome, HIV, and cancer of the head/neck), as well as bone marrow transplant recipients	Reduced dilutional and cleansing effect caused by low secretion rate and low pH in saliva: saliva and mucosa secretions have defense factors, such as lactoferrin, sialoperoxidase, isozyme, histidine-rich polypeptide, secretory IgA antibodies, specific anti-*Candida* antibodies that help prevent adhesion and overgrowth of *Candida* species
Smoking	
Disruption of oral mucosa caused by chemotherapy and radiotherapy, ulcers, endotracheal intubation trauma, and burns	Oral mucositis induced by radiation and breaks in the physical barrier of the oral epithelium, which is protective against invasion by microorganisms; altered rate of mucosa regeneration by cancer chemotherapy, which increases vulnerability to infection.
Systemic factors	**Potential mechanisms**
Drugs (e.g., cytotoxic agents, corticosteroids, and immunosuppressants after organ transplant), omeprazole, and environmental chemicals (e.g., benzene and pesticides)	Reduced immunity because of drug-induced neutropenia or cell-mediated immunity; potent inhibition of gastric acid by PPIs can facilitate the growth of *Candida* species; PPIs also can inhibit the cytotoxic effect of lymphocytes and reduce salivary secretion
Neonates or the elderly	Immature immune system of neonates who usually acquire infection during birth to a mother with vaginal candidiasis or from exposure to infected bottle nipples or to skin of adult caregiver
	Elderly—unclear if this is the direct effect of age per se or contribution from dentures or underlying comorbidity
HIV infection/AIDS	Depletion of CD4 T lymphocytes especially below 200–300 cells/mm^3; anti-*Candida* protective mechanism of T lymphocytes at a mucosal level is unclear but can be caused by altered cytokines, especially interferon-γ, that inhibit transformation of *Candida* blastoconidia to the more invasive hyphal phase
Diabetes	Higher than normal numbers of *Candida albicans* cultured from saliva of diabetic patients; can be related to the elevated glucose levels and reduced chemotactic factor in saliva, altered neutrophil function, and reduced saliva volume and flow
Malignancies (e.g., leukemia and head/neck cancer)	Use of intensive radiotherapy and chemotherapy can disrupt oral mucosa and cause xerostomia; prolonged use of broad-spectrum antibiotics in neutropenic patients can alter the normal oral flora; because of the prolonged neutropenia, the principal immune defect, seen especially in leukemic patients, the initial oropharyngeal candidiasis can become systemic or invasive
Nutritional deficiencies (e.g., iron, folate, and vitamins B$_1$, B$_2$, B$_6$, B$_{12}$, and C)	Can be related to dietary restriction or GI absorption problems; deficiencies can serve to enhance the pathogenic potential of the *Candida* inhabitants, alter host defense mechanisms, or change epithelial barrier integrity

AIDs = acquired immunodeficiency syndrome, GI = gastrointestinal, HIV = human immunodeficiency virus, IgA = immunoglobulin A, PPI = proton pump inhibitor.

a protective threshold, and protection against infection becomes dependent on secondary or local immune mechanisms.[27,28] When the number of CD4 T cells drops too low, recruitment of these cells to the oral cavity is impaired. The CD4 T-cell count has been considered as the hallmark predictor for development of OPC. However, HIV viral load may have a stronger association with OPC than CD4 cell number.[34] This requires further confirmation by larger cohort studies. The possibility that HIV plays a strong role in susceptibility to infection is supported clinically by the observation that OPC is more common in HIV-infected persons than in those with similar immunosuppression, such as lymphoma and bone marrow transplant. When the primary line of defense fails, the secondary host defenses become crucial. These include the CD8 T cells, salivary cytokines, and other innate immune cells, such as the neutrophils, macrophages, and epithelial cells (with anti-*Candida* activity). Deficiencies or dysfunction in any of these can result in susceptibility to OPC. The problem with the CD8 T cells is caused more by a dysfunction of the microenvironment, specifically, reduction in the E-cadherin adhesion molecule that promotes migration of the cells through mucosal tissues.[28] The role of humoral immunity by antibodies as a protective mechanism is unclear and controversial. The changeover of the role of *Candida* species from commensal to pathogenic in the human host usually occurs when breakdown in these host defenses occurs. The pathogenesis of OPC is still not completely understood. It is important to develop a better understanding of the pathogenesis and role of host defenses, including

the mechanism of CD8 T-cell activity, reduced adhesion molecules, and whether other cofactors, such as HIV viral load, HAART, and injection drug use (IDU), play a role. Immunotherapeutic modalities can then be developed to eliminate the susceptibility factors and significantly reduce OPC in the at-risk populations.

Significant differences exist in the virulence among *Candida* species in mucosal candidiasis. One virulence factor is the ability of the organism to adapt and survive in response to changes in the host environment.[29] The genes required for virulence are regulated in response to the environmental signals indigenous to the host environment (e.g., temperature, pH, osmotic pressure, iron and calcium ion concentrations, oxygenation, and carbon and nitrogen availability). The ability of *C. albicans* to undergo reversible morphologic transition between the budding pseudohyphal and the more invasive hyphal growth forms is also a determinant of virulence, and genes are recognized to play a role.[29] Other virulence factors are the adhesive ability of *C. albicans* to epithelial cells and proteins and its ability to invade host cells by means of phospholipase and proteinase enzymes. This may be one of the factors leading to OPC in non-HIV-infected individuals. Other components of the pathogenesis in the absence of HIV that have been postulated are the ability of the *Candida* species to adhere to buccal epithelial cells. A close correlation between adhesion of *Candida* species and their ability to cause infection has been demonstrated in animal model studies.[35] This is hypothesized to be a key element in the development of OPC in patients with altered microflora, including those receiving broad-spectrum antimicrobial therapy.

TABLE 129-4 Clinical Classification of Oropharyngeal Candidiasis

Types	Population at Risk	Clinical Signs and Appearance
Pseudomembranous (thrush)	Neonates, patients with HIV or cancer, the debilitated elderly, patients on broad-spectrum antibiotics or steroid inhalers, patients with dry mouth from various causes, and smokers	Classic "cottage cheese" appearance, yellowish white, soft plaques (or milk curds) overlying areas of erythema on the buccal mucosa, tongue, gums, and throat; plaques are easily removed by vigorous rubbing but can leave red or bleeding sites when removed; lesions on the tongue dorsum give it a bald, depapillated appearance
Erythematous (acute atrophic)	Patients with HIV, patients on broad-spectrum antibiotics or steroid inhalers	Sensitive and painful erythematous mucosa with few, if any, white plaques; lesions are generally on the dorsal surface of the tongue or the hard palate, occasionally on the soft palate, but any part of the mucosa can be involved; appear as flat red patches on the palate or atrophic patches on the tongue dorsum with loss of papillae
Hyperplastic (candidal leukoplakia)	Smokers; uncommon in patients with HIV	Thick white and adherent keratotic plaques commonly seen on the buccal mucosa and lateral border of the tongue; can also be seen on the lips and the bottom of the mouth; plaques cannot be easily scraped off or only partially removed; this condition is distinct from oral hairy leukoplakia, and it can progress to severe dysplasia or malignancy
Angular cheilitis	Patients with HIV, denture wearers	Painful red, ulcerative, cracking, or fissuring lesion at one or both corners of the mouth because of an inflammatory reaction; usually lesions are small and rather punctate, but occasionally they can extend in a linear fashion from the angles onto the facial skin
Denture stomatitis (chronic atrophic)	Denture wearers who tend to be elderly and have poor oral hygiene	Red, flat lesions on the mucosa beneath the denture and extend right up to the denture border; more commonly located beneath a maxillary denture, although they can be encountered beneath a mandibular denture

HIV = human immunodeficiency virus.

RISK FACTORS

❹ Several host and exogenous factors contribute to the ability of *Candida* species to cause infection (see Table 129–3). Local and systemic factors, as well as characteristics of the organism itself, can increase the susceptibility of an individual to *Candida* infections.[27,29,31] Endocrine disorders besides diabetes mellitus, such as hypothyroidism, hypoparathyroidism, and hypoadrenalism, also can predispose patients to *Candida* species overgrowth. Patients with primary immune deficiencies such as lymphocytic abnormalities, phagocytic dysfunction, immunoglobulin A (IgA) deficiency, viral-induced immune paralysis, and severe congenital immunodeficiencies are also at risk for oropharyngeal candidiasis as well as disseminated candidiasis. Oral mucosal disease, such as lichen planus, can be preexistent causes of candidiasis. Smoking has been suggested as a predisposing risk factor. In many cases, multiple concurrent predisposing factors to candidiasis can exist, for example, xerostomia with mucositis and a break in the epithelial surface or immunosuppression, such as might occur in a leukemic patient receiving radiation and chemotherapy. The severity and extent of *Candida* infections increase with the number and severity of predisposing risk factors.

CLINICAL PRESENTATION AND DIAGNOSIS

Oropharyngeal candidiasis can manifest in several major forms (Table 129–4).[27,29,31] The clinical signs and symptoms of OPC and the locations of the lesions can be quite diverse (Table 129–5). A presumptive diagnosis of OPC usually is made by the characteristic appearance on the oral mucosa, with resolution of signs and symptoms after antifungal therapy. Pseudomembranous candidiasis, commonly known as *oral thrush*, is the classic and most common

TABLE 129-5 Clinical Presentation of Oropharyngeal and Esophageal Candidiasis

Oropharyngeal Candidiasis	Esophageal Candidiasis
General	**General**
The clinical features can be quite diverse (see Table 129–4)	This usually occurs as an extension of OPC; however, the esophagus can be the only site involved; the distal two-thirds, rather than the proximal one-third, is the most common site
Symptoms	**Symptoms**
Symptoms are diverse and range from none to sore, painful mouth, burning tongue, metallic taste, and dysphagia and odynophagia with involvement of the hypopharynx	Typically, the symptoms are dysphagia, odynophagia, and retrosternal chest pain but can be asymptomatic in some patients; although rare, epigastric pain can be the dominant symptom
Signs	**Signs**
Signs are variable and can include diffuse erythema and white patches on the surfaces of the buccal mucosa, throat, tongue, or gums; constitutional signs are absent	Constitutional signs, including fever, occasionally occur; physical findings can range from a few to numerous white or beige plaques of variable size
Laboratory tests	Plaques can be hyperemic or edematous, with ulceration in more severe cases
Scraping of an active lesion for microscopic examination can help confirm the diagnosis (presence of pseudohyphae and budding yeast) but is usually not necessary	Most advanced cases can occur with increased mucosal friability and narrowing of lumen
Cultures are not necessary because isolation of *Candida* species does not distinguish between colonization and true infection; cultures can be taken in patients responding poorly to therapy to determine the infecting species and to predict likely drug resistance	Uncommon complications include perforation and aortic–esophageal fistula formation
	Laboratory tests
	The best test is upper GI endoscopy (more useful than barium swallow); helps exclude other causes of esophagitis (e.g., viral, aphthous ulcers); diagnosis is confirmed by the histologic presence of *Candida* species in biopsy lesions taken during endoscopy
	Cultures to look for drug-resistant *Candida* species are warranted in patients who require endoscopy

GI = gastrointestinal, OPC = oropharyngeal candidiasis.

form seen in immunosuppressed and immunocompetent hosts. Erythematous and hyperplastic candidiasis and angular cheilitis occur less commonly in the HIV-infected population. Dysphagia, odynophagia, and retrosternal chest pain are common complaints of esophageal candidiasis, which is usually, but not always, accompanied by the presence of OPC. Clinical symptomatology, along with a therapeutic trial of antifungal, can provide a reliable presumptive diagnosis of esophageal candidiasis. If antifungal therapy does not lead to resolution, more invasive tests such as upper GI endoscopy can be undertaken.

TREATMENT

Oropharyngeal and Esophageal Candidiasis

■ DESIRED OUTCOMES

The primary desired outcome in the management of OPC is a clinical cure, that is, elimination of clinical signs and symptoms. Even when the patient is relatively asymptomatic, it is important to treat the initial episode of OPC to avoid progression to more extensive disease. In the most severe cases, the patient's quality of life can be impaired; this can result in decreased fluid and nutritional intake. Lack of appropriate treatment of OPC can lead to more extensive oral disease, especially in patients who are immunocompromised. The most serious complication of untreated OPC is extension of the infection to esophageal candidiasis. Because esophageal candidiasis is more debilitating, the patient's quality of life is more affected. It is important to initiate appropriate antifungal therapy for both OPC and esophageal candidiasis. Preventing or minimizing the number of future recurrences of both types of candidiasis is an equally important outcome. The approach depends largely on the underlying predisposing conditions. Mycologic cure is not a necessary treatment outcome because it may not be feasible or realistic, given that *Candida* species exist commonly as part of the normal mouth flora.

Minimizing toxicities and drug–drug interactions of systemic antifungal agents, as well as maximizing adherence by ensuring that the patient understands the importance of therapy and the directions to take the medication appropriately, are important secondary outcomes of therapy.

■ GENERAL APPROACH TO TREATMENT

The management of OPC should be individualized for each patient, taking into consideration the underlying immune status, other concurrent mucosal and medical diseases, concomitant medications, and exogenous infectious sources. In HIV-infected patients with inadequately controlled disease, antifungal treatment produces only a transient clinical response, and the relapse rates are higher than in other patient populations. These patients usually require frequent courses of antifungal treatment. Therefore, in patients with HIV disease, treatment with effective HAART is paramount because this would provide the best prophylaxis against recolonization and recurrence of symptoms.[29,31,33]

Whenever feasible, it is desirable to minimize all predisposing factors, such as administration of corticosteroids, chemotherapeutic agents, and antimicrobials, as well as institute proper oral hygiene and resolve concurrent conditions, such as denture stomatitis. Selection of an appropriate antifungal agent for treatment of candidiasis requires consideration of several factors, including the patient's drug adherence, adequate saliva for dissolution of

solid topical medications, risk of caries from sucrose- or dextrose-containing preparations, potential drug interactions, coexisting medical conditions (e.g., liver disease), location and severity of the infection, and the need for long-term maintenance therapy. Another factor that could affect drug selection is overuse of fluconazole, leading to the emergence of fluconazole-resistant species of *C. albicans,* and in some cases to all azoles, and other intrinsically more resistant species, such as *C. krusei, C. glabrata,* and *C. tropicalis.*

❺ Topical therapies should be the first choice for milder forms of infections.[37] The efficacy of antifungal agents for OPC varies in different patient populations. Until the polyene antifungal agents became available in the 1950s, gentian violet, an aniline dye, was used to treat OPC. Problems with gentian violet include fungal resistance, skin irritation, and especially the unaesthetic staining of the oral mucosa. Topical agents, such as nystatin and clotrimazole, have been the standard of treatment for uncomplicated OPC and generally are effective for treatment in otherwise healthy adults and infants with no underlying immunodeficiencies. Topical agents are available in an assortment of formulations, including oral rinses (suspension), troches, powder, vaginal tablets, and creams. The two most common types of formulations currently used are suspension and troches (Table 129–6).

Topical agents require frequent applications because of the short contact time with the oral mucosa; the ideal contact time is 20 to 30 minutes. Sufficient saliva is needed to dissolve clotrimazole troches, and this can be problematic for patients with xerostomia. Also, the rough surface of the tablet can become irritating to the oral soft tissue. Troches also contain dextrose, which has cariogenic potential. Nystatin suspension might be a better choice for patients with xerostomia, but it is difficult to maintain adequate contact time with the oral mucosa. Some patients complain of the unpleasant taste of nystatin, which can cause nausea and vomiting; this is especially problematic in cancer patients experiencing chemotherapy-induced nausea. The high sucrose content of nystatin suspension is cariogenic in dentate patients, and it should be used with caution in diabetic patients. Topical creams, such as clotrimazole, ketoconazole, miconazole, and nystatin (usually mixed with a steroid), are more appropriate for application three times daily to the corners of the mouth in treating angular cheilitis.[38]

Systemic therapy is necessary in patients with OPC that is refractory to topical treatment, those who cannot tolerate topical agents, moderate to severe disease, and those at high risk for disseminated systemic or invasive candidiasis. Effective treatment of esophageal candidiasis generally requires the use of systemic antifungal agents. However, these agents have the disadvantage of producing more side effects (see Table 129–6) and drug–drug interactions (see Chapter 130). Fluconazole is inexpensive and generally well tolerated, and its absorption is unaffected by food or gastric acidity. Ketoconazole requires gastric acidity for absorption, which can be problematic in AIDS patients with achlorhydria; hence, it is best given with an acidic beverage. It is not recommended today with the availability of more effective triazoles. Itraconazole capsules also have the same absorption problem and are no longer recommended. In contrast, itraconazole solution has enhanced absorption and is best taken in a fasting state; in addition, the solution provides the benefit of both topical effects to the oral mucosa and systemic effects and is beneficial to patients with mucositis or swallowing problems. Whenever possible, it is generally beneficial to limit the use of systemic azole agents to prevent unnecessary drug exposure and to minimize the potential for occurrence of drug-resistant candidiasis, particularly from fluconazole resistance.

When patients become unresponsive to topical agents or fluconazole and itraconazole, alternative agents are available.[32,33,37] These include amphotericin B and newer triazoles (voriconazole and

TABLE 129-6 Therapeutic Options for Mucosal Candidiasis

	Common/significant side effects
Initial episodes of OPC:[a] Treat for 7–14 days	**Common/significant side effects**
Clotrimazole 10 mg troche: hold 1 troche in mouth for 15–20 minutes for slow dissolution 5 times daily (B-2)	Altered taste, mild nausea, vomiting
Nystatin 100,000 units/mL suspension: 5 mL swish and swallow 4 times daily (B-2)	Mild nausea, vomiting, diarrhea
Fluconazole100 mg tablets:[b] 100–200 mg daily (A-1)	GI upset, hepatitis not common
Itraconazole 10 mg/mL solution:[c] 200 mg daily (A-2)	GI upset, not common: hepatotoxicity, CHF, pulmonary edema with long-term use[e]
Posaconazole 40 mg/mL suspension: 400 mg daily with a full meal (A-2)	GI upset, fever, headache, increased hepatic transaminases not common
Fluconazole-refractory OPC: Treat for ≥ 14 days	**Common/significant side effects**
Itraconazole 10 mg/mL solution: 200 mg daily (A-3)	See above
Voriconazole 200 mg tablets: 200 mg twice daily (>40 kg), taken on empty stomach (A-3)	GI upset, rash, reversible visual disturbance (altered light perception, photopsia, chromatopsia, photophobia), increased hepatic transaminases, hallucinations, or confusion
Posaconazole 40 mg/mL suspension: 400 mg twice daily × 3 days, then 400 mg daily × 28 days (A-2)	See above
Amphotericin B 100 mg/mL suspension:[d] 1–5 mL swish and swallow 4 times daily (B-2)	Oral: nausea, vomiting, diarrhea with higher dose
Amphotericin B deoxycholate 50 mg injection: 0.3–0.7 mg/kg/day IV daily (B-2)	IV: fever, chills, sweats, nephrotoxicity, electrolyte disturbances, bone marrow suppression
Caspofungin 50 mg IV daily (B-2)	Fever, headache, infusion-related reactions (<5%) (e.g., rash, facial swelling, pruritus, vasodilation), hypokalemia, increased hepatic transaminases, anemia, neutropenia
Micafungin 150 mg IV daily (B-2)	Similar to caspofungin
Anidulafungin 200 mg IV daily (B-2)	Similar to caspofungin
Esophageal candidiasis:[a] Treat for 14–21 days	**Common/significant side effects**
Fluconazole 100 mg tablets: 200–400 mg (3–6 mg/kg) daily (A-1)	See above
Echinocandin: see above (B-2)	See above
Amphotericin B deoxycholate 50 mg injection: 0.3–0.7 mg/kg/day IV daily (B-2)	See above
Posaconazole 40 mg/mL suspension: 400 mg twice daily (A-3)	See above
Itraconazole 10 mg/mL solution:[c] 200 mg daily (A-3)	See above
Voriconazole 200 mg tablets: 200 mg twice daily (>40 kg) (A-3)	See above
Voriconazole and echinocandins (A-1): generally reserved for refractory cases	See above
Fluconazole-refractory EC: Treat for 21–28 days	**Common/significant side effects**
Itraconazole 10 mg/mL solution: 200 mg daily. (A-2)	See above
Posaconazole 40 mg/mL suspension: 400 mg twice daily (A-3)	See above
Voriconazole 200 mg tablets: 200 mg twice daily (>40 kg), taken on empty stomach (A-3)	See above
Caspofungin 50 mg IV daily (B-2)	See above
Micafungin 150 mg IV daily (B-2)	Similar to caspofungin
Anidulafungin 100 mg IV on day 1, then 50 mg IV daily (B-2)	Similar to caspofungin
Amphotericin B deoxycholate: 0.3–0.7 mg/kg/day IV, or lipid-based amphotericin 3–5 mg/kg/day IV (B-2)	See above

CHF = congestive heart failure, GI = gastrointestinal, IV = intravenous.

[a]Initial episodes of OPC can be adequately treated first with topical agents before resorting to systemic therapy (B-2), but systemic therapy is required for effective treatment of esophageal candidiasis. (A-2) Suppressive therapy is recommended for patients with frequent or severe recurrences (A-1).

[b]Fluconazole is more effective than ketoconazole (A-1).

[c]Solution is more effective than capsule (A-1); solution is better taken on an empty stomach.

[d]Suspension is not marketed; can be prepared extemporaneously by pharmacy.[50]

[e]See discussion under onychomycosis.

Recommendation grades:

Strength of recommendation: **A**–Both strong evidence for efficacy and substantial clinical benefit to support recommendation for use. *Should always be offered.* **B**–Moderate evidence for efficacy but only limited clinical benefit, to support recommendation for use. *Should generally be offered.* **C**–Evidence for efficacy is insufficient to support recommendation for or against use; or evidence for efficacy might not outweigh adverse consequences or cost of the treatment under consideration. *Optional.* **D**–Moderate evidence for lack of efficacy or adverse outcome supports a recommendation against use. *Should generally not be offered.*

Quality of evidence: **1**–Evidence from at least one properly designed randomized, controlled trial. **2**–Evidence from at least one well-designed trial without randomization, from cohort or case-controlled analytic studies (preferably from more than one center), or from multiple time-series studies, or dramatic results from uncontrolled experiments. **3**–Evidence from opinions of respected authorities based on clinical experience, descriptive studies, or reports of expert committees. (UR) Evidence currently unrated.

posaconazole) and echinocandins (caspofungin, micafungin, and anidulafungin) (see discussion below).

Oropharyngeal Candidiasis: HIV-Infected Patients

It is appropriate to start therapy with topical agents for initial or recurrent episodes of OPC, provided that clinical symptoms are not severe and that there is minimal risk of esophageal involvement.[32,37] Clinical responses with the resolution of signs and symptoms generally occur within 5 to 7 days of initiating treatment. Clotrimazole appears to be the most effective topical agent and demonstrates comparable clinical response rates with both fluconazole and itraconazole.[30,33] However, topical therapy is associated with more frequent relapses than with fluconazole.[32,33] This may be of limited clinical significance in patients receiving effective HAART because of their decreased susceptibility to opportunistic infection. In practice, nystatin suspension is still used frequently in initial episodes of OPC, although it is the least effective agent and is associated with frequent treatment failures and early relapses, especially in patients with advanced HIV disease or neutropenia.[30,33]

Systemic oral azoles should be reserved for use in the more severe episodes of OPC unresponsive to topical agents or in patients with concurrent esophageal involvement.[30,32,33] In clinical practice, fluconazole usually is the systemic azole agent of choice because of its proven efficacy, favorable absorption, safety, and drug-interaction profiles, and it is relatively inexpensive. Fluconazole is superior to ketoconazole and itraconazole capsules.[30,32,33] Current guidelines suggest a regimen of 100 to 200 mg/day for 7 to 14 days.[37] There is evidence from one study showing a single dose of fluconazole 750 mg orally is as effective as fluconazole 150 mg orally for 14 days, which warrants further evaluation, given the potential advantages of adherence and cost-effectiveness.[38] Itraconazole oral solution with an improved absorption profile compared with the capsule formulation is as effective as fluconazole, with comparable clinical and mycologic response and relapse rates.[30,32,33] However, it carries a higher risk of drug interactions because it is a potent inhibitor of the cytochrome P450 enzymes, and it is associated with more nausea than fluconazole. Posaconazole is a new extended-spectrum triazole with potent in vitro activity against both *C. albicans* and non–*C. albicans* species. It is equivalent to fluconazole in terms of efficacy, safety, and tolerability.[37] Posaconazole has joined itraconazole solution and voriconazole as the azole alternatives to fluconazole in the management of moderate to severe OPC. Other agents that are effective are amphotericin B and the echinocandins (caspofungin, micafungin, and anidulafungin). They are better reserved for refractory OPC, however, because of their greater toxicity. They are also more expensive and are less convenient to use.

Oropharyngeal Candidiasis: Non-HIV-Infected Patients

This patient population includes patients with hematologic malignancy (e.g., leukemias) or blood and marrow transplantation (BMT) with a long duration of neutropenia and chronic graft-versus-host disease, patients with solid tumors, patients with solid-organ transplants who are receiving immunosuppressive therapy, and patients with diabetes mellitus, as well as patients on prolonged courses of antibiotics or corticosteroids and the debilitated elderly. Factors to consider in deciding whether to use topical or systemic antifungal therapy include the severity and extent of mucosal involvement (oropharyngeal vs esophageal), predisposing risk factors, and risk for dissemination. Patients who develop neutropenia (e.g., leukemic and BMT patients) are usually at high risk for disseminated and invasive fungal disease, and treatment of oral candidiasis is more aggressive. Patients with cell-mediated immune deficits but normal or near-normal granulocyte function and number (e.g., solid tumors, solid-organ transplants, or diabetic patients) are at low risk for dissemination of infection.

Specific antifungal therapy can be unnecessary for asymptomatic patients at relatively low risk for disseminated candidiasis, such as those who are not granulocytopenic or who are expected to have a short duration of granulocytopenia.[39] Many of these infections will clear spontaneously after recovery of the granulocytes or discontinuation of antibiotic and/or immunosuppressive therapy. However, antifungal therapy usually is required for patients who have persistent infection or significant symptoms, usually pain, or who are granulocytopenic with a relatively high risk of fungal dissemination. Topical agents first can be given a therapeutic trial depending on the severity of infection and the degree of immunosuppression. Although both nystatin and clotrimazole can be effective in treating OPC, nystatin suspension does not effectively reduce the incidence of either oropharyngeal or systemic *Candida* infections in immunocompromised patients receiving chemotherapy or radiation; its use often is associated with treatment failures and early relapses.[39,40] Clotrimazole appears to be more effective in reducing colonization and treating acute episodes in cancer patients who are immunocompromised.

Systemic azole agents are used for treating OPC in patients who have failed or who are unable to take topical therapy.[33,39]

The preceding discussion on the relative efficacy of fluconazole, itraconazole, and ketoconazole in HIV-infected patients can be extrapolated to the non-HIV-infected population. Fluconazole 100 to 200 mg daily is used more commonly because of more extensive experience with its use, and it is more effective and has a more favorable absorption and side effect profile compared with other available azoles.[30] If the oral route is not feasible for reasons such as severe chemotherapy-induced mucositis, fluconazole can be administered intravenously. In patients unresponsive to azoles, IV amphotericin B in relatively low doses of 0.1 to 0.3 mg/kg/day can be tried.[39] Because of the higher risk for dissemination in patients who are severely neutropenic ($<0.1 \times 10^9$ neutrophils/L) or clinically unstable (hypotensive or febrile), some clinicians prefer to initiate therapy with IV amphotericin B at 0.6 mg/kg/day, with therapy continued until the neutropenia has resolved.[39] The echinocandins caspofungin, micafungin, and anidulafungin have all been studied for the treatment of OPC and found to be effective, thus offering another option in the patient with refractory disease.[37]

Topical therapy with clotrimazole or nystatin for 7 days is usually adequate for treating mucocutaneous candidiasis in most solid-organ transplant patients.[36] Use of topical therapy will reduce the number of systemic drugs that these patients receive and hence minimize the risk of drug–drug interactions. Failure to respond to topical agents warrants the use of fluconazole. Low-dose amphotericin B solution as swish and swallow (100 mg/mL, 1 mL four times daily) for 7 to 10 days is reserved for the unusual cases of treatment failure.

Patients who develop OPC because of prolonged antibiotic use or aerosolized corticosteroids use can be managed successfully by discontinuation of the offending agent, and the infection usually will resolve. If there is a strong desire to treat because of discomfort or need to hasten symptom resolution or an inability to stop the offending agent, therapy with a topical agent, either clotrimazole or nystatin, is effective in most cases. The advantage of systemic azoles is the convenience of less frequent dosing. Symptoms usually improve in 3 or 4 days. Infants should be given smaller amounts more frequently (e.g., nystatin 100,000 units every 2–3 hours) to ensure better contact time. For denture-related OPC, or candidal stomatitis, effective therapy requires treatment of both the mouth and the dentures to avoid relapse. The dentures must be brushed vigorously and disinfected every night by soaking in antiseptic solution, such as chlorhexidine gluconate 0.25% or a product such as Polident or Efferdent.[31,33] Topical antifungal therapy of the oral cavity is required. Consistent proper oral hygiene and care of the dentures can help prevent relapse.

Esophageal Candidiasis: HIV-Infected Patients

⑥ Treatment of esophageal candidiasis has not been as well studied as OPC. Because of the significant morbidity of esophageal candidiasis and the absence of evidence supporting the efficacy of topical antifungals, treatment requires systemic antifungal agents.[32,33,37] Fluconazole is superior to ketoconazole and itraconazole capsules with respect to endoscopic cure and clinical response and usually produces a more rapid onset of action and resolution of symptoms.[30,32,33,37] Fluconazole is as effective as itraconazole solution, with reported response rates of >80% to 90%.[33] However itraconazole solution causes more nausea and drug interactions because of inhibition of the cytochrome P450 enzymes. Amphotericin B, voriconazole, posaconazole, and the echinocandins are also effective in esophageal candidiasis, but they are generally reserved for patients with advanced or inadequately controlled HIV disease where the candidiasis tends to recur or becomes refractory to azole therapy.[43–46]

Esophageal Candidiasis: Non–HIV-Infected Patients

As in the case of HIV-infected patients, treatment of esophageal candidiasis requires systemic therapy. Patients can be started on fluconazole 200 to 400 mg/day for 14 to 21 days.[37] Higher fluconazole doses (up to 400 mg/day) have been suggested for patients with severe symptoms or those who are neutropenic.[36] Other agents currently recommended if fluconazole is not an option are an echinocandin or amphotericin B at 0.3 to 0.7 mg/kg. Itraconazole solution, posaconazole, and voriconazole are effective alternatives that may be considered for those not responding adequately to fluconazole. An echinocandin or IV amphotericin B may be selected over fluconazole for initial therapy in neutropenic patients who present with severe symptoms or who are at high risk for dissemination of Candida species, such as those receiving other aggressive immunosuppressive therapy (e.g., corticosteroids, total-body irradiation, or antithymocyte globulin) and who have documented evidence of esophageal candidiasis or who have failed an initial empirical trial of oral nonabsorbable agents or systemic azoles.[40] Therapy should be continued until at least the neutropenia resolves. For patients whose symptoms have resolved and who are afebrile and clinically stable, therapy should be discontinued, and the patients should be monitored closely for infection recurrence. In high-risk patients, particularly those with persistent fever and neutropenia, the potential presence of clinically occult, diffuse GI or disseminated candidiasis should be considered. The echinocandins and newer azole agents (voriconazole and posaconazole) offer less toxic alternatives or oral agents and are preferred in patients who are intolerant of amphotericin B deoxycholate or who have preexisting renal impairment.[29,47,48] There are limited data on the clinical efficacy of anidulafungin compared with fluconazole, 95% versus 89% cure rates, respectively, in the non-HIV-infected patients.[49]

Antifungal-Refractory Oral Mucosal Candidiasis

Treatment failure is generally defined as persistence of signs and symptoms of OPC or esophageal candidiasis after an appropriate trial of antifungal therapy.[28] Treatment of refractory oral mucosal candidiasis is frequently unsatisfactory, and clinical response is usually short-lived, with rapid and periodic recurrences. The key risk factors for occurrence of refractory candidiasis are advanced stage of AIDS with low CD4 cell counts (<50 cells/mm^3) and repeated or prolonged courses of various systemic antifungal agents, in particular systemic azoles.[29,33,37] Frequent or prolonged use of fluconazole can be associated with fluconazole-refractory candidiasis because of selection of more resistant non–C. albicans species. An important initial management strategy is to assess and optimize the antiretroviral therapy of the patient with refractory OPC to help improve the immune function. With the widespread use of HAART, fluconazole-refractory OPC is now less commonly encountered. It is also important to identify and rectify potentially correctable causes of clinical failures of mucosal candidiasis, such as poor drug adherence, adequate dosing, reduced drug absorption associated with hypochlorhydria, and drug–drug interactions.

There have been few controlled studies that assess the effectiveness of antifungals. Doubling of the fluconazole dosage to 400 or 800 mg/day can be effective in some patients with infection caused by Candida species of intermediate resistance, although the response may be only transient.[29] Fluconazole oral suspension can be beneficial in some patients because of increased salivary concentrations obtained when the suspension is taken with the swish-and-swallow technique.[37] Patients with fluconazole-refractory mucosal candidiasis can be treated with itraconazole oral suspension because it can be effective in 64% to 80% of patients; however, the benefit is short-lived if chronic suppressive therapy is not maintained.[28,37] Posaconazole suspension has been reported to be successful in ~74% of patients with refractory oral or esophageal candidiasis; voriconazole may also be efficacious in these patients. Amphotericin B oral suspension is another alternative for azole-refractory patients.[32,37] It has broad-spectrum activity against many fungal species and low likelihood of Candida species resistance. There are limited data and experience on its use in immunosuppressed patients, and results from small studies have yielded mixed results.[50] Amphotericin B suspension is no longer available commercially in the United States, but it can be prepared extemporaneously by the pharmacy.[50]

Until recently, IV amphotericin B deoxycholate has been the alternative for patients with endoscopically proven disease who have failed fluconazole or itraconazole therapy.[29] Patients with severe disease unresponsive to other agents require IV amphotericin B 0.3 to 0.7 mg/kg/day for 7 to 10 days to achieve clinical response; higher dose or longer treatment duration can be needed in more severe disease.[29,32,33,37] After response, suppressive therapy with amphotericin B is required to increase disease-free intervals. Patients who fail to respond to amphotericin B and require >1 mg/kg/day might be candidates for liposomal amphotericin B preparations because of renal and/or bone marrow toxicities, although at a markedly higher cost. Flucytosine usually is not used as monotherapy because of rapid development of resistance but can be used in combination with an azole or amphotericin B.[29] Less toxic agents that are also effective are voriconazole and the echinocandins.[47–49] Voriconazole, a triazole antifungal available in both oral and IV preparations, appears to be as effective as fluconazole for esophageal candidiasis, and it has shown success in treatment of fluconazole-refractory disease.[46] However, voriconazole has more side effects and multiple pharmacokinetic drug interactions compared to fluconazole.[29,48] Caspofungin is the first of the echinocandins to be approved for esophageal candidiasis; more recently, micafungin and anidulafungin have been approved for this indication. All three echinocandins have similar efficacy and tolerability profile as fluconazole, although higher relapse has been reported with caspofungin and anidulafungin compared with fluconazole.[33,49] Because the echinocandins require IV administration and are expensive, they are primarily used in patients who are refractory to the triazoles or have serious triazole-related adverse effects. As a class, the echinocandins have a favorable adverse effect profile. They are less toxic than amphotericin B (see Table 129–6) and have less impact on the cytochrome P450 enzymes than either itraconazole or voriconazole. Immunmodulation with adjunctive granulocyte-macrophage colony-stimulating factor and interferon have been used for refractory oral candidiasis in very limited numbers of patients.[37]

Antifungal Prophylaxis

❼ Ensuring that the HIV-infected patient is receiving appropriate antiretroviral therapy to enhance the immune system is perhaps the most important measure in preventing future episodes of mucosal candidiasis (oropharyngeal, esophageal, and vulvovaginal).[33,37] Initial success of treatment often is followed by symptomatic recurrences, especially in patients with advanced or poorly controlled HIV disease. Long-term suppressive therapy with fluconazole is effective in preventing recurrences or new infections of OPC in AIDS and in patients with cancer.[33,37] However, the indications for antifungal prophylaxis and the best long-term management strategy still have not been well established. Fluconazole does not provide complete protection, and breakthrough infections can occur.[29] The reduced risk of recurrence of OPC also has not been demonstrated to improve survival. In addition, chronic exposure to azole therapy is a concern in that it might lead to the development of refractory disease or emergence of azole resistance.[33,37] However, in a randomized trial of continuous versus episodic fluconazole therapy, continuous therapy did not result in a higher rate of refractory OPC or esophageal disease.[49] Currently, HIV specialists do not recommend primary or secondary prophylaxis for OPC.[32] The rationale includes effectiveness of therapy for acute episodes of OPC, low incidence of serious invasive fungal disease, low mortality associated with mucosal candidiasis, potential for drug interactions, potential for emergence of drug resistance, and the prohibitive long-term cost of prophylaxis.

CLINICAL CONTROVERSY

The optimal strategy for the management of recurrent oral mucosal candidiasis is unclear. Specific criteria for use of secondary prophylaxis are not well defined, and a wide range of approaches can be seen in clinical practice.

❽ The decision to use secondary prophylaxis should be individualized for each patient. Secondary prophylaxis can be considered in patients with multiple recurrent episodes of symptomatic OPC or when the disease is sufficiently severe and affecting the quality of life.[32] Patients with a history of one or more episodes of documented esophageal candidiasis and a CD4 T-cell count still <200 cells/mm³ despite being on HAART are candidates for secondary prophylaxis. Fluconazole 100 mg daily is the usual regimen recommended for OPC and esophageal candidiasis,[32,33,37] although 200 mg three times weekly also appears to be effective.[51] Once-weekly fluconazole (200 mg) is also effective for preventing OPC recurrences in those with less advanced AIDS.[29] Itraconazole solution 200 mg daily is an alternative as suppressive therapy for OPC.[37]

Patients with malignant neoplastic diseases who are receiving irradiation, cytotoxic, and/or immunosuppressive therapy are at high risk for fungal infections in addition to bacterial and viral infections. Prophylaxis of *Candida* infection is controversial, and the results of studies have been conflicting and difficult to evaluate. In the hematopoietic stem cell transplant (HSCT) population, fluconazole prophylaxis is recommended prior to engraftment. Cross-resistance to other azoles may occur among *Candida* species; this should be a treatment consideration in a patient who develops a breakthrough fungal infection. Micafungin is an alternative to fluconazole prophylaxis of candidiasis.[52] The value of antifungal prophylaxis in these patients needs to be considered in the broader context of not only reducing colonization and the risk of superficial candidiasis but also, more importantly, reducing the risk for invasive candidiasis and improving survival. Management of these infections in this patient population is discussed further in Chapter 131.

CLINICAL CONTROVERSY

Several new antifungal agents, in both the triazole and echinocandin class, are now available for the treatment of oral mucosal candidiasis. Although they have demonstrated efficacy, their place in therapy remains to be defined. It is not established which specific agent should be used next after failing fluconazole or itraconazole, and current guidelines now suggest an echinocandin or amphotericin. Factors to consider in the selection can include the underlying clinical condition, the risk for drug, and side effect profiles.

TABLE 129-7	Patient Counseling Tips for Managing Oropharyngeal Candidiasis

1. Clean the oral cavity prior to administering the topical antifungal agent. Daily fluoride rinses can help reduce the risk of caries when using an agent containing sucrose or dextrose.
2. Use the topical antifungal agent after meals, as saliva flow and mouth movements can reduce the contact time.
3. Troches should be slowly dissolved in the mouth, not chewed or swallowed whole, over 15 to 30 minutes, and the saliva swallowed.
4. Suspension should be swished around the mouth in the oral cavity to cover all areas for as long as possible, ideally at least 1 minute, then gargled and swallowed.
5. Remove dentures while medication is being applied to the oral tissues.
6. Use a suspension instead of a troche if xerostomia is present; if a troche is preferred, the patient should rinse or drink water prior to dosing. For xerostomia, suggest nonpharmacologic measures for symptomatic relief (e.g., ice chips, sugarless gum or hard candy, citrus beverages).
7. Dentures should be removed and disinfected overnight using an antiseptic solution (e.g., chlorhexidine 0.12–0.2%). Disinfect oral tissues in addition to dental prosthesis.
8. Complete treatment course even though symptomatic improvement can occur in 48–72 hours.
9. Maintain good oral hygiene. Brush teeth daily (twice daily) and floss, rinse mouth, or brush teeth after eating sweets.
10. Stop smoking; avoid alcohol.

From Akpan A, Morgan R. Oral candidiasis. Postgrad Med J 2002;78:455–459.

EVALUATION OF THERAPEUTIC OUTCOMES

Efficacy end points for oropharyngeal and esophageal candidiasis include rapid relief of symptoms and prevention of complications without early relapse after completion of the course of therapy.[32,37] Sterilization of the oral cavity is not a feasible end point because mycologic eradication is rarely achievable, especially in HIV-positive patients. Symptomatic relief of presenting signs and symptoms (see Table 129–5) generally occurs within 48 to 72 hours of starting therapy, with complete resolution by 7 to 10 days. Patients should be advised about the time course and told to return for reassessment when signs and symptoms recur. It is usually unnecessary for the patient to be reassessed soon after finishing the treatment course. However, HIV patients should be questioned and examined for the occurrence of mucosal candidiasis as part of their regular follow-up. The frequency of monitoring can be more often in neutropenic patients because of concern for dissemination of candidiasis. During the period of neutropenia, temperature should be monitored daily, as well as signs of dissemination.

Efficacy of the antifungal agent is partly influenced by patient adherence to the medication regimen. Patients must be counseled on proper administration and dosing, in particular for topical agents (Table 129–7).[36] Safety end points include monitoring for occurrence of the relevant drug side effects and drug interactions (Table 129–6). Mild GI intolerance can occur with topical therapy, but serious adverse effects are rare. It is still prudent to monitor for hypersensitivity reactions, especially rash and pruritus, that might occur with any medication. GI intolerance is more associated with the oral azoles. Hepatotoxicity can occur when azole therapy is prolonged beyond 7 to 10 days or high doses are used. Periodic monitoring of liver enzymes (alanine transaminase and aspartate amino-transferase) should be considered, especially if prolonged therapy (longer than 21 days) is anticipated. Patients who are receiving IV amphotericin B require daily monitoring by the pharmacist.

MYCOTIC INFECTIONS OF THE SKIN, HAIR, AND NAILS

Superficial mycotic infections of the skin are referred to as *dermatophytoses*. They are common infections that usually are caused by dermatophytes classified by genera: *Trichophyton, Epidermophyton,* and *Microsporum*.[53] Dermatophytes have the ability to penetrate keratinous structures of the body. These infections affect both male and female genders and all races. Reservoirs of mycotic infections include humans, animals, and soil.[53] Individuals can develop an infection if they come in contact with a reservoir in addition to having a conducive environment for mycotic growth (i.e., moist conditions).[54] Risk factors for the development of an infection include prolonged exposure to sweaty clothes, failure to bathe regularly, many skinfolds, sedentariness, and confinement to bed.[54]

Mycotic infections of the skin have a classic appearance that consists of a central clearing surrounded by an advancing red, scaly, elevated border.[54] Infections of the nail can appear chalky and dull yellow or white and become brittle and crumbly.

Diagnosis usually is based on patient history, as well as the physical examination.[55] Diagnostic tests include direct microscopic examination of a specimen after the addition of KOH or fungal cultures. The KOH test is quick, inexpensive, and easy to perform, whereas cultures are more expensive and take longer to obtain results. Diagnostic tests are recommended when systemic therapy is likely to be prescribed.[55]

❾ A general approach to treatment of superficial mycotic infections includes keeping the infected area dry and clean and limiting exposure to the infected reservoir. Topical agents generally are considered to be first-line therapy for infections of the skin. Oral therapy is preferred when the infection is extensive or severe or when treating tinea capitis or onychomycosis.[56-58] Table 129–8 lists specific treatments for each mycotic infection. Superficial mycotic infections are categorized by the pattern and site of infection.[53] The most commonly occurring infections in North America are detailed in the following sections.

CLINICAL CONTROVERSY

Evidence for the treatment of superficial mycotic infections of the skin and hair comes from a small number of trials with relatively small numbers of subjects.

TINEA PEDIS

Tinea pedis is the most common dermatophytoses (affecting ~70% of adults). It is better known as "athlete's foot" and occurs in hot weather, with exposure to surface reservoirs (locker room floors), and with use of occlusive footwear.[54] Treatment with topical therapy for 2 to 4 weeks often is adequate for mild infections; however,

TABLE 129-8 Treatment of Mycoses of the Skin, Hair, and Nails

	Topical[a,b]	Oral[c]
Tinea pedis	Butenafine, daily	Fluconazole 150 mg 1 per week × 1–4 weeks
Tinea manuum	Ciclopirox, twice daily	Ketoconazole 200 mg daily × 4 weeks
Tinea cruris	Clotrimazole, twice daily	Itraconazole 200–400 mg/day × 1 week
Tinea corporis	Econazole, daily	Terbinafine 250 mg/day × 2 weeks
	Haloprogin, twice daily	
	Ketoconazole cream, daily	
	Miconazole, twice daily	
	Naftifine cream, daily; gel, twice daily	
	Oxiconazole, twice daily	
	Sulconazole, twice daily	
	Terbinafine, twice daily	
	Tolnaftate, twice daily	
	Triacetin cream, solution, 3 times daily	
	Undecylenic acid, various preparations: apply as directed	
Tinea capitis	Shampoo only in conjunction with oral therapy or for treatment of asymptomatic carriers	Terbinafine 250 mg/day × 4–8 weeks
Tinea barbae		Ketoconazole 200 mg daily × 4 weeks
	Ketoconazole 2 per week × 4 weeks	Itraconazole 100–200 mg/day × 4–6 weeks
	Selenium sulfide daily × 2 weeks	Griseofulvin 500 mg/day × 4–6 weeks
Pityriasis versicolor	Clotrimazole, twice daily	Ketoconazole
	Econazole, daily	
	Haloprogin, twice daily	
	Ketoconazole, daily	Fluconazole
	Miconazole, twice daily	
	Oxiconazole cream only, twice daily	Itraconazole 200 mg daily × 3–7 days
	Sulconazole, twice daily	
	Tolnaftate, three times daily	
Onychomycosis	Ciclopirox 8% nail lacquer: apply solution at night for up to 48 weeks	Terbinafine 250 mg/day × 6 weeks (finger), 12 weeks (toe)
Fingernail		Itraconazole 200 mg twice daily × 1 week per month; repeat for total of two pulses (finger) or three pulses (toe)
Toenail		Itraconazole 200 mg daily for 6 weeks (finger) or 12 weeks (toe)
		Fluconazole 50 mg daily or 300 mg once weekly for ≥6 months (finger) or 12 months (toe)

[a]Other products are available, including combination products.
[b]Length of therapy depends on mycotic sensitivity and severity of infection.
[c]Only capsule formulation studied; give with food for increased absorption.

severe infections or involvement of the nails requires oral therapy[54] (see Table 129–8). Recurrence of infection occurs in up to 70% of individuals. Prolonged treatment with either topical or systemic therapy may be required.[55,56]

TINEA MANUUM

Tinea manuum usually involves the palmar surface of the hands, is unilateral, and can involve the feet. Treatment of this infection is similar to tinea pedis (see Table 129–8). Emollients that contain lactic acid also can be useful.[54]

TINEA CRURIS

Tinea cruris is an infection of the proximal thighs and buttocks.[57] It is referred to as "jock itch" and is more common in males. The scrotum and penis often are spared from infection. Treatment with topical therapy is recommended and should continue for 1 to 2 weeks after symptom resolution. Severe infections can require oral therapy (see Table 129–8). Relief of pruritus and burning can be facilitated by the use of short-term (2 or 3 days) topical steroids (2.5% hydrocortisone).[54]

TINEA CORPORIS

Tinea corporis is an infection of the glabrous skin of the trunk and extremities.[57] Therapy is similar to that for tinea pedis, tinea manuum, and tinea cruris (see Table 129–8).

TINEA CAPITIS

Tinea capitis is a mycotic infection involving the scalp, hair follicles, and adjacent skin[58,59] that primarily affects children. Treatment should consist of oral therapy, as well as the cleaning of combs and brushes, which can be contaminated (see Table 129–8). Daily shampooing is recommended for removal of scales. Some children and adults can be asymptomatic carriers, thereby facilitating spread of the infection.[58] Family members who culture positive for Trichophyton tonsurans should be treated with an antifungal shampoo (e.g., ketoconazole, selenium sulfide, or povidone-iodine).[58]

TINEA BARBAE

Tinea barbae affects the hairs and follicles of beards and mustaches.[58] Treatment is similar to that for tinea capitis (see Table 129–8). Removal of the beard or mustache is recommended.[54]

PITYRIASIS VERSICOLOR

Hyper- and hypopigmented scaly patches characterize pityriasis versicolor which is also known as Dermatomycosis furfuracea and is caused by Malassezia globosa and M. fur. These patches are found on the trunk and extremities.[60] It is more common in adults and in areas with tropical ambient temperatures. Topical treatment usually is adequate unless there is extensive involvement, recurrent infections, or failure of topical therapy.[60] A study of 100 subjects treated with either ketoconazole 2% shampoo or selenium sulfide 2.5% shampoo showed that ketoconazole was significantly more effective that selenium sulfide (89% vs. 35% cure rate).[61]

ONYCHOMYCOSIS (TINEA UNGUIUM)

Onychomycosis is a fungal infection of the nail apparatus and is the most common single cause of nail dystrophy, affecting up to 8% of the general population and accounting for up to 50% of all nail problems.[62–64] Onychomycosis more commonly affects the toenails (2% to 14% of adults), ~4 to 19 times more frequently than fingernails, with prevalence increasing with age.[64] This can be because of the slower growth of toenails (three times slower than fingernails), making it easier for fungi to establish infection. Onychomycosis has a significant impact on quality of life, both functional and psychosocial. In addition, the affected nails can disrupt the integrity of the surrounding skin, potentially increasing the risk of secondary bacterial infections.[64]

Dermatophytes are the most frequent causes of onychomycois (~90% in toenail and ~50% in fingernail infections).[65] The dermatophytes responsible for causing >90% of cases of onychomycosis are Trichophyton rubrum (71%) and Trichophyton mentagrophytes (20%).[58,59] Less common fungi causing onychomycosis are the nondermatophytic molds (2.3% to 11%) and yeasts (5.6%). C. albicans is the most commonly isolated yeast and typically affects fingernails rather than toenails.[62,66] Risk factors for dermatophytic onychomycosis are increasing age (especially older than 40 years), family history and genetic factors, immunodeficiency (e.g., HIV, renal transplant, immunosuppressive therapy, and defective polymorphonuclear chemotaxis), diabetes mellitus, psoriasis, peripheral vascular disease, smoking, prevalence of tinea pedis, frequent nail trauma, and sporting activities such as swimming.[66,67] These risk factors also appear to apply to recurrence of onychomycosis. Mold onychomycosis does not seem to be associated with systemic or local predisposing factors, but there is a risk of systemic dissemination in immunosuppressed patients.[66] Candida onychomycosis seems to always occur in immunosuppressed patients.[66]

Onychomycosis can present in four or five different major clinical forms, of which lateral distal subungual onychomycosis (DSO) is the most common type.[62,66,68] In DSO, the nail plate, the nail bed, and, in advanced cases, the matrix are all affected, and T. rubrum is the most common etiologic cause. The worst case of onychomycosis is progression of the infection to total dystrophic onychomycosis, characterized by almost complete destruction of the nail plate. White superficial onychomycosis (WSO) is usually caused by T. mentagrophytes, where the infection is localized to the surface of the nail plate. In proximal subungual onychomycosis (PSO), the fungi (usually T. rubrum) invade the nail through the proximal nail fold and spread to the nail plate and matrix. Although PSO is relatively uncommon in the general population, it occurs most frequently in severely immunocompromised patients and is often considered a marker for AIDS.[66,68] Because of the multifactorial etiology of onychomycosis, it is important to differentiate onychomycosis from other causes of nail dystrophies so that the patient receives appropriate therapy and is not subjected to prolonged treatment with unnecessary drugs. Besides clinical history and physical examination, proper diagnosis of onychomycosis can include the combination of direct microscopy of scrapings from the appropriate nail area to look for fungal hyphae and fungal cultures, and, if necessary, histologic examination.[63,69,70] Table 129–9 provides a differential diagnosis for fungal nail diseases.[71]

TABLE 129-9	Differntial Diagnosis of Fungal Nail Infections
Diagnosis	**Features Consistent with Diagnosis**
Psoriasis	Nail pitting, rash elsewhere on body, family history of psoriasis
Lichen planus	Nail atrophy, scarring at proximal aspect of the nail
Periungual squamous cell carcinoma	Single nail affected, pain, warty nail fold change, or ooze from the edge of nail
Yellow nail syndrome	Multiple nails turn yellow, grow slowly, increased longitudinal and transverse curvature, intermittent pain and shedding, associated with chronic sinusitis, bronchiectasis, lymphadema
Trauma	Single nail affected, homogeneous alteration of nail color and altered shape of nail

TREATMENT

■ GENERAL APPROACH

Onychomycosis merits proper assessment and treatment consideration because it is a debilitating disease and can exert a negative impact on quality of life (e.g., cosmetic and psychosocial effects, pain, discomfort, and decreased ambulation).[63,66,72] It is reasonable to not treat persons with minimal toenail involvement and no associated symptoms.[71] Although definitive data are lacking regarding the risk of progression of untreated disease, it can lead to complications such as cellulitis or reduced mobility, which can further compromise peripheral circulation in those with diabetes or peripheral vascular disease; additionally, infected nails can serve as a source of transmission of fungi to other areas of the body, as well as to other people, such as close household contacts, or in communal bathing places.[63,66,72,73] Treatment decisions should be made on an individual basis. The primary end point of treatment is eradication of the organism, with secondary end points being clinical cure and improvement.[63] Assessment of clinical success (cure or improvement) requires followup for several months after the end of treatment because of the slow growth rate of nails, especially toenails (1 mm/month).[63,66] Successful eradication of the fungus does not always result in normalization of the nails because they can have been dystrophic prior to infection. This can cause patient dissatisfaction, especially if this is not explained before starting treatment.[68] There are several factors that must be taken into account on a patient-by-patient basis to ensure appropriate treatment decisions (Table 129–10). The impact of patient adherence on the success of treatment cannot be overemphasized. Patients need to be educated about their disease, expectations of treatment, and prevention of recurrence, and various strategies have been suggested to improve treatment success.[70]

In general, onychomycosis of the toenail is more difficult to treat than fingernails, requires longer treatment duration, and is associated with a higher recurrence. The treatment options for onychomycosis include oral and topical therapies, mechanical or chemical nail avulsion, or a combination of these. Mechanical or chemical nail avulsion is used primarily as adjunct to oral therapy in patients with total dystrophic onychomycosis, in whom there is severe onycholysis and extensive nail thickening or longitudinal spikes. This is to enhance penetration of the antifungal agent to the entire nail plate and unit.[63,70,73]

TABLE 129-10	Factors that may Impact Treatment Decisions and Outcomes

- Type and severity of onychomycosis
- Causative organism—dermatophyte versus molds or yeast
- Infection of the finger versus toenail
- Extent of disease—involvement of matrix, one or two lateral edges, number of nails
- Thickness of nail plate
- Other sites of mycotic infection (palms, soles, toe webs)
- Other nail alterations affecting outcome (onycholysis, paronychia, dermatophytoma, etc.)
- Other nail diseases and symptoms
- Age and underlying medical conditions (diabetes, poor perfusion, immunocompromised)
- Drug interactions and adverse effects
- Cost of therapy

Data from Effendy I, Lecha M, Feuilhade de Chauvin M, et al. Epidemiology and clinical classification of onychomycosis. J Eur Acad Dermatol Venereol 2005;19(Supp1 1):8–12; Gupta AK, Tu LQ. Onychomycosis therapies: Strategies to improve efficacy. Dermatol Clin 2006;24:381–386; Lecha M, Effendy I, Feuilhade de Chauvin M, et al. Treatments options–Development of consensus guidelines. J Euro Acad Dermatol Venereol 2005;19(Suppl 1):25–33; and Gupta AK, Tu LQ. Therapies for onychomycosis: a review. Dermatol Clin 2006;24:375–379.

CLINICAL CONTROVERSY

Treatment of onychomycosis is associated with a high failure rate of 20% to 50%. There appears to be a sound pharmacologic rationale behind the use of combination therapy, which has been used to improve overall efficacy. However, the best combination of agents for use in treating onychomycosis is unclear, and there is no consensus on when to use such agents.

■ TOPICAL THERAPY

⑩ Conventional topical antifungal products are available as creams, ointments, powders, and solutions. Because these formulations do not penetrate through the nail plate to the nail bed, they are most appropriately used when the nail plate has been removed.[73] Even then cure rates are still low and variable and are influenced by patient adherence.[66,73] Nail lacquer represents the latest advance in topical formulation. The volatile vehicle, used to deliver the drug, evaporates and leaves an occlusive film with a high drug concentration on the nail surface.[66,73] There are only two marketed nail lacquers, amorolfine 5% and ciclopirox 8% solution (Penlac), the latter being the only one approved in North America for the treatment of mild to moderate onychomycosis caused by *T. rubrum* without lunula involvement.[66,72,73] Ciclopirox, a hydroxypyridine, has a broad spectrum of antifungal activity (dermatophytes, *Candida* species, and some molds) and requires treatment for 1 year. Although ciclopirox was significantly better than vehicle alone, the mycologic cure rate was only 32% with ciclopirox versus 10% for vehicle alone after 48 weeks of treatment; the overall treatment cure (mycologic cure with 0% to 10% involvement of the target nail) was 9% versus 0.9% for drug and vehicle, respectively.[66,73] However, higher mycologic cure rates of 45% to 65% have been reported in a variety of open-label trials involving 6 to 12 months of treatment.[66] Amorolfine appears to produce higher mycologic and treatment cure rates than ciclopirox.[66,72] Most experts consider topical therapy a feasible option when the infection is superficial involving the nail plate without matrix involvement, such as WSO, involves a partial area of the nail plate not exceeding 50% (owing to difficulty of applying treatment to the margin of the nail), is limited to a few (three or four) nails, is in the very early stages of DSO when infection is still confined to the distal edge of the nail, or when systemic therapy is contraindicated.[63,66,72] Combining topical therapy with debridement of the affected nail (thus diminishing the amount of nail requiring treatment) may increase the likelihood of successful treatment, although there is no strong supporting evidence.[71] Topical therapy is not associated with systemic adverse effects or drug interactions. Any adverse effect will be localized to the application site, such as mild erythema in the adjacent skin area.

■ SYSTEMIC THERAPY

Oral antifungal therapy is considered to be more effective than topical for treating onychomycosis. Terbinafine and itraconazole (capsule), the current first-line agents for treatment, have yielded higher efficacy rates using shorter treatment periods (generally 3 months or shorter) for toenail and fingernail onychomycosis compared with the traditional agents, such as griseofulvin and ketoconazole, which are rarely used nowadays. Terbinafine, an allylamine, exerts fungicidal activity and demonstrates the greatest in vitro activity against dermatophytes compared with the other oral antifungals; it has good activity against nondermatophyte molds and only marginal activity against *Candida* species.[63,73] Like other azoles, itraconazole is fungistatic, has a broad antifungal spectrum, and is very active against dermatophytes, nondermatophytes, and *Candida* species.[63,73] Both agents have lipophilic and keratinophilic properties, which explains their excellent penetration (appearing in the nail plate within days of treatment initiation) and accumulation in the nails, achieving concentrations far exceeding the minimal inhibitory concentration (MIC) of most dermatophytes. Nail terbinafine concentrations are detected within 1 week of starting therapy, whereas itraconazole can be detected 1 (fingernails) to 2 weeks (toenails) after starting therapy.[66] Both drugs are slowly eliminated from the nail, with effective drug concentrations persisting in nails for 30 to 36 weeks after completion of treatment with terbinafine and for 27 weeks with itraconazole.[68] The persistence of drug in the nails explains in part the long-term protection against relapses after the end of treatment and also permits use of intermittent (pulse) dosing.

The treatment of toenail onychomycosis requires a 12-week course, whereas a 6-week course is adequate for fingernail onychomycosis with either drug.[63,68] In general, cure rates of 80% to 90% for fingernail infection and 70% to 80% for toenail infection can be expected.[63] Terbinafine is licensed for daily dosing (see Table 129–8).[63,68,74] Various terbinafine pulse regimens have been evaluated;[73] in some trials, pulse dosing was less effective than continuous dosing, and it did not provide clear safety advantages.[69,70] One trial demonstrated similar efficacy of pulse terbinafine compared with continuous therapy and better outcomes compared with pulse itraconazole treatment.[75] Itraconazole pulse therapy is the preferred method over continuous dosing for fingernail infections, and it is licensed as twice-daily dosing for a 1-week cycle per month for 2 consecutive months (i.e., two pulses), or as daily therapy for 6 weeks (see Table 129–8).[68,74] Although itraconazole pulse therapy is not approved by the US Food and Drug Administration (FDA), three or four pulses are effective for toenail infections; otherwise, half the dose is taken daily for 3 months (see Table 129–8).[68,74] In addition to lower drug cost, the potential advantages of itraconazole pulse therapy compared with continuous therapy are a lower risk of adverse drug effects and improved patient adherence.

Terbinafine is generally considered by most experts as the first-line agent for onychomycosis; itraconazole is the alternative. Direct comparative trials generally have shown that terbinafine is more effective than itraconazole either by continuous or pulse dosing.[63,72,73] Mycologic cure rates for terbinafine range from 77% to 100% depending on the study.[66] In a cumulative meta-analysis of randomized, controlled trials, mycologic cure rates for terbinafine, itraconazole pulse, itraconazole continuous, fluconazole, and griseofulvin were 76% ± 3%, 63% ± 7%, 59% ± 5%, 60% ± 6%, and 48% ± 5%, respectively.[78] An earlier meta-analysis and systematic review also reported that continuous terbinafine was the most effective therapy for toenail onychomycosis.[72,73] In addition, terbinafine was reported to achieve high cure rates in high-risk immunosuppressed patients, such as diabetics and organ transplant recipients, comparable to the immunocompetent population, with no significant adverse effects or drug interactions. It also appears to be effective in HIV patients and nondermatophyte infections.[74,81] A pharmacoeconomic analysis of oral and topical (ciclopirox) therapies showed that from a managed care perspective, terbinafine was the most cost-effective therapy in terms of highest success rate, lowest relapse rate, and highest number of disease-free days for both fingernail and toenail infections.[82] An analysis that looked only at oral therapy estimated that the cost per cure with the use of terbinafine (based on cure rates from clinical trials) ranged from $2,439 to $7,944, depending on disease severity.[83] Compared with the amount of money a patient would consider reasonable to spend on treatment, the current charges for a course of systemic therapy are considerably higher.[83,84]

CLINICAL CONTROVERSY

There is controversy regarding the cost–benefit ratio of treating onychomycosis. People commonly receive treatment without a proper diagnosis of onchymycosis. These patients are not accounted for in any pharmacoeconomic analysis as such this inappropriate treatment will markedly increase the cast per cure. Also relevant to decision making are the risks of treatment and the effects of treatment on quality of life. A study translating these considerations into an amount of money a patient would consider reasonable to spend on treatment found the current costs of a course of therapy are much greater than this sum.[84]

Both terbinafine and itraconazole generally are well tolerated. The more common adverse effects reported with terbinafine are GI (e.g., diarrhea, dyspepsia, nausea, and abdominal pain), dermatologic (e.g., rash, urticaria, and pruritus), and headache; less common adverse effects are taste disturbances, fatigue, inability to concentrate, and asymptomatic liver enzyme abnormalities.[68,72,74] Terbinafine can cause transient decrease in absolute lymphocyte counts; hence, monitoring of complete blood counts can be useful, especially in immunocompromised patients.[74] Although uncommon, severe adverse effects have been reported with terbinafine, including erythema multiforme, Stevens-Johnson syndrome, toxic epidermal necrolysis, pancytopenia, lupus erythematosus, psoriasis, hair loss, and hepatotoxicity. Although the incidence of severe hepatotoxicity is considered rare, the FDA issued a public health advisory in 2001 regarding the association of terbinafine tablets with 16 possible cases of liver failure, including 2 liver transplants and 11 deaths.[85] Terbinafine thus is not recommended for patients with chronic or active liver disease, although hepatotoxicity can occur in patients with no preexisting liver disease or serious underlying medical condition. Prior to initiating terbinafine treatment, it is recommended to obtain appropriate nail specimens for laboratory testing to confirm the diagnosis of onychomycosis. Liver function parameters (serum transaminases) should be assessed at baseline and periodically during treatment with terbinafine.[74,85]

The common adverse effects of itraconazole are similar to those of terbinafine, such as GI disturbance, dermatologic disorders, and headache; less common adverse effects include dizziness, fatigue, fever, decreased libido, and asymptomatic liver enzyme abnormalities (1% to 5% with continuous dosing and ~2% with pulse dosing).[68,72,86] Although still considered rare, 24 serious cases of liver failure, including transplantation and death, have been reported with the use of itraconazole, resulting in an FDA public health advisory warning.[85] Some of these patients did not have preexisting liver disease or serious underlying medical conditions, and some developed within the first week of treatment. Itraconazole should be avoided in patients with elevated liver enzymes or active liver disease or in those who have experienced other drug-induced liver toxicity. Liver function parameters (serum transaminases) should be assessed prior to and periodically during treatment. However, some experts have suggested that frequent monitoring is not as necessary if pulse therapy is used because symptomatic hepatotoxicity has not been reported with pulse therapy.[86] In addition, there is an FDA warning on the risk of developing congestive heart failure (CHF) associated with the use of itraconazole, possibly related to its potential negative inotropic effect.[63,76] Therefore, itraconazole should not be used in patients with evidence of ventricular dysfunction, such as CHF. Symptomatic assessment for the development of CHF also should be included as part of therapy monitoring. Before a patient is subjected to several months of itraconazole treatment, it is important to confirm the diagnosis of onychomycosis.

In contrast to the azoles, terbinafine does not inhibit the cytochrome P450 (CYP) 3A4 isoenzymes, but it is a potent inhibitor of the CYP2D6 isoenzymes, which are responsible for metabolism of tricyclic antidepressants and other psychotropic drugs.[63,68,74] The most significant drug interactions with terbinafine are decreased clearance of 33% by cimetidine and increased clearance of 100% by rifampin. Other drug interactions of variable clinical significance are tricyclic antidepressants, cyclosporine, caffeine, theophylline, and terfenadine. Itraconazole and its major metabolite can inhibit the CYP3A4 isoenzymes and result in numerous clinically significant drug interactions where coadministration with several drugs are contraindicated (e.g., alprazolam, midazolam, triazolam, pimozide, lovastatin, simvastatin, cisapride, and terfenadine).[63,68,74]

Fluconazole is also active against dermatophytes, *Candida* species, and some nondermatophytes;[68,72] however, it does not have current FDA-approved indication for treatment of onychomycosis. The overall mycologic cure rate of fluconazole is 48%, which is lowest compared with all other oral agents.[78] The most effective dose and treatment duration have not been clearly established, with a variety of dosing regimens used, ranging from 50 mg daily to 300 mg once weekly for 6 to 12 months (see Table 129–8).[68,74] The advantages of fluconazole include a relatively good safety profile and fewer drug interactions compared with itraconazole.[68,74]

These three oral antifungal agents have superseded the use of griseofulvin and ketoconazole as treatments of choice for onychomycosis.[63,72,73] Griseofulvin has a narrow antifungal spectrum, low clinical efficacy, especially for toenail infections, high relapse rates, and the need for prolonged treatment duration (up to 12 to 18 months for toenails). Use of ketoconazole is also associated with high relapse rates, and the prolonged treatment duration carries an increased risk of hepatotoxicity.

■ TREATMENT RESPONSE AND RECURRENCE

Treatment failures and recurrence rates of infection following initial cure are high, ranging from 20% to 50%.[63,71] Recurrence could be either a relapse (original infection not completely cured) or reinfection (new infection after achieving a cure of the original). Factors associated with poor response to systemic therapy include a compromised immune system (AIDS), reduced blood flow (diabetes, peripheral vascular disease, vasculitis, connective tissue disease, and CHF), coexisting nail disease (psoriasis), nail factors (slow growth, thick nails, and severe disease), drug-resistant organisms because of extensive prior drug exposure, and reduced bioavailability (absorption problems, poor compliance, and drug interactions).[68,71] To improve treatment outcomes and reduce recurrence, patients should be counseled on the importance of proper foot hygiene, for example, wearing breathable footwear and 100% cotton socks with frequent changes, keeping the nails short and clean, keeping the feet dry, protecting the feet in shared bathing areas, treating tinea pedis, and controlling other predisposing medical conditions.[71]

The use of combination therapy (topical–oral or oral–oral agents) can improve cure rates and shorten treatment duration, as this approach provides complementary mechanisms of attack.[71,72] Studies in Europe have reported favorable results achieved with itraconazole or terbinafine combined with amorolfine.[71,72] To date no specific combination has been approved or endorsed for use. Other novel approaches include giving supplemental therapy and use of boosted therapy.[71,72] The efficacy and role of either approach remain to be defined.

ABBREVIATIONS

ACOG: American College of Obstetricians and Gynecologists

AIDS: acquired immune deficiency syndrome

BMT: Bone marrow transplantation

CHF: Congestive heart failure

CMI: Cell-mediated immunity

CYP: Cytochrome P450

DSO: Distal subungual onychomycosis

HAART: Highly active antiretroviral therapy

HIV: Human immunodeficiency virus

HSCT: Hematopoietic stem cell transplant

IgA: Immunoglobulin A

KOH: Potassium hydroxide

MIC: Minimum inhibitory concentration

OPC: Oropharyngeal candidiasis

PSO: Proximal subungual onychomycosis

RVVC: Recurrent vulvovaginal candidiasis

VVC: Vulvovaginal candidiasis

WSO: White superficial onychomycosis

REFERENCES

1. Sobel JD, Faro S, Force R, et al. Vulvovaginal candidiasis: Epidemiologic, diagnostic and therapeutic considerations. Am J Obstet Gynecol 1998;178:203–211.

2. Center for Disease Control and Prevention. Vaginal Discharge-STD Treatment Guidelines. 2006. *www.cdc.gov/std/treatment/2006/vaginaldischarge.htm.*

3. Haefner HK. Current evaluation and management of vulvovaginitis. Clin Obstet Gynecol 1999;42:184–195.

4. Foxman B, Barlow R, D'arcy H, et al. *Candida* vaginitis self-reported incidence and associated costs. Sex Transm Dis 2000;27:230–235.

5. Lipsky MS, Waters T, Sharp LK. Impact of vaginal antifungal products on utilization of health care services: Evidence from physician visits. J Am Board Fam Pract 2000;13:178182.

6. Clinical Effectiveness Group. National guideline for the management of vulvovaginal candidiasis. Sex Transm Infect 1999;75(Suppl 1): S19-S20.

7. Larsen B. Vaginal flora in health and disease. Clin Obstet Gynecol 1993;36:107–121.

8. Sobel JD. Clinical vulvovaginitis. Clin Obstet Gynecol 1993;36: 153–165.

9. Barbone F, Austin H, Louv WC, Alexander WJ. A follow-up study of the methods of contraception, sexual activity, and rates of trichomoniasis, candidiasis, and bacterial vaginosis. Am J Obstet Gynecol 1990;163:510–514.

10. Ferris DG, Dekle C, Litaker MS. Women's use of over-the-counter antifungal pharmaceutical products for gynecologic symptoms. J Fam Pract 1996;42:595–600.

11. ACOG practice bulletin: Clinical management guidelines for obstetrician-gynecologists. Obstet Gynecol 2006;107:1195–1206.

12. Watson MC, Bond CM, Grimshaw J, Johnston M. Factors predicting the guideline compliant supply (or non-supply) of non-prescription medicines in the community pharmacy setting. Qual Safe Health Care 2006;15:53–57.

13. Hilton E, Isenberg HD, Alperstein P, et al. Ingestion of yogurt containing *Lactobacillus acidophilus* as prophylaxis for candidal vaginitis. Ann Intern Med 1992;116:353–357.

14. Tooley PJ. Patient and doctor preferences in the treatment of vaginal candidiasis. Practitioner 1985;229:655–662.

15. Nurbhai M, Grimshaw J, Watson M, Bond CM, Mollison JA, Ludbrook A. Oral versus intravaginal imidazole and triazole antifungal treatment of uncomplicated vulvovaginal candidiasis (thrush). Cochrane Database Syst Rev 2007;(4). Art. No.: CD002845. DOI: 10.1002/14651858.CD002845.pub2.

16. Edelman DA, Grant S. One-day therapy for vaginal candidiasis a review. J Reprod Med 1999;44:543–547.

17. Mendling W, Plempel M. Vaginal secretion levels after 6 days, 3 days and 1 day of treatment with 100-, 200-, 500-mg vaginal tablets of clotrimazole and their therapeutic efficacy. Chemotherapy 1982;28(Suppl 1): 43–47.

18. Sobel JD, Kapernick PS, Zervos M, et al. Treatment of complicated candida vaginitis: Comparison of single and sequential doses of fluconazole. Am J Obstet Gynecol 2001;185:363–369.

19. Young G, Jewell D. Topical treatment for vaginal candidiasis (thrush) in pregnancy. Cochrane Database Sys Rev 2001; (4). Art. No.: CD000225. DOI: 10.1002/14651858.CD000225.

20. Mastroiacovo P, Mazzone T, Botto L, et al. Prospective assessment of pregnancy outcomes after first-trimester exposure to fluconazole. Am J Obstet Gynecol 1996;175:1645–1650.

21. Pursley TJ, Blomquist IK, Abraham J, Andersen HF, Bartley JA. Fluconazole-induced congenital anomalies in three infants. Clin Infect Dis 1996;22:336–340.

22. Sobel JD, Wiesenfeld HC, Martens M, et al. Maintenance fluconazole therapy for recurrent vulvovaginal candidiasis. N Engl J Med 2004;351:363–369.

23. Pappas PG, Kauffman CA, Andes DA, et al. Clinical practice guidelines for the management of candidiasis: 2009 update by the infectious diseases society of America. Clinical InfectDis 2009;48:503–535.

24. Sobel JD, Chiam W, Nagappan V, Leaman D. Treatment of vaginitis caused by *Candida glabrata*: Use of topical boric acid and flucytosine. Am J Obstet Gynecol 2003;189:1297–1300.

25. Sobel JD, Chaim W. Treatment of *Torulopsis glabrata* vaginitis: Retrospective review of boric acid therapy. Clin Infect Dis 1996;22: 336–340.

26. Ray D, Goswami R, Banerjee U, Dadhawl V, et al. Prevalence of *Candida glabrata* and its response to boric acid vaginal suppositories in comparison with oral fluconazole in patients with diabetes and vulvovaginal candidiasis. Diabetes Care 2007;30:312–317.

27. Leigh JE, Shetty K, Fidel Jr PL. Oral opportunistic infections in HIV-positive individuals: Review and role of mucosal immunity. AIDS Patient Care STDS 2004;18:443–456.

28. Delgado ACD, de Jesus PR, Aoki FH, et al. Clinical and microbiological assessment of patients with long-term diagnosis of human immunodeficiency virus infection and *Candida* oral colonization. Clin Microbiol Infect 2009;15:364–371.

29. Vasquez JA. Invasive oesophageal candidiasis: Current and developing treatment options. Drugs 2003;63:971–989.

30. Darouiche RO. State-of-the-art clinical article—Oropharyngeal and esophageal candidiasis in immunocompromised patients: Treatment issues. Clin Infect Dis 1998;26:259–274.

31. Oropharyngeal candidiasis. 2005. *www.doctorfungus.org/mycoses/human/candida*.

32. Benson CA, Kaplan JE, Masur H, et al. Treating opportunistic infections among HIV-infected adults and adolescents: Recommendations from CDC, the National Institutes of Health, and the HIV Medicine Association/Infectious Diseases Society of America. Clin Infect Dis 2004;40:S131–S235.

33. Kauffman CA. Treatment of oropharyngeal and esophageal candidiasis. 2010. *www.uptodate.com*.

34. Mercante DE, Leigh JE, Lilly EA, et al. Assessment of the association between HIV viral load and CD4 cell count on the occurrence of oropharyngeal candidiasis in HIV-infected patients. J Acquir Immune Defic Syndr 2006;42:578–583.

35. Soysa NS, Samaranayake LP, Ellepola ANB. Antimicrobials as a contributory factor in oral candidosis: A brief overview. Oral Dis 2008;14:138–143.

36. Akpan A, Morgan R. Oral candidiasis. Postgrad Med J 2002;78:455–459.

37. Pappas PG, Kauffman CA, Andes D, et al. Guidelines for management of candidiasis: 2009 update by the Infectious Diseases Society of America. Clin Infect Dis 2009;48:503–535.

38. Hamza OJM, Matee MIN, Bruggemann RJM, et al. Single-dose fluconazole versus standard 2-week therapy for oropharyngeal candidiasis in HIV-infected patients: A randomized, double-blind, double-dummy trial. Clin Infect Dis 2008;47:1270–1276.

39. Vasquez JA, Skiest DJ, Nieto L, et al. A multicenter randomized trial evaluating posaconazole versus fluconazole for the treatment of oropharyngeal candidiasis in subjects with HIV/AIDS. Clin Infect Dis 2006;42:1179–1186.

40. Freifeld AG, Walsh TJ, Pizzo PA. Clinical approaches to infections in the compromised host. In: Hoffman R, Benz EJ Jr, Shattil SJ, et al, eds. Hematology: Basic Principles and Practice. 3rd ed. New York: Churchill-Livingstone, 2000.

41. Gotzsche PC, Johansen HK. Nystatin prophylaxis and treatment in severely immunodepressed patients. Cochrane Database Syst Rev 2003;4:1–15.

42. International Conference for the Development of a Consensus on the Management and Prevention of Severe Candidal Infections. Clin Infect Dis 1997;25:43–59.

43. Villanueva A, Arathoon EG, Gotuzzo E, et al. A randomized double-blind study of caspofungin versus amphotericin for the treatment of candidal esophagitis. Clin Infect Dis 2001;33:1529–1535.

44. Arathoon EG, Gotuzzo E, Noriega LM, et al. Randomized, double-blind, multicenter study of caspofungin versus amphotericin B for treatment of oropharyngeal and esophageal candidiasis. Antimicrob Agents Chemother 2002;46:451–457.

45. Villanueva A, Gotuzzo E, Arathoon EG, et al. A randomized, double-blind study of caspofungin versus fluconazole for the treatment of esophageal candidiasis. Am J Med 2002;113:294–299.

46. Ally R, Schurmann D, Kreisel W, et al. A randomized, double-blind, double-dummy, multicenter trial of voriconazole and fluconazole in the treatment of esophageal candidiasis in immunocompromised patients. Clin Infect Dis 2001;33:1447–1454.

47. Deresinski SC, Stevens DA. Caspofungin. Clin Infect Dis 2003;36: 1445–1457.

48. Johnson LB, Kauffman CA. Voriconazole: A new triazole antifungal agent. Clin Infect Dis 2003;36:630–637.

49. Morris MI, Villmann. Echinocandins in the management of invasive fungal infections, part 1. Am J Health Syst Pharm 2006;63:1693–1703.

50. Grim SA, Smith KM, Romanelli F, Ofotokun I. Treatment of azole-resistant oropharyngeal candidiasis with topical amphotericin B. Ann Pharmacother 2002;36:1383–1386.

51. Goldman M, Cloud GA, Wade KD, et al. A randomized study of the use of fluconazole in continuous versus episodic therapy in patients with advanced HIV infection and a history of oropharyngeal candidiasis: AIDS clinical trials group study 323/mycoses study group 40. Clin Infect Dis 2005;41:1473–1480.

52. Marr KA, Bow E, Chiller T, et al. Fungal infection prevention after hematopoietic cell transplantation. Bone Marrow Transplant 2009;44:483–487.

53. Nowak MA, Brodell RT. Rapid diagnosis of superficial fungal infections. Postgrad Med 1999;2:179–180.

54. Goldstein AO, Smith KM, Ives TJ, Goldstein B. Mycotic infections. Effective management of conditions involving the skin, hair, and nails. Geriatrics 2000;55:40–52.

55. Drake LA, Dinehart SM, Farmer ER, et al. Guidelines of care for superficial mycotic infections of the skin: Tinea corporis, tinea cruris, tinea faciei, tinea manuum, and tinea pedis. J Am Acad Dermatol 1996;34:282–286.

56. Gupta AK, Chow M, Daniel CR, Aly R. Treatments of tinea pedis. Dermatol Clin 2003;21:431–462.

57. Gupta AK, Chaudhry M Elewski B. Tinea corporis, tinea cruris, tinea nigra, and piedra. Dermatol Clin 2003;21:395–400.

58. Drake LA, Dinehart SM, Farmer ER, et al. Guidelines of care for superficial mycotic infections of the skin: Tinea capitis and tinea barbae. J Am Acad Dermatol 1996;34:290–294.

59. Higgins EM, Fuller LC, Smith CH. Guidelines for the management of tinea capitis. Br J Dermatol 2000;143:53–58.

60. Gupta AK, Batra R, Bluhm R, Faergemann J. Pityriasis versicolor. Dermatol Clin 2003;21:413–429.

61. Ansarun H, Ghaffarpour G. Comparison of effectiveness between ketoconazole 2% and selenium sulfide 2% shampoos in the treatment of tinea versicolor. Iranian J Derm 2005;8:21–25.

62. Effendy I, Lecha M, Feuilhade de Chauvin M, et al. Epidemiology and clinical classification of onychomycosis. J Eur Acad Dermatol Venereol 2005;19(Suppl 1):8–12.

63. Roberts DT, Taylor WD, Boyle J. Guidelines for treatment of onychomycosis. Br J Dermatol 2003;148:402–410.

64. Nunley KS, Cornelius L. Current management of onchymycosis. J Hand Surg 2008;33A:1211–1214.

65. Kaur R, Kashyap B, Bhalla P. Oncychomycosis—Epidemiology, diagnosis and management. Ind J Med Micro 2008;26(2):108–116.

66. Baran R, Kaoukhov A. Topical antifungal drugs for the treatment of onychomycosis: An overview of current strategies for monotherapy and combination therapy. J Eur Acad Dermatol Venereol 2005;19:21–29.

67. Tosti A, Hay R, Arenas-Guzman R. Patients at risk of onychomycosis—Risk factor identification and active prevention. J Eur Acad Dermatol Venereol 2005;19(Suppl 1):13–16.

68. Iorizzo M, Piraccini BM, Rech G, Tosti A. Treatment of onychomycosis with oral antifungal agents. Expert Opin Drug Deliv 2005;2:435–440.

69. Feuilhade de Chauvin M. New diagnostic techniques. J Eur Acad Dermatol Venereol 2005;19(Suppl 1):20–24.

70. Gupta AK, Tu LQ. Onychomycosis therapies: Strategies to improve efficacy. Dermatol Clin 2006;24:381–386.

71. de Berker D. Fungal nail disease. N Engl J Med 2009;360:2108–2116.

72. Lecha M, Effendy I, Feuilhade de Chauvin M, et al. Treatment options—Development of consensus guidelines. J Euro Acad Dermatol Venereol 2005;19(Suppl 1):25–33.

73. Gupta AK, Tu LQ. Therapies for onychomycosis: a review. Dermatol Clin 2006;24:375–379.

74. Gupta AK, Ryder JE, Skinner AR. Treatment of onychomycosis: Pros and cons of antifungal agents. J Cutan Med Surg 2004;8:25–30.

75. Gupta AK, Lynch LE, Kogan N, et al. The use of intermittent terbinafine for the treatment of dermatophyte toenail onychomycosis. JEADV 2009;23:2562–62.

76. Sigurgeirsson B, Elewski EE, Rich PA, et al. Intermittent versus continuous terbinafine in the treatment of toenail onychomycosis: A randomized, double-blind, comparison. J Dermatolog Treat 2006;17:38–44.

77. Warshaw EM, Fett DD, Bloomfield HE, et al. Pulse verus continuous terbinafine for onychomycosis: A randomized, double-blind, controlled trial. J Am Acad Dermatol 2005;53:578–584.

78. Gupta AK, Ryder JE, Johnson AM. Cumulative meta-analysis of systemic antifungal agents for the treatment of onychomycosis. Br J Dermatol 2004;150:537–544.

79. Haugh M, Helou S, Boissel JP, Cribier BJ. Terbinafine in fungal infections of the nails: A meta-analysis of randomized clinical trials. Br J Dermatol 2002;147:118–121.

80. Crawford F, Young P, Godfrey C, et al. Oral treatments for toenail onychomycosis: A systematic review. Arch Dermatol 2002;138:811–816.

81. Cribier BJ, Bakshi R. Terbinafine in the treatment of onychomycosis: A review of its efficacy in high-risk populations and in patients with nondermatophyte infections. Br J Dermatol 2004;150:414–420.

82. Casciano J, Amaya K, Doyle J, et al. Economic analysis of oral and topical therapies for onychomycosis of the toenails and fingernails. Manag Care 2003;12:47–54.

83. Schram SE, Warshaw EM. Costs of pulse versus continuous terbinafine for onychomycosis. J Am Acad Dermatol 2007;56:525–527.

84. Cham PM, Chen SC, Grill JP, et al. Reliability of self-reported willingness-to-pay and annual income in patients treated for toenail onychomycosis Br J Dermatol 2007;156:922–928.

85. Food and Drug Administration. FDA issues health advisory regarding the safety of Sporanox products and Lamisil tablets to treat finger nail infections. 2001. *www.fda.gov/cder/drug/advisory/sporanox-lamisil/advisory.htm*.

86. Gupta AK, Chwetzoff, Del Rosso J, Baran R. Hepatic safety of itraconazole. J Cutan Med Surg 2002;6:210–213.

CHAPTER 130

Invasive Fungal Infections

PEGGY L. CARVER

KEY CONCEPTS

❶ Systemic mycoses can be caused by pathogenic fungi and include histoplasmosis, coccidioidomycosis, cryptococcosis, blastomycosis, paracoccidioidomycosis, and sporotrichosis, or infections by opportunistic fungi such as *Candida albicans*, *Aspergillus* species, *Trichosporon*, *Candida glabrata*, *Fusarium*, *Alternaria*, and *Mucor*.

❷ The diagnosis of fungal infection generally is accomplished by careful evaluation of clinical symptoms, results of serologic tests, and histopathologic examination and culture of clinical specimens.

❸ Histoplasmosis is caused by *Histoplasma capsulatum* and is endemic in parts of the central United States along the Ohio and Mississippi River valleys. Although most patients experience asymptomatic infection, some can experience chronic, disseminated disease.

❹ Asymptomatic patients with histoplasmosis are not treated, although patients who do not have acquired immune deficiency syndrome (AIDS) patients with evident disease are treated with either oral ketoconazole or intravenous amphotericin B; AIDS patients are treated with amphotericin B and then receive lifelong suppression.

❺ Blastomycosis is caused by *Blastomyces dermatitidis* and generally is an asymptomatic, self-limited disease; however, reactivation can lead to chronic disease. Although treatment for self-limited disease is controversial, patients with chronic pulmonary disease or extrapulmonary disease should be treated with ketoconazole, and those with central nervous system (CNS), progressive, or life-threatening disease should receive amphotericin B.

❻ Coccidioidomycosis is caused by *Coccidioides immitis* and is endemic in some parts of the southwestern United States. It can cause nonspecific symptoms, acute pneumonia, or chronic pulmonary or disseminated disease. Primary pulmonary disease (unless severe) frequently is not treated, whereas extrapulmonary disease is treated with amphotericin B, and meningitis is treated with fluconazole.

❼ Cryptococcosis is caused by *Cryptococcus neoformans* and occurs primarily in immunocompromised patients. Patients

with acute meningitis are treated with amphotericin B with flucytosine. Patients infected with human immunodeficiency virus (HIV) often require long-term suppressive therapy with fluconazole or itraconazole.

❽ A variety of *Candida* species (including *C. albicans*, *C. glabrata*, *Candida tropicalis*, *Candida parapsilosis*, and *Candida krusei*) can cause diseases such as mucocutaneous, oral, esophageal, vaginal, and hematogenous candidiasis, as well as candiduria. Candidemia can be treated with a variety of antifungal agents; the optimal choice depends on previous patient exposure to antifungal agents, potential drug interactions and toxicities of each agent, and local epidemiology of intensive care unit or hematology-oncology centers.

❾ Aspergillosis can be caused by a variety of *Aspergillus* species that can cause superficial infections, pneumonia, allergic bronchopulmonary aspergillosis, or invasive infection. Treatment with amphotericin B or voriconazole generally is instituted but often is not successful. Combination therapy, while widely used, lacks clinical trial data to support its use.

Learning objectives, review questions, and other resources can be found at **www.pharmacotherapyonline.com**.

For many years, fungal infections were classified as either superficial "nuisance diseases," such as athlete's foot or vulvovaginal candidiasis, or as relatively rare infections confined primarily to endemic areas of the country. When invasive fungal infections were encountered, amphotericin B was the only consistently effective, systemically active agent available for the treatment of systemic mycoses. ❶ Advances in medical technology, including organ and bone marrow transplantation, cytotoxic chemotherapy, the widespread use of indwelling intravenous (IV) catheters, and the increased use of potent broad-spectrum antimicrobial agents all have contributed to the dramatic increase in the incidence of fungal infections worldwide.

Fungal infections have emerged as a major cause of death among cancer patients and transplant recipients.[1–4] In addition, patients with AIDS experience substantially more frequent and severe forms of cryptococcosis, histoplasmosis, coccidioidomycosis, and mucocutaneous (esophageal, oral, and vulvovaginal) candidiasis.

Problems remain in the diagnosis, prevention, and treatment of fungal infections. Unlike the available diagnostic techniques for most bacterial pathogens, there remains a host of unresolved issues regarding standardization of susceptibility testing methods, in vitro and in vivo models of infection, the usefulness of monitoring antifungal plasma concentrations, and the development and identification of resistant pathogens.[1,5,6] The Infectious Diseases Society of America published guidelines for the treatment of many commonly encountered fungal infections. These guidelines provide summaries of the literature and a consensus of expert opinions regarding the treatment of these difficult infections.[6]

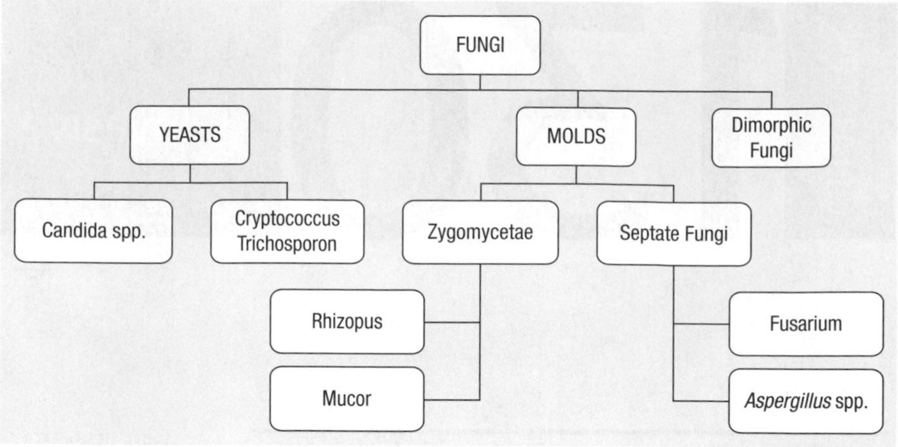

FIGURE 130-1. Morphologically, pathogenic fungi can be grouped as either filamentous molds or unicellular yeasts. *Molds* grow as multicellular branching, thread-like filaments (hyphae) that are either septate (divided by transverse walls) or coenocytic (multinucleate without cross walls).

MYCOLOGY

Fungi are eukaryotic organisms with a defined nucleus enclosed by a nuclear membrane; a cytoplasmic membrane containing lipids, glycoproteins, and sterols, mitochondria, Golgi apparatus, and ribosomes bound to endoplasmic reticulum; and a cytoskeleton with microtubules, microfilaments, and intermediate filaments. Fungi have rigid cell walls composed of chitin, cellulose, or both that stain with Gomori methenamine silver or periodic acid–Schiff reagent. Most fungi, except *Candida* species, are too weakly gram-positive to be seen well on Gram stain. *Cryptococcus neoformans* has a polysaccharide capsule surrounding the cell wall.[6]

Morphologically, pathogenic fungi can be grouped as either filamentous molds or unicellular yeasts (Fig. 130–1). *Molds* grow as multicellular branching, threadlike filaments (hyphae) that are either septate (divided by transverse walls) or coenocytic (multi-nucleate without cross walls). On agar media, molds grow outward from the point of inoculation by extension of the tips of filaments and then branch repeatedly, interweaving to form fuzzy, matted growths called *mycelia*. Yeasts are oval or spherically shaped unicellular forms that generally produce pasty or mucoid colonies on agar medium similar to those observed with bacterial cultures. Yeasts have rigid cell walls and reproduce by budding, a process in which daughter cells arise from pinching off a portion of the parent cell.

Fungi reproduce by forming spores asexually through mitosis to produce motile sporangiospores or nonmotile conidia (singular, conidium), or they reproduce sexually through meiosis to produce ascospores, basidiospores, oospores, or zygospores. Although terms such as *spore* and *conidia* should no longer be used interchangeably, some newer literature and much of the older medical literature continue to confuse these terms.

Many pathogenic fungi, termed *dimorphic fungi*, exist as either a yeast or a mold, depending on pathogen, site of growth (in the host or in the laboratory setting), and temperature. Usually yeasts are the parasitic form that invades human or animal host tissue, whereas molds are the free-living form found in the environment. For example, *Histoplasma capsulatum* exists as a yeast in humans and as a mold in the laboratory.[1]

SUSCEPTIBILITY TESTING OF ANTIFUNGAL AGENTS

Most laboratories do not routinely perform susceptibility tests on fungal isolates, but standardized methods for performing these tests are being developed and are now available for testing selected yeasts. To date, reference broth macrodilution and microdilution methods have been established for *Candida* and *Cryptococcus* species, whereas the broth microdilution method has been standardized for filamentous fungi. Additionally, minimal inhibitory concentration (MIC) reference ranges for American Type Culture Collection (ATCC) quality control strains have been established against various antifungal agents, as well as interpretive breakpoints for fluconazole, itraconazole, and flucytosine against *Candida* species[5] (Tables 130–1 and 130–2). For further detail, refer to the section outlining treatment of *Candida* infections. Reliable and convincing interpretive breakpoints are not yet available for amphotericin B. The National Committee for Clinical Laboratory Standards' (NCCLS) M27-A methodology does not reliably identify amphotericin B–resistant isolates; variations of the methodology using different media appear to enhance detection of resistant isolates.[5,7] The breakpoints should be used following testing with the standardized, reproducible laboratory methodology (NCCLS 27-A) used to develop the test and they should be interpreted in the context of the delivered dose of the antifungal agent.

Because in vitro correlations with in vivo outcomes in patients are not yet known, the role of routine susceptibility testing is unknown at this time. Several concerns need to be considered as the use of MIC breakpoints is incorporated into the clinical practice setting. First, MICs are not actual physical measurements; rather, they provide estimates of drug activity. Because the MICs obtained can span greater than three twofold dilutions for the same isolate despite meticulous technique, MICs must be interpreted with caution. Second, host factors contribute greatly to clinical outcome. The same isolate in an immunocompetent patient might not result in the same outcome as in an immunocompromised patient. Thus, in vitro susceptibility does *not* necessarily equate with in vivo clinical success, and in vitro resistance might *not* always correlate with treatment failure. Susceptibility testing occasionally is indicated, for example, in a patient with prolonged fungemia with a presumed susceptible isolate. Because of wide interlaboratory variability in test results, isolates should be tested at specialty laboratories that routinely perform these specialized tests. Susceptibility testing is most helpful in dealing with infections caused by non-*albicans* species of *Candida*.[5,7]

RESISTANCE TO ANTIFUNGAL AGENTS

It is important to distinguish between clinical resistance and microbial resistance. *Clinical resistance* refers to failure of an antifungal agent in the treatment of a fungal infection that arises from factors other than microbial resistance, such as failure of the antifungal agent to reach the site of infection or inability of a patient's immune system to eradicate a fungus whose growth is retarded by an antifungal agent.[8]

TABLE 130-1 General Patterns of Susceptibility and Interpretive Breakpoints of *Candida* Species[a]

	Patterns of Susceptibility							
	Azoles				Echinocandins			Amphotericin
Candida Species	Fluconazole	Itraconazole	Voriconazole	Posaconazole	Caspofungin	Micafungin	Anidulafungin	Amphotericin B
C. albicans	+++ S	+++ S	+++ S	S	+++	+++	+++	+++
C. tropicalis	+++ S	+++ S	+++ S	+++ S	+++ S	+++ S	+++ S	+++ S
C. parapsilosis	S	S	S	S	S[d]	S[d]	S[d]	S
C. glabrata	++ S-DD to R[b]	++ S-DD to R[c]	++	S	S	S	S	S-I[e]
C. krusei	R	S-DD to R[c]	S	S	S	S	S	S-I[e]
C. lusitaniae	S	S	S	S	S	S	S	S to R[f]
Interpretive breakpoints								
Sensitive	≤8	≤0.125	≤0.1	NA	NA	NA	NA	NA
S-DD or I	S-DD: 16–32	S-DD: 0.25–0.5	2	NA	NA	NA	NA	NA
R	>32	>0.5	≤4	NA	NA	NA	NA	NA

[a]Except for amphotericin B, interpretations are based on the use of a broth sensitivity test.
[b]Approximately 15% of *C. glabrata* isolates are resistant to fluconazole.
[c]Approximately 46% of *C. glabrata* isolates and 31% of *C. krusei* isolates are resistant to itraconazole.
[d]Most isolates of *C. parapsilosis* have reduced susceptibility to echinocandins.
[e]A significant proportion of *C. glabrata* and *C. krusei* isolates has reduced susceptibility to amphotericin B.
[f]Although frank resistance to amphotericin B is not observed in all isolates, it is well described for isolates of *C. lusitaniae*.
For antifungal drugs and pathogens for which susceptibility breakpoints have been established (fluconazole, itraconazole, voriconazole):
S = susceptible; S-DD = susceptible-dose dependent (see text); I = intermediate; R = resistant; NA = not available (has not been established for this antifungal against this pathogen).
For antifungal drugs and pathogens for which susceptibility breakpoints have not been established, an estimate of relative activity:
+++ = reliable activity with occasional resistance
++ = moderate activity but resistance is noted
+ = occasional activity
0 = no meaningful activity
Data from NCCLS,[5] Pappas et al.,[7] and Eschenauer et al.[12]

Microbial resistance can refer to *primary* or *secondary* resistance, as determined by in vitro susceptibility testing using standardized methodology. NCCLS resistance breakpoints are based on data relating treatment outcomes and fungal MICs and indicate the MIC at which clinical responses demonstrate a marked decline.[8] However, they do not serve as absolute predictors of therapeutic success or failure.

Primary or *intrinsic resistance* refers to resistance recorded prior to drug exposure in vitro or in vivo. *Secondary* or *acquired resistance* develops on exposure to an antifungal agent and can be either reversible, owing to transient adaptation, or acquired as a result of one or more genetic alterations. The clinical consequences of antifungal resistance can be observed in treatment failures and in changes in the prevalences of *Candida* species

TABLE 130-2 General Patterns of In Vitro Susceptibility of Non-*Candida* Fungal Pathogens[a]

	Patterns of Susceptibility							
	Azoles				Echinocandins			Amphotericin B
Pathogen	Fluconazole	Itraconazole	Voriconazole	Posaconazole	Caspofungin	Micafungin	Anidulafungin	Amphotericin B
Aspergillus								
A. fumigatus	No	Yes	Yes	Yes	Yes	Yes	Yes	Yes
A. flavus	No	Yes	Yes	Yes	Yes	Yes	Yes	Yes
A. terreus	No	Yes	Yes		Yes			No
Fusarium	No	No	Yes (but breakthrough infections are seen)	Conflicting data (species dependent)	No	No	No	Yes but occasional resistance
Scedosporium	No	No	Yes	Yes (apiospermum)	No	No	No	No
Zygomycetes[b]	No	No	No	Yes	No	No	No	Yes
Trichosporon	No	No	Yes	Yes	No	No	No	No
Cryptococcus	Yes	Yes	Yes	Yes	No	No	No	Yes
Histoplasma	Yes	Yes	Yes	Yes	No[c]	No[c]	No[c]	Yes
Coccidioides	Yes	Yes	Yes	Yes	No[c]	No[c]	No[c]	Yes

[a]No = has minimal or no in vitro activity versus the pathogen; Yes = possesses adequate in vitro activity versus the pathogen.
[b]Includes *Rhizopus, Mucor, Absidia* species.
[c]While the echinocandins display activity against the mycelial forms of endemic fungi such as *Histoplasma* spp., *Blastomyces* spp., and *Coccidioides* spp., they display significantly higher MIC values against the yeast forms of these organisms, and should not be used to treat these infections.
Data from Eschenauer et al.[12] and Dodds.[78]

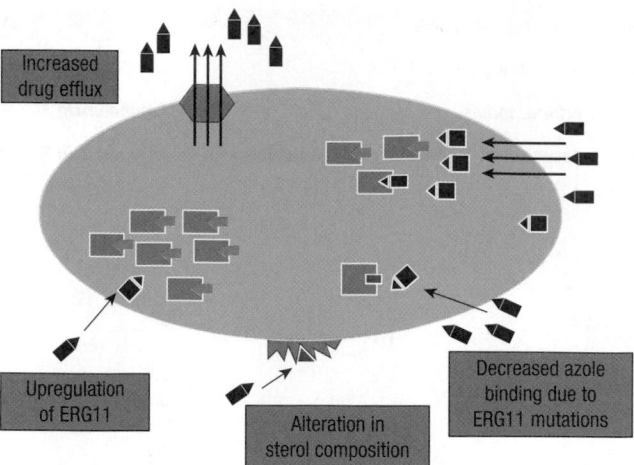

FIGURE 130-2. Mechanisms of azole resistance. Four different mechanisms result in azole resistance: (a) mutations or upregulation of *ERG11*, the target enzyme of azoles, (b) expression of multidrug efflux transport pumps that decrease antifungal drug accumulation within the fungal cell, (c) alteration of the structure or concentration of antifungal drug target proteins, and (d) alteration of membrane sterol proteins.

causing disease. The evidence for the emergence of antifungal-resistant yeasts in patients other than those with HIV infection is confounded by the lack of standardized susceptibility testing methods and definitions of resistance. Large-scale surveys of yeasts from blood cultures, tested by standardized methodology, do not yet suggest that antifungal resistance is a significant or growing therapeutic problem.[8]

A patient may respond clinically to treatment with an antifungal agent despite resistance to that agent in vitro because the patient's own immune system may eradicate the infection, or the agent may reach the site of infection in high concentrations.[8] Resistance to azole antifungal agents has been studied intensively, partly because of the increased number of fluconazole-resistant *Candida* strains isolated from AIDS patients. Resistance can be acquired (i.e., transferred from other organisms or developed during therapy as a result of exposure to the antifungal agent) or intrinsic (innate lack of susceptibility of the antifungal agent to a pathogen). This issue has been reviewed extensively.

The most exhaustive and definitive accounts of antifungal resistance have been described in *Candida* species, in particular *Candida albicans* and, to a lesser extent, *C. glabrata*, *C. tropicalis*, and *C. krusei*, as well as in a few *Cryptococcus neoformans* isolates.[9–11] There are four different mechanisms that result in azole resistance: (a) mutations or upregulation of *ERG11* (an enzyme involved in the ergosterol biosynthesis pathway), (b) expression of multidrug efflux transport pumps that decrease antifungal drug accumulation within the fungal cell, (c) alteration of the structure or concentration of antifungal drug target proteins, and (d) alteration of membrane sterol proteins (Fig. 130–2). It is beyond the scope of this chapter to provide a complete discussion of the biochemical mechanisms of fungal resistance. Interested readers are referred to several excellent reviews concerning this topic.[8–11] Efflux pumps have been identified in *C. albicans*, *C. glabrata*, *C. tropicalis*, and *Candida dubliniensis* and appear to be the most common mechanism of resistance encountered in clinical isolates. Some of these mechanisms (efflux pumps in particular) appear to be reversible when selective pressure of antifungal agents is withdrawn.

Even though ketoconazole was used widely for the treatment of mucocutaneous candidiasis, resistant strains appeared very rarely. In patients with the uncommon syndrome of chronic mucocutaneous

candidiasis, however, the chronic use of ketoconazole was associated with the emergence of ketoconazole-resistant *C. albicans*. Resistance likely developed in this specific population of patients because of two factors: the chronic use of ketoconazole and the inability of patients with this syndrome to eradicate the organism by normal host defense mechanisms. Fluconazole-resistant *C. albicans* have been noted primarily in AIDS patients, usually after CD4 counts are less than 50 cells/mm[3] and after fluconazole has been used chronically for repeated episodes of thrush over months to years. Resistance develops in a stepwise progression in patients who have repeated episodes of thrush with one or several persisting strains of *C. albicans*.

Among hospitalized patients, there is increasing evidence for a shift toward isolation of other resistant species, such as *C. glabrata* and *C. krusei*, that have moderate or high-level resistance to fluconazole. This phenomenon has been especially common among patients in whom fluconazole has been used extensively.[3]

Resistance has not been described widely with itraconazole. This can be partly related to the fact that the drug has been used primarily for the treatment of endemic mycoses and not candidiasis. Even in patients never treated with itraconazole, however, *C. albicans* strains that are resistant to fluconazole also show decreased susceptibility to itraconazole.

The most commonly reported mechanisms of azole resistance among *C. albicans* isolates include reduced permeability of the fungal cell membrane to azoles, alteration in the target fungal enzymes (cytochrome P450) resulting in decreased binding of the azole to the target site, and overproduction of the fungal cytochrome P450 (CYP) enzymes. Studies also suggest the presence of efflux pumps capable of actively pumping azoles from the target pathogen, thereby conferring multidrug resistance to azole antifungals.[8–11]

C. glabrata is intrinsically more resistant than *C. albicans* to ketoconazole. Several strains of *C. glabrata* have been well characterized in terms of the mechanism of ketoconazole resistance. Decreased permeability to azoles has been described, but other strains show enhanced activity of the P450 cell membrane enzymes as well. *C. krusei* is inherently resistant to fluconazole, but it appears to be more susceptible to the other azoles. Decreased uptake of fluconazole into the fungal cell has been noted for several *C. krusei* strains.[8–11]

Although rare, in vitro intrinsic resistance to amphotericin B is described, mainly in *Candida lusitaniae*, *Candida guilliermondii*, and some molds (*Fusarium* spp. and *Pseudallescheria boydii*).[11] However, the current in vitro M27-A methodology discriminates poorly between rates of susceptibility of *Candida* species to amphotericin B. Although the rate of apparent resistance to amphotericin B appears to be quite low, breakthrough bacteremias in patients treated with amphotericin B have been observed. *C. glabrata*, *C. guilliermondii*, *C. krusei*, and *C. lusitaniae* appear to have a higher propensity than other *Candida* species to develop resistance to amphotericin B; this point should be kept in mind when treating patients with infections caused by one of these pathogens.[8] Because polyenes target ergosterol in the membranes of fungal cells, it is not surprising that amphotericin B–resistant strains of *Candida* generally have a marked decrease in ergosterol content compared with amphotericin B–susceptible strains. Resistant isolates of *Cryptococcus neoformans* have been reported to have a mutation in the C8 isomerization step of ergosterol synthesis.[11]

Although spontaneous resistance of *C. albicans* to echinocandins has been documented in vitro, the specific mechanisms of resistance have not been fully elucidated and prospective worldwide surveillance of clinical *Candida* isolates has revealed no evidence of emerging caspofungin resistance.[12]

PATHOGENESIS AND EPIDEMIOLOGY

Systemic mycoses caused by primary or pathogenic fungi include histoplasmosis, coccidioidomycosis, cryptococcosis, blastomycosis, paracoccidioidomycosis, and sporotrichosis. Primary pathogens can cause disease in both healthy and immunocompromised individuals, although disease generally is more severe or disseminated in the immunocompromised host. In contrast, mycoses caused by opportunistic fungi such as *C. albicans*, *Aspergillus* species, *Trichosporon*, *Torulopsis (Candida) glabrata*, *Fusarium*, *Alternaria*, and *Mucor* generally are found only in the immunocompromised host.[1]

Most fungal infections are acquired as a result of accidental inhalation of airborne conidia. For example, *Histoplasma capsulatum* is found in soil contaminated by bat, chicken, or starling excreta, and *C. neoformans* is associated with pigeon droppings. Although some fungi, including *C. albicans*, *C. neoformans*, and *Aspergillus* species, are ubiquitous pathogens with worldwide distribution, other fungi have regional distributions associated with specific geographic environments.[1]

Systemic fungal infections are a major cause of morbidity and mortality in the immunocompromised patient. Fungal infections account for 20% to 30% of fatal infections in patients with acute leukemia, 10% to 15% of fatal infections in patients with lymphoma, and 5% of fatal infections in patients with solid tumors. The frequency of fungal infections among transplant recipients ranges from 0% to 20% for kidney and bone marrow transplant recipients, to 10% to 35% for heart transplant recipients, and 30% to 40% for liver transplant recipients.[4]

Approximately 2% to 4% of all hospitalized patients develop a nosocomial infection. Of these, bacteria comprise the most common etiologic agent.[1] Fungi, however, are becoming increasingly significant nosocomial pathogens. Fungi account for 10% of all bloodstream isolates. *Candida* species (primarily *C. albicans*) are the fourth most commonly isolated bloodstream isolate and account for 78% of all nosocomial fungal infections.[13]

Nosocomially acquired fungal infections can arise from either exogenous or endogenous flora. Endogenous flora can include normal commensal organisms of the skin, gastrointestinal (GI), genitourinary, or respiratory tract. *C. albicans* is found as a normal commensal of the GI tract in 20% to 30% of humans.

A complex interplay of host and pathogen factors influences the acquisition and development of fungal infections. Intact skin or mucosal surfaces serve as primary barriers to infection. Desiccation, epithelial cell turnover, fatty acid content, and low pH of the skin are believed to be important factors in host resistance. Bacterial flora of the skin and mucous membranes compete with fungi for growth. Alterations in the balance of normal flora caused by the use of antibiotics or alterations in nutritional status can allow the proliferation of fungi such as *Candida*, increasing the likelihood of systemic invasion and infection.[1]

The growth of fungi within tissues is restrained by a number of mechanisms. For example, serum has fungistatic activity against *Candida*, in part because of transferrins, the human iron-binding proteins that deprive microbes of the iron needed for synthesis of respiratory enzymes. Serum also contains globulins, which cause a nonimmunologic clumping of *Candida*, facilitating their elimination by inflammatory cells.[1]

Tissue reaction in the presence of fungi varies with fungal species, site of proliferation, and duration of infection. Phagocytosis by neutrophils and macrophages is the earliest mechanism that prevents the establishment of fungi. Consequently, patients with decreased neutrophil counts or decreased neutrophil function are at higher risk of infections, particularly infections caused by *Candida* and *Aspergillus* species. Some mycoses are characterized by a low-grade inflammatory response that does not eliminate the fungi. Fungal cells sometimes can persist within macrophages without being killed, perhaps because of resistance to the effects of lysosomal enzymes.[1]

DIAGNOSIS

❷ The diagnosis of invasive fungal infections generally is accomplished by careful evaluation of clinical symptoms, results of serologic tests, and histopathologic examination and culture of clinical specimens. Skin tests generally are not useful diagnostically because they do not distinguish between active and past infection. They remain useful as screening tools and in epidemiologic studies to determine endemic areas. It is beyond the scope of this chapter to discuss the relative merits of each of the immunologic tests used in the diagnosis of invasive fungal infections. Interested readers, however, are referred to several excellent reviews concerning this topic.[14]

TREATMENT

Invasive Mycoses

Strategies for the prevention or treatment of invasive mycoses can be classified broadly as prophylaxis, early empirical therapy, empirical therapy, and secondary prophylaxis or suppression.[1] In patients undergoing cytotoxic chemotherapy, antifungal therapy is directed primarily at the prevention or treatment of infections caused by *Candida* and *Aspergillus* species. Prophylactic therapy with topical, oral, or intravenous antifungal agents is administered prior to and throughout periods of granulocytopenia (absolute neutrophil count <1,000 cells/L). The potential benefits of prophylactic therapy must be weighed against the potential risks inherent in each regimen, including safety, efficacy, cost, the prevalence of infection, and the potential consequences (e.g., resistance) of widespread use.

Early empirical therapy is the administration of systemic antifungal agents at the onset of fever and neutropenia. Empirical therapy with systemic antifungal agents is administered to granulocytopenic patients with persistent or recurrent fever despite the administration of appropriate antimicrobial therapy.

Secondary prophylaxis (or suppressive therapy) is the administration of systemic antifungal agents (generally prior to and throughout the period of granulocytopenia) to prevent relapse of a documented invasive fungal infection that was treated during a previous episode of granulocytopenia.

Although these treatment classifications also have been applied to the treatment of fungal infections in AIDS, patients with AIDS rarely acquire systemic infections caused by *Candida* or *Aspergillus* species unless they become granulocytopenic because of disease or drugs. The use of antifungal prophylaxis is much less widely studied in this population, although studies suggest that early antifungal prophylaxis with fluconazole or itraconazole decreases the incidence of invasive cryptococcal disease among adult patients who have advanced HIV disease and severe immune suppression (CD4 count <50 cells/mm^3). However, neither of these interventions showed a clear effect on mortality.[15] Suppressive therapy generally is necessary following acute therapy for histoplasmosis, coccidioidomycosis, and cryptococcosis because of the high rates of relapse when antifungal therapy is discontinued.

■ PROPHYLAXIS OF FUNGAL INFECTION IN THE HIV-INFECTED PATIENT

The use of antifungal prophylaxis to prevent fungal infections in HIV-infected patients has been assessed. Fluconazole prevented cryptococcosis and local *Candida* infections, including esophagitis, in HIV-infected patients, but overall mortality was not improved. Because of the high costs of long-term prophylaxis, improved therapeutic regimens available for treating cryptococcal meningitis, and increasing reports of fluconazole resistance among *Candida* isolates from AIDS patients, many clinicians prefer not to use fluconazole prophylaxis in AIDS patients. For some patients with very low CD4 counts (<50 cells/microliter), however, some clinicians feel that it is cost-effective to use fluconazole prophylaxis (100 to 200 mg daily) to prevent cryptococcosis. In endemic areas where the incidence of histoplasmosis is 110 cases per 100 patient-years, prophylaxis with itraconazole (200 mg daily orally) is recommended in HIV-infected patients with CD4 cell counts <150 cells/mm³.

HISTOPLASMOSIS

In humans, histoplasmosis is caused by inhalation of dust-borne microconidia of the dimorphic fungus *H. capsulatum*. Although there exist two dimorphic varieties of *H. capsulatum*, the small-celled (2–5 microns) form (var. *capsulatum*) occurs globally, whereas the large-celled (8–15 microns) form (var. *duboisii*) is confined to the African continent and Madagascar. In tissues stained by conventional techniques, *H. capsulatum* appears as an oval or round, narrow-pore, budding, unencapsulated yeast.[16]

EPIDEMIOLOGY

❸ Although histoplasmosis is found worldwide, certain areas of North and Central America are recognized as endemic areas. In the United States, most disease is localized along the Ohio and Mississippi River valleys, where more than 90% of residents may be affected. Precise reasons for this endemic distribution pattern are unknown but are thought to include moderate climate, humidity, and soil characteristics. *H. capsulatum* is found in nitrogen-enriched soils, particularly those heavily contaminated by avian or bat guano, which accelerates sporulation. Blackbird or pigeon roosts, chicken coops, and sites frequented by bats, such as caves, attics, or old buildings, serve as "microfoci" of infections; once contaminated, soils yield *Histoplasma* for many years. Although birds are not infected because of their high body temperature, bats (mammals) may be infected and can pass yeast forms in their feces, allowing the spread of *H. capsulatum* to new habitats. Air currents carry the spores for great distances, exposing individuals who were unaware of contact with the contaminated site.[16–18]

PATHOPHYSIOLOGY

At ambient temperatures, *H. capsulatum* grows as a mold. The mycelial phase consists of septate branching hyphae with terminal micro- and macroconidia that range in size from 2 to 14 microns in diameter. When soil is disturbed, these conidia become aerosolized and reach the bronchioles or alveoli.[16]

Animal studies demonstrate that within 2 to 3 days after reaching lung tissue, the conidia germinate, releasing yeast forms that begin multiplying by binary fission. During the next 9 to 15 days, organisms are ingested but not destroyed by large numbers of macrophages that are recruited to the infected site, resulting in small infiltrates. Infected macrophages migrate to the mediastinal lymph nodes and other sites within the mononuclear phagocyte system, particularly the spleen and liver. At this time, the onset of specific T-cell immunity in the nonimmune host activates the macrophages, rendering them capable of fungicidal activity. Tissue granulomas form, many of which develop central caseation and necrosis over the next 2 to 4 months. Over a period of several years, these foci become encapsulated and calcified, often with viable yeast trapped within the necrotic tissue.[16,19]

Cellular immunity, as measured by histoplasmin skin-test reactivity, wanes in the absence of occasional reexposure. Although exposure to heavy inocula can overcome these immune mechanisms, resulting in severe disease, reinfection occurs frequently in endemic areas. In the immune individual, the reactions of acquired immunity begin 24 to 48 hours after the appearance of yeast forms, resulting in milder forms of illness and little proliferation of organisms. Although viable organisms can be found within granulomas years after initial infection, the organisms appear to have little ability to proliferate within the fibrous capsules, except in immunocompromised patients.[16,19]

CLINICAL PRESENTATION[15,16,18,19]

General

The outcome of infection with *H. capsulatum* depends on a complex interplay of host, pathogen, and environmental factors. Host factors include the degree of immunosuppression and the presence of immunity (from prior infection). Environmental factors include inoculum size, exposure within an enclosed area, and duration of exposure. Hematogenous dissemination from the lungs to other tissues probably occurs in all infected individuals during the first 2 weeks of infection before specific immunity has developed but is nonprogressive in most cases, which leads to the development of calcified granulomas of the liver and/or spleen. Progressive pulmonary infection is common in patients with underlying centrilobular emphysema.

Acute and chronic manifestations of histoplasmosis appear to result from unusual inflammatory or fibrotic responses to the pathogen, including pericarditis and rheumatologic syndromes during the first year after exposure, with chronic mediastinal inflammation or fibrosis, broncholithiasis, and enlarging parenchymal granulomas later in the course of disease.

Acute Pulmonary Histoplasmosis

In the vast majority of patients, low-inoculum exposure to *H. capsulatum* results in mild or asymptomatic pulmonary histoplasmosis. The course of disease generally is benign, and symptoms usually abate within a few weeks of onset. Patients exposed to a higher inoculum during an acute primary infection or reinfection can experience an acute, self-limited illness with flu-like pulmonary symptoms, including fever, chills, headache, myalgia, and a nonproductive cough. Patients with diffuse pulmonary histoplasmosis can have diffuse radiographic involvement, become hypoxic, and require ventilatory support. A low percentage of patients present with arthritis, erythema nodosum, pericarditis, or mediastinal granuloma.

Chronic Pulmonary Histoplasmosis

Chronic pulmonary histoplasmosis generally presents as an opportunistic infection imposed on a preexisting structural abnormality, such as lesions resulting from emphysema. Patients demonstrate chronic pulmonary symptoms and apical lung lesions that progress with inflammation, calcified granulomas, and fibrosis. Patients with early, noncavitary disease often recover without treatment. Progression of disease over a period of years, seen in 25% to 30% of patients, is associated with cavitation, bronchopleural fistulas, extension to the other lung, pulmonary insufficiency, and often death.

Disseminated Histoplasmosis

In patients exposed to a large inoculum and in immunocompromised hosts, successful containment of the organism within macrophages may not occur, resulting in a progressive illness characterized by yeast-filled phagocytic cells and an inability to produce granulomas. This disease, termed *disseminated histoplasmosis*, is characterized by persistent parasitization of macrophages. The clinical severity of the diverse forms of disseminated histoplasmosis (Table 130–3) generally parallels the degree of macrophage parasitization observed.

Acute (infantile) disseminated histoplasmosis is characterized by massive involvement of the mononuclear phagocyte system by yeast-engorged macrophages. Classically, this severe type of infection is seen in infants and young children and (rarely) in adults with Hodgkin disease or other lymphoproliferative disorders. In infants or children, acute disseminated histoplasmosis is characterized by unrelenting fever, anemia, leukopenia or thrombocytopenia, enlargement of the liver, spleen, and visceral lymph nodes, and GI symptoms, particularly nausea, vomiting, and diarrhea. The chest roentgenogram often demonstrates remnants of the initiating acute pulmonary lesion. Untreated disease is uniformly fatal in 1 to 2 months. A less severe "subacute" form of the disease, which occurs in both infants and immunocompetent adults, is characterized by focal destructive lesions in various organs, weight loss, weakness, fever, and malaise. Untreated disease generally is fatal in approximately 10 months.

Most adults with disseminated histoplasmosis demonstrate a mild, chronic form of the disease. Untreated patients often are ill for 10 to 20 years, demonstrating long asymptomatic periods interrupted by relapses of clinical illness characterized primarily by weight loss, weakness, and fatigue. Chronic disseminated histoplasmosis can be seen in patients with lymphoreticular neoplasms (Hodgkin disease) and patients undergoing immunosuppressant chemotherapy for organ transplantation or for rheumatic diseases. Although CNS involvement occurs in 10% to 20% of patients with severe underlying immunosuppressive conditions, focal organ involvement is uncommon. The disease is characterized by the development of focal granulomatous lesions, often with bone marrow involvement resulting in thrombocytopenia, anemia, and leukemia. Fever, hepatosplenomegaly, and GI ulceration are common.

Histoplasmosis in HIV-Infected Patients

Adult patients with AIDS demonstrate an acute form of disseminated disease that resembles the syndrome seen in infants and children. Progressive disseminated histoplasmosis (PDH), which is defined as a clinical illness that does not improve after at least 3 weeks of observation and that is associated with physical or radiographic findings and/or laboratory evidence of involvement of extrapulmonary tissues, can occur as the direct result of initial infection or because of the reactivation of dormant foci. In endemic areas, 50% of AIDS patients demonstrate PDH as the first manifestation of their disease. PDH is characterized by fever (75% of patients), weight loss, chills, night sweats, enlargement of the spleen, liver, or lymph nodes, and anemia. Pulmonary symptoms occur in only one third of patients and do not always correlate with the presence of infiltrates on chest roentgenogram. A clinical syndrome resembling septicemia is seen in approximately 25% to 50% of patients.[19]

DIAGNOSIS

Detection of single, yeastlike cells 2 to 5 microns in diameter with narrow-based budding by direct examination or by histologic study of blood smears or tissues should raise strong suspicion of infection with *H. capsulatum* because colonization does not occur as with *Aspergillus* or *Candida* infection. Identification of mycelial isolates from clinical cultures can be made by conversion of the mycelium to the yeast form (requires 3 to 6 weeks) or through a rapid (2-hour) and 100% sensitive chemiluminescent DNA probe that recognizes ribosomal DNA. In patients with suspected disseminated or chronic cavitary histoplasmosis, 2 to 3 blood, sputum, and bone marrow cultures and stains should be obtained using the lysis centrifugation (Isolator tube) technique, and the cultures should be held for 14 to 21 days for optimal yield of *H. capsulatum*. In patients with acute self-limited histoplasmosis, extensive testing to verify the diagnosis may not be necessary.

In most patients, serologic evidence remains the primary method in the diagnosis of histoplasmosis. Results obtained from commercially available complement fixation (CF), immunodiffusion (ID), and latex agglutination (LA) antibody tests are used alone or in combination. In general, the use of histoplasmin skin tests is of little value except in epidemiologic studies because histoplasmin reactivity waxes in the absence of occasional reexposure. In addition, histoplasmin skin testing can result in a false increase in the CF titer for mycelial antigen (CF-M) to *H. capsulatum*. A fourfold rise in the CF titer is usually indicative of recent infection, although some patients with severe disease or profound immunosuppression can demonstrate a weaker antibody response. CF titers remain positive for many years, since CF antibodies persist after infection. Because the ID test is more specific but less sensitive than CF, it should be used to assess the importance of weakly reactive results obtained by CF rather than as a screening procedure.

In the AIDS patient with PDH, the diagnosis is best established by bone marrow biopsy and culture, which yield positive cultures in more than 90% of patients, although blood cultures and histopathologic examination and culture of pulmonary tissue, sputum, skin, and lymph nodes also can be helpful. Detection of *H. capsulatum* polysaccharide antigen (HPA) in urine, blood, or cerebrospinal fluid (CSF) by enzyme-linked immunosorbent assay (ELISA) or by modified RIA offer promising new techniques for the rapid diagnosis of histoplasmosis. The HPA (RIA) levels also have been used successfully to monitor the course of therapy and to detect relapses in patients with AIDS, and the clearance of antigen from serum and urine correlates with clinical efficacy during maintenance therapy with itraconazole.[19]

TREATMENT

Histoplasmosis

■ NON–HIV-INFECTED PATIENT

❹ Table 130–3 summarizes the recommended therapy for the treatment of histoplasmosis. In general, asymptomatic or mildly ill patients and patients with sarcoid-like disease do not benefit from antifungal therapy. In the vast majority of patients, low-inoculum exposure to *H. capsulatum* results in *mild* or *asymptomatic* pulmonary histoplasmosis. The course of disease generally is benign, and symptoms usually abate within a few weeks of onset. Therapy can be helpful in symptomatic patients whose conditions have not improved during the first month of infection. Fever persisting more than 3 weeks can indicate that the patient is developing progressive disseminated disease, which can be aborted by antifungal therapy. Whether antifungal therapy hastens recovery or prevents complications is unknown because it has never been studied in prospective trials.

Fluconazole remains a second-line agent for the treatment of histoplasmosis. Clinical data regarding the use of newer azoles such as voriconazole and posaconazole are limited. While both

TABLE 130-3 Clinical Manifestations and Therapy of Histoplasmosis

Type of Disease and Common Clinical Manifestations	Approximate Frequency (%)[a]	Therapy/Comments
Nonimmunosuppressed host		
Acute pulmonary histoplasmosis		
Asymptomatic or mild-moderate disease	50–99	*Asymptomatic, mild, or symptoms <4 weeks:* No therapy generally required. Itraconazole (200 mg 3 times daily for 3 days and then 200 mg once or twice daily for 6–12 weeks) is recommended for patients who continue to have symptoms for 11 months
		Symptoms >4 weeks: Itraconazole 200 mg once daily × 6–12 weeks[b]
Self-limited disease	1–50	*Self-limited disease:* Amphotericin B[c] 0.3–0.5 mg/kg/day × 2–4 weeks (total dose 500 mg) or ketoconazole 400 mg orally daily × 3–6 months can be beneficial in patients with severe hypoxia following inhalation of large inocula; Antifungal therapy generally not useful for arthritis or pericarditis; NSAIDs or corticosteroids can be useful in some cases
Mediastinal granulomas	1–50	Most lesions resolve spontaneously; surgery or antifungal therapy with amphotericin B 40–50 mg/day × 2–3 weeks or itraconazole 400 mg/day orally × 6–12 months can be beneficial in some severe cases; mild to moderate disease can be treated with itraconazole for 6–12 months
Moderately severe-severe diffuse pulmonary disease		Lipid amphotericin B 3–5 mg/kg/day followed by itraconazole 200 mg twice daily for 3 days then twice daily for a total of 12 weeks of therapy; Alternatively, in patients at low risk for nephrotoxicity, amphotericin B deoxycholate 0.7–1 mg/kg/day can be utilized; Methylprednisolone (0.5–1.0 mg/kg daily IV) during the first 1–2 weeks of antifungal therapy is recommended for patients who develop respiratory complications, including hypoxemia or significant respiratory distress
Inflammatory/fibrotic disease	0.02	*Fibrosing mediastinitis:* The benefit of antifungal therapy (itraconazole 200 mg twice daily × 3 months) is controversial but should be considered, especially in patients with elevated ESR or CF titers ≤1:32; surgery can be of benefit if disease is detected early; late disease cannot respond to therapy
		Sarcoid-like: NSAIDs or corticosteroids[d] can be of benefit for some patients
		Pericarditis: Severe disease: corticosteroids 1 mg/kg/day or pericardial drainage procedure
Chronic cavitary pulmonary histoplasmosis	0.05	Antifungal therapy generally recommended for all patients to halt further lung destruction and reduce mortality
		Mild–moderate disease: Itraconazole (200 mg 3 times daily for 3 days and then 1 or 2 times daily for at least 1 year; Some clinicians recommend therapy for 18–24 months due to the high rate of relapse; Itraconazole plasma concentrations should be obtained after the patient has been receiving this agent for at least 2 weeks
		Severe disease: Amphotericin B 0.7 mg/kg/day for a minimum total dose of 25-35 mg/kg is effective in 59–100% of cases and should be used in patients who require hospitalization or are unable to take itraconazole because of drug interactions, allergies, failure to absorb drug, or failure to improve clinically after a minimum of 12 weeks of itraconazole therapy
Histoplasma endocarditis		Amphotericin B (lipid formulations may be preferred, due to their lower rate of renal toxicity) plus a valve replacement is recommended; If the valve cannot be replaced, lifelong suppression with itraconazole is recommended
Central nervous system histoplasmosis		Amphotericin B should be used as initial therapy (lipid formulations at 5 mg/kg/day, for a total dosage of 175 mg/kg may be preferred, due to their lower rate of renal toxicity) for 4–6 weeks, followed by an oral azole (fluconazole or itraconazole 200 mg 2 or 3 times daily) for at least a year; Some patients may require lifelong therapy; Response to therapy should be monitored by repeat lumbar punctures to assess *Histoplasma* antigen levels, WBC, and CF antibody titers; Blood levels of itraconazole should be obtained to ensure adequate drug exposure
Immunosuppressed host		
Disseminated histoplasmosis	0.02 – 0.05	*Disseminated histoplasmosis:* Untreated mortality 83–93%; relapse 5– 23% in non-AIDS patients; therapy is recommended for all patients
Acute (Infantile)		*Nonimmunosuppressed patients:* Ketoconazole 400 mg/day orally × 6–12 months or amphotericin B 35 mg/kg IV
Subacute		*Immunosuppressed patients (non-AIDS) or endocarditis or CNS disease:* Amphotericin B >35 mg/kg × 3 months followed by fluconazole or itraconazole 200 mg orally twice daily × 12 months
Progressive histoplasmosis (immunocompetent patients and immunosuppressed patients without AIDS)		*Moderately severe to severe:* Liposomal amphotericin B (3.0 mg/kg daily), amphotericin B lipid complex (5.0 mg/kg daily), or deoxycholate amphotericin B (0.7–1.0 mg/kg daily) for 1–2 weeks, followed by itraconazole (200 mg twice daily for at least 12 months)
		Mild to moderate: Itraconazole (200 mg twice daily for at least 12 months)
Progressive disease of AIDS	25–50[e]	Amphotericin B 15–30 mg/kg (1–2 g over 4–10 weeks)[f] or itraconazole 200 mg three times daily for 3 days then twice daily for 12 weeks, followed by lifelong suppressive therapy with itraconazole 200–400 mg orally daily; Although patients receiving secondary prophylaxis (chronic maintenance therapy) might be at low risk for recurrence of systemic mycosis when their CD4+ T-lymphocyte counts increase to >100 cells/microliter in response to HAART, the number of patients who have been evaluated is insufficient to warrant a recommendation to discontinue prophylaxis

AIDS, acquired immunodeficiency syndrome; CF, complement fixation; ESR, erythrocyte sedimentation rate; HAART, highly active antiretroviral therapy; NSAIDs, nonsteroidal antiinflammatory drugs; PO, orally.

[a]As a percentage of all patients presenting with histoplasmosis.

[b]Itraconazole plasma concentrations should be measured during the second week of therapy to ensure that detectable concentrations have been achieved. If the concentration is below 1 mcg/mL, the dose may be insufficient or drug interactions can be impairing absorption or accelerating metabolism, requiring a change in dosage. If plasma concentrations are greater than 10 mcg/mL, the dosage can be reduced.

[c]Desoxycholate amphotericin B.

[d]Effectiveness of corticosteroids is controversial.

[e]As a percentage of AIDS patients presenting with histoplasmosis as the initial manifestation of their disease.

[f]Liposomal amphotericin B (AmBisome) may be more appropriate for disseminated disease.

Data from Deepe,16 Wheat et al.,[18] and Wheat and Kauffman.[19]

have activity against *Histoplasma*, posaconazole appears to be more active than itraconazole in the immune compromised and nonimmune compromised mouse model of infection, while voriconazole has not been tested in animal models. Both agents have been used successfully in a few patients. Of note, the echinocandins have no activity against *Histoplasma*.

Patients with mild, self-limited disease, chronic disseminated disease, or chronic pulmonary histoplasmosis who have no underlying immunosuppression usually can be treated with either oral itraconazole or IV amphotericin B. The goals of therapy are resolution of clinical abnormalities, prevention of relapse, and eradication of infection whenever possible, although chronic suppression of infection can be adequate in immunosuppressed patients, including those with HIV disease.[18,19] Patients with arthritis, erythema nodosum, pericarditis, or mediastinal granuloma can require the addition of a 2-week course of corticosteroids to their therapy.[16]

■ HIV-INFECTED PATIENT

In AIDS patients, intensive 12-week primary antifungal therapy (induction and consolidation therapy) is followed by lifelong suppressive (maintenance) therapy with itraconazole. Amphotericin B dosages of 50 mg/day (up to 1 mg/kg per day) should be administered intravenously to a cumulative dose of 15 to 35 mg/kg (1 to 2 g) in patients who require hospitalization. Amphotericin B can be replaced with itraconazole 200 mg orally twice daily when the patient no longer requires hospitalization or intravenous therapy to complete a 12-week total course of induction therapy. In patients who do not require hospitalization, itraconazole therapy for 12 weeks can be used.

Fluconazole 800 mg/day orally as induction, followed by 400 mg/day, was effective in 88% of patients, but relapses occurred in approximately one third of patients, and in vitro resistance developed in approximately 50% of patients who relapsed.

In regions experiencing high rates of histoplasmosis (>5 cases/100 patient years), itraconazole 200 mg/day is recommended as prophylactic therapy in HIV-infected patients. Fluconazole is not an acceptable alternative because of its inferior activity against *H. capsulatum* and its lower efficacy for the treatment of histoplasmosis.[18]

Although patients receiving secondary prophylaxis (chronic maintenance therapy) might be at low risk for recurrence of systemic mycosis when their CD4+ T lymphocyte counts increase to >100 cells/microliter in response to highly active antiretroviral therapy (HAART), the number of patients who have been evaluated is insufficient to warrant a recommendation to discontinue prophylaxis.

EVALUATION OF THERAPEUTIC OUTCOMES

Response to therapy should be measured by resolution of radiologic, serologic, and microbiologic parameters and by improvement in signs and symptoms of infection. Although investigators are limited by the lack of standardized criteria to quantify the extent of infection, degree of immunosuppression, or treatment response, response rates (based on resolution or improvement in presenting signs and symptoms) of greater than 80% have been reported in case series in AIDS patients receiving varied dosages of amphotericin B. Rapid responses are reported, with the resolution of symptoms in 25% and 75% of patients by days 3 and 7 of therapy, respectively.

After the initial course of therapy for histoplasmosis is complete, lifelong suppressive therapy with oral azoles or amphotericin B (1 to 1.5 mg/kg weekly or biweekly) is recommended because of the frequent recurrence of infection.[20] Relapse rates in AIDS patients not receiving maintenance therapy range from 50% to 90%.[18]

Antigen testing can be useful for monitoring therapy in patients with disseminated histoplasmosis. Antigen concentrations decrease with therapy and increase with relapse. Some investigators recommend that treatment should continue until antigen concentrations revert to negative or less than 4 units. If treatment is discontinued before antigen concentrations in serum and urine revert to negative, patients should be followed closely for relapse, and antigen levels should be monitored every 3 to 6 months until they become negative.[18]

BLASTOMYCOSIS

North American blastomycosis is a systemic fungal infection caused by *Blastomyces dermatitidis*, a dimorphic fungus that infects primarily the lungs. Patients, however, can present with a variety of pulmonary and extrapulmonary clinical manifestations. Pulmonary disease can be acute or chronic and can mimic infection with tuberculosis, pyogenic bacteria, other fungi, or malignancy. Blastomycosis can disseminate to virtually every other body organ, and approximately 40% of patients with blastomycosis present with skin, bone and joint, or genitourinary tract involvement without any evidence of pulmonary disease.[21]

Pulmonary infection probably occurs by inhalation of conidia, which convert to the yeast form in the lung. A vigorous inflammatory response ensues, with neutrophilic recruitment to the lungs followed by the development of cell-mediated immunity and the formation of noncaseating granulomas.

EPIDEMIOLOGY

Blastomycosis was renamed *North American blastomycosis* in 1942, when Conant and Howell named a similar fungus endemic to South America, *Blastomyces braziliensis*, and the disease it caused *South American blastomycosis*. Although the disease is now recognized to be endemic to the southeastern and south central states of the United States (especially those bordering on the Mississippi and Ohio River basins) and the midwestern states and Canadian provinces bordering the Great Lakes, numerous cases of North American blastomycosis have been diagnosed in Africa, northern parts of South America, India, and Europe. Endemic areas have been defined primarily by analysis of sporadic cases and epidemics or clusters of disease because the lack of a dependable skin or laboratory test makes wide-scale epidemiologic testing to determine the incidence of infection unfeasible at present.[19,20] Although initial review of sporadic cases suggested that males with outdoor occupations that exposed them to soil were at greatest risk for blastomycosis, there is no sex, age, or occupational predilection for blastomycosis.[19,21]

Although *B. dermatitidis* generally is considered to be a soil inhabitant, attempts to isolate the organism in nature frequently have been unsuccessful. *B. dermatitidis* has been isolated from soil containing decayed vegetation, decomposed wood, and pigeon manure, frequently in association with warm, moist soil of wooded areas that is rich in organic debris.[19,21]

PATHOPHYSIOLOGY AND CLINICAL PRESENTATION[13,19,21]

General

Colonization does not occur with *Blastomyces*. *Acute pulmonary blastomycosis* generally is an asymptomatic or self-limited disease characterized by fever, shaking chills, and productive, purulent cough, with or without hemoptysis, in immunocompetent individuals. The clinical presentation can be difficult to differentiate from other respiratory infections, including bacterial pneumonia, on the basis of clinical symptoms alone.

Sporadic (nonepidemic) pulmonary blastomycosis can present as a more chronic or subacute disease, with low-grade fever, night sweats, weight loss, and productive cough that resembles tuberculosis rather than bacterial pneumonia. *Chronic pulmonary blastomycosis* is characterized by fever, malaise, weight loss, night sweats, chest pain, and productive cough. Patients often are thought to have tuberculosis and frequently have evidence of disseminated disease that can appear 1 to 3 years after the primary pneumonia has resolved. Reactivation of disease can occur in the lungs or as the focus of new infection in other organs.

In approximately 40% of patients, dissemination is not accompanied by reactivation of pulmonary disease. The most common sites for disseminated disease include the skin and bony skeleton, although less commonly the prostate, oropharyngeal mucosa, and abdominal viscera are involved. CNS disease, while exceedingly uncommon, is associated with the highest mortality rate.

Laboratory and Diagnostic Tests

The simplest and most successful method of diagnosing blastomycosis is by direct microscopic visualization of the large, multinucleated yeast with single, broad-based buds in sputum or other respiratory specimens following digestion of cells and debris with 10% potassium hydroxide. Histopathologic examination of tissue biopsies and culture of secretions also should be used to identify *B. dermatitidis*, although it can require up to 30 days to isolate and identify a small inoculum.

No reliable skin test exists to determine the incidence and prevalence of disease in endemic populations, and reliable serologic diagnosis of blastomycosis has long been hampered by the lack of specific and standardized reagents. Serologic response does not always correlate with clinical improvement, although some investigators have noted that a decline in the number of precipitins or CF titers can offer evidence of a favorable prognosis in patients with established disease.

Acute pulmonary blastomycosis generally is an asymptomatic or self-limited disease characterized by fever, shaking chills, and productive, purulent cough, with or without hemoptysis, in immunocompetent individuals. The clinical presentation can be difficult to differentiate from other respiratory infections, including bacterial pneumonia, on the basis of clinical symptoms alone. Sporadic (nonepidemic) cases of pulmonary blastomycosis can present as a more chronic or subacute disease with low-grade fever, night sweats, weight loss, and productive cough that resembles tuberculosis rather than bacterial pneumonia.

TREATMENT

Blastomycosis

■ NON–HIV-INFECTED PATIENT

❺ In patients with mild pulmonary blastomycosis, the clinical presentation of the patient, the immune competence of the patient, and the toxicity of the antifungal agents are the main determinants of whether or not to administer antifungal therapy. All immunocompromised patients and patients with progressive pulmonary disease or with extrapulmonary disease should be treated (Table 130–4). In the case of disease limited to the lungs, cure might have occurred without treatment before the diagnosis is made. Regardless of whether or not the patient receives treatment, however, he or she

TABLE 130-4 Therapy of Blastomycosis

Type of Disease	Preferred Treatment	Comments
Pulmonary[a]		
Life-threatening	Amphotericin B[b] IV 0.7–1 mg/kg/day IV (total dose 1.5–2.5 g)	Patients can be initiated on amphotericin B and changed to oral itraconazole 200–400 mg orally daily once patient is clinically stabilized and a minimum dose of 500 mg of amphotericin B has been administered
Mild to moderate	Itraconazole 200 mg orally twice daily × ≥ 6 months[c]	*Alternative therapy:* Ketoconazole 400–800 mg orally daily × ≥6 months or fluconazole 400–800 mg orally daily × ≥6 months[d] *In patients intolerant of azoles or in whom disease progresses during azole therapy:* Amphotericin B 0.5–0.7 mg/kg/day IV (total dose 1.5–2.5 g)
Disseminated or extrapulmonary		
CNS	Amphotericin B 0.7–1 mg/kg/day IV (total dose 1.5–2.5 g)	For patients unable to tolerate a full course of amphotericin B, consider lipid formulations of amphotericin B or fluconazole ≥ 800 mg orally daily
Non-CNS		
Life-threatening	Amphotericin B 0.7–1 mg/kg/day IV (total dose 1.5–2.5 g)	Patients can be initiated on amphotericin B and changed to oral itraconazole 200–400 mg orally daily once stabilized
Mild to moderate	Itraconazole 200–400 mg orally daily × ≥ 6 months	Ketoconazole 400–800 mg orally daily or fluconazole 400–800 mg orally daily × ≥ 6 months *In patients intolerant of azoles or in whom disease progresses during azole therapy:* Amphotericin B 0.5–0.7 mg/kg/day IV (total dose 1.5–2.5 g) *Bone disease:* Therapy with azoles should be continued for 12 months
Immunocompromised host (including patients with AIDS, transplants, or receiving chronic glucocorticoid therapy)		
Acute disease	Amphotericin B 0.7–1 mg/kg/day IV (total dose 1.5–2.5 g)	Patients without CNS infection can be switched to itraconazole once clinically stabilized and a minimum dose of 1 g of amphotericin B has been administered; long-term suppressive therapy with an azole is advised
Suppressive therapy	Itraconazole 200–400 mg orally daily	For patients with CNS disease or those intolerant of itraconazole, consider fluconazole 800 mg orally daily

AIDS, acquired immunodeficiency syndrome.
[a]Some patients with acute pulmonary infection can have a spontaneous cure. Patients with progressive pulmonary disease should be treated.
[b]Desoxycholate amphotericin B.
[c]In patients not responding to 400 mg, dosage should be increased by 200 mg increments every 4 weeks to a maximum of 800 mg daily.
[d]Therapy with ketoconazole is associated with relapses, and fluconazole therapy achieves a lower response rate than itraconazole.
Data from Wheat and Kauffman[19] and O'Shaughnessy et al.[21]

must be followed carefully for many years for evidence of reactivation or progressive disease.[19,21]

Some authors recommend ketoconazole therapy for the treatment of self-limited pulmonary disease, with the hope of preventing late extrapulmonary disease; however, data supporting the efficacy of these regimens are lacking.[19,21] Itraconazole 200 to 400 mg/day demonstrated 90% efficacy as a first-line agent in the treatment of non–life-threatening non-CNS blastomycosis, and for compliant patients who completed at least 2 months of therapy, a success rate of 95% was noted. No therapeutic advantage was noted with the higher (400 mg) dosage as compared with patients treated with 200 mg.

All patients with disseminated blastomycosis, as well as those with extrapulmonary disease, require therapy. Ketoconazole 400 mg/day orally for 6 months cures more than 80% of patients with chronic pulmonary and nonmeningeal disseminated blastomycosis. Amphotericin B is more efficacious but more toxic and therefore is reserved for noncompliant patients and patients with overwhelming or life-threatening disease, CNS infection, and treatment failures. Cumulative amphotericin B dosages of more than 1 g have resulted in cure without relapse in 70% to 91% of patients with blastomycosis. Relapse rates depend on the total dosage of amphotericin B administered.[19,21] Patients with genitourinary tract disease should be treated initially with 600–800 mg/day of ketoconazole because of the low concentrations of drug achieved in the urine and prostate tissue.

Patients should be monitored carefully for signs of clinical failure, and those who fail or are unable to tolerate itraconazole therapy or who develop CNS disease should be treated with amphotericin B for a total cumulative dose of 1.5 to 2.5 g.[19,21]

Lipid preparations of amphotericin B are effective in animal models of blastomycosis, but they have not been evaluated adequately in humans. Limited clinical experience suggests that these preparations can provide an alternative for patients unable to experience standard therapy with amphotericin B because of toxicity. Surgery has only a limited role in the treatment of blastomycosis.

■ HIV-INFECTED PATIENT

For unclear reasons, blastomycosis is an uncommon opportunistic disease among immunocompromised individuals, including AIDS patients; however, blastomycosis can occur as a late (CD4 lymphocytes <200 cells/mm^3) and frequently fatal complication of HIV infection. In this population, overwhelming disseminated disease with frequent involvement of the CNS is common.[19] Following induction therapy with amphotericin B (total cumulative dose of 1 g), HIV-infected patients should receive chronic suppressive therapy with an oral azole antifungal. Despite its higher cost, itraconazole has become the drug of choice for non–life-threatening histoplasmosis (mild to moderate disease) in HIV-infected patients.[21]

COCCIDIOIDOMYCOSIS

EPIDEMIOLOGY

Coccidioidomycosis is caused by infection with *Coccidioides immitis*, a dimorphic fungus found in the southwestern and western United States, as well as in parts of Mexico and South America. In North America, the endemic regions encompass the semiarid areas of the southwestern United States from California to Texas known as the Lower Sonoran Zone, where there is scant annual rainfall, hot summers, and sandy, alkaline soil. *Coccidioides immitis* grows in the soil as a mold, and mycelia proliferate during the rainy season.

TABLE 130-5 Risk Factors for Severe, Disseminated Infection with Coccidioidomycosis

Race (Filipinos > African-Americans > Native Americans > Hispanics > Asians)
Pregnancy (especially when infection is acquired or reactivated in the second or third trimester)
Compromised cellular immune system, including
  AIDS patients
  Patients receiving
    Corticosteroids
    Immunosuppressive agents
    Chemotherapy
Male gender
Neonates
Patients with B or AB blood types

AIDS, acquired immune deficiency syndrome.
Data from Galgiani JM, Ampel NM, Blair JE, Catanzaro A, et al. Practice guidelines for the treatment of coccidioidomycoses. Clin Infect Dis 2005;30:658–661.

During the dry season, resistant arthroconidia form and become airborne when the soil is disturbed.

Although generally considered to be a regional disease, coccidioidomycosis has increased in importance in recent years because of the increased tourism and population in endemic areas, the increased use of immunosuppressive therapy in transplantation and oncology, and the AIDS epidemic. Although there is no racial, hormonal, or immunologic predisposition for acquiring primary disease, these factors affect the risk of subsequent dissemination of disease (Table 130–5).[20]

PATHOPHYSIOLOGY

When individuals come in contact with contaminated soil during ranching, dust storms, or proximity to construction sites or archaeologic excavations, arthroconidia are inhaled into the respiratory tree, where they transform into spherules, which reproduce by cleavage of the cytoplasm to produce endospores. The endospores are released when the spherules reach maturity. Similar to histoplasmosis, an acute inflammatory response in the tissue leads to infiltration of mononuclear cells, ultimately resulting in granuloma formation.[20]

CLINICAL PRESENTATION OF COCCIDIOIDOMYCOSIS[11,19–22]

Coccidioidomycosis encompasses a spectrum of illnesses ranging from primary uncomplicated respiratory tract infection that resolves spontaneously to progressive pulmonary or disseminated infection. Initial or primary infection with *C. immitis* almost always involves the lungs. Although approximately one third of the population in endemic areas is infected, the average incidence of symptomatic disease is only approximately 0.43%.

Signs and Symptoms

In *asymptomatic disease* (60% of patients), patients have nonspecific symptoms that are often indistinguishable from ordinary upper respiratory infections, including fever, cough, headache, sore throat, myalgias, and fatigue. A fine, diffuse rash can appear during the first few days of the illness. Primary pneumonia can be the first manifestation of disease, characterized by a productive cough that can be blood-streaked, as well as single or multiple soft or dense homogeneous hilar or basal infiltrates on chest roentgenogram. Chronic, persistent pneumonia or persistent pulmonary coccidioidomycosis (primary disease lasting more than 6 weeks) is complicated by hemoptysis, pulmonary scarring, and the formation of cavities or bronchopleural fistulas.

Necrosis of pulmonary tissue with drainage and cavity formation occurs commonly. Most parenchymal cavities close spontaneously or form dense nodular scar tissue that can become superinfected with bacteria or spherules of *C. immitis*. These patients often have persistent cough, fevers, and weight loss.

Valley fever occurs in approximately 25% of patients and is characterized by erythema nodosum and erythema multiforme of the upper trunk and extremities in association with diffuse joint aches or fever. More commonly, a diffuse, mild erythroderma or maculopapular rash is observed. Patients can have pleuritic chest pain and peripheral eosinophilia.

Disseminated disease occurs in less than 1% of infected patients. The most common sites for dissemination are the skin, lymph nodes, bone, and meninges, although the spleen, liver, kidney, and adrenal gland also can be involved. Occasionally, miliary coccidioidomycosis occurs, with rapid, widespread dissemination, often in concert with positive blood cultures for *C. immitis*. Patients with AIDS frequently present with miliary disease. Coccidioidomycosis in AIDS patients appears to be caused by reactivation of disease in most patients.

CNS infection occurs in approximately 16% of patients with disseminated coccidioidomycosis. Patients can present with meningeal disease without previous symptoms of primary pulmonary infection, although disease usually occurs within 6 months of the primary infection. The signs and symptoms are often subtle and nonspecific, including headache, weakness, changes in mental status (lethargy and confusion), neck stiffness, low-grade fever, weight loss, and occasionally, hydrocephalus. Space-occupying lesions are rare, and the main areas of involvement are the basilar meninges.

DIAGNOSIS

Laboratory Tests

Recovery of *C. immitis* from infected tissues or secretions for direct examination and culture provides an accurate and rapid method of diagnosis. For the safe isolation of *Coccidioides* spp., the laboratory should maintain a biological safety level 2 or 3. Direct microscopic examination and histopathologic studies of infected tissues will reveal the large, mature endosporulating spherules. Young spherules without endospores can be confused, however, with other fungi. Silver stains of body fluids or tissue biopsies are also helpful.

With chronic, persistent pneumonia, *C. immitis* often can be cultured from the sputum for a period of several years. Chest radiographs usually demonstrate apical fibronodular lesions or slowly progressive cavitation. With CNS infection, analysis of the CSF generally reveals a lymphocytic pleocytosis with elevated protein and a decreased glucose concentration. Although serum usually is positive for coccidioidal CF antibodies, the coccidioidal skin test is often negative.

Other Diagnostic Tests

Most patients develop a positive skin test within 3 weeks of the onset of symptoms. Baseline evaluation of skin test reactivity and serology is essential to assess cell-mediated immunity. Patients who develop early positive skin-test reactivity or whose coccidioidin skin-test reactivity turns from negative to positive during therapy have an improved prognosis compared with patients whose skin-test reactivity develops later or does not change during therapy. Patients with disseminated coccidioidomycosis whose skin tests are persistently negative are more likely to require prolonged therapy, and they are more likely to relapse after completion of therapy.

Antibody production can be used to follow the course of disease because most patients produce antibodies in response to infection with *C. immitis*. Early infection is characterized by the development of the IgM antibody, which peaks within 2 to 3 weeks of infection and then declines rapidly. The IgM antibody can be detected by either tube precipitin or immunodiffusion techniques.

The IgG antibody levels increase between 4 and 12 weeks after infection and decrease slowly over months to years, and IgG can be detected in many body fluids, including serum, CSF, and pleural fluid, by CF and ID techniques. Higher titers (>1:16 or 1:32) occur more frequently with severe disease. Titers can be followed serially to evaluate the efficacy of antifungal therapy.

Radiographic features tend to be quite variable; hilar adenopathy with alveolar infiltrates, tissue excavation of an infiltrate (resulting in a thin-walled cavity), or small pleural effusions are all seen commonly. With chronic persistent pneumonia, chest radiographs usually demonstrate apical fibronodular lesions or slowly progressive cavitation.[21,22]

TREATMENT

Coccidioidomycosis

■ GENERAL GUIDELINES

❻ Therapy for coccidioidomycosis is difficult, and the results are unpredictable. Guidelines are available for treatment of this disease; however, optimal treatment for many forms of this disease still generates debate.[20] The efficacy of antifungal therapy for coccidioidomycosis is often is less certain than that for other fungal etiologies, such as blastomycosis, histoplasmosis, or cryptococcus, even when in vitro susceptibilities and the sites of infections are similar. The refractoriness of coccidioidomycosis can relate to the ability of *C. immitis* spherules to release hundreds of endospores, maximally challenging host defenses.[20,22] Fortunately, only approximately 5% of infected patients require therapy.[22]

■ GOALS OF THERAPY

Desired outcomes of treatment are resolution of signs and symptoms of infection, reduction of serum concentrations of anticoccidioidal antibodies, and return of function of involved organs. It would also be desirable to prevent relapse of illness on discontinuation of therapy, although current therapy is often unable to achieve this goal.

■ SPECIFIC AGENTS USED FOR THE TREATMENT OF COCCIDIOIDOMYCOSIS

Azole antifungals, primarily fluconazole and itraconazole, have replaced amphotericin B as initial therapy for most chronic pulmonary or disseminated infections. Amphotericin B is now usually reserved for patients with respiratory failure because of infection with *Coccidioides* species, those with rapidly progressive coccidioidal infections, or women during pregnancy. Therapy often ranges from many months to years in duration, and in some patients, lifelong suppressive therapy is needed to prevent relapses. Specific antifungals (and their usual dosages) for the treatment of coccidioidomycosis include intravenous amphotericin B (0.5 to 1.5 mg/kg per day), ketoconazole (400 mg/day orally), intravenous or oral fluconazole (usually 400 to 800 mg/day, although dosages as high as 1200 mg/day have been used without complications), and itraconazole (200 to 300 mg orally twice daily or three times daily, as either capsules or solution).[20,22] If itraconazole is used, measurement of serum concentrations can be helpful to ascertain whether oral bioavailability is adequate.

Amphotericin B generally is preferred as initial therapy in patients with rapidly progressive disease, whereas azoles generally are preferred in patients with subacute or chronic presentations. The lipid formulations of amphotericin B have not been studied extensively in coccidioidal infection but can offer a means of giving more drug with less toxicity. Fluconazole probably is the most frequently used medicine given its tolerability, although high relapse rates have been reported in some studies. Relapse rates with itraconazole therapy can be lower than with fluconazole.[20,22]

The usefulness of newly available antifungal agents of possible benefit for the treatment of refractory coccidioidal infections has not been adequately assessed and they are not yet FDA approved for use in this population. Case reports have suggested that voriconazole can be effective in selected patients. Caspofungin has been effective in treating experimental murine coccidioidomycosis, but in-vitro susceptibility of isolates varies widely, and there is only one report regarding its value. Posaconazole was shown to be an effective treatment in a small clinical trial and in patients with refractory infections. Its efficacy relative to other triazole antifungals is unknown.

Combination therapy with members of different classes of antifungal agents has not been evaluated in patients, and there is a hypothetical risk of antagonism. However, some clinicians feel that outcome in severe cases is improved when amphotericin B is combined with an azole antifungal. If the patient improves, the dosage of amphotericin B can be slowly decreased while the dosage of azole is maintained.[20,22]

CLINICAL CONTROVERSY

Because of the lack of prospective, controlled trials, there is continued disagreement among experts in endemic areas whether patients with coccidioidomycosis should be treated, and if so, which ones and for how long. The excellent tolerability of oral azoles has lowered the threshold for deciding to treat primary infection, and some clinicians treat all primary infections. Rationales for treating a primary self-limiting infection include the ability to lessen the morbidity associated with the acute infection and the possible ability to reduce the development of more serious complications. However, there is currently no evidence that treatment of the primary infection accomplishes either of these goals.[22]

■ PRIMARY RESPIRATORY INFECTION

Although most patients with symptomatic primary pulmonary disease recover without therapy, management should include follow-up visits for 1 to 2 years to document resolution of disease or to identify as early as possible evidence of pulmonary or extrapulmonary complications.

Patients with a large inoculum, severe infection, or concurrent risk factors (e.g., HIV infection, organ transplant, pregnancy, or high doses of corticosteroids) probably should be treated, particularly those with high CF titers, in whom incipient or occult dissemination is likely. Because some racial or ethnic populations have a higher risk of dissemination, some clinicians advocate their inclusion in the high-risk group. Common indicators used to judge the severity of infection include weight loss (>10%), intense night sweats persisting more than 3 weeks, infiltrates involving more than one half of one lung or portions of both lungs, prominent or persistent hilar adenopathy, CF antibody titers of greater than 1:16, failure to develop dermal sensitivity to coccidial antigens, inability to work, or symptoms that persist for more than 2 months.[20,22]

Commonly prescribed therapies include currently available oral azole antifungals at their recommended doses for courses of therapy ranging from 3 to 6 months.[20,22] In patients with diffuse pneumonia with bilateral reticulonodular or miliary infiltrates, therapy usually is initiated with amphotericin B; several weeks of therapy generally are required to produce clear evidence of improvement. Consolidation therapy with oral azoles can be considered at that time. The total duration of therapy should be at least 1 year, and in patients with underlying immunodeficiency, oral azole therapy should be continued as secondary prophylaxis. Although HIV-infected patients receiving secondary prophylaxis might be at low risk for recurrence of systemic mycosis when their CD4+ T-lymphocyte counts increase to >100 cells/microliter in response to HAART, the number of patients who have been evaluated is insufficient to warrant a recommendation to discontinue prophylaxis.

■ INFECTIONS OF THE PULMONARY CAVITY

Many pulmonary infections that are caused by *C. immitis* are benign in their course and do not require intervention. In the absence of controlled clinical trials, evidence of the benefit of antifungal therapy is lacking, and asymptomatic infections generally are left untreated. Symptomatic patients can benefit from oral azole therapy, although recurrence of symptoms can be seen in some patients once therapy is discontinued. Surgical resection of localized cavities provides resolution of the problem in patients in whom the risks of surgery are not too high.[20,22]

■ EXTRAPULMONARY (DISSEMINATED) DISEASE

Nonmeningeal Disease

Almost all patients with disease located outside the lungs should receive antifungal therapy; therapy usually is initiated with 400 mg/day of an oral azole. Amphotericin B is an alternative therapy and can be necessary in patients with worsening lesions or with disease in particularly critical locations such as the vertebral column. Approximately 50% to 75% of patients treated with amphotericin B for nonmeningeal disease achieve a sustained remission, and therapy usually is curative in patients with infections localized strictly to skin and soft tissues without extensive abscess formation or tissue damage. The efficacy of local injection into joints or the peritoneum, as well as intraarticular or intradermal administration, remains poorly studied. Amphotericin B appears to be most efficacious when cell-mediated immunity is intact (as evidenced by a positive coccidioidin or spherulin skin test or low CF antibody titer). Controlled trials that document these clinical impressions are lacking, however.[20,22]

Meningeal Disease

Fluconazole has become the drug of choice for the treatment of coccidioidal meningitis. A minimum dose of 400 mg/day orally leads to a clinical response in most patients and obviates the need for intrathecal amphotericin B. Some clinicians will initiate therapy with 800 or 1,000 mg/day, and itraconazole dosages of 400 to 600 mg/day are comparably effective. It is also clear, however, that fluconazole only leads to remission rather than cure of the infections; thus suppressive therapy must be continued for life. Ketoconazole cannot be recommended routinely for the treatment of coccidioidal meningitis because of its poor CNS penetration following oral administration. Patients who do not respond to fluconazole or itraconazole therapy are candidates for intrathecal amphotericin B therapy with or without continuation of azole therapy. The intrathecal dose of amphotericin B ranges from 0.01 to 1.5 mg given at intervals ranging from daily to weekly. Therapy is initiated with a low dosage and is titrated upward as patient tolerance develops.[20,22]

CRYPTOCOCCOSIS

EPIDEMIOLOGY

Cryptococcosis is a noncontagious, systemic mycotic infection caused by the ubiquitous encapsulated soil yeast *Cryptococcus neoformans*, which is found in soil, particularly in pigeon droppings, although disease occurs throughout the world, even in areas where pigeons are absent. Infection is acquired by inhalation of the organism. The incidence of cryptococcosis has risen dramatically in recent years, reflecting the increased numbers of immunocompromised patients, including those with malignancies, diabetes mellitus, chronic renal failure, and organ transplants and those receiving immunosuppressive agents. The AIDS epidemic also has contributed to the increased numbers of patients; cryptococcosis is the fourth most common infectious complication of AIDS and the second most common fungal pathogen.[23]

Although *C. neoformans* produces no toxins and evokes only a minimal inflammatory response in tissue, the polysaccharide capsule appears to allow the organism to resist phagocytosis by the host. The capsular polysaccharide of *C. neoformans* appears to comprise the major virulence factor for this pathogen. Four serotypes of *C. neoformans* (A through D) have been identified; they vary in their polysaccharide content, virulence, geographic foci, and response to antifungal therapy. Serotypes A and D are commonly associated with pigeon droppings and other environmental sites and generally require shorter therapy than do infections caused by serotypes B or C, which have been found only in infected humans and animals. Serotypes B and C appear more resistant to antifungal agents in vitro. Patients with AIDS are almost always infected with serotypes A and D, even in areas endemic for serotypes B and C. There is no particular geographic area of endemic focus for *C. neoformans*.

Cell-mediated immunity appears to play a major role in host defense against infection with *C. neoformans;* 29% to 55% of patients with cryptococcal meningitis have a predisposing condition. Many patients with disseminated cryptococcosis demonstrate defects in cell-mediated immunity. The predilection of *C. neoformans* for the CNS appears to be caused by the lack of immunoglobulins and complement and the excellent growth medium afforded by CSF.[23]

Disease can remain localized in the lungs or can disseminate to other tissues, particularly the CNS, although the skin also can be affected. Hematogenous spread generally occurs in the immunocompromised host, although it also has been seen in individuals with intact immune systems. Cryptococcemia is the most common symptomatic extraneural infection associated with *C. neoformans*. Cryptococcemia can be documented in 5% to 22% of non-AIDS patients, and CNS involvement of *C. neoformans* can be found in 18% to 50% of AIDS patients. Cryptococcal disease is present in 7.5% to 10% of AIDS patients. Therefore, patients with evidence of extraneural cryptococcosis should be evaluated for CNS disease.

CLINICAL PRESENTATION OF CRYPTOCOCCOSIS[11,23,24]

Primary cryptococcosis in humans almost always occurs in the lungs, although the pulmonary focus usually produces a subclinical infection. Symptomatic infections usually are manifested by cough, rales, and shortness of breath that generally resolve spontaneously. In non-AIDS patients, the symptoms of cryptococcal meningitis are nonspecific. Headache, fever, nausea, vomiting, mental status changes, and neck stiffness generally are observed. Less common symptoms include visual disturbances (photophobia and blurred vision), papilledema, seizures, and aphasia. In AIDS patients, fever and headache are common, but meningismus and photophobia are much less common than in non-AIDS patients. Approximately 10% to 12% of AIDS patients have asymptomatic disease, similar to the rate observed in non-AIDS patients.[24]

Laboratory Tests

With cryptococcal meningitis, the CSF opening pressure generally is elevated. There is a CSF pleocytosis (usually lymphocytes), leukocytosis, a decreased glucose concentration, and an elevated CSF protein concentration. There is also a positive cryptococcal antigen (detected by LA). The test is rapid, specific, and extremely sensitive, but false-negative results can occur. False-positive tests can result from cross-reactivity with rheumatoid factor and *Trichosporon beigelli*. *C. neoformans* can be detected in approximately 60% of patients by India ink smear of CSF, and it can be cultured in more than 96% of patients. Occasionally, large volumes of CSF are required to confirm the diagnosis.

The CSF parameters in patients with AIDS are similar to those seen in non-AIDS patients, with the exception of a decreased inflammatory response to the pathogen, resulting in a strikingly low number of leukocytes in CSF and extraordinarily high cryptococcal antigen titers.

TREATMENT

Cryptococcosis

The choice of treatment for disease caused by *C. neoformans* depends on both the anatomic sites of involvement and the host's immune status.

■ NONIMMUNOCOMPROMISED PATIENTS

For asymptomatic immunocompetent hosts with isolated pulmonary disease and no evidence of CNS disease, careful observation can be warranted; in the case of symptomatic infection, fluconazole or amphotericin B is warranted (Table 130–6). In individuals with non-CNS cryptococcemia, a positive serum cryptococcal antigen titer (>1:8), cutaneous infection, a positive urine culture, or prostatic disease, the clinician must decide whether to follow the regimen for isolated pulmonary disease or the more aggressive regimen for patients with CNS (disseminated) disease.[15]

❼ Prior to the introduction of amphotericin B, cryptococcal meningitis was an almost uniformly fatal disease; approximately 86% of patients died within 1 year. The use of large (1 to 1.5 mg/kg) daily doses of amphotericin B resulted in cure rates of approximately 64%. When amphotericin B is combined with flucytosine, a smaller dose of amphotericin B can be employed because of the in vitro and in vivo synergy between the two antifungal agents. Resistance develops to flucytosine in up to 30% of patients treated with flucytosine alone, limiting its usefulness as monotherapy.[24,25] Combination therapy with amphotericin B and flucytosine will sterilize the CSF within 2 weeks of treatment in 60% to 90% of patients, and most immunocompetent patients will be treated successfully with 6 weeks of combination therapy.[23] However, because of the need for prolonged IV therapy and the potential for renal and hematologic toxicity with this regimen, alternative regimens have been advocated. Despite a lack of clinically controlled trials in this population, amphotericin B induction therapy for 2 weeks, followed by consolidation therapy with fluconazole for an additional 8 to 10 weeks, is

TABLE 130-6 Therapy of Cryptococcosis[a,b]

Type of Disease and Common Clinical Manifestations	Therapy/Comments
Nonimmunocompromised host	Comparative trials for amphotericin B[c] versus azoles not available
Isolated pulmonary disease (without evidence of CNS infection)	*Asymptomatic disease:* Drug therapy generally not required; observe carefully or fluconazole 400 mg orally daily × 3–6 months
	Mild to moderate symptoms: Fluconazole 200–400 mg orally daily × 3–6 months
	Severe disease or inability to take azoles: Amphotericin B 0.4–0.7 mg/kg/day (total dose of 1–2 g)
Cryptococcemia with positive serum antigen titer (>1:8), cutaneous infection, a positive urine culture, or prostatic disease	Clinician must decide whether to follow the pulmonary therapeutic regimen or the CNS (disseminated) regimen
Recurrent or progressive disease not responsive to amphotericin B; Isolated pulmonary disease (without evidence of CNS infection)	Amphotericin B[d] IV 0.5–0.75 mg/kg/day ± IT amphotericin B 0.5 mg 2–3 times weekly
	Mild to moderate symptoms or asymptomatic with a positive pulmonary specimen: Fluconazole 200–400 mg orally daily × lifelong
	or
	Itraconazole 200–400 mg orally daily × lifelong
	or
	Fluconazole 400 mg orally daily + flucytosine 100–150 mg/kg/day orally × 10 weeks
	Severe disease: Amphotericin B until symptoms are controlled, followed by fluconazole
CNS disease	
Acute (induction/consolidation therapy) (follow all regimens with suppressive therapy)	Amphotericin B[d] IV 0.7–1 mg/kg/day + flucytosine 100 mg/kg/day orally × ≤ 2 weeks, then fluconazole 400 mg orally daily × ≤ 8 weeks[e]
	or
	Amphotericin B[d] IV 0.7–1 mg/kg/day + flucytosine 100 mg/kg/day orally × 6–10 weeks[e]
	or
	Amphotericin B[d] IV 0.7–1 mg/kg/day × 6–10 weeks[e]
	or
	Fluconazole 400–800 mg orally daily × 10–12 weeks
	or
	Itraconazole 400–800 mg orally daily × 10–12 weeks
	or
	Fluconazole 400–800 mg orally daily + flucytosine 100–150 mg/kg/day orally × 6 weeks[e]
	or
	Lipid formulation of amphotericin B IV 3–6 mg/kg/day × 6–10 weeks
	Note: Induction therapy with azoles alone is discouraged.
CNS disease	Amphotericin B[d] IV 0.7–1 mg/kg/day + flucytosine 100 mg/kg/day orally × 2 weeks, followed by fluconazole 400 mg orally daily for a minimum of 10 weeks (in patients intolerant to fluconazole, substitute itraconazole 200–400 mg orally daily)
	or
	Amphotericin B[d] IV 0.7–1 mg/kg/day + 5-flucytosine 100 mg/kg/day orally × 6–10 weeks
	or
	Amphotericin B[d] IV 0.7–1 mg/kg/day × 10 weeks
	Refractory disease: Intrathecal or intraventricular amphotericin B
Immunocompromised patients	
Non-CNS pulmonary and extrapulmonary disease	Same as nonimmunocompromised patients with CNS disease
CNS disease	Amphotericin B[d] IV 0.7–1 mg/kg/day × 2 weeks, followed by fluconazole 400–800 mg orally daily 8–10 weeks, followed by fluconazole 200 mg orally daily × 6–12 months (in patients intolerant to fluconazole, substitute itraconazole 200–400 mg orally daily)
	Refractory disease: Intrathecal or intraventricular amphotericin B
HIV-infected patients	
Suppressive/maintenance therapy	Fluconazole 200–400 mg orally daily × lifelong
	or
	Itraconazole 200 mg orally twice daily × lifelong
	or
	Amphotericin B IV 1 mg/kg 1–3 times weekly × lifelong

HIV, human immunodeficiency virus; IT, intrathecal.
[a]When more than one therapy is listed, they are listed in order of preference.
[b]See text for definitions of induction, consolidation, suppressive/maintenance therapy, and prophylactic therapy.
[c]Deoxycholate amphotericin B.
[d]In patients with significant renal disease, lipid formulations of amphotericin B can be substituted for deoxycholate amphotericin B during the induction.
[e]Or until cerebrospinal fluid (CSF) cultures are negative
Data from Bennett et al.,[23] Francis and Walsh,[24] Powderly et al.,[25] Saag et al.,[26] and van der Horst et al.[27]

frequently recommended based on data extrapolated from studies conducted in HIV-infected patients. Suppressive therapy with fluconazole 200 mg/day for 6 to 12 months after the completion of induction and consolidation therapy is optional.[15,25–27]

Pilot studies evaluating combination therapy with fluconazole plus flucytosine as initial therapy yielded unsatisfactory results, and this approach is discouraged even in "low-risk" patients.

Ketoconazole has been used successfully in the treatment of cutaneous cryptococcosis, but it is not useful in the treatment of CNS disease, probably because of its poor penetration into the CNS.[15]

Despite low CSF concentrations of amphotericin B (2% to 3% of those observed in plasma), the use of intrathecal amphotericin B is not recommended for the treatment of cryptococcal meningitis except in very ill patients or in patients with recurrent or progressive disease despite aggressive therapy with IV amphotericin B. The dosage of amphotericin B employed is usually 0.5 mg administered through the lumbar, cisternal, or intraventricular (through an Ommaya reservoir) route 2 or 3 times weekly. Side effects of intrathecal amphotericin B include arachnoiditis and paresthesias. Intrathecal amphotericin B therapy should be administered in combination with IV amphotericin B.[27]

■ IMMUNOCOMPROMISED PATIENTS

Immunocompromised hosts with isolated pulmonary and extrapulmonary disease without CNS disease should be treated similarly to nonimmunocompromised patients with CNS disease. Immunocompromised patients with CNS infection require more prolonged therapy; treatment regimens are based on those used in the HIV-infected population and follow induction and consolidation therapy with 6 to 12 months of suppressive therapy with fluconazole.[15]

HIV-Infected Patients

There are no controlled clinical trials evaluating the therapy of isolated pulmonary infection; thus the specific treatment of choice is unclear. However, because these patients are at high risk for disseminated infection, antifungal therapy is warranted in all patients. Lifelong therapy with fluconazole is recommended; in patients for whom fluconazole is not an option, itraconazole can be used.

Fluconazole is beneficial for both acute and chronic maintenance therapy for cryptococcal meningitis. Amphotericin B 0.4 to 0.5 mg/kg IV daily was compared with oral fluconazole 200 mg/day. Although the overall 10-week mortality was the same in both groups, the time until the CSF culture became negative was longer, and there were more deaths in the first 2 weeks of therapy in the fluconazole group.[26] In later trials,[27] amphotericin B 0.7 mg/kg IV daily for 2 weeks (with or without oral flucytosine 100 mg/kg per day), followed by consolidation therapy with either itraconazole 400 mg/day orally or fluconazole 400 mg/day orally, led to markedly improved outcomes in comparison with earlier regimens. This study confirmed the benefit of early high-dose (0.7 mg/kg per day) amphotericin B use, the usefulness of flucytosine added to amphotericin B for induction therapy, and the slight superiority of fluconazole over itraconazole for consolidation therapy.

Amphotericin B combined with flucytosine is the initial treatment of choice. In patients who cannot tolerate flucytosine, amphotericin B alone is an acceptable alternative. After the initially successful 2-week induction period, consolidation therapy with fluconazole can be administered for 8 weeks or until CSF cultures are negative. In patients in whom fluconazole cannot be given, itraconazole is an acceptable, albeit less effective, alternative. Combination therapy with fluconazole plus flucytosine is effective; however, it is recommended as an alternative to the preceding therapies because of its potential for toxicity. Lipid formulations of amphotericin B are effective, but the optimal dosage is unknown.[15]

In HIV-infected patients, mortality is highly associated with elevated intracranial pressure (CSF opening pressure >250 mm). At the initiation of antifungal therapy, lumbar drainage should remove enough CSF to reduce the opening pressure by 50%. Patients initially should undergo daily lumbar punctures to maintain CSF opening pressure in the normal range. When the CSF pressure is normal for several days, the procedure can be suspended. Adjunctive steroid treatment is not recommended because therapy has resulted in mixed results and its impact on outcome is unclear. Similarly, neither mannitol nor acetazolamide therapy provides any clear benefit in the management of elevated intracranial pressure.[15]

Suppressive (Maintenance) Therapy for Cryptococcal Meningitis in the HIV-Infected Patient

Relapse of *C. neoformans* meningitis occurs in approximately 50% of AIDS patients after completion of primary therapy. Persistence of asymptomatic urinary *C. neoformans* has been documented in a high percentage of AIDS patients despite seemingly adequate courses of therapy for primary meningeal disease. The prostate appears to act as a sequestered reservoir of infection in these patients, resulting in systemic relapse. Fluconazole is recommended for chronic suppressive therapy of cryptococcal meningitis in AIDS patients. The AIDS Clinical Trials Group's (ACTG) 026 study demonstrated that oral fluconazole 200 mg/day was superior to IV administration of amphotericin B 1 mg/kg weekly in preventing relapse. In addition, the fluconazole-treated group showed a lower incidence of adverse drug reactions and bacterial infections.[27] Randomized comparative trials also demonstrated the superiority of fluconazole versus itraconazole as maintenance therapy. Thus itraconazole should be reserved for patients intolerant to fluconazole. Ketoconazole is not effective as maintenance therapy.

Although the numbers of patients who have been evaluated remain limited and recurrences can occur, patients are at low risk for recurrence of cryptococcosis when they have successfully completed a course of initial therapy for cryptococcosis, remain asymptomatic with regard to signs and symptoms of cryptococcosis, and have a sustained increase (e.g., >6 months) in their CD4+ T-lymphocyte counts to >100 to 200 cells/microliter and an HIV viral load of fewer than 50 copies/mL.[15,25–28]

EVALUATION OF THERAPEUTIC OUTCOMES

Once the CNS is involved, the usual course is weeks to months of progressive deterioration, with 80% of untreated patients dying within the first year. The prognosis of cryptococcal meningitis depends largely on the underlying predisposing factors of the host. Although cryptococcal antigen is positive in 90% of patients with cryptococcal meningitis, fewer than one half of the patients with cryptococcal meningitis develop antibody to capsular polysaccharide. Those who produce antibody have a slightly improved prognosis. In contrast, the presence of headache is a favorable symptom, presumably because it leads to an earlier diagnosis. A favorable outcome is also associated with a normal mental status on diagnosis and a CSF white blood cell (WBC) count of less than 20 cells/mm³. A poor outcome is predicted, however, by the presence of one or more underlying diseases (including hematopoietic disorders and AIDS), corticosteroid or immunosuppressive therapy, pretreatment serum cryptococcal antigen titers of 1:32, and posttherapy serum antigen titers of 1:8. In non-AIDS patients, the cryptococcal antigen titer can be followed during therapy to assess response to antifungal therapy. In AIDS patients, decreasing titers are not necessarily predictive of success, and titers rarely become negative at the completion of therapy.

CANDIDA INFECTIONS

Candida species are yeasts that exist primarily as small (4 to 6 microns), unicellular, thin-walled, ovoid cells that reproduce by budding. On agar medium, they form smooth, white, creamy colonies resembling staphylococci. Although there are more than 150 species of *Candida*, eight species—*C. albicans, C. tropicalis, Candida parapsilosis, C. krusei, Candida stellatoidea, C. guilliermondii, C. lusitaniae,* and *C. glabrata*—are regarded as clinically important pathogens in human disease.[13] Yeast forms, hyphae, and pseudohyphae can be found in clinical specimens.

PATHOPHYSIOLOGY

8 *C. albicans* is a normal commensal of the skin, female genital tract, and entire GI tract of humans. Therefore, the mere presence of hyphae or pseudohyphae in a clinical specimen is insufficient for the diagnosis of invasive disease. The majority of infections with *C. albicans* are acquired endogenously, although human-to-human transmission also can occur. Oral candidiasis in the newborn probably is acquired during passage through the birth canal, and balanitis in the uncircumcised male can be acquired through contact with a female with vaginal candidiasis. Although the term *fungemia* refers to the presence of fungi in the blood, the most commonly isolated organism is *C. albicans*. Candidiasis can cause mucocutaneous or systemic infection, including endocarditis, peritonitis, arthritis, and infection of the CNS. (Mucocutaneous infections caused by *Candida* are discussed in further detail in Chap. 129.)

The role of an intact integument is crucial in the prevention of mucocutaneous or hematogenous candidiasis. After *Candida* invades the dermis or enters the bloodstream, polymorphonuclear (PMN) leukocytes play a major role in the defense of the patient because PMN leukocytes are capable of damaging pseudohyphae and can phagocytize and kill blastoconidia. In addition to neutrophils, lymphocytes, monocytes, macrophages, complement, and eosinophils play a role in the prevention of infection. Adherence of *C. albicans* is important in the pathogenesis of oral candidiasis and subsequent colonization of the GI tract. Because evidence suggests that the GI tract is often the portal of entry for *Candida* in disseminated disease, factors that alter the adherence of *Candida* are crucial in the development of local and systemic infection. *Candida tropicalis* adheres to intravascular catheters at a higher rate than *C. albicans*, a factor that may help to account for the increased incidence of systemic infections caused by this pathogen.

HEMATOGENOUS CANDIDIASIS

EPIDEMIOLOGY

The incidence of fungal infections caused by *Candida* species has increased substantially in the past three decades, and *Candida* infections currently constitute a significant cause of morbidity and mortality among severely ill patients. *Candida* species now constitute the fourth most common cause of bloodstream infections (BSIs) for patients hospitalized in intensive care units (ICUs) in the United States, following coagulase-negative staphylococci, *Staphylococcus aureus*, and enterococci. The Centers for Disease Control and Prevention's (CDC) National Nosocomial Infection Survey implicated fungi as the cause of 8% of nosocomial infections. Although *C. albicans* accounted for approximately 50% of *Candida* species, non-*albicans* species of *Candida*, including *C. glabrata*, *C. tropicalis*, *C. krusei*, and *C. parapsilosis*, are increasingly frequent causes of invasive candidal infections.[29–31] *Candida lusitaniae* infections are a cause of breakthrough fungemia in cancer patients; *C. parapsilosis* has emerged as the second most common pathogen, following *C. albicans*, in neonatal ICU patients, where it is often associated with central lines and parenteral nutrition, and fungemias in patients outside the United States, in particular in South America. Fungemia caused by *C. glabrata* is observed more commonly in adults older than 65 years of age.[29,32] The change in species is of concern clinically because certain pathogens, such as *C. krusei* and *C. glabrata*, are intrinsically more resistant to commonly used triazole drugs (see Table 130–1).

PATHOPHYSIOLOGY

Candida generally is acquired via the GI tract, although organisms also can enter the bloodstream via indwelling IV catheters. Immunosuppressed patients, including those with lymphoreticular or hematologic malignancies, diabetes, and immunodeficiency diseases and those receiving immunosuppressive therapy with high-dose corticosteroids, immunosuppressants, antineoplastic agents, or broad-spectrum antimicrobial agents, are at high risk for invasive fungal infections. However, a number of prospective, randomized, controlled trials have validated the efficacy of antifungal prophylaxis and the use of antifungal agents for the treatment of persistently febrile patients with neutropenia who do not respond to antibiotics, and in the prophylaxis of patients undergoing hematopoietic stem cell transplantation (HSCT), in particular in HSCT patients with graft-versus-host disease (GVHD).[33] These efforts have resulted in a reduction in the frequency of bloodstream infections caused by *Candida* species and systemic candidiasis in patients with neutropenia. In fact, most bloodstream infections caused by *Candida* species now occur in patients who have been hospitalized in ICUs, especially adult and neonatal ICUs. Retrospective studies have identified a number of risk factors for candidal bloodstream infections in ICU patients, most of which have been verified in multiple studies, although some remain controversial[34] (Table 130–7). Major risk factors include the use of central venous catheters, total parenteral nutrition, receipt of multiple antibiotics, extensive surgery and burns, renal failure and hemodialysis, mechanical ventilation, and prior fungal colonization. Patients who have undergone surgery (particularly surgery of the GI tract) are increasingly susceptible to disseminated candidal infections.[34,35]

CLINICAL PRESENTATION OF HEMATOGENOUS CANDIDIASIS[11,13]

Dissemination of *C. albicans* can result in infection in single or multiple organs, particularly the kidney, brain, myocardium, skin, eye, bone, and joints. In most patients, multiple micro- and macro-abscesses are formed. Infection of the liver and spleen is becoming recognized as a particularly common and difficult-to-treat site of infection that characteristically occurs in patients undergoing chemotherapy for acute leukemia or lymphoma.

Diagnosis

Signs and Symptoms Several distinct presentations of disseminated *C. albicans* have been recognized:[10]

1. Patients present with the acute onset of fever, tachycardia, tachypnea, and occasionally, chills or hypotension. The clinical presentation generally is indistinguishable from that seen with sepsis of bacterial origin.

2. Patients develop intermittent fevers and are ill only when febrile.

3. Patients manifest progressive deterioration of their conditions with or without fever.

4. Hepatosplenic candidiasis often is manifested only as fever while the patient remains neutropenic (<1,000 WBCs/mm³).

Laboratory Tests Although a variety of serologic tests have been proposed for the detection of *Candida* protein antigens, serum antibodies to *Candida*, and antibodies to cell wall components such as mannan, no test has demonstrated reliable accuracy in the clinical setting for the diagnosis of disseminated infection with *Candida*. Only 25% to 45% of neutropenic patients with disseminated candidiasis at autopsy had a positive blood culture with *C. albicans*

TABLE 130-7 Risk Factors for Invasive Candidiasis

Colonization
Corrected colonization index (CCI) ≥ 0.4[a]
Colonization index (CI) ≥ 0.8[a]
Candida spp. cultured from sites other than blood
Candiduria

Antibiotic use
Number of antibiotics prior to infection (per additional antibiotics)
Use of 2 or more antibiotics
Use of broad spectrum antibiotics in previous 10 days

Surgery
Surgery on ICU admission
Gastro-abdominal surgery
Abdominal drainage
Elective surgery
Cardiopulmonary bypass time > 120min
Hickman catheter

Foreign devices
Central venous catheter
Triple lumen catheter in patients who have undergone surgery
Bladder catheter

Renal failure and dialysis
Prior hemodialysis
Hemofiltration procedures
Increased serum creatinine[b]
New onset hemodialysis within 3 days of admission to ICU
Acute renal failure

Underlying disease/baseline characteristics
Total parenteral nutrition
Diabetes mellitus
Apache II (per point)
Signs of severe sepsis
Diarrhea at any time
Mechanical ventilation ≥ 10 days
Hospital acquired bacterial infection
Bacterial peritonitis by ICU day 11
Gastrointestinal disease
ICU length of stay
Transferred from other hospital
Use of corticosteroids
Profound neutropenia (ANC < 100/mm³)

[a]CI = the ratio of number of nonblood distinct body sites (dbs) heavily colonized with identical strains to total number of dbs; CCI = the product of the CI and the ratio of the number of dbs showing heavy growth (≥10⁵ CFU/mL) to the total of dbs growing *Candida* spp.
[b]Serum creatinine >1.2 mg/dl in females, >1.6 mg/dl in males
Data from Lam et al.[34] and Wey et al.[35]

prior to death. The interpretation of positive surveillance cultures of the skin, mouth, sputum, feces, or urine is hampered by their occurrence as commensal pathogens and in distinguishing colonization from invasive disease.

Until recently, a rapid presumptive identification of *C. albicans* could be made by incubation of the organism in serum; formation of a germ tube (the beginning of hyphae, which arise as perpendicular extensions from the yeast cell, with no constriction at their point of origin) within 1 to 2 hours offered a positive identification of *C. albicans*. Unfortunately, *C. dubliniensis*, a new species of *Candida* that was identified recently as an important cause of mucosal colonization and infection in HIV-infected individuals, also can produce a germ tube. A negative germ tube test does not rule out the possibility of *C. albicans*, but further biochemical tests must be performed to differentiate between other non-*albicans* species.[36]

In patients with hepatosplenic candidiasis, as the WBC count increases to >1,000 cells/mm³, imaging studies can detect the presence of abscess or microabscesses in the liver and spleen, often found with acute suppurative and granulomatous reactions.

A new peptide nucleic acid (PNA) fluorescence in situ hybridization (FISH) method uses fluorescein-labeled PNA probes that target *C. albicans* 26S rRNA for the identification of *C. albicans* directly from blood culture bottles that test positive, and in which yeasts observed by Gram staining have been developed. The probe is added to smears made directly from the contents of blood culture bottles and is hybridized for 90 minutes, and the smears are subsequently examined by fluorescence microscopy. The test has excellent sensitivity (99% to 100%) and specificity (100%) in the direct identification of *C. albicans* from blood cultures.[14]

TREATMENT

Hematogenous Candidiasis

Fraser and colleagues[34] documented the high rate of mortality in nonneutropenic patients with fungal blood cultures. Mortality was highest in patients with sustained positive blood cultures, those who did not receive antifungal therapy, and those infected with non-*albicans* strains of *Candida*. This study clearly documented the importance of early recognition and treatment of positive fungal blood cultures. Prompt initiation of therapy is important. Delays in empiric antifungal treatment greater than 12 hours after obtaining a positive blood sample are associated with greater hospital mortality.[37,38,39] Despite increased awareness of the importance of treating patients with positive blood cultures, mortality associated with candidemia remains high.[40]

Treatment of candidiasis should be guided by knowledge of the infecting species; the clinical status of the patient; when available, the antifungal susceptibility of the infecting isolate; and whether the patient has received antifungal therapy previously (Table 130–8). Therapy should be continued for 2 weeks after the last positive blood culture and resolution of signs and symptoms of infection. All patients should undergo an ophthalmologic examination to exclude the possibility of candidal endophthalmitis.[7] Amphotericin B can be switched to fluconazole (intravenous or oral) for the completion of therapy. Susceptibility testing of the infecting isolate is a useful adjunct to species identification during selection of a therapeutic approach because it can be used to identify isolates that are unlikely to respond to fluconazole or amphotericin B. However, this is not currently available at most institutions.

■ NONIMMUNOCOMPROMISED PATIENT

Prophylaxis

In ICUs, the use of fluconazole for prophylaxis or empirical therapy has increased exponentially in the past decade. However, studies that demonstrated benefit in the prevention of invasive candidal bloodstream infections did so either by using highly selective criteria or by studying patients in an unusually high-risk ICU setting, and the role of antifungal prophylaxis in the surgical ICU remains extremely controversial. Rex and colleagues[7] have suggested that for a study to demonstrate efficacy in clinical trials, the baseline rate of invasive candidiasis must be >10%, and that prophylaxis must result in > fourfold reduction of disease. Although ICU-specific, a >10% rate of invasive candidiasis is generally found only in the setting of high-risk transplant patients (e.g., patients undergoing liver transplantation), or in patients with one or more of the following risk factors by day 3 of their ICU stay: new onset dialysis, receipt of broad-spectrum antibiotics, the presence of diabetes, and in patients receiving parenteral nutrition.[41–43]

TABLE 130-8 Therapy of Invasive Candidiasis[7,34]

Type of Disease and Common Clinical Manifestations	Therapy/Comments
Prophylaxis of candidemia	
Nonneutropenic patients[a]	Not recommended except for severely ill/high-risk patients in whom fluconazole IV/PO 400 mg daily should be used (see text)
Neutropenic patients[a]	The optimal duration of therapy is unclear but at a minimum should include the period at risk for neutropenia: Fluconazole IV/PO 400 mg daily *or* itraconazole solution 2.5 mg/kg every 12 hours PO *or* micafungin 50 mg (1 mg/kg in patients under 50 kg) intravenously daily
Solid-organ transplantation, liver transplantation	*Patients with two or more key risk factors[b]:* Amphotericin B IV 10–20 mg daily *or* liposomal amphotericin B (AmBisome) 1 mg/kg/day *or* fluconazole 400 mg orally daily
Empirical antifungal therapy (unknown *Candida* species)	
Suspected disseminated candidiasis in febrile nonneutropenic patients	None recommended; data are lacking defining subsets of patients who are appropriate for therapy (see text)
Febrile neutropenic patients with prolonged fever despite 4–6 days of empirical antibacterial therapy	*Treatment duration:* Until resolution of neutropenia. An echinocandin[d] is a reasonable alternative; Voriconazole can be used in selected situations (see text)
Less critically ill patients with no recent azole exposure	An echinocandin[d] or fluconazole (loading dose of 800 mg [12 mg/kg], then 400 mg [6 mg/kg] daily)
Additional mold coverage is desired	Voriconazole
Empirical therapy of candidemia and acute hematogenously disseminated candidiasis	
Nonimmunocompromised host[c]	*Treatment duration:* 2 weeks after the last positive blood culture and resolution of signs and symptoms of infection. *Remove existing central venous catheters when feasible plus* fluconazole (loading dose of 800 mg [12 mg/kg], then 400 mg [6 mg/kg] daily) or an echinocandin[d]
Patients with recent azole exposure, moderately severe or severe illness, or who are at high risk of infection due to *C. glabrata* or *C. krusei*	An echinocandin[d]. Transition from an echinocandin to fluconazole is recommended for patients who are clinically stable and have isolates (eg, *C. albicans*) likely to be susceptible to fluconazole
Patients who are less critically ill and who have had no recent azole exposure	Fluconazole
Therapy of specific pathogens	
Candida albicans, Candida tropicalis, Candida parapsilosis	Fluconazole IV/PO 6 mg/kg/day *or* an echinocandin[d] *or* amphotericin B IV 0.7 mg/kg/day plus fluconazole IV/PO 800 mg/day; Amphotericin B deoxycholate 0.5–1.0 mg/kg daily or a lipid formulation of amphotericin B (3–5 mg/kg daily) are alternatives in patients who are intolerant to other antifungals; Transition from Amphotericin B deoxycholate or a lipid formulation of amphotericin B to fluconazole is recommended in patients who are clinically stable and whose isolates are likely to be susceptible to fluconazole (eg *C. albicans*); Voriconazole (400 mg [6 mg/kg] twice daily x 2 doses then 200 mg [3mg/kg] twice daily thereafter is efficacious, but offers little advantage over fluconazole; It may be utilized as stepdown oral therapy for selected cases of candidiasis due to *C. krusei* or voriconazole-susceptible *C. glabrata*. *Patients intolerant or refractory to other therapy[e]:* Amphotericin B lipid complex IV 5 mg/kg/day; Liposomal amphotericin B IV 3–5 mg/kg/day; Amphotericin B colloid dispersion IV 2–6 mg/kg/day
Candida krusei	Amphotericin B IV ≤1 mg/kg/day *or* an echinocandin[d]
Candida lusitaniae	Fluconazole IV/PO 6 mg/kg/day
Candida glabrata	An echinocandin[d] (Transition to fluconazole or voriconazole therapy is not recommended without confirmation of isolate susceptibility)
Neutropenic host[f]	*Treatment duration:* Until resolution of neutropenia. *Remove existing central venous catheters when feasible, plus:* Amphotericin B IV 0.7–1 mg/kg/day (total dosages 0.5–1 g) *or Patients failing therapy with traditional amphotericin B:* Lipid formulation of amphotericin B IV 3–5 mg/kg/day
Chronic disseminated candidiasis (hepatosplenic candidiasis)	*Treatment duration:* Until calcification or resolution of lesions. *Stable patients:* Fluconazole IV/PO 6 mg/kg/day. *Acutely ill or refractory patients:* Amphotericin B IV 0.6–0.7 mg/kg/day
Urinary candidiasis	*Asymptomatic disease:* Generally no therapy is required. *Symptomatic or high-risk patients[g]:* Removal of urinary tract instruments, stents, and Foley catheters, +7–14 days therapy with fluconazole 200 mg orally daily *or* amphotericin B IV 0.3–1 mg/kg/day

PO, orally.

[a]Patients at significant risk for invasive candidiasis include those receiving standard chemotherapy for acute myelogenous leukemia, allogeneic bone marrow transplants, or high-risk autologous bone marrow transplants. However, among these populations, chemotherapy or bone marrow transplant protocols do not all produce equivalent risk, and local experience should be used to determine the relevance of prophylaxis.

[b]Risk factors include retransplantation, creatinine of more than 2 mg/dL, choledochojejunostomy, intraoperative use of 40 units or more of blood products, and fungal colonization detected within the first 3 days after transplantation.

[c]Therapy is generally the same for acquired immunodeficiency syndrome (AIDS)/non-AIDS patients except where indicated and should continued for 2 weeks after the last positive blood culture and resolution of signs and symptoms of infection. All patients should receive an ophthalmologic examination. Amphotericin B can be switched to fluconazole (intravenous or oral) for the completion of therapy. Susceptibility testing of the infecting isolate is a useful adjunct to species identification during selection of a therapeutic approach because it can be used to identify isolates that are unlikely to respond to fluconazole or amphotericin B. However, this is not currently available at most institutions.

[d]Echinocandin = caspofungin 70 mg loading dose, then 50 mg IV daily maintenance dose, or micafungin 100 mg daily, or anidulafungin 200 mg loading dose, then 100 mg daily maintenance dose.

[e]Often defined as failure of ≥500 mg amphotericin B, initial renal insufficiency (creatinine ≥2.5 mg/dL or creatinine clearance <25 mL/min), a significant increase in creatinine (to 2.5 mg/dL for adults or 1.5 mg/dL for children), or severe acute administration-related toxicity.

[f]Patients who are neutropenic at the time of developing candidemia should receive a recombinant cytokine (granulocyte colony-stimulating factor or granulocyte-monocyte colony-stimulating factor) that accelerates recovery from neutropenia.

[g]Patients at high risk for dissemination include neutropenic patients, low-birth-weight infants, patients with renal allografts, and patients who will undergo urologic manipulation.

Data from NCCLS,[5] Pappas et al.[7,40]

TABLE 130-9 Treatment of Candidemia in the Nonneutropenic Host

Year Published	Study Drugs and Dosages	Study Design	Results and Comments
1994	Fluconazole vs. amphotericin B	Randomized, non-blinded, multicenter	Similar outcomes but higher rate of nephrotoxicity in the amphotericin B group
2002	Caspofungin (70 mg IV × 1 loading dose; then 50 mg IV daily) vs. amphotericin B (0.6–0.7 mg/kg/day IV) each antifungal agent was changed to fluconazole after ≥10 days to complete therapy	Randomized, multicenter	Successful outcome was achieved in 73.9% and 61.7% of patients receiving caspofungin and amphotericin B, respectively, but there was a higher rate of nephrotoxicity in the amphotericin B group
2003	Fluconazole 800 mg/day + placebo vs. fluconazole 800 mg/d + amphotericin B 0.7 mg/kg/day	Randomized, blinded, multicenter	The study was confounded by differences in the severity of illness of the two study populations (the fluconazole group had more severe illness). The regimens were comparable and noted a trend toward better response (based principally on more effective bloodstream clearance) in the group receiving combination therapy
2005	Voriconazole (6 mg/kg IV every 12 hours on day 1; 3 mg/kg every 12 hours IV on days 2 and 3; then 200 mg PO every 12 hours) vs. amphotericin B (≤0.7 mg/kg/day) followed by fluconazole (≥400 mg PO/ IV daily)	Randomized, non-blinded, multicenter	Voriconazole was as effective as the regimen of amphotericin B followed by fluconazole in the clearing of blood cultures; Treatment discontinuations cased by all-cause adverse events were more frequent in the voriconazole group, although most discontinuations were caused by non–drug-related events, and there were significantly fewer serious adverse events and cases of renal toxicity than in the amphotericin B/fluconazole group
2005	Anidulafungin (200 mg loading dose × 1, then 100 mg/day) vs. IV fluconazole (800 mg loading dose × 1, then 400 mg/day)	Randomized, double-blind	A statistically significantly greater response was observed with anidulafungin in the microbiologic intent-to-treat arm at the end of IV therapy, and at the 2-week and 6-week follow-ups in patients with APACHE II scores of >20; Survival was improved with anidulafungin
2005	Micafungin (100 mg/day IV) vs. liposomal amphotericin B (3 mg/kg/day) × 2–4 weeks	Randomized, double-blind	Micafungin treatment was considered effective (clinical plus mycological response) in 89.6% of patients (181:202), compared to 89.5% (170:190) in the amphotericin B group. The amphotericin B group had a significantly higher incidence of side effects, including infusion-related reactions and increases in serum creatinine.
2006	Caspofungin (70 mg IV × 1 loading dose; then 50 mg IV daily) vs. micafungin 100 mg/day vs. micafungin 150 mg/day	Randomized, double-blind	Micafungin was found noninferior to caspofungin; Higher dosages of micafungin (150 mg/day vs. 100 mg/day) were not more efficacious; The safety profiles for the three treatments were similar

APACHE, Acute Physiology and Chronic Health Evaluation; PO, orally.
Data from Rex et al.,[44] Reboli et al.,[45] Mora-Duarte et al.,[46] Rex et al.,[47] Kullberg et al.,[48] Ruhnke et al.,[49] and Betts et al.[50]

Empirical Therapy

Few data are available for assessing the role of fluconazole as empirical therapy for suspected fungemia or for isolates other than *C. albicans*. Because fluconazole has poor activity against *Aspergillus* species and some non-*albicans* strains of *Candida*, many clinicians advocate amphotericin B as the therapy of choice in patients with suspected fungemia. If therapy is given, its use should be limited to patients with (a) *Candida* colonization at multiple sites, (b) multiple other risk factors, and (c) the absence of any other uncorrected causes of fever.[7]

Specific Therapy

Several large randomized studies in nonneutropenic patients have demonstrated that azoles (fluconazole or voriconazole) and deoxycholate amphotericin B are similarly effective; however, fewer adverse effects are observed with azole therapy (Table 130–9). Similarly, echinocandins are at least as effective as amphotericin B or fluconazole in (mainly nonneutropenic) adult patients with candidemia with fewer drug-related adverse events. Although the use of combination therapy (high-dose fluconazole plus amphotericin B) was demonstrated recently to be superior to treatment with fluconazole alone, it was associated with a higher rate of nephrotoxicity, and the routine use of combination therapy in this patient population is not yet recommended. Alternatives to fluconazole should be considered when patients have a history of recent exposure to fluconazole or other azoles, when a broader spectrum is desirable (e.g., persistently neutropenic patient), when non-*albicans* species are isolated during or immediately following azole therapy, and in unstable or severely immunocompromised patients.[44–50]

Neonates with disseminated candidiasis usually are treated with amphotericin B because of its low toxicity in this patient population and because of the lack of experience with other agents in this population; however, micafungin or caspofungin may offer safe, effective alternatives.[7,12,40] Treatment should continue until 2 weeks following the last positive blood culture and resolution of signs and symptoms of infection.

C. krusei infections should be treated with large doses of amphotericin B (≥1 mg/kg per day) or with caspofungin (70-mg IV loading dose, followed by 50 mg/day IV).[7] *C. tropicalis*, and *C. parapsilosis* can be treated with either amphotericin B at 0.6 mg/kg per day or fluconazole at 6 mg/kg per day. Amphotericin B resistance remains relatively rare despite more than 45 years of clinical use, although it has been reported in *C. lusitaniae* (now *Clavispora lusitaniae*) and *C. guilliermondii. Candida rugosa* often is considered to be "polyene tolerant," and these isolates are believed to be selected owing to the wide use of amphotericin B.

Among the lipid-associated formulations of amphotericin B, only liposomal amphotericin B (AmBisome) and amphotericin B lipid complex (Abelcet) have been approved for use in proven cases of candidiasis; however, patients with invasive candidiasis also have been treated successfully with amphotericin B colloid dispersion (Amphotec or Amphocil). The lipid-associated formulations are less toxic but as effective as amphotericin B deoxycholate.

■ IMMUNOCOMPROMISED PATIENTS

In immunocompromised patients, the presence of candidemia is associated with evidence of disseminated disease in more than 70% of patients and with a 70% to 80% fatality rate. Therapy should include removal of the catheter and administration of systemic antifungal therapy.[7] The optimal agent, dose, and duration of therapy are unclear, and patients must be monitored carefully with serial blood cultures and careful physical examinations, particularly of the retina. Patients who are neutropenic at the time of developing candidemia should receive a recombinant cytokine (granulocyte colony-stimulating factor or granulocyte-monocyte colony-stimulating factor) that accelerates recovery from neutropenia.[7]

Prophylaxis

Recognition of the role of the GI tract in invasive *Candida* infections has led to efforts to decrease infections by prophylactic administration of topical or systemically absorbed antifungal agents in immunocompromised patients. The use of systemically absorbable agents such as azole antifungal agents appears to decrease the risk of invasive fungal infections.[7,51,52]

Fluconazole (400 mg/day), posaconazole (200 mg 3 times daily), or micafungin (50 mg daily) from the start of the conditioning regimen until day 75, can reduce the frequency of invasive *Candida* infections and decrease mortality at day 110 in patients undergoing allogeneic bone marrow transplantation.[7,52,53] Intravenous caspofungin (50 mg daily) was compared with intravenous itraconazole (200 mg twice daily for 2 days, then 200 mg once daily). Mortality was similar in both groups. Micafungin 50 mg daily was compared to intravenous fluconazole 400 mg daily in patients undergoing HSCT. Significantly fewer patients in the micafungin arm versus the fluconazole arm required empiric antifungal therapy, and mortality was decreased, although not significantly, in the micafungin arm. Based on this limited data, micafungin and caspofungin may provide options for prophylaxis in patients undergoing HSCT. However, more compelling data have been demonstrated with posaconazole.[12] In a double-blinded, multi-center clinical trial of the prophylaxis of invasive fungal infections in patients who had undergone HSCT with GVHD, posaconazole (200 mg every 8 hours), was superior to fluconazole (400 mg daily) in preventing aspergillosis and comparable to fluconazole in preventing other breakthrough invasive fungal infections.[56,57]

In less risk-selected patients with hematologic malignancies who are undergoing remission-induction chemotherapy, fluconazole (400 mg/day), posaconazole (200 mg 3 times daily), or caspofungin (50 mg daily), during induction chemotherapy for the duration of neutropenia, are effective in preventing systemic infection and death caused by *Candida* species.[7,54,55] Itraconazole cyclodextrin (2.5 mg/kg orally twice daily) is an option for less risk-selected patients, but it offers little advantage over other agents and is less well tolerated.

For solid-organ transplant recipients, fluconazole (200–400 mg [3–6 mg/kg] daily) or liposomal amphotericin B (1 to 2 mg/kg daily for 7 to 14 days) is recommended as postoperative antifungal prophylaxis for liver, pancreas, and small bowel transplant recipients at high risk of candidiasis.[7,35]

The use of prophylactic fluconazole (400 mg [6 mg/kg] daily) can decrease the incidence of fungal infections in select high-risk groups of patients. However, despite decreases in the rate of invasive candidiasis, to date, no mortality benefit has been demonstrated in any clinical trial. Widespread use of prophylactic fluconazole in all ICU patients is not warranted and may lead to an increase in resistance and adverse events. If utilized, prophylactic fluconazole should target high-risk patients with a presumed risk of invasive candidiasis of 10% to 15%.[7,34]

Empirical Therapy for Febrile Neutropenic Patients

Many clinicians advocate early institution of empirical IV amphotericin B in patients with neutropenia and persistent (>5 to 7 days) fever.[57] However, the potential toxicities (particularly nephrotoxicity) of this agent preclude its routine use in all patients. Suggested criteria for the empirical use of amphotericin B include (a) fever of 5 to 7 days' duration that is unresponsive to antibacterial agents, (b) neutropenia of more than 7 days' duration, (c) no other obvious cause for fever, (d) progressive debilitation, (e) chronic adrenal corticosteroid therapy, and (f) indwelling intravascular catheters. In patients who fail therapy with amphotericin B, lipid formulations of amphotericin B can be used (3 to 5 mg/kg per day). Comparative trials have indicated that lipid formulations of amphotericin B can be used as alternatives to amphotericin B deoxycholate for empirical therapy. Although they do not appear to be substantially more effective, there is less drug-related toxicity (Table 130–10).[57]

TABLE 130-10	Comparative Trials for Empiric Therapy in the Febrile Neutropenic Host		
Year Published	**Study Drugs**	**Study Design**	**Results and Comments**
1982	Placebo vs. amphotericin B	Randomized	Favored amphotericin B
1989	Placebo vs. amphotericin B	Randomized	Favored amphotericin B
1996	Fluconazole vs. amphotericin B	Randomized	Defervescence: equivalence; safety analysis favored fluconazole
1998	Fluconazole vs. amphotericin B	Randomized	Composite: equivalence; secondary analysis favored fluconazole
2000	Fluconazole vs. amphotericin B	Randomized	Composite: equivalence; safety analysis favored fluconazole
1999	liposomal amphotericin B vs. amphotericin B	Randomized, double blind	Composite: equivalence; secondary analysis favors liposomal amphotericin B
2000	liposomal amphotericin B vs amphotericin B lipid complex	Randomized, double blind	Liposomal amphotericin B had superior safety vs. amphotericin B lipid complex and a similar therapeutic success rate
2001	Itraconazole vs. amphotericin B	Randomized, open label	Composite: equivalence; secondary analysis favors itraconazole
2002	Voriconazole vs. liposomal amphotericin B	Randomized, open label	Composite: equivalence; secondary analysis variable (voriconazole failed to meet criteria for noninferiority); Fewer breakthrough infections with voriconazole.
2004	Caspofungin vs. liposomal amphotericin B	Randomized, double blind	Composite: equivalence; secondary analysis favored caspofungin for treatment of baseline infections
2005	Liposomal amphotericin B loading regimen (10 mg/kg/ day ×14 day) vs. standard dosing (3 mg/kg/day)	Randomized, prospective, double blind	Loading regimen did not demonstrate any benefit in overall response or survival and was associated with higher rates of nephrotoxicity and hypokalemia

Data from Boogaerts et al.,[58] Winstan et al.,[59] Marr,[60] Walsh et al.,[61] Cornely et al.,[80] and Walsh et al.[86]

Itraconazole and fluconazole have demonstrated efficacy equivalent to that of deoxycholate amphotericin B in patients with hematologic malignancy (not treated with allogeneic hematopoietic stem cell transplantation).[58-60] However, as fluconazole is not active against filamentous fungi, its use in patients at high risk for these pathogens should be avoided. If itraconazole is used, the intravenous formulation should be used because the bioavailability of the oral formulations (including the solution) is unreliable, however it is no longer available. Voriconazole and caspofungin were compared with liposomal amphotericin B in large randomized, multicenter trials of empirical antifungal therapy in febrile neutropenic patients. Voriconazole did not fulfill the protocol-defined criteria for noninferiority (a difference in success rates between voriconazole and amphotericin B of no more than 10 percentage points) to liposomal amphotericin; however, it was superior in reducing documented breakthrough infections, infusion-related toxicity, and nephrotoxicity. Patients who received voriconazole had more frequent episodes of transient visual disturbances and hallucinations. Caspofungin demonstrated equivalent efficacy but was superior in the successful treatment of baseline invasive fungal infections.[12,61]

Specific Therapy

Amphotericin B, the azoles, and the echinocandins have roles in the treatment of hematogenous candidiasis, and the choice of therapy is guided by weighing the greater activity of amphotericin B for some non-*albicans* species (e.g., *C. krusei*) against the lower toxicity and ease of administration of fluconazole and the echinocandins.[7]

Most clinicians recommend amphotericin B in total dosages of 0.5 to 1 g administered over approximately 1 to 2 weeks in patients with *Candida* endophthalmitis and in all neutropenic patients with candidemia.[13] Longer courses of therapy can be needed in some patients.[13] Fluconazole and amphotericin B appear similarly effective for the treatment of *C. albicans* bloodstream infections in the neutropenic patient; controlled data, however, are lacking. In patients with uncomplicated *C. albicans* fungemia who have not received systemic prophylaxis with antifungal azoles, therapy with fluconazole 400 to 800 mg/ day IV can be considered.[62] However, in patients who have undergone allogeneic HSCT, the role of fluconazole is becoming more limited because of its widespread use for antifungal prophylaxis. In this setting, particularly if the patient has been treated previously with an azole antifungal agent, the possibility of microbiologic resistance must be considered.[7] Infections with fluconazole-resistant *Candida* species, including *C. glabrata*, *C. krusei*, and fluconazole-resistant *C. albicans*, or with *Aspergillus* species, are more likely.

CLINICAL CONTROVERSY

Because *C. glabrata* demonstrates reduced susceptibility in vitro to both fluconazole and amphotericin B, optimal therapy is unclear. Larger doses of fluconazole (800 mg/ day in a 70-kg patient) have been used in less critically ill patients or amphotericin B (≥0.7 mg/kg per day). However, observational studies demonstrated no difference in mortality in nonneutropenic patients administered fluconazole versus amphotericin B for bloodstream infections caused by *C. glabrata*.[40] In vitro, echinocandin antifungal agents appear very active against *C. glabrata*. Current guidelines recommend the use of echinocandins, instead of fluconazole, for the treatment of fungemia caused by *C. glabrata;* however, their usefulness in vivo has not been adequately assessed in controlled trials.[7,40]

In patients intolerant to amphotericin B or fluconazole, one of the lipid formulations can be used. In a randomized trial, amphotericin B lipid complex (ABLC) was found to be equivalent to 0.6 to 1 mg/kg per day of amphotericin B, and open-label therapy with amphotericin B colloid dispersion (ABCD) has been successful.

CANDIDURIA

Within the urinary tract, most common lesions are either *Candida* cystitis or hematogenously disseminated renal abscesses. *Candida* cystitis often follows catheterization or therapy with broad-spectrum antimicrobial agents. The diagnosis of *Candida* cystitis can be problematic because of the frequent presence of *Candida* pseudohyphae and yeast cells in urine specimens secondary to urethral colonization. The usefulness of urine colony counts or antibody coating techniques is questionable. The recovery of 10,000 organisms or visualization of both yeast and pseudohyphae from fresh midstream urine or from bladder urine obtained by single catheterization (not indwelling) is suggestive of genitourinary candidiasis. In most patients, the infection is asymptomatic and clears spontaneously without specific antifungal therapy.

Initial therapy of candidal cystitis should focus on removal of urinary catheters whenever possible. Changing the catheter will eliminate candiduria in only 20% of patients, whereas discontinuation will eradicate *Candida* in 40% of patients. Asymptomatic candiduria rarely requires therapy. Therapy should be used in symptomatic patients and in neutropenic patients, as well as in patients with renal allografts and those who will undergo urologic manipulation, because of the risk of dissemination.[63,64]

Fluconazole 200 mg/day for 14 days hastens the time to a negative urine culture as compared with placebo treatment, but 2 weeks after the end of therapy, the frequency of a negative urine culture remains the same with both treatments.[64] Short courses of therapy are not recommended; treatment should include removal of catheters and stents whenever possible plus 7 to 14 days of therapy. Bladder irrigation with amphotericin B (50 mg in 500 mL sterile water instilled twice daily into the bladder via a three-way catheter) is only transiently effective. Minimal quantities (<3%) of amphotericin B are absorbed systemically from the bladder.[17,64]

ROLE OF CATHETER REMOVAL

Although it is common practice in today's standard of care to place indwelling catheters in patients for the administration of medications and parenteral nutrition (PN), catheter-related infections are a common complication. These foreign bodies (especially triple-lumen catheters) double as entry ports for normal skin flora or other nosocomial pathogens, and they provide a readily available site for the binding of pathogens through microbiotic biofilms. Their subsequent role as a source of bloodstream infections is facilitated by frequent use, PN, and the potential for contamination of catheters by medical staff who are colonized with *Candida* species.

Most consensus recommendations urge that, if feasible, initial non-medical management should include removal of all existing tunneled central venous catheters (CVCs) and implantable devices, particularly in patients with fungemia caused by *C. parapsilosis*, which is very frequently associated with catheters.[7] Arguments against the removal of all catheters in patients with candidemia include the prominent role of the gut as a source for disseminated candidiasis, the significant cost and potential for complications, and the problems that can be encountered in patients with difficult vascular access.[65] However, in an individual patient it is often difficult to determine the relative contribution of gut versus catheter as the primary source of fungemia. The evidence for this recommendation is weakest in cancer patients with severe neutropenia and mucositis (e.g., acute leukemia, stem cell transplant), in whom candidemia is almost always primarily of gut origin, and removal of CVCs is least likely to have an impact on mortality. Nucci and Anaissie[62] have proposed that CVCs be removed in nonneutropenic patients without a short life expectancy who have one of the following criteria: (a) otherwise unexplained hemodynamic instability, (b) lack of clinical improvement or resolution of candidemia after more than 72 hours of an optimal dose of an appropriate antifungal agent, (c) established or at high risk for endocarditis or septic thrombophlebitis, or (d) a pocket infection or cellulitis. In patients with more than one CVC, they recommend removal if one tunneled or implanted CVC is the likely source of infection and the patient meets the preceding criteria.[62]

ASPERGILLOSIS

EPIDEMIOLOGY

Aspergillus is a ubiquitous mold that grows well on a variety of substrates, including soil, water, decaying vegetation, moldy hay or straw, and organic debris. Although more than 300 species of *Aspergillus* have been characterized, three species are most commonly pathogenic: *Aspergillus fumigatus, Aspergillus flavus,* and *Aspergillus niger.* The varying degrees of pathogenicity of each species depend on their relative geographic prevalence, conidial size and shape, thermotolerance, and production of mycotoxins. For example, transport of *A. fumigatus* conidia into the lungs is facilitated by their smaller diameter in comparison with *A. flavus* and *A. niger.*

❾ The term *aspergillosis* may be broadly defined as a spectrum of diseases attributed to allergy, colonization, or tissue invasion caused by members of the fungal genus *Aspergillus.* A single satisfactory classification system for these disease entities is difficult because different populations of patients can develop the same type of infection. For example, osteomyelitis can result from local trauma or hematogenous dissemination in an immunocompromised host. Colonization in normal hosts can lead to allergic diseases ranging from asthma to allergic bronchopulmonary aspergillosis or, rarely, invasive disease.[66]

PATHOPHYSIOLOGY

Aspergillosis generally is acquired by inhalation of airborne conidia that are small enough (2.5 to 3 microns) to reach alveoli or the paranasal sinuses. Each conidiophore releases 10^4 conidia that remain suspended for long periods and are viable for months in dry locations. Although some authors advocate monitoring of hospital air for *Aspergillus* conidia, guidelines for interpreting results do not exist. The use of high-efficiency particulate air (HEPA) filters in operating rooms and laminar flow rooms and removal of immunocompromised patients from hospital renovation sites can be helpful in preventing infection in this population. Although the fate of *Aspergillus* conidia in the GI tract has not been closely studied, limited evidence suggests that this route may provide an important portal of entry for disseminated infections in humans.[67]

Superficial Infection

Superficial or locally invasive infections of the ear, skin, or appendages often can be managed with topical antifungal therapy. Skin infections in patients with burn wounds, although uncommon, can progress to deep-tissue invasion despite the use of topical or parenteral antifungal agents. Risk factors for deep infection include extensive thermal injuries, malnutrition, cirrhosis, and previous infection with *Pseudomonas aeruginosa.*[67]

Allergic Bronchopulmonary Aspergillosis

Allergic manifestations of *Aspergillus* range in severity from mild asthma to allergic bronchopulmonary aspergillosis (BPA). BPA, which is almost always caused by *A. fumigatus,* is characterized by severe asthma with wheezing, fever, malaise, weight loss, chest pain, and a cough productive of blood-streaked sputum. Following recurrent episodes of severe asthma, the disease usually progresses to fibrosis and bronchiectasis with granuloma formation. When *Aspergillus* conidia become trapped in the viscous mucus of asthmatic patients, BPA develops. The fungus grows, releasing toxins and antigens. The resulting host sensitization results in a variety of immune reactions. Early in the course of disease, an immunoglobulin E (IgE)-mediated (type I) immune reaction results in bronchospasm, eosinophilia, and immediate skin reactivity. The ensuing fibrosis and pulmonary infiltrates appear to be mediated by circulating or precipitating antibody complexes of IgG antibody, followed by granuloma formation and mononuclear infiltration because of a type IV delayed hypersensitivity reaction. Therapy is aimed at minimizing the quantity of antigenic material released in the tracheobronchial tree. Management of acute asthma attacks minimizes trapping of *Aspergillus* by bronchial secretions, and administration of parenteral corticosteroids clears lung infiltrates.[67] Antifungal therapy generally is not indicated in the management of allergic manifestations of aspergillosis, although some patients have demonstrated a decrease in their corticosteroid dose following therapy with itraconazole. A double-blind, randomized, placebo-controlled trial showed that itraconazole 200 mg orally twice daily for 16 weeks resulted in significant differences in the amelioration of disease, as measured by the reduction in corticosteroid dose and improvement in exercise tolerance and pulmonary function.[66]

Aspergilloma

In the nonimmunocompromised host, *Aspergillus* infections of the sinuses most commonly occur as saprophytic colonization (aspergillomas or "fungus balls") of previously abnormal sinus tissue. An aspergilloma is composed of intertwined *Aspergillus* hyphae matted together with fibrin, mucus, and cellular debris. Infection usually is localized in the maxillary sinus and rarely is associated with local invasion of adjacent bone or brain tissue. Sinus aspergillosis also can present as allergic sinusitis with nasal drainage of brownish mucous plugs. Therapy with corticosteroids and surgery generally is successful. In the immunocompromised host, subacute, chronic, or fulminant invasive disease can be seen, and a combination of antifungal and surgical therapy generally is required.[67,68]

Pulmonary aspergillomas are fungus balls arising in preexisting cavities because of tuberculosis, histoplasmosis, lung tumors, or radiation fibrosis, although occasionally no previous pulmonary disease is present. The diagnosis of aspergilloma generally is made on the basis of chest radiographs, on which aspergillomas appear as a solid rounded mass, sometimes mobile, of water density within a spherical or ovoid cavity and separated from the wall of the cavity by an airspace of variable size and shape. Patients generally experience chest pain, dyspnea, and sputum production. Hemoptysis is observed in 50% to 80% of patients, probably because of ulceration of the epithelial lining of the cavity with formation of granulation tissue, and hemoptysis is the cause of death in up to 26% of patients with aspergilloma. A poor prognosis is associated with increasing size or number of aspergillomas, immunosuppression (including corticosteroids), increasing *Aspergillus*-specific titers, underlying sarcoidosis, and HIV infection. Although *Aspergillus* can be cultured in only 50% to 60% of patients, precipitating antibodies are positive in virtually 100% of patients.

Invasive disease occurs rarely, and therapy therefore is controversial. There are no controlled clinical trials with which to guide therapy, and recommendations for treatment have been generated from uncontrolled trials and case reports.[68] Concern regarding the risk of severe hemorrhage has led some clinicians to use aggressive surgical excision of aspergillomas or pulmonary resection in patients with hemoptysis. Complications, including bronchopulmonary fistulas, hemorrhage, empyema, and persistent airspace problems, have led to the recommendation that surgical intervention be reserved for patients with severe (>500 mL/24 h) hemoptysis, however. Bronchial artery embolization (BAE) has been used to occlude the vessel that supplies the bleeding site in patients experiencing hemoptysis. Unfortunately, BAE generally is unsuccessful or only temporarily effective. Collateral circulation eventually develops, supplying blood flow to the affected area, and hemoptysis often recurs; consequently, reembolization is often unsuccessful. BAE should be used as a temporizing procedure in a patient with life-threatening disease who might respond to more definitive therapy if hemoptysis is stabilized. Mild to moderate hemoptysis should be managed conservatively. Although IV amphotericin B generally is not useful in eradicating aspergillomas, inhaled or intracavitary instillation of amphotericin B has been employed successfully in a limited number of patients. Itraconazole has been efficacious in uncontrolled studies; however, the dose and duration of therapy have not been standardized. Hemoptysis generally ceases when the aspergilloma is eradicated.[67,68]

Invasive Aspergillosis

Although exposure to *Aspergillus* conidia is nearly universal, impaired host defenses are required for the development of invasive disease. Phagocytes (neutrophils, monocytes, and macrophages) rather than antibodies or lymphocytes constitute the primary host defense system against invasive disease with aspergillosis. Macrophages prevent germination of conidia and also eradicate conidia, providing the first line of defense against invasive disease. Administration of corticosteroids appears to impair the killing of conidia by macrophages and to impair mobilization of neutrophils. Neutrophils halt hyphal growth and dissemination and kill mycelia, constituting a second line of defense. Prolonged neutropenia appears to be the most important predisposing factor to the development of invasive aspergillosis, accounting for the high frequency of disease in patients with acute leukemia. Complement provides a source of chemotactic factor and facilitates neutrophil damage to hyphae and monocyte killing of conidia. Complement is not necessary for the attachment or ingestion of conidia by human alveolar macrophages.[67,69]

Aspergillosis is an uncommon fungal infection in patients with AIDS. AIDS patients may be at less risk for aspergillosis than other fungal infections because the primary cellular defect in AIDS patients is in the T-lymphocytes, whereas neutrophils and macrophages constitute the primary lines of defense to infection with aspergillosis. Aspergillosis was reported as a late complication of disease in AIDS patients with additional risk factors for aspergillosis, such as corticosteroid use, neutropenia, previous *Pneumocystis carinii* or cytomegalovirus pneumonia, marijuana smoking, or the use of broad-spectrum antibiotics. However, approximately 50% of patients with aspergillosis have no classic risk factors. The majority of these patients had CD4 counts < 50 cells/mm³. Although some patients diagnosed early in their infection responded to treatment, most patients do not respond to therapy with amphotericin B 0.5 mg/kg per day or itraconazole 200 to 600 mg/day.[70]

Invasive disease with *Aspergillus* can arise de novo or from any of the allergic or colonizing forms of aspergillosis. Predisposing factors to the development of invasive aspergillosis include glucocorticoid therapy, particularly following chronic administration or with higher dosages (30 to 200 mg/day of prednisone), cytotoxic agents, and recent or concurrent therapy with broad-spectrum antimicrobial agents. Patients with chronic hepatitis, alcoholism, diabetes mellitus, chronic granulomatous disease, leukopenia (<1000 cells/mm³), leukemia (particularly acute lymphocytic or myelogenous leukemia), lymphoma, and acute rejection of an organ transplant are also at a higher risk of invasive disease. Although rare, invasive aspergillosis has been reported in apparently normal hosts.[67]

CLINICAL PRESENTATION[67,68]

The lung is the most common site of invasive disease. In the immunocompromised host, aspergillosis is characterized by vascular invasion leading to thrombosis, infarction, necrosis of tissue, and dissemination to other tissues and organs in the body. Survival beyond 2 or 3 weeks is uncommon. If bone marrow function returns, cavitation of the pulmonary lesion generally occurs, and the spread of infection can be halted. The progressive nature of the disease and its refractoriness to therapy are, in part, caused by the organism's rapid growth and its tendency to invade blood vessels.

Signs and Symptoms

Patients often present with classic signs and symptoms of acute pulmonary embolus: pleuritic chest pain, fever, hemoptysis, and friction rubs. The CNS, liver, spleen, heart, GI tract, pericardium, and other body sites are involved in a substantial minority of cases. In neutropenic patients with *Aspergillus* pneumonia, hyphae invade the walls of bronchi and surrounding parenchyma, resulting in an acute necrotizing, pyogenic pneumonitis. As a result, patients often present with classic signs and symptoms of acute pulmonary embolus: pleuritic chest pain, fever, hemoptysis, and friction rubs.

Diagnosis

The diagnosis of aspergillosis is complicated by the presence of *Aspergillus* as a normal commensal in the human GI tract and respiratory secretions, and establishment of a definitive diagnosis of disease is difficult. Although suggestive of infection, the presence of hyphae in a smear or biopsy specimen is not diagnostic. Demonstration of *Aspergillus* by repeated culture and microscopic examination of tissue provides the most firm diagnosis. The appearance of *Aspergillus* in tissues varies with increasing host resistance from the normal vegetative hyphae found with necrotic tissue and exudate in the alveoli of immunocompromised hosts to the compact, tangled filaments (*granules*) observed in fungal balls. Identification of *Aspergillus* generally is based on the appearance of 2- to 4-micron-wide septate hyphae that are dichotomously branched at 45-degree angles. Sporulation is observed rarely in tissue. Although growth on Sabouraud dextrose or brain-heart infusion agar can be used for primary culture, bronchoscopy or bronchoalveolar lavage cultures are positive in only 40% of histopathologically identified specimens. Blood, CSF, and bone marrow cultures are rarely positive for *Aspergillus*.

Many clinicians treat positive respiratory cultures of *Aspergillus* as a common contaminant and argue that a minimum of two to three positive cultures is necessary before antifungal therapy is indicated. Any positive culture, however, can be indicative of true infection in the immunocompromised host, and the positive predictive value can be as high as 80% to 90% in patients with leukemia or bone marrow transplants.

Diagnostic Tests Galactomannan is a cell-wall polysaccharide specific to *Aspergillus* species that is detectable in serum and other body fluids during invasive aspergillosis (IA). Galactomannan levels, reported as optical density values, can be measured in body fluids by means of a double-sandwich enzyme immunosorbent assay (EIA).

The Platelia *Aspergillus* EIA test (Bio-Rad Laboratories) is FDA-approved for use in the diagnosis of invasive aspergillosis in HSCT recipients and in patients with leukemia; its usefulness in solid-organ transplant and pediatric populations need to be established. The use of mold-active antifungals can decrease the sensitivity of the test. In most patients, circulating antigen can be detected at a mean of 8 days before diagnosis by other means. However, false-positive galactomannan assay results have been reported for patients receiving piperacillin-tazobactam and amoxicillin-clavulanate, those with bifidobacteria infections, and in neonates.[14]

The BG test (Fungitell; Associates of Cape Cod) detects (1,3)-β-D glucan (BG) in the serum of patients with symptoms of or medical conditions predisposing to invasive fungal infections and aids in the diagnosis of deep-seated mycoses and fungemia. BG is a cell-wall constituent of many pathogenic fungi, including *Aspergillus* and *Candida* species, and is detectable in patients' serum during invasive disease due to these organisms. In addition to patients with IA and candidiasis, BG is also detectable in patients with infections caused by species of *Fusarium, Trichosporon, Saccharomyces,* and *Acremonium,* which are less common but very important fungal pathogens, especially in immunocompromised hosts. Detection of BG in serum uses a chromogenic variant of the limulus amoebocyte lysate assay. Although a positive test result for the presence of BG does not identify the infecting fungus, the practical application of this test includes its use as a screening assay (presumptive marker) for invasive fungal infection to allow the earlier initiation of antifungal therapy. Other tests are necessary for the confirmation and identification of the fungal pathogen.[14]

Late findings on radiographic studies include wedge-shaped pleural-based infiltrates or cavities on chest radiographs. Findings on computed tomographic (CT) scans include the halo sign (an area of low attenuation surrounding a nodular lung lesion) initially (caused by edema or bleeding surrounding an ischemic area) and, later, the crescent sign (an air crescent near the periphery of a lung nodule caused by contraction of infarcted tissue). CT abnormalities are best documented in neutropenic marrow transplant recipients and commonly precede plain chest radiograph abnormalities.

TREATMENT

Invasive Aspergillosis

Therapy for invasive aspergillosis is far from optimal at this time in part because of the difficulties in establishing a diagnosis and in part because of a lack of truly effective antifungal agents. Administration of amphotericin B appears to decrease mortality from more than 90% to approximately 45%. These data, however, are difficult to interpret because many patients were diagnosed postmortem, or amphotericin B therapy was not administered until the patient had very advanced disease. Mortality from pulmonary aspergillosis in bone marrow transplant recipients exceeds 94% regardless of therapy.[67] Although early diagnosis and administration of antifungal therapy can result in higher response rates, correction of underlying immune deficits (in particular, return of neutrophil counts) is of paramount importance in eradication of infection.[68]

Until the diagnosis of aspergillosis can be determined more rapidly and definitively, empirical therapy must be instituted when invasive disease is suspected. In patients at highest risk for invasive disease (acute leukemia and bone marrow transplant recipients), the most important predisposing factors include prolonged severe neutropenia (<100 cell/microliter for more than 1 week), graft rejection, chronic administration of corticosteroids, and tissue damage from preexisting infection. In these patients, antifungal therapy should be instituted in any of these conditions: (a) persistent fever or progressive sinusitis unresponsive to antimicrobial therapy, (b) an eschar over the nose, sinuses, or palate, (c) the presence of characteristic radiographic findings, including wedge-shaped infarcts, nodular densities, and new cavitary lesions, or (d) any clinical manifestation suggestive of orbital or cavernous sinus disease or an acute vascular event associated with fever. Isolation of *Aspergillus* species from nasal or respiratory tract secretions should be considered confirmatory evidence in any of the previously mentioned clinical settings.[67]

◼ NON–HIV-INFECTED PATIENT

Prophylaxis

Unfortunately, effective chemoprophylaxis against infections by *Aspergillus* species has not been demonstrated thus far.[7] As noted above in the discussion of prophylaxis for *Candida* infections in immunocompromised hosts, prophylaxis with azoles or echinocandins can reduce the incidence of fungal infections in select high-risk populations.

Specific Therapy

Even though older azole antifungal agents (miconazole and ketoconazole) possess poor in vitro activity against *Aspergillus* species, newer triazoles demonstrate improved activity both in vitro and in animal models of infection.[71] Voriconazole has emerged as the drug of choice of most clinicians for primary therapy of most patients with invasive aspergillosis.[72] A randomized trial, which compared voriconazole with amphotericin B (followed by other licensed antifungal therapy) for primary therapy of aspergillosis, noted better responses, improved survival, and fewer severe side effects with voriconazole.[73]

In patients who are unable to tolerate voriconazole, amphotericin B can be used. Because *Aspergillus* is only moderately susceptible to amphotericin B, full doses (1 to 1.5 mg/kg/day) are generally recommended, with response measured by defervescence and radiographic clearing. To treat microfoci, therapy should be continued after resolution of clinical and radiographic abnormalities until cultures (if they can be obtained) are negative, and reversible underlying predispositions have abated. Clinical response rather than any arbitrary total dose should guide duration of therapy. The optimal dosage or duration of amphotericin B therapy for the treatment of invasive disease is unknown and dependent on the extent of disease, the response to therapy, and the patient's underlying disease(s) and immune status. Unfortunately, the response rate averages only 37% (range, 14% to 83%), and the response to therapy is largely related to the extent of aspergillosis at the time of diagnosis, and host factors, such as resolution of neutropenia and the return of neutrophil function, lessening immunosuppression, and the return of graft function from a bone marrow or organ transplant.

Lipid formulations of amphotericin B can be indicated in patients with impaired renal function, and in those patients who develop nephrotoxicity while receiving deoxycholate amphotericin B. The lipid-based formulations may be preferred as initial therapy in patients with marginal renal function or in patients receiving other nephrotoxic drugs. Although these preparations appear less toxic than standard preparations, only limited data regarding their relative efficacy for invasive aspergillosis are available at this time, as the studies with the lipid preparations have been open-label or with historical conventional amphotericin B controls.[70,74]

Caspofungin was approved by the FDA for use as salvage therapy in patients who are intolerant or who fail therapy with one of the amphotericin B formulations.[12] Caspofungin has in vitro activity against *Aspergillus* species and is indicated for the treatment of invasive aspergillosis in patients who are refractory to or intolerant of other therapies such as conventional amphotericin B, lipid formulations of amphotericin B, and/or itraconazole. Caspofungin has not yet been studied as first-line therapy for patients with aspergillosis. Because of the high risk of mortality from invasive aspergillosis even following treatment with standard therapy such as amphotericin B or itraconazole, caspofungin can offer a new mechanism for salvage therapy for patients with this disease.

The use of adjuvant therapies, such as granulocyte transfusions or recombinant colony-stimulating factors, remains controversial, and controlled trials are lacking at this time. Although some authors advocate combination therapy with azoles, flucytosine, or rifampin plus amphotericin B, controlled clinical studies verifying the efficacy of these combination therapies are lacking.

Secondary Prophylaxis

The use of prophylactic antifungal therapy to prevent primary infection or reactivation of aspergillosis during subsequent courses of chemotherapy is controversial.[18] Studies assessing the utility of IV administration of amphotericin B in low doses (0.1 mg/kg per day) as prophylactic therapy or with higher dosages (0.5 to 0.6 mg/kg per day) as empirical therapy for invasive fungal infections in patients with granulocytopenia have not included sufficient numbers of patients to enable detection of differences in the number of *Aspergillus* infections.

The prophylactic use of intranasal amphotericin B aerosol sprays (5 or 10 mg/day in three divided doses) appeared beneficial in small studies in human and animal models. A larger randomized trial found, however, that amphotericin B sprays reduced colonization of the nasal mucosal without any reduction in the frequency of invasive pulmonary infections with aspergillosis. Because failure of amphotericin B sprays can be a result of the ability of small airborne conidia to access the alveolar spaces directly and to establish infection, use of aerosolized forms of amphotericin B capable of reaching the alveolar spaces can be required.

In granulocytopenic patients who recover from an episode of invasive aspergillosis, the risk of relapse of aspergillosis during subsequent courses of chemotherapy is greater than 50%. Secondary prophylaxis of aspergillosis with empirical administration of high-dose amphotericin B decreases the risk of relapse. Amphotericin B 1 mg/kg per day is started 24 to 48 hours prior to the start of chemotherapy and continued throughout the period of granulocytopenia. Some investigators recommend the addition of flucytosine (dosed to achieve peak serum concentrations of 30 to 60 mcg/mL) to the amphotericin B regimen. Although the use of itraconazole (alone or in combination with amphotericin B or flucytosine) can be beneficial in this patient population, little is known regarding its efficacy in this setting. If itraconazole is administered, serum levels should be monitored to assess absorption because poor absorption of drug has been documented in this patient population.[12]

EMERGING PATHOGENS

The increased frequency of fungal pathogens that were once rare is gaining attention from the medical community. Permissive environmental conditions, selective antifungal pressure, and increased numbers of immunosuppressed patients have led to increased numbers of infections caused by the Zygomycetes (e.g., *Mucor*, *Rhizopus* spp., or *Absidia*) or filamentous fungi such as *Scedosporium* or *Fusarium* species. Unfortunately, the early presentation of *Fusarium* and *Scedosporium* infections often mimics that of aspergillosis. On histopathology, *Scedosporium* species resembles *Aspergillus* species with dichotomously branching, septate hyphae and has a tendency for invasion of vascular structures.[75] These pathogens often demonstrate intrinsic resistance to amphotericin B and are associated with high mortality rates.[73] For example, mortality caused by *Scedosporium prolificans*, previously known as *Scedosporium inflatum*, exceeds 85%; *Scedosporium apiospermum* (the asexual state of *P. boydii*), was uniformly fatal in 23 solid-organ transplant recipients with disseminated disease.[75] However, in vitro data suggest that *S. prolificans* is more sensitive to voriconazole than to amphotericin B or itraconazole.[75,76] Voriconazole recently received FDA approval for the treatment of serious fungal infections caused by *S. apiospermum* and *Fusarium* species, including *Fusarium solani*, in patients intolerant of or refractory to other therapy.[77] Posaconazole appears promising for the treatment of zygomycoses infections.

ANTIFUNGAL THERAPY

The antifungal armamentarium for the treatment of invasive fungal infections includes (a) inhibitors of the fungal cell membrane, such as polyenes (e.g., amphotericin B) and azole antifungals, (b) inhibitors of DNA (5-flucytosine), and more recently, (c) inhibitors of cell wall biosynthesis (echinocandins).[78]

Antifungal therapy generally uses one or more of these agents, depending on the severity of infection and the patients' immune status. Rarely are the agents used in combination. Often therapy is initiated with an intravenous agent such as amphotericin B, and therapy is changed to an oral (azole) regimen as the patient's clinical status improves and oral therapy is tolerated. The most widely used combination therapy consists of flucytosine plus amphotericin B. The role of combination therapy is unclear at this time; controlled trials are lacking and the possibility of therapeutic antagonism when using azoles in combination with amphotericin B remains debated. Controlled trials are needed to define the role of azoles plus amphotericin B and azoles or amphotericin B plus an echinocandin.

AMPHOTERICIN B

Amphotericin B remains the therapy of choice for many systemic fungal infections despite a lack of controlled clinical trials documenting the optimal dosage, duration of therapy, or relative efficacy of this agent in comparison with newer azole antifungal agents. During pregnancy, amphotericin B remains the treatment of choice for most fungal infections because azole antifungals are teratogenic.[17,79]

The side effects of amphotericin B generally are categorized as acute (infusion-related) or long term. Gallis and Drew[17] recently reviewed the side effects and clinical uses of amphotericin B.

LIPID FORMULATIONS OF AMPHOTERICIN B

The use of deoxycholate amphotericin B frequently is associated with the development of induced nephrotoxicity. In an attempt to decrease the incidence of nephrotoxicity, three lipid formulations of amphotericin B have been developed and approved for use in humans: amphotericin B lipid complex (ABLC, Abelcet; Enzon Pharmaceuticals), amphotericin B colloidal dispersion (ABCD, Amphotec; Intermune Pharmaceuticals), and liposomal amphotericin B (AmBisome; Gilead Pharmaceuticals). In these preparations, amphotericin B is incorporated into the phospholipid bilayer membrane rather than in the enclosed aqueous phase.

The various lipid formulations of amphotericin B exhibit markedly different pharmacokinetics; however, the clinical implications of these differences remain unclear. Although larger doses of these preparations are required to achieve similar pharmacologic effects as the deoxycholate form of amphotericin B, the toxicity appears to be much lower.[79] Although the FDA-approved dosages of these agents are 5 mg/kg per day (amphotericin B lipid complex), 3 to 6 mg/kg per day (amphotericin B colloid dispersion), and 3 to 5 mg/kg per day (liposomal amphotericin B), the agents appear generally equipotent. The optimal dose of these compounds for serious *Candida* infections is unknown; however, dosages of 3 to 5 mg/kg per day appear reasonable. Liposomal amphotericin B administered at 3 mg/kg per day was equally as effective but less toxic than a dosage of 10 mg/kg per day as initial therapy for invasive mold infections.[80] The relative efficacy of these agents is unknown; whether differences in pharmacokinetic features result in different outcomes in the treatment of specific types of infections (e.g., CNS infections) is unclear.[7]

Lipid formulations of amphotericin B are indicated for patients intolerant of, refractory to, or at high risk of being intolerant to conventional antifungal therapy.[7,81] Intolerance generally is defined as initial renal insufficiency (creatinine >2.5 mg/dL or creatinine clearance <25 mL/min), a significant increase in creatinine (to 2.5 mg/dL for adults or 1.5 mg/dL for children), or severe acute administration-related toxicity, whereas refractory infections are defined as therapeutic failure of more than 500 mg amphotericin B.

Only ABLC and liposomal amphotericin B have been approved for use in proven candidiasis. Both in vivo and clinical studies indicate that these compounds are less toxic but as effective as amphotericin B when used in appropriate dosages. Nevertheless, their higher cost and the paucity of randomized trials in proven invasive candidiasis limit their front-line use in these infections.[81]

CLINICAL CONTROVERSY

Owing to the higher cost and paucity of randomized trials showing the efficacy of lipid-associated formulations of amphotericin B against proven invasive candidiasis, many clinicians limit their first-line use for the treatment of these infections to individuals who are intolerant to, at high risk of intolerance to, or refractory to amphotericin B deoxycholate. However, the data demonstrating up to a 6.6-fold increase in mortality in patients with amphotericin B–induced nephrotoxicity have convinced other clinicians that high-risk patients (e.g., residence in an ICU care or intermediate care unit at the time of initiation of amphotericin B therapy) warrant first-line therapy with these agents.

CLINICAL CONTROVERSY

Should lipid formulations of amphotericin B be used rather than the traditional deoxycholate formulation? Many clinicians feel that lipid formulations have shown clear superiority in the treatment of aspergillosis and histoplasmosis and are "at least as good" as deoxycholate amphotericin B for the treatment of *Candida*, cryptococcosis, and febrile neutropenia. However, they lack FDA approval for these infections except (in some cases) as salvage therapy and their costs can be prohibitive.[81]

FLUCYTOSINE

Flucytosine (also known as 5-flucytosine) is a fluorinated pyrimidine analogue that is highly water-soluble. Patients with creatinine clearances of less than 40 mL/min should receive 100 to 150 mg/kg daily in four divided doses. The dosage should be reduced by 50% in patients with a creatinine clearance of 25 to 50 mL/min and by 75% in patients with a clearance of 13 to 25 mL/min. Peak serum concentrations (2 hours after an oral dose) should be monitored in all patients (particularly those with a creatinine clearance of less than 10 mL/min) to maintain peak serum concentrations of more than 100 mg/L.[24,25]

Flucytosine generally is associated with few side effects in patients with normal renal, GI, and hematologic function, although rash, GI discomfort, diarrhea (5% to 10%), and reversible elevations in hepatic enzymes are observed occasionally. In patients with renal dysfunction or concomitant amphotericin B therapy, leukopenia, thrombocytopenia, and (rarely) enterocolitis can occur. Although studies have suggested that little or no conversion of flucytosine to fluorouracil occurs in vitro, serum concentrations of greater than 1,000 ng/mL (therapeutic for the treatment of malignancies) have been documented in some patients. Investigators have theorized that flucytosine may be secreted into the GI tract, deaminated by intestinal bacteria, and reabsorbed as 5-fluorouracil.[24,25]

Flucytosine is used in combination with amphotericin B or fluconazole in the treatment of cryptococcosis or (less commonly) candidiasis. The rapid development of resistance to flucytosine, however, precludes its use as single-agent therapy. Mechanisms for drug resistance can include loss of deaminase and decreased permeability to the drug.[24,25]

ECHINOCANDINS

The echinocandins (caspofungin, micafungin, and anidulafungin) are a new class of antifungal agents that act as concentration-dependent, noncompetitive inhibitors of β(1,3)-D-glucan synthase, an essential component of the cell wall of susceptible filamentous fungi that is absent in mammalian cells.[12]

All echinocandins display linear pharmacokinetics following administration of intravenous dosages, and are degraded primarily by the liver (also in the adrenals and spleen) by hydrolysis and N-acetylation. Following initial distribution, echinocandins are taken up by red blood cells (micafungin) and the liver (caspofungin and micafungin) where they undergo slow degradation to mainly inactive metabolites, although two uncommon metabolites of micafungin possess antifungal activity. Degradation products are excreted slowly over many days, primarily through the bile. Among the echinocandins, anidulafungin is unique in being eliminated almost exclusively by slow chemical degradation rather than undergoing hepatic metabolism.[12]

Echinocandins are available only as parenteral formulations, are not dialyzable, and do not require dosage adjustment in patients with renal insufficiency. They have minimal CSF penetration, largely because of their high protein binding and large molecular weights, although the clinical relevance of these findings can be disputed, given that several other antifungal agents (amphotericin B and itraconazole) are effective for the treatment of fungal meningitis despite low CSF concentrations.

Adverse effects of echinocandins include histamine release resulting in rash, facial swelling, and itchiness. Limited experience suggests that caspofungin and micafungin are safe to use in pediatric patients; the safety and effectiveness of anidulafungin in pediatric patients has not been established. At the time of FDA approval, there were concerns regarding the safety of caspofungin when combined with cyclosporine. However, three retrospective analyses of the use of caspofungin and cyclosporine in patients do not support a risk of clinically relevant hepatotoxicity.[12]

AZOLE ANTIFUNGAL AGENTS

The introduction of the azole antifungal agents has rapidly expanded the armamentarium of agents useful in the treatment of systemic fungal infections.[9] Adverse effects of azoles include GI disturbances (primarily nausea, vomiting, epigastric pain, and diarrhea), which appear to be more common in patients receiving ketoconazole and the solution formulation of itraconazole. Although cyclodextrin is not absorbed following oral administration, use of the IV formulations of itraconazole and voriconazole is limited to 2 weeks because of concerns for potential nephrotoxicity secondary to accumulation of the cyclodextrin vehicle.[82] Fluconazole is well tolerated; intestinal complaints are the most frequently reported, followed by headaches and rash. Unlike ketoconazole, fluconazole does not inhibit testicular or adrenal steroidogenesis in healthy volunteers or hospitalized patients. Reversible alopecia occurs not infrequently and usually appears after several months of treatment with higher doses of fluconazole. Azoles are potentially teratogenic and should be avoided in pregnant women.[82]

Itraconazole

Itraconazole is triazole antifungal with a broad spectrum of antifungal activity. Despite its marked structural similarity to ketoconazole, itraconazole differs in several important respects. Itraconazole appears to have greater specificity against fungal versus mammalian CYP, resulting in greater potency and a decrease in CYP-mediated side effects. In addition, itraconazole possesses excellent in vitro activity against *Aspergillus* and *Sporothrix* species.

Like ketoconazole, the capsule formulation of itraconazole depends on the availability of low gastric pH for dissolution and absorption. Administration with food appears to enhance significantly the bioavailability of itraconazole capsules, whereas it decreases the bioavailability of the oral solution. Because itraconazole exhibits pH-dependent dissolution and absorption, absorption of the capsule formulation is impaired in patients receiving antacids or H_2-receptor antagonists and in patients with achlorhydria.[82] Plasma concentrations of itraconazole following a single oral dose (capsules) in HIV-infected patients are approximately 50% lower than concentrations observed in healthy volunteers. The capsule formulation of itraconazole exhibits unpredictable oral bioavailability, particularly in subjects with hypochlorhydria and in patients with enteropathy caused by mucositis or graft-versus-host gut disease. An oral suspension formulation of itraconazole is available; that uses cyclodextrin as a solubilizing vehicle to increase the solubility of the drug. The oral bioavailability of the solution is unaffected by alterations in gastric pH or in patients with enteropathy.[7,82]

Fluconazole

Fluconazole is a triazole antifungal agent with markedly different pharmacologic features than other marketed azole antifungals. The small molecular weight, low protein binding, and increased water solubility of fluconazole result in rapid, essentially complete absorption of drug following oral administration. Because fluconazole is excreted primarily (>80%) as unchanged drug in the urine, dosage adjustments are necessary in patients with renal dysfunction.[71]

Voriconazole

The hepatic biotransformation of voriconazole is fairly complex and involves CYP2C19, CYP3A4, and CYP2C9, with most metabolism mediated through CYP2C19. Two of the CYPs involved in voriconazole metabolism (CYP2C19 and CYP2C9) exhibit genetic polymorphism; variability in the CYP2C19 genotype accounts for approximately 30% of the overall between-subject variability in voriconazole pharmacokinetics. About 3% to 5% of white and African human populations are poor metabolizers, while 15% to 20% of Asian populations are poor metabolizers. Drug levels can be as much as fourfold greater in poor metabolizers than in individuals who are homozygous extensive metabolizers. Coadministration of voriconazole with drugs that are potent CYP450 enzyme inducers can significantly reduce voriconazole levels. Voriconazole drug interactions are dose-dependent, as they exhibit unpredictable nonlinear pharmacokinetics; thus, drug interactions are more difficult to predict and manage.

The most common side effect of voriconazole is a reversible disturbance of vision (photopsia), which occurs in approximately 30% of patients but rarely leads to discontinuation of the drug. Symptoms tend to occur during the first week of therapy and decrease or disappear despite continued therapy. Patients experience altered color discrimination, blurred vision, the appearance of bright spots and wavy lines, and photophobia. Patients should be cautioned that driving can be hazardous because of the risk of visual disturbances. The visual effects are associated with changes in electroretinogram tracings, which revert to normal when treatment with the drug is stopped; no permanent damage to the retina has been demonstrated.[71]

CLINICAL CONTROVERSY

Controversy has arisen about whether single-drug therapy or combination therapy (e.g., voriconazole plus an echinocandin or voriconazole plus a lipid formulation of amphotericin B) is optimum therapy. At present, the highest interest concerns combination therapy in the treatment of aspergillosis, given the continued high mortality of these infections.[84] However, in vitro and animal data have produced conflicting results. Several retrospective studies have suggested an improvement in mortality with combination therapy with two or three antifungal agents; however, prospective, controlled human studies are lacking. Thus, there are as yet no firm recommendations regarding the use of such combinations in humans.[12]

Posaconazole

Posaconazole has a broad spectrum of antifungal activity, including *Aspergillus* and *Candida* species and zygomycetes. In vitro studies demonstrate that posaconazole is an inhibitor but not a substrate of hepatic (but not total) CYP3A4, and both a substrate and an inhibitor of P-glycoprotein (Pgp), suggesting that it may exhibit a drug interaction profile similar to other azoles. In addition, posaconazole undergoes glucuronidation by uridine diphosphate (UDP)-glucuronosyltransferase enzymes.[71]

DRUG INTERACTIONS WITH ANTIFUNGAL AGENTS

Drug interactions with azole antifungals generally can be placed into three broad categories: (a) decreases in azole bioavailability because of chelation or secondary to increases in gastric pH, (b) interactions with other CYP–metabolized drugs, and (c) interactions caused by inhibition of Pgp. Drug interactions in the latter two categories can result in increases or decreases in the azole antifungal, in the interacting drug, or in both drugs.

TABLE 130-11 Plasma Concentration Monitoring of Antifungal Agents[78,83,85]

	Serum Concentration Monitoring Necessary?	Target Concentration Range	Timing of Sample
Echinocandins	No	NA	NA
Amphotericin B (including lipids)	No	NA	NA
Fluconazole	No	NA	NA
Itraconazole	Yes, to ensure absorption and efficacy	>0.5 mcg/mL	Trough after 7 days of therapy
Voriconazole	Yes, (a) metabolism is variable, (b) low concentrations are associated with poor outcome, (c) high concentrations are associated with adverse effects (hepatotoxicity, visual disturbances)	Troughs >1 mcg/mL; concentrations >2.05 mcg/mL have been associated with improved outcomes; the likely therapeutic range is ~2–6 mcg/mL	Trough after 7 days of therapy
Posaconazole	Unclear; perhaps to ensure absorption	>0.25 mcg/mL ?	Trough after 7 days of therapy
Flucytosine	Yes–high concentrations (>100 mcg/mL) are associated with bone marrow suppression and hepatotoxicity	Peak concentration <100 mcg/mL	2-hour post-dose peak

NA, not applicable.

The interaction of azole antifungal agents with other CYP–metabolized drugs is well recognized. The azoles appear to be metabolized almost entirely via the CYP3A4 subfamily. As expected, they interact with other drugs metabolized partly or wholly through this enzyme pathway. In addition, fluconazole and voriconazole use the CYP2C19 pathway. Numerous clinically significant interactions have been documented with azole antifungals and a variety of other drugs. In most cases, the azole interferes with the metabolism of the other CYP–metabolized drug.[71]

The interaction between ketoconazole and cyclosporine has been exploited to reduce drug costs associated with administration of cyclosporine following organ transplantation. Relative to ketoconazole and itraconazole, fluconazole appears to be intermediate in its ability to inhibit human cytochromes P450. The magnitude of fluconazole-induced inhibition of cyclosporine metabolism appears, however, to depend on the dosage of fluconazole.

Predictably, drugs such as rifampin, rifabutin, isoniazid, phenytoin, and carbamazepine, which are known to induce the activity of cytochromes P450, result in increased metabolism of the azole antifungals and can result in therapeutic failures. Increased dosages of azole antifungals can be required in patients receiving these combinations of drugs.

Itraconazole is an inhibitor of intestinal Pgp. Significant increases in digoxin (a Pgp substrate) have been observed in patients receiving both agents concurrently. Interactions with other substrates of Pgp would be expected to occur.

Echinocandins are not inducers of cytochrome P450 enzymes, nor do they interact with Pgp, and are considered poor substrates of CYP3A4. Nevertheless, cyclosporine increases the area under the curve (AUC) of caspofungin by ~35%, and tacrolimus AUC, peak, and 12-hour concentrations are decreased by approximately 20% during concomitant administration with caspofungin. Additionally, when caspofungin was administered concurrently with tacrolimus, tacrolimus levels were reduced by 20% compared to administration with tacrolimus alone. The mechanism for these interactions is not yet known. Rifampin both inhibits (acutely) and induces (after chronic administration) caspofungin metabolism. A dosage increase is recommended in patients receiving other enzyme inducers, such as efavirenz, nevirapine, phenytoin, dexamethasone, and carbamazepine. Although micafungin does not significantly affect the clearance (or AUC) of tacrolimus, it increases the AUC of sirolimus by 21%, and of nifedipine by 18%, and decreases clearance of cyclosporine by 16%. Monitoring of cyclosporine levels during combination therapy with micafungin is recommended. Administration of cyclosporine and anidulafungin revealed only a clinically insignificant 22% increase in the AUC of anidulafungin following 4 days of concomitant cyclosporine therapy, and concurrent administration of rifampin or a variety of other substrates, inhibitors, or inducers of CYP450 with anidulafungin does not affect its clearance.[12]

PLASMA CONCENTRATION MONITORING OF ANTIFUNGAL AGENTS

Routine monitoring of plasma concentrations of antifungal agents to assess efficacy or toxicity of these agents generally is not available. Correlations between plasma concentrations of antifungal agents and therapeutic outcomes have been poorly studied. Under certain circumstances, serum or plasma concentration monitoring is warranted, for example, in patients susceptible to flucytosine toxicity or to document adequate oral absorption of ketoconazole, itraconazole, or voriconazole in cases of suspected treatment failure, concern about compliance or absorption, or when drug interactions that might reduce the solubility or accelerate the metabolism of azoles are suspected (Table 130–11).[83]

CLINICAL CONTROVERSY

Although "therapeutic" levels have not been defined, some investigators recommend maintenance of serum concentrations of itraconazole (2 to 4 hours after administration) of 1 mcg/mL, measured by bioassay, and voriconazole.[18] Among AIDS patients, those receiving itraconazole dosages of 200 mg once or twice daily achieved median plasma concentrations of 3 or 6 mcg/mL, respectively.[18] Although pharmacokinetic-pharmacodynamic analysis of early clinical trials of voriconazole did not reveal an association between voriconazole concentration and efficacy, they did suggest a trend toward worse outcome in those patients with voriconazole concentrations of <0.5 mcg/mL. This lack of association is likely because the antifungal exposure far exceeded the MICs of most pathogens (MIC_{90}, ≤0.5 mcg/mL). However, in a recent study, favorable responses were observed in 10:10 patients with voriconazole plasma concentrations >2.05 mcg/mL, whereas disease progressed in 44% of patients with concentrations <2.05 mcg/mL.[85]

COMBINATION ANTIFUNGAL THERAPY FOR ASPERGILLOSIS

Based on extensive experience in the management of bacterial, and more recently, retroviral infections, the use of combination agents for synergistic or additive effects is now common practice, particularly for the treatment of invasive aspergillosis.[84] High-dose fluconazole, alone or in combination with amphotericin B, in non-immunocompromised patients with candidemia demonstrated no antagonism and a trend toward improved success and more rapid clearance of *Candida* from the bloodstream.[47]

ABBREVIATIONS

AIDS: acquired immunodeficiency syndrome

ACTG: AIDS Clinical Trials Group

ATCC: American Type Culture Collection

ABCD: amphotericin B colloid dispersion

ABLC: amphotericin B lipid complex

BG: (13)-β-D-Glucan

BPA: bronchopulmonary aspergillosis

BSI: bloodstream infection

CDC: Centers for Disease Control and Prevention

CNS: central nervous system

CVC: central venous catheter

CSF: cerebrospinal fluid

CF-M: CF titer for mycelial antigen

CF: complement fixation

ELISA: enzyme-linked immunosorbent assay

FISH: fluorescence in-situ hybridization

GI: gastrointestinal

GVHD: graft-versus-host disease

HEPA: high-efficiency particulate air

HAART: highly active antiretroviral therapy

HSCT: hematopoietic stem cell transplantation

ID: immunodiffusion

IgM: immunoglobulin M

ICUs: intensive care units

IV: intravenous

LA: latex agglutination

NCCLS: National Committee for Clinical Laboratory Standards

PMN: polymorphonuclear leukocytes

PDH: progressive disseminated histoplasmosis

PN: total parenteral nutrition

PNA: peptide nucleic acid

RIA: radioimmunoassay

WBC: white blood cell

REFERENCES

1. Bennett JE. Introduction to mycoses. In: Mandell GL, Bennett JE, Dolin R, eds. Principles and Practice of Infectious Diseases, 6th ed. Philadelphia, PA: Churchill Livingstone, 2005:2935–2938.
2. Pfaller MA, Jones RN, Messer SA, et al. National surveillance of nosocomial blood stream infection due to *Candida* albicans: Frequency of occurrence and antifungal susceptibility in the SCOPE program. Diagn Microbiol Infect Dis 1998;31:327–332.
3. Pfaller MA, Jones RN, Doern GV, et al. International surveillance of blood stream infections due to *Candida* species in the European SENTRY Program: Species distribution and antifungal susceptibility including the investigational triazole and echinocandin agents. SENTRY Participant Group (Europe). Diagn Microbiol Infect Dis 1999;35:19–25.
4. Singh N. Invasive mycoses in organ transplant recipients: Controversies in prophylaxis and management. J Antimicrob Chemother 2000;45:749–755.
5. National Committee for Clinical Laboratory Standards (NCCLS). Reference method for broth dilution antifungal susceptibility testing of yeasts: Approved Standard. Wayne, PA: NCCLS, 1997. NCCLS document M27-A.
6. Sobel JD. Practice guidelines for the treatment of fungal infections. Clin Infect Dis 2000;30:652.
7. Pappas PG, Kauffman CA, Andes D, et al. Clinical practice guidelines for the management of candidiasis: 2009 update by the Infectious Diseases Society of America. Clin Infect Dis 2009;48(5):503–35.
8. Sanglard D, Odds FC. Resistance of *Candida* species to antifungal agents: Molecular mechanisms and clinical consequences. Lancet Infect Dis 2002;2:73185.
9. White TC, Marr KA, Bowden RA. Clinical, cellular, and molecular factors that contribute to antifungal drug resistance. Clin Microbiol Rev 1998;11:382–402.
10. Lupetti A, Danesi R, Campa M, et al. Molecular basis of resistance to azole antifungals. Trends Mol Med 2002;8:76–81.
11. Bille J. Mechanisms and clinical significance of antifungal resistance. Int J Antimicrob Agents 2000;16:331–333.
12. Eschenauer G, DePestel DD, Carver PL. Comparison of Echinocandin Antifungals. Therapeutics and Clinical Risk Management, 2007;3(1):71–97.
13. Edwards JE. *Candida* species. In: Mandell GL, Bennett JE, Dolin R, eds. Principles and Practice of Infectious Diseases, 6th ed. Philadelphia, PA: Churchill Livingstone, 2005:2938–2953.
14. Alexander BD, Pfaller MA. Contemporary tools for the diagnosis and management of invasive mycoses. Clin Infect Dis 2006; 43:S15–27.
15. Saag MS, Graybill RJ, Larsen RA, et al. Practice guidelines for the management of cryptococcal disease. Clin Infect Dis 2000;30:710–718.
16. Deepe GS. Histoplasma capsulatum. In: Mandell GL, Bennett JE, Dolin R, eds. Principles and Practice of Infectious Diseases, 6th ed. Philadelphia, PA: Churchill Livingstone, 2005:3012–3026.
17. Gallis HA, Drew RH, Pickard WW. Amphotericin B: 30 years of clinical experience. Rev Infect Dis 1990;12:308–329.
18. Wheat LJ, Freifeld AG, Kleiman MB, et al. Clinical practice guidelines for the management of patients with histoplasmosis: 2007 update by the Infectious Diseases Society of America. Clin Infect Dis 2007;45(7):807–825.
19. Kauffman CA. Histoplasmosis: a clinical and laboratory update. Clin Microbiol Rev 2007;20(1):115–132.
20. Galgiani JN, Ampel NM, Blair JE, et al. Practice guidelines for the treatment of coccidioidomycoses. Clin Infect Dis 2005;41:1217–1223.
21. O'Shaughnessy EM, Shea YM, Witebsky FG. Laboratory diagnosis of invasive mycoses. Infect Dis Clin North Am 2003;17(1):135–158.
22. Parish JM, Blair JE. Coccidioidomycosis Mayo Clin Proc 2008;83(3):343–348.
23. Bennett JE, Dismukes WE, Duma RJ, et al. A comparison of amphotericin B alone and combined with flucytosine in the treatment of cryptococcal meningitis. N Engl J Med 1979;301:126–131.
24. Francis P, Walsh TJ. Evolving role of flucytosine in immunocompromised patients: New insights into safety, pharmacokinetics, and antifungal therapy. Clin Infect Dis 1992;15:1003–1018.
25. Powderly WG, Saag MS, Cloud GA, et al. A controlled trial of fluconazole or amphotericin B to prevent relapse of cryptococcal meningitis in patients with the acquired immunodeficiency syndrome. N Engl J Med 1992;326:793–798.
26. Saag MS, Powderly WG, Cloud GA, et al. Comparison of amphotericin B with fluconazole in the treatment of acute AIDS-associated cryptococcal meningitis: The NIAID Mycoses Study Group and the AIDS Clinical Trials Group. N Engl J Med 1992;326:83–89.
27. van der Horst CM, Saag MS, Cloud GA, et al. Treatment of cryptococcal meningitis associated with the acquired immunodeficiency syndrome. N Engl J Med 1997;37:15–21.
28. Vibhagool A, Sungkanuparph S, Mootsikapun P, et al. Discontinuation of secondary prophylaxis for cryptococcal meningitis in human immunodeficiency virus-infected patients treated with highly active

antiretroviral therapy: A prospective, multicenter, randomized study. Clin Infect Dis 2003;36:1329–1331.

29. Minari A, Hachem R, Raad I. *Candida lusitaniae:* A cause of breakthrough fungemia in cancer patients. Clin Infect Dis 2001;32: 186–190.

30. Pfaller MA, Jones RN, Doern GV, et al. International surveillance of bloodstream infections due to *Candida* species: Frequency of occurrence and antifungal susceptibilities of isolates collected in 1997 in the United States, Canada, and South America for the SENTRY program. J Clin Microbiol 1998;36:1886–1889.

31. Winston DJ, Chandrasekar PH, Lazarus HM, et al. Fluconazole prophylaxis of fungal infections in patients with acute leukemia: Results of a randomized placebo-controlled, double-blind, multicenter trial. Ann Intern Med 1993;118:495–503.

32. Rangel-Frausto MS, Wiblin T, Blumberg HM, et al. National Epidemiology of Mycoses Survey (NEMIS): Variations in rates of blood stream infections due to *Candida* species in seven surgical intensive care units and six neonatal intensive care units. Clin Infect Dis 1999;29:253–258.

33. Edmond MB, Wallace SE, McClish DK, et al. Nosocomial bloodstream infections in United States hospitals: A three-year analysis. Clin Infect Dis 1999;29:239–244.

34. Lam SW, Eschenauer GA, Carver PL. Evolving role of early antifungals in the adult intensive care unit. Crit Care Med 2009;37(5):1580–1593.

35. Eschenauer GA, Lam SW, Carver PL. Antifungal prophylaxis in liver transplant recipients. Liver Transpl 2009;15(8):842–858.

36. Sullivan DJ, Moran GP, Coleman DC. Candida dubliniensis: Ten years on. FEMS Microbiol Lett 2005;253(1):9–17.

37. Morrell M, Fraser VJ, Kollef MH. Delaying the empiric treatment of candida bloodstream infection until positive blood culture results are obtained: A potential risk factor for hospital mortality. Antimicrob Agents Chemother 2005;49:3640–3645.

38. Gudlaugsson O, Gillespie S, Lee K, et al. Attributable mortality of nosocomial candidemia, revisited. Clin Infect Dis 2003;37:1172–1177.

39. Garey KW, Rege M, Pai MP, et al. Time to initiation of fluconazole therapy impacts mortality in patients with candidemia: A multi-institutional study. Clin Infect Dis 2006;43(1):25–31.

40. Pappas, PG, Rex JH, Lee J, et al. A prospective observational study of candidemia: Epidemiology, therapy, and influences on mortality in hospitalized adult and pediatric patients. Clin Infect Dis 2003;37:634–643.

41. Eggimann P, Francioli P, Bille J, et al. Fluconazole prophylaxis prevents intraabdominal candidiasis in high-risk surgical patients. Crit Care Med 1999;27:1066–1072.

42. Rocco TR, Reinert SE, Simms H. Effect of fluconazole administration in critically ill patients. Arch Surg 2000;135:160–165.

43. Sobel JD, Rex JH. Invasive candidiasis: Turning risk into a practical prevention policy? Clin Infect Dis 2001;33:187–190.

44. Rex JH, Bennett JE, Sugar AM, et al. A randomized trial comparing fluconazole with amphotericin B for the treatment of candidemia in patients without neutropenia. N Engl J Med 1994;331:1325–1330.

45. Reboli AC, Rotstein C, Pappas PG, et al. Anidulafungin versus fluconazole for invasive candidiasis. N Engl J Med 2007;356(24):2472–2482.

46. Mora-Duarte J, Betts R, Rotstein C, et al. Comparison of caspofungin and amphotericin B for invasive candidiasis. N Engl J Med 2002;347:2020–2029.

47. Rex JH, Pappas PG, Karchmer AW, et al. A randomized and blinded multicenter trial of high-dose fluconazole plus placebo versus fluconazole plus amphotericin B as therapy for candidemia and its consequences in nonneutropenic subjects. Clin Infect Dis 2003;36:1221–1228.

48. Kullberg BJ, Sobel JD, Ruhnke M, et al. Voriconazole versus a regimen of amphotericin B followed by fluconazole for candidemia in nonneutropenic patients: A randomised non-inferiority trial. Lancet 2005;366(9495):1435–1442.

49. Kuse ER, Chetchotisakd P, da Cunha CA, et al. Micafungin versus liposomal amphotericin B for candidaemia and invasive candidosis: a phase III randomised double-blind trial. Lancet 2007 May 5;369(9572):1519–1527

50. Pappas PG, Rotstein CM, Betts RF, et al. Micafungin versus caspofungin for treatment of candidemia and other forms of invasive candidiasis. Clin Infect Dis 2007;45(7):883–893.

51. Goodman JL, Winston DJ, Greenfield RA, et al. A controlled trial of fluconazole to prevent fungal infections in patients undergoing bone marrow transplantation. N Engl J Med 1992;326:845–851.

52. Slavin MA, Osborne B, Adams R, et al. Efficacy and safety of fluconazole prophylaxis for fungal infections after marrow transplantation: A prospective, randomized, double-blind study. J Infect Dis 1995;171:1545–1552.

53. Marr KA, Seidel K, Slavin MA, et al. Prolonged fluconazole prophylaxis is associated with persistent protection against candidiasis-related death in allogeneic marrow transplant recipients: Long-term follow-up of a randomized, placebo-controlled trial. Blood 2000;96: 2055–2061.

54. Menichetti F, Del Favero A, Martino P, et al. Itraconazole oral solution as prophylaxis for fungal infections in neutropenic patients with hematologic malignancies: A randomized, placebo-controlled, double-blind, multicenter trial. GIMEMA Infection Program. Gruppo Italiano Malattie Ematologiche dell' Adulto. Clin Infect Dis 1999;28:250–255.

55. Rotstein C, Bow EJ, Laverdiere M, et al. Randomized placebo-controlled trial of fluconazole prophylaxis for neutropenic cancer patients: Benefit based on purpose and intensity of cytotoxic therapy. Clin Infect Dis 1999;28:331–340.

56. Ullmann AJ, Lipton JH, Vesole DH, et al. A multicenter trial of oral posaconazole vs. fluconazole for the prophylaxis of invasive fungal infections in recipients of allogeneic hematopoietic stem cell transplantation with graft-vs.-host disease. Mycoses 2005;48(Suppl 2):26a–27a.

57. McCoy D, DePestel DD, Carver PL. Primary antifungal prophylaxis in adult hematopoietic stem cell transplant recipients: current therapeutic concepts. Pharmacotherapy 2009;29(11)1306–1325.

58. Boogaerts M, Winston DJ, Bow EJ, et al. Intravenous and oral itraconazole versus intravenous amphotericin B as empirical antifungal therapy for persistent fever in neutropenic patients with cancer who are receiving broad-spectrum antibacterial therapy. Ann Intern Med 2001;135:412–422.

59. Winston DJ, Hathorn JW, Schuster MG, et al. A multicenter, randomized trial of fluconazole versus amphotericin B for empiric antifungal therapy of febrile neutropenic patients with cancer. Am J Med 2000;108:282–289.

60. Marr KA. Empirical antifungal therapy—New options, new tradeoffs. N Engl J Med, 2002;346:278–280.

61. Walsh TJ, Pappas P, Winston DJ, et al. Voriconazole compared with liposomal amphotericin B for empirical antifungal therapy in patients with neutropenia and persistent fever. N Engl J Med 2002;346: 225–234.

62. Anaissie EJ, Darouiche RO, Abi-Said D, et al. Management of invasive candidal infections: Results of a prospective, randomized, multicenter study of fluconazole versus amphotericin B and review of the literature. Clin Infect Dis 1996;23:964–972.

63. Kauffman CA, Vazquez JA, Sobel JD, et al. Prospective multicenter surveillance study of funguria in hospitalized patients. Clin Infect Dis 2000;30:14–18.

64. Sobel JD, Kauffman CA, McKinsey D, et al. Candiduria: A randomized, double-blind study of treatment with fluconazole and placebo. Clin Infect Dis 2000;30:19–24.

65. Nucci M, Anaissie E. Should vascular catheters be removed from all patients with candidemia? An evidence-based review. Clin Infect Dis 2002;34:591–599.

66. Stevens DA, Schwartz HJ, Lee JT, et al. A randomized trial of itraconazole in allergic bronchopulmonary aspergillosis. N Engl J Med 2000;342:756–762.

67. Steinbach WJ, Stevens DA. Review of newer antifungal and immunomodulatory strategies for invasive aspergillosis. Clin Infect Dis 2003;37(Suppl 3):S157–187.

68. Walsh TJ, Anaissie EJ, Denning DW, et al. Treatment of aspergillosis: clinical practice guidelines of the Infectious Diseases Society of America. Clin Infect Dis 2008;46(3):327–360.

69. Lin SJ, Schranz J, Teutsch SM. Aspergillus case fatality rate: Systematic review of the literature. Clin Infect Dis 2001;32:358–366.

70. Holding KJ, Dworkin MS, Wan PCT, et al. Aspergillosis among people infected with human immunodeficiency virus: Incidence and survival. Clin Infect Dis 2000;31:1253–1257.

71. Saad A, DePestel DD, Carver PL. Factors influencing the magnitude and clinical significance of drug interactions between azole antifungals and select immunosuppressants. Pharmacotherapy 2006;26: 1730–1744.

72. Dismukes, WE. Antifungal therapy: Lessons learned over the past 27 years. Clin Infect Dis 2006;42:1289–1296.

73. Herbrecht R, Denning DW, Patterson TF, et al. Voriconazole versus amphotericin B for primary therapy of invasive aspergillosis. N Engl J Med 2002;347:408–415.

74. Ellis M, Spence D, de Pauw B, et al. An EORTC international multicenter randomized trial (EORTC no. 19923) comparing two dosages of liposomal amphotericin B for treatment of invasive aspergillosis. Clin Infect Dis 1998;27:1406–1412.

75. Castiglioni B, Sutton DA, Rinaldi MG, et al. *Pseudallescheria boydii* (anamorph *Scedosporium apiospermum*) infection in solid organ transplant recipients in a tertiary medical center and review of the literature. Medicine 2002;81:333–348.

76. Lamaris, GA, Chamilos G, Lewis, RE, et al. Scedosporium infection in a tertiary care cancer center: A review of 25 cases from 1989–2006. Clin Infect Dis 2000;43:1580–1584.

77. Vfend (voriconazole). Package insert. New York: Pfizer, 2002.

78. Dodds Ashley ES, Lewis R, Lewis JS, Martin C, Andes D. Pharmacology of Systemic Antifungal Agents. Clin Infect Dis 2006;43:S28–39.

79. King CT, Rogers PD, Cleary JD, et al. Antifungal therapy during pregnancy. Clin Infect Dis 1998;27:1151–1160.

80. Cornely OA, Maertens J, Bresnik M, et al. Liposomal amphotericin B as initial therapy for invasive mold infection: a randomized trial comparing a high-loading dose regimen with standard dosing (AmBiLoad trial). Clin Infect Dis 2007;44(10):1289–1297.

81. Ostrosky-Zeichner L, Marr KA, Rex JH, Cohen SH. Amphotericin B. Time for a new "gold standard." Clin Infect Dis 2003;37: 415–425.

82. Stevens DA. Itraconazole in cyclodextrin solution. Pharmacotherapy 1999;19:603–611.

83. Smith J, Andes D. Therapeutic drug monitoring of antifungals: pharmacokinetic and pharmacodynamic considerations. Ther Drug Monit 2008;30(2):167–172.

84. Marr KA, Boeckh M, Carter RA, et al. Combination antifungal therapy for invasive aspergillosis. Clin Infect Dis 2004;39:797–802.

85. Smith J, Safdar N, Knasinski V, et al. Voriconazole therapeutic drug monitoring. Antimicrob Agents Chemother 2006;50(4): 1570–1572.

86. Walsh TJ, Teppler H, Donowitz GR, et al. Caspofungin versus liposomal amphotericin B for empirical antifungal therapy in patients with persistent fever and neutropenia. N Engl J Med 2004;351: 1391–1402.

131

Infections in Immunocompromised Patients

DOUGLAS N. FISH

KEY CONCEPTS

❶ An *immunocompromised host* is a patient with defects in host defenses that predispose to infection. Risk factors include neutropenia, immune system defects (from disease or immunosuppressive drug therapy), compromise of natural host defenses, environmental contamination, and changes in normal flora of the host.

❷ Immunocompromised patients are at high risk for a variety of bacterial, fungal, viral, and protozoal infections. Bacterial infections caused by gram-positive cocci (staphylococci and streptococci) occur most frequently, followed by gram-negative bacterial infections caused by Enterobacteriaceae and *Pseudomonas aeruginosa*. Fungal infections caused by *Candida* and *Aspergillus*, as well as certain viral infections (herpes simplex virus, Cytomegalovirus), are also important causes of morbidity and mortality.

❸ Risk of infection in neutropenic patients is associated with both the severity and duration of neutropenia. Patients with severe neutropenia (ANC <500 cells/mm^3) for greater than 7 to 10 days are considered to be at high risk of infection.

❹ Fever (single oral temperature of ≥38.3°C [101°F], or a temperature of ≥38°C [100.4°F] for ≥1 hour) is the most important clinical finding in neutropenic patients and is usually the stimulus for further diagnostic workup and initiation of antimicrobial treatment. Infection should be considered as the cause of fever until proven otherwise. Usual signs and symptoms of infection may be altered or absent in neutropenic patients. Appropriate empiric broad-spectrum antimicrobial therapy must be rapidly instituted to prevent excessive morbidity and mortality.

❺ Empiric antimicrobial regimens for neutropenic infections should take into account patients' individual risk factors, as well as institutional infection and susceptibility patterns. The significant morbidity and mortality associated with gram-negative infections require that initial empiric regimens for treatment of febrile neutropenia have good activity against *P. aeruginosa* and Enterobacteriaceae. Inpatient parenteral regimens most commonly recommended for initial treatment include monotherapy with an antipseudomonal cephalosporin or carbapenem, or a combination regimen consisting of an antipseudomonal cephalosporin or carbapenem, plus an aminoglycoside. Low-risk patients may be successfully treated with oral antibiotics (ciprofloxacin plus amoxicillin/clavulanate), with the treatment setting determined by the patient's clinical status.

❻ Neutropenic patients who remain febrile after 3 to 5 days of initial antimicrobial therapy should be reevaluated to determine whether treatment modifications are necessary. Common regimen modifications include addition of vancomycin (if not already administered) and antifungal therapy (amphotericin B or fluconazole). Therapy should be directed at causative organisms, if identified, but broad-spectrum regimens should be maintained during neutropenia.

❼ The optimal duration of therapy for febrile neutropenia is controversial. The decision to discontinue antimicrobials is based on resolution of neutropenia, defervescence, culture results, and clinical stability of the patient.

❽ Prophylactic antimicrobials are administered to cancer patients expected to experience prolonged neutropenia, as well as to both hematopoietic stem cell and solid-organ transplant recipients. Prophylactic regimens may include antibacterial, antifungal, antiviral, or antiprotozoal agents, or a combination of these, selected according to risk of infection with specific pathogens. Optimal prophylactic regimens should take into account individual patient risk for infection and institutional infection and susceptibility patterns.

❾ Patients undergoing hematopoietic stem cell transplantation are at an extremely high risk of infection because of prolonged neutropenia following intensive chemotherapy ± irradiation, while solid-organ transplant recipients are at high risk because of prolonged administration of immunosuppressive drugs. Fungal *(Aspergillus)* and viral (Cytomegalovirus) infections are particularly troublesome in these populations, and prophylactic regimens directed against these pathogens are commonly used. When documented, these infections must be treated aggressively in order to optimize patient outcomes. Nevertheless, mortality rates are often high despite appropriate and aggressive antimicrobial therapy.

❿ Immunocompromised patients must be continuously assessed for evidence of infection and response to antimicrobial therapy. Because a large number of antimicrobials may potentially be used, the occurrence of drug-related adverse effects must also be carefully assessed. Efforts should be directed at designing cost-effective treatment strategies that promote optimal patient outcomes.

Learning objectives, review questions, and other resources can be found at **www.pharmacotherapyonline.com**.

An immunocompromised host is a patient with intrinsic or acquired defects in host immune defenses that predispose to infection. Advances in modern medicine have created more immunocompromised hosts than ever before. Historically, many of these patients died of their underlying diseases. Dramatic improvements in survival have been achieved by more aggressive therapy of underlying diseases and improved supportive care. However, because such aggressive therapy often renders patients profoundly immunosuppressed for long periods, opportunistic infections remain important causes of morbidity and mortality. This chapter focuses on risk factors for infection, common pathogens and infection sites, and prevention and management of suspected or documented infections in cancer patients (including hematopoietic stem cell transplantation [HSCT] patients) and solid-organ transplant recipients. Chapter 134 discusses infectious complications associated with human immunodeficiency virus (HIV) infection.

RISK FACTORS FOR INFECTION/EPIDEMIOLOGY

Many factors influence the degree of immunosuppression and also influence the epidemiology of the associated infections.

NEUTROPENIA

①②③ Neutropenia is defined as an abnormally reduced number of neutrophils circulating in peripheral blood. Although exact definitions of neutropenia can vary, an absolute neutrophil count (ANC) of less than 1,000 cells/mm³ indicates a reduction sufficient to predispose patients to infection.[1] ANC is the sum of the absolute numbers of both mature neutrophils (polymorphonuclear cells [PMNs], also called *polys* or *segs*) and immature neutrophils (*bands*). The absolute number of PMNs and bands is determined by dividing the total percentage of these cells (obtained from the white blood cell [WBC] differential) by 100 and then multiplying the quotient obtained by the total number of WBCs.

The degree or severity of neutropenia, rate of neutrophil decline, and duration of neutropenia are important risk factors for infection.[1-5] All neutropenic patients are considered to be at risk for infection, but those with ANC less than 500 cells/mm³ are at greater risk than those with ANCs of 500 to 1,000 cells/mm³. Most treatment guidelines use ANC less than 500 cells/mm³ as the critical value in making therapeutic decisions regarding the management of suspected or documented infections.[1-5] Risk of infection and death are greatest among patients with less than 100 neutrophils/mm³ ("profound neutropenia").[1,2] In patients with chemotherapy-induced neutropenia, the risk of infection is also increased according to the rapidity of ANC decline. Infection risk also increases as the duration of neutropenia increases; patients with severe neutropenia of more than 7 to 10 days' duration are considered to be at especially high risk for serious infections.[3] The duration of chemotherapy-induced neutropenia varies considerably among subsets of cancer patients according to the specific chemotherapeutic agents used and the intensity of treatment. Patients undergoing HSCT may have no detectable granulocytes in peripheral blood for up to 3 to 4 weeks and are at particular risk for severe infections with a variety of pathogens.[6]

Bacteria and fungi commonly cause infections in neutropenic patients. Gram-positive cocci (*Staphylococcus aureus*, *Staphylococcus epidermidis*, streptococci, and enterococci) have emerged as the most common cause of acute bacterial infections among neutropenic patients. Gram-negative bacilli (*Escherichia coli*, *Klebsiella pneumoniae*, *Pseudomonas aeruginosa*) traditionally were the most common causes of bacterial infection and remain frequent pathogens.[4,7-9] Although not now as common as gram-positive bacteria,

the incidence of gram-negative infections may again be increasing.[3,8] Gram-negative infections are associated with significant morbidity and mortality, in large part due to increasing antibiotic resistance.[7-9] Patients who are neutropenic for extended periods and who receive broad-spectrum antibiotics are at high risk for fungal infections, usually due to *Candida* or *Aspergillus* spp.[2,3,10,11] Viral infections, although not as common as bacterial and fungal infections, also may cause severe infection in neutropenic patients.[2,3,5,12] Successful treatment of infections in neutropenic patients depends on resolution of neutropenia.[1-3,5]

Although not readily quantifiable, abnormalities may exist in granulocyte function as well as in cell numbers. Defects in phagocyte function may be caused by underlying disease (e.g., leukemia) or its treatment (e.g., corticosteroids, antineoplastic agents, and radiation).[3,13,14]

IMMUNE SYSTEM DEFECTS

In addition to neutropenia, defects in T lymphocyte and macrophage function (cell-mediated immunity), B-cell function (humoral immunity), or both predispose patients to infection. Cellular immune dysfunction is the result of underlying disease or immunosuppressive drug therapy; these defects result in a reduced ability of the host to defend against intracellular pathogens. Patients with Hodgkin's disease and transplant patients receiving a wide variety of immunosuppressive drugs, such as cyclosporine, tacrolimus, sirolimus, mycophenolate, corticosteroids, azathioprine, and antineoplastic agents, are at risk for a variety of bacterial, fungal, viral, and protozoal infections (Table 131–1). Although some of these pathogens are associated with asymptomatic or mild disease in normal hosts, they may cause disseminated, life-threatening infections in immunocompromised hosts.

Underlying disease also frequently causes defects in humoral immune function. Patients with multiple myeloma and chronic lymphocytic leukemia have progressive hypogammaglobulinemia that results in defective humoral immunity. Splenectomy performed as a part of the staging process for Hodgkin's disease places patients at risk for infectious complications. Disease states with humoral immune dysfunction predispose the patient to serious, life-threatening infection with encapsulated organisms such as *Streptococcus pneumoniae*, *Haemophilus influenzae*, and *Neisseria meningitidis*.

DESTRUCTION OF PROTECTIVE BARRIERS

Loss of protective barriers is a major factor predisposing immunocompromised patients to infection. Damage to skin and mucous membranes by surgery, venipuncture, intravenous (IV) and urinary catheters, radiation, and chemotherapy disrupts natural host defense systems, leaving patients at high risk for infection. Chemotherapy-induced mucositis may erode mucous membranes of the oropharynx and gastrointestinal (GI) tract and establish a portal for subsequent infection by bacteria, herpes simplex virus (HSV), and *Candida*.[3,15] Medical and surgical procedures, such as transplant surgery, indwelling IV catheter placement, bone marrow aspiration, biopsies, and endoscopy, further damage the integument and predispose patients to infection. Infections resulting from disruption of protective barriers usually are a result of skin flora, such as *S. aureus*, *S. epidermidis*, and various streptococci.[1,3,5,13,15]

ENVIRONMENTAL CONTAMINATION/ ALTERATION OF MICROBIAL FLORA

Infections in immunocompromised patients are caused by organisms either colonizing the host or acquired from the environment.

TABLE 131-1 Risk Factors and Common Pathogens in Immunocompromised Patients

Risk Factor	Patient Conditions	Common Pathogens
Neutropenia	Acute leukemia Chemotherapy	Bacteria: *Staphylococcus aureus, Staphylococcus epidermidis, Escherichia coli, Klebsiella pneumoniae, Pseudomonas aeruginosa*, streptococci, enterococci Fungi: *Candida, Aspergillus, Zygomycetes* Viruses: Herpes simplex
Impaired cell-mediated immunity	Lymphoma Immunosuppressive therapy (steroids, cyclosporine, chemotherapy)	Bacteria: *Listeria, Nocardia, Legionella*, Mycobacteria Fungi: *Cryptococcus neoformans, Candida, Aspergillus, Histoplasma capsulatum* Viruses: Cytomegalovirus, varicella-zoster, herpes simplex Protozoal: *Pneumocystis jiroveci*
Impaired humoral immunity	Multiple myeloma Chronic lymphocytic leukemia Splenectomy Immunosuppressive therapy (steroids, chemotherapy)	Bacteria: *S. pneumoniae, H. influenzae, N. meningitidis*
Loss of protective skin barriers	Venipuncture, bone marrow aspiration, urinary catheterization, vascular access devices, radiation, biopsies	Bacteria: *S. aureus, S. epidermidis, Bacillus* spp, *Corynebacterium jeikeium* Fungi: *Candida*
Mucous membranes	Respiratory support equipment, endoscopy, chemotherapy, radiation	Bacteria: *S. aureus, S. epidermidis*, streptococci, Enterobacteriaceae, *P. aeruginosa, Bacteroides* spp Fungi: *Candida* Viruses: Herpes simplex
Surgery	Solid-organ transplantation	Bacteria: *S. aureus, S. epidermidis*, Enterobacteriaceae, *P. aeruginosa, Bacteroides* spp Fungi: *Candida* Viruses: Herpes simplex
Alteration of normal microbial flora	Antimicrobial therapy Chemotherapy Hospital environment	Bacteria: Enterobacteriaceae, *P. aeruginosa, Legionella, S. aureus, S. epidermidis* Fungi: *Candida, Aspergillus*
Blood products, donor organs	Bone marrow transplantation Solid-organ transplantation	Fungi: *Candida* Viruses: Cytomegalovirus, Epstein-Barr virus, hepatitis B, hepatitis C Protozoal: *Toxoplasma gondii*

Data from references 1, 3, 4, 5, 7, 13, 19, 22, 27, 28, and 33.

Microorganisms may be transferred easily from patient to patient on the hands of hospital personnel unless strict infection control guidelines are followed. Contaminated equipment, such as nebulizers or ventilators, and contaminated water supplies have been responsible for outbreaks of *P. aeruginosa* and *Legionella pneumophila* infections, respectively. Foods, such as fruits and green leafy vegetables, which often are colonized with gram-negative bacteria and fungi, are sources of microbial contamination in immunocompromised hosts.[3,16]

Most infections in cancer patients are caused by organisms colonizing body sites, such as the skin, oropharynx, and GI tract.[1,3,15,16] Approximately 80% of infecting bacterial pathogens are from the patient's own endogenous flora.[1,3] The GI tract is the most common site from which infections in immunocompromised hosts originate. Periodontitis, pharyngitis, esophagitis, colitis, perirectal cellulitis, and bacteremias are caused predominantly by normal flora of the gut; bloodstream infections are thought to arise from microbial translocation across injured GI mucosa.[1,15,16] Normal flora may be significantly disrupted and altered; oropharyngeal flora rapidly change to primarily gram-negative bacilli in hospitalized patients. Many cancer patients may already be colonized with gram-negative bacilli on admission as a result of frequent prior hospitalizations and clinic visits. In hospitalized cancer patients, however, up to 50% of infections are caused by colonizing organisms acquired after admission.[1,3]

Although hospitalization and severity of illness are important risk factors for colonization by gram-negative bacilli, administration of broad-spectrum antimicrobial agents has the greatest impact on flora of immunocompromised hosts. Use of these agents disrupts GI tract flora and predisposes patients to infection with more virulent pathogens. Antineoplastic drugs (e.g., cyclophosphamide, doxorubicin, and fluorouracil) and acid-suppressive therapy (e.g.,

H_2-receptor antagonists, proton pump inhibitors, and antacids) also may result in changes in GI flora and possibly predispose patients to infection.[1,3,16]

Numerous factors, such as underlying disease, immunosuppressive drug therapy, and antimicrobial administration, determine the immunocompromised host's risk of developing infection. Several risk factors are present concomitantly in many patients (see Table 131–1).

ETIOLOGY OF INFECTIONS IN NEUTROPENIC CANCER PATIENTS

❷ Infection remains a significant cause of morbidity and mortality in neutropenic cancer patients. More than 50% of febrile neutropenic patients have an established or occult infection.[1,5] Patients with profound neutropenia are at greatest risk for systemic infection, with at least 20% of these individuals developing bacteremia. Areas of impaired or damaged host defenses, such as the oropharynx, lungs, skin, sinuses, and GI tract, are common sites of infection. These local infections may progress to cause systemic infection and bacteremia.[15] Febrile episodes in neutropenic cancer patients can be attributed to microbiologically documented infection in approximately 30% to 40% of cases, about half of which are due to bacteremia. Further, infections can be documented clinically (but not microbiologically) in another 30% to 40% of patients, with the remaining 30% of patients manifesting infection only by fever.[3,4,8,13]

Table 131–1 lists organisms commonly infecting immunocompromised patients. Approximately 45% to 70% of bacteremic episodes in cancer patients are the result of gram-positive organisms compared with less than 30% of episodes documented during the 1970s and 1980s.[1,4,7,13,17,18] This shift is attributed to the frequent use of indwelling central and peripheral IV catheters, frequent use of broad-spectrum antibiotics with excellent gram-negative activity but relatively poor gram-positive coverage, higher rates of mucositis caused by aggressive cancer treatments, and prophylaxis with trimethoprim–sulfamethoxazole or quinolones.[1,4,7,13] S. aureus and coagulase-negative staphylococci (especially S. epidermidis) account for most infections, but Bacillus spp and Corynebacterium jeikeium are also important pathogens.[1,5,13,18] Data from the U.S. Centers for Disease Control and Prevention's (CDC) National Nosocomial Infection Surveillance System (NNIS) indicate increasing rates of infection due to methicillin-resistant Staphylococcus aureus (MRSA) in the hospital setting.[19] Resistance is also common in community-acquired staphylococcal infections.[20,21] Viridans streptococci, which may be resistant to β-lactams, also have emerged as important pathogens, particularly in patients with chemotherapy-induced mucositis of the oropharynx.[4,13,22] Enterococci, including vancomycin-resistant strains, also may be problematic in many institutions.[2,7] Bacteremia caused by vancomycin-resistant enterococci (VRE) in neutropenic patients is associated with a mortality rate exceeding 70%.[4,23]

Gram-positive infections do not always cause immediately life-threatening infections and are associated with somewhat lower mortality rates (approximately 5%–10%) compared with gram-negative infections.[1,13,18] However, increasing rates of antibiotic resistance have made treatment of gram-positive infections in immunocompromised patients more challenging.[7,13] MRSA infections are associated with increased morbidity and mortality and hospital costs compared with susceptible organisms.[24] Methicillin resistance among coagulase-negative staphylococci, which may cause 40% to 80% of infections in certain populations, is very common (70%–90% of isolates).[7,25] Organisms that are intrinsically resistant to vancomycin (e.g., Lactobacillus) are increasing in importance.[7] Thus, prevention and timely diagnosis and treatment of gram-positive infections are clearly of great importance in the management of neutropenic cancer patients.

Gram-negative infections remain important causes of morbidity and mortality (approximately 20%) in immunocompromised cancer patients.[13,18] However, the relative frequency of infection owing to specific pathogens has been shifting among gram-negative infections. E. coli and Klebsiella spp remain the most common isolates at many centers.[18] Strains of Klebsiella spp producing plasmid-mediated extended-spectrum β-lactamases that hydrolyze extended-spectrum cephalosporins have emerged and are cause for concern.[1,7] The frequency of infections resulting from other gram-negative organisms, such as Enterobacter, Serratia, and Citrobacter, has been increasing.[7] Enterobacter spp are also important causes of bacteremias; use of broad-spectrum antibiotics, particularly third-generation cephalosporins, is thought to have played a major role in this trend. Infections with Enterobacter, Serratia, and Citrobacter may be difficult to treat because of the ease of β-lactamase induction and the more frequent development of resistance to multiple antibiotics.[3,7,13]

P. aeruginosa has long been an important pathogen in cancer patients. P. aeruginosa infection rates are decreasing in patients with solid tumors but not in patients with hematologic malignancies.[4,7] Infections caused by P. aeruginosa are associated with significant morbidity and mortality in neutropenic patients, with mortality rates of 31% to 75% reported.[13,18] The frequency of infection caused by difficult-to-treat organisms such as Stenotrophomonas maltophilia and Burkholderia cepacia appears to be increasing at many centers, probably because of selective pressures of broad-spectrum antimicrobial use.[4,13] As with gram-positive organisms, antibiotic resistance among gram-negative organisms has continued to increase at alarming rates and has made appropriate antibiotic selection for treatment of febrile neutropenia more difficult.[1,7,19] Although the GI tract is a common site of bacterial infection, severe infections

caused by anaerobic organisms are relatively infrequent. Anaerobes are found most frequently in mixed infections, such as perirectal cellulitis and mucositis-associated oropharyngeal infections.[13]

In addition to bacterial infections, neutropenic cancer patients are at risk for invasive fungal infections. Patients with extended periods of profound neutropenia who have been receiving broad-spectrum antibiotics, corticosteroids, or both are at the highest risk for invasive fungal infection. Up to one third of febrile neutropenic patients who do not respond to 1 week of broad-spectrum antibiotic therapy will have a systemic fungal infection.[1,13] Large autopsy studies have documented that up to 40% of patients with hematologic malignancies had deep fungal infections, fully 75% of which were undiagnosed prior to death. Causative pathogens were usually either Candida spp (35%) or Aspergillus spp (55%).[26]

Candida albicans is the most common fungal pathogen in neutropenic cancer patients.[4,13,27] However, non-albicans species of Candida including C. glabrata, C. tropicalis, C. parapsilosis, and C. krusei are being isolated with increasing frequency and are more common than C. albicans infections in some studies.[11,27] Increased infections caused by pathogens such as Trichosporon spp, Fusarium spp, and Curvularia have also been reported.[27–31] The shift toward more frequent infection with non-albicans Candida is important because of significantly decreased rates of susceptibility among many of these strains.[32] Because Candida spp are normal flora, alteration of body host defenses is an important risk factor for the development of these infections. Oral thrush is the most common clinical manifestation of fungal infection. Mucous membranes damaged from chemotherapy and radiation serve as areas of Candida surface colonization and subsequent entry into the bloodstream; disease then may disseminate throughout the body. Organs such as the liver, spleen, kidney, and lungs are commonly involved in disseminated disease.[14,26,28] Hepatosplenic candidiasis is a particularly important infection in patients with hematologic malignancies.[3,26,28] Diagnosis of candidal infections is difficult and often requires invasive tissue sampling.[6] Overall mortality attributed to candidal infections in patients with invasive candidiasis is as high as 35% to 50%.[4,11,27]

Invasive infections caused by Aspergillus spp are a serious complication of neutropenia, with mortality approaching 80% in patients with prolonged neutropenia and/or patients undergoing allogeneic HSCT.[4,13] These infections are particularly prevalent in patients with hematologic malignancies and in patients undergoing HSCT.[4,28,31,33] Infections resulting from Aspergillus spp (including A. fumigatus, A. terreus, A. flavus, and A. niger) usually are acquired via inhalation of airborne spores. After colonizing the lungs, Aspergillus invades the lung parenchyma and pulmonary vessels, resulting in hemorrhage, pulmonary infarcts, and a high mortality rate. Invasive pulmonary disease is the dominant manifestation of infection in patients with neutropenia. However, Aspergillus spp also may cause other infections, including sinusitis, cutaneous infection, and disseminated disease involving multiple organs, including the central nervous system (CNS).[33] Prolonged neutropenia is the primary risk factor for invasive pulmonary aspergillosis in neutropenic patients with acute leukemia; use of corticosteroids also may predispose patients to disease.[33] Invasive aspergillosis should be suspected in neutropenic cancer patients colonized with Aspergillus (in sputum and/or nasal cultures) who remain persistently febrile despite at least 1 week of broad-spectrum antibiotic therapy.[1,33]

Chemotherapy-induced mucous membrane damage may predispose neutropenic cancer patients to the reactivation of HSV, manifesting as gingivostomatitis or recurrent genital infections. Untreated oropharyngeal HSV infections may spread to involve the esophagus and often coexist with candidal infections. Clinical disease resulting from HSV occurs most often in patients with serologic evidence (e.g., serum antibodies to HSV) of prior infection. Both HSV-seropositive HSCT patients and HSV-seropositive leukemics receiving intensive chemotherapy are at high risk for recurrent HSV disease during periods of immunosuppression.[3,4,6,13]

Pneumocystis jiroveci and *Toxoplasma gondii* are the most common parasitic pathogens found in immunocompromised cancer patients. Patients with hematologic malignancies (i.e., acute lymphocytic leukemia, lymphoma, and Hodgkin's disease) and those receiving high-dose corticosteroids as part of chemotherapy regimens are at the greatest risk of infection.[3,4,6,13] Routine use of trimethoprim–sulfamethoxazole prophylaxis has reduced substantially the incidence of these infections.[1,6]

Because the majority of infecting organisms in cancer patients are from the host's own flora, some centers have used routine surveillance cultures in an attempt to prospectively identify causes of fever and suspected infection. In a typical surveillance culture program, cultures of the nose, mouth, axillae, and perirectal area are performed twice weekly, and culture results are correlated with the clinical status of the patient. Because these cultures are costly and have low diagnostic yield, the utility of surveillance culture programs is believed to be limited.[1] However, surveillance cultures are useful as research tools and in certain clinical situations, including patients with prolonged profound neutropenia and in institutions that have high rates of antimicrobial resistance or have problems with virulent pathogens such as *P. aeruginosa* or *Aspergillus* spp. Surveillance cultures should be limited to the anterior nares for detecting colonization with MRSA, *Aspergillus*, and penicillin-resistant pneumococci and to the rectum for detecting *P. aeruginosa*, multiple-antibiotic-resistant gram-negative rods, and VRE.[1,13]

Knowledge of infection rates and local susceptibility patterns is essential for guiding optimal management of febrile neutropenia. These parameters must be monitored closely because the spectrum of infectious complications is related to multiple factors, including cancer chemotherapy regimens and antimicrobial therapy used for treatment and prophylaxis.

CLINICAL PRESENTATION

❹ The most important clinical finding in the neutropenic cancer patient is fever. Because of the potential for significant morbidity and mortality associated with infection in these patients, fever should be considered to be the result of infection until proved otherwise.[1–3,8,13] At the appearance of fever, the patient should be evaluated carefully for other signs and symptoms of infection.

CLINICAL PRESENTATION OF FEBRILE NEUTROPENIA[1,3,4,6,12]

General

- Because neutropenic cancer patients are at high risk for serious infections, frequent (at least daily) careful clinical assessments must be performed to search for possible evidence of infection.
- Physical assessment should include examination of all common sites of infection, including mouth/pharynx, nose and sinuses, respiratory tract, GI tract, urinary tract, skin, soft tissues, perineum, and intravascular catheter insertion sites.

Symptoms

- Usual signs and symptoms of infection may be absent or altered in neutropenic patients owing to low numbers of leukocytes and an inability to mount an inflammatory response (e.g., no infiltrate on chest x-ray film, urinary tract infection without pyuria).
- Pain may be present at the infection site(s).

Signs

- Fever in this setting is defined as a single oral temperature ≥38.3°C (≥101°F) in the absence of other causes or temperature ≥38°C (≥100.4°F) for 1 hour or more. Other causes of fever unrelated to infection in this patient population include reactions to blood products, chemotherapeutic agents (and other drugs, including biologics), cell lysis, and underlying malignancy.
- Usual signs of infection may be absent or altered; patients with bacteremia commonly exhibit no signs of infection other than fever.

Laboratory Tests

- Neutropenia (ANC ≤1,000 cells/mm³).
- Blood cultures (two or more sets, including vascular access devices) for bacteria and fungi; cultures of other suspected infection sites (infection can be documented microbiologically in only about 30% of cases, about half of which are due to bacteremia).
- Other cultures should be obtained as indicated clinically according to the presence of signs or symptoms.
- Recent surveillance cultures (nasal, rectal) should be reviewed, if available.
- Complete blood count and blood chemistries should be obtained frequently to monitor neutropenia, plan supportive care, guide drug dosing, and assess patient's overall status.

Other Diagnostic Tests

- Chest x-ray film
- Aspiration, biopsy of skin lesions
- Other diagnostic tests as indicated clinically on the basis of physical examination and other assessments

TREATMENT

Infections in Cancer Patients

Management of patients with febrile neutropenia, including both treatment and prophylaxis of infectious complications, can be extremely challenging. Although published guidelines are available, the most optimal clinical management of these patients remains unclear in many aspects.

■ FEBRILE EPISODES IN NEUTROPENIC CANCER PATIENTS

❹ ❺ The goals of antimicrobial therapy in neutropenic patients (including HSCT recipients) are (a) to protect the neutropenic patient from early death caused by undiagnosed infection; (b) to prevent breakthrough bacterial, fungal, viral, and protozoal infections during periods of neutropenia; and (c) to treat established infections effectively, all aimed at reducing patient morbidity and mortality and allowing for administration of optimal antineoplastic therapy. All these goals must be achieved at the lowest possible toxicity and cost.

Approach to Treatment

General guidelines for management of febrile episodes and documented infections in neutropenic patients are shown in Figure 131–1 (from the Infectious Diseases Society of America [IDSA],

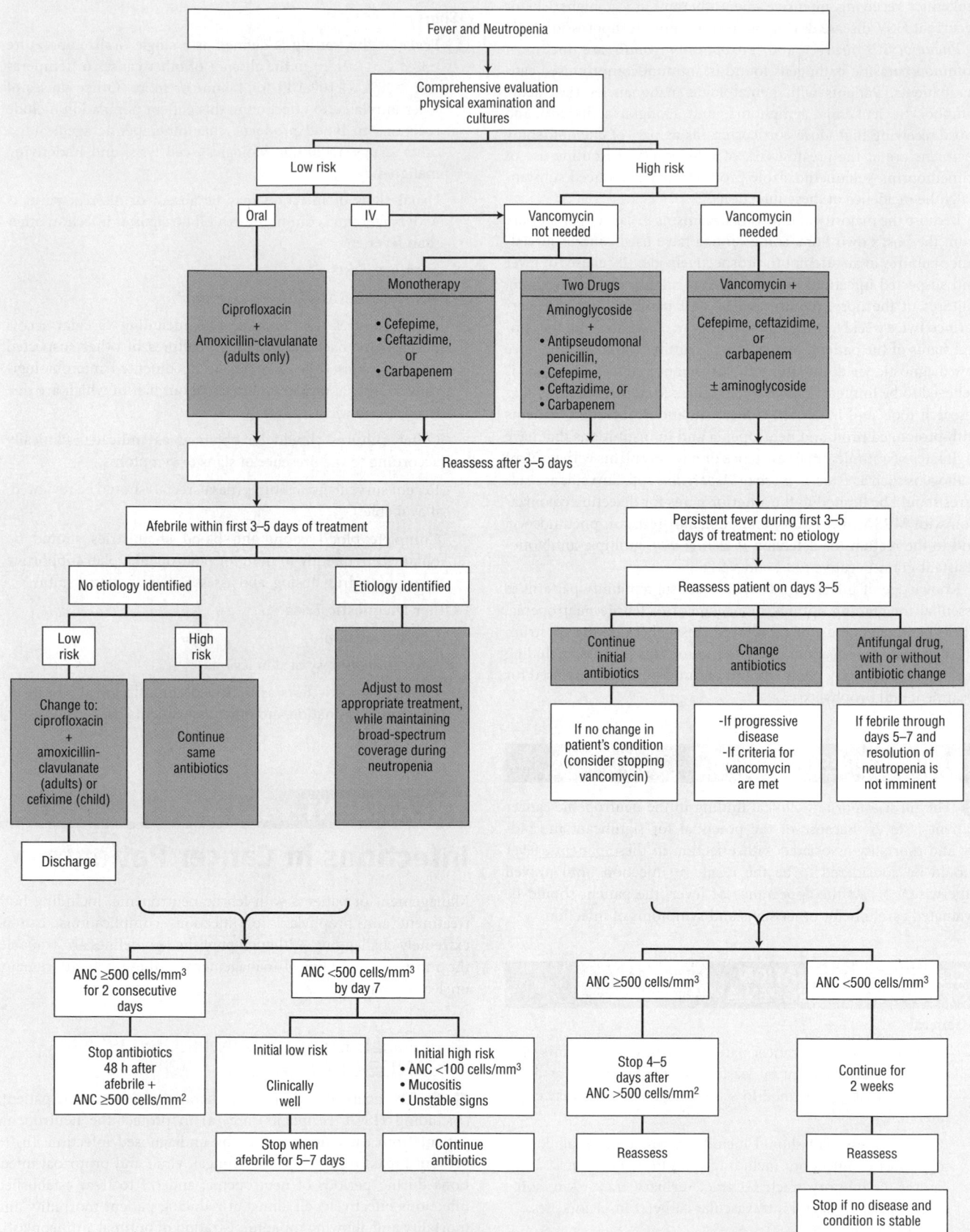

FIGURE 131-1. Management of febrile episodes in neutropenic cancer patients. (ANC, absolute neutrophil count; carbapenem, imipenem–cilastatin, meropenem.) *(Adapted from Hughes WT, Armstrong D, Bodey GP, et al. 2002 guidelines for the use of antimicrobial agents in neutropenic patients with cancer. Clin Infect Dis 2002;34:730–751. © 2002 by the Infectious Diseases Society of America. Used with permission of the University of Chicago Press.)*

TABLE 131-2 Summary of Evidence-Based Recommendations for Management of Febrile Episodes in Neutropenic Patients

Recommendations	Recommendation Grades[a]
Use of oral antibiotics for outpatient management	
Oral antibiotics are feasible for treatment of carefully selected patients at low risk for complications.	A-1
Use of monotherapy	
Monotherapy with appropriate antibiotics is as effective as combination regimens for initial empirical treatment of febrile neutropenic episodes.	A-1
Route of antibiotic administration for initial treatment	
Patients at high risk for serious life-threatening infections must be initially treated with intravenous antibiotics. Patients at low risk can be treated with either intravenous or oral drugs (see text for risk stratification criteria).	A-2
Management of patients who become afebrile	
Patients who become afebrile within 3–5 days of beginning initial empirical antibiotic therapy and in whom specific organisms have been identified should be treated for ≥7 days (until cultures are negative and patient has clinically recovered). Low-risk patients in whom no organism is identified can be switched to oral antibiotics if desired, whereas patients originally classified as high risk should continue on intravenous antibiotics.	B-2
Management of patients with persistent fever during first 3–5 days of treatment	
In patients initially receiving monotherapy or a two-drug regimen *not* including vancomycin, addition of vancomycin can be considered if any criteria for use of vancomycin are present (see text for specific criteria).	C-3
In patients *already* receiving vancomycin as part of the initial empirical regimen, withdrawal of vancomycin should be considered in the absence of a documented pathogen requiring continued therapy. Other initial antibiotics can be continued if the disease has not progressed, or switched to oral therapy if the patient was classified as low risk even in the presence of continued fever.	C-3
Management of patients with fever persisting for more than three days after initial treatment	
Reassess patient after 3 days of treatment. If still febrile by day 5, then continue the same antibiotics if clinically stable; change antibiotics if any evidence of disease progression or antibiotic toxicities; or add an antifungal drug if the duration of neutropenia is expected to be more than 5–7 additional days.	B-2
Continuation of antibiotics in afebrile patients with no identified infection	
Antibiotic therapy can be discontinued after 3 days of treatment if patient is afebrile for ≥48 hours and absolute neutrophil count (ANC) is ≥500 cells/mm³ for 2 consecutive days.	C-3
If patient remains neutropenic, continue intravenous or oral antibiotics.	B-2
Antibiotics should be continued in patients with profound neutropenia (ANC <100 cells/mm³), mucous membrane lesions of mouth or gastrointestinal tract, unstable vital signs, or other identified risk factors.	C-3
Antibiotics can be stopped after 2 weeks in patients with prolonged neutropenia of unclear continued duration, no identified site of infection, and who can be closely observed.	C-3
Alternatively, antibiotics can be discontinued after 4 days if no infection is documented and the patient shows no response to therapy.	C-3
Management of Fungal infections	
Suspected candidiasis:	
Lipid-formulated amphotericin B or caspofungin	A-1
Voriconazole	B-1
Fluconazole or itraconazole	B-1
Candidemia:	
An echinocandin or lipid-formulated ampohotericin B	A-2
Fluconazole or voriconazole	B-3
Granulocyte transfusions	
There are no specific indications for routine use of granulocyte transfusions.	C-2
Colony-stimulating factors	
Colony-stimulating factors are not indicated for routine treatment of neutropenia in either febrile or afebrile patients.	D-2
Antimicrobial prophylaxis in neutropenic patients	
Prophylaxis with trimethoprim-sulfamethoxazole should be administered to all patients at risk for *Pneumocystis jiroveci* pneumonia, regardless of whether they are neutropenic.	A-1
Prophylaxis with fluconazole, posaconazole, or caspofungin is recommended with induction chemotherapy and continued for duration of neutropenia; itraconzole is an effective alternative agent.	A-1 for all agents except caspofungin (B-2)
In HSCT, prophylaxis with fluconazole, posaconazole, or micafungin is recommended during the period of risk of neutropenia.	A-1
In HSCT patients with graft-versus-host disease, or neutropenic patients with hematologic malignancies, prophylaxis with posaconazole is recommended for prevention of invasive fungal infections.	A-1

[a]Strength of recommendations: A, B, C = good, moderate, and poor evidence to support recommendation for use, respectively; D = moderate evidence to support a recommendation against use.
Quality of evidence: 1 = evidence from ≥1 properly randomized, controlled trial; 2 = evidence from ≥1 well-designed clinical trial without randomization, from cohort or case-control analytic studies, from multiple time series, or from dramatic results from uncontrolled experiments; 3 = evidence from opinions of respected authorities, based on clinical experience, descriptive studies, or reports of expert committees.
Data from references 1, 5, 27, and 33.

revised in 2002).[1] Updated guidelines from the IDSA are expected in 2010. Although many controversies remain regarding optimal management of these patients, the IDSA guidelines and those of other expert panels, such as the National Comprehensive Cancer Network (NCCN),[5] offer an evidence-based consensus approach to the management of febrile neutropenia. Selected specific recommendations as discussed in the following sections of this chapter, and their associated evidence-based rankings are summarized in Table 131–2.

Fever in the neutropenic cancer patient is considered to be caused by infection until proved otherwise. High-dose broad-spectrum bactericidal, usually parenteral, empirical antibiotic therapy should

TABLE 131-3 Risk-Based Therapy for Febrile Patients with Neutropenia

Risk Group	Patient Characteristics	Treatment Strategies
High risk	*Neutropenia:* Severe (absolute neutrophil count <100/mm³) and/or prolonged (≥14 days) *Malignancy/treatment:* Hematologic malignancy or allogeneic HSCT *Comorbidities:* Substantial comorbidity; poor performance status *Clinical status:* Clinical or hemodynamic instability (e.g., shock) and/or complex infection (e.g., pneumonia, bacteremia) *Response to initial therapy:* Slow response	*Therapy/setting:* Broad-spectrum, parenteral (IV) therapy, hospital-based for duration of febrile neutropenia
Moderate risk	*Neutropenia:* Moderate duration (7–14 days) *Malignancy/treatment:* Solid tumor treated with autologous HSCT *Comorbidities:* Minimal medical comorbidity *Clinical status:* Clinically stable *Response to initial therapy:* Favorable (e.g., early defervescence)	*Therapy/setting:* Initial parenteral, hospital-based therapy, followed by early discharge on a parenteral or oral regimen (sequential)
Low risk	*Neutropenia:* Short duration (≤7 days) *Malignancy/treatment:* Solid tumor treated with conventional chemotherapy *Comorbidities:* None *Clinical status:* Clinically stable at onset of fever; no identified focus of infection, or simple infection (e.g., urinary tract infection)	*Therapy/setting:* Broad-spectrum outpatient therapy (parenteral, sequential, or oral) for the entire episode

HSCT, hematopoietic stem cell transplantation.

Data from Hughes et al.,[1] Ellis,[4] National Comprehensive Cancer Network Practice Guidelines,[5] Antoniadou and Giamarellou,[13] Kern,[35] Moores,[36] and Carstensen and Sorensen.[37]

thus be initiated at the onset of fever or at the first signs or symptoms of infection. Withholding antibiotic therapy until an organism is isolated results in unacceptably high mortality rates. Undiagnosed infection in immunocompromised patients can rapidly disseminate and result in death if left untreated or if treated improperly. Failure to initiate appropriate antibiotic therapy for *P. aeruginosa* bacteremia at the onset of fever in neutropenic cancer patients resulted in mortality rates of 15% and 70% within 12 and 48 hours, respectively.[1] Empirical antibiotic therapy is 70% to 90% effective at reducing early morbidity and mortality.[13] Therapy must be appropriate and initiated promptly. Antimicrobial therapy also should be initiated promptly in afebrile cancer patients with clinical signs and symptoms of infection.

When designing optimal empirical antibiotic regimens, clinicians must consider infection patterns and antimicrobial susceptibility trends in their respective institutions. Patient factors such as risk for infection, drug allergies, concomitant nephrotoxins, and previous antimicrobial exposure (including prophylaxis) must be considered.[1,4,5] Assessment of the patient's risk of infection will help determine the appropriate route and setting for antibiotic administration. Patients with neutropenia can be divided into low-, moderate-, and high-risk groups based on the projected duration of neutropenia and other risk factors for serious infection (Table 131–3).[3,4,9,11,13] Patients with neutropenia of short duration (≤7 days), clinically stable, and without significant co-morbidities are often considered to be at relatively low risk of severe infection. Patients with neutropenia lasting 7 to 14 days are considered to be at moderate risk for severe infection. High-risk patients are those with profound neutropenia, neutropenia for 14 or more days, and/or clinically unstable with systemic signs of infection; these patients are at increased risk for severe bacterial infection as well as from fungal, viral, and parasitic infection.[1,13]

Oral empirical antimicrobial therapy may be appropriate for certain low-risk patients, such as those without a focus of infection and no systemic signs of infection other than fever.[1,5,34–37] The patient's overall clinical condition and other risk factors for infection determine whether oral therapy is administered on an inpatient or outpatient basis. If therapy is administered on an outpatient basis, the patient must be compliant with treatment and have prompt access to medical care around the clock, should his or her condition worsen. Patients considered at moderate risk of infection should receive at least the first few days of therapy administered

parenterally in the hospital setting.[1,4,13] High-risk patients generally are treated with hospital-based parenteral therapy for the entire course of their treatment.

The optimal antibiotic regimen for empirical therapy in febrile neutropenic cancer patients remains controversial, but it is clear that no single regimen can be recommended for all patients. Because of their frequency and relative pathogenicity, *P. aeruginosa* and other gram-negative bacilli and staphylococci remain the primary targets of empirical antimicrobial therapy.[1,13] Although *P. aeruginosa* is documented in fewer than 5% of bloodstream infections in the population of hospitalized patients, adequate antipseudomonal antibiotic coverage still must be included in empirical regimens because of the significant morbidity and mortality associated with this pathogen.[1,4,13,19]

At least four different types of empirical parenteral antibiotic regimens are in use: (a) monotherapy with an antipseudomonal cephalosporin (cefepime or ceftazidime) or antipseudomonal carbapenem (imipenem–cilastatin or meropenem); (b) combination therapy with an aminoglycoside plus an antipseudomonal penicillin (piperacillin–tazobactam or ticarcillin–clavulanate), an antipseudomonal cephalosporin, or an antipseudomonal carbapenem; (c) vancomycin plus an antipseudomonal cephalosporin or antipseudomonal carbapenem, with or without an aminoglycoside; and (d) a fluoroquinolone (ciprofloxacin or levofloxacin) in combination with an antipseudomonal cephalosporin, antipseudomonal carbapenem, aminoglycoside, or vancomycin.[1,3–5,13] Each of these regimens has advantages and disadvantages, which are summarized in Table 131–4. There is no overwhelming evidence that any one of these regimens is superior to the others. The overall response to empirical antibiotic regimens in febrile neutropenic cancer patients is approximately 70% to 90% regardless of whether a pathogen is isolated or which antimicrobial regimen is used.[4,13]

Regardless of initial antibiotic selection, all empirical regimens must be monitored appropriately and revised on the basis of documented infections, susceptibilities of bacterial isolates, development of more defined clinical signs and symptoms of infection, or a combination of these factors. Consensus guidelines recommend three general empirical parenteral antibiotic regimens: monotherapy with an antipseudomonal cephalosporin or carbapenem; two-drug therapy without vancomycin (aminoglycoside plus antipseudomonal penicillin, cephalosporin, or carbapenem); or vancomycin plus one to two other drugs (antipseudomonal cephalosporin

TABLE 131-4 Comparative Advantages and Disadvantages of Various Antibiotic Regimens for Empiric Therapy of Febrile Neutropenic Cancer Patients

Regimen	Potential Advantages	Potential Disadvantages
β-Lactam monotherapy (ceftazidime 1–2 g every 8 h, cefepime 1–2 g every 12 h, piperacillin–tazobactam 4.5 g every 6 h, imipenem–cilastatin 0.5 g every 6 h, or meropenem 1 g every 8 h)[a]	Efficacy comparable to combination regimens; decreased drug toxicities; ease of administration; possibly less expensive	Possibly less efficacy in profound neutropenia or prolonged neutropenia; limited gram-positive activity; no potential for additive/synergistic effects; increased selection of resistant organisms; increased colonization and superinfection rates
Antipseudomonal β-lactam plus aminoglycoside (e.g., cefepime 1–2 g every 12 h or ceftazidime 1–2 g every 8 h + gentamicin or tobramycin)[a,b]	Traditional regimen, broad-spectrum coverage; optimal therapy of Pseudomonas aeruginosa; rapidly bactericidal; synergistic activity; decreased bacterial resistance; reduction of superinfections	Limited gram-positive activity; potential for nephrotoxicity; need for therapeutic monitoring of aminoglycoside concentrations
Empirical regimens containing vancomycin[c] (ceftazidime 1–2 g every 8 h + vancomycin 0.5–1 g every 6–12 h)[a] ± gentamicin or tobramycin[b]	Early effective therapy of gram-positive infections	No demonstrated benefit of vancomycin empirical therapy vs addition of vancomycin if needed later; increased risk of selection for vancomycin-resistant enterococci; risk of toxicities; excessive cost; need for therapeutic monitoring of vancomycin concentrations
Empirical regimens containing fluoroquinolones (ciprofloxacin 0.4 g every 8–12 h + ceftazidime 1–2 g every 8 h, aminoglycoside, or vancomycin[c] 0.5–1 g every 6–12 h)[a]	Efficacy similar to other regimens when used in combination therapy; no cross-resistance with β-lactams; possibility for oral administration; may be useful in patients with renal impairment in whom aminoglycosides are undesirable	Marginal gram-positive activity; fluoroquinolones not recommended as monotherapy; resistance may develop rapidly
Oral antibiotic regimens (e.g., ciprofloxacin 0.75 g every 12 h or levofloxacin 0.75 g every 24 h + amoxicillin–clavulanate 0.875 g every 12 h or clindamycin 0.6–0.9 g every 8 h)[d]	Efficacy comparable with parenteral therapy in low-risk patients; less expensive; reduced exposure of patients to nosocomial pathogens	Least studied treatment approach; less potent than parenteral antibiotics; requires compliant patient with 24-h access to medical care should clinical instability develop

[a]Dosing guidelines in patients with normal renal function.
[b]Gentamicin or tobramycin 2 mg/kg loading dose, followed by maintenance dose determined by serum concentrations. Choice of specific agent determined according to institutional susceptibilities to individual drugs.
[c]Vancomycin dosing may be guided by serum concentrations.
[d]Clindamycin recommended for patients with β-lactam allergy.
Data from reference 1, 3, 4, 5, and 13.

or carbapenem, with or without an aminoglycoside; Fig. 131–1).[1,5] However, other alternative regimens also may be appropriate, based on specific patient characteristics.

Prompt initiation of broad-spectrum empirical antibiotic therapy is essential to prevent early morbidity and mortality in febrile neutropenic patients with cancer. Choice of empirical regimens should take into account the patient's risk of infection and clinical status as well as patterns of hospital infections and susceptibility.

β-Lactam Monotherapy

Several β-lactam antibiotics in current use have been evaluated as monotherapy for management of febrile episodes in neutropenic cancer patients, including antipseudomonal cephalosporins (ceftazidime and cefepime), antipseudomonal penicillins (ticarcillin–clavulanic acid and piperacillin–tazobactam), and antipseudomonal carbapenems (imipenem–cilastatin and meropenem).[1,3,5,13,17] Three different meta-analyses assessing as many as 46 clinical trials involving more than 7,600 patients found no significant differences overall between monotherapy and combination therapy (β-lactam/aminoglycoside) in rates of survival, treatment response, and bacterial/fungal superinfections.[38–40] One study also found a higher rate of adverse effects in aminoglycoside-containing combination regimens.[39] In addition, one analysis found that cefepime monotherapy was associated with a significantly higher risk of mortality compared with the other β-lactams evaluated.[40] Significantly lower response rates for ceftazidime (but not cefepime) monotherapy have been reported in another review of the clinical literature.[41] However, until the results of these conflicting studies can be validated, both ceftazidime and cefepime still are among the monotherapy regimens routinely recommended as appropriate initial therapy of febrile neutropenic patients.[1,5,12,13,40,41]

At least seven clinical studies have documented the efficacy of piperacillin–tazobactam monotherapy for the empirical treatment of febrile neutropenic patients.[17,39–41] Piperacillin–tazobactam has an appropriate overall spectrum of antibacterial activity with good activity against P. aeruginosa and other gram-negative organisms as well as many gram-positive pathogens. The 2002 IDSA consensus guidelines did not recommend piperacillin–tazobactam as appropriate for monotherapy due to a relative lack of supportive clinical evidence at the time the guidelines were written.[1] Piperacillin-tazobactam monotherapy is, however, recommended in the 2009 NCCN guidelines and is considered by many clinicians to be appropriate for this use.[5]

Use of monotherapy has several potential advantages and disadvantages (see Table 131–4). Perhaps the most common concerns are those regarding the selection of resistant strains of organisms, such as P. aeruginosa, Enterobacter spp, and Serratia spp, through extended-spectrum β-lactamases and type 1 β-lactamases, especially with ceftazidime.[1,5,7,13] Activity against gram-positive organisms, such as coagulase-negative staphylococci, MRSA, enterococci (including VRE), penicillin-resistant S. pneumoniae, and some strains of viridans streptococci is poor with some single β-lactams, but cefepime and antipseudomonal carbapenems have good activity against viridans streptococci and pneumococci.[1] Although ceftazidime has been studied widely and used for treatment of febrile neutropenia, newer agents may be more effective owing to ceftazidime's susceptibility to β-lactamase induction and lower activity against gram-positive organisms.[1,7,41] Doripenem, a newer carbapenem antibiotic, has an appropriate spectrum of activity for empirical treatment of febrile neutropenia but has not been formally studied in this setting. Ertapenem, a carbapenem, and tigecycline, a glycylcycline antibiotic, have excellent activity against many gram-negative organisms but should not be used in the empirical treatment of febrile neutropenia due to their weaker activity against *P. aeruginosa*.

As with all empirical antibiotic regimens, patients receiving monotherapy should be monitored closely for treatment failure, secondary infections, and development of resistance. Use of monotherapy may not be appropriate in institutions with high rates of gram-positive infections or infections caused by relatively resistant gram-negative pathogens such as *P. aeruginosa* and *Enterobacter* spp. Imipenem–cilastatin and meropenem are less susceptible to inducible β-lactamases and often may be used effectively in these institutions. Overall, similar efficacy has been observed with monotherapy with antipseudomonal β-lactams and aminoglycoside combination therapy for treatment of *P. aeruginosa* infections.[1,13,39–41]

Aminoglycoside Plus Antipseudomonal β-Lactam

Regimens consisting of an aminoglycoside plus an antipseudomonal penicillin, antipseudomonal cephalosporin, or antipseudomonal carbapenem traditionally have been the most commonly used for empirical treatment of febrile neutropenia, although many such regimens may lack adequate gram-positive activity (see Table 131–4).[1] This relative lack of activity remains a concern because of the increasing frequency of gram-positive infections. The choice of aminoglycoside and β-lactam for inclusion in empirical regimens should be based on institutional epidemiology and antimicrobial susceptibility patterns. Use of empirical tobramycin or amikacin may be strongly considered because these agents are generally more active than gentamicin against *P. aeruginosa*. However, gentamicin still is an appropriate choice in many institutions based on known susceptibility patterns in those locations. Similar efficacy is observed with an antipseudomonal penicillin, antipseudomonal cephalosporin, or antipseudomonal carbapenem in combination with an aminoglycoside.[1]

Combinations of broad-spectrum β-lactams and aminoglycosides often provide synergistic activity against bacteria commonly infecting neutropenic patients. The exact role of synergy in the outcome of febrile neutropenic patients treated with empirical antibiotic therapy is somewhat controversial, particularly in light of the efficacy of single-drug regimens. Nevertheless, synergistic combinations of antibiotics appear to be beneficial in patients with persistent profound neutropenia. Moreover, administration of antipseudomonal β-lactams in combination with an aminoglycoside may result in a lower rate of drug resistance.[4]

Aminoglycoside toxicity may be a concern in patients receiving these regimens who are already receiving other nephrotoxic drugs, such as cisplatin and cyclosporine. Administration of aminoglycosides in large single daily doses (once-daily dosing) may be as effective, less costly, and no more toxic than conventional dosing methods.[41] Although once-daily aminoglycoside dosing regimens appear to be safe and effective in these patients, however, data are not sufficient to recommend once-daily dosing for routine use in this population.[1,5,13]

Empirical Regimens Containing Vancomycin

The inclusion of vancomycin in initial empirical therapy of febrile neutropenic cancer patients remains an ongoing debate. This controversy continues because of the increasing incidence of gram-positive infections in this population, particularly MRSA. One approach is to include vancomycin in the initial empirical antibiotic regimen, thereby providing early effective treatment of possible gram-positive infections. Decreased mortality from penicillin-resistant viridans streptococcal infections has been observed when vancomycin was included in initial therapy.[1,13]

A second approach is to withhold vancomycin from initial empirical regimens, later adding the drug if gram-positive organisms are isolated from cultures or if there is no response to initial therapy. Support for both these approaches can be found in the medical literature.[1,5,7,13,42,43] Prospective studies and at least two meta-analyses have failed to document increased response rates or decreased mortality with the routine addition of vancomycin to initial empirical regimens, provided that vancomycin can be added later as needed.[1,5,13,42,43] In addition to increased costs of therapy, vancomycin was also associated with increased adverse effects, including nephrotoxicity.[42,43] Finally, concerns remain regarding selection of resistant gram-positive bacteria such as VRE with excessive vancomycin use.[1,5,13]

Inclusion of vancomycin in initial empirical regimens may be more appropriate today because of higher rates of MRSA infections as well as aggressive chemotherapy regimens causing significant mucosal damage that increases the risk for streptococcal infections. Vancomycin is recommended for inclusion in initial empirical regimens in patients at high risk for gram-positive infection, particularly due to MRSA and coagulase-negative staphylococci (including patients with evidence of infection of central venous catheters and other indwelling lines), high risk for viridans streptococcal infection due to severe mucositis, or pneumonitis or soft tissue infection in hospitals with high rates of MRSA infections.[1,3,5,7,13,42,43] Rates of β-lactam resistance among viridans streptococci range from 18% to 29%.[5] Empirical vancomycin use may be justified in institutions using empirical or prophylactic antibiotic regimens without good activity against streptococci (e.g., ciprofloxacin) and in patients known to be colonized with MRSA or β-lactam–resistant pneumococci. In patients with preliminary culture results indicating gram-positive infection, empirical vancomycin is appropriate while the susceptibility results are pending. Lastly, empirical use of vancomycin may be recommended in patients with hypotension or other evidence of cardiovascular impairment or sepsis without an identified pathogen.[1,5,42,43] If empirical vancomycin therapy is initiated and no evidence of gram-positive infection is found after 48 to 72 hours, the drug should be discontinued.[1,4,5] Continuing vancomycin when not warranted results in higher costs, more toxicities, and greater risk of development of VRE.[1,5]

If vancomycin is to be used, vancomycin plus carbapenem regimens may have advantages over vancomycin plus cephalosporin regimens because of lower rates of carbapenem resistance to gram-negative bacilli.[1] Newer antimicrobial agents, such as quinupristin–dalfopristin, linezolid, daptomycin, and telavancin, should be reserved for documented infections caused by multiresistant gram-positive pathogens such as VRE. The role of these drugs in the routine treatment of fever in neutropenic patients is undetermined, and linezolid is associated with myelosuppression.[1,5]

CLINICAL CONTROVERSY

Inclusion of vancomycin into empirical antimicrobial regimens for febrile neutropenia remains controversial. Although the incidence of bacterial infections caused by gram-positive pathogens has increased significantly over the past 2 decades, the benefits of adding vancomycin or other agents with specific gram-positive activity to initial treatment regimens have not been conclusively demonstrated. Although published reviews and meta-analyses recommend against routine initial use of vancomycin, the practice remains widespread in actual clinical practice.

Fluoroquinolones as a Component of Empirical Regimens

Because the fluoroquinolone antibiotics have broad-spectrum activity (particularly against gram-negative pathogens), rapid bactericidal activity, and favorable pharmacokinetic and toxicity profiles, these agents have been investigated as empirical therapy for febrile neutropenic patients. Ciprofloxacin is the preferred quinolone for use in this clinical setting because of its relatively better activity against *P. aeruginosa* and more extensive evidence-based support for its use.[1,13] Response rates to quinolone-containing combination regimens are comparable to those obtained with the other regimens described previously.[1,4,5] Ciprofloxacin is not recommended for monotherapy, however, because of its relatively poor activity against gram-positive pathogens, particularly streptococci, and variable response rates in clinical studies.[1] Quinolones should also not be used as empirical therapy in patients who have received quinolones as infection prophylaxis because of the risk of drug resistance.[1,5,13] Rates of fluoroquinolone resistance are increasing, and streptococcal treatment failures are a concern.[19,44] Although fluoroquinolones are not generally considered first-line empirical therapy, they may be useful as one component of combination regimens in patients with allergies or other contraindications to first-line agents.[1,5]

Oral Antibiotic Therapy for Management of Febrile Neutropenia

An individual patient's risk of severe infection determines appropriate antibiotic therapy and the setting for administration (see Table 131–3).[1,4,5] Risk stratification is based on several parameters, including duration and degree of neutropenia, type of cancer and its management (including history of HSCT), clinical status, comorbidities, and response to empirical antimicrobial therapy.[1] Because of the excellent spectrum of activity and favorable pharmacokinetics of relatively newer oral antibiotics, particularly the fluoroquinolones, oral antibiotics have an important role in the management of selected patients. In patients at low risk for severe or complicated bacterial infection, empirical therapy with broad-spectrum oral antibiotic agents achieves similar patient outcomes as parenteral antibiotics, with response rates of 77% to 95%.[1,4,13,34–37] The availability of oral antibiotics with broad-spectrum activity has made possible the treatment of febrile neutropenia in low-risk patients completely in the outpatient setting. Patients with solid tumors undergoing conventional chemotherapy with an expected duration of neutropenia of less than 7 to 10 days and who are clinically stable may be appropriate candidates for oral antibiotic therapy administered on an outpatient basis.[1,4,5,13,34–37] Fluoroquinolones, either as monotherapy or in combination with amoxicillin–clavulanate (or clindamycin for penicillin-allergic patients) for enhanced gram-positive coverage, have been most commonly studied for outpatient therapy in low-risk patients. IDSA and NCCN guidelines recommend oral antibiotic therapy with ciprofloxacin plus amoxicillin–clavulanate in clinically stable low-risk adults (particularly those with recovering neutrophils) with no focus of bacterial infection and no signs of infection other than fever.[1,5] Oral cephalosporins such as cefixime also may be suitable for outpatient treatment.[1] Careful patient selection obviously is required for such management strategies. Important patient characteristics include a history of medication compliance, good caregiver support, and close proximity to medical care in the event of failure to respond to outpatient antibiotic therapy. Benefits of oral therapy on an outpatient basis include increased convenience and quality of life for patients and caregivers and reduced exposure to multidrug-resistant institutional pathogens.[1,5] Outpatient therapy of low-risk patients now is common practice in most institutions.

In patients at moderate risk for severe bacterial infection, oral antibiotics may play a role in step-down therapy. Carefully selected neutropenic patients may be safely switched from broad-spectrum parenteral therapy to oral antibiotic regimens (e.g., ciprofloxacin plus amoxicillin–clavulanate) with response rates comparable to patients remaining on IV therapy.[13,34–37] Patient selection criteria generally include defervescence within 72 hours of initiation of parenteral therapy, hemodynamic stability, absence of positive cultures or a discernible site of infection, and ability to take oral medications. Many of these patients are able to complete their course of therapy at home.[1,13,35–37] Changing parenteral antimicrobials to oral regimens in carefully selected patients is now relatively common practice and allows for less expensive hospitalizations and earlier patient discharges.

ANTIMICROBIAL THERAPY AFTER INITIATION OF EMPIRICAL THERAPY

6 After initiation of empirical antimicrobial therapy, judicious assessment of febrile neutropenic cancer patients is mandatory to evaluate response, clinical status, laboratory data, and potential need for therapy adjustments. After 72 hours or more of empirical antimicrobial therapy, the clinical status and culture results of febrile neutropenic patients should be reevaluated to determine whether therapeutic modifications are necessary. Additions or modifications to the initial antimicrobial regimen likely will be required for patients with ANC less than 500 cells/mm³ for more than 1 week. Modifications of antimicrobial therapy should be based on clinical and laboratory data; antibiotic therapy should be optimized based on culture results. However, during periods of neutropenia, patients generally should continue to receive broad-spectrum therapy because of risk of secondary infections or breakthrough bacteremias when antimicrobial coverage is too narrow.[1,5,13]

In patients who become afebrile after 3 to 5 days of therapy with no infection identified, it is generally optimal to continue antibiotic therapy until neutropenia has resolved (ANC ≥500 cells/mm³). Some clinicians switch therapy to an oral regimen (e.g., ciprofloxacin plus amoxicillin-clavulanate) after 2 days of IV therapy in low- to moderate-risk patients who become afebrile and have no evidence of infection. This approach may facilitate earlier hospital discharge. In high-risk patients, the parenteral antibiotic regimen should be continued for at least 7 days.[1,5] However, in afebrile patients with prolonged neutropenia but no signs or symptoms of infection, consideration can be given to discontinuing antibiotic therapy, provided patients can be observed carefully and have ready access to medical care.

The optimal management of patients who remain febrile in the absence of microbiologic or clinical documentation of infection remains highly controversial. Persistently febrile patients should be evaluated carefully, but modifications generally are not made to initial antimicrobial regimens within the first 3 to 5 days of therapy unless there is evidence of clinical deterioration (see Fig. 131–1).[1,4,5] It is important to note that the persistence of fever does not necessarily mean failure of a given antimicrobial regimen; up to 25% of neutropenic patients have fever due to noninfectious causes.[8] This is particularly true if patients are otherwise clinically stable. Fever after 3 or more days of antibiotic therapy can be due to a number of causes, including nonbacterial infection, resistant bacterial infection or infection slow to respond to therapy, emergence of a secondary infection, inadequate drug concentrations, drug fever, fever at an avascular site (e.g., catheter infection or abscess), or noninfectious causes such as tumor or administration of blood products.[1,4,5,13] Patients with documented infection who are receiving appropriate antimicrobial therapy (based on in vitro susceptibility tests) often remain febrile until resolution of neutropenia occurs.

Therefore, the same antibiotic regimen can be continued in patients who remain febrile despite 3 to 5 days of antibiotic therapy but are otherwise clinically stable, especially if neutropenia is expected to resolve within 1 week. However, antibiotic regimens may require modification in patients experiencing toxicities as well as in patients with evidence of progressive disease or documentation of an organism not covered by the initial regimen. When a causative organism is identified, specific therapy directed at the organism should be included; however, patients should continue to receive broad-spectrum therapy while they remain neutropenic.[1,3,4,5,13] Need for addition of vancomycin should be considered as warranted by clinical and laboratory findings; however, if vancomycin was included in the initial empirical regimen and the patient is still febrile after 3 days of therapy, discontinuation of vancomycin should be considered to reduce the risk of toxicities or resistance.

Initiation of Antifungal Therapy

Neutropenic patients who remain febrile despite 5 or more days of broad-spectrum antibiotic therapy are candidates for antifungal therapy. A high percentage of febrile patients who die during prolonged neutropenia have evidence of invasive fungal infection on autopsy, even though many had no evidence of fungal disease before death.[26] Persistence of fever or development of a new fever during broad-spectrum antibiotic therapy may indicate the presence of a fungal infection, most commonly due to *Candida* or *Aspergillus* spp.[13,26] Blood cultures are positive in fewer than 50% of neutropenic patients with invasive fungal infections.[13,31] Rapid, sensitive diagnostic tests for fungi such as serum β–D-glucan assay are not yet in common usage and waiting for isolation of fungal organisms is associated with high morbidity and mortality; the empirical addition of antifungal therapy is thus justified in this clinical setting.[1,13,31] Therefore, empirical antifungal therapy should be initiated after 5 to 7 days of broad-spectrum antibiotic therapy at adequate doses to treat undiagnosed fungal infection and prevent fungal superinfection in high-risk febrile neutropenic patients.[27]

Evidence-based recommendations from published guidelines for management of suspected or documented fungal infections in neutropenic patients are summarized in Table 131–2.[27,33] Empirical coverage for both *Candida* spp and *Aspergillus* should be considered because these organisms are responsible for more than 90% of fungal infections in neutropenic cancer patients.[6,26] *Aspergillus* is particularly common in patients with hematologic malignancies and in patients with hematologic malignancies undergoing HSCT; therefore, amphotericin B traditionally has been preferred for these patients.[13,45,46] In the setting of febrile neutropenia, lipid-associated amphotericin B (LAMB) products are similar in efficacy to conventional amphotericin B while causing fewer toxicities. LAMB products are thus almost exclusively recommended over conventional amphotericin B despite the significantly higher cost without clear improvement in efficacy.[27,33,45–47] Although the use of higher doses of LAMB has been advocated in an effort to improve efficacy, one study demonstrated that lower doses (3 mg/kg) of liposomal amphotericin B were as efficacious as higher doses (10 mg/kg) with lower cost and fewer toxicities.[48]

The azole compounds fluconazole, itraconazole, and voriconazole are also used in the management of febrile neutropenia.[27,33,49] Despite the increased cost and toxicities of LAMB, concerns regarding the emergence of *Candida* strains with decreased azole susceptibility and unclear efficacy advantages relative to other agents have prevented these agents from replacing amphotericin B as the gold standard in persistently febrile neutropenic patients.[32,33,45,46] Fluconazole has good efficacy against *C. albicans* but lacks activity against molds such as *Aspergillus*. The use of fluconazole as

an alternative to amphotericin B for empirical antifungal therapy is thus perhaps most appropriate in hospitals in which infections due to *Aspergillus* or non-*albicans* strains of *Candida* are not common.[1,45,46] If fluconazole is used as antifungal prophylaxis in cancer patients, it should not be included in empirical antifungal regimens. Voriconazole has shown efficacy in the treatment of documented invasive fungal infections but may be less desirable for empirical therapy in febrile neutropenic patients due to lack of improved efficacy compared to amphotericin B.[31,45,46] Voriconazole is recommended as appropriate for empirical antifungal therapy in neutropenic patients,[33] but is often limited to allogeneic HSCT patients and patients with relapsed leukemia who are at very high risk of invasive *Aspergillus* infections.[31,49–51] Itraconazole has similar efficacy as amphotericin B, with fewer toxicities. However, current lack of a parenteral dosage form, sometimes erratic oral absorption which often necessitates the use of serum concentration monitoring, numerous potential drug-drug interactions, and availability of many other antifungal options has limited the use of itraconazole as a preferred treatment option.[49–51]

The echinocandin antifungals (caspofungin, micafungin, and anidulafungin) are attractive agents for treatment of febrile neutropenia because of their broad spectrum of antifungal activity and favorable adverse effect profiles. Caspofungin is as effective as, and also generally better tolerated than, liposomal amphotericin B for empirical treatment of neutropenic patients with persistent fever.[49–51] Therefore, caspofungin is considered an appropriate alternative to LAMB and voriconazole.[5,27,31,33,45,46,50] Micafungin and anidulafungin have not been as well studied specifically in neutropenic patients and are not routinely recommended for routine empirical use at this time.[5,27,33]

As with antibiotic therapy, the optimal duration of antifungal therapy remains controversial. Most clinicians agree that antifungal therapy can be discontinued when neutropenia has resolved in clinically stable patients with no evidence of fungal infection. In neutropenic patients, antifungal therapy generally should be continued for at least 2 weeks in the absence of signs and symptoms of active fungal disease, but many experts advocate continuing therapy until resolution of the neutropenia.[4,13,27,45,46] In neutropenic patients with documented fungal disease, antifungal therapy should be directed at the causative organism, and therapy should be continued for at least 2 weeks after clinical and culture data indicate resolution of the infection.[27] In addition to fungal infections, other causes of persistent fever of unknown origin include resistant bacterial infection, tissue necrosis as a result of underlying tumor, nonbacterial and nonfungal infection (e.g., viral, mycobacterial, or parasitic), and drug or blood product administration. The persistence of fever should not be considered the sole indication for modification of antifungal regimens, assuming that an agent active against *Aspergillus* was initially selected.[31,45,46] Treatment recommendations for specific fungal infections are given in Table 131–5.

Initiation of Antiviral Therapy

Febrile neutropenic patients with vesicular or ulcerative skin or mucosal lesions should be evaluated carefully for infection due to HSV or varicella-zoster virus (VZV). Mucosal lesions from viral infections provide a portal of entry for bacteria and fungi during periods of immunosuppression. If viral infection is presumed or documented, neutropenic patients should receive aggressive antiviral therapy to aid healing of primary lesions and prevent disseminated disease. Acyclovir traditionally has been used in this population. However, the newer antivirals valacyclovir and famciclovir have better oral absorption and more convenient dosing schedules. Routine use of antiviral agents in the management of patients without mucosal lesions or other evidence of viral infection

TABLE 131-5 Infectious Complications after Bone Marrow and Solid-Organ Transplantation: Syndromes of Disease and Treatment Guidelines

Pathogen	Syndromes of Disease	Treatment
Bacterial		
Gram-negative aerobic bacilli (Enterobacteriaceae, *Pseudomonas aeruginosa, Haemophilus influenzae*)	Blood, urinary tract, pulmonary, abdomen	*Empiric:* Ceftazidime 1–2 g every 8 h + aminoglycoside,[a,b] cefepime 1–2 g every 12 h + aminoglycoside[a,b]; piperacillin–tazobactam 3.375–4.5 g every 4–6 h; imipenem–cilastatin 0.25–0.5 g every 6 h ± aminoglycoside[a,b] *Definitive:* According to culture and sensitivity results
Gram-positive cocci (*Staphylococcus aureus, Staphylococcus epidermidis, Streptococcus pneumoniae, Enterococcus faecalis*)	Skin, blood, urinary tract, pulmonary, abdomen	*Empiric:* Nafcillin 1–2 g every 4–6 h; vancomycin 0.5–1 g every 6–12 h[c] *Definitive:* According to culture and sensitivity results
Legionella spp	Pulmonary	Erythromycin 0.5–1 g every 6 h; ciprofloxacin 0.4 g every 8–12 h; levofloxacin 0.75 g every 24 h
Listeria monocytogenes	Central nervous system	Ampicillin 1–2 g every 4–6 h with gentamicin[a]; trimethoprim–sulfamethoxazole 4 mg/kg every 12 h[d]
Nocardia spp	Skin, pulmonary, central nervous system	Sulfadiazine 1 g every 4–6 h; trimethoprim–sulfamethoxazole 4 mg/kg every 12 h[d]
Fungal		
Candida spp[e]	Blood, urinary tract, mucous membranes, skin	Clotrimazole 10 mg 5 times daily; nystatin 100,000 units every 6 h; fluconazole 100–800 mg daily; itraconazole 200–400 mg daily; amphotericin B 0.3–0.7 mg/kg/day ± 5-flucytosine 100–150 mg/kg/day divided every 6 h; lipid-associated amphotericin B 3–5 mg/kg daily; caspofungin 50 mg daily; micafungin 100 mg daily; anidulafungin 100 mg daily
Aspergillus spp[f]	Skin, pulmonary, central nervous system	Voriconazole 4 mg/kg every 12 h; lipid-associated amphotericin B 3–5 mg/kg daily; caspofungin 50 mg daily; micafungin 100–150 mg daily; posaconazole 400 mg every 12 h; itraconazole 400 mg daily
Cryptococcus neoformans	Skin, pulmonary, central nervous system	Lipid-associated amphotericin B 3-5 mg/kg/day + 5-flucytosine 100 mg/kg/day; fluconazole 400 mg daily
Zygomycetes (*Mucor*)	Rhinocerebral disease	Lipid-associated amphotericin B 4–5 mg/kg daily; posaconazole 200 mg every 8 h[e]
Viral		
Herpes simplex virus	Skin, central nervous system, mucous membranes, pulmonary	Acyclovir 5–10 mg/kg every 8 h; foscarnet 60 mg/kg every 8 h
Cytomegalovirus	Pulmonary, blood, urinary tract, gastrointestinal tract	Ganciclovir 5 mg/kg every 12 h; foscarnet 60 mg/kg every 8 h; hyperimmune globulins 100–500 mg/kg every 1–2 wk
Varicella-zoster virus	Skin, disseminated disease	Acyclovir 10 mg/kg every 8 h; foscarnet 60 mg/kg every 8 h
Epstein-Barr virus	Lymphoproliferative disease	No effective treatment
Papovaviruses (BK, JC)	Skin, central nervous system	No effective treatment
Protozoal/parasitic		
Pneumocystis jiroveci	Pulmonary	Trimethoprim–sulfamethoxazole 15–20 mg/kg/day divided every 6 h[d]; atovaquone 750 mg every 12 h; pentamidine 4 mg/kg daily; dapsone 100 mg daily + trimethoprim 15–20 mg/kg/day divided every 6 h; clindamycin 450–600 mg every 6 h + primaquine 15 mg daily
Toxoplasma gondii	Central nervous system	Pyrimethamine 50–100 mg daily + sulfadiazine 1 g every 4–6 h[g]; pyrimethamine 50–100 mg daily + clindamycin 450–600 mg every 6 h[g]
Strongyloides stercoralis	Pulmonary, central nervous system	Thiabendazole 25 mg/kg every 12 h (maximum 3 g/day)

[a]Gentamicin or tobramycin 2 mg/kg loading dose, followed by maintenance dose determined by serum concentrations. Choice of specific agent determined according to institutional susceptibilities to individual drugs.
[b]For penicillin-allergic adults, use ciprofloxacin 0.4 g every 8–12 h plus an aminoglycoside.
[c]Vancomycin dosing may be guided by serum concentrations.
[d]Based on the trimethoprim component of the combination.
[e]Refer to the Clinical Practice Guidelines of the Infectious Diseases Society of America (*reference 27*) for selection and dosing of antifungal agents for specific infections.
[f]Refer to the Clinical Practice Guidelines by the Infectious Diseases Society of America (*reference 33*) for selection and dosing of antifungal agents for specific infections.
[g]Folinic acid (5–10 mg/day) often recommended in conjunction with pyrimethamine-containing regimens for prevention of bone marrow toxicity.

generally is not recommended.[1,5] Treatment recommendations for viral infections are given in Table 131–5.

Duration of Antimicrobial Therapy

❼ The optimal duration of antimicrobial therapy in the neutropenic cancer patient remains controversial. Decisions regarding discontinuation of empirical antimicrobial therapy often are more difficult and complex than those regarding initiation of therapy (see Fig. 131–1). One point on which experts agree, however, is that the most important determinant of the total duration of antibiotic therapy is the patient's ANC.[1,3,5,13] If ANC is ≥500 cells/mm³ for 2 consecutive days, if the patient is afebrile and clinically stable for 48 to 72 hours or more, and if no pathogen has been isolated,

then antibiotics can be discontinued. Some clinicians advocate that patients with ANC less than 500 cells/mm³ be maintained on antibiotic therapy until resolution of neutropenia, even if they are afebrile. However, prolonged antibiotic use has been associated with superinfections resulting from resistant bacteria and fungi and increases the risk of antibiotic-related toxicities.[1,5,13] If low-risk patients are stable clinically but the ANC still is less than 500 cells/mm³, antibiotics may be discontinued after a total of 5 to 7 afebrile days. However, patients with profound neutropenia (ANC <100 cells/mm³), mucosal lesions, or unstable vital signs or other risk factors should continue to receive antibiotics until ANC has increased to 500 cells/mm³ or greater or the patient is stable clinically.[1,5,13]

Patients who are persistently neutropenic and febrile, but who are stable clinically with no active site of infection, often can be successfully discontinued from antimicrobials after at least 2 weeks of therapy. However, these patients must be monitored carefully because reinstitution of antibiotics may be necessary.[1,5,13] An alternative approach is to place these patients on antimicrobial prophylaxis (discussed below in Prophylaxis of Infections in Neutropenic Cancer Patients). Patients with documented infections should receive antimicrobial therapy until the infecting organism is eradicated and signs and symptoms of infection have resolved (at least 10–14 days of therapy).

Consensus guidelines provide useful information regarding the management of febrile episodes in cancer patients with neutropenia.[1,5] However, therapy (including initial empirical regimens, modifications, and duration of treatment) must be individualized based on individual patient parameters and response to therapy.

CLINICAL CONTROVERSY

The optimal time to stop empirical antimicrobial therapy in patients who remain persistently febrile remains a key controversy in the overall management of febrile neutropenia in cancer patients. One unresolved issue is whether the patient's neutropenia must be resolved prior to discontinuing antimicrobial therapy. The patient's individual risk of severe infection (determined by extent and duration of neutropenia as well as other risk factors) helps to guide treatment decisions in this setting.

Colony-Stimulating Factors

Because resolution of neutropenia is arguably the most important determinant of patient outcome from both febrile episodes and documented infections, numerous studies have evaluated hematopoietic colony-stimulating factors (CSFs) (sargramostim [granulocyte-macrophage colony-stimulating factor] and filgrastim [granulocyte colony-stimulating factor]) as adjunct therapy to antimicrobial treatment of febrile neutropenic cancer patients.[52] These studies consistently found that use of CSFs reduces the total duration and severity of chemotherapy-related neutropenia; some studies have also shown fewer hospitalizations and decreased hospital length of stay.[52,53] However, these studies have failed to demonstrate consistent benefits of CSFs compared with placebo in relation to important outcomes such as decreased overall mortality or infection-related mortality.[52,53] Evidence-based guidelines from the American Society of Clinical Oncology (ASCO) and the NCCN recommend that CSFs should not be routinely used in patients with uncomplicated fever and neutropenia.[52,54] However, CSFs should be considered in patients who are at high risk for infection–associated complications, or who have factors that are predictive of poor clinical outcomes.[52,54] These factors are summarized in Table 131-6. Patients with prolonged neutropenia and documented severe infections who are not responding to appropriate antimicrobial therapy may also benefit from treatment with CSFs.[52,54] Clinical judgment must be exercised in determining which patients may benefit from judicious use of these expensive agents.

Direct transfusion of neutrophils has also been studied for treatment of febrile neutropenia or documented infections.[55,56] Routine use of neutrophil transfusions is not generally supported by data demonstrating improved clinical outcomes. However, use may be considered in patients with profound prolonged neutropenia with severe documented infections and in whom causative organisms have not been eradicated with appropriate antimicrobial therapy in

TABLE 131-6	Recommendations for Use of Colony-Stimulating Factors in the Management of Neutropenic Cancer Patients and Those Undergoing Hematopoietic Stem Cell Transplantation

A. Primary prophylaxis of febrile neutropenia

1. Colony-stimulating factors (CSFs) (filgrastim, pegfilgrastim, or sargramostim) may be considered in patients who have a high risk of FN (>20% incidence) based on myelotoxicity of the planned chemotherapy regimen.
2. When risk of febrile neutropenia is 10%–20%, CSFs may be considered in the presence of certain patient and clinical factors predisposing to increased complications from prolonged neutropenia, including: patient age >65 years; poor performance status; extensive prior treatment including large radiation ports; administration of combined chemoradiotherapy; cytopenias due to bone marrow involvement by tumor; poor nutritional status; presence of open wounds or active infections; previous surgery; poor renal function; liver dysfunction, particularly when evidenced by increased bilirubin; and lack of antibiotic prophylaxis.

B. Secondary prophylaxis of febrile neutropenia

1. CSFs (filgrastim, pegfilgrastim, or sargramostim) recommended for patients who experienced neutropenic complications from prior cycles of chemotherapy, and in which a reduced dose may compromise disease-free or overall survival or treatment outcome.

C. Therapeutic use in febrile neutropenia

1. CSFs should not be routinely used for patients with neutropenia who are afebrile.
2. CSFs (filgrastim or sargramostim only) may be considered in patients with febrile neutropenia who are at high risk for infection-associated complications, or who have prognostic factors that are predictive of poor clinical outcomes, including: profound neutropenia (absolute neutrophil count <100 cells/mm³); expected prolonged period of neutropenia (>10 days); patient age >65 years; uncontrolled primary disease; sepsis syndrome, or severe infection manifest by hypotension and multiorgan dysfunction; pneumonia; invasive fungal infection; other clinically documented infection; hospitalized at the time of the development of fever; or severe complications during previous episode of febrile neutropenia.

D. Reduction in duration of neutropenia in HSCT

1. CSFs are recommended to mobilize peripheral-blood progenitor cells (PBPC) prior to chemotherapy and to reduce the duration of neutropenia after autologous PBPC transplantation.

Data from references 52–54 and 59.

combination with CSFs.[1,5,55] At present, the use of neutrophil transfusions is considered investigational and is not recommended for routine management of febrile neutropenic patients.[55]

■ PROPHYLAXIS OF INFECTIONS IN NEUTROPENIC CANCER PATIENTS

❽ Owing to the potential morbidity and mortality of infections in neutropenic cancer patients, environmental modifications and prophylactic antimicrobial regimens have been implemented to prevent these complications. The overall goal of antimicrobial prophylaxis in cancer patients is to decrease the number and severity of systemic infections during prolonged periods of neutropenia.

General Measures

Because approximately 50% of pathogens infecting neutropenic cancer patients are acquired in the hospital, reducing acquisition of infectious organisms from the environment is a basic component in controlling nosocomial infections.[1,2,5,6,13] Neutropenic patients should be placed in reverse isolation (isolation to protect patients from contracting infections after exposure to others), with strict adherence to infection control guidelines by hospital personnel.[1,5,13] Proper meticulous handwashing by hospital personnel is a simple yet very effective infection control measure. To reduce the risk of infection caused by airborne pathogens, such as *Aspergillus* spp, laminar airflow rooms are used at some cancer centers performing HSCT. Laminar airflow rooms work by directing filtered air away from the patient, thus minimizing the risk of infection from airborne or environmental pathogens. Laminar airflow rooms are expensive, and use of these protective environments does not improve overall survival in HSCT recipients.[6,13]

Bacterial Infections

Combinations of oral nonabsorbable antibiotics, such as gentamicin, nystatin, vancomycin, polymyxin B, and colistin, have been widely studied as a means of reducing colonization of the GI tract with virulent pathogens, such as *P. aeruginosa*, and their translocation into the bloodstream. Although clinical trials have demonstrated that selective intestinal decontamination with oral nonabsorbable antibiotics successfully reduces infections, these regimens are not routinely recommended for prophylaxis because of problems that include unpalatability, high cost, and frequent adverse effects (e.g., nausea, vomiting, diarrhea).[1,2,4–6,13] Use of nonabsorbable antibiotic regimens has been associated with the development of resistance to aminoglycosides among gram-negative bacilli, rendering the aminoglycosides useless as treatment alternatives for ensuing infections.[1,2,13] Owing to concerns regarding development of resistance, prophylaxis with aminoglycosides and vancomycin should be avoided.[1,5]

Selective decontamination with systemic antimicrobial prophylaxis has been combined with oral agents, particularly the fluoroquinolones.[1,2,57] Prospective clinical trials have shown that orally absorbed prophylactic antibiotics, including trimethoprim–sulfamethoxazole and fluoroquinolones, are more effective and better tolerated than nonabsorbable antibiotics.[1,5] Most placebo-controlled studies indicate that trimethoprim–sulfamethoxazole significantly reduces infection rates in cancer patients.[1,5] Although trimethoprim–sulfamethoxazole is effective as prophylaxis against *P. jiroveci*, its lack of activity against *P. aeruginosa* is worrisome, particularly in institutions where pseudomonal infections are frequent.[1] Other concerns with trimethoprim–sulfamethoxazole prophylaxis include selection of resistant organisms, predisposition to development of oral fungal infections, and delay in bone marrow recovery resulting in prolonged neutropenic episodes.[1,5,6]

Numerous studies have shown that oral fluoroquinolones are more effective than placebo, nonabsorbable antibiotics, or trimethoprim–sulfamethoxazole in preventing gram-negative infections in neutropenic cancer patients.[57,58] Fluoroquinolone prophylaxis during periods of neutropenia decreases the incidence of fever and microbiologically documented gram-negative infections and may decrease the risk of death in these patients.[57,58] However, there are several potential limitations to their use. In particular, ciprofloxacin may lack adequate gram-positive activity. As a result, combination of ciprofloxacin with a second agent providing enhanced gram-positive activity (e.g., rifampin, penicillin, or a macrolide) may be required for effective prophylaxis.[1,5] Although fluoroquinolone prophylaxis has been associated with the development of resistant gram-negative organisms, two meta-analysis reports suggest that the risk of infection with resistant pathogens is not significantly increased.[57,58] Also the risk of colonization or infection with strains resistant to the prophylactic agent is lower with fluoroquinolones than with trimethoprim–sulfamethoxazole. However, patients experiencing breakthrough infection during fluoroquinolone prophylaxis should not be subsequently placed on a fluoroquinolone-containing empirical antibiotic regimen.[1,5]

Although studies have concluded that the benefits of prophylaxis with fluoroquinolones outweigh the potential risks, antibacterial prophylaxis in general remains somewhat controversial due to continued concerns regarding the potential for development of resistant

bacteria, high cost, and lack of impact on patient survival.[1,2,5] Therefore, antibacterial prophylaxis is not recommended routinely for all neutropenic patients. Prophylaxis (with trimethoprim–sulfamethoxazole or quinolone plus penicillin) generally is indicated for patients expected to be profoundly neutropenic for more than 1 week, such as HSCT patients.[1,6] Additional risk factors that may provide justification for prophylaxis include mucous membrane or skin lesions, presence of indwelling catheters, need for instrumentation or severe periodontal disease.[1,5] Neutrophil recovery eliminates the need for continued prophylaxis, and recovery may be facilitated by use of CSFs.[52] CSFs have also been formally recommended by the ASCO and the European Organisation for Research and Treatment of Cancer (EORTC) for primary prevention of febrile neutropenia in high-risk patients (see Table 131–6).[52,59]

Fungal Infections

Because neutropenic patients are at risk for mucocutaneous and invasive fungal infections that are difficult to diagnose and treat in this population, antifungal prophylaxis can be considered during high-risk periods at institutions where fungal infections in cancer patients occur frequently.[60] The goal of antifungal prophylaxis is to prevent development of invasive fungal infections during periods of risk, thereby reducing morbidity and mortality. A meta-analysis of antifungal prophylaxis in 38 trials involving more than 7,000 cancer patients reported a decrease in the use of parenteral antifungal therapy, superficial and invasive systemic fungal infections, and fungal infection–related mortality rate.[61] Antifungal prophylaxis in these studies resulted in decreased mortality in patients with prolonged neutropenia and HSCT but no effect on rates of invasive *Aspergillus* infections.

Although the choice of antifungal prophylaxis agents remains controversial, fluconazole prophylaxis (400 mg/day) has been particularly well studied and reduces the incidence of both superficial and systemic fungal infections; it also significantly decreases mortality from fungal infections in patients with leukemia and HSCT recipients.[60,61] However, use of fluconazole prophylaxis has contributed to the emergence of infections caused by *C. krusei* and *C. glabrata*, pathogens that frequently are resistant to fluconazole and other azole-type antifungal agents.[32,60] Therefore, routine antifungal prophylaxis with oral fluconazole (400 mg/day), itraconazole oral solution (200 mg/day), posaconazole (200 mg 3 times daily), or caspofungin (50 mg/day) are now routinely recommended starting with induction chemotherapy.[27] The choice of a specific agent should be determined by the types of fungal isolates at individual institutions.[27,62] After initiation, antifungal prophylaxis should be continued until resolution of neutropenia or the need for institution of antifungal therapy for suspected/documented infection.[27]

Itraconazole, low to moderate doses of amphotericin B, intranasal and aerosolized amphotericin B, lipid-associated amphotericin B products, voriconazole, and the echinocandin agents have been investigated for *Aspergillus* prophylaxis in neutropenic patients.[6,33,63] Posaconazole (200 mg suspension 3 times daily) was more effective than either fluconazole 400 mg/day or itraconazole 200 mg twice daily in the prevention of *Aspergillus* and other invasive fungal infections in patients with hematologic malignancies and prolonged neutropenia.[33,63] However, outside of the HSCT setting, posaconazole is currently only recommended for routine prevention of *Aspergillus* infections in neutropenic patients with hematologic malignancies.[33]

Other Infections

Use of trimethoprim–sulfamethoxazole in cancer patients at risk for *P. jiroveci* pneumonia has substantially reduced the incidence of this protozoal infection.[1] Antiviral prophylaxis with acyclovir, valacyclovir, or famciclovir is used in most centers to reduce the risk of HSV reactivation in patients with acute leukemia undergoing intensive chemotherapy. Varicella vaccine provides good protection (90%) in leukemic children and may be useful in seronegative adults, although the vaccine has been less well studied in this population.

When considering use of antimicrobial (antibacterial, antifungal, antiprotozoal, and antiviral) prophylaxis in neutropenic patients with cancer, the risks and benefits of prophylaxis must be weighed against issues with development of resistance, toxicities, and other concerns.

PHARMACOECONOMIC CONSIDERATIONS

❿ As in all areas of modern healthcare, attention has been directed increasingly toward providing cost-effective management of febrile neutropenia in cancer patients. Use of oral and/or outpatient antimicrobial therapy in low-risk patients is an effective, less costly alternative that is preferred by patients.[1,5,65] Potent oral antimicrobials facilitate conversion from IV antibiotics to oral therapy when appropriate. Judicious use of antimicrobials also helps to contain costs. In the situation of febrile neutropenia in a cancer patient, clinicians often are tempted to treat suspected/documented infections extremely aggressively; however, following guidelines such as those published by the IDSA and NCCN helps to assure the most appropriate use of available antimicrobials. Future consequences of antimicrobial overuse, such as resistance and limited treatment options, must be considered when choosing antimicrobial therapy for any indication, including management of febrile neutropenia. Each institution should examine its own infection and susceptibility patterns and use this information to guide empirical treatment decisions while individualizing therapy for each patient.

EVALUATION OF THERAPEUTIC OUTCOMES

❿ Close monitoring of febrile neutropenic patients, including both clinical and laboratory parameters, is essential for early detection and treatment of infectious complications. Three general therapeutic outcomes have been defined in the setting of febrile neutropenia: (a) success (survival during the febrile episode until resolution of neutropenia by judicious selection of empirical antimicrobial therapy), (b) success with modification (same as (a) but with additions/ modifications to empirical therapy), and (c) failure (death during febrile neutropenia).[13] Because many of the drugs that can be used in this setting (e.g., aminoglycosides and amphotericin B) have significant toxicity potential, careful attention must be paid to prevention and management of drug-related adverse effects. Evaluations of the parameters given in the Clinical Presentation are appropriate to help monitor and guide therapy. In addition, the NCCN guidelines for febrile neutropenia provide comprehensive recommendations on clinical/laboratory monitoring parameters, including schedules.[5] The reader is referred to individual chapters within this book for more detailed discussions of monitoring parameters related to specific types of infections (e.g., pneumonia and urinary tract infections).

INFECTIONS IN PATIENTS UNDERGOING HSCT

❶ Infection remains a major barrier to successful HSCT.[66,67] Recipients of HSCT are at enhanced risk for infection because of prolonged periods of neutropenia. In addition, patients receiving allogeneic or matched unrelated donor transplants have immune system insults imposed by prolonged immunosuppressive drug therapy for prevention and treatment of graft-versus-host disease (GVHD). Intensive pre-transplant conditioning regimens (high-dose chemotherapy and total-body irradiation), as well as GVHD itself, often disrupt protective barriers, such as mucous membranes, skin, and the GI tract, placing patients at further risk of infection. Patients experiencing failure to engraft have extended periods of profound neutropenia often resulting in death from infectious causes. The U.S. Food and Drug Administration (FDA) approved sargramostim for marrow graft failure in both autologous and allogeneic transplants.

ETIOLOGY AND CLINICAL PRESENTATION OF INFECTIONS

❷ ❿ The timing with which specific types of infections typically occur following HSCT is shown in Figure 131–2, but the relative incidence and importance of specific pathogens vary greatly according to the specific type of HSCT performed. Patients receiving allogeneic transplants are at greatest risk for infection after HSCT and are predisposed to earlier and more severe infections with opportunistic pathogens such as *Aspergillus*. The presence of GVHD also has an impact on the incidence and timing of various infections, including invasive fungal infections.

After administration of intensive conditioning regimens to eliminate malignant cells and prevent rejection of donor cells, patients may remain profoundly neutropenic for 3 to 4 weeks. During this pre-engraftment period, patients are at risk for the same types of infectious complications that occur in other granulocytopenic cancer patients (e.g., bacterial and fungal infections) and should be managed accordingly (see Table 131–1). Table 131–5 lists regimens for treatment of specific infections.

Patients undergoing HSCT are at significant risk for serious bacterial infections.[66-68] The risk of bacterial infection is particularly increased in patients undergoing allogeneic transplantation and those with GVHD. Gram-negative bacteremia occur in approximately 20% of patients, and mortality rates may reach 25%.[68]

Fungal infections, especially those caused by *Candida* and *Aspergillus* spp, are serious and often result in fatal complications associated with HSCT. Fungi remain a serious cause of infection, particularly in allogeneic HSCT recipients, for up to 1 to 2 years following transplantation and may occur in as many as 10% of patients.[66,67,69] Mortality rates associated with invasive aspergillosis infections may be as high as 90%.[66,67,69,70]

In addition to bacterial and fungal infections, HSCT recipients are at risk for serious HSV infections including gingivostomatitis, esophagitis, genital lesions, and, rarely, pneumonia during the first month after transplant.[66,67,71] Clinical disease is more common in patients with serologic evidence (e.g., serum antibodies) of prior exposure and latent HSV infection pretransplant. Therefore, reactivation of latent disease during periods of immunosuppression is the most common etiology of HSV infection. Without prophylaxis, as many as 80% of HSV-seropositive patients experience mucocutaneous disease after intensive chemotherapy compared with less than 25% of seronegative patients.[66,67,71,72] HSV infections often coexist with candidal infection and mucositis secondary to chemotherapy, radiation, or both.[71,72] Acyclovir-resistant HSV infections occur following HSCT but are not common.[71] Painful swallowing associated with these conditions often makes it difficult for patients to take oral medications and maintain adequate nutritional intake. Because of the considerable morbidity associated with reactivation of HSV after transplantation, the HSV serologic status of patients should be determined prior to transplant.

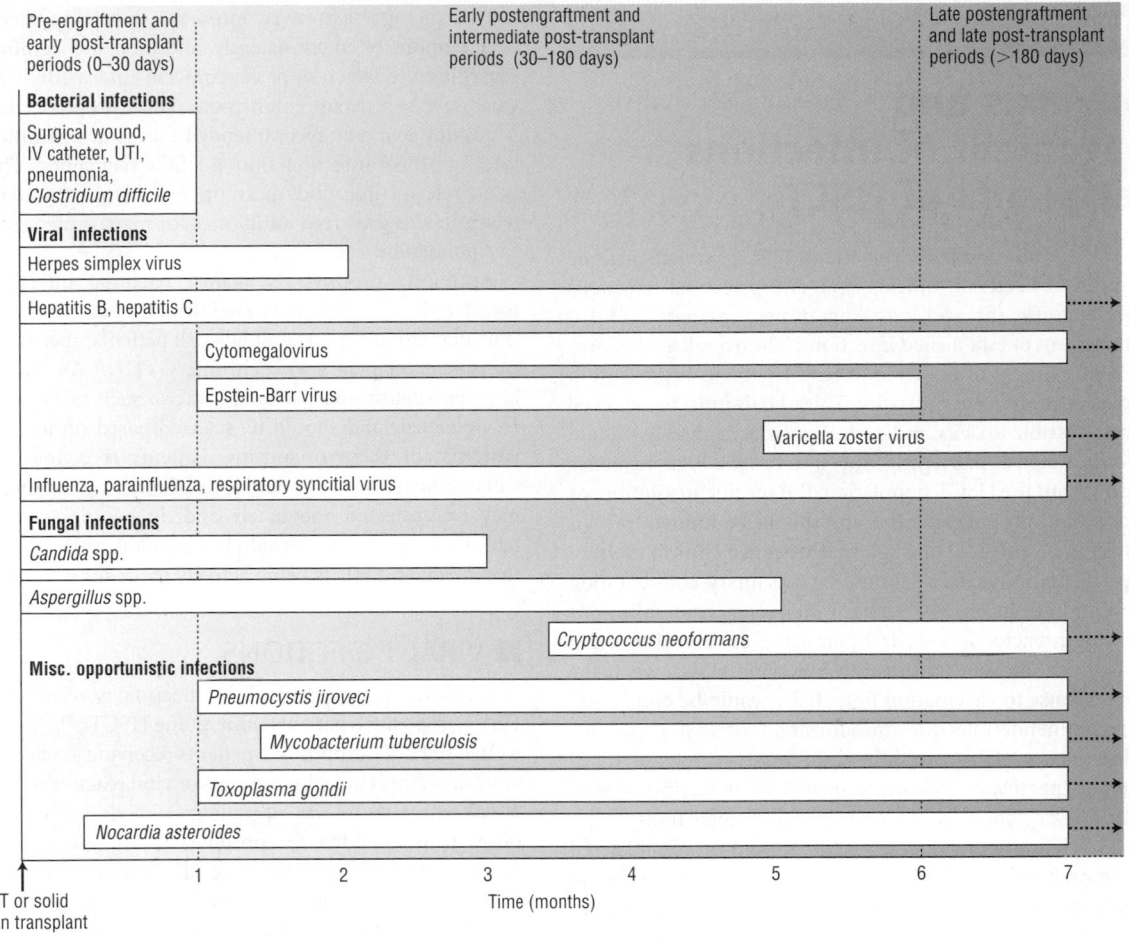

FIGURE 131-2. Timetable for the occurrence of infections in hematopoietic stem cell transplantation HSCT and solid organ-transplant patients. (IV, intravenous; UTI, urinary tract infection.)

HSCT recipients remain at high risk for infection after bone marrow engraftment has occurred.[66,67,71] Significant defects in neutrophil function and cell-mediated and humoral immunity, persisting for several months after transplantation, predispose patients to infectious complications. Acute and chronic GVHD also result in prolonged periods of immunosuppression and increased infection rates.

Bone marrow transplant patients are at high risk for Cytomegalovirus (CMV) infections during the early post-engraftment period. They range in severity from asymptomatic viral shedding (urine, throat, lungs) to life-threatening disseminated disease and interstitial pneumonia.[66,67,71,72]

As with HSV, patients seropositive for CMV before transplantation are at high risk for recurrent disease during periods of immunosuppression; approximately 70% of seropositive patients develop recurrent CMV disease after transplantation compared with only 3% of seronegative patients.[66,67,71,72] Other risk factors for CMV disease in HSCT patients include advanced age, human lymphocyte antigen mismatch, total-body irradiation, multiagent conditioning regimens, and presence of GVHD.[66,71] Patients without evidence of latent CMV infection (CMV seronegative) before transplantation may develop primary CMV disease after receiving bone marrow or blood products from CMV-seropositive donors. Although the typical onset of both primary and recurrent CMV infection is 1 to 2 months after transplantation, late-onset infections may occur more than 100 days after transplantation.[66,67,71,72] Patients receiving allogeneic transplants are at highest risk for CMV disease.[67,71,72]

The most serious clinical manifestation of CMV disease and the leading cause of infectious death in HSCT recipients is interstitial pneumonia, which is associated with an 85% mortality rate if left untreated.[66,67,71] This clinical syndrome manifests as fever, dyspnea, hypoxia, nonproductive cough, and diffuse pulmonary infiltrates. As many as 40% of allogeneic HSCT patients will develop interstitial pneumonia; of the patients with interstitial pneumonia, up to 40% of cases are caused by CMV.[67,71] Interstitial pneumonia also may result from other infectious (P. jiroveci, VZV) and noninfectious causes (pulmonary damage by radiation and chemotherapy).[67,71]

During the late post-engraftment period (beginning approximately 100 days after transplantation), infections remain a major problem in patients suffering from chronic GVHD. Additional immunosuppressive therapy for treatment of GVHD places these patients at added risk for infection. Infections common during the late post-engraftment period include those caused by encapsulated bacteria, such as S. pneumoniae and H. influenzae, fungi, and viruses, including CMV and VZV.[66,67,71] Patients not undergoing allogeneic transplantation or suffering from chronic GVHD generally have few infections in this period.

Up to 50% of all patients surviving up to 10 months after transplantation develop an infection caused by VZV.[67,71] Infection with VZV is most common in patients receiving allogeneic transplants with acute or chronic GVHD.[71,72] Both primary (varicella) or recurrent disease (herpes zoster) usually present as skin lesions, most of which remain contained to local areas; however, 30% to 45% of these infections may disseminate to other cutaneous areas or body organs, causing mortality as high as 50%.[71,72]

TREATMENT

Prophylaxis and Management of Infections in Recipients of HSCT

8 9 Goals of antimicrobial drug use in HSCT patients include (a) prevention of bacterial, fungal, viral, and protozoal infections during pre-engraftment and post-engraftment periods and (b) effective treatment of established infections. The overall goal of prophylaxis and treatment of infection in HSCT patients is prevention of infectious morbidity and mortality. These goals must be achieved at the lowest possible toxicity and cost. Prophylactic therapy should be specifically aimed at pathogens known to cause a high incidence of infection within the HSCT population, the specific institution, or both. In addition, prophylactic therapy should be limited to regimens proved to be effective through well-designed clinical trials.

Appropriate immunizations should be a primary consideration in the prevention of infections in HSCT recipients. Immunizations against common bacterial and viral pathogens are timed to avoid periods of severe immunosuppression following HSCT when the protective response to vaccination potentially would be decreased.[6] Current recommendations for immunization of HSCT patients include three doses each of diphtheria-pertussis-tetanus or diphtheria-tetanus, inactivated polio, conjugated *H. influenzae* type b, and hepatitis B vaccines at 12, 14, and 24 months after transplantation. The 23-valent pneumococcal vaccine should be administered at 12 and 24 months after HSCT, and the influenza vaccine should be administered prior to HSCT, resumed at least 6 months after transplantation, and continued for life. Family members, close contacts, and healthcare providers of HSCT patients also should be vaccinated annually against influenza. Finally, the measles-mumps-rubella vaccine should be administered no sooner than 24 months after HSCT when the patient is considered to be immunocompetent. The varicella vaccine is contraindicated for administration to HSCT patients owing to the live-attenuated nature of the product and the risk of VZV infection.[6]

■ BACTERIAL INFECTIONS

Prophylaxis of infections in HSCT patients is similar in many ways to that used in other neutropenic patients. Selective decontamination with oral antimicrobials is used commonly; considerations are the same as those discussed previously in the "Prophylaxis of Infections in Neutropenic Cancer Patients" section. Although some studies have shown decreased rates of bacteremia and other bacterial infections after HSCT, overall mortality rates were not reduced.[6,71] Therefore, routine use of prophylactic antibiotics in HSCT is still controversial. Fluoroquinolones have become the most frequently used agents, often combined with another agent (e.g., macrolides or rifampin), for enhanced gram-positive activity.[6,71] These regimens usually are started either within 72 hours of beginning the chemotherapy conditioning regimens or on the day of hematopoietic stem cell infusion and continued throughout the neutropenic period. Patients who become febrile while receiving prophylaxis should be managed according to general guidelines for febrile neutropenic patients.

Routine use of parenteral vancomycin for prophylactic therapy is not recommended. Prophylaxis with vancomycin has been studied because of the high incidence of gram-positive infections following transplantation. Vancomycin prophylaxis appears to decrease the overall incidence of gram-positive bacterial infections, number of days of empirical antimicrobial therapy, and

cost of therapy.[6] However, important mortality benefits have not been demonstrated consistently, and there are significant concerns regarding the selection of vancomycin-intermediate *S. aureus* and vancomycin-resistant enterococci. Thus, prophylactic vancomycin use is not generally recommended except in institutions with high rates of MRSA infection among HSCT recipients.[6] There currently is no role for linezolid, quinupristin–dalfopristin, daptomycin, or telavancin as preferred antibiotics for management of infections in this population.

Antibiotic prophylaxis against bacterial infection is recommended in the late post-engraftment period (>100 days after transplantation) in certain high-risk patients, specifically allogeneic transplant recipients with chronic GVHD.[6] Antibiotics should be targeted against encapsulated bacteria such as *S. pneumoniae* and *H. influenzae* and should be selected based on local susceptibility patterns for these organisms. Patients receiving trimethoprim–sulfamethoxazole for prophylaxis of other opportunistic infections may be protected adequately and do not necessarily require an additional antibiotic.[6] Prophylaxis should be continued as long as the chronic GVHD is being actively treated.

■ VIRAL INFECTIONS

Prophylaxis of recurrent HSV infection is recommended for all HSV-seropositive patients undergoing HSCT.[6,71] Approximately 0% to 10% of HSV-seropositive patients receiving acyclovir experienced viral shedding, clinical symptoms of viral reactivation, or both compared with 60% to 80% of patients receiving placebo.[6,71] Acyclovir doses recommended for prophylaxis are 250 mg/m^2 (5 mg/kg) IV every 12 hours or 200 mg orally 3 times daily.[6,71] Intravenous therapy eventually is necessary in most patients because of the development of severe mucositis from conditioning regimens. Oral acyclovir is effective and considerably less expensive in patients who can take oral medications. Valacyclovir in doses of 500 to 1,000 mg/day is also commonly used and has replaced acyclovir as first-line therapy in many institutions.[6,71] Although the duration of antiviral prophylaxis differs among centers, acyclovir usually is started at the time of the conditioning regimen and continued until bone marrow engraftment or resolution of mucositis (approximately 30 days after HSCT).[6,71] In addition to preventing recurrence of HSV disease, acyclovir prophylaxis may reduce the incidence of CMV reactivation.[6] Patients developing active HSV or VZV infection should be treated with high-dose acyclovir (10 mg/kg IV every 8 hours).[71]

Although high-dose oral acyclovir given for 6 months after transplantation significantly reduces reactivation of VZV infections, routine use of long-term acyclovir is controversial and not generally recommended for this indication.[6,71] Patients who received HSCT within the previous 24 months or those more than 24 months after HSCT who have chronic GVHD or are undergoing immunosuppressive therapy should receive varicella-zoster immunoglobulin 625 units intramuscularly within 48 to 96 hours after close contact with persons with chickenpox or shingles for prevention of VZV-related disease.[6]

Acyclovir-resistant HSV has been reported occasionally in HSCT patients receiving acyclovir prophylaxis. Foscarnet is the drug of choice for treatment of acyclovir-resistant HSV. Foscarnet for HSV prophylaxis has not been well studied.[6,71]

Prevention of CMV disease has been studied extensively in HSCT patients and is a well-accepted indication for prophylaxis because of the high associated infectious morbidity and mortality. If possible, CMV-seronegative patients should receive donor cells and supportive blood products from seronegative donors only; however, CMV-seropositive patients are not at significant additional risk by receiving blood or donor cells from seropositive donors.[71] Although acyclovir has relatively poor in vitro activity against CMV, a decrease in CMV infection and an improvement in overall survival were reported in HSV- and CMV-seropositive allogeneic HSCT recipients receiving IV acyclovir.[6]

Ganciclovir has been well studied for prophylaxis because of its superior activity against CMV compared with acyclovir.[6] Although administration of prophylactic ganciclovir to CMV-seropositive patients may significantly decrease the occurrence of CMV disease, studies have found no clear survival benefit, and ganciclovir-related bone marrow suppression frequently was problematic. Therefore, ganciclovir prophylaxis is only recommended routinely among allogeneic HSCT recipients for the first 100 days after transplantation.[6,71] The recommended dose of ganciclovir in these patients is 5 mg/kg IV every 12 hours for the first 5 to 7 days, followed by 5 to 6 mg/kg IV once daily 5 times per week until day 100 after HSCT.[6]

Perhaps a more appropriate role for ganciclovir is early or preemptive therapy, in which ganciclovir is administered at first isolation of CMV from the blood or bronchoalveolar lavage fluid. Detection of CMV can be accomplished by use of either a monoclonal antibody–based test for viral antigens or by detection of viral DNA through polymerase chain reaction (PCR)–based tests. Preemptive therapy has been evaluated in several studies.[71] It significantly reduced the occurrence of CMV disease (including CMV pneumonia) and improved survival significantly up to 180 days after transplantation.[71] Because CMV viremia and bronchoalveolar lavage cultures are highly predictive of subsequent CMV disease, preemptive ganciclovir therapy should be considered for autologous HSCT recipients within the first 100 days after transplantation or in allogeneic HSCT recipients at any time after transplantation.[6,71] The dose of ganciclovir for preemptive therapy is the same as that used for prophylaxis. Foscarnet can be used for either prophylaxis or preemptive therapy of CMV disease in patients intolerant of ganciclovir. The recommended foscarnet dose is 60 mg/kg IV every 12 hours for 7 days, followed by 90 to 120 mg/kg IV daily.[6,71] Oral valganciclovir 900 mg every 12 hours has not been well studied in the setting of HSCT.[73] However, oral valganciclovir has excellent pharmacokinetics and produces serum levels of ganciclovir which are at least similar to those achieved after intravenous administration.[74] Although not routinely recommended, valganciclovir is nevertheless used in many centers based on the favorable pharmacokinetic properties and convenience of oral dosing in certain patients.[71,73,74] CSFs are beneficial in this setting (Table 131–6), providing benefits similar to those noted in neutropenic patients with acquired immunodeficiency syndrome receiving ganciclovir therapy for CMV retinitis.[52,54]

Pharmacologic prevention of CMV disease with either intravenous immunoglobulin (IVIG) or CMV hyperimmune globulin (CMVIG) produced variable and inconclusive results.[75,76] The benefits of immunoglobulins for CMV prophylaxis in HSCT patients have not been demonstrated conclusively, and their use is not currently recommended.[75,76]

Ganciclovir is the drug of choice for treatment of active CMV infection in HSCT patients (see Table 131–5). Foscarnet also may be of benefit for treatment or prevention of infections in HSCT patients and may be used as an alternative to ganciclovir because of its relative lack of bone marrow toxicity. Foscarnet-related nephrotoxicity may be problematic, however, especially in the posttransplant period when patients may be receiving other nephrotoxic agents. Use of cidofovir is limited by the risk of nephrotoxicity, and this agent has not been well studied in HSCT patients.

Numerous single-agent treatments, such as vidarabine, interferon, and ganciclovir, have been used unsuccessfully as treatment for CMV pneumonitis. However, the combination of high-dose IVIG and ganciclovir may decrease the mortality of the syndrome from 85% to only 30% to 50%.[71,75,77] Ganciclovir plus hyperimmune

CMVIG also is considered effective for treatment of CMV disease, although this regimen has not been studied as extensively in the HSCT population in a controlled fashion. The potential for ganciclovir-associated bone marrow suppression prior to marrow engraftment and in patients who are just recovering from granulocytopenia remains a concern, especially in patients with unstable renal function. Ganciclovir plus CMVIG is used widely as the treatment regimen of choice for severe or life-threatening CMV disease, this use being based on benefit-versus-risk considerations more than definitive clinical data. Ganciclovir plus IVIG also is used frequently, although CMVIG has replaced IVIG in many institutions.[75,77]

CLINICAL CONTROVERSY

Use of CMVIG for prophylaxis and/or treatment of CMV infections in HSCT and solid-organ transplantation patients is advocated by many clinicians. However, the clinical benefits of this expensive adjunct therapy have not been clearly demonstrated in these patients. Although CMVIG often is recommended in combination with ganciclovir for treatment of CMV pneumonia in transplant patients due to high mortality risk and few treatment options, its role in other types of infections is not clear.

■ FUNGAL INFECTIONS

Prophylaxis with antifungal agents is efficacious and generally recommended for prevention of mucocutaneous and disseminated candidal infections in high-risk HSCT patients (Table 131–2).[6,27,31,63,71,78–81] Patients specifically recommended for prophylaxis include all allogeneic transplant recipients and autologous recipients who are expected to have prolonged neutropenia, have received intensive conditioning regimens associated with extensive mucositis, or have recently received fludarabine.[6,27,31,63,71,78,79] Fluconazole 400 mg IV or orally once daily is the most commonly used regimen; it is started on the day of transplantation and continued until engraftment or resolution of neutropenia.[6,27,71,79] The variable activity of fluconazole against non-albicans species of Candida may be problematic in this population, as is lack of activity against Aspergillus.[31,63,32,79] Prophylaxis with fluconazole (as well as itraconazole), although effectively reducing colonization and infection with yeasts, has not been consistently demonstrated to reduce overall mortality or invasive infections such as aspergillosis in HSCT recipients.[31,63,71,78–81] Two newer antifungal agents have also shown efficacy in the prevention of fungal infections in patients undergoing HSCT. Micafungin 50 mg IV once daily was demonstrated to be more efficacious than fluconazole in the prevention of early-onset Candida infections in patients with neutropenia prior to engraftment. Posaconazole 200 mg suspension three times daily was also more effective than fluconazole 400 mg orally once daily in the late prevention of invasive Aspergillus and other fungal infections in HSCT patients with GVHD. Fluconazole, posaconazole, and micafungin are all recommended for prophylaxis of fungal infections in HSCT. In high-risk HSCT patients with GVHD, posaconazole is the preferred agent with micafungin recommended as an alternative agent along with itraconazole (Table 131–2).[31,33,63,78–80]

Fluconazole, posaconazole, and other azole antifungals may cause significant elevations in serum cyclosporine concentrations and pre-dispose to cyclosporine toxicities; this interaction should be monitored closely in HSCT patients receiving these agents concurrently.[27,33,80]

■ PROTOZOAL INFECTIONS

Pulmonary infection with *P. jiroveci* is a relatively infrequent complication of HSCT. However, mortality rates in this population are approximately 60% and are especially high in patients with GVHD.[6,67] Prophylactic trimethoprim–sulfamethoxazole (one double-strength tablet 3 times per week or one single-strength tablet daily) is given commonly in this setting. Toxoplasmosis is not a common infection in HSCT patients but is associated with mortality rates of approximately 70%.[82] Toxoplasmosis should be prevented by trimethoprim–sulfamethoxazole prophylaxis.[6]

■ USE OF COLONY-STIMULATING FACTORS

A number of studies have evaluated the use of filgrastim, pegfilgrastim, and sargramostim in HSCT patients in an effort to speed bone marrow recovery, reduce the period of neutropenia, and decrease infectious complications. CSFs appear effective as well as safe following autologous transplantation, although increased rates of GVHD and mortality have been reported with use of CSFs following allogeneic transplantation.[52] The use of CSFs is now routinely recommended to mobilize blood progenitor cells and reduce the period of neutropenia in autologous transplants (Table 131–6).[52,54]

EVALUATION OF THERAPEUTIC OUTCOMES

❿ Close monitoring of HSCT patients, including clinical and laboratory data, is essential for early detection and treatment of infectious complications. In addition, because many of the drugs commonly used in this setting (e.g., ganciclovir, amphotericin B, and trimethoprim–sulfamethoxazole) have significant toxicity potential in HSCT patients, careful attention must be paid to prevention and management of drug-related adverse effects. Monitoring parameters related to specific types of infections (e.g., pneumonia and urinary tract infections) should be applied as appropriate. The reader is referred to other chapters within this book for more specific information.

INFECTIONS IN SOLID-ORGAN TRANSPLANT RECIPIENTS

Since the introduction of cyclosporine in 1980, solid-organ transplantation has become an established mode of treatment for end-stage diseases of the heart, lungs, kidney, liver, pancreas, and small bowel. Patient and allograft survival rates greatly exceed those of the past. Reasons for improved survival include continuous improvements in immunosuppressive drug therapy, candidate selection, and transplant surgery techniques and more experience in the management of complications (including infection) in these patients. Despite advances in diagnostic techniques and antimicrobial therapy, infectious complications remain important causes of morbidity and mortality after solid-organ transplantation.

RISK FACTORS

❶ Many of the risk factors for infection are present in solid-organ transplant patients (see Table 131–1). The most important risk factor in this population is immunosuppressive drug therapy for prevention and treatment of allograft rejection. Risk of infection depends on specific immunosuppressive drug regimens as well as the intensity (dose) and duration of immunosuppression. Most opportunistic infections in transplant patients occur during the first 6 months after transplantation, when the intensity and total cumulative doses of immunosuppressive therapy are very high.[83,84]

Immunosuppressive drugs, often in escalated doses, are used to treat episodes of graft rejection. Drugs used to treat rejection include immunoglobulins directed against T cells (e.g., antithymocyte globulin), murine monoclonal antibodies (muromonab), antibodies against interleukin 2 receptors (daclizumab and basiliximab), T-cell-depleting antibodies (alemtuzumab), and high-dose IV or oral corticosteroids. Rejection episodes often occur during the post-transplant period when the overall cumulative dose or net state of immunosuppression is highest (2–4 months post-transplant).[83,85] Therefore, patients already at risk for infection are placed at even higher risk if additional immunosuppressive therapy is needed to treat one or more episodes of graft rejection. Immunosuppressive drug therapy must be evaluated carefully when infections occur because, in many cases, immunosuppression may have to be reduced to allow patients to survive the infectious episode, at the expense of increased risk of graft rejection. Risk of increased infectious complications from immunosuppressive therapy used to treat rejection episodes is determined, at least in part, by the specific therapy used.[83–85]

ETIOLOGY

❷ As with cancer patients, microorganisms infecting solid-organ transplant patients are present before transplantation or are acquired from exogenous sources. All transplant recipients are at risk for mucocutaneous candidiasis from species colonizing body sites. Invasive fungal infection is less common following kidney and pancreas transplantation (5%–15%) but also may occur in 30% to 60% of heart, lung, liver, and small bowel transplant recipients. Rates are highest following liver and small bowel transplantation and are associated with mortality rates up to 60% to 70%.[83,86,87] Approximately 50% to 90% of all systemic fungal infections in transplant recipients are caused by *Candida* spp.[83,86,87] Abdominal surgery, especially the more complex procedures required for liver and small bowel transplantation, predispose patients to serious fungal disease, most likely as a consequence of entering an area already colonized with *Candida* spp.[86] Lung and heart transplant recipients are particularly at risk for invasive aspergillosis; these infections may occur in up to 10% of patients.[86] Liver and lung transplant recipients are at high risk for serious gram-negative bacterial infections as a result of the technically difficult surgical procedures.[83]

Organisms present as latent tissue infections may reactivate and cause clinical disease after transplantation with administration of immunosuppressive drug therapy. Disease resulting from infection reactivation has been noted with viral (HSV-1 and HSV-2, CMV, VZV, Epstein-Barr virus), protozoal (*Toxoplasma gondii, P. jiroveci*), and mycobacterial (*Mycobacterium tuberculosis*) pathogens.[88,89] Serologic or immunologic tests are performed prior to transplantation to assess the risk for infection because of reactivation and identify other subclinical infections (e.g., hepatitis B, hepatitis C, *Legionella*). Many patients with reactivated disease have no clinical symptoms; often the only evidence of active infection is a rise in antibody titer from the pre-transplant baseline, positive culture, or histologic evidence. Reactivation of latent infection may result in severe life-threatening disease in immunosuppressed hosts.[89]

Exogenous sources of infection in transplant patients include environmental contamination and transmission of microorganisms via transplanted organs and blood products. Environmental sources of infection are similar to those noted in other immunocompromised hosts, such as cancer patients. Airborne pathogens, especially fungi, such as *Aspergillus* and *Cryptococcus neoformans*, may cause infections in transplant patients; this is thought to be a direct cause of increased *Aspergillus* infections among lung transplant patients.[83,86] Transplant patients are at risk for common nosocomial infections and infections occurring as hospital outbreaks (*P. aeruginosa, Acinetobacter*, and *Legionella*). Optimal prevention and management of nosocomial infections in transplant patients require knowledge of the current epidemiology of infections and susceptibility patterns in the institution.

Infections transmitted via donor organs or blood products are major causes of morbidity and mortality in transplant patients and may include HSV, *T. gondii*, and hepatitis B and C. The most important infections transmitted from the donor, however, are caused by CMV. These infections may cause serious disease (e.g., pneumonia, hepatitis, hematologic disorders, and chorioretinitis). They also may predispose patients to other opportunistic infections and contribute to acute and chronic allograft dysfunction or rejection, post-transplant lymphoproliferative disorders, and cardiac complications and atherosclerosis in heart transplant recipients.[83,90] In contrast to reactivation disease, transplant patients contracting primary CMV disease are at increased risk for serious life-threatening infections.[83,91–93] The most important source of primary CMV infection in transplant patients is the donor organ. Efforts are made to avoid transplanting organs from CMV-seropositive donors into CMV-seronegative recipients because of the potentially severe consequences. With the relative scarcity of suitable organs and the rapidity with which transplant decisions often must be made, however, this is not always possible. The consequences of transplanting an organ from a CMV-seropositive donor into an already CMV-seropositive recipient are less clear. CMV reinfection (as well as reactivation) syndromes may occur in these patients.[83,84,93] In addition to transmission from donor organs, primary CMV disease may be transmitted from seropositive blood products, although this is a much less common mode of transmission.

Organs from donors seropositive for *T. gondii* or HSV generally are not withheld from seronegative patients. Organs from known HIV-infected donors, however, are not used for transplantation. Asymptomatic HIV-seropositive individuals with CD4+ lymphocyte count greater than 400 cells/mm^3 may be considered for solid-organ transplantation (as well as HSCT) without prohibitively high risk for acceleration of HIV disease.[92,94] However, this practice is not widespread because of the shortage of donor organs. The impact of protease inhibitors and highly active antiretroviral therapy on long-term outcome of HIV-infected patients following transplantation is not precisely known but is believed to have improved the overall feasibility of transplanting these individuals.[94]

Table 131–5 provides information on microbiology, clinical presentation, and treatment of infections in HSCT and solid-organ transplant recipients. Although opportunistic viral, fungal, and protozoal infections may occur commonly, bacterial infections remain the most frequent infectious complications after transplantation in all allograft recipients.

TIMING OF INFECTIONS AFTER TRANSPLANTATION

Although risk of infection with specific pathogens varies with the type of transplant, the time course of infections is similar in all transplant recipients. The overall risk of infection is greatest during the first 6 months after transplantation, when the greatest number of risk factors are present. Both daily and cumulative doses of immunosuppressive drugs are at high levels, and additional agents may be necessary for treatment of acute rejection episodes.[83,84]

As with HSCT, the overall time course for infections can be divided into three general periods after transplantation (see Fig. 131–2). During the early post-transplant period (within the first month after transplantation), patients are at risk for infections already present and brought forward from the pre-transplant period (e.g., hepatitis B); postoperative infections, such as surgical wound and catheter infections; infection resulting from colonized donor organs (pneumonia following lung transplant); and reactivation of HSV.[83,84,89] In the intermediate post-transplant period (2–6 months after transplant), risk is highest for viral infections, including CMV, Epstein-Barr virus, and hepatitis B and C. The combination of these "immunomodulating" viruses plus sustained immunosuppressive therapy leads to a high risk for opportunistic infections with pathogens such as *P. jiroveci*, *Aspergillus*, and *Nocardia asteroides*.[83,84,86,89] In the late post-transplant period (>6 months after transplant), patients are at risk for persistent infections (particularly viral) from earlier post-transplant periods, reactivation of VZV and *C neoformans*, and routine infections affecting the general population.[83] In addition, patients who required additional immunosuppression therapy for acute or chronic rejection are at continued high risk for opportunistic infections (*Aspergillus* and *P. jiroveci*).[83,84,86] Although Figure 131–2 illustrates infection patterns common to all solid-organ transplants, the relative incidence and importance of a particular pathogen vary according to the type of transplant.

TYPES OF INFECTIONS AND CLINICAL PRESENTATION

❿ Transplant patients are at risk for infections occurring at a variety of sites, including skin, surgical wound, urinary tract, lungs, blood, abdomen, and CNS. However, most infections occur at or near the site of the transplanted organ. For example, heart transplant and heart and lung transplant recipients most often are infected within the lungs or thoracic cavity. Urinary tract infections remain an important cause of morbidity in renal transplant patients, especially in the early post-transplant period. Administration of prophylactic antibiotics (e.g., trimethoprim–sulfamethoxazole) to these patients has reduced the incidence and severity of urinary tract infections.[83,84] Serious bacterial and fungal infections originating from the abdomen and GI tract are most common after liver transplantation and are related to variables such as length of surgery and surgical procedures performed. Risk of bacteremia, usually originating from the gut, is highest in liver transplant patients. Renal transplant recipients are at the lowest risk for infections and infectious deaths, whereas patients receiving heart, lung, and liver transplants are at the highest risk for infection-related morbidity and mortality.[83,84,86]

CLINICAL PRESENTATION OF INFECTIONS IN SOLID-ORGAN TRANSPLANT PATIENTS

General

- Because transplant patients are at high risk for serious infections, frequent (at least daily), careful clinical assessments must be performed to search for evidence of infection.

- Clinical presentation of infection is variable and depends on the type and site of infection, type of transplant, time after transplantation, immune status of the host, and dose and duration of immunosuppressive therapy.

- Primary viral disease usually is more symptomatic and severe than disease caused by reactivation.

- Physical assessment should include examination of all common sites of infection, including mouth/pharynx, nose and sinuses, respiratory tract, GI tract, urinary tract, skin, soft tissues, perineum, and intravascular catheter insertion sites.

Symptoms

- Usual signs and symptoms of infection may be absent or altered in patients receiving intensive immunosuppressive regimens owing to an inability to mount a typical inflammatory response (e.g., no infiltrate on chest x-ray film, urinary tract infection without pyuria).

- Pain may be present at infection site(s).

Signs

- Fever is the single most important clinical sign indicating the presence of infection. Other causes of fever unrelated to infection in this patient population include reactions to blood products, drugs, embolic events, and ischemic injury.

- Usual signs of infection may be absent or altered.

- Signs of allograft dysfunction may be related to infection. Distinguishing fever caused by allograft rejection from that caused by infection often is difficult and frequently requires allograft biopsy.

Laboratory Tests

- Blood cultures (at least two sets, including vascular access devices) for bacteria and fungi; cultures of other suspected or potential infection sites (urine, lungs, surgical wounds, and soft tissue infections).

- Other cultures should be obtained as clinically indicated according to the presence of signs or symptoms.

- Complete blood count and chemistries should be obtained frequently to monitor allograft function, plan supportive care, guide drug dosing, and assess patient's overall status.

- Surveillance cultures for CMV and HSV may be useful during first 3 months after transplantation for early detection of infection.

Other Diagnostic Tests

- Chest x-ray film

- Aspiration, biopsy of skin lesions

- Other diagnostic tests as indicated clinically on the basis of physical examination and other assessments

In contrast to febrile neutropenic patients, the threshold for initiating empirical antimicrobial therapy is higher in febrile transplant patients. Appropriate therapy for the large numbers of pathogens that may cause infections in transplant patients varies greatly from organism to organism (Table 131–5). Therefore, careful attempts at definitive diagnosis of suspected infections must be made. If comprehensive workup reveals no source of infection, careful observation of the febrile transplant patient (rather than empirical therapy) is common practice. Surveillance cultures may be useful during the first 3 months for detecting CMV and HSV infections.[83,86,91,92,95] Management and monitoring of documented infections are similar to that in other types of patients.

Prevention of Infection in Solid-Organ Transplantation

❽ The goals of antimicrobial drug use in solid-organ transplant recipients are (a) prevention of infectious complications in the immediate postoperative period, (b) prevention of late infectious complications associated with prolonged periods of immunosuppression, and (c) effective treatment of established infections in order to prevent graft dysfunction and rejection and decrease patient morbidity and mortality. All of these goals must be achieved at the lowest possible toxicity and cost.

Prevention of infection in the transplant patient can be accomplished in a number of ways. First, risk of environmental contamination should be minimized.[96] Patients should be protected from institutional infectious outbreaks. Transplant patients should receive the pneumococcal vaccine once and the influenza vaccine yearly; however, their immunologic responses to these vaccines may be blunted by immunosuppressive therapy.[83]

Because the most important source of primary CMV disease is an infected donor organ, CMV-seronegative patients should not receive organs or blood products from seropositive donors if possible. A number of pharmacologic strategies have been studied in an attempt to prevent CMV infection. Prophylactic ganciclovir (administered as either 5 mg/kg IV every 12 hours or oral valganciclovir in doses ranging from 900 mg once daily to 1,000 mg 3 times daily) is effective in reducing the incidence of both primary and reactivated CMV disease in solid-organ transplantation.[73,77,83,84,90–93] Ganciclovir prophylaxis also may reduce reactivation of CMV disease significantly in seropositive patients receiving antithymocyte globulin or muromonab for treatment of acute rejection.[84,92,93] High-dose oral acyclovir effectively reduces the incidence of CMV infection and disease following renal transplantation. However, acyclovir is less efficacious in high-risk renal transplant patients (donor positive, recipient negative for CMV serum antibodies) and other nonrenal transplant types.[83,84,90–93,97] Preemptive ganciclovir or valganciclovir (initiated after actual isolation of CMV from blood, urine, bronchoalveolar lavage fluid, or other site) is more effective than acyclovir in preventing both primary and reactivation disease in liver transplant recipients. Preemptive ganciclovir effectively prevents CMV disease in other types of solid-organ transplants as well.[91,92,95] Ganciclovir-related bone marrow suppression is not as problematic in solid-organ transplant recipients as in HSCT patients; most studies report the drug is reasonably well tolerated.[77,83,91,92,95,97]

Whether prophylaxis or preemptive therapy is the best approach to preventing CMV disease is controversial.[77,83,91–93,95] Prophylaxis is effective and easy to administer without the need for careful discrimination among suitable patients. However, universal prophylaxis results in unnecessary exposure of low-risk individuals to adverse effects of drugs, and there are concerns that prolonged exposure may increase the risk of viral resistance to drugs.[91,92,97] Preemptive therapy is effective and results in exposure of fewer patients to drugs. However, this strategy requires the availability and routine use of sensitive and specific diagnostic tests in order to identify high-risk individuals at an early stage of CMV infection. Although currently available PCR-based methods make this latter consideration less of an issue, PCR testing is not available at all centers. Prophylactic therapy should be used primarily in patients at highest risk of disease (i.e., seronegative patients receiving organs from seropositive donors), whereas other lower-risk patients should receive only preemptive therapy.[83,91,92,95] However, these recommendations are not universally accepted or practiced.

CMVIG is valuable in decreasing the incidence and severity of CMV disease following kidney, heart, lung, and liver transplantation.[77,83,91] Although prophylaxis with CMVIG has been strongly recommended for CMV-seronegative transplant recipients receiving organs from seropositive donors, the benefits of CMVIG relative to other therapies (e.g., prophylactic or preemptive ganciclovir) are not well known, and available studies have conflicting results. Whether the combination of CMVIG plus ganciclovir offers advantages over the use of either agent alone, either for primary prophylaxis or for treatment of established CMV disease, in solid-organ transplantation is unclear.[83,91] However, some authorities recommend use of CMVIG in combination with ganciclovir for treatment of severe, life-threatening CMV pneumonitis in solid-organ transplant recipients.[75,77]

Although use of prophylactic acyclovir in HSV-seropositive patients undergoing HSCT is well accepted, prophylaxis in solid-organ transplant recipients remains controversial. Reactivation disease caused by HSV occurs in approximately 25% of HSV-seropositive patients who are not receiving prophylaxis.[83] Oral or genital mucocutaneous disease is the most common presentation, but HSV pneumonitis also is seen occasionally and is associated with a mortality rate of approximately 75%.[83] Acyclovir is used at some centers because of the high incidence of clinical HSV infection, including pneumonias, after transplantation.

Prophylactic antimicrobial agents are of benefit to transplant patients in certain clinical situations. Antibiotic prophylaxis, with agents such as cefazolin started perioperatively and continued for less than 24 hours, is considered to reduce wound infection rates effectively following renal transplantation.[83,96] Although the benefits of perioperative prophylaxis have not been well demonstrated in other types of transplantation procedures, surgical prophylaxis usually is considered mandatory for liver, heart, lung, or small bowel transplant patients because of the high risk of perioperative bacterial infections.[83,96] Pulmonary infections are particularly common in lung and heart-lung transplant recipients. They often are caused by bacteria colonizing the airways of the diseased organs prior to transplantation. Therefore, perioperative antibiotics for lung and heart and lung procedures often are selected based on pre-transplant sputum cultures.[83,96] In addition, post-transplant antibiotic prophylaxis is effective in decreasing the number of bacterial infections in renal transplant patients. Prophylactic trimethoprim–sulfamethoxazole traditionally has been used because it is inexpensive and well tolerated; other antibiotics, such as the fluoroquinolones, also have been evaluated.[83] Administration of oral low-dose trimethoprim–sulfamethoxazole (one double-strength tablet daily) for 6 to 12 months for prevention of *P. jiroveci* infection following heart and lung transplantation is common, although the efficacy and optimal duration are somewhat controversial.[83,98] Selective bowel decontamination with nonabsorbable antibiotics in combination with a low-bacterial diet (no fresh fruits and vegetables) effectively reduces oropharyngeal and GI colonization with gram-negative aerobes and *Candida* in liver transplant patients. However, selective bowel contamination is less efficacious when administered for a period of less than 1 week prior to transplantation.[96] Because liver transplantation usually is performed without advance notice as organs become emergently available, the practice of selective bowel decontamination remains controversial and is not recommended routinely.[83,96]

Because immunosuppressed transplant recipients are at risk for mucocutaneous fungal infections, prophylactic oral or topical antifungal agents may be indicated in these patients. Liver, pancreas, and small bowel transplant recipients are clearly at high risk for invasive fungal infections and should receive prophylaxis with fluconazole (400 mg/day).[27,83,86,99] Prophylaxis has also been suggested for lung and heart-lung transplant recipients with high-dose fluconazole, itraconazole, or voriconazole; however, data supporting either this general recommendation or choice of specific agent are lacking.[27,86] Concentrations of immunosuppressant drugs should be monitored closely in transplant patients receiving azole-type antifungal agents (fluconazole, itraconazole, voriconazole).

Transplant patients, especially heart and heart and lung recipients, without serologic evidence of prior exposure to *T. gondii* who receive organs from seropositive donors are at high risk for toxoplasmosis.[83] Many of these patients will be receiving trimethoprim–sulfamethoxazole for prophylaxis of *P. jiroveci* infection; this agent will also provide effective prophylaxis against *T. gondii* as well as *N. asteroides*. Although prophylaxis is not given routinely at all centers, this therapy may be justified in high-risk patients because of the delays in diagnosis and serious infections associated with toxoplasmosis.[83]

EVALUATION OF THERAPEUTIC OUTCOMES

Close monitoring of transplant recipients, including both clinical and laboratory data, is essential for early detection and treatment of potentially severe opportunistic infections.

ABBREVIATIONS

ANC: absolute neutrophil count

ASCO: American Society for Clinical Oncology

CDC: U.S. Centers for Disease Control and Prevention

CMV: Cytomegalovirus

CMVIG: Cytomegalovirus hyperimmune globulin

CSF: colony-stimulating factor

EORTC: European Organisation for Research and Treatment of Cancer

GVHD: graft-versus-host disease

HSCT: hematopoietic stem cell transplantation

HSV: herpes simplex virus

IDSA: Infectious Diseases Society of America

LAMB: lipid-associated amphotericin B

MRSA: methicillin-resistant *Staphylococcus aureus*

NCCN: National Comprehensive Cancer Network

NNIS: National Nosocomial Infection Surveillance

PCR: polymerase chain reaction

PMN: polymorphonuclear leukocyte

VRE: vancomycin-resistant enterococci

VZV: varicella-zoster virus

WBC: white blood cell

REFERENCES

1. Hughes WT, Armstrong D, Bodey GP, et al. 2002 guidelines for the use of antimicrobial agents in neutropenic patients with cancer. Clin Infect Dis 2002;34:730–751.

2. Bow EJ. Management of the febrile neutropenic cancer patient: Lessons from 40 years of study. Clin Microbiol Infect 2005;11(Suppl 5): 24–29.

3. Viscoli C, Varnier O, Machetti M. Infections in patients with febrile neutropenia: Epidemiology, microbiology, and risk stratification. Clin Infect Dis 2005;40(Suppl 4):S240–S245.

4. Ellis M. Febrile neutropenia. Evolving strategies. Ann NY Acad Sci 2008;1138:329–350.

5. National Comprehensive Cancer Network. Prevention and treatment of cancer-related infections. Practice Guidelines in Oncology v.2.2009; August 28, 2009. http://www.nccn.org/professionals/physician_gls/f_guidelines.asp.

6. Sullivan KM, Dykewicz CA, Longworth DL, et al. Preventing opportunistic infections after hematopoietic stem cell transplantation: The Centers for Disease Control and Prevention, Infectious Diseases Society of America, and American Society for Blood and Marrow Transplantation practice guidelines and beyond. Hematology Am Soc Hematol Educ Program 2001;392–421.

7. Rolston KVI. Challenges in the treatment of infections caused by Gram-positive and Gram-negative bacteria in patients with cancer and neutropenia. Clin Infect Dis 2005;40(Suppl 4):S246–S252.

8. Toussaint E, Bahel-Ball E, Vekemans M, et al. Causes of fever in cancer patients (prospective study over 477 episodes). Support Care Cancer 2006;14:763–769.

9. Feld R. Bloodstream infections in cancer patients with febrile neutropenia. Int J Antimicrob Agents 2008;32(Suppl):S30–S33.

10. Neuburger S, Maschmeyer G. Update on the management of infections in cancer and stem cell transplant patients. Ann Hematol 2006;85:345–356.

11. Horn DL, Neofytos D, Anaissie EJ, et al. Epidemiology and outcomes of candidemia in 2019 patients: data from the prospective antifungal therapy alliance registry. Clin Infect Dis 2009;48:1695–1703.

12. Hicks KL, Chemaly RF, Kontoyiannis DP. Common community respiratory viruses in patients with cancer: More than just "common colds." Cancer 2003;97:2576–2587.

13. Antoniadou A, Giamarellou H. Fever of unknown origin in febrile leukopenia. Infect Dis Clin N Am 2007;21:1055–1090.

14. Safdar A. Managing opportunistic infections against the odds of neutropenia. Abstr Hematol Oncol 2003;6:20–26.

15. O'Brien SN, Blijlevens NMA, Mahfouz TH, Anaissie EJ. Infections in patients with hematological cancer: Recent developments. Hematology Am Soc Hematol Educ Program 2003;438–472.

16. Pascoe J, Cullen M. The prevention of febrile neutropenia. Curr Opin Hematol 2006;18:325–329.

17. Viscoli C, Cometta A, Kern WV, et al. Piperacillin-tazobactam monotherapy in high-risk febrile neutropenic cancer patients. Clin Microbiol Infect 2006;12:212–216.

18. Klastersky J, Ameye L, Maertens J, et al. Bacteraemia in febrile neutropenic cancer patients. Int J Antimicrob Agents 2007;30(Suppl 1):S51–S59.

19. U.S. Department of Public Health and Human Services, Public Health Service. National Nosocomial Infections Surveillance (NNIS) System Report, data summary from January 1992 through June 2004, issued October 2004. Am J Infect Control 2004;32:470–485.

20. Moran GJ, Amil RN, Abrahamian FM, Talan DA. Methicillin-resistant Staphylococcus aureus in community-acquired skin infections. Emerg Infect Dis 2005;11:928–930.

21. King MD, Humphrey BJ, Wang YF, et al. Emergence of community-acquired methicillin-resistant Staphylococcus aureus USA 300 clone as the predominant cause of skin and soft-tissue infections. Ann Intern Med 2006;144:309–317.

22. Reilly AF, Lange BJ. Infections with viridans group streptococci in children with cancer. Pediatr Blood Cancer 2007;49:774–780.

23. Avery R, Kalaycio M, Pohlman B, et al. Early vancomycin-resistant enterococcus (VRE) bacteremia after allogeneic bone marrow transplantation is associated with a rapidly deteriorating clinical course. Bone Marrow Transplant 2005;35:497–499.

24. Engemann JJ, Carmeli Y, Cosgrove SE, et al. Adverse clinical and economic outcomes attributable to methicillin resistance among patients with Staphylococcus aureus surgical site infection. Clin Infect Dis 2003;36:592–598.

25. Bissinger AL, Einsele H, Hamprecht K, et al. Infectious pulmonary complications after stem cell transplantation or chemotherapy: Diagnostic yield of bronchoalveolar lavage. Diagn Microbiol Infect Dis 2005;52:275–280.

26. Chamilos G, Luna M, Lewis RE, et al. Invasive fungal infections in patients with hematologic malignancies in a tertiary care cancer center: an autopsy study over a 15-year period (1989–2003). Haematologica 2006; 91:986–989.

27. Pappas PG, Kauffman CA, Andes D, et al. Clinical practice guidelines for the management of candidiasis: 2009 update by the Infectious Diseases Society of America. Clin Infect Dis 2009;48:503–535.

28. Pagano L, Caira M, Candoni A, et al. The epidemiology of fungal infections in patients with hematologic malignancies: the SEIFEM-2004 study. Haematologica 2006;91:1068–1075.

29. Nucci M, Marr KA. Emerging fungal diseases. Clin Infect Dis 2005;41:521–526.

30. Malani A, Hmoud J, Chiu L, et al. Candida glabrata fungemia: Experience in a tertiary care center. Clin Infect Dis 2005;41:975–981.

31. Segal BH, Almyroudis NG, Battiwalla M, et al. Prevention and early treatment of invasive fungal infection in patients with cancer and neutropenia and in stem cell transplant recipients in the era of newer broad-spectrum antifungal agents and diagnostic adjuncts. Clin Infect Dis 2007;44:402–409.

32. Ruan S-Y, Chu C-C, Hsueh P-R. In vitro susceptibilities of invasive isolates of Candida species: rapid increase in rates of fluconazole susceptible-dose dependent Candida glabrata isolates. Antimicrob Agents Chemother 2008;52:2919–2922.

33. Walsh TJ, Anaissie EJ, Denning DW, et al. Treatment of aspergillosis: clinical practice guidelines of the Infectious Diseases Society of America. Clin Infect Dis 2008;46:327–360.

34. Vidal L, Paul M, Ben dor I, et al. Oral versus intravenous antibiotic treatment for febrile neutropenia in cancer patients: A systematic review and meta-analysis of randomized trials. J Antimicrob Chemother 2004;54:29–37.

35. Kern WV. Risk assessment and treatment of low-risk patients with febrile neutropenia. Clin Infect Dis 2006;42:533–540.

36. Moores KG. Safe and effective outpatient management of adults with chemotherapy-induced neutropenic fever. Am J Health Syst Pharm 2007;64:717–722.

37. Carstensen M, Sorensen JB. Outpatient management of febrile neutropenia: time to revise the present treatment strategy. J Support Onc 2008;6:199–208.

38. Furno P, Bucaneve G, Del Favero A. Monotherapy or aminoglycoside-containing combinations for empirical antibiotic treatment of febrile neutropenic patients: A meta-analysis. Lancet Infect Dis 2002;2:231–242.

39. Paul M, Soares-Weiser K, Grozinsky S, Leibovici L. β-Lactam versus β-lactam-aminoglycoside combination therapy in cancer patients with neutropaenia. Cochrane Database Syst Rev 2003;3:CD003038.

40. Paul M, Yahava D, Fraser A, Leibovici L. Empirical antibiotic monotherapy for febrile neutropenia: Systematic review and meta-analysis of randomized controlled trials. J Antimicrob Chemother 2006;57:176–189.

41. Glasmacher A, von Lilienfeld-Toal M, Schulte S, et al. An evidence-based evaluation of important aspects of empirical antibiotic therapy in febrile neutropenic patients. Clin Microbiol Infect 2005;11(Suppl 5):17–23.

42. Paul M, Borok S, Fraser A, et al. Additional anti-Gram-positive antibiotic treatment for febrile neutropenic cancer patients. Cochrane Database Syst Rev 2005(3);CD003914.

43. Paul M, Borok S, Fraser A, et al. Empirical antibiotics against Gram-positive infections for febrile neutropenia: Systematic review and meta-analysis of randomized controlled trials. J Antimicrob Chemother 2005;55:436–444.

44. Scheld WM. Maintaining fluoroquinolone class efficacy: Review of influencing factors. Emerging Infectious Diseases; 2004. http://www.cdc.gov/ncidod/eid/vol9no1/02-0277.htm.

45. Martino R, Viscoli C. Empirical antifungal therapy in patients with neutropenia and persistent of recurrent fever of unknown origin. Br J Haematol 2005;132:138–154.

46. Goldberg E, Gafter-Gvili A, Robenshtok E, et al. Empirical antifungal therapy for patients with neutropenia and persistent fever: Systematic review and meta-analysis. Eur J Cancer 2008;44:2192–2203.

47. Moen MD, Lyseng-Williamson KA, Scott LJ. Liposomal amphotericin B: a review of its use as empirical therapy in febrile neutropenia and in the treatment of invasive fungal infections. Drugs 2009;69:361–392.

48. Cornely OA, Maertens J, Bresnik M, et al. Liposomal amphotericin B as initial therapy for invasive mold infection: a randomized trial comparing a high-loading dose regimen with standard dosing (AmBiLoad trial). Clin Infect Dis 2007;44:1289–1297.

49. Zonios DI, Bennett JE. Update on azole antifungals. Sem Resp Crit Care Med 2008;29:198–210.

50. Rogers TR, Frost S. Newer antifungal agents for invasive fungal infections in patients with haematological malignancy. Br J Haematol 2009;144:629–641.

51. Naeger-Murphy N, Pile JC. Clinical indications for newer antifungal agents. J Hosp Med 2009;4:102–111.

52. Smith TJ, Khatcheressian J, Lyman GH, et al. 2006 update of recommendations for the use of white blood cell growth factors: an evidence-based clinical practice guideline. J Clin Oncol 2006;24:3187–3205.

53. Clark OA, Lyman G, Castro AA, et al. Colony-stimulating factors for chemotherapy-induced febrile neutropenia. Cochrane Database Syst Rev 2003;3:CD003039.

54. National Comprehensive Cancer Network. Myeloid growth factors. National Comprehensive Cancer Network. Fever and neutropenia. Practice Guidelines in Oncology v.1.2010; December 7, 2009. http://www.nccn.org/professionals/physician_gls/f_guidelines.asp.

55. Atallah E, Schiffer CA. Granulocyte transfusion. Curr Opin Hematol 2006;13:45–49.

56. Seidel MG, Peters C, Wacker A, et al. Randomized phase III study of granulocyte transfusions in neutropenic patients. Bone Marrrow Transplant 2008;42:679–684.

57. Gafter-Gvili A, Paul M, Fraser A, Leibovici L. Effect of quinolone prophylaxis in afebrile neutropenic patients on microbial resis-

tance: Systematic review and meta-analysis. J Antimicrob Chemother 2007;59:5–22.

58. Leibovici L, Paul M, Cullen M, et al. Antibiotic prophylaxis in neutropenic patients: new evidence, practical decisions. Cancer 2006;107:1743–1751.

59. Aaproa MS, Cameron DA, Pettengell R, et al. EORTC guidelines for the use of granulocyte-colony stimulating factor to reduce the incidence of chemotherapy-induced febrile neutropenia in adult patients with lymphomas and solid tumours. Eur J Cancer 2006;42:2433–2453.

60. Cornely OA, Ullmann AJ, Karthaus M. Evidence-based assessment of primary antifungal prophylaxis in patients with hematologic malignancies. Blood 2003;101:3365–3372.

61. Bow EJ, Laverdiere M, Lussier N, et al. Antifungal prophylaxis for severely neutropenic chemotherapy recipients: A meta-analysis of randomized-controlled clinical trials. Cancer 2002;94:3230–3246.

62. Rotstein C, Bow EJ, Laverdiere M, et al. Randomized placebo-controlled trial of fluconazole prophylaxis for neutropenic cancer patients: Benefit based on purpose and intensity of cytotoxic therapy. Clin Infect Dis 1999;28:331–340.

63. Ullmann AJ, Cornely OA. Antifungal prophylaxis for invasive mycoses in high risk patients. Curr Opin Infect Dis 2006;19:571–576.

64. Stokes ME, Muehlenbein CE, Marciniak MD, et al. Neutropenia-related costs in patients treated with first-line chemotherapy for advanced non-small cell lung cancer. J Manag Care Pharm 2009;15:669–682.

65. van Tiel FH, Harbers MM, Kessels AG, Schouten HC. Home care versus hospital care of patients with hematological malignancies and chemotherapy-induced cytopenia. Ann Oncol 2005;16:195–205.

66. Gratwohl A, Brand R, Frassoni F, et al. Cause of death after allogeneic hematopoietic stem cell transplantation (HSCT) in early leukemias: An EBMT analysis of lethal infectious complications and changes over calendar time. Bone Marrow Transplant 2005;36:757–769.

67. Afessa B, Peters SG. Major complications following hematopoietic stem cell transplantation. Semin Respir Crit Care Med 2006;27:297–309.

68. Mitchell AE, Derrington P, Turner P, et al. Gram-negative bacteraemia (GNB) after 428 unrelated donor bone marrow transplants (UDBMT): Risk factors, prophylaxis, therapy, and outcome. Bone Marrow Transplant 2004;33:303–310.

69. Camps IR. Risk factors for invasive fungal infections in haematopoietic stem cell transplantation. Int J Antimicrob Agents 2008;32(Suppl 2):S119–S123.

70. Bhatti Z, Shaukat A, Almyroudis NG, Segal BH. Review of epidemiology, diagnosis, and treatment of invasive mould infections in allogeneic hematopoietic stem cell transplant recipients. Mycopathologia 2006;162:1–15.

71. Angarone M. Ison MG. Prevention and early treatment of opportunistic viral infections in patients with leukemia and allogeneic stem cell transplantation recipients. J Nat Comprehens Cancer Net 2008;6:191–201.

72. Neuburger S, Maschmeyer G. Update on management of infections in cancer and stem cell transplant patients. Ann Hematol 2006;85:345–356.

73. Razonable RR, Paya CV. Valganciclovir for the prevention and treatment of cytomegalovirus disease in immunocompromised hosts. Expert Rev Anti Infect Ther 2004;2:27–42.

74. Einsele H, Reusser P, Bornhaeuser M, et al. Oral valganciclovir leads to higher exposure to ganciclovir than intravenous ganciclovir in patients following allogeneic stem cell transplantation. Blood 2006;107:3002–3008.

75. Orange JS, Hossny EM, Weiler CR, et al. Use of intravenous immunoglobulin in human disease: A review of evidence by members of the Primary Immunodeficiency Committee of the American Academy of Allergy, Asthma, and Immunology. J Allergy Clin Immunol 2006;117:S525–S553.

76. Raanani P, Gafter-Gvili A, Paul M, et al. Immunoglobulin prophylaxis in hematopoietic stem cell transplantation: systematic review and meta-analysis. J Clin Oncol 2008;27:770–781.

77. Crumpacker CS, Wadhwa S. Cytomegalovirus. In: Mandell GL, Bennett JE, Dolin R, eds. Principles and Practice of Infectious Diseases, 6th ed. New York: Churchill Livingstone, 2005:1786–1801.

78. Strasfeld L, Weinstock DM. Antifungal prophylaxis among allogeneic hematopoietic stem cell transplant recipients: Current issues and new agents. Expert Rev Anti Infect Ther 2006;4:457–468.

79. Michallet M, Ito JI. Approaches to the management of invasive fungal infections in hematological malignancy and hematopoietic cell transplantation. J Clin Oncol 2009;27:3398–3409.

80. Nucci M, Anaissie E. Fungal infections in hematopoietic stem cell transplantation and solid-organ transplantation – focus on aspergillosis. Clin Chest Med 2009;30:295–306.

81. Winston DJ, Maziarz RT, Chandrasekar PH, et al. Intravenous and oral itraconazole versus intravenous and oral fluconazole for long-term antifungal prophylaxis in allogeneic hematopoietic stem-cell transplant recipients: A multicenter, randomized trial. Ann Intern Med 2003;138:705–713.

82. Mele A, Paterson PJ, Prentice HG, et al: Toxoplasmosis in bone marrow transplantation: A report of two cases and systematic review of the literature. Bone Marrow Transplant 2002;29:691–698.

83. Fishman JA. Infection in solid-organ transplant recipients. N Engl J Med 2007;357:2601–2614.

84. Varon NF, Alangaden GJ. Emerging trends in infections among renal transplant recipients. Expert Rev Anti Infect Ther 2004;2:95–109.

85. Issa NC, Fishman JA. Infectious complications of antilymphocyte therapies in solid organ transplantation. Clin Infect Dis 2009;48:772–786.

86. Singh N. Fungal infections in the recipients of solid organ transplantation. Infect Dis Clin North Am 2003;17:113–134.

87. San Juan R, Aguado JM, Lumbreras C, et al. Incidence, clinical characteristics and risk factors of late infection in solid organ transplant recipients: data from the RESITRA study group. Am J Transplant 2007;7:964–971.

88. Kotton CN. Zoonoses in solid-organ and hematopoietic stem cell transplant recipients. Clin Infect Dis 2007;44:857–866.

89. Kotton CN, Fishman JA. Viral infection in the renal transplant recipient. J Am Soc Nephrol 2005;16:1758–1774.

90. Pescovitz MD. Benefits of cytomegalovirus prophylaxis in solid organ transplantation. Transplantation 2006;82:S4–S8.

91. Jancel T, Penzak SR. Antiviral therapy in patients with hematologic malignancies, transplantation, and aplastic anemia. Semin Hematol 2009;46:230–247.

92. Kalil AC, Levitsky J, Lyden E, et al. Meta-analysis: the efficacy of strategies to prevent organ disease by cytomegalovirus in solid organ transplant recipients. Ann Intern Med 2005;143:870–880.

93. Torres-Madriz G, Boucher HW. Immunocompromised hosts: perspectives in the treatment and prophylaxis of cytomegalovirus disease in solid-organ transplant recipients. Clin Infect Dis 2008;47:702–711.

94. Roland ME, Adey D, Carlson LL, Terrault NA. Kidney and liver transplantation in HIV-infected patients: Case presentations and review. AIDS Patient Care STDs 2003;17:501–507.

95. Strippoli GFM, Hodson EM, Jones C, Craig JC. Preemptive treatment for cytomegalovirus viremia to prevent cytomegalovirus disease in solid organ transplant recipients. Transplantation 2006;81:139–145.

96. Hanson K, Alexander B. Strategies for the prevention of infection after solid organ transplantation. Expert Rev Anti Infect Ther 2006;4:837–852.

97. Infectious Diseases Community of Practice of the American Society of Transplantation. Cytomegalovirus. Am J Transplant 2004;4(Suppl 10):51–58.

98. Green H, Paul M, Vidal L, Leibovici L. Prophylaxis for Pneumocystis pneumonia (PCP) in non-HIV immunocompromised patients. Cochrane Database Syst Rev 2007(3);CD005590.

99. Bassetti M, Righi E, Bassetti D. Antimicrobial prophylaxis in solid-organ transplantation. Expert Rev Antiinfect Ther 2004;2:761–769.

132

Antimicrobial Prophylaxis in Surgery

SALMAAN KANJI

KEY CONCEPTS

❶ Prophylactic antibiotic therapy differs from presumptive and therapeutic antibiotic therapy in that the latter two involve treatment regimens for documented or presumed infections, whereas the goal of prophylactic therapy is to prevent infections in high-risk patients or procedures.

❷ The risk of a surgical site infection (SSI) is determined from both the type of surgery and the patient-specific risk factors; however, most commonly used classification systems account for only procedure-related risk factors.

❸ The timing of antimicrobial prophylaxis is of paramount importance. Antibiotics should be administered within 1 hour before surgery to ensure adequate drug levels at the surgical site prior to the initial incision.

❹ Antimicrobial agents with short half-lives (e.g., cefazolin) may require intraoperative redosing during long (>3 hours) procedures.

❺ The type of surgery, intrinsic patient risk factors, most commonly identified pathogenic organisms, institutional antimicrobial resistance patterns, and cost must be considered when choosing an antimicrobial agent for prophylaxis.

❻ Single-dose prophylaxis is appropriate for many types of surgery. First-generation cephalosporins (e.g., cefazolin) are the mainstay for prophylaxis in most surgical procedures because of their spectrum of activity, safety, and cost.

❼ Vancomycin as a prophylactic agent should be limited to patients with a documented history of life-threatening β-lactam hypersensitivity or those in whom the incidence of infections with organisms resistant to cefazolin (e.g., methicillin-resistant *Staphylococcus aureus*) is high enough to justify use.

According to the National Center for Health Statistics, some 46 million surgical procedures are performed annually in the United States, the majority of which are done in an outpatient setting.[1] Infection is the most common complication of surgery.[2] Surgical site infections (SSIs) occur in ~3% to 6% of patients and prolong hospitalization by an average of 7 days at a direct annual cost of $5

billion to $10 billion.[3,4] SSIs are the third (14–16%) most frequent cause of nosocomial infections among hospitalized patients and the primary (40%) cause of nosocomial infection in surgical patients.[3] Prophylactic administration of antibiotics decreases the risk of infection after many surgical procedures and represents an important component of care for this population.

Antibiotics administered prior to the contamination of previously sterile tissues or fluids are called prophylactic antibiotics. The goal of therapy is to prevent an infection from developing. Although eradication of distal (preexisting, unrelated to surgery) infections lowers the risk for subsequent postoperative infections, it does not per se constitute a prophylactic regimen. In fact, surgical prophylaxis often is prescribed concurrently under these circumstances because of important antimicrobial spectrum- and timing-related concerns. Both SSIs and infections not directly related to the surgical site (e.g., urinary tract infections and pneumonia) are termed *nosocomial*. Prevention of hospital-acquired infections is a major goal of antibiotic prophylaxis.

❶ Presumptive antibiotic therapy is administered when an infection is suspected but not yet proven. Clinical scenarios where presumptive therapy is used commonly include acute cholecystitis, open compound fractures, and acute appendicitis of less than 24 hours' duration. In these situations, if signs of perforation or infection are absent during surgery, then routine prophylactic treatment rather than presumptive therapy is warranted. An operative finding of a gangrenous gallbladder or a perforated appendix, however, is suggestive of an established infectious process, and a therapeutic antibiotic regimen is required.[3]

According to the Centers for Disease Control and Prevention's (CDC) National Nosocomial Infections Surveillance System (NNIS),[3] SSIs can be categorized as either incisional (e.g., cellulitis of the incision site) or organ/space (e.g., meningitis; Fig. 132–1). Incisional SSIs are subcategorized into superficial (involving only the skin or subcutaneous tissue) and deep (fascial and muscle layers) infections. Organ/space SSIs can involve any anatomic area other than the incision site. For example, a patient who develops bacterial peritonitis after bowel surgery has an organ/space SSI. By definition, SSIs must occur within 30 days of surgery. If a prosthetic implant is involved, a deep incisional or organ/space SSI can be reported up to 1 year from the date of surgery. Although microbiologic testing of surgical drainage material or sites may help to guide care, the specificity of a negative culture is poor and generally does not rule out an SSI.[3]

RISK FACTORS FOR SURGICAL SITE INFECTIONS

❷ SSI incidence depends on both procedure- and patient-related factors. Traditionally, the risk for SSIs has been stratified by surgical procedure in a classification system developed by the National

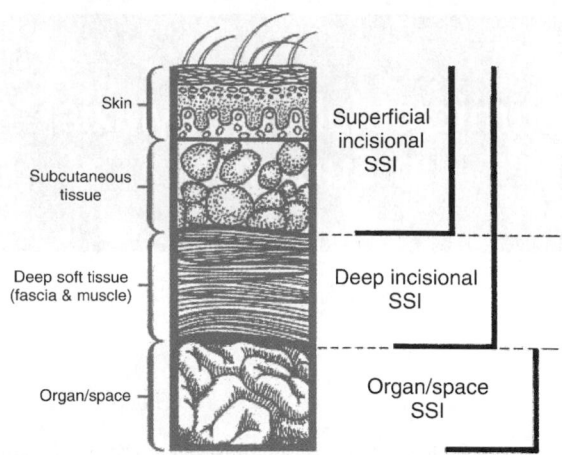

FIGURE 132-1. Cross section of abdominal wall depicting Centers for Disease Control and Prevention classifications of surgical site infections (SSI). *(Reprinted from Mangram AJ, Horan TC, Pearson ML, et al. Guideline for prevention of surgical site infection. Am J Infect Control 1999;27:97–132 with permission from Elsevier. Centers for Disease Control and Prevention (CDC) Hospital Infection Control Practices Advisory Committee, Copyright 1999, with permission from the Association for Professionals in Infection Control and Epidemiology.)*

Research Council (NRC; Table 132–1).[5] The NRC classification system proposes that the risk of an SSI depends on the microbiology of the surgical site, the presence of a preexisting infection, the likelihood of contaminating previously sterile tissue during surgery, and the events during and after surgery.[5,6] A patient's NRC procedure classification is the primary determinant of whether antibiotic prophylaxis is warranted. However, because a patient's NRC wound classification is influenced by surgical findings (e.g., gangrenous gallbladder) and perioperative events (e.g., major technique breaks), categorization generally occurs intraoperatively.[7]

INHERENT PATIENT RISK

The NRC classification system does not account for the influence of underlying patient risk factors for SSI development, instead categorizing the risks for SSIs simply based on a specific surgical procedure. Disease states and conditions known to increase SSI risk are listed in Table 132–2. Preexisting distal infections increase SSI rates and should be resolved prior to surgery whenever possible. Diabetic patients have an increased risk for SSIs, especially those with uncontrolled perioperative blood sugars. Preoperative smoking has been identified as an independent risk factor for SSI because

of the deleterious effects of nicotine on wound healing. Preoperative immunosuppression, including corticosteroid use, may increase infection risk. Patients co-infected with human immunodeficiency virus (HIV) and hepatitis C are at approximately double the risk of SSI as the general population.[8] Malnutrition is a well-described risk factor for postoperative complications, including SSI, impaired wound and colonic anastomosis healing, and prolonged hospital stay. Although enteral feeding during the perioperative period can reduce bacterial translocation by maintaining the integrity of the intestinal mucosa, nutritional supplementation does not decrease the incidence of infection.[9]

Colonization of the nares with *Staphylococcus aureus* is a well-described SSI risk factor.[3] Although intranasal application of mupirocin ointment reduces the rate of nasal carriage of *S. aureus*, one large, randomized, double-blind study of 4,030 surgical patients found that prophylactic intranasal mupirocin did not reduce the rate of *S. aureus* SSI, although it did reduce the rate of nosocomial *S. aureus* infections among patients who were *S. aureus* carriers.[10] Other factors shown to increase the risk of SSI are age, length of preoperative hospital stay, and obesity.[3]

IDENTIFYING SSI RISK

Two large epidemiologic studies have objectively quantified SSI risk based on specific patient- and procedure-related factors. The Study on the Efficacy of Nosocomial Infection Control (SENIC) analyzed more than 100,000 surgery cases to identify and validate risk factors for SSI.[11] Abdominal operations, operations lasting longer than 2 hours, contaminated or "dirty" procedures (as per NRC classification), and more than three underlying medical diagnoses each was associated with an increased incidence of SSI. When NRC classification was stratified by number of SENIC risk factors present, SSI incidence varied by as much as a factor of 15 within the same NRC operative category (Table 132–3).[12]

In a subsequent analysis of more than 84,000 surgical cases, the NNIS attempted to simplify and refine the SENIC system by quantifying intrinsic patient risk using the American Society of Anesthesiologists' (ASA) preoperative assessment score (Table 132–4).[14,15] An ASA score ≥3 was a strong predictor for the development of an SSI. Other factors associated with increased SSI incidence are contaminated or "dirty" operations (NRC criteria) and surgical procedures lasting longer than average. As in the SENIC study, the SSI rate was linked to the number of risk factors present and varied considerably within NRC class. The NNIS basic SSI risk index is composed of the following criteria: ASA score = 3, 4, or 5; wound class; and duration of surgery. Overall, for 34 of the 44 NNIS procedure categories, SSI rates increased proportionally

TABLE 132-1	National Research Council Wound Classification, Risk of Surgical Site Infection, and Indication for Antibiotics

| | SSI Rate (%) | | | |
Classification	Preoperative Antibiotics	No Preoperative Antibiotics	Criteria	Antibiotics
Clean	5.1	0.8	No acute inflammation or transection of GI, oropharyngeal, genitourinary, biliary, or respiratory tracts; elective case, no technique break	Not indicated unless high-risk procedure[a]
Clean–contaminated	10.1	1.3	Controlled opening of aforementioned tracts with minimal spillage/minor technique break; clean procedures performed emergently or with major technique breaks	Prophylactic antibiotics indicated
Contaminated	21.9	10.2	Acute, nonpurulent inflammation present; major spillage/technique break during clean–contaminated procedure	Prophylactic antibiotics indicated
Dirty	N/A	N/A	Obvious preexisting infection present (abscess, pus, or necrotic tissue present)	Therapeutic antibiotics required

[a]High-risk procedures include implantation of prosthetic materials and other procedures where surgical site infection is associated with high morbidity (see text).
GI = gastrointestinal; N/A = not applicable; SSI = surgical site infection.
Adapted from National Academy of Sciences, National Research Council. Postoperative wound infections: The influence of ultraviolet irradiation of the operating room and of various other factors. Ann Surg 1964;160:32–135; and Haley RW, Culver DH, Morgan WM, et al. Identifying patients at high risk of surgical wound infection: A simple multivariate index of patient susceptibility and wound contamination. Am J Epidemiol 1985;127:206–215.

TABLE 132-2	Patient and Operation Characteristics That May Influence the Risk of Surgical Site Infection
Patient	**Operation**
Age	Duration of surgical scrub
Nutritional status	Preoperative skin preparation
Diabetes	Preoperative shaving
Smoking	Duration of operation
Obesity	Antimicrobial prophylaxis
Coexisting infections at distal body sites	Operating room ventilation
Colonization with resistant microorganisms	Sterilization of instruments
Altered immune response	Implantation of prosthetic materials
Length of preoperative stay	Surgical drains
	Surgical technique

Reprinted from Mangram AJ, Horan TC, Pearson ML, et al. Guideline for prevention of surgical site infection. Am J Infect Control 1999;27,97–132 with permission from Elsevier. Centers for Disease Control and Prevention (CDC) Hospital Infection Control Practices Advisory Committee, Copyright 1999, with permission from the Association for Professionals in Infection Control and Epidemiology.

with the number of risk factors present.[13] The SSI rate was generally lower when the procedure was done laparoscopically.

Although evidence-based recommendations for antimicrobial prophylaxis during surgery are best established using the results of randomized clinical trials, many studies have small sample sizes and do not stratify patients according to overall SSI risk. Future studies, particularly those involving clean procedures, should be stratified by SSI risk so that the subset of high-risk patients who might benefit the most from prophylaxis is clearly established.

BACTERIOLOGY

The most important consideration when choosing antibiotic prophylaxis is the bacteriology of the surgical site. Organisms involved in an SSI are acquired by one of two ways: endogenously (from the patient's own normal flora) or exogenously (from contamination during the surgical procedure). Based on the type and anatomic location of the procedure and the NRC classification (see Table 132-1), resident flora can be predicted and appropriate antibiotic choices made. According to NNIS data, *S. aureus,* coagulase-negative staphylococci, enterococci, *Escherichia coli,* and *Pseudomonas aeruginosa* are the pathogens most commonly isolated (Table 132-5).[14] With the widespread use of broad-spectrum antibiotics, however, *Candida* species and methicillin-resistant *S. aureus* (MRSA) are becoming more prevalent.[14]

Factors affecting the ability of an organism to induce an SSI depend on organism count, organism virulence, and host immunocompetency. Organisms in the commensal flora generally are

TABLE 132-3	Surgical Site Infection Incidence (%) Stratified by NRC Wound Classification and SENIC Risk Factors[a]

No. of SENIC Risk Factors	Clean	Clean–Contaminated	Contaminated	Dirty
0	1.1	0.6	N/A	N/A
1	3.9	2.8	4.5	6.7
2	8.4	8.4	8.3	10.9
3	15.8	17.7	11.0	18.8
4	N/A	N/A	23.9	27.4

[a]Study on the Efficacy of Nosocomial Infection Control (SENIC) risk factors include abdominal operation, operations lasting >2 hours, contaminated or dirty procedures by National Research Council (NRC) classification, and more than three underlying medical diagnoses.
N/A = not applicable.
Reprinted from Gaynes RP, Culver DH, Horan TC, et al. Surgical site infection (SSI) rates in the United States, 1992–1998: The national nosocomial infections surveillance system basic SSI risk index. Clin Infect Dis 2001;33(Suppl 2):S69–S77 with permission.

TABLE 132-4	American Society of Anesthesiologists' Physical Status Classification

Class	Description
1	Normal healthy patient
2	Mild systemic disease
3	Severe systemic disease that is not incapacitating
4	Incapacitating systemic disease that is a constant threat to life
5	Not expected to survive 24 hours with or without operation

From Owens WD, Felts JA, Spitznagel EL: ASA physical status classifications: A study of consistency of ratings. Anesthesiology 1978;49:239–243.

not pathogenic. These organisms often serve the host as a form of protection against invasive organisms that otherwise would colonize the surgical site. Opportunistic organisms usually are kept in check by normal flora and rarely are problematic unless they are present in large numbers. The loss of normal flora through the use of broad-spectrum antibiotics can destabilize homeostasis, allowing pathogenic bacteria to proliferate and infection to occur.[4]

Normal flora translocated to a normally sterile tissue site or fluid during a surgical procedure can become pathogenic. For example, *S. aureus* or *Staphylococcus epidermidis* may be translocated from the surface of the skin to deeper tissues or *E. coli* from the colon to the peritoneal cavity, bloodstream, or urinary tract. Studies in animals and healthy volunteers have shown bacterial virulence to be an important determinant in the development of secondary infections.[16,17] Whereas more than one million *S. aureus* per square centimeter or gram of tissue are required to produce infection in animals, less than 100,000 *Streptococcus pyogenes* per square centimeter or gram of tissue are required at the same site.[17,18]

Impaired host defense reduces the number of bacteria required to establish an infection. A breach of normal host defenses through surgical intervention (e.g., insertion of a prosthetic device) may enable organisms to cause infection. In addition, the loss of specific immune factors, such as complement activation, tissue-derived inhibitors (e.g., proinflammatory cytokines), cell-mediated response (e.g., T-cell function), and granulocytic or phagocytic function (e.g., neutrophils or macrophages) can greatly increase the risk for SSI development.[19] Vascular occlusive states related to the surgical procedure or those occurring from hypovolemic shock can greatly affect blood flow to the surgical site, thus diminishing host defense mechanisms against microbial invasion. Traumatized

TABLE 132-5	Major Pathogens in Surgical Wound Infections

Pathogen	Percent of Infections[a]
Staphylococcus aureus	20
Coagulase-negative staphylococci	14
Enterococci	12
Escherichia coli	8
Pseudomonas aeruginosa	8
Enterobacter species	7
Proteus mirabilis	3
Klebsiella pneumoniae	3
Other *Streptococcus* species	3
Candida albicans	3
Group D streptococci	2
Other gram-positive aerobes	2
Bacteroides fragilis	2

[a]Data reported by the National Nosocomial Infections Surveillance System from January 1992 through June 2004.

Adapted from National Academy of Sciences, National Research Council. Postoperative wound infections: The influence of ultraviolet irradiation of the operating room and of various other factors. Ann Surg 1964;160:32–135.

tissue, hematomas, and the presence of foreign material also lead to more infections. When a foreign body is introduced during a surgical procedure, fewer than 100 bacterial colony-forming units are required to cause an SSI.[20] Studies examining *S. aureus*–contaminated wound infections on the skin of healthy volunteers demonstrate a 10,000-fold reduction in the number of organisms required to establish a wound infection if sutures are not present.[16]

ANTIMICROBIAL RESISTANCE

Colonization of the host with antibiotic-resistant hospital flora prior to or during surgery may lead to an SSI that is unresponsive to routine antibiotic therapy. The most common cause of nosocomially acquired multiresistant organisms is transmission from hospital personnel.[21] Patients treated with broad-spectrum antibiotic therapy are at increased risk for colonization with hospital flora.

With cephalosporins established as first-line agents for prophylaxis over the past decade, organisms resistant to cephalosporins represent the majority of pathogens causing SSIs. The CDC has reported an alarming increase in the incidence of vancomycin-resistant enterococci (VRE) infections, particularly those with *Enterococcus faecium*.[3] Risk factors for VRE colonization include severe concomitant diseases, immunosuppression, admission to the intensive care unit (ICU), previous intraabdominal or cardiothoracic surgery, placement of indwelling catheters, and prolonged courses of antimicrobials, ❼ particularly vancomycin.[22,23] In an effort to control the spread of VRE, the CDC has published recommendations that include strict criteria for use of vancomycin as surgical prophylaxis.[23] The guidelines suggest vancomycin substitution for cefazolin as SSI prophylaxis only in cases with a high suspicion of MRSA or in patients with a documented history of a life-threatening allergy to penicillins or cephalosporins. Other limitations to vancomycin use, other than risk of inducing resistant organisms, are the drug's narrow spectrum of activity, its poor penetration into some tissues, and the potential for infusion-related reactions.

The emergence of *S. aureus* displaying intermediate resistance (minimum inhibitory concentration [MIC] ≥ 8 mcg/mL) further underscores the need to limit routine use of vancomycin for prophylaxis. Methicillin resistance not only limits the options available to treat these infections but is associated with mortality rates twice that of patients with infections caused by methicillin-sensitive *S. aureus* (MSSA).[24] Postoperative factors associated with MRSA include discharge to a long-term care facility and duration of postoperative antibiotic treatment for more than 1 day.[25] Although the use of vancomycin for prophylaxis may be appropriate for some operations performed in hospitals with a high rate of infection due to MRSA, there is little guidance on what constitutes a "high rate" of MRSA infection and whether providing prophylaxis with vancomycin alone will result in fewer SSIs.[26]

Although cefazolin remains a mainstay in cardiovascular SSI prophylaxis, its failure has been reported in cases involving MSSA. In a comparison trial between cefamandole and cefazolin, significantly more failures were attributed to cefazolin, even though the primary pathogen was MSSA.[27] However, a similar trial comparing cefazolin and cefuroxime did not show any difference in SSI incidence between the two regimens.[27] It has been proposed that the β-lactamase expressed by some MSSA is capable of hydrolyzing cefazolin more readily than cefuroxime or cefamandole. Although this trend is disturbing, the overall incidence of cefazolin failure remains low, and cefazolin remains the drug of choice for SSI prophylaxis in cardiovascular surgery.[27]

The increase in frequency of fungal infections in surgical patients has drawn concern. In hospitalized patients, the incidence of nosocomial *Candida* infections nearly doubled from 1992 to 2004.[14,28]

Overzealous use of broad-spectrum antibiotics is the most likely cause for this increase. A study of patients undergoing cardiovascular surgery identified sex (female), length of stay in the ICU, and duration of central venous catheterization as risk factors for postoperative *Candida* infections.[29] Although presurgical *Candida* colonization is associated with a higher risk of fungal SSIs, routine preoperative use of prophylactic antifungal agents is not being advocated at this time.[28,30]

SCHEDULING ANTIBIOTIC ADMINISTRATION

❸ ❹ The following principles must be considered when providing antimicrobial surgical prophylaxis: (a) the agents should be delivered to the surgical site prior to the initial incision, and (b) bactericidal antibiotic concentrations should be maintained at the surgical site throughout the surgical procedure. Although animal and human models have demonstrated the efficacy of a single dose of an antibiotic administered just prior to bacterial contamination, long operations often require intraoperative doses of antibiotics to maintain adequate concentrations at the surgical site for the duration of surgery.[31] Antibiotics should be administered with anesthesia just prior to the initial incision. Administration of antibiotics too early may result in concentrations below the MIC toward the end of the operation, and administration too late leaves the patient unprotected at the time of initial incision. In a study examining the timing of antibiotic administration to 2,847 patients receiving prophylaxis, Classen et al[31] evaluated patients who received prophylaxis early (2–24 hours before surgery), preoperative prophylaxis (0–2 hours prior to surgery), perioperative prophylaxis (up to 3 hours after first incision), and postoperative prophylaxis (>3 hours after first incision). The risk of infection was lowest (0.6%) for patients who received preoperative prophylaxis, moderate (1.4%) for those who received perioperative antibiotics, and greatest for those who received postoperative antibiotics (3.3%) or preoperative antibiotics too early (3.8%). The risk for an SSI increases dramatically with each hour from the time of initial incision to the time when antibiotics are eventually administered. For these reasons, prophylactic antibiotics should not be prescribed to be given "on call to the operating room (OR)," which can occur 2 or more hours prior to the initial incision, nor should concurrent therapeutic antibiotics be relied on to provide adequate protection. In both situations, the chance for improperly timed doses is high. Although the landmark study by Classen et al.[31] confirmed that antimicrobial prophylaxis should be administered within 2 hours prior to the initial incision, administration immediately prior to the incision may not allow enough time for the drug to distribute throughout the tissues involved in the surgery.

In a large prospective observational study of 3,836 visceral, trauma, and vascular surgeries where antimicrobial prophylaxis with cefuroxime and metronidazole was employed, the incidence of SSIs was analyzed according to the timing of antimicrobial administration. When antimicrobial prophylaxis was administered within 30 minutes or between 1 and 2 hours before the initial incision, the risk of SSI was greater when compared to antimicrobial prophylaxis administered 30 to 59 minutes prior to the initial incision. The authors conclude that the optimal window for antimicrobial (cefuroxime and metronidazole) is between 30 and 59 minutes prior to the initial incision.[32] This effect may be a function of the pharmacodynamics and pharmacokinetics of the antimicrobial chosen for the prophylactic regimen. A larger study of 4,472 patients undergoing cardiac, orthopedic, and gynecologic surgery with a variety of antimicrobial prophylactic regimens also evaluated the temporal relationship between SSI occurrence and the timing of antibiotics. After excluding patients who received drugs with prolonged infusion times (i.e., fluoroquinolones and vancomycin), there was a statistically nonsignificant trend toward fewer SSIs in patients who received their prophylactic regimen within the 30 minutes prior to incision as compared with those who received the regimen 31 to 60 minutes prior to incision (odds ratio, OR: 1.74; 95% confidence interval: 0.98–3.04).[33]

Despite the importance of appropriately timed prophylactic antibiotic therapy, few patients receive antibiotics at the optimal time in relation to surgery. Potential barriers include antibiotics ordered after the patient has arrived in the OR, delayed antibiotic preparation or delivery, and use of antibiotics that require long infusion times. One study assessed the timing of prophylactic antibiotics in 100 patients and found that only 26% of patients received an antibiotic dose within 2 hours of the initial surgical incision.[34]

Although most studies comparing single versus multiple doses of prophylactic antibiotics have failed to show a benefit of multidose regimens, the duration of operations in these studies may not be as long as that frequently observed in clinical practice. Proponents of administering a second antibiotic dose during lengthy operations suggest that the risk for SSI is just as great at the end of surgery (during wound closing) as it is during the initial incision. One study of patients undergoing clean-contaminated operations suggests that procedures longer than 3 hours require a second intraoperative dose of cefazolin or substitution of cefazolin with a longer-acting antimicrobial agent.[4] A second study of patients undergoing elective colorectal surgery suggests that low serum antimicrobial concentrations at the time of surgical closure is the strongest predictor of postoperative SSI.[35] Studies of patients undergoing cardiac surgery also have demonstrated a higher infection rate among patients with undetectable antibiotic serum concentrations at the conclusion of the procedure.[36]

One strategy to ensure appropriate redosing of prophylactic antibiotics during long operations is use of a visual or auditory reminder system. One hospital reported its experience with such a system, finding that an automated reminder improved compliance and reduced SSIs. However, even with the reminder system, intraoperative redosing was done in only 68% of eligible patients.[37] Another strategy currently being evaluated is the role of continuous infusions of cefazolin, which one pilot study has found to be a feasible way to ensure adequate serum concentrations of antibiotic during prolonged surgeries.[38] Further trials are required before such an intervention can be recommended.

Underlying disease states that may affect antibiotic metabolism and/or elimination should be considered when developing a prophylactic regimen. For example, patients with thermal burn and spinal cord injuries eliminate certain classes of antibiotics, primarily the aminoglycosides and β-lactams, at unusually high rates compared with controls.[39] Individuals undergoing cardiac bypass may have altered antibiotic disposition related to increased volume of distribution and reduced total body clearance and thus require special dosing consideration.[40]

ANTIMICROBIAL CHOICE

⑤ The choice of prophylactic antibiotic depends on the type of surgical procedure, the most frequent pathogens seen with this procedure, safety and efficacy profiles of the antimicrobial agent, current literature evidence supporting its use, and cost. Although most SSIs involve the patient's normal flora, antimicrobial selection also must take into account the susceptibility patterns of nosocomial pathogens within each institution. Typically, gram-positive coverage should be included in the choice of surgical prophylaxis because organisms such as S. aureus and S. epidermidis are encountered commonly as skin flora. The decision to broaden antibiotic prophylaxis to agents

with gram-negative and anaerobic spectra of activity depends on both the surgical site (e.g., upper respiratory, gastrointestinal (GI), or genitourinary tract) and whether the operation will transect a hollow viscous or mucous membrane that may contain resident flora.[3]

Although antimicrobial prophylaxis can be administered through a variety of routes (e.g., oral, topical, or intramuscular), the parenteral route is favored because of the reliability by which adequate tissue concentrations may be acheived.[41] Cephalosporins are the most commonly prescribed agents for surgical prophylaxis because of their broad antimicrobial spectrum, favorable pharmacokinetic profile, low incidence of adverse side effects, and low cost. First-generation cephalosporins, such as cefazolin, are the preferred choice for surgical prophylaxis, particularly for clean surgical procedures.[3,4,7] In cases where broader gram-negative and anaerobic coverage is desired, antianaerobic cephalosporins, such as cefoxitin and cefotetan, are appropriate choices. Although third-generation cephalosporins (e.g., ceftriaxone) have been advocated for prophylaxis because of their increased gram-negative coverage and prolonged half-lives, their inferior gram-positive and anaerobic activity and high cost have discouraged the widespread use of these agents.[3,4,7]

Allergic reactions are the most common side effects associated with cephalosporin use. Reactions can range from minor skin manifestations at the site of infusion to rash, pruritus, and rarely anaphylaxis (<0.02%). The structural similarity between penicillins and cephalosporins (each contains a β-lactam ring) has led to considerable confusion about the cross-allergenicity between these two classes of drugs. Twenty percent of the general population is labeled "penicillin allergic," yet these patients, only 10% to 20% have positive results of a penicillin skin test.[42] The rate of cross-reactivity is ~2%, but as only 20% of all "penicillin-allergic" patients truly are penicillin allergic, the true incidence of cross-reactivity likely is less than 1%. Routine penicillin skin testing is not cost-effective.[42] In summary, the administration of cephalosporins is both safe and cost-effective for many patients who are labeled "penicillin allergic," and they can be used by patients who have not experienced an immediate or type I penicillin allergy.

Vancomycin can be considered for prophylactic therapy in surgical procedures involving implantation of a prosthetic device in which the rate of MRSA is high.[23,43] If the risk of MRSA is low, and a β-lactam hypersensitivity exists, clindamycin can be used for many procedures instead of cefazolin to limit vancomycin use. Infusion-related side effects, such as thrombophlebitis and hypotension, particularly with vancomycin, usually can be controlled by adequate dilution and slower administration rates.[44]

Pseudomembranous colitis secondary to cephalosporins is uncommon and generally easily treated with a short course of oral metronidazole. Although infrequent, bleeding abnormalities related to cephalosporin use have been reported.[45] The primary hematologic effect appears to be inhibition of vitamin K–dependent clotting factors that results in prolongation of the prothrombin time. The mechanism for this effect, most commonly seen with cefotetan, is related to the methylthiotetrazole side chain of the β-lactam molecule. Patients at greatest risk for this hypoprothrombinemic effect have received a prolonged course of these agents and have underlying risk factors for vitamin K deficiency, such as malnutrition.[46]

Because inappropriate prophylactic antibiotic use not only can induce antibiotic resistance but also can negatively affect an institution's antibiotic budget, initiatives to curtail inappropriate antibiotic use have become the focus of many drug use evaluation efforts. Potential sources of inappropriate antibiotic prophylaxis include the use of broad-spectrum antimicrobials when a narrow-spectrum agent is warranted, extending prophylaxis for durations beyond that recommended in published guidelines, and using expensive antibiotics when equivalent, less expensive agents are available. The most effective tools for ensuring appropriate prophylactic antibiotic prescribing are knowledge of the institutional postoperative infection rate for each type of surgical procedure and familiarity with the bacterial epidemiology patterns for each surgical population. Individualized institutional guidelines that take into account the best literature evidence, institution-based antibiotic susceptibility data, and surgeon preference are important tools for rationalizing antibiotic prophylaxis use.[47]

RECOMMENDATIONS FOR SPECIFIC TYPES OF SURGERY

Guidelines for surgical prophylaxis usually are structured according to the tissues affected during an operation. Although many different surgical procedures may be performed at any one anatomic site, this method of categorization still is optimal because the factors related to the success of a prophylactic regimen, such as the endogenous flora that are expected and the pharmacokinetics, pharmacodynamics, and spectrum of selected antimicrobials, generally are constant for a particular surgical site (see the discussion above). The choice of antimicrobial prophylaxis is always best evaluated using the results of properly conducted clinical trials. In the absence of studies specific to the procedure in question, extrapolation from data on regimens for different procedures in the same anatomic site in question usually can be made. Subsequent modifications to each prophylactic regimen should be based on intraoperative findings or events.

❻ A comprehensive review of the surgical prophylaxis literature is beyond the scope of this chapter, but important factors are reviewed here for each type/site of surgery. Specific recommendations are summarized in Table 132–6. The reader is referred to published guidelines and review articles.[3,7,4,41,48]

GI SURGERY

GI surgery can be categorized according to surgical site and infectious risk. Gastroduodenal surgery and hepatobiliary surgery generally are considered to be clean or clean-contaminated surgeries, with SSI rates generally less than 5%. Colorectal surgery, including appendectomies, is considered contaminated because of the large quantities and polymicrobial nature of bacterial flora within the colon. SSI rates for these types of surgeries generally range from 15% to 30%. Emergent abdominal surgery involving bowel perforation or peritonitis is considered a dirty surgical procedure, associated with a greater than 30% risk of SSI, and should be treated with therapeutic rather than prophylactic antibiotics.[3]

Gastroduodenal Surgery

Insignificant numbers of bacteria usually are found in the stomach and duodenum because of their acidity. The rate of SSIs in gastroduodenal surgery generally is low, so procedures in this region can be classified as clean. The risk for an SSI in this population increases with any condition that can lead to bacterial overgrowth, such as obstruction, hemorrhage, or malignancy, or increasing the pH of gastroduodenal secretions with concomitant acid suppression therapy. Antimicrobial prophylaxis is of clinical benefit only in this high-risk population. In most cases, a single dose of intrauenous (IV) cefazolin will provide adequate prophylaxis.[48] For patients with a β-lactam allergy, oral ciprofloxacin is as efficacious as parenteral cefuroxime as prophylactic therapy for gastroduodenal surgery.[49] Antimicrobial prophylaxis is indicated in esophageal surgery only in the presence of obstruction. Postoperative therapeutic antibiotics may be indicated if perforation is detected during surgery, depending on whether an established infection is present.

Use of antibiotic prophylaxis for percutaneous endoscopic gastrostomy placement is controversial.[50] Although postoperative peristomal infection can occur in up to 30% of patients, clinical trials with cefazolin given 30 minutes preoperatively in this population are conflicting.[50] A pharmacoeconomic study that incorporated a meta-analysis of available studies to determine efficacy suggested that antibiotic prophylaxis was cost-effective for patients undergoing percutaneous endoscopic gastrostomy placements.[51]

Hepatobiliary Surgery

Although bile normally is sterile, and the SSI rate after biliary surgery is low, antibiotic prophylaxis is of benefit in this population. Bile contamination (bactobilia) can increase the frequency of SSIs and is present in many patients (e.g., those with acute cholecystitis or biliary obstruction and those of advanced age).[48] In general, however, the correlation between bactobilia in surgical specimens and the subsequent pathogens implicated in an SSI is poor. The most frequently encountered organisms are *E. coli, Klebsiella* species, and enterococci. *Pseudomonas* is an uncommon finding in the absence of cholangitis. Trials comparing first-, second-, and third-generation cephalosporins have not demonstrated benefit over single-dose cefazolin prophylaxis even in high-risk patients (e.g., age >60 years, previous biliary surgery, acute cholecystitis, jaundice, obesity, diabetes, and common bile duct stones).[52] Ciprofloxacin and levofloxacin are effective alternatives for β-lactam-allergic patients undergoing open cholecystectomy.[53,54] In fact, orally administered levofloxacin appears to provide similar intraoperative gallbladder tissue concentrations.[54] For low-risk patients undergoing elective laparoscopic cholecystectomy, antibiotic prophylaxis is not of benefit and is not recommended.[55] The risk for SSIs in cirrhotic patients undergoing transjugular intrahepatic portosystemic shunt surgery may be reduced with a single prophylactic dose of ceftriaxone[56] but not with single doses of shorter-acting cephalosporins.[57]

Although surgeons may use presumptive antibiotic therapy for patients with acute cholecystitis or cholangitis and defer surgery until the patient is afebrile in an effort to decrease the risk of subsequent infections, this practice is controversial. Detection of an active infection during surgery (e.g., gangrenous gallbladder and suppurative cholangitis) is an indication for a course of postoperative therapeutic antibiotics. In either case, antibiotics with additional antianaerobic activity (e.g., cefoxitin or cefotetan) are indicated.[58]

Appendectomy

Suspected appendicitis is a frequent cause of abdominal surgery. Numerous antibiotic regimens, all with activity against gram-positive and gram-negative aerobes and anaerobic pathogens, are effective in reducing SSI incidence.[48] A cephalosporin with antianaerobic activity, such as cefoxitin or cefotetan, is recommended as first-line therapy; however, a comparative trial of cefoxitin and cefotetan suggests that cefotetan may be superior, possibly because of its longer duration of action.[59] In patients with β-lactam allergy, metronidazole in combination with gentamicin is an effective regimen. Broad-spectrum antibiotics covering nosocomial pathogens (e.g., *Pseudomonas*) do not further reduce SSI risk and instead may increase the cost of therapy and promote bacterial resistance.[60] Although single-dose therapy with cefotetan is adequate, prophylaxis with cefoxitin may require intraoperative dosing if the procedure extends beyond 3 hours. Established intraabdominal infections (e.g., gangrenous or perforated appendix) require an appropriate course of postoperative therapeutic antibiotics. Laparoscopic appendectomy produces lower postoperative infection rates than open appendectomy; however, antimicrobial prophylaxis was used for all patients in these studies; thus, the role for prophylaxis in this population remains poorly studied.[61]

TABLE 132-6 Most Likely Pathogens and Specific Recommendations for Surgical Prophylaxis

Type of Operation	Likely Pathogens	Recommended Prophylaxis Regimen[a]	Comments	Grade of Recommendation[b]
GI surgery				
Gastroduodenal	Enteric gram-negative bacilli, gram-positive cocci, oral anaerobes	Cefazolin 1 g × 1 (see text for recommendations for percutaneous endoscopic gastrostomy)	High-risk patients only (obstruction, hemorrhage, malignancy, acid suppression therapy, morbid obesity)	IA
Cholecystectomy	Enteric gram-negative bacilli, anaerobes	Cefazolin 1 g × 1 for high-risk patients Laparoscopic: none	High-risk patients only (acute cholecystitis, common duct stones, previous biliary surgery, jaundice, age >60 years, obesity, diabetes mellitus)	IA
Transjugular intrahepatic portosystemic shunt (TIPS)	Enteric gram-negative bacilli, anaerobes	Ceftriaxone 1 g × 1	Longer-acting cephalosporins preferred	IA
Appendectomy	Enteric gram-negative bacilli, anaerobes	Cefoxitin or cefotetan 1 g × 1	Second intraoperative dose of cefoxitin may be required if procedure lasts longer than 3 hours	IA
Colorectal	Enteric gram-negative bacilli, anaerobes	Orally: neomycin 1 g + erythromycin base 1 at 1 PM, 2 PM, and 11 PM 1 day preoperatively plus mechanical bowel preparation IV: cefoxitin or cefotetan 1 g × 1	Benefits of oral plus IV is controversial except for colostomy reversal and rectal resection	IA
GI endoscopy	Variable, depending on procedure, but typically enteric gram-negative bacilli, gram-positive cocci, oral anaerobes	Orally: amoxicillin 2 g × 1 IV: ampicillin 2 g × 1 or cefazolin 1 g × 1	Recommended only for high-risk patients undergoing high-risk procedures (see text)	IA
Urologic surgery				
Prostate resection, shock-wave lithotripsy, ureteroscopy	*Escherichia coli*	Ciprofloxacin 500 mg orally or trimethoprim-sulfamethoxazole 1 DS tablet	All patients with positive pre-operative urine cultures should receive a course of antibiotic treatment	IA–IB
removal of external urinary catheters, cystography, urodynamic studies, simple cystourethroscopy	*E. coli*	Ciprofloxacin 500 mg orally or trimethoprim-sulfamethoxazole 1 DS tablet	Should be considered only in patients with risk factors (see text)	IB
Gynecological surgery				
Cesarean section	Enteric gram-negative bacilli, anaerobes, group B streptococci, enterococci	Cefazolin 2 g × 1	Can be given before initial incision or after cord is clamped	IA
Hysterectomy	Enteric gram-negative bacilli, anaerobes, group B streptococci, enterococci	Vaginal: cefazolin 1 g × 1 Abdominal: cefotetan 1 g × 1 or cefazolin 1 g × 1	Metronidazole 1 g IV × 1 is recommended alternative for penicillin allergy	IA
Head and neck surgery				
Maxillofacial surgery	*Staphylococcus aureus*, streptococci oral anaerobes	Cefazolin 2 g or clindamycin 600 mg	Repeat intraoperative dose for operations longer than 4 hours	IA
Head and neck cancer resection	*S. aureus*, streptococci oral anaerobes	Clindamycin 600 mg at induction and every 8 hours × 2 more doses	Add gentamicin for clean–contaminated procedures	IA
Cardiothoracic surgery				
Cardiac surgery	*S. aureus, Staphylococcus epidermidis, Corynebacterium*	Cefazolin 1 g every 8 hours × 48 h	Patients >80 kg (176 lb) should receive 2 g of cefazolin instead; in areas with high prevalence of *S. aureus* resistance, vancomycin should be considered	IA
Thoracic surgery	*S. aureus, S. epidermidis, Corynebacterium*, enteric gram-negative bacilli	Cefuroxime 750 mg IV every 8 hours × 48 hours	First-generation cephalosporins are deemed inadequate, and shorter durations of prophylaxis have not been adequately studied	IA
Vascular surgery				
Abdominal aorta and lower extremity vascular surgery	*S. aureus, S. epidermidis*, enteric gram-negative bacilli	Cefazolin 1 g at induction and every 8 hours × 2 more doses	Although complications from infections may be infrequent, graft infections are associated with significant morbidity	IB
Orthopedic surgery				
Joint replacement	*S. aureus, S. epidermidis*	Cefazolin 1 g × 1 preoperatively, then every 8 hours × 2 more doses	Vancomycin reserved for penicillin-allergic patients or where institutional prevalence of methicillin-resistant *S. aureus* warrants use	IA

(continued)

TABLE 132-6 Most Likely Pathogens and Specific Recommendations for Surgical Prophylaxis (continued)

Type of Operation	Likely Pathogens	Recommended Prophylaxis Regimen[a]	Comments	Grade of Recommendation[b]
Hip fracture repair	S. aureus, S. epidermidis	Cefazolin 1 g × 1 preoperatively, then every 8 hours for 48 hours	Compound fractures are treated as if infection is presumed	IA
Open/compound fractures	S. aureus, S. epidermidis, gram-negative bacilli, polymicrobial	Cefazolin 1 g × 1 preoperatively, then every 8 hours for a course of presumed infection	Gram-negative coverage (i.e., gentamicin) often indicated for severe open fractures	IA
Neurosurgery				
CSF shunt procedures	S. aureus, S. epidermidis	Cefazolin 1 g every 8 h × 3 doses or ceftriaxone 2 g × 1	No agents have been shown to be better than cefazolin in randomized comparative trials.	IA
Spinal surgery	S. aureus, S. epidermidis	Cefazolin 1 g × 1	Limited number of clinical trials comparing different treatment regimens	IB
CSF shunt procedures	S. aureus, S. epidermidis	Cefazolin 1 g every 8 h × 3 doses or ceftriaxone 2 g × 1	No agents have been shown to be better than cefazolin in randomized comparative trials.	IA
Craniotomy	S. aureus, S. epidermidis	Cefazolin 1 g × 1 or cefotaxime 1 g × 1	IV × 1 can be substituted for patients with penicillin allergy Trimethoprim-sulfamethoxazole (160/800 mg)	IA

[a]One-time doses are optimally infused at induction of anesthesia except as noted. Repeat doses may be required for long procedures. See text for references.
[b]Strength of recommendations:
Category IA: Strongly recommended and supported by well-designed experimental, clinical, or epidemiologic studies.
Category IB: Strongly recommended and supported by some experimental, clinical, or epidemiologic studies and strong theoretical rationale.
Category II: Suggested and supported by suggestive clinical or epidemiologic studies or theoretical rationale.
CSF = cerebrospinal fluid, DS = double strength, GI = gastrointestinal, IV = intravenous(ly).

Colorectal Surgery

In the absence of adequate prophylactic therapy, the risk for SSI after colorectal surgery is high because of the significant bacterial counts in fecal material present in the colon (frequently >10⁹ per gram). Anaerobes and gram-negative aerobes predominate, but gram-positive aerobes also may play an important role. Reducing this bacterial load with a thorough bowel preparation regimen (4 L of polyethylene glycol solution or 90 mL of sodium phosphate solution administered orally the day before surgery) is controversial; however, 99% of surgeons in a survey routinely use mechanical preparation.[62] Risk factors for SSIs include age over 60 years, hypoalbuminemia, poor preoperative bowel preparation, corticosteroid therapy, malignancy, and operations lasting longer than 3.5 hours.[7]

Antimicrobial prophylaxis reduced mortality from 11.2% to 4.5% in a pooled analysis of trials comparing antimicrobial prophylaxis with no prophylaxis for colon surgery.[65] Effective antibiotic prophylaxis reduces even further the risk for an SSI. Several oral regimens designed to reduce bacterial counts in the colon have been studied.[48] The combination of 1 g neomycin and 1 g erythromycin base given orally 19, 18, and 9 hours preoperatively is the regimen most commonly used in the United States.[66] Neomycin is poorly absorbed but provides intraluminal concentrations that are high enough to effectively kill most gram-negative aerobes. Oral erythromycin is only partially absorbed but still produces concentrations in the colon that are sufficient to suppress common anaerobes. If surgery is postponed, the antibiotics must be readministered to maintain efficacy. Optimally, the bowel preparation regimen should be completed prior to starting the oral antibiotic regimen. This is of particular concern because most procedures now are performed electively on a "same-day surgery" basis. In this case, the bowel preparation regimen is self-administered by the patient at home on the day prior to hospital admission, and compliance cannot be monitored carefully.

Patients who cannot take oral medications should receive parenteral antibiotics. Cefoxitin or cefotetan is used most commonly, but other second- and some third-generation cephalosporins also are effective.[67] The role of metronidazole in combination with cephalosporin therapy is unclear. Only retrospective evidence suggests that the addition of metronidazole to a cephalosporin or extended-spectrum penicillin provides additional benefit.[68] Until this finding is confirmed in prospective studies, metronidazole should be reserved for combination therapy with cephalosporins with poor anaerobic coverage (e.g., cefazolin). At this time, the evidence recommending the addition of metronidazole to cephalosporins with anaerobic activity (e.g., cefotaxime, cefoxitin, and ceftriaxone) is insufficient.[69] For β-lactam-allergic patients, perioperative doses of gentamicin and metronidazole have been used. Combination therapy (i.e., oral and IV therapy) is controversial. A Cochrane review suggests that combination therapy is superior to either oral or IV antibiotics alone.[69] However, the largest study (491 patients) comparing combination therapy with only IV therapy, which showed no benefit with combination therapy, was not included in the meta-analysis.[70] Postoperative antibiotics generally are unnecessary in the absence of any untoward events or findings during surgery. IV antibiotics are required for colostomy reversal and rectal resection because enterally administered antibiotics will not reach the distal segment that is to be reanastomosed or resected.[71]

CLINICAL CONTROVERSY

A randomized trial of 380 patients undergoing elective colorectal surgery suggests that SSIs are not reduced by preoperative mechanical bowel preparation.[63] This finding was confirmed in a meta-analysis showing that mechanical bowel preparation does not reduce the risk of anastomotic leakage or other complications, including postoperative infection.[64] Despite this new evidence, mechanical bowel preparations continue to be a standard of practice prior to elective bowel surgery.

Gastrointestinal Endoscopy

Despite the large number of endoscopic procedures performed each year, the rate of postprocedural infection is relatively low. The highest bacteremia rates have been reported in patients undergoing esophageal dilation for stricture or sclerotherapy for management of esophageal varices. Although postprocedural bacteremia can occur in as many as 22% of patients, the bacteremia usually is transient (<30 minutes) and rarely results in clinically significant infection. Therefore, antimicrobial prophylaxis is routinely recommended only for high-risk patients (e.g., patients with prosthetic heart valves, a history of endocarditis, systemic-pulmonary shunt, synthetic vascular graft <1 year old, complex cyanotic congenital heart disease, obstructed bile duct, or liver cirrhosis, as well as immunocompromised patients) undergoing high-risk procedures (e.g., stricture dilation, variceal sclerotherapy, and endoscopic retrograde cholangiopancreatography).[72] Single-dose preprocedural regimens similar to those for endocarditis prophylaxis are most common (amoxicillin for patients who can tolerate oral premedication or either IV ampicillin or cefazolin). A meta-analysis of antimicrobial prophylaxis for endoscopic placement of percutaneous feeding tubes also suggests that a single preoperative dose of antibiotics reduces the risk of postoperative infection compared with no antibiotic (6.4% vs 24%).[73] Consensus guidelines have adopted this recommendation and suggest a single dose of cefazolin within 30 minutes prior to the procedure.[72]

UROLOGIC SURGERY

Preoperative bacteriuria is the most important risk factor for development of an SSI after urologic surgery. All patients should have a preoperative urinalysis and should receive therapeutic antibiotics if bacteriuria is detected. Patients with sterile urine preoperatively are at low risk for developing an SSI, and the benefit of prophylactic antibiotics in this setting is controversial. Antibiotic prophylaxis is recommended for all patients undergoing transurethral resection of the prostate or bladders tumors, shock-wave lithotripsy, percutaneous renal surgery, or ureteroscopy.[74] The exact incidence of SSIs in this population is obscured by the frequent use of postoperative urinary catheters and the subsequent risk of bacteriuria. E. coli is the most frequently encountered organism. Routine use of broad-spectrum antibiotics, such as third-generation cephalosporins and fluoroquinolones, does not decrease SSI rates more than cefazolin, but the ability to administer fluoroquinolones orally rather than intravenously makes antimicrobial prophylaxis with ciprofloxacin easier and less expensive.[75] First- or second-generation cephalosporins are considered the antimicrobial agents of choice for patients undergoing open or laparoscopic procedures involving entry into the urinary tract and any urologic surgical procedures involving the intestine, rectum, vagina, or implanted prosthesis.[74] The evidence for antimicrobial prophylaxis for the removal of external urinary catheters, cystography, urodynamic studies, simple cystourethroscopy, and open or laparoscopic urologic procedures that do not involve entry into the urinary tract is not as evident. Only patients considered to have risk factors (patients of advanced age; those with anatomic anomalies; poor nutritional history, externalized catheters, colonized endogenous/exogenous material, or distant coexistent infection; smokers; immunocompromised patients; and those who are hospitalized for a prolonged stay) should receive antimicrobial prophylaxis.[74]

OBSTETRIC AND GYNECOLOGIC SURGERIES

Cesarean Section

Cesarean section is the most frequently performed surgical procedure in the United States.[7] Prophylactic antibiotics are given to prevent endometritis, the most commonly occurring SSI. In the past, antibiotics were recommended for only high-risk patients, including those with premature membrane rupture or those not receiving prenatal care. Several large trials, as well as a meta-analysis of 81 trials, have shown benefit in administering prophylactic antibiotics to all women undergoing emergent or elective cesarean section regardless of their underlying risk factors.[76] Cefazolin remains the drug of choice despite the wide spectrum of potential pathogens, and a single 2 g dose appears to be superior to single or multiple 1 g doses.[77] Providing a broader spectrum of coverage with cefoxitin (for anaerobes) or piperacillin (for Pseudomonas or enterococci) does not further reduce postoperative infection rates. For patients with a β-lactam allergy, preoperative metronidazole is an acceptable alternative.[76]

CLINICAL CONTROVERSY

During a cesarean section, unlike other surgical procedures, the most appropriate timing of antibiotic administration is controversial. Traditionally, antimicrobials were administered after the initial incision and when the umbilical cord was clamped in an attempt to minimize infant drug exposure, which theoretically could mask the signs of neonatal sepsis and select resistant organisms in infants who develop infections. Recent studies and systematic reviews, however, suggest that preincision antibiotics are more effective at preventing postoperative endometritis and other SSIs but are underpowered to evaluate the impact on neonatal infectious complications.[78]

Hysterectomy

The most important factor affecting the incidence of SSI after hysterectomy is the type of procedure performed. Vaginal hysterectomies are associated with a high rate of postoperative infection when performed without the benefit of prophylactic antibiotics because of the polymicrobial flora normally present at the operative site.[79] As with cesarean sections, cefazolin is the drug of choice for vaginal hysterectomies despite the wide spectrum of possible pathogens.[79] The American College of Obstetricians and Gynecologists (ACOG) recommends a single dose of either cefazolin or cefoxitin.[80] For patients with a β-lactam allergy, a single preoperative dose of either metronidazole or doxycycline also is effective.[80]

Prophylactic antibiotics are recommended for abdominal hysterectomy despite the lack of bacterial contamination from the vaginal flora. Both cefazolin and antianaerobic cephalosporins (e.g., cefoxitin and cefotetan) have been studied extensively. Single-dose cefotetan is superior to single-dose cefazolin,[81] and the investigators suggest that cefotetan should be the drug of choice for abdominal hysterectomies. However, other investigators suggest that either agent is appropriate, provided 24 hours of antimicrobial coverage is not exceeded.[7] The ACOG guidelines suggest that first-, second-, or third-generation cephalosporins can be used for prophylaxis.[80] Metronidazole also is effective and can be used if patients are allergic to β-lactam antibiotics.[79] Antibiotic prophylaxis may not be required in laparoscopic gynecologic surgery or tubal microsurgery.[82] As with other surgical procedures, perioperative events and findings may require the use of therapeutic antibiotics after surgery.

HEAD AND NECK SURGERY

The use of prophylactic antibiotics during head and neck surgery depends on the procedure type. Clean procedures (per NRC definition), such as parotidectomy and simple tooth extraction, are associated with a low incidence of SSI. Head and neck procedures involving an incision through a mucosal layer are associated with a higher risk for SSI. The normal flora of the mouth is polymicrobial; both anaerobes and gram-positive aerobes predominate. Although typical doses of cefazolin usually are ineffective for anaerobic infections, a 2 g dose produces concentrations high enough to inhibit these organisms. A pharmacokinetic study suggested that a single dose of clindamycin is adequate for prophylaxis in maxillofacial surgery unless the procedure lasts longer than 4 hours, when a second dose should be administered intraoperatively.[83] For most head and neck cancer resection surgeries, including free-flap reconstruction, 24 hours of clindamycin is appropriate, and no additional benefit of extending therapy beyond 24 hours is seen. A combination of clindamycin and gentamicin to cover aerobic, anaerobic, and gram-negative bacteria in clean-contaminated oncologic surgery is recommended.[84] Topical therapy with clindamycin, amoxicillin–clavulanate, and ticarcillin–clavulanate has been described in small trials, but the exact role of topical antibiotics is not defined.[85] Antimicrobial prophylaxis is not indicated for endoscopic sinus surgery without nasal packing.[41]

CARDIOTHORACIC SURGERY

Although cardiac surgery generally is considered a clean procedure, antibiotic prophylaxis lowers SSI incidence.[48] The substantial morbidity related to an SSI in this population, coupled with the routine implementation of prosthetic devices, further justifies the routine use of prophylaxis.[86] Patients who develop SSIs after coronary artery bypass graft surgery have a mortality rate of 22% at 1 year compared with 0.6% for those who do not develop an SSI.[87] Risk factors for developing an SSI after cardiac surgery include obesity, renal insufficiency, connective tissue disease, reexploration for bleeding, and poorly timed administration of antibiotics.[86] Skin flora pathogens predominate; gram-negative organisms are rare.

Cefazolin has been studied extensively and is considered the drug of choice. Although several studies and a meta-analysis advocate the use of second-generation cephalosporins (e.g., cefuroxime) rather than cefazolin, various methodologic flaws in these studies have limited the extrapolation of these results to practice. Cefazolin was as effective as cefuroxime in a large randomized trial of 702 patients undergoing open heart surgery and thus remains the standard of care.[88] Both patient weight and timing of cefazolin administration relative to surgery must be considered when developing a dosing strategy. Patients weighing >80 kg (176 lb) should receive 2 g cefazolin rather than 1 g. Doses should be administered no earlier than 60 minutes before the first incision and no later than the beginning of induction.[84] Extending therapy beyond 48 hours does not further reduce SSI rates. Single-dose cefazolin therapy may be sufficient but is not recommended by the Society of Thoracic Surgeons at this time pending further study.[89]

Routine vancomycin administration may be justified in hospitals having a high incidence of MRSA or when sternal wounds are to be explored surgically for possible mediastinitis. However, a large comparative trial enrolling almost 900 patients in a single center with a high prevalence of MRSA infections found that both cefazolin and vancomycin had similar efficacy in preventing SSI in patients undergoing cardiac surgery that required sternotomy.[90] Mediastinitis constitutes a failure of a prior prophylactic regimen. Continued postoperative vancomycin should be guided by culture and sensitivity data.[42] Subsequent antibiotic therapy is guided by intraoperative findings.

Pulmonary resection is associated with significant SSI risk, and prophylactic antibiotics have an established role in preventing postoperative infectious morbidity. Pleuropulmonary infections are much more common than wound infections, and pathogenic organisms likely migrate from the oral cavity or pharynx.[91] First-generation cephalosporins are inadequate; 48 hours of cefuroxime is preferred. A regimen of ampicillin–sulbactam is superior to first-generation cephalosporins, but further studies are required before this agent can be recommended as first-line prophylactic therapy.[92]

VASCULAR SURGERY

Vascular surgery, like cardiac surgery, generally is considered clean by NRC criteria. Although vascular graft infections occur infrequently (3%–5%), the associated morbidity and mortality are extensive because treatment often requires surgical graft removal along with therapeutic antibiotic therapy.[93] Prophylactic antibiotics are of benefit, particularly for procedures involving the abdominal aorta and the lower extremities. Cefazolin is regarded as the drug of choice.[94] Twenty-four hours of prophylaxis with cefazolin is adequate; longer courses may lead to bacterial resistance.[95] For patients with β-lactam allergy, 24 hours of oral ciprofloxacin has been shown to be effective.[93]

ORTHOPEDIC SURGERY

Most orthopedic surgery is clean by definition; thus, prophylactic antibiotics generally are indicated only when prosthetic materials (e.g., pins, plates, and artificial joints) are implanted.[20] A late-occurring infectious complication in this surgical population can result in substantial morbidity and may lead to prosthesis failure and subsequent removal. Staphylococci are the most frequently encountered pathogens; gram-negative aerobes are infrequent. The use of cefazolin is supported by substantial evidence in the literature and therefore is the prophylactic agent of choice. Vancomycin, although effective, is not recommended for routine use unless a patient has a documented history of a serious allergy to β-lactams, or the propensity for MRSA infections at a particular institution necessitates its use. The current recommended duration of prophylaxis for joint replacement and hip fracture surgery is 24 hours.[7] Antibiotic-impregnated cement and beads have been used to lower SSI rates, but conclusive data regarding their efficacy are lacking.[20]

Patients suffering open (compound) fractures are particularly susceptible to infection because bacterial contamination almost always has occurred already. Under these circumstances, the use of antibiotics is presumptive. In this setting, cefazolin often is combined with an aminoglycoside, but controlled trials are lacking.[96] A clinical trial comparing clindamycin and cloxacillin suggests that clindamycin is superior and may be appropriate as monotherapy for Gustilo type I and II open fractures but not for type III fractures, for which added gram-negative activity is recommended.[97] Duration of antibiotic therapy is highly variable and depends on surgical findings during debridement, results of intraoperative cultures, and clinical status. A prospective trial comparing short (<24 hours) and long (>24 hours) courses of antimicrobial prophylaxis for severe trauma suggests that longer courses of antibiotics do not offer additional benefit and may be associated with the development of resistant infections.[98] However, established joint infections and osteomyelitis require an extended course of therapeutic antibiotics.

NEUROSURGERY

Definitive recommendations on the role of antibiotic prophylaxis in neurosurgery cannot be made at this time.[99] Although the rates of SSI after these generally clean operations are low, the morbidity and mortality of SSI, should they occur, are high. Procedures involving cerebrospinal fluid (CSF) shunt placement should be considered separately because this procedure involves placement of a foreign body and is associated with higher infection rates. When choosing an antibiotic, considerations include not only the spectrum of activity but also the penetration of the agent into the site of action (CSF). A meta-analysis suggested that single doses of cefazolin or, where required, vancomycin appear to lower SSI risk after craniotomy.[100] The largest prospective randomized trial to date of 826 patients undergoing clean neurosurgical procedures suggested that a single dose of ceftizoxime was as effective as a combination regimen of single-dose vancomycin and gentamicin. The authors also reported that ceftizoxime was better tolerated and more consistently achieved adequate CSF levels to inhibit the most common organisms.[101] A study of 780 patients undergoing neurosurgical procedures that included shunt surgery reported that single doses of cefotaxime and trimethoprim–sulfamethoxazole were equally effective in preventing SSIs.[102] Most studies of procedures involving a shunt have been small in size and do not consistently show lower infection rates with antibiotic prophylaxis, although the results of a systematic review and meta-analysis suggest that a significant improvement in the incidence of shunt infection with 24 hours of systemic antibiotics (i.e., cefazolin) and the use of antibiotic-impregnated catheters independently.[103]

SSIs associated with spinal surgery are rare but devastating when they occur. The use of antimicrobial prophylaxis in this setting is warranted and recommended by a meta-analysis.[104] Large randomized, controlled trials are lacking, but cefazolin is the antibiotic recommended most commonly. Cephalosporin penetration into the vertebral disk has been questioned. Some small studies suggest that the addition of gentamicin, which has better penetration, might be warranted; however, there is a paucity of clinical trials comparing these two regimens.[105]

MINIMALLY INVASIVE AND LAPAROSCOPIC SURGERY

Laparoscopic surgeries are being performed more frequently for a variety of different operations, including gynecologic, orthopedic, and biliary surgeries. This minimally invasive technique is associated with smaller wounds, fewer infectious complications, smaller inflammatory response, and therefore a better-preserved immune response to infection compared with the open surgical approach.[106] The role of antimicrobial prophylaxis in this setting depends on the type of surgery performed and preexisting risk factors for infection. Unfortunately, few large prospective, placebo-controlled trials have determined in which patients and surgeries antimicrobial prophylaxis is warranted.

In addition to the recommendations for previously mentioned laparoscopic procedures, there is a variety of levels of evidence for prophylaxis in other laparoscopic and endoscopic procedures. Patients undergoing endoscopic retrograde cholangiopancreatography do not need antimicrobial prophylaxis unless biliary obstruction is evident. In these situations, a single 1 g dose of cefazolin will suffice.[107] The role of antimicrobial prophylaxis for transurethral resection of the prostate is better established. A third-generation cephalosporin such as ceftriaxone (or cotrimoxazole for severely β-lactam-allergic patients) can be recommended as single-dose prophylaxis, especially for patients with nonsterile urine preoperatively or indwelling catheters.[107] Insertion of peritoneal dialysis catheters by laparoscopic technique is associated with significantly lower rates of postoperative infection. With SSI rates less than 5%, prophylactic antimicrobial therapy may not be warranted, but this has not been studied in a sufficiently large placebo-controlled trial. If the decision to provide antimicrobial prophylaxis is made, a single dose of cefazolin will suffice.[107]

NONPHARMACOLOGIC INTERVENTIONS

Strategies other than antimicrobial and aseptic technique for reducing postoperative infections have been investigated in different types of surgeries. The most commonly cited and practiced interventions include intraoperative maintenance of normothermia, provision of supplemental oxygen in the perioperative period, and aggressive perioperative glucose control.

CLINICAL CONTROVERSY

Several studies have investigated the role of specialized enteral formulas fortified with a variety of immunomodulating micronutrients thought to enhance the immune response and gut function after trauma or surgery. Although many clinicians are exploring the role of supplements such as glutamine, arginine, omega fatty acids, and nucleotides, no study to date has shown a significant reduction in postoperative infection rates using these formulations.

CLINICAL CONTROVERSY

Although interventions to maintain normothermia intraoperatively, provide supplemental oxygen in the perioperative period, and aggressively control perioperative glucose show a significant reduction in SSI, they cannot be generalized to all types of surgeries. However, given the simplicity and low cost of these interventions, many clinicians consider applying these measures outside of the studied population(s). At this time, pending further research, these interventions can be recommended for routine use only in the type of patient or surgery for which they were studied.

Core body temperature can fall by 1°C to 1.5°C (33.8–34.7°F) intraoperatively in patients under general anesthesia. Intraoperative hypothermia has been associated with impaired immune function, decreased blood flow to the surgical site, decreased tissue oxygen tension, and an increased risk of SSI. Efforts to maintain intraoperative normothermia should be exercised and may include the use of warming blankets and IV fluid warmers to maintain core body temperature above 36°C (97°F). One prospective trial of 200 patients undergoing colorectal surgery found that maintenance of normothermia reduced postoperative infection rates along with other morbidity parameters, including length of stay.[108]

Low oxygen tension in the tissues that make up the surgical site increases the risk of bacterial colonization and subsequent SSI by decreasing the efficiency of neutrophil activity. Administration of high concentrations of oxygen (80% via ventilator or 12 L/min via a nonrebreather mask) reduced postoperative infection rates significantly in a multicenter randomized trial of 500 patients undergoing colorectal surgery.[109]

Diabetes and poor glucose control are well-known risk factors for SSI. The increased risk of infection is thought to be due to both macrovascular (vasculopathy and venoocclusive disease) and microvascular (subtle immunologic deficiencies, including neutrophil dysfunction and reduced complement and antibody activity) complications. Aggressive control of perioperative blood glucose level decreases the incidence of SSI in diabetics undergoing cardiac surgery and is being evaluated in other types of surgery and in nondiabetic patients.[110]

QUALITY ASSURANCE AND PHARMACOECONOMIC IMPLICATIONS

The recommendations and literature reviewed in this chapter indicate that SSIs are preventable with appropriately chosen and timed prophylactic therapy in combination with meticulous aseptic technique and a variety of nonantimicrobial methods. Despite this practice, infection is the most common complication seen postoperatively. For this reason, many organizations, including the Centers for Medicare and Medicaid Service (CMS), CDC, and Joint Commission on Accreditation of Healthcare Organizations (JCAHO), have mandated a formalized approach to improving patient safety and reducing SSIs. Quality assurance data collected from Medicare inpatients found that two of the three performance measures of the National Surgical Infection Project (SIP), implemented by the CMS and the CDC in 2002, are not consistently being met.[111] Although 92.6% of patients were given a prophylactic antimicrobial regimen consistent with published guidelines, only 55.7% of these surgical patients had parenteral antimicrobial prophylaxis initiated within 1 hour prior to incision, and the prophylactic antimicrobial was discontinued within 24 hours after surgery end time in only 40.7% of patients.[111] Strategies have been investigated and shown to improve surgical antibiotic prophylaxis practices for these three outcomes as part of the SIP. These three performance outcomes have been adopted as core measures by the JCAHO as publicly reported quality measure by the Hospital Quality Alliance. However, in light of a lack of clear guidance on what constitutes "high rates" of MRSA in published SIP guidelines, the national shortage of antibiotics recommended for patients undergoing general abdominal colorectal surgery (e.g., cefotetan, cefoxitin), and conflicting recommendations for prevention of endocarditis in patients undergoing surgery who have coexisting valvular heart disease, the CMS and the JCAHO have temporarily suspended the public reporting of these SIP quality measures.[112] Standardized institutional guidelines can effectively ensure appropriate prophylactic antimicrobial therapy and ultimately reduce SSIs at individual institutions. Strategies for improving such programs are outlined in Table 132–7.[113]

It is paramount to consider the cost implications of pharmacotherapy guidelines that affect a large number of patients. Although investigators have incorporated basic financial analysis into the results of antibiotic prophylaxis comparative trials,[42,47,50,87] robust pharmacoeconomic studies of various regimens of antimicrobial prophylaxis in surgery are lacking. Most of these are cost minimization studies because only drug acquisition costs are considered. Studies that incorporate all relevant drug and treatment costs in relation to pertinent patient outcomes, such as incidence of SSIs, hospital length of stay, and antibiotic-related adverse events, are needed.

TABLE 132-7	Strategies for Implementing an Institutional Program to Ensure Appropriate use of Antimicrobial Prophylaxis in Surgery

1. Educate

Develop an educational program that enforces the importance and rationale of timely antimicrobial prophylaxis.

Make this educational program available to all healthcare practitioners involved in the patient's care.

2. Standardize the ordering process

Establish a protocol (e.g., a preprinted order sheet) that standardizes antibiotic choice according to current published evidence, formulary availability, institutional resistance patterns, and cost.

3. Standardize the delivery and administration process

Use system that ensures antibiotics are prepared and delivered to the holding area in a timely fashion.

Standardize the administration time to less than 1 hour preoperatively.

Designate responsibility and accountability for antibiotic administration.

Provide visible reminders to prescribe/administer prophylactic antibiotics (e.g., checklists).

Develop a system to remind surgeons/nurses to readminister antibiotics intraoperatively during long procedures.

4. Provide feedback

Follow up with regular reports of compliance and infection rates.

EVALUATION OF THERAPEUTIC OUTCOMES

When evaluating the outcome of surgical antibiotic prophylaxis, it is important to differentiate any potential SSI from other postoperative infection or complication. Although fever and leukocytosis are common in the immediate postoperative period, they typically resolve with prompt ambulation, timely removal of invasive devices, prevention and/or resolution of atelectasis through optimal respiratory care, and effective analgesia. It is important to remember that the emergence of distal infections, such as pneumonia, does not constitute a failure of surgical prophylaxis. Prophylaxis should be as short as possible because prolonged prophylactic regimens may contribute to the selection of resistant organisms and may make any infection more difficult to treat.

Surgical site appearance is the most important determinant of the presence of an infection. Drainage of pus from the incision accompanied by redness, warmth, and pain or tenderness is highly suggestive of an SSI. By definition, any surgical site that requires incision and drainage by the surgeon is considered infected regardless of appearance. Failure to heal and wound dehiscence also are seen with SSIs, although surgical technique and nutritional status may be important contributing factors.

The presentation of signs and symptoms consistent with an SSI in relation to previous surgery is an important consideration when evaluating therapeutic outcomes after surgical prophylaxis. Many SSIs will not be evident during acute hospitalization. In fact, SSIs may not become evident until up to 30 days later or, in the case of prosthesis implantation, up to 1 year later. Thus, the true incidence of SSI can be determined only by completing comprehensive postdischarge surveillance. All studies investigating the efficacy of surgical prophylaxis must include adequate postdischarge follow-up to be able to thoroughly assess the success of any prophylactic regimen.

ABBREVIATIONS

ACOG: American College of Obstetricians and Gynecologists

ASA: American Society of Anesthesiologists

CDC: Centers for Disease Control and Prevention

CSF: Cerebrospinal fluid

JCAHO: Joint Commission on Accreditation of Healthcare Organizations

MIC: Minimum inhibitory concentration

MRSA: Methicillin-resistant *Staphylococcus aureus*

MSSA: Methicillin-sensitive *Staphylococcus aureus*

NNIS: National Nosocomial Infections Surveillance System

NRC: National Research Council

SENIC: Study on the Efficacy of Nosocomial Infection Control

SSI: Surgical site infection

VRE: Vancomycin-resistant enterococci

REFERENCES

1. Mitka M. Preventing surgical infection is more important than ever. JAMA 2000;283:44–45.
2. de Lalla F. Antimicrobial chemotherapy in the control of surgical infectious complications. J Chemother 1999;11:440–445.
3. Mangram AJ, Horan TC, Pearson ML, et al. Guideline for prevention of surgical site infection, 1999. Centers for Disease Control and

Prevention (CDC) Hospital Infection Control Practices Advisory Committee. Am J Infect Control 1999;27:97–132.

4. Hendrick TL, Anastacio MM, Sawyer RG. Prevention of surgical site infection. Expert Rev Anti Infect Ther 2006;4:223–233.

5. National Academy of Sciences, National Research Council. Postoperative wound infections: The influence of ultraviolet irradiation of the operating room and of various other factors. Ann Surg 1964;160:32–135.

6. Cruse PJE, Foord R. A five-year prospective study of 23,649 surgical wounds. Arch Surg 1973;107:206–210.

7. ASHP Commission on Therapeutics. ASHP therapeutic guidelines on antimicrobial prophylaxis in surgery. In: Deffenbaugh J, ed. Best Practices for Health System Pharmacy. Bethesda, MD: ASHP, 1999;349–396.

8. Drapeau CMJ, Pan A, Bellacosa C, et al. Surgical site infections in HIV-infected patients: Results from an Italian prospective multicenter observational study. Infection 2009;37:455–460.

9. Dionigi R, Rovera F, Dionigi G, et al. Risk factors in surgery. J Chemother 2001;13:6–11.

10. Perl TM, Cullen JJ, Wenzel RP, et al. Intranasal mupirocin to prevent postoperative Staphylococcus aureus infections. N Engl J Med 2002;346:1871–1817.

11. Haley RW, Culver DH, Morgan WM, et al. Identifying patients at high risk of surgical wound infection: A simple multivariate index of patient susceptibility and wound contamination. Am J Epidemiol 1985;127:206–215.

12. Wilson AP, Hodgson B, Liu M, et al. Reduction in wound infection rates by wound surveillance with postdischarge follow-up and feedback. Br J Surg 2006;93:630–638.

13. Gaynes RP, Culver DH, Horan TC, et al. Sugical site infection (SSI) rates in the United States, 1992–1998: The national nosocomial infections surveillance system basic SSI risk index. CID 2001;33(Suppl 2):S69–S77.

14. National Nosocomial Infections Surveillance (NNIS) System Report, data summary from January 1992 through June 2004 issued October 2004. Am J Infect Control 2004;32:470–485.

15. Owens WD, Felts JA, Spitznagel EL. ASA physical status classifications: A study of consistency of ratings. Anesthesiology 1978;49:239–243.

16. Elek SD, Conen PE. The virulence of Staphylococcus pyogenes for man: A study of the problems of wound infection. Br J Exp Pathol 1958;38:573–586.

17. Burke JF. Identification of the sources of staphylococci contaminating the surgical wound during operation. Ann Surg 1963;158:898–904.

18. Kaiser AB, Kernodle DS, Parker RA. Low-inoculum model of surgical wound infection. J Infect Dis 1992;166:393–399.

19. Esposito S. Immune system and surgical site infection. J Chemother 2001;13:12–16.

20. De Lalla F. Antibiotic prophylaxis in orthopedic prosthetic surgery. J Chemother 2001;13:48–53.

21. Halwani M, Solaymani-Dodaran M, Grundman H, et al. Cross transmission of nosocomial pathogens in an adult intensive care unit: Incidence and risk factors. J Hosp Infect 2006;63:39–46.

22. Murray BE. Vancomycin-resistant enterococcal infections. N Engl J Med 2000;342:710–721.

23. Hospital Infection Control Practices Advisory Committee. Recommendations for preventing the spread of vancomycin resistance. MMWR 1995;44:1–13.

24. Cosgrove SE, Qi Y, Kaye KS, et al. The impact of methicillin resistance in Staphylococcus aureus bacteremia on patient outcomes: Mortality, length of stay, and hospital charges. Infect Control Hosp Epidemiol 2005;26:166–174.

25. Manian FA, Meyer PL, Setzer J, et al. Surgical site infections associated with methicillin-resistant Staphylococcus aureus: Do postoperative factors play a role? Clin Infect Dis 2003;36:863–868.

26. Falagas ME, Alexiou VG, Peppas G, Makris GC. Do changes in antimicrobial resistance necessitate reconsideration of surgical antimicrobial prophylaxis strategies? Surg Infect (Larchmt) 2009;10:557–562.

27. Lowy FD, Waldhausen JA, Miller M, et al. Report of the National Heart, Lung and Blood Institute–National Institute of Allergy and Infectious Diseases working group on antimicrobial strategies and cardiothoracic surgery. Am Heart J 2004;147:575–581.

28. Munoz P, Burrillo A, Bouza E. Criteria used when initiating antifungal therapy against Candida spp. in the intensive care unit. Int J Antimicrob Agents 2000;15:83–90.

29. Lipsett PA. Surgical critical care: Fungal infections in surgical patients. Crit Care Med 2006;34:S25–S24.

30. McKinnon PS. Goff DA, Kern JW, et al. Temporal assessment of Candida risk factors in the surgical intensive care unit. Arch Surg 2001;136:1401–1408.

31. Classen DC, Evans RS, Pestotnik SL, et al. The timing of prophylactic administration of antibiotics and the risk of surgical wound infection. N Engl J Med 1992;326:281–286.

32. Weber WP, Marti WR, Zwahlen M, et al. The timing of surgical antimicrobial prophylaxis. Ann Surg 2008;247:918–926.

33. Steinberg JP, Braun BI, Hellinger WC, et al. Timing of antimicrobial prophylaxis and the risk of surgical site infections: Results from the trial to reduce antimicrobial prophylaxis errors. Ann Surg 2009;250:10–16.

34. Bratzler DW, Houck PM, Richards C, et al. Use of antimicrobial prophylaxis for major surgery: Baseline results from the National Surgical Infection Prevention Project. Arch Surg 2005;140:174–182.

35. Zelenitzky SA, Ariano RE, Harding GKM, et al. Antibiotic pharmacodynamics in surgical prophylaxis: An association between intraoperative antibiotic concentrations and efficacy. Antimicrob Agents Chemother 2002;46:3026–3030.

36. Goldman DA, Hopkins CC, Karchmer AW. Cephalothin prophylaxis in cardiac valve surgery: A prospective, double-blind comparison of two-day and six-day regimen. J Thorac Cardiovasc Surg 1977;73:470–479.

37. Zanetti G, Flanagan HL Jr, Cohn LH, et al. Improvement of intraoperative antibiotic prophylaxis in prolonged cardiac surgery by automated alerts in the operating room. Infect Control Hosp Epidemiol 2003;24:7–9.

38. Waltrip T, Lewis R, Young V, et al. A pilot study to determine the feasibility of continuous cefazolin infusion. Surg Infect 2002;3:5–9.

39. Weinbren MJ. Pharmacokinetics of antibiotics in burn patients. J Antimicrob Chemother 1999;44:319–327.

40. Caffarelli AD, Holden JP, Baron EJ, et al. Plasma cefazolin during cardiovascular surgery: Effects of cardiopulmonary bypass and profound hypothermic circulatory arrest. J Thorac Cardiovasc Surg 2006;131:1338–1343.

41. Weed HG. Antimicrobial prophylaxis in the surgical patient. Med Clin North Am 2003;27:59–75.

42. Salkind AR, Cuddy PG, Foxworth JW. The rational clinical examination: Is this patient allergic to penicillin? An evidence-based analysis of the likelihood of penicillin allergy. JAMA 2001;285:2498–2505.

43. Gemmel CG, Edwards DI, Fraise AP, et al. Guidelines for the prophylaxis and treatment of methicillin Staphylococcus aureus (MRSA) infections in the UK. J Antimicrob Chemother 2006;57:589–608.

44. Hadaway L, Chamallas SN. Vancomycin: New perspectives on an old drug. J Infus Nurs 2003;26:278–284.

45. Wong RS, Cheng G, Chang NP, et al. Use of cefoperazone still needs a caution for bleeding from induced vitamin K deficiency. Am J Hematol 2006;81:76.

46. Williams KJ, Bax RP, Brown H, Machin SJ. Antibiotic treatment and associated prolonged prothrombin time. J Clin Pathol 1991;44:738–741.

47. Frighetto L, Marra CA, Stiver HG, et al. Economic impact of standardized orders for antimicrobial prophylaxis program. Ann Pharmacother 2000;34:154–160.

48. Bratzler DW, Houck PM. Antimicrobial prophylaxis for surgery: An advisory statement from the National Surgical Infection Prevention Project. Clin Infect Dis 2004;38:1706–1715.

49. McArdle CS, Morran CG, Anderson JR, et al. Oral ciprofloxacin as prophylaxis in gastroduodenal surgery. J Hosp Infect 1995;30:211–216.

50. Sharma VK, Howden CW. Meta-analysis of randomized, controlled trials of antibiotic prophylaxis before percutaneous endoscopic gastrostomy. Am J Gastroenterol 2000;95:3133–3136.

51. Kulling D, Sonnenberg A, Fried M, Bauerfeind P. Cost analysis of antibiotic prophylaxis for PEG. Gastrointest Endosc 2000;51:152–156.

52. Jewesson PJ, Stiver G, Wai A, et al. Double-blind comparison of cefazolin and ceftizoxime for prophylaxis against infections following elective biliary tract surgery. Antimicrob Agents Chemother 1996;40:70–74.

53. Agrawal CS, Sehgal R, Singh RK, Gupta AK. Antibiotic prophylaxis in elective cholecystectomy: A randomized, double-blinded study comparing ciprofloxacin and cefuroxime. Ind J Physiol Pharmacol 1999; 43:501–504.

54. Swoboda S, Oberdorfer K, Klee F, et al. Tissue and serum concentrations of levofloxacin 500 mg administered intravenously or orally for antibiotic prophylaxis in biliary surgery. J Antimicrob Chemother 2003;51:459–462.

55. Koc M, Zulfikaroglu B, Kece C, et al. A prospective, randomized study of prophylactic antibiotics in elective laparoscopic cholecystectomy. Surg Endosc 2003;17:1716–1718.

56. Gulberg V, Deibert P, Ochs A, et al. Prevention of infectious complications after transjugular intrahepatic portosystemic shunt in cirrhotic patients with a single dose of ceftriaxone. Hepatogastroenterology 1999;46:1126–1130.

57. Deibert P, Schwartz S, Olschewski M, et al. Risk factors and prevention of early infection after implantation or revision of transjugular intrahepatic portosystemic shunts: Results of a randomized study. Dig Dis Sci 1998;43:1708–1713.

58. Sheen-Chen SM, Chen WJ, Eng HL, et al. Bacteriology and antimicrobial choice in hepatolithiasis. Am J Infect Control 2000;28:298–301.

59. Liberman MA, Greason KL, Frame S, Ragland JJ. Single-dose cefotetan or cefoxitin versus multiple-dose cefoxitin as prophylaxis in patients undergoing appendectomy for acute nonperforated appendicitis. J Am Coll Surg 1995;180:77–80.

60. Colliza S, Rossi S. Antibiotic prophylaxis and treatment of surgical abdominal sepsis. J Chemother 2001;13:193–201.

61. Chung RS, Rowland DY, Li P, Diaz J. A meta-analysis of randomized, controlled trials of laparoscopic versus conventional appendectomy. Am J Surg 1999;177:250–256.

62. Zmora O, Wexner SD, Hajjar L, et al. Trend in preparation for colorectal surgery: Survey of the members of the American Society of Colon and Rectal Surgeons. Am Surg 2003;69:150–154.

63. Zmora O, Mahajna A, Bar-Zakai B, et al. Colon and rectal surgery without mechanical bowel preparation: A randomized, prospective trial. Ann Surg 2003;237:363–367.

64. Guenaga KF, Matos D, Castro AA, et al. Mechanical bowel preparation for elective colorectal surgery. Cochrane Database Syst Rev 2005;1:CD001544.

65. Baum ML, Anish DS, Chalmers TC, et al. A survey of clinical trials of antibiotic prophylaxis in colon surgery: Evidence against further use of no-treatment controls. N Engl J Med 1981;305:795–799.

66. Solla JA, Rothenberger DA. Preoperative bowel preparation: A survey of colon and rectal surgeons. Dis Colon Rectum 1990;33:154–159.

67. Fujita S, Saito N, Yamada T, et al. Randomized, multicenter trial of antibiotic prophylaxis in elective colorectal surgery: Single dose vs 3 doses of a second-generation cephalosporin without metronidazole and oral antibiotics. Arch Surg 2007;142:657–661.

68. Mittelkotter U. Antimicrobial prophylaxis for abdominal surgery: Is there a need for metronidazole? J Chemother 2001;13:27–34.

69. Kobayashi M, Mohri Y, Tonouchi H, et al. Randomized clinical trial comparing intravenous antimicrobial prophylaxis alone with oral and intravenous antimicrobial prophylaxis for the prevention of a surgical site infection in colorectal cancer surgery. Surg Today 2007;37:383–388.

70. Nelson RL, Glenny AM, Song F. Antimicrobial prophylaxis for colorectal surgery. Cochrane Database Syst Rev 2009;1:CD001181.

71. Ghorra SG, Rzeczycki TP, Natarajan R, Pricolo VE. Colostomy closure: Impact of preoperative risk factors on morbidity. Am Surg 1999;65:266–269.

72. Hirota WK, Petersen K, Baron TH, et al. Guidelines for antibiotic prophylaxis for GI endoscopy. Gastrointest Endosc 2003;58:475–482.

73. Sharma VK, Howden CW. Meta-analysis of randomized, controlled trials of antibiotic prophylaxis before percutaneous endoscopic gastrostomy. Am J Gastroenterol 2001;96:1951–1952.

74. Wolf Jr JS, Bennett CJ, Dmochowski RR, Hollenbeck BK, Pearles MS, Schaeffer AJ. Best practice policy statement on urologic surgery antimicrobial prophylaxis. J Urol 2008;179:1379–1390.

75. Christiano AP, Hollowell CM, Kim H, et al. Double-blind, randomized comparison of single-dose ciprofloxacin versus intravenous cefazolin in patients undergoing outpatient endourologic surgery. Urology 2000;55:182–185.

76. Smaill F, Hofmeyr GJ. Antibiotic prophylaxis for cesarean section. Cochrane Database Syst Rev 2002;2:CD000933.

77. Rouzi AA, Khalifa F, Ba'aqeel H, et al. The routine use of cefazolin in cesarean section. Int J Gynaecol Obstet 2000;69:107–112.

78. Tita ATN, Rouse DJ, Blackwell S, Saade GR, Spong CY, Andrews WW. Emerging concepts in antibiotic prophylaxis for cesarean delivery: A systematic review. Obstet Gynecol 2009;113:675–682.

79. Guaschino S, De Santo D, De Seta F. New perspectives in antibiotic prophylaxis for obstetric and gynaecological surgery. J Hosp Infect 2002;50(Suppl A):S13–S16.

80. American College of Obstetricians and Gynecologists. Antibiotic prophylaxis for gynecologic procedures. Obstet Gynecol 2006;108: 225–234.

81. Hemsell DL, Johnson ER, Hemsell PG, et al. Cefazolin is inferior to cefotetan as single dose prophylaxis for women undergoing elective total abdominal hysterectomy. Clin Infect Dis 1995;20: 677–684.

82. Sturlese E, Retto G, Pulia A, et al. Benefits of antibiotic prophylaxis in laparoscopic gynaecological surgery. Clin Exp Obstet Gynecol 1999;26:217–218.

83. Meuller SC, Henkel KO, Neumann J, et al. Perioperative antibiotic prophylaxis in maxillofacial surgery: Penetration of clindamycin into various tissues. J Craniomaxillofac Surg 1999;27:172–176.

84. Simo R, French G. The use of prophylactic antibiotics in head and neck oncological surgery. Curr Opin Otolaryngol Head Neck Surg 2006;14:55–61.

85. Grandis JR, Vickers RM, Rihs JD, et al. Efficacy of topical amoxicillin plus clavulanate-ticarcillin plus clavulanate and clindamycin in contaminated head and neck surgery: Effect of antibiotic spectra and duration of therapy. J Infect Dis 1994;170:729–732.

86. Roy MC. Surgical-site infections after coronary artery bypass graft surgery: Discriminating site-specific risk factors to improve prevention efforts. Infect Control Hosp Epidemiol 1998;19:229–233.

87. Hollenbeak CS, Murphy DM, Koenig S, et al. The clinical and economic impact of deep chest surgical site infections following coronary artery bypass graft surgery. Chest 2000;118:397–402.

88. Curtis JJ, Boley TM, Walls JT, et al. Randomized, prospective comparison of first- and second-generation cephalosporins as infection prophylaxis for cardiac surgery. Am J Surg 1993;166:734–737.

89. Edwards FH, Egleman RM, Houck P, et al. The Society of Thoracic Surgeons Practice Guidelines Series: Antibiotic prophylaxis in cardiac surgery, part 1: duration. Ann Thorac Surg 2006;81:397–404.

90. Finkelstein R, Rabino G, Masiah T, et al. Vancomycin versus cefazolin prophylaxis for cardiac surgery in the setting of a high prevalence of methicillin-resistant staphylococcal infections. J Thorac Cardiovasc Surg 2002;123:326–332.

91. Sok M, Dragas AZ, Erzen J, et al. Sources of pathogens causing pleuropulmonary infections after lung cancer resection. Eur J Cardiothorac Surg 2002;22:23–27.

92. Boldt J, Piper S, Uphus D, et al. Preoperative microbiologic screening and antibiotic prophylaxis in pulmonary resection operations. Ann Thorac Surg 1999;68:208–211.

93. Pratesi C, Russo D, Dorigo W, et al. Antibiotic prophylaxis in clean surgery: Vascular surgery. J Chemother 2001;13:123–128.

94. Marroni M, Cao P, Fiorio M, et al. Prospective, randomized, double-blind trial comparing teicoplanin and cefazolin as antibiotic prophylaxis in prosthetic vascular surgery. Eur J Clin Microbiol Infect Dis 1999;18:175–178.

95. Terpstra S, Noorkhoek GT, Voesten HG, et al. Rapid emergence of resistant coagulase-negative staphylococci on the skin after antibiotic prophylaxis. J Hosp Infect 1999;43:195–202.

96. Gillespie WJ, Walenkamp G. Antibiotic prophylaxis for surgery for proximal femoral and other closed long bone fractures. Cochrane Database Syst Rev 2001;1:CD000244.

97. Vasenius J, Tulikoura I, Vainionpaa S, Rokkanen P. Clindamycin versus cloxacillin in the treatment of 240 open fractures: A randomized, prospective study. Ann Chir Gynaecol 1998;87:224–228.

98. Velmahos GC, Toutouzas KG, Sarkisyan G, et al. Severe trauma is not an excuse for prolonged antibiotic prophylaxis. Arch Surg 2002;137: 537–541.

99. Hosein IK, Hill DW, Hatfield RH. Controversies in the prevention of neurosurgical infection. J Hosp Infect 1999;43:5–11.

100. Barker FG. Efficacy of prophylactic antibiotics for craniotomy: A meta-analysis. Neurosurgery 1994;35:484–492.

101. Pons VG, Denlinger SL, Guglielmo BJ, et al. Ceftizoxime versus vancomycin and gentamicin in neurosurgical prophylaxis: A randomized, prospective, blinded clinical trial. Neurosurgery 1993;33:416–422.

102. Whitby M, Johnson BC, Atkinson RL, et al. The comparative efficacy of intravenous cefotaxime and trimethoprim/sulfamethoxazole in preventing infection after neurosurgery: A prospective, randomized study. Brisbane Neurosurgical Infection Group. Br J Neurosurg 2000;14:13–18.

103. Ratilal B, Costa J, Sampaio C. Antibiotic prophylaxis for surgical introduction of intracranial ventricular shunts: A systematic review. J Neurosurg Pediatr 2008;1:48–56.

104. Barker FG. Efficacy of prophylactic antibiotic therapy in spinal surgery: A meta-analysis. Neurosurgery 2002;51:391–400.

105. Riley LH 3d. Prophylactic antibiotics for spine surgery: Description of a regimen and its rationale. J South Orthop Assoc 1998;7:212–217.

106. Balague Ponz C, Trias M. Laparoscopic surgery and surgical infection. J Chemother 2001;13:17–22.

107. Wilson APR. Antibiotic prophylaxis in endoscopic and minimally invasive surgery. J Chemother 2001;13:102–107.

108. Kurz A, Sessler DI, Lenhardt R. Perioperative normothermia to reduce the incidence of surgical-wound infection and shorten hospitalization. Study of Wound Infection and Temperature Group. N Engl J Med 1996;334:1209–1215.

109. Greif R, Akca O, Horn EP, et al. Supplemental perioperative oxygen to reduce the incidence of surgical-wound infection. Outcomes Research Group. N Engl J Med 2000;342:161–167.

110. Kao LS, Meeks D, Moyer VA, Lally KP. Peri-operative glycaemic control regimens for preventing surgical site infections in adults. Cochrane Database Syst Rev 2009;3:CD006806.

111. Braztler DW, Houck PM, Richards C, et al. Use of antimicrobial prophylaxis for major surgery: Baseline results from the National Surgical Infection Prevention Project. Arch Surg 2005;190:9–15.

112. Braztler DW, Hunt DR. The surgical infection prevention and surgical care improvement projects: National initiatives to improve outcomes for patients having surgery. Clin Infect Dis 2006;43: 322–330.

113. Joint Commission on Accreditation of Healthcare Organizations. Surgical infection prevention core performance measures for national implementation. http//www.jcaho.org/pms/core+measures/10asipmeaslistpop.pdf.

MARY S. HAYNEY

CHAPTER 133

Vaccines, Toxoids, and Other Immunobiologics

KEY CONCEPTS

❶ Live vaccines may confer life long immunity but cannot be administered to the immunosuppressed individual.

❷ Inactivated and subunit vaccines and toxoids often require multiple doses to protect from infection and generally booster doses are needed following the primary series.

❸ Children younger than 2 years of age are unable to mount a T-cell–independent immune responses that are elicited by polysaccharide vaccines.

❹ Severely immunocompromised individuals should not receive live vaccines; and their responses to inactivated, polysaccharide, toxoid, and recombinant vaccines may be poor.

❺ The childhood and adolescent immunization schedule are updated frequently and published annually. These documents can be used to develop an immunization plan for children.

❻ Pneumococcal immunization is done with two different types of vaccines with the conjugate 13 valent vaccine used in infants and the pneumococcal polysaccharide vaccine used in the elderly and other individuals with high risk medical conditions.

❼ Immunoglobulin (Ig) provides rapid post-exposure protection from measles, hepatitis A, varicella, and other infections that wane over time.

❽ Ig adverse effects are often secondary to infusion rate. Slowing the intravenous infusion rate ameliorates chills, nausea, and fever that may develop during administration.

❾ $Rh_o(D)$ Ig prevents Rh-negative mothers from mounting an immune response against hemolytic disease of the newborn. Hemolytic disease of the newborn results when Rh-negative mothers are sensitized to the Rh(D) antigen on the red blood cells of their fetuses.

Immunization is defined as rendering a person protected from an infectious agent. Immunity to an infectious agent can be acquired by exposure to the disease, by transfer of antibodies from mother to fetus, through administration of immunoglobulin (Ig), and from

Learning objectives, review questions, and other resources can be found at **www.pharmacotherapyonline.com**.

vaccination. Immunization is the process of introducing an antigen into the body to induce protection against the infectious agent without causing disease. An *antigen* is a substance that induces an immune response. An *antibody* produced by the humoral arm of the immune system usually is the response that is measured as evidence of successful vaccination. However, the cellular immune response, which is much more difficult to measure, is also an important aspect of vaccine response.

This chapter introduces three groups of agents: vaccines, toxoids, and immune sera (together known as *immunobiologics*). Agents with a limited scope of use, such as agents for bioterrorism or travel, are beyond the scope of this chapter.

PRODUCTS USED TO IMMUNIZE

Vaccines and toxoids are separate and distinct products. However, both types of products induce active immunity—that is, immunity generated by a natural immunologic response to an antigen. Vaccines can be live attenuated or inactivated. Inactivated vaccines may consist of whole or split particles derived from the pathogen. Bacterial vaccines generally are killed whole bacteria or specific bacterial antigens or conjugates. Live-attenuated vaccines induce an immunologic response more consistent with that occurring with natural infection. ❶ Because the organisms in live-attenuated vaccines undergo limited replication in the vaccinated individual after administration, they may confer lifelong immunity with one dose (as does a primary natural infection). ❷ Multiple doses of killed vaccines usually are needed to induce long-lasting, effective immunity. Additional doses at varying time intervals (booster doses) often are required to maintain immunity. Booster doses of such vaccines elicit memory responses from the B cells that produce immunoglobulin G (IgG). The immune system already has developed an array of antibodies to the antigen. Upon restimulation with a booster dose, the B cells, which produce the most specific antibodies against the antigen, are activated. Restimulation allows the most active antibodies against the antigen to be selected and maintained in the "immunologic memory." Thus, the booster dose results in a rapid, intense antibody response that is long lasting. Inactivated vaccines also can differ in immunity potential, depending on their composition. For example, polysaccharide vaccines tend to be poorly immunogenic in infants, whereas protein–polysaccharide conjugated vaccines of the same antigen tend to be highly immunogenic (e.g., pneumococcal polysaccharide vaccine vs pneumococcal conjugated vaccine). ❸ A T cell–independent immune response is made to polysaccharide antigens that stimulate B cells directly.[1] There is no maturation or booster response with a T-cell–independent immune response, and children younger than 2 years cannot make this type of response. Protein–polysaccharide conjugate vaccines stimulate T cells and promote interactions between T cells and B cells when producing the protective immune responses consisting of immunologic memory and high-affinity IgG.

Toxoids are inactivated bacterial toxins that generally are combined with aluminum salts to enhance their antigenicity by prolonging antigen absorption and exposure. These adjuvants also increase local tissue irritation when injected. Toxoids stimulate the production of antibodies against the bacterial toxins rather than the infecting bacterial pathogens.

Immune sera are sterile solutions containing antibody derived from human (immunoglobulin) sources. Immunoglobulins are derived from donor pools of blood plasma and are processed using cold ethanol fractionation in order to inactivate known potential pathogens. These sera are indicated for induction of passive immunity (temporary immunity to infection as a result of administration of antibodies not produced by the host; see Other Immunobiologics below).

In addition to the active component in an immunobiologic, other active and inert ingredients are often present. Suspending agents, such as water, saline, or complex fluids containing proteins (e.g., albumin), are used as the vehicle for the immunobiologic agent. Preservatives, stabilizers, and antibiotics may be added to help maintain the integrity of the product. Immunized individuals may respond with allergic reactions not to the immunobiologic agent itself but to the other components of the pharmaceutical preparation. Different manufacturers of the same immunobiologic may have different active and inert ingredients or different quantities of these ingredients in their products.

Certain vaccines manufactured by various companies are considered interchangeable. Hepatitis A, hepatitis B, and *Haemophilus influenzae* type b (Hib) conjugate vaccines for the primary series of three doses are considered interchangeable. It is preferable to use diphtheria, tetanus toxoids, and acellular pertussis (DTaP) vaccine from the same manufacturer to complete the entire primary series. However, immunization should not be delayed if the particular type of vaccine administered for the initial doses cannot be ascertained easily.[1]

In general, vaccines and toxoids must be kept refrigerated because breaking the "cold chain" may result in loss of potency. Varicella vaccine and zoster vaccines must be stored frozen. Immune sera generally should be kept refrigerated and not frozen except for lyophilized human intravenous immunoglobulin (IVIG), which can be stored at room temperature. Careful attention to appropriate storage of all vaccines and immunobiologics is absolutely imperative. Directions for appropriate storage can be found in the package inserts.

FACTORS AFFECTING RESPONSE TO IMMUNIZATION

Various factors are known to affect response to vaccines and toxoids. Viability of the antigen is an important factor (live attenuated vs inactivated), as discussed previously. Total dose also is important because there seems to exist a threshold dose above which no further increase in antibody titer is seen. The interval between immunization doses, number of doses given, or both may change immune response to an agent. Among hepatitis B vaccine nonresponders, a significant proportion of individuals mount a vaccine response when given additional doses of vaccine.[2] In contrast, additional doses of influenza vaccine are minimally effective in individuals with chronic illness.[3,4] Generally, intervals longer than those recommended between vaccine doses do not reduce immune response.[1]

The route and site of administration of the immunobiologic are important. This is best illustrated by the hepatitis B vaccine, which elicits a satisfactory antibody response when given in the deltoid muscle but not a consistent response when administered in the gluteal area. Injections should be administered at a site with little likelihood of site damage. Immunobiologics containing adjuvants should be given into a muscle mass because they can cause irritation when given subcutaneously or intradermally.[1]

Host factors influence vaccine response. Immunocompromise, increasing age, underlying disease, and genetic background have been associated with poor response rates.[5-8]

VACCINE ADMINISTRATION

Subcutaneous injections should be administered into the thigh of infants and in the upper arm area of older children and adults. A ⅝-inch, 25-gauge needle should be used, taking care not to administer the dose intradermally or intramuscularly (IM). For IM injection, the anterolateral aspect of the upper thigh (infants and toddlers) or the deltoid muscle of the upper arm (children and adults) should be used. When giving an IM injection to an adult, at least a 1-inch needle should be used for persons weighing less than 90 kg and a 1.5-inch needle for persons weighing more than 90 kg to ensure injection in the muscle.[1] The buttock should not be used because of the potential for inadequate immunologic response and the potential risk of injury to the sciatic nerve. When the buttock must be used (as for large doses of Ig), only the upper outer quadrant should be used, with the needle inserted anteriorly.

The rotavirus vaccines are administered orally. The tube of vaccine should be squeezed inside the infant's mouth toward the inner cheek until the dosing tube is empty. If the infant regurgitates or spits out the vaccine, readministration is not recommended.[9]

Live-attenuated influenza vaccine is administered intranasally. A specially designed sprayer is inserted just inside the nostril, and the dose is sprayed by depressing the plunger of the sprayer. The clip is removed from the plunger so that the second half of the dose can be administered into the other nostril. The vaccinated individual should breathe normally. The dose does not need to be repeated if the individual sneezes during or shortly after administration.[4]

Questions often arise concerning the simultaneous administration of vaccines. In general, inactivated and live-attenuated vaccines can be administered simultaneously at separate sites. If two or more inactivated vaccines cannot be administered simultaneously, they can be administered without regard to spacing between doses. Inactivated and live vaccines can be administered simultaneously or, if they cannot be administered simultaneously, at any interval between doses, except for cholera (killed) and yellow fever (live) vaccines, which should be given at least 3 weeks apart. If live vaccines are not administered simultaneously, their administration should be separated by at least 4 weeks. Live viral vaccines may interfere with purified protein derivative response; thus, tuberculin testing should be postponed 4 to 6 weeks after administration of live-virus vaccine.[1]

Simultaneous administration of Ig and live-attenuated vaccines may inhibit host antibody response because of impairment of viral replication. A dose relationship exists between administration of Ig and inhibition of immune response to a vaccine (Table 133-1). Whole blood and other blood products containing antibodies may interfere with the response to the measles, mumps, and rubella (MMR) and varicella vaccines. In any patient, if vaccination with MMR or varicella is followed by emergency Ig administration, the vaccine can be repeated or seroconversion to viral antigens can be confirmed after sufficient time has elapsed (see Table 133-1). Immunoglobulin does not interfere with the response to oral vaccines, zoster vaccine, or yellow fever vaccine.[1,10]

Simultaneous administration of inactivated vaccines along with immunoglobulins is not contraindicated. However, different sites are recommended for killed vaccine and Ig administration.

TABLE 133-1	Suggested Intervals Between Administration of Immunoglobulin and Measles- or Varicella-Containing Vaccine	
Product/Indication	**Dose, Including mg Immunoglobulin G (IgG)/kg Body Weight**	**Recommended Interval Before Measles or Varicella-Containing[a] Vaccine Administration**
RSV monoclonal antibody (Synagis®)[b]	15 mg/kg intramuscularly (IM)	None
Tetanus IG (TIG)	250 units (10 mg IgG/kg) IM	3 months
Hepatitis A IG		
Contact prophylaxis	0.02 mL/kg (3.3.mg IgG/kg) IM	3 months
International travel	0.06 mL/kg (10 mg IgG/kg) IM	3 months
Hepatitis B IG (HBIG)	0.06 mL/kg (10 mg IgG/kg) IM	3 months
Rabies IG (RIG)	20 IU/kg (22 mg IgG/kg) IM	4 months
Measles prophylaxis IG		
Standard (i.e., nonimmunocompromised) contact	0.25 mL/kg (40 mg IgG/kg) IM	5 months
Immunocompromised contact	0.50 mL/kg (80 mg IgG/kg) IM	6 months
Blood tranfusion		
Red blood cells (RBCs), washed	10 mL/kg negligible IgG/kg intravenously (IV)	None
RBCs, adenine-saline added	10 mL/kg (10 mg IgG/kg) IV	3 months
Packed RBCs (Hct 65%)[c]	10 mL/kg (60 mg IgG/kg) IV	6 months
Whole blood (Hct 35%-50%)[c]	10 mL/kg (80-100 mg IgG/kg) IV	6 months
Plasma/platelet products	10 mL/kg (160 mg IgG/kg) IV	7 months
Cytomegalovirus intravenous immune globulin (IGIV)	150 mg/kg maximum	6 months
IGIV		
Replacement therapy for immune deficiencies[d]	300-400 mg/kg IV[c]	8 months
Immune thrombocytopenic purpura	400 mg/kg IV	8 months
Immune thrombocytopenic purpura	1000 mg/kg IV	10 months
Postexposure varicella prophylaxis[e]	400 mg/kg IV	8 months
Kawasaki's disease	2 g/kg IV	11 months

This table is not intended for determining the correct indications and dosages for using antibody-containing products. Unvaccinated persons might not be fully protected against measles during the entire recommended interval, and additional doses of immune globulin or measles vaccine might be indicated after measles exposure. Concentrations of measles antibody in an immune globulin preparation can vary by manufacturer's lot. Rates of antibody clearance after receipt of an immune globulin preparation also might vary. Recommended intervals are extrapolated from an estimated half-life of 30 days for passively acquired antibody and an observed interference with the immune response to measles vaccine for 5 months after a dose of 80 mg IgG/kg.

[a]Varicella-containing vaccine, as used here, does not include zoster vaccine. Zoster vaccine may be given with antibody-containing blood products.
[b]Contains antibody only to respiratory syncytial virus.
[c]Assumes a serum IgG concentration of 16 mg/mL.
[d]Measles and varicella vaccinations are recommended for children with asymptomatic or mildly symptomatic human immunodeficiency virus (HIV) infection but are contraindicated for persons with severe immunosuppression from HIV or any other immunosuppressive disorder.
[e]The investigational product VariZIG, similar to licensed VZIG, is a purified human immune globulin preparation made from plasma containing high levels of anti-varicella antibodies (immunoglobulin class G [IgG]). When indicated, health care providers should make every effort to obtain and administer VariZIG. In situations in which administration of VariZIG does not appear possible within 96 hours of exposure, administration of immune globulin intravenous (IGIV) should be considered as an alternative. IGIV also should be administered within 96 hours of exposure. Although licensed IGIV preparations are known to contain anti-varicella antibody titers, the titer of any specific lot of IGIV that might be available is uncertain because IGIV is not routinely tested for antivaricella antibodies. The recommended IGIV dose for postexposure prophylaxis of varicella is 400 mg/kg, administered once. For a pregnant woman who cannot receive VariZIG within 96 hours of exposure, clinicians can choose either to administer IGIV or closely monitor the woman for signs and symptoms of varicella and institute treatment with acyclovir if illness occurs. (CDC. A new product for postexposure prophylaxis available under an investigational new drug application expanded access protocol. MMWR 2006;55:209–210.)

Increasing the dose or number of vaccines in this circumstance is not recommended.

VACCINE STORAGE

Appropriate storage is critical to maintaining the integrity of vaccines because improperly stored vaccines can fail to protect the individuals to whom they are administered. Refrigerator temperature is defined as between 2°C and 8°C (36°F–46°F) and freezer temperature as −15°C (5°F) or colder. Inactivated vaccines are stored refrigerated. Varicella and zoster vaccines must be stored frozen. Measles-mumps-rubella vaccine can be stored in either the freezer or refrigerator. Live attenuated influenza vaccine is stored in the refrigerator. Specific storage conditions for individual vaccines can be found in the package insert.

IMMUNIZATION OF SPECIAL POPULATIONS

INFANTS

The age of the recipient is an important determining factor in vaccine and toxoid response. In the first few months of life, maternal antibodies acquired via transplacental transfer during the third trimester of gestation protect an infant. However, the maternal antibodies also inhibit the immune response to live vaccines because the circulating antibodies neutralize the vaccine before the infant has the opportunity to mount an immune response. For this reason, live vaccines are not administered until maternal antibodies have waned, generally by infant age 12 months.[1]

Premature infants should be vaccinated at the same chronologic age using the same schedule and precautions for full-term infants. The full recommended doses of vaccines should be used, regardless of age or birth weight. Breastfed infants should be vaccinated according to standard pediatric schedules.

PREGNANT WOMEN AND POST-PARTUM IMMUNIZATION

Most vaccines are pregnancy category C. As with most drugs, the vaccines are given this category assignment not because of a known risk to the fetus but because of lack of information. No birth defect has ever been attributed to vaccine exposure.[1] For example, no cases of congenital rubella syndrome from inadvertent administration of rubella vaccine to a pregnant woman have ever been reported. Universal influenza immunization is recommended for women who will be or are pregnant during influenza season. Tetanus-diphtheria (Td) vaccine is recommended for pregnant women who have not received a Td booster in the past 10 years or requires tetanus prophylaxis with a tetanus prone wound (see Tetanus section). Although live vaccines generally are avoided because of the theoretical risk of transmission of the vaccine organism to the fetus, inactivated vaccines may be administered to pregnant women when the benefits outweigh the risks.[1] Hepatitis B, hepatitis A, meningococcal, inactivated polio, and pneumococcal polysaccharide vaccines should be administered to pregnant women who are at risk for contracting these infections.[11]

Administration of live vaccines, such as rubella or varicella, are deferred until post-partum and are routinely recommended for new mothers who do not have evidence of immunity prior to hospital discharge. These live vaccines can be administered without regard to administration of $Rh_o(D)$ Ig in the postpartum period. Additionally, Tdap is recommended for all new mothers who have not received a tetanus dose in the past two years because household contacts are frequently implicated as the source of pertussis infection in a young infant.[12]

IMMUNOCOMPROMISED HOSTS

Vaccination in compromised hosts (e.g., those with chronic disease, such as diabetes or connective tissue disease, alcoholics, or those with cancer or HIV disease) must be individualized based on the disease state and its treatment. ❹ In general, severely immunocompromised individuals should not receive live vaccines. Administration of other vaccines may be indicated, but responses may be lower than those mounted by healthy individuals, but may still confer protection.[6,8]

Patients with chronic pulmonary, renal, hepatic, or metabolic disease who are not receiving immunosuppressants can receive both live-attenuated and killed vaccines and toxoids to induce active immunity. These patients often need higher doses of vaccines or more frequent dosing to induce immunity. Generally, immunization should be considered early in the course of the disease in an attempt to induce immunity at a point when the disease is less severe.

Patients with active malignant disease can receive killed vaccines or toxoids but should not be given live vaccines. The MMR vaccine is not contraindicated for close contacts, however. Live-virus vaccines can be administered to persons with leukemia who have not received chemotherapy for at least 3 months. Vaccines should be timed so that they do not coincide with the start of chemotherapy or radiation therapy. Zoster vaccine should be administered at least 2 weeks prior to the start of immunosuppressing therapy.[10] Annual influenza vaccine should be administered 2 weeks prior to chemotherapy or between cycles.[6] If vaccines cannot be given at least 2 weeks before the start of these therapies, immunization should be postponed until 3 months after the therapy has been completed. Passive immunization with Ig can be used in place of active immunization regardless of the history of immunization.

Glucocorticoids may cause suppressed responses to vaccines. For the purposes of immunization, the immunosuppressing dose of corticosteroids is prednisone 20 mg or more daily or 2 mg/kg daily, or an equivalent dose of another steroid, for at least 2 weeks. Patients receiving long-term, alternate-day steroid therapy with short-acting agents, administration of maintenance physiologic doses of steroids (e.g., 5–10 mg/day of prednisone) topical, aerosol, intraarticular, bursal, or tendon steroid injections require no special consideration for immunization. If patients have been receiving high-dose corticosteroids or have had a course lasting longer than 2 weeks, then at least 1 month should pass before immunization with live-virus vaccines.[1]

Patients with HIV infection require special consideration. Responses to live and inactivated vaccines generally are suboptimal and decrease as the disease progresses because HIV produces defects in cell-mediated immunity and humoral immunity. The routinely recommended vaccines should be administered to children. Two doses of MMR vaccine should be administered at least 1 month apart as soon as possible after the first birthday. MMR and varicella virus should be administered only to children who have no or only moderate evidence of immunosuppression.[1] Two doses of varicella vaccine separated by 3 months are recommended only for children with no evidence of immunosuppression. Adults should receive routinely recommended vaccines. Zoster vaccine may be administered to individuals with HIV infection who do not have clinical manifestations of AIDS and have CD4 counts $>200/mm^3$.[1,10]

TRANSPLANT PATIENTS

Solid-Organ Transplant Patients

Organ transplantation has become routine treatment of end-stage organ disease of many causes. Although the number of organ transplants performed is severely limited by the availability of donor organs, survival of transplant recipients is increasing. Solid-organ transplant patients remain on immunosuppressive regimens for the rest of their lives. These immunosuppressive regimens result in a higher risk of infection and decrease the protection conferred by immunization.[13]

Whenever possible, transplant patients should be immunized prior to transplantation. Live vaccines generally are not given after transplantation. Post-transplantation diphtheria, tetanus, pneumococcal, and influenza vaccine responses are unpredictable. Decreased immune response has been documented following hepatitis B vaccine.

Hematopoietic Stem Cell Transplant Patients

Reimmunization of patients with hematopoietic stem cell transplantation is necessary because antibody concentrations wane rapidly. Annual influenza immunization may begin as soon as 6 months after successful engraftment. Reimmunization with inactivated vaccines should begin approximately 12 months after hematopoietic stem cell transplantation. Hematopoietic stem cell transplant recipients are at increased risk for fulminant infection with encapsulated bacteria so PPSV23 and Hib vaccines are recommended. Less evidence exists in support of meningococcal conjugate vaccine or pneucmococcal conjugate vaccine administration. MMR can be administered at 24 months. Varicella vaccine is not routinely recommended but can be considered on a case-by-case basis. Immunization of household contacts and healthcare workers also is necessary.[1]

CONTRAINDICATIONS AND PRECAUTIONS

There are few contraindications to the use of vaccines except those outlined earlier. The contraindications include a history of anaphylactic reactions to the vaccine or a component of the vaccine. Unexplained encephalopathy occurring within 7 days of a dose of pertussis vaccine is a contraindication to future doses of pertussis vaccines. Immunosuppression and pregnancy are temporary contraindications to live vaccines. An interval of time must elapse based on the dose of Ig before a live vaccine can be administered (see Table 133–1). Precautions for DTaP administration include hypotonic hyporesponsive episode, fever of 40.5°C (104.9°F) or greater, crying lasting more than 3 hours within 48 hours of a previous dose, and seizures with or without fever within 3 days after a dose.[1] Generally, mild to moderate local reactions, mild acute illnesses, concurrent antibiotic use, prematurity, family history of adverse events, diarrhea, and lactation or breastfeeding are not contraindications to immunization.

OBTAINING AN IMMUNIZATION HISTORY

An immunization history should be obtained from every patient, regardless of the reason for the healthcare visit. Ideally, any history provided by the patient from memory should be verified by reviewing the patient's personal written immunization record or a database that contains the complete immunization history. State-based or other public health jurisdiction-based immunization registries has been developed to improve immunization coverage by allowing healthcare providers access to records at any contact with the healthcare system. Registries are aimed primarily at facilitation of childhood immunization records.[14] If an official written record is not available, patient characteristics (e.g., military service, travel history, and occupation) may provide clues to the immunization history. Serologic testing for immunity against certain diseases can provide specific information but is used routinely for only a few selected diseases (e.g., measles, rubella, hepatitis A and B, and varicella) and selected circumstances (e.g., employment in a healthcare facility). If a written record does not exist, one should be generated at the time of initiation of immunization. Patients without a written record should be considered susceptible, and an immunization program started and completed unless a serious adverse reaction occurs. As a general rule, the risks associated with overimmunization are minimal relative to the risks associated with contracting vaccine-preventable diseases.[1]

Every healthcare visit, regardless of its purpose, should be viewed as an opportunity to review a patient's immunization status and to administer needed vaccines. Immunization is perhaps the most cost-effective health intervention available. Each visit should include assessment of individuals' vaccine needs, administration of indicated agents, and documentation of immunization histories. The outcome measurement of what percentage of patients in a particular practice site is completely immunized is extremely important because the benefits of optimal vaccine use extend beyond the individual patient to the public as a whole.

NATIONAL VACCINE INJURY COMPENSATION PROGRAM

The National Childhood Vaccine Injury Act of 1986 was passed by the U.S. Congress in response to reports of vaccine side effects and liability concerns of vaccine manufacturers and healthcare providers. With vaccine safety being questioned and manufacturers ceasing the development and marketing of vaccines, the National Vaccine Injury Compensation Program was implemented to offer a no-fault alternative means to compensate victims for injury following vaccination. The program offers liability protection to manufacturers and an efficient means of recovering damages for individuals potentially injured by vaccines. Compensation for vaccine-related injuries is outlined in the Health Resources and Services Administration's Vaccine Injury Table (*http://www.hrsa. gov/vaccinecompensation/table.htm*). Healthcare providers must report all events requiring medical attention within 30 days of vaccination to the Vaccine Adverse Event Reporting System (VAERS), which serves as a central depot for vaccine-related adverse effects. Only a temporal association between the adverse event and vaccine administration needs to be made. No adverse event rates can be determined because only the number of adverse events reported is known; the number of vaccines administered is not known. This database can be used to determine changes in the frequencies of adverse events, to evaluate risk factors for adverse events, and to find rare adverse events.[15] VAERS report forms can be obtained by calling 1-800-822-7967, or reports can be made online at *https:// vaers.hhs.gov/esub/index*.

USE OF VACCINES AND TOXOIDS

❺ The Appendices show the recommended schedules for routine immunization of children and adults. All states require children to be fully immunized prior to entering elementary school; however, optimal protection is achieved by immunizing at the recommended ages, which requires special attention to children younger than 2 years. Adults and adolescents also require vaccination and often are unaware of this need. An early adolescent preventive health visit is recommended. This visit is an opportunity to catch up on missed immunizations and to administer meningococcal conjugate, Tdap, and, for females, human papillomavirus (HPV) vaccines. Adults should receive routine Td or Tdap boosters and be immune to measles, mumps, rubella, and varicella by either immunization or history of infection. Older adults need an annual influenza vaccine after age 50 years, zoster vaccine after age 60 years, and pneumococcal polysaccharide vaccine after age 65 years. Certain individuals with conditions or lifestyles that put them at high risk for vaccine-preventable diseases also should be immunized as described in the following text and outlined in the immunization schedules in the appendices.

TOXOIDS

DIPHTHERIA TOXOID ADSORBED

Diphtheria is an acute illness caused by the toxin released by a *Corynebacterium diphtheriae* infection. The toxin inhibits cellular protein synthesis, and membranes form on mucosal surfaces. Systemic toxemia can result in myocarditis, neuritis, and thrombocytopenia. Membrane formation can cause respiratory obstruction, and significant toxin absorption can lead to severe illness and death.

Diphtheria toxoid adsorbed is a sterile suspension of modified toxins of *C. diphtheriae* that induces immunity against the exotoxin of this organism. Two strengths of diphtheria toxoid are available in the United States: pediatric strength (D) and adult strength (d), which contains less antigen. The widespread use of diphtheria toxoid essentially has eliminated diphtheria from the United States.

Primary immunization with diphtheria toxoid (D) is indicated for children older than 6 weeks. The toxoid is given in combination with tetanus toxoid and acellular pertussis vaccine (as DTaP or in combination with additional childhood vaccines that have been licensed to decrease the number of injections required to complete the childhood immunization recommendations) at age 2, 4, and 6 months. Additional doses are given at age 15 to 18 months and again at age 4 to 6 years.[16] Completing the primary diphtheria toxoid immunization series usually induces immunity of at least 10 years' duration in 90% of persons. Booster doses should be given every 10 years.

For unimmunized adults, a complete three-dose series of diphtheria toxoid should be administered, with the first two doses given at least 4 weeks apart and the third dose given 6 to 12 months after the second. The combined Td preparation is recommended for adults because it contains less diphtheria toxoid than the pediatric dose and is associated with fewer reactions to the diphtheria component. If the adult is 64 years of age or younger, one of the vaccine doses in this series should be Tdap.[17] All adults should receive booster doses of Td every 10 years. Adverse effects of diphtheria toxoid include mild to moderate tenderness, erythema, and induration at the injection site. Systemic reactions occur very rarely.

TETANUS TOXOID, TETANUS TOXOID ADSORBED, AND TETANUS IMMUNOGLOBULIN

Tetanus is a severe acute illness caused by the exotoxin of *Clostridium tetani*. Tetanus is the only vaccine-preventable disease that is not contagious. It is acquired from the environment. Sustained muscle contractions are characteristic of tetanus. Tetanus toxin interferes with neurotransmitters that promote muscle relaxation, leading to continuous muscle spasms.[17] Death can be due to the tetanus toxin itself or secondary to a complication such as aspiration pneumonia, dysregulation of the autonomic nervous system, or pulmonary embolism.

Tetanus toxoid and tetanus toxoid adsorbed (adsorbed onto aluminum hydroxide, phosphate, or potassium sulfate to increase antigenicity) are sterile suspensions of the toxoid derived from *C. tetani*. Both toxoids are used to promote active immunity against tetanus; however, tetanus toxoid adsorbed is the preferred agent because it elicits a greater immune response and is associated with fewer adverse reactions.

A series of three 0.5-mL doses of tetanus toxoid elicits protection in virtually all individuals. Primary vaccination provides protection for at least 10 years.[12,17,18] Additional doses of tetanus toxoid (combined with diphtheria toxoid, i.e., Td) are recommended as part of wound management if a patient has not received a dose of tetanus toxoid within the preceding 5 years. For minor or clean wounds, no dose is given. Table 133-2 summarizes these recommendations. Tetanus Ig should be given to individuals who have received fewer than three doses of tetanus toxoid and have more serious wounds. It can be administered with tetanus toxoid, provided that separate syringes and separate injection sites are used.

In children, primary immunization against tetanus usually is offered in conjunction with diphtheria and pertussis vaccination (using DTaP or a combination vaccine that includes other antigens used to decrease the number of injections to complete the childhood immunization schedule). A 0.5-mL dose is recommended at age 2, 4, 6, and 15 to 18 months, but the first dose can be administered as early as age 6 weeks.[16] In children 7 years and older and in adults who have not been immunized previously, a series of three 0.5-mL doses of Td is administered IM initially. The first two doses are given 1 to 2 months apart, and the third dose is recommended at 6 to 12 months after the second dose. Boosters are recommended every 10 years, and unless there is contraindication to diphtheria toxoid, Td should be used. Tetanus toxoid can be given simultaneously with other killed and live vaccines, and, if indicated, it can be given to immunosuppressed patients.

Adverse reactions to tetanus toxoid include mild to moderate local reactions at the injection site, such as warmth, erythema, and induration. Rarely, fever, malaise, aches and pains, or neurologic disorders have been reported. In general, major local reactions occur within 2 to 8 hours of administration to patients with high serum tetanus antitoxin levels. This type of reaction is indicative of high preexisting antibody concentrations, and additional doses of toxoid should not be given any sooner than 10 years. Local reactions do not limit the use of the toxoid for further dosing.

TABLE 133-2 Tetanus Prophylaxis				
Vaccination History	**Clean, Minor**		**All Other**	
	Td[a]	TIG	Td[a]	TIG
Unknown or fewer than three doses	Yes	No	Yes	Yes
Three or more doses	No[a,b]	No	No[a,c]	No

[a]A single dose of Tdap should be used for the next dose of tetanus-diphtheria toxoid for individuals aged 10 or 11 years to 64 years.
[b]Yes, if more than 10 years since last dose.
[c]Yes, if more than 5 years since last dose.

Tetanus immunoglobulin is a sterile, concentrated, nonpyrogenic solution of immunoglobulins prepared from hyperimmunized humans. It is used to provide passive immunity to tetanus after the occurrence of traumatic wounds in nonimmunized or suboptimally immunized persons (see Table 133-2). A dose of 250 to 500 units IM should be administered. When administered with tetanus toxoid, separate sites for administration should be used. Tetanus immunoglobulin also is used for treatment of tetanus. In this setting, a single dose of 3,000 to 6,000 units IM is administered.

Adverse effects of tetanus immunoglobulin include pain, tenderness, erythema, and muscle stiffness at the injection site, which may persist for several hours. Systemic reactions occur rarely. IV administration has been associated with severe adverse reactions and is not recommended.

VACCINES

HAEMOPHILUS INFLUENZAE TYPE B VACCINES

Before 1995, Hib was responsible for thousands of cases of serious illnesses (e.g., meningitis, epiglottitis, pneumonia, sepsis, and septic arthritis). The incidence of Hib disease has declined more than 99% since introduction of the conjugate vaccines based on the organism's capsular substance, polyribosylribitol phosphate (PRP).[19]

The Hib vaccines used are conjugate products consisting of either a polysaccharide or an oligosaccharide of PRP covalently linked to a protein carrier. The protein carrier is important because it provides for T-lymphocyte–dependent immunologic response, whereas earlier Hib vaccines that consisted of only unconjugated PRP elicited a response that was T-cell independent. T-cell involvement in the response provides for (a) a greater antibody response regardless of the age of the patient receiving the vaccine, (b) immunologic response at an earlier age (including infants), and (c) a booster effect on subsequent exposure to the Hib capsule, whether through revaccination or natural exposure. The protein carrier is not considered a vaccine and should not be substituted for immunization against tetanus, diphtheria, or *Neisseria meningitidis*.

Hib conjugate vaccines are indicated for routine use in all infants and children younger than 5 years. Additionally, these three products differ in their immunogenicity and schedule of administration (Table 133-3). The primary series of Hib vaccination consists of a 0.5-mL IM dose at ages 2, 4, and 6 months if HbOC (HibTITER) or PRP-T (ActHIB) is used. If PRP-OMP is being used, the primary series consists of doses given at ages 2 and 4 months. The series should not be initiated in an infant younger than 6 weeks. Although use of one product for the entire primary series is desirable, adequate protection is achieved even when different products are used during the initial doses. Following the primary series, a booster dose is recommended at age 12 to 15 months. Any of the Hib conjugate vaccines are suitable for the booster dose regardless of which conjugate was used for the primary series of doses.[16]

TABLE 133-3 *Haemophilus influenzae* Type b Conjugate Vaccine Products

Vaccine	Trade Name	Protein Carrier
PRP-T	ActHIB (Sanofi Pasteur)	Tetanus toxoid
PRP-OMP	PedvaxHIB (Merck)	*Neisseria meningitides* serogroup B outer membrane protein
PRP-T	Hiberix (Glaxo Smith Kline)	Tetanus toxoid (booster only)

The polysaccharide is polyribosylribitol-phosphate (PRP).

Schedules are more complex for infants who do not begin Hib immunization at the recommended age or who have fallen behind in the immunization schedule. For infants 7 to 11 months of age who have not been vaccinated, three doses of HbOC, PRP-OMP, or PRP-T should be given: two doses spaced 4 weeks apart and then a booster dose at age 12 to 15 months (but at least 8 weeks since the second dose). For unvaccinated children ages 12 to 14 months, two doses should be given, with an interval of 2 months between doses. In a child older than 15 months, a single dose of any of the four conjugate vaccines is indicated.[16] The American Academy of Pediatrics has made recommendations for children with lapsed immunization. For infants 7 to 11 months who have received one or two doses of Hib vaccine, one dose of vaccine with a booster dose at least 8 weeks later at age 12 to 15 months should be given. For children 12 to 14 months who received two doses, a single dose is indicated. If the child received only one dose before age 12 months, two additional doses separated by 8 weeks should be given. A single dose of vaccine is needed for a child 15 to 59 months old who has received any incomplete schedule.[16]

Vaccines for Hib are recommended for routine use only for patients up to age 59 months; beyond this age, most individuals will have natural immunity to Hib infection. Patients with certain underlying conditions (e.g., HIV infection, IgG$_2$ subclass deficiency, sickle cell disease, splenectomy, and hematopoietic stem cell transplants and those receiving chemotherapy for malignancies) are at higher than normal risk for Hib infection, and use of at least one dose of vaccine in these patients should be considered, although efficacy data in most of these situations are lacking.[1,20]

Adverse reactions to the Hib vaccine are uncommon. Erythema and induration at the injection site occur in approximately 25% of children and resolve within 24 hours. Fever, diarrhea, and vomiting are reported occasionally. Fever greater than 38°C (100.4°F) is reported in 2.4% of children.

HEPATITIS VACCINES

Information on vaccination for viral hepatitis is given in Chapter 47.

HUMAN PAPILLOMAVIRUS VACCINE

HPV infections are the most common sexually transmitted infections, with the highest prevalence of infection in sexually active young adults.[21] Although more than 120 different HPV types have been identified, at least 40 different types of HPV infect the anogenital tract. These 40 different viruses are grouped into low-risk and high-risk types. Low-risk types can cause genital warts and mild abnormalities on Papanicolaou (Pap) tests. Ninety percent of all cases of genital warts are caused by types 6 and 11. As many as 18 types are considered high risk. They cause abnormal Pap test results and may lead to cancer of the cervix, vulva, vagina, anus, or penis. Types 16 and 18 cause about 70% of all cervical cancers. High-risk HPV infections are necessary but not sufficient for the development of cervical cancer and for the majority of other anogenital and oral squamous cell cancers.

A bivalent human papillomavirus vaccine (Cervarix, GSK) containing virus-like particles for types 16 and 18 was licensed in late 2009. The quadrivalent vaccine (Gardasil, Merck Vaccines) is directed against cervical cancer-causing types 16 and 18 and types 6 and 11. ACIP recommends either of these HPV vaccine preparations for the prevention of cervical cancer and precancerous lesions. No head-to-head comparison of these vaccines is available, but both vaccines are very efficacious for the prevention of precancerous lesions caused by types 16 and 18.[22] Both vaccines offer some protection against oncogenic nonvaccine strains too.[23-25] Both vaccines are administered as a three dose series using a harmonized schedule of 0, 1 to 2, and 6 months. The vaccines are recommended for females aged 11 to 12 years and for all females aged 13 to 26 years. Although administration of these vaccines before sexual debut is preferable, the vaccines can be administered without regard to history of sexual activity.

The quadrivalent HPV vaccine is licensed for the prevention of genital warts in males aged 9 to 26 years. Types 6 and 11 cause approximately 90% of genital warts. Although not considered a serious disease, the direct medical cost of genital warts is about $200 million annually, and genital warts have an impact on quality of life.[26] Additionally, approximately one fourth to one third of oropharyngeal cancers are associated with a high risk HPV infection.[27] No data on the usefulness of the vaccine for the prevention of these cancers are available yet. ACIP stated that HPV4 may be given to males aged 9-26 years of age but stopped short of a recommendation for it. The vaccine is effective for the prevention of genital warts, but the cost-effectiveness of the vaccine series for males is a major hurdle.

The vaccines are well tolerated, with injection-site reactions and systemic reactions (e.g., headache and fatigue) occurring as commonly in immunized individuals as in the groups receiving placebo. Although syncope is possible with any immunization, the target population of young women have a higher incidence of syncope, including with administration of the HPV vaccine.[27,28]

These effective vaccines is an important advance, but the need for a Pap test for cervical cancer screening remains. Surveillance for duration of protection conferred by the vaccine series is ongoing; the need for future booster doses is not yet known.

INFLUENZA VIRUS VACCINE

Information on vaccination for influenza is given in Chapter 118.

MEASLES VACCINE

Measles (rubeola) is a highly contagious viral illness characterized by rash and high fever. Complications of measles infections include severe diarrhea, otitis media, pneumonia, and encephalitis. Measles results in one to two deaths per 1,000 cases, with a much higher death rate in developing countries. With widespread vaccination, measles is on the verge of elimination from the Western Hemisphere.

The measles vaccine is a live-attenuated viral vaccine that produces a subclinical, noncommunicable infection. Approximately 95% of vaccine recipients seroconvert after a single dose, and most individuals are protected for life.[25] Most persons who do not respond to the initial dose of measles vaccine will seroconvert after receiving a second dose, and this forms the basis for the two-dose vaccine strategy that was implemented in the United States in 1989.

The measles vaccine is administered subcutaneously as a 0.5-mL dose in the arm (or in the thigh if the patient is younger than 15 months). The vaccine is administered routinely for primary immunization to persons 12 to 15 months of age, usually as the MMR vaccine. The measles vaccine is not administered earlier than 12 months (except in certain outbreak circumstances) because persisting maternal antibody that was acquired transplacentally late in gestation can neutralize the vaccine virus before the vaccinated person can mount an immune response. A second dose of MMR or MMRV is recommended when children are 4 to 6 years old.[16] The second dose of vaccine results in seroconversion in 95% of individuals who were first-dose nonresponders.

Measles-containing vaccine should not be given to pregnant women or immunosuppressed patients. The one exception is HIV-infected patients, who are at very high risk for severe complications if they develop measles.[26] Persons with HIV infection who have never had measles or have never been vaccinated against it should be given measles-containing vaccine unless there is evidence of severe immunosuppression. The second dose should be given 1 month later rather than waiting for entry to school.

Recent administration of Ig interferes with measles vaccine response, so the recommended interval between the Ig and vaccine is determined by the dose of Ig (see Table 133–1).[1] Live vaccines not administered during the same visit must be delayed for at least 30 days following measles or MMR vaccine. Live measles vaccine may suppress a positive tuberculin skin test for up to 6 weeks postadministration.[1] Persons with a history of anaphylactic reaction to egg protein were considered to be at high risk for serious reactions to measles vaccine, a product derived from chick embryo fibroblasts. However, the risk of measles vaccination to egg-allergic patients is exceedingly low. Therefore, individuals requiring the measles vaccine should receive it regardless of a history of egg allergy.[25] A history of serious neomycin hypersensitivity remains a contraindication to measles vaccine use because each 0.5-mL dose contains 25 mcg neomycin. Finally, mild febrile illness and upper respiratory tract infections are not contraindications to vaccination.[25]

Measles vaccination is indicated in all persons born after 1956 or in those who lack documentation of wild virus infection by either history or antibody titers. Persons who received killed measles vaccine alone, who were given live vaccine within 3 months of receiving killed vaccine, or who received a vaccine of unknown type between 1963 and 1967 should be revaccinated. Two doses of a measles-containing vaccine are required for college students and healthcare workers who were born in 1957 or later. If two doses are needed (the person has never been vaccinated), the doses should be given at least 1 month apart.[27]

The measles vaccine has an excellent safety record. The most common side effect following vaccination is fever, which occurs in 5% to 15% of vaccinees. Transient generalized rash may occur in approximately 5% of vaccine recipients. These reactions generally appear 5 to 12 days postvaccination and last 2 to 5 days. Other adverse effects, such as headache, cough, sore throat, eye pain, malaise, and transient thrombocytopenia, occur less frequently. Local reactions at the injection site are rare but may occur in subjects who have been vaccinated previously with killed vaccine. After extensive study, no association between MMR vaccination and the development of autism has been made.[28]

MENINGOCOCCAL POLYSACCHARIDE AND CONJUGATE VACCINES

N. meningitidis is a leading cause of meningitis and sepsis in children and young adults in the United States. College freshmen, particularly those living in dormitories or residence halls, are at modestly increased risk for invasive meningococcal disease compared with the rest of the population in this age group.[29]

Two meningococcal conjugate vaccines combining the same serotypes are licensed for use in individuals aged 2 to 55 years old (Menaetra®, Sanofi-Pasteur) or 11 to 55 years old (Menveo®,

Novartis). A quadrivalent vaccine containing capsular polysaccharides for serotypes A, C, Y, and W-135 has been available since the early 1970s. A conjugate vaccine containing the same serotypes was licensed for use in individuals 2 to 55 years old. Although serogroup B causes approximately one third of all cases, it has not been incorporated into the vaccine because group B polysaccharide is not immunogenic. Either meningococcal conjugate vaccine is recommended for all children 11 to 12 years old and others at high risk for invasive meningococcal infection, including high school students and college freshmen who live in dormitories. The meningococcal polysaccharide vaccine is indicated in high-risk populations, such as those exposed to the disease, those in the midst of uncontrolled outbreaks, travelers to areas with epidemic or hyperendemic meningococcal disease, and individuals who have terminal complement component deficiencies or asplenia. The polysaccharide preparation can be used for the immunization of college students and adults between 20 and 55 years of age, but the conjugate vaccine is preferred.[29]

Meningococcal polysaccharide vaccine is administered subcutaneously as a 0.5-mL dose. Meningococcal conjugate vaccine is administered by IM injection. Reimmunization at 5-year intervals should be considered for individuals who remain at high risk for invasive meningococcal disease.[30]

Injection-site reactions are the most common adverse effects following administration of either the meningococcal conjugate or polysaccharide vaccine.

MUMPS VACCINE

Mumps is a viral illness that classically causes bilateral parotitis 16 to 18 days after exposure. Fever, headache, malaise, myalgia, and anorexia may precede the parotitis. Serious complications are rare but more common in adults.

The mumps vaccine is a lyophilized live-attenuated vaccine prepared from chick embryo cultures. Each 0.5-mL dose of the vaccine also contains neomycin 25 mcg. The vaccine is available alone or in combinations with measles, rubella (as MMR), and varicella (MMRV) vaccines.

The vaccine is administered as a 0.5-mL subcutaneous injection in the upper arm. Dosing recommendations coincide with those for measles vaccine, with the first dose administered at age 12 to 15 months and the second dose prior to the child's entry into elementary school. Two doses of mumps-containing vaccine are recommended for school-aged children, international travelers, students in post-high school educational institutions, and healthcare workers born after 1956.[31] A single dose of vaccine is acceptable documentation of immunity to mumps for other adults considered at lower risk of mumps infection, including adults born after 1956 and those with an uncertain history of wild virus infection.

Mumps vaccine should not be given to pregnant women or immunosuppressed patients.[1] Anaphylactic reactions to mumps-containing vaccines are very rare and generally not associated with hypersensitivity to eggs. Therefore, egg allergy is not a contraindication to vaccination. The effect of Ig preparations on mumps vaccine response is unknown, but the response to measles, rubella, and varicella is compromised if the vaccine is administered after immunoglobulins. The recommended interval between the Ig and vaccine is determined by the dose of Ig (see Table 133–1).[1] The vaccine should not be given to individuals with anaphylactic reactions to neomycin.

Serious adverse reactions to the vaccine are reported rarely. Parotitis, rash, pruritus, and purpura occur rarely. Local reactions, including soreness, burning, and stinging, may occur at the injection site.

PERTUSSIS VACCINE

Pertussis is caused by a bacterial infection with *Bordetella pertussis*. The illness is characterized by paroxysms of coughing to expel thick mucus. At the end of every burst, a long inspiratory effort results in the traditional "whooping" sound. Children will often become cyanotic during the coughing spasm and be exhausted or vomit at the end of the attack. It is during this stage when pertussis is usually diagnosed. Adolescents and adults with pertussis experience similar symptoms, though typically not nearly as severe as infants and young children. Adults are less likely to "whoop" in the paroxysmal stage; in fact their cough can be so minor that it is difficult to distinguish from other common respiratory infections. Prior to the availability of a vaccine, pertussis was a common childhood infection and was a significant cause of childhood mortality. Pertussis is most contagious in the early stage of the disease, can infect people of all ages, but is most serious in infants and young children.[17,18]

Acellular pertussis vaccines contain components of the *B. pertussis* organism. All acellular vaccines contain pertussis toxin, and some contain one or more additional bacterial components (e.g., filamentous hemagglutinin, pertactin [a 69-kDa outer membrane protein], and fimbriae types 2 and 3). Acellular pertussis vaccine is recommended for all doses of the pertussis schedule at 2, 4, 6, and 15 to 18 months of age. A fifth dose of pertussis vaccine is given to children 4 to 6 years of age.[16] Pertussis vaccine is administered in combination with diphtheria and tetanus (DTaP). Administration of an acellular pertussis–containing vaccine is also recommended for adolescents once between ages 11 and 18 years. Also, adults up to age 64 years should receive a pertussis-containing vaccine with their next dose of Td toxoids.[17,18]

Local administration site reactions are relatively common. Systemic reactions, such as moderate fever, occur in 3% to 5% of vaccinees. Very rarely, high fever, febrile seizures, persistent crying spells, and hypotonic hyporesponsive episodes occur following vaccination. Allergy to a vaccine component and encephalopathy without known cause within 7 days of a pertussis vaccine are contraindications to future doses of vaccine.

PNEUMOCOCCAL VACCINES

Streptococcus pneumoniae is a common pathogen with a range of manifestations, including asymptomatic upper respiratory tract colonization, sinusitis, acute otitis media, pharyngitis, pneumonia, meningitis, and bacteremia. Rates of invasive infections are highest in children younger than 2 years and in the elderly.[32] Invasive pneumococcal infections cause approximately 40,000 deaths annually. Most of the deaths occur in the elderly or in those with underlying medical conditions.[33] Approximately half the deaths could be preventable by vaccine. Two pneumococcal vaccine preparations, PCV13 and 23-valent pneumococcal polysaccharide vaccine (PPV23) are available. The vaccines have different indications and are not interchangeable.

Pneumococcal Polysaccharide Vaccine

Pneumococcal polysaccharide vaccine (Pneumovax 23) is a mixture of highly purified capsular polysaccharides from 23 of the most prevalent or invasive types of *S. pneumoniae* seen in the United States. Serotypes included are 1, 2, 3, 4, 5, 6B, 7F, 8, 9N, 9V, 10A, 11A, 12F, 14, 15B, 17F, 18C, 19A, 19F, 20, 22F, 23F, and 33F. These 23 types represent 85% to 90% of all blood isolates and 85% of pneumococcal isolates from other generally sterile sites seen in the United States. The vaccine is administered IM or subcutaneously as a single 0.5-mL dose. Each 0.5-mL dose of vaccine contains 25 mcg of each polysaccharide type dissolved in isotonic saline solution (for a total of 575 mcg polysaccharide) and 0.25% phenol as preservative.[33]

❻ PPSV23 is recommended for the following individuals:[33]

- Persons 65 years and older (if an individual received vaccine more than 5 years earlier and was younger than 65 years at the time of administration, revaccination should be given)

- Persons aged 2 to 64 years with a chronic illness (congestive heart failure, cardiomyopathy, chronic pulmonary disease, diabetes, alcoholism, liver disease)

- Persons aged 2 to 64 years with functional or anatomic asplenia (when splenectomy is planned, PPSV23 should be given at least 2 weeks before surgery; a single revaccination is recommended at 5 years in subjects older than 10 years and at 3 years in subjects younger than 10 years)

- Persons aged 2 to 64 years of age living in environments where the risk of invasive pneumococcal disease or its complications is increased (this does not include daycare center employees and children)

- Persons aged 19 to 64 years who smoke cigarettes or have asthma[34]

- Persons with cochlear implants[35]

PPSV23 is recommended for immunocompromised persons 2 years and older with (a) HIV infection, (b) leukemia, (c) lymphoma, (d) Hodgkin disease, (e) multiple myeloma, (f) generalized malignancy, (g) chronic renal failure or nephrotic syndrome, (h) patients receiving immunosuppressive therapy including corticosteroids, and (i) organ and bone marrow transplant recipients. A single revaccination should be given if 5 years or more have passed since the first dose in subjects older than 10 years. In subjects 10 years of age and younger, revaccination should be given 3 years after the previous dose.

PPSV23 induces type-specific antibodies (T-cell–independent mechanisms) with a twofold rise within 2 to 3 weeks in 80% of young healthy adults. No correlation of antibody levels and protection has been determined. Antibody levels to these strains remain elevated for at least 5 years. In certain individuals, these levels decline within 10 years. Children may be protected for only 3 to 5 years. Elderly individuals and patients with chronic disease may have lower antibody levels produced with the vaccine. Children younger than 2 years do not respond adequately to the vaccine.

A number of other groups, including immunocompromised patients (e.g., leukemia, lymphoma, and multiple myeloma), dialysis patients, and patients with acquired immune deficiency syndrome, have reduced antibody production with the vaccine. Asymptomatic HIV-infected patients respond sufficiently to the vaccine. Patients with Hodgkin disease respond to the vaccine better before splenectomy, chemotherapy, or radiation therapy.

PPSV23 vaccine efficacy has been debated in the literature. Although prelicensure trials in young, healthy gold miners in South Africa showed a reduction in nonbacteremic disease rates, randomized clinical trials performed in the postmarketing period on elderly persons with chronic disease did not confirm these findings.[33] A large study of elderly individuals demonstrated a decreased risk of pneumonia caused by *S. pneumoniae* in vaccinated individuals but showed no change in the risk of community-acquired pneumonia even though most community-acquired pneumonias are caused by *S. pneumonia*.[36] For invasive disease, reduction rates of 56% to 81% with the vaccine have been shown. Adults hospitalized with community-acquired pneumonia are significantly less likely to die if they have been immunized. In addition, immunized patients were less likely to have respiratory failure and had hospitalization stays that were shorter by 2 days.[37]

A meta-analysis of nine randomized controlled trials concluded that the vaccine was efficacious in reducing the frequency of bacteremic pneumococcal disease among adults in low-risk groups and that the vaccine was cost-effective.[33]

PPSV23 safety is well documented. Local reactions occur frequently within the first 48 hours and generally are mild. Local erythema and induration (30%), local discomfort (40%), and local swelling (3%) are the side effects observed most commonly. Revaccination has been associated with self-limited injection-site reactions more commonly than after the first dose.[38] Severe systemic reactions occur rarely and consist of weakness, myalgia, headache, photophobia, chills, and fever.

Pneumococcal Conjugate Polysaccharide Vaccine

Invasive pneumococcal disease occurs even more frequently in children younger than 2 years than in those older than 65 years. The infection ranges goes from nasopharyngeal carriage to bacteremia and meningitis. Because of the lack of immune responsiveness in children younger than 2 years when exposed to polysaccharide vaccines, a conjugate vaccine was developed to protect young children from certain strains of S. pneumoniae.

A 13 valent vaccine (Prevnar-13) is available for use in children. This vaccine contains the conjugated capsular polysaccharides of serotypes 1, 3, 4, 5, 6A, 6B, 7F, 9V, 14, 18C, 19A, 19F, and 23F, which cause the vast majority of pediatric pneumococcal bacteremias in the United States.[39,40] The vaccine elicits a primary T-cell–dependent antibody response with the first dose and an immunologic memory effect after four doses. In clinical use, the vaccine is associated with a dramatic decline in invasive disease not only in immunized young children but also in individuals in all age groups.[32]

❽ PCV13 is administered as a 0.5-mL IM injection at 2, 4, and 6 months of age and between 12 and 15 months of age. PCV13 also should be used in older children aged 24 to 59 months who are at high risk. Children with sickle cell disease or splenic dysfunction, HIV infection, immunocompromising conditions, or chronic illnesses should be immunized. PPV23 can be used in conjunction with PCV13. PPV23 should be administered after age 2 years and at least 2 months after the last dose of PCV13.

The vaccine series generally is well tolerated. Injection-site reactions and fever are the most commonly reported adverse effects.[52] Widespread use of conjugated pneumococcal vaccines in infants and young children has resulted in a decreased incidence of invasive pneumococcal disease in the entire population.[39]

POLIOVIRUS VACCINES

Poliomyelitis is a contagious viral infection that usually causes asymptomatic infection; however, in its serious form it causes acute flaccid paralysis. Poliovirus is spread via the fecal–oral route. The virus replicates in the upper respiratory tract, gastrointestinal tract, and local lymphatics. The vast majority of polio infections are subclinical and asymptomatic. Indigenous polio has been absent from the United States since 1979, and the last case in Western Hemisphere was reported in 1991. Global eradication efforts are entering the final stages, and the eradication of polio should be accomplished in the next few years.

An inactivated trivalent vaccine developed by Jonas Salk was licensed for use in 1955. In 1987, an enhanced-potency IPV was introduced and has replaced the original inactivated vaccine. A live-attenuated oral polio vaccine (OPV) was developed by Albert Sabin in 1962. OPV was the primary immunizing agent for poliovirus infection. Widespread OPV use is responsible for eradication of wild-type polio in most of the world. However, with no poliovirus circulation in the United States for years, IPV is the recommended

vaccine for the primary series and booster dose for children. OPV will continue to be used in areas of the world that have circulating poliovirus. The CDC maintains a stockpile of OPV to be used only in case of an outbreak.[42]

The IPV series is administered routinely to children at ages 2, 4, and 6 to 18 months, and 4 to 6 years. Protective antibodies to all three serotypes develop in 90% to 100% of children after two doses of vaccine. After three doses, 99% to 100% develop protective immunity, and the fourth dose results in long-term immunity.[42]

Primary poliomyelitis immunization is recommended for all children up to age 18 years. Primary immunization of adults over age 18 years is not recommended routinely because a high level of immunity already exists in this age group and the risk of exposure in developed countries is exceedingly small. However, unimmunized adults who are at increased risk for exposure because of travel, residence, or occupation should receive IPV series. Incompletely immunized adults or children should complete the series of IPV regardless of the interval since initiation of primary immunization. Adults do not need a booster dose routinely unless they are at increased risk of exposure (travel), in which case a single dose of IPV can be given.[55]

Allergies to any component of IPV, including streptomycin, polymyxin B, and neomycin, are contraindications to vaccine use. No serious side effects are attributable to IPV. Pregnant women should be given IPV only if there is a clear need, such as women who will be traveling or living in an area with endemic or epidemic poliovirus. IPV is recommended for immunodeficient individuals and their household contacts. Although the response may be lower, some protection against infection may be conferred.

The routine use of OPV in the United States has been discontinued because OPV is rarely associated with vaccine-associated paralytic poliomyelitis in vaccinees (1 in 6.2 million doses) or contacts (1 in 7.6 million doses). Because individuals with primary immune deficiency are at increased risk for this adverse reaction, OPV is not recommended for persons who are immunodeficient or for normal individuals who reside in a household with an immunocompromised person. The use of OPV is reserved for polio outbreak control.[42]

RABIES VACCINE

Rabies is a virtually universally fatal infection in humans. Although all mammals are susceptible to rabies, carnivorous mammals are reservoirs of the virus and responsible for persistence of the virus in nature. In the United States, most human cases of rabies are from exposure to rabid bats, but raccoons, foxes, skunks, and coyotes are also associated with possible exposure. Worldwide, canines are the primary vectors. Transmission of rabies can occur via percutaneous, permucosal, or airborne exposure to the rabies virus. Circumstances favoring such transmission include animal bites and attacks and contamination of scratches, cuts, abrasions, and mucous membranes with saliva or other infectious material (brain tissue). Unprovoked attacks and daytime attacks by nocturnal animals are considered highly suspect. A few cases of person-to-person transmission have been reported.[43]

Symptoms of rabies are nonspecific during the prodomal stage—fever, headache, malaise, irritability, nausea, and vomiting. The acute neurologic phase is characterized by hyperexcitability, hyperactivity, hallucinations, salivation, a fear of water and air. A minority of patients present with limp paralysis. Patients die within 5 days of presentation with these neurologic symptoms.

Human diploid cell vaccine (HDCV), and purified chick embryo cell (PCECV) rabies vaccine are killed vaccines used for preexposure and postexposure rabies virus prophylaxis. Preexposure indications for using HDCV, RVA, or PCECV rabies vaccine include persons whose vocation or avocation place them at high risk for rabies exposure, such as veterinarians, animal handlers, laboratory workers in rabies research or diagnostic laboratories, cavers, wildlife officers where animal rabies is common, and anyone who handles bats. Travelers who will be in a country or area of a country where there is a constant threat of rabies, whose stay is likely to extend beyond 1 month, and who may not have readily available medical services (e.g., Peace Corps workers and missionaries) should be considered for preexposure prophylaxis.[43] Rabies immunization of immunocompromised individuals should be postponed until the immunosuppression has resolved, or activities should be modified to minimize the potential exposure to rabies. If the vaccine is used in immunocompromised persons, antibody titers should be checked postimmunization. Pregnancy is not a contraindication if the risk of rabies is great. A rabies immunization series should be completed with the same product because no data exist on interchangeability of products. Both vaccine preparations can be administered for preexposure prophylaxis as a three-dose series of 1 mL IM on days 0 and 7 and once between days 21 and 28.

Individuals with ongoing risk of exposure—either continuous risk (e.g., research laboratory staff or those involved in rabies biologics production) or individuals with frequent exposures (e.g., those involved with rabies diagnosis, spelunkers, veterinarians, animal control workers, and wildlife workers in rabies-enzootic areas)—should undergo serologic testing every 6 months and 2 years, respectively, to monitor rabies antibody concentrations. A booster dose is recommended if the complete virus neutralization is <1:5 serum dilution by the rapid fluorescent focus inhibition test.

Preexposure prophylaxis does not eliminate the need for postexposure therapy. Persons previously immunized with HDCV or PCECV rabies vaccine or those who previously received postexposure prophylaxis should receive two 1-mL IM doses of HDCV or PCECV rabies vaccine on postexposure days 0 and 3. Rabies Ig should not be given to this group.

Postexposure prophylaxis should be given after percutaneous or permucosal exposure to saliva or other infectious material from a high-risk source. Each case must be considered individually. Consideration needs to be given to the geographic area, species of animal, circumstances of the incident, and type of exposure. Local or state health departments should be contacted for assistance. Thorough cleansing of the wound with soap and water followed by irrigation with a virucidal agent such as povidone–iodine solution is an extremely important part of the management of rabies-prone wounds. Individuals who have not been immunized previously should receive the recommended regimen of rabies Ig (see Rabies Immunoglobulin below) and four doses of HDCV or PCECV rabies vaccine 1 mL IM on days 0, 3, 7, and 14 after exposure. However, a fifth dose in a series should be considered if the exposed individual is immunocompromised. Vaccine response for these individuals should be checked.[44] Rabies vaccine must be administered in the deltoid muscle in adults and in the anterolateral thigh in children. The gluteal region should not be used.[1,43]

Adverse reactions to rabies biologicals are less common and less serious with the currently available vaccines compared with previously used preparations. Local or mild systemic symptoms can typically be managed with antiinflammatory medications or antihistamines. Systemic allergic reactions ranging from hives to anaphylaxis occur in a very small number of subjects. Given the lack of alternative therapy and the fact that rabies infection is almost always fatal, persons exposed to rabies who do have adverse reactions should continue the vaccine series in a setting with medical support services.[43]

Rabies Immunoglobulin

Human rabies Ig is used in conjunction with rabies vaccine as part of postexposure rabies management for previously unvaccinated individuals. The product is derived from plasma obtained from donors who have been hyperimmunized with rabies vaccine and have high titers of circulating antibody.

In persons who previously have not been immunized against rabies, rabies Ig is given simultaneously with HDCV or PCECV rabies vaccine to provide optimal coverage in the interval before immune response to the vaccine occurs. The efficacy of this regimen has been clearly demonstrated. In situations where a vaccine has been used alone, mortality rates of 50% to 60% have been observed. Mortality after the combination vaccine and rabies Ig regimens is exceedingly rare; however, deaths have been reported when the wound was not infiltrated with rabies Ig.[45]

Rabies Ig does not interfere with vaccine-induced antibody formation. Its use is not recommended beyond 8 days after initiation of the vaccine series nor in persons previously immunized to rabies.

Human rabies Ig is administered in a dose of 20 international units/kg (0.133 mL/kg). If anatomically feasible, the entire dose should be infiltrated around the wound(s). Any remaining volume should be administered IM at a site distant from the rabies vaccination site. This product should never be administered by the intravenous route. Because other antibodies in the rabies Ig may interfere with the response to live-virus vaccines (MMR and varicella), it is recommended that these immunizations be delayed for 3 months.[1]

Side effects are rare but may include local soreness at the wound or IM injection site and mild temperature elevations. Caution is advised when administering the product to persons with known systemic allergies to immunoglobulin or thimerosal. Pregnancy is not a contraindication to its use.

RUBELLA VACCINE

Rubella (German measles) is characterized by an erythematous rash, lymphadenopathy, arthralgia, and low-grade fever. As many as 20% to 50% of rubella infections are asymptomatic.[25] The most important consequence of rubella infection occurs during pregnancy, particularly during the first trimester. Congenital rubella syndrome is associated with auditory, ophthalmic, cardiac, and neurologic defects. Rubella infection during pregnancy also can result in miscarriage or stillbirth. The primary goal of rubella immunization is to prevent congenital rubella syndrome. Rubella is no longer endemic in the United States, but high immunization rates are necessary to prevent rubella outbreaks from imported cases.

Rubella vaccine contains lyophilized live-attenuated rubella virus grown in human diploid cell culture. The vaccine is available in combination with measles vaccine, mumps vaccine, and varicella vaccine. Each 0.5-mL dose also contains 25 mcg neomycin and is administered subcutaneously.

Rubella vaccine induces antibodies that are protective against wild-virus infection. The duration of immunity has not been established. A second dose is recommended, however, at the same time measles vaccine is administered (as a second dose of MMR). The vaccine is indicated for children older than 1 year of age. Individuals born before 1957 are assumed to be immune to rubella except for women who could become pregnant. Therefore, all women of childbearing potential should have documentation of receiving at least one dose of a rubella-containing vaccine or laboratory evidence of immunity.[25] Recent administration of Ig interferes with rubella vaccine response for at least 3 months and depends on the dose of Ig that is administered.[1,25,46] Table 133–1 can be used as a guide for the recommended interval. The vaccine should not be given to immunosuppressed individuals, although MMR vaccine should be administered to young children with HIV infection without severe immunosuppression as soon as possible after their first birthday.[26] The vaccine should not be given to individuals who have experienced anaphylactic reactions to neomycin.

Adverse effects of the rubella virus vaccine tend to increase with the age of the recipient. Mild symptoms are similar to wild-virus infection and include lymphadenopathy, rash, urticaria, fever, malaise, sore throat, headache, myalgias, and paresthesias of the extremities. These symptoms occur 7 to 12 days after vaccination and last 1 to 5 days. Joint symptoms occur more often in susceptible postpubertal females. Arthralgia occurs in 25% of vaccinees, and 10% have arthritis-like symptoms. These symptoms usually begin 1 to 3 weeks after vaccination and persist for 1 day to 3 weeks. A very small excess risk of chronic arthropathy exists.[25] The vaccine may cause suppression of tuberculin skin tests for up to 6 weeks after vaccination. The vaccine virus may be excreted in nose and throat secretions, but it is not contagious.

The rubella vaccine has never been associated with congenital rubella syndrome, but its use during pregnancy is contraindicated. However, routine pregnancy testing prior to vaccination is not recommended. Women should be counseled not to become pregnant for 4 weeks following vaccination.[46] Termination of pregnancy is not indicated in women who are accidentally given the vaccine or who become pregnant during the month after vaccination.

VARICELLA AND ZOSTER VACCINES

Varicella is a highly contagious disease caused by varicella-zoster virus. The clinical illness is characterized by the appearance of successive waves of pruritic vesicles that rapidly crust over. Malaise and fever are common and last for 2 to 3 days. The virus remains dormant in the dorsal ganglia and reactivates as herpes zoster, also known as *shingles*. Although the exact stimulus for reactivation is unknown, a decrease in varicella-specific cell-mediated immunity associated with age or immunosuppression appears to be necessary but not sufficient for reactivation.

Varicella Vaccine

Live-attenuated varicella vaccine contains the Oka/Merck strain of varicella virus, which was attenuated by propagation through several different cell culture lines. Varicella vaccine is a lyophilized product that must be kept frozen and protected from light. Once reconstituted, it must be administered subcutaneously within 30 minutes. Each 0.5-mL dose contains a minimum of 1,350 plaque-forming units of virus as well as 12.5 mg of hydrolyzed gelatin and trace amounts of neomycin, fetal bovine serum, and residual components from cell culture.[47]

The varicella vaccine is safe and immunogenic in healthy children and adults. In clinical studies, varicella vaccine has been 70% to more than 95% effective in preventing chickenpox. Vaccinated individuals who develop chickenpox typically experience milder disease, with low or no fever and fewer skin lesions, many of which do not vesiculate. Similarly, vaccinated individuals who develop breakthrough infections transmit the varicella virus to others at a lower rate.[14]

The varicella vaccine is recommended for all children at 12 to 18 months of age, with a second dose prior to entering school between ages 4 and 6 years.[16] A second dose is also recommended for patients older than this age if they have not already had chickenpox. Varicella vaccine can be used for postexposure prophylaxis. The vaccine is effective in the prevention or modification of varicella infection when given within 3 days and possibly 5 days of exposure. Because the varicella vaccine is a live vaccine, it is contraindicated

in pregnant women and in immunocompromised individuals. An exception is children with asymptomatic or mildly symptomatic HIV infection, who should receive two doses of varicella vaccine 3 months apart. Also, children with humoral immune deficiencies may be immunized. Varicella vaccination is contraindicated in individuals with a history of anaphylactic reaction to any component of the vaccine. Persons who have received blood, plasma, or Ig products in the recent past should not receive varicella vaccine because of concern that passively acquired antibody will interfere with response to the vaccine. The recommended time interval between antibody-containing products and varicella vaccine depends on the dose of immunoglobulin (see Table 133–1). Although no adverse events associated with salicylate use after vaccination have been reported, salicylates should be avoided for 6 weeks after vaccination because of the association of salicylate use and Reye syndrome following varicella infection.[47]

The varicella vaccine has an excellent safety record. Pain, local swelling, and erythema at the injection site occur in up to 32% of patients and fever in 10% to 15%. A varicella-like rash occurs in approximately 4% of vaccinees, accompanied by few, if any, systemic symptoms. The rash may be localized at the injection site or generalized. Lesions usually are few in number (2–10) and often papular rather than vesicular. Transmission of vaccine virus to susceptible close contacts has occurred but is rare and believed to occur only when the vaccinee develops a rash. Because the risk of vaccine virus transmission is very low and primary infection can be very severe, vaccination of household contacts of immunocompromised patients is recommended to prevent introduction of varicella into the household.[47]

Zoster Vaccine

After the primary infection with varicella-zoster virus manifested as chicken pox, the virus remains latent in the dorsal ganglia. Herpes zoster, more commonly known as *shingles*, occurs upon reactivation of varicella-zoster virus replication. Herpes zoster can occur at any age, but the incidence dramatically increases with increasing age. The rate of disease increases sharply beginning in the after age 50 years. The disease rate in individuals older than 80 years of age is 11 cases per 1,000 person-years.[48] Patients with HIV, cancer, or other conditions associated with immunosuppression are at increased risk for disease.[10] The development of the disease is associated with declining cellular immunity to varicella-zoster virus.

The clinical presentation of herpes zoster usually is a vesicular eruption limited to one dermatome. The most common complication is postherpetic neuralgia, which is pain that persists after the skin lesions have healed. The duration and severity of the pain varies. Postherpetic neuralgia can persist for weeks to years. The risk of postherpetic neuralgia increases dramatically with age. Virtually no risk of developing postherpetic neuralgia with herpes zoster exists prior to age 50 years, but the risk increases to 50% to 75% after ages 60 and 75 years, respectively. The pain can be so severe as to limit activities of daily living and quality of life.[10]

The zoster vaccine contains 19,000 plaque-forming units of Oka/Merck strain live varicella-zoster virus. Although the same strain of vaccine virus is contained in the childhood varicella vaccines, the doses of vaccine virus are dramatically different, and the vaccines are *not* interchangeable. Zoster vaccine reduces the burden of disease by 60%. The burden of disease is a composite measure considering incidence, severity, and duration of herpes zoster. The incidence of zoster is cut in half and the development of postherpetic neuralgia can be decreased by 67%.[49]

The zoster vaccine is recommended for immunocompetent individuals older than 60 years. This live vaccine should not be used in immunocompromised individuals, including those on high dose

- Immunize patients with a history of shingles
- Screening patients for a history of chickenpox is not necessary. Assume anyone born before 1980 is immune to varicella[47]
- Zoster vaccine may be administered to individuals on inhaled, topical or intra-articular steroids or low dose oral steroids
- Zoster vaccine may be administered to individuals treated with low-dose methotrexate (<0.4 mg/kg/wk) or 6-mercaptopurine (<1.5 mg/kg/day). These therapies are often used for autoimmune diseases
- The vaccine may be administered to individuals anticipating immunosuppressive therapy. The minimum duration between immunization and initiation of immunosuppressive therapy is 14 days, and some clinicians recommend 1 month
- Stop antiviral therapy at least 24 hours before immunization and restart it at least 14 days after immunization
- Zoster vaccine can be administered without regard to blood product or immunoglobulin administration
- Do not administer zoster vaccine to
  - Individuals with AIDS or clinical manifestations of HIV, such as a CD4+ count less than 200 per mm³
  - Patients on high doses of steroids (prednisone or its equivalent of 20 mg daily or more for more than 2 weeks)
- Risks and benefits of administering zoster vaccine to individuals on immune modulators, such as tumor necrosis factor agents, must be determined on a case-by-case basis. Immunize prior to initiating therapy if possible. A recent study observed a rate of 11 cases per 1000 person-years which is similar to the zoster rate in people older than 80 years of age[59,60]

corticosteroids or with HIV (CD4 cell count <200/mm³) or malignancies.[10] Immunization of some special populations can be done (see Table 133–4). No evidence of transmission of the live vaccine virus exists, but transmission of the varicella vaccine virus has been documented. Postmarketing surveillance will be used to establish if the theoretical risk is a small clinical problem. The duration of protection is unknown but immunized participants from clinical trials are being followed for immunological markers and clinical efficacy.[49] Future doses may be required for continued protection.

Varicella-Zoster Immunoglobulin

Varicella-zoster Ig is used after exposure to varicella for passive immunization of susceptible immunodeficient patients or other susceptible individuals at particularly high risk for complications of varicella infection. Varicella-zoster Ig is available only under an investigational new drug protocol.[50]

Postexposure prophylaxis with varicella-zoster Ig is indicated for the following susceptible individuals: (a) immunocompromised patients, (b) neonates whose mothers develop varicella within 5 days before or 2 days after delivery, (c) preterm infants (<28 weeks' gestation or weight <1,000 g) who are exposed to varicella while hospitalized, and (d) susceptible pregnant women.[50] If varicella is prevented, vaccination should be offered at a later date. Exposure to varicella is defined as direct indoor contact for more than 1 hour with an infectious person. A negative history of clinical disease is not a reliable indicator of varicella susceptibility. Most people with a negative clinical history will have detectable antibody on laboratory testing. Caution is warranted when interpreting a low positive result in an immunosuppressed patient who has received blood products or Ig because the circulating antibody may be acquired passively.

For maximum effectiveness, varicella-zoster Ig must be given as soon as possible and not more than 96 hours following exposure. Because this agent may only attenuate infection, patients who receive varicella-zoster Ig still may have a period of communicability, and varicella-zoster Ig may prolong the incubation period to 28 days. Antiviral therapy can be initiated if signs and symptoms of varicella infection become apparent.

Administration of varicella-zoster Ig is by the IM route at doses of 125 plaque-forming units per 10 kg of body weight up to 625 units (five vials) for patients weighing more than 40 kg. The dose for newborn infants is 125 units.

OTHER IMMUNOBIOLOGICS

IMMUNOGLOBULIN

Immunoglobulin is available as both an intramuscular (IMIG) and an intravenous (IVIG) preparation. The IMIG preparation, or the Cohn fraction II, is prepared from pooled plasma of several thousand donors by cold ethanol fractionation. It typically contains greater than 95% IgG and trace amounts of IgM, IgA, and other plasma proteins. Because Ig is harvested from a large donor pool, it contains a wide spectrum of IgG antibodies to the pathogens prevalent in the area from which the donors were obtained. In the fractionation process, high-molecular-weight IgG aggregates are formed, which can activate complement in the absence of antigen and precipitate anaphylactoid reactions. For this reason, IMIG is unsuitable for IV administration. IMIG typically contains 15% to 18% protein and not less than 90% IgG. A number of IVIG preparations are available commercially in the United States. Generally, these preparations contain greater than 90% IgG monomers and trace to small amounts of IgA. These products are available as lyophilized powders or solutions.

When administered either IV or IM, Ig distributes in approximately 5% of the body weight of the recipient. The plasma half-life of Ig ranges from 18 to 32 days. This range of half-life probably is attributable to the variation in the half-life of IgG subclasses. Peak serum concentrations occur immediately with IVIG but within 2 days with IMIG. After the initial period of equilibration, circulating IgG levels are superimposable between IV and IM equivalent dosages. No dosage adjustment is necessary in patients with renal insufficiency, hepatic insufficiency, or both, dialysis patients, or geriatric patients.

❽ Immunoglobulin is indicated in a wide variety of circumstances to provide passive immunity to individuals. The indications for IMIG differ from those for IVIG. IMIG is indicated for providing passive immunity in patients with hepatitis A infections in those <1 year and older than 39 years, hepatitis B exposures (however, hepatitis B Ig is significantly more effective), measles, varicella, and primary immunodeficiency diseases. Although IMIG is indicated for treatment of primary immunodeficiency, IVIG is better tolerated and is more effective. IMIG is not indicated for prevention of rubella, mumps, or poliomyelitis. Table 133–5 lists the suggested dosages of IMIG for prevention or attenuation of various infectious diseases.

There are many licensed indications, as well as off-label uses, for IVIG.[51] The therapeutic dose of IVIG is set empirically at 2 g/kg,[52] often given as five daily doses of 400 mg/kg each. However, it may be preferable to divide the total dose into two daily doses of 1 g/kg if the patient can tolerate the volume of the infusion. Mechanisms of IVIG action for treatment of these conditions have been hypothesized.

- *Primary Immunodeficiency States.*[53] In primary immunodeficiency states, monthly doses of between 100 and 800 mg/kg are administered; the average dose is 200 to 400 mg/kg. The immunodeficiency states for which IVIG is indicated include both antibody deficiencies and combined immune deficiencies. Significant reactions can occur in patients with low intrinsic levels of IgA given IVIG with greater amounts of IgA. An IVIG product with very low amounts of IgA should be used for these patients.

TABLE 133-5 Indications and Dosage of Intramuscular Immunoglobulin in Infectious Diseases

Primary immunodeficiency states	1.2 mL/kg IM then 0.6 mL/kg every 2–4 weeks
Hepatitis A exposure	0.02 mL/kg IM within 2 weeks if <1 year or >39 years of age
Hepatitis A prophylaxis	0.02 mL/kg IM for exposure <3 months' duration
	0.06 mL/kg IM for exposure up to 5 months' duration
Hepatitis B exposure	0.06 mL/kg (HBIG preferred in known exposures)
Measles exposure	0.25 mL/kg (maximum dose 15 mL) as soon as possible
	0.5 mL/kg (maximum dose 15 mL) as soon as possible for immunocompromised individuals
Varicella exposure	0.6–1.2 mL/kg as soon as possible when VZIG not available

- *Idiopathic (Immune) Thrombocytopenic Purpura.*[54] For treatment of hemorrhage associated with idiopathic (immune) thrombocytopenic purpura (ITP), doses of 1 g/kg daily for 2 to 3 days plus high-dose methylprednisolone are indicated. Adults tend to respond less well to IVIG than do children. IVIG is acceptable for treatment of both chronic and acute ITP, and IVIG has been used for ITP associated with pregnancy without adverse effects on the fetus. Corticosteroids remain the drugs of choice for adult ITP. In thrombotic thrombocytopenia purpura, IVIG is reported to be effective in patients who do not respond to plasmapheresis. Other platelet disorders in which IVIG may be useful include neonatal immune thrombocytopenia, perinatal autoimmune thrombocytopenia, drug-induced thrombocytopenia, thrombocytopenia secondary to infection, and transfusion-refractory thrombocytopenia; however, the data supporting these uses are minimal.

- *Chronic Lymphocytic Leukemia.* IVIG is used as a prophylactic measure in patients with chronic lymphocytic leukemia who have had a serious bacterial infection. Doses of 400 mg/kg every 3 to 4 weeks are used.

- *Kawasaki's Disease (Mucocutaneous Lymph Node Syndrome).* This disease, which generally occurs in children, carries the hallmark of development of coronary artery abnormalities. Generally, the American Academy of Pediatrics recommends that if the strict criteria for Kawasaki's disease are met, an IVIG dose of 400 mg/kg/day for 4 consecutive days be used or, preferably, 2 g/kg as a single dose. The dose should be administered within 10 days of disease onset. Aspirin therapy also should be initiated.[55]

- *Varicella-Zoster.* Another licensed indication for IVIG is for prophylaxis of varicella-zoster if varicella-zoster Ig is not available.

A number of other proposed uses of IVIG have been identified. It is important to note that these uses are off-label but may be generally accepted in the medical community for routine treatment.[51,52,56] Off-label uses include the following:

- *Neonatal Sepsis.* Neonatal sepsis can cause significant morbidity within 24 hours of birth. Group B *Streptococcus* and *Escherichia coli* are the primary infecting organisms, but other bacteria and fungi may be associated with sepsis. IVIG appears to be effective in neonates older than 34 weeks' gestational age or who weigh

less than 1,500 g. Routine use is not recommended; however, IVIG may be useful in neonates with recurrent infections.

- *Guillain-Barré Syndrome.* IVIG is effective and is considered an alternative to plasmapheresis.[56]

- *Autoimmune Diseases.* IVIG may be effective in self-limited immunoregulatory diseases but less effective in chronic diseases such as systemic lupus erythematosus. Overall, little evidence indicates that IVIG is useful for management of autoimmune diseases, except for patients with severe active disease who have not responded to or tolerated other interventions.[56]

- *Intractable Epilepsy.* IVIG may be useful for patients with confirmed IgG deficiency. IVIG may be considered for certain syndromes, such as West or Lennox-Gastaut's syndrome.[56]

- *Chronic Inflammatory Demyelinating Polyneuropathy.* Although steroids are the first-line therapy, IVIG may be used in patients who do not respond to or do not tolerate steroids.[56]

Adverse effects of Ig vary with the route of administration. Following IMIG, pain, tenderness, and muscle stiffness persisting for hours or days are common. Repeat courses may cause sensitization with resulting allergic reactions. ❾ With IVIG, adverse effects occur in fewer than 1% of immunocompetent patients and in fewer than 10% of other patients. Chills, fever, nausea, and vomiting often are related to the rate of the infusion. Infusion should be given at a rate of 0.01 to 0.02 mL/kg/min for 30 minutes. If no reactions occur, then the rate can be increased to 0.02 to 0.04 mL/kg/min. If reactions do occur, the infusion should be stopped for 30 minutes and restarted at a lower rate. Although recommendations for infusion rate vary slightly depending on the preparation, the guidelines presented can be followed for the various IV preparations.

Most adverse reactions are mild and transient. Arthralgia, myalgia, fever, pruritus, nausea, vomiting, chest tightness, palpitations, diaphoresis, dizziness, pallor, and respiratory distress have been reported. Rarely, aseptic meningitis has occurred from a few hours to 2 days after high-dose infusion. The syndrome resolves within days without sequelae. Acute renal failure has been reported, primarily in individuals with underlying renal dysfunction, diabetes, sepsis, volume depletion, or other nephrotoxic drugs or in patients older than 65 years. To minimize the risk, ensure adequate hydration prior to infusion and choose an IVIG product that does not contain high sucrose concentrations for individuals at high risk.[57,58]

Immunoglobulin products are derived from human blood. Precautions such as donor screening and fractionation procedures and solvent-detergent treatment during the manufacturing process render the IVIG products free of HIV and hepatitis B and C viruses. Although no manufacturing process can guarantee no viral contamination, the potential infection risk from Ig preparations is very small.[57]

RH$_o$(D) IMMUNOGLOBULIN

Second only to the ABO blood group system, Rhesus antigen D [Rh$_o$(D)] is an important antigen in human blood. The Rh$_o$(D) locus encodes this antigen, but this locus is absent in approximately 15% of the population. ❿ Individuals lacking the Rh$_o$(D) locus are Rh$_o$(D) negative and have the potential to mount an antibody response to erythrocytes with the Rh$_o$(D) present. Rh$_o$(D) incompatibility during pregnancy can lead to sensitization of the mother. The maternal antibodies developed following normal fetal leakage of erythrocytes to the mother can cause hemolytic disease of the newborn during subsequent pregnancies.

Rh$_o$(D) Ig is a sterile solution of immunoglobulins prepared from human sera with high titers of Rh$_o$(D) antibody. Rh$_o$(D) Ig suppresses the antibody response and formation of anti-Rh$_o$(D) in Rh$_o$(D)-negative women exposed to Rh$_o$(D)-positive blood. Administration of Rh$_o$(D) Ig prevents hemolytic disease of the newborn in subsequent pregnancies with a Rh$_o$(D)-positive fetus. When administered within 72 hours of delivery of a full-term infant, Rh$_o$(D) Ig reduces active antibody formation from 12% to 1% to 2%. The reduction in antibody formation is lower when Rh$_o$(D) Ig is given beyond 72 hours postpartum. Smaller doses of Rh$_o$(D) Ig are used after abortion, miscarriage, amniocentesis, or abdominal trauma. In addition, Rh$_o$(D) Ig is used in the case of a premenopausal woman who is Rh$_o$(D) negative and has inadvertently received Rh$_o$(D)-positive blood or blood products.

The dosage of Rh$_o$(D) Ig varies with the indication. A standard dose of 300 mcg is given within 72 hours of a term delivery. Occasionally, when the fetus is known to be Rh$_o$(D) positive, a 300-mcg dose is given at 28 weeks' gestation and within 72 hours after delivery. For postpregnancy termination occurring up to 13 weeks' gestation, one microdose (50 mcg) vial is given within 72 hours. For pregnancy termination after 13 weeks, one standard dose (300 mcg) is given within 72 hours. In other circumstances, such as in abdominal trauma, amniocentesis, or transfusion accidents, the dosage (number of standard dose vials) is based on the estimated packed red blood cell volume of fetal/maternal hemorrhage divided by 15. Rh$_o$(D) Ig is administered IM only.

When considering use of Rh$_o$(D) Ig use, the mother's Rh$_o$(D) antigen status must be known with certainty. Rh$_o$(D) Ig should not be given to individuals positive for this antigen or to those with anti-Rh$_o$(D) antibodies. Occasionally, a large fetal bleed of Rh$_o$(D)-positive blood may make cross-matching of the mother difficult. In these cases, Rh$_o$(D) Ig should be given only if previous tests have shown that the mother is Rh$_o$(D) negative with no anti-Rh$_o$(D) antibody.

Adverse reactions to Rh$_o$(D) Ig include injection-site tenderness and fever. Rh$_o$(D) does not interfere with response to rubella vaccine. Rubella-seronegative women should be immunized at hospital discharge even if they received Rh$_o$(D) Ig postpartum.

CYTOMEGALOVIRUS IMMUNOGLOBULIN

Cytomegalovirus (CMV) causes a generally mild infection in immunocompetent individuals. However, immunocompromised individuals are at risk for serious complications, including pneumonia, retinitis, gastrointestinal manifestations, and hepatitis. CMV causes a latent infection that can be transmitted from a previously infected solid organ donor to a seronegative recipient. CMV-IVIG contains IgG antibodies obtained from healthy persons with high titers of antibodies to CMV.

Attenuation of primary CMV disease associated with solid-organ transplantation in seronegative recipients of seropositive organs is the indication for CMV-IVIG. It is dosed using a tapering schedule that varies depending on the type of transplant. CMV-IVIG is administered intravenously every 2 weeks, with the final dose administered 16 weeks post-transplantation. Use of CMV-IVIG has resulted in a significant decrease in CMV-related syndromes.

Adverse effects of CMV-IVIG are seen in fewer than 5% of recipients and include flushing, chills, muscle cramps, back pain, chest tightness, fever, nausea, vomiting, hypotension, and tachycardia. These adverse events may be related to the infusion rate and can be managed by temporarily discontinuing the infusion. The infusion can be restarted at a decreased rate. Anaphylaxis occurs rarely and should be considered if hypotension develops during the infusion. Because CMV-IVIG contains other antibodies, live-virus vaccines should be withheld until 3 months after CMV-IVIG administration.

TABLE 133-6	Web Resources for Vaccine Information
Recommended Internet Sites for Vaccine Information	
http://www.cdc.gov/vaccines/	Vaccines & Immunizations Centers for Disease Control and Prevention
www.immunize.org	Immunization Action Coalition
www.nfid.org/	National Foundation for Infectious Diseases
www.cdc.gov/mmwr/	Morbidity and Mortality Weekly Report
www.iom.edu/	Institute of Medicine of the National Academies
http://www.hrsa.gov/ vaccinecompensation/	Vaccine Injury Compensation Program
http://www.chop.edu/service/ vaccine-education-center/	Vaccine Education Center Children's Hospital of Philadelphia
http://vaers.hhs.gov/index	Vaccine Adverse Event Reporting System
Recommended Electronic Newsletters	
www.immunize.org/express	The Immunization Action Coalition's newsletter
www.cdc.gov/mmwr/	Morbidity and Mortality Weekly Report

VACCINE INFORMATION RESOURCES

The field of vaccinology is developing ever more rapidly, with numerous changes in recommendations for vaccine use made each year. Keeping up to date with the current recommendations can be a challenge. The childhood, adolescent, and adult immunization schedules are updated frequently and published annually. Recommendations for the use of influenza vaccine are issued annually. Healthcare providers involved in primary care and immunization delivery must keep themselves abreast of these changes in a systematic way. Reading electronic newsletters and browsing reliable Websites are efficient methods for obtaining information (Table 133–6). Although several excellent, reliable, and timely Websites exist, hundreds of sites with misleading and incorrect information also exist. Many of these sites are targeted at parents.

Vaccines are the only class of medications to which nearly every patient is exposed. Knowledge of these agents is critical to providing pharmaceutical care. Dramatic progress in public health has been made through the appropriate use of immunization. Additional improvements in quality of life and mortality can be made through continued increases in vaccination coverage with careful attention to this aspect of care by all healthcare providers.

ABBREVIATIONS

ACIP: Advisory Committee on Immunization Practices

CDC: U.S. Centers for Disease Control and Prevention

CMV-IVIG: Cytomegalovirus intravenous immunoglobulin

DTaP: diphtheria-tetanus-acellular pertussis

HDCV: human diploid cell rabies vaccine

Hib: *Haemophilus influenzae* type b

HPV: human papilloma virus

Ig: immunoglobulin

IMIG: intramuscular immunoglobulin

IPV: inactivated polio vaccine

ITP: idiopathic (immune) thrombocytopenic purpura

IVIG: intravenous immunoglobulin

MMRV: measles-mumps-rubella vaccine

OPV: oral polio vaccine

PCECV: purified chick embryo cell rabies vaccine

PCV: pneumococcal conjugate vaccine

PPSV23: pneumococcal polysaccharide vaccine 23 valent

PRP: polyribosylribitol phosphate

Td: tetanus-diphtheria

Tdap: tetanus-diphtheria-acellular pertussis

VAERS: Vaccine Adverse Event Reporting System

REFERENCES

1. Centers for Disease Control and Prevention. General recommendations on immunization. Recommendations of the Advisory Committee on Immunization Practices (ACIP). MMWR Morb Mortal Wkly Rep 2006;55(No. RR-15):1–47.

2. Centers for Disease Control and Prevention. A comprehensive immunization strategy to eliminate transmission of hepatitis B virus infection in the United States. Recommendations of the Advisory Committee on Immunization Practices (ACIP) Part II: Immunization of adults. MMWR Morb Mortal Wkly Rep 2006;55(No.RR-16):1–33.

3. Arrowood JR, Hayney MS. Immunization recommendations for adults with cancer. Ann Pharmacother 2002;36(7–8):1219–1229.

4. Centers for Disease Control and Prevention. Prevention and control of seasonal influenza with vaccines. Recommendations of the Advisory Committee on Immunization Practices (ACIP), 2009. MMWR Morb Mortal Wkly Rep 2009;58(No. RR-8):1–51.

5. Davis MM, Taubert K, Benin AL, et al. Influenza vaccination as secondary prevention for cardiovascular disease: a science advisory from the American Heart Association/American College of Cardiology. J Am Coll Cardiol 2006;48(7):1498–1502.

6. Pearce C, O'Laughlin J, Hayney M. Optimal cancer management includes influenza vaccination. J Am Pharm Assoc (2003) 2008;48(6): 813–814.

7. Poland G, Ovsyannikova I, Jacobson R. Application of pharmacogenomics to vaccines. Pharmacogenomics 2009;10(5):837–852.

8. Sester M, Gärtner BC, Girndt M, Sester U. Vaccination of the solid organ transplant recipient. Transplant Rev 2008;22(4):274–284.

9. Centers for Disease Control and Prevention. Prevention of rotavirus gastroenteritis among infants and children. Recommendations of the Advisory Committee on Immunization Practices (ACIP). MMWR Morb Mortal Wkly Rep 2009;58(No. RR-2):1–24.

10. Centers for Disease Control and Prevention. Prevention of herpes zoster. Recommendations of the Advisory Committee on Immunization Practices (ACIP). MMWR Morb Mortal Wkly Rep 2008;57(No. RR-5):1–30.

11. Centers for Disease Control and Prevention. Guidelines for vaccinating pregnant women from the Recommendation of the Advisory Committee on Immunization Practices (ACIP). In: U.S. Department of Health & Human Services; 1998 (updated October 2003):1–11.

12. Centers for Disease Control and Prevention. Prevention of pertussis, tetanus, and diphtheria among pregnant and postpartum women and their infants. MMWR Morb Mortal Wkly Rep 2008;57(No. RR-4): 1–51.

13. Masters J, Thomsen A, Hayney M. Vaccinations in solid-organ transplant patients: what a health professional should know. J Am Pharm Assoc (2003) 2009;49(3):458–459.

14. Centers for Disease Control and Prevention. Immunization information systems progress–United States, 2006. MMWR Morb Mortal Wkly Rep 2008;57(11):289–291.

15. Centers for Disease Control and Prevention. Surveillance for safety after immunization: Vaccine Adverse Event Reporting System (VAERS)–United States, 1991–2001. MMWR Morb Mortal Wkly Rep 2003;52(No. SS-1):1–24.

16. Centers for Disease Control and Prevention. Recommended childhood and adolescent immunization schedule–United States, 2009. MMWR Morb Mortal Wkly Rep 2009;57(51):Q1–Q4.

17. Centers for Disease Control and Prevention. Preventing tetanus, diphtheria, and pertussis among adults: Use of tetanus toxoid, reduced diphtheria toxoid and acellular pertussis vaccines. Recommendations fo the Advisory Committee on Immunization Practices (ACIP) and Recommendation of ACIP, supported by the Healthcare Infection

Control Practices Advisory Committee (HIPAC), for the Use of Tdap Among Health-Care Personnel. MMWR Morb Mortal Wkly Rep 2006;55(No. RR-17):1–37.

18. Centers for Disease Control and Prevention. Preventing tetanus, diphtheria, and pertussis among adolescents: Use of tetanus toxoid, reduced diphtheria toxoid and acellular pertussis vaccines. Recommendations fo the Advisory Committee on Immunization Practices (ACIP). MMWR Morb Mortal Wkly Rep 2006;55(No. RR-3):1–42.

19. Centers for Disease Control and Prevention. Progress toward elimination of Haemophilus influenzae type b invasive disease among infants and children–United States, 1998–2000. MMWR Morb Mortal Wkly Rep 2002;51(11):234–237.

20. Centers for Disease Control and Prevention. Recommended adult immunization schedule–United States, October 2007-September 2008. MMWR Morb Mortal Wkly Rep 2007;56(41):Q1–Q4.

21. Dunne EF, Unger ER, Sternberg M, et al. Prevalence of HPV Infection Among Females in the United States. JAMA 2007;297(8):813–819.

22. Centers for Disease Control and Prevention. FDA licensure of bivalent human papillomavirus vaccine (HPV2, Cervarix) for use in females and updated HPV vaccination recommendations from the Advisory Committee on Immunization Practices (ACIP). MMWR Morb Mortal Wkly Rep 2010;59(20):626–629.

23. Brown DR, Kjaer Susanne K, Sigurdsson K, et al. The impact of quadrivalent human papillomavirus (HPV; Types 6, 11, 16, and 18) L1 virus-like particle vaccine on infection and disease due to oncogenic nonvaccine HPV types in generally HPV-naive women aged 16-26 years. The Journal of Infectious Diseases 2009;199(7):926–935.

24. Wheeler Cosette M, Kjaer Susanne K, Sigurdsson K, et al. The impact of quadrivalent human papillomavirus (HPV; Types 6, 11, 16, and 18) L1 virus-like particle vaccine on infection and disease due to oncogenic nonvaccine HPV types in sexually active women aged 16-26 years. The Journal of Infectious Diseases 2009;199(7):936–944.

25. Paavonen J, Naud P, Salmerón J, et al. Efficacy of human papillomavirus (HPV)-16/18 AS04-adjuvanted vaccine against cervical infection and precancer caused by oncogenic HPV types (PATRICIA): final analysis of a double-blind, randomised study in young women. The Lancet 2009;374(9686):301–314.

26. Centers for Disease Control and Prevention. FDA licensure of quadrivalent human papillomavirus vaccine (HPV4, Gardasil) for use in males and guidance from the Advisory Committee on Immunization Practices (ACIP). MMWR Morb Mortal Wkly Rep 2010;59(20):630–632.

27. Centers for Disease Control and Prevention. Syncope after vaccination–United States, January 2005-July 2007. MMWR Morb Mortal Wkly Rep 2008;57(17):457–460.

28. Driscoll DJ, Jacobsen SJ, Porter CJ, Wollan PC. Syncope in children and adolescents. J Am Coll Cardiol 1997;29(5):1039–1045.

29. Centers for Disease Control and Prevention. Measles, mumps, and rubella–Vaccine use and strategies for elimination of measles, rubella, and congenital rubella syndrome and control of mumps: recommendations of the Advisory Committee on Immunization Practices (ACIP). MMWR Morb Mortal Wkly Rep 1998;47(No. RR-8):1–57.

30. Mofenson L, Brady M, Danner S, et al. Guidelines for the Prevention and Treatment of Opportunistic Infections among HIV-exposed and HIV-infected children: recommendations from CDC, the National Institutes of Health, the HIV Medicine Association of the Infectious Diseases Society of America, the Pediatric Infectious Diseases Society, and the American Academy of Pediatrics. MMWR Morb Mortal Wkly Rep 2009;58(No. RR-11):1–166.

31. Centers for Disease Control and Prevention. Recommended adult immunization schedule–United States, 2010. MMWR Morb Mortal Wkly Rep 2010;59(1):01–04.

32. Institute of Medicine. Immunization Safety Review. Measles-Mumps-Rubella Vaccine and Autism. Washington, DC: National Academy Press; 2001.

33. Centers for Disease Control and Prevention. Prevention and control of meningococcal disease. Recommendations of the Advisory Committee on Immunization Practices (ACIP). MMWR Morb Mortal Wkly Rep 2005;54(No. RR-7):1–21.

34. Centers for Disease Control and Prevention. Updated recommendation from the Advisory Committee on Immunization Practices (ACIP) for

revaccination of persons at prolonged increased risk for meningococcal disease MMWR Morb Mortal Wkly Rep 2009;58(37):1042–1043.

35. Centers for Disease Control and Prevention. Updated recommendations of the Advisory Committee on Immunization Practices (ACIP) for the control and elimination of mumps. MMWR Morb Mortal Wkly Rep 2006;55:629–630.

36. Centers for Disease Control and Prevention. Direct and indirect effects of routine vaccination of children with 7-valent pneumococcal conjuage vaccine on incidence of invasive pneumococcal disease–United States, 1998–2003. MMWR Morb Mortal Wkly Rep 2005;54(36):893–897.

37. Centers for Disease Control and Prevention. Prevention of pneumococcal disease: Recommendations of the Advisory Committee on Immunization Practices (ACIP). MMWR Morb Mortal Wkly Rep 1997;46(RR-8):1–24.

38. ACIP provisional recommendations for the use of pneumococcal vaccines. Centers for Disease Control and Prevention; 2008. *http://www.cdc.gov/vaccines/recs/provisional/downloads/pneumo-oct-2008-508.pdf.*

39. Centers for Disease Control and Prevention. Notice to readers: Pneumococcal vaccination for cochlear implant recipients. MMWR Morb Mortal Wkly Rep 2002;51(41):931.

40. Jackson LA, Neuzil KM, Yu O, et al. Effectiveness of pneumococcal polysaccharide vaccine in older adults. N Engl J Med 2003;348(18):1747–1755.

41. Fisman DN, Abrutyn E, Spaude KA, Kim A, Kirchner C, Daley J. Prior pneumococcal vaccination is associated with reduced death, complications, and length of stay among hospitalized adults with community-acquired pneumonia. Clin Infect Dis 2006;42(8):1093–1101.

42. Jackson LA, Benson P, Sneller VP, et al. Safety of revaccination with pneumococcal polysaccharide vaccine. JAMA 1999;281(3):243–248.

43. Centers for Disease Control and Prevention. Preventing pneumococcal disease among infants and young children: recommendations of the Advisory Committee on Immunization Practices (ACIP). MMWR Morb Mortal Wkly Rep 2000;49(No. RR-9):1–35.

44. Kaplan SL, Barson WJ, Lin PL, et al. Serotype 19A is the most common serotype causing invasive pneumococcal infections in children. Pediatrics 2010;125:429–436.

45. Huang SS, Hinrichsen VL, Stevenson AE, et al. Continued impact of pneumococcal conjugate vaccine on carriage in young children. Pediatrics 2009;124(1):e1–11.

46. Centers for Disease Control and Prevention. Poliomyelitis prevention in the United States: updated recommendations of the Advisory Committee on Immunization Practices (ACIP). MMWR Morb Mortal Wkly Rep 2000;49(No. RR-5):1–22.

47. Centers for Disease Control and Prevention. Human rabies prevention–United States, 2008. Recommendations of the Advisory Committee on Immunization Practices. MMWR Morb Mortal Wkly Rep 2008;57(No.RR-3):1–28.

48. Centers for Disease Control and Prevention. Use of a reduced (4-dose) vaccine schedule for postexposure prophylaxis to prevent human rabies. Recommendations of the advisory Committee on Immunization Practices. MMWR Morb Mortal Wkly Rep. 2010;50(No. RR–2).

49. Wilde H, Sirikawin S, Sabcharoen A, et al. Failure of postexposure treatment of rabies in children. Clin Infect Dis 1996;22(2):228–232.

50. Centers for Disease Control and Prevention. Revised ACIP recommendation for avoiding pregnancy after receiving a rubella-containing vaccine. MMWR Morb Mortal Wkly Rep 2001;50(49):1117.

51. Centers for Disease Control and Prevention. Prevention of varicella. Recommendations of the Advisory Committee on Immunization Practices (ACIP). MMWR Morb Mortal Wkly Rep 2007;56(No. RR-4):1–39.

52. Yawn BP, Saddier P, Wollan PC, St Sauver JL, Kurland MJ, Sy LS. A population-based study of the incidence and complication rates of herpes zoster before zoster vaccine introduction. Mayo Clin Proc 2007;82(11):1341–1349.

53. Oxman MN, Levin MJ, Johnson GR, et al. A vaccine to prevent herpes zoster and postherpetic neuralgia in older adults. N Engl J Med 2005;352(22):2271–2284.

54. Centers for Disease Control and Prevention. A new product (VariZIG™) for postexposure prophylaxis of varicella available under an investigational new drug application expanded access protocol. MMWR Morb Mortal Wkly Rep 2006;55(8):209–210.

55. Leong H, Stachnik J, Bonk ME, Matuszewski KA. Unlabeled uses of intravenous immune globulin. Am J Health Syst Pharm 2008;65(19):1815–1824.

56. Chen C, Danekas LH, Ratko TA, Vlasses PH, Matuszewski KA. A multicenter drug use surveillance of intravenous immunoglobulin utilization in US academic health centers. Ann Pharmacother 2000;34(3):295–299.

57. Durandy A, Wahn V, Petteway S, Gelfand EW. Immunoglobulin replacement therapy in primary antibody deficiency diseases–maximizing success. Int Arch Allergy Immunol 2005;136(3):217–229.

58. Stasi R, Evangelista M, Stipa E, Buccisano F, Venditti A, Amadori S. Idiopathic thrombocytopenic purpura: current concepts in pathophysiology and management. Thromb Haemost 2008;99(1):4–13.

59. Freeman AF, Shulman ST. Kawasaki's disease: summary of the American Heart Association guidelines. Am Fam Physician 2006;74(7):1141–1148.

60. Dalakas MC. Intravenous immunoglobulin in autoimmune neuromuscular diseases. JAMA 2004;291(19):2367–2375.

61. Carbone J. Adverse reactions and pathogen safety of intravenous immunoglobulin. Curr Drug Saf 2007;2(1):9–18.

62. Centers for Disease Control and Prevention. Renal insufficiency and failure associated with immune globulin intravenous therapy–United States, 1985–1998. MMWR Morb Mortal Wkly Rep 1999;48(24):581–521.

63. Strangfeld A, Listing J, Herzer P, et al. Risk of herpes zoster in patients with rheumatoid arthritis treated with anti-TNF-α agents. JAMA 2009;301(7):737–744.

64. Whitley RJ, Gnann JW, Jr. Herpes zoster in the age of focused immunosuppressive therapy. JAMA 2009;301(7):774–775.

Appendix 133-1
2010 Childhood and Adolescent Immunization Schedules

Recommended Immunization Schedule for Persons Aged 0 Through 6 Years—United States • 2010
For those who fall behind or start late, see the catch-up schedule

Vaccine ▼ Age ▶	Birth	1 Month	2 Month	4 Month	6 Month	12 Month	15 Month	18 Month	19–23 Month	2–3 Years	4–6 Years
Hepatitis B[1]	HepB	HepB			HepB						
Rotavirus[2]			RV	RV	RV[2]						
Diphtheria, tetanus, pertussis[3]			DTaP	DTaP	DTaP	See footnote[3]	DTaP				DTaP
Haemophilus influenzae type b[4]			Hib	Hib	Hib[4]	Hib					
Pneumococcal[5]			PCV	PCV	PCV	PCV					PPSV
Inactivated poliovirus[6]			IPV	IPV		IPV					IPV
Influenza[7]						Influenza (yearly)					
Measles, mumps, rubella[8]						MMR		See footnote[8]			MMR
Varicella[9]						Varicella		See footnote[9]			Varicella
Hepatitis A[10]						HepA (2 doses)				HepA series	
Meningococcal[11]										MCV	

■ Range of recommended ages for all children except certain high-risk groups ■ Range of recommended ages for certain high-risk groups

This schedule includes recommendations in effect as of December 15, 2009. Any dose not administered at the recommended age should be administered at a subsequent visit, when indicated and feasible. The use of a combination vaccine generally is preferred over separate injections of its equivalent component vaccines. Considerations should include provider assessment, patient preference, and the potential for adverse events. Providers should consult the relevant Advisory Committee on Immunization Practices statement for detailed recommendations: **http://www.cdc.gov/vaccines/pubs/acip-list.htm**. Clinically significant adverse events that follow immunization should be reported to the Vaccine Adverse Event Reporting System (VAERS) at **http://www.vaers.hhs.gov** or by telephone, **800-822-7967**.

1. **Hepatitis B vaccine (HepB).** (Minimum age: birth)
   At birth:
   - Administer monovalent HepB to all newborns before hospital discharge.
   - If mother is hepatitis B surface antigen (HBsAg)-positive, administer HepB of hepatitis B immune globulin (HBIG) within 12 hours of birth.
   - If mother's HBsAg status is unknown, administer HepB within 12 hours of birth. Determine mother's HBsAg status as soon as possible and, if HBsAg-positive, administer HBIG (no later than age 1 week).
   After the birth dose:
   - The HepB series should be completed with either monovalent HepB or a combination vaccine containing HepB. The second dose should be administered at age 1 or 2 months. Monovalent HepB vaccine should be used for doses administered before age 6 weeks. The final dose should be administered no earlier than age 24 weeks.
   - Infants born to HBsAg-positive mothers should be tested for HBsAg and antibody to HBsAg 1 to 2 months after completion of at least 3 doses of the HepB series, at age 9 through 18 months (generally at the next well-child visit).
   - Administration of 4 doses of HepB to infants is permissible when a combination vaccine containing HepB is administered after the birth dose. The fourth dose should be administered no earlier than age 24 weeks.
2. **Rotavirus vaccine (RV).** (Minimum age: 6 weeks)
   - Administer the first dose at age 6 through 14 weeks (maximum age: 14 weeks 6 days). Vaccination should not be initiated for infants aged 15 weeks 0 days or older.
   - The maximum age for the final dose in the series is 8 months 0 days.
   - If Rotarix is administered at ages 2 and 4 months, a dose at 6 months is not indicated.
3. **Diphtheria and tetanus toxoids and acellular pertussis vaccine (DTaP).** (Minimum age: 6 weeks)
   - The fourth dose may be administered as early as age 12 months, provided at least 6 months have elapsed since the third dose.
   - Administer the final dose in the series at age 4 through 6 years.
4. *Haemophilus influenzae* **type b conjugate vaccine (Hib).** (Minimum age: 6 weeks)
   - If PRP-OMP (PedvaxHIB or Comvax [HepB-Hib]) is administered at ages 2 and 4 months, a dose at age 6 months is not indicated.
   - TriHiBit (DTaP/Hib) and Hiberix (PRP-T) should not be used for doses at ages 2, 4, or 6 months for the primary series but can be used as the final dose in children aged 12 months through 4 years.
5. **Pneumococcal vaccine.** (Minimum age: 6 weeks for pneumococcal conjugate vaccine [PCV]; 2 years for pneumococcal polysaccharide vaccine [PPSV])
   - PCV is recommended for all children aged younger than 5 years. Administer 1 dose of PCV to all healthy children aged 24 through 59 months who are not completely vaccinated for their age.
   - Administer PPSV 2 or more months after last dose of PCV to children aged 2 years or older with certain underlying medical conditions, including a cochlear implant. See *MMWR* 1997;46(No. RR-8).

6. **Inactivated poliovirus vaccine (IPV)** (Minimum age: 6 weeks)
   - The final dose in the series should be administered on or after the fourth birthday and at least 6 months following the previous dose.
   - If 4 doses are administered prior to age 4 years a fifth dose should be administered at age 4 through 6 years. See *MMWR* 2009;58(30):829–30.
7. **Influenza vaccine (seasonal).** (Minimum age: 6 months for trivalent inactivated influenza vaccine [TIV]; 2 years for live, attenuated influenza vaccine [LAIV])
   - Administer annually to children aged 6 months through 18 years.
   - For healthy children aged 2 through 6 years (i.e., those who do not have underlying medical conditions that predispose them to influenza complications), either LAIV or TIV may be used, except LAIV should not be given to children aged 2 through 4 years who have had wheezing in the past 12 months.
   - Children receiving TIV should receive 0.25 mL if aged 6 through 35 months or 0.5 mL if aged 3 years or older.
   - Administer 2 doses (separated by at least 4 weeks) to children aged younger than 9 years who are receiving influenza vaccine for the first time or who were vaccinated for the first time during the previous influenza season but only received 1 dose.
   - For recommendations for use of influenza A (H1N1) 2009 monovalent vaccine see *MMWR* 2009;58(No. RR-10).
8. **Measles, mumps, and rubella vaccine (MMR).** (Minimum age: 12 months)
   - Administer the second dose routinely at age 4 through 6 years. However, the second dose may be administered before age 4, provided at least 28 days have elapsed since the first dose.
9. **Varicella vaccine.** (Minimum age: 12 months)
   - Administer the second dose routinely at age 4 through 6 years. However, the second dose may be administered before age 4, provided at least 3 months have elapsed since the first dose.
   - For children aged 12 months through 12 years the minimum interval between doses is 3 months. However, if the second dose was administered at least 28 days after the first dose, it can be accepted as valid.
10. **Hepatitis A vaccine (HepA).** (Minimum age: 12 months)
    - Administer to all children aged 1 year (i.e., aged 12 through 23 months). Administer 2 doses at least 6 months apart.
    - Children not fully vaccinated by age 2 years can be vaccinated at subsequent visits.
    - HepA also is recommended for older children who live in areas where vaccination programs target older children, who are at increased risk for infection, or for whom immunity against hepatitis A is desired.
11. **Meningococcal vaccine.** (Minimum age: 2 years for meningococcal conjugate vaccine [MCV4] and for meningococcal polysaccharide vaccine [MPSV4])
    - Administer MCV4 to children aged 2 through 10 years with persistent complement component deficiency, anatomic or functional asplenia, and certain other conditions placing tham at high risk.
    - Administer MCV4 to children previously vaccinated with MCV4 or MPSV4 after 3 years if first dose administered at age 2 through 6 years. See *MMWR* 2009; 58:1042–3.

The Recommended Immunization Schedules for Persons Aged 0 through 18 Years are approved by the Advisory Committee on Immunization Practices (**http://www.cdc.gov/vaccines/recs/acip**), the American Academy of Pediatrics (**http://www.aap.org**), and the American Academy of Family Physicians (**http://www.aafp.org**).
Department of Health and Human Services • Centers for Disease Control and Prevention

Recommended immunization schedule for persons aged 7 through 18 years — United States • 2010
For those who fall behind or start late, see the schedule below and the catch-up schedule

Vaccine ▼ Age ▶	7–10 years	11–12 years	13–18 years
Tetanus, diphtheria, pertussis[1]		Tdap	Tdap
Human papillomavirus[2]	see footnote 2	HPV (3 doses)	HPV series
Meningococcal[3]	MCV	MCV	MCV
Influenza[4]	Influenza (yearly)		
Pneumococcal[5]	PPSV		
Hepatitis A[6]	Hep A series		
Hepatitis B[7]	Hep B series		
Inactivated poliovirus[8]	IPV series		
Measles, mumps, rubella[9]	MMR series		
Varicella[10]	Varicella series		

Range of recommended ages for all children except certain high-risk groups

Range of recommended ages for catch-up immunization

Range of recommended ages for certain high-risk groups

This schedule includes recommendations in effect as of December 15, 2009. Any dose not administered at the recommended age should be administered at a subsequent visit, when indicated and feasible. The use of a combination vaccine generally is preferred over separate injections of its equivalent component vaccines. Considerations should include provider assessment, patient preference, and the potential for adverse events. Providers should consult the relevant Advisory Committee on Immunization Practices statement for detailed recommendations: **http://www.cdc.gov/vaccines/pubs/acip-list.htm.** Clinically significant adverse events that follow immunization should be reported to the Vaccine Adverse Event Reporting System (VAERS) at **http://www.vaers.hhs.gov** or by telephone, **800-822-7967.**

1. **Tetanus and diphtheria toxoids and acellular pertussis vaccine (Tdap).** (Minimum age: 10 years for boostrix and 11 years for Adacel)
   - Administer at age 11 or 12 years for those who have completed the recommended childhood DTP/DTaP vaccination series and have not received a tetanus and diphtheria toxoid (Td) booster dose.
   - Persons aged 13 through 18 years who have not received Tdap should receive a dose.
   - A 5-year interval from the last Td dose is encouraged when Tdap is used as a booster dose; however, a shorter interval may be used if pertussis immunity is needed.
2. **Human papillomavirus vaccine (HPV).** (Minimum age: 9 years)
   - Two HPV vaccines are licensed: a quadrivalent vaccine (HPV4) for the prevention of cervical, vaginal and vulvar cancers (in females) and genital warts (in females and males), and a bivalent vaccine (HPV2) for the prevention of cervical cancers in females.
   - HPV vaccines are most effective for both males and females when given before exposure to HPV through sexual contact.
   - HPV4 or HPV2 is recommended for the prevention of cervical precancers and cancers in females.
   - HPV4 is recommended for the prevention of cervical, vaginal and vulvar precancers and cancers and genital warts in females.
   - Administer the first dose to females at age 11 or 12 years.
   - Administer the second dose 1 to 2 months after the first dose and the third dose 6 months after the first dose (at least 24 weeks after the first dose).
   - Administer the series to females at age 13 through 18 years if not previously vaccinated.
   - HPV4 may be administered in a 3-dose series to males aged 9 through 18 years to reduce their likelihood of acquiring genital warts.
3. **Meningococcal conjugate vaccine (MCV4).**
   - Administer at age 11 or 12 years, or at age 13 through 18 years if not previously vaccinated.
   - Administer to previously unvaccinated college freshmen living in a dormitory.
   - Administer MCV4 to children aged 2 through 10 years with persistent complement component deficiency, anatomic or functional asplenia, or certain other conditions placing them at high risk.
   - Administer to children previously vaccinated with MCV4 or MPSV4 who remain at increased risk after 3 years (if first dose administered at age 2 through 6 years) or after 5 years (if first dose administered at age 7 years or older). Persons whose only risk factor is living in on-campus housing are not recommended to receive an additional dose. See *MMWR* 2009;58:1042–3.
4. **Influenza vaccine (seasonal)**
   - Administer annually to children aged 6 months through 18 years.
   - For healthy nonpregnant persons aged 7 through 18 years (i.e., those who do not have underlying medical conditions that predispose them to influenza complications), either LAIV or TIV may be used.
   - Administer 2 doses (separated by at least 4 weeks) to children aged younger then 9 years who are receiving influenza vaccine for the first time or who were vaccinated for the first time during the previous influenza season but only received 1 dose.
   - For recommendations for use of influenza A (H1N1) 2009 monovalent vaccine. See *MMWR* 2009;58(No. RR-10).
5. **Pneumococcal polysaccharide vaccine (PPSV).**
   - Administer to children with certain underlying medical conditions, including a cochlear implant. A singlerevaccination should be administered after 5 years to children with functional or anatomic asplenia or an immunocompromising condition. See *MMWR* 1997;46(No. RR-8).
6. **Hepatitis A vaccine (HepA).**
   - Administer 2 doses at least 6 months apart.
   - HepA is recommended for children aged older than 23 months who live in areas where vaccination programs target older children, who are at increased risk for infection, or for whom immunity against hepatitis A is desired.
7. **Hepatitis B vaccine (HepB).**
   - Administer the 3-dose series to those not previously vaccinated.
   - A 2-dose series (separated by at least 4 months) of adult formulation Recombivax HB is licensed for children aged 11 through 15 years.
8. **Inactivated poliovirus vaccine (IPV).**
   - The final dose in the series should be administered on or after the fourth birthday and at least 6 months following the previous dose.
   - If both OPV and IPV were administered as part of a series, a total of 4 doses should be administered, regardless of the child's current age.
9. **Measles, mumps, and rubella vaccine (MMR).**
   - If not previously vaccinated, administer 2 doses or the second dose for those who have received only 1 dose, with at least 28 days between doses.
10. **Varicella vaccine.**
   - For persons aged 7 through 18 years without evidence of immunity (see *MMWR* 2007;56[No. RR-4]), administer 2 doses if not previously vaccinated or the second dose if only 1 dose has been administered.
   - For persons aged 7 through 12 years, the minimum interval between doses is 3 months. However, if the second dose was administered at least 28 days after the first dose, it can be accepted as valid.
   - For persons aged 13 years and older, the minimum interval between doses is 28 days.

CS207330-A

The Recommended Immunization Schedules for Persons Aged 0 through 18 Years are approved by the Advisory Committee on Immunization Practices (**http://www.cdc.gov/vaccines/recs/acip**), the American Academy of Pediatrics (**http://www.aap.org**), and the American Academy of Family Physicians (**http://www.aafp.org**). Department of Health and Human Services • Centers for Disease Control and Prevention

Catch-up Immunization Schedule for Persons Aged 4 Months Through 18 Years Who Start Late or Who Are More Than 1 Month Behind—United States • 2010

The table below provides catch-up schedules and minimum intervals between doses for children whose vaccinations have been delayed. A vaccine series does not need to be restarted, regardless of the time that has elapsed between doses. Use the section appropriate for the child's age.

		Minimum interval between doses			
Persons aged 4 months through 6 years					
Vaccine	Minimum age for dose 1	Dose 1 to dose 2	Dose 2 to dose 3	Dose 3 to dose 4	Dose 4 to dose 5
Hepatitis B[1]	Birth	4 weeks	**8 weeks** (and at least 16 weeks after first dose)		
Rotavirus[2]	6 wks	4 weeks	4 weeks[2]		
Diphtheria, tetanus, pertussis[3]	6 wks	4 weeks	4 weeks	6 months	6 months[3]
Haemophilus influenzae type b[4]	6 wks	**4 weeks** if first dose administered at younger than age 12 months **8 weeks (as final dose)** if first dose administered at age 12–14 months **No further doses needed** if first dose administered at age 15 months or older	**4 weeks[4]** if current age is younger than 12 months **8 weeks (as final dose)[4]** if current age is 12 months or older and first dose administered at younger than age 12 months and second dose administered at younger than 15 months **No further doses needed** if previous dose administered at age 15 months or older	**8 weeks (as final dose)** This dose only necessary for children aged 12 months through 59 months who received 3 doses before age 12 months	
Pneumococcal[5]	6 wks	**4 weeks** if first dose administered at younger than age 12 months **8 weeks (as final dose for healthy children)** if first dose administered at younger than age 12 months or current age 24 through 59 months **No further doses needed** if first dose administered at age 12–14 months administered at age 24 months or older	**4 weeks** if current age is younger than 12 months **8 weeks (as final dose for healthy children)** if current age is 12 months or older **No further doses needed** for healthy children if previous dose administered at age 24 months or older	**8 weeks (as final dose)** This dose only necessary for children aged 12 months through 59 months who received 3 doses before age 12 months or for high-risk children who received 3 doses at any age	
Inactivated poliovirus[6]	6 wks	4 weeks	4 weeks	6 months	
Measles, mumps, rubella[7]	12 mos	4 weeks			
Varicella[8]	12 mos	3 months			
Hepatitis A[9]	12 mos	6 months			
Persons aged 7 through 18 years					
Tetanus, diphtheria/tetanus, diphtheria, pertussis[10]	7 yrs[10]	4 weeks	**4 weeks** if first dose administered at younger than age 12 months **6 months** if first dose administered at 12 months or older	**6 months** if first dose administered at younger than age 12 months	
Human papillomavirus[11]	9 yrs	**Routine dosing intervals are recommended[11]**			
Hepatitis A[9]	12 mos	6 months			
Hepatitis B[1]	Birth	4 weeks	**8 weeks** (and at least 16 weeks after first dose)		
Inactivated poliovirus[6]	6 wks	4 weeks	4 weeks	6 months	
Measles, mumps, rubella[7]	12 mos	4 weeks			
Varicella[8]	12 mos	**3 months** if person is younger than age 13 years **4 weeks** if person is aged 13 years or older			

1. **Hepatitis B vaccine (HepB).**
   • Administer the 3-dose series to those not previously vaccinated.
   • A 2-dose series (separated by at least 4 months) of adult formulation Recombivax HB is licensed for children aged 11 through 15 years.
2. **Rotavirus vaccine (RV).**
   • The maximum age for the first dose is 14 weeks 6 days. Vaccination should not be initiated for infants aged 15 weeks 0 days or older.
   • The maximum age for the final dose in the series is 8 months 0 days.
   • If Rotarix was administered for the first and second doses, a third dose is not indicated.
3. **Diphtheria and tetanus toxoids and acellular pertussis vaccine (DTaP).**
   • The fifth dose is not necessary if the fourth dose was administered at age 4 years or older.
4. **Haemophilus influenzae type b conjugate vaccine (Hib).**
   • Hib vaccine is not generally recommended for persons aged 5 years or older. No efficacy data are available on which to base a recommendation concerning use of Hib vaccine for older children and adults. However, studies suggest good immunogenicity in persons who have sickle cell disease, leukemia, or HIV infection, or who have had a splenectomy; administering 1 dose of Hib vaccine to these persons who have not previously received Hib vaccine is not contraindicated.
   • If the first 2 doses were PRP-OMP (PedvaxHIB or Comvax), and administered at age 11 months or younger, the third (and final) dose should be administered at age 12 through 15 months and at least 8 weeks after the second dose.
   • If the first dose was administered at age 7 through 11 months, administer the second dose at least 4 weeks later and a final dose at age 12 through 15 months.
5. **Pneumococcal vaccine.**
   • Administer 1 dose of pneumococcal conjugate vaccine (PCV) to all healthy children aged 24 through 59 months who have not received at least 1 dose of PCV on or after age 12 months.
   • For children aged 24 through 59 months with underlying medical conditions, administer 1 dose of PCV if 3 doses were received previously or administer 2 doses of PCV at least 8 weeks apart if fewer than 3 doses were received previously.
   • Administer pneumococcal polysaccharide vaccine (PPSV) to children aged 2 years or older with certain underlying medical conditions, including a cochlear implant, at least 8 weeks after the last dose of PCV. See MMWR 1997;46(No. RR-8).
6. **Inactivated poliovirus vaccine (IPV).**
   • The final dose in the series should be administered on or after the fourth birthday and at least 6 months following the previous dose.

• A fourth dose is not necessary if the third dose was administered at age 4 years or older and at least 6 months following the previous dose.
• In the first 6 months of life, minimum age and minimum intervals are only recommended if the person is at risk for imminent exposure to circulating poliovirus (i.e., travel to a polio-endemic region or during an outbreak).
7. **Measles, mumps, and rubella vaccine (MMR).**
   • Administer the second dose routinely at age 4 through 6 years. However, the second dose may be administered before age 4, provided at least 28 days have elapsed since the first dose.
   • If not previously vaccinated, administer 2 doses with at least 28 days between doses.
8. **Varicella vaccine.**
   • Administer the second dose routinely at age 4 through 6 years. However, the second dose may be administered before age 4, provided at least 3 months have elapsed since the first dose.
   • For persons aged 12 months through 12 years, the minimum interval between doses is 3 months. However, if the second dose was administered at least 28 days after the first dose, it can be accepted as valid.
   • For persons aged 13 years and older, the minimum interval between doses is 28 days.
9. **Hepatitis A vaccine (HepA).**
   • HepA is recommended for children aged older than 23 months who live in areas where vaccination programs target older children, who are at increased risk for infection, or for whom immunity against hepatitis A is desired.
10. **Tetanus and diphtheria toxoids vaccine (Td) and tetanus and diphtheria toxoids and acellular pertussis vaccine (Tdap).**
    • Doses of DTaP are counted as part of the Td/Tdap series.
    • Tdap should be substituted for a single dose of Td in the catch-up series or as a booster for children aged 10 through 18 years; use Td for other doses.
11. **Human papillomavirus vaccine (HPV).**
    • Administer the series to females at age 13 through 18 years if not previously vaccinated.
    • Use recommended routine dosing intervals for series catch-up (i.e., the second and third doses should be administered at 1 to 2 and 6 months after the first dose). The minimum interval between the first and second doses is 4 weeks. The minimum interval between the second and third doses is 12 weeks, and the third dose should be administered at least 24 weeks after the first dose.

Information about reporting reactions after immunization is available online at **http://www.vaers.hhs.gov** or by telephone, **800-822-7967.** Suspected cases of vaccine-preventable diseases should be reported to the state or local health department. Additional information, including precautions and contraindications for immunization, is available from the National Center for Immunization and Respiratory Diseases at **http://www.cdc.gov/vaccines** or telephone, **800-CDC-INFO** (800-232-4636).

Department of Health and Human Services • Centers for Disease Control and Prevention

Appendix 133-2
2010 Adult Immunization Schedule

Figure 2. Vaccines that might be indicated for adults based on medical and other indications

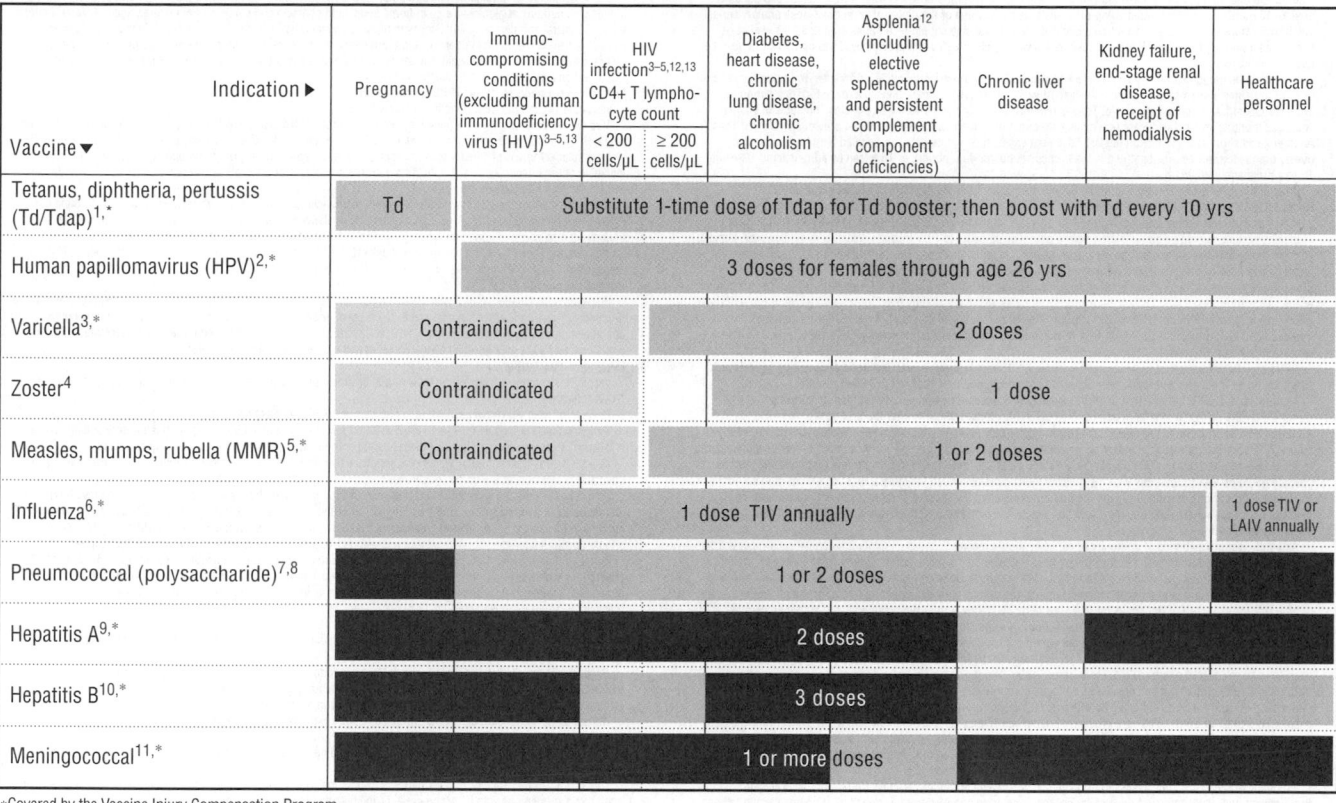

Vaccine ▼ / Indication ▶	Pregnancy	Immuno-compromising conditions (excluding human immunodeficiency virus [HIV])[3–5,13]	HIV infection[3–5,12,13] CD4+ T lymphocyte count < 200 cells/µL	HIV infection[3–5,12,13] CD4+ T lymphocyte count ≥ 200 cells/µL	Diabetes, heart disease, chronic lung disease, chronic alcoholism	Asplenia[12] (including elective splenectomy and persistent complement component deficiencies)	Chronic liver disease	Kidney failure, end-stage renal disease, receipt of hemodialysis	Healthcare personnel
Tetanus, diphtheria, pertussis (Td/Tdap)[1,*]	Td	Substitute 1-time dose of Tdap for Td booster; then boost with Td every 10 yrs							
Human papillomavirus (HPV)[2,*]		3 doses for females through age 26 yrs							
Varicella[3,*]	Contraindicated			2 doses					
Zoster[4]	Contraindicated			1 dose					
Measles, mumps, rubella (MMR)[5,*]	Contraindicated			1 or 2 doses					
Influenza[6,*]	1 dose TIV annually								1 dose TIV or LAIV annually
Pneumococcal (polysaccharide)[7,8]		1 or 2 doses							
Hepatitis A[9,*]		2 doses							
Hepatitis B[10,*]		3 doses							
Meningococcal[11,*]		1 or more doses							

*Covered by the Vaccine Injury Compensation Program.

For all persons in this category who meet the age requirements and who lack evidence of immunity (e.g., lack documentation of vaccination or have no evidence of prior infection)

Recommended if some other risk factor is present (e.g., on the basis of medical, occupational, lifestyle, or other indications)

No recommendation

These schedules indicate the recommended age groups and medical indications for which administration of currently licensed vaccines is commonly indicated for adults ages 19 years and older, as of January 1, 2010. Licensed combination vaccines may be used whenever any components of the combination are indicated and when the vaccine's other components are not contraindicated. For detailed recommendations on all vaccines, including those used primarily for travelers or that are issued during the year, consult the manufacturers' package inserts and the complete statements from the Advisory Committee on Immunization Practices (www.cdc.gov/vaccines/pubs/acip-list.htm).

The recommendations in this schedule were approved by the Centers for Disease Control and Prevention's (CDC) Advisory Committee on Immunization Practices (ACIP), the American Academy of Family Physicians (AAFP), the American College of Obstetricians and Gynecologists (ACOG), and the American College of Physicians (ACP).

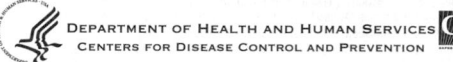

DEPARTMENT OF HEALTH AND HUMAN SERVICES
CENTERS FOR DISEASE CONTROL AND PREVENTION
CDC

Footnotes

Recommended Adult Immunization Schedule—UNITED STATES · 2010

For complete statements by the Advisory Committee on Immunization Practices (ACIP), visit www.cdc.gov/vaccines/pubs/ACIP-list.htm.

1. **Tetanus, diphtheria, and acellular pertussis (Td/Tdap) vaccination**
Tdap should replace a single dose of Td for adults aged 19 through 64 years who have not received a dose of Tdap previously.
Adults with uncertain or incomplete history of primary vaccination series with tetanus and diphtheria toxoid-containing vaccines should begin or complete a primary vaccination series. A primary series for adults is 3 doses of tetanus and diphtheria toxoid-containing vaccines; administer the first 2 doses at least 4 weeks apart and the third dose 6–12 months after the second; Tdap can substitute for any one of the doses of Td in the 3-dose primary series. The booster dose of tetanus and diphtheria toxoid-containing vaccine should be administered to adults who have completed a primary series and if the last vaccination was received <10 years previously. Tdap or Td vaccine may be used, as indicated.
If a woman is pregnant and received the last Td vaccination ≥10 years previously, administer Td during the second or third trimester. If the woman received the last Td vaccination <10 years previously, administer Tdap during the immediate postpartum period. A dose of Tdap is recommended for postpartum women, close contacts of infants aged <12 months, and all healthcare personnel with direct patient contact if they have not previously received Tdap. An interval as short as 2 years from the last Td is suggested; shorter intervals can be used. Td may be deferred during pregnancy and Tdap substituted in the immediate postpartum period, or Tdap can be administered instead of Td to a pregnant woman.
Consult the ACIP statement for recommendations for giving Td as prophylaxis in wound management.

2. **Human papillomavirus (HPV) vaccination**
HPV vaccination is recommended at age 11 or 12 years with catch-up vaccination at ages 13 through 26 years.
Ideally, vaccine should be administered before potential exposure to HPV through sexual activity; however, females who are sexually active should still be vaccinated consistent with age-based recommendations. Sexually active females who have not been infected with any of the four HPV vaccine types (types 6, 11, 16, 18 all of which HPV4 prevents) or any of the two HPV vaccine types (types 16 and 18 both of which HPV2 prevents) receive the full benefit of the vaccination. Vaccination is less beneficial for females who have already been infected with one or more of the HPV vaccine types. HPV4 or HPV2 can be administered to persons with a history of genital warts, abnormal Papanicolaou test, or positive HPV DNA test, because these conditions are not evidence of prior infection with all vaccine HPV types.
HPV4 may be administered to males aged 9 through 26 years to reduce their likelihood of acquiring genital warts. HPV4 would be most effective when administered before exposure to HPV through sexual contact.
A complete series for either HPV4 or HPV2 consists of 3 doses. The second dose should be administered 1–2 months after the first dose; the third dose should be administered 6 months after the first dose.
Although HPV vaccination is not specifically recommended for persons with the medical indications described in Figure 2, "Vaccines that might be indicated for adults based on medical and other indications," it may be administered to these persons because the HPV vaccine is not a live-virus vaccine. However, the immune response and vaccine efficacy might be less for persons with the medical indications described in Figure 2 than in persons who do not have the medical indications described or who are immunocompetent. Healthcare personnel are not at increased risk because of occupational exposure, and should be vaccinated consistent with age-based recommendations.

3. **Varicella vaccination**
All adults without evidence of immunity to varicella should receive 2 doses of single-antigen varicella vaccine if not previously vaccinated or the second dose if they have received only 1 dose, unless they have a medical contraindication. Special consideration should be given to those who (1) have close contact with persons at high risk for severe disease (e.g., healthcare personnel and family contacts of persons with immunocompromising conditions) or (2) are at high risk for exposure or transmission (e.g., teachers; child-care employees; residents and staff members of institutional settings, including correctional institutions; college students; military personnel; adolescents and adults living in households with children; nonpregnant women of childbearing age; and international travelers).
Evidence of immunity to varicella in adults includes any of the following: (1) documentation of 2 doses of varicella vaccine at least 4 weeks apart; (2) U.S.-born before 1980 (although for healthcare personnel and pregnant women, birth before 1980 should not be considered evidence of immunity); (3) history of varicella based on diagnosis or verification of varicella by a healthcare provider (for a patient reporting a history of or presenting with an atypical case, a mild case, or both, healthcare providers should seek either an epidemiologic link with a typical varicella case or to a laboratory-confirmed case or evidence of laboratory confirmation, if it was performed at the time of acute disease); (4) history of herpes zoster based on diagnosis or verification of herpes zoster by a healthcare provider; or (5) laboratory evidence of immunity or laboratory confirmation of disease.
Pregnant women should be assessed for evidence of varicella immunity. Women who do not have evidence of immunity should receive the first dose of varicella vaccine upon completion or termination of pregnancy and before discharge from the healthcare facility. The second dose should be administered 4–8 weeks after the first dose.

4. **Herpes zoster vaccination**
A single dose of zoster vaccine is recommended for adults aged ≥60 years regardless of whether they report a prior episode of herpes zoster. Persons with chronic medical conditions may be vaccinated unless their condition constitutes a contraindication.

5. **Measles, mumps, rubella (MMR) vaccination**
Adults born before 1957 generally are considered immune to measles and mumps.
Measles component: Adults born during or after 1957 should receive 1 or more doses of MMR vaccine unless they have (1) a medical contraindication; (2) documentation of vaccination with 1 or more doses of MMR vaccine; (3) laboratory evidence of immunity; or (4) documentation of physician-diagnosed measles.
A second dose of MMR vaccine, administered 4 weeks after the first dose, is recommended for adults who (1) have been recently exposed to measles or are in an outbreak setting; (2) have been vaccinated previously with killed measles vaccine; (3) have been vaccinated with an unknown type of measles vaccine during 1963–1967; (4) are students in postsecondary educational institutions; (5) work in a healthcare facility; or (6) plan to travel internationally.
Mumps component: Adults born during or after 1957 should receive 1 dose of MMR vaccine unless they have (1) a medical contraindication; (2) documentation of vaccination with 1 or more doses of MMR vaccine; (3) laboratory evidence of immunity; or (4) documentation of physician-diagnosed mumps.
A second dose of MMR vaccine, administered 4 weeks after the first dose, is recommended for adults who (1) live in a community experiencing a mumps outbreak and are in an affected age group; (2) are students in postsecondary educational institutions; (3) work in a healthcare facility; or (4) plan to travel internationally.
Rubella component: 1 dose of MMR vaccine is recommended for women who do not have documentation of rubella vaccination, or who lack laboratory evidence of immunity. For women of childbearing age, regardless of birth year, rubella immunity should be determined and women should be counseled regarding congenital rubella syndrome. Women who do not have evidence of immunity should receive MMR vaccine upon completion or termination of pregnancy and before discharge from the healthcare facility.
Healthcare personnel born before 1957: For unvaccinated healthcare personnel born before 1957 who lack laboratory evidence of measles, mumps, and/or rubella immunity or laboratory confirmation of disease, healthcare facilities should consider vaccinating personnel with 2 doses of MMR vaccine at the appropriate interval (for measles and mumps) and 1 dose of MMR vaccine (for rubella), respectively. During outbreaks, healthcare facilities should recommend that unvaccinated healthcare personnel born before 1957, who lack laboratory evidence of measles, mumps, and/or rubella immunity or laboratory confirmation of disease, receive 2 doses of MMR vaccine during an outbreak of measles or mumps, and 1 dose during an outbreak of rubella. Complete information about evidence of immunity is available at www.cdc.gov/vaccines/recs/provisional/default.htm.

6. **Seasonal Influenza vaccination**
Vaccinate all persons aged ≥50 years and any younger persons who would like to decrease their risk of getting influenza. Vaccinate persons aged 19 through 49 years with any of the following indications.
Medical: Chronic disorders of the cardiovascular or pulmonary systems, including asthma; chronic metabolic diseases, including diabetes mellitus; renal or hepatic dysfunction, hemoglobinopathies, or immunocompromising conditions (including immunocompromising conditions caused by medications or HIV); cognitive, neurologic or neuromuscular disorders; and pregnancy during the influenza season. No data exist on the risk for severe or complicated influenza disease among persons with asplenia; however, influenza is a risk factor for secondary bacterial infections that can cause severe disease among persons with asplenia.
Occupational: All healthcare personnel, including those employed by long-term care and assisted-living facilities, and caregivers of children aged <5 years.
Other: Residents of nursing homes and other long-term care and assisted-living facilities; persons likely to transmit influenza to persons at high risk (e.g., in-home household contacts and caregivers of children aged <5 years, persons aged ≥50 years, and persons of all ages with high-risk conditions). Healthy, nonpregnant adults aged <50 years without high-risk medical conditions who are not contacts of severely immunocompromised persons in special-care units may receive either intranasally administered live, attenuated influenza vaccine (FluMist) or inactivated vaccine. Other persons should receive the inactivated vaccine.

7. **Pneumococcal polysaccharide (PPSV) vaccination**
Vaccinate all persons with the following indications.
Medical: Chronic lung disease (including asthma); chronic cardiovascular diseases; diabetes mellitus; chronic liver diseases, cirrhosis; chronic alcoholism; functional or anatomic asplenia (e.g., sickle cell disease or splenectomy [if elective splenectomy is planned, vaccinate at least 2 weeks before surgery]); immunocompromising conditions including chronic renal failure or nephrotic syndrome; and cochlear implants and cerebrospinal fluid leaks. Vaccinate as close to HIV diagnosis as possible.
Other: Residents of nursing homes or long-term care facilities and persons who smoke cigarettes. Routine use of PPSV is not recommended for American Indians/Alaska Natives or persons aged <65 years unless they have underlying medical conditions that are PPSV indications. However, public health authorities may consider recommending PPSV for American Indians/Alaska Natives and persons aged 50 through 64 years who are living in areas where the risk for invasive pneumococcal disease is increased.

8. **Revaccination with PPSV**
One-time revaccination after 5 years is recommended for persons with chronic renal failure or nephrotic syndrome; functional or anatomic asplenia (e.g., sickle cell disease or splenectomy); and for persons with immunocompromising conditions. For persons aged ≥65 years, one-time revaccination is recommended if they were vaccinated ≥5 years previously and were younger than aged <65 years at the time of primary vaccination.

9. **Hepatitis A vaccination**
Vaccinate persons with any of the following indications and any person seeking protection from hepatitis A virus (HAV) infection.
Behavioral: Men who have sex with men and persons who use injection drugs.
Occupational: Persons working with HAV–infected primates or with HAV in a research laboratory setting.
Medical: Persons with chronic liver disease and persons who receive clotting factor concentrates.
Other: Persons traveling to or working in countries that have high or intermediate endemicity of hepatitis A (a list of countries is available at wwwn.cdc.gov/travel/contentdiseases.aspx).
Unvaccinated persons who anticipate close personal contact (e.g., household contact or regular babysitting) with an international adoptee from a country of high or intermediate endemicity during the first 60 days after arrival of the adoptee in the United States should consider vaccination. The first dose of the 2-dose hepatitis A vaccine series should be administered as soon as adoption is planned, ideally ≥2 weeks before the arrival of the adoptee.
Single-antigen vaccine formulations should be administered in a 2-dose schedule at either 0 and 6–12 months (Havrix), or 0 and 6–18 months (Vaqta).If the combined hepatitis A and hepatitis B vaccine (Twinrix) is used, administer 3 doses at 0, 1, and 6 months; alternatively, a 4-dose schedule, administered on days 0, 7, and 21–30 followed by a booster dose at month 12 may be used.

10. **Hepatitis B vaccination**
Vaccinate persons with any of the following indications and any person seeking protection from hepatitis B virus (HBV) infection.
Behavioral: Sexually active persons who are not in a long-term, mutually monogamous relationship (e.g., persons with more than one sex partner during the previous 6 months); persons seeking evaluation or treatment for a sexually transmitted disease (STD); current or recent injection-drug users; and men who have sex with men.
Occupational: Healthcare personnel and public-safety workers who are exposed to blood or other potentially infectious body fluids.
Medical: Persons with end-stage renal disease, including patients receiving hemodialysis; persons with HIV infection; and persons with chronic liver disease.
Other: Household contacts and sex partners of persons with chronic HBV infection; clients and staff members of institutions for persons with developmental disabilities; and international travelers to countries with high or intermediate prevalence of chronic HBV infection (a list of countries is available at wwwn.cdc.gov/travel/contentdiseases.aspx).
Hepatitis B vaccination is recommended for all adults in the following settings: STD treatment facilities; HIV testing and treatment facilities; facilities providing drug-abuse treatment and prevention services; healthcare settings targeting services to injection-drug users or men who have sex with men; correctional facilities; end-stage renal disease programs and facilities for chronic hemodialysis patients; and institutions and nonresidential daycare facilities for persons with developmental disabilities.
Administer or complete a 3-dose series of HepB to those persons not previously vaccinated. The second dose should be administered 1 month after the first dose; the third dose should be administered at least 2 months after the second dose (and at least 4 months after the first dose). If the combined hepatitis A and hepatitis B vaccine (Twinrix) is used, administer 3 doses at 0, 1, and 6 months; alternatively, a 4-dose schedule, administered on days 0, 7, and 21–30 followed by a booster dose at month 12 may be used.
Adult patients receiving hemodialysis or with other immunocompromising conditions should receive 1 dose of 40 μg/mL (Recombivax HB) administered on a 3-dose schedule or 2 doses of 20 μg/mL (Engerix-B) administered simultaneously on a 4-dose schedule at 0, 1, 2 and 6 months.

11. **Meningococcal vaccination**
Meningococcal vaccine should be administered to persons with the following indications.
Medical: Adults with anatomic or functional asplenia, or persistent complement component deficiencies.
Other: First-year college students living in dormitories; microbiologists routinely exposed to isolates of *Neisseria meningitidis*; military recruits; and persons who travel to or live in countries in which meningococcal disease is hyperendemic or epidemic (e.g., the "meningitis belt" of sub-Saharan Africa during the dry season [December through June]), particularly if their contact with local populations will be prolonged. Vaccination is required by the government of Saudi Arabia for all travelers to Mecca during the annual Hajj.
Meningococcal conjugate vaccine (MCV4) is preferred for adults with any of the preceding indications who are aged ≤55 years; meningococcal polysaccharide vaccine (MPSV4) is preferred for adults aged ≥56 years. Revaccination with MCV4 after 5 years is recommended for adults previously vaccinated with MCV4 or MPSV4 who remain at increased risk for infection (e.g., adults with anatomic or functional asplenia). Persons whose only risk factor is living in on-campus housing are not recommended to receive an additional dose.

12. **Selected conditions for which *Haemophilus influenzae* type b (Hib) vaccine may be used**
Hib vaccine generally is not recommended for persons aged ≥5 years. No efficacy data are available on which to base a recommendation concerning use of Hib vaccine for older children and adults. However, studies suggest good immunogenicity in patients who have sickle cell disease, leukemia, or HIV infection or who have had a splenectomy. Administering 1 dose of Hib vaccine to these high-risk persons who have not previously received Hib vaccine is not contraindicated.

13. **Immunocompromising conditions**
Inactivated vaccines generally are acceptable (e.g., pneumococcal, meningococcal, influenza [inactivated influenza vaccine]) and live vaccines generally are avoided in persons with immune deficiencies or immunocompromising conditions. Information on specific conditions is available at www.cdc.gov/vaccines/pubs/acip-list.htm.

134

Human Immunodeficiency Virus Infection

PETER L. ANDERSON, THOMAS N. KAKUDA, AND COURTNEY V. FLETCHER

KEY CONCEPTS

❶ Infection with human immunodeficiency virus (HIV) occurs through three primary modes: sexual, parenteral, and perinatal. Sexual intercourse, primarily receptive anal and vaginal intercourse, is the most common method for transmission.

❷ HIV infects cells expressing cluster of differentiation 4 (CD4) receptors, such as T-helper lymphocytes, monocytes, macrophages, dendritic cells, and brain microglia. Infection occurs via an interaction between glycoprotein 120 on HIV with CD4 (primary interaction) and chemokine co-receptors (secondary interactions) present on the surfaces of these cells.

❸ The hallmark of untreated HIV infection is profound CD4 T-lymphocyte depletion and severe immunosuppression that puts patients at significant risk for infectious diseases caused by opportunistic pathogens. Opportunistic infections in settings without access to antiretroviral drugs are the chief cause of morbidity and mortality associated with HIV infection.

❹ General principles for the management of opportunistic infections include preventing or reversing immunosuppression with antiretroviral therapy, preventing exposure to pathogens, vaccination, prospective immunologic monitoring, primary chemoprophylaxis, treatment of acute episodes, secondary chemoprophylaxis, and discontinuation of such prophylaxes following antiretroviral therapy and subsequent immune recovery.

❺ Eradication of HIV is not possible at this time. Therefore, the goal of antiretroviral therapy is to achieve maximal and durable suppression of HIV replication, interpreted to be a sustained plasma viral load less than the lower limit of quantitation. Another equally important outcome is an increase in CD4 lymphocytes because this closely correlates with the risk for developing opportunistic infections.

❻ Current recommendations for the initial treatment of HIV advocate a minimum of three active antiretroviral agents from at least two drug classes. The typical regimen consists of two nucleoside analogs with either a protease inhibitor (pharmacologically enhanced with low-dose ritonavir), a nonnucleoside reverse transcriptase inhibitor, or an integrase inhibitor.

❼ Clinical use of antiretroviral agents is complicated by drug–drug interactions. Some interactions are beneficial and used

purposely; others may be harmful, leading to dangerously elevated or inadequate drug concentrations. For these reasons, clinicians involved in the pharmacotherapy of HIV infection must exercise constant vigilance and maintain a current knowledge of drug interactions.

❽ Inadequate suppression of viral replication allows HIV to select for antiretroviral-resistant HIV variants, the major factor limiting the ability of antiretroviral drugs to inhibit virus replication and delay disease progression.

❾ Current recommendations for treating drug-resistant HIV include choosing at least two drugs (preferably three) to which the patient's virus is susceptible. Susceptibility can be assessed using either (virtual) genotypic or phenotypic resistance testing.

❿ The longer life span conferred by antiretroviral treatment has given rise to new medical issues. First, a wide spectrum of early aging complications have become common, some of which are adverse effects from antiretroviral drugs. Second, hepatitis C virus coinfection has emerged as an important cause of morbidity and mortality. Medical management of these contemporary HIV complications is constantly evolving.

Acquired immune deficiency syndrome (AIDS) was first recognized in a cohort of young, previously healthy homosexual men with new-onset profound immunologic deficits, *Pneumocystis carinii* (now *P. jiroveci*) pneumonia (PCP), and/or Kaposi's sarcoma. A retrovirus, human immunodeficiency virus type 1 (HIV-1), is the major cause of AIDS. A second retrovirus, HIV-2, also is recognized to cause AIDS, although it is less virulent, transmissible, and prevalent than HIV-1. These retroviruses are transmitted primarily by sexual contact and by contact with infected blood or blood products. Several risk behaviors for the acquisition of HIV infection have been identified in the United States, most notably the practice of anorectal intercourse and the sharing of blood-contaminated needles by injection-drug users. In many resource-limited countries, the majority of HIV transmission occurs via heterosexual intercourse and from childbearing women to their offspring. Initially, the medical management of HIV consisted of repeated treatments for opportunistic infections (OIs) and eventual palliative care. Single and dual antiretroviral therapies with nucleoside reverse transcriptase inhibitors (NRTIs) followed, but were not highly effective when compared with contemporary therapies. In the mid 1990s, a new era in the pharmacotherapy for HIV, known as *combination antiretroviral therapy* (ART), was born. ART consists of combinations of antiretroviral agents with different mechanisms of action that potently and durably suppress HIV replication, delay the onset of AIDS, reverse HIV-associated immunologic deficits, and significantly prolong survival. Modern antiretroviral drugs and ART regimens have improved upon tolerability and efficacy. Unfortunately, therapeutic challenges remain in the ART era and include the need for continuous adherence to medication and care, drug–drug interactions, drug-resistant HIV, acute and long-term drug toxicities, and other complications associated with a prolonged life span. Progress has been made in the treatment access for this disease, but the worldwide picture remains grim. No strategies to date have been successful in curing HIV, and no viable vaccine is available.

HUMAN IMMUNODEFICIENCY VIRUS

EPIDEMIOLOGY

The epidemiologic characteristics of HIV infection differ according to geographic region and depend upon the mode of transmission, governmental prevention efforts and resources, and cultural factors.[1]

❶ Infection with HIV occurs through three primary modes: sexual, parenteral, and perinatal. Sexual intercourse, primarily anal and vaginal intercourse, is the most common method for transmission. The probability of HIV transmission depends upon the type of sexual exposure. The highest risk appears to be from receptive anorectal intercourse at about 0.5% to 3% per sexual act.[2] Transmission risk is lower for receptive vaginal or oral intercourse and each is lower for insertive versus receptive sex acts.[3] Condom use reduces risk of transmission by approximately 20-fold.[3] Other factors that affect the probability of infection include the stage of HIV disease in the index partner. For example, transmission is higher when the index partner has early or late HIV compared with asymptomatic HIV, as these disease stages are associated with higher viral loads.[4] Individuals with genital ulcers or sexually transmitted diseases are at greater risk for contracting HIV. HIV incidence and prevalence are lower in cultures that advocate male circumcision, which is estimated to reduce risk of male acquisition of HIV during heterosexual intercourse by 60%.[4] However, male circumcision may not have the same protective effects for anal intercourse or for the female partner.[5] Casual contact with patients with AIDS or HIV infection is not a significant risk factor for HIV transmission.

Prevention of sexual transmission has focused primarily on education that encourages abstinence (especially for adolescents), use of condoms, and reduction of high-risk behavior (anal intercourse and promiscuity).[1] A combined approach has been advocated for optimal prevention. Prevention strategies under investigation include HIV vaccines, topical vaginal microbicides, and pre-exposure prophylaxis (PrEP) with antiretroviral agents.[6]

Parenteral transmission of HIV broadly encompasses infections due to infected blood exposure from needle sticks, intravenous injection with used needles, receipt of blood products, and organ transplants. Use of contaminated needles or other injection-related paraphernalia by drug abusers has been the main cause of parenteral transmissions. The risk of HIV transmission from sharing needles is approximately 0.67% per episode.[7] Prevention strategies include stopping drug abuse, obtaining needles from credible sources (e.g., pharmacies), never reusing any paraphernalia, using sterile procedures in all injecting activities, and safely disposing of used paraphernalia.[3]

Before widespread screening, HIV was readily transmitted in blood products. However, blood and tissue products in the healthcare system are now rigorously screened for HIV. The estimated risk for receiving tainted blood or blood products in the United States is approximately 1:2,000,000 and that for receiving a tainted tissue transplant is 1:55,000.[8,9] Healthcare workers have a small but definite occupational risk of contracting HIV through accidental injury. Most cases of occupationally acquired HIV have been the result of a percutaneous needle stick injury, which carries an estimated 0.3% risk of transmitting HIV. Mucocutaneous exposures (e.g., tainted blood splash in eyes, mouth, nose) carries a transmission risk of approximately 0.09%.[10] Significant risk factors for seroconversion with a needle stick include deep injury, injury with a device visibly contaminated with blood, and advanced HIV disease in the index patient (high viral load). The risk of transmission from an HIV-infected healthcare worker to a patient is extremely remote. Comprehensive medical guidelines have been developed to minimize the hazard of HIV transmission for healthcare workers and for persons exposed by rape or other means.[7,10]

Perinatal infection, or vertical transmission, is the most common cause of pediatric HIV infection.[11] Most infections occur during or near to the time of birth, although a fraction can occur in utero. The risk of mother-to-child transmission is approximately 25% in the absence of antiretroviral therapy. Factors that increase the likelihood of vertical transmission include prolonged rupture of membranes, chorioamnionitis, genital infection during pregnancy, preterm delivery, vaginal delivery, birth weight less than 2.5 kg, illicit drug use during pregnancy, and high maternal viral load. Breastfeeding also can transmit HIV. The estimated frequency of breast milk transmission is approximately 4% to 16%, with the majority of infections developing within the first 6 months.[12] High levels of virus in breast milk and in the mother are associated with higher risk of transmission.[12] Formula feeding prevents breast milk transmission of HIV but may not improve mortality from other causes early in life in some settings.[13] Whenever formula feeding is acceptable, feasible, affordable, sustainable, and safe, HIV-infected mothers are recommended not to breast-feed. A separate and comprehensive set of medical guidelines have been developed to minimize the hazard of mother-to-child HIV transmission.[11] Prevention guidelines are discussed in the Treatment of Special Population section.

Persons with HIV infection are broadly categorized as those living with HIV and those with an AIDS diagnosis. An AIDS diagnosis is made when the presence of HIV is laboratory-confirmed and the cluster of differentiation 4 (CD4; T-helper cell) count drops below 200 cells/mm^3 or after an AIDS indicator condition is diagnosed.[14] Further distinctions regarding the stage of HIV and AIDS are given in the Revised Centers for Disease Control and Prevention (CDC) surveillance case definition (Table 134–1).[14] In the United States, new HIV/AIDS cases are reported by healthcare providers to a public health department.[15] The cumulative number of reported HIV/AIDS diagnoses in the US is approximately 1.7 million; more than 550,000 persons have already died.[16] The estimated prevalence of HIV infections including AIDS cases in the United States is about 1.2 million individuals. Each year the CDC estimates that 55,000 new cases of HIV infection occur in the United States.[16] Approximately 25% of persons with HIV are unaware of their infection. The epidemic in the United States initially was established in white men who have sex with men (MSM), and the prevalence of HIV in this population still is high. New trends in transmission include more cases in women (currently ~25%) and African Americans and Hispanics, a proportion of whom are not well linked to appropriate prevention, care, and treatment services.[16] Approximately half of new cases occur in African Americans (who make up only 12% of the general population), about one third in Caucasians, and less than one fourth in Hispanics.[15] The main risk factor for transmission in women is heterosexual intercourse (~80% of cases) and injection-drug use (~20% of cases). For men the main risks are men who have sex with men (~65%), heterosexual sex (~15%), and injection-drug use (~15%).[17]

Today, the estimated number of individuals living with HIV/AIDS worldwide has stabilized at approximately 33.4 million persons, including 2.1 million children (younger than 15 years).[18,19] The new infection rate is approximately 2.7 million per year, including 430,000 children.[19] About 2 million people succumbed to AIDS in 2008. Globally, the highest concentration of HIV/AIDS cases is in sub-Saharan Africa, where approximately 22.4 million people are infected. Some African countries have HIV prevalence rates of up to 26% (e.g., Swaziland); however, other African areas have declining

	Laboratory evidence	
Stage	**(laboratory-confirmed HIV infection *plus*)**	**Clinical evidence**
Stage 1	CD4+ cell count ≥500 cells/mm³ or CD4+ percentage ≥29	None required (but no AIDS-defining condition)
Stage 2	CD4+ cell count 200-499 cells/mm³ or CD4+ percentage 14–28	None required (but no AIDS-defining condition)
Stage 3 (AIDS)	CD4+ cell count <200 cells/mm³ or CD4+ percentage <14	or documentation of an AIDS-defining condition (with laboratory-confirmed HIV infection)
Stage unknown	no information on CD4+ counts	and no information on presence of AIDS-defining conditions

TABLE 134-1 Surveillance Case Definition for HIV Infection among Adults and Adolescents (≥13 years) – United States, 2008

AIDS indicator conditions

Candidiasis of bronchi, trachea, or lungs	Lymphoma, Burkitt
Candidiasis, esophageal	Lymphoma, immunoblastic
Cervical cancer, invasive	Lymphoma, primary, for brain
Coccidioidomycosis, disseminated or extrapulmonary	*Mycobacterium avium* complex or *Mycobacterium kansasii*, disseminated or extrapulmonary
Cryptococcosis, extrapulmonary	*Mycobacterium tuberculosis*, any site (pulmonary or extrapulmonary)
Cryptosporidiosis, chronic intestinal (duration >1 month)	*Mycobacterium*, other species or unidentified species, disseminated or extrapulmonary
Cytomegalovirus disease (other than liver, spleen, or nodes)	*Pneumocystis jirovecii* pneumonia
Cytomegalovirus retinitis (with loss of vision)	Pneumonia, recurrent
Encephalopathy, HIV related	Progressive multifocal leukoencephalopathy
Herpes simplex: chronic ulcer(s) (duration >1 month); or bronchitis, pneumonitis, or esophagitis	*Salmonella* septicemia, recurrent
Histoplasmosis, disseminated or extrapulmonary	Toxoplasmosis of brain
Isosporiasis, chronic intestinal (duration >1 month)	Wasting syndrome due to HIV
Kaposi sarcoma	

From reference 14.

prevalence rates (e.g., Eastern Africa) due to successful prevention strategies.[18,19] Heterosexual transmission is the most common mode of transmission in sub-Saharan Africa and worldwide (85% of cases). Women in sub-Saharan Africa and resource-limited countries are at disproportionately high risk for acquiring HIV because of biologic and cultural factors that foster HIV transmission, such as limited ability to refuse sex.[19] Other important epidemiologic features of the HIV epidemic include relatively high prevalence in Eastern Europe (e.g., Russian Federation), central Asia (e.g., Ukraine), and growing prevalence in Bangladesh and China.[18] Injection-drug use is fueling several of these epidemics.

ETIOLOGY

HIV is an enveloped single-stranded RNA virus and a member of the *Lentivirinae* (*lenti*, meaning "slow") subfamily of retroviruses. Lentiviruses are characterized by their indolent infectious cycle. There are two related but distinct types of HIV: HIV-1 and HIV-2. HIV-2, found mostly in western Africa, consists of seven phylogenetic lineages designated as subtypes (clades) A through G. HIV-1 also can be categorized based on phylogeny.[20] Three groups of HIV-1 are recognized: M (main or major), N (non-M, non-O), and O (outlier). More recently, a new HIV-1 virus was classified as group P (pending the identification of further cases).[21] The nine subtypes of HIV-1 group M are identified as A through D, F through H, and J and K. Mixtures of subtypes are referred to as *circulating recombinant forms* (CRFs). Group M, subtype B, is primarily responsible for the epidemic in North America and Western Europe.[20]

The origin of HIV is of considerable interest. The accumulated evidence suggests that HIV in humans was the result of a cross-species transmission (zoonosis) from primates infected with simian immunodeficiency virus (SIV). Phylogenetic and geographic relationships suggest that HIV-2 arose from SIV that infects sooty mangabeys and HIV-1 group M and N arose from SIVcpz, a virus that infects chimpanzees (*Pan troglodytes troglodytes*). Group O may have arisen from an SIV variant that infects wild gorillas. Cultural practices, such as preparation and eating of bush meat or keeping animals as pets, may have allowed the virus to jump from primates

to humans. The earliest known human infection with HIV has been traced to central Africa in 1959, but cross-species transmissions probably date back to the early 1900s.[22] Modern transportation, promiscuity, and drug abuse have caused the rapid spread of the virus within the United States and throughout the world.[1,22] This chapter focuses on HIV-1 group M, which is the predominant strain likely to be encountered in the Western world.

DETECTION OF HIV AND SURROGATE MARKERS OF DISEASE PROGRESSION

The preferred method for diagnosing HIV-1 infection is an enzyme-linked immunosorbent assay (ELISA), which detects antibodies against HIV-1.[17] ELISA is both highly sensitive (>99%) and highly specific (>99%), but rare false-positive results can occur in multiparous women; recent recipients of hepatitis B, HIV, influenza, or rabies vaccine; patients with multiple blood transfusion, liver disease, and renal failure; or those undergoing chronic hemodialysis. False-negative results may occur and most commonly are attributed to new infection where antibody production is not yet adequate. The minimum time to develop antibodies is 3 to 4 weeks from initial exposure, with greater than 95% of individuals developing antibodies after 6 months. Convenient methods for obtaining an ELISA sample from blood or saliva have been developed, including a rapid (20–40 minutes) turnaround test.

Positive ELISA results are repeated in duplicate, and if one or both tests are reactive, a confirmatory test is performed for final diagnosis. Western blot is the most commonly used confirmatory test, although an indirect immunofluorescence assay is available. A reactive ELISA test and a positive confirmatory test indicate an established HIV infection. If the confirmatory test is indeterminate, the individual should be retested 4 weeks later.[17]

HIV testing is recommended when HIV infection is suspected because of symptoms and/or high-risk behavior. Additionally, the CDC now recommends routine HIV screening in all healthcare settings in persons 13 to 64 years, a new policy called "opt-out" testing.[17] The policy states that consent for medical care will imply consent for HIV testing; however, the person must be informed of the test and can opt out of taking it. Because states may have different

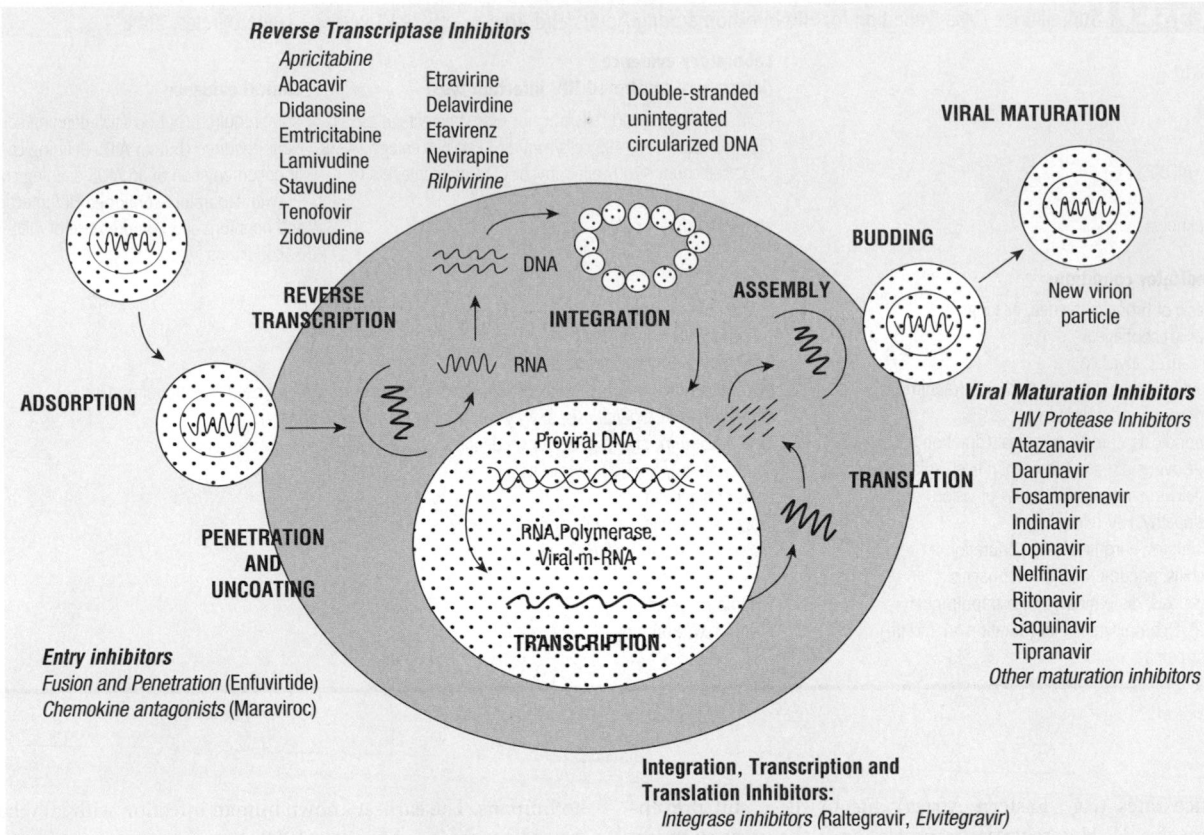

FIGURE 134-1. Life cycle of human immunodeficiency virus with potential targets where replication may be interrupted. Italicized compounds were in development at the time of this writing. *(Reprinted with permission, Courtney V. Fletcher, 2009.)*

HIV consent laws, the local requirements for HIV testing should be consulted. The rationale for the opt-out strategy is to diagnose those who unknowingly carry HIV so as to improve their prognosis and reduce further transmission.

Once diagnosed, HIV disease is monitored primarily by two surrogate biomarkers, viral load and CD4 cell count.[23] The viral load test quantifies the degree of viremia by measuring the number of copies of viral RNA (HIV RNA) in the plasma. Methods for determining HIV RNA include reverse-transcription polymerase chain reaction (RT-PCR), branched-chain DNA, transcription-mediated amplification, and nucleic acid sequence–based assay. RT-PCR is used more widely than the other techniques. Irrespective of the method used, viral load is reported as the number of viral RNA copies per milliliter of plasma. Each assay has its own lower limit of sensitivity to viral subtypes, and results can vary from one assay method to the other; therefore, it is recommended that the same assay method be used consistently within patients. Reductions in viral load often are reported in base 10 logarithm. For example, if a patient presents initially with a viral load of 100,000 copies/mL (10^5 copies/mL) and subsequently has a viral load of 10,000 copies/mL (10^4 copies/mL), the decrease in viral load is 1 $\log_{10}$. Given that HIV RNA varies within patients, a clinical response is generally considered when the decline in viral load is more than 0.5 $\log_{10}$.[23] Viral load is a major prognostic factor for monitoring disease progression and the effects of treatment.

Because HIV attacks and leads to the destruction of cells bearing the CD4 receptor, the number of CD4 lymphocytes (T-helper cells) in the blood is a critical surrogate marker of disease progression. The normal adult CD4 lymphocyte count ranges from 500 to 1,600 cells/mm³, or 40% to 70% of total lymphocytes. CD4 counts in children are age dependent, with younger children having higher CD4 counts. The hallmark of HIV disease is depletion of CD4 cells and the associated development of OIs and malignancies.

PATHOGENESIS

❷ Understanding the life cycle of HIV (Fig. 134–1) is necessary because the current strategies used for treatment of HIV target various points in this cycle. Once HIV enters the human body, the outer glycoprotein (gp160) on its surface, which is composed of two subunits (gp120 and gp41) has affinity for CD4 receptors, proteins present on the surface of T-helper lymphocytes, monocytes, macrophages, dendritic cells, and brain microglia.[24] The gp120 subunit is responsible for CD4 binding. Once initial binding occurs, the intimate association of HIV with the cell is enhanced by further binding to chemokine co-receptors. The two major chemokine receptors used by HIV are CCR5 and CXCR4. HIV isolates may contain a mixture of viruses that target one or the other of these co-receptors, and some viral strains may be dual-tropic (i.e., can use both co-receptors). The HIV strain that preferentially uses CCR5, R5 viruses, are macrophage-tropic and typically implicated in most cases of sexually transmitted HIV. Individuals with a common 32-base-pair deletion in the CCR5 gene are protected from progression of HIV disease.[25] The HIV strain that targets CXCR4, designated X4 virus, is T-cell–tropic and often is predominant in the later stage of disease. Other chemokine co-receptors and galactosyl ceramide may also serve as a binding site for HIV. CD4 and co-receptor attachment of HIV to the cell promotes membrane fusion, which is mediated by gp41, and finally internalization of the viral genetic material and enzymes necessary for replication.

After internalization, the viral protein shell surrounding the nucleic acid (capsid) is uncoated in preparation for replication.[24] The genetic material of HIV is two molecules of positive-sense (5′ to 3′) single-stranded RNA; the virus must transcribe this RNA into DNA (transcription normally occurs from DNA to RNA; HIV works backward, hence the name *retrovirus*). To do so,

HIV is equipped with the unique enzyme RNA-dependent DNA polymerase (reverse transcriptase). HIV reverse transcriptase first synthesizes a complementary strand of DNA using the viral RNA as a template. The RNA portion of this DNA–RNA hybrid is then partially removed by ribonuclease H (RNase H), allowing HIV reverse transcriptase to complete the synthesis of a double-stranded DNA molecule. The fidelity of HIV reverse transcriptase is poor, and many mistakes are made during the process. These errors in the final DNA product contribute to the rapid mutation of the virus, which enables the virus to evade the immune response (thus complicating vaccine development), and promotes the evolution of drug resistance. Following reverse transcription, the final double-stranded DNA product migrates into the nucleus and is integrated into the host cell chromosome by integrase, another enzyme unique to HIV.

The integration of HIV into the host chromosome is troublesome. Most notably, HIV can establish a persistent, latent infection, particularly in long-lived cells of the immune system such as memory T lymphocytes. The virus is effectively hidden in these cells, and this characteristic has greatly inhibited the ability to cure HIV infection. Second, random integration of HIV may cause cellular abnormalities and induce apoptosis.

After integration, HIV preferentially replicates in activated cells. Activation by antigens, cytokines, or other factors stimulates the cell to produce nuclear factor kappa B (NF-κB), an enhancer-binding protein. NF-κB normally regulates the expression of T-lymphocyte genes involved in growth but also can inadvertently activate replication of HIV. HIV encodes six regulatory and accessory proteins: Tat, Nef, Rev, Vpu, Vif, and Vpr, which enhance replication and inhibit innate immunity. For example, the Tat protein is a potent amplifier of HIV gene expression; it binds to a specific RNA sequence of HIV that initiates and stabilizes transcription elongation. Vif is a viral protein that binds human APOBEC 3G, a deoxycytidine deaminase that converts viral DNA cytosine to uracil and thereby provides innate cellular immunity.[26] Vpu inhibits tetherin, a human cellular membrane protein that prevents diffusion of virus particles after budding from infected cells, thereby allowing HIV to detach from the infected cell.[27] Assembly of new virion particles occurs in a stepwise manner beginning with the coalescence of HIV proteins beneath the host cell lipid bilayer. The nucleocapsid subsequently is formed with viral single-stranded RNA and other components packaged inside. Once packaged, the virion then buds through the plasma membrane, acquiring the characteristics of the host lipid bilayer. After the virus buds, the maturation process begins. Within the virion, protease, another enzyme unique to HIV, begins cleaving a large precursor polypeptide (gag-pol) into functional proteins that are necessary to produce a complete virus. Without this enzyme, the virion is immature and unable to infect other cells.

The characteristics of viral replication and pathogenesis exhibit three general phases, acute, chronic, and terminal (AIDS).[28,29] Recent evidence suggests that initial rounds of HIV replication during acute infection take place largely in the mucosal CD4+ CCR5+ T-cell pools in the gut resulting in a massive CD4 T-cell depletion in these tissues.[28,29] Cells are destroyed by a number of mechanisms, including cell lysis from newly budding virions, cytotoxic T-lymphocyte–induced cell killing, and induction of apoptosis. Following this destruction of the mucosal CD4 T cell pool, which lasts for 2 to 3 weeks, a state of heightened immune activation ensues during the chronic infection phase, which can last for several years. The activated state is characterized by high levels of activation markers on circulating T cells and pro-inflammatory cytokines and may result from HIV antigen as well as translocation of microbial antigens from the T-cell–depleted gut mucosa. Heightened activation enables further HIV replication and ultimately leads to continued depletion of CD4+ CCR5+ T cells. HIV-1 exhibits a very high turnover rate during this chronic phase, with an estimated 10 billion new viruses produced each day. More than 99% of these viruses are produced in newly infected activated cells. Nevertheless, the immune system is able to operate well enough during the chronic phase to prevent overt opportunistic infections that herald AIDS. Eventually, the depletion of CD4 cells and the continuous cellular activation leads to a final collapse of the immune system, or AIDS. HIV may use CXCR4 co-receptor during this last phase of infection and these viruses infect a broader range of CD4 cells (naïve and central-memory) speeding the disease progression. It is this unrelenting destruction of CD4 cells that causes the profoundly compromised immune system and AIDS.[28,29]

| TABLE 134-2 | Clinical Presentation of HIV Infection |

Symptoms

Fever, sore throat, fatigue, weight loss, myalgia

40% to 80% of patients exhibit a morbilliform or maculopapular rash usually involving the trunk

Diarrhea, nausea, vomiting

Lymphadenopathy, night sweats

Aseptic meningitis (fever, headache, photophobia, stiff neck) may be present in 25% of presenting cases

Other

High viral load (may exceed 1,000,000 copies per milliliter)

Persistent decrease in CD4 lymphocytes

CLINICAL PRESENTATION

❸ Clinical presentation of primary HIV infection varies, but most patients (40%–90%) have an acute retroviral syndrome or mononucleosis-like illness (Table 134–2).[30] Symptoms often last 2 weeks, and hospitalization may be required for 15% of patients. Primary infection is associated with a high viral load (>10[6] copies/mL) and a precipitous drop in CD4 cells. After several weeks an immune response is mounted, the amount of HIV RNA in plasma falls substantially, and symptoms resolve gradually. However, as described above, this clinically latent period is not virologically latent because HIV replication is continuous (~10 billion viruses per day) and immune system destruction is ongoing. A steady decrease in CD4 cells is the most measurable aspect of this immune system deterioration. Plasma viral load, on the other hand, will appear to have stabilized at a particular level or "set point." The set point that is established correlates directly with the time to AIDS and morbidity. The Multicenter AIDS Cohort Study measured viral load in 181 HIV-positive men and followed them for as long as 11 years. The mortality rates within 5 years for those with a viral load below 4530 copies/mL was 5% compared with 49% for those with a viral load above 36,270 copies/mL.[31] Thus, a higher viral set point is associated with poorer prognosis. Not all individuals infected with HIV progress to AIDS—these so-called "long-term non-progressors" may be infected with a defective virus (e.g., nef-deficient HIV) or may have an intrinsic ability to resist infection (e.g., CCR5 mutation).[25]

Most children born with HIV are asymptomatic. On physical examination, children often present with nonspecific signs, such as lymphadenopathy, hepatomegaly, splenomegaly, failure to thrive, weight loss or unexplained low birth weight (in prenatally exposed infants), and fever of unknown origin.[32] Laboratory findings include anemia, hypergammaglobulinemia (primarily immunoglobulin [Ig] A and IgM), altered mononuclear cell function, and altered T-cell subset ratios. Of note, the normal range for CD4 cell counts in young children is much different from the range in adults (Table 134–3).[33] Children have different susceptibility and/or exposures to OIs compared with adults.[32] Bacterial infections, including *Streptococcus pneumoniae*, *Salmonella* spp, and *Mycobacterium tuberculosis*,

TABLE 134-3 Centers for Disease Control and Prevention 1994 Revised Classification System for Human Immunodeficieny Virus Infection in Children Younger Than 13 Years

Immunologic Categories	12 Month CD4 Cells/mm³ (%ᵃ)	1–5 Years CD4 Cells/mm³ (%ᵃ)	6–12 Years CD4 Cells/mm³ (%ᵃ)	
1. No evidence of suppression	≥1,500 (≥25%)	≥1,000 (≥25%)	≥500 (≥25%)	
2. Evidence of moderate suppression	750–1,499 (15%–24%)	500–999 (15%–24%)	200–499 (15%–24%)	
3. Severe suppression	<750 (<15%)	<500 (<15%)	<200 (<15%)	
Immunologic Categories	N: No Signs/Symptoms	A: Mild Signs/Symptoms	B: Moderate Signs/Symptoms	C: Severe Signs/Symptoms
1. No evidence of suppression	N1	A1	B1	C1
2. Evidence of moderate suppression	N2	A2	B2	C2
3. Severe suppression	N3	A3	B3	C3

ᵃPercentage of total lymphocytes.
From reference 33.

may be more prevalent in children with AIDS than in adults with the disease. Kaposi sarcoma is rare in children. Children with HIV infection may develop lymphocytic interstitial pneumonitis without evidence of *P. jiroveci* or other pathogens on lung biopsy. Some children (~25%) will progress to AIDS rapidly within the first year of life. A presentation of serious opportunistic infections such as *P. jiroveci* pneumonia, encephalopathy, failure to thrive, and a precipitous drop in CD4 cells are common in these infants.[32] The current CDC pediatric AIDS surveillance definition (see Table 134–3) excludes children with congenital or perinatally acquired cytomegalovirus or other identified causes of congenital immunodeficiency; laboratory-confirmed HIV-infection is required.[14,33] General management of the HIV-infected child involves principles similar to those used for the adult: antiretroviral therapy, treatment and prophylaxis of OIs, and supportive care.[34,35]

TREATMENT

■ DESIRED OUTCOME

❺ The central goals of antiretroviral therapy are to decrease morbidity and mortality, improve quality of life, restore and preserve immune function, and prevent further transmission. The most important and effective way to achieve these goals is maximal suppression of HIV replication, which is interpreted as plasma HIV RNA less than the lower limit of quantitation (i.e., undetectable; usually <50 copies/mL).[23] Such a profound reduction in HIV RNA is associated with long-term response to therapy (i.e., durability) as well as increases in CD4 lymphocytes, which closely correlates with the risk for developing OIs. While undetectable HIV RNA almost always corresponds with a rise in CD4 lymphocytes, some patients respond virologically or immunologically without the other.[23]

■ GENERAL APPROACH TO TREATMENT

❹ Prior to 1996, HIV infection was treated with one or two nucleoside analog reverse transcriptase inhibitors, which were generally not effective at controlling viremia. Thus, the mainstay of treatment was pharmacologic management of OIs and palliative care. At that time, the prognosis for HIV infection was dire and most patients were disabled and eventually died. In 1995, HIV protease inhibitors (PIs) were introduced followed by non-nucleoside analog reverse transcriptase inhibitors (NNRTIs), and a new paradigm in HIV treatment was born. Combinations of three active antiretroviral agents from two pharmacologic classes were shown to profoundly inhibit HIV replication, prevent and reverse immune deficiency, and substantially decrease morbidity and mortality—constituting the ART era.[36] At the same time, multiple other major medical

advances were introduced, such as the discovery that HIV establishes a long-lived reservoir in chronically infected cells, and the viral load test (plasma HIV-RNA). With this backdrop of dramatic changes, in 1997 the National Institutes of Health Office of AIDS Research convened a panel to define the scientific principles that might serve as a guide for the clinical use of antiretroviral agents.[37] The 11 principles presented here are an amalgamation of knowledge of the life cycle of HIV, the consequences of HIV replication, clinical trials of antiretroviral agents, and scientific opinion. These foundational principles are still relevant today.

1. Ongoing HIV replication leads to immune system damage and progression to AIDS. HIV infection is always harmful, and true long-term survival free of clinically significant immune dysfunction is unusual.

2. Plasma HIV RNA levels indicate the magnitude of HIV replication and its associated rate of CD4 cell destruction, whereas CD4 cell counts indicate the extent of HIV-induced immune damage already suffered. Regular periodic measurement of plasma HIV RNA levels and CD4 cell counts is necessary to determine the risk of disease progression in an HIV-infected individual and to determine when to initiate or modify antiretroviral treatment regimens.

3. Because rates of disease progression differ among individuals, treatment decisions should be individualized by level of risk indicated by plasma HIV RNA levels and CD4 cell counts.

4. Use of potent combination antiretroviral therapy to suppress HIV replication to below the levels of detection of sensitive plasma HIV RNA assays limits the potential for selection of antiretroviral-resistant HIV variants, the major factor limiting the ability of antiretroviral drugs to inhibit virus replication and delay disease progression. Therefore, maximum achievable suppression of HIV replication should be the goal of therapy.

5. The most effective means for accomplishing durable suppression of HIV replication is simultaneous initiation of combinations of effective anti-HIV drugs with which the patient has not been treated previously and that are not cross-resistant with antiretroviral agents with which the patient has been treated previously.

6. Each of the antiretroviral drugs used in combination therapy regimens always should be used according to optimal schedules and dosages.

7. The available effective antiretroviral drugs are limited in number and mechanism of action, and cross-resistance between specific drugs has been documented. Therefore, any change in antiretroviral therapy increases future therapeutic constraints.

8. Women should receive optimal antiretroviral therapy regardless of pregnancy status.

9. The same principles of antiretroviral therapy apply to both HIV-infected children and adults, although treatment of HIV-infected children involves unique pharmacologic, virologic, and immunologic considerations.

10. Persons with acute primary HIV infections should be treated with combination antiretroviral therapy to suppress virus replication to levels below the limit of detection of sensitive plasma HIV RNA assays.

11. HIV-infected persons, even those with viral loads below detectable limits, should be considered infectious and should be counseled to avoid sexual and drug-use behaviors that are associated with transmission or acquisition of HIV and other infectious pathogens.

The extent to which these 11 principles will continue to stand the test of time is unknown; new information on the pathogenesis and treatment of HIV accrues constantly. One continuing source of controversy is whether to treat patients with acute HIV infection. As of December 2009, 25 distinct antiretroviral compounds have been approved by the U.S. Food and Drug Administration (FDA); one (zalcitabine) has since been removed from the market. Table 134–4 presents the state of the art for treatment of HIV-infected individuals as of December 2009.[23] Treatment is recommended for all HIV-infected persons with a history of an AIDS-defining event, symptomatic disease, or a CD4 lymphocyte count below 350 cells/mm³. Therapy is also recommended for asymptomatic patients with CD4 counts between 350 and 500 cells/mm³, and some clinicians would also favor starting therapy in those with >500 CD4 cells/mm³. Other indications for therapy at any CD4 count include pregnancy, HIV-associated nephropathy, or when treatment is needed for hepatitis B co-infection.

CLINICAL CONTROVERSY

Treatment of persons with acute primary HIV infection with combination antiretroviral therapy to suppress virus replication to levels below the limit of detection of sensitive plasma HIV RNA assays is controversial. Well-designed trials with clinical end points that define the long-term safety and efficacy of initiating combination antiretroviral therapy during acute HIV infection are lacking. Theoretical benefits are decreasing the severity of acute disease; perhaps lowering the initial viral load setpoint, which affects progression rates; preserving immune function; and reducing the risk for viral transmission. However, these potential benefits must be weighed against the issues imposed by early intervention of chronic therapy, which would be many years ahead of normal initiation of therapy (discussed below).

The optimal time to initiate therapy in chronic HIV infection has also been a matter of debate over the last 10 years. The relative risk of death in asymptomatic HIV-infected individuals is higher when antiretroviral therapy is delayed. Among individuals with a CD4 count of 351 to 500 cells/mm³ prior to therapy, a 69% increase in the risk of death was found if treatment was deferred until their CD4 cell count fell below 350 cells/mm³ compared to those initiating immediate treatment; similarly, deferring therapy until the CD4 cell count fell below 500 cells/mm³ was associated with a 94% increase in the risk of death.[38] Healthcare professionals involved in the care of HIV-infected persons must consult the most current literature on the principles and strategies for therapy. Better patient outcomes are demonstrated when clinicians have significant HIV expertise. Likewise, the patient must be ready and willing to commit to life-long treatment including an understanding of its risks and benefits and the need to maintain a high level of adherence. An excellent source for information on treatment guidelines, which is regularly updated, is available at *www.AIDSinfo.NIH.gov*. Additional guidelines and electronic resources for HIV clinicians are provided in reference 17.

CLINICAL CONTROVERSY

The precise time to start therapy is controversial. Early in the ART era, the mantra was "hit early and hit hard," with hopes that the drugs would be well tolerated and the virus could be eradicated. When it became clear that treatment was long term and that these earlier drugs had potential long-term side effects, the mantra changed to a drug-sparing paradigm where therapy was initiated as late as possible. Newer agents have improved upon tolerability, but lack long-term safety data. The benefits of early therapy include preventing the known detriments of unchecked viral replication, including irreversible immune damage and increased likelihood of viral transmission. The potential risks of initiating combination antiretroviral therapy include the lifestyle demands of continuous therapy, drug toxicities, and development of antiretroviral drug resistance.

■ PHARMACOLOGIC THERAPY

Conceptually the four primary methods of therapeutic intervention against HIV are inhibition of viral replication, microbicides to prevent HIV infection, vaccination to stimulate a more effective immune response, and restoration of the immune system with immunomodulators; the latter three approaches are mostly investigational. Several approaches for an HIV vaccine are in development, including whole killed virus, subunit and peptide vaccination, recombinant live vector, and naked DNA delivery. A randomized placebo-controlled trial demonstrated a modest 30% reduction in HIV transmission in a modified-intention to treat analysis of ALVAC-HIV plus AIDSVAX vaccine in 16,402 volunteers ($P=0.04$).[39] The modified analysis excluded subjects who were found to be HIV-infected prior to randomization. However, the efficacy difference was not significant in the per-protocol analysis ($P=0.16$). Therefore, the findings must be considered tentative until more definitive data become available. Overall, progress has been slow for the vaccine field. Genetic variability in HIV and a nascent understanding of the role of the immune system in suppressing viral replication are significant barriers to the development of an effective HIV vaccine with long-lasting and protective immunity. Immunomodulators, such as aldesleukin (interleukin 2), provide mild benefits in terms of increased CD4 cells, however, aldesleukin is also associated with significant toxicities and no apparent clinical benefit.[40] Additional immunotherapies are in earlier phases of study. Microbicides for use vaginally or rectally to prevent sexual transmission of HIV are in various phases of development.[41]

Antiretroviral Agents

❻ Inhibiting viral replication with combinations of potent antiretroviral agents has been the most clinically successful strategy. Four general classes of drugs are used today: entry inhibitors, reverse transcriptase inhibitors, integrase strand transfer inhibitors and HIV protease inhibitors (Table 134–5).[23,42,43] Reverse transcriptase inhibitors consist of two classes: those that are chemical derivatives

TABLE 134-4 Treatment of Human Immunodeficiency Virus Infection: Antiretroviral Regimens Recommended in Antiretroviral-Naïve Persons

	Preferred Regimens	Limitation
NNRTI based	Efavirenz + tenofovir + emtricitabine (AI)	Not in first trimester of pregnancy or in women without adequate contraception
PI based	Darunavir + ritonavir + tenofovir + emtricitabine (AI)	Caution in HCV–HBV co-infection, rash
	Atazanavir + ritonavir + tenofovir + emtricitabine (AI)	Not with high doses of proton-pump-inhibitors, rash
	Raltegravir + tenofovir + emtricitabine (AI)	Twice daily (not once daily)
Alternative regimens (some potential disadvantages versus preferred regimens)		
	Efavirenz + (abacavir or zidovudine) + lamivudine (BI)	Possible reduced efficacy for high viral loads (abacavir), more subcutaneous fat loss (zidovudine)
	Nevirapine + zidovudine + lamivudine (BI)	Not in moderate to severe hepatic disease or in women with CD4 >250 cells/mm³ or men with CD4 >450 cells/mm³
PI based	Atazanavir-ritonavir + (abacavir or zidovudine) + lamivudine (BI)	See above
	Lopinavir-ritonavir (once or twice daily) either with (abacavir or zidovudine) + lamivudine or (tenofovir+ emtricitabine) (BI)	Gastrointestinal intolerance, lipids
	Fosamprenavir/ritonavir (once or twice daily) either with (abacavir or zidovudine) + lamivudine or (tenofovir + emtricitabine) (BI)	Rash
	Saquinavir-ritonavir (twice daily) + tenofovir + emtricitabine (BI)	High number of pills/complexity
Acceptable regimens (potential additional disadvantages or pending additional data)		
	Efavirenz + didanosine + (lamivudine or emtricitabine) (CI)	Mitochondrial toxicities with didanosine
	Atazanavir + (abacavir or zidovudine) + lamivudine (CI)	Lower atazanavir concentrations compared with atazanavir-ritonavir
	Maraviroc + zidovudine + lamivudine (CIII)	Lower virologic activity versus efavirenz, need tropism test
	Raltegravir + abacavir or zidovudine + lamivudine	See above
	(Darunavir-ritonavir or saquinavir-ritonavir) + (abacavir or zidovudine) + lamivudine	See above
Regimens or components that should not be used		
Regimen or component		**Comment**
Any all NRTI regimen (EI)		Inferior virologic efficacy
Abacavir + didanosine or abacavir + tenofovir (DIII)		Insufficient data
Didanosine + tenofovir (EII)		Inferior virologic efficacy, CD4 declines
Stavudine (EI)		Toxicity including subcutaneous fat loss, peripheral neuropathy, and lactic acidosis
Darunavir or tipranavir or saquinavir without ritonavir (EI)		Insufficient plasma concentrations and efficacy or not studied
Delavirdine (EII)		Inferior virologic efficacy and inconvenient dosing
Enfuvirtide (DIII)		Not studied in naïve patients, inconvenient injections
Etravirine (DIII)		Not studied in naïve patients
Indinavir with or without ritonavir (EIII)		Nephrolithiasis, fluid requirements and inconvenient
Nelfinavir (without ritonavir) (EI)		Inferior virologic efficacy
Ritonavir at virologic doses (EIII)		Gastrointestinal intolerance
Tipranavir-ritonavir (EI)		Inferior virologic efficacy

NRTI, nucleoside reverse transcriptase inhibitor.

Evidence-based Rating Definition

Rating Strength of Recommendation:

A: Both strong evidence for efficacy and substantial clinical benefit support recommendation for use; should always be offered.

B: Moderate evidence for efficacy or strong evidence for efficacy but only limited clinical benefit, supports recommendation for use; should usually be offered.

C: Evidence for efficacy is insufficient to support a recommendation for or against use, or evidence for efficacy might not outweigh adverse consequences (e.g., drug toxicity, drug interactions) or cost of treatment under consideration; use is optional.

D: Moderate evidence for lack of efficacy or for adverse outcome supports recommendation against use; should usually not be offered.

E: Good evidence for lack of efficacy or for adverse outcome supports a recommendation against use; should never be offered.

Rating Quality of Evidence Supporting the Recommendation:

I: Evidence from at least one correctly randomized, controlled trial with clinical outcomes and/or validated laboratory endpoints.

II: Evidence from at least one well-designed clinical trial without randomization or observational cohorts with long-term clinical outcomes.

III: Evidence from opinions of respected authorities based on clinical experience, descriptive studies, or reports of consulting committees.

*a*Lamivudine and emtricitabine are considered interchangeable.

Adapted from Department of Health and Human Services (DHHS) Panel on Antiretroviral Guidelines for Adults and Adolescents. Guidelines for the use of antiretroviral agents in HIV-infected adults and adolescents. December 1, 2009. http://AIDSinfo.NIH.gov.

of purine- and pyrimidine-based nucleosides and nucleotides (nucleoside/nucleotide reverse transcriptase inhibitors [NRTIs]) and those that are not (nonnucleoside reverse transcriptase inhibitors [NNRTIs]). NRTIs include the thymidine analogs stavudine (d4T) and zidovudine (AZT or ZDV); the deoxycytidine analogs emtricitabine (FTC) and lamivudine (3TC); the deoxyguanosine analog abacavir sulfate (ABC); and the deoxyadenosine analogs

of which didanosine (ddI) is an inosine derivative and tenofovir disoproxil fumarate (TDF) is a deoxyadenosine-monophosphate nucleotide analog (a nucleotide is a nucleoside with one or more phosphates). **Note that drug abbreviations are provided here and below for reference, but their use is discouraged because they may lead to prescribing or administration errors.** As a class, the NRTIs require phosphorylation to the 5′-triphosphate moiety to become

TABLE 134-5 Selected Pharmacologic Characteristics of Antiretroviral Compounds

Drug	F (%)	$t_{1/2}(h)^a$	Adult Dose^b (doses/day)	Plasma $C_{max}/$ $C_{min}(\mu M)$	Distinguishing Adverse Effect
Integrase inhibitors (InSTI)					
Raltegravir	?	9	400 mg (2)	1.74/0.22	Increased creatine kinase
Nucleoside (Nucleotide) reverse transcriptase inhibitors (NRTIs)					
Abacavir	83	1.5/20	300 mg (2)	5.2/0.03	Hypersensitivity
			or		
			600 mg (1)	7.4^c	
Didanosine	42	1.4/24	200 mg (2)	2.8/0.03	Peripheral neuropathy, pancreatitis
			or		
			400 mg (1)	5.6^c	
Emtricitabine	93	10/39	200 mg (1)	7.3/0.04	Pigmentation on soles and palms in non-whites
Lamivudine	86	5/22	150 mg (2)	6.3/1.6	Headache, pancreatitis (children)
			or		
			300 mg (1)	10.5/0.5	
Stavudine	86	1.4/7	40 mg (2)	2.4/0.04	Lipoatrophy, peripheral neuropathy
Tenofovir	40	17/150	300 mg (1)	1.04/0.4	Renal toxicity (proximal tubule)
Zidovudine	85	2/3.5	200 mg (3)	0.2	Anemia, neutropenia, myopathy
			or		
			300 mg (2)	3^c	
Nonnucleoside reverse transcriptase inhibitors (NNRTIs)					
Delavirdine	85	5.8	400 mg (3)	35/14	Rash, elevated liver function tests
			or		
			600 mg (2)		
Efavirenz	43	48	600 mg (1)	12.9/5.6	Central nervous system disturbances and teratogenicity
Etravirine	?	41	200 mg (2)	1.69/0.86	Rash, nausea
Nevirapine	93	25	200 mg (2)^d	22/14	Potentially serious rash and hepatotoxicity
Protease inhibitors (PIs)					
Amprenavir^e	?	9	1,400 mg (2)^e	9.5/0.7	Rash
	or		or		
Forsamprenavir^e			1,400 mg (1)^{ef}	14.3/2.9	
Atazanavir	68	7	400 mg (1)	3.3/0.23	Unconjugated hyperbilirubinemia
			or		
			300 mg (1)^f	6.2/0.9	
Darunavir	82	15	800 mg (1) or 600 mg (2)^f	11.9/6.5	Hepatitis, rash
Indinavir	60	1.5	800 mg (3)	13/0.25	Nephrolithiasis
			or		
			400–800 mg (2)^f		
Lopinavir^g	?	5.5	800 mg (1) or 400 mg (2)	13.6/7.5	Hyperlipidemia/GI intolerance
Nelfinavir	?	2.6	750 mg (3)	5.3/1.76	Diarrhea
			or		
			1,250 mg (2)	7/1.2	
Ritonavir	60	3–5	600 mg (2)^d	16/5	Gastrointestinal intolerance
			or		
			"Boosting doses"		
Saquinavir	4	3	1,000 mg (2)^f	3.9/0.55	Mild nausea, bloating
Tipranavir	?	6	500 mg (2)^f	77.6/35.6	Hepatoxocity, intracranial hemorrhage
Entry inhibitorsFusion inhibitor					
Enfuvirtide	84	3.8	90 mg (2)	1.1/0.73	Injection-site reactions
Co-receptor inhibitor					
Maraviroc	33	15	300 mg (2)	1.2/0.066	Hepatitis, allergic reaction

C_{max}, maximum plasma concentration; C_{min}, minimum plasma concentration; F, bioavailability; $t_{1/2}$, elimination half-life.
^{a}NRTIs: Plasma NRTI $t_{1/2}$/intracellular (peripheral blood mononuclear cells) NRTI-triphosphate $t_{1/2}$; plasma $t_{1/2}$ only for other classes.
^{b}Dose adjustment may be required for weight, renal or hepatic disease, and drug interactions.
^{c}C_{min} concentration typically below the limit of quantification.
^{d}Initial dose escalation recommended to minimize side effects.
^{e}Fosamprenavir is a tablet phosphate prodrug of amprenavir. Amprenavir is available only as oral solution.
^{f}Must be boosted with low doses of ritonavir (100–200 mg).
^{g}Available as coformulation 4:1 lopinavir to ritonavir.
Data from Department of Health and Human Services (DHHS) Panel on Antiretroviral Guidelines for Adults and Adolescents. Guidelines for the use of antiretroviral agents in HIV-infected adults and adolescents; December 1, 2009; references 42 and 43, and product information for agents.

pharmacologically active. Intracellular phosphorylation occurs by cytoplasmic or mitochondrial kinases and phosphotransferases (not viral kinases). The 5′-triphosphate moiety acts in two ways: (a) it competes with endogenous deoxyribonucleotides for the catalytic site of reverse transcriptase, and (b) it prematurely terminates DNA elongation as it lacks the requisite 3′-hydroxyl for sugar-phosphate linking.[42] Although NRTI tri-phosphates (or diphosphate for tenofovir) are specific for HIV reverse transcriptase, their adverse effects may be caused in part by inhibition of mitochondrial DNA or RNA synthesis.[44] Toxicities include peripheral neuropathy, pancreatitis, lipoatrophy (subcutaneous fat loss), myopathy, anemia, and rarely life-threatening lactic acidosis with fatty liver.[45] Use of stavudine and didanosine has declined in favor of more tolerable NRTIs (e.g., emtricitabine, lamivudine and tenofovir).[23] With some exceptions, NRTIs are mainly eliminated by the kidney and dose adjustments are required for renal insufficiency. Resistance has been reported for all NRTIs, including cross-resistance within the class as multiple and/or specific mutations accrue.[46]

NNRTIs are a chemically heterogeneous group of agents that bind noncompetitively to reverse transcriptase adjacent to the catalytic site. Unlike NRTIs, NNRTIs do not require intracellular activation, do not compete against endogenous deoxyribonucleotides, and do not have potent antiviral activity against HIV-2. Given the different site of binding to reverse transcriptase, NNRTIs can be used with NRTIs effectively. Available NNRTIs include efavirenz (EFV), delavirdine (DLV), nevirapine (NVP) and etravirine (ETR).[23] As a class, the NNRTIs are generally associated with rash and elevated liver function tests, including life-threatening cases rarely, particularly for nevirapine.[44] NNRTIs tend to have long plasma half-lives and are mainly cleared by liver and/or gut-mediated metabolism through the cytochrome P450 enzyme system. The NNRTIs are unique in that a single mutation is needed to confer high-level cross-resistance for the class (except etravirine), which has been termed a *low-genetic barrier* to resistance.[46]

The HIV protease inhibitors (PIs) include amprenavir (APV) and its prodrug fosamprenavir (FPV), atazanavir (ATV), darunavir (DRV), indinavir (IDV), lopinavir (LPV), nelfinavir (NFV), ritonavir (RTV), saquinavir (SQV), and tipranavir (TPV). PIs competitively inhibit the cleavage of the gag-pol polyprotein, which is a crucial step in the viral maturation process, thereby resulting in the production of immature, noninfectious virions. PIs are generally associated with gastrointestinal distress and metabolic changes, such as increased lipids, insulin insensitivity, and changes in body fat distribution.[45] PIs are cleared by liver- and gut-mediated metabolism (mainly CYP3A). PIs are almost always used with small doses of ritonavir, a CYP3A inhibitor, to enhance the plasma concentrations of the PI of interest. CYP3A-mediated drug interactions are important considerations for PIs. Resistance to the PIs generally requires the buildup of multiple mutations, termed a *high-genetic barrier*. Multiple mutations can lead to cross-resistance.[46]

There are currently two types of entry inhibitors: fusion inhibitors and CCR5 antagonists. Enfuvirtide (ENF) is the only fusion inhibitor available at this time. Enfuvirtide is a synthetic 36-amino-acid peptide that binds gp41, which inhibits fusion of HIV with the target cell. Because of the peptide nature of enfuvirtide, oral delivery is impossible, and subcutaneous injection is the preferred route of administration. Injection-site reactions are the most common adverse effect. Enfuvirtide is cleared via protein catabolism and amino acid recycling. Enfuvirtide appears to have a low genetic barrier to resistance.[46] Maraviroc is CCR5 antagonists. Unlike the other available antiretrovirals which target a viral protein (i.e., enzyme), CCR5 antagonists block a human receptor. The long-term consequences of blocking CCR5 are unknown but may include increased susceptibility to infection by flavivirus (e.g., West Nile virus and tickborne encephalitis virus).[47] One advantage of targeting a human receptor is that resistance to CCR5 antagonists may be more difficult to develop. Because CCR5 antagonists are only effective against R5 virus and not X4 virus, a viral tropism assay should be performed prior to using a CCR5 antagonist. Whether long-term use of CCR5 antagonists shifts viral tropism from predominantly R5 to the more pathogenic X4 strain remains to be determined. Maraviroc is a CYP3A substrate; a substrate of P-glycoprotein, thus it is susceptible to drug–drug interactions.

Raltegravir is the first integrase strand transfer inhibitor (InSTIs) to be FDA approved and marketed with elvitegravir and other compounds under development. InSTIs bind to HIV integrase while it is in a specific complex with viral DNA. As a result, viral DNA cannot become incorporated into the human genome and cellular enzymes degrade unincorporated viral DNA. Alternatively, recombination and repair mechanisms may form long-terminal repeat (LTR) circular DNA from the unincorporated viral DNA. Raltegravir is primarily glucuronidated by UGT1A1 and is not broadly susceptible to CYP-mediated drug interactions. Elvitegravir is first metabolized by CYP3A then glucuronidated and is thus susceptible to CYP3A drug interactions. Higher elvitegravir plasma concentrations are achieved when coadministered with either low-dose ritonavir or the novel CYP3A inhibitor, cobicistat under development.[48]

Novel antiviral agents in the classes listed above and novel agents in new drug classes that exploit other steps in the HIV life cycle (see Fig. 134–1) are in development, with a focus on activity against drug-resistant virus.[49] For example, drugs that block steps in the maturation or assembly of HIV other than protease cleavage are under development. New drugs including cobicistat that increase the plasma concentrations of CYP3A substrates such as PIs are also in development.[48]

Interestingly, the antimalarials chloroquine and hydroxychloroquine exert anti–HIV-1 and anti–HIV-2 activity through interference with gp120 (HIV envelope glycoprotein) during assembly.[50] The antivirals acyclovir and foscarnet exhibit modest anti-HIV activity via inhibition of HIV reverse transcriptase.[51,52]

Drug Interactions

❼ Medical use of antiretroviral agents is complicated by clinically significant drug–drug interactions that can occur with many of these agents.[23,53] Some interactions are beneficial and used purposely (e.g., ritonavir); others may be harmful, leading to dangerously elevated or inadequate drug concentrations. Clinicians involved in the pharmacotherapy of HIV must understand the mechanistic basis for these interactions and maintain a current knowledge of drug interactions for these reasons.

Many clinically significant antiretroviral-associated drug interactions involve CYP3A-mediated metabolism and clearance. The PIs, except nelfinavir, the NNRTIs delavirdine and etravirine, the CCR5 antagonist maraviroc, and the InSTI elvitegravir are metabolized by CYP3A. In general, efavirenz, etravirine and nevirapine are inducers of CYP3A, whereas delavirdine and the PIs inhibit CYP3A. Ritonavir is a potent inhibitor of CYP3A-mediated metabolism and is now used almost exclusively at lower doses as a pharmacokinetic enhancer of other PIs.[48] Darunavir, lopinavir, saquinavir, and tipranavir must be taken with ritonavir to achieve optimal plasma concentrations. Atazanavir, fosamprenavir, and indinavir are also primarily used with ritonavir for the same reason. Nelfinavir is not effectively boosted by ritonavir given its CYP2C19-mediated metabolism. Many potential concomitant drugs on the market are also metabolized by CYP3A and therefore susceptible to clinically relevant drug interactions with PIs and NNRTIs.[23,53] Agents with narrow therapeutic indices and/or that exhibit major changes in pharmacokinetics with CYP3A inhibition are most important in this regard. Examples include, but are not limited to, simvastatin, lovastatin, corticosteroids, ergot derivatives, and some antiarrhythmics. The drug interaction potential of antimycobacterium agents, specifically the rifamycins, are particularly relevant given the high potential for such infections in HIV-infected patients.[53] Rifampin, a potent inducer of CYP3A metabolism and conjugation enzymes, is contraindicated with use of most PIs, etravirine, and maraviroc because concentrations are reduced substantially even with ritonavir enhancement. Raltegravir dose should be doubled in the presence of rifampin; efavirenz is an alternative agent. Ritonavir enhancement generally allows coadministration of PIs and rifabutin.[53] In such cases, the rifabutin dose will require adjustment given its CYP3A-mediated clearance.

The herbal product St. John's wort (*Hypericum perforatum*) is a potent inducer of metabolism and is contraindicated with PIs, NNRTIs, and maraviroc.[23] It must be stressed that the pharmacology of CYP3A interactions may be complicated by simultaneous induction/inhibition of drug transporter-mediated (e.g., P-glycoprotein) clearance and or other phase I or phase II enzymes. Clinicians who treat HIV must stay abreast of antiretroviral drug interaction data. The Department of Health and Human Services guidelines for antiretroviral use provide, and regularly update, excellent summaries of known clinically relevant drug interactions.[23,53]

NRTIs are not metabolized by CYP3A, but other drug interaction considerations are important. Generally, NRTIs of the same nucleobase should not be coadministered. For example, zidovudine and stavudine are both thymidine analogs and phosphorylated by the same cellular enzymes. Antagonism occurs between these two drugs both in vitro and in vivo; thus, the two should never be given together. Similarly, deoxycytidine analogs should not be coadministered. The deoxyadenosine analogs didanosine and tenofovir exhibit a plasma drug interaction whereby didanosine concentrations are significantly increased.[23] Furthermore, the two adenosine analogs are less effective together compared with other recommended NRTI regimens and there is concern for CD4 lymphotoxicity, a troubling effect that appears unique to this NRTI combination. Coadministration of didanosine and tenofovir is not recommended for initial therapy.[23]

Landmarks in the Evolution of Antiretroviral Therapy

Antiretroviral therapy has undergone major changes over the past decades. Illustrating these changes is important for a thorough understanding of current treatment strategies. The fundamental landmarks in the use of antiretroviral agents are as follows:

- An early study demonstrated that zidovudine monotherapy confers a survival benefit in persons who have AIDS.[54] This study showed that a single drug provided moderate clinical benefit.

- Further investigation showed that combination regimens of two NRTIs (e.g., zidovudine and didanosine or zalcitabine) were superior to zidovudine monotherapy in immunologic and virologic parameters, particularly in patients with no previous antiretroviral therapy, and conferred a superior survival benefit.[55] This established that NRTI monotherapy was inferior to dual NRTI therapy.

- A pivotal study showed that dual NRTI therapy was inferior to triple therapy consisting of 2 NRTIs and the PI indinavir.[56] Use of triple therapy with combinations of two NRTIs with NNRTIs or PIs was associated with a durable response as well as significantly reduced incidence of OIs and improved survival, thus establishing the current paradigm of ART. [57]

- Evolution of triple-therapy regimens with a boosted PI or efavirenz showed superior virologic efficacy versus unboosted PIs and triple NRTI regimens.[58,59] Further studies demonstrated that certain ART regimens provided slightly better virologic efficacy, safety/tolerability, and or dosing convenience compared with other three-drug regimens.

❻ Taken together, the pivotal studies described above established that HIV should not be treated with single or dual NRTIs. Current recommendations for initial treatment of HIV infection advocate a minimum of three active antiretroviral agents: Tenofovir disoproxil fumarate plus emtricitabine with either a ritonavir-enhanced PI (darunavir or atazanavir), the NNRTI

efavirenz, or the InSTI raltegravir.[23] Multiple alternative regimens are also safe and effective, but have one or two disadvantages compared with the preferred regimens, such as weaker virologic responses with high viral loads, lower tolerability, or greater risk of long-term toxicities such as subcutaneous fat loss. Preferred and alternative antiretroviral regimens are listed in Table 134–4.[23] The World Health Organization (WHO) also updated its treatment recommendations for resource-limited settings. The main updates to the WHO guidelines are the recommendation to treat at higher CD4 count thresholds (350 cell/mm^3) and not to include stavudine as initial therapy.[60]

A great number of considerations go into choosing the optimal drug regimen for a given patient. A resistance test is generally recommended when the patient enters HIV care and the results should help guide therapy. Other considerations include avoidance of PIs in patients taking contraindicated concomitant medications such as rifampin (efavirenz would be an alternative), avoidance of tenofovir in patients with pre-existing renal dysfunction (abacavir would be an alternative), and avoidance of efavirenz in fertile women not on stable and reliable contraception (PIs would be an alternative). The most convenient regimen is a once-daily fixed-dose combination formulation of efavirenz–tenofovir disoproxil fumarate–emtricitabine. Other antiretrovirals are also available in fixed-dose combinations to minimize the number of pills required per dose. Several factors contribute to whether the patient will mount a durable response to initial therapy, including adherence, pharmacologic effectiveness, and tolerability.

The simplest definition of adherence is the patient's ability to take medication as directed. Antiretroviral therapy is complex and long term, and the risk for virologic failure increases as adherence decreases.[61] As clinicians, it is critical to establish a relationship of trust with the patient and to communicate to the patient the importance of proper medication taking. Education should be aimed at understanding the disease process, monitoring, and goals of therapy. An individual's "readiness" to take medications should be clearly established before any treatment is initiated.[23] Help from caregivers, friends, and/or family members should be leveraged by the patient because social and psychological support are among the most important factors that influence adherence in this patient population.

Based on clinical trial data, approximately 70% to 90% of patients will achieve undetectable viral loads with modern ART regimens. Tenofovir disoproxil fumarate and emtricitabine (tenofovir-emtricitabine) has emerged as the preferred NRTI combination.[62-65] An open-labeled trial of 517 antiretroviral naïve patients randomized to tenofovir-emtricitabine versus zidovudine-lamivudine both with efavirenz demonstrated that significantly more patients in the tenofovir-emtricitabine arm achieved less than 400 copies/mL of HIV-RNA at 48 weeks (84%) compared with patients randomized to zidovudine-lamivudine (73%).[63] CD4 increases were also significantly greater in the tenofovir-emtricitabine versus zidovudine-lamivudine group. Part of this difference was attributed to more patients discontinuing zidovudine-lamivudine due to adverse events compared with tenofovir-emtricitabine. Subcutaneous fat loss and lipid elevations were also higher in the zidovudine- lamivudine group through 48 weeks. A slight decrease in glomerular filtration rate was observed in the tenofovir-emtricitabine group versus a slight increase in the zidovudine-lamivudine group. Another randomized study compared abacavir-lamivudine to tenofovir-emtricitabine in a blinded manner in combination with either efavirenz or atazanavir/ritonavir (open labeled) in 1858 antiretroviral naïve adults. Among subjects with >100,000 copies/mL of plasma HIV-RNA at screening, those randomized to abacavir-lamivudine experienced twice the virologic failure rate and significantly more adverse events compared with those randomized to tenofovir-emtricitabine.[66] Other studies have also evaluated virologic efficacy and safety of abacavir-lamivudine in subjects with >100,000 copies/mL at baseline and have found high rates of efficacy and safety regardless of baseline viral load.[67] Taken together, these studies have solidified tenofovir-emtricitabine as the first line NRTI combination, as well as efavirenz-tenofovir-emtricitabine as a first line regimen for antiretroviral naïve patients.

The STARTMRK study was a randomized, placebo-controlled, multi-center comparison of efavirenz versus raltegravir, both with tenofovir-emtricitabine, in 566 antiretroviral naïve adults.[62] In the intent-to-treat analysis, 86% of subjects had <50 copies/mL at 48 weeks in the raltegravir group versus 82% of subjects in the efavirenz group (noninferiority $P<0.0001$). The mean CD4 increase at week 48 was 189 and 163 cells/mm^3, respectively ($P=0.02$), and the time to reach <50 copies/mL was faster in the subjects randomized to raltegravir. About half as many subjects randomized to raltegravir had an adverse effect of moderate-to-severe intensity compared with those randomized to efavirenz. This study led to the inclusion of raltegravir-tenofovir-efavirenz as a preferred regimen for initial treatment of HIV-infection.

The ARTEMIS trial was a noninferiority, open-labeled, randomized study of darunavir-ritonavir once daily versus lopinavir-ritonavir either once or twice daily all in combination with tenofovir-emtricitabine in 689 antiretroviral naïve adults.[64] At week 48, 84% versus 78% of subjects had HIV-RNA levels <50 copies/mL in the darunavir-ritonavir and lopinavir-ritonavir groups, respectively (noninferiority $P<0.001$). CD4 responses were similar between the two groups, however, the virologic response was higher for darunavir-ritonavir in those with >100,000 copies/mL of HIV-RNA at baseline. More subjects in the lopinavir-ritonavir group experienced gastrointestinal intolerance and lipid elevations. The CASTLE study was another noninferiority, open-labeled, randomized trial that compared atazanavir-ritonavir to lopinavir-ritonavir (twice daily) both with tenofovir-emtricitabine in 883 antiretroviral-naïve adults.[65] At 48 weeks, 78% and 76% of subjects in the respective groups achieved <50 copies/mL (noninferiority $P<0.001$). CD4 responses were similar in the two groups as were responses in subjects with high viral loads at baseline. More subjects in the lopinavir-ritonavir group experienced gastrointestinal intolerance and high lipids whereas more subjects in the atazanavir-ritonavir group experienced asymptomatic hyperbilirubinemia from atazanavir's inhibition of UGT1A1. These studies established darunavir-ritonavir and atazanavir-ritonavir both with tenofovir-efavirenz as preferred first-line regimens for HIV-infection and, along with other studies, moved lopinavir-ritonavir to an alternative regimen.[68]

Patients with sustained undetectable HIV-RNA taking out-of-date drug regimens may be candidates to simplify to one of the preferred regimens or a more desirable alternative regimen based on past treatment history and other variables. If abacavir is to be used in any regimen, a test for the presence of human leukocyte antigen (HLA) B*5701 should be done as its presence has been strongly correlated with the development of abacavir hypersensitivity. Should this test be positive, an abacavir allergy should be added to the patient's chart and abacavir should not be used in the patient. Similarly, a tropism test is required prior to using maraviroc to establish that the patient's virus uses the CCR5 co-receptor.[23]

Finally, because of the risk of side effects and resistance associated with NRTIs and NNRTIs, several trials have assessed ritonavir boosted PI monotherapy. In general, this strategy is inferior to three drug regimens unless the patient has been virologically suppressed for at least 6 months.[69] Ritonavir-boosted PI monotherapy cannot be advocated at this time.[23]

Resistance

❽ Regimen failure is commonly associated with antiretroviral resistance, and testing for such resistance is a useful clinical tool.[46] The two types of resistance tests available are phenotype and genotype. A phenotype test determines the concentration of antiretroviral necessary to inhibit 50% replication of the patient's viral isolate (inhibitory concentration of 50% [IC_{50}]) in a recombinant in vitro viral assay. Results usually are expressed as a fold change in susceptibility (IC_{50}) compared with a wild-type laboratory strain virus. Generally, the fold-change in IC_{50} increases as HIV accumulates additional mutations that confer resistance to a particular drug. However, a single mutation may confer a very high fold-change in IC_{50} for some drugs (e.g., lamivudine, emtricitabine, efarvirenz, nevirapine) rendering them ineffective after a single mutation. Although small to moderate increases in the fold change suggests reduced susceptibility to that antiretroviral agent, resistance may not be absolute, and partial susceptibility may remain. Theoretically, drug levels may be increased to overcome reduced susceptibility; this strategy is currently under evaluation. The strengths of phenotypic testing is to provide resistance information for complex mutation patterns, but it is also associated with higher cost, limited number of commercial providers, and slower turnaround time for results. Genotyping assesses genetic mutations and associated codon changes in gp41, reverse transcriptase, integrase or protease in the patient's virus and compares it to the wild-type sequence. Mutations, when present, are listed by the wild-type amino acid followed by the position in the genetic sequence of the protein or enzyme and end with the mutation found in the patient. For example, a common mutation caused by lamivudine and emtricitabine is the M184V mutation: a substitution of valine (V) for methionine (M) at the 184 position of reverse transcriptase. Mutations can confer varying degrees of antiretroviral drug resistance and in some cases, weighting algorithms have been developed to predict the relative impact of mutation combinations on antiretroviral activity. Algorithms have also been developed to predict a phenotype from a genotype test (i.e., virtual phenotype). Not all mutations, however, are only detrimental — for example, while M184V confers significant resistance to lamivudine and emtricitabine, it is also associated with a less fit virus.[70] New genetic mutations are discovered occasionally and interpretation of genotypes resistance tests is complex, therefore the reader is encouraged to consult the most recent guidelines on HIV resistance testing.[46]

Treatment of Special Populations

■ PREGNANCY

Several considerations are relevant to the treatment of pregnant women, including the health of the mother, prevention of HIV transmission to the fetus, potential for teratogenicity, and dosing issues based on pharmacokinetic changes during pregnancy. Treatment recommendations should be consulted to address the specific requirements for HIV-infected pregnant women and the prevention of vertical transmission.[11] Generally, pregnant women should be treated as would nonpregnant women, with some exceptions. For example, efavirenz should not be used, particularly in the first trimester, because of potential teratogenicity. Zidovudine prophylaxis is generally recommended as part of treatment regimens based on early studies demonstrating clear prophylactic effectiveness as well as extensive familiarity with the side-effect profile.[11] Infants also receive zidovudine prophylaxis for 6 weeks after birth. Lopinavir-ritonavir has also been studied extensively in pregnant women, and is recommended in this population. Currently, HIV transmission rates have been reduced to <2% for women who are treated with ART and when zidovudine prophylaxis is used.[11]

In resource-limited settings or when HIV infection is detected very close to delivery, an abbreviated course of zidovudine (i.e., given during labor or in the first 48 hours of the baby's life) also can reduce transmission substantially and may be easier for the patient to take. Alternatively, single-dose nevirapine given to the mother during labor and to the baby within 3 days of birth can reduce transmission of HIV; however, the risk of nevirapine resistance in the mother is considerable (and in infants who become HIV-infected), occurring in nearly 60% of cases.[71] The high risk likely is due to the low genetic barrier to resistance for nevirapine coupled with the long decay half-life and subsequent prolonged suboptimal concentrations. Resistance from single-dose nevirapine in mothers can be reduced from approximately 60% to 9% with the addition of 4 to 7 days of zidovudine-lamivudine.[71]

■ POSTEXPOSURE PROPHYLAXIS

Protection of healthcare workers from accidental exposure to HIV and in cases of rape or high-risk postcoital and postinjection drug-use episodes are important concerns. The CDC has issued guidelines governing treatment of occupational and other high risk HIV exposures.[7,10] These guidelines should be consulted for updates as the knowledge in this field evolves. The principles of the guidelines are to grade the exposure risk and treat as soon as possible after high-risk exposures to prevent HIV infection. The makeup of the treatment depends upon the risk. Postexposure prophylaxis (PEP) with a triple-drug regimen consisting of two NRTIs and a boosted-PI is recommended for percutaneous blood exposure involving significant risk (e.g., large-bore needle, visible blood from patients with advanced AIDS). Two NRTIs may be offered to the healthcare worker with lower risk of exposure, such as cases involving superficial exposures to the mucous membrane or broken skin. Urine, saliva, nasal secretions, stool, and sputum are not considered infectious unless visibly contaminated with blood. The optimal duration of treatment is unknown, but at least 4 weeks of therapy is advocated. Treatment ideally should be initiated within 1 to 2 hours of exposure, but treatment is recommended up to 72 hours postexposure. Expert consultation is needed when exposure to drug-resistant virus is suspected or confirmed, but this should not delay initiation of postexposure prophylaxis.[7,10]

Preexposure prophylaxis (PrEP) is under phase III study for reducing HIV transmission. The concept is to prevent HIV infection by treating persons at high risk for HIV exposure with antiretrovirals before they are actually exposed. Tenofovir-emtricitabine are the agents under most study at this time. However, this strategy cannot be recommended until safety and efficacy information become available.

EVALUATION OF THERAPEUTIC OUTCOMES

Two laboratory tests are used to evaluate response to antiretroviral therapy: the plasma HIV RNA and the CD4 count.[23] After therapy is initiated, patients are generally monitored at 3-month intervals, although an assessment at 2 to 8 weeks is warranted to document early response. The two main indications for a change in therapy are significant toxicity and treatment failure. Should a single agent be responsible for an intolerable side effect, that agent often can be singly changed out of the regimen; for example, the patient who experiences intolerable central nervous system disturbances during initiation of efavirenz can switch to a boosted PI without changing the dual NRTI backbone. Caution must be exercised when drugs

in the regimen have overlapping toxicities, which makes changing a single agent problematic. Serious and life-threatening toxicities warrant cessation of the whole regimen before deciding upon a subsequent therapy.

As a general guide, the following events indicate treatment failure and should prompt consideration for changing therapy:

1. Less than 1 $\log_{10}$ reduction in HIV RNA 1 to 4 weeks after initiation of therapy or a failure to achieve less than 400 copies/mL by 24 weeks or less than 50 copies/mL by 48 weeks.

2. After HIV RNA suppression, repeated detection of HIV-RNA.

3. Failure to achieve a rise in CD4 of 25 to 50 cells/mm³ by 48 weeks.

4. Clinical disease progression, usually the development of a new OI.

THERAPEUTIC FAILURE

❾ Therapeutic failure can be defined by suboptimal suppression of viral replication, inadequate immunological recovery, or the development of AIDS-defining conditions. Many reasons may underlie therapeutic failure such as nonadherence to medication, development of drug resistance, intolerance to one or more medications, adverse drug–drug or drug–food interactions, or pharmacokinetic–pharmacodynamic variability.[23] In cases of therapeutic failure, these potential causes should be investigated and addressed, if possible. As a general rule, drug resistance develops for regimens that do not maximally suppress HIV replication. Drug resistance testing is recommended while the patient is undergoing the failing regimen or within 4 weeks after stopping the regimen as long as the HIV RNA count is greater than 500 copies/mL, which is the threshold for resistance assays (~500–1,000 copies/mL).[46] Most clinicians use the genotype assay because it is less expensive and results typically are available sooner compared with the phenotype assay. Resistance results usually require expert interpretation. Treating patients with drug resistant HIV utilizes many of the same general treatment approaches described for initial therapy above. Patients should be treated with at least two (preferably three) fully active antiretroviral drugs based on medication history, resistance tests, and new mechanistic drug classes (e.g., maraviroc, enfuvirtide, raltegravir). The goal of therapy is to suppress HIV-RNA to <50 copies/mL. In cases when <50 copies/mL cannot be attained, maintenance on the regimen is preferred over drug discontinuation so as to prevent rapid immunological and clinical decline.

Several recently approved drugs are active against highly resistant HIV.[23] For example, the two newest PIs darunavir and tipranavir and the newest NNRTI, etravirine are active against multidrug-resistant HIV in controlled trials. The drugs in the newer drug classes, raltegravir, maraviroc, and enfuvirtide are also active against NRTI, NNRTI, and PI resistant viruses in highly treatment experienced patients in controlled trials.

Previous strategies for therapeutic failure have proven largely ineffective, including drug holidays, structured or strategic treatment interruptions, and structured intermittent therapy. The overall premise of these strategies was similar: stop all antiretrovirals and allow the patient time off medication. Reinitiation of therapy was intended to reestablish control of viral replication, as wild-type virus would be expected to predominate, although the resistant virus is likely archived in long-lived cells. A landmark clinical trial tested the hypothesis that episodic antiretroviral therapy guided by the CD4 count would lower morbidity and mortality, including that associated with drug toxicity compared with continuous therapy.[72] However, the patients randomized to episodic therapy (drug-sparing) experienced significantly increased risk of opportunistic disease or death from any cause, including non-AIDS causes.[73] Most morbidity and mortality were consequences of lowering the CD4 count and increasing the viral load, but increased drug-related toxicity was also observed. Thus, episodic drug sparing did not reduce the risk of adverse events that have been associated with antiretroviral therapy, and drug-sparing approaches are generally not advocated. Finally, it is important to consider the implications of stopping all drugs simultaneously for regimens containing drugs with short half-lives (e.g., zidovudine) as well as drugs with long half-lives (e.g., efavirenz and nevirapine). The result may be functional monotherapy for the drug with a long half-life once the shorter half-life drugs are cleared, which can lead to resistance mutations especially for drugs with low genetic barriers (e.g., NNRTIs).[74] At this time, the optimal time sequence for staggered component discontinuation has not been determined.

CLINICAL CONTROVERSY

There is a compelling theoretical rationale for therapeutic drug monitoring in the experienced patient, but this approach is currently controversial. Drug susceptibility is founded on the premise that increasing drug concentration corresponds with stronger inhibition of replication up to a maximal effectiveness. This principle holds for drug-resistant variants, except higher drug concentrations are needed for the same levels of inhibition. Therefore, drug concentration monitoring could guide dose adjustments needed to attain the higher target drug concentrations required for optimal viral inhibition. Currently, therapeutic drug monitoring is suggested as a consideration for patients with multidrug-resistant HIV as well as in other select clinical situations. However, limitations to therapeutic drug monitoring include the lack of established target concentrations, intrapatient pharmacokinetic variability, lack of randomized clinical trials proving benefit or cost effectiveness, and few analytical laboratories and experts available for interpretation. Most antiretrovirals are not suitably formulated for minor dose adjustments.

COMPLICATIONS OF HIV INFECTION AND AIDS

❸ In the pre-ART era, the major therapeutic focus was prevention and treatment of opportunistic infections associated with uncontrolled HIV replication and a steady decline in CD4 cells.[36] Uncontrolled HIV is an insidious disease; persons infected often present with OIs, a consequence of the weakened immune system rather than HIV per se. Most OIs are caused by organisms that are common in the environment and often represent the reactivation of quiescent, hidden infections common in the population. The probability of developing specific OIs is closely related to CD4 count thresholds (Fig. 134–2). These CD4 thresholds serve as a basis for initiating primary OI chemoprevention.

❹ In the ART era, the main principle in the management of OIs is treating HIV infection to enable CD4 cell recovery and maintenance above safe levels.[53] Additional important principles regarding management of OIs are as follows:

1. Prevent exposure to opportunistic pathogens

2. Vaccinations to prevent first-episode disease (consult HIV-specific guidelines)

3. Primary chemoprophylaxis at certain CD4 thresholds to prevent first-episode disease

4. Treat emergent OI

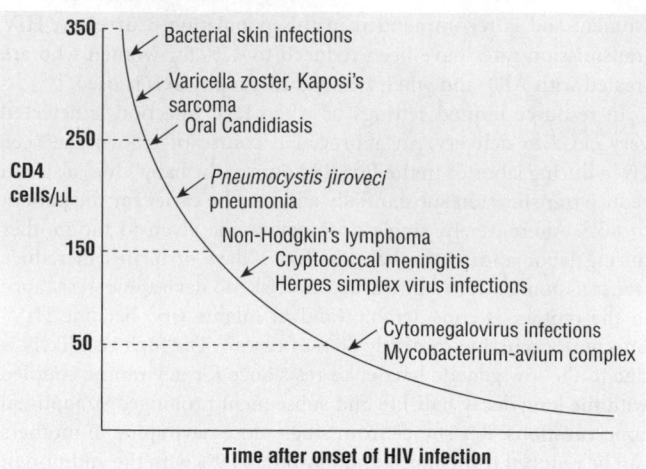

FIGURE 134-2. Natural history of opportunistic infections associated with human immunodeficiency virus infection. (*Reprinted with permission, © Courtney V. Fletcher, 2009.*)

5. Secondary chemoprophylaxis to prevent disease recurrence

6. Discontinuation of certain prophylaxes with sustained ART-associated immune recovery

Several considerations are required for the patient who presents with an OI and is simultaneously diagnosed with HIV and who thus needs both OI and ART treatment.[53] Immediate initiation of ART is indicated for OIs that respond to CD4 recovery, such as cryptosporidiosis, progressive multifocal leukoencephalopathy, and Kaposi sarcoma. However, for other OIs such as tuberculosis, *Mycobacterium avium* complex (MAC), and PCP, several potential problems complicate the timing of when to initiate ART relative to OI therapy. First, drug–drug interactions and the complexity of adhering to concomitant regimens can be daunting. Second, potentially overlapping drug toxicities can hand-tie clinicians trying to stop specific drugs thought to be eliciting the toxicity event. Third, an immune reconstitution syndrome (IRIS) has been associated with initiation of ART in the presence of underlying OIs. Although the reaction has not been systematically defined, IRIS is generally characterized by fever and worsening of OI manifestations in the initial 4 to 8 weeks after ART, and the reaction may take weeks to months to resolve.[53] Risk factors for IRIS are a low CD4 count, a rapid virologic response to ART, and a high antigenic burden.[75] An ART-associated rapid-onset immune reconstitution against the smoldering OI infection is thought to be the mechanism of IRIS. Treatment of IRIS is supportive, but may also include interruption of ART or antiinflammatory drugs.[75]

The AIDS Clinical Trials A5164 study compared immediate versus deferred ART in subjects treated for an acute OI (63% PCP, 12% Cryptococcal meningitis, 12% bacterial infections). Subjects had advanced HIV infection with an average CD4 count of 29 cells/mm³ and viral load >100,000 copies/mL. Subjects with tuberculosis were excluded. The immediate ART arm (n=141) initiated ART within 12 days after OI treatment was started versus within 45 days for the deferred ART arm (n=141). The rate of AIDS progression or death was significantly greater in the deferred ART arm compared with early ART arm (14% vs 24%; *P*=0.035). IRIS was reported in only 7% of subjects; 8 in the early ART arm and 12 in the deferred ART arm. On the basis of these findings, clinicians should consider early initiation of ART in subjects in the setting of these OIs provided there are no contraindications.[76] However, clinicians must make such decisions on a case-by-case basis.

The three major OIs (PCP, MAC, and Cytomegalovirus retinitis) all have decreased substantially in incidence with the

TABLE 134-6 Therapies for Common Opportunistic Pathogens in HIV-Infected Individuals

Clinical Disease	Preferred Initial Therapies for Acute Infection in Adults (Strength of Recommendation in Parentheses)	Common Drug- or Dose-Limiting Adverse Reactions
Fungi		
Candidiasis, oral	Fluconazole 100 mg orally for 7–14 days (AI)	Elevated liver function tests, hepatotoxicity, nausea and vomiting
	or	
	Nystatin 500,000 units oral swish (~5 mL) 4 times daily for 7–14 days (BII)	Taste, patient acceptance
Candidiasis, esophageal	Fluconazole 100–400 mg orally or IV daily for 14–21 days (AI)	Same as above
	or	
	Itraconazole 200 mg/day orally for 14–21 days (AI)	Elevated liver function tests, hepatotoxicity, nausea and vomiting
Pneumocystis jiroveci pneumonia	Trimethoprim–sulfamethoxazole IV or orally 15–20 mg/kg/day as trimethoprim component in 3–4 divided doses for 21 days[a] (AI) moderate or severe therapy should be started IV	Skin rash, fever, leucopenia, thrombocytopenia
	or	
	Pentamidine IV 4 mg/kg/day for 21 days[a] (AI)	Azotemia, hypoglycemia, hyperglycemia, arrhythmias
	Mild episodes	
	Atovaquone suspension 750 mg (5 mL) orally twice daily with meals for 21 days[a] (BI)	Rash, elevated liver enzymes, diarrhea
Cryptococcal meningitis	Amphotericin B 0.7 mg/kg/day IV for a minimum of 2 weeks with flucytosine 100 mg/kg/day orally in four divided doses (AI) *followed by*	Nephrotoxicity, hypokalemia, anemia, fever, chills, Bone marrow suppression, Elevated liver enzymes
	Fluconazole 400 mg/day, orally for 8 weeks or until CSF cultures are negative (AI)[a]	Same as above
Histoplasmosis	Liposomal amphotericin B 3 mg/kg/day IV for 3–10 days (AI) *followed by*	Same as above
	Itraconazole 200 mg orally thrice daily for 3 days, then twice daily for 12 months[a] (AII)	
Coccidioidomycosis	Amphotericin B 0.7–1 mg/kg/day IV until clinical improvement (usually after 500–1,000 mg) then switch to azole (AII)[a]	Same as above
	followed by	
	Fluconazole 400–800 mg once daily (meningeal disease) (AII)[a]	Same as above
Protozoa		
Toxoplasmic encephalitis	Pyrimethamine 200 mg orally once, then 50–75 mg/day	Bone marrow suppression
	plus	
	Sulfadiazine 1–1.5 g orally 4 times daily	Allergy, rash, drug fever
	and	
	Leucovorin 10–25 mg orally daily for 6 weeks (AI)[a]	
Isosporiasis	Trimethoprim and sulfamethoxazole: 160 mg trimethoprim and 800 mg sulfamethoxazole orally or IV 4 times daily for 10 days (AII)[a]	Same as above
Bacteria		
Mycobacterium avium complex	Clarithromycin 500 mg orally twice daily, *plus* ethambutol 15 mg/kg/day orally (AI), *and*	Gastrointestinal intolerance, optic neuritis, peripheral neuritis
	For advanced disease, rifabutin 300 mg/day (dose may need adjustment with ART) (AI)[a]	Rash, gastrointestinal intolerance, Neutropenia, discolored urine, uveitis
Salmonella enterocolitis or bacteremia	Ciprofloxacin 500–750 mg orally (or 400 mg IV) twice daily for 14 days (longer duration for bacteremia or advanced HIV) (AIII)	Gastrointestinal intolerance
Campylobacter enterocolitis	Ciprofloxacin 500 mg orally twice daily	Same as above
	or	
	Azithromycin 500 mg orally daily for 7 days (or 14 days with bacteremia) (BIII)	
Shigella enterocolitis	Ciprofloxacin 500 mg orally twice daily for 5 days (or 14 days for bacteremia) (AIII)	Same as above
Viruses		
Mucocutaneous herpes simplex	Acyclovir 5 mg/kg IV every 8 hours until lesions regress, then acyclovir 400 mg orally 3 times daily until complete healing (famciclovir or valacyclovir is alternative) (AII)	Gastrointestinal intolerance, crystalluria
Primary varicella-zoster	Acyclovir 10–15 mg/kg every 8 hours IV for 7–10 days, then switch to oral acyclovir 800 mg 5 times daily after defervescence (famciclovir or valacyclovir is alternative) (AIII)	Obstructive nephropathy, central nervous system symptomatology
Cytomegalovirus (retinitis)	Ganciclovir intraocular implant *plus* valganciclovir 900 mg twice daily for 14–21 days then once daily until immune recovery from ART (AI)[a]	Neutropenia, thrombocytopenia
Cytomegalovirus esophagitis or colitis	Ganciclovir 5 mg/kg IV every 12 hours for 21 to 28 days (BII)	Same as above

ART, antiretroviral therapy; CSF, cerebrospinal fluid; HIV, human immunodeficiency virus.

[a]Maintenance therapy is recommended.

See Table 134–4 for levels of evidence-based recommendations.

From reference 53.

advent of ART.[36,53] Furthermore, primary and secondary chemoprophylaxes for OIs have contributed to the same decreases. Nevertheless, opportunistic diseases continue to be complications of HIV disease and occur at low CD4 lymphocyte counts in patients who are unaware of their HIV infection, or who have not responded to ART therapy or OI prophylaxis because of adherence issues or inadequate engagement with the healthcare system.[53]

The spectrum of OIs observed in HIV-infected individuals and recommended first-line regimens for treatment are given in Table 134–6. Recommended therapies for primary prophylaxis are given in Table 134–7.[53] These lists of recommendations are not as

TABLE 134-7 Therapies for Prophylaxis of Select First-Episode Opportunistic Diseases in Adults and Adolescents

Pathogen	Indication	First Choice (Strength of Recommendation in Parentheses)
I. Standard of care		
Pneumocystis jiroveci	CD4$^+$ count <200/mm^3 *or* oropharyngeal candidiasis	Trimethoprim–sulfamethoxazole, one double-strength tablet orally once daily (AI) or 1 single-strength tablet orally once daily (AI)
Mycobacterium tuberculosis Isoniazid sensitive	(Active TB should be ruled out): + test for latent TB infection with no prior TB treatment history *or* - test for latent TB infection, but close contact with case of active tuberculosis *or* history of untreated or inadequately treated healed TB regardless of latent TB infection test results	Isoniazid 300 mg orally plus pyridoxine, 50 mg orally once daily for 9 months (AII)
		or Isoniazid 900 mg orally twice weekly (BII) plus pyridoxine 50 mg orally daily for 9 months (BIII)
For exposure to drug resistant TB	Consult public health authorities	
Toxoplasma gondii	Immunoglobulin G antibody to *Toxoplasma* and CD4$^+$ count <100/mm^3	Trimethoprim–sulfamethoxazole, one double-strength tablet orally once daily (AII)
Mycobacterium avium complex	CD4$^+$ count <50/mm^3	Azithromycin 1,200 mg orally once weekly (AI) or 600 mg orally twice weekly (BIII) or clarithromycin 500 mg orally twice daily (AI)
Varicella zoster virus (VZV)	Pre-exposure: CD4 ≥200/mm^3, no history of varicella infection, or, if available, negative antibody to VZV	Varicella vaccination; two doses, three months apart (CIII)
	Postexposure: Significant exposure to chicken pox or shingles for patients who have no history of either condition or, if available, negative antibody to VZV	Varicella-zoster immune globulin, 125 IU per 10 kg (maximum of 625 IU) IM, within 96 hours after exposure to a person with active varicella or herpes zoster (AIII)
Streptococcus pneumoniae	CD4 count ≥200 cells/mm^3 or no receipt of vaccination in past 5 years. Consider for those with CD4 <200/mm^3 and those with an CD4 increase to >200/mm^3 on ART (CIII)	23-valent polysaccharide vaccine, 0.5 mL intramuscularly (BII) revaccination every 5 years may be considered (CIII)
Hepatitis B virus	All susceptible patients	Hepatitis B vaccine, three doses (AII). Anti-HBs should be obtained one month after the vaccine series completion (BIII)
Influenza virus	All patients (annually, before influenza season)	Inactivated trivalent influenza virus vaccine (annual): 0.5 mL intramuscularly (AIII)
Hepatitis A virus	All susceptible (anti–hepatitis A virus–negative) patients at increased risk for hepatitis A infection (e.g., chronic liver disease, illegal drug users, men who have sex with men)	Hepatitis A vaccine: two doses (AII) antibody response should be assessed 1 month after vaccination; with revaccination as needed (BIII)
Human papillomavirus (HPV) infection	15–26 year old women	HPV quadrivalent vaccine months 0, 2, and 6 (CIII)
Bacteria	Neutropenia	Granulocyte colony-stimulating factor (G-CSF), 5–10 mcg/kg subcutaneously once daily for 2–4 weeks; or granulocyte-macrophage colony-stimulating factor (GM-CSF), 250 mcg/m^2 subcutaneously for 2–4 weeks (CII)
Histoplasma capsulatum	CD4$^+$ count <150/mm^3, endemic geographic area and high risk for exposures	Itraconazole 100–200 mg orally once daily (CI)

See Table 134–4 for levels of evidence-based recommendations.
From reference 53.

extensive as in the published guidelines, which include multiple additional alternatives and cover other less common OIs.[53] The following brief discussion of PCP provides an overview of the epidemiology, diagnosis, clinical manifestations, and results of treatment and serves as an illustration for the principles discussed earlier.

PNEUMOCYSTIS CARINII (PNEUMOCYSTIS JIROVECI) PNEUMONIA

PCP has been and continues to be the most common life-threatening OI in patients with AIDS.[77] *P. jiroveci* was formerly named *P carinii*; the name change was made to distinguish the organism that infects humans (*P. jiroveci*) from the strain that infects rodents (*P carinii*). The acronym PCP is still used today. Early in the AIDS epidemic 80% of patients experienced PCP at some point during their lifetime.[53,78] Although the incidence of PCP has fallen substantially since the advent of ART and effective prophylaxis for PCP, it still occurs in persons unaware of their HIV infection, and breakthrough PCP can occur in those with variable adherence to ART and/or prophylaxis.[53]

P. jiroveci is a fungus that has protozoan characteristics as well.[77,78] Exposure to *P. jiroveci* is widespread; two thirds of the population

has developed serum antibodies by age 2 to 4 years.[53] The organism appears to reside without consequence in humans unless the host becomes immunologically impaired.[79] Disease associated with immunosuppression probably occurs from both new acquisition and reactivation. Ninety percent of PCP cases in AIDS patients occurred in those with CD4 counts less than 200 cells/mm^3.[53] Other risk factors include oral thrush, recurrent bacterial pneumonia, unintentional weight loss, and high plasma HIV RNA. Past episodes of PCP increase risk for future episodes, which provides the basis for secondary chemoprophylaxis, as described below.[53]

The presentation of PCP in AIDS often is insidious.[53,77] Characteristic symptoms include fever and dyspnea. Clinical signs are tachypnea with or without rales or rhonchi and a nonproductive or mildly productive cough occurring over a period of weeks, although more fulminant presentations can occur. Chest radiographs may show florid or subtle infiltrates but occasionally are normal. Infiltrates usually are interstitial and bilateral, however. Arterial blood gases may show minimal hypoxia (Pao$_2$ 80–95 mm Hg) but in more advanced disease may be markedly abnormal. The diagnosis of PCP usually is made by identification of the organism in induced sputum or in specimens obtained from bronchoalveolar lavage. Less commonly, transbronchial or open lung biopsy is used to locate the organism. Diagnostic PCR tests are available in some institutions.[77]

Untreated PCP has a mortality rate of nearly 100%. Several potential treatments are available for PCP, but the treatment of choice is trimethoprim–sulfamethoxazole (or cotrimoxazole), which is associated with a response rate of 60% to 100%.[53] Parenteral pentamidine is equally efficacious but significantly more toxic. Trimethoprim–sulfamethoxazole is also the regimen of choice for primary and secondary prophylaxis of PCP in patients with and without HIV.[53,77]

When used for treatment of PCP, the dose of trimethoprim–sulfamethoxazole is 15 to 20 mg/kg/day (based on the trimethoprim component) as three to four divided doses.[53,77] Treatment duration typically is 21 days but also must be based on clinical response. Trimethoprim–sulfamethoxazole usually is initiated by the intravenous route, although oral therapy may suffice in mildly ill and reliable outpatients or for completion of a course of therapy after a response has been achieved with intravenous administration. Patients with moderate to severe PCP should be treated with corticosteroids as soon as possible after starting PCP therapy and certainly within 72 hours, in order to blunt the deterioration seen just after initiation of PCP therapy. Alternative regimens include pentamadine for moderate to severe disease and dapsone with trimethoprim, primaquine with clindamycin, and atovaquone for mild to moderate PCP.[53] Early initiation of ART is also generally recommended as long as there are no contraindications.[76]

Adverse reactions to trimethoprim–sulfamethoxazole and pentamidine are common, occurring in 20% to 85% of patients in this setting.[53] The more common adverse reactions seen with trimethoprim–sulfamethoxazole are rash (including Stevens-Johnson syndrome), fever, leukopenia, elevated serum transaminase levels, and thrombocytopenia. The incidence of these adverse reactions is higher in HIV-infected individuals than in those not infected with HIV.[80] Mild rashes should be watched closely for progression to more severe reactions but are not an absolute contraindication to continuing therapy.[53] This highlights the need for thoughtful consideration of ART components because of overlapping toxicities with some antiretrovirals such as abacavir and nevirapine, which also are associated with rash and hypersensitivity, including life-threatening cases. For pentamidine, side effects are pronounced and include hypotension, tachycardia, nausea, vomiting, severe hypoglycemia or hyperglycemia, pancreatitis, irreversible diabetes mellitus, elevated serum transaminase levels, nephrotoxicity, leukopenia, and cardiac arrhythmias. Some of these reactions appear to be related to the infusion rate (e.g., hypotension and tachycardia) and can be minimized by infusing pentamidine over 1 hour or more.[78] Dosage modification or pharmacokinetic monitoring can reduce the toxicity of both pentamidine and trimethoprim–sulfamethoxazole.[81] Dose reduction of pentamidine from 4 to 3 mg/kg/day appears to be successful in minimizing further rises in serum creatinine levels.[78] Maintenance of serum trimethoprim concentrations between 5 and 8 mcg/mL may help to prevent severe myelosuppression.[81] Early addition of adjunctive corticosteroid therapy to anti-PCP regimens decreases the risk of respiratory failure and improves survival in patients with AIDS and moderate to severe PCP ($Pao_2 \leq 70$ mm Hg or alveolar-arterial gradient ≥ 35 mm Hg).[53,77] The adverse effects associated with corticosteroid therapy in these patients were minimal, primarily an increased incidence of herpetic lesions, although some concerns exist about the potential for reactivation of tuberculosis or cytomegalovirus and/or long-term effects on bones.[78,82]

Prevention of PCP is clearly a preferable treatment strategy. Primary prophylaxis is recommended for any HIV-infected person who has a CD4 lymphocyte count less than 200 cells/mm³ (or CD4 percentage of total lymphocytes <14%) or a history of oropharyngeal candidiasis.[53,77] Secondary PCP prophylaxis is recommended for all HIV-infected individuals who have had a previous episode of PCP.

Trimethoprim–sulfamethoxazole is the most effective and least expensive agent and is the preferred therapy for both primary and secondary prophylaxis of PCP in adults and adolescents.[53,77] It also appears to confer cross-protection against toxoplasmosis and many bacterial infections. The recommended dose in adults and adolescents is one double-strength tablet daily, although other regimens, such as one double-strength tablet thrice weekly or one single-strength tablet daily and gradual dose escalation using liquid trimethoprim–sulfamethoxazole, have been used in an attempt to reduce the incidence of adverse reactions and improve compliance. Alternative prophylactic regimens are available if trimethoprim–sulfamethoxazole cannot be tolerated.

In the ART era, the profound reduction in HIV replication and restoration in CD4 cell count to levels rarely associated with the development of OIs provides a basis for the discontinuation of primary and secondary prophylaxis.[53] For PCP, primary prophylaxis should be discontinued in patients receiving and responding to ART who have a CD4 cell count greater than 200 cells/mm³ sustained for at least 3 months, but should be reinstated if the CD4 count drops to less than 200 cells/mm³. The same criteria apply for both discontinuation and reinitiation of secondary prophylaxis of PCP. However, continued secondary prophylaxis should be considered when the original PCP episode occurred at a CD4 count greater than 200 cells/mm³.[53]

In summary, comprehensive recommendations are available for management of PCP and other OIs in the context of HIV infection including prevention and treatment.[53] Readers are advised that data continue to emerge on new OI therapies, the safety of stopping primary and secondary prophylaxis, as well as criteria for when to restart secondary prophylaxes. The most current guidelines always should be consulted. Similar OI guidelines have been developed and are updated regularly that are specific to children.[34]

COMPLICATIONS IN THE ART ERA

❿ As with any medication, adverse reactions occur with antiretroviral agents that can range from life-threatening to minor intolerances. Characteristic side effects for each antiretroviral agent are listed in Table 134–5. A comprehensive discussion of all the adverse effects during antiretroviral therapy is beyond the scope of this chapter, but can be found in various other sources.[23,44,45] The purpose of this section is to highlight certain medical issues that have emerged in the ART era as HIV-infected patients live longer and are exposed to antiretroviral drugs for many years.

A broad spectrum of complications usually associated with aging appear to occur earlier in HIV-infected patients in the ART era.[73] These complications include osteoporosis and osteopenia, renal insufficiency, metabolic syndrome, neurocognitive decline, atherosclerotic disease, frailty, and malignancy. The cause of the early manifestation of these complications is not entirely clear, but evidence suggests that immune-dysregulation (e.g., a state of persistent heightened cellular activation) and viral replication play a role, as well as adverse events from antiretroviral medications.[73,82]

While contemporary antiretroviral therapy has reduced the incidence of some HIV-related cancers such as Kaposi sarcoma and non-Hodgkin lymphoma, other non–AIDS–related malignancies are beginning to plague HIV-infected individuals at significantly elevated rates such as Hodgkin lymphoma and anal-, lung-, skin- and hepato-carcinoma.[83] Part of, but not all, this increased risk in HIV-infected patients may be attributed to elevated exposures to human papillomavirus (anal cancer), smoking (lung carcinoma), and chronic hepatitis B and/or C co-infection (liver cancer). Some concern has been raised that antiretroviral drugs may contribute directly to these increased cancer rates, as some agents have caused cancers in laboratory animals as well as genotoxicity in vitro.[11] However, studies have shown similar cancer rates in organ transplant recipients with medication-induced immunosuppression, which suggests that it is the impairment to the immune system associated with HIV infection that is driving these higher cancer rates.[84] While the approach to treatment of malignancies in HIV-infected patients is similar to that in non-HIV–infected patients, treatment is complicated by drug–drug interactions that may exist between the antiretrovirals and the oncolytics.[83]

Antiretroviral drugs may contribute to several complications. Tenofovir has been associated with renal proximal tubulopathy (including rare cases of Fanconi syndrome and renal failure) as well as osteopenia.[85] Protease inhibitors and zidovudine-lamivudine have also been associated with osteopenia, although the precise mechanism for these effects is not clear.[86,87] Relationships exist between protease inhibitors, efavirenz, and the thymidine analog NRTIs and dyslipidemia (increased triglycerides and low-density lipoproteins [LDLs] and decreased high-density lipoproteins), abnormal glucose homeostasis (insulin resistance and impaired glucose tolerance), body fat abnormalities (lipoatrophy of the face and extremities and central lipoaccumulation), and lactic acidosis with hepatosteatosis (for all the NRTIs).[88,89] These metabolic abnormalities often occur in combination. Notably, some of the same abnormalities are also associated with the HIV infection itself, such as hypertriglyceridemia and insulin resistance.[88] Distinguishing the contribution of disease versus drug and ascertaining whether one abnormality precipitates the development of other abnormalities is difficult.[89,90] Various mechanistic hypotheses have been put forward, including NRTI-induced mitochondrial toxicity, and PI/NNRTI interactions with various cellular processes, such as glucose uptake, altered apolipoprotein degradation or synthesis, adipocyte differentiation, and lipolysis.[88,90] Some agents within these classes are less associated with these complications, including atazanavir for the PIs, nevirapine for NNRTIs, and tenofovir and abacavir for the NRTIs.[88] Early evidence also suggests that raltegravir and maraviroc are less associated with metabolic complications as well.[62,91]

Metabolic complications create several challenges and concerns. First, the metabolic abnormalities may increase the risk of adverse cardiovascular events, and some evidence gives credence to this concern.[88] A large observational prospective cohort study of 23,468 HIV-infected patients applied the Framingham cardiovascular risk algorithm and compared the estimated cardiovascular event rate with the actual event rate.[92] The algorithm takes into account known risk factors, many of which are associated with ART, such as diabetes and dyslipidemia as well as sex, age, smoking, and blood pressure. The estimated event rate paralleled the actual event rate, and both increased with years on ART. This finding suggests that increased cardiovascular risk can be explained by conventional risk factors, which are aggravated by ART. Therefore, the metabolic abnormalities precipitated by ART and HIV should be treated as cardiovascular disease risk factors and may warrant medical intervention. Finally, some observational studies have found an association between myocardial infarction and abacavir and didanosine use.[93] However, these associations have not been duplicated in other datasets, so these findings are tentative at this time.[94]

A second concern and challenge is how to manage the changes in body fat distribution, which can be disfiguring and upsetting to patients.[90] Some strategies have led to a mild return of subcutaneous fat for those with severe peripheral lipoatrophy. Controlled trials of antiretroviral substitution have demonstrated that patients randomized to switch away from stavudine to either abacavir or tenofovir have had small gains in subcutaneous fat.[95] Small controlled studies have demonstrated modest but inconsistent gains in subcutaneous fat with thiazolidinedione therapy.[96] Central fat accumulation is difficult to treat. Metformin reduces central fat accumulation, but lean body mass and subcutaneous fat may exhibit unwanted declines.[96] Lifestyle changes, such as reducing calorie intake and increasing aerobic exercise, may reduce central fat. Unfortunately, both lipoatrophy and fat accumulation eventually may lead to reconstructive surgery strategies in severe or refractory cases. Perhaps the best management of body fat changes is prevention through initiation of regimens less likely to cause such changes (see current recommendations for initial therapy).[23]

ART-associated hyperlipidemia can create several therapeutic challenges. Antiretroviral substitution studies have shown lipid improvements after switching away from PIs to either NNRTIs or atazanavir, but direct pharmacologic intervention may be required.[96] Elevated LDL may respond to β-hydroxy-β-methylglutaryl-coenzyme A (HMG-CoA) reductase inhibitor (statin) therapy. However, serious concerns exist regarding drug–drug interactions between PIs and statins, including lovastatin and simvastatin.[23,96] The plasma area under the concentration time curve of these statins can be increased >10-fold and may increase the risk for rhabdomyolysis. Generally, fluvastatin, pravastatin, atorvastatin, or rosuvastatin are recommended for ART-associated LDL elevations. Guidelines generally recommend starting with low doses with careful monitoring. Other HIV-specific recommendations exist for lifestyle modifications, and the use of fibrates, niacin, ezetimibe, and/or fish oil for isolated hypertriglyceridemia.[23] Current guidelines should always be consulted, as new information regarding the special concerns and challenges associated with HIV associated metabolic abnormalities continue to accrue.[88,96]

Many HIV-infected patients are co-infected with hepatitis C (HCV), which poses another challenge in the ART-era. HIV–HCV coinfection is common because of the shared blood-borne route of transmission.[97,98] Approximately 30% of HIV-infected patients in the United States have HIV–HCV (approximately 300,000 individuals). Up to 90% of injection-drug users and 90% of hemophiliacs with HIV are coinfected with HCV.[97]

Medical management of HIV–HCV-infected patients is complicated. First, HIV worsens the prognosis of HCV by reducing the chance of HCV clearance and accelerating HCV progression. After acute HCV infection, approximately 20% of patients without HIV will clear HCV compared with only 5% to 10% of those who also have HIV. With chronic HCV infection, progression to fibrosis, cirrhosis, and liver failure is several-fold faster in HIV–HCV patients versus HCV-monoinfected patients.[98] Whether HCV alters HIV disease is unclear, as the evidence to date is mixed. However, it is clear that end-stage liver disease from HCV has become an important cause of morbidity and death in HIV–HCV-infected patients.[23]

Randomized controlled trials have demonstrated lower response rates to standard-of-care HCV therapy (ribavirin and pegylated interferon-α) in HIV–HCV-infected patients compared with similar studies in HCV-monoinfected patients.[97,98] HIV–HCV patients in these studies had high levels of CD4 cells (average ~500 cells/mm³) and either were taking ART or had stable HIV disease. Sustained virologic responses for HCV were only 27% to 44% overall (14%–29% for HCV genotype 1), which compares poorly with response rates in HCV-monoinfected patients (>50% overall and >40% for HCV genotype 1). In HCV monoinfection, genotype 2 and 3 can be treated for 24 weeks, whereas HIV–HCV patients may need 48 weeks of treatment for the same genotypes.[98] Generally, HIV-induced immunologic defects may worsen HCV disease and response, but the precise underlying mechanism(s) of this attenuated HCV response in HIV–HCV patients has not been fully elucidated.[97,98]

Another challenge in HIV–HCV patients is the potential for liver toxicity to ART. Coinfected patients have several-fold higher risk of ART-associated transaminase elevations versus patients infected with HIV but not HCV.[97,98] Nevirapine and full-dose ritonavir appear to carry the highest risk of transaminase elevations, whereas stavudine has been linked with steatosis. Ritonavir-boosted PIs generally do not carry the same elevated risk as full-dose ritonavir with the exception of tipranavir-ritonavir or darunavir-ritonavir, which are associated with risk of clinical hepatitis and hepatic decompensation in those with HCV or hepatitis B infections. Liver function must be monitored with extra vigilance if tipranavir or darunavir are used in this population.[23] Stavudine and didanosine (also see below) are generally not recommended in combination with HCV therapy owing to risk of mitochondrial toxicity.[97,98] Other than these examples, the general threat of major liver toxicity is low overall, and this concern should not dissuade the use of ART in HIV–HCV-coinfected persons given the known benefits of therapy.[97,98]

Finally, two potentially dangerous drug–drug interactions exist between ART and HCV therapies. Didanosine should not be used with HCV therapy because of increased risk for pancreatitis and/or lactic acidosis.[97,98] The mechanism for this increase risk is not entirely clear, but may involve an intracellular interaction. Ribavirin inhibits inosine 5′-monophosphate dehydrogenase in vitro, which increases the phosphate donor pool available such that higher intracellular levels of dideoxyadenosine triphosphate (the active anabolite of didanosine) are produced with potentially more mitochondrial toxicity.[99] The other potentially dangerous interaction is severe anemia when zidovudine is used with ribavirin and interferon.[97,98] This appears to be a pharmacodynamic interaction, as zidovudine reduces red blood cell output and ribavirin causes hemolysis. At this time, zidovudine is not contraindicated with ribavirin and interferon, but close hematologic monitoring is needed.[97,98] It is likely that the list of drug–drug interactions among ART and HCV therapies will lengthen as therapeutic options for HCV expand.

As with the many other special circumstances and considerations that apply in the management of HIV-infected patients discussed in this chapter, specific guidelines have been established for managing HCV in HIV–HCV-coinfected patients, including recommendations for managing ART-associated liver toxicity.[23,100] The most current recommendations should always be consulted, as new knowledge and treatment strategies accrue continuously.

CONCLUSIONS

Irrefutable progress has been made in the management of HIV. Disease progression can be delayed, survival can be prolonged, and the risk of maternal-to-fetal HIV transmission can be reduced substantially. However, a cure and an effective vaccine remain elusive. Twenty-four distinct antiretroviral agents are available now for clinical use, and additional compounds will follow. There continues to be progress in our understanding of the virologic and immunologic processes associated with HIV infection and the clinical pharmacology of anti-HIV compounds, but deficits remain. Particular issues include the ever-present need for simpler and more tolerable and potent regimens, strategies for drug-resistant viral isolates, and better understanding of the inexorably progressive nature of HIV infection in some patients despite antiretroviral therapy. The medical management of OIs associated with HIV disease has changed dramatically since the recognition of AIDS early in the 1980s and changes continue today. The approach to PCP is illustrative. Chronologic landmarks in the evolution of PCP management include treatment of only established PCP disease to treatment in which primary and secondary prophylaxis based on CD4 lymphocyte count are standards of care, and finally to treatment where prophylaxis should be discontinued with sustained CD4 recovery on ART. Such evolution reflects progress in both understanding the risk factors for OIs and pharmacologic therapy. Collectively, three important general lessons have been learned from the treatment of HIV and associated OIs: the need for prospective immunologic and virologic monitoring and early recognition of HIV infection, the use of potent combinations of antiretroviral agents to maximally inhibit viral replication and restore immune function, and the primary and secondary prophylaxis of OIs. Observance of these principles, coupled with carefully controlled investigations of novel agents and therapeutic strategies, will continue to offer definite benefit and improve the quality and duration of life for HIV-infected individuals and yield an advantage over this pernicious virus that causes AIDS.

ACKNOWLEDGMENTS

Supported by Grants RO1 AI64029, UO1 AI84735, AI68636, and AI68632, and PO1 AI74340 from the National Institute of Allergy and Infectious Disease.

DISCLOSURES

Thomas Kakuda is an employee of Tibotec, Inc, a Johnson & Johnson company and a stock holder of Johnson & Johnson.

ABBREVIATIONS

ACTG: AIDS Clinical Trials Group

AIDS: acquired immunodeficiency syndrome

ART: combination antiretroviral therapy

CD: cluster of differentiation

CCR5: chemokine (C-C motif) receptor 5

CDC: Centers for Disease Control and Prevention

CRFS: circulating recombinant forms

CXCR4: chemokine (C-X-C motif) receptor 4

CYP: cytochrome P450

ELISA: enzyme-linked immunosorbent assay

FDA: Food and Drug Administration

gp: glycoprotein

HCV: hepatitis C virus

HIV: human immunodeficiency virus

IC_{50}: concentration of antiretroviral agent necessary to inhibit 50% of viral replication in vitro

InSTIs: integrase strand transfer inhibitor

IRIS: immune reconstitution syndrome

LDL: low-density lipoprotein

LTR: long-term repeat

MAC: *Mycobacterium avium* complex

NNRTI: non-nucleoside analog reverse transcriptase inhibitor

NRTI: nucleoside/nucleotide analog reverse transcriptase inhibitor

OI: opportunistic infection

PCP: *Pneumocystis jiroveci (carinii)* pneumonia

PI: protease inhibitor

PEP: postexposure prophylaxis

PrEP: preexposure prophylaxis

RT-PCR: reverse-transcription polymerase chain reaction

SIV: simian immunodeficiency virus

WHO: World Health Organization

REFERENCES

1. Simon V, Ho DD, Abdool Karim Q. HIV/AIDS epidemiology, pathogenesis, prevention, and treatment. Lancet 2006;368(9534):489–504.

2. DeGruttola V, Seage GR 3rd, Mayer KH, Horsburgh CR Jr. Infectiousness of HIV between male homosexual partners. J Clin Epidemiol 1989;42(9):849–856.

3. Incorporating HIV prevention into the medical care of persons living with HIV. Recommendations of CDC, the Health Resources and Services Administration, the National Institutes of Health, and the HIV Medicine Association of the Infectious Diseases Society of America. MMWR Recomm Rep 2003;52(RR-12):1–24.

4. Boily MC, Baggaley RF, Wang L, Masse B, et al. Heterosexual risk of HIV-1 infection per sexual act: systematic review and meta-analysis of observational studies. Lancet Infect Dis 2009;9(2):118–129.

5. Wawer MJ, Makumbi F, Kigozi G, Serwadda D, et al. Circumcision in HIV-infected men and its effect on HIV transmission to female partners in Rakai, Uganda: a randomised controlled trial. Lancet 2009;374(9685):229–237.

6. Rotheram-Borus MJ, Swendeman D, Chovnick G. The past, present, and future of HIV prevention: integrating behavioral, biomedical, and structural intervention strategies for the next generation of HIV prevention. Annu Rev Clin Psychol 2009;5:143–167.

7. Smith DK, Grohskopf LA, Black RJ, Auerbach JD, et al. Antiretroviral postexposure prophylaxis after sexual, injection-drug use, or other nonoccupational exposure to HIV in the United States: recommendations from the U.S. Department of Health and Human Services. MMWR Recomm Rep 2005;54(RR-2):1–20.

8. Stramer SL, Glynn SA, Kleinman SH, Strong DM, et al. Detection of HIV-1 and HCV infections among antibody-negative blood donors by nucleic acid-amplification testing. N Engl J Med 2004;351(8):760–768.

9. Zou S, Dodd RY, Stramer SL, Strong DM. Probability of viremia with HBV, HCV, HIV, and HTLV among tissue donors in the United States. N Engl J Med 2004;351(8):751–759.

10. Panlilio AL, Cardo DM, Grohskopf LA, Heneine W, et al. Updated U.S. Public Health Service guidelines for the management of occupational exposures to HIV and recommendations for postexposure prophylaxis. MMWR Recomm Rep 2005;54(RR-9):1–17.

11. Public Health Services Task Force. Recommendations for Use of Antiretroviral Drugs in Pregnant HIV-1-Infected Women for Maternal Health and Interventions to Reduce Perinatal HIV-1 Transmission in the United States – Living Document; April 29, 2009. http://www. AIDSinfo.NIH.gov.

12. Shapiro RL, Smeaton L, Lockman S, Thior I, et al. Risk factors for early and late transmission of HIV via breast-feeding among infants born to HIV-infected women in a randomized clinical trial in Botswana. J Infect Dis 2009;199(3):414–418.

13. Thior I, Lockman S, Smeaton LM, Shapiro RL, et al. Breastfeeding plus infant zidovudine prophylaxis for 6 months vs formula feeding plus infant zidovudine for 1 month to reduce mother-to-child HIV transmission in Botswana: a randomized trial: the Mashi Study. JAMA 2006;296(7):794–805.

14. Schneider E, Whitmore S, Glynn KM, Dominguez K, et al. Revised surveillance case definitions for HIV infection among adults, adolescents, and children aged <18 months and for HIV infection and AIDS among children aged 18 months to <13 years–United States, 2008. MMWR Recomm Rep 2008;57(RR-10):1–12.

15. Hall HI, Song R, Rhodes P, Prejean J, et al. Estimation of HIV incidence in the United States. JAMA 2008;300(5):520–529.

16. Lubinski C, Aberg J, Bardeguez AD, Elion R, et al. HIV policy: the path forward–a joint position paper of the HIV Medicine Association of the Infectious Diseases Society of America and the American College of Physicians. Clin Infect Dis 2009;48(10):1335–1344.

17. Aberg JA, Kaplan JE, Libman H, Emmanuel P, et al. Primary care guidelines for the management of persons infected with human immunodeficiency virus: 2009 update by the HIV medicine association of the infectious diseases society of America. Clin Infect Dis 2009;49(5):651–681.

18. Kilmarx PH. Global epidemiology of HIV. Curr Opin HIV AIDS 2009;4(4):240–246.

19. UNAIDS. 09 AIDS epidemic report; November 2009. http://data. unaids.org/pub/Report/2009/2009_epidemic_update_en.pdf.

20. Robertson DL, Anderson JP, Bradac JA, Carr JK, et al. HIV-1 nomenclature proposal. Science 2000;288(5463):55–56.

21. Plantier JC, Leoz M, Dickerson JE, De Oliveira F, et al. A new human immunodeficiency virus derived from gorillas. Nat Med 2009;15(8):871–872.

22. Kallings LO. The first postmodern pandemic: 25 years of HIV/ AIDS. J Intern Med 2008;263(3):218–243.

23. Panel on Antiretroviral Guidelines for Adults and Adolescents. Guidelines for the use of antiretroviral agents in HIV-1-infected adults and adolescents. Department of Health and Human Services. December 1, 2009; 1-161. http://www.aidsinfo.nih.gov/ContentFiles/ AdultandAdolescentGL.pdf.

24. Tang H, Kuhen KL, Wong-Staal F. Lentivirus replication and regulation. Annu Rev Genet 1999;33:133–170.

25. Stewart GJ, Ashton LJ, Biti RA, Ffrench RA, et al. Increased frequency of CCR-5 delta 32 heterozygotes among long-term non-progressors with HIV-1 infection. The Australian Long-Term Non-Progressor Study Group. AIDS 1997;11(15):1833–1838.

26. Cullen BR. Role and mechanism of action of the APOBEC3 family of antiretroviral resistance factors. J Virol 2006;80(3):1067–1076.

27. Neil SJ, Zang T, Bieniasz PD. Tetherin inhibits retrovirus release and is antagonized by HIV-1 Vpu. Nature 2008;451(7177):425–430.

28. Derdeyn CA, Silvestri G. Viral and host factors in the pathogenesis of HIV infection. Curr Opin Immunol 2005;17(4):366–373.

29. Grossman Z, Meier-Schellersheim M, Paul WE, Picker LJ. Pathogenesis of HIV infection: what the virus spares is as important as what it destroys. Nat Med 2006;12(3):289–295.

30. Kahn JO, Walker BD. Acute human immunodeficiency virus type 1 infection. N Engl J Med 1998;339:33–39.

31. Mellors JW, Rinaldo CR, Jr, Gupta P, White RM, et al. Prognosis in HIV-1 infection predicted by the quantity of virus in plasma. Science 1996;272:1167–1170.

32. Khoury M, Kovacs A. Pediatric HIV infection. Clin Obstet Gynecol 2001;44(2):243–275.

33. Centers for Disease Control and Prevention. 1994 revised classification system for human immunodeficiency virus infection in children less than 13 years of age. MMWR 1994;43(RR-12):1–10.

34. Mofenson LM, Brady MT, Danner SP, Dominguez KL, et al. Guidelines for the Prevention and Treatment of Opportunistic Infections among HIV-exposed and HIV-infected children: recommendations from CDC, the National Institutes of Health, the HIV Medicine Association of the Infectious Diseases Society of America, the Pediatric Infectious Diseases Society, and the American Academy of Pediatrics. MMWR Recomm Rep 2009;58(RR-11):1–166.

35. Working Group on Antiretroviral Therapy and Medical Management of HIV-Infected Children. Guidelines for the Use of Antiretroviral Agents in Pediatric HIV Infection. February 23, 2009; pp 1-139. http:// aidsinfo.nih.gov/ContentFiles/PediatricGuidelines.pdf.

36. Walensky RP, Paltiel AD, Losina E, Mercincavage LM, et al. The survival benefits of AIDS treatment in the United States. J Infect Dis 2006;194(1):11–19.

37. NIH Panel to Define Principles of Therapy of HIV Infection. Report of the NIH panel to define principles of therapy of HIV infection. MMWR 1998;47(RR-5);1–41.

38. Kitahata MM, Gange SJ, Abraham AG, Merriman B, et al. Effect of early versus deferred antiretroviral therapy for HIV on survival. N Engl J Med 2009;360(18):1815–1826.

39. Rerks-Ngarm S, Pitisuttithum P, Nitayaphan S, Kaewkungwal J, et al. Vaccination with ALVAC and AIDSVAX to prevent HIV-1 infection in Thailand. N Engl J Med 2009;361(23):2209–2220.

40. Abrams D, Levy Y, Losso MH, Babiker A, et al. Interleukin-2 therapy in patients with HIV infection. N Engl J Med 2009;361(16):1548–1559.

41. Hendrix CW, Cao YJ, Fuchs EJ. Topical microbicides to prevent HIV: clinical drug development challenges. Annu Rev Pharmacol Toxicol 2009;49:349–375.

42. Anderson PL, Kakuda TN, Lichtenstein KA. The cellular pharmacology of nucleoside- and nucleotide-analogue reverse-transcriptase inhibitors and its relationship to clinical toxicities. Clin Infect Dis 2004;38(5):743–753.

43. Anderson MS, Kakuda TN, Hanley W, Miller J, et al. Minimal pharmacokinetic interaction between the human immunodeficiency virus nonnucleoside reverse transcriptase inhibitor etravirine and the integrase inhibitor raltegravir in healthy subjects. Antimicrob Agents Chemother 2008;52(12):4228–4232.

44. Calmy A, Hirschel B, Cooper DA, Carr A. A new era of antiretroviral drug toxicity. Antivir Ther 2009;14(2):165–179.

45. Carr A. Toxicity of antiretroviral therapy and implications for drug development. Nat Rev Drug Discov 2003;2:624–634.

46. Hirsch MS, Gunthard HF, Schapiro JM, Brun-Vezinet F, et al. Antiretroviral drug resistance testing in adult HIV-1 infection: 2008 recommendations of an International AIDS Society-USA panel. Clin Infect Dis 2008;47(2):266–285.

47. Telenti A. Safety concerns about CCR5 as an antiviral target. Curr Opin HIV AIDS 2009;4(2):131–135.

48. Xu L, Desai MC. Pharmacokinetic enhancers for HIV drugs. Curr Opin Investig Drugs 2009;10(8):775–786.

49. Stellbrink HJ. Novel compounds for the treatment of HIV type-1 infection. Antivir Chem Chemother 2009;19(5):189–200.

50. Romanelli F, Smith KM, Hoven AD. Chloroquine and hydroxychloroquine as inhibitors of human immunodeficiency virus (HIV-1) activity. Curr Pharm Des 2004;10(21):2643–2648.

51. McMahon MA, Siliciano JD, Lai J, Liu JO, et al. The antiherpetic drug acyclovir inhibits HIV replication and selects the V75I reverse transcriptase multidrug resistance mutation. J Biol Chem 2008;283(46):31289–31293.

52. Canestri A, Ghosn J, Wirden M, Marguet F, et al. Foscarnet salvage therapy for patients with late-stage HIV disease and multiple drug resistance. Antivir Ther 2006;11(5):561–566.

53. Kaplan JE, Benson C, Holmes KH, Brooks JT, et al. Guidelines for prevention and treatment of opportunistic infections in HIV-infected adults and adolescents: recommendations from CDC, the National Institutes of Health, and the HIV Medicine Association of the Infectious Diseases Society of America. MMWR Recomm Rep 2009;58(RR-4):1-207; quiz CE1-4.

54. Fischl MA, Richman DD, Grieco MH, Gottlieb MS, et al. The efficacy of azidothymidine (AZT) in the treatment of patients with AIDS and AIDS-related complex. N Engl J Med 1987;317:185–191.

55. Hammer SM, Katzenstein DA, Hughes MD, Gundacker H, et al. A trial comparing nucleoside monotherapy with combination therapy in HIV-infected adults with CD4 cell counts from 200 to 500 per cubic millimeter. N Engl J Med 1996;335:1081–1090.

56. Hammer SM, Squires K, Hughes M, Grimes JM, et al. A controlled trial of two nucleoside analogues plus indinavir in persons with human immunodeficiency virus infection and CD4 cell counts of 200 per cubic millimeter or less. AIDS Clinical Trials Group 320 Study Team. N Engl J Med 1997;337:725–733.

57. Palella FJ, Jr, Delaney KM, Moorman AC, Loveless MO, et al. Declining morbidity and mortality among patients with advanced human immunodeficiency virus infection. N Engl J Med 1998;338:853–860.

58. Walmsley S, Bernstein B, King M, Arribas J, et al. Lopinavir-ritonavir versus nelfinavir for the initial treatment of HIV infection. N Eng J Med 2002;346:2039–2046.

59. Gulick RM, Ribaudo HJ, Shikuma CM, Lustgarten S, et al. Triple-nucleoside regimens versus efavirenz-containing regimens for the initial treatment of HIV-1 infection. N Engl J Med 2004;350(18):1850–1861.

60. World Health Organization. Rapid advice: Antiretroviral therapy for HIV infection in adults and adolescents; November 2009. http://www.who.int/hiv/pub/arv/advice/en/index.html.

61. Gardner EM, Burman WJ, Steiner JF, Anderson PL, et al. Antiretroviral medication adherence and the development of class-specific antiretroviral resistance. AIDS 2009;23(9):1035–1046.

62. Lennox JL, DeJesus E, Lazzarin A, Pollard RB, et al. Safety and efficacy of raltegravir-based versus efavirenz-based combination therapy in treatment-naive patients with HIV-1 infection: a multicentre, double-blind randomised controlled trial. Lancet 2009;374(9692):796–806.

63. Gallant JE, DeJesus E, Arribas JR, Pozniak AL, et al. Tenofovir DF, emtricitabine, and efavirenz vs. zidovudine, lamivudine, and efavirenz for HIV. N Engl J Med 2006;354(3):251–260.

64. Ortiz R, Dejesus E, Khanlou H, Voronin E, et al. Efficacy and safety of once-daily darunavir/ritonavir versus lopinavir/ritonavir in treatment-naive HIV-1-infected patients at week 48. AIDS 2008;22(12):1389–1397.

65. Molina JM, Andrade-Villanueva J, Echevarria J, Chetchotisakd P, et al. Once-daily atazanavir/ritonavir versus twice-daily lopinavir/ritonavir, each in combination with tenofovir and emtricitabine, for management of antiretroviral-naive HIV-1-infected patients: 48 week efficacy and safety results of the CASTLE study. Lancet 2008;372(9639):646–655.

66. Sax PE, Tierney C, Collier AC, Fischl MA, et al. Abacavir-lamivudine versus tenofovir-emtricitabine for initial HIV-1 therapy. N Engl J Med 2009;361(23):2230–2240.

67. Ha B, Liao QM, Dix LP, Pappa KA. Virologic response and safety of the abacavir/lamivudine fixed-dose formulation as part of highly active antiretroviral therapy: analyses of six clinical studies. HIV Clin Trials 2009;10(2):65–75.

68. Riddler SA, Haubrich R, DiRienzo AG, Peeples L, et al. Class-sparing regimens for initial treatment of HIV-1 infection. N Engl J Med 2008;358(20):2095–2106.

69. Bierman WF, van Agtmael MA, Nijhuis M, Danner SA, et al. HIV monotherapy with ritonavir-boosted protease inhibitors: a systematic review. AIDS 2009;23(3):279–291.

70. Turner D, Brenner BG, Routy JP, Petrella M, et al. Rationale for maintenance of the M184V resistance mutation in human immunodeficiency virus type 1 reverse transcriptase in treatment experienced patients. New Microbiol 2004;27(2 Suppl 1):31–39.

71. McIntyre JA, Hopley M, Moodley D, Eklund M, et al. Efficacy of short-course AZT plus 3TC to reduce nevirapine resistance in the prevention of mother-to-child HIV transmission: a randomized clinical trial. PLoS Med 2009;6(10):e1000172.

72. El-Sadr WM, Lundgren JD, Neaton JD, Gordin F, et al. CD4+ count-guided interruption of antiretroviral treatment. N Engl J Med 2006;355(22):2283–2296.

73. Phillips AN, Neaton J, Lundgren JD. The role of HIV in serious diseases other than AIDS. AIDS 2008;22(18):2409–2418.

74. Taylor S, Boffito M, Khoo S, Smit E, et al. Stopping antiretroviral therapy. AIDS 2007;21(13):1673–1682.

75. Beishuizen SJ, Geerlings SE. Immune reconstitution inflammatory syndrome: immunopathogenesis, risk factors, diagnosis, treatment and prevention. Neth J Med 2009;67(10):327–331.

76. Zolopa A, Andersen J, Powderly W, Sanchez A, et al. Early antiretroviral therapy reduces AIDS progression/death in individuals with acute opportunistic infections: a multicenter randomized strategy trial. PLoS One 2009;4(5):e5575.

77. Krajicek BJ, Thomas CF, Jr., Limper AH. Pneumocystis pneumonia: current concepts in pathogenesis, diagnosis, and treatment. Clin Chest Med 2009;30(2):265–278, vi.

78. Santamauro J, Stover D. Pneumocystis carinii pneumonia. Med Clin North America 1997;81:299–318.

79. Kovacs JA, Masur H. Evolving health effects of Pneumocystis: one hundred years of progress in diagnosis and treatment. JAMA 2009;301(24):2578–2585.

80. Wofsy C. Use of trimethoprim-sulfamethoxazole in the treatment of Pneumocystis carinii pneumonitis in patients with acquired immunodeficiency syndrome. Rev Infect Dis 1987;9(Suppl 2):S184-S194.

81. Wharton J, Coleman D, Wofsy C, Luce JM, et al. Trimethoprim-sulfamethoxazole or pentamidine for Pneumocystis carinii pneumonia in the acquired immunodeficiency syndrome. Ann Intern Med 1986;105:37–44.

82. Morse CG, Kovacs JA. Metabolic and skeletal complications of HIV infection: the price of success. JAMA 2006;296(7):844–854.

83. Spano JP, Costagliola D, Katlama C, Mounier N, et al. AIDS-related malignancies: state of the art and therapeutic challenges. J Clin Oncol 2008;26(29):4834–4842.

84. Grulich AE, van Leeuwen MT, Falster MO, Vajdic CM. Incidence of cancers in people with HIV/AIDS compared with immunosuppressed transplant recipients: a meta-analysis. Lancet 2007;370(9581):59–67.

85. Izzedine H, Harris M, Perazella MA. The nephrotoxic effects of HAART. Nat Rev Nephrol 2009;5(10):563–573.

86. van Vonderen MG, Lips P, van Agtmael MA, Hassink EA, et al. First line zidovudine/lamivudine/lopinavir/ritonavir leads to greater bone loss compared to nevirapine/lopinavir/ritonavir. AIDS 2009;23(11):1367–1376.

87. Brown TT, Qaqish RB. Antiretroviral therapy and the prevalence of osteopenia and osteoporosis: a meta-analytic review. AIDS 2006;20(17):2165–2174.

88. Kotler DP. HIV and antiretroviral therapy: lipid abnormalities and associated cardiovascular risk in HIV-infected patients. J Acquir Immune Defic Syndr 2008;49(Suppl 2):S79–S85.

89. Koutkia P, Grinspoon S. HIV-associated lipodystrophy: pathogenesis, prognosis, treatment, and controversies. Annu Rev Med 2004;55:303–317.

90. Grinspoon S, Carr A. Cardiovascular risk and body-fat abnormalities in HIV-infected adults. N Engl J Med 2005;352(1):48–62.

91. Vandekerckhove L, Verhofstede C, Vogelaers D. Maraviroc: perspectives for use in antiretroviral-naive HIV-1-infected patients. J Antimicrob Chemother 2009;63(6):1087–1096.

92. Law MG, Friis-Moller N, El-Sadr WM, Weber R, et al. The use of the Framingham equation to predict myocardial infarctions in HIV-infected patients: comparison with observed events in the D:A:D Study. HIV Med 2006;7(4):218–230.

93. Sabin CA, Worm SW, Weber R, Reiss P, et al. Use of nucleoside reverse transcriptase inhibitors and risk of myocardial infarction in HIV-infected patients enrolled in the D:A:D study: a multi-cohort collaboration. Lancet 2008;371(9622):1417–1426.

94. Brothers CH, Hernandez JE, Cutrell AG, Curtis L, et al. Risk of myocardial infarction and abacavir therapy: no increased risk across 52 GlaxoSmithKline-sponsored clinical trials in adult subjects. J Acquir Immune Defic Syndr 2009;51(1):20–28.

95. Moyle GJ, Sabin CA, Cartledge J, Johnson M, et al. A randomized comparative trial of tenofovir DF or abacavir as replacement for a thymidine analogue in persons with lipoatrophy. AIDS 2006;20(16):2043–2050.

96. Wohl DA, McComsey G, Tebas P, Brown TT, et al. Current concepts in the diagnosis and management of metabolic complications of HIV infection and its therapy. Clin Infect Dis 2006;43(5):645–653.

97. Lo Re V, 3rd, Kostman JR, Amorosa VK. Management complexities of HIV/hepatitis C virus coinfection in the twenty-first century. Clin Liver Dis 2008;12(3):587–609, ix.

98. Matthews GV, Dore GJ. HIV and hepatitis C coinfection. J Gastroenterol Hepatol 2008;23(7 Pt 1):1000–1008.

99. Balzarini J, Lee CK, Herdewijn P, De Clercq E. Mechanism of the potentiating effect of ribavirin on the activity of 2′,3′-dideoxyinosine against human immunodeficiency virus. J Biol Chem 1991;266(32):21509–21514.

100. Tien PC. Management and treatment of hepatitis C virus infection in HIV-infected adults: recommendations from the Veterans Affairs Hepatitis C Resource Center Program and National Hepatitis C Program Office. Am J Gastroenterol 2005;100(10):2338–2354.

CHAPTER

135

Cancer Treatment and Chemotherapy

PATRICK J. MEDINA AND STACY S. SHORD

KEY CONCEPTS

❶ Carcinogenesis is a multistep process that includes initiation, promotion, conversion, and progression. The growth of both normal and cancerous cells is genetically controlled by the balance or imbalance of oncogene, proto-oncogene, and tumor suppressor gene protein products. Multiple genetic mutations are required to convert normal cells to cancerous cells. Apoptosis and cellular senescence (aging) are normal mechanisms for cell death.

❷ Because patients with clinically evident metastatic cancer can rarely be cured, early detection is critical. Screening programs are designed to detect cancers in asymptomatic people who are at risk of a specific type of cancer. Knowing the early warning signs of cancer is also important in early detection, when cancers are most likely to be localized.

❸ Treatment for cancer should not begin until the presence of cancer is confirmed by a tissue (e.g., histologic) diagnosis. Clinical cancer staging provides prognostic information, and in conjunction with the patient's treatment goals, guides the selection of cancer treatment. The goals of cancer treatment include cure, prolongation of life, and relief of symptoms. Surgery and radiation therapy provide the best chance of cure for patients with localized cancers, but systemic treatment methods are required for disseminated cancers.

❹ Adjuvant therapy is systemic therapy that is administered to treat any existing micrometastases remaining after surgical excision of localized disease. Because adjuvant therapy is given to patients with no remaining clinical evidence of cancer, the benefit of the treatment cannot be proven for an individual patient, but only for patient populations. Treatment decisions are based largely on an assessment of the presence of risk

factors in an individual patient and the patient's estimated risk for cancer recurrence. The effectiveness of adjuvant therapies is measured by the relative and absolute reduction in the risk of recurrence.

❺ Traditional chemotherapy agents target rapidly proliferating cells. Agents can be either "cell-cycle phase-specific," targeting one specific phase of the cell cycle, or "cell-cycle phase-nonspecific," targeting all proliferating cells regardless of their place in the cell cycle. Cell-cycle phase-specific agents are generally given more frequently or as continuous infusions while cell-cycle phase-nonspecific agents are usually given as a single dose.

❻ Monoclonal antibodies recognize an antigen that is expressed preferentially on cancer cells or target growth factors responsible for cancer growth. These agents can vary in the amount of foreign component that can be used to predict tolerability of the agents. Monoclonal antibodies that target cellular antigens induce cell death by a variety of mechanisms that involve the host immune system. These agents can also be used to deliver drugs or radioisotopes to the antigen-expressing cells.

❼ The HER (human epidermal growth factor receptor) family contains four known receptor subtypes that regulate cell proliferation pathways through signal transduction. The HER family is dysregulated in many common tumors. Several agents have been developed to prevent signal transduction through this pathway. Monoclonal antibodies, which competitively bind to extracellular receptors, and small molecular inhibitors, which target intracellular signal transduction pathways, are commercially available for several malignancies.

❽ Tumors must develop new blood vessels through the process of angiogenesis in order to grow. This process, regulated by proangiogenic and antiangiogenic factors, becomes dysregulated in several malignancies and can lead to tumor growth, invasion, and metastasis. New anticancer agents can target this process and decrease tumor growth.

❾ Understanding the mechanism of chemotherapy toxicities can lead to more effective prevention and treatment of these toxicities. Prospective dose modification of some chemotherapeutic agents and targeted therapies are essential in patients

Learning objectives, review questions, and other resources can be found at **www.pharmacotherapyonline.com**.

with impaired renal or hepatic function, to reduce the risk of severe toxicities. Identification of genetic variations that affect activation and metabolism may permit the development of individualized therapy that optimize effectiveness and minimize toxicity.

⑩ Myelosuppression is the acute dose-limiting toxicity for most nonspecific chemotherapeutic agents. Anemia can cause fatigue in cancer patients, whereas risk of infection in patients is related to the depth and duration of neutropenia. Unexplained fever in neutropenic patients requires prompt initiation of empiric antibiotic therapy. Colony-stimulating factors are available to improve fatigue in patients with anemia and reduce the risk of febrile neutropenia. Evidence-based clinical guidelines should direct the use of these supportive care measures.

Cancer is a group of more than 100 different diseases that are characterized by uncontrolled cellular growth, local tissue invasion, and distant metastases.[1] It is now the leading cause of mortality in Americans younger than age 85 years. About 1.5 million cases of cancer will be diagnosed in 2009, and cancer will claim an estimated 562,340 lives in the United States.[2] Figure 135–1 illustrates the estimated incidence of common cancers and cancer-related deaths. The four most common cancers are prostate, breast, lung, and colorectal cancer. The most common cause of cancer-related deaths in the United States is lung cancer, which accounts for about 160,000 deaths each year. These cancers are discussed in further detail in the chapters that follow.

The roles of healthcare professionals in the management of cancer patients can be very diverse. Thorough knowledge of anticancer drug pharmacology and pharmacokinetics is essential to prevent and manage drug-induced toxicities. Supportive care issues, such as nutritional support, pain management, infection, and nausea and vomiting, require application of clinical, pharmacologic, and economic principles. Provision of drug information to other healthcare professionals and to patients and their families is another critical role. Experienced healthcare professionals are able to fulfill these roles and to make valuable contributions to patient care in the oncology setting.

Estimated new cases*

			Males	Females			
Prostate	217,730	28%		Breast	207,090	28%
Lung & bronchus	116,750	15%		Lung & bronchus	105,770	14%
Colon & rectum	72,090	9%		Colon & rectum	70,480	10%
Urinary bladder	52,760	7%		Uterine corpus	43,470	6%
Melanoma of the skin	38,870	5%		Thyroid	33,930	5%
Non-Hodgkin lymphoma	35,380	4%		Non-Hodgkin lymphoma	30,160	4%
Kidney & renal pelvis	35,370	4%		Melanoma of the skin	29,260	4%
Oral cavity & pharynx	25,420	3%		Kidney & renal pelvis	22,870	3%
Leukemia	24,690	3%		Ovary	21,880	3%
Pancreas	21,370	3%		Pancreas	21,770	3%
All sites	**789,620**	**100%**		**All sites**	**739,940**	**100%**

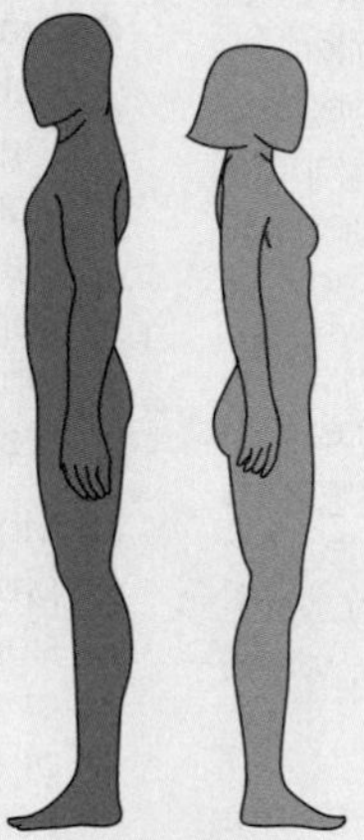

Estimated deaths

			Males	Females			
Lung & bronchus	86,220	29%		Lung & bronchus	71,080	26%
Prostate	32,050	11%		Breast	39,840	15%
Colon & rectum	26,580	9%		Colon & rectum	24,790	9%
Pancreas	18,770	6%		Pancreas	18,030	7%
Liver & intrahepatic bile duct	12,720	4%		Ovary	13,850	5%
Leukemia	12,660	4%		Non-Hodgkin lymphoma	9,500	4%
Esophagus	11,650	4%		Leukemia	9,180	3%
Non-Hodgkin lymphoma	10,710	4%		Uterine corpus	7,950	3%
Urinary bladder	10,410	3%		Liver & intrahepatic bile duct	6,190	2%
Kidney & renal pelvis	8,210	3%		Brain & other nervous system	5,720	2%
All sites	**299,200**	**100%**		**All sites**	**270,290**	**100%**

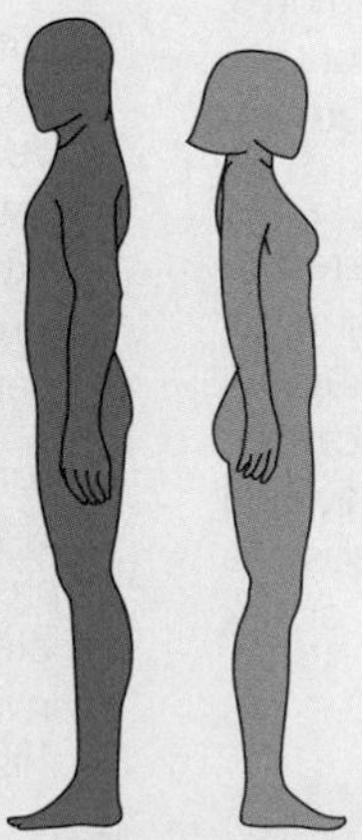

FIGURE 135-1. Estimated 2010 cancer incidences (*top*) and deaths (*bottom*) in the United States for males and females. (*Reproduced with permission from Jemal et al.[2]*)

This chapter introduces the basic concepts of carcinogenesis, tumor growth, and cancer treatment, provides general information on the pharmacology and clinical use of the antineoplastic agents, and presents an overview of supportive care issues in the oncology patient.

ETIOLOGY OF CANCER

CARCINOGENESIS

❶ The mechanisms by which cancers occur are incompletely understood. A cancer, or neoplasm, is thought to develop from a cell in which the normal mechanisms for control of growth and proliferation are altered. Current evidence supports the concept of carcinogenesis as a multistage process that is genetically regulated.[3-6] The first step in this process is *initiation*, which requires exposure of normal cells to carcinogenic substances. These carcinogens produce genetic damage that, if not repaired, results in irreversible cellular mutations. This mutated cell has an altered response to its environment and a selective growth advantage, giving it the potential to develop into a clonal population of neoplastic cells. During the second phase, known as *promotion*, carcinogens or other factors alter the environment to favor growth of the mutated cell population over normal cells. The primary difference between initiation and promotion is that promotion is a reversible process. Because it is reversible, the promotion phase may be the target of future chemoprevention strategies, including changes in lifestyle and diet. At some point, however, the mutated cell becomes cancerous (*conversion* or *transformation*). Depending on the type of cancer, 5 to 20 years may elapse between the carcinogenic phases and the development of a clinically detectable cancer. The final stage of neoplastic growth, called *progression*, involves further genetic changes leading to increased cell proliferation. The critical elements of this phase include tumor invasion into local tissues and the development of metastases.

Substances that may act as carcinogens or initiators include chemical, physical, and biologic agents.[5] Exposure to chemicals may occur by virtue of occupational and environmental means, as well as lifestyle habits. The association of aniline dye exposure and bladder cancer is one such example. Benzene is known to cause leukemia. Some drugs and hormones used for therapeutic purposes are also classified as carcinogenic chemicals (Table 135–1). Physical agents

that act as carcinogens include ionizing radiation and ultraviolet light. These types of radiation induce mutations by forming free radicals that damage DNA and other cellular components. Viruses are biologic agents that are associated with certain cancers. The Epstein-Barr virus is believed to be an important factor in the initiation of Burkitt lymphoma. Likewise, infection with human papilloma virus is known to be a major cause of cervical cancer. All the previously mentioned carcinogens, as well as age, gender, diet, growth factors, and chronic irritation, are among the factors considered to be promoters of carcinogenesis.

GENETIC AND MOLECULAR BASIS OF CANCER

❶ In recent years there has been marked progress in our understanding of the genetic changes that lead to the development of cancer, largely because of improvements in research techniques and new genomic information.[3,5-7] Two major classes of genes are involved in carcinogenesis: oncogenes and tumor suppressor genes. Figure 135–2 illustrates the acquired capabilities of cancer cells that differ from normal cellular function.[8] Oncogenes develop from normal genes, called proto-oncogenes, and may have important roles in all phases of carcinogenesis. Proto-oncogenes are present in all cells and are essential regulators of normal cellular functions, including the cell cycle. Genetic alteration of the proto-oncogene through point mutation, chromosomal rearrangement, or gene

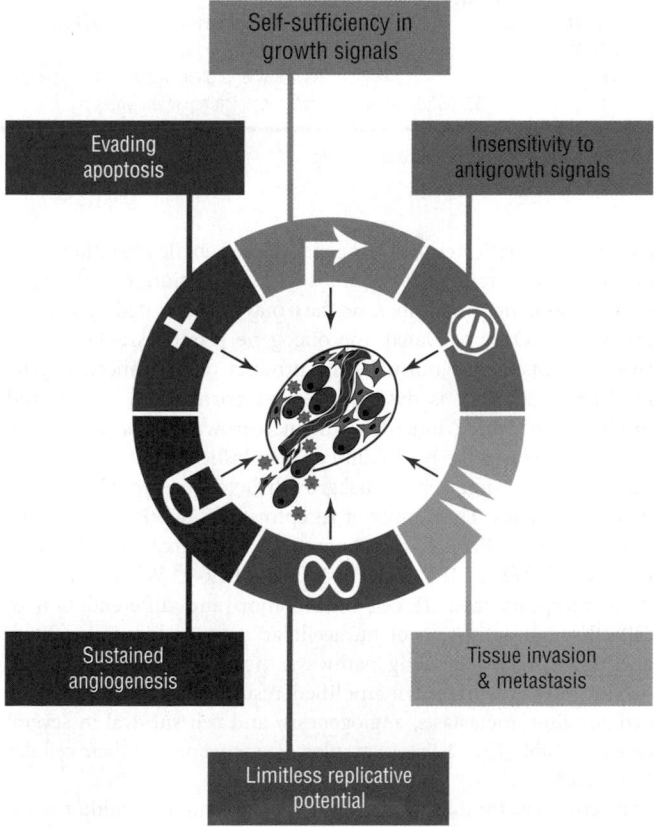

FIGURE 135-2. Functional capabilities acquired by cancer cells including angiogenesis, self-proliferation, insensitivity to antigrowth signals and limitless growth potential, metastasis; and antiapoptotic effects. It is thought that most, if not all cancer cells acquire these functions through a variety of mechanisms, including activation of oncogenes and mutations in tumor suppressor genes. (*Reprinted from Cell, Vol 100(1), Hanahan D, Weinberg RA, The Hallmarks of Cancer, pages 57–70, Copyright © 2000, with permission from Elsevier.*)

TABLE 135-1	Selected Drugs and Hormones Known to Cause Cancer in Humans
Drug or Hormone	**Type of Cancer Caused**
Alkylating agents (e.g., chlorambucil, mechlorethamine, melphalan, nitrosoureas)	Leukemia
Anabolic steroids	Liver
Analgesics containing phenacetin	Renal, urinary bladder
Anthracyclines (e.g., doxorubicin)	Leukemia
Antiestrogens (tamoxifen)	Endometrium
Coal tars (topical)	Skin
Estrogens	
Nonsteroidal (diethylstilbestrol)	Vagina/cervix, endometrium, breast, testes
Steroidal (estrogen replacement therapy, oral contraceptives)	Endometrium, breast, liver
Epipodophyllotoxins (etoposide, teniposide)	Leukemia
Immunosuppressive drugs (cyclosporine, azathioprine)	Lymphoma, skin
Oxazaphosphorines (cyclophosphamide, ifosfamide)	Urinary bladder, leukemia

Adapted from Compagni and Christofori[4] and Cotran et al.[6]

TABLE 135-2 Examples of Oncogenes and Tumor Suppressor Genes

Gene	Function	Associated Human Cancer
Oncogenes		
Genes for growth factors or their receptors		
EGFR or Erb-B1	Codes for epidermal growth factor (EGFR) receptor	Glioblastoma, breast, head and neck, and colon cancers
HER-2/neu or Erb-B2	Codes for a growth factor receptor	Breast, salivary gland, prostate, bladder, and ovarian cancers
RET	Codes for a growth factor receptor	Thyroid cancer
Genes for cytoplasmic relays in stimulatory signaling pathways		
K-RAS and N-RAS	Code for guanine nucleotide-proteins with GTPase activity	Lung, ovarian, colon, pancreatic binding cancers Neuroblastoma, acute leukemia
Genes for transcription factors that activate growth-promoting genes		
c-MYC		Leukemia and breast, colon, gastric, and lung cancers
N-MYC		Neuroblastoma, small cell lung cancer, and glioblastoma
Genes for cytoplasmic kinases		
BCR-ABL	Codes for a nonreceptor tyrosine kinase	Chronic myelogenous leukemia
Genes for other molecules		
BCL-2	Codes for a protein that blocks apoptosis	Indolent B-cell lymphomas
BCL-1 or PRAD1	Codes for cyclin D_1, a cell-cycle clock stimulator	Breast, head, and neck cancers
MDM2	Protein antagonist of p53 tumor suppressor protein	Sarcomas
Tumor-suppressor genes		
Genes for proteins in the cytoplasm		
APC	Step in a signaling pathway	Colon and gastric cancer
NF-1	Codes for a protein that inhibits the stimulatory Ras protein	Neurofibroma, leukemia, and pheochromocytoma
NF-2	Codes for a protein that inhibits the stimulatory Ras protein	Meningioma, ependymoma, and schwannoma
Genes for proteins in the nucleus		
MTS1	Codes for p16 protein, a cyclin-dependent kinase inhibitor	Involved in a wide range of cancers
RB1	Codes for the pRB protein, a master brake of the cell cycle	Retinoblastoma, osteosarcoma, and bladder, small cell lung, prostate, and breast cancers
p53	Codes for the p53 protein, which can halt cell division and induce apoptosis	Involved in a wide range of cancers
Genes for protein whose cellular location is unclear		
BRCA1	DNA repair, transcriptional regulation	Breast and ovarian cancers
BRCA2	DNA repair	Breast cancer
VHL	Regulator of protein stability	Renal cell cancer
MSH2, MLH1, PMS1, PMS2, MSH6	DNA mismatch repair enzymes	Hereditary nonpolyposis colorectal cancer

Data from Liotta et al,[3] Cotran et al,[6] and Weinberg.[7]

amplification activates the oncogene. These genetic alterations may be caused by carcinogenic agents such as radiation, chemicals, or viruses (somatic mutations), or they may be inherited (germ-line mutations). Once activated, the oncogene produces either excessive amounts of the normal gene product or an abnormal gene product. The result is dysregulation of normal cell growth and proliferation, which imparts a distinct growth advantage to the cell and increases the probability of neoplastic transformation. An example is the human epidermal growth factor receptor (HER) family of oncogenes. This family of receptor tyrosine kinases contains four members: ErbB-1, also known as epidermal growth factor receptor (EGFR), HER-2, HER-3, and HER-4. When activated, these receptors mediate cell proliferation and differentiation of cells through activation of intracellular tyrosine kinase receptors and downstream signaling pathways. As an oncogene, the gene product is overexpressed or amplified, resulting in excessive cellular proliferation, metastasis, angiogenesis, and cell survival in several cancers. Table 135–2 lists examples of oncogenes by their cellular function.[9]

In contrast, tumor suppressor genes regulate and inhibit inappropriate cellular growth and proliferation.[3,6,7] Gene loss or mutation results in loss of control over normal cell growth. Two common examples of tumor suppressor genes are the retinoblastoma and p53 genes. Mutation of p53 is one of the most common genetic changes associated with cancer, and is estimated to occur in half of all malignancies.[7] The normal gene product of p53 is responsible for negative regulation of the cell cycle, allowing the cell cycle to halt for repairs, corrections, and responses to other external signals. Inactivation of p53 removes this checkpoint, allowing mutations to occur. Mutation of p53 is linked to a variety of malignancies, including brain tumors (astrocytoma); carcinomas of the breast, colon, lung, cervix, and anus; and osteosarcoma. Another important function of p53 may be modulation of cytotoxic drug effects. Loss of p53 is associated with anticancer drug resistance.

Another group of genes important in carcinogenesis are the DNA repair genes. The normal function of these genes is to repair DNA that is damaged by environmental factors, or errors in DNA that occur during replication.[6] If not corrected, these errors can result in mutations that activate oncogenes or inactivate tumor suppressor genes. As more mutations in the genome occur, the risk for malignant transformation increases. The DNA repair genes have been classified as tumor suppressor genes because a loss in their function results in increased risk for carcinogenesis. Deficiencies in DNA repair genes have been discovered in familial colon cancer (hereditary nonpolyposis colon cancer) and breast cancer syndromes.

❶ Oncogenes and tumor suppressor genes provide the stimulatory and inhibitory signals that ultimately regulate the cell cycle.[3,7] These signals converge on a molecular system in the nucleus known as the cell-cycle clock. The function of the clock in normal tissue is to integrate the signal input and to determine if the cell cycle should proceed. The clock is composed of a series of interacting proteins, the most important of which are cyclins and cyclin-dependent kinases. Cyclins (especially cyclin D_1) and cyclin-dependent kinases promote entry into the cell cycle and are overexpressed in several cancers, including breast cancer. Cyclin-dependent kinase inhibitors have been identified as important negative regulators of the cell cycle.

The cell cycle proceeds from one cell division to the next. The cycle involves five phases: DNA replication (S phase), cell division (M phase), two resting phases (G_1, G_2), and a nondividing state (G_0 phase). In the first resting phase G_1, the cell grows in size and decides to commit to the cell cycle or remain in a resting state. If the cell is healthy, the cell will move into the S phase to synthesize its DNA. Next, the cell enters the second resting phase G_2, in which the cell prepares to divide. In the M phase, the cell enters mitosis and yields two daughter cells. If the cell is not healthy, the cell can stop dividing and initiate apoptosis.

Four checkpoints exist within the cell cycle, one in each phase of the cell cycle and serve as quality control checkpoints. The cell will not proceed to the next phase if all requirements for the current phase are not met. Complexes of cyclin and cyclin-dependent kinases (CDK) regulate these checkpoints. These complexes lead to the activation of other proteins that are responsible for the specific events of each phase of the cell cycle. The first checkpoint is called the restriction site. The restriction site is controlled by retinoblastoma (Rb) complexed to a transcription factor called E2F. The presence of this complex prevents cell cycle progression. A cell can proceed beyond the G_1 restriction site and continue into the S phase, when cyclin-CDK complexes phosphorylate Rb and target it for degradation. A cell may alternatively withdraw into the G_0 phase in the presence of anti-mitogenic or the absence of mitogenic factors.[10]

❶ When the normal regulatory mechanisms for cellular growth fail, backup defense systems may be activated. The secondary defenses include apoptosis (programmed cell death or suicide) and cellular senescence (aging). Apoptosis is a normal mechanism of cell death required for tissue homeostasis.[3,7,11] This process is regulated by oncogenes and tumor suppressor genes and is also a mechanism of cellular death after exposure to cytotoxic agents. Overexpression of oncogenes responsible for apoptosis may produce an "immortal" cell, which has increased potential for malignancy. The *bcl-2* oncogene is an example. The most common chromosomal abnormality found in lymphoid malignancies is the t(14;18) translocation. The *bcl-2* proto-oncogene is normally located on chromosome 18. Translocation of this proto-oncogene to chromosome 14 in proximity to the immunoglobulin heavy chain gene leads to overexpression of *bcl-2*, which decreases apoptosis and confers a survival advantage to the cell. Studies show that *p53* is also a regulator of apoptosis. Loss of *p53* disrupts normal apoptotic pathways, imparting a survival advantage to the cell. Apoptosis may also play an important role as a mechanism of inherent resistance to chemotherapy.[11]

Cellular senescence is another important defense mechanism.[6,7] Laboratory studies demonstrate that once a cell population has undergone a preset number of doublings, growth stops and cells die. This is known as senescence, a process that is regulated by telomeres. Telomeres are the DNA segments or caps at the ends of chromosomes. They are responsible for protecting the end of the DNA from damage. With each replication, the length of the telomeres is shortened. After the telomeres are shortened to a critical length, senescence is triggered. In this way, telomeres tally and limit the number of cell doublings. In cancer cells, the function of telomeres is overcome by overexpression of an enzyme known as telomerase. Telomerase replaces the portion of the telomeres that is lost with each cell division, thereby avoiding senescence and permitting an infinite number of cell doublings. Telomerase is a target for anticancer drug development.

❶ As information regarding the role of oncogenes and tumor suppressor genes accumulated, it became evident that a single mutation is probably insufficient to initiate cancer.[4–7] Scientists postulate that combinations of mutations are required for carcinogenesis and that each mutation is inherited by the next generation of cells. Thus, several detectable genetic mutations may be present in an established tumor. Early mutations are found in both premalignant lesions and in established tumors, whereas later mutations are found only in the established tumor. This theory of sequential genetic mutations resulting in cancer has been demonstrated in colon cancer. In colon cancer, the initial genetic mutation is believed to be loss of the adenomatous polyposis coli gene, which results in formation of a small benign polyp. Oncogenic mutation of the *ras* gene is often the next step, leading to enlargement of the polyp. Loss of function of DNA mismatch repair enzymes may occur at many points in the progression of malignant transformation. Loss of the *p53* gene and another gene, believed to be the "deleted in colorectal cancer" (DCC) gene, complete the transformation into a malignant lesion. Loss of *p53* is thought to be a late event in the development and progression of the malignancy.

Identification of genes and other proteins involved in carcinogenesis has several important clinical implications. They may be used in cancer screening to identify individuals at increased risk for cancer and are being used to design new anticancer agents and gene therapies, several of which have recently been approved for use. Specific genetic abnormalities are so commonly associated with some types of cancers that the presence of that abnormality may aid in the diagnosis of that cancer. If the presence of these genes (i.e., gene expression profile) can reliably predict the clinical course of a cancer or response to certain cancer therapies, then genetic analysis may also become an important prognostic and treatment decision tool. An example of this is overexpression of HER-2 predicting response to trastuzumab.[9]

EPIGENETICS

Epigenetics refers to changes in gene expression that occur without altering the DNA sequence.[12] The two most common mechanisms of epigenetic regulation include methylation and histone modification. DNA methylation commonly occurs at CpG dinucleotides (or islands) and is catalyzed by DNA methyltransferases (DNMT). Histones are basic proteins associated with DNA in the nucleosome. These proteins may be modified by acetylation, methylation or phosphorylation on their N-terminal tail. These modifications play a role in transcriptional regulation. For example, histone deacetylases (HDAC) repress transcription, whereas histone acetylases activate transcription. Epigenetic changes may be involved in the development of cancer by either priming the cell and making it susceptible to genetic changes associated with the development of cancer or initiating malignant transformation. As an example, hypermethylation at CpG dinucleotides found near tumor suppressor genes can switch these genes off and promote the development of cancer. New anticancer agents, classified as DNMT inhibitors or HDAC inhibitors, target these modifications.

PATHOLOGY OF CANCER

TUMOR ORIGIN

Tumors may arise from any of four basic tissue types: epithelial tissue, connective tissue (i.e., muscle, bone, and cartilage), lymphoid tissue, and nerve tissue. Although some malignant cells are atypical of their cells of origin, the involved cells usually retain enough of their parent's traits to identify their origin. Benign tumors are named by adding the suffix *-oma* to the name of the cell

TABLE 135-3 Tumor Classification by Tissue Type

Tissue of Origin	Benign	Malignant
Epithelial		
Surface epithelium	Papilloma	Carcinoma (squamous, epidermoid)
Glandular tissue	Adenoma	Adenocarcinoma
Connective tissue		
Fibrous tissue	Fibroma	Fibrosarcoma
Bone	Osteoma	Osteosarcoma
Smooth muscle	Leiomyoma	Leiomyosarcoma
Striated muscle	Rhabdomyoma	Rhabdomyosarcoma
Fat	Lipoma	Liposarcoma
Lymphoid tissue and hematopoietic cells		
Bone marrow elements		
Lymphoid tissue		Hodgkin and non-Hodgkin lymphoma
Plasma cell		Multiple myeloma
Neural tissue		
Glial tissue	"Benign" gliomas	Glioblastoma multi-forme, astrocytoma
Nerve sheath	Neurofibroma	Neurofibrosarcoma
Melanocytes	Pigmented nevus (mole)	Malignant melanoma
Mixed tumors		
Gonadal tissue	Teratoma	Teratocarcinoma

Adapted from Cotran et al.[6]

type. Hence, adenomas are benign growths of glandular origin, or growths that exhibit a glandular pattern. Table 135–3 lists common tumor nomenclature by tissue type.[6]

Some cancers are preceded by cellular changes that are abnormal, but not yet malignant. Correction of these early changes could potentially prevent the occurrence of a cancer. Precancerous lesions may be described as consisting of either hyperplastic or dysplastic cells. Hyperplasia is an increase in the number of cells in a particular tissue or organ, which results in an increased size of the organ. It should not be confused with hypertrophy, which is an increase in the size of the individual cells. Hyperplasia occurs in response to a stimulus and reverses when the stimulus is removed. Dysplasia is defined as an abnormal change in the size, shape, or organization of cells or tissues. Hyperplasia and dysplasia may precede the appearance of a cancer by several months or years.

Malignant cells are divided into those of epithelial origin or the other tissue types. Carcinomas are malignant growths arising from epithelial cells. Malignant growths of muscle or connective tissue are called sarcomas. An adenocarcinoma is a malignant tumor arising from glandular tissue. When the cancer is limited to the epithelial cells of origin, it is labeled *carcinoma in situ*. Carcinoma in situ is a preinvasive stage of malignancy, and most tumors have progressed well beyond this stage at diagnosis. Like all classification systems, there are exceptions to these rules. Malignancies of hematologic origin, such as leukemias and lymphomas, are classified separately. Leukemias and lymphomas are discussed in later chapters.

TUMOR CHARACTERISTICS

Tumors may be either benign or malignant. Benign tumors are noncancerous growths that are often encapsulated, localized, and indolent. Cells of benign tumors resemble the cells from which they developed. These masses seldom metastasize, and once removed they rarely recur. In contrast, malignant tumors invade and destroy the surrounding tissue. The cells of malignant tumors are genetically unstable, and loss of normal cell architecture results in cells that are atypical of their tissue or cell of origin. These cells lose the ability to perform their usual functions. This loss of structure and function is defined as anaplasia. In contrast to benign tumors, malignant tumors tend to metastasize, and consequently, recurrences are common after removal or destruction of the primary tumor.

INVASION AND METASTASIS

❷ Metastasis is the spread of neoplastic cells from the primary tumor site to distant sites.[5,13] Despite advances in diagnostic techniques and screening for cancer, many patients have detectable metastatic disease at diagnosis. Once clinically evident distant metastases are present, cancers are seldom curable. Newly diagnosed cancer patients may also have microscopic cancer metastases (i.e., micrometastases). Although clinically undetectable, these small clusters of diseased cells must be present, because many patients subsequently relapse at distant sites despite removal of the primary tumor. Some patients with micrometastatic disease may be cured with systemic chemotherapy.

The two primary pathways of metastasis are hematogenous and lymphatic. Other less common modes of disease spread include dissemination via cerebrospinal fluid and transabdominal spread within the peritoneal cavity. Tumors are constantly shedding neoplastic cells into the systemic circulation or surrounding lymphatics. This process may begin early in the life of the tumor and often increases with time. The time course for metastasis depends largely on the biology of the tumor. Breast cancer, for example, tends to metastasize very early. Not all of the shed cancer cells, or "seeds," result in a metastatic lesion. The "seed" must first find the appropriate "soil," or an environment suitable for growth.[13] This process is illustrated in the diverse patterns of metastasis that are characteristic of individual types of cancer. An example is prostate cancer, which commonly metastasizes to bone, but rarely to the brain.

The process of invasion and metastasis involves several essential steps. After neoplastic transformation, the malignant cells and surrounding host tissue secrete substances that stimulate the formation of new blood vessels to provide oxygen and nutrients. This process is known as *angiogenesis* or *neovascularization*.[14] Tumor cells must then detach from the primary mass and invade surrounding blood and lymph vessels. The tumor cells or cell aggregates detach and embolize through these vessels, but most do not survive circulation. The disseminated cells must then attach to the vascular endothelium. The cells may proliferate within the lumen of the vessel, but most commonly extravasate into the surrounding tissue. The local microenvironment may provide growth factors that can serve as "fertilizer" to potentiate the proliferation of the metastasis. At every step of the way, the potential metastatic cell must fight the host immune system. Last, the metastasis must again initiate angiogenesis to ensure continued growth and proliferation. Because angiogenesis has been recognized as a critical element in primary tumor growth as well as metastasis, it has become a target for development of new anticancer agents, which will be described later in the chapter. Figure 135–3 summarizes the functions acquired by a cell to survive as well as mechanisms by which the cancer cell achieves this function.[8]

DIAGNOSIS AND STAGING

SCREENING

❷ Because cancers are most curable with surgery or radiation before they have metastasized, early detection and treatment

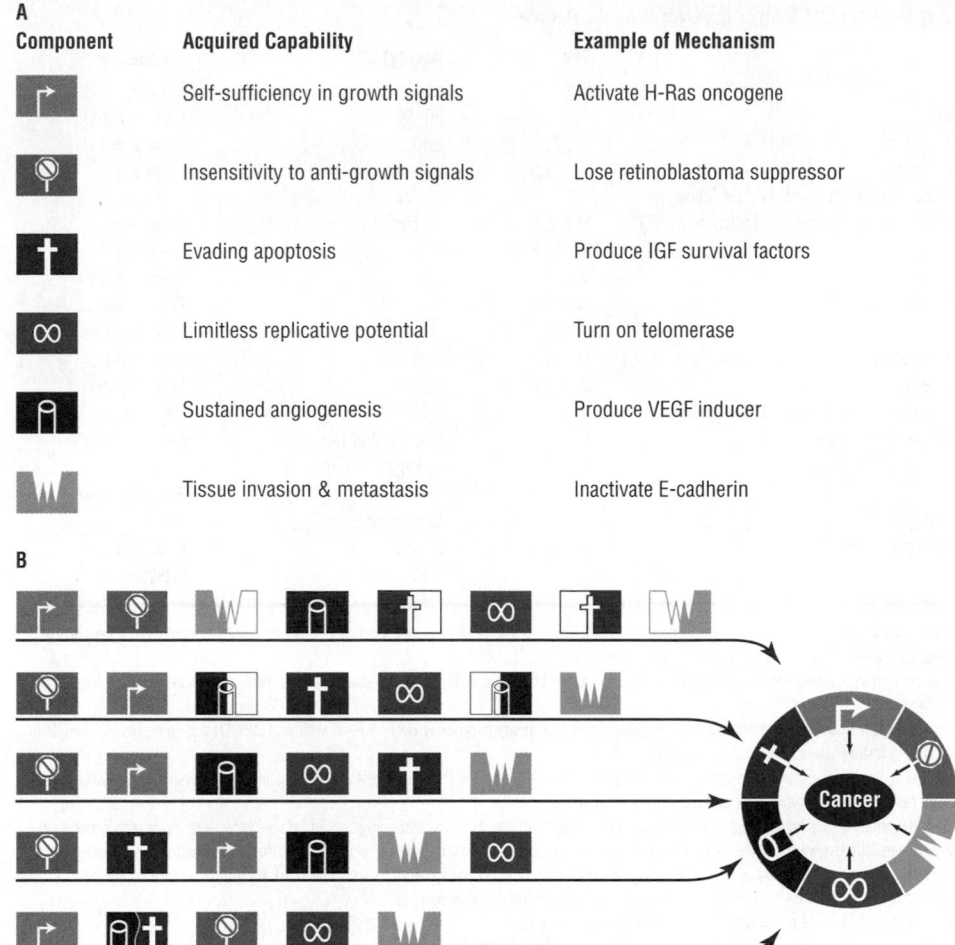

A

Component	Acquired Capability	Example of Mechanism
	Self-sufficiency in growth signals	Activate H-Ras oncogene
	Insensitivity to anti-growth signals	Lose retinoblastoma suppressor
	Evading apoptosis	Produce IGF survival factors
	Limitless replicative potential	Turn on telomerase
	Sustained angiogenesis	Produce VEGF inducer
	Tissue invasion & metastasis	Inactivate E-cadherin

B

FIGURE 135-3. The mechanisms of tumorigenesis exhibited by most cancers. (IGF, insulin-like growth factor; VEGF, vascular endothelial growth factor.) *(Reprinted from Cell, Vol 100(1), Hanahan D, Weinberg RA, The Hallmarks of Cancer, pages 57–70, Copyright © 2000, with permission from Elsevier.)*

have obvious potential benefits. In addition, small tumors are more responsive to chemotherapy, as discussed previously. Early diagnosis is difficult for many cancers because they do not produce clinical signs or symptoms until they have become large or have metastasized. Cancer screening programs are designed to detect signs of cancer in people who have not yet developed symptoms from cancer. Lack of effective screening methods for some cancers and inaccessibility of some anatomic sites further complicate the process. Other limitations of screening methods include false-negatives (related to the sensitivity of the test), false-positives (related to the specificity), and overdiagnosis (true positives that will not become clinically significant). For example, most abnormal tests identified by a screening mammography are false-positives, although the specificity of this screening method exceeds 90%. Education of the public on the early warning signs of common cancers is extremely important for facilitating early detection. Effective screening procedures exist for some cancers. The Papanicolaou (Pap) smear test, for example, is an effective tool to detect cervical cancer in its early stages. The American Cancer Society has published guidelines for routine screening examinations (Table 135–4).[15]

DIAGNOSIS

The presenting signs and symptoms of cancer vary widely and depend on the type of cancer. The presentation in adults may include any of cancer's seven warning signs (Table 135–5), as well as pain or loss of appetite.[16] The warning signs of cancer in children are different, and reflect the types of tumors more common in this

patient population (Table 135–6).[16] Even with increased public awareness, the fear of a cancer diagnosis can deter patients from seeking medical attention. The definitive diagnosis of cancer relies on the procurement of a sample of the tissue or cells suspected of malignancy and pathologic assessment of this sample. This sample can be obtained by numerous methods, including biopsy, exfoliative cytology, or fine-needle aspiration. A tissue diagnosis is essential, because many benign conditions can masquerade as cancer. Definitive treatment should not begin without a pathologic diagnosis.

STAGING AND WORKUP

❸ In addition to tissue diagnosis, tumors should be staged to determine the extent of disease before any definitive treatment is initiated. The process is dictated by knowledge of the biology of the tumor and by the signs and symptoms elicited in the history and physical examination. Staging provides information on prognosis and guides treatment selection. After treatment is implemented, the staging workup is usually repeated to evaluate the effectiveness of the treatment. Uniform staging criteria are important in clinical trials that evaluate cancer treatment regimens. Staging has been valuable in learning more about the biology of various tumor types. A staging workup may involve radiographs, computed tomography scans, magnetic resonance imaging, positron emission tomography scans, ultrasonograms, bone-marrow biopsies, bone scans, lumbar puncture, and a variety of laboratory tests, including appropriate tumor markers. Some cancers produce antigens or other substances that are characteristic of that particular cancer. These

TABLE 135-4 Screening Guidelines for Early Detection of Cancer in Asymptomatic People

Disease	Test or Procedure	Sex	Age (y)	Frequency
Breast cancer	Breast self-examination	F	≥20	Monthly[a]
	Clinical breast examination	F	20–39	Every 3 years
			≥40	Every year
	Mammography	F	≥40	Every year[b]
Colorectal cancer	One of the following examination schedules should be followed:			
	Fecal occult blood test (FOBT) or fecal immunochemical test (FIT)	M and F	50 and over	Every year
	Stool DNA test	M and F	≥50	Uncertain
	Flexible sigmoidoscopy	M and F	≥50	Every 5 years
	Annual FOBT or FIT and flexible sigmoidoscopy[c]	M and F	≥50	Every 5 years
	Colonoscopy	M and F	≥50	Every 10 years
	Computed tomography colonography	M and F	≥50	Every 5 years
	Double contrast barium enema	M and F	≥50	Every 5 years
Prostate cancer	Digital rectal exam and prostate-specific antigen (PSA) blood test	M	≥50	Every year[d]
Cervical cancer	Conventional pap test or liquid-based pap test	F	3 years after beginning vaginal intercourse	Every year[e]
				Every 2-3 years
Endometrial cancer	Information on risks and symptoms	F	Menopause	Once[f]
Cancer-related check-up	Health counseling and physical examination[g]	M and F	20–40	Every 3 years
			≥40	Every year

[a]Beginning in their early 20s, women should be told about the benefits and limitations of breast self-examination (BSE). The importance of prompt reporting of any new breast symptoms to a healthcare professional should be emphasized. It is acceptable for women to choose not to do BSE or to do BSE irregularly.

[b]Women at increased risk (e.g., family history, genetic tendency, or past breast cancer) should talk with their physician about benefits and limitations of starting earlier, having additional tests, or more frequent examinations.

[c]Flexible sigmoidoscopy together with FOBT or FIT is preferable to either test alone, although annual FOBT/FIT alone and flexible sigmoidoscopy every 5 years without FOBT/FIT has some benefit. People at moderate-to-high risk for colorectal cancer should discuss a different testing schedule with their physician.

[d]Healthcare providers should discuss the potential benefits and limitations of prostate cancer early detection testing with men and offer the PSA blood test and the digital rectal examination annually, beginning at age 50, to men who are at average risk of prostate cancer, and who have a life expectancy of at least 10 years.

[e]Cervical cancer screening should begin approximately 3 years after a woman begins having vaginal intercourse, but no later than age 21 years. Screening should be performed every year with conventional Pap tests or every 2 years using liquid-based Pap tests. At or after age 30 years, women who have had three normal test results in a row may get screened every 2 to 3 years with cervical cytology (either conventional or liquid-based Pap test) alone, or every 3 years with a human papillomavirus DNA test plus cervical cytology. Women aged 70+ years who have had three or more normal Pap tests and no abnormal Pap tests within the last 10 years and women who have undergone a total hysterectomy may choose to stop cervical cancer screening.

[f]Women with or at risk for hereditary nonpolyposis colon cancer should begin annual endometrial biopsy starting at age 35 years.

[g]To include examination for cancers of the mouth, thyroid, testicles, skin, lymph nodes, and ovaries, as well as health counseling about tobacco, sun exposure, diet and nutrition, risk factors, sexual practices, and environmental and occupational exposures.

From Smith et al.[15]

tumor markers are often nonspecific and may be elevated in many different cancer types, or in patients with nonmalignant diseases. As a result, tumor markers are generally more useful for monitoring response and detecting recurrence than as diagnostic tools. Examples are human chorionic gonadotropin and alfa-fetoprotein in patients with testicular cancer, or prostate-specific antigen in prostate cancer.[6]

The most commonly applied staging system for solid tumors is the TNM classification, where T = tumor, N = node, and M = metastases. A numerical value is assigned to each letter to indicate the size or extent of disease. The designated rating for tumor describes the size of the primary mass and ranges from T_1 to T_4. Carcinoma in situ is designated T_{is}. Nodes are described in terms of the extent of the spread of regional lymph nodal involvement (N_0 to N_3). Metastases are generally scored depending on their presence or absence (M_0 or M_1). To simplify the staging process, most cancers are classified according to the extent of disease by a numerical system involving stages I through IV. Stage I usually indicates localized tumor, stages II and III represent local and regional spread of disease, and stage IV denotes the presence of distant metastases. The assigned TNM rating translates into a particular stage classification. For example, $T_3 N_1 M_0$ describes a moderate-to-large-sized primary mass, with regional lymph node involvement and no distant metastases, and for most cancers is stage III. The criteria for classifying disease extent are quite specific for each different type of cancer.[17] For some tumors, such as prostate cancer, alternative alphabetical systems (stage A, B, C, or D) are used in clinical practice.

TABLE 135-5 Cancer's Seven Warning Signs

Change in bowel or bladder habits
A sore that does not heal
Unusual bleeding or discharge
Thickening or lump in breast or elsewhere
Indigestion or difficulty in swallowing
Obvious change in wart or mole
Nagging cough or hoarseness
If YOU have a warning signal, see your doctor!

American Cancer Society Study Communicating Cancer Information Through Mass Distribution Leaflets—an American Cancer Society Study. CA Cancer J Clin 1967;17:291–293.

TABLE 135-6 Cancer's Warning Signs in Children

Continued, unexplained weight loss
Headaches with vomiting in the morning
Increased swelling or persistent pain in bones or joints
Lump or mass in abdomen, neck, or elsewhere
Development of a whitish appearance in the pupil of the eye
Recurrent fevers not caused by infections
Excessive bruising or bleeding
Noticeable paleness or prolonged tiredness

Data from American Cancer Society. http://www.cancer.org/docroot/CRI/content/CRI_2_2_3x_Can_Childhood_Cancers_Be_Detected_Early.asp?sitearea=CRI.

TREATMENT

Modalities of Cancer Treatment

Four primary modalities are employed in the approach to cancer treatment: surgery, radiation, chemotherapy, and biologic therapy. The oldest of these is surgery, which plays a major role in the diagnosis and treatment of cancer. Surgery remains the treatment of choice for most solid tumors diagnosed in the early stages. Radiation therapy was first used for cancer treatment in the late 1800s and remains a mainstay in the management of cancer. Although very effective for treating many types of cancer, surgery and radiation are local treatments. These modalities are likely to produce a cure in patients with truly localized disease. But because most patients with cancer have micrometastatic or metastatic disease at diagnosis, localized therapies often fail to completely eliminate the cancer. In addition, systemic diseases such as leukemia cannot be treated with a localized modality. Chemotherapy and endocrine therapy access the systemic circulation and can theoretically treat the primary tumor and any metastatic disease. Biologic therapies (i.e., immunotherapy) are made from a living organism or its products and include antibodies, vaccines, growth factors and cytokines.

❹ Many solid tumors or lymphomas appear to be eliminated by surgery or radiation. However, the high incidence of later recurrence implies that the primary tumor began to metastasize before it was removed. Adjuvant therapy is defined as the use of systemic agents to eradicate micrometastatic disease following localized modalities such as surgery and/or radiation. The goal of adjuvant therapy is to reduce subsequent recurrence rates and prolong long-term survival. Thus, adjuvant therapy is given to patients with potentially curable malignancies who have no clinically detectable disease after surgery or radiation. Because adjuvant therapy is given at a time when the cancer is undetectable (i.e., no measurable disease), its effectiveness cannot be measured by response rates; instead, it is evaluated by recurrence rates and survival. The value of adjuvant therapy is best established in colorectal and breast cancers. Drug therapy may also be given in the neoadjuvant or preoperative setting. The goals in this instance are to make other treatment modalities more effective by reducing tumor burden and to destroy micrometastases. It is often used to reduce the size of the primary tumor and allow for a less invasive surgical procedure. Early stage breast cancer is a good example of the use of a combined-modality approach. The primary tumor is removed surgically, and radiation therapy is delivered to the remaining breast (after lumpectomy) or to the axilla (if there is marked lymph node involvement). Adjuvant therapy is then administered to eradicate any micrometastatic disease. Neoadjuvant therapy may sometimes be administered before definitive surgery to increase the likelihood of a tumor resection compared to a mastectomy.

The management of hematological malignancies also involves the use of combined modalities, but the terminology is different. Chemotherapy that is administered to eradicate the tumor cells from the bone marrow is called induction therapy. Once a complete remission (the disappearance of all signs of the cancer) is documented, additional therapy is administered. This therapy is called post-remission or consolidation therapy and is designed to eradicate any remaining disease, similar to adjuvant therapy for solid tumors. The additional therapy may include chemotherapy, a stem cell transplant or radiation therapy. Some treatment protocols also include maintenance therapy. This therapy is given to prevent the cancer from recurring and may include a combination of anticancer agents.

When anticancer therapy is administered to patients with local or regional disease, the treatment is often administered to cure the patient and may be labeled curative therapy. However, once the cancer has metastasized to distant sites, cure is usually not possible. Anticancer therapy administered to patients with metastatic disease can often slow the progression of cancer and prolong survival by months to years. Anticancer therapy administered to patients with terminal cancer with the goal of reducing symptoms is called palliative therapy. This therapy can lead to a prolongation in overall survival.

Principles of Drug Therapy

■ PURPOSES OF CHEMOTHERAPY

The era of modern cancer chemotherapy was born in 1941, when Goodman and Gilman first administered nitrogen mustard to patients with lymphoma.[18] Since then, numerous anticancer agents have been developed, and a variety of chemotherapy regimens have been investigated in every type of cancer. Table 135–7 lists tumors and their responsiveness to chemotherapy.[6,19] Cancer chemotherapy may be indicated as a curative or palliative. Treatment with chemotherapeutic agents is the primary curative modality for a few diseases, including leukemias, lymphomas, choriocarcinomas, and testicular cancer. Most solid tumors are not curable with chemotherapy alone, either because of the biology of the tumor or because of advanced disease at presentation. Chemotherapy in this setting is often initiated for palliative purposes. It is often possible to decrease tumor size or to retard growth enough to reduce untoward symptoms caused by the tumor.

TABLE 135–7	The Role of Chemotherapy in the Treatment of Cancer
Chemotherapy used alone with curative intent	
Acute lymphocytic leukemia	Acute myelogenous leukemia
Burkitt lymphoma	Diffuse large B-cell lymphoma
Hodgkin lymphoma	Testicular cancer
Choriocarcinoma (gestational trophoblastic neoplasm)	
Chemotherapy used as adjuvant therapy with curative intent	
Breast cancer	Colorectal cancer
Ewing sarcoma	Osteosarcoma
Wilms tumor	Ovarian cancer
Chemotherapy used as neoadjuvant therapy	
Anal carcinoma[a]	Bladder cancer
Breast cancer (locally advanced)[a]	Cervical cancer
Esophageal cancer	Head and neck cancers[a]
Osteosarcoma[a]	Rectal cancer
Soft tissue sarcoma[a]	
Chemotherapy used to palliate symptoms in advanced disease	
Bladder cancer[a]	Brain tumors
Breast cancer[a]	Carcinoid tumors
Cervical cancer	Chronic lymphocytic leukemia
Chronic myelogenous leukemia[a]	Colorectal cancer[a]
Endometrial cancer	Esophageal cancer
Gastric cancer	Head and neck cancers
Hairy cell leukemia[a]	Kaposi sarcoma
Indolent non-Hodgkin lymphomas	Metastatic melanoma
Multiple myeloma[a]	Mycosis fungoides
Neuroblastoma[a]	Non-small-cell lung cancer
Osteosarcoma	Ovarian cancer[a]
Pancreatic cancer	Prostate cancer
Small cell lung cancer[a]	Soft-tissue sarcoma
Chemotherapy has little or no effect on palliation	
Hepatocellular cancer	Renal cell carcinoma
Thyroid cancer	

[a]Significant increase in survival is achieved.
Data from Cotran et al.[6] *and Buick.*[19]

MOLECULAR AND CELLULAR BASIS FOR DRUG THERAPY

PRINCIPLES OF TUMOR GROWTH

The study of tumor growth forms the foundation for many of the basic principles of modern cancer chemotherapy. The growth of most tumors is illustrated by the gompertzian tumor growth curve (Fig. 135–4).[6,19,20] Gompertz was an insurance actuary who described the relationship between age and expected death. This mathematical model also approximates tumor cell proliferation. In the early stages, tumor growth is exponential, which means that the tumor takes a constant amount of time to double its size. During this early phase, a large portion of the tumor cells is actively dividing. This population of cells is called the *growth fraction*. The doubling time, or time required for the tumor to double in size, is very short. Because most anticancer agents have greater effect on rapidly dividing cells, tumors are most sensitive to the effects of chemotherapy when the tumor is small and the growth fraction is high. However, as the tumor grows, the doubling time is slowed.[19,20] The growth fraction is decreased, probably owing to the tumor outgrowing its blood and nutrient supply or the inability of blood and nutrients to diffuse throughout the tumor mass. Wide variability exists in measured doubling times for different cancers. The doubling time of most solid tumors is about 2 to 3 months. However, some tumors have doubling times of only days (e.g., aggressive non-Hodgkin lymphomas) and others have even longer doubling times (e.g., some salivary gland tumors).[6]

Figure 135–4 also illustrates the impact of tumor burden. It takes about 10^9 cancer cells (1-g mass, 1 cm in diameter) for a tumor to be clinically detectable by palpation or radiography. Such a tumor has undergone about 30 doublings in cell number. It only takes 10 additional doublings for this 1 g mass to reach 1 kg in size. A tumor possessing 10^{12} cancer cells (1-kg mass) is considered lethal. Thus, a tumor is clinically undetectable for most of its life span. Tumor burden also impacts response to chemotherapy. The cell kill hypothesis states that a certain percentage of cancer cells (not a certain number of cells) will be killed with each course of chemotherapy. For example, if a tumor consists of 1,000 cancer cells and

the chemotherapy regimen kills 90% of the cells, then 10% or 100 cancer cells remain. The second chemotherapy course kills another 90% of cells, and again only 10% or 10 cells remain. According to this hypothesis, the tumor burden will never reach zero. Tumors consisting of less than 10^4 cells are believed to be small enough for elimination by host factors, including immunologic mechanisms, and these factors must be in place for a cure to be possible. The limitations of this theory are that it assumes all cancers are equally responsive and that resistance to anticancer agents and metastases do not occur.[1,6,19,20]

TUMOR PROLIFERATION

Both cancer cells and normal cells reproduce in a series of steps known as the cell cycle as described earlier in the chapter. Figure 135–5 depicts the cell cycle and the phases of activity for commonly used anticancer agents.[19,20]

5 All cancer cells do not proliferate faster than normal cells; some cancer cells reproduce more rapidly while others are more indolent. Many anticancer agents target rapidly proliferating cells (both normal and cancerous cells), and these agents may act at selective or multiple sites of the cell cycle. Agents with major activity in a particular phase of the cell cycle are known as cell-cycle phase-specific agents. For example, antimetabolites exert their major effect during the S phase. Cell-cycle phase-specific agents may also be active to a lesser extent in other phases of the cycle. Cell-cycle phase-nonspecific agents are those with significant activity in multiple phases. Alkylating agents, such as nitrogen mustards, are examples of a cell-cyle non-specific agent. In many cases, the cytotoxic effects of an agent may result from interactions with other intracellular activities and are not related to specific cell-cycle events. Hormones are an example of this type of anticancer drug.

Knowledge of cell-cycle specificity has been applied to the scheduling of chemotherapy administration. By definition, cell-cycle phase-specific agents exert their major activity when cells are in a particular phase of the cell cycle. At any given time, the heterogeneous cell populations within a tumor are at various phases in the cell cycle. By giving cell-cycle phase-specific agents as a continuous infusion or in multiple repeated fractions, clinicians can theoretically target

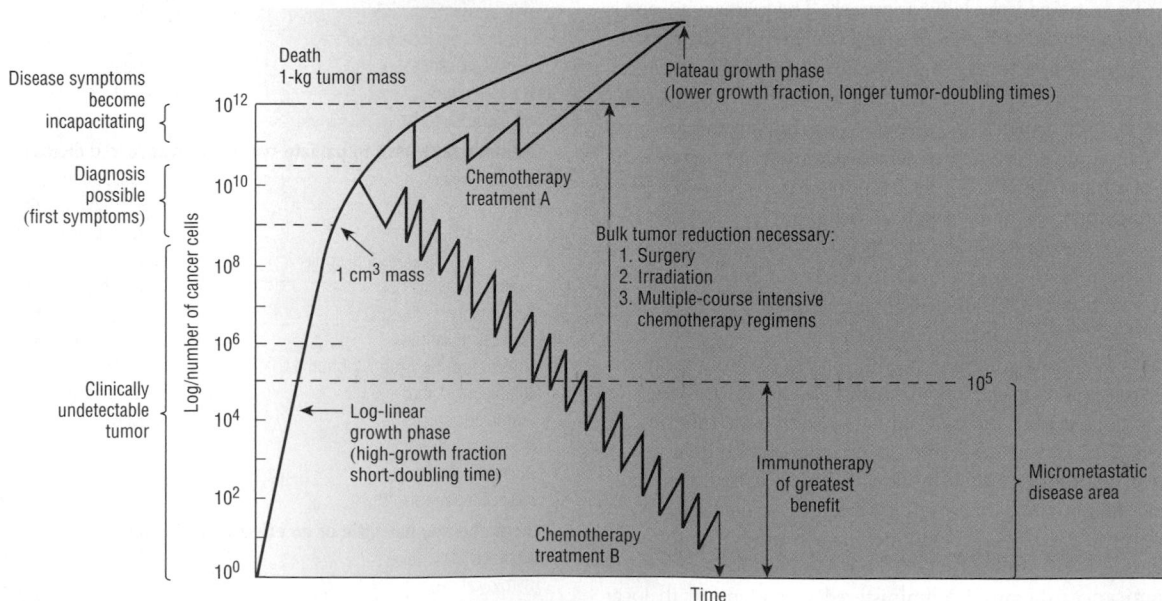

FIGURE 135-4. Gompertzian kinetics tumor-growth curve: relationship to symptoms, diagnosis, and various treatment regimens. (*Reproduced with permission from Buick.[19]*)

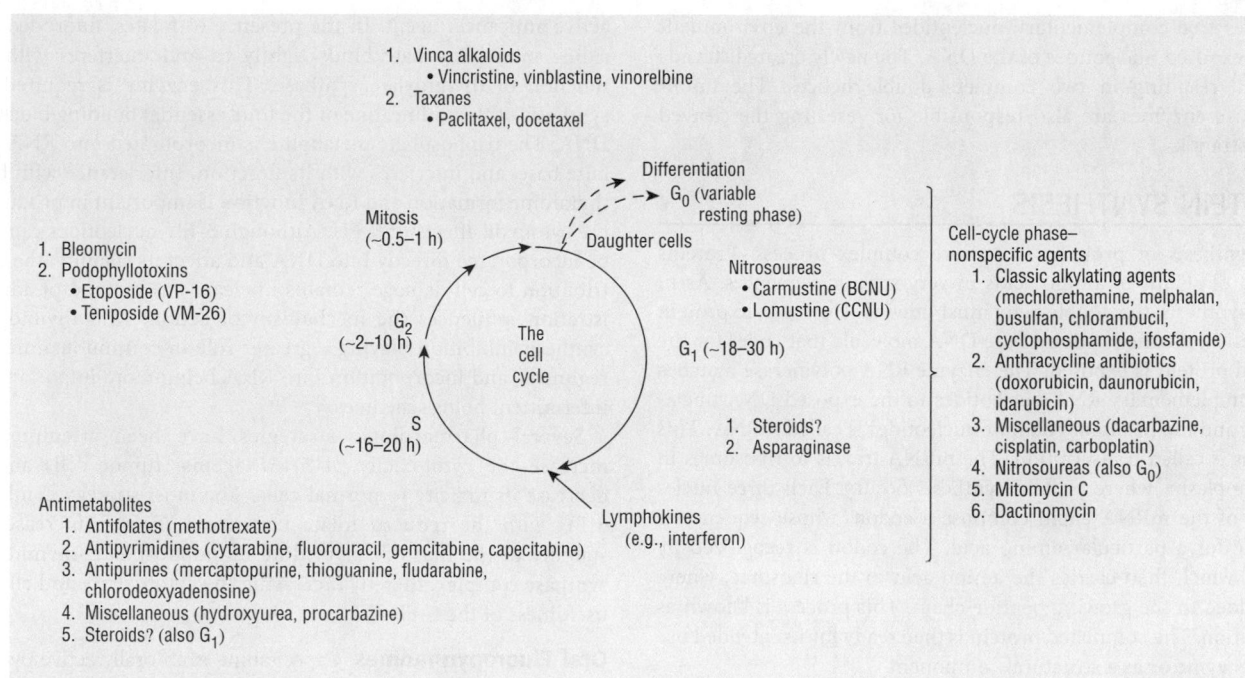

1. Vinca alkaloids
   • Vincristine, vinblastine, vinorelbine
2. Taxanes
   • Paclitaxel, docetaxel

Mitosis (~0.5–1 h)

Differentiation

G_0 (variable resting phase)

Daughter cells

1. Bleomycin
2. Podophyllotoxins
   • Etoposide (VP-16)
   • Teniposide (VM-26)

G_2 (~2–10 h)

The cell cycle

G_1 (~18–30 h)

S (~16–20 h)

Nitrosoureas
   • Carmustine (BCNU)
   • Lomustine (CCNU)

1. Steroids?
2. Asparaginase

Cell-cycle phase–nonspecific agents
1. Classic alkylating agents (mechlorethamine, melphalan, busulfan, chlorambucil, cyclophosphamide, ifosfamide)
2. Anthracycline antibiotics (doxorubicin, daunorubicin, idarubicin)
3. Miscellaneous (dacarbazine, cisplatin, carboplatin)
4. Nitrosoureas (also G_0)
5. Mitomycin C
6. Dactinomycin

Antimetabolites
1. Antifolates (methotrexate)
2. Antipyrimidines (cytarabine, fluorouracil, gemcitabine, capecitabine)
3. Antipurines (mercaptopurine, thioguanine, fludarabine, chlorodeoxyadenosine)
4. Miscellaneous (hydroxyurea, procarbazine)
5. Steroids? (also G_1)

Lymphokines (e.g., interferon)

FIGURE 135-5. Cell-cycle activity for anticancer drugs. Cell-cycle phase-specific agents appear to be most active during a particular phase, but may also be active in another phase. Cell-cycle phase-nonspecific agents may have greater activity in one phase than another, but not to the degree of cell-cycle (phase)-specific agents. In many cases, it is likely that drug cytotoxicity involves multiple intracellular sites of action and may not be linked to specific cell-cycle events.

more cells as they progress into the agent's sensitive phase. Thus cell-cycle phase-specific agents are also termed *schedule dependent*. In contrast, cell-cycle phase-nonspecific agent are active in many phases, and consequently are not schedule dependent. The activity of these agents depend on the dose, and these agent are termed *dose dependent*.

MOLECULAR BIOLOGY

Because many anticancer agents interfere with the cellular synthesis of DNA, RNA, and proteins, it is important to review the basic principles of molecular biology.[3] Each normal human cell contains 46 chromosomes, which are composed of DNA (deoxyribonucleic acid). DNA carries hereditary information in units called genes. A single chromosome can contain 20,000 or more genes. Genes code for specific proteins that regulate cellular activity and inherited traits (some of which affect carcinogenesis and cancer growth, as well as the efficacy and metabolism of anticancer drugs). The genetic information is encoded in DNA by precise sequencing of subunits known as nucleotides. Each nucleotide consists of a sugar (deoxyribose), phosphoric acid, and a base. Four bases exist in DNA: adenine, thymine, guanine, and cytosine. Adenine and guanine are purine-type bases; thymine and cytosine are pyrimidine-type bases (Fig. 135–6). These nucleotides are connected linearly to form a chain. Each DNA molecule is made up of two chains of nucleotides, which wind around each other to form a double helix. The two strands are held together by chemical bonding between the bases. The bonding process is very specific—adenine binds only with thymine, and guanine binds only with cytosine. This is known as complementary base pairing. RNA is important in the DNA-directed synthesis of proteins or enzymes. RNA differs from DNA in that it is composed of a single strand of nucleotides, the sugar is ribose, and the base uracil is substituted for thymine. There are three known types of RNA: messenger RNA (mRNA), transfer RNA (tRNA), and ribosomal RNA (rRNA).

DNA SYNTHESIS

During the DNA synthesis phase, which takes place in the cell nucleus, the DNA unwinds and exposes its nucleotides. When DNA unwinds for replication or protein synthesis, only the portion of the molecule containing the needed nucleotides needs to be exposed. Rather than unwinding the entire strand, topoisomerase I and II enzymes cleave the DNA strands to facilitate unwinding of the section that is needed. The enzyme DNA polymerase

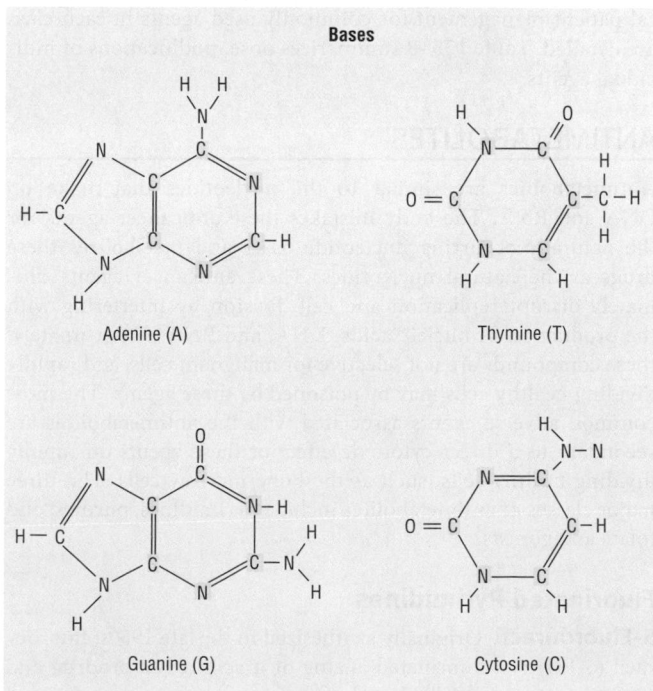

Bases

Adenine (A)

Thymine (T)

Guanine (G)

Cytosine (C)

FIGURE 135-6. Structures of DNA constituents.

matches free complementary nucleotides from the environment to the exposed nucleotides of the DNA. The newly created strands rewind, resulting in two complete double helices. The topoisomerase enzymes are also responsible for resealing the cleaved DNA strands.

PROTEIN SYNTHESIS

The synthesis of proteins is a more complex process. Proteins consist of chains of amino acids in very specific sequences. As in DNA synthesis, the double helix must unwind. However, in protein synthesis, only the portion of the DNA molecule that codes for the desired protein is exposed. The enzyme RNA polymerase matches free complementary RNA nucleotides to the exposed DNA nucleotides, and the resultant chain of nucleotides is called mRNA. This process is called transcription. The mRNA travels to ribosomes in the cytoplasm, where protein synthesis occurs. Each three nucleotides of the mRNA chain compose a codon, whose sequence is specific for a particular amino acid. The codon is recognized by tRNA, which then carries the amino acid to the ribosome, where it is added to the growing peptide chain. This process is known as translation. The completed protein is then ready for its intended use as an enzyme or as a structural component.

CLINICAL PHARMACOLOGY OF CHEMOTHERAPY AND ENDOCRINE AGENTS

Anticancer agents are commonly categorized by their mechanism of action or by their origin. Alkylating agents exert their effects on DNA and protein synthesis by binding to DNA and preventing the unwinding of the DNA molecule. Antimetabolites resemble naturally occurring nuclear structural components ("metabolites"), such as the nucleotide bases, or inhibit enzymes involved in the synthesis of DNA and proteins. Antitumor antibiotics derive their name from their source; they are fermentation products of *Streptomyces* species. Figure 135–7 shows the sites of action of common categories of anticancer agents. The following section addresses these and other classes of agents used in the treatment of cancer. The clinical uses, mechanisms, side effects, and practical patient management for commonly used agents in each class are detailed. Table 135–8 summarizes dose modifications of individual agents.

ANTIMETABOLITES

Antimetabolites are similar to the nucleotides that make up DNA and RNA. The body mistakes these anticancer agents for the naturally occurring nucleotide bases and metabolizes these drugs as the natural nucleotides. These anticancer agents ultimately disrupt replication and cell division by interfering with the production of nucleic acids, DNA, and RNA. Unfortunately, these compounds are not selective for malignant cells, and rapidly dividing healthy cells may be poisoned by these agents. The most common adverse events associated with the antimetabolites are secondary to a direct cytotoxic effect of these agents on rapidly dividing healthy cells, such as the bone marrow cells. The three major classes of antimetabolites include pyrimidines, purines, and folate antagonists.

Fluorinated Pyrimidines

5-Fluorouracil Originally synthesized in the late 1950s, fluorouracil (5-FU) is a fluorinated analog of uracil. It is a prodrug and undergoes sequential phosphorylation to a mono-, di- and triphsophate similar to natural nucleotide bases to become an active anticancer agent. In the presence of folates, fluorodeoxyuridine monophosphate binds tightly to and interferes with the function of thymidylate synthase. This enzyme is required for synthesis of thymidine, one of the four essential building blocks of DNA. The triphosphate metabolite is incorporated into RNA as a false base, and interferes with its function. Interference with both thymidine formation and RNA function is important in producing the cytotoxic effects of 5-FU. Although 5-FU nucleotides can also be incorporated directly into DNA and affect its stability, the contribution to cell damage remains unclear. The method of administration influences the mechanism of action, with thymidylate synthesis inhibition playing a greater role in continuous-infusion regimens, and incorporation into RNA being more important for intermittent bolus schedules.[21]

Several pharmacologic strategies have been attempted to increase the cytotoxicity of 5-FU against tumor cells and to decrease its toxicity to normal cells. The most strategy combines 5-FU with the reduced folate leucovorin. Folates increase the stability of the fluorodeoxyuridine monophosphate–thymidylate synthase complex, thereby increasing the cytotoxicity and clinical usefulness of the 5-FU.[21]

Oral Fluoropyrimidines Capecitabine is an orally active pyrimidine analog of uracil and is a prodrug of 5-FU. Because capecitabine is enzymatically converted to 5-FU, it shares the same mechanisms of action. It generates higher levels of 5-FU selectively within some tumors compared with healthy tissues. Because chronic twice-daily oral dosing of capecitabine produces sustained 5-FU levels similar to continuous intravenous infusions of 5-FU, the toxicity pattern is similar to that of 5-FU infusions.[21,22]

The most common toxicities of fluoropyrmidines include neutropenia, thrombocytopenia, and anemia when administered as an IV bolus administration and hand–foot syndrome and diarrhea when administered as a continuous IV infusion.[21,22]

Cytidine Analogs

Cytarabine Cytarabine (ara-C) is an arabinose analog of cytosine. Ara-C is phosphorylated to its active triphosphate form (ara-CTP) within tumor cells and ara-CTP inhibits DNA polymerase, an enzyme responsible for strand elongation. It is also incorporated directly into DNA, where it inhibits the replication of DNA and acts as a chain terminator to prevent DNA elongation. Deaminase enzymes, particularly cytidine deaminase, degrades ara-C to an inactive form ara-U.[21,23]

Cytidine deaminase levels are very low in the CNS. Cytotoxic concentrations are maintained in the CNS for several hours after intrathecal administration of traditional cytarabine formulations, and for more than 2 weeks following administration of a depot formulation.

The toxicity of cytarabine is dose dependent. The most characteristic toxicity of high-dose ara-C (>1 g/m^2 per dose) is a cerebellar syndrome of dysarthria, nystagmus, and ataxia. Risk of CNS toxicity is strongly correlated with advanced age and renal dysfunction. Renal insufficiency permits accumulation of high levels of ara-CTP, which is believed to be neurotoxic. Hepatic dysfunction, high cumulative doses, and bolus dosing may also increase the risks of neurotoxicity.[21,23]

Gemcitabine Gemcitabine is a fluorine-substituted deoxycytidine analog related structurally to cytarabine. Its activation and mechanism of action are similar to those of cytarabine. Gemcitabine is incorporated into DNA, where it inhibits DNA polymerase activity. It also inhibits ribonucleotide reductase, which is the enzyme required to convert ribonucleotides into the deoxyribonucleotide forms needed for both DNA synthesis and

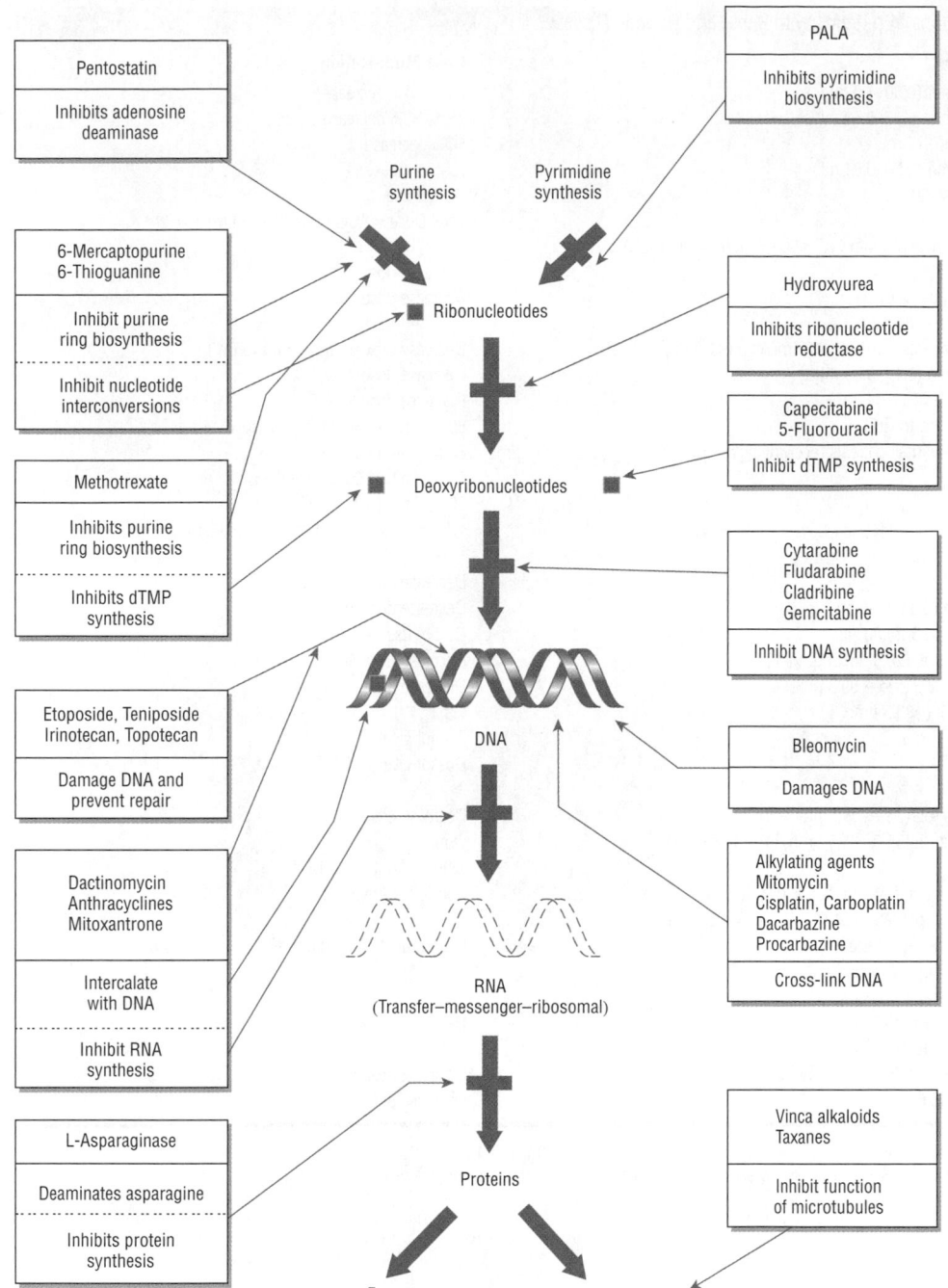

FIGURE 135-7. Mechanisms of action of commonly used anticancer agents. (dTMP, deoxythymidylic acid; PALA, N-phosphonacetyl-ʟ-aspartate.) *(From Chabner BA, Amrein PC, Druker BJ, et al. Antineoplastic agents. In: Brunton LL, Lazo JS, Parker KL, eds. Goodman & Gilman's The Pharmacologic Basis of Therapeutics, 11th ed. New York: McGraw-Hill, 2006:1319.)*

repair. Compared with cytarabine, gemcitabine achieves intracellular concentrations about 20 times higher than does ara-C, secondary to increased penetration of cell membranes, and greater affinity for the activating enzyme deoxycytidine kinase. Gemcitabine that is incorporated into DNA has a prolonged intracellular half-life. Its stereoconfiguration causes another normal base pair to be added next to the fraudulent gemcitabine base pair in the DNA strand. This "masked chain termination" protects the gemcitabine from excision and elimination.[21,23]

Azacytidine and Decitabine Azacytidine was approved in 2004 and decitabine in 2006 for the treatment of patients with myelodysplastic syndrome, a disorder of hematopoietic cell maturation that can progress to acute myeloid leukemia. Both of these agents are nucleoside analogs, and they are believed to exert their pharmacodynamic effects by direct incorporation into DNA and inhibition of DNA methyltransferase, which cause hypomethylation of DNA.[24] Cellular differentiation, and apoptosis are believed to result from this effect. The cytotoxicity of these agents may also be attributed to the formation of covalent adducts between DNA methyltransferase and active drug being incorporated into DNA, particularly in cells actively dividing. Hypomethylation of DNA also appears to normalize the function of genes that control cell differentiation and proliferation, promoting normal cell maturation.[24]

These agents have demonstrated efficacy in slowing the progression of myelodysplastic syndrome to acute myelogenous leukemia, reducing transfusion requirements and allowing for the improvement of normal hematopoiesis over time. The primary toxicity is myelosuppression, particularly during early phases of treatment

TABLE 135-8 Empiric Dose Modifications in patients with Renal and Hepatic Disease[a]

Agent	Organ Dysfunction	Dose Modification
Bleomycin	CrCl = 30–60 mL/min (0.50–1.0 mL/s)	25%–50% decrease
	CrCl = 10–30 mL/min (0.17–0.50 mL/s)	25%–50% decrease
	CrCl <10 mL/min (<0.17 mL/s)	50% decrease
Capecitabine	CrCl = 30–50 mL/min (0.50–0.84 mL/s)	25% decrease
	CrCl <30 ml/min (<0.50 mL/s)	Do not use
Carboplatin	Renal insufficiency	Total Dose = AUC × (CrCl [in mL/min] + 25)
Cisplatin	Use with caution in patients with CrCl <50 mL/min (<0.84 mL/s)	
Cyclophosphamide	Renal failure	Decrease dose 25%
Etoposide	Decrease in proportion to CrCl:	Decrease dose 25%
	15–50 mL/min (0.25–0.84 mL/s)	
Fludarabine, hydroxyurea	Use in caution in patients with CrCl <60 mL/min (<1.0 mL/s)	Decrease dose in proportion to CrCl
Ifosfamide	CrCl = 10–50 mL/min (0.17–0.84 mL/s)	Decrease dose 25%
	CrCl = <10 mL/min (<0.17 mL/s)	Decrease dose 50%
Methotrexate	Decrease in proportion to CrCl	80 mL/min (1.34 mL/s)–full dose
	Monitor levels closely in all patients receiving high-dose therapy (e.g., ≥150 mg/m²)	80 mL/min (1.34 mL/s)–75%
		60 mL/min (1.00 mL/s)–63%
		50 mL/min (0.84 mL/s)–56%
		< 50 mL/min (< 0.84 mL/s)–use alternative chemotherapy
Pentostatin	Dose in proportion to CrCl	
Streptozocin	Renal Failure	Decrease dose 50%–75%
Topotecan	CrCl 20–39 mL/min (0.33–0.65 mL/s)	Decrease dose 50%
	CrCl <20 ml/min (<0.33 mL/s)	Do not use
Anthracyclines	Bilirubin 1.2–3.0 mg/dL (20.5– 51.3 μmol/L)	Decrease dose 50%
	Bilirubin 3.1–5.0 mg/dL (53.0– 85.5 μmol/L)	Decrease dose 75%
	Bilirubin >5.0 mg/dL (>85.5 μmol/L)	Omit
Docetaxel	Bilirubin > ULN	Do not give
	AST or ALT >1.5 ULN and	Do not give
	Alk Phos >2.5 ULN	
Etoposide	Bilirubin 1.5–3.0 mg/dL (25.7– 51.3 μmol/L)	Decrease dose 50%
	Bilirubin 3.1–5.0 mg/dL (53.0– 85.5 μmol/L)	Omit
Imatinib	Bilirubin >3 × ULN	Withhold until <1.5 ULN
Ixabepilone	As a monotherapy agent if AST or ALT >10 × ULN or bilirubin >3 × ULN	Contraindicated
	In combination with capecitabine AST or ALT >2.5 × ULN or bilirubin >1 × ULN	
Lapatinib	Child–Pugh class C hepatic dysfunction	Dose reduction to 750 mg/day
Paclitaxel	Use with caution in hepatic failure	
Thiotepa	Use with caution in hepatic failure	
Vinblastine, vincristine	Bilirubin 1.5–3.0 mg/dL (25.7–51.3 μmol/L)	Decrease dose 50%
	Bilirubin 3.1–5.0 mg/dL (53.0–85.5 μmol/L)	Omit
Vinorelbine	Bilirubin 2.1–3.0 mg/dL (35.9–51.3 μmol/L)	Decrease dose 50%
	Bilirubin >3 mg/dL (51.3 μmol/L)	Decrease dose 75%

CrCl, creatinine clearance; ULN, upper limit of normal laboratory values. Renal failure: creatinine clearance <25 mL/min (<0.42 mL/s).

[a]Only approximate guidelines can be given. See text for explanations and limitations. Consult current references prior to dispensing as not all dose adjustments are provided in the table.

Adapted from Chabner[1] and Prescribing Information package inserts.

as the malignant clone driving myelodysplastic syndrome is cleared from the bone marrow and normal hematopoiesis is slowly restored. As a result, infectious complications occur frequently.

Purines and Purine Antimetabolites

Mercaptopurine and Thioguanine 6-Mercaptopurine (MP) was the first purine analog to be used in cancer chemotherapy. Thioguanine is the two-amino analog of 6-MP. Both agents are rapidly converted to ribonucleotides that inhibit purine biosynthesis. They also undergo purine interconversion reactions needed to supply purine precursors for synthesis of nucleic acids. Clinical cross-resistance is generally observed.[21] Both anticancer agents are metabolized by thiopurine methyltransferase (TPMT) and hypoxanthine phosphoribosyl transferase to produce multiple metabolites responsible for the efficacy, hepatic toxicity and myelosuppression associated with these agents. Genetic polymorphsims of TPMT are associated with reduced enzyme activity and decreased tolerance of standard doses of 6-MP.

MP depends on xanthine oxidase for an initial oxidation step. Its metabolism is markedly decreased by concomitant administration of the xanthine oxidase inhibitor allopurinol, and serious toxicity may result. Oral MP doses must be reduced when allopurinol is administered together with 6-MP.[21]

Fludarabine Monophosphate Fludarabine monophosphate is an analog of the purine adenine. Like cytarabine, fludarabine interferes with DNA polymerase, causing chain termination. Fludarabine also incorporates into RNA, resulting in inhibited transcription. The usual dose-limiting toxicity is myelosuppression. Fludarabine is also immunosuppressive, with associated opportunistic infections resulting from fludarabine's effect on T cells and a subsequent decrease in CD4 counts; prophylactic antibiotics and antiviral medications are recommended and should continue until CD4 counts normalize.[21,25]

Cladribine and Pentostatin Cladribine and pentostatin are purine nucleoside analogs with slightly different mechanisms of action. Cladribine is resistant to inactivation by adenosine deaminase and triphosphorylated to an active form that is incorporated into DNA, resulting in inhibition of DNA synthesis and early chain termination. Cladribine's antitumor activity is unusual for an antimetabolite in that it affects both actively dividing and resting cancer cells. Pentostatin is a potent inhibitor of adenosine deaminase. Adenosine deaminase is an enzyme critical in purine base metabolism and is found in high concentrations in lymphatic tissue. Like fludarabine, these agents possess immunosuppressive effects that place patients at risk for serious opportunistic infections.[21,23]

Antifolates

Folate vitamins are essential cofactors in DNA synthesis. They carry one-carbon groups in transfer reactions that are required for purine and thymidylic acid synthesis, and, in turn, for formation of DNA and for cell division. Natural folates circulating in the blood have a single glutamic acid group, but within cells they are converted to polyglutamates, which are more efficient cofactors and preferentially retained inside the cells.[26]

Dietary folates must be chemically reduced to their tetrahydro forms, with four hydrogens on the pteridine ring, to be active. The enzyme responsible for this reduction is dihydrofolate reductase (DHFR), a key enzyme whose actions are inhibited by methotrexate and other antifolates. The result of this inhibition is depletion of intracellular pools of reduced folates (tetrahydrofolates) essential for thymidylate and purine synthesis. Lack of either thymidine or purines prevents synthesis of DNA. The DHFR-mediated effects of antifolate drugs on normal and probably also on cancerous cells may be neutralized by supplying reduced folates exogenously. The reduced folate used clinically for "rescue" is leucovorin (folinic acid), which bypasses the metabolic block induced by DHFR inhibitors.[26]

Methotrexate The folic acid analog methotrexate (MTX) is the best understood of all drugs in the broad category of antimetabolites. It has been in clinical use for more than 50 years. Like physiologic folates, MTX is transported intracellularly by an active transport system. In high doses, passive diffusion may overcome tumor cell resistance caused by saturated active transport systems. Resistance to the antifolates can also be caused by amplification of DHFR. Other potential causes of resistance are slow rates of thymidylate synthesis, decreased affinity of DHFR for MTX, and lack of polyglutamation within tumor cells. Polyglutamated forms of folates are better retained within cells. Malignant cells may achieve greater MTX polyglutamate levels than normal cells, which may, in part, explain the selective effects of MTX on malignant versus normal cells.[26]

Accurate and readily available assays for serum MTX levels have made therapeutic drug monitoring of MTX a valuable clinical tool. The threshold for cytotoxic effects of MTX is approximately 0.02 mg/L (50 nmol/L). Toxicity and efficacy relates not only to peak concentrations, but more importantly, to time that concentrations remain above this threshold level. For MTX doses requiring leucovorin rescue (generally doses greater than 1,000 mg/m^2), leucovorin must be administered until levels fall below 0.02 mg/L (50 nmol/L). Therapeutic drug monitoring is also an effective means of increasing the likelihood of therapeutic success, by individualizing doses based on target levels.[26]

Pemetrexed Pemetrexed is a multitargeted antifolate that inhibits at least three biosynthetic pathways in thymidine and purine synthesis. In addition to inhibition of DHFR, it also inhibits thymidine synthase and glycinamide ribonucleotide formyltransferase, decreasing the risk of the development of drug resistance. Severe hematologic toxicity and deaths associated with neutropenic sepsis have been reported in clinical trials with pemetrexed. Elevated baseline cystathionine or homocysteine concentrations correlated with this unexpected toxicity. Routine supplementation of folic acid and vitamin B$_{12}$ lowers levels of these substances and lowers the risk of mortality related to neutropenic sepsis. The approved labeling of pemetrexed requires administration of folic acid and vitamin B$_{12}$ throughout the duration of treatment.[18,26]

Antifolates are associated with neutropenia and thrombocytopenia, mucositis, and nausea and vomiting. Renal tubular necrosis is seen with high-dose MTX therapy and vigorous hydration with or without alkalinization of the urine necessary to decrease risk of renal failure.

MICROTUBULE-TARGETING DRUGS

Vinca Alkaloids

Vincristine, vinblastine, and vinorelbine are natural alkaloids derived from the periwinkle (vinca) plant. They act as mitotic inhibitors, or "spindle poisons." Although the alkaloids are very similar structurally, they have different activities and patterns of toxicity. Vinorelbine and vinblastine are associated with dose-limiting myelosuppression, whereas vincristine causes mild myelosuppressive effects but is more neurotoxic.

Vinca alkaloids bind to tubulin, the structural protein that polymerizes to form microtubules. These are the hollow tubes that make up the mitotic spindle and that are also important in nerve conduction and neurotransmission. Vinca alkaloids disrupt the normal balance between polymerization and depolymerization of microtubules, inhibiting assembly of microtubules and disrupting microtubule dynamics. This interferes with formation of the mitotic spindle and causes cells to accumulate in mitosis. They also disturb a variety of microtubule-related processes in cells, and induce apoptosis. Resistance to the vinca alkaloids develops primarily from P-glycoprotein (Pgp)–mediated multidrug resistance, which decreases drug accumulation and retention within tumor cells.[27]

Taxanes

Paclitaxel and docetaxel are taxane plant alkaloids with antimitotic activity. Paclitaxel was isolated from the bark of the Pacific yew tree, *Taxus brevifolia*, but is now produced semisynthetically from the needles of the European yew, *Taxus baccata*. Docetaxel is a semisynthetic taxoid extracted from 10-deacetyl baccatin III, a noncytotoxic precursor found in the renewable needle biomass of yew plants.[27]

Paclitaxel and docetaxel both act by binding to tubulin, but unlike the vincas, they do not interfere with tubulin assembly. Instead, the taxanes promote microtubule assembly and therefore interfere with microtubule disassembly. They induce tubulin polymerization, resulting in formation of inappropriately stable, nonfunctional microtubules. The stability of the microtubules damages cells, because the dynamics of microtubule-dependent structures required for mitosis and other cellular functions are disrupted. Taxanes also have some nonmitotic actions that can promote cancer cell death, such as inhibition of angiogenesis. Resistance to the antitumor effects of the taxanes is attributable to alterations in tubulin or tubulin binding sites, or to Pgp multidrug resistance. Although paclitaxel and docetaxel have very similar mechanisms of action, cross-resistance between the two agents is incomplete.[27] Myelosuppression is common with both agents but other adverse effects can differ. Increased fluid retention is seen with docetaxel, whereas increased neurotoxicity and hypersensitivity reactions are seen with paclitaxel.[18,27] Both agents require premedications with corticosteroids; paclitaxel also requires antihistamines to decrease the likelihood of allergic reactions.

To circumvent the hypersensitivity reactions with paclitaxel, and possibly increase its efficacy, paclitaxel was formulated to be bound to albumin (nab-paclitaxel). This new dosage form is devoid of the Cremophor excipient that is believed to mediate the hypersensitivity reactions and exacerbate myelosuppression with the conventional formulation. This formulation appears to be selectively activated by tumor cells to the active paclitaxel compound.[28] In comparative clinical trials, this novel compound has shown comparable activity to the conventional formulation of paclitaxel with a lower incidence of hypersensitivity reactions. Peripheral neuropathies remain a common adverse effect with this formulation.

Epothilones

Similar to the taxanes, the epothilones work in the M phase of the cell cycle. Epothilone binding to microtubules is distinct from taxanes with activity demonstrated in paclitaxel-resistant cell lines.[29] Epothilones appear to be poor substrates for Pgp and their cytotoxicity is not affected by its overexpression. Natural epothilones are macrolide derivatives that have stability and pharmacokinetic problems. Synthetic agents have been developed with the first agent, ixabepilone, approved for the treatment of metastatic breast cancer. Toxicities are similar to taxanes; premedication with antihistamines are required, although no corticosteroid is administered unless the patient experiences an allergic reaction to a previous dose.

Estramustine

Estramustine is an unusual drug because it structurally combines the alkylating agent nor-nitrogen mustard with the hormone estradiol.[18] It was designed with the intent that the estradiol portion of the molecule would facilitate uptake of the alkylating agent into hormone-sensitive prostate cancer cells. Despite the inclusion of an alkylator, estramustine does not function in vivo as an alkylating agent. Estrogens are released after its administration and are responsible for most of the toxicity of estramustine, but are not believed to contribute to its cytotoxic effect. In the mid 1980s, estramustine was redefined as an antimicrotubule agent. It binds covalently to microtubule-associated proteins that are part of the structural support for microtubules. The binding causes the separation of microtubule-associated proteins from the microtubules, inhibiting microtubule assembly and eventually causing their disassembly.[18]

TOPOISOMERASE INHIBITORS

Topoisomerases are essential enzymes involved in maintaining DNA topologic structure during replication and transcription. DNA topoisomerase enzymes relieve torsional strain during DNA unwinding by producing strand breaks. They cleave DNA strands and form intermediates with the strands, producing a gap through which DNA strands can pass, then reseal the strand breaks. Topoisomerase I produces single-strand breaks; topoisomerase II produces double-strand breaks.[30] Several important anticancer agents target topoisomerase enzymes: camptothecins, anthracyclines, and the epipodophyllotoxins.

Camptothecin Derivatives

The camptothecin analogs irinotecan and topotecan were synthesized to reduce toxicity and improve therapeutic effects of camptothecin, a plant alkaloid derived from *Camptotheca acuminata*. Both topotecan and irinotecan, through its active metabolite SN-38, inhibit topoisomerase I enzyme activity. Topoisomerase I enzymes stabilize DNA single-strand breaks and inhibit strand resealing.[30,31] Irinotecan undergoes metabolism to SN-38 by the polymorphic enzyme uridine diphosphate glucosyltransferase and variant tandem repeats in the promoter of this gene are associated with a higher risk of diarrhea and neutropenia.

Etoposide And Teniposide

Etoposide and teniposide are semisynthetic podophyllotoxin derivatives that bind to tubulin and interfere with microtubule formation. Etoposide and teniposide also damage tumor cells by causing strand breakage through inhibition of topoisomerase II.[30] Resistance may be caused by differences in topoisomerase II levels, increased cell ability to repair strand breaks, or increased levels of Pgp. Etoposide and teniposide are usually clinically cross-resistant. They are cell-cycle phase-specific and arrest cells in the S or early G_2 phase. As a result, activity is much greater when they are administered in divided doses over several days, rather than in large single doses.

Anthracene Derivatives

The most widely used and best understood anthracene derivative is doxorubicin, also commonly known by its earliest trade name, Adriamycin or "Adria." Other members of the anthracene group include daunorubicin (daunomycin), idarubicin, epirubicin, and mitoxantrone. All of these agents, except mitoxantrone, are anthracyclines and share a common, four-membered anthracene ring complex with an attached aglycone or sugar portion. The ring complex is a chromophore and accounts for the intense colors of these compounds. Doxorubicin differs from its parent compound daunorubicin by the addition of a hydroxyl group on the attached sugar, and it is sometimes referred to as hydroxydaunorubicin. A hydroxyl group on epirubicin is in the *epi* conformation compared with doxorubicin (epidoxorubicin), and idarubicin is demethoxydaunorubicin. Mitoxantrone is an anthracenedione rather than an anthracycline, and has no sugar group attached to the three-membered, anthracene ring complex.[30,32]

Doxorubicin, Daunorubicin, Idarubicin, and Epirubicin

Anthracyclines are classified as antitumor antibiotics, but it is more accurate to refer to them as intercalating topoisomerase inhibitors. Intercalating agents are compounds that insert or stack between base pairs of DNA. Although it is well established that the planar groups of the anthracene ring complex do intercalate with DNA, causing structural changes that interfere with DNA and RNA synthesis, this is not their primary mechanism of cytotoxicity. The anthracyclines are primarily topoisomerase II inhibitors, producing double-strand DNA breaks.[18,30,32]

The anthracyclines also undergo electron reductions to reactive compounds that can damage DNA and cell membranes. Free radicals formed from reduction of the anthracyclines first donate electrons to oxygen to make superoxide, which can react with itself to make hydrogen peroxide. Cleavage of hydrogen peroxide produces the highly reactive and destructive hydroxyl radical. This last step requires iron, and the anthracyclines are potent iron binders. Iron–anthracycline complexes can bind to DNA and react rapidly with hydrogen peroxide to produce the hydroxyl radicals that actually cleave DNA. Human cells have natural defenses against oxygen radical damage, in the form of enzymes that can convert the radicals to less reactive compounds, or that can repair DNA damage. Differences in distribution of these defensive enzymes may account for the cardiotoxicity of the anthracyclines. For example, cardiac muscle has low levels of defensive enzymes and high levels of enzymes that activate anthracyclines. Oxygen free-radical formation is firmly established as a cause of cardiac damage and extravasation injury, but is not a major mechanism of tumor-cell killing. Resistance to the anthracyclines is usually secondary to Pgp–dependent multidrug resistance, causing the anthracyclines to be actively pumped out of tumor cells. Altered topoisomerase II activity may contribute to the development of resistance.[18,32]

Mitoxantrone The anthracenedione mitoxantrone was synthesized in an attempt to develop agents with comparable antitumor activity to doxorubicin, but with an improved safety profile. Like the anthracyclines, mitoxantrone is an intercalating topoisomerase II inhibitor, but its potential for free-radical formation is much less than that of the anthracyclines. This decreased tendency for free-radical formation may explain the reduced risks of cardiac toxicity and ulceration after extravasation.[18,32]

ALKYLATING AGENTS

The alkylating agents are among the oldest and most useful classes of anticancer agents. Their clinical use evolved from the observation of bone marrow suppression and lymph node shrinkage in soldiers exposed to sulfur mustard gas warfare during World War I.[18] In an effort to develop similar agents that might be useful in treating cancerous overgrowths of lymphoid tissues, less-reactive derivatives were synthesized. Their effectiveness as anticancer agents was confirmed by clinical trials in the middle 1940s.

All of the alkylating agents work through the covalent bonding of highly reactive alkyl groups or substituted alkyl groups with nucleophilic groups of proteins and nucleic acids. Some alkylating agents react directly with biologic molecules; others form an intermediate compound that reacts with the targets. The most common binding site for alkylating agents is the seven-nitrogen group of guanine. These covalent interactions result in cross-linking between two DNA strands or between two bases in the same strand of DNA. Reactions between DNA and RNA and between drug and proteins may also occur, but the main insult that results in cell death is inhibition of DNA replication, because the interlinked strands do not separate as required. Because the alkylating agents can damage DNA during any phase of the cell cycle, they are not cell-cycle phase-specific. However, their greatest effect is seen in rapidly dividing cells.

As a class, alkylators are cytotoxic, mutagenic, teratogenic, carcinogenic, and myelosuppressive. Resistance to these agents can occur from increased DNA repair capabilities, decreased entry into or accelerated exit from cells, increased inactivation of the agents inside cells, or lack of cellular mechanisms to result in cell death following DNA damage. They react with water and are inactivated by hydrolysis, making spontaneous degradation an important component of their elimination.[33]

Nitrogen Mustards

Cyclophosphamide and ifosfamide are nitrogen mustard derivatives, and are widely used alkylating agents in the treatment of solid tumors and hematologic malignancies. They are closely related in structure, clinical use, and toxicity. Neither agent is active in its parent form and must be activated by mixed hepatic oxidase enzymes including the cytochrome P450 (CYP) 2B6 and CYP3A4 enzymes. The active metabolite of cyclophosphamide is phosphoramide mustard. Another metabolite, 4-hydroxycyclophosphamide is cytotoxic, but is not an alkylating agent. Ifosfamide is hepatically activated to ifosfamide mustard. Acrolein, a metabolite of both cyclophosphamide and ifosfamide, has little antitumor activity, but is responsible for the hemorrhagic cystitis associated with ifosfamide and sometimes high-dose cyclophosphamide.[33]

Encephalopathy following ifosfamide can occur within 48 to 72 hours following the infusion and is reversible. The increased production of dechloroethylated metabolites following administration of ifosfamide compared with cyclophosphamide may explain the increased risk of central nervous system toxicity associated with ifosfamide.[34]

Bendamustine is an alkylating agent (nitrogen mustard derivative) with a benzimidazole ring (purine analog) that demonstrates only partial cross-resistance (in vitro) with other alkylating agents.[35] It leads to cell death via single and double strand DNA cross-linking. Bendamustine is active against quiescent and dividing cells. The primary cytotoxic activity is due to bendamustine rather than its metabolites. It is used primarily to treat lymphoid malignancies such as chronic lymphocytic leukemia and non-Hodgkin lymphoma.

Nitrosoureas

The nitrosoureas are alkylating agents characterized by lipophilicity and ability to cross the blood–brain barrier. Carmustine or bischloroethylnitrosourea (BCNU) and lomustine (CCNU) are commercially available. BCNU is available as an intravenous preparation and as a drug-impregnated biodegradable wafer (Gliadel) for direct application to residual tumor tissue following surgical resection of brain tumors. The nitrosoureas decompose to reactive alkylating metabolites and to isocyanate compounds that have several effects on reproducing cells.[33]

Nonclassic Alkylating Agents

Several other cytotoxic agents appear to act as alkylators, although their structures do not include the classic alkylating groups. They are capable of binding covalently to cellular components and include procarbazine, dacarbazine, temozolomide, the heavy metal compounds, and some antitumor antibiotics.[33]

Dacarbazine and Temozolomide Dacarbazine (DTIC) and temozolomide are nonclassic alkylating agents. Both compounds undergo demethylation to the same active intermediate (monomethyl triazeno-imidazole-carboxamide [MTIC]) that interrupts DNA replication by causing methylation of guanine. Unlike dacarbazine, temozolomide does not require the liver for activation, and is chemically degraded to MTIC at physiologic pH. Both agents inhibit DNA, RNA, and protein synthesis.[18,33]

Important pharmacokinetic differences exist between the two agents. Dacarbazine is poorly absorbed, and must be administered by intravenous infusion. Temozolomide is rapidly absorbed after oral administration, and is nearly 100% bioavailable when given on a completely empty stomach. Dacarbazine penetrates the CNS poorly, but temozolomide readily crosses the blood–brain barrier, achieving therapeutically active concentrations in cerebrospinal fluid and brain tumor tissues.[18,33]

HEAVY METAL COMPOUNDS

Cisplatin, Carboplatin, and Oxaliplatin

The platinum derivatives—cisplatin, carboplatin, and oxaliplatin— are anticancer agents with remarkable usefulness in cancer treatment. Recognition of cisplatin's cytotoxic activity was the result of a serendipitous observation that bacterial growth in culture was altered when an electric current was delivered to the media through platinum electrodes. The growth change was noted to be similar to that produced by alkylating agents and radiation. It was found that a platinum–chloride complex, now known as cisplatin, generated by the current was responsible for the changes. Carboplatin is a structural analog of cisplatin in which the chloride groups of the parent compound are replaced by a carboxycyclobutane moiety. It shares a similar spectrum of clinical activity with cisplatin, and cross-resistance is common. Oxaliplatin is an organoplatinum compound in which the platinum is complexed with an oxalate ligand as the leaving group and to diaminocyclohexane. Its spectrum of activity differs substantially from the other platinum compounds, and includes notable activity against colorectal cancers.[18,33]

The cytotoxicity of the platinum derivatives depends on platinum binding to DNA and the formation of intrastrand cross-links or adducts between neighboring guanines. These intrastrand links cause a major bending of the DNA. They may cause cellular damage by distorting the normal DNA conformation and preventing bases that are normally paired from lining up with each other. Interstrand cross-links also occur.[18,33]

The cytotoxic form of cisplatin is the aquated species, in which hydroxyl groups or water molecules replace the two chloride groups. This reaction occurs readily in low concentrations of chloride, such as the concentrations present within cells, and produces a positively charged compound that can react with DNA. The aquated species is responsible for both the efficacy and toxicity of cisplatin. Carboplatin also undergoes aquation, but at a slower rate. Oxaliplatin becomes active when the oxalate ligand is displaced in physiologic solutions.[18,33]

Resistance to the therapeutic effects of platinum compounds may occur through several mechanisms. The ability to repair platinum-induced DNA damage may be increased, or the agents may be inactivated by increased levels of intracellular glutathione, metallothioneins, or other thiol-containing proteins. Altered uptake into cells may also affect sensitivity to platinum compounds.[18,33]

Cisplatin is a highly toxic anticancer agent that can cause serious nephrotoxicity, ototoxicity, peripheral neuropathy, emesis, and anemia. The significant efficacy of cisplatin against many tumor types makes it a valuable agent despite these toxicities, most of which can be prevented or managed with aggressive supportive care measures.[18] In contrast, carboplatin administration is limited by hematologic toxicity. Patients with compromised renal function require dose reductions to limit myelosuppressive toxicity.[18,33] The most widely used dosage schema, the Calvert formula (Table 135–9), uses a target area-under-the-curve and renal function parameters to estimate the carboplatin dose. Carboplatin's potential to cause renal damage, peripheral neuropathy, ototoxicity, and nausea and vomiting is much less than that of comparable cisplatin doses.[33] Oxaliplatin is not nephrotoxic or ototoxic, is moderately emetogenic, but can cause peripheral neuropathies and unique cold-induced neuropathies.[36] All of the platinum derivatives have potential to cause hypersensitivity reactions, including anaphylaxis, after a threshold exposure is reached.

TABLE 135-9 Dosing Formulas for Chemotherapy Agents[a]

DuBois and DuBois
BSA (m^2) = Wt (kg)$^{0.425}$ × Ht (cm)$^{0.725}$ × 0.007184

Mosteller
BSA (m^2) = $\sqrt{}$(Ht (cm) × Wt (kg)/3600)

Calvert (for carboplatin)
Dose (mg)^a = AUC^b × (CrCl^c + 25)

AUC, area-under-the-curve; BSA, body surface area; CrCl, creatinine clearance in mL/min; Ht, height; Wt, weight.
^{a}Note that the dose is in total milligrams to be administered, not mg/m^2.
^{b}AUC needs to be stated in the dosing protocol.
^{c}Cockcroft and Gault equation often clinically used.
Data from Haskell CM. Principles of cancer chemotherapy. In: Haskell CM, ed. Cancer Treatment, 5th ed. Philadelphia, PA: WB Saunders; 2001:62–86.

ENDOCRINE THERAPIES

Perhaps the earliest successful approach to target the growth processes of cancerous cells was the use of endocrine therapies. Endocrine manipulation is an option for management of cancers from tissues whose growth is under gonadal hormonal control, especially breast, prostate, and endometrial cancers. These cancers may regress if the "feeding" hormone is eliminated or antagonized. Major organ system toxicity is uncommon from hormonal treatment, making it the least toxic of systemic anticancer therapies. Increasingly specific agents such as the selective estrogen receptor modulators and aromatase inhibitors have increased the utility of hormonal therapies in the treatment of cancer.[37–39] These agents are discussed in detail in Chapters 136 and 139.

Corticosteroid hormones are also useful anticancer agents because of their lymphotoxic effects. Their primary use is in management of hematologic malignancies, especially lymphoid malignancies such as lymphomas, lymphocytic leukemias, and multiple myeloma. In addition to their cytotoxic effects, corticosteroids have many other applications in supportive care of cancer patients. Corticosteroids have diverse toxicities in chronic or high-dose use, but are generally well tolerated in the short-term therapies usually used in cancer patient care.[40]

MISCELLANEOUS AGENTS

Bleomycin

Bleomycin is an antitumor antibiotic. It is a mixture of peptides from fungal *Streptomyces* species, and its strength is expressed in units of drug activity.[18] One unit is roughly equal to 1 mg of polypeptide protein. The predominant peptide is bleomycin A2, which makes up approximately 70% of the commercial drug product. Bleomycin's cytotoxicity is secondary to DNA strand breakage, or scission, which it produces via free-radical formation. Cytotoxicity depends on binding of the bleomycin–iron complex to DNA. The bleomycin–iron complex then reduces molecular oxygen to free oxygen radicals that cause primarily single-strand breaks in DNA. Bleomycin has greatest effect on cells in the G$_2$ phase of the cell cycle and in mitosis.[18]

Bleomycin is inactivated within cells by the enzyme aminohydrolase. This enzyme is widely distributed, but is present in only low concentrations in the skin and the lungs, explaining the predominant toxicities of bleomycin to those sites. Baseline pulmonary function tests and monitoring for pulmonary toxicity is necessary during bleomycin therapy. The presence of hydrolase enzymes in tumor cells is the primary mechanism of resistance to bleomycin. Cells can also become resistant by repairing the DNA breaks produced by bleomycin.[18]

Hydroxyurea

Hydroxyurea is a unique drug that inhibits ribonucleotide reductase. Cells accumulate in the S phase because DNA synthesis is inhibited, and only abnormally short DNA strands are produced.[21] This drug is often used to cause a rapid decline in a patient's white blood cells prior to initiating more potent chemotherapy agents.

L-Asparaginase

L-Asparaginase is unique among anticancer agents in its unusual mechanism of action, patterns of toxicity, and source. It is an enzyme produced by *Escherichia coli* and other bacteria. L-Asparagine is a nonessential amino acid that can be synthesized by most mammalian cells, except for those of certain lymphoid human malignancies, which lack or have very low levels of the synthetase enzyme required for L-asparagine formation.[18] L-Asparagine is degraded by the enzyme L-asparaginase, which depletes existing supplies and inhibits protein synthesis. Increased L-asparagine synthetase activity within tumor cells causes resistance to L-asparaginase treatment.[18]

Arsenic Trioxide

Arsenic is an organic element and a well-known poison that is an effective treatment for acute promyelocytic leukemia.[41] As an anticancer agent, arsenic trioxide acts as a differentiating agent, inducing the growth progression of cancerous cells into mature, more normal cells. It also induces programmed cell death or apoptosis.

Mitomycin C

Mitomycin C is a natural product that is sometimes classified as an antitumor antibiotic.[33,42] It has similarities to nitrogen mustard compounds and may function as an alkylating agent, although its toxicity pattern differs from conventional alkylating agents.

Vorinostat

Vorinostat belongs to a new class of anticancer agents referred to as HDAC inhibitors. As described in the section on epigenetics, HDAC catalyzes the removal of acetyl groups from the lysine residues of proteins, including histones and transcription factors.[12,43] By inhibiting HDAC activity, vorinostat causes the accumulation of acetylated histones and induces cell cycle arrest and apoptosis of cancer cells. Pulmonary embolism and deep vein thrombosis have been reported along with dose-related thrombocytopenia and anemia.

CLINICAL PHARMACOLOGY OF BIOLOGIC AND TARGETED AGENTS

Biologic agents include cytokines, monoclonal antibodies, growth factors, and vaccines. The newer biologic therapies (e.g., monoclonal antibodies) are frequently termed "targeted therapies" because they target specific tumor antigens. These newer therapies are designed to target pathways critical for the survival and growth of cancer cells. Several anticancer agents that target malignant cells or the biochemical processes that control cancerous cell growth are available to treat both solid and hematologic malignancies. These agents are designed to improve outcomes while minimizing adverse effects. Small molecules (-nibs) typically interfere with downstream intracellular signaling by binding to the target proteins within the cell. In comparison, the monoclonal antibodies (-mabs) bind to the extracellular receptor or to its natural ligand and prevent the activation of the downstream intracellular signaling. Well-described intracellular signaling pathways include PI3K and MAPK pathways and when activated, promote cell proliferation and survival. The downstream effectors of these pathways also initiate cell cycle progression by promoting the expression of cyclins and repressing the expression of CDK inhibitors. The small molecules and monoclonal antibodies ultimately suppress cell cycle progression, cell proliferation and survival by stopping the relay of the intracellular signals.

MONOCLONAL ANTIBODIES

6 Monoclonal antibodies have become established agents in the treatment of cancer. Monoclonal antibodies (MoABs) consist of immunoglobulin sequences that are known to recognize a specific antigen or protein on the surface of cells. There are five classes of immunoglobulins (IgA, IgD, IgE, IgG, and IgM), with IgG the most commonly used therapeutically. The fundamental structure of all antibodies is identical and consists of two heavy and two light chains joined to form a molecule that resembles the letter Y. The variable region (Fab fragment) of antibodies differs greatly and is composed of three complementary determining regions. The Fab portion is composed of heavy (V_H) and light chains (V_L) that are responsible for binding to antigens. The constant region (Fc fragment) determines the effector function of the antibody.[44]

Two main classes of MoABs are used in the treatment of cancer, the most common of which are unconjugated or naked MoABs. The other class is immunoconjugates, which are MoABs conjugated to a toxin (immunotoxin), chemotherapy agent, or radioactive particle (radioimmunoconjugate). MoABs may also be divided into agents that target cell surface antigens and induce cell death and those that target growth factor receptors or ligands.[44] Standardized nomenclature exists for naming MoABs and can provide information to the clinician.[45] The suffix -mab is used for all MoABs and fragments and is always preceded by the identification of the animal source of the product. The letters *o*, *u*, *xi*, and *zu* before the -mab suffix indicate a murine, human, chimeric, and humanized source, respectively. The general disease state the MoAB is treating precedes the source and is identified using a code. Currently, most approved MoABs used in cancer have the code syllabus -tu(m) that designates it for use against miscellaneous tumors. If the product is conjugated to another chemical, such as a toxin, or is radiolabeled, a separate word is added for this designation. In addition, the name of the isotope, element symbol, and isotope number should precede the name of the MoAB. For example, iodine I-131-tositumomab is a murine MoAB designated for use in cancer that is conjugated to the radioisotope iodine 131.

6 The first MoABs used in humans were murine, but most of the MoABs used today are chimeric, humanized, or fully human. These agents differ in the amount of foreign component. Hypersensitivity and infusion-related reactions, with or without the development of human antimouse antibodies (HAMAs), are generally greatest with murine antibodies and least with humanized antibodies.[44,46] Human antibodies would not be expected to cause HAMA reactions. However, clinicians should be careful when administering any MoAB as rare HAMA-like reactions have occurred to chimeric and humanized MoABs. The severity of these reactions can range from mild (e.g., fever, chills, nausea, and rash) to severe, life-threatening anaphylaxis with cardiopulmonary collapse. Many patients also experience chest or back pain during the infusion. Patients with circulating tumor cells in the bloodstream are at highest risk for more severe reactions. For these reasons, patients must be monitored closely during infusion. The reactions tend to be more severe with the initial infusion, and subside with subsequent treatment. Most agents require premedication with antihistamines and acetaminophen. Recommended infusion rates are usually lower for the initial dose, with incremental increases as tolerated by the patient. For patients experiencing signs or symptoms of infusion-related reactions, the infusion should be interrupted and prompt treatment with antihistamines, corticosteroids, and other supportive measures should be initiated. Pulmonary toxicity may occur as part of the infusion-related reaction or may occur as a distinct entity.[44,46,47]

HAMA reactions can also increase the clearance of the MoAB from the body by targeting the murine portion of the antibody as foreign. This will decrease the half-life of the MoAB and may decrease the ability of the MoAB to bind to its target antigen and potentially decrease its efficacy over time.

Additionally, the toxicities of the MoABs will be determined by the selectivity of the target antigen. Antibodies against antigens found on normal and tumor cells will have increased toxicity compared to tumor-specific antigens found only on tumor tissues. For example, gemtuzumab targets CD33⁺ antigen, which is found on tumor and early myeloid cells. As a result, prolonged myelosuppression is an anticipated adverse effect of gemtuzumab.[44]

❻ There are several mechanisms by which MoABs may induce death of cancer cells. Unconjugated MoABs that target antigens on the cell surface of cancer cells may directly mediate cell killing through complement activation (complement-dependent cytotoxicity [CDC]), antibody-dependent cellular toxicity (ADCC), or signaling the cascade of events that lead to tumor cell apoptosis.[44,46,48] CDC results when the Fc portion of the MoAB activates the complement system leading to tumor cell lysis. In ADCC, effector cells that contain Fc receptors bind to the Fc portion of the MoAB and either lyses or phagocytosizes the antibody-containing cell. Natural killer cells, monocytes, and macrophages are all capable of mediating ADCC. Finally, antibody binding may result in the transmission of signals that induce apoptosis, or programmed cell death in the targeted cell.

❻ In addition to the mechanisms of cell death above, immunoconjugates deliver a chemotherapy agent or radioactive particle to the site of disease. Once bound to target antigens, the chemotherapy drug conjugated to the MoAB is internalized by the target cell and kills tumor cells through traditional mechanisms of action.[49] MoABs conjugated to radiation deliver radiation targeted to the site of tumor involvement, resulting in cell death. In addition to killing the target cell, radioimmunoconjugates are capable of killing antigen-negative cancer cells through radiation crossfire sometimes termed the "innocent bystander" effect. Both types of immunoconjugates are able to deliver therapy to specific sites of disease while limiting systemic exposure to the chemotherapy agent or radiation.

Finally, MoABs have been developed that target the underlying mechanism of cell growth and proliferation. These agents are discussed later in the chapter but have similar structure, nomenclature, and potential adverse effects as agents that target antigens present on malignant cells.

MONOCLONAL ANTIBODIES THAT TARGET CELL SURFACE GLYCOPROTEINS

Gemtuzumab Ozogamicin

Gemtuzumab ozogamicin consists of a recombinant humanized anti-CD33 MoAB conjugated to the calicheamicin derivative N-acetyl-gamma calicheamicin, a cytotoxic antitumor antibiotic, by the linker ozogamicin.[44,46] The myeloid cell-surface antigen CD33 is expressed on the surface of leukemic blasts in more than 80% of patients with acute myelogenous leukemia.[44,46] The binding of the Fab fragment of gemtuzumab ozogamicin to the CD33 antigen results in the formation of a complex that is internalized into CD33⁺ cells. Upon internalization, the calicheamicin derivative is cleaved from the antibody and released inside the cell. The released calicheamicin derivative binds to DNA in the minor groove resulting in DNA double-strand breaks and cell death.[46,50]

Gemtuzumab ozogamicin was indicated in elderly patients with CD33⁺ acute myelogenous leukemia and who have failed at least one chemotherapy regimen. Gemtuzumab has been voluntarily withdrawn from the United States market because of concerns over efficacy and safety. Some of the adverse events reported with gemtuzumab ozogamicin are myelosuppression, tumor lysis syndrome, and hepatotoxicity. Myelosuppression is the most severe toxicity associated with gemtuzumab ozogamicin.[44,51] Tumor lysis

syndrome including secondary renal failure secondary has been reported in association with the use of gemtuzumab ozogamicin. Leukoreduction with hydroxyurea or leukapheresis prior to administration of gemtuzumab ozogamicin and appropriate preventive measures may be considered to decrease the likelihood of tumor lysis syndrome. Hepatotoxicity, including severe venoocclusive disease, has also been reported in association with the use of gemtuzumab ozogamicin.[50,51] Risk factors include receiving gemtuzumab before or after hematopoietic stem cell transplantation, underlying hepatic disease or abnormal liver function, and patients receiving gemtuzumab ozogamicin in combination with chemotherapy.

Rituximab

Rituximab was the first MoAB approved as an anticancer agent by the FDA (November 1997). Rituximab is a chimeric MoAB directed against the CD20 antigen found on the surface of normal and malignant B cells.[52] The Fab domain of Rituximab binds to the CD20 antigen on B lymphocytes and the Fc domain recruits immune effector functions to mediate B-cell lysis.[52] Possible explanations for its antitumor effect include CDC- and ADCC-mediated killing of malignant B cells along with a direct apoptotic effect.[52]

Rituximab is approved for the treatment of patients with relapsed or refractory, low-grade or follicular, CD20-positive, B-cell non-Hodgkin's lymphomas and as first-line therapy for patients with aggressive and indolent non-Hodgkin lymphomas in combination with chemotherapy. It is also approved for use in patients with other malignancies with CD20-antigen expression (e.g., chronic lymphocytic leukemia) in combination with standard chemotherapy.[52,53] Rituximab is also approved for the treatment of refractory rheumatoid arthritis and has an evolving role in a variety of immune-mediated diseases such as Waldenström macroglobulinemia, aplastic anemia, and others.

Most of rituximab's adverse events occur during the first infusion and are components of an infusion-related complex secondary to the amount of circulating B cells. After the first infusion, the incidence and the severity of these reactions decrease dramatically.[52,53] The most common events in the infusion-related complex are transient fever, chills, nausea, asthenia, and headache. Infection and severe hematologic events with rituximab are infrequent with neutropenia, anemia, and thrombocytopenia occurring in less than 1% of patients.[52]

Ibritumomab Tiuxetan

Ibritumomab tiuxetan is an immunoconjugate that consists of the murine anti-CD20 MoAB ibritumomab and tiuxetan, a linker-chelator, that allows the attachment of indium-111 (used for imaging and dosimetry) and yttrium-90 (active radiotherapy).[55] The ibritumomab therapeutic regimen consists of two steps.[50,55] Y-90–ibritumomab is the therapeutic radiation isotope and selectively delivers radiation to B cells that express the CD20 antigen.

The radiation-induced cytotoxicity delivered by Y-90–ibritumomab not only affects the tumor cells it binds to, but also other cells that are within the pathlength of the radioisotope's emissions (innocent bystander effect).[49,50,55] Consequently, Y-90–ibritumomab can induce cell death in CD-20–positive and –negative tumors and eradicate a large number of tumor cells. Ibritumomab also induces ADCC, CDC, and apoptosis in target cells.[49,50,55]

Ibritumomab tiuxetan is indicated for the treatment of relapsed or refractory low-grade, follicular, or transformed B-cell non-Hodgkin lymphoma, including rituximab-refractory non-Hodgkin lymphoma. Because ibritumomab is derived from murine sources, only one course of therapy is recommended to prevent the development of HAMA reactions.

Adverse reactions associated with the ibritumomab tiuxetan treatment regimen include severe infusion-related reactions, including life-threatening anaphylaxis.[49,50,55] Unlike rituximab, myelosuppression is common with ibritumomab as a consequence of the radioisotope component of the antibody.[49,55] Ibritumomab tiuxetan results in prolonged thrombocytopenia and neutropenia and dose modifications are necessary based on baseline neutrophil and platelet blood counts.[55] The median durations of thrombocytopenia and neutropenia were 24 and 22 days, respectively, and monitoring and management of cytopenias, along with their complications (e.g., febrile neutropenia, bleeding) is necessary for up to 3 months after the completion of treatment.[50,55]

Tositumomab

Tositumomab is another murine anti-CD20 radioimmunoconjugate, similar to ibritumomab. One important difference is that tositumomab is combined with the radioisotope iodine I-131 which has therapeutic and safety implications. The tositumomab therapeutic regimen also consists of two steps.[49] The mechanisms of cell death are similar to ibritumomab as is the indication for use in patients with refractory non-Hodgkin lymphoma.

Most adverse effects are similar to ibritumomab with infusion-related reactions requiring appropriate premedications along with prolonged myelosuppression, primarily neutropenia and thrombocytopenia. Complete blood counts should be obtained weekly for 10 to 12 weeks to assess recovery of normal blood counts. To prevent iodine uptake by the thyroid gland, and subsequent delivery of ionizing radiation to the thyroid gland, thyroid protective agents such as saturated solution of potassium iodide should be initiated prior to the start of the tositumomab regimen and continued for 14 days after the therapeutic dose.[49,56]

Alemtuzumab

Alemtuzumab is a recombinant humanized MoAB that is directed against CD52. CD52 is expressed on the surface of B and T lymphocytes, natural killer cells, monocytes, and macrophages.[57] Alemtuzumab's therapeutic effect comes from binding to the CD52 antigen present on leukemic lymphocytes in chronic lymphocytic leukemia and inducing cell lysis and death.[57]

Alemtuzumab is indicated for the treatment of B-cell chronic lymphocytic leukemia in patients who have been treated with alkylating agents and who have failed fludarabine therapy. It is also being investigated as part of conditioning regimens for hematopoietic stem cell transplants, treatment of autoimmune hematologic disorder, indolent non-Hodgkin lymphomas, and treatment of graft-versus-host disease.[50,57]

Alemtuzumab is associated with severe infusion-related reactions, hematologic toxicity, and opportunistic infections that are severe enough to warrant a black box warning in the package insert.[44,57] Hematologic toxicity consisting of severe prolonged neutropenia and thrombocytopenia occur in most patients. Clinicians should monitor blood counts prior to alemtuzumab administration to determine if the dose needs to be delayed or reduced.[44,50,57]

Because CD52 is expressed on lymphocytes, alemtuzumab can induce profound lymphopenia including a decrease in CD4 and CD8 counts.[44,50,57] Patients should receive prophylaxis for *Pneumocystis jirovecii* pneumonia and herpes virus which should be continued for up to six months after alemtuzumab therapy or until recovery of CD4 counts to prevent complications.[44,57]

AGENTS THAT TARGET GROWTH FACTOR RECEPTORS AND LIGANDS

Recent advances in molecular biology have identified a number of pathways and potential targets related to cancer cell growth and survival. Targeting the HER pathway is currently used to treat a variety of solid tumor malignancies. MoABs have been developed to target the extracellular receptors of the HER family. In addition, small molecular inhibitors that target intracellular signal transduction pathways are available to clinicians for several malignancies. Additional agents target the vascular endothelial growth factor (VEGF) ligand or receptor and other downstream signaling targets.

❼ As mentioned previously, the HER family of receptors contains four known members, which upon binding to growth factor ligands result in intracellular phosphorylation of transcription factors and cell proliferation (Fig. 135–8).[9,58,59] HER-1 (more commonly called EGFR) and HER-2 are known to be overexpressed in several cancers, including breast, lung, and colon cancers.

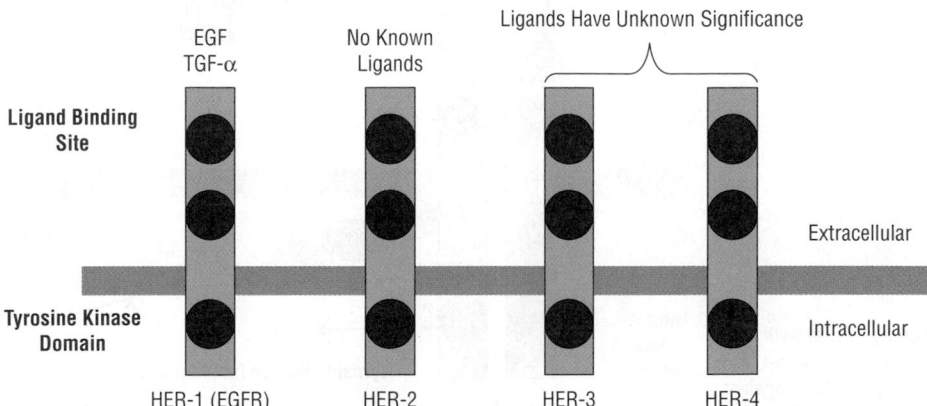

FIGURE 135-8. The HER family of growth factor receptors. All members of the human epidermal growth factor receptor (HER) contain a transmembrane glycoprotein, an extracellular ligand binding site, and a hydrophobic intracellular portion with a tyrosine kinase domain. HER-1 (or more commonly called EGFR [epidermal growth factor receptor]) has several known ligands (commonly implicated in cancer are EGF [epidermal growth factor] and TGF-α [transforming growth factor-α]); HER-2 has no known ligands; while the significance of ligands for HER-3 and HER-4 are unknown at this time. Once the molecule binds to another member of the HER family the tyrosine kinase domain is phosphorylated and genes regulating proliferation, antiapoptosis, and cell transformation are turned on.

Activation of these receptors leads to uncontrolled cellular growth and proliferation, tumor metastasis, and the prevention of apoptosis in malignant cells.[58] The roles of HER-3 and HER-4 in cancer growth and proliferation are still under investigation. All members of this family contain a transmembrane glycoprotein extracellular ligand binding site, a transmembrane domain, and a cytosolic tyrosine kinase tail. Members of the HER family are inactive by themselves, and must form a dimer (a molecule composed of two subunits), either with a member of the same family (homodimer), or with a member of a different subtype of the HER family (heterodimer).[59] Dimerization of the receptor leads to tyrosine kinase phosphorylation and subsequent activation of downstream pathways required to activate signal transduction and cell growth.

Based on these identified cellular targets, several agents have been developed to prevent signal transduction through this pathway. MoABs which competitively bind to extracellular receptors of the HER family and prevent ligand binding and subsequent dimerization of receptors are available to clinicians. In addition, small molecules that target intracellular tyrosine kinase receptors are approved for use in a variety of tumors. These agents allow growth factor receptors to dimerize but prevent the phosphorylation of tyrosine kinase domains. The net effect of both strategies is to prevent downstream activation of the signal transduction resulting in a decrease in cell proliferation (Fig. 135–9).

Human Epidermal Growth Factor Receptor Family

Cetuximab and Panitumumab Cetuximab is a chimeric MoAB that binds specifically to the extracellular domain of EGFR.[44,46,60] Cetuximab binds to EGFR on both normal and tumor cells and competitively inhibits the binding of epidermal growth factor and other ligands, such as transforming growth factor-α.[46,60] Binding of cetuximab to the EGFR results in inhibition of cell growth, induction of apoptosis, and inhibition of VEGF production. Cetuximab is primarly given as monotherapy or in combination with other anticancer agents in the treatment of metastatic colorectal cancer.[60,61]

Cetuximab is also approved for use in head and neck cancer either by itself or in combination with radiation.[62]

The most serious adverse events associated with cetuximab are infusion-related reactions and development of an acne-like rash.[44,61,63] Skin reactions occur in most patients receiving cetuximab and can be severe. This reaction is similar between all EGFR inhibitors regardless of the site of action (extracellular or intracellular) and appears to be related to the function of EGFR in skin follicles.[64] Skin reactions appear most commonly on the face, upper chest, and back, but can extend to the extremities. These reactions are characterized by multiple follicular or pustular appearing lesions that generally appear within the first 2 weeks of therapy. Although the reactions usually resolve following cessation of treatment, resolution can be slow, continuing beyond 28 days in nearly one half of cases. In patients who develop severe rash, dose modifications may be necessary. Interestingly, a trend for improved responses with increasing severity of skin reactions has been reported and requires further follow-up to assess the clinical importance of these reactions.[61,64] Other common adverse events with cetuximab include fatigue, gastrointestinal complaints (nausea, vomiting, diarrhea, and constipation), and abdominal pain.[61]

Panitumumab is a MoAB that also binds to the cell surface EGFR. It is an IgG2 antibody, and the first fully human MoAB approved to treat cancer.[65] Panitumumab is approved as a single agent in refractory metastatic colon cancer. Adverse reactions are similar to cetuximab though severe reactions appear to be rare because it does not have a murine component.[65]

Trastuzumab Trastuzumab is a humanized MoAB that selectively binds to HER-2.[53,56] HER-2 is overexpressed in about one third of patients with breast cancer and to varying degrees in a variety of other malignancies (e.g., ovarian, lung, prostate).[9,53] Trastuzumab inhibits cell-cycle progression by decreasing cells entering the S phase of the cell cycle, leading to downregulation of HER-2 receptors on tumor cells and decreased cell proliferation.[66] Trastuzumab also leads to ADCC and CDC, along with

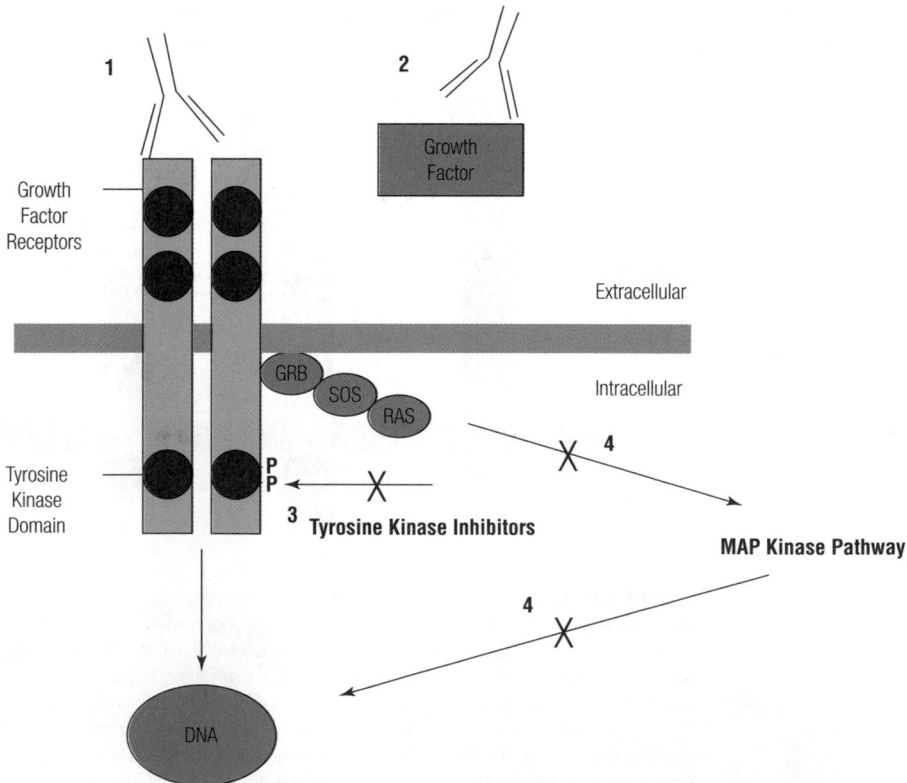

FIGURE 135-9. Strategies against growth factor receptors include (1) MoABs against the growth factor receptor; (2) MoABs against the growth factor itself; (3) molecules that target intracellular tyrosine kinases and prevent phosphorylation of tyrosine residues and subsequent activation of downstream signals; and (4) targeting downstream signals such as the MAP (mitogen activation protein) kinase pathway. All of these targets have the same goal of decreasing cell proliferation and increasing cell death of tumor cells.

directly inducing apoptosis in cells overexpressing the HER-2 protein.[66] In addition, synergy between trastuzumab and traditional chemotherapeutic agents has been demonstrated, resulting in trastuzumab often being used in combination with traditional chemotherapy agents.

Trastuzumab is approved in the treatment of metastatic breast cancer as a single agent or in combination with paclitaxel. Trastuzumab has also demonstrated a benefit in the adjuvant treatment of HER-2 positive breast cancer and is given for 1 year in combination with chemotherapy.[67] The combination of trastuzumab with other chemotherapy agents including vinorelbine, carboplatin, and others has shown synergistic effects and is under clinical investigation.[53] The addition of trastuzumab to anthracycline therapy is not recommended because of concerns of additive cardiotoxicity.

Trastuzumab is administered as a loading dose followed by weekly infusions as a single-agent or in combination with chemotherapy.[66] Trastuzumab has been administered every 3 weeks in combination with various chemotherapy agents to simplify the chemotherapy regimen; response rates and safety appear similar to those seen in the approved weekly trastuzumab regimen.[68]

The most serious adverse reactions caused by trastuzumab include cardiomyopathy, infusion-related reactions, hypersensitivity reactions (including anaphylaxis), and increased myelosuppression. An evaluation of cardiac function should be performed prior to administration and extreme caution should be exercised in patients with preexisting cardiac dysfunction and in those who have received prior anthracyclines. In patients who develop a clinically significant decrease in left ventricular function (ejection fraction <50% or greater than 10% decrease), discontinuation of therapy should be considered. Similar to most MoABs, the symptoms associated with a hypersensitivity reaction are most common with the initial infusions of trastuzumab and occur infrequently thereafter.

Myelosuppression is infrequent following the administration of trastuzumab as a single agent, but the incidence of neutropenia and febrile neutropenia is higher when trastuzumab is given with myelosuppressive chemotherapy as compared to giving the chemotherapy alone.[66]

Erlotinib Erlotinib is an orally active, selective EGFR-tyrosine kinase inhibitor that blocks signal transduction pathways involved in proliferation, survival, and metastases of cancer cells.[69,70] It inhibits EGFR activity by competing with adenosine triphosphate for its binding site on the EGFR tyrosine kinase cytosolic domain, which blocks the tyrosine kinase cascade of downstream signaling, and ultimately interferes with the proliferation and growth of cancer cells.

Erlotinib is indicated for the treatment of patients with locally advanced or metastatic non-small-cell lung cancer as a second-line agent.[70] Erlotinib is also approved for use in pancreatic cancer in combination with gemcitabine. Erlotinib has also demonstrated activity in a variety of other tumors such as head and neck and brain tumors.

Rash and diarrhea are the most common adverse events reported with erlotinib. Some studies suggest that the development of a rash may be predictive of a response to therapy and correlates with clinical benefit.[64] The rash that develops is similar to cetuximab and is treated similarly. Interstitial lung disease is a rare adverse effect reported in patients taken erlotinib. Drug interactions include increased international normalized ratio for patients on concomitant warfarin and increased or decreased erlotinib drug levels with inhibitors or inducers of CYP3A4, respectively.

Lapatinib Lapatinib is a small molecule 4-anilinoquinazoline kinase inhibitor that inhibits the intracellular kinase domains of both EGFR and HER-2.[72] It has demonstrated clinical activity in combination with capecitabine in breast cancer patients who have overexpression of HER-2 and who have previously received therapy with trastuzumab, an anthracycline and a taxane.[72] Toxicity for lapatinib was notable for an increased incidence of diarrhea, hepatoxicity, rash, and QT interval prolongation. Lapatinib has significant CYP450 mediated drug–drug interactions.

Vascular Endothelial Growth Factor

8 Angiogenesis, the development of new blood vessels, is a process important for normal physiologic processes but becomes unregulated in several malignancies and can lead to tumor growth, invasion, and metastasis. This process is regulated by pro- and antiangiogenic growth factors, which are released in response to hypoxia and other stresses to the cell.[80] Proangiogenic growth factors include VEGF, fibroblast growth factors, platelet-derived growth factor, tumor necrosis factor-α, and keratinocyte growth factor. Antiangiogenic growth factors include interleukin (IL) 12, interferons, platelet factor 4, and tissue inhibitors of metalloproteinase.[73]

The best studied proangiogenic factor is VEGF, whose elevated levels have been associated with a poor prognosis and an increased risk of metastases in a variety of malignancies, including acute myeloid leukemia, breast cancer, hepatocellular carcinoma, non-small cell lung cancer, ovarian cancer, and colon cancer.[73] Similar to other growth factors, VEGF binds to specific receptors located on the extracellular domain of growth factor receptors. Three known receptors of VEGF have been identified: VEGFR-1, −2, and −3.[73] The VEGFR-1 and VEGFR-2 receptors are expressed primarily in endothelial cells and in some tumor cells, and mediate the biologic effects of VEGF. Each of the receptors induces a different signal transduction pathway. These pathways eventually result in the generation of proteases that are necessary for the breakdown of the extracellular matrix, the first step of angiogenesis. Interference with their ability to develop new blood vessels by means of antiangiogenic agents can limit or prevent tumor growth.[73]

Anticancer agents can interfere with angiogenesis in many different ways. Examples are targeting vascular growth factors, or the production and control of the endothelial cells that make up the vessel linings. Most antiangiogenic agents are cytostatic rather than truly cytotoxic, as they prevent new vessel growth and thus cause growth delay of the tumors. Some vascular targeting agents, however, can destroy existing blood vessels and may have cytotoxic properties.[73]

Bevacizumab Bevacizumab is a humanized MoAB directed against circulating VEGF.[73] It binds to all biologically active circulating isoforms of VEGF and prevents the activation and promotion of angiogenesis.[73]

Bevacizumab is approved, in combination with 5-FU–based chemotherapy, for the initial treatment of metastatic colorectal cancer[74] and for first-line treatment, in combination with carboplatin and paclitaxel, of patients with unresectable, locally advanced, recurrent or metastatic nonsquamous non-small cell lung cancer. Additional FDA approved uses include breast, renal cell, and glioblastoma malignancies with off-labeled use in ovarian, pancreatic, head and neck, and cervical cancers.

The three most frequent adverse effects associated with bevacizumab are hypertension, bleeding episodes, and thrombotic events.[74,75] Hypertension associated with bevacizumab is more common in patients with a previous history of hypertension and responds to oral antihypertensive medications. The most common type of bleeding associated with bevacizumab is transient nosebleeds. However, fatal CNS and gastrointestinal hemorrhages have been reported. The manufacturer has issued a black box warning regarding the risk of gastrointestinal perforation, wound dehiscence, and fatal hemoptysis.[75] Bevacizumab is not recommended for use within 28 days of major surgery and patients should be instructed to report abdominal pain (an initial sign of gastrointestinal hemorrhage) to their healthcare provider immediately. Paradoxically, bevacizumab also has been found to cause thrombotic events, including deep vein thrombosis, pulmonary embolism, and myocardial infarction, especially in elderly patients with a history of cardiac events. Another rare adverse effect associated with bevacizumab is proteinuria and patients should be monitored for the development or worsening of proteinuria by checking urine dipsticks for protein. Patients with a 2+ or greater urine dipstick reading should undergo further assessment to determine if bevacizumab is safe to administer.

Sunitinib and Sorafenib

Most targeted agents approved to date have been developed against a single target associated with either the tumor or its growth and survival. Two similar agents—sunitinib and sorafenib—inhibit multiple tyrosine kinases, with the goal of enhanced antitumor activity. These agents are inhibitors of VEGFR-2 and platelet-derived growth factor receptor, which are involved in angiogenesis; c-KIT involved in gastrointestinal stromal tumors; and FLT3 involved in leukemia. In addition, sorafenib inhibits several isoforms of the serine/threonine kinase Raf, which is part of the mitogen-activated protein kinase-signaling pathway involved in cell proliferation.[76]

Gastrointestinal adverse effects such as diarrhea are common with both agents, as is rash, fatigue, and hypertension. Unique adverse events include congestive heart failure with sunitinib and hand–foot syndrome with sorafenib.

Both of these agents are approved for use in advanced renal cell cancers and sunitinib is also approved for gastrointestinal stromal tumors after imatinib failures. Ongoing trials are evaluating both of these agents in other tumors.

MISCELLANEOUS BIOLOGIC AND TARGETED AGENTS

Imatinib, Dasatinib, and Nilotinib

Imatinib is a selective inhibitor of the tyrosine kinase activity of BCR-ABL fusion gene, the product of the Philadelphia chromosome.[77] The Philadelphia chromosome is the hallmark finding of chronic myeloid leukemia and is a translocation of genetic material between chromosomes 9 and 22. Imatinib binds to the kinase binding site of the BCR-ABL gene, competitively blocking access to adenosine triphosphate. This prevents tyrosine-kinase phosphorylation of the gene and downstream activation of cellular proliferation.[84] Imatinib also causes apoptosis or arrest of growth in hematopoietic cells expressing BCR-ABL. An additional effect of imatinib is its ability in blocking the tyrosine kinase activity of c-KIT (stem-cell factor receptor) and platelet-derived growth factor receptor.[46,77]

Imatinib is a standard treatment option for newly diagnosed Philadelphia chromosome-positive (Ph+) chronic myeloid leukemia and for c-KIT (CD117)-positive gastrointestinal stromal tumors. A major advance observed with imatinib therapy is its ability to eliminate the Philadelphia chromosome in patients receiving therapy resulting in cytogenetic responses (elimination of the genetic defect), thus achieving the goal of all targeted therapies; the attack and elimination of the underlying cancer biology.

Adverse effects to imatinib are usually mild to moderate in severity. Severe fluid retention (pleural effusion, pericardial effusion, and ascites) occurs in less than 10% of patients taking imatinib. Patients should be monitored regularly for early signs and symptoms of fluid retention (leg swelling, shoes no longer fitting, and shortness of breath) and instructed to call their healthcare

clinicians when symptoms first develop. Additional adverse effects for imatinib include mild or moderate superficial edema, elevation of liver enzymes, nausea, muscle cramps, headache, and rash.[78] Rash may require early intervention as rare cases of Stevens-Johnson syndrome have been reported with imatinib and may require permanent discontinuation of therapy.[78]

Imatinib is metabolized by and is an inhibitor of the CYP3A4 enzyme system and caution should be exercised when substrates, inducers, or inhibitors of CYP3A4 are used concomitantly with imatinib.[78] Imatinib is also an inhibitor of CYP2D6 and levels of CYP2D6 substrates can increase.

Dasatinib and nilotinib are next-generation tyrosine kinase inhibitors that share the same binding site on the BCR-ABL tyrosine kinase adenosine triphosphate-binding domain with imatinib.[79] In contrast, dasatinib and nilotinib maintain clinical activity in chronic myeloid leukemia patients with mutations in the BCR-ABL binding site that confer imatinib resistance with the exception of one polymorphism (T135I) in which all three anti-cancer agents appear resistant. Nilotinib and dasatinib received FDA-approval for the treatment of patients with chronic myeloid leukemia resistant or intolerant to imatinib. Nilotinib and dasatinib recently received FDA approval for first-line treatment of newly diagnosed chronic myeloid leukemia. Dasatinib also inhibits a family of tyrosine kinases called SRC kinases that are believed to mediate cellular differentiation, proliferation, and survival; SRC kinases have been implicated in modulating multiple oncogenic signal transduction pathways.[84]

Dasatinib and nilotinib have a toxicity profile similar to that of imatinib with myelosuppression, nausea and vomiting, headache, and fluid retention being commonly reported. Dasatinib has also been reported to cause hypocalcemia and pleural effusions. Similar to other tyrosine kinase inhibitors, these anticancer drugs have extensive drug–drug interactions with substrates, inducers and inhbitors of CYP3A4, as well as other CYP enzymes.

Bortezomib

The proteasome is an enzyme complex that is responsible for degrading proteins that control the cell cycle. Some of the proteins degraded by proteosomes regulate critical functions for cancer growth, such as regulation of the cell cycle, transcription factors, apoptosis, angiogenesis, and cell adhesion.[80] One proteosome inhibitor, bortezomib, is commercially available. Bortezomib has very specific affinity for the catalytic portion of the proteosome. It can induce apoptosis in cancer cells indirectly. Bortezomib is a specific inhibitor of the 26S proteasome; one consequence of 26S proteasome inhibition is the accumulation of IκB, an inhibitor of the major transcription factor NF-κB. NF-κB induces transcription of genes that block cell death pathways and promote cell proliferation. Its activity depends on its release from its inhibitory partner protein, IκB, in the cytoplasm and move to the nucleus. When IκB fails to degrade, through the actions of bortezomib, NF-κB remains in the cytoplasm, preventing it from transcribing the genes that promote cancer growth. Bortezomib is approved for the treatment of patients with multiple myeloma and mantle cell lymphoma.[80]

The most commonly reported adverse events are asthenia (fatigue, malaise, and weakness), nausea, and diarrhea occurring in over half of patients. Additional adverse effects include decreased appetite, nausea, constipation, myelosuppression, peripheral neuropathies, and fever.[80] Most of these adverse effects are mild to moderate and managed with supportive care measures. Of these common adverse effects, severe adverse effects were limited to thrombocytopenia, neutropenia, asthenia, and peripheral neuropathies. Bortezomib is administered every 72 hours to minimize cumulative toxicity, by permitting the restoration of proteasome function between doses.

Temsirolimus and Everolimus

Mammalian target of rapamycin (mTOR) is a component of intracellular signaling pathways involved in the growth and proliferation of cells. mTOR receives input from upstream signaling pathways, including growth factors and hormones. Once activated, mTOR stimulates protein synthesis by phosphorylating translation regulators. mTOR also contributes to protein degradation and angiogenesis.[81]

Temsirolimus binds to FKBP-12 and the protein–drug complex inhibits the activity of mTOR by blocking its kinase activity.[81] mTOR inhibition suppresses the production of proteins that regulate progression through the cell cycle and angiogenesis. mTOR inhibition also results in reduced levels of cell growth factors involved in angiogenesis such as VEGF. Temsirolimus is approved for metastatic renal cell carcinoma, in which angiogenesis is a prominent clinical feature.

The most common adverse reactions with temsirolimus are rash, fatigue, mucositis, nausea, edema, and loss of appetite. The most common laboratory abnormalities are increases in serum creatinine and liver function tests, thrombocytopenia, and neutropenia. Additionally, hyperglycemia and hyperlipidemia that require monitoring of glucose and lipid profiles should be expected.[81] Rare, but potentially serious adverse effects include interstitial lung disease, immunosuppression (and infection), and renal failure. Temsirolimus is metabolized by CYP3A4, and possible drug interactions requiring dosage adjustments may be necessary.

Everolimus is an oral inhibitor of mTOR that is approved for the treatment of patients with advanced renal cell carcinoma after failure of treatment with sunitinib or sorafenib.[81] Adverse reactions and potential drug interactions are similar to temsirolimus.

Thalidomide and Lenalidomide

Thalidomide, the infamous drug that caused severe limb deformities (phocomelia or "seal limbs") when used by pregnant women as a nonprescription sedative in the 1960s, is approved for treatment of leprosy and has orphan drug status for multiple myeloma. It also has documented clinical activity in several other types of cancer. Thalidomide is a glutamic acid derivative, and is broadly classed as an immunomodulatory agent. Lenalidomide, is a novel 4-aminoglutarimide analog of thalidomide with similar therapeutic activity, but a different adverse effect profile.[82] These agents have many potential mechanisms of action, with the main hypothesis thought to be through angiogenesis inhibition, an action also linked to its teratogenic effects. Other possible mechanisms include direct inhibition of cancer cells, free radical oxidative damage to DNA, interfering with adhesion of cancer cells, inhibiting tumor necrosis factor-production, or altering secretion of cytokines that affect the growth of cancer cells.[82]

The most common adverse events for thalidomide include somnolence, constipation, dizziness, orthostatic hypotension, rash, and peripheral neuropathies. Neutropenia is extremely rare. In contrast, lenalidomide is associated with much less somnolence and neuropathies compared to thalidomide.[82] Neutropenia, thrombocytopenia, and thrombotic issues are most prevalent with lenalidomide use. Because thalidomide is teratogenic, great care must be taken to prevent their use during pregnancy and several members of the healthcare team are required by the FDA to assist in this goal. All pharmacies and prescribers must be enrolled in the System for Thalidomide Education and Prescribing Safety (S.T.E.P.S.) program to dispense thalidomide and lenalidomide is only available under a special restricted distribution program called RevAssist.

Retinoids

Vitamin A and its metabolites, collectively referred to as the retinoids, play important roles in numerous biologic processes, including normal cellular differentiation. Because cancerous growth is characterized by abnormal cellular differentiation, retinoids may play important therapeutic roles in the treatment and perhaps in the prevention of cancers. Tretinoin (all-*trans*-retinoic acid) is a naturally occurring derivative of vitamin A (retinol). Other retinoids indicated for treatment of cancers include alitretinoin (9-*cis*-retinoic acid), available in gel form for topical management of Kaposi sarcoma lesions, and bexarotene (Targretin) gel or capsules for treatment of cutaneous T-cell lymphoma.[18,83]

Retinoids are classed as morphogens, small molecules released from one type of cell that can affect the growth and differentiation of neighboring cells. Their normal roles in the human body are to induce differentiation of some cells, stop the differentiation of others, and both suppress and induce apoptosis in different cell types. Their diverse actions come from the diversity of their receptors. The two classes of retinoid receptors are retinoid X receptors (RXRs) and retinoic acid receptors (RARs), each with α, β, and γ subclasses. RXRs are versatile; they bind to RARs and to other nuclear receptors such as thyroid hormone receptors. Once activated, the receptors act as transcription factors that, in turn, regulate the expression of genes that control cellular growth and differentiation.[18,83]

Tretinoin binds primarily to the RAR-α receptors. Alitretinoin is considered a panagonist, which means that it binds to all known retinoid receptors, producing diverse regulatory effects. Bexarotene is synthetic and is classed as a rexinoid. It is the first RXR-selective retinoid agonist. The exact mechanism of action of alitretinoin and bexarotene as anticancer agents is unknown.[18,83]

Interferons

The interferons (IFNs) are a family of proteins produced by nucleated cells and by recombinant DNA technology, with antiviral, antiproliferative, and immunoregulatory activities. They are classified as α, β, or γ interferons based on antigenic, biologic, and pharmacologic properties. Many subtypes of IFN-α are known. IFN-α_{2a} and IFN-α_{2b}, approved for anticancer indications, are very similar single-species recombinant products.

The mechanisms of IFN-α's antitumor action are complex. IFN increases the activity of cytotoxic cells within the immune system, but they also have direct antiproliferative effects. IFNs prolong the cell cycle, which results in cytostasis, an increase in cell size, and apoptosis. They can inhibit new blood vessel formation in tumors and can increase the expression of antigens on tumor cell surfaces, making the cancerous cells more easily recognized by immune effector cells. They also inhibit or block certain oncogenes that can direct the unregulated cell growth that is characteristic of cancerous cells. Alterations in gene expression may change the levels of receptors for other cytokines, or the concentration of regulatory proteins on immune cells, or may activate enzymes that alter cellular growth and function.[84]

The most frequent adverse effects are flu-like symptoms. Other adverse events include psychiatric symptoms (e.g., depression, anxiety), insomnia and sleep disturbances, myelosuppression, and alopecia.

Interleukin-2 (Aldesleukin)

Interleukin-2 (IL-2) is a cytokine produced by recombinant DNA technology that promotes B- and T-cell proliferation and differentiation and initiates a cytokine cascade with multiple interacting immunologic effects. The IL-2 receptor is expressed in increased amounts on activated T cells and mediates most of the effects of aldesleukin. Antitumor effects depend on proliferation of cytotoxic immune cells that can recognize and destroy tumor cells without damaging normal cells. Some of these cytotoxic cells are natural killer cells, lymphokine-activated killer (LAK) cells, and tumor-infiltrating lymphocytes.[85]

The toxicity of aldesleukin is related to dose, route, and duration of therapy, but aldesleukin is toxic therapy that requires vigorous supportive care. The most common dose-limiting toxicities are hypotension, fluid retention, and renal dysfunction. Aldesleukin decreases peripheral vascular resistance, producing peripheral vasodilation, tachycardia, and hypotension. A characteristic vascular- or capillary-leak syndrome produces fluid retention, which, in turn, can cause respiratory compromise. These toxicities require administration of vasopressors in most patients, judicious use of fluid support and diuretics, and supplemental oxygen. Patients with underlying cardiovascular or renal abnormalities are more susceptible to these adverse effects, making careful patient selection important.[85] Most patients treated with aldesleukin experience thrombocytopenia, anemia, eosinophilia, reversible cholestasis, and skin erythema with burning and pruritus, and some have neuropsychiatric changes, hypothyroidism, and bacterial infections.[85] In general, the toxicities from aldesleukin therapy reverse quickly once therapy is stopped, and can be managed or prevented by careful prospective monitoring and pharmacologic supportive care.

Denileukin Diftitox

Denileukin diftitox is a recombinant fusion protein that combines the active sections of both IL-2 and diphtheria toxin. Unconjugated diphtheria toxin is much too toxic to administer to humans. As the "payload" of the fusion protein, however, its cytotoxic effects are directed toward cells that express the high-affinity form of the IL-2 receptor, such as cancer cells of some patients with cutaneous T-cell lymphoma. Once denileukin diftitox interacts with the IL-2 receptors, the toxin inhibits protein synthesis in the cancer cells and causes cell death.[86]

Although denileukin diftitox is directed therapy, its targeting of cells that express high-affinity IL-2 receptors is not specific because these receptors are expressed on cells other than cancer cells. Denileukin diftitox produces acute hypersensitivity reactions, flu-like symptoms, sometimes with prominent diarrhea, and vascular-leak syndrome. It differs from the vascular-leak syndrome produced by high-dose aldesleukin in that it occurs in fewer patients, is delayed in onset, is usually self-limited, and does not consistently recur on retreatment.[85,86] Patients with an albumin less than 3 g/dL (30 g/L) are at increased risk for vascular-leak syndrome and use in these patients is not recommended.

RESPONSE CRITERIA

The response to anticancer agents and other treatment modalities may be described as a cure, complete response, partial response, stable disease, or progression.[87] A cure implies that the patient is entirely free of disease and has the same life expectancy as a cancer-free individual. Because of our inability to detect small numbers of tumor cells, we can never be absolutely certain that an individual patient is cured. Cancers that are curable with treatment are characterized by a stable plateau in the survival curve where the risk of relapse is very low. For most of these curable cancers, the survival curve has plateaued by about 5 years. Therefore, patients with one of these curable cancers who are alive 5 years from the time of diagnosis without disease recurrence are often considered "cured" of their cancer. However, patients with some malignancies, such as breast cancer and melanoma, are still at significant risk for relapse after 5 years.

In an attempt to simply and unify response definitions in both clinical practice and published reports, the RECIST (Response Evaluation Criteria in Solid Tumors) criteria were developed in 2000 and revised in 2009.[87] *Complete response* (CR) means complete disappearance of all cancer without evidence of new disease for at least 1 month after treatment. The terms *cure* and *CR* are not synonymous. Although an individual must have a CR to be cured, many individuals who achieve a CR will eventually relapse. A *partial response* is defined as a 30% or greater decrease in the tumor size or other objective disease markers, and no evidence of any new disease for at least 1 month. Overall objective response rates for a given treatment are calculated by adding the CR and partial response rates. *Progressive disease* is defined as a 20% increase in the tumor size or the development of any new lesions while receiving treatment. A patient whose tumor size neither grows nor shrinks by the above criteria is termed to have *stable disease*. Some patients may experience subjective improvement in the symptoms caused by their cancer without a defined response. Although clinically important, this does not indicate an objective response. The term *clinical benefit response* was recently developed to document these subjective responses; it refers to patients who have clinical benefit as measured by decreases in pain or analgesic consumption, or improved quality of life or performance status.

These response definitions are applicable to solid tumors, but diseases such as leukemias and multiple myeloma are not characterized by discrete, measurable masses. Responses in these diseases are measured by elimination of abnormal cells (e.g., return to normal hematology parameters and normal bone marrow in leukemia), return of tumor markers to normal levels (e.g., normal serum protein electrophoresis in multiple myeloma), or improved function of affected organs (e.g., improved renal function after obstructive uropathy). Cytogenetic markers and molecular techniques have an increasingly important role in determining whether all cancer has been truly eliminated. For example, in chronic myelogenous leukemia, the Philadelphia chromosome can be detected by polymerase chain reaction techniques, even when no leukemia is evident in the bone marrow or bloodstream. Patients without evidence of the Philadelphia chromosome are classified as a *complete cytogenetic response*. Measuring cytogenetic responses is increasingly common in patients with known cytogenetic abnormalities and absence of complete cytogenetic responses may predict disease relapse.

Finally, different survival endpoints may be used to assess treatment response. Overall survival is considered as the gold standard but increasing emphasis is being placed on other survival endpoints that consider quality of life. These endpoints include disease-free survival and progression-free survival, which measure the time the patient "survives" free of disease (e.g., cancer) or progression, respectively.

The U.S. FDA publishes guidance for industry to facilitate the drug development process.[88] New therapies must demonstrate a favorable risk benefit ratio in adequate and well controlled clinical trials. Overall survival and symptom improvement is considered an appropriate measure of effectiveness. Accelerated approval promulgated in 1992 supported the approval of therapies intended to treat life-threatening or serious illnesses in which the new therapy demonstrated improvement compared to current therapies or provided therapy in the absence of current therapy, based on surrogate endpoints that are likely to predict clinical benefit. Common surrogate endpoints include disease-free survival, progression-free survival, objective response rates and complete response rates; overall response rate is the most common surrogate endpoint used to support accelerated approval. Biomarkers have not been used as primary endpoints to support approval. A clinical trial following accelerated approval must be conducted with due diligence and demonstrate clinical benefit, or the product may be removed from the market. In the time elapsed from 1990 to 2003, 75% of the new therapies for cancer were approved based on endpoints other than survival.[88]

FACTORS AFFECTING RESPONSE TO CHEMOTHERAPY

These include tumor burden, tumor-cell heterogeneity, drug resistance, dose intensity, and patient-specific factors. The significance of tumor burden was discussed earlier in the Principles of Tumor Growth section. Tumors consist of a heterogeneous population of cell types. Because of the genetic instability of cancer cells as compared to normal cells, mutations commonly occur during cell division. Large tumors have undergone many cell divisions and express multiple cell mutations resulting in genetically varied cell populations.[6,19] In 1979, Goldie and Coldman proposed that these cytogenetic changes were not completely random and were highly associated with the development of the ability of tumors to develop drug resistance.[1,6,19] The probability of developing resistant cell populations increases as tumor size increases. It is believed that a small percentage of resistant cancer cells may survive initial chemotherapy. Resistant populations later proliferate and eventually become the dominant cell types, which may explain the common pattern of an initial response to chemotherapy, followed by progressive tumor regrowth despite continuing the same treatment regimen.

Drug resistance may be either an acquired or inherited property of a cancerous cell. Mechanisms of drug resistance include decreased activation of prodrugs, decreased uptake of drugs secondary to alterations in drug transport systems, changes in target enzymes, alterations in the ability to repair drug-induced damage, increased drug inactivation, and decreased apoptosis.[6,11,19] One focus of research is in the area of multidrug resistance.[19,89] When some cancer cells are exposed to increasing concentrations of a specific anticancer agent in vitro, they become resistant to that agent. Surprisingly, these same cells also become resistant to other structurally unrelated anticancer agents and are therefore considered multidrug resistant. Cytotoxic agents derived from natural products, such as the anthracyclines, actinomycin D, mitomycin C, the vinca alkaloids, the epipodophyllotoxins, and the taxanes, produce multidrug resistance. The resistant cancer cells possess a membrane-associated protein known as Pgp, which appears to enhance the export of toxins, such as chemotherapy agents, out of the cell (Fig. 135–10). The gene that encodes for Pgp is known as the *mdr-1* gene. Expression of this gene is amplified in cells that are resistant to the natural products listed previously. Pgp is also found in high concentrations in tumors that are traditionally resistant to chemotherapy (e.g., renal cell cancer and non-small cell lung cancer) and thus may also be an important mechanism of intrinsic or inherited drug resistance. Several drugs have been investigated as possible inhibitors of this efflux pump, such as the calcium channel blockers, quinidine, cyclosporine, and the phenothiazines. Another efflux pump, known as the multidrug resistance-associated protein (MRP), was also recently identified. Other potential mechanisms of drug resistance include inactivation of chemotherapy agents by glutathione metabolism, upregulation of target enzymes such as topoisomerases or dihydrofolate reductase, and decreased apoptosis after exposure to chemotherapy. The last mechanism can be mediated by *bcl-2* oncogene overexpression or loss of the *p53* gene, as discussed in the oncogene section. The interplay between apoptosis and resistance is an area of intense research.

The relationship between dose and response has been extensively explored in cancer chemotherapy.[1] Dose is believed to be a critical factor in determining response for many types of cancers. *Dose intensity* is defined as the dose delivered to the patient over a specified period of time. The three main variables that determine delivered dose intensity are the dose per course, the interval between doses, and the total cumulative dose. *Dose density* refers

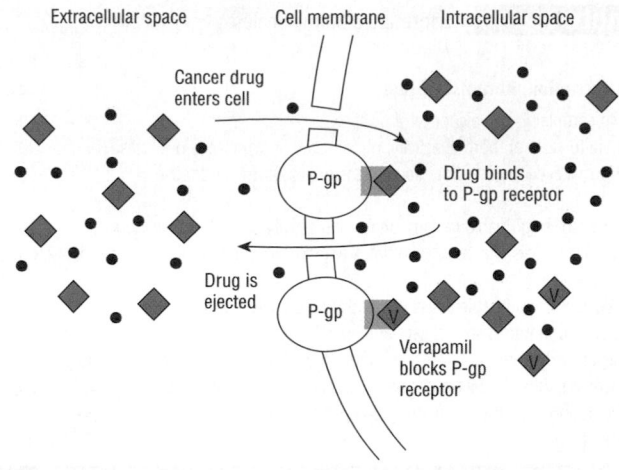

FIGURE 135-10. P-glycoprotein (P-gp) is a membrane-associated protein that acts as a drug efflux pump. Anticancer agents enter the cell, bind to the P-gp receptor, and are ejected. Some agents that modify multidrug resistance, like verapamil, block the P-gp receptor, allowing the anticancer agent to remain in the cell.

to shortening of the usual interval between doses (e.g., every 2 weeks instead of every 3 weeks) and is designed to maximize the drugs' effects on tumor growth kinetics. This strategy has been most extensively studied in breast cancer, with positive results from adjuvant therapy given to patients with high-risk node-positive disease. The delivery of optimal dose intensity is often compromised by the toxicities of the anticancer agent. Treatment cycles are commonly delayed because of inadequate recovery from toxicity, especially myelosuppression. Subsequent doses of chemotherapy are often reduced to prevent or reduce the severity of these toxicities. The impact of this issue on patient outcome has been proven in studies showing reduced rates of response and survival in individuals receiving less-than-optimal chemotherapy doses.[1] Understanding the pathophysiology of toxicities has led to the development of more effective agents for prevention and management of these toxicities. The development of agent- and toxicity-specific chemo protective agents has facilitated application of dose-intensity principles.[1] The colony-stimulating factors avert neutropenia and permit delivery of dose-intensive or dose-dense regimens that are myelosuppressive. The issue of dose intensity is particularly important in the setting of high-dose chemotherapy with autologous hematopoietic stem cell support. Although lethal myelosuppression is avoided by administering hematopoietic stem cells, other severe end-organ toxicities emerge as doses of the anticancer agents are increased.

Patient-specific factors create unpredictable variability in response to chemotherapy. The biology of cancer is strongly affected by host characteristics and genetics. The pathway of genetic mutations that resulted in malignancy can also affect response to therapy. For example, breast cancers that overexpress the HER-2 oncogene are often sensitive to anthracycline-based regimens.[66] Interindividual variations in absorption, distribution, elimination, or metabolism may lead to sub- or supratherapeutic levels of anticancer agents and their metabolites. As a result, both drug efficacy and drug toxicity can be affected. Until recently, healthcare professionals in oncology have modified dose based on variations in body size, blood counts, and renal and hepatic function. Prospective dose modifications based on these parameters are still very important to optimize the effectiveness of therapy and minimize toxicity. But more specific tools are becoming available, as we learn how to identify and apply differences in people's genetic makeup to their anticancer therapy. *Pharmacogenomics* is the study

TABLE 135-10 Performance Status Scales

Description: Karnofsky Scale	Karnofsky Scale (%)	Zubrod Scale (ECOG)	Description: ECOG Scale
No complaints; no evidence of disease	100	0	Fully active, able to carry on all predisease activity
Able to carry on normal activity; minor signs or symptoms of disease	90		
Normal activity with effort, some signs or symptoms of disease	80	1	Restricted in strenuous activity, but ambulatory and able to carry out work of a light or sedentary nature
Cares for self; unable to carry on normal activity or to do active work	70		
Requires occasional assistance but is able to care for most personal needs	60	2	Out of bed more than 50% of time; ambulatory and capable of self-care, but unable to carry out any work activities
Requires considerable assistance and frequent medical care	50		
Disabled; requires special care and assistance	40	3	In bed more than 50% of time; capable of only limited self-care
Severely disabled; hospitalization indicated, although death not imminent	30		
Very sick; hospitalization necessary; requires active supportive treatment	20	4	Bedridden; cannot carry out any self-care; completely disabled
Moribund; fatal processes progressing rapidly	10		
Dead	0		

ECOG, Eastern Cooperative Oncology Group.
Adapted from reference 91.

of the role of inheritance in individual variation in drug response.[90] In oncology, several clinically relevant genetic polymorphisms, or variations, have been identified that can affect pharmacokinetics and pharmacodynamics. Examples include polymorphisms in genes responsible for the activity of the enzymes dihydropyrimidine dehydrogenase (responsible for 5-fluorouracil metabolism), thiopurine *S*-methyltransferase (responsible for thiopurine metabolism), and uridine diphosphate-glucuronosyltransferase 1A1 (responsible for irinotecan metabolism).[90] Patients with deficiencies in these enzymes can experience significant, and possibly life-threatening, toxicity. Screening for these genetic variants might permit individualization of regimens to avoid toxicity and maximize antitumor effects. Monitoring of anticancer agents drug concentrations may also improve the therapeutic index. For example, pharmacokinetic and pharmacodynamic modeling is associated with improved responses and decreased toxicity in children with acute lymphoblastic leukemia.

The presence of other disease states (e.g., comorbidities) may also affect response to treatment by limiting treatment options. The overall functional status of a patient may be assessed using performance status scales, such as the Karnofsky and Eastern Cooperative Oncology Group scales (Table 135–10).[91] These scales can be used to predict patient tolerance of chemotherapy and to assess the effects of chemotherapy on the patient's level of activity and quality of life. For many cancers, performance status at diagnosis is the most important prognostic indicator.

Today's oncology clinician has a wealth of information to consider when designing a treatment approach for an individual patient. Patient-specific factors (e.g., performance status, comorbidities, renal and hepatic function, and pharmacogenomics), tumor-specific factors (e.g., pathology, stage, and molecular profile), and treatment goals (e.g., palliation and cure) are all considered when determining the best treatment option. Treatment cost can also be an important consideration.

COMBINATION CHEMOTHERAPY

Although single agents are sometimes employed, the more common approach to anticancer therapy involves administration of multiple agents to overcome factors for decreased patient response noted previously.[1,18,91] Initially, this approach was based on the Goldie-Coldman hypothesis, which addresses the issue of tumor cell heterogeneity and the inevitable development of drug resis-

tance. Combination chemotherapy is given to target as many types of cells in the tumor as possible. Selection of agents for combination chemotherapy regimens involves consideration of drug-specific factors such as mechanism of action, antitumor activity, and toxicity profile. Drugs that possess minimally overlapping mechanisms of action and toxicities are combined, when possible. Myelosuppressive combinations are sometimes alternated with nonmyelosuppressive combinations to allow bone marrow recovery, while gaining additive antitumor effects. The selected agents should each have significant activity against the tumor that is to be treated. If a synergistic reaction is known to exist for two agents, they may be combined in various treatment regimens.

With the availability of new targeted therapies, one area of research is to determine the optimal ways to combine these agents, both with traditional anticancer agents and other targeted agents. In theory, these therapies make ideal combination agents because they target the underlying cancer biology while usually avoiding typical chemotherapy adverse effects. Clinicians must be careful in combining these agents based on clinical data that demonstrate additive or synergistic benefit. Combinations of chemotherapy and targeted agents have proven successful in breast and colon cancer. Predictive markers are needed to identify which patients may benefit from combinations of chemotherapy and targeted agents and how best to give them.

ADMINISTRATION OF CHEMOTHERAPY

DOSING AND ADMINISTRATION

Healthcare practitioners should monitor several clinical and laboratory values prior to the administration of chemotherapy. In general, a white blood cell (WBC) count $\geq$3,000 cells/mm^3 (3×10^9/L) or an absolute neutrophil count (ANC) $\geq$1,500 cells/mm^3 ($\geq$1.5 $\times$ 10^9/L) and a platelet count of $\geq$100,000 cells/mm^3 ($\geq$100 $\times$ 10^9/L) are usually required prior to administering chemotherapy. In addition, a chemistry panel is drawn to assess renal and hepatic function, especially for agents eliminated via those routes. Table 135–8 lists agents that require dosing adjustments and require specific laboratory tests prior to administration; failure to do so may result in overdosing and excessive toxicity from the agent.

Once it is determined that it is safe to administer, chemotherapy is generally dosed based on body surface area (BSA).[93] BSA is commonly used as an estimate of cardiac output and subsequent distribution to the liver and kidneys, the primary determinants of drug elimination. The most common methods used to determine BSA are the Mosteller and DuBois formulas, which are listed in Table 135–9.

CLINICAL CONTROVERSY

The use of actual versus ideal body weight for calculating BSA is a source of debate in oncology. Although actual body weight is most often used, some clinicians prefer to use an adjusted body weight in obese patients. Clinicians need to clearly state the weight used in the BSA calculation. New methods of dosing using individual patient- and tumor-specific factors are an area of active research.

When determining the dose to be administered, healthcare practitioners should use with caution extreme values in BSA (values greater than 2 m²) and assess patient clinical factors. New dosing methods are being developed to improve the accuracy of chemotherapy dosing and prevent both over- and underdosing. Carboplatin is now commonly dosed based on the patient's estimated glomerular filtration rate. This method, listed in Table 135–9, is known as the Calvert formula and has been demonstrated to achieve adequate levels of carboplatin without excessive toxicity.[94] Chemotherapy may also be dosed based on weight or drug levels and clinicians should be proficient in these calculations prior to dosing and administering any chemotherapy. Additional methods using pharmacogenomic testing are being studied to individualize chemotherapy doses.

SAFETY AND HANDLING ISSUES

The cytotoxic drugs used to treat cancer are carcinogenic, mutagenic, and teratogenic. Consequently, these drugs should be handled with care to avoid inadvertent exposure of healthcare professionals.[95] All pharmacies should have written procedures for handling these drugs safely, and all personnel should be oriented to these procedures. The United States Pharmacopeia (USP) chapter 797 regulates the preparation of extemporaneously compounded sterile preparations and should be used by centers that prepare chemotherapy.[95]

The most common avenue of exposure is via inhalation of aerosolized drug. Individuals preparing chemotherapy should work in a class II biologic safety cabinet and wear gowns and powder-free disposable latex gloves. The gowns should be made of lint-free, low-permeability fabric with a solid front, long sleeves, and tight-fitting elastic cuffs. Negative-pressure techniques should be employed in drug preparation to minimize aerosolization. Healthcare workers administering these agents should take similar precautions to avoid exposure. Kits for cleaning up chemotherapy spills should be located in all areas of the institution in which chemotherapy is handled. Cytotoxic waste should be disposed of properly, and patients should be informed of proper methods of disposing of potentially contaminated body excreta and cytotoxic waste.

GENERAL SUPPORTIVE CARE ISSUES

⑨ The treatment of cancer with most anticancer agents is complicated by the risk of multiple serious toxicities, many of which are life-threatening. Adverse events are commonly graded on a scale from no toxicity to death; a common scale used in clinical trials is the common toxicity criteria (CTC) for adverse events developed by the National Cancer Institute and the standard adverse event reporting classification system used in the United States for all drugs is the Medical Dictionary for Regulatory Activities (med-DRA). Specific toxicities, such as doxorubicin-induced cardiotoxicity and bleomycin-related pulmonary toxicity, were summarized earlier. Several adverse effects are common to many anticancer agents. These include nausea and vomiting, myelosuppression, mucositis, alopecia, infertility, and carcinogenesis. With the addition of targeted therapies, new toxicities such as rash have become issues for healthcare practitioners to address. Nutritional support and pain management are also important supportive care issues, although malnutrition and pain are not usually direct results of toxicity. The management of chemotherapy-induced nausea and vomiting and the basic principles of nutritional support and pain management are discussed in detail in other chapters.

Because many anticancer agents affect DNA synthesis, all rapidly proliferating cells are more sensitive to the toxic effects of chemotherapy. Normal tissues such as the bone marrow, intestinal mucosa, and hair follicles are such tissue sites where drug effects are manifested.

MYELOSUPPRESSION

⑩ Although not seen with all anticancer agents, myelosuppression is the most common dose-limiting side effect of cytotoxic agents. Myelosuppression is increased when chemotherapy is administered concurrently with radiation to the chest or pelvic region. Bone marrow suppression does not usually occur immediately after chemotherapy administration. Blood components that have already been produced must be consumed before the effect is evident. WBCs, especially neutrophil precursors, are most significantly affected because of their rapid proliferation and short life span (6 to 12 hours). Platelets (5- to 10-day life span) are also affected, but to a much less degree than neutrophils. Erythrocytes, with a 120-day life span, are affected the least. Usual nadirs, or lowest blood cell counts, occur at 10 to 14 days following chemotherapy administration, with recovery by 3 to 4 weeks. There are some exceptions to this general rule. The nitrosoureas, mitomycin C, and radiolabeled antibodies exhibit a delayed pattern of nadir (4 to 6 weeks) and recovery (6 to 8 weeks). Planned courses of chemotherapy may have to be delayed while waiting for the granulocyte count to return to normal. Patients with leukemia or receiving a stem cell transplant may have a more rapid nadir of about 5 to 7 days. A guide for suggested blood counts for a patient to safely receive myelosuppressive chemotherapy is listed in the previous section on chemotherapy administration.

Myelotoxicity is a desired therapeutic effect in patients with acute myeloid leukemia during induction chemotherapy. However, myelosuppression, particularly with fever, is an undesirable side effect during chemotherapy for other malignancies. If significant myelosuppression has occurred with prior courses of chemotherapy, the doses of the offending agent(s) in subsequent courses may be reduced. The magnitude of dose reduction is dictated by the degree of myelosuppression incurred and the incidence and severity of infection or bleeding. Empiric dosage reductions may be made for the first chemotherapy treatment if the patient has a low baseline WBC or platelet count, has diminished bone marrow reserve, has impaired drug-elimination, or is to receive a combination of several drugs that cause myelosuppression. Patients who have received multiple prior courses of other myelotoxic chemotherapy regimens or extensive radiation therapy, especially to the pelvis or chest, may have a decreased bone marrow reserve. They are more sensitive to the myelosuppressive effects of chemotherapy, and normal doses may produce profound marrow toxicity. The pharmacokinetic profile of a myelosuppressive agent is also important in determining the appropriate dose. For example, the anthracyclines produce bone marrow suppression as an acute dose-limiting toxicity, and these agents depend on biliary excretion as their primary route of elimination. A patient with biliary obstruction may have compromised elimination of anthracyclines and is at increased risk for severe bone marrow suppression if the dose is not appropriately adjusted (Table 135–8).

However, in some tumors (e.g., breast cancer or lymphoma) dosage reduction may compromise antitumor response, leading to worse patient outcomes.[1] In patients who are responding well to treatment, some degree of myelosuppression is accepted by most healthcare practitioners if it is not compromising the patient's quality-of-life and the tumor is responding to therapy. In these patients, empiric use of hematopoietic growth factors provides an alternative to dose reduction.

Anemia

⑩ Although usually not life-threatening, anemia is the most common hematologic complication of cancer chemotherapy.[96] The incidence of anemia depends on several factors, including the type and duration of therapy and the type and stage of the underlying malignancy. For example, carboplatin is more commonly associated with anemia than many other chemotherapeutic agents. Multiple conditions are known to cause anemia in cancer patients, including chronic gastrointestinal blood loss, nutrient deficiency (e.g., iron and folate), chemotherapy and radiation therapy, bone marrow invasion by the tumor, hemolysis, renal dysfunction, and anemia of chronic disease. Of all the signs and symptoms of anemia, fatigue is most common in cancer patients.[96] In fact, fatigue is the most commonly reported symptom overall in patients undergoing chemotherapy. The presence of fatigue is correlated with the severity of anemia; treatment of anemia may result in improvement in fatigue and quality-of-life. Anemia is only one of many possible causes of fatigue in patients with cancer. Other common causes of fatigue include insomnia, depression, unrelieved pain, and the underlying malignancy.

Previously, the only option for the treatment of chemotherapy-related anemia was red blood cell transfusions. This intervention is still the mainstay of acute management, but the availability of the recombinant human erythropoietic products—epoetin alfa and darbepoetin alfa—has provided another therapeutic option.[96] Several studies have documented the efficacy of these agents in the anemia associated with chemotherapy. Both epoetin alfa and darbepoetin alfa increase hemoglobin and hematocrit and decrease transfusion requirements. Improvements in other outcomes such as fatigue and quality-of-life are under further investigation. One difference between the products is that darbepoetin has a threefold longer half-life, which allows for less-frequent administration of darbepoetin in the clinical setting.[97]

Clinical practice guidelines to guide the appropriate use of erythropoietic agents have been developed.[96] The first step is to evaluate the underlying cause of the anemia and initiate specific therapy as indicated. For example, patients with iron-deficiency anemia should receive iron supplementation. Patients with chronic bleeding or hemolysis should not receive erythropoietic therapy, as this does not target the underlying cause of their anemia. Epoetin alfa and darbepoetin alfa may be considered for chemotherapy- or cancer-related anemia only after otherwise treated causes of anemia have been ruled out. The 2010 National Comprehensive Cancer Network guidelines suggest starting symptomatic patients when their hemoglobin is less than 10 g/dL (100 g/L; 6.21 mmol/L) with a target hemoglobin of 10 to 12 g/dL (100 to 120 g/L; 6.21 to 7.45

mmol/L) to achieve maximum benefit.[96] Several early indicators of response have been proposed, including an increase in hemoglobin of 1 g/dL (10 g/L; 0.62 mmol/L) above baseline, a decline in ferritin, or an increase in the absolute reticulocyte count after 2 to 4 weeks of therapy. These surrogate endpoints can be used to identify non-responders early, so that therapy may be modified or discontinued, as indicated. Serum erythropoietin levels have minimal utility in predicting response or monitoring therapy and are often not measured in clinical practice.

Patients should only receive the labeled doses of the drugs, which are epoetin alfa 40,000 units once, each week or darbepoetin alfa at a dose of 2.25 mcg every other week or 500 mcg every 3 weeks. After 4 to 6 weeks, the hemoglobin should be reassessed. In patients who do not achieve at least a 1 g/dL (10 g/L; 0.62 mmol/L) rise in hemoglobin, the 2010 National Comprehensive Cancer Network guidelines recommend to increase the epoetin alfa dose to 60,000 units once a week and the darbepoetin alfa dose to 4.5 mcg every other week.[96] Iron stores should be checked to rule out iron deficiency as a cause of treatment failure. Supplemental intravenous iron may be administered to increase the response to erythropoietic therapy. Treatment should be discontinued in patients who do not respond after 8 weeks at the higher dose.

Several serious outcomes have been reported with the use of these agents that have resulted in significant changes to their approved labeling and have drastically decreased their use.[96] Recent studies in advanced breast, cervical, head and neck, lymphoma, and non-small-cell lung cancers reported decreased survival in cancer patients receiving erythropoietic drugs for correction of anemia resulting in a black box warning in the package insert. This warning restricts the use of these agents to patients receiving myelosuppressive chemotherapy without curative intent and requires that the minimal dose to reduce blood transfusions be used. Most of these studies had target hemoglobin levels of >12 g/dL (>120 g/L; >7.45 mmol/L), therefore use of these agents in patients with hemoglobin levels >12 g/dL (>120 g/L; >7.45 mmol/L) should be avoided. Agents should be stopped when the chemotherapy-related anemia resolves and these agents should not be used on patients with cancer-related anemia. Patients are also required to be given a medication guide that warns them of this risk without conclusive benefits outside of decreased blood transfusions.

Other serious adverse effects related to erythropoietic products include thrombosis and pure red cell aplasia, which may result in an increased mortality from use. These events have generally occurred when the target hemoglobin of 12 g/dL (120 g/L; 7.45 mmol/L) is exceeded or the hemoglobin rises too quickly. The 2010 National Comprehensive Cancer Network guidelines recommend that if hemoglobin increases by more than 1 g/dL (10 g/L; 0.62 mmol/L) in a 2-week period, the dose of either product should be reduced by 25% or by the amount needed to avoid blood transfusions. If hemoglobin levels exceed 12 g/dL (120 g/L; 7.45 mmol/L) while on therapy, healthcare practitioners should hold therapy and reinitiate therapy at dose to avoid transfusions if the patient's hemoglobin falls below 10 g/dL (100 g/L; 6.21 mmol/L).[96]

Other rare and generally mild adverse effects include pain at injection site, rash, flu-like symptoms, seizures, and hypertension.

Neutropenia

⑩ When the ANC falls below 500 cells/mm³ (0.5 × 10⁹/L), infection risk increases.[98] The ANC may be calculated by multiplying the percentage of neutrophils (segmented plus banded neutrophils) by the total WBC count. The risk of infection is also directly proportional to the duration of neutropenia. Other risk factors for infection include alteration in the integrity of physical defense barriers and the functional integrity of WBCs. The patient's underlying cancer and treatment with cytotoxic drugs and radiation can affect neutrophil function. The diagnosis of infection in the neutropenic patient is complicated by the lack of WBCs. Usual signs and symptoms of infection, such as pus, abscesses, and infiltrates on chest radiography, are often absent as a result of the lack of WBCs. Clinicians must rely on fever as an indication of infection in these patients. Definitive culture results may take days, and a septic neutropenic cancer patient can die within hours if not treated. Therefore, the basic approach to the management of the febrile neutropenic cancer patient is prompt initiation of empiric antibiotics. The antibiotics are chosen based on reliable coverage of the most likely organisms, antibiotic sensitivities at the institution, the patient's signs and symptoms (if present), side-effect profiles, and cost.[98] The most common source of infection in these patients is self-infection with body flora, which includes both gram-positive and gram-negative bacteria. Specific treatment of infections in immunocompromised hosts is discussed in Chapter 131.

Numerous methods have been explored to prevent infections in cancer patients. Colony-stimulating factors (CSFs) are commonly employed for this purpose.[98] These hormones are naturally

occurring proteins that are essential for the normal growth and maturation of blood cell components (Fig. 135–11). The CSFs have the ability to enhance the production and also the function of their target cells. Two agents, G-CSF (granulocyte colony-stimulating factor) and GM-CSF (granulocyte-macrophage colony-stimulating factor) are commercially available in the United States. G-CSF (filgrastim) specifically stimulates the production of neutrophilic granulocytes. GMCSF (sargramostim) promotes the proliferation of granulocytes (neutrophils and eosinophils) and monocytes/macrophages.[99] Although GM-CSF stimulates megakaryocytes, no consistent effect on platelet production has been observed in clinical trials. Both agents initially enhance demargination and mobilization of mature cells from the marrow and then provide constant stimulation of stem cell progenitors. CSFs are produced by recombinant DNA technology, and several host cells are used to produce CSFs, including bacteria (*E coli*), yeast, and mammalian cells (Chinese hamster ovary cells). Products derived from yeast or mammalian sources are glycosylated to varying degrees, as are naturally occurring CSFs, while those derived from *E coli* are nonglycosylated.[99] This difference does not result in any clinically

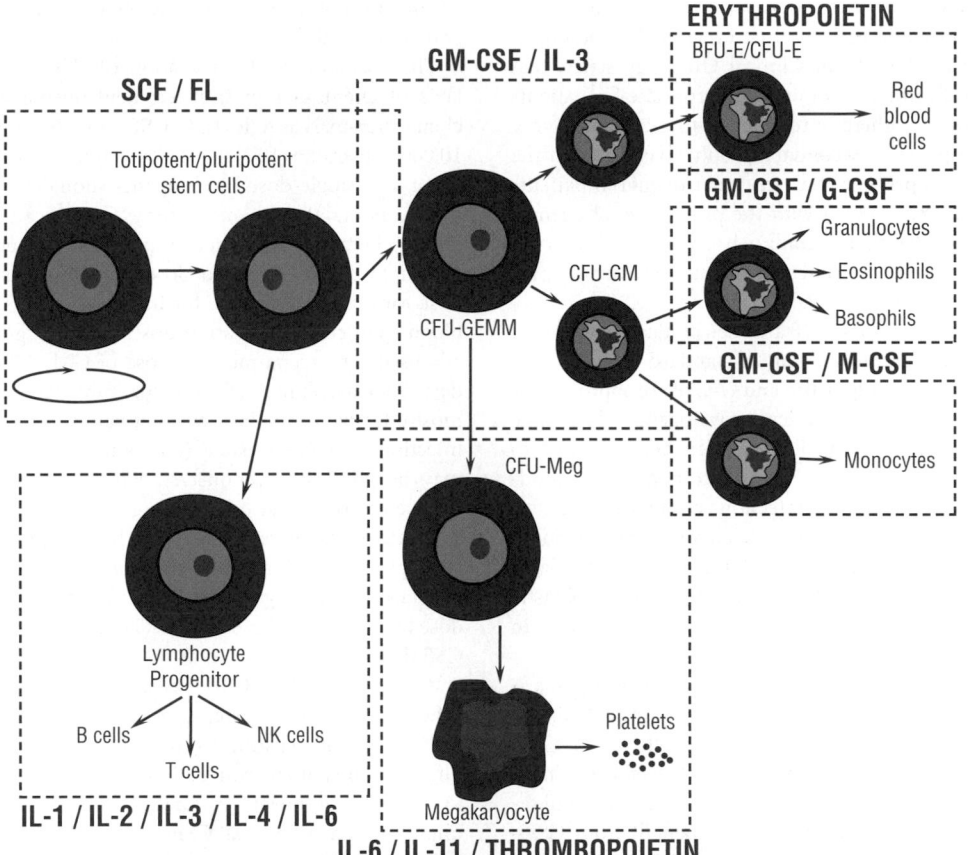

FIGURE 135-11. Sites of action of hematopoietic growth factors in the differentiation and maturation of marrow cell lines. A self-sustaining pool of marrow stem cells differentiates under the influence of specific hematopoietic growth factors to form a variety of hematopoietic and lymphopoietic cells. Stem cell factor (SCF), FTL- 3 ligand (FL), interleukin-3 (IL- 3), and granulocyte/macrophage colony-stimulating factor (GM-CSF), together with cell–cell interactions in the marrow, stimulate stem cells to form a series of burst-forming units (BFU) and colony-forming units (CFU): CFU-GEMM, CFU-GM, CFU-Meg, BFU-E, and CFU-E (GEMM, granulocyte, erythrocyte, monocyte, and megakaryocytes; GM, granulocyte and macrophage; Meg, megakaryocyte; E, erythrocyte). After considerable proliferation, further differentiation is stimulated by synergistic interactions with growth factors for each of the major cell lines—granulocyte colony-stimulating factor (G-CSF), monocyte/macrophage-stimulating factor (M-CSF), thrombopoietin, and erythropoietin. Each of these factors also influences the proliferation, maturation, and, in some cases, the function of the derivative cell line. (*Adapted from Kaushansky K and Kipps TJ. Hematopoietic agents: Growth factors, minerals and vitamins. In: Brunton LL, Lazo JS, Parker KL, eds. Goodman & Gilman's The Pharmacologic Basis of Therapeutics, 11th ed. New York: McGraw-Hill, 2006: 1435.*)

significant effects on neutrophil production. Pegfilgrastim is a long-acting CSF, created by addition of a polyethylene glycol molecule to G-CSF.[100] Clinical trials have demonstrated that a single dose of pegfilgrastim provides equivalent effects to 10 to 11 days of daily G-CSF, with similar side-effect profiles.

The CSFs reduce the incidence, magnitude, and duration of neutropenia when used as preventive therapy following a variety of myelosuppressive chemotherapy regimens.[98,101] These effects have been accompanied by a modest decrease in febrile days, infections, and days on antibiotics. In some studies, use of CSFs also resulted in a decrease in the incidence of mucositis. Growth factors have also permitted the administration of subsequent chemotherapy courses on schedule, resulting in enhanced dose intensity. However, the increased dose intensity provided by the CSFs has not consistently translated into improved tumor response or survival. Because of lack of impact on response rates and survival, decisions regarding appropriate use of growth factors should be based on weighing proven clinical benefits against economic considerations. The American Society of Clinical Oncology has developed evidence-based clinical practice guidelines to promote appropriate use of the CSFs.[101]

Growth factors may be used in either primary or secondary prophylaxis of neutropenia. Primary prophylaxis refers to the use of CSFs to prevent neutropenia with the first cycle of chemotherapy. Recently, the American Society of Clinical Oncology stated that this strategy is clinically and economically appropriate for patients who are receiving a chemotherapy regimen with a 20% or higher risk of febrile neutropenia.[108] Secondary prophylaxis refers to the use of growth factors to prevent recurrent neutropenia in patients who had experienced neutropenia with the prior cycle of chemotherapy. It is recommended that secondary prophylaxis be reserved for patients with chemosensitive cancers where dose reduction may affect disease-free or overall survival.[101]

Pegfilgrastim, G-CSF, and GM-CSF are used clinically to prevent febrile neutropenia after administration of standard doses of chemotherapy although only pegfilgrastim and G-CSF are approved for this indication. One exception is in acute myelogenous leukemia, in which both G-CSF and GM-CSF have been demonstrated to reduce the duration of neutropenia, often accompanied by modest decreases in hospitalization and infectious complications, after induction chemotherapy. Benefits have been most clearly documented in patients older than age 55 years. Similar data are available for G-CSF in the treatment of patients with acute lymphoblastic leukemia. These beneficial effects, however, have not resulted in improved response rates or overall survival.[101]

The role of CSFs in the treatment of established neutropenia is less-well defined. Most studies suggest no or only minimal clinical benefit from use of CSFs in treating neutropenia; therefore, CSFs should not be routinely employed in patients with established neutropenia, regardless of the presence of fever. However, certain high-risk patients with fever and neutropenia may benefit from CSFs: neutropenia >10 days, ANC <100 cells/mm³ (>0.1 × 10⁹/L), age <65 years, infectious complications (pneumonia, sepsis, or invasive fungal infections), and patients who are hospitalized at the time of the development of neutropenic fever.[98,101]

Both G-CSF and GM-CSF have also proven effective in acceleration of hematopoietic engraftment and in treatment of graft failure following hematopoietic stem cell transplantation. Other uses for the CSFs include peripheral blood stem cell mobilization, neutropenia in patients with acquired immune deficiency syndrome, myelodysplastic syndromes, congenital neutropenia, and aplastic anemia. Growth factors should not be used in patients receiving concomitant chemotherapy and radiotherapy, especially if the radiation involves the mediastinum. These patients appear to experience more significant thrombocytopenia when administered CSFs.

At currently recommended doses, the CSFs are well tolerated. Side effects are more commonly seen with GM-CSF and may be related to the drug's ability to enhance binding of neutrophils to endothelial cells or to activation of monocytes/macrophages, which may stimulate the release of cytokines such as IL-1 and tumor necrosis factor.[99] The most common toxicity of the CSFs is bone pain (20% to 25% of patients), which can be treated with acetaminophen. Other side effects of G-CSF include an increase in lactate dehydrogenase, alkaline phosphatase, and uric acid levels. Additional toxicities of GM-CSF include constitutional symptoms, such as low-grade fever, myalgia, arthralgia, lethargy, and mild headache. GM-CSF may also produce an elevation in liver transaminases. At higher doses of GM-CSF, pleural and pericardial effusions, capillary-leak syndrome, and thrombus formation may occur. A first-dose reaction described after GM-CSF administration has been reported more commonly with the *E coli*-derived product (molgramostim), which is not commercially available in the United States. This reaction is more common after intravenous infusion and consists of dyspnea, facial flushing, hypotension, hypoxia, and tachycardia. Both G-CSF and GM-CSF may produce mild erythema at subcutaneous injection sites, as well as a generalized maculopapular rash with either subcutaneous or intravenous administration. Pegfilgrastim adverse effects are similar to G-CSF and are treated the same.[100]

The dosing and administration of CSFs approved for prophylaxis of chemotherapy-induced neutropenia after standard dose chemotherapy is as follows: G-CSF 5 mcg/kg until the ANC reaches 10,000 cells/mm³ (10 × 10⁹/L) (or clinically safe) or pegfilgrastim 6 mg as a single dose. Both agents should be started between 24 and 72 hours after chemotherapy; G-CSF can be stopped the day before chemotherapy whereas pegfilgrastim needs to be stopped within 14 days of the next dose because of its long half-life. The dose for other uses varies, for instance in the setting of peripheral blood stem cell mobilization doses of 10 mcg/kg per day are usually used. The recommended dose of GM-CSF is 250 mcg/m² per day. Pharmacokinetic data favor subcutaneous injection as the most effective route. However, in patients in whom subcutaneous injections are not feasible (e.g., anasarca), G-CSF and GM-CSF may be given intravenously. Pegfilgrastim should not be given intravenously. Because of the high cost associated with CSF use, alternative dosing regimens have been explored. These regimens attempt to decrease the total amount of CSF used by either delaying the start of CSFs (e.g., to day 3 after chemotherapy), decreasing the dose (e.g., to 3 mcg/kg/day of G-CSF), or decreasing the duration of CSF therapy. Standardized doses of 300 mcg or 480 mcg of G-CSF and 500 mcg of GM-CSF, based on product vial sizes, are often used to minimize waste. Specifically, the posttreatment target ANC of 10,000 cells/mm³ (10 × 10⁹/L) recommended by product information is often reduced in clinical practice to 5,000 cells/mm³ (5 × 10⁹/L) or lower. For patients receiving pegfilgrastim, it is important that additional CSFs not be administered for the 10 days following administration, as additional benefit is not realized.[100]

Thrombocytopenia

Chemotherapy-induced thrombocytopenia puts the patient at risk for significant bleeding. To date, platelet transfusions remain the mainstay of management. At most centers, platelet transfusions are reserved for patients with a platelet count of <10,000 cells/mm³ (<10 × 10⁹/L) unless they are actively bleeding, must undergo a surgical procedure, or have documented infections or fever in which the threshold is higher. For patients with nonmyeloid malignancies who experienced significant thrombocytopenia with a prior cycle of chemotherapy, oprelvekin (IL-11) may be considered as secondary prophylaxis.[102] When used after chemotherapy regimens associated with a high risk of thrombocytopenia, oprelvekin decreased the need for platelet transfusions, as well as the numbers of platelets required for transfusion. Unfortunately, oprelvekin is associated with some significant adverse effects, mostly related to fluid retention (e.g., edema, dilutional anemia, dyspnea, and pleural effusions). Cardiac toxicity, especially tachycardia, and atrial fibrillation and flutter also have been observed. Prophylactic oprelvekin also is significantly more expensive than platelet transfusions.[103] Considering the modest clinical benefit, the adverse effects, and the high cost, oprelvekin use should be reserved for patients who are at high risk for severe thrombocytopenia from chemotherapy where dose reduction is known to compromise disease response. Other CSFs, such as IL-1, −3, and −6, have also been studied, but significant impact on platelet counts with an acceptable adverse effect profile has not been demonstrated.[85,102] The discovery and development of thrombopoietin, a megakaryocyte-stimulating factor, may represent the most significant factor in the future of thrombocytopenia treatment.

MUCOSITIS

The gastrointestinal mucosa is composed of epithelial cells with a high mitotic index and rapid turnover rate, making it a common site of chemotherapy-induced toxicity.[104] The subsequent inflammation, or mucositis, can lead to painful ulcerations, local infection, and inability to eat, drink, or swallow. Disruption of the gastrointestinal mucosal barrier may also provide an avenue for systemic microbial invasion. The time course for development and resolution of mucositis often parallels that of neutropenia. Agents most commonly associated with mucositis include 5-FU, doxorubicin, and methotrexate. Currently, the most effective means of preventing mucositis is through good oral hygiene. Patients who are at high risk for this toxicity (those with poor dentition, high-dose chemotherapy, or radiation therapy involving the oropharynx) should be evaluated by a dentist prior to chemotherapy and should be instructed to rinse their mouths frequently with baking soda and salt water or plain saline rinses during and between courses of chemotherapy. Clinical practice guidelines for the prevention and treatment of cancer therapy-induced mucositis were recently published.[104] The benefit of chlorhexidine rinses over saline rinses is unclear. In patients undergoing radiation therapy to the head and neck region, chlorhexidine rinses have detrimental effects on the oral mucosa. For patients receiving 5-FU treatment, the use of ice (oral cryotherapy) may decrease the risk for mucositis by decreasing drug delivery to the oral mucosa. A better understanding of the pathophysiology of mucositis has resulted in identification of promising new agents to better prevent mucositis. The keratinocyte growth factor palifermin is approved for use in patients receiving high-dose chemoradiotherapy prior to hematopoietic stem cell transplantation. Palifermin is given intravenously at a dose of 60 mcg/kg/day for 3 consecutive days immediately before the initiation of conditioning therapy and then again for 3 days after hematopoietic stem cell transplantation.[105] The effect of palifermin on solid tumor growth is unknown and its use in nonhematologic cancers is not recommended.

After mucositis has developed, treatment is mainly supportive, including use of topical or systemic analgesics and oral hygiene (including the rinses described).[104] Viscous lidocaine, diphenhydramine liquid, and dyclonine are topical anesthetics commonly employed. Severe cases of mucositis may lead to dehydration and require intravenous hydration and pain medications including patient-controlled analgesia pumps. Local infections caused by *Candida* species and reactivation of herpes simplex viruses are common in these patients. Suspicious lesions should be cultured, and appropriate antifungal and/or antiviral treatment should then

be instituted. Antifungal therapy may be delivered topically for mild infections (thrush) with clotrimazole troches or nystatin oral suspension. For more severe oral or esophageal fungal infections, systemic treatment with oral fluconazole or intravenous antifungals is indicated.

Mucosal damage can occur at any point along the entire length of the gastrointestinal tract. In the lower portion of the gastrointestinal tract, this damage is usually manifested as diarrhea (mild to life-threatening in nature) and abdominal pain. Support with intravenous fluids and electrolyte supplementation should be initiated promptly in severe cases. After infectious causes have been ruled out, diarrhea can safely be treated with antispasmodics such as Lomotil or loperamide. The somatostatin analog octreotide has also been used successfully to treat severe cases of chemotherapy-induced diarrhea; guidelines exist to assist practitioners in treating this toxicity.[104,106]

CUTANEOUS REACTIONS

Cutaneous reactions to chemotherapy are generally reversible and self-limiting upon chemotherapy dose reductions or delays. Common reactions include localized rash, photosensitivity, skin hyperpigmentation, nail changes, and hand–foot syndrome, but can be associated with severe hypersensitivity reactions. Common agents known to cause rash in patients include cytarabine, 5-FU, and bleomycin.

In targeted therapies, particularly those that target the EGFR receptor, rash is often the most common adverse effect associated with therapy and requires prompt recognition by healthcare professionals to prevent drug discontinuation. Some studies suggest that the rash may be a surrogate marker of response to these agents, perhaps indicating a genetic predisposition to response with EGFR targeted agents. Rash occurs in up to two thirds of patients on EGFR inhibitors, most commonly in the first month on treatment with the typical site of presentation being the face and upper torso. Although no clear guidelines exist for the treatment of this rash, patients should be supported based on their presentation.[64] Anecdotal reports indicate that emollients help if patients complain of dry skin, topical and systemic antibiotics may help if the rash becomes infected, and steroids may help prevent itching and inflammation.[64]

ALOPECIA

Although not a life-threatening side effect of chemotherapy, the toxicity that many patients find most distressing is alopecia. Alopecia from chemotherapy is usually temporary, and the degree of hair loss varies widely.[107] Loss of hair is not limited to the scalp; any area of the body may be affected. Patients receiving a taxane as part of their chemotherapy regimen are especially prone to total body alopecia. Hair loss usually begins 1 to 2 weeks after chemotherapy, and regrowth may begin before the chemotherapy courses are completed. Cryotherapy (local application of ice) and scalp tourniquets have both been investigated as methods of preventing alopecia. Both techniques produce vasoconstriction, resulting in decreased exposure of hair follicles to the chemotherapy agents. These techniques are not uniformly effective and are contraindicated in patients with cancers that may metastasize to the scalp, such as leukemia and lymphoma.

EXTRAVASATION

Vesicants are agents that may cause severe tissue damage if they escape from the vasculature.[108] These agents include the anthracyclines, actinomycin D, the vinca alkaloids, mitomycin C, nitrogen mustard, and the taxanes. The anthracyclines are the most notorious agents, and the most extensively investigated. The tissue damage may result in prolonged pain, tissue sloughing, infection, and loss of mobility. Prompt initiation of the appropriate interventions is important to minimize morbidity. Unfortunately, most information on extravasation management is anecdotal; few controlled clinical trials have been conducted to determine optimal intervention strategies. Consequently, prevention is the focus of extravasation management. The most important method of prevention is good administration technique, but extravasations may occur despite good administration technique.[108] The vein selected for administration should be on the distal portion of the arm. The large veins of the forearm are desirable because if a drug does extravasate, there is adequate soft-tissue coverage to protect crucial structures like nerves and tendons, and joint function is not put at risk. Peripherally administered vesicants should be given slowly via intravenous injection (IV push) through the side arm of a running intravenous line. The person administering the vesicant should verify needle stability and adequate blood return after each 1 to 2 mL of drug is injected. Vesicants should not be administered by intravenous infusion unless the patient has a central venous catheter. For extravasation of vesicants, one of the most important interventions is the application of ice packs to the affected area. One exception to this rule is the vinca alkaloids, which are better managed with application of heat. Only a few antidotes to vesicant agents are employed clinically. Sodium thiosulfate is used to neutralize nitrogen mustard extravasations, and hyaluronidase (if available) can improve the outcome after extravasation of vinca alkaloids, etoposide, and taxanes. Topical application of dimethyl sulfoxide may be an effective method for managing anthracycline and mitomycin C extravasations.[108] A new packaging of dexrazoxane, marketed as Totect®, has been approved to treat anthracycline extravasation and is given as an intravenous infusion.[109]

INFERTILITY

Advances in the treatment of some cancers, such as Hodgkin disease and testicular cancer, have produced long-term survivors and the opportunity to examine the late consequences of chemotherapy administration. Infertility and secondary cancers have emerged as important late effects. The gonadal toxicities of chemotherapy have not received much attention in the past because they are not life-threatening. High rates of fertility deficits and sexual dysfunction have been noted for both men and women.[110] In men, antitumor drugs produce severe oligospermia or azoospermia as well as infertility. Serum testosterone levels are only rarely altered. The recovery of spermatogenesis after completion of chemotherapy is unpredictable. Men receiving combination chemotherapy appear to sustain more long-lasting adverse effects on fertility than do men receiving single-agent therapy. Age, total dose, duration of therapy, and type of drug are other important variables. In women, toxic effects on the ovaries result clinically in amenorrhea, vaginal epithelial atrophy, and menopausal symptoms. These effects are related to dose and age. Younger patients are more resistant to the effects on the ovaries. As with men, the recovery of fertility is unpredictable, but women younger than 25 years of age appear to have the best outcomes. The effects of the alkylating agents on fertility have been extensively studied. This group of drugs exerts profound and consistently detrimental effects on reproductive function.[110] The impact of this drug-induced amenorrhea on patient survival has been less clear with some trials demonstrating a benefit to those patients who achieve chemotherapy-induced amenorrhea. Trial results have been mixed though and conclusive statements cannot be made at this time. Less is known about commonly used agents such as doxorubicin, taxanes, and platinum compounds. The risk of infertility should be discussed with all patients prior to receiving chemotherapy and they should be informed about options for fertility preservation.

SECONDARY MALIGNANCIES

Secondary cancers induced by chemotherapy and radiation are a serious long-term complication.[111] Although many types of solid tumors have been reported as chemotherapy-induced malignancies, acut myelogenous leukemia or myelodysplastic syndromes are the most common secondary cancers. Acute myelogenous leukemia or myelodysplastic syndrome has been reported following successful treatment of Hodgkin and non-Hodgkin lymphoma, acute leukemias, multiple myeloma, breast cancer, and advanced ovarian cancer. For curable cancers, the relatively small risk for occurrence of secondary malignancies is far outweighed by the benefits of survival in large numbers of patients. However, for cancers such as ovarian cancer, the risk of leukemia is not offset by improved survival in patients treated with chemotherapy. The issue of secondary malignancies is of particular concern in patients receiving adjuvant chemotherapy. As with the late complication of infertility, the anticancer agents primarily associated with secondary cancers are the alkylating agents. Etoposide, teniposide, radionucleotides, and the anthracyclines also are linked to secondary leukemias. Solid tumors as secondary malignancies occur more commonly after treatment with radiation than with chemotherapy.

ABBREVIATIONS

ADCC: antibody dependent cellular cytotoxicity

ANC: absolute neutrophil count

ara-C: cytarabine

ara-CTP: active triphosphate form of cytarabine

BCNU: carmustine

BSA: body surface area

CCNU: lomustine

CDC: complement-dependent cytotoxicity

CR: complete response

CSF: colony-stimulating factor

DHFR: dihydrofolate reductase

DNA: deoxyribonucleic acid

DNMT: DNA methyltransferase

EGFR: epidermal growth factor receptor

5-FU: fluorouracil

G_0: dormant phase of the cell cycle

G_1: first gap phase of the cell cycle

G_2: second gap or premitotic phase of the cell cycle

G-CSF: granulocyte colony-stimulating factor

GM-CSF: granulocyte-macrophage colony-stimulating factor

HAMA: human antimouse antibodies

HER: human epidermal growth factor receptor

HDAC: histone deacetylases

IL: interleukin

IFN: interferon

6-MP: 6-mercaptopurine

M: mitosis

MoAB: monoclonal antibody

mRNA: messenger RNA

MTIC: monomethyl triazeno imidazole carboxamide

mTOR : mammalian target of rapamycin

MTX: methotrexate

NF-κB: nuclear factor-κB

Pgp: p-glycoprotein

RAR: retinoic acid receptor

RNA: ribonucleic acid

rRNA: ribosomal RNA

RXR: retinoid X receptor

S: DNA synthesis phase of the cell cycle

tRNA: transfer RNA

VEGF: vascular endothelial growth factor

WBC: white blood cell

REFERENCES

1. Chabner BA. Clinical strategies for cancer treatment: The role of drugs. In: Chabner BA, Longo DL, eds. Cancer Chemotherapy and Biotherapy: Principles and Practice, 4th ed. Philadelphia: Lippincott Williams & Wilkins, 2006: 1–14.
2. Jemal A, Siegel R, Xu J, Ward E, et al. Cancer statistics, 2010. CA Cancer J Clin 2010; 60:277–300.
3. Liotta LA, Liotta LA, Petricoin EF. Genomics and proteomics. In: DeVita VT, Hellman S, Rosenberg SA, eds. Cancer: Principles and Practice of Oncology, 8th ed. Philadelphia, PA: Lippincott Williams & Wilkins, 2008: 13–34.
4. Compagni A, Christofori G. Recent advances in research on multistage tumorigenesis. Br J Cancer 2000;83:1–5.
5. Weston A, Harris CC. Chemical carcinogenesis. In: Kufe DW, Bast RC, Hait WN, et al., eds. Cancer Medicine, 7th ed. Hamilton, Ont: BC Decker, 2006: 246–258.
6. Cotran RS, Kumar V, Collins T. Neoplasia. In: Cotran RS, Kumar V, Collins T, eds. Robbins' Pathologic Basis of Disease. Philadelphia, PA: WB Saunders, 1999: 260–328.
7. Weinberg RA. How cancer arises. Sci Am 1996;275:62–71.
8. Hanahan D, Weinberg RA. The hallmarks of cancer. Cell 2000;100(1):57–70.
9. Gross ME, Shazer RL, Agus DB. Targeting the HER-kinase axis in cancer. Semin Oncol 2004;31(Suppl 3):9–20.
10. Hartwell LH, Kastan MB. Cell cycle control and cancer. Science 1994;266:1821–1828.
11. Johnstone RW, Ruefli AA, Lowe SW. Apoptosis: A link between cancer genetics and chemotherapy. Cell 2002;108:153–164.
12. Esteller M, Garcia-Foncillas J, Andion E, et al. Inactivation of the DNA-repair gene MGMT and the clinical response of gliomas to alkylating agents. N Engl J Med 2008;358:1148–1159.
13. Minn AJ, Massave J. Invasion and Metastases. In: DeVita VT, Hellman S, Rosenberg SA, eds. Cancer: Principles and Practice of Oncology, 8th ed. Philadelphia, PA: Lippincott Williams & Wilkins, 2008: 117–134.
14. Folkman J, Heymach J, Kalluri R. Tumor angiogenesis. In: Kufe DW, Bast RC, Hait WN, et al, eds. Cancer Medicine, 7th ed. Hamilton, Ont: BC Decker, 2006: 157–191.
15. Smith RA, Cokkinides V, Brawley OW. Cancer screening in the United States, 2009: A review of current American Cancer Society guidelines and issues in cancer screening. CA Cancer J Clin 2009;59:27–41.
16. American Cancer Society. Warning Signs of Cancer. Atlanta, GA: American Cancer Society, 2007.
17. Fleming ID, et al., eds. AJCC Cancer Staging Manual, 6th ed. New York: Springer-Verlag, 2002: 209–217.
18. Chabner BA, Amrein PC, Druker BJ, et al. Antineoplastic agents. In Brunton LL, Lazo JS, Parker KL, eds. Goodman & Gilman's The Pharmacological Basis of Therapeutics, 11th ed. New York: McGraw-Hill, 2006: 1315–1403.
19. Buick RN. Cellular basis of chemotherapy. In: Dorr RT, Von Hoff DD, eds. Cancer Chemotherapy Handbook, 2nd ed. New York: Elsevier, 1994: 3–14.
20. Gilweski TA, Norton L. Chemotherapy: Cytokinetics. In: Kufe DW, Bast RC, Hait WN, et al, eds. Cancer Medicine, 7th ed. Hamilton, Ont: BC Decker, 2006: 570–589.
21. Pizzorno G, Diasio RB, Cheng Y-C. Pyrimidines and purine antimetabolites. In: Kufe DW, Bast RC, Hait WN, et al, eds. Cancer Medicine, 7th ed. Hamilton, Ont: BC Decker, 2006: 661–674
22. Wagstaff AJ, Ibbotson T, Goa KL. Capecitabine: A review of its pharmacology and therapeutic efficacy in the management of advanced breast cancer. Drugs 2003;63:217–236.
23. Johnson SA. Clinical pharmacokinetics of nucleoside analogues: Focus on haematological malignancies. Clin Pharmacokinet 2000;39:5–26.
24. Fandy TE. Development of DNA methyltransferase inhibitors for the treatment of neoplastic diseases. Curr Med Chem 2009;16:2075–2085.
25. Plosker GL, Figgitt DP. Oral fludarabine [see comment]. Drugs 2003;63:2317–2323.
26. Cole PD, Kamen BA, Bertino JR. Folate antagonists. In: Kufe DW, Bast RC, Hait WN, et al, eds. Cancer Medicine, 7th ed. Hamilton, Ont: BC Decker, 2006:648–660.
27. Rowinsky E. Microtubule-targeting natural products. In: Kufe DW, Bast RC, Hait WN, et al, eds. Cancer Medicine, 7th ed. Hamilton, Ont: BC Decker, 2006: 699–721.
28. Gradishar WJ, Tjulandin S, Davidson N, et al. Phase III trial of nanoparticle albumin-bound paclitaxel compared with polyethylated castor oil-based paclitaxel in women with breast cancer. J Clin Oncol 2005;23:7794–7803.
29. Goodin S. Ixabepilone: A novel microtubule-stabilizing agent for the treatment of metastatic breast cancer. Am J Health Syst Pharm 2008;65:2017–2026.
30. Rubin EH, Hait WN. Drugs that target DNA topoisomerase. In: Kufe DW, Bast RC, Hait WN, et al, eds. Cancer Medicine, 7th ed. Hamilton, Ont: BC Decker, 2006: 688–699.
31. Ulukan H, Swaan PW. Camptothecins: A review of their chemotherapeutic potential. Drugs 2002;62:2039–2057.
32. Danesi R, Fogli S, Gennari A, et al. Pharmacokinetic-pharmacodynamic relationships of the anthracycline anticancer drugs. Clin Pharmacokinet 2002;41:431–444.
33. Colvin M. Alkylating agents and platinum antitumor compounds. In: Kufe DW, Bast RC, Hait WN, et al, eds. Cancer Medicine, 7th ed. Hamilton, Ont: BC Decker, 2006: 674–687.
34. Ajlthkumar T, Parkinson C, Shamshad F, et al. Ifosfamide. Encephalopathy. Clin Oncol 2007;19:108–114.
35. Cheson BD, Rummel MJ. Bendamustine: rebirth of an old drug. J Clin Oncol 2009;27:1492–1501.
36. Grothey A, Goldberg RM. A review of oxaliplatin and its clinical use in colorectal cancer. Expert Opin Pharmacother 2004;5:2159–2170.
37. Buzdar AU, Harvey HA, Jordan VC. Antiestrogens and aromatase inhibitors. In: Kufe DW, Bast RC, Hait WN, et al, eds. Cancer Medicine, 7th ed. Hamilton, Ont: BC Decker, 2006: 828–842.
38. Osborne CK, Zhao H, Fuqua SA. Selective estrogen receptor modulators: Structure, function, and clinical use. J Clin Oncol 2000;18:3172–3186.
39. Denmeade SR. Androgens. In: Kufe DW, Bast RC, Hait WN, et al, eds. Cancer Medicine, 7th ed. Hamilton, Ont: BC Decker, 2006: 850–859.
40. McKay LI, Cidlowski JA. Corticosteroids. In: Kufe DW, Bast RC, Hait WN, et al, eds. Cancer Medicine, 7th ed. Hamilton, Ont: BC Decker, 2006: 817–827.
41. Soignet SL, Frankel SR, Douer D, et al. United States multicenter study of arsenic trioxide in relapsed acute promyelocytic leukemia. J Clin Oncol 2001;19:3852–3860.
42. Bradner WT. Mitomycin C. A clinical update. Cancer Treat Rev 2001;27:35–50.
43. Bolden JE, Peart MJ, Johnstone RW. Anticancer activities of histone deacetylase inhibitors. Nat Rev Drug Discov 2006;5:769–784.
44. Toma MB, Medina PJ. Update on Targeted Therapy-Focus on Monoclonal Antibodies. J Pharm Pract 2008;21:4–16.
45. American Medical Association. Monoclonal antibodies. *http://www.ama-assn.org/ama/pub/about-ama/our-people/coalitions-consortiums/united-states-adopted-names-council/naming-guidelines/naming-biologics/monoclonal-antibodies.shtml.*

46. Rotea W Jr, Saad ED. Targeted drugs in oncology: New names, new mechanisms, new paradigm. Am J Health Syst Pharm 2003;60:1233-1243; quiz 1244–1245.

47. Harris M. Monoclonal antibodies as therapeutic agents for cancer. Lancet Oncol 2004;5:292–302.

48. Villamor N, Montserrat E, Colomer D. Mechanism of action and resistance to monoclonal antibody therapy. Semin Oncol 2003;30:424–433.

49. Cheson BD. Radioimmunotherapy of non-Hodgkin's lymphomas. Blood 2003;101:391–398.

50. Cersosimo RJ. Monoclonal antibodies in the treatment of cancer, Part 2. Am J Health Syst Pharm 2003;60:1631-1641; quiz 1642–1643.

51. Mylotarg (gemtuzumab). Prescribing information. Philadelphia, PA: Wyeth Pharmaceuticals; 2008.

52. Plosker GL, Figgitt DP. Rituximab: A review of its use in non-Hodgkin's lymphoma and chronic lymphocytic leukaemia. Drugs 2003;63:803–843.

53. Cersosimo RJ. Monoclonal antibodies in the treatment of cancer, Part 1. Am J Health Syst Pharm 2003;60:1531–1548.

54. Zahrani AA, Ibrahim N, Eid AA. Rapid infusion rituximab changing practice for patient care. J Oncol Pharm Pract 2009;15:183–186.

55. Hernandez MC, Knox SJ. Radiobiology of radioimmunotherapy with 90Y ibritumomab tiuxetan (Zevalin). Semin Oncol 2003;30 (Suppl 17):6–10.

56. Kaminski MS, Zelenetz AD, Press OW, et al. Pivotal study of iodine I 131 tositumomab for chemotherapy-refractory low-grade or transformed low-grade B-cell non-Hodgkin's lymphomas [see comment]. J Clin Oncol 2001;19:3918–3928.

57. Gribben JG, Hallek M. Rediscovering alemtuzumab: Current and emerging therapeutic roles. Br J Haematol 2009;144:818–831.

58. Syed S, Rowinsky E. The new generation of targeted therapies for breast cancer. Oncology (Williston Park) 2003;17:1339-1351; discussion 52.

59. Rowinsky EK. Signal events: Cell signal transduction and its inhibition in cancer. Oncologist 2003;2006;8(Suppl 3):5–17.

60. Finley RS. Overview of targeted therapies for cancer. Am J Health Syst Pharm 2003;60(Suppl 9):S4-S10.

61. Cunningham D, Humblet Y, Siena S, et al. Cetuximab monotherapy and cetuximab plus irinotecan in irinotecan-refractory metastatic colorectal cancer [see comment]. N Engl J Med 2004;351:337–345.

62. Bonner JA, Harari PM, Giralt J, et al. Radiotherapy plus cetuximab for squamous-cell carcinoma of the head and neck [see comment]. N Engl J Med 2006;354:567–578.

63. Chung CH, Mirakhur B, Chan E, et al. Cetuximab-induced anaphylaxis and IgE specific for galactose-1,3-galactose. N Engl J Med 2008;358:1109–1117.

64. Li T, Perez-Soler R, Saltz L. Skin toxicities associated with epidermal growth factor inhibitors. Target Oncol 2009;4:107–119.

65. Hoy SM, Wagstaff AJ. Panitumumab in the treatment of metastatic colorectal cancer. Drugs 2006;66:2005–2014.

66. Treish I, Schwartz R, Lindley C. Pharmacology and therapeutic use of trastuzumab in breast cancer. Am J Health Syst Pharm 2000;57:2063-2076; quiz 2077–2079.

67. Romond EH, Perez EA, Bryant J, et al. Trastuzumab plus adjuvant chemotherapy for operable HER2-positive breast cancer. N Engl J Med 2005;353:1673–1684.

68. Leyland-Jones B, Gelmon K, Ayoub JP, et al. Pharmacokinetics, safety, and efficacy of trastuzumab administered every three weeks in combination with paclitaxel [see comment]. J Clin Oncol 2003;21:3965–3971.

69. Cersosimo RJ. Gefitinib: A new antineoplastic for advanced non-small-cell lung cancer [see comment]. Am J Health Syst Pharm 2004;61:889–898.

70. Tang PA, Tsao M-S, Moore MJ. A review of erlotinib and its clinical use. Expert Opin Pharmacother 2006;7:177–193.

71. Janne PA, Johnson BE. Effect of epidermal growth factor receptor tyrosine kinase domain mutations on the outcome of patients with non-small cell lung cancer treated with epidermal growth factor receptor tyrosine kinase inhibitors. Clin Cancer Res 2006;12(Pt 2):4416s-4420s.

72. Medina PJ, Goodin S. Lapatinib: a dual inhibitor of human epidermal growth factor receptor tyrosine kinases. Clin Ther 2008;30:1426–1447.

73. Zondor SD, Medina PJ. Bevacizumab: An angiogenesis inhibitor with efficacy in colorectal and other malignancies. Ann Pharmacother 2004;38:1258–1264.

74. Hurwitz H, Fehrenbacher L, Novotny W, et al. Bevacizumab plus irinotecan, fluorouracil, and leucovorin for metastatic colorectal cancer [see comment]. N Engl J Med 2004;350:2335–2342.

75. Avastin (bevacizumab). Prescribing information. San Francisco, CA: Genentech; 2009.

76. Rini BI, Campbell SC, Escdier B. Renal cell carcinoma. Lancet 2009;373:1119–1132.

77. Deininger M, Buchdunger E, Druker BJ. The development of imatinib as a therapeutic agent for chronic myeloid leukemia. Blood 2005;105:2640–2653.

78. Gleevec (imatinib mesylate). Prescribing information. East Hanover, NJ: Novartis Pharmaceutical Corporation; January 2009.

79. McFarland KL, Wetzstein GA. Chronic myeloid leukemia therapy: focus of second-generation tyrosine-kinase inhibitors. Cancer Control 2009;16:132–140.

80. Curran MP, McKeage K. Bortezomib: a review of its use in patients with multiple myeloma. Drugs 2009;69:859–888.

81. Kapoor A, Figlin RA. Targeted inhibition of mammalian target of rapamycin for the treatment of advanced renal cell carcinoma. Cancer 2009;115:3618–3630.

82. Rajkumar SV, Kyle RA. Multiple myeloma: Diagnosis and treatment. Mayo Clin Proc 2005;80:1371–1382.

83. Altucci L, Leibowitz MD, Oglivie KM, et al. RAR and RXR modulation in cancer and metabolic disease. Nat Rev Drug Discov 2007;6:793–810.

84. Borden EC. Interferons. In: Kufe DW, Bast RC, Hait WN, et al, eds. Cancer Medicine, 7th ed. Hamilton, Ont: BC Decker, 2006: 733–743.

85. Ekmekcioglu S, Grimm EA, Kurzrock R. Cytokines and hematopoietic growth factors. In: Kufe DW, Bast RC, Hait WN, et al, eds. Cancer Medicine, 7th ed. Hamilton, Ont: BC Decker, 2006: 744–769.

86. Foss F. Clinical experience with denileukin diftitox (ONTAK). Semin Oncol 2006;33(Suppl 3):S11–S16.

87. Therasse P, Arbuck SG, Eisenhauer EA, et al. New guidelines to evaluate the response to treatment in solid tumors. J Natl Cancer Inst 2000;92:205–216.

88. Johnson JR, Williams G, Pazdur R. End points and United States Food and Drug Administration approval of oncology drugs. J Clin Oncol 2003;21:1404–1411.

89. Kellen JA. The reversal of multidrug resistance: An update. J Exp Ther Oncol 2003;3:5–13.

90. Lee W, Lockhart AC, Kim RB, Rothenberg ML. Cancer Pharmacogenomics: Powerful tools in cancer chemotherapy and drug development. Oncologist 2005;10:104–111.

91. Haskell CM. Principles of cancer chemotherapy. In: Haskell CM, ed. Cancer Treatment, 5th ed. Philadelphia, PA: WB Saunders, 2001: 62–86.

92. Johnson DH. Targeted therapies in combination with chemotherapy in non-small cell lung cancer. Clin Cancer Res 2006;12(Pt 2): 4451s-4457s.

93. Vu TT. Standardization of body surface area calculations. J Oncol Pharm Pract 2002;8:49–54.

94. Calvert AH, Newell DR, Gumbrell LA, et al. Carboplatin dosage: Prospective evaluation of a simple formula based on renal function. J Clin Oncol 1989;7:1748–1756.

95. American Society of Hospital Pharmacists. ASHP guidelines on handling hazardous drugs. Am J Health Syst Pharm 2006;63:1172–1193.

96. The NCCN Cancer- and Chemotherapy-Induced Anemia Clinical Practice Guidelines in Oncology (Version 2.2010). 2009 National Comprehensive Cancer Network, Inc.; 2009. *http://www.nccn.org*.

97. Siddiqui MAA, Keating GM. Darbepoetin alfa: A review of its use in the treatment of anaemia in patients with cancer receiving chemotherapy. Drugs 2006;66:997–1012.

98. Hughes WT, Armstrong D, Bodey GP, et al. 2002 Guidelines for the use of antimicrobial agents in neutropenic patients with cancer [see comment]. Clin Infect Dis 2002;34:730–751.

99. Nemunaitis J. A comparative review of colony-stimulating factors. Drugs 1997;54:709–729.

100. Wolf T, Densmore JJ. Pegfilgrastim use during chemotherapy: Current and future applications. Curr Hematol Rep 2004;3:419–423.

101. Smith TJ, Khatcheressian J, Lyman GH, et al. 2006 Update of recommendations for the use of white blood cell growth factors: An evidence-based clinical practice guideline. J Clin Oncol 2006;24:3187–3205.

102. Demetri GD. Pharmacologic treatment options in patients with thrombocytopenia. Semin Hematol 2000;37(Suppl 4):11–18.

103. Cantor SB, Elting LS, Hudson DV Jr, Rubenstein EB. Pharmacoeconomic analysis of oprelvekin (recombinant human interleukin-11) for secondary prophylaxis of thrombocytopenia in solid tumor patients receiving chemotherapy. Cancer 2003;97:3099–3106.

104. Keefe DM, Schubert MM, Elting LS, et al. Updated clinical practice guidelines for the prevention and treatment of mucositis. Cancer 2007;109:820–831.

105. Spielberger R, Stiff P, Bensinger W, et al. Palifermin for oral mucositis after intensive therapy for hematologic cancers. N Engl J Med 2004;351:2590–2598.

106. Benson AB, III, Ajani JA, Catalano RB, et al. Recommended guidelines for the treatment of cancer treatment-induced diarrhea. J Clin Oncol 2004;22:2918–2926.

107. Karakunnell J, Berger AM. Hair loss. In: DeVita V, Hellman S, Rosenberg SA, eds. Cancer Principles and Practice of Oncology, 8th ed. Philadelphia, PA: Lippincott Williams & Wilkins, 2008: 2688–2691.

108. Albanell J, Baselga J. Systemic therapy emergencies. Semin Oncol 2000;27:347–361.

109. Reeves D. Management of anthracycline extravasation injuries. Ann Pharmacother 2007;41:1238–1242.

110. Lee SJ, Schover LR, Partridge AH, et al. American Society of Clinical Oncology recommendations on fertility preservation in cancer patients. J Clin Oncol 2006;24:2917–2931.

111. Travis LB, Hodgson D, Allan JM, et al. Second cancers. In: DeVita VT, Hellman S, Rosenberg SA, eds. Cancer Principles and Practice of Oncology, 8th ed. Philadelphia, PA: Lippincott Williams & Wilkins, 2008: 2718–2743.

CHAPTER 136

Breast Cancer

LAURA BOEHNKE MICHAUD, CHAD M. BARNETT, AND FRANCISCO J. ESTEVA

KEY CONCEPTS

❶ Breast cancer is usually diagnosed in early stages, when it is a highly curable malignancy.

❷ Local therapy of early-stage breast cancer consists of modified radical mastectomy or lumpectomy plus external beam radiation therapy. The surgical approach to the ipsilateral axilla may consist of a full level I/II axillary lymph node dissection or a lymph node mapping procedure with sentinel lymph node biopsy.

❸ Adjuvant endocrine therapy reduces the rates of relapse and death in patients with hormone receptor-positive early breast cancer tumors. Adjuvant chemotherapy reduces the rates of relapse and death in all patients with early stage breast cancer.

❹ The choice of chemotherapy regimen, dose, schedule and duration of therapy, and the choice of endocrine therapy are controversial and rapidly changing as results from ongoing randomized clinical trials are reported.

❺ Neoadjuvant chemotherapy is appropriate for patients with locally advanced breast cancer, inflammatory breast cancer, and selected patients with early breast cancer followed by local therapy and further adjuvant systemic therapy.

❻ Initial therapy of metastatic breast cancer in most women with hormone receptor-positive tumors should consist of hormonal therapy.

❼ Women with metastatic breast cancer who have hormone receptor-positive tumors and respond to an initial hormonal manipulation will usually respond to a second hormonal manipulation.

❽ Approximately 60% of women with metastatic breast cancer will respond to chemotherapy regimens; anthracycline- and taxane-containing regimens are the most active.

❾ The goal of adjuvant chemotherapy is curative, whereas the goal of chemotherapy in the metastatic setting is palliative.

❿ Although controversial, annual screening mammography in women younger than 50 years of age is clearly beneficial

The complete chapter, learning objectives, and other resources can be found at
www.pharmacotherapyonline.com.

and many national and international studies demonstrate a reduction in breast cancer mortality from annual or biennial screening mammography in women ages 50 to 70 years.

Breast cancer is the most common site of cancer and is second only to lung cancer as a cause of cancer death in American women. It is estimated that 207,090 new cases of breast cancer will be diagnosed and that 39,840 women will die of breast cancer in 2010.[1] In addition to invasive breast cancers, it is estimated that 54,010 cases of noninvasive, or in situ, cancer will be diagnosed among women in the United States in 2010.

Female breast cancer incidence rates vary considerably across racial and ethnic groups. The average annual age-adjusted incidence rate from 2001 to 2005 was 130.6 cases per 100,000 among white females, 117.5 cases among African Americans, 90.1 cases in Hispanics, 89.6 cases among Asian-Americans/Pacific Islanders, and 75.0 cases in American Indians/Alaska Natives.[2] Reasons for the higher incidence rates in whites than in other racial and ethnic groups may include differences in reproductive and lifestyle factors, and access to and use of screening.[3]

Female breast cancer incidence rates have increased for all women combined since 1980, although the rate of increase slowed in the 1990s, and has decreased by approximately 2% per year from 1999 to 2006. Factors that may explain the decrease in incidence include a slight reduction in the use of screening mammography and decreased use of postmenopausal hormone-replacement therapy (HRT).[2] The incidence of ductal carcinoma in situ (DCIS) also increased rapidly between the early and late 1980s, and continues to increase. The increase in DCIS is largely attributed to increased use of screening mammography, because most cases of DCIS manifest solely as clustered microcalcifications seen on mammography.[3]

❶ For all racial and ethnic groups, most breast cancers are diagnosed at an early stage, when tumors are small and localized. However, a higher proportion of disease is diagnosed at more advanced stages in African American and other minority women than in white women. The death rate is also higher among African American women than white women despite the lower incidence. From 2001 to 2005, the breast cancer death rate was highest in African Americans (33.5 cases per 100,000 women), followed by whites (24.4), American Indians/Alaska Natives (17.1), Hispanics (15.8), and Asian-Americans/Pacific Islanders (12.6).[2] The cause of this disparity between white and African American women is controversial, with possible explanations including access to care, socioeconomic status, cultural differences, higher stage at diagnosis, and more aggressive biologic features. Despite these differences, overall mortality rates from breast cancer in the United States have declined since 1990. These declines have been attributed to increased use of screening and effectiveness of adjuvant treatment.[4,5] Figure 136–1 shows the temporal trends in incidence and mortality by race.

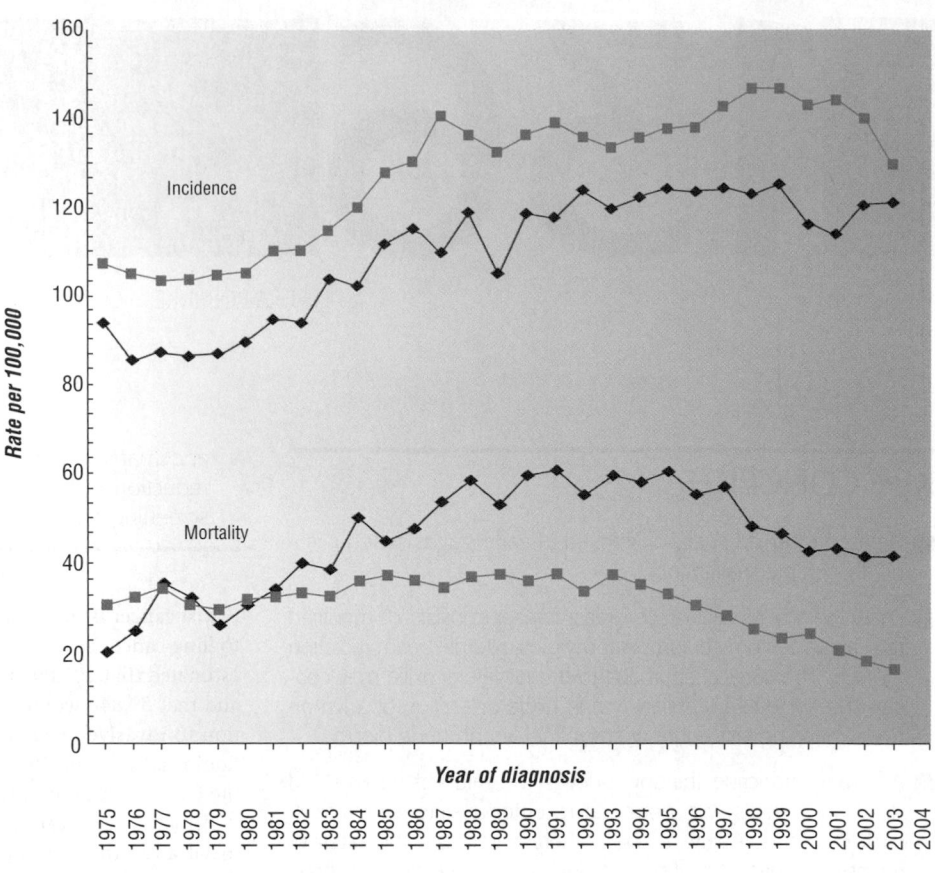

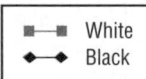

FIGURE 136-1. Breast cancer incidence and mortality rates by race, 1975–2004. *(From reference 2.)*

The median age at diagnosis for breast cancer is between the ages of 60 and 65 years.[2] Although lung cancer is the leading cause of cancer deaths for women regardless of age, breast cancer is the leading cause of cancer deaths for females between the ages of 20 and 59 years.[1]

EPIDEMIOLOGY AND ETIOLOGY

The two variables most strongly associated with the occurrence of breast cancer are gender and age. Although one commonly thinks of breast cancer as a disease confined to women, about 1,970 cases of male breast cancer will be diagnosed in the United States in 2010.[1] Male gender had been considered a poor prognostic factor in some investigations, but it is now believed that higher mortality rates in men are attributable to more advanced disease at the time of diagnosis. When stage and other known prognostic factors are controlled for, the clinical outcome for men with breast cancer is comparable to women.[6] Likewise, treatment of male breast cancer is similar to treatment of breast cancer in females.

The incidence of breast cancer increases with advancing age. A frequently quoted breast cancer statistic is that 1 in 8 women will develop breast cancer during their lifetime. It should be emphasized that this is a cumulative lifetime risk of developing the disease from birth to death. The 1-in-8-women figure is often misinterpreted by women who assume that it translates into 1 in 8 women being diagnosed with breast cancer each year. A more useful method of presenting the risk data is based on age intervals.[7] Table 136–1 shows that the risk of a woman developing breast cancer before the age of 40 years is about 1 in 206, and more than half the risk occurs after age 60 years.

An understanding of the relationship between age and the incidence of breast cancer is particularly relevant when one discusses "risk factors" or factors other than age that increase a woman's probability of developing breast cancer. The relative risk (RR) of developing breast cancer for an individual woman in a defined risk group is usually multiplied by the probability of a woman developing breast cancer during her lifetime, and this figure is taken as the cumulative lifetime risk of that individual developing breast cancer. However, the risk of developing breast cancer depends on age. Therefore, a more meaningful way to counsel patients regarding their risk of developing breast cancer based on the presence of a known risk factor incorporates an age-specific incidence rate, not cumulative lifetime risk. For example, if a 40-year-old woman with a strong family history of breast cancer has a RR ratio of 2.0, her risk of developing breast cancer by the age of 50 is only 7.6% (2 × 3.8) not 24% (2 × 12) (Table 136–1). It is also important to note that recognized risk factors are not additive in a simple mathematical sense.

TABLE 136-1	Risk of Developing Breast Cancer, Women, All Races 2004–2006
Age Interval (years)	**Probability (%) of Developing Invasive Breast Cancer during the Interval**
Birth–39	0.49 or 1 in 206
40–59	3.75 or 1 in 27
60–69	3.40 or 1 in 29
70 and older	6.50 or 1 in 15
From birth to death	12.08 or 1 in 8

SEER, Surveillance Epidemiology and End Results.
(From reference 1.)

Finally, it should be emphasized that most women with breast cancer have no identifiable major risk factor, indicating that the search for the etiology of this disease is largely incomplete.

A number of calculators are available to estimate a patient's risk of developing breast cancer. The National Cancer Institute has an online version of the Breast Cancer Risk Assessment Tool (*www.cancer.gov/bcrisktool/Default.aspx*). This tool is based on a statistical model known as the Gail Model, derived from data from the Breast Cancer Detection and Demonstration Project, a mammography screening project conducted in the 1970s. The Breast Cancer Risk Assessment Tool was designed for healthcare professionals to project a woman's individualized risk for invasive breast cancer over a 5-year period and over her lifetime. This model has been shown to provide accurate estimates in white women, but it has not been validated for other racial and ethnic groups, and other subgroups including those with genetic risk factors. Other risk assessment models also exist, each taking into account different risk factors. Gail and colleagues have developed a similar model for assessing the risk of developing breast cancer in African-American women.[8] These empiric models may not be as useful for women with a history suggestive of hereditary breast cancer. Thus, no one model is appropriate for every patient.

ENDOCRINE FACTORS

A number of endocrine factors have been linked to the incidence of breast cancer.[9,10] Many of these relate to the total duration of menstrual life. Early menarche, generally defined as menstruation beginning before age 12 years, increases the cumulative lifetime risk of breast cancer development. Similarly, most studies demonstrate an increased risk in women with a late age of natural menopause (age 55 years or later). Conversely, bilateral oophorectomy prior to age 40 years reduces the relative risk of developing breast cancer.

Nulliparity and a late age at first birth (≥30 years) are reported to increase the lifetime risk of developing breast cancer. It is suggested that the period between the onset of menses and the age of first pregnancy provides a "window of initiation" for the development of breast cancer. This is a time when an unbalanced hormonal environment reacts with the abundant and highly responsive breast tissue. Investigators postulate that international differences in age of menarche, age at menopause, and childbearing may account for a substantial part of the international differences in the incidence of breast cancer.

Many studies have evaluated the relationship between exogenous hormones and development of breast cancer. Postmenopausal estrogen replacement therapy has been the subject of several epidemiologic studies and meta-analyses, with conflicting results. The NCI-sponsored Women's Health Initiative (WHI) is a set of clinical trials designed to investigate the risks and benefits of treatment strategies that could affect women's health issues, such as breast cancer. The WHI trials of hormone therapy were two large parallel, randomized, double-blind, placebo-controlled trials that evaluated estrogen plus progestin in combination or estrogen alone in post-menopausal women. The estrogen plus progestin trial randomized more than 16,000 postmenopausal women to take conjugated equine estrogen combined with medroxyprogesterone or a placebo.[11] This study reported an increased risk of breast cancer (38 vs 30 cases per 10,000 person-years [RR = 1.26; 95% confidence interval (CI), 1.00-1.59]) in women taking combined estrogen/progestin for an average of 5.2 years when compared to those receiving placebo. Analysis of the National Cancer Institute's Surveillance, Epidemiology, and End Results (SEER) registries showed that the age-adjusted incidence rate of breast cancer in women in the United States in 2003 fell by 6.7% compared to 2002.[12] This decrease in breast cancer incidence seems to be temporally associated with the first report of the WHI study and subsequent decrease in estrogen and progestin hormone replacement therapy use among postmenopausal women. In the estrogen alone trial, over 10,000 women who had a hysterectomy and therefore did not require progestin therapy due to a decreased risk of endometrial carcinoma, were randomized to estrogen alone or placebo.[13] The risk of breast cancer was not increased in women who received estrogen alone as compared to placebo. Differences in dosages, formulations, and routes of administration of various hormonal preparations available make interpretation of these studies complex. However, most of the current evidence does show a causal relationship between HRT and breast cancer.[14] Unresolved issues remain as to whether lower doses or short-term use for menopausal symptoms can be safe and effective. Longer duration of use of HRT and concurrent use of progestins appear to contribute to breast cancer risk.

The use of postmenopausal HRT in women with a history of breast cancer is generally contraindicated. Because of the association of estrogen and risk of breast cancer, many clinicians believe that patients with a strong family history or other risk factors for breast cancer should not receive postmenopausal HRT. Women who are considering HRT should carefully consider the risks versus benefits (see Chap. 91 for a detailed discussion of hormone replacement therapy).

Epidemiologic studies of oral contraceptives do not show a consistent relationship between use of birth control pills and breast cancer risk. Results are conflicting and assessment of the studies should consider the particular oral contraceptive products involved, daily and cumulative doses of the hormones administered, and the latency for development of breast cancer. Newer formulations of oral contraceptives contain lower hormone concentrations, with different routes of administration (e.g., patch, injections, etc.). Reassuring data that oral contraceptives do not increase breast cancer risk later in life have recently been published.[15,16] It is also important to note that oral contraceptives are known to reduce the risk of ovarian and endometrial cancers. Although it is not entirely possible to rule out a promotional effect of oral contraceptives on breast cancer development in young patients, most experts believe that the safety and benefits of low-dose oral contraceptives currently outweigh the potential risks.

GENETIC FACTORS

Both personal and family histories influence a woman's risk of developing breast cancer. A past medical history of breast cancer is associated with an increased risk of contralateral breast cancer. Cancer of the uterus and ovary is also associated with an increased risk for the development of breast cancer. Breast cancer is also observed as part of cancer family syndromes in association with other tumors.

Many women have "lumpy breasts" and have a clinical diagnosis of fibrocystic breast disease or benign breast disease. Fibrocystic disease encompasses a heterogeneous group of processes with various degrees of breast cancer risks, and therefore is not clinically meaningful for counseling patients regarding individual risk of breast cancer. Benign breast conditions are classified as nonproliferative, proliferative without atypia, or atypical hyperplasia. Nonproliferative lesions, such as cysts or simple fibroadenomas, do not increase the risk of breast cancer. Proliferative lesions without atypia, such as intraductal papillomatosis, are associated with a mildly elevated breast cancer risk of about 1.5 to 2.0 times the general population. Atypical hyperplasias are classified as either ductal or lobular units, and these lesions may increase a woman's risk for breast cancer to about 4.5 to 5.0 times the general population.[17]

Dense breast tissue reduces the sensitivity of mammography for detecting breast cancer, and is also associated with an increased risk of breast cancer. Genetic factors may play a role in this finding because mammographic breast density has been shown to have high heritability and is also strongly associated with a positive family history of breast cancer. Many variables including age, weight, menopausal status, HRT, and parity can influence mammographic breast density. The risk of breast cancer in women with dense breasts (defined by mammography) has been estimated to be between 2 and 6 times that of women of the same age with little density.[18]

It has been recognized for some time that a family history of breast cancer is associated with a woman's own risk for developing the disease. The percentage of all breast cancers in the population that can be attributed to family history is approximately 10%. Empirical estimates of the risks associated with particular patterns of family history of breast cancer indicate the following:[19]

1. Having any first-degree relative with breast cancer increases a woman's risk of breast cancer about 1.5- to 3-fold. Risk increases with increasing numbers of affected first-degree relatives.

2. The risk is affected by both a woman's own age and the age of the relative when diagnosed. A higher RR is seen when a woman and her relative at diagnosis are younger than 50 years.

3. The risk associated with having any second-degree relative with breast cancer is complex, and depends on other family history patterns. However, the risk is generally lower than that of first-degree relatives.

4. Affected family members on both the maternal and the paternal sides are important to consider in evaluation of risk.

Although women with a family history of breast cancer are at increased risk for the disease, the diagnosis of breast cancer is still uncommon in young women, even with a positive family history. Although family history is an important risk factor to consider, other risk factors should also be considered as most women who develop breast cancer do not have a family history. Nonetheless, increasing knowledge about the genetics of the disease continues to add to our understanding.

In the early 1990s, pedigree analysis of 23 high-risk families for breast and ovarian cancer provided evidence for a rare autosomal dominant allele.[20] Further studies identified an abnormal gene on the long arm of chromosome 17 (17q21) in a large percentage of these hereditary breast and ovarian cancer patients. Isolation of the *BRCA1* gene was initially reported in 1994. A second breast cancer gene, called *BRCA2*, has been mapped to chromosome 13. These genes function as tumor suppressor genes, maintaining genomic integrity and DNA repair. Germ-line mutations in either *BRCA1* or *BRCA2* are associated with an increased risk for breast and ovarian cancer. Compared to an average woman's 13% lifetime risk of developing breast cancer, the probability of developing breast or ovarian cancer by the age of 70 years in women with a *BRCA1* or *BRCA2* mutation is estimated to be 35% to 84% for breast cancer and 10% to 50% for ovarian cancer.[21,22] The risk of ovarian cancer is considered higher among carriers of *BRCA1* mutations than for carriers of *BRCA2* mutations.

The probability of being a *BRCA* gene-mutation carrier is related to ethnicity and family history. Particular family history patterns are associated with an increased risk, including the number of unaffected and affected family members who had breast and/or ovarian cancer, including first- and second-degree relatives; younger age (<50 years) at which breast cancer is diagnosed; the presence of bilateral breast cancer; and a history of breast cancer in a male relative. Both maternal and paternal family histories are relevant. Specific gene mutations can also be seen more often among certain ethnic groups. Jewish people of Eastern European decent (Ashkenazi Jews)

have an unusually high (2.5%) carrier rate of germ-line mutations in *BRCA1* and *BRCA2* as compared to the rest of the U.S. population. Three particular *BRCA* founder mutations are most often identified in women of Jewish ancestry, obviating the need to sequence entire genes and making genetic testing less complicated.[20] For this reason, some clinicians have advocated for *BRCA1* and *BRCA2* screening for all patients of Jewish descent regardless of personal or family history of breast or ovarian cancer, although current national guidelines do not recommend this broad approach.

Since the discovery of *BRCA1* and *BRCA2*, genetic testing for mutations in these genes has become available. The question of who should receive screening for *BRCA* gene mutations is unresolved. It is estimated that clinically significant *BRCA* mutations occur at a frequency of about 1 in 500 persons in the general, non-Jewish U.S. population.[22] Risk tools to predict for the presence of a clinically significant *BRCA* mutation exist. Because many of these tools were developed from data in previously tested women with existing cancer, their applicability and effectiveness for screening in the general population are unknown. Several organizations have published recommendations on genetic susceptibility testing for individuals who meet the criteria for increased risk.[21,23,24] Testing for *BRCA1* and *BRCA2* mutations is now widely available, can be accomplished through varying methodologies, and has been directly marketed to the public.[25] Nonetheless, testing is generally recommended only when there is personal or family history suggestive of hereditary cancer, when the test can be adequately interpreted, and when results will assist with diagnosis and management. Genetic counseling is highly recommended with all genetic tests to assist individuals in making informed decisions.

The clinical significance of other unclassified variant gene mutations is unknown. Testing negative for a *BRCA* gene mutation does not necessarily rule out a hereditary form of breast cancer. In cases where there is significant personal or family history, a negative test may be considered an uninformative negative, as it may be a result of mutations undetected by currently available screening techniques, or a result of mutations in other, unidentified genes. *BRCA1* and *BRCA2* account for at least 30% of all hereditary breast cancer.[26] Other genes that have been identified as being associated with hereditary breast cancer include *TP53, CHK2, PTEN,* and *ATM*.[20]

ENVIRONMENTAL AND LIFESTYLE FACTORS

Breast cancer incidence rates vary considerably between countries, which suggests that environmental and lifestyle factors play an important role in the etiology. Compelling evidence is derived from studies of Asian women who migrated to the United States. Although the incidence of breast cancer in Asian women is quite low, the incidence of breast cancer in Asian women who were born in the United States, or who migrated from Asia to the United States, gradually increases to equal that of the white population in the same geographic area.[10]

Diet is an obvious environmental factor, and possible relationships between fat intake and steroid hormone metabolism have led to an emphasis on dietary fat as a possible etiologic agent for breast cancer. Epidemiologic data show a positive correlation between higher dietary fat intake and breast cancer risk. The correlation is stronger in postmenopausal than in premenopausal women. A low-fat diet is linked to low blood estrogen levels and lower breast cancer risk. Studies in laboratory animals provide further evidence of a relationship between dietary fat intake and breast cancer. Despite these compelling indirect data, case control and cohort studies report mixed results. In a meta-analysis of 31 case-control and 14 cohort studies on dietary fat and breast cancer, Boyd et al. reported a small but significant RR of 1.13 (95% CI, 1.03- 1.25) when comparing highest and lowest fat intake categories.[27]

Additional investigated dietary factors include food-derived heterocyclic amines, which are known carcinogens found commonly in cooked meat. Experimental and epidemiologic data suggest an association between breast cancer and the Western diet, which typically includes a large amount of cooked meats and fat. In the meta-analysis by Boyd et al., saturated fat and meat intake were also associated with a small, but significant increased risk in breast cancer.[27] Other studies have found no significant association between breast cancer and the Western diet. Effects may depend on menopausal status, as studies of premenopausal women suggest a possible increased risk.[28]

Many studies have also examined the association between breast cancer and intake of dietary fiber and micronutrients, including β-carotene, and vitamins A, C, and E. The relationship between vitamins and breast cancer is unclear. Studies of breast cancer risk in relation to fruit and vegetable intake suggest some protective effect, as they are food sources of micronutrients and fiber. A meta-analysis of 21 case-control and 5 cohort studies reported a significant reduction in breast cancer risk with higher vegetable consumption, with no significant difference seen with fruit intake.[29] Additional reviews of prospective, cohort studies reported no significant associations with either vegetable or fruit intake and breast cancer risk.[30] Thus, results of studies investigating the effects of fruit, vegetable, fiber, and meat consumption on breast cancer incidence are inconclusive.

One dietary factor that deserves mention is the possible effect of phytoestrogens on breast cancer risk. Phytoestrogens are natural plant estrogens found in soybean products, seeds, berries, and nuts. The two most studied classes of dietary phytoestrogens are isoflavones and ligands; isoflavones are richer in Asian diets and ligands are the main source of phytoestrogens in the Western diet.[31] Interest in the study of these compounds has largely been based on observational studies showing lower rates of breast cancer in Asian countries, where soy consumption is high.[32] Because these compounds exhibit weak estrogenic properties, some experts believe that they may function as relative antiestrogens by displacing natural estradiol. However, studies have also reported a potential stimulatory effect on breast tissue. A meta-analysis of observational studies which evaluated phytoestrogen use and the risk of breast cancer suggests that the associated risk reduction may be limited to postmenopausal patients.[33] Nonetheless, the effect of phytoestrogens on breast cancer is very controversial, and further research is needed.

The hypothesis that low dietary fat intake reduces breast cancer risk was tested in the WHI Randomized Controlled Dietary Modification Trial.[34] This study is the first large-scale, prospective, controlled trial to study the relationship between diet and breast cancer. It randomized more than 48,000 postmenopausal women to a dietary intervention that consisted of reducing total fat intake to 20% of energy, consuming at least five servings of fruits and vegetables daily and six servings of grains daily, versus a comparison group without any dietary interventions. Risk factors for breast cancer were evenly balanced between groups. Over an 8-year mean follow-up period, 3.35% of women in the intervention group developed invasive breast cancer versus 3.66% of women in the comparison group (annualized incidence rate, 0.42% vs 0.45%; hazard ratio [HR], 0.91; 95% CI, 0.83-1.01). Although the difference was not statistically significant, a trend toward a decreased incidence over time was seen, suggesting the need for longer follow-up. Limitations from this study include the inability to separate out the effects on breast cancer attributed to dietary fat reduction as compared to that attributed to increased fruit, vegetable, and grain intake. Because the WHI trial only evaluated women who adopted dietary changes after menopause, it is unknown what the effects would be in younger women or girls who make these dietary interventions sooner in life. Although there is still much to be learned about the effects of diet

on the risk of developing breast cancer, a low-fat diet seems to be a reasonable approach to potentially reduce the risk of breast cancer.

Both body weight and height are associated with developing breast cancer. High body mass index and obesity are related to breast cancer risk in a complex way that differs by age and menopausal status. Most studies of premenopausal women show either no relationship with body weight, or slightly declining breast cancer risks with increasing body weight. One plausible biologic mechanism to explain this observation is reduced ovarian activity in obese women. Most studies in postmenopausal women, however, show increasing breast cancer risks with increasing body weight. Accordingly, a recent meta-analysis found that an increase in body mass index was associated with an increase in the risk of breast cancer for postmenopausal women (RR, 1.12; 95% CI 1.08–1.16; $P < 0.0001$), but had the opposite effect in premenopausal women (RR, 0.92; 95% CI 0.88–0.97; $P < 0.001$).[35] In addition to obesity, the distribution of body fat also may play an independent role in the development of breast cancer. Upper body (central or abdominal) adiposity increases the risk of breast cancer independent of overall obesity. This association may be related to the excess levels of free-circulating estrogen resulting from the conversion of androstenedione to estradiol in peripheral adipose tissue.[36] Although height is not a modifiable risk factor, weight and body composition are modifiable and should be studied further.

Many studies report an inverse association between physical activity and breast cancer risk.[37] A review of 19 cohort and 29 case-control studies suggests that the association is stronger for postmenopausal breast cancer than for premenopausal breast cancer. Exercise may provide modest protection against breast cancer, but the relationship is complex. Possible explanations include the effects of physical activity on menstrual characteristics (in premenopausal women), body size, weight, and serum hormone levels. Thus estrogen-related pathways or other metabolic hormones such as insulin or insulin-like growth factors may play a role.

Many epidemiologic studies have evaluated the relationship between alcohol and breast cancer. Alcohol is the only dietary factor that has shown consistent results in clinical trials. Studies indicate both a modest positive association between alcohol and breast cancer and a dose–response relationship.[38,39] The risk increases with consumption of alcohol in general, regardless of the beverage type or woman's menopausal status. Potential biologic mechanisms for this association include increased levels of estrogen or other reproductive steroid hormones; increased production of insulin-like growth factors by the liver; and altered hepatic metabolism of carcinogens. Although a causal relationship between alcohol consumption and breast cancer has not been proven in a prospective trial, the weight of the evidence suggests that a relationship, direct or indirect, may exist. As alcohol consumption is a modifiable risk factor, use in moderation is a sensible approach.

Radiation is associated with an increased risk of breast cancer, particularly with exposure at a young age (<20 years), which again suggests that a "window of initiation" for breast cancer occurs at a relatively early age. Much of the knowledge about radiation-related breast cancer comes from epidemiologic studies of patients exposed to diagnostic or therapeutic radiation, and of survivors of the Japanese atomic bombs.[40] Women treated with chest irradiation for childhood and adolescent Hodgkin lymphoma, as well as survivors of other childhood cancers (where radiation is used as a mainstay of therapy) are among the populations at greater risk for secondary breast cancers. The risk increases linearly with radiation dose. Exposure to diagnostic x-rays including annual screening mammography does not impart a sufficient dose of radiation for clinical concern in the general population. The risk of breast cancer after radiation exposure in those with genetic risk factors is unclear and is an ongoing area of research.

In conclusion, numerous studies have been performed to investigate potential causative factors in the etiology of breast cancer. Several endocrine, genetic, environmental, and lifestyle factors are associated with the development of breast cancer to varying degrees. Some factors are modifiable, whereas others are not. Additionally, the impact of individual risk factors may vary depending on other confounding variables such as age, family history, estrogen use, and menopausal status. Although epidemiologic studies provide a large body of the current evidence, each has its limitations and results are varied. Meta-analyses can summarize the numerous study results, but heterogeneity of studies can be a limitation. Additional prospective, randomized controlled trials will add to our knowledge of factors that affect the risk of developing breast cancer.

CLINICAL PRESENTATION

CLINICAL PRESENTATION

General

☐ The patient may not have any symptoms, as breast cancer may be detected in asymptomatic patients though routine screening mammography.

Local Signs and Symptoms

☐ A painless, palpable lump is most common.

☐ Less common: pain; nipple discharge, retraction or dimpling; skin edema, redness or warmth.

☐ Palpable local–regional lymph nodes may also be present.

Signs and Symptoms of Systemic Metastases

☐ Depends on the site of metastases, but may include bone pain, difficulty breathing, abdominal pain or enlargement, jaundice, mental status changes.

Laboratory Tests

☐ Tumor markers such as cancer antigen (CA 27.29) or carcinoembryonic antigen (CEA) may be elevated.

☐ Alkaline phosphatase or liver function tests may be elevated in metastatic disease.

Other Diagnostic Tests

☐ Mammogram (with or without ultrasound, breast MRI, or both).

☐ Biopsy for pathology review and determination of tumor estrogen/progesterone receptor (ER/PR) status and *HER2* status.

☐ Systemic staging tests may include: chest x-ray, chest CT, bone scan, abdominal CT or ultrasound, or MRI.

A painless lump is the initial sign of breast cancer in most women. The typical malignant mass is solitary, unilateral, solid, hard, irregular, and nonmobile. In small numbers of cases, stabbing or aching pain is the first symptom. Less commonly, nipple discharge, retraction, or dimpling may herald the onset of the disease. In more advanced cases, prominent skin edema, redness, warmth, and induration of the underlying tissue may be observed.

The breast is a complex organ composed of skin, subcutaneous tissue, fatty tissue, and branching ductal and glandular structures (Fig. 136–2). Various diseases that affect these structures can produce a palpable mass. In addition, the physiologic changes associated with the menstrual cycle can cause breast abnormalities. Common causes of breast masses in young women are fibroadenoma, fibrocystic disease, carcinoma, and fat necrosis.

Many women will detect some breast abnormality themselves, underscoring the importance of breast self-examination. But in the United States, it is increasingly common for breast cancer to be detected during routine screening mammography in asymptomatic women. It is widely accepted that the smaller the mass, the higher the likelihood of cure. Thus as the number of breast cancer cases found by screening mammography increases, overall survival of breast cancer patients has improved, albeit this decreasing mortality is also related to improved systemic therapy.

Breast cancer that is confined to a localized breast lesion is often referred to as *early*, *primary*, *localized*, or *curable*. Breast cancer that has spread to local-regional lymph nodes is still considered early stage (Fig. 136–3). Unfortunately, breast cancer cells often spread by contiguity, lymph channels, and through the blood to distant sites. This often occurs early in breast cancer growth, and deposits of tumor cells form in distant sites that cannot be detected with current diagnostic methods and equipment (micrometastases). When breast cancer cells can be detected clinically or radiologically in sites distant from the breast, the disease is referred to as *advanced* or *metastatic* breast cancer. Tissues most commonly involved with metastases are lymph nodes (other than local–regional lymph nodes), skin, bone, liver, lungs, and brain. Symptoms of bone pain, difficulty breathing, abdominal enlargement, jaundice, and mental status changes may herald the clinical presentation of metastatic breast cancer. A small percentage of women have signs and symptoms of distant metastases when they first seek treatment. In virtually all of them, a breast mass has been present for several months to years. In addition, about one half of all patients who initially are treated for localized disease will eventually develop signs and symptoms of metastatic breast cancer.

DIAGNOSIS

Initial workup for a woman presenting with a lesion or symptoms suggestive of breast cancer should include a careful history, physical examination of the breast, 3-D mammography, and possibly other breast imaging techniques such as ultrasonography or MRI. Most breast cancers can be visualized on a mammogram as a mass, a cluster of calcifications, or a combination. Specific mammographic features associated with the highest risk of malignancy include masses with spiculated margins and/or irregular shape, and calcifications with a linear and/or segmental distribution.[41] Factors that affect the ability of mammography to detect cancer include breast density (the fat-to-glandular tissue ratio of the breast) which may be affected by age, menopausal status, and HRT. Ultrasonography, MRI, and digital mammography are alternate breast imaging methods that are being investigated for women with dense breasts or other specific subsets of patients with breast cancer (e.g., MRI in patients with inflammatory breast cancer).[42] The technical quality of the examination and the expertise of the radiologist are also important factors.

The Breast Imaging Reporting and Data System (BI-RADS) was developed by the American College of Radiology to standardize mammographic reporting.[43] Table 136–2 lists the BI-RADS classifications for standardized reporting for mammography. There are seven assessment categories with four possible recommendations: (a) additional imaging evaluation, (b) routine interval screening, (c) short-term follow-up, and (d) biopsy. The probability of a biopsy positive for malignancy increases from <2% for BI-RADS category 3 mammograms to 20% to 30% for category 4 mammograms, to >95% for category 5 mammograms. Similar categories for reporting have also been developed for breast MRI and ultrasonography.

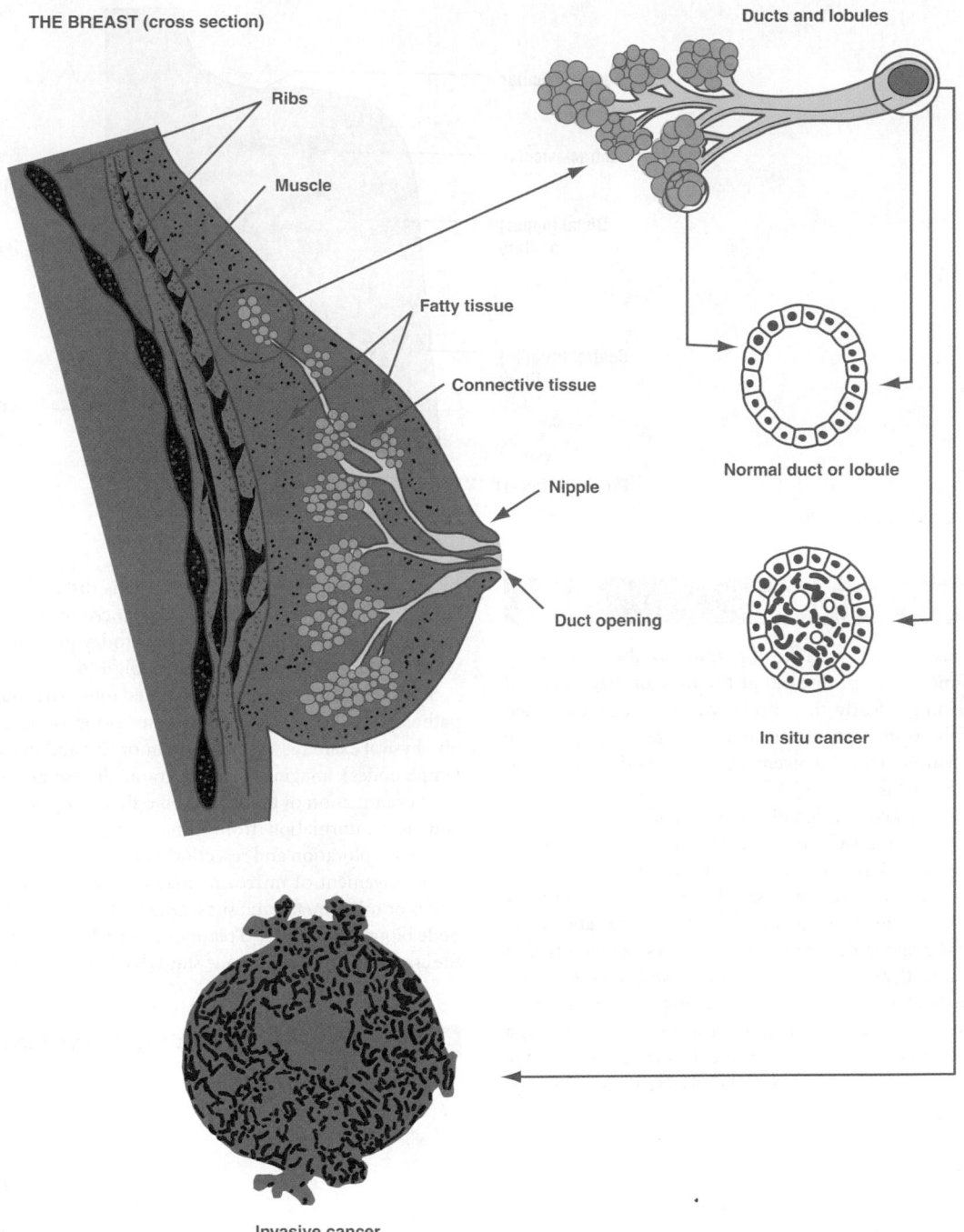

FIGURE 136-2. Breast anatomy.

Breast biopsy is indicated for a mammographic abnormality that suggests malignancy or for a palpable mass on physical examination. Three techniques are available: fine-needle aspiration, core-needle biopsy, and excisional biopsy.[44] Excisional biopsy, which completely removes the abnormal tissue, is performed with either a local or general anesthetic, and is usually done as an outpatient operative procedure. Needle biopsies are performed percutaneously, and include both core-needle biopsy (which removes a core of tissue) and fine-needle aspiration (which removes cells from the suspicious site). These are generally office procedures that are associated with minimal discomfort and anxiety, few complications, no disfigurement, and decreased costs when compared to surgical excisional biopsy. The accuracy of fine-needle aspiration is good in experienced hands, but its limitations include false negatives, specimens with insufficient material for diagnosis, and the inability to distinguish invasive from in situ cancer. Core-needle biopsy is the preferred biopsy method for mammographically detected, nonpalpable abnormalities.[42] Core-needle biopsy offers a more definitive histologic diagnosis, avoids inadequate samples, and can distinguish invasive from in situ breast cancer. Following confirmation of malignancy via core-needle biopsy, subsequent surgical procedures are performed to assure complete removal of the abnormal tissue.

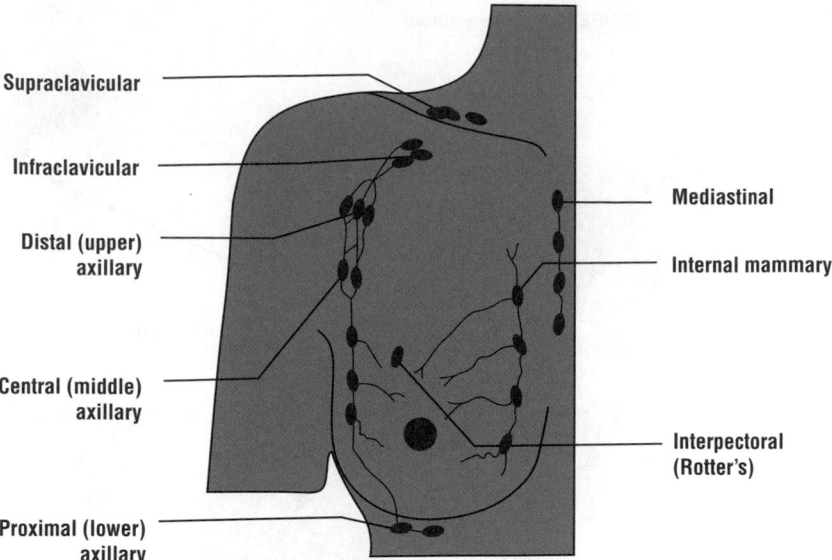

FIGURE 136-3. Lymph node anatomy.

STAGING AND PROGNOSIS

Few malignant diseases illustrate the importance of the relationship of stage (anatomic extent of disease) at the time of diagnosis and overall survival more clearly than breast cancer. Stage is defined on the basis of the primary tumor extent and size (T_{1-4}), presence and extent of lymph node involvement (N_{1-3}), and presence or absence of distant metastases (M_{0-1}) (Table 136–3 and Fig. 136–4). Although many possible combinations of T and N are possible within a given stage, simplistically, stage 0 represents carcinoma in situ (T_{is}) or disease that has not invaded the basement membrane of the breast tissue. Stage I represents a small primary invasive tumor without lymph node involvement or with micrometastatic nodal involvement, and stage II disease usually involves regional lymph nodes. Stages I and II are often referred to as *early breast cancer*. It is in these early stages that the disease is highly curable. Stage III, also referred to as *locally advanced disease*, usually represents a large tumor with extensive nodal involvement in which either node or tumor is fixed to the chest wall. Stage IV disease is characterized by the presence of metastases to organs distant from the primary tumor and is often referred to as *advanced or metastatic disease* as described earlier. Most breast cancer today presents in early stages where the prognosis is favorable (Table 136–4).

Staging for breast cancer is separated into two groups, clinical and pathologic. Clinical staging is assigned prior to surgery and is based on physical exam (assessment of tumor size and presence of axillary lymph nodes), imaging (mammogram, ultrasound, etc.), and pathologic examination of tissues. Pathologic staging occurs after surgery and uses information from clinical staging, but adds data from surgical exploration and resection, such as tumor size at surgery and the involvement of micro- or macro-invasive tumor in the lymph nodes or other metastatic sites. Due to the advent of sentinel lymph node biopsy (SLNB; see Treatment of Early Breast Cancer section), the assessment of lymph node status has become more complex. The

TABLE 136-2	Breast Imaging Reporting and Database System (BI-RADS®) Assessment Categories for Mammography
Category	**Assessment**
a. Assessment is Incomplete	
0	Need Additional Imaging Evaluation and/or Prior Mammograms for Comparison
b. Assessment is Complete – Final Categories	
1	Negative
2	Benign Finding(s)
3	Probably Benign Finding – Initial Short-Interval Follow-Up Suggested
4	Suspicious Abnormality – Biopsy Should Be Considered
5	Highly Suggestive of Malignancy – Appropriate Action Should Be Taken
6	Known Biopsy-Proven Malignancy – Appropriate Action Should Be Taken

American College of Radiology (ACR). ACR BI-RADS® – Mammography. 4th ed. In: ACR Breast Imaging Reporting and Data System, Breast Imaging Atlas. Reston, VA: American College of Radiology; 2003:193–198. Reprinted with permission of the American College of Radiology. No other representation of this material is authorized without expressed, written permission from the American College of Radiology.

TABLE 136-3	TNM Stage Grouping for Breast Cancer		
Stage Grouping			
0	T_{is}	N_0	M_0
IA	$T_1{}^a$	N_0	M_0
IB	T_0	N_1mi	M_0
	$T_1{}^a$	N_1mi	M_0
IIA	T_0	$N_1{}^b$	M_0
	$T_1{}^a$	$N_1{}^b$	M_0
	T_2	N_0	M_0
IIB	T_2	N_1	M_0
	T_3	N_0	M_0
IIIA	T_0	N_2	M_0
	$T_1{}^a$	N_2	M_0
	T_2	N_2	M_0
	T_3	N_1	M_0
	T_3	N_2	M_0
IIIB	T_4	N_0	M_0
	T_4	N_1	M_0
	T_4	N_2	M_0
IIIC	Any T	N_3	M_0
IV	Any T	Any N	M_1

TNM, tumor, node, metastasis.

$^a T_1$ includes T_1mi.

$^b T_0$ and T_1 tumors with nodal micrometastasis only are excluded from stage IIa and are classified as stage Ib

(Used with the permission of the American Joint Committee on Cancer (AJCC), Chicago, Illinois. The original source for this material is the AJCC Cancer Staging Manual, 7th ed. (2010) published by Springer Science and Business Media LLC, www.springer.com.)

Tumor (T)

T_x Primary tumor cannot be assessed
T_0 No evidence of tumor
T_{is} Carcinoma in situ
T_1 ≤2 cm
   T_1 mic ≤0.1 cm
   T_{1a} > 0.1–0.5 cm
   T_{1b} > 0.5–1 cm
   T_{1c} > 1–2 cm
T_2 >2–5 cm
T_3 >5 cm
T_4 Any size; with direct extension to chest wall
   or skin
T_{4a} Extension to chest wall (not including pectoralis muscle)
T_{4b} Edema (including peau d'orange) or ulceration of skin or
   satellite skin nodules
T_{4c} Both T_{4a} and T_{4b}
T_{4d} Inflammatory carcinoma

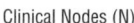

Clinical Nodes (N)

N_x Regional lymph nodes cannot be assessed (e.g., previously removed)
N_0 No regional lymph node metastasis
N_1 Metastasis in movable ipsilateral axillary lymph node(s)
N_2 Metastases in ipsilateral axillary lymph nodes fixed or matted, or in clinically detected ipsilateral internal
   mammary nodes in the absence of clinically evident axillary lymph node metastasis
   N_{2a} Metastasis in ipsilateral axillary lymph nodes fixed to one another (matted) or to other structures
   N_{2b} Metastasis only in clinically detected ipsilateral internal mammary nodes and in the absence of clinically
      evident axillary lymph node metastasis
N_3 Metastasis in ipsilateral infraclavicular lymph node(s), or in clinically detected ipsilateral internal mammary
   lymph node(s) and in the presence of clinically evident axillary lymph node metastasis; or metastasis in
   ipsilateral supraclavicular lymph node(s) with or without axillary or internal mammary lymph node
   involvement
   N_{3a} Metastasis in ipsilateral infraclavicular lymph node(s) and axillary lymph node(s)
   N_{3b} Metastasis in ipsilateral internal mammary lymph node(s) and axillary lymph node(s)
   N_{3c} Metastasis in ipsilateral supraclavicular lymph node(s)

Pathologic Nodes (pN)†

pN0   No regional lymph node metastasis histologically
pN1mi Micrometastasis (>0.2 mm but none >2.0 mm)
pN1   Metastasis in one to three axillary lymph nodes and/or internal mammary
   nodes with microscopic disease detected by sentinel lymph node
   dissection but not clinically detected
pN2   Metastasis in four to nine axillary lymph nodes, or in clinically detected
   internal mammary lymph nodes in the absence of axillary lymph node
   metastasis
pN3   Metastasis in 10 or more axillary lymph nodes, or in infraclavicular lymph
   nodes, or in clinically detected ipsilateral internal mammary lymph nodes
   in the presence of one or more positive axillary lymph nodes; or in more
   than three axillary lymph nodes with clinically negative microscopic
   metastasis in internal mammary lymph nodes; or in ipsilateral
   supraclavicular lymph nodes

†Based on axillary lymph node dissection with or without sentinel lymph node dissection

Metastasis (M)

M_x Distant metastasis cannot be assessed
M_0 No distant metastases
M_1 Distant metastasis

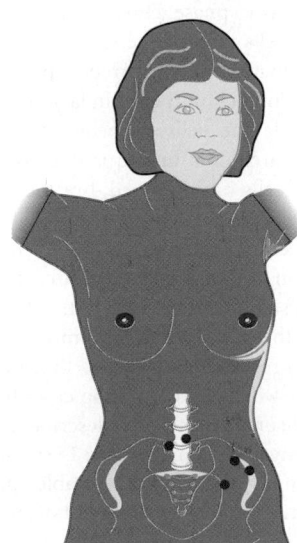

FIGURE 136-4. TNM (tumor, node, metastasis) staging system for breast cancer. *(Used with the permission of the American Joint Committee on Cancer (AJCC), Chicago, Illinois. The original source for this material is the AJCC Cancer Staging Manual, 7th ed. (2010) published by Springer Science and Business Media LLC, www.springer.com.).*

TABLE 136-4	Estimated Stage at Diagnosis and 5-Year Relative Survival Rates		
Stage at Diagnosis	**Percentage of Cases**	**5-Year Survival**[d]	
Localized[a]	60%	98%	
Regional[b]	33%	84%	
Distant[c]	5%	23%	
Unstaged	2%	58%	

[a]Confined to primary site. Includes stages I and II.
[b]Regional spread to lymph nodes or directly beyond primary site. Includes stages II and III.
[c]Distant metastasis. Stage IV.
[d]With conventional local and systemic therapy.
From Horner MJ, Ries LAG, Krapcho M, eds. SEER Cancer Statistics Review, 1975–2006, National Cancer Institute. Bethesda, MD. Based on November 2008 SEER data submission, posted to the SEER Website, 2009. http://seer.cancer.gov/csr/1975_2006/.

American Joint Committee for Cancer (AJCC) publishes staging criteria for cancers and the breast cancer criteria were updated and officially implemented in January 2010.[45] Tumor staging systems are periodically updated to incorporate new diagnostic and therapeutic advances that affect risk of disease recurrence and survival. One of the major changes in the 2010 staging system updated from the 2003 version is the designation of new substages, IA and IB. Other subtle, yet important differences are noted. However, these are complex and well beyond the scope of this chapter. The reader is referred to the AJCC manual for details.[45] This staging system is widely accepted and used in all breast cancer patients to determine prognosis and assist with treatment decisions.

PATHOLOGY

The pathologic evaluation of breast lesions serves to establish the histologic diagnosis and to confirm the presence or absence of other factors believed to influence prognosis.

INVASIVE CARCINOMA

Invasive breast cancers are a histologically heterogeneous group of lesions. Most breast cancers are adenocarcinomas and are classified on the basis of their microscopic appearance as ductal or lobular, corresponding to the ducts and lobules of the normal breast (Fig. 136–2). The various histologic types of breast cancer have different prognoses, but it is unknown whether their response to therapy differs, because patients in therapeutic trials are not typically stratified according to histologic type. The five most common types of invasive breast cancer are briefly described.[46]

Invasive or *infiltrating ductal carcinoma* is the most common histology. These tumors are generally referred to as infiltrating ductal carcinoma "not otherwise specified," and account for approximately 75% of all invasive breast cancers. These tumors commonly spread to the axillary lymph nodes and their prognosis is poorer than for other histologic types (specifically tubular, medullary, and mucinous). *Invasive or infiltrating lobular carcinoma* accounts for 5% to 10% of breast tumors. Both clinical and radiologic findings for these tumors may be quite subtle. Typical presentation is an area of ill-defined thickening in the breast, in contrast to a prominent lump characteristic of infiltrating ductal carcinoma. *Infiltrating lobular carcinoma* can also be more difficult to detect by mammography. Overall, *infiltrating lobular carcinoma* and *infiltrating ductal carcinoma* have similar likelihoods of axillary node involvement and disease recurrence and death, yet the sites of metastases tend to differ. *Infiltrating ductal carcinoma* more frequently metastasizes to the bone or to the liver, lung, or brain, whereas *infiltrating lobular carcinoma* tends to metastasize to the leptomeninges, peritoneal

surfaces, retroperitoneum, gastrointestinal tract, reproductive organs, and other unusual sites.

The three most common special types of invasive cancer are *medullary*, *mucinous*, and *tubular*. Prognosis may be more favorable with these unusual histologies. *Medullary carcinoma* accounts for less than 7% of all breast carcinomas, *mucinous (or colloid) carcinoma* constitutes approximately 3%, *and tubular carcinoma* accounts for approximately 2% of all breast cancers. Histologies rarely reported include adenocystic carcinoma, carcinosarcomas, metaplastic, cribriform, and papillary carcinoma.

Special situations seen clinically and histologically include Paget's disease of the breast, phyllodes tumors, and inflammatory breast cancer. Paget's disease of the breast occurs in 1% to 4% of all patients with breast cancer, and is characterized by neoplastic cells in the nipple areolar complex. The patient presents clinically with eczematous changes in the nipple with itching, burning, oozing, bleeding, or some combination of these. In most cases, the nipple changes are associated with an underlying carcinoma in the breast that is usually palpable.

Phyllodes tumors of the breast (also known as cystosarcoma phyllodes) are rare tumors with subtypes that range from benign to malignant. These tumors often enlarge rapidly, are painless, and can appear radiographically as fibroadenomas.[47]

Inflammatory breast cancer is characterized clinically by prominent skin edema, redness and warmth, and induration of the underlying tissue. Biopsies of the involved skin reveal cancer cells in the dermal lymphatics. Inflammatory breast cancer typically has a very rapid onset and is often mistaken for an infectious cellulitis or mastitis. Although it may look somewhat similar to a neglected mass, its presentation with rapid onset and progression of local symptoms distinguishes it from other cases of locally advanced breast cancer. Prognosis of patients with inflammatory breast cancer is poor, even if the disease is apparently localized.[48]

NONINVASIVE CARCINOMA

As with invasive carcinoma, the noninvasive lesions may be divided broadly into ductal and lobular categories. Evidence supports that the development of malignancy is a multistep process and that invasive breast cancer has a preinvasive phase. During the carcinoma in situ phase, normal epithelial cells undergo genetic alterations that result in malignant transformation. Transformed epithelial cells proliferate and pile up within lobules or ducts, but lack the required genetic alterations that enable the cells to penetrate the basement membrane. Therefore carcinoma in situ is diagnosed when malignant transformation of cells has occurred, but the basement membrane is intact.

The widespread use of screening mammography and subsequent biopsy and greater recognition of noninvasive breast carcinoma by pathologists has resulted in a significant increase in the diagnosis of in situ breast cancer during the past decade. Assuming consistent incidence and survival rates, researchers estimate that the prevalence of breast in situ cancers will exceed 1 million cases by 2016.[49] The natural history of these disorders is not well described, and thus the debate continues regarding carcinoma in situ: Is carcinoma in situ preinvasive cancer or simply a marker of unstable epithelium that represents an increased risk for the development of subsequent aggressive cancer?[50,51]

DCIS is more frequently diagnosed than lobular carcinoma in situ (LCIS). Most cases of DCIS today are found by biopsies performed for clustered microcalcifications seen on screening mammography. Five distinct histologic patterns of DCIS have been identified: comedo, cribriform, micropapillary, papillary, and solid.

The ultimate goal of treatment for noninvasive carcinomas is to prevent the development of invasive disease. If left untreated, it is estimated that 14% to 50% of DCIS lesions will progress to invasive breast cancer.[52] Treatment of DCIS depends on its location, size, and pathology.[47] Treatment options include: (1) local excision alone with negative margins; (2) local excision (with negative margins) followed by breast irradiation; and (3) traditional total mastectomy with or without reconstruction. Whole breast irradiation is recommended following excision to significantly decrease the risk of local recurrence, although there is no evidence that survival differs between the previously mentioned options.[47] Excision with negative margins alone, without radiation may be considered in patients with small and low-grade DCIS. Mastectomy had been the standard treatment of DCIS for several decades, but long-term survival appears to be equivalent with mastectomy versus excision and irradiation, and the latter option allows for breast conservation. If more than one area of the breast is involved with DCIS, a mastectomy is the preferred option. It has also been suggested that breast conservation may not be appropriate for younger women whose lifetime risk of breast cancer is high given a diagnosis of DCIS, including *BRCA1* or *BRCA2* mutation carriers. Axillary lymph node dissection is generally not indicated, although sentinel lymph node biopsy (see Early Breast Cancer section) may be considered in selected patients.[47] Patients with invasive disease found at the time of surgery should be treated according to guidelines for patients with early stage invasive breast cancer.[47] Currently cytotoxic chemotherapy has no role in the treatment of patients with pure DCIS. It is important to determine tumor hormone receptor status because tamoxifen treatment for 5 years may be considered in some women with DCIS. The National Surgical Adjuvant Breast and Bowel Project (NSABP) B-24 trial, which randomized women with DCIS to lumpectomy with radiation plus either tamoxifen or placebo, showed a benefit with tamoxifen in reducing ipsilateral breast cancer recurrence (44% reduction; $P = 0.03$).[53] Further subgroup analyses of this trial suggest a benefit for those patients with estrogen receptor-positive DCIS. Ongoing clinical trials are evaluating the role of aromatase inhibitors in the treatment of postmenopausal DCIS. Follow-up of women who have been treated for DCIS should be as comprehensive as that of a woman with invasive carcinoma to facilitate early detection of subsequent malignancy.[51]

LCIS is a microscopic diagnosis because there is no palpable mass and no specific clinical abnormality. Unlike DCIS, LCIS does not generally demonstrate calcifications on mammography, and in fact is usually undetectable by mammography. Consequently, the diagnosis of LCIS is usually an incidental finding in biopsy specimens obtained because of symptoms or mammography findings consistent with benign lesions. It is unclear whether LCIS is a precursor lesion to invasive carcinoma or serves as a marker of risk for invasive carcinoma developing somewhere in the breast. The risk for developing invasive carcinoma is approximately 0.5% to 1% per year, and both invasive ductal carcinoma and invasive lobular carcinoma can occur. In approximately 30% to 50% of patients, there are multiple foci of LCIS in the ipsilateral breast, and the contralateral breast is also affected. Thus the risk for the development of breast cancer is equally high in either breast, which makes the management of LCIS very controversial.[50] Some experts favor a program of observation, with semiannual physical examination and annual mammography.[47] In selected patients with high-risk genetic mutations or strong family history, or in women who are particularly anxious about the development of cancer, bilateral mastectomies with or without reconstruction may be considered.[54] Radiation and systemic chemotherapy have no role in the management of LCIS. The use of chemoprevention with tamoxifen in premenopausal women or tamoxifen or raloxifene in postmenopausal women can be considered as an option for risk reduction. Patients with LCIS were included in both the NSABP Breast Cancer Prevention Trial (P1) and the Study of Tamoxifen and Raloxifene (P2) trials.[55,56]

Both trials showed approximately a 50% reduction in the risk of developing invasive breast cancer for women with LCIS receiving either tamoxifen or raloxifene (see Prevention and Early Detection below).

PROGNOSTIC FACTORS

The natural history of breast cancer varies between patients, with some having an extremely aggressive disease that progresses rapidly, whereas others follow a more indolent course. The ability to predict prognosis is extremely important in designing treatment recommendations to maximize quantity and quality of life. A number of pathologic prognostic and predictive factors have been identified. Prognostic factors are characteristics or measurements available at diagnosis or time of surgery, that in the absence of adjuvant therapy are associated with recurrence rate, death rate, or other clinical outcomes. Predictive factors are measurements available at diagnosis that are associated with response to a specific therapy. Prognostic and predictive factors fall into three categories: patient characteristics that are independent of the disease such as age; disease characteristics such as tumor size or histologic type; and biomarkers that are measurable parameters in tissues, cells, or fluids, such as hormone receptor status.[51,52] Ideally, the use of prognostic and predictive factors can limit a specific treatment to patients who are most likely to derive benefit, thus sparing unwanted toxicities in those who are unlikely to benefit.

Age at diagnosis and ethnicity are patient characteristics that may affect prognosis. Some younger patients, particularly those younger than 35 years of age, have more aggressive forms of disease and a worse prognosis. Younger patients are more likely to present with poor prognostic features, such as affected lymph nodes, large tumor size, and tumors negative for hormone receptors. Race and ethnicity may also play a role in breast cancer prognosis. African American women have decreased survival compared to white women. The cause of this racial disparity is widely debated, with possible explanations including access to care, socioeconomic status, cultural differences, higher stage at diagnosis, and more aggressive biologic features.

Potentially modifiable prognostic factors include alcohol use, dietary factors, and exercise. Kwan and colleagues found that alcohol use (>6 g/day) increases the risk of recurrence and breast cancer death in patients with a personal history of breast cancer, primarily in postmenopausal and obese women.[57] Diet may also play an important role in breast cancer recurrence. In the Women's Healthy Eating and Living (WHEL) trial, 3,088 pre- and postmenopausal women previously treated for early stage breast cancer were randomized to: group 1, a diet rich in vegetables (five servings of vegetables plus 16 oz vegetable juice), fruits (three servings), and fiber (30 g) and low in fat (15%–20% of energy intake from fat) or; group 2, a five-a-day diet (five servings of fruits and vegetables, more that 20 g of fiber, and less than 30% of total energy intake from fat).[58] After a 7.3 year follow-up period, the group 1 diet did not reduce breast cancer events or mortality compared to the group 2 diet. In a second trial by Chlebowski and colleagues, a low-fat diet (goal of reducing percentage of fat to 15%) improved relapse-free survival in women with early stage, resected breast cancer compared to a control group, although the results were not statistically significant (HR, 0.76; 95% CI, 0.60-0.98; $P = 0.077$). Interestingly, in women with ER-negative breast cancer, a low-fat diet significantly improved relapse-free survival compared to the control group (HR 0.58; 95% CI, 0.37-0.91; $P = 0.018$). Although there is still much to be learned about the effects of diet on the risk of developing breast cancer, a low-fat diet may reduce the risk of recurrence and improve relapse-free survival in women with early stage, resected breast

TABLE 136-5 Five-Year Survival Rates (%) According to Tumor Size and Axillary Lymph Node Status

Lymph Node Status	Tumor Size		
	<2 cm	2–5 cm	>5 cm
Negative	96	89	82
1–3 positive	87	80	73
≥4 positive	66	59	46

Data from Schnitt SJ, Guidi AJ. Pathology of invasive breast cancer. In: Harris JR, Lippman ME, Morrow M, Osborne CK, eds. Diseases of the Breast, 3rd ed. Philadelphia, PA: Lippincott Williams & Wilkins, 2004:567.

cancer, especially in patients with ER negative disease.[59] Exercise in women following a diagnosis of breast cancer may also increase the likelihood of overall survival.[60] Based on these data, agencies such as the American Cancer Society have recognized that physical activity, weight control, and diet are potentially modifiable risk factors for reducing the risk of recurrent breast cancer and other comorbidities (e.g., heart disease, diabetes).[61]

Disease characteristics that have been shown to provide important prognostic information include lymph node status, tumor size, histologic subtype, nuclear or histologic grade, lymphatic and vascular invasion, and proliferation indices.

Tumor size and the presence and number of involved lymph nodes are established primary factors in assessing the risk for breast cancer recurrence and subsequent metastatic disease. Table 136–5 shows 5-year survival rates according to size of the primary tumor and axillary node involvement. The major factor that influences the likelihood of recurrence is the presence of positive lymph nodes. However, regardless of lymph node status, the size of the primary tumor remains an independent prognostic factor for disease recurrence.

The number of affected lymph nodes is directly related to disease recurrence. The revised staging system for breast cancer recognizes the absolute number of positive nodes as a prognostic factor: N_1 represents 1 to 3 positive nodes, N_2 represents 4 to 9 positive nodes, and N_3 represents 10 or more positive nodes in its pathologic staging system.[45]

Certain histologic subtypes and clinical presentation of breast cancer have prognostic importance. As mentioned earlier, because women with pure *tubular* or *mucinous* tumors have more favorable outcomes than *invasive ductal carcinomas*, treatment recommendations may differ.[47] Inflammatory breast cancer, although a clinical designation and not a distinct histologic subtype, is associated with a poor prognosis.

Nuclear grade and tumor (histologic) differentiation are known independent prognostic indicators. Several histologic grading systems have been developed, most of which grade tumors with a score from 1 to 3: grade 1 (well differentiated); grade 2 (moderately differentiated); grade 3 (poorly differentiated). Higher-grade tumors are associated with higher rates of distant metastasis and poorer survival. This factor aids in making treatment decisions, particularly for patients with small tumors and negative lymph nodes.

Lymphatic and vascular invasion, defined as evidence of tumor emboli in lymphatic or vascular spaces, has emerged in recent years as having prognostic significance for the risk of recurrence. This factor helps identify node-negative patients who are at increased risk for lymph node involvement and metastases. However, in at least one prospective evaluation of more than 15,000 patients with early stage breast cancer, lymphovascular invasion was not associated with shorter disease-free interval or overall survival in patients categorized as low-risk for the development of breast cancer recurrence.[62]

The rate of tumor cell proliferation also has prognostic significance for breast cancer recurrence. Rate of cell proliferation can be evaluated with various techniques, including mitotic index, which counts the number of mitotic bodies; thymidine-labeling index or S-phase fraction with DNA flow cytometry, which determines the percentage of tumor cells actively dividing; or through the use of monoclonal antibodies to antigens present on proliferating cells, such as Ki-67. In a meta-analysis which included 85 studies and nearly 33,000 patients, proliferation markers (including Ki-67, mitotic index, proliferating cell nuclear antigen, and thymidine or bromodeoxyuridine labeling index) were associated with significantly shorter disease-free and overall survival.[63] These proliferation indices are additional factors that may be useful in decision making, and may also be predictive markers for responsiveness to chemotherapy, although this is still controversial.

Hormone receptors are not strong prognostic markers, but are used clinically to predict response to hormone therapy. Hormone receptors are nuclear transcription factors that, upon ligand binding, activate a variety of signal transduction pathways that result in cell growth and proliferation. The hormone receptors clinically useful in discussions of breast cancer include the estrogen receptor (ER) and the progesterone receptor (PR). Determination of both ER and PR status is an established procedure that is important in the management of breast cancer. Immunohistochemistry is used to determine the level (i.e., quantity) of hormone receptors, which is important for predictive ability. A more recent method of determining ER and PR status involves using gene-based assays which measure mRNA expression and is able to quantitate the amount of ER (or PR) protein present on cancer cells. These new methods have not been validated as predictive tools for treatment decisions. However, a great deal of investigation is ongoing looking into this type of application. Although the ER has received the most attention, presence of the PR protein is important for the functional effects of the ER protein to occur. Hormone receptors are most valuable in predicting response to hormone therapy. Approximately 60% to 70% of patients with ER-positive and PR-positive tumors will respond to hormonal manipulation. Patients with ER-negative and PR-negative tumors rarely respond to hormonal manipulation. The response rate in patients with ER-positive and PR-negative or ER-negative and PR-positive tumors is somewhere in between, but significant benefit may still be gained with hormonal therapy in these patients.

Approximately 50% to 70% of patients with primary or metastatic breast cancer have hormone receptor-positive tumors. Hormone receptor positivity, more common in postmenopausal women, is associated with a superior response to hormone therapy and a longer disease-free survival.

The *HER2/neu (HER2)* gene is located on chromosome 17q21 and encodes a 185-kilodaton transmembrane tyrosine kinase growth factor receptor. The *HER2* protein is normally expressed at low levels in the epithelial cells of normal breast tissue. *HER2* is a member of the erbB (or HER) growth factor receptor family and its overexpression is associated with transmission of growth signals that control aspects of normal cell growth and division. *HER2* overexpression occurs in approximately 20% to 30% of breast cancers, and is associated with increased tumor aggressiveness, increased rates of recurrence, and increased mortality. In some studies, *HER2* gene amplification and protein overexpression, measured by fluorescence in situ hybridization (FISH) and immunohistochemistry (IHC), respectively, correlates with factors associated with a poor prognosis. Clearly, a *HER2*-positive status predicts response to trastuzumab therapy, which is a monoclonal antibody directed against the extracellular domain of the *HER2* receptor. A final controversy surrounds the testing method employed to determine *HER2* status. Although there are many methods, *HER2* gene amplification measured by FISH (reported as either positive, equivocal, or negative) and overexpression of the *HER2* protein product measured by IHC (reported as 0, 1+, 2+, or 3+) are the most commonly used methods.

HER2 status should be determined for all invasive breast cancers, and guidelines for testing are available.[64] Tumors that are either IHC 3+ or FISH positive for gene amplification are considered to be positive for HER2. Some have argued that HER2 testing by FISH should be the primary method of determining HER2 positivity, based on technical limitations of IHC testing as well as other reasons.[65] However, FISH testing is not always available and may require sending tissue to an outside laboratory. Therefore, both methods are acceptable for predicting response to HER2-targeted therapy. For equivocal results of IHC (2+) or FISH, confirmatory testing with the alternate test is recommended. HER2 gene amplification or protein overexpression has traditionally been considered a poor prognostic factor. However, in a recent retrospective analysis, patients with HER2-positive metastatic breast cancer treated with first-line trastuzumab had improved 1-year survival rates compared to patients with HER2-negative metastatic breast cancer or patients with HER2-positive metastatic breast cancer who did not receive trastuzumab.[66] These results demonstrate the powerful impact trastuzumab therapy has made on improving patient outcomes. The outcomes of patients with HER2-positive breast cancer may continue to change with the advent of new targeted therapies being used in the treatment of all stages of breast cancer.

Although there is a growing understanding of the prognostic significance of individual factors, it is not clear how each contributes to the overall prognosis for an individual patient. Computer-aided models, including Adjuvant! (www.adjuvantonline.com) are available that combine patient- and tumor-related variables to estimate overall prognosis for individual patients with early stage breast cancer and aid in decisions regarding adjuvant systemic therapy.[67] Such programs have limitations, and should be used by healthcare professionals and not directly by patients because of the importance of accurate data entry, selection of different treatment options, and appropriate interpretation of results (see Systemic Adjuvant Therapy below).

Genetic profiling is also being used to provide prognostic and predictive information on clinical outcomes of breast cancer. The Oncotype DX assay uses a reverse-transcription polymerase chain reaction assay of 21 genes to predict the likelihood of distant recurrence in lymph node-negative and ER-positive breast cancer patients treated with tamoxifen.[68] A recurrence score is calculated to categorize patients into low-, intermediate-, or high-risk groups. MammaPrint is another molecular prognostic test that uses DNA microarray analysis to measure the activity of a set of 70 genes to determine the likelihood of breast cancer recurrence in women with stage I or II breast cancer, tumor size 5 cm or less, and no lymph node involvement. To predict the risk of breast cancer metastasis, an algorithm is used to issue a score that indicates whether the patient is at low or high risk.[69] These tools provide additional prognostic information to aid in decision making regarding treatment for these subgroups of patients with otherwise favorable prognostic features. Prospective validation of these assays is required, and clinical trials such as TAILORx and MINDACT are ongoing. Genetic profiling is also being studied for predicting responsiveness or resistance to treatment, and has immense potential for improving prognostic and predictive accuracy.

Novel molecular markers that have shown prognostic and predictive significance include urokinase-type plasminogen activator and its inhibitor, plasminogen activator inhibitor type 1, cyclin E, and presence of tumor cells in bone marrow and/or circulating blood.[70] Completion of prospective validation studies will provide further information as to whether these tests are suitable for use in making treatment decisions in individual patients.

In summary, lymph node status and tumor size are two significant prognostic factors that assist clinicians in estimating prognosis and making treatment recommendations for most breast cancer

patients (see also Systemic Adjuvant Therapy below). Although the risk of recurrence is clearly high in patients with large primary tumors or lymph node-positive disease, many patients with small primary tumors and lymph node-negative disease will still develop metastases, yet our ability to accurately identify these individual patients is limited. Evaluation of additional prognostic factors can help identify which patients will have a good outcome with local therapy alone, as well as those patients with aggressive features who would benefit from more aggressive, multimodality treatment.

TREATMENT

■ EARLY BREAST CANCER (STAGE I AND II)

Local–Regional Therapy

❷ Most patients presenting with breast cancer today have either an in situ tumor, a small invasive tumor with negative lymph nodes (stage I), or a small invasive tumor with axillary lymph node involvement (stage II). Surgery alone can cure most, if not all, patients with in situ cancers, 70% to 80% of patients with stage I, and about one half of all patients with stage II cancers. The choice of surgical procedures has changed drastically over the past 50 years. This is partly a result of changes in our understanding of the biology of breast cancer, and is partly a result of a series of well-conducted clinical trials performed over this time period.

The Halstedian theory and concept of tumor growth, formulated at the end of the 19th century, held that breast cancer was a local–regional disease that spread to involve larger contiguous areas of the breast, chest wall, and adjacent lymph nodes. This hypothesis gave rise to the Halsted radical mastectomy, a surgical approach based on the rationale that cure of early disease could best be achieved with expansive, meticulously performed surgical procedures. *Radical mastectomy* involves removal of the breast and both major and minor pectoralis muscles. The axillary nodes on the same side (ipsilateral) as the breast lesion are also removed. Substantial morbidity is associated with this procedure. Muscle resection decreases strength and range of motion, and removal of axillary lymph nodes can produce edema of the arm and resected breast area. This procedure was often followed by external beam radiation therapy to the involved area.

During the 1960s, it was recognized that breast cancer is often microscopically disseminated at the time of initial diagnosis. This evolutionary concept that breast cancer is not only a local, but also a systemic disease, resulted in major changes in local and systemic therapy. The modified radical mastectomy, also termed *total mastectomy with axillary lymph node dissection*, became the standard surgical approach in the 1970s and was not as precisely defined or standardized as the radical mastectomy. The pectoralis minor muscle may be excised, divided, or left intact, and more importantly, there may be variation in the extent of axillary lymph node dissection, ranging from sampling to full dissection (including levels I and II ipsilateral axillary lymph nodes). Despite the lack of standardization, the modified radical mastectomy procedure is associated with significantly less morbidity and long-term complications compared to its radical counterpart.

Results of several large trials have since repudiated the Halsted theory and supported the alternative systemic hypothesis. Over the years these trials have investigated reducing the amount of surgery required to maintain acceptable cosmetic results and rates of local and distant recurrence and mortality. Breast-conserving therapy (BCT) includes removal of part of the breast, surgical evaluation of the axillary lymph node basin, and radiation therapy to the breast. The amount of breast tissue removed as a part of BCT varies from just removing the cancerous "lump" (a lumpectomy) with a small margin of adjacent normal-appearing tissue, to removing the "lump" with a wider excision of adjacent normal-appearing tissue (a wide local excision), to removing the entire quadrant of the breast that includes the cancerous "lump" (a quadrantectomy). All of these techniques are referred to as a *segmental or partial mastectomy*. In 1990, the National Institutes of Health Consensus Development Conference reviewed six trials comparing modified radical mastectomy with BCT.[71] Those patients who underwent BCT had removal of only part of the breast, and an axillary lymph node dissection followed by radiation therapy to the whole breast. From this analysis, the National Institutes of Health conference concluded that "BCT is an appropriate method of primary therapy for the majority of women with stage I and stage II breast cancer and is preferable because it provides survival equivalent to total mastectomy and axillary dissection while preserving the breast."[71] The median follow-up for these trials was 6.5 years at the time the National Institutes of Health conference was convened and this recommendation was made.

In a meta-analysis of updated information from these same six trials with a median follow-up of 14.7 years, the authors concluded that no difference in overall survival between mastectomy and BCT remained.[72] However, with longer follow-up it does appear that local recurrence rates are significantly higher with BCT (pooled data odds ratio [OR], 1.56; 95% CI, 1.29-1.89; P <0.001). This observation was also demonstrated in previous meta-analyses, including one by Morris et al. reported in 1997,[73] the Early Breast Cancer Trialists' Collaborative Group (EBCTCG) overview completed in 2000,[74] and one by Yang et al. reported in 2008.[75] Although local–regional recurrences are concerning, it is not clear what impact they have on overall survival. In the Jatoi meta-analysis, no impact on overall survival was seen with more than 4,000 patients included in the analysis.[72] But in the EBCTCG meta-analysis, which included 25,000 women, increased locoregional recurrences were associated with increased breast cancer mortality.[74] Collectively, these data indicate that any negative impact on survival, if present, is probably very small, and competing causes of death from adverse effects related to cancer therapy and comorbid diseases must be considered to determine the overall risks associated with BCT for an individual patient. These risks should be weighed against the potential benefits of any local therapy. Also, most patients with early stage breast cancer receive systemic adjuvant therapy (to be discussed later; see Systemic Adjuvant Therapy below), which further reduces the risk of recurrence and death from breast cancer, possibly negating any potential increase in recurrence attributed to BCT. Because the studies included in all of these meta-analyses are quite heterogeneous and of varying quality, it is difficult to draw sound conclusions. Other clinical trials have investigated methods to better identify patients at high risk for recurrence to better define who might be appropriate candidates for BCT compared with mastectomy. Some clinical trials suggest that young age (<35 years) is predictive for ipsilateral breast recurrences, but these trials also indicate a similar survival with BCT compared with mastectomy in this same population.[76,77] Women with a family history of breast cancer or an identified mutation in *BRCA1* or *BRCA2* are more likely to exist in this younger population, which may confound the independent contribution of age and treatment on clinical outcome.[78] This may be a result of the high risk of another cancer developing in the remaining breast tissue rather than a recurrence of the previously diagnosed cancer. However, despite the lack of sound clinical evidence to support the recommendation, the National Comprehensive Cancer Network (NCCN) recommends that women who are 35 years of age or younger, or who are premenopausal and a carrier of a known *BRCA1* or *BRCA2* mutation, undergo mastectomy and

consider additional risk reduction strategies (e.g., bilateral mastectomies).[47] Bilateral total mastectomy and/or oophorectomy reduce the risk of breast cancer occurrence in patients with *BRCA1* or *BRCA2* mutations, but both breast and ovarian cancers have been reported in patients who have had prophylactic removal of these organs. Most experts agree that BCT is an appropriate option for local therapy of early stage breast cancer. BCT is appropriate for most women, but full disclosure of the risks and benefits should be made and thoroughly discussed, and the patient's clinical situation and preferences should be carefully considered prior to undergoing any such procedure.

Most patients diagnosed today with breast cancer can be treated with BCT. Several factors should be considered in selecting patients for BCT. Multiple sites of cancer within the breast and the inability to attain negative pathologic margins on the excised breast specimen are predictive for an increased risk of recurrence with BCT and are indications for mastectomy. Some preexisting collagen vascular diseases (e.g., scleroderma and systemic lupus erythematosus) are relative contraindications for the use of BCT because of an increased risk of radiation-related adverse effects. Although local recurrence following BCT has not been consistently associated with increased mortality, it is distressing to the patient and requires surgical removal of the breast. In addition, reconstructive therapy is often not feasible in a breast that has previously received irradiation. Another major consideration in selecting patients for BCT is the expected cosmetic result. Although tumor size is not an important consideration for breast cancer recurrence if negative margins can be achieved, the relationship of the size of the tumor to the total breast volume is an important cosmetic consideration. If the volume of the tissue removed encompasses a significant portion of the breast, better results may be obtained with mastectomy and reconstruction. Additionally, for some patients, preservation of a limited amount of breast tissue may not justify the inconvenience of radiation therapy. Another approach to therapy for these patients is primary (neoadjuvant) systemic therapy to potentially shrink the tumor and minimize surgery (see sections on Systemic Adjuvant Therapy and Locally Advanced Breast Cancer for further details). Aside from the probability of local recurrence and the ability to achieve a satisfactory cosmetic result, consideration must be given to the availability of an external beam radiation facility and the patient's willingness to comply with the prescribed course of radiotherapy. In most instances, external beam radiation therapy used in conjunction with breast-conserving procedures involves 4 to 6 weeks of radiation therapy directed to the entire breast tissue (typically a total of 50 Gy [5000 Rad] administered in 25 daily doses Mondays through Fridays, with an optional boost of radiation) to eradicate residual disease. Complications associated with radiation therapy to the breast are minor and include reddening and erythema of the breast tissue and subsequent shrinkage of total breast mass beyond that predicted on the basis of breast tissue removal.

Although the current standard of care is to include local radiation therapy to the whole breast as a required component of BCT, current clinical trials are investigating the use of accelerated partial breast irradiation, intraoperative radiotherapy, or no radiation after segmental mastectomy for certain patient populations with a very low risk of recurrence.[79] Potential advantages of partial breast irradiation include decreased volume of breast tissue irradiated and shorter duration of treatment. Partial breast irradiation can be delivered with brachytherapy (such as with the Mammosite device) or external beam irradiation (with 3-D conformational radiation or intensity modulated radiation therapy). Others are investigating a single dose of radiation intraoperatively. None of these newer methods are considered standard of care, but may be included as part of a clinical trial. The underlying goal of local therapy is to minimize complications while maximizing outcomes that are relevant to the patient (e.g., cosmetic results, local and distant recurrence rates, mortality).

Postmastectomy radiation therapy to the chest wall may also be required in certain situations where tumors are large or the number of positive axillary lymph nodes is high (see section on Locally Advanced Breast Cancer). However, these criteria are also widely debated and are the subject of several meta-analyses. Despite the controversy, it is clear that some women may benefit from local radiation therapy even after removal of the entire breast (i.e., total mastectomy). The NCCN Guidelines state that women with the following criteria should undergo postmastectomy radiation therapy: (a) positive surgical margins, (b) a tumor larger than 5 cm in greatest dimension, or (c) four or more positive axillary lymph nodes.[47] Patients with close margins (<1 mm of normal adjacent tissue) or one to three positive ipsilateral axillary lymph nodes should consider postmastectomy chest wall radiation therapy, but the benefits are controversial. Patients with surgical margins of at least 1 mm, tumor size of 5 cm or less and negative axillary lymph nodes do not require postmastectomy chest wall radiation therapy. The optimal sequence of radiation therapy and chemotherapy is somewhat controversial. Concurrent administration of chemotherapy and radiation therapy is usually avoided because of an increase in local adverse effects. Most clinicians administer systemic chemotherapy immediately following surgery (if chemotherapy was not administered prior to surgery) given the hypothetical presence of systemic micrometastases that cannot be eradicated by local radiation therapy. Radiation therapy is then administered after chemotherapy, leaving hormone therapy (which is given for many years) for the end (see section on Adjuvant Biologic Therapy for discussion of sequencing trastuzumab).

Accurate assessment of the spread of breast cancer cells to the axillary lymph nodes is critical for prognosis and the determination of the utility of both local and systemic treatments. Axillary lymph node dissection with histopathologic study of the full axillary specimen, including level I and II lymph nodes, was the gold standard for detecting axillary nodal involvement and determining the number of lymph nodes containing tumor. The number of positive axillary lymph nodes remains the most powerful predictor of breast cancer recurrence and survival, but other benefits may include a therapeutic effect of removing the lymph nodes and obtaining information to guide treatment selection. However, axillary dissection is associated with significant morbidity, with an acute complication rate as high as 20% to 30% and rates of chronic lymphedema as high as 20% to 30%.[80,81] Recent studies indicate that approximately 60% of patients with early stage breast cancer present with lymph node–negative disease, which indicates that many women would derive no therapeutic benefit, but would be exposed to the complications from the procedure.

For these reasons, a procedure involving lymphatic mapping and sentinel lymph node biopsy (SLNB) is increasingly accepted at many centers across the United States and guidelines regarding recommendations for this procedure are now available.[82–84] The sentinel lymph node(s) is the first lymph node(s) that receives lymph drainage from the primary tumor. Injection of a vital blue dye, a radiocolloid, or both around the primary breast tumor identifies the sentinel lymph node(s) in most patients, and the status of this lymph node(s) may predict the status of the remaining nodes in the nodal basin. Patients with lymph nodes that are suspicious for cancer involvement either by physical exam or imaging should have a biopsy performed to exclude lymph node involvement. SLNB has become the standard of care for patients with clinically negative axillary lymph nodes.[47,85] Patients with a positive sentinel node or in cases where the sentinel node is not identified should proceed to a level I and II axillary lymph node dissection, although the definition of sentinel lymph node positivity is also controversial.

Many uncontrolled studies support the use of sentinel lymph node biopsy. Despite differences in the mapping technique, the experience of the surgeon, or the patient populations studied, recent studies show that the technique identified the sentinel lymph node(s) in more than 90% of patients.[84] In studies that incorporated completed axillary dissections for comparison, the SLNB procedure accurately predicted the status of the remaining axillary nodes in more than 90% of patients. Considerable controversy exists over the use of this procedure in women with large tumors (>5 cm) or locally advanced disease, palpable axillary lymph nodes, a multifocal or multicentric breast tumor, prior neoadjuvant (preoperative) chemotherapy, or prior surgery involving the breast and/or axilla. Patients who are pregnant or lactating are generally not considered candidates for this procedure due to concerns regarding the effects of the blue dye and/or the radiocolloid on the fetus.

Another factor that should be considered is the experience and mastery of the procedure by the surgical team. It has been shown that an individual surgeon must perform at least 20 procedures to attain competency, and the American Society of Breast Surgeons has incorporated this caveat into its *2005 Consensus Statement on Guidelines for Performing Sentinel Lymph Node Dissection for Breast Cancer.*[86] The false-negative rate with this procedure appears to inversely correlate with the rate of identification of the sentinel lymph node and may also be an early indicator of accuracy within an institution.[84]

The long-term outcome of patients who are undergoing this procedure alone (without axillary dissection) is unknown. Ongoing clinical trials will hopefully provide answers to these questions. A recent meta-analysis of 48 studies involving nearly 15,000 patients with a clinically negative axilla and a SLNB (without subsequent ALND) showed a median weighted axillary recurrence rate of 0.3% and a median weighted sensitivity for SLNB to detect axillary cancer cells of 100% (range, 97%–100%).[87] These results are reassuring, albeit with a relatively short median follow-up of less than 3 years. Despite the absence of long-term data, total mastectomy with SLNB (without ALND) can spare patients from the morbidities associated with an axillary lymph node dissection while providing critical information about breast cancer prognosis to guide local and systemic treatment decisions. The decision of whether to use the sentinel lymph node procedure or a full axillary dissection is complex and the reader is referred to excellent reviews and guidelines for further information.[82–84,86]

Simple or *total mastectomy* involves removal of the entire breast without dissection of the underlying muscle or axillary nodes. The major disadvantage of this procedure is that axillary nodal status is not determined, and therefore important prognostic information may be lost. This procedure is used in patients with carcinoma in situ, in whom there is a 1% incidence of axillary node involvement, or in cases of in-breast recurrences following BCT.

The early trials investigating less-extensive surgical approaches to breast cancer are widely credited with the finding that BCT is an appropriate primary therapy for most women with stages I and II disease, and is preferable because it arguably provides survival rates equivalent to those of modified radical mastectomy. But these trials provided valuable information regarding the natural history of the disease and identified pathologic prognostic factors associated with early cancer spread. The preponderance of information available regarding selection of women most likely to benefit from systemic adjuvant therapy was derived from pathologic evaluation of tissues archived from these early trials. It is hoped that further investigation into less-extensive local therapy (now focused on the surgical approach to the axilla and radiation therapy) will continue to provide valuable information for the future.

TABLE 136-6 Laboratory Findings, Clinical Observations, and Biologic Hypothesis of Breast Cancer as a Systemic Disease and the Value of Adjuvant Chemotherapy

- By the time cancer becomes clinically detectable, it is advanced (about 30 doublings) and has had ample opportunity to establish distant micrometastases.
- There is no orderly pattern of tumor cell dissemination, and the bloodstream is of considerable importance in tumor spread.
- Operable breast cancer is often a systemic disease and variations in local–regional therapy have not substantially affected survival. Only by control of distant disease can there be an improvement in the outcome of breast cancer patients.
- Likelihood of disease recurrence is related to size of tumor mass and axillary node involvement at diagnosis.
- Recurrence of breast cancer following local–regional therapy is most commonly at sites distant from the breast.
- Tumor growth fraction is inversely related to tumor population. Therefore, optimal kinetic conditions to achieve cure with chemotherapy exist in the setting of micrometastatic disease.
- Efficacy of chemotherapy is dose dependent and optimal doses of combination chemotherapy can be more safely and effectively administered in the adjuvant setting as opposed to the setting of advanced disease.

Systemic Adjuvant Therapy

❸ *Systemic adjuvant therapy* is defined as the administration of systemic therapy following definitive local therapy (surgery, radiation, or a combination of these) when there is no evidence of metastatic disease, but a high likelihood of disease recurrence. The concept of breast cancer being a systemic disease and the rationale of adjuvant chemotherapy was based on a series of laboratory and clinical investigations conducted during the 1960s and 1970s that were directed primarily toward achieving a better understanding of tumor metastases. Table 136–6 illustrates the laboratory findings, clinical abnormalities, and biologic hypotheses that lead to recognition of breast cancer as a systemic disease and documented the value of adjuvant chemotherapy. The earliest adjuvant trials in breast cancer consisted of perioperative administration of alkylating agents with the intent of eradicating micrometastases that were disseminated at the time of surgical excision of the tumor. Many collaborative research groups have conducted stepwise series of studies designed to identify appropriate candidates for systemic adjuvant therapy, and the optimal regimens and duration of therapy. Several hundred randomized clinical trials evaluating various systemic adjuvant modalities have been reported. Most published results confirm that chemotherapy, hormonal therapy, or both, result in improved disease-free survival (DFS) and/or overall survival (OS) for all treated patients, or more commonly for patients in specific prognostic subgroups (e.g., nodal involvement, menopausal status, hormonal receptor status, or *HER2* status). The huge amounts of data generated by these trials have resulted in a great deal of controversy, with different conclusions being reached by various experts.

Interpretation of results of systemic adjuvant therapy is difficult because of differences in the patient populations studied, the variation in natural history of breast cancer, the absence of information regarding pathologic prognostic factors in many studies, and differences in treatment approach and methods of analysis. It is important to remember that because the goal of systemic adjuvant therapy is cure, patients in these studies must be followed for long periods of time before results can be determined. In addition, because most patients with early breast cancer (50%–90%) in the various trials are cured with local–regional therapy alone, large numbers of patients are required to show a statistically significant difference that can be attributed to systemic adjuvant therapy. For these reasons, several groups around the world have conducted

meta-analyses of similar breast cancer trials in hopes of gaining more insight regarding adjuvant systemic therapy than a single study can provide. One such effort, organized by the EBCTCG, is based on a worldwide collaboration involving multiple randomized trials and is continually updated with results from new clinical trials.[5] The EBCTCG overview analyses are updated every 5 years and have been published in 1988, 1992, 1998, and 2005. The most recent update, published in 2005 as a result of analyses that took place in 2000, reflects the 10-year and 15-year effects on breast cancer recurrence and survival, respectively. Many important questions regarding the optimal way to administer adjuvant chemotherapy and hormonal therapy, and the magnitude of benefit as measured by DFS or OS to clinically relevant subsets of patients, have been answered by these overview analyses. Simply stated, the results of these analyses support the use of adjuvant hormonal therapy in all patients with positive hormone receptor status, regardless of age, menopausal status, involvement of axillary lymph nodes, or tumor size. The results of these overview analyses also support the use of adjuvant chemotherapy in most women with lymph node metastases or with primary breast cancers larger than 1 cm in diameter (both node-negative and node-positive).[5] It is important to note that data from clinical trials incorporating the taxanes, modern aromatase inhibitors, or trastuzumab into adjuvant chemotherapy regimens were not included in these analyses, as trials with these agents were not started by 1995, the cut-off for data inclusion.[5] Results from these more recent clinical trials are discussed later (see sections on Adjuvant Chemotherapy, Adjuvant Biologic Therapy, and Adjuvant Endocrine Therapy).

It is important to understand the relative and absolute magnitude of benefit associated with adjuvant systemic therapy in breast cancer. Table 136–7 shows the proportional reduction in the annual odds of recurrence and death by age for adjuvant polychemotherapy and adjuvant tamoxifen given for 5 years in women with tumors that are positive for hormone receptors based on the results of these overview analyses. Throughout these reports, the results are presented as they are in Table 136–7, as proportional benefits that compare the effects of two groups, in this case, chemotherapy or hormonal therapy versus no chemotherapy or hormonal therapy. A proportional reduction of 25% might equivalently be described as an OR, RR, or HR of 0.75; a RR or odds reduction of 25%; or a 25% reduction in the risk of death or death rate. For a given proportional reduction in death rate, the absolute improvement in 15-year survival will depend on the baseline risk of death with no treatment, which varies based on prognostic factors that include patient characteristics, disease characteristics and biomarkers identified earlier in this chapter. Table 136–8 shows the number of deaths avoided per 100 patients treated in several hypothetical subsets of patients with different estimated 15-year survivals without adjuvant therapy,

TABLE 136-7 Fifteen-Year Results of the Overview Analysis

Age (years)	Tamoxifen vs None[a] Reduction in Annual Odds		Polychemotherapy vs None Reduction in Annual Odds	
	Recurrence (%)	*Death (%)*	*Recurrence (%)*	*Death (%)*
All patients	39 ± 3	32 ± 4	23 ± 2	17 ± 2
<40	44 ± 10	39 ± 12	40 ± 6	29 ± 7
40–49	29 ± 7	24 ± 9	36 ± 4	30 ± 5
50–59	34 ± 5	24 ± 7	23 ± 3	15 ± 4
60–69	45 ± 5	35 ± 6	13 ± 3	9 ± 4
≥70	51 ± 12	37 ± 15	12 ± 11	13 ± 12

[a]Estrogen-receptor positive or unknown disease with about 5 years of tamoxifen versus no adjuvant therapy.
(Adapted from reference 5.)

TABLE 136-8 Absolute Reduction in Mortality at 10 Years per 100 Patients Treated

Estimated 10-year Death Rate with No Therapy	Hypothetical Proportional Reduction in Mortality as a Result of Treatment				
	50%	40%	30%	20%	10%
50% (5-cm tumor, one positive node)	25	20	15	10	5
30% (4-cm tumor, negative nodes)	15	12	9	6	3
10% (1.5-cm tumor, negative nodes)	5	4	3	2	1

TABLE 136-9 Absolute Benefits of Adjuvant Chemotherapy by Age and Nodal Status

	With Polychemotherapy (%)	With No Polychemotherapy (%)	Absolute Benefit (%)
Disease-free survival			
Age <50 years			
Node-negative	82.5	72.6	9.9
Node-positive	59.4	44.8	14.6
Age 50–69 years			
Node-negative	85.7	80.4	5.3
Node-positive	63.3	57.4	5.9
Survival[a]			
Age <50 years	67.6	57.6	10
Age 50–69 years	52.6	49.6	3

[a]Younger women, 35% node positive; older women, 70% node positive.
(Adapted from reference 5.)

as a function of different estimates of treatment benefit shown as the proportional reductions in mortality if they did receive adjuvant therapy. About 15 of every 100 patients benefited at 15 years from adjuvant therapy when a 30% proportional reduction in mortality is observed in the highest-risk subgroups (50% death rate with no adjuvant therapy). In contrast, the same 30% proportional reduction in mortality translated into a benefit for only 3 of 100 patients in the lowest-risk subset (10% death rate with no adjuvant therapy). Thus the absolute benefit of adjuvant therapy depends on both the proportional reduction in mortality and the risk of disease recurrence, with the greatest benefit observed in the highest-risk treatment groups. Table 136–9 uses data from the overview analyses to show the absolute benefits of adjuvant chemotherapy in terms of age and nodal status. In the highest-risk group, node-positive women younger than 50 years of age, only 42.8% were alive at 10 years with no polychemotherapy as compared to 54.2% with polychemotherapy, which translates into an absolute survival benefit of 11.4%. However, in the node-negative group, patients younger than 50 years old where survival with no polychemotherapy was highest (i.e., 76.3%), the addition of polychemotherapy produced an absolute benefit of only 4.8%. It should be pointed out that all of these differences in survival are clearly statistically significant and form the basis for national and international guidelines that recommend offering cytotoxic chemotherapy to most women with early stage breast cancer.[47,88] However, the absolute benefit in node-positive women 50 to 69 years old is quite small (2.7%), and depending on other disease characteristics and comorbid conditions, patients may elect not to pursue treatment. Although a 2% absolute reduction in death attributable to polychemotherapy may appear small, at least two investigators report that most patients with breast cancer would accept severe toxicity from treatment to achieve as little as a 1% to 5% absolute improvement in survival.[89,90]

Several international and national groups have developed guidelines for treatment of early stage breast cancer based on specific patient and disease characteristics and the results of the overview analyses. The two most commonly referenced guidelines are the St. Gallen International Expert Consensus Conference and the NCCN guidelines.[47,88] The St. Gallen guidelines are updated every 2 years by an international group of researchers that meet in St. Gallen, Switzerland to review available evidence and create consensus recommendations for selection of adjuvant systemic therapies in specific patient populations outside of the framework of clinical trials. The NCCN has also developed practice guidelines for the treatment of breast cancer which are updated annually or more often based on the available evidence. Recommendations from the NCCN for patients with tumors 1 cm or larger or positive lymph nodes are summarized in Figure 136–5. For patients with tumors less than 1 cm, micrometastatic lymph node involvement, or negative lymph nodes, treatment is highly individualized and based on multiple patient- and tumor-related factors, including hormone receptor status, *HER2* status, concomitant comorbidities, and patient preference. Specific treatment recommendations are complex and the reader is referred to the guideline for further details.

Intensive research efforts are directed toward identifying those characteristics of the primary tumor (e.g., pathologic or molecular prognostic factors) that may predict for a higher or lower likelihood of distant metastases and death in node-negative patients. Although many prognostic factors are being investigated, no single factor or combination of factors sufficiently identifies those at risk of metastases or is sufficiently standardized to be reproducibly applicable to all patients. Currently, two commercially available genetic tests are being prospectively validated as decision-support tools for adjuvant chemotherapy. Oncotype DX is one of these tests which screens for expression of 21 genes using reverse-transcription polymerase chain reaction and results in a recurrence score that can be used to determine the risk of distant recurrence and/or death from breast

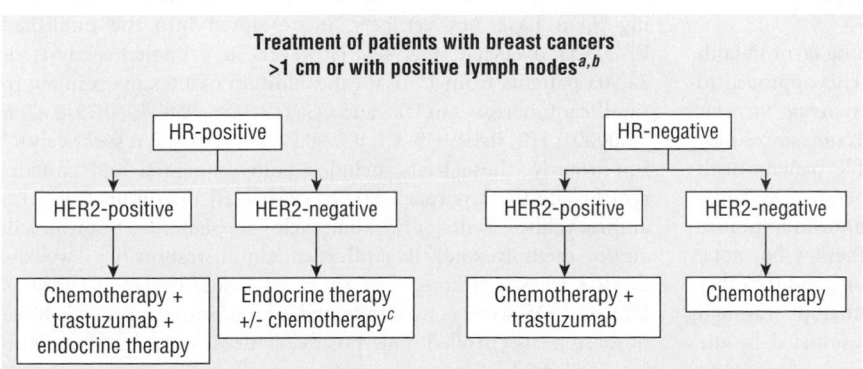

FIGURE 136-5. Treatment of patients with breast cancers >1 cm or with positive lymph nodes. HR, hormone receptor; HER2, human epidermal growth factor receptor-2. [a]Refer to text for definitions of HR and HER2 positivity. [b]Refer to text for management of patients with tumors <1 cm, micrometastatic lymph node involvement, or negative lymph nodes. [c]Oncotype DX may identify patients who derive little benefit from chemotherapy (lymph node negative patients only) (see Systemic Adjuvant Therapy section for details).

cancer in women with ER-positive, node-negative, invasive breast cancer.[68] The tumor tissue used for this test is paraffin-embedded tumor from archived samples. A low recurrence score (<18) indicates a low risk of recurrence with endocrine therapy alone indicating that perhaps adjuvant chemotherapy could be avoided. A high recurrence score (≥31) would indicate a high risk of recurrence despite endocrine therapy, suggesting a need for adjuvant chemotherapy followed by endocrine therapy. The utility of chemotherapy in patients with an intermediate score (18–30) is unclear, and ongoing clinical trials hope to further elucidate the role of Oncotype DX in this patient population. A second test, MammaPrint, was approved to estimate prognosis in breast cancer patients with early-stage disease, regardless of hormone receptor status. MammaPrint screens the tumor for 70 genes using microarray technology. The assay requires fresh-frozen tissue and reports the predicted rates of recurrence as high or low. This information has been shown to accurately predict for recurrence in a subset of patients not receiving systemic adjuvant therapy.[69] The MINDACT (Microarray In Node-negative Disease may Avoid ChemoTherapy) trial, ongoing in Europe, will compare the predictive capabilities of MammaPrint against the standard prognostic factors to assess which patients with node-negative, ER-positive breast cancer will benefit from adjuvant chemotherapy. We await further information to guide the use of these novel pharmacogenomic tools.

A clinical tool that is gaining favor is an Internet-based tool called Adjuvant! (www.adjuvantonline.com), which helps clinicians and patients make informed decisions regarding adjuvant therapy for breast, colon, and lung cancers. The tool allows healthcare professionals to estimate the risks of negative outcomes (e.g., cancer recurrence and/or death), and the potential benefits of therapy (e.g., reductions in risks of recurrence and/or death). This is a validated, evidence-based tool which incorporates multiple prognostic and predictive factors into a mathematical model in which each factor is weighted based on established evidence from clinical trials and is placed in the background of the Surveillance, Epidemiology, and End Results (SEER) database for patients living in the United States.[91,92] By entering the patient's age, comorbidities, ER status, tumor grade, tumor size, and nodal status, the clinician can use the tool to estimate the breast cancer mortality and/or recurrence risk at 10 years and determine the impact of chemotherapy, hormone therapy or both on these risks. The results are then projected in a graphic format which is easy to understand and explain to patients. Some of the limitations of Adjuvant! include the limited information regarding outcome in patients with tumors that are smaller than 1 cm and no axillary lymph node involvement; it does not incorporate proliferation markers or *HER2* status of the primary tumor; and it does not consider potential adverse effects of therapy. Estimates of outcome with the Adjuvant! program may also vary in specific subgroups of patients, such as women who are diagnosed with breast cancer at a younger age. For a more in-depth discussion of the issues and controversies regarding adjuvant therapy of breast cancer, the reader is referred to two excellent reviews.[93,94]

The use of preoperative systemic therapy is gaining favor in both early stage and locally advanced breast cancers. This approach to therapy, referred to as *neoadjuvant* or *primary systemic therapy*, usually consists of chemotherapy, but in special circumstances may also include hormonal therapy (e.g., in inoperable patients with significant comorbidities). Advantages of preoperative systemic therapy include (a) a decrease in the size of the tumor to minimize surgery; (b) determining the response to chemotherapy/hormone therapy in vivo (an important prognostic indicator); and (c) other theoretical advantages (e.g., delivery of chemotherapy through an intact vascular system). In a pivotal study conducted by the NSABP (Trial B18), preoperative chemotherapy was compared to traditional chemotherapy given after surgery (same chemotherapy and same number of cycles).[95,96] Although no difference was found in DFS or OS, rates of BCT were higher in the group receiving preoperative chemotherapy (67.8% vs 59.8%).[96] This study also identified a small subset of patients (13%) who had a pathologic complete response (no tumor left at surgery) after chemotherapy. These patients went on to have a significantly longer DFS as compared with patients who did not achieve a pathologic complete response (P <0.0001).[96] Importantly, even after 16 years of follow-up, patients who achieved a pCR continued to have superior DFS and OS compared with patients who did not achieve a pCR.[97] While this approach to therapy was historically reserved for patients with inoperable tumors (locally advanced), the use of preoperative systemic therapy in patients with early-stage breast cancer is increasing in popularity due to the ability to assess the response to therapy in vivo as well as the potential to decrease the size of the tumor, allowing for less radical surgery and better cosmetic results.

❹ Adjuvant Chemotherapy Cytotoxic drugs that have been used alone and in combination as adjuvant therapy in breast cancer include doxorubicin, epirubicin, cyclophosphamide, methotrexate, fluorouracil, paclitaxel, docetaxel, melphalan, prednisone, vinorelbine, and vincristine. Table 136–10 lists some of the most common combination chemotherapy regimens employed in the adjuvant setting.

The basic principle of adjuvant therapy for any cancer type is that the regimen with the highest response rate in advanced disease should be the optimal regimen for use in the adjuvant setting. However, results from individual clinical trials investigating specific regimens in the adjuvant setting are required to identify the benefits and risks in a specific patient population. Early administration of effective combination chemotherapy at a time when the tumor burden is low should increase the likelihood of cure and minimize the emergence of drug-resistant tumor cell clones. Historically, combination chemotherapy regimens (polychemotherapy) have been more effective than single-agent chemotherapy. Anthracyclines (doxorubicin and epirubicin) and more recently taxanes (paclitaxel and docetaxel) have become the cornerstones of modern chemotherapy for the adjuvant treatment of breast cancer. The overview analysis of polychemotherapy (discussed previously) analyzed results from 17 trials that directly compared an anthracycline-containing regimen with a cyclophosphamide, methotrexate, fluorouracil (CMF)-type regimen and demonstrated a significant advantage with the anthracycline regimens.[5] In that meta-analysis, anthracycline-containing regimens were modestly superior in reducing recurrence and death as compared to regimens without anthracyclines. An 11% ± 3% reduction in annual odds of recurrence and a 15% ± 3% reduction in annual odds of death were reported in the 2005 update, which translated into an absolute difference in OS of 3% at 5 years and 4% at 10 years.[5] None of the clinical trials included in this meta-analysis contained a taxane.

Because the taxanes are relatively new, adjuvant studies including them have not yet been incorporated into the published EBCTCG overview analyses. However, in a pooled analysis of 22,903 patients from 13 trials, the addition of a taxane resulted in significant increases in DFS and OS (HR, 0.83; 95% CI, 0.79-0.87; P <0.00001; HR, 0.85; 95% CI, 0.79-0.91; P <0.00001; respectively).[98] Importantly, these trials included both sequential and concurrent taxane therapy (paclitaxel or docetaxel) in conjunction with anthracyclines (with or without cyclophosphamide, fluorouracil, and/or methotrexate). Regardless of administration (e.g., weekly, every 3 weeks, prolonged or short infusions) or type of taxane, DFS and OS were consistently and significantly improved. Most of these trials enrolled node-positive patients only, but some also included high-risk node-negative patients. Taxane-containing,

TABLE 136-10 Selected Adjuvant Chemotherapy Regimens for Breast Cancer

AC[a,b]	TC[a,c]
Doxorubicin 60 mg/m² IV, day 1	Docetaxel 75 mg/m² IV, day 1
Cyclophosphamide 600 mg/m² IV, day 1	Cyclophosphamide 600 mg/m² IV, day 1
Repeat cycles every 21 days for 4 cycles	Repeat cycles every 21 days for 4 cycles
FAC[d,m]	**TAC[a,e]**
Fluorouracil 500 mg/m² IV, days 1 and 4	Docetaxel 75 mg/m² IV, day 1
Doxorubicin 50 mg/m² IV continuous infusion over 72 hours	Doxorubicin 50 mg/m² IV bolus, day 1
Cyclophosphamide 500 mg/m² IV, day 1	Cyclophosphamide 500 mg/m² IV, day 1
Repeat cycles every 21–28 days for 6 cycles	(Doxorubicin should be given first) Repeat cycles every 21 days for 6 cycles (must be given with growth factor support)
AC → Paclitaxel[a,f]	**Paclitaxel → FAC[g,m]**
Doxorubicin 60 mg/m² IV, day 1	Paclitaxel 80 mg/m² per week IV over 1 hour every week for 12 weeks
Cyclophosphamide 600 mg/m² IV, day 1	Followed by:
Repeat cycles every 21 days for 4 cycles	Fluorouracil 500 mg/m² IV, days 1 and 4
Followed by:	Doxorubicin 50 mg/m² IV continuous infusion over 72 hours
Paclitaxel 80 mg/m² IV weekly	Cyclophosphamide 500 mg/m² IV, day 1
Repeat cycles every 7 days for 12 cycles	Repeat cycles every 21–28 days for 4 cycles[g]
FEC[h]	**CEF[i]**
Fluorouracil 500 mg/m² IV, day 1	Cyclophosphamide 75 mg/m² per day orally on days 1–14
Epirubicin 100 mg/m² IV bolus, day 1	Epirubicin 60 mg/m² IV, days 1 and 8
Cyclophosphamide 500 mg/m² IV, day 1	Fluorouracil 600 mg/m² IV, days 1 and 8
Repeat cycle every 21 days for 6 cycles	Repeat cycles every 21 days for 6 cycles (requires prophylactic antibiotics or growth factor support)
CMF[j,k]	**Dose-Dense AC → Paclitaxel[a,l,n]**
Cyclophosphamide 100 mg/m² per day orally, days 1–14	Doxorubicin 60 mg/m² IV bolus, day 1
Methotrexate 40 mg/m² IV, days 1 and 8	Cyclophosphamide 600 mg/m² IV, day 1
Fluorouracil 600 mg/m² IV, days 1 and 8	Repeat cycles every 14 days for 4 cycles (must be given with growth factor support)
Repeat cycles every 28 days for 6 cycles	Followed by:
or	Paclitaxel 175 mg/m² IV over 3 hours
Cyclophosphamide 600 mg/m² IV, day 1	Repeat cycles every 14 days for 4 cycles (must be given with growth factor support)
Methotrexate 40 mg/m² IV, day 1	
Fluorouracil 600 mg/m² IV, days 1 and 8	
Repeat cycles every 21 days for 6 cycles	

AC, Adriamycin (doxorubicin), Cytoxan (cyclophosphamide); CAF, Cytoxan (cyclophosphamide), Adriamycin (doxorubicin), 5-fluorouracil; CEF, cyclophosphamide, epirubicin, 5-fluorouracil; CMF, cyclophosphamide, methotrexate, 5-flourouracil; FAC, 5-fluorouracil, Adriamycin (doxorubicin), cyclophosphamide; FEC, 5-fluorouracil, epirubicin, cyclophosphamide; TAC, Taxotere (docetaxel), Adriamycin (doxorubicin) cyclophosphamide; TC, Taxotere (docetaxel), cyclophosphamide.

[a]Designated as a preferred regimen in the NCCN Breast Cancer Guidelines.
[b]From Fisher B, Brown AM, Dimitrov NV, et al. J Clin Oncol 1990;8:1483.
[c]From Jones SE, Savin MA, Holmes FA, et al. J Clin Oncol 2006;24:5381.
[d]From Buzdar AU, Hortobagyi GN, Singletary SE, et al. In: Salmon S, ed. Adjuvant Therapy of Cancer, VIII. Philadelphia, PA: Lippincott-Raven, 1997:93–100.
[e]From Martin M, Dienkowski T, Mackey J, et al. N Engl J Med 2005;352:2302.
[f]From Sparano JA, Wang M, Martino S, et al. N Engl J Med 2008;358:1663–1671.
[g]From Green MC, Buzdar AU, Smith T, et al. J Clin Oncol 2005;23:5983.
[h]From French Adjuvant Study Group. J Clin Oncol 2001;19:602.
[i]From Levine MN, Bramwell VH, Pritchard KI, et al. J Clin Oncol 1998;16:2651.
[j]From Bonadonna G, Brusamolino E, Valagussa P, et al. N Engl J Med 1976;294:405.
[k]From Fisher B, Redmond C, Dimitrov NV, et al. N Engl J Med 1989;320:473.
[l]From Citron ML, Berry DA, Cirrincione C, et al. J Clin Oncol 2003;21:1431–1439.
[m]FAC may also be given with bolus doxorubicin administration, and the fluorouracil dose is then given on days 1 and 8.
[n]Another way to give these agents in a dose-dense manner is A → P → C as sequential single agents, in the same doses indicated above, every 14 days for 4 cycles each with growth factor support.

non-anthracycline regimens may be appropriate for some patients with a low risk of disease recurrence. However, this subject remains widely debated.

CLINICAL CONTROVERSY

Although incorporation of taxanes into many different adjuvant chemotherapy regimens, both sequentially and concurrently, has led to a shift in therapy for node-positive breast cancer patients, the use of taxane-containing regimens in node-negative patients remains controversial. The use of an anthracycline-containing regimen is established for both node-negative and node-positive breast cancer patients.

There is no apparent biologic reason why node-negative disease should respond differently to the taxanes than node-positive disease. However, the absolute benefits for this population may not be large enough to warrant a change from the standard of care. Further follow-up from these trials will continue to address this issue. Since the addition of a taxane may predispose patients to some transient peripheral neuropathy, myelosuppression, and alopecia, adverse events should also be considered. The long-term adverse events related to these regimens are yet to be determined. Also, the cost-effectiveness of adding a taxane to an adjuvant regimen is still largely debated given the paucity of reliable information addressing this issue.

Cytotoxic chemotherapy is a particularly important treatment modality for patients with tumors that do not express ER or PR and do not overexpress *HER2* (so called triple-negative breast cancers, TNBC). Patients with TNBC treated with anthracycline and taxane-based chemotherapy have significantly decreased survival compared to patients with other breast cancer subtypes. Ironically, this subgroup of patients is more likely to respond to neoadjuvant chemotherapy. Therefore, patients with TNBC who achieve a pCR have an excellent long-term survival, but those who have residual disease at the time of surgery have a worse prognosis than non-TNBC patients.[99] The optimal type and duration of chemotherapy for patients with TNBC is unknown. Because none of the previously identified molecular targets are present in TNBC, incorporation of non-traditional chemotherapy (e.g., platinum agents) into these regimens is under investigation. Identification of meaningful molecular targets is much needed and is where most research is ongoing. Molecular targets of interest include epidermal growth factor receptor (EGFR), vascular endothelial growth factor (VEGF), and poly-ADP ribose polymerase (PARP).

No validated predictive factors exist for response to chemotherapy, but some studies suggest that *HER2* status and ER negativity may be useful predictors of response. Some retrospective studies suggest that the benefit of anthracycline-containing regimens over CMF-like regimens is limited to those tumors that overexpress *HER2* or are topoisomerase II (*TOP2A*) amplified. This concept is theoretically plausible, since *HER2* and *TOP2A* are closely located on chromosome 17 and *TOP2A* is a known target for anthracycline therapy. However, data supporting these relationships are contradictory, and therefore should not influence chemotherapy treatment decisions at this time. ER status has also been evaluated as a predictor of response to chemotherapy. Several clinical trials have attempted to correlate ER-negative status with response to adjuvant chemotherapy, but the results of these studies are inconsistent and decisions concerning chemotherapy should not be based on ER status at this time. Several investigators have attempted to predict response to specific chemotherapy regimens (e.g., taxane-containing regimens) with microarray technology, which uses DNA from the tumor to test for thousands of genetic mutations. Although these types of genetic tests need to be validated in prospective clinical trials, they may serve in the future to help determine what chemotherapy regimen a patient should receive to gain the most benefit. For the time being, chemotherapy options are chosen based on the prescriber's experience with the regimen and current evidence from clinical trials.

Although the optimal duration of adjuvant chemotherapy administration is unknown, it appears to be on the order of 12 to 24 weeks and depends on the regimen being used. Chemotherapy should be initiated within 12 weeks of surgical removal of the primary tumor.[100] "Dose intensity" and "dose density" appear to be critical factors in achieving optimal outcomes in adjuvant breast cancer therapy. *Dose intensity* is defined as the amount of drug administered per unit of time and is typically reported in milligrams per square meter of body surface area per week (mg/m²/week). Increasing dose, decreasing time between doses, or both can increase dose intensity. *Dose density* is one way of achieving dose intensity, but not by increasing the amount of drug given, as occurs with dose escalation, but instead by decreasing the time between treatment cycles. The importance of dose intensity first received wide attention in 1981, when the Milan group reported in a retrospective analysis of their original CMF adjuvant study that only those patients who received at least 85% of their planned CMF dose benefited significantly from adjuvant therapy, while those receiving less than 65% of the planned dose had the same DFS and OS as the group of control patients treated with surgery alone.[101] Therefore, dose reductions for standard treatment regimens should be avoided, unless necessitated by severe toxicity. But increasing doses beyond those contained in standard treatment regimens does not appear to be beneficial and may be harmful.

Several studies investigating the impact of *dose density* have now been reported. Interest in this approach to adjuvant therapy was stimulated when the CALGB reported results from their trial 9741 which tested not only dose density, but also the question of using sequential versus combination chemotherapy regimens. Using a 2 × 2 factorial design, investigators randomized node-positive breast cancer patients after surgery to compare sequential versus concurrent chemotherapy, and standard dose versus dose density.[102] The arms of the study were (group 1) sequential doxorubicin (A) for four cycles, followed by paclitaxel (P) for four cycles, followed by cyclophosphamide (C) for four cycles, with all cycles given every 3 weeks; (group 2) sequential A for four cycles, followed by P for four cycles, followed by C for four cycles, with all cycles given every 2 weeks with filgrastim; (group 3) concurrent AC for four cycles, followed by P for four cycles, with all cycles given every 3 weeks; and (group 4) concurrent AC for four cycles, followed by P for four cycles, with all cycles given every 2 weeks with filgrastim. After a median follow-up of 36 months, the patients receiving chemotherapy every 2 weeks had a significantly prolonged DFS (at 3 years: 85% vs 81%; RR, 0.74; *P* = 0.01) and OS (92% vs 90%; RR, 0.69; *P* = 0.013) as compared with every 3-week chemotherapy.[102] The use of sequential versus concurrent chemotherapy did not show a benefit for one over the other in terms of DFS or OS, but sequential therapy did appear to be less toxic. Patients in the concurrent every 2-week group (group 4) had significantly more regimen-related toxicity, including a very high rate of red blood cell transfusions for anemia (13% of cycles).[102] Red blood cell transfusions are rarely required with most other standard adjuvant chemotherapy regimens used for breast cancer.

Dose intensity appears to be important for some drugs but not for others. Many studies with anthracyclines (without taxanes) appear to indicate no benefit from a dose-dense approach to drug administration. These data seem to contradict the CALGB 9741 data. However, data with the taxanes, especially paclitaxel, appear to support a dose-dense (not intense) approach, with weekly therapy producing optimal outcomes.[102] Data with paclitaxel given weekly versus every 3 weeks indicates that this drug is more effective when given weekly in the adjuvant, neoadjuvant, and metastatic

settings.[103,104] Thus some speculate that the different paclitaxel schedule is the primary reason for the success with this approach to therapy. A direct comparison between taxane dosing intervals was evaluated in the North American Breast Cancer Intergroup Trial E1199 which randomized patients in a 2 × 2 factorial design to receive doxorubicin and cyclophosphamide for four cycles every 3 weeks followed by either weekly or 3-weekly paclitaxel or docetaxel.[103] While this study does not directly address the question of dose density because of the lower doses given in the weekly arms, it appears to support the pharmacologic advantage of a taxane given more frequently as the essential factor driving the beneficial outcomes seen with "dose density" in the CALGB 9741 trial. Although no differences in DFS or OS were observed between the weekly or 3-weekly schedule or the different taxanes in the E1199 trial, a subgroup analysis indicated that the weekly paclitaxel arm resulted in improved DFS (OR, 1.27; 95% CI, 1.03-1.57; *P* = 0.006) and OS (OR, 1.32; 95% CI, 1.02-1.72; *P* = 0.01) compared to paclitaxel administered every 3 weeks. Docetaxel, when administered every 3 weeks, resulted in improved DFS (OR, 1.23; 95% CI, 1.00-1.52; *P* = 0.02) but not OS (OR, 1.13; 95% CI, 0.88-1.46; *P* = 0.25) when compared to paclitaxel administered every 3 weeks. DFS and OS with weekly docetaxel was not significantly different from paclitaxel administered every 3 weeks. Although other trials have attempted to investigate dose-dense regimens, they also have other variables that were altered that could potentially impact the outcomes. Consequently, they do not directly address the question and their results may be influenced by factors other than dose density. A detailed discussion of these nuances is beyond the scope of this chapter and the reader is referred to excellent references on this topic for further information.[105,106] Nonetheless, despite a relatively short follow-up, unclear overall benefit compared to conventional regimens, and potentially more toxicity, the dose-dense regimens may be considered as options for adjuvant therapy for node-positive breast cancer. Thorough discussion regarding the risks and benefits each individual patient may face is imperative given the uncertainty surrounding these regimens.

A major focus of clinical investigations in the past was the use of high-dose chemotherapy regimens as adjuvant therapy. Because bone marrow suppression is the dose-limiting toxicity for most chemotherapeutic agents, high-dose chemotherapy regimens followed by colony-stimulating factors or reinfusion of autologous hematopoietic stem cells were developed. Several cooperative groups have conducted trials of high-dose chemotherapy with stem cell support versus conventional adjuvant therapy. None of the trials showed a significant difference in DFS or OS. Based on the available evidence, this approach to therapy is currently not recommended outside the context of a clinical trial.

The short-term toxic effects of chemotherapy used in the adjuvant setting are generally well tolerated. Although a number of investigators have demonstrated a reduction in quality-of-life, most patients are able to maintain a reasonable level of function and emotional and social well-being during treatment.[107,108] Supportive therapy of the patient receiving systemic adjuvant chemotherapy has improved over the past decades. Increased attention to the impact of symptoms on quality-of-life may account for some of this improvement. In addition, more effective antiemetics have become available to assist in managing chemotherapy-induced nausea and vomiting, and colony-stimulating factors are often helpful in preventing febrile neutropenia, particularly in elderly patients or patients receiving dose-dense chemotherapy regimens. Despite the use of newer antiemetics for prevention of nausea and vomiting, many women still have difficulty with this side effect and delayed nausea and vomiting remains problematic in some patients. Aprepitant, a novel neurokinin-1 antagonist, may be considered in addition to serotonin receptor antagonists and dexamethasone to improve outcomes for some patients receiving anthracycline-based chemotherapy, but clinicians should be aware of the potential for clinically significant drug–drug interactions between aprepitant and other drugs, including some chemotherapy. The use of growth factors to support some adjuvant chemotherapy regimens may be required (e.g., with dose-dense regimens), but should also be used with caution. Myeloid growth factors and erythropoietic stimulating agents (ESAs) have potential effects on cancer cells and the cellular environment that may negatively impact the antitumor effects of chemotherapy or enhance adverse effects related to the chemotherapy.[109] Although these effects are very controversial, the addition of growth factors to a regimen should be undertaken only after all risks and benefits are thoroughly considered.

Many other side effects are common with the chemotherapy regimens employed for treatment of early stage breast cancer and patients should be appropriately counseled regarding the likelihood of alopecia, weight gain, and fatigue. Patients who are menstruating will often experience a cessation of menses that may not return; cessation of menses may be accompanied by signs and symptoms of menopause. Deep vein thrombosis has been reported in women receiving combination chemotherapy regimens.[110] Leukemia and other hematologic disorders have long been associated with the alkylating agents (e.g., cyclophosphamide) and the topoisomerase II inhibitors (e.g., doxorubicin and epirubicin). Several studies have estimated a 0% to 1.5% cumulative incidence of leukemia and/or myelodysplasia after adjuvant chemotherapy with median follow-up of 3 to 11 years.[111] To date, the dose-dense regimens have not been associated with an excess rate of leukemias, but the follow-up on these trials is relatively short.

Cardiomyopathy induced by doxorubicin occurs in less than 1% of women whose total dose of doxorubicin is less than 320 mg/m^2.[112] This risk may be further decreased by use of continuous infusion doxorubicin. It should be noted that epirubicin in the adjuvant setting is usually given at a dose of 100 to 120 mg/m^2.[113] At this dose, epirubicin has an equal chance of causing cardiomyopathy as standard doxorubicin doses when both agents are given as bolus or short infusions. Taxanes are often associated with hypersensitivity reactions, peripheral neuropathy and/or myalgias and arthralgias for several days following the infusion.

It is important to note that the magnitude of survival benefit for adjuvant chemotherapy in stages I and II breast cancer is modest, with an absolute reduction in mortality of only 5% at 10 years for patients with negative axillary lymph nodes and 10% for patients with positive axillary lymph nodes. In addition, it is currently not possible to accurately predict who will attain this survival benefit. The advent of genetic prognostic tools, such as Oncotype DX, can help to identify patients who may derive little or no benefit from chemotherapy. However, these tests are only appropriate in specific subsets of patients. Studies have reported that most breast cancer patients would accept severe toxicity from treatment to achieve as little as a 1% to 5% improvement in survival.[89,90] Thus in the absence of the ability to predict who will benefit, it is likely that most patients with stage I and stage II breast cancer would choose adjuvant chemotherapy.

The optimal chemotherapy regimen for use in the adjuvant setting has yet to be identified and the choice of chemotherapy regimen for a specific patient is complex. Many adjuvant chemotherapy regimens are available, and the majority of these regimens have not been directly compared in randomized clinical trials. In some cases the choice of chemotherapy regimen may be geographic, particularly if a regimen has been developed and studied by a particular institution. Based on data from clinical trials and the previously mentioned pooled analysis, the concomitant or sequential addition of a taxane to an anthracycline-based chemotherapy regimen has

become the standard of care for women with node-positive breast cancer. The use of taxanes in combination with anthracyclines is more controversial in patients with node-negative disease, and therefore taxanes may or may not be utilized in this patient population. Results from a single trial which evaluated a taxane-containing (non-anthracycline) regimen are available and this regimen may be an appropriate treatment in a subset of patients at low risk of disease recurrence. NCCN recommendations are purposefully vague, and they do not differentiate between patients with node positive or negative breast cancer. The NCCN has designated preferred chemotherapy regimens, as listed in Table 136–10, although detailed information is not provided regarding the rationale behind these designations.

Adjuvant Biologic Therapy As biologic agents continue to demonstrate significant activity against metastatic breast cancer, they are subsequently tested in the adjuvant setting. Trastuzumab is a monoclonal antibody targeted against the *HER2*-receptor protein. It has demonstrated significant survival benefits when administered with chemotherapy in women with metastatic, *HER2*-positive breast cancer. Several published or presented studies support the use of trastuzumab in combination with or sequentially following adjuvant chemotherapy for patients with early-stage, *HER2*-positive breast cancer (Table 136–11).[114-118] Results from these trials report up to a 50% reduction in the risk of recurrence with the addition of trastuzumab to an adjuvant chemotherapy regimen. While similar benefits are seen in the published trials to date, the chemotherapy regimens, sequence of administration and duration of trastuzumab differ (Table 136–11).

A meta-analysis of five clinical trials involving 9,739 women revealed superior DFS (RR, 0.62; 95% CI, 0.56-0.68; *P* <0.0001) and OS (RR, 0.66; 95% CI, 0.57-0.77; *P* <0.0001) in patients with *HER2*-positive breast cancer who received trastuzumab with chemotherapy compared to those that received chemotherapy alone.[119] This difference in DFS translated into a 38% overall lower relative risk for disease progression or death from any cause for patients who received trastuzumab.

Most of the regimens investigated in these adjuvant trials included an anthracycline and a taxane given concurrently with trastuzumab or sequentially prior to trastuzumab. From the available evidence, it appears that administration of a taxane with trastuzumab may be more effective than trastuzumab administered after chemotherapy. The benefit of sequential administration of trastuzumab has come into question since only one study (Herceptin Adjuvant Trial, HERA) has demonstrated a significant benefit with trastuzumab administered in this manner. The adjuvant use of trastuzumab without an anthracycline has been reported in one trial (Breast Cancer International Research Group 006) and from preliminary analyses appears to provide similar benefit with diminished adverse effects as compared with traditional anthracycline-containing adjuvant trastuzumab regimens. The duration of trastuzumab therapy in these adjuvant trials ranges from 9 to 52 weeks in the published studies. The optimal duration of trastuzumab therapy is unknown. In the United States, trastuzumab has been approved for adjuvant therapy of early-stage, *HER2*-positive breast cancer when given in combination with doxorubicin and cyclophosphamide followed by paclitaxel or docetaxel and the trastuzumab is initiated with the taxane and continued for 1 year (total duration of trastuzumab is 52 weeks). Trastuzumab has also been approved by the U.S. Food and Drug Administration (FDA) in combination with docetaxel and carboplatin followed by trastuzumab (for a total of 1 year), as well as administered alone for 1 year following anthracycline-based chemotherapy. These approvals are based on results from the NSABP/NCCTG (North Central Cancer Treatment Group) combined analysis, the HERA (Herceptin Adjuvant) trial, and the BCIRG 006 trial.[120] One year of trastuzumab, either concomitantly

TABLE 136-11 Selected Trastuzumab-based Regimens for Breast Cancer

		Adjuvant		
Regimen	**Drugs**	**Doses**	**Frequency**	**Cycles**
$AC \Rightarrow PH \Rightarrow H^a$	Doxorubicin	60 mg/m^2 IV	q 21 days	4
	Cyclophosphamide	600 mg/m^2 IV	q 21 days	4
	followed by			
	Paclitaxel	175 mg/m^2 IV over 3 h	q 21 days	4
	or			
	Paclitaxel	80 mg/m^2 IV over 1 h	q 7 days	12 wk
	with Trastuzumab	4 mg/kg IV → 2 mg/kg IV	q 7 days	12 wk
	followed by			
	Trastuzumab	2 mg/kg IV or 6 mg/kg IV	q 7 days or q 21 days	Complete 1 year
TCH^b	Docetaxel	75 mg/m^2 IV	q 21 days	6
	Carboplatin	AUC 6 IV	q 21 days	6
	Trastuzumab	4 mg/kg IV → 2 mg/kg IV	q 7 days	18 wk
	followed by			
	Trastuzumab	6 mg/kg IV	q 21 days	Complete 1 year
$Chemo \Rightarrow H^c$	Chemotherapy	See reference for details		At least 4
	followed by			
	Trastuzumab	8 mg/kg IV → 6 mg/kg IV	q 21 days	1 year
$AC \Rightarrow TH^b$	Doxorubicin	60 mg/m^2 IV	q 21 days	4
	Cyclophosphamide	600 mg/m^2 IV	q 21 days	4
	followed by			
	Docetaxel	100 mg/m^2 IV	q 21 days	4
	Trastuzumab	4 mg/kg IV → 2 mg/kg IV	q 7 days	12 wk
	followed by			
	Trastuzumab	6 mg/kg IV	q 21 days	Complete 1 year
		Neoadjuvant		
Regimen	**Drugs**	**Doses**	**Frequency**	**Cycles**
$PH \Rightarrow FEC/H^d$	Paclitaxel	225 mg/m^2 IV over 24 h	q 21 days	4
	or			
	Paclitaxel	80 mg/m^2 IV over 1 h	q 7 days	12 wk
	with Trastuzumab	4 mg/kg IV → 2 mg/kg IV	q 7 days	12 wk
	followed by			
	Fluorouracil	500 mg/m^2 IV (days 1 and 4)	q 21 days	4
	Epirubicin	75 mg/m^2 IV	q 21 days	4
	Cyclophosphamide	500 mg/m^2 IV	q 21 days	4
	with Trastuzumab	2 mg/kg IV	q 7 days	12 wk

AC, Adriamycin (doxorubicin), Cytoxan (cyclophosphamide); FEC, fluorouracil, epirubicin, cyclophosphamide; H, Herceptin (trastuzumab); PH, paclitaxel, Herceptin (trastuzumab); TH, Taxotere (docetaxel), Herceptin (trastuzumab); TCH, Taxotere (docetaxel), carboplatin, Herceptin (trastuzumab).
[a]From Romond EH, Perez EA, Bryant J, et al. N Engl J Med. 2005;353:1673-1684.
[b]From Slamon D, Eiermann W, Robert N, et al. 32nd Annual CTRC-AACR San Antonio Breast Cancer Symposium; 2009. Abstract 62.
[c]From Smith I, Procter M, Gelber RD et al. Lancet 2007;369:29–36.
[d]From Buzdar AU, Ibrahim NK, Francis D, et al. J Clin Oncol. 2005;23:3676.

with chemotherapy or sequentially after chemotherapy has become the standard duration of therapy in the United States and many other countries.

The incidence of adverse cardiac effects associated with the addition of trastuzumab appears to increase when an anthracycline is included in the regimen prior to administration of trastuzumab. In the previously mentioned meta-analysis, trastuzumab use resulted in an increased risk of class III/IV heart failure (RR, 7.60; 95% CI, 4.07-14.18; P <0.0001) compared with chemotherapy alone.[119] However, the higher risk of cardiac complications may be acceptable given the significant reductions in breast cancer recurrence and death rates. Sequential administration of trastuzumab after chemotherapy (as in the HERA trial) appears to produce a lower incidence of cardiac toxicity (severe congestive heart failure = 2% with trastuzumab). However, the definition of cardiac events in each trial was different. Concurrent administration of trastuzumab with an anthracycline is very controversial, potentially associated with higher rates of cardiac dysfunction (although not yet proven in this clinical setting), and should not be done outside the context of a clinical trial or an institution with extensive experience with this approach to trastuzumab dosing. Rare cases of interstitial pneumonitis were reported in the trastuzumab arm (nine patients) in the combined NSABP/NCCTG trial only. The causality of these events is unclear, but may be related to trastuzumab. Chemotherapy-related adverse effects are slightly more frequent with the addition of concurrent trastuzumab therapy, including neutropenia, infection and diarrhea, but these toxicities are easily managed and do not preclude the use of trastuzumab in patients with early stage breast cancer.

All of these adjuvant trials continued trastuzumab administration during adjuvant radiation therapy and hormonal therapy. The administration of trastuzumab during radiation therapy was evaluated in patients that participated in the N9831 clinical trial. Patients that received concurrent radiation therapy with adjuvant trastuzumab did not experience a significant increase in cardiac events or acute radiation-related adverse events with the exception of transient leukopenia.[121] Therefore, if radiation therapy is clinically indicated, trastuzumab is typically administered concomitantly with radiation.

CLINICAL CONTROVERSY

Trastuzumab clearly has improved the outcome for women with early-stage, *HER2*-positive breast cancer. However, the optimal trastuzumab-containing regimen remains unknown. Questions remain regarding optimal concurrent chemotherapy; optimal dose, schedule, and duration of trastuzumab therapy; and use of other concurrent therapeutic modalities. Many ongoing clinical trials hope to answer these questions. Also, while the addition of trastuzumab has improved DFS and OS, it is not effective for all women and issues regarding trastuzumab resistance are becoming more complex.

Many questions remain regarding the optimal use of trastuzumab in the adjuvant therapy of early stage breast cancer. The use of trastuzumab with chemotherapy in the adjuvant setting is now considered to be the standard of care for patients with node-positive and high-risk node negative *HER2*-positive breast cancer. A retrospective analysis of patients with tumors smaller than 1 cm demonstrated that patients with *HER2*-positive tumors have a lower recurrence free survival at 5 years as compared to patients with *HER2*-negative tumors (HR, 2.68; 95% CI, 1.44-5; *P* = 0.002).[122] Therefore, treatment with trastuzumab in patients with small, *HER2*-positive, node negative tumors may be considered. In the United States, only one study has analyzed the cost-effectiveness of adjuvant trastuzumab administration. Hillner estimated an incremental cost of about $50,000 per life-year gained based on data from the NCCTG/NSABP and HERA trials combined.[123] This figure is well below what has typically been considered acceptable for other therapeutic advances in the United States (e.g., dialysis, adjuvant chemotherapy for early-stage breast cancer), but borders on unacceptable for other countries with nationalized healthcare. While this type of discussion is far beyond the scope of this chapter, the reader is referred to the following reviews for further discussion regarding this topic.[124,125] Nonetheless, trastuzumab is a very effective, but costly, addition to adjuvant therapy, with apparent risks that should be discussed in detail with all patients with *HER2*-positive breast cancer prior to undergoing therapy. A similar approach has been used in the neoadjuvant treatment of *HER2*-positive breast cancer as well (see section on Locally Advanced Breast Cancer). Clinical trials involving other novel *HER2*-directed therapies, such as lapatinib, in the adjuvant and neoadjuvant settings are ongoing.

Adjuvant Endocrine Therapy ❹ Hormonal therapies that have been studied in the treatment of primary or early stage breast cancer include tamoxifen, toremifene, oophorectomy, ovarian irradiation, luteinizing hormone-releasing hormone (LHRH) agonists and aromatase inhibitors. Choice of agent(s) depends on menopausal status and is based on a multitude of clinical trials completed in this setting that establish different roles for different therapies.

Tamoxifen was traditionally the gold standard adjuvant hormonal therapy and has been used in the adjuvant setting for more than three decades. Tamoxifen is antiestrogenic in breast cancer cells, but it appears to have estrogenic properties in other tissues and organs.[126,127] More recent studies show that tamoxifen and other similar drugs have many estrogenic and antiestrogenic effects that depend on the tissue and the gene in question, and they are more appropriately called selective estrogen receptor modulators (SERMs). Women receiving adjuvant tamoxifen therapy have reduced risk of recurrence and mortality as compared with women not receiving adjuvant tamoxifen therapy.[5] This observation, coupled with evidence of tolerability for tamoxifen, including beneficial estrogenic effects on the lipid profile and bone density,

led to tamoxifen being the hormonal agent of choice for both pre- and postmenopausal women when compared with older, more toxic therapies (e.g., megestrol acetate). Premenopausal patients may derive equivalent benefit from ovarian ablation via surgery or administration of LHRH agonists when compared with tamoxifen.[5] In the United States, tamoxifen is generally considered the adjuvant hormonal therapy of choice for premenopausal women. However, many ongoing clinical trials are investigating the use of the LHRH agonists or oophorectomy instead of tamoxifen or in addition to tamoxifen or aromatase inhibitors in this group of women.

The optimal dose of tamoxifen is unclear. The EBCTCG overview showed that more (up to 40 mg/day) is not necessarily better for response rates.[5] Lower doses of tamoxifen (less than 20 mg/day) may be effective, but no clinical trials have addressed this question. Therefore the current recommended dose for tamoxifen in the adjuvant, metastatic, and preventive settings is 20 mg/day. Because tamoxifen has a long biologic half-life, it can be administered as a single daily dose. Adjuvant tamoxifen therapy is generally initiated shortly after surgery or as soon as pathology results are known and the decision to administer tamoxifen as adjuvant therapy is made.

When adjuvant tamoxifen is given with chemotherapy, it should be given after chemotherapy is completed. This recommendation is based on laboratory and clinical evidence from a phase III trial suggesting tamoxifen administered concurrently with chemotherapy may antagonize the beneficial effect of chemotherapy.[128] In the phase III clinical trial, administration of sequential tamoxifen resulted in a marginally superior DFS as compared to concurrent use of tamoxifen with chemotherapy (HR, 0.84; 95% CI, 0.70-1.01; *P* = 0.061).[128] Some clinicians also advocate the initiation of tamoxifen following completion of radiation therapy, but this subject is very controversial and few trials have addressed the issue of concurrent versus sequential hormone therapy and radiation therapy.

The optimal duration of tamoxifen therapy in the adjuvant setting is currently 5 years. Studies of prolonged administration (e.g., 10 years) have failed to demonstrate any advantage and in fact may be associated with a slightly worse survival.[129] Other clinical trials investigating durations of tamoxifen use longer than 5 years are ongoing.

The pharmacologic disposition of tamoxifen in humans is very complex and has only recently been elucidated (Fig. 136–6). Tamoxifen is now considered to be a prodrug. Although the parent compound has significant clinical activity, tamoxifen is metabolized through multiple enzymes including CYP3A4, CYP2C19, CYP2D6, and others to metabolites which appear to be more active than the parent compound.[130] The active metabolites 4-hydroxytamoxifen (4OH-TAM) and 4-hydroxy-N-desmethyltamoxifen (endoxifen) have nearly a 100-fold higher affinity for the estrogen receptor compared to tamoxifen. Endoxifen is present in the serum at a 6- to 12-fold higher concentration compared to 4OH-TAM, hence endoxifen is thought to be the most important metabolite for the clinical activity of tamoxifen. The formation of endoxifen is highly dependent on the enzymatic activity of CYP2D6. However, multiple other pathways may also be important for determining activity, including deactivation pathways (e.g., SULT-1-A1, UGT). Polymorphisms in CYP2D6 can lead to increased or decreased formation of endoxifen and may be related to improved or diminished clinical outcomes, respectively. Although there are clinical data to suggest that certain polymorphisms in CYP2D6 may result in poorer disease-free or relapse-free survival in patients receiving tamoxifen, these analyses are based mostly on retrospective analyses and contradictory studies also exist to refute these claims. Multiple commercially available assays for CYP2D6 are available, but widespread testing for patients receiving tamoxifen is not currently recommended based on available evidence.[47,88] Excellent reviews

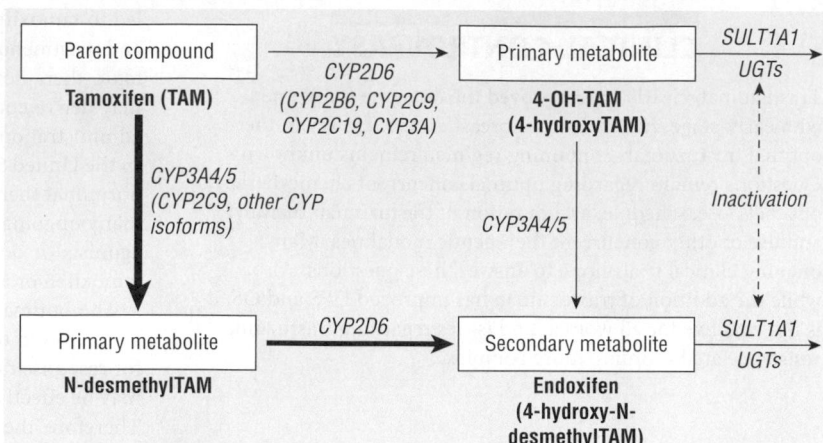

FIGURE 136-6. Tamoxifen metabolism.[131] Widths of the arrows approximate allocation of parent compound to various metabolites. See text for further explanation.

on this subject are available.[130] Potent inhibitors of CYP2D6, such as paroxetine and fluoxetine, may decrease levels of endoxifen in patients receiving tamoxifen.[131] The clinical outcomes related to such drug-drug interactions in an individual patient are largely unknown and depend on their underlying CYP2D6 genetic status (e.g., poor metabolizer, extensive metabolizer). However, common sense would dictate avoiding known strong inhibitors of CYP2D6, if possible, in patients receiving tamoxifen.

The most reliable information regarding the side effects of tamoxifen comes from the NSABP Breast Cancer Prevention Trial (P1).[55] This trial randomized 13,388 women 35 years of age or older who were at increased risk for breast cancer to placebo (n = 6,707) or to 20 mg/day of tamoxifen (n = 6,681) for 5 years. Although the primary finding of this study is that tamoxifen reduces the risk of invasive breast cancer by 49%, this study also provides an excellent opportunity to determine the risk of side effects associated with tamoxifen. Information was prospectively collected with regard to the occurrence of hot flashes, vaginal discharge, irregular menses, fluid retention, nausea, skin changes, diarrhea, and weight gain or loss. The self-administered depression scale and a global quality-of-life and a sexual function scale were administered at each follow-up visit. The only symptomatic differences noted between the placebo and tamoxifen group were related to hot flashes and vaginal discharge, both of which occurred more often in the tamoxifen group. No important differences between the two groups were observed in the various self-reporting instruments. Tamoxifen did not increase the risk of ischemic heart disease, but reduced the risk of hip radius and spine fractures. Of note, the rates of stroke, pulmonary embolism, and deep vein thrombosis were elevated in the tamoxifen group (stroke: RR, 1.59; pulmonary embolism: RR, 3.01; and deep vein thrombosis: RR, 1.60), particularly in women age 50 years or older. The rate of endometrial cancer was increased in the tamoxifen group (RR, 2.53), and this increased risk occurred predominantly in women age 50 years or older. The increased risk of endometrial carcinoma is similar in magnitude to that associated with postmenopausal estrogen replacement therapy and is likely a consequence of an estrogenic effect of tamoxifen on the endometrium. Some experts argue that this risk is acceptable because the endometrial cancer induced by tamoxifen is low stage, low grade, and easily treated with surgery or other means and does not pose a life-threatening risk to women. Tamoxifen was also associated with an increased risk of uterine sarcomas (a more aggressive form of endometrial cancer), but this risk appears to be lower than the more common endometrial cancers identified in the NSABP P-1 study.[132] Routine endometrial biopsy is not currently recommended for women receiving tamoxifen therapy. However, women receiving tamoxifen therapy

should be counseled to have regular gynecologic examinations and immediately report unusual vaginal bleeding to their primary clinicians for further evaluation.

Toremifene is another marketed antiestrogen whose primary advantage is a lower estrogenic-to-antiestrogenic ratio as compared to tamoxifen (based on laboratory data).[133] Toremifene (60 mg orally daily) has been found to have efficacy similar to that of tamoxifen in metastatic disease and a generally similar side-effect profile.[134] Toremifene is currently indicated as an alternative to tamoxifen in patients with metastatic breast cancer, but studies are ongoing to evaluate its safety and efficacy in the adjuvant setting. Preliminary results from these trials indicate similar efficacy and safety, with possibly inferior bone protection with toremifene.[135,136] However, further follow-up is required to determine the long-term effects of toremifene in the adjuvant setting.

In premenopausal women, the use of LHRH-agonists or other means of ovarian ablation provides benefit in the adjuvant setting. In the EBCTCG overview analysis published in 2005, the overall benefit of ovarian ablation or suppression was significant compared with no treatment, but smaller than previously reported in 1996 (reduction in annual odds of recurrence = 25% ± 12% in women <40 years old and 29% ± 6% in women 40–49 years old).[5] Many of the ongoing trials with the LHRH agonists were not yet included in this analysis and most of the clinical trials analyzed included patients with hormone receptor-positive, -negative, and unknown status. In an update of this analysis, study inclusion was restricted to patients treated with ovarian suppression with LHRH agonists (not ovarian oblation or oophorectomy) and those patients with tumors known to be hormone receptor-positive.[137] The addition of a LHRH agonist reduced the rates of recurrence by 25%, deaths after recurrence by 28%, and all deaths by 27% in women younger than 40 years; no significant reductions in recurrence or death were noted in patient older than 40 years. Also, a similar benefit was observed with goserelin as compared with CMF chemotherapy in hormone-sensitive premenopausal breast cancer patients, but not in patients with hormone receptor-negative tumors.[137] It is not clear whether the benefit of chemotherapy in this population is a result of the actual effects of chemotherapy or a result of the endocrine effects of chemotherapy-induced menopause. Consequently, some studies have investigated the benefits of adding ovarian ablation or suppression to chemotherapy, either with or without tamoxifen. Results from these studies clearly indicate a benefit from ceasing menses, regardless of whether this is caused by chemotherapy or ovarian ablation or suppression.[137] It is not clear whether the addition of an LHRH agonist to tamoxifen is advantageous in women with hormone receptor-positive tumors who continue to menstruate after chemotherapy. The optimal duration of adjuvant

LHRH agonist use is unknown, with trials ranging from 18 months to 5 years of treatment. Multiple ongoing trials are attempting to answer this question; these trials include an LHRH agonist alone, with tamoxifen or with an aromatase inhibitor. Currently, the only trial with available results is a study by the Austrian Breast and Colorectal Cancer Study Group (ABCSG-12) which randomized premenopausal patients with hormone receptor-positive early stage breast cancer to 3 years of tamoxifen or anastrozole, both concomitantly with goserelin for ovarian suppression.[138] After a median follow-up of 48 months, there was no significant difference in DFS between the two groups. However, a tamoxifen-only arm was not included in this trial.

In postmenopausal women, aromatase inhibitors (AI) are gradually replacing tamoxifen in the adjuvant setting. Four different approaches to therapy have been undertaken with these new agents: (a) direct comparison with tamoxifen for adjuvant hormonal therapy, (b) sequential use after 5 years of adjuvant tamoxifen therapy, (c) sequential use after 2 to 3 years of adjuvant tamoxifen, and (d) 2 years of treatment with an AI followed by 3 years of adjuvant tamoxifen. Anastrozole and letrozole have been directly compared with tamoxifen as initial therapy in postmenopausal women with hormone receptor-positive, early stage breast cancer (ATAC [Arimidex, Tamoxifen, Alone or in Combination] Trial and BIG [Breast International Group] 1–98 Trial).[139,140] These comparisons show an advantage with the aromatase inhibitors over tamoxifen in terms of DFS. Other approaches to adjuvant hormonal therapy with AIs include sequential use of newer agents after either 5 years or 2 to 3 years of tamoxifen. In the MA-17 study, 5 additional years of letrozole was compared with placebo in postmenopausal breast cancer patients who had completed 5 years of tamoxifen therapy.[141] After a median follow-up of 2.4 years, letrozole was associated with superior estimated 4-year DFS as compared with placebo (93% vs 87%; P <0.001). Because of this difference, patients were unblinded and allowed to crossover to the active arm of therapy. In a pooled analysis of trials investigating a switch to an AI, 9,015 patients who had completed 2 to 3 years of adjuvant tamoxifen therapy were randomized to continue tamoxifen or crossover to anastrozole or exemestane for the remainder of 5 years.[142] The results of this analysis show a decreased risk of recurrence at 6 years following randomization in patients who switched to an AI as compared to those who continued with tamoxifen alone (12.6% vs 16.0%; P <0.00001). The BIG 1–98 trial which compared letrozole with tamoxifen also included two separate arms which investigated the value of switching from tamoxifen to an AI or vice versa. With 71 months of follow-up, the sequential arms did not improve estimated 5-year DFS compared to letrozole alone in either comparison.[143] Clinical trials are also investigating longer durations of AI use to assess the benefits and harms of continued estrogen deprivation, the results of which are greatly anticipated.

Most national and international guidelines currently recommend incorporation of an AI into the adjuvant hormonal therapy regimen for all postmenopausal, hormone-sensitive breast cancers.[47] The current NCCN guidelines for breast cancer management state that any of the following are acceptable endocrine therapy regimens for these women: (a) an AI for 5 years (or longer, based on expert opinion); (b) tamoxifen for 2 to 3 years followed by an AI for a total of 5 years of endocrine therapy; or (c) tamoxifen for 5 years followed by an AI for another 5 years (total of 10 years of endocrine therapy).[47] The NCCN panel believes that the three available AIs (anastrozole, letrozole, and exemestane) have similar antitumor efficacy and toxicity profiles and many other clinicians agree. Therefore, the optimal hormonal therapy regimen in the adjuvant setting has yet to be determined, and results from ongoing trials are eagerly awaited to more clearly define a treatment strategy for women facing this clinical dilemma.

AIs are generally well tolerated. Adverse effects include bone loss/osteoporosis, hot flashes, myalgia/arthralgia, vaginal dryness/atrophy, mild headaches, and diarrhea. Although concerns surrounding loss of bone density and an increased risk of osteoporosis are evident in these adjuvant trials, the overall impact on quality-of-life and long-term survival are still being evaluated. Bisphosphonates are coadministered with the AI in many patients in the metastatic setting and may also be beneficial in the adjuvant setting. Other adverse events that are worrisome include questionable effects on the cardiovascular system (e.g., hypercholesterolemia), cognitive functioning and joint health. Longer follow-up from these trials will continue to provide valuable information to guide treatment decisions and side-effect management.

CLINICAL CONTROVERSY

The optimal use of antiaromatase agents in the adjuvant setting for postmenopausal women with hormone receptor-positive tumors is controversial. Multiple studies have been published with results indicating a benefit to regimens that include an aromatase inhibitor as initial therapy or after tamoxifen. However, many questions remain as to the optimal drug, dose, sequence, and duration of therapy for these agents.

In summary, tamoxifen has been used in the adjuvant setting for nearly 30 years and has a very well-defined safety and efficacy profile in this setting. Although it is difficult to define the role of new therapies given the lengthy history of tamoxifen, the role of tamoxifen in the adjuvant setting is changing with the incorporation of newer agents either concurrently (e.g., LHRH agonists) or sequentially (e.g., AIs).

■ LOCALLY ADVANCED BREAST CANCER (STAGE III)

❺ *Locally advanced breast cancer* generally refers to breast carcinomas with significant primary tumor and nodal disease, but in which distant metastases cannot be documented. A wide variety of clinical scenarios can be seen within this group of patients, including neglected tumors that have spread locally, to inflammatory breast cancers that are a unique clinical entity. Inflammatory breast cancer is associated with similar clinical findings as compared to other neglected, locally advanced breast tumors (e.g., erythema representing skin involvement). The distinction between the two diagnoses lies in the rapidity of onset of symptoms. Many locally advanced breast cancers are diagnosed in patients who have had symptoms for months to years and have neglected to seek medical attention. Although these women have a poor prognosis because of the delay in diagnosis, they are not classified as inflammatory breast cancer. The hallmark of inflammatory breast cancers is the rapid onset of symptoms within weeks to months, including erythema of the skin with or without a detectable underlying breast mass. These patients are often inappropriately treated for cellulitis with antibiotics for several weeks to months. Because of the aggressive nature of this disease, a delay in diagnosis can be fatal for some of these women.

The natural history of locally advanced breast cancer shows that even when local-regional control is accomplished, systemic relapse and death from breast cancer eventually occur in most patients if systemic therapy is not utilized.[144] That observation led to interest in the use of neoadjuvant or primary chemotherapy in locally advanced breast cancer, which renders inoperable tumors resectable, and can increase rates of BCT. Other potential benefits related to early initiation of systemic therapy include delivery of drugs through an intact vasculature, in vivo assessment of response to therapy, and the opportunity to study the biologic effects of the systemic treatment. However, this approach to therapy also results in a loss of standard, well-validated pathologic prognostic markers, such as initial tumor size (measured by pathologic examination) and the number of axillary lymph nodes involved. Also, as discussed earlier, OS with adjuvant as compared with neoadjuvant chemotherapy is similar. However, in light of other benefits gained with neoadjuvant therapy, these two factors may not be enough to continue to drive the practice of primary surgery. The topic of adjuvant versus neoadjuvant systemic therapy is fraught with controversy, but the many advantages of neoadjuvant, primary systemic therapy are continuing to drive an increase in the number of operable patients offered this treatment modality.[145] For patients with inoperable breast cancer, including inflammatory breast cancer, the initial approach to therapy should be chemotherapy with the goal of achieving resectability. The NCCN guidelines addressing the management of locally advanced disease recommend primary chemotherapy with an anthracycline-containing regimen with or without a taxane.[47]

After neoadjuvant chemotherapy, most tumors respond with more than a 50% decrease in tumor size; approximately 70% of patients experience a reduction in their stage of disease. The chemotherapy regimens used in this setting are similar to those used in the adjuvant setting, but the regimens usually include an anthracycline, incorporate a taxane in some manner, and may have higher dose density or dose intensity. For patients with *HER2*-positive tumors, the incorporation of trastuzumab with chemotherapy is appropriate.[146] For more detailed information regarding the specific regimen-related information, the reader is referred to the referenced review.[147] Neoadjuvant endocrine therapy may be an option for patients who have unresectable hormone receptor-positive tumors who are unable to receive chemotherapy (e.g., multiple comorbid conditions).[148]

Local therapy usually follows chemotherapy, and the extent of surgery is determined by response to chemotherapy, the wishes of the patient, and the cosmetic results likely to be achieved. However, many patients may be able to have BCT if an acceptable response to chemotherapy is achieved. Adjuvant radiation therapy should be administered to all locally advanced breast cancer patients to minimize local recurrences, regardless of the type of surgery used for that individual patient (e.g., mastectomy or segmental mastectomy). Inoperable tumors that are unresponsive to systemic chemotherapy may require radiation therapy for local management and may not be eligible for surgical resection after radiation. These patients are not commonly seen, but have a very poor prognosis. For most patients in this category, cure is still the primary goal of therapy and can be achieved in a large number of patients when all treatment modalities are employed.

■ METASTATIC BREAST CANCER (STAGE IV)

❻ The goal of therapy with early and locally advanced breast cancer is to cure the disease. After it has advanced beyond local–regional disease, breast cancer is currently incurable. However, some patients live for many years with metastatic disease, making this a chronic disease requiring long-term management strategies that incorporate improvements and/or maintenance of quality of life. The goals of treatment of metastatic breast cancer are to improve symptoms and quality-of-life and extend survival. Thus it is important to choose therapy with optimal activity while minimizing toxicities. Treatment of metastatic breast cancer with cytotoxic, biologic, or endocrine therapy often results in regression of disease and improvements in quality-of-life. In patients who respond to therapy, duration of survival is also increased. The choice of therapy for metastatic disease is based on the site of disease involvement and

presence or absence of certain characteristics. The most important factor predicting response to endocrine therapy is the presence of estrogen and progesterone receptors in the primary tumor tissue. Fifty percent to 60% of patients with ER-positive tumors and 75% to 80% of patients with ER- and PR-positive tumors will respond to hormonal therapy, whereas those with ER- and PR-negative tumors have a less than 10% response rate. Thus the most important factor determining choice of endocrine versus cytotoxic chemotherapy is the presence of hormone receptors in the primary breast tumor. Site of disease is also important because endocrine therapy is more likely to be effective in patients with bone and soft-tissue metastases. Patients with asymptomatic visceral involvement (e.g., liver or lung) may be candidates for hormonal therapy, depending on the clinical circumstance (hormones usually work more slowly than chemotherapy). Patients with symptomatic visceral and/or central nervous system involvement generally have more rapidly growing cancers that require chemotherapy. Endocrine therapy is the treatment of choice for patients with hormone receptor-positive tumors who exhibit the first sign of metastatic disease in soft tissue, bone, or pleura, because of the equal probability of response to hormonal therapy as compared to chemotherapy, and a preferable toxicity profile with endocrine therapy.

❼ Patients who respond to initial endocrine therapy often respond to a second (or even third) hormonal manipulation. But the response rate is lower and duration of response is shorter with second (and third) hormonal manipulations. Patients are sequentially treated with endocrine therapy until their tumors cease to respond or the patient ceases to benefit from endocrine therapy, at which time cytotoxic chemotherapy can be administered. Concurrent administration of different hormonal therapies or chemotherapy plus hormones is generally not used in the setting of metastatic breast cancer because of lack of increased efficacy and evidence of increased toxicity. Women with hormone receptor-negative tumors, with rapidly progressive or symptomatic lung, liver, or bone marrow involvement, and those with progressive disease while on initial endocrine therapy are usually treated initially with cytotoxic chemotherapy. Patients with tumors that have *HER2* protein overexpression or gene amplification should be considered for treatment with *HER2*-targeted therapy alone or with chemotherapy or endocrine therapy. All breast cancer patients with metastases to the bone should be considered for treatment with an intravenous bisphosphonate (e.g., pamidronate or zoledronic acid) as these agents have been shown to decrease the rates of skeletal-related events (SREs) such as fractures, spinal cord compression, pain, and/or the need for radiation to the bones or surgery.[149] These agents do not act as anticancer agents and should be coadministered with chemotherapy, endocrine therapy and/or *HER2*-targeted therapy.

Endocrine Therapy

❻ The pharmacologic goal of endocrine therapy for breast cancer is to either (a) decrease circulating levels of estrogen or (b) prevent the effects of estrogen at the breast cancer cell (targeted therapy) by blocking the hormone receptors or downregulating the presence of those receptors. Achievement of the first goal depends on the menopausal status of the patient, but achievement of the second goal is independent of menopausal status. Many endocrine therapies are available to target either goal of therapy, and combinations of drugs with different mechanisms of action have also been investigated. Unfortunately, most combinations have not demonstrated any efficacy benefits over single-agent hormone therapy, but have increased toxicity. Therefore, combinations of endocrine agents for breast cancer are generally not recommended outside the context of a clinical trial. One exception to this statement is the combination of LHRH agonist with an AI or SERM (as discussed below). Sequential

TABLE 136-12 Endocrine Therapies Used for Metastatic Breast Cancer

Class	Drug	Dose	Side Effects
Aromatase inhibitors			
Nonsteroidal	Anastrozole	1 mg orally daily	Hot flashes, bone loss/osteoporosis, arthralgias, myalgias, headaches, diarrhea,
	Letrozole	2.5 mg orally daily	mild nausea
Steroidal	Exemestane	25 mg orally daily	
Antiestrogens			
SERMs	Tamoxifen	20 mg orally daily	Hot flashes, vaginal discharge, mild nausea, thromboembolism, endometrial
	Toremifene	60 mg orally daily	hyperplasia/cancer
SERDs	Fulvestrant	250 mg IM every 28 days	Hot flashes, injection site reactions, possibly thromboembolism
LHRH analogs	Goserelin	3.6 mg SC every 28 days	Hot flashes, amenorrhea, menopausal symptoms, injection site reactions
	Leuprolide	3.75 mg IM every 28 days	(extended formulations of more than 28 days are not recommended for
	Triptorelin	3.75 mg IM every 28 days	the treatment of breast cancer)
Progestins	Megestrol acetate	40 mg orally 4 times a day	Weight gain, hot flashes, vaginal bleeding, edema, thromboembolism
	Medroxyprogesterone	400–1,000 mg IM every week	
Androgens	Fluoxymesterone	10 mg orally twice a day	Deepening voice, alopecia, hirsutism, facial/truncal acne, fluid retention,
			menstrual irregularities, cholestatic jaundice
Estrogens	Diethylstilbestrol	5 mg orally 3 times a day	Nausea/vomiting, fluid retention, anorexia, thromboembolism, hepatic
	Ethinyl estradiol	1 mg orally 3 times a day	dysfunction, myocardial infarction
	Conjugated estrogens	2.5 mg orally 3 times a day	

LHRH, luteinizing hormone-releasing hormone; SC, subcutaneous; SERD, selective estrogen receptor downregulator SERM, selective estrogen receptor modulator.

use of endocrine agents is now becoming popular in the adjuvant setting and may play a role in the metastatic setting when a patient is progressing on one agent after an initial response. These patients are often treated with a series of endocrine agents, usually over several years, before chemotherapy is considered.

Until recently, there was little evidence that the response or survival benefit from one endocrine therapy was clearly superior to that achieved with other therapies. Randomized controlled trials showed that antiestrogens, progestins, aminoglutethimide, estrogens, and androgens; and surgical procedures including oophorectomy, adrenalectomy, and hypophysectomy were equivalent in patients with metastatic breast cancer. Consequently, the choice of a particular endocrine therapy was based primarily on toxicity and patient preference (Table 136–12). Based on these criteria, tamoxifen was the preferred initial agent when metastases were present, except when the patient received adjuvant tamoxifen at the same time or within 1 year of occurrence of metastatic disease. In these cases, other agents were generally employed.

Over the past decade, results of clinical trials of third-generation AIs have changed the treatment of metastatic breast cancer, as well as of early-stage breast cancer (as was noted previously). In postmenopausal and castrated women, the main source of estrogen is derived from the peripheral conversion of androstenedione, produced by the adrenal gland, into estrone and estradiol. This conversion requires the enzyme aromatase. Aromatase also catalyzes the conversion of androgens to estrogens in the ovary in premenopausal women and in extraglandular tissue, including the breast and breast cancer cells, in postmenopausal women. Therefore, AIs effectively reduce the levels of circulating estrogens and estrogens in the target organ. Aminoglutethimide was the prototype aromatase inhibitor, but was a nonspecific, weak enzyme inhibitor associated with many toxicities and is no longer available in the United States. Several analogs and derivatives of aminoglutethimide, as well as novel endocrine compounds, have been tested over the years to try and improve on the therapeutic ratio of this agent. Third-generation AIs now available include anastrozole, letrozole, and exemestane. These agents have far greater selectivity and higher potency for the aromatase enzyme than aminoglutethimide. A major advantage of these newer compounds is their preferable toxicity profile, which consists mainly of bone loss/osteoporosis, mild nausea, hot flashes, arthralgias/myalgias, and mild fatigue. Anastrozole and letrozole are nonsteroidal compounds that exhibit reversible, competitive inhibition of aromatase. These are triazole compounds and have no intrinsic hormonal activity. Exemestane is a steroidal compound which binds irreversibly to aromatase, forming a covalent bond. While this mechanism may have theoretical advantages to the reversible binding seen with the nonsteroidal agents, there is no clinical evidence that this drug is superior to other agents in this class. Exemestane does possess some androgenic properties at doses that are much higher than those used clinically and may have some unique toxicities in some patients.

These third-generation AIs have been compared with megestrol acetate (MA) as second-line therapy in postmenopausal women with positive or unknown hormone receptor status who have progressed while on tamoxifen therapy. Although response rates with these agents have not been significantly better time-to-progression, and OS are significantly better than MA with at least two of the three AIs (anastrozole and exemestane).[150] Rates of clinical benefit (objective response + stabilization of disease for 24 weeks) are also improved with the AIs. Clinical benefit, a category of response used in metastatic breast cancer clinical trials, is another clinically relevant endpoint because it is associated with similar OS compared with patients who have objective responses.[151] Tolerability is also improved with the AIs as compared with MA. Toxicity patterns showed more nausea, vomiting, and hot flashes with the AI and more weight gain, fluid retention, and thromboembolism with MA. All three agents are approved for second-line therapy of advanced breast cancer in postmenopausal women, and have largely replaced MA for second-line therapy.

Both anastrozole and letrozole are also approved for first-line therapy of advanced breast cancer in postmenopausal women. Large randomized trials have compared these agents to tamoxifen and found similar response rates and a longer median time to progression for patients receiving the selective AI.[150] A consistent finding in these trials was a lower incidence of thromboembolic events and vaginal bleeding in patients who received selective AIs. Based on these results, many experts have concluded that the new AIs are superior to tamoxifen as first-line therapy for advanced breast cancer in postmenopausal women. Although not FDA approved for this indication, exemestane has been compared with tamoxifen as front-line therapy for hormone-sensitive metastatic breast cancer. In one, large randomized phase III trial, exemestane demonstrated a modest advantage over tamoxifen in terms of progression-free survival (PFS) (9.9 vs 5.8 months; $P = 0.121$).[152] While this difference failed to reach statistical significance, the numerical difference is quite large confirming the advantage of exemestane as first-line therapy for metastatic breast cancer. Use of a steroidal aromatase inhibitor (exemestane) after a patient progresses on a nonsteroidal inhibitor (anastrozole or letrozole) may provide some benefit and is a common practice based on limited data. The opposite sequence also has shown some benefit; thus patients may receive two AIs (first line and second line, sequentially), especially those patients who progress while on adjuvant tamoxifen therapy.

The AIs should only be used in postmenopausal women. Pre- or perimenopausal women, whose ovaries are functioning, are inappropriate candidates for these therapies, at least based on the available evidence. Use of the AIs in addition to ovarian ablation (e.g., oophorectomy or LHRH agonists) is under investigation. Interestingly, the use of AIs in men with advanced breast cancer is controversial due to concerns that the pituitary feedback loop may be activated, increasing the levels of FSH, LH, and possibly testosterone. Therefore, while objective responses are seen with single-agent AI therapy in men with breast cancer, consensus has yet to be reached regarding the clinical utility of these agents in men and some clinicians are investigating the combination of an LHRH agonist with an AI in this population.[153] Until further clinical trials are completed, the efficacy and safety of this treatment approach are unknown.

Antiestrogens bind to estrogen receptors, which inhibit receptor-mediated gene transcription and therefore block the effect of estrogen on the end target. This class of agents is now subdivided into two pharmacologic categories, SERMs and pure antiestrogens. SERMs include tamoxifen and toremifene (and raloxifene for breast cancer risk reduction in high-risk women) and demonstrate tissue-specific activity, both estrogenic and antiestrogenic, as described previously. The agonistic activity is thought to be responsible for many of the adverse reactions seen with these agents, including the increased risk of endometrial cancer, and has led to the development of pure estrogen receptor antagonists that lack estrogen agonist activity. Pure antiestrogens are a new class of agents and are also referred to as selective estrogen receptor downregulators (SERDs). These molecules bind to the ER, inhibit estrogen binding, and degrade the drug-ER complex, thus decreasing the amount of ER on the tumor cell surface. Fulvestrant is currently the only pure antiestrogen commercially available in the United States.

Tamoxifen is generally considered to be the antiestrogen of choice in premenopausal women with metastatic breast cancer who have hormone receptor-positive tumors. Tamoxifen is usually administered in 20 mg once-daily doses. A tamoxifen dose of 20 mg/day reaches a steady-state concentration after about 4 months of therapy. The half-life of tamoxifen during chronic dosing is 7 days. Serum tamoxifen concentrations can be detected 6 weeks after discontinuation of therapy. Thus the maximum beneficial effects of tamoxifen are not observed for at least 2 months following initiation of therapy, and it is unlikely that symptoms of metastatic disease will return, even if patients miss several doses. The toxicities of tamoxifen are described in the Adjuvant Endocrine Therapy section above. The only additional toxicity that may be observed in the setting of metastatic breast cancer (specifically bone metastases) is a tumor flare and/or hypercalcemia, which occurs in approximately 5% of patients following the initiation of any SERM therapy and is not an indication to discontinue SERM therapy. It is generally accepted that this reaction is associated with response to endocrine therapy, but patients who do not experience such a reaction may still respond. This reaction is seen less frequently with the concurrent use of bisphosphonates as a result of

their inhibition of osteoclasts, subsequently preventing the release of calcium from the bone.

Toremifene is another commercially available SERM for the treatment of breast cancer. It exhibits similar efficacy and tolerability compared with tamoxifen in the metastatic setting and is given at a dose of 60 mg daily. The same issues apply to toremifene as were discussed with tamoxifen. Cross-resistance to toremifene has been demonstrated in patients with tamoxifen-refractory disease.[154] Thus at the current time, toremifene appears to be an alternative to tamoxifen in postmenopausal patients with positive or unknown hormone receptor status with metastatic breast cancer. Raloxifene, another SERM, received approval in December 1997 for prevention of osteoporosis in postmenopausal women. Available data with raloxifene as a treatment for breast cancer show very low response rates and no clinical benefit. Consequently, use of this agent for breast cancer treatment should be discouraged. Investigation into the use of raloxifene for breast cancer risk reduction in high-risk women has recently been reported (see Prevention and Early Detection).

Fulvestrant is approved for the second-line therapy of postmenopausal metastatic breast cancer patients with hormone receptor-positive tumors. It is given as an intramuscular injection every 28 days and is marketed as a single injection of 5 mL. Studies have compared this agent to anastrozole, exemestane and tamoxifen in the treatment of postmenopausal women with metastatic breast cancer. Biologically, fulvestrant should produce similar outcomes in premenopausal women, but no data exist to confirm the safety or efficacy in premenopausal women. In the comparative trials with fulvestrant and an AI (anastrozole or exemestane), similar efficacy and safety were demonstrated with both agents when given after patients progressed on tamoxifen therapy.[155] When compared directly with tamoxifen, time-to-progression was slightly shorter in the fulvestrant arm but the difference did not reach statistical significance.[155] That trial failed to confirm statistical noninferiority, which indicates that the trial could not show that fulvestrant was equivalent to tamoxifen. Adverse events related to fulvestrant include injection-site reactions, hot flashes, asthenia, and headaches. The FDA-approved dose of fulvestrant is 250 mg given intramuscularly every 28 days. This agent is covered by Medicare and is a good option for patients who are unable to take an oral medication. Other dosing strategies have been investigated and appear to be safe and effective. The optimal dose of fulvestrant is widely debated and many strategies exist. Often reimbursement or insurance coverage dictates which dose is used.

Another goal of hormonal therapy in premenopausal women is to reduce estrogen production with surgery, irradiation, or medication. No difference in the overall response rate has been found in two randomized trials of tamoxifen and oophorectomy in premenopausal women. However, the secondary response rate to oophorectomy after tamoxifen treatment was somewhat higher than the response to tamoxifen after primary oophorectomy (33% vs 11%).[156,157] Based on this finding, some experts suggest that tamoxifen does not completely antagonize available estrogen, particularly in premenopausal women. Ovarian ablation (surgically or chemically) is still commonly used in some parts of the United States and is considered by many specialists to be the endocrine therapy of choice in premenopausal women. The mortality rate with surgical oophorectomy is low, usually less than 3% in appropriately selected patients. Irradiation of the ovaries was a means of castration many years ago, but was associated with multiple complications and is no longer performed for these purposes. Chemical castration with LHRH analogs is increasingly used instead of oophorectomy in premenopausal women.

Medical castration with LHRH analogs induce remission in about one third of unselected premenopausal metastatic breast cancer cases. The mechanism of action of LHRH analogs in breast cancer is downregulation of LHRH receptors in the pituitary. Decreased levels of luteinizing hormone subsequently lead to a decrease in estrogen to castrated levels. Thus the effect of LHRH analogs on circulating estrogen levels in premenopausal breast cancer simulates oophorectomy. The three agents available and utilized in the United States are leuprolide, goserelin, and triptorelin, but only goserelin is approved for the treatment of metastatic breast cancer. These agents are administered as an injection every 4 weeks (all products have extended formulations, lasting 3 months to 1 year, but they are not recommended for the treatment of breast cancer) and are associated with minimal side effects including amenorrhea, bone loss/osteoporosis, hot flashes, and occasional nausea (Table 136–12). LHRH agonists may also produce a flare response because of an initial surge in luteinizing hormone and estrogen production for the first 2 to 4 weeks of LHRH agonist administration. This flare response is similar to that seen with tamoxifen and patients with high volume disease should be monitored for increasing pain and/or hypercalcemia during the initiation period. A meta-analysis was conducted of several trials that combined tamoxifen and LHRH agonists versus LHRH agonists alone in premenopausal patients with metastatic breast cancer.[158] With a median follow-up of 6.8 years, there was a significant survival benefit and PFS benefit in favor of the combined treatment. The overall response rate was significantly higher with combined endocrine treatment. However, this analysis did not compare tamoxifen alone to the combination of an LHRH agonist with tamoxifen. Therefore if an LHRH agonist is used as first-line therapy for metastatic breast cancer, it should be used in combination with tamoxifen. But if tamoxifen is used as first-line therapy for metastatic breast cancer, the addition of a LHRH agonist is controversial because of the lack of clinical data to support any additional benefit.

Progestins such as MA and medroxyprogesterone acetate have been compared with tamoxifen in randomized trials and have been found to yield equivalent response rates. Medroxyprogesterone acetate is more frequently used in Europe, while MA is more frequently used in the United States. Based on efficacy and tolerability, these agents are generally reserved as third-line therapy after patients have failed an AI and an antiestrogen (tamoxifen, toremifene, or fulvestrant). The most common dose used for megestrol acetate is 160 mg/day. The most common side effect is weight gain, occurring in 20% to 50% of patients. Patients experiencing weight gain may also have fluid retention, but fluid retention is not totally responsible for the weight gain. In cachectic cancer patients, the weight gain may be desirable, but this is not uniformly true of all patients with metastatic breast cancer. Other side effects associated with progestins include vaginal bleeding in 5% to 10% of patients either while taking the progestational agent or when it is discontinued, and less than a 10% incidence of hot flashes. Thromboembolic complications are also associated with these agents.

High-dose estrogens and androgens are rarely used today because of their side effect profile and the availability of better tolerated alternatives (e.g., AIs). About one third of patients placed on high-dose estrogens will discontinue them because of side effects, the most important of which are thromboembolic events, vomiting, and fluid retention. Less common side effects include areolar hyperpigmentation, breast tenderness and engorgement, vaginal discharge, incontinence, hot flashes, and phlebitis. All the effective androgens cause masculinizing effects, including hirsutism and acne, in more than 50% of patients. The mechanism by which these agents exert a therapeutic effect in breast cancer is unknown. However, these agents may inhibit aromatase among other pharmacologic effects that antagonize estrogen. Approximately 20% response rates were reported in clinical trials conducted in the 1960s and 1970s in unselected groups of breast cancer patients treated with androgens.

Cytotoxic Therapy

❽ Cytotoxic chemotherapy is eventually required in most patients with metastatic breast cancer. Patients with hormone receptor-negative tumors require chemotherapy as initial therapy of metastases. Patients with hormone-sensitive tumors who initially respond to hormonal manipulations eventually cease to respond and go on to require chemotherapy. Combination chemotherapy results in an objective response in approximately 60% of patients previously unexposed to chemotherapy. Most patients have partial responses, and complete disappearance of disease occurs in fewer than 10% of patients treated. The median duration of response is 5 to 12 months, but some patients will have an excellent response to an initial course of chemotherapy and may live 5 to 10 years or longer without evidence of disease. Median survival of patients after treatment with commonly used drug combinations for metastatic breast cancer ranges between 14 and 33 months. The median time to response ranges from 2 to 3 months in most studies, but this period depends on the site of measurable disease and can range from 3 weeks (skin and lymph node metastases) to 18 weeks (bone metastases). Once a chemotherapy regimen has been initiated, it is usually continued until there is unequivocal evidence of progressive disease or intolerable side effects. Table 136–13 lists some selected chemotherapy agents employed in the metastatic setting.

Factors associated with an increased likelihood of response include a good performance status, a limited number (one to two) of disease sites (or involved organ systems), and a prolonged previous response to chemotherapy or hormonal therapy (i.e., long disease-free interval). Patients who have progressive disease during chemotherapy have a lower likelihood of response to a different type of chemotherapy. However, this is not necessarily true for patients who are given chemotherapy after some interval during which they have received no chemotherapy. Patients may actually be retreated with a regimen they received earlier if some time has passed since receiving the similar drugs (e.g., several years), but this is rarely done because of the large number of agents now available to treat breast cancer. Patients who do not respond to endocrine therapy are as likely to respond to chemotherapy as patients who are treated with chemotherapy as their initial treatment modality. Age, menopausal status, and receptor status do not appear to be directly associated with response to chemotherapy. There continues to be much debate surrounding the potential association between hormone receptor status and response to chemotherapy (e.g., ER status and anthracyclines).

A number of chemotherapeutic agents have demonstrated activity in the treatment of breast cancer, including doxorubicin, epirubicin, paclitaxel (conventional and protein bound), docetaxel, capecitabine, fluorouracil, cyclophosphamide, methotrexate, vinblastine, vinorelbine, gemcitabine, mitoxantrone, mitomycin-C, thiotepa, and melphalan. The most active classes of chemotherapy in metastatic breast cancer are the anthracyclines and the taxanes, producing response rates as high as 50% to 60% in patients who have not received prior chemotherapy for metastatic disease.[159] Paclitaxel was FDA approved in 1994 for single-agent treatment of metastatic breast cancer for patients who had relapsed following therapy with a doxorubicin-containing regimen. Weekly administration of paclitaxel results in higher response rates, time-to-progression, and survival in addition to a more favorable side-effect profile as compared with every 3-week administration.[160] The most useful weekly dose in the metastatic setting appears to be 80 mg/m²/week with no breaks in therapy. With this approach, the toxicity profile of paclitaxel changes with less myelosuppression and delayed onset of peripheral

TABLE 136-13 Selected Chemotherapy Regimens for Metastatic Breast Cancer

Single-Agent Chemotherapy

Paclitaxel[a,b]

Paclitaxel 175 mg/m^2 IV over 3 hours
Repeat cycles every 21 days
or
Paclitaxel 80 mg/m^2/week IV over 1 hour
Repeat dose every 7 days

Vinorelbine[c]

Vinorelbine 30 mg/m^2 IV, days 1 and 8
Repeat cycles every 21 days
or
Vinorelbine 25–30 mg/m^2/week IV
Repeat cycles every 7 days (adjust dose based on absolute neutrophil count; see product information)

Docetaxel[d,e]

Docetaxel 60–100 mg/m^2 IV over 1 hour
Repeat cycles every 21 days
or
Docetaxel 30–35 mg/m^2/week IV over 30 minutes
Repeat dose every 7 days

Gemcitabine[f]

Gemcitabine 600–1,000 mg/m^2/week IV, days 1, 8, and 15
Repeat cycles every 28 days (may need to hold day 15 dose based on blood counts)[g]

Protein-bound Paclitaxel[g,h]

Protein-bound Paclitaxel 260 mg/m^2 IV over 30 minutes
Repeat cycles every 21 days
or
Protein-bound Paclitaxel 100–150 mg/m^2 IV over 30 minutes on days 1, 8, and 15
Repeat cycle every 28 days

Ixabepilone[i]

Ixabepilone 40 mg/m^2 IV over 3 hours
Repeat cycles every 21 days

Capecitabine[j]

Capecitabine 2,000–2,500 mg/m^2 per day orally, divided twice daily for 14 days
Repeat cycles every 21 days

Liposomal doxorubicin[k]

Liposomal doxorubicin 30–50 mg/m^2 IV over variable duration
Repeat cycles every 28 days

Combination Chemotherapy Regimens

Docetaxel + capecitabine[l]

Docetaxel 75 mg/m^2 IV over 1 hour, day 1
Capecitabine 2,000–2,500 mg/m^2 per day orally divided twice daily for 14 days
Repeat cycles every 21 days

Paclitaxel + Gemcitabine[m]

Paclitaxel 175 mg/m^2 IV over 3 hours, day 1
Gemcitabine 1250 mg/m^2 IV days 1 and 8
Repeat cycles every 21 days

Ixabepilone + capecitabine[i]

Ixabepilone 40 mg/m^2 IV over 3 hours, day 1
Capecitabine 1,750–2,000 mg/m^2/day orally divided twice daily for 14 days
Repeat cycles every 21 days

Paclitaxel + bevacizumab[n]

Paclitaxel 90 mg/m^2 IV over 1 hour, days 1, 8, and 15
Bevacizumab 10 mg/kg IV over 30–90 minutes, days 1 and 15
Repeat cycles every 28 days

[a]From Taxol (paclitaxel) product information. Princeton, NJ: Bristol-Myers Squibb; July 2007.
[b]From Perez EA, Vogelci, Irwin DH, et al. Clin Oncol 2001;19:4216.
[c]From Zelek L, Bartheir S, Riofrio M, et al. Cancer 2001;92:2267.
[d]From Taxotere (docetaxel) product information. Bridgewater, NJ: Sanofi-aventis; 2008.
[e]From Hainsworth JD, Burris HA 3rd, Erlaud JB, et al. J Clin Oncol 1998;16:2164.
[f]From Carmichael J, Possinger K, Philip P, et al. J Clin Oncol 1995;13:2731.
[g]From Abraxane (paclitaxel protein-bound particles for injectable suspension) product information. Bridgewater, NJ: Abraxis Bioscience; September 2009.
[h]From Gradishar WJ, Krasnojon D, Cheporov S, et al. J Clin Oncol 2009;27:3611–3619.
[i]From Boehnke Michaud L. J Oncol Pharm Pract 2009;15(2):95–106.
[j]From Gralow, JR. Breast Cancer Res Treat 2005;89 Suppl 1: S9–S15.
[k]From O'Brien ME, Wigler N, Inbar M, et al. Ann Oncol 2004;15(3):440–449.
[l]From O'Shaughnessy J, Miles D, Vukelja S, et al. J Clin Oncol 2002;20(12):2812–2823.
[m]From Gemzar (gemcitabine) product information. Indianapolis, IN: Eli Lilly and Company; May 2007.
[n]From Miller K, Wang M, Gralow J, et al. N Engl J Med 2007;357(26):2666–2676.

neuropathy, but slightly more fluid retention and skin and nail changes. Although the incidence of hypersensitivity reactions is also slightly less at these lower doses (requiring fewer premedications) it remains at approximately 3%, despite incorporation of all available preventive measures.

Docetaxel has also demonstrated high single-agent activity against metastatic breast cancer. It received FDA approval in 1995 for treatment of metastatic breast cancer for patients with relapse following therapy with doxorubicin-containing regimens. Impressive overall response rates of 54% to 68% were reported in four studies of docetaxel 100 mg/m^2 as first-line chemotherapy. As compared with paclitaxel (175 mg/m^2 over 3 hours every 3 weeks), docetaxel (100 mg/m^2 every 3 weeks) was associated with longer time-to-progression (HR, 1.64; P <0.0001) and OS (HR, 1.41; P = 0.03).[161] As noted above, this is not the most effective dose or schedule of paclitaxel. Nonetheless, this difference appears to be real, although clinically irrelevant at this time. Myelosuppression is the major dose-limiting toxicity of docetaxel. Nonhematologic toxicities include fatigue, mucosal toxicity, mild-to-moderate nausea and vomiting, diarrhea, and neurosensory complaints. Results from the comparative randomized trial mentioned above show that although docetaxel is associated with less neuropathy, myalgia, and hypersensitivity than paclitaxel given every 3 weeks, febrile neutropenia, fluid retention, and skin reactions appear to occur more frequently with docetaxel.[161]

A new formulation of paclitaxel has been approved by the FDA. This protein-bound paclitaxel (Abraxane®) is covalently bound to albumin, then microemulsified into nanoparticles to improve solubility of the chemotherapeutic agent. In a randomized trial of protein-bound paclitaxel versus conventional paclitaxel (each given every 3 weeks), the protein-bound paclitaxel was associated with improved response rates and time-to-progression in patients with taxane-naive metastatic breast cancer.[162] Myelosuppression was more pronounced in the conventional paclitaxel arm, whereas peripheral neuropathy was more frequently observed in the protein-bound paclitaxel arm. Weekly administration of the protein-bound paclitaxel also has been reported to be efficacious and safe. Final results from phase III comparative studies with docetaxel or weekly conventional paclitaxel have yet to be reported. Many ongoing clinical trials will help to further elucidate the role of protein-bound paclitaxel in the clinical management of both metastatic and early breast cancer.

After patients have been treated with an anthracycline and a taxane, single-agent capecitabine, vinorelbine or gemcitabine have resulted in response rates of 20% to 25%.[163] Of these agents, only capecitabine is FDA approved as a single agent for metastatic breast cancer. Gemcitabine is only FDA approved in combination with paclitaxel for metastatic breast cancer. However, all of these are included in most national and international guidelines as appropriate therapy for metastatic breast cancer. Decisions regarding which agent to choose are based on patient characteristics, expected toxicities and previous exposure to chemotherapy. An increasing number of patients diagnosed with metastatic breast cancer have been exposed to adjuvant chemotherapy consisting of an anthracycline and a taxane. If metastases are found within 6 to 12 months of completing treatment with these agents, many clinicians will choose treatment from a different chemotherapy class. If it has been longer since their adjuvant therapy, then retreating with the same agents may be considered. However, given the cardiotoxicity associated with the anthracyclines, the use of these agents in the metastatic setting has been generally avoided until the availability of the liposomal anthracyclines. Pegylated liposomal doxorubicin is associated with less cardiotoxicity and similar efficacy compared to conventional doxorubicin and is a viable option for women who recur more than 1 year after their adjuvant anthracycline regimen.[164]

Anthracyclines, taxanes and capecitabine are all approved for metastatic breast cancer and have very specific indications for their use. Patients who initially respond to these classic agents progress later, are usually in fairly good health and have few effective options at this juncture in the course of their disease. One class of drugs that shows promise in this resistant population is the epothilones. Epothilones are natural compounds first identified from soil-derived *Sorangium cellulosum* myxobacterium. They are classified as microtubule stabilizing agents (MSAs). The mechanism of action of the epothilones is similar to but distinct from the taxanes, binding to β-microtubulin in a unique manner but ultimately leading to microtubule stabilization and cell death in similar manner compared to the taxanes. These natural compounds are very lipophilic and unstable in solution, leading to development of semisynthetic analogues. One of these analogues, ixabepilone, has shown significant activity in patients with metastatic breast cancer who have received a taxane, anthracycline and capecitabine and is FDA approved in this setting. Single agent data with ixabepilone demonstrated a 22% to 57% objective response rate in patients who were heavily to minimally pretreated, respectively.[165] In combination with capecitabine, ixabepilone was found to increase response rates (35% vs 14%; *P* <0.0001) and time-to-progression (5.8 months vs 4.2 months; *P* = 0.0003) compared to capecitabine alone in metastatic breast cancer patients who had received a prior taxane and ananthracycline.[165] Ixabepilone is also FDA approved in combination with capecitabine for this indication as well. Adverse effects associated with ixabepilone include myelosuppression, peripheral neuropathy, myalgias/arthralgias, alopecia, mild nausea, and skin/nail changes.[165] Other epothilones are currently in clinical trials and could lead to significant advances in many other cancers.

Combination chemotherapy regimens are associated with higher response rates than are single-agent therapies in the treatment of metastatic breast cancer, but the higher response rates have not usually translated into significant differences in time-to-progression and OS. The use of sequential single-agent chemotherapies versus the combination regimens is widely debated for metastatic breast cancer.

One trial investigating the combination of doxorubicin with paclitaxel versus each single agent with crossover to the other agent upon progression set out to help answer the question of which approach is more effective.[166] While response rates were higher with the combination regimen, time-to-progression and OS were similar between all arms of the study. This was probably because most patients who progressed on their first single agent went on to receive the second-line single agent, thereby negating any potential survival benefits seen with improved response rates. In another study comparing single-agent docetaxel to the combination of docetaxel with capecitabine, the combination arm produced higher response rates, time-to-progression, and OS than did the single agent.[167] However, because only 15% of patients in the docetaxel-alone arm received capecitabine after progression, this study does not answer the question of whether combination therapy is better than sequential single-agent therapy. Other studies also have demonstrated similar results, but none of them adequately answer the question of whether sequential administration of single-agent chemotherapy or concurrent combination chemotherapy is optimal. Recently published international guidelines reflect this assertion with recommendations which favor sequential single agents over combination regimens unless the patient has rapidly progressive disease, life-threatening visceral disease, or the need for rapid symptom control.[168]

Combination regimens are associated with greater toxicity. In the palliative metastatic setting, the least toxic approach is preferred when efficacy is considered equal. In clinical practice, patients who require a rapid response to chemotherapy (e.g., those with symptomatic bulky metastases) often receive combination therapy despite the added toxicity. This decision is complex and should be made on an individual patient basis.

Biologic or Targeted Therapy

Therapies that focus on molecular targets through novel mechanisms are often referred to as biologic or targeted therapy. These agents, while using the biologic knowledge gained from decades of research, are designed to specifically target cancer cells while generally sparing normal tissues. For breast cancer, several agents that focus on a myriad of targets that are differentially expressed in breast cancer cells and play a critical role in their proliferation and survival are available in this class.

HER2-Targeted Agents Trastuzumab and lapatinib are the only *HER2*-targeted agents currently available in the United States, while many others are under investigation. Trastuzumab is a humanized monoclonal antibody that binds with a specific epitope of the *HER2* protein. Mechanisms of action of trastuzumab include disruption of HER receptor dimerization, disruption of downstream signaling pathways (e.g., PI3K/Akt), G_1 arrest and reduced proliferation, induction of apoptosis, suppression of angiogenesis, induction of immune-mediated responses (e.g., antibody-dependent cellular cytotoxicity), inhibition of *HER2* extracellular domain proteolysis and inhibition of DNA repair. These biologic effects lead to inhibition of cellular growth, decreased malignant potential, and possibly reversal of resistance to certain chemotherapies and endocrine therapy. Single-agent treatment with trastuzumab has a response rate of 15% to 20% and a clinical benefit rate of nearly 40% in patients with *HER2*-overexpressing cancers.[169] Moreover, the results of a large randomized trial demonstrated that trastuzumab has at least additive, and perhaps synergistic, activity with other chemotherapeutic agents.[170] In this pivotal trial comparing chemotherapy in combination with trastuzumab versus chemotherapy alone, the addition of trastuzumab increased response rates, time-to-progression, and OS when compared to chemotherapy alone. Patients who were anthracycline naive were treated with an anthracycline (mostly doxorubicin, some epirubicin) plus cyclophosphamide, and patients who had received an adjuvant anthracycline regimen were treated with paclitaxel. During this trial, patients who received the anthracycline-trastuzumab combination had a very high incidence of cardiotoxicity (27%), leading to discontinuation of this arm of the study and a black box warning regarding this contraindication in the product information for trastuzumab. Many investigators are attempting to circumvent this toxicity while giving these two classes of agents together (e.g., liposomal doxorubicin, continuous-infusion doxorubicin, lower-dose epirubicin). However, until further information regarding the safety of these approaches becomes available, anthracyclines administered concurrently with trastuzumab should not be given outside the context of a clinical trial in patients with metastatic breast cancer.

Many other chemotherapy agents have successfully been administered with trastuzumab. Only two other phase III trials have been published comparing chemotherapy alone versus chemotherapy plus trastuzumab. Marty et al. compared docetaxel alone versus docetaxel with trastuzumab in patients with previously untreated *HER2*-positive metastatic breast cancer.[171] That trial demonstrated significant advantages to the combination over chemotherapy alone in terms of response rates, time-to-progression, and OS. von Minckwitz et al. randomized patients who were progressing on front-line trastuzumab-containing regimen to receive either capecitabine alone or capecitabine with continued trastuzumab therapy.[172] Median time-to-progression was 5.6 months with capecitabine alone and 8.2 months with capecitabine plus trastuzumab (HR, 0.69; 95% CI, 0.48-0.97; *P* = 0.034). While there were methodological problems with this trial (e.g., slow accrual led to early closure, open-label design, etc.), results support the decade-long clinical practice of continuing trastuzumab beyond progression, but raise other questions as to the comparative benefit with this approach versus a lapatinib-based regimen (see discussion below).

Other chemotherapy agents that have been evaluated in several phase II trials in combination with trastuzumab include vinorelbine, gemcitabine, and the platinum agents (cisplatin and carboplatin). In phase II trials, vinorelbine in combination with trastuzumab has shown very high response rates, even in heavily pretreated patients.[173] In another phase III trial, the triplet combination of paclitaxel, carboplatin, and trastuzumab was compared with paclitaxel and trastuzumab as dual therapy.[174] This study demonstrated superior response rates and time-to-progression with the triplet regimen versus the doublet regimen. A similar trial designed to confirm this data using docetaxel instead of paclitaxel failed to demonstrate any advantage with the addition of carboplatin to a taxane-trastuzumab regimen.[175] These conflicting results indicate that the benefit of adding a platinum compound to these regimens remains questionable. Toxicities with the addition of carboplatin are significantly greater in terms of myelosuppression and nausea, which should be considered when making treatment decisions in the setting of metastatic breast cancer where quality-of-life is paramount.

Significant cross-talk exists between the growth factor pathways (e.g., HER2) and the hormone receptor pathways (e.g., ER). This has generated a hypothesis that combining endocrine therapies with HER2-targeted therapies may be synergistic or at least additive in their anticancer effects. The TAnDEM trial randomized patients with HER2-positive MBC to anastrozole with or without trastuzumab.[176] The addition of trastuzumab improved PFS from 2.4 months to 4.8 months ($P = 0.0016$) and overall response rate and clinical benefit rate were also significantly improved. Many other trials are seeking to confirm this information. While confirming information is awaited, these combinations are frequently utilized in current clinical practice for patients with hormone-receptor-positive, HER2-positive metastatic breast cancer.

Trastuzumab is generally well tolerated. The most common adverse effects are infusion-related (primarily fever and chills), occur in approximately 40% of patients during the initial infusion and generally go unrecognized by patients. Other infusion-related reactions include mild nausea, pain at tumor sites, rigors, headaches, dizziness, hypotension, rash, and asthenia, which are much less common.[177] These reactions are generally mild to moderate and last about 1 to 2 hours after the infusion is started and usually do not recur with subsequent infusions. Acetaminophen and diphenhydramine may be given and/or the infusion rate reduced to help alleviate the symptoms related to these reactions. If infusion-related symptoms occur, subsequent doses should be infused over 90 minutes. Infusion over 30 minutes is appropriate if symptoms subside. A rare, but more severe reaction consisting of severe hypersensitivity and/or pulmonary reactions has been reported. It is important to educate patients regarding the pulmonary reactions, as these may occur up to 24 hours after the infusion and can be fatal if not promptly treated. Trastuzumab may increase the incidence of infection, diarrhea, and/or other adverse events slightly when given with chemotherapy, but most of these increases are not clinically significant for an individual patient.

The most serious adverse effect of trastuzumab is cardiotoxicity. As mentioned earlier, the incidence of heart failure is approximately 5% with single-agent trastuzumab and the risk is unacceptably high when trastuzumab is given with an anthracycline. Fortunately, heart failure seen with trastuzumab is somewhat reversible with pharmacologic management and some patients have continued therapy with trastuzumab after their left ventricular ejection fraction has returned to normal with medical management. Although there are no guidelines for cardiac monitoring with this agent, close monitoring for clinical signs and symptoms of heart failure is recommended in order to intervene with appropriate cardiac treatments.

Trastuzumab may be administered as an initial loading dose of 4 mg/kg, followed by a 2-mg/kg dose administered weekly or every 3 weeks utilizing a loading dose of 8 mg/kg followed by 6 mg/kg. Both of these dose/schedules are FDA approved. Every 3-week administration is more convenient than weekly administration, but comparative data with this dose schedule versus the weekly dose schedule are not available at this time. The schedule of chemotherapy often dictates which trastuzumab dosing regimen will be utilized. When patients progress on therapy with trastuzumab, many clinicians will continue the trastuzumab and change the chemotherapy regimen. With the capecitabine data (mentioned previously) now available, this practice seems effective and reasonable. This practice has changed with the availability of lapatinib, which is effective in trastuzumab-resistant disease (see below). However, upon progression on a lapatinib-containing regimen, clinicians often resume therapy with trastuzumab in combination with a different chemotherapy regimen. There are no data to support this practice, but in light of the other available evidence this approach also seems reasonable.

Lapatinib is a tyrosine kinase inhibitor that dually targets HER2 and the epidermal growth factor receptor (EGFR or HER1). This small molecule works intracellularly to actively shut down the signaling pathway from these two receptors and thus inhibit cell growth and division. Lapatinib is an oral agent with modest activity against breast cancer as a single agent. In metastatic breast cancer patients as first-line therapy, response rates to single agent lapatinib have been reported to be 24% in one phase II study and were generally confined to a HER2-positive subset of patients. This benefit is similar to what is seen with single agent trastuzumab administered as first-line therapy for metastatic breast cancer. In combination with capecitabine in women with HER2-positive metastatic breast cancer who were previously treated with an anthracycline, a taxane, and trastuzumab, it improves response rates (22% vs 14%; $P = 0.09$) and time-to-progression (8.4 vs 4.4 months; HR, 0.49; 95% CI, 0.34-0.71; $P <0.001$) as compared to capecitabine alone.[178] Based on this evidence, the FDA approved lapatinib in this setting only. In combination with paclitaxel as first-line therapy for metastatic breast cancer (HER2-positive and -negative), the addition of lapatinib did not appear to improve outcomes for patients with HER2-negative disease. However, for patients with HER2-positive metastatic breast cancer, the addition of lapatinib significantly improved time-to-progression, event-free survival, objective response rates and clinical benefit rate, although the HER2-positive patients on the paclitaxel/placebo arm did not receive any HER2-directed therapy.[179]

Lapatinib has also been combined with endocrine therapy in hopes of taking advantage of the cross-talk between the growth factor receptor and the hormone receptor pathways as mentioned previously. In a large, randomized phase III study, letrozole was administered with either lapatinib or placebo in hormone-receptor-positive patients with metastatic breast cancer (HER2-negative and -positive).[180] The addition of lapatinib in HER2-positive patients improved PFS from 3 months to 8.2 months (HR, 0.71; 95% CI, 0.53-0.96; $P = 0.019$). In HER2-negative patients, no significant benefit was observed with the addition of lapatinib. Another interesting approach to HER2-positive metastatic breast cancer has been to combine HER2-targeted agents with differing mechanisms of action. O'Shaughnessy and colleagues compared lapatinib alone to lapatinib plus trastuzumab in patients with metastatic breast cancer progressing on trastuzumab therapy. PFS was significantly improved with the combination (12 vs 8.4 weeks; $P = 0.029$).[181] However, the clinical significance of this small difference (less than 1 month) is debatable and the expense of this regimen is obvious.

Because lapatinib is a small molecule and can readily cross the blood-brain barrier, investigation has ensued to ascertain its effects on brain metastases. Trastuzumab does not cross the blood–brain barrier and the central nervous system is often a sanctuary site for progressive metastases, representing the first site of recurrence in a relatively large number of patients. Phase II trials investigating the efficacy of lapatinib in patients with treated brain metastases failed to demonstrate any significant response. However, in the large randomized trial with capecitabine ± lapatinib, the addition of lapatinib was associated with a lower rate of the central nervous system as a site of first progression (2% with lapatinib vs 6% with capecitabine alone; $P = 0.045$).[178] Ongoing adjuvant trials with lapatinib will continue to evaluate this relationship and determine the value of lapatinib for prevention of central nervous system metastases.

Adverse events associated with the addition of lapatinib are primarily rash and diarrhea. These adverse effects appear to be more significant when combined with chemotherapy (e.g., capecitabine, paclitaxel), but are generally manageable with aggressive antidiarrheal therapy and/or dose reductions. Other rare effects have been reported (QT prolongation, hepatotoxicity, and interstitial lung disease) and patients should be counseled regarding these effects. Because of concerns regarding the role of *HER2* in normal cardiac functioning, lapatinib may also increase the risk for cardiac dysfunction. However, in a review of more than 3,689 patients who received lapatinib in phase I to III trials, cardiotoxicity occurred in only 1.6% of patients.[182] Although these data are reassuring, it does not rule out the possibility of expanded toxicity when this agent is used in patients not included in the clinical trials such as those with underlying cardiac risks. Drug–drug and/or drug–food interactions are particularly important with lapatinib due to its metabolism through the cytochrome P450 system (3A4) and other pharmacokinetic/pharmacodynamic issues. Many of the adverse effects listed previously may be exacerbated due to drug or food interactions and careful review of patients' medication lists and education regarding these issues are extremely important. Lapatinib is currently being investigated in numerous clinical trials, the results of which will further elucidate the role of this agent in the management of both early and late stages of the disease.

It should be noted that only 20% to 30% of patients with metastatic breast cancer overexpress *HER2*, and commercially available IHC tests that are reported as 2+ for *HER2* are often negative by the more sensitive and specific FISH technique. To date, there is no benefit associated with the administration of trastuzumab to patients with *HER2*-negative tumors (IHC score of 0 to 1+, or FISH-negative), and a very questionable benefit associated with administration of trastuzumab to women with tumors that are 2+ for *HER2* by IHC staining alone. The patients who benefit most from trastuzumab therapy include those whose tumors express *HER2* protein at the 3+ level or who clearly demonstrate gene amplification by FISH testing. Further analyses investigating what other predictive markers for response to trastuzumab and lapatinib may be clinically useful are currently ongoing.

Other Targeted Agents Targeting tumor blood vessels is another strategy to fight breast cancer. One of the most important growth factors that regulate the development of new blood vessels (angiogenesis) is vascular endothelial growth factor. Bevacizumab is a monoclonal antibody targeted against vascular endothelial growth factor and is FDA approved for use with chemotherapy for the management of a variety of malignancies. Bevacizumab has also been tested in clinical trials with capecitabine and paclitaxel in metastatic breast cancer patients. In the first clinical trial reported in breast cancer patients, bevacizumab was given every 3 weeks in combination with capecitabine in women who had failed both anthracycline- and taxane-containing regimens.[183] While response rates were significantly higher in the bevacizumab arm of this trial, time-to-progression and OS remained

the same as with capecitabine alone. In a subsequent trial, newly diagnosed metastatic breast cancer patients were randomized to receive weekly paclitaxel with or without bevacizumab (given every other week).[184] That trial demonstrated significantly better response rates and time-to-progression with the addition of bevacizumab, but failed to demonstrate a survival benefit with the addition of bevacizumab. These two trials differed in their patient populations, choice of chemotherapy and bevacizumab dose and schedule. Other trials with bevacizumab include the AVADO trial, which randomized newly diagnosed metastatic breast cancer patients to docetaxel or docetaxel plus bevacizumab (both administered every 3 weeks).[185] This trial also demonstrated a similar although smaller advantage with bevacizumab in terms of PFS. Other clinical trials confirm the benefits of bevacizumab in combination with other chemotherapy agents (e.g., RIBBON I and II trials conducted in metastatic breast cancer patients as first-line and second-line therapy, respectively).[186,187] Adverse events attributable to bevacizumab in these combination regimens include hypertension, proteinuria (which can lead to renal tubular necrosis), thrombosis, bleeding, and cardiotoxicity. The addition of bevacizumab may also increase the incidence of neuropathy, fatigue and neutropenia associated with the chemotherapy. Based on these conflicting results, the relatively small differences in beneficial outcomes, and the questionable tolerability, the role of bevacizumab is not clearly defined for the management of metastatic breast cancer. Nonetheless, the NCCN has incorporated the bevacizumab/paclitaxel regimen into their guidelines as one option for the management of metastatic breast cancer and the FDA has approved its use with paclitaxel in the first-line setting.[47]

Many other biologic or targeted agents are being investigated and may end up changing the overall management of breast cancer for both early and metastatic disease.

Radiation Therapy

Radiation is an important modality in the treatment of symptomatic metastatic disease. The most common indication for treatment with radiation therapy is painful bone metastases or other localized sites of disease refractory to systemic therapy. Radiation therapy provides significant pain relief to approximately 90% of patients who are treated for painful bone metastases. Radiation is also an important modality in the palliative treatment of metastatic brain lesions and spinal cord lesions, which respond poorly to systemic therapy, as well as eye or orbit lesions and other sites where significant accumulation of tumor cells occurs. Skin and/or lymph node metastases confined to the chest wall area may also be treated with radiation therapy for palliation (e.g., open wounds or painful lesions). Chemotherapy may also be added to radiation for sensitization purposes.

PREVENTION AND EARLY DETECTION

Current efforts at breast cancer prevention are directed toward the identification and removal of risk factors often referred to as risk reduction strategies. Unfortunately, a number of risk factors associated with development of breast cancer, such as family history of breast cancer or personal history of breast or other gynecologic malignancies, cannot be modified. Isolation and cloning of breast cancer susceptibility genes now allows screening of women with histories suggestive of "breast cancer families" and identification of appropriate candidates for prophylactic bilateral mastectomies and/or bilateral salpingo oophorectomy. These surgeries are considered for women who are at very high risk for the development

TABLE 136-14 Current National Guidelines on Risk Reduction (Prevention) Strategies for Breast Cancer in Women Desiring Risk Reduction Therapy

Risk Category/Strategy	NCCN[42]	ASCO[189]
Average Risk		
Mastectomy[a]	Not recommended	Not addressed
Oophorectomy[b]	Not recommended	Not addressed
Tamoxifen[c]	Not recommended for women with: • Gail 5-year risk < 1.7%[f]	Not recommended for women with: • Gail 5-year risk < 1.66%[f] • Limited data women < 35 years old
Raloxifene[d]	Not recommended for women with: • Gail 5-year risk < 1.7%[f] • Premenopausal status	Not recommended for women with: • Gail 5-year risk < 1.66%[f] • Premenopausal status
High Risk		
Mastectomy[a,e]	Consider in the following women: • BRCA 1/2 carriers • Pedigree suggestive of genetic predisposition	Not addressed
Oophorectomy[b]	Limited to women with: • Known or strongly suspected BRCA 1/2 mutations	Not addressed
Tamoxifen[c,h]	Consider in the following women: • Prior thoracic RT or LCIS • Gail 5-year risk ≥ 1.7%[f] • Lifetime risk > 20% (using models based largely on family history)[g] • Pre- or postmenopausal	May offer to the following women: • LCIS • Gail 5-year risk ≥ 1.66%[f] • Pre- or postmenopausal
Raloxifene[d,h]	Consider in the following women: • Prior thoracic RT or LCIS • Gail 5-year risk ≥ 1.7%[f] • Lifetime risk > 20% (using models based largely on family history)[g] • ONLY postmenopausal	May offer to the following women: • LCIS • Gail 5-year risk ≥ 1.66%[f] • ONLY postmenopausal

NCCN = National Comprehensive Cancer Network; ACSO = American Society of Clinical Oncology; RT = radiotherapy; LCIS = lobular carcinoma in situ.
[a]Mastectomy = bilateral total mastectomy ± reconstruction.
[b]Oophorectomy = bilateral salpingo oophorectomy with peritoneal washings; pathologic assessment should include fine sectioning of the ovaries and fallopian tubes.
[c]Tamoxifen = 20 mg orally daily for 5 years.
[d]Raloxifene = 60 mg orally daily for 5 years; may continue for longer in women with osteoporosis.
[e]There are no data to support the use of pharmacologic risk reduction after bilateral mastectomies and the likely benefit would be very small, since the breast tissue at risk has largely been removed.
[f]The National Cancer Institute (NCI) Breast Cancer Risk Assessment Tool is a computer-based version of the modified Gail model and can be accessed via the NCI website (www.nci.nih.gov).
[g]Including but not limited to the Clause and BRCAPRO models.
[h]Contraindications to tamoxifen/raloxifene include: (1) history of thromboembolism (including venous thromboembolism, pulmonary embolism, thrombotic stroke, and/or transient ischemic attack); (2) pregnancy or pregnancy potential without adequate contraception. Endometrial hyperplasia has been reported with both agents; however, risk of endometrial cancer appears to be greater with tamoxifen. Therefore, adequate monitoring for gynecologic changes is paramount with both therapies.

of breast and/or ovarian cancer, particularly if the women's breasts are difficult to evaluate by both physical examination and mammography and if they have persistent disabling fears that they will be diagnosed with cancer. Guidelines for the incorporation of surgical risk reduction strategies are largely based on genetics and other known risk factors for development of breast (or ovarian) cancer (Table 136–14).

In the past 15 years, there has been increasing interest in pharmacologic risk reduction for breast cancer. Three important classes of agents being studied in this setting are the retinoids, SERMs, and aromatase inhibitors. Retinoids (all vitamin A and its isomer derivatives and synthetic analogs) are biologic regulators of orderly epithelial cell development, and are therefore potentially ideal agents for controlling abnormal epithelial proliferation that occurs in carcinogenesis. Because only preclinical data are available to suggest a benefit with these types of therapies, clinical trials are needed to further investigate the role of the retinoids in prevention of breast cancer.

The drugs with the most clinical information as risk reduction agents for breast cancer are the SERMs, tamoxifen and raloxifene. As previously described, tamoxifen is useful as an adjunct after treatment of primary breast cancer. In randomized trials of tamoxifen as an adjuvant treatment for breast cancer, women who received tamoxifen were also found to have a reduced incidence of contralateral primary breast carcinomas.[5] In a large, randomized, placebo-controlled study, the NSABP demonstrated significant reductions in risk of invasive and noninvasive breast cancers with 5 years of

tamoxifen therapy (20 mg/day) in women at high risk for developing the disease.[55] Although this study is controversial, other studies from around the world also have been reported that investigated the role of tamoxifen as a risk reduction strategy. A meta-analysis of these trials indicates a consistent benefit with tamoxifen in reducing the incidence of ER-positive breast cancers (48% reduction; 95% CI, 36%–58%; P <0.0001).[188] Tamoxifen has been repeatedly shown to be a relatively safe drug with an acceptable toxicity profile when used to treat patients with breast cancer. However, its estrogenic effects on the uterus and the coagulation system increase the risk of serious adverse effects that may be critical for patients taking this agent as a risk reduction strategy. Toxicities associated with tamoxifen were previously described in the Adjuvant Endocrine Therapy section above. Any decision to use tamoxifen for risk reduction should be made after a thorough discussion of the woman's risk of breast cancer, the potential benefits of tamoxifen, and the potential serious adverse events associated with tamoxifen.

A second trial has been reported that compared tamoxifen to raloxifene in a similar population of high-risk women. The Study of Tamoxifen and Raloxifene (STAR or P2) was published in 2006 and demonstrated a similar rate of invasive breast cancers with the two drugs.[56] However, the rates of noninvasive breast cancer were numerically higher in the raloxifene arm of the trial, although this difference did not reach statistical significance. It is not clear what long-term outcome will be related to this difference, but further follow-up will be required to draw any sound conclusions. Rates of endometrial cancer and deep venous thromboses were more frequent in the tamoxifen arm, but overall quality-of-life was similar between the two agents.[56] Based on these results, the FDA approved raloxifene for breast cancer risk reduction in women at high risk of the disease. A similar reduction in the incidence of contralateral primary breast cancers was demonstrated with anastrozole in the adjuvant ATAC study (discussed previously), leading to the premise that AIs may also play a role in risk reduction of breast cancer.[139] No data are yet available investigating the AIs in this setting, but clinical trials are underway.

The NCCN has established guidelines for risk reduction strategies, including mastectomy, oophorectomy, and/or pharmacologic agents.[54] These guidelines are based on risk assessment tools such as the Gail model, BRCAPRO, or Claus models (discussed earlier) as well as other established risk factors. Much of the guideline is dependent on a woman's wishes for intervention. The American Society of Clinical Oncology (ASCO) recently published recommendations guiding the use of the pharmacologic agents for breast cancer risk reduction.[189] These guidelines are similar to the NCCN guidelines in that they recommend the use of tamoxifen or raloxifene for postmenopausal women at high risk (as defined by the Gail or other models) and tamoxifen for premenopausal women at high risk based on the woman's wishes (Table 136–14).

🔟 The rationale for early detection of breast cancer is based on the relationship between stage of breast cancer at diagnosis and the probability for cure. If all breast cancer cases could be detected at a very early stage of the disease (i.e., small primary tumor and negative lymph nodes), then more patients theoretically could be cured of their disease. Screening guidelines for early detection of breast cancer in women at average risk have been developed by several organizations, including but not limited to the American Cancer Society (ACS), the United States Preventive Services Task Force (USPTF), and the NCCN.[42,190,191] The American Cancer Society guidelines are most commonly cited. However, it is important to note that the expert panels developing these guidelines often differ in their approach and analysis of the available data, as is evident in the controversies that currently exist.

The ACS currently recommends that all women 20 years and older be informed of the benefits and limitations of breast self-examinations (BSEs).[190] Several studies have investigated the benefits of BSE. These trials were primarily conducted prior to the routine use of mammographic screening and demonstrated an inferential benefit in diagnosis of earlier stages of breast cancer. One trial, the Shanghai trial, appeared to indicate no benefit, but there was a higher rate of biopsies in women who were taught BSE than in women who were not taught BSE.[192] The investigators from this trial caution that this was a study of BSE instruction and not BSE performance. Compliance and competency with the BSE were neither guaranteed nor evaluated in this trial. Because of the lack of direct evidence to support or refute a benefit with BSE and the apparent associated increase in biopsy rates, the ACS has taken the position that it is optional, but women of all ages should be encouraged to be aware of their breasts in order to recognize any changes and promptly report these to a health professional.[190] Other organizations have taken a similar approach to their recommendations regarding BSE or simply state that there is insufficient evidence to recommend this practice.

Recommendations for breast examination by a healthcare professional (clinical breast examination) vary among the screening guidelines most often cited. The rate of breast cancer detection using clinical breast examination (CBE) alone is low, with even lower rates in younger women and women with higher body weight.[190] Randomized clinical trials have reported inconsistent results and often evaluated CBE in conjunction with mammograms. The ACS recommends CBE in conjunction with mammography for women ages 40 years and older.[190] For younger patients (in their 20s and 30s), it is recommended as part of a periodic health examination every 3 years, but this recommendation is based on weak evidence. The USPTF concluded that there is insufficient evidence to assess the benefits/risks of CBE beyond screening mammography in women over the age of 40 years.

The most controversial screening recommendation for breast cancer is related to annual mammography. It is clear that screening mammography decreases mortality from breast cancer. The controversies surround the balance of benefits and harms associated with a less than perfect screening test in women at average risk of developing breast cancer but of differing ages. Multiple clinical trials have been completed over the years and multiple meta-analyses of these trials have been conducted as well. Most of the trials included women 50 to 74 years of age and the interval between testing ranged from 12 to 33 months. The most recent meta-analysis of these data estimated a "number needed to invite for screening to extend one woman's life" (NNI) as 1,339 for women aged 50 to 59 years.[193] Some trials also included women aged 40 to 49 years, albeit significantly fewer women in this age group were included in the meta-analyses. The estimated NNI for women aged 40 to 49 years was reported as 1,904. The largest benefit was found in women ages 60 to 69 years with an estimated NNI of 377. None of the trials included women 75 years of age or older, thus there are no data to support or refute the benefit of screening mammography in this population.[193]

Incorporation of this new information into national guidelines differs with each organization. The ACS continues to recommend annual screening mammography for women ages 40 and older (as long as they are in good health).[190] This recommendation allows for individualized decisions to be made based on the overall health of the woman, but does not limit access to younger or older women who may benefit from screening. The USPTF has taken a different approach, recommending against routine screening mammography for women ages 40 to 49 and 75 years or older.[191] These recommendations are based on the available evidence, but do not allow for individualization based on a woman's overall health and make an arbitrary judgment that the NNI of 1,904 for women 40 to 49 years is not acceptable compared to 1,339 for women aged 50 to 59 years. For women 50 to 74 years of age, the USPTF recommends biennial screening mammography. This interval recommendation was based on assumptions of risks and benefits based on the available studies. While the upper limit for screening varies among guidelines, most experts agree that mammograms in women over the age of 74 are not supported by the current body of evidence, but some women may benefit if they are otherwise in good health and have a life expectancy of 10 years or more. There are also many other debates within this controversial area and the reader is referred to these references for further details.[42,190,191,193]

Other radiologic methods of breast imaging are also being investigated (e.g., digital mammography, ultrasonography, and MRI) and minimal data exist to support these methods in some high risk populations. Recommendations for women with a high risk of breast cancer are not fully established and definitions of "high risk" vary between different guidelines. The ACS include breast screening MRI as an adjunct to mammography for the following groups of high-risk women: (1) known *BRCA* mutation carriers; (2) untested individuals with a first-degree relative with a *BRCA* mutation; (3) women with a 20% or greater lifetime risk of breast cancer based on models that largely depend on family history; (4) women who had radiation to the chest between the ages of 10 and 30 years of age; (5) women with LiFraumeni syndrome, Cowden syndrome, Bannayan-Riley-Ruvalcaba syndrome, or have a first-degree relative with one of these syndromes.[190,194] The NCCN also has adopted consensus guidelines for women at high risk of breast cancer, incorporating breast MRI with other established screening tools for women as young as 25 years old (Table 136–15).[42]

TABLE 136-15 Breast Cancer Screening Guidelines

Risk Category	ACS[189]	USPTF[190]	NCCN[54]
Average risk			
BSE	Age ≥20 y: optional (discuss benefits/limitations)	Not recommended	Age ≥20 y: breast awareness
CBE	Age ≥20–39 y: every 3 years	Insufficient evidence	Age ≥20–39 y: every 1–3 years
	Age ≥40 y: annually (as long as in good health)		Age ≥40 y: annually
Mammography	Age ≥40 y: annually (as long as in good health)	Age 50–74 y: biennial	Age ≥40 y: annually
High risk[a,b]			
BSE	NA	NA	All ages: breast awareness
CBE	NA	NA	All ages: every 6–12 months
Mammography	Annually w/ MRI	NA	Prior RT or strong family Hx or genetic predisposition, age ≥25: annually (+ CBE)
			All other categories: annually (+ CBE)
Breast MRI	Annually w/ mammogram	NA	Consider annually w/ mammogram + CBE for: (1) prior RT, age ≥25 y; (2) lifetime risk >20%; (3) strong family history or genetic predisposition, age ≥25 y; (4) history of LCIS
	Consider in moderate risk women as well		

ACS, American Cancer Society; USPTF, United States Preventive Task Force; NCCN, National Comprehensive Cancer Network; BSE, breast self-exam; CBE, clinical breast exam by a health care professional; MRI, magnetic resonance imaging; NA, not addressed; RT, thoracic radiation therapy; LCIS, lobular carcinoma in situ.

[a]High risk is defined by the ACS as women with (1) a known *BRCA1/2* gene mutation; (2) untested woman with first-degree relative with a known *BRCA1/2* gene mutation; (3) lifetime risk of breast cancer of 20%–25% or greater using a risk assessment tool based largely on family history; (4) radiation therapy to the chest between the ages of 10 and 30 years; (5) LiFraumeni syndrome, Cowden syndrome, Bannayan-Riley-Ruvalcaba syndrome, or have first-degree relatives with one of these syndromes. Moderately increased risk is defined as a woman with (1) a lifetime risk of breast cancer of 15%–20% using a risk assessment tool based largely on family history; (2) personal history of breast cancer, DCIS, LCIS, or AH; (3) extremely dense breasts or unevenly dense breasts when viewed by mammograms.

[b]High risk is defined by the NCCN as women with (1) prior thoracic radiation therapy; (2) 5-year risk of ≥1.7% of invasive breast cancer in women ≥35 years old; (3) lifetime risk of >20% as defined by models that are largely based on family history; (4) strong family history or genetic predisposition; (5) LCIS/atypical hyperplasia; (6) prior history of breast cancer.

It should also be noted that there are risks associated with any screening procedure and they should be discussed with each patient so they are able to make an informed decision regarding these procedures. The risks involved with screening mammograms include false-negative results, false-positive results, overdiagnosis (true positives that will not become clinically significant), and radiation risk. The rate of false-negative results with the current technology is approximately 20%, which explains why CBE is an important adjunct to screening for many women. Although the specificity of mammography is quite high (90%), most abnormal examinations are false positives, leading to additional biopsies and psychological distress. The issue of overdiagnosis refers primarily to the growth in detection of DCIS from screening mammography. The biologic significance of these tumors is unknown because only some of them would become invasive if left in place. So the question remains: Are we treating women who do not require treatment? Experts in the field continue to debate this issue. Radiation exposure also has been discussed in the context of screening mammography, but the small doses of radiation exposure with mammograms (2 to 4 mGy [0.2 to 0.4 Rad] per standard two-view examination) appears to be overshadowed by other benefits in terms of reduction in mortality as a consequence of early cancer detection.[191]

Significant advances in the safety and efficacy of screening mammography have occurred during the past two decades. These advances have enabled superior visualization of breast and breast tissue with a lower dose of radiation being delivered. Despite these advances, approximately 10% of all palpable masses are not detected by mammography. This is most commonly observed in premenopausal women, and may be directly related to the increased density of breast tissue in this estrogen-rich environment.

Although the safety and efficacy of screening mammography in terms of image quality and dosimetry are very acceptable, the need for greater quality control in mammography was recognized for some time. The Mammography Quality Standards Act (MQSA) of 1992 assures that all mammographic facilities achieve a common high standard of quality assurance. Responsibility for operation of the act was given to the FDA and all facilities that offer mammography must be FDA certified to remain open. The MQSA has now been updated to also include full field digital mammography

as well, although the use of this new technology has not yet been incorporated into national screening guidelines. Passage of this landmark legislation, as well as provision of appropriate levels of funding to conduct this program, represents an important contribution to the health of women. Similar quality assurance measures will need to be implemented for breast MRIs and ultrasonography, given the recommendations to utilize these imaging methods for early detection and diagnosis, respectively, in high-risk women and those with suspicious masses. All women should be aware that breast MRIs and ultrasounds are not currently regulated and should choose to have these tests performed at a reputable facility to insure quality. The American College of Radiology has developed reporting guidelines to standardize the way these images are interpreted. These are referred to as the Breast Imaging Reporting and Data System (BI-RADS) and are available for mammography, breast ultrasonography and breast MRIs.[43] This reporting method allows for uniformity between facilities and better comparisons over time. Nonetheless, differences remain between breast imaging quality and interpretation and it is best to have imaging conducted at the same facility over time if possible.

EVALUATION OF THERAPEUTIC OUTCOMES

❾ The desired therapeutic outcome of adjuvant therapy of breast cancer differs significantly from that of metastatic disease. Adjuvant therapy—chemotherapy, biologic therapy, and hormonal therapy—is administered with curative intent. The rationale for adjuvant therapy is that breast cancer, even when diagnosed in early stages when clinical evidence of distant spread is not apparent, is a systemic disease that spreads early to distant sites. Adjuvant therapy is intended to eradicate micrometastases and thus cure the patient of breast cancer. Therefore, the overall goal of adjuvant therapy is to cure the disease, which is something that cannot be fully evaluated for years following initial diagnosis and treatment. In addition, because disease cannot be detected at the time adjuvant therapy is started, assessment of disease response is not possible. Instead, a predetermined number of cycles of adjuvant therapy and/or years of biologic or hormonal therapy are administered. Adjuvant chemotherapy is often associated with significant toxicity. Maintaining dose intensity has been demonstrated to be important in the cure of disease, and therefore optimizing supportive care measures such as antiemetics and growth factors is highly recommended. The concept of dose density, using growth factors to maintain blood counts while decreasing the interval between chemotherapy administrations, is very controversial in the management of early-stage breast cancer. Multiple studies investigating this approach to adjuvant chemotherapy have been conducted with conflicting results and many more trials continue to be analyzed in hopes of determining the long-term outcomes related to this approach to therapy. The goals of therapy with neoadjuvant chemotherapy are slightly different. These goals focus on earlier end points of tumor response so as to minimize surgery, determine prognosis, and potentially conserve the breast tissue for a better cosmetic result. The other outcomes discussed with adjuvant therapy also apply to this scenario, in terms of improving survival and decreasing recurrences as compared to no systemic therapy.

Palliation is the therapeutic outcome in treatment of metastatic breast cancer. In general, the least-toxic therapies are used initially, with increasingly aggressive therapies applied in a sequential fashion and in a manner that does not significantly compromise the quality of the patient's life. Tumor response to a particular treatment regimen may be measured by clinical chemistry such as liver enzyme elevation in a patient with hepatic metastases or tumor markers, or imaging techniques such as bone scans or chest radiographs. However, assessment of the patient's clinical status and symptom control is often adequate to evaluate response to the therapy administered. In the patient with metastatic breast cancer, it is common to initiate hormonal therapy or chemotherapy and continue administration until signs and symptoms of disease progression or new signs and symptoms present. Optimizing quality-of-life is the therapeutic end point in the treatment of patients with metastatic breast cancer. A number of valid and reliable tools are available for objective assessment of quality-of-life in patients with breast cancer.

CONCLUSIONS

Breast cancer is the most commonly occurring cancer in women in the United States, and is second only to lung cancer as the most common cancer cause of death. The etiology of breast cancer is unknown, but a number of factors that increase a woman's chances of developing the disease have been identified. These risk factors suggest a complex interplay between hormones, genetic factors, environment, and lifestyle. The identification of the *BRCA1* and *BRCA2* genes, tumor suppressor genes important in the development of inherited and perhaps sporadic breast and ovarian cancer, has been instrumental in identifying patients who are at high risk, as well as improving our basic understanding of the causes of breast and ovarian cancer.

Most breast cancers are diagnosed in early stages before the disease has disseminated to sites distant from the breast. Treatment of early-stage breast cancer consists of local management, as well as systemic adjuvant therapy with chemotherapy, biologic and hormonal therapy, or a combination of these. BCT, which consists of complete removal of the tumor (lumpectomy), combined with breast irradiation and axillary lymph node staging, is currently the preferred method of treatment for most patients with localized breast cancer. Patients who are not candidates for breast conservation or who do not choose this local therapy will generally receive a modified radical mastectomy.

It is apparent from clinical and laboratory experiments and observation that spread of breast cancer via the bloodstream occurs early in the course of the disease, which can result in patients relapsing with systemic metastatic disease following local curative therapy.

The likelihood of later development of metastatic disease is related to the size of the primary tumor, presence of lymph node involvement and number of nodes affected, and a number of additional pathologic prognostic factors, which include proliferative capacity, nuclear grade, hormone receptor status, and presence or absence of oncogenes and other protein products. Systemic adjuvant therapy is commonly administered to patients with localized breast cancer following surgical procedures to diminish the risk of or delay disease recurrence. The NCCN and other groups have developed guidelines for adjuvant systemic therapy for early stage breast cancer based on expert consensus and evidence, and these treatment recommendations continue to evolve as new data become available.

Advanced breast cancer includes locally advanced breast cancer (stage III) and metastatic breast cancer (stage IV). Treatment of stage III breast cancer generally consists of a combination of surgery, radiation, and chemotherapy administered in an aggressive approach. Although response rates and survival have improved, there is still much progress to be made in stage III breast cancer. Metastatic breast cancer is usually incurable with available therapies, and patients should be encouraged to participate in clinical trials of novel agents or therapeutic approaches. It is interesting to note that some long-term responses have been observed in a subset of patients with metastatic disease who have a complete or near complete response to conventional chemotherapy. Unfortunately, this represents a small number of the total population of patients with metastatic breast cancer. Metastatic breast cancer is treated with endocrine therapy, chemotherapy or biologic therapy depending on receptor status. Patients who are hormone receptor-positive will generally receive initial endocrine therapy followed by chemotherapy when endocrine therapy fails. Patients who are hormone receptor-negative or who have symptomatic disease involving the liver, lung, or central nervous system will generally receive chemotherapy as first-line therapy of metastatic disease. Chemotherapy will result in an objective response in approximately 50% to 60% of patients previously unexposed to chemotherapy. Most patients have partial responses, and complete disappearance of disease occurs in fewer than 10% of patients treated. Median duration of response is 5 to 12 months; although some patients will have an excellent response to an initial course of chemotherapy and may live 5 to 10 years without evidence of disease. In general, median survival of patients after treatment with commonly used drug regimens for metastatic breast cancer ranges from 14 to 33 months. The response rate to second- and third-line chemotherapy varies from 20% to 40%, depending on the previous chemotherapy regimens the patient has received. Development of novel targeted agents (e.g., trastuzumab, lapatinib) has also changed the outlook for patients whose tumors overexpress *HER2*. Through continued research, other biologic or targeted agents may also improve outcomes for breast cancer patients.

Current efforts at breast cancer prevention are directed toward the identification and removal of risk factors and risk reduction with surgery or drug therapy. Three classes of agents, the retinoids, SERMs, and AIs, are being evaluated for their ability to reduce the risk of breast cancer. Tamoxifen and raloxifene have demonstrated efficacy in decreasing rates of invasive breast cancer in women who are at high risk of developing the disease. Early detection of breast cancer remains important for decreasing breast cancer mortality. The rationale for early detection of breast cancer is based on the clear relationship between stage of breast cancer at diagnosis and the probability of a cure. The ACS and other groups have developed screening guidelines for early detection of breast cancer. Although these guidelines differ, the overall benefits of screening mammography are apparent in their recommendations. Incorporation of newer screening methods (e.g., MRI) into these guidelines has occurred and will continue to evolve as new data become available.

Intensive research efforts are ongoing in all aspects of breast cancer etiology, detection, prevention, and treatment. Thanks to the thousands of patients who volunteered for these clinical trials, a substantial reduction in mortality has been seen in select patient subsets. It is hoped that the information obtained in the next decade will result in the knowledge required to significantly reduce mortality from breast cancer for all women. Only through these continued efforts and participation of patient volunteers will advances be made in the management of this disease.

ABBREVIATIONS

ACS: American Cancer Society

AI: aromatase inhibitor

ASCO: American Society of Clinical Oncology

BCT: breast-conserving therapy

BSE: breast self-examination

CALGB: Cancer and Leukemia Group B

CBE: clinical breast examination

CMF: cyclophosphamide, methotrexate, fluorouracil (regimen)

DCIS: ductal carcinoma in situ

DFS: disease-free survival

ER: estrogen receptor

FISH: fluorescence in situ hybridization

HR: hazard ratio

IHC: immunohistochemistry

LCIS: lobular carcinoma in situ

LHRH: luteinizing hormone-releasing hormone

MA: megestrol acetate

NCCN: National Comprehensive Cancer Network

NNI: number needed to invite for screening to extend one woman's life

NSABP: National Surgical Adjuvant Breast and Bowel Project

OS: overall survival

PFS: progression-free survival

PR: progesterone receptor

RR: relative risk

SERD: selective estrogen receptor downregulator

SERM: selective estrogen receptor modulators

USPSTF: United States Preventive Services Task Force

REFERENCES

1. Jemal A, Siegel R, Xu J, Ward E, et al. Cancer statistics 2010. CA Cancer J Clin 2010;60:277–300.
2. Cancer Facts & Figures 2009. 2009 [cited 2010 January 19]; Available from: http://www.cancer.org/acs/groups/content/@nho/documents/document/bcfffinalpdf.pdf.
3. Ghafoor A, Jemal A, Ward E, et al. Trends in breast cancer by race and ethnicity. CA Cancer J Clin 2003;53:342–355.
4. Berry DA, Cronin KA, Plevritis SK, et al. Effect of screening and adjuvant therapy on mortality from breast cancer. N Engl J Med 2005;353:1784–1792.
5. Effects of chemotherapy and hormonal therapy for early breast cancer on recurrence and 15-year survival: An overview of the randomised trials. Lancet 2005;365:1687–1717.
6. Fentiman IS, Fourquet A, Hortobagyi GN. Male breast cancer. Lancet 2006;367:595–604.
7. Fay MP, Pfeiffer R, Cronin KA, et al. Age-conditional probabilities of developing cancer. Stat Med 2003;22:1837–1848.
8. Gail MH, Costantino JP, Pee D, et al. Projecting individualized absolute invasive breast cancer risk in African American women. J Natl Cancer Inst 2007;99(23):1782–1792.
9. Clemons M, Goss P. Estrogen and the risk of breast cancer. N Engl J Med 2001;344:276–285.
10. Velie EM, Nechuta S, Osuch JR. Lifetime reproductive and anthropometric risk factors for breast cancer in postmenopausal women. Breast Dis 2005;24:17–35.
11. Rossouw JE, Anderson GL, Prentice RL, et al. Risks and benefits of estrogen plus progestin in healthy postmenopausal women: Principal results From the Women's Health Initiative randomized controlled trial. JAMA 2002;288:321–333.
12. Ravdin PM, Cronin KA, Howlader N, et al. The decrease in breast-cancer incidence in 2003 in the United States. N Engl J Med 2007;356(16):1670–1674.
13. Anderson GL, Limacher M, Assaf AR, et al. Effects of conjugated equine estrogen in postmenopausal women with hysterectomy: The Women's Health Initiative randomized controlled trial. JAMA 2004;291:1701–1712.
14. Colditz GA. Estrogen, estrogen plus progestin therapy, and risk of breast cancer. Clin Cancer Res 2005;11(Pt 2):909s–917s.
15. Marchbanks PA, McDonald JA, Wilson HG, et al. Oral contraceptives and the risk of breast cancer. N Engl J Med 2002;346:2025–2032.
16. Vessey M, Painter R. Oral contraceptive use and cancer. Findings in a large cohort study, 1968-2004. Br J Cancer 2006;95:385–389.
17. Meisner AL, Fekrazad MH, Royce ME. Breast disease: benign and malignant. Med Clin North Am 2008;92(5):1115–1141, x.
18. McCormack VA, dos Santos Silva I. Breast density and parenchymal patterns as markers of breast cancer risk: A meta-analysis. Cancer Epidemiol Biomarkers Prev 2006;15:1159–1169.
19. Collaborative Group on Hormonal Factors in Breast Cancer. Familial breast cancer: Collaborative reanalysis of individual data from 52 epidemiological studies including 58,209 women with breast cancer and 101,986 women without the disease. Lancet 2001;358:1389–1399.
20. Narod SA, Foulkes WD. BRCA1 and BRCA2: 1994 and beyond. Rev Cancer 2004;4:665–676.
21. U.S. Preventive Services Task Force. Genetic risk assessment and BRCA mutation testing for breast and ovarian cancer susceptibility: Recommendation statement. Ann Intern Med 2005;143:355–361.
22. Nelson HD, Huffman LH, Fu R, et al. Genetic risk assessment and BRCA mutation testing for breast and ovarian cancer susceptibility: Systematic evidence review for the US Preventive Services Task Force. Ann Intern Med 2005;143:362–379.
23. ASCO Working Group on Genetic Testing for Cancer Susceptibility. American Society of Clinical Oncology policy statement update: Genetic testing for cancer susceptibility. J Clin Oncol 2003;21: 2397–2406.
24. NCCN Clinical Practice Guidelines in Oncology: Genetic/Familial High-Risk Assessment: Breast and Ovarian v.1.2009. NCCN Clinical Practice Guidelines in Oncology 2009. http://www.nccn.org/professionals/physician_gls/PDF/genetics_screening.pdf.
25. BRACAnalysis product information. Salt Lake City, UT: Myriad Genetic Laboratories, Inc.; 2010. http://www.myriadtests.com/index.php?page_id=68.
26. Lynch HT, Silva E, Snyder C, Lynch JF. Hereditary breast cancer: part I. Diagnosing hereditary breast cancer syndromes. Breast J 2008;14: 3–13.
27. Boyd NF, Stone J, Vogt KN, et al. Dietary fat and breast cancer risk revisited: A meta-analysis of the published literature. Br J Cancer 2003;89:1672–1685.
28. Taylor VH, Misra M, Mukherjee SD. Is red meat intake a risk factor for breast cancer among premenopausal women? Breast Cancer Res Treat 2009;117:1–8.
29. Gandini S, Merzenich H, Robertson C, et al. Meta-analysis of studies on breast cancer risk and diet: The role of fruit and vegetable consumption and the intake of associated micronutrients. Eur J Cancer 2000;36:636–646.

30. van Gils CH, Peeters PH, Bueno-de-Mesquita HB, et al. Consumption of vegetables and fruits and risk of breast cancer. JAMA 2005;293:183–193.

31. Velentzis LS, Woodside JV, Cantwell MM, et al. Do phytoestrogens reduce the risk of breast cancer and breast cancer recurrence? What clinicians need to know. Eur J Cancer 2008;44(13):1799–1806.

32. Trock BJ, Hilakivi-Clarke L, Clarke R. Meta-analysis of soy intake and breast cancer risk. J Natl Cancer Inst 2006;98:459–471.

33. Velentzis LS, Cantwell MM, Cardwell C, et al. Lignans and breast cancer risk in pre- and post-menopausal women: meta-analyses of observational studies. Br J Cancer 2009;100(9):1492–1498.

34. Prentice RL, Caan B, Chlebowski RT, et al. Low-fat dietary pattern and risk of invasive breast cancer: The Women's Health Initiative Randomized Controlled Dietary Modification Trial. JAMA 2006;295:629–642.

35. Renehan AG, Tyson M, Egger M, Heller RF, Zwahlen M. Body-mass index and incidence of cancer: a systematic review and meta-analysis of prospective observational studies. Lancet 2008;371(9612):569–578.

36. Connolly BS, Barnett C, Vogt KN, et al. A meta-analysis of published literature on waist-to-hip ratio and risk of breast cancer. Nutr Cancer 2002;44:127–138.

37. Monninkhof EM, Elias SG, Vlems FA, et al. Physical activity and breast cancer: A systematic review. Epidemiology 2007;18:137–157.

38. Key J, Hodgson S, Omar RZ, et al. Meta-analysis of studies of alcohol and breast cancer with consideration of the methodological issues. Cancer Causes Control 2006;17:759–770.

39. Hamajima N, Hirose K, Tajima K, et al. Alcohol, tobacco and breast cancer—collaborative reanalysis of individual data from 53 epidemiological studies, including 58,515 women with breast cancer and 95,067 women without the disease. Br J Cancer 2002;87:1234–1245.

40. Ronckers CM, Erdmann CA, Land CE. Radiation and breast cancer: A review of current evidence. Breast Cancer Res 2005;7:21–32.

41. Helvie MA. Imaging analysis: Mammography, In: Harris JR, Lippman ME, Morrow M, et al., eds. Diseases of the Breast, 3rd ed. Philadelphia, PA: Lippincott Williams & Wilkins, 2004:131–148.

42. NCCN Clinical Practice Guidelines in Oncology: Breast Cancer Screening and Diagnosis Guidelines v.1.2010. NCCN Clinical Practice Guidelines in Oncology 2010. http://www.nccn.org/professionals/physician_gls/PDF/breast-screening.pdf.

43. D'Orsi C, Bassett BL, Berg W, et al. ACR Breast Imaging Reporting and Data System (BI-RADS Atlas), 4th ed. Reston, VA: American College of Radiology, 2003.

44. Brenin DR. Management of the palpable breast mass. In: Harris JR, Lippmann ME, Morrow M, et al., eds. Diseases of the Breast, 3rd ed. Philadelphia, PA: Lippincott Williams & Wilkins, 2004:33–46.

45. American Joint Committee on Cancer (AJCC), Chicago, Illinois. The original source for this material is the AJCC Cancer Staging Manual, 7th ed. (2010) published by Springer Science and Business Media LLC, www.springer.com.

46. Schnitt SJ, Guidi AJ. Pathology of invasive breast cancer. In: Harris JR, Lippman ME, Morrow M, et al., eds. Diseases of the Breast, 3rd ed. Philadelphia, PA: Lippincott Williams & Wilkins, 2004:541–584.

47. NCCN Clinical Practice Guidelines in Oncology: Breast Cancer v.1.2010. NCCN Clinical Practice Guidelines in Oncology; 2010. http://www.nccn.org/professionals/physician_gls/PDF/breast.pdf.

48. Merajver SD, Sabel MS. Inflammatory breast cancer. In: Harris JR, Lippman ME, Marrow M, et al., eds. Diseases of the Breast, 3rd ed. Philadelphia, PA: Lippincott Williams & Wilkins, 2004:971–982.

49. Sprague BL, Trentham-Dietz A. Prevalence of breast carcinoma in situ in the United States. JAMA 2009;302(8):846–848.

50. Newman LA. Lobular carcinoma in situ: Clinical management. In: Harris JR, Lippman ME, Morrow M, et al., eds. Diseases of the Breast, 3rd ed. Philadelphia, PA: Lippincott Williams & Wilkins, 2004;497–506.

51. Morrow M, Harris JR. Ductal carcinoma in situ and microinvasive carcinoma. In: Harris JR, Lippman ME, Morrow M, et al., eds. Diseases of the Breast, 3rd ed. Philadelphia, PA: Lippincott Williams & Wilkins, 2004;521–540.

52. Kuerer HM, Albarracin CT, Yang WT, et al. Ductal carcinoma in situ: state of the science and roadmap to advance the field. J Clin Oncol 2009;27(2):279–288.

53. Fisher B, Dignam J, Wolmark N, et al. Tamoxifen in treatment of intraductal breast cancer: National Surgical Adjuvant Breast and Bowel Project B-24 randomised controlled trial. Lancet 1999;353:1993–2000.

54. NCCN Clinical Practice Guidelines in Oncology: Breast Cancer Risk Reduction v.2.2009. NCCN Clinical Practice Guidelines in Oncology 2009. http://www.nccn.org/professionals/physician_gls/PDF/breast_risk.pdf.

55. Fisher B, Costantino JP, Wickerham DL, et al. Tamoxifen for prevention of breast cancer: Report of the National Surgical Adjuvant Breast and Bowel Project P-1 Study. J Natl Cancer Inst 1998;90:1371–1388.

56. Vogel VG, Costantino JP, Wickerham DL, et al. Effects of tamoxifen vs raloxifene on the risk of developing invasive breast cancer and other disease outcomes: The NSABP Study of Tamoxifen and Raloxifene (STAR) P-2 trial. JAMA 2006;295:2727–2741.

57. Kwan ML, Kushi LH, Weltzien E, Castillo A, Caan BJ. Alcohol and breast cancer survival in a prospective cohort study. Abstract presented at: 32nd Annual CTRC-AACR San Antonio Breast Cancer Symposium; December 9-13, 2009; San Antonio, TX.

58. Pierce JP, Natarajan L, Caan BJ, et al. Influence of a diet very high in vegetables, fruit, and fiber and low in fat on prognosis following treatment for breast cancer: the Women's Healthy Eating and Living (WHEL) randomized trial. JAMA 2007;298(3):289–298.

59. Chlebowski RT, Blackburn GL, Thomson CA, et al. Dietary fat reduction and breast cancer outcome: Interim efficacy results from the Women's Intervention Nutrition Study. J Natl Cancer Inst 2006;98:1767–1776.

60. Irwin ML, Smith AW, McTiernan A, et al. Influence of pre- and postdiagnosis physical activity on mortality in breast cancer survivors: the health, eating, activity, and lifestyle study. J Clin Oncol 2008;26(24):3958–3964.

61. Doyle C, Kushi LH, Byers T, et al. Nutrition and physical activity during and after cancer treatment: an American Cancer Society guide for informed choices. CA Cancer J Clin 2006;56(6):323–353.

62. Ejlertsen B, Jensen MB, Rank F, et al. Population-based study of peritumoral lymphovascular invasion and outcome among patients with operable breast cancer. J Natl Cancer Inst 2009;101(10):729–735.

63. Stuart-Harris R, Caldas C, Pinder SE, Pharoah P. Proliferation markers and survival in early breast cancer: a systematic review and meta-analysis of 85 studies in 32,825 patients. Breast 2008;17(4):323–334.

64. Wolff AC, Hammond ME, Schwartz JN, et al. American Society of Clinical Oncology/College of American Pathologists guideline recommendations for human epidermal growth factor receptor 2 testing in breast cancer. J Clin Oncol 2007;25:118–145.

65. Sauter G, Lee J, Bartlett JM, et al. Guidelines for human epidermal growth factor receptor 2 testing: biologic and methodologic considerations. J Clin Oncol 2009;27(8):1323–1333.

66. Dawood S, Broglio K, Buzdar AU, et al. Prognosis of women with metastatic breast cancer by HER2 status and trastuzumab treatment: an institutional-based review. J Clin Oncol 2010;28(1):92–98.

67. Ravdin PM, Siminoff LA, Davis GJ, et al. Computer program to assist in making decisions about adjuvant therapy for women with early breast cancer. J Clin Oncol 2001;19:980–991.

68. Paik S, Shak S, Tang G, et al. A multigene assay to predict recurrence of tamoxifen-treated, node-negative breast cancer. N Engl J Med 2004;351:2817–2826.

69. Buyse M, Loi S, van't Veer L, et al. Validation and clinical utility of a 70-gene prognostic signature for women with node-negative breast cancer. J Natl Cancer Inst 2006;98:1183–1192.

70. Harris L, Fritsche H, Mennel R, et al; American Society of Clinical Oncology. American Society of Clinical Oncology 2007 update of recommendations for the use of tumor markers in breast cancer. J Clin Oncol 2007;25(33):5287–5312.

71. NIH Consensus Development Conference on the Treatment of Early-Stage Breast Cancer. Bethesda, MD, June 18–21. J Natl Cancer Inst Monogr 1992:1–187.

72. Jatoi I, Proschan MA. Randomized trials of breast-conserving therapy versus mastectomy for primary breast cancer: A pooled analysis of updated results. Am J Clin Oncol 2005;28:289–294.

73. Morris AD, Morris RD, Wilson JF, et al. Breast-conserving therapy vs mastectomy in early-stage breast cancer: A meta-analysis of 10-year survival. Cancer J Sci Am 1997;3:6–12.

74. Clarke M, Collins R, Darby S, et al. Effects of radiotherapy and of differences in the extent of surgery for early breast cancer on local recurrence and 15-year survival: An overview of the randomised trials. Lancet 2005;366:2087–2106.

75. Yang SH, Yang KH, Li YP, et al. Breast conservation therapy for stage I or stage II breast cancer: a meta-analysis of randomized controlled trials. Ann Oncol 2008;19(6):1039–1044.

76. Komoike Y, Akiyama F, Iino Y, et al. Ipsilateral breast tumor recurrence (IBTR) after breast-conserving treatment for early breast cancer: Risk factors and impact on distant metastases. Cancer 2006;106: 35–41.

77. Zhou P, Gautam S, Recht A. Factors affecting outcome for young women with early stage invasive breast cancer treated with breast-conserving therapy. Breast Cancer Res Treat 2007;10151–10157.

78. Golshan M, Miron A, Nixon AJ, et al. The prevalence of germline BRCA1 and BRCA2 mutations in young women with breast cancer undergoing breast-conservation therapy. Am J Surg 2006;192: 58–62.

79. Buchholz TA. Radiation therapy for early-stage breast cancer after breast-conserving surgery. N Engl J Med 2009;360(1):63–70.

80. Ivens D, Hoe AL, Podd TJ, et al. Assessment of morbidity from complete axillary dissection. Br J Cancer 1992;66:136–138.

81. Keramopoulos A, Tsionou C, Minaretzis D, et al. Arm morbidity following treatment of breast cancer with total axillary dissection: A multivariated approach. Oncology 1993;50:445–449.

82. Lyman GH, Giuliano AE, Somerfield MR, et al. American Society of Clinical Oncology guideline recommendations for sentinel lymph node biopsy in early-stage breast cancer. J Clin Oncol 2005;23: 7703–7720.

83. Quan ML, McCready D. The evolution of lymph node assessment in breast cancer. J Surg Oncol 2009;99(4):194–198.

84. Kim T, Giuliano AE, Lyman GH. Lymphatic mapping and sentinel lymph node biopsy in early-stage breast carcinoma: A metaanalysis. Cancer 2006;106:4–16.

85. Surgical guidelines for the management of breast cancer. Association of Breast Surgery at Baso 2009. Eur J Surg Oncol 2009;35(Suppl 1): 1–22.

86. Consensus Statement on Guidelines for Performing Sentinel Lymph Node Dissection in Breast Cancer October 19, 2003; 2005. *http://www. breastsurgeons.org/slnd.shtml.*

87. van der Ploeg IM, Nieweg OE, van Rijk MC, et al. Axillary recurrence after a tumour-negative sentinel node biopsy in breast cancer patients: A systematic review and meta-analysis of the literature. Eur J Surg Oncol 2008;34(12):1277–1284.

88. Goldhirsch A, Ingle JN, Gelber RD, et al. Thresholds for therapies: highlights of the St Gallen International Expert Consensus on the primary therapy of early breast cancer 2009. Ann Oncol 2009;20(8): 1319–1329.

89. Ravdin PM, Siminoff IA, Harvey JA. Survey of breast cancer patients concerning their knowledge and expectations of adjuvant therapy. J Clin Oncol 1998;16:515–521.

90. Lindley C, Vasa S, Sawyer WT, et al. Quality of life and preferences for treatment following systemic adjuvant therapy for early-stage breast cancer. J Clin Oncol 1998;16:1380–1387.

91. Mook S, Schmidt MK, Rutgers EJ, et al. Calibration and discriminatory accuracy of prognosis calculation for breast cancer with the online Adjuvant! program: a hospital-based retrospective cohort study. Lancet Oncol 2009;10(11):1070–1076.

92. Campbell HE, Taylor MA, Harris AL, Gray AM. An investigation into the performance of the Adjuvant! Online prognostic programme in early breast cancer for a cohort of patients in the United Kingdom. Br J Cancer 2009;101(7):1074–1084.

93. Bedard PL, Cardoso F. Recent advances in adjuvant systemic therapy for early-stage breast cancer. Ann Oncol 2008;19(Suppl 5):v122–v127.

94. Lopez-Tarruella S, Martin M. Recent advances in systemic therapy: advances in adjuvant systemic chemotherapy of early breast cancer. Breast Cancer Res 2009;11(2):204.

95. Fisher B, Brown A, Mamounas E, et al. Effect of preoperative chemotherapy on local-regional disease in women with operable breast cancer: Findings from National Surgical Adjuvant Breast and Bowel Project B-18. J Clin Oncol 1997;15:2483–2493.

96. Fisher B, Bryant J, Wolmark N, et al. Effect of preoperative chemotherapy on the outcome of women with operable breast cancer. J Clin Oncol 1998;16:2672–2685.

97. Rastogi, P., et al., Preoperative chemotherapy: updates of National Surgical Adjuvant Breast and Bowel Project Protocols B-18 and B-27. J Clin Oncol, 2008. 26(5):778–85.

98. De Laurentiis M, Anderson SJ, Bear HD, et al. Taxane-based combinations as adjuvant chemotherapy of early breast cancer: a meta-analysis of randomized trials. J Clin Oncol 2008;26(1):44–53.

99. Gluz O, Liedtke C, Gottschalk N, et al. Triple-negative breast cancer–current status and future directions. Ann Oncol 2009;20(12): 1913–1927.

100. Lohrisch C, Paltiel C, Gelmon K, et al. Impact on survival of time from definitive surgery to initiation of adjuvant chemotherapy for early-stage breast cancer. J Clin Oncol 2006;24(30):4888–4894.

101. Bonadonna G, Valagussa P, Moliterni A, et al. Adjuvant cyclophosphamide, methotrexate, and fluorouracil in node-positive breast cancer: The results of 20 years of follow-up. N Engl J Med 1995;332:901–906.

102. Citron ML, Berry DA, Cirrincione C, et al. Randomized trial of dosedense versus conventionally scheduled and sequential versus concurrent combination chemotherapy as postoperative adjuvant treatment of node-positive primary breast cancer: First report of Intergroup Trial C9741/Cancer and Leukemia Group B Trial 9741. J Clin Oncol 2003;21:1431–1439.

103. Sparano JA, Wang M, Martino S, et al. Weekly paclitaxel in the adjuvant treatment of breast cancer. N Engl J Med 2008;358(16): 1663–1671.

104. Seidman AD, Berry D, Cirrincione C, et al. Randomized phase III trial of weekly compared with every-3-weeks paclitaxel for metastatic breast cancer, with trastuzumab for all HER-2 overexpressors and random assignment to trastuzumab or not in HER-2 nonoverexpressors: final results of Cancer and Leukemia Group B protocol 9840. J Clin Oncol 2008;26(10):1642–1649.

105. Kummel S, Rezai M, Kimmig R, et al. Dose-dense chemotherapy for primary breast cancer. Curr Opin Obstet Gynecol 2007;19:75–81.

106. McArthur HL, Hudis CA. Breast cancer chemotherapy. Cancer J 2007;13(3):141–147.

107. Moore HC. Impact on quality of life of adjuvant therapy for breast cancer. Curr Oncol Rep 2007;9:42–46.

108. Groenvold M, Fayers PM, Petersen MA, et al. Breast cancer patients on adjuvant chemotherapy report a wide range of problems not identified by healthcare staff. Breast Cancer Res Treat 2007;103:185–195.

109. Orzano JA, Swain SM. Concepts and clinical trials of dose-dense chemotherapy for breast cancer. Clin Breast Cancer 2005;6:402–411.

110. Levine MN, Gent M, Hirsh J, et al. The thrombogenic effect of anticancer drug therapy in women with stage II breast cancer. N Engl J Med 1988;318:404–407.

111. Matesich SM, Shapiro CL. Second cancers after breast cancer treatment. Semin Oncol 2003;30:740–748.

112. Henderson IC, Sloss LJ, Jaffe N, et al. Serial studies of cardiac function in patients receiving Adriamycin. Cancer Treat Rep 1978;62:923–929.

113. Ellence (epirubicin) product information. New York: Pharmacia & Upjohn Company; Pfizer, Inc.; 2007. *http://www.pfizer.com/pfizer/ download/uspi_ellence.pdf.*

114. Perez EA, Romond EH, Suman VJ, et al. Updated results of the combined analysis of NCCTG N9831 and NSABP B-31. Adjuvant chemotherapy with or without trastuzumab (H) in patients with HER2-positive breast cancer. Presented at: ASCO Annual Meeting 2007. June 1–5, 2007; Chicago, IL. Abstract 511.

115. Smith I, Procter M, Gelber RD et al. 2-year follow-up of trastuzumab after adjuvant chemotherapy in HER2-positive breast cancer: a randomised controlled trial. Lancet 2007;369(9555):29–36.

116. Joensuu H, Kellokumpu-Lehtinen PL, Bono P, et al. Adjuvant docetaxel or vinorelbine with or without trastuzumab for breast cancer. N Engl J Med 2006;354:809–820.

117. Slamon D, Eiermann W, Robert N, et al. Phase III randomized trial comparing doxorubicin and cyclophosphamide followed by docetaxel (AC→T) with doxorubicin and cyclophosphamide followed by docetaxel and trastuzumab (AC→TH) with docetaxel, carboplatin and trastuzumab (TCH) in Her2neu positive early breast cancer patients: BCIRG 006 study. Paper presented at: 32nd Annual CTRC-

AACR San Antonio Breast Cancer Symposium; December 9-13, 2009; San Antonio, TX. Abstract 62.

118. Spielmann M, Roché H, Delozier T, et al. Trastuzumab for patients with axillary-node-positive breast cancer: results of the FNCLCC-PACS 04 trial. J Clin Oncol 2009;27(36):6129–6134.

119. Dahabreh IJ, Linardou H, Siannis F, et al. Trastuzumab in the adjuvant treatment of early-stage breast cancer: a systematic review and meta-analysis of randomized controlled trials. Oncologist 2008;13(6):620–630.

120. Herceptin (trastuzumab) product information. San Francisco, CA: Genetech, Inc.; 2009. *http://www.gene.com/gene/products/information/oncology/herceptin/insert.jsp.*

121. Halyard MY, Pisansky TM, Dueck AC, et al. Radiotherapy and adjuvant trastuzumab in operable breast cancer: tolerability and adverse event data from the NCCTG Phase III Trial N9831. J Clin Oncol 2009;27(16):2638–2644.

122. Gonzalez-Angulo AM, Litton JK, Broglio KR, et al. High risk of recurrence for patients with breast cancer who have human epidermal growth factor receptor 2-positive, node-negative tumors 1 cm or smaller. J Clin Oncol 2009;27(34):5700–5706.

123. Hillner B. Clinical and cost-effectiveness implications of the adjuvant trastuzumab in HER2+ breast cancer trials. Paper presented at: 28th Annual San Antonio Breast Cancer Symposium; December 10, 2005; San Antonio, TX. Abstract 5040.

124. Norum J. The cost-effectiveness issue of adjuvant trastuzumab in early breast cancer. Expert Opin Pharmacother 2006;7:1617–1625.

125. Chan AL, Leung HW, Lu CL, Lin SJ. Cost-effectiveness of trastuzumab as adjuvant therapy for early breast cancer: a systematic review. Ann Pharmacother 2009;43(2):296–303.

126. Love RR, Wiebe DA, Newcomb PA, et al. Effects of tamoxifen on cardiovascular risk factors in postmenopausal women. Ann Intern Med 1991;115:860–864.

127. Love RR, Mazess RB, Barden HS, et al. Effects of tamoxifen on bone mineral density in postmenopausal women with breast cancer. N Engl J Med 1992;326:852–856.

128. Albain KS, Barlow WE, Ravdin PM, et al. Adjuvant chemotherapy and timing of tamoxifen in postmenopausal patients with endocrine-responsive, node-positive breast cancer: a phase 3, open-label, randomised controlled trial. Lancet 2009;374(9707):2055–2063.

129. Fisher B, Dignam J, Bryant J, et al. Five versus more than five years of tamoxifen for lymph node-negative breast cancer: Updated findings from the National Surgical Adjuvant Breast and Bowel Project B-14 randomized trial. J Natl Cancer Inst 2001;93:684–690.

130. Higgins MJ, Rae JM, Flockhart DA, et al. Pharmacogenetics of tamoxifen: Who should undergo CYP2D6 genetic testing? J Natl Compr Canc Netw 2009;7(2):203–213.

131. Jin Y, Desta Z, Stearns V, et al. CYP2D6 genotype, antidepressant use, and tamoxifen metabolism during adjuvant breast cancer treatment. J Natl Cancer Inst 2005;97(1):30–39.

132. Nolvadex (tamoxifen) product information; 2003. *http://www.fda.gov/medwatch/SAFETY/2003/03Jan_labels/Nolvadex_01-03.PDF.*

133. Fareston (toremifene) product information. Memphis, TN: GTx, Inc.; 2004. *http://www.fareston.com/pdfs/Prescribing_Info.pdf.*

134. Hayes DF, Van Zyl JA, Hacking A, et al. Randomized comparison of tamoxifen and two separate doses of toremifene in postmenopausal patients with metastatic breast cancer. J Clin Oncol 1995;13:2556–2566.

135. Pagani O, Gelber S, Price K, et al. Toremifene and tamoxifen are equally effective for early-stage breast cancer: First results of International Breast Cancer Study Group Trials 12–93 and 14–93. Ann Oncol 2004;15:1749–1759.

136. Holli K. Tamoxifen versus toremifene in the adjuvant treatment of breast cancer. Eur J Cancer 2002;38(Suppl 6):S37–S38.

137. LHRH-agonists in Early Breast Cancer Overview group, Cuzick J, Ambroisine L, Davidson N, et al. Use of luteinising-hormone-releasing hormone agonists as adjuvant treatment in premenopausal patients with hormone-receptor-positive breast cancer: a meta-analysis of individual patient data from randomised adjuvant trials. Lancet 2007;369(9574):1711–1723.

138. Gnant M, Mlineritsch B, Schippinger W, et al. Endocrine therapy plus zoledronic acid in premenopausal breast cancer. N Engl J Med 2009; 360(7):679–691.

139. Howell A, Cuzick J, Baum M, et al. Results of the ATAC (Arimidex, Tamoxifen, Alone or in Combination) trial after completion of 5 years' adjuvant treatment for breast cancer. Lancet 2005;365:60–62.

140. Coates AS, Keshaviah A, Thurlimann B, et al. Five years of letrozole compared with tamoxifen as initial adjuvant therapy for postmenopausal women with endocrine-responsive early breast cancer: Update of study BIG 1–98. J Clin Oncol 2007;25:486–492.

141. Goss PE, Ingle JN, Martino S, et al. A randomized trial of letrozole in postmenopausal women after five years of tamoxifen therapy for early-stage breast cancer. N Engl J Med 2003;349:1793–1802.

142. Dowsett M, Cuzick J, Ingle J, et al. Meta-analysis of breast cancer outcomes in adjuvant trials of aromatase inhibitors versus tamoxifen. J Clin Oncol 2009;28(3):509–518.

143. BIG 1-98 Collaborative Group, Mouridsen H, Giobbie-Hurder A, Goldhirsch A, et al. Letrozole therapy alone or in sequence with tamoxifen in women with breast cancer. N Engl J Med 2009;361(8): 766–776.

144. Giordano SH. Update on locally advanced breast cancer. Oncologist 2003;8:521–530.

145. Kaufmann M, Hortobagyi GN, Goldhirsch A, et al. Recommendations from an international expert panel on the use of neoadjuvant (primary) systemic treatment of operable breast cancer: An update. J Clin Oncol 2006;24:1940–1949.

146. Buzdar AU, Ibrahim NK, Francis D, et al. Significantly higher pathologic complete remission rate after neoadjuvant therapy with trastuzumab, paclitaxel, and epirubicin chemotherapy: Results of a randomized trial in human epidermal growth factor receptor 2-positive operable breast cancer. J Clin Oncol 2005;23:3676–3685.

147. Hanrahan EO, Hennessy BT, Valero V. Neoadjuvant systemic therapy for breast cancer: An overview and review of recent clinical trials. Expert Opin Pharmacother 2005;6:1477–1491.

148. Macaskill EJ, Renshaw L, Dixon JM. Neoadjuvant use of hormonal therapy in elderly patients with early or locally advanced hormone receptor-positive breast cancer. Oncologist 2006;11:1081–1088.

149. Gralow JR, Biermann JS, Farooki A, et al. NCCN Task Force Report: Bone health in cancer care. J Natl Compr Canc Netw 2009;7(Suppl 3):S1–S32; quiz S33–S35.

150. Altundag K, Ibrahim NK. Aromatase inhibitors in breast cancer: An overview. Oncologist 2006;11:553–562.

151. Robertson J LD. Static disease of long duration (greater than 24 weeks) is an important remission criterion in breast cancer patients treated with the aromatase inhibitor "Arimidex" (anastrozole). Breast Cancer Res Treat 1997;46:214.

152. Paridaens RJ, Dirix LY, Beex LV, et al. Phase III study comparing exemestane with tamoxifen as first-line hormonal treatment of metastatic breast cancer in postmenopausal women: the European Organisation for Research and Treatment of Cancer Breast Cancer Cooperative Group. J Clin Oncol 2008;26(30):4883–4890.

153. Doyen J, Italiano A, Largillier R, et al. Aromatase inhibition in male breast cancer patients: biological and clinical implications. Ann Oncol 2009;21(6):1243–1245.

154. Stenbygaard LE, Herrstedt J, Thomsen JF, et al. Toremifene and tamoxifen in advanced breast cancer—a double-blind cross-over trial. Breast Cancer Res Treat 1993;25:57–63.

155. Valachis A, Mauri D, Polyzos NP, et al. Fulvestrant in the treatment of advanced breast cancer: A systematic review and meta-analysis of randomized controlled trials. Crit Rev Oncol Hematol 2009;73(3): 220–227.

156. Hackshaw A. Luteinizing hormone-releasing hormone (LHRH) agonists in the treatment of breast cancer. Expert Opin Pharmacother 2009;10(16):2633–2639.

157. Ingle JN, Krook JE, Green SJ, et al. Randomized trial of bilateral oophorectomy versus tamoxifen in premenopausal women with metastatic breast cancer. J Clin Oncol 1986;4:178–185.

158. Klijn JG, Blamey RW, Boccardo F, et al. Combined tamoxifen and luteinizing hormone-releasing hormone (LHRH) agonist versus LHRH agonist alone in premenopausal advanced breast cancer: A meta-analysis of four randomized trials. J Clin Oncol 2001;19: 343–353.

159. Michaud LB, Valero V, Hortobagyi G. Risks and benefits of taxanes in breast and ovarian cancer. Drug Saf 2000;23:401–428.

160. Mauri D, Kamposioras K, Tsali L, et al. Overall survival benefit for weekly vs. three-weekly taxanes regimens in advanced breast cancer: A meta-analysis. Cancer Treat Rev 2009;36(1):69–74.

161. Jones SE, Erban J, Overmoyer B, et al. Randomized phase III study of docetaxel compared with paclitaxel in metastatic breast cancer. J Clin Oncol 2005;23:5542–5551.

162. Gradishar WJ, Tjulandin S, Davidson N, et al. Phase III trial of nanoparticle albumin-bound paclitaxel compared with polyethylated castor oil-based paclitaxel in women with breast cancer. J Clin Oncol 2005;23:7794–7803.

163. Gralow JR. Optimizing the treatment of metastatic breast cancer. Breast Cancer Res Treat 2005;89(Suppl 1):S9–S15.

164. O'Brien ME, Wigler N, Inbar M, et al. Reduced cardiotoxicity and comparable efficacy in a phase III trial of pegylated liposomal doxorubicin HCl (CAELYX/Doxil) versus conventional doxorubicin for first-line treatment of metastatic breast cancer. Ann Oncol 2004;15:440–449.

165. Boehnke Michaud L. The optimal therapeutic use of ixabepilone in patients with locally advanced or metastatic breast cancer. J Oncol Pharm Pract 2009;15(2):95–106.

166. Sledge GW, Neuberg D, Bernardo P, et al. Phase III trial of doxorubicin, paclitaxel, and the combination of doxorubicin and paclitaxel as front-line chemotherapy for metastatic breast cancer: An intergroup trial (E1193). J Clin Oncol 2003;21:588–592.

167. O'Shaughnessy J, Miles D, Vukelja S, et al. Superior survival with capecitabine plus docetaxel combination therapy in anthracyclinepretreated patients with advanced breast cancer: Phase III trial results. J Clin Oncol 2002;20:2812–2823.

168. Cardoso F, Bedard PL, Winer EP, et al. International guidelines for management of metastatic breast cancer: combination vs sequential single-agent chemotherapy. J Natl Cancer Inst 2009;101(17):1174–1181.

169. Cobleigh MA, Vogel CL, Tripathy D, et al. Multinational study of the efficacy and safety of humanized anti-HER2 monoclonal antibody in women who have HER2-overexpressing metastatic breast cancer that has progressed after chemotherapy for metastatic disease. J Clin Oncol 1999;17:2639–2648.

170. Slamon DJ, Leyland-Jones B, Shak S, et al. Use of chemotherapy plus a monoclonal antibody against HER2 for metastatic breast cancer that overexpresses HER2. N Engl J Med 2001;344:783–792.

171. Marty M, Cognetti F, Maraninchi D, et al. Randomized phase II trial of the efficacy and safety of trastuzumab combined with docetaxel in patients with human epidermal growth factor receptor 2-positive metastatic breast cancer administered as first-line treatment: The M77001 study group. J Clin Oncol 2005;23:4265–4274.

172. von Minckwitz G, du Bois A, Schmidt M, et al. Trastuzumab beyond progression in human epidermal growth factor receptor 2-positive advanced breast cancer: a german breast group 26/breast international group 03-05 study. J Clin Oncol 2009;27(12):1999–2006.

173. Burstein HJ, Harris LN, Marcom PK, et al. Trastuzumab and vinorelbine as first-line therapy for HER2-overexpressing metastatic breast cancer: Multicenter phase II trial with clinical outcomes, analysis of serum tumor markers as predictive factors, and cardiac surveillance algorithm. J Clin Oncol 2003;21:2889–2895.

174. Robert N, Leyland-Jones B, Asmar L, et al. Phase III comparative study of trastuzumab and paclitaxel with and without carboplatin in patients with HER2/neu positive advanced breast cancer. Paper presented at: 25th Annual San Antonio Breast Cancer Symposium; December 10-14, 2005; San Antonio, TX. Abstract 35.

175. Forbes JF, Kennedy J, Pienkowski T, et al. BCIRG 007: Randomized phase III trial of trastuzumab plus docetaxel with or without carboplatin first line in HER2 positive metastatic breast cancer (MBC) (meeting abstract). Paper presented at: ASCO Annual Meeting Proceeding; J Clin Oncol 2006;24(18S). Abstract LBA516.

176. Kaufman B, Mackey JR, Clemens MR, et al. Trastuzumab plus anastrozole versus anastrozole alone for the treatment of postmenopausal women with human epidermal growth factor receptor 2-positive, hormone receptor-positive metastatic breast cancer: results from the randomized phase III TAnDEM study. J Clin Oncol 2009;27(33):5529–5537.

177. Ross JS, Slodkowska EA, Symmans WF, et al. The HER-2 receptor and breast cancer: ten years of targeted anti-HER-2 therapy and personalized medicine. Oncologist 2009;14(4):320–368.

178. Geyer CE, Forster J, Lindquist D, et al. Lapatinib plus capecitabine for HER2-positive advanced breast cancer. N Engl J Med 2006;355:2733–2743.

179. Di Leo A, Gomez HL, Aziz Z, et al. Phase III, double-blind, randomized study comparing lapatinib plus paclitaxel with placebo plus paclitaxel as first-line treatment for metastatic breast cancer. J Clin Oncol 2008;26(34):5544–5552.

180. Johnston S, Pippen J Jr, Pivot X, et al. Lapatinib combined with letrozole versus letrozole and placebo as first-line therapy for postmenopausal hormone receptor-positive metastatic breast cancer. J Clin Oncol 2009;27(33):5538–5546.

181. O'Shaughnessy JB, Blackwell KL, Burstein H, et al. A randomized study of lapatinib alone or in combination with trastuzumab in heavily pretreated HER2+ metastatic breast cancer progressing on trastuzumab therapy. J Clin Oncol 2008;26(May 20 Suppl). Abstract 1015.

182. Perez EA, Koehler M, Byrne J, et al. Cardiac safety of lapatinib: pooled analysis of 3689 patients enrolled in clinical trials. Mayo Clin Proc 2008;83(6):679–686.

183. Miller KD, Chap LI, Holmes FA, et al. Randomized phase III trial of capecitabine compared with bevacizumab plus capecitabine in patients with previously treated metastatic breast cancer. J Clin Oncol 2005;23:792–799.

184. Miller K, Wang M, Gralow J, et al. Paclitaxel plus bevacizumab versus paclitaxel alone for metastatic breast cancer. N Engl J Med 2007;357(26):2666–2676.

185. Miles DC, Chan A, Romieu G, et al. Randomized, double-blind, placebo-controlled, phase III study of bevacizumab with docetaxel or docetaxel with placebo as first-line therapy for patients with locally recurrent or metastatic breast cancer (mBC): AVADO. J Clin Oncol 2008;26(May 20 Suppl). Abstract LBA1011.

186. Robert NJ, Dieras V, Glaspy J, et al. RIBBON-1: Randomized, double-blind, placebo-controlled, phase III trial of chemotherapy with or without bevacizumab (B) for first-line treatment of HER2-negative locally recurrent or metastatic breast cancer (MBC). J Clin Oncol 2009;27(May 20 Suppl). Abstract 1005.

187. Brufsky AB, Bondarenko IN, Smirnov, V, et al. RIBBON-2: A randomized, double-blind, placebo-controlled, phase iii trial evaluating the efficacy and safety of bevacizumab in combination with chemotherapy for second-line treatment of HER2-negative metastatic breast cancer. Paper presented at: 32nd Annual San Antonio Breast Cancer Symposium; December 10-13, 2009; San Antonio, TX. Abstract 42.

188. Cuzick J, Powles T, Veronesi U, et al. Overview of the main outcomes in breast-cancer prevention trials. Lancet 2003;361:296–300.

189. Visvanathan K, Chlebowski RT, Hurley P, et al. American Society of Clinical Oncology clinical practice guideline update on the use of pharmacologic interventions including tamoxifen, raloxifene, and aromatase inhibition for breast cancer risk reduction. J Clin Oncol 2009;27(19):3235–3258.

190. Smith RA, Cokkinides V, Brawley OW. Cancer screening in the United States, 2009: A review of current American Cancer Society guidelines and issues in cancer screening. CA Cancer J Clin 2009;59(1):27–41.

191. Screening for breast cancer: U.S. Preventive Services Task Force recommendation statement. Ann Intern Med 2009;151(10):716–726, W–236.

192. Thomas DB, Gao DL, Self SG, et al. Randomized trial of breast self-examination in Shanghai: Methodology and preliminary results. J Natl Cancer Inst 1997;89:355–365.

193. Nelson HD, Tyne K, Naik A, et al. Screening for breast cancer: an update for the U.S. Preventive Services Task Force. Ann Intern Med 2009;151(10):727–737, W237–242.

194. Saslow D, Boetes C, Burke W, et al. American Cancer Society guidelines for breast screening with MRI as an adjunct to mammography. CA Cancer J Clin 2007;57:75–89.

137

Lung Cancer

DEBORAH A. FRIEZE AND VAL R. ADAMS

KEY CONCEPTS

❶ Lung cancer is the leading cause of cancer deaths in both men and women in the United States. The overall 5-year survival rate for all types of lung cancer is approximately 15%.

❷ Cigarette smoking is responsible for most lung cancers. Smoking cessation should be encouraged, particularly in those receiving curative treatment (i.e., stages I to IIIA non–small cell lung cancer and limited-stage small cell lung cancer).

❸ Non–small cell lung cancer (NSCLC) is diagnosed in most (~80%) lung cancer patients. NSCLC typically has a slower growth rate and doubling time than small cell lung cancer (SCLC).

❹ No screening test is currently recommended to identify lung cancer. However, several studies are evaluating different methods of screening in an attempt to diagnose lung cancer at an earlier stage, when it should be more curable.

❺ Treatment decisions are guided by the stage of disease, which is characterized by tumor size and spread. Patient-specific factors (i.e., performance status, co-morbid conditions, etc.) must also be considered when developing a treatment plan.

❻ The treatment goals in lung cancer are cure (early-stage disease), prolongation of survival, and maintenance or improvement of quality of life through alleviation of symptoms.

❼ Early-stage lung cancer has the highest cure rates when surgical resection of the tumor is used with or without chemotherapy for NSCLC and chemoradiotherapy for SCLC.

❽ Advanced-stage lung cancer is primarily treated with systemic therapy. Doublet chemotherapy regimens are superior in response to single-agent regimens and should be used when the patient can tolerate the associated toxicity. Platinum-containing doublets are first-line treatment in most cases of NSCLC and SCLC.

❾ Optimal patient care needs to include prevention and treatment of adverse events from chemotherapy. Adverse events may cause delays in chemotherapy administration, increase morbidity, and contribute to treatment failure.

Lung cancer is a major cause of morbidity and mortality. It has reached epidemic proportions in many industrialized countries and is the most frequently fatal malignancy in the world. It is estimated that 222,520 new cases of lung cancer were diagnosed in the United States in 2010.[1] Despite major advances in the understanding and management of lung cancer, the overall 5-year survival rate for all types of lung cancer remains a dismal 15%. In the United States, lung cancer is estimated to account for approximately 15% of all newly diagnosed cancer in adults.[2] ❶ It remains the leading cause of cancer death in both adult men and women, with about 157,300 deaths in 2010.[1] The incidence and death rate caused by lung cancer are declining in men, but the incidence recently plateaued and mortality continues to increase in women. Since 1987, lung cancer has surpassed breast cancer as the primary cause of cancer death in American women. In comparison to whites, the incidence of lung cancer is greater in African Americans, and the mortality rate is greater in African American men, but lower in African American women.[1]

The incidence of lung cancer increases with age, with peak age of diagnosis being between 55 and 65 years.[1] Among patients 40 years of age and older, the likelihood that a solitary pulmonary nodule seen on chest radiography is carcinoma is high, and this probability increases proportionately with age. Patients with lung cancer may undergo surgery, chemotherapy, radiation, or multimodality therapy, depending on the histological type of the tumor, its size and location, and the presence of metastases at diagnosis. Two leading oncology groups representing leading clinicians in the United States have published clinical practice guidelines for the treatment of lung cancer. The National Comprehensive Cancer Network (NCCN) has developed consensus-based guidelines that provide recommendations regarding the screening, staging, and treatment of both small cell lung cancer (SCLC) and non–small cell lung cancer (NSCLC).[3,4] The American Society of Clinical Oncology first published evidence-based guidelines regarding the staging and treatment of NSCLC in 1997, which were subsequently updated in 2003; they updated the stage IV NSCLC guideline in 2009.[5] In addition, the Agency for Healthcare Research and Quality has published an evidence report regarding the management of SCLC.[6] The American College of Chest Physicians (ACCP) also recently published evidence-based clinical practice guidelines.[7]

ETIOLOGY

Lung carcinomas arise from normal bronchial epithelial cells that have acquired multiple genetic lesions and are capable of expressing a variety of phenotypes.[2] Recently, significant advances have been made in understanding the molecular genetic changes involved in lung cancer pathogenesis.[2] A large variety of molecular lesions result in abrogation of key cellular regulatory and growth control pathways. Activation of a proto-oncogene, inhibition or mutation of tumor suppressor genes, and production of autocrine (self-stimulatory) growth factors contribute to cellular proliferation and malignant transformation.[2] Many of the autocrine loops and proto-oncogene and tumor suppressor gene changes are common to both SCLC and NSCLC, but certain mutations are found more frequently in each subtype of lung cancer. These unique tumor characteristics may offer more targeted interventions to prevent or treat lung cancer. For example, of the autocrine loops, SCLC frequently overexpresses c-KIT, whereas NSCLC frequently overexpresses epidermal growth factor receptor (EGFR).[2,8] EGFR inhibitors, such as erlotinib, are used clinically to treat NSCLC (see Human Epidermal Growth Factor Receptor Inhibitors) and offer a potential method of lung cancer chemoprevention. Properly designed clinical trials are necessary, however, as demonstrated by the lack of efficacy of imatinib in the treatment of SCLC. Although imatinib inhibits c-KIT kinase in several SCLC lines, no responses occurred in patients with SCLC overexpressing c-KIT.[9]

❷ Smoking is a major cause of lung cancer, with approximately 80% of lung cancer deaths in the United States directly attributed to tobacco use. Tobacco smoke contains many substances, including tumor promoters, carcinogens, and co-carcinogens.[2,10] Many of these carcinogens cause lung tumors in laboratory animals or humans and are likely to be involved in induction of lung cancer. Most cases of NSCLC and SCLC are caused by cigarette smoking, although cigars and pipes are also carcinogenic.[2,10] Smoking cessation is associated with a gradual decrease in the risk, but more than 5 years is necessary before an appreciable decline in risk occurs.[2,10] Although smoking cessation substantially reduces the risk of lung cancer, the risk is never lowered to that of a nonsmoker. Because of the public health implications, the United States has several, mainly state-led, tobacco control efforts, including antismoking campaigns, increased tobacco taxes, and smoke-free areas in many public areas. Continued efforts are needed as the prevalence of cigarette smoking has slowly decreased but was estimated to be approximately 18% in 2008.[11] The association between environmental tobacco smoke (ETS, also referred to as passive smoking) and lung cancer risk in nonsmokers in not as clear. Most studies have consistently found that spouses of smokers have higher rates of lung cancer than spouses of nonsmokers (~25% higher risk). Additionally, data from workplace exposure to environmental smoke seems to increase the risk of lung cancer by ~17%. The current estimates are that ETS contributes to approximately 3,000 lung cancers annually. Although many of these studies have flaws, the data seem consistent and seem to indicate a dose–risk relationship, with no safe level of exposure.[12]

Although most cases of lung cancer are attributable to cigarette smoking, less than 20% of smokers develop lung cancer, which suggests that other risk factors are relevant. An increased risk of lung cancer has been associated with exposure to other environmental respiratory carcinogens (e.g., asbestos, benzene). Genetic risk factors are also important, with an increased risk of lung cancer observed in those with first-degree relatives diagnosed with the disease. Lung cancer risk is associated with polymorphisms that affect the expression and/or function of enzymes regulating metabolism of tobacco carcinogens, DNA repair, or inflammation. Patients with a history of chronic obstructive airway disease and adults with asthma are at an increased risk for lung cancer.[1,2,7,12] Gathering data to better identify which patients are at highest risk of developing lung cancer will be key for new lung cancer screening trials and in chemoprevention trials.

HISTOLOGIC CLASSIFICATION

Before treatment begins, it is critical that an experienced lung cancer pathologist reviews the pathological material because of the different treatment regimens for NSCLC and SCLC. ❸ NSCLC is

---

TABLE 137-1 The World Health Organization/International Association for the Study of Lung Cancer Histologic Classification of Non-Small Cell Lung Carcinomas

1. Squamous cell carcinoma
   - Papillary
   - Clear cell
   - Small cell
   - Basaloid
2. Adenocarcinoma
   - Acinar
   - Papillary
   - Bronchioloalveolar carcinoma
     - Nonmucinous
     - Mucinous
     - Mixed mucinous and nonmucinous or indeterminate cell type
   - Solid adenocarcinoma with mucin
   - Adenocarcinoma with mixed subtypes
   - Variants
     - Well-differentiated fetal adenocarcinoma
     - Mucinous (colloid) adenocarcinoma
     - Mucinous cystadenocarcinoma
     - Signet ring adenocarcinoma
     - Clear cell adenocarcinoma
3. Large cell carcinoma
   - Variants
     - Large cell neuroendocrine carcinoma
     - Combined large cell neuroendocrine carcinoma
     - Basaloid carcinoma
     - Lymphoepithelioma-like carcinoma
     - Clear cell carcinoma
     - Large cell carcinoma with rhabdoid phenotype
4. Adenosquamous carcinoma
5. Carcinomas with pleomorphic, sarcomatoid, or sarcomatous elements
   - Carcinomas with spindle and/or giant cells
   - Spindle cell carcinoma
   - Giant cell carcinoma
   - Carcinosarcoma
   - Pulmonary blastoma
6. Carcinoid tumor
   - Typical carcinoid
   - Atypical carcinoid
7. Carcinomas of salivary gland type
   - Mucoepidermoid carcinoma
   - Adenoid cystic carcinoma
   - Others
8. Unclassified carcinoma

Adapted from references 13 and 14.

---

diagnosed in most (80%) lung cancer patients. NSCLC typically has a slower growth rate and doubling time than SCLC. The World Health Organization Classification of Lung Cancer is widely accepted (Table 137–1). In the most recent update of this classification, adenocarcinoma was further subclassified, the definition of bronchioalveolar carcinoma was restricted to noninvasive tumors, and large cell neuroendocrine carcinoma was recognized histologically as a high-grade NSCLC.[2,4]

Four major cell types of carcinomas (squamous cell, adenocarcinoma, large cell, and small cell) account for more than 90% of all lung tumors. Because squamous cell, adenocarcinoma, and large cell carcinomas have a similar overall prognosis and treatment strategy, they are frequently grouped together and referred to as NSCLC. Historically, NSCLC's treatment regimens did not differ between histology, but clinical trials with newer agents have shown differences in efficacy and toxicity with regard to histology. Consequently, knowledge concerning the histology is essential in optimizing drug therapy.[2,4]

Squamous cell carcinoma was once the most common histology but is now estimated to constitute less than 30% of all lung cancers. Squamous cell carcinomas have a much higher incidence in smokers and among males and appear to have a strong dose-response relationship to tobacco exposure. The majority of these tumors occur centrally, but the incidence of peripheral presentation is increasing. Although they can grow rapidly, most squamous cell carcinomas tend to be slow growing and confined to the lungs (especially early in the disease course). Such tumors may eventually metastasize to the hilar and mediastinal lymph nodes, liver, adrenal glands, kidneys, bone, and gastrointestinal tract.[2,4]

Adenocarcinoma accounts for about one-half of lung cancers and is increasing in frequency. As outlined in Table 137–1, there are several subclassifications of adenocarcinoma, and mixed histologies predominate. The importance of these subtypes to treatment is currently limited, but newer targeted therapies may work best in certain subtypes, thus allowing more individualized treatment selection. For example, erlotinib is generally effective in adenocarcinoma, but it appears to be most effective in patients with the bronchioloalveolar subtype of adenocarcinoma. Adenocarcinoma is the most common subtype in nonsmoking lung cancer patients. Patients with adenocarcinoma can present with a single nodule, multifocal nodules, or rapidly progressing, bilateral, diffuse processes. This histology is likely to metastasize at an early stage (often before the diagnosis of the primary tumor) and spread widely to distant sites, including the contralateral lung, liver, bone, adrenal glands, kidneys, and central nervous system. As a result, adenocarcinoma has a worse prognosis than squamous cell carcinoma; however, the prognosis is similar when controlled for stage.[2,4]

Large cell carcinomas are undifferentiated epithelial tumors, which are often a diagnosis of exclusion. These tumors tend to be large and bulky tumors arising in the periphery of the lung, have a propensity to metastasize in a pattern quite similar to adenocarcinomas, and are associated with a similar poor prognosis.[2,4]

Small cell carcinomas account for approximately 15% of all lung tumors. Nearly all SCLCs are immunoreactive for keratin, epithelial membrane antigen, and thyroid transcription factor 1, and many stain positively for markers of neuroendocrine differentiation. They are distinguished by a proliferation of neoplastic cells with round to oval nuclei. These tumors occur in both the major bronchi and the periphery of the lung. SCLC is a very aggressive and rapidly growing tumor, with approximately 60% to 70% of patients initially presenting with disseminated disease outside of the hemithorax. These tumors commonly express neuroendocrine differentiation, which may account for some of the paraneoplastic syndromes frequently associated with this disease. SCLC secretes gastrin-releasing peptide that acts as an autocrine growth factor. Secretion of other peptide hormones, cytogenetic abnormalities, and amplification and increased expression of oncogenes are also common. This disease has a propensity to metastasize to the lymph nodes, opposite lung, liver, adrenal glands and other endocrine organs, bone, bone marrow, and central nervous system.[2,3]

Lung can exhibit more than one histological cell type (e.g., adenosquamous), which may impact therapy. Occasionally, patients can also have multiple lung nodules arising in different lobes or the contralateral lung. They can be the same or different histology. This is referred to as synchronous tumors, and the nodules may be of similar or different cell types. This usually worsens the patient's overall prognosis.

CLINICAL PRESENTATION

At the time of diagnosis, 16% of lung cancers are localized, 25% have regional spread, and 51% have distant metastases (the remaining were not staged).[1] Location and extent of the tumor determine the presenting signs and symptoms. A lesion in the central portion of the bronchial tree is more likely to cause symptoms at an earlier stage as compared with a lesion in the periphery of the lung, which may remain asymptomatic until the lesion is large or has spread to other areas. The most common initial signs and symptoms include cough, dyspnea, and chest pain or discomfort, with or without hemoptysis.[2] Unfortunately, many patients with lung cancer also have chronic pulmonary and/or cardiovascular diseases (usually related to smoking), and such symptoms may go unnoticed or be attributed to the concomitant disease. Many patients also exhibit systemic symptoms of malignancy such as anorexia, weight loss, and fatigue. Disseminated disease can cause extrapulmonary signs and symptoms such as neurological deficits resulting from CNS metastases, bone pain or pathological fractures secondary to bone metastases, or liver dysfunction resulting from tumor involvement in the liver.[2]

CLINICAL PRESENTATION OF LUNG CANCER

Local Signs and Symptoms Associated with Primary Tumor or Regional Spread within the Thorax

- Cough
- Hemoptysis
- Dyspnea
- Rust-streaked or purulent sputum
- Chest, shoulder, or arm pain
- Wheeze and stridor
- Superior vena cava obstruction
- Pleural effusion or pneumonitis
- Dysphagia (secondary to esophageal compression)
- Hoarseness (secondary to laryngeal nerve paralysis)
- Horner's syndrome
- Phrenic nerve paralysis
- Pericardial effusion/tamponade
- Tracheal obstruction

Extrapulmonary Signs and Symptoms Associated with Metastatic Involvement

- Bone pain and/or pathologic fractures
- Liver dysfunction
- Neurologic deficits
- Spinal cord compression

Paraneoplastic Syndromes

- Weight loss
- Cushing's syndrome
- Hypercalcemia (most commonly in squamous cell lung cancer)
- Syndrome of inappropriate secretion of antidiuretic hormone (most commonly in SCLC)
- Pulmonary hypertrophic osteoarthropathy
- Clubbing
- Anemia
- Eaton-Lambert's myasthenic syndrome
- Hypercoagulable state

Paraneoplastic syndromes are signs and symptoms that occur at sites away from the primary tumor or its metastases and are not associated with direct tumor involvement. They may be caused by the production of biologically active substances (e.g., peptide hormones) or antibodies, or by other undefined mechanisms. Paraneoplastic syndromes occur more frequently with lung cancer than with any other tumor, and more frequently with SCLC than with NSCLC. These syndromes may be the first signs of a tumor and may prompt the search for an underlying malignancy.[2]

SCREENING AND PREVENTION

❹ Most lung cancer patients are diagnosed with advanced disease, which is a key factor in the poor prognosis associated with this disease. Surgery (NSCLC) and radiation (SCLC) are the most effective treatment modalities, which generally limits curative intent to patients diagnosed at an early clinical stage.[2-4] Therefore, it is important to diagnose lung cancer earlier through screening and identify early signs and symptoms. Several screening techniques, including computed tomography (CT) and positron emission tomography (PET) scanning, are being investigated to detect lung cancer at an earlier stage.[13] However, screening is not part of the current recommendations. The current approach is based on diagnosing lung cancer in patients who present with signs and symptoms. Patients interested in screening should be enrolled in a clinical trial.

The term *chemoprevention* refers to the use of prophylactic medications to prevent the development of cancer. Many studies of potential chemopreventive agents, including nonsteroidal anti-inflammatory drugs (NSAIDs), retinoids, inhaled glucocorticoids, vitamin E, selenium, and green tea extracts, have been conducted, but none have been successful.[14] Large randomized clinical trials have evaluated β-carotene as a lung cancer chemopreventive agent in high-risk patients (older smokers). Rather than prevent lung cancer, the trials clearly show that older people who smoke have a higher risk of developing and dying of lung cancer if they take a β-carotene supplement. Nonsmokers do not appear to have an altered risk of lung cancer with β-carotene consumption.[8] The impact of selenium and/or vitamin E supplementation was evaluated in older men as part of a large prostate cancer prevention study (SELECT trial).[15] Unfortunately, no benefit was seen with selenium or vitamin E supplementation.[8,15]

Since screening and chemoprevention trials have not yet proven to provide a survival benefit, the current recommendation is to avoid smoking and maintain a healthy diet with high amounts of fruits and vegetables.[16]

DIAGNOSIS

A patient suspected of have lung cancer should undergo a diagnostic evaluation. Diagnosis of lung cancer requires both visualization of the cancerous lesion and tissue sampling for pathological assessment. All patients must have a thorough history and physical examination with emphasis on detecting signs and symptoms of the primary tumor, regional spread of the tumor, distant metastases, and paraneoplastic syndromes. The patient's performance status should be assessed to determine whether or not a patient may be able to tolerate surgery and/or chemotherapy.[2-4]

Visualization of the suspected tumor provides the clinician with the information necessary to choose the most appropriate sampling technique. Chest radiographs, endobronchial ultrasound, CT scans, and PET scans are among the most valuable diagnostic tests.[17] Chest radiography is the primary method of lung cancer detection and may also be used to measure tumor size, establish gross lymph node enlargement, and detect other tumor-related findings, such as pleural effusion, lobar collapse, and metastatic bone involvement of ribs, spine, and shoulders. In addition, CT may be helpful in the evaluation of parenchymal lung abnormalities, detection of masses only

suspected on the chest radiography, and assessment of mediastinal and hilar lymph nodes. PET scans are more accurate than CT scans in distinguishing malignant from benign lesions, detecting mediastinal lymph node metastases, and identifying metastatic spread. Most recently, the use of integrated CT-PET technology has been reported to improve the diagnostic accuracy in the staging of NSCLC over either CT or PET technology alone.[18]

Once the tumor has been located, pathological examination of tumor tissue is necessary to establish the diagnosis of lung cancer. Tissue is typically obtained through the least invasive method likely to result in an adequate sample; methods include sputum cytology, tumor biopsy by bronchoscopy, mediastinoscopy, percutaneous needle biopsy, or open-lung biopsy. The tissue sample not only confirms malignancy but is also necessary to determine the histology (i.e., squamous cell, adenocarcinoma, large cell, or small cell). Once the diagnosis is established, additional radiologic tests may be required to evaluate lymph nodes and potential metastatic sites for accurate staging. Surgical candidates will have additional sampling of their mediastinal nodes to determine those with stage IIIB (N_3) disease (Table 137–2).[2-4,18]

STAGING

❺ Once the diagnosis of lung cancer is confirmed, the extent of disease must be determined to estimate prognosis and guide therapy. For NSCLC, tumor growth and spread are staged with the American Joint Committee on Cancer (AJCC) tumor, node, and metastasis (TNM) staging system. Small cell lung cancer is typically staged with the Veterans Administration Lung Cancer Study Group method.[2-4,18]

NON–SMALL CELL LUNG CANCER

Clinical staging of NSCLC with the TNM system evaluates the size of the tumor, extent of nodal involvement, and presence of metastatic sites. The TNM criteria have recently been updated,[19] and went into effect in January 2010.[4] The combination of these three evaluations determines the stage. Clinical stages and associated survival rates are described in Table 137–2. For comparison of various therapeutic modalities, a simpler stage grouping system is used in which stage I refers to tumors confined to the lung without lymphatic spread; stage II refers to large tumors with ipsilateral peribronchial or hilar lymph node involvement; stage III includes other lymph node and regional involvement; and stage IV includes tumor with distant metastases. Local disease is associated with the highest cure and survival rates, whereas those with advanced disease have less than a 10% 5-year survival rate.

SMALL CELL LUNG CANCER

The most commonly used system of staging SCLC was developed originally by the Veterans Administration Lung Cancer Study Group. This system categorizes SCLC into two stages: limited and extensive disease. When evidence of the tumor is confined to a single hemithorax and can be encompassed by a single radiation port, the disease is considered limited. Any progression beyond this point is extensive disease. Approximately 60% to 70% of patients initially present with extensive stage disease. The initial pretreatment evaluation of an SCLC patient should include a medical history, a clinical examination, and laboratory survey, as well as a CT scan of the chest, abdomen, and head. Typically the approach is to identify tumor spread that would demonstrate extensive stage, at which time the workup can stop. For patients without extrathoracic disease identified by these tests, a bone scan and bone marrow biopsy should be performed to confirm limited-stage disease.[2,3]

TABLE 137-2 Tumor (T), Node (N), Metastasis (M) Staging for Non-Small Cell Lung Cancer

Primary Tumor		Description
T_1		Tumor ≤3 cm diameter, surrounded by lung or visceral pleura, without invasion more proximal than lobar bronchus
	T_{1a}	Tumor ≤2 cm in diameter
	T_{1b}	Tumor >2 cm but ≤3 cm in diameter
T_2		Tumor >3 cm but ≤7 cm, or tumor with any of the following features: – Involves main bronchus, ≥2 cm distal to carina – Invades visceral pleura – Associated with atelectasis or obstructive pneumonitis that extends to the hilar region but does not involve the entire lung
	T_{2a}	Tumor >3 cm but ≤5 cm
	T_{2b}	Tumor >5 cm but ≤7 cm
T_3		Tumor >7 cm or any of the following: – Directly invades any of the following: chest wall, diaphragm, phrenic nerve, mediastinal pleura, parietal pericardium, main bronchus <2 cm from carina (without involvement of carina) – Atelectasis or obstructive pneumonitis of the entire lung – Separate tumor nodules in the same lobe
T_4		Tumor of any size that invades the mediastinum, heart, great vessels, trachea, recurrent laryngeal nerve, esophagus, vertebral body, carina, or with separate tumor nodules in a different ipsilateral lobe
Regional lymph nodes (N)		
N_0		No regional lymph node metastases
N_1		Metastasis in ipsilateral peribronchial and/or ipsilateral hilar lymph nodes and intrapulmonary nodes, including involvement by direct extension
N_2		Metastasis in ipsilateral mediastinal and/or subcarinal lymph node(s)
N_3		Metastasis in contralateral mediastinal, contralateral hilar, ipsilateral or contralateral scalene, or supraclavicular lymph node(s).
Distant metastasis (M)		
M_0		No distant metastasis
M_1		Distant metastasis
	M_{1a}	Separate tumor nodule(s) in a contralateral lobe; tumor with pleural nodules or malignant pleural or pericardial effusion
	M_{1b}	Distant metastasis

Stage	T	N	M	5 Yr Survival
Stage IA:	T_{1a}-T_{1b}	N_0	M_0	73%
Stage IB:	T_{2a}	N_0	M_0	58%
Stage IIA:	$T_{1a'}$ $T_{1b'}$ T_{2a}	N_1	M_0	46%
	T_{2b}	N_0	M_0	
Stage IIB:	T_{2b}	N_1	M_0	36%
	T_3	N_0	M_0	
	$T_{1a'}$ $T_{1b'}$ $T_{2a'}$ T_{2b}	N_2	M_0	
Stage IIIA:	T_3	N_1, N_2	M_0	24%
	T_4	N_0, N_1	M_0	
Stage IIIB:	T_4	N_2	M_0	9%
	Any T	N_3	M_0	
Stage IV:	Any T	Any N	M_{1a} or M_{1b}	13%

TREATMENT

❻ The treatment of lung cancer depends on tumor histology, stage of disease, and patient characteristics such as age, history, and performance status.[2] These aspects must be assessed before appropriate treatment can be recommended. In the development of a patient care plan, keep in mind the ultimate goals of therapy. In patients with early-stage disease, a definitive cure is the primary goal of treatment, although this end point is not always met. Additional goals of treating lung cancer patients include prolongation of survival and improvement of quality of life through alleviation of symptoms. The goals of treatment must be considered when selecting a therapeutic plan. Delivering a treatment that may prolong survival by a few months but at the expense of toxicity that significantly decreases patient quality of life may not be the best approach. Treatment decisions must include both the healthcare team and an informed and well-counseled patient.

■ NON–SMALL CELL LUNG CANCER

If left untreated, most patients with NSCLC will die within 1 year of diagnosis. Surgery, radiation therapy, and systemic therapy with cytotoxic chemotherapy or targeted therapies are all used in the management of NSCLC patients. The applications of these treatment modalities are determined by stage and other patient-specific factors (e.g., age, performance status).[2,4] A list of commonly used chemotherapy regimens including doses and schedules can be seen in Table 137–3.[4,5]

Local Disease (Stages 1A, 1B, and IIA)

❼ Local disease is associated with a favorable prognosis, and the goal of therapy is cure. Surgery is the mainstay of treatment and may be used alone or in some situations with radiation and/or chemotherapy. Patients who have comorbid conditions preventing them from being surgical candidates can be treated with radiation in place of surgery with curative intent, although the cure rates are lower. Stage IA tumors are treated with surgery alone; adjuvant therapy has not been studied adequately to know if it is beneficial. If surgical margins are positive, re-resection is recommended, alternatively patients may receive radiotherapy with or without chemotherapy.[2,4,5]

CLINICAL CONTROVERSY

The benefit of adjuvant cytotoxic chemotherapy for patients with stage I NSCLC is unclear. Adjuvant cytotoxic chemotherapy improves overall survival in patients with later stages (i.e., stage II to IIIA) NSCLC. However, limited numbers of patients with stage IA are enrolled in these trials, and the data do not suggest a survival benefit. Additional clinical trials are needed to clarify the role of adjuvant chemotherapy for patients with stage IA NSCLC.

Stage IB, IIA, and IIB disease is primarily treated with surgery, which should be followed by adjuvant chemotherapy. Although trials evaluated patients with stage IB tumors (Table 137–4), the benefit in this subset of patients is unclear. A recent guideline recommends that patients with IB tumors and high-risk features (poorly differentiated tumors, vascular invasion, wedge resection, minimal margins, tumors > 4 cm, or visceral pleural involvement) should receive chemotherapy. Patients who have positive or questionable margins may receive radiation therapy, which is typically administered with the adjuvant chemotherapy. The adjuvant treatment regimen of choice is not clear, but the positive clinical trials used platinum-based regimens, with arguably the best data coming from cisplatin-vinorelbine (Table 137–4).[4,20–26] The benefit in terms of 5-year overall survival in large randomized trials ranges from

TABLE 137-3 Common Chemotherapy Regimens Used to Treat Lung Cancer

Non-small cell lung cancer[3]

Carboplatin/Paclitaxel/Bevacizumab	Carboplatin AUC 6 IV mg/mL/min on day 1 Paclitaxel 200 mg/m2 IV on day 1 Bevacizumab 15 mg/kg IV on day 1 Repeat cycle every 3 weeks – Continue bevacizumab until progression	Vinorelbine/cisplatin (VC)	Vinorelbine 25 mg/m² IV weekly Cisplatin 100 mg/m² IV day 1 repeat cycle every 28 days[43] or Vinorelbine 30 mg/m² IV days 1 and 8
Carboplatin/Pemetrexed	Carboplatin AUC 5 mg/mL/min IV day 1 Pemetrexed 500 mg/m² IV day 1 Repeat cycle every 3 weeks		Cisplatin 80 mg/m² IV day 1 repeat cycle every 21 days[88]
Cetuximab/cisplatin/vinorelbine	Cetuximab 400 mg/m² IV 1st dose day 1, then 250 mg/m² IV weekly Cisplatin 80 mg/m² IV on day 1 Vinorelbine 25 mg/m² IV on day 1 and day 8 Repeat cycle every 3 weeks	Etoposide/cisplatin (EP)	Etoposide 100 mg/m² IV days 1, 2, and 3 Cisplatin 100 mg/m² IV day 1 repeat cycle every 28 days[32]
Cisplatin/paclitaxel (CP)	Cisplatin 75 mg/m² IV day 1 Paclitaxel 175 mg/m² over 24 hours IV day 1 repeat cycle every 21 days[42] or Cisplatin 80 mg/m² IV day 1 Paclitaxel 175 mg/m² IV over 3 hours day 1 repeat cycle every 21 days[87]	Vinorelbine/gemcitabine (VG)	Vinorelbine 25 mg/m² IV days 1 and 8 Gemcitabine 1,000 mg/m² days 1 and 8 Repeat cycle every 21 days[88,90]
		Paclitaxel/gemcitabine (PG)	Paclitaxel 175 mg/m² IV over 3 hours day 1 Gemcitabine 1,250 mg/m² days 1 and 8 repeat cycle every 21 days[87]
Gemcitabine/cisplatin (GC)	Gemcitabine 1,000 mg/m² IV days 1, 8, 15 Cisplatin 100 mg/m² IV day 1 repeat cycle every 28 days[42]	Gemcitabine/docetaxel (GD)	Gemcitabine 1,000 mg/m² IV days 1 and 8 Docetaxel 100 mg/m² IV day 8 repeat cycle every 21 days[91]
Gemcitabine/cisplatin (GCq21)	Gemcitabine 1,200 mg/m² days 1 and 8 Cisplatin 80 mg/m² IV day 1 repeat cycle every 21 days[88] or Gemcitabine 1,250 mg/m² days 1 and 8 Cisplatin 80 mg/m² IV day 1 repeat cycle every 21 days[87]	Paclitaxel/vinorelbine (PV)	Paclitaxel 135 mg/m² IV day 1 Vinorelbine 25 mg/m² IV day 1 repeat cycle every 14 days for 9 cycles[89]
		Small cell lung cancer[4]	
		Etoposide/cisplatin (EP)	Cisplatin 80 mg/m² IV day 1 Etoposide 100 mg/m² IV days 1, 2, and 3 repeat cycle every 3 weeks[83,92] or Cisplatin 60 mg/m² IV day 1 Etoposide 120 mg/m² IV days 1, 2, and 3 repeat cycle every 3 weeks[84]
Docetaxel/cisplatin (DC)	Docetaxel 75 mg/m² IV day 1 Cisplatin 75 mg/m² IV day 1 repeat cycle every 21 days[42]		
Paclitaxel/carboplatin (PCb)	Paclitaxel 225 mg/m² over 3 hours IV day 1 Carboplatin AUC 6 mcg*h/mL IV day 1 repeat cycle every 21 days[42,43] or Paclitaxel 175 mg/m² IV over 3 hours day 1 Carboplatin AUC 6 mcg*h/mL IV day 1 repeat cycle every 21 days for 6 cycles[89]	Cisplatin/irinotecan (IP)	Cisplatin 60 mg/m² IV day 1 Irinotecan 60 mg/m² IV days 1, 8, and 15 repeat cycle every 4 weeks[83,92] or Cisplatin 30 mg/m² IV day 1 Irinotecan 65 mg/m² IV days 1 and 8 repeat cycle every 3 weeks[84]

TABLE 137-4 Adjuvant Chemotherapy for Early Stage Lung Cancer

Trial	Stage	Number of Participants	Treatment Arms	Number of Cycles	Postoperative Radiotherapy	5-Year Survival	P Value
BLT[23,25]	I–IV	381	Observation Cisplatin plus vindesine; mitomycin/ifosfamide; mitomycin/vinblastine; or vinorelbine	 3	Per individual institutional policy	60% (2-year) 74% (2-year)	0.90
IALT[20]	I–III	1,867	Observation Cisplatin-based doublet (etoposide, vindesine, vinorelbine, vinblastine)		Per individual institutional policy	40.4% 44.5%	0.03
ALPI[23,25]	I–IIIA	1,209	Observation Cisplatin, mitomycin, and vindesine	 3	Per individual institutional policy	No difference in overall survival	0.585
ANITA[21]	I–IIIA	840	Observation Vinorelbine/cisplatin	 4	Per individual institutional policy	43% 51%	0.017
JBR.10[26]	IB–II	482	Observation Vinorelbine/cisplatin	 4	None	54% 69%	0.002
CALGB 9633[27]	IB	344	Observation Paclitaxel/carboplatin	 4	None	57% 60%	0.32

ALPI, Adjuvant Lung Cancer Project Italy; ANITA, Adjuvant Novelbine International Trialist Association; BLT, Big Lung Trial; CALGB, Cancer and Leukemia Group B; IALT, International Adjuvant Lung Cancer Trial; JBR.10, National Cancer Institute of Canada JBR10.10.

no benefit to 15%, with a recent systematic review reporting an absolute difference of 5%.[2,4,27] Adjuvant radiation should be avoided in patients who have clean margins, because it appears to have a detrimental effect.[2,4,22,28]

Locally Advanced Disease (Stages IIB and IIIA)

❼ Patients with more advanced local disease should still be considered for surgery.[2,4] Adjuvant chemotherapy (Table 137–4) has become the standard and appears to improve overall survival.[20,27] In some situations, chemotherapy with concurrent radiotherapy can be used prior to surgery.[2,4] Although small studies have shown a survival benefit with neoadjuvant treatment, large definitive studies have not been performed. Consequently, this practice is not standardized and varies from institution to institution. Nonresectable locally advanced disease may be treated with both an active platinum-containing regimen and radiotherapy. Responding patients may then become surgical candidates. Patients who are not surgical candidates should be treated with concurrent chemotherapy and radiation. Adjuvant radiotherapy for patients with N_2 disease may be used; it decreases the incidence of local recurrence but has not been shown to prolong overall survival.[2,4,28]

Unresectable Stage IIIB or Stage IV Disease

❽ About two-thirds of NSCLC patients present with advanced disease (unresectable stage IIIB or IV) at the time of diagnosis.[1,2] Most of these advanced tumors are not surgically resectable as a result of disseminated (multiple sites) metastatic disease or metastatic sites that are not amenable to surgery. Patients with single metastatic sites may undergo surgical resection of both the primary tumor and the metastatic site.[4]

Chemotherapy is the first-line therapy for most patients with advanced NSCLC. The intent of chemotherapy is to palliate symptoms, improve quality of life, and increase the duration of survival. Improved response rates, a modest increase in survival, and decreased toxicity profiles observed with many of the newer chemotherapy agents and combination regimens have led experts to agree that most patients with stage IV disease should receive at least one chemotherapy regimen.[2,4,5]

In the setting of advanced NSCLC, the benefits of cytotoxic chemotherapy—as measured by overall survival and quality of life—were not clearly established until the 1990s. The Non–Small Cell Lung Cancer Collaborative Group reported the pivotal results of a large meta-analysis encompassing more than 25 years and 52 clinical trials of chemotherapy in the management of NSCLC.[29] The results of this meta-analysis and other evidence suggest that chemotherapy, when combined with surgery or radiotherapy or both, improves median survival for patients with advanced stage NSCLC by 2 to 4 months and increases the 1-year absolute survival rate by 10% to 20%.[29,30] Several studies have compared chemotherapy to the best supportive care and have shown consistently better outcomes for chemotherapy.[2,30]

Both the NCCN[4] and American Society of Clinical Oncology guidelines[5] recommend first-line chemotherapy consisting of a doublet with a platinum (i.e., cisplatin or carboplatin) and a newer agent (i.e., gemcitabine, paclitaxel, docetaxel, vinorelbine, and premetrexed) (Table 137–3). Older non-platinum-containing regimens and regimens containing alkylating agents generally produce inferior outcomes.[30] For patients with a contraindication to a platinum agent, the guidelines recommend gemcitabine in combination with paclitaxel or docetaxel.[4,5]

The results of first-line chemotherapy in patients with advanced NSCLC depend on the patient's current performance status (ECOG performance status of 0–2), which appears to be the most consistent predictor of a better response and improved survival after chemotherapy. All patients with a good performance status without significant comorbidities, including elderly patients, should receive first-line doublet chemotherapy. Single-agent chemotherapy should be considered in those patients with an ECOG performance status 2 (PS-2) or significant comorbidities. Patients with poor ECOG performance status ($\geq$ PS-3) do not respond well to chemotherapy. Patients with an unfavorable prognosis (poor performance status or significant concomitant diseases) should receive best supportive care and palliative radiation when necessary.[4,5,7,30]

First-line platinum-based doublet chemotherapy is usually administered for a total of four to six cycles in those patients whose NSCLC is stable or responding to chemotherapy. The optimal number of cycles remains controversial. Response rates and quality of life were not improved with administration of six as compared to three cycles of mitomycin, cisplatin, and vinblastine.[31] For those receiving paclitaxel-carboplatin (PCb), administration of chemotherapy until disease progression had no clinically significant benefit in survival, response rate, or quality of life, but increased toxicity as compared to administration of four cycles.[32] However, pemetrexed was recently approved as maintenance therapy in patients responding to a first-line platinum-containing regimen. The registry trial was performed in 663 patients randomized (2:1) to pemetrexed maintenance or no further therapy until relapse. The results show that pemetrexed maintenance therapy prolonged median overall survival (13.4 months vs. 10.6 months, $P = 0.012$).[33] Interestingly, the benefit was only seen in patients with nonsquamous histology, and the best results occurred in patients with adenocarcinoma (median survival 16.8 months vs. 11.5 for placebo, hazard ratio 0.73, 95% CI 0.56–0.96). This histology specificity is consistent with pemetrexed as first-line with cisplatin and also as second-line as monotherapy.[33] Another recently reported randomized phase III trial shows that maintenance therapy with erlotinib prolongs disease-free survival versus placebo (SATURN Study).[34] Interestingly, this study also appeared most effective in patients with adenocarcinoma histology. Although only one of these studies has been through the peer review process, both are compelling and will likely change the current practice of limiting treatment to four or six cycles of therapy in nonsquamous histology.[5,35]

Second-line chemotherapy is usually offered to those patients with an ECOG performance status of 0–2 who experience disease progression to or after first-line chemotherapy. Third-line therapy can be offered if disease progression continues in a patient with adequate performance status. Best supportive care is recommended by the NCCN guidelines for those patients with disease progression and ECOG performance status worse than 2.[4,5]

Single-Agent Chemotherapy Single-agent chemotherapy is an alternative in elderly patients or those with an ECOG performance status of 2.[4,5] First-line, single-agent chemotherapy has objective response rates of 5% to 25% with no significant effect on overall survival. Complete responses are rare and responses that do occur are of brief duration (i.e., 2 to 4 months months).[2,36] Among the most active cytotoxic chemotherapy agents in NSCLC are cisplatin, carboplatin, docetaxel, paclitaxel, etoposide, gemcitabine, ifosfamide, irinotecan, topotecan, mitomycin, vinblastine, vinorelbine, and pemetrexed.[4,5] The EGFR inhibitor erlotinib is also active as a single agent, as discussed later under Human Epidermal Growth Factor Receptor Inhibitors.[37]

Combination Chemotherapy **❽** Response rates for combination chemotherapy regimens are generally higher than for single-agent therapy, but improvement in overall survival rates has not been consistently observed.[2,36] Combination chemotherapy regimens that have consistently reported response rates exceeding 30% have used various combinations of cisplatin, carboplatin, gemcitabine, ifosfamide, or mitomycin, and vinblastine, vindesine, or vinorelbine (Tables 137–3 and 137–5). Some studies show that cisplatin dose may have an impact on tumor response, and the most widely recommended first-line regimens now include a platinum—either cisplatin or carboplatin—with a newer cytotoxic chemotherapy agent.

Until the mid-1990s, first-line chemotherapy with etoposide and cisplatin (EP) was regarded as the most active regimen in the treatment of advanced NSCLC. Subsequently, numerous randomized, controlled clinical trials demonstrated that a platinum-based doublet with a newer cytotoxic chemotherapy agent had superior response rates or median survival rates.[2,38] Each of these newer chemotherapeutic agents had single-agent activity of greater than 20% in NSCLC and include plant alkaloids (i.e., vinorelbine), taxanes (i.e., paclitaxel and docetaxel), antimetabolites (i.e., gemcitabine), antifolates (i.e., pemetrexed), and topoisomerase I inhibitors (i.e., topotecan and irinotecan).[39] Results from many published trials combining these new chemotherapy agents with platinum-based regimens suggest improved 1-year survival rates in advanced NSCLC of 30% to 40% versus 15% to 25% with older cisplatin-based combination regimens.[38,40,41] A pivotal intergroup study[38] compared four of these newer, more effective regimens, cisplatin-paclitaxel (CP) to gemcitabine-cisplatin (GC), docetaxel-cisplatin (DC), and carboplatin-paclitaxel (PCb). When considering survival, they were all deemed equivalent, but time-to-disease progression was highest with GC. When considering all grade 4 and 5 toxic effects, the PCb regimen was lowest at 57%. The investigators concluded that all four regimens are acceptable, but ECOG chose the PCb regimen for future studies due to the lower grade 4 and 5 toxicity.[38] Table 137–5 shows the outcomes of this study and other selected phase III trials of chemotherapy in patients with advanced NSCLC.[38,40,42–46]

A number of trials and meta-analyses have been performed to determine if carboplatin and cisplatin are equally effective or if one is more effective in NSCLC.[47–49] Individual clinical trials have produced equivocal data; even meta-analyses evaluating both agents disagree.[47,49] However, cisplatin appears to be slightly superior. In one meta-analysis of doublet regimens with a "newer" agent, cisplatin improved survival by 11% (P = 0.039).[48] Clinical trials comparing the two agents have also demonstrated a different toxicity profile; cisplatin is associated with more gastrointestinal (severe nausea and vomiting) and renal toxicity than carboplatin. However, carboplatin is associated with more hematologic toxicity (thrombocytopenia) than cisplatin.[49] Although neither is clearly superior to the other, many clinicians historically used carboplatin because of its more tolerable gastrointestinal toxicity, but over the past few years there seems to be a reversal toward increased use of cisplatin, which could be attributed to improved antiemetics (i.e., the neurokinin-1 receptor antagonist aprepitant).

Nonplatinum doublets (e.g., gemcitabine-paclitaxel and gemcitabine-docetaxel) have been evaluated in the setting of first-line therapy of advanced NSCLC. The results of a meta-analysis comparing platinum-based regimens with either the same regimen without the platinum or with the platinum replaced by another agent demonstrated that platinum provides a modest benefit.[50,51] One meta-analysis[51] evaluated 17 trials with a total of 4,792 patients and found a small but significant 1-year survival benefit with a platinum-based combination regimen compared with nonplatinum combination regimens (relative risk = 1.08, 95% CI 1.01–1.16). Further analysis of carboplatin regimens and cisplatin regimens demonstrated that benefit was only seen with cisplatin-based regimens.[51] Although platinum-based combination regimens remain the preferred treatment, non-platinum-based combinations are acceptable and recommended in patients with a contraindication to a platinum agent.

Addition of a third drug to a platinum doublet has been extensively studied. The combination of three cytotoxic agents has produced equivocal data when it comes to overall survival; however, most increase response rates and toxicity.[52] Because the goal of treatment for advanced-stage disease is to prolong life and improve quality of life, the use of three cytotoxic agents has not become a standard of care. However, the addition of a targeted agent to a platinum doublet appears to improve survival with acceptable increases in toxicity.[4,5,37,53] This is seen with both an EGFR inhibitor and a VEGF inhibitor, which are discussed later in separate sections.

TABLE 137-5	First-Line Combination Regimens in Stage IIIB or IV Non-Small Cell Lung Cancer					
Reference	**Number Evaluable/ Performance Status**	**Regimen**	**Overall Response Rate (%)**	**Median Survival Duration**	**Median 1-Year Survival (%)**	**Time to Disease Progression**
Scagliotti et al.[44]	1725	GC	28.2%	10.3 mo	41.9%	5.1 mo
	All PS 0-1	Pem/C	30.6%	10.3 mo	43.5%	4.8 mo
Schiller et al. (ECOG 1594)[38]	1,155	CP	21%	7.8 mo	31%	3.4 months
	1,083 PS-0-1, 63 PS-2	GC	22%	8.1 mo	36%	4.2 months[a]
		DC	17%	7.4 mo	31%	3.7 months
		PCb	17%	8.1 mo	34%	3.1 months
Kelly et al. (SWOG)[40]	408	PCb	PR 27%	8 mo	36%	NR
	All PS-0-1	VC	PR 27%	8 mo	33%	NR
		EP	22%	7.2 mo	NR	7.2 months
Gridelli et al.[43]	503	VG	25%	8 mo	31%	4.3 months
	PS-0-2	GCq21	30%	9.5 mo	38%	5.8 months
		VCq21				
Smit et al. (EORTC)[45]	458	CP	32%	8.1 mo	36%	4.2 months
	PS-0-2	GCq21	37%	8.9 mo	33%	5.1 months
		PG	28%	6.7 mo	27%	3.5 months[b]
Georgeoulias et al.[42]	389	GD	30%	9 mo	34%	4 months
	PS-0-2	VC	39%	9.7 mo	41%	5 months
Stathopoulos et al.[46]	360	PV	43%	10 mo	38%	6 months
	PS-0-2	PCb	46%	11 mo	43%	7 months

Pem/C, pemetrexed and cisplatin; CP, cisplatin and paclitaxel; DC, docetaxel and cisplatin; ECOG, Eastern Cooperative Oncology Group; EORTC, European Organization for Research and Treatment of Cancer; EP, etoposide and cisplatin; GC, gemcitabine and cisplatin; GCq21, gemcitabine and cisplatin repeated every 21 days; GD, gemcitabine and docetaxel; NR, not reported; PCb, paclitaxel and carboplatin; PG, paclitaxel and gemcitabine; PR, partial response; PS, performance status; PV, paclitaxel and vinorelbine; SWOG, Southwest Oncology Group; VC, vinorelbine and cisplatin; VG, vinorelbine and gemcitabine.

[a]Statistically significant difference.
[b]Statistically significant difference between CP and PG, but not CP and GCq21.

Historically, ECOG PS-2 patients were excluded from NSCLC trials because of excessive toxicity with minimal benefit from combination cytotoxic therapy. A recent randomized phase III trial[54] comparing single-agent weekly docetaxel (n = 171) to docetaxel/gemcitabine (n = 174) in elderly or poor performance status (35% of patients) had disappointing results. No survival differences were observed with docetaxel/gemcitabine versus weekly docetaxel in the 122 poor performance status patients (3.8 months vs. 2.9 months, respectively), and the median survival is short compared with good performance patients.[54] Another recent randomized phase III trial[55] compared single-agent gemcitabine (n = 85) to gemcitabine/carboplatin (n = 85) in PS-2 patients. The median overall survival was not different between gemcitabine and gemcitabine/carboplatin (5.1 months vs. 6.7 months, respectively). The authors concluded that single-agent therapy is still the standard in this setting.[55] The updated ASCO guidelines state that available data support the use of single-agent chemotherapy and data are insufficient to recommend combination therapy.[5] A recent meta-analysis shows that PS-2 patients benefit from treatment.[56]

In summary, cisplatin-based doublets improve survival and quality of life as compared with best supportive care or single-agent chemotherapy in patients with advanced NSCLC. The optimal combination regimen has not yet been identified. Non-platinum-based combination regimens are reasonable options and are recommended for patients with a contraindication to platinums.

Second-Line Chemotherapy Monotherapy with docetaxel, pemetrexed, or erlotinib are options for second-line therapy in patients with a good performance status who progress during or after first-line chemotherapy.[2,4,5] Erlotinib is a relatively nontoxic agent that targets the EGFR and is discussed later in the EGFR inhibitors section. Docetaxel was the first to receive FDA approval for the treatment of advanced NSCLC after failure of a platinum-based chemotherapy regimen. The initial docetaxel dose of 100 mg/m^2 IV over 1 hour every 21 days was decreased to 75 mg/m^2 after an interim analysis showed a greater risk of severe neutropenia with the higher dose. Docetaxel, at the 75 mg/m^2 dose, was superior to best supportive care in terms of time-to-disease progression (10.6 weeks vs. 6.7 weeks, P = 0.001), median survival (7.5 months vs. 4.6 months; P = 0.047), and 1-year survival (37% vs. 11%; P = 0.003).[57] Both doses had a statistically significant improvement in 1-year survival when compared with a control regimen of vinorelbine or ifosfamide (32%, 21%, and 19%, respectively).[58]

Subsequently, pemetrexed (Alimta) was FDA approved for second-line treatment of advanced NSCLC based on results of a phase III trial.[59] In that trial, 571 patients were randomized to receive either pemetrexed 500 mg/m^2 with folate and cyanocobalamin supplementation or docetaxel 75 mg/m^2. No significant differences in overall response rate, stable disease, or median survival between the pemetrexed and docetaxel arms were observed. Docetaxel had significantly more hematologic toxicities as compared with pemetrexed, leading to more hospitalizations and use of growth factors and erythropoiesis-stimulating agents. Patients receiving docetaxel had a significantly higher rate of alopecia, while patients receiving pemetrexed had a significantly higher elevation of alanine aminotransferase.[59]

CLINICAL CONTROVERSY

There is no consensus regarding the optimal second-line treatment of patients with NSCLC. Pemetrexed and docetaxel have similar response and survival rates. These two cytotoxic chemotherapy agents have differing toxicity profiles, which may help choose treatment for an individual patient.

Human Epidermal Growth Factor Receptor Inhibitors The human epidermal growth factor receptor (HER) family consists of four receptors that homo- or heterodimerize upon cytokine binding, enabling them to trigger cellular signaling events (i.e., proliferation, antiapoptosis, etc.). The EGFR (also known as HER1) was the first tyrosine kinase receptor within the HER family to be discovered. EGFR amplification or mutations lead to increased and/or aberrant signaling through downstream pathways, which are commonly observed in NSCLC. The signals most commonly studied and documented in cancer cells and tumors include proliferation and survival of cancer cells. Due to its apparent role in cancer, it quickly became a target for drug development. Today we have three EGFR-targeted agents that have a role in treating NSCLC. Gefitinib and erlotinib are small-molecule tyrosine kinase inhibitors. They bind to the intracellular ATP binding site on the receptor, preventing the receptor from stimulating signal transduction pathways. Cetuximab is a monoclonal antibody that binds to the extracellular portion of the receptor, blocking ligands from binding to the receptor; it also downregulates receptor expression and signaling through the receptor.[2]

Gefitinib (Iressa) was the first EGFR-targeted agent approved for NSCLC. The FDA approved the agent via fast-track designation to be used as monotherapy in patients who had failed a platinum-based combination regimen and docetaxel. However, the Iressa Survival Evaluation in Lung Cancer (ISEL) postmarketing trial (mandated by the FDA), failed to demonstrate a survival advantage for those receiving gefitinib as compared with best supportive care.[60] Thus the FDA has restricted the use of gefitinib to patients who continue to benefit from the medication or who are enrolled in a clinical trial.[61]

Erlotinib, which is structurally and functionally similar to gefitinib, was approved in November 2004 (after gefitinib) with the indication as a single agent for patients with advanced NSCLC whose disease progressed after at least one prior chemotherapy regimen. Its approval was based on an international, multicenter, randomized, double-blind phase III trial (BR.21)[37] in 731 patients with locally advanced or metastatic NSCLC who had failed at least one prior chemotherapy regimen. Patients were randomized to receive either erlotinib 150 mg or placebo orally once daily. Patients in the erlotinib group had a significantly higher objective response rate (9% vs. 1%, P < 0.001) and longer median progression-free and overall survival (9.9 weeks vs. 7.9 weeks, P < 0.001 and 6.7 months vs. 4.7 months [hazard ratio = 0.73], P < 0.001, respectively) than those in the placebo group. Patients in the erlotinib group also had significantly improved symptom control, specifically time to deterioration of cough, dyspnea, and pain.[37]

The potential benefit of adding erlotinib or gefitinib to doublet platinum-based chemotherapy has been studied. Both agents have been studied in two large, randomized, controlled trials, with each enrolling more than 1,000 patients.[62-65] Unfortunately, the results of all four trials showed that adding an EGFR inhibitor to platinum-based doublet therapy in first-line treatment of NSCLC did not improve efficacy.

Although these agents provide relatively modest benefits, some individual patients show a profound response. This has led researchers to investigate patient and/or tumor-specific factors that can be used to select patients likely to respond to an EGFR inhibitor. Consistent epidemiology findings show that patients who have the following characteristics are most likely to respond to EGFR inhibitors: never smokers, women, Asians, and those with adenocarcinoma histology, particularly the bronchial alveolar carcinoma subset of adenocarcinoma.[66] A recent study conducted in an Asian advanced lung cancer population compared first-line gefitinib to the combination of carboplatin and paclitaxel in patients with adenocarcinoma that were former light smokers (stopped > 15 years prior and < 10 pack-year history) or never smokers.[67] Although median progression-free survival was similar for gefitinib and carboplatin-paclitaxel (5.7 vs. 5.8 months), the 1-year progression-free survival rates were 24.9% versus 6.7%. This trial found gefitinib to be noninferior to carboplatin-paclitaxel and superior based on progression-free survival. Additionally, less grade 3 or 4 toxicity occurred in the gefitinib arm (28.7% vs. 61%). A subset analysis of this study showed the greatest benefit occurred in patients with EGFR mutations.[67] This population does not represent the United States lung cancer patient population, and access to gefitinib is restricted to study patients in the United States, making its practical application unreasonable in general practice.[61] However, it validates that individualizing treatment can produce better results and has stimulated research in this area.

Preclinical and clinical data demonstrate that certain mutations in the kinase domain of EGFR (L858R and del746-750) are associated with significant responses to such agents.[68–70] The presence of other mutations in EGFR (T790M) is associated with resistance to such inhibitors through decreased drug binding to the receptor.[71] Finally, the presence of activating mutations in *K-Ras*, another oncogene which is known to play a role in lung cancer, is also associated with clinical resistance to EGFR inhibitors.[72] These findings have prompted some experts to suggest that patients should have their tumor assessed for EGFR and KRAS mutations to determine the appropriateness of an EGFR inhibitor therapy.[73] However, these molecular tests are not routinely used due to the lack of FDA-approved test kits, which limits the likelihood of third party reimbursement.

Cetuximab is a monoclonal antibody that binds to the extracellular portion of the EGFR receptor. The properties of cetuximab, an IgG1 antibody, include complement fixation and participation in antibody-dependent cellular cytotoxicity. These additional mechanisms of action suggest that it could be more effective than the small-molecule EGFR inhibitors. Recently, the results of adding cetuximab to cisplatin and vinorelbine as first-line treatment of advanced NSCLC have been reported. The primary end point in the study involving 1,125 patients showed that cetuximab prolonged median overall survival by 1.2 months (11.3 months vs. 10.1 months [hazard ratio for death 0.87, 95% CI 0.762–0.996; *P* = 0.044).[53] Although the study met the primary end point, some have questioned whether the survival advantage is large enough to justify an expensive drug that has toxicity, especially since the quality of life during the additional month has not been evaluated.[74]

Vascular Endothelial Growth Factor Inhibitors Vascular endothelial growth factor (VEGF) is important for the development of vasculogenesis required for tumor cell growth and metastasis, thus making it a key therapeutic target. Bevacizumab (Avastin®) is the recombinant, humanized monoclonal antibody that neutralizes VEGF. Preclinical trials demonstrate synergy when bevacizumab is combined with cytotoxic chemotherapy in a number of malignancies without untoward adverse effects. A phase II trial randomized 99 chemotherapy-naïve patients with advanced or recurrent NSCLC to bevacizumab 7.5 mg/kg or 15 mg/kg plus PCb or PCb alone.[75] Patients with CNS metastases, nonhealing wounds, significant cardiovascular disease, significant peripheral vascular disease, active secondary malignancy, pregnancy, or major surgery within 4 weeks of starting therapy, and those requiring anticoagulation were excluded from the trial because of concern over excessive toxicity to the angiogenesis inhibitor. An independent review faculty evaluated the data and found a response rate of 40%, 22%, and 31% and a median survival of 17.7 months, 11.6 months, and 14.9 months for the high-dose bevacizumab arm, the low-dose bevacizumab arm, and the control arm, respectively. Nineteen patients in the control arm crossed over to the bevacizumab monotherapy upon disease progression.

Five patients had disease stabilization, and 12-month survival was 47% following crossover. Adverse effects of chemotherapy were not statistically different with the addition of bevacizumab. However, leucopenia, diarrhea, fever, headache, rash, and chills were slightly more common in the bevacizumab-containing arms. In addition, several patients in the bevacizumab arms developed hypertension, proteinuria, and bleeding. Bleeding events included minor mucocutaneous hemorrhage (most commonly grade 1 or 2 epistaxis) and major hemoptysis. Four patients died as a result of hemoptysis or hematemesis, two others experienced life-threatening bleeding complications. All six patients had centrally located tumors, five had vacitation or necrosis of tumors, and four of the patients had squamous cell carcinoma. A prospective, randomized trial evaluating the addition of bevacizumab 15 mg/kg to PCb was conducted by ECOG.[76] As a result of bleeding complications seen in the phase II trial, patients with squamous cell carcinoma or brain metastases were excluded. The addition of bevacizumab led to an improvement of progression-free survival from 4.5 months to 6.2 months (*P* < 0.001), median survival from 10.3 months to 12.3 months (*P* = 0.003), and 1-year survival from 44% to 51%. The risk of bleeding events was significantly higher in the bevacizumab-containing arm (4.4% vs. 0.7%, *P* < 0.001). Seventeen treatment-related deaths occurred during the study: 2 in the PCb group and 15 in the PCb-bevacizumab group. Other adverse events seen more frequently in the PCb-bevacizumab group include hypertension, neutropenia, febrile neutropenia, thrombocytopenia, hyponatremia, rash, and headache (*P* < 0.05).[76] NCCN guidelines recommend the addition of bevacizumab to chemotherapy for patients with advanced NSCLC of non–squamous cell histology, no history of hemoptysis, no CNS metastasis, and not receiving therapeutic anticoagulation.[4] Interestingly, a later study that randomized patients to cisplatin and gemcitabine with or without bevacizumab did not find any survival benefit with the addition of bevacizumab.[77] This trial indicates that bevacizumab is not synergistic with all chemotherapy regimens and consequently should only be used in combination with carboplatin and paclitaxel for lung cancer at this time.

Radiation Therapy Palliative radiotherapy with chemotherapy may be helpful in selected patients to control local and systemic disease and to reduce disease-related symptoms. Brain metastases are also commonly treated with radiotherapy; in the case of a solitary brain lesion, surgical resection may be used in conjunction with whole-brain radiation.[2,4,78]

Adverse effects of radiotherapy frequently result in severe esophagitis, pneumonitis, skin desquamation, myelopathies, cardiac abnormalities, and pulmonary toxicity in surrounding normal tissues. Improved radiotherapy delivery techniques, such as multiple daily radiation fractions (hyperfractionated accelerated radiation therapy) and three-dimensional treatment planning, allow delivery of greater dosage fractions specifically to the tumor site while decreasing the toxicity to surrounding normal tissues, as compared to standard radiotherapy. A phase III trial randomized patients with unresectable NSCLC to receive two cycles of PCb followed by either once daily radiation 64 Gy (6400 rad) delivered in 32 2-Gy (200 rad) fractions or hyperfractionated accelerated radiation therapy delivered three times a day for 15 days with a total dose of 57.6 Gy (5760 rad).[78] Of the 14 patients, the median survival for hyperfractionated accelerated radiation therapy arm was 20.3 months as compared to 14.9 months in the daily radiation arm (*P* = 0.28). Only 42% of the target accrual was met as a consequence of low patient accrual, difficulty in delivering hyperfractionated accelerated radiation therapy, mucosal toxicity, and data from other trials demonstrating the benefit of concurrent over the sequential radiotherapy.

Concurrent radiotherapy plus chemotherapy with radiosensitizing agents, such as cisplatin, paclitaxel, and gemcitabine, improves survival but further complicate the risks for severe toxicity, especially esophagitis.[79] Several trials have evaluated the use of sequential and concurrent chemoradiation, but the results of only one trial have been published. In that trial, Furuse et al. randomized 320 patients to chemotherapy (cisplatin, vindesine, and mitomycin) and radiation (56 Gy [5600 rad] delivered in 28 fractions) beginning on either day 2 of chemotherapy or following the completion of chemotherapy.[80] After a median followup of 5 years, median survival was significantly improved with concurrent chemoradiation when compared to sequential chemotherapy followed by radiotherapy (16.5 vs. 13.3 months, $P = 0.04$). Myelosuppression was increased in the concurrent arm as opposed to the sequential arm, while nonhematologic toxicities were similar between the two groups. Numerous randomized, combined modality trials continue to evaluate the optimal delivery method, schedule, and dosages for radiotherapy in concert with cisplatin and the newer chemotherapy agents.

■ EVALUATION OF THERAPEUTIC OUTCOMES

For patients who have undergone surgical resection with or without chemotherapy, radiation, or both, a physical examination and chest radiography are recommended every 3 to 4 months for the first 2 years, then every 6 months for 3 years, and then annually. In addition, a low-dose spiral chest CT scan is recommended annually to monitor for evidence of local recurrence. Suspicious symptoms or physical findings (e.g., bone pain, visual abnormalities, or headache, or elevated liver function tests) should prompt an evaluation to rule out distant metastases.[2,4,5]

Tumor response to chemotherapy is generally evaluated at the end of the second or third cycle and at the end of every second cycle thereafter. Patients with stable disease, with objective response, or with measurable decrease in tumor size (complete or partial response) should continue until four to six cycles have been administered. Responding patients with nonsquamous histology should be considered for maintenance therapy with pemetrexed. Following initial therapy for NSCLC, patients must be monitored for evidence of disease progression.[2,4,5]

TREATMENT

Small Cell Lung Cancer

SCLC is a rapidly dividing malignancy that spreads early in the disease course. Consequently, most patients present with extensive-stage disease (approximately 60% to 70% of new cases). When patients with SCLC are not treated, the disease quickly becomes fatal. Fortunately, small cell carcinomas are very responsive to chemotherapy and radiation. In the vast majority of patients, chemotherapy with or without radiotherapy is the treatment of choice. Even after a complete response to therapy, the cancer usually recurs within 6 to 8 months, and survival time following recurrence is typically short (~4 months). With treatment, median survival rates for patients with limited and extensive disease are 14 to 20 months and 9 to 11 months, respectively. Treatment planning starts with stage of disease (i.e., limited vs. extensive-stage), but must also take into account other factors, including: performance status (treatment usually restricted to PS-0 or PS-1 patients), patient age, comorbid conditions (e.g., renal failure), and patient desire to receive treatment.[2,3]

■ LIMITED DISEASE

❼ When a single SCLC mass is found, local therapy with radiation or surgery would be considered. One of the factors differentiating SCLC and NSCLC is the fact that local disease is treated most commonly with radiation instead of surgery. Radiotherapy became the standard in 1969, when a randomized trial showed that it offered the potential for cure.[81] With improved radiologic imaging, there has been renewed interest in identifying patients who would benefit from surgery. There is currently no clear role for surgery in SCLC treatment. Due to the low cure rate with radiation alone, several studies have evaluated the addition of systemic chemotherapy to radiation. The regimen of choice for limited-disease SCLC is etoposide-cisplatin (EP). Carboplatin may be substituted for cisplatin to reduce nausea and vomiting, nephrotoxicity, or neurotoxicity,[82] although increased myelosuppression in the form of thrombocytopenia may result.[83] In patients who are able to tolerate combined therapy, concomitant chemoradiotherapy offers the most substantial survival benefit. In European countries, a three-drug combination containing an anthracycline has been the mainstay of therapy, but mounting clinical evidence shows that these regimens are inferior to EP plus concurrent radiation and have more toxicity.[84] Consequently, the guidelines recommend that the EP regimen be used with concurrent radiotherapy.[85] Since patients with SCLC commonly have a recurrence in the CNS, trials have been performed to evaluate the benefit of prophylactic cranial irradiation (PCI). A pivotal study showed that PCI reduces the incidence of brain metastasis and increases 3-year survival from 15% to 21%.[86,87] Therefore, patients who achieve a complete response with treatment should be offered PCI.

■ EXTENSIVE DISEASE

❽ Platinum regimens are also the treatment of choice in extensive disease, and many studies have failed to show superiority to the EP regimen as first-line treatment. A combination of irinotecan and cisplatin in one Japanese study demonstrated an increased median survival time by approximately 3 months over the EP regimen. This regimen showed a lower incidence of severe neutropenic side effects but exhibited higher rates of moderate- to high-grade diarrhea.[88] However, this study was repeated in the United States and did not show a similar improvement over the EP regimen.[89] Therefore, EP remains the regimen of choice for treating extensive SCLC in the United States, with irinotecan and cisplatin being an acceptable alternative. Concurrent radiotherapy is not used routinely in extensive disease. However, a recent study that randomized extensive-stage patients responding to chemotherapy to observation or PCI reported that PCI decreased the 1-year risk of brain metastasis (14.6% vs. 40.4%), and prolonged survival (27.1% vs. 13.3% at 1 year).[90] This study led to guideline revisions recommending PCI for patients with extensive disease responding to chemotherapy.[3]

■ RECURRENT DISEASE

SCLC patients who relapse or progress after first-line chemotherapy have a median survival of 4 to 5 months. Unfortunately, when disease recurs, it is usually less sensitive to chemotherapy. The decision of whether or not to use second-line chemotherapy is often based on the length of time between completion of the induction chemotherapy regimen and relapse. If this interval is less than 3 months, the patient has refractory SCLC and is unlikely to respond to second-line therapy, hence they should receive best supportive care or be enrolled in a clinical trial. For those with greater than a 3-month time interval between first-line chemotherapy and relapse, the expected response rate to treatment is approximately

25%, and they should be treated.[2,3] Topotecan (intravenous and oral) are the only FDA-approved second-line therapy for SCLC. The pivotal trial[91] leading to the approval randomized patients to IV topotecan or the CAV regimen. The response rates (24% vs. 18%), time-to-progression (13 vs. 12 weeks), and overall survival (25 weeks vs. 25 weeks) were not different between groups. Interestingly, the proportion of patients experiencing symptom improvement was higher in the topotecan arm. The hematologic toxicity was similar between arms; there was slightly more neutropenia in the CAV arm and more anemia and thrombocytopenia in the topotecan arm. Nonhematologic toxicity appears to be higher in the CAV arm; 11% of patients required a dose reduction compared to 1% in the topotecan arm.[91] Oral topotecan appears to be equally effective and similar in terms of dosing, toxicity, and effectiveness as IV topotecan.[92] Based on these studies, one could consider topotecan the second-line treatment of choice, but due to the modest efficacy other agents warrant consideration. Agents that are recommended in national guidelines[3] include single-agent topotecan, irinotecan, gemcitabine, paclitaxel, docetaxel, and vinorelbine, as well as the CAV (cyclophosphamide, doxorubicin, and vincristine) regimen. These patients could also be enrolled in a clinical trial.

■ EVALUATION OF THERAPEUTIC OUTCOMES

The effectiveness of first-line therapy is evaluated after two to three cycles of treatment. At this point, therapy is continued for patients with a complete or partial response or stable disease, and discontinued or changed to a non-cross-resistant regimen in patients demonstrating evidence of progressive disease. The induction chemotherapy regimen is administered for four to six cycles if the SCLC is responsive. In those with a response, PCI should be offered. After recovery from first-line therapy, followup visits should occur every 3 months for years 1, 2, and 3, then every 4 to 6 months for years 4 and 5, then annually for patients with either a partial or complete response.[3]

COMPLICATIONS AND SUPPORTIVE CARE

Patients with lung cancer frequently have numerous concurrent medical problems. Such problems may be related to invasion of the primary tumor and its metastases, paraneoplastic syndromes (see clinical presentation earlier), chemotherapy and radiotherapy toxicity, or concomitant disease states (e.g., cardiac disease, renal dysfunction, chronic obstructive pulmonary disease, asthma, or diabetes). Depression is also common and sometimes persistent in patients with SCLC and NSCLC and should be treated. Identification, diagnosis, and treatment of the patient as a whole may improve the patient's overall quality of life and tolerance to cancer treatments.

❾ The chemotherapy regimens used in the management of lung cancer are intensive and are associated with a wide variety of toxic effects. Nausea and vomiting may be severe. Cisplatin-containing regimens require the use of aggressive acute and delayed antiemetic regimens containing a serotonin antagonist, dexamethasone, and aprepitant.[93] Patients experiencing protracted nausea and vomiting may require intravenous hydration and nutritional support. Myelosuppression is often the dose-limiting toxicity associated with chemotherapy. Granulocytopenia places patients at a high risk for serious infections. Other toxic effects associated with these chemotherapy regimens include mucositis, anemia, nephrotoxicity, peripheral neuropathies, and ototoxicity.

Approximately 30% to 65% of advanced-stage NSCLC patients will develop bone metastases, which may lead to significant bone pain, pathological fractures, spinal cord compression, and hypercalcemia.[94] Zoledronic acid, an intravenously administered bisphosphonate, has been shown to reduce skeletal-related events in patients with bone metastases at a dose of 4 mg over 15 minutes infused every 3 weeks. Although the data do not show a significant reduction in skeletal-related events, time to first event is significantly increased (230 vs. 163 days for placebo, $P = 0.023$), thereby making zoledronic acid a viable therapy for patients with bone metastases.

Patients receiving radiation therapy may experience complications including severe esophagitis, fatigue, radiation pneumonitis, and cardiac toxicity. These toxicities are usually more common and severe when radiation is combined with chemotherapy. The patient's baseline performance status and the degree of pulmonary dysfunction (e.g., chronic obstructive pulmonary disease from years of tobacco use) must be considered in decisions concerning radiation dosage and fractionation.

It is readily apparent that many lung cancer patients receive complex pharmacologic regimens that may include chemotherapeutic agents, antiemetics, antibiotics, analgesics, anticoagulants, bronchodilators, corticosteroids, anticonvulsants, and cardiovascular agents. Such regimens necessitate intensive therapeutic monitoring in order to avoid drug-related and radiotherapy-related toxic effects and to optimize therapeutic outcome for individual patients.

ABBREVIATIONS

ACCP: American College of Chest Physicians

AJCC: American Joint Committee on Cancer

ASCO: American Society of Clinical Oncology

ATP: adenosine triphosphate

BR.21: National Cancer Institute of Canada non-small cell lung cancer trial evaluating erlotinib

CAV: cyclophosphamide, doxorubicin, vincristine

c-KIT: A protein tyrosine kinase receptor that is specific for stem cell factor (aka, CD117)

CNS: central nervous system

CT: computed tomography

ECOG: Eastern Cooperative Oncology Group

EGFR: epidermal growth factor receptor

EP: etoposide, cisplatin

ETS: environmental tobacco smoke

FDA: Food and Drug Administration

HER: human epidermal growth factor receptor

ISEL: Iressa Survival Evaluation in Lung cancer – trial

IV: Intravenous

KRAS: Kirsten rat sarcoma viral oncogene homolog (italicized refers to the gene – non-italicized refers to the protein)

NCCN: National Comprehensive Cancer Network

NSAIDs: nonsteroidal anti-inflammatory drugs

NSCLC: non small cell lung cancer

PCI: prophylactic cranial irradiation

PET: positron emission tomography

PS: performance status

SATURN: Sequential Tarceva in Unresectable NSCLC - trial

SCLC: small cell lung cancer

SELECT: the Selenium and Vitamin E Cancer Prevention Trial

TNM: tumor, node, and metastasis – part of staging

VEGF: vascular endothelial-derived growth factor

REFERENCES

1. Jemal A, Siegel R, Xu J, Ward E. Cancer statistics, 2010. CA Cancer J Clin 2010;60:277–300.

2. Johnson DH, Blot WJ, Carbone DP, Gonzalez A, Hallahan D, Massion PP, Putnam JB, Sandler AB. Cancer of the lung: Non–small cell lung cancer and small cell lung cancer. In: Abeloff MD, Armitage JO, Niederhuber JE, Kastan MB, McKenna WG, eds. Abeloff's Clinical Oncology. 4th ed. Philadelphia: Churchill Livingstone Elsevier; 2008.

3. NCCN Clinical Practice Guidelines in Oncology: Small Cell Lung Cancer. National Comprehensive Cancer Network, 2010, *http://www.nccn.org/professionals/physician_gls/PDF/sclc.pdf.*

4. NCCN Clinical Practice Guidelines in Oncology: Non–Small Cell Lung Cancer. National Comprehensive Cancer Network, 2010, *http://www.nccn.org/professionals/physician_gls/PDF/nscl.pdf.*

5. Azzoli CG, Baker S Jr., Temin S, et al. American Society of Clinical Oncology Clinical Practice Guideline update on chemotherapy for stage IV non-small-cell lung cancer. J Clin Oncol 2009;27:6251–6266.

6. Seidenfeld J, Samson DJ, Bonnell C, Ziegler KM, Aronson N. Mangement of small cell lung cancer. In: Agency for Healthcare Research and Quality; 2006. *http://www.ahrq.gov/clinic/tp/lungcantp.htm.*

7. Alberts WM. Diagnosis and management of lung cancer executive summary: ACCP evidence-based clinical practice guidelines (2nd edition). Chest 2007;132:1S–19S.

8. Kim ES, Lippman SM, Hong WK. Chemoprevention of lung cancer. In: Pass HI, Carbone DP, Johnson DH, et al., eds. Lung Cancer: Principles and Practice. 3rd ed. Philidelphia: Lippincott, Williams & Wilkins; 2005:220–228.

9. Dy GK, Miller AA, Mandrekar SJ, et al. A phase II trial of imatinib (ST1571) in patients with c-kit expressing relapsed small-cell lung cancer: A CALGB and NCCTG study. Ann Oncol 2005;16:1811–1816.

10. Schottenfeld D, Searle JG. The etiology and epidemiology of lung cancer. In: Pass HI, Carbone DP, Johnson DH, Minna JD, Turrisi AT, eds. Lung Cancer: Principles and Practice. 3rd ed. Philidelphia: Lippincott, Williams & Wilkins; 2005:3–24.

11. State-specific secondhand smoke exposure and current cigarette smoking among adults—United States, 2008. MMWR Morb Mortal Wkly Rep 2009;58:1232–1235.

12. Alberg AJ, Ford JG, Samet JM. Epidemiology of lung cancer: ACCP evidence-based clinical practice guidelines (2nd edition). Chest 2007;132:29S–55S.

13. Black WC. Computed tomography screening for lung cancer: review of screening principles and update on current status. Cancer 2007;110:2370–2384.

14. Keith RL. Chemoprevention of lung cancer. Proc Am Thorac Soc 2009;6:187–193.

15. Lippman SM, Klein EA, Goodman PJ, et al. Effect of selenium and vitamin E on risk of prostate cancer and other cancers: The Selenium and Vitamin E Cancer Prevention Trial (SELECT). JAMA 2009;301:39–51.

16. Kushi LH, Byers T, Doyle C, et al. American Cancer Society Guidelines on Nutrition and Physical Activity for Cancer Prevention: Reducing the Risk of Cancer With Healthy Food Choices and Physical Activity. CA Cancer J Clin 2006;56:254–281.

17. Silvestri GA, Gould MK, Margolis ML, et al. Noninvasive staging of non-small cell lung cancer: ACCP evidenced-based clinical practice guidelines (2nd edition). Chest 2007;132:178S–201S.

18. Kligerman S, Digumarthy S. Staging of non-small cell lung cancer using integrated PET/CT. AJR Am J Roentgenol 2009;193:1203–1211.

19. Goldstraw P, Crowley J, Chansky K, et al. The IASLC Lung Cancer Staging Project: Proposals for the revision of the TNM stage groupings in the forthcoming (seventh) edition of the TNM Classification of malignant tumours. J Thorac Oncol 2007;2:706–714.

20. Arriagada R, Bergman B, Dunant A, Le Chevalier T, Pignon JP, Vansteenkiste J. Cisplatin-based adjuvant chemotherapy in patients with completely resected non-small-cell lung cancer. N Engl J Med 2004;350:351–360.

21. Douillard JY, Rosell R, De Lena M, et al. Adjuvant vinorelbine plus cisplatin versus observation in patients with completely resected stage IB-IIIA non-small-cell lung cancer (Adjuvant Navelbine International Trialist Association [ANITA]): A randomised controlled trial. Lancet Oncol 2006;7:719–727.

22. Dunant A, Pignon JP, Le Chevalier T. Adjuvant chemotherapy for non–small cell lung cancer: contribution of the International Adjuvant Lung Trial. Clin Cancer Res 2005;11:5017s–5021s.

23. Scagliotti GV. The ALPI Trial: The Italian/European experience with adjuvant chemotherapy in resectable non–small lung cancer. Clin Cancer Res 2005;11:5011s–5016s.

24. Visbal AL, Leighl NB, Feld R, Shepherd FA. Adjuvant Chemotherapy for early-stage non–small cell lung cancer. Chest 2005;128:2933–2943.

25. Waller D, Peake MD, Stephens RJ, et al. Chemotherapy for patients with non–small cell lung cancer: The surgical setting of the Big Lung Trial. Eur J Cardiothorac Surg 2004;26:173–182.

26. Winton T, Livingston R, Johnson D, et al. Vinorelbine plus cisplatin vs. observation in resected non-small-cell lung cancer. N Engl J Med 2005;352:2589–2597.

27. Pignon JP, Tribodet H, Scagliotti GV, et al. Lung adjuvant cisplatin evaluation: A pooled analysis by the LACE Collaborative Group. J Clin Oncol 2008;26:3552–3559.

28. Postoperative radiotherapy in non-small-cell lung cancer: Systematic review and meta-analysis of individual patient data from nine randomised controlled trials. PORT Meta-analysis Trialists Group. Lancet 1998;352:257–263.

29. Chemotherapy in non–small cell lung cancer: A meta-analysis using updated data on individual patients from 52 randomised clinical trials. Non–small Cell Lung Cancer Collaborative Group. BMJ 1995;311:899–909.

30. Spira A, Ettinger DS. Multidisciplinary management of lung cancer. N Engl J Med 2004;350:379–392.

31. Smith IE, O'Brien ME, Talbot DC, et al. Duration of chemotherapy in advanced non-small-cell lung cancer: A randomized trial of three versus six courses of mitomycin, vinblastine, and cisplatin. J Clin Oncol 2001;19:1336–1343.

32. Socinski MA, Schell MJ, Peterman A, et al. Phase III trial comparing a defined duration of therapy versus continuous therapy followed by second-line therapy in advanced-stage IIIB/IV non-small-cell lung cancer. J Clin Oncol 2002;20:1335–1343.

33. Alimta prescribing information, Eli Lilly and Company. 2009.

34. Cappuzzo F, Ciuleanu T, Stelmakh L, et al. SATURN: A double-blind, randomized, phase III study of maintenance erlotinib versus placebo following nonprogression with first-line platinum-based chemotherapy in patients with advanced NSCLC. J Clin Oncol 2009;27:15s (suppl; abstr 8001).

35. Mok TS, Ramalingam SS. Maintenance therapy in nonsmall-cell lung cancer: A new treatment paradigm. Cancer 2009;115:5143–5154.

36. Lilenbaum RC, Herndon JE 2nd, List MA, et al. Single-agent versus combination chemotherapy in advanced non-small-cell lung cancer: The cancer and leukemia group B (study 9730). J Clin Oncol 2005;23:190–196.

37. Shepherd FA, Rodrigues Pereira J, Ciuleanu T, et al. Erlotinib in previously treated non-small-cell lung cancer. N Engl J Med 2005;353:123–132.

38. Schiller JH, Harrington D, Belani CP, et al. Comparison of four chemotherapy regimens for advanced non-small-cell lung cancer. N Engl J Med 2002;346:92–98.

39. Bonomi P, Kim K, Fairclough D, et al. Comparison of survival and quality of life in advanced non-small-cell lung cancer patients treated with two dose levels of paclitaxel combined with cisplatin versus etoposide with cisplatin: Results of an Eastern Cooperative Oncology Group trial. J Clin Oncol 2000;18:623–631.

40. Kelly K, Crowley J, Bunn PA Jr., et al. Randomized phase III trial of paclitaxel plus carboplatin versus vinorelbine plus cisplatin in the treatment of patients with advanced non–small-cell lung cancer: A Southwest Oncology Group trial. J Clin Oncol 2001;19:3210–3218.

41. Kosmidis P, Mylonakis N, Nicolaides C, et al. Paclitaxel plus carboplatin versus gemcitabine plus paclitaxel in advanced non-small-cell lung cancer: A phase III randomized trial. J Clin Oncol 2002;20:3578–3585.

42. Georgoulias V, Ardavanis A, Tsiafaki X, et al. Vinorelbine plus cisplatin versus docetaxel plus gemcitabine in advanced non-small-cell lung cancer: A phase III randomized trial. J Clin Oncol 2005;23:2937–2945.

43. Gridelli C, Gallo C, Shepherd FA, et al. Gemcitabine plus vinorelbine compared with cisplatin plus vinorelbine or cisplatin plus gemcitabine for advanced non-small-cell lung cancer: A phase III trial of the Italian GEMVIN Investigators and the National Cancer Institute of Canada Clinical Trials Group. J Clin Oncol 2003;21:3025–3034.

44. Scagliotti GV, Parikh P, von Pawel J, et al. Phase III study comparing cisplatin plus gemcitabine with cisplatin plus pemetrexed in chemotherapy-naive patients with advanced-stage non-small-cell lung cancer. J Clin Oncol 2008;26:3543–3551.

45. Smit EF, van Meerbeeck JP, Lianes P, et al. Three-arm randomized study of two cisplatin-based regimens and paclitaxel plus gemcitabine in advanced non-small-cell lung cancer: A phase III trial of the European Organization for Research and Treatment of Cancer Lung Cancer Group–EORTC 08975. J Clin Oncol 2003;21:3909–3917.

46. Stathopoulos GP, Veslemes M, Georgatou N, et al. Front-line paclitaxel-vinorelbine versus paclitaxel-carboplatin in patients with advanced non-small-cell lung cancer: A randomized phase III trial. Ann Oncol 2004;15:1048–1055.

47. Ardizzoni A, Boni L, Tiseo M, et al. Cisplatin-versus carboplatin-based chemotherapy in first-line treatment of advanced non-small-cell lung cancer: An individual patient data meta-analysis. J Natl Cancer Inst 2007;99:847–857.

48. Hotta K, Matsuo K, Ueoka H, Kiura K, Tabata M, Tanimoto M. Meta-analysis of randomized clinical trials comparing cisplatin to carboplatin in patients with advanced non-small-cell lung cancer. J Clin Oncol 2004;22:3852–3859.

49. Jiang J, Liang X, Zhou X, Huang R, Chu Z. A meta-analysis of randomized controlled trials comparing carboplatin-based to cisplatin-based chemotherapy in advanced non-small cell lung cancer. Lung Cancer 2007;57:348–358.

50. D'Addario G, Pintilie M, Leighl NB, Feld R, Cerny T, Shepherd FA. Platinum-based versus non-platinum-based chemotherapy in advanced non-small cell lung cancer: A meta-analysis of the published literature. J Clin Oncol 2005;23:2926–2936.

51. Rajeswaran A, Trojan A, Burnand B, Giannelli M. Efficacy and side effects of cisplatin- and carboplatin-based doublet chemotherapeutic regimens versus non-platinum-based doublet chemotherapeutic regimens as first line treatment of metastatic non-small cell lung carcinoma: A systematic review of randomized controlled trials. Lung Cancer 2008;59:1–11.

52. Delbaldo C, Michiels S, Syz N, Soria JC, Le Chevalier T, Pignon JP. Benefits of adding a drug to a single-agent or a 2-agent chemotherapy regimen in advanced non-small-cell lung cancer: A meta-analysis. JAMA 2004;292:470–484.

53. Pirker R, Pereira JR, Szczesna A, et al. Cetuximab plus chemotherapy in patients with advanced non-small-cell lung cancer (FLEX): An open-label randomised phase III trial. Lancet 2009;373:1525–1531.

54. Hainsworth JD, Spigel DR, Farley C, et al. Weekly docetaxel versus docetaxel/gemcitabine in the treatment of elderly or poor performance status patients with advanced nonsmall cell lung cancer: A randomized phase 3 trial of the Minnie Pearl Cancer Research Network. Cancer 2007;110:2027–2034.

55. Reynolds C, Obasaju C, Schell MJ, et al. Randomized phase III trial of gemcitabine-based chemotherapy with in situ RRM1 and ERCC1 protein levels for response prediction in non-small-cell lung cancer. J Clin Oncol 2009;27:5808–5815.

56. Non-Small Cell Lung Cancer Collaborative Group, Chemotherapy for non-small cell lung cancer. Cochrane Database of Systematic Reviews 2009.

57. Shepherd FA, Dancey J, Ramlau R, et al. Prospective randomized trial of docetaxel versus best supportive care in patients with non-small-cell lung cancer previously treated with platinum-based chemotherapy. J Clin Oncol 2000;18:2095–2103.

58. Fossella FV, DeVore R, Kerr RN, et al. Randomized phase III trial of docetaxel versus vinorelbine or ifosfamide in patients with advanced non-small-cell lung cancer previously treated with platinum-containing chemotherapy regimens. The TAX 320 Non-Small Cell Lung Cancer Study Group. J Clin Oncol 2000;18:2354–2362.

59. Hanna N, Shepherd FA, Fossella FV, et al. Randomized phase III trial of pemetrexed versus docetaxel in patients with non-small-cell lung cancer previously treated with chemotherapy. J Clin Oncol 2004;22:1589–1597.

60. Thatcher N, Chang A, Parikh P, et al. Gefitinib plus best supportive care in previously treated patients with refractory advanced non-small-cell lung cancer: Results from a randomised, placebo-controlled, multicentre study (Iressa Survival Evaluation in Lung Cancer). Lancet 2005;366:1527–1537.

61. Stinchcombe TE, Socinski MA. Gefitinib in advanced non–small cell lung cancer: does it deserve a second chance? Oncologist 2008;13:933–944.

62. Gatzemeier U, Pluzanska A, Szczesna A, et al. Phase III study of erlotinib in combination with cisplatin and gemcitabine in advanced non-small-cell lung cancer: The Tarceva Lung Cancer Investigation Trial. J Clin Oncol 2007;25:1545–1552.

63. Giaccone G, Herbst RS, Manegold C, et al. Gefitinib in combination with gemcitabine and cisplatin in advanced non-small-cell lung cancer: A phase III trial–INTACT 1. J Clin Oncol 2004;22:777–784.

64. Herbst RS, Giaccone G, Schiller JH, et al. Gefitinib in combination with paclitaxel and carboplatin in advanced non-small-cell lung cancer: A phase III trial–INTACT 2. J Clin Oncol 2004;22:785–794.

65. Herbst RS, Prager D, Hermann R, et al. TRIBUTE: A phase III trial of erlotinib hydrochloride (OSI-774) combined with carboplatin and paclitaxel chemotherapy in advanced non-small-cell lung cancer. J Clin Oncol 2005;23:5892–5899.

66. Tokumo M, Toyooka S, Kiura K, et al. The relationship between epidermal growth factor receptor mutations and clinicopathologic features in non–small cell lung cancers. Clin Cancer Res 2005;11:1167–1173.

67. Mok TS, Wu YL, Thongprasert S, et al. Gefitinib or carboplatin-paclitaxel in pulmonary adenocarcinoma. N Engl J Med 2009;361:947–957.

68. Sequist LV, Martins RG, Spigel D, et al. First-line gefitinib in patients with advanced non-small-cell lung cancer harboring somatic EGFR mutations. J Clin Oncol 2008;26:2442–2449.

69. Inoue A, Suzuki T, Fukuhara T, et al. Prospective phase II study of gefitinib for chemotherapy-naive patients with advanced non-small-cell lung cancer with epidermal growth factor receptor gene mutations. J Clin Oncol 2006;24:3340–46.

70. Eberhard DA, Johnson BE, Amler LC, et al. Mutations in the epidermal growth factor receptor and in KRAS are predictive and prognostic indicators in patients with non-small-cell lung cancer treated with chemotherapy alone and in combination with erlotinib. J Clin Oncol 2005;23:5900–5909.

71. Pao W, Miller VA, Politi KA, et al. Acquired resistance of lung adenocarcinomas to gefitinib or erlotinib is associated with a second mutation in the EGFR kinase domain. PLoS Med 2005;2:e73.

72. Pao W, Wang TY, Riely GJ, et al. KRAS mutations and primary resistance of lung adenocarcinomas to gefitinib or erlotinib. PLoS Med 2005;2:e17.

73. Non-small cell lung cancer guidelines. NCCN, 2008, www.nccn.org.

74. Herbst RS, Hirsch FR. Patient selection criteria and the FLEX Study. Lancet 2009;373:1497–1498.

75. Johnson DH, Fehrenbacher L, Novotny WF, et al. Randomized phase II trial comparing bevacizumab plus carboplatin and paclitaxel with carboplatin and paclitaxel alone in previously untreated locally advanced or metastatic non-small-cell lung cancer. J Clin Oncol 2004;22:2184–2191.

76. Sandler A, Gray R, Perry MC, et al. Paclitaxel-carboplatin alone or with bevacizumab for non-small-cell lung cancer. N Engl J Med 2006;355:2542–2550.

77. Reck M, von Pawel J, Zatloukal P, et al. Phase III trial of cisplatin plus gemcitabine with either placebo or bevacizumab as first-line therapy

for nonsquamous non-small-cell lung cancer: AVAil. J Clin Oncol 2009;27:1227–1234.

78. Belani CP, Wang W, Johnson DH, et al. Phase III study of the Eastern Cooperative Oncology Group (ECOG 2597): Induction chemotherapy followed by either standard thoracic radiotherapy or hyperfractionated accelerated radiotherapy for patients with unresectable stage IIIA and B non-small-cell lung cancer. J Clin Oncol 2005;23:3760–3767.

79. Johnson DH. Locally advanced, unresectable non-small cell lung cancer: new treatment strategies. Chest 2000;117:123S–126S.

80. Furuse K, Fukuoka M, Kawahara M, et al. Phase III study of concurrent versus sequential thoracic radiotherapy in combination with mitomycin, vindesine, and cisplatin in unresectable stage III non-small-cell lung cancer. J Clin Oncol 1999;17:2692–2699.

81. Miller AB, Fox W, Tall R. Five-year follow-up of the Medical Research Council comparative trial of surgery and radiotherapy for the primary treatment of small-celled or oat-celled carcinoma of the bronchus. Lancet 1969;2:501–505.

82. Kosmidis PA, Samantas E, Fountzilas G, Pavlidis N, Apostolopoulou F, Skarlos D. Cisplatin/etoposide versus carboplatin/etoposide chemotherapy and irradiation in small cell lung cancer: A randomized phase III study. Hellenic Cooperative Oncology Group for Lung Cancer Trials. Semin Oncol 1994;21:23–30.

83. Simon GR, Wagner H. Small cell lung cancer. Chest 2003;123:259S–271S.

84. Johnson DH. "The guard dies, it does not surrender!" Progress in the management of small-cell lung cancer? J Clin Oncol 2002;20:4618–4620.

85. Small cell lung cancer guidelines. NCCN, 2008, *www.nccn.org.*

86. Auperin A, Arriagada R, Pignon J-P, et al. Prophylactic cranial irradiation for patients with small-cell lung cancer in complete remission. N Engl J Med 1999;341:476–484.

87. Christodoulou C, Skarlos DV. Treatment of small cell lung cancer. Semin Respir Crit Care Med 2005;26:333–341.

88. Noda K, Nishiwaki Y, Kawahara M, et al. Irinotecan plus cisplatin compared with etoposide plus cisplatin for extensive small-cell lung cancer. N Engl J Med 2002;346:85–91.

89. Hanna NH, Einhorn L, Sandler A, et al. Randomized, phase III trial comparing irinotecan/cisplatin (IP) with etoposide/cisplatin (EP) in patients (pts) with previously untreated, extensive-stage (ES) small cell lung cancer (SCLC). J Clin Oncol 2005;23:622s.

90. Slotman BJ, Mauer ME, Bottomley A, et al. Prophylactic cranial irradiation in extensive disease small-cell lung cancer: Short-term health-related quality of life and patient reported symptoms: Results of an international phase III randomized controlled trial by the EORTC Radiation Oncology and Lung Cancer Groups. J Clin Oncol 2009;27:78–84.

91. von Pawel J, Schiller JH, Shepherd FA, et al. Topotecan versus cyclophosphamide, doxorubicin, and vincristine for the treatment of recurrent small-cell lung cancer. J Clin Oncol 1999;17:658–667.

92. Eckardt JR, von Pawel J, Pujol JL, et al. Phase III study of oral compared with intravenous topotecan as second-line therapy in small-cell lung cancer. J Clin Oncol 2007;25:2086–2092.

93. Kris MG, Hesketh PJ, Somerfield MR, et al. American Society of Clinical Oncology guideline for antiemetics in oncology: Update 2006. J Clin Oncol 2006;24:2932–2947.

94. Rosen LS, Gordon D, Tchekmedyian S, et al. Zoledronic acid versus placebo in the treatment of skeletal metastases in patients with lung cancer and other solid tumors: A phase III, double-blind, randomized trial—the Zoledronic Acid Lung Cancer and Other Solid Tumors Study Group. J Clin Oncol 2003;21:3150–3157.

95. Fukuoka M, Furuse K, Saijo N, et al. Randomized trial of cyclophosphamide, doxorubicin, and vincristine versus cisplatin and etoposide versus alternation of these regimens in small-cell lung cancer. J Natl Cancer Inst 1991;83:855–861.

96. Furuse K, Fukuoka M, Kuba M, et al. Randomized study of vinorelbine (VRB) versus vindesine (VDS) in previously untreated stage IIIB or IV non-small-cell lung cancer (NSCLC). The Japan Vinorelbine Lung Cancer Cooperative Study Group. Ann Oncol 1996;7:815–820.

97. Oken MM, Creech RH, Tormey DC, et al. Toxicity and response criteria of the Eastern Cooperative Oncology Group. Am J Clin Oncol 1982;5:649–655.

98. Scagliotti GV, De Marinis F, Rinaldi M, et al. Phase III randomized trial comparing three platinum-based doublets in advanced non-small-cell lung cancer. J Clin Oncol 2002;20:4285–4291.

CHAPTER 138

Colorectal Cancer

LISA E. DAVIS, WEIJING SUN, AND PATRICK J. MEDINA

KEY CONCEPTS

❶ Maintaining a diet with high fiber and low fat intake has not been proven to reduce colorectal cancer risk but is beneficial for reducing risk of other chronic diseases.

❷ Regular use of aspirin and other nonsteroidal antiinflammatory drugs, estrogen replacement therapy, and calcium and vitamin D supplementation may reduce risk of colorectal cancer in certain selected populations, but they are not currently recommended for routine cancer prevention.

❸ Effective colorectal cancer screening programs incorporate regular examination of the entire colon starting at age 50 years for average-risk individuals. Colorectal adenomas can progress to cancer and should be removed.

❹ The histologic stage of colorectal cancer upon diagnosis— determined by depth of bowel invasion, lymph node involvement, and presence of metastases—is the most important prognostic factor for disease recurrence and survival.

❺ The treatment goal for stages I, II, and III colon cancer is cure; surgery should be offered to all eligible patients for this purpose.

❻ Adjuvant therapy consisting of fluoropyrimidine-based chemosensitized radiation therapy should be offered to patients with stage II or III cancer of the rectum. Adjuvant fluoropyrimidine-based chemotherapy plus radiation decreases risk of local and distant disease recurrence as compared to observation alone.

❼ Six months of fluoropyrimidine and oxaliplatin-based adjuvant chemotherapy significantly reduces the risk of cancer recurrence and overall mortality as compared with fluoropyrimidine alone in patients with stage III colon cancer.

❽ Chemotherapy is palliative for metastatic disease. Fluoropyrimidine-based chemotherapy regimens, administered in a variety of schedules, provide a modest improvement in survival and can be highly beneficial in reducing patient symptoms.

❾ Bevacizumab plus chemotherapy as initial therapy for metastatic disease is considered standard of care and provides a survival benefit compared with combination chemotherapy alone. A fluoropyrimidine with oxaliplatin or irinotecan improves survival compared to fluoropyrimidine monotherapy and should be offered to patients who are candidates for aggressive treatment. The ability for patients to receive all active cytotoxic agents (e.g., fluoropyrimidine, oxaliplatin, irinotecan) during the course of their disease improves their overall survival.

❿ Capecitabine is an acceptable alternative to intravenous fluorouracil both in adjuvant therapy and in the setting of metastatic disease, as it provides similar efficacy and its oral dosing may offer greater patient convenience.

⓫ Individuals whose disease progresses or is refractory to chemotherapy may benefit from cetuximab, either alone or combined with continuing irinotecan. Patients with chemotherapy-refractory disease may also benefit from single-agent panitumumab. However, patients with codon 12 or 13 KRAS gene mutations should not receive cetuximab or panitumumab as these tumor mutations predict lack of treatment response. Tumor epidermal growth factor receptor (EGFR) immunohistochemistry test results do not predict tumor response to these agents.

Colorectal cancer involves the colon, rectum, and anal canal. It is one of the three most common cancers occurring in adult men and women in the United States and accounts for about one in nine cancer diagnoses. In 2010, an estimated 142,570 new cases will be diagnosed, of which 102,900 will involve the colon and 39,670 the rectum.[1] An additional 5,260 new cases of cancer involve the anus, anal canal, or anorectum.[1]

For both adult men and women, colorectal cancer is the third leading cause of cancer-related deaths in the United States. An estimated 51,370 deaths will occur during 2010.[1]

Mortality and incidence rates associated with colorectal cancer in the United States have decreased over the past 2 decades. Incidence rates vary worldwide, with recent increasing incidence rates in newer economically developed countries in eastern Europe, while incidence rates are relatively stable in longstanding economically developed countries in North America, western Europe, Australia, and Japan.[2] Colorectal cancer mortality rates are comparable between the United States, western Europe, and Japan.[2]

Multiple factors are associated with the development of colorectal cancer, including acquired and inherited genetic susceptibility, environmental elements, and lifestyle choices. Overall, approximately 39% of affected individuals undergo a surgical procedure alone intended for cure. An additional 37% of individuals can potentially be cured by undergoing surgery followed by adjuvant radiation therapy (XRT), chemotherapy, or both. Curability is influenced primarily by depth of tumor penetration into adjacent tissues or organs, involvement of lymph nodes, and presence of metastatic disease. Five-year survival rates are close to 92% and 89% for persons with early stages of colon and rectal cancer, respectively.[3] After the tumor has spread regionally to adjacent lymph nodes or tissues, 5-year survival rates drop to 70% for colon cancer and to 67% for cancer of the rectum; 5-year survival for individuals with metastatic disease is approximately 12%.

Treatment modalities for colorectal cancer include surgery, XRT, chemotherapy, and other targeted molecular therapies (e.g., angiogenesis inhibitors, epidermal growth factor receptor inhibitors). Surgery is the important and definitive procedure associated with cure; XRT can improve curability following surgical resection in rectal cancer and may reduce symptoms and complications associated with advanced disease. Chemotherapy is used in adjuvant treatment regimens and in treatment for advanced stages of disease. Selected patients with advanced disease who receive aggressive preoperative chemotherapy experience higher resection rates and can be potentially cured. Much progress has been made in the treatment of advanced disease, in the ability to identify candidates for potentially curative surgical procedures, and the availability of active drug regimens that can improve patients' survival.

EPIDEMIOLOGY

Colorectal cancer is the third most common malignancy worldwide, accounting for an estimated 1,023,256 new cases annually.[4] The variation in colorectal cancer occurrence worldwide is at least 25-fold.[2] The highest incidence rates occur in the most highly developed areas such as Australia, New Zealand, North America, Japan, and western and northern Europe. Most recently, incidence rates have increased in newer economically developed countries in eastern Europe such as the Czech Republic and Slovakia.[2] The lowest incidence rates are seen in less-developed areas such as Africa, South Central Asia, and Central America. The influence

of environmental factors (e.g., increased intake of caloric-dense foods and physical inactivity) on colorectal cancer risk has become evident through studies of migrants, where the incidence of colorectal cancer increases rapidly within first-generation immigrants who migrate from low- to high-risk areas.[2] However, colorectal cancers are known to develop more frequently in certain families, and genetic predisposition to this disease is also well recognized.

The incidence of invasive colon cancer is greatest among males, who have an age-adjusted incidence rate of 34.59 per 100,000, as compared with females for whom the rate is 29.72 per 100,000.[3] Invasive cancer of the rectum occurs less frequently; the incidence rate is 16.30 and 9.83 per 100,000 for males and females, respectively. Differences in colorectal cancer incidence exist among ethnic groups in American men and women. Although cancer of the colon and rectum is the third most frequent malignancy among white, African American, Asian American/Pacific Islander, and American Indian/Alaska Native males, it ranks second among Hispanic/Latino males.[1] In women, cancer of the colon and rectum is the second most frequent malignancy in African American, Asian American/Pacific Islander, American Indian/Alaska Native, and Hispanic/Latino females, but the third most common cancer in white females.[1] Cultural and genetic factors, as well as disparities in access to healthcare services, may influence risk among population groups.[1]

The overall incidence of colon and rectal cancers in the United States continues to decline, with an annual percent decrease of 2.6% from 1998 to 2007.[3] In almost every ethnic group, the decline in cancer incidence accelerated from 1999 to 2007. An increase in screening and polyp removal may contribute to a part of this trend. Figure 138–1 displays trends for incidence and mortality rates among white and African American males and females in the United States.

The median age at diagnosis is 70 years, with fewer than 20% of patients diagnosed younger than age 54 years.[3] An individual's risk increases with increasing age, and about 40% of cases develop in adults older than 75 years of age. The stage of disease at presentation is similar among different ethnic groups, although the tendency to present with later-stage disease is slightly higher for African Americans than in whites.

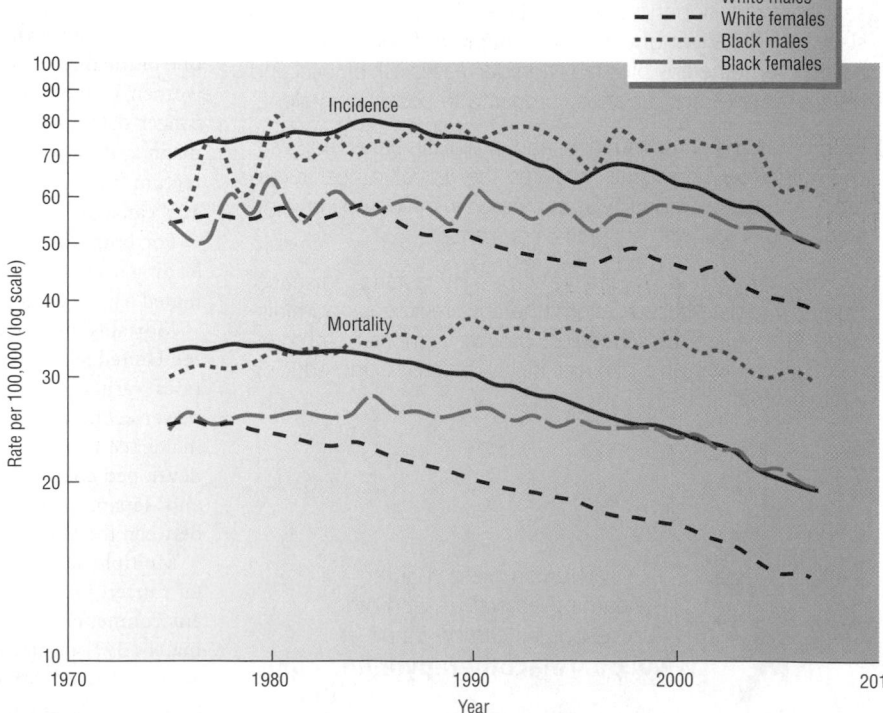

FIGURE 138-1. SEER incidence and mortality rates for invasive colon and rectum cancer, 1975-2007. Rates are per 100,000 and age-adjusted to the 2000 U.S. standard population. (*From reference* 3.)

Cancer of the colon and rectum accounts for approximately 10% of all cancer deaths in the United States. The median age for death from cancer of the colon or rectum is 75 years.[3] It is estimated that 51,370 individuals will die of colorectal cancer in the United States in 2010, which represents a continued decline in overall combined mortality for both colon and rectal cancer observed during the last 20 years. For women, the decline in colorectal cancer mortality rates has been evident since 1950, whereas death rates among men did not start to decline until the late 1970s.[3] Overall mortality rates are also higher among African American males and females, and the rates of decline are lower as compared to those among white, American Indian/Alaska Native, Asian/Pacific Islander, and Hispanic males and females.[3] Factors contributing to the overall decline in colorectal cancer mortality include decreasing incidence rates, screening programs with early polyp removal, and more effective and better tolerated treatments. Differences among different world geographic regions, and in population groups in the United States, may also reflect variations in underlying tumor biology, stage at diagnosis, access to screening programs, and availability of effective treatments.[2,4]

ETIOLOGY AND RISK FACTORS

Numerous studies suggest that the development of colorectal cancer is related to dietary or environmental factors that affect the bowel, lifestyle choices, and certain comorbid conditions, in addition to physical and genetic susceptibilities.

DIETARY INTAKE AND NUTRIENTS

❶ Epidemiologic studies of worldwide incidence of colorectal cancer suggest that economic development and dietary habits strongly influence its development. Although findings based on epidemiologic data are subject to potential biases and inconsistencies in how dietary factors are categorized and measured, numerous studies have attempted to ascertain the true contribution of dietary habits as independent risk factors for colorectal cancer development.

Fiber, Fruit, and Vegetables

❶ Dietary fiber is composed of remnants of plant cells that are not processed by normal human digestive enzymes.[5] Fibers are frequently classified as either water soluble (pectins, gums, agar, and mucilages) or insoluble (celluloses, hemicellulose, and lignins). The insoluble fibers are most likely to protect against cancer.[5] Foods that are high in fiber include vegetables, fruits, grains, and cereals. Dietary fiber is postulated to reduce colonic mucosal cell exposure to carcinogens through the dilution or reduced absorption of carcinogens in the bowel, reduced fecal pH, reduced bowel transit time, alterations in bile acid metabolism, or increased production of short-chain fatty acids, such as butyrate, which possesses known anticarcinogenic properties.[5,6] A protective effect from a diet high in fruits and vegetables is biologically plausible because certain constituents may reduce oxidative damage to DNA and lipids, induce drug-metabolizing enzymes, or enhance DNA repair processes.[7]

Results from numerous population-focused and epidemiologically based studies that have focused on various forms of dietary fiber intake (e.g., fruit, cruciferous vegetables, wheat bran, whole grains, etc.) have suggested a variety of associations, but recent large, controlled studies do not show an inverse relationship between total fiber intake and risk of colorectal adenomas or carcinoma.[5,7] Although fruit and vegetable intake may be protective against colorectal cancer, there is no consistent evidence to support this effect.[5]

Red Meat and Fat

❶ Epidemiologic studies suggest that a relationship exists between dietary fat intake and colorectal cancer risk, although this has not been consistently seen.[5,6] This may have resulted from the use of dietary evaluations that focused on the quantity, origin, or type (saturated, monounsaturated, and polyunsaturated) of fat rather than on the source of dietary fat ingested. Dietary fat may promote cancer development as a result of its effect on fecal bile acid concentrations. The release of bile acids is stimulated following ingestion of dietary fat. These acids are then converted by colonic flora to secondary bile acids, which are associated with bowel mucosal irritation and cell proliferation responses and may promote tumor growth.[8]

The association between red but not white meat consumption and colorectal cancer is strongest, which may be related to the heterocyclic amines and polycyclic aromatic hydrocarbons formed during cooking, or the presence of specific fatty acids in red meat such as arachidonic acid.[9] Processed meat products containing certain preservatives may increase exogenous exposure to carcinogenic N-nitroso compounds.[9] Although data support associations between red and processed meat and high saturated fat intake with increased risk of colorectal cancer, the exact nature and magnitude of these risks have not been determined.

Calcium and Vitamin D

❷ Inverse associations between dietary calcium, vitamin D intake, and serum 25-hydroxyvitamin D_3 levels, and colorectal cancer risk have been reported in several observational studies.[5,6] Calcium may exert antiproliferative effects by binding to bile and fatty acids in the small intestine, thereby reducing colonic epithelial cell exposure to mutagens.[5,10] In addition, calcium induces differentiating, pro-apoptotic, and direct growth-restraining activities on both normal and tumor cells in the gastrointestinal tract.[5,10] Vitamin D has antiproliferative and differentiation and pro-apoptotic effects on colonic epithelial cells and on a variety of tumor cells.[10,11] Most of its actions are mediated through a high-affinity nuclear vitamin D receptor (VDR), and the expression of this receptor is altered during different phases of colon cancer development.[11] Other genes involved in key signaling pathways that influence colorectal cancer development, such as Wnt/β-catenin, are also regulated by the VDR transcription factor.[11] Thus cellular responsiveness to vitamin D and associated cancer risk is unlikely limited to dietary intake alone. Vitamin D and calcium appear to interact synergistically to protect against adenoma recurrence and colorectal cancer.[5]

Folate and Other Micronutrients

Folate intake has been linked to colorectal cancer risk through epidemiologic and experimental studies in cell lines, animals, and humans.[5,6] However, the underlying basis for this is complex, particularly since alcohol use, smoking, genetic variants of the methylenetetrahydrofolate reductase (MTHFR) gene, and other factors can interfere with folate metabolism.[5,6,12] Folate is a key constituent of dark-green vegetables, citrus fruits, and dried beans, and the contribution of these dietary components is considered beneficial. Cellular folates act to accept and donate methyl groups in cellular processes that influence DNA synthesis and methylation of DNA, RNA, and proteins.[12] Variations in DNA methylation of gene promoter regions influence gene expression and DNA stability. Inappropriate hypermethylation leads to inactivation of tumor suppressor gene function and hypomethylation can result in oncogene activation.[12]

These effects as mechanisms of oncogenic transformation and tumor progression have been described in colon cancer, but the relationship between the timing of folate exposure to the development of neoplastic foci may influence what appears to be a bimodal impact of folate on tumorigenesis.[6,12] Moderate folate supplementation, if initiated prior to the establishment of neoplastic foci, may be protective, whereas excessive or increased intake might enhance growth of established early neoplastic lesions.[5,6,12] Thus an adequate dietary folate intake may be enough to lower the risk of colorectal cancer, and exceeding normal intake may not be beneficial.

Epidemiologic and animal model data suggest that deficiencies in other dietary micronutrients, including selenium, vitamin C, vitamin E, and carotenoids, may increase colorectal cancer risk, but there is no convincing evidence that the incidence of colorectal cancer is greater in patients with low serum levels than in patients with adequate levels.[6]

LIFESTYLE FACTORS

Nonsteroidal Antiinflammatory Drug and Aspirin Use

❷ Several lifestyle factors are known to affect colorectal cancer risk (Table 138-1). Observational studies have demonstrated that regular (at least 2 doses per week) nonsteroidal antiinflammatory drug (NSAID) and aspirin use is associated with a reduced risk of colorectal cancer. In an average-risk individual, regular aspirin use is associated with a 13% to 28% reduction in the risk of colorectal adenoma, and the pooled relative risk reduction in colorectal cancer from cohort studies is approximately 22%.[13] The reduction in risk appears greater for individuals with a history of adenoma. The dose of aspirin may be important, as low-dose aspirin was not beneficial in reducing colorectal cancer incidence in either the Physician's Health Study or the Women's Health Study.[14]

Benefit has also been seen with NSAID and cyclooxygenase-2 inhibitor (COX-2) use. NSAID use over a 10- to 15-year period is associated with protection against adenomas and colorectal cancer, with a 30% to 50% reduction in the risk of colorectal cancer.[5,14,15] Although COX-2 inhibitors reduce the incidence of colorectal

adenoma recurrence, there is no evidence to show that they reduce colorectal cancer risk or mortality.[14]

The protective effects of these agents appear to be related to their inhibition of COX-2 and free radical formation. COX-2 overexpression is seen in precancerous and cancerous lesions in the colon and is associated with decreased colon cancer cell apoptosis and increased production of angiogenesis-promoting factors.[15] Up to 50% of colorectal adenomas and 85% of sporadic colon carcinomas have elevated levels of COX-2; COX-2 overexpression in colorectal cancer is associated with a worse survival.[15] COX-2 appears to play a role in polyp formation, and COX-2 inhibition suppresses polyp growth, restores apoptosis, and decreases expression of proangiogenic factors. In contrast, cyclooxygenase-1 (COX-1) levels remain normal in both normal and malignant tissue, although COX-1 inhibition may also be important.[16]

Postmenopausal Hormone-Replacement Therapy

❷ Exogenous postmenopausal oral hormone-replacement therapy is associated with a significant reduction in colorectal cancer risk.[17–19] Risk reduction is seen in postmenopausal women receiving both estrogen only and combined estrogen and progestin therapy, and persists for about 10 years after therapy is discontinued.

Several mechanisms for a protective effect of estrogens on the bowel have been identified.[18] Declining estrogen levels associated with aging are associated with estrogen receptor hypermethylation, resulting in reduced expression of the estrogen receptor gene and dysregulated colonic mucosal cell growth. Estrogen may also interact with bile acids, or alter levels of insulin and insulin-like growth factor-1 (IGF-1), an important mitogen that influences cell-cycle progression in certain cells.

Obesity and Physical Inactivity

Physical inactivity and elevated body mass index (BMI), independent of level of physical activity, are associated with an elevated risk of colon adenoma, colon cancer, and rectal cancer.[20,21] Individuals with a total higher level of activity throughout life have the lowest risk. Hypotheses for these relationships include the observation that physical activity stimulates bowel peristalsis, resulting in decreased bowel transit time, and the possibility that exercise-induced alterations in body glucose, insulin resistance, hyperinsulinemia, and perhaps other hormones may reduce tumor cell growth.[20,22]

In most studies, a 5-unit increase above a healthy BMI was associated with increased risk of colorectal cancer in men, but the relationship is weaker and less consistent for women, possibly because of interactions with age or hormone-replacement therapy.[20] Differences in body composition and distribution of fat weight among men and women could contribute to this discrepancy.[23] Several mechanisms that link body size to colorectal cancer risk have been proposed, including insulin resistance, chronic inflammation, and alterations in growth factors or steroid hormones.[24]

Alcohol and Tobacco Use

Alcohol consumption increases the risk of colorectal cancer, but stronger associations have been observed for men than for women, possibly because alcohol consumption is generally greater in men than in women.[25] Lifetime and baseline alcohol consumption increase risk of cancer of the colon and rectum, and an alcohol intake greater than 30 g/day is associated with a greater apparent increase in risk.[25]

Cigarette smoking is associated with an increased risk of colorectal cancer and mortality, with a stronger association for cancer of the rectum than for cancer of the colon.[26] A dose relationship with

TABLE 138-1	Lifestyle Factors Associated with Colorectal Cancer Risk
Factor	**Comments**
Elevated risk	
Obesity and physical inactivity	Elevated BMI, waist circumference, waist-to-hip ratio, and physical inactivity associated with increased risk
Alcohol intake	Colorectal cancer risk increased with alcohol intake greater than 30 g/day
Tobacco use	Use of tobacco products contributes to approximately 12% of colorectal cancer deaths annually; higher colorectal cancer risk and mortality with cigarette smoking
Type 2 diabetes mellitus	Associated with 30% increase in risk of colorectal cancer and increased risk of mortality
Western diet	High saturated fat, red, and processed meat consumption; role of low dietary fiber intake less established
Reduced risk	
Aspirin and nonaspirin NSAID use	Regular aspirin or NSAID use associated with 30–50% reduction in colorectal cancer risk
Postmenopausal hormone use	Exogenous hormone intake decreases risk of colon and rectal cancer by about 20%
Calcium and vitamin D intake	Vitamin D 400 international units and calcium intake of 1,000 mg/day (adults < 50 years) or 1,200 mg/day (adults > 50 years) may be sufficient to reduce colorectal cancer risk

BMI, body mass index; NSAID, nonsteroidal antiinflammatory drug.

increasing number of pack-years and cigarettes smoked per day was also statistically significant but only among patients who had smoked for at least 30 years. Compared to never-smokers, the relative risks of colorectal cancer and mortality in smokers were 18% and 25% higher, respectively.[26] Participants in the Prostate, Lung, Colorectal, and Ovarian Trial who were current tobacco users had a greater risk of having hyperplastic polyps, adenomas, or concurrent hyperplastic and adenomatous polyps detected when they underwent flexible sigmoidoscopy.[27]

HMG-CoA Reductase Inhibitor Use

Preclinical findings and epidemiologic studies have evaluated the association between HMG-CoA reductase inhibitor (statin) use and colorectal cancer risk.[28,29] Despite two large trials of pravastatin and simvastatin that found a reduction in colon cancer incidence and one report of a reduced risk of stage IV cancer among statin users, more recent epidemiologic studies show no association between chronic statin use and risk of colorectal cancer.[28,29]

Coffee and Tea Consumption

The association between coffee and tea consumption and colorectal cancer risk is controversial, despite findings from several small studies.[30,31] Coffee and tea contain several constituents that have anticarcinogenic properties in vitro and in animal studies, but evidence in humans is limited. In a meta-analysis of studies that addressed black and green tea consumption and colorectal cancer risk, there was inadequate evidence that either type of tea is protective against colorectal cancer.[31] A meta-analysis of studies of coffee consumption and colorectal cancer risk showed no significant effect on cancer risk.[32]

CLINICAL RISK FACTORS

Chronic Inflammatory Diseases

Chronic ulcerative colitis, particularly when it involves the entire large intestine, predisposes individuals to colorectal cancer at a rate that is 5- to 10-fold greater than average.[33] The risk is even greater for young individuals and increases for all affected individuals with increasing extent of bowel involvement and disease duration. The cumulative risk of colorectal cancer is low early in life, but increases from 2% at 10 years after diagnosis to 8% and 18% at 20 and 30 years, respectively.[33] Chronic underlying inflammation, oxidative stress, and release of various cytokines, including nuclear factor-kappaB (NF-κB) and tumor necrosis factor-alpha (TNF-α), appear to promote tumorigenesis.[34] The progressive dysplastic changes that bowel mucosa undergo are similar to those observed in adenomatous polyps. Similarly, patients with Crohn disease are also at increased risk, and the risk is believed to be about that of patients with ulcerative colitis.[33] As compared with sporadic colon cancer or cancer associated with ulcerative colitis, colon cancer in patients with Crohn disease tends to arise in the proximal colon.[33] This is most likely related to the area of bowel affected by the chronic inflammatory process in individuals with Crohn disease. Overall, persons diagnosed with either disease constitute approximately 1% to 2% of all new cases of colorectal cancer each year.

Type 2 Diabetes Mellitus

Type 2 diabetes mellitus, independent of body mass size and physical activity level, is associated with increased colorectal cancer risk, although previous findings have been heterogeneous with regard to sex and cancer subsite.[35] In a meta-analysis of 15 studies, diabetes was associated with a 30% increase in risk of colorectal cancer and increased risk of colorectal cancer mortality.[35] Features associated with type 2 diabetes, such as hyperinsulinemia and elevated levels of free IGF-1 promote tumor cell proliferation.[36] Evidence is also accumulating that supports an association between metabolic syndrome and an elevated risk of colorectal cancer.[37]

GENETIC SUSCEPTIBILITY

Hereditary

Three specific patterns of colon cancer occurrence are generally observed: sporadic, inherited, and familial. Although most cases of colon cancer are sporadic in nature, as many as 10% of cases are thought to be hereditary.[38,39] The two most common forms of hereditary colon cancer are familial adenomatous polyposis (FAP) and hereditary nonpolyposis colorectal cancer (HNPCC). Both forms result from a specific germline mutation. FAP is a rare autosomal dominant trait caused by inactivating mutations of the adenomatous polyposis coli (APC) gene and accounts for 0.2% to 1% of all colorectal cancers. The disease is manifested by hundreds to thousands of tiny sessile adenomatous polyps that carpet the colon and rectum, typically arising during adolescence.[39] The polyps continue to proliferate throughout the colon, with eventual transformation to malignancy. The risk of developing colorectal cancer for individuals with untreated FAP is virtually 100%; most will develop colorectal cancer between the fourth and fifth decades of life.[38] Several variants of FAP exist and are associated with different extracolonic manifestations.[40]

HNPCC, also referred to as Lynch syndrome, is an autosomal dominant inherited syndrome that accounts for up to 5% of colon cancer cases.[38] Germline mutations in one of the DNA mismatch-repair (MMR) genes, most commonly MLH1, MSH2, or MSH6, are responsible for HNPCC.[41] Carriers of a germline mutation have an 80% lifetime risk of developing colorectal cancer.[41] Multiple generations within a family are affected, and colorectal cancer develops early in life, with a mean age at time of diagnosis of about 45 years of age.[38] In contrast to FAP, adenomatous polyps are not a primary manifestation of the HNPCC. Polyps that do form tend to be located primarily in the right-sided, or proximal colon. Because the clinical presentation of HNPCC is difficult to distinguish from "sporadic" forms of colorectal cancer, the diagnosis of HNPCC can be confirmed by the presence of germline mutations in a family of genes responsible for DNA MMR. Criteria for diagnosis of HNPCC have been established, and it is important to identify carriers of these MMR mutations so that they can be counseled and followed appropriately.[42] In addition, these individuals have a moderately increased risk of developing cancers in other organs.

Familial colon cancer represents the least-understood pattern of colorectal cancer. Approximately 20% of patients who develop colorectal cancer will have a family history of colorectal cancer.[38] In these families, the frequency of colorectal cancer is too high to be considered sporadic, but the pattern is not consistent with an inherited syndrome. First-degree relatives of patients diagnosed with colorectal cancer have an increased risk of the disease that is at least two to four times that of persons in the general population without a family history.[39]

Enzyme Polymorphisms

Increasing evidence suggests that genetic polymorphisms in drug-metabolizing enzymes, such as N-acetyltransferases (NAT1 and NAT2), cytochrome P450 (CYP) isoenzymes, glutathione-S-transferase (GST) enzymes, methylenetetrahydrofolate reductase (MTHFR), and hemochromatosis gene mutations may confer genetic susceptibility to colorectal cancer.[43] Individuals with certain variations in NAT1, NAT2, CYP1A2, CYP1A1, and CYP2E1 enzyme genotypes may be particularly susceptible to carcinogenic effects of a high dietary intake of meat, tobacco smoke, or other environmental factors.[43,44]

SUMMARY OF RISK FACTORS

In summary, multiple factors are associated with colorectal cancer risk. Lifestyle factors associated with economically developed countries, such as obesity, physical inactivity, chronic hyperinsulinemia, and alcohol and tobacco use, increase risk of colorectal cancer. Observational studies suggest associations between high dietary intake of processed and red meats and saturated fat with increased risk of colorectal cancer, but the majority of evidence does not indicate that low dietary fiber intake plays a role in the development of colorectal cancer. Regular aspirin and NSAID use and postmenopausal hormone replacement therapy decrease risk, but recommendations have not been made because of unresolved issues regarding risk-to-benefit considerations. Inherited genetic susceptibilities and clinical risk factors, such as inflammatory bowel disease, are well known risks for colon cancer.

PATHOPHYSIOLOGY

ANATOMY AND BOWEL FUNCTION

The large intestine consists of the cecum; the ascending, transverse, descending, and sigmoid colon; and the rectum (Fig. 138–2). In adults, it extends about 1.5 m and has a diameter ranging from 8 cm in the cecum to 2 cm in the sigmoid colon. The function of the large intestine is to receive 500 to 2,000 mL of ileal contents per day. Absorption of fluid and solutes occurs in the right colon or the segments proximal to the middle of the transverse colon, with movement and storage of fecal material in the left colon and distal segments of the colon. Mucus secretion from goblet cells into the intestinal lumen lubricates the mucosal surface and facilitates movement of the dehydrated feces. It also serves to protect the luminal wall from bacteria and colonic irritants such as bile acids.

Four major tissue layers, from the lumen outward, form the large intestine: the mucosa, submucosa, muscularis externa, and serosa (Fig. 138–3). Embedded in the submucosa and muscularis externa is a rich lymphatic capillary system. Lymphatic channels do not extend into the mucosa. The muscularis externa consists of circular

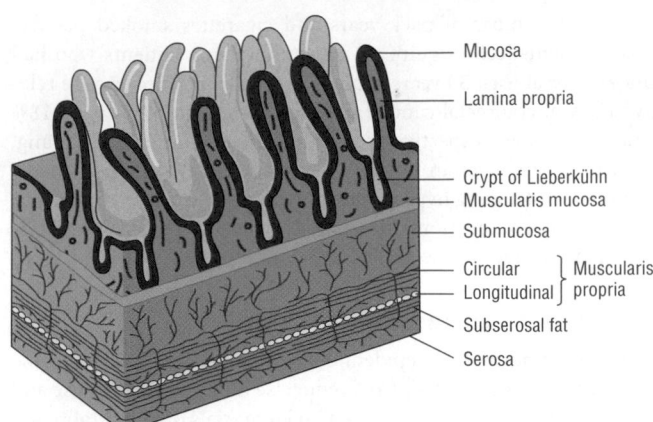

FIGURE 138-3. Cross-section of bowel wall.

smooth muscle and three outer longitudinal smooth muscle bands. Contraction of these muscle groups moves colonic material toward the anal canal. The outermost layer of the colon, the serosa, secretes a fluid that allows the colon to slide easily over nearby structures within the peritoneum. The serosa covers only the anterior and lateral aspects of the upper third of the rectum. The lower third lies completely extraperitoneal and is surrounded by fibrofatty tissue as well as adjacent organs and structures.

The surface epithelium of the colonic mucosa undergoes continual renewal, and complete replacement of epithelial cells occurs every 4 to 8 days. Cell replication normally takes place within the lower third of the crypts, the tubular glands located within the intestinal mucosa. The cells then mature and differentiate to either goblet or absorptive cells as they migrate toward the bowel lumen. The total number of epithelial cells remains relatively constant as the number of cells migrating from the crypts is balanced by the rate of exfoliation of cells from the mucosal surface. This two-phase process is critical to the malignant transformation of the epithelial cells. The number of dysplastic and hyperplastic aberrant crypt foci increases with increasing age; as the mass of abnormal cells accumulates at the top of the crypt and starts to protrude into the stream of fecal matter, their contact with fecal mutagens can lead to further cell mutations and eventual adenoma formation.

COLORECTAL TUMORIGENESIS

The development of a colorectal neoplasm is a multistep process involving several genetic and phenotypic alterations of normal bowel epithelium structure and function, leading to dysregulated cell growth, proliferation, and tumor development. Because most colorectal cancers develop sporadically, with no inherited or familial disposition, efforts have been directed toward identifying these alterations and learning whether detection of such changes may lead to improved cancer detection and/or treatment outcomes.

Features of colorectal tumorigenesis includes genomic instability, activation of oncogene pathways, mutational inactivation of tumor-suppressor genes, and activation of growth factor pathways.[41] A genetic model has been proposed for colorectal tumorigenesis that describes a process of transformation from adenoma to carcinoma. Figure 138–4 is an overview of the adenoma–carcinoma model. The adenoma–carcinoma sequence of tumor development reflects an accumulation of mutations within colonic epithelium that confers a selective growth advantage to the affected cells. Key elements of this process include hyperproliferation of epithelial cells to form a small benign neoplasm or adenoma in conjunction with acquisition of various genetic mutations.[41] These mutations occur early and frequently in sporadic cases of both adenomas and colorectal cancer. Somatic mutations must occur in multiple genes to produce

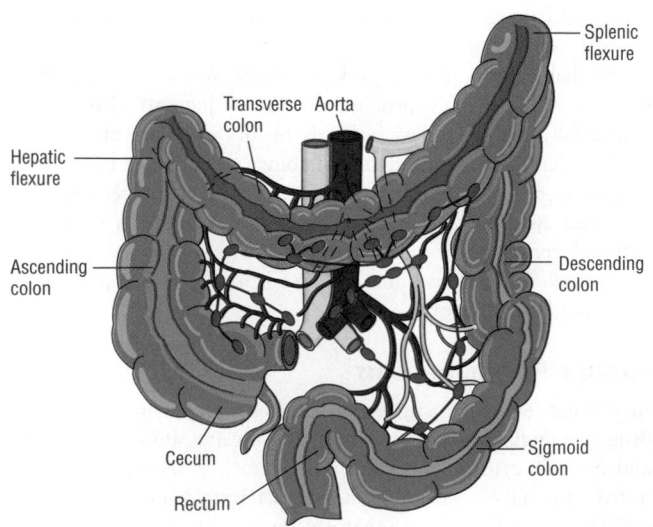

FIGURE 138-2. Colon and rectum anatomy.

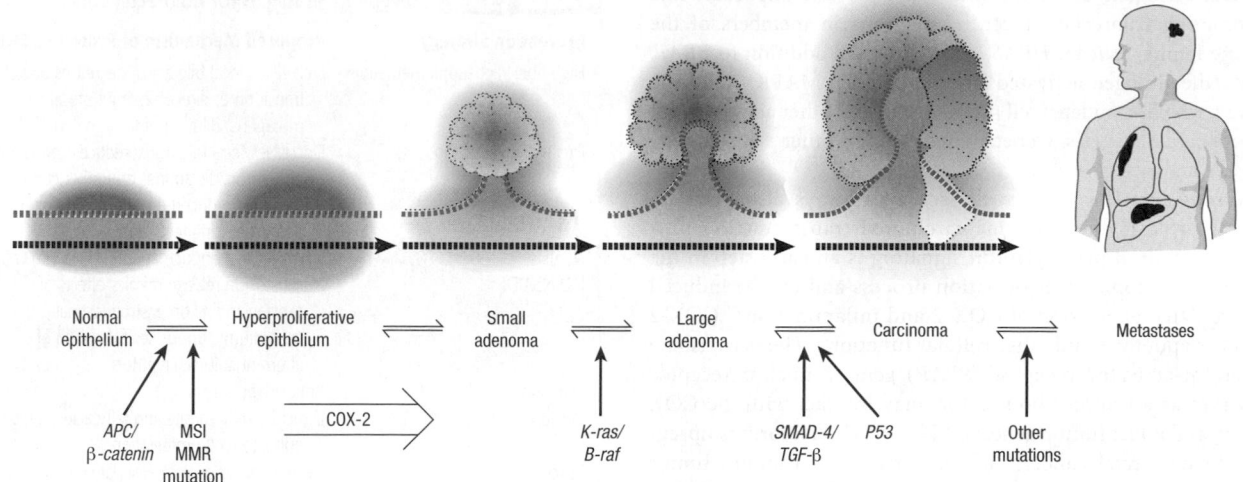

FIGURE 138-4. Genetic changes associated with the adenoma–carcinoma sequence in colorectal cancer. The accumulation of genetic changes in the pathogenesis of colorectal cancer includes DNA hypomethylation across the genome, mutation in the adenomatous polyposis coli *(APC)* gene or abnormalities in β-catenin; microsatellite instability (MSI) initiated by mismatch repair (MMR) gene mutation or methylation defects; mutational activation of cyclooxygenase-2 (COX-2); *KRAS* or *BRAF* oncogene activation; tumor suppressor gene deletions in chromosome 18q (SMAD-4 mutations) and disruption of transforming growth factor-β receptor type II signaling; and defects in *P53* function. *(Data from references 39, 41, and 45.)*

the malignant transformation. Table 138–2 lists important genetic mutations that are associated with colorectal cancers.

Several patterns of genomic instability may be present in colorectal cancer; the most common type of genomic instability is chromosomal instability, which leads to alterations in chromosomal structure and copy number.[41] An important consequence of chromosomal instability is loss of a wild-type allele of a tumor-suppressor gene, also referred to as loss of heterozygosity (LOH). Up to 85% of sporadic colorectal cancers exhibit chromosomal instability and the tumor suppressor genes *APC*, *P53*, and *SMAD-4* are commonly affected.[41] Other forms include somatic or germline defects in DNA MMR genes, germline inactivation of *MYH*, a base excision repair gene, and aberrant DNA methylation that results in epigenetic silencing of tumor suppressor gene expression.

Mutation or loss of the *APC* tumor suppressor gene is a key factor involved in tumor formation through activation of the Wnt signaling pathway, a mediator of cell proliferation, differentiation,

and survival.[41] The *APC* gene encodes for APC protein that binds to and degrades α- and β-catenin, which belong to a family of proteins associated with intracellular adhesion.[41] β-catenin, a downstream component of the Wnt signaling pathway, influences cell–cell communication, cell–cycle regulation, or apoptosis, and may contribute to abnormal epithelial proliferation and differentiation of cells.[11,41] In the absence of functional APC, β-catenin accumulates in the cytoplasm, then enters the nucleus and activates transcription of various genes, leading to constitutive activation of the Wnt signaling pathway. Inactivation of the *APC* gene is the single gene defect responsible for FAP, and is frequently an early event in the development of sporadic colorectal cancer cases.[41] A specific *APC* mutation, I1307K, is a factor in the development of familial colon cancer in individuals of Ashkenazi Jewish ancestry.[39]

Mutational inactivation of *P53* represents a second key step in colorectal tumorigenesis.[41] Normal *P53* gene expression is important for G_1 cell-cycle arrest to facilitate DNA repair during replication, and to induce apoptosis, an irreversible cell process resulting in cell death. *P53* is inactivated in up to 55% of sporadic colorectal cancers.[41] A third step in tumor progression is the mutational inactivation of the transforming growth factor-β (TGF-β) signaling pathway, which facilitates adenoma transition to high-grade dysplasia or carcinoma and also inactivates *SMAD-4*.[41] In normal epithelium, TGF-β has an antiproliferative role and induces growth arrest and apoptosis. Alterations in *SMAD-4* or TGF-β receptors lead to a loss of the normal growth inhibitory response to TGF-β. The frequency of *SMAD-4* mutations in colorectal cancer is reported to range from 10% to 35%.[41]

A distinct group of genetic traits has also been identified for individuals with HNPCC, but they also occur in sporadic cases of colorectal cancer. Replication errors occur frequently and represent widespread alterations in the length of a series of repeated nucleotides, or microsatellites, within tumor DNA. Mutations of the MMR genes that recognize and regulate DNA mismatch-repair errors contribute to microsatellite instability and colorectal tumorigenesis.[41] Failure to repair DNA mismatches results in microsatellite instability, which accelerates further gene mutations, leading to oncogene activation or tumor suppressor gene inactivation. Tumor progression is then facilitated through a link between DNA repair defects and mutations of critical growth regulatory genes.

TABLE 138-2	Genetic Mutations Associated with Colorectal Cancer	
Type of Mutation	**Disease**	**Genes**
Germline	Familial adenomatous polyposis (FAP)	*APC*
	MYH-associated polyposis (MAP)	*MYH*
	Hereditary nonpolyposis colorectal cancer (HNPCC)	DNA mismatch-repair genes:
		MSH2
		MLH1
		MSH6
Somatic	Sporadic colorectal cancer	Oncogenes:
		KRAS
		BRAF
		Tumor suppressor genes:
		P53
		SMAD-4
		APC
		TGFβR2

APC, adenomatous polyposis coli; TGFβR2, transforming growth factor-β receptor type II. Data from references 39, 41, and 45.

Several oncogene activating mutations play an important role in promoting colorectal cancer.[41] Mutations in members of the Ras gene family—*KRAS*, *HRAS*, and *NRAS*—in addition to *BRAF*, activate the mitogen-activated protein kinase (MAPK) signaling pathway, which stimulates cell proliferation and other activities that promote carcinogenesis. Genetic alterations in other cell signaling pathways may occur, as well.

Aberrant signaling of growth factor pathways also plays an important role in the adenoma-carcinoma transformation process. Activation of prostaglandin signaling is an early step in the adenoma-carcinoma transformation process and can be induced by upregulated expression of COX-2 and inflammation.[41] COX-2 influences apoptosis and other cellular functions. The peroxisome proliferator-activated receptor (*PPAR*) gene, a nuclear receptor that serves as a transcription factor, may interact with the COX pathway and affect tumorigenesis.[45] The PPARd isoform is upregulated in colorectal cancer, and its activation promotes tumor growth. COX-derived prostaglandins indirectly activate PPARd, which further enhances adenoma growth. The protooncogene *C-erbB* is activated in a high percentage of human tumors, including colorectal cancer, and encodes for expression of epidermal growth factor receptor (EGFR), a transmembrane glycoprotein involved in signaling pathways that affect cell growth, differentiation, proliferation, and angiogenesis. EGFR, which is overexpressed in a high proportion (72% to 82%) of colorectal cancers, is associated with increased cell proliferation and metastasis.[46] These mechanisms are potentially important because of the availability of pharmacologic agents that can influence these processes and affect cell growth.

HISTOLOGY

Adenocarcinomas account for more than 90% of tumors of the large intestine.[47] Other histologic types such as mucinous adenocarcinoma, signet-ring adenocarcinoma, carcinoid simplex, and carcinoid tumors occur less frequently. Adenocarcinomas are assigned one of three tumor grade designations based on the degree of cellular differentiation, the degree to which the tumor resembles the structure, and function of its cell of origin. The most differentiated adenocarcinomas are grade I tumors, whereas grade III tumors are considered "high grade," the most undifferentiated, and have frequently lost the characteristics of mature normal cells. Poorly differentiated tumors are associated with a worse prognosis than those that are better differentiated.[47]

Mucinous adenocarcinomas possess the same basic structure as adenocarcinomas but differ in that they secrete an abundant quantity of extracellular mucus. They account for only approximately 10% of colorectal carcinomas but tend to be frequent in patients with HNPCC and patients with coexisting ulcerative colitis.[47] Signet-ring adenocarcinomas have a characteristic appearance because of the displacement of the nucleus to one side by large vacuoles of intracellular mucin. Patients tend to present with a more advanced stage of disease and have a highly invasive tumor. Both mucinous and signet-ring adenocarcinoma histologies confer a poor prognosis.[48]

PREVENTION AND SCREENING

Cancer prevention efforts can be considered as either primary or secondary. Primary prevention strategies aim to prevent the development of colorectal cancer in a population at risk. Secondary prevention approaches are undertaken to prevent malignancy in a population that has already manifested an initial disease process. The basis for primary prevention depends on identification of

TABLE 138-3 Prevention Strategies for Colorectal Cancer

Prevention Strategy	Proposed Mechanism of Protective Effect
High-fiber diet supplementation[a]	Decreases fecal bile acids; decreases bowel transit time; direct binding to fecal mutagens; dilution of fecal material
Dietary fat reduction[a]	Decreases fecal bile acids; reduces consumption of heterocyclic amines and other carcinogens that are produced through meat preparation and processing techniques
NSAIDs[b,c]	Inhibit COX-2; induce apoptosis via 15-LOX-1
NO-NSAIDSs	Nitrous-oxide release mimics effects of prostaglandins on gastrointestinal epithelium; suppresses formation of aberrant colonic crypt foci
Selenium	Antioxidant effects
Calcium	Direct binding to bile and fatty acids; inhibits epithelial cell proliferation
Estrogens[c]	Decrease synthesis of secondary bile acids; decrease production of IGF-1; direct antiproliferative effects on colorectal epithelium
5-Aminosalicylic acids	Induce apoptosis via caspase 3 induction; inhibit TNF-α-mediated intestinal cell proliferation and MAPK activation
Bile salts	Reduce concentration of deoxycholic acid in colon; modulate phospholipase A2 expression and protein kinase C; antioxidant effects
HMG-CoA reductase inhibitors	Induce intestinal cell apoptosis and inhibit cell proliferation; suppress angiogenesis; synergistic COX-2 inhibition with NSAIDs
Difluoromethylornithine	Inhibits cellular proliferation through alterations in polyamine metabolism via inhibition of ornithine decarboxylase
Curcumin	Induces glutathione S-transferase (GST) enzymes; inhibits COX-2 expression
Omega-3 fatty acids	Inhibit COX-2 expression
PPAR-γ agonists	Epigenetic modulation
Resveratrol	Antioxidant effects
Green tea polyphenols	Antioxidant effects

COX-2, cyclooxygenase-2; 15-LOX-1, 15-lipoxygenase-1; NSAIDs, nonsteroidal antiinflammatory drugs; NO-NSAIDs, nitrous oxide donating nonsteroidal antiinflammatory drugs; IGF-1, insulin-like growth factor 1; TNF-α, tumor necrosis factor-alpha; MAPK, mitogen-activated protein kinase

[a]To date, findings from randomized trials have failed to demonstrate a protective effect of low-fat high-fiber fruit and vegetable dietary intake in reducing risk of recurrence of colorectal adenomas or colorectal cancer.

[b]Includes COX-2 inhibitors.

[c]Risk of use may outweigh benefit.

Data from references 5, 6, 51, and 52.

risk factors followed by eradication or alteration of their effects on carcinogenesis. Primary prevention also includes lifestyle and diet modification. Several primary preventive measures have undergone or are currently undergoing study (Table 138–3).

DIET

❶ Although early studies suggest that a substantial increase in daily dietary fiber and/or decrease in dietary fat intake might significantly reduce colorectal cancer risk, results from recent randomized trials are inconsistent. As such, there is insufficient evidence to support the use of fiber supplementation as a colorectal cancer prevention strategy at this time.

CHEMOPREVENTION

❷ The most widely studied agents for the chemoprevention of colorectal cancer are aspirin, nonaspirin NSAIDs, and COX-2 inhibitors, but their use as chemopreventive agents in the general population has not been established. Nonaspirin NSAIDs and COX-2 inhibitors were associated with reduced risk of colorectal adenomas in cohort and case-control studies, and COX-2 inhibitors were also effective in controlled trials.[14] However, the United States Preventive Services Task Force has concluded that potential harms associated with their use outweigh the benefits of aspirin and NSAIDs for prevention of colorectal cancer in the general population.[49]

In randomized studies of individuals with FAP, sulindac and celecoxib reduced the size and number of adenomatous polyps, but they are not viewed as alternatives to surgery. Sulindac can induce regression of existing adenomas, but in a randomized study of newly diagnosed patients with FAP it did not prevent new adenoma formation.[50] In 1999, the FDA approved the use of celecoxib to reduce the number of adenomatous colorectal polyps in FAP as an adjunct to usual care. This approval was based primarily on results from a trial of 77 patients with FAP who received celecoxib, 400 mg orally twice daily, or placebo, for 6 months. Celecoxib administration significantly reduced the mean polyp number (28% vs. 4.5%) and polyp burden (30.7% vs. 4.9%) as compared with placebo.[51] Recently, celecoxib was shown to decrease sporadic adenoma formation by more than 30% as compared with placebo, but the risk of cardiovascular events was increased in the treatment group, and its use in the general population cannot be recommended at this time.[51] In addition, its benefits are likely to be transient, because patients receiving sulindac experienced an increase in size and number of polyps within 3 months after the sulindac was discontinued.[50]

The use of aspirin as both a primary and a secondary chemopreventive agent remains controversial. Regular use of aspirin reduced the incidence of colorectal cancer in cohort studies by 22%, and it reduced the incidence of adenomas in randomized controlled trials, case-control studies, and cohort studies.[13] The benefits appear greatest with high-dose rather than low-dose (325- vs. 81-mg) aspirin and with administration for periods longer than 10 years, but the risk of bleeding complications is also greater.[13] In addition, aspirin use appears to reduce the risk of colorectal cancers that overexpress COX-2 but not those with absent or weak COX-2 expression.[52]

Randomized trials of calcium and folate supplementation as chemoprevention have also been conducted, and findings do not support their use at this time. In the placebo-controlled Calcium Polyp Prevention Study, patients with a previous colorectal adenoma who received calcium carbonate supplementation for 5 years experienced a moderate reduction in risk of recurrent colorectal adenomas.[5] In another randomized trial, protection was limited to individuals with higher serum vitamin D levels. These findings are in contrast with results from a large, randomized trial of calcium plus vitamin D supplementation for 7 years in 36,282 women from the Women's Health Initiative, which did not demonstrate any difference in the incidence of invasive colorectal cancer between treatment or placebo.[51] Because of the long latency period associated with cancer development, the 7-year duration of this trial may have been too short. However, there is no evidence that calcium intake greater than that recommended to reduce osteoporosis is protective against colorectal cancer. Although calcium intake appears to be inversely related to colon cancer, its role as a chemopreventive agent has not been defined.[51]

Additional intervention trials of various micronutrients, including selenium, folic acid, ursodiol, curcumin, difluoromethylornithine (DFMO), epigenetic modulators (e.g., PPAR agonists, histone deacetylase inhibitors), and other chemopreventive agents have been completed or are ongoing.[5,12,51,52] A randomized, placebo-controlled trial of folate 1 mg daily for up to 6 years as primary prevention of colorectal adenomas did not show reduced adenoma

risk.[12] Furthermore, folate supplementation was associated with a nonsignificant increase in adenoma recurrence in two studies.[12] Therefore until the efficacy and safety of folate supplementation to reduce colorectal cancer risk can be evaluated, it is not recommended at this time. Several trials of DFMO, an irreversible inhibitor of the polyamine synthetic pathway, show promising activity as a chemopreventive agent.[53]

SURGICAL RESECTION

Surgical resection remains an option to prevent colon cancer in individuals at extremely high risk for its development. Despite the potential for NSAIDs to reduce adenoma development and to induce adenoma regression in individuals with FAP, their effects are incomplete and their use cannot replace surgical resection as an important means of cancer prevention for these high-risk individuals. Individuals with FAP who are found to have polyposis on lower endoscopy screening examinations should undergo total proctocolectomy and ileal pouch–anal anastomosis or subtotal colectomy with an ileorectal anastomosis.[54] Because of the high incidence of metachronous cancers (45%) in patients with HNPCC, prophylactic subtotal colectomy with an ileorectal anastomosis is recommended for those individuals.[54] Colonoscopic polypectomy, removal of polyps detected during screening colonoscopy, is considered the standard of care for all individuals to prevent the progression of premalignant adenomatous polyps to adenocarcinomas.

SCREENING

❸ Based on the recognized incidence of colorectal cancer, identification of high-risk individuals, and the high rate of curability associated with localized lesions, screening recommendations for early detection of colorectal cancer have been established.[55–58] Some tests effectively detect early cancer, whereas others detect colorectal polyps and cancer. Differences exist in specific screening guidelines published by various organizations. This section reviews available screening techniques for colon cancer.

Fecal Occult Blood Testing

❸ The use of fecal occult blood tests (FOBTs) annually or biannually, results in an increased number of asymptomatic individuals diagnosed with early stages of disease. Results from randomized, controlled trials where standard FOBTs were administered annually or biennially show a reduction in colorectal cancer mortality by 15% to 33%.[55] Two main methods are available to detect occult blood in the feces: guaiac dye or derivative, and immunochemical methods. The Hemoccult II is a standard guaiac-based test that detects peroxidase activity of heme when hemoglobin comes in contact with a guaiac-impregnated paper. When a solution containing hydrogen peroxide is poured over the paper, a blue color appears if the test is positive. The testing process is complex and requires specific patient counseling to avoid inaccurate results (Table 138–4).

The Hemoccult Sensa, another guaiac-based test, is preferred by some organizations because it may have increased sensitivity and specificity as compared with the Hemoccult II. Clinical guidelines have been developed for performing and interpreting results of FOBT.[59] The limitations associated with fecal occult blood screening remain an issue of active concern. Many early-stage tumors do not bleed, and therefore the false-negative rates are approximately 70% for cancer and 90% for polyps. In addition, the test results may not be valid because the test is often poorly performed both in the home and in physician office settings.[55] However, these concerns are addressed through continued

TABLE 138-4 Patient Counseling Points Prior to Hemoccult II Testing

To Avoid False Positives	To Avoid False Negatives

1. Dietary restrictions
  • Avoid rare red meat and vegetables with peroxidase activity (turnips, broccoli, cauliflower, and radishes) for 3 days prior to testing
2. Medical restrictions
  • Avoid iron products, rectal administration of medications, and digital rectal examinations for 3 days prior to testing
  • Avoid nonsteroidal antiinflammatory drugs for up to 7 days prior to testing
	• Avoid vitamin C for 3 days prior to testing
	• Avoid testing dehydrated samples (rehydrating of samples is not recommended)

Procedure for Hemoccult II testing

Patient applies two separate samples of three different stools to six test card windows.

serial screening with FOBT. In addition, approximately 1% to 5% of randomly selected individuals will have a positive test result, and approximately 2% to 17% of those individuals will be found to have colorectal cancer.[55,59] False-positive results can prove to be very expensive and inconvenient for a patient because of the followup tests required to confirm a positive result. Nevertheless, studies evaluating the effects of FOBT as a screening modality have established that their annual use reduces colorectal cancer mortality by up to 33%.[55,59]

Newer tests, such as immunochemical assays, were developed to reduce the rate of false-positive results associated with the guaiac-based tests. Fecal immunochemical tests (FIT) (InSure and others) use antibodies to detect the globin protein portion of human hemoglobin. These FITs have the advantage of improved specificity and sensitivity.[55] A potential increase in patient compliance is expected because these tests do not react with dietary factors or medications, but performance varies among different available tests. To date, these FITs have not found widespread use in the United States because of commercial and technical reasons, although they, along with guaiac-based tests, are recommended in some screening protocols.[57,58] They are preferred over FOBT by the American College of Gastroenterology.[56]

Flexible Sigmoidoscopy

❸ Sigmoidoscopy can examine the lower 35% to 60% of the bowel, depending on the instrument, and thus increases the detection rate by about two- to threefold.[56] Unlike FOBT, sigmoidoscopy detects polyps as well as early cancer. A 60-cm flexible sigmoidoscope can be used to reach the splenic flexure so as to detect 50% to 60% of cancers, but it requires more operator training, is associated with increased risk, and is not tolerated as well as the 35-cm instrument. The combination of sigmoidoscopy plus FOBT appears to improve sensitivity for lesions that will be missed by sigmoidoscopy alone, but the true benefit of this approach to general practice has not been established.[57,58] Because the entire colon cannot be examined with sigmoidoscopy, many clinicians prefer to perform a colonoscopy.[55]

Total Colonic Examination

❸ Total colonic examination can be accomplished with colonoscopy or double-contrast barium enema. A colonoscope facilitates examination of the whole bowel to the cecum in most patients, and allows for simultaneous removal of premalignant lesions. Although it allows for greater visualization of the colon, colonoscopy involves greater risk and inconvenience to patients. However, it is the preferred screening method based on its superior ability to detect

lesions in the proximal colon as compared with sigmoidoscopy.[55,56] This may become increasingly important, as the proportion of tumors occurring in the proximal or right (cecum, ascending, and transverse colon) side of the colon has increased over the past 30 years, with fewer occurring in the rectum and distal or left (descending and sigmoid colon) side. It remains somewhat controversial whether this observation reflects a change in the biology of the disease or the nature of screening techniques. Most lesions, however, still occur in the distal colon.

A double-contrast barium enema produces an image of the entire colon in most examinations, and the retained barium outlines small polyps and mucosal lesions. This approach is the least-expensive method of examining the entire colon, but is considered inferior to colonoscopy for detecting polyps and colorectal cancer.[55] In addition, a supplemental colonoscopy is required if suspicious lesions are identified. Because of these limitations, the combination of double-contrast barium enema with flexible sigmoidoscopy could be used to increase the sensitivity for detecting a colorectal malignancy compared with a double-contrast barium enema alone. However, it is generally reserved for use if other tests are not available.[55]

Novel Screening Strategies

Molecular screening strategies analyze stool samples for presence of potential markers of malignancy in cells that are shed from premalignant polyps or adenocarcinomas in the bowel.[55–57] These include abnormalities or mutations in DNA, RNA expression patterns that are characteristic of malignancy, and the presence of proteins or other molecular cellular components. Of these, DNA testing has undergone the most testing. In a large-scale comparison of fecal DNA analysis to FOBT in asymptomatic individuals at average risk, neither test was able to identify most of the neoplastic lesions found with colonoscopy, but fecal DNA analysis detected a greater proportion of lesions than did FOBT without compromising specificity.[60] Additional work is ongoing to identify the role of novel molecular markers in colorectal cancer detection, but none to date have shown improvement over FIT. Genetic testing is an important cancer-screening approach for family members of individuals diagnosed with FAP or HNPCC and is appropriate for selected individuals, but it should only be offered in conjunction with genetic counseling.

Computed tomography (CT) colonography (virtual colonoscopy) is an imaging procedure that creates two- or three-dimensional images of the colon by combining multiple helical CT scans. Initial tests are promising, although patients still require bowel cleansing, and many will be referred for colonoscopy to remove detected lesions.[55]

Screening Summary

Table 138–5 outlines current U.S. guidelines for screening and surveillance for early detection of colorectal cancer. Men and women who are 50 years of age and are at average risk (their only risk factor is age >50 years) should be screened annually using a sensitive FOBT or FIT or undergo examination of the colon every 5 to 10 years, depending on the type of test used.[55] Although several methods for examining the colon are available, there is no evidence that one test should be chosen over another.[55] However, colonoscopy is the preferred modality of the American College of Gastroenterology.[56] More rigorous (usually starting at an earlier age) screening recommendations are recommended for moderate- to high-risk individuals.[56,57] The United States Preventive Services Task Force recommends routine screening for individuals age 50 to 75 years with different consideration given to adults 76 to 85 years and those older than 85 years.[58]

TABLE 138-5 Guidelines for Colorectal Cancer Screening in the United States for Individuals at Average Risk, 50 Years of Age and Older

ACS	ACG	USPSTF	ACS-USMSTF-ACR
gFOBT[a,f]	Colonoscopy[d]	gFOBT[a,f]	gFOBT[a,f]
Or	Or	Or	Or
FIT[a,f]	FIT[a]	gFOBT[b,f] + FSIG[c]	FIT[a,f]
Or	Or	Or	Or
sDNA[e]	FSIG[c-d]	Colonoscopy[d]	sDNA[e]
Or	Or		Or
FSIG[c]	CTC[c]		FSIG[c]
Or	Or		Or
gFOBT[a] + FSIG[c]	gFOBT[a,f]		Colonoscopy[d]
Or	Or		Or
DCBE[c]	sDNA[b]		DCBE[c]
Or			Or
Colonoscopy[d]			CTC[c]
Or			
CTC[c]			

ACS, American Cancer Society; ACG, American College of Gastroenterology; USPSTF, U.S. Preventive Services Task Force; USMSTF, U.S. Multi-Society Task Force on Colorectal Cancer; ACR, American College of Radiology; DCBE, double-contrast barium enema; gFOBT, guaiac-based fecal occult blood testing; FIT, fecal immunochemical testing; sDNA, stool DNA test; FSIG, flexible sigmoidoscopy; CTC, CT colonography

[a]Annually
[b]Every 3 years
[c]Every 5 years
[d]Every 10 years
[e]Interval uncertain
[f]If >50% sensitivity for colorectal cancer
Data from references 55–58.

DIAGNOSIS

SIGNS AND SYMPTOMS

The signs and symptoms associated with colorectal cancer can be extremely varied, subtle, and nonspecific. Patients with early stage colorectal cancer are often asymptomatic, and lesions are usually found as a result of screening studies. Any change in bowel habits (e.g., constipation, diarrhea, or alteration in size or shape of stool), vague abdominal discomfort, abdominal pain, or distension may all be warning signs of a malignant process. Obstructive symptoms and changes in bowel habits frequently develop with tumors located in the transverse and descending colon. Bleeding may be acute or chronic and most commonly appears as bright red blood mixed with stool. Iron-deficiency anemia, presenting as weakness and occasionally as high-output congestive heart failure, frequently develops as a result of chronic occult blood loss.

PRESENTATION OF COLORECTAL CANCER

General

☐ Patient symptoms are usually nonspecific and can vary drastically among patients.

Symptoms

☐ Change in bowel habits (generally an increase in frequency) or rectal bleeding.

☐ Constipation, depending on the location of the tumor.

☐ Nausea, vomiting, and abdominal discomfort.

☐ Fatigue may be present if anemia is severe.

Signs

☐ Blood in the stool is the most common sign.

☐ Hepatomegaly and jaundice in advanced disease.

☐ Leg edema as a consequence of lymph node involvement, thrombophlebitis, fistula formation, weight loss, and pain in the lower back or radiating down the legs are indicative of widespread disease.

Laboratory Tests

☐ Positive guaiac stool test and anemia (iron deficiency) from blood loss.

☐ Elevated carcinoembryonic antigen (most patients).

☐ Elevated liver enzymes may be present with metastatic disease.

Approximately 19% of patients with colorectal cancer present with metastatic disease.[3] Metastatic spread occurs as a result of direct tumor invasion of adjacent tissues or by lymphatic or hematogenous spread. The venous drainage of the colon and rectum influences the pattern of metastases most commonly seen. The most common site of metastasis is the liver, often the only site of metastatic disease in 40% of patients, followed by the lungs and then bones, specifically the sacrum, coccyx, pelvis, and lumbar vertebrae. Liver metastases are present in 5% to 10% of patients at presentation.

WORKUP

When a patient is suspected of having colorectal carcinoma, a careful history and physical examination should be performed. The patient history should include a past medical history and family history, especially noting the presence of inflammatory bowel disease, colorectal cancer, polyps, and cancers of the breast, ovary, and endometrium. A complete physical examination includes careful abdominal examination for the presence of masses or ascites, a rectal examination, and an assessment for possible hepatomegaly and lymphadenopathy. A breast and pelvic examination is recommended in all women, especially in women with a history of breast, ovarian, or endometrial cancer.

An unexplained anemia in an older patient requires surveillance of the entire large bowel, especially the right colon. Red blood cell indices (e.g., hemoglobin, hematocrit, mean corpuscular volume, and reticulocyte count) and a workup of iron status (e.g., serum ferritin, serum iron, and total iron-binding capacity) may be useful to confirm acute or chronic blood loss and/or iron-deficiency anemia. An evaluation of the entire large bowel is undertaken with either colonoscopy or sigmoidoscopy and a double-contrast barium enema. A barium enema may be preferred in situations in which a partially obstructing lesion prohibits passage of the endoscope, but it should be avoided if complete obstruction or perforation of the bowel is suspected. A characteristic finding indicative of colon cancer seen on barium enema is an apple core–shaped lesion with tumor involving the circumference of the bowel. When possible, the endoscope is used to collect tissue for a histologic evaluation and provide a preliminary diagnosis following the procedure.

Baseline laboratory tests should be obtained and include a complete blood cell count, platelet count, international normalized ratio (INR), prothrombin time, activated partial thromboplastin time, liver chemistries, and renal function tests. Abnormal liver chemistry test results may suggest liver involvement with tumor. However, patients with metastatic disease to the liver may have normal liver chemistries, and abnormal liver test results are not always indicative of metastatic disease.

Additional laboratory tests may include a baseline carcinoembryonic antigen (CEA) level if it is likely to augment staging and treatment plans.[61] CEA belongs to a group of cell-surface glycoproteins termed *oncofetal proteins*, which are expressed during embryonic development and reexpressed on the cell surfaces of many carcinomas, particularly those originating from the gastrointestinal tract. CEA concentrations can be measured in the blood and can therefore potentially serve as a marker for colorectal cancer. But not all colorectal cancers produce CEA, and elevated concentrations are more frequent in patients with metastatic disease. It is important to recognize, however, that several concomitant disease states are associated with an elevated CEA: liver diseases, gastritis, peptic ulcer disease, diverticulitis, chronic obstructive pulmonary disease, chronic or acute inflammatory conditions, and diabetes.[61] Most commercially available assays list a value of less than 5 ng/mL (5 mcg/L) as the upper limit of normal. Although CEA measurement is too insensitive and nonspecific to be used as a screening test for early-stage colorectal cancer, it is the surrogate marker of choice for monitoring colorectal cancer response to treatment, particularly if the pretreatment concentration is elevated.[61] The CEA test may have preoperative prognostic implications because it has been shown to correlate with the size and degree of differentiation of the carcinoma. Elevated preoperative CEA levels correlate with a poor survival and may predict likelihood of recurrence, regardless of tumor stage at diagnosis. However, it should not be used to determine whether a patient should receive adjuvant therapy. After a potentially curative resection, CEA levels should return to normal within 4 to 6 weeks. Persistently elevated CEA levels may indicate residual disease, while elevations after normalization may indicate relapsed disease.

Radiographic imaging studies evaluate the extent of disease involvement. Although a chest radiograph is recommended to rule out the presence of metastatic spread to the lungs, a CT scan of the chest is preferred. A CT scan of the abdomen and pelvis is often performed to evaluate hepatic and retroperitoneal involvement and occult abdominal and pelvic disease, and to determine the depth of tumor penetration into the bowel wall and/or invasion to adjacent organs. Detection of lymph node involvement with either study is limited by the difficulty of distinguishing inflammatory or reactive lymph nodes from those infiltrated with tumor. Because CT scans may not adequately detect peritoneal seeding, small distant lymph node metastasis, or liver metastasis in colon cancer, an occasional patient may need to undergo a laparotomy, spiral CT, magnetic resonance imaging, or glucose analog [^{18}F]-fluorodeoxyglucose-positron emission tomography (PET) scan in order to confirm metastatic disease. PET imaging can provide functional information to discriminate between benign and malignant disease by detecting tumor-related metabolic alterations in affected tissues. PET scans are commonly used for the detection of recurrent colorectal cancer in patients with rising CEA levels and inconclusive findings on standard imaging studies. A PET scan is often combined with or followed by a CT scan because anatomical localization of a lesion using PET alone can be difficult.

Endoscopic ultrasound is a technique that is becoming more widely available for the evaluation of patients with rectal cancer. It is useful for detecting the depth of tumor penetration, and like pelvic CT scans, is fair to good in determining lymph node involvement. Cystoscopy or IV pyelography studies are rarely indicated except for very large rectal tumors found on examination, if the patient exhibits symptoms, or if a CT scan suggests bladder involvement. Intraluminal and hepatic magnetic resonance imaging studies may also provide useful information.

Radioimmunoscintigraphy uses tumor-directed antibodies labeled with γ-producing radionuclides such as ^{99m}technetium or ^{111}indium to detect malignant cells.[62] Several tumor-associated proteins have been identified within or on the surface membrane of colorectal malignant cells to which monoclonal antibodies have been targeted. Of these, TAG-72 and CEA are commonly used. Radiolabeled monoclonal antibodies directed against these antigens are used in clinical studies for both external immunoscintigraphy as well as intraoperative localization of tumor. OncoScint, an ^{111}indium-labeled B72.3 monoclonal antibody targeted to the TAG-72 cell-surface antigen, is an FDA-approved diagnostic imaging agent available for determining the location and extent of extrahepatic disease in patients with colorectal cancer. CEA-Scan is a ^{99m}Tc-labeled fragment of the anti-CEA antibody for the assessment of recurrent colorectal carcinoma. The use of these tests is generally reserved for those patients who have completed standard diagnostic imaging tests, but may still require additional information regarding the extent of disease. They may also play an important role in identifying metastatic or recurrent disease in individuals with rising CEA levels and negative standard radiographic studies.

STAGING

❹ The purpose of the staging examinations is to determine the extent of disease, which allows the oncologist to develop treatment options and estimate overall prognosis. Traditionally, the Dukes classification, originally published in 1932, was used in the staging of colorectal cancers.[47] Since its original publication, it has undergone several modifications; a modified Astler-Coller version is now used more commonly. In an effort to standardize the staging system for colorectal cancer, the American Joint Committee on Cancer and the Union for International Cancer Control (UICC) jointly recommend the TNM classification system. This classification takes three aspects of cancer growth: T (tumor size), N (lymph node involvement), and M (presence or absence of metastases) into account. The TNM classification also allows for various subdivisions within each of the three categories, which is then used for determining the disease stage. Table 138–6 summarizes the staging definitions using the TNM system and corresponding SEER 5-year survival rates.[63,64] Figure 138–5 shows the relationship between the modified Astler-Coller and American Joint Committee on Cancer/Union for International Cancer Control staging systems.

PROGNOSIS

❹ The stage of colorectal cancer upon diagnosis is the most important independent prognostic factor for survival and disease recurrence. Five-year relative survival is approximately 92% for individuals who present with a localized tumor stage at diagnosis as compared with about 11% for individuals with metastatic disease at diagnosis.[3]

Clinical factors present at the time of diagnosis that are associated with a poor prognosis and decreased survival include bowel obstruction or perforation, rectal bleeding, high preoperative CEA level, distant metastases, and location of the primary tumor in the rectum or rectosigmoid area.[47] Along with resection of the primary tumor, a minimum of 12 lymph nodes must be examined to accurately determine regional lymph node involvement and predict lymph node-negative disease.[48] The pathologic assessment also includes determination of TNM stage, tumor type and histologic grade, presence of vascular invasion, and whether the resected margins are free of tumor. Consideration of these factors plays an important role in determining optimal strategies for treatment and appropriate follow-up.

Additional stage-independent pathologic variables that have negative prognostic or predictive value with regard to adjuvant therapy include presence of lymphatic or perineural invasion; mucinous or signet-ring histology; high tumor proliferation indices; tumor

TABLE 138-6 Colon Cancer by TNM Classification and Associated 5-Year Relative Survival

Stage	T	N	M	Dukes[a]	MAC[a]	Survival (%)
0	T_{is}	N_0	M_0	–	–	
I	T_1	N_0	M_0	A	A	} 97.4
	T_2	N_0	M_0	A	B_1	
IIA	T_3	N_0	M_0	B	B_2	87.5
IIB	T_{4a}	N_0	M_0	B	B_2	79.6
IIC	T_{4b}	N_0	M_0	B	B_3	58.4
IIIA	$T_1–T_2$	N_1/N_{1c}	M_0	C	C_1	} 79.0–90.7
	T_1	N_{2a}	M_0	C	C_1	
IIIB	$T_3–T_{4a}$	N_1/N_{1c}	M_0	C	C_2	
	$T_2–T_3$	N_{2a}	M_0	C	C_1/C_2	53.4–79.0
	$T_1–T_2$	N_{2b}	M_0	C	C_1	
IIIC	T_{4a}	N_{2a}	M_0	C	C_2	
	$T_3–T_{4a}$	N_{2b}	M_0	C	C_2	15.7–40.9
	T_{4b}	$N_1–N_2$	M_0	C	C_3	
IVA	Any T	Any N	M_{1a}	–	–	} 11.5
IVB	Any T	Any N	M_{1b}	–	–	

T_{is}: Carcinoma in situ: intraepithelial or invasion of lamina propia[b]

T_1: Tumor invades submucosa

T_2: Tumor invades muscularis propria

T_3: Tumor invades through the muscularis propria into pericolorectal tissues

T_{4a}: Tumor penetrates to the surface of the visceral peritoneum[c]

T_{4b}: Tumor directly invades or is adherent to other ogans or structures[c,d]

[a]Dukes B is a composite of better ($T_3 N_0 M_0$) and worse ($T_4 N_0 M_0$) prognostic groups, as is Dukes C (Any T $N_1 M_0$ and Any T $N_2 M_0$). MAC is the modified Astler-Coller classification.

[b]T_{is} includes cancer cells confined within the glandular basement membrane (intraepithelial) or mucosal lamina propria (intramucosal) with no extension through the muscularis mucosae into the submucosa.

[c]Direct invasion in T_4 includes invasion of other organs or other segments of the colorectum as a result of direct extension through the serosa, as confirmed on microscopic examination (for example, invasion of the sigmoid colon by a carcinoma of the cecum) or, for cancers in a retroperitoneal or subperitoneal location, direct invasion of other organs or structures by virtue of extension beyond the muscularis propria (i.e., respectively, a tumor on the posterior wall of the descending colon invading the left kidney or lateral abdominal wall; or a mid or distal rectal cancer with invasion of prostate, seminal vesicles, cervix, or vagina).

[d]Tumor that is adherent to other organs or structures, grossly, is classified cT_{4b}. However, if no tumor is present in the adhesion, microscopically, the classification should be pT_{1-4a} depending on the anatomical depth of wall invasion. The V and L classifications should be used to identify the presence or absence of vascular or lymphatic invasion whereas the PN site-specific factor should be used for perineural invasion.

Data from references 3, 63, and 64.

aneuploidy; absence of host immune response to the tumor; and presence of certain molecular markers (18q/*DCC* mutation or loss of heterozygosity, microsatellite stability [MSS], *RAS* mutations, elevated thymidylate synthase [TS] expression, and *P53* mutation or loss).[47,48,65] Of these, the highest level of evidence supports the consideration of lymphatic invasion as a prognostic factor. The next level of evidence, which is supporting but requires additional validation, is for 18q/*DCC* mutation or loss of heterozygosity and MSS.

Colorectal cancers with allelic loss of heterozygosity on chromosome 18q or absent DCC protein are associated with a worse prognosis within stage II disease and may predict response to adjuvant chemotherapy, but data are insufficient to warrant its use at this time.[61,66] MSS can be determined through DNA sequencing or by immunohistochemistry staining for protein products of the *MSH2* or *MLH1* genes. Colorectal cancers that demonstrate high-frequency MSS appear to be associated with a more favorable outcome and may predict the benefit of fluorouracil.[67] Although findings from several studies suggest that MSS status may predict efficacy of adjuvant fluoropyrimidine therapy, this finding must be confirmed in a prospective study before its use can be recommended.[61] Trials that account for MSS are ongoing.

Tumors that overexpress mutant *P53* demonstrate a high degree of resistance to radiation, fluorouracil, and certain other chemotherapeutic agents and are associated with a less-favorable prognosis. However, because of heterogeneous and conflicting results of reported studies, often attributable to methodologies that do not address the functional status of both *P53* alleles, *P53* status does not appear useful as a guide for treatment decisions.[61]

Tumors that overexpress TS, an enzyme that converts deoxyuridine monophosphate to deoxythymidine monophosphate, an essential step for DNA synthesis, are less sensitive to fluorouracil chemotherapy. Patients whose colon cancers have higher levels of TS appear to have a significantly worse overall 5-year survival than patients whose cancers have a low level of TS.[47] The importance of elevated TS and type of therapeutic interventions is unclear. No large cooperative group trial has identified a subgroup of patients who failed to benefit from fluorouracil plus leucovorin therapy based on tumor TS levels. Consideration of tumor TS expression in several adjuvant therapy trials is ongoing.

Tumors that have a high rate of proliferation are generally associated with a poor prognosis. Ki-67 is expressed in cells actively engaged in the cell cycle and has also been used as a measure of colon cancer proliferation. Interestingly, for unknown reasons, high levels of Ki-67 were associated with an increase in overall survival in patients with early-stage colon cancer. EGFR testing of colorectal tumor cells with immunohistochemistry has been a standard component of pathologic analysis, but the value of EGFR positive staining in predicting response to anti-EGFR treatment is still unclear. Although EGFR overexpression may be linked to more advanced disease or predict risk of metastasis, its relationship to overall survival is controversial.[46] Other methods to assess EGFR status are being evaluated.

Evaluation of these factors may predict which patients will benefit most from more aggressive therapy, individuals who may not in the future require systemic chemotherapy, and new therapeutic targets for the treatment of colorectal cancer, but further study is required. The current American Society of Clinical Oncology (ASCO) guidelines do not recommend the use of DNA ploidy, DNA flow cytometric proliferation analysis, *P53* expression or mutation analysis, *RAS* oncogene testing, MSS markers, or 18q loss of heterozygosity/DCC determination to determine prognosis or response to therapy.[61]

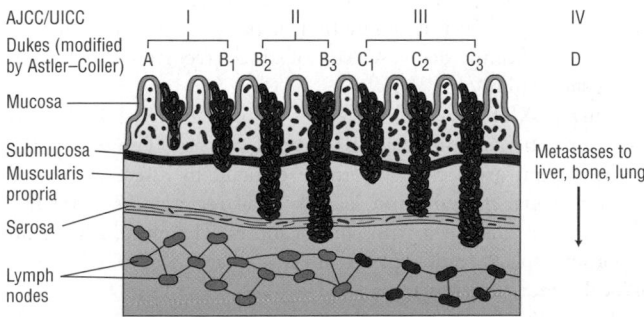

AJCC/UICC — I, II, III, IV
Dukes (modified by Astler–Coller) — A, B_1, B_2, B_3, C_1, C_2, C_3, D
Mucosa
Submucosa
Muscularis propria
Serosa
Lymph nodes
Metastases to liver, bone, lung

FIGURE 138-5. Staging systems for colorectal cancer. (Used with the permission of the American Joint Committee on Cancer (AJCC), Chicago, Illinois. The original source for this material is the AJCC Cancer Staging Manual, Seventh Edition (2010) published by Springer Science and Business Media LLC, www.springer.com; UICC, Union for International Cancer Control.)

TREATMENT

Colorectal Cancer

◼ DESIRED OUTCOME

Treatment goals for cancer of the colon or rectum are based on the stage of disease at presentation. Stages I, II, and III disease are considered potentially curable and are managed with the intent of eradicating micrometastases that may be present. Based on the numbers and site(s) of metastases, approximately 20% to 30% of patients with metastatic colorectal cancer may be cured, if their metastases are considered resectable. Most patients with stage IV disease are not curable, and treatments for metastatic disease are considered palliative to reduce symptoms, avoid disease-related complications, and prolong survival.

■ GENERAL APPROACH TO TREATMENT

Although advanced age is not an absolute contraindication for aggressive therapies, the age of the patient, concomitant disease states, lifestyle factors, performance status, and the patient's preferences must be considered in the treatment planning process. Special or emergent conditions, such as bowel perforation, spinal cord compression, and severe pain, anemia, or other symptomatic problems, need to be addressed acutely, after which time a more long-term disease-specific plan can be developed. The treatment approaches for colorectal cancer reflect two primary treatment goals: curative therapy for localized disease and palliative therapy for metastatic cancer.

For patients for whom treatment intent is curative, surgical resection of the primary tumor is the most important component of therapy. Depending on the extent of disease and whether the tumor originated in the colon or rectum, further adjuvant chemotherapy or chemotherapy plus XRT may be appropriate. For selected patients with resectable metastases, surgical resection may be an option. However, for most patients with metastases, systemic chemotherapy is the mainstay of treatment; XRT may also be useful for disease palliation of localized symptoms or when chemotherapy is no longer effective. Patients with metastatic disease who are asymptomatic may benefit from initiation of therapy, and treatment should not be withheld until they develop symptoms.

■ OPERABLE DISEASE

Surgery

❺ Individuals with operable—stages I, II, and III—colorectal cancer should undergo complete surgical resection of the primary tumor mass with regional lymphadenectomy as a curative approach for their disease.[47] The surgical approach for colon cancer generally involves complete resection of the tumor with an appropriate margin of tumor-free bowel and a regional lymphadenectomy. A total colectomy is rarely needed in colon cancer but may be indicated for selected patients with FAP or chronic ulcerative colitis.

Surgery for rectal cancer depends on the region of tumor involvement. A low anterior resection is the procedure of choice in patients with lesions in the middle to upper rectum.[68] Patients with lesions in the lower portion of the rectum may require an abdominoperineal resection if the amount of unaffected bowel is insufficient for a resection far enough away from the tumor, or if the affected bowel is too close to areas that cannot permit an anastomosis. Excision of the mesorectum, the surrounding tissue that contains perirectal fat and draining lymph nodes, has also been advocated. Newer surgical techniques have been developed in an attempt to retain function of the rectal sphincter and still achieve complete tumor resection. Individuals who are not candidates for sphincter-sparing resections or have extensive local spread of tumor will require an abdomino-perineal resection. This involves removal of the distal sigmoid, rectosigmoid, rectum, and anus with the establishment of a permanent sigmoid colostomy. Less than one-third of patients will require a permanent colostomy for rectal cancer.[68] Other complications that occur frequently with surgery for rectal cancer include urinary retention, incontinence, impotence, and locoregional recurrence.

Overall, surgery for colorectal cancer is associated with a morbidity and mortality rate of 8% to 15% and 1% to 2%, respectively, depending on the type and extent of procedure.[47,68] Common complications associated with colorectal surgery include infection, anastomotic leakage, obstruction, adhesion formation, and malabsorption syndromes. Laparoscopic colectomy has become an accepted procedure for colon cancer, and there are limited data for patients with rectal cancer.[69] This technique appears to produce similar results to conventional surgery, with the benefits of a smaller surgical incision, shorter hospital stay, and reduced pain.

Adjuvant Therapy for Colon Cancer

Adjuvant therapy in colorectal cancer is administered to selected individuals after complete tumor resection in an attempt to eliminate residual micrometastatic disease, thereby decreasing tumor recurrence and improving survival rates. Because more than 90% of patients with stage I colon or rectal cancer are cured by surgical resection alone, adjuvant therapy is not indicated.[47] The role of adjuvant chemotherapy for stage II colon cancer is less clear because the results of studies in patients with stage II disease are conflicting. Adjuvant chemotherapy for patients with stage II disease has not been shown to be superior to surgery alone, with the exception of some high-risk patients. The ASCO guideline does not recommend routine use of adjuvant chemotherapy in patients with stage II disease unless it is administered in conjunction with a clinical trial.[70] Stage II patients who are at higher risk for relapse include those with inadequate lymph node sampling, perforation of the bowel at presentation, poorly differentiated tumors, and T_4 lesions. Adequate examination of the lymph nodes for tumor involvement is most important for appropriate staging of the patient with colorectal cancer. Various tumor molecular genetic factors (e.g., chromosome 18q deletion, tumor ploidy, mutations of protooncogenes or tumor suppressor genes, tumor TS expression, and MSS) are also being studied in an effort to identify subsets of patients with stage II disease who have an increased risk of relapse. Despite the lack of a consensus regarding the use of adjuvant chemotherapy for individuals with high-risk stage II colon cancer, many practitioners offer this therapy to selected patients, with a detailed discussion with patients regarding the potential benefits versus treatment-related toxicities. Optimal dosing, administration schedule, and duration of therapy have yet to be determined, but most practitioners use the same treatment approach as that used for patients with stage III colon cancer.

Adjuvant chemotherapy is standard therapy for patients with stage III colon cancer. The presence of lymph node involvement with tumor places patients with stage III colon cancer at high risk for recurrence, and the risk of death within 5 years of surgical resection alone is as high as 70%, depending on the number of lymph nodes involved.[47] In this population of patients, adjuvant chemotherapy significantly decreases risk of cancer recurrence and death and is standard of care.

Adjuvant XRT plus chemotherapy is considered standard treatment for patients with stage II/III rectal cancer.[68] Tumors arising in the rectum are technically more difficult to resect with wide circumferential margins and lead to local recurrences more frequently than those seen with colon cancers. Therefore, XRT is an important aspect of adjuvant therapy for rectal cancer to reduce risk of local tumor recurrence.

Adjuvant Radiation Therapy ❻ Adjuvant XRT has no definite role in colon cancer because most recurrences are extrapelvic and occur in the abdomen.[47] Although local recurrence and debilitating pelvic pain are uncommon, a subset of patients with T_3 or T_4 tumors located in the cecum and in hepatic and splenic flexures are at increased risk of local recurrence and may benefit from postoperative XRT and chemotherapy. Early trials with whole-abdominal XRT were limited by considerable toxicity.[68] However, results from studies combining abdominal XRT plus fluorouracil are promising. To date, postoperative local XRT may reduce the risk of local recurrence and improve survival compared to adjuvant chemotherapy alone but should only be considered for select patients with colon cancer.[47] Additionally, intraoperative radiation should be considered for patients with T_4 lesions that are fixed to an adjacent lesion.[71]

In patients undergoing surgery for rectal cancer, XRT is used to reduce risk of local tumor recurrence. Radiation therapy is given prior to or following surgery and can be delivered with a variety of dosing regimens, administration schedules, and techniques.[68] Preoperative XRT may be used to reduce the initial size of the tumor to such an extent that the tumor can be reclassified to a lower stage, or "down-staged," and therefore rendered more resectable. This might lead to improved patient survival or result in the need for a less-extensive surgical procedure. Preoperative XRT is also administered to reduce the amount of tumor seeding that can occur during surgery, but this approach is more likely to affect a greater area than is necessary.[68] Postoperative administration of XRT may more adequately treat a defined area but is associated with more toxicity because of a greater amount of bowel being present in the treatment field.

Adverse effects associated with XRT in colorectal cancer can be acute or chronic. Acute effects primarily include hematologic depression, dysuria, diarrhea, abdominal cramping, and proctitis. Chronic symptoms that sometimes persist for months following discontinuation of XRT include persistent diarrhea, proctitis or enteritis, small bowel obstruction, perineal tenderness, and impaired wound healing.

Adjuvant Chemotherapy For more than 40 years, fluorouracil has been the most widely used chemotherapeutic agent for the adjuvant treatment of colorectal cancer, both as a single agent and in combination with other agents. Newer agents such as oxaliplatin and capecitabine have been incorporated into combination chemotherapy regimens for the adjuvant treatment of colon cancer.[72,73] Investigational chemotherapy agents, biologic therapies that target the underlying tumor biology, and new administration methods are also being developed. Current adjuvant trials focus on combination chemotherapy regimens with newer targeted agents added.

Based on their activity for metastatic colon cancer, fluorouracil and floxuridine were investigated as single-agent chemotherapy agents for use after surgery. In 1988, a meta-analysis of phase III trials showed a small, statistically insignificant improvement in survival with fluorouracil-based regimens as compared with surgery alone.[74] Since then, most trials focused on improving the efficacy of fluorouracil in the adjuvant treatment of colon cancer.

Subsequently, clinicians identified strategies that modified the pharmacology of fluorouracil to increase its antitumor activity. The addition of leucovorin increases the binding affinity of the active fluorouracil metabolite to TS, thus enhancing its cytotoxic activity. Combinations of fluorouracil plus leucovorin have been studied extensively in the adjuvant setting, based on the observation that fluorouracil plus leucovorin substantially improves response rates as compared with fluorouracil alone for metastatic disease.

Schedules of fluorouracil and leucovorin administration vary among the different regimens. In the United States, the Roswell Park regimen and the Mayo Clinic regimen were most commonly used, while in Europe, treatments such as the de Gramont regimen favored a continuous intravenous schedule of fluorouracil (Table 138–7).

Clinical studies comparing the efficacy of bolus and continuous infusion schedules generally favor continuous infusion of

TABLE 138-7 Chemotherapy Regimens for the Adjuvant Treatment of Colorectal Cancer

Regimen	Agents	Comment
FOLFOX4[72]	Oxaliplatin 85 mg/m² IV day 1 Folinic acid 200 mg/m² per day IV over 2 hours days 1 and 2 Fluorouracil 400 mg/m² IV bolus, after folinic acid then 600 mg/m² CIV over 22 hours days 1 and 2 • Repeat every 14 days	Improved OS and DFS as compared with infusional fluorouracil-leucovorin–based regimens.
FLOX[73]	Oxaliplatin 85 mg/m² IV administered on weeks 1, 3, and 5 Fluorouracil 500 mg/m² IV bolus weekly × 6 Folinic acid 500 mg/m² IV weekly × 6 • Each cycle lasts 8 weeks and is repeated for 3 cycles	Improved DFS as compared with bolus fluorouracil-leucovorin–based regimens. Increased toxicity compared to FOLFOX4.
Capecitabine	Capecitabine 1,250 mg/m² PO twice daily on days 1 through 14 every 21 days	Equivalent DFS as compared with the Mayo Clinic regimen with improved tolerability.
Fluorouracil-based regimens		
Roswell Park regimen[75]	Fluorouracil 600 mg/m² per day IV, day 1 Folinic acid 500 mg/m² per day IV over 2 hours • Repeat weekly for 6 of 8 weeks	
Mayo Clinic regimen[76]	Fluorouracil 425 mg/m² per day IV, days 1–5 Folinic acid 20 mg/m² per day IV, days 1–5 • Repeat every 4 to 5 weeks	
de Gramont regimen[77]	Fluorouracil 400 mg/m² per day IV bolus, followed by 600 mg/m² CIV over 22 hours, days 1 and 2 for 2 consecutive days Folinic acid 200 mg/m² per day IV over 2 hours days 1 and 2 • Repeat every 2 weeks	Improved safety as compared with the Mayo Clinic regimen.

CIV, continuous intravenous infusion; OS, overall survival; DFS, disease-free survival.

fluorouracil, which is probably related to its short plasma half-life and S-phase specificity for optimal TS inhibition. Continuous intravenous (IV) infusions also permit increased fluorouracil dose intensity, which may account for the higher response rates observed with prolonged infusions of fluorouracil. In most common combination regimens, fluorouracil is administered by both IV bolus injection and continuous IV infusion.

Clinically significant differences in toxicity occur based on the dose, route, and schedule of fluorouracil administration. Leukopenia is the primary dose-limiting toxicity of IV bolus fluorouracil, although diarrhea, stomatitis, and nausea and vomiting can also occur.[78] The incidence and severity of stomatitis can be significantly reduced with the use of oral cryotherapy. In this approach, the patient is instructed to chew and hold ice chips in the mouth during the period between 5 minutes prior to and 30 minutes following the bolus injection of fluorouracil. The protective effects of this procedure are probably related to the local vasoconstriction caused by the ice chips, which temporarily reduces blood flow to the oral mucosa, thereby reducing drug exposure to the oral mucosa.

Although continuous IV infusion fluorouracil is generally well tolerated, dose-limiting toxicities can be substantial. A distinct toxicity, palmar–plantar erythrodysesthesia ("hand–foot syndrome" or PPE), and stomatitis occur most frequently with this route of administration.[78] Hand–foot syndrome occurs in 24% to

40% of patients receiving extended continuous IV infusions and is characterized by painful swelling and erythroderma of the soles of the feet, palms of the hands, and distal fingers. The skin toxicity is fully reversible upon interruption of therapy or dose reduction and is not life threatening, but it can be significant and acutely disabling. The incidence of stomatitis, diarrhea, and hematologic toxicity is not substantial at standard doses, but it increases with increasing fluorouracil doses. No significant difference is noted in the incidence of mucositis, diarrhea, nausea and vomiting, or alopecia between continuous and bolus IV fluorouracil administration.[78]

An additional determinant of fluorouracil toxicity, regardless of the method of administration, is related to its catabolism and pharmacogenomic factors. Dihydropyrimidine dehydrogenase (DPD) is the main enzyme responsible for the catabolism of fluorouracil to inactive metabolites. A rare pharmacogenetic disorder characterized by complete or near-complete deficiency of this enzyme has been identified in patients with cancer. Patients with this enzyme deficiency develop severe toxicity, including death, after fluorouracil administration. Molecular studies have identified a relationship between allelic variants in the *DPYD* gene (the gene that encodes DPD) and a deficiency in DPD activity.[79] Approximately 3% of patients may be genotypically heterozygous for a mutant DPYD allele, although differences between sex and races are unknown at this time.

In summary, fluorouracil and leucovorin can be administered in a variety of treatment schedules, but none has proven superior with regard to overall patient survival. Table 138–7 lists examples of some of these regimens.

❼ Fluorouracil Plus Oxaliplatin. The role of oxaliplatin in adjuvant chemotherapy was evaluated based on its activity in metastatic disease. In the Multicenter International Study of Oxaliplatin/5-Fluorouracil/Leucovorin in the Adjuvant Treatment of Colon Cancer (MOSAIC) trial, 2,246 patients with stage II or III colon cancer were randomized to receive fluorouracil plus leucovorin or FOLFOX4 (fluorouracil/leucovorin plus oxaliplatin) postoperatively.[80] The addition of oxaliplatin resulted in a 20% risk reduction in disease recurrence and increased 5-year disease-free survival (DFS) (73.3% vs. 67.4%) as compared with fluorouracil plus leucovorin alone. With a median follow up of 81.9 months, the addition of oxaliplatin resulted in an absolute 6-year overall survival (OS) difference of 2.5%, which was statistically significant. Overall, the relative risk of death was reduced by 16%, with the benefit limited to stage III patients. The addition of oxaliplatin was associated with increased risk of paresthesia, neutropenia, and gastrointestinal toxicity (nausea, vomiting, diarrhea) that were manageable with supportive care. Further supporting the role of oxaliplatin in the adjuvant setting are the results of the recently reported National Surgical Adjuvant Breast and Bowel Project C-07 trial, which compared the Roswell Park regimen of bolus fluorouracil/leucovorin with or without oxaliplatin. A 20% risk reduction in disease recurrence was seen with oxaliplatin (hazard ratio [HR] = 0.80, P = 0.0034) added to the fluorouracil backbone. As expected, neurotoxicity was increased with oxaliplatin.[81] This method of administration is associated with increased diarrhea and neuropathies as compared with the aforementioned regimen used in the MOSAIC trial. FLOX, a oxaliplatin-containing regimen with bolus fluorouracil and leucovorin, was more toxic as compared to FOLFOX.[73]

The 2010 National Comprehensive Cancer Network (NCCN) guidelines recommend oxaliplatin-based regimens as the first-line option for patients with stage III colon cancer who can tolerate combination therapy, and most practitioners incorporate oxaliplatin into adjuvant treatment regimens.[71]

Further modifications of the FOLFOX4 regimen may also improve tolerability. Capecitabine, an oral prodrug of fluorouracil, and other oral pyrimidines are also being evaluated in adjuvant studies as a replacement for fluorouracil in an attempt to improve the safety and ease of administration of the chemotherapy regimens.

Capecitabine. In addition to being investigated as a replacement for fluorouracil in combination regimens, capecitabine is FDA approved as a single agent in the adjuvant setting. The Xeloda in Adjuvant Colon Cancer Therapy (X-ACT) trial compared capecitabine to the Mayo Clinic regimen of bolus fluorouracil/leucovorin in the adjuvant treatment of 1,987 patients with stage III colon cancer.[82] Both regimens were given for 6 months. This trial was designed to show noninferiority of capecitabine to bolus fluorouracil. DFS between the groups was found to be equivalent. Secondary end points of relapse-free survival (HR 0.86; 95% CI 0.74 to 0.99; P = 0.04) and safety were improved with capecitabine. In particular, the incidence of diarrhea, stomatitis, and neutropenia was decreased with capecitabine, but the incidence of hand–foot syndrome was increased with capecitabine.

Investigational Approaches. Despite its proven benefit in the metastatic setting, irinotecan has not shown a benefit in the adjuvant setting and should not be used outside of clinical trials at this time. Three trials have evaluated the addition of irinotecan to bolus or continuous infusion fluorouracil/leucovorin, and all have failed to demonstrate a DFS benefit. Cancer and Leukemia Group B 89803 compared with the irinotecan plus fluorouracil/leucovorin (IFL) regimen to bolus fluorouracil/leucovorin; not only was there no DFS benefit but the IFL regimen was associated with significant toxicity.[83] The Third Pan-European Trial in Adjuvant Colon Cancer (PETACC-3) and ACCORD studies, which used infusional regimens similar to folinic acid, fluorouracil, and irinotecan (FOLFIRI), also found no difference in DFS as compared with infusional fluorouracil/leucovorin.[84,85]

The combination of capecitabine and oxaliplatin (XELOX) as adjuvant therapy for stage III colon cancer has been compared to fluorouracil/leucovorin (either Mayo Clinic or Roswell Park regimens).[86] Efficacy data showed a significantly improved DFS with XELOX as compared to bolus fluorouracil/leucovorin (P = 0.0024), with a trend toward improved OS with XELOX, even in patients age 70 years and older.

With the success of cetuximab and bevacizumab in the metastatic setting, adjuvant trials evaluating monoclonal antibodies in combination with the previously mentioned regimens have been conducted. FOLFOX ± bevacizumab or cetuximab are part of large phase III trials currently enrolling or recently completed in cooperative groups to assess the benefit of these monoclonal antibodies in this setting. The final results of the NSABP-C08 trial that compared FOLFOX with or without bevacizumab was recently completed and did not meet its primary end point of DFS.[87] Also, recent results showed no benefit in 3-year DFS (P = 0.33) from the addition of cetuximab to the combination of infusional fluorouracil plus oxaliplatin (mFOLFOX6) as adjuvant therapy for patients with *KRAS* wild-type stage III colon cancer.[88] As such, there is no clear role for these agents in the adjuvant treatment setting at this time.

Approach to Selecting an Adjuvant Regimen. Selecting a specific regimen from those listed in Table 138–7 requires an assessment of several patient-specific factors, including the performance status of the patient, comorbid conditions that may exist, and patient preferences for treatment based on lifestyle factors that are important to the patient. If a clinical trial is not an option, most patients with a good performance status will receive oxaliplatin in combination with fluorouracil/leucovorin. Single-agent capecitabine may be the preferred option for patients with preexisting neuropathies, such as diabetic patients, or those patients wishing not to receive IV chemotherapy for any other reason. Fluorouracil/leucovorin has limited use at this time but is an acceptable option for patients who cannot receive oxaliplatin and are unable to tolerate or take oral capecitabine. For example, patients who develop severe hand–foot syndrome may tolerate bolus fluorouracil/leucovorin because this toxicity is minimal with this administration method.

Adjuvant Therapy for Rectal Cancer

6 Rectal cancer involves those tumors found below the peritoneal reflection in the most distal 15 cm of the large bowel, and as such is distinct from colon cancer in that it has a propensity for both local and distant recurrence. The higher incidence of local failure and overall poorer prognosis associated with rectal cancer is a result of anatomic limitations in excising adequate radial margins around the rectal tumor. Although an abdominoperineal resection of the tumor and adjacent tissues results in a high probability of local control and long-term survival, the sequelae, including need for a permanent colostomy and high incidence of sexual and genitourinary dysfunction, has led to investigation of approaches that use multimodal therapies that preserve the integrity of the anal sphincter.[89] In addition, adjuvant therapy after surgical resection is an important aspect of treatment of the primary tumor. The effectiveness of postoperative XRT and fluorouracil-based chemotherapy for stage II or III rectal cancer is well established. Although T_1 tumors with a favorable histology may be treated successfully with local excision alone, adjuvant XRT plus chemotherapy should be offered for larger lesions. Similar to adjuvant therapy for colon cancer, fluorouracil provides the basis for chemotherapy regimens for rectal cancer. The XRT decreases the rate of local pelvic recurrences, whereas the fluorouracil decreases the risk of distant tumor recurrence and enhances the effectiveness of the XRT. The optimal delivery schedule for these two therapies is the subject of ongoing investigation, but many trials have demonstrated improved local control and survival for patients who receive a combination of postoperative XRT and chemotherapy as compared with surgery alone.[90] The use of concurrent chemotherapy and XRT significantly affects local recurrence, relapse-free survival, and OS as compared with XRT alone and have established fluorouracil plus XRT as the foundation for adjuvant therapy in stages II and III rectal cancer. Treatment with the combined approach should total 6 months.

Many treatment centers now administer continuous-infusion fluorouracil throughout the 5- or 6-week schedule of postoperative XRT for rectal cancer. Several schedules for combining fluorouracil with postoperative XRT provide similar relapse-free survival and OS but differ with regard to toxicity profile and catheter requirements for drug administration.[91] Alternative regimens including FOLFOX and capecitabine may be used in place of fluorouracil.

Preoperative (Neoadjuvant) Therapy **6** Interest in preoperative or neoadjuvant therapy has increased based on advances in imaging techniques to more accurately stage rectal tumors preoperatively and the success of combined XRT plus fluoropyrimidine-based chemotherapy administered in the postoperative setting. By shrinking and thereby downstaging the tumor prior to surgical resection, preoperative XRT improves sphincter preservation, but the primary concern with this approach is potential overtreatment with XRT in some patients.

Neoadjuvant chemoradiotherapy may further enhance tumor shrinkage and improve the rate of tumor resectability with rectal sphincter preservation. The European Organization for Research and Treatment of Cancer 22921 trial evaluated the addition of fluorouracil plus leucovorin to preoperative XRT and showed an improvement in tumor shrinkage with lower lymph node

involvement.[92] The 2010 NCCN guidelines for rectal cancer indicate that preoperative infusional fluorouracil-based chemotherapy plus XRT is the preferred treatment for resectable $T_3 N_0$ or any T, N_{1-2} lesions (category 1 recommendation).[90] This should be followed by additional adjuvant chemotherapy after surgery to total 6 months of chemotherapy (combined total from preoperative and postoperative regimens). Neoadjuvant fluorouracil or capecitabine chemoradiation followed by abdominoperineal resection or low anterior resection should be considered for locally unresectable tumors (T_4). Postoperative therapy should be administered to all patients who received preoperative chemotherapy for rectal cancer, regardless of whether the disease was initially resectable.[90]

■ METASTATIC DISEASE

Initial Therapy

8 Several advances have been made in developing efficacious treatment options for metastatic colorectal cancer. Although surgery and XRT are usually used to manage isolated sites of tumor, chemotherapy is most useful for patients with disseminated disease and is the primary treatment modality for unresectable metastatic colorectal cancer.

Surgery Complete surgical resection of discrete hepatic, pulmonary, abdominal, or brain metastases in patients with colorectal cancer, if possible, may extend DFS in selected patients. Patients who have from one to three small nodules isolated to the liver, lungs, or abdomen have the most favorable outcomes. Up to 25% of patients will present with hepatic metastases at time of diagnosis, and 60% of patients with colorectal cancer will develop hepatic metastases sometime during the course of their disease. Approximately 35% of patients who undergo resection of hepatic-limited metastases can be cured.[93] These results are substantially better than those in patients with unresectable metastatic colorectal cancer, in whom 5-year survival is uncommon. Patients with no significant general medical risk factors, fewer than four hepatic lesions, CEA levels less than 200 ng/mL (200 mcg/L), small tumor size, lack of extrahepatic tumor, and adequate surgical margins have the best opportunity for an improved long-term outcome. The primary site of tumor should also be completely resected. Ablative therapies that involve destroying the tumor through freezing and thawing (cryoablation), heat (radiofrequency), or alcohol injection may be useful for patients who have very small hepatic lesions and are unable to undergo liver resection surgery but are less successful than surgical interventions. Outcomes associated with resection of isolated pulmonary, abdominal, and brain metastases have been less studied, but this approach is potentially curative and should be considered for patients with resectable disease who are appropriate surgical candidates.

Because about two-thirds of patients who undergo resection of hepatic metastases will have disease recurrence, postoperative treatments (e.g., adjuvant systemic and hepatic arterial infusion chemotherapy) have been studied in an attempt to improve long-term outcomes. A randomized trial that compared 6 months of hepatic floxuridine and dexamethasone plus IV fluorouracil with leucovorin to IV fluorouracil with leucovorin alone following resection of hepatic metastases in 156 patients showed improved 2-year DFS (86% vs. 72%) and hepatic recurrence-free survival at 2 years (90% vs. 60%) with the combined therapy.[94] Many practitioners offer adjuvant chemotherapy to selected patients following potentially curative hepatic resection, but further studies, especially those involving more active agents, are needed to determine an optimal treatment regimen.[95]

Neoadjuvant (Conversional) Chemotherapy. Patients that present with metastatic disease isolated to the liver and who undergo resection of all metastatic and primary lesions have an increased probability of survival compared with those whose liver lesions remain unresected.[96] Therefore, strategies to increase the success rate of these resections (or convert unresectable lesions to resectable) is the primary goal in patients with liver metastasis. Administration of neoadjuvant chemotherapy, also referred to as conversional chemotherapy, is the primary method to increase complete resection rates in both patients with resectable or unresectable liver lesions.

Patients with initially resectable disease should receive 2 to 3 months of preoperative chemotherapy. The choice of agents depends on patient-specific factors but may include regimens such as FOLFOX, FOLFIRI, or CapeOx. Biologic agents have been added to the foregoing regimens. If patients receive bevacizumab, surgery should not occur within 6 weeks of the last dose of therapy, and bevacizumab should not be restarted until 6 to 8 weeks after surgery. EGFR inhibitors should be considered only in patients that have tumors with wild-type *KRAS*. Postoperative chemotherapy should be administered to patients to complete a total of 6 months of chemotherapy (pre- and postoperative).[71]

Patients with unresectable lesions are eligible for the same chemotherapy regimens already noted. However, since the primary goal is surgical resection whenever possible, patients should be evaluated for possible resection after every 2 months of therapy. If resection occurs, adjuvant chemotherapy should be administered to complete a total of 6 months of chemotherapy.

Radiation Symptom control is the primary goal of XRT for patients with advanced or metastatic colorectal cancer.

Chemotherapy ❽ Accepted initial chemotherapy regimens for metastatic colorectal cancer consist of oxaliplatin plus fluorouracil and leucovorin, irinotecan plus fluorouracil and leucovorin, bevacizumab plus a fluorouracil-based regimen, capecitabine alone, or fluorouracil plus leucovorin alone (Table 138–8). The site(s) of tumor involvement and history of prior chemotherapy help to define an appropriate management strategy. In general, treatment options are similar for metastatic cancer of the colon and rectum.

Currently, most metastatic colorectal cancers are incurable, and treatment goals are to reduce patient symptoms, improve quality-of-life, and extend survival. Two recent meta-analyses have estimated the magnitude of benefit and harm associated with palliative chemotherapy for metastatic colorectal cancer. In a pooled analysis of randomized trials comparing chemotherapy to observation or supportive care alone, a total of nine trials that included 614 patients were evaluated.[106] All trials used fluorouracil-based chemotherapy, but three trials in which hepatic arterial or portal vein administration was used were also included. Several trials allowed delayed or discretionary use of chemotherapy in patients assigned to observation or supportive care alone; 12% to 57% of control patients received at least one course of chemotherapy. Despite these discrepancies, chemotherapy was associated with a significant reduction in mortality at 1 year (relative risk [RR] 0.69) but not at 2 years (RR 0.93). The second meta-analysis analyzed individual patient data and summary statistics from 13 randomized trials that included 1,365 patients.[107] Eligible trials compared palliative chemotherapy given via any route of administration to supportive care alone or treatments not involving chemotherapy. Trials that allowed chemotherapy use in control patients were not excluded. In the analysis of seven trials in which individual patient data were available, palliative chemotherapy was shown to reduce the risk of death by 35%, which translates to a prolongation of median survival by 3.7 months. The investigators were unable to determine the effect of treatment on toxicities or quality-of-life because of inadequate data. However, the results of both analyses suggest that palliative chemotherapy is beneficial and improves survival in metastatic colorectal cancer. Because many patients assigned to control arms eventually received chemotherapy, the magnitude of survival benefit associated with chemotherapy could be underestimated.

Fluorouracil continues to be incorporated into current first-line chemotherapy regimens used for metastatic colorectal cancer. The addition of irinotecan to fluorouracil plus leucovorin significantly improves response rates, progression-free survival (PFS), and median survival. Oxaliplatin in combination with fluorouracil and leucovorin has been shown to be equivalent to the combination of irinotecan plus fluorouracil and leucovorin in the initial treatment of metastatic colon cancer when administered in a similar schedule. The addition of bevacizumab to fluorouracil-based regimens improves efficacy compared with chemotherapy alone. Either of these three- or four-drug combinations may be considered as first-line therapy for metastatic colorectal cancer. Ongoing trials are evaluating the sequencing of these regimens and comparing the efficacy of combinations of fluorouracil plus leucovorin, to investigational treatments with capecitabine, oral fluoropyrimidines, and newer agents, such as cetuximab. Table 138–9 summarizes comparative outcome data from potentially useful chemotherapeutic treatments for metastatic colorectal cancer.

Fluorouracil-Based Regimens. ❽ Fluorouracil has been administered as a single agent by IV bolus injection but response rates are only 10% to 20%. As such, IV bolus fluorouracil as a single agent is considered ineffective for metastatic colorectal cancer. A variety of continuous IV infusion fluorouracil regimens have been developed to increase the duration of drug exposure during the S-phase of the cell cycle and increase cytotoxicity. Despite differences in dose intensity among the different regimens, no clear survival advantages or trends are observed for any particular regimen. However, in comparison to IV bolus fluorouracil, response rates with continuous infusion fluorouracil are about doubled. However, these effects are generally considered as marginal. Additional clinical benefit with continuous infusion fluorouracil has been demonstrated when fluorouracil is administered with other agents and is becoming commonplace in clinical practice.

Numerous studies have evaluated various doses and administration schedules of fluorouracil plus leucovorin in an attempt to improve treatment response rates and survival in metastatic colorectal cancer. Response rates of 14% to 58% have been observed with a variety of doses of fluorouracil in combination with leucovorin at doses ranging from 20 to 500 mg/m^2.[47] The administration sequence and timing of leucovorin may be important factors in the efficacy of biochemical modulation with leucovorin. Leucovorin administration prior to fluorouracil is the most effective approach to enable intracellular-reduced folates to accumulate prior to fluorouracil administration. Despite significantly higher response rates and improved PFS achieved with leucovorin-modulated fluorouracil regimens, their effect on OS is modest.

The Mayo Clinic regimen was the reference regimen in metastatic colon cancer for many years, but the limitations of this regimen (increased toxicity and no survival advantage) have made it largely obsolete.[76] Weekly bolus regimens such as the Roswell Park regimen may also be used but are also associated with significant toxicity.[75]

Bimonthly and weekly regimens of infusional fluorouracil are most commonly administered in the metastatic setting. Increased response rates are noted in bimonthly regimens of fluorouracil administered first as an IV bolus infusion followed by a 22-hour continuous infusion in combination with high-dose leucovorin administered over 2 hours (de Gramont regimen).[100] Although this did not translate to improved median survival as compared with the Mayo Clinic schedule, it was associated with a lower incidence

TABLE 138-8 Chemotherapeutic Regimens for Metastatic Colorectal Cancer

	Regimen	Major Dose-Limiting Toxicities/Comments
Initial therapy		
Oxaliplatin plus fluorouracil plus leucovorin		
Oxaliplatin plus bimonthly infusional fluorouracil; FOLFOX4[72]	Oxaliplatin 85 mg/m² IV day 1 plus bolus fluorouracil 400 mg/m² IV plus leucovorin 200 mg/m² IV followed by fluorouracil 600 mg/m² IV in 22-hour infusion on days 1 and 2, every 2 weeks	Sensory neuropathy, neutropenia
mFOLFOX6[97]	Oxaliplatin 85 mg/m² IV day 1 plus leucovorin 400 mg/m² IV on day 1 followed by fluorouracil 400 mg/m² IV bolus on day 1, then 1200 mg/m²/day × 2 days (total 2,400 mg/m² over 46–48 hours) continuous infusion, repeat every 2 weeks	Sensory neuropathy, neutropenia; easier administration as compared to FOLFOX4
Irinotecan plus fluorouracil plus leucovorin		
Irinotecan plus infusional fluorouracil; FOLFIRI[77]	Irinotecan 180 mg/m² IV plus leucovorin 400 mg/m² IV plus bolus fluorouracil 400 mg/m² IV, followed by fluorouracil 2,400 mg/m² continuous IV infusion over 46 hours on day 1, repeated every 2 weeks	Nausea, diarrhea, mucositis, neutropenia
Biweekly irinotecan plus infusional fluorouracil[98]	Irinotecan 180 mg/m² IV day 1 plus leucovorin 400 mg/m² then fluorouracil 400 mg/m² IV, followed by fluorouracil 600 mg/m² continuous IV infusion over 22 hours, days 1 and 2, repeated every 2 weeks	Neutropenia, diarrhea
Bevacizumab		
Bevacizumab plus fluorouracil-based regimens	Bevacizumab 5 mg/kg IV every 2 weeks plus fluorouracil and leucovorin (given in any schedule below)	Hypertension, thrombosis, proteinuria from bevacizumab added to toxicities of regimen chosen
	or FOLFOX or CapeOx or FOLFIRI	
Capecitabine		
Capecitabine monotherapy[99]	See Table 138-7[a]	Diarrhea, hand–foot syndrome
CapeOx[97]	Oxaliplatin 130 mg/m² day 1 plus capecitabine 850 mg/m² twice a day for 14 days, repeat every 3 weeks	Diarrhea, hand–foot syndrome, neuropathies
Fluorouracil plus leucovorin only		
Bolus plus infusional fluorouracil; (LV5FU2)[100]; de Gramont regimen	See Table 138-7[a]	Neutropenia, mucositis
Salvage therapy[b]		
Irinotecan		
Weekly irinotecan[101]	Irinotecan 125 mg/m² IV every week for 4 of 6 weeks	Neutropenia, diarrhea
Every 3-weeks irinotecan[102]	Irinotecan 350 mg/m² IV every 3 weeks	Neutropenia, diarrhea (less-than-weekly irinotecan)
Oxaliplatin plus fluorouracil plus leucovorin		
Oxaliplatin plus bimonthly infusional fluorouracil; FOLFOX4[103]	Same as FOLFOX4 above; CapeOx may be used in place of FOLFOX4	Sensory neuropathy, neutropenia
Cetuximab		
Cetuximab plus irinotecan[c,104]	Continue irinotecan as previously dosed, plus cetuximab 400 mg/m² IV loading dose, then cetuximab 250 mg/m² IV weekly thereafter; if cetuximab is used with FOLFIRI the dose is the same	Asthenia, diarrhea, nausea, acneiform rash, vomiting
Cetuximab[d,104]	Cetuximab 400 mg/m² IV loading dose, then cetuximab 250 mg/m² IV weekly thereafter	Papulopustular and follicular rash, asthenia, constipation, diarrhea, allergic reactions, hypomagnesemia
Panitumumab		
Rash, hypomagnesemia, rare allergic reactions	6 mg/kg IV over 60 minutes every 2 weeks	
Fluorouracil		
Protracted continuous infusion[105]	Fluorouracil 250–300 mg/m² per day continuous IV infusion until disease progression	Mucositis, hand–foot syndrome

[a]Doses and schedule the same as in the adjuvant setting.
[b]See Figure 138–6 for comments on salvage regimens.
[c]If irinotecan-refractory disease.
[d]If patient cannot tolerate irinotecan.

of severe granulocytopenia, diarrhea, and mucositis.[100] Similar increases in response rate and lower toxicity rates have been seen in patients receiving weekly fluorouracil as a continuous 24-hour IV infusion in combination with high-dose leucovorin given over 2 to 24 hours.[115]

In summary, a weekly or bimonthly schedule of leucovorin plus fluorouracil (either bolus or continuous infusion) may be more convenient for the patient in terms of fewer scheduled clinic appointments, less interference with work schedules, and ease of dose adjustments based on toxicity. However, the incorporation of

newer agents into treatment regimens rather than continual adjustments of fluorouracil and leucovorin doses and administration schedules have led to the greatest advances in drug therapy for metastatic colorectal cancer and will be discussed in the following sections.

Fluorouracil and Leucovorin Plus Irinotecan ❽ Based on irinotecan's activity against untreated and fluorouracil-resistant colorectal cancer, several investigations have been completed to determine whether the addition of irinotecan to fluorouracil

TABLE 138-9 Comparative Outcomes from Selected Trials in Metastatic Colorectal Cancer

Trial	Number	Outcome Measures	Results
First-line			
Goldberg[108]	795	Primary: TTP; secondary: OS, ORR, time to treatment discontinuation	Median TTP: IFL vs. FOLFOX 6.9 vs. 8.7 months ($P = 0.0014$). Median survival 15.0 months with IFL vs. 19.5 months with FOLFOX ($P = 0.001$). ORR with FOLFOX (45%) higher compared to IFL (31%; $P = 0.002$) and IROX (35%, $P = 0.03$). TTP and OS with IROX (6.5 and 17.4 months) no different from FOLFOX.
de Gramont[103]	420	Primary: PFS; secondary: ORR, OS, tolerability, QOL	Median PFS: 9.0 vs. 6.2 months ($P = 0.0003$); ORR: 50.7 vs. 22.3% ($P = 0.0001$), oxaliplatin plus LV5FU2 vs. LF5FU2 alone; no difference in OS (16.2 vs. 14.7 months) or QOL between oxaliplatin plus LV5FU2 vs. LV5FU2 alone.
Saltz[101]	683	Primary: PFS; secondary: ORR, OS	Median PFS longer with IFL (7.0 months) vs. FU/LV (4.3 months; $P = 0.004$); PFS similar with irinotecan alone (4.2 months) compared with FU/LV; ORR higher with IFL vs. FU/LV (50 vs. 28%; $P < 0.001$); median survival longer with IFL (14.8 months) vs. 12.6 months with FU/LV ($P = 0.04$), which was similar to irinotecan (12.0 months).
Douillard[98]	387	Primary: ORR; secondary: TTP, response duration, TTF, OS, QOL	Significantly higher ORR with infusional IFL vs. infusional FU/LV alone (35 vs. 22%; $P < 0.005$) by ITT; TTP longer with IFL (6.7 vs. 4.4 months; $P < 0.001$) and OS longer with IFL vs. infusional FU/LV alone (17.4 vs. 14.1 months; $P = 0.031$).
Tournigand[77]	226	Test the best sequence of FOLFIRI vs. FOLFOX6; primary: second PFS; secondary: PFS, OS, ORR, safety	Median survival 21.5 months with FOLFIRI then FOLFOX6 vs. 20.6 months with FOLFOX6 then FOLFIRI; median PFS also no different (14.2 vs. 10.9 months), or ORR or median PFS with first treatment: FOLFOX6 54% and 8.0 months, vs. 56% and 8.5 months with FOLFIRI.
Hurwitz[109]	925	Primary: OS; secondary: PFS, ORR, response duration, QOL	Bevacizumab plus IFL increased median survival (20.3 months) vs. IFL alone (15.6 months; $P = 0.00003$), PFS (10.6 vs. 6.24 months; $P < 0.00001$), ORR (45% vs. 35%; $P = 0.0029$), and duration of response (10.4 vs. 7.1 months; $P = 0.0014$).
Twelves[99]	1,207	Primary: ORR; secondary: TTP, OS, response duration	Tumor response to capecitabine greater than with FU/LV (25.7 vs. 16.7%; $P < 0.0002$), but no difference in median TTP (4.6 vs. 4.7 months) or median survival (392 vs. 391 days).
Hochster[97]	360	Primary: toxicity; secondary ORR, TTP, OS	Grade 3/4 toxicity not increased with bevacizumab. TTP, ORR, and OS all greater when bevacizumab added to CapeOx, FOLFOX, or bolus fluorouracil/leucovorin. Median survival with bevacizumab-containing regimens was 24.4 months vs. 18.4 months without bevacizumab (not a randomized trial).
Saltz[110]	1,401	Primary: PFS; Secondary ORR, OS	PFS increased from 8 to 9.4 months with bevacizumab added to oxaliplatin-containing regimens (XELOX or FOLFOX). ORR and OS not different between groups.
Fuchs[111]	547	Primary: PFS; Secondary ORR, OS, toxicity	PFS increased with FOLFIRI compared with IFL (7.6 vs. 5.9 months, $P = 0.004$); addition of bevacizumab improved OS (28 months for FOLFIRI + bevacizumab vs. 19.2 months for IFL + bevacizumab; $P = 0.037$). Cape Iri equivalent to IFL and not included in final analysis.
Bokemeyer[112]	337	Primary: ORR; Secondary PFS, OS, toxicity	ORR and PFS increased in patients with wild-type *KRAS* treated with FOLFOX + cetuximab compared with FOLFOX alone; *KRAS* mutant patients had no benefit with cetuximab (ORR 33 vs. 49%, $P = 0.106$ in cetuximab + FOLFOX and FOLFOX treated patients, respectively).
Van Cutsem[113]	1,198	Primary: PFS	FOLFIRI + cetuximab increased PFS by 0.9 months and ORR by 8% compared with FOLFIRI alone. Similar to FOLFOX + cetuximab in that benefit limited to *KRAS* wild-type patients.
Second-line			
Rougier[105]	267	Primary: OS; secondary: PFS, ORR, symptom-free survival, adverse effects, QOL	Irinotecan improved median PFS (4.2 vs. 2.9 months; $P = 0.030$) compared with infusion fluorouracil and 1-year survival (45% vs. 35%; $P = 0.035$) but not median OS (10.8 vs. 8.5 months). Median pain-free survival was similar ($P = 0.06$; 10.3 vs. 8.5 months) between irinotecan and fluorouracil, as was QOL.
Cunningham[102]	279	Primary: OS; secondary: performance status, body weight, tumor-related symptoms, QOL	Compared to best supportive care, OS was improved with irinotecan (13.8% 1-year survival vs. 36.2%; $P = 0.0001$); survival without deterioration in performance status, weight loss greater than 5%, and pain-free survival were also improved with irinotecan.
Cunningham[104]	329	Primary: PFS; secondary: ORR, OS, safety	Panitumumab plus BSC prolonged PFS compared to BSC alone, with a median PFS of 8 weeks with panitumumab (hazard ratio 0.54; 95% CI, 0.44–0.66).
Giantonio[72]	829	Primary: ORR; secondary: TTP, OS	Addition of cetuximab to continuing irinotecan associated with 22.9% ORR compared with 10.9% with cetuximab alone ($P = 0.0074$); median survival with cetuximab plus irinotecan similar to cetuximab alone (8.6 vs. 6.9 months; $P = 0.48$), but TTP was longer with cetuximab plus irinotecan (4.1 vs. 1.5 months; hazard ratio 0.54; 95% CI, 0.42–0.71).
Van Cutsem[114]	463	Primary: OS; secondary: PFS, ORR, toxicity	Addition of bevacizumab to FOLFOX4 in patients previously treated with irinotecan and a fluoropyrimidine improved median OS (12.2 vs. 10.8 months; P = 0.001), PFS (7.3 vs. 4.7 months; P < 0.0001), and ORR (22.7% vs. 8.6%, P < 0.0001) compared with FOLFOX4 alone.

BSC, best supportive care; FU5LV2, bolus plus infusional fluorouracil and leucovorin; FU/LV, fluorouracil plus leucovorin; IFL, irinotecan plus fluorouracil plus leucovorin; IROX, irinotecan plus oxaliplatin; ITT, intention to treat; OS, overall survival; PFS, progression-free survival; QOL, quality-of-life; ORR, overall response rate; TTF, time-to-treatment failure; TTP, time-to-tumor progression.

plus leucovorin as initial therapy for metastatic disease could further improve survival. In a randomized trial of 387 previously untreated patients with advanced colorectal cancer, irinotecan plus fluorouracil and leucovorin was compared to fluorouracil plus leucovorin with regard to tumor response, survival, and quality-of-life (see Table 138–9).[98] Patients randomized to fluorouracil plus leucovorin could receive weekly fluorouracil (2,600 mg/m²) as a 24-hour IV infusion plus leucovorin (500 mg/m²), or the de

Gramont regimen of IV bolus and infusional fluorouracil. For the three-drug treatment, a weekly regimen of irinotecan (80 mg/m²) with a 24-hour infusion of fluorouracil (2,300 mg/m²) plus leucovorin 500 mg/m², or an every-2-week regimen consisting of irinotecan (180 mg/m²) on day 1 with IV bolus fluorouracil (400 mg/m²) followed by a 22-hour IV infusion (600 mg/m²) plus leucovorin (200 mg/m² given on days 1 and 2) can be used. Tumor response, median time-to-disease progression, and OS were all greater in the irinotecan group. Diarrhea and neutropenia were the most common toxicities and were worse in the irinotecan-containing groups. Diarrhea was the most common reason for dose reduction or treatment discontinuation with the weekly regimens and led to hospital admission for 32% of patients receiving irinotecan as compared with 12% of patients who received only fluorouracil plus leucovorin. Neutropenia was the most common cause of dose reductions with the every-2-weeks regimens. Results from questionnaires indicated that quality-of-life consistently declined later in the irinotecan group.

A second randomized trial compared the addition of irinotecan (125 mg/m²) to weekly fluorouracil plus leucovorin (fluorouracil 500 mg/m² IV bolus plus leucovorin 20 mg/m² IV bolus, each given weekly for 4 weeks, repeated every 6 weeks; IFL regimen) to the Mayo Clinic regimen and to irinotecan alone (125 mg/m² IV weekly for 4 weeks, repeated every 6 weeks) as first-line therapy in 683 patients with metastatic colorectal cancer.[101] The combination of irinotecan, fluorouracil, and leucovorin resulted in significantly increased tumor response rates and improved PFS and OS as compared with fluorouracil plus leucovorin and irinotecan alone, respectively. The combined incidence of grade 3 or 4 diarrhea was 22.7% with the three-drug combination, as compared with 13.2% with fluorouracil plus leucovorin and 31% with irinotecan alone. However, the incidence of grade 3 diarrhea was almost threefold greater with triple-drug therapy as compared with the two-drug regimen. Midcycle dose reductions caused by neutropenia, which were more common with the three-drug treatment, could potentially have lowered subsequent risk of grade 4 diarrhea. Mucositis was more frequent in the fluorouracil plus leucovorin group. Quality-of-life analyses did not indicate that the addition of irinotecan to fluorouracil plus leucovorin compromised quality of life.

Modifications of the original IFL regimen have been made to give irinotecan on an every-2-weeks schedule with fluorouracil as a continuous infusion (FOLFIRI regimen). The median OS is improved by 5.7 months with decreased toxicity by this method of administration, and irinotecan administered as IFL is no longer recommended.[71,116]

The most common adverse effects of irinotecan in these regimens are diarrhea, neutropenia, nausea and vomiting, asthenia, abdominal pain, and alopecia; diarrhea and neutropenia are dose limiting.[98,101] Two distinct patterns of diarrhea have been described. Early-onset diarrhea occurs during or within 2 to 6 hours after irinotecan administration and is characterized by lacrimation, diaphoresis, abdominal cramping, flushing, and/or diarrhea. These cholinergic symptoms, thought to be caused by inhibition of acetylcholinesterase, respond to atropine 0.25 to 1 mg given intravenously or subcutaneously. Approximately 10% of patients experience the acute symptoms during or shortly following the irinotecan. More commonly, late-onset diarrhea occurs 1 to 12 days after irinotecan administration and may last for 3 to 5 days. Late-onset diarrhea may require hospitalization or discontinuation of therapy, and fatalities have been reported. The incidence of late-onset diarrhea was as high as 39% in some studies but is now much lower with aggressive antidiarrheal intervention.[47] Aggressive intervention with high-dose loperamide therapy should consist of 4 mg taken at the first sign of soft or watery stools, followed by 2 mg orally every 2 hours until symptom-free for 12 hours; this regimen can be modified to 4 mg taken orally every 4 hours during the night.

The severity of delayed diarrhea has been correlated with the systemic exposure (i.e., area under the concentration-versus-time curve) of irinotecan and SN-38 (irinotecan's active metabolite) and with genetic polymorphisms in the enzyme uridine diphosphate-glucuronosyltransferase (UGT1A1), which is responsible for the glucuronidation of SN-38 to inactive metabolites. Reduced or deficient levels of the UGT1A1 enzyme are observed in Gilbert syndrome, a familial hyperbilirubinemia disorder, and correlate with irinotecan-induced diarrhea and neutropenia.[117] An FDA-approved test for deficiency in this enzyme is available, and clinicians can consider obtaining these results for individual patients prior to initiating irinotecan-based therapy to see if a dose-reduction is warranted.

Based on these studies, the addition of irinotecan to fluorouracil plus leucovorin (FOLFIRI or IFL) increases survival when compared to fluorouracil plus leucovorin in the first-line treatment of metastatic colorectal cancer. These data support the current consensus that the three-drug treatment regimen be considered a first-line option for metastatic colorectal cancer. Accordingly, irinotecan is FDA-approved as first-line therapy for metastatic colorectal cancer in combination with fluorouracil and leucovorin. FOLFIRI is preferred for most patients because it has fewer toxicities and improved OS compared to IFL.

Fluorouracil and Leucovorin Plus Oxaliplatin. ❾ Oxaliplatin, a 1,2-diaminocyclohexane platinum carrier ligand with a mechanism of action similar to cisplatin, in combination with infusional fluorouracil plus leucovorin, is FDA-approved for use in first-line and salvage regimens for metastatic colorectal cancer (see Table 138–8). Oxaliplatin differs from cisplatin in that the DNA damage induced by oxaliplatin may not be as easily recognized by the DNA MMR complex.[118] Thus oxaliplatin-induced DNA damage may play a particularly important role in colorectal cancers that are associated with defects in MMR genes, which are common in HNPCC. Oxaliplatin's incorporation into fluorouracil-based regimens as first-line therapy for metastatic colorectal cancer is associated with higher response rates and improved PFS, with variable effects on OS.[103]

Intergroup Trial N9741, a comparison of oxaliplatin plus fluorouracil and leucovorin (FOLFOX4) to weekly irinotecan plus IV bolus fluorouracil and leucovorin (IFL), and a combination of irinotecan plus oxaliplatin (IROX) in 795 patients with previously untreated metastatic colorectal cancer showed superior efficacy with FOLFOX4.[108] The IROX arm showed no advantage over either of the other two arms. Significant improvements in response rates, PFS, and median survival were seen with FOLFOX4 as compared with IFL (see Table 138–9).[108] The study design allowed patients who failed either regimen to cross over to irinotecan or oxaliplatin, depending on their initial treatment assignment. Sixty percent of patients who failed FOLFOX4 received salvage irinotecan, whereas 24% of IFL failures received salvage oxaliplatin. The impact that this crossover had on survival is unknown but may have resulted in improved survival for the FOLFOX4 arm. In addition, the method of fluorouracil administration, and its impact on study results, has been called into question. Patients on the IFL arm received weekly IV bolus fluorouracil, while patients on the FOLFOX4 arm were administered fluorouracil as IV bolus followed by continuous-infusion IV, which is known to increase response rates. Consequently, it is not possible to evaluate the true contributions of oxaliplatin and irinotecan combined with fluorouracil plus leucovorin in this study. The deletion of fluorouracil (or any fluorinated pyrimidine) from a first-line regimen may be undesirable.

In a phase III cooperative group study, a simplified combined bolus and infusional fluorouracil regimen with irinotecan (FOLFIRI) was compared with oxaliplatin combined with the same fluorouracil plus leucovorin schedule (FOLFOX6) in previously untreated patients with advanced colorectal cancer to determine whether the sequence of administration of both regimens differed with regard to efficacy and toxicities.[77] Patients were randomized to receive initial treatment with FOLFIRI or FOLFOX6, and at disease progression the patients then received the alternate regimen. Both sequences resulted in similar response rates, PFS, and median survival, but the grade 3 or 4 toxicity profiles were different.

Neurotoxicity, neutropenia, and thrombocytopenia were more common with FOLFOX6, while febrile neutropenia, nausea/vomiting, mucositis, and fatigue were significantly more frequent with FOLFIRI.

Oxaliplatin has minimal renal toxicity, myelosuppression, and nausea and vomiting when compared with other platinum-based drugs. Oxaliplatin is associated with both acute and persistent neuropathies.[119] The acute neuropathies occur within 1 to 2 days of dosing and resolve within 2 weeks. The neuropathies usually occur peripherally, but may also occur in the jaw and tongue. A rare acute syndrome of pharyngolaryngeal dysesthesia (1% to 2% of patients) is characterized by subjective sensations of difficulty in swallowing and shortness of breath. Overall, acute neuropathies occur in approximately 90% of patients, and are precipitated or exacerbated by exposure to cold temperatures or cold objects. Thus patients should be instructed to avoid cold drinks and use of ice, and to cover skin before exposure to cold or cold objects. Several prophylactic and treatment strategies have been studied with varying degrees of success. Carbamazepine, gabapentin, amifostine, and calcium and magnesium infusions have been used to both prevent and treat oxaliplatin-induced neuropathies. Persistent neuropathy is typically a cumulative adverse effect, occurring after 8 to 10 cycles, and is seen mostly in patients who are responding to therapy.[108] The neuropathy is characterized by paresthesia, dysesthesia, and hypoesthesia, but may also include deficits in proprioception that can interfere with daily activities (e.g., writing, buttoning, swallowing, and difficulty walking as a result of impaired proprioception), and occur in half of patients receiving oxaliplatin with infusional fluorouracil plus leucovorin, but usually resolve with dosage reductions or cessation of oxaliplatin therapy.[119,120]

CLINICAL CONTROVERSY

The results of N9741 have been debated among clinicians since their presentation. Whether an irinotecan-containing regimen (IFL or FOLFIRI) or FOLFOX4 should be the first regimen used in metastatic colon cancer is an unanswered question. Sequencing trials suggest that it does not matter, and most patients should receive both irinotecan- and oxaliplatin-containing regimens at some point during treatment for their disease.

Capecitabine. ⑩ Capecitabine (Xeloda®) is an oral, tumor-activated and tumor-selective fluoropyrimidine carbamate. Capecitabine is converted to fluorouracil through a three-step activation process, the final step being activation by thymidine phosphorylase, which is present in greatest concentrations at the tumor site. These activation steps lead to about a 3-fold increase in tumor and 1.4-fold increase in hepatic fluorouracil levels. Capecitabine was compared to fluorouracil plus leucovorin as first-line therapy for metastatic colorectal cancer in two randomized phase III trials. In a pooled analysis of 1,207 patients randomized to capecitabine (1,250 mg/m^2 orally twice daily for 14 days, repeated every 3 weeks) or the Mayo Clinic regimen, tumor response to capecitabine was superior to that of fluorouracil plus leucovorin (25.7% vs. 16.7%).[99] Time-to-tumor-progression and median survival, however, were no different. Hand–foot syndrome was more common with capecitabine, whereas grade 3 or 4 neutropenia and stomatitis were more common with fluorouracil plus leucovorin. The convenience of oral administration and different toxicity profile make capecitabine a useful alternative to IV fluorouracil regimens in the setting of metastatic disease. However, because the IV treatment arm in these comparative studies could be con-

sidered more toxic than the weekly IV fluorouracil plus leucovorin treatment schedule, it is premature to conclude that capecitabine is as efficacious as and less toxic than all parenteral fluorouracil-based regimens. Infusional fluorouracil is generally considered to be superior to bolus administration, and oral capecitabine may mimic this method of fluorouracil administration. These data, along with capecitabine's ease of administration, and data that irinotecan and oxaliplatin appear to have a greater effect when combined with infusional fluorouracil has led to capecitabine being evaluated as a replacement for infusional fluorouracil.

Both irinotecan and oxaliplatin have been combined with capecitabine. In a study of over 2,000 patients with metastatic colon cancer, FOLFOX was compared with the combination of CapeOx (capecitabine/fluorouracil/leucovorin) and found to have equivalent OS and PFS. Toxicity was as expected with increased grade 3/4 neutropenia (including neutropenic fever) and increased diarrhea and hand–foot syndrome seen with oxaliplatin and capecitabine-based regimens, respectively.[120] Based on these results, CapeOx is an acceptable first-line option for the treatment of metastatic colorectal cancer.[71]

The combination of capecitabine with irinotecan resulted in no survival benefit compared with IFL and showed inferior results when compared with FOLFIRI in a randomized trial of 430 patients. Additionally, the combination of capecitabine with irinotecan had higher rates of nausea, vomiting, and dehydration and is not recommended for use outside of clinical trials.[116]

The current FDA-approved indication for capecitabine in metastatic colon cancer is when therapy with a fluoropyrimidine alone is desired. Replacement of fluorouracil-leucovorin with capecitabine in other regimens is not currently approved, although completed trials demonstrate that capecitabine is a suitable replacement for infusional fluorouracil in combination with oxaliplatin.

Biologic Therapy. ❾ Bevacizumab is a recombinant, humanized monoclonal antibody that inhibits vascular endothelial growth factor. Bevacizumab, in combination with intravenous fluorouracil-based chemotherapy, was FDA approved in 2004 for initial treatment of patients with metastatic colorectal cancer. This represents the third available combination regimen for first-line treatment. Results from two randomized trials show increased benefit as compared with chemotherapy alone.

A phase III trial of bevacizumab in combination with IFL as first-line therapy in patients with metastatic colorectal cancer has also been completed. Patients were randomized to receive IFL plus placebo or IFL plus bevacizumab 5 mg/kg every 2 weeks.[109] The addition of bevacizumab to IFL therapy resulted in an increase in response rate (34.7% vs. 44.9%) and median survival (15.6 vs. 20.3 months) and PFS (6.24 vs. 10.6 months) as compared with IFL alone. The frequency of typical adverse effects associated with IFL chemotherapy was not increased with the addition of bevacizumab. Grade 3 hypertension was significantly increased in the bevacizumab group. The incidence of other safety concerns with bevacizumab, such as bleeding, thromboembolism, and proteinuria, were not increased in the bevacizumab group as compared with placebo. The hypertension is easily managed with oral antihypertensive agents. The risk of gastrointestinal perforation was increased by the addition of bevacizumab to IFL, and patients complaining of abdominal pain associated with vomiting or constipation should be considered for this rare but potentially fatal complication. Bevacizumab is also associated with a twofold increased risk of arterial thrombotic events, with patients who are older than age 65 or who have a prior history of arterial thrombotic events at greatest risk. Nevertheless, because these individuals derive the same survival benefits with bevacizumab as do other patients, they may be appropriate candidates to receive bevacizumab.

Similar to what was noted previously when IFL was compared with FOLFIRI without bevacizumab, infusional fluorouracil should be administered in combination with bevacizumab and irinotecan. A randomized phase III trial demonstrated a median survival of 28 months compared with 19.2 months with FOLFIRI and IFL, respectively (HR for death 1.79; $P = 0.037$) when given in combination with bevacizumab.[111]

Bevacizumab has also been combined with oxaliplatin in a variety of chemotherapy regimens for the initial treatment of metastatic colon cancer. In contrast to irinotecan-containing regimens, the method of fluorouracil administration (or substitution with capecitabine) does not appear to significantly affect outcomes. One trial, randomized one cohort of patients to one of three oxaliplatin-based regimens (TREE-1 [arm 1: oxaliplatin plus infusional 5-FU; arm 2: oxaliplatin plus bolus 5-FU; arm 3: oxaliplatin plus oral capecitabine]) while the second cohort of patients (TREE-2) received the same chemotherapy regimens plus bevacizumab as their first-line treatment for metastatic colon cancer. The addition of bevacizumab was associated with increased overall response rate and longer time-to-progression and median survival, although these differences were not significant as a consequence of the small sample size. Overall median survival was 18.2 months in the TREE-1 cohort and 23.7 months in the TREE-2 cohort with the addition of bevacizumab.[97] In a separate phase III trial, the addition of bevacizumab to oxaliplatin-based chemotherapy (XELOX or FOLFOX) significantly improved PFS but not OS.[110] Studies that compare the addition of bevacizumab to FOLFOX4 to irinotecan-based combinations of bevacizumab are ongoing.

CLINICAL CONTROVERSY

Currently, continuation of bevacizumab after disease progression is not recommended. Some clinicians have taken retrospective data that demonstrate improved survival with duration of bevacizumab use and applied it to clinical practice, but insurance coverage for patients may be difficult to obtain.

Investigational First-Line Approaches

Targeted Agents Results with cetuximab in the first-line metastatic setting combined with either FOLFOX or FOLFIRI suggest that the combination improves response rates and PFS to either chemotherapy regimen without adding substantial toxicity.[112,113]

The benefit in either of these combinations is limited to patients with wild-type *KRAS* tumors and should not be used in patients with tumor *KRAS* mutations. Cetuximab combined with FOLFIRI demonstrated an increase in PFS of 1.2 months and improved median OS from 21 to 24.9 months (HR 0.84, $P = NS$) compared with FOLFIRI alone in the subset of patients with wild-type *KRAS*.[113] No benefit is seen in patients with mutant *KRAS*. Similar results have been reported with cetuximab in combination with FOLFOX.[112] Cetuximab in combination with FOLFOX demonstrated an increased response rate and a decreased PFS (HR 0.57; $P = .0163$) as compared with FOLFOX-4 alone in patients with wild-type *KRAS*.

Panitumumab was also combined with FOLFIRI or IFL in a phase II trial and demonstrated activity without substantially increasing toxicity of FOLFIRI but not IFL.[121] The effect of *KRAS* status on response was not evaluated.

For reasons that are not well understood, the addition of panitumumab or cetuximab to bevacizumab plus irinotecan- or oxaliplatin-containing chemotherapy *reduces* PFS and is currently not recommended. The Panitumumab Advanced Colorectal Cancer

Evaluation Study (PACCE) trial and the CAIRO2 demonstrated a decrease in PFS of 1.4 months when panitumumab and 1.3 months when cetuximab was added to bevacizumab-containing chemotherapy, respectively.[122,123] Both of these results were clinically and statistically significant. The results from these trials demonstrate the potential pitfalls of treating patients with multiple biologic agents outside of the setting of a clinical trial and why this practice should be avoided.

Hepatic Artery Infusion. Although hepatic chemotherapy infusion for metastatic colorectal cancer remains an area of investigation, it has not been shown to be superior to systemic chemotherapy. The rationale for hepatic artery infusion (HAI) is based on the principle that normal liver hepatocytes and early micrometastases obtain their primary blood supply from the portal vein. In contrast, tumors in the liver are thought to receive most of their blood supply via the hepatic artery.[124] Consequently, drug administration via the hepatic artery should result in delivery of high drug concentrations to the tumor cells with a much lower exposure to normal liver tissue.

Because the liver is a common site of colorectal cancer metastasis, and the only site of metastatic involvement in up to one-third of patients, hepatic-directed therapies continue to be explored. Historically, floxuridine and fluorouracil have undergone the most study for hepatic artery infusion, but other active agents such as irinotecan and oxaliplatin have also been studied. Trials involving HAI have been conducted in patients with unresectable liver metastases and as adjuvant therapy following curative resection of isolated metastases.

Regional HAI can be accomplished using a hepatic arterial port, a totally implantable pump, or a percutaneously placed catheter into the hepatic artery that is connected to an external pump. Early trials of HAI revealed objective response rates ranging from 30% to 88%, many of which were observed in previously treated patients, and increased survival rates as compared with historic controls. Because supportive care alone is no longer considered standard of care for metastatic disease, when HAI was compared with systemic chemotherapy, most comparisons did not yield a survival benefit.[124] Furthermore, most studies allowed patients in the systemic therapy treatment groups to cross over to HAI upon tumor progression; therefore, the impact of these treatments on survival is difficult to interpret. Most recently, HAI was compared with systemic fluorouracil plus leucovorin in patients with hepatic-only metastasis.[125] HAI was associated with significantly longer OS (median: 24.4 vs. 20 months, $P = 0.003$) and time-to-hepatic-progression (median: 9.8 vs. 7.3 months, $P = 0.034$) as compared with systemic chemotherapy. As expected, time-to-extrahepatic-progression was longer with systemic chemotherapy. This study has been criticized for the systemic chemotherapy treatment arm, which is considered less-than-optimal therapy by current standards.

Given the significant improvements with systemic chemotherapy for metastatic disease achieved with systemic chemotherapy over the past several years, attention has been directed to HAI with nonfluoropyrimidines, including irinotecan, oxaliplatin, and biologic agents. Early studies show promising results, but it is not clear whether this approach offers any advantage compared with systemic therapy.

Because of toxicities associated with HAI, most patients require some transient interruption of therapy, a decrease in dosage, or discontinuation of therapy. Furthermore, extrahepatic disease progression with HAI therapy alone remains a clinical problem. Although increased response rates and a trend toward improved survival have been reported, the costs and toxicities with this approach are significant. Therefore, for the minority of patients who present with unresectable disease to the liver only, HAI may represent a reasonable therapeutic option, but it is not considered standard therapy at this time.

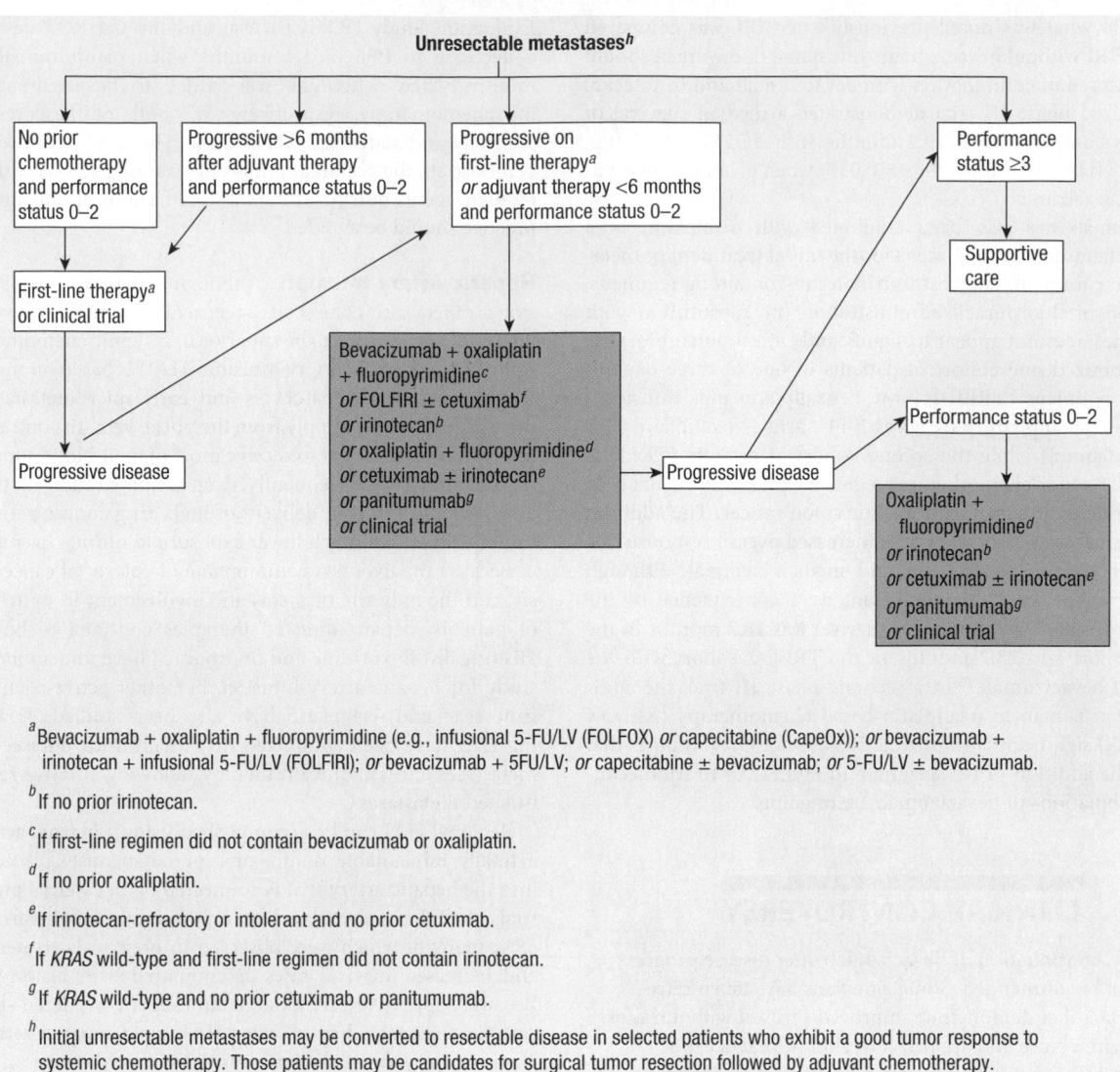

FIGURE 138-6. Algorithm for treatment of unresectable or refractory metastatic colorectal cancer.

Footnotes for figure:

a Bevacizumab + oxaliplatin + fluoropyrimidine (e.g., infusional 5-FU/LV (FOLFOX) or capecitabine (CapeOx)); or bevacizumab + irinotecan + infusional 5-FU/LV (FOLFIRI); or bevacizumab + 5FU/LV; or capecitabine ± bevacizumab; or 5-FU/LV ± bevacizumab.

b If no prior irinotecan.

c If first-line regimen did not contain bevacizumab or oxaliplatin.

d If no prior oxaliplatin.

e If irinotecan-refractory or intolerant and no prior cetuximab.

f If KRAS wild-type and first-line regimen did not contain irinotecan.

g If KRAS wild-type and no prior cetuximab or panitumumab.

h Initial unresectable metastases may be converted to resectable disease in selected patients who exhibit a good tumor response to systemic chemotherapy. Those patients may be candidates for surgical tumor resection followed by adjuvant chemotherapy.

Approach to Selecting an Initial Metastatic Regimen

Practitioners can select first-line treatment for metastatic colorectal cancer from among four main options: oxaliplatin plus fluorouracil plus leucovorin (FOLFOX); irinotecan plus fluorouracil plus leucovorin (FOLFIRI); capecitabine plus oxaliplatin (CapeOx); or fluorouracil plus leucovorin.[71] The most important factor in patient survival is not the initial regimen but whether or not the patient is able to receive all three active cytotoxic drugs (fluorouracil, irinotecan, and oxaliplatin) at some point in the treatment course.[126] Based on the comparable results of FOLFIRI versus FOLFOX6, combined with the inferiority of IFL to FOLFOX4, either of these regimens (FOLFOX or FOLFIRI) are considered the reference standard in metastatic colorectal cancer. The IFL regimen is no longer recommended in clinical practice. Similar to the adjuvant setting, patient-specific factors may lead practitioners to choose between FOLFOX and FOLFIRI. Preexisting neuropathies may lead to FOLFIRI being chosen initially, whereas increased bilirubin or known UGT1A1 deficiency (known risk factors for delayed diarrhea) may lead to FOLFOX as the initial choice. The 2010 NCCN guidelines recommend the addition of bevacizumab to any initial fluorouracil-based regimen unless its use is contraindicated in an individual patient.[71] Cetuximab may be added to FOLFIRI, FOLFOX, or CapeOx in patients with wild-type KRAS tumors only.

Capecitabine may be an appropriate substitute for intravenous fluorouracil in oxaliplatin combination regimens; the 2010 NCCN guidelines list CapeOx plus bevacizumab as an acceptable initial regimen based on data that demonstrated its equivalence to oxaliplatin plus continuous infusion 5-FU.[97] Fluorouracil plus leucovorin alone or capecitabine monotherapy is also appropriate first-line treatment for those individuals who cannot tolerate three-drug combination regimens.

Second-Line Therapy

Systemic chemotherapy represents the mainstay of therapy for patients whose disease progresses following initial treatment for metastatic disease. Figure 138–6 depicts an algorithm for treatment of refractory metastatic disease. Treatment options are based on the type of and response to prior treatments, the site and extent of disease, and patient factors and treatment preferences.

Systemic Chemotherapy Upon disease progression following standard initial therapy, appropriate treatment options may include oxaliplatin plus fluorouracil and leucovorin with or without bevacizumab, irinotecan plus cetuximab, cetuximab, panitumumab irinotecan, continuous-infusion fluorouracil, capecitabine plus oxaliplatin, capecitabine, intrahepatic therapy for selected patients, supportive care, or participation in a clinical trial. The choice of specific agents depends primarily on the type of prior therapy received. Because most patients will have received a combination of a fluoropyrimidine with either irinotecan or oxaliplatin, second-line therapy with the alternate regimen should be considered. Patient survival can exceed 2 years.

Irinotecan. Two important trials have delineated an appropriate standard of care for patients who experience disease progression with fluorouracil therapy for metastatic colorectal cancer.[102,105] The results of these trials demonstrate a survival benefit associated with irinotecan, which was FDA approved in 1996 as second-line therapy for recurrent or progressive disease following fluorouracil. In phase II studies of previously treated patients with metastatic colorectal cancer, objective response rates of 13% to 27% have been observed.[102,105]

In a phase III trial of 189 patients with metastatic colorectal cancer that had progressed within 6 months of treatment with fluorouracil, irinotecan was compared to supportive care alone with regard to survival, quality-of-life, and other clinical variables.[102] Irinotecan was administered as 350 mg/m^2 IV every 3 weeks; the dose was reduced to 300 mg/m^2 for individuals who were 70 years of age or older, who had a World Health Organization performance status of 2, or who had clinical risk factors for developing excessive treatment-related toxicity. Supportive care could include any symptomatic therapy with the exception of irinotecan or any other topoisomerase I inhibitor. With the exception of more patients with poor performance status in the supportive care group, baseline patient characteristics were similar between groups. Median survival was 9.2 months with irinotecan, as compared to 6.5 months with supportive care alone. One-year survival was significantly greater with irinotecan (36.2% vs. 13.8%) and was not associated with significantly worse quality-of-life scores except for diarrhea. Clinical variables such as cognitive functioning, pain, dyspnea, and appetite loss were in favor of irinotecan therapy. The most common grade 3 or 4 side effects with irinotecan included leukopenia and neutropenia (22%), diarrhea (22%), nausea (14%), and vomiting (14%). Seventy-two percent of patients receiving irinotecan required hospital admission for adverse events, as compared with 63% of supportive care patients. Thus irinotecan was associated with an improved survival and quality-of-life as compared with supportive care alone that appeared to balance treatment-related toxicities.

A comparison of irinotecan to continuous-infusion fluorouracil in a similar population of 267 patients allocated patients to irinotecan, 300 to 350 mg/m^2 IV every 3 weeks, or one of three continuous-infusion fluorouracil regimens: leucovorin 200 mg/m^2 IV over 2 hours followed by IV bolus fluorouracil (400 mg/m^2) and 22-hour continuous-infusion fluorouracil (600 mg/m^2), given the first 2 days of every 2-week period; fluorouracil 250 to 300 mg/m^2 as prolonged continuous IV infusion until disease progression; or fluorouracil 2,600 to 3,000 mg/m^2 per day IV over 24 hours, with or without leucovorin (20 to 500 mg/m^2 IV), given weekly for 6 weeks, with a 2-week rest period between cycles.[105] Median follow up after 15 months revealed a longer 1-year survival (45% vs. 32%) and median survival (10.8 months vs. 8.5 months) with irinotecan, as compared with fluorouracil. Sixty-nine percent of patients receiving irinotecan experienced at least one grade 3 or 4 toxicity, as compared with 54% of patients receiving fluorouracil. The most common toxicities with irinotecan were diarrhea, neutropenia, pain, vomiting, and asthenia, while pain, asthenia, diarrhea, and dermatologic toxicities were most common with fluorouracil. The hospitalization requirement for adverse effects did not differ between treatments.

Finally, the use of the FOLFIRI regimen after progression with first-line FOLFOX demonstrated an objective response rate of 4% with a median PFS of 2.5 months.[77] These results are consistent with the meta-analysis that demonstrated improved outcomes in those patients who are able to receive all active cytotoxic agents during the course of their disease.[126]

Based on these results, irinotecan should be considered standard second-line therapy for patients who have failed prior treatment with oxaliplatin and fluorouracil-based regimens. Initial administration of irinotecan at the lower dose should be considered for patients who have received significant prior pelvic or abdominal irradiation. Protracted continuous-infusion fluorouracil (FOLFIRI) or single-agent irinotecan should be considered the regimen of choice with or without cetuximab as will be explained in the following section on cetuximab.

Oxaliplatin. Oxaliplatin plus fluorouracil and leucovorin should be considered for patients who received primary treatment with irinotecan plus fluorouracil. Despite the low activity of single-agent oxaliplatin against fluorouracil-refractory disease, when oxaliplatin has been administered in a bimonthly regimen with high-dose leucovorin and continuous fluorouracil infusion, a 20.6% response rate with a median survival in excess of 10 months has been reported.[127] The combination of oxaliplatin plus fluorouracil and leucovorin is also effective as salvage therapy after initial treatment with irinotecan plus fluorouracil and leucovorin, with a response rate of approximately 20%.[128] Although irinotecan can be used effectively as a single agent in colorectal cancer, it should be noted that oxaliplatin does not have substantial activity alone, and should only be given in combination with a fluoropyrimidine.

In patients who did not receive bevacizumab in their initial treatment, FOLFOX plus bevacizumab is recommended based on phase III data. Results from Eastern Cooperative Group 3200 demonstrated that bevacizumab, in combination with FOLFOX4, improved survival in patients with previously treated advanced colorectal cancer.[72] It should be noted that patients were excluded if they received prior oxaliplatin or bevacizumab and the dose of bevacizumab was 10 mg/kg instead of 5 mg/kg. Median survival was improved from 10.7 to 12.5 months ($P = 0.0018$). Data to support the use of bevacizumab after progression on first-line bevacizumab is retrospective, and its use beyond initial progression is not recommended at this time.

Biologic Therapy. ⑪ Cetuximab is a chimeric monoclonal antibody directed against an EGFR that received FDA approval in 2004. Cetuximab may be administered in combination with irinotecan but can be used as a single agent in patients who cannot tolerate irinotecan-based chemotherapy.

In a phase II study, patients with EGFR-expressing metastatic colorectal cancer who experienced disease progression with an irinotecan-based regimen received open-label cetuximab, 400 mg/m^2 IV as a loading dose, followed by weekly infusions of 250 mg/m^2 IV until disease progression.[129] Of 57 patients treated, five achieved a partial response, with a minor response or stable disease developing in 21 additional patients. The median survival was 6.4 months. The most common grade 3 or 4 adverse events were papulopustular, follicular skin rash (18% grade 3), and adverse effects characterized as asthenia, lethargy, malaise, or fatigue (9% grade 3).

The combination of cetuximab plus irinotecan was also compared with cetuximab as a single agent in patients with EGFR-positive colorectal cancer that had progressed on irinotecan.[104] Three hundred and twenty-nine patients were randomized in a 2:1 ratio to receive cetuximab plus continuation of the irinotecan or cetuximab alone. The objective response rates, 22.9% and 10.8% with cetuximab plus irinotecan and cetuximab alone, respectively, were very encouraging, and resulted in the endorsement of cetuximab by the FDA via accelerated approval. Median survival was 8.6 months for the combination and 6.9 months with monotherapy ($P = 0.48$). Time-to-disease-progression was significantly longer with cetuximab plus irinotecan than with cetuximab alone (4.1 vs. 1.5 months;

HR 0.54), even among patients who also had oxaliplatin-refractory disease. The incidence of grade 3 or 4 adverse effects was as anticipated based on previous trials; asthenia and a follicular rash occurred most commonly with cetuximab alone, and in addition to typical irinotecan-related side effects (e.g., nausea, vomiting, and diarrhea) with combination treatment. Interestingly, tumor response was not associated with the intensity of EGFR-positive staining. Because patients who experienced disease progression on monotherapy were allowed to cross over to combination treatment, any difference in OS between the two groups is difficult to ascertain.

Cetuximab should be considered in patients with irinotecan- and oxaliplatin-refractory colorectal cancer. As a single agent, cetuximab is associated with a 23% improvement in OS compared with best supportive care. Current evidence does not support restricting the use of cetuximab to patients with immunohistochemical evidence of EGFR-positive staining.[130]

An important caveat for most of these initial trials is that KRAS testing was not initially performed. Retrospective analysis on subsets of patients with known KRAS testing has been performed in limited patients with tumor samples available. One study tested 394 of 572 patient tumor samples for KRAS mutations.[131] These patients were treated with cetuximab plus best supportive care versus best supportive care. Patients with KRAS mutations had a shorter PFS and OS compared with those with wild-type KRAS. Overall survival was improved by 4.7 months (HR 0.55; $P < 0.001$) and PFS by 1.8 months (HR 0.40; $P < 0.001$) when treated with cetuximab. No benefit was seen with cetuximab in patients with mutant KRAS.

These results stress the influence of KRAS mutations on the efficacy of EGFR inhibitors, including cetuximab and panitumumab, in treating colorectal cancer. KRAS is located downstream from the EGFR receptor and is involved in the EGFR signaling cascade by activating the MAP kinase pathway that influences cellular proliferation. Activating mutations in exon 2 are able to activate KRAS independent of EGFR receptor activation.[131] Therefore, EGFR receptor inhibition strategies are not effective in controlling cancer proliferation and growth. Several studies have demonstrated that KRAS mutational status predicts response to EGFR inhibitors used in colorectal cancer and its status should be determined prior to starting therapy directed at the EGFR receptor. Therapy with an EGFR inhibitor is not recommended in patients with mutant KRAS.[71]

Tumors harboring BRAF mutations are also associated with a poor prognosis and a poor response to EGFR inhibitors in patients with wild-type KRAS.[132] Although BRAF mutation testing is not routinely recommended at this time, BRAF mutation status may be considered in patients with wild-type KRAS. Individuals with BRAF mutations should not receive EGFR inhibitors.

Panitumumab is a fully human monoclonal antibody targeted to the EGFR that was FDA approved for use in patients with metastatic colorectal cancer that no longer responds to previous therapy. The approval was based on a comparison of panitumumab to best supportive care in patients who had experienced disease progression after standard chemotherapy, including a fluoropyrimidine, irinotecan, and oxaliplatin. Patients received best supportive care or panitumumab (6 mg/kg IV every 2wo weeks) until tumor progression.[114] Those patients who received panitumumab showed a 46% decrease in the rate of tumor progression compared with those who only received best supportive care (HR 0.54, 95% CI 0.44 to 0.66). Retrospective analysis of KRAS testing demonstrated that the benefit was limited to patients with wild-type KRAS in that a 0% overall response rate and decreased PFS was reported in patients with KRAS mutations treated with panitumumab.[133] As expected, dermatologic toxicities were observed in patients receiving panitumumab, as well as fatigue, abdominal pain, nausea, and diarrhea. Only one hypersensitivity reaction was reported. As with cetuximab, EGFR-positivity with immunohistochemistry should

not be used to determine appropriate candidates for panitumumab but KRAS mutational status should be determined.[134]

Neither of the EGFR inhibitors should be used in the second-line setting if they were part of a patient's initial treatment regimen.

Miscellaneous Salvage Chemotherapy Similar to initial treatment of metastatic colon cancer, capecitabine is being investigated as a replacement for infusional fluorouracil in salvage regimens in combination with irinotecan or oxaliplatin.

One interesting subject of debate is whether treatment could be suspended once disease stabilization occurs, and restarted upon disease progression. In the OPTIMOX study, patients were randomized to receive continuous FOLFOX4 until disease progression, or a simplified regimen, FOLFOX7, with intermittent oxaliplatin.[135] The results of this study demonstrated that oxaliplatin could be stopped after six cycles of chemotherapy, but that an appropriate strategy to reintroduce chemotherapy needed to be developed. Ongoing studies are evaluating various agents as maintenance treatments in conjunction with a similar intermittent treatment regimen. Patients whose disease progresses following standard treatment for metastatic colorectal cancer should be encouraged to participate in a clinical trial evaluating new treatment approaches for this incurable disease.

Hepatic-Directed Therapies Patients with hepatic-predominant disease whose disease progresses with systemic therapy may be candidates for chemoembolization, cryotherapy, or radiofrequency ablation. Percutaneous ethanol injection can be performed but is considered relatively ineffective against colorectal hepatic metastases.[136] Response rates to HAI therapy in patients who are refractory to fluorouracil-based therapy may be as high as 33%.

The largest experience with hepatic arterial chemoembolization has been seen in patients with metastatic carcinoid tumors or primary hepatocellular carcinomas. Most recently, small trials have been expanded to include hepatic metastases caused by colorectal cancer. Hepatic arterial chemoembolization delivers high concentrations of cytotoxic agents directly to the tumor and results in the embolization or devascularization of the liver, which blocks perfusion of the tumor and eliminates its blood supply. This procedure involves the instillation of a mixture that incorporates chemotherapeutic agents, radioactive contrast dye, and/or an embolic agent directly into the hepatic artery. Agents and doses most commonly studied include doxorubicin (40 to 60 mg), mitomycin (10 to 20 mg), and cisplatin (100 to 150 mg), which are usually dissolved in about 10 to 15 mL of a radiographic contrast dye.[137] Addition of an embolic agent to the mixture results in either a temporary or permanent occlusion of the hepatic artery. Although approximately 80% of patients in one trial experienced a response, the number of patients with colorectal cancer who have undergone this procedure thus far is relatively low, and patients still experience eventual disease progression. However, preliminary results from small series suggest that the high tumor responses might be associated with a survival benefit, and randomized trials comparing systemic therapy to hepatic chemoembolization for unresectable disease are ongoing.

Cryosurgery involves placement of a cryoprobe into the tumor, either percutaneously or intraoperatively, and then lowering the probe temperature to −100°C (− 148°F).[136] This is repeated in cycles, resulting in formation of an ice ball that causes tumor destruction. Cryosurgery may be used alone or in conjunction with other localized procedures, such as radiofrequency ablation, which is becoming increasingly used for colorectal liver metastases. The technique involves placement of a chilled perfusion electrode needle into the tumor with subsequent application of alternating electrical current through the electrode, resulting in thermal coagulative necrosis of the tumor.[136] Laser interstitial thermal therapy represents an alternate method for causing tumor coagulative necrosis using a laser. Radiofrequency ablation is also being evaluated in conjunction with HAI, in an effort to reduce local recurrence of metastatic tumors. Procedure-related complications can include bleeding, coagulopathy, liver abscess, biliary stricture, and pleural effusion.[136] Although these approaches represent potential treatment strategies for patients with unresectable, yet limited hepatic metastases, additional experience is needed to determine long-term outcomes. Furthermore, extrahepatic sites of disease continue to be a problem even for those individuals in whom the liver tumors can be eradicated.

New Strategies and Agents in Development

At present, fluorouracil plus leucovorin, bevacizumab, capecitabine, irinotecan, oxaliplatin, and cetuximab are the most frequently used chemotherapeutic agents for cancer of the colon and rectum. New chemotherapy agents have been studied in an attempt to further improve antitumor efficacy and reduce treatment toxicities. Oral fluorinated pyrimidines and TS inhibitors, such as fluorouracil prodrugs and inhibitors of fluorouracil catabolism, can prolong in vivo fluorouracil exposure and enhance antitumor effects without the use of continuous IV infusions. But traditional chemotherapy agents, which target rapidly dividing cells, kill both malignant and nonmalignant cells, and new cancer therapies are needed to improve therapeutic outcomes. In particular, targeted therapies aimed at the underlying cancer pathology are increasingly being developed and used in colorectal cancer treatment. A variety of agents targeted toward augmenting the host immune system response have undergone, or are currently undergoing, study for colorectal cancer, including monoclonal antibodies and tumor vaccines. Another potential strategy is regulating tumor growth through the inhibition of various cell signal-transduction pathways. Agents that can alter microenvironmental factors which support angiogenesis and tumor metastases may also be of benefit.

In addition, observations that various tumor characteristics (e.g., TS expression), patient drug-metabolizing enzymes (e.g., DPD and plasma uracil-to-dihydrouracil ratio), and molecular markers (e.g., chromosome 18q allelic loss, microsatellite instability, and *P53* mutation or loss) may predict prognosis and response to certain therapies and provide the rationale for pharmacogenomic strategies to select first-line therapies for individual patients.[138–140] Although patients who are deficient in DPD experience severe and potentially life-threatening toxicities with conventional doses of fluorouracil, determination of DPD activity is relatively time consuming and the techniques are not amenable to routine clinical practice. As an alternative, plasma ratio determinations of uracil and dihydrouracil, which are more easily obtainable, can identify individuals with DPD deficiency who are at risk of developing significant toxicities. Of factors predictive for tumor sensitivity to fluorouracil, TS expression has been most studied. Results from in vitro studies demonstrate that pretreatment intratumoral TS levels are inversely correlated to tumor response to fluorouracil. Whether increased tumor TS expression reflects a biologically more aggressive tumor or is directly related to fluorouracil resistance is unknown. Studies are under way to use this and other information to identify rational therapeutic approaches for select patients.

One of these strategies involves measuring plasma fluorouracil concentrations and adjusting individual patient dosing regimens to achieve fluorouracil concentrations within an established therapeutic range to optimize efficacy and minimize side effects. Published data suggest that only 20% to 30% of patients treated with fluorouracil achieve therapeutic concentrations.[141] A prospective study that compared pharmacokinetically guided fluorouracil dosing with conventional dosing in patients with metastatic colorectal cancer demonstrated that pharmacokinetically guided dose adjustments reduced grade 3/4 toxicities, increased the objective tumor

response rate, and provided a higher yet not significantly increased survival rate.[142] Valid assay methods that facilitate therapeutic drug monitoring are now available and are being used in some centers. Whether clinicians adopt this strategy and if it will indeed advance therapeutic outcomes have yet to be established. For those patients with tumors that have *KRAS* mutations or *BRAF* mutations, more studies are needed.

PHARMACOECONOMIC CONSIDERATIONS

The estimated expenditures for colorectal cancer in the United States alone are between $5.3 and $6.5 billion per year.[143] The total lifetime cost for managing a patient with cancer of the colon based on North American data is close to $100,000.[143] Costs for patients with rectal cancer are approximately 15% higher because of the added expense of XRT. The highest treatment costs are incurred during the initial and terminal phases of care. Thus a long-term approach is needed to accurately estimate the cost of treating patients diagnosed with colorectal cancer. In addition, long-term cancer-related excess costs were calculated with the Surveillance, Epidemiology, and End Results (SEER)-Medicare–linked database as $33,700 and $36,500 for colon and rectal cancer, respectively.[143] The impact of changes in clinical practice on treatment costs, such as increased use of adjuvant therapy, changes in duration of hospital stay and outpatient delivery of health services, and incorporation of costly agents into standard treatment regimens, must also be continually considered.

The cost of the drugs alone (based on 95% of average wholesale price in 2004) were estimated for a 70-kg, 170-cm tall patient with colorectal cancer for a typical treatment period of 8 weeks.[143] The cost of biweekly infusional fluorouracil plus leucovorin (LV5FU2) is only about $263, but the incorporation of irinotecan (FOLFIRI) or oxaliplatin (FOLFOX) increases drug costs to $9,381 and $11,889, respectively. Total drug costs are about $21,000 with the addition of bevacizumab; an 8-week treatment course of standard cetuximab-containing regimens costs about $31,000. Thus, while the availability of these newer cytotoxic and biologic agents has extended median survival of patients with metastatic colorectal cancer, the economic impact of drug therapy alone on the healthcare system is of increasing importance.

Most recently, an observational registry of patients receiving chemotherapy for colorectal cancer at clinics across the United States was used to determine actual costs associated with eight commonly prescribed treatment regimens.[144] The costs were determined by adding the cost of each chemotherapeutic agent, as well as other commonly prescribed drugs. The costs associated with regimens varied widely. FOLFOX, the most common regimen, cost $2,931 per cycle; patients receiving this regimen also had the greatest utilization of white blood cell growth factors and erythropoiesis-stimulating agents. Depending on the regimen, total cost of chemotherapy for a full course of treatment could vary by as much as $36,999.

The cost-effectiveness of therapeutic regimens in various treatment settings has also been evaluated. The addition of irinotecan to fluorouracil and leucovorin as first-line therapy for metastatic disease was supported in the United Kingdom based on an incremental cost-effectiveness ratio of £14,794 per life-year gained.[145] A comparison of the costs and effects of FOLFOX compared with IFL, based on the perspective of a United States payer, showed total costs of $94,693 for FOLFOX and $66,231 for IFL, with a gain in survival of 4.4 months with FOLFOX at an incremental cost-effectiveness ratio of $80,410 per life-year gained.[145] The associated $11,890 per quality-adjusted life-year gained is considered an acceptable oncology intervention within the United States.

In adjuvant treatment, a cost-effectiveness analysis of FOLFOX4 compared to LV5FU2 from a Medicare perspective showed an incremental cost-effectiveness ratio with FOLFOX4 of $20,603 per life-year gained and $22,804 per quality-adjusted life-year gained.[146] At a threshold of $50,000 per quality-adjusted life-year, FOLFOX4 would be viewed as cost-effective adjuvant therapy for stage III colon cancer. Substitution of intravenous fluorouracil with oral capecitabine may have positive economic effects, but data are limited.[145] Reduced costs for capecitabine with regard to drug administration and drug-related adverse effects offset its higher acquisition cost as compared with fluorouracil plus leucovorin in adjuvant therapy for stage III colon cancer, but a cost-effectiveness analysis was not reported.[147]

The cost-effectiveness of combination chemotherapy with cetuximab, bevacizumab, or panitumumab in the United States has not been established. A report by the National Institute for Health and Clinical Excellence (NICE) suggests that neither first-line bevacizumab nor second-line or subsequent treatment cetuximab would be considered cost-effective.[145]

Colorectal cancer screening is regarded as cost-effective, but only approximately 35% of the population age 50 years and older undergoes regular screening.[148] The cost-effectiveness of standard methods varies. Base-case estimates, adjusted to year 2000 dollars, were $6,300 to $19,700 per life-year saved, $13,600 to $36,300 per life-year saved, and $7,300 to $22,000 per life-year saved for FOBT, sigmoidoscopy, and colonoscopy, respectively.[148] When adjusted average cost-effectiveness ratios were calculated and compared among FOBT, colonoscopy, and sigmoidoscopy, colonoscopy was the most cost-effective screening strategy when performed every 10 years. Based on an average estimated adherence rate with FOBT or sigmoidoscopy of approximately 50%, the ability to offer patients a choice of screening alternatives has been proposed in an attempt to increase acceptance of screening.[148] A base-rate estimate of the cost-effectiveness of offering a choice of cancer screening options to individuals age 50 years and older is $11,900 per life-year gained.[148] Because most accepted screening strategies have cost-effectiveness ratios that are well below the accepted benchmark of $50,000 per life-year saved, this strategy is considered cost-effective. As many as 12,000 deaths each year might be prevented if all individuals who were candidates for colorectal screening participated in a regular program.[148]

EVALUATION OF THERAPEUTIC OUTCOMES

The goal of monitoring is to evaluate whether the patient is receiving any benefit from the management of the disease or to detect recurrence. Similarly, examinations help to determine whether preventive interventions or screening studies effectively reduce an individual's risk for developing colorectal cancer or presenting with an advanced stage of disease. During treatment for active disease, patients should undergo monitoring for measurable tumor response, progression, or new metastases; these tests may include chest CT scans or radiographs, abdominal or pelvic CT scans or radiographs, depending on the site of disease being evaluated for response, and CEA measurements every 3 months if the CEA is or was previously elevated. In addition, a complete blood cell count should be obtained prior to each course of chemotherapy administration to ensure that hematologic indices are adequate. Baseline liver function tests and an assessment of renal function should be evaluated prior to and periodically during therapy. These tests and other selected serum chemistries should also be evaluated with the development of any new symptoms or significant change in disease status. Patients should be evaluated during every treatment visit for the presence of anticipated side effects, which generally include loose stools or diarrhea, nausea or vomiting, mouth sores, fatigue, and fever, as well as other side effects such as neuropathy and skin rash that are typically associated with oxaliplatin and cetuximab, respectively. Patients receiving bevacizumab should be evaluated for hypertension and proteinuria.

Symptoms of recurrence such as pain syndromes, changes in bowel habits, rectal or vaginal bleeding, pelvic masses, anorexia, and weight loss develop in less than 50% of patients. A greater percentage of recurrences are detected in asymptomatic patients because of increased serum CEA levels that lead to further examination. Although the value of CEA monitoring for asymptomatic disease recurrence is questioned by some because of the related expense and emotional stress associated with false-positive elevations, CEA monitoring plays an important role in postoperative followup studies for most individuals. A PET scan can be considered to identify localized sites of metastatic disease when a rising CEA level suggests metastatic disease but CT scans and other imaging studies are negative.

Patients who undergo curative surgical resection, with or without adjuvant therapy, require close follow up based on the premise that early detection and treatment of recurrence could still render them cured. In addition, early treatment for asymptomatic metastatic colorectal cancer appears superior to delayed therapy. Specific practice guidelines for postoperative surveillance examinations were developed by ASCO and include: history and physical examination every 3 to 6 months for the first 3 years, every 6 months during the fourth and fifth years, and then at the discretion of the physician; annual chest and abdominal CT scan for 3 years following primary therapy; and colonoscopy at 3 years after operative treatment. These guidelines also recommend against routinely monitoring liver function tests, complete blood cell count, FOBT, annual chest radiographs in asymptomatic patients.[149]

Recent advances in the treatment for cancer of the colon and rectum now offer the potential to improve patient survival, but for many patients, improved DFS and PFS represent equally important therapeutic outcomes. Although treatment approaches for metastatic colorectal cancer have been historically assessed by their ability to produce a measurable objective tumor response, which is generally believed necessary for any treatment to improve survival, the effects of therapies on survival are clinically more meaningful than their ability to induce a tumor response. However, with the availability of multiple active treatments for metastatic disease, and the likelihood that patients will receive more than one during the course of their treatment, improvements in OS with new therapies will be increasingly difficult to determine.

In the absence of the ability of a specific treatment to demonstrate improved survival, important outcome measures should include the effects of the treatment on patient symptoms, daily activities and performance status, and other quality-of-life indicators, as well as PFS and time-to-treatment failure. Because most metastatic colorectal cancers are incurable, a specific decision regarding an individual patient's care will ultimately be required. This decision should be based on a careful assessment of the balance between risks associated with treatment (or lack thereof) and benefits of treatment. Effort should also be made to ensure that the costs of screening, diagnostic tests, treatments, and procedures for colorectal cancer are consistent with their value in improving patient outcomes.

ABBREVIATIONS

APC: adenomatous polyposis coli (gene)

ASCO: American Society of Clinical Oncology

BMI: body mass index

CAPEOX: capecitabine, oxaliplatin

CEA: carcinoembryonic antigen

COX: cyclooxygenase

CT: computed tomography

CYP: cytochrome P450 isoenzyme

DFMO: difluoromethylornithine

DFS: disease-free survival

DPD: dihydropyrimidine dehydrogenase

EGFR: epidermal growth factor receptor

FAP: familial adenomatous polyposis

FIT: fecal immunochemical test

FOBT: fecal occult blood test

FOLFIRI: fluorouracil, leucovorin, irinotecan

FOLFOX: fluorouracil, leucovorin, oxaliplatin

5-FU: fluorouracil

HAI: hepatic artery infusion

HNPCC: hereditary nonpolyposis colorectal cancer

HR: hazard ratio

IFL: irinotecan plus fluorouracil plus leucovorin

IGF-1: insulin-like growth factor-1

MMR: mismatch-repair (gene)

MTHFR: methylenetetrahydrofolate reductase

MSS: microsatellite stability

NCCN: National Comprehensive Cancer Network

NF-κB: nuclear factor kappa B

NSAID: nonsteroidal antiinflammatory drug

OS: overall survival

PET: positron emission tomography

PFS: progression-free survival

RR: relative risk

TGF-β: transforming growth factor-β

TNF-α: tumor necrosis factor-alpha

TS: thymidylate synthase

UGT1A1: uridine diphosphate-glucuronosyltransferase

UICC: Union for International Cancer Control

VDR: vitamin D receptor

XELOX: capecitabine, oxaliplatin

XRT: radiation therapy

REFERENCES

1. Jemal A, Siegel R, Xu J, Ward E. Cancer statistics, 2010. CA Cancer J Clin 2010;60:277–300.
2. Center MM, Jemal A, Smith RA, Ward E. Worldwide variations in colorectal cancer. CA Cancer J Clin 2009;59:366–378.
3. Altekruse SF, Kosary CL, Krapcho M, et al (eds). SEER Cancer Statistics Review, 1975–2007, National Cancer Institute. Bethesda, MD, http://seer.cancer.gov/csr/1975_2007/, based on November 2009 SEER data submission, posted to the SEER web site, 2010.
4. Kamangar F, Dores G, Anderson W. Patterns of cancer incidence, mortality, and prevalence across five continents: Defining priorities to reduce cancer disparities in different geographic regions of the world. J Clin Oncol 2006;24:2137–2150.
5. Das D, Arber N, Jankowski JA. Chemoprevention of colorectal cancer. Digestion 2007;76:51–67.
6. Marshall JR. Nutrition and colon cancer prevention. Curr Opin Clin Nutr Metab Care 2009;12:539–543.
7. Schatzkin A, Mouw T, Park Y, et al. Dietary fiber and whole-grain consumption in relation to colorectal cancer in the NIH-AARP Diet and Health Study. Am J Clin Nutr 2007;85:1353–1360.
8. Kim YS, Milner JA. Dietary modulation of colon cancer risk. J Nutr 2007;137(11 suppl):2576S–2579S.
9. Zheng W, Lee SA. Well-done meat intake, heterocyclic amine exposure, and cancer risk. Nutr Cancer 2009;61:437–446.
10. Huncharek M, Muscat J, Kupelnick B. Colorectal cancer risk and dietary intake of calcium, vitamin D, and dairy products: A meta-analysis of 26,335 cases from 60 observational studies. Nutr Cancer 2009;61:47–69.
11. Pend's-Franco N, Aguilera Ó, Pereira F, et al. Vitamin D and Wnt/β-catenin pathway in colon cancer: Role and regulation of *DICKKOPF* genes. Anticancer Res 2008;28:2613–2624.
12. Hubner RA, Houlston RS. Folate and colorectal cancer prevention. Br J Cancer 2009;100:233–239.
13. Dube C, Rostom A, Lewin G, et al. The use of aspirin for primary prevention of colorectal cancer: A systematic review prepared for the U.S. Preventive Services Task Force. Ann Intern Med 2007;146:365–375.
14. Rostom A, Dube C, Lewin G, et al. Nonsteroidal anti-inflammatory drugs and cyclooxygenase-2 inhibitors for primary prevention of colorectal cancer: A systematic review prepared for the U.S. Preventive Services Task Force. Ann Intern Med 2007;146:376–389.
15. Wang D, Dubois RN. The role of COX-2 in intestinal inflammation and colorectal cancer. Oncogene 2010;29:781–788.
16. Flossmann E, Rothwell PM. Effect of aspirin on long-term risk of colorectal cancer: Consistent evidence from randomised and observational studies. Lancet 2007;369:1603–1613.
17. Chan JA, Meyerhardt JA, Chan AT, Giovannucci EL, Colditz GA, Fuchs CS. Hormone replacement therapy and survival after colorectal cancer diagnosis. J Clin Oncol 2006;24:5680–5686.
18. Chlebowski RT, Wactawski-Wende J, Ritenbaugh C, et al. Estrogen plus progestin and colorectal cancer in postmenopausal women. N Engl J Med 2004;350:991–1004.
19. Rennert G, Rennert HS, Pinchey M, et al. Use of hormone replacement therapy and the risk of colorectal cancer. J Clin Oncol 2009;27:4542–4547.
20. Larsson SC, Wolk A. Obesity and colon and rectal cancer risk: A meta-analysis of prospective studies. Am J Clin Nutr 2007;86:556–565.
21. Campbell PT, Jacobs ET, Ulrich CM, et al. Case-control study of overweight, obesity, and colorectal cancer, overall and by tumor microsatellite instability status. J Natl Cancer Inst 2010;102:391–400.
22. Harriss DJ, Cable NT, George K, et al. Physical activity before and after diagnosis of colorectal cancer: disease risk, clinical outcomes, response pathways, and biomarkers. Sports Med 2007;37:947–960.
23. Pischon T, Lahmann PH, Boeing H, et al. Body size and risk of colon and rectal cancer in the European Prospective Investigation Into Cancer and Nutrition (EPIC). J Natl Cancer Inst 2006;98:920–931.
24. Gunter MJ, Leitzmann MF. Obesity and colorectal cancer: Epidemiology, mechanisms and candidate genes. J Nutr Biochem 2006;17:145–156.
25. Ferrari P, Jenab M, Norat T, et al. Lifetime and baseline alcohol intake and risk of colon and rectal cancers in the European prospective investigation into cancer and nutrition (EPIC). Int J Cancer 2007;121:2065–2072.
26. Botteri E, Iodice S, Bagnardi V, et al. Smoking and colorectal cancer: A meta-analysis. JAMA 2008;300:2765–2778.
27. Ji B-T, Weissfeld JL, Chow W-H, et al. Tobacco smoking and colorectal hyperplastic and adenomatous polyps. Cancer Epidemiol Biomarkers Prev 2006;15:897–901.
28. Bonovas S, Filioussi K, Flordellis CS, Sitaras NM. Statins and the risk of colorectal cancer: A meta-analysis of 18 studies involving more than 1.5 million patients. J Clin Oncol 2007;25:3462–3468.
29. Coogan PF, Smith J, Rosenberg L. Statin use and risk of colorectal cancer. J Natl Cancer Inst 2007;99:32–40.
30. Michels KB, Willett WC, Fuchs CS, Giovannucci E. Coffee, tea, and caffeine consumption and incidence of colon and rectal cancer. J Natl Cancer Inst 2005;97:282–292.

31. Sun C-L, Yuan J-M, Koh W-P, Yu MC. Green tea, black tea and colorectal cancer risk: A meta-analysis of epidemiologic studies. Carcinogenesis 2006;27:1301–1309.

32. Je Y, Liu W, Giovannucci E. Coffee consumption and risk of colorectal cancer: A systematic review and meta-analysis of prospective cohort studies. Int J Cancer 2009;124:1662–1668.

33. Collins P, Mpofu C, Watson A, Rhodes J. Strategies for detecting colon cancer and/or dysplasia in patients with inflammatory bowel disease. Cochrane Database Syst Rev 2006;(2):CD000279.

34. Triantafillidis JK, Nasioulas G, Kosmidis PA. Colorectal cancer and inflammatory bowel disease: Epidemiology, risk factors, mechanisms of carcinogenesis and prevention strategies. Anticancer Res 2009;29:2727–2737.

35. Larsson SC, Orsini N, Wolk A. Diabetes mellitus and risk of colorectal cancer: A meta-analysis. J Natl Cancer Inst 2005;97:1679–1687.

36. Berster JM, Göke B. Type 2 diabetes mellitus as risk factor for colorectal cancer. Arch Physiol Biochem 2008;114:84–98.

37. Pais R, Silaghi H, Silaghi AC, et al. Metabolic syndrome and risk of subsequent colorectal cancer. World J Gastroenterol 2009;15:5141–5148.

38. Lynch HT, de la Chapelle A. Hereditary colorectal cancer. N Engl J Med 2003;348:919–932.

39. Chapelle ADL. Genetic predisposition to colorectal cancer. Nat Rev Cancer 2004;4:769–780.

40. Galiatsatos P, Foulkes WD. Familial adenomatous polyposis. Am J Gastroenterol 2006;101:385–398.

41. Markowitz SD, Bertagnolli MM. Molecular basis of colorectal cancer. N Engl J Med 2009;361:2449–2460.

42. Vasen HFA, Moslein G, Alonso A, et al. Guidelines for the clinical management of Lynch syndrome (hereditary non-polyposis cancer). J Med Genet 2007;44:353–362.

43. Reszka E, Wasowicz W, Gromadzinska J. Genetic polymorphism of xenobiotic metabolising enzymes, diet and cancer susceptibility. Br J Nutr 2006;96:609–619.

44. Goode EL, Potter JD, Bamlet WR, Rider DN, Bigler J. Inherited variation in carcinogen-metabolizing enzymes and risk of colorectal polyps. Carcinogenesis 2007;28:328–341.

45. Calvert PM, Frucht H. The genetics of colorectal cancer. Ann Intern Med 2002;137:603–612.

46. Italiano A. Targeting the epidermal growth factor receptor in colorectal cancer: Advances and controversies. Oncology 2006;70:161–167.

47. Libutti KS, Saltz LB, Tepper JE. Cancers of the gastrointestinal tract: Colon cancer. In: DeVita VT, Lawrence TS, Rosenberg SA, eds. Cancer: Principles and Practice of Oncology. 8th ed. Philadelphia: Lippincott Williams & Wilkins; 2008:1232–1285.

48. Compton CC. Colorectal carcinoma: Diagnostic, prognostic, and molecular features. Mod Pathol 2003;16:376–388.

49. U.S. Preventive Services Task Force. Routine aspirin or nonsteroidal anti-inflammatory drugs for the primary prevention of colorectal cancer: U.S. Preventive Services Task Force Recommendation Statement. Ann Intern Med 2007;146:361–364.

50. Giardiello FM, Yang VW, Hylind LM, et al. Primary chemoprevention of familial adenomatous polyposis with sulindac. N Engl J Med 2002;346:1054–1059.

51. Half E, Arber N. Colon cancer: Preventive agents and the present status of chemoprevention. Expert Opin Pharmacother 2009;10:211–219.

52. Takayama T, Goji T, Taniguchi T, Inoue A. Chemoprevention of colorectal cancer-experimental and clinical aspects. J Med Invest 2009;56:1–5.

53. Chan AT, Ogino S, Fuchs CS. Aspirin and the risk of colorectal cancer in relation to the expression of COX-2. N Engl J Med 2007;356:2131–2142.

54. Kwak E, Chung D. Hereditary colorectal cancer syndromes: An overview. Clin Colorectal Cancer 2007;6:340–344.

55. Lieberman DA. Screening for colorectal cancer. N Engl J Med 2009;361:1179–1187.

56. Rex DK, Johnson DA, Anderson JC, et al. American College of Gastroenterology Guidelines for Colorectal Cancer Screening 2008. Am J Gastroenterol 2009;104:739–750.

57. Smith RA, Cokkinides V, Brooks D, et al. Cancer Screening in the United States, 2010: A review of current American Cancer Society guidelines and issues in cancer screening. CA Cancer J Clin 2010;60:99–119.

58. U.S. Preventive Services Task Force. Screening for colorectal cancer: U.S. Preventive Services Task Force recommendation statement. Ann Intern Med 2008;149:627–637.

59. Hewitson P, Glasziou P, Irwig L, et al. Screening for colorectal cancer using the faecal occult blood test, Hemoccult. Cochrane Database Syst Rev 2007. Issue 1. Art. No.: CD001216. DOI: 10.1002/14651858.CD001216.pub 2.

60. Imperiale TF, Ransohoff DF, Itzkowitz SH, Turnbull BA, Ross ME, the Colorectal Cancer Study Group. Fecal DNA versus fecal occult blood for colorectal-cancer screening in an average-risk population. N Engl J Med 2004;351:2704–2714.

61. Locker GY, Hamilton S, Harris J, et al. ASCO 2006 update of recommendations for the use of tumor markers in gastrointestinal cancer. J Clin Oncol 2006;24:5313–5327.

62. Saunders TH, Mendes Ribeiro HK, Gleeson FV. New techniques for imaging colorectal cancer: The use of MRI, PET and radioimmunoscintigraphy for primary staging and follow-up. Br Med Bull 2002;64:81–99.

63. Colon and rectum. In: Edge SB, Byrd DR, Compton CC, et al., eds.: American Joint Committee on Cancer. AJCC Cancer Staging Manual. 7th ed. New York: Springer; 2010:143–159.

64. Gunderson LL, Jessup JM, Sargent DJ, Greene FL, Stewart AK. Revised TN categorization for colon cancer based on national survival outcomes data. J Clin Oncol 2010;28:264–271.

65. Pages F, Berger A, Camus M, et al. Effector memory T cells, early metastasis, and survival in colorectal cancer. N Engl J Med 2005;353:2654–2666.

66. Ogino S, Nosho K, Irahara N, et al. Prognostic significance and molecular associations of 18q loss of heterozygosity: A cohort study of microsatellite stable colorectal cancers. J Clin Oncol 2009;27:4591–4598.

67. Ribic CM, Sargent DJ, Moore MJ, et al. Tumor microsatellite-instability status as a predictor of benefit from fluorouracil-based adjuvant chemotherapy for colon cancer. N Engl J Med 2003;349:247–257.

68. Libutti SK, Tepper JE, Saltz LB. Cancers of the gastrointestinal tract: rectal cancer. In: DeVita VT, Lawrence TS, Rosenberg SA, eds. Cancer: Principles and Practice of Oncology. 8th ed. Philadelphia: Lippincott Williams & Wilkins; 2008:1285–1301.

69. Kahnamoui K, Cadeddu M, Farrokhyar F, Anvari M. Laparoscopic surgery for colon cancer: A systematic review. Can J Surg 2007;50:48–57.

70. Benson AB III, Schrag D, Somerfield MR, et al. American Society of Clinical Oncology recommendations on adjuvant chemotherapy for stage II colon cancer. J Clin Oncol 2004;22:3408–3419.

71. The NCCN Clinical Practice Guidelines in Oncology v.2.2010 Colon Cancer, 02/08/10 Copyright 2010. National Comprehensive Cancer Network, http://www.nccn.org.

72. Giantonio BJ, Catalano PJ, Meropol NJ, et al. Bevacizumab in combination with oxaliplatin, fluorouracil, and leucovorin (FOLFOX4) for previously treated metastatic colorectal cancer: Results from the Eastern Cooperative Oncology Group Study E3200. J Clin Oncol 2007;25:1539–1544.

73. Kuebler JP, Wieand HS, O'Connell MJ, et al. Oxaliplatin combined with weekly bolus fluorouracil and leucovorin as surgical adjuvant chemotherapy for stage II and III colon cancer: Results from NSABP C-07. J Clin Oncol 2007;25:2198–2204.

74. Buyse M, Zeleniuch-Jacquotte A, Chalmers T. Adjuvant therapy of colorectal cancer. Why we still don't know. JAMA 1988;259:3571–3578.

75. Wolmark N, Rockette H, Fisher B, et al. The benefit of leucovorin-modulated fluorouracil as postoperative adjuvant therapy for primary colon cancer: Results from National Surgical Adjuvant Breast and Bowel Project protocol C-03. J Clin Oncol 1993;11:1879–1887.

76. O'Connell MJ, Mailliard JA, Kahn MJ, et al. Controlled trial of fluorouracil and low-dose leucovorin given for 6 months as postoperative adjuvant therapy for colon cancer. J Clin Oncol 1997;15:246–250.

77. Tournigand C, Andre T, Achille E, et al. FOLFIRI Followed by FOLFOX6 or the reverse sequence in advanced colorectal cancer: A randomized GERCOR Study. J Clin Oncol 2004;22:229–237.

78. Meta-Analysis Group in Cancer. Toxicity of fluorouracil in patients with advanced colorectal cancer: Effect of administration schedule and prognostic factors. J Clin Oncol 1998;16:3537–3541.

79. van Kuilenburg ABP, Haasjes J, Richel DJ, et al. Clinical implications of dihydropyrimidine dehydrogenase (DPD) deficiency in patients with severe 5-fluorouracil-associated toxicity: Identification of new mutations in the DPD gene. Clin Cancer Res 2000;6:4705–4712.

80. Andre T, Boni C, Navarro M, et al. Improved overall survival with oxaliplatin, fluorouracil, and leucovorin as adjuvant treatment in stage II or III colon cancer in the MOSAIC trial. J Clin Oncol 2009;27:3109–3116.

81. Kuebler JP, Wieand HS, O'Connell MJ, et al. Oxaliplatin combined with weekly bolus fluorouracil and leucovorin as surgical adjuvant chemotherapy for stage II and III colon cancer: results from NSABP C-07. J Clin Oncol 2007;25:2198–2204.

82. Twelves C, Wong A, Nowacki MP, et al. Capecitabine as adjuvant treatment for stage III colon cancer. N Engl J Med 2005;352:2696–2704.

83. Saltz LB, Niedzwiecki D, Hollis D, et al. Irinotecan fluorouracil plus leucovorin is not superior to fluorouracil plus leucovorin alone as adjuvant treatment for stage III colon cancer: results of CALGB 89803. J Clin Oncol 2007;25:3456–3461.

84. Van Cutsem E, Labianca R, Bodoky G, et al. Randomized phase III trial comparing biweekly infusional fluorouracil/leucovorin alone or with irinotecan in the adjuvant treatment of stage III colon cancer: PETACC-3. J Clin Oncol 2009;27:3117–3125.

85. Ychou M, Raoul J, Douillard J, et al. A phase III randomized trial of LV5FU2+CPT-11 vs. LV5FU2 alone in adjuvant high risk colon cancer (FNCLCC Accord02/FFCD9802). Ann Oncol 2009;20:674–680.

86. Haller DG, Cassidy J, Tabernero J, et al. Efficacy finding from the randomized phase III trial of capecitabine plus oxaliplatin versus bolus 5-FU/LV for stage III colon cancer (NO16968): impact of age on disease-free survival (DFS). J Clin Oncol 2010;28:15s (supplement:abstract 3521).

87. Wolmark N, Yothers G, O'Connell MJ, et al. A phase III trial comparing mFOLFOX6 to mFOLFOX6 plus bevacizumab in stage II or III carcinoma of the colon: Results of NSABP Protocol C-08. ASCO Annual Meeting Proceedings (Post-Meeting Edition). J Clin Oncol 2009;27(18S):LBA4.

88. Alberts SR, Sargent DJ, Smyrk TC, et al. Adjuvant mFOLFOX6 with or without cetuximab (Cmab) in KRAS wild-type (WT) patients (pts) with resected stage III colon cancer (CC): results from NCCTG Intergroup Phase III Trial N0147. J Clin Oncol 2010;28:18s (supplement; abstr CRA3507).

89. Baxter NN, Garcia-Aguilar J. Organ preservation for rectal cancer. J Clin Oncol 2007;25:1014–1020.

90. The NCCN Clinical Practice Guidelines in Oncology v.2.2010 Rectal Cancer, 02/08/10 Copyright 2010. National Comprehensive Cancer Network, http://www.nccn.org.

91. Smalley SR, Benedetti JK, Williamson SK, et al. Phase III trial of fluorouracil-based chemotherapy regimens plus radiotherapy in postoperative adjuvant rectal cancer: GI INT 0144. J Clin Oncol 2006;24:3542–3547.

92. Bosset J-F, Collette L, Calais G, et al. Chemotherapy with preoperative radiotherapy in rectal cancer. N Eng J Med 2006;355:1114–1123.

93. Gill S, Blackstock AW, Goldberg RM. Colorectal cancer. Mayo Clin Proc 2007;82:114–129.

94. Kemeny N, Huang Y, Cohen AM, et al. Hepatic arterial infusion of chemotherapy after resection of hepatic metastases from colorectal cancer. N Engl J Med 1999;341:2039–2048.

95. Cohen AD, Kemeny NE. An update on hepatic arterial infusion chemotherapy for colorectal cancer. Oncologist 2003;8:553–566.

96. Simmonds PC, Primrose JN, Colquitt JL, et al. Surgical resection of hepatic metastases from colorectal cancer: A systematic review of published studies. Br J Cancer 2006;94:982–999.

97. Hochster HS, Hart LL, Ramanathan RK, et al. Safety and efficacy of oxaliplatin and fluoropyrimidine regimens with or without bevacizumab as first-line treatment of metastatic colorectal cancer: Results of the TREE study. J Clin Oncol 2008;26:3523–3529.

98. Douillard J, Cunningham D, Roth A, et al. Irinotecan combined with fluorouracil compared with fluorouracil alone as first-line treatment for metastatic colorectal cancer: A multicentre randomised trial. Lancet 2000;355:1041–1047.

99. Twelves C. Capecitabine as first-line treatment in colorectal cancer. Eur J Cancer 2002;38:15–20.

100. de Gramont A, Bosset JF, Milan C, et al. Randomized trial comparing monthly low-dose leucovorin and fluorouracil bolus with bimonthly high-dose leucovorin and fluorouracil bolus plus continuous infusion for advanced colorectal cancer: A French intergroup study. J Clin Oncol 1997;15:808–815.

101. Saltz LB, Cox JV, Blanke C, et al. Irinotecan plus fluorouracil and leucovorin for metastatic colorectal cancer. N Engl J Med 2000;343:905–914.

102. Cunningham D, Pyrhönen S, James R, et al. Randomised trial of irinotecan plus supportive care versus supportive care alone after fluorouracil failure for patients with metastatic colorectal cancer. Lancet 1998;352:1413–1418.

103. de Gramont A, Figer A, Seymour M, et al. Leucovorin and fluorouracil with or without oxaliplatin as first-line treatment in advanced colorectal cancer. J Clin Oncol 2000;18:2938–2947.

104. Cunningham D, Humblet Y, Siena S, et al. Cetuximab monotherapy and cetuximab plus irinotecan in irinotecan-refractory metastatic colorectal cancer. N Engl J Med 2004;351:337–345.

105. Rougier P, Van Cutsem E, Bajetta E, et al. Randomised trial of irinotecan versus fluorouracil by continuous infusion after fluorouracil failure in patients with metastatic colorectal cancer. Lancet 1998;352:1407–1412.

106. Jonker D, Maroun J, Kocha W. Survival benefit of chemotherapy in metastatic colorectal cancer: A meta-analysis of randomized controlled trials. Br J Cancer 2000;82:1789–1794.

107. Colorectal Cancer Collaborative Group. Palliative chemotherapy for advanced colorectal cancer: Systematic review and meta-analysis. BMJ 2000;321:531–535.

108. Goldberg RM, Sargent DJ, Morton RF, et al. A randomized controlled trial of fluorouracil plus leucovorin, irinotecan, and oxaliplatin combinations in patients with previously untreated metastatic colorectal cancer. J Clin Oncol 2004;22:23–30.

109. Hurwitz H, Fehrenbacher L, Novotny W, et al. Bevacizumab plus irinotecan, fluorouracil, and leucovorin for metastatic colorectal cancer. N Engl J Med 2004;350:2335–2342.

110. Saltz L, Clark S, Diaz-Rubio E, et al. Bevacizumab in combination with oxaliplatin-based chemotherapy as first-line therapy in metastatic colorectal cancer: A randomized phase III study. J Clin Oncol 2008;26:2013–2039.

111. Fuchs CS, Marshall J, Barrueco J. Randomized, controlled trial of irinotecan plus infusional, bolus, or oral fluoropyrimidines in first-line treatment of metastatic colorectal cancer: Updated results from the BICC-C study. J Clin Oncol 2008;26:689–690.

112. Bokemeyer C, Bondarenko I, Makhson A, et al. Fluorouracil, leucovorin, and oxaliplatin with and without cetuximab in the first-line treatment of metastatic colorectal cancer. J Clin Oncol 2009;27:663–667.

113. Van Cutsem E, Kohne C-H, Hitre E, et al. Cetuximab and chemotherapy as initial treatment for metastatic colorectal cancer. N Engl J Med 2009;360:1408–1417.

114. Van Cutsem E, Peeters M, Siena S, et al. Open-label phase III trial of panitumumab plus best supportive care compared with best supportive care alone in patients with chemotherapy-refractory metastatic colorectal cancer. J Clin Oncol 2007;25:1658–1664.

115. Kohne CH, Wils J, Lorenz M, et al. Randomized phase III study of high-dose fluorouracil given as a weekly 24-hour infusion with or without leucovorin versus bolus fluorouracil plus leucovorin in advanced colorectal cancer: European Organization of Research and Treatment of Cancer Gastrointestinal Group Study 40952. J Clin Oncol 2003;21:3721–3728.

116. Fuchs CS, Marshall J, Mitchell E, et al. Randomized, controlled trial of irinotecan plus infusional, bolus, or oral fluoropyrimidines in first-line treatment of metastatic colorectal cancer: Results from the BICC-C Study. J Clin Oncol 2007;25:4779–4786.

117. O'Dwyer PJ, Catalano RB. Uridine diphosphate glucuronosyltransferase (UGT) 1A1 and irinotecan: Practical pharmacogenomics arrives in cancer therapy. J Clin Oncol 2006;24:4534–4538.

118. Raymond E, Faivre S, Chaney S, Woynarowski J, Cvitkovic E. Cellular and molecular pharmacology of oxaliplatin. Mol Cancer Ther 2002;1:227–235.

119. Grothey A. Oxaliplatin-safety profile: Neurotoxicity. Semin Oncol 2003;30:5–13.

120. Cassidy J, Clarke S, Diaz-Rubio E, et al. Randomized phase III study of capecitabine plus oxaliplatin compared with fluorouracil/folinic acid plus oxaliplatin as first-line therapy for metastatic colorectal cancer. J Clin Oncol 2008;26:2006–2012.

121. Berlin J, Posey J, Tchekmedyian S, et al. Panitumumab with irinotecan/leucovorin/5-fluorouracil for first-line treatment of metastatic colorectal cancer. Clin Colorectal Cancer 2007;6:427–432.

122. Hecht JR, Mitchell E, Chidiac T, et al. A randomized phase IIIB trial of chemotherapy, bevacizumab, and panitumumab compared with chemotherapy and bevacizumab alone for metastatic colorectal cancer. J Clin Oncol 2009;27:672–680.

123. Tol J, Koopman M, Cats A, et al. Chemotherapy, bevacizumab, and cetuximab in metastatic colorectal cancer. N Engl J Med 2009;360:563–572.

124. Cohen AD, Kemeny NE. An update on hepatic arterial infusion chemotherapy for colorectal cancer. Oncologist 2003;8:553–566.

125. Kemeny NE, Niedzwiecki D, Hollis DR, et al. Hepatic arterial infusion versus systemic therapy for hepatic metastases from colorectal cancer: A randomized trial of efficacy, quality of life, and molecular markers (CALGB 9481). J Clin Oncol 2006;24:1395–1403.

126. Grothey A, Sargent D. Overall survival of patients with advanced colorectal cancer correlates with availability of fluorouracil, irinotecan, and oxaliplatin regardless of whether doublet or single-agent therapy is used first line. J Clin Oncol 2005;23:9441–9442.

127. Andre T, Bensmaine MA, Louvet C, et al. Multicenter phase II study of bimonthly high-dose leucovorin, fluorouracil infusion, and oxaliplatin for metastatic colorectal cancer resistant to the same leucovorin and fluorouracil regimen. J Clin Oncol 1999;17:3560–3568.

128. Kouroussis C, Souglakos J, Mavroudis D, et al. Oxaliplatin with high-dose leucovorin and infusional 5-fluorouracil in irinotecan-pretreated patients with advanced colorectal cancer (ACC). Am J Clin Oncol 2002;25:627–631.

129. Saltz LB, Meropol NJ, Loehrer PJ Sr, et al. Phase II trial of cetuximab in patients with refractory colorectal cancer that expresses the epidermal growth factor receptor. J Clin Oncol 2004;22:1201–1208.

130. Jonker DJ, O'Callaghan CJ, Karapetis CS, et al. Cetuximab for the treatment of colorectal cancer. N Engl J Med 2007;357:2040–2048.

131. Karapetis CS, Khambata-Ford S, Jonker DJ, et al. K-RAS mutations and benefit from cetuximab in advanced colorectal cancer. N Engl J Med 2008;359:1757–1765.

132. Kohne C, Rougier P, Stroh C, et al. Cetuximab with chemotherapy (CT) as first-line treatment for metastatic colorectal cancer (mCRC): a meta-analysis of CRYSTAL and OPUS studies according to KRAS and BRAF mutation status. Am Soc Clin Oncol 2010 Gastrointestinal Cancers Symposium, abstr 406.

133. Amado RG, Wolf M, Peeters M, et al. Wild-type KRAS is required for panitumumab efficacy in patients with metastatic colorectal cancer. J Clin Oncol 2008;26:1626–1634.

134. Chung KY, Shia J, Kemeny NE, et al. Cetuximab shows activity in colorectal cancer patients with tumors that do not express the epidermal growth factor receptor by immunohistochemistry. J Clin Oncol 2005;23:1803–1810.

135. Tournigand C, Cervantes A, Figer A, et al. OPTIMOX1: A randomized study of FOLFOX4 or FOLFOX7 with oxaliplatin in a stop-and-go fashion in advanced colorectal cancer—a GERCOR study. J Clin Oncol 2006;24:394–400.

136. Dick EA, Taylor-Robinson SD, Thomas HC, Gedroyc WMW. Ablative therapy for liver tumours. Gut 2002;50:733–739.

137. Fraker D, Soulen M. Regional therapy of hepatic metastases. Hematol Oncol Clin North Am 2002;16:947–967.

138. Marsh S. Pharmacogenetics of colorectal cancer. Expert Opin Pharmacother 2005;6:2607–2616.

139. Ruzzo A, Graziano F, Loupakis F, et al. Pharmacogenetic profiling in patients with advanced colorectal cancer treated with first-line FOLFOX-4 chemotherapy. J Clin Oncol 2007;25:1247–1254.

140. Del Rio M, Molina F, Bascoul-Mollevi C, et al. Gene expression signature in advanced colorectal cancer patients select drugs and response for the use of leucovorin, fluorouracil, and irinotecan. J Clin Oncol 2007;25:773–780.

141. Saif MW, Choma A, Salamone SJ, Chu E. Pharmacokinetically guided dose adjustment of 5-fluorouracil: A rational approach to improving therapeutic outcomes. J Natl Cancer Inst 2009;101:1543–1552.

142. Gamelin E, Delva R, Jacob J, et al. Individual fluorouracil dose adjustment based on pharmacokinetic follow-up compared with conventional dosage: Results of a multicenter randomized trial of patients with metastatic colorectal cancer. J Clin Oncol 2008;26:2099–3105.

143. Jansman FGA, Postma M, Brouwers JRBJ. Cost considerations in the treatment of colorectal cancer. Pharmacoeconomics 2007;25:537–562.

144. Ferro SA, Myer BS, Wolff DA, et al. Variation in the cost of medications for the treatment of colorectal cancer. Am J Manag Care 2008;14:717–725.

145. Krol M, Koopman M, Uyl-de Groot C, Punt CJA. A systematic review of economic analyses of pharmaceutical therapies for advanced colorectal cancer. Expert Opin Pharmacother 2007;8:1313–1328.

146. Aballea S, Chancellor JVM, Raikou M, et al. Cost-effectiveness analysis of oxaliplatin compared with 5-fluouracil/leucovorin in adjuvant treatment of stage III colon cancer in the US. Cancer 2007;109:1082–1089.

147. Twelves C. Xeloda in Adjuvant Colon Cancer Therapy (X-ACT) trial: Overview of efficacy, safety, and cost-effectiveness. Clin Colorectal Cancer 2006;6:278–287.

148. Maciosek MV, Solberg LI, Coffield AB, Edwards NM, Goodman MJ. Colorectal cancer screening: Health impact and cost effectiveness. Am J Prev Med 2006;31:80–89.

149. Desch CE, Benson AB, III, Somerfield MR, et al. Colorectal cancer surveillance: 2005 update of an American Society of Clinical Oncology practice guideline. J Clin Oncol 2005;23:8512–8519.

CHAPTER

139

Prostate Cancer

LEANN B. NORRIS AND JILL M. KOLESAR

KEY CONCEPTS

❶ Prostate cancer is the most frequent cancer in U.S. men. African American ancestry, family history, and increased age are the primary risk factors for prostate cancer.

❷ Prostate-specific antigen is a useful marker to detect prostate cancer at early stages, predict outcome for localized disease, define disease-free status, and monitor response to androgen-deprivation therapy or chemotherapy for advanced-stage disease.

❸ The prognosis for prostate cancer patients depends on the histologic grade, the tumor size, and the disease stage. More than 85% of patients with stage A_1 disease but less than 1% of those with stage D_2 can be cured.

❹ Androgen deprivation therapy with a luteinizing hormone–releasing hormone (LH-RH) agonist plus an antiandrogen should be used prior to radiation therapy for patients with locally advanced prostate cancer to improve outcomes over radiation therapy alone.

❺ Androgen deprivation therapy, with either orchiectomy, an LH-RH agonist alone or an LH-RH agonist plus an antiandrogen (combined hormonal blockade), can be used to provide palliation for patients with advanced (stage D_2) prostate cancer. The effects of androgen deprivation seem most pronounced in patients with minimal disease at diagnosis.

❻ Antiandrogen withdrawal, for patients having progressive disease while receiving combined hormonal blockade with an LH-RH agonist plus an antiandrogen, can provide additional symptomatic relief. Mutations in the androgen receptor have been documented that cause antiandrogen compounds to act like receptor agonists.

❼ Chemotherapy, with docetaxel and prednisone improves survival in patients with hormone-refractory prostate cancer. Patients with hormone-refractory prostate cancer should be considered for entry into clinical trials investigating new therapies for prostate cancer.

Learning objectives, review questions,
and other resources can be found at
www.pharmacotherapyonline.com.

Prostate cancer is the most commonly diagnosed cancer in American men.[1] For most men, prostate cancer has an indolent course, and treatment options for early disease include expectant management, surgery, or radiation. With expectant management, patients are monitored for disease progression or development of symptoms. Localized prostate cancer can be cured by surgery or radiation therapy, advanced prostate cancer is not yet curable. Treatment for advanced prostate cancer can provide significant disease palliation for many patients for several years after diagnosis. The endocrine dependence of this tumor is well documented, and hormonal manipulation to decrease circulating androgens remains the basis for the treatment of advanced disease.

EPIDEMIOLOGY

❶ Prostate cancer is the most frequent cancer among American men and represents the second leading cause of cancer-related deaths in all males.[1] In the United States alone, it is estimated that 217,730 new cases of prostatic carcinoma were diagnosed and more than 32,050 men died from this disease in 2010.[1] Although prostate cancer incidence increased during the late 1980s and early 1990s owing to widespread prostate-specific antigen (PSA) screening, deaths from prostate cancer have been declining since 1995.[1]

ETIOLOGY

Table 139–1 summarizes the possible factors associated with prostate cancer.[2,3] The widely accepted risk factors for prostate cancer are age, race-ethnicity, and family history of prostate cancer.[2,3] The disease is rare under the age of 40, but the incidence sharply increases with each subsequent decade, most likely because the individual has had a lifetime exposure to testosterone, a known growth signal for the prostate.[3]

RACE AND ETHNICITY

The incidence of clinical prostate cancer varies across geographic regions. Scandinavian countries and the United States report the highest incidence of prostate cancer, while the disease is relatively rare in Japan and other Asian countries.[4] African American men have the highest rate of prostate cancer in the world, and in the United States, prostate cancer mortality in African Americans is more than twice that seen in Caucasian populations.[1] Hormonal, dietary, and genetic differences, and differences in access to healthcare may contribute to the altered susceptibility to prostate cancer in these populations.[2,3] Testosterone, commonly implicated in the pathogenesis of prostate cancer, is 15% higher in African American men compared with Caucasian males. Activity of 5-α-reductase,

TABLE 139-1 Risk Factors Associated with Prostate Cancer

Factor	Possible Relationship
Probable risk factors	
Age	More than 70% of cases are diagnosed in men greater than 65 years old
Race	African Americans have higher incidence and death rate
Genetic	Familial prostate cancer inherited in an autosomal dominant manner
	Mutations in *p53*, *Rb*, E-cahedrin, *α*-catenin, androgen receptor, *KAI1*, microsatellite instability, loss of heterozygocity at 1, 2q, 12p, 15q, 16p, and 16q, *BRCA1* and *BRCA2* mutation
	Candidate prostate cancer gene locus identified on chromosome 1
Possible risk factors	
Environmental	Clinical carcinoma incidence varies worldwide
	Latent carcinoma similar between regions
	Nationalized males adopt intermediate incidence rates between those of the United States and their native country
Occupational	Increased risk associated with cadmium exposure
Diet	Increased risk associated with high-meat and high-fat diets
	Decreased intake of 1,25-dihydroxyvitamin D, lycopene, and *β*-carotene increases risk
Hormonal	Does not occur in eunuchs
	Low incidence in cirrhotic patients
	Up to 80% are hormonally dependent; African Americans have 15% increased testosterone
	Japanese have decreased 5-*α*-reductase activities
	Polymorphic expression of the androgen receptor

the enzyme that converts testosterone to its more active form, dihydrotestosterone (DHT), in the prostate, is decreased in Japanese men compared with African Americans and Caucasians.[2,3] In addition, genetic variations in the androgen receptor exist. Activation of the androgen receptor is inversely correlated with CAG repeat length. Shorter CAG repeat sequences have been found in African Americans. Therefore the combination of increased testosterone and increased androgen receptor activation may account for the increased risk of prostate cancer for African American men.[2,3] The Asian diet is generally considered to be low in fat and high in fiber with a high concentration of phytoestrogens, potentially explaining their decreased risk.[4,5]

FAMILY HISTORY

Men with a brother or father with prostate cancer have twice the risk for prostate cancer as compared with the rest of the population.[5] There appears to be a familial clustering of a prostate cancer syndrome, and genomewide scans have identified potential prostate cancer susceptibility candidate genes. Male carriers of germline mutations of *BRCA1* and *BRCA2* are known to have an increased risk for developing prostate cancer.[6] Common exposure to environmental and other risk factors may also contribute to increased risk among patients with first-degree relatives with prostate cancer.[5,7]

DIET

A number of epidemiologic studies support an association between high fat intake and risk of prostate cancer. A strong correlation between national per capita fat consumption and national prostate cancer mortality has been reported, and prospective case-control studies suggest that a high-fat diet doubles the risk of prostate cancer.[5,8] This relationship between high fat intake and prostate cancer may explain differences in insulin-like growth factor-1 (IGF-1). High calorie and high fat diets stimulate hepatic production of IGF-1, which is involved in the regulation of proliferation

and apoptosis of cancer cells.[5,8] High levels of IGF-1 are associated with an increased risk for prostate cancer.[5]

Other dietary factors implicated in the development or prevention of prostate cancer include retinol, carotenoids, lycopene, and vitamin D consumption.[5,7,9] Retinol, or vitamin A, intake, especially in men older than 70, is correlated with an increased risk of prostate cancer, whereas intake of its precursor, *β*-carotene, has a protective or neutral effect. Lycopene, obtained primarily from tomatoes, decreases the risk of prostate cancer in small cohort studies. Men who developed prostate cancer in one cohort study had lower levels of 1,25(OH)$_2$-vitamin D than matched controls, although a prospective study did not support this. Clearly, dietary risk factors require further evaluation, but because fat and vitamins are modifiable risk factors, dietary intervention may be promising in prostate cancer prevention. Investigations of selenium and vitamin E supplementation are discussed further in the section titled chemoprevention.

OTHER FACTORS

Benign prostatic hyperplasia (BPH) is a common problem among elderly men, affecting more than 40% of men over the age of 70 (see Chapter 93). BPH results in the urinary symptoms of hesitancy and frequency. Since prostate cancer affects a similar age group and often has similar presenting symptoms, the presence of BPH often complicates the diagnosis of prostate cancer, although it does not appear to increase the risk of developing prostate cancer.[2,7]

Smoking has not been associated with an increased risk of prostate cancer, but smokers with prostate cancer have an increased mortality resulting from the disease when compared with nonsmokers with prostate cancer (relative risk 1.5 to 2).[2,7] In addition, in a prospective cohort analysis, alcohol consumption was not associated with the development of prostate cancer.

CHEMOPREVENTION

Currently, the most promising agents for the prevention of prostate cancer are the 5-*α* reductase inhibitors, finasteride and dutasteride.[7,10,11] These medications inhibit 5-*α* reductase, an enzyme that converts testosterone to its more active form, dihydrotestosterone (DHT), which is involved in prostate epithelial proliferation. There are two types of 5-*α* reductase, type I and type II; both are implicated in the development of prostate cancer. Finasteride selectively inhibits the 5-*α* reductase type II isoenzyme, whereas dutasteride inhibits both isoenzymes.[11] Both finasteride and dutasteride falsely lower the PSA by approximately 50% in patients, and this needs to be adjusted for when measuring the PSA in patients on these medications.[7,11]

The Prostate Cancer Prevention Trial (PCPT) compared finasteride 5 mg daily for 7 years to placebo for the prevention of prostate cancer.[7] When compared with placebo, the point prevalence of prostate cancer was reduced for those on finasteride by 25% (hazard ratio [HR] = 0.75, 95% confidence interval [CI], 18.6-30.6%). However, in those that did develop prostate cancer, there was an increase in the number of high-grade (Gleason grade 7–10) tumors detected at biopsy in the finasteride group. Overall, finasteride did reduce the frequency of prostate cancer, but the prostate cancers that were diagnosed in the finasteride group were more aggressive. Since the original trial was reported, a number of biases in cancer detection caused by finasteride have been proposed, including improved detection of overall and high-grade prostate cancer, increased sensitivity of digital rectal examination, and increased sensitivity of biopsy for high-grade cancer detection. Redman and colleagues recently reevaluated the data from the PCPT trial to determine what effect these potential biases had on the diagnosis of aggressive prostate cancer in the finasteride group.[12] The analysis had an additional 3 months of follow-up, with unadjusted prostate cancer rates of 23% (4.8% with high grade) in the placebo group compared to 17% (5.8% with high grade) in the finasteride group. When the results were adjusted for these biases, prostate cancer rates were estimated to be 21% (4.2% high-grade) in the placebo group compared to 15% (4.8% high-grade), corresponding to a 30% risk reduction in prostate cancer (relative risk [RR] = 0.70, 95% CI, 0.64–0.76; P < 0.0001) and a nonsignificant, 14% increase in high-grade cancer (RR, 1.14; 95% CI, 0.96-1.35; P = 0.12) with finasteride.[12]

Following this reanalysis, the American Society of Clinical Oncology and the American Urological Association published a joint practice guideline for prostate cancer chemoprevention.[13] While dutasteride is still being investigated for prostate cancer prevention, preliminary reports from REDUCE suggest that effects of dutasteride and finasteride are similar, and both agents were considered in the guideline.[13]

The guideline recommends that asymptomatic men with a prostate-specific antigen (PSA) ≤3.0 ng/mL (3.0 mcg/L) who are regularly screened with PSA for early detection of prostate cancer may benefit from a discussion of both the benefits of dutasteride or finasteride for 7 years for the prevention of prostate cancer and the potential risks.[13]

The guideline does not recommend the use of finasteride or dutasteride for prostate cancer chemoprevention and noted that, while most panel members believed the higher risk of high-grade cancer in the finasteride group seen in the PCPT is most likely related to biases, cancer induction or promotion by finasteride cannot be excluded with certainty. Additionally, while finasteride reduces the prevalence of prostate cancer, the impact of finasteride on prostate cancer morbidity and mortality has not been demonstrated. Patients considering finasteride or dutasteride for prostate cancer chemoprevention or taking it for benign conditions such as BPH must weigh the risks and benefits of treatment. The primary benefit is that these agents reduce the incidence of prostate cancer by approximately 25%, and improve lower urinary tract symptoms of BPH, but the risks include the potential for more high-grade prostate cancers; the long-term benefit of these agents is not known; and reversible sexual adverse effects can occur.[13]

Selenium and vitamin E alone or in combination were evaluated in the *Selenium and Vitamin E Cancer Prevention Trial* (SELECT), a clinical trial investigating their effects on the incidence of prostate cancer. The data and safety monitoring committee found that after 5 years selenium and vitamin E taken alone or together did not prevent prostate cancer. Based on these data and safety concerns, the trial was halted.[14] Other agents, including vitamin D, lycopene, green tea, nonsteroidal antiinflammatory agents, isoflavones, and statins are under investigation for prostate cancer and show promise, however, none are currently recommended for routine use outside of a clinical trial.[15]

SCREENING

Digital rectal examination (DRE) has been recommended since the early 1900s for the detection of prostate cancer. The primary advantage of DRE is its specificity, reported at greater than 85%, for prostate cancer. Other advantages of DRE include low cost, safety, and ease of performance. However, DRE is relatively insensitive and is subject to interobserver variability. DRE as a single screening method has poor compliance and has had little effect on preventing metastatic prostate cancer in one large case-control study.[16]

❷ Prostate-specific antigen (PSA) is a useful marker for detecting prostate cancer at early stages, predicting outcome for localized disease, defining disease-free status, and monitoring response to androgen-deprivation therapy or chemotherapy for advanced-stage disease. PSA is used widely for prostate cancer screening in the United States, with simplicity its major advantage and low specificity its primary limitation.[17] PSA may be elevated in men with acute urinary retention, acute prostatitis, and prostatic ischemia or infarction, as well as BPH, a nearly universal condition in men at risk for prostate cancer. PSA elevations between 4.1 (4.1 mcg/L) and 10 ng/mL (10 mcg/L) cannot distinguish between BPH and prostate cancer, limiting the utility of PSA alone for the early detection of prostate cancer. Additionally, only 38% to 48% of men with clinically significant prostate cancer have a serum PSA outside the reference range.[18]

Early detection of potentially curable prostate cancers is the goal of prostate cancer screening. For cancer screening to be beneficial, it must reliably detect cancer at an early stage, when intervention would decrease mortality. Whether prostate cancer screening, with PSA, DRE or a combination fits these criteria has generated considerable controversy, and two recent studies have done little to resolve the controversy.[19–21] The European Randomized Study of Screening for Prostate Cancer (ERSPC) evaluated the effect of PSA screening on prostate cancer mortality. More than 182,000 men from seven different European countries were randomized between being offered screening with PSA to no screening. The frequency of screening and PSA threshold for a biopsy varied by country. Most centers used a PSA cutoff of 3 ng/mL (3 mcg/L), but Belgium allowed up to 10 ng/mL (10 mcg/L). Most centers screened every 4 years, although Sweden screened every 2 years. Eighty-two percent of men in the screening group had at least one PSA performed. With a median follow-up of 9 years, the cumulative incidence of prostate cancer was 8.2% in the screening group and 4.8% in the control group.[20] The rate ratio for death from prostate cancer in the screening group, compared with the control group, was 0.80 (95% CI, 0.65 to 0.98; adjusted P = 0.04), which corresponds to about one less death in the screened group compared with the nonscreened group. Of the 126,462 PSA tests performed, 16.2% of the tests were positive. Biopsies were performed for elevated PSAs, with 75.9% having a false-positive result.[20]

In the United States, clinicians believe that neither DRE nor PSA is sensitive or specific enough to be used alone as a screening test. Although the relative predictability of DRE and PSA is similar, the tumors identified by each method are different. Catalona and associates[22] confirmed that the combination of a DRE plus PSA determination is a better method of detecting prostate cancer than DRE alone.

In the United States, the Prostate, Lung, Colon and Ovarian Screening study (PLCO) randomized 76,693 men to receive either annual screening (38,343 subjects) or usual care as the control (38,350 subjects). In the screening group, men were offered annual PSA testing for 6 years and DRE for 4 years with compliance with screening was 85%. Men in the usual care group were able to receive screening, with the rate of PSA testing ranging from 40% to 52% and DRE from 41% to 46%. After 7 years of follow-up, the incidence of death per 10,000 person-years was not significantly different between the two groups with 2.0 (50 deaths total) in the screening group and 1.7 (44 deaths total) in the control group (rate ratio, 1.13; 95% CI, 0.75 to 1.70).[21]

The common approach to prostate cancer screening today involves offering a baseline PSA and DRE at age 40 with annual evaluations beginning at age 50 to all men of normal risk with a 10-year or greater life expectancy. Men with an increased risk of prostate cancer, including men of African American ancestry and men with a family history of prostate cancer, may begin screening earlier, at age 40 to 45.

Despite this common practice, the benefits of prostate cancer screening remain controversial.[23] The ERSPC demonstrated that PSA testing every 4 years was better than no PSA testing, decreasing prostate cancer deaths in the screened group by approximately

1 per 1,000 men screened compared with the unscreened group, but the false-positive rate was 76%, resulting in more than 13,000 unnecessary biopsies. The PLCO screening study showed no reduction in prostate cancer death between the annual (PSA and DRE) screening group and the usual care group, which is not surprising given the small reduction in death expected and that about one-half of the patients in the usual screening groups had PSA and DRE screening performed. Both studies demonstrated that screening identifies more prostate cancers than not screening.[19-23] PSA measurements can identify small, subclinical prostate cancers, where no intervention may be required. Detecting prostate cancer in those not needing therapy not only increases the cost of care through unnecessary screening and workups, but also increases the toxicity of therapy, by subjecting some patients to unnecessary therapy.[24,25] The American College of Physicians currently recommends that rather than screening all men for prostate cancer as a matter of routine, physicians should describe the potential benefits and known risks of screening, diagnosis, and treatment, listen to the patient's concerns, and then decide on an individual's screening method. That recommendation is based on the uncertain benefit of prostate cancer screening on prostate cancer mortality, and the well-established risks, including pain, drug toxicity and psychological distress of unnecessary screening, biopsies, and treatment.

PATHOPHYSIOLOGY

The prostate gland is a solid, rounded, heart-shaped organ positioned between the neck of the bladder and the urogenital diaphragm (Fig. 139–1). The normal prostate is composed of acinar secretory cells arranged in a radial shape and surrounded by a foundation of supporting tissue. The size, shape, or presence of acini is almost always altered in the gland that has been invaded by prostatic carcinoma. Adenocarcinoma, the major pathologic cell type, accounts for more than 95% of prostate cancer cases.[26,27] Much rarer tumor types include small cell neuroendocrine cancers, sarcomas, and transitional cell carcinomas.

Prostate cancer can be graded systematically according to the histologic appearance of the malignant cell and then grouped into well, moderately, or poorly differentiated grades.[27,28] Gland architecture is examined and then rated on a scale of 1 (well differentiated) to 5 (poorly differentiated). Two different specimens are examined, and the score for each specimen is added. Groupings for total Gleason score are 2 to 4 for well differentiated, 5 or 6 for moderately

differentiated, and 7 to 10 for poorly differentiated tumors. Poorly differentiated tumors grow rapidly (poor prognosis), while well-differentiated tumors grow slowly (better prognosis).

Metastatic spread can occur by local extension, lymphatic drainage, or hematogenous dissemination.[28,29] Lymph node metastases are more common in patients with large, undifferentiated tumors that invade the seminal vesicles. The pelvic and abdominal lymph node groups are the most common sites of lymph node involvement (Fig. 139–1). Skeletal metastases from hematogenous spread are the most common sites of distant spread. Typically, the bone lesions are osteoblastic or a combination of osteoblastic and osteolytic. The most common site of bone involvement is the lumbar spine. Other sites of bone involvement include the proximal femurs, pelvis, thoracic spine, ribs, sternum, skull, and humerus. The lung, liver, brain, and adrenal glands are the most common sites of visceral involvement, although these organs are not usually initially involved. About 25% to 35% of patients will have evidence of lymphangitic or nodular pulmonary infiltrates at autopsy. The prostate is rarely a site for metastatic involvement from other solid tumors.

Normal growth and differentiation of the prostate depend on the presence of androgens, specifically DHT.[29,30] The testes and the adrenal glands are the major sources of circulating androgens. Hormonal regulation of androgen synthesis is mediated through a series of biochemical interactions between the hypothalamus, pituitary, adrenal glands, and testes (Fig. 139–2). Luteinizing hormone–releasing hormone (LH-RH) released from the hypothalamus stimulates the release of luteinizing hormone (LH) and follicle-stimulating hormone (FSH) from the anterior pituitary gland. LH complexes with receptors on the Leydig cell testicular membrane and stimulates the production of testosterone and small amounts of estrogen. FSH acts on the Sertoli cells within the testes to promote the maturation of LH receptors and to produce an androgen-binding protein. Circulating testosterone and estradiol influence the synthesis of LH-RH, LH, and FSH by a negative feedback loop operating at the hypothalamic and pituitary level.[31] Prolactin, growth hormone, and estradiol appear to be important accessory regulators for prostatic tissue permeability, receptor binding, and testosterone synthesis.

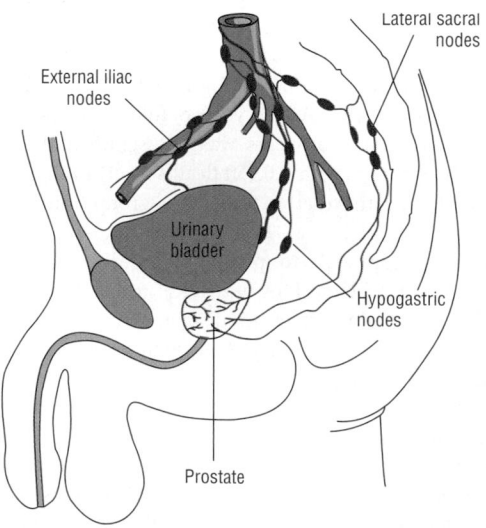

FIGURE 139-1. The prostate gland.

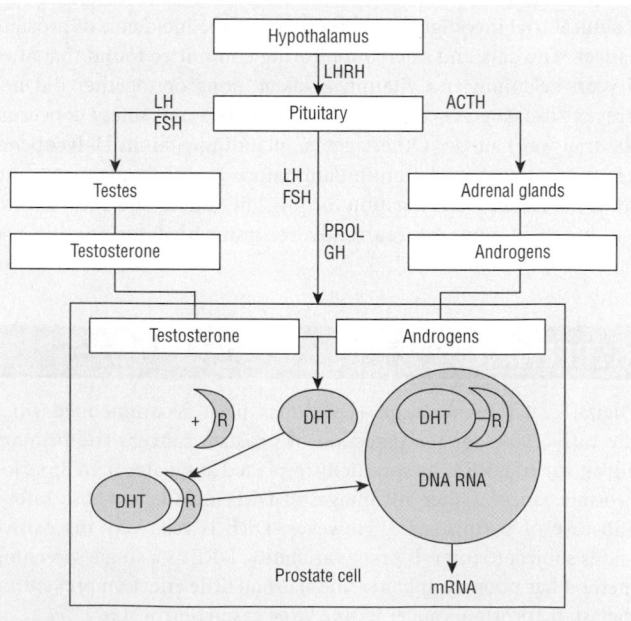

FIGURE 139-2. Hormonal regulation of the prostate gland. (ACTH, adrenocorticotropic hormone; DHT, dihydrotestosterone; FSH, follicle-stimulating hormone; GH, growth hormone; LH, luteinizing hormone; LH-RH, luteinizing hormone–releasing hormone; PROL, prolactin; R, receptor).

TABLE 139-2 Hormonal Manipulations in Prostate Cancer

Androgen source ablation	Antiandrogens
Orchiectomy	Flutamide
Adrenalectomy	Bicalutamide
Hypophysectomy	Nilutamide
LH-RH or LH inhibition	Cyproterone acetate[b]
Estrogens	Progesterones
LH-RH agonists	5-α-Reductase inhibition
Progesterones[a]	Finasteride[b]
Cyproterone acetate[b]	
Androgen synthesis inhibition	
Aminoglutethimide	
Ketoconazole	
Progesterones[a]	

[a]Minor mechanisms of action.
[b]Investigational compounds or use.
LH, luteinizing hormone; LH-RH, luteinizing hormone–releasing hormone.

Testosterone, the major androgenic hormone, accounts for 95% of the androgen concentration. The primary source of testosterone is the testes; however, 3% to 5% of the testosterone concentration is derived from direct adrenal cortical secretion of testosterone or C19 steroids such as androstenedione.[28–30]

In early-stage prostate cancers, aberrant tumor cell proliferation is promoted by the presence of androgens. For these tumors, blockade of androgens induces tumor regression in most patients. Hormonal manipulations to ablate or reduce circulating androgens can occur through several mechanisms[29,30] (Table 139–2). The organs responsible for androgen production can be removed surgically (orchiectomy, hypophysectomy, or adrenalectomy). Hormonal pathways that modulate prostatic growth can be interrupted at several steps (see Fig. 139–2). Interference with LH-RH or LH can reduce testosterone secretion by the testes (estrogens, LH-RH agonists, progestogens, and cyproterone acetate). Estrogen administration reduces androgens by directly inhibiting LH release, by acting directly on the prostate cell, or by decreasing free androgens by increasing steroid-binding globulin levels.[28–30]

Isolation of the naturally occurring hypothalamic decapeptide hormone luteinizing hormone–releasing hormone or LH-RH has provided another group of effective agents for advanced prostate cancer treatment. The physiologic response to LH-RH depends on both the dose and the mode of administration. Intermittent pulsed LH-RH administration, which mimics the endogenous release pattern, causes sustained release of both LH and FSH, whereas high-dose or continuous intravenous administration of LH-RH inhibits gonadotropin release due to receptor downregulation.[23] Structural modification of the naturally occurring LH-RH and innovative delivery have produced a series of LH-RH agonists that cause a similar downregulation of pituitary receptors and a decrease in testosterone production.[31]

Androgen synthesis can also be inhibited in the testes or in the adrenal gland. Aminoglutethimide inhibits the desmolase-enzyme complex in the adrenal gland, thereby preventing the conversion of cholesterol to pregnenolone. Pregnenolone is the precursor substrate for all adrenal-derived steroids, including androgens, glucocorticoids, and mineralocorticoids. Ketoconazole, an imidazole antifungal agent, causes a dose-related reversible reduction in serum cortisol and testosterone concentration by inhibiting both adrenal and testicular steroidogenesis.[32] Megestrol is a synthetic derivative of progesterone that exhibits a secondary mechanism of action by inhibiting the synthesis of androgens. This inhibition appears to occur at the adrenal level, but circulating levels of testosterone are also reduced, suggesting that inhibition at the testicular level may also occur.[32]

Antiandrogens inhibit the formation of the DHT-receptor complex and thereby interfere with androgen-mediated action at the cellular level.[32] Megestrol acetate, a progestational agent, is also available and has antiandrogen actions.[32] Finally, the conversion of testosterone to DHT may be inhibited by 5-α-reductase inhibitors.[7]

In advanced stages of disease, prostate cancer cells may be able to survive and proliferate without the signals normally provided by circulating androgens.[33] When this occurs, the tumors are no longer sensitive to therapies that are dependent on androgen blockade. These tumors are often referred to as hormone refractory or androgen independent.

CLINICAL PRESENTATION

Localized Disease

☐ Asymptomatic

Locally Invasive Disease

☐ Ureteral dysfunction, frequency, hesitancy, and dribbling

☐ Impotence

Advanced Disease

☐ Back pain

☐ Cord compression

☐ Lower extremity edema

☐ Pathologic fractures

☐ Anemia

☐ Weight loss

Prior to the implementation of routine screening, prostate cancers were frequently identified on the investigation of symptoms, including urinary hesitancy, retention, painful urination, hematuria, and erectile dysfunction. With the introduction of screening techniques, most prostate cancers are now identified prior to the development of symptoms.[34]

The information obtained from the diagnostic tests is used to stage the patient (Table 139–3). There are two commonly recognized staging classification systems (Table 139–4). The formal international classification system (tumor, node, metastases; TNM), adopted by the International Union Against Cancer in 1974, was last updated in 2002. The AUS classification is the most commonly used staging system in the United States. Patients are assigned to stages

TABLE 139-3 Diagnostic and Staging Workup for Prostate Cancer

Initial tests	Digital rectal examination (DRE)
	Prostate-specific antigen (PSA) Transrectal ultrasonography (TRUS) if either DRE is positive or PSA is elevated
	Biopsy
Staging tests	Gleason score on biopsy specimen
	Bone scan
	Complete blood count
	Liver function tests
	Serum phosphatases (acid/alkaline)
	Excretory urogram
	Chest x-ray
Additional staging tests (depends on tumor classification, PSA, and Gleason score)	Skeletal films
	Lymph node evaluation
	Pelvic computed tomography
	111In-labeled capromab pendetide scan
	Bipedal lymphangiogram
	Transrectal magnetic resonance imaging

TABLE 139-4 Staging and Classification Systems for Prostate Cancer

AUS[a] Stage (A–D)	AJCC-UICC[b] Classification (TNM)
A (occult, nonpalpable)	$T_xN_xM_x$ (cannot be assessed)
A_1: Focal	$T_0N_0M_0$ (nonpalpable)
A_2: Diffuse	T_0: Focal or diffuse
B (confined to prostate)	$T_1N_0M_0$, $T_2N_0M_0$
B_1: Single nodule in one lobe, less than 1.5 cm	T_1 (Clinically inapparent tumor not palpable or visible by imaging)
	T_{1a}: Tumor incidental histologic finding in 5% or less of tissue resected
	T_{1b}: Tumor incidental histologic finding in 5% or more of tissue resected
	T_{1c}: Tumor identified by needle biopsy (e.g., because of elevated PSA)
B_2: Diffuse involvement of whole gland, greater than 1.5 cm	T_2: (Tumor confined within the prostate[c])
	T_{2a}: Tumor involves half of a lobe or less
	T_{2b}: Tumor involves more than half a lobe, but not both lobes
	T_{2c}: Tumor involves both lobes
C (localized to periprostatic area)	$T_3N_0M_0$, $T_4N_0M_0$
C_1: No seminal vesicle involvement, less than 70 g	T_3: (Tumor extends through the prostatic capsule[d])
	T_{3a}: Unilateral extracapsular extension
	T_{3b}: Bilateral extracapsular extension
	T_{3c}: Tumor invades the seminal vesicle(s)
C_2: Seminal vesicle involvement, greater than 70 g	T_4: (Tumor is fixed or invades adjacent structures other than the seminal vesicles)
	T_{4a}: Tumor invades any of bladder neck, external sphincter, or rectum
	T_{4b}: Tumor invades levator muscles and/or is fixed to the pelvic wall
D (metastatic disease)	Any T, N_{1-4}, M_0, or N_{0-4}, M_1
D_1: Pelvic lymph nodes or ureteral obstruction	N_1: Metastasis in a single lymph node, 2 cm or less in greatest dimension
D_2: Bone, distant lymph node, organ, or soft tissue metastases	N_2: Metastasis in single lymph node more than 2 cm but not more than 5 cm in greatest dimension; or multiple lymph node metastases, none more than 5 cm in greatest dimension
	N_3: Metastasis in lymph node more than 5 cm in greatest dimension
	M_{1a}: Nonregional lymph node(s)
	M_{1b}: Bone(s)
	M_{1c}: Other site(s)

[a]American Urologic System.
[b]American Joint Committee on Cancer–International Union Against Cancer.
[c]Note: Tumor found in one or both lobes by needle biopsy, but not palpable or visible by imaging, is classified as T_{1c}.
[d]Note: Invasion into the prostatic apex or into (but not beyond) the prostatic capsule is not classified as T_3 but as T_2.

A through D and corresponding subcategories based on size of the tumor (T), local or regional extension, presence of involved lymph node groups (N), and presence of metastases (M). Some studies classify patients who have progressed after hormonal therapy as stage D_3.[35] Based on men diagnosed with prostate cancer at Walter Reed Army Medical Center from 1988 to 1998, including over 2,042 prostate cancer diagnoses, localized prostate cancer (stage T_1 and T_2) was diagnosed more frequently (89% vs. 68%), and advanced disease (stages T_3, T_4, and D) was diagnosed less frequently (11% vs. 32%) when comparing the 1998 to the 1988 incidence rates.

❸ The prognosis for patients with prostate cancer depends on the histologic grade, the tumor size, and the local extent of the primary tumor.[27] The most important prognostic criterion appears to be the histologic grade, because the degree of differentiation

ultimately determines the stage of disease. Poorly differentiated tumors are highly associated with both regional lymph node involvement and distant metastases.[27]

From 1999 to 2005, 5-year overall survival rates were estimated at 100% for whites and 97% for African Americans.[1] For this same period, the survival rates for localized or regional disease (100%), and distant disease (30%) in white males were about the same as the survival rates for localized or regional disease (100%), and distant disease (29%) in African American males.[1] A 4.1% decline in age-adjusted mortality has been observed for the period 1994 to 2006. Ten-year cancer-specific survival is estimated as 95% for stage A_1, 80% for stages A_2 to B_2, 60% for stage C, 40% for stage D_1, and 10% for stage D_2.[36] It is estimated that more than 85% of patients with stage A_1 can be cured, whereas fewer than 1% of patients with stage D_2 will be cured.

TREATMENT

Prostate Cancer

■ DESIRED OUTCOME

The desired outcome in early-stage prostate cancer is to minimize morbidity and mortality due to prostate cancer.[37] The most appropriate therapy of early-stage prostate cancer is a matter of debate. Early-stage disease may be treated with surgery, radiation, or expectant management. While surgery and radiation are curative, they are associated with significant morbidity and mortality. Since the overall goal is to minimize morbidity and mortality associated with the disease, watchful waiting is appropriate in selected individuals. Advanced prostate cancer (stage D) is not currently curable, and treatment should focus on providing symptom relief and maintaining quality of life.[38] The mainstay of treatment for advanced prostate cancer is androgen deprivation therapy, with a goal of reducing testosterone to castrate levels, with either an orchiectomy or an LH-RH agonist.

■ GENERAL APPROACH TO TREATMENT

The initial treatment for prostate cancer depends primarily on the disease stage, the Gleason score, the presence of symptoms, and the life expectancy of the patient.[37] Prostate cancer is usually initially diagnosed by PSA and DRE and confirmed by a biopsy, where the Gleason score is assigned. Asymptomatic patients with a low risk of recurrence, those with a T_1 or T_{2a}, with a Gleason score of 2 through 6, and a PSA of less than 10 ng/mL (10 mcg/L) may be managed by expectant management, radiation, or radical prostatectomy (Table 139–5). As patients with asymptomatic early-stage disease generally have an excellent 10-year survival, immediate morbidities of treatment must be balanced with the lower likelihood of dying from prostate cancer. In general, more aggressive treatments of early-stage prostate cancer are reserved for younger men, although patient preference is a major consideration in all treatment decisions. In a patient with a normal life expectancy of less than 10 years, expectant management or radiation therapy may be offered. In those with a normal life expectancy of equal to or greater than 10 years, either expectant management, radiation (external beam or brachytherapy), or radical prostatectomy with a pelvic lymph node dissection may be offered. Radiation and radical prostatectomy therapy are generally considered therapeutically equivalent for localized prostate cancer, although neither has been proven to be better than observation alone.[38,39] Wilt and colleagues conducted a systematic review of 18 randomized trials and 473 observational studies to compare the effectiveness and

TABLE 139-5 Management of Prostate Cancer with Low and Intermediate Recurrence Risk

Recurrence Risk	Expected Survival	Initial Therapy
Low	Less than 10	Expectant management or radiation therapy
T_1–T_{2a} and Gleason 2–6 and PSA less than 10 ng/mL (10 mcg/L) and less than 5% tumor in specimen	Greater than or equal to 10	Expectant management or radical prostatectomy with or without pelvic lymph node dissection or radiation therapy
	Less than 10	Expectant management or radical prostatectomy with or without pelvic lymph node dissection or radiation therapy with or without 4–6 months of androgen deprivation therapy
Intermediate		
T_{2b}–T_{2c} or Gleason 7 or PSA 10–20 ng/mL (10–20 mcg/L)	Greater than or equal to 10	Radical prostatectomy with or without pelvic lymph node dissection or radiation therapy with or without 4–6 months of androgen deprivation therapy

potential complications from treatment options from prostate cancer. This study showed that superiority between radiation, radical prostatectomy, and androgen deprivation therapy could not be determined because of the paucity of high-quality evidence available for analysis. Side effect profiles were found to be similar, although severity varied among the treatments.[40] Complications from radical prostatectomy include blood loss, stricture formation, incontinence, lymphocele, fistula formation, anesthetic risk, and impotence. Nerve-sparing radical prostatectomy can be performed in many patients; 50% to 80% regain sexual potency within the first year. Although a recent prospective study found that even in patients with good preoperative sexual health, many do not return to baseline after surgery even with the assistance of erectile dysfunction treatments.[41] Acute complications from radiation therapy include cystitis, proctitis, hematuria, urinary retention, penoscrotal edema, and impotence (30% incidence).[27] Chronic complications include proctitis, diarrhea, cystitis, enteritis, impotence, urethral stricture, and incontinence.[27] In addition to possibly intensifying these problems, androgen deprivation can also cause cognitive impairment, mood disturbances, and lack of initiative.[40] Since radiation and prostatectomy have significant and immediate mortality when compared with expectant management alone, many patients may elect to postpone therapy until symptoms develop.

Individuals with T_{2b} and T_{2c} disease or a Gleason score of 7 or a PSA ranging from 10 to 20 ng/mL (10 to 20 mcg/L) are considered at intermediate risk for prostate cancer recurrence.[37] Individuals with less than a 10-year expected survival may be offered expectant management, radiation therapy, or radical prostatectomy with or without a pelvic lymph node dissection, and those with a greater than or equal to 10-year life expectancy may be offered either radical prostatectomy with or without a pelvic lymph node dissection or radiation therapy (Table 139-6).

TABLE 139-6 Management of Prostate Cancer with High and Very High Recurrence Risk

Recurrence Risk	Initial Therapy
High	ADT (2–3 years) and radiation therapy, or short-term ADT and radiation therapy for those with a single high risk factor or radical prostatectomy with or without pelvic lymph node dissection
T_{3a}, Gleason 8–10, PSA greater than 20 ng/mL (20 mcg/L)	
Locally Advanced, Very High	ADT (2–3 years) or radiation therapy + ADT (4–6 months) or radical prostatectomy
T_{3b}–T_4	
Very High	ADT (2–3 years) or radiation therapy + ADT (4–6 months)
Any T, N_1	
Very High	ADT 2–3 years
Any T, Any N, M_1	

ADT= androgen deprivation therapy to achieve serum testosterone levels less than 50 ng/dL (1.7 nmol/L)

LHRH agonist (medical castrations or surgical are equivalent)

The treatment of patients at high risk of recurrence (stage T_3, a Gleason score ranging from 8 to 10, or a PSA value greater than 20 ng/mL [20 mcg/L]) should be treated with androgen ablation for 2 to 3 years combined with radiation therapy (see Table 139–6). Select individuals with a low tumor volume may receive a radical prostatectomy with or without a pelvic lymph node dissection.

Patients with T_{3b} and T_4 disease have a very high risk of recurrence and are not candidates for radical prostatectomy because of extensive local spread of disease.[37] ❹ Androgen deprivation therapy with a LH-RH agonist plus an antiandrogen should be used prior to radiation therapy for patients with locally advanced prostate cancer to improve outcomes over radiation therapy alone. Recent evidence suggests that androgen ablation should be instituted at diagnosis rather than waiting for symptomatic disease or progression to occur. In a randomized clinical trial enrolling 500 men with locally advanced prostate cancer who were randomized to either immediate initiation of androgen ablation with either orchiectomy or androgen ablation, or deferred hormonal therapy, individuals with immediate therapy had a median actuarial cause-specific survival duration of 7.5 years for immediate treatment and 5.8 years for deferred treatment.[42]

❺ Androgen deprivation therapy, with either orchiectomy, an LH-RH agonist alone, or an LH-RH agonist plus an antiandrogen (combined androgen blockade), can be used to provide palliation for patients with advanced (stage D_2) prostate cancer. Estrogens were once widely used, but the primary estrogen, diethylstilbestrol (DES), was withdrawn from the U.S. market in 1997 due to increased cardiovascular risk. Secondary hormonal manipulations, cytotoxic chemotherapy, or supportive care is used for the patient who progresses after initial therapy.[43]

■ NONPHARMACOLOGIC THERAPY

Expectant Management

Expectant management, also known as observation or watchful waiting, involves monitoring the course of disease and initiating treatment if the cancer progresses or the patient becomes symptomatic. A PSA and DRE are performed every 6 months, with a repeat biopsy at any sign of disease progression. The advantages of expectant management are avoiding the adverse effects associated with definitive therapies such as radiation and radical prostatectomy, and minimizing the risk of unnecessary therapies. The major disadvantage of expectant management is the risk that the cancer progresses and requires a more intensive therapy.[37]

Orchiectomy

Bilateral orchiectomy, or removal of the testes, is a form of androgen deprivation therapy that rapidly reduces circulating androgens to castrate levels (less than 50 ng/dL [1.7 nmol/L]).[22] However, many patients are not surgical candidates owing to their advanced age, and other patients find this procedure psychologically unacceptable.[26] Orchiectomy is the preferred initial treatment in patients with impending spinal cord compression or ureteral obstruction.

Radiation

The two commonly used methods for radiation therapy are external beam radiotherapy, and brachytherapy.[37] In external beam radiotherapy, doses of 70–75 Gy (7000–7500 rad) are delivered in 35–41 fractions in patients with low-grade prostate cancer and 75–80 Gy (7500–8000 rad) for those with intermediate or high-grade prostate cancer. Brachytherapy involves the permanent implantation of radioactive beads of 145 Gy (14500 rad) [125]Iodine or 124 Gy (12400 rad) of [103]Palladium and is generally reserved for individuals with low-risk cancers. Radiation therapy may also be given after surgery in patients with localized disease. In a recent study in men with early-stage prostate cancer, radiation therapy administered after radical prostatectomy was found to reduce the risk of prostate cancer by 29% with a 28% increase in survival.[44]

Radical Prostatectomy

Complications from radical prostatectomy include blood loss, stricture formation, incontinence, lymphocele, fistula formation, anesthetic risk, and impotence. Nerve-sparing radical prostatectomy can be performed in many patients; 50% to 80% regain sexual potency within the first year. Acute complications from radiation therapy include cystitis, proctitis, hematuria, urinary retention, penoscrotal edema, and impotence (30% incidence).[16] Chronic complications include proctitis, diarrhea, cystitis, enteritis, impotence, urethral stricture, and incontinence.[26] Since radiation and prostatectomy have significant and immediate mortality when compared with observation alone, many patients may elect to postpone therapy until symptoms develop.

■ PHARMACOLOGIC THERAPY

Drug Treatments of First Choice

Luteinizing Hormone-Releasing Hormone Agonists Luteinizing hormone–releasing hormone (LH-RH) agonists are a reversible method of androgen ablation and are as effective as orchiectomy in treating prostate cancer.[45] Currently available LH-RH agonists include leuprolide, leuprolide depot, leuprolide implant, treptorelin depot, treptorelin implant, and goserelin acetate implant. Leuprolide acetate is administered once daily, whereas leuprolide depot and goserelin acetate implant can be administered either once monthly, once every 12 weeks, or once every 16 weeks (leuprolide depot, every 4 months). The leuprolide depot formulation contains leuprolide acetate in coated pellets. The dose is administered intramuscularly, and the coating dissolves at different rates to allow sustained leuprolide levels throughout the dosing interval. Goserelin acetate implant contains goserelin acetate dispersed in a plastic matrix of D, L-lactic and glycolic acid copolymer and is administered subcutaneously. Hydrolysis of the copolymer material provides continuous release of goserelin over the dosing period. A recently approved leuprolide implant is a mini-osmotic pump that delivers 120 mcg of leuprolide daily for 12 months. After 12 months the implant is removed, and a different implant can be placed. Triptorelin LA is administered as an intramuscular injection of 11.25mg every 84 days. Triptorelin depot is 3.75 mg once every 28 days.

Several randomized trials have demonstrated that leuprolide, goserelin, and triptorelin are effective agents when used alone in patients with advanced prostate cancer.[30] Response rates around 80% have been reported, with a lower incidence of adverse effects compared with estrogens.[30] The currently available LH-RH agonists or the dosage formulations have not been directly compared in clinical trials, but a recent meta-analysis showed no significant differences in efficacy or toxicity between leuprolide and goserelin. Triptorelin is a more recent addition but is generally considered equally effective. Therefore the choice between the three agents is usually made based on cost and patient and physician preference for a dosing schedule.

The most common adverse effects reported with LH-RH agonist therapy include a disease flare-up during the first week of therapy, hot flashes, erectile impotence, decreased libido, and injection-site reactions.[30] The disease flare-up is caused by an initial induction of LH and FSH by the LH-RH agonist leading to an initial phase of increased testosterone production, and manifests clinically as either increased bone pain or increased urinary symptoms.[30] This flare reaction usually resolves after 2 weeks and has a similar onset and duration pattern for the depot LH-RH products.[46,47] Initiating an antiandrogen prior to the administration of the LH-RH agonist and continuing for 2 to 4 weeks is a frequently employed strategy to minimize this initial tumor flare.[31]

LH-RH agonist monotherapy can be used as initial therapy, with response rates similar to those for orchiectomy. The incidence of cardiovascular-related adverse effects is lower with LH-RH therapy than with estrogen administration. Patients should be counseled to expect worsening symptoms during the first week of therapy. Appropriate pain and symptom management is required during this period, and a short course of concomitant antiandrogen therapy may need to be considered prior to initiating the LHRH agonist. Caution should be exercised if initiating LH-RH agonist therapy in patients with widely metastatic disease involving the spinal cord or having the potential for ureteral obstruction because irreversible complications may occur.

Another potentially serious complication of androgen deprivation therapy (ADT) is a resultant decrease in bone-mineral density leading to an increased risk for osteoporosis, osteopenia, and an increased risk for skeletal fractures. During initial therapy, bone mineral density of the hip and spine decreases by 2% to 3%.[48] Additionally, ADT has been associated with a 21% to 45% relative increase in fracture risk.[49–51] Therefore, most clinicians recommend that men starting long-term ADT should have a baseline bone mineral density and be initiated on a calcium and vitamin D supplement.[31,37]

Several agents are being tested in clinical trials to prevent bone loss and fractures during ADT therapy. Zoledronic acid, an intravenous bisphosphonate, has been studied in patients receiving ADT at a dose of 4 mg every 3 weeks for 1 year in several randomized trials. Although the use of this agent increases bone mineral density in the spine (3.3% to 5.6%) and hip (0.7% to 1.6%), long-term data regarding the impact on reducing the incidence of fractures are lacking.[52] A promising agent is denosumab, a human monoclonal antibody targeted against receptor activator of nuclear factor-κB ligand (RANKL). In previous studies, denosumab increased bone mineral density at multiple skeletal sites in breast cancer patients receiving aromatase inhibitor therapy.[53] In a large randomized trial, nonmetastatic prostate cancer patients on ADT therapy received denosumab 60 mg subcutaneously every 6 months versus placebo. The results revealed that denosumab increased bone mineral density at all sites and reduced new vertebrae fractures at 36 months (1.5% vs 3.9% with placebo).[54]

ADT has also been associated with a higher incidence of metabolic effects. In a landmark population-based trial, patients treated with ADT and a GnRH agonist were found to have a greater risk of new-onset diabetes, coronary artery disease, and myocardial infarctions.[55] A subsequent study found that concomitant use of ADT and a GnRH agonist was associated with cardiovascular mortality. However, retrospective studies have shown conflicting results.[56-61] Based on these results, screening for and interventions to prevent and standard medical management to treat cardiovascular disease and diabetes are recommended for patients receiving ADT.[37]

Gonadotropin-Releasing Hormone (GnRH) Antagonists An alternative to LH-RH agonists is the recently approved GnRH antagonist, degarelix. Degarelix works by binding reversibly to GnRH receptors in the pituitary gland, reducing the production of testosterone to castrate levels. The major advantage of degarelix over LH-RH agonists is the rapidity at which it can reduce testosterone levels; castrate levels are achieved in 7 days or less with degarelix, as compared with 28 days with leuprolide, eliminating the tumor flare seen and the need for antiandrogens, with LH-RH agonists.

In a trial of 610 men with advanced prostate cancer, degarelix was shown to be equivalent to leuprolide in lowering testosterone levels for up to 1 year and is FDA-approved for the treatment of advanced prostate cancer. Degarelix is available as a 40 mg/mL and a 20 mg/mL vial for subcutaneous injection, and the starting dose is 240 mg followed by 80 mg every 28 days. The starting dose should be split into two 120 mg injections.[62] Degarelix has not been studied in combination with antiandrogens, and routine use of the combination cannot be recommended.

The most frequently reported adverse reactions were injection site reactions, including pain (28%), erythema (17%), swelling (6%), induration (4%), and nodule (3%). Most were transient and mild to moderate, leading to discontinuation in less than 1% of study subjects. Other adverse effects included elevations in lever function tests, which occurred in approximately 10% of study subjects. Like other methods of androgen supplementation therapy, osteoporosis may develop and calcium and vitamin D supplementation should be considered.[62]

Like degarelix, abarelix is a GnRH antagonist, with the same advantage of reducing testosterone to castrate levels rapidly and avoiding the tumor flare associated with LH-RH agonists. Unfortunately, abarelix is also associated with severe allergic reactions, including syncope and hypotension, which occur in approximately 1% of initial doses and an increased frequency with repeat doses, for an incidence approaching 5% overall. Therefore, abarelix is available only through a restricted distribution program (Plenaxis PLUS Program) and is only indicated for men with advanced prostate cancer who can not tolerate LH-RH agonist therapy and who refuse surgical castration and have one or more of the following: (1) risk of neurological compromise due to metastases, (2) ureteral or bladder outlet obstruction due to local encroachment or metastatic disease, or (3) severe bone pain from skeletal metastases persisting on narcotic analgesia. The recommended dose of abarelix is 100 mg administered intramuscularly to the buttock on days 1, 15, 29 (week 4), and every 4 weeks thereafter.

Antiandrogens Three antiandrogens, flutamide, bicalutamide,[46] and nilutamide,[45] are currently available (Table 139–7). Cyproterone is another agent with antiandrogen activity, but it is not available in the United States. Antiandrogens have been used as monotherapy in previously untreated patients, but a recent meta-analysis determined that monotherapy with antiandrogens is less effective than LH-RH agonist therapy.[47] Therefore, for advanced prostate cancer, all currently available antiandrogens are indicated only in combination with androgen-ablation therapy; flutamide and bicalutamide are indicated in combination with an LH-RH agonist, and nilutamide is indicated in combination with orchiectomy.[43]

The most common antiandrogen-related adverse effects are listed in Table 139–7. In the only randomized comparison of

TABLE 139-7 Antiandrogens

Antiandrogen	Usual Dose	Adverse Effects
Flutamide	750 mg/day	Gynecomastia Hot flushes Gastrointestinal disturbances (diarrhea) Liver function test abnormalities Breast tenderness Methemoglobinemia
Bicalutamide	50 mg/day	Gynecomastia Hot flushes Gastrointestinal disturbances (diarrhea) Liver function test abnormalities Breast tenderness
Nilutamide	300 mg/day for first month then 150 mg/day	Gynecomastia Hot flushes Gastrointestinal disturbances (nausea or constipation) Liver function test abnormalities Breast tenderness Visual disturbances (impaired dark adaptation) Alcohol intolerance Interstitial pneumonitis

bicalutamide plus an LH-RH agonist versus flutamide plus an LH-RH agonist, diarrhea was more common in flutamide-treated patients. Antiandrogens can reduce the symptoms from the flare phenomenon associated with LH-RH agonist therapy.[31]

Combined Androgen Blockade Although up to 80% of patients with advanced prostate cancer will respond to initial hormonal manipulation, almost all patients will progress within 2 to 4 years after initiating therapy.[26] Two mechanisms have been proposed to explain this tumor resistance. The tumor could be heterogeneously composed of cells that are hormone-dependent and hormone-independent, or the tumor could be stimulated by extratesticular androgens that are converted intracellularly to DHT. The rationale for combination hormonal therapy is to interfere with multiple hormonal pathways to completely eliminate androgen action. In clinical trials, combination hormonal therapy, sometimes also referred to as maximal androgen deprivation or total androgen blockade, or *combined androgen blockade (CAB)*, has been used. The combination of LH-RH agonists or orchiectomy with antiandrogens is the most extensively studied combined androgen blockade approach.

Many studies comparing CAB with conventional medical or surgical castration have been performed.[35,63,64] In studies with LH-RH agonists, the results have varied, with no consistent benefit demonstrated for CAB. A recently completed National Cancer Institute Intergroup trial involving 1,387 evaluable stage D_2 prostate cancer patients failed to show any significant survival benefits for the combination of orchiectomy plus flutamide over orchiectomy alone.[65] Like other studies of CAB, overall survival was longest in patients with minimal disease. Diarrhea, elevated liver function tests, and anemia were more common in those patients who received flutamide.

A meta-analysis of 27 randomized trials in 8,270 patients (4,803 treated with flutamide, 1,683 treated with nilutamide, and 1,784 treated with cyproterone) comparing CAB with conventional medical or surgical castration showed a small survival benefit at 5 years for those treated with flutamide or nilutamide (27.6%) compared to those with castration alone (24.7%; $P = .0005$).[63]

In one of the few combination androgen-deprivation studies comparing two different antiandrogens (bicalutamide vs. flutamide), the time-to-treatment failure (the main study end point), time-to-progression (as defined by appearance of new or worsening bone or extraskeletal lesions), and time-to-death were equivalent, suggesting that the two treatments are equally effective.[66]

Although some investigators now consider CAB to be the initial hormonal therapy of choice for newly diagnosed patients, the clinician is left to weigh the costs of combined therapy against potential benefits in light of conflicting results in the randomized trials[43] and the modest benefit seen in the meta-analysis.[63] For those trials that did show an advantage for CAB, whether these effects are specific to the testosterone-deprivation method (orchiectomy vs. leuprolide vs. goserelin), the antiandrogen, the duration of therapy, or patient selection is not clear. Until further carefully designed studies that use survival, time to progression, quality of life, patient preference, and cost as end points are conducted, it is appropriate to use either LH-RH agonist monotherapy or CAB as initial therapy for metastatic prostate cancer. CAB may be most beneficial for improving survival in patients with minimal disease and for preventing tumor flare, particularly in those with advanced metastatic disease. All other patients may be started on LH-RH monotherapy, and an antiandrogen may be added after several months if androgen ablation is incomplete.

CLINICAL CONTROVERSY

The use of CAB is controversial. Meta-analysis shows a small survival advantage when comparing combined androgen blockade to orchiectomy or LH-RH agonist alone. However, this modest benefit is achieved at significant financial cost and with additional toxicities.

It is not clear when to start hormonal-deprivation therapy in patients with advanced prostate cancer.[30] The original recommendation to start therapy when symptoms appeared was based on the Veterans Administration Cooperative Urologic Research Group (VACURG) trials, in which no overall survival difference was demonstrated in patients who either started DES initially or crossed over to active treatment when symptoms appeared; the excess mortality was attributed to estrogen administration.[66] Because LH-RH agonists and antiandrogens are viable therapies with less cardiovascular toxicity, it is not clear whether delaying therapy is justified with these agents. Reanalysis of the original VACURG data[67] and recent combined androgen-deprivation trials[67,68] demonstrate a survival advantage for young, good-performance-status, minimal-disease patients treated initially with hormonal therapy, suggesting that early intervention before symptoms appear may be appropriate.[67] The issue of when best to start hormonal therapy is the subject of several ongoing clinical trials.[67]

CLINICAL CONTROVERSY

Older data, using DES, showed that initiation of hormonal therapy at symptom onset yielded equivalent survival to starting hormonal therapy at initial diagnosis. With equivalent survival, decreased costs, and decreased toxicity from DES, the standard of practice was to delay initiation of hormonal therapy until symptoms developed. The favorable toxicity profile of LH-RH agonists led to the re-evaluation of the starting time for therapy; current research shows that younger men with a good performance status may benefit from initiation of hormonal therapy at diagnosis, rather than waiting for symptoms to develop.

Alternative Drug Treatments

Secondary or salvage therapies for patients who progress after their initial therapy depend on what was used for initial management.[37] For patients initially diagnosed with localized prostate cancer, radiotherapy can be used in the case of failed radical prostatectomy. Alternatively, androgen ablation can be used in patients who progress after either radiation therapy or radical prostatectomy.

Secondary Hormonal Manipulations In patients treated initially with one hormonal modality, secondary hormonal manipulations may be attempted. This may include adding an antiandrogen to a patient who incompletely suppresses testosterone secretion with an LH-RH agonist. In patients that have progression while receiving CAB, withdrawing antiandrogens, or using agents that inhibit androgen synthesis may be attempted. Supportive care, chemotherapy, or local radiotherapy can be used in patients who have failed all forms of androgen-ablation manipulations because these patients are considered to have hormone-refractory prostate cancer.

For patients who initially received an LH-RH agonist alone, castration testosterone levels should be documented. Patients with inadequate testosterone suppression (greater than 20 ng/dL [0.7 nmol/L]) can be treated by adding an antiandrogen or performing an orchiectomy. If castration testosterone levels have been achieved, the patient is considered to have androgen-independent disease, and palliative androgen-independent salvage therapy can be used.

6 Antiandrogen withdrawal, for patients having progressive disease while receiving combined hormonal blockade with an LH-RH agonist plus an antiandrogen, can provide additional symptomatic relief. Mutations in the androgen receptor have been documented that cause antiandrogen compounds to act like receptor agonists.

If the patient initially received combined androgen blockade with an LH-RH agonist with an antiandrogen, then androgen withdrawal is the first salvage manipulation.[37] Objective and subjective responses have been noted following the discontinuation of flutamide,[67] bicalutamide,[68] or nilutamide[69] in patients receiving these agents as part of combined androgen ablation with an LH-RH agonist. Mutations in the androgen receptor have been demonstrated that allow antiandrogens such as flutamide, bicalutamide, and nilutamide (or their metabolites) to become agonists and activate the androgen receptor.[70] Patient responses to androgen withdrawal manifest as significant PSA reductions and improved clinical symptoms. Androgen withdrawal responses lasting 3 to 14 months have been noted in up to 35% of patients, and predicting response seems to be most closely related to longer androgen exposure times.[66] Incomplete cross-resistance has been noted in some patients who received bicalutamide after they had progressed while receiving flutamide.[71] Adding an agent that blocks adrenal androgen synthesis, such as aminoglutethimide, at the time that androgens are withdrawn may produce a better response than androgen withdrawal alone.[70] Because of the potential for response immediately after antiandrogen withdrawal, a sufficient observation and assessment period (usually 4 to 6 weeks) is usually required before a patient can be enrolled on a clinical trial evaluating a new agent or therapy for advanced prostate cancer.

Androgen synthesis inhibitors, such as aminoglutethimide or ketoconazole, can provide symptomatic relief for a short time in approximately 50% of patients with progressive disease despite previous androgen-ablation therapy.[43] Adverse effects during aminoglutethimide therapy occur in approximately 50% of patients.[43] Central nervous system effects that include lethargy, ataxia, and dizziness are the major adverse reactions. A generalized morbilliform, pruritic rash has been reported in up to 30% of patients treated. The rash is usually self-limiting and resolves within 5 to 8 days with continued

TABLE 139-8 First-Line Chemotherapy Regimens for Metastatic Hormone-Independent Prostate Cancer

Regimen	Usual Dose	Adverse Effects	Dose Adjustments
Docetaxel	75 mg/m² every 3 weeks	Fluid retention, alopecia, mucositis, myelosuppression, hypersensitivity	Hepatic Aspartate transaminase/Alanine transaminase greater than 1.5 times the upper limit of normal and alkaline phosphatase greater than 2.5 times the upper limit of normal do not administer Hematologic Assure complete blood count recovered
Estramustine	280 mg three times daily days 1–5	Edema, gynecomastia, leucopenia, increased risk of thromboembolic events	Hematologic Assure complete blood count recovered

therapy. Adverse effects from ketoconazole include gastrointestinal intolerance, transient rises in liver and renal function tests, and hypoadrenalism. Ketoconazole is combined with replacement doses of hydrocortisone to prevent symptomatic hypoadrenalism.[43]

Supportive Care After all hormonal manipulations are exhausted, the patient is considered to have androgen-independent disease, also known as hormone-refractory prostate cancer. At this point, either chemotherapy or palliative supportive therapy is appropriate. Palliation can be achieved by pain management, using radioisotopes such as strontium-89[72] or samarium-153 lexidronam[73] for bone-related pain, analgesics, corticosteroids, bisphosphonates,[74] or local radiotherapy.[37]

Skeletal metastases from hematogenous spread are the most common sites of distant spread of prostate cancer. Typically, the bone lesions are osteoblastic or a combination of osteoblastic and osteolytic. Bisphosphonates or denosumab may prevent skeletal-related events and improve bone mineral density. A randomized, controlled trial of zoledronic acid at a dose of 4 mg every 3 weeks reduced the incidence of skeletal-related events by 25% ($P = 0.021$) compared with placebo.[75] The usual dose of pamidronate is 90 mg every month and the usual dose of zoledronic acid is 4 mg every 3 to 4 weeks. Renal function should be monitored as bisphosphonates should not be administered to patients with a CrCl < 30 mL/min (0.5 mL/s).[37] A trial of pamidronate or zoledronic acid can be initiated in prostate cancer patients with bone pain; if no benefit is observed, the drug may be discontinued.[74]

Chemotherapy ❼ Chemotherapy with docetaxel and prednisone improves survival in patients with hormone-refractory prostate cancer. Patients with hormone-refractory prostate cancer should be considered for entry into clinical trials investigating new therapies for prostate cancer.

Docetaxel 75 mg/m² every 3 weeks combined with prednisone 5 mg twice a day improves survival in hormone-refractory metastatic prostate cancer.[76] The most common adverse events reported with this regimen are nausea, alopecia, and bone marrow suppression. Other adverse effects of docetaxel include fluid retention and peripheral neuropathy. Docetaxel is hepatically eliminated; patients with hepatic impairment may not be eligible for treatment with docetaxel because of an increased risk for toxicity.

The combination of estramustine (280 mg three times a day, days 1–5) and docetaxel 60 mg/m² on day 2, every 3 weeks also improves survival in hormone refractory metastatic prostate cancer.[77] Estramustine causes a decrease in testosterone and a corresponding increase in estrogen; therefore, the adverse effects of estramustine include an increase in thromboembolic events, gynecomastia, and decreased libido (Table 139–8). Estramustine is an oral capsule and should be refrigerated. Calcium inhibits the absorption or estramustine. While both the docetaxel/prednisone and the docetaxel/estramustine regimens are effective in hormone refractory prostate cancer, most clinicians prefer the docetaxel/prednisone regimen because of the cardiovascular adverse effects associated with estramustine. In addition, androgen ablation is usually continued when chemotherapy is initiated.[37]

The regimen of mitoxantrone plus prednisone has been shown to be effective in reducing pain from bone metastasis. The effectiveness of mitoxantrone after failure of docetaxel-based therapy has not been evaluated. Many clinicians will treat patients with radiation therapy for palliation of symptoms after failure of docetaxel-based chemotherapy.[37] Cabazitaxel, a new taxane, recently received FDA approval for use with prednisone in the treatment of patients with hormone-refractory metastatic prostate cancer after failure of doxetaxel-based chemotherapy.

Immunotherapy Sipuleucel-T is a novel autologous cellular immunotherapy that was FDA-approved in April 2010 for the treatment of asymptomatic or minimally symptomatic metastatic hormone-refractory prostate cancer. Each patient undergoes leukapheresis on day 1 to collect peripheral blood mononuclear cells, the cellular fraction that includes immune effector cells. These cells are incubated with a prostatic acid phosphatase - granulocyte-macrophage colony-stimulating factor (PAP-GM-CSF) fusion protein; PAP is the specific tumor antigen and GM-CSF is the immune cell activator. The cellular product is then infused intravenously into the patient on day 3 or 4, providing an autologous infusion of activated cells. Each course of sipuleucel-T consists of three infusions of activated cells, given every 2 weeks. In the pivotal trial, sipuleucel-T prolonged median survival by 4.1 months and reduced the risk of death by 22% (HR = 0.78, 95% CI, 0.61-0.98; $P = 0.03$).[78] Adverse effects related to sipuleucel-T were generally mild and nearly all patients were able to receive the entire course (i.e. 3 infusions). A course of sipuleucel-T costs about $93,000, and some insurers have questioned the value of the therapy.

PHARMACOECONOMIC CONSIDERATIONS

The main economic concerns for prostate cancer focus on prostate cancer screening for asymptomatic men, initial therapy of clinically localized disease, surgical vs. medical castration, and the use of combined hormonal blockade as treatment for advanced disease. Unfortunately, the paucity of high-quality evidence to determine the most appropriate therapy reduces the usefulness of economic modeling.

Prostate cancer screening remains highly controversial because the survival benefits and the associated costs are not well defined. Krahn and colleagues[79] determined that annual screening of all eligible Canadian men would cost 45 million Canadian dollars, or 0.15% of total health care expenditures. Available cost-utility studies estimate that the cost per crude or quality-adjusted life-year gained from prostate cancer screening ranges from $3,000 to $729,000.[78–82] Since the cost-effectiveness of prostate cancer screening cannot be determined until the benefits are documented, it is important to incorporate economic analysis into the large ongoing screening studies.

Treatment options for clinically localized prostate cancer include radiation therapy, surgery, or watchful waiting. There is currently no evidence to suggest which therapy is the most clinically effective, and treatment choice is often made by patient or physician preference. However, there are large economic differences in the therapies, with the cost of a radical prostatectomy $12,000 more expensive than watchful waiting, and radiation therapy $15,000 more expensive than watchful waiting.[82]

Surgical castration (by removal of the testes) and medical castration with LH-RH agonists yield similar clinical results, although the majority of patients prefer medical castration. In two economic analysis comparisons, the primary cost of the surgical castration was hospital length of stay and medical castration drug costs. Both analyses found that in patients surviving 18 to 24 months, a surgical castration was more cost effective.[81]

Table 139–9 lists the costs for the initial hormonal therapies for stage D_2 prostate cancer. Using a societal perspective and data from the original leuprolide plus flutamide versus leuprolide alone trial to calculate the incremental cost per life-year gained, Hillner and colleagues[80] concluded that CAB has an incremental cost-effectiveness ratio of $25,300 per life-year gained, which is within current accepted benchmarks. The cost dropped to $13,700 per life-year gained in patients with minimal disease.

In a follow-up study, this same group used physician focus group estimates to generate quality-of-life factors and incorporated these factors into an economic model.[82] The incremental cost per quality-adjusted life-year gained seemed reasonable when data from the original CAB were used: $25,000 for patients with minimal disease and $18,000 for patients with severe disease. However, these incremental costs increased dramatically to $53,700 for patients with minimal disease and $41,000 for patients with severe disease when the same model was applied to survival data from a meta-analysis.

Because there is considerable debate about the value of using CAB for advanced prostate cancer, continued economic assessments of this therapy will be crucial to help policymakers and clinicians decide on the most appropriate therapy. It will also become very important to incorporate economic analyses into chemotherapy trials because these efforts move toward including clinical benefit response as a main end point.

A cost report from the United Kingdom National Institute for Health and Clinical Excellence estimated the cost of docetaxel plus prednisone to be approximately $16,800 compared with $8,900 for patients treated with mitoxantrone. Based on the median survival advantage provided by docetaxel, they estimated an incremental cost of $40,000 per life-year gained.[83]

EVALUATION OF THERAPEUTIC OUTCOMES

Monitoring of prostate cancer depends on the stage of the cancer.[33] When definitive, curative therapy is attempted, objective parameters to assess tumor response include assessment of the primary tumor size, evaluation of involved lymph nodes, and the response of tumor markers such as PSA to treatment. PSA may continue to rise before declining, leading to an interruption or discontinuation of therapy. Therefore, treatment decisions are often difficult, and more research about end points is needed to facilitate prostate cancer treatment, continued enrollment in clinical trials, and drug development.[84] Following definitive therapy, the PSA level is checked every 6 months for the first 5 years, then annually. Local recurrence in the absence of a rising PSA may occur, so the DRE is also performed. In the metastatic setting, clinical benefit responses can be documented by evaluating performance status changes, weight changes, quality of life, and analgesic requirements, in addition to the PSA or DRE at 3-month intervals.

ABBREVIATIONS

ACS: American Cancer Society

ADT: Androgen deprivation therapy

AUS: American Urologic System

BPH: benign prostatic hyperplasia

CAB: combined androgen blockade

DES: diethylstilbestrol

DHT: dihydrotestosterone

DRE: digital rectal examination

EGF: epidermal growth factor

FSH: follicle-stimulating hormone

IGF-1: insulin-like growth factor

LH: luteinizing hormone

LH-RH: luteinizing hormone–releasing hormone

NCCN: National Comprehensive Cancer Network

NCI: National Cancer Institute

PCPT: Prostate Cancer Prevention Trial

PSA: prostate-specific antigen

TRUS: transrectal ultrasound

VACURG: Veterans Administration Cooperative Urologic Research Group

TABLE 139-9	Comparative Costs of Hormonal Therapy for Advanced Prostate Cancer	
Drug	**Dose**	**Average Wholesale Price per Month of Therapy**
Leuprolide depot	7.5 mg/mo	$781.90
Leuprolide depot	22.5 mg/12 wk	$781.89
Leuprolide depot	30 mg/16 wk	$781.89
Goserelin implant	3.6 mg every 28 days	$451.19
Goserelin implant	10.8 mg/12 wk	$451.19
Flutamide	750 mg/day	$390.79
Bicalutamide	50 mg/day	$523.92
Nilutamide	300 mg/day for first mo then 150 mg/day	$830.28 then $415.14
Combined Androgen Blockade		**Average Wholesale Price per 3 Months of Therapy**
Leuprolide depot 22.5 mg/12 wk		
+ flutamide	750 mg/day	$3,518.03
+ bicalutamide	50 mg/day	$3,917.42
+ nilutamide	150 mg/day	$3,591.08 ($3,175.94 1st month)
Goserelin depot 10.8 mg/12 wk		
+ flutamide	750 mg/day	$2,525.95
+ bicalutamide	50 mg/day	$2,925.34
+ nilutamide	150 mg/day	$2,599.00 ($2,183.86 1st month)

Compiled from Drug Topics, Annual Pharmacists' Reference (Redbook). Montvale, NJ, Thomson Healthcare, 2008.

REFERENCES

1. Jemal A, Siegel R, Xu J, Ward E. Cancer statistics, 2010. CA Cancer J Clin 2010;60:277–300.
2. Hsieh K, Albertsen PC. Populations at high risk for prostate cancer. Urol Clin North Am 2003;30:669–676.

3. Odedina FT, Ogunbiyi JO, Ukoli FA. Roots of prostate cancer in African-American men. J Natl Med Assoc 2006;98:539–543.

4. Denis L, Morton MS, Griffiths K. Diet and its preventive role in prostatic disease. Eur Urol 1999;35:377–387.

5. Crawford ED. Epidemiology of prostate cancer. Urology 2003;62:3–12.

6. Liede A, Karlan BY, Narod SA. Cancer risks for male carriers of germline mutations in BRCA1 or BRCA2: A review of the literature. J Clin Oncol 2004;22:735–742.

7. Thompson IM, Goodman PJ, Tangen CM, et al. The influence of finasteride on the development of prostate cancer. N Engl J Med 2003349:215–224.

8. Gurel B, Iwata T, Koh CM, et al. Molecular alterations in prostate cancer as diagnostic, prognostic, and therapeutic targets. Adv Anat Pathol 2008;15:319–331.

9. Marberger M, Adolfsson J, Borkowski A, et al. The clinical implications of the prostate cancer prevention trial. BJU Int 2003;92:667–671.

10. Musquera M, Fleshner NE, Finelli A, et al. The REDUCE trial: Chemoprevention in prostate cancer using a dual 5alpha-reductase inhibitor, dutasteride. Expert Rev Anticancer Ther 2008;8:1073–1079.

11. Thorpe JF, Jain S, Marczylo TH, et al. A review of phase III clinical trials of prostate cancer chemoprevention. Ann R Coll Surg Engl 2007;89:207–211.

12. Redman MW, Tangen CM, Goodman PJ, Lucia MS, Coltman CA Jr, Thompson IM. Finasteride does not increase the risk of high-grade prostate cancer: A bias-adjusted modeling approach. Cancer Prev Res (Phila Pa). 2008 Aug;1(3):174–181.

13. Kramer BS, Hagerty KL, Justman S, et al. Use of 5-alpha-reductase inhibitors for prostate cancer chemoprevention: American Society of Clinical Oncology/American Urological Association 2008 Clinical Practice Guideline. J Urol 2009 Apr;181(4):1642–1657.

14. Annonymous. Selenium and Vitamin E Cancer Prevention Trial (SELECT) http://www.cancer.gov/newscenter/pressreleases/SELECTQ andA.

15. Neill MG, Fleshner NE. An update on chemoprevention strategies in prostate cancer for 2006. Curr Opin Urol 2006;16:132–137.

16. Galic J, Karner I, Cenan L, et al. Role of screening in detection of clinically localized prostate cancer. Coll Antropol 2003;27(suppl 1): 49–54.

17. Wilson SS, Crawford ED. Screening for prostate cancer: Current recommendations. Urol Clin North Am 2004;31:219–226.

18. Gohagan JK, Prorok PC, Kramer BS, et al. The Prostate, Lung, Colorectal, and Ovarian-Cancer Screening Trial of the National-Cancer-Institute. Cancer 1995;75:1869–1873.

19. Schmid HP, Prikler L, Semjonow A. Problems with prostate-specific antigen screening: A critical review. Recent Results Cancer Res 2003;163:226–231.

20. Schröder FH, Hugosson J, Roobol MJ, et al; ERSPC Investigators. Screening and prostate-cancer mortality in a randomized European study. N Engl J Med 2009 Mar 26;360(13):1320–1328.

21. Andriole GL, Crawford ED, Grubb RL 3rd, et al; PLCO Project Team. Mortality results from a randomized prostate-cancer screening trial. N Engl J Med. 2009 Mar 26;360(13):1310–1319.

22. Catalona WJ, Smith DS, Ratliff TL, et al. Measurement of prostate-specific antigen in serum as a screening test for prostate cancer. N Engl J Med 1991;324:1156–1161.

23. Screening for prostate cancer: U.S. Preventive Services Task Force recommendation statement. Ann Intern Med 2008.149:185–191.

24. Harris R, Lohr KN. Screening for prostate cancer: An update of the evidence for the U.S. Preventive Services Task Force. Ann Intern Med 2002;137:917–929.

25. Ross KS, Carter HB, Pearson JD, et al. Comparative efficiency of prostate-specific antigen screening strategies for prostate cancer detection. JAMA 2000;284:1399–1405.

26. Khauli RB. Prostate cancer: Diagnostic and therapeutic strategies with emphasis on the role of PSA. J Med Liban 2005;53:95–102.

27. Iczkowski KA. Current prostate biopsy interpretation: Criteria for cancer, atypical small acinar proliferation, high-grade prostatic intra-epithelial neoplasia, and use of immunostains. Arch Pathol Lab Med 2006;130:835–843.

28. De Marzo AM, Meeker AK, Zha S, et al. Human prostate cancer precursors and pathobiology. Urology 2003;62:55–62.

29. Culig Z. Role of the androgen receptor axis in prostate cancer. Urology 2003;62:21–26.

30. Marks LS. Luteinizing hormone-releasing hormone agonists in the treatment of men with prostate cancer: Timing, alternatives, and the 1-year implant. Urology 2003;62:36–42.

31. Sharifi N, Gulley JL, Dahut WL. Androgen deprivation therapy for prostate cancer. JAMA 2005;294:238–244.

32. Anderson J. The role of antiandrogen monotherapy in the treatment of prostate cancer. BJU Int 2003;91:455–461.

33. Nieto M, Finn S, Loda M, et al. Prostate cancer: Re-focusing on androgen receptor signaling. Int J Biochem Cell Biol 2007;39: 1562–1568.

34. Cooperberg MR, Moul JW, Carroll PR. The changing face of prostate cancer. J Clin Oncol 2005;23:8146–8151.

35. Labrie F, Dupont A, Cusan L, et al. Combination therapy with flutamide and medical (LHRH agonist) or surgical castration in advanced prostate cancer: 7-year clinical experience. J Steroid Biochem Mol Biol 1990;37:943–950.

36. Leach FS, Koh MS, Chan YW, et al. Prostate specific antigen as a clinical biomarker for prostate cancer: What's the take home message? Cancer Biol Ther 2005;4:371–375.

37. National Comprehensive Cancer Network. National Comprehensive Cancer Network guidelines for the management of prostate cancer, www.nccn.org. Prostate Cancer v.2.2009.

38. Schroder FH, de Vries SH, Bangma CH. Watchful waiting in prostate cancer: Review and policy proposals. BJU Int 2003;92:851–859.

39. Scher HI. Prostate carcinoma: Defining therapeutic objectives and improving overall outcomes. Cancer 2003;97:758–771.

40. Wilt TJ, Macdonald R, Rutks I, et al. Systematic review: Comparative effectiveness and harms of treatments for clinically localized prostate cancer. Ann Intern Med 2008;148:435–448.

41. Dalkin BL, Christopher BA. Potent men undergoing radical prostatectomy: A prospective study measuring sexual health outcomes and the impact of erectile dysfunction treatments. Urol Oncol 2008;26: 281–285.

42. Immediate versus deferred treatment for advanced prostatic cancer: Initial results of the Medical Research Council Trial. The Medical Research Council Prostate Cancer Working Party Investigators Group. Br J Urol 1997;79:235–246.

43. Oh WK. Secondary hormonal therapies in the treatment of prostate cancer. Urology 2002;60:87–92.

44. Thompson IM, Tangen CM, Paradelo J, et al. Adjuvant radiotherapy for pathological T3N0M0 prostate cancer significantly reduces risk of metastases and improves survival: Long-term follow up of a randomized clinical trial. J Urolo 2009;181:956–962.

45. Maximum androgen blockade in advanced prostate cancer: An overview of the randomised trials. Prostate Cancer Trialists' Collaborative Group. Lancet 2000;355:1491–1498.

46. Hedlund PO, Henriksson P. Parenteral estrogen versus total androgen ablation in the treatment of advanced prostate carcinoma: Effects on overall survival and cardiovascular mortality. The Scandinavian Prostatic Cancer Group (SPCG)-5 Trial Study. Urology 2000;55: 328–333.

47. Seidenfeld J, Samson DJ, Hasselblad V, et al. Single-therapy androgen suppression in men with advanced prostate cancer: A systematic review and meta-analysis. Ann Intern Med 2000;132:566–577.

48. Smith MR, Finkelstein JS, McGovern FJ, et al. Changes in body composition during androgen deprivation therapy for prostate cancer. J Clin Endocrinol Metab 2002;87:599–603.

49. Shahinian VB, Kuo YF, Freeman JL, Goodwin JS. Risk of fracture after androgen deprivation for prostate cancer. N Engl J Med 2005;352: 154–164.

50. Smith MR, Boyce SP, Moyneur E, Duh MS, Raut MK, Brandman J. Risk of clinical fractures after gonadotropin-releasing hormone agonist therapy for prostate cancer. J Urol 2006;175:136–139.

51. Smith MR, Lee WC, Brandman W, Wang Q, Botteman M, Pashos CL. Gonadotropin-releasing hormone agonist and fracture risk: A claims-based cohort study of men with nonmetastatic prostate cancer. J Clin Oncol 2005;23:7897–7903.

52. Saad F, Adachi JD, Brown JP, et al. Cancer treatment—induced bone loss in breast and prostate cancer. J Clin Oncol 2008;26:5465–5476.

53. Ellis GK, Bone HG, Chlebowski R, et al. Randommmized trial of denosumab in patients receiving adjuvant aromatase inhibitors for nonmetastatic breast cancer. J Clin Oncol 2008;26:4875–4882.

54. Smith MR, Egerdie B, Toriz NH, et al. Denosumab in men receiving androgen deprivation therapy for prostate cancer. N Engl J Med 2009;361:745–755.

55. Keating NL, O'Malley AJ, Smith MR. Diabetes and cardiovascular disease during androgen deprivation therapy for prostate cancer. J Clin Oncol 2006;24:4448–4456.

56. Saigal S, Gore JL, Krupski TL, et al. Androgen deprivation therapy increases cardiovascular morbidity in men with prostate cancer. Cancer 2007;110:1493–1500.

57. D'Amico AV, Denham JW, Crook J, et al. Influene of androgen suppression therapy for prostate cancer on the frequency and timing of fatal myocardial infarctions. J Clin Oncol 2007;25:2420–2425.

58. Efstathiou JA, Bae K, Shipley WU. Cardiovascular mortality following androgen deprivation therapy for locally advanced prostate cancer. Analysis of RTOG 92-02. Eur Urol 2008;54:816–823.

59. Roach M, Bae K, Speight J, et al. Short-term neoadjuvant androgen deprivation therapy and external-beam radiotherapy for locally advanced prostate cancer. Long-term results of RTOG 8610. J Clin Oncol 2008;26:585–591.

60. Studer UE, Whelan P, Albrecht W, et al. Immediate or deferred androgen deprivation for patients with prostate cancer not suitable for local treatment with curative intent: European Organization for Research and Treatment of Cancer (EORTC) Trial 30891. J Clin Oncol 2006;24:1868–1876.

61. Tsai HK, D'Amica AV, Sadetsky N, et al. Androgen deprivation therapy for localized prostate cancer and the risk of cardiovascular mortality. J Natl Cancer Inst 2007;99:1516–1524.

62. Klotz L, Boccon-Gibod L, Shore ND, et al. The efficacy and safety of degarelix: A 12-month, comparative, randomized, open-label, parallel group phase III study in patients with prostate cancer. BJU Int 2008 102(11):1531–1538.

63. Moul JW, Fowler JE Jr. Evolution of therapeutic approaches with luteinizing hormone-releasing hormone agonists in 2003. Urology 2003;62:20–28.

64. Tyrrell CJ, Altwein JE, Klippel F, et al. Comparison of an LH-RH analogue (Goeserelin acetate, "Zoladex") with combined androgen blockade in advanced prostate cancer: Final survival results of an international multicentre randomized-trial. International Prostate Cancer Study Group. Eur Urol 2000;37:205–211.

65. Eisenberger MA, Blumenstein BA, Crawford ED, et al. Bilateral orchiectomy with or without flutamide for metastatic prostate cancer. N Engl J Med 1998;339:1036–1042.

66. Carcinoma of the prostate: Treatment comparisons. J Urol 1967;98:516–522.

67. Scher HI, Kelly WK. Flutamide withdrawal syndrome: Its impact on clinical trials in hormone-refractory prostate cancer. J Clin Oncol 1993;11:1566–1572.

68. Small EJ, Srinivas S. The antiandrogen withdrawal syndrome: experience in a large cohort of unselected patients with advanced prostate cancer. Cancer 1995;76:1428–1434.

69. Huan SD, Gerridzen RG, Yau JC, et al. Antiandrogen withdrawal syndrome with nilutamide. Urology 1997;49:632–634.

70. Sartor O, Cooper M, Weinberger M, et al. Surprising activity of flutamide withdrawal, when combined with aminoglutethimide, in treatment of "hormone-refractory" prostate cancer. J Natl Cancer Inst 1994;86:222–227.

71. Scher HI, Liebertz C, Kelly WK, et al. Bicalutamide for advanced prostate cancer: The natural versus treated history of disease. J Clin Oncol 1997;15:2928–2938.

72. Crawford ED, Kozlowski JM, Debruyne FM, et al. The use of strontium 89 for palliation of pain from bone metastases associated with hormone-refractory prostate cancer. Urology 1994;44:481–485.

73. Resche I, Chatal JF, Pecking A, et al. A dose-controlled study of 153Sm-ethylenediaminetetramethylenephosphonate (EDTMP) in the treatment of patients with painful bone metastases. Eur J Cancer 1997;33:1583–1591.

74. Posadas EM, Dahut WL, Gulley J. The emerging role of bisphosphonates in prostate cancer. Am J Ther 2004;11:60–73.

75. Saad F, Gleason DM, Murray R, et al. Long-term efficacy of zoledronic acid for the prevention of skeletal complications in patients with metastatic hormone-refractory prostate cancer. J Natl Cancer Inst 2004;96:879–882.

76. Tannock IF, de Wit R, Berry WR, et al. Docetaxel plus prednisone or mitoxantrone plus prednisone for advanced prostate cancer. N Engl J Med 2004;351:1502–1512.

77. Petrylak DP, Tangen CM, Hussain MH, et al. Docetaxel and estramustine compared with mitoxantrone and prednisone for advanced refractory prostate cancer. N Engl J Med 2004;351:1513–1520.

78. Kantoff PW, Higano CS, Shore ND, et al. Sipuleucel-T immunotherapy for castration-resistant prostate cancer. N Engl J Med 2010;363:411–442.

79. Krahn MD, Coombs A, Levy IG. Current and projected annual direct costs of screening asymptomatic men for prostate cancer using prostate-specific antigen. CMAJ 1999;160:49–57.

80. Hillner BE, McLeod DG, Crawford ED, et al. Estimating the cost effectiveness of total androgen blockade with flutamide in M1 prostate cancer. Urology 1995;45:633–640.

81. Hummel S, Paisley S, Morgan A, et al. Clinical and cost-effectiveness of new and emerging technologies for early localised prostate cancer: A systematic review. Health Technol Assess 2003;7:1–157.

82. Turini M, Redaelli A, Gramegna P, et al. Quality of life and economic considerations in the management of prostate cancer. Pharmacoeconomics 2003;21:527–541.

83. Zeliadt SB, Penson DF. Pharmacoeconomics of available treatment options for metastatic prostate cancer. Pharmacoeconomics 2007;25:309–327.

84. Scher HI, Halabi S, Tannock I, et al. Design and end points of clinical trials for patients with progressive prostate cancer and castrate levels of testosterone: Recommendations of the prostate cancer clinical trials working group. J Clin Oncol 2008;26:1148–1159.

CHAPTER

140

Lymphomas

ALEXANDRE CHAN AND GARY C. YEE

KEY CONCEPTS

❶ Patients with Hodgkin lymphoma present with a painless, rubbery lymph node, which most commonly resides in the neck (cervical or supraclavicular nodes).

❷ Patients with early-stage Hodgkin lymphoma should be treated with combination chemotherapy with or without involved-field radiation

❸ Combination chemotherapy with doxorubicin (Adriamycin), bleomycin, vinblastine, and dacarbazine (ABVD) is the primary treatment for patients with advanced-stage Hodgkin lymphoma. Patients with advanced unfavorable disease may be treated with more aggressive regimens that have greater activity, but are associated with a higher risk of secondary malignancies.

❹ Some patients with Hodgkin lymphoma will be refractory to initial therapy or will have a recurrence following a complete remission. Response to salvage therapy depends on the extent and site of recurrence, previous therapy, and duration of initial remission. High-dose chemotherapy and autologous hematopoietic stem cell transplantation should be considered in patients with refractory or relapsed disease.

❺ The current classification system for non-Hodgkin lymphoma is the World Health Organization classification system, which is based on the principle that non-Hodgkin lymphomas can be classified into specific disease entities, defined by a combination of morphology, immunophenotype, genetic features, and clinical features.

❻ As compared with Hodgkin lymphoma, the clinical presentation of non-Hodgkin lymphoma is more variable because of disease heterogeneity and more frequent extranodal involvement.

❼ The Ann Arbor staging system correlates poorly with prognosis in non-Hodgkin lymphoma because the disease does not spread through contiguous lymph nodes and often involves extranodal sites.

❽ Several prognostic models have been developed to estimate prognosis in patients with non-Hodgkin lymphoma. The

International Prognostic Index (IPI) score is a well-established model for patients with aggressive non-Hodgkin lymphoma. The Follicular Lymphoma International Prognostic Index (FLIPI) is a similar model used for patients with follicular and other indolent lymphomas.

❾ The clinical behavior and degree of aggressiveness can be used to categorize non-Hodgkin lymphoma into indolent and aggressive lymphomas. Patients with an indolent lymphoma usually have a relatively long survival, with or without aggressive chemotherapy. Although these lymphomas respond to a wide range of therapeutic approaches, few if any of these patients are cured of their disease. In contrast, aggressive lymphomas are rapidly growing tumors and patients have a short survival if appropriate therapy is not initiated. Most patients with aggressive lymphomas respond to intensive chemotherapy and many are cured of their disease.

❿ Patients with localized follicular lymphoma can be cured with radiation therapy alone. Advanced follicular lymphoma is not curable, and there are many treatment options, including watchful waiting, extended-field radiation therapy, single-agent alkylating agents, anthracycline-containing combination chemotherapy, purine analogs, interferon-α, anti-CD20 monoclonal antibodies, and high-dose chemotherapy with hematopoietic stem cell transplantation.

⓫ Patients with localized aggressive lymphomas can be cured with several cycles of R-CHOP (rituximab, cyclophosphamide, doxorubicin, Oncovin, prednisone) chemotherapy and involved-field irradiation. Patients with bulky stage II, stage III, or stage IV aggressive lymphomas can be cured of their disease with R-CHOP chemotherapy.

⓬ Conventional-dose salvage therapy can induce responses in patients with aggressive lymphomas who relapse, but long-term survival and cure is uncommon. Some patients with aggressive lymphoma who relapse and respond to salvage therapy can be cured with high-dose chemotherapy and autologous hematopoietic stem cell transplantation.

Lymphomas are a heterogeneous group of malignancies that arise from malignant transformation of immune cells that reside predominantly in lymphoid tissues. They most commonly present as a solid tumor, but can sometimes present as circulating tumor cells in peripheral blood. The differing histology of lymphoma cells has led to classification of Hodgkin lymphoma (Reed–Sternberg cells) or non-Hodgkin lymphoma (B- or T-cell lymphocyte markers). Non-Hodgkin lymphomas (NHLs) are further classified into distinct clinical entities, which are defined by a combination of morphology, immunophenotype, genetic features, and clinical

Learning objectives, review questions, and other resources can be found at **www.pharmacotherapyonline.com**.

features. Chemotherapy is the mainstay of treatment in patients with lymphoma, especially those with widespread disease. Overall cure rates are high for many subtypes of lymphomas, even when patients present with advanced disease.

HODGKIN LYMPHOMA

Hodgkin lymphoma is a form of lymphoma, named after Thomas Hodgkin who first described seven cases of a mysterious disease of the lymph system over 150 years ago. Hodgkin lymphoma is fatal in more than 90% of the patients who are untreated for two to three years, and the cause is still unknown. The prognosis with treatment is generally good, but is not well predicted by stage alone. The International Prognostic Score was created to better predict an individual's risk of recurrence, which in turn influences treatment decisions. Patients with Hodgkin lymphoma can be categorized into four prognostic groups: early favorable disease, early unfavorable disease, advanced favorable disease, and advanced unfavorable disease. These groups are defined by patient age, gender, tumor size and spread (tumor stage), presence or absence of systemic symptoms, and laboratory test results. When appropriate therapy is given, more than 75% of all newly diagnosed Hodgkin lymphoma patients can be cured. However, the success of treatment has not been without cost. The treatment programs are intense, technically demanding, and associated with considerable acute toxicity and long-term complications. The long-term effects, particularly secondary malignancies, account for a higher cumulative mortality than Hodgkin lymphoma 15 to 20 years after treatment. Long-term toxicities with standard chemotherapy regimens have been more fully documented in recent years and are shaping future therapies.[1-3]

EPIDEMIOLOGY AND ETIOLOGY

Hodgkin lymphoma represents less than 1% of all known cancers in the United States. It is estimated that 8,490 new cases of Hodgkin lymphoma will be diagnosed in the United States in 2010, and there will be 1,320 deaths associated with Hodgkin lymphoma during this same period.[4] This disease occurs slightly more frequently in males than in females. Once thought to be a disease of the young, it is now recognized that Hodgkin lymphoma exhibits bimodal distribution in industrialized countries. The first peak occurs in the third decade of life, with a small peak occurring after age 50.[2,3] The five-year overall survival for all stages of Hodgkin lymphoma is approximately 85%.[5] Death rates as a consequence of recurrent Hodgkin lymphoma are less than those from other causes 15 years after treatment.[6]

The etiology of Hodgkin lymphoma is currently unknown but there is laboratory evidence to support infectious exposure as a potential cause.[7,8] Studies suggest an increased risk of Hodgkin lymphoma in patients who have been infected with the Epstein–Barr virus (EBV); and many patients experience EBV activation even before the onset of Hodgkin lymphoma. EBV is found in approximately 40% of all classical Hodgkin lymphoma cases, and it is frequently observed in cases of mixed cellularity and lymphocyte-depleted Hodgkin lymphoma.[9] Reed–Sternberg cells (large, bilobate, multinuclear cells), the malignant cells in Hodgkin lymphoma, are linked to EBV. Immunosuppressed individuals are also at much higher risk to develop Hodgkin lymphoma. Such individuals include patients with congenital immunosuppression, solid-organ transplantation recipients, and human immunodeficiency virus (HIV)-infected patients. Although the risk of developing Hodgkin lymphoma is approximately sevenfold greater in patients with HIV, the level of CD4 may vary depending on the subtype of Hodgkin lymphoma.[8]

Genetic factors are also shown to be associated with an increased risk of Hodgkin lymphoma. The strongest evidence suggesting that genes are important in the etiology of Hodgkin lymphoma comes from identical twin studies, which show that the unaffected identical twin has almost a 100-fold increase in risk.[10]

PATHOPHYSIOLOGY

Hodgkin lymphoma is a clonal malignant lymphoid disease of transformed lymphocytes. The malignant cell in Hodgkin lymphoma is known as the *Reed–Sternberg* cell named after Drs. Dorothy Reed and Carl Sternberg, who were credited with the first definitive microscopic description of Hodgkin lymphoma.[2,3,11] Procedures to isolate and analyze Reed–Sternberg cells remain a challenge to scientists, due to the relatively small percentage (1% to 2%) of Reed–Sternberg cells that are found in the Hodgkin lymphoma mass.[9] Fortunately, new laboratory techniques have led to significant progress in identifying the origin of the Reed–Sternberg cell. Single-cell polymerase chain reaction and DNA microarray analyses indicate that nearly all classic Hodgkin lymphoma cases and all nodular lymphocyte-predominant Hodgkin lymphomas have immunoglobulin gene rearrangements, which indicates a germinal center or postgerminal center B-cell origin (Table 140–1).[9,12] Interestingly, nearly all Reed–Sternberg cells fail to express B-cell specific cell surface proteins.

B-cell transcriptional processes are disrupted during malignant transformation, which prevents B-cell surface marker expression and production of immunoglobulin messenger ribonucleic acid. The normal cellular consequence of failure to express immunoglobulin is apoptosis, but because of alterations in the normal apoptotic pathways, cell survival and proliferation are favored. Reed–Sternberg cells overexpress nuclear factor-κB, which is associated with cell proliferation and antiapoptotic signals. Infections with viral and bacterial pathogens upregulate nuclear factor-κB and consequently are hypothesized to be involved with the etiology of Hodgkin lymphoma.[2,9,12] This hypothesis is supported by the presence of EBV in many Hodgkin lymphoma tumors, but it is important to note that not all tumors are associated with EBV. Another signaling pathway, Janus Kinase–signal transduction and transcription (JAK–STAT), has also been found to be active in Hodgkin lymphoma.[2,9] As molecular techniques continue to improve, our understanding of the pathophysiology of Hodgkin lymphoma will also improve.

The histopathologic classification of Hodgkin lymphoma has undergone numerous changes over the last three decades. The

TABLE 140-1	B-Cell Development and the Corresponding Neoplasm Derived at Each Stage		
		B Cells	**Corresponding Neoplasm**
Foreign antigen independent	Bone marrow	Stem cell	
		Pro-B cell	
		Pre-B cell	B-LBL/ALL
		Immature B cell	
Foreign antigen dependent	Peripheral lymphoid tissue	Mature naïve B cell	B-CLL, MCL
		Germinal center	BL, FL, LPHL, DLBCL, cHL
		Memory B cell	MZL, B-CLL
Terminal differentiation		Plasma cell	Plasmacytoma/ myeloma

ALL, acute lymphocytic leukemia; BL, Burkitt lymphoma; B-CLL, B-cell chronic lymphocytic leukemia; B-LBL, B-cell lymphoblastic lymphoma; cHL, classical Hodgkin lymphoma; DLBCL, diffuse large B-cell lymphoma; FL, follicular lymphoma; LPHL, lymphocyte-predominant Hodgkin lymphoma; MCL, mantle cell lymphoma; MZL, marginal zone B-cell lymphoma.
Adapted from Harris NL, Stein H, Coupland SE, et al. New approaches to lymphoma diagnosis. Hematology (Am Soc Hematol Educ Program) 2001:194–220.

TABLE 140-2 WHO Classification of the Mature B-Cell, T-Cell, and NK-Cell Neoplasms (2008)

B Cell	T Cell	Hodgkin Lymphoma
B-cell chronic lymphocytic leukemia/small lymphocytic lymphoma	T-cell prolymphocytic leukemia	Nodular lymphocyte-predominant Hodgkin lymphoma
B-cell prolymphocytic leukemia	T-cell large granular lymphocytic leukemia	Classical Hodgkin lymphoma
Splenic marginal zone lymphoma	Aggressive NK cell leukemia	Nodular sclerosis classical Hodgkin lymphoma
Hairy cell leukemia	Systemic EBV-positive T-cell lymphoproliferative disorder of childhood	Lymphocyte-rich classical Hodgkin lymphoma
Lymphoplasmacytic lymphoma	Hydroa vacciniforme-like lymphoma	Mixed cellularity classical Hodgkin lymphoma
Waldenström macroglobinemia	Adult T-cell leukemia/lymphoma	Lymphocyte-depleted classical Hodgkin lymphoma
Heavy chain diseases	Extranodal NK/T-cell lymphoma, nasal type	
Plasma cell myeloma	Enteropathy-associated T-cell lymphoma	
Solidtary plasmacytoma of bone	Hepatosplenic T-cell lymphoma	
Extraosseous plasmacytoma	Subcutaneous panniculitis-like T-cell lymphoma	
Extranodal marginal zone B-cell lymphoma of MALT type	Mycosis fungoides	
Nodal marginal zone B-cell lymphoma	Sézary syndrome	
Follicular lymphoma	Primary cutaneous CD30+ T-cell lymphoproliferative disorders	
Primary cutaneous follicle center lymphoma	Primary cutaneous gamma-delta T-cell lymphoma	
Mantle cell lymphoma	Peripheral T-cell lymphoma, not otherwise specified (NOS)	
Diffuse large B-cell lymphoma (DLBCL), not otherwise specified (NOS)	Angioimmunoblastic T-cell lymphoma	
DLBCL associated with chronic inflammation	Anaplastic large cell lymphoma, ALK positive	
Lymphamatoid granulomatosis		
Primary mediastinal (thymic) large B-cell lymphoma		
Intravascular large B-cell lymphoma		
ALK positive large B-cell lymphoma		
Plasmablastic lymphoma		
Large B-cell lymphoma arising in HHV8-associated multicentric Castleman disease		
Primary effusion lymphoma		
Burkitt lymphoma		
B-cell lymphoma, unclassifiable, with features intermediate between DLBCL and Burkitt lymphoma		
B-cell lymphoma, unclassifiable, with features intermediate between DLBCL and classical Hodgkin lymphoma		

HTLV, human T-cell lymphotropic virus; MALT, mucosa-associated lymphoid tissue; NK, natural killer; HHV8, human herpesvirus 8; EBV, Epstein-Barr virus; ALK, anaplastic lymphoma kinase; WHO, World Health Organization.

current classification system is the 2008 World Health Organization (WHO) classification (Table 140–2).[13] This classification divides Hodgkin lymphoma into two major groups: classical Hodgkin lymphoma and nodular lymphocyte-predominant Hodgkin lymphoma, which constitute approximately 95% and 5% of cases, respectively. Classic Hodgkin lymphoma is further divided into four subtypes: nodular sclerosis, mixed cellularity, lymphocyte-depletion, and lymphocyte-rich. The subtypes in these classifications are based on characteristics of the Reed–Sternberg cell, the surrounding cells, and the connective tissue. Nodular sclerosis has features that make it distinct from the other three subtypes, which represent a continuum of background cellularity, with lymphocyte-predominance being the most cellular and lymphocyte-depletion being the least cellular. Nodular lymphocyte-predominant Hodgkin lymphoma is separated because of its distinct immunophenotype: CD15−, CD20+, CD30−, and CD45+ (the opposite of classical Hodgkin lymphoma). With the introduction of extensive staging, sophisticated radiotherapy, and effective combination chemotherapy, the prognostic value of these subtypes is becoming less clear. The true value of understanding these subtypes is likely tied to the pathogenesis of the disease and its potential prevention in the future.

CLINICAL PRESENTATION

❶ Most patients with Hodgkin lymphoma present with a painless, rubbery, enlarged lymph node in the supradiaphragmatic area and commonly have mediastinal nodal involvement.[14] Hodgkin lymphoma is occasionally diagnosed in an asymptomatic patient who has a mediastinal mass found with chest radiography or another imaging procedure. Asymptomatic adenopathy of the inguinal and axillary regions may be present at diagnosis but is less common (Fig. 140–1).[2] Patients can also present with constitutional symptoms (B symptoms) before the discovery of lymph node enlargement, and these symptoms include fever, drenching night sweats, and weight loss. At diagnosis, these symptoms may appear in approximately 25% of all patients and up to 50% of patients with advanced disease. Patients may also experience other nonspecific symptoms including pruritus, fatigue, and development of pain after alcohol consumption at sites where nodes are involved.[3] Extranodal manifestations, such as bowel and hepatic involvements, are much less common in Hodgkin lymphoma than non-Hodgkin lymphoma.[2]

DIAGNOSIS, STAGING, AND PROGNOSTIC FACTORS

Diagnostic and staging procedures are based on recommendations made at the Ann Arbor and Cotswolds conferences and new scientific advances, as described in the National Comprehensive Cancer Network (NCCN) guidelines.[15] The diagnosis and pathologic classification of Hodgkin lymphoma can only be made by review of a biopsy (preferably an excisional biopsy) of the enlarged node by an expert hematopathologist.

In addition to a careful physical examination and routine laboratory tests, chest radiography and computed tomography (CT) scans of the chest, abdomen, and pelvis are routinely performed.

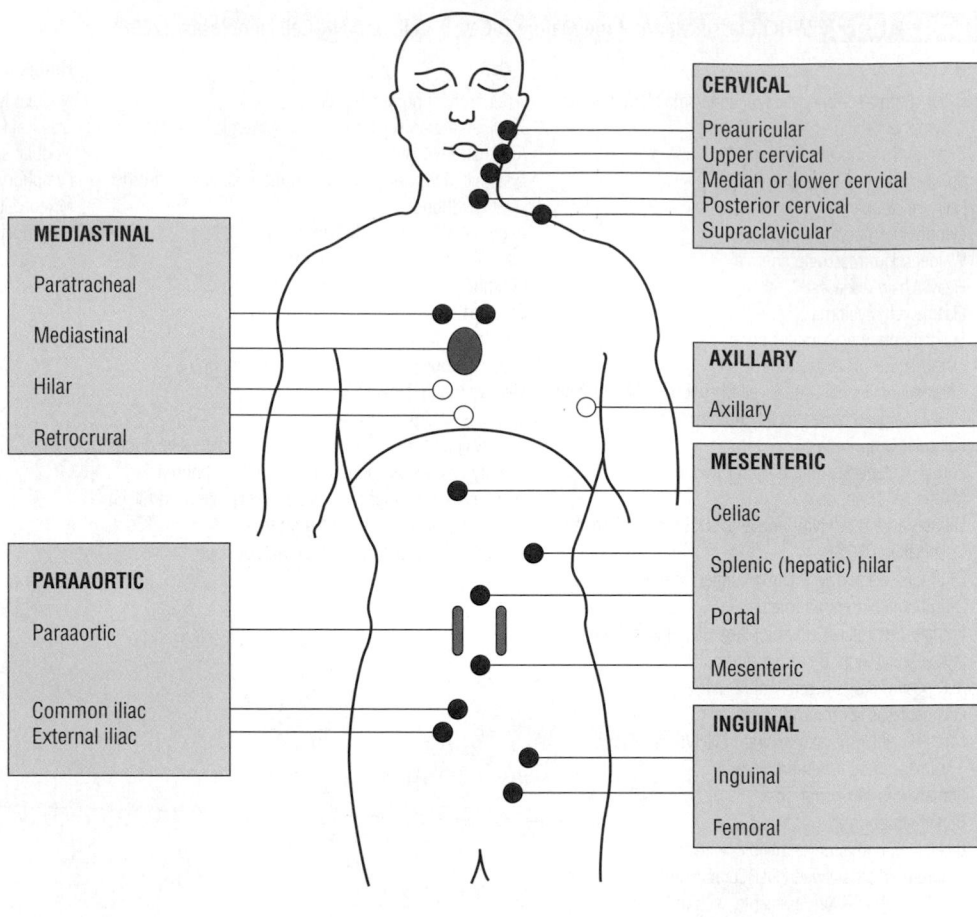

FIGURE 140-1. Areas of lymph nodes used in the staging of Hodgkin and non-Hodgkin lymphoma. Each rectangle corresponds to a nodal area. *(This research was originally published and modified from Blood. Solal-Celigny P, Roy P, Colombat P, et al. Follicular lymphoma international prognostic index. Blood 2004;104:1258–1265. Copyright © American Society of Hematology.)*

Furthermore, positron emission tomography (PET) plays an important role in the initial staging of Hodgkin lymphoma, as it has shown high sensitivity and specificity in the staging of the disease.[16] The use of integrated PET-CT has further improved the staging of Hodgkin lymphoma given that it can provide more sensitive and specific imaging as compared with each imaging alone. Currently, the NCCN guideline recommends either an integrated PET-CT scan (preferred) or a PET scan with diagnostic CT for initial staging.[15] Bone marrow biopsy is also recommended in patients with advanced-stage disease.

Staging can be based on clinical or pathologic findings. The clinical stage is based on all non-invasive procedures (history, physical examination, laboratory tests, and radiologic findings), whereas the pathologic stage is based on the biopsy findings of strategic sites (muscle, bone, skin, spleen, and abdominal nodes) with an invasive procedure such as a laparoscopy or laparotomy. Patients with extranodal disease (muscle, skin, bone, or Waldeyer ring) contiguous to involved nodes are classified with the subscript "E" in the Cotswolds staging system.[3,15] As a result of improved imaging techniques, pathologic workup and staging that can be associated with toxicity is rarely performed.

The Ann Arbor staging classification, which was developed at the 1970 Ann Arbor conference, has proven to be a good workable scheme. At the Cotswolds meeting in 1989, the Ann Arbor classification was modified to account for new diagnostic techniques (e.g., CT and magnetic resonance imaging), and the understanding that prognosis is associated with the bulk of the disease and the number of involved nodal sites (Table 140–3).[3] After careful staging, about one

TABLE 140-3	The Cotswolds Staging Classification of Hodgkin Lymphoma
Stage I	Involvement of a single lymph node region or structure (I) or of a single extralymphatic organ or site (I_E)
Stage II	Involvement of two or more lymph node regions on the same side of the diaphragm (II) or localized involvement of an extralymphatic organ or site and of one or more lymph node regions on the same side of the diaphragm (II_E). The number of nodal regions involved should be indicated by a subscript (e.g., II_2)
Stage III	Involvement of lymph node regions on both sides of the diaphragm (III), which may also be accompanied by localized involvement of an extralymphatic organ or site (III_E) or by involvement of the spleen (IIIS) or both ($IIIS_E$). III_1: with or without splenic, hilar, celiac, or portal node involvement. III_2: with paraaortic, iliac, or mesenteric node involvement
Stage IV	Diffuse or disseminated involvement of one or more extralymphatic organs or tissues with or without associated lymph node enlargement

A–No symptoms
B–Fever, night sweats, weight loss (>10%)
X–Bulky disease
>One-third the width of the mediastinum
>10 cm maximal dimension of nodal mass
E–Involvement of extralymphatic tissue on one side of the diaphragm by limited direct extension from an adjacent, involved lymph node region
S–Involvement of the spleen
CS–Clinical stage
PS–Pathologic stage

TABLE 140-4	The International Prognostic Factors Project Score for Advanced Hodgkin Lymphoma

Risk Factors

Serum albumin (<4 g/dL [<40 g/L])
Hemoglobin (<10.5 g/dL [<105 g/L; 6.52 mmol/L])
Male gender
Stage IV disease
Age (≥45 years)
White blood cell (WBC) count (≥15,000 cells/mm³ [≥15 x 10⁹/L])
Lymphocytopenia (<600 cells/mm³ [<0.6 x 10⁹/L] or <8% of WBC count)

Number of Factors	Freedom from Progression[a]	Overall Survival[a]
0	84 ± 4	89 ± 2
1	77 ± 3	90 ± 2
2	67 ± 2	81 ± 2
3	60 ± 3	78 ± 3
4	51 ± 4	61 ± 4
≥5	42 ± 5	56 ± 5

[a]Percentage of patients at 5 years.
Data from Hasenclever D, Diehl V. A prognostic score for advanced Hodgkin's disease. International Prognostic Factors Project on Advanced Hodgkin's Diease. N Engl J Med 1998;339:1506–1514.

half of patients have localized disease (stages I, II, and II_E) and the remainder have advanced disease (stage III or IV). Approximately 10% to 15% present with metastatic disease (stage IV). It is important to note that Hodgkin lymphoma appears to follow a predictable pattern of nodal spread that is not seen with the NHLs.[14,15]

Patient prognosis is predominately driven by age and tumor stage. Patients older than ages 65 to 70 have a lower cure rate than younger patients. The difference in cure rates may be related to the high rate of comorbid diseases and decreased organ function, which impairs the patient's ability to tolerate intensive chemotherapy.[17] Stage is the other dominant factor in predicting survival; patients with limited-stage disease (stages I to II) have a 90% to 95% cure rate, whereas those with advanced disease (stages III to IV) have only a 60% to 80% cure rate.[3,15]

Seven adverse prognostic factors with similar impact on survival (each factor reduced survival by 7% to 8% per year) have been identified through an international collaborative effort. These factors can be combined to generate an International Prognostic Score (IPS) that can be used to predict progression-free and overall survival (Table 140–4).[18]

TREATMENT

Hodgkin Lymphoma

The current goal in the treatment of Hodgkin lymphoma is to maximize curability while minimizing short- and long-term treatment-related complications. According to the SEER database, the five-year age-adjusted relative survival is greater than 80%.[5] Therefore, the treatment goal of all stages of Hodgkin lymphoma should be cure.

Although multiple treatment modalities are used to treat Hodgkin lymphoma, surgery has a limited therapeutic role regardless of stage. It is, however, important for diagnosis (excisional biopsy), and on certain occasions, such as placement of a central line.

Combination chemotherapy is the primary treatment modality for most patients with Hodgkin lymphoma. In general, patients with early-stage Hodgkin lymphoma are treated with combination chemotherapy and radiation, whereas patients with advanced-stage disease are treated with combination chemotherapy with or without radiation therapy. For patients with refractory or recurrent disease, salvage therapy consists of multiagent chemotherapy with or with-

out high-dose chemotherapy and autologous hematopoietic stem cell transplantation (HSCT), which can be curative.[2,3,19]

Radiation is often an integral part of the treatment plan. Selected patients with early-stage disease (usually nodular lymphocyte-predominant histology) can receive radiation as the only treatment modality, whereas most patients will receive chemotherapy and radiation. Although radiation is a local therapy, many patients with advanced disease will also receive radiation therapy to residual or bulky disease sites after chemotherapy. The major concern with radiation therapy is its long-term effects, such as cardiovascular disease and secondary malignancies, which commonly occur in the lung, breast, gastrointestinal tract, and connective tissue.[20] To avoid these toxicities, several studies have been completed and others are ongoing to determine the optimal extent (radiation field) and dose of radiation.[21] Radiation to a single field that contains Hodgkin lymphoma is called *involved-field radiation*; radiation to the involved field and a second uninvolved area is termed *extended-field radiation* or *subtotal nodal irradiation*; and radiation of all areas is called *total nodal irradiation*.[22] When given with chemotherapy (the most common scenario), involved-field radiation is usually used to avoid the increased toxicity associated with extended-field radiation.[21] The following sections review treatment of early-stage favorable disease, early-stage unfavorable disease, advanced-stage favorable disease, advanced-stage unfavorable disease, and salvage therapy.

TREATMENT OF EARLY-STAGE FAVORABLE DISEASE

Patients with early-stage favorable disease have stage IA or IIA disease and no adverse risk factors (extranodal disease, bulky disease, three or more sites of nodal involvement, or an erythrocyte sedimentation rate of ≥50 mm/h [≥13.9 μm/s]). In the past, extended-field radiation was considered to be the treatment of choice for stages IA and IIA disease. This treatment strategy produces disease-free survival rates ranging from 65% to 85% and overall survival rates ranging from 75% to 93%. However, there is a potential for long-term toxicities due to large radiation fields, such as increased risk for heart disease, pulmonary dysfunction, and secondary malignancies.[3,23]

In an effort to avoid the long-term effects of extended-field radiation and improve treatment results, several studies have evaluated a combined modality approach that involves the use of short-duration chemotherapy and involved-field radiation. Based on favorable results of these studies, most patients with early-stage favorable disease are no longer treated with radiation alone.[21,23,24]

Clinical trials comparing radiation alone to radiation plus chemotherapy show lower relapse rates in patients treated with combined modality therapy (radiation and chemotherapy), but no change in overall survival.[21] Current trials focus on questions such as the optimal number of chemotherapy cycles and the volume of radiation that must be used to obtain optimal patient outcomes. Emerging data also suggests that as few as two cycles of chemotherapy followed by involved-field radiation is sufficient in favorable, early-stage disease patients. Different combination chemotherapy regimens have been used in these studies, and no one regimen is clearly superior to another.[21,23]

The current NCCN guidelines recommend that patients with early-stage favorable disease be treated with two cycles of the Stanford V regimen (doxorubicin, vinblastine, mechlorethamine, etoposide, vincristine, bleomycin, and prednisone) or four cycles of the ABVD (doxorubicin [Adriamycin], bleomycin, vinblastine, and dacarbazine) regimen, followed by consolidative involved-field radiation.[15] With this approach, five-year progression-free and overall survival rates of >90% can be achieved.

Nodular lymphocyte-predominant Hodgkin lymphoma has been described as more indolent in nature, and better prognosis can be achieved when compared with classic Hodgkin lymphoma. The use of radiation alone for nodular lymphocyte-predominant Hodgkin lymphoma patients who choose to omit chemotherapy, or who cannot tolerate chemotherapy, does not appear to adversely affect survival.[15] The disadvantage of radiation therapy alone as compared with combination chemotherapy and radiation is the higher relapse rate. The lack of difference in survival rates is a result of the fact that patients who relapse after radiation alone (20% to 25%) can be successfully salvaged with chemotherapy. If the decision is made to use radiation alone, extended-field radiation appears to be superior to involved-field radiation.[25] It is shown that more extensive radiation reduces the risk of treatment failure at ten years (31% vs. 43%), although it does not improve ten-year overall survival. However, the risk of long-term complications (such as secondary malignancies) is increased with the use of extended-field radiotherapy when compared with less extensive radiation fields.

TREATMENT OF EARLY-STAGE UNFAVORABLE DISEASE

Patients with early-stage disease who have certain features associated with a poor prognosis (B symptoms, extranodal disease, bulky disease, three or more sites of nodal involvement, or an erythrocyte sedimentation rate >50 mm/h [≥13.9 μm/s]) are defined as having unfavorable disease. Current guidelines recommend combined modality therapy (combination chemotherapy and involved-field radiation) to reduce the relapse rate and avoid the toxicity associated with extended-field radiation.[15]

❷ Although randomized trials show that combined modality therapy reduces the relapse rate in patients with early-stage unfavorable disease, questions concerning the appropriate radiation volume, most effective chemotherapy regimen, and number of chemotherapy cycles remain.[23] A number of studies have compared extended-field radiation to involved-field radiation. In one large trial conducted by the German Hodgkin Study Group (GHSG), patients with early-stage unfavorable Hodgkin lymphoma treated with chemotherapy and involved-field radiation had similar freedom from treatment failure and overall survival as those treated with the same chemotherapy regimen and extended-field radiation.[26] Because toxicity was greater with extended-field radiation, the accepted standard is chemotherapy and involved-field radiation.

Different chemotherapy regimens and number of chemotherapy cycles were also compared in clinical trials. Mechlorethamine, vincristine, procarbazine, and prednisone (MOPP) was one of the first highly effective regimens introduced to treat Hodgkin lymphoma. MOPP or MOPP-like regimens were then given alternately or hybridized with a combination of ABVD. In advanced disease, ABVD was found to be less toxic than alternating MOPP/ABVD, and both were found to be superior to MOPP alone. Consequently, ABVD has now become the standard regimen used to treat patients with early-stage unfavorable disease. It has established effectiveness in patients with advanced-stage disease and a favorable toxicity (both acute and chronic) profile.

Despite excellent results from treatment with ABVD and radiation, approximately 5% of patients do not respond to initial treatment and another 15% of patients will relapse following an initial response. Several studies have evaluated more aggressive regimens or more cycles of therapy. However, none of these regimens has proven to be more effective than ABVD, and each is associated with more toxicity. The current NCCN guideline lists the Stanford V regimen as an acceptable option, which also uses more drugs than the ABVD regimen.[15]

In summary, most patients with early-stage disease will be treated with two to four cycles of ABVD chemotherapy and involved-field radiation. The number of cycles administered is based on the classification of favorable versus unfavorable disease. For patients who have unfavorable disease, six cycles of ABVD are recommended when radiation is completely omitted.[15] Although this approach results in excellent outcomes, studies are still ongoing to maximize the efficacy in this regimen while minimizing acute and long-term toxicity.

TREATMENT OF ADVANCED-STAGE DISEASE

Advanced-stage disease consists of stages III and IV disease. In some studies, stage IIB with a large mediastinal mass or extranodal disease is also considered advanced-stage disease (Table 140–3). By definition, patients with stages III and IV disease have tumors on both sides of the diaphragm, which almost always precludes the use of radiation alone as a therapeutic modality. Intensive combination chemotherapy is the mainstay of treatment, although some patients will benefit from radiation following chemotherapy. The prognosis of advanced-stage disease is excellent with five-year overall survival rates ranging from less than 56% to 90%. Prognostic factors have been identified and standardized to provide a more accurate individual prognosis (Table 140–4).[18]

Combination Chemotherapy

One of the initial combination chemotherapy regimens introduced in the early 1960s that was shown to cure advanced Hodgkin lymphoma was the MOPP regimen (Table 140–5). MOPP chemotherapy was a mainstay of treatment for patients with stages III and IV advanced Hodgkin lymphoma. It produced complete remissions in 84% of patients and has a ten-year cure rate of 54%.[27]

Ever since MOPP therapy was introduced and its efficacy confirmed, researchers have tried to modify the regimen in an attempt to improve efficacy and decrease toxicity.[19] Some MOPP variations, including MVPP (vinblastine substituted for vincristine), CVPP (cyclophosphamide substituted for mechlorethamine), and ChlVPP (chlorambucil substituted for mechlorethamine, and vinblastine substituted for vincristine) were attractive alternatives to MOPP because they offered equal efficacy and differing or less severe toxicities.

❸ The development of ABVD by Bonnadonna et al. at the Milan Cancer Institute approximately a decade later represents the next important step in the evolution of therapy for Hodgkin lymphoma (Table 140–5). ABVD was initially shown to be effective in treating MOPP failures and was later compared directly to MOPP in advanced disease, where it produced an 82% complete response rate, as compared to a 67% complete response rate with MOPP. Improved failure-free survival was demonstrated with ABVD, but no significant differences in five-year overall survival were noted.[28] Since ABVD was less toxic and provided similar or better outcomes than MOPP, it eventually replaced MOPP as the standard regimen for advanced-stage Hodgkin lymphoma.[3]

In the early 1980s, the Goldie–Coldman hypothesis proposed that chemotherapy resistance was related to spontaneous mutation rates and the development of resistant clones. To test that hypothesis, researchers designed several clinical trials to evaluate the efficacy of alternating non–cross-resistant drug combinations in patients with Hodgkin lymphoma.[29] The initial approach adopted by investigators was to alternate or combine the MOPP and ABVD regimens. When MOPP and ABVD (or ABV) are combined in a monthly cycle, it is referred to as a hybrid regimen. Besides a potential benefit in efficacy, another potential benefit of alternating or

TABLE 140-5 Combination Chemotherapy Regimens for Hodgkin Lymphoma

Drug	Dosage (mg/m²)	Route	Days
MOPP			
Mechlorethamine	6	IV	1, 8
Vincristine	1.4	IV	1, 8
Procarbazine	100	Oral	1–14
Prednisone	40	Oral	1–14
Repeat every 21 days			
ABVD			
Adriamycin (doxorubicin)	25	IV	1, 15
Bleomycin	10	IV	1, 15
Vinblastine	6	IV	1, 15
Dacarbazine	375	IV	1, 15
Repeat every 28 days			
MOPP/ABVD			
Alternating months of MOPP and ABVD			
MOPP/ABV hybrid			
Mechlorethamine	6	IV	1
Vincristine	1.4	IV	1
Procarbazine	100	Oral	1–7
Prednisone	40	Oral	1–14
Doxorubicin	35	IV	8
Bleomycin	10	IV	8
Vinblastine	6	IV	8
Repeat every 28 days			
Stanford V			
Doxorubicin	25	IV	Weeks 1, 3, 5, 7, 9, 11
Vinblastine	6	IV	Weeks 1, 3, 5, 7, 9, 11
Mechlorethamine	6	IV	Weeks 1, 5, 9
Etoposide	60	IV	Weeks 3, 7, 11
Vincristine	1.4ᵃ	IV	Weeks 2, 4, 6, 8, 10, 12
Bleomycin	5	IV	Weeks 2, 4, 6, 8
Prednisone	40	Oral	Every other day for 12 weeks; begin tapering at week 10
One course (12 weeks)			
BEACOPP (standard-dose)			
Bleomycin	10	IV	8
Etoposide	100	IV	1–3
Adriamycin (doxorubicin)	25	IV	1
Cyclophosphamide	650	IV	1
Oncovin (vincristine)	1.4ᵃ	IV	8
Procarbazine	100	Oral	1–7
Prednisone	40	Oral	1–14
Repeat every 21 days			
BEACOPP (escalated-dose)			
Bleomycin	10	IV	8
Etoposide	200	IV	1–3
Adriamycin (doxorubicin)	35	IV	1
Cyclophosphamide	1250	IV	1
Oncovin (vincristine)	1.4ᵃ	IV	8
Procarbazine	100	Oral	1–7
Prednisone	40	Oral	1–14
Granulocyte colony-stimulating factor		Subcutaneously	8+
Repeat every 21 days			

ᵃVincristine dose capped at 2 mg.

hybrid regimens is the decreased risk of long-term toxicities. In the alternating MOPP/ABVD regimen, the cumulative doses of procarbazine and mechlorethamine are reduced by 50% and the cumulative doxorubicin dose is reduced by 50%. In the hybrid regimen, the cumulative doxorubicin dose is reduced by 33% and the cumulative bleomycin dose is reduced by 50%.

Several clinical trials have been performed to evaluate the efficacy of alternating or hybrid MOPP/ABVD regimens. The results of these trials show that alternating and hybrid regimens are superior to MOPP but not to ABVD.[28] Another approach adopted by researchers was the administration of sequential cycles of MOPP and ABVD (MOPP → ABVD). Results of an intergroup

trial showed sequential MOPP and ABVD to be inferior to the MOPP/ABV hybrid regimen in terms of response and survival.[30] In another randomized comparison trial of the MOPP/ABV hybrid regimen and ABVD, the complete remission rate, failure-free survival, and overall survival were similar between the two regimens.[31] The latter trial was closed prematurely because of an increased number of treatment-related deaths and secondary malignancies in the patients who received the MOPP/ABV hybrid regimen.

More aggressive regimens such as Stanford V and BEACOPP have been evaluated as alternatives to MOPP or ABVD.[19] The Stanford V regimen generated significant interest because of the results of phase II trials.[23,32] Stanford V, ABVD, and a MOPP/ABV hybrid-like regimen (MOPPEBVCAD) were compared in a randomized trial to determine the best regimen to support a reduced radiotherapy program.[33] Five-year failure-free and progression-free survival were significantly worse for the Stanford V regimen as compared to the other two regimens. However, no significant differences in projected five-year progression-free and overall survival were observed between Stanford V and ABVD in a recently published randomized trial of patients with advanced Hodgkin lymphoma.[34] The investigators speculated that differences in the application of radiotherapy may explain the divergent results in the two randomized trials. More pulmonary toxicity occurred in the ABVD group, but other toxicities occurred more frequently in the Stanford V group.

The GHSG developed the BEACOPP regimens based on principles of dose density, dose intensity, and mathematical modeling. BEACOPP uses similar drugs as in the COPP/ABVD regimen (a combination of bleomycin, etoposide, doxorubicin, cyclophosphamide, vincristine, procarbazine, and prednisone), but rearranges the drugs in a shorter three-week cycle. Several different versions of BEACOPP have been developed: standard-dose BEACOPP, escalated-dose BEACOPP, and dose-dense BEACOPP (BEACOPP-14).[35] Granulocyte colony-stimulating factor support is required for the escalated-dose BEACOPP and BEACOPP-14 regimens.

Several randomized trials have compared BEACOPP to other regimens.[3,19] The GHSG conducted a randomized comparison of COPP/ABVD (alternating), BEACOPP, or an escalated-dose BEACOPP regimen in 1,201 patients with advanced Hodgkin lymphoma.[36] Most patients had advanced favorable disease and after chemotherapy, all patients received radiation to sites of bulky or residual disease. Escalated-dose BEACOPP appears to be the best regimen in this study with ten-year freedom from treatment failure at 82% and overall survival at 86%, but this regimen also appeared to be more toxic.[37] Despite filgrastim support, 90% of patients in the escalated-dose BEACOPP group had grade IV leukopenia, as compared with 19% in patients in the COPP/ABVD arm and 37% in the standard-dose BEACOPP arm. The higher rate of acute toxicity did not translate into a difference in acute treatment-related fatalities (<2% for all three regimens). The risk of toxic deaths due to sepsis or acute cardiac events was higher in elderly patients receiving BEACOPP.[38] Furthermore, the higher rates of leukemia among patients receiving escalated-dose BEACOPP (2.5% at 5 years follow up, and 3% at 10 years followup) as compared with those in the COPP/ABVD arm (0.4%) are of concern. Some experts recommend that these more intensive regimens should only be considered in patients with high-risk disease because of the potentially higher risk of secondary malignancies.

In a recently published study, the HD2000 trial compared three regimens in the treatment of advanced Hodgkin lymphoma: ABVD, BEACOPP, and CEC (cyclophosphamide, lomustine, vindesine, melphalan, prednisone, epirubicin, vincristine, procarbazine, vinblastine, bleomycin).[39] In this study, 370 patients were randomized to receive six cycles of ABVD, six cycles of CEC, or four cycles of escalated-dose BEACOPP with two cycles of standard-dose BEACOPP. The results of this trial showed that BEACOPP was superior to ABVD for five-year failure-free survival (78% vs. 65%, $P = 0.036$) and progression-free survival (81% vs. 68%, $P = 0.038$). However, five-year overall survival was not significantly different between ABVD and BEACOPP. It appears that BEACOPP may be superior to ABVD in patients with high-risk advanced Hodgkin lymphoma (IPS ≥3). Higher rates of neutropenia and severe infections were observed with BEACOPP as compared with ABVD. Further data is needed to determine whether BEACOPP is superior to ABVD in the treatment of advanced Hodgkin lymphoma.

CLINICAL CONTROVERSY

Some clinicians believe that escalated-dose BEACOPP is superior to ABVD in the treatment of patients with advanced-stage Hodgkin lymphoma. Escalated-dose BEACOPP has been shown to be superior to COPP/ABVD, which is similar to MOPP/ABVD. Other experts believe that ABVD is still the treatment of choice because escalated-dose BEACOPP has not been tested directly against it. They also express concern over the long-term toxicity with escalated-dose BEACOPP.

Risk-Adapted Therapy

Patients with advanced-stage Hodgkin lymphoma can be classified into two groups based on the number of prognostic factors present from the International Prognostic Index (Table 140–4). Advanced-stage patients with three or fewer poor prognostic factors are considered to have favorable disease and an approximately 60% likelihood of being failure-free at five years with traditional combination chemotherapy.[31] Advanced-stage patients with four or more poor prognostic factors are considered to have unfavorable disease and a less than 50% likelihood of being failure-free at five years with traditional combination chemotherapy. Due to the high treatment failure rate, the therapeutic goal for this group of high-risk patients is to improve antitumor control.

One recently published study has reported the feasibility of a risk-adapted treatment approach based on the IPS, with the goal of reducing cumulative doses of chemotherapy in patients with low-risk Hodgkin lymphoma.[40] Patients at low risk with early unfavorable disease and standard-risk patients with IPS of 2 or less were treated with two cycles of standard-dose BEACOPP, and high-risk patients with an IPS of 3 or higher were treated with two cycles of escalated-dose BEACOPP. After an interim gallium or PET/CT scan, patients with positive disease were given escalated-dose BEACOPP while patients who had negative disease were given standard-dose BEACOPP. For all patients, the complete remission rate, five-year event-free survival, and overall survival were 97%, 85%, and 90%, respectively. Although this was not a randomized study, the results suggested the feasibility of using a risk-adapted treatment modality in the treatment of advanced-stage Hodgkin lymphoma.

Currently, the NCCN guidelines suggest that escalated-dose BEACOPP be considered for patients with unfavorable disease because of the increase in efficacy. It is recommended that patients in advanced-stage disease with an IPS less than 4 should be treated with ABVD because of less-acute toxicity, the absent of sterility, and a low risk of secondary acute myeloid leukemia/myelodysplastic syndrome.[15]

Radiation

The role of low-dose consolidative radiation when added to chemotherapy for the treatment of advanced-stage Hodgkin lymphoma is controversial.[23] The rationale for its use is based on the radiosensitivity of Hodgkin lymphoma, a 20% to 40% relapse rate, and the tendency of Hodgkin lymphoma to relapse at sites of initial involvement.[41] Many clinical trials have been conducted to evaluate the benefit of additional radiation in patients who have a complete response to combination chemotherapy. The results of these studies are inconsistent, and a meta-analysis of 14 randomized trials showed a modest improvement in disease control at ten years, but no difference in overall survival.[42] In one study, patients with advanced disease were randomized to receive either involved-field radiation after MOPP/ABV hybrid chemotherapy or no further therapy. Eight-year event-free survival reported for patients achieving a complete response randomized to receive radiation, no radiation, and a group of partial responders who received radiation were 73%, 77% and 76%, respectively. These results suggest that radiation provides no benefit for patients who achieve a complete remission with chemotherapy. Furthermore, radiation was also associated with a higher risk of secondary cancers (12.9% vs. 5.6% in the radiation and no radiation arms, respectively). It does, however, show a significant role for consolidative radiation in patients who have a partial response after chemotherapy.[43]

Summary

In summary, the standard treatment of advanced-stage favorable Hodgkin lymphoma is six to eight cycles of ABVD chemotherapy. BEACOPP should be considered for patients with unfavorable disease. This risk-adapted approach should result in approximately 70% to >90% of patients achieving a complete remission and approximately 60% to 80% of patients being cured of their disease. No further treatment is needed for patients attaining a complete remission. Patients achieving a partial remission should receive consolidative radiation to residual sites of disease.

■ TREATMENT OF REFRACTORY OR RELAPSED DISEASE

④ The goal of salvage therapy is cure regardless of the site(s) of recurrence or primary therapy. With the increasing use of chemotherapy with or without radiation, regardless of disease extent, the rate of primary refractory disease is decreasing. Patients who do not achieve a complete remission with the initial regimen are considered to have primary refractory disease. These patients have a poor prognosis when treated with salvage chemotherapy, and therefore should be offered autologous HSCT as a treatment option.[44,45]

Patients who relapse after an initial complete response can be treated with the same regimen, a different potentially non–cross-resistant regimen, radiation, or high-dose chemotherapy and autologous HSCT (often preceded by conventional-dose chemotherapy). There is no data available from randomized trial comparing the cytoreductive regimens that are utilized before transplantation. However, as most patients are now treated with ABVD, doxorubicin should be avoided in salvage chemotherapy regimens if the cumulative dose has reach >400 mg/m^2, particularly in those patients who have received mediastinal radiotherapy because they are at much higher risk of cardiotoxicities.

The response to salvage therapy depends on the extent and site of recurrence, previous therapy, and duration of initial remission. Patients who relapse after radiation therapy alone have a good chance of being cured with combination chemotherapy, although fewer patients are being treated with radiation alone. High response rates (60% to 87%) have been observed with salvage chemotherapy regimens.[19,46] Other patient groups who have a favorable prognosis following salvage therapy include patients who experience a local recurrence in a nonirradiated location and those who relapse more than 1 year after completion of their initial chemotherapy. Patients who experience late relapses can be cured with retreatment with the same chemotherapy regimen, treatment with a different, potentially non–cross-resistant regimen, or high-dose chemotherapy and autologous HSCT.

Patients who have an early relapse (less than one year after treatment) generally respond poorly to standard-dose salvage chemotherapy. High-dose chemotherapy and autologous HSCT is more effective, but also produces a higher risk of treatment-related mortality. Therefore, the choice of salvage treatment should consider the patient's tolerance for a particular set of chemotherapeutic agents and treatment approach (standard-dose chemotherapy vs. high-dose chemotherapy and autologous HSCT).[45]

High-dose therapy should be considered in patients who relapse within 12 months of initial remission and in those who are refractory to first-line chemotherapy.[45] Although no single preparative regimen has been shown to be superior to another, most regimens do not include total-body irradiation because of its potential pulmonary toxicity. Most patients are already at higher risk for pulmonary toxicity because of previous exposure to one or more of the following: bleomycin, thoracic radiation, and nitrosoureas. Long-term effects of high-dose chemotherapy and autologous HSCT were elucidated in a recent study. Among 218 Hodgkin lymphoma patients who were treated with high-dose chemotherapy and autologous HSCT, 70% survived over two years. A total of 15 patients were diagnosed with a second malignancy and the median time from autologous HSCT to secondary malignancy diagnosis was nine years. The risk of secondary malignancy is possibly caused by high-dose etoposide in the rescue regimen, as well as those patients who were initially treated with MOPP chemotherapy.[47] Chapter 148 provides more details about high-dose chemotherapy and HSCT.

■ LONG-TERM COMPLICATIONS

A variety of acute and chronic toxicities may occur as a result of treatment for Hodgkin lymphoma. Long-term complications of radiation therapy, chemotherapy, and combined modality therapy have become more evident as the curability and long-term survival of Hodgkin lymphoma patients has improved.[2,3] Gonadal dysfunction (including sterility and hypothyroidism), secondary malignancies, and cardiopulmonary diseases have become important considerations in the treatment of this malignancy. Almost all men and up to 50% of premenopausal women treated with six cycles of regimens containing alkylating agents become sterile. This appears to be a dose-related phenomenon. For men, even a single dose of nitrogen mustard or chlorambucil can cause sterility, so if fertility is a major concern, ABVD may be the best alternative.[48]

The risk of secondary malignancies is increased about threefold in long-term survivors of Hodgkin lymphoma. The risk of developing leukemia carries the highest increase in risk and is seen with radiotherapy, chemotherapy, and chemoradiotherapy. Solid tumors, including breast cancers, gastrointestinal cancers and lung cancers are also likely to develop more than 10 years after the completion of treatment.[49-51] However, studies that evaluate the risk of secondary malignancies (and other complications) must be interpreted cautiously because many factors probably contribute to the development of secondary malignancies.[52] In addition, much of the long-term complication data is derived from patients who were treated with older regimens and extensive field radiotherapy, which are no longer commonly used in clinical practice. Furthermore, as minimal data is currently available on the appropriate follow-up duration and procedures to monitor for long-term effects, many of the recommendations in the NCCN guideline are based on clinical practice but not evidence-based information. Nonetheless, follow-up schedule should be personalized and patient-specific, after assessing a patient's potential risks for long-term complications.[15]

NON-HODGKIN LYMPHOMA

The NHLs are a heterogeneous group of lymphoproliferative disorders that affect individuals from early childhood to late adulthood. Advances in molecular biology techniques and our understanding of the human immune system have led to major progress in understanding the pathogenesis and treatment of the lymphomas. NHLs are classified into distinct clinical entities that are defined by a combination of morphology, immunophenotype, genetic features, and clinical features. These differences influence the natural history, and approach and response to treatment. The use of extensive combination chemotherapeutic regimens shows dramatic improvement in survival and cure in patients with a disease that was once considered incurable. The five-year survival rate for patients with NHL has increased from 48% to 71% over the past 25 years, and the mortality rate actually *declined* from 1997 to 2004.[4,5] Further improvement in survival is anticipated with the continued expansion of our therapeutic armamentarium, including high-dose chemotherapy and biologic therapy.

EPIDEMIOLOGY AND ETIOLOGY

NHL is the fifth most common cause of newly diagnosed cancer in the United States and accounts for approximately 4% of all cancers. An estimated 65,540 new cases will be diagnosed in 2010, and it is estimated that 20,210 people will die from NHL during this same period.[4] Although the average age of patients at the time of diagnosis is about 67 years, NHL can occur at any age. The incidence rate generally increases with age, and is higher in men than in women and in whites than in blacks.[5] The age-adjusted incidence rate of NHL increased by more than 80% in the United States since the early 1970s, from about 11 cases per 100,000 in 1975 to approximately 20 cases per 100,000 in 2003 and 2004.[5] The incidence of NHL increased by 3% to 4% from 1975 to 1991, but appears to have stabilized since reaching its peak in 1994. The increased incidence of NHL over the past three decades is second only to melanoma and has been referred to as an epidemic of NHL. Although the increase has been noted particularly among the elderly and patients with acquired immune deficiency syndrome (AIDS), much of it cannot be explained by known risk factors.

The etiology of NHL is unknown, although several genetic diseases, environmental agents, and infectious agents are associated with the development of NHL.[53-55] An increased incidence of NHL is seen in many congenital and acquired immunodeficiency states, supporting the role of immune dysregulation in the etiology of NHL.[54] Patients with congenital immunodeficiency disorders such as Wiskott-Aldrich syndrome and ataxia telangiectasia, acquired immunodeficiency disorders such as AIDS, and those receiving chronic pharmacologic immunosuppression in the setting of solid-organ transplantation are predisposed to the development of NHL. Autoimmune diseases (Hashimoto thyroiditis, Sjögren's syndrome) cause chronic inflammation in the mucosa-associated lymphoid tissue (MALT), which predisposes patients to subsequent lymphoid malignancies. Other autoimmune diseases, such as systemic lupus erythematosus and rheumatoid arthritis, are also associated with the development of NHL, but the use of immunosuppressive agents in these diseases makes the pathologic cause less clear.

Certain infections are associated with the development of lymphoma.[53,55] EBV was discovered in cell lines from tumors of patients with African (endemic) Burkitt lymphoma, and EBV DNA is associated with nearly all cases of endemic Burkitt lymphoma. However, EBV is associated with sporadic Burkitt lymphoma in 15% to 85% of cases. EBV is also associated with posttransplant lymphoproliferative disorders and some lymphomas in patients with AIDS or congenital immunodeficiencies. The human T-cell lymphotropic virus type 1 was the first human retrovirus associated with a malignancy. Infection with human T-cell lymphotropic virus type 1, especially in early childhood, is strongly associated with an aggressive form of T-cell lymphoma, known as adult T-cell leukemia/lymphoma. Human T-cell lymphotropic virus type 1 is endemic in parts of southern Japan, Africa, South America, and the Caribbean. In endemic areas, more than 50% of all NHL cases are adult T-cell leukemia/lymphoma. A third virus associated with NHL is human herpes virus 8 (also referred as

Kaposi sarcoma–associated herpesvirus [KSHV]). This virus was originally isolated from Kaposi sarcoma lesions in AIDS patients. Gastric infection with *Helicobacter pylori*, a gram-negative bacteria that leads to chronic gastritis, is associated with gastric MALT lymphomas. Finally, hepatitis C virus has been associated with splenic and nodal marginal zone lymphomas.

A number of physical agents are also associated with the development of NHL.[53,54] Exposure to herbicides, particularly phenoxyl herbicides, is associated with the development of NHL. These observations may explain why certain occupations, such as farmers, forestry workers, and agricultural workers, are associated with a higher risk of NHL. Exposure to lawn-care pesticides is also increasing in the general population. A higher risk of NHL is also associated with exposure to other chemical solvents and dyes, exposure to radiation from nuclear explosions, and high intake of meats and dietary fats. Smoking or alcohol consumption is not strongly associated with an increased risk of NHL.

MOLECULAR ABNORMALITIES

Chromosomal translocations have become a hallmark of many lymphoid malignancies.[56,57] The presence of these specific translocations can be helpful in the diagnosis and classification of lymphoid malignancies. The mechanisms leading to the translocations are unknown, but they usually involve the antigen receptor loci. In contrast to most myeloid and some lymphoid leukemias, NHLs usually place a structurally intact cellular protooncogene under the regulatory influence of highly expressed immunoglobulin or T-cell receptor genes, leading to effects on cell growth, cellular differentiation, or apoptosis. The most common chromosomal translocations involve t(8;14), t(14;18), and t(11;14); each translocation involves the immunoglobulin heavy-chain gene locus on chromosome 14 at 14q32. The translocation t(8;14) that involves c-*MYC*, a well-characterized oncogene clearly associated with malignancy, is implicated in nearly all cases of Burkitt lymphoma. The translocation t(14;18) that involves *BCL*-2, one of several putative B-cell lymphoma–associated oncogenes, is found in approximately 90% of cases of follicular B-cell lymphomas. The translocation t(11;14) that involves *BCL*-1 is found in about 70% of patients with mantle cell lymphoma. Another putative B-cell lymphoma–associated oncogene, *BCL*-6, is found in about one third of diffuse large B-cell lymphomas.

Although mutations in the *p53* tumor suppressor gene have been recognized in many human neoplasms, such mutations have not been consistently found in patients with lymphoma, which suggests that it may occur late in malignant evolution.

Because of their role in the pathogenesis of lymphoma, oncogenes are attractive molecular targets for the development of new and novel therapies.[58]

PATHOLOGY AND CLASSIFICATION

NHLs are neoplasms derived from the monoclonal proliferation of malignant B or T lymphocytes and their precursors. Approximately 85% to 90% of NHLs in the United States are of B-cell origin.[54] Proliferation of malignant cells results in the replacement of the normal cells and architecture of lymph nodes or bone marrow with a relatively uniform population of lymphoid cells. The classification of NHLs has evolved over the last five decades, as advances in immunology and genetics have allowed scientists to recognize a number of previously unrecognized subtypes of NHLs (Table 140–6).[11,59] The current classification schemes characterize the NHLs according to the cell of origin (B cell vs. T cell), clinical features, and morphologic features. Additional immunohistochemical markers, cytogenetic features, and genotypic characteristics may also be of help to further classify NHL into subtypes.

TABLE 140-6	Evolution in the Classification of Non-Hodgkin Lymphomas	
Time	**Classification System**	**Basis for Classification**
1950s–1960s	Rappaport	Morphology
1970s–1980s	Luke–Collins	Morphology and immunophenotype
1970s–1980s	Kiel	Morphology and immunophenotype
1980s–1990s	International Working Formulation	Morphology and clinical behavior
1990s	REAL	Disease entities
2001	WHO	Disease entities

REAL, Revised European–American Classification of Lymphoid Neoplasms developed by the International Lymphoma Study Group; WHO, World Health Organization.

Morphology

The macroscopic and microscopic appearance of the involved tissue remains one of the most important factors in the diagnosis and classification of NHLs.[11,59] In the 1950s, Rappaport et al. proposed a morphologic classification of malignant lymphomas based on two features: that the malignant cell would disrupt the nodal architecture in a *nodular* or *diffuse* manner, and that lymphomas of histiocytic origin existed. The Rappaport classification gained rapid acceptance in the United States because of its precision, simplicity, and prognostic significance. Application of the system divided NHLs into those with large (i.e., incorrectly called "histiocytes") or small cells, with or without a nodular (i.e., follicular) growth pattern.

Immunology

In the 1970s, it became apparent that NHLs were tumors of the immune system and were derived from B or T lymphocytes. The availability of techniques using antibodies to antigens on the surface of lymphoid cells (i.e., immunophenotype) and cytochemical assays led to the following conclusions: most NHLs were of B-cell origin; all follicular or nodular lymphomas were of follicle center cell origin; and most lymphomas previously classified as reticulum cell sarcoma, clasmatocytic lymphoma, or histiocytic lymphoma had the immunologic characteristics of transformed lymphocytes. Using this new information, expert pathologists independently developed new classification schemes for NHL in the 1970s and 1980s.[11,59] The Kiel classification was based primarily on the work of Lennert in Germany and became widely used in Europe. In North America, the Lukes and Collins classification scheme was used briefly, but was soon superseded by the Working Formulation. Like the Rappaport classification, divisions within the Working Formulation were based largely on cell size (large [histiocytic] vs. small [lymphocytic]), cell shape (round vs. not round), and growth pattern (follicular [nodular] vs. diffuse). Both the Kiel and Working Formulation classification schemes considered the histologic grade of the tumor, but only the Working Formulation considered actual survival curves of patients with the various subtypes of NHL. *Low-grade* indicated longer median survival (i.e., indolent) whereas *intermediate-grade* and *high-grade* indicated shorter median survival (i.e., aggressive). In the 1980s and early 1990s, the Working Formulation became the most widely used classification scheme in North America, whereas the Kiel classification was widely used in Europe and Asia. It was based on the premise that NHL was a single disease with a range of histologic grades and clinical aggressiveness.

New Disease Entities

In the 1980s and early 1990s, rapid advances in immunology and genetics allowed scientists to recognize a number of previously unrecognized subtypes of NHLs. Cytogenetic and molecular genetic analyses identified the presence of many chromosomal translocations, oncogenes, and their gene products in patients with NHL (see Molecular Abnormalities later in this chapter). In addition, diseases that would have been lumped together as low-grade or intermediate/high grade in the Working Formulation showed marked differences in survival, which prompted scientists to reevaluate lymphoma classification schemes.

Information from these studies allowed scientists to further classify B-cell lymphomas as malignant expansions of cells from the germinal center, mantle zone, or marginal zone of normal lymph nodes (Table 140–1).[11,60,61] Germinal centers are complex structures that form in the spleen and lymph nodes in response to antigenic challenge. In addition to B cells, germinal centers contain antigen-presenting cells and helper T cells that cooperate in mediating the B-cell changes that result in a more potent secondary immune response. Malignant transformation often occurs or is initiated in germinal center B cells. Follicular, Burkitt, and most large cell lymphomas are believed to be tumors of germinal center B cells. Three histologically distinct microenvironments have been described within the germinal center: a mantle zone surrounding interior, dark, and light zones. The mantle zone contains small resting B cells that have not been exposed to antigens (naïve). Tumors of cells from the mantle zone are usually clinically indolent and histologically low grade. Antigen-triggered activation of the densely packed B cells of the dark zone causes cells to proliferate and subjects genomic DNA to somatic hypermutation. Surviving clones from within the dark zone then enter the light zone where proliferation slows and affinity selection occurs. During affinity selection, only cells with surface immunoglobulin receptors with high affinity for the antigen survive. Antigen-specific B cells generated in the germinal center reaction leave the follicle and reappear in the outer mantle zone, to form a marginal zone. Marginal zones are particularly prominent in mesenteric lymph nodes, Peyer patches, and the spleen. These post-germinal center B cells include memory B cells of the marginal zone and plasma cells. Marginal cell B-cell lymphomas tend to be indolent and may be either extranodal or nodal; extranodal marginal cell B-cell lymphomas are also referred to as MALT lymphomas.

T-cell lymphomas can be classified on the basis of antigen expression as either precursor (thymic) or mature (peripheral) in origin. These classifications clinically translate to precursor lymphoblastic lymphomas or to a heterogeneous group of peripheral T-cell lymphomas. Tumors of natural killer or natural killer-like T cells are uncommon.

The International Lymphoma Study Group, an informal group of 19 hematopathologists from the United States, Europe, and Asia, adopted a new approach to lymphoma classification in 1993. Because it represented a revision of current or prior European and American lymphoma classifications, it was called the Revised European–American Classification of Lymphoid Neoplasms (REAL). The REAL classification system is based on the principle that a classification is a list of "real" disease entities, which are defined by a combination of morphology, immunophenotype, genetic features, and clinical features.[11,59] The relative importance of each of these criteria for both definition and diagnosis differs among different diseases. Morphology is always important, and some diseases are primarily defined by morphology alone (e.g., follicular lymphoma), although immunophenotype can be helpful in difficult cases. Some diseases have a specific immunophenotype (e.g., mantle cell lymphoma, small lymphocytic lymphoma) that is virtually diagnostic of that disease. A specific genetic abnormality is important in some lymphomas—t(11;14) in mantle cell lymphoma, t(8;14) in Burkitt lymphoma, and t(14;18) in follicular lymphoma—whereas other lymphomas lack specific genetic abnormalities (e.g., MALT lymphoma, diffuse large B-cell lymphoma). Finally, other lymphomas consider clinical features (e.g., extranodal vs. nodal presentation in marginal zone lymphoma and peripheral T-cell lymphoma).

Since 1995, members of the European and American Hematopathology societies have worked to develop a new WHO classification of hematologic malignancies. The final classification was published in 2001 and revised in 2008.[13] The WHO classification uses an updated version of the REAL classification and expands the principles of the REAL classification to the classification of myeloid and lymphoid malignancies.

❺ The 2008 WHO classification categorizes lymphoid malignancies into two major categories: B-cell lymphomas and T-cell (and natural killer cell) lymphomas (Table 140–2).[11,13,59] B-cell lymphomas represent about 85% to 90% of all NHLs. Lymphomas within each category can be divided into malignancies of precursor or mature cells. Hodgkin lymphoma and multiple myeloma are now recognized as mature B-cell neoplasms. The WHO classification uses the term *grade* to refer to histologic parameters such as cell and nuclear size, density of chromatin, and proliferation fraction, and the term *aggressiveness* to denote clinical behavior of a tumor. This classification scheme includes both lymphomas and lymphoid leukemias because there is no distinction between the solid and circulating forms of these diseases. The WHO classification includes several previously unrecognized types of lymphomas, and new entities not specifically recognized in the Working Formulation account for approximately 20% to 25% of the cases.

The WHO classification has broad clinical implications. The WHO Clinical Advisory Committee has agreed that clinical groupings of lymphoid neoplasms into prognostic categories are neither necessary nor desirable because such arbitrary groupings are of no practical value and may be misleading.[62] Treatment of a specific patient should be determined not by the broad prognostic group into which the patient's neoplasm falls but by the specific type of neoplasm, with the addition of grade *within* the tumor type (if applicable), and clinical prognostic factors.

CLINICAL PRESENTATION

❻ Patients with NHL present with a wide variety of symptoms, depending on the site of involvement and whether tumor involvement is nodal or extranodal.[63] Sites of involvement and dissemination of the malignant cells can sometimes be predicted based on the cell of origin and the tendency of tumors to frequently disseminate to areas where the normal counterparts of the lymphoma cells are located. For example, B-cell lymphomas involve areas of the lymphoid system normally populated by B-lymphocytes, such as lymph nodes, spleen, and bone marrow. T-cell lymphomas commonly disseminate to various extranodal sites, such as the skin and lungs.

Most patients present with peripheral lymphadenopathy.[63] The lymphadenopathy may be either localized or generalized, and the involved nodes are often painless, rubbery, and discrete, and usually located in the cervical and supraclavicular regions as in Hodgkin lymphoma (Fig. 140–1). Rapid and progressive lymphadenopathy is more characteristic of aggressive lymphomas. Waxing and waning of lymph nodes, including their complete disappearance and reappearance, is more characteristic of indolent lymphomas. Massive lymphadenopathy can sometimes lead to organ dysfunction. For example, patients with NHL may present with acute renal failure from retroperitoneal adenopathy causing ureteral obstruction or from metabolic abnormalities such as hyperuricemia with uric acid nephropathy.

Approximately 40% of patients with NHL present with fever (temperature >38°C [100.4°F]), weight loss (unexplained weight loss of 10% of body weight over the past 6 months), or night sweats (drenching night sweats). If one or more of these symptoms is present, the patient is noted to have B symptoms, and a B is added to the stage of disease (discussed in the Diagnosis, Staging, and Prognostic Factors section under Hodgkin Lymphoma earlier in this chapter). B symptoms are more commonly observed in patients with aggressive NHLs.

CLINICAL PRESENTATION OF NON-HODGKIN LYMPHOMA

General

- Patients with NHL present with a wide variety of symptoms, depending on the site of involvement and whether tumor involvement is nodal or extranodal.

Symptoms

- Approximately 40% of patients present with fever, night sweats, and weight loss (i.e., B symptoms).
- Fatigue, malaise, and pruritus.

Signs

- More than two thirds of patients present with peripheral lymphadenopathy.

Laboratory Tests

- A complete blood count, tests of renal and liver function, and serum electrolytes should be obtained.
- Serum β_2-microglobulin and lactate dehydrogenase levels may be useful as prognostic factors and for monitoring response to therapy.

Other Diagnostic Tests

- Varies depending on sites of involvement.

Patients with Hodgkin lymphoma rarely present with extranodal (i.e., extralymphatic) disease, but 10% to 35% of patients with NHL have primary extranodal disease at the time of diagnosis.[63] The frequency of extranodal presentation varies dramatically among different subtypes. The most common extranodal sites are the gastrointestinal tract followed by the skin. The liver or spleen may be enlarged in patients with generalized adenopathy. Patients with mesenteric or gastrointestinal involvement may present with signs and symptoms of nausea, vomiting, obstruction, abdominal pain, a palpable abdominal mass, or gastrointestinal bleeding. Patients with bone marrow involvement may have symptoms related to anemia, neutropenia, or thrombocytopenia. Other sites of extranodal disease include the testes and bone. The incidence of solitary brain lymphoma is increasing, especially in patients with AIDS.

DIAGNOSIS, STAGING, AND PROGNOSTIC FACTORS

As with Hodgkin lymphoma, the diagnosis of NHL must be established by pathologic review of tissue obtained by biopsy.[63] The preferred procedure is an excisional biopsy, where the entire involved lymph node is removed for review by an experienced hematopathologist. This procedure should be done carefully to prevent distortional artifact of the architecture, which could lead to an inaccurate diagnosis. Needle biopsy of the node can sometimes provide adequate tissue for pathologic diagnosis, if an excisional biopsy cannot be performed. When adenopathy is not present, diagnosis may be established by biopsy of cutaneous lesions, bone marrow biopsy and aspiration in patients with unexplained myelosuppression, liver biopsy in patients with hepatomegaly or elevated liver function tests, or biopsy of involved extranodal organs, such as bone, Waldeyer ring, lung, and testis.

After the diagnosis is established, further workup is required to determine the extent of involvement.[56,63,64] Clinical staging always begins with a thorough history and physical examination. Patients should be questioned about the presence or absence and extent of fever, night sweats, and weight loss. A detailed history of lymphadenopathy should also be obtained, including when and where the lymph nodes were first noted, and their rate of growth. A complete physical examination is performed to assess the extent

TABLE 140-7 Clinical Characteristics of Patients with Common Types of Non-Hodgkin Lymphomas

Disease	Median Age (Years)	Frequency in Children	% Male	Stage I/II vs. III/IV (%)	B Symptoms (%)	BM Involvement (%)	GI Tract Involvement (%)	% Surviving 5 years
B-cell chronic lymphocytic leukemia/small lymphocytic lymphoma	65	Rare	53	9 vs. 91	33	72	3	51
Mantle cell lymphoma	63	Rare	74	20 vs. 80	28	64	9	27
Extranodal marginal zone B-cell lymphoma of MALT type	60	Rare	48	67 vs. 33	19	14	50	74
Follicular lymphoma	59	Rare	42	33 vs. 67	28	42	4	72
Diffuse large B-cell lymphoma	64	≈25% of childhood NHL	55	54 vs. 46	33	16	18	46
Burkitt lymphoma	31	≈30% of childhood NHL	89	62 vs. 38	22	33	11	45
Precursor T-cell lymphoblastic lymphoma	28	≈40% of childhood NHL	64	11 vs. 89	21	50	4	26
Anaplastic large T-/null cell lymphoma	34	Common	69	51 vs. 49	53	13	9	77
Peripheral T-cell non-Hodgkin lymphoma	61	≈5% of childhood NHL	55	20 vs. 80	50	36	15	25

BM, bone marrow; GI, gastrointestinal; MALT, mucosa-associated lymphoid tissue; NHL, non-Hodgkin lymphoma

From Longo DL. Malignancies of Lymphoid Cells. In: Fauci AS, Braunwald E, Kasper DL, et al. eds. Harrison's Principles of Internal Medicine. 17th ed. New York, NY: McGraw-Hill, 2008.

of disease involvement, with special attention given to all nodal areas (Fig. 140–1). All patients should have a complete blood count, serum chemistries including liver and renal profiles, a chest radiograph, and bone marrow aspiration and biopsy. The likelihood of bone marrow involvement varies among the different histologic types of lymphoma (Table 140–7). Lumbar puncture to evaluate the cerebrospinal fluid is recommended in patients who have histologic types of lymphoma that often spread to the CNS.

Imaging studies are usually important in the staging workup.[63,64] CT scanning can identify both nodal and extranodal sites of disease, and has largely replaced lymphangiography for the evaluation of retroperitoneal lymphadenopathy. The abdominal and pelvic CT scan can identify mesenteric and retrocrural node involvement. CT scans can also detect tumor involvement of organs, including the kidneys, ovary, spleen, and liver. PET is currently not used routinely for staging of NHL.[64,65] Magnetic resonance imaging is of limited usefulness in the staging of NHL. Gallium scans are sometimes used as part of the staging work up. Other tests, such as liver–spleen scan, bone scan, upper gastrointestinal series, and intravenous pyelogram, are sometimes useful in patients with organ symptomatology or serum chemistry abnormalities.

Although staging laparotomy was widely used in the late 1960s and 1970s as part of the staging workup in patients with lymphoma, it is rarely used today because of technical improvements in imaging studies and the morbidity and potential mortality associated with the procedure.

The Ann Arbor staging classification developed for the clinical staging of Hodgkin lymphoma is also used to stage patients with NHL (see Table 140–3). After completion of the staging workup, most patients will be found to have advanced disease (stages III and IV). The frequency of localized disease at the time of diagnosis varies depending on the histologic type of lymphoma (Table 140–7). Stage is a more important prognostic factor in Hodgkin lymphoma than in NHL.

❼ The Ann Arbor system emphasizes the distribution of nodal disease sites because Hodgkin lymphoma usually spreads through contiguous lymph nodes and does not involve extranodal sites. But NHL is a disease with tremendous heterogeneity that does not spread through contiguous lymph nodes and that often involves extranodal sites. As a result of these clinical differences between Hodgkin lymphoma and NHL, Ann Arbor stage correlates poorly with prognosis.

❽ This lack of accuracy with the Ann Arbor staging system in NHL has led to several international projects to develop prognostic models for the most common types of NHLs—diffuse large B-cell

lymphomas and follicular lymphomas. The International Non-Hodgkin Lymphoma Prognostic Factors Project was based on more than 2,000 patients with diffuse aggressive lymphomas treated with an anthracycline-containing combination chemotherapy regimen in the United States, Europe, and Canada.[66] The Project identified five risk factors that correlated with low response to chemotherapy and poor survival: age >60 years, reduced performance status ≥2, abnormal serum lactate dehydrogenase (LDH) levels, two or more extranodal sites of disease, and advanced tumor stage (Ann Arbor stages III or IV) (Table 140–8). In patients ≤60 years old, three risk factors correlated with low response to chemotherapy and poor survival: reduced performance status, abnormal serum LDH levels, and Ann Arbor stage. It is unclear whether the effect of serum LDH level is related to a tumor or a host event. LDH likely measures cellular catabolism (the enzyme is released from injured cells), or the product of tumor

TABLE 140-8 Risk Factors and Survival According to the International Non-Hodgkin Lymphoma Prognostic Factors Project

All Patients	Patients ≤ 60 Years of Age
Age >60 years	Abnormal LDH level
Abnormal LDH level	Performance status ≥2
Performance status ≥2	Ann Arbor stage III or IV
Ann Arbor stage III or IV	
Extranodal involvement ≥2 sites	

Risk Group	Number of Risk Factors	Complete Response Rate (%)	5-Year Survival Rate (%)
Patients of all ages (% of patients)			
Low (35)	0, 1	87	73
Low intermediate (27)	2	67	51
High intermediate (22)	3	55	43
High (16)	4, 5	44	26
Patients ≤60 years of age (% of patients)			
Low (22)	0	92	83
Low intermediate (32)	1	78	69
High intermediate (32)	2	57	46
High (14)	3	46	32

LDH, lactic dehydrogenase

Data from The International Non-Hodgkin's Lymphoma Prognostic Factors Project. A predictive model for aggressive non-Hodgkin's lymphoma. N Engl J Med 1993;329:987–994. Copyright © 1993 Massachusetts Medical Society.

burden and proliferation. Because each of the factors has about the same impact (e.g., relative risk) on prognosis, the number of adverse risk factors is summed to provide the International Prognostic Index (IPI). Patients could, therefore, have a score of 0 to 5. Table 140–8 shows the correlation between four risk groups based on the IPI score and complete response rate and five-year survival. For patients ≤60 years old, a simplified IPI score can be developed based on Ann Arbor stage, serum LDH level, and performance status.

As prognosis improves as a result of more effective therapy, it is important to reevaluate prognostic factors. The IPI was based on patients treated from 1982 to 1987 with anthracycline-based combination chemotherapy; none of the patients received rituximab. In a reexamination of the IPI in a cohort of patients treated with rituximab-containing chemotherapy, Sehn et al. found that the IPI remained predictive but it only identified two, rather than four, risk groups.[67] When the number of risk factors is redistributed, three risk groups are identified that correlate with prognosis. This revised IPI score may more accurately predict prognosis in patients treated with rituximab-containing combination chemotherapy, but needs to be validated in a larger group of patients.

Although the IPI is often used to predict prognosis in patients with other NHL subtypes, the IPI has several shortcomings when applied to patients with indolent lymphomas. Because only patients with diffuse aggressive lymphomas were used to develop the IPI system, some important prognostic factors may have been missed. Furthermore, the IPI system has limited discriminating power in follicular lymphoma because only approximately 10% of patients are categorized as high-risk in the IPI system. To address these concerns, an international cooperative study was designed to develop a prognostic model similar to the IPI in patients with follicular lymphoma. The results of that study, which was based on more than 4,000 patients with follicular lymphoma diagnosed between 1985 and 1992, were recently published.[68] Five factors were identified that correlated with poor survival: age >60 years, advanced tumor stage (Ann Arbor stage III or IV), low hemoglobin level (<12 g/dL [<120 g/L; 7.45 mmol/L]), five or more nodal sites of disease (Fig. 140–1), and an abnormal serum LDH level. Analogous to the IPI, the number of adverse risk factors is summed to provide the Follicular Lymphoma International Prognostic Index (FLIPI). Three prognostic groups were identified: low-risk (0 to 1 factors), intermediate-risk (2 factors), and high-risk (≥3 factors). The new system appeared to have higher discriminating power among groups as compared with the IPI system. Table 140–9 shows the correlation between the FLIPI score and overall survival. The survival data may not reflect current figures because none of the patients used to derive the FLIPI were treated with rituximab.

Although IPI and FLIPI are clinically useful tools to estimate prognosis, the factors used to calculate these scores probably represent clinical surrogates for the biologic heterogeneity among NHLs and many researchers are interested in determining the prognostic importance of certain phenotypic and molecular characteristics of NHLs. For example, markers of apoptosis, cell-cycle regulation, cell lineage, and cell proliferation are being evaluated as potentially clinically useful prognostic factors.[69]

Gene expression profiling with microarrays may also correlate with survival. Using gene expression profiling, investigators identified at least two molecularly distinct forms of diffuse large B-cell lymphomas based on gene expression patterns indicative of different stages of B-cell differentiation: germinal center B-cell–like (GCB) and activated B-cell–like (ABC).[70] The GCB subtype of diffuse large B-cell lymphoma probably arises from normal germinal center B-cells while the ABC subtype may arise from post-germinal center B-cells. Many oncogenic pathways are different for the GCB and ABC subtypes, and these differences may lead to the development of targeted therapies for each subtype.[61] Patients with the germinal center B-cell profile had significantly better overall survival independent of IPI score after treatment with CHOP (cyclophosphamide, doxorubicin, Oncovin, prednisone) or CHOP-like chemotherapy. In a recently published study of patients with diffuse large B-cell lymphoma treated with either CHOP or rituximab and CHOP (R-CHOP), Lenz et al. identified several gene expressions signatures that predicted survival in both CHOP and R-CHOP cohorts: GCB, stromal-1, and stromal-2.[71] The GCB and stromal-1 signatures were associated with a favorable prognosis while the stromal-2 signature was associated with an unfavorable prognosis. The stromal-1 signature reflects extracellular matrix deposition and histiocytic infiltration whereas the stromal-2 signature reflects tumor blood vessel density. The authors speculated that diffuse large B-cell lymphomas that express the stromal-2 signature may respond to antiangiogenic agents.

Two molecularly distinct profiles of follicular lymphoma also have been identified; the first included genes encoding for T-cell markers and genes highly expressed in macrophages, and the second included genes that are preferentially expressed in macrophages, dendritic cells, or both.[72] Patients with the first molecular signature had a more favorable outcome than those with the second signature. These results suggest that molecular classification of tumors on the basis of gene expression may allow identification of clinically significant subtypes of cancer.

TREATMENT

Non-Hodgkin Lymphoma

■ GENERAL TREATMENT PRINCIPLES

The primary goals in the treatment of NHL are to relieve symptoms, cure the patient of the disease whenever possible, and minimize the risk of serious toxicities. The treatment strategy depends on many factors, including the patient's age, concomitant disease, disease type, stage of disease, site of disease, and patient preference.

❾ Historically, both the clinical behavior and degree of aggressiveness are often used to describe NHLs. Indolent lymphomas, which make up approximately 25% to 40% of all NHLs, are characterized by their slow-growth behavior. Patients with an indolent lymphoma usually have a relatively long survival (measured in years), with or without aggressive chemotherapy. Although these lymphomas respond to a wide range of therapeutic approaches, there is no convincing evidence of a survival plateau, which indicates that patients are rarely cured of their disease. In contrast,

TABLE 140–9	Risk Factors and Survival According to the Follicular Lymphoma International Prognostic Index

All Patients

Age >60 years
Ann Arbor stage III or IV
Number of nodal sites ≥5
Abnormal lactate dehydrogenase level
Hemoglobin <12 g/dL [<120 g/L; 7.45 mmol/L]

Risk Group (% of Patients)	Number of Risk Factors	5-Year Overall Survival (%)	10-Year Overall Survival (%)
Low (36)	0–1	91	71
Intermediate (37)	2	78	51
High (27)	≥3	53	36

Adapted from Solal-Celigny P, Roy P, Colombat P, et al. Follicular lymphoma international prognostic index. Blood 2004;104:1258–1265.

aggressive lymphomas, which make up approximately 60% to 75% of all NHLs, are characterized by rapid growth rate and short survival (measured in weeks to months), if appropriate therapy is not initiated. Despite their more aggressive nature, many patients with aggressive lymphomas who respond to chemotherapy can experience prolonged disease-free survival and some are cured of their disease. Therefore, the terminology for the NHLs represents a paradox, where "indolent" is bad and "aggressive" is good in terms of the likelihood for cure.

Therapeutic approaches to NHL include radiation therapy, chemotherapy, and biologic agents. The role of radiation therapy in the treatment of NHL differs from its role in the treatment of Hodgkin lymphoma. Although the disease responds to radiation therapy, only a small percentage of patients with NHL present with truly localized disease that can be treated with local or regional radiation therapy. Radiation therapy is used more commonly in advanced disease, primarily as a palliative measure to control local bulky disease.

Effective chemotherapy for NHL ranges from single-agent therapy in indolent lymphomas to aggressive, complex chemotherapy regimens in aggressive lymphomas. The most active agents used in the treatment of NHL include the alkylating agents (e.g., cyclophosphamide, chlorambucil), bleomycin, doxorubicin, purine analogs, etoposide, methotrexate, vincristine, and corticosteroids (e.g., prednisone, dexamethasone). The most aggressive chemotherapy approaches are dose-dense chemotherapy or high-dose chemotherapy followed by autologous or allogeneic HSCT.

B-cell lymphomas have served as a model for immunotherapy with monoclonal antibodies for more than 20 years, beginning with the successful use of custom-made monoclonal antibodies targeted against the idiotype present on the patient's cancer cells.[73,74] These encouraging results lead to the development of monoclonal antibodies against a more generic target, a molecule on the surface of B cells that would be present on tumor cells. One potential target, the CD20 molecule, is present only on cells in the B-lymphocyte lineage. It is expressed on the surface of both normal and malignant B cells, but not on other normal tissues. Rituximab (Rituxan®) is a chimeric monoclonal antibody directed at the CD20 molecule. Its antitumor activity is mediated through complement-dependent cytotoxicity, antibody-dependent cytotoxicity, and induction of apoptosis.[74] Since rituximab was approved in November 1997 to treat relapsed or refractory indolent or follicular CD20+ lymphomas, it has become one of the most widely used therapies for NHL. More recently, two radiolabeled monoclonal antibodies (i.e., radioimmunoconjugates) targeted against the CD20 antigen were approved. With the availability of monoclonal antibodies and radioimmunoconjugates for the therapy of lymphoma, nearly all patients with NHL will receive one or more biologic agents during the course of their disease.

Objective response to therapy for NHL should be defined according to the International Workshop to Standardize Response Criteria for Non-Hodgkin Lymphoma, which was recently updated to incorporate the results of newer tests to monitor response such as PET, immunohistochemistry, and flow cytometry.[65] The revised guidelines describe criteria for response (e.g., complete response, partial response, and stable disease) and survival (e.g., overall, disease-free, event-free, progression-free).

Appropriate therapy for NHL depends on the patient's age, histologic type, stage of disease, site of disease, and presence of adverse prognostic factors (as measured by IPI or FLIPI score), and patient preferences. In general, treatment of lymphoma can be divided into limited disease and advanced disease. Limited disease includes those patients with localized disease (Ann Arbor stages I and II). Advanced disease is defined as all Ann Arbor stage III or IV patients, and also frequently includes Ann Arbor stage II patients with poor prognostic features (Tables 140–8 and 140–9).[66,68]

The following section discusses the clinical characteristics and therapy of the most common disease entities.

■ INDOLENT LYMPHOMAS

Follicular Lymphomas

The combined group of follicular lymphomas makes up the second most common histologic type of NHL in the United States, comprising approximately 20% of all NHLs worldwide and up to 70% of indolent lymphomas reported in American and European clinical trials.[75] The WHO classification includes criteria for grading follicular lymphoma based on the number of centroblasts per high-power field: grade 1 to 2 (0 to 15 centroblasts/high-power field) and grade 3 (>15 centroblasts/high-power field).[13] The clinical behavior and treatment outcome of grades 1 and 2 follicular lymphoma are similar, and they are usually treated as indolent lymphomas. In contrast, grade 3 follicular lymphoma is synonymous with what is often referred to as follicular large cell lymphoma and is usually treated as an aggressive lymphoma.

Follicular lymphomas tend to occur in older adults, with a slight female predominance (Table 140–7). Most patients have advanced disease at diagnosis, but approximately 25% to 33% of patients have localized disease (clinical stage I or II) at diagnosis.[76] Extranodal disease, bulky disease, and B symptoms are uncommon features at diagnosis. Most patients with follicular lymphoma have the chromosomal translocation t(14;18) at the time of diagnosis.

The clinical course is generally indolent, with median survivals of eight to ten years. But the natural history of follicular lymphoma can be unpredictable. Spontaneous regression of objective disease has been noted in as many as 20% to 30% of patients.[77] There is also a high conversion rate of follicular lymphoma to a more aggressive histology over time that steadily increases after diagnosis and reaches approximately 30% at ten years.[78] At autopsy, most patients with follicular lymphoma have some evidence of diffuse large B-cell lymphoma. Patients with transformed indolent lymphoma should be treated in the same way as patients with an aggressive lymphoma.

Most patients have dramatic responses to initial therapy, and their disease course is characterized by multiple relapses, with responses to salvage therapy becoming progressively shorter after every relapse, eventually leading to death from disease-related causes.[77] This pattern of constant relapses over time without evidence of a survival plateau and the failure of randomized controlled trials to show a survival benefit with aggressive chemotherapy led to the conclusion that therapy does not prolong overall survival and patients are not cured of their disease. However, several recently published studies suggest that the use of biologic agents, particularly rituximab, has changed the natural history of the follicular lymphoma. In a study of patients enrolled in Southwest Oncology Group (SWOG) trials over a period of more than 20 years, patients treated with CHOP and a monoclonal antibody had a significantly longer four-year overall survival than those treated with CHOP alone (91% vs. 69%).[79] Similar results were reported in patients treated over a 30-year period at the M.D. Anderson Cancer Center.[80] That study also showed an apparent plateau in the failure-free survival curve.

Certain subsets of patients with follicular lymphoma have a much better or worse prognosis.[69] Some studies suggest that the natural history of follicular large cell lymphoma (i.e., grade 3 follicular lymphoma) is similar to that of other aggressive lymphomas and that treatment with intensive combination chemotherapy regimens may result in long-term disease-free survival, including a possible plateau in the survival curve.[75] The recent development of the FLIPI prognostic model should help clinicians to identify patients in different prognostic groups based on disease characteristics at the time of diagnosis.[68] Patients who are predicted to have a poor prognosis (i.e., high-risk) could then be offered aggressive or experimental therapy, whereas those who are predicted to have a good prognosis (i.e., low-risk) would be treated with standard therapy, avoiding unnecessary toxicity.

Treatment of Localized Disease (Stages I and II) Radiation therapy is the standard treatment for early-stage follicular lymphoma. Involved-field, extended-field, and total nodal irradiation have been used. Carefully staged patients with either stage I or contiguous stage II disease treated with radiation therapy alone can achieve disease-free survival rates of 40% to 50% and overall survival rates of 60% to 70% at ten years.[75] Late relapses are uncommon; only 10% of patients who reached ten years without relapse subsequently experienced a recurrence.

Chemotherapy is not usually given in most patients with localized follicular lymphoma, but it may be helpful in some patients with high-risk stage II disease (e.g., multiple sites of involvement or bulky disease).[81]

❿ Approximately 40% to 60% of patients with clinical stage I or II follicular lymphoma are cured of their disease with radiation therapy alone.[75] Most centers use radiation at a dose of 30 to 40 Gy (3000 to 4000 rad) to either involved (i.e., local) or regional fields, which would consist of irradiation to the involved nodal region plus one additional uninvolved region on each side of the involved nodes. Extended-field irradiation is not usually used because of the absence of a survival benefit and possible increased risk of secondary malignancies. In addition, previous use of extended-field irradiation compromises the ability of that patient to receive subsequent chemotherapy. The current NCCN guidelines state that locoregional radiation therapy is preferred for most patients with early-stage follicular lymphoma.[64] Immunotherapy (i.e., rituximab) with or without chemotherapy or radiation therapy is also listed as an option (category 2B).

Treatment of Advanced Disease (Stages III and IV) ❿ The management of stages III and IV indolent lymphomas remains controversial because until recently, no therapeutic approaches had been shown to prolong overall survival despite the high complete remission rates to initial therapy. However, the results of recently published studies suggest that the initial use of biologic therapy such as rituximab is associated with longer overall survival.[79,80] More than 80% of patients with stage III or IV follicular lymphoma are alive at five years, and the median survival ranges between seven and ten years.

Therapeutic options for these patients are diverse and include watchful waiting, radiation therapy, single-agent chemotherapy, combination chemotherapy, biologic therapy, radioimmunotherapy, and combined-modality therapy.[75,82] Although complete remission can be achieved in 50% to 80% of patients with various treatments, the median time to relapse is usually only 18 to 36 months. Approximately 20% of patients who have a complete response remain in remission for longer than ten years. After relapse, patients are retreated, and high remission rates can be achieved. Unfortunately, response rates and duration of response both decrease with each retreatment.

Several different approaches can be used to treat follicular lymphoma. Carefully selected patients may receive no initial therapy followed by single-agent chemotherapy, rituximab, or radiation therapy when treatment is needed. Candidates for the conservative approach are usually older, asymptomatic, and have minimal tumor burden. Patients with symptoms, extensive extranodal involvement, bulky disease, cytopenia due to bone marrow involvement, or impaired end-organ function at the time of diagnosis are not candidates for conservative treatment. Alternatively, patients can be treated aggressively with combination chemotherapy, with or without rituximab, or radioimmunotherapy early in the disease course. Both conservative and aggressive approaches are listed as possible options in the current NCCN guidelines, but the guidelines

recommend that initial therapy should include rituximab unless contraindicated.[64] Patients who respond to induction therapy may receive maintenance therapy with single-agent rituximab.

A recently published observational study of 2,728 patients with newly diagnosed follicular lymphoma treated in the United States from March 2004 to March 2007 showed that approximately two thirds of patients were treated with rituximab, either alone (14%) or combined with chemotherapy (52%).[83] Approximately 18% of patients were treated with observation.

At the time of relapse, many of the same treatment options are available, and the following factors must be considered: age, symptomatic status of the patient, tumor burden, rate of regrowth (based on previous assessment of active disease sites), presence or absence of characteristics suggesting transformation or biologic progression, prior therapy, degree and duration of response to prior therapy, availability of clinical trials, and patient preferences.[64,75]

No Initial Therapy. Because there are no convincing data that standard treatment approaches have improved survival, some clinicians have adopted a "watch-and-wait" approach for asymptomatic patients where therapy is delayed until the patient experiences systemic symptoms or disease progression such as rapidly progressive or bulky adenopathy, anemia, thrombocytopenia, or disease in threatening sites such as the orbit or spinal cord.[82] The median time until treatment is required is 3 to 5 years, and approximately 20% of patients do not require therapy for up to ten years. The ten-year survival is 73%, which is not significantly different from patients who received therapy at the time of diagnosis. In a randomized study of asymptomatic patients with indolent lymphomas (mostly follicular), patients who underwent watchful waiting had similar cause-specific and overall survival as compared with those who received immediate chlorambucil.[84] With a median length of followup of 16 years, approximately 17% of patients who were randomized to the watchful waiting group died of other causes without receiving chemotherapy and an additional 9% are alive and have not yet had chemotherapy. As described above, patients with follicular lymphoma who are followed without therapy sometimes have spontaneous regressions that can be complete while the disease in other patients can convert to a more aggressive histology. If the watchful waiting approach is chosen, the patient should be evaluated at least every 2 months for the first year and quarterly thereafter, so that intervention can occur before serious problems occur.

Chemotherapy. Oral alkylating agents, given either alone or combined with prednisone, have been the mainstay of treatment for follicular lymphoma. More intensive chemotherapy has not been shown to improve patient outcome. In a randomized trial of oral chlorambucil, oral cyclophosphamide, or CVP (cyclophosphamide, vincristine, and prednisone) in patients with indolent lymphoma, no significant difference in overall survival or freedom-from-relapse between the three groups was observed.[77] In a more recently published randomized trial of single-agent cyclophosphamide vs. CHOP-B (CHOP and bleomycin), no significant difference in overall time-to-failure or overall survival was observed at ten years.[85] The dosage of single-agent chlorambucil or cyclophosphamide is usually adjusted to maintain a platelet count above 100,000 cells/mm^3 (100×10^9/L) and a white blood cell count above 3,000 cells/mm^3 (3×10^9/L). Although single-agent alkylating agents have a high initial complete remission rate, the time required to achieve a complete response is slow (median time is 9 to 12 months). Complete responses occur more rapidly with combination chemotherapy, particularly with doxorubicin-containing regimens. Many clinicians will therefore give CHOP or CHOP-like chemotherapy when a rapid response is necessary. The development of the CHOP regimen is described in more detail in the Aggressive Lymphomas section later in this chapter. Table 140–10 shows the CHOP

TABLE 140-10	CHOP Regimen		
Drug	**Dose (mg/m²)**	**Route**	**Treatment Days**
Cyclophosphamide	750	IV	1
Doxorubicin	50	IV	1
Vincristine	1.4	IV	1
Prednisone	100	Oral	1–5
One cycle is 21 days			

Another name for doxorubicin is hydroxydaunorubicin.

regimen that is widely used in the treatment of NHL. In those who achieve a complete response, the duration of response is relatively short (about 2.5 years). There is no benefit of maintenance therapy with chemotherapy. After the "best" response is achieved, many experts will discontinue therapy and observe.

Both single-agent alkylating agents and CVP are well tolerated by most patients. The advantages of oral chlorambucil are no hair loss, little or no nausea, and minimal myelosuppression. Because of its mild side effect profile, oral chlorambucil is usually recommended for older patients who are minimally symptomatic or who have other comorbidities. There are some concerns with the risk of secondary acute leukemia in patients receiving continuous exposure to alkylating agents.

Bendamustine. Bendamustine is an alkylating agent with structural similarities to both alkylating agents and purine analogs.[86] The mechanism of action of bendamustine appears to be different from other alkylating agents and it does not show cross-resistance to other alkylating agents. When used as a single agent, bendamustine shows antitumor activity in relapsed or refractory indolent lymphomas. Overall and complete response rates of 70% to 80% and 30% to 35% have been reported, respectively, in phase II trials. Bendamustine received FDA approval for relapsed or refractory indolent NHL in October 2008.

Purine Analogs. Several studies report encouraging results with two adenosine analogs, fludarabine phosphate and cladribine (2-chlorodeoxyadenosine), in previously untreated and relapsed advanced follicular lymphoma.[87] The mechanism of action for both drugs is not well understood, but both agents accumulate in lymphocytes and are resistant to adenosine deaminase. In patients with relapsed or refractory indolent lymphoma, single-agent fludarabine has an overall response rate of almost 50% and a complete response rate of 10% to 15%. Response rates are higher in previously untreated patients, with overall and complete response rates of 70% and almost 40%, respectively. The median time to progression is less than 6 months for relapsed disease and more than 12 months for previously untreated patients. Although the response rates to 2-chlorodeoxyadenosine in previously untreated patients is similar to those with fludarabine, the duration of response appears to be shorter with 2-chlorodeoxyadenosine.

Combination regimens that include one of these purine analogs are also being investigated.[87] Fludarabine and mitoxantrone (FN) and fludarabine, mitoxantrone, and dexamethasone (FND), given with or without rituximab, are examples of fludarabine-containing regimens that show encouraging results in patients with indolent lymphoma. Fludarabine plus rituximab and FND plus rituximab are listed as acceptable first-line options for follicular lymphoma (Category 2A).[64]

Purine analogs usually do not cause nausea and vomiting or hair loss, but they are associated with cumulative and prolonged myelosuppression and profound immunosuppression, which increases the risk of opportunistic infections, such as fungal infections, *Pneumocystis jiroveci* pneumonia, and viral infections. Because the use of fludarabine-based regimens may impair stem cell mobilization

and collection, some experts avoid fludarabine-based regimens for patients who are potential candidates for autologous HSCT.

Interferon-α. Single-agent interferon-α (IFN-α) is active in the treatment of follicular lymphoma, but is not curative. Several randomized controlled trials have evaluated the potential benefit of adding IFN-α to combination chemotherapy. Based on the results of one of these trials, IFN-α_{2b} (Intron® A) was granted FDA approval as initial treatment for patients with clinically aggressive follicular lymphoma and a large tumor burden, in combination with an anthracycline-containing regimen. Its approval was based on the Groupe d'Etude des Lymphomes Folliculaires (GELF) trial, which compared CHVP (cyclophosphamide, doxorubicin, teniposide, and prednisone) to CHVP and IFN-α_{2b}.[88] CHVP was given monthly for six cycles, then every two months for six more cycles, whereas IFN-α_{2b} was given at a dose of 5 million units three times a week for 18 months. Patients who received concurrent IFN-α_{2b} had a significantly higher response rate (85% vs. 69%), which translated into significant differences in median progression-free survival (2.9 years vs. 1.5 years) and overall survival (not reached vs. 5.6 years).

At least 10 randomized controlled trials in the United States and Europe have evaluated the role of IFN-α either during induction, as maintenance therapy, or in both settings. The results of these trials have been inconsistent.[89] In a meta-analysis of more than 1,500 newly diagnosed patients from the various randomized trials, the efficacy of IFN-α depended on the intensity of the initial chemotherapy regimen and the IFN-α dose.[90] The major conclusion of the meta-analysis was that IFN-α was probably beneficial in patients receiving relatively intensive initial chemotherapy (anthracycline or anthracene-containing regimen) and at a dose of ≥5 million units (≥36×10^6 units per month).

In the most recent randomized controlled trial, 571 patients with stage III or IV indolent NHL (mostly follicular) were studied as part of a SWOG trial. Patients who responded to intensive chemotherapy that consisted of six to eight cycles of prednisone, methotrexate, doxorubicin, cyclophosphamide, and etoposide/mechlorethamine, vincristine, procarbazine, and prednisone (ProMACE-MOPP) or chemotherapy plus irradiation therapy were randomized to receive either consolidation IFN-α_{2b} (2 million units/m² given subcutaneously three times weekly) for two years or observation.[91] With a median follow-up of more than six years, no difference in progression-free or overall survival was observed.

The reasons for the divergent results cannot be easily explained.[89] Based on these negative results, the significant cost and toxicities associated with this agent and the recent availability of other treatment options, most clinicians no longer use IFN-α in patients with indolent lymphomas.

Rituximab. The approval of rituximab is arguably the most important recent development in the treatment of NHL. Its initial approval in 1997 was based on an open-label multicenter study that enrolled 166 patients with relapsed or recurrent indolent lymphoma.[92] Rituximab, given intravenously at a dose of 375 mg/m² weekly for four weeks, resulted in an overall response of 48% (complete response: 6%, partial response: 42%). Median time to progression for responders was 13.2 months and median duration of response was 11.6 months. Other studies of single-agent rituximab in patients with relapsed or refractory indolent NHL have reported overall response rates of 40% to 60% and complete response rates of 5% to 10%.[93]

Based on the activity of rituximab in relapsed or refractory patients, it is currently being used as first-line therapy, either alone or in combination with chemotherapy.[74,83,93,94] When given as a single agent to patients with previously untreated indolent NHL, the overall response rate is 60% to 70% and the complete response rate is 20% to 30%. It is interesting to note that many of these patients remain in molecular remission (i.e., polymerase chain reaction–negative) at 12 months. Single-agent rituximab is listed as an acceptable option for first-line therapy of follicular lymphoma, particularly for patients who cannot tolerate more intensive chemotherapy regimens.[64]

The rationale for the use of rituximab in combination with conventional agents is based on clinical activity of both agents/ regimens, non–cross-resistant mechanisms of action, nonoverlapping toxicities, and synergistic antitumor activity in vitro. Many clinical trials have evaluated the use of rituximab in combination with other chemotherapy agents. In a phase II trial of six courses of R-CHOP, the overall and complete response rate in 40 patients with previously untreated or relapsed indolent lymphoma was 95% and 55%, respectively.[95] More than 70% of patients were progression-free after 4 years of followup. In an updated analysis, median time-to-progression was reached at 82 months.[96] Based on these encouraging results, several randomized controlled trials have evaluated rituximab in combination with various chemotherapy regimens in first-line therapy for follicular or other indolent lymphomas.[74,94] In the R-CHOP vs. CHOP trial, patients who were randomized to receive R-CHOP as initial therapy had significantly higher overall response rates (96% vs. 90%), reduced risk for treatment failure (relative risk 0.4), and longer time-to-treatment failure and overall survival.[97] In another randomized trial of R-CHOP versus CHOP in relapsed or resistant follicular lymphoma, patients treated with R-CHOP had higher overall and complete response rates (85% vs. 72% and 30% vs. 16%, respectively) and lower risk of treatment failure (hazard ratio [HR] 0.65), but no significant difference in overall survival was observed.[98] Similar results were reported when rituximab was added to other combination regimens.[74,94] In a meta-analysis of all randomized controlled trials, patients with indolent lymphoma treated with rituximab and chemotherapy had a significantly higher overall response rate and reduced risk of treatment failure (HR 0.62) and death (HR 0.65).[99] In 2006, rituximab was FDA-approved for first-line therapy for follicular lymphoma in combination with CVP chemotherapy. R-CHOP is listed as an acceptable option for first-line therapy of follicular lymphoma (Category 1).[64]

Rituximab and CHOP chemotherapy can be combined in many different ways.[100] In the R-CHOP regimen developed by Czuczman et al., two doses of rituximab are given before the start of CHOP therapy; two more doses are given in the middle of the six cycles of CHOP; and two additional doses are given at the end of CHOP therapy.[95] However, in most NHL protocols and in clinical practice, rituximab is given on day 1 of CHOP chemotherapy.[100] In some protocols, rituximab is given on the day before chemotherapy (i.e., day 0) or rituximab is given on day 1 and the other drugs are given on day 3.

Although R-CHOP is the most commonly used chemoimmunotherapy regimen, other regimens may have similar antitumor activity. Bendamustine and rituximab (BR) has been evaluated in rituximab-refractory NHL. In a phase II trial, the overall and complete response rate to BR was 92% and 55%, respectively.[101] In a randomized controlled trial of first-line therapies for advanced indolent NHL, patients who received BR had a higher complete response rate (40% vs. 30%) and longer median progression-free survival (55 vs. 35 mos) as compared with those who received R-CHOP.[102] The BR regimen was tolerated better than R-CHOP. Based on these results, BR is listed as an acceptable option for first-line therapy of follicular lymphoma (Category 2A).[64]

In patients who respond to rituximab, either alone or combined with chemotherapy, maintenance therapy with single-agent rituximab is often given to prolong the duration of remission. In a phase II study, patients with indolent lymphoma who responded to first-line single-agent rituximab received maintenance rituximab, given at a dose of 375 mg/m² weekly for 4 weeks every 6 months, in an attempt to improve the initial therapeutic response and prolong

duration of remission.[103] With continued maintenance therapy, the final response rate increased to 73%, with 37% complete responses. Median progression-free survival was 34 months. Based on these encouraging results, several randomized controlled trials were initiated in previously untreated or chemotherapy-treated patients with indolent lymphoma.[74,82,94] Patients in these trials received induction therapy with either single-agent rituximab or combination chemotherapy with or without rituximab. Several different maintenance rituximab schedules have been used in these trials: 375 mg/m² weekly for 4 weeks every 6 months for 2 years; 375 mg/m² weekly × 4 in months 3 and 9 following induction therapy; 375 mg/m² every 2 to 3 months for 1 to 2 years; and 375 mg/m² every 2 months for 8 months.[74,94,100] Administration every 2 to 3 months is supported by the observation that therapeutic rituximab levels are maintained for about 3 months.[100] A meta-analysis of five randomized controlled trials of maintenance rituximab showed that the effect on overall survival depended on the treatment setting.[104] Patients with refractory or relapsed follicular lymphoma who received maintenance rituximab had a significant improvement in overall survival (hazard ratio 0.58, 95% CI [confidence interval] 0.42 – 0.79) while patients with previously untreated disease had no significant overall survival benefit.[104]

CLINICAL CONTROVERSY

Maintenance rituximab is often used in patients with indolent lymphoma who respond to induction chemoimmunotherapy. While maintenance rituximab has been shown to prolong overall survival in patients with refractory or relapsed disease, no consistent survival benefit has been observed in newly diagnosed patients. Various dosing schedules have been used.

Although rituximab is FDA approved as maintenance therapy for patients with stable disease or who achieve a partial or complete response following induction chemotherapy, its use in patients with newly diagnosed follicular lymphoma is controversial.[105,106] The FDA approval was based on a randomized controlled trial in previously untreated patients with advanced-stage follicular lymphoma treated with maintenance rituximab after CVP chemotherapy.[107] Three-year progression-free survival was significantly longer in the maintenance rituximab group as compared with the observation group (68% vs. 33%). However, only approximately 3% of patients with newly diagnosed follicular lymphoma are treated with chemotherapy alone in the United States.[83] No consistent overall survival benefit has been observed with maintenance rituximab and none of the trials used rituximab combined with CHOP (or CHOP-like) as induction therapy. Furthermore, maintenance rituximab is expensive and associated with adverse effects, including an increased risk of grades 3 or 4 infections.[104] The NCCN guideline lists rituximab maintenance as an option in both first- and second-line therapy, but the strength of the recommendation depends on the treatment setting.[64] The recommendation in refractory or relapsed patients (i.e., second-line therapy) is considerably stronger (category 1, based on high-level evidence) than the recommendation in previously untreated patients (i.e. first-line therapy [category 2B, based on lower-level evidence]).

Most of the adverse effects of rituximab are infusion-related, particularly after the first infusion, and consist of fever, chills, respiratory symptoms, fatigue, headache, pruritus, and angioedema.[94] Premedication with oral acetaminophen 650 mg and diphenhydramine 50 mg is usually given 30 minutes before rituximab infusion. Reactivation of hepatitis B has been reported in patients receiving chemotherapy, either alone or combined with rituximab.[108] Hepatitis B testing is recommended in patients who are considering rituximab therapy.[64]

Radioimmunotherapy. The recent approval of the anti-CD20 radioimmunoconjugates—[131]I-tositumomab (Bexxar) and ^{90}Y-ibritumomab tiuxetan (Zevalin)—has provided clinicians with a novel treatment option for patients with indolent NHLs.[74,109,110] Both ^{131}I-tositumomab and ^{90}Y-ibritumomab tiuxetan are mouse antibodies linked to a radioisotope, either iodine-131 (^{131}I) or yttrium-90 (^{90}Y). Indolent lymphomas are known to be responsive to radiation therapy (i.e., radiosensitive), and the rationale of radioimmunotherapy is that the antibody will act as a guided missile to deliver its payload (i.e., radiation) to its target (i.e., lymphoma cells that express the CD20 antigen). The specificity of the monoclonal antibody allows delivery of the radiation selectively to the tumor (and adjacent normal tissues).

Radioimmunoconjugates have some advantages and disadvantages over unlabeled ("naked") monoclonal antibodies such as rituximab. Tumor cell kill following rituximab depends on binding of the antibody to the tumor cell and the host immune system. Therefore, tumor cells that do not express the target antigen are not accessible to the antibody, or those that are resistant to immune-mediated attacks may escape treatment. Radioimmunoconjugates, because of their ability to deliver radiation over a distance from a source, can not only kill tumor cells that are in contact with the antibody, but also adjacent tumor cells which may not have been in contact with the antibody or may not express the target antigen. This effect is sometimes referred to as the relevant bystander or crossfire effect. However, one disadvantage of radioimmunotherapy is that it can also damage adjacent normal tissues, such as bone marrow cells.

Both ^{131}I-tositumomab and ^{90}Y-ibritumomab tiuxetan have shown activity in relapsed and refractory patients with indolent or transformed lymphomas.[109,110] In patients who respond to radioimmunotherapy, the duration of remission can be more than several years. Although radioimmunotherapy is usually reserved for second-line therapy of follicular lymphoma, some clinicians consider radioimmunotherapy earlier in the disease course, including for patients with previously untreated disease. In a phase II study, patients with previously untreated follicular lymphoma were treated with six cycles of CHOP chemotherapy followed 4 to 8 weeks later by ^{131}I-tositumomab.[111] The overall response rate to the entire treatment regimen was 91%, including 69% complete remissions, and the five-year progression-free survival is estimated to be 67%. Similar results were reported in a phase II trial of ^{131}I-tositumomab given without induction CHOP chemotherapy in previously untreated patients with advanced-stage follicular lymphoma.[112] A current multicenter cooperative group study (SWOG S0016) randomizes previously untreated patients with advanced indolent lymphomas to either CHOP or rituximab (given concurrently, based on the Czuczman regimen[95]) or CHOP and ^{131}I-tositumomab (given sequentially).

Radioimmunotherapy is generally well-tolerated. The major acute toxicities with both radioimmunoconjugates are infusion-related reactions and myelosuppression. ^{131}I-tositumomab can also cause thyroid dysfunction. The primary concern with radioimmunotherapy is the development of treatment-related myelodysplastic syndrome or acute myelogenous leukemia.[113]

The decision to use radioimmunotherapy must be made carefully because of the complexity, risks, and costs of the treatment regimen. Because of safety concerns related to delivery of radiation to bone marrow, candidates for radioimmunotherapy usually have limited bone marrow involvement and adequate absolute neutrophil and platelet counts. Although medical oncologists usually select patients for therapy, the radioimmunotherapy regimen must be administered at a radiation oncology or nuclear medicine facility.

Hematopoietic Stem Cell Transplantation. High-dose chemotherapy, followed by autologous or allogeneic HSCT, is another option for patients with relapsed follicular lymphoma.[75,114,115] In patients who are transplanted at the time of initial treatment failure, five-year event-free survival is approximately 40% to 50%. Although the rate of recurrence is lower after allogeneic HSCT as compared with autologous HSCT, that benefit is offset by increased treatment-related mortality after allogeneic HSCT. The presence of a survival plateau after allogeneic HSCT suggests that some patients may be cured of their disease.

A panel of follicular lymphoma experts recently published their recommendations, which stemmed from an evidence-based review.[115] Their recommendations are: (1) autologous HSCT is recommended as salvage therapy based on pre-rituximab data, with a significant improvement in progression-free and overall survival; (2) autologous HSCT is not recommended as consolidation therapy after first-line chemotherapy for most patients because of no significant improvement in overall survival; (3) autologous HSCT is recommended for transformed follicular lymphoma patients; (4) reduced-intensity conditioning before allogeneic HSCT appears to be an acceptable alternative to myeloablative regimens; and (5) an HLA-matched unrelated donor appears to be as effective as an HLA-matched related donor for reduced intensity conditioning allogeneic HSCT. There are insufficient data to make a recommendation on the use of autologous HSCT after rituximab-based salvage therapy.

Rituximab is being evaluated in the setting of autologous HSCT.[93,116] It is given pretransplant as an in vivo purging agent prior to stem cell collection. In other studies, rituximab is given as posttransplant consolidation.

■ AGGRESSIVE LYMPHOMAS

Diffuse Large B-Cell Lymphoma

Diffuse large B-cell lymphomas (DLBCLs) are the most common lymphoma in the International NHL Classification Project, accounting for approximately 30% of all NHLs.[76,117] DLBCLs are characterized by the presence of large cells, which are similar in size to or larger than tissue macrophages and usually more than twice the size of normal lymphocytes. The median age at the time of diagnosis is in the seventh decade, but DLBCL can affect individuals of all ages, from children to the elderly. Patients often present with a rapidly enlarging symptomatic mass, with B symptoms in approximately 30% to 40% of cases.[63,117] Approximately 30% to 40% of patients with DLBCL present with extranodal disease; common sites include the head and neck, gastrointestinal tract, skin, bone, testis, and CNS. DLBCL is the most common type of diffuse aggressive lymphomas, which are characterized by an aggressive clinical behavior that leads to death within weeks to months if the tumor is not treated. Diffuse aggressive lymphomas are also sensitive to many chemotherapeutic agents, and some patients treated with chemotherapy can be cured of their disease.

Several factors have been shown to correlate with response to chemotherapy and survival in patients with aggressive lymphoma.[69] Because the IPI was originally developed based on patients with aggressive lymphoma, IPI score correlates with prognosis (Table 140–8).[66] As described above, the revised IPI score may more accurately predict prognosis in patients receiving rituximab-containing combination chemotherapy.[67]

Therapy of DLBCL is based on the Ann Arbor stage, IPI (or revised IPI) score, and other prognostic factors.[117] About one half of patients present with localized (stage I or II) disease. However, many patients present with large bulky masses (i.e., larger than 10 cm), and patients with bulky stage II disease are treated with the same approach used for patients with advanced disease (stage III or IV).

Treatment of Localized Disease (Stages I and II) Before 1980, radiation therapy was the primary treatment for patients with localized DLBCL. Five-year disease-free survival with radiation therapy alone was approximately 50% and 20% in patients with stage I and stage II disease, respectively.[117,118] Randomized trials in the 1980s showed that radiation therapy followed by chemotherapy resulted in significantly longer disease-free and overall survival as compared with radiation therapy alone. Other studies reported excellent results with a short course of chemotherapy (three cycles) followed by involved-field radiotherapy or six to eight cycles of CHOP chemotherapy, with or without consolidation radiotherapy. With either of these approaches, five-year progression-free survival was >90% for patients with stage I disease and approximately 70% for patients with stage II disease.[117,118]

Because the more effective approach was not clear, the SWOG performed a randomized trial that compared three cycles of CHOP and involved-field radiotherapy or eight cycles of CHOP in patients with stage I and nonbulky stage II aggressive lymphoma.[119] Patients treated with three cycles of CHOP plus radiotherapy had significantly better 5-year progression-free (77% vs. 64%) and overall (82% vs. 72%) survival than did patients treated with CHOP alone. The incidence of life-threatening toxicity was higher in patients who received CHOP alone. But with longer followup, more patients who received abbreviated chemotherapy experienced late relapses and the differences in progression-free or overall survival were no longer significant between the two arms. Further subgroup analysis of that trial identified several prognostic factors that led to the development of the stage-modified IPI score.[118] Four adverse risk factors comprise the score: nonbulky stage II disease (bulky stage II disease is considered advanced disease), age >60 years, elevated LDH levels, or performance status ≥2.

The stage-modified IPI score is often used to identify patients with localized aggressive NHL who may have a poor prognosis. Based on the results of this trial, the current standard for therapy of most patients with localized nonbulky aggressive lymphoma without any adverse risk factors is three to four cycles of R-CHOP followed by locoregional radiation therapy (30 to 40 Gy [3000 to 4000 rad]).[64,117] Five-year median survival in this favorable group of patients exceeds 90%.[118]

Five-year median survival is reduced to approximately 70% in patients with at least one adverse risk factor in the stage-modified IPI score.[118] Patients in this high-risk subgroup may benefit from more aggressive chemotherapy (six to eight cycles of R-CHOP) followed by locoregional radiation therapy.[64]

Treatment of Advanced Disease (Bulky Stage II, Stages III and IV) It has been known since the late 1970s that intensive combination chemotherapy can cure some patients with disseminated DLBCL.[117] Initial studies with COP (same as CVP) produced a plateau on the survival curve of just 10%, with a median survival of less than one year. Based on the activity of single-agent doxorubicin, McKelvey et al. developed the CHOP regimen (Table 140–10).[120] A few years later, a SWOG study showed that CHOP was more active than COP, and CHOP chemotherapy rapidly became the treatment of choice for patients with aggressive lymphomas.[121] Studies in larger numbers of patients showed that approximately 50% of patients had a complete remission to CHOP chemotherapy, and 50% to 75% of the patients who had a complete response (about one third of all patients) experienced long-term disease-free survival and cure of their disease.

In an effort to improve these results, many investigators used several general approaches to develop second- and third-generation regimens in the 1980s.[117] Results of phase II trials suggested that these second- and third-generation regimens were more active than CHOP, with slightly higher complete response rates and improved disease-free survival rates. However, they were also more difficult to administer, more toxic, and more expensive. Based on these results, many oncologists adopted one of these second- or third-generation combination regimens as their standard regimen for patients with advanced aggressive lymphomas.

Many randomized studies have compared different combination regimens in patients with aggressive lymphoma.[56,117] Although the results of these studies show that no one regimen is clearly superior to another, they demonstrate the superiority of anthracycline-containing regimens over those that do not contain an anthracycline. In the largest and most widely quoted study, the SWOG initiated a randomized trial in 1986 that compared CHOP to three of the most commonly used third-generation regimens in nearly 900 patients with bulky stage II, stage III, or stage IV aggressive NHL. At the time of the initial publication (median followup: 35 months), no differences in disease-free and overall survival were observed between the four groups.[122] Furthermore, no significant differences in disease-free or overall survival were observed in any subgroup of patients. But the risk of treatment-related mortality was higher in patients receiving one of the third-generation regimens. Extended followup of that trial shows that approximately 35% of patients who participated in that trial are probably cured of their disease, regardless of the initial combination chemotherapy regimen.[118] Interestingly, the overall survival is approximately 10% higher than the disease-free survival, which probably reflects the effectiveness of salvage high-dose chemotherapy with autologous HSCT (see the Treatment of Refractory or Relapsed Disease section later in this chapter).

Based on the lack of survival benefit with the newer combination chemotherapy regimens, the less complicated and less expensive CHOP regimen was considered as the treatment of choice for most patients with DLBCL and other aggressive NHLs for many years. Even with CHOP chemotherapy, however, less than 50% of patients with DLBCL were cured of their disease and most patients who relapse after an initial response do so in the first two years. New treatment approaches were clearly needed.

Several studies attempted to improve treatment results by increasing chemotherapy dose (i.e., dose-intensity), shortening the interval between chemotherapy cycles (i.e., dose-density), or both. Because of the increased risk of severe neutropenia, these approaches require growth factor support. Although results of these studies have not consistently shown improved survival, encouraging results from several recently published studies suggest that these approaches be evaluated in future randomized trials.[123,124]

Based on the encouraging results of R-CHOP in indolent lymphomas, several studies evaluated this combination in aggressive lymphomas.[94,118] The first randomized controlled trial that established the efficacy of R-CHOP in advanced-stage DLBCL showed that R-CHOP significantly increased complete response rates and overall survival in elderly (≥60 years old) patients as compared with CHOP alone (discussed in the Treatment of Elderly Patients with Advanced Disease section later in this chapter).[125] Although the results of that study established R-CHOP as standard therapy in older patients, the role of R-CHOP in the treatment of younger patients was not clear. That issue was recently addressed in the MabThera International Trial, which enrolled younger (18 to 60 years old) patients with good-prognosis DLBCL.[126] Patients randomized to receive rituximab plus CHOP-like chemotherapy had significantly higher complete response rates (86% vs. 68%) and longer three-year event-free and overall survival (79% vs. 59% [HR 0.44] and 93% vs. 84% [HR 0.40], respectively). Furthermore, in a population-based study conducted in British Columbia, institution of a policy recommending R-CHOP for all patients with newly diagnosed advanced-stage DLBCL resulted in significant improvements in progression-free and overall survival.[127] Based on these trial results, rituximab received FDA approval for first-line treatment in combination with CHOP or CHOP-like chemotherapy and R-CHOP is recommended for all patients with advanced-stage DLBCL in the current NCCN guideline.[64]

Treatment outcomes for high-risk patients according to the IPI (or revised IPI) score are unsatisfactory. High-risk groups generally include all patients older than 60 years and those with an IPI score of ≥3 (or an age-adjusted IPI score of ≥2). Because progression-free survival is only approximately 50% in these high-risk patients treated with R-CHOP,[67,128] other more aggressive treatments, preferably as part of a clinical trial, should be considered in these patients. Examples of more aggressive approaches include dose-intense or dose-dense chemotherapy with growth factor support, usually combined with rituximab, or high-dose chemotherapy with autologous HSCT.[117,118,129]

One approach is to give high-dose chemotherapy with autologous HSCT as intensive consolidation in high-risk patients with DLBCL who achieve a remission with standard chemotherapy.[117,130] Several randomized controlled trials have been conducted in patients with aggressive NHLs, and no consistent survival advantage has been reported. A recently published meta-analysis of all randomized controlled trials of autologous HSCT as intensive consolidation in aggressive NHL concluded that there was no evidence that autologous HSCT improved outcomes in good-risk patients.[131] The evidence for high-risk patients was inconclusive.

<hr>

CLINICAL CONTROVERSY

Because of high relapse rate in patients who have a complete response to R-CHOP, some experts believe that high-dose chemotherapy with autologous HSCT should be considered as consolidation therapy in high-risk patients with aggressive NHLs who have a complete remission to R-CHOP chemotherapy. Other experts, however, believe that the evidence supporting high-dose chemotherapy with autologous HSCT in this setting is inconclusive and that autologous HSCT should be reserved for patients who relapse.

⓫ In summary, all patients with bulky stage II, stage III, or stage IV disease should be treated with R-CHOP or rituximab and CHOP-like chemotherapy until a complete response is achieved (usually four cycles).[64] Clinicians are encouraged to adopt the revised response criteria proposed by the International Working Group.[65] In patients who have a positive pretreatment PET scan, PET scanning can be useful in response assessment. A rapid response to chemotherapy (i.e., a complete response achieved in the first three treatment cycles) is associated with a more durable remission compared with patients requiring longer treatment cycles. Two or more cycles of chemotherapy should be given following attainment of a complete response (total of six to eight cycles). The use of long-term maintenance therapy following a complete response has not been shown to improve survival. Treatment outcomes for high-risk patients according to the IPI (or revised IPI) score are unsatisfactory and alternative treatment approaches, preferably as part of a clinical trial, should be considered in these patients.[64] High-dose chemotherapy with autologous HSCT should be considered in high-risk patients who respond to standard chemotherapy and are candidates for autologous HSCT.

Treatment of Elderly Patients with Advanced Disease More than one half of patients with NHL are older than 60 years of age at diagnosis, and about one third are older than age 70 years. The International Non-Hodgkin Lymphoma Prognostic Factors Project showed that patients older than 60 years of age had a significantly lower complete response rate and overall survival.[66] The reasons for the poorer outcome in elderly patients are not clear. Older patients do not tolerate intensive chemotherapy as well as younger patients, and some studies report that older patients have a higher risk of treatment-related mortality. As a result, many clinicians treat elderly patients with reduced dose or less-aggressive chemotherapy regimens. In general, these less-intensive regimens have used anthracyclines with less cardiotoxicity than doxorubicin, have substituted mitoxantrone for doxorubicin, or have used short-duration weekly therapy.[117]

Over the past few years, several nonrandomized and randomized trials have evaluated different treatment approaches in older patients with aggressive NHL.[117] The results of these studies suggest that carefully selected elderly patients with good performance status and without significant comorbidities can tolerate aggressive anthracycline-containing regimens as well as younger patients. These patients should be treated initially with full-dose R-CHOP or similar regimens; dosages can be reduced later if severe toxicity occurs. Hematopoietic growth factors may allow elderly patients to maintain dose intensity.

The combination of rituximab and CHOP (R-CHOP) has replaced CHOP as standard treatment for elderly patients with aggressive lymphoma, based on the results of the Groupe d'Etude des Lymphomes de l'Adulte (GELA) study.[125] In that study of 399 elderly patients with DLBCL, patients who were randomized to receive R-CHOP had a significantly higher complete response rate (76% vs. 63%) and longer event-free and overall survival as compared with those who received CHOP. In an updated analysis of that trial, significant differences in five-year event-free survival (47% vs. 29%) and overall survival (58% vs. 45%) were observed between the two treatment groups.[128] In another randomized controlled trial conducted primarily in the United States (Eastern Cooperative Group 4494), elderly (≥ 60 years old) patients who received rituximab, either as induction or maintenance with CHOP chemotherapy, had significantly longer failure-free survival as compared with those not given rituximab during their treatment course.[132] Maintenance therapy with single-agent rituximab did not provide any additional benefit in patients who received R-CHOP as induction therapy. It is important to note that rituximab is given differently in the two studies. In the GELA study, rituximab is given on day 1 (the same day that cyclophosphamide, doxorubicin, and vincristine are administered) with each cycle of CHOP chemotherapy.[125] In the Eastern Cooperative Group 4494 study,[132] R-CHOP was modeled after the regimen developed by Czuczman et al: two doses of rituximab are given before cycle 1, and one dose is given before cycles 3, 5, and 7 (if administered).[95] In most NHL protocols and in clinical practice, rituximab is given on day 1 of CHOP chemotherapy.[100]

Dose-dense CHOP, where the interval between cycles is shortened from three weeks to two weeks, has been evaluated in elderly patients (61 to 75 years old) with advanced-stage aggressive NHL by the German High-Grade NHL Study Group. In the first study, patients who were randomized to receive biweekly CHOP (CHOP-14) had significantly longer five-year event-free and overall survival than patients who received standard CHOP every 21 days (CHOP-21).[133] All patients in the CHOP-14 group received prophylactic growth factors starting from day 4. Toxicity was similar between the two groups. In the next study, the same group of investigators evaluated the addition of rituximab (CHOP-14 vs. R-CHOP-14) and the number of treatment cycles (six vs. eight cycles).[134] Patients who received rituximab did better than those who did not, and eight cycles were not better than six cycles. The addition of rituximab to the CHOP-14 regimen resulted in significantly longer three-year event-free and overall survival (67% vs. 47% and 78% vs. 68%, respectively). A higher risk of *Pneumocystis jirovecii* has been recently reported in patients treated with R-CHOP-14.[135] Dose-dense R-CHOP (R-CHOP-14) is listed as a first-line option in the NCCN guideline (Category 2B).

Treatment of Refractory or Relapsed Disease Although many patients with aggressive NHL experience long-term survival and cure with intensive chemotherapy, approximately 10% to 20% of patients fail to achieve a complete remission and, of those patients who do achieve a complete remission, approximately 20% to 30% subsequently relapse. Therefore, approximately 30% to 40% of all patients with aggressive NHL will require salvage therapy at some point during their disease course. Response to salvage therapy depends on the initial responsiveness of the tumor to chemotherapy. Patients who achieve an initial complete remission and then relapse generally have a better response to salvage therapy than those who are primarily or partially resistant to chemotherapy.

Many conventional-dose salvage chemotherapy regimens have been used in patients with relapsed or refractory NHL. Many patients who respond to salvage therapy (i.e., chemosensitive relapse) will then receive high-dose chemotherapy with autologous HSCT. In an effort to avoid cross-resistance, most salvage regimens incorporate drugs not used in the initial therapy. Some of the more commonly used salvage regimens include DHAP (dexamethasone, cytarabine, cisplatin), ESHAP (etoposide, methylprednisolone, cytarabine, cisplatin), and MINE (mesna, ifosfamide, mitoxantrone, etoposide), and no one regimen appears to be clearly superior to any other regimen.[116,117] Rituximab is sometimes added to these salvage regimens. With these salvage regimens, approximately 30% to 50% of patients achieve a complete response, with a median duration of remission of 1 to 2 years. Only approximately 5% to 10% of patients will have long-term disease-free survival.

ICE (ifosfamide, carboplatin, and etoposide) chemotherapy is a newer regimen that has been used in patients with refractory disease. Some clinicians believe that ICE is better tolerated than older cisplatin-based regimens, particularly in older patients. The combination of ICE and rituximab (RICE) is currently being evaluated as a salvage regimen, and early results are encouraging.[116] Rituximab is given before the first dose of ICE and then weekly during the regimen.

⓬ To improve the cure rate, many studies have evaluated high-dose chemotherapy with autologous HSCT as intensive consolidation therapy in patients who respond to salvage therapy.[117,130] In the PARMA study, 215 patients with relapsed aggressive NHL who had a response to DHAP salvage therapy were randomized to receive either high-dose chemotherapy or continued DHAP therapy.[136] Patients who received high-dose chemotherapy had significantly longer five-year disease-free survival (46% vs. 12%) and overall survival (53% vs. 32%) than those treated with conventional salvage therapy. Further analysis of that study showed that patients who relapsed within 12 months of their initial diagnosis were less likely to benefit from high-dose chemotherapy than patients who relapsed after 12 months. Based on a review of the available evidence, including the PARMA study, high-dose chemotherapy with autologous HSCT is considered to be the treatment of choice in younger patients with chemotherapy-sensitive relapse.[64,117] High-dose chemotherapy with autologous HSCT is not recommended in patients with untested or chemotherapy-refractory relapse.

Rituximab is being evaluated in the setting of autologous HSCT.[116,130] It can be given pretransplant as an in vivo purging agent prior to stem cell collection and as posttransplant consolidation.

Other Aggressive Lymphomas

Mantle cell lymphoma (MCL) is one of the new disease entities that was previously unrecognized by other classification systems.[118,137] This histologic type was found in 6% of cases in the International Lymphoma Classification Project.[76] The chromosomal translocation t(11;14) occurs in most cases of MCL. MCL usually occurs in older adults, particularly in men, and most patients have advanced disease at the time of diagnosis (Table 140–7). Extranodal involvement is found in approximately 90% of cases. The course of the disease is moderately aggressive; the median overall survival is about three years, with no evidence of a survival plateau.

Patients with disseminated MCL are usually treated with the same intensive combination chemotherapy regimens that are used in diffuse aggressive lymphomas. One widely used combination regimen is HyperCVAD (cyclophosphamide, vincristine, doxorubicin, dexamethasone alternating with methotrexate and cytarabine) with or without rituximab. Overall response rates to these regimens is approximately 90%, with about two thirds of patients achieving a complete response.[137] Because MCL usually expresses CD20, rituximab, either alone or combined with CHOP, has been used with some success in patients with newly diagnosed and relapsed MCL.[94,118,137] In a meta-analysis of randomized controlled trials, the addition of rituximab to combination chemotherapy was associated with improved overall survival (HR 0.60).[99] Despite the high response rates, MCL is not considered curable with standard chemotherapy. Consequently, younger patients who have an initial response to chemotherapy often undergo autologous or allogeneic HSCT as consolidation therapy.[137] The NCCN guideline recommends that patients with advanced-stage MCL be treated initially with rituximab and combination chemotherapy, followed by autologous HSCT as first-line consolidation therapy.[64] Unfortunately, most patients with MCL eventually relapse and are treated with salvage therapy or enrolled in trials of investigational agents, some of which are aimed at molecular targets. Bortezomib (Velcade®) received FDA approval in 2006 for treatment of relapsed or refractory MCL based on the results of a phase II study that showed a 33% response rate.[138]

◼ NON-HODGKIN LYMPHOMA IN ACQUIRED IMMUNE DEFICIENCY SYNDROME

The risk of NHL for patients with AIDS is increased more than 100-fold as compared with the general population.[139,140] AIDS-related lymphoma arises as a consequence of long-term stimulation and proliferation of B lymphocytes from HIV and the reactivation of prior EBV infection as a consequence of HIV-induced immunosuppression. AIDS-related lymphoma usually occurs late in the course of HIV infection and is the cause of death in approximately 15% of HIV-infected individuals. Although HIV infects T cells, more than 95% of AIDS-related lymphomas are B-cell neoplasms. Most cases of AIDS-related lymphomas are classified as Burkitt or DLBCL.

The clinical presentation is similar to that observed in other immunocompromised states. Most patients with AIDS-related lymphoma present with B symptoms and have advanced-stage (III or IV) disease at the time of diagnosis.[139] Involvement of extranodal sites is common. The clinical course of AIDS-related lymphoma is usually aggressive and has improved with the availability of highly active antiretroviral therapy (HAART). Improved survival has been observed, primarily in patients with DLBCL. Patients with AIDS-related lymphoma treated with intensive therapy have a median survival that is similar to the survival of patients with HIV-negative NHLs.[140] In the post-HAART era, many of the prognostic factors have also changed and only lymphoma-related factors such as the IPI remain as independent predictors of prognosis.

The treatment of patients with AIDS-associated lymphomas is difficult because the immunocompromised state of these patients increases their risk of significant toxicity as a consequence of myelosuppressive therapy. Except for primary CNS lymphoma, AIDS-related lymphoma is never considered truly localized and systemic chemotherapy is indicated. For patients with adequate immune function and without a history of an opportunistic infection, chemotherapy regimens similar to that used for aggressive lymphomas may be used.[64,139,140] However, many patients with AIDS-related lymphoma were previously treated with less-intensive regimens because of the increased risk of treatment-related toxicity. In the post-HAART era, however, most clinicians believe that standard doses of chemotherapy can be safely administered to patients who achieve a virologic response to HAART.

The results of treatment with standard chemotherapy regimens have been disappointing, particularly in patients with Burkitt lymphoma. In patients with DLBCL, the complete response rate with combination chemotherapy is approximately 40% to 50%, with 5-year overall survival rates of approximately 20% to 30%. Newer approaches, such as the dose-adjusted EPOCH (etoposide, prednisone, vincristine, cyclophosphamide, and doxorubicin) regimen developed at the National Cancer Institute, appear promising. The role of rituximab in the treatment of AIDS-related DLBCL is not clear. In a randomized trial of CHOP versus R-CHOP, no significant differences in progression-free and overall survival were observed.[141] However, 14% of patients treated with R-CHOP died of treatment-related infection as compared with only 2% of those in the CHOP group.

The optimal timing for HAART is not clear in patients with AIDS-related lymphoma.[139,140] If HAART is given concurrently with chemotherapy, patients should be monitored closely for possible pharmacokinetic interactions between HAART and chemotherapy. Some experts suggest that HAART should be withheld until the completion of chemotherapy to allow administration of full chemotherapy doses and to avoid the risk of pharmacokinetic interactions. Prophylactic antibiotics should be continued during chemotherapy and intrathecal chemotherapy should be administered to prevent CNS relapses.

EVALUATION OF THERAPEUTIC OUTCOMES

Hodgkin and non-Hodgkin lymphomas tend to respond well to radiation, chemotherapy, and biologic therapy. The goal of therapy for patients with Hodgkin lymphoma and aggressive NHL is long-term survival and cure. The therapeutic goal in patients with indolent NHLs is less clear because of the indolent nature of the disease and the lack of convincing evidence showing that therapy prolongs survival. Therapeutic responses should be evaluated based on physical examination, radiologic evidence, PET/CT scanning, and other positive findings at baseline. Patients with Hodgkin lymphoma and aggressive NHLs are usually evaluated for response at the end of four cycles of therapy or at the end of treatment if fewer than four cycles of therapy are planned. If patients are treated with chemotherapy alone, two additional cycles of chemotherapy are given after the patient has achieved a complete remission. Recent studies have also shown that early interim PET scans may possess prognostic value in patients with advanced Hodgkin lymphoma. The rapidity of response to therapy in patients with indolent NHL depends on the choice of therapy. Responses occur slowly with therapy with oral alkylating agents, but occur much more rapidly with aggressive therapies such as combination chemotherapy with or without rituximab. If radiation alone is used, then a therapeutic evaluation should occur at the end of treatment.

CONCLUSIONS

Several decades ago, lymphomas were considered a fatal disease. Today, most patients with Hodgkin lymphoma and many patients with aggressive NHLs can be cured with radiation therapy, chemotherapy, or a combination of radiation and chemotherapy. Our ability to achieve long-term survival and cure in these patients is the result of many factors, including development of accurate and reproducible classification systems; a more uniform approach to the staging of lymphoma; and advances in treatment strategies, especially the use of intensive combination chemotherapy. The routine use of hematopoietic growth factors allows oncologists to maintain dose intensity, which may be important for the treatment of aggressive lymphomas. The use of high-dose chemotherapy with autologous HSCT as intensive consolidation therapy for selected patients with aggressive NHLs who respond to initial induction therapy or as salvage therapy after relapse for patients with Hodgkin lymphoma or aggressive NHLs has also contributed to increased cure rates.

New treatment approaches are needed, particularly for indolent NHLs. One of the most exciting therapies is biologic therapy with anti-CD20 monoclonal antibodies. The recent approval of radio-labeled anti-CD20 antibodies (i.e., radioimmunoconjugates) provides another therapeutic option for these patients. There is some evidence that these new therapies have changed the natural history of the disease. It is important to better understand how to use these new agents, either alone or combined with standard chemotherapy. Although approximately one half of patients with aggressive lymphomas can be cured of their disease, many patients will relapse and eventually die of their disease. More effective induction chemotherapy regimens are needed for newly diagnosed patients, and more active salvage therapy is needed for patients with relapsed aggressive NHLs.

The goal for the future is to develop treatment modalities to achieve cure in a larger number of patients. But the acute and chronic toxicities associated with treatment must also be considered, particularly in elderly patients and those with significant comorbidities. Consideration of long-term toxicities is of particular concern to patients with Hodgkin lymphoma because of the high cure rate.

Finally, a better understanding of the pathogenesis of NHL through continued research in molecular biology and immunology will hopefully lead to the development of specific therapies aimed at molecular targets. In addition, gene expression profiling may also allow researchers to identify new clinically important subtypes of NHL and to identify subgroups of patients who do respond poorly to standard therapy.

REFERENCES

1. Josting A, Heidecke C, Dieh V. Overview of the Sixth International Symposium on Hodgkin's disease–recent advances in basic and clinical trials. Eur J Haematol Suppl 2005:1–5.
2. Diehl V, Re D, Harris NL, Mauch PM. Hodgkin Lymphoma. In: DeVita VT, Jr., Hellman S, Rosenberg SA, eds. Cancer: Principles & Practice of Oncology. Philadelphia, PA: Lippincott Williams & Wilkins; 2008:2167–2220.
3. Horning SJ. Hodgkin's lymphoma. In: Abeloff MD, Armitage JO, Niederhuber JE, Kastan MB, McKenna WG, eds. Abeloff's Clinical Oncology. 4th ed. Philadelphia, PA: Elsevier Churchill Livingstone; 2008:2353–2370.
4. Jemal A, Siegel R, Xu J, Ward E. Cancer statistics, 2010. CA Cancer J Clin 2010;60:277–300.
5. SEER Cancer Statistics Review. National Cancer Institute. Bethesda, MD, 1975-2006. 2009, *http://seer.cancer.gov/csr/1975_2006/*.
6. Ng AK, Bernardo MP, Weller E, et al. Long-term survival and competing causes of death in patients with early-stage Hodgkin's disease treated at age 50 or younger. J Clin Oncol 2002;20:2101–2108.
7. Hjalgrim H, Engels EA. Infectious aetiology of Hodgkin and non-Hodgkin lymphomas: A review of the epidemiological evidence. J Intern Med 2008;264:537–5348.
8. Ambinder RF. Epstein-Bar virus and Hodgkin lymphoma. Hematology (Am Soc Hematol Educ Program) 2007:204–209.

9. Kuppers R. The biology of Hodgkin's lymphoma. Nat Rev Cancer 2009; 9:15–27.

10. Mack TM, Cozen W, Shibata DK, et al. Concordance for Hodgkin's disease in identical twins suggesting genetic susceptibility to the young-adult form of the disease. N Engl J Med 1995;332:413–418.

11. Jaffe ES, Harris NL, Stein H, Isaacson PG. Classification of lymphoid neoplasms: The microscope as a tool for disease discovery. Blood 2008;112:4384–4399.

12. Papadaki T, Stamatopoulos K. Hodgkin disease immunopathogenesis: Long-standing questions, recent answers, further directions. Trends Immunol 2003;24:508–511.

13. Swerdlow SH, Campo E, Harris NL, et al. WHO Classification of Tumours of Haematopoietic and Lymphoid Tissues. 4th ed. Lyon, France: IARC Press, 2008.

14. Mauch PM, Kalish LA, Kadin M, Coleman CN, Osteen R, Hellman S. Patterns of presentation of Hodgkin disease. Implications for etiology and pathogenesis. Cancer 1993;71:2062–2071.

15. NCCN Clinical Practice Guidelines in Oncology. Hodgkin Disease/ Lymphoma. (version 1.2010). 2010, *http://www.nccn.org*.

16. Seam P, Juweid ME, Cheson BD. The role of FDG-PET scans in patients with lymphoma. Blood 2007;110:3507–3516.

17. Proctor SJ, Wilkinson J, Sieniawski M. Hodgkin lymphoma in the elderly: A clinical review of treatment and outcome, past, present and future. Crit Rev Oncol Hematol 2009;71:222–232.

18. Hasenclever D, Diehl V. A prognostic score for advanced Hodgkin's disease. International Prognostic Factors Project on Advanced Hodgkin's Disease. N Engl J Med 1998;339:1506–1514.

19. Kuruvilla J. Standard therapy of advanced Hodgkin lymphoma. Hematology (Am Soc Hematol Educ Program) 2009:497–506.

20. Gustavsson A, Osterman B, Cavallin-Stahl E. A systematic overview of radiation therapy effects in Hodgkin's lymphoma. Acta Oncol 2003;42: 589–604.

21. Radford J. Limited-stage disease: Optimal use of chemotherapy and radiation treatment. Hematology (Am Soc Hematol Educ Program) 2008:321–325.

22. Lee CK. Evolving role of radiation therapy for hematologic malignancies. Hematol Oncol Clin North Am 2006;20:471–503.

23. Evens AM, Hutchings M, Diehl V. Treatment of Hodgkin lymphoma: The past, present, and future. Nat Clin Pract Oncol 2008;5:543–556.

24. Gospodarowicz MK, Meyer RM. The management of patients with limited-stage classical Hodgkin lymphoma. Hematology (Am Soc Hematol Educ Program) 2006:253–258.

25. Specht L, Gray RG, Clarke MJ, Peto R. Influence of more extensive radiotherapy and adjuvant chemotherapy on long-term outcome of early-stage Hodgkin's disease: A meta-analysis of 23 randomized trials involving 3,888 patients. International Hodgkin's Disease Collaborative Group. J Clin Oncol 1998;16:830–843.

26. Engert A, Schiller P, Josting A, et al. Involved-field radiotherapy is equally effective and less toxic compared with extended-field radiotherapy after four cycles of chemotherapy in patients with early-stage unfavorable Hodgkin's lymphoma: Results of the HD8 trial of the German Hodgkin's Lymphoma Study Group. J Clin Oncol 2003;21: 3601–3608.

27. Longo DL, Duffey PL, Young RC, et al. Conventional-dose salvage combination chemotherapy in patients relapsing with Hodgkin's disease after combination chemotherapy: The low probability for cure. J Clin Oncol 1992;10:210–218.

28. Canellos GP, Anderson JR, Propert KJ, et al. Chemotherapy of advanced Hodgkin's disease with MOPP, ABVD, or MOPP alternating with ABVD. N Engl J Med 1992;327:1478–1484.

29. Goldie JH, Coldman AJ, Gudauskas GA. Rationale for the use of alternating non-cross-resistant chemotherapy. Cancer Treat Rep 1982;66: 439–449.

30. Glick JH, Young ML, Harrington D, et al. MOPP/ABV hybrid chemotherapy for advanced Hodgkin's disease significantly improves failure-free and overall survival: The 8-year results of the intergroup trial. J Clin Oncol 1998;16:19–26.

31. Duggan DB, Petroni GR, Johnson JL, et al. Randomized comparison of ABVD and MOPP/ABV hybrid for the treatment of advanced Hodgkin's disease: Report of an intergroup trial. J Clin Oncol 2003; 21:607–614.

32. Horning SJ, Hoppe RT, Breslin S, Bartlett NL, Brown BW, Rosenberg SA. Stanford V and radiotherapy for locally extensive and advanced Hodgkin's disease: Mature results of a prospective clinical trial. J Clin Oncol 2002;20:630–637.

33. Gobbi PG, Levis A, Chisesi T, et al. ABVD versus modified Stanford V versus MOPPEBVCAD with optional and limited radiotherapy in intermediate- and advanced-stage Hodgkin's lymphoma: Final results of a multicenter randomized trial by the Intergruppo Italiano Linfomi. J Clin Oncol 2005;23:9198–207.

34. Hoskin PJ, Lowry L, Horwich A, et al. Randomized comparison of the Stanford V regimen and ABVD in the treatment of advanced Hodgkin's lymphoma: United Kingdom National Cancer Research Institute Lymphoma Group Study ISRCTN 64141244 J Clin Oncol 2009;27:5390–5396.

35. Klimm B, Diehl V, Pfistner B, Engert A. Current treatment strategies of the German Hodgkin Study Group (GHSG). Eur J Haematol 2005;75(Suppl):125–134.

36. Diehl V, Franklin J, Pfreundschuh M, et al. Standard and increased-dose BEACOPP chemotherapy compared with COPP-ABVD for advanced Hodgkin's disease. N Engl J Med 2003;348:2386–2395.

37. Engert A, Diehl V, Franklin J, Lohri A, Dorken B. Escalated-dose BEACOPP in the treatment of patients with advanced-stage Hodgkin's Lymphoma: 10 Years of Follow-Up of the GHSG HD9 Study. J Clin Oncol 2009;27.

38. Ballova V, Ruffer JU, Haverkamp H, et al. A prospectively randomized trial carried out by the German Hodgkin Study Group (GHSG) for elderly patients with advanced Hodgkin's disease comparing BEACOPP baseline and COPP-ABVD (study HD9elderly). Ann Oncol 2005;16:124–131.

39. Federico M, Luminari S, Iannitto E, et al. ABVD compared with BEACOPP compared with CEC for the initial treatment of patients with advanced Hodgkin's lymphoma: results from the HD2000 Gruppo Italiano per lo Studio dei Linfomi Trial. J Clin Oncol 2009;27: 805–811.

40. Dann EJ, Bar-Shalom R, Tamir A, et al. Risk-adapted BEACOPP regimen can reduce the cumulative dose of chemotherapy for standard and high-risk Hodgkin lymphoma with no impairment of outcome. Blood 2007;109:905–909.

41. Prosnitz LR. Consolidation radiotherapy in the treatment of advanced Hodgkin's disease: Is it dead? Int J Radiat Oncol Biol Phys 2003;56: 605–608.

42. Loeffler M, Brosteanu O, Hasenclever D, et al. Meta-analysis of chemotherapy versus combined modality treatment trials in Hodgkin's disease. International Database on Hodgkin's Disease Overview Study Group. J Clin Oncol 1998;16:818–829.

43. Aleman BM, Raemaekers JM, Tomisic R, et al. Involved-field radiotherapy for patients in partial remission after chemotherapy for advanced Hodgkin's lymphoma. Int J Radiat Oncol Biol Phys 2007;67:19–30.

44. Majhail NS, Weisdorf DJ, Defor TE, et al. Long-term results of autologous stem cell transplantation for primary refractory or relapsed Hodgkin's lymphoma. Biol Blood Marrow Transplant 2006;12: 1065–1072.

45. Brice P. Managing relapsed and refractory Hodgkin lymphoma. Br J Haematol 2008;141:3–13.

46. Seyfarth B, Josting A, Dreyling M, Schmitz N. Relapse in common lymphoma subtypes: salvage treatment options for follicular lymphoma, diffuse large B-cell lymphoma and Hodgkin disease. Br J Haematol 2006;133:3–18.

47. Goodman KA, Riedel E, Serrano V, Gulati S, Moskowitz CH, Yahalom J. Long-term effects of high-dose chemotherapy and radiation for relapsed and refractory Hodgkin's lymphoma. J Clin Oncol 2008;26:5240–5247.

48. Kulkarni SS, Sastry PS, Saikia TK, Parikh PM, Gopal R, Advani SH. Gonadal function following ABVD therapy for Hodgkin's disease. Am J Clin Oncol 1997;20:354–357.

49. Dores GM, Metayer C, Curtis RE, et al. Second malignant neoplasms among long-term survivors of Hodgkin's disease: A population-based evaluation over 25 years. J Clin Oncol 2002;20:3484–3494.

50. Franklin J, Pluetschow A, Paus M, et al. Second malignancy risk associated with treatment of Hodgkin's lymphoma: Meta-analysis of the randomised trials. Ann Oncol 2006;17:1749–17460.

51. Swerdlow AJ, Barber JA, Hudson GV, et al. Risk of second malignancy after Hodgkin's disease in a collaborative British cohort: The relation to age at treatment. J Clin Oncol 2000;18:498–509.

52. Travis LB. Evaluation of the risk of therapy-associated complications in survivors of Hodgkin lymphoma. Hematology (Am Soc Hematol Educ Program) 2007:192–196.

53. Vose JM, Chiu BC-H, Cheson BD, Dancey J, Wright J. Update on epidemiology and therapeutics for non-Hodgkin's lymphoma. Hematology (Am Soc Hematol Educ Program) 2002:241–2462.

54. Wang SS, Hartge P. Epidemiology. In: Armitage JO, Mauch PM, Harris NL, Coiffier B, Dalla-Favera R, eds. Non-Hodgkin Lymphoma. 2nd ed. Philadelphia, PA: Lippincott Williams & Wilkins, 2010:64–82.

55. Ambinder RF. Infectious etiology of lymphoma. In: Armitage JO, Mauch PM, Harris NL, Coiffier B, Dalla-Favera R, eds. Non-Hodgkin Lymphoma. 2nd ed. Philadelphia, PA: Lippincott Williams & Wilkins, 2010:83–101.

56. Wilson WH, Armitage JO. Non-Hodgkin's lymphoma. In: Abeloff MD, Armitage JO, Niederhuber JE, Kastan MB, McKenna WG, eds. Abeloff's Clinical Oncology. 4th ed. New York, NY: Churchill Livingstone, 2008:2371–2404.

57. Dalla-Favera R, Pasqualucci L. Molecular genetics of lymphoma. In: Armitage JO, Mauch PM, Harris NL, Coiffier B, Dalla-Favera R, eds. Non-Hodgkin Lymphoma. 2nd ed. Philadelphia, PA: Lippincott Williams & Wilkins, 2010:115–130.

58. Hachem A, Gartenhaus RB. Oncogenes as molecular targets in lymphoma. Blood 2005;106:1911–1923.

59. Harris NL. History and classification of lymphoid malignancies. In: Armitage JO, Mauch PM, Harris NL, Coiffier B, Dalla-Favera R, eds. Non-Hodgkin Lymphoma. Philadelphia, PA: Lippincott Williams & Wilkins, 2010:xv–xxix.

60. Harris NL, Stein H, Coupland SE, et al. New approaches to lymphoma diagnosis. Hematology (Am Soc Hematol Educ Program) 2001: 194–220.

61. Lenz G, Staudt LM. Aggressive lymphomas. N Engl J Med 2010;362:1417–1429.

62. Harris NL, Jaffe ES, Diebold J, et al. World Health Organization Classification of neoplastic diseases of the hematopoietic and lymphoid tissues: report of the Clinical Advisory Committee meeting – Airlie House, Virginia, November 1997. J Clin Oncol 1999;17: 3835–3849.

63. Freedman AS, Friedberg JW. Approach to the diagnosis of non-Hodgkin's lymphoma. In: Rose BD, ed. UpToDate. Waltham, MA; 2009.

64. NCCN Clinical Practice Guidelines in Oncology. Non-Hodgkin's Lymphoma. (Version 1.2010). 2010, *http://www.nccn.org*.

65. Cheson BD, Pfistner B, Juweid ME, et al. Revised response criteria for malignant lymphoma. J Clin Oncol 2007;25:579–586.

66. The International Non-Hodgkin's Lymphoma Prognostic Factors Project. A predictive model for aggressive non-Hodgkin's lymphoma. N Engl J Med 1993;329:987–994.

67. Sehn LH, Berry B, Chhanabhai M, et al. The revised International Prognostic Index (R-IPI) is a better predictor of outcome than the standard IPI for patients with diffuse large B-cell lymphoma treated with R-CHOP. Blood 2007;109:1857–1861.

68. Solal-Celigny P, Roy P, Colombat P, et al. Follicular lymphoma international prognostic index. Blood 2004;104:1258–1265.

69. Sehn LH. Optimal use of prognostic factors in non-Hodgkin's lymphoma. Hematology (Am Soc Hematol Educ Program) 2006: 295–302.

70. Rosenwald A, Wright G, Chan WC, et al. The use of molecular profiling to predict survival after chemotherapy for diffuse large-B-cell lymphoma. N Engl J Med 2002;346:1937–1947.

71. Lenz G, Wright G, Dave SS, et al. Stromal gene signatures in large-B-cell lymphomas. N Engl J Med 2008;359:2313–2323.

72. Dave SS, Wright G, Tan B, et al. Predicton of survival in follicular lymphoma based on molecular features of tumor-infiltrating immune cells. N Engl J Med 2004;351:2159–2169.

73. Maloney DG. Immunotherapy for non-Hodgkin's lymphoma: Monoclonal antibodies and vaccines. J Clin Oncol 2005;23: 6421–6428.

74. Cheson BD, Leonard JP. Monoclonal antibody therapy for B-cell non-Hodgkin's lymphoma. N Engl J Med 2008;359:613–626.

75. Freedman AS, Friedberg JW, Mauch PM, Dalla-Favera R, Harris NL. Follicular lymphoma. In: Armitage JO, Mauch PM, Harris NL, Coiffier B, Dalla-Favera R, eds. Non-Hodgkin's Lymphoma. 2nd ed. Philadelphia, PA: Lippincott Williams & Wilkins, 2010:266–283.

76. The Non-Hodgkin's Lymphoma Classification Project. A clinical evaluation of the International Lymphoma Study Group classification of non-Hodgkin's lymphoma. Blood 1997;89:3909–3918.

77. Horning SJ. Natural history of and therapy for the indolent non-Hodgkin's lymphomas. Semin Oncol 1993;20 (suppl 5):75–88.

78. Bernstein SH, Burack WR. The incidence, natural history, biology, and treatment of transformed lymphoma. Hematology (Am Soc Hematol Educ Program) 2009:532–541.

79. Fisher RI, LeBlanc M, Press OW, Maloney DG, Unger JM, Miller TP. New treatment options have changed the survival of patients with follicular lymphomas. J Clin Oncol 2005;23:8477–52.

80. Liu Q, Fayad L, Cabanillas F, et al. Improvement of overall and failure-free survival in stage IV follicular lymphoma: 25 years of treatment experience at The University of Texas M.D. Anderson Cancer Center. J Clin Oncol 2006;24:1582–1589.

81. Seymour JF, Pro B, Fuller LM, et al. Long-term follow-up of a prospective study of combined modality therapy for stage I-II indolent non-Hodgkin's lymphoma. J Clin Oncol 2003;21:2115–2122.

82. Gribben JG. How I treat indolent lymphoma. Blood 2007;109: 4617–4626.

83. Friedberg JW, Taylor MD, Cerhan JR, et al. Follicular lymphoma in the United States: first report of the National LymphoCare Study. J Clin Oncol 2009;27:1202–1208.

84. Ardeshna KM, Smith P, Norton A, et al. Long-term effect of a watch and wait policy versus immediate systemic treatment for asymptomatic advanced-stage non-Hodgkin's lymphoma: A randomised controlled trial. The Lancet 2003;362:516–522.

85. Peterson BA, Petroni GR, Frizzera G, et al. Prolonged single-agent versus combination chemotherapy in indolent follicular lymphomas: A study of the Cancer and Leukemia Group B. J Clin Oncol 2003;21: 5–15.

86. Cheson BD, Rummel MJ. Bendamustine: rebirth of an old drug. J Clin Oncol 2009;27:1492–1501.

87. Di Bella N, Ravandi F. Purine analogue combinations for indolent lymphomas. Semin Hematol 2006;43 (suppl 2):S11–S21.

88. Solal-Celigny P, Lepage E, Brousse N, et al. Doxorubicin-containing regimen with or without interferon alfa-2b for advanced follicular lymphoma: Final analysis of survival and toxicity in the Groupe d'Etude des Lymphomes Folliculaires 86 Trial. J Clin Oncol 1998;16: 2332–2338.

89. Cheson BD. The curious case of the baffling biological. J Clin Oncol 2000;18:2007–2009.

90. Rohatiner AZS, Gregory WM, Peterson B, et al. Meta-analysis to evaluate the role of interferon in follicular lymphoma. J Clin Oncol 2005;34:2215–2223.

91. Fisher RI, Dana BW, LeBlanc M, et al. Interferon alfa consolidation after intensive chemotherapy does not prolong the progression-free survival of patients with low-grade non-Hodgkin's lymphoma: Results of the Southwest Oncology Group Randomized Phase III Study 8809. J Clin Oncol 2000;18:2010–2016.

92. McLaughlin P, Grillo-Lopez AJ, Link BK, et al. Rituxumab chimeric anti-CD20 monoclonal antibody therapy for relapsed indolent lymphoma: Half of patients respond to a four-dose treatment program. J Clin Oncol 1998;16:2825–2833.

93. Cohen Y, Solal-Celigny P, Polliack A. Rituximab therapy for follicular lymphoma: A comprehensive review of its efficacy as primary treatment, treatment for relapsed disease, re-treatment and maintenance. Haematologica 2003;88:811–823.

94. Cvetkovic RS, Perry CM. Rituximab: A review of its use in non-Hodgkin's lymphoma and chronic lymphocytic leukemia. Drugs 2006;66:791–820.

95. Czuczman MS, Grillo-Lopez AJ, White CA, et al. Treatment of patients with low-grade B-cell lymphoma with the combination of chimeric anti-CD20 monoclonal antibody and CHOP chemotherapy. J Clin Oncol 1999;17:268–276.

96. Czuczman MS, Weaver R, Alkuzweny B, Berlfein J, Grillo-Lopez AJ. Prolonged clinical and molecular remission in patients with low-grade or

follicular non-Hodgkin's lymphoma treated with rituximab plus CHOP chemotherapy: 9-year follow-up. J Clin Oncol 2004;22:4711–4716.

97. Hiddemann W, Kneba M, Dreyling M, et al. Frontline therapy with rituximab added to the combination of cyclophosphamide, doxorubicin, vincristine, and prednisone (CHOP) significantly improves the outcome for patients with advanced-stage follicular lymphoma compared with therapy with CHOP alone: Results of a prospective randomized study of the German Low-Grade Lymphoma Study Group. Blood 2005;106:3725–3732.

98. van Oers MHJ, Klasa R, Marcus RE, et al. Rituximab maintenance improves clinical outcome of relapsed/resistant follicular lymphoma non-Hodgkin's lymphoma in patients both with and without rituximab during induction: Results of a prospective randomized phase 3 intergroup trial. Blood 2006;108:3295–3301.

99. Schulz H, Bohlius JF, Trelle S, et al. Immunochemotherapy with rituximab and overall survival in patients with indolent or mantle cell lymphoma: A systematic review and meta-analysis. J Natl Cancer Inst 2007;99:706–714.

100. Ghielmini M. Multimodality therapies and optimal schedule of antibodies: rituximab in lymphoma as an example. Hematology (Am Soc Hematol Educ Program) 2005:321–328.

101. Robinson KS, Williams ME, van der Jagt RH, et al. Phase II multicenter study of bendamustine plus rituximab in patients with relapsed indolent B-cell and mantle cell non-Hodgkin's lymphoma. J Clin Oncol 2008;26:4473–4479.

102. Rummel MJ, Niederle N, Maschmeyer G, et al. Bendamustine plus rituximab is superior to CHOP plus rituximab as first-line treatment of patients with advanced follicular, indolent, and mantle cell lymphomas: Final results of a randomized phase III study of the StiL (Study Group Indolent Lymphomas, Germany). Blood 2009.

103. Hainsworth JD, Litchy S, Burris HA, et al. Rituximab as first-line and maintenance therapy for patients with indolent non-Hodgkin's lymphoma. J Clin Oncol 2002;20:4261–4267.

104. Vidal L, Gafter-Gvili A, Leibovici L, et al. Rituximab maintenance for the treatment of patients with follicular lymphoma: Systematic review and meta-analysis of randomized trials. J Natl Cancer Inst 2009;101:248–255.

105. Cheson BD. The case against rituximab maintenance. Nature Rev Clin Oncol 2009;6:622–624.

106. Seymour JF. Follicular lymphoma: maintenance therapy is (often) indicated. Nature Rev Clin Oncol 2009;6:624–626.

107. Hochster H, Weller E, Gascoyne RD, et al. Maintenance rituximab after cyclophosphamide, vincristine, and prednisone prolongs progression-free survival in advanced indolent lymphoma: Results of the randomized phase III ECOG1496 study J Clin Oncol 2009;27:1607–1614.

108. Yeo W, Chan TC, Leung NWY, et al. Hepatitis B virus reactivation in lymphoma patients with prior resolved hepatitis B undergoing anticancer therapy with or without rituximab. J Clin Oncol 2009;27:605–611.

109. Cheson BD. Radioimmunotherapy of non-Hodgkin lymphomas. Blood 2003;101:391–698.

110. Goldsmith SJ. Radioimmunotherapy of lymphoma: Bexxar and Zevalin. Semin Nuclear Med 2010;40:122–135.

111. Press OW, Unger JM, Braziel RM, et al. Phase II trial of CHOP chemotherapy followed by tositumomab/iodine I-131 tositumomab for previously untreated follicular non-Hodgkin's lymphoma: Five-year follow-up of Southwest Oncology Group Protocol S9911. J Clin Oncol 2006;24:4143–4149.

112. Kaminski MS, Tuck M, Estes J, et al. ^{131}I-tositumomab therapy as initial treatment for follicular lymphoma. N Engl J Med 2005;352:441–449.

113. Armitage JO, Carbone PP, Connors JM, Levine AM, Bennett JM, Kroll S. Treatment-related myelodysplasia and acute leukemia in non-Hodgkin's lymphoma patients. J Clin Oncol 2003;21:897–906.

114. van Besien KW. Allogeneic stem cell transplantation in follicular lymphoma: Recent progress and controversy. Hematology (Am Soc Hematol Educ Program) 2009:610–618.

115. Oliansky DM, Gordon LI, King J, et al. The role of cytotoxic therapy with hematopoietic stem cell transplantation in the treatment of follicular lymphoma: An evidence-based review. Biol Blood Marrow Transplant 2010;16:443–468.

116. Gisselbrecht C. Use of rituximab in diffuse large B-cell lymphoma in the salvage setting. Br J Haematol 2008;143:607–621.

117. Armitage JO, Mauch PM, Harris NL, Dalla-Favera R, Bierman PJ. Diffuse large B-cell lymphoma. In: Armitage JO, Mauch PM, Harris NL, Coiffier B, Dalla-Favera R, eds. Non-Hodgkin Lymphoma. 2nd ed. Philadelphia, PA: Lippincott Williams & Wilkins, 2010:304–326.

118. Fisher RI, Miller TP, O'Connor OA. Diffuse aggressive lymphoma. Hematology (Am Soc Hematol Educ Program) 2004:221–236.

119. Miller TP, Dahlberg S, Cassady JR, et al. Chemotherapy alone compared with chemotherapy plus radiotherapy for localized intermediate- and high-grade non-Hodgkin's lymphoma. N Engl J Med 1998;339:21–26.

120. McKelvey EM, Gottlieb JA, Wilson HE, et al. Hydroxyldaunomycin (Adriamycin) combination chemotherapy in malignant lymphoma. Cancer 1976;38:1484–1493.

121. Jones SE, Grozea PN, Metz EN, et al. Superiority of Adriamycin containing combination chemotherapy in the treatment of diffuse lymphoma: A Southwest Oncology Group study. Cancer 1979;43:417–425.

122. Fisher RI, Gaynor ER, Dahlberg S, et al. Comparison of a standard regimen (CHOP) with three intensive chemotherapy regimens for advanced non-Hodgkin's lymphoma. N Engl J Med 1993;328:1002–1006.

123. Blayney DW, LeBlanc ML, Grogan T, et al. Dose-intense chemotherapy every 2 weeks with dose-intense cyclophosphamide, doxorubicin, vincristine, and prednisone may improve survival in intermediate- and high-grade lymphoma: A phase II study of the Southwest Oncology Group (SWOG 9349). J Clin Oncol 2003;21:2466–2473.

124. Coiffier B. Increasing chemotherapy intensity in aggressive lymphoma: A renewal? J Clin Oncol 2003;21:2457–2459.

125. Coiffier B, Lepage E, Briere J, et al. CHOP chemotherapy plus rituximab compared with CHOP alone in elderly patients with diffuse large-B-cell lymphoma. N Engl J Med 2002;346:235–242.

126. Pfreundschuh M, Trumper L, Osterborg A, et al. CHOP-like chemotherapy plus rituximab versus CHOP-like chemotherapy alone in young patients with good-prognosis diffuse large B-cell lymphoma: A randomised controlled trial by the MabThera International Trial (MInT) Group. Lancet Oncol 2006;7:379–391.

127. Sehn LH, Donaldson J, Chhanabhai M, et al. Introduction of combined CHOP plus rituximab therapy dramatically improved outcome of diffuse large B-cell lymphoma in British Columbia. J Clin Oncol 2005;23:5027–5033.

128. Feugier P, Van Hoof A, Sebban C, et al. Long-term results of the R-CHOP study in the treatment of elderly patients with diffuse large B-cell lymphoma: A study by the Groupe d'Etude des Lymphomes de l'Adulte. J Clin Oncol 2005;23:4117–4126.

129. Held G, Schubert J, Reiser M, Pfreundschuh M. Dose-intensified treatment of advanced-stage diffuse large B-cell lymphomas. Semin Hematol 2006;43:221–229.

130. Nademanee A, Forman SJ. Role of hematopoietic stem cell transplantation for advanced-stage diffuse large B-cell lymphoma. Semin Hematol 2006;43:240–250.

131. Greb A, Bohlius J, Trelle S, et al. High-dose chemotherapy with autologous stem cell support in first-line treatment of aggressive non-Hodgkin lymphoma: Results of a comprehensive meta-analysis. Cancer Treat Rev 2007;33:338–346.

132. Habermann TM, Weller EA, Morrison VA, et al. Rituximab-CHOP versus CHOP alone or with maintenance rituximab in older patients with diffuse large B-cell lymphoma. J Clin Oncol 2006;24:3121–3127.

133. Pfreundschuh M, Trumper L, Kloess M, et al. Two-weekly or 3-weekly CHOP chemotherapy with or without etoposide for the treatment of elderly patients with aggressive lymphomas: Results of the NHL-B2 trial of the DSHNHL. Blood 2004;104:634–641.

134. Pfreundschuh M, Schubert J, Ziepert M, et al. Six versus eight cycles of bi-weekly CHOP-14 with or without rituximab in elderly patients with aggressive CD20$^+$ B-cell lymphomas: a randomised controlled trial (RICOVER-60). Lancet Oncol 2008;9:105–116.

135. Tadmor T, McLaughlin P, Polliack A. A resurgence of *Pneumocystis* in aggressive lymphoma treated with R-CHOP-14: The price of a dose-dense regimen? Leukemia & Lymphoma 2010;51:737–738.

136. Philip T, Guglielmi C, Hagenbeek A, et al. Autologous bone marrow transplantation as compared with salvage chemotherapy in relapses of chemotherapy-sensitive non-Hodgkin's lymphoma. N Engl J Med 1995;333:1540–1545.

137. Zain J, Bhagat G, O'Connor OA. Mantle cell lymphoma. In: Armitage JO, Mauch PM, Harris NL, Coiffier B, Dalla-Favera R, eds. Non-Hodgkin Lymphoma. 2nd ed. Philadelphia, PA: Lippincott Williams & Wilkins, 2010:284–303.

138. Fisher RI, Bernstein SH, Kahl BS, et al. Multicenter phase II study of bortezomib in patients with relapsed or refractory mantle cell lymphoma. J Clin Oncol 2006;24:4867–4874.

139. Levine AM, Said JW. Management of acquired immunodeficiency syndrome-related lymphoma. In: Armitage JO, Mauch PM, Harris NL, Coiffier B, Dalla-Favera R, eds. Non-Hodgkin Lymphoma. 2nd ed. Philadelphia, PA: Lippincott Williams & Wilkins, 2010:507–526.

140. Mounier N, Spina M, Gisselbrecht C. Modern management of non-Hodgkin's lymphoma in HIV-infected patients. Br J Haematol 2007;136:685–698.

141. Kaplan LD, Lee JY, Ambinder RF, et al. Rituximab does not improve clinical outcome in a randomized phase III trial of CHOP with or without rituximab in patients with HIV associated non-Hodgkin's lymphoma: AIDS Malignancy Consortium trial 010. Blood 2005;106:1538–1543.

141

Ovarian Cancer

JUDITH A. SMITH AND JUDITH K. WOLF

KEY CONCEPTS

❶ Ovarian cancer is denoted "the silent killer" because of the nonspecific signs and symptoms that contribute to the delay in diagnosis. The few patients who present with disease still confined to the ovary will have a 5-year survival rate greater than 90%, but most patients present with advanced disease and have a 5-year survival rate of 10 to 30%.

❷ Ovarian cancer is a sporadic disease with less than 10% of cases of ovarian cancer attributed to heredity. However, a history of two or more first-degree relatives with ovarian cancer increases a woman's risk of developing ovarian cancer by greater than 50%.

❸ CA-125 is a nonspecific antigen used as a tumor marker for diagnosis and monitoring epithelial ovarian carcinoma. If CA-125 is positive at the time of diagnosis, changes in CA-125 levels correlate with disease response and progression.

❹ Although most patients will achieve a complete response to initial treatment, over 50% will have recurrence within the first 2 years. If recurrence is less than 6 months after completion of chemotherapy, tumor is defined to be platinum-resistant. The antitumor activity of second-line chemotherapy regimens is similar, and the choice of treatment for recurrent platinum-resistant ovarian cancer depends on residual toxicities, physician preference, and patient convenience. Participation in a clinical trial is also a reasonable option for these patients.

❺ Ovarian cancer is staged surgically with the International Federation of Gynecology and Obstetrics (FIGO) staging algorithm. Tumor debulking and total abdominal hysterectomy–bilateral oophorectomy surgery are the primary surgical interventions for ovarian cancer. After the completion of the staging and primary surgical treatment, the current standard of care is six cycles of a taxane/platinum-containing chemotherapy regimen.

Ovarian cancer is a gynecologic cancer that usually arises from disruption or mutations in the epithelium of the ovary.[1] It is associated with the highest mortality among the gynecologic cancers, primarily because most patients present with advanced

disease. ❶ Ovarian cancer is denoted "the silent killer" because of the nonspecific signs and symptoms that often lead to a delay in diagnosis. Ovarian cancers often metastasize via the lymphatic and blood systems to the liver and/or lungs. Common complications of advanced and progressive ovarian cancer include ascites and small bowel obstruction. The few patients who present with disease still confined to the ovary will have a 5-year survival rate greater than 90%, but most patients present with advanced disease and have a 5-year survival rate of 10% to 30%. Primary treatment includes tumor-debulking surgery followed by six cycles of a taxane-platinum chemotherapy regimen. Although 70% of patients achieve an initial complete response to chemotherapy, more than 50% of these patients will have recurrence within the first 2 years from diagnosis.[2]

ETIOLOGY AND EPIDEMIOLOGY

It is estimated that 21,880 new cases of ovarian cancer were diagnosed, and 13,850 women died of the disease in 2010.[3] Ovarian cancer is associated with the highest mortality rate among the gynecologic cancers and is the fifth leading cause of cancer-related deaths in women. The mortality rate associated with ovarian cancer has not changed significantly over the past 3 decades. The high mortality rate is related to the insidious onset of nonspecific symptoms and the lack of adequate screening tools, which allows the disease to go undiagnosed until it has progressed beyond the pelvic cavity.

As with many other cancers, the risk of ovarian cancer increases with increasing age. A woman's risk increases from 15.7 to 54 per 100,000 as her age advances from 40 to 79 years, and the median age at diagnosis is 59.[3] Most cases of ovarian cancer are diagnosed during the peri- and postmenopausal phase of women's reproductive life span.[4]

❷ Heredity accounts for less than 10% of all ovarian cancer cases. Family history is an important risk factor in the development of ovarian cancer. If one family member has a diagnosis of ovarian cancer, the associated lifetime risk is 9%, but this risk increases to greater than 50% if there are two or more first-degree relatives (e.g., her mother and sister) with a diagnosis of ovarian cancer or multiple cases of ovarian and breast cancer within the same family.[1,2]

BRCA1 and BRCA2 are the tumor suppressor genes thought to be involved in one or more pathways of DNA damage recognition and repair. The BRCA1 gene is located on chromosome 17q12–21, and the BRCA2 gene is located on chromosome 13q12–13. Both BRCA1 and BRCA2 mutations are associated with ovarian cancer. However, BRCA1 is more prevalent, being associated with 90% of inherited and 10% of sporadic cases of ovarian cancer.[5] Patients with BRCA1-associated ovarian cancer are usually considerably younger than patients with BRCA2 mutations, with a mean age of 54 years.[6] Patients usually present with advanced stage at diagnosis, and the *BRCA1*-linked ovarian cancers are more aggressive tumors that typically are serous histology, moderate to high grade. As *BRCA1* and *BRCA2* are thought to be involved in DNA damage or repair, their inactivation/mutations may be associated with an increased resistance of ovarian cancer cells to cytotoxic agents.

Hereditary breast and ovarian cancer syndrome is one of the two different forms of hereditary ovarian cancer and is associated with germline mutations in *BRCA1* and *BRCA2*.[5,7] The hereditary nonpolyposis colorectal cancer or Lynch syndrome is a familial syndrome with germline mutations causing defects in enzymes involved in DNA mismatch repair, which is associated with up to 12% of hereditary ovarian cancer cases.[5] This syndrome is associated with mutations in DNA mismatch repair genes such as *MSH2, MLH1, PMS1,* and *PMS2* and leads to microsatellite instability.

Hormone exposure, specifically estrogen, and reproductive history are also associated with the risk of developing ovarian cancer. Conditions that increase the total number of ovulations in women's reproductive history, such as nulliparity, early menarche, or late menopause, are associated with an increasing risk for epithelial ovarian cancers.[8,9] Conversely those conditions that limit ovulations are associated with a protective effect. Each time ovulation occurs, the ovarian epithelium is broken, followed by cellular repair. According to the *incessant ovulation hypothesis*, the risk of mutations and, ultimately, cancer increases each time the ovarian epithelium undergoes cell repair.

Finally, ovarian cancer is associated with certain dietary and environmental factors. A diet that is high in galactose, animal fat, and meat may increase the risk of ovarian cancer, whereas a vegetable-rich diet may decrease the risk of ovarian cancer.[7,10] Although controversial, exogenous factors such as asbestos and talcum powder use in the perineal area are also associated with an increased risk of ovarian cancer.[7,10]

PATHOLOGY AND CLASSIFICATION

Ovarian carcinomas can be separated into three major entities: epithelial carcinomas, germ cell tumors, and stromal carcinomas. Most ovarian tumors (85% to 90%) are derived from the epithelial surface of the ovary.[11] The classification of common epithelial tumors has been developed by the World Health Organization and the International Federation of Gynecology and Obstetrics.[12] The nomenclature considers cell type, location of the tumor, and the degree of the malignancy, which ranges from benign tumors to tumors of low malignancy to invasive carcinomas. Epithelial tumors classified as low malignancy ("borderline malignancy") are characterized by epithelial papillae with atypical cell clusters, cellular stratification, nuclear atypia, and increased mitotic activity, and have a much better prognosis than those classified as invasive carcinomas. Malignant tumors are characterized by an infiltrative destructive growth pattern with malignant cells growing in a disorganized manner and dissection into stromal planes.

Invasive epithelial adenocarcinomas are characterized by histologic subtype and grade, which measures the degree of cellular differentiation. Although the histologic type of the tumor is not a significant prognostic factor, with the exception of clear cell, the histopathologic grade is an important prognostic factor. Undifferentiated tumors are associated with a poorer prognosis than those lesions that are considered to be well or moderately differentiated. A universal grading system for ovarian cancer was developed that combines mitotic score, nuclear atypia score, and architectural score based on the histologic pattern.[13]

The histologic subtypes of adenocarcinomas include papillary serous, mucinous, endometrioid, clear cell, mixed epithelial, transition-cell, and undifferentiated.[2,4,13] Papillary serous adenocarcinoma is the most common type of epithelial ovarian cancer and accounts for approximately 46% of cases. The peak age of diagnosis ranges from 45 to 65 years with 63 years as the median age of diagnosis.[14] Serous carcinomas typically display complex papillary and solid patterns and qualify as high-grade carcinomas. Endometrioid carcinomas are seen in women 40 to 50 years of age and comprise approximately 8% of ovarian carcinomas, of which approximately 6% are surface epithelial neoplasms.[14] Endometrioid tumors are usually diagnosed as stage I disease and have a better prognosis than tumors with serous histology. Mucinous carcinomas occur in women between 40 and 70 years of age and account for approximately 36% of all ovarian cancers. The overall prognosis for mucinous carcinoma is better than for serous carcinoma because most patients present with stage I disease. Clear cell carcinoma comprises approximately 3% of ovarian carcinomas in women, with a mean age of 57 years. Although clear cell carcinoma is the least common ovarian neoplasm, it is most commonly associated with paraneoplastic-related hypercalcemia.[14]

Germ cell tumors of the ovary, including malignant teratoma and dysgerminomas, are rare, comprising approximately 2% to 3% of all ovarian cancers in Western countries with an increased incidence in black and Asian women.[15,16] These tumors are highly curable and affect primarily young women. In contrast to epithelial tumors, approximately 60% to 70% of germ cell tumors are stage I at diagnosis, which is related to earlier detection and response to symptoms in this younger patient population.[16] Serum markers (human β-chorionic gonadotropin and α-fetoprotein) are helpful to confirm the diagnosis and monitor response to treatment.

Finally, ovarian sex cord-stromal tumors account for 7% of all ovarian cancers and tend to be diagnosed at stage I.[12] Sex cord-stromal tumors are associated with hormonal effects, such as precocious puberty, amenorrhea, and postmenopausal bleeding. Because these tumors are rare, the optimal treatment of ovarian sex cord-stromal tumors is not clear. The current recommended standard of care is surgery followed by treatment with a platinum-based chemotherapy regimen.

Ovarian cancer is usually confined to the abdominal cavity, but spread can occur to the lung, liver, and, less commonly, the bone or brain. Disease is spread by direct extension, peritoneal seeding, lymphatic dissemination, or bloodborne metastasis. Lymphatic seeding is the most common pathway and frequently causes ascites.

SCREENING AND PREVENTION

SCREENING

Ovarian cancer is an uncommon disease with no known preinvasive component, which has made it difficult to screen patients to detect early disease. In addition, the risk factors for developing ovarian cancer are not well understood, which also makes it difficult to identify a high-risk group of individuals. At the present time, there are no effective screening tools for early detection of ovarian cancer.

Pelvic examinations are noninvasive and well accepted and can detect large tumors with a sensitivity of 67% for detecting all tumors.[15] However, because pelvic examinations cannot detect minimal or microscopic disease, they do not usually detect ovarian cancer until it is in an advanced stage. As a result of these limitations, routine pelvic examinations are not an effective screening tool and do not decrease overall mortality.[15]

Transvaginal ultrasound (TVUS) creates an image of the ovary by releasing sound waves. It can be used to evaluate the size and shape and to detect the presence of cystic or solid masses or abdominal fluid. TVUS can also evaluate blood flow within an ovarian mass. Normal ovarian size cutoff parameters range from 1.25 cm^2 for women 55 to 59 years of age to 1.0 cm^2 for women older than age 65 to 69 years.[17,18] TVUS is sensitive in identifying ovarian lesions and abnormalities, but its use as a routine screening test is limited by a lack of specificity and an inability to detect peritoneal cancer or cancer in normal-size ovaries.[19,20]

Serum cancer antigen-125 (CA-125) is a nonspecific inflammatory antigen that can be elevated in numerous conditions associated with inflammation in the abdominal cavity. CA-125 has been extensively studied as a potential tumor marker for ovarian cancer based on the observation that CA-125 levels in a woman without ovarian cancer tend to stay the same or decrease over time, whereas levels associated with malignancy tend to gradually increase over time.[19] However, CA-125 is a nonspecific test that can be elevated in a number of benign conditions, including other gynecologic conditions, such as endometriosis, and many nongynecologic conditions, such as diverticulitis and peptic ulcer disease. Because of these limitations, CA-125 levels are not recommended as a routine screening test for detection of ovarian cancer. Numerous other serologic markers such as carcinoembryonic antigen and lipid-associated sialic acid have been evaluated but cannot be recommended for routine screening for ovarian cancer.

The United States Preventive Services Task Force found fair evidence to support screening with CA-125 or TVUS and concluded that earlier detection would likely have a small effect, at best, on mortality from ovarian cancer.[21] Unfortunately, because of the low prevalence of ovarian cancer and the invasive nature of diagnostic testing after a positive screening test, the United States Preventive Services Task Force also found fair evidence that screening could likely lead to important harms. The United States Preventive Services Task Force concluded that the potential harms outweigh the potential benefits and recommended against any form of routine screening with CA-125 or TVUS for ovarian cancer.

In high-risk women, as defined by family history, most clinicians use a multimodality approach for ovarian cancer screening that includes an annual TVUS in combination with a CA-125 blood test every 6 months. Changes in CA-125 are monitored over time, and changes such as a persistent elevation or consistent increases in CA-125 levels in conjunction with TVUS abnormalities are evaluated further.

PREVENTION

It is difficult to make recommendations for prevention for the general population because ovarian cancer is a sporadic disease with no established risk factors. Noninvasive measures, such as chemoprevention, have demonstrated some benefit in decreasing the risk of developing ovarian cancer. Ovulation itself is considered a potential insult to the ovarian epithelium, increasing its susceptibility to damage and, ultimately, to cancer. Interventions or reproductive conditions associated with decreasing the number of ovulations, including multiparity, may have a protective effect for the prevention of ovarian cancer. However, the more invasive prevention interventions, such as prophylactic surgery and genetic screening, should be reserved for those women identified to be at high risk based on their heredity for developing ovarian cancer.

Chemoprevention

Although a number of agents have been investigated as chemoprevention of ovarian cancer, including oral contraceptives, aspirin, nonsteroidal antiinflammatory agents, and retinoids, none of these agents is currently accepted as standard treatment for the prevention of ovarian cancer. Oral contraceptives inhibit ovulation, which reduces the opportunity for potential for damage to the ovarian epithelium. Oral contraceptives decrease the relative risk to less than 0.4 in women who used oral contraceptives for longer than 10 years.[22,23] Because oral contraceptive use is associated with an increased risk of breast cancer, women with a family history of breast cancer are not candidates for this use of oral contraceptives as chemoprevention of ovarian cancer.[22,23]

Nonsteroidal antiinflammatory drugs, aspirin, and acetaminophen also have been suggested for use in the chemoprevention of different cancers, especially hereditary nonpolyposis colon cancer.[24] Although the results of observational studies show that the use of nonsteroidal antiinflammatory drugs, aspirin, and acetaminophen reduces the risk of ovarian cancer, these findings have not been confirmed in prospective clinical studies. The proposed mechanism of these agents is the antiinflammatory effect on normal ovulation and inhibition of ovulation.[24,25]

Prophylactic Surgery

Prophylactic surgical interventions for the prevention of ovarian cancer are reserved for patients with a significant family history and/or with known genetic mutations such as BRCA1 and should be postponed until after childbearing is completed. The goal is to remove healthy, at-risk organs before any carcinogenic activity is initiated, ultimately reducing the risk of developing cancer. These surgeries include prophylactic oophorectomy or bilateral salpingo-oophorectomy and tubal ligation. These procedures will cause surgical menopause, which can be associated with severe hot flashes, vaginal dryness, sexual dysfunction, and increased risk for development of osteoporosis and heart disease in these women. Because of the potential impact on quality of life and increased health risks, prophylactic surgery is not recommended as a general prevention intervention for the general population.

Although prophylactic surgical interventions are associated with significant reduction in risk of developing ovarian cancer, patients who choose to have a prophylactic oophorectomy/bilateral salpingo-oophorectomy completed need to be informed that complete protection is not guaranteed.[15,23,26] Although a 67% risk reduction has been shown, a potential 2% to 5% risk of primary peritoneal cancer remains.[27,28] Primary peritoneal cancers have identical histology of ovarian tumors with diffuse involvement of peritoneal surfaces. Often primary peritoneal cancers can result from "seeding" during the prophylactic surgery. It is recommended for peritoneal washings to be completed during the prophylactic surgery to check for presence of peritoneal surfaces. If positive, then prophylactic surgery would change to staging and treatment surgery to determine extent of disease and remove any other possible lesions.

Tubal ligation is another procedure that can potentially reduce the risk for developing ovarian cancer. In a case-control study, Narod et al. reported that tubal ligation in BRCA-positive women was associated with a 63% reduction in risk of developing ovarian cancer.[29] However, it is not recommended as a sole procedure in prophylaxis. The mechanism for its protective effect is not clear, but it has been proposed that tubal ligation may limit exposure of the ovary to environmental carcinogens.

GENETIC SCREENING

Genetic screening should be considered for those women with a significant family history of ovarian cancer. Patients should be evaluated for the presence of genes such as BRCA1, BRCA2, or other genes such as those associated with hereditary nonpolyposis colorectal cancer or the hereditary breast ovarian cancer (hereditary breast and ovarian cancer syndrome) syndrome.[29–32] Prior to genetic screening, appropriate patient/family counseling and genetic counseling should be available to help women prepare and deal with the health and psychosocial implications of the genetic screening results.

CLINICAL PRESENTATION

Patients with early ovarian cancer are often asymptomatic and the ovarian mass is often detected incidentally during their annual pelvic examinations. Patients with ovarian cancer often present with non-specific, vague symptoms such as abdominal bloating, indigestion, or change in bowel movements.[2,4,33] These symptoms can easily be confused with symptoms of common benign gastrointestinal disorders. Patients will often not seek medical attention until these symptoms become unrelenting and bothersome, which allows the disease to progress undetected. Patients with advanced disease may report symptoms such as pain, abdominal distension, and ascites.[2,33]

Several groups have partnered together to educate women about early signs and symptoms of ovarian cancer. Goff et al. recently developed a symptom index, based on a comparison of symptoms experienced in patients with ovarian cancer and a matched control group.[34] Symptoms that were correlated with ovarian cancer were persistent or recurrent bloating, pelvic or abdominal pain, difficulty eating or feeling full quickly, and urinary symptoms (either urgency or frequency). The Gynecologic Cancer Foundation, Society of Gynecologic Oncologists, and American Cancer Society recommend that women who have any of those problems nearly every day for more than 2 or 3 weeks should see a gynecologist, especially if the symptoms are new and quite different from her usual state of health.

CLINICAL PRESENTATION OF OVARIAN CANCER

GENERAL

- Ovarian cancer is sometimes referred to as "the silent killer" because of the vague nonspecific signs and symptoms that contribute to the delay in diagnosis.

SYMPTOMS

- The patient may complain of abdominal discomfort, nausea, dyspepsia, flatulence, bloating, fullness, early satiety, urinary frequency, change in bowel function (diarrhea or constipation), weight change, and digestive disturbances.

SIGNS

- Abdominal or pelvic mass may be palpable.
- Lymphadenopathy may be present.
- Vaginal bleeding may be irregular.
- Patient may have signs of ascites (abdominal distension, shifting, and dullness to percussion—may present like "pregnant abdomen").

LABORATORY TESTS

- CA-125 may be elevated (normal level is less than 35 units/mL [35 kU/L]).
- Abnormalities in liver function tests may suggest hepatic involvement.
- Abnormalities in renal function tests may suggest compression of the renal system by the tumor.

DIAGNOSIS

The diagnostic workup for suspected ovarian cancer includes a careful physical examination including a Papanicolaou (Pap) smear and a pelvic and rectovaginal examination.[7] The presence of a pelvic mass that is unilateral or bilateral, solid, irregular, fixed, or nodular is highly suggestive of ovarian cancer. Unfortunately, by the time a pelvic mass can be palpitated on physical exam, the disease is already advanced beyond the pelvic cavity. A detailed family history should be taken, especially noting the number and pattern of first-degree relatives with malignancies.

A complete blood count, chemistry profile (including liver and renal function tests), and CA-125, carcinoembryonic antigen, and CA19–9 levels should be performed. ❸ Although CA-125 is a nonspecific antigen, it is the best current tumor marker for epithelial ovarian carcinoma. A normal CA-125 value is less then 35 units/mL (35 kU/L). If CA-125 is elevated at the time of diagnosis, changes in CA-125 levels correlate with tumor burden. Rising CA-125 levels are often associated with disease progression, but CA-125 can be elevated in various other conditions such as different phases of the menstrual cycle, diverticulitis, endometriosis, as well as other nongynecologic cancers. When a patient presents with an abdominal mass, it is important to rule out other cancers in the abdominal cavity. Carcinoembryonic antigen and CA19–9 are markers for other gastrointestinal cancers and may be helpful in the differential diagnosis.

Other diagnostic tests should include a transvaginal or abdominal ultrasonography, chest radiography, computed tomography, magnetic resonance imaging, or positron emission tomography scan. An upper GI series, intravenous pyelogram, cystoscopy, proctoscopy, or barium enema is sometimes indicated to confirm diagnosis and extent of disease.

TREATMENT

Ovarian Cancer

❹ A multimodality approach that includes comprehensive surgery and chemotherapy is used for the initial treatment of ovarian cancer with curative intent. Although most patients will initially achieve a complete response, more than 50% will recur within the first 2 years.[2,35] A clinical complete response to treatment is defined as no evidence of disease by physical examination or diagnostic tests and a normal CA-125 level.

Chemotherapy regimens for ovarian cancer have evolved over the past few decades. Treatment regimens began with single-agent melphalan followed by single-agent cyclophosphamide. Shortly after cisplatin was introduced into clinical practice, it was added to cyclophosphamide, and this combination was the "standard of care" for over a decade until the introduction of paclitaxel in the 1980s. Paclitaxel soon replaced cyclophosphamide and paclitaxel plus cisplatin became the standard of care. Carboplatin was then substituted for cisplatin because of its improved toxicity profile, and paclitaxel plus carboplatin was adopted. During this same period, many researchers have conducted numerous clinical trials of intraperitoneal (IP) chemotherapy. In 2006, Armstrong and colleagues published the first IP therapy clinical trial to demonstrate a survival advantage over the standard IV regimen.[36] However, these advances in chemotherapy for the treatment of ovarian cancer have not translated into major changes in overall 5-year survival, which remains less then 20%.

Certain subgroups of patients have a better or worse response to chemotherapy. The histologic subtype of the tumor is a prognostic factor; clear cell histology is more likely to be poorly differentiated, faster growing, and have intrinsic drug resistance.[2,37] However, the extent of residual disease, size larger than 1 cm, and tumor grade are better predictors of response to chemotherapy and overall survival.[2]

In general, younger patients have a better performance status and tolerate chemotherapy better than elderly patients. For unknown reasons, white women tend to have a worse prognosis and response to therapy as compared with women of other ethnic backgrounds.[2,6,7]

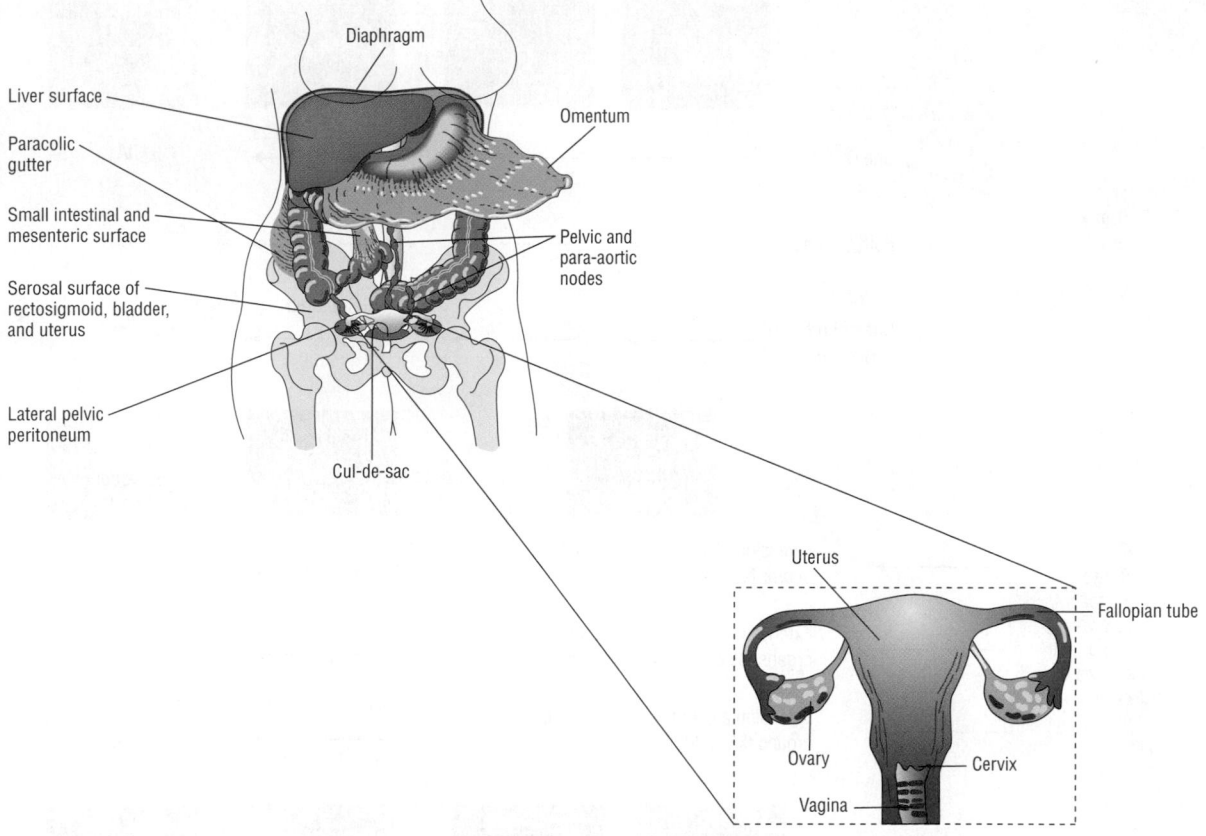

FIGURE 141-1. Staging laparotomy for ovarian cancer with diagram of female reproductive tract (uterus, fallopian tubes, ovaries, vagina). Dashed line box outlines what is removed during the total abdominal hysterectomy with bilateral salpingo-oophorectomy.

In patients with recurrent ovarian cancer, the goals of treatment are to relieve symptoms such as pain or discomfort from ascites, slow disease progression, and prevent serious complications such as small bowel obstructions.

■ SURGERY

Surgery is the primary treatment intervention for ovarian cancer.[37–41] Surgery may be curative for selected patients with limited stage IA disease.

Primary surgical treatment includes a total abdominal hysterectomy with bilateral salpingo-oophorectomy, omentectomy, and lymph node dissection (Fig. 141–1).[37–41] The primary objective of the surgery is to optimally debulk the tumor to less than 1 cm of residual disease.[42] Long-term follow-up studies confirm that residual disease smaller than 1 cm correlates with higher complete response rates to chemotherapy and longer overall survival as compared to patients with bulky residual disease (larger than 1 cm).[40,41]

A comprehensive exploratory laparotomy is vital for the accurate confirmation of diagnosis and staging of ovarian cancer.[37–39] ❺ Unlike other cancers that are typically diagnosed by biopsy or laboratory results and clinically staged by results from imaging tests, gynecologic cancers, such as ovarian cancer, are surgically diagnosed and then staged according to the International Federation of Gynecology and Obstetrics (FIGO) staging algorithm (Fig. 141–2). The FIGO staging system requires a fairly extensive surgery by an experienced gynecologic oncologist. The skill of the surgeon has a significant impact on prognosis, with definitive benefit of a trained gynecologic oncologist performing surgery as compared with a gynecologist or general surgeon.[43] The reasons for this approach include (a) pelvic tumors cannot be readily biopsied without risk of "tumor seeding," which can increase the risk of recurrence, and (b) surgical staging takes

into account the presence of microscopic disease in samples obtained by pelvic washing and lymph node dissection and read by a pathologist during the surgical procedure. It is recommended that the initial surgical staging and tumor-debulking surgery be completed by a trained gynecologic oncology surgeon when ovarian cancer is suspected to prevent understaging and to optimize overall outcome.[44]

Secondary cytoreduction or interval debulking is when surgery is performed after completion of some or all chemotherapy to remove residual disease. Some protocols include additional cycles of chemotherapy after the surgical procedure. The importance of cytoreduction before, during, or after chemotherapy is still controversial, but it has been recommended to facilitate response to chemotherapy and improve overall survival. Randomized trials of secondary surgical cytoreduction have reported conflicting results. In an older randomized trial, van der Burg et al. performed interval debulking surgery on 140 stage IIB to stage IV suboptimally debulked (less than 1 cm of residual disease) ovarian cancer patients after receiving three cycles of cisplatin plus cyclophosphamide.[45] Patients then received an additional three cycles of these same drugs after surgery. Patients randomized to the nonsurgical treatment arm received six cycles of chemotherapy. Interval debulking surgery significantly prolonged overall and progression-free survival and reduced the risk of death by 33%. However, in a recently published study of 550 women with stage III or IV disease treated with primary cytoreductive surgery and three cycles of paclitaxel and cisplatin, patients randomized to receive secondary cytoreductive surgery followed by three more cycles of chemotherapy had similar progression-free survival and overall survival as compared with those randomized to receive three more cycles of chemotherapy alone.[46]

The overall effect of interval debulking is influenced by several factors, including initial response to chemotherapy, the amount of residual disease before and after second-look surgery, and the presence of microscopic residual disease. The results of recent trials

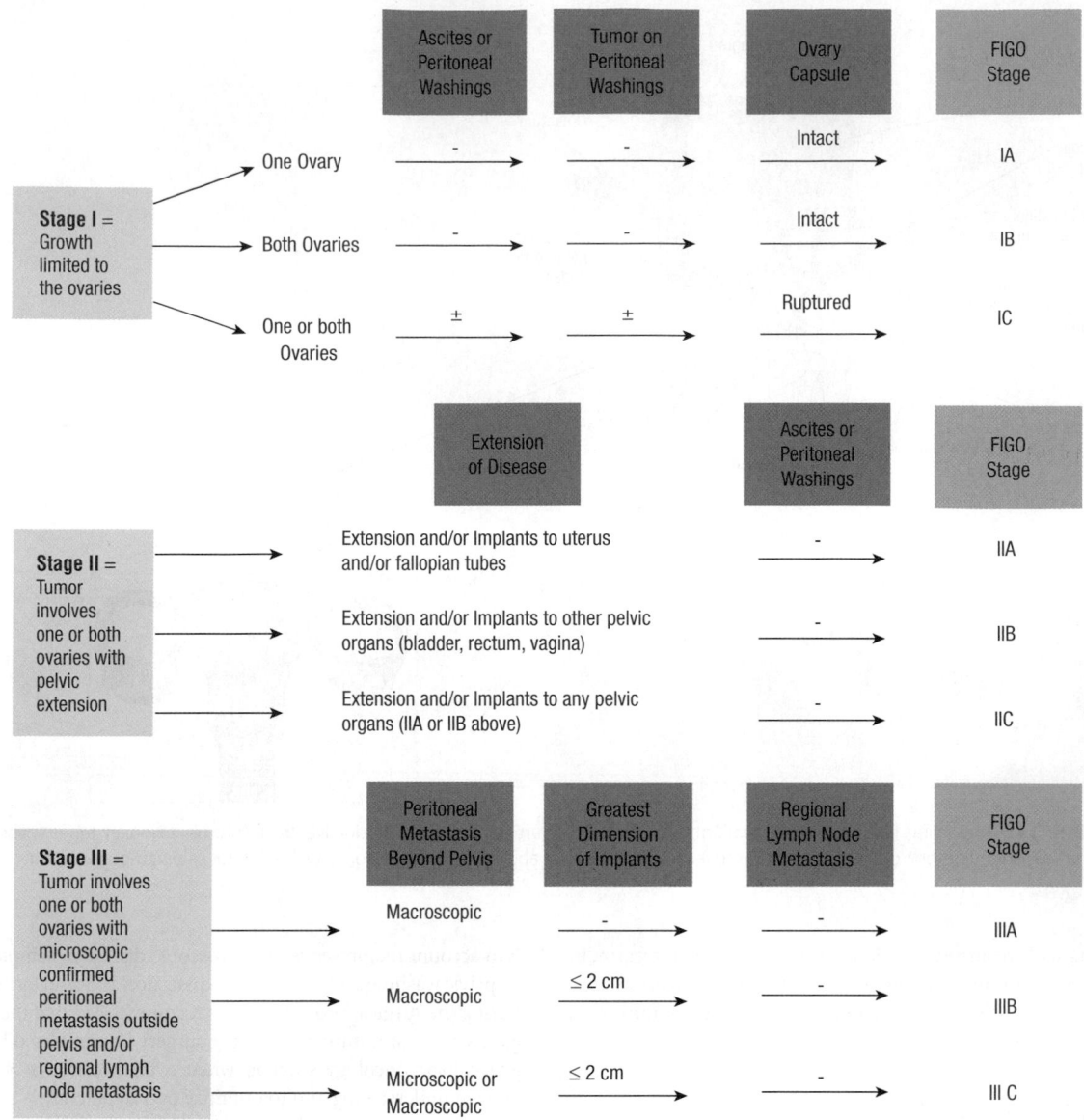

FIGURE 141-2. International Federation of Gynecology and Obstetrics (FIGO) staging algorithm.

suggest that secondary surgical cytoreduction does not prolong survival in patients who are treated with maximal primary cytoreductive surgery followed by appropriate postoperative chemotherapy.

"Second-look surgery" is an elective surgical procedure performed in patients who achieve a clinical complete response after primary chemotherapy to determine if any visible or microscopic disease is present in the peritoneal cavity. The benefit of "second-look laparotomy" to evaluate residual disease after completing chemotherapy remains controversial because it has been difficult to establish any impact on overall survival. It has questionable benefit because approximately 50% of those with a negative second look still relapsed.[3] If visible or microscopic disease is detected during second look, then the clinician may decide to give additional chemotherapy. But if no visible or microscopic disease is detected during second look, the clinician may decide to observe and monitor

the patient. Use of laparoscopic surgical techniques is controversial for initial surgery but is sometimes considered in debulking of recurrent or advanced disease when the intent is palliative rather than curative.[40] In patients with recurrent disease, the goal of debulking surgery is to relieve symptoms associated with complications such as small bowel obstructions and to help improve the patient's quality of life.

■ **RADIATION**

Radiation has a limited role in the management of ovarian cancer. Use of radiation for treatment of early-stage disease has had no benefit or impact on overall survival.[47] Radiation therapy is most beneficial for palliation of symptoms in patients with recurrent pelvic disease, often associated with small bowel obstructions. The two

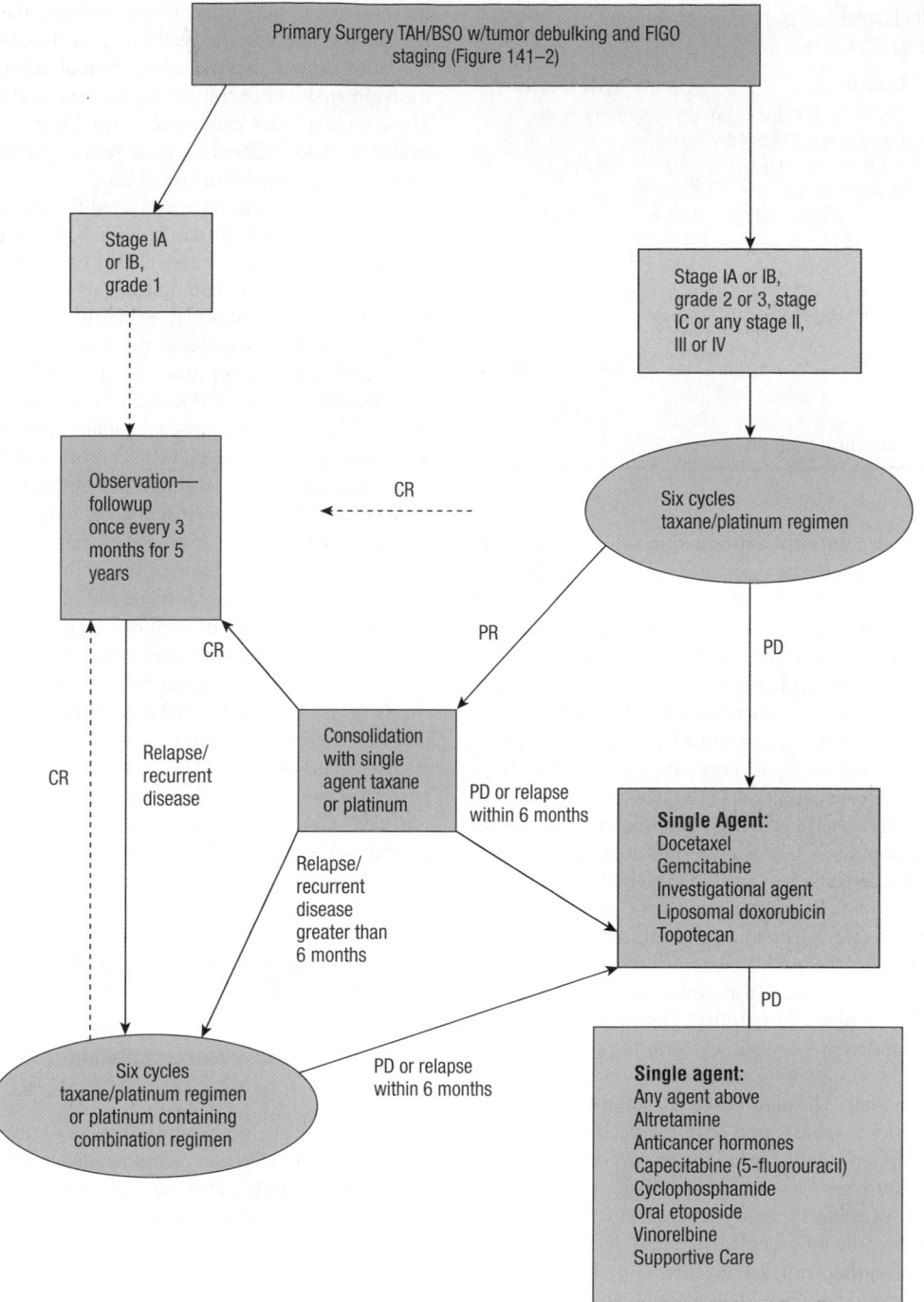

FIGURE 141-3. Management of newly diagnosed, refractory, and progressive epithelial ovarian cancer. All recommendations are category 2A unless otherwise indicated. (BSO, bilateral salpingo-oophorectomy; CR, complete response; PD, progression of disease; PR, partial response; TAH, total abdominal hysterectomy; USO, unilateral salpingo-oophorectomy.)

forms of radiation therapy used in ovarian cancer are external beam whole-abdominal irradiation and intraperitoneal isotopes such as ^{32}P. Alleviation of symptoms with external beam whole-abdominal irradiation is associated with a significant improvement in the patient's quality of life. The recommended dose ranges from 35 to 45 Gy (3500 to 4500 rad), depending on the treatment history and ability to tolerate radiation treatments.

■ CHEMOTHERAPY

The mainstay of ovarian cancer treatment is chemotherapy. It is used as a component of first-line treatment after completion of surgery and is the primary modality of treatment for recurrent ovarian cancer.

First-Line Treatment

Systemic chemotherapy with a taxane and platinum regimen following optimal surgical debulking is the standard of care for treatment of epithelial ovarian cancer (Fig. 141-3). Table 141-1 summarizes the chemotherapeutic regimens used as the initial treatment of newly diagnosed epithelial ovarian cancer. More than 60 randomized, controlled clinical trials have evaluated combination chemotherapy regimens for the treatment of advanced ovarian cancer, and a meta-analysis of these trials confirmed the efficacy of platinum and taxane regimens over other regimens.[48,49]

Historically, single-agent alkylating agents such as melphalan, and later cyclophosphamide, were used for the treatment of

TABLE 141-1 Initial Chemotherapeutic Regimens of Epithelial Ovarian Cancer

Drug(s)	Dose(s)	Cycle Frequency
Paclitaxel + carboplatin	175 mg/m² IV (3-h infusion) day 1 Dosed to AUC 5–7.5 IV day 1	Every 21 days
Paclitaxel + cisplatin (IV)	135 mg/m² IV (24-h infusion) day 1 75 mg/m² IV day 1	Every 21 days
Paclitaxel + cisplatin (IP)	Day 1: Paclitaxel 135 mg/m² IV infused over 24 hours + Day 2: Cisplatin 100 mg/m² IP infused over 1 hour + Day 8: Paclitaxel 60 mg/m² IP infused over 1 hour.	Every 21 days
Cisplatin + cyclophosphamide	50–100 mg/m² IV day 1 500–1,000 mg/m² IV day 1	Every 21–28 days
Docetaxel + carboplatin	75 mg/m² IV day 1 Dosed to AUC 5 IV day 1	Every 21 days

advanced ovarian cancer until the introduction of cisplatin in the 1970s. Combination chemotherapy regimens containing cisplatin and cyclophosphamide achieved higher response rates and overall survival than regimens without cisplatin in patients with advanced ovarian cancer.[50] Based on the results of these trials, the combination of cisplatin plus cyclophosphamide remained the standard of care for the treatment of ovarian cancer until the early 1990s.

The next major advance in the therapy of advanced ovarian cancer occurred with the introduction of paclitaxel into chemotherapy regimens. McGuire et al. reported the results of a Gynecologic Oncology Group (GOG)-111 study that found the combination of paclitaxel 135 mg/m² over 24 hours and cisplatin 75 mg/m² achieved higher response rates and longer survival than did cyclophosphamide 750 mg/m² and cisplatin 75 mg/m² in patients with newly diagnosed, suboptimally debulked, stages III and IV ovarian cancer.[51] Survival improved significantly in the paclitaxel arm, with an increase in median progression-free survival (18 months vs. 13 months) and overall survival (38 months vs. 24 months). Neutropenia, alopecia, and peripheral neuropathy were more severe in the paclitaxel plus cisplatin group. Similar results were reported in a large European-Canadian Intergroup Phase III randomized trial study (OV10) that also confirmed superior response rates with the paclitaxel 135 mg/m² over 24 hours with cisplatin 75 mg/m² regimen as compared with cyclophosphamide 750 mg/m² with cisplatin 75 mg/m² regimen.[52] Based on the results of these studies, paclitaxel plus cisplatin was widely adopted and became the accepted standard of care.

The availability of carboplatin led to clinical trials to evaluate whether carboplatin could be substituted for cisplatin, which would spare patients from the significant neurotoxicity and nephrotoxicity associated with cisplatin. Several prospective randomized comparisons of carboplatin plus paclitaxel versus cisplatin plus paclitaxel in patients with advanced ovarian cancer have been conducted.[53–56] The results of these trials show that carboplatin plus paclitaxel is equally efficacious and better tolerated than cisplatin and paclitaxel. In the GOG-158 study, 840 previously untreated patients with optimally resected stage III disease (no residual tumor nodule >1 cm) were randomized to carboplatin (area-under-the-curve = 7.5) plus paclitaxel 175 mg/m² over 3 hours, or cisplatin 75 mg/m² plus paclitaxel 135 mg/m² over 24 hours administered every 21 days for six cycles.[53,55] The results of that trial showed no difference in progression-free survival between the two treatment arms with a median time-to-progression of 19.4 months in the paclitaxel plus cisplatin arm versus 20.7 months in the paclitaxel plus carboplatin arm. As expected, the incidence of leukopenia, fever, gastrointestinal toxicity, and metabolic toxicity was higher in patients in the cisplatin arm, whereas patients the carboplatin arm experienced more thrombocytopenia and pain. Although

the incidence of neurotoxicity was similar in the two treatment arms, it was more severe in the paclitaxel plus cisplatin arm. The results of this study showed that the substitution of carboplatin for cisplatin in the regimen does not compromise efficacy and improves tolerability. These findings were confirmed in two other large randomized, controlled studies.[55,56] Based on these results, paclitaxel plus carboplatin became the accepted standard of care.

Other clinical trials have evaluated the use of docetaxel as a substitute for paclitaxel. In the Scottish Randomized Trial in Ovarian Cancer (SCOTROC), Vasey et al. compared carboplatin (area-under-the-curve = 5) combined with either docetaxel (75 mg/m² over 1 hour) or paclitaxel (175 mg/m² over 3 hours) administered every 21 days for six cycles as first-line chemotherapy for stages IC to IV epithelial ovarian cancer.[57] The results of this study showed that the substitution of docetaxel for paclitaxel does not compromise efficacy and improves tolerability, particularly neurotoxicity. These findings have not yet been confirmed in another randomized, controlled trial. Based on the results of this study, the combination of docetaxel plus carboplatin is considered a reasonable treatment option for patients with advanced ovarian cancer. Six cycles of paclitaxel plus carboplatin following tumor debulking surgery remain the current standard of care for treatment of advanced ovarian cancer.

Although the choice of taxane or platinum agent does not appear to have a major effect on antitumor activity, weekly paclitaxel administration ("dose density") may be superior to administration every 3 weeks.[58–60] In a phase III trial conducted in Japan, Katsumata et al. reported that patients randomized to six cycles of dose-dense weekly paclitaxel plus carboplatin every 3 weeks had longer progression-free survival as compared to the standard paclitaxel plus carboplatin every 3 weeks.[60] Overall survival at 3 years was also significantly longer in patients who received the dose-dense regimen (72% vs. 65%, P = 0.03). However, more patients who received the dose-dense regimen dropped out of the study because of treatment-related toxicities. A confirmatory Gynecologic Oncology Group (GOG) phase III trial is ongoing to confirm these results and address concerns regarding the feasibility of the dose-dense regimen in a larger group of patients.

CLINICAL CONTROVERSY

The use of IP chemotherapy as first-line treatment of advanced ovarian cancer has been recommended by the NCCN guidelines. Most clinical trials have used platinum agents given IP until the GOG172 trial that incorporated IP paclitaxel. Many clinicians are concerned about how to manage hypersensitivity reactions to either platinum or taxane agents when administered IP.

Intraperitoneal (IP) chemotherapy was initially employed as palliative care in the management of ascites and uncontrolled intraabdominal tumors. In the late 1970s, IP chemotherapy administration as a primary treatment intervention was initiated based on the rationale that exposure of the tumor to high drug concentrations would increase tumor drug uptake by passive diffusion and ultimately cancer cell death.[61] The increase in area-under-the-curve exposure in the peritoneal cavity was demonstrated, but the correlative increase in drug uptake in tumor tissue has yet to be validated in any preclinical or clinical study.

IP chemotherapy has demonstrated a benefit in the first-line treatment of patients with optimally debulked advanced-stage ovarian cancer.[49,62–64] In the most recent trial, Armstrong et al. reported the results of the GOG-172 study, which evaluated 415 patients randomized to receive either the combination regimen of paclitaxel 135 mg/m² over 24 hours and cisplatin 75 mg/m² or a new combination regimen that included paclitaxel 135 mg/m² IV infused over 24 hours followed by cisplatin 100 mg/m² IP infused over 1 hour on day 2, and then paclitaxel 60 mg/m² IP infused over 1 hour on day 8.[36] Both treatment regimens were given once every 21 days for a total of six cycles. Patients randomized to the IP chemotherapy arm had a 5.5-month increase in the median progression-free survival and a 15.9-month increase in overall survival.[36]

Since the publication of this study, there has been a resurgence of interest in the use of IP chemotherapy despite the limitation that only 42% of the patients on the IP treatment arm were able to complete the planned six cycles as a result of significantly more toxicity, including pain, fatigue, myelosuppression, gastrointestinal, metabolic, and neurotoxicity.[36,63,65,66] Because only 42% of patients were able to complete the planned six courses of IP chemotherapy, some experts have questioned whether the route of administration was an important contributing factor in the observed differences in overall survival.[36] The significant increase in systemic toxicity, primarily neurotoxicity, has led to the question of whether IP carboplatin could be substituted for IP cisplatin. Although these platinum agents have demonstrated equal efficacy when administered intravenously to ovarian cancer patients, based on the concept that drug passively diffuses into the tumor, the difference in molecular size of cisplatin versus carboplatin makes it difficult to extrapolate IP activity of cisplatin to carboplatin.

The NCCN 2010 guidelines recommend that IP chemotherapy be considered and offered to patients as appropriate first-line treatment of optimally debulked, ≥1 cm residual disease, ovarian cancer.[67] The National Cancer Institute also released a position statement in January 2006 supporting the role of IP chemotherapy as first-line treatment for advanced ovarian cancer.[68] Because of the significant toxicities associated with IP therapy, only carefully selected patients should receive IP therapy. Ideal candidates for IP therapy are younger patients with good performance status, minimal comorbidities, adequate renal and liver function, and optimally debulked disease without significant bowel resection.[62,66]

In patients who are poor surgical candidates because of comorbidities or bulky tumors, neoadjuvant chemotherapy can be given prior to any surgical interventions.[69] In patients with bulky disease, the goal of neoadjuvant chemotherapy is to reduce tumor burden to make surgery more feasible and optimal tumor debulking more likely. The typical regimen used in neoadjuvant chemotherapy is three cycles of a taxane combined with a platinum agent followed by surgery. After surgery, patients usually receive another three to six cycles, depending on their response to chemotherapy. In patients who are poor candidates for surgery because of comorbidities, the, primary intent of neoadjuvant chemotherapy is to relieve symptoms and slow disease progression. In this setting, palliative chemotherapy alone has not been curative for patients with advanced ovarian cancer.[69] If tolerated, these patients will receive the standard taxane plus platinum chemotherapy regimen once every 3 to 4 weeks. Another option for palliative neoadjuvant chemotherapy, especially in elderly patients, is single-agent carboplatin once every 4 weeks.

Consolidation Therapy

If patients do not achieve a clinical complete response after completion of six cycles of taxane-platinum regimen, then consolidation chemotherapy should be considered in an attempt to achieve a complete response (Fig. 141–3). If the patient has a partial response to first-line chemotherapy, as measured by a greater than 50% decline in CA-125 (as compared with the presurgery level) or tumor regression, the cancer is still considered sensitive to the regimen. The typical regimens for consolidation chemotherapy are the taxane plus platinum regimen or single-agent therapy with either a taxane or platinum agent.[70] If the patient had a poor response to taxane and platinum, then alternative second-line agents can be considered.[67] Additional cycles of chemotherapy are given until

complete response is achieved. Another alternative in the setting of no or minimal measurable disease after completion of primary chemotherapy is to just observe the patient and provide supportive care as indicated until disease progresses, then reinitiate chemotherapy at that time.[67]

Because the initial clinical complete response observed in first-line treatment has not been durable, optimization of first-line therapy is under investigation. Numerous options have been evaluated, including the use of additional cycles or maintenance chemotherapy and dose intensity.

Maintenance Chemotherapy Maintenance chemotherapy is similar to consolidation chemotherapy except maintenance chemotherapy is given to those patients who have achieved a clinically complete response. The primary differences between consolidation and maintenance chemotherapy are the types of agents used and duration of therapy. Consolidation therapy usually consists of more aggressive combination regimens, whereas maintenance chemotherapy usually consists of single agents given less frequently (i.e., once monthly) to minimize adverse effects. The goal of maintenance chemotherapy is to eradicate any residual microscopic disease that may be present to extend progression-free and overall survival.

Maintenance chemotherapy has gained popularity after the publication of the results of the collaborative Southwest Oncology Group and GOG 178 study that compared single-agent paclitaxel 175 mg/m² over 3 hours once every 21 days for three additional cycles versus an additional 12 cycles.[71,72] Eligible patients had to have been in complete clinical remission after at least five to six cycles of a taxane-platinum regimen. This study was closed after the interim analysis by the Southwest Oncology Group Safety Monitoring Committee because patients receiving the additional 12 cycles had longer progression-free survival than those receiving three cycles of single-agent paclitaxel (28 vs. 21 months). After the results were reported, many patients randomized to the three-cycle arm chose to receive nine additional cycles of paclitaxel, which reduced the ability of the trial to show a difference in overall survival.[73] Because this study was closed early and did not demonstrate an overall survival benefit, another randomized, controlled trial through the GOG was initiated to confirm the improvement in progression-free survival and to attempt to determine the impact on overall survival. Until these confirmatory trials are completed, the role of maintenance chemotherapy is controversial in the management of advanced ovarian cancer patients. Maintenance chemotherapy is listed as an option in the 2010 NCCN guidelines (2B recommendation).[67]

High-Dose Chemotherapy with Hematopoietic Stem Cell Rescue High-dose chemotherapy with autologous or allogeneic hematopoietic stem cell transplantation (HSCT) is an option for selected patients with chemosensitive disease, few comorbidities, and good performance status. Although high response rates have been reported in patients with recurrent ovarian cancer treated with autologous HSCT, the duration of response is usually short and few patients have experienced long-term progression-free survival.[74,75] Allogeneic HSCT has also been evaluated in recurrent ovarian cancer to induce an immune response against the tumor ("graft-versus-tumor" effect).

Based on the activity of autologous HSCT in recurrent ovarian cancer, Goncalves et al. evaluated the modality for first-line treatment of patients with optimally debulked ovarian cancer. In this multicenter phase II study, 34 patients received two cycles of high-dose cyclophosphamide-epirubicin once every 21 days followed by two cycles of high-dose carboplatin (days 42 and 98).[76] Each dose of high-dose carboplatin was followed by hematopoietic stem cell infusion. The results of this study failed to show an improvement in the rate of pathologic complete response with upfront autologous HSCT as compared with standard taxane plus platinum

TABLE 141-2 Single-Agent Chemotherapeutic Regimens for Recurrent or Refractory Ovarian Cancer

Drug(s)	Dose(s)	Cycle Frequency
Docetaxel	75 mg/m^2 IV day 1	Every 21 days
Pegylated-liposomal doxorubicin	40 mg/m^2 IV day 1	Every 28 days
Gemcitabine	800–1000 mg/m^2 IV days 1, 8, and 15	Every 28 days
Paclitaxel	60–80 mg/m^2 IV (1-h infusion) day 1	Every week
Paclitaxel	135–175 mg/m^2 IV day 1	Every 21 days
Carboplatin	AUC 5 IV day 1	Every 21–28 days
Cisplatin	75 mg/m^2 IV day 1	Every 21–28 days
Topotecan	1.3–1.5 mg/m^2 IV once daily for 5 days	Every 21 days
Topotecan	4 mg/m^2 IV once a week × 3 weeks, then 1 week off	Every 21 days
Etoposide	50 mg/m^2 orally once daily days 1–10 repeat every 21 days	Every 28 days
Capecitabine	1800–2000 mg/m^2 in divided dose twice a day for 2 weeks on, 1 week off	Every 21 days
Altretamine	260 mg/m^2 orally (total daily dose divided in four doses) for 14–21 days	Every 28 days
Tamoxifen	20 mg orally twice a day	Continuous
Letrozole	2.5 mg orally once daily	Continuous

TABLE 141-3 Combination Chemotherapy Regimens for Platinum-Sensitive Recurrent Ovarian Cancer

Drug(s)	Dose(s)	Cycle Frequency
Gemcitabine + carboplatin	800 mg/m^2 IV day 1 & 8	Every 21 days
Gemcitabine + cisplatin	Dosed to AUC 5 IV day 1	Every 21 days
Liposomal doxorubicin + carboplatin	Day 1 & Day 8: Gemcitabine 800 mg/m^2 & Cisplatin 40 mg/m^2	Every 28 days
Cyclophosphamide + bevacizumab	30 mg/m^2 IV over 1–3 hr & carboplatin AUC 5	Every 28 days
	50 mg PO once daily + bevacizumab 15 mg/kg q 3 weeks	

chemotherapy. Additional studies are ongoing to determine the role of autologous or allogeneic HSCT in the treatment of advanced ovarian cancer.

Treatment of Recurrent Disease

❹ Although most patients will achieve a complete response to initial treatment, most patients will eventually have recurrence of their disease. When a patient relapses, the prognostic factors are similar to the factors after initial surgery except that the disease-free interval—defined as the length of time that has lapsed since the completion of chemotherapy—should be considered to determine if the tumor is likely to be drug resistant. If recurrence occurs less than 6 months after completion of chemotherapy, or if the patient progresses during platinum-based chemotherapy, the tumor is defined as platinum-resistant. Patients with platinum-sensitive disease generally have a better prognosis than platinum-resistant patients.

Because the chemotherapy agents used for second-line treatment of recurrent or refractory platinum-resistant disease have similar response rates that average less than 30%, the selection of the agent depends on the toxicity profile of the agent, physician preference, patient performance status, residual toxicities, and patient convenience (Fig. 141–3). Participation in a clinical trial of an investigational agent is also a reasonable option for these patients. If the patient has a clinical complete response to first-line chemotherapy and the recurrence occurs more than 6 months after chemotherapy is completed, the tumor is considered platinum-sensitive. Table 141–2 summarizes some of the chemotherapeutic regimens used in the treatment of recurrent or refractory ovarian cancer.

CLINICAL CONTROVERSY

In patients with recurrent ovarian cancer that is platinum-sensitive, some clinicians will recommend re-treatment with a chemotherapy regimen including a platinum agent. Other clinicians suggest that the platinum-free interval for these patients should be extended and will recommend that recurrent disease first be treated with a nonplatinum regimen (i.e., liposomal doxorubicin) and reserving the platinum agent until the next relapse.

Platinum-Sensitive Disease Re-treatment with a platinum-containing regimen should be considered in patients with platinum-sensitive disease. The International Collaborative Ovarian Neoplasm 4 and Arbeitsgemeinschaft Gynaekologische randomized 802 patients with recurrent platinum-sensitive ovarian cancer to either single-agent platinum, a non–taxane-platinum combination, or a taxane plus platinum combination.[75] Patients treated with the paclitaxel plus platinum regimen had significantly longer progression-free (29 vs. 24 months) and overall survival (hazard ratio = 0.82 [95% CI 0.69 to 0.97]) as compared with the other two treatment arms.[77,78] Although the taxane–platinum combination was clearly superior in this European study, it is difficult to extrapolate these results to patients treated in the United States because of differences in first-line treatment. At the time that International Collaborative Ovarian Neoplasm (ICON) 4 was conducted, the standard of care in Europe for first-line treatment was single-agent carboplatin, so most patients enrolled in this study had no prior exposure to a taxane agent.[77] However, the standard of care in the United States has been a taxane-platinum combination since the early 1990s. Confirmatory data is needed to evaluate whether combination regimens would also be more beneficial in these patients for treatment of recurrent ovarian cancer.

The 2010 NCCN guidelines recommend the combination of carboplatin with gemcitabine, liposomal doxorubicin, or paclitaxel for treatment of platinum-sensitive recurrent ovarian cancer[67] (Table 141–3). In addition, the combination of gemcitabine plus cisplatin has demonstrated improvement in progression-free survival[78] (Table 141–3). Carboplatin alone or any of the second-line agents is recommended for patients with platinum-sensitive disease who are unable to tolerate additional combination chemotherapy regimens because of residual toxicity or poor performance status.[67,79]

Platinum-Resistant Disease Frequently patients present with recurrent drug-resistant disease after initial platinum-based therapy and cytoreductive surgery.[80,81] Patients who progress on a platinum agent or have no response are considered "platinum-refractory," whereas those patients who have recurrence within 6 months of completing a platinum-containing regimen are considered "platinum-resistant."[79] The 2010 NCCN guidelines list many possible treatment options for recurrent platinum-resistant or -refractory ovarian carcinoma.[67] The optimal chemotherapeutic agent or regimen in the treatment of platinum-resistant disease is currently unclear. Ideally, the agent should be active in ovarian cancer and non–cross-resistant with taxanes or platinum agents. Regrettably, the response rate is low for all of the agents in platinum-refractory or -resistant ovarian cancer.[82] Patients should typically be evaluated for response after treatment with at least three cycles of the chemotherapy agent or regimen. Because partial responses are rare, stable disease is considered a treatment success. If no response is observed, then an alternative chemotherapy regimen may be selected.

Topotecan, an analog of the plant alkaloid 20(S)-camptothecin, is active in patients with metastatic ovarian cancer and is non–cross-resistant with platinum-based chemotherapy.[83] Preclinical studies suggest that protracted schedules of administration with low doses achieve the greatest antitumor response.[84] Topotecan has demonstrated activity in phase II trials as second-line and salvage therapy in patients who have relapsed after, or progressed during, platinum-based therapy.[83–85] A randomized phase III trial compared topotecan and paclitaxel in patients with advanced ovarian cancer who had failed one platinum-based regimen.[86] Patients were randomized to receive topotecan 1.5 mg/m^2 per day as a 30-minute infusion for 5 days repeated every 21 days or paclitaxel 175 mg/m^2 as a 3-hour infusion every 21 days. The overall response rate was 21% and 13% for the topotecan- and paclitaxel-treated groups, respectively. The median time-to-progression for topotecan-treated patients (32 weeks) was not significantly different from that for paclitaxel-treated patients (20 weeks). Median survival was 61 weeks in the topotecan-treated group and 43 weeks in the paclitaxel-treated group. Topotecan was well tolerated with minimal nonhematologic toxicities.[83,85,86]

Pegylated liposomal doxorubicin is one of the primary agents used for second-line therapy of recurrent ovarian cancer.[87–89] The drug tends to be better tolerated than topotecan, which is important for heavily pretreated patients with advanced disease. A large, randomized phase III study compared pegylated liposomal doxorubicin 50 mg/m^2 every 4 weeks to topotecan 1.5 mg/m^2 per day for 5 days repeated every 21 days in patients who failed first-line platinum therapy.[86] A total of 474 patients were randomized, 239 to pegylated liposomal doxorubicin and 235 to topotecan. The overall response rates for the pegylated liposomal doxorubicin and topotecan groups were 20% and 17%, respectively. Overall survival tended to favor pegylated liposomal doxorubicin, with a median of 108 weeks versus 71 weeks for topotecan. Differences in toxicity were observed between the arms, with more hematologic toxicity occurring in the topotecan arm and more palmar-plantar erythrodysesthesia (PPE) in the pegylated liposomal doxorubicin arm. However, the incidence of PPE has decreased in current clinical practice because the standard dose of pegylated liposomal doxorubicin used currently, 40 mg/m^2, is less than the dose that was used in the initial clinical trials and approved by the FDA.[90,91]

Gemcitabine, a novel pyrimidine antimetabolite, is also widely used in the treatment of recurrent platinum-resistant ovarian cancer. Although the overall response rate is only approximately 13% to 22% with single-agent gemcitabine in patients with platinum-refractory recurrent ovarian cancer, an additional 16% to 50% of patients have stable disease for a median of 7 months.[92,93] The main toxicities include myelosuppression, fatigue, myalgia, and skin rash. Because of its non–cross-resistant activity and in vivo synergy with platinum agents, gemcitabine is being evaluated in doublet regimens in patients with refractory disease and with carboplatin/taxane regimens in previously untreated patients.[93] The combination of gemcitabine with taxanes has demonstrated response rates from 36% to 90%, which if confirmed, are extremely encouraging.[93]

Other agents that have shown an overall response rate of 10% to 25% in patients with recurrent ovarian cancer include altretamine, etoposide, capecitabine, tamoxifen, letrozole, vinorelbine, and oxaliplatin.[94] Response rates tend to be higher in the platinum-sensitive subgroups. Most of these agents are available in oral formulations, which allows for outpatient administration in the palliative care setting.

Although there are no therapeutic guidelines for the selection of agents for the treatment of recurrent platinum-resistant ovarian cancer, the three most commonly used agents in clinical practice include pegylated liposomal doxorubicin, gemcitabine, and topotecan. These agents have demonstrated efficacy when used as a single agent and in combination with other agents. A phase II GOG study is ongoing to help define the optimal chemotherapy combination for treatment of recurrent or refractory platinum-resistant ovarian cancer.

Additional research continues to identify new agents and new targets for the treatment of ovarian cancer. Because platinum agents and taxanes have been identified as the most active classes of agents for treatment of ovarian cancer, drug development has focused on new platinum derivatives, taxanes and taxane analogs, and agents that exert cytotoxic activity by interacting with DNA directly. Specifically, new cytotoxic agents such as Yondelis, TLK-286, pemetrexed, and epothilones are currently being evaluated in clinical trials.

Biologic and Targeted Agents

Monoclonal antibodies such as bevacizumab and cetuximab and small-molecule tyrosine kinase inhibitors such as sunitinib, gefitinib, or sorafenib, are being incorporated into first-line and recurrent treatment regimens for ovarian cancer.[95–99] Although the biological agents as single agents have not demonstrated significant activity, the results of several clinical trials support the incorporation of agents such as bevacizumab into first-line and maintenance regimens to improve progression-free survival.

Bevacizumab Bevacizumab is a recombinant humanized monoclonal antibody that targets vascular endothelial growth factor (VEGF), a key mediator of angiogenesis. In the setting of recurrent disease, single-agent bevacizumab produces a response rate similar to other therapies of 16% to 21%.[100,101] Response rates with combinations of bevacizumab range from 15% to 80%.[98,100–110] However, these phase II trials have also reported a higher risk of bowel perforation in patients treated with bevacizumab-containing regimens.[100,101,111] Bevacizumab should therefore not be given to patients who have had recent bowel surgery or a history of significant bowel resections. Recent efforts have focused on the integration of bevacizumab into first-line treatment regimens. Phase II studies confirmed the safety and feasibility of six cycles of paclitaxel, carboplatin plus bevacizumab, given every 3 weeks, followed by maintenance bevacizumab once every 3 weeks for 1 year.[107,108] Based on these encouraging results, the GOG initiated a confirmatory phase III study comparing six cycles of standard paclitaxel plus carboplatin to six cycles of the same regimen with bevacizumab to determine whether bevacizumab improves the efficacy of paclitaxel plus carboplatin. The duration of maintenance bevacizumab remains controversial. The results of these trials should determine the role of bevacizumab in the treatment of ovarian cancer.

CLINICAL CONTROVERSY

Although bevacizumab has demonstrated some progression-free survival advantages when used in combination, its impact on overall survival is not clear. There are concerns regarding the high cost of bevacizumab with potential minimal or no benefit. As a result, health insurance companies do not consistently reimburse providers for bevacizumab when used for the treatment of ovarian cancer.

Targeted Agents Tyrosine kinase inhibitors such as sorafenib, sunitinib, pazopanib, and cediranib inhibit angiogenesis by specifically targeting the VEGF receptor (VEGFR). When given as single agents, tyrosine kinase inhibitors have demonstrated some antitumor activity in ovarian cancer.[112,113] Ongoing trials have focused on combination regimens with cytotoxic agents for first-line treatment and also treatment of recurrent ovarian cancer. Another interesting targeted agent is VEGF Trap (aflibercept), a fusion protein that targets VEGF-A. Aflibercept has been beneficial in the treatment of malignant ascites and is currently being incorporated into first-line regimens. Epidermal growth factor receptor (EGFR) inhibitors such as erlotinib have not demonstrated activity either alone or combined with chemotherapy or bevacizumab for the treatment of ovarian cancer.[109] The newer classes of targeted therapies such as platelet-derived growth factor (PDGF) inhibitors and poly-ADP-ribose polymerase (PARP) inhibitors are being investigated in ongoing clinical trials.[114]

PHARMACOECONOMIC CONSIDERATIONS

Healthcare at the end of life is associated with higher costs than at any other time, and, unfortunately, most patients with ovarian cancer will eventually die from the disease.[115] In the past, cost-to-benefit analyses have demonstrated palliative care, despite the limited benefit, is cost-effective based on patients' expectations and "willingness to pay."[116,117] Economic analyses of new chemotherapy agents usually measure cost-effectiveness, where effectiveness is measured as changes in survival (i.e., overall survival, progression-free survival) or quality-adjusted life-years.[118]

The paclitaxel plus platinum regimen is the current accepted standard of care for first-line treatment of advanced ovarian cancer. When paclitaxel was initially evaluated as first-line treatment, several economic analyses showed that the cost-effectiveness ratio of paclitaxel and cisplatin was within the range of other accepted medical interventions and supported its adoption as first-line treatment of advanced ovarian cancer.[118,119] In another cost-benefit study, Dranitsaris et al. reported that patients were willing to pay a mean of $64, which was marginally lower than the incremental cost of $87 to receive docetaxel rather than paclitaxel to reduce their risk of toxicity, primarily neuropathy.[120]

In the setting of recurrent ovarian cancer, Smith et al. performed a retrospective cost minimization analysis of pegylated liposomal doxorubicin versus topotecan.[121] The results of that analysis showed that pegylated liposomal doxorubicin was the preferred second-line agent, based on lower costs because of reduced toxicities as compared with topotecan.[121]

Finally the other pharmacoeconomic struggle is the use of biologically targeted agents such as bevacizumab in the maintenance and recurrent ovarian treatment settings. Since neither the dose nor optimal regimen have been defined yet for treatment of ovarian cancer, this issue will remain unresolved until more long-term data are available.

EVALUATION OF THERAPEUTIC OUTCOMES

Patients receiving a taxane or platinum chemotherapy regimen should be monitored for signs of hypersensitivity or infusion-related reactions. Patients treated with paclitaxel often experience infusion-related reactions, which have been attributed to the cremophor diluent. Premedications including an H_1-blocker, H_2-blocker, and steroid should be administered prior to each chemotherapy administration to prevent hypersensitivity reactions. If a patient has a reaction, increasing the duration of the infusion from 3 to 6 hours may help with infusion-related reactions. For patients with a true taxane allergy, paclitaxel desensitization can be attempted with 24 hours of premedications (H_1-blocker, H_2-blocker, and steroids) followed by paclitaxel given as a titrated infusion (1:1000 → 1:100 →1:10 → full dose) over 8 hours. With repeated exposure (i.e., seven cycles or more) to carboplatin, patients can develop a delayed hypersensitivity reaction. A similar protocol can be used for carboplatin desensitization.

Ovarian cancer patients receive multiple courses of chemotherapy that can have varying effects on kidney and liver function. Appropriate laboratory tests should be ordered to assess organ function so that chemotherapy doses can be adjusted as indicated. Patients on platinum-containing regimens can often experience electrolyte wasting, so patients should be monitored for electrolyte replacement, intravenous or oral, as indicated. The use of myeloid growth factors should be considered to prevent treatment delays and/or dose reductions. Prevention of nausea and vomiting, both acute and delayed, is critical for patients receiving emetogenic chemotherapy regimens such as paclitaxel plus carboplatin.

During initial taxane plus platinum chemotherapy, a CA-125 level should be obtained with each cycle and monitored for at least a 50% reduction in CA-125 after completion of four cycles, which is related to an improved prognosis. Patients who achieve a complete response after completion of first-line treatment should have follow-up once every 3 months, including CA-125, physical examination, pelvic examination, and appropriate diagnostic scans (i.e., computed tomography, magnetic resonance imaging, or positron emission tomography), which should be evaluated for presence of disease. In addition to routine follow-up examinations, clinicians should monitor for resolution of any residual chemotherapy-related side effects, including neuropathies, nephrotoxicity, ototoxicity, myelosuppression, and nausea/vomiting.

In the progressive disease or recurrent setting, CA-125 levels can still be used to monitor for response and should be checked with each cycle, although no change in therapy is recommended until after completion of at least three cycles of the second-line chemotherapy. In addition to laboratory monitoring, appropriate diagnostic scans (i.e., computed tomography, magnetic resonance imaging, or positron emission tomography) should be done once every three cycles. Patients need to be monitored with each cycle of chemotherapy to evaluate for new or persistent toxicities such as neuropathies, fluid retention, PPE, myelosuppression, and nausea/vomiting. Another precaution to keep in mind for patients with significant ascites, the "dry weight" or an adjusted body weight should be used for dosing chemotherapy.

Eventually, most ovarian cancer patients will progress through all chemotherapy regimens and investigational treatment options, after which the best supportive care measures should be provided to maintain patient comfort and quality of life. A plan to treat common complications of progressive ovarian cancer, including thrombosis, ascites, uncontrollable pain, and small bowel obstruction should be developed. The primary goal at the end of life for patients with progressive ovarian cancer is to provide any measures necessary to maintain patient comfort and quality of life.

CONCLUSIONS

Despite gallant research efforts, ovarian cancer remains one of the major challenges in gynecologic oncology. One of the key issues for improving outcome is to educate patients as to the signs and symptoms of ovarian cancer. Earlier diagnosis is associated with a significant improvement in prognosis and overall survival. Although some milestones have been reached in extending progression-free and overall survival over the past few decades, there are still many unresolved issues. More data are needed to determine the role of biological agents to be used in first-line and recurrent treatment regimens and their impact on overall survival. Research needs to identify and develop new approaches to the treatment of advanced primary and recurrent or refractory ovarian cancer, such as agents to modulate or overcome drug resistance, new molecular targets, and optimized chemotherapy regimens.

ABBREVIATIONS

AUC: area-under-the-curve

BRCA1: breast cancer activator gene 1

BRCA2: breast cancer activator gene 2

BSO: bilateral sphingo-oophorectomy

CA125: cancer antigen 125

CA-19: cancer antigen 19

CEA: carinoembroynic antigen

CR: complete response

DLT: dose limiting toxicity

FIGO: International Federation of Gynecology and Obstetrics

GFR: glomerular filtration rate

GOG: Gynecologic Oncology Group

HBOC: hereditary breast ovarian cancer

HNPCC: Hereditary Nonpolyposis Colorectal Cancer

IP: intraperitoneal

NCCN: National Comprehensive Cancer Network

NR: not reported

PD: progressive disease

PR: partial response

SBO: small bowel obstruction

SWOG: Southwest Oncology Group

VEGF: vascular endothelial growth factor

VEGFR: vascular endothelial growth factor receptor

REFERENCES

1. Bast RC, Brewer M, Zou, C, et al. Prevention and early detection of ovarian cancer: Mission impossible? *Recent Results Cancer Res.* 2007;174:91–100.

2. Heintz APM, Odicino F, Maisonneuve P, et al. Carcinoma of the ovary. FIGO 6th annual report on the results of treatment in gynecological cancer. Int J Gynaecol Obstet 2006; 95(suppl): S161–S192.

3. Jemal A, Siegel R, Xu J, Ward E. Cancer statistics, 2010 CA Cancer J Clin 2010;60:277–300.

4. Colomob N, VanGorp T, Parma G, et al. Ovarian cancer. Crit Rev Oncol Hematol 2006;60:159–179.

5. Lux MP, Fashing PA, Beckmann MW. Hereditary breast and ovarian cancer: Review and future perspectives. J Mol Med 2006;84:16–28.

6. Prat J, Ribe A, Gallarda A. Hereditary ovarian cancer. Hum Pathol. 2005;36:861–870.

7. Lancaster JM, Powell CB, Kauff ND, et al. Society of Gynecologic Oncologists Education Committee statement on risk assessment for inherited gynecologic cancer predispositions. Gynecol Oncol 2007;107:159–162.

8. Riman T, Persson I, Nilsson S. Hormonal aspects of epithelial ovarian cancer: review of epidemiological evidence. Clin Endocrinol 1998;49:695–707.

9. Aletti GC, Gallenberg MM, Cliby WA, et al. Current management strategies for ovarian cancer. Mayo Clin Proc 2007;82(6):751–770.

10. Edmondson RJ, Monaghan JM. The epidemiology of ovarian cancer. Int J Gynecol Cancer 2001;11:423–429.

11. Bhoola S, Hoskins WJ. Diagnosis and management of epithelial ovarian cancer. Obstet Gynecol 2006;107:1399–1410.

12. Cannistra SA, Gershenson, DM, Recht A. Ovarian cancer, fallopian tube carcinoma, and peritoneal carcinoma. In: Devita VT, Hellman S, Rosenberg SA, eds. Cancer: Principles and Practice of Oncology. 8th ed. Philadelphia: Lippincott Williams & Wilkins; 2008: 1568–1592.

13. Silverberg SG, Histopathologic grading of ovarian carcinoma: A review and proposal. Int J Gynecol Pathol 2000;19:7–15.

14. Seidman JD, Kuman RJ. Pathology of ovarian carcinoma. Hematol Oncol Clin North Am 2003;17:909–925.

15. Krygiou M, Tsoumpou I, Martin-Hirsch P, et al. Ovarian cancer screening. Anticancer Res 2006;26:4793–4801.

16. Patterson DM, Rustin GJS. Controversies in the management of germ cell tumours of the ovary. Curr Opin Oncol 2006;18:500–506.

17. Sherman ME, Lacey JV, Buys SS, et al. Ovarian volume: Determinants and associations with cancer among postmenopausal women. Cancer Epidemiol Biomarkers Prev 2006;15:1550–1554.

18. Pavlik EJ, DePriest PD, Gallion HH, et al. Ovarian volume related to age. Gynecol Oncol 2000;77:410–412.

19. Edwards BK, Brown ML, Wingo PA, et al. Annual report to the nation on the status of cancer 1975–2002 featuring population-based trends in cancer treatment. J Natl Cancer Inst 2005;97:1407–1427.

20. Munkarah A, Chatterjee M, Tainsky MA. Update on ovarian cancer screening. Curr Opin Obstet Gynecol 2007;19:22–26.

21. U.S. Preventive Services Task Force. Screening for ovarian cancer: Recommendation statement. Ann Fam Med 2004;2:260–262.

22. Chu CS, Rubin SC. Screening for ovarian cancer in the general population. Best Pract Res Clin Obstet Gynaecol 2006;20:307–320.

23. Dann JL, Zorn KK. Strategies for ovarian cancer prevention. Obstet Gynecol Clin N Am 2007;34:667–686.

24. Harris RE, Beebe-Donk J, Doss H, et al. Aspirin, ibuprofen, and other non-steroidal anti-inflammatory drugs in cancer prevention: A critical review of non-selective COX-2 blockade. Oncol Rep 2005;13: 559–583.

25. Tavani A, Gallus S, La Vecchia C, Cont E, Montella M, Franceschi S. Aspirin and ovarian cancer: An Italian case-control study. Ann Oncol 2000;11:1171–1173.

26. Domchek SM, Rebbeck TR. Prophylactic oophorectomy in women at increased cancer risk. Curr Opin Obstet Gynecol 2007;19:27–30.

27. Meeuwissen PAM, Seynaeve C, Brekelmans CTM, Meijers-Heijboer HJ, Klijn JGM, Burger CW. Outcome of surveillance and prophylactic salpingo-oophorectomy in asymptomatic women at high risk for ovarian cancer. Gynecol Oncol 2005;97:476–482.

28. Finch A, Beiner M, Lubinski J, et al. Salpingo-oophorectomy and the risk of ovarian, fallopian tube, and peritoneal cancers in women with a *BRCA1* or *BRCA2* mutation. JAMA 2006;296:185–192.

29. Narod SA, Sun P, Ghadirian P, et al. Tubal ligation and risk of ovarian cancer in carriers of *BRCA1* and *BRCA2* mutations: A case control study. Lancet 2001;357:1467–1470.

30. Lux MP, Fashing PA, Beckmann MW. Hereditary breast and ovarian cancer: Review and future perspectives. J Mol Med 2006;84(1): 16–28.

31. Coukos, G. Gene therapy for ovarian cancer. Oncology 2001;15: 1197–1208.

32. Tait DL, Obermiller PS, Hatmaker AR, Relin-Frazier S, Holt JT. Ovarian cancer *BRCA1* gene therapy: Phase I and II trial differences in immune response and vector stability. Clin Cancer Res 1999;5:1708–1714.

33. Goff BA, Mandel LS, Melancon CH, Muntz HG. Frequency of symptoms of ovarian cancer in women presenting to primary care clinics. JAMA 2004;291:2705–2712.

34. Goff BA, Mandel LS, Drescher CW, et al. Development of an ovarian cancer symptom index. Cancer 2007;109:221–227.

35. Salzberg M, Thurlimann B, Bonnefois H, et al. Current concepts of treatment strategies in advanced or recurrent ovarian cancer. Oncology 2005;68:293–298.

36. Armstrong DK, Bundy B, Wenzel L, et al. Intraperitoneal cisplatin and paclitaxel in ovarian cancer. N Engl J Med 2006;354:34–43.

37. Cooper A, DePriest P. Surgical management of women with ovarian cancer. Semin Oncol 2007;34:226–233.

38. Dauplat J, Le Bouedec G, Pomel C, Scherer C. Cytoreductive surgery for advanced stages of ovarian cancer. Semin Surg Oncol 2000;19:42–48.

39. Stratton JF, Tidy JA, Paterson MEL. The surgical management of ovarian cancer. Cancer Treat Rev 2001;27;111–118.

40. Bristow RE, Tomacruz RS, Armstrong DK, Trimble EL, Montz FJ. Survival effect of maximal cytoreductive surgery for advanced ovarian carcinoma during platinum era: A meta analysis. J Clin Oncol 2002;20:1248–1259.

41. Hoffman MS, Griffin D, Tebes S, et al. Sites of bowel resected to achieve optimal ovarian cancer cytoreduction: Implications regarding surgical management. Am J Obstet Gynecol 2005;193:582–588.

42. Bhoola S, Hoskins WJ. Diagnosis and management of epithelial ovarian cancer. Obstet Gynecol 2006;107:1399–1410.

43. Mayer AR, Chambers SK, Graves E, et al. Ovarian cancer staging: Does it require a gynecologic oncologist? Gynecol Oncol 1992;47:223–227.

44. Nguyen HN, Averette HE, Hoskins W, et al. National survey of ovarian carcinoma, V: The impact of physician's specialty on patients' survival. Cancer 1993;72:3663–3670.

45. van der Burg ME, van Lent M, Buyse M, et al. The effect of debulking surgery after induction chemotherapy on the prognosis in advanced epithelial ovarian cancer. Gynecological Cancer Cooperative Group of the European Organization for Research and Treatment of Cancer [see comments]. N Engl J Med 1995;332:629–634.

46. Rose PG, Nerenstone S, Brady MF, et al. Secondary surgical cytoreduction for advanced ovarian carcinoma. N Engl J Med 2004;351:2489–2497.

47. Berek JS, Trope C, Vergote I. Surgery during chemotherapy and at relapse of ovarian cancer. Ann Oncol 1999;10(suppl 1):3–7.

48. Marsden DE, Friedlander M, Hacker NF. Current management of epithelial ovarian carcinoma: A review. Semin Surg Oncol 2000;19:11–19.

49. Kyrgiou M, Salanti G, Pavlidis N, Paraskevaidis E, Ioannidis JPA. Survival benefits with diverse chemotherapy regimens for ovarian cancer: Meta-analysis or multiple treatments. J Natl Cancer Inst 2006;98:1655–1663.

50. Ozols R. Systemic therapy for ovarian cancer: Current status and new treatments. Semin Oncol 2006;33(suppl 6):S3–S11.

51. McGuire WP, Hoskins WJ, Brady MF, et al. Cyclophosphamide and cisplatin compared with paclitaxel and cisplatin in patients with stage III and stage IV ovarian cancer. N Engl J Med 1996;334:1–6.

52. Piccart MJ, Bertelsen K, Stuart G, et al. Long-term follow-up confirms a survival advantage of the paclitaxel-cisplatin regimen over the cyclophosphamide-cisplatin combination in advanced ovarian cancer. Int J Gynecol Cancer 2003;13(suppl 2):144–148.

53. Bookman MA, Greer BE, Ozols RF. Optimal therapy of advanced ovarian cancer: Carboplatin and paclitaxel vs. cisplatin and paclitaxel (GOG 158) and an update on GOG0 182-ICON5. Int J Gynecol Cancer 2003;136:735–740.

54. Ozols RF, Bundy BN, Green BE, et al. Phase III trial of carboplatin and paclitaxel compared with cisplatin and paclitaxel in patients with optimally resected stage III ovarian cancer: A Gynecologic Oncology Group Study. J Clin Oncol 2003;21:3194–3200.

55. du Bois A, Luck HJ, Meier W, et al. A randomized clinical trial of cisplatin/paclitaxel versus carboplatin/paclitaxel as first-line treatment of ovarian cancer. J Natl Cancer Inst 2003;3;95:1320–1329.

56. Neijt JP, Engelholm SA, Tuxen MK, et al. Exploratory phase III study of paclitaxel and cisplatin versus paclitaxel and carboplatin in advanced ovarian cancer. J Clin Oncol 2000;18:3084–3092.

57. Vasey PA, Jayson GC, Gordon A, et al. Phase III randomized trial of docetaxel-carboplatin versus paclitaxel-carboplatin as first-line chemotherapy for ovarian carcinoma. J Natl Cancer Inst 2004;1796:1682–1691.

58. Fennelly D, Aghajanian C, Shapiro F, et al. Phase I and pharmacologic study of paclitaxel administered weekly in patients with relapsed ovarian cancer. J Clin Oncol 1997;15:187–192.

59. Markman M, Blessing J, Rubin SC, et al. Phase II trial of weekly paclitaxel (80 mg/m²) in platinum and paclitaxel-resistant ovarian and primary peritoneal cancers: A Gynecologic Group Study. Gynecol Oncol 2006;101:436–440.

60. Katsumata N, Yasuda M, Takahashi F, et al. Dose-dense paclitaxel once a week in combination with carboplatin every 3 weeks for advanced ovarian cancer: A phase 3, open-label, randomized controlled trial. Lancet 2009;374:1331–1338.

61. Fujiwara K, Armstrong D, Morgan M, Markman M. Principles and practice of intraperitoneal chemotherapy for ovarian cancer. Int J Gynecol Cancer 2007;17:1–20.

62. Jaaback K, Johnson N. Intraperitoneal chemotherapy for the initial management of primary epithelial ovarian cancer. Cochrane Database Syst Rev 2006;3:1–28.

63. Markman M, Bundy BN, Alberts DS, et al. Phase III trial of standard-dose intravenous cisplatin in small-volume stage III ovarian carcinoma: An intergroup study of the gynecologic oncology group, southwestern oncology group, and eastern cooperative oncology group. J Clin Oncol 2001;19:1001–1007.

64. Alberts DS, Liu PY, Hannigan EV, et al. Intraperitoneal cisplatin plus intravenous cyclophosphamide versus intravenous cisplatin plus intravenous cyclophosphamide for stage III ovarian cancer. N Engl J Med 1996;335:1950–1955.

65. Walker JL, Armstrong DK, Huang HQ, et al. Intraperitoneal catheter outcomes in a phase III trial of intravenous versus intraperitoneal chemotherapy in optimal stage III ovarian and primary peritoneal cancer: A Gynecologic Oncology Group Study. Gynecol Oncol 2006;100:27–32.

66. Markman M, Walker JL. Intraperitoneal chemotherapy of ovarian cancer: A review, with a focus on practical aspects of treatment. J Clin Oncol 2006;24:988–994.

67. National Comprehensive Cancer Network (NCCN) Practice Guidelines in Oncology—Ovarian Cancer, V1.2010. 2010, http://www.nccn.org.

68. NCI Clinical Announcement. Intraperitoneal Chemotherapy for Ovarian Cancer. Released on January 5, 2006, http://ctep.cancer. gov/highlights/clin_annc_010506.pdf.

69. Salzberg M, Thurlimann B, Bonnefois H, et al. Current concepts of treatment strategies in advanced or recurrent ovarian cancer. Oncology 2005;68:293–298.

70. Gadducci A, Cosio S, Conte PF, Genazzani AR. Consolidation and maintenance treatments for patients with advanced epithelial ovarian cancer in complete response after first-line chemotherapy: A review of the literature. Crit Rev Oncol Hematol 2005;55:153–166.

71. Markman M, Liu PY, Wilczynski S, et al. Phase III randomized trial of 12 versus 3 months of maintenance paclitaxel in patients with advanced ovarian cancer who attained a clinically-defined complete response to platinum/paclitaxel-based chemotherapy: A Southwest Oncology Group and Gynecology Oncology Group trial. J Clin Oncol 2003;21:2460–2465.

72. Gadducci A, Cosio S, Conte PF, Genazzani AR. Consolidation and maintenance treatments for patients with advanced epithelial ovarian cancer in complete response after first-line chemotherapy: A review of the literature. Crit Rev Oncol Hematol 2005;55:153–166.

73. Markman M. Unresolved issues in the chemotherapeutic management of gynecologic malignancies. Semin Oncol 2006;33(suppl 6):S33–S38.

74. Mulder PO, Willemse PH, Aalders JG, et al. High-dose chemotherapy with autologous bone marrow transplantation in patients with refractory ovarian cancer. Eur J Cancer Clin Oncol 1989;25:645–649.

75. Stiff PJ, Veum-Stone J, Lazarus HM, et al. High-dose chemotherapy and autologous stem cell transplantation for ovarian cancer: An autologous blood and marrow transplant registry report. Ann Intern Med 2000;133:504–515.

76. Goncalves A, Delva R, Fabbro M, et al. Post-operative sequential high-dose chemotherapy with haematopoietic stem cell support as front-line treatment in advanced ovarian cancer: A multicenter study. Bone Marrow Transplant 2006;37:651–659.

77. ICON and AGO Collaborators. Paclitaxel plus platinum-based chemotherapy versus conventional platinum-based chemotherapy in women with relapsed ovarian cancer: The ICON4/AGO-OVAR-2.2 trial. Lancet 2003;361:2099–2106.

78. Bozas G, Bamias A, Koutsoukou, et al. Biweekly gemcitabine and cisplatin in platinum resistant/refractory, paclitaxel pre-treated, ovarian and peritoneal carcinoma. Gyncel Oncol 2007;104:580–585.

79. Gronlund B, Hogdall C, Hansen HH, Engelholm SA. Performance status rather than age is the key prognostic factor in second-line treatment of elderly patients with epithelial ovarian carcinoma. Cancer 2002;94:1961–1967.

80. Fung-Kee-Fung M, Oliver T, Elit L, et al. Optimal chemotherapy treatment for women with recurrent ovarian cancer. Curr Oncol 2007;14:195–208.

81. Inciura A, Simavicius A, Juozaityte E, et al. Comparison of adjuvant and neoadjuvant chemotherapy in the management of advanced ovarian cancer: A retrospective study of 574 patients. BMC Cancer 2006;6:153.

82. Herzog TJ, Pothuri B. Ovarian cancer: A focus on management of recurrent disease. Nat Clin Pract Oncol 2006;3:604–611.

83. Swisher EM, Mutch DG, Rader JS, et al. Topotecan in platinum- and paclitaxel-resistant ovarian cancer. Gynecol Oncol 1997;66:480–486.

84. Markman M. Topotecan: An important new drug in the management of ovarian cancer. Semin Oncol 1997;24:S5–S11.

85. ten Bokkel Huinink W, Gore M, Carmichael J, et al. Topotecan versus paclitaxel for the treatment of recurrent epithelial ovarian cancer. J Clin Oncol 1997;15:2183–2193.

86. Creemers GJ, Bolis G, Gore M, et al. Topotecan, an active drug in the second-line treatment of epithelial ovarian cancer: Results of a large European phase II study. J Clin Oncol 1996;14:3056–3061.

87. Muggia FM, Hainsworth JD, Jeffers S, et al. Phase II study of liposomal doxorubicin in refractory ovarian cancer: Antitumor activity and toxicity modification by liposomal encapsulation. J Clin Oncol 1997;15:987–993.

88. Gordon AN, Cranai CO, Rose PG, et al. Phase II study of liposomal doxorubicin in platinum- and paclitaxel refractory epithelial ovarian cancer. J Clin Oncol 2000;18:3093–3100.

89. Gordon AN, Fleagle JT, Guthrie D, et al. Recurrent epithelial ovarian carcinoma: A randomized phase III trial of pegylated liposomal doxorubicin versus topotecan. J Clin Oncol 2001;19:3312–3322.

90. Wilailk S, Linasmita V. A study of pegylated liposomal doxorubicin in platinum-refractory epithelial ovarian cancer. Oncology 2004;67:183–186.

91. Drake RD, Lin WM, King M, Farrar D, Miller DS, Coleman RL. Oral dexamethasone attenuates Doxil-induced palmer-plantar erythrodysesthesias in patients with recurrent gynecologic malignancies. Gynecol Oncol 2004;94:320–324.

92. Lund B, Hansen P, Theilade K, et al. Phase II study of gemcitabine (2x, 2xdilfuorodeoxycytidine in previously treated ovarian cancer patients. J Natl Cancer Inst 1994;6:1530–1533.

93. Poveda A. Gemcitabine in patients with ovarian cancer. Cancer Treat Rev 2005;31(suppl 4):S29–S37.

94. Cannistra SA, Bast RC, Berek JS, et al. Progress in the management of gynecologic cancer: Consensus summary statement. J Clin Oncol 2003;21(suppl):129S–132S.

95. Ozols RF. Systemic therapy for ovarian cancer: Current status and new treatments. Semin Oncol 2006;33(suppl 6):S3–S11.

96. Kurzeder C, Sauer G, Deissler H. Molecular targets of ovarian carcinomas with acquired resistance to platinum/taxane chemotherapy. Curr Cancer Drug Targets 2006;6:207–227.

97. Cannistra SA, Bast RC, Berek JS, et al. Progress in the management of gynecologic cancer: Consensus summary statement. J Clin Oncol 2003;21(suppl):129s–132s.

98. Garcia AA, Hirte H, Fleming G, et al. Phase II Clinical Trial of Bevacizumab and Low-Dose Metronomic Oral Cyclophosphamide in Recurrent Ovarian Cancer: A Trial of the California, Chicago, and Princess Margaret Hospital Phase II Consortia. Journal of Clinical Oncology 2008;26(1):76–82.

99. Cohn DE, Valmadre S, Resnick KE, et al. Bevacizumab and weekly taxane chemotherapy demonstrates activity in refractory ovarian cancer. Gynecol Oncol 2006;102(2):134–139.

100. Cannistra SA, Matulonis UA, Penson RT, et al. Phase II study of bevacizumab in patients with platinum-resistant ovarian cancer or peritoneal serous cancer. J Clin Oncol 2007;25:5180–5186.

101. Burger RA, Sill MW, Monk BJ, Greer BE, Sorvosky JI. Phase II trial of bevacizumab in persistent or recurrent epithelial ovarian cancer or primary peritoneal cancer:a gynecologic oncology group study. J Clin Oncol 2007;25:5165–5171.

102. Monk BJ, Han E, Josephs-Cowan CA, Pugmire G, Burger RA. Salvage bevacizumab (rhuMAB VEGF)-based therapy after multiple prior cytotoxic regimens in advanced refractory epithelial ovarian cancer. Gynecol Oncol 2006;102(2):140–144.

103. Wright JD, Hagemann A, Rader JS, et al. Bevacizumab combination therapy in recurrent, platinum-refractory, epithelial ovarian carcinoma. Cancer 2006;107(1):83–89.

104. Chura JC, Van Iseghem K, Downs LS Jr, Carson IF, Judson PI. Bevacizumab plus cyclophosphamide in heavily pretreated patients with recurrent ovarian cancer. Gynecol Oncol 2007;107(2):326–330.

105. Simpkins F, Belinson JI, Rose PG, et al. Avoiding bevacizumab related gastrointestinal toxicity for recurrent ovarian cancer by careful patient screening. Gynecol Oncol 2007;107(1):118–123.

106. McGonigle KF, Muntz HG, Vuky Ji, et al. A phase II prospective study of weekly topotecan and bevacizumab in platinum refractory ovarian cancer or peritoneal cancers. J Clin Oncol 2008;26:abstract 5551.

107. Penson RT, Dizon DS, Cannistra SA, et al. Phase II study of carboplatin, paclitaxel, and bevacizumab with maintenance bevacizumab as first-line chemotherapy for advanced mullerian tumors. J Clin Oncol 2009;28:154–159.

108. Micha JP, Goldstein BH, Rettenmaier MA, et al. A phase II study of outpatient first-line paclitaxel, carboplatin, and bevacizumab for advanced-stage epithelial ovarian, peritoneal, and fallopian tube cancer. Int J Gynecol Cancer 2007;17:771–776.

109. Nimeiri HS, Oza AM, Morgan RJ, et al. Efficacy and safety of bevacizumab plus erlotinib for patients with recurrent ovarian, primary peritoneal, and fallopian tube cancer: A trial of the Chicago, PMH, and California Phase II consortia. Gynecol Oncol 2008;110:49–55.

110. Azad NS, Posadas EM, Kwitkowski, et al. Combination targeted therapy with sorafenib and bevacizumab results in enhanced toxicity and antitumor activity. J Clin Oncol 2008;26(22):3709–3714.

111. Richardson DL, Backes FJ, Seamon LG, et al. Combination gemcitabine, platinum, and bevacizumab for the treatment of recurrent ovarian cancer. Gynecol Oncol 2008;111:461–466.

112. Matulonis UA, Berlin S, Ivy P, et al. Cediranib, an inhibitor of vascular endothelial growth factor receptor kinases, in an active drug in recurrent epithelial ovarian, fallopian tube and peritoneal cancer. J Clin Oncol 2009;27(33):5601–5606.

113. Buckstein R, Meyer RM, Seymour L, et al. Phase II testing of sunitinib: The National Cancer Institute of Canada Clinical Trials Group IND Program. Current Oncolog 2007;14(4):154–161.

114. Campos SM, Ghosh S. A current review of targeted therapeutics for ovarian cancer. J Oncol 2010. [Epub 149362].

115. Higginson IJ, Edmonds P. Services, costs and appropriate outcomes in end of life care. Ann Oncol 1999;10:135–136.

116. Patnaik A, Doyle C, Oza AM. Palliative therapy in advanced ovarian cancer: Balancing patient expectations, quality of life and cost. Anti-cancer Drugs 1998;9:869–878.

117. Ferguson JS, Summerhayes M, Masters S, Schey S, Smith IE. New treatments for advanced cancer: An approach to prioritization. Br J Cancer 2000;83:1268–1273.

118. Cowens A, Boucher S, Roche, et al. Is paclitaxel and cisplatin a cost effective first line therapy for advanced ovarian carcinoma. Cancer 1996;77:2086–2091.

119. Young M, Plosker GL. Paclitaxel: A pharmacoeconomic review of its use in the treatment of ovarian cancer. Pharmacoeconomics 2001;19:1227–1259.

120. Dranitsaris G, Elia-Pacitti J, Cottrell W. Measuring treatment preferences and willingness to pay for docetaxel in advanced ovarian cancer. Pharmacoeconomics 2004;22:375–387.

121. Smith DH, Adam JR, Johnston SRD, Gordan A, Drummond MF, Bennett CL. A comparative economic analysis of pegylated liposomal doxorubicin versus topotecan in ovarian cancer in the USA and the UK. Ann Oncol 2002;13:1590–1597.

142

Acute Leukemias

BETSY BICKERT POON AND DIANNE M. BRUNDAGE

KEY CONCEPTS

❶ Acute leukemias are the most common malignancies in children and the leading cause of cancer-related death in patients younger than age 35 years.

❷ To establish a definitive diagnosis of acute leukemia, the following diagnostic components are required: bone marrow biopsy and aspirate (with ≥20% blasts), cytogenetics, and immunophenotyping.

❸ Several risk factors correlate with prognosis for acute lymphoblastic leukemia (ALL). Poor prognostic factors include high white blood cell count at presentation, very young or very old age at diagnosis, delayed remission induction and presence of certain cytogenetic abnormalities (e.g., Philadelphia [Ph+] chromosome).

❹ For children with ALL, remission induction therapy includes vincristine, a corticosteroid, and asparaginase, with or without an anthracycline. For adults with ALL, vincristine, prednisone, and an anthracycline are given, and asparaginase is sometimes added.

❺ All patients with ALL require prophylactic therapy to prevent CNS disease because of the high risk of central nervous system relapse. The choice for therapy includes a combination of the following: cranial irradiation, intrathecal chemotherapy, or high-dose systemic chemotherapy with drugs that cross the blood–brain barrier.

❻ Long-term maintenance therapy for 2 to 3 years is essential to eradicate residual leukemia cells and prolong the duration of remission in patients with ALL. Maintenance therapy consists of oral methotrexate and mercaptopurine, with or without monthly pulses of vincristine and a corticosteroid.

❼ Disease-free survival is lower in adults with ALL and has been attributed to greater drug resistance, poor side-effect tolerance with subsequent nonadherence, and possibly less-effective therapy. This population is also more likely to have Ph+ ALL, which is associated with a worse outcome.

❽ Colony-stimulating factors can be safely and effectively used with myelosuppressive chemotherapy for acute leukemias. The benefits can include reduced incidence of serious infections, reduced hospital stays, and fewer treatment delays, but do not include prolonged disease-free survival or overall survival.

❾ There are several poor prognostic factors for adult acute myeloid leukemia (AML): older age, organ impairment, certain FAB subtypes, presence of extramedullary disease, and presence of certain cytogenetic and molecular abnormalities.

❿ Therapy of AML usually includes induction therapy with an anthracycline and cytarabine. Postremission therapy is required in all patients and can include either consolidation chemotherapy with or without maintenance therapy, or hematopoietic stem cell transplantation.

⓫ It is estimated that up to 10^8 to 10^9 malignant cells remain following attainment of a complete remission. Postremission therapy with either chemotherapy or hematopoietic stem cell transplantation is essential in AML.

⓬ Treatment of acute promyelocytic leukemia consists of induction therapy, followed by consolidation and maintenance therapy. Induction includes tretinoin and an anthracycline; consolidation therapy consists of two to three cycles of anthracycline-based therapy; maintenance consists of pulse doses of tretinoin, mercaptopurine, and methotrexate for 2 years.

The leukemias are heterogeneous hematologic malignancies characterized by unregulated proliferation of the blood-forming cells in the bone marrow. These immature proliferating leukemia cells (blasts) physically "crowd out" or inhibit normal cellular maturation in bone marrow, resulting in anemia, neutropenia, and thrombocytopenia. Leukemic blasts may also infiltrate a variety of tissues such as lymph nodes, skin, liver, spleen, kidney, testes, and the central nervous system.

Historically, leukemia has been classified as acute or chronic based on differences in cell of origin and cell line maturation, clinical presentation, rapidity of progression of the untreated disease, and response to therapy. Four major leukemias are recognized: acute lymphoblastic (or lymphocytic) leukemia (ALL), acute myeloid leukemia (AML), chronic lymphocytic leukemia, and chronic myeloid leukemia. Undifferentiated immature cells that proliferate autonomously characterize acute leukemias. Chronic leukemias also proliferate autonomously, but the cells are more differentiated and mature. Untreated, acute leukemia is fatal within months.

EPIDEMIOLOGY

It is estimated that 17,660 new cases of acute leukemia—12,330 cases of AML and 5,330 cases of ALL—will be diagnosed in the United States in 2010, accounting for 1.2% of the total cancer incidence.[1] The incidence has been relatively stable for two decades. An estimated 10,400 deaths per year, representing about 2% of all cancer deaths, are caused by acute leukemias.[1] ❶ Leukemia is the leading cause of cancer-related deaths in persons younger than age 20 years, but an uncommon cause of cancer-related death after age 40 years.[1] Among adults, acute and chronic leukemias occur at equal rates. More than 90% of the cases of acute and chronic leukemia occur in adults. AML accounts for most cases of acute leukemia in adults, and occurs with increasing frequency in elderly patients. There are about 3.5 cases of AML and 1.6 cases of ALL per 100,000 individuals.[2] The median age at diagnosis of patients with AML is about 67 years, whereas the median age for ALL patients is about 13 years.[1,2] The incidence of AML rises with age from 1.7 per 100,000 in individuals younger than age 65 years to 16 per 100,000 in those 65 years or older.[2,3] Acute leukemia is slightly more common in males than in females. In the United States, acute leukemia is more common among whites than among African Americans, American Indians, and Hispanic ethnicities.[2]

Despite the low incidence rate, the acute leukemias are the most common malignancy in persons younger than 20 years of age, accounting for 27% of all childhood malignancies.[4] The lifetime risk of developing ALL is 1 in 810 Americans and 1 in 272 Americans for AML.[2] Approximately 77% of children with leukemia have ALL and 18% AML.[4] Childhood ALL is 30% more common in males than in females, peaks at 2 to 5 years of age, and is twice as likely to affect white children as African American children.[4,5] The incidence of childhood AML is highest in the Hispanic population and occurs throughout childhood without any peak age period. Acute leukemia during the first year of life (infant leukemia) slightly favors ALL over AML.[4,6]

Chemotherapy has dramatically improved the outlook of patients with acute leukemia. More than 85% of children and young adults with acute leukemia achieve an initial complete remission (CR) of their disease. Overall, 65% to 85% of adults achieve an initial CR.[3] For persons younger than 15 years of age, the 5-year survival rate is 88% for ALL and 55% for AML.[2] The prognosis of adult acute leukemia is generally worse than that of childhood leukemia, with only 30% to 40% of patients becoming long-term survivors. When all ages are included, the 5-year relative survival rate in 2004 for ALL was 65% and 23% for AML.[2]

ETIOLOGY

The exact cause of the acute leukemias is unknown. A multifactorial process involving genetics, environmental and socioeconomic factors, toxins, immunologic status, and viral exposures is likely. Table 142–1 summarizes the major factors that have been linked to acute leukemias. Infectious and genetic factors have the strongest associations to date.[5] In pediatric ALL, a number of environmental factors are inconsistently linked to the disease: exposure to ionizing radiation, toxic chemicals, herbicides and pesticides; maternal use of contraceptives, diethylstilbestrol, or cigarettes; parental exposure to drugs (amphetamines, diet pills, and mind-altering medications), diagnostic radiographs, alcohol consumption, or chemicals before and during pregnancy; and chemical contamination of groundwater.[7,8] A growing body of evidence indicates that high birthweight is a risk factor for ALL.[5,9] Ionizing radiation and benzene exposure are the only environmental risk factors strongly associated with ALL or AML.[8] A few studies have reported a possible link between electromagnetic fields of high-voltage power lines and the development of leukemia, but larger studies could not confirm this association. In most patients who develop leukemia, a cause cannot be identified.

Childhood AML is associated with Hispanic ethnicity, prior exposure to alkylating agents or epipodophyllotoxins, and in utero

TABLE 142-1 Risk Factors for Acute Leukemia

Drugs	**Chemical**
Alkylating agents	Benzene
Epidopophyllotoxins	**Pesticides**
Genetic conditions	**Pyrethroid-based shampoo**
Amegakaryocytic thrombocytopenia	**Radiation**
Ataxia telangiectasia	Ionizing radiation
Bloom syndrome	**Virus**
Diamond-Blackfan anemia	Epstein-Barr virus
Down syndrome	Human T-lymphocyte virus
Dyskeratosis congenita	(HTLV-1 and HTLV-2)
Familial monosomy 7	**Social habits**
Fanconi anemia	Cigarette smoking
Klinefelter syndrome	Maternal marijuana use
Kostmann syndrome	Maternal ethanol use
Langerhans cell histiocytosis	
Li Fraumeni syndrome	
Neurofibromatosis type 1	
Noonan syndrome	
Schwachman syndrome	
Severe combined immunodeficiency syndrome	
Wiskott-Aldrich syndrome	

exposure to ionizing radiation.[6,8] Maternal alcohol consumption, parental and child organophosphate pesticide exposure, and parental benzene exposure are also associated with childhood AML.[6] AML has been associated with both low and high birth weight.[9]

PATHOPHYSIOLOGY

A basic understanding of normal hematopoiesis is needed before one can understand the pathogenesis of leukemia (see Chap. 95). Normal hematopoiesis consists of multiple well-orchestrated steps of cellular development. A pool of pluripotent stem cells undergoes differentiation, proliferation, and maturation, to form the mature blood cells seen in the peripheral circulation. These pluripotent stem cells initially differentiate to form two distinct stem cell pools. The myeloid stem cell gives rise to six types of blood cells (erythrocytes, platelets, monocytes, basophils, neutrophils, and eosinophils), while the lymphoid stem cell differentiates to form circulating B and T lymphocytes and natural killer cells. Leukemia may develop at any stage and within any cell line.

Two features are common to both AML and ALL: first, both arise from a single leukemic cell that expands and acquires additional mutations, culminating in a monoclonal population of leukemia cells. Second, the relative balance between proliferation and differentiation is not maintained, so that the cells do not differentiate past a particular stage of hematopoiesis. Cells (lymphoblasts or myeloblasts) then proliferate uncontrollably. Proliferation, differentiation, and apoptosis are under genetic control, and leukemia can occur when the balance between these processes is altered.

AML probably arises from a defect in the pluripotent stem cell or a more committed myeloid precursor, resulting in partial differentiation and proliferation of immature precursors of the myeloid blood-forming cells. In older patients, trilineage leukemic involvement occurs suggesting that the cell of origin is probably a stem or very early progenitor cell. In younger patients, a more differentiated progenitor becomes malignant, allowing maturation of some granulocytic and erythroid populations. These two forms of AML exhibit different patterns of resistance to chemotherapy, with resistance more evident in the older adults with AML. ALL is a disease characterized by proliferation of immature lymphoblasts. In

TABLE 142-2 Morphologic (FAB) Classification of Acute Myeloid Leukemia

Subtype		Frequency of FAB Subtype[a]		
		Adults (%)	Children <2 years (%)	Children >2 years (%)
M0	Acute myeloblastic leukemia, without maturation	5	Low	Low
M1	Acute myeloblastic leukemia with minimal maturation	15	17	25
M2	Acute myeloblastic with maturation	25		27
M3	Acute promyelocytic leukemia	10		5
M4	Acute myelomonocytic leukemia	25	30	26
M5a	Acute monoblastic leukemia, poorly differentiated	5	52	16
M5b	Acute monoblastic leukemia, well differentiated	5		
M6	Acute erythroleukemia	5		2
M7	Acute megakaryoblastic leukemia	10		5–7

FAB, French-American-British.
[a]Percentages should be compared vertically, not horizontally.

this type of acute leukemia, the defect is probably at the level of the lymphopoietic stem cell or a very early lymphoid precursor.

Leukemic cells have growth and/or survival advantages over normal cells, leading to a "crowding out" phenomenon in the bone marrow. This growth advantage is not caused by more rapid proliferation as compared with normal cells. Some studies suggest that it is caused by factors produced by leukemic cells that either inhibit normal cellular proliferation and differentiation, or reduce apoptosis as compared with normal blood cells.

The types of genetic alterations that lead to leukemia have only recently become evident. The genetic defects may include (a) activation of a normally suppressed gene (protooncogene) to create an oncogene that produces a protein product that signals increased proliferation; (b) loss of signals for the blood cell to differentiate; (c) loss of tumor suppressor genes that control normal proliferation; and (d) loss of signals for apoptosis. Most normal cells are programmed to die eventually through apoptosis, but the appropriate programmed signal is often interrupted in cancer cells, leading to continued survival, replication, and drug resistance. Signal transduction, RNA transcription, cell-cycle control factors, cell differentiation, and programmed cell death may all be affected.

LEUKEMIA CLASSIFICATION

The French-American-British (FAB) classification system identifies eight different subtypes of AML based on granulocytic differentiation and maturation (Table 142–2), and this system is used to determine prognosis and choice of therapy. However, it does not consider clinical characteristics, clonal cytogenetic abnormalities, immunophenotyping, or response to therapy. In 2001, the World Health Organization (WHO), in collaboration with the Society for Hematopathology and the European Association of Haematopathology, proposed a new classification system for myeloid neoplasms. This new classification system incorporates not only morphologic findings, but also genetic, immunophenotypic, cytochemical, and clinical features. It has long been known that certain cytogenetic abnormalities have prognostic significance, but did not always correlate well with the FAB classification system. About 40% to 50% of adult patients with AML have no detectable chromosomal abnormality on standard cytogenetic analysis, but the percent increases with age.[10] The WHO classification attempts to formally incorporate the relationship between AML and myelodysplastic syndrome (MDS). In 2008, this classification was revised (Table 142–3) and is being used routinely in pediatric studies, but not in adults.[11]

A number of factors may affect the cytogenetics of acute myeloid leukemia in adults. First, in about 5% of adult AML patients, simultaneous blood and marrow samples demonstrate normal cytogenetics versus abnormal cytogenetics, respectively.[10] Second, central cytogenetic analysis is done in multi-center trials because of variability in specimen examination. A small number of patients may have a normal karyotype on standard review, but carry fusion genes, which are identical to those of translocations or inversions. These insertions of very small chromosome segments do not alter chromosome morphology but may affect outcome.

Lymphoblast analysis is used to classify ALL. Immunophenotype is determined by flow cytometry that analyzes specific antigens, known as clusters of differentiation (often abbreviated "CD"), present on the surface of hematopoietic cells. Although no leukemia-specific antigens have been identified, the pattern of cell-surface antigen expression reliably distinguishes between lymphoid and myeloid leukemia. The immunophenotype defines the cell of origin. The major phenotypes are mature B-cell, precursor B-cell, and T-cell disease. Eighty percent of childhood ALL derives from precursor B cells and about 15% from T cells. The remainder is either mixed lineage or from mature B cells.

TABLE 142-3 World Health Organization Classification of Acute Myeloid Leukemia

Acute myeloid leukemia (AML) with recurrent genetic abnormalities
　AML with t(8;21)(q22;q22), (AML1/ETO)
　AML with abnormal bone marrow eosinophils and inv(16)(p13;q22) or t(16;16)(p13;q22), (CBFβ/MYH11)
　Acute promyelocytic leukemia with t(15;17)(q22;q12), (PML/RAR-α) and variants
　AML with 11q23 (MLL) abnormalities
Acute myeloid leukemia with multilineage dysplasia
　Following MDS or MDS/MPD disorder
　Without antecedent MDS or MDS/MPD, but with dysplasia in at least 50% of cells or two or more lineages
Acute myeloid leukemia and MDS, therapy-related
　Alkylating agent/radiation-related type
　Topoisomerase II inhibitor-related type (some may be lymphoid)
　Others
Acute myeloid leukemia, not otherwise categorized, classify as
　Acute myeloid leukemia, minimally differentiated
　Acute myeloid leukemia without maturation
　Acute myeloid leukemia with maturation
　Acute myelomonocytic leukemia
　Acute monoblastic/acute monocytic leukemia
　Acute erythroid leukemia (erythroid/myeloid and pure erythroleukemia)
　Acute megakaryocytic leukemia
　Acute basophilic leukemia
　Acute panmyelosis with myelofibrosis
　Myeloid sarcoma

MDS, myelodysplastic syndrome; MLL, mixed lineage leukemia; MPD, myeloproliferative disease; PML, promyelocytic leukemia; RAR, retinoic acid receptor-α.

ALL may also be described by cytogenetic abnormalities. Chromosome alterations include numerical (hyperdiploidy and hypodiploidy), and structural abnormalities due to exchanges of genetic information within (inversion) or between (translocation) chromosomes.[12]

ACUTE LYMPHOBLASTIC LEUKEMIA

CLINICAL PRESENTATION

Common signs and symptoms at presentation result from malignant cells that replace and suppress normal hematopoietic progenitor cells and infiltrate into extramedullary spaces. In addition to clinical presentation, laboratory and pathology evaluations are required for a definitive diagnosis of leukemia. An abnormal complete blood count is usually the diagnostic test that initiates a leukemia diagnostic workup. The most important test is a bone marrow biopsy and aspirate, which is submitted to hematopathology for numerous evaluations. A lumbar puncture is performed to determine if there are blasts in the central nervous system (CNS). A chest radiograph is performed to screen for a mediastinal mass (most common in T-cell disease).

❷ Leukemia is suspected if the bone marrow contains greater than 5% blasts. Cytochemical stains are helpful to determine if the acute leukemia is of myeloid or lymphoid lineage. Cytogenetic analysis of the marrow to determine the presence of nonrandom numerical and structural chromosomal abnormalities in leukemic cells is also helpful for diagnosis, establishing prognosis, and evaluating response to therapy.[5,7] Chromosome translocations can result in abnormal expression and/or function of cellular oncogenes. Unique translocations can identify specific subtypes of acute leukemia. Twenty-five percent of children with precursor B-cell ALL have the *TEL-AML1* (translocation ETS leukemia-acute myeloid leukemia-1) fusion gene generated by the t(12;21)(p13;q22) chromosomal translocation.[5] This translocation gives the preleukemic cell altered self-renewal and survival properties. The most common translocation in adult ALL is the t(9;22) or Philadelphia chromosome which causes fusion of the BCR signaling protein to the ABL non-receptor tyrosine kinase, resulting in constitutive tyrosine kinase activity. More than 50% of childhood T-cell ALL have activating mutations of the *NOTCH1* gene that encodes for a transmembrane receptor implicated in regulation of T-cell development.[5]

CLINICAL PRESENTATION

General

- Recent history of vague symptoms such as tiredness, lack of exercise tolerance, and "feeling unwell," but in no obvious distress.

Symptoms

- Patient's commonly report fever, pallor, weight loss, malaise, fatigue, palpitations, and bone pain. Other possible symptoms include epistaxis, palpitations, dyspnea on exertion, seizures, headache, or diplopia.

Signs

- Temperature is often elevated and may be caused by disease or infection; ecchymoses or petechiae; painless testicular enlargement; splenomegaly, hepatomegaly, and/or lymphadenopathy; and, rarely, small, blue-green collections of leukemia cells under the skin (chloromas).

Laboratory Tests

- Complete blood count with differential. Anemia (43% <7 g/dL) is normochromic and normocytic (without a compensatory increase in reticulocytes). Thrombocytopenia (severe, <20,000 cells/mm³) is present in 28% of cases. Leukopenia/leukocytosis: 17% of patients will present with a white blood cell (WBC) count ≥50,000 cells/mm³ and 53% with a WBC <10,000 cells/mm³.

- Uric acid may be elevated because of rapid cellular turnover and is more common in patients presenting with elevated WBC count.

- Electrolytes: potassium and phosphate may be elevated with a compensatory decrease in calcium.

Other Diagnostic Tests

- Bone marrow aspirate and biopsy: send for morphologic examination, cytochemical staining, immunophenotyping, and cytogenetic (chromosome) analysis. All patients should have a screening lumbar puncture performed to assess CNS involvement.

RISK CLASSIFICATION

Many clinical and biologic features at diagnosis are associated with response to treatment, as measured by the complete remission rate, duration of remission, and long-term survival. Identification of these risk factors allows the clinician to better understand the disease and to tailor treatment according to risk of disease recurrence (i.e., risk-adapted therapy). For example, if a patient has many clinical and laboratory features that are associated with a good response to chemotherapy ("standard-risk"), then the clinician may choose to give less intensive therapy to reduce the risk of long-term side effects. Conversely, if a patient is unlikely to respond well to standard therapy ("high-risk" or "very-high-risk" disease), then the clinician may choose to give more intensive chemotherapy.

❸ The National Cancer Institute developed an ALL risk stratification to create a standard for comparison in children.[13] Induction therapy is initially selected based on this classification, which divides children into standard- or high-risk categories based on age and initial WBC count (Fig. 142–1). Karyotype is also considered if the results are available. Age remains an independent predictor of outcome with children aged 1 to 9 years having the best event-free survival (EFS). This is mostly explained by the more frequent occurrence of the *TEL-AML1* translocation and hyperdiploidy (>51 chromosomes) in addition to increased drug sensitivity in this age group.[14] Recently, more sophisticated biologic studies have allowed more refined risk stratification.[15] For example, the current algorithm incorporates treatment response through the measurement of subclinical minimal residual disease (MRD) by either flow cytometry or polymerase chain reaction.

The strongest prognostic factor for outcome for ALL is response to therapy, which traditionally was measured morphologically in bone marrow specimens. More recently molecular measurement of MRD has enabled detection of leukemic cells not visible on morphologic examination to assess treatment response and detect relapse in children and adults.[16] This technique allows detection of 1 leukemia cell in 10,000 normal cells, which is about 100-fold more sensitive than morphologic examination.[16] If MRD is detected at the end of induction therapy, the clinician may decide to give more intensive therapy to decrease the risk of relapse.

The Children's Oncology Group utilizes a risk- and response-based classification of childhood ALL (Fig. 142–1).[15] This classification system uses the National Cancer Institute risk assignment

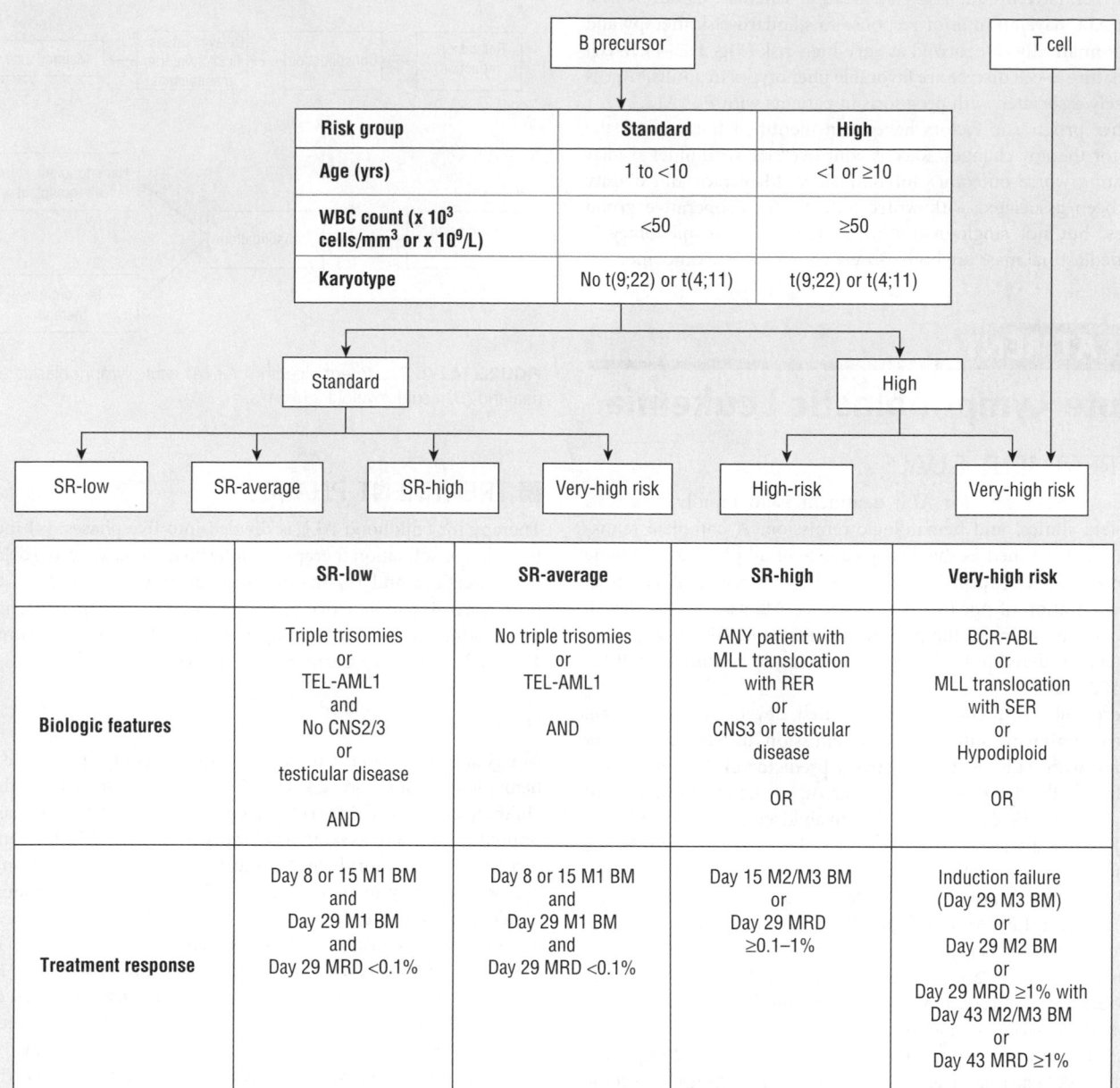

FIGURE 142-1. Risk- and response-based classification of childhood ALL. *Note:* Patients with T-cell ALL are automatically categorized as very-high-risk regardless of other factors. (BM, bone marrow; CNS2, lymphoblasts with <5 cells/microliter [<5 × 10⁶/L]; CNS3, lymphoblasts with ≥5 cells/microliter [≥5 × 10⁶/L] or clinical signs of CNS disease; M1, <5% blasts, M2, 5%–25% blasts, M3, >25% blasts; MLL, mixed lineage leukemia; MRD, minimal residual disease; RER, rapid early response; SER, slow early response; SR, standard risk; TEL-AML1, translocation ETS leukemia-acute myeloid leukemia-1; WBC, white blood cell.)

to initially categorize patients into standard- or high-risk groups. Patients categorized as high-risk usually receive more intensive remission induction therapy. Following remission induction therapy, risk is reclassified based on the biologic features (the presence or absence of molecular or cytogenetic abnormalities, and CNS or testicular involvement) and the rapidity and completeness of response to therapy (Fig. 142–1). Standard-risk patients are then classified as standard-risk-low, standard-risk-average, standard-risk-high, or very-high-risk. Patients who are initially high-risk remain in the high-risk category, unless they have biologic features or slow early response, as defined in the very-high-risk category.

Children who are initially classified as standard-risk and have three copies of chromosomes 4, 10, and 17 (triple trisomies) or the *TEL-AML1* fusion gene and less than 5% blasts in the bone mar-

row (M1) on days 15 and 29 of induction and MRD less than 0.1% on day 29 are reclassified as standard-risk-low and will have their therapy reduced. Children with the same rapid treatment response but without triple trisomies or the *TEL-AML1* fusion gene are reclassified as standard-risk-average. Children with certain biologic features (evidence of CNS or testicular disease, MLL translocation with a rapid early response to therapy), delayed treatment response (>5% blasts in the bone marrow (M2/M3) by day 15 or MRD ≥ 0.1% but <1% on day 29), or who received steroids prior to diagnosis are reclassified as standard-risk-high and have post-induction therapy intensified. Childhood precursor B-ALL with the Philadelphia chromosome [Ph⁺ disease, t(9;22)], hypodiploidy (<44 chromosomes), induction failure, mixed lineage leukemia (MLL) gene rearrangement with a slow response to therapy are considered very-high-risk and have therapy intensified. Infant ALL and childhood

T-cell ALL have unique risk classification schemas. Children with T-cell ALL have an inferior response to standard-risk therapy and are automatically categorized as very-high-risk (Fig. 142–1). T-cell and mature B-cell disease are favorable phenotypes in adults.[5] Age is inversely associated with prognosis in patients with Ph+ ALL.[5]

Other prognostic factors have been identified but are not the basis for therapy changes. Race is controversial, with older studies indicating worse outcomes for minorities. Male race and obesity have been associated with worse outcome in cooperative group studies, but not single-institution studies.[5] Hepatosplenomegaly and mediastinal mass are both associated with worse outcomes.

TREATMENT

Acute Lymphoblastic Leukemia

■ TREATMENT GOALS

The short-term goal for ALL treatment is to rapidly achieve a complete clinical and hematologic remission. A complete remission (CR) is defined as the disappearance of all physical and bone marrow evidence (normal cellularity with <5% blasts) of leukemia, with restoration of normal hematopoiesis. After a CR is achieved, the goal is to maintain the patient in continuous CR. In general, a child is considered to be "cured" after being in continuous CR for at least 5 years.

Successful treatment of ALL was first developed in children. Current regimens induce clinical remission in 96% to 99% of children with ALL.[5] MRD is a strong predictor of relapse in ALL. Children with MRD in the bone marrow at the end of induction have a 5-year EFS of 59% versus 88% in children without.[17] Children with low-risk disease have a 5-year EFS of 97%.[17] The 5-year EFS is 71% for high-risk childhood B-precursor and T-cell ALL including rapid and slow responders.[18] Children with very-high-risk disease have a 5-year EFS of less than 45%.[19] Response to treatment is determined by intrinsic drug sensitivity in concert with the patient's pharmacogenomics and pharmacodynamics, treatment received, and treatment adherence. Cure rates in children have risen from less than 5% with treatments used in the 1960s to about 90% by 2005.[12] The reason for this improvement lies largely in improved scheduling of existing drugs, as relatively few new drugs have come to the market since the 1960s.

Although treatment results with adult ALL are worse than those with childhood ALL, recent use of aggressive chemotherapy in adult ALL has increased the CR rate to 60% to 85%. Long-term EFS in this population, however, remains low (between 30% and 40%) because a higher proportion of adults present with poor-risk disease. CR rates and EFS vary according to a number of poor prognostic factors and certain types of ALL are associated with a very poor outcome.

CLINICAL CONTROVERSY

Which corticosteroid is superior for the treatment of ALL? Prednisone/prednisolone has been the steroid of choice for many years. Dexamethasone was recently shown to have better CNS penetration than prednisone with a consequent decrease in CNS relapse rate. However, the incidence of debilitating side effects such as osteonecrosis is higher with dexamethasone. Many investigators have difficulty weighing the quality-of-life decrease from the side effects against the small increase in survival.

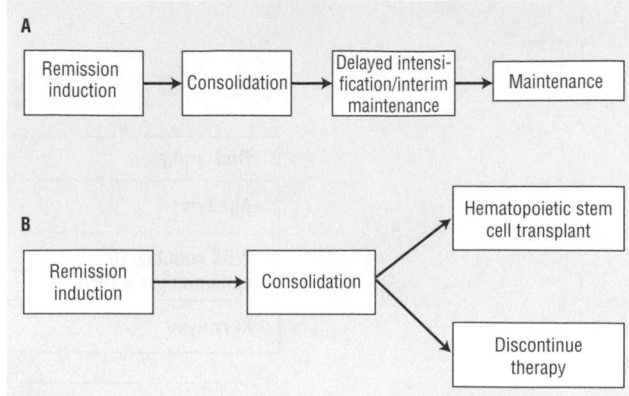

FIGURE 142-2. Treatment algorithm for (A) acute lymphoblastic leukemia and (B) acute myeloid leukemia.

■ TREATMENT PHASES

Therapy for childhood ALL is divided into five phases: (a) induction; (b) consolidation therapy; (c) interim maintenance; (d) delayed intensification; and (e) maintenance therapy (Fig. 142–2). CNS prophylaxis is a mandatory component of ALL treatment regimens and is administered longitudinally during all phases of treatment. The total duration of treatment is 2 to 3 years.

Induction

The goal of induction is to rapidly induce a complete clinical and hematologic remission. ❹ The CR rate is 98% for standard-risk children treated with vincristine, a glucocorticoid (dexamethasone or prednisone), and asparaginase or pegaspargase.[12] Most treatment protocols add daunorubicin to induction (four-drug induction) for high-risk or very-high-risk ALL, while others add cyclophosphamide, methotrexate, or cytarabine. Most children achieve a CR in 4 weeks and are considered rapid early responders. Those who have a M2 (5%–25% blasts) or M3 (>25% blasts) marrow on day 15 of induction or have positive MRD at day 29 are considered slow early responders and receive intensified therapy. Half of the induction failures die from toxicity and half receive intensified therapy.[14]

Historically, prednisone has been the primary glucocorticoid used in pediatric ALL regimens. Dexamethasone is now being used in most standard-risk protocols because of its longer duration of action and higher cerebrospinal fluid penetration compared to prednisone.[5,12] Dexamethasone, when used in place of prednisone during induction, consolidation, and maintenance improves EFS 8% to 9% and decreases the risk of CNS relapse by about 3%.[14,20] However, dexamethasone increases the risk of side effects such as osteonecrosis, steroid myopathy, hyperglycemia, and infections.[20,21] Patients older than 10 years of age are particularly prone to osteonecrosis and receive prednisone instead of dexamethasone to minimize this side effect. Dexamethasone exposure is prolonged in children with ALL who have low serum albumin and may contribute to increased toxicity.[14] Patients with Down syndrome have increased infections and mortality with dexamethasone; therefore these patients receive prednisone.

The incidence of transient hyperglycemia during pediatric ALL induction therapy has increased. In a recent study where transient hyperglycemia was defined as at least two random serum glucose levels greater than or equal to 200 mg/dL (11.1 mmol/L), the overall incidence was 20%.[22] This increased to 42% for children over 10 years of age. The risk was higher for patients with a BMI greater than or equal to the 95th percentile and those receiving native l-asparaginase in comparison to pegaspargase.

Asparaginase is available in three forms. Asparaginase and pegaspargase are isolated from *Escherichia coli* while crisantaspase (investigational agent available if allergic to the other products) is isolated from *Erwinia chrysanthemi*. Pegaspargase is pegylated *E coli* asparaginase; pegylation prolongs its duration of activity and allows it to be given less frequently. Pegaspargase is used in the majority of protocols and is preferred over asparaginase because of fewer intramuscular injections, decreased antibody formation, and superior response rates. Pegaspargase is also approved for intravenous administration. Asparaginase products are the chemotherapeutic agents most likely to cause hypersensitivity reactions (10%–40%). The reaction is delayed with pegaspargase and usually occurs 6 to 12 hours following a dose. The hypersensitivity reaction to pegaspargase may also be prolonged and frequently requires hospitalization for 5 to 7 days.

Ph+ ALL has historically been associated with a poor long-term outcome and is treated as very-high-risk disease. This includes a four-drug induction and a matched related-donor allogeneic hematopoietic stem cell transplant (HSCT) if available. The addition of continuous imatinib mesylate, a signal transduction inhibitor that inhibits BCR-ABL kinase, through all phases of treatment resulted in a 3-year EFS of 80% in comparison to 35% for historical controls.[19] The results for patients receiving chemotherapy with imatinib were equivalent to those receiving stem cell transplantation. Imatinib is currently incorporated into childhood treatment trials for Ph+ ALL in Europe and the United States. Trials are ongoing with the more potent tyrosine kinase inhibitors, nilotinib and dasatinib.

Central Nervous System Prophylaxis

CNS prophylaxis is incorporated throughout all phases of therapy. The rationale for CNS prophylaxis is based on two observations. First, many chemotherapeutic agents do not readily cross the blood–brain barrier. Second, results from early clinical trials of ALL showed that 50% to 85% of patients with ALL and no CNS involvement at diagnosis experienced a CNS relapse.[7] These observations indicate that the CNS is a potential sanctuary for leukemic cells and that undetectable leukemic cells are present in the CNS in many patients at the time of diagnosis. Detectable CNS involvement at the time of diagnosis occurs in 3% of children with ALL.[14] Factors that are associated with an increased risk of CNS involvement at diagnosis in children include a high initial WBC count, T-cell phenotype, mature B-cell phenotype, age ≤1 year, African American race, thrombocytopenia, lymphadenopathy, and hepatomegaly or splenomegaly.[12]

The goal of CNS prophylaxis is to eradicate undetectable leukemic cells from the CNS while minimizing neurotoxicity and late effects. Leukemic meningitis is more easily prevented than treated. Once CNS relapse has occurred, patients are at increased risk of bone marrow relapse and death from refractory leukemia. Initial trials of childhood ALL in the 1960s established craniospinal irradiation as the standard for prevention of CNS relapse.[12] However, this approach was associated with long-term sequelae including neuropsychological deficits, precocious puberty, osteoporosis, decreased intellect, thyroid dysfunction, an increased risk of brain tumors, short stature, and obesity. Subsequent trials have demonstrated that irradiation may be replaced by frequent administration of intrathecal chemotherapy in most children with ALL.[12] Only patients with T-cell disease or very-high-risk disease receive prophylactic cranial radiation in the United States as a consequence of the long-term sequelae. Most children with CNS disease at diagnosis receive cranial radiation, but current research is aimed at eliminating this if possible.

❺ The selection of a CNS prophylaxis regimen must consider efficacy, toxicity, and risk of CNS disease. Intrathecal chemotherapy, cranial irradiation, dexamethasone, and high-dose intravenous methotrexate or cytarabine can be used to treat or prevent CNS disease. Current treatment approaches have reduced isolated CNS relapses to less than 5% among children.[23] Risk factors for CNS relapse include male sex, hepatomegaly, T-cell phenotype, CNS2 disease (the presence of leukemic blasts in a cerebrospinal fluid sample that contains <5 WBC/mm³ [<5 × 10⁶/L]), age younger than 2 years or older than 6 years, and a bloody diagnostic lumbar puncture.[5,23] Intrathecal therapy consists of methotrexate and cytarabine, given either alone or in combination. When given together, hydrocortisone is commonly added (triple intrathecal therapy) to decrease the incidence of arachnoiditis. For standard-risk ALL, triple intrathecal therapy reduces CNS relapse rates by 2.5% in comparison to intrathecal methotrexate, but has no effect on overall survival.[23] The doses of intrathecal chemotherapy used for childhood ALL are age-based because of differences in the volume of cerebrospinal fluid at various ages. For example, intrathecal methotrexate is dosed as 8 mg if <2 years, 10 mg for 2 to 2.99 years, 12 mg for 3 to 8.99 years, and 15 mg for ≥9 years. Liposomal cytarabine induces CNS remission in 57% of relapsed patients, but is associated with a high incidence of arachnoiditis and other CNS-related side effects.[24] Currently its use is limited to refractory or relapsed CNS disease in children.

Patients with T-cell leukemia have an increased incidence of CNS disease and benefit from systemic therapy that penetrates the CNS such as high-dose methotrexate.[21] A WBC count greater than 100,000 cells/mm³ (100 × 10⁹/L) have an increased risk of CNS relapse.[5] Patients with T-cell disease have lower methotrexate polyglutamate accumulation and addition of high-dose methotrexate results in fewer CNS relapses and improves EFS.[14]

Consolidation Therapy

Consolidation therapy in ALL is started after a CR has been achieved, and refers to continued intensive chemotherapy in an attempt to eradicate clinically undetectable disease in order to secure (consolidate) the remission. Regimens usually incorporate either non–cross-resistant drugs that are different from the induction regimen, or more dose-intensive use of the same drugs.

Randomized trials show that consolidation therapy clearly improves patient outcome in children, but its benefit in adults is less clear.[12] The relative benefit of individual components of treatment regimens is difficult to demonstrate because of the overall complexity of therapy in ALL. Standard consolidation lasts 4 weeks and usually consists of vincristine, mercaptopurine, and intrathecal methotrexate. Children with testicular disease usually receive radiation during this phase of therapy if a complete clinical response in the testes is not achieved by the end of induction. In children, the intensity of consolidation therapy is based on the child's risk classification and rate of cytoreduction during induction. Patients who respond slowly to induction therapy are at higher risk of relapse if they are not treated on more aggressive regimens. Children who are slow early responders or have high-risk disease benefit from intensified consolidation that includes the addition of vincristine and pegaspargase to standard therapy (cyclophosphamide, low-dose cytarabine, mercaptopurine).[18]

Imatinib has been incorporated into consolidation for children with Ph+ disease. Children with Ph+ ALL, infants with mixed lineage leukemia (MLL), or children who only achieve a partial remission may receive an allogeneic HSCT in first remission if a suitable donor is available. Nelarabine is a prodrug of ara-G that preferentially accumulates in T-lymphoblasts as ara-GTP. Children and young adults in first bone marrow relapse had a 55% complete or partial response in the phase II trial.[25] Nelarabine is currently incorporated into a high-risk backbone for initial therapy of childhood T-cell ALL.

Reinduction (Delayed Intensification/Interim Maintenance)

One or two delayed intensification phases separated by low-intensity interim maintenance cycles have been added to maintain remission and to decrease cumulative toxicity. Delayed intensification usually consists of drugs used during induction and consolidation or agents that lack cross-resistance with those already received. This includes cyclophosphamide, methotrexate, and limited amounts of doxorubicin. The dose of methotrexate is variable. Standard-risk children generally receive 1 to 2 g/m^2 while those with T-cell disease generally receive 5 g/m^2. Interim maintenance usually consists of dexamethasone, vincristine, weekly methotrexate, mercaptopurine, and intrathecal methotrexate. Delayed intensification improves EFS for standard-risk children.[14,18] Intensified delayed intensification improved EFS and decreased late relapses for high-risk childhood ALL, but there was no additional benefit for two delayed intensification cycles.[18] Children on the intensified arms of the study received significantly more antifungals, antibacterials, blood products and parenteral nutrition but had no increase in mortality.[18] The antimetabolite-based regimens may have a reduced risk of late toxicities, but the more intensive regimens appear to result in better survival for some patients, especially those with higher-risk disease.

Maintenance Therapy

6 Maintenance therapy allows long-term drug exposure to slowly dividing cells, allows the immune system time to eradicate leukemia cells, and promotes apoptosis (programmed cell death). The goal of maintenance therapy is to further eradicate residual leukemic cells and prolong remission duration. Although maintenance therapy is clearly beneficial in childhood ALL, the possible benefit in adults has only recently been demonstrated.

Maintenance therapy usually consists of daily mercaptopurine and weekly methotrexate for 12-week courses, at doses that produce relatively little myelosuppression, with monthly "pulses" of vincristine and a steroid for 5 days per month. In an effort to determine the long-term outcome of the duration and intensity of maintenance therapy, the Childhood ALL Collaborative Group published findings from a large meta-analysis involving 12,000 randomized children from 42 trials initiated prior to 1987.[26] The analysis revealed that longer maintenance, pulses of vincristine and prednisone, and the inclusion of one or two delayed intensification courses significantly reduced the total number of deaths or relapse. However, only delayed intensification improved survival.

Based on the results of studies that show a trend toward an increase in late relapse (excluding isolated testicular relapse) among male children treated for 2 years versus 3 years, some centers treat female children for 2 years while males receive maintenance to complete a total of 3 years of therapy.

Interpatient variability in the pharmacokinetics of oral methotrexate and mercaptopurine may also be an important determinant of the effectiveness and toxicity of maintenance therapy. Patients who take oral methotrexate and mercaptopurine on an evening versus a morning schedule appear to have a superior outcome. Mercaptopurine cannot be given with milk or milk products because of the presence of xanthine oxidase. To account for the interpatient variability, most clinicians will titrate the dose of either agent to maintain an absolute neutrophil count of 500 to 1,500 cells/mm^3 (0.5 to 1.5 × 10^9/L).[5] Some protocols circumvent bio-availability and poor adherence issues by administering methotrexate intravenously or intramuscularly. The importance of these pharmacokinetic issues in adults is less well defined.

ACUTE LYMPHOBLASTIC LEUKEMIA IN INFANTS

ALL and AML in infants younger than 1 year of age accounts for less than 5% of the reported acute leukemias in childhood, but they are associated with poor outcomes. Overall survival (OS) in infant ALL is 30% to 50%.[27] Seventy percent to 80% of infants with acute leukemia have MLL gene rearrangements.[27] MLL gene rearrangements are associated with worse outcome, with only 18% to 34% 4- to 8-year EFS.[27] Infants with ALL are more likely to present with a high WBC count, hepatosplenomegaly, and CNS disease.[27] Age less than 6 months at diagnosis and poor response to a prednisone prophase are poor prognostic indicators.[27] Infants with MLL gene rearrangements are more likely to overexpress FLT3, a tyrosine kinase implicated in leukemogenesis. Current research is testing the efficacy of lestaurtinib, a FLT3 inhibitor, following chemotherapy against infant ALL.[14]

Patients with infant ALL may have greater drug resistance to asparaginase, vincristine, and corticosteroids, but increased sensitivity to cytarabine and cladribine.[27] Although intensive regimens such as high-dose methotrexate and high-dose cytarabine have improved survival rates, unacceptably high mortality rates have also been observed with some regimens. Lack of pharmacokinetic data for chemotherapy in infants has contributed to toxicity from inappropriate dosing of doxorubicin and vincristine. To reduce neuropsychological complications, most protocols avoid cranial irradiation. The use of allogeneic HSCT for infants with ALL remains controversial due to a lack of donors, concerns over the long-term toxicity of total body irradiation, and excessive mortality in some series.

ACUTE LYMPHOBLASTIC LEUKEMIA IN ADULTS

Complete remission is achieved in 70% to 90% of adults with a four-drug regimen containing daunorubicin or doxorubicin, vincristine, asparaginase, and prednisone.[7] EFS is considerably lower and is achieved in 30% to 40% of patients. Recent comparison of 5-year EFS for adolescents and young adults found approximately 30% improvement when treated on pediatric versus adult protocols in the United States and Europe.[14]

The value of adding more drugs to the basic three- or four-drug induction regimen is unclear. Equally unclear is the value of higher doses of standard combinations of drugs for remission induction. Some studies suggest that high-dose methotrexate and cytarabine alternating with fractionated cyclophosphamide plus vincristine, doxorubicin, and dexamethasone (HyperCVAD) may improve response and survival in adults with ALL.[28] Intrathecal chemotherapy during the first cycle of HyperCVAD is held until blasts disappear from the peripheral differential in order to prevent seeding of the central nervous system. **7** Poorer outcomes in adults have been attributed to greater drug resistance, poor side-effect tolerance with subsequent nonadherence, and possibly less-effective therapy.

A considerable number of ALL cases occur in patients older than age 60 years, and treatment of this group of patients is an even greater challenge. The response to therapy and durability of response seem less than in younger adults or children. Treatment-related mortality rates during remission induction therapy are also higher in this population. Older patients are more likely to be Ph$^+$ positive, with the Ph$^+$ present in most patients age 55 years and older. Older patients are less likely to have T-cell ALL.[7] Based on data demonstrating improved and sustained responses in Ph$^+$ chronic myeloid leukemia with the tyrosine kinase inhibitor imatinib, several groups have evaluated the addition of imatinib to conventional chemotherapy in Ph$^+$ ALL patients.[29–32] Although no randomized trials have compared imatinib and conventional chemotherapy versus conventional chemotherapy alone, several single-center uncontrolled trials have reported improved OS with the addition of imatinib.[29,30] This approach also appears to be tolerated in the elderly.[31] Two other tyrosine kinase inhibitors, dasatinib and nilotinib, have also been evaluated in imatinib-resistant Ph⁺ leukemias. Responses are achieved, although are short lived, with relapses occurring within 6 months.[33,34] A primary concern with the tyrosine kinase inhibitors is the emergence of resistance, specifically T315I mutations. A prospective study of adult patients with Ph⁺ ALL demonstrated a modest benefit of allogeneic transplantation over chemotherapy, but the study was conducted before the availability of imatinib.[35] The CR was 82%, with an OS of 22% at 5 years. Age and presenting WBC were the factors predicting achievement of CR. Currently a study adding imatinib into the intensification and induction phases is underway.

TREATMENT OF RELAPSED ACUTE LYMPHOBLASTIC LEUKEMIA

Approximately 20% of children with ALL will relapse.[36] The most common site for relapse is the bone marrow (53%), although isolated relapses can occur in the CNS (19%) or testicles (5%), in addition to multiple sites of disease.[36] Because marrow relapse usually follows isolated CNS or testicular relapses, patients with isolated extramedullary relapses are treated with localized radiation (cranial or testicular) and aggressive systemic chemotherapy similar to that given to patients with a marrow relapse.[37]

Children who fail to achieve a CR by day 29 of induction therapy at initial diagnosis receive an additional 2 weeks of four-drug induction therapy. If the child does not achieve a CR with the additional therapy, they are usually treated for bone marrow relapse. This includes an intensive induction therapy consisting of at least three cycles of chemotherapy. Such cycles may include vincristine, pegaspargase, corticosteroid, and doxorubicin; etoposide, cyclophosphamide, and high-dose methotrexate; and high-dose cytarabine and asparaginase.[38]

Patients who have completed treatment and who have stayed in remission for longer periods are more likely to be reinduced into remission again. Patients with more favorable risk factors initially, and those who received less intensive initial treatments, are likely to respond well to reinduction/salvage regimens. A second remission with anthracycline, corticosteroid, vincristine, and asparaginase/pegaspargase occurs in 38% of children whose initial remission lasts less than 18 months, 80% if 18 to 36 months, and 95% if more than 36 months.[36] The 3-year OS following bone marrow (28%), CNS (60%), and testicular relapse (60%) is not optimal.[37] With the three cycle reinduction protocol described above, 68% of patients achieved CR if relapsed within 36 months and 96% if greater than 36 months.[38] For extramedullary relapse, overall survival is improved if relapse is at least 18 months after initial remission.[36] Survival is only 8% for children achieving a third remission after a second bone marrow relapse.[37] Clofarabine, a purine antimetabolite, achieves a 12.5% complete response rate, but the duration of response is less than 6 months. Current research is assessing clofarabine in combination with cytarabine.

Allogeneic HSCT (alloHSCT) is the treatment of choice for early bone marrow relapse (first CR less than 36 months).[37] Children who relapse more than 36 months after completion of initial therapy have reasonable outcomes with chemotherapy alone.[12,39] For patients with initial remissions less than 36 months, alloHSCT performed while in second CR is associated with a 8-year EFS of 41%, versus 23% with chemotherapy.[40] Patients who undergo alloHSCT are less likely to relapse, but are more likely to experience treatment-related morbidity and mortality if total-body irradiation is included in the conditioning regimen.[41]

Historically high-risk adult patients with a human leukocyte antigen (HLA)-matched sibling have been offered alloHSCT, but recent data suggest that there is no benefit to alloHSCT in this population (with the exception of Ph⁺ ALL). High treatment-related mortality in this group may offset any benefit from a lower relapse rate.[42] Most elderly patients are not candidates for standard alloHSCT but are candidates for nonmyeloablative alloHSCT. Whether this approach will reduce treatment-related mortality and result in more favorable outcomes is currently unknown. The National Marrow Donor Program and the American Society for Blood and Marrow Transplantation have developed guidelines for transplant consultation based on current clinical practice and evidence-based medicine. The following groups of ALL patients are at risk for progression and should be referred for transplant evaluation: high-risk ALL, including patients with high-risk cytogenetics (i.e., Ph⁺), high WBC count (>30,000–50,000 cells/mm³ [>30 × 10⁹ to 50 × 10⁹/L]) at diagnosis, CNS or testicular leukemia, no CR within 4 weeks of initial treatment, remission induction failures, and those patients in second CR and beyond.[43,44]

PHARMACOGENOMICS

Genetic polymorphisms may affect drug metabolism, receptor expression, drug transportation, drug disposition, and pharmacologic response. These alterations may contribute to acute and chronic toxicity from ALL therapy as well as differences in treatment outcome. The most studied polymorphism involves thiopurine metabolism. Cellular thiopurine S-methyltransferase (TPMT) catalyzes S-methylation of thiopurines such as mercaptopurine and thioguanine resulting in inactivation. Approximately 10% of the population has intermediate TPMT activity as a result of heterozygous polymorphisms in the gene encoding for TPMT, and 1 in 300 has extremely low activity as a result of homozygous presence of this TPMT polymorphism.[5] Deficiency of TPMT activity results in excessive myelosuppression from thiopurines. Patients with low activity (homozygous mutant TPMT genotype) require 85% to 90% dose reductions.[45] Approximately half of the heterozygous patients will require dose reductions.[5] TPMT deficiency also confers an increased risk of developing secondary AML and radiation-induced brain tumors.[5] Prospective evaluation of TPMT status was complicated in the past, as many ALL patients receive transfusions prior to definitive diagnosis. TPMT status can now be determined directly by DNA-based testing, which may become a standard of care in the near future.

LATE EFFECTS OF ACUTE LYMPHOBLASTIC LEUKEMIA

Certain late effects associated with cranial or craniospinal irradiation and/or corticosteroids were discussed earlier. The Childhood Cancer Survivor Study tracks the health status of adults treated for childhood cancer between 1970 and 1986 and has yielded invaluable information on how to monitor adult survivors.[46] Leukemia survivors are 3.7 times more likely to develop a severe or life-threatening chronic health condition as compared with healthy siblings, and 2.8 times more likely to report multiple chronic conditions.[46] Former ALL regimens that incorporated intensive use of topoisomerase II inhibitors (etoposide and teniposide) are associated with unacceptably high risks of development of secondary leukemia.[12] High cumulative doses of anthracyclines used in high-risk or relapsed patients can cause cardiomyopathy. Cranial irradiation has also been found to cause learning deficits, especially in patients younger than 5 years of age at the time of treatment. Patients who received cranial radiation as children also have higher unemployment rates and lower marital rates among females 2 decades after diagnosis.[46] The Children's Oncology Group has developed long-term, follow-up guidelines for survivors of childhood, adolescent, and young adult cancers (*www.survivorshipguidelines.org*).

ACUTE MYELOID LEUKEMIA

CLINICAL PRESENTATION

Common signs and symptoms at presentation are described below. In addition to clinical presentation, laboratory and pathology evaluations are required for a definitive diagnosis of leukemia. The most important test is a bone marrow aspirate and biopsy, which is submitted to hematopathology for testing and evaluation. The WHO classification defines acute leukemias as >19% blasts in the marrow or blood; previous and ongoing trials may use the criteria of >29% blasts until study completion. Cytochemical stains are helpful to determine if the acute leukemia is of myeloid or lymphoid lineage. Immunophenotyping is necessary and was described in the ALL clinical presentation above. Cytogenetic analysis of the marrow to determine the presence of nonrandom numerical and structural chromosomal abnormalities in leukemic cells is also helpful for diagnosis, establishing prognosis, and evaluating response to therapy.[47] Chromosome translocations can result in abnormal expression and/or function of cellular oncogenes. Unique translocations can identify specific subtypes of acute leukemia. For example, acute promyelocytic leukemia (APL) is characterized by a specific translocation between chromosomes 15 and 17: t(15;17). Recently, technically difficult cytogenetic analysis has been supplemented with fluorescent in situ hybridization that allows for quick, sensitive analysis of samples that might be inadequate for karyotyping. Molecular tests may be used to identify products of specific translocations, such as promyelocytic leukemia (PML) retinoic acid receptor-α (RARα) in APL and AML1-ETO and CBF-β/MYH 11 in other subtypes of AML. The results of some of these molecular tests correlate with prognosis and are discussed in Risk Classification below. Testing for FLT3-ITD, c-KIT and NPM1 are not commonly available in the community so samples may be frozen for testing at a later point if it becomes relevant.[48]

CLINICAL PRESENTATION

General

- Recent history of vague symptoms such as tiredness, lack of exercise tolerance, chest pain, and "feeling unwell" but in no obvious distress.

Symptoms

- The patient may report weight loss, malaise, fatigue, and palpitations and dyspnea on exertion. They may also present with fever, chills, and rigors suggestive of infection; bruising (excessive vaginal bleeding, epistaxis, ecchymoses, and petechiae); gum hypertrophy (AML M4 and AML M5 subtypes); bone pain; seizures; headache; and diplopia.

Signs

- Temperature may be elevated because of low neutrophil count; petechiae.

Laboratory Tests

- Complete blood cell count (with differential). Anemia is usually present and is normochromic and normocytic (without a compensatory increase in reticulocytes). Thrombocytopenia (severe, <50,000 cells/mm³) is present in approximately 50% of cases. Leukopenia/leukocytosis: approximately 20% of patients will present with an elevated WBC count, 20% with a low WBC count, and the rest with normal counts. Even patients with elevated counts can be considered functionally neutropenic.

- Uric acid may be elevated as a result of rapid cellular turnover (more common in patients presenting with elevated WBC counts).

- Electrolytes: potassium and phosphate are usually elevated.

- Coagulation: elevated prothrombin time, partial thromboplastin time, D-dimers; hypofibrinogenemia.

Other Diagnostic Tests

- Bone marrow biopsy and aspirate: send for morphologic examination, cytochemical staining, immunophenotyping, and cytogenetic (chromosome) analysis. At diagnosis the marrow is typically hypercellular, with normal erythropoiesis being replaced by leukemic blasts. To be diagnosed with AML, there needs to be more than 20% blasts. Molecular testing for FMS-like tyrosine kinase 3 (FLT3) mutations is warranted.

- For patients presenting with CNS signs, a diagnostic lumbar puncture should be performed. This is typically performed once there is clearance of blasts from the peripheral blood. CNS involvement is common with AML M4 and M5 subtypes.

RISK CLASSIFICATION

Many clinical and laboratory features at diagnosis are associated with response to treatment, as measured by the CR rate, duration of remission, and long-term survival. Identification of these risk factors may allow the clinician to better understand the disease and to tailor treatment according to risk of disease recurrence. For example, if a patient has many clinical and laboratory features that are associated with a good response to chemotherapy ("good-risk"), then the clinician may choose to give less-intensive therapy to reduce the risk of long-term toxic effects. Conversely, if a patient is unlikely to respond well to therapy ("high-risk"), then the clinician may choose to give more intensive chemotherapy that might include HSCT.

Several prognostic factors have been identified for adults with AML. ❾ The most important patient factor is age, with younger patients more likely to achieve a CR than patients older than age 60 years.[3,49] The lower CR rate in older patients results from an increased frequency of fatal infection and bleeding complications and resistance to conventional chemotherapy. The duration of remission is also shorter in older patients as compared to younger patients. Other patient-specific prognostic factors include concurrent infection and any major organ impairment.[3] FAB morphologic subtype may be important, with some subtypes associated with a worse outcome. Patients with extramedullary disease, CNS involvement, or underlying MDS have a worse prognosis. Other unfavorable prognostic factors in adult AML include: age >60 years, multidrug resistance gene expression, WBC >100,000 cells/mm³ (>100 × 10⁹/L), and therapy-related AML.[50] Age must be evaluated as a continuous variable when looking at prognostic factors. The clinical difference between a patient 61 years old and one 71 years old, is much greater than a 59 year old and a 61 year old. Certain cytogenetic abnormalities are also known to worsen the response rate and survival of patients with AML (Table 142–4).[3,47] Chromosome 16 or translocations between chromosome 8 and 21 alter core binding factor. Core binding factor is associated with sensitivity to cytarabine, gemtuzumab, and ozogamicin[51] In addition, patients who develop a "secondary" leukemia after treatment of another malignancy usually have a very poor response to antileukemic chemotherapy (i.e. therapy-related AML). Another factor that needs consideration for any cancer treatment is performance status. A bedridden patient with a new diagnosis of AML would not be a good candidate for treatment because of high

TABLE 142-4 Risk Category According to Cytogenetic Abnormalities Present

Disease	Risk Category		
	Good-Risk	*Intermediate-Risk*	*High-Risk*
AML	t(8;21); inv(16)/t(16;16); t(15;17);	Normal karyotype; trisomy 6, 8; −Y, del(12p)	Complex abn(3q), (9q), (11q),(21q) −5/del(5q), −7, t(6;9), t(9;22), add(5q), add (7q), −17, and abn(17p)
4-Year survival	≥70%	40%–50%	≤20%
ALL	Hyperdiploidy; t(10;14); or 6q		t(9;22); t(8;14); t(4;11); t(1;9)

ALL, acute lymphoblastic leukemia; AML, acute myeloid leukemia; abn, abnormal.
Data from Jemel et al.[1] and Grimwade and Hills.[52]

treatment-related morbidity and mortality. Patients with poor performance status are excluded from protocols or treatment.

Cytogenetics may be the most important prognostic factor for a newly diagnosed patient with AML.[52] Patients with core binding factor with t(8;21)(q22;q22) or inv(16)(p13q22)/t(16;16)(p13;q22) treated with a cytarabine based regimen have a relatively favorable prognosis. Adults with 3q(abn(3q)], deletions of 5q [del(5q)], monosomies of chromosome 5 and/or 7(−5/−7) have a poor prognosis with standard chemotherapy for AML, and may benefit from experimental treatments. The limitations to karyotype as a risk stratification tool include: failed cytogenetic analysis, presence of cryptic chromosomal rearrangements, and about 40% of cases have a normal karyotype. Genomic mutations, such as FLT3, nucleophosmin, and CCAAT/enhancer–binding protein alpha, have helped distinguish subsets of patients with differing outcome who have normal karyotypes. FLT3 is a receptor tyrosine kinase which is mutated in about 33% of AML, including those with normal karyotype, and is associated with higher presenting WBC and a poorer prognosis. Nucleophosmin is present in about 30% of AML, even in patients with normal karyotype, and commonly coexists with FLT3, and is associated with a higher CR and reduced relapse risk compared to patients without the mutation. CCAAT/enhancer binding protein alpha is present in about 10% of AML, and is associated with a favorable outcome. The area of cytogenetics is complex and still evolving.

Prognostic factors associated with pediatric AML have been reported but few have been shown to consistently predict treatment outcome. Poor prognostic factors include an FAB subtype M0 and M7, monosomy 7, age older than 10 years, black race, internal tandem duplications of FLT3, and having AML secondary to prior chemotherapy or radiation therapy.[6] Inversion of chromosome 16, trisomy 21, and t(8;21) are associated with a favorable outcome.[6]

More recently, several genetic molecular abnormalities have been identified in adults with AML that have prognostic significance. Abnormalities that are associated with a poor outcome include FLT3 abnormalities; MLL; brain and acute leukemia gene, cytoplasmic (*BAALC*) and Wilms tumor gene (*WT-1*).[10] Nucleophosmin mutations, member 1 (*NPM1*) (in the absence of FLT3 abnormalities) are associated with an improved relapse-free survival and OS.[10] The future of AML treatment may lie in targeted therapy based on molecular classification. Treatment algorithms based on the presence or absence of these abnormalities have been proposed but they are not currently incorporated into standard practice.[10]

TREATMENT

Acute Myeloid Leukemia

■ TREATMENT GOALS

The short-term goal of treatment for AML is to rapidly achieve a complete clinical and hematologic remission. In the absence of a

CR, a rapid and fatal outcome is inevitable. CR is defined as the disappearance of all clinical and bone marrow evidence (normal cellularity >20% with <5% blasts) of leukemia, with restoration of normal hematopoiesis (neutrophils ≥1,000 cells/mm³ [≥1 × 10⁹/L] and platelets >100,000/mm³ [>100 × 10⁹/L]).[53] Partial remission is a significant response to treatment (a decrease of at least 50% of blasts), but evidence of residual disease in the bone marrow remains (5%–25% blasts) and is considered a treatment failure requiring additional therapy. The definition of response for adult AML was reevaluated in 2003, and changes in the definition of response were proposed to include not only CR (morphologic CR with restoration of normal hematopoiesis), but also CR with incomplete blood count recovery (CRi), cytogenetic CR ([CRc] patient with normal cytogenetics in which cytogenetics were previously abnormal), and molecular CR ([CRm] molecular studies negative).[53] If there is a question of residual leukemia on bone marrow biopsy in adults, a bone marrow aspirate/biopsy should be repeated in 1 week.

After a CR is achieved, the goal is to maintain the patient in continuous CR. As discussed later, the occurrence of leukemic relapse in the bone marrow significantly reduces the likelihood of cure. Most patients who will die from acute leukemia die within the first 6 years; the survival curve (percentage alive versus time) beyond the 6th year after therapy does not continue to decline as rapidly ("survival plateau"), and at this time patients can be considered "cured."

With recent advances in chemotherapy and supportive care, 65% to 85% of all patients with AML achieve a CR, and 20% to 40% become long-term survivors.[3] Overall, the median duration of remission is 1 to 2 years. In patients older than 60 years of age, the percentage of patients achieving a CR is lower (39%–64%), and the median duration of remission is shorter than 1 year.[54] In contrast to ALL, effective therapies used in AML cause severe and often prolonged myelosuppression, with the exception of tretinoin. As a result, patients with AML, particularly patients older than 60 years of age, are at greater risk for treatment-related fatal infectious and bleeding complications.

The 5-year survival in children with AML has increased from 17% in 1976 to 50% in 2005.[6,21] Children with Down syndrome and AML receive less-intense therapy and have a 83% EFS.[6,21] Treatment of childhood AML, unlike that of ALL, usually only consists of induction and intensive postremission therapy (Fig. 142–2). CNS prophylaxis is not routinely given to patients with AML.

■ TREATMENT PHASES

Remission Induction

As with ALL, the goal of remission induction for AML is to rapidly induce a CR with associated restoration of normal hematopoiesis. Compared to ALL, however, fewer patients with AML achieve CR. Because the CR rate in AML is related to the intensity of the remission induction regimen, the drugs used in AML are given at doses that uniformly cause severe myelosuppression (except tretinoin).

One reason for the lower CR rate in AML as compared to ALL is the inability to give optimal doses of chemotherapy because of marrow toxicity. With continued improvement of supportive care for patients undergoing chemotherapy, more intensive treatment regimens are being given in an effort to reduce the high rate of leukemic relapse and increase the proportion of long-term survivors. Most patients achieve a CR after one or two courses of chemotherapy. Patients who require additional chemotherapy to achieve a CR have been reported to have a poor prognosis, even if remission is ultimately achieved.

❿ The most active single agents in AML are the anthracycline antibiotics (daunorubicin, doxorubicin, and idarubicin), anthracenediones (mitoxantrone), and the antimetabolite cytarabine. The most common regimen ("7+3") combines daunorubicin administered as a short infusion of 45 to 60 mg/m²/day on days 1 to 3, along with cytarabine administered as a continuous 24-hour infusion of 100 to 200 mg/m²/day on days 1 to 7.[3,55,56] The CR rate with the 7+3 regimen is 65% to 75% in patients 18 to 60 years old. Several trials have attempted to improve upon conventional 7+3 therapy, but have shown no improvement by (a) increasing cytarabine to 10 days, (b) shortening cytarabine to 5 days, (c) substituting doxorubicin for daunorubicin, (d) adding thioguanine, or (e) increasing cytarabine dosage to 200 mg/m²/day (given by continuous infusion).[3] Results of a recently published study showed that increasing the daunorubicin dose may improve treatment outcome. In that study, adults ≤60 years old with AML who were randomized to receive higher daunorubicin dosages (90 mg/m² given over 3 days) in combination with 7 days of standard-dose cytarabine (100 mg/m²/day) had a significantly higher CR rate (71% vs 57%) and increased overall median survival (23.7 vs 15.7 months) as compared with those who received the standard 7+3 regimen of daunorubicin (45 mg/m² given over 3 days) and cytarabine.[57]

Idarubicin or mitoxantrone has been evaluated as alternatives to daunorubicin in combination with standard-dose continuous infusion cytarabine. Trials in younger patients reported improved CR rates with these newer anthracyclines/anthracenediones and one trial demonstrated prolonged survival. Among older adults, the CR rate and OS does not appear to be different among the different anthracyclines/anthracenediones.[55,56] Thus the anthracycline of choice for the standard 7+3 regimen remains controversial, with many centers adopting idarubicin into the induction regimen in younger AML patients, and the choice in the elderly is based on individual clinician preference and institutional acquisition costs. The anthracycline of choice is now more controversial given the results of the recent studies of treatment of newly diagnosed AML.[57,58]

CLINICAL CONTROVERSY

Is there a superior anthracycline to use as part of the induction regimen for AML? Some clinicians believe that idarubicin is superior in attaining a complete remission following one cycle of induction compared to alternative anthracyclines or anthracenediones. Randomized trials in the elderly show similar remission rates with all anthracyclines and anthracenediones. Whether there is a difference in younger patient's remains to be seen.

Other strategies that have been evaluated include adding another agent such as etoposide to the induction regimen.[3,55,56] A comparison of the standard 7+3 regimen with or without etoposide on days 1 to 7 ("7+3+7") in newly diagnosed AML patients ages 15 to 70 years demonstrated no difference in CR rates or OS. A subset analysis of patients younger than 55 years of age demonstrated a doubling of the duration of remission and OS in the etoposide-containing arm. The 7+3+7 regimen was more toxic in patients older than 55 years of age. These results have been confirmed in other studies, but as yet are to be adopted in the United States as part of standard therapy.

Based on experimental tumor models that showed a steep dose–response curve for cytarabine, higher doses of cytarabine have also been evaluated as a means to enhance the outcome of remission induction therapy. Several groups, including the Southwest Oncology Group and the Australian Leukemia Study Group, have evaluated the impact of adding high-dose cytarabine to induction therapy. This strategy does not improve the CR rate or OS, but does improve EFS. A retrospective study conducted by the European Group for Blood and Marrow Transplantation demonstrated that the cytarabine dose administered during induction and/or consolidation did not influence the outcome in patients who ultimately went on to receive allogeneic or autologous HSCT.[59] These data suggest that high doses of cytarabine during induction may not be needed in patients who receive HSCT as postremission therapy. In summary, the role of high-dose cytarabine during induction remains controversial. If used during induction, high-dose cytarabine is more appropriate in younger patients than in elderly patients because of poor tolerance by elderly patients.

The National Comprehensive Cancer Network (NCCN) has published guidelines for the treatment of AML.[44] The classic 7+3 regimen may be inadequate in adults younger than 60 years of age because the duration of remission is less than that reported in some studies that employed high-dose cytarabine during induction.[44] The NCCN guideline recommends that adults younger than 60 years of age without an antecedent hematologic disorder (i.e., no preexisting hematologic malignancy such as MDS) be treated with either the 7+3 regimen or more aggressive chemotherapy including high-dose cytarabine with an anthracycline or anthracenedione. In patients ≥60 years of age with good performance status, the conventional 7+3 regimen should be used or the patient should be enrolled in available clinical trials. The approach in patients with an antecedent hematologic disorder differs, and younger patients (<60 years) should be offered available clinical trials or proceed to alloHSCT (provided a suitable donor is available). Older patients (≥60 years) with an antecedent hematologic disorder or those with significant comorbidities unrelated to leukemia should be offered a clinical trial or best supportive care because of the dismal outcomes associated with conventional chemotherapy. All adult patients who present with CNS symptoms, and all AML M4 and AML M5 patients who are not symptomatic, should have a diagnostic lumbar puncture, and if it is positive, should be treated for disease. Methotrexate 12 to 15 mg, with or without cytarabine, should be administered intrathecally twice a week until clearance of leukemic blasts from the cerebrospinal fluid, and then monthly for about 6 months.

Intensive Postremission Therapy

Although most adults with AML achieve a CR, the duration of remission is short (4–8 months) if no further treatment is given. Relapse is presumably a consequence of the presence of residual, but clinically undetectable, leukemic cells after remission induction therapy. The goal of intensive postremission therapy is to eradicate these residual leukemic cells and to prevent the emergence of drug-resistant disease. ⓫ The need for postremission therapy is based on postmortem analysis and cell kinetic data suggesting that nearly 10⁹ residual leukemic cells remain after effective remission induction therapy. Strategies evaluated as postremission therapy include (a) low-dose, prolonged maintenance therapy, (b) short-course intensive chemotherapy-alone regimens and (c) high-dose chemotherapy with or without radiation therapy followed by alloHSCT or autologous HSCT.

Chemotherapy In the treatment of AML, intensive postremission therapy is often referred to as consolidation therapy. Results of randomized trials in adults clearly show that intensive postremission therapy following remission induction therapy prolongs survival versus no therapy, although the exact duration of postremission therapy is controversial.[3,55,56]

The intensity of postremission therapy is important. In a large Cancer and Leukemia Group B (CALGB) trial, all patients who achieve a CR after standard 7+3 induction, were randomized to receive one of three cytarabine-based consolidation regimens: 100 mg/m²/day or 400 mg/m²/day as a continuous 24-hour infusion, or 3,000 mg/m² every 12 hours on days 1, 3, and 5.[60] For adults younger than age 60 years, the probability of remaining in CR after 4 years was significantly higher in patients who received high-dose cytarabine (25% vs 29% vs 44%, respectively).[60] Elderly patients had lower response rates in all arms and did not benefit from the administration of higher doses of cytarabine, probably because they were unable to tolerate the high-dose regimen. Dose-limiting neurotoxicity in the high-dose arm was greater in elderly patients and those patients with impaired kidney function.[60]

It is not clear whether the same agents (cytarabine and an anthracycline) given for remission induction should be used for postremission therapy in higher doses, or whether different agents should be given. If leukemic relapse is caused by a resistant cell line, then the use of different agents that are non–cross-resistant with drugs used in induction might be beneficial.

High-dose cytarabine appears to be a key part of postremission therapy, particularly if not used in induction therapy. However, many questions remain, such as the optimal dose (g/m²), number of doses per cycle, and number of cycles of high-dose cytarabine. Among patients with core-binding factor AML, defined as the presence of either t(8;21) or inv(16), it is clear that multiple cycles are beneficial, generally three to four cycles.[61] The NCCN guideline recommends four cycles of high-dose cytarabine for adults younger than 60 years of age and with good cytogenetics or, alternatively, one cycle of high-dose cytarabine followed by autologous HSCT.[48] Patients with intermediate-risk cytogenetics should receive four cycles of high-dose cytarabine or undergo either an autoHSCT or an allogeneic (sibling) HSCT.[48] If a patient is 60 years of age or older, standard-dose cytarabine with or without anthracycline for one to two cycles, a reduced-dose high-dose cytarabine regimen (1–1.5 g/m²/day for four to six doses) for one to two cycles, or enrollment in a clinical trial is recommended. Patients with high-risk cytogenetics, underlying MDS, or secondary AML should either be enrolled in a clinical trial or be referred for either a matched sibling or alternative donor alloHSCT.[48]

CLINICAL CONTROVERSY

Intensive postremission therapy is clearly necessary to prevent relapse and those regimens containing high-dose cytarabine appear to be a key part of postremission therapy. However, the optimal dose of high-dose cytarabine, the number of doses per cycle, and the number of cycles to give remain unknown.

Allogeneic Hematopoietic Stem Cell Transplantation

AlloHSCT represents the most aggressive approach to postremission therapy in the management of AML. Much controversy surrounds this treatment approach, specifically the appropriateness, timing, treatment design, and donor selection.

The antileukemic activity of alloHSCT is based on the administration of pretransplant high-dose chemotherapy (or chemoradiotherapy) and the development of a posttransplant immune-based antileukemic response. The immune-based response, referred to as a graft-versus-leukemia (GVL) effect, often accompanies the graft-versus-host disease (GVHD) reaction. The immune-based benefit of alloHSCT has been demonstrated through the observation of consistently lower relapse rates with alloHSCT as compared to autologous or syngeneic HSCT. This potential benefit of alloHSCT can be offset by the risk of posttransplant complications such as GVHD, sinusoidal obstruction syndrome, graft failure, and infections.

AlloHSCT was first evaluated as a treatment modality for AML in refractory patients, but because of initial success in small numbers of patients, it has also been evaluated as intensive postremission therapy in AML patients in first or subsequent remission. Nonrandomized trials of HLA-identical sibling alloHSCT performed in AML patients in first CR (CR1) reported 5-year survival rates of 45% to 60% with relapse rates of 10% to 20%.[3,55,56] Transplant-related mortality following HLA-matched sibling alloHSCT is 15% to 25% in most series. As clinicians have gained more experience in this intensive form of therapy and been provided with more effective immunosuppressive and antibiotic regimens, transplant-related mortality rates have decreased and survival rates have increased. Bone marrow registry data indicate that long-term survival rates in AML patients who receive a matched sibling alloHSCT while in first remission have increased from about 45% in the early 1980s to about 60% in the mid-1990s.

AlloHSCT from an HLA-matched sibling donor for AML patients in CR1 results in long-term EFS in 43% to 55% of patients. Although the results vary, some of the studies show longer EFS and lower relapse rates with alloHSCT in AML in CR1 as compared to chemotherapy-alone postremission regimens.

AlloHSCT is generally restricted to patients younger than 60 years of age, which limits the number of patients eligible for treatment of a disease that primarily affects older adults. One new approach, termed nonmyeloablative stem cell transplant (NST), uses reduced intensity preparative regimens and is now being evaluated in AML patients, particularly in older patients and those with comorbid illnesses that would limit their eligibility for conventional alloHSCT. NST is designed to provide enough immunosuppression in the preparative regimen to allow for engraftment of donor cells, and depends heavily on the development of a GVL effect as a means to treat and prevent relapse of AML. Initial results of NST in AML indicate that the procedure is well tolerated in a wide age range of patients, and that it is associated with low rates of regimen-related toxicity.[62,63] Evaluations in larger numbers of patients are necessary to determine the comparative impact of NST on GVHD, EFS, and OS. Because only 30% of patients have an HLA-matched sibling donor, alloHSCT is further restricted as a treatment alternative for AML patients.[64] Matched unrelated donor transplantation with a phenotypically HLA-matched donor identified from bone marrow registries is also a treatment option in young adults and pediatric AML patients. This approach is associated with long-term EFS rates of 30% to 40%, which are slightly lower than in AML patients undergoing HLA-matched sibling alloHSCT because of a higher risk of treatment-related mortality with the procedure.[3,56]

The decision to transplant a patient depends a great deal on which biological risk group the patient belongs. Among patients with favorable risk AML, alloHSCT does not result in better outcomes as compared to high-dose cytarabine-based therapy. All patients with high-risk AML, including those with an antecedent

TABLE 142-5 Comparative Trials of Allogeneic HSCT (AlloHSCT) or Autologous HSCT (AutoHSCT) or Chemotherapy (Chemo) Alone as Postremission Therapy for AML in First Complete Remission

	Disease-Free Survival at 4 Years (%)			Overall Survival at 4 Years (%)		
	AlloHSCT	**AutoHSCT**	**Chemo**	**AlloHSCT**	**AutoHSCT**	**Chemo**
Zittoun et al. (EORTC-GIMEMA)	55%[a]	48%[b]	30%	59%	56%	46%
Harousseau et al. (GOELAM)	44%	44%	40%	53%	50%	54%
Cassileth et al. (Intergroup)	43%	35%	35%	46%	43%	52%[c]
Burnett et al. (UK MRC)	47%	50%	40%–58%	53%	52%	46%–52%

AML, acute myeloid leukemia; HSCT, hematopoietic stem cell transplantation.
[a]$p < 0.01$ (vs chemo)
[b]$p = 0.05$ (vs chemo)
[c]$p = 0.05$ (vs autoHSCT), $p = 0.04$ (vs alloHSCT)
Data from references 4 and 51.

hematologic disorder, treatment-related MDS, or induction failure, should undergo evaluation for HSCT. Similarly patients in CR1 with high-risk cytogenetics and patients in second CR (CR2) and beyond should undergo evaluation for alloHSCT.[44]

Autologous Hematopoietic Stem Cell Transplantation

Compared to alloHSCT, autologous HSCT (autoHSCT) has the advantage of a lower risk of posttransplant complications because of lack of immunosuppression and GVHD, and more broad applicability because of a lack of donor limitations and fewer age restrictions. Although the preparative regimen still provides antileukemic activity, autoHSCT is associated with a higher risk of relapse because of a lack of a GVL effect and potential tumor contamination with autologous stem cells. EFS following autoHSCT for AML in CR1 ranges from 40% to 60%, with treatment-related mortality of 5% to 15% and relapse rates of 30% to 50%.[65] Long-term response rates decrease proportionally as autoHSCT is employed in second or subsequent CR. Controversies in autoHSCT include the optimal timing of therapy, the amount of consolidation therapy needed prior to HSCT, the dose of stem cells needed, and the impact of posttransplant therapy.[65]

Comparisons of Postremission Therapy Options Several randomized trials in AML patients in CR1 have compared outcomes following alloHSCT, autoHSCT, and/or intensive consolidation chemotherapy (Table 142-5).[56] In most trials, eligible patients based on age and donor availability received an alloHSCT and the remaining patients were randomized between autoHSCT and chemotherapy alone. The European Organization for Research and Treatment of Cancer-GIMEMA (Gruppo Italiano Malattie Ematologiche Maligne dell'Adulto) trial observed a EFS advantage and reduced relapse risk for alloHSCT or autoHSCT as compared to chemotherapy alone, but no differences in OS.[3,56] Survival rates were comparable because of a higher relapse rate in the chemotherapy group as compared to a higher treatment-related mortality rate in the alloHSCT group. This is the only trial that has demonstrated superior 4-year EFS with transplantation versus chemotherapy. Interestingly, the response rates in the conventional chemotherapy arm in this trial were lower than those reported in other studies, which may account for the survival benefit in the transplant group. Several other trials have shown no difference in EFS or OS between autoHSCT, alloHSCT, and conventional chemotherapy. In aggregate, these trials show that either autoHSCT or alloHSCT can reduce the risk of relapse, although this has not translated into a survival benefit. One trial design issue that might explain this lack of survival benefit was the low percentage of patients who progressed to transplantation when randomized, thus diluting the effect of transplantation. The effect of stem cell source on EFS and OS is controversial. Several comparative trials of bone marrow versus peripheral blood have been completed

in patients with hematologic malignancies, and a meta-analysis of nine randomized trials demonstrated a lower relapse rate for those patients receiving peripheral blood stem cells.[66]

Most transplant centers base their decision to transplant on cytogenetic risk category.[3] Patients with high-risk cytogenetics do poorly with conventional chemotherapy or autoHSCT (EFS <15%), making alloHSCT the treatment of choice in this population. Patients with good-risk cytogenetics should not proceed to transplant in CR1, as neither auto- nor alloHSCT is superior to conventional chemotherapy. The optimal treatment of choice in patients with intermediate-risk cytogenetics is not clear and is based on clinician preference. Many centers consider a relapse probability of 40% to 50% sufficiently high so as to warrant the risk of transplantation-related mortality. The decision to proceed with HSCT in this group may rest on the results of molecular testing. As discussed in Risk Classification above, several genetic molecular abnormalities have been identified in adults with AML that have prognostic significance. Abnormalities that are associated with a poor outcome include FLT3 abnormalities, myeloid/lymphoid or MLL abnormalities, BAALC, and WT-1.

According to the NCCN guidelines, the decision to proceed to HSCT depends on cytogenetics.[48] If the patient has a good-risk cytogenetic profile and is younger than age 60 years, then high-dose cytarabine for four cycles or one cycle of high-dose cytarabine-based therapy followed by autoHSCT is preferred over alloHSCT. If the patient has a high-risk cytogenetic profile and is younger than 60 years of age, then alloHSCT should be considered early after remission induction. Patients with intermediate-risk cytogenetics should be entered into a clinical trial, but if a clinical trial is not available, either a matched sibling alloHSCT or an autoHSCT should be considered. AutoHSCT can be used if a hematologic and cytogenetic remission is achieved. For patients 60 years and older, the NCCN guidelines do not favor HSCT and recommend either enrollment into a clinical trial, or consideration of conventional dose cytarabine with or without an anthracycline or intermediate-dose cytarabine. Clinicians increasingly consider autoHSCT as a treatment option, and for selected patients older than 60 years of age, NST is being used more frequently.[62,63] For the AML patient who relapses early after induction therapy, if a sibling or matched related donor is available, then alloHSCT is the primary reinduction therapy because conventional chemotherapy offers little benefit. If the relapse occurs late, then HSCT can be used as postremission consolidation after conventional induction therapy.[48]

■ CHILDHOOD ACUTE MYELOID LEUKEMIA

The most effective induction regimens for children include an anthracycline, cytarabine, and etoposide, yielding a CR rate of

80% to 90%.[6] Five-year OS is 36% to 66%.[6] The use of risk-adapted therapy is not as prevalent with AML as with ALL. Intensified therapy regimens, which include more antileukemic agents, higher doses of agents, or compression of the time in which the agents are delivered, improve survival rates. The Children's Cancer Group used a compressed regimen, whereby the second course of therapy was given 6 to 10 days after the first instead of 14 days, without waiting for marrow recovery to occur. Although intensive therapy is associated with an increased mortality rate as compared with standard chemotherapy in children with AML, the long-term EFS is significantly better in the intensive-therapy group (49% vs 35%).[67] The use of intrathecal CNS prophylaxis varies by cooperative group, due to the low CNS relapse rate (2%).[6] Cranial radiation is only rarely used in the United States for patients with refractory CNS disease.

Gemtuzumab ozogamicin is an immunoconjugate that consists of a monoclonal antibody to CD33 which is expressed on >80% of AML blasts linked to calicheamicin, a potent antineoplastic agent. Following the binding of the antibody to the myeloblasts, the antibody-antigen complex is internalized causing the release of the calicheamicin inside the cell. The Children's Oncology Group has established a dose for gemtuzumab when given in combination with chemotherapy and is assessing the benefit of adding gemtuzumab to frontline therapy in a current phase III clinical trial.[68] As of October 1, 2010, gemtuzumab ozogamicin is no longer commercially available. Future access may be available only through clinical trials.

Following induction therapy, patients should be evaluated for a response. Those not achieving a CR will require additional chemotherapy called *reinduction*. A bone marrow biopsy is usually performed 7 to 10 days after the completion of chemotherapy to document disease eradication. If there is persistent disease, a second course of therapy is administered. The second course may be identical to the initial induction regimen, or include high-dose cytarabine and asparaginase, or mitoxantrone and cytarabine. If the marrow is aplastic, a repeat marrow biopsy should be performed upon hematologic recovery to document a CR.

Following induction, children proceed onto consolidation therapy. An evidence-based review of the role of HSCT in the treatment of pediatric AML concluded that HSCT was indicated in the following settings: (a) initial CR: matched sibling alloHSCT is superior to autoHSCT and chemotherapy, but are only available in 25% of children; (b) second CR: alloHSCT is preferable to chemotherapy and autoHSCT.[6,69] Children with no suitable donor should receive consolidation chemotherapy including high-dose cytarabine, which yields results similar to those seen with autoHSCT.[6] Maintenance chemotherapy is not used in children in the United States.

Infant AML is usually myelomonoblastic or monoblastic in morphology. Poor prognostic factors include t(1;22), high WBC count, and CNS disease. Neonates with Down syndrome may develop transient myeloproliferative disease that usually spontaneously resolves without treatment within a few months. Infants with AML receive the same therapy as children of other ages, with the dosing per kilogram and not per body surface area.

■ ACUTE MYELOID LEUKEMIA IN THE ELDERLY

As the median age at diagnosis is in the range of 65 to 70 years, AML is a disease of the elderly. Unfortunately, long-term EFS is lower in older patients, ranging from 5% to 15%, as compared with 40% in younger patients.[54] In patients older than age 55 years, a review of ECOG studies reported the median duration of survival to be 6 to 9 months, as compared with 11 months in patients younger than age 55 years. The actual response and survival rates

may be even lower, as many elderly patients with AML are not included in clinical trials because of a lack of eligibility and poor performance status.[3,54]

Elderly patients with AML have a poor outcome as a result of the frequent presence of unfavorable prognostic factors, including high-risk cytogenetic features, preceding myelodysplasia, and a higher incidence of inherent drug resistance.[3] More than 70% of de novo AML patients older than age 55 years will express the multidrug resistance phenotype associated with chemotherapy resistance, including resistance to the leukemia-active anthracyclines and etoposide.[54] Older patients with AML may also have poor outcome because of the inability to withstand aggressive therapy as a result of poor organ function, poor performance status, or existing comorbidities. Although older patients with AML may be able to tolerate aggressive remission induction therapy, they often cannot tolerate intensive postremission therapy, which increases their likelihood of leukemic relapse. Despite newer therapies, the prognosis of AML in the elderly has not changed significantly over the last several decades.

The potential therapeutic strategies in elderly AML patients include (a) no chemotherapy (i.e., best supportive care or palliative care therapy), (b) attenuated chemotherapy, (c) investigational therapy, or (d) standard-dose chemotherapy.[3] The palliative approach is most appropriate in patients with slowly progressive leukemia ("smoldering leukemia"). The difficulty lies in the ability to reliably identify these patients at diagnosis. Although initially accepted in older patients, palliative care approaches in older patients with AML with moderate-to-good performance status and organ function are now considered inappropriate. An ECOG-CALGB study randomized patients to either conventional chemotherapy or to observation in which patients could receive modest doses of chemotherapy for symptom palliation. Survival was twice as long in the chemotherapy group. The quality-of-life of each group was similar, with patients in each group spending approximately 50% of the study time in the hospital.[70]

These results show that chemotherapy prolongs survival without significantly decreasing the quality-of-life for elderly patients. Thus chemotherapy is a viable treatment option for elderly patients, although the best chemotherapy regimen and overall treatment approach are controversial. One approach is to attenuate the dose of chemotherapy, preferably with oral agents where possible, or lower doses of intravenous agents. Agents used in this strategy include oral etoposide, low-dose subcutaneous cytarabine, and other oral agents such as thioguanine and idarubicin (oral idarubicin is not currently commercially available in the United States). The United Kingdom AML Study Group recently published a comparative trial of low-dose subcutaneous cytarabine twice daily versus hydroxyurea. Low-dose cytarabine produced a greater number of complete remissions compared to placebo, and prolonged 1-year survival.[71]

Another approach is to use the same remission induction regimens that would be used in younger adults. With this approach, the complete remission rate in older AML patients ranges from 41% to 62%, as compared with 65% to 73% in adults younger than 60 years of age, and are very short-lived (5–10 months). Treatment-related mortality ranges from 15% to 20%. More elderly patients than younger patients will require two courses of remission induction therapy to achieve a complete remission. In an effort to improve response rates, some trials have attempted to determine the optimal anthracycline and the appropriate dose. Unlike younger patients, results of clinical trials in elderly patients do not suggest any efficacy or toxicity advantages of idarubicin or mitoxantrone over daunorubicin for AML induction therapy.[72] Older patients with AML also do not experience added benefit when etoposide is incorporated into an anthracycline and cytarabine-containing regimen, or when etoposide is substituted for cytarabine in induction.[73,74] The combination of clofarabine 30 mg/m^2/day for 5 days and cytarabine was found to be an effective first-line regimen for patients over 59 years with AML and high-risk MDS by achieving a CR rate of 56%.[75] Recently, a randomized trial of daunorubicin 30 mg/m^2/day on days 1 through 3 with cytarabine 200 mg/m^2/day as a continuous 7-day infusion in patients older than 60 years demonstrated a more rapid response with a higher response rate (64% vs 54%) as compared with the conventional dose of daunorubicin (45 mg/m^2 over 3 days) with cytarabine. While there was no difference in toxicity, 30-day mortality or life-threatening events, overall survival was only improved in the subgroup of patients aged 60 to 65 years (38% vs 23%).[58]

Postremission strategies in elderly AML patients are less-well defined.[3] Although high-dose cytarabine is a standard component of postremission therapy in younger patients, it has not been shown to be beneficial in elderly AML patients. In the elderly, attenuated-dose cytarabine during remission induction decreases remission and survival rates while decreasing treatment-related mortality rates, which raises the concern that attenuated-dose cytarabine during postremission therapy may cause similar outcomes. In the CALGB trial that compared postremission cytarabine doses, higher doses of cytarabine (3,000 mg/m^2) was not as effective in patients older than age 60 years as it was in younger patients.[60] Serious toxicities, particularly neurotoxicity, were more frequent in elderly patients, and these toxicities limited the ability to deliver the planned four courses of therapy. An ECOG review concluded that lower doses of cytarabine (1,500 mg/m^2 for 6 to 12 doses) in older AML patients are well tolerated, with a treatment-related mortality rate of only 2% and median survival at 2 years of 30%.[76] Based on these data, some clinicians suggest that attenuated high-dose regimens (such as 1,500 mg/m^2) may be sufficient for elderly AML patients. The appropriate number of cycles of postremission consolidation therapy is unknown and currently under investigation in a randomized ECOG trial. An alternative approach to intensive postremission therapy is the administration of multiple courses of chemotherapy in the ambulatory setting. The Acute Leukemia French Association recently demonstrated improved overall survival among patients receiving 6 monthly courses of outpatient chemotherapy (daunorubicin or idarubicin day 1; low-dose subcutaneous cytarabine for 5 days) compared to intensive consolidation (daunorubicin or idarubicin days 1 to 4; cytarabine continuous infusion).[77]

Although maintenance therapy is considered inferior to intensive consolidation chemotherapy in younger patients, its role in older patients with AML is still undefined. Some studies suggest that maintenance therapy following consolidation prolongs EFS but not OS as compared to no maintenance therapy.[78] Because older patients may not be able to tolerate more aggressive postremission strategies such as HSCT, maintenance therapy may play an important role in improving outcomes.

Several FLT3 inhibitors are in clinical development, including ABT-869, lestaurtinib (CEP-701), and midostaurin (PKC 412). Inhibition of farnesyl transferase is another treatment target. Tipifarnib has been the most extensively evaluated, demonstrating CR rates of 14%.[79] Other approaches include antiangiogenic therapies (e.g., lenalidomide, semaxanib [SU5416], axitinib [AG013736], bevacizumab, arsenic trioxide), proteasome inhibition and antiapoptotic therapies (e.g., bortezomib, oblimersen), epigenetic therapies (e.g., azacitidine, decitabine), and novel alkylating agents such as cloretazine. Response rates with these new approaches in the elderly range from 0% to 59%. Whether they can modify the course of disease resulting in prolonged survival is unclear.

NST is another therapeutic option in elderly patients with AML and MDS. Two small studies suggest this is a feasible option, with actuarial OS and EFS rates of 44% to 69% and 37% to 56%, respectively.[62,63] The advantage of this approach is less toxicity as a result of less-intensive chemotherapy, with the immune system providing the major antileukemic effect via GVHD/GVL mechanisms (see Chap. 148).

■ TREATMENT OF RELAPSED OR REFRACTORY ACUTE MYELOID LEUKEMIA

The most common cause of treatment failure in AML patients receiving chemotherapy alone or undergoing HSCT is relapse. In addition, many patients, particularly elderly patients, have refractory disease as defined by the inability to achieve a CR after two courses of induction therapy. In most cases, the preferred method of treatment for relapsed or refractory disease is HSCT. Prolonged EFS is observed in 30% to 40% of patients receiving allo- or autoHSCT in first relapse or CR2. Unfortunately, only a small percentage of relapsed or refractory adult patients will be eligible for HSCT, particularly alloHSCT, because of age and donor restrictions. The role of NST is also being evaluated in this setting.

The timing of HSCT to treat relapse is controversial. Some studies suggest that outcomes of HLA-matched, related alloHSCT are similar regardless of whether the transplant is performed at the time of early first relapse or in CR2. The difficulty with this approach is identifying a patient in "early relapse," as often the patient will present in a florid relapse. While performing the alloHSCT in first relapse eliminates the need for and toxicity of salvage chemotherapy, the feasibility of this approach is limited by the lead time required to activate a donor search. An International Bone Marrow Transplant Registry study demonstrated that alloHSCT was superior to chemotherapy for treatment of relapse occurring 1 to 2 years following induction.[80] Prolonged leukemia-free survival occurred in at least twofold more alloHSCT recipients as compared to patients receiving chemotherapy. In the treatment of refractory disease, alloHSCT is superior to autoHSCT in adults younger than age 55 years.

Patients who relapse following alloHSCT have a poor outcome, with a median survival of about 3 to 4 months.[81] In this setting, treatment options depend on performance status, clinical condition, and the time since alloHSCT. Patients relapsing less than 100 days following alloHSCT are unlikely to respond to current therapies, and salvage attempts are often associated with a high treatment-related mortality. For selected patients relapsing more than 1 year after alloHSCT, a second alloHSCT may be an alternative, but the likelihood of prolonged survival is generally less than 10% with a second transplant. Other strategies being investigated for the treatment of relapse after alloHSCT include immune manipulation to stimulate a GVL effect through donor lymphocyte infusions, and premature discontinuation of calcineurin inhibitors and other immunosuppressants.

AutoHSCT is an option at the time of first relapse if cells have been previously collected and stored during first remission. If such cells were not collected, then it is necessary to achieve a second CR in order to proceed to autoHSCT. Prolonged EFS of 30% and 20% are reported when autoHSCT is performed in CR2 and CR3, respectively. The advantages of autoHSCT are the lack of donor limitations and fewer age-based restrictions; the disadvantage is the need to achieve a CR, which requires exposure to more cytotoxic chemotherapy. If patients relapse following autoHSCT, alloHSCT from a related or unrelated donor is preferred in selected younger patients. NST or other investigational therapies can be considered for older patients who relapse after autoHSCT.

If patients with relapsed or refractory disease are not candidates for HSCT, until recently the primary mode of treatment was salvage chemotherapy. The ability to achieve a second CR with salvage chemotherapy is related to the duration of the first remission. About 50% to 60% of patients who relapse longer than 2 years after induction therapy will achieve a second CR, often with the same induction regimen.[3,56] If the patient relapses 1 to 2 years after induction therapy, the second CR rate decreases to 40%, and only 10% to 20% of patients who relapse within 6 to 12 months following induction are able to achieve a second CR with alternate salvage chemotherapy regimens. Long-term survival at 3 years ranges from zero in patients who relapse early to 20% to 25% in those who experience a prolonged duration of initial remission. Based on these data, a risk-adapted approach should be taken when considering treatment options.

The most commonly used salvage regimens include high-dose cytarabine given at doses of 2,000 to 3,000 mg/m² every 12 hours for 8 to 12 doses. High-dose cytarabine schedules that use once-daily doses or alternate-day doses have also been used in an attempt to minimize toxicity.[56] Cytarabine has been administered alone or in combination with various agents, including etoposide, fludarabine, topotecan, clofarabine, and an anthracycline, as treatment of relapsed or refractory AML. Response rates to such salvage regimens range from 30% to 50%, but are often short-lived. Patients who received high-dose cytarabine during remission induction may be less likely to benefit from such a regimen for treatment of relapse, and thus require alternate salvage strategies. Patients with remission duration of longer than 1 year appear to benefit most from high-dose cytarabine regimens.[3,56]

About 70% of relapsed or refractory AML express the multidrug resistance phenotype, which confers a high degree of chemotherapy resistance because of its encoding and overexpression of P-glycoprotein. P-glycoprotein is a membrane protein capable of removing certain antineoplastics from the intracellular to extracellular space. Monoclonal antibodies have the potential to deliver targeted therapy to the malignant cell. Patients with AML in first untreated relapse treated with gemtuzumab (9 mg/m² for two doses separated by 14 days) attained a CR in 16% of patients, with an additional 13% of patients having normalization of blood counts with the exception of persistent platelet counts <100,000/mm³ (<100 × 10⁹/L).[82] Toxicity can be problematic with gemtuzumab. Common adverse effects include infusion-related reactions (fever and chills), prolonged neutropenia and thrombocytopenia, and transient elevations in hepatic enzymes. A more serious adverse event associated with gemtuzumab therapy is sinusoidal obstruction syndrome. It was initially thought that this only occurred in patients receiving gemtuzumab following HSCT, but has now been described in several patients who never underwent HSCT. Patients treated with gemtuzumab should have their weight and liver function tests, particularly bilirubin, monitored. Because gemtuzumab lacks specific dose-limiting organ toxicities, it has also been investigated in combination with other chemotherapy agents. In a salvage regimen consisting of gemtuzumab 9 mg/m² on day 4, cytarabine 1,000 mg/m² every 12 hours on days 1 through 5, and mitoxantrone 12 mg/m² on days 1 through 3, the 2-year EFS was 33% making gemtuzumab an attractive addition to salvage therapy.[83] The future role of gemtuzumab ozogamicin will need to be determined by clinical trials since its withdrawal from the commercial market in fall 2010.

Several classes of new agents are being investigated as alternate treatment approaches for relapsed or refractory AML, including the ubiquitin-proteasome pathway inhibitors (bortezomib), new novel nucleoside analogs (troxacitabine), hypomethylating agents (decitabine and 5-azacitidine), histone deacetylase inhibitors (phenylbutyrate, vorinostat), and angiogenesis modulators (bevacizumab and thalidomide).[84] Arsenic trioxide, which is effective in the treatment of APL, is being investigated for the treatment of AML via its modulation of apoptotic and chromatin remodeling pathways.

In children with AML, the duration of first CR predicts response to salvage chemotherapy. The BFM (Berlin-Frankfurt-Munster) group reported that patients who relapse within 1.5 years of initial diagnosis have a 5-year survival of 10%, versus 40% for those who relapse later than 1.5 years after initial diagnosis.[85] In children with relapsed or refractory AML, a regimen of mitoxantrone 12 mg/m²/day for 4 days starting on the third day of treatment and cytarabine 1,000 mg/m² per dose every 12 hours for eight doses can achieve a second CR rate of 76% with only a 3% mortality rate.[86] However, the 2-year OS rate was only 24%. Patients were eligible to receive intensification with high-dose cytarabine and etoposide at the investigator's discretion, and this arm was closed as a consequence of a toxic death rate of 10%. Currently, most pediatric patients in CR2 receive alloHSCT if a suitable donor is available with 30% OS.[6]

LATE EFFECTS OF THERAPY FOR ACUTE MYELOID LEUKEMIA

Because of the intense therapy received by children with AML, they are at risk for a variety of long-term sequelae. A recent study reported that more than 50% of survivors have growth abnormalities.[87] Other findings include neurocognitive deficits, transfusion-associated hepatitis, endocrine disorders, cataracts, and cardiomyopathy (median cumulative anthracycline dose: 335 mg/m²). The 20-year cumulative risk for a second malignancy is estimated to be 1.8%.

TREATMENT

Acute Promyelocytic Leukemia

APL is a subclass of AML (FAB M3) that accounts for about 10% of all cases, and is the most curable of the AML subtypes. Most patients are diagnosed between the ages of 15 and 60 years. Five-year EFS rates of 70% to 80% are reported with APL.[88] APL is clinically unique from the other subclasses because of the common occurrence of severe coagulopathy (characterized by disseminated intravascular coagulation) at diagnosis and during induction therapy, which frequently resulted in intracerebral hemorrhage. In APL, differentiation and maturation arrest are caused by alterations in the RAR because of the translocation of chromosomes 15 and 17. The discovery of t(15;17) now provides a cytogenetic marker of the disease and is predictive of response to differentiation therapy with tretinoin (commonly referred to as all-*trans* retinoic acid or ATRA). This translocation leads to a fusion protein of the PML gene on chromosome 15 and the RAR-α on chromosome 17.

Prior to the availability of tretinoin in the late 1980s, treatment of APL consisted of the same combination chemotherapy regimens used in the treatment of other subclasses of AML. Such standard regimens produced CR rates of 50% to 60%, but were associated with a high treatment-related mortality rate caused by hemorrhagic complications. The introduction of molecularly targeted therapy with tretinoin allows for high CR rates with a significant reduction in life-threatening bleeding complications. Arsenic trioxide targets the PML moiety, resulting in apoptosis, and appears to be synergistic with tretinoin.

The WBC count at initial presentation is the most important prognostic factor in patients with APL. Abnormal creatinine, increased peripheral blast count and presence of coagulopathy are prognostic factors that predict for early death due to hemorrhage.[89]

■ TREATMENT PHASES

Induction

Tretinoin, an oral vitamin A analog, is given orally in a dose of 45 mg/m²/day, as a single dose or divided into two doses, given after a meal. Tretinoin-based regimens achieve CR rates as high as 95% in APL patients within 1 to 3 months. Because tretinoin does not cross the blood–brain barrier, leukemic meningitis should be treated with conventional intrathecal chemotherapy.

Although devoid of myelosuppressive effects, tretinoin therapy is associated with headache, skin and mucous membrane reactions, bone pain, nausea, and the retinoic acid syndrome. When tretinoin is started, rapid onset of differentiation of promyelocytes occurs, which can lead to leukocytosis and retinoic acid syndrome. The retinoic acid syndrome (fever, respiratory distress, interstitial pulmonary infiltrates, pleural effusions, and weight gain) is now referred to as the APL differentiation syndrome or APL hyperleukocytosis syndrome, because it is associated with other treatment modalities in the management of APL. Among tretinoin-treated patients, this syndrome is fatal in 5% to 29% of cases. A combination of chemotherapy with tretinoin induction decreases the risk of APL differentiation syndrome, and rapid initiation of dexamethasone 10 mg (0.2 mg/kg per dose in children) twice daily for 3 days upon development of symptoms decreases associated mortality.[88]

A number of clinical trials have evaluated treatment regimens for APL since the discovery of tretinoin.[88] These trials demonstrated that tretinoin induction therapy, followed by consolidation chemotherapy, produced similar CR rates but decreased relapse and increased EFS and OS as compared to chemotherapy alone for remission induction and consolidation. However, a significant proportion of patients receiving tretinoin in that study relapsed by 4 years, and 25% of patients experienced the APL differentiation syndrome. In an effort to extend the duration of remission and decrease tretinoin-associated toxicity, other trials have evaluated the sequential and concurrent administration of tretinoin with chemotherapy during remission induction therapy. The United Kingdom Medical Research Council trial compared concurrent administration of tretinoin with chemotherapy to sequential tretinoin during induction (given 5 days before anthracycline-based remission induction chemotherapy) with the hope of reducing coagulopathy-related complications. Concurrent administration was superior in terms of CR rates, early death, and EFS and OS at 3 years. The French study demonstrated similar CR rates with concurrent or sequential tretinoin and standard induction chemotherapy, but noted a better EFS and EFS at 2 years in the concurrent administration group (suggesting a synergistic or additive effect for the combination).[88] ⑫ Based on these data, the current NCCN guideline for induction therapy for newly diagnosed APL patients include tretinoin 45 mg/m²/day until a CR is achieved, in combination with an anthracycline (either daunorubicin 50–60 mg/m² per dose for 3 days, or idarubicin 12 mg/m² per dose every other day for four doses) or tretinoin plus arsenic trioxide for patients unable to tolerate anthracycline therapy.[48] Similar CR rates are observed with daunorubicin or idarubicin. APL cells appear to be more sensitive to anthracyclines, perhaps as a consequence of decreased P-glycoprotein expression.

It is important to note that chemotherapy regimens used in combination with tretinoin differ from standard AML regimens, primarily as a result of the lack of cytarabine. Several studies have evaluated the role of cytarabine in remission induction regimens for APL. In earlier trials, the addition of cytarabine did not improve the CR rate.[88] Children should also be treated with tretinoin and an anthracycline, with results similar to those achieved in adults.

Another difference in the treatment of APL is the timing of bone marrow biopsy. Assessment of response to treatment of APL is done at the time of count recovery after induction therapy. A day 10 to 14 day bone marrow biopsy, which is usually done for monitoring the effect of induction chemotherapy for other types of AML, is not long enough because leukemic promyelocytes need more time for differentiation. Assessment of molecular remission should be made after consolidation.

Arsenic trioxide is a compound with demonstrated efficacy in relapsed APL. It has been evaluated as part of remission induction therapy in several small studies. The concept of a "chemotherapy-free" regimen in this disease is attractive. Administration of arsenic trioxide with or without tretinoin (± chemotherapy) results in high initial CR rates and molecular response rates.[90] Larger studies are needed before this can be adopted as a standard of care.

Consolidation Therapy

Consolidation chemotherapy should be administered to patients with APL because of the high relapse rate. Consolidation therapy usually consists of an idarubicin or daunorubicin-based regimen in combination with tretinoin. Arsenic trioxide has also been evaluated in consolidation therapy. The CALGB recently released the results of a randomized trial that compared standard chemotherapy plus tretinoin followed by arsenic trioxide to standard chemotherapy plus tretinoin followed by standard postremission therapy. The addition of arsenic trioxide resulted in longer EFS and OS.[91]

Post-Consolidation Therapy

Unlike other subtypes of AML, maintenance therapy is an important component of therapy for APL. Before the advent of tretinoin, nonrandomized trials suggested a benefit of continuous low-dose methotrexate and mercaptopurine in prevention of relapse of APL. Larger prospective randomized trials have demonstrated decreased relapse rates in patients who received maintenance therapy (either tretinoin or combination chemotherapy), and some trials have demonstrated increased EFS and OS.[88] In a study that compared maintenance with tretinoin, chemotherapy, or tretinoin plus chemotherapy versus observation, observation was associated with the highest relapse rate and tretinoin plus chemotherapy with the lowest relapse rate.[88] Current recommendations for maintenance therapy in adult APL patients include tretinoin 45 mg/m²/day for 15 days every 3 months, in addition to mercaptopurine 100 mg/m² orally daily and methotrexate 10 mg/m²/week, for 2 years in all patients.[88] The NCCN guidelines also recommend tretinoin maintenance therapy with or without mercaptopurine and methotrexate.[48]

■ TREATMENT OF RELAPSED ACUTE PROMYELOCYTIC LEUKEMIA

Relapsed APL can also be effectively treated with tretinoin therapy. Patients relapsing after tretinoin-based therapy can achieve a second CR with tretinoin-based reinduction. For patients resistant to induction or reinduction with tretinoin-based regimens, alternative strategies include arsenic trioxide, and allo- or autoHSCT. Outcomes with autoHSCT depend on the disease status of the patient at the time of transplant. AutoHSCT in CR2 (versus CR1) is associated with a lower OS, leukemia-free survival, and increased treatment-related mortality. Based on the sensitive nature of patients to chemotherapy, autoHSCT in CR1 is currently not warranted, but offers an excellent option for polymerase chain reaction PML/RAR-α–negative patients in CR2. AlloHSCT should not be offered to patients in CR1, as the mortality associated with alloHSCT outweighs the risks of conventional chemotherapy. However, it is an appropriate choice in CR2 as consolidation after reinduction with either arsenic trioxide or tretinoin.[92]

Arsenic trioxide has induced clinical remissions in relapsed APL through its induction of apoptosis and differentiation.[93,94] The recommended dose is 0.15 mg/kg/day intravenously until bone marrow remission, not to exceed 60 doses, followed by consolidation beginning 3 to 6 weeks after completion of induction at the same dose for a total of 25 doses over a period up to 5 weeks. Arsenic trioxide therapy is associated with two specific toxicities. First, it can cause the APL hyperleukocytosis syndrome, similar to that seen with tretinoin. Management is similar: corticosteroids at first signs of pulmonary distress or a rapidly rising WBC count. The second toxicity is a prolongation of the QT_c interval. Consequently, it is important to obtain a baseline 12-lead electrocardiogram prior to starting therapy with arsenic trioxide, and correct any electrolyte abnormalities, including potassium, calcium, and magnesium. Other medications known to prolong the QT_c interval should be avoided, if possible, during arsenic trioxide therapy. The QT_c interval should not exceed 500 milliseconds at baseline, and if it increases to >500 milliseconds during therapy, the patient should be reevaluated. Do not reintroduce the arsenic trioxide until the QT_c is <460 milliseconds. Following induction of a second CR with arsenic trioxide in relapsed patients, postremission therapy with combination arsenic trioxide and chemotherapy can result in molecular remissions and improved EFS, as compared to chemotherapy or arsenic trioxide alone following remission.[94] Additional investigations are underway to evaluate the role of arsenic trioxide in multidrug postremission regimens.

Gemtuzumab ozogamicin was recommended by the NCCN panel for patients who have relapsed within 6 months of arsenic trioxide therapy as second-line therapy after tretinoin and arsenic trioxide therapy, until gemtuzumab ozogamicin was withdrawn from the market. Caution should be exercised if the patient is a potential candidate for either auto- or alloHSCT because of the apparent increased risk for sinusoidal obstruction syndrome.[48]

■ PATIENT MONITORING

In comparison to non-APL AML, molecular and cytogenetic testing at the end of remission induction therapy in APL has no prognostic value. Clinicians should not make decisions based on the presence or absence of any genetic abnormalities at this time. Because terminal differentiation of blasts in APL requires more than 40 days, results of a bone marrow biopsy obtained at the end of remission induction can be misleading because insufficient time has elapsed to determine response. Molecular and cytogenetic response assessment should occur after the completion of consolidation treatment.

Detection of residual PML/RAR-α transcripts in the bone marrow at the end of consolidation therapy is strongly associated with subsequent hematologic relapse. Achievement of PML/RAR-α–negative status is associated with a higher probability of cure. The use of this molecular technique allows the clinician to assess response to therapy and also detect relapse earlier, which might prevent the development of overt disease recurrence and is associated with improved outcome compared with delaying treatment until overt morphologic relapse.[88] Most experts recommend that APL patients should be routinely evaluated for continuous remission status. Suggested followup includes polymerase chain reaction for PML/RAR-α every 3 to 6 months for 2 years, and then every 6 months for 2 years.[88]

ROLE OF COLONY-STIMULATING FACTORS IN ACUTE MYELOID LEUKEMIA

8 Colony-stimulating factors have been evaluated in AML patients to enhance chemotherapy cytotoxicity, shorten the duration of neutropenia, and reduce the incidence and severity of infection following induction and consolidation chemotherapy. Most studies show limited benefit with the use of colony-stimulating factors as "priming" agents administered during remission induction therapy in an effort to recruit leukemia cells into the cycle to enhance susceptibility to cell-cycle–specific chemotherapy agents, leading to increased cell kill. A recent trial demonstrated similar response rates, but those patients in CR following remission induction chemotherapy had a higher EFS if they received filgrastim.[95] No effect on OS was observed. Subgroup analysis demonstrated improved OS and EFS for patients with standard-risk AML receiving filgrastim. Results from the French Association (ALFA)-9000 trial were recently published. In that trial, the addition of sargramostim to induction and consolidation courses resulted in higher CR rates and EFS, but no effect on OS was observed.[96] Use of colony-stimulating factors concurrently during chemotherapy administration is discouraged outside the setting of a clinical trial and is not recommended for this use in the American Society of Clinical Oncology guidelines.[97]

Both filgrastim and sargramostim are FDA approved to prevent neutropenic complications in adult AML patients receiving intensive chemotherapy. The original package inserts listed myeloid malignancies as a contraindication to the use of filgrastim or sargramostim. Myeloid blast cells have receptors for granulocyte colony-stimulating factor and granulocyte-macrophage colony-stimulating factor, and there was initial concern that the use of these factors would stimulate regrowth of the myeloid leukemia. Although subsequent studies have addressed these concerns, many pediatric clinicians do not initiate filgrastim until an initial remission is achieved.

A number of randomized trials, primarily in elderly patients, consistently demonstrate that filgrastim or sargramostim reduces the duration of neutropenia following AML induction chemotherapy.[97] While neutropenia can be reduced from 2 to 12 days depending on the trial, results vary in terms of improvements in infectious morbidity and mortality, resource use, and disease response rates. The American Society of Clinical Oncology Guidelines for the Use of White Blood Cell Growth Factors considers the use of colony-stimulating factors after initial induction therapy reasonable, with the understanding that the effects on length of hospitalization and incidence of severe infection are modest.[97] Patients older than age 55 years appear to derive the greatest benefit, and use is appropriate in this population where more rapid marrow recovery might decrease the duration of hospitalization.[97] Following consolidation therapy, patients receiving colony-stimulating factors have a more profound shortening of the duration of severe neutropenia resulting in a reduction in infection rates and an associated reduction in the use of antibiotic therapy.[97] Growth factor use after consolidation does not affect CR duration or OS. Further pharmacoeconomic data are required in this setting, but the body of evidence supports their use following consolidation therapy in adults. Other controversial issues surrounding colony-stimulating factor use in AML include which colony-stimulating factor to use, what dose, which day to start after chemotherapy, how long to continue, and should the marrow be examined for leukemia prior to starting a colony-stimulating factor. All growth factors have been evaluated in patients with AML, including sargramostim, filgrastim, and pegfilgrastim. Although pegfilgrastim is not FDA approved for this indication, research supports its use in this setting.[98] The use of colony-stimulating factors can also interfere with the interpretation of the day 14 bone marrow examination. Growth factors should be discontinued at least 7 days prior to a bone marrow aspirate and biopsy to avoid interfering with the interpretation of the results (i.e., may see immature myeloid forms that would suggest residual disease).

SUPPORTIVE CARE

The most common and significant toxic effect of antileukemic agents is marrow suppression. With the exception of corticosteroids, tretinoin, asparaginase/pegaspargase, and vincristine, antineoplastic agents used to treat acute leukemia cause myelosuppression. During AML remission and postremission therapy, daily monitoring of the complete blood count and the absolute neutrophil count is necessary to determine when red cell and platelet transfusions are needed and when neutropenia is achieved. Less-frequent monitoring may be sufficient during ALL induction. Marrow hypoplasia from the myelosuppressive regimens usually reaches its lowest point (nadir) after 1 to 2 weeks of therapy and lasts for another 1 to 2 weeks. During this period of hypoplasia, infectious and bleeding complications are major causes of death in leukemic patients. As typical signs and symptoms of infection may be absent in the neutropenic host, frequent monitoring of vital signs (especially fever) and daily physical examination are important.[99] Infection control strategies often include routine hand washing; dietary restrictions; reverse isolation and laminar-air flow rooms; fungal, Pneumocystis, and bacterial prophylaxis; and the empiric use of broad-spectrum antibiotics when fever occurs (see Chap. 131).[99] In contrast to the practice at many institutions, the NCCN guidelines do not recommend prophylactic antimicrobials or gut decontamination during induction or consolidation, and leave the choice to the discretion of the treating facility based on local infection patterns and concerns.[48] Several groups have analyzed the literature surrounding the use of prophylactic antibacterials. In general, prophylactic antibacterials should be reserved for patients who are expected to have prolonged (more than 7 days) and profound (absolute neutrophil count <100 cells/mm³ [<0.1 × 10⁹/L]) neutropenia. Based on these criteria, prophylaxis following induction chemotherapy is warranted and postconsolidation therapy is warranted on a case-by-case basis.

In children, prophylactic antibiotics have not proven useful and have resulted in increased resistance. Pediatric ALL patients on standard induction regimens, which generally are minimally myelosuppressive, often have recovered blood counts earlier and do not require very aggressive measures. However, they do require close monitoring of vital signs and blood counts until their counts recover. Pediatric AML patients are usually admitted for at least 1 month during induction and again for consolidation. Infectious complications, especially fungal, are a major cause of morbidity and mortality. The incidence of viridans streptococci has increased with the intensity of therapy and is most associated with high-dose cytarabine. These infections can lead to meningitis or delayed acute respiratory distress syndrome.

Pneumocystis jiroveci prophylaxis (usually trimethoprim-sulfamethoxazole) is begun in all adults and children with ALL by the end of induction and continues until 6 months after therapy is discontinued. Infants are at high-risk for developing Pneumocystis jiroveci pneumonia early in therapy, so should start prophylaxis immediately.[27] These infants can receive trimethoprim-sulfamethoxazole despite the risk of kernicterus with careful monitoring.

Acute leukemia patients, particularly those patients with an initial elevated WBC count, are at risk for tumor lysis syndrome. Preventive measures include allopurinol or rasburicase, and adequate hydration (with or without sodium bicarbonate) prior to and during chemotherapy to prevent the development of urate nephropathy from rapid destruction of WBCs. Rasburicase, a recombinant urate-oxidase enzyme produced by genetic modification of Saccharomyces cerevisiae, catalyzes the enzymatic oxidation of uric acid into the inactive soluble metabolite, allantoin. In children, rasburicase more rapidly reduces uric acid levels in patients with aggressive malignancies compared to allopurinol, and reduces the need for dialysis.[100] Rasburicase has been evaluated in adults, and some studies in adults show that fixed dosing produces equivalent outcomes to a mg/kg dosing strategy.[101] Because of its cost, this product is usually limited to patients with ALL who have a high WBC count or bulky extramedullary disease, aggressive non-Hodgkin lymphoma, or patients with AML with a high presenting WBC. Most institutions also include an elevated uric acid as part of the criteria for use. Rasburicase has a rapid onset of action and long duration of action, so many institutions also limit its use to a single dose and allow repeat doses when the criteria for use are met again. Rasburicase is contraindicated in patients with glucose-6-phosphate dehydrogenase deficiency. Tumor lysis syndrome may lead not only to hyperuricemia, but also to hyperkalemia, hyperphosphatemia, and hypocalcemia.[100]

Hematologic support consists primarily of platelet and packed red blood cell transfusions. Platelet transfusions are often given for peripheral counts below 10,000 cells/mm³ (10 × 10⁹/L) or clinical signs of bleeding. Transfusions of packed red cells may also be indicated for a hemoglobin less than 8 gm/dL (80 g/L; 4.97 mmol/L), profound fatigue, shortness of breath, tachycardia, or chest pain. APL can release procoagulants that can cause disseminated intravascular coagulation, necessitating close monitoring and replacement of coagulation factors with cryoprecipitate. Because of the gastrointestinal toxic effects of chemotherapy, parenteral nutrition may be required. Patients are frequently receiving infusions of antibiotics, fluids, hyperalimentation, and blood products simultaneously. To provide the total support needed for these patients, a multiple-lumen central venous access device should be considered at the start of therapy.

EVALUATION OF THERAPEUTIC OUTCOMES

Appropriate development of a pharmaceutical care plan for the acute leukemia patient begins with establishing the diagnosis and prognosis for the patient. Long-term therapeutic goals for the patient may include long-term EFS, although palliative care is a possibility in some patients. The desired short-term outcome is the establishment of remission. The return of hematologic values to normal and a repeat bone marrow biopsy that demonstrates no evidence of disease serve as documentation that remission has been achieved. Monitoring guidelines for induction or consolidation are similar (Table 142–6). After the appropriate post-remission therapy has been completed, the patient may return monthly for 1 year, and then every 3 months, to check hematologic values. If no evidence of disease exists after 5 years from the diagnosis and the patient has been in continuous CR, the patient is considered cured.

Intense monitoring of fevers, hematologic and chemistry laboratory values, microbiology reports, and the patient's physical condition are necessary to identify infection, risk of bleeding, and tumor lysis syndrome early. A coagulation screening panel will identify patients with ongoing disseminated intravascular coagulation, a particular risk with APL.

During therapy, the pharmacist can be an important provider of patient education. Patients should receive information regarding acute and chronic toxicities of the chemotherapy being administered, as well as possible treatments for those toxicities. Pharmacists should follow patients during consolidation therapy for dosing adjustments and toxicities due to chemotherapy. For

TABLE 142-6 Acute Myeloid Leukemia Assessment and Monitoring

Baseline Workup	Monitoring during Therapy	Postremission Monitoring
History and physical examination	Daily physical examination	Routine physical examination at clinic visit
CBC with differential, platelets	CBC with differential, platelets	CBC with differential, platelets
Serum chemistries (creatinine, bilirubin, AST, ALT to assess organ function)	Serum chemistries (including uric acid, K⁺, Ca⁺², PO₄, S_cr during tumor lysis syndrome risk period^a)	Bone marrow biopsy and aspirate at set intervals to evaluate ongoing remission and if peripheral blood counts are abnormal or if they fail to recover within 5 weeks of treatment
Coagulation (PT, PTT, D-dimers, fibrinogen)	Coagulation (PT, PTT, D-dimers, fibrinogen [if APL])	PML/RARα monitoring [if APL]
Bone marrow biopsy and aspirate with cytogenetics	Bone marrow biopsy and aspirate 7–10 days after end of chemotherapy. Repeat bone marrow biopsy and aspirate upon hematologic recovery to document complete response (with cytogenetics if initially abnormal)	
Immunophenotyping and cytochemistry		
Human leukocyte antigen (HLA) typing		
Cardiac workup (MUGA or echocardiogram; ECG)		
Intravascular access	Temperature curve (initiate antibiotics when febrile)	
Lumbar puncture (if symptomatic or AML M4 or M5)	Lumbar puncture (with intrathecal chemotherapy) if initial lumbar puncture was positive for leukemia	
Chest radiography		
Height and weight		
Molecular testing for genetic aberrations (FLT3, NPM1)		

ALT, alanine aminotransferase; APL, acute promyelocytic leukemia; AST, aspartate aminotransferase; CBC, complete blood cell count; ECG, electrocardiogram; FLT3, FMS-related tyrosine kinase 3; MUGA, multiple-gated acquisition (blood pool scan); NMP1, nucleophosmin; PML/RARα, promyelocytic-leukemia retinoic acid receptor-α; PT, prothrombin time; PTT, partial thromboplastin time; S_cr, serum creatinine.

^{a}Risk for tumor lysis syndrome during induction therapy only.

example, the pharmacist should make sure the patient is receiving corticosteroid and saline eye drops 4 times daily while the patient is receiving high-dose cytarabine to prevent the ocular toxicity of cytarabine. The pharmacist can also be an important resource for information regarding antibiotics, antiemetics, nutritional support, colony-stimulating factors, and other supportive care issues.

Pharmacists should be involved in checking drug doses and any dose modifications for organ dysfunction or prior toxicity. Pharmacists are often in the best position to recognize the potential for medication errors and drug interaction and to help avoid them. Similarly, pharmacists are often able to identify the possibility that patient problems are secondary to drug treatments.

Numerous late sequelae from leukemia therapy have been recognized and should be included in the monitoring plan after therapy is completed. Chapter 148 discusses the long-term consequences of HSCT.

ABBREVIATIONS

ALL: acute lymphoblastic leukemia

AML: acute myeloid leukemia

APML: acute promyelocytic leukemia

alloHSCT: allogeneic hematopoietic stem cell transplantation

autoHSCT: autologous hematopoietic stem cell transplantation

CALGB: Cancer and Leukemia Group B

CNS: central nervous system

CR: complete remission

ECOG: Eastern Cooperative Oncology Group

EFS: event-free survival

FAB: French-American-British classification system

HSCT: hematopoietic stem cell transplantation

MDS: myelodysplastic syndrome

MLL: mixed lineage leukemia

MRD: minimal residual disease

NCCN: National Comprehensive Cancer Network

OS: overall survival

Ph⁺: Philadelphia chromosome

TPMT: thiopurine methyltransferase

WBC: white blood cell

REFERENCES

1. Jemel A, Siegel R, Xu J, Ward E. Cancer statistics, 2010. CA Cancer J Clin 2010;60:277–300.
2. Horner M, Ries L, Krapcho M, Neyman N, Aminou R, Howlader N. SEER Cancer Statistics Review, 1975-2006. Bethesda, MD: National Cancer Institute; 2009. *http://seer.cancer.gov/csr/1975_2006*.
3. Estey E, Dohner H. Acute myeloid leukemia. Lancet 2006;368: 1894–907.
4. Linabery AM, Ross JA. Trends in childhood cancer incidence in the U.S. (1992-2004). Cancer 2008;112:416–432.
5. Pui C-H, Robison LL, Look AT. Acute lymphoblastic leukemia. Lancet 2008;371:1030–1043.
6. Rubnitz JE, Gibson B, Smith FO. Acute myeloid leukemia. Pediatr Clin N Am 2008;55:21–51.
7. Faderl S, Jeha S, Kantarjian H. The biology and therapy of adult acute lymphoblastic leukemia. Cancer 2003;98:1337–1354.
8. Belson M, Kingsley B, Holmes A. Risk factors for acute leukemia in children: A review. Environ Health Perspect 2007;115:138–145.
9. Caughey RW, Michels KB. Birth weight and childhood leukemia: A meta-analysis and review of the current evidence. Int J Cancer 2009;124:2658–2670.
10. Mrozek K, Marcucci G, Paschka P, Whitman S, Bloomfield C. Clinical relevance of mutations and gene-expression changes in adult acute myeloid leukemia with normal cytogenetics: are we ready for a prognostically prioritized molecular classification. Blood 2007;109:431–448.
11. Vardiman JW, Thiele J, Arber DA, Brunning RD. The 2008 revision of the World Health Organization (WHO) classification of myeloid neoplasms and acute leukemia:rationale and important changes. Blood 2009;114(5):937–951.
12. Pui C-H, Evans WE. Treatment of acute lymphoblastic leukemia. N Engl J Med 2006;354:166–178.
13. Smith M, Arthur D, Camitta B, Carroll AJ, Crist W, Gaynon P, Gelber R, Heerema N. Uniform approach to risk classification and treatment assignment for children with acute lymphoblastic leukemia. J Clin Oncol 1996;14:18–24.
14. Seibel NL. Treatment of acute lymphoblastic leukemia in children and adolescents: Peaks and pitfalls. Hematology 2008;2008:374–380.
15. Schultz KR, Pullen DJ, Sather HN, et al. Risk- and response-based classification of childhood B-precursor acute lymphoblastic leukemia: a combined analysis of prognostic markers from the Pediatric

Oncology Group (POG) and Children's Cancer Group (CCG). Blood 2007;109(3):926–935.

16. Campana D. Minimal residual disease in acute lymphoblastic leukemia. Sem Hematol 2009;46(1):100–106.

17. Borowitz MJ, Devidas M, Hunger SP, et al. Clinical significance of minimal residual disease in childhood acute lymphoblastic leukemia and its relationship to other prognostic factors: a Children's Cancer Group study. Blood 2008;111:5477–5485.

18. Seibel NL, Steinherz PG, Sather HN, Nachman JB, Cynthia D. Early postinduction intensification therapy improves survival for children and adolescents with high-risk acute lymphoblastic leukemia: a report from the Children's Oncology Group. Blood 2008;111:2548–2555.

19. Schultz KR, Bowman WP, Aledo A, Slayton WB, Sather H, Devidas M. Improved early event-free survival with imatinib in Philadelphia chromosome-positive acute lymphoblastic leukemia: A Children's Oncology Group study. J Clin Oncol 2009;27(31):5175–5181.

20. Mitchell CD, Richards S, Kinsey S, Lilleyman J, Vora A, Eben T. Benefit of dexamethasone compared with prednisolone for childhood lymphoblastic Leukaemia: results of the UK Medical Research Council ALL97 randomised trial. Br J Haematol 2005;129:734–745.

21. Ravindranath Y. Recent advances in pediatric acute lymphoblastic and myeloid leukemia. Curr Opin Oncol 2003;15:23–35.

22. Lowas SR, Marks D, Malempati S. Prevalence of transient hyperglycemia during induction chemotherapy for pediatric acute lymphoblastic leukemia. Pediatr Blood Cancer 2009;52:814–818.

23. Matloub Y, Lindemulder S, Gaynon PS, et al. Intrathecal triple therapy decreases central nervous system relapse but fails to improve event-free survival when compared with intrathecal methotrexate: results of the Children's Cancer Group (CCG) 1952 study for standard-risk acute lymphoblastic leukemia, reported by the Children's Oncology Group. Blood 2006;108:1165–1173.

24. Bomgaars L, Geyer JR, Franklin JL, et al. Phase I trial of intrathecal liposomal cytarabine in children with neoplastic meningitis. J Clin Oncol 2004;22(19):3916–3921.

25. Berg SL, Blaney SM, Devidas M. Phase II study of nelarabine (Compound 506U78) in children and young adults with refractory T-cell malignancies: A report from the Children's Oncology Group. J Clin Oncol 2005;23:3376–3382.

26. Richards S, Gray R, Peto R. Duration and intensity of maintenance chemotherapy in acute leukemia: Overview of 42 trials involving 12,000 randomised children. Childhood ALL Collaborative Group. Lancet 1996;347:1783–1788.

27. Silverman LB. Acute lymphoblastic leukemia in infancy. Pediatr Blood Cancer 2007;49:1070–1073.

28. Kantarjian H, O'Brien S, Smith T. Results of treatment with hyper-CVAD, a dose-intensive regimen, in adult acute lymphocytic leukemia. J Clin Oncol 2000;18:547–561.

29. Thomas D, Faderl S, Cortes J. Treatment of Philadelphia chromosome-positive acute lymphocytic leukemia with hyper-CVAD and imatinib mesylate. Blood 2004;103:4396–4407.

30. Yanada M, Takeuchi J, Sugiura I. High complete remission rate and promising outcome by combination imatinib and chemotherapy for newly diagnosed BCR-ABL-positive acute lymphoblastic leukemia: A phase II study by the Japan Adult Leukemia Study Group. J Clin Oncol 2006;24:460–466.

31. Delannoy A, Delabesse E, Lheritier V. Imatinib and methylprednisolone alternated with chemotherapy improve the outcome of elderly patients with Philadelphia-positive acute lymphoblastic leukemia: Results of the GRAALL AFR09 study. Leukemia 2006;20:1526–1532.

32. Wassmann B, Pfeifer H, Goekbuget N. Alternating versus concurrent schedules of imatinib and chemotherapy as front-line therapy for Philadelphia-positive acute lymphoblastic leukemia (PH+ ALL). Blood 2006;108:1469–1477.

33. Talpaz M, Shah N, Kantarjian H. Dasatinib in imatinib-resistant Philadelphia chromosome-positive leukemias. N Engl J Med 2006;354:2531–2541.

34. Kantarjian H, Giles F, Wunderle L. Nilotinib in imatinib-resistant CML and Philadelphia chromosome-positive ALL. N Engl J Med 2006;354:2542–2551.

35. Fielding A, Rowe J, Richards S. Prospective outcome data on 267 unselected adult patients with Philadelphia chromosome-positive acute lymphoblastic leukemia confirms superiority of allogeneic transplantation over chemotherapy in the pre-imatinib era: results from the International ALL Trial MRC UKALLXII/ECOG2993. Blood 2009;19:4489–4496.

36. Harned TM, Gaynon PS. Relapsed acute lymphoblastic leukemia: Current status and future opportunities. Curr Opin Oncol 2008;10:453–458.

37. Gaynon PS. Childhood acute lymphoblastic leukemia and relapse. Br J Haematol 2005;131:579–587.

38. Raetz EA, Borowitz MJ, Devidas M, et al. Reinduction platform for children with first marrow relapse of acute lymphoblastic leukemia: A Children's Oncology Group Study. J Clin Oncol 2008;26(24):3971–3978.

39. Gaynon PS. Childhood acute lymphoblastic leukaemia and relapse. Br J Haematol 2005;131:579–587.

40. Eapen M, Raetz E, Zhang M-J, et al. Outcomes after HLA-matched sibling transplantation or chemotherapy in children with B-precursor acute lymphoblastic leukemia in a second remission: a collaborative study of the Children's Oncology Group and the Center for International Blood and Marrow Transplant Research. Blood 2006;107:4961–4967.

41. Hahn T, Wall D, Camitta BM. The role of cytotoxic therapy wtih hematopoietic stem cell transplantation in the therapy of acute lymphoblastic leukemia in children: An evidence-based review. Biol Blood Marrow Transplant 2005;11:823–861.

42. Goldstone AH, Richards S, Lazarus H. In adults with standard-risk acute lymphoblastic leukemia (ALL) the greatest benefit is achieved from matched sibling allogeneic transplant in first complete remission (CR) and an autologous transplant is less effective than conventional consolidation/maintenance chemotherapy in ALL patients: Final results of the international ALL trial (MRC UKALL XII/ECOG E2993). Blood 2008;111:1827–1833.

43. Hahn T, Wall D, Camitta BM. The role of cytotoxic therapy with hematopoietic stem cell transplantation in the therapy of acute lymphoblastic leukemia in adults: An evidence-based review. Biol Blood Marrow Transplant 2006;12:1–30.

44. National Marrow Donor Program. *http://www/nmdp.org*.

45. Wall AM, Rubnitz JE. Pharmacogenomic effects on therapy for acute lymphoblastic leukemia in children. Pharmacogenomics J 2003;3:128–135.

46. Mody R, Li S, Dover DC, Sallan S, et al. Twenty-five-year follow-up among survivors of childhood acute lymphoblastic leukemia: A report from the Childhood Cancer Survivor Study. Blood 2008;111:5515–5523.

47. Byrd JC, Mrozek K, Dodge RK. Pretreatment cytogenetic abnormalities are predictive of induction success, cumulative incidence of relapse, and overall survival in adult patients with de novo acute myeloid leukemia: Results from Cancer and Leukemia Group B(CALGB 8461). Blood 2002;100:4325–4336.

48. National Comprehensive Cancer Network Clinical Practice Guidelines in Oncology. Acute Myeloid Leukemia. Version 1.2009. *http://www.nccn.com/physician_gls/f_guidelines.html*.

49. Deschler B, Lübbert M. Acute myeloid leukemia: Epidemiology and etiology. Cancer 2006;107:2099–2107.

50. Kolitz JE. Acute leukemias in adults. Dis Mon 2008;54:226–241.

51. Estey EH. Treatment of acute myeloid leukemia. Haematologica 2009;94(1):10–16.

52. Grimwade D, Hills R. Independent prognostic factors for AML outcome. Hematology Am Soc Hematol Educ Program 2009:385–395.

53. Cheson B, Bennett J, Kopecky K. Revised recommendations of the International Working Group for diagnosis, standardization or response criteria, treatment outcomes, and reporting standards for therapeutic trials in acute myeloid leukemia. J Clin Oncol 2003;21:4642–4649.

54. Buchner T, Berdel W, Wormann B. Treatment of older patients with acute myeloid leukemia. Crit Rev Oncol Hematol 2005;56:247–259.

55. Kolitz JE. Current therapeutic strategies for acute myeloid leukemia. Br J Haematol 2006;134:555–572.

56. Milligan DW, Grimwade D, Cullis J. Guidelines on the management of acute myeloid leukemia in adults. Br J Haematol 2006;135:450–474.

57. Fernandez HF, Sun Z, Yao X, et al. Anthracycline Dose Intensification in Acute Myeloid Leukemia. N Engl J Med 2009 September 24, 2009;361(13):1249–1259.

58. Lowenberg B, Ossenkoppele GJ, van Putten W, et al, the Dutch-Belgian Cooperative Trial Group for Hemato-Oncology GASG, Swiss Group for Clinical Cancer Research Collaborative Group. High-Dose Daunorubicin in Older Patients with Acute Myeloid Leukemia. N Engl J Med 2009;361(13):1235–1248.

59. Cahn JY, Labopin M, Sierra J. No impact of high-dose cytarabine on the outcome of patients transplanted for acute myeloblastic leukaemia in first remission. Acute Leukemia Working Party of the European Group for Blood and Marrow Transplant (EBMT). Br J Haematol 2000;110:308–314.

60. Mayer RJ, Davis RB, Schiffer CA. Intensive post-remission chemotherapy in adults with acute myeloid leukemia. Cancer and Leukemia Group B. N Engl J Med 1994;331:896–903.

61. Byrd JC, Ruppert AS, Mrozek K. Repetitive cycles of high-dose cytarabine benefit patients with acute myeloid leukemia and inv(16) (p13q22) or t(16;16)(p13;q22): Results from CALGB 8461. J Clin Oncol 2004;22:1087–1094.

62. Alyea EP, Kim HT, Ho V. Comparative outcome of nonmyeloablatic and myeloablative allogeneic hematopoietic cell transplantation for patients older than 50 years of age. Blood 2005;105:1810–1814.

63. Aoudjhane M, Labopin M, Gorin NC. Comparative outcome of reduced intensity and myeloablative conditioning regimen in HLA identical sibling allogeneic haematopoietic stem cell transplantation for patients older than 50 years of age with acute myeloblastic leukaemia: A retrospective survey from the Acute Leukemia Working Party (ALWP) of the European Group for Blood and Marrow Transplantation (EBMT). Leukemia 2005;18:2304–2312.

64. Estey E, de Lima M, Tibes R. Prospective feasibility analysis of reduced-intensity conditioning (RIC) regimens for hematopoietic stem cell transplantation (HSCT) in elderly patients with acute myeloid leukemia (AML) and high-risk myelodysplastic syndrome (MDS). Blood 2007;109:1395–1400.

65. Breems DA, Lowenberg B. Autologous stem cell transplantation in the treatment of adults with acute myeloid leukemia. Br J Haematol 2005;2005:825–833.

66. Group SCTC. Allogeneic peripheral blood stem-cell compared with bone marrow transplantation in the management of hematologic malignancies: An individual patient data meta-analysis of nine randomized trials. J Clin Oncol 2005;23:5074–5087.

67. Woods WG. Curing childhood acute myeloid leukemia (AML) at the half-way point: Promises to keep and miles to go before we sleep. Pediatr Blood Cancer 2006;46:565–569.

68. Aplenc R, Alonzo TA, Gerbing RB, et al. Safety and Efficacy of Gemtuzumab Ozogamicin in Combination With Chemotherapy for Pediatric Acute Myeloid Leukemia: A Report From The Children's Oncology Group. J Clin Oncol 2008;26(14):2390–2395.

69. Oliansky DM, Rizzo JD, Aplan PD. The role of cytotoxic therapy with hematopoietic stem cell transplantation in the therapy of acute myeloid leukemia in children: An evidence-based review. Biol Blood Marrow Transplant 2007;13:1–25.

70. Lowenberg B, Zittoun R, Kerkhofs H. On the value of intensive remission-induction chemotherapy in elderly patients of 65+ years with acute myeloid leukemia: A randomized phase III study of the European Organization for Research and Treatment of Cancer Leukemia Group. J Clin Oncol 1989;7:1268–1274.

71. Burnett A, Milligan DW, Prentice A. A comparison of low-dose cytarabine and hydroxyurea with or without all-trans-retinoic acid for acute myeloid leukemia and high-risk myelodysplastic syndrome in patients not considered fit for intensive treatment on behalf of the National Cancer Research Institute Haemotological Oncology Study Group. Cancer 2007;109:1114–1124.

72. Group AC. A systematic collaborative review of randomized trials comparin idarubicin with daunorubicin (or other anthracyclines) as induction therapy for acute myeloid leukemia. Br J Haematol 1998;103:100–109.

73. Bishop JF, Lowenthal RM, Joshua D. Etoposide in acute nonlymphocytic leukemia. Australian Leukemia Study Group. Blood 1990;75:27–32.

74. Anderson JE, Kopecky K, Willman CL. Outcome after induction chemotherapy for older patients with acute myeloid leukemia is not improved with mitoxantrone and etoposide compared to cytarabine and daunorubicin: A Southwest Oncology Group study. Blood 2002;100:3869–3876.

75. Faderl S, Ravandi F, Huang X. A randomized study of clofarabine versus clofarabine plus low-dose cytarabine as front-line therapy for patients aged 60 years and older with acute myeloid leukemia andhigh-risk myelodysplastic syndrome.. Blood 2008;112:1638–1645.

76. Rowe JM, Andersen JW, Mazza JJ. Randomized placebo-controlled phase III study of granulocyte-macrophage colony stimulating factor in adult patients (>55–70 years) with acute myelogenous leukemia: A study of the Eastern Cooperative Oncology Group (E1490). Blood 1995;96:457–462.

77. Gardin C, Turlure P, Fagot T. Postremission treatment of elderly patients with acute myeloid leukemia in first complete remission after intensive induction chemotherapy: Results of the multicenter randomized Acute Leukemia French Association (ALFA) 9803 trial. Blood 2007;109:5129–5135.

78. Buchner T, Berdel W, Schoch C. Double induction containing either one course of high-dose cytarabine plus mitoxantrone and postremission therapy by either autologous stem cell transplantation or by prolonged maintenance for acute myeloid leukemia. J Clin Oncol 2006;24:2480–2489.

79. Lancet JE, Gojo I, Grotlib J. A phase 2 study of the farnesyltransferase inhibitor tipifarnib in poor-risk and elderly patients with previously untreated acute myelogenous leukemia. Blood 2007;109:1387–1394.

80. Gale RP, Horowitz MM, Rees JKH. Chemotherapy versus transplants for acute myelogenous leukemia in second remission. Leukemia 1996;10:13–19.

81. Michallet M, Thomas X, Vernant J-P. Long-term outcome after allogeneic hematopoietic stem cell transplantation for advanced stage acute myeloblastic leukemia: A retrospective study of 379 patients reported to the Societe Francaise de Greffe de Moelle (SFGM). Bone Marrow Transplant 2000;26:1157–1163.

82. Larson RA, Sievers EL, Stadmauer EA. Final reports of the efficacy and safety of gemtuzumab ozogamicin (Mylotarg) in patients with CD33-positive acute myeloid leukemia in first recurrence. Cancer 2005;104:1442–1152.

83. Chevallier P, Delaunay J, Turlure P. Long-term disease-free survival after gemtuzumab, intermediate-dose cytarabine, and mitoxantrone in patients with CD33(+) primary resistant or relapsed acute myeloid leukemia. J Clin Oncol 2008;26(32):5192–5197.

84. Brune M, Castaigne S, Catalano J. Improved leukemia-free survival after postconsolidation immunotherapy with histamie dihydrochloride and interleukin-2 in acute myeloid leukemia: Results of a randomized phase 3 trial. Blood 2006;108:88–96.

85. Stahnke K, Boos J, Bender-Gotze C. Duration of first remission predicts rates and long-term survival in children with relapsed acute myelogenous leukemia. Leukemia 1998;12:1534–1538.

86. Wells RJ, Adams MT, Alonzo TA. Mitoxantrone and cytarabine induction, high-dose cytarabine, and etoposide intensification for pediatric patients with relapsed or refractory acute myeloid leukemia: Children's Cancer Group Study 2951. J Clin Oncol 2003;21:2940–2947.

87. Leung W, Hudson MM, Strickland DK. Late effects of treatment in survivors of childhood acute myeloid leukemia. J Clin Oncol 2000;18:3273–3279.

88. Ades L, Sanz MA, Chevret S. Treatment of newly diagnosed acute promyelocytic leukemia (APL): a comparison of French-Belgian-Swiss and PETHEMA results Blood 2008;111:1078–1084.

89. DelaSerna J, Montesinos J, Vellenga E. Causes and prognostic factors of remission induction failure in patients with acute promyelocytic leukemia treated with all-trans retinoic acid and idarubicin. Blood 2008;111:3395–3402.

90. Ghavamzadeh A, Alimoghaddam K, Ghaffari SH. Treatment of acute promyelocytic leukemia with arsenic trioxide without ATRA and/or chemotherapy. Ann Oncol 2006;17:131–134.

91. Powell BL, Moser B, Stock W. Effect of consolidation with arsenic trioxide on event-free survival and overall survival among patients

with newly diagnosed acute promyelocytic leukemia: North American Intergroup Protocol C9710 [abstract]. J Clin Oncol 2007 ASCO Annual Meeting Proceedings (Part 1) 2007;25:2.

92. Nabhan C, Mehta J, Tallman MS. The role of bone marrow transplantation in acute promyelocytic leukemia. Bone Marrow Transplant 2001;28:219–226.

93. Soignet S, Maslak P, Wang Z. Complete remission after treatment of acute promyelocytic leukemia with arsenic trioxide. N Engl J Med 1998;339:1341–1348.

94. Soignet S, Frankel S, Douer D. United States multicenter study of arsenic trioxide in relapsed acute promyelocytic leukemia. J Clin Oncol 2001;19:3852–3860.

95. Lowenberg B, van Putten W, Theobald M. Effect of priming with granulocyte colony-stimulating factor on the outcome of chemotherapy for acute myeloid leukemia. N Engl J Med 2003;349:743–752.

96. Thomas X, Raffoux E, de Botton S. Effect of priming with granulocyte-macrophage colony-stimulating factor in younger adults with newly diagnosed acute myeloid leukemia: A trial by the Acute Leukemia French Association (ALFA) Group. Leukemia 2007;21:453–461.

97. Smith TJ, Khatcheressian J, Lyman GH, et al. 2006 Update of Recommendations for the Use of White Blood Cell Growth Factors: An Evidence-Based Clinical Practice Guideline. J Clin Oncol 2006;24(19):3187–3205.

98. Sierra J, Szer J, Kassis J, et al. A single dose of pegfilgrastim compared with daily filgrastim for supporting neutrophil recovery in patients treated for low-to-intermediate risk acute myeloid leukemia: results from a randomized, double-blind, phase 2 trial. BMC Cancer 2008;8(1):195.

99. Hughes WT, Armstrong D, Bodey GP. 2002 Guidelines for the use of antimicrobial agents in neutropenic patients with cancer. Clin Infect Dis 2002;34:730–751.

100. Coiffier B, Altman A, Pui C-H, Younes A, Cairo MS. Guidelines for the Management of Pediatric and Adult Tumor Lysis Syndrome: An Evidence-Based Review. J Clin Oncol 2008;26(16): 2767–2778.

101. Trifilio S, Gordon L, Singhal S. Reduced-dose rasburicase (recombinant xanthine oxidase) in adult cancer patients with hyperuricemia. Bone Marrow Transplant 2006;37:997–1001.

CHAPTER

143

Chronic Leukemias

CHRISTOPHER A. FAUSEL AND PATRICK J. KIEL

KEY CONCEPTS

❶ Chronic myelogenous leukemia (CML) is defined by the presence of the Philadelphia chromosome (Ph), a translocation between chromosomes 9 and 22. The resulting abnormal fusion protein, p210 *BCR-ABL*, phosphorylates tyrosine kinase residues and is constitutively active, resulting in uncontrolled hematopoietic cell proliferation.

❷ The disease course of CML is characterized by a progressive increase in white blood cells over a period of years that ultimately transforms to an acute leukemia.

❸ Imatinib is a tyrosine kinase inhibitor and is the most commonly used therapy in the treatment of chronic phase CML. Second-generation tyrosine kinase inhibitors, dasatinib and nilotinib, are active in most patients that have resistance or intolerance to imatinib.

❹ Interferon alfa (IFN-α) plays a minor role in the current treatment of CML and is reserved for patients who fail tyrosine kinase inhibitors and are ineligible for allogeneic hematopoietic stem cell transplant (HSCT).

❺ Allogeneic HSCT is the only known curative treatment option for CML and is reserved for patients with a suitable donor and progression after treatment with tyrosine kinase-based therapy.

❻ The management of CLL is highly individualized and includes observation in patients with early stage disease and treatment with chemotherapy, biologic therapy or both in patients with more advanced disease.

❼ Alemtuzumab is a monoclonal antibody against CD52, which is expressed on B and T cells. It has proven activity in first-line treatment and relapsed disease. Routine use must be balanced against the known risks of opportunistic infections.

❽ Regimens such as fludarabine, cyclophosphamide, and rituximab are considered as first-line therapy for patients with CLL who are younger or have more aggressive disease, such as the presence of chromosome 17 deletion.

❾ Allogeneic HSCT in patients with CLL appears to achieve long-term disease-free survival in some patients, but the older

Learning objectives, review questions,
and other resources can be found at
www.pharmacotherapyonline.com.

patient population diagnosed with the disease and donor availability preclude widespread use.

The chronic leukemias include chronic myeloid leukemia (CML), chronic lymphocytic leukemia (CLL), hairy cell leukemia, and prolymphocytic leukemia. The typical clinical presentation of the chronic leukemias is an indolent course in contrast to patients with acute leukemia who will die of their disease within weeks to months if not treated. The introduction of tyrosine kinase inhibitor therapy has dramatically changed the clinical course of CML where patients can now expect to maintain disease control for many years. This chapter focuses on the two most common types of chronic leukemia, CML and CLL.

CHRONIC MYELOID LEUKEMIA

Chronic myeloid leukemia is a myeloproliferative disease that results from malignant transformation of a subpopulation of pluripotent hematopoietic stem cells. Bone marrow hyperplasia and accumulation of differentiated myeloid cells in the peripheral blood are the initial presenting features of the disease. The terminal stage of CML develops over a period of years and is characterized by rapid accumulation of blast cells in the bone marrow and suppression of normal hematopoiesis that will ultimately become fatal. Chronic myeloid leukemia was the first malignant disease to be identified with a consistent cytogenetic abnormality, namely the Philadelphia chromosome (Ph) that codes for the *BCR-ABL* oncogene. This dominant cytogenetic abnormality has allowed CML to become the template for development of molecular targeted drug therapies.

EPIDEMIOLOGY AND ETIOLOGY

It is estimated that 4,870 new cases of CML will be diagnosed in the United States in 2010, representing 11% of all leukemias.[1] Median age at diagnosis is 65 years and incidence increases with age.[2] There are no currently known associations between the development of CML and hereditary, familial, geographic, ethnic, or economic status. An increased risk of CML has been noted with ionizing radiation exposure and in atomic bomb survivors from Hiroshima and Nagasaki.[3,4]

PATHOPHYSIOLOGY

Chronic myeloid leukemia was first described in 1845, but extensive research into the genetic and molecular characteristics of the disease began with the discovery of the Philadelphia chromosome (Ph) in 1960 by Nowell and Hungerford.[5] Research in the 1980s

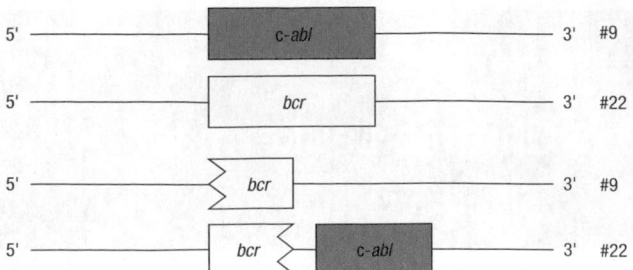

FIGURE 143-1. Diagram of the chromosomal translocation that results in the Philadelphia chromosome. *(Reprinted with permission from Fishleder AJ. Oncogenes and cancer: Clinical applications. Cleve Clin J Med 1990; 57:721–726. Copyright © 1990 Cleveland Clinic. All rights reserved.)*

identified the molecular changes that occur as a result of the Ph when an oncogenic protein was identified and implicated in the pathophysiology of CML.[5,6]

Ph is the first karyotypic abnormality specifically implicated in the pathogenesis of cancer, and its discovery has resulted in extensive research into the molecular biology of CML.[7] This chromosomal abnormality is characteristic of CML and is present in approximately 95% of patients with the disease.[8,9]

❶ Ph, identified as a shortened long arm of chromosome 22, is found in granulocyte and erythrocyte progenitors, macrophages, megakaryocytes, and lymphocytes. The Ph is the consequence of breaks in chromosomes 9 and 22 resulting in a transposition that relocates the 3' end of *ABL* (Abelson proto-oncogene) from its normal site on chromosome 9 at band 34 to the 5' end of *BCR* (breakpoint cluster region) on chromosome 22 at band 11 [symbolized as t(9;22)(q34;q11)].[9,10] This results in the formation of the hybrid *BCR-ABL* fusion gene (Fig. 143–1). Through this chromosomal translocation, the *ABL* protooncogene is able to escape the normal genetic controls on its senescence and is activated into a functional oncogene, directing the transcription of an 8.5-kilobase messenger ribonucleic acid (mRNA) molecule. The mRNA is translated into a 210-kDa protein—p210$^{BCR-ABL}$—that is constitutively (constantly) activated compared to the 145-kDa protein translated by the normal *ABL* gene.[8,9] Although p210$^{BCR-ABL}$ is the most common tyrosine kinase found in CML, variations in the breakpoints in the *ABL* gene encode different size proteins. For example, a smaller protein, p190 *BCR-ABL*, is involved in two thirds of adults with Ph-positive acute lymphoblastic leukemia, although rarely found in patients with CML.[9]

Since CML begins with the malignant transformation of a single cell, it is considered a clonal disease. The progeny from this transformed primitive hematopoietic stem cell results in a proliferative advantage over normal hematopoietic cells that displaces normal hematopoiesis. The Ph can be found in both myeloid and lymphoid cells, which suggests that the transformed cell of CML is a pluripotent stem cell.[10] This alteration gives the transformed progenitor cell an inheritable growth advantage, leading to the proliferation of a neoplastic, monoclonal population of cells.[9] Disrupted maturation leads to additional divisions by CML progenitor cells before reaching a nonproliferative stage; the resulting number of circulating granulocytes may be many times higher than normal. In the advanced stages of CML, cytopenias may occur in association with fibrotic changes in the bone marrow.[9]

The *BCR-ABL* fusion gene encodes for a constitutively active tyrosine kinase that is involved in both the increased proliferation of the CML clone and the reduction in FAS-mediated apoptosis. Characterization of the adenosine triphosphate binding site on the *BCR-ABL* tyrosine kinase has provided a target for inhibition of tyrosine kinase activity. The first FDA-approved tyrosine kinase inhibitor, imatinib mesylate (Gleevec®), was indicated for patients in chronic phase who had failed interferon alfa (IFN-α) or for those with advanced disease. Imatinib received additional FDA approval in 2002 for first-line treatment in newly diagnosed CML. Second-generation tyrosine kinase inhibitors with a higher binding affinity and selectivity for *ABL* kinase have been developed and approved for use in patients who are intolerant or resistant to imatinib.

CLINICAL PRESENTATION

CLINICAL PRESENTATION OF CML[1]

General

- 90% of patients are diagnosed in chronic phase
- 50% are asymptomatic in chronic phase and often diagnosed following abnormal complete blood count

Signs and Symptoms

- Fatigue
- Left upper quadrant pain
- Abdominal pain or distension
- Weight loss
- Night sweats

Physical Examination

- Splenomegaly
- Hepatomegaly

Laboratory Tests

- Peripheral blood
  - Leukocytosis
  - Thrombocytosis
  - Basophilia
  - Low or undetectable leukocyte alkaline phosphatase
  - Elevated uric acid and lactate dehydrogenase
- Molecular testing
  - Presence of *bcr-abl* by reverse-transcription polymerase chain reaction
- Bone marrow
  - Hypercellular
  - Fully mature myeloid cells
  - Increased megakaryocytes
  - <10% blasts in chronic phase
- Cytogenetics
  - Presence of the Ph chromosome
  - Additional abnormalities

CLINICAL COURSE

❷ Three clinical phases of CML are recognized: chronic phase (CP), accelerated phase (AP), and blast crisis (BC). Nearly 90% of patients present with chronic phase at the time of diagnosis. Often the diagnosis of CML is found incidentally during routine examination or if a complete blood count is obtained for unrelated reasons because patients are often asymptomatic upon presentation. Signs and symptoms include fatigue, sweating, bone pain, weight loss, abdominal discomfort, and early satiety secondary to splenomegaly. Leukocytosis is the hallmark of CP, which can be as high as 1,000,000 cells/mm³ (1,000 × 10⁹/L) placing patients at risk for complications of leukostasis. Symptoms secondary to leukostasis include acute abdominal pain resulting from splenic infarctions, priapism, retinal hemorrhage, cerebrovascular accidents, confusion, hyperuricemia, and gouty arthritis.[9] CP has an approximately three to 5-year survival without treatment.

Initial laboratory workup includes complete blood count with differential, complete metabolic panel, and serum uric acid. A bone marrow aspiration and biopsy is required to confirm the diagnosis of CML. The differential diagnosis of CML includes infection, myeloproliferative disorders (i.e., polycythemia vera, essential thrombocythemia, myelofibrosis), and chronic myelomonocytic leukemia. Bone marrow is markedly hypercellular (75%–90%) with increased granulocyte/erythroid ratio increased (10–30:1), erythropoiesis increased megakaryocytes normal. Karyotyping (cytogenetic analysis) is required for a diagnosis. The bone marrow aspiration is analyzed with Fluorescent in situ hybridization (FISH) to determine the presence of the Ph chromosome. Quantitative real time polymerase chain reaction (RT-PCR) is also performed to assess the baseline BCR-ABL transcript levels.

Accelerated phase is characterized by progressive myeloid maturation arrest and loss of efficacy of drug therapy directed to attenuate the increase in white blood cells. Clinical findings of AP include anemia, increasing peripheral blood and bone marrow blasts and basophils, clonal cytogenetic evolution, extramedullary disease sites (bone, breast, CNS, mucosal tissue, lymph nodes, and skin), exacerbation of splenomegaly, and either thrombocytosis or thrombocytopenia. Nonspecific findings such as bone pain, fever, night sweats, and weight loss may occur. The most commonly observed cytogenetic changes with disease progression are an additional Ph chromosome, trisomy 8, and isochrome I(17q). Survival typically will not exceed several months. The World Health Organization (WHO) classification defines AP CML as one or more of the following changes: 10% to 19% of blasts in the peripheral blood or bone marrow, persistent thrombocytopenia less than 100,000 cells/mm³ (100 × 10⁹/L) (not related to drug therapy), thrombocytosis greater than 1,000,000 cells/mm³ (1,000 × 10⁹/L) despite drug therapy, peripheral basophilia >20%, increasing spleen size and white blood cell count despite drug therapy, bone marrow evidence of progression of the leukemic clone or new cytogenetic abnormalities (Table 143–1).[11]

Blast crisis is the terminal stage of disease and clinically resembles acute leukemia where the leukemic clone overwhelmingly dominates the bone marrow at the expense of normal hematopoiesis. The WHO classification defines BC CML as the presence of one or more of the following: >20% blasts in the peripheral blood or bone marrow, extramedullary disease, or large clusters of blasts in the bone marrow (Table 143–1).[11] A minority of patients present with BC without an apparent AP. One third of patients present with BC of lymphoid lineage, whereas two thirds present with BC of myeloid lineage or undifferentiated like phenotype. The increased proliferative rate in BC CML is the consequence of a number of factors in addition to BCR-ABL, such as the activation of the RAC- and RAS-signaling pathways and loss of tumor suppressors such as p53. Duration of BC is typically days to weeks before death.

PROGNOSIS

Several models have been proposed for estimating prognosis in patients with CML, but the one proposed by Sokal et al. has become the most widely used.[13] The Sokal algorithm uses spleen size, percentage of circulating blasts, platelet count, and age as prognostic factors for patients in CP. However, this scoring system was developed prior to the advent of tyrosine kinase inhibitor therapy and may have limited predictive value in the era of imatinib. The median overall survival for patient diagnosed with CP, AP, and BC CML was reported to be 47 months, 12 to 24 months, and 3 to 6 months respectively in the era prior to the introduction of tyrosine kinase inhibitors.[13,14]

TREATMENT

■ GOALS OF TREATMENT

Without effective treatment, CML disease progression leads inexorably to a fatal outcome within five years. The overriding treatment goals for CML include the eradication of the leukemic clone from the bone marrow and maintenance of CP with minimal toxicity from treatment. The only proven therapy to eradicate the malignant clone from the bone marrow is a hematopoietic stem cell transplant (HSCT). Both immunotherapy with IFN-α and tyrosine kinase inhibitor based therapies have demonstrated the ability to extend CP beyond the expected period of several years, but data to confirm the curative ability of these agents are lacking. The current standard of practice is to institute imatinib therapy for newly diagnosed CML patients. Long-term follow-up from phase III trials have documented a response in excess of 85% of patients that receive imatinib as primary treatment.[15,16] Table 143–2 shows the effect of various treatment modalities on survival in CP CML.

Clinical response in CML is measured by hematologic, cytogenetic, and molecular indices all of which have standardized criteria.[17] Hematologic response is defined as the normalization of peripheral blood counts and is the earliest type of response observed in CML patients. Cytogenetic responses are based on the percentage of cells positive for Ph in a bone marrow biopsy.

TABLE 143-1	Criteria for Defining Phases of Chronic Myelogenous Leukemia	
Chronic Phase	**Accelerated Phase**	**Blast Crisis**
• <10% blasts in peripheral blood or bone marrow	• 10%–29% blasts in peripheral blood or bone marrow • Platelets <100,000 cells/mm³ or >1,000,000 cells/mm³ Additional findings • Cytogenetic evolution • Progressive splenomegaly	• >30% blasts in peripheral blood or bone marrow • Large clusters of blasts on bone marrow biopsy • Presence of extramedullary infiltrates Additional findings • Fever • Malaise • Splenomegaly

Data from Cortes JE, Talpaz M, O'Brien S, et al. Staging of chronic myeloid leukemia in the imatinib era. Cancer 2006;106:1306–1315.

TABLE 143-2	Effect of Therapy on Survival in Patients with Early Chronic-Phase Chronic Myelogenous Leukemia	
Therapy	**5-Year Survival (%)**	**Median Survival (Months)**
Busulfan[25]	30–40	40–50
Hydroxyurea[25]	40–50	50–60
IFN-α[1]	50–70	60–80
IFN-α + ara-C[1]	60–80	NR
Allogeneic transplantation		
Matched sibling[1,55]	60–80	NR
Matched unrelated[1,7]	40–70	NR
Imatinib[21]	89	NR

NR, not yet reached.

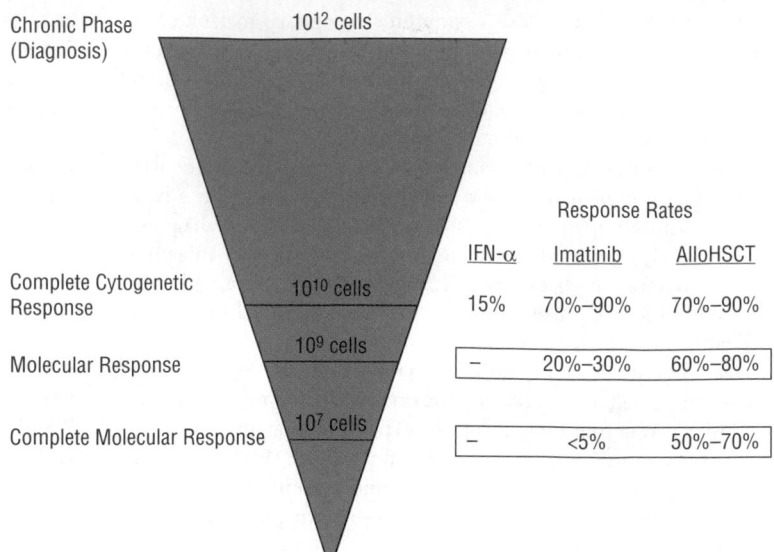

FIGURE 143-2. Type and frequency of response associated with common CML therapies. (AlloHSCT, allogeneic hematopoietic stem cell transplantation; IFN, interferon.) *(Adapted from Lowenberg B. Minimal residual disease in chronic myeloid leukemia. N Engl J Med 2003;349(15): 1399–1401. Copyright © 2003 Massachusetts Medical Society. All rights reserved.)*

Complete cytogenetic response is defined as the elimination of Ph from all cells in the marrow sample whereas *major cytogenetic response* is defined as fewer than 35% Ph-positive cells. Patients who have a major or complete cytogenetic response have an improved survival compared to those who fail to achieve a cytogenetic response.[18]

Because most patients on imatinib achieve a complete cytogenetic response, more sensitive tests to monitor disease status have become more prominently used. *Molecular responses* are determined by quantitative reverse-transcriptase polymerase chain reactions (RT-PCR), which are several logs more sensitive than methods used to measure cytogenetic responses. A *complete molecular response* is the absence of *BCR-ABL* transcripts by RT-PCR. RT-PCR assays should be interpreted carefully because they have varying sensitivities and may show a complete molecular remission even when low levels of *BCR-ABL* transcripts are present.[18] Quantitative RT-PCR should be performed on every patient prior to initiating therapy and throughout therapy to monitor residual disease. Because bone marrow and peripheral blood *BCR-ABL* mRNA levels are correlated, peripheral blood can often be used for this analysis.[17,18] Figure 143–2 illustrates the residual disease that remains after various types of responses and the response rates obtained with the common therapies for CML.

■ CONVENTIONAL CHEMOTHERAPY

Conventional cytotoxic chemotherapy is used in CP CML to reduce and temporarily control high peripheral white blood cell (WBC) counts. Historically, the two agents used for leukoreduction are busulfan (Myleran®) and hydroxyurea (Hydrea®). Busulfan is no longer used because randomized trials have shown that hydroxyurea treatment provides a modest survival advantage and busulfan has a risk of potentially life-threatening pulmonary fibrosis.[19]

Hydroxyurea rapidly lowers high circulating WBCs in CP CML by inhibiting ribonucleotide reductase, which inhibits DNA synthesis, eliminating cells in the S phase of the cell cycle, and synchronizing cells in the G_1 or pre-DNA synthesis phase. Hydroxyurea is initiated at 40 to 50 mg/kg/day in divided doses until the WBC count falls to approximately 10,000 cells/mm³ (10×10^9/L). Hydroxyurea may be discontinued once adequate control of the WBC count is achieved and imatinib has been initiated. Hydroxyurea is not specifically active against Ph and will not alter the natural progression of the disease to BC.

■ IMATINIB MESYLATE (GLEEVEC®)

A transformative discovery in cancer therapeutics was the characterization of the adenosine triphosphate binding site on the *BCR-ABL* tyrosine kinase. This specific receptor established a novel drug discovery platform for molecular targeted therapy in CML. Numerous tyrosine kinase inhibitors were in development in the 1990s and STI571 (STI stands for signal transduction inhibitor), subsequently named imatinib (Gleevec®), emerged as the drug with the best oral bioavailability and high binding affinity for the *BCR-ABL* tyrosine kinase.[20,21] In 2001, imatinib mesylate received FDA approval for patients in CP who had failed IFN-α treatment and in patients with AP or BC based on phase II studies. In 2002, it received FDA approval for first-line treatment in newly diagnosed CML on the basis of the 2-year follow-up in the International Randomized Interferon vs STI571 (IRIS) phase III trial.[22]

Imatinib inhibits several other tyrosine kinases including *BCR-ABL*, c-KIT, and platelet-derived growth factor receptor. Imatinib competitively binds to the adenosine triphosphate (ATP)-binding site on *BCR-ABL*, which inhibits the phosphorylation of proteins involved with CML clone proliferation.[23] Table 143–3 summarizes the clinical results of imatinib in CML patients in CP, AP, and BC. Early phase I and phase II studies of imatinib, designed to determine maximum tolerated dose and safety, showed higher than expected response rates in all stages of CML.[24]

TABLE 143-3	Cytogenetic Response Associated with Tyrosine Kinase Inhibitor Therapy in Chronic Myelogenous Leukemia			
Drug (Disease Status)	**Daily Dose**	**MCyR**	**CCyR**	**Median Follow-up**
Imatinib (CP)[21]	400 mg	92%	87%	60 months
	800 mg	96%	90%	30 months
Imatinib (AP)[38]	600 mg	49%	43%	12 months
	400 mg	16%	11%	
Imatinib (BC)[20,39]	400–800 mg	16%	7.4%	–
Dasatinib (CP)	100 mg	59%	41%	6 months
Dasatinib (AP)	140 mg	39%	32%	15 months
Nilotinib (AP)	800 mg	29%	16%	12 months

CCyR, complete cytogenetic response; CML, chronic myelogenous leukemia; AP, accelerated phase; BC, blast crisis; CP, chronic phase; MCyR, major cytogenetic response.

Chronic Phase

The IRIS study (N = 1,106) compared imatinib 400 mg orally daily to IFN-α plus low-dose subcutaneous cytarabine.[22] After a median follow-up of 19 months, patients who received imatinib achieved a complete hematologic response of 96%, major cytogenetic response of 85%, and complete cytogenetic response of 69%. Six percent of patients had progressed to AP or BC and only 4% discontinued imatinib due to an adverse event. The study was designed to allow crossover to the opposite treatment arm for lack of response or intolerance. After 60 months of follow-up, only 3% of patients who were originally randomized to receive IFN-α remained on their initial regimen compared with 69% of patients in the imatinib arm. The 5-year follow-up data from the IRIS trial was published in December 2006 and 6-year follow-up data in March 2009.[15,25] The estimated 5-year and 6-year overall survival of the 553 patients who were originally randomized to receive imatinib is 89% and 88%, respectively. At 60 months, the best observed rate of a major cytogenetic response and complete cytogenetic response while on imatinib was 89% and 82%, respectively. When the Sokal prognostic scoring system was used the complete cytogenetic response rates were 89%, 82%, and 69% in low-risk, intermediate-risk, and high-risk patients, respectively.

Cytogenetic and molecular responses secondary to imatinib are associated with event-free survival and risk of progression to AP or BC. Patients that do not achieve a hematologic response by 3 months, cytogenetic response by 6 months, or a major cytogenetic response by 12 months fare significantly worse compared to responders. Additionally, patients with a complete cytogenetic response and at least a 3-log reduction in *BCR-ABL* levels via RT-PCR correlated with a 100% survival without disease progression at 18 months. The risk of disease progression according to the Sokal scoring system estimated the rates of disease progression to be 3%, 8%, and 17% in low-risk, intermediate-risk, and high-risk patients, respectively. However, the Sokal score was not associated with disease progression in patients who achieved a complete cytogenetic response.[15]

❸ Although most patients attain a complete cytogenetic response on imatinib, very few patients achieve a complete molecular remission. In a study of patients enrolled in the IRIS study, Hughes et al. reported that less than 5% of patients on imatinib have undetectable levels of *BCR-ABL* when analyzed by RT-PCR.[26] Recent data suggest that the level of residual disease is predictive of progression-free survival. A decline in *BCL-ABL* mRNA by 3-log within 3 months after achieving a complete cytogenetic response is reported to be a predictor of longer progression-free survival.[27] Careful monitoring of *BCR-ABL* levels by RT-PCR is necessary to guide clinician decision making for therapy modification.

The 2011 National Comprehensive Cancer Network (NCCN) guidelines recommend imatinib 400 mg orally daily as one of several options for patients in CP.[16] Most newly diagnosed patients in CP will be started on imatinib 400 mg daily and nearly 90% of these patients will achieve a complete cytogenetic response (see Table 143–3).

Higher imatinib doses are being evaluated in clinical trials. The European LeukemiaNet conducted a randomized phase II trial in high-risk patients defined by the Sokol scoring system to imatinib 400 mg daily (n = 108) vs 800 mg daily (n = 108) and evaluated the proportion of patients achieving a complete cytogenetic response at 12 months.[28] Patients receiving the higher dose of imatinib achieved a 64% complete cytogenetic response compared to 58% of patients receiving standard dose with a median follow-up period of 12 months (P = 0.435). These study results do not justify the routine use of imatinib 800 mg daily as front-line therapy in high-risk patients with CP CML. A phase II trial evaluated imatinib 400 mg daily for 2 weeks, then titrated to 400 mg twice daily in patients with

an intermediate-risk Sokol score appeared to have benefit with 88% and 91% of patients achieving a complete cytogenetic response at 12 and 24 months.[29] These data require validation with a phase III clinical trial before a widespread use of a higher dose can become standard of care in CP CML.

Accelerated Phase/Blast Crisis

Response rates for patients with AP or BC CML are reduced compared with those in CP. A phase II study evaluating imatinib 600 mg daily in patients with AP CML yielded complete hematologic and complete cytogenetic response rates of 71% and 19%, respectively.[30] Prior to protocol amendments, patients were able to receive imatinib 400 mg daily, but the rates of hematologic response, cytogenetic response, disease progression, and overall survival were inferior to imatinib 600 mg. The toxicity profile between imatinib 400 mg and 600 mg daily was similar.

Traditional therapy for BC has focused on administering cytotoxic chemotherapy in treatment programs similar to acute leukemia induction. Etoposide (VP-16) cytarabine (Ara-C), and carboplatin (VAC-regimen) has demonstrated efficacy in patients with BC CML with a median overall survival of 7 months.[31] Imatinib has demonstrated modest benefit in BC. An open-label, non-randomized trial evaluated imatinib 400 mg daily with dose escalation to 600 mg daily and 400 mg twice daily (for patients not achieving a hematologic response after 1 month).[32] The primary objectives were to assess hematologic response, complete cytogenetic response, and the return to CP CML. Fifteen percent developed a complete hematologic response, 7.4% achieved a complete cytogenetic response, and 18% achieved a second CP. Imatinib 600 mg was an independent predictive factor for the likelihood of a sustained hematologic response. The median overall survival was 6.9 months.

Imatinib Resistance

Despite having high cytogenetic response rates, some patients treated with imatinib will not respond to therapy or will relapse after primary response.[33] The most prominent mechanism of imatinib resistance is the presence of point mutations in one or more areas on the ABL kinase. More than 100 different mutations have been discovered thus far. Many of these mutations can cause a conformational change in the ATP binding site, which greatly decreases the ability of imatinib to bind and inhibit kinase activity.[34] Imatinib binds to *BCR-ABL* by establishing a series of hydrogen bonds with side changes of amino acids within the kinase domain. Mutations which alter this surface can decrease the affinity of imatinib for *BCR-ABL*, potentially preventing binding entirely. The kinase domain of *BCR-ABL*, which encompasses amino acids 225–400, can be subdivided into ATP and imatinib binding site (P loop), the catalytic site where the phosphate from ATP is transferred to the substrate protein, and the activation domain which determines the state of the kinase (open or closed). The imatinib binding site is located in the region of amino acids 300–325. Resistance is caused by point mutations in one or more of several areas on the Abl kinase. The T315I mutation occurs directly within the imatinib binding site and completely disrupts imatinib binding.[35] This mutation has gained notoriety by conferring resistance not only to imatinib but also to second-generation *BCR-ABL* kinase inhibitors.

The other known clinically relevant mechanism of resistance is *BCR-ABL* gene amplification. The *BCR-ABL* gene is overexpressed to such an extent that the typical 400 mg daily dose of imatinib is insufficient to inhibit the activity of the kinase. Reports of clinically significant resistance have been published owing to *BCR-ABL* gene amplification, multiple copies of Ph, or both. The largest series published this far included 66 patients, in whom only two had confirmed *BCR-ABL* genomic amplification.[35] Other proposed mechanisms of resistance to imatinib include differential binding to alpha-1 acid glycoprotein in serum, overexpression of p-glycoprotein induced drug efflux and clonal evolution to acquisition of additional cytogenetic abnormalities.[36]

Imatinib Monitoring

Imatinib therapy should be frequently monitored to assess response or disease progression. Recommendations for monitoring include baseline molecular and cytogenetic assessment. A complete hematologic response is expected within 3 months of starting imatinib in patients with CP CML. *BCR-ABL* transcripts should be evaluated by RT-PCR every 3 months and bone marrow cytogenetics performed at 6 and 12 months following the start of therapy.[16–18] If the patient has achieved a cytogenetic response at 6 months, then it is not necessary to repeat bone marrow cytogenetics at 12 months. However, if a patient has not yet achieved a cytogenetic response at 12 months then bone marrow cytogenetic should be repeated at 18 months and as clinically indicated.

If a patient develops an increase in *BCR-ABL* transcripts (a 1-log increase) the following measures should be implemented: assess patient adherence, repeat *BCR-ABL* in 1 to 3 months for patients with a prior major molecular response, obtain bone marrow cytogenetics in patients without a previous major molecular response and consider mutation analysis for the *BCR-ABL* tyrosine kinase.[16]

Side Effects and Drug Interactions

Imatinib-induced myelosuppression is one of the most common adverse events. Moderate-to-severe myelosuppression occurs in approximately 5% to 10% of patients with CP CML and in 50% to 60% of patients in AP or BC.[12] The myelosuppression typically occurs within the first 4 weeks of therapy and is more common in patients with advanced disease (i.e., high blastic involvement of the bone marrow) and those with a low hemoglobin. Hematopoiesis in patients with CML depends on the amount of Ph-positive progenitors, although some degree of myelosuppression should be expected when the malignant clone is suppressed. However, imatinib also suppresses normal hematopoiesis, which suggests that myelosuppression associated with imatinib is probably related to effects on the Ph clone and normal hematopoietic cells.[4] Patients should have complete blood counts drawn every 1 to 2 weeks to assess for myelosuppression while receiving imatinib. Appropriate initial management of myelosuppression is to interrupt imatinib treatment, not dose reduce, as dose reductions below 300 mg daily do not fully inhibit *BCR-ABL* and may lead to the emergence of imatinib resistance.[16]

Nonhematologic toxicities associated with imatinib include gastrointestinal complications, fluid retention, mylagias/arthralgias, rash, and hepatotoxicity. Nausea and vomiting is the event most commonly reported and can be managed by administering the drug with food. Higher doses of imatinib may be split in half and taken twice daily to reduce gastrointestinal side effects. Diarrhea may be dose related and can be controlled with antidiarrheal medications such as loperamide or diphenoxylate/atropine. Fluid retention most often manifests as periorbital swelling or peripheral edema. Rarely, fluid retention can be severe, leading to pulmonary and cerebral edema. Risk factors for edema include female gender, age older than 65 years, and a history of heart or kidney disease. Approximately 20% to 40% of patients complain of musculoskeletal symptoms, which tend to occur during the first month of therapy and decline in severity over time. Calcium and magnesium supplementation may provide symptomatic relief. Drug rash frequently occurs but is usually mild and can be managed with antihistamines or topical steroids. Severe rash, while uncommon, has been reported as an important cause for discontinuation of therapy. Algorithms for desensitization for patients that have experienced serious imatinib-associated rash have been published.[37] Hepatotoxicity can occur with imatinib, and the drug should be withheld if liver function tests exceed 5 times the upper limits of normal. After the liver function tests normalize, imatinib can be restarted at a reduced dose of not less than 300 mg per day. Imatinib is then dose escalated to the initial dose if liver function tests do not rise during 6 to 12 weeks of treatment. Death as a consequence of liver failure has been reported in a patient receiving large doses of acetaminophen concomitantly with imatinib. It is recommended that patients on imatinib limit their use of acetaminophen to 1,300 mg daily.[16] Use of other medications that are known to be hepatotoxic should be used with caution while patients are treated with imatinib.

Imatinib is metabolized primarily via CYP3A4 and inducers of this enzyme may decrease imatinib concentrations. Other isoenzymes CYP1A2, CYP2D6, CYP2C9, CYP2C19 play a minor role in metabolism. During the phase I trial of imatinib, a patient who received concurrent phenytoin therapy developed a suboptimal response and was found to have a 75% reduction in plasma imatinib concentrations as compared to patients not receiving phenytoin. The clinical significance of this interaction was confirmed when disease control was acquired with the discontinuation of phenytoin.[24] Imatinib may increase the concentrations of other drugs that are substrates or inhibitors of CYP3A4, 3A5, 2D6, and 2C9. Imatinib has been reported to increase blood levels of cyclosporine and simvastatin. Other agents that should be closely monitored include aprepitant, dexamethasone, St. John's wort, voriconazole, and warfarin.

■ SECOND-GENERATION TYROSINE KINASE INHIBITORS

Dasatinib (Sprycel®) and nilotinib (Tasigna®) are approved second-generation tyrosine kinase inhibitors used for the treatment of CML in patients who are resistant or intolerant to imatinib therapy; both drugs are also approved for first-line treatment of CP CML. Dasatinib is an oral *BCR-ABL* tyrosine kinase inhibitor that was FDA approved in 2006 for the treatment of imatinib-resistant CML. Dasatinib is an oral tyrosine kinase inhibitor of *BCR-ABL,* the SRC family (SRC, LKC, YES, FYN), c-KIT, EPHA2, and platelet-derived growth factor receptor. Preclinical data show that dasatinib is 300 times more potent than imatinib and has inhibitory activity in imatinib-resistant clones, with the exception of the T315I.[38] Dasatinib received accelerated approval based on hematologic and cytogenetic responses seen in imatinib-resistant or imatinib-intolerant patients.

Dasatinib has been evaluated in patients with imatinib-resistant or -intolerant CP, AP, and BC CML. In a phase II trial of 186 patients in CP CML receiving dasatinib 70 mg orally twice daily a hematologic response and major cytogenetic response were noted in 90% and 52% of patients, respectively.[39] Kantarjian et al. evaluated imatinib 400 mg twice daily compared to dasatinib 70 mg twice daily in patients who developed resistance or were intolerant to imatinib 400 mg daily dosing. At 2 years' follow-up, patients receiving dasatinib were more likely to achieve a complete hematologic response (93% vs 82%; P = 0.034), major cytogenetic response (53% vs 33%; P = 0.023), and an increased estimated progression-free survival at 2 years, suggesting that dasatinib is superior to imatinib dose escalation in disease progression.[40] A trial evaluating different dosing strategies of dasatinib showed that 100 mg given once daily was as efficacious as dasatinib 70 mg twice daily, 50 mg twice daily or 140 mg once daily but with decreased adverse events such as pleural effusions.[41] Standard dose dasatinib for patients with CP CML is now accepted to be 100 mg daily.

Dasatinib is able to induce responses in patients who are resistant or intolerant to imatinib with advanced disease CML. Patients with AP CML were administered dasatinib 70 mg twice daily with 45% achieving a complete hematologic response, 39% achieved a complete cytogenetic response, 66% had progression-free survival, and 82% were alive 2 years.[42] A phase III trial comparing dasatinib 70 mg twice daily to 140 mg once daily resulted in similar efficacy at 15 months follow-up, but an improved safety profile that established dasatinib 140 mg once daily is the preferred dosing in AP CML.[43] Dasatinib induced a hematologic response in 35% and a major cytogenetic response in 33% of patients with BC CML. Median overall survival for patients receiving dasatinib in BC CML is 11.8 months.[44]

Dasatinib has been evaluated as first-line therapy in a phase III trial of 519 patients with CP CML.[45] Patients were randomized to dasatinib 100 mg once daily or imatinib 400 mg once daily. The rate of complete cytogenetic response at 12 months was significantly higher with dasatinib as compared with imatinib (77% vs. 66%, $P = 0.007$). The rate of major molecular response was also significantly higher in the dasatinib group (46% vs. 28%, $P < 0.0001$). Toxicities were similar between the two treatment groups, with the exception that 10% of dasatinib-treated patients developed grade 1 or 2 pleural effusions.

Nilotinib has 20 to 30 times the inhibitory activity of the BCR-ABL tyrosine kinase with activity against c-KIT and platelet-derived growth factor receptor (but not SRC kinases) due to a modification of the methylpiperazinyl structure of imatinib. Nilotinib has inhibitory activity against imatinib-resistant mutants with the exception of T315I. In a phase II trial of 280 patients with imatinib-resistant or -intolerant CP CML, nilotinib 400 mg twice daily resulted in 48% of patients achieving a major cytogenetic response.[46] In AP CML, nilotinib achieved a complete hematologic response of 26% and major cytogenetic responses of 29% were achieved with nilotinib 400 mg or 600 mg twice daily.[47] For front-line treatment of CML, results of a randomized trial in 846 patients comparing nilotinib at two doses (300 or 400 mg twice daily) to imatinib 400 mg once daily have been published.[48] The primary endpoint of the trial was major molecular response at 12 months. Both nilotinib arms had a significantly higher major molecular response rate at 12 months (43% and 44% for nilotinib 300 and 400 mg twice daily, respectively) as compared to imatinib (22%, $P < 0.001$ for both comparisons). The nilotinib arms also had a significant improvement in the time-to-progression to the AP or BC, as compared to the imatinib arm. The number of patients discontinued from treatment was similar in all three treatment arms. Nilotinib provides an alternative to dasatinib in patients with imatinib-resistant or -intolerant CP or AP CML and is one of several options in front-line treatment of CP CML.[16]

The side-effect profile of the second tyrosine kinase inhibitors is similar to imatinib. Reversible myelosuppression is the most common side effect seen with dasatinib and nilotinib, and may require interruption of therapy. Side effects unique to dasatinib include fluid retention and pleural effusions, which appear to be related to peak drug concentrations.[39,44] Edema and plural effusions can be managed by dasatinib drug holiday, diuretics, or short courses of steroids. Nilotinib can be associated with indirect bilirubin elevations in 10% to 15% of patients.[46,47] Nilotinib may prolong the QTc interval (block box warning) and patients should have an electrocardiogram at baseline, at 7 days following initiation of therapy, and periodically thereafter.

Like imatinib, dasatinib and nilotinib are metabolized by CYP3A4. Clinicians need to be aware of possible drug interactions with inducers and inhibitors of the CYP3A4 pathway such as phenytoin, azole antifungals, or macrolide antibiotics. Dasatinib and nilotinib may prolong the QTc interval and patients should avoid concomitant therapy with other drugs that are known to prolong the QTc interval, such as antiarrhythmics, macrolide antibiotics, azole antifungals, and fluoroquinolones. In vitro data also suggest that long-term suppression of gastric acid decreases dasatinib absorption; therefore, patients should refrain from taking concomitant H_2-blockers or proton pump inhibitors, if clinically feasible. The bioavailability of nilotinib is increased when given with a meal and should be taken on an empty stomach, whereas dasatinib should be taken with food.

Dasatinib and nilotinib have an established role in patients who have failed imatinib either because of disease resistance or drug intolerance. The 2011 NCCN guidelines recommend dasatinib or nilotinib as viable treatment options for patients who do not achieve a complete hematologic response in 3 months or cytogenetic response in 6 months. If patients continue to have a partial response or have disease progression while on imatinib, then a change in therapy to dasatinib or nilotinib is warranted in the absence of an immediate allogeneic HSCT option.[16] Limited treatment data are available with the use of a third tyrosine kinase inhibitor due to disease progression and patients should be considered for a HSCT.[49]

■ INTERFERON ALFA

Prior to the introduction of imatinib, IFN-α was the preferred agent in the treatment of CML. The role of IFN-α has since been relegated to patients who fail tyrosine kinase inhibitor therapies and are not candidates for HSCT.

The interferons are a family of glycoproteins involved in many of the functional aspects of the hematopoietic system. Two recombinant forms of IFN-α are currently marketed: IFN-α_{2a} (Roferon® A) and IFN-α_{2b} (Intron® A). Two polyethylene glycol conjugated products of IFN-α (PEG-IFN-α_{2b} and PEG-IFN-α_{2a}) can be administered weekly as compared with daily administration for the non-pegylated formulation.[50,51] The pegylated dosage forms of IFN have similar efficacy and toxicity profiles relative to the conventional formulation.

❹ Use of IFN-α in the treatment of CP CML was based on reports that 20% to 50% of patients achieve a major cytogenetic response, which led to prolonged survival.[7] In the 10% to 15% of patients achieving a complete cytogenetic response, the median survival was more than 10 years.[16] Patients enrolled on the IFN-α arm in the IRIS trial had a complete cytogenetic response of 14%, as compared with 76% of patients treated with imatinib.[15] Historically, those who achieved a cytogenetic response with IFN-α typically continue to receive the drug as maintenance therapy. The 2011 NCCN guidelines recommend IFN-α only for post-transplant relapse.

IFN-α use is also limited by its toxicity profile because it is associated with both short-term constitutional toxicities and potentially dose-limiting long-term toxicities.[52] In the IRIS trial, 26% of patients discontinued IFN-α as a result of intolerable side effects.[15] The most predictable early toxicity is a flu-like syndrome characterized by fever, chills, myalgia, headache, and anorexia. These dose-dependent effects may be a result of IFN-α–induced leukocytosis and release of inflammatory cytokines. This acute flu-like syndrome can be ameliorated by starting IFN-α dosing at 50% of the final dose during the first week, giving the drug at bedtime, and co-administering acetaminophen or indomethacin with each IFN-α dose.[52] Reduction of initial WBC counts to below 10,000 cells/mm³ (10×10^9/L) with hydroxyurea may also reduce these symptoms. Despite supportive care approaches to ameliorate the flu-like syndrome, it remains a formidable morbidity occasionally requiring termination of the drug. Cardiovascular toxicities (tachycardia, hypotension) are seen in approximately 15% of patients in the first few weeks. Long-term adverse effects include weight loss, alopecia, neurologic effects (paresthesia, cognitive impairment, depression), and immune-mediated complications (hemolysis, thrombocytopenia, nephrotic syndrome, systemic lupus erythematosus, hypothyroidism) are documented in approximately 5% to 20% of patients.

Despite falling out of clinical favor, IFN-α still remains a disease-modifying agent and ongoing clinical trials are investigating the use of imatinib and IFN-α in combination for the treatment of CML.[53]

■ HEMATOPOIETIC STEM CELL TRANSPLANTATION

⑤ Allogeneic HSCT remains the only therapy proven to cure patients with CML, with many patients alive and disease-free decades after transplant. Patients undergoing allogeneic HSCT from a human leukocyte antigen (HLA)-matched sibling donor have 5-year survival rates ranging from 60% to 80% and long-term survival of approximately 50%.[54,55] In most long-term survivors, the *BCR-ABL* translocation is absent in all diagnostic tests including RT-PCR. Prognostic risk factors associated with survival outcomes include age, phase of disease and disease duration. Increasing age is associated with poorer prognosis, with higher transplant-related mortality in patients older than age 50 years. Patients with early disease who receive transplantations have better outcomes than those in accelerated phase or blast crisis. The time from diagnosis to transplantation also affects outcomes. Patients who undergo matched-sibling allogeneic HSCT within the first year of diagnosis have a better 5-year survival rate than those who undergo transplantation more than 1 year after their diagnosis (70%–80% vs 50%–60%).[54,55] This data was reported prior to the use of imatinib as first-line therapy for CML.

The major impediment for broad application of HSCT is that fewer than 30% of patients who are transplant-eligible will have an HLA-matched sibling donor. The most practical approach is to utilize an HLA-matched unrelated donor, if available. Matched unrelated donor HSCT has an overall 5-year survival reported to be 40% to 70%, which approaches overall survival data results reported for matched-sibling donor transplantations.[9,54,55]

The advent of imatinib as first-line therapy has resulted in fewer transplants for CML and has stimulated debate as to which, if any, subgroup should be treated with allogeneic HSCT as primary therapy. The difficulty lies in identifying those patients who will have suboptimal responses and might benefit from early transplantation. A recent study by the German CML Study Group reported that survival with drug therapy (IFN-α or imatinib) is superior to early allogeneic HSCT for low-risk patients, but no difference in survival was observed in high-risk patients.[56] Recent studies show that imatinib use prior to transplantation does not negatively affect transplant-related mortality.[57,58]

Patients who should be considered candidates for allogeneic HSCT are those who are healthy enough to tolerate the procedure and who have an HLA-matched related or unrelated donor; patients who have not achieved a hematologic remission within 3 months of therapy; patients who do not achieve a cytogenetic response after 6 to 12 months; and patients who are in AP or BC CML. With the median age of onset for CML being in the seventh decade of life and the high risk of mortality in patients older than 50 years of age, more than half of CML patients will be excluded from allogeneic HSCT based on age alone. Even when all the criteria are met (matched donor and younger age), 100-day mortality from allogeneic HSCT is between 10% and 20% in established transplant centers. Historically, improved outcomes have been observed when a patient undergoes transplantation within the first 2 years of diagnosis. Consequently, with HSCT being relegated to salvage therapy after primary treatment with tyrosine kinase inhibitors, long-term follow-up is needed to ascertain if delayed HSCT adversely affects outcomes.

Treatment options in patients who relapse after transplantation are limited. Graft-versus-leukemia (GVL) effect, tyrosine kinase inhibitors, IFN-α, or a clinical trial are reasonable options. The infusion of donor lymphocytes function as a form of adoptive immunotherapy can induce a GVL effect. In relapsed CML, donor lymphocytes induce durable responses and these responses strongly correlate with the development of graft-versus-host disease (GVHD).[59] Tumor burden also predicts the likelihood of response to donor lymphocyte infusion in relapsed CML. A study by Raiola et al. stratified the response rate of donor lymphocyte infusion according to relapse type. The response rate to donor lymphocytes was 100% in patients with molecular relapse, 90% in patients with cytogenetic relapse, 75% with relapsed CP CML, and 35% in patients with relapsed AP or BC CML.[60] The dose, timing, and method of administration of donor lymphocytes may also impact effectiveness. In one study, a significantly lower incidence of GVHD was observed with escalating doses of donor lymphocyte infusion (fractionated dosing) rather than single-dose donor lymphocytes while maintaining a similar 70% to 90% complete cytogenetic remission rate.[61] The optimal method of administering donor lymphocytes remains unclear, but these data suggest it may be possible to partially separate the GVL effect from GVHD.

Imatinib has been used in patients who have residual disease after allogeneic HSCT. Most patients respond to imatinib with complete molecular response of 70% without development of acute GVHD, which is often associated with donor lymphocyte infusions.[62] Use of imatinib or other tyrosine kinase inhibitor therapies require further study to determine the magnitude of benefit when applied in the post-HSCT setting.

The role of nonmyeloablative transplants in CML is evolving, but preliminary results suggest comparable outcomes to myeloablative transplants. The experience of German registry data suggests that 17% of all transplants for CML are using a reduced intensity conditioning regimen.[63]

CLINICAL CONTROVERSY

The controversy of whether to use allogeneic HSCT or second-generation tyrosine kinase inhibitor therapy as second-line treatment for patients that have progression or are intolerant to imatinib is ongoing. Dasatinib keeps 90% of CP patients treated first-line with imatinib free from disease progression with a median follow-up of 15 months. For patients that have progressed to AP, dasatinib and nilotinib can produce hematologic response in approximately half of patients and major cytogenetic responses in close to one-third of patients. At one year, three out of four patients will still be alive. It is unknown what efficacy of second-generation tyrosine kinase inhibitors will confer as a long-term treatment option. Allogeneic HSCT remains an option for patients with a suitable donor, younger age, and good performance status.

EVALUATION OF THERAPEUTIC OUTCOMES

Current standard of care is for patients with newly diagnosed CP CML to receive imatinib or one of the second-generation tyrosine kinase inhibitors. The goal of disease monitoring in CML is to differentiate patients who have optimally responded to an initial course of imatinib or one of the second-generation tyrosine kinase inhibitors from those at high risk for treatment failure. A suboptimal response is defined as no complete hematologic response at 3 months or lack of a complete cytogenetic response at 9 to 12 months. Recently published guidelines suggest that monitoring of *BCR-ABL* transcripts at 3-month intervals is currently the best available test to monitor disease response.[17,18] An escalation in *BCR-ABL* transcripts allows practitioners to identify patients who have progressive disease and may need a therapy adjustment. Imatinib dose escalation, dasatinib, nilotinib, or allogeneic HSCT are therapy options in patients who do not respond or fail to maintain a molecular response.[16]

CHRONIC LYMPHOCYTIC LEUKEMIA

EPIDEMIOLOGY AND ETIOLOGY

CLL is a lymphoproliferative disorder characterized by accumulation of functionally incompetent clonal B lymphocytes.[64] CLL is the most common form of leukemia in the United States, but is rare in other countries, such as Japan and China. It is estimated that 14,990 new cases of CLL will be diagnosed in the United States in 2010 with 4,390 deaths.[1] Occasional family clusters have been recognized, and first-degree relatives of patients with CLL are at 3 times the risk of developing a lymphoid malignancy as compared with the general population. CLL is a disease of the elderly, with a median age of 72 years, although 20% to 30% of CLL occurs in patients who are younger than 55 years of age.[2] Male sex, Caucasian race, family history, and advanced age are known risk factors for the disease.

CLINICAL PRESENTATION OF CLL

Constitutional Symptoms

Fever, fatigue, weight loss

Physical Examination

Lymphadenopathy (87%)

Splenomegaly (54%)

Hepatomegaly (14%)

Laboratory Tests

Peripheral blood

Lymphocytosis

Coombs-positive autoimmune hemolytic anemia

Hyper- or hypogammaglobulinemia

Monoclonal gammopathy

Anemia

Thrombocytopenia

Bone marrow

Hypercellular

Increased mature lymphocytes

Increased megakaryocytes

Molecular markers

Cytogenetics (17p-)

ZAP-70 mutations

PATHOPHYSIOLOGY

CLL cells are believed to be a neoplastic clone of CD5+ cells, which express low levels of surface-membrane IgM and IgD compared to normal peripheral blood B cells. Normal CD5+ B lymphocytes are present in the lymph nodes and in the blood. Neoplastic CD5+ cells accumulate in the lymph nodes and spleen because of the loss of apoptosis by either the overexpression of an oncogene, such as *bcl-1*

or -2, or loss of a tumor suppressor gene, such as *RB1*.[64] The bcl-2 protein is a major regulator of apoptosis or programmed cell death. Evidence is emerging that antigenic stimulation and cytokines drive the proliferation of the CLL cells.

A monoclonal population of B cells with a similar surface antigen phenotype as CLL cells has been recently identified in patients up to several years prior to diagnosis of the disease.[65] This phenomena, termed monoclonal B-cell lymphocytosis (MBL) appears to be predictive as to whether a patient is at risk for developing CLL over time. In a population of 77,000 patients enrolled in a cancer screening trial, 45 patients were diagnosed with CLL throughout the duration of the study. Baseline blood samples collected upon enrollment of the screening trial were analyzed for the patients that developed CLL. MBL was present in 44 of 45 of the patients by either flow cytometric or molecular analysis (i.e., RT-PCR assay) and confirmed in 41 of 45 of these patients by both methods. Samples predated the diagnosis of CLL in a time period ranging from 6 months to 6.4 years. This finding opens the door for potentially earlier diagnosis and intervention for CLL.

Cytogenetic abnormalities correlate with disease progression in CLL. Approximately 80% of patients with CLL have a karyotypic abnormality. The chromosomes that are most frequently involved include chromosomes 13, 12, 11, and 17.[66] Additional cytogenetic abnormalities may be acquired during therapy, particularly with deletions of chromosome 17, which have an adverse effect on survival.[67]

Four percent of patients with CLL have a risk of developing an aggressive histology non-Hodgkin lymphoma (diffuse large B cell), which is termed Richter syndrome. Richter syndrome may be triggered by accumulation of additional cytogenetic abnormalities in the malignant clone of lymphocytes or by viral infections, such as Epstein-Barr virus.[68]

STAGING AND PROGNOSIS

Survival times for patients with CLL are widely variable, with some patients dying within 3 years and others living into a second decade from the time of diagnosis. The Rai and the Binet staging systems are commonly used in CLL with the Rai being favored in the United States and the Binet in Europe. The Rai staging system has been combined into a risk classification scheme: low risk (stage 0), intermediate risk (stages I and II), and high risk (stages III and IV) with median survivals of greater than 10 years, 7 years, and 2 to 4 years, respectively.[69]

The disease course for CLL varies within each stage such that one patient may have an indolent course with long survival time, while another patient may have more aggressive disease and a relatively short survival time. The Rai and Binet staging systems incompletely predict for individual patients who may experience more rapid disease progression. Patients with Richter syndrome will have a rapidly advancing disease course that mimics diffuse large B-cell non-Hodgkin lymphoma. However, successful treatment of the diffuse large B-cell non-Hodgkin lymphoma with combination chemotherapy will not eradicate the underlying clone of CLL cells and patients will ultimately relapse.[68]

Biomarkers such as CD38 expression and ZAP-70 expression have been explored as prognostic factors for CLL. CD38 is a cell-surface antigen that is associated with early progression, significantly shorter overall survival and a poor response to fludarabine.[70-72] ZAP-70 is an intracellular protein with tyrosine kinase activity. Once considered as simply a surrogate marker for the unmutated variable region of the immunoglobulin heavy chain gene (IgVH), elevated ZAP-70 expression appears to predict for rapid CLL disease progression and independently correlates with prognosis.[70,73,74]

Cytogenetic changes such as deletion of the short arm of chromosome 17 (17p-), which corresponds to p53 silencing, are a robust determinant of patients with disease that is poorly responsive to therapy. A prospective study showed that newly diagnosed patients with 17p- had a median time to progression following first-line therapy with either fludarabine or fludarabine/cyclophosphamide of 10 to 12 months.[67] Patients with chromosomal abnormalities of 13, 12, 11, and 17 have reported median survivals of 133 months, 114 months, 79 months, and 32 months, respectively.[66]

CLINICAL CONTROVERSY

Certain molecular and cellular markers have been identified that may predict CLL disease progression. ZAP-70 expression, CD38 expression, IgVH mutations, and 17p- are associated with a more aggressive clinical course of CLL. Controversy surrounds whether or not treatment should be based on these biologic markers alone. 17p- is the most consistent poor prognostic marker and results in a loss of the tumor suppressor gene, *p53*. Consensus guidelines now delineate treatment options for patients based on the presence of 17p-. If a patient has 17p- more aggressive regimens that contain immunotherapy and purine analogues (e.g., fludarabine, cyclophosphamide, and rituximab) are recommended as first-line treatments. For second-line therapy, regimens with multiagent chemotherapy combined with immunotherapy (e.g., oxaliplatin, fludarabine, cytarabine, and rituximab) are considered standard therapy.

TREATMENT

■ GOALS OF TREATMENT

6 The primary goals of treatment for CLL are to improve survival duration and minimize treatment-related toxicity. The management of patients with CLL is highly individualized with some patients receiving therapy upon diagnosis, while other patients with early-stage disease are managed expectantly. Indications for starting treatment include disease-related symptoms (fatigue, night sweats, weight loss, fever), threatened end-organ function, bulky disease, doubling of lymphocyte doubling time in less than 6 months, progressive anemia and platelet count less than 100,000 /mm³ (100 × 10⁹/L).[75,76,77] Consideration of initial treatment options is based on several factors including age of the patient, disease stage, and high-risk prognostic factors, such as 17p-.

Most stage 0 patients do not require treatment and can be managed with observation. In patients with stage I disease, treatment is controversial. A consistent survival benefit from early therapy has not been reported in asymptomatic patients.[76,78] Cytotoxic chemotherapy in early stage CLL is usually reserved for patients who have disease characteristics consistent with a more aggressive course, such as short lymphocyte doubling times and presence of biologic markers such as ZAP-70 or high-risk cytogenetics. In stages II through IV disease, treatment is required, with the goal of achieving a partial or complete remission. Overall survival is improved in patients that achieve a complete response with initial treatment. Table 143–4 reviews the regimens used to treat newly diagnosed and previously treated CLL.[69,70,72,73]

■ CYTOTOXIC CHEMOTHERAPY

Orally administered alkylating agents such as chlorambucil and cyclophosphamide either given alone or with corticosteroids historically have been used as primary treatment for CLL. Results from a meta-analysis involving 2,048 patients from six randomized controlled studies evaluated low-dose alkylating agents in CLL.[78]

TABLE 143-4 Treatment for Newly Diagnosed and Previously Treated Chronic Lymphocytic Leukemia

Treatment	Overall Response	Complete Response
Chlorambucil		
Untreated	37%	4%
Fludarabine alone		
Untreated	60%–80%	20%–30%
Previously treated	13%–59%	3%–37%
Fludarabine + cyclophosphamide		
Untreated	80%–90%	25%–40%
Previously treated	60%–70%	10%–15%
Rituximab alone		
Untreated	50%–60%	10%–20%
Previously treated	80%–90%	20%–40%
Fludarabine + rituximab		
Untreated	80%–100%	30%–50%
Previously treated	80%–90%	20%–40%
Fludarabine + cyclophosphamide + rituximab		
Untreated	95%	70%
Previously treated	73%	25%
Alemtuzumab alone		
Untreated	80%–90%	20–30%
Previously treated	30%–50%	0–20%
Alemtuzumab + fludarabine		
Previously treated	83%	17%–30%
Oxaliplatin + fludarabine + cytarabine + rituximab		
Previously treated	33%	6%

Adapted from Abbott,[69] Zenz et al.,[75] Robak et al.,[81] and Tsimberidou.[99]

That analysis showed that delayed treatment with alkylating agents in asymptomatic patients did not adversely affect 10-year survival. More importantly, if only deaths caused by CLL were considered, significantly longer survival was observed when treatment was deferred. Chlorambucil continues to be widely used in elderly, symptomatic patients as initial treatment for CLL, but its use is based on a small number of studies with no demonstrable survival advantage.[69] Commonly used dosing schedules for chlorambucil are intermittent pulse dosing of 15 to 40 mg/m² orally every 28 days or daily doses of 4 to 8 mg/m²/day.[79] The dose of chlorambucil is often titrated to circumvent myelosuppression.

Cyclophosphamide produces a similar response rate as chlorambucil (overall response rate: 40%–60%; complete response: 4%) and can be used in patients who cannot tolerate chlorambucil or in whom response is not optimal. Some patients who do not respond to chlorambucil will respond to single-agent cyclophosphamide. Cyclophosphamide is typically given orally at a daily dose of 1 to 3 mg/kg. Oral cyclophosphamide is less commonly used compared to chlorambucil because of the risk of hemorrhagic cystitis and bladder cancer with prolonged treatment.

Fludarabine-based therapy is a common initial treatment in CLL. It is particularly useful in younger patients and in those patients who can tolerate immunosuppressive chemotherapy. Fludarabine, along with the other purine analogs, 2-chlorodeoxyadenosine (cladribine) and 2-deoxycoformycin (pentostatin), are highly active in CLL, with fludarabine being the most widely studied agent in the class in the treatment of CLL.[79,80] Most patients receive fludarabine 20 mg/m² intravenously daily for 5 days when used as a single agent. Cladribine and pentostatin have similar activity, although head-to-head trials comparing these three nucleosides have not been conducted.[79,81,82]

Fludarabine was initially studied in CLL patients who were refractory to chlorambucil. Several trials reported overall response rates to fludarabine in previously treated patients ranging from 13% to 59% and complete response rates of 3% to 37%.[83] Based on these encouraging results in patients with refractory disease, fludarabine was studied in chemotherapy-naïve patients. Three large phase II trials conducted in symptomatic, untreated CLL patients confirmed the efficacy of fludarabine. In these trials, fludarabine produced higher overall response rates and complete remissions than did alkylating-based therapies. In one of the randomized studies that compared fludarabine to chlorambucil in chemotherapy-naïve patients, fludarabine-treated patients had a higher complete remission rate as compared with chlorambucil (20% vs 5%).[84] However, the higher complete remission rate did not translate into a significant difference in overall survival and patients treated with fludarabine had a higher rate of severe neutropenia and infection. The study allowed chlorambucil failures to cross over to fludarabine, which may have hampered the ability to show a survival advantage in the fludarabine arm. A recent review of younger patients enrolled in a large phase III trial showed that 33% of patients receiving fludarabine or fludarabine-based therapy had infectious complications.[85] An increase in *Pneumocystis* infections was not observed, but a 6% increase in herpes and varicella zoster infection was documented. Dose reductions occurred frequently as a result of the infectious episodes. Based on the increased risk of infectious complications, some practitioners recommend antiviral and antibacterial prophylaxis be given with treatment.[77,85]

Bendamustine is an alkylating agent that contains a purine-derivative benzimidazole ring in its chemical structure that yields a compound that is non–cross-resistant with other alkylating agents. Bendamustine induces cell death via single and double-stranded cross-links.[86] It was approved for treatment of CLL and relapsed indolent non-Hodgkin lymphoma in 2008. Efficacy for bendamustine was established as first-line agent in Binet stage B or C CLL in a phase III trial that randomized 319 patients to bendamustine or chlorambucil.[87] Complete response rates of 31% vs 2% and an overall response rate for 68% vs 31% were observed for bendamustine and chlorambucil respectively. The median progression-free survival was 21.6 vs 8.3 months favoring bendamustine. Adverse events reported for bendamustine includes hematologic toxicity in approximately 25% of patients, gastrointestinal and cutaneous toxicity.

■ BIOLOGIC THERAPY

Monoclonal antibodies, such as rituximab and alemtuzumab, are increasingly being used in the treatment of CLL. Rituximab is a chimeric monoclonal antibody that targets the CD20 antigen expressed on B lymphocytes. Rituximab was initially approved for patients with indolent non-Hodgkin lymphoma and later for aggressive non-Hodgkin lymphoma. Rituximab received FDA approval for the treatment of CD20-positive CLL in 2010. The results from early trials of rituximab in CLL showed limited efficacy, with a 10% to 15% partial response rate.[88] This finding was attributed to the lower CD20 expression on the surface of the CLL cells as compared to non-Hodgkin lymphoma and a more rapid clearance of rituximab in CLL, possibly through shedding of CD20.[89] When rituximab was used as the sole therapy in CLL, higher doses than those used in indolent non-Hodgkin lymphoma had to be given to overcome these biologic features. Subsequent studies with higher rituximab doses (up to 2,250 mg/m²) have reported increased overall response rates to 40% to 75% in previously treated patients.[75,88,89]

❼ Alemtuzumab is a monoclonal antibody that targets the CD52 antigen found on both B and T lymphocytes. It was FDA approved in 2001 for the treatment of patients with CLL who had been treated with alkylating agents and had failed fludarabine therapy. Alemtuzumab has generally been reserved for CLL patients who are refractory to other available therapies, although data as first-line therapy are accumulating.[90] Alemtuzumab is titrated to a maintenance dose of 30 mg intravenously given 3 times a week for 12 weeks. As a single agent, alemtuzumab has produced response rates from 33% to 53% in patients with refractory disease, but complete response rates are infrequent.[90,91]

Results from a randomized phase III trial comparing alemtuzumab to chlorambucil in chemotherapy-naïve patients with symptomatic CLL showed higher complete response rates with alemtuzumab than with chlorambucil, 24% vs 2%, respectively.[91] These differences in response rate translated into a significant difference in progression-free survival (hazard ratio, 0.58; 95% confidence interval, 0.43-0.77, P < 0.0001). Based on these results, alemtuzumab received FDA approval in 2007 as first-line treatment for CLL.

Infusion-related reactions are one of the most frequently reported toxicities with alemtuzumab. The reactions experienced with intravenous administration include fever, rigors, and hypotension. Alemtuzumab is associated with serious, potentially life-threatening toxicities, including pancytopenia, infusion reactions, and opportunistic infections. Because of alemtuzumab's profound immunosuppression, the 2010 NCCN guidelines recommend antibacterial and antiviral prophylaxis to prevent *Cytomegalovirus* reactivation and *Pneumocystis* infections.[77] Prophylaxis with trimethoprim-sulfamethoxazole and famciclovir or valacyclovir is recommended with the use of alemtuzumab.[92] Alemtuzumab is FDA approved for intravenous administration, although the use of subcutaneous alemtuzumab has been explored to reduce the frequency of these reactions. In a study by Lundin et al., 41 patients received 30 mg of subcutaneous alemtuzumab 3 times a week for 12 weeks which yielded a response rate of 87%.[93] Major adverse event were grades 1 and 2 skin reactions in 90% of patients; fever, rigors, and hypotension were infrequent. Approximately 10% of patients had reactivation of *Cytomegalovirus* and required ganciclovir treatment. Similar to intravenous administration, antiviral and antibacterial prophylaxis is warranted when alemtuzumab is given via the subcutaneous route.[93]

Ofatumumab is a fully human monoclonal antibody to CD20 that was approved as single-agent therapy in 2009 for patients with CLL that is refractory to fludarabine and alemtuzumab. The drug was granted accelerated approved based on 54 patients who had either failed to response to or had progressed within 6 months of both fludarabine and alemtuzumab.[94] Ofatumumab is administered as an IV infusion with an initial dose of 300 mg then 4 weekly doses followed by 4 monthly doses of 2,000 mg. An overall response rate was reported of 42% (no complete responses) with patients achieving a median time-to-progression of 6.5 months. Adverse events reported in greater than 10% of patients included anemia, bronchitis, cough, diarrhea, dyspnea, fatigue, nausea, neutropenia, pneumonia, pyrexia, rash, and upper respiratory infections. Infusion-related events were reported in 44% of patients with the first infusion and 29% with the second infusion which is less than most literature reports of infusion-related hypersensitivity events with rituximab. Serious toxicities such as fatal infections, progressive multifocal leukoencephalopathy, and hepatitis B reactivation have been reported.

■ COMBINATION THERAPY

The single-agent activity of fludarabine has led to incorporation of fludarabine in combination regimens in patients with CLL. The most widely studied combination is fludarabine with cyclophosphamide, which produces complete response rates between 25% and 40% in treatment-naïve patients as compared with 20% to 30% for single-agent fludarabine.[75,81] Although improved response rates and progression-free survival have been reported with fludarabine and cyclophosphamide combinations compared with fludarabine alone, no benefit in overall survival has yet been observed.

8 The combination of fludarabine and rituximab has promising activity. In vitro studies suggest that rituximab is synergistic with fludarabine and cyclophosphamide and has led investigators to evaluate this combination in clinical trials. Results from an uncontrolled trial of fludarabine, cyclophosphamide, and rituximab (FCR) reported a complete remission rate of 70% in previously untreated CLL patients.[95] FCR has documented a complete remission rate of 25% in previous treated patients Preliminary results of two phase III trials comparing FCR with fludarabine and cyclophosphamide documented a progression-free survival benefit (30 vs 20 months with 26 months' median follow-up) in patients treated with FCR in patients with refractory disease and an overall survival benefit (87.2% vs 82.5% with 38 months' median follow-up) in patients with newly diagnosed disease.[96,97] The results of these phase III trials led to FDA approval of rituximab with fludarabine and cyclophosphamide in CLL.

Combinations with alemtuzumab have also been studied. The combination of fludarabine and alemtuzumab achieved an overall response rate of 83% in heavily pretreated patients.[98] Patient selection is critical given the high risk of serious infection. Younger patients will be candidates for fludarabine-monoclonal antibody–based combination therapy. Symptomatic elderly patients with aggressive disease who can tolerate immunosuppressive therapy may also be candidates for this regimen.[76]

The novel combination of oxaliplatin, fludarabine, cytarabine, and rituximab was piloted in a phase I/II trial in 55 patients with either fludarabine-refractory CLL or Richter syndrome.[99] This regimen was developed on the basis of preclinical work that oxaliplatin produced synergistic cell kill when given with fludarabine plus cytarabine and that fludarabine administered prior to cytarabine increases the intracellular concentrations of the active metabolite of cytarabine, cytarabine triphosphate. The overall response rate and 6-month overall survival was 33% vs 50% and 59% vs 89% in fludarabine-refractory and Richter syndrome patients, respectively, with a median follow-up of 9 months. Virtually all patients developed neutropenia, anemia, thrombocytopenia, and fatigue with five treatment-related deaths reported.

■ HEMATOPOIETIC STEM CELL TRANSPLANTATION

9 There is limited experience with the use of HSCT in CLL. Patients treated with allogeneic HSCT achieve higher remission rates and appear to have a longer disease-free survival, but at the expense of high treatment-related mortality which approaches 40%. Contrary to the high mortality reported in most studies, a randomized phase II study of high-risk CLL patients comparing allogeneic and autologous HSCT reported 100-day mortality of 4% in both arms. After 6 years of follow-up, no difference in overall survival (58% autologous and 55% allogeneic) was observed.[100] This low early mortality must be interpreted carefully, given that only 25 carefully selected patients received allogeneic HSCT as compared with 137 who received autologous transplantation. T-cell depletion was performed on the allogeneic grafts, which may reduce 100-day mortality at the cost of increased relapse, infectious complications, or post-transplant lymphoproliferative disorders as a consequence of reduced GVL effect.[100]

Although allogeneic HSCT may offer the potential of cure in CLL, the advanced age of most patients, limited donor availability and the high treatment-related mortality precludes the routine application in the management of this disease. Allogeneic HSCT is a more viable option for younger patients with aggressive disease. Older patients who are not candidates for full-intensity allogeneic HSCT may be candidates for nonmyeloablative allogeneic HSCT.

EVALUATION OF THERAPEUTIC OUTCOMES

CLL is an incurable disease and the goal of therapy is to optimize remission duration while minimizing the burden of treatment-related adverse effects. The 2010 NCCN guidelines segregate treatment options based on the presence of 17p-, age older than 70 years, and first- and second-line regimens.[77] Preferred first-line therapy options for patients younger than 70 years without 17p- are aggressive chemoimmunotherapy regimens such as fludarabine, cyclophosphamide, rituximab; and pentostatin, cyclophosphamide, and rituximab. Patients who are older than 70 years without 17p- may be treated with chemotherapy (bendamustine, chlorambucil, and cyclophosphamide/vincristine/prednisone) or immunotherapy (rituximab) or milder chemoimmunotherapy (fludarabine/rituximab). Second-line therapeutic options for patients without 17p- are again divided by the age of 70 years. Regimens recommended for younger patients consist of chemoimmunotherapy (fludarabine/cyclophosphamide/rituximab, pentostatin/cyclophosphamide/rituximab, and oxaliplatin/fludarabine/cytarabine/rituximab) or traditional regimens used for aggressive non-Hodgkin lymphoma (cyclophosphamide/doxorubicin/vincristine/prednisone) with rituximab. For patients who have 17p-, first-line therapy options consist primarily of more aggressive chemoimmunotherapy (fludarabine/cyclophosphamide/rituximab) regimens. Second-line regimens are similar to those outlined above for patients younger than 70 years.

Supportive care for patients undergoing active treatment for CLL is crucial for ensuring a successful outcome. Patients may become hypogammaglobinemic as a consequence of disease progression or treatment will need routine monitoring of serum IgG. If the serum IgG falls below 500 mg/dL (5 g/L), then monthly replacement doses of 300 to 500 mg/kg of intravenous immune globulin is warranted. Antibiotic prophylaxis for patients receiving fludarabine-based regimens or chemoimmunotherapy should be considered for herpes virus and *Pneumocystis*. Patients that are treated with alemtuzumab will require monitoring for CMV antigen every 1 to 2 weeks while on therapy and for 2 months after or be given prophylaxis with valganciclovir.

TREATMENT SUMMARY OF CHRONIC LEUKEMIA

The treatments used for CML and CLL are strikingly different with tyrosine kinase inhibitors use expanding in CML and monoclonal antibodies, either with or without chemotherapy, playing an increasingly important role in CLL. Front-line treatment for CML is imatinib or one of the other second-generation tyrosine kinase inhibitors with second-line options including dasatinib, nilotinib, and allogeneic HSCT being selected on the basis of patient-specific factors. Allogeneic HSCT is distinguished among other therapies as the only known treatment intervention in CML that achieves long-term cure. IFN-α is now used sparingly for CML and can be considered a treatment option for patients who are intolerant of tyrosine kinase inhibitors without an HSCT option.

The goal in the treatment of CLL is to prospectively identify patients with poor prognostic features and individualize intensity of therapy based on the likelihood of rapid disease progression. Observation is appropriate in asymptomatic patients with early-stage disease. In patients with advanced disease, stratification by presence of 17p- and age will help to decide whether to initiate treatment with chemoimmunotherapy compared to chemotherapy or immunotherapy alone. Monitoring for hypogammaglobinemia and instituting appropriate infectious prophylaxis is critical to prevent the emergence of opportunistic infections during and for months following treatment.

ABBREVIATIONS

AP: accelerated phase

BC: blast crisis

CLL: chronic lymphocytic leukemia

CML: chronic myelogenous leukemia

CP: chronic phase

FCR: fludarabine, cyclophosphamide, rituximab

GVHD: graft-versus-host disease

GVL: graft-versus-leukemia (effect)

HLA: human leukocyte antigen

HSCT: hematopoietic stem cell transplantation

IgVH: immunoglobulin heavy chain gene

IFN-α: interferon alfa

IFN-α_{2a}: interferon alfa$_{2a}$

IFN-α_{2b}: interferon alfa$_{2b}$

IRIS: International Randomized study of Interferon vs STI571 trial

MBL: monoclonal B-cell lymphocytosis

NCCN: National Comprehensive Cancer Network

Ph: Philadelphia chromosome

RT-PCR: reverse transcriptase-polymerase chain reaction

WBC: white blood cell

ZAP-70: zeta-associated protein 70

REFERENCES

1. Jemal A, Siegel R, Xu J, Ward E, et al. Cancer statistics, 2010. CA Cancer J Clin 2010;60:277–300.
2. Ries LAG, Harkins D, Krapcho M, et al., eds. SEER Cancer Statistics Review, 1975-2006. Based on November 2008 SEER data submission. Bethesda, MD: National Cancer Institute; 2009. *http://seer.cancer.gov/csr/1975_2006/*.
3. Corso A, Lazzarino M, Morra E, et al. Chronic myelogenous leukemia and exposure to ionizing radiation—a retrospective study of 443 patients. Ann Hematol 1995;70:79–82.
4. Ichimaru M, Ishimaru T, Belsky JL. Incidence of leukemia in atomic bomb survivors belonging to a fixed cohort in Hiroshima and Nagasaki, 1950-71. Radiation dose, years after exposure, age at exposure, and type of leukemia. J Radiat Res (Tokyo) 1978;19:262–282.
5. Druker BJ. Translation of the Philadelphia chromosome into therapy for CML. Blood 2008;112:4808–4817.
6. Borgaonkar DS. Philadelphia-chromosome translocation and chronic myeloid leukaemia. Lancet 1973;1:1250.
7. Stam K, Heisterkamp N, Grosveld G, et al. Evidence of a new chimeric bcr/c-abl mRNA in patients with chronic myelocytic leukemia and the Philadelphia chromosome. N Engl J Med 1985;313:1429–1433.
8. Goldman JM, Melo JV. Chronic myeloid leukemia—Advances in biology and new approaches to treatment. N Engl J Med 2003;349:1451–1464.
9. Quintas-Cardama A, Cortes JE. Chronic myelogenous leukemia: Diagnosis and treatment. Mayo Clin Proc 2006;81:973–988.
10. Fialkow PJ, Jacobson RJ, Papayannopoulou T. Chronic myelocytic leukemia: clonal origin in a stem cell common to the granulocyte, erythrocyte, platelet, and monocyte/macrophage. Am J Med 1977;63:125–130.
11. Vardiman JW, Harris NL, Brunning RD. The World Health Organization (WHO) classification of myeloid neoplasms. Blood 2002;100:2292–2302.
12. Alvarez RH, Kantarjian H and Cortes JE. The biology of chronic myelogenous leukemia: Implications for imatinib therapy. Semin Hematol 2007;44(Suppl 1):S4–S14.
13. Sokal JE, Cox EB, Baccarani M, et al. Prognostic discrimination in "good-risk" chronic granulocytic leukemia. Blood 1984;63:789–799.
14. Cortes JE, Talpaz M, O'Brien S, et al. Staging of chronic myeloid leukemia in the imatinib era. Cancer 2006;106:1306–1315.
15. Druker BJ, Guilhot F, O'Brien S, et al. Five-year follow-up of patients receiving imatinib for chronic myelogenous leukemia. N Engl J Med 2006;355:2408–2417.
16. National Comprehensive Cancer Network. The NCCN Chronic Myelogenous Leukemia Clinical Practice Guideline (Version 2.2011). *http://www.nccn.org*.
17. Baccarani M, Pane F, Saglio G. Monitoring treatment for CML. Haematologica 2008;93:161–169.
18. Radich JP. How I monitor residual diseases in chronic myeloid leukemia. Blood 2009;114:3376–3381.
19. Hehlmann R, Heimpel H, Hasford J, et al. Randomized comparison of busulfan and hydroxyurea in chronic myelogenous leukemia: Prolongation of survival by hydroxyurea. The German CML Study Group. Blood 1993;82:398–407.
20. Deininger MWN, Druker BJ. Specific targeted therapy at chronic myelogenous leukemia with imatinib. Pharmacol Rev 2003;55:401–423.
21. Deininger M, Buchdunger E, Druker BJ. The development of imatinib as a therapeutic agent for chronic myeloid leukemia. Blood 2005;105:2640–2653.
22. O'Brien SG, Guilhot F, Larson RA, et al. Imatinib compared with interferon and low-dose cytarabine for newly diagnosed chronic-phase chronic myeloid leukemia. N Engl J Med 2003;348:994–1004
23. Kurzrock R, Kantarjian HM, Druker BJ, Talpaz M. Philadelphia chromosome-positive leukemias: From basic mechanisms to molecular therapeutics. Ann Intern Med 2003;138:819–830.
24. Druker BJ, Talpaz M, Resta DJ, et al. Efficacy and safety of a specific inhibitor of the *BCR-ABL* tyrosine kinase in chronic myeloid leukemia. N Engl J Med 2001;344:1031–1037.
25. Hochhaus A, O'Brien SG, Guilhot F, et al. Six-year follow-up of patients receiving imatinib for the first-line treatment of chronic myeloid leukemia. Leukemia 2009;23:1054–1061.
26. Hughes TP, Kaeda J, Branford S, et al. Frequency of major molecular responses to imatinib or interferon alfa plus cytarabine in newly diagnosed chronic myeloid leukemia. N Engl J Med 2003;349:1423–1432.
27. Press RD, Love Z, Tronnes AA, et al. *BCR-ABL* mRNA levels at and after the time of a complete cytogenetic response (CCR) predict the duration of CCR in imatinib mesylate-treated patients with CML. Blood 2006;107:4250–4256.
28. Baccarani M, Rosti G, Castagnetti F, et al. Comparison of imatinib 400mg and 800mg daily in the front-line treatment of high-risk, Philadelphia-positive chronic myeloid leukemia: a European LeukemiaNet study. Blood 2009;113:4497–4504.
29. Castagnetti F, Palandri F, Amabile M, et al. Results of high-dose imatinib mesylate in intermediate Sokal risk chronic myeloid leukemia in early chronic phase: a phase 2 trial of the GIMEMA CML Working Party. Blood 2009;113:3428–3434.
30. Talpaz M, Silver RT, Druker BJ, et al. Imatinib induces durable hematologic and cytogenetic responses in patients with accelerated phase chronic myeloid leukemia: Results of a phase 2 study. Blood 2002;99:1928–1937.
31. Amadori S, Picardi A, Fazi P, et al. A phase II study of VP-16, intermediate-dose Ara-C and carboplatin (VAC) in advanced acute myelogenous leukemia and blastic chronic myelogenous leukemia. Leukemia 1996;10:766–768.
32. Sawyers CL, Hochhaus A, Feldman E, et al. Imatinib induces hematologic and cytogenetic responses in patients with chronic myelogenous leukemia in myeloid blast crisis: results of a phase II study. Blood 2002;99:3530–3539.
33. Quintas-Cardama A, Cortes J. Molecular biology of bcr-abl1 positive chronic myeloid leukemia. Blood 2009;113:1619–1630.
34. Milojkovic D, Apperly J. Mechanisms of resistance to imatinib and second-generation tyrosine kinase inhibitors in chronic myeloid leukemia. Clin Cancer Res 2009;15:7519–7527.
35. Apperly JF. Part I: Mechanisms of resistance to imatinib in chronic myeloid leukemia. Lancet Oncol 2007;8:1018–1029.
36. Krause DS, Van Etten RA. Tyrosine kinases as targets for cancer therapy. N Engl J Med 2005;353:172–187.

37. Nelson RP, Cornetta K, Ward KE, Ramanaju S, Fausel C, Cripe L. Desensitization to imatinib in patients with leukemia. Ann Allergy Asthma Immunol 2006;97:216–222.

38. Talpaz M. Shah NP, Kantarjian H, et al. Dasatinib in imatinib-resistant Philadelphia chromosome-positive leukemias. N Engl J Med 2006;354:2531–2541.

39. Hochhaus A, Kantarjian HM, Baccarani M, et al. Dasatinib induces notable hematologic and cytogenetic responses in chronic-phase chronic myeloid leukemia after failure of imatinib therapy. Blood 2007;109:2303–2309.

40. Kantarjian HM, Pasquini R, Levy V, et al. Dasatinib or high-dose imatinib for chronic-phase chronic myeloid leukemia restant to imatinib at a dose of 400 to 600 milligrams daily. Cancer 2009;115:4136–4147.

41. Shah NP, Kantarjian HM, Kim DW, et al. Intermittent target inhibition with dasatinib 100 mg once daily preserves efficacy and improves tolerability in imatinib-resistant and –intolerant chronic-phase chronic myeloid leukemia. J Clin Oncol 2008;26:3204–3212.

42. Apperley JF, Cortes JE, Kim DW, et al. Dasatinib in the treatment of chronic myeloid leukemia in accelerated phase after imatinib failure: The START A trial. J Clin Oncol 2009;24:3472–3479.

43. Kantarjian HM, Cortes J, Kim DW, et al. Phase 3 study of dasatinib 140 mg once daily versus 70 mg twice daily in patients with chronic myeloid leukemia in accelerated phase resistant or intolerant to imatinib: 15-month median follow-up. Blood 2009;113:6322–6329.

44. Cortes J, Kim DW, Martinelli G, et al. Efficacy and safety of dasatinib in imatinib-resistant or –intolerant patients with chronic myeloid leukemia in blast phase. Leukemia 2008;22:2176–2183.

45. Kantarjian HM, Shah NP, Hochhaus A, et al. Dasatinib versus imatinib in newly diagnosed chronic phase chronic myeloid leukemia. N Engl J Med 2010;362:2260–2270.

46. Kantarjian HM, Giles F, Gattermann N, et al. Nilotinib (formerly AMN107), a highly selective BCR-ABL tyrosine kinase inhibitor, is effective in patients with Philadelphia chromosome-positive chronic myelogenous leukemia in chronic phase following imatinib resistance and intolerance. Blood 2007;110:3540–3546.

47. Le Coutre P, Ottmann OG, Giles F, et al. Nilotinib (formerly AMN107), a highly selective BCR-ABL tyrosine kinase inhibitor, is active in patients with imatinib-resistant or -intolerant accelerated phase chronic myelogenous leukemia. Blood 2008;111:1834–1839.

48. Saglio G, Kim DW, Issaragrisil S, et al. Nilotinib demonstrates superior efficacy compared with imatinib in patients with newly diagnosed Chronic Myeloid Leukemia in Chronic Phase: Results from the ENESTnd Trial. N Engl J Med 2010;362:2251–2259.

49. Garg RJ, Kantarjian H, O'Brien S, et al. The use of nilotinib or dasatinib after failure to two prior tyrosine kinase inhibitors (TKI): long-term follow-up. Blood 2009;114:4361–4368.

50. Michallet M, Maloisel F, Delain M, et al. Pegylated recombinant interferon alpha-2b vs recombinant interferon alpha-2b for the initial treatment of chronic-phase chronic myelogenous leukemia: A phase III study. Leukemia 2004;18:309–315.

51. Bukowski RM, Tendler C, Cutler C, et al. Treating cancer with PEG Intron. Cancer 2002;95:389–396.

52. Jonasch E, Haluska FG. Interferon in oncologic practice: Review of interferon biology, clinical applications and toxicities. Oncologist 2001;6:34–55.

53. Baccarani M, Martinelli G, Rosti G, et al. Imatinib and pegylated human recombinant interferon-a2b in early chronic-phase chronic myeloid leukemia. Blood 2004;104:4245–4251.

54. Gratwohl A, Brand R, Apperley J, et al. Allogeneic hematopoietic stem cell transplantation for chronic myeloid leukemia in Europe 2006: Transplant activity, long-term data and current results. An analysis by the Chronic Leukemia Working Party of the European Group for Blood and Marrow Transplantation (EBMT). Haematologica 2006;91:513–521.

55. van Rhee F, Szydlo RM, Hermans J, et al. Long-term results after allogenic bone marrow transplantation for chronic myelogenous leukemia in chronic phase: A report from the Chronic Leukemia Working Party of the European Group for Blood and Marrow Transplantation. Bone Marrow Transplant 1997;20:553–560.

56. Hehlmann R, Berger U, Pfirrmann M, et al. Drug treatment is superior to allografting as first-line therapy in chronic myeloid leukemia. Blood 2007;109:4686–4692.

57. Deininger M, Schleuning M, Greinix H, et al. The effect of prior exposure to imatinib on transplant-related mortality. Haematologica 2006;91:452–459.

58. Oehler VG, Gooley T, Snyder DS, et al. The effects of imatinib treatment with allogeneic transplant for chronic myelogenous leukemia. Blood 2007;109:1782–1789.

59. Porter D, Levine JE. Graft-versus host disease and graft-versus leukemia after donor leukocyte infusion. Semin Hematol 2006;43:53–61.

60. Raiola AM, Van Lint MT, Valbonesi M, et al. Factors predicting response and graft-versus-host disease after donor lymphocyte infusions: A study on 593 infusions. Bone Marrow Transplant 2003;31:687–693.

61. Dazzi F, Szydlo RM, Craddock C, et al. Comparison of single-dose and escalating-dose regimens of donor lymphocyte infusion for relapse after allografting for chronic myeloid leukemia. Blood 2000;95:67–71.

62. Hess G, Bunjes D, Siegert W, et al. Sustained complete molecular remissions after treatment with imatinib mesylate in patients with failure after allogeneic stem cell transplantation for chronic myelogenous leukemia: Results of a prospective phase II open label multicenter study. J Clin Oncol 2005;23:7583–7593.

63. Bacher U, Klyuchnikov E, Zabelina T, et al. The changing scene of allogeneic stem cell transplantation for chronic myeloid leukemia: a report from the German Registry covering the period from 1998-2004. Ann Hematol 2009;88:1237–1247.

64. Chiorazzi N, Rai KR, Ferarini M. Chronic lymphocytic leukemia. N Engl J Med 2005;352:804–815.

65. Landgren O, Albitar M, Ma W, et al. B-cell clones as early markers for chronic lymphocytic leukemia. N Engl J Med 2009;360:659–667.

66. Dohner H, Stilgenbauer S, Benner A, et al. Genetic aberrations and survival in chronic lymphocytic leukemia N Engl J Med 2000;343:1910–1916.

67. Tam CS, Shanafelt TD, Wierda WG, et al. De novo deletion of 17p13.1 chronic lymphocytic leukemia shows significant clinical heterogeneity: the MD Anderson and Mayo Clinic experience. Blood 2009;114:957–964.

68. Tsimberidou AS, O'Brien S, Khouri I, et al. Clinical outcomes and prognostic factors in patients with Richter's syndrome treated with chemotherapy or chemoimmunotherapy with or without stem cell transplantation. J Clin Oncol 2006;24:2343–2351.

69. Abbott BL. Chronic lymphocytic leukemia: Recent advances in diagnosis and treatment. Oncologist 2006;11:21–30.

70. Eisele L, Haddad T, Sellmann L, Durhsen U, Durig J. Expression of CD38 on leukemic B-cells but not on non-leukemic T-cells are comparably stable over time and predict the course of disease in chronic lymphocytic leukemia. Leuk Res 2009;33:775–778.

71. Vroblova V, Smolej L, Vrbacky F, et al. Biological prognostic markers in chronic lymphocytic leukemia. Acta Medica 2009;52:3–8.

72. Deaglio S, Vaisitti T, Aydin S, Ferrero E, Malavasi F. In-tandem insight from basic science combined with clinical research: CD38 as both marker and key component of the pathogenetic network underlying chronic lymphocytic leukemia. Blood 2006;108:1135–1144.

73. Rassenti LZ, Huynh L, Toy TL, et al. ZAP-70 compared with immunoglobulin heavy-chain gene mutation status as a predictor of disease progression in chronic lymphocytic leukemia. N Engl J Med 2004;351:893–901.

74. Orchard J, Ibbotson R, Best G, Parker A, Oscier D. ZAP-70 in B cell malignancies. Leuk Lymphoma 2005;46:1689–1698.

75. Zenz T, Mertens D, Kuppers R, Dohner H, Stilgenbauer S. From pathogenesis to treatment of chronic lymphocytic leukemia. Nat Rev Cancer 2010;10:37–50.

76. Shanafelt TD, Byrd JC, Call TG, Zent CS, Kay NE. Narrative review: Initial management of newly diagnosed, early-stage chronic lymphocytic leukemia. Ann Intern Med 2006;145:435–447.

77. National Comprehensive Cancer Network. The NCCN non-Hodgkin's Lymphoma Clinical Practice Guideline (Version 1.2010). http://www.nccn.org.

78. Chemotherapeutic options in chronic lymphocytic leukemia: A meta-analysis of the randomized trials. CLL Trialists' Collaborative Group. J Natl Cancer Inst 1999;91:861–868.

79. Lamanna N, Weiss MA. Purine analogue-based chemotherapy regimens for second-line therapy in patients with chronic lymphocytic leukemia. Semin Hematol 2006;43:S44-S49.

80. Gribben JG. How I treat CLL up front. Blood 2010;115:187–197.

81. Robak T, Blonski JZ, Kasznicki M, et al. Cladribine with or without prednisone in the treatment of previously treated and untreated B-cell chronic lymphocytic leukaemia—Updated results of the multicentre study of 378 patients. Br J Haematol 2000;108:357–368.

82. Sorensen JM, Vena DA, Fallavollita A, et al. Treatment of refractory chronic lymphocytic leukemia with fludarabine phosphate via the group C protocol mechanism of the National Cancer Institute: Five-year follow-up report. J Clin Oncol 1997;15:458–465.

83. Rai KR, Peterson BL, Appelbaum FR, et al. Fludarabine compared with chlorambucil as primary therapy for chronic lymphocytic leukemia. N Engl J Med 2000;343:1750–1757.

84. Eichhorst BF, Busch R, Schweighofer C, et al. Due to the low infection rates no routine anti-infective prophylaxis is required in younger patients with chronic lymphocytic leukemia during fludarabine-based first line therapy. Br J Haematol 2007;136:63–72.

85. Keating MJ, O'Brien S, Kontoyiannis D, et al. Results of first salvage therapy for patients refractory to a fludarabine regimen in chronic lymphocytic leukemia. Leuk Lymphoma 2002;43:1755–1762.

86. Cheson BD, Rummel MJ. Bendamustine: Rebirth of an old drug. J Clin Oncol 2009;27:1492–1501.

87. Knauf WU, Lissichkov T, Aldaoud A, et al. Phase III randomized study of bendamustine compared with chlorambucil in previously untreated patients with chronic lymphocytic leukemia. J Clin Oncol 2009;27:4378–4384.

88. Keating M, O'Brien S, Albitar M. Emerging information on the use of rituximab in chronic lymphocytic leukemia. Semin Oncol 2002;29(Suppl 2):70–74.

89. Hillmen P. Advancing therapy for chronic lymphocytic leukemia—The role of rituximab. Semin Oncol 2004;31(Suppl 2):22–26.

90. Ravandi F, O'Brien S. Alemtuzumab in CLL and other lymphoid neoplasms. Cancer Invest 2006;24:718–725.

91. Hillmen P, Skotnicki AB, Robak T, et al. Alemtuzumab compared with chlorambucil as first-line therapy for chronic lymphocytic leukemia. J Clin Oncol 2007;35:5616–5623.

92. Osterborg A, Karlsson C, Lundin J, Kimby E, Mellstedt H. Strategies in the management of alemtuzumab-related side effects. Semin Oncol 2006;33(Suppl 5):S29–S35.

93. Lundin J, Kimby E, Bjorkholm M, et al. Phase II trial of subcutaneous anti-CD52 monoclonal antibody alemtuzumab (Campath-1H) as first-line treatment for patients with B-cell chronic lymphocytic leukemia (B-CLL). Blood 2002;100:768–773.

94. Coiffier B, Leprette S, Pederson L, et al. Safety and efficacy of ofatumumab, a fully human monoclonal anti-CD20 in patients with relapsed or refractory B-cell chronic lymphocytic leukemia: a Phase I/II study. Blood 2008;111:1094–1100.

95. Keating MJ, O'Brien S, Albitar M, et al. Early results of a chemoimmunotherapy regimen of fludarabine, cyclophosphamide, and rituximab as initial therapy for chronic lymphocytic leukemia. J Clin Oncol 2005;23:4079–4088.

96. Robak T, Dmoszynska A, Solal-Céligny P, et al. Rituximab plus fludarabine and cyclophosphamide prolongs progression-free survival compared with fludarabine and cyclophosphamide alone in previously treated chronic lymphocytic leukemia. J Clin Oncol 2010;28:1756–1765.

97. German CLL Study Group. CLL8 survival results: First-line treatment with fludarabine, cyclophosphamide, and rituximab improves overall survival in previously untreated patients with advanced CLL: Results of a randomized phase III trial on behalf of an international group of investigators and the German CLL Study Group. Proc Am Soc Hematol 2009. Abstract 535.

98. Elter T, Borchmann P, Schulz H, et al. Fludarabine in combination with alemtuzumab is effective and feasible in patients with relapsed or refractory B-cell chronic lymphocytic leukemia: Results of a phase II trial. J Clin Oncol 2005;23:7024–7031.

99. Tsimerberidou AS, Wierda WG, Plunkett W, et al. Phase I-II study of oxaliplatin, fludarabine, cytarabine and rituximab combination therapy in patients with Richter's syndrome or fludarabine-refractory chronic lymphocytic leukemia. J Clin Oncol 2008;26:196–203.

100. Delgado J, Milligan DW, Dreger P. Allogeneic hematopoietic cell transplantation for chronic lymphocytic leukemia: ready for prime time? Blood 2009;114:2581–2588.

144

Multiple Myeloma

TIMOTHY R. MCGUIRE AND CASEY B. WILLIAMS

KEY CONCEPTS

❶ Multiple myeloma (MM) is a cancer that develops in plasma cells leading to excessive production of a monoclonal immunoglobulin (M protein).

❷ Most patients have skeletal involvement at the time of diagnosis with associated bone pain and fractures. Anemia, hypercalcemia, and renal failure may also be present. A bone marrow biopsy with 10% or more plasma cells and a M-protein spike on plasma or urine electrophoresis confirm the diagnosis.

❸ Most patients will require treatment after diagnosis but treatment can be deferred in patients with smoldering (asymptomatic) MM. In patients with symptomatic disease, treatment produces benefits in various measures of survival and quality of life.

❹ Thalidomide, lenalidomide, or bortezomib plus dexamethasone are commonly used induction regimens. They produce higher complete remission rates as compared with the classic regimen of melphalan plus prednisone and vincristine, doxorubicin, dexamethasone. The increased response is at the risk of significant grades III and IV toxicity which can include venous thromboembolism and neuropathy depending on the regimen used.

❺ Bortezomib is commonly used to treat relapsed MM and increasingly as initial therapy combined with dexamethasone or chemotherapy. Bortezomib activity is maintained in patients with high-risk cytogenetics.

❻ Lenalidomide is more potent and better tolerated than thalidomide and is becoming the most common drug used in induction regimens.

❼ Melphalan plus prednisone is not used in transplant candidates as part of induction but commonly used in transplant ineligible patients combined with thalidomide, lenalidomide, or bortezomib.

❽ Autologous hematopoietic stem cell transplantation (autoHSCT) is used after induction in patients with reasonably good performance status to maximize complete remissions and prolong survival.

❾ The quality of induction responses may be important, including in those receiving autoHSCT to maximize clinical benefit.

❿ The use of myeloablative allogeneic hematopoietic stem cell transplantation (alloHSCT) produces high early mortality, but the use of nonmyeloablative alloHSCT may offer a chance for long-term disease-free survival.

⓫ Bisphosphonates are used to treat bone disease associated with MM, which results in decreased pain and skeletal-related events and improvement in quality of life.

⓬ Salvage therapy for patients with relapsed or refractory MM can include any of the prior listed therapies, depending on performance status of the patient, risk category of the patient, and prior treatments used for induction.

Multiple myeloma (MM) is a relatively common hematologic malignancy that develops in plasma cells or immunoglobulin-producing B lymphocytes.[1,2] The plasma cells produce excessive monoclonal immunoglobulins that can be measured in the plasma or urine. Because of the various bone-mobilizing cytokines secreted from the MM clone and bone marrow stromal cells, patients often have skeletal involvement at diagnosis. MM is initially sensitive to chemotherapy but drug resistance develops relatively rapidly. Although therapy is not curative, several new agents have been developed that have improved the duration and quality of life of MM patients. Disease progression is influenced by cytokines and adhesion molecules which are part of an abnormal bone marrow microenvironment. Cytokines are able to stimulate plasma cell growth and angiogenesis. Several of these cytokines, including interleukin 6 (IL-6), basic fibroblast growth factor (bFGF), tumor necrosis factor alfa (TNF-α), and vascular endothelial growth factor (VEGF), have become targets for therapies such as thalidomide, its congener lenalidomide, and bortezomib.

EPIDEMIOLOGY AND ETIOLOGY

In the United States, it is estimated that 20,180 cases of MM will be diagnosed in 2010, with 10,650 deaths. It is a disease that affects older adults with a median age at diagnosis of 70 years. MM occurs more frequently in males and African Americans.[1–3]

No cause can be identified in most patients. Exposure to high doses of radiation increases the risk of developing MM.[1,2] Although not proven, there may be a hereditary component to MM, given the reports of familial associations. The relationship between viral infection and risk of MM is controversial. Human herpes virus 8 is often reported to be a likely candidate virus for development of MM.[1] However, investigators were unable to isolate human herpes virus 8 from patients with MM and it is unlikely that this virus is an etiologic agent in MM.[4] Patients with HIV-1 infections have 4.5 times the risk of developing MM, which suggests a role for HIV-1 as a viral cofactor. HIV-1–positive patients develop MM at an earlier age and with disease that has aggressive characteristics leading to poorer outcomes.[5]

PATHOPHYSIOLOGY

MM presents a very complex picture of multistep malignant transformation. A precursor condition called monoclonal gammopathy of undetermined significance (MGUS) is associated with monoclonal immunoglobulin in the blood (≤3 g/dL [≤30 g/L]) without clinical manifestations of the complications of MM.[6,7] The conversion rate of MGUS to MM is approximately 1% per year. The molecular changes associated with the conversion of MGUS to MM are not clear, but genome-wide studies have identified several candidate genes associated with disease progression.[8] Distinct from MGUS, which is a pre-malignant syndrome, smoldering MM is asymptomatic disease with low tumor burden and an indolent course.[1,9] In patients with smoldering MM, the risk of progression is approximately 10% per year for the first 5 years after diagnosis, approximately 3% per year for the next 5 years, and approximately 1% per year for the next 10 years.[9]

In early MM, the balance between apoptotic and antiapoptotic genes is disrupted with overexpression of antiapoptotic genes.[10] As the disease progresses, a greater number of gene products that confer resistance, such as mutated *p53*, are over expressed.[11] Molecules such as IL-6 and the transcriptional regulator nuclear factor kappa B (NF-κB) also stimulate clonal growth and promote resistance to therapy. Given their imprecise but important role in initiation and progression of MM, IL-6 and NF-κB are targets for both old and new therapies.[12,13]

❶ MM is characterized by the accumulation of malignant plasma cells in the bone marrow and the production of a monoclonal immunoglobulin (M protein). These proteins, secreted by the malignant clone, are frequently referred to as paraproteins.[1,2] Both MM and normal plasma cells are produced from differentiated B cells after antigen stimulation. Normal plasma cells will die within days to weeks after differentiation, whereas MM plasma cells are immortalized.[1,2] MM cells are seldom seen in large quantities in the peripheral blood because of their interaction with bone marrow stromal cells. This interaction between MM cells and bone marrow stroma is mediated by adhesion molecules within an abnormal bone marrow microenvironment and is required for growth and disease progression.[13] Figure 144–1 shows several of the factors involved in disease pathogenesis and progression and potential targets for the newer agents thalidomide, lenalidomide, and bortezomib.

One of the major targets for the newer therapies is NF-κB. The effects of NF-κB are pleiotropic and integral to MM progression. NF-κB is activated in MM and results in the production of MM growth factors such as IL-6 and adhesion molecules in the bone marrow. Thalidomide is a potent inhibitor of TNF-α, which is a cytokine with important NF-κB–inducing activity. Thalidomide also directly inhibits NF-κB by conserving the inhibitor of NF-κB (IκB) in the cytosol. Lenalidomide has similar mechanisms of action as thalidomide but is significantly more potent. Thalidomide and lenalidomide also activate important antimyeloma immune responses. Bortezomib is the most specific of the NF-κB inhibitors. Through its inhibition of the protease complex, the proteasome, bortezomib prevents IκB degradation and terminates the NF-κB signal. Understanding the targets of these newer agents has led to a better understanding of the pathophysiology of MM.[13]

CLINICAL PRESENTATION

❷ Most patients with MM present with complaints of bone pain and fatigue at diagnosis. Approximately 10% to 20% of patients are asymptomatic at the time of diagnosis, and have what is called smoldering MM.[14,15] Most patients show evidence of end-organ damage at the time of diagnosis. Initial laboratory evaluation often reveals hypercalcemia, renal insufficiency, anemia, and abnormalities in various disease markers, such as albumin and β_2-microglobulin. Skeletal evaluation shows gross abnormalities in most patients. Bone scans show abnormalities that often include lytic lesions, osteoporosis, and fractures. This group of findings (hypercalcemia, renal insufficiency, anemia, and bone lesions) is often referred by the acronym CRAB.[6] A bone marrow biopsy with 10% or more plasma cells and an M-protein spike on plasma or urine electrophoresis confirms the diagnosis.[14] Immunofixation is more sensitive and identifies the M-protein isotype being secreted. In a minority of patients, no M protein can be detected in the plasma but is found in the urine, requiring that urine be examined as part of a complete diagnostic workup. Approximately 60% of patients will have intact monoclonal immunoglobulin G (IgG), 20% will have monoclonal IgA, and the remaining 20% will secrete only monoclonal light chains. Antibodies are composed of two light chains where antigen binds and two heavy chains. Light-chain immunoglobulin alone can be secreted by the MM clone. Free monoclonal light chains in the urine are called Bence Jones proteins because they were first described by Dr. Henry Bence Jones and are primarily responsible for MM-associated renal failure.[1,14] In addition, serum IgG light chain can be measured with an FLC assay (Freelite). This new assay may have certain advantages compared to serum protein and urine electrophoresis particularly increased sensitivity and light chain ratio which may add valuable information on likelihood of disease progression.[16]

As discussed above, the skeleton is involved at the time of diagnosis in most patients with MM.[17] The effects of MM on the skeleton result from abnormal production of cytokines including IL-1, IL-6, TNF-α, and the receptor for activation of NF-κB ligand (RANK-L). Bone disease is the net effect of the activation of osteoclasts and inhibition of osteoblastogenesis.[18] In addition, patients are frequently anemic from infiltration of the bone marrow with the MM clone and poor erythropoietin response. Patients can have clinically important hypercalcemia, which results from calcium mobilization from the bone. Renal failure can occur as a result of high protein load from the monoclonal protein secretion as well as dehydration.

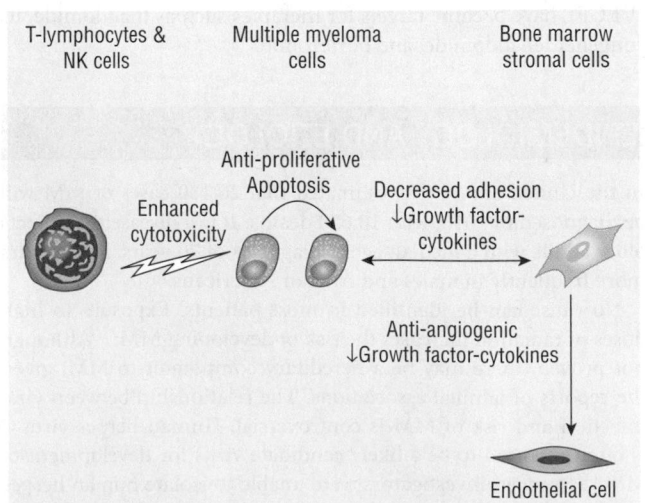

FIGURE 144-1. Sites of action for thalidomide, lenalidomide, and bortezomib.

CLINICAL PRESENTATION OF MULTIPLE MYELOMA

General Criteria
▪ 80% of patients present with symptomatic disease

Signs and Symptoms
▪ Bone pain (fractures, lytic lesions)
▪ Fatigue (anemia)
▪ Infection (reduced polyclonal response)
▪ Neurologic symptoms (nerve compression)
▪ Polyuria (hypercalcemia)
▪ Nausea and vomiting (hypercalcemia)

Laboratory Parameters
▪ Elevated paraproteins
  ▪ Plasma electrophoresis
  ▪ Urine electrophoresis
  ▪ Immunofixation
▪ Elevated serum creatinine
▪ Hypercalcemia
▪ Low hemoglobin
▪ Low albumin
▪ Elevated β_2-microglobulin
▪ Elevated C-reactive protein

Bone Marrow
▪ ≥10% plasma cells

Cytogenetics
▪ Chromosome 13 deletion
▪ Translocation (4;14)
▪ Del (17p)

TABLE 144-1 The International Staging System (ISS) for Multiple Myeloma

Stage	Characteristics	Median Survival (Months)
I	Serum β_2-microglobulin <3.5 mcg/mL (<3.5 mg/L) Serum albumin ≥3.5 g/dL (≥35 g/L)	62
II	Not stage I or stage III	44
III	Serum β_2-microglobulin ≥5.5 mcg/mL (≥5.5 mg/L)	29

From Greipp PR, Miguel JS, Durie BG, et al. International staging system for multiple myeloma. J Clin Oncol 2005;23:3412–3420.

including genetic damage (chromosome 13 deletion), proinflammatory changes (C-reactive protein), tumor load (β_2-microglobulin) and dysregulated cellular growth (labeling index and marrow microvessel density).

TREATMENT

■ OVERVIEW OF INITIAL THERAPY

❸ MM is not currently a curable disease. The role of therapy is to prolong progression-free and overall survival and improve quality of life. Patients with more active (symptomatic) or advanced disease (stages II and III) require therapy.[1,14,20] In patients with smoldering MM, watchful waiting is the general practice despite a systematic review that suggests early treatment with chemotherapy slows disease progression and may decrease vertebral compression.[21] These benefits are offset by the absence of convincing evidence that early treatment improves overall survival and important toxicities associated with therapy. The National Comprehensive Cancer Network (NCCN) guidelines recommend watchful waiting for smoldering MM.[14]

Initial management of symptomatic MM depends on the presence or absence of high-risk features of the disease (cytogenetics), patient age, renal function, performance status, and whether autoHSCT is planned. Although current treatments are not curative, median survival has increased significantly from about 7 months to 24 to 36 months, primarily as a result of improved treatment of symptomatic MM and supportive care.[1] There is no standard initial or induction therapy for the treatment of symptomatic MM. Table 144–2 lists commonly used regimens, which are categorized based on whether or not the patient is an autoHSCT candidate. The age restriction for autoHSCT has changed because of low transplant-related mortality, but autoHSCT is generally reserved for patients ≤65 years of age.

The choice of induction therapy in autoHSCT candidates include VAD (vincristine, doxorubicin, and dexamethasone) or VAD-like chemotherapy, dexamethasone combined with thalidomide, lenalidomide, or bortezomib, and bortezomib combined with lenalidomide or thalidomide and dexamethasone. The practice of using VAD chemotherapy prior to autoHSCT has become largely obsolete given data which suggest superior outcomes in those patients receiving newer drug combinations.[22,23] Melphalan should be avoided in patients who are eligible for autoHSCT because of its adverse effect on stem cell mobilization. When autoHSCT is not an option, melphalan plus prednisone has been an acceptable choice for induction therapy but now thalidomide (MPT) or bortezomib (MPB) is frequently added to the melphalan and prednisone backbone. Based on the results of randomized controlled trials that show significantly higher response rates and longer progression-free survival with MPT or MPB when compared with MP, these new combinations are listed as acceptable first-line therapies in the

STAGING AND PROGNOSTIC FACTORS

Some patients with MM are asymptomatic and have no evidence of end-organ damage at the time of diagnosis. These patients are categorized as having smoldering (asymptomatic) MM.[1,9] Most patients will have evidence of end-organ damage (hypercalcemia [>10.5 g/dL (>2.63 mmol/L)], renal impairment [>2.0 mg/dL (>177 μmol/L)], anemia [<10 g/dL (<100 g/L; 6.21 mmol/L) or >2 g/dL (>20 g/L; 1.24 mmol/L) below normal], or bone disease) at the time of diagnosis and are categorized as having active (symptomatic) disease. Patients with asymptomatic disease have an indolent course, with a median survival of approximately 5 years.[9]

The International Staging System (ISS) uses serum β_2-microglobulin and albumin concentrations to stage patients.[19] These two routine laboratory tests are powerful prognostic discriminators. The ISS predicts survival in patients treated with either conventional treatment or autologous hematopoietic stem cell transplantation (autoHSCT). An older staging system, Durie-Salmon, uses hemoglobin, serum calcium, bone involvement, and M protein to categorize patients in one of three stages. Table 144–1 describes the ISS and median survival for each of the three ISS stages.

Several adverse prognostic factors have been proposed for MM, including chromosome 13 deletion and other cytogenetic abnormalities, elevated β_2-microglobulin, elevated C-reactive protein, high plasma cell labeling index, low albumin, and high bone marrow microvessel density.[1] These prognostic factors generally represent the underlying pathologic changes associated with MM

TABLE 144-2 Drug Therapy in Newly Diagnosed Multiple Myeloma

Induction Regimen	Level of Evidence
Regimens in non-autoHSCT candidates	**Category**
Dexamethasone	2B
Vincristine + doxorubicin + dexamethasone (VAD)	2B
Lenalidomide + low-dose dexamethasone	1
Lipo doxorubicin/vincristine/dexamethasone (DVD)	2B
Thalidomide + dexamethasone	2B
Melphalan + prednisone (MP)	2A
Melphalan + prednisone + thalidomide (MPT)	1
Melphalan + prednisone + bortezomib (MPB)	1
Regimens in autoHSCT candidates	
Dexamethasone	2B
Thalidomide + dexamethasone	2B
Liposomal doxorubicin + vincristine + dexamethasone (DVD)	2B
Bortezomib + dexamethasone	1
Lenalidomide + dexamethasone	1
Bortezomib + doxorubicin + dexamethasone	1
Bortezomib + thalidomide + dexamethasone	1
Bortezomib + lenalidomide + dexamethasone	2B

Category 1: Uniform NCCN consensus based on high-level evidence.
Category 2A: Uniform NCCN consensus based on lower evidence, including clinical experience.
Category 2B: Nonuniform NCCN consensus but no major disagreement.
Data from NCCN Guidelines NCCN. Clinical Practice Guidelines in Oncology. Multiple myeloma (Version 1.2011). http://www.NCCN.org.

TABLE 144-3 Definition of Clinical Response in Multiple Myeloma

Type of Response	Definition[a]
Partial response (PR)	• ≥50% decrease in serum M protein
	• Reduction in 24-hour urine light chain by ≥90%
Very good partial remission (vgPR)	• Serum and urine M protein detected on immunofixation but not electrophoresis
Complete remission (CR)	• Negative immunofixation on serum and urine
	• No soft-tissue plasmacytomas
Stringent complete response	• <5% plasma cells in the bone marrow
	• CR definition
	• Normal free light chain ratio
	• Absence of clonal cells in the bone marrow

[a]Maintained for a minimum of 6 weeks.

NCCN guidelines (category 1 evidence). In addition, lenalidomide plus low-dose dexamethasone has been given a category 1 recommendation based on a phase III study showing high response rates and acceptable toxicity in MM patients, including some who were too old to receive autoHSCT.[14,20]

Clinical response to therapy is generally defined by a reduction in paraprotein in blood and urine.[1] Clinical complete response is defined as elimination of plasma paraprotein, as measured by electrophoresis and immunofixation, and plasma cells (≤5%) in the bone marrow. A specialized type of complete remission (CR), called stringent CR, is defined by negative-free light chain and immunofixation. Complete remissions are uncommon in MM and lesser responses, including, partial response (PR), near complete response (nCR), and very good partial response (vgPR), are more commonly attained. While the nCR term is less commonly used in current trials, it was used in several important studies. These lesser responses can be important because they may correlate with improved survival. Table 144–3 describes the most common types of responses that are used clinically.[14]

■ DRUGS USED IN THE MANAGEMENT OF MULTIPLE MYELOMA

Conventional Chemotherapy

Two of the common conventional chemotherapy regimens used historically to treat MM are melphalan plus prednisone (MP) and VAD.[1,2] Despite more active combinations, MP and VAD remain listed as options as initial therapy in patients with MM.[14] Since conventional-dose melphalan has an adverse effect on stem cell mobilization and subsequent autoHSCT, the use of melphalan is limited to patients ineligible for autoHSCT. Melphalan may also lead to the development of myelodysplastic syndrome.[24] The use of VAD chemotherapy as initial treatment became more common because of these concerns with melphalan. However, the slightly higher response rates with VAD and similar combination chemotherapy did not translate into improved survival as compared with MP, and VAD is now rarely used in MM.[25]

Dexamethasone accounts for most of the antimyeloma activity of VAD (Table 144–4), which led to the use of dexamethasone alone as initial therapy. However, one study reported that MP produced similar response rates and survival as compared to dexamethasone. The higher rate of infection and CNS toxicity in patients treated with dexamethasone led these investigators to conclude that high-dose dexamethasone be used with caution as initial therapy, particularly in older patients who are not eligible for autoHSCT and who would usually receive MP.[26] Increasingly, patients receive newer agents (thalidomide, bortezomib, lenalidomide) combined with dexamethasone or the MP backbone to maximize initial response rates.[27]

Thalidomide (Thalomid®)

Thalidomide was first used clinically in Europe in the late 1950s as a sedative and antiemetic but its use was largely abandoned when teratogenicity was reported. Its immunomodulatory effects became evident with its use in Hansen disease (or leprosy), and it continues to be used for this rare indication. These clinical benefits are thought to be related to the anti-TNF activity of thalidomide. Because of the role of inflammatory cytokines in the pathophysiology of MM, thalidomide was first studied in refractory MM in 1999. The observation that thalidomide had activity against myeloma rejuvenated it as an important therapeutic agent.[28]

Thalidomide has multiple immune effects including inhibition of inflammatory mediators, antiangiogenic activity, and T-cell modulating activity.[29] Thalidomide destabilizes TNF-α messenger RNA, which leads to increased destruction of the transcripts and reduction in TNF-α production. One potential explanation for thalidomide's antimyeloma activity is inhibition of TNF-mediated NF-κB activation, which results in increased apoptosis of the MM clone. Thalidomide also has TNF-independent effects on NFκB; it protects the cytosolic inhibitor of NFκB (IκB) and prevents signal transduction to the nucleus, resulting in a decline in MM growth factors.[28,29]

Myeloma bone marrow has a high rate of neovascularization, which makes it susceptible to antiangiogenic therapy. Bone marrow microvessel density has been identified as an independent prognostic factor in MM.[30] One explanation for the angiogenesis that occurs in MM is the paracrine release of TNF-α by the myeloma clone and bone marrow stromal cells, which leads to the release of angiogenic factors, including VEGF, IL-8, bFGF, and IL-1, through NF-κB induction. Thalidomide treatment can reduce bone marrow microvessel density, which may contribute to its antimyeloma activity.

The role of TNF-α inhibition is supported by the observation that TNF-α polymorphisms may predict for thalidomide response in patients with MM.[31] High producers of TNF-α had significantly higher response rates and improved survival with thalidomide therapy as compared to patients without the hypersecretory phenotype. These results may be explained by inhibition of TNF-α as

TABLE 144-4	Initial Therapies for Multiple Myeloma		
	Type of Response (%)		
Regimen	**OR**	**CR**	**CR + nCR or VgPR**
Melphalan + prednisone[26,37–39]	40–50	1–2	5–10
Dexamethasone[26,36]	40–50	1	
Thalidomide[34]	34–40		
Thalidomide + dexamethasone[34,35]	50–70	5	
Melphalan, prednisone, and thalidomide[34,37–39]	70–80	15–30	20–40
VAD chemotherapy[64,67]	50–60		
Doxorubicin combinations + thalidomide[35,40]	70–90	10–30	40–50
Single autoHSCT[63,67]	80–90	10–40	40–50
Tandem autoHSCT[74–76]	80–90	20–40	30–50
AutoHSCT followed by RI-alloHSCT[88–90]	80–90	50–60	60
Bortezomib[50]	40–50	3	12
Bortezomib + dexamethasone[50,51]	80–90	5–20	20–30
Bortezomib + chemotherapy[52,53]	89	32	43
Lenalidomide + dexamethasone[57–59]	90	6	38
Lenalidomide + chemotherapy[60,61]	85	17	41

alloHSCT, allogeneic hematopoietic stem cell transplantation; autoHSCT, autologous hematopoietic stem cell transplantation; CR, complete response; OR, overall response (at least PR); RI, reduced intensity; VAD, vincristine, doxorubicin, and dexamethasone.

a required growth factor in patients with the TNF-α hypersecretory phenotype. The authors commented that larger studies are required to confirm and explain these results. Figure 144–1 shows that thalidomide inhibits proliferation and angiogenesis, stimulates T lymphocytes, and modifies the cytokine-secreting ability of bone marrow stromal cells.

Single-agent thalidomide has been extensively evaluated in refractory MM where it produces overall response rates (includes minor responses) in about 30% of patients.[32] Although minor and partial responses are the most common types of responses, these endpoints result in improvement in survival.[33]

❹ With the activity of thalidomide in refractory MM established, subsequent studies evaluated its activity in newly diagnosed patients and in combination with other therapies, including dexamethasone and chemotherapy. Partial response rates with single-agent thalidomide in untreated patients are approximately 30% to 40%.[34] When dexamethasone is added to thalidomide in untreated patients, response rates (≥PR) increase to approximately 70% to 80%.[35] The higher response rate with thalidomide plus dexamethasone makes this an attractive combination for initial therapy. However, the higher rate of thromboembolism with this combination (15%–20%) when used in newly diagnosed patients is a concern.[35,36]

The addition of thalidomide to chemotherapy also increases response rates (Table 144–4). Two published randomized controlled trials in newly diagnosed MM showed that the addition of thalidomide to MP improved response.[37,38] In the first randomized trial, the overall complete response rate with MPT was about 15% as compared to 4% with MP. With a median follow-up of about 3 years, patients in the MPT group had significantly improved progression-free survival but not overall survival.[37] The second randomized trial was stopped early because MPT showed clear improvements over the other treatment arms. Results of that trial also showed significantly improved median progression-free (27.5 vs 17.8 months) and overall survival (51.6 vs 33.2 months) with MPT.[38] A third trial was recently published where MPT was compared with MP in patients older than 75 years of age. Patients on MPT had superior progression-free and overall survival at the cost of increased peripheral neuropathy and neutropenia.[39] Based on these impressive results, some have recommended that MPT be the new standard induction therapy in older patients ineligible for

autoHSCT. However, it is not possible to define a single standard regimen in this setting because of the number of highly active combination regimens and the lack of head-to-head comparative trials. The increased response rate of MPT is at the expense of higher rates of grades III and IV toxicity, particularly venous thromboembolism (VTE), peripheral neuropathy, and infection.[38,39]

The combination of thalidomide, dexamethasone, and pegylated liposomal doxorubicin produces a high overall response rate of 98% and a complete remission rate of 34%. The major grades III and IV toxicities were VTE (14%) and infection (22%). Toxicity was acceptable, even in patients older than 65 years of age.[40] Although the activity of doxorubicin plus thalidomide compares favorably with other combinations, one disadvantage of this regimen is that pegylated liposomal doxorubicin requires intravenous administration. The high response rate of thalidomide plus pegylated liposomal doxorubicin combinations needs to be confirmed in a randomized trial that compares it with an accepted standard.

Thalidomide dose correlates with response and toxicity. In one large trial of single-agent thalidomide, a higher response rate was observed when more than 42 g of thalidomide was administered over a 3-month period, which is equivalent to a daily dose of about 450 mg.[33] As expected, the higher dose was associated with higher rates of thalidomide-related toxicity. When thalidomide is combined with chemotherapy, thalidomide doses of 100 mg/day are associated with high complete remission rates.[37,40] Neuropathy, one of the important dose-limiting toxicities, may correlate with cumulative thalidomide doses. Thalidomide-induced neuropathy is usually, but not always, reversible and is associated with demyelinating changes in peripheral neurons. Approximately 10% to 20% of patients are unable to tolerate thalidomide and neuropathy is often the toxicity associated with discontinuation of therapy.[33,39] Unfortunately, no effective methods have been identified to prevent or treat thalidomide-induced neuropathy.

Other common toxicities associated with thalidomide include constipation, sedation, and rash. While these toxicities can be problematic, they rarely require discontinuation of thalidomide treatment. Stimulant laxatives can be used to prevent severe constipation. The severity of constipation and sedation declines over time in many patients.[41]

The rate of VTE with single-agent thalidomide is relatively low (<5%) and may not exceed the baseline incidence for MM patients. VTE prophylaxis is not recommended in patients receiving single-agent thalidomide.[42] When thalidomide is combined with dexamethasone, MP, or doxorubicin, the risk of thrombosis is elevated. The underlying mechanism for thrombosis in these patients is unknown but rates in several studies of combination therapy were as high as 10% to 30%.[37–39,43] VTE prophylaxis is recommended and preventive strategies include therapeutic doses of warfarin or low-molecular-weight heparin (LMWH). Warfarin is associated with bleeding complications particularly in patients with thrombocytopenia and should be reserved for patients unable to adhere to LMWH therapy.[43] Aspirin (81 mg or 325 mg) may be beneficial in preventing thrombosis, but large, well-controlled studies are required. Aspirin should be reserved for those patients at high risk of bleeding on warfarin or LMWH and low-to-moderate risk of developing VTE.[43,44]

Bortezomib (Velcade®)

❺ Bortezomib is a proteasome inhibitor approved for use in newly diagnosed and relapse/refractory MM. The proteasome is a protease complex responsible for degrading cytosolic proteins that are conjugated to ubiquitin. Ubiquitin is a 8.5-kilodalton polypeptide that tags various proteins for destruction.[45] By reversibly binding to the chymotrypsin site in the catalytic core of the 26S proteasome, bortezomib inhibits the degradation of these targeted proteins.

In MM, NF-κB activity is increased, resulting in increased transcription of inflammatory cytokines such as IL-6 and TNF-α, which are involved in the pathogenesis and progression of MM. In the cytosol, NF-κB is bound to and inhibited by IκB. The proteasome degrades IκB. When the proteasome is inhibited with bortezomib, cytosolic concentrations of IκB remain high and NF-κB is retained in the cytosol as an inactive complex. The resulting inhibition of the NF-κB signal leads to a reduction in cytokine production and growth inhibition of the MM clone. Other proteins involved in cell-cycle regulation and apoptotic signaling that may be affected by bortezomib include p53, JNK proteins, and capase 3.[45]

In phase I studies in patients with refractory hematologic malignancies, bortezomib was administered twice weekly for two consecutive weeks followed by a week of rest. The responses observed in those studies included a complete response in 1 of 8 patients who completed the first course of therapy and minor responses in two patients. These responses were impressive for a phase I trial and confirmed the promising activity in preclinical studies.[46]

Patients with refractory MM were then enrolled into a phase II trial and received 1.3 mg/m^2 of bortezomib twice weekly for 2 weeks followed by a week of rest. Patients received up to eight cycles. The overall response rate was 35% (includes minor responses) with 7 (3.6%) patients achieving a complete response.[47] Based on the phase I and II studies, bortezomib was approved in May 2003 under the FDA's accelerated approval process for relapsed or refractory MM in patients who had failed at least two prior therapies.

Subsequently, a large phase III study (Assessment of Proteasome Inhibition for Extending Remissions [APEX] trial) demonstrated that bortezomib had superior activity as compared with high-dose dexamethasone in relapsed MM.[48] Bortezomib-treated patients had higher complete and partial response rates (38% vs 18%), longer median time-to-progression (6.2 vs 3.5 months), and improved 1-year overall survival (80% vs 66%) as compared to patients receiving dexamethasone. The differences in each of these endpoints were statistically significant. The results from this study led to expanded FDA approval in 2005 to include patients who had relapsed after one therapy.

Combination therapy with bortezomib has shown promising results in relapsed MM. It was reported that relapsed patients who had suboptimal response to bortezomib alone may respond after the addition of dexamethasone. Subsequent studies reported improved results with the combination of bortezomib and corticosteroids with the complete and nCR rate ranging between 5% and 15%.[49] The inclusion of bortezomib in three to four drug combinations which may include doxorubicin, melphalan, thalidomide, and lenalidomide produce CR and nCR rates of 10% to 50% in relapsed MM.[45,49]

There are a number of studies investigating bortezomib in newly diagnosed patients (Table 144–4). Bortezomib alone produces about a 40% response rate (complete remission plus partial response) with approximately 3% of patients obtaining a complete remission. When combined with dexamethasone, the overall response rate increases to approximately 90% (complete remission plus partial response) with complete remissions of 5% to 20%.[50,51] In a phase II study of bortezomib combined with MP (MPB) in newly diagnosed elderly MM patients, the overall response rates of 89% and complete remission rates of 32% are among the highest reported with induction therapies.[52] Subsequently MPB was compared with MP in the large phase III VISTA (Velcade as Initial Standard Therapy in multiple myeloma) trial. The overall response and CR rates, time-to-progression, and overall survival were significantly better in the MPB group. Based on these results, bortezomib received FDA approval in 2008 as first-line therapy in newly diagnosed patients with MM. The improvement in response came at the expense of greater serious adverse effects including neuropathy, gastrointestinal toxicity,

and herpes zoster. However, treatment-related mortality was not different between MPB and MP groups.[53]

Bortezomib can cause significant toxicity the most common being mild-to-moderate fatigue and gastrointestinal toxicities. Neuropathy occurs frequently and is the most common cause for discontinuation of therapy. In the VISTA trial, the rate of neuropathy was 44% in the MPB group vs 5% in the MP group.[53] However, MPB and MP groups had similar rates of therapy discontinuation at about 15%. Other important toxicities included thrombocytopenia, fever, neutropenia, and infection. An increased risk of shingles has been reported in bortezomib-treated patients, and the NCCN guidelines recommend that herpes zoster prophylaxis be considered.[14] VTE prophylaxis is not required with bortezomib when it is combined with MP, based on the results of the VISTA trial which reported low rates of VTE and nearly identical rates in the MPB versus MP group.[53]

Lenalidomide (Revlimid®)

6 Lenalidomide is a thalidomide analog that shares a similar mechanism of action with thalidomide, but is significantly more potent than thalidomide. Because of differences in the toxicity profile, the use of lenalidomide is likely to increase. In phase I studies, patients with relapsed, refractory MM were found to have a maximum tolerated dose of lenalidomide of 25 mg/day and this dose was the most commonly used dose in subsequent phase II and III studies.[54]

The addition of lenalidomide to high-dose dexamethasone has been shown to increase response rate and prolong survival in patients with relapsed MM. In 2006, lenalidomide received FDA approval in relapsed-refractory MM based on the results of two recently published randomized controlled trials.[55,56] One trial was conducted in North America while the other trial was conducted outside of North America. In both trials, patients were randomized to receive a combination of either lenalidomide (25 mg/day on days 1 to 21 of a 28-day cycle) and high-dose dexamethasone or an identical lenalidomide placebo and high-dose dexamethasone. In the North American trial, patients in the lenalidomide and dexamethasone group had overall (complete, near-complete, or partial) and complete response rates of 61% and 14%, as compared with 20% and 0.6% in the dexamethasone alone group (P <0.001).[55] These improved response rates translated into longer median overall survival in the lenalidomide and dexamethasone group (29.6 vs 20.5 months). Similar results were reported in the trial conducted outside of the United States.[56]

Lenalidomide has been studied as initial therapy in newly diagnosed MM (Table 144–4). Preliminary results of phase I and phase II studies of lenalidomide plus dexamethasone report an overall response rate of 90% and a complete response rate of 18%.[41,57] These rates may be higher than those reported with thalidomide plus dexamethasone. Lenalidomide causes less neurotoxicity and constipation but more myelosuppression than thalidomide.[42,58] When used as part of combination therapy, the risk of VTE with lenalidomide is similar to that observed with thalidomide and VTE prophylaxis is recommended. Results from a phase III trial in newly diagnosed MM reported that patients randomized to lenalidomide plus high-dose dexamethasone had a 26% incidence of VTE as compared with a 12% rate in those randomized to the lenalidomide plus low-dose dexamethasone arm.[59] That trial also reported a superior 2-year overall survival in the lenalidomide plus low-dose dexamethasone group (87% vs 75%) and this regimen could become the new standard induction regimen for older patients ineligible for autoHSCT. The improved survival in the low-dose dexamethasone arm comes from a lower mortality from adverse events, particularly VTE. Excess deaths in the high-dose dexamethasone group usually occurred in the first 4 months and in elderly patients. The low risk of VTE in the lenalidomide plus low-dose dexamethasone arm may allow for VTE prophylaxis with aspirin alone.[59] These results have led to a category 1 NCCN recommendation. A reasonable strategy is to use high-dose dexamethasone plus lenalidomide in younger patients who are transplant candidates and use low-dose dexamethasone plus lenalidomide in older patients ineligible for transplant.[14]

Summary of Newer Therapy Combinations as Initial Therapy

7 In patients ineligible for autoHSCT, thalidomide, lenalidomide, or bortezomib is being added to chemotherapy as initial therapy. MP can be the backbone to which these newer drugs are added if the patient is not a candidate for autoHSCT. As previously discussed, MPT produces high response rates and bortezomib added to MP (MPB) produces similar results.[37,38] Based on the results of phase III trials demonstrating superiority of MPT over MP, many experts suggested that MPT was the preferred induction regimen in patients who are ineligible for autoHSCT. However, the results of the recently published VISTA trial support the addition of MPB as another preferred induction regimen. Both MPB and MPT are listed as NCCN category 1 recommendations.[53,14] MPB may be particularly useful in MM patients with high-risk cytogenetics (chromosome 13 deletion, t(4;14), and 17p-).

A phase II study has reported good activity with MP combined with lenalidomide (MPR) in newly diagnosed patients.[60] Results from randomized controlled trials for MP combined with lenalidomide are not available in full form but a recent abstract of a phase III study demonstrated superiority of MPR over MP alone.[61] The preferred combination (MPT, MPB, or MPR) is currently unclear and will require head-to-head comparisons between these combinations.

If autoHSCT is planned after induction therapy, melphalan should be avoided, and thalidomide, bortezomib, or lenalidomide can be added to dexamethasone or VAD-like chemotherapy. The NCCN guidelines lists several induction therapies (Table 144–2). Because there is no standard induction regimen, clinicians can select from a wide range of possible induction regimens. Many clinicians recommend lenalidomide and dexamethasone or bortezomib, lenalidomide, and dexamethasone in patients who are autoHSCT candidates. Patients with chromosome 13 or 17p deletion, which are adverse prognostic factors, may benefit from bortezomib-containing induction regimens because of its activity in these high-risk patients.[20,14] Because patients with high-risk cytogenetics may have poorer outcomes after autoHSCT, bortezomib-containing regimens should be considered in this group of patients, regardless of their eligibility for autoHSCT.[20,14]

CLINICAL CONTROVERSY

For patients who are autoHSCT candidates, induction therapy has historically involved the administration of four months of VAD. High-dose dexamethasone alone was also an option, given that most of the activity of VAD resides with dexamethasone. Newer agents, such as thalidomide, bortezomib, or lenalidomide combined with dexamethasone are now routinely used as induction therapy. There is growing evidence that the higher response rates associated with these newer regimens improve outcomes in patients undergoing autoHSCT. There is no standard choice for induction and choices are made based on individual characteristics of the patient. For example, a patient with high-risk cytogenetics may benefit from a bortezomib-containing induction regimen and may not respond as well to thalidomide-based therapy. Lenalidomide may remain an option in patients with high risk cytogenetics

but may also negatively effect stem cell collections. This has led to recommendations that lenalidomide induction be limited to four months to reduce the chance of this negative effect on stem cell mobilization an effect not seen with thalidomide or bortezomib. Patients with renal dysfunction, a relatively common diagnosis in myeloma patients, require dose adjustment of lenalidomide to avoid severe myelosuppression. To better guide the selection of induction prior to autoHSCT studies need to be performed on the above described subgroups.

■ AUTOLOGOUS HEMATOPOIETIC STEM CELL TRANSPLANTATION

Although MM is a chemosensitive tumor with significant response rates after treatment with conventional chemotherapy, complete remission rates have historically been low and response durations have been short. In an attempt to improve outcomes with chemotherapy, high-dose chemotherapy regimens with stem cell support have been used after initial induction therapy. The intent of the induction therapy prior to transplant is to reduce tumor load. With the newer combinations being used as induction, high rates of quality responses (CR, VgPR) can be obtained and recent data suggest that obtaining quality responses during induction improves the outcomes associated with autoHSCT.[62]

8 Several well-designed, randomized, controlled trials have evaluated the role of high-dose chemotherapy followed by autoHSCT. In these trials, previously untreated patients were randomized to induction therapy alone versus the same induction therapy followed by high-dose chemotherapy and autoHSCT. The results generally showed that autoHSCT improved progression-free survival with a more variable effect on overall survival.[63–65] No survival plateau was observed in the group treated with autoHSCT, which suggests that few, if any, patients are cured of their disease. Despite these variable effects on overall survival, MM has become the leading indication for autoHSCT worldwide.

A systematic review of autoHSCT in newly diagnosed MM was published in 2007.[65] The review pooled results from nine studies comprising 2,411 patients randomized to either autoHSCT or standard dose chemotherapy. The combined hazard ratio for overall survival with autoHSCT was 0.92 (95% confidence interval [CI], 0.74-1.13) and for progression-free survival was 0.75 (95% CI, 0.59-0.96). These results indicate that high-dose therapy with autoHSCT significantly improves progression-free survival but does not significantly improve overall survival. This benefit in progression-free survival was at the risk of greater transplant-related mortality. Patients who received autoHSCT had a 3-fold higher risk of treatment-related death as compared to conventional dose chemotherapy. The authors concluded that for every 26 patients who received a transplant, there would be one excess death from autoHSCT as compared to conventional chemotherapy. It should be noted that these trials used an induction of VAD or VAD-like chemotherapy which is inferior to the modern induction therapies described previously.

Two of the randomized trials comparing autoHSCT to standard therapy in newly diagnosed MM included in the systematic review were updated and illustrates the divergent results seen with autoHSCT. Barlogie et al. reported that progression-free and overall survival were equivalent between high-dose and conventional-dose groups.[66] This is different than the conclusions of the systematic review, which reported a significant improvement in progression-free survival. The Barlogie study has been criticized for using total-body irradiation plus melphalan rather than the more commonly used high-dose melphalan alone. However, several other studies that used total-body irradiation in addition to melphalan have reported variable results, which suggest that the differences in the preparative regimen do not fully explain these negative results. In the second updated study, Fermand et al. reported a benefit in event-free survival but no benefit in overall survival. These results were consistent with the systematic review. This study used standard high-dose melphalan and compared it with conventional therapy in previously untreated patients.[67]

Although the use of autoHSCT as consolidation therapy has become standard of care in patients younger than age 65 years, it is associated with higher treatment-related mortality and there is no convincing evidence that it improves overall survival. The widespread adoption of autoHSCT as standard therapy is related to the significant improvement in progression-free survival. But as conventional therapy continues to improve, response rates and progression-free survival are likely to approach those seen with autoHSCT without the low but present elevated risk of transplant-related mortality.

The role of autoHSCT as consolidation therapy has been questioned because newer combinations such as lenalidomide plus dexamethasone produce results similar to transplantation without the risk of mortality. However, many investigators believe that the use of autoHSCT as a scheduled sequential therapy after induction therapy, even in those patients who achieve a CR, is a logical next step in the evolving approach to treating MM. This controversy will continue until the results of several ongoing trials comparing these new combinations to autoHSCT have been completed.[68]

9 Preliminary results have shown that induction regimens containing at least one of the novel agents can make a significant difference in outcomes after autoHSCT. Also the use of these novel agents in induction may reduce the number of patients who require a second transplant because of the higher proportion of patients achieving major responses (CR, nCR, or VgPR) after the combination of novel induction regimen and the first transplant. A randomized phase III trial performed by the French group compared bortezomib in combination with dexamethasone with VAD as induction prior to autoHSCT.[69] Patients were randomized to one of four arms which included either bortezomib plus dexamethasone or VAD. All arms underwent autoHSCT with melphalan preparation (200 mg/m[2]). Post-induction CR/nCR rates were 15% in the bortezomib-containing arms as compared to 6% in those receiving VAD. The progression-free survival was superior in the patients where autoHSCT was preceded by bortezomib plus dexamethasone induction. Also, the proportion of patients requiring a second transplant was significantly lower in the bortezomib plus dexamethasone arm due to the higher rates of acquiring at least a VgPR in the bortezomib plus dexamethasone group.

Most patients are treated with autoHSCT as consolidation therapy after a short course of induction chemotherapy. However, a smaller number of patients receive autoHSCT as salvage therapy after patients have failed conventional treatments. A study in the early 1990s compared autoHSCT with chemotherapy in previously treated MM patients.[70] The results of that study showed that high-dose therapy was no better then VAD alone. However, more recent studies report benefit from autoHSCT in both primary treatment failures and relapsed MM.[71,72] The NCCN guidelines list autoHSCT as one of the acceptable options in the salvage setting. Responses to autoHSCT in the salvage setting can occur even in patients who have relapsed after prior successful autoHSCT.[14]

The optimal timing of autoHSCT (early vs late) in MM was investigated in a randomized controlled trial. Patients were randomized to early (n = 91) or late transplantation (n = 94) and no significant difference in 5-year overall survival was observed between the groups.[73] Event-free survival, however, was significantly longer in the early transplantation group (39 months vs 13 months). In an analysis that factors in the time without symptoms, treatment, or treatment toxicity (TWisTT), patients receiving early transplantation had a longer time in a state associated with good quality of life (27.8 vs 22.3 months). The results of this study support early autoHSCT because of its effects on event-free survival and quality of life. The often long period of disease response after autoHSCT without ongoing treatment must be considered as newer combinations are considered as upfront therapy to replace autoHSCT. While these new combinations may produce equivalent responses, they require prolonged treatment which may lead to decline in quality of life and can make these therapies more expensive than autoHSCT.

A specialized form of autoHSCT, tandem transplantation, involves the use of two separate autoHSCT procedures separated by a rest period of several months. In a recent meta-analysis, six randomized controlled trials (N = 1,803) were included and the authors concluded that while overall response was superior with tandem transplant, overall survival was not superior compared to single transplant. Higher transplant related mortality was observed in patients receiving tandem transplant.[74]

Transplant-related mortality is generally low for autoHSCT but is higher in patients receiving tandem transplants (2.7% vs 4.8%). Approximately 10% to 15% of patients who did not achieve a complete remission with the first transplant attained it with the second transplant.[75] Because of this increased risk of mortality with tandem transplants, it would be helpful to identify those patients who would benefit most. Two French studies reported that patients who did not achieve at least a very good partial response after the first transplant benefited most from the second transplant.[76,77] One of these studies reported an estimated 7-year overall survival of 21% in the single-transplant arm and a 42% survival in the double-transplant arm.[76]

The primary conclusion from the current data on autoHSCT as consolidation therapy in MM is that it should be used in younger patients with good performance status.[14] Prior to transplant, all patients should receive induction therapy to reduce tumor burden. Because of higher transplant-related mortality, a second autoHSCT should only be considered in patients who do not achieve a very good partial response or better with the first autoHSCT.

Maintenance

Even with recent advances in induction therapy and autoHSCT, most patients will eventually progress within 3 to 5 years, suggesting that effective maintenance therapy is needed to control or delay disease progression. Variable results and high toxicities have been reported with interferon-α (IFN-α) and dexamethasone and neither drug can be recommended outside of a clinical trial.[78] IFN-α at one time was considered to be maintenance of choice after autoHSCT, based on data from a randomized trial showing superior progression-free and overall survival after autoHSCT.[79] A later meta-analysis supported the benefit of IFN-α maintenance.[80] The major limitation of IFN-α is its high toxicity, which has limited its widespread use in maintenance. A randomized trial conducted by the Southwest Oncology Group evaluated the benefit of prednisone maintenance therapy in 125 patients.[81] Patients who received high-dose steroids had significantly longer progression-free and overall survival. While IFN-α or corticosteroids maintenance has not been widely adopted due to toxicity, these therapies served as proof of principle and led to phase III trials evaluating thalidomide.

Thalidomide has also been studied as maintenance after autoHSCT. To date, results of three separate phase III studies show that thalidomide improves overall survival. In the largest study to date, 597 patients were randomized to receive either no maintenance, pamidronate alone, or the combination of thalidomide plus pamidronate. Patients randomized to the thalidomide group had significantly longer event-free and overall survival as compared with those who received no thalidomide.[82] The median duration of thalidomide maintenance was 15 months and the average dose was 200 mg/day. Nearly 40% of patients had to discontinue thalidomide as a consequence of toxicity. In a subgroup analysis, patients with deletion of chromosome 13 did not benefit and other maintenance therapies may need to be evaluated for this high-risk group.

In another approach, investigators at the University of Arkansas used thalidomide in both induction and maintenance as part of the Total Therapy II trial.[83,84] Thalidomide increased CR and VgPR rates. In addition, event-free survival was improved in the thalidomide arm, including patients with adverse cytogenetics. An update by this group indicated that outcome with thalidomide was not related to cumulative dose, which may allow clinicians to limit the duration of thalidomide therapy and therefore reduce toxicity.[84]

Thalidomide maintenance has also been used after induction in elderly patients who were not candidates for autoHSCT. The results in this setting are not clear and remain controversial. Despite evidence that thalidomide maintenance after autoHSCT can improve outcomes, it is not widely used due to the adverse toxicity profile.[85]

Maintenance with bortezomib and lenalidomide may be more effective, particularly in high-risk MM patients. Bortezomib and lenalidomide are likely to be better tolerated than thalidomide. The NCCN guidelines indicate that there is no consensus on the use of dexamethasone and IFN-α maintenance. Thalidomide is given a category 1 recommendation in the NCCN guidelines.[14] Lenalidomide maintenance is given a category 2A recommendation, based on preliminary results of randomized trials showing that lenalidomide maintenance is superior to placebo. Recommendations for bortezomib maintenance will require completion of ongoing trials.

■ ALLOGENEIC HEMATOPOIETIC STEM CELL TRANSPLANTATION

AlloHSCT uses a stem cell source other than the patient themselves and is therefore a transplant across immunologic barriers. The major post-transplant complications associated with transplanting across these barriers are graft failure and acute and chronic graft-versus-host disease. Acute or chronic graft-versus-host disease may be associated with a graft-versus-myeloma effect. The graft-versus-myeloma effect, which is mediated by antitumor effector cells from the graft-versus-host disease reaction, reduces relapse risk and may offer the patient the best chance for long-term disease-free survival.[86] Unlike autoHSCT, which is simply a method of increasing the dose-intensity of chemotherapy, alloHSCT is a form of immune therapy. This is best illustrated by nonmyeloablative alloHSCT where reduced-intensity preparation provides immunosuppression so the graft is not rejected but little or no antitumor activity yet cures can be achieved as a result of graft-versus-tumor effect.[87]

⑩ Despite data reporting lower relapse rates in MM patients, myeloablative alloHSCT produces high transplant-related mortality (20%–50%), leading to overall survival rates similar to autoHSCT.[72] The reasons for the high transplant-related mortality in alloHSCT are not entirely clear. One possible explanation is that MM patients come to transplantation heavily pretreated, at an older age, and with greater existing organ damage as compared to other cancers. However, a study was closed prematurely in MM patients younger than 55 years of age with minimal pretreatment because of unacceptably high transplant-related mortality (~50%) suggesting these explanations do not completely account for the high mortality.[75]

With the high transplant-related mortality associated with myeloablative alloHSCT, the use of nonmyeloablative alloHSCT is an attractive option to reduce early post-transplant mortality. Several conclusions can be made based on the available data regarding the use of nonmyeloablative alloHSCT in MM patients. First,

the transplant-related mortality associated with nonmyeloablative alloHSCT is lower than that reported with myeloablative alloHSCT. Second, the cytoreductive activity of the reduced-intensity preparation may be insufficient for the graft-versus-myeloma effect to have its full impact. Most immune therapies, including the graft-versus-myeloma reaction, are most effective when patients have minimal residual disease and nonmyeloablative alloHSCT may have insufficient antitumor activity to achieve important tumor reduction. The need for cytoreduction may be accomplished by autoHSCT preceding the reduced-intensity alloHSCT procedure. The trials investigating this novel approach have produced conflicting results. These studies compared tandem autoHSCT with single autoHSCT followed by reduced-intensity alloHSCT. Garban et al. reported no differences in event-free or overall survival between tandem autoHSCT and single autoHSCT followed by reduced-intensity alloHSCT.[88] A more recent trial reported significantly improved event-free and overall survival when autoHSCT was combined with reduced-intensity alloHSCT.[89] These conflicting results may relate to the inclusion of particularly high-risk patients and the use of more aggressive immunosuppression in the negative trial. In both trials, transplant-related mortality was not higher in the combined autoHSCT and reduced-intensity alloHSCT arm when compared with tandem autoHSCT.[88,89] More recently, Rosinol et al. found a nonsignificant improvement in progression-free survival and no improvement in overall survival in patients receiving combined autoHSCT and nonmyeloablative alloHSCT. The lack of benefit on overall survival may be explained by higher transplant-related mortality in the nonmyeloablative arm.[90] Because of the variability of these results, the combined use of auto and alloHSCT should be performed as part of an investigational protocol.

■ SUPPORTIVE CARE

Bisphosphonates

Along with anti-MM therapy, supportive care measures are aggressively used to stabilize skeletal abnormalities. Bisphosphonates have been used for more than a decade in the management of MM. Once a well-accepted standard of care, the optimal use of bisphosphonates is more controversial because of reports of osteonecrosis of the jaw (ONJ), a rare but serious adverse effect of bisphosphonate use.

⑪ Bisphosphonates have a major role in the treatment of bone-related complications associated with MM. Bone resorption is a manifestation of the disease process and is mediated in part by inflammatory molecules including IL-6, IL-1, and TNF-α.[1] Bone disease is not seen in MGUS but occurs in approximately 80% of MM patients at diagnosis. Although the classic cytokine mediators of bone loss are important, a newer view involves excessive production of RANK-L, which activates NF-κB through its receptor (RANK).[91] As previously stated, NF-κB is a transcriptional regulator that increases the production of various inflammatory molecules. Normally, RANK-L mediated activation is in equilibrium with osteoprotegerin, which inhibits NF-κB by serving as a decoy receptor for RANK-L.[91] In the bone marrow of MM patients, excess RANK-L is produced particularly from stromal cells, which, when coupled with a decline in osteoprotegerin from both stromal cells and osteoblasts, leads to osteoclast activation and bone destruction. Macrophage inflammatory protein α_1, macrophage colony-stimulating factor, and VEGF may also play important roles in MM bone disease by stimulating the production and activation of osteoclasts.[92] Macrophage inflammatory protein α_1 is also an important chemotactic factor released by MM cells; it attracts osteoclast precursors, enabling myeloma cells to influence the maturation and activation of osteoclasts, which suggests that antimyeloma drugs can have a beneficial effect on MM bone disease.[92,93] Although MM bone disease may involve many cell types and many soluble and cell-bound molecules, it is useful to simplify its pathophysiology and consider it to be an imbalance between RANK-L and osteoprotegerin.

Activation of osteoclasts leads to a net loss of bone mass and to many of the common clinical features of MM, including fractures, hypercalcemia, and bone pain. The bone resorption is influenced by the MM cells in proximity to the osteolytic lesions and is associated with recruitment of osteoclasts.[94] The disruptive effect on skeletal integrity can lead to direct mortality, but more commonly has a major impact on morbidity and quality of life.[1]

Bisphosphonates are analogs of endogenous pyrophosphate but are more resistant to hydrolysis than pyrophosphate. Like endogenous pyrophosphate, the bisphosphonates bind to crystalline calcium in the bone and are then phagocytized by osteoclasts.[95] The best described effect of the bisphosphonates is the inhibition of osteoclast activity, which likely occurs by direct osteoclast cytotoxicity.[96] In addition to osteoclast inhibition, bisphosphonates may also promote apoptosis in MM cells. This effect may result from the inhibition of the mevalonic acid pathway, which produces several molecules required for growth of the MM clone.[97] In addition, other potential antimyeloma effects of bisphosphonates may include modifying the cytokine microenvironment, inhibiting the adhesion of MM cells to bone marrow matrix cells, and inhibiting angiogenesis.[98] Although it is possible that bisphosphonates have an antimyeloma effect, there is little direct clinical evidence to support this activity.

The use of bisphosphonates in MM is based on the results from two large, randomized, controlled trials. In the pamidronate study, the drug was compared to placebo in a group of MM patients undergoing their first or second course of chemotherapy.[99] Several clinical end points were found to be positively impacted by pamidronate therapy. The investigators reported that patients in the pamidronate group had a lower risk of skeletal-related events, lower pain scores, and improved quality of life. Importantly, a survival advantage was observed in the pamidronate-treated patients who had already received one or more courses of antimyeloma chemotherapy. This finding of improved survival in subgroup analysis is part of the circumstantial evidence to propose an antimyeloma effect for the bisphosphonates.

Guidelines for the use of zoledronic acid in MM are based largely on a randomized study in MM and breast cancer. In patients with bone metastases, zoledronic acid was compared to pamidronate with the intent of demonstrating clinical equipoise.[100] The study did show equivalence between pamidronate and zoledronic acid. The lack of a placebo arm because of ethical concerns complicates interpretation of this study. Despite this limitation, pamidronate and zoledronic acid appear to have equivalent clinical benefit in stabilizing the skeleton.

Other randomized, controlled trials have been conducted, and the results of these trials were pooled in a systematic review.[101] Eleven randomized trials were included, which accounted for 1,113 MM patients receiving bisphosphonate therapy along with 1,070 MM patients in a control arm who received no bisphosphonate therapy. The risk of vertebral fractures was significantly lower in the bisphosphonate-treated patients as compared to controls (odds ratio = 0.59; 95% CI, 0.45–0.78). Pain scores were also reduced (odds ratio = 0.59; 95% CI, 0.46–0.76). Given that the aggregate data in the systematic review agreed with the large controlled studies described above, the effect on vertebral fractures and pain are well-supported benefits of bisphosphonate therapy.

Clinical practice guidelines for the use of bisphosphonates in MM were updated by an expert panel under the auspices of the American Society of Clinical Oncology Health Services Research Committee.[17] The evidence-based guidelines recommend that symptomatic MM patients be placed on bisphosphonate therapy at the time of diagnosis to reduce pain and skeletal-related events, and

to improve quality of life. No firm recommendation was made on the duration of bisphosphonate therapy and which of the two agents should be used. However, the expert panel suggested a duration of bisphosphonate use of 2 years in those patients with responsive or stable disease. Reinstituting bisphosphonate therapy at relapse or progression is at the discretion of the clinician.[17]

CLINICAL CONTROVERSY

Although bisphosphonates are indicated in MM patients with bone disease, controversies surrounding the selection of the best agent and duration of therapy remain. Because of recent reports of ONJ in MM patients, a more cautious approach on bisphosphonate use is being considered. ONJ is associated with patients undergoing dental procedures, those receiving the more potent bisphosphonates, and those receiving longer than two years of bisphosphonate therapy. Clinical practice guidelines developed by clinicians at the Mayo Clinic recommend that all dental procedures be performed prior to the administration of bisphosphonates, that therapy be given for no more than 2 years, and that pamidronate rather than zoledronic acid be used in newly diagnosed patients. Given the benefit of bisphosphonates on skeletal-related events, limiting therapy to 2 years remains controversial. The preference of pamidronate over zoledronic acid is also controversial given that ONJ has also been reported with pamidronate and the higher risk of ONJ with zoledronic acid is based on observational studies and not head-to-head randomized comparisons. Because of effects on the bone marrow microenvironment including effects on osteoblastogenesis, ostoclast inhibition, and differentiation of mesenchymal stem cells, bortezomib and lenalidomide combinations may be an alternative for or supplement to bisphosphonate therapy to prevent progression of myeloma bone disease. While markers of bone formation are positively affected by bortezomib, studies are required to describe this potential clinical benefit on MM bone disease.

Although a good case can be made for the use of bisphosphonates early after the diagnosis of MM, many controversies remain, including whether an antimyeloma effect exists, how long patients should remain on this expensive therapy, and, most importantly, the risk of ONJ. The association between bisphosphonates and ONJ suggests a more cautious approach with bisphosphonate therapy.

ONJ is characterized by an area of exposed necrotic bone and often affects the mandible and the maxilla, but can also affect the soft palate. The development of ONJ may be related to dental disease and tooth extraction, and appears to be more common with zoledronic acid than with pamidronate. The relationship with zoledronic acid is sufficiently strong to lead the Mayo Clinic to recommend that pamidronate be used in newly diagnosed MM patients.[102] The incidence of ONJ is unknown but may be as high as 10% in MM patients receiving zoledronic acid for extended periods of time. Because the risk of ONJ during the first 2 years of pamidronate appears to be very low, the Mayo Clinic guidelines recommend monthly infusions of pamidronate for 2 years after diagnosis.

A recent longitudinal cohort study supported many of the conclusions of the Mayo Clinic recommendations. These investigators concluded that ibandronate and pamidronate were safer alternatives and that dental procedures and dentures were risk factors for the development of ONJ. They recommended a comprehensive dental exam with management of dental problems prior to initiating bisphosphonate therapy but made no recommendation on which agent is preferred.[103]

Pamidronate and zoledronic acid are usually well tolerated. Flu-like symptoms can occur following the administration of bisphosphonates. Acute renal impairment can occur with both agents and is related to both infusion time and dose. For zoledronic acid, the risk of acute renal impairment is higher with the 8-mg dose (vs 4 mg) and when the duration of infusion is 5 minutes (vs 15 minutes). Patients with moderate renal impairment (creatinine clearance: 30–60 mL/min [0.5 to 1.0 mL/s]) should have their dose of zoledronic acid adjusted downward by 25% (3 mg). This recommendation was included in the zoledronic acid package insert and is based on a greater renal toxicity in patients with preexisting renal impairment.[17] Randomized studies suggest that renal effects are similar between pamidronate and zoledronic acid, and patients on bisphosphonate therapy should have serum creatinine measured at baseline and then periodically thereafter.[17,104]

■ SALVAGE THERAPY

⓬ A variety of factors must be considered when determining the most appropriate therapy for an individual who relapses including the type and duration of previous therapies, presence or absence of adverse prognostic factors, toxicity of prior therapies, and how much time has elapsed from initial response to relapse. The same drugs used to treat MM initially can also be used as salvage therapy in MM patients who have relapsed. Patients who relapse more than six months after initial induction therapy can have that induction therapy repeated. Bortezomib is an effective salvage therapy. When bortezomib was compared to high-dose dexamethasone, response rates were 38% versus 18%, respectively.[48] The activity of bortezomib in patients with high-risk cytogenetics is particularly useful because these high-risk patients are more likely to relapse and require salvage therapy. Lenalidomide plus dexamethasone is also approved for treating patients in the salvage setting, based on the results of two phase III trials.[55,56] Thalidomide can also be used at relapse with overall response rates that appear somewhat lower than bortezomib and lenalidomide.[33] Thalidomide, bortezomib, and lenalidomide can be combined with chemotherapy in the salvage setting to improve responses.

The combination of bortezomib and pegylated liposomal doxorubicin is another active regimen in relapsed or refractory MM. In a published phase III trial, patients randomized to the bortezomib and pegylated liposomal doxorubicin arm had significantly longer median time-to-progression (9.3 vs 6.5 months; hazard ratio = 0.55; 95% CI, 0.43- 0.71) and 15-month survival (76% vs 65%) as compared with patients randomized to receive bortezomib alone.[105] It is interesting to note that the overall (complete and partial) response rate was only slightly higher in the bortezomib and pegylated liposomal doxorubicin group (44% vs 41%). Based on the results of this study, the combination of bortezomib and pegylated liposomal doxorubicin received FDA approval in 2007 for patients with previously treated MM and is listed as a category 1 recommendation in the NCCN guidelines.[14] As expected, patients who received the combination experienced more adverse effects. A recent phase III trial suggests that bortezomib with or without dexamethasone had activity in relapse/refractory disease even in patients with prior thalidomide therapy or autoHSCT.[106]

As previously discussed, questions remain on the optimal timing for autoHSCT. For patients who are eligible for autoHSCT and did not receive transplant as part of initial therapy, it is appropriate to offer autoHSCT at first relapse. It is important to emphasize that while higher quality of life was realized when autoHSCT was used as consolidation therapy, there was no difference in overall survival based on timing of transplant. In patients with relapsed or refractory MM, autoHSCT followed by nonmyeloablative alloHSCT has potential benefit but at the expense of increased transplant-related

TABLE 144-5	Salvage Therapy in Multiple Myeloma
Regimen	**Level of Evidence** **Category**
Bendamustine	2B
Bortezomib	1
Bortezomib + dexamethasone	2A
Bortezomib + lenalidomide + dexamethasone	2B
Bortezomib + liposomal doxorubicin	1
Cyclophosphamide-VAD	2A
Dexamethasone	2A
Dexamethasone + cyclophosphamide + etoposide + cisplatin (DCEP)	2A
Dexamethasone + thalidomide + cisplatin + doxorubicin + cyclophosphamide + etoposide (DT-PACE)	2A
High-dose cyclophosphamide	2A
Lenalidomide + dexamethasone	1
Lenalidomide	2A
Repeat primary induction therapy (if relapse at > 6 months)	2A
Thalidomide	2A
Thalidomide + dexamethasone	2A

Category 1: Uniform NCCN consensus based on high-level evidence.
Category 2A: Uniform NCCN consensus based on lower evidence, including clinical experience.
Category 2B: Nonuniform NCCN consensus but no major disagreementç.
Data from NCCN Guidelines NCCN. Clinical Practice Guidelines in Oncology. Multiple myeloma (Version 1.2011). http://www.NCCN.org.

mortality requiring treatment only be performed as part of a clinical protocol.

One of the most important questions that remain in the treatment of the relapsed-refractory patient is whether to use multiple active agents at the same time or to use agents sequentially. As an example, the combined use of bortezomib with lenalidomide has not been proven to be superior to each agent combined with chemotherapy or dexamethasone. Until combined bortezomib and lenalidomide is found to be a superior treatment, sequential use of these agents may be able to extend the duration of effective therapy.

Treatment decisions for individual patients with relapsed disease may potentially be improved by taking into account patient-specific information such as the type of previous therapies, adverse cytogenetics, and end-organ dysfunction. For example, in patients with relapsed MM, combined bortezomib and liposomal doxorubicin has shown improved time to progression compared to bortezomib alone including patients who had received prior anthracyclines, lenalidomide, and thalidomide.[105] In contrast, treatment with lenalidomide and dexamethasone resulted in a significantly shorter time to progression in patients that had previously been treated with thalidomide than in thalidomide-naïve patients.[56]

The NCCN guidelines offer many options for salvage, including thalidomide, lenalidomide, or bortezomib with or without dexamethasone or chemotherapy (Table 144–5). In addition, autoHSCT or nonmyeloablative alloHSCT also have a role as salvage therapy in some patients.[14] Careful selection of therapy based on disease and patient risk factors and previous treatment will allow for maximal clinical benefit.

EVALUATION OF THERAPEUTIC OUTCOMES

Because MM is currently not a curable disease, the goals of therapy are to prolong survival and to improve quality of life. Patients with asymptomatic MM are usually followed and not treated. Asymptomatic patients are assessed every 3 to 6 months for disease progression, which would then require therapy. Assessment involves measurement of M protein in blood and urine and laboratory tests that include complete blood count, serum creatinine, and calcium. Patients are treated as the disease produces symptoms. Disease response is defined by a decline in M protein. After completion of the initial course of therapy and response is obtained, patients should be monitored every 3 months. Bone surveys are performed yearly or as required because of changes in symptoms. Various other tests are performed on an as-needed basis to evaluate disease status, including bone marrow biopsy, magnetic resonance imaging, and positron emission tomography, or computed tomography scan.

CONCLUSIONS

MM remains an incurable disease despite significant therapeutic advances. Lenalidomide plus dexamethasone is a reasonable upfront regimen for both autoHSCT eligible and ineligible patients. Patients who are not candidates for autoHSCT are often older with lower performance status and lenalidomide combined with low dose dexamethasone may be a better tolerated option. Bortezomib plus dexamethasone or chemotherapy may be particularly valuable in patients with MM who have high-risk cytogenetics. Younger patients with good performance status should receive autoHSCT after a short course of induction. The use of maintenance therapy after autoHSCT should be considered as part of a clinical trial. Nonmyeloablative alloHSCT may produce long-term disease-free survival but may require that the patient achieve a minimal residual disease state prior to the transplant procedure. When patients progress after initial therapy, salvage therapy may include regimens that contain thalidomide, lenalidomide, or bortezomib; autoHSCT and alloHSCT may be used in patients who are able to tolerate transplantation. Although there now are multiple therapies that can be used and there has been improvement in survival times and quality of life, MM remains a fatal disease that requires continued treatment advances.

ABBREVIATIONS

alloHSCT: allogeneic hematopoietic stem cell transplantation

autoHSCT: autologous hematopoietic stem cell transplantation

bFGF: basic fibroblast growth factor

IFN: interferon

IL: interleukin

IκB: inhibitor of NF-κB

ISS: International Staging System

LMWH: low-molecular-weight heparin

MGUS: monoclonal gammopathy of undetermined significance

MM: multiple myeloma

MP: melphalan plus prednisone

MPB: melphalan, prednisone, plus bortezomib

MPR: melphalan, prednisone, plus lenalidomide (Revlimid®)

MPT: melphalan, prednisone, plus thalidomide

NF-κB: nuclear factor kappa B

ONJ: osteonecrosis of the jaw

RANK-L: receptor for activation of NF-κB ligand

TNF-α: tumor necrosis factor alfa

VAD: vincristine, doxorubicin, plus dexamethasone

VEGF: vascular endothelial growth factor

VTE: venous thromboembolism

REFERENCES

1. Munshi NC, Anderson KC. Plasma cell neoplasms. In: Devita VT, Hellman S, Rosenberg SA, eds. Cancer Principles and Practice of Oncology, 8th ed. Philadelphia, PA: Lippincott Williams & Wilkins, 2008: 2305–2342.
2. Barlogie B, Shaughnessy J, Epstein J, et al. Plasma cell myeloma. In: Lichtman MA, Beutler E, Kipps TJ, et al. Hematology, 7th ed. New York: McGraw-Hill, 2006: 1501–1533.
3. Jemal A, Siegel R, Xu J, Ward E. Cancer statistics, 2010. CA Cancer J Clin 2010;60:277-300.
4. Brander C, Raje N, O'Connor PG, et al. Absence of biologically important Kaposi sarcoma associated herpesvirus gene products and virus-specific cellular responses in multiple myeloma. Blood 2002;100:698–700.
5. Cheung MC, Pantanowitz L, Dezube BJ. AIDS-related malignancies: Emerging challenges in the era of highly active anti-retroviral therapy. Oncologist 2005;10:412–426.
6. Kyle RA, Rajkumar S. Multiple myeloma. N Engl J Med 2004;351: 1860–1873.
7. Kyle RA, Therneau TM, Rajkumar SV, et al. Prevalence of monoclonal gammopathy of undetermined significance. N Engl J Med 2006;354: 1362–1369.
8. Walker BA, Leone PE, Jenner MW, et al. Integration of global SNP-based mapping and expression arrays reveals key regions, mechanisms, and genes important to the pathogenesis of multiple myeloma. Blood 2006;108:1733–1743.
9. Kyle RA, Remstein ED, Thereau TM, et al. Clinical course and prognosis of smoldering (asymptomatic) multiple myeloma. N Engl J Med 2007;356:2582–2590.
10. Spets H, Stromberg T, Georgii-Hemming P, et al. Expression of the bcl-2 family of pro- and anti-apoptotic genes in multiple myeloma and normal plasma cells. Eur J Haematol 2002;69:76–89.
11. Liebisch P, Dohner H. Cytogenetics and molecular cytogenetics in multiple myeloma. Eur J Cancer 2006;42:1520–1529.
12. Gertz MA, Ghobrial I, Luc-Harousseau J. Multiple myeloma: Biology, standard therapy, and transplant therapy. Biol Blood Marrow Transplant 2009;15:46–52.
13. Podar K, Chauhan D, Anderson KC. Bone marrow microenvironment and the identification of new targets for myeloma therapy. Leukemia 2009;23:10–24.
14. National Comprehensive Cancer Network. The NCCN Multiple Myeloma Clinical Practice Guidelines in Oncology (Version 1.2011). *http://www.NCCN.org.*
15. Kyle RA, Rajkumar SV. Monoclonal gammopathy of undetermined significance and smoldering multiple myeloma. Hematol Oncol Clin N Am 2007;21:1093–1113.
16. Dispenzieri A, Kyle R, Merlini G, et al. International myeloma working group guidelines for serum light chain analysis in multiple myeloma and related disorders. Leukemia 2009;23:215–224.
17. Kyle RA, Yee GC, Somerfield MR, et al. American Society of Clinical Oncology 2007 Clinical Practice Guideline update on the role of bis-phosphonates in multiple myeloma. J Clin Oncol 2007;25:2462–2472.
18. Roodman GD. Pathogenesis of myeloma bone disease. Leukemia 2009;23:435–441.
19. Greipp PR, Miguel JS, Durie BG, et al. International staging system for multiple myeloma. J Clin Oncol 2005;23:3412–3420.
20. Palumbo A, Rajkumar SV. Treatment of newly diagnosed myeloma. Leukemia 2009;23:449–456.
21. He Y, Wheatley K, Clark O, et al. Early versus deferred treatment for early stage multiple myeloma. Cochrane Database Syst Rev 2003(1):CD004023.
22. Raab MS, Podar K, Breitkreutz I, et al. Multiple myeloma. Lancet 2009;374:324–339.
23. Ludwig H, Beksac M, Blade J, et al. Current multiple myeloma treatment strategies with novel agents: A European perspective. Oncologist 2010;15:6–25.
24. Ishii Y, Hsiao HH, Sashida G, et al. Derivative (1;7)(q10;p10) in multiple myeloma. A sign of therapy-related hidden myelodysplastic syndrome. Cancer Genet Cytogenet 2006;167:131–137.
25. Kumar A, Loughran T, Alsina M, et al. Management of multiple myeloma: A systematic review and critical appraisal of published studies. Lancet Oncol 2003;4:293–304.

26. Facon T, Mary JY, Pegourie B, et al. Dexamethasone-based regimens versus melphalan prednisone for elderly multiple myeloma patients ineligible for high dose therapy. Blood 2006;107:1292–1298.

27. Palumbo A, Rajkumar SV. Treatment of newly diagnosed myeloma. Leukemia 2009;23:449–456.

28. Gordan JN, Goggin PM. Thalidomide and its derivative emerging from the wilderness. Postgrad Med J 2003;79:127–132.

29. Kotla V, Gold S, Nischal S, et al. Mechanism of action of lenalidomide in hematological malignancies. J Hematol Oncol 2009;2:36.

30. Rajkumar SV, Leong T, Roche PC, et al. Prognostic value of bone marrow angiogenesis in multiple myeloma. Clin Cancer Res 2000;6:3111–3116.

31. Neben K, Mytilineos J, Moehler TM, et al. Polymorphisms of the TNF-α gene promoter predict for outcome after thalidomide therapy in relapsed and refractory multiple myeloma. Blood 2002;100: 2263–2265.

32. Reece DE, Leitch HA, Atkins H, et al. Treatment of relapsed and refractory myeloma. Leuk Lymphoma 2008;49:1470–1485.

33. Barlogie B, Desikan R, Eddlemon P, et al. Extended survival in advanced and refractory multiple myeloma after single-agent thalidomide: Identification of prognostic factors in a phase 2 study of 169 patients. Blood 2001;98:492–494.

34. Cavallo F, Boccadoro M, Palumbo A. Review of thalidomide in the treatment of newly diagnosed multiple myeloma. Ther Clin Risk Management 2007;3:543–552.

35. Harousseau JL. Induction therapy in multiple myeloma. Hematology Am Soc Hematol Educ Program 2008:306–312.

36. Rajkumar SV, Blood E, Vesole D, et al. Phase III clinical trial of thalidomide plus dexamethasone compared with dexamethasone alone in newly diagnosed multiple myeloma: A clinical trial coordinated by Eastern Cooperative Oncology Group. J Clin Oncol 2006;24:431–436.

37. Palumbo A, Bringhen S, Liberati AM, et al. Oral melphalan with prednisone and thalidomide in elderly patients with multiple myeloma: Updated results of a randomized controlled trial. Blood 2008;112:3107–3114.

38. Facon T, Mary JY, Hulin C, et al. Melphalan and prednisone plus thalidomide versus melphalan and prednisone alone or reduced-intensity autologous stem cell transplantation in elderly patients with multiple myeloma (IFM 99–06): a randomised trial. Lancet 2007;370:1209–1218.

39. Hulin C, Facon T, Rodon P, et al. Efficacy of melphalan and prednisone plus thalidomide in patients older than 75 years with newly diagnosed multiple myeloma: IFM 01/01 Trial. J Clin Oncol 2009;27:3664–3670.

40. Offidani M, Corvatta L, Piersantelli M, et al. Thalidomide, dexamethasone, and pegylated liposomal doxorubicin for patients older than 65 years with newly diagnosed multiple myeloma. Blood 2006;108:2159–2164.

41. Laubach JP, Mitsiades CS, Mahindra A, et al. Novel therapies in the treatment of multiple myeloma. J Natl Compr Canc Netw 2009;7:947–960.

42. Gleason C, Nooka A, Lonial S. Supportive therapies in multiple myeloma. J Natl Compr Canc Netw 2009;7:971–979.

43. Palumbo A, Rajkumar SV, Dimopoulos MA, et al. Prevention of thalidomide and lenalidomide associated thrombosis in myeloma. Leukemia 2008;22:414–423.

44. Lyman GH, Khorana AA, Falanga A, et al. ASCO Guideline: Recommendations for venous thromboembolism prophylaxis and treatment in patients with cancer. J Clin Oncol 2007;25:5490–5505.

45. Shah JJ, Orlowski RZ. Proteasome inhibitors in the treatment of multiple myeloma. Leukemia 2009;23:1964–1979.

46. Orlowski RZ, Stinchcombe TE, Mitchell BS, et al. Phase 1 trial of the proteasome inhibitor PS341 in patients with refractory hematologic malignancies. J Clin Oncol 2002;20:4420–4427.

47. Richardson P, Barlogie B, Berenson J, et al. A phase II study of bortezomib in relapsed, refractory myeloma. N Engl J Med 2003;348:2609–2617.

48. Richardson PG, Sonneveld P, Schuster MW, et al. Bortezomib or high dose dexamethasone in relapsed multiple myeloma. N Engl J Med 2005;352:2487–2498.

49. Richardson PG, Mitsiades C, Ghobrial I, Anderson K. Beyond single agent bortezomib: Combination regimens in relapsed multiple myeloma. Curr Opin Oncol 2006;18:598–608.

50. Jagannath S, Durie BG, Wolf J, et al. Bortezomib therapy alone and in combination with dexamethasone for previously untreated symptomatic multiple myeloma. Br J Haematol 2005;129:776–783.

51. Harousseau JL, Attal M, Leleu X, et al. Bortezomib plus dexamethasone as induction treatment prior to autologous stem cell transplant in patients with newly diagnosed multiple myeloma: Results of an IFM Phase II study. Haematologica 2006;91:1498–1505.

52. Mateos MV, Hernandez JM, Hernandez MT, et al. Bortezomib plus melphalan and prednisone in elderly untreated patients with multiple myeloma: Results of a multivariate phase I/II study. Blood 2006;108:2165–2172.

53. San Miguel JF, Schlag R, Khuageva NK, et al. Bortezomib plus melphalan and prednisone for initial treatment of multiple myeloma. N Engl J Med 2008;359:906–917.

54. Armoiry X, Auglagner G, Facon T. Lenalidomide in the treatment of multiple myeloma: A review. J Clin Pharm Ther 2008;33:219–226.

55. Weber DM, Chen C, Niesvizky R, et al. Lenalidomide plus dexamethasone for relapsed multiple myeloma in North America. N Engl J Med 2007;357:2133–2142.

56. Dimopoulous M, Spencer A, Attal M, et al. Lenalidomide plus dexamethasone for relapsed or refractory multiple myeloma. N Engl J Med 2007;357:2123–2132.

57. Lacy MQ, Gertz MA, Dispenzieri A, et al. Long-term results of response to therapy, time to progression, and survival with lenalidomide plus dexamethasone in newly diagnosed myeloma. Mayo Clin Proc 2007;82:1179–1184.

58. Rajkumar SV, Hayman SR, Lacy MQ, et al. Combination therapy with lenalidomide plus dexamethasone for newly diagnosed myeloma. Blood 2005;106:4050–4053.

59. Rajkumar SV, Jacobus S, Callander NS, et al. Lenalidomide plus high-dose dexamethasone versus lenalidomide plus low-dose dexamethasone as initial therapy for newly diagnosed multiple myeloma: an open-labeled randomized control trial. Lancet Oncol 2010;11:29–37.

60. Palumbo A, Falco P, Corradini P, et al. Melphalan, prednisone, lenalidomide treatment for newly diagnosed myeloma: A report from the GIMEMA Italian Multiple Myeloma Network. J Clin Oncol 2007;25:4459–4465.

61. Palumbo A, Dimopoulous MA, Delforge M, et al. A phase III study to determine the efficacy and safety of lenalidomide in combination with melphalan and prednisone in elderly patients with newly diagnosed multiple myeloma. Presented at: 51st American Society of Hematology Annual Meeting and Exposition; December 5–8, 2009; New Orleans, LA.

62. Harousseau JL. Integrating novel therapies in the transplant paradigm. Cancer J 2009;15:479–484.

63. Child JA, Morgan GJ, Davies FE, et al. High-dose chemotherapy with hematopoietic stem cell rescue for multiple myeloma. N Engl J Med 2003;348:1875–1883.

64. Attal M, Harousseau JL, Stoppa AM, et al. A prospective, randomized trial of autologous bone marrow transplantation and chemotherapy in multiple myeloma. N Engl J Med 1996;335:91–97.

65. Koreth J, Cutler CS, Djulbegovic B, et al. High-dose therapy with single autologous transplantation versus chemotherapy for newly diagnosed multiple myeloma: A systematic review and meta-analysis of randomized controlled trials. Biol Blood Marrow Transplant 2007;12:183–196.

66. Barlogie B, Kyle RA, Anderson KC, et al. Standard chemotherapy compared with high dose chemotherapy for multiple myeloma: Final results of phase III US Intergroup Trial S9321. J Clin Oncol 2006;24:929–936.

67. Fermand JP, Katsahian S, Divine M, et al. High dose therapy and autologous blood stem cell transplantation compared with conventional treatment in multiple myeloma patients aged 55 to 65 years: Long-term results of a randomized control trial from the Group Myeloma-Autograffe. J Clin Oncol 2005;23:9227–9233.

68. San-Miguel JF, Mateos MV. How to treat a newly diagnosed young patient with multiple myeloma. Hematology Am Soc Hematol Educ Program 2009:555–565.

69. Harousseau JL, Avet-Loiseau H, Attal M, et al. High complete and very good partial response rates with bortezomib-dexamethasone as induction prior to autologous stem cell transplant in newly diagnosed patients with high risk multiple myeloma: Results of IFM 2005-01 phase III trial. Blood 2009;114 [abstract 353].

70. Alexanian R, Dimopoulos M, Smith T, et al. Limited value of myeloablative therapy for late multiple myeloma. Blood 1994;83:512-516.

71. Kumar S, Lacy MQ, Dispenzieri A, et al. High-dose therapy and autologous stem cell transplantation for multiple myeloma poorly responsive to initial therapy. Bone Marrow Transplant 2004;34:161-167.

72. Pant S, Copeland EA. Hematopoietic stem cell transplantation in multiple myeloma. Biol Blood Marrow Transplant 2007;13:877-885.

73. Fermand JP, Ravaud P, Chevaer S, et al. High dose therapy and autologous peripheral blood stem cell transplantation in multiple myeloma: Up-front or rescue treatment? Results of a multicenter sequential randomized clinical trial. Blood 1998;92:3131-3136.

74. Kumar A, Kharfan-Dabaja MA, Glasmacher A, Djulbegovic B. Tandem versus single autologous hematopoietic cell transplantation for treatment of multiple myeloma: A systematic review and meta-analysis. J Natl Cancer Instit 2009;101:100-106.

75. Vesole DH, Simic A, Lazarus HM. Controversy in multiple myeloma transplants: Tandem autotransplants and mini-allografts. Bone Marrow Transplant 2001;28:725-735.

76. Attal M, Harousseau JL, Facon T, et al. Single versus double autologous stem cell transplantation for multiple myeloma. N Engl J Med 2003;349:2495-2502.

77. Harousseau JL, Avet-Loiseau H, Attal M, et al. Achievement of at least very good partial response is a simple and robust prognostic factor in patients with multiple myeloma treated with high-dose therapy: Long-term analysis of the IFM 99-02 and 99-04 trials. J Clin Oncol 2009;34:5720-5726.

78. Mihelic R, Kaufman JL, Lonial S. Maintenance therapy in multiple myeloma. Leukemia 2007;21:1150-1158.

79. Mandelli F, Avvisati G, Amadori S, et al. Maintenance treatment with recombinant interferon-alpha 2b in patients with multiple myeloma responding to conventional induction chemotherapy. N Engl J Med 1990;322:1430-1434.

80. Fritz E, Ludwig H. Interferon-alpha treatment in multiple myeloma: Meta-analysis of 30 randomized trials among 3948 patients. Ann Oncol 2000;11:1427-1436.

81. Berenson JR, Crowley JJ, Grogan TM, et al. Maintenance therapy with alternate-day prednisone improves survival in multiple myeloma patients. Blood 2002;99:3163-3168.

82. Attal M, Harousseau JL, Leyvraz S, et al. Maintenance therapy with thalidomide improves survival in patients with multiple myeloma. Blood 2006;108:3289-3294.

83. Barlogie B, Tricot G, Anaisse E, et al. Thalidomide and hematopoietic-cell transplantation for multiple myeloma. N Engl J Med 2006;354:1021-1030.

84. Barlogie B, Pineda-Roman M, vanRhee F, et al. Thalidomide arm of total therapy II improve complete response duration and survival in myeloma patients with metaphase cytogenetic abnormalities. Blood 2008;112:3115-3121.

85. Ghobrial IM, Stewart AK. ASH evidence-based guidelines: What is the role of maintenance therapy in treatment of multiple myeloma? Hematology Am Soc Hematol Educ Program 2009;587-589.

86. Laterveer L, Verdonck LF, Peeters T, et al. Graft-versus-myeloma may overcome the unfavorable effect of deletion of chromosome 13 in multiple myeloma. Blood 2003;101:1201-1202.

87. Champlin R, Khouri I, Anderlini P, et al. Nonmyeloablative preparative regimens for allogeneic hematopoietic transplantation. Oncology 2003;17:94-100.

88. Garban F, Attal M, Michallet M, et al. Prospective comparison of autologous stem cell transplantation followed by dose reduced allograft with tandem autologous stem cell transplant in high risk de novo multiple myeloma. Blood 2006;107:3474-3480.

89. Bruno B, Rotta M, Patriarcia F, et al. A comparison of allografting with autografting for newly diagnosed myeloma. N Engl J Med 2007;356:1110-1120.

90. Rosinol L, Perez-Simon JA, Sureda A, et al. A prospective study of tandem autologous transplant versus autologous transplant followed by reduced intensity conditioning allogeneic transplant in newly diagnosed multiple myeloma. Blood 2008;112:3591-3593.

91. Sezer O, Heider U, Zavrski, et al. RANK ligand and osteoprotegerin in myeloma bone disease. Blood 2003;101:2094-2098.

92. Roodman GD. Pathogenesis of myeloma bone disease. Leukemia 2009;23:435-441.

93. Terpos E, Dimopoulos MA. Myeloma bone disease: Pathophysiology and management. Ann Oncol 2005;16:1223-1231.

94. Andersen TL, Soe K, Sondergaard TE, et al. Myeloma cell-induced disruption of bone remodeling compartments leads to osteolytic lesions and generation of osteoclast-myeloma hybrid cells. Br J Hematol 2009;148:551-561.

95. Russell RG. Bisphosphonates: From bench to bedside. Ann N Y Acad Sci 2006;1068:367-401.

96. Papapoulos SE. Bisphosphonate actions: Physical chemistry revisited. Bone 2006;38:613-616.

97. Baulch-Brown C, Molloy TJ, Yeh SL, et al. Inhibitor of the mevalonate pathway as potential therapeutic agents in multiple myeloma. Leuk Res 2007;31:341-352.

98. Neville-Webbe HL, Holen I, Coleman RE. The anti-tumor activity of bisphosphonates. Cancer Treat Rev 2002;28:305-319.

99. Berenson JR, Lichtenstein A, Porter L, et al. Long-term pamidronate treatment of advanced multiple myeloma patients reduces skeletal events. Myeloma Aredia Study Group. J Clin Oncol 1998;16:593-602.

100. Rosen LS, Gordon D, Antonio BS, et al. Zoledronic acid versus pamidronate in the treatment of skeletal metastases in patients with breast cancer or osteolytic lesions of multiple myeloma: A phase III, double blind, comparative trial. Cancer J 2001;7:377-387.

101. Djulbegovic B, Wheatley K, Ross J, et al. Bisphosphonates in multiple myeloma. Cochrane Database Syst Rev 2002(4):CD003188.

102. Lacy MQ, Dispenzieri A, Gertz MA, et al. Mayo clinic consensus statement for the use of bisphosphonates in multiple myeloma. Mayo Clin Proc 2006;81:1047-1053.

103. Vahtsevanos K, Kyrgidis A, Verrou F, et al. Longitudinal cohort study of risk factors in cancer patients of bisphosphonate-related osteonecrosis of the jaw. J Clin Oncol 2009;27:5356-5362.

104. Guarueri V, Donati S, Nicolini M, et al. Renal safety and efficacy of intravenous bisphosphonates in patients with skeletal metastases treated for up to ten years. Oncologist 2005;10:842-848.

105. Orlowski RZ, Nagler A, Sonnveld P, et al. Randomized phase III study of pegylated liposomal doxorubicin plus bortezomib compared with bortezomib alone in relapsed or refractory multiple myeloma: Combination therapy improves time to progression. J Clin Oncol 2007; 25:3892-3901.

106. Mikhael JR, Belch AR, Prince HM, et al. High response rates to bortezomib with or without dexamethasone in patients with relapsed or refractory multiple myeloma: Results of a global phase IIIb expanded access programs. Br J Hematol 2009;144:169-175.

CHAPTER 145

Myelodysplastic Syndromes

JULIANNA A. BURZYNSKI AND TRACEY WALSH-CHOCOLAAD

KEY CONCEPTS

❶ Myelodysplastic syndromes (MDS) primarily occur in the elderly, with median age at diagnosis between 75 and 84 years.

❷ MDS are associated with environmental, occupational, and therapeutic exposures to chemicals or radiation.

❸ The manifestations of MDS are due to immune dysregulation and genomic instability, which creates a dysplastic, clonal population of cells in a milieu unable to support normal hematopoiesis.

❹ Most patients with MDS present with fatigue and lethargy or symptoms related to anemia-induced tissue hypoxia.

❺ The prognosis of patients with MDS is variable. Overall survival ranges from a few months to several years and can be estimated with the International Prognostic Scoring System (IPSS) or World Health Organization Classification-based Scoring System.

❻ Palliation of symptoms and improvement in quality of life are the goals of therapy for most patients.

❼ Current guidelines recommend erythropoietin or darbepoetin for management of anemia in patients with MDS.

❽ Allogeneic hematopoietic stem cell transplantation (HSCT) offers potentially curative therapy to patients with MDS who have a donor and are healthy enough for the procedure.

❾ Hypomethylating agents are appropriate for patients with transfusion-dependent or symptomatic MDS who are not candidates for allogeneic HSCT.

❿ Antithymocyte globulin is appropriate treatment for low or intermediate-1 IPSS risk, human leukocyte antigen DR15 positive expressing MDS in patients with symptomatic anemia that is unlikely to respond to erythropoietic agents.

⓫ Lenalidomide is the recommended initial treatment for low-risk 5q syndrome accompanied by symptomatic anemia.

Myelodysplastic syndromes (MDS) encompass a spectrum of clonal myeloid disorders characterized by ineffective hematopoiesis that results in anemia, thrombocytopenia, leukopenia, or a combination of peripheral cytopenias.[1-3] The hallmark feature of MDS is bone marrow dysplasia in at least 10% of cells of a single myeloid lineage.[3] MDS are frequently associated with clonal chromosomal abnormalities, qualitative disorders of blood cells, and a variable propensity for progression to acute myeloid leukemia (AML). The clinical course of patients with MDS varies along a continuum from a rapid progression to AML to years of slowly progressive bone marrow failure.[4]

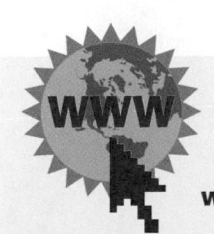

146

Renal Cell Carcinoma

CHRISTINE M. WALKO, NINH M. LA-BECK, AND MARK D. WALSH

KEY CONCEPTS

❶ Renal cell carcinoma (RCC) predominantly occurs later in life, with 70% of all cases diagnosed between the ages of 55 and 84.

❷ The most established risk factors for RCC are smoking, obesity, and hypertension.

❸ Genetic factors contribute to ~15% of cases of RCC; the remaining 85% are believed to be sporadic.

❹ Inactivation of the von Hippel-Lindau (VHL) tumor suppressor gene is the hallmark of the most common type of RCC, the clear cell subtype.

❺ More than 50% of RCC cases are diagnosed by incidental findings on routine imaging for unrelated reasons.

❻ The Memorial Sloan-Kettering Cancer Center Prognostic Factors Model for Survival classifies patients into low-, intermediate- and high-risk groups based on five clinical factors and can predict survival in untreated patients and those treated with immunotherapy and targeted agents.

❼ Surgical removal of the primary tumor, either by total or partial nephrectomy, is the preferred initial treatment for all stages of RCC.

❽ Immunotherapy used to be considered first-line therapy for metastatic RCC but has largely been replaced by targeted agents because of their improved efficacy and tolerability.

❾ Sunitinib is an oral small molecule inhibitor of vascular endothelial growth factor (VEGF) and platelet-derived growth factor (PDGF) and is recommended as first-line therapy for metastatic RCC.

❿ Sorafenib is an oral small molecular inhibitor of VEGF, PDGF, and c-kit and is recommended as second-line therapy for metastatic RCC.

⓫ Temsirolimus is an intravenously administered mTOR (mammalian target of rapamycin) inhibitor indicated for first-line therapy in patients with high-risk metastatic RCC.

⓬ Ongoing trials with approved and novel targeted therapies either alone or in combination with immunotherapy will elucidate optimal treatment options for RCC.

Renal cell carcinoma (RCC) is a less common malignancy that, until recently, had few treatment options that were poorly tolerated and resulted in few positive outcomes for patients. However, treatment for the disease has been revolutionized by an increased understanding of the pathophysiology of RCC. Clear cell is the predominant subtype of RCC and is the result of inactivation of the von Hippel-Lindau (VHL) tumor suppressor gene on chromosome 3p25, which leads to increased production of growth factors such as vascular endothelial growth factor (VEGF), transforming growth factor (TGF), platelet-derived growth factor (PDGF), and others responsible for angiogenesis and cell growth.[1] Before 2005, the primary therapy option for patients with advanced RCC following nephrectomy was immunotherapy with few responses and high toxicity. However, six new drugs were approved recently either as first- or second-line therapy for RCC: sorafenib, sunitinib, temsirolimus, bevacizumab (in combination with interferon-α), everolimus, and pazopanib.[2–7] Each is an example of targeted therapy against growth factors important in the pathophysiology of RCC and has yielded much needed progress in a disease with few therapeutic options. RCC serves as an example of rational development of targeted agents based on knowledge of tumor biology for the treatment of other malignancies.

CHAPTER

147

Melanoma

CINDY L. O'BRYANT AND JAMIE C. POUST

KEY CONCEPTS

❶ Cutaneous melanoma is an increasingly common malignancy, but it is a cancer that can be cured if detected early. Public education about screening and early detection is one strategy for controlling the increase in incidence and the mortality associated with cutaneous melanoma.

❷ Surgical resection can cure patients with early-stage melanoma.

❸ The toxicities associated with interferon-α_{2b} therapy are significant and require patient education, close patient monitoring, and appropriate dose modification based on toxicity.

❹ Patients with locally advanced disease should be evaluated for adjuvant therapy; recommended options include interferon α_{2b} or participation in a clinical trial.

❺ High-dose aldesleukin (interleukin 2) is an option for some individuals with metastatic melanoma. The toxicities associated with this regimen are significant and warrant close patient selection. Individuals receiving high-dose aldesleukin require close monitoring and management by an experienced healthcare team. A small subset of patients experience a durable response with this therapy, although the question of risk versus benefit should be assessed on an individualized basis.

❻ Metastatic melanoma remains a clinical challenge. At this time, there is not a single standard treatment approach for individuals with metastatic disease. Dacarbazine and temozolomide are considered the most active chemotherapies and can be used as single agents. Combination chemotherapy has not been shown to be superior to single-agent therapy with dacarbazine.

❼ As the biology of melanoma has been further delineated, a growing number of potential targets for drug therapy have been identified. Recent work has focused on drugs that target specific pathways of melanoma development and progression.

Melanoma is the sixth most common cancer in the United States. The incidence of melanoma steadily increased from the 1970s to the 1990s and has remained relatively stable since 2000. While nonmelanoma skin cancers (NMSCs) are the most common malignancies of the skin, cutaneous melanoma accounts for up to 75% of all skin cancer-related deaths. With the rise in the number of

melanoma skin cancer and the associated mortality, it is essential to consider issues of care beyond that of disease treatment. Skin cancer prevention and screening have a major impact on public health and on the success of treatment for those individuals diagnosed with both NMSC and melanoma. Skin cancers tend to occur more frequently in older individuals. Therefore, as the population continues to age, effective strategies to prevent, detect, and treat individuals with these cancers are needed.

The incidence of melanoma varies worldwide with the highest rates found in Australia, New Zealand, North America, and Northern Europe. In the United States, the lifetime risk of developing melanoma is greater in men (2.6%) than women (1.7%) and varies with ethnicity, whites 2%, Hispanics 0.5 %, and blacks 0.1%.[1] The median age at diagnosis is 59 years old.[2] In 2010 it was estimated that approximately 68,130 new cases of melanoma would be diagnosed in the United States. Unfortunately, this estimate may not be accurate because many superficial and in situ melanomas are managed in facilities that do not routinely report their cases to cancer registries.[1] Childhood and adolescent melanoma is rare with 2% of cases being diagnosed in individuals <20 years old. The incidence in this age group is increasing by 2.9% per year. Young adults between the ages of 15 and 19 years account for approximately three quarters of childhood melanomas. Different than the adult population, the incidence of melanoma appears to be the same between genders except in the 10- to 19-year-old age group where the incidence is higher in girls than boys.[3]

The estimated number of individuals expected to die of melanoma in 2010 in the United States is approximately 8,700. While the 5-year survival rates for melanoma have increased from 82% in 1975 to 92% in 2004, the overall mortality rate has remained stable.[1] Men >65 years old have the highest mortality rates from melanoma. Death rates have declined in younger patients. The stabilization of mortality rates appears to be related to efforts at both primary and secondary prevention of melanoma in addition to advances in the treatment and management of melanoma patients.

ETIOLOGY AND EPIDEMIOLOGY

The etiology of melanoma, like most other malignancies, is not fully understood. A number of patient-specific factors and environmental factors have been identified (Table 147–1), and it is likely that these factors alone or in combination increase the occurrence of cutaneous melanomas.

Individual physical characteristics can determine responses to UV radiation. White persons with fair-colored hair (red or blond), light-colored eyes (blue or green), high degrees of freckling and those who have a tendency to burn and rarely tan with exposure to sunlight appear especially at risk.[4,5] Clinical and epidemiologic research show a higher rate of melanoma in those who have

TABLE 147-1 Risk Factors for Melanoma

Patient-specific risk factors
Adulthood (age >15 years)
History of cutaneous melanoma
Dysplastic nevi
High density of common nevi and atypical nevi
Cutaneous melanoma in first-degree relative
Immunodeficiency/immunosuppression
High degree of freckling
Sunburns easily/tans rarely
Blonde or red hair
Blue, green, or gray eyes
Socioeconomic status (higher > lower)
Race (white > Hispanics > black)

External risk factors
Intense intermittent sun exposures
History of sunburn
More than four painful sunburns before age 15 years
Recreational sun exposure

extensive or repeated intense sun exposure.[6] Intermittent intense sun exposure, blistering sunburns, and the time of life of exposure to the sun now are believed to be critical factors for development of cutaneous melanoma and individuals with a history of these are at this highest risk. Individuals who have had chronic sun exposure without a history of burning and those with occupational exposure have a lower risk. The risk with sunlight and UV radiation seems to be greatest during childhood and adolescence and is more hazardous than exposure during adult life.

One of the most important risk factors for melanoma is the number of melanocytic nevi (pigmented lesions or moles) on the body. The formation of these nevi has been shown to be directly related to cumulative sun exposure. The relative risk of developing melanoma increases with the greater the number of typical nevi an individual has. A second risk factor is the presence of atypical melanocytic nevi.[4] Atypical nevi may progress from a normal nevus or be dysplastic from the onset. Up to one fifth of melanomas develop from atypical nevi and individuals with these have an increased risk of developing melanoma as compared to the general population. Small congenital melanocytic nevi may be present at birth or within the first few months after birth. Approximately 1% to 3% of newborns are born with pigmented lesions, and the lifetime risk of developing melanoma is related to the size of the nevus.[3]

Immunocompromised patients are at an increased risk for development of cutaneous melanoma.[3,5] Immunodeficiency includes individuals with ataxia telangiectasia, chronic lymphocytic leukemia, Hodgkin lymphoma, and immunosuppression following organ transplant. Acquired immunodeficiency syndrome has been shown to increase the risk of developing cutaneous melanoma, and the disease often is more aggressive.[7] Personal history of nonmelanoma or melanoma skin cancers is a risk factor for subsequent melanoma and may be associated with a poor prognosis. Xeroderma pigmentosum is a rare skin disorder but does carry an increased risk for melanoma.

A rare but important risk for melanoma is maternal–fetal transfer of melanoma. Although melanoma is not the most common cancer in pregnancy, it is the cancer most likely to metastasize to the placenta and the fetus.[3] Maternal–fetal transmission of melanoma is commonly lethal. However, neonates delivered with concomitant placental involvement but without clinical evidence of disease still are considered to be at increased risk for development of disease.

A number of genes have been implicated in melanoma development and progression, and molecular profiling studies have identified several distinct molecular subclasses of melanoma.[8] Familial atypical multiple mole syndrome (FAMMS) or dysplastic nevus syndrome is

a hereditary disease characterized by a predisposition to develop dysplastic nevi and cutaneous melanoma. Approximately 8% to 10% of cases of melanoma are associated with a family history or hereditary dysplastic nevus syndrome. Patients with familial atypical multiple mole syndrome suggest a risk for melanoma of 400- to 1,000-fold higher than that seen in the general population. The mode of inheritance is somewhat controversial and is believed to be polygenic.

Genetic studies of this heritable trait in families led to the identification of *CDKN2A* as the familial melanoma gene, located at chromosome 9p21. *CDKN2A* encodes two distinct proteins: inhibitor of cyclin-dependent kinase 4 (INK4A or p16^{INK4a}) and ARF (p14ARF). INK4A regulates cell cycle progression at the G_1/S checkpoint by inhibiting the G_1 cyclin-dependent kinases that phosphorylate and inactivate the retinoblastoma protein. ARF inhibits p53 degradation; therefore, loss of ARF inactivates p53. The frequency of *CDKN2A* mutations vary in melanoma but are found more commonly in individuals with familial inheritance patterns and are associated with multiple cases of melanoma in a family, young age at diagnosis, multiple primary melanomas amongst family members, and pancreatic cancer.[9]

One of the major signaling pathways found to be associated with the development of melanoma is the mitogen-activated protein kinase pathway (MAPK) which mediates receptor tyrosine kinases resulting in activation of RAS and downstream BRAF. Activating *BRAF* mutations are the most common somatic genetic event in human melanoma, occurring in 25% to 70% of melanoma patients and primarily noted by a single point mutation *BRAF* (V600E). *BRAF* does not appear to be an inherited disposition gene, but the high prevalence of *BRAF* mutations in cutaneous melanoma appear to be an epidemiologic link between ultraviolet (UV) radiation and melanoma. *BRAF* mutations are common in melanomas arising from skin with intermittent sun exposure and not as common in melanomas in chronically sun-exposed areas. This may be an early event in the damage to the melanocytes as these mutations are also found in benign and dysplastic nevi.[5]

Other genetic alterations involved with the development of melanoma include *MITF* (microphthalmia-associated transcription factor), a gene that is important to the survival of melanocytes and has been shown to play a key role in melanoma signaling. The melanocortin 1 receptor gene (*MC1R*), which is associated with the red hair/fair skin phenotype, is involved in melanin synthesis and is more prevalent in individuals with melanoma. *NEDD9* modulates metastatic activity and has been found to be unregulated in melanoma. These melanoma-specific pathways give better understanding of the biology of the disease and may lead to better more directed treatment. A variety of other molecular pathways and receptor tyrosine kinases are also being studied to identify their role in the development of melanoma.[5]

Sunlight is one of the most important environmental factors in the pathogenesis of melanoma, and the incidence of melanoma has been associated with latitude and the intensity of solar exposure among susceptible populations. Radiation in the ultraviolet B (UVB) range (280 nm to 320 nm) is historically considered to be the critical factor linking sunlight and melanoma, although prolonged exposure to ultraviolet A (UVA) radiation (320 nm to 400 nm) also may be important. Use of older UVB-blocking sunscreens may not be as protective as once thought because they allow more sustained sun exposure without any clinical symptoms of burn (e.g., erythema or pain), ultimately resulting in intense irradiation of the skin by UVA light.

PATHOGENESIS

Melanomas most often arise within epidermal melanocytes of the skin, although they also can arise from noncutaneous melanocytes. Human melanocytes are dendritic pigmented cells that arise from the neural crest tissue during early fetal development and migrate over a predictable route to a variety of sites within the body, including the skin, uveal tract, meninges, and ectodermal mucosa. In adults, most melanocytes are located at the epidermal–dermal junction of the skin and the choroid of the eye, but they can be found in other tissues such as the meninges and the alimentary and respiratory tract. Primary melanoma can arise in any area of the body with melanocytes. The skin is the most frequent site of melanoma; cutaneous melanoma constitutes 90% of all melanoma. Primary melanoma can arise in the eye (ocular melanoma) and less frequently the mucosa and metastatic disease with unknown primary site.[5]

Normal melanocytes arise from melanoblasts. They undergo a series of differentiation events before reaching a final end-cell differentiation state and can be arrested in their differentiation process at any given state of maturation without loss of their proliferation capacity. Melanocytes adhere to the basement membrane of the epidermis and, despite a resting state, maintain a lifelong proliferation potential. The existence of melanoma stem cells has been suggested from work with cells from melanoma lines.[8]

Melanocytes synthesize melanin to protect various tissues, such as the skin, from UV radiation–induced damage and reach the keratinocytes in the upper layers of the epidermis via dendrites. Tyrosinase is an essential enzyme within melanosomes that synthesizes melanin. They are resistant to severe UV radiation, unlike keratinocytes, and their survival leads to the proliferation of mutated genes.[6]

Skin melanocytes transform from preexisting nevocellular nevi in the development of melanoma. A series of distinct steps are involved in the development and progression of melanoma from melanocytes. The pathologic components of the progression in human melanoma involve a series of morphologic stages: melanocytic atypia, atypical melanocytic hyperplasia, radial growth phase in which limited growth and radial expansion of the nevi may occur without metastatic competence, primary melanoma in the vertical growth phase with or without in-transit metastases, regional lymph node metastatic melanoma, and distant metastatic melanoma.[4] Primary melanoma is characterized by radial growth and limited vertical thickness (<0.75 mm). Primary melanoma demonstrates little tendency to metastasize. Melanoma has a potential for metastasis formation with the onset of a vertical growth phase. Therefore, the thickness of a primary melanoma is an important prognostic factor and is used in the staging classification of cutaneous melanoma. Of note, melanomas can skip steps in this development pathway.

Normal melanocytes require growth factors for proliferation, but melanoma cells can proliferate without growth factors. Melanoma cells secrete a variety of growth autocrine and paracrine factors that may facilitate proliferation. Additionally, with disease progression, melanoma cells increase production of certain growth factors and cytokines. The phosphatidylinositol 3-kinase (PI3K)–AKT pathway often is overactive in melanoma. Integrins and growth factors promote growth and survival of melanoma through these pathways.

Basic fibroblast growth factors (bFGFs) are thought to be important mediators of growth stimulation and cell survival and act as motility factors for melanoma cells as well as upregulate serine proteinases and metalloproteinases. Melanoma cells are strong producers of chemoattractive proteins such as interleukin 8. Vascular endothelial growth factor can be triggered in the vertical growth phase.[10] Most of these changes occur between the radial growth phase and vertical growth phase of primary melanoma, and metastatic cells often show the highest cytokine production.

Understanding the biology of melanoma has provided potential targets for drug therapy.[11,12] For example, the role of bFGF in the pathogenesis of melanoma has led to investigation of antisense oligonucleotides to block bFGF. Other pathways, such as mitogen-activated protein kinase pathway has been targeted by RAF and MEK inhibitors and the PI3K/AKT pathway by mTOR inhibitors. As pathways are identified and as agents that inhibit these pathways enter clinical trials and practice, there is growing excitement about the opportunities to impact treatment of melanoma in new and effective ways.

Immune factors appear to be involved in the progression of melanoma more often than in most other solid tumors.[3,5] Spontaneous cancer regressions are rare but are a well-documented phenomenon seen in melanoma. Focal regression in primary melanoma has been reported. Tumor regression appears to be associated with host immunity.

A number of different tumor antigens have been identified in the cellular membrane and cytoplasm of melanoma cells and are referred to as melanoma-associated antigens. Ganglioside antigens have been of particular interest in the development of immunotherapy for melanoma. A large number of monoclonal antibodies to melanoma-associated antigens have been developed and are being evaluated in clinical trials for diagnosis of and therapy for melanoma.

The humoral and cellular responses of individuals with melanoma who express melanoma-associated antigen have been described and provide the rationale for immunotherapy in the management of metastatic melanoma.[5] Melanoma-directed antibodies have been isolated in the sera of patients with melanoma. The presence of antimelanoma antibodies in the sera of patients correlates with the clinical status of the patients, and the antibodies gradually disappear from the serum as the disease progresses. This phenomenon may be explained by the possible formation of anti-idiotype antibodies directed against the antimelanoma antibodies, an increase in the circulation of soluble tumor antigens that saturate all antibody combining sites, increased levels of immunosuppression, or absorption of antibodies on the tumor mass.

Interest has focused on the role of cell-mediated immune response in melanoma. Specific cell-mediated responses may play a role in tumor regression, but the role of specific cells, such as cytotoxic T lymphocytes (CTLs), is not fully understood. Tumor-infiltrating lymphocytes (TILs) have been shown in vivo and in vitro to possess antitumor reactivity. TILs contain a large number of mature tumor-specific lymphocytes and have been a target for manipulation in immunotherapeutic approaches for melanoma.[5] Two identified targets are cytotoxic T lymphocyte antigen 4 (CTLA-4) and toll-like receptor 9 (TLR9). CTLA-4 is a glycoprotein expressed on the surface of activated T cells that appears to have an inhibitory effect on T cells. Blocking the effect of CTLA-4 could be an effective strategy for increasing the T-cell antitumor response.[13]

HISTOLOGIC SUBTYPES

Cutaneous melanomas are categorized by growth patterns. Four major histologic subtypes or growth patterns of primary cutaneous melanoma have been identified: superficial spreading melanoma, nodular melanoma, lentigo maligna melanoma, and acral lentiginous melanoma. Clinical outcomes of the four major melanoma subtypes are similar, if the comparison controls for depth of penetration or tumor thickness. Any of the four subtypes can present as an amelanotic variant. Amelanotic melanomas appear to be devoid of clinically apparent pigmentation. Two less common types of melanoma include desmoplastic melanoma and lentiginous melanoma. Desmoplastic melanoma is more commonly seen in older individuals and its clinical presentation is similar to that seen in nonmelanoma skin cancers. If a biopsy of the lesion is not obtained, the disease may be mismanaged. Lentiginous melanoma is histologically different than the four major subtypes. Uveal melanoma is considered a separate disease from cutaneous melanoma.

Superficial spreading melanoma is the most common morphologic type of cutaneous melanoma, accounting for approximately 70% of all melanomas.[5] The lesions usually arise from a preexisting nevus, known as a *precursor lesion*, and evolve slowly over 1 to 5 years. At some point, superficial spreading melanoma may progress to a more rapid growth phase. Early in lesion development, the superficial spreading melanoma is flat, but the surface becomes irregular and asymmetrical as the lesion progresses. The lesion enlarges when it enters into a rapid growth phase, and the edges appear notched or lacy. The lesions can be blue, black, or pink. Areas within the lesion may be hypopigmented. These patches of color variation, specifically the hypopigmented areas, are thought to be associated with tumor regression within the lesion or pigment inconsistency. The clinical differential diagnosis of superficial spreading melanoma includes both benign and malignant skin disease. This subtype is sometimes confused with seborrheic keratoses or pigmented basal cell carcinoma. Superficial spreading melanoma may occur at any anatomic site on the body, but they are more commonly seen on the back in men and on the legs in women. This subtype of melanoma is more common in women. The mean age of diagnosis of superficial spreading melanoma is 50 years, which is earlier than that seen for other subtypes. Superficial spreading melanoma usually occurs after puberty.

Lentigo maligna melanoma represents 10% to 20% of melanomas and is commonly found on the head and neck. It is unique from other histologic subtypes because due to its prolonged radial growth phase it does not have the same propensity to metastasize.[5] Lentigo maligna melanoma arises on chronically sun-exposed sites in older individuals and presents as a freckle-like lesion. Lentigo maligna melanomas are generally large (>3 cm), flat, and tan-colored lesions with shades of brown and black. The lesions gradually grow and develop darker, with asymmetric flecks in areas. Lentigo maligna melanoma is uncommon before age 50 years and may have been present for more than 5 years. Only approximately 5% to 8% of lentigo maligna melanoma evolve into invasive melanoma, which is characterized by nodular development within the flat precursor lesion. Lentigo maligna melanoma can be difficult to distinguish from solar lentigo, which typically is a smaller and evenly pigmented flat-appearing lesion.

Nodular melanoma is the second most common growth pattern of melanoma, occurring in 15% to 30% of patients. Nodular melanoma is a pure vertical growth phase disease. In nodular melanoma, a small expansive nodule in the papillary dermis invades the reticular dermis and subcutis. The radial growth phase is absent at all times. Nodular melanomas are more aggressive and develop more rapidly than superficial spreading melanoma. Nodular melanomas are dark blue–black and often uniform in color with a shiny surface, although a small percentage of nodular melanomas are amelanotic and have a fleshy appearance. Nodular melanomas are raised and often symmetric. They can occur at any age, typically around 50 years of age, and are most common on the trunk, head, and neck. Nodular melanomas are more common in men. Of note, nodular melanomas can resemble traumatized nevi.

Acral lentiginous melanoma makes up approximately 5% of melanomas and is most likely not related to UV exposure. It presents as three distinct clinical subtypes: melanoma on the palms of the hands or soles of the feet, subungual melanoma, and mucosal melanoma.[5] Most acral lentiginous melanomas are located on the soles of the feet and look like a large tan or brown stain. The lesions often have irregular convoluted borders. The initial macular component of palmar/plantar melanomas can be masked by the thickened stratum corneum at these sites. Many of these lesions look verrucous in appearance, making them difficult to distinguish from warts by the untrained eye. Suspicious lesions on the palms or soles of the feet should be evaluated. Acral lentiginous melanoma includes subungual melanoma, which arises in the nail matrix or nail bed. The most common presentation is a brown or black line in the great toe or the thumbnail. Mucosal melanoma is rare but can occur on any mucosal surface. Mucosal melanoma occurs most commonly in the oropharyngeal mucosa, followed by the anal/rectal mucosa, genital mucosa, and urinary mucosa. Unfortunately, mucosal melanoma often does not become clinically apparent until the mass is large or the lesion bleeds. Acral lentiginous melanoma occurs in less than 10% of white people with melanoma but is the most common type of melanoma reported in individuals with a dark complexion (e.g., African Americans, Asians, and Hispanics). Like lentigo maligna melanomas, this subtype is characterized by a protracted radial growth phase.

Uveal melanoma is the most common primary intraocular malignancy seen in adults but is an uncommon tumor.[14] Unlike cutaneous melanoma, the frequency and mortality of uveal melanoma have remained steady. This melanoma arises from the pigmented epithelium of the choroid. Iris melanoma is a subset of uveal melanoma and tends to have a more benign course. The risk of metastasis varies with the histologic type and size of the tumor as well as the location in the eye. Metastases occur most frequently in the liver but have been documented in a variety of tissues.

The ability to predict the metastatic potential of melanomas would be a valuable prognostic tool. An attempt to predict the likelihood for metastasis is based on radial and vertical growth phases. Radial growth phase describes the early stage of melanoma when the tumor is thin and primarily intraepidermal in location. By definition, malignant melanoma in situ is a form of radial growth phase melanoma. Vertical growth phase is the stage of melanoma with clear metastatic potential.

CLINICAL PRESENTATION

Benign nevi often occur in sun exposed areas and typically are 4 to 6 mm in diameter (about the size of a pencil eraser), raised or flat, are uniform in color and round in shape. Dysplastic nevi are believed to be a link between benign nevi and melanoma. Dysplastic nevi tend to be larger that the common nevi (>5 mm), appear as flat macules with asymmetry, have a fuzzy or ill-defined shape, and vary in color. Compared to melanoma lesions, dysplastic nevi appear less evolved.

The initial clinical presentation of melanoma often is a cutaneous lesion and is dependent on the histologic subtype as well as the stage of development of the lesion. The lesion can be located anywhere on the body but is most commonly discovered on the lower extremities in women and on the back and trunk in men. The cardinal clinical feature of a cutaneous melanoma is a pigmented skin lesion that changes over a period of time. The clinical features used to describe or evaluate a questionable lesion are highlighted by the mnemonic "ABCDE." Unlike benign pigmented lesions, the shape of a melanoma lesion is often (A) *asymmetric*. Benign lesions tend to have regular margins, whereas melanoma lesions often have irregular (B) *borders*. The (C) *color* of melanoma lesions is often variegated, ranging in color from tan to blue-black, and at times the lesion is intermingled with colors of red, purple, and white. The size or (D) *diameter* of a melanoma lesion is frequently 6 mm or greater when identified, whereas benign lesions usually are smaller. Early melanoma lesions may be diagnosed at a smaller size, and size of a lesion should not be used as "the trigger" to have a suspicious lesion evaluated. Another warning sign of a potential melanoma is the *enlargement* or *evolution* (E) in preexisting nevi. Changes such as a sudden or continuous enlargement of a lesion, an elevation of a lesion, or any change in the skin surrounding a nevus, including redness or swelling, are important clinical signs. Uncommonly, the sensation of the lesion may become itchy or tender and painful. Friability of the lesion resulting in bleeding or oozing is a danger sign. Perhaps the most important warning sign of danger is the evolution in any characteristic of a lesion.

The diagnosis of melanoma is complicated by the number of pigmented moles (melanocytic nevi) and nonmelanocytic lesions that resemble melanoma. An average of 10 to 40 ordinary nevi can be found on the skin of white adults. Nonmelanocytic pigmented lesions such as seborrheic keratoses, pigmented basel cell carcinoma, and vascular lesions, also can appear similar to a melanoma lesion. In childhood melanoma, commonly the lesions are thicker at the time of diagnosis. This may be in part to the low level of suspicion by pediatricians, the fact that many melanomas associated with congenital nevi develop in the dermis rather than the epidermis, and histological uncertainty.[3]

❶ Improved survival rates for melanoma have been attributed to the identification and treatment of disease at an early stage, when the disease is limited and has not yet metastasized. It follows that one strategy to improve survival rates would be to increase efforts to identify early-stage melanoma. The cost-effectiveness of massive screening for all adults by a physician has never been demonstrated. However, routine examination of the skin by physicians is recommended for individuals, adults, or children who are at high risk. The entire cutaneous surface, including the scalp, should be examined.

It has been estimated that approximately 50% of the initial melanoma lesions found are discovered by self-examination. Therefore, one of the most direct strategies to improve early detection would be a method to increase effective skin self-examination (SSE) by the individual, the individual's partner, and/or a caregiver. Identification of early melanoma allows the opportunity to treat the lesions when they are thin and curable. Persons who perform SSE present for care at an earlier stage in the disease process and have 50% less advanced melanoma and lower mortality from the disease.[15] Healthcare individuals who routinely work with the public, such as community pharmacists, have an opportunity to increase public awareness concerning the benefits and appropriate methods for SSE. Educational pamphlets describing SSE (Table 147–2) for the public are widely available through the American Cancer Society, American Academy of Dermatology, and Skin Cancer Foundation. If a newly discovered pigmented lesion is identified or if a preexisting pigmented lesion changes, the individual should be evaluated by a physician immediately.

SSE is of special interest in the elderly. As the population of older adults (≥65 years of age) increases, it is expected that the mortality from melanoma also will increase. Barriers to successful SSE in the elderly, such as failing eyesight, lack of partners, and poor memory, impact the older adult in detecting new or changing lesions. These barriers, coupled with the higher incidence of melanoma in males, present a challenge and an opportunity for the healthcare professional to target education on this growing segment of our population.

A biopsy of the lesion is critical to establish diagnosis of melanoma. Subsequent pathologic interpretation of the biopsy will help provide information on prognosis and treatment options. An excisional biopsy with a 1 to 2 mm margin of normal-appearing skin is recommended for a suspicious lesion and should include a portion of underlying subcutaneous fat for microstaging. For larger lesions where an excisional biopsy is impractical, an incisional or punch biopsy can be performed and should include a core of full-thickness skin and subcutaneous tissue. When excisional biopsies are not appropriate, as with the face or palmar surface of the hands, a full-thickness incisional or punch biopsy is preferred. A shave biopsy is never appropriate because it can underestimate the thickness of the lesion and may not fully remove the lesion, and the scarring may mask the remaining tumor.

Evaluation of any individual with a suspected melanoma includes a complete history and total body skin examination. The focus of the patient history is identifying potential risk factors. Risk-related questions include an assessment of family history of melanoma, personal history of skin cancer and/or nevus excisions, sun exposure, and phenotype. Total dermatologic examination is necessary to determine melanoma risk factors (e.g., mole pattern, mole type, or freckling) and for staging. Melanoma commonly spreads to the lymph nodes, therefore individuals suspicious for advanced disease should have their lymph nodes examined for lymphadenopathy. Any clinical indication of regional lymph node involvement should be confirmed with fine-needle aspiration or on biopsy of the enlarged lymph node. Laboratory and imaging studies (chest x-ray, computed tomography (CT) with or without positron emission tomography (PET) or magnetic resonance imaging (MRI)) can be used in the workup for melanoma. These tests may not be sensitive in detecting occult disease in early-stage (stages I and II) patients and may be optional if an individual is low risk or asymptomatic.[16] Lactate dehydrogenase should be measured as elevated serum levels have been shown to be an independent predictor of decreased survival.[17] Additionally, any other signs or symptoms suggestive of metastatic disease should be completely evaluated.

STAGING AND PROGNOSTIC FACTORS

The size of a primary melanoma lesion is associated with the likelihood of metastases. The prognostic factor originally used to determine survival was based on the cross-sectional profile of the primary tumor. The cross-sectional profile could be evaluated if the deepest invasive tumor cells lay above or below the sweat glands. This assessment was further clarified by Clark,[18] who described the relationship of depth of invasion of the cancer cells to the standard anatomic landmarks of the skin (Table 147–3). Clark's classification is a practical approach for patients with more superficial tumors, because tumors classified as Clark levels I through III seldom metastasize. The classification system has been criticized because of problems associated with practical measurements. Melanoma lesions that occur in the presence of lymphoid infiltration, fibrosis, or even the cells of preexisting nevi are difficult to assess with classic reference landmarks.

Breslow[19] replaced Clark's classification of reference landmarks with the use of thickness of the primary melanoma lesion. Tumor thickness is quantified to the nearest tenth of a millimeter with an

---

TABLE 147-2 Self-Examination of Suspicious Moles

1. Examine your body front and back in the mirror, and then right and left sides with arms raised.
2. Bend the elbows and look carefully at the forearms and upper arms and palms.
3. Look at the backs of the legs and feet. Look specifically in the spaces between toes and at the soles of the feet.
4. Examine the back of the neck and scalp with the help of a hand-held mirror; part hair (or use a blow dryer) to lift hair and give yourself a closer look.
5. Check the back and buttocks with a hand-held mirror.

Derived from publications of the American Academy of Dermatology.

TABLE 147-3 Clark's Classification

Clark Level	Anatomic Landmark
N	Epidermis
I	Dermal-epidermal junction
II	Papillary dermis
III	Interface between papillar dermis and reticular dermis
IV	Reticular dermis and subcutaneous fat

ocular micrometer, measuring from the top of the granular layer of the overlying epidermis to the deepest contiguous invasive melanoma cell. The correlation between tumor thickness and probability of tumor metastases is strong but does not include aspects such as tumor satellites, defined rather arbitrarily as skin involvement within 2 cm of the primary lesion, and vascular invasion. It was once thought that the presence of satellite nodule(s) had the same impact on prognosis as a high-risk primary lesion (tumor thickness >4 mm). It is now known that patients with satellitosis have a worse prognosis than patients with thick primary lesions, and prognosis is more similar to that of patients with nodal metastases. A number of prognostic factors, in addition to tumor thickness and level of invasion, are associated with the risk for developing metastatic disease.[20]

The American Joint Committee on Cancer (AJCC) developed a staging system for melanoma that divides patients with localized melanoma into four stages according to microstaging criteria of Breslow and Clark.[21] In addition to consideration of the primary lesion, the AJCC staging system includes aspects of the tumor satellite, extent of lymph node involvement, and presence of metastatic disease.[21] Analysis of several large databases worldwide identified areas in which the AJCC staging system, which was published in 1997, did not reflect the natural history of melanoma. Issues such as the appropriate cutoff values for primary tumor thickness, ulceration of the melanoma, and satellite lesions of the primary tumor should be considered when making decisions about therapy.[20] The cutoff values initially proposed by Breslow for primary tumor thickness were initially used in the AJCC staging system, but it appears that cutoff depths of 1, 2, and 4 mm of thickness may better predict overall survival. Melanoma ulceration is associated with increased mitotic rate within a primary melanoma. The presence of ulceration of the primary lesion has been correlated with poorer survival for patients with very thin or thick lesions, but ulceration of the melanoma was not included in the 1997 AJCC staging system.

The revised AJCC staging system for cutaneous melanoma was published in 2002 and has been used for several years.[21] It is important to carefully examine older clinical trials to determine which staging system was used to determine patient inclusion and exclusion criteria, as results may differ based on these patient criteria. Revisions of the new melanoma staging system include (a) melanoma thickness and ulceration for all tumors (except T_1 tumors); (b) number of metastatic lymph nodes versus gross dimensions and delineation of clinically occult versus clinically apparent nodal metastases; (c) site of distant metastases and presence of elevated serum lactate dehydrogenase for metastatic disease; (d) upstaging of all patients with stage I, II, or III disease when a primary melanoma is ulcerated; and (e) new convention for separating clinical and pathologic staging to include information obtained from intraoperative lymphatic mapping and sentinel node biopsy. Clinical staging includes microstaging of the primary melanoma and clinical and radiologic evaluation. It is used after complete excision of the primary melanoma with clinical assessment for regional and distant metastasis. Pathologic staging includes microstaging of the primary melanoma and pathologic information about the regional nodes after partial or complete lymphadenectomy. At this time, it appears that patients with very limited disease (in situ or stage 0) do not require pathologic evaluation of lymph nodes (Tables 147–4 and 147–5). As with other solid tumors, the presence of regional lymph node involvement is a powerful predictor of tumor burden and patient outcome. In the past, the primary method for determining nodal status was surgical resection and analysis of the lymph nodes via a regional lymph node dissection. The extent of lymph node dissection was determined by the anatomy of the area of the lesion. In recent years, preoperative lymphoscintigraphy and intraoperative sentinel node mapping have become more widely used methods for

TABLE 147-4 Melanoma TNM Classification

T Classification	Thickness	Ulcerative Status
T_X	Primary tumor cannot be addressed (e.g., shave biopsy)	
T_0	No evidence of primary tumor	
T_{is}	Melanoma in situ	
T_1	≤1 mm	A: No ulceration and level II/III
		B: With ulceration or level IV/V
T_2	1.01–2 mm	A: No ulceration
		B: With ulceration
T_3	2.01–4 mm	A: No ulceration
		B: With ulceration
T_4	>4 mm	A: No ulceration
		B: With ulceration

N Classification	No. of Metastatic Nodes	Nodal Metastatic Mass
N_X	Regional lymph nodes cannot be assessed	
N_0	No regional lymph nodes	
N_1	1 node	A: Micrometastasis
		B: Macrometastasis
N_2	2–3 nodes	A: Micrometastasis
		B: Macrometastasis
		C: In-transit metastases/ satellite(s) without metastatic nodes
N_3	≥4 metastatic regional lymph nodes, matted metastatic nodes, metastatic lymph nodes, or intransit metastatic or satellite lesions in regional nodes	

M Classification	Site	Serum Lactate Dehydrogenase
M_X	Distant metastases cannot be assessed	
M_0	No distant metastasis	
M_1	Any distant metastasis	
M_{1a}	Distant skin, subcutaneous tissue, or nodal metastatic disease	Normal
M_{1b}	Lung metastases	Normal
M_{1c}	All other visceral metastases or distant metastasis at any site associated with elevated serum lactic dehydrogenase	Elevated

Micrometastases are diagnosed after sentinel or elective lymphadenectomy.
Macrometastases are defined as clinically detectable lymph node metastases confirmed by therapeutic lymphadenectomy or when any lymph node metastasis exhibits extracapsular extension.
Data from Barch CM, Buzaid AC, Soong SJ, et al. Final version of the American Joint Committee on cancer staging system for cutaneous melanoma. J Clin Oncol 2001;19:3635–3648.

identifying the first or sentinel lymph node in the direct pathway of lymph drainage from the primary cutaneous melanoma. Sentinel lymph node biopsy (SLNB) is a minimally invasive procedure that determines if a patient is a candidate for a complete lymph node dissection. The rationale for lymphatic mapping and subsequent sentinel node biopsy is based on the observation that regions of the skin have patterns of lymphatic drainage to specific lymph nodes in the regional lymphatic basin. The sentinel lymph node is believed to be the first node in the lymphatic basin into which the primary melanoma drains. Unlike other solid tumors, melanoma appears to progress in an orderly nodal distribution. Evaluation of sentinel nodes has been used for detection of micrometastases in breast cancer and in melanoma. SLNB allows for more thorough examination

TABLE 147-5 American Joint Committee on Cancer Tumor (T), Node (N), Metastasis (M) Stage Grouping for Cutaneous Melanoma

Pathologic Stage	T	N	M	Clinical Stage	T	N	M
0	T_{is}	N_0	M_0	0	T_{is}	N_0	M_0
IA	T_{1a}	N_0	M_0	IA	T_{1a}	N_0	M_0
IB	T_{1b}	N_0	M_0	IB	T_{1b}	N_0	M_0
	T_{2a}	N_0	M_0		T_{2a}	N_0	M_0
IIA	T_{2b}	N_0	M_0	IIA	T_{2b}	N_0	M_0
	T_{3a}	N_0	M_0		T_{3a}	N_0	M_0
IIB	T_{3b}	N_0	M_0	IIB	T_{3b}	N_0	M_0
	T_{4a}	N_0	M_0		T_{4a}	N_0	M_0
IIC	T_{4b}	N_0	M_0	IIC	T_{4b}	N_0	M_0
IIIA	T_{1-4a}	N_{1a}	M_0	III	Any	N_{1-3}	M_0
	T_{1-4a}	N_{2a}	M_0				
IIIB	T_{1-4a}	N_{1a}	M_0				
	T_{1-4a}	N_{2a}	M_0				
	T_{1-4b}	N_{1b}	M_0				
	T_{1-4b}	N_{2b}	M_0				
	$T_{1-4a/b}$	N_{2c}	M_0				
IIIC	T_{1-4b}	$N_{2b}-N_{2c}$	M_0				
	Any T	N_3	M_0				
IV	Any T	Any N	M_1	IV	Any T	Any N	M_1

of a single sentinel node than is possible when examining multiple lymph nodes with a lymph node dissection and may be most useful for melanomas located in ambiguous drainage sites such as the head and neck areas. SLNB is associated with low false-negative rates and low complication rates.[22] Detection of clinically undetectable disease in a lymph node basin that is not directly adjacent to the primary lesion may allow for upstaging of patients who initially are believed to have node-negative disease.

Reverse-transcription polymerase chain reaction (RT-PCR) is another method used to detect occult micrometastases in biopsied lymph nodes. This technique identifies submicroscopic levels of melanoma-specific genetic material. Initial studies with RT-PCR suggested that individuals who were RT-PCR negative had increased survival. Since these data have not been confirmed in a larger prospective trial, the prognostic value of RT-PCR remains unclear.[5,23] Strategies that combine RT-PCR with other newer detection methods are being evaluated.

The stage of melanoma at the time of diagnosis is one of the primary indicators of natural history of the disease and contributes to prognosis. Tumor thickness, level of tumor invasion and ulceration all contribute to the stage of a patient and their overall outcome. Other factors such as tumor growth pattern or histological subtype, mitotic rate, density of TILs infiltrating the tumor tissue, elevated lactate dehydrogenase, satellite lesions, angiolymphatic invasion, gender, and age also have been reported to have an impact on survival (Table 147–6). The location of the primary tumor on the skin

is also important as individuals with tumors of the extremities have an increased survival as compared to those with axial, neck, head, and trunk tumors. In addition, a number of additional prognostic factors have been identified in patients with advanced disease. The number of metastatic sites, disease involvement of the gastrointestinal tract, liver, pleura, or lung, Eastern Cooperative Oncology Group (ECOG) performance status ≥1, male sex, and prior immunotherapy have been associated with poor prognosis.[20]

TREATMENT

Melanoma

Treatment of cutaneous melanoma depends on the stage of disease. Local disease is managed, and often cured, with surgical ablation. Regional disease is treated with surgical resection of the primary lesion and, depending on the risk of recurrence, possibly adjuvant therapy. Use of adjuvant therapy after surgical resection and the role of interferon-α as adjuvant therapy remain controversial. Treatment of disseminated melanoma continues to be a challenge. Although numerous clinical trials have evaluated single-agent and combination chemotherapy, immunotherapy, targeted therapy, and biochemotherapy regimens, there is not a single standard approach for management of the individual with metastatic melanoma.[4,5,16,24]

■ SURGERY

❷ Patients who present with a suspicious pigmented lesion should undergo a full-thickness excisional biopsy, if possible. Sites at which excisional biopsy is inappropriate include the face, palm of the hand, sole of the foot, distal digit, and subungual lesions. A full-thickness incisional or punch biopsy is preferred in these cases to provide microstaging and ultimately to determine therapy.

Localized cutaneous melanoma can often be cured with surgical excision. The cure rates for melanomas <1 mm are as high as 98%.[5] The extent of the excision margin is important in preventing local recurrence and ultimate survival. For melanoma in situ, excision of the visible lesion or biopsy site with a 0.5 to 1 cm border of clinically normal skin and a layer of subcutaneous tissue with confirmation

TABLE 147-6 Prognostic Factors for Cutaneous Melanoma

Tumor-related factors
Tumor thickness
Level of tumor invasion
Ulceration
Histologic subtype
Anatomic site of primary tumor
Mitotic rate
Lymphangitic invasion
Occurrence of microsatellites
Presence of tumor-infiltrating lymphocytes

Patient-related factors
Age
Gender

of histologically negative peripheral margins is recommended. The recommended clinical margin for invasive melanoma depends on the tumor thickness. Excision with a 1 cm margin of clinically normal skin and underlying subcutaneous tissue is recommended for invasive melanomas ≤1 mm thick.[16,25] The appropriate margin of excision for melanomas between 1 and 2 mm in thickness is controversial. A study suggests the risk of locoregional recurrence is higher when melanomas that are at least 2 mm thick are excised with a 1 cm margin rather than a 2 cm margin.[26] Current National Comprehensive Cancer Network (NCCN) guidelines recommend a 1 to 2 cm margin for melanoma with tumor thickness of 1.01 to 2 mm.[16] Lesions that are 2 to 4 mm thick should be excised with a 2 cm margin. Primary tumors more than 4 mm thick require at least a 2 cm margin, but whether a larger margin is beneficial is not clear. Surgical management of lentigo maligna melanoma is problematic, as subclinical extension of atypical junctional melanocytic hyperplasia may extend beyond the visible margins. Complete excision of these lesions is important.

When isolated regional lymph nodes are detected via physical examination in the absence of distant disease, therapeutic lymphadenectomy is recommended. The extent of therapeutic lymph node dissection often is modified according to the anatomic area of the lymphadenopathy. Prophylactic lymphadenectomy in all patients is not recommended. Although a subgroup of patients with early-stage melanoma will have microscopic metastatic disease in nonpalpable lymph nodes, prophylactic regional lymph node dissection does not prolong survival or decrease time to relapse in randomized clinical trials.[5,27,28] Selective regional lymphadenectomy performed after scintigraphic and dye lymphographic identification of the affected sentinel draining lymph node(s) is the standard of care for melanomas >1 mm thick. If the sentinel node is found to have micrometastatic melanoma, regional dissection of the involved nodal basin is performed. If the lesion is 0.75 to 1 mm in thickness with ulceration or is Clark level IV or V, lymphatic mapping with sentinel node biopsy may be considered based on patient characteristics such as ulceration of the tumor.[24] Of note, the likelihood of detecting metastatic disease in the sentinel lymph node depends on tumor thickness. The likelihood of detecting metastatic disease is approximately 1% in tumors that are less than 0.8 mm but increases to more than 30% in tumors 4 mm thick.[24] Sentinel lymph node biopsy results are important for accurate staging, therapeutic lymphadenectomy, and to aid in the decision to offer adjuvant treatment.[22,27]

One of the most important aspects of surgical management of cutaneous melanoma is the role of patient followup.[4,16] Postsurgical followup of patients who have had a melanoma excised is essential to monitor for undetected metastatic disease and the development of a second primary cutaneous melanoma or nonmelanoma primary malignancy. Scheduled screening in addition to routine surgical followup are required for any patient with a melanoma; the recommended frequency and duration depend on the stage of melanoma. The optimal duration of followup remains controversial. Most patients who develop recurrent disease will do so in the first 5 years after treatment, but late recurrences more than ten years after surgery have been observed. The increased lifetime risk of developing a second primary melanoma supports lifetime dermatologic surveillance for all patients.

Curative surgery usually is limited to patients with early-stage disease. A patient with stage III melanoma usually has lymph node involvement, but in-transit metastases also may occur. In-transit metastasis is the clinical manifestation of tumor that develops in lymphatics between the primary melanoma and the regional lymph node basin.[5] In-transit metastases are more than 2 cm from the original lesion. In-transit metastases are more common in individuals with thick ulcerated lesion. Surgery is used for management of in-transit lesions, and the goal is complete resection. Unfortunately, subsequent recurrence in the same extremity often occurs after initial resection of in-transit metastases.

The role of surgery beyond that of cure is less clear, although surgery may offer palliation for patients with isolated metastases.[27] Resection of isolated lesions in the brain and lungs may be appropriate in certain cases and should be evaluated based on individual patient criteria. Surgery can be an option in situations where the lesion is accessible and where the lesion may cause problems if not removed. Surgery can extend survival in select patients with metastatic disease. Patients whose metastases can be completely resected may experience improved quality of life, improved overall survival, and occasionally long-term disease control.[27]

Brain metastasis is a frequent complication of advanced melanoma. Approximately 20% to 50% of patients with stage IV disease will develop clinically apparent central nervous system involvement. Surgical resection, with or without radiation, has been used in select individuals. More recently, high control rates of brain metastases have been achieved with focal radiation therapy such as linear accelerator-based stereotactic radiosurgery or gamma-knife technologies.[29,30] Melanoma in the gastrointestinal tract can lead to bowel obstruction, and appropriate resection or bypass may allow the patient significant relief of symptoms. Despite the lack of controlled clinical trials, the impact on palliative surgery should be evaluated in the context of a patient's comfort and quality of life. Surgery may be an appropriate option if the perceived outcome is to provide patient comfort. On the other hand, surgery may constitute a significant physical challenge or financial burden to a patient with a limited life expectancy. The clinical scenarios involving surgical resection should be fully evaluated in terms of overall quality of life.

The risk of relapse and death after resection of a local or regional cutaneous melanoma is the primary determinant for use of adjuvant therapy after primary resection. Adjuvant trials have focused on patients at intermediate or high risk for recurrence.

■ IMMUNOTHERAPY

Melanoma is considered one of the most immunogenic solid tumors, and it appears to interact with and respond to the immune system of the host in which it arises. Spontaneous regressions of melanoma suggest the importance of the immune system in disease modulation. Lymphoid infiltration into the primary melanoma also suggests that immunomodulation may impact the biology of melanoma. Early work showed that nonspecific immunomodulators, such as levamisole and bacillus Calmette-Guérin, for treatment of melanoma were associated with some regression of the tumor, although many of these responses were limited and short lived. Because melanoma is one of the cancers most resistant to traditional treatment modalities such as radiation and chemotherapy, immunotherapy offers an avenue of treatment. Although the complete response rate seen in patients with melanoma treated with biotherapy is relatively low, the durability of responses in individuals who respond can be significant. Remaining unanswered questions include what is the best approach to biotherapy in a patient with melanoma and can biotherapy be combined with other available and emerging antineoplastic therapy.

Interferon

One of the oldest, and most controversial, immunotherapy approaches for the treatment of melanoma is the use of interferons (IFN).[4] The *interferons* are a group of proteins with diverse immunomodulatory and antiangiogenic properties. A number of studies have evaluated various doses and schedules of recombinant interferon for treatment of metastatic melanoma. Response rates in metastatic melanoma range from 10% to 30%, and overall response rates are approximately 15% for IFN-α. Unfortunately, the optimal dose, treatment schedule, and treatment combinations/regimens have not been established for management of metastatic melanoma.[5]

In clinical trials of interferon therapy for patients with metastatic melanoma, response rates were highest in patients with minimal disease. Responses were seen at all sites of disease but were most frequent in subcutaneous, lymph node, and pulmonary metastases. The success of interferon in patients with minimal disease encouraged investigators to evaluate the role of adjuvant interferon after curative surgical resection in patients who were at high risk for recurrent disease (bulky disease or regional lymph node involvement). Early trials of short-term or low-dose regimens of IFN-α did not demonstrate a survival benefit in the adjuvant setting. In an attempt to optimize response in the adjuvant setting, maximum tolerated doses of IFN-α were administered for 1 month, followed by prolonged therapy of IFN-α at more tolerable doses for 48 weeks. The rationale for the intensive induction phase was to provide peak interferon levels sufficient to inhibit tumor growth and avoid the development of anti-interferon antibodies. A large, multicenter cooperative group trial (E1684) of adjuvant IFN-α_{2b} versus observation was designed for 287 patients with high-risk (stages IIB and III disease based on the 1997 AJCC staging criteria) melanoma following curative surgical resection.[31] IFN-α_{2b} was given intravenously as an induction therapy at maximum tolerated doses of 20 million international units/m^2 per dose 5 days per week for 4 weeks in an outpatient setting; treatment was continued for 48 weeks with subcutaneous IFN-α_{2b} 10 million international units/m^2 per dose 3 times per week at home. This therapy now is often referred to as *high-dose interferon* (HDI). With a median followup of 6.9 years, patients treated with HDI had significantly longer relapse-free and overall survival compared to patients who were observed following surgical resection (1.72 vs. 0.98 years and 3.8 vs. 2.8 years, respectively).[31] Table 147–7 shows 5-year relapse-free and overall survival results. With longer followup (median, 12.6 years), however, the difference in overall survival was no longer significant.[32] Further analysis showed that the greatest reduction in melanoma recurrence occurred during the first few months of treatment. Subgroup analysis of this study indicated that patients with large primary tumors and node-negative disease ($T_4N_0M_0$) did not receive the same benefit from therapy, but the small number of patients in this group made it difficult to draw definite conclusions about the role of interferon for adjuvant therapy in this subgroup.

HDI treatment is associated with multiple toxicities, including flu-like syndrome. Other toxicities include depression, nausea, weight loss, fatigue, myelosuppression, elevations in liver function tests, and renal insufficiency. Toxicities of interferon therapy in the adjuvant HDI trials were common and severe, and most patients required dose reductions and/or delays at some point during treatment. Dose modifications were required for dose-limiting constitutional symptoms, myelosuppression, and hepatic toxicities, but 74% of patients were able to complete the year of therapy in an outpatient setting.

One of the strategies for reducing the toxicities associated with interferon was to modify the dose and duration. A subsequent ECOG trial (E1690) of low-dose interferon (LDI; 3 million units per dose given subcutaneously 3 times weekly) for 24 months compared with the HDI regimen described above versus observation did not demonstrate an overall survival advantage of HDI versus observation.[33] At median followup of 52 months, the 5-year estimated relapse-free survival rates for HDI, LDI, and observation were 44%, 40%, and 35%, respectively. Relapse-free survival was significantly longer in the HDI group, prolonging the median time to relapse by 10 months compared to observation and LDI. With longer followup, however, the difference in relapse-free survival was no longer significant.[32] A significant overall survival benefit was not seen for HDI or LDI compared to observation, although the investigators speculated that this analysis of survival was affected by the number of patients in the observation arm who received interferon therapy after disease progression.[33]

The use of interferon in the adjuvant setting remains controversial. Although the HDI regimen is used in the United States, the LDI strategy remains standard in many European countries.[4] In a pooled analysis of 713 patients who participated in two randomized controlled trials (E1684 and E1690), HDI was associated with a significant reduction in relapse-free survival compared with observation ($P <0.006$).[32] No benefit in overall survival was observed in the pooled analysis. The results of nine randomized clinical trials of adjuvant HDI or LDI versus observation in melanoma were included in a systematic review. The systematic review observed a trend toward reduction of risk of recurrence of melanoma and of death among the interferon-treated patients in nearly all studies.[34] Adjuvant IFN-α has been evaluated in a number of clinical trials in patients with intermediate- to very-high-risk melanoma after surgical resection. A systematic review evaluated nine randomized controlled trials of high- and low-dose regimens.[34] Due to differences in dose, frequency, and duration of IFN-α treatment in the various trials, the review was not able to compare LDI versus HDI. Furthermore, the wide variability in number of patients enrolled, endpoints, patient selection, quality, type of therapy, duration of treatment, and followup precluded statistical analysis of the pooled results. Although the differences in overall survival were not always statistically significant, HDI remains the only adjuvant treatment shown to prolong survival in prospective randomized trials. IFN-α_{2b} is approved by the U.S. Food and Drug Administration (FDA) for treatment of patients with primary melanomas larger than 4 mm (stages IIB and IIC) and in patients with melanoma involving regional lymph nodes who are disease-free following lymph node dissection (stage III).

Although interferon is widely used in the adjuvant setting, there are concerns over the considerable treatment toxicities and the lack of consistent overall survival advantage of a toxic and expensive regimen. In addition, whether the results from the HDI trials should be extrapolated to patients with local recurrences, satellite lesions, or in-transit metastases is not clear. Remaining questions include the following: (a) Are the toxicities associated with HDI treatment worth the potential benefits for patients? (b) What are the mechanism(s) and best approaches to managing interferon toxicity?

TABLE 147-7	Results of Eastern Cooperative Oncology Group Trials of Adjuvant High-Dose Interferon-α_{2b} Therapy in Melanoma Patients at High Risk for Recurrence			
Trial	Regimen	5-Year Relapse-Free Survival	5-Year Overall Survival	Reference
E1684	High-dose IFN[a]	37%	46%	Kirkwood et al.[31]
	Observation	26%	37%	
E1690	High-dose IFN[b]	44%	52%	Kirkwood et al.[32]
	Low-dose IFN	40%	53%	
	Observation	35%	55%	

[a]High-dose interferon (IFN) 20 million international units/m^2/day IV for 1 month and 10 million international units/m^2 3 times per week subcutaneously (SC) for 48 weeks.
[b]High-dose IFN 20 million international units/m^2/day 5 days per week IV for 4 weeks and 10 million international units/m^2 three times per week subcutaneously (SC) for 48 weeks.

(c) Is the regimen/schedule of interferon used in the initial positive trial (HDI) necessary to achieve the benefits seen in this study? Aggressive toxicity evaluation and individualized management are essential to help preserve quality of life in individuals receiving interferon therapy.

❸ A mechanism for optimizing the care of patients receiving interferon is to effectively prevent and manage treatment-related toxicities. A common syndrome seen with IFN-α therapy is a diverse group of side effects referred to as *constitutional symptoms*, which can include acute symptoms such as fever, chills, myalgia, and fatigue, and can encompass some of the more chronic toxicities such as fatigue, anorexia, and depression.[35] Acetaminophen can be used to prevent or minimize acute dose-related symptoms such as fever, myalgia, and chills. Opiates, such as meperidine, are often required when patients experience severe chills or rigors, most commonly during the initial month of the HDI induction phase. Nonsteroidal antiinflammatory drugs (NSAIDs) have been used to manage interferon-related myalgia but may have overlapping side effects with interferon, such as a decrease in renal blood flow. NSAIDs, like acetaminophen, may mask fevers that occur in patients who experience neutropenia while undergoing therapy. Additionally, NSAIDs may add to the risk of bleeding in the setting of thrombocytopenia caused by interferon. Fatigue is one of the most frequently observed dose-limiting toxicities seen with interferon therapy occurring in 70% to 100% of patients.[35] The mechanisms of interferon-induced fatigue are not fully understood and may be multifactorial in individual patients. Interferon-induced fatigue appears to be dose related and may worsen with continued therapy. Pharmacologic (e.g., methylphenidate) and nonpharmacologic interventions (e.g., exercise, psychosocial techniques, distraction, energy management, and dietary modifications) for treatment of cancer-related fatigue and now interferon-related fatigue are being evaluated.[35] Depression is common and should be fully evaluated. Contributing factors such as interferon-induced hypothyroidism and/or concomitant interferon symptoms (e.g., nausea and fatigue) should be evaluated concurrently with depression symptoms to optimize treatment decisions.[36] Antidepressants, such as selective serotonin-reuptake inhibitors, have been studied in interferon-induced depression with notable benefit.[35] Anorexia was reported in approximately 70% of patients receiving adjuvant interferon therapy for melanoma and is thought to be mediated through direct effects on hypothalamic neurons, modification of normal hypothalamic neurotransmitters/neuropeptides, or effects from stimulation of other cytokines.[35] Taste alterations may contribute to anorexia. Investigational strategies for ameliorating interferon-induced anorexia include nutritional intervention, use of appetite stimulants such as megestrol acetate, and patient education. Glucocorticoids should not be used for appetite stimulation or as part of an antiemetic therapy because they may adversely impact the immunomodulatory effects of interferon. Other toxicities such as hematologic or hepatic toxicities require monitoring and appropriate dose modification.

Because of the associated toxicity and adverse effects seen with IFN-α therapy, many experts have questioned the usefulness of intensive adjuvant therapy for melanoma despite the possible benefits in relapse-free and overall survival.[37] A subsequent report from the cooperative group study demonstrated a quality-of-life benefit with interferon therapy based on the quality-of-life–adjusted survival analysis.[38] This analysis calculates the quality-of-life–adjusted years gained as a result of IFN-α treatment or the clinical benefit of time without toxicities and without disease. Another approach that has been investigated is the use of a pegylated product. Unfortunately, pegylated interferon has been evaluated in an attempt to improve the benefit-toxicity ratio without much success.[39]

❹ The role of interferon as adjuvant therapy is not clear at this time. If adjuvant interferon is given, it is not clear what product (e.g., pegylated interferon), dose, and duration of therapy should be used. The issues of patient side effects and cost must be carefully weighed against the potential disease-free survival benefit. Because HDI is the only therapy to demonstrate benefit in large comparative trials, it should be considered for patients with high-risk disease. The 2010 NCCN guidelines for melanoma list IFN-α as one of several options for select patients with high-risk disease.[16] Other options include observation and probably, most importantly, clinical trials. Individuals should be prescreened for potential problems associated with therapy; relative contraindications to HDI therapy include autoimmune diseases, immunosuppression, decompensated liver disease, severe neuropsychiatric diseases, and life-threatening infection.[35] Efforts continue to better define the optimal treatment regimen for HDI versus other strategies in well-designed clinical trials.

The role of interferon in advanced disease is even less clear, especially for patients who have recurred after treatment with adjuvant interferon therapy. IFN-α has been used as a single agent in patients with metastatic disease who have not received adjuvant therapy and in combination with chemotherapy and/or other biotherapy for metastatic melanoma. The challenges of combination therapy are that many of the toxicities seen with interferon can be exacerbated by concomitant chemotherapy (e.g., nausea, vomiting, and neutropenia).

CLINICAL CONTROVERSY

The role of IFN-α as adjuvant therapy for high-risk patients after surgical resection of melanoma is controversial. Assessment of patient risk factors, availability of clinical trials, and cost of therapy should be evaluated prior to initiation of therapy.

Interleukin 2

Interleukin 2 (IL-2) is a glycoprotein produced by activated lymphocytes.[41] IL-2 was first identified as a T-cell growth factor, but now IL-2 clearly is a growth factor for a variety of cells including lymphocytes, T cells, and natural killer (NK) cells. IL-2 also may be immunosuppressive. The role of each of these effects of IL-2 on disease control in melanoma is not clear.

The precise mechanism of cytotoxicity of IL-2 is unknown. High concentrations of IL-2 have not been shown to have a direct antitumor effect on cancer cells in vitro. In vitro and in vivo, IL-2 stimulates the production and release of many secondary monocyte-derived and T-cell–derived cytokines, including IL-4, IL-5, IL-6, IL-8, tumor necrosis factor (TNF)-α, granulocyte-macrophage colony-stimulating factor, and interferon-γ, which may have direct or indirect antitumor activity. In addition, IL-2 stimulates the cytotoxic activities of NK cells, monocytes, lymphokine-activated killer (LAK) cells, and CTLs. IL-2 also appears to activate endothelial cells, which results in increased expression of adhesion molecules.[41]

❺ Based on preclinical studies that demonstrated a dose–response relationship between recombinant IL-2 (aldesleukin) and tumor response, initial clinical trials of aldesleukin in patients with melanoma used relatively high doses of the drug as a single agent or in combination with LAK cells. The response rates seen in these trials ranged from 15% to 25%, and 2% to 5% of patients achieved complete responses, some of which were durable (median response = 70 months).[41] Responses were seen at a number of metastatic sites such as lung, liver, bone, lymph nodes, and subcutaneous tissue. Based on reevaluation of early clinical trials, aldesleukin received FDA approval for treatment of metastatic melanoma. Overall, objective response rates were approximately 16%, but 4% to 6% of responses were durable and were observed in patients with large tumor burdens.[42] The high doses of aldesleukin used in the initial clinical trials and recommended in the labeling of the drug are associated with serious toxicities and may limit the practicality of therapy for individual patients and broad application in certain healthcare systems. The high-dose aldesleukin regimen used for treatment of metastatic melanoma is 600,000 international units/kg per dose every 8 hours for 14 doses maximum in a 5-day period given for two cycles, with a 10- to 14-day rest period between cycles. At these doses, cytokine-induced capillary leak syndrome is a common problem and often is accompanied by significant hypotension, visceral edema, dyspnea, tachycardia, and arrhythmias. Increased permeability of capillary walls allows for a fluid shift from the intravascular space into tissue. As the patient becomes intravascularly dehydrated, hypotension may occur, resulting in reflex tachycardia and arrhythmias. In addition, the decrease in blood volume may result in decreased renal blood flow and urine output, manifesting as an increase in blood urea nitrogen, serum creatinine, edema, weight gain, and a decrease in urine output (input greater than output). Visceral edema can result in pulmonary congestion, pleural effusions, and edema. The management of patients receiving high-dose aldesleukin requires extensive supportive care medications, careful monitoring, and a staff trained in aspects of critical care such as hypotension management. Although patients initially receiving high-dose aldesleukin are treated in an intensive care unit, most patients can be managed on a designated oncology unit if the staff is familiar with the toxicities and management strategies of the toxicities. Constitutional symptoms are a frequent complication of aldesleukin therapy and become more intense as therapy progresses. Additional side effects seen with aldesleukin include pruritus, eosinophilia, bone marrow suppression including thrombocytopenia, increased liver function tests, neurological disturbances, diarrhea, and nausea.[43]

In an attempt to reduce treatment-related toxicities, a number of studies have evaluated continuous-infusion aldesleukin and lower doses of aldesleukin, given either alone or combined with chemotherapy and interferon therapy. Although initial reports were encouraging, survival has not been significantly affected. At this time, direct head-to-head comparisons of various dosing schedules and regimens are needed to determine the optimum approach to aldesleukin therapy in metastatic melanoma. Coadministration of LAK cells with aldesleukin does not appear to significantly improve clinical response.[44]

One of the greatest treatment challenges in treatment of metastatic melanoma is determining the role of aldesleukin therapy for each patient. Pre-treatment factors such as performance status, site of metastases, and LDH may play a role in who will respond and are currently being assessed in clinical trials. Based on reports of long-term responses (>10 years) experienced by some patients, the risk certainly is worth the benefit for those individuals. Unfortunately, at this time it is difficult to determine which individuals will respond to aldesleukin therapy, as no biologic or immunologic parameters have been found to correlate with response. The decision to treat an individual with high-dose aldesleukin should be based on an analysis of an individual patient's risk versus potential benefit. Patients with inadequate pulmonary function, cardiac function, renal insufficiency, active infection, or poor performance status are poor candidates for this therapy. Aldesleukin can be safely administered with a properly trained healthcare team and is one of only two approved therapies for treatment of metastatic melanoma.

CLINICAL CONTROVERSY

Although aldesleukin has been associated with long-term durable responses in a small subset of patients with metastatic melanoma, the toxicity profile, intensity of therapy, and cost have limited its acceptance in the United States. Patients should be evaluated for treatment prior to initiation of therapy.

■ CHEMOTHERAPY

A number of antineoplastic agents have demonstrated in vitro activity against melanoma, but only a few drugs have consistently shown a response rate greater than 10% in individuals with metastatic melanoma. Most clinical trials that evaluate new agents in melanoma measure activity in terms of response rates, which often include partial response rates in addition to complete response. It is important to understand that these response rates do not always correlate with survival and do not evaluate benefit to the patient. Complete responses can be durable in a small number of patients.

❻ *Dacarbazine*, a cytotoxic drug thought to exert its antitumor effect through alkylation, currently is the most effective single agent for treatment of melanoma. Dacarbazine remains the only FDA-approved chemotherapeutic agent for treatment of metastatic melanoma in the United States.[45] Prospective controlled clinical trials have observed response rates of 10% to 25%, with an average duration of response of 5 to 7 months. Recent randomized trials in large numbers of patients have confirmed that response rates are closer to 7%.[46] Complete responses are uncommon, with less than 5% of patients treated with single-agent dacarbazine sustaining long-term complete responses. There does not appear to be a survival benefit for dacarbazine relative to other treatments or supportive care. Patients with skin, subcutaneous tissue, and lymph node involvement respond most frequently, whereas patients with metastatic disease to the liver, bone, and central nervous system often are unresponsive. The optimum dose schedule of dacarbazine has never been determined; therefore, single-dose regimens are often preferred for patient convenience. Doses of 250 mg/m$_2$/day for 5 days or 800 to 1,000 mg/m^2 every 3 weeks are seen in practice. Common side effects of dacarbazine therapy include myelosuppression, severe nausea and vomiting, and a flu-like syndrome after large doses. Nausea and vomiting can be prevented and managed with available antiemetics and is not a major complication. At this time, dacarbazine has no defined role in the adjuvant setting.

Temozolomide is one of a series of imidazole tetrazine derivatives that was developed as a potential alternative to dacarbazine.[45] Temozolomide is an oral prodrug of the active metabolite of dacarbazine. Dacarbazine requires hepatic transformation to its active intermediate, whereas at physiologic pH, temozolomide chemically degrades to the cytotoxic monomethyltriazenoimidazole carboxamide (MTIC). Temozolomide is administered orally and appears to be less emetogenic than dacarbazine, although nausea can be a challenging chronic toxicity. Temozolomide appears to cross into the central nervous system and so initially was thought to have benefit for patients with central nervous system metastases. In a phase III trial of chemotherapy-naïve individuals with metastatic melanoma, temozolomide showed efficacy at least equivalent to that of dacarbazine in terms of objective response rates, time to progression, and overall and disease-free survival.[47] Temozolomide appeared to be associated with improvement in some aspects of quality of life, although overall disease control was similar to dacarbazine.[48]

A potential advantage of temozolomide is the convenience of oral dosing, which allows a potentially more effective dosing schedule. Low-dose intermittent dosing schedules with a rest period are being evaluated. This schedule allows for a threefold increase in drug exposure and may overcome some drug resistance mechanisms. The active metabolite of dacarbazine and temozolomide, MTIC, methylates guanine residues in DNA at the O^6 position. Resistance to agents that produce O^6 methylation is partly due to increased levels of O^6-alylguanine-DNA alkyltransferase. Temozolomide administration results in the depletion of the DNA repair protein O^6-methylguanine-DNA methyltransferase (MGMT), which is a major mechanism of tumor resistance.[49] Clinical evaluations of prolonged administration of temozolomide are ongoing, often in combination with other agents such as interferon.

The *nitrosoureas* are active against melanoma. Nitrosoureas, such as carmustine and lomustine, have antitumor activity similar to that of dacarbazine, with reported response rates between 10% and 20%. Sites of responses are similar to those seen with dacarbazine. It was initially hoped that use of the lipophilic nitrosoureas would provide added benefit against a malignancy that can metastasize to the brain. Unfortunately, despite the ability of these agents to cross the blood–brain barrier, the commercially available nitrosoureas have not been shown to have increased activity against melanoma in the central nervous system. Fotemustine, a nitrosourea available in Australia and some European countries, appears to cross the blood–brain barrier more rapidly than do other nitrosoureas. Response rates of 30% have been reported in previously untreated patients, with response rates of 25% of patients who had cerebral metastases. Fotemustine is considered standard therapy in some countries.[50] The most common toxicities of the nitrosoureas are nausea and vomiting, delayed myelosuppression, particularly thrombocytopenia. Leukopenia and thrombocytopenia may be seen as long as 3 to 5 weeks after drug administration and may limit the inclusion of these agents to multidrug regimens.

Cisplatin and related compounds have been evaluated in the management of metastatic melanoma. The effectiveness of platinum compounds as single agents is limited, with reported response rates of 10% to 15% with a short median duration. The activity of cisplatin in melanoma may be dose dependent, and higher response rates have been seen with higher doses of cisplatin in single-institution studies.[51] The toxicities of cisplatin can be problematic, especially in higher doses, and include acute and delayed nausea and vomiting, renal toxicity, and neurotoxicity. Carboplatin, another platinum analog, has been evaluated in small trials for treatment of melanoma. Results demonstrated similar response rates to cisplatin with differing toxicities.[47] Carboplatin is currently being studied in combination regimens for treatment of melanoma.

Taxanes have demonstrated encouraging results in initial trials of metastatic melanoma. Response rates of 15% to 17% have been seen in initial phase II trials with paclitaxel and docetaxel. Abraxane, the albumin-bound nanoparticle formulation of paclitaxel, has shown encouraging results in a very small phase II trial and is being evaluated in a randomized phase III trial.[52] At this time, these agents are not routinely used as single-agent therapy for melanoma but are being incorporated into multidrug strategies undergoing evaluation for use against metastatic melanoma.

In an attempt to improve the limited responses seen with single-agent chemotherapy, a variety of combination chemotherapy regimens (Table 147–8) have been evaluated in both small and large clinical trials. Response rates as high as 30% to 50% were reported in single-institution phase II trials of patients with metastatic melanoma. The combination of dacarbazine with other chemotherapy, most commonly cisplatin, increased the response rates reported with dacarbazine alone, but the survival benefit has been minimal. Responses often were limited to metastases in soft tissue, lymph nodes, and the lung, the sites most likely to respond to single-agent dacarbazine therapy. The concern with combination chemotherapy is increased toxicity, and any reports of increased

TABLE 147-8	Combination Chemotherapy Regimens for Metastatic Melanoma

Dartmouth regimen (CDBT): Repeated every 3–4 weeks
Cisplatin 25 mg/m² IV daily × 3 (days 1, 2, and 3)
Dacarbazine 220 mg/m² IV daily × 3 (days 1, 2, and 3)
Carmustine 150 mg/m² IV daily × 1 (day 1)
Tamoxifen 10 mg orally twice a day

CVD
Cisplatin 20 mg/m² IV daily × 4 (days 2, 3, 4, 5)
Vinblastine 1.6 mg/m² IV daily × 5 (days 1, 2, 3, 4, 5)
Dacarbazine 800 mg/m² IV daily × 1 (day 1)

response rates should be weighed against the effect of toxicities on overall quality of life. The initial reports with the cisplatin, vinblastine, and dacarbazine (CVD) regimen were exciting, with reported response rates greater than 50%, 4% complete response rate, median response duration of nine months, and acceptable toxicities.[53] Comparisons of this regimen to dacarbazine alone have been conflicting. Subsequent reports showed no difference in response rates or survival.

The Dartmouth regimen is a combination that includes carmustine, dacarbazine, cisplatin, and tamoxifen. Initial reports from uncontrolled phase II trials of this combination have demonstrated high response rates of 20% to 50%, but few patients achieve long-term survival. The benefit of tamoxifen to this regimen has been controversial, but a controlled clinical trial from the National Cancer Institute of Canada demonstrated no benefit in response or survival from tamoxifen in this combination.[54] Careful analysis of the initial studies demonstrates that the criteria used to measure response were not consistent with standards used in large multicenter studies. Phase III trials have shown no benefit of the Dartmouth regimen compared to single-agent dacarbazine.[55,56] Response rates were 15%, and median survival was approximately 7 months in both studies. Of concern, toxicities were higher with the combination study and included bone marrow suppression, nausea, vomiting, and fatigue.

■ BIOCHEMOTHERAPY

Low overall response rates and toxicity have limited the routine use of chemotherapy alone or immunotherapy alone in the management of metastatic disease. Over the past decade, the strategy of a combination of chemotherapy (dacarbazine, platinum agents, or vinka alkaloids) and cytokines, aldesleukin, and/or interferon, often termed *biochemotherapy*, has been a major focus of investigation in the management of metastatic melanoma and more recently in the adjuvant setting. The primary rationale is to combine two therapies with some biologic activity to increase overall activity and perhaps response rates. Additionally, some preclinical trials suggest potential synergistic interactions between cytokines and some chemotherapy agents. As with other treatment strategies in melanoma, the results from initial trials suggested a higher response rate with biochemotherapy than the rates seen with either chemotherapy or biotherapy alone. Although several studies have suggested an increase in response rate with the addition of IFN-α to chemotherapy, results of most studies have shown that the addition of IFN-α does not increase the antitumor effect of dacarbazine but does increase toxicity and cost. Similarly, the combination of aldesleukin to chemotherapy has not been consistently shown to increase response or survival. The most encouraging results have been seen with combination chemotherapy and combination biotherapy, but the results of phase III studies have not demonstrated a clear advantage of biochemotherapy compared with chemotherapy alone.[57] A recently published meta-analysis of 18 randomized trials of chemotherapy versus biochemotherapy showed that biochemotherapy was associated with a significantly higher response rate in treatment of metastatic melanoma.[58] However, these differences in response rates did not translate into a significant difference in overall survival. Toxicities can be severe and are consistent with the individual agents in the regimen. A more recent strategy for biochemotherapy is substitution of newer agents into the combination. For example, a small phase II trial of patients with metastatic melanoma evaluated the substitution of temozolomide for dacarbazine.[59,60]

One of the problems with most studies of biochemotherapy is the relatively short duration of response. Recurrence rates among patients who respond to therapy are as high as 50% within 18 to 24 months. Strategies such as subcutaneous low-dose aldesleukin are being investigated in an effort to prolong overall survival and time to progression in patients who do respond to treatment. Initial response rates, durable complete remission, and activity in patients in whom HDI therapy was not successful have stimulated interest in evaluating biochemotherapy in the adjuvant setting for high-risk patients with node-positive disease as compared to HDI.

Biochemotherapy is also being evaluated in the adjuvant setting. Phase II data of neoadjuvant provided promising results in terms of response rates, relapse-free survival, and overall survival.[57] Currently, phase III studies are evaluating biochemotherapy compared to interferon as adjuvant therapy in stage III disease.

ENDOCRINE THERAPY

The role of endocrine therapy in the management of melanoma has been debated over the last decade.[5] Initial reports that described high-affinity cytoplasmic estrogen receptors in patients with metastatic melanoma caused some experts to speculate about the possibility that antiestrogens or other hormonal manipulation may be beneficial in modulating the biology of melanoma. Additionally, estrogens have been shown to suppress T-lymphocyte activity and to suppress or stimulate the activities of B lymphocytes, macrophages, and NK cells, supporting a hypothesis that estrogens influence the immunologic mechanisms that appear to be important in melanoma.

In a randomized trial, tamoxifen was shown to have a response and survival benefit when combined with dacarbazine in patients with metastatic melanoma; this benefit was most pronounced in women.[61] Well-designed prospective randomized studies demonstrate that tamoxifen does not significantly enhance the antitumor effect of dacarbazine alone or the combination of dacarbazine with cisplatin and carmustine.[5] As discussed previously, subsequent trials have not been able to confirm the initial reported benefit of the antiestrogen when combined with chemotherapy, and tamoxifen is no longer routinely included in chemotherapy regimens.[45]

VACCINES

The rationale for vaccination as a therapeutic modality is based on the observation that antigens expressed on the surface of tumor cells differ from normal cells and the hope that vaccines might induce effective tumor-specific immune responses with fewer toxicities than conventional chemotherapy or other immunotherapies. Greater knowledge about tumor antigens and the mechanism of antigen presentation and immune response to antigens has led to the development of several vaccination strategies for treatment of early and advanced melanoma.

A variety of melanoma vaccines based on whole tumor cells, peptides, proteins, and tumor lysates have been evaluated for treatment of patients with metastatic disease and for intermediate- and high-risk patients after surgical resection of disease.[62,63] Although tumor responses with some of these approaches have been observed in phase I and II trials, none of the vaccine responses have been confirmed in phase III trials.[63] These early trials have focused on safety, feasibility, and immunogenicity of the vaccine. Vaccines are a promising but still experimental approach in the treatment of melanoma.

Vaccination is a form of active specific immunotherapy directed against a particular cellular target or specific membrane antigen. The ideal tumor vaccine would generate an active, systemic, long-lived immune response in the cancer-bearing host against tumors; protect against primary development or subsequent relapse of cancer; or induce regression of established cancer. Obstacles in the development of a vaccine include identifying appropriate antigens to target and generating immune responses against tumor antigens to which the immune system has been already exposed.

Whole-cell tumor vaccines can be derived from cell lines that are already established (allogeneic vaccines) or from the patient's own tumor cells (autologous). Whole-cell vaccines are challenging to produce for several reasons: a new vaccine must be prepared for each patient, patients must have sufficient tumor available to provide adequate material, and considerable delay may exist between time of tumor removal and vaccine administration. In addition, there are technical challenges to producing the vaccine in the laboratory.[62] Currently, no autologous tumor cell vaccine has been successfully studied in a phase III randomized clinical trial. An example of a whole-cell tumor vaccine that is being studied is Canvaxin. Canvaxin (CancerVax®, Carlsbad, CA) is an allogeneic whole-cell vaccine that uses bacillus Calmette-Guérin as an immune adjuvant. Small trials have shown improvements in survival compared with historical controls, and some objective clinical responses have been seen in patients with metastatic melanoma. The results from two large phase III trials that compared Canvaxin to observation in stage III and IV melanoma demonstrated a survival disadvantage for patients that received the vaccine.[64]

Antigen vaccines use individual antigens to stimulate immune responses, as compared with whole-cell vaccines, which contain many thousands of antigens.[63] These antigens usually are proteins or pieces of proteins called *peptides*. Antigen vaccines may be specific for a certain type of cancer, but they are not made for a specific patient. Vaccines against GM2 ganglioside, a glycolipid expressed on most melanomas, are examples of vaccines targeted against an antigen. Two randomized controlled trials with anti-GM2 vaccines have failed to show any benefit with the vaccine.[63]

Peptide antigen vaccines match the patient's haplotype with the spectrum of immunity that he or she expresses. T cells recognize antigens as peptide epitopes on the surface of major histocompatibility complex (MHC) molecules. Antigenic peptides can be mixed with an immunologic adjuvant and administered with the goal of loading empty MHC molecules in vivo. To date, the most commonly used peptides have shown activity only in patients who express human leukocyte antigen (HLA)-A2. However, many patients would not be eligible for this vaccine because not all patients express this HLA antigen. Additional peptide antigens that are compatible in other haplotypes have been identified, and eventually this disadvantage may be overcome. Peptide vaccination can generate quantifiable and functional tumor-reactive T cells, but clinical responses are rare and do not consistently correlate with CTL response.

Because protein antigen vaccines have a slightly broader spectrum of antigen diversity, all patients with melanoma potentially could be eligible for vaccination with this particular type of vaccine. Proteins intrinsically produced by the cell are presented only to CD8+ T cells, whereas proteins taken up by antigen-presenting cells are presented only to CD4+ T cells. Under certain conditions, antigen-presenting cells can present protein-derived antigens to both CD4+ and CD8+ in a process known as *cross-presentation*.[63]

Tumor lysates can be generated from tumor cells by mechanical disruption or enzymatic digestion. Tumor cells that shed antigens in culture can be purified and used as an antigen source for vaccines. Production of a vaccine from these sources raises concern because standardization of production and verification of purity and biological activity are more difficult.

Vaccines in combination with other biologic therapies are being evaluated. In a randomized trial of 604 patients with resected stage III cutaneous melanoma, LDI combined with an allogeneic melanoma lysate vaccine (2 years) was compared with HDI alone (1 year).[65] Median overall survival was not significantly different between the two treatment arms. Five-year relapse-free and overall survival were similar in the two treatment arms. The incidence of serious treatment-related adverse events was similar in the two arms, but more severe neuropsychiatric toxicity was observed in patients receiving HDI. Although the results of this trial suggest that the vaccine has some activity in melanoma, the study was not powered sufficiently to show either equivalency or small differences in efficacy. HLA typing was optional based on whether the centers were able to perform the typing. With ongoing research additional trials performed with this vaccine, specifically in patients with certain HLA types, may prove promising.

Occasional clinical responses have been observed in clinical trials of melanoma vaccines, which demonstrate the potential of this form of treatment. Many clinical trials with vaccine therapy in melanoma patients are ongoing. The results of completed clinical trials have not yet shown definitive evidence of improved survival. Further research is needed to improve vaccine responses and to determine how to apply treatment to melanoma patients.

■ TARGETED THERAPY

❼ The role of protein kinases in the regulation and proliferation signals in cancer cells is becoming a key focus for anticancer agents. The role of protein kinase inhibitors has emerged as standard therapy for malignancies such as renal cell carcinoma, chronic myelogenous leukemia, and gastrointestinal stromal tumors. As the biology of melanoma continues to unfold, there is increasing excitement about the development of targeted therapies against targets important for the development and progression of melanoma.[13,66] There now is greater interest in identifying potential targets in melanoma and determining the applicability in specific patients and/ or patient subsets.

The mitogen-activated protein kinase (MAPK) pathway and the Akt pathway are involved in tumor cell growth and differentiation and are activated in melanoma. BRAF is downstream in the MAPK pathway. Mutations of BRAF have been described in melanoma cell lines, and it appears that approximately 70% of melanomas exhibit BRAF alteration.[67] Sorafenib is a multikinase inhibitor that inhibits both wild-type and mutant BRAF, in addition to other tyrosine kinases involved in angiogenesis and tumor progression. Preclinical studies demonstrated activity against human melanoma tumor xenografts in preclinical trials, but minimal activity was observed in phase I-II clinical trials in refractory metastatic melanoma. However, sorafenib may be active when given in combination with chemotherapy. In phase I-II studies, 27% of patients responded to sorafenib when given in combination with carboplatin and paclitaxel, and 73% of patients maintained a response at a 6-month followup.[67] Although a phase III trial with this same combination failed to show an improvement in progression-free survival, an ECOG phase III trial is currently evaluating carboplatin, paclitaxel, and sorafenib as first-line treatment for metastatic melanoma.[67] In this study, it will be important to evaluate the efficacy of the addition of sorafenib to the "untested" combination of carboplatin and paclitaxel for treatment of metastatic melanoma.

Other drugs targeted to mutated BRAF have reported encouraging results. In a phase I/II trial, PLX4032, an investigational orally available inhibitor of mutated BRAF, showed activity in patients with melanoma that had BRAF with the V600E mutation. Among the 16 patients with melanoma that had BRAF with the V600E mutation and who received 240 mg or more of PLX4032 twice daily, 10 had a partial response and one had a complete response.[68]

Another agent of interest is imatinib mesylate, an oral agent that inhibits c-*Kit* and PDGFR. c-*Kit* and PDGFR are highly expressed on melanoma cells. Imatinib has been shown to suppress melanoma cell growth in preclinical studies. In phase II trials, imatinib was shown to be inactive in metastatic melanoma despite the downregulation of phosphorylated c-*Kit*, the biologic target, in the tumor.[67]

The anti-apoptotic protein Bcl-2 is overexpressed in melanoma and has been linked to chemotherapy resistance. In a large phase III trial comparing oblimersen, a Bcl-2 antisense, in combination with dacarbazine compared to dacarbazine alone, demonstrated a significant increase in the overall response rate (13.5% vs. 7.5%; $P = 0.007$) but this did not translate into a significant difference in overall survival (9 months vs. 7.8 months; $P = 0.077$) and as a result was not approved by the FDA for the treatment of metastatic melanoma. Other targeted therapies such as toll-like receptor agonists, antiangiogenic agents, heat shock protein 90 inhibitors and m-TOR inhibitors have also been studied in early clinical trials for the treatment of metastatic melanoma and all have modest activity.[67]

■ OTHER APPROACHES

Dendritic cells are potent antigen-presenting cells that initiate antigen-specific immune responses. Dendritic cells express high levels of MHC class I and class II molecules, which are essential in antigen presentation. Activation of T cells and recruitment of non–antigen-specific effectors, such as NK cells and macrophages, result in a broad immune response. One strategy that uses dendritic cells for inducing antitumor immune responses is peptide-pulsed dendritic cells. Antimelanoma CTLs can be generated from healthy donors and patients with melanoma with dendritic cells pulsed with melanoma-derived peptides. A number of clinical trials are evaluating dendritic cell–based immunotherapy.[62,63]

Monoclonal antibodies have been used for diagnosis and treatment of melanoma. Monoclonal antibodies can be used to target biologic pathways that are associated with tumor progression and as a delivery system for antineoplastic drugs. Monoclonal antibodies have been conjugated to cytotoxic agents, radioisotopes, and toxins such as ricin A.[5,13] More recently, monoclonal antibodies have been developed to target processes that are involved in the host immune response to melanoma. Cytotoxic T-lymphocyte antigen 4 (CTLA-4) is a transmembrane protein expressed on T lymphocytes that is a homodimer which functions as an inhibitory receptor for the costimulatory molecule B7. Crosslinking of CTLA-4 by B7 inhibits T-cell activation, transcription, translation, and transduction. CTLA-4 blockage sustains activation and proliferation of T cells.[69] CTLA-4 blockade may represent a novel approach to enhance the immune response against melanoma antigens. Ipilimumab (MDX-010) and tremelimumab (CP-675206) are two fully human monoclonal antibodies against CTLA-4 currently in phase III clinical trials. Preliminary results of clinical trials show promising activity in malignant melanoma. Results from phase I and II trials with ipilimumab and tremelimumab demonstrate up to 20% response rates in advanced disease.[70] In a phase III trial of 676 HLA-A*0201-positive patients with refractory metastatic melanoma, ipilimumab plus a glycoprotein 100 (gp100) peptide vaccine was compared with ipilimumab alone or gp100 alone.[71] Median overall survival was significantly longer in patients treated with ipilimumab either alone or combined with gp100 as compared with patients treated with gp100 alone (10.0 or 10.1 months vs. 6.4 months). No difference in overall survival was observed between the two ipilimumab groups. Unfortunately, recent phase III data with tremelimumab showed no difference in overall survival when compared with dacarbazine or temozolamide.[69] CTLA-4 antibodies produce several immune-mediated adverse events that are distinct from the typical adverse events associated with conventional cancer treatments. Many of these adverse effects are autoimmune in nature and can occur in up to 40% of patients.[69] Antibodies against CTLA-4 may cause autoimmune-mediated adverse events by promoting the activation of self-reactive T cells. The most common serious adverse events included dermatitis, enterocolitis, and diarrhea. Less common adverse effects include autoimmune thyroiditis, adrenal disease, or hepatitis.[70,71] Early administration of corticosteroids is important in the management of immune-related adverse effects. In the clinical studies reported to date, patients who have experienced grade III or grade IV autoimmune toxicities have also been the most likely to exhibit tumor regression and increased time to relapse.[69–71] The timing of adverse effects is variable and may occur several months after the cessation of treatment.

Gene therapy of human melanoma is in its infancy but suggests several exciting approaches to management of metastatic melanoma. Several strategies for gene therapy are under investigation for treatment of melanoma. One approach to gene therapy for melanoma is modification of melanoma cells with insertion of one or more cytokine genes and then administration of these altered allogeneic or autologous cells as a vaccine. Cytokine gene transduction has been accomplished with a number of cytokines, including aldesleukin (IL-2), TNF-α, IL-4, and interferon. It is hoped that insertion of cytokine genes into melanoma cells will significantly increase the cells' immunogenicity.

Genes can be transferred in vitro into TILs associated with melanoma in an attempt to potentiate the cytotoxicity of these cells. Rosenberg et al. were the first to attempt to transduce the gene coding for resistance to neomycin into human TILs.[72] This approach has since been used to transfer the tumor necrosis factor gene into TILs.

Thalidomide and thalidomide analogs are being evaluated for management of melanoma. Thalidomide, given either as a single agent or in combination with chemotherapy or cytokines, is being evaluated in a variety of studies. Thalidomide analogs also are being evaluated in an attempt to avoid toxicities associated with the parent compound. The thalidomide analogs are grouped into two classes: selective cytokine inhibitory drugs and immunomodulatory derivatives. Both classes appear to have antiangiogenic and antiinflammatory properties, but the selective cytokine inhibitory drugs are phosphodiesterase inhibitors. Immunomodulatory derivatives also have effects on T-cell stimulation and inhibition of TNF-α. Several of these agents are being evaluated in clinical trials of metastatic melanoma.[45]

■ RADIATION

The role of radiation for the adjuvant treatment of melanoma is being investigated, based on retrospective data that suggest that patients at high risk for reoccurrence benefit from postoperative adjuvant radiation to the nodal basins. Overall these data demonstrate improvement in locoregional control with reasonable toxicity but with no impact on overall survival. This has been substantiated in one phase II trial. As a result, a phase III trial is currently underway to further elucidate the benefit of radiation in this setting.[5,73] For patients with metastatic melanoma, radiation is limited to the palliative setting to symptomatic areas of disease progression.

■ LIMB PERFUSION AND LIMB INFUSION

Isolated limb perfusion is a surgical procedure of regional intravascular delivery of chemotherapy and/or biotherapy into an extremity with cutaneous melanoma.[74] When in-transit metastases occur in extremities, local therapy with isolated limb perfusion or isolated limb infusion has been used.[5] Isolated limb perfusion is a method for escalating the dose of chemotherapeutic drugs to a specific region of the body while limiting the systemic toxicities of the agent. Most perfusions can be performed with drug exposures of less than 2%. The most significant side effect of isolated limb perfusion is regional toxicity; all of the skin, subcutaneous tissue, and tissue of the extremity receives the same dose and is subjected to the same perfusion conditions as the tumor located within the extremity. After regional perfusions, objective response rates greater than 50% in treated limbs have been reported, with overall response rates possibly as high as 80%. The role of hyperthermia (39°C to 40°C [102°F to 104°F]) with regional isolated perfusion is not clearly defined. Although most clinical trials have used melphalan, whether the combination of melphalan with other agents may improve results is not known.[75] Agents that have been combined with melphalan include actinomycin D, nitrogen mustard, thiotepa, and cisplatin. Work with biologic response modifiers, such as TNF-α, have been encouraging.[76] A simplified form of isolated limb perfusion, called isolated limb infusion, is a low-flow isolated limb perfusion performed under hypoxic conditions via small-caliber arterial and venous catheters. It has been proposed that the hypoxia that develops during isolated limb infusion may be beneficial with certain cytotoxic agents such as melphalan.

■ TREATMENT BY STAGE

Treatment of cutaneous melanoma is determined by many factors, including disease-related and patient-related issues. Most available reviews and guidelines provide treatment recommendations based on stage of disease.[16] Most patients present with localized disease.[16] Treatment of localized disease is surgical excision, with the extent of excision based on the tumor size. Wide excision is recommended for in situ melanoma and wide excision with SLNB for stage IA, IB, and II disease. Long-term survival of individuals with early-stage disease and thin tumors (<1 mm) is good, but survival is negatively impacted as tumor thickness increases.

The role of adjuvant therapy in the management of individuals at high risk for recurrence remains controversial. One controversy is determination of which patients are appropriate candidates for treatment after resection of the primary tumor. Although adjuvant therapy has been considered historically in patients with locally advanced disease (stages II and III), it is increasingly being considered after surgical resection of an isolated distant metastases.

Another controversy with adjuvant therapy is the choice of therapy. HDI has the most evidence supporting its use and is FDA approved for this indication. The challenges with this therapy have been discussed, and the therapy has limited worldwide acceptance. The most appropriate option is a clinical trial, if available. New therapies and combinations must be evaluated to help answer the questions that remain about adjuvant therapy in melanoma. Clinical trials of chemotherapy, immunotherapy, vaccines, and emerging therapies are ongoing.

Another treatment challenge is the management of patients with advanced disease. The 2010 NCCN guidelines list a variety of systemic therapies for advanced or metastatic melanoma, including dacarbazine, temozolomide, high-dose aldesleukin, and combination therapies of biochemotherapy that include dacarbazine or temozolomide.[16] Of note, the preferred treatment is participation in a clinical trial. Best supportive care is also an option in some

TABLE 147-9 Options for Sun Protection Sunscreens

Behavioral	Sunscreens	
	Physical Blockers (Reflectants)	Chemical Absorbers
Protective clothing and accessories	Zinc oxide	Ultraviolet B absorbers
Seek shade (avoid peak sun hours)	Talc	Salicylates
Avoid tanning equipment	Titanium dioxide	Cinnamates
	Red petrolatum	Camphor derivatives
		Aminobenzoates
		Ultraviolet A absorbers
		Benzopehnone-6
		Dibenzoylmethanes

individuals. Data suggest that surgical treatment of metastatic melanoma should be considered in select individuals based on the extent and location of disease and performance status.

An important consideration for treatment of melanoma is the presentation of the disease. As discussed, treatment of melanoma isolated to the limb may be most appropriately treated with regional therapy. Treatment options for metastatic uveal melanoma include strategies for managing hepatic metastasis, such as chemoembolization to the liver and intrahepatic chemotherapy.[77]

PREVENTION AND DETECTION

The results of early treatment emphasize the role of early detection and prevention. There are three different strategies for chemoprevention for melanoma. Primary chemoprevention is used to prevent occurrences of melanoma in healthy individuals. Secondary chemoprevention is used to prevent premalignant melanoma precursors from becoming melanoma. Tertiary chemoprevention is used to prevent melanoma recurrence in individuals who were treated for melanoma and have no evidence of disease. The mainstay of melanoma prevention remains strategies to protect individuals from harmful effects of the sun[78] (Table 147–9).

UV light exposure plays a major role in melanoma development. Childhood sunburns and intermittent sun exposure correlate positively with melanoma risk. Studies have shown that a decrease in recreational sun exposure is associated with a reduction of a second primary melanoma in individuals diagnosed with primary melanoma.[79] Education and reeducation about the importance of sun protection have the potential to help decrease the rising incidence of this disease. Strategies, such as sun avoidance, especially during peak hours of sun intensity (10 AM to 4 PM), and staying in the shade when outdoors, are important education concepts for individuals who are in the sun for prolonged periods and/or who are at high risk for burning. Skiers and winter sports enthusiasts should be cautioned about exposure to UV radiation, as the reflection off snow and high altitude contribute to increased UV exposure. There is also the use of protective clothing to minimize damage to the skin for individuals who spend time in the sun. Clothing designed to protect an individual from sun exposure but allows for physical activities such as water sports and hiking are widely available. The clothes are designed for skin protection, but it is important to realize that not all clothing provides sufficient protection from UV radiation. Clothes with tight weaves provide the greatest protection. In addition to protective clothing, wide brimmed hats to protect ears, neck, and nose as wells as sunglasses with both UVA and UVB protection are important. Additionally, the use of tanning beds over the last three decades have led to an increased exposure of individuals to UVA light. Observational studies have shown individuals who spent time in tanning devices before the age of 35 have a 75% increase in risk of melanoma.[80] As a result, the World Health Organization International

Agency for Research on Cancer declared in 2009 that ultraviolet light emitted from tanning beds was a human carcinogen.[81]

It is important to counsel patients about the appropriate use of sunscreens to optimize benefits from these products. Sunscreens should be applied 15 to 30 minutes before going into the sun and should be reapplied every 2 hours, after swimming, and after perspiring heavily. About 1 ounce of sunscreen (a "palmful") should be used to cover the arms, legs, neck, and face of the average adult. Sun protection must be used regularly and not limited to times of recreation or anticipated "prolonged" exposure. Times of season changes, when the potential for sun exposure can be perceived as erratic, are possible times for the "first-of-the-season sunburn."

Historically, patients have been counseled that the risk of skin cancer can be limited by the use of sunscreens with a sun protection factor (SPF) of 15 or greater. SPF is a measure of protection from UVB radiation only. Although some studies have found a decreased risk of melanoma in sunscreens users, others have demonstrated no association and even increased melanoma risk with sunscreen use. Methodologic difficulties may explain the discrepancy in study results. Factors that include variables in sun exposure, sunscreen use, and sun sensitivity are very difficult to control in these trials. In addition, all sunscreens are not the same. It is important that people understand that no sunscreen provides complete protections and that the SPF scale is not linear, the higher the SPF, the smaller the difference in sun protection. For example, SPF 15 sunscreens filter out about 93% of UVB rays, while SPF 30 sunscreens filter out about 97%, SPF 50 sunscreens about 98%, and SPF 100 about 99%.

Sunscreens traditionally have been designed to prevent erythema by blocking UVB, leaving users relatively unprotected from wavelengths such as UVA. As a result, the use of sunscreens, especially those with higher SPFs, may lead to the ability of individuals to increase their time in the sun without clinical indication of sunburn. Newer forms of sunscreens combine protection for UVA and UVB. Unfortunately, no currently approved system rates products for UVA protective capabilities; however, the FDA has proposed new sunscreen rules that will establish an UVA testing and labeling system. It is unclear when this system will be put into place. The impact of the use of high-potency sunscreens on the incidence of melanoma is not clear at this time, because the lag time for melanoma is approximately two decades and high-potency sunscreens have only been popular for approximately 10 years.

Thickness and stage of the disease are inversely related to melanoma survival. Early detection can play a large part in the secondary prevention of melanoma. Many healthcare organizations and skin cancer groups recommend monthly self-examination of skin to serve as a mechanism for recognizing moles or marks on the skin that may be melanoma. Patients with a strong family history should additionally have a clinical examination and, in some cases, screening photography to document the size, shape, and location of moles. Both patients and clinicians need to be properly educated in the clinical features of the disease to ensure more appropriate diagnosis. Currently there are no consistent recommendations for the screening and early detection of melanoma.

EVALUATION OF THERAPEUTIC OUTCOMES

The outcome of patients treated with melanoma depends on the stage of disease at presentation. The prognosis of patients with thin tumors (<1 mm in thickness) and localized disease is good, with long-term survival in more than 90% of patients. The risk of regional nodal involvement increases with increasing tumor thickness, so survival rates decrease in patients with nodal involvement. Long-term survival in patients with distant metastases is even lower. Therefore, early diagnosis and appropriate treatment of early disease are essential. Patients with suspicious pigmented lesions should be evaluated and the lesion excised whenever possible. Treatment is determined by patient factors and stage of disease.

Clinical practice guidelines published by the NCCN and ESMO provide some guidance for followup of patients with melanoma.[16,82] Intensive surveillance has the benefit of early detection of recurrent disease, which may lead to better options of surgical resection. Emphasis on evaluation of locoregional areas is important. For patients with in situ melanoma, periodic skin examinations for life are recommended, although frequency is determined based on patient risk factors. Local recurrence is associated with aggressive tumor biology and frequently is a manifestation of an aggressive primary tumor. If a local recurrence occurs after inadequate primary disease, the patient should undergo a workup based on the lesion thickness of the original melanoma. Patients with nodal recurrence should be evaluated for lymph node metastases. Patients with systemic recurrence should be evaluated and treated in a fashion similar to patients presenting with systemic disease.

ABBREVIATIONS

AJCC: American Joint Committee on Cancer

ARF: alternative reading frame

bFGF: basic fibroblast growth factor

CTL: cytotoxic T lymphocyte

CTLA-4: cytotoxic T lymphocyte antigen 4

ECOG: Eastern Cooperative Oncology Group

ESMO: European Society of Clinical Oncology

HDI: high-dose interferon

HLA: human leukocyte antigen

IFN: inteferon

IL-2: interleukin 2

INK4A: inhibitor of cyclin-dependent kinase 4

LAK: lymphokine-activated killer

LDI: low-dose interferon

NCCN: National Comprehensive Cancer Network

NMSC: nonmelanoma skin cancer

NSAID: nonsteroidal antiinflammatory drug

SLNB: sentinel lymph node biopsy

SPF: sun protection factor

TNF: tumor necrosis factor

TIL: tumor-infiltrating lymphocyte

TLR9: toll-like receptor 9

UVA: ultraviolet A

UVB: ultraviolet B

REFERENCES

1. Jemal A, Siegel R, Xu J, Ward E. Cancer statistics, 2010. CA Cancer J Clin 2010;60:277–300.
2. U.S. National Center for Health Statistics (NCHS) and the Surveillance, Epidemiology, and End Results (SEER) database. http://seer.cancer.gov/canques/.
3. Jen M, Murphy M, Grant-Kels J. Childhood melanoma. Clin Dermatol 2009;27:529–536.
4. Garbe C, Eigentler TK. Diagnosis and treatment of cutaneous melanoma: State of the art 2006. Melanoma Res 2007;17:117–127.
5. Slinluff CL, Flaherty K, Rosenberg SA, Read PW. Cutaneous melanoma. In: DeVita VT, Hellman S, Rosenberg SA, eds. Cancer: Principles and Practice of Oncology, 8th ed. Philadelphia, PA: Lippincott Williams & Wilkins, 2008: 1897–1951.
6. Gilchrest BA, Eller MS, Geller AC, Yaar M. The pathogenesis of melanoma induced by ultraviolet radiation. N Engl J Med 1999;340:1341.
7. Wilkins K, Turner R, Dolev JC, et al. Cutaneous malignancy and human immunodeficiency virus disease. J Am Acad Dermatol 2006;54:189–206.
8. Chin L, Garraway LA, Fisher DE. Malignant melanoma: Genetics and therapeutics in the genomic era. Genes Dev 2006;20:2149–2182.
9. Goldstein AM, Cahn M, Harland M, et al. Features associated with germline CDKN2A mutations: a GenoMEL study of melanoma-prone families from three continents. J Med Genet 2007;44:99.
10. Mahabeleshwar GH, Byzova TV. Angiogenesis in melanoma. Semin Oncol 2007;34:555–565.
11. Gray-Schopfer V, Wellbrock C, Marais R. Melanoma biology and new targeted therapy. Nature 2007;445:851–857.
12. Lejeune FJ, Rimoldi D, Speiser D. New approaches in metastatic melanoma: Biological and molecular targeted therapies. Expert Rev Anticancer Ther 2007;7:701–713.
13. Queirolo P, Acquati M. Targeted therapies in melanoma. Cancer Treat Rev 2006;32:524–531.
14. Albert DM, Van Buren JJ. Intraocular melanoma. In: DeVita VT, Hellman S, Rosenberg SA, eds. Cancer: Principles and Practice of Oncology, 8th ed. Philadelphia, PA: Lippincott Williams & Wilkins, 2008: 1952–1965.
15. Berwick M, Begg CM, Fine JA, Roush CG, Barnhill RL. Screening for cutaneous melanoma by skin self-examination. J Natl Cancer Inst 1996;88:17–23.
16. National Comprehensive Cancer Network. NCCN Melanoma Clinical Practice Guidelines in Oncology (Version 2.2010). http://www.nccn.org.
17. Balch CM, Soong SJ, Buzaid AC, et al. The new melanoma staging system and factors predicting melanoma survival. Clin Oncol Update 2002;5:3.1–19.
18. Clark WH Jr. A classification of malignant melanoma in man correlated with histogenesis and biologic behavior. In: Montagna W, Hu F, eds. Advances in Biology of the Skin. The Pigmentary System. London: Pergamon, 1967: 621–645.
19. Breslow A. Thickness, cross-sectional areas and depth of invasion in the prognosis of cutaneous melanoma. Ann Surg 1970;172:1902–1908.
20. Balch CM, Soong SJ, Gershenwald JE, et al. Prognostic factors analysis of 17,600 melanoma patients: Validation of the American Joint Committee on Cancer melanoma staging system. J Clin Oncol 2001;19:3622–3634.
21. Greene FL, Page DL, Flemming ID, et al., eds. AJCC Cancer Staging Manual, 6th ed. Philadelphia, PA: Lippincott-Raven, 2002:209.
22. Morton DL, Thompson JF, Cochran AJ, et al. Sentinel-node biopsy or nodal observation in melanoma. N Engl J Med 2006;355:1307–1317.
23. Mocellin S, Hoon DSB, Pilati P, et al. Sentinel lymph node molecular ultrastaging in patients with melanoma: A systematic review and meta-analysis of prognosis. J Clin Oncol 2007;25:1588–1595.
24. Tsao H, Atkins MB, Sober AJ. Management of cutaneous melanoma. N Engl J Med 2004;351:998–1012.
25. Balch CM, Urist MM, Karakousis CP, et al. Efficiency of 2-cm surgical margins for intermediate-thickness melanomas (1–4 mm): Results of a multi-institutional randomized surgical trial. Ann Surg 1993;218: 262–269.
26. Meirion Thomas K, Newton-Bishop J, A'Hern R, Coombes G, et al. Excision margins in high-risk malignant melanoma. N Engl J Med 2004;350:757–766.
27. Wargo JA, Tanabe K. Surgical management of melanoma. Hematol Oncol Clin North Ame 2009;23:565–581.
28. Testori A, Rutkowski P, Marsden J, et al. Surgery and radiotherapy in the treatment of cutaneous melanoma. Ann Oncol 2009;20(Suppl 6):vi22–29.
29. Ulm AJ, Friedman WA, Bova FJ, et al. Linear accelerator radiosurgery in the treatment of brain metastases. Neurosurgery 2004;55:1076–1085.
30. Kondziolka D, Martin JJ, Flickinger JC, et al. Long-term survivors after gamma knife radiosurgery for brain metastases. Cancer 2005;104:2784–2791.

31. Kirkwood JM, Straderman MH, Ernstoff MS, et al. Interferon alfa-2b adjuvant therapy of high-risk resected cutaneous melanoma: The Eastern Cooperative Oncology Group Trial EST 1684. J Clin Oncol 1996;14:7–17.

32. Kirkwood JM, Manola J, Ibrahim J, et al. A pooled analysis of Eastern Cooperative Oncology Group and Intergroup trials of adjuvant high-dose interferon for melanoma. Clin Cancer Res 2004;10:1670–1677.

33. Kirkwood JM, Ibrahim JG, Sondak VK, et al. High- and low-dose interferon alfa-2b in high risk melanoma: First analysis of intergroup trial E1690/S9111/C9190. J Clin Oncol 2000;18:2444–2458.

34. Lens MB, Dawes M. Interferon alfa therapy for malignant melanoma: A systematic review of randomized controlled trials. J Clin Oncol 2002;20:1818–1825.

35. Hauschild A, Gogas H, Tarhini A, et al. Practical guidelines for the management of interferon-alpha-2b side effects in patients receiving adjuvant treatment for melanoma. Cancer 2008;112:982–994.

36. Myint AM, Schwarz MJ, Steinbusch HW, et al. Neuropsychiatric disorders related to interferon and interleukins treatment. Metab Brain Dis 2009;24:55–68.

37. Moschos SJ, Kirkwood JM. Present status and future prospects for adjuvant therapy of melanoma: Time to build upon the foundation of high-dose interferon alfa-2b. J Clin Oncol 2004;22:11–14.

38. Cole BF, Gelber RD, Kirkwood JM, et al. A quality-of-life-adjusted survival analysis of interferon alfa-2b adjuvant treatment for high-risk resected cutaneous melanoma: An Eastern Cooperative Oncology Group Study (E1684). J Clin Oncol 1996;14:2666–2673.

39. Bottomley A, Coens C, Suciu S, et al. Adjuvant therapy with pegylated interferon alfa-2b versus observation in resected stage III melanoma: a phase III randomized controlled trial of health-related quality of life and symptoms by the European Organisation for Research and Treatment of Cancer Melanoma Group. J Clin Oncol 2009;27:2916–2923.

40. Bukowski RM, Tannenbaum CS, Finke JH. Clinical pharmacokinetics of interleukin 1 interleukin 2 interleukin 4 tumor necrosis factor, interleukin 12 and macrophage colony-stimulating factor. In: Chabner B, Longo DL, eds. Cancer Chemotherapy & Biotherapy: Principles and Practice, 3rd ed. Philadelphia, PA: Lippincott Williams & Wilkins, 2001:779–828.

41. Petrella T, Quirt I, Verma S, et al. Single-agent interleukin-2 in the treatment of metastatic melanoma: a systematic review. Cancer Treat Rev 2007;33:484–496.

42. Schadendorf D, Algarra SM, Bastholt L, et al. Immunotherapy for distant metastatic disease. Ann Oncol 2009;20(Suppl 6):41–50.

43. Schwartz RN, Stover L, Dutcher J. Managing toxicities of high-dose interleukin-2. Oncology 2002;16(Suppl 13):11–20.

44. Law TM, Motzer RJ, Mazumdar M, et al. Phase III randomized trial of interleukin-2 with or without lymphokine-activated killer cells in the treatment of patient with advanced renal-cell carcinoma. Cancer 1995;76:824–832.

45. Gogas HJ, Kirkwood JM, Sondak VK. Chemotherapy for metastatic melanoma. Time for a change? Cancer 2007;109:455–464.

46. Agarwala SS. Metastatic melanoma: an AJCC review. Community Oncol 2008;5(8)441–445.

47. Yang AS, Chapman PB. The history and future of chemotherapy for melanoma. Hematol Oncol Clin North Am 2009;23:583–597.

48. Quirt I, Verma S, Petrella T, et al. Temozolomide for the treatment of metastatic melanoma: a systematic review. Oncologist 2007;12:1114–1123.

49. Trinh VA. Current management of metastatic melanoma. Am J Health Syst Pharm 2008;65(24 Suppl 9):S3–S8.

50. Jacquillat C, Khayat D, Banzet P, et al. Final report of the French multicenter phase II study of the nitrosourea fotemustine in 153 evaluable patients with disseminated malignant melanoma including patients with cerebral metastases. Cancer 1990;66:1873–1878.

51. Glover D, Ibrahim J, Kirkwood J, et al. Phase II randomized trial of cisplatin and WR-2721 versus cisplatin alone for metastatic melanoma: An Eastern Cooperative Oncology Group study (E1686). Melanoma Res 2003;13:619–626.

52. Hersch E, O'Day S, Gonzales R, et al. Phase II trial of ABI-007 (Abraxane) in previously treated and chemotherapy naïve patients with metastatic melanoma [abstract]. Melanoma Res 2006;16:S78.

53. Legha SS, Ring S, Papadopoulos N, et al. A prospective evaluation of a triple-drug regimen containing cisplatin, vinblastine and DTIC (CVD) for metastatic melanoma. Cancer 1989;64:2024–2029.

54. Rusthoven JJ, Quirt IC, Iscoe NA, et al. Randomized, double-blind, placebo-controlled trial comparing the response rates of carmustine, dacarbazine, and cisplatin with and without tamoxifen in patients with metastatic melanoma. National Cancer Institute of Canada clinical trials group. J Clin Oncol 1996;14:2083–2090.

55. Chapman PB, Einhorm L, Meyeres ML, et al. Phase III multicenter randomized trial of the Dartmouth regimen versus dacarbazine in patients with metastatic melanoma. J Clin Oncol 1999;17:2745–2751.

56. Middleton MR, Lorigan P, Owen J, et al. A randomized phase III study comparing dacarbazine, BCNU, cisplatin and tamoxifen with dacarbazine and interferon in advanced melanoma. Br J Cancer 2000;82:1158–1162.

57. Hamm C, Verna S, Petrella T, et al. Biochemotherapy for the treatment of metastatic melanoma: a systemic review. Cancer Treat Rev 2007;34:145–156.

58. Ives NJ, Stowe RL, Lorigan P, Whearley K. Chemotherapy compared with biochemotherapy for the treatment of metastatic melanoma. A meta-analysis of 18 trials involving 2,621 patients. J Clin Oncol 2007;25:5426–5434.

59. Gonazalez Cao M, Malvehy J, Marti R, et al. Biochemotherapy with temozolomide, cisplatin, vinblastine, subcutaneous interleukin-2 and interferon-α in patients with metastatic melanoma. Melanoma Res 2006;16:59–64.

60. Majer M, Jensen RL, Shrieve DS, et al. Biochemotherapy of metastatic melanoma in patients with recently diagnosed brain metastases. Cancer 2007;110:1329–1337.

61. Cocconi G, Bella M, Calabresi F, et al. Treatment of metastatic malignant melanoma with dacarbazine plus tamoxifen. N Engl J Med 1992:327:516–523.

62. Terando AM, Faries MB, Morton DL. Vaccine therapy for melanoma: Current status and future directions. Vaccine 2007;25(Suppl 2):B4–16.

63. Chapman PB. Melanoma vaccines. Semin Oncol 2007;34:516–523.

64. Kirkwood JM, Tarhini AA, Panelli MC, et al. Next generation of immunotherapy for melanoma. J Clin Oncol 2008;26:3445–3455.

65. Mitchell MS, Abrams J, Thompson JA, et al. Randomized trial of allogeneic melanoma lysate vaccine with low-dose interferon alfa-2b compared with high-dose interferon alfa-2b for resected stage III cutaneous melanoma. J Clin Oncol 2007;25:2078–2085.

66. Becker JC, Kirkwood JM, Agarwala SS, et al. Molecularly targeted therapy for melanoma. Cancer 2006;107:2317–2327.

67. Jilaveanu LB, Aziz S, Kluger HM. Chemotherapy and biologic therapies for melanoma: do they work? Clin Dermatol. 2009;27:614–625.

68. Flaherty KT, Puzanov I, Kim KB, et al. Inhibition of mutated, activated BRAF in metastatic melanoma. N Engl J Med 2010;363:809–819.

69. Sarnaik AA, Weber JS. Recent advances using anti-CTLA-4 for the treatment of melanoma. Cancer J 2009;15:169–173.

70. O'Day SJ, Hamid O, Urba WJ. Targeting cytotoxic T-lymphocyte antigen-4 (CTLA-4): A novel strategy for the treatment of melanoma and other malignancies. Cancer 2007;110:2614–2627.

71. Hodi FS, O'Day SJ, McDermott DF, et al. Improved survival with ipilimumab in patients with metastatic melanoma. N Engl J Med 2010;363:711–723.

72. Rosenberg SA, Yannelli JR, Yang JC, et al. Treatment of patients with metastatic melanoma with autologous tumor-infiltrating lymphocytes and interleukin 2. J Natl Cancer Inst 1994;86:1159–1166.

73. Burmeister BH, Smither BM, Burmeister E, et al. A prospective phase II study of adjuvant postoperative radiation therapy following nodal surgery in malignant melanoma – Trans Tasman Radiation Oncology Group (TROG) Study 96.06. Radiother Oncol 2006;81:136.

74. Coleman A, Augustine CK, Beasely G, et al. Optimizing regional infusion treatment strategies for melanoma extremites. Expert Rev Anticancer Ther 2009;9:1599–1609.

75. Sanki A, Kam PCA, Thompson JF. Long-term results of hyperthermic isolated limb perfusion for melanoma. Ann Surg 2007;245:591–596.

76. Lejeune FJ, Eggermont AMM. Hyperthermic isolated limb perfusion with tumor necrosis factor is a useful therapy for advanced melanoma of the limbs. J Clin Oncol 2007;25:1449–1450.

77. Feldman ED, Finkpank JF, Alexander HR. Regional treatment options for patients with ocular melanoma metastatic to the liver. Ann Surg Oncol 2004;11:290–297.

78. Francis SO, Mahlberg MJ, Johnson KR, et al. Melanoma chemoprevention. J Am Acad Dermatol 2006;55:849–861.

79. Kricker A, Armstrong BK, Goumas C, et al. Ambient UV, personal sun exposure and risks of multiple primary melanomas. Cancer Causes Control 2007;18:295.

80. The International Agency for Research on Cancer Working Group on artificial ultraviolet (UV) light and skin cancer. The association of use of sunbeds with cutaneous malignant melanoma and other skin cancers: A systematic review. Int J Cancer 2007;120: 1116–1122.

81. El Ghissassi F, Baan R, Straif K, et al. A review of human carcinogens-part D: radiation. Lancet Oncol 2009;10:751.

82. Dummer R, Hauschild A, Jost L. Cutaneous malignant melanoma: ESMO Clinical Recommendations for diagnosis, treatment and follow-up. Ann Oncol 2008;19:ii86–ii88.

JANELLE B. PERKINS AND GARY C. YEE

CHAPTER 148

Hematopoietic Stem Cell Transplantation

KEY CONCEPTS

❶ Hematopoietic stem cell transplantation (HSCT) is a process that involves intravenous infusion of hematopoietic stem cells from a donor into a recipient, after the administration of chemotherapy with or without radiation. The rationale is to increase tumor cell kill by increasing the dose of chemotherapy. Immune-mediated effects contribute to the tumor cell kill observed after allogeneic HSCT.

❷ Hematopoietic stem cells used for transplantation can come from the recipient (autologous) or from a related or unrelated donor (allogeneic). If the related donor is a twin, the transplant is referred to as a syngeneic transplant.

❸ Human leukocyte antigen (HLA) mismatching of allogeneic donor/recipient pairs at either a class I or class II locus correlates with the risk of graft failure, graft-versus-host disease (GVHD), and survival. The ideal donor is matched at HLA-A, HLA-B, HLA-C, and HLA-DRB1.

❹ Hematopoietic stem cells are found in the bone marrow, peripheral blood, and umbilical cord blood. Because of their rarity and their similarity to other cells, hematopoietic stem cells are difficult to isolate and measure. These stem cells express the CD34 antigen, and quantification of the number of CD34+ cells has become a clinically useful measure of the number of hematopoietic stem cells.

❺ Because of clinical and economic advantages, peripheral blood has replaced bone marrow as the source of hematopoietic stem cells in the autologous and adult allogeneic HSCT setting. Bone marrow continues to be the primary graft source in children undergoing allogeneic HSCT.

❻ The purpose of the preparative (or conditioning) regimen in traditional myeloablative transplants is twofold: (a) maximal tumor cell kill and (b) immunosuppression of the recipient to reduce the risk of graft rejection (allogeneic HSCT only).

❼ Reduced-intensity conditioning regimens (including those that are nonmyeloablative) reduce early posttransplant morbidity and mortality while maximizing the graft-versus-malignancy (GVM) effect of the allogeneic graft. The advantage of this approach is that patients who otherwise would not be eligible for allogeneic HSCT can be offered a potentially curative therapy.

❽ Posttransplant immunotherapy is based on the GVM effect caused by certain subsets of T cells responsible for eradication of malignant cells. Posttransplant immunotherapy includes the use of donor lymphocyte infusions, immunomodulatory cytokines, monoclonal antibodies, or antitumor vaccines.

❾ Transplant-related mortality associated with allogeneic HSCT ranges from 10% to 80%, depending on age, donor, and disease status. Major causes of death include infection, organ toxicity, and GVHD. The most common cause of death after autologous HSCT is disease relapse. Transplant-related mortality usually is less than 5%, depending on the conditioning regimen, age, and disease status.

❿ Treatment of acute GVHD often is unsuccessful, and the resulting complications can be fatal. Patients undergoing allogeneic HSCT are given prophylactic immunosuppressive therapy, which inhibits T-cell activation and/or proliferation. The most commonly used GVHD prophylaxis regimen is cyclosporine or tacrolimus and methotrexate.

⓫ Initial treatment of both acute and chronic GVHD consists of prednisone, either alone or combined with cyclosporine or tacrolimus. Treatment of patients with steroid-refractory GVHD is problematic.

Learning objectives, review questions, and other resources can be found at **www.pharmacotherapyonline.com**.

❶ Hematopoietic stem cell transplantation (HSCT) is a process that involves intravenous infusion of hematopoietic stem cells from a compatible donor into a recipient, usually after administration of high-dose chemotherapy. Hematopoietic stem cells can be derived from the bone marrow, peripheral blood, or umbilical cord blood. The original rationale for HSCT for treatment of malignant disease is based on studies showing that most anticancer drugs have a steep dose–response relationship and that bone marrow suppression limits the chemotherapy dosage that can be safely administered. Although standard-dose chemotherapy can prolong survival in many cancer patients, most patients are not cured of their disease (Fig. 148–1). Infusion of hematopoietic stem cells allows administration of very high doses of chemotherapy (as much as 10-fold higher). If tumor cells that are resistant to standard doses are sensitive to higher doses of chemotherapy, then tumor cell kill will be greatly increased, and the likelihood of cure would be higher with HSCT. However, the chemotherapy dose cannot be escalated indefinitely because of the risk for death caused by nonhematopoietic toxicity. The success and increasing use of reduced-intensity regimens (including those that are nonmyeloablative) show that immune-mediated effects also contribute to the antitumor effect of allogeneic HSCT.

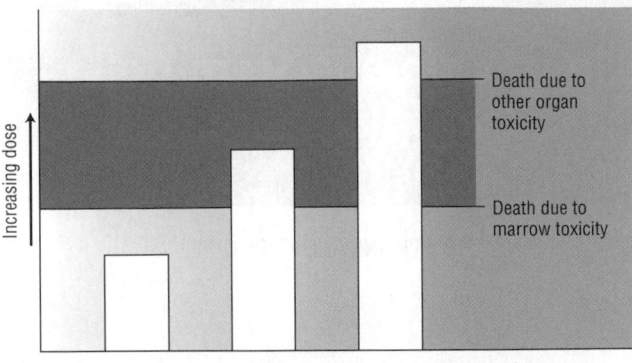

FIGURE 148-1. Patients represented by the middle column are the best candidates for hematopoietic stem cell transplantation because the technique allows for administration of chemotherapy or radiation in doses that otherwise would be intolerable because of severe myelosuppression.

High-dose chemotherapy followed by HSCT has become an important modality for treatment of a variety of malignant and nonmalignant diseases. It is estimated that 50,000 to 60,000 transplants are performed worldwide each year, primarily for malignant diseases.[1] Approximately 40% of these transplants are performed in North America. The number of transplants has grown steadily over the last decade due to an increase in the number of patients receiving umbilical cord blood (UCB) transplants and patients older than 60 years being transplanted after reduced-intensity conditioning regimens.

Historically, the most common type of donor was a genetically nonidentical individual, such as a histocompatible sibling (referred to as allogeneic HSCT). However, the number of autologous transplants in which the patient serves as his or her own donor has increased dramatically, and the number of autologous transplants performed (approximately 35,000) currently exceeds the number of allogeneic HSCTs (approximately 25,000) performed each year.[1] This chapter focuses on the application of HSCT for treatment of malignant disease, but it is important to note that many nonmalignant diseases—including aplastic anemia, thalassemia, sickle cell anemia, immunodeficiency disorders, and other genetic disorders—are potentially curable with allogeneic HSCT. Transplantation is also being investigated as a treatment modality for patients with life-threatening autoimmune diseases, such as rheumatoid arthritis, systemic and multiple sclerosis, and systemic lupus erythematosus.

This chapter summarizes the procedures involved in HSCT and the common complications associated with HSCT. More detailed information on HSCT can be found in published reviews and books.[2-5] Information on HSCT also can be found on several websites, including *http://www.cibmtr.org* (Center for International Blood and Marrow Transplant Research) and *http://www.marrow. org* (National Marrow Donor Program).

DONORS AND HISTOCOMPATIBILITY TESTING

❷ Different types of donors are used in HSCT. In *autologous* transplants, patients receive their own hematopoietic stem cells, which were collected and stored before intensive cytotoxic therapy. In *syngeneic* transplants, an identical twin serves as the donor. In *allogeneic* transplants, the donor is genetically not identical to the recipient but shares some common tissue antigens. Immunologic compatibility is evaluated by studies of cell surface antigens

(human leukocyte antigens [HLAs]) encoded by genes of the major histocompatibility complex (MHC), which is located on the sixth chromosome.[6] The genes of the HLA system are clustered in three distinct regions designated as class I, class II, and class III. Class I and class II genes encode for antigens that function as major transplantation antigens; products of class III genes have other important roles in the immune system. The major class I loci in humans are referred to as HLA-A, HLA-B, and HLA-C. The one major class II locus is HLA-D. Class II genes encode for the α and β polypeptide chains of the class II molecules. The designation of class II genes consists of three letters: the first (D) indicates the class, the second (M, O, P, Q, or R) the family, and the third (A or B) the chain (α and β, respectively). Class I and class II antigens differ in their tissue distribution, structure, and function. Class I antigens are expressed on virtually all nucleated cells and serve as the primary targets for cytotoxic T lymphocytes. Class II antigens normally are expressed only on macrophages, B lymphocytes, and activated T lymphocytes, and they serve as the primary targets for helper T lymphocytes.

HLA genes are closely linked to one another within the MHC and generally are inherited together. The series of HLA alleles occurring on a single chromosome is termed a *haplotype*. The combination of two parental haplotypes inherited by an individual determines an individual's *genotype*. For a given HLA locus, an individual generally has two different corresponding antigens expressed in their genotype (e.g., HLA-A2 and HLA-A3; HLA-B44 and HLA-B7; HLA-DR4 and HLA-DR2).

Historically, the most important HLA loci in allogeneic HSCT were HLA-A, HLA-B, and HLA-D (or HLA-DR [D-Related]). Typing for HLA-A and HLA-B traditionally was performed by serologic typing with standard microcytotoxicity assays having panels of antisera containing HLA molecules.[7] HLA types determined by this method were reported as the locus (A or B), followed by a number that designated the cell surface HLA antigen (e.g., HLA-A2). Typing for the HLA-D was performed with cellular typing methods, such as the mixed lymphocyte reaction (MLR) or mixed lymphocyte culture (MLC). A "positive" MLR or MLC indicated incompatibility somewhere in the HLA-D region. Individuals who had a low degree of reactivity in the MLR or MLC (expressed as a low percent relative response), and who met other selection criteria, could serve as donors.

Serologic methods of HLA typing have been replaced by DNA-based techniques that use polymerase chain reaction (PCR) amplification of specific HLA genes from genomic DNA. DNA typing methods are categorized by the level of discrimination they provide in defining the sequence of an HLA gene. *Low-resolution* methods provide limited sequence information about a particular HLA gene and allow identification only to the antigen level, much like older serologic methods. Results of low-resolution typing are given in the form HLA-A*02, where the asterisk denotes DNA-based typing and the corresponding serologic equivalent of the antigen is labeled as a two-digit number. Low-resolution typing typically is used to identify sibling donors. However, neither serologic nor low-resolution techniques can distinguish the extremely polymorphic nature of many of the HLA antigens. HLA antigens are characterized by thousands of allelic variations, and each allele may correspond to a unique HLA molecule. Different alleles can be distinguished only by *high-resolution* typing techniques. Results of high-resolution techniques are reported as the corresponding HLA antigen, followed by an asterisk and a four-digit number identifying the allele. For example, the HLA-A*02 antigen may be encoded by alleles HLA-A*0201, A*0202, A*0203, etc. In some cases, the four-digit allele name includes several alleles. For example, HLA-B*4006 includes B*40060101 and B*40060102. Methods that define the HLA type A beyond the serologic level but short of the allele level are termed *intermediate-resolution*. This method might identify the presence of either HLA-A*0201 or A*0205 but may not be able to discriminate one allele from the other.

❸ The degree of HLA mismatching correlates with the risk of graft failure, graft-versus-host disease (GVHD), and survival.[7] In an analysis of 1,874 patients who received HLA-matched unrelated bone marrow donor transplants under the auspices of the National Marrow Donor Program (NMDP), low-resolution mismatches at HLA-A, HLA-B, HLA-C, and HLA-DRB1 were similarly associated with increased risk of GVHD and mortality.[8] The observation concerning the prognostic value of HLA-C was particularly important since until that time the locus was omitted from most matching algorithms. Based on these results, HLA-C typing is now included in standard typing protocols. High-resolution mismatches, particularly at HLA-A and HLA-DRB1, also were associated with increased mortality. In addition, among patients who received transplants from "6 antigen-matched" (HLA-A, HLA-B, and HLA-DRB1 matched) donors, the number of allele mismatches correlated with the risk of grades III to IV acute GVHD and survival. These findings were confirmed in an analysis of over 3,800 unrelated bone marrow donor–recipient pairs in which high-resolution matching for HLA-A, -B, -C, and DRB1 was associated with the best overall survival.[9] That study also showed that mismatches at HLA-DQ or -DP had no effect on survival.

The most common donor for allogeneic HSCT is an HLA-identical sibling. The odds that any one full sibling will match a patient are 1:4. Approximately 30% of Americans have an HLA-identical sibling. In an effort to offer allogeneic HSCT to patients who lack an HLA-identical sibling donor, alternative donors are being used. Rarely, a parent is HLA identical with his or her child. A relative can be a zero- (rare), one-, two-, or three-loci antigen mismatch (assuming testing for HLA-A, HLA-B, and HLA-DR antigens). Although some patients who receive transplants from mismatched related donors experience long-term survival, their risks of graft failure and acute GVHD are higher than for recipients of matched-sibling transplants. It is estimated that only another 10% of patients will have a closely HLA-matched related donor.

The most common type of alternative donor is an individual unrelated to the recipient who is fully or closely HLA-matched. To facilitate identification of these donors, the NMDP (*http://www.marrow.org*) was started in 1986 with initial funding from a U.S. Navy contract. To date, the NMDP has registered more than eight million donors in the United States, and the NMDP has facilitated approximately 40,000 HLA-matched unrelated donor transplants. Patients searching NMDP also have access to an additional four million donors through agreements with international cooperative registries. Approximately one third of the allogeneic HSCTs performed worldwide are from unrelated donors.[1] The NMDP currently requires that the recipient be typed by high-resolution methodology at HLA-A, -B, -C, and -DRB1. The NMDP also suggests typing other DR and DQ alleles when developing a search strategy. Although it is the transplant center's responsibility to select the donor, the NMDP *recommends* that selected donor and recipient be matched at HLA-A, -B, -C, and -DRB1 by high-resolution typing, when possible. To permit an NMDP donor as a source for transplant, the NMDP *requires* a high-resolution match for at least five of six HLA antigens at HLA-A, -B, and -DR for marrow or peripheral blood transplants and four of six for UCB transplants. The following guidelines should be used for unrelated donor selection: (a) assume that HLA-A, -B, -C, and -DRB1 are equally important; (b) avoid antigen mismatches, if possible; (c) accept one allele mismatch over one antigen mismatch; and (d) minimize the number of allele mismatches.[10] If more than one suitable HLA matched unrelated donor is identified, other factors can be used to select the donor, such as younger age, male or nulliparous female, and negative CMV serostatus.

The likelihood of any one unrelated individual being an antigen-level match ranges from 1:100 to 1:1,000,000, depending on the prevalence of the patient's HLA type, race, and ethnic background. With the current size of the NMDP registry, the matching likelihood is higher than 80% for Caucasians. Because most minorities are not as well represented in the program, the likelihood of finding a donor for patients from certain racial or ethnic groups is lower. Agreements between NMDP and international registries may improve the likelihood of finding donors for these patients. Another limitation is the time needed to search for a potential donor. Some donor searches take up to three to four months, and many patients with acute leukemia may relapse while waiting for completion of the search. Cost is also a concern, with the cost for donor search and procurement ranging from $25,000 to $50,000. The clinical results of allogeneic HSCT with unrelated donors are encouraging. With improved HLA typing techniques and better supportive care, most reported outcomes are no longer significantly different than with related sibling donors.[7,11,12]

COLLECTION OF HEMATOPOIETIC STEM CELLS

Hematopoietic stem cells serve as "mother" cells for all blood cells, including erythrocytes, leukocytes, and platelets (see Chap. 95). Stem cells have varying degrees of "stemness." True *pluripotent* stem cells are capable of replicating indefinitely and can give rise to stem and progenitor cells of *all* tissues. *Multipotent* stem cells, such as hematopoietic stem cells, have the capacity for self-renewal and can differentiate into more than one cell type in a particular tissue lineage. Because of their capacity for self-renewal, hematopoietic stem cells are capable of repopulating the recipient's marrow which has been "emptied" by administration of high-dose chemotherapy, either alone or combined with radiation.

❹ Hematopoietic stem cells are rare cells, composing less than 0.01% of all bone marrow cells. Isolation and quantitative measurement of hematopoietic stem cells are extremely difficult because of their rarity and their similar appearance to other cells. For these reasons, surrogate markers are used to measure the number of stem cells. Determination of the number of cells expressing the CD34 antigen (CD34⁺ cells), as determined by flow cytometry, has become the standard method of measuring hematopoietic stem cell content.[13] CD34 is an antigen expressed on hematopoietic stem cells and other early progenitor cells.

Hematopoietic stem cells are found in the bone marrow, peripheral blood, and UCB. Hematopoietic stem cells from the bone marrow are obtained by multiple aspirations from the anterior and posterior iliac crests while the donor is under general anesthesia. The procedure takes approximately one hour and yields 200 to 1,500 mL, depending on the size of the donor. The marrow is transferred into tissue culture medium containing preservative-free heparin. The pooled marrow is passed through a series of stainless steel screens to break up aggregated particles, resulting in an essentially single-cell suspension. In allogeneic HSCT, the marrow stem cells are given to the recipient 12 to 24 hours after harvest. In autologous HSCT, the marrow is frozen and stored until needed. After intravenous infusion, the marrow stem cells enter the systemic circulation and find their way to the bone marrow cavity, where they reseed and grow in the bone marrow microenvironment. Although the donor experiences local soreness for a few days, the procedure usually is well tolerated, with no delayed complications resulting from the marrow aspiration. The major risk of serving as a marrow donor is the risk of undergoing general anesthesia.

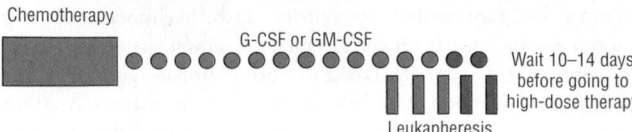

FIGURE 148-2. Schema for collection of peripheral blood progenitor cells after hematopoietic growth factor administration (top) or after chemotherapy and hematopoietic growth factor administration (bottom). Symbols with darker shading represent procedures performed only if adequate numbers of CD34+ cells have not been collected. (G-CSF, granulocyte colony-stimulating factor; GM-CSF, granulocyte-macrophage colony-stimulating factor.)

Hematopoietic stem cells in peripheral blood (peripheral blood progenitor cells or peripheral blood stem cells [PBSCs]) are found in the mononuclear fraction of white blood cells (lymphocytes and monocytes) and are collected by a procedure called *leukapheresis* (or *apheresis*). In this outpatient procedure, approximately 9 to 14 L of blood are processed over several hours during each daily apheresis session. Most of the blood cells are returned to the donor, and each apheresis yields approximately 200 mL of cells.

The number of hematopoietic stem cells that circulate in peripheral blood normally is too low for this approach to be technically feasible. Without mobilization techniques, at least six aphereses usually are required to collect a sufficient number of PBSCs. Several methods have been used clinically to "mobilize" hematopoietic stem cells from the bone marrow into peripheral blood for use in autologous transplantation.[14,15] Figure 148-2 shows representative schemas for mobilization and collection of PBSCs. With current mobilization techniques, most HSCT centers collect sufficient PBSCs with three or fewer aphereses. One type of mobilization method is administration of chemotherapy, which can briefly increase the number of PBSCs as much as 100-fold. The more commonly used method is administration of a recombinant hematopoietic growth factor such as granulocyte colony-stimulating factor (G-CSF; filgrastim) or granulocyte-macrophage colony-stimulating factor (GM-CSF; sargramostim). Each agent has its own potential advantages and disadvantages.[16] Both agents are FDA-approved for this indication, but G-CSF is the most commonly used growth factor. Dosages are 10 mcg/kg/day (5 to 32 mcg/kg/day) for G-CSF and 250 mcg/m²/day for GM-CSF. The combination of chemotherapy followed by a hematopoietic growth factor increases the number of PBSCs to a greater extent than either method alone. This approach is more expensive and is associated with more adverse effects than a growth factor alone, but the number of aphereses is reduced and the additional chemotherapy may further reduce the tumor burden before transplant, which may reduce the likelihood of tumor cell contamination in the apheresis collection. Pegfilgrastim has also been evaluated in the mobilization setting, either alone (12 mg) or combined with chemotherapy (6 mg). It appears to be safe and at least as effective as G-CSF. Further studies are needed to evaluate the functional characteristics of cells mobilized by pegfilgrastim as preliminary data suggest that there may be important biologic differences between cells mobilized by pegfilgrastim versus G-CSF.[17]

Plerixafor (AMD3100) is a novel inhibitor of the CXCR4 chemokine receptor that received FDA approval in 2008 as a mobilizing agent. Its approval was based on two multicenter randomized double-blinded trials that compared G-CSF plus plerixafor or placebo as primary mobilization in patients with multiple myeloma or non-Hodgkin lymphoma.[18,19] In both studies, patients received G-CSF 10 mcg/kg/day daily for four days; on the evening of the fourth day, they received either 240 mcg/kg of plerixafor or placebo. Starting on day 5, patients began daily apheresis for up to four days, continuing G-CSF and plerixafor or placebo until at least 5 × 10⁶ CD34+ cells/kg were collected (a minimum of 6 × 10⁶ CD34+ cells/kg were used in the myeloma study). In both studies, a significantly larger proportion of the G-CSF plus plerixafor–treated patients were able to collect the target number of CD34+ cells in no more than two aphereses procedures as compared with the G-CSF plus placebo–treated group. In addition, more patients with both diagnoses were able to reach the target with just one apheresis when given plerixafor. The most common adverse events related to plerixafor were gastrointestinal complaints and injection site reactions. Neutrophil and platelet engraftment posttransplant were similar between treatment groups in both studies. Due to the high cost of plerixafor, many transplant centers are developing mobilization protocols to define its appropriate role. The general trend is to evaluate peripheral blood CD34+ counts after 4–5 days of G-CSF (but prior to apheresis); if this count does not meet a pre-specified level, plerixafor is initiated. Patients who are identified as high risk for primary mobilization failure are often given plerixafor in combination with G-CSF as initial mobilization therapy.

Several studies show that the number of CD34+ cells infused correlates significantly with the rate of neutrophil and platelet recovery after high-dose chemotherapy.[13–15] Rapid neutrophil recovery usually is observed in patients who receive at least 2 × 10⁶ CD34+ cells/kg (body weight of recipient). More rapid platelet recovery is observed when at least 5 × 10⁶ CD34+ cells/kg are transplanted compared to lower cell doses. As a result, most transplant centers use 2 × 10⁶ CD34+ cells/kg as a minimum number to collect for autologous transplant, with an optimal target of 5 × 10⁶ CD34+ cells/kg. For patients with multiple myeloma undergoing tandem transplants, cells for both transplants are collected prior to the first transplant. A minimum of 4 × 10⁶ CD34+ cells/kg are required and generally the entire cell dose collected is divided into two approximately equal aliquots, one for each transplant.

There may be clinical and economic benefits associated with infusion of higher CD34+ cell doses.[20–21] Although the difference in the *median* number of days to neutrophil or platelet recovery usually is no more than 1 to 2 days in patients who receive more than 5 × 10⁶ CD34+ cells/kg compared with those who receive less than 5 × 10⁶ CD34+ cells/kg, fewer patients who receive more than 5 × 10⁶ CD34+ cells/kg have delayed engraftment. This small effect may be important because patients with delayed engraftment consume a disproportionate share of healthcare resources, such as additional transfusions, hospital days, and drugs (e.g., antibiotics and growth factors).

In some otherwise-eligible transplant candidates, an optimal number of CD34+ cells will not be obtained with standard mobilization methods. Risk factors associated with poor mobilization include the amount (greater than six cycles) and type of prior chemotherapy (alkylating agents), lenalidomide use, and prior radiation therapy.[14,15,22] Older age and some diagnoses also are associated with poor mobilization. Several strategies for overcoming the obstacle of poor mobilization have been evaluated, including remobilization with the same or higher doses of the same hematopoietic growth factor, a combination of hematopoietic growth factors, or a combination of chemotherapy and a hematopoietic growth factor. Bone marrow harvest is an option but often is of limited value. Plerixafor has also been evaluated in patients who have failed primary mobilization. In a study of 115 patients who had failed at least one previous mobilization attempt, plerixafor and G-CSF were given with the objective of collecting at least 2×10^6 CD34[+] cells/kg.[23] Depending on diagnosis, aproximately 60% to 75% of patients successfully mobilized with this regimen, which compares favorably with other secondary mobilization strategies.

❺ Use of peripheral blood instead of bone marrow as a source of hematopoietic stem cells offers several clinical and economic advantages. The most clinically important advantage is that patients who receive mobilized PBSCs experience more rapid hematopoietic engraftment. Although engraftment of all lineages is more rapid when PBSCs are used, the most significant effect is observed with platelet recovery. Patients who receive mobilized PBSCs experience platelet recovery as much as two to three weeks earlier and require fewer platelet transfusions than those who receive bone marrow stem cells. As a result, patients usually are discharged earlier from the hospital, so the overall cost of autologous HSCT is reduced with the use of PBSCs. Another advantage is that the donor does not experience the discomfort associated with marrow aspirations and is not exposed to the risk associated with general anesthesia. PBSCs may be less likely to be contaminated with malignant cells as compared with marrow stem cells. Finally, because PBSCs are collected from the mononuclear cell fraction, a fraction that also contains immunocompetent cells (e.g., natural killer [NK] cells and T lymphocytes), some investigators believe that infusion of PBSCs represents a form of "adoptive immunotherapy." In this model, NK cells and lymphocytes targeted against tumor cells help to kill residual tumor cells. As a result of these clinical and economic advantages, peripheral blood has replaced bone marrow as the source of stem cells in the autologous setting.

Peripheral blood has also become the predominant source of hematopoietic stem cells in adult allogeneic HSCT.[1,24] Approximately 75% of allogeneic HSCTs performed in adults currently come from PBSCs harvested from normal donors, despite early concerns that the increased numbers of T lymphocytes found in peripheral blood could increase the risk of GVHD. Concerns also were raised over the safety and ethics of administering G-CSF to normal individuals volunteering as donors. G-CSF is generally well tolerated. Short-term effects are similar to those seen in cancer patients (e.g., bone pain, headache, fever, arthralgias, malaise). Although there are concerns about increased risk of acute leukemia in healthy subjects given G-CSF, no higher risk has been observed.[25]

Randomized controlled trials and large registry studies show that patients who received allogeneic PBSC transplants from HLA-identical siblings experienced more rapid hematopoietic recovery and required fewer transfusions compared with patients receiving bone marrow.[24,26,27] The difference in the rate of engraftment may be related to the threefold higher numbers of CD34[+] cells infused in recipients of PBSC transplants. Although most of these studies did not report an increased risk of acute GVHD or transplant-related mortality in patients receiving allogeneic PBSC transplants, a higher incidence of chronic GVHD has been observed. In a meta-analysis of nine randomized trials evaluating HLA-matched sibling donor transplants in adult patients, the risk of chronic GVHD was nearly twofold higher for patients who received allogeneic PBSC transplants compared with those who received bone marrow transplantation (BMT). However, the risk of relapse was higher in the patients receiving BMT and no significant difference in overall survival was observed. When patients were analyzed based on disease status at the time of transplant, patients with hematologic malignancies at high risk of relapse had a better overall survival when transplanted with PBSC as compared to those who received BMT, which may be related in part to the lower risk of relapse in patients who received PBSC transplants.[27] A randomized comparison of BMT versus PBSC transplants from matched unrelated donors has been completed by the NMDP and data analysis is ongoing.

In addition to bone marrow and peripheral blood, hematopoietic stem cells are found in UCB. UCB is an attractive source for several reasons.[28,29] Because the stem cells are collected from placental blood, there is no risk to the mother or the baby and a very low risk of transmissible infectious diseases, such as cytomegalovirus and Epstein-Barr virus. As most UCB units are banked, the cells are available immediately because the donor does not have to be located and the material harvested. UCB initially was obtained from siblings, but now recipients of transplants from unrelated donors account for almost all patients who receive UCB transplants. More than 450,000 UCB grafts are available in over 100 UCB banks and greater than 20,000 unrelated UCB transplants have been performed worldwide.

Results of uncontrolled studies show that recipients of UCB transplantation have a lower risk of GVHD but a higher risk of graft failure as compared with recipients of BMT.[28] Recipients of UCB transplantation usually receive a CD34[+] cell dose more than one log lower than that given to recipients of BMT, and this difference in CD34[+] cell dose may explain the delayed engraftment in recipients of UCB transplantation. The number of infused total nucleated and CD34[+] cells correlates with outcomes following UCB transplantation. Although no randomized comparisons have been performed, analysis of data from the CIBMTR and the New York Blood Center showed similar survival in children with acute leukemia who underwent either unrelated HLA-mismatched UCB transplantation or unrelated HLA-matched BMT. Children who received an HLA-matched UCB transplant had better outcomes than those who received an HLA-matched BMT. However, higher transplant-related mortality was observed in children transplanted with a low UCB cell dose and a mismatched UCB graft.[30]

A major limitation of UCB transplants is the small volume of blood collected, usually 60 to 150 mL with resultant low numbers of CD34[+] cells. Although the relatively low numbers of hematopoietic cells may be adequate for hematopoietic engraftment in children and small adults, it may not be adequate for larger recipients. Efforts to expand the number of hematopoietic stem cells include culturing them ex vivo with combinations of hematopoietic growth factors or "pooling" several units of UCB for one recipient. Retrospective reviews and registry data with unrelated UCB transplants following both myeloablative and reduced-intensity regimens in adult recipients show similar outcomes as compared to BM and PBSC transplants. UCB transplants are now considered an acceptable alternative if an HLA-matched donor is not available.[28,29]

APPROACHES TO ERADICATE MALIGNANT CELLS

CONDITIONING REGIMENS

❻ Traditionally, the role of the pretransplant conditioning regimen has been to eradicate malignant cells and thus these regimens contained very high doses of chemotherapy with or without radiation. Due to the severe myelosuppression caused by these regimens, these types of regimens are classified as "myeloablative" conditioning (MAC). All patients undergoing autologous HSCT receive MAC. These regimens are also commonly used in allogeneic transplantation but over the last 15 years, reduced-intensity conditioning (RIC) regimens have emerged in the allogeneic setting. These regimens consist of lower doses of chemotherapy, with or without radiation, or different drugs. The primary goal of RIC is to suppress the recipient's immune system to allow for donor engraftment; malignant cells are primarily eradicated by the graft-versus-malignancy effect.

Myeloablative Regimens

MAC regimens usually include anticancer drugs which have a relatively steep dose-response curve and bone marrow suppression as their dose-limiting toxicity. As part of the conditioning regimen, they are given at very high doses, which would be associated with severe and life-threatening bone marrow suppression if hematopoietic stem cells were not infused. In patients undergoing allogeneic HSCT, another purpose of the conditioning regimen is to suppress the immune system of the recipient so that the graft is not rejected.

Cyclophosphamide, a drug with both immunosuppressive and cytotoxic effects, is commonly used in MAC regimens. Because of the inadequate antitumor activity of cyclophosphamide in some types of cancers, other drugs are often added or substituted. Examples include cytarabine (ara-C), busulfan, thiotepa, etoposide (VP-16), carboplatin, cisplatin, carmustine (BCNU), melphalan, and ifosfamide.

Total-body irradiation (TBI) is sometimes used in pretransplant conditioning regimens. In patients with malignant disease, the rationale of TBI is to eradicate malignant cells located in areas inaccessible to the systemic circulation and thus to the cytotoxic agents. TBI also has significant immunosuppressive activity. Historically, the standard TBI regimen involved administration of a midline tissue dose of approximately 10 Gy (1,000 rad), which is more than twice the lethal dose of radiation for a normal person. Many centers currently give fractionated (split over several days, once or twice a day) rather than single-dose TBI to patients with malignant disease. The rationale for this approach is an improved therapeutic ratio, that is, destruction of more leukemic cells and marrow stem cells while sparing other normal tissues. The acute toxicities of TBI consist of fever, nausea, vomiting, diarrhea, mucositis, and tender swelling of the parotid gland. Long-term complications of TBI-containing regimens include cataract formation, growth retardation, carcinogenesis, permanent reproductive sterility, and secondary malignancies.

Two of the most commonly used MAC regimens (especially for allogeneic HSCT) are cyclophosphamide and TBI (CyTBI) or busulfan and cyclophosphamide (BuCy). When given with TBI, cyclophosphamide is usually given first as two doses of 60 mg/kg/day, followed by TBI. In the original BuCy regimen, busulfan was given orally at a dosage of 1 mg/kg orally every six hours for 16 doses on days −9 to −6 (4 mg/kg/day for four days), followed by four doses of cyclophosphamide given intravenously once daily at a dosage of 50 mg/kg on days −5 to −2. In one widely used modification of the regimen (BuCy2), the total cyclophosphamide dosage is reduced from 200 (50 × 4) to 120 (60 × 2) mg/kg. Plasma busulfan concentrations are monitored at some centers because studies suggest that systemic exposure correlates with outcome, and use of a targeted busulfan and cyclophosphamide preparative regimen may improve patient outcome.[31] A commercially available intravenous form of busulfan (Busulfex®) reduces some of the interpatient variability in systemic exposure and may also reduce the risk of sinusoidal obstruction syndrome. The dose of intravenous busulfan approved for pretransplant conditioning regimens is 0.8 mg/kg every six hours for four days, although once daily dosing regimens have also been developed.

Several prospective randomized studies have compared CyTBI to BuCy in patients with acute or chronic myelogenous leukemia undergoing allogeneic HSCT.[32–34] Results of these studies show that BuCy has similar or greater antileukemic activity than CyTBI in patients with chronic myelogenous leukemia (CML). However, some studies suggest that the CyTBI regimen in patients with acute myelogenous leukemia (AML) was associated with slightly better disease-free survival rates than BuCy. However, none of the patients in these studies who were randomized to BuCy received busulfan doses adjusted on the basis of plasma concentrations, which may explain the differences between CyTBI and BuCy.[31] Long-term toxicities between the two regimens appear to be comparable.

Most preparative regimens used in autologous HSCT include an alkylating agent (either cyclophosphamide or melphalan), with other agents added that may have specific activity against the tumor type being treated. TBI usually is not included in the conditioning regimen in patients who have received prior radiotherapy. One commonly used regimen in autologous HSCT for lymphoma is the CBV regimen, which consists of cyclophosphamide (1.5 g/m² on days −6 to −3), carmustine (BCNU; 300 mg/m² on day −6), and etoposide (VP-16; 100 mg/m² every 12 hours for six doses on days −6 to −4). Other examples of lymphoma conditioning regimens are BEAC (BCNU, etoposide, ara-C, and cyclophosphamide) and BEAM (BCNU, etoposide, ara-C, and melphalan). The availability of anti-CD20–radiolabeled monoclonal antibodies offers the potential to deliver targeted radiation to CD20 positive tumor cells and less to normal organs. ^{131}I-tositumomab has been given, either alone or combined with high-dose cyclophosphamide and etoposide, or with the BEAM regimen followed by autologous HSCT to patients with non-Hodgkin lymphoma.[35,36] With this approach, very high radiation doses could be delivered to sites of disease. Preliminary results with this approach are encouraging and a Blood and Marrow Clinical Trials Network study that randomized patients with non-Hodgkin lymphoma to BEAM conditioning with or without ^{131}I-tositumomab has been completed; analysis of the data is ongoing. No single preparative regimen is clearly superior to other regimens for treatment of lymphoma. Single agent melphalan (200mg/m²) is the standard conditioning regimen for patients undergoing autologous HSCT for myeloma. Studies are ongoing evaluating the addition of newer agents (e.g., bortezomib).

Reduced-Intensity Conditioning Regimens

❼ Donor T cells contribute to the tumor cell kill and prevention of relapse observed after allogeneic HSCT, an effect referred to as the *graft-versus-malignancy* (GVM) *effect*. Evidence for the GVM effect is based on retrospective studies showing that patients who developed GVHD had a lower risk of leukemic relapse than those who did not develop GVHD. However, the overall survival rate was not different because of the increased nonrelapse mortality associated with GVHD. Other anecdotal evidence supporting a T-cell–mediated GVM effect was the increased risk of relapse found with T-cell–depleted transplants compared with unmodified transplants and the difference in relapse rates between recipients of syngeneic and HLA-identical sibling transplants.

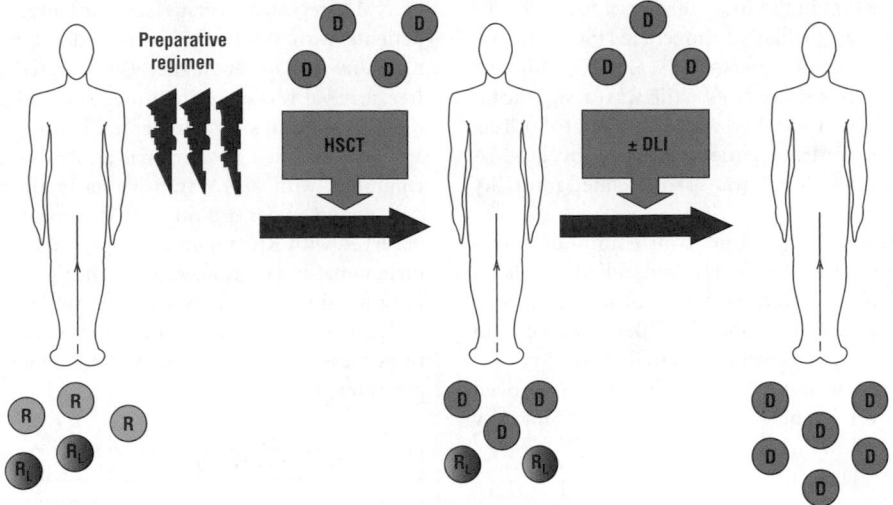

FIGURE 148-3. Schema for nonmyeloablative transplantation for hematologic malignancy. Recipients (R) receive a reduced-intensity conditioning regimen and an allogeneic hematopoietic stem cell transplant (HSCT). Initially, mixed chimerism is present with the coexistence of donor (D) cells and recipient-derived normal and leukemia/lymphoma (R_L) cells. Donor-derived T cells mediate a graft-versus-host hematopoietic effect that eradicates residual recipient-derived normal and malignant hematopoietic cells. Donor lymphocyte infusions (DLI) can be administered to enhance graft-versus-malignancy effects.

In the early 1990s, researchers began to evaluate RIC regimens as a method to take advantage of the GVM effect. The rationale for RIC is based on the assumption that much of the tumor cell kill associated with allogeneic HSCT is the result of the GVM effect and not only an effect of the myeloablative doses of chemotherapy or radiation (Fig. 148–3).[37,38] If this assumption is correct, a major role of the conditioning regimen is to suppress the host immune system, thus allowing engraftment of donor hematopoietic stem cells and donor T-cell cytotoxicity. A major advantage of RIC is that potentially curative transplants are being offered to patients who typically would not be considered for allogeneic HSCT because of their unacceptably high risk of transplant-related complications (e.g., increased age or moderately compromised organ function). More than 60% of patients receiving RIC regimens are older than 50 years compared to less than 20% of those receiving MAC regimens.[1] In addition, because of the lower rate of toxicity, allogeneic HSCT with RIC can be offered to patients who have relapsed after traditional myeloablative autologous or allogeneic transplants. Approximately 30% of allogeneic transplants are now being performed with RIC regimens.[1]

Because RIC regimens may not be completely myeloablative, host hematopoiesis can persist and lead to mixed chimerism (blood cells from both donor and recipient are present; see Fig. 148–3).[37] Several studies have reported significant correlations between donor T-cell chimerism levels and the risk of graft rejection, GVHD, and relapse. For example, a low percentage of donor T and NK cells present on day 14 has been associated with graft rejection, whereas high T-cell donor chimerism on day 28 has been associated with acute GVHD. Achievement of full donor chimerism was associated with better progression-free survival. These data suggest that monitoring donor chimerism posttransplant may allow early interventions to prevent graft rejection or relapse.

A number of RIC regimens that vary in their cytotoxic, myelosuppressive, and immunosuppressive activity have been developed.[37,38] Most regimens include fludarabine (125–240 mg/m²) because of its potent immunosuppressive activity, combined with either low-dose TBI (at doses up to 8 Gy [800 rad]) or an alkylating agent, such as cyclophosphamide (2–3.6 g/m² or 120–200 mg/kg), busulfan (up to 10 mg/kg), or melphalan (up to 180 mg/m²). Antithymocyte globulin or alemtuzumab is sometimes given for additional immunosuppression, and other purine analogs (e.g., pentostatin or clofarabine) are sometimes used instead of fludarabine. Rituximab has also been included in patients with CD20-positive lymphoid malignancies.[39] Many of these regimens are myeloablative but are defined as RIC because of the reduced doses of chemotherapy used resulting in a lower transplant-related mortality.

Some RIC regimens are considered nonmyeloablative (NMA). These regimens generally result in minimal myelosuppression (not requiring hematopoietic cell support) and very little regimen-related toxicity but, like other RIC regimens, are immunosuppressive enough to result in full engraftment of important donor immune effector cells.[40] Two of the most common NMA regimens are fludarabine (25 mg/m²/day for 3 to 5 days) combined with cyclophosphamide (60 mg/kg/ day × two days) or with TBI (≤2 Gy [<200 rad]). Although regimen-related toxicity is reduced with RIC and NMA regimens, GVHD remains a significant cause of morbidity and mortality similar to that seen after MAC regimens.[41]

Several clinical studies have reported the results of RIC regimens from HLA-matched related or unrelated donors.[37,38] Two hundred and fifty-three patients received HLA-matched related allogeneic HSCT with an NMA regimen at one of several transplant centers that are part of an international consortium of transplant centers led by the Fred Hutchinson Cancer Research Center. All patients had a hematologic malignancy. The source of hematopoietic stem cells was G-CSF–mobilized PBSCs. The median age was 54 years; the oldest patient was 73 years. The median followup was at 13 months. The first 58 patients were conditioned with TBI alone (2 Gy [200 rad]); 17% of these patients experienced nonfatal graft rejection. Fludarabine was added to the conditioning regimen in the remaining patients and the incidence of graft rejection decreased to less than 5%. A combination of cyclosporine and mycophenolate mofetil was given as GVHD prophylaxis. Most patients did not require platelet transfusions, and only approximately two thirds of patients required RBC transfusions. Most of the transplants were performed entirely in the ambulatory care setting. Typical side effects, such as mucositis, diarrhea, and organ toxicities, were absent.

Although the risk of infection in the first 100 days appeared to be lower than that seen with myeloablative allogeneic HSCT, the risk of late viral and fungal infections persisted.[41] GVHD, although delayed compared to historical controls, still was a significant problem. Transplant-related mortality was only 5% at day 100. Compared with matched controls, patients who received NMA conditioning had significantly lower transplant-related mortality at day 100 and at one year.[42]

Under a similar protocol, the same consortium of transplant centers treated 89 patients with HLA-matched unrelated NMA transplant.[43] Durable engraftment was observed in 85% of patients who received G-CSF–mobilized PBSCs but only in 56% of marrow recipients. Transplant-related mortality was 11% at day 100. Patients who received PBSCs had improved progression-free and overall survival compared with marrow recipients.

CLINICAL CONTROVERSY

Although RIC regimens reduce transplant-related mortality, whether this approach results in improved survival compared with MAC regimens is not clear. Also unclear is whether this approach improves survival compared with conventional chemotherapy. Direct comparison of the results of NMT versus myeloablative transplants is difficult because patients undergoing NMT tend to be older and have more comorbidities. Randomized controlled trials addressing these questions are ongoing, and the results of these studies should better define the role of RIC regimens and NMT.

Progression-free and overall survival varies depending on the specific RIC regimen, disease type and status at the time of transplant, donor type, and patient age and comorbidities. Patients with indolent lymphoid malignancies had the lowest relapse rate after NMA transplants, whereas those with advanced myeloid and lymphoid malignancies had the highest relapse rate.[44] Patients transplanted while in remission had lower relapse rates than those who were not in remission at the time of transplant. Direct comparison of the results of NMA versus myeloablative transplants is difficult because patients receiving NMA regimens tend to be older and have more comorbidities. In two retrospective comparisons of NMA regimens versus standard myeloablative transplants in patients with AML who were older than 50 years, nonrelapse mortality was lower in the NMA-treated patients, but leukemia-free survival was equivalent due to the higher relapse rate seen in the NMA groups.[45,46] Studies evaluating "disease-targeted" therapy (radiolabeled monoclonal antibody, imatinib, or rituximab) combined with NMA transplants to improve outcomes in specific malignancies are ongoing.[37] Antitumor responses have been observed with RIC regimens in patients with renal cell carcinoma, melanoma, breast cancer, and other solid tumors.[37,47] In order to improve the efficacy seen in this setting, some investigators are evaluating novel approaches that enhance allogeneic immune responses against tumor-associated antigens (if available), such as posttransplant vaccination.

PURGING THE STEM CELL PRODUCT

One disadvantage of autologous HSCT is that the stem cell product (graft) may be contaminated with malignant cells. Infusion of these malignant cells may contribute to tumor relapse. Many approaches have been developed to eliminate ("purge") the marrow of these tumor cells. The most common approach is addition of substances, such as chemicals or monoclonal antibodies, to the stem cell product while it is outside of the body (ex vivo; Fig. 148–4). Because the substances are removed before the stem cells are infused, nonhematopoietic tissues are not exposed to the substances and therefore are not damaged. However, these substances can remove or damage hematopoietic stem cells, which are essential for complete and rapid engraftment, and purging has been associated with delayed marrow recovery. Ex vivo marrow purging has also been performed in allogeneic HSCT in an attempt to eliminate T lymphocytes believed to be responsible for acute GVHD (Fig. 148–4). Results with this approach are discussed in the section on Graft-Versus-Host Disease.

One approach is the addition of one or more monoclonal antibodies that are directed against specific antigens present on the tumor cells but are absent on nearly all other cells.[35] Although this approach is theoretically attractive, it is limited because not all cells from patients with the same type of cancer express a specific antigen. Furthermore, for some types of cancers, identifying antigens distinct from those present on normal hematopoietic stem cells is difficult. To date, this strategy has been used most commonly in patients with lymphoid malignancies, such as acute lymphoblastic leukemia (ALL), chronic lymphocytic leukemia, or non-Hodgkin lymphoma.

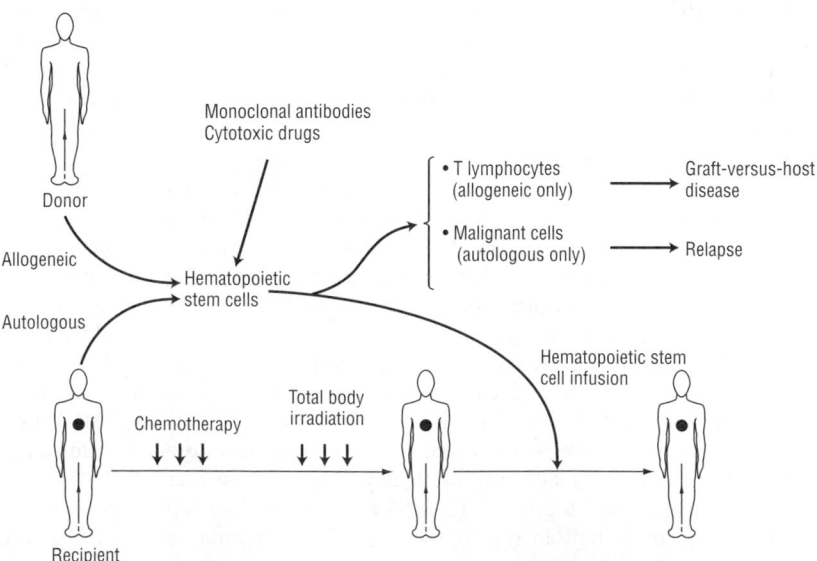

FIGURE 148-4. Use of ex vivo marrow purging to remove or destroy T cells (allogeneic only) or residual malignant cells (autologous only).

Rituximab has been used pretransplant for in vivo purging of the stem cell graft prior to autologous HSCT in patients with non-Hodgkin lymphoma.[35,39] When used for in vivo purging, rituximab usually is given before apheresis. Although use of rituximab was effective in reducing the number of tumor cells in the stem cell graft, whether this approach improves disease-free survival after autologous HSCT is not clear.

POSTTRANSPLANT THERAPY

8 Relapse of primary disease remains the most common cause of death for both allogeneic and autologous transplant patients. Several posttransplant therapies have been evaluated including immunotherapy, conventional chemotherapy, and targeted therapy. Relapse following autologous transplant can often be treated with standard doses of chemotherapy, a second autologous transplant. or even an allogeneic transplant, depending on the diagnosis, disease status, and side effects, response and duration of response to the first transplant. Options for treatment of relapse after an allogeneic transplant, however, are limited by GVHD and regimen-related toxicities caused by the conditioning regimen.

Immunotherapy

Donor Lymphocyte Infusions The rationale for posttransplant immunotherapy after allogeneic HSCT is based on the GVM effect. To take advantage of the GVM effect in patients who relapse after allogeneic HSCT, immunosuppressive therapy being used for GVHD is withdrawn as quickly as possible without inducing a serious GVHD flare. In rare cases, this is enough to reinduce a remission but in the majority of cases, further therapy is required.

Perhaps the most commonly used form of posttransplant immunotherapy is donor lymphocyte infusions (DLI).[48,49] Lymphocytes are collected from the same donor who provided hematopoietic stem cells. Most experiences with DLI have been in patients with CML. More than 80% of patients who are in cytogenetic or molecular relapse respond to DLI. The response rate of patients in more advanced phases is approximately 15% to 30%. Although the time to response is delayed (median 3 to 4 months), patients often have a durable molecular remission to DLI.

Response rates to DLI of patients with other myeloid malignancies, such as AML and myelodysplasia, are generally lower (25% to 30%) than the rates of patients with CML.[48,49] This may be related to the rapid proliferation of acute leukemia within the often prolonged time to response after DLI or to the lack of suitable target antigens on non-CML cells for recognition by donor cytotoxic T cells. Patients with relapsed AML post-HSCT are more likely to achieve a complete response to DLI if they had a longer remission period after transplant and had some GVHD after the DLI; low tumor burden, remission at the time of DLI, and good-risk cytogenetics have also been shown to be favorable characteristics. Administration of induction chemotherapy prior to DLI administration may improve the antitumor activity of DLI in patients with AML, but this method has not been tested in a randomized study. DLI has been shown to have limited benefit in patients with relapsed ALL after transplant.

DLI appears to be effective in patients with multiple myeloma who relapse after allogeneic HSCT, with reported response rates of 40% to 50%. Unfortunately, these responses tend to be transient and associated with the occurrence of GVHD. Anecdotal evidence suggests a graft-versus-lymphoma effect in patients with indolent non-Hodgkin lymphoma and chronic lymphocytic leukemia

DLI is sometimes given posttransplant for treatment of residual or progressive disease in patients with mixed chimerism after NMA conditioning. Preliminary results show that DLI in this setting is effective and is associated with acceptable toxicity (mostly GVHD) in patients with early signs of disease persistence or progression.[50] Prophylactic DLI to eradicate residual disease and reduce the risk of relapse is being investigated.

The most serious complications of DLI are pancytopenia and GVHD, and DLI is not usually given to patients with GVHD. The cytopenias generally are transient and can be treated with hematopoietic growth factors. A small percentage of patients may have a more prolonged course of aplasia with associated risk of infection, bleeding, and anemia. These patients may benefit from another infusion of donor stem cells. Acute GVHD (grade II or greater) occurs in 40% to 60% of patients receiving DLI. Although the severity of GVHD has been correlated with the GVM effect, complete responses have been seen in the absence of GVHD, suggesting that the effects can be separated. DLI is associated with 10% to 15% nonrelapse mortality at one year.

Because of the potential of DLI to cure some patients with certain hematologic malignancies, investigators are evaluating strategies to separate the GVM effect from the GVH effect, which would make DLI more tolerable. Other investigators are developing methods that would expand the efficacy of DLI to other malignancies. Some of these strategies include T-cell depletion from the stem cells, followed by delayed T-cell add-back transplant for patients with evidence of residual disease approximately three months posttransplant; selective depletion of CD8+ cells from the DLI; in vivo or in vitro T-cell activation with interleukin (IL)-2; and infusion of T cells that are selected to recognize tumor-specific antigens.[49]

Immunomodulatory Cytokines Another approach to inducing a GVM effect in patients who relapse after HSCT is posttransplant administration of a cytokine with immunomodulatory activity, such as IL-2.[51] Some benefit in terms of effects on NK cells and other important antitumor immune responses has been observed with the use of IL-2. Toxicities have been tolerable in most patients but can be serious and life-threatening. Studies that will define the role of these cytokines in prolonging relapse-free survival after HSCT are necessary.

Monoclonal Antibodies Rituximab is being evaluated as adjuvant therapy in patients with non-Hodgkin lymphoma treated with autologous HSCT.[35,39] The timing and number of doses of rituximab therapy vary. The Stanford program reported promising results with two four-week courses starting at day 42 and 6 months posttransplant.[52] Neutropenia was observed in approximately 50% of the patients treated.

Chemotherapy or Targeted Therapy

Imatinib has been evaluated for the treatment of posttransplant relapse of CML in several studies.[53] These reports suggest that imatinib may be an effective therapy with up to 70% of patients achieving a complete molecular response, which is maintained in some patients even after discontinuation of imatinib. There was no indication that GVHD was exacerbated and imatinib appeared to be well tolerated posttransplant. Based on these data, imatinib may be considered an alternative to DLI in selected patients. There are less data to support the use of second-generation tyrosine kinase inhibitors but these agents may play a role in this setting because most CML patients who currently undergo allogeneic HSCT have imatinib-resistant disease. Patients may also benefit from combining one of these agents with DLI. Patients with Philadelphia chromosome positive ALL who relapse posttransplant may also respond favorably to tyrosine kinase inhibitors. Ongoing clinical trials are evaluating tyrosine kinase inhibitors as remission maintenance therapy to prevent relapse after transplant.

Based on its activity in AML and MDS, 5-azacitidine is being evaluated in the posttransplant setting to prevent or treat relapse. Investigators at the M.D. Anderson Cancer Center reported their experience with low-dose 5-azacitidine (16 to 40 mg/m^2/day subcutaneously for five days) in 17 patients.[54] That study demonstrated that administration of these lower doses is feasible without extramedullary toxicity or exacerbation of GVHD. Durable remissions were seen in some patients who were treated for posttransplant relapse but those with rapidly progressing disease were less likely to respond. A randomized controlled trial for posttranplant maintenance therapy is underway at that institution.

Finally, posttransplant therapy is being evaluated in multiple myeloma. Previous studies have shown a potential benefit of thalidomide to prevent relapse posttransplant but questions remain regarding which patients would benefit the most from this approach. In addition, the use of thalidomide is limited by its neurotoxicity and other bothersome side effects. Combinations of newer agents such as lenalidomide and bortezomib are now being evaluated in this setting.[55]

TRANSPLANT-RELATED COMPLICATIONS

⑨ Although many patients with cancer who are treated with high-dose chemotherapy and autologous or allogeneic HSCT experience long-term survival and cure of their disease, this modality is associated with many serious and potentially life-threatening complications. In the early 1970s, posttransplant mortality was extremely high, and most allogeneic HSCT patients did not survive beyond 100 days because of infection, GVHD, organ toxicities, and leukemic relapse. Today, largely because of the availability of improved broad-spectrum antiinfective agents, immunosuppressive drugs, and hematopoietic growth factors, transplant-related mortality after allogeneic HSCT with HLA-matched sibling donors has been reduced to less than 30%. Mortality is even lower with the use of RIC regimens. Causes of death are still related to transplant-related organ toxicity, GVHD, or immunosuppression. Until recently, allogeneic HSCT usually was restricted to patients younger than 50 years with an HLA-identical sibling donor and younger than 40 years with an HLA-matched unrelated donor. With advances in the prevention and treatment of transplant-related complications and the availability of RIC regimens, allogeneic HSCT now is being offered to patients up to the age of 70. The risk of transplant-related mortality after high-dose chemotherapy with autologous HSCT generally is less than 5%, depending on patient population and conditioning regimen. Mortality is lower with autologous transplants because of the lack of GVHD and associated complications of immunosuppression. Transplant-related mortality in autologous HSCT usually is caused by conditioning regimen organ toxicity or infection.

Table 148-1 lists the dose-limiting nonhematologic toxicities for several drugs that are commonly included in MAC regimens. These toxicities may be uncommon or rare with administration of conventional doses of specific drugs. When these agents are given in high doses, the toxicities seen with conventional doses (e.g., mucositis, enteritis, nausea, vomiting, hematuria) can be more frequent and/or severe. Several unusual and severe manifestations of regimen-related toxicities are discussed in this section.

SINUSOIDAL OBSTRUCTION SYNDROME

Sinusoidal obstruction syndrome (SOS), formerly known as hepatic venoocclusive disease (VOD), occurs as a result of chemotherapy-induced dilation of hepatic sinusoids, necrosis of perivenular hepatocytes, and collagenization of the hepatic sinusoids and

| TABLE 148-1 | Dose-Limiting Nonhematologic Toxicities for Selected Chemotherapeutic Agents Included in Myeloablative Conditioning Regimens in Hematopoietic Stem Cell Transplantation |

Drug	Conventional Dose^a (mg/m^2)	HSCT Dose (mg/m^2)	Dose-Limiting Toxicity
Busulfan (oral)	2	450	Hepatic
Carboplatin	400	2,000	Hepatic, renal
Carmustine	200	1,200	Pulmonary, hepatic
Cisplatin	100	200	Renal, peripheral neuropathy
Cyclophosphamide	1,000	7,500	Cardiomyopathy
Etoposide	300–600	2,400	Mucositis
Ifosfamide	5,000	18,000	Renal
Melphalan	40	225	Mucositis
Thiotepa	20–50	1125	Mucositis, central nervous system

HSCT, hematopoietic stem cell transplantation.

^{a}Doses are approximate and are for drugs used as single agents. When combinations are used, doses may need to be decreased.

Eder JP, Elias A, Shea TC, et al. A phase I–II study of cyclophosphamide, thiotepa, and carboplatin with autologous bone marrow transplantation in solid tumor patients. J Clin Oncol 1990;8:1242. Reprinted with permission. © 1990 American Society of Clinical Oncology. All right reserved.

venules. These histologic changes can lead to obstruction of sinusoidal flow, portal hypertension, and hepatic failure.[53] Clinical signs of SOS include fluid retention (resulting in sudden weight gain and ascites), hepatomegaly (sometimes painful), and hyperbilirubinemia/jaundice. SOS usually occurs within the first three weeks after transplant. The incidence of SOS ranges from 5% to 20% in most published series. Severe SOS is fatal in 50% to 75% of cases. Factors that reportedly increase the risk of SOS include use of TBI-containing conditioning regimens (dose-dependent), increased systemic exposure to busulfan, individual variability in cyclophosphamide metabolism, chronic viral hepatitis, and elevated liver function tests pretransplant. Pretransplant exposure to gemtuzumab ozogamicin (Mylotarg®) has been implicated in the development of SOS in patients undergoing allogeneic HSCT, especially when given within a few months of transplant.

The pharmacokinetics of busulfan or cyclophosphamide may correlate with the risk of SOS.[56] Because busulfan concentrations have been correlated with the risk of SOS, many HSCT centers adjust busulfan doses based on plasma concentrations. Exposure to the O-carboxyethyl-phosphoramide mustard metabolite of cyclophosphamide has been reported to correlate with the risk of SOS and nonrelapse mortality. In addition, when busulfan and cyclophosphamide are given in combination, the order in which they are given may contribute to the risk of SOS. Presumably because of the effect of busulfan on cyclophosphamide pharmacokinetics (increased exposure to active and/or toxic metabolites), liver toxicity appears to be worse when busulfan is given first, as traditionally given in the BuCy regimen. This effect appears to be ameliorated by reversing the order or delaying cyclophosphamide administration to 24 to 48 hours after busulfan.

Some studies suggest that prostaglandin E$_1$, unfractionated low-molecular-weight heparin, or ursodiol may be partially effective in preventing SOS.[56] In a systematic review of three randomized trials comparing prophylactic ursodiol versus no treatment, Tay et al.[57] found a reduced risk of SOS (relative risk 0.34, 95% confidence interval 0.17–0.66) with prophylactic ursodiol. These studies were conducted in patients undergoing myeloablative transplants. Transplant-related mortality was reduced (relative risk 0.58, 95% confidence interval 0.35–0.95). Other outcomes, such as relapse and overall survival, were not affected. Prophylactic defibrotide may also be effective.[56]

Treatment is generally supportive, including fluid and electrolyte management. Mild-to-moderate disease generally resolves without specific therapy. Recombinant tissue plasminogen activator has been given to patients with severe SOS because of the possible role of the coagulation cascade in the pathogenesis of SOS. Responses have been reported, but patients also experienced a higher risk of bleeding.[56] Defibrotide has been evaluated in a randomized phase II study as therapy of severe SOS.[58] Patients received either 25 mg/kg/day or 40 mg/kg/day. Overall response rate and posttransplant day 100 survival rates were 46% and 42%, respectively, with no difference between the two doses. There was also no significant difference in adverse events. Defibrotide 25 mg/kg/day was selected for ongoing phase III trials in patients with SOS.

PULMONARY COMPLICATIONS

Pulmonary complications following HSCT can be categorized as infectious and noninfectious (infectious complications are discussed in Chap. 131). Noninfectious complications can be caused by direct damage to the pulmonary tissue by chemotherapy or radiation used in the conditioning regimen, immune effects of the graft, or other causes not clearly understood. Early complications include diffuse alveolar hemorrhage, engraftment syndrome, and idiopathic interstitial pneumonitis. Diffuse alveolar hemorrhage is characterized by dyspnea, hypoxia, dry cough, and fever; chest x-ray usually shows diffuse infiltrates in an alveolar pattern. Diffuse alveolar hemorrhage is diagnosed by examination of bronchoalveolar lavage fluid via bronchoscopy, which reveals progressively bloodier fluid with each instilled aliquot, and negative findings on microbiologic analysis. Although the condition can be life-threatening or fatal, prompt treatment with high doses of corticosteroids is sometimes beneficial. A few patients have been treated successfully with recombinant human activated factor VIIa, desmopressin, or aminocaproic acid.[59]

Engraftment syndrome is characterized by fever, erythrodermatous skin rash, and noncardiogenic pulmonary edema can occur during neutrophil recovery after HSCT.[60] The incidence of engraftment syndrome is not known because of the lack of uniform diagnostic criteria, although some series report that approximately 10% of patients who receive autologous HSCT develop the syndrome. Engraftment syndrome can progress to life-threatening respiratory failure with or without multiple organ failure. Corticosteroids are effective in some patients.

Idiopathic interstitial pneumonitis (also called idiopathic pneumonia syndrome) is defined as widespread alveolar injury in the absence of active lower respiratory tract infection following HSCT. Patients with idiopathic interstitial pneumonitis are clinically indistinguishable from patients with interstitial pneumonitis related to infection. Idiopathic interstitial pneumonitis is postulated to have a multifactorial etiology, including toxic effects of myeloablative conditioning, immunologic cell-mediated injury, inflammatory cytokine-induced lung damage, and occult pulmonary infections. The risk is similar in recipients of autologous HSCT or allogeneic HSCT but appears to be higher in patients who are conditioned with a TBI-containing regimen or who have acute GVHD. The incidence of idiopathic interstitial pneumonitis may be lower after RIC compared to conventional regimens.[61] Mortality as high as 70% has been reported, and treatment consists of supportive care only. Etanercept has been beneficial in some patients with idiopathic interstitial pneumonitis.[62]

Late pulmonary complications cover a wide spectrum of disorders and include both obstructive and restrictive lung diseases. The most well-described of these disorders is bronchiolitis obliterans with or without organizing pneumonia.[63] While bronchiolitis obliterans is thought to be a result of chronic GVHD affecting the lungs, its pathogenesis has not been completely elucidated. Therapy consists of corticosteroids, which are approximately 50% effective. Patients with mild-to-moderate airflow impairment appear to have the best response. Survival at five years from diagnosis of bronchiolitis obliterans is less than 20%.

GRAFT FAILURE

Initial engraftment after high-dose chemotherapy conditioning regimens usually occurs in the first two to four weeks posttransplant. Engraftment is evidenced by rising peripheral blood counts and the presence of hematopoietic precursor cells in the marrow. In allogeneic HSCT, the presence of donor cells (i.e., chimerism) is confirmed by fluorescent in situ hybridization of sex chromosomes and PCR-based analysis of polymorphic DNA sequences. Full chimerism is defined as greater than 95% of T cells of donor origin. In most patients, engraftment is sustained with complete recovery of hematopoiesis.

Graft failure can occur after autologous, syngeneic, and allogeneic HSCT. It can be the result of an immunologic reaction between donor and host, heavy pretreatment with chemotherapy and/or radiation therapy, infusion of insufficient numbers of hematopoietic stem cells, viral infection, recurrence of primary hematologic malignancy, drug reaction (e.g., to ganciclovir), or development of a secondary myelodysplasia. Two syndromes have been observed. Early graft failure occurs when the rate of hematopoietic recovery is delayed (primary graft failure or delayed engraftment), whereas late graft failure is characterized by a decline in peripheral blood counts after initial engraftment (secondary graft failure). With widespread use of PBSCs and posttransplant growth factors, primary graft failure is rare after autologous and HLA-matched related allogeneic HSCT but is not uncommon after UCB transplant. Graft failure that occurs after allogeneic HSCT, characterized by regrowth of immunocompetent host cells and a simultaneous loss of donor cells, is referred to as *graft rejection*. Graft rejection occurs rarely after HLA-matched related allogeneic HSCT. An increased risk of graft rejection has been observed in recipients of hematopoietic stem cells from HLA-mismatched related or unrelated donors, recipients of T cell–depleted marrow, and patients with severe aplastic anemia. The long-term prognosis of patients with graft failure is poor. Despite supportive care, death may result from infection or bleeding. In some patients with an allogeneic donor, a second infusion of stem cells can be attempted. The most effective therapy for graft failure is G-CSF or GM-CSF.

Hematopoietic growth factors usually are given posttransplant to patients who receive autologous HSCT, although some clinicians believe that posttransplant G-CSF or GM-CSF is unnecessary because of the already rapid engraftment seen after mobilized PBSC transplants.[64,65] The usual dosage of GM-CSF is 250 mcg/m²/day. Many different dosages and schedules of G-CSF have been used after autologous HSCT. Originally, G-CSF was given at a dose of 5 to 10 mcg/kg/day beginning on the day of or the day after infusion of stem cells and continued until neutrophil recovery to greater than an arbitrary number of neutrophils (500 to 1,000 cells/mm³ [0.5×10^9 to 1.0×10^9]). In one study of three different G-CSF dosages (5, 10, and 16 mcg/kg/day), no significant difference in the rate of hematopoietic recovery between the different dosages was observed.[66] In another study, delayed initiation of G-CSF at a dosage of 5 mcg/kg/day until day five posttransplant did not impair hematopoietic recovery after autologous HSCT.[67] Pegfilgrastim in the posttransplant setting has been evaluated in several uncontrolled trials and one randomized, controlled trial.[17] Although pegfilgrastim appears to be equally efficacious to filgrastim, more data is needed to justify the added cost of pegfilgrastim in this setting.

Hematopoietic growth factors accelerate the rate of hematopoietic recovery in patients undergoing allogeneic HSCT. However, laboratory studies show that growth factors can modify T-cell and dendritic cell function, and one retrospective study of patients with acute leukemia reported that G-CSF use after allogeneic BMT was associated with significantly increased risk of acute GVHD and death.[68] No detrimental effects of G-CSF were noted in patients receiving allogeneic PBSC transplants. In a meta-analysis of 34 randomized controlled trials, no increased risk of acute GVHD or treatment-related mortality was observed when G-CSF or GM-CSF was used after allogeneic HSCT.[69] In another retrospective analysis of 2,719 patients from the CIBMTR, no association between G-CSF use and acute or chronic GVHD, transplant-related mortality, or survival was observed in recipients of HLA-identical sibling bone marrow, recipients of HLA-identical sibling peripheral blood, and recipients of HLA-matched unrelated donor bone marrow.[70] The use of growth factors after allogeneic HSCT remains controversial, except in patients receiving UCB transplants who are at increased risk for delayed engraftment and graft failure.

Results of studies with platelet growth factors, such as thrombopoietin and IL-11, given posttransplant have been disappointing. Platelet transfusions remain the standard of care in patients with thrombocytopenia below a given threshold (e.g., 10,000 cells/mm³ [10×10^9]) or in patients with significant bleeding.

Anemia may be problematic in the posttransplant setting, especially in patients receiving allogeneic HSCT. The etiology is unclear and most likely is multifactorial. Although erythropoietin administration may be useful in reducing the need for red blood cell transfusions, its use in cancer patients is associated with an increased risk of adverse events and is limited by FDA warnings and restrictions.

GRAFT-VERSUS-HOST DISEASE (GVHD)

GVHD is caused by immunocompetent allogeneic donor T cells reacting against recipient/host antigens presented by antigen-presenting cells. In that setting, donor T cells recognize unmatched major or minor histocompatibility antigens of the host as genetically foreign, become activated, proliferate, and attack recipient tissue, thereby producing the clinical syndrome of GVHD.

Two different clinical GVHD syndromes (acute and chronic) are recognized, depending on the time of onset and clinical presentation.[71,72] *Acute* GVHD usually presents prior to day 100 posttransplant (*classic* acute GVHD), but it can be *persistent, recurrent,* or *late-onset* with clinical manifestations occurring after day 100. Acute GVHD observed after day 100 usually is the result of immunosuppression withdrawal for relapsed or persistent malignancy or administration of DLI, or occurs in the setting of RIC. *Chronic* GVHD usually occurs after day 100, either with or without concurrent acute GVHD. Chronic GVHD without characteristics of acute GVHD (*classic* chronic GVHD) occurs after resolution of acute GVHD or de novo (no prior acute GVHD). An "overlap syndrome" may occur in which features of both acute and chronic GVHD are present simultaneously, usually when chronic GVHD develops prior to resolution of acute GVHD (progressive onset). Acute GVHD usually is limited to the gastrointestinal tract, skin, and liver, whereas signs and symptoms of chronic GVHD resemble an autoimmune disorder and can affect many organ systems.

A "hyperacute" form of GVHD may occur in patients with multiple HLA mismatches and in patients who receive T-cell–replete transplants without adequate GVHD prophylaxis, especially in myeloablative regimens.[73] Descriptions of hyperacute GVHD vary but usually include fever, generalized erythroderma, desquamation, and edema. More severe forms with accompanying organ failure have been seen in haploidentical donors. Hyperacute GVHD typically occurs approximately one week after transplant before engraftment of neutrophils. The response rate to first-line therapy appears to be lower in patients with hyperacute GVHD compared with patients who develop GVHD later posttransplant, but no difference in survival has been observed.

Acute Graft-Versus-Host Disease

The pathophysiology of acute GVHD has been described as a three-step process.[74] In step 1, the conditioning regimen causes damage to the intestinal mucosa leading to release of lipopolysaccharides into the systemic circulation. This stimulates secretion of inflammatory cytokines such as IL-1 and tumor necrosis factor-α (TNF-α). These cytokines upregulate MHC gene products and host antigen-presenting cells such as dendritic cells, which play a critical role in this immune response. In step 2, donor T cells are activated, and secretion of other cytokines (IL-2 and interferon-γ) by activated T cells results in recruitment of macrophages and alteration of target cells in the gastrointestinal tract and skin so that they are more susceptible to damage. In step 3, multiple cytotoxic effector cells (T cells and macrophages) are generated and contribute to target tissue injury by secreting more inflammatory cytokines that cause target cell apoptosis. The term *cytokine storm* is sometimes used to describe the critical role of inflammatory cytokines in this process.

Based on this three-step model, three general approaches can be used to prevent GVHD in humans. The first is to reduce host tissue damage with the use of RIC regimens. The second and most widely used approach is to modulate donor T cells by reducing T-cell numbers (T-cell depletion), activation (most immunosuppressive agents), or proliferation (antiproliferative agents). The third approach is to block inflammatory stimulation and effectors (e.g. TNF-α inhibition, IL-1 receptor blockade).

The principal target organs in acute GVHD are the skin, liver, and gastrointestinal tract.[74] Acute GVHD is classified into four grades, depending on the number of organs involved and the degree of involvement of each organ (Table 148–2). Grade I disease involves only the skin. Grades II through IV involve the skin and either the liver, gastrointestinal tract, or both. The initial sign of acute skin GVHD usually is a generalized maculopapular rash that initially involves the face, ears, palms, soles, and upper trunk. The skin rash can spread to the rest of the body and, if untreated or refractory to treatment, will progress to bullae formation and desquamation, much like a burn injury. Gastrointestinal GVHD is manifested as diarrhea but may progress to abdominal pain/cramping and ileus. GVHD of the upper intestinal tract has been described presenting as nausea, vomiting, anorexia, and dyspepsia. The diagnosis of gastrointestinal GVHD should be made by biopsy of the intestinal tract (stomach, duodenum, or rectum). Hepatic GVHD usually is asymptomatic, consisting of hyperbilirubinemia and elevated alkaline phosphatase levels; increases in serum transaminases occur less consistently. The diagnosis can be made by biopsy, although many patients cannot provide biopsy samples because of the inherent risk of hemorrhage.

The overall incidence of moderate to severe (grades II to IV) acute GVHD ranges from 10% to more than 80%.[74] Mortality directly attributable to acute GVHD or its treatment occurs in 10% to 20% of patients. The incidence of GVHD is related to the degree of histocompatibility, number of T cells in the graft, donor and recipient age and gender, intensity of the conditioning regimen, source of hematopoietic cells (bone marrow versus peripheral blood), and prophylactic regimen. The risk of acute GVHD is lower in recipients of UCB transplants.[28] The most severe acute GVHD is

TABLE 148-2 Consensus Grading of Acute Graft-Versus-Host Disease

Organ/Extent of Involvement

Stage	Skin	Liver	Intestinal Tract
1	Rash on <25% of skin[a]	Bilirubin 2–3 mg/dL (34.2–51.3 μmol/L)[b]	Diarrhea >500 mL/day[c] or persistent nausea[d]
2	Rash on 25–50% of skin	Bilirubin 3–6 mg/dL (51.3–102.6 μmol/L)	Diarrhea >1,000 mL/day
3	Rash on >50% of skin	Bilirubin 6–15 mg/dL (102.6–256.5 μmol/L)	Diarrhea >1,500 mL/day
4	Generalized erythroderma with bulla formation	Bilirubin >15 mg/dL (>256.5 μmol/L)	Severe abdominal pain with or without ileus

Grade			
0	None	None	None
I	Stage 1–2	None	None
II	Stage 3	or Stage 1	or Stage 1
III	–	Stage 2–3	or Stage 2–4
IV[e]	Stage 4	or Stage 4	–

[a]Use the "rule of nines" to determine body surface area involvement.

[b]Range given as total bilirubin. Downgrade one stage if an additional cause of elevated bilirubin has been documented.

[c]Volume of diarrhea applies to adults. For pediatric patients, the volume of diarrhea should be based on body surface area.

[d]Persistent nausea with histologic evidence of graft-versus-host disease in the stomach or duodenum.

[e]Grade IV may include lesser organ involvement but with extreme decrease in performance status.

Reprinted from Semin Hematol, Vol. 43, Deeg HJ, Artin JH. The clinical spectrum of acute graft-verus-host disease, pages 24–31. Copyright © Elsevier 2006 with permission from Elsevier.

observed in allogeneic HSCT with non–HLA-identical donors. In these settings, the incidence of grades II to IV acute GVHD exceeds 50% despite aggressive GVHD prophylaxis.

Multiorgan acute GVHD and the drugs given to prevent or treat the disease are associated with delayed immunologic recovery and increased susceptibility to infections. Infection is often the primary cause of death in patients with GVHD. Patients with GVHD treated with an immunosuppressive regimen should receive prophylactic antiviral, antibacterial, and antifungal therapy and be monitored routinely for the occurrence of these infections.

❿ Because treatment of established acute GVHD often is unsatisfactory, aggressive preventive measures usually are taken. The most common strategy used to prevent acute GVHD is blocking the activation of T cells by administration of immunosuppressive agents.[74] Several immunosuppressive agents have been used, including methotrexate, cyclosporine, tacrolimus, mycophenolate mofetil, antithymocyte globulin, corticosteroids, and monoclonal antibodies directed at T cells. Most GVHD prophylaxis regimens combine two or more immunosuppressive agents that affect different stages of T-cell activation. Another strategy is removing or depleting most T cells from donor bone marrow ex vivo prior to transplant by physical separation (i.e., lectin agglutination) or by treatment with monoclonal antibodies directed at T cells (Fig. 148–4).[74]

In allogeneic HSCT with HLA-matched donors, the combination of cyclosporine or tacrolimus and either methotrexate or corticosteroids reduces the incidence of grades II to IV acute GVHD to 25% to 40%. Intravenous cyclosporine or tacrolimus usually is started a few days before or on day 0. Cyclosporine is given at an initial dosage of 3 to 5 mg/kg/day and tacrolimus at 0.02 to 0.03 mg/kg/day. Dosages are adjusted based on trough concentrations. Patients are converted to oral formulations when they can be tolerated. Cyclosporine and tacrolimus typically are given at full doses until days 50 to 100, gradually tapered in the absence of GVHD, and discontinued by day 180. Methotrexate

is given intravenously on days 1, 3, 6, and 11 posttransplant. The methotrexate dosage is 10 mg/m², except for the first dose given on day 1 (15 mg/m²). Alternatively, some centers use 5 mg/m² (same schedule). The day 11 dose is sometimes omitted because of the drug's myelosuppressive effects, severe mucositis or other toxicities, or development of conditions that may prolong methotrexate systemic exposure (e.g., renal failure or third spacing). When corticosteroids are used, methylprednisolone or prednisone usually is started during the first two weeks posttransplant, given at full dosages for several weeks, and gradually tapered in the absence of GVHD. Although the efficacy of methotrexate-based regimens and corticosteroid-based regimens appears to be similar, use of methotrexate may increase the risk of delayed engraftment and is associated with significant mucositis, and corticosteroid administration is associated with a higher incidence of infections. Three-drug regimens composed of cyclosporine, methotrexate, and corticosteroids have been studied but have not been shown to be more efficacious in HLA-matched transplants.

Two large multicenter randomized trials compared cyclosporine and methotrexate with tacrolimus and methotrexate. One study was performed in patients undergoing HLA-identical sibling allogeneic HSCT,[75] and the other study was performed in patients undergoing matched unrelated allogeneic HSCT.[76] Both studies found the tacrolimus combination to be significantly superior to the cyclosporine combination in preventing grades II to IV acute GVHD. The incidence of renal impairment was higher in patients receiving tacrolimus, and more tacrolimus-treated patients in the HLA-identical sibling allogeneic HSCT trial required hemodialysis. The incidence of hypertension was significantly higher in cyclosporine-treated patients in the HLA-matched sibling allogeneic HSCT trial. No difference in the overall or relapse-free survival rate was reported in the two trials. However, in the subgroup of patients with advanced disease in the HLA-identical sibling allogeneic HSCT trial, cyclosporine-treated patients had significantly better overall and disease-free survival rates at two years compared to patients who received tacrolimus. The authors explained that lowering the target blood levels to less than 20 ng/mL (20 mcg/L; 24.8 nmol/L) might reduce the renal toxicity of tacrolimus and most centers currently use target trough tacrolimus levels of 5 to 15 ng/mL (5–15 mcg/L; 6.2–18.6 nmol/L). Based on the results of these two studies, many transplant centers use tacrolimus and methotrexate as first-line acute GVHD prophylaxis.

With alternative donors, the risk of moderate-to-severe (grades II–IV) acute GVHD is 50% or higher with conventional two-drug prophylaxis. Several approaches are used to reduce the risk of acute GVHD in this high-risk group of patients: three-drug GVHD prophylaxis, pretransplant administration of antithymocyte globulin, or ex vivo T-cell depletion of donor bone marrow (Fig. 148–4). Encouraging results have been reported with the addition of novel immunosuppressive agents, such as sirolimus, to two-drug prophylaxis regimens.[77] The addition of antilymphocyte or antithymocyte globulin to the pretransplant conditioning regimen reduced the risk of acute and chronic GVHD but increased the risk of serious infections.[78]

Because of the gastrointestinal and hematologic toxicities of methotrexate, other prophylactic regimens have been evaluated. One of these regimens, developed by investigators at the Dana-Farber Cancer Institute, uses sirolimus in place of methotrexate in combination with tacrolimus. In an uncontrolled study of 53 patients receiving myeloablative allogeneic HSCT, the combination of sirolimus and tacrolimus was associated with rapid engraftment and low incidences of grades II to IV acute GVHD and treatment-related mortality.[79] A randomized trial comparing this regimen to standard methotrexate in combination with tacrolimus is being conducted by the Blood and Marrow Clinical Trials Network. Another drug that has been substituted for methotrexate is mycophenolate mofetil. The results of two small randomized trials have shown less toxicity with mycophenolate mofetil but little to no improvement in the rate of acute GVHD or overall survival.[80,81] Acute GVHD prophylaxis regimens used with RIC or NMA conditioning regimens generally consist of cyclosporine and mycophenolate mofetil. Single agent cyclophosphamide (50 mg/kg on days 3 and 4 posttransplant) also has been tested in patients undergoing RIC or NMA conditioning.[82]

The role of ex vivo T-cell depletion from donor grafts is controversial (Fig. 148–4).[74] Although use of T-cell–depleted marrow can reduce the incidence and severity of acute GVHD, it is associated with an increased risk of graft failure, delayed immune reconstitution, leukemic relapse, cytomegalovirus reactivation, and Epstein-Barr virus–related lymphoproliferative disorders. As a result, this approach does not improve the survival rate in recipients of HLA-identical sibling donor marrow. These observations suggest that important cell populations are being eliminated in the depletion process. Various approaches that selectively remove the T cells responsible for GVHD while leaving those cells that mediate engraftment, antileukemic effect, and suppression of Epstein-Barr virus–transformed lymphocytes are being investigated. Another approach is infusion of the T cells originally depleted from the graft later in the posttransplant period to prevent leukemic relapse. Because of the higher risk of GVHD in allogeneic HSCT with HLA-mismatched donors, T-cell depletion is sometimes included as part of the GVHD prophylaxis regimen in that setting.

Patients with mild skin-only acute GVHD (grade I) can be treated with topical corticosteroid preparations and counseled on the appropriate use of sunscreen. If a patient develops grades II to IV GVHD, prophylactic agents are continued and high-dose corticosteroids in the form of intravenous methylprednisolone are given.[74] The usual dosage is 1 to 2 mg/kg/day, given in two divided doses; higher dosages have not been shown to be more efficacious. Approximately 25% to 40% of patients with established acute GVHD respond to high-dose corticosteroids. If the patient responds, the corticosteroid dose is tapered gradually over several weeks to months, depending on response. In patients who experience a flare in GVHD during the taper phase, therapy consists of increasing the corticosteroid dose and then tapering more slowly. Oral beclomethasone dipropionate, a topically active corticosteroid, has been shown to reduce the frequency of gastrointestinal GVHD relapses when continued after prednisone taper.[83] Administration of beclomethasone has been associated with a better survival at 200 days and 1 year after transplant. Budesonide, another nonabsorbable corticosteroid, has also been evaluated in uncontrolled studies.[84] GVHD-associated mortality is strongly correlated to response to initial treatment and ranges from approximately 25% in patients who had a complete response to approximately 80% in patients who had no response or progressive disease.

Several randomized trials have evaluated other agents combined with methylprednisolone as initial therapy for acute GVHD.[74] In particular, the addition of anti–T-cell antibodies, such as antithymocyte globulin or monoclonal antibodies (e.g., daclizumab), has not been shown to improve patient outcome.[85] Similarly, the combination of methylprednisolone and the anti–TNF-α monoclonal antibody infliximab has not been shown to increase response rate compared to methylprednisolone alone.[86] The Blood and Marrow Transplant Clinical Trials Network conducted a randomized phase II trial designed to identify the most promising agent for initial therapy of acute GVHD in combination with 2 mg/kg/day of methylprednisolone.[87] One hundred and eighty patients were randomized to etanercept, mycophenolate mofetil, denileukin diftitox, or pentostatin. After 28 days of treatment, complete response rates were 60% for mycophenolate mofetil, 53% for denileukin diftitox, 38% for penotstatin, and 26% for etanercept. Efficacy and toxicity data suggest the use of mycophenolate

mofetil plus corticosteroids is the most promising regimen to compare with corticosteroids alone in a definitive phase III trial.

While different centers may have varying criteria for corticosteroid-refractory acute GVHD, in general, if the manifestations of acute GVHD in any organ worsen over three days of treatment or symptoms do not improve by five days, the patient likely will not respond to corticosteroids and secondary therapy should be considered.[88] Most clinicians continue administration of corticosteroids and add another immunosuppressant agent, such as antithymocyte globulin, mycophenolate mofetil, sirolimus, or pentostatin. One approach that has shown benefit as corticosteroid-sparing therapy is extracorporeal photopheresis. During this procedure, the patient's blood is exposed extracorporeally to 8-methoxypsoralen followed by ultraviolet A radiation, and then returned to the patient. This process is thought to result in suppression of T-cell reactivity and induction of regulatory T cells. Clinical results have been positive, especially in patients with skin GVHD.[89] In addition, a variety of humanized monoclonal antibodies or fusion proteins, such as denileukin diftitox (Ontak®), daclizumab (Zenapax®), infliximab (Remicade®), rituximab (Rituxan) and etanercept (Enbrel®), are being evaluated for treatment of corticosteroid-refractory acute GVHD.[88] There is no standard treatment of patients with corticosteroid-refractory acute GVHD and the prognosis is dismal. New agents continue to be evaluated.

CLINICAL CONTROVERSY

Optimal treatment of steroid-refractory GVHD is unclear. Comparative trials are needed to determine a standard approach to this difficult condition.

Chronic Graft-Versus-Host Disease

Chronic GVHD is the major determinant of late transplant-related morbidity and mortality.[71,90] The pathophysiology of chronic GVHD is poorly understood but is generally thought to be a result of pathogenic donor T cells that proliferate unchecked by normal mechanisms. These T cells are responsible for tissue damage through direct cytolytic attack, stimulation of inflammatory cytokines, or B-cell activation and antibody production. Chronic GVHD is often considered an autoimmune disease because of its similarity to other autoimmune disorders.

The incidence of chronic GVHD in patients who survive more than 150 days ranges from 20% to 70%.[90] The risk of chronic GVHD increases with increasing donor and recipient age and is higher in patients who receive transplants from HLA-nonidentical donors and in patients who receive PBSC transplants (especially with higher CD34+ cell doses). The incidence of chronic GVHD is rising because of increasing use of alternative donors, use of PBSCs as the graft source, use of DLI for treatment of recurrence, and older recipient age. Previous acute GVHD increases the risk of chronic GVHD, but approximately 20% to 30% of patients who develop chronic GVHD after HLA-matched allogeneic HSCT have no history of acute GVHD. Unlike acute GVHD, prophylactic immunosuppression does not appear to reduce the incidence or severity of chronic GVHD.

Chronic GVHD resembles autoimmune diseases and can affect any organ or tissue of the body.[91] The most common sites involved are the skin, mouth, liver, and eye but other sites include the gastrointestinal tract, joints, muscles, and lungs. The National Institutes of Health Consensus Development Project developed standardized criteria for the diagnosis of chronic GVHD and proposed a new clinical scoring system for the evaluation of patients with chronic GVHD.[72] The Working Group recommends that the diagnosis of chronic GVHD be made with the presence of at least one *diagnostic* clinical sign of chronic GVHD (e.g., poikiloderma or esophageal web) or a *distinctive* manifestation (e.g. keratoconjunctivitis sicca) confirmed by biopsy or other test (e.g., Schirmer test).

The most widely used staging system for chronic GVHD prior to the National Institutes of Health Consensus Development Project was the limited/extensive classification proposed by the Seattle HSCT program. In that system, chronic GVHD is classified as limited or extensive, depending on pathologic findings and the extent of systemic involvement. *Limited* chronic GVHD indicates localized skin involvement, mild hepatic dysfunction, or both. Most patients have *extensive* disease, with involvement of the skin, liver, eyes, mouth, esophagus, or other organs. Many patients with extensive chronic GVHD will die of infections or become disabled.

The National Institutes of Health Consensus Working Group recommended a global staging system that categorizes chronic GVHD into mild, moderate, and severe.[72] *Mild* chronic GVHD involves only one or two organs or sites (except the lung) with no clinically significant functional impairment (maximum score of one in all affected organs or sites). *Moderate* chronic GVHD involves at least one organ or site with clinically significant but no major disability (maximum score of two in any affected organ or site), or three or more organs or sites with no clinically significant functional impairment (maximum score of one in all affected organs or sites), or lung score of one. *Severe* chronic GVHD indicates major disability caused by chronic GVHD (score of three in any organ or site) or lung score of two or greater.

⓫ If no functional impairment is present, patients with mild skin-only disease can be treated with a variety of topical preparations, such as clobetasol, tacrolimus, and pimecrolimus.[92] Initial treatment of patients with more severe or systemic involvement of chronic GVHD consists of prednisone 1 mg/kg/day.[90] Prospective randomized trials evaluating the addition of cyclosporine or mycophenolate mofetil have shown limited to no benefit compared to prednisone alone.[92] If patients are on tapering doses of prednisone for treatment of acute GVHD, the dose is generally increased and/or another immunosuppressive agent is added. Treatment is continued until signs and symptoms of the disease have resolved and then are tapered gradually, usually over a period of several months to years. Approximately 50% of patients will require long-term immunosuppression to control chronic GVHD.

In addition to topical therapy for skin manifestations, other treatments can be applied to lessen the symptoms of chronic GVHD.[93] Patients should be educated on the use of sunscreens (and/or avoidance of sun exposure) to reduce skin injury and exacerbation of GVHD skin lesions. Nonsclerotic skin lesions without erosions or ulcerations may respond well to topical corticosteroids and emollients. Patients should be advised to maintain good oral hygiene with routine dental care. Saliva substitutes can be given for dry mouth symptoms, and topical corticosteroid gels can be used for localized and symptomatic oral lesions. Artificial tears or, if necessary for more severe symptoms, cyclosporine or corticosteroid eye drops are useful for patients with chronic GVHD manifesting as dry eyes or conjunctivitis. Physical therapy is recommended to reduce functional loss as a result of steroid myopathy, joint contractures, and deconditioning.

Patients who do not respond to initial therapy have a very poor prognosis. Noncomparative trials have investigated several therapies with varying degrees of success, including thalidomide, extracorporeal photophoresis, tacrolimus, sirolimus, pentostatin, mycophenolate mofetil, hydroxychloroquine, rituximab, imatinib and others.[90,91,94,95] The Blood and Marrow Clinical Trials Network has initiated a randomized phase II/III trial comparing the following three treatment strategies: sirolimus and prednisone; sirolimus, extracorporeal photophoresis, and prednisone; and sirolimus, a calcineurin inhibitor, and prednisone. Eligible subjects must have chronic GVHD, as diagnosed by National Institutes of Health consensus criteria, and must be either untreated and high risk or not responding to standard therapy. Sirolimus and extracorporeal photophoresis were chosen due to favorable response rates seen in phase II studies and because of laboratory data suggesting a positive effect on regulatory T cells which are thought to mitigate GVHD.

Infection is the primary cause of death in patients with chronic GVHD, and antimicrobial prophylaxis is an important component of the care of patients being treated for chronic GVHD. Patients should receive oral trimethoprim–sulfamethoxazole, penicillin, an antifungal azole agent, and acyclovir to prevent infections commonly seen in immunocompromised patients.[90-92] Routine monitoring for cytomegalovirus reactivation should be performed. Some HSCT centers also administer intravenous immunoglobulin to patients with low serum immunoglobulin G levels.

INFECTION

Patients undergoing high-dose chemotherapy with autologous HSCT or allogeneic HSCT are severely immunocompromised and therefore are at high risk for bacterial, fungal, and viral infection. Management of these infections is discussed in detail in Chap. 131.

LATE COMPLICATIONS

With the success of HSCT, the number of long-term survivors has grown. Many survivors experience delayed complications of transplantation, including restrictive and obstructive pulmonary disease; bone and joint disease (including osteoporosis and avascular necrosis); cataract formation; endocrine dysfunction (including sterility and thyroid dysfunction); impaired growth and development; infections; cardiovascular disease; chronic renal and hepatic dysfunction; and secondary malignancies.[96,97] Physical recovery tends to occur earlier than psychological or work recovery. Full recovery usually takes several years, and approximately two thirds of patients are without major limitations by five years. The Bone Marrow Transplant Survivor Study compared late mortality (two years after HSCT) in allogeneic and autologous patients with that of the general population.[98,99] Both types of transplants were associated with a several-fold increase in risk of premature death; relative mortality decreased with time but remained significantly elevated even ten years posttransplant. The leading cause of death was relapse of primary disease in both allogeneic and autologous patients but allogeneic HSCT patients also continued to die from complications of chronic GVHD while autologous HSCT patients frequently succumbed to secondary malignancies.

ABBREVIATIONS

ALL: acute lymphoblastic leukemia

AML: acute myelogenous leukemia

BMT: bone marrow transplant

BuCy: busulfan and cyclophosphamide

CIBMTR: Center for International Blood and Marrow Transplant Research

CML: chronic myelogenous leukemia

DLI: donor lymphocyte infusion

G-CSF: granulocyte colony-stimulating factor

GM-CSF: granulocyte-macrophage colony-stimulating factor

GVHD: graft-versus-host disease

GVM: graft-versus-malignancy (effect)

HLA: human leukocyte antigen

HSCT: hematopoietic stem cell transplantation

MAC: myeloablative conditioning

MHC: major histocompatibility complex

MLC or MLR: mixed lymphocyte culture or reaction

MMF: mycophenolate mofetil

NK: natural killer (cells)

NMDP: National Marrow Donor Program

NMA: nonmyeloablative

PBSC: peripheral blood stem cell

RIC: reduced-intensity conditioning

SOS: sinusoidal obstruction syndrome

TBI: total-body irradiation

TNF-α: tumor necrosis factor-α

UCB: umbilical cord blood

REFERENCES

1. Pasquini MC and Wang Z. Current use and outcome of hematopoietic stem cell transplantation: Parts I and II - CIBMTR Summary Slides. 2009, *http://www.cibmtr.org/ReferenceCenter/Newsletters/PDF/Newsletter_Aug2009.pdf* and *http://www.cibmtr.org/ReferenceCenter/Newsletters/PDF/Newsletter_Dec2009.pdf.*

2. Wingard JA, Gastineau DA, Leather HL, Szczepiorkowski ZM, and Snyder EL, eds. Hematopoietic Stem Cell Transplantation: A Handbook for Clinicians. Bethesda, MD: AABB, 2009.

3. Appelbaum F, Forman S, Negrin R, Blume K, eds. Thomas' Hematopoietic Cell Transplantation. Oxford, UK: Wiley-Blackwell, 2009.

4. Appelbaum FR. The current status of hematopoietic cell transplantation. Annu Rev Med 2003;54:491–512.

5. Copelan EA. Hematopoietic stem-cell transplantation. N Engl J Med 2006;354:1813–1826.

6. Klein J, Sato A. The HLA system. N Engl J Med 2000;343:702–709.

7. Nowak J. Role of HLA in hematopoietic SCT. Bone Marrow Transplant 2008;42:S71–S76.

8. Flomenberg N, Baxter-Lowe LA, Confer D, et al. Impact of HLA class I and class II high resolution matching on outcomes of unrelated donor bone marrow transplantation: HLA-C mismatching is associated with a strong adverse effect on transplant outcome. Blood 2004;104:1923–1930.

9. Lee SJ, Kline J. Haagenson M, et al. High resolution donor-recipient HLA matching contributes to the success of unrelated donor marrow transplantation. Blood 2007; 110:4576–4583.

10. Hurley CK, Lowe LB, Logan B, et al. National Marrow Donor Program HLA-matching guidelines for unrelated marrow transplants. Biol Blood Marrow Transplant 2003;9:610–615.

11. Ringden O, Pavletic SZ, Anasetti C, et al. The graft-versus-leukemia effect using matched unrelated donors is not superior to HAL-identical siblings for hematopoietic stem cell transplantation. Blood 2009;113:3110–3118.

12. Moore J, Nivison-Smith I, Goh K, et al. Equivalent survival for sibling and unrelated donor allogeneic stem cell transplantation for acute myelogenous leukemia. Biol Blood Marrow Transplant 2007;13:601–607.

13. Siena S, Schiavo R, Pedrazzoli P, Carlo-Stella C. Therapeutic relevance of CD34+ cell dose in blood cell transplantation for cancer therapy. J Clin Oncol 2000;18:1360–1377.

14. Kessinger A, Sharp JG. The whys and hows of hematopoietic progenitor and stem cell mobilization. Bone Marrow Transplant 2003;31:319–329.

15. Fruehauf S, Seggewiss R. It's moving day: Factors affecting peripheral blood stem cell mobilization and strategies for improvement. Br J Haematol 2003;122:360–375.

16. Cashen AF, Lazarus HM, Devine SM. Mobilizing stem cells from normal donors: Is it possible to improve upon G-CSF? Bone Marrow Transplant 2007;39:577–588.

17. Kobbe G, Bruns I, Fenk R, Czibere A, Haas R. Pegfilgrastim for PBSC mobilization and autologous haematopoietic SCT. Bone Marrow Transplant 2009;43:669–677.

18. DiPersio JF, Stadtmauer EA, Nademanee A, et al. Plerixafor and G-CSF versus placebo and G-CSF to mobilize hematopoietic stem cells for autologous stem cell transplantation in patients with multiple myeloma. Blood 2009;113:5720–5726.

19. DiPersio, Micallef IV, Stiff PJ, et al. Phase III prospective randomized double-blind placebo-controlled trial of plerixafor plus granulocyte colony stimulating factor compared with placebo plus granulocyte colony stimulating factor for autologous stem cell mobilization and transplantation for patients with non-Hodgkin's lymphoma. J Clin Oncol 2009;27:4767–4773.

20. Glaspy JA. Economic considerations in the use of peripheral blood progenitor cells to support high-dose chemotherapy. Bone Marrow Transplant 1999;23(Suppl 2):S21–S27.

21. Schulman KA, Birch R, Zhen B, Pania N, Weaver CH. Effect of CD34+ cell dose on resource utilization in patients after high-dose chemotherapy with peripheral blood stem cell support. J Clin Oncol 1999;17:1227–1233.

22. Popat U, Saliba R, Thandi R, et al. Impairment of filgrastim-induced stem cell mobilization after prior lenalidomide in patients with multiple myeloma. Biol Blood Marrow Transplant 2009;15:718–723.

23. Calandra G, McCarty J, McGuirk J, et al. AMD3100 plus G-CSF can successfully mobilize CD34+ cells from non-Hodgkin's lymphoma, Hodgkin's disease and multiple myeloma patients previously failing mobilization with chemotherapy and/or cytokine treatment: compassionate use data. Bone Marrow Transplant 2008;41:331–338.

24. Koca E and Champlin RE. Peripheral blood progenitor cell or bone marrow transplantation; controversy remains. Curr Opin Oncol 2008;20:220–226.

25. Tigue CC, McKoy JM, Evens AM, Trifilio SM, Tallman MS, Bennett CL. Granulocyte-colony stimulating factor administration to healthy individuals and persons with chronic neutropenia or cancer: An overview of safety considerations from the Research on Adverse Drug Effects and Reports project. Bone Marrow Transplant 2007;40:185–192.

26. Schmitz N, Eapen M, Horowitz M, et al. Long-term outcome of patients given transplants of mobilized blood or bone marrow: A report from the International Bone Marrow Transplant Registry and the European Group for Blood and Marrow Transplantation. Blood 2006;108:4288–4290.

27. Group SCTsC. Allogeneic peripheral blood stem-cell compared with bone marrow transplantation in the management of hematologic malignancies: An individual patient data meta-analysis of nine randomized trials. J Clin Oncol 2005;23:5074–5087.

28. Smith AR and Wagner JE. Alternative haematopoietic stem cell sources for transplantation: Place of umbilical cord blood. Br J Haematol 2009;147:246–261.

29. Cutler C and Ballen D. Reduced-intensity conditioning and umbilical cord blood transplantation in adults. Bone Marrow Transplant 2009;44:667–671.

30. Eapen M, Rubinstein P, Zhang MJ, et al. Outcomes of transplantation of unrelated donor umbilical cord blood and bone marrow in children with acute leukaemia: A comparison study. Lancet 2007;369:1947–1954.

31. Ciurea SO and Andersson BS. Busulfan in hematopoietic stem cell transplantation. Biol Blood Marrow Transplant. 2009;15:523–536.

32. Socie G, Clift RA, Blaise D, et al. Busulfan plus cyclophosphamide compared with total-body irradiation plus cyclophosphamide before marrow transplantation for myeloid leukemia: Long-term follow-up of 4 randomized studies. Blood 2001;98:3569–3574.

33. Ferry C, Socie G. Busulfan-cyclophosphamide versus total body irradiation-cyclophosphamide as preparative regimen before allogeneic hematopoietic stem cell transplantation for acute myeloid leukemia: What have we learned? Exp Hematol 2003;31:1182–1186.

34. Gupta V, Lazarus HM, Keating A. Myeloablative conditioning regimens for AML allografts: 30 years later. Bone Marrow Transplant 2003;32:969–978.

35. Fernandez HF, Escalon MP, Pereira D, Lazarus HM. Autotransplant conditioning regimens for aggressive lymphoma: Are we on the right road? Bone Marrow Transplant 2007; 40:505–513.

36. Gopal AK, Gooley TA, Maloney DG, et al. High-dose radioimmunotherapy versus conventional high-dose therapy and autologous hematopoietic stem cell transplantation for relapsed follicular non-Hodgkin's lymphoma: A multivariate cohort analysis. Blood 2003;102:2351–2357.

37. Sandmaier BM, Mackinnon S, Childs RW. Reduced intensity conditioning for allogeneic hematopoietic cell transplantation: Current perspectives. Biol Blood Marrow Transplant 2007;13:87–97.

38. Barrett AJ, Savani BN. Stem cell transplantation with reduced-intensity conditioning regimens: A review of ten years experience with new transplant concepts and new therapeutic agents. Leukemia 2006;20:1661–1672.

39. Kharfan-Dabaja MA, Barzarbachi A. Emerging role of CD20 blockade in allogeneic hematopoietic cell transplantation. Biol Blood Marrow Transplant 2010 Oct;16(10):1347–1354. Epub 2010 Jan 18.

40. Bacigalupo A, Ballen K, Rizzo D, et al. Defining the intensity of conditioning regimens: Working definitions. Biol Blood Marrow Transplant 2009;15:1628–1633.

41. Mielcarek M, Martin PJ, Leisenring W, et al. Graft-versus host disease after nonmyeloablative versus conventional hematopoietic stem cell transplantation. Blood 2003;102:756–762.

42. Diaconescu R, Flowers CR, Storer B, et al. Morbidity and mortality with nonmyeloablative compared to myeloablative conditioning before hematopoietic cell transplantation from HLA matched related donors. Blood 2004;104:1550–1558.

43. Maris MB, Niederwieser D, Sandmaier BM, et al. HLA-Matched unrelated donor hematopoietic cell transplantation after nonmyeloablative conditioning for patients with hematologic malignancies. Blood 2003;102:2021–2030.

44. Kahl C, Storer BE, Sandmaier BM, et al. Relapse risk in patients with malignant disease given allogeneic hematopoietic cell transplantation after nonmyeloablative conditioning. Blood 2007;110:2744–2748.

45. Alyea EP, Kim HT, Ho V. Comparative outcomes of nonmyeloablative and myeloablative allogeneic hematopoietic cell transplantation for patients older than 50 years of age. Blood 2005;105:1810–1814.

46. Aoudjhane M, Labopin M, Gorin N-C, et al. Comparative outcome of reduced intensity and myeloablative conditioning regimen in HLA identical sibling allogeneic haematopoietic stem cell transplantation for patients older than 50 years of age with acute myeloblastic leukaemia: A retrospective survey from the Acute Leukemia Working Party (ALWP) of the European group for Blood and Marrow Transplantation (EBMT). Leukemia 2005;19:2304–2312.

47. Bregni M, Ueno NT, Childs R. The second international meeting on allogeneic transplantation in solid tumors. Bone Marrow Transplant 2006;38:527–537.

48. Tomblyn M, Lazarus HM. Donor lymphocyte infusions: the long and winding road: should it be traveled? Bone Marrow Transplantation 2008;42:569–579.

49. Kolg HJ. Graft-versus leukemia effects of transplantation and donor lymphocytes. Blood 2008;112:4371–4383.

50. Bethge A, Hegenbart U, Stuart MJ, et al. Adoptive immunotherapy with donor lymphocyte infusions after allogeneic hematopoietic cell transplantation following nonmyeloablative conditioning. Blood 2004;103:790–795.

51. Stein AS, O'Donnell MR, Slovak ML, et al. Interleukin-2 after autologous stem cell transplantation for adult patients with acute myeloid leukemia in first complete remission. J Clin Oncol 2003;21:615–623.

52. Horwitz SM, Negrin RS, Blume KG, et al. Rituximab as adjuvant to high-dose therapy and autologous hematopoietic cell transplantation for aggressive non-Hodgkin's lymphoma. Blood 2004;103:777–783.

53. Klyuchnidov E, Kroger N, Brummendorf TH, Wiedemann B, Zander AR, Bacher U. Current status and perspectives of tyrosine kinase inhibitor treatment in the posttransplant period in patients with chronic myelogenous leukemia. Biol Blood Marrow Transpln 2010;16:301–310.

54. Jabbour E, Giralt S, Kantarjian H, et al. Low-dose azacitidine after allogeneic stem cell transplantation for acute leukemia. Cancer 2009;115:1899–1905.

55. Harousseau JL. Hematopoietic stem cell transplantation in multiple myeloma. JNCCN 2009;7:961–970.

56. Ho VT, Revta C, Richardson PG. Hepatic veno-occlusive disease after hematopoietic stem cell transplantation: Update on defibrotide

and other current investigational therapies. Bone Marrow Transplant 2008;41:229–237.

57. Tay J, Timmouth A, Fergusson D, Huebsch L, Allan DS. Systematic review of controlled clinical trials on the use of ursodeoxycholic acid for the prevention of hepatic venoocclusive disease in hematopoietic stem cell transplant. Biol Blood Marrow Transplant 2007;13:206–217.

58. Richardson PG, Soiffer RJ, Antin JH, et al. Defibrotide for the treatment of severe hepatic veno-occlusive disease and multi-organ failure post stem cell transplantation: A multi-center, randomized, dose-finding trial. Biol Blood Marrow Transplant 2010 Feb 15. [Epub ahead of print].

59. Gupta S, Jain A, Warneke CL, et al. Outcome of alveolar hemorrhage in hematopoietic stem cell transplant. Bone Marrow Transplant 2007;40:71–78.

60. Gorak E, Geller N, Srinivasan R, et al. Engraftment syndrome after nonmyeloablative allogeneic hematopoietic stem cell transplantation: Incidence and effects on survival. Biol Blood Marrow Transplant 2005;11:542–550.

61. Fukuda T, Hackman RC, Guthrie KA, et al. Risks and outcomes of idiopathic pneumonia syndrome after nonmyeloablative compared to conventional conditioning regimens for allogeneic hematopoietic stem cell transplantation. Blood 2003;102:2777–2785.

62. Yanik GA, Ho VT, Levine JE, et al. The impact of sulubel tumor necrosis factor receptor etanercept on the treatment of idiopathic pneumonia syndrome after allogeneic hematopoietic stem cell transplantation. Blood 2008;112:3073–3081.

63. Williams KM, Chien JW, Gladwin MT, Pavletic SZ. Bronchiolitis obliterans after allogeneic hematopoietic stem cell transplantation. JAMA 2009;302:306–314.

64. Trivedi M, Martinez S, Corringham S, Medle K, Ball ED. Optimal use of G-CSF administration after hematopoietic SCT. Bone Marrow Transplant 2009;43:895–908.

65. Smith TJ, Khatcheressian J, Lyman GH, et al. 2006 update of recommendations for the use of white blood cell growth factors: An evidence-based clinical practice guidelines. J Clin Oncol 2006;24:3187–3205.

66. Bolwell B, Goomastic M, Dannley R, et al. G-CSF post-autologous progenitor cell transplantation: A randomized study of 5, 10 and 16 mcg/kg/day. Bone Marrow Transplant 1997;19:215–219.

67. Bolwell B, Pohlman B, Andresen S, et al. Delayed G-CSF after autologous progenitor cell transplantation: Prospective randomized trial. Bone Marrow Transplant 1998;21:369–373.

68. Ringden O, Labopin M, Gorin N-C, et al. Treatment with granulocyte colony-stimulating factor after allogeneic bone marrow transplantation for acute leukemia increases the risk of graft-versus-host disease and death: A study from the Acute Leukemia Working Party of the European Group for Blood and Marrow Transplantation. J Clin Oncol 2004;22:416–423.

69. Dekker A, Bulley S, Beyene J, et al. Meta-analysis of randomized controlled trials of prophylactic granulocyte colony-stimulating factor and granulocyte-macrophage colony-stimulating factor after autologous and allogeneic stem cell transplantation. J Clin Oncol 2006;24:5207–5215.

70. Khoury HJ, Loberiza FR, Ringden O, et al. Impact of posttransplantation G-CSF on outcomes of allogeneic hematopoietic stem cell transplantation. Blood 2006;107:1712–1716.

71. Reddy P., Arora M, Guimond M, Mackall CL. GVHD: A continuing barrier to the safety of allogeneic transplantation. Biol Blood Marrow Transplant 2009;15:162–168.

72. Filipovich AH, Weisdorf DJ, Pavletic S, et al. National Institutes of Health Consensus Development Project on Criteria for Clinical Trials in Chronic Graft-versus-Host Disease: I. Diagnosis and Staging Working Group Report. Biol Blood Marrow Transplant 2005;11:945–955.

73. Saliba RM, deLima M, Giralt S, et al. Hyper-acute GVHD. Risk factors, outcomes, and clinical applications. Blood 2007;109:2751–2758.

74. Ferrara JLM, Levine JE, Reddy P, Holler E. Graft-versus-host disease. Lancet 2009;373:1550–1561.

75. Ratanatharathorn V, Nash RA, Przepiorka D, et al. Phase III study comparing methotrexate and tacrolimus (Prograf, FK506) with methotrexate and cyclosporine for graft-versus-host disease prophylaxis after HLA-identical sibling bone marrow transplantation. Blood 1998;92:2303–2314.

76. Nash RA, Antin JH, Karanes C, et al. Phase 3 study comparing methotrexate and tacrolimus with methotrexate and cyclosporine for prophylaxis of acute graft-versus-host disease after marrow transplantation from unrelated donors. Blood 2000;96:2062–2068.

77. Antin JH, Kim HT, Cutler C, et al. Sirolimus, tacrolimus, and low-dose methotrexate for graft-versus-host disease prophylaxis in mismatched related donor or unrelated donor transplantation. Blood 2003;102:1601–1605.

78. Bacigalupo A. Antilymphocyte/thymocyte globulin for graft-versus-host disease prophylaxis: Efficacy and side effects. Bone Marrow Transplant 2006;35:225–231.

79. Cutler C, Li S, Ho VT, et al. Extended follow-up of methotrexate-free immunosuppression using sirolimus and tacrolimus in related and unrelated donor peripheral blood stem cell transplantation. Blood 2007;109:3108–3114.

80. Perkins J, Field T, Kim J, et al. A randomized phase II trial comparing tacrolimus and mycophenolate mofetil to tacrolimus and methotrexate for acute graft-versus-host disease prophylaxis. Biol Blood Marrow Transplant 2010 Jan 23 [Epub ahead of print].

81. Bolwell B, Sobecks R, Pohlman B, et al. A prospective randomized trial comparing cyclosporine and short course methotrexate with cyclosporine and mycophenolate mofetil for GVHD prophylaxis in myeloablative allogeneic bone marrow transplantation. Bone Marrow Transplant 2004;34:621–625.

82. Luznik L, Bolanos-Meade J, Zahurak M, et al. High-dose cyclophosphamide as single agent, short-course prophylaxis of graft-versus-host disease. Blood 2010 Feb 2 [Epub ahead of print].

83. Hockenbery DM, Cruickshank S, Rodell TC, et al. A randomized, placebo-controlled trial of oral beclomethasone dipropionate as a prednisone-sparing therapy for gastrointestinal graft-versus-host disease. Blood 2007;109:4557–4563.

84. Ibrahim RB, Abidi MH, Cronin SM, et al. Nonabsorbable corticosteroid use in the treatment of gastrointestinal graft-versus-host disease. Biol Blood Marrow Transplant 2009;15:395–405.

85. Lee SJ, Zahrieh D, Agura E, et al. Effect of up front daclizumab when combined with steroids for the treatment of acute graft versus host disease: Results of a randomized trial. Blood 2004;104:1559–1564.

86. A phase III study of infliximab and corticosteroids for the initial treatment of acute graft-versus-host disease. Biol Blood Marrow Transplant 2009;15:1555–1562.

87. Alousi AM, Weisdorf DJ, Logan BR, et al. Etanercept, mycophenolate, denileukin, or pentostatin plus corticosteroids for acute graft-versus-host disease: a randomized phase 2 trial from the Blood and Marrow Transplant Clinical Trials Network. Blood 2009;114: 511–517.

88. Deeg HJ. How I treat refractory acute GVHD. Blood 2007;109: 4119–4126.

89. Knobler R, Barr ML. Couriel DR, et al. Extracorporeal photopheresis: Past, present, and future. J Am Acad Dermatol 2009;61:652–665.

90. Lee SJ. New approaches for preventing and treating chronic graft-versus-host disease. Blood 2005;105:4200–4206.

91. Lee SJ, Vogelsang G, Flowers MED. Chronic graft-versus-host disease. Biol Blood Marrow Transplant 2003;9:215–233.

92. Martin PJ, Storer BE, Rowley SD, et al. Evaluation of mycophenolate mofetil for initial treatment of chronic graft-versus-host disease. Blood 2009;113:5074–5082.

93. Couriel D, Carpenter PA, Cutler C, et al. Ancillary Therapy and Supportive Care of Chronic Graft-versus-Host Disease: National Institutes of Health Consensus Development Project on Criteria for Clinical Trials in Chronic Graft-versus Host Disease: V. Ancillary Therapy and Supportive Care Working Group Report. Biol Blood Marrow Transplant 2006;12:375–396.

94. Cutler C, Miklos D, Kim HT, et al. Rituximab for steroid-refractory chronic graft-versus-host disease. Blood 2006;108:756–762.

95. Magro L, Mohty M, Catteau, et al. Imatinib mesylate as salvage therapy for refractory sclerotic chronic graft-versus-host disease. Blood 2009;114:719–722.

96. Socie G, Salooja N, Cohen A, et al. Nonmalignant late effects after allogeneic stem cell transplantation. Blood 2003;101:3373–3385.

97. Syrjala KL, Langer SL, Abrams JR, et al. Recovery and long-term function after hematopoietic cell transplantation for leukemia and lymphoma. JAMA 2004;291:2335–2343.

98. Bhatia S, Robison LL, Francisco L, et al. Late mortality in survivors of autologous hematopoietic cell transplantation: Report from the Bone Marrow Transplant Survivor Study. Blood 2005;105: 4215–4222.

99. Bhatia S, Francisco L, Carter A, et al. Late mortality after allogeneic hematopoietic cell transplantation and functional status of long-term survivors: Report from the Bone Marrow Transplant Survivor Study. Blood 2007;110:3784–3792.

CHAPTER

149

Assessment of Nutrition Status and Nutrition Requirements

KATHERINE HAMMOND CHESSMAN AND VANESSA J. KUMPF

KEY CONCEPTS

❶ Classification of nutrition status is often desired as a means to identify those who are nutritionally at risk due to over- or undernutrition.

❷ Nutrition screening programs should identify those at risk for poor nutrition-related outcomes as a consequence of either over- or undernutrition.

❸ Comprehensive nutrition assessment is the first step in formulating a patient-specific nutrition care plan for a patient who is found to be nutritionally at risk.

❹ A nutrition-focused medical, surgical, and dietary history and a nutrition-focused physical examination are key components of nutrition assessment and will reveal risk factors for and the likelihood of malnutrition and nutrient deficiencies or toxicities.

❺ Appropriate anthropometric measurements are essential in a complete nutrition assessment and should be evaluated based on published standards.

❻ Biochemical (laboratory) tests are essential for nutrition assessment but must be interpreted in the context of the physical findings, medical and surgical history, and clinical status of the patient, as well as specific test limitations.

❼ Nutrient deficiencies and toxicities involving micronutrients (e.g., vitamins or trace elements) or macronutrients (e.g., fat, protein, or carbohydrate) are possible, and a comprehensive nutrition assessment will identify the presence of these.

❽ When determining patient-specific nutrition requirements, goals should be established based on the patient's clinical condition and the need for maintenance or repletion in adults, as well as for continued growth and development in children.

❾ Drug-nutrient interactions can affect an individual's nutrition status as well as the response to and adverse effects seen with drug therapy and must be considered when evaluating a patient's nutrition care plan.

❿ An initial nutrition assessment and determination of nutrition requirements only defines an empirical starting point for a nutrition care plan. Close monitoring is required so that timely adjustments to the nutrition care plan can be made based on patient-specific responses to ensure appropriate nutrition-related outcomes.

Nutrition care is a vital component of quality patient care. This chapter reviews the tools most commonly used for nutrition screening and accurate, relevant, and cost-effective nutrition assessment. Determination of patient-specific macro- and micronutrient requirements and potential drug–nutrient interactions are also discussed.

CLASSIFICATION OF NUTRITION DISEASE

❶ Undernutrition usually results from starvation (inadequate nutrient intake), impaired absorption of nutrients, or altered metabolism (inappropriate use of ingested nutrients). An alteration in nutrient metabolism exists when the cell has altered substrate demands or use, such as cachexia associated with inflammatory or neoplastic conditions. In such situations, enhancing nutritional intake may not be sufficient to meet the increased demand.[1] Regardless of the cause, undernutrition results in changes in subcellular, cellular, and/or organ function that expose the individual to increased risks of morbidity and mortality. In general, deficiency states can be categorized as those involving protein and calories or single nutrients such as individual vitamins or trace elements. Protein-calorie malnutrition can be classified as marasmus, kwashiorkor, or mixed marasmus/kwashiorkor.

Marasmus is a chronic condition resulting from prolonged inadequate intake or utilization of protein and calories. Somatic protein (skeletal muscle) and adipose tissue (subcutaneous fat) wasting occurs, but visceral protein (e.g., albumin [ALB] and transferrin [TFN]) production is usually preserved. Weight loss typically exceeds 10% of usual body weight (UBW; typical weight). When severe, cell-mediated immunity, measured by delayed cutaneous hypersensitivity (DCH), and muscle function are impaired. Patients with wasting diseases such as cancer commonly have marasmus and a prototypical starved, wasted appearance.[1,2]

Kwashiorkor develops when there is inadequate protein and anti-oxidant micronutrient intake and usually develops in geographic areas where there is famine, limited food supply, and low levels of education. This condition has rarely been reported in the United States but can be seen in children who are abused or neglected and has been reported in elderly individuals. While these patients may appear well nourished due to relative adipose tissue preservation, especially with mild undernutrition, there is depletion of visceral (and to some degree somatic) protein stores with severe hypoalbuminemia and edema commonly seen in more advanced cases.[2]

Mixed marasmus/kwashiorkor is a form of severe protein-calorie malnutrition that develops in chronically ill, starved patients during periods of hypermetabolic stress, such as trauma, infection, and burns. There is reduced visceral protein synthesis superimposed on wasting of somatic protein and energy (adipose tissue) stores. Immunocompetence is lowered, increasing the incidence of infection, and wound healing is compromised.

Obesity (overnutrition) is a major healthcare concern in the United States. It is estimated that 66% of American adults are overweight (defined as a body mass index [BMI] ≥ 25 kg/m^2), while 32.9% of American adults are obese (BMI ≥ 30 kg/m^2).[3] In 2008, only one state (Colorado) had a prevalence of obesity less than 20%.[4] Additionally, many children and adolescents (age 2–19 years) are obese with approximately 11.3% having a BMI at or above the 97th percentile for age, and 16.3% having a BMI at or above the 95th percentile for age[5] on the gender-appropriate BMI-for-age growth chart published by the Centers for Disease Control National Center for Health Statistics [NCHS]).[6] Many more children (31.9%) are considered to be overweight (BMI at or above the 85th percentile for age).[5] Nutrition assessment allows identification of obese individuals or those at risk of becoming obese. The consequences of obesity are numerous and include type 2 diabetes mellitus, cardiovascular disease, and stroke (see Chap. 154).

NUTRITION SCREENING

❷ Because it is neither practical nor warranted to conduct a comprehensive nutrition assessment on every patient, nutrition screening provides a rapid systematic way to identify individuals for whom a more detailed nutrition assessment is needed. A nutrition screen can be used to detect those who are overweight, obese, malnourished, or at risk for malnutrition, predict the probability of their outcome as a result of nutritional factors, and provide an indication as to whether nutritional treatment is likely to influence the patient's outcome.[7-10] The nutrition screen should be a rapid and simple process that can be done in homes by patients, caregivers, or home healthcare professionals, in long-term care facilities, in ambulatory care clinics, or in hospitals. Nutrition screening using simple tools in the community or outpatient setting, especially in young children and the elderly, can identify potential nutrition issues early before they become significant problems. Because the Joint Commission includes nutrition screening and assessment in its performance standards for accredited institutions, each entity must define in writing the process by which a nutrition screen is done and criteria that determine when a more in-depth assessment needs to be performed. For inpatients, these screenings typically must be completed within 24 hours of admission. For outpatients, nutrition screening should occur at the first visit with a provider and thereafter as warranted by the patient's condition.[11] By identifying at-risk individuals, nutrition screening can be a cost-effective way to decrease complications and length of hospital stays.

Appropriate screening is based on risk factor identification. Risk factors for undernutrition include any disease state, complicating condition, treatment, or socioeconomic condition that may result in a decreased nutrient intake, altered metabolism or nutrient utilization, and/or malabsorption. Risk factors for obesity include family history of obesity, certain medical diagnoses, poor dietary habits, lack of exercise, and some drug therapies. Various rating and classification systems have been proposed to assess nutrition risk and guide subsequent interventions.[7,8,12,13] Checklists are used in many clinical settings to quantify a person's food and alcohol consumption habits; ability to buy, prepare, and eat food; weight history; diagnoses; and medical/surgical procedures. Depending on the specific criteria evaluated, the presence of three to four risk factors may increase a person's risk for malnutrition. Pediatric screening programs most often evaluate growth parameters against the NCHS growth charts and medical conditions known to increase nutrition risk. Screening programs must also identify patients receiving specialized nutrition support (enteral or parenteral nutrition). In any setting, patients determined to be at "nutrition risk" should receive a comprehensive nutrition assessment to verify nutrition-related risk and to formulate a nutrition care plan.

ASSESSMENT OF NUTRITION STATUS

❸ A comprehensive nutrition assessment is the first step in formulating a patient-specific nutrition care plan. Nutrition assessment has four major goals: (a) identification of the presence of factors associated with an increased risk of developing malnutrition, including disorders resulting from macro- or micronutrient deficiencies (undernutrition), obesity (overnutrition), or impaired metabolism or utilization; (b) determination of risk of malnutrition-associated complications; (c) establishment of estimated nutrition needs; and (d) establishment of baseline nutrition status with parameters against which to measure nutrition therapy outcomes.

Nutrition assessment should include a nutrition-focused medical, surgical, and dietary history, a nutrition-focused physical examination including anthropometrics, and laboratory measurements. A comprehensive nutrition assessment provides a basis for determining the patient's nutrition requirements and the optimal type and timing of nutrition intervention.

CLINICAL EVALUATION

❹ Clinical or bedside evaluation of nutrition status correlates well with objective evaluations (e.g., laboratory and anthropometric measurements). The medical, surgical, and dietary history components of the clinical evaluation provide information regarding those factors that predispose to malnutrition (e.g., prematurity, chronic diseases, gastrointestinal [GI] malfunction, and alcohol abuse) and overnutrition (e.g., poor dietary habits, limited exercise, chronic diseases, and family history). The clinician should direct the interview to elicit any history of weight gain or loss, anorexia, vomiting, diarrhea, and decreased or unusual food intake (Table 149–1).

The nutrition-focused health history and physical examination takes a systems approach to assess lean body mass (LBM) and findings of vitamin, trace element, or essential fatty acid deficiencies or excesses. The assessment should include documentation of the presence and degree of muscle wasting, edema, loss of subcutaneous fat, dermatitis, glossitis, cheilosis, jaundice, or other findings suggestive of malnutrition (Table 149–2).

Since the 1980s, the Subjective Global Assessment, a simple, reproducible, cost-effective, bedside approach to nutrition assessment, has been used by many practitioners in a variety of patient populations.[2,8,14,15] Five aspects of the medical and dietary history make up the Subjective Global Assessment: weight changes in the previous

TABLE 149-1	Pertinent Data from Nutrition-Focused Medical, Surgical, and Dietary History

Nutrition intake and dietary habits
Anorexia
Unusual or absent taste
Dietary intake and special diets, including enteral or parenteral nutrition
Supplemental vitamin, mineral, or herbal intake
Food allergies or intolerance

Underlying pathology with nutritional effects
Chronic infections or inflammatory states
Neoplastic diseases
Endocrine disorders
Chronic illness, including pulmonary disease, cirrhosis, and kidney failure
Hypermetabolic states, such as trauma, burns, and sepsis
Digestive or absorptive disease, nausea, vomiting, diarrhea, and constipation
Hyperlipidemia

End-organ effects
Weight changes
Skin or hair changes
Exercise intolerance or fatigue
Gastrointestinal tract symptoms such as diarrhea, vomiting, and constipation

Gastrointestinal surgery
Bariatric surgery
Small bowel and/or colon resection
Gastrectomy

Miscellaneous
Catabolic medications or therapies, including corticosteroids, immunosuppressive agents, radiation, or chemotherapy
Other medications, including diuretics, laxatives, or anabolic steroids
Genetic background, including body habitus of parents, siblings, and family
Alcohol or drug abuse

Data from references 7 to 16.

TABLE 149-2	Physical Findings Suggestive of Malnutrition

General appearance
Edema (especially ankle and sacral)
Cachexia or obesity
Ascites
Signs and symptoms of dehydration, including poor skin turgor, sunken eyes, orthostasis, or dry mucous membranes
Muscle wasting or loss of subcutaneous fat

Skin and mucous membranes
Thin, shiny, dry, or scaly skin
Decubitus ulcers
Ecchymoses or perifollicular petechiae
Poor healing of surgical or traumatic wounds
Pallor or redness of gums or fissures at mouth edge
Glossitis, stomatitis, or cheilosis

Musculoskeletal
Retarded growth/short stature
Bone pain or tenderness or epiphyseal swelling
Muscle mass less than expected for habitus, genetic history, and level of exercise

Neurologic
Ataxia, positive Romberg test[a], or decreased vibratory or position sense
Nystagmus
Seizures or paralysis
Encephalopathy
Failure to meet age-appropriate developmental milestones

Hepatic
Jaundice
Hepatomegaly

[a]The Romberg test is a neurologic test used to detect problems with balance.
Data from references 7 to 16.

6 months, dietary intake changes, GI symptoms, functional capacity of the GI tract, and the presence of disease states known to affect nutrition status. Weight loss of less than 5% of UBW is considered a "small" loss, 5% to 10% loss is "potentially significant," and more than a 10% loss is "definitely significant." Dietary intake is characterized as either normal or abnormal, and the length of time and degree of abnormal intake is noted. The presence of GI symptoms (e.g., anorexia, nausea, vomiting, or diarrhea) on a daily basis for longer than 2 weeks is significant. Functional capacity assesses the patient's energy level and whether the patient is active or bedridden. Finally, disease states present are assessed as to their impact on metabolic demands (i.e., no stress, low, moderate, or high stress). Four physical examination findings are rated as normal, mild, moderate, or severe: loss of subcutaneous fat (triceps and chest), muscle wasting (quadriceps and deltoids), edema (ankle and sacral), and ascites. The clinician then ranks the patient's nutrition status as adequately nourished, moderately malnourished or suspected of being malnourished, or severely malnourished. Critics of the Subjective Global Assessment find it time-consuming and complex.[2] Another tool, the Mini Nutritional Assessment has been used extensively in geriatric patients and found to be useful for community-living elderly, residents in subacute care facilities, and those in nursing homes.[2,16]

ANTHROPOMETRIC MEASUREMENTS

❺ Anthropometric measurements, physical measurements of the size, weight, and proportions of the human body, are often used to assess nutrition status. The most common measurements are weight, stature (standing height or recumbent length, depending on age), head circumference (for children younger than 3 years of age), waist circumference, and measurements of limb size, such as skinfold thickness, midarm muscle circumference, and wrist circumference. Bioelectrical impedance analysis (BIA) is also an anthropometric assessment tool. These parameters are used to compare an individual with normative standards for a population and as repeated measurements in an individual to monitor response to a nutrition care plan. In adults, nutrition-related changes in anthropometric measurements occur slowly; several weeks or more are usually required before detectable changes are noted. In infants and young children, however, changes may occur more quickly. Acute changes in weight and skinfold thickness usually reflect changes in hydration status, which must be considered when interpreting these parameters, particularly in hospitalized patients.

WEIGHT, STATURE, AND HEAD CIRCUMFERENCE

Body weight is a nonspecific measure of body cell mass, representing skeletal mass, body fat, and the energy-using component referred to as LBM. Change in weight over time, particularly in the absence of edema, ascites, and voluntary losses, is an important indicator of altered LBM. Interpretation of actual body weight (ABW) should take into consideration ideal weight-for-height, also referred to as the ideal body weight (IBW), UBW, fluid status, and age (Table 149–3). The UBW is intended to describe an individual's typical weight and is generally more useful when assessing weight loss or gain than comparing the current weight to the estimated IBW. Dehydration will result in decreased ABW but not a loss in LBM. Once the patient is rehydrated, rechecking the weight is important to establish the baseline weight to use for nutrition evaluation. The presence of edema or ascites increases total body water (TBW), thus increasing ABW. Weights of patients with severe edema and ascites should not be used for nutrition assessment without taking the extra water weight into consideration. Thus, acute and chronic changes in fluid status can affect the ABW; these changes often can be detected by monitoring the patient's daily fluid intake and output.

TABLE 149-3 Evaluation of Body Weight

ABW compared to IBW	
ABW <69% IBW	Severe malnutrition
ABW 70%–79% IBW	Moderate malnutrition
ABW 80%–89% IBW	Mild malnutrition
ABW 90%–120% IBW	Normal
ABW >120% IBW	Overweight
ABW ≥150% IBW	Obese
ABW ≥200% IBW	Morbidly obese
ABW compared to UBW	
ABW 85%–95% UBW	Mild malnutrition
ABW 75%–84% UBW	Moderate malnutrition
ABW <75% UBW	Severe malnutrition
BMI (kg/m²) or (lb/in²)	**Interpretation**
Adults	
<16	Severe malnutrition
16–16.9	Moderate malnutrition
17–18.9	Mild malnutrition
19–24.9	Healthy
25–29.9	Overweight
30–40	Moderate obesity
>40	Severe or morbid obesity
Children	
BMI-for-age <5th percentile	Underweight
BMI-for-age 5th–84th percentile	Healthy
BMI-for-age 85th–94th percentile	Overweight
BMI-for-age ≥95th percentile	Obese

ABW, actual body weight; BMI, body mass index; IBW, ideal body weight; UBW, usual body weight.
Data from references 5, 6, and 8.

TABLE 149-4 Expected Growth Velocities in Term Infants and Children

Age	Weight (g/day)	Height (cm/month)[a]
0–3 months	24–35	2.8–3.4
4–6 months	15–21	1.7–2.4
7–12 months	10–13	1.3–1.6
1–3 years	5–9	0.6–1
4–6 years	5–6	0.5–0.6
7–10 years	7–11	0.4–0.5

Example of growth assessment:
Age: 2 months; weight: 3.9 kg; weight at 1 month of age, 3.1 kg; days since last wt: 30
Growth velocity = [(3.9 kg–3.1 kg) × 1,000 g/kg]/30 days = 26.7 g/day
Interpretation: normal growth

[a]Growth velocity of 1 cm/month is equivalent to 0.4 inches/month.
Data from reference 6.

The IBW provides one population reference standard against which the ABW can be compared to detect both over- and undernutrition states. Numerous IBW-for-height reference tables have been generated based on various populations. In clinical practice, mathematical equations based on gender and height (Hamwi method) are used commonly. IBW is calculated as 48 kg + [2.7 × (inches over 5 feet)] for adult men, and for adult women as 45 kg + [2.3 × (inches over 5 feet)]. For both equations, a range of ± 4.5 kg for large or small frame size is used for interpretation purposes.[8] For obese adults, use of an adjusted IBW has been recommended for nutrition-related calculations: adjusted IBW = [(ABW − IBW) × 0.25] + IBW. However, there is no evidence that supports the use of adjusted body weight, and its use can result in overfeeding; thus this practice has largely been abandoned. The IBW of children can be calculated as {[(height in cm)² × 1.65]/1,000}. Alternatively, IBW-for-height in children can be determined by identifying the weight corresponding to the same growth percentile as the child's measured stature on the appropriate NCHS growth chart.

Change in weight over time can be calculated as the percentage of UBW, where percent change = [(ABW/UBW) × 100] (see Table 149–3). Use of the UBW as a reference point provides a more accurate reflection of clinically and nutritionally significant weight changes. Determining a patient's UBW, however, depends on patient or family recall, which may be inaccurate. The use of UBW avoids the problems of normative tables and documents comparative changes in body weight. Any change in weight also should be interpreted relative to time. Unintentional weight loss, especially rapid weight loss (e.g., 5% of UBW in 1 month or 10% of UBW in 6 months), may increase the risk of poor clinical outcomes.[8]

Stature is determined by both genetics and nutrition intake. In infants, recumbent length is measured, while in older children and adults, a standing height is preferred. If a standing height cannot be measured, the measurement of demispan can be used to project height. Demispan is determined by measuring the distance from the sternal notch to the web between the middle and ring fingers along a horizontally outstretched arm with the wrist in neutral rotation and zero extension or flexion while the patient is seated. Demispan may more accurately assess height in the elderly, especially those with kyphosis and/or vertebral collapse. Once the demispan is measured, height can be estimated using the following equations: women: height (cm) = 1.35 × demispan (cm) + 60.1; men: height (cm) = 1.4 × demispan (cm) + 57.8.[17] Knee height may also be used to estimate stature and is especially helpful in patients with limb contractures, such as patients with cerebral palsy.[17–20] In one method, the knee height is measured from just under the heel to the anterior surface of the thigh just proximal to the patella. Using the average of two measurements rounded to the nearest 0.1 cm, height is estimated using the following equations: women: height (cm) = 84.88 (0.24 × age [years]) + (1.83 × knee height [cm]); men: height (cm) = 64.19 (0.04 × age [years]) + (2.02 × knee height [cm]).[19]

The best indicator of adequate nutrition in a child is an appropriate rate of growth. At each medical encounter, weight, stature, and head circumference should be plotted on the appropriate NCHS gender- and age-specific growth curve. These charts were developed in 1977 from a large population of healthy, primarily white children and revised in 2002 to better reflect the ethnic mix of the United States' population. Special growth charts are available for assessment of short- and long-term growth of premature infants,[21,22] children with Down syndrome,[23] and other specific conditions. For premature infants with corrected postnatal age of 40 weeks or more, the NCHS growth charts can be used; however, weight-for-age and length-for-age should be plotted according to corrected postnatal age until 2 years and 3.5 years of age, respectively.

Recommended intervals between measurements are weight, 7 days; length, 4 weeks; height, 8 weeks; and head circumference, 7 days in infants and 4 weeks in children up to 3 years of age. Growth velocity can be used to assess growth at intervals too close to plot accurately on a growth chart (Table 149–4). In newborns, average weight gain is 10 to 20 g/kg/day (24–35 g/day in term infants and 10–25 g/day in preterm infants). Weight gain declines considerably after 2 to 3 months of age. Head growth (measured by head circumference), which is usually 0.5 cm/week (0.2 inches/week) during the first year of life, can be compromised during periods of critical illness or malnutrition. Sustained head growth during these periods, especially at a rate above expected, suggests hydrocephalus.

Growth failure or failure-to-thrive is defined as weight-for-age or weight-for-height (or length) below the 5th percentile or a falloff of two or more major percentiles (major percentiles are defined as 97th, 95th, 90th, 75th, 50th, 25th, 10th, 5th, and 3rd). Weight-for-height evaluation is age-independent and helps differentiate the stunted child (chronic malnutrition) from the wasted child (acute malnutrition). Short stature, which is associated with many chronic diseases, is a manifestation of chronic undernutrition. Short stature in the absence of malnutrition suggests an endocrinopathy, such as growth hormone deficiency, but may also be a normal variant (e.g., constitutional growth delay).

BODY MASS INDEX

In general, a healthy weight is one associated with a reduction in disease risk. BMI, which is most commonly defined as body weight in kilograms divided by the square of the patient's height in meters (kg/m^2), is another index of the appropriateness of weight-for-height. Using pounds and inches, BMI (lb/in^2) can also be estimated as (weight [pounds] × 703/height^2 [inches^2]). A BMI of 25 kg/m^2 or higher is considered a risk factor for premature death and disability as a consequence of being overweight or obese (see Chap. 154). These health risks increase as the BMI increases. Although BMI correlates strongly with total body fat, individual variation, especially in very muscular persons, may lead to erroneous classification of either obesity or malnutrition when BMI alone is used to assess nutrition status. BMI should be interpreted based on an individual's characteristics, including gender, frame size, and age. For example, at the same BMI, a woman tends to have more body fat than a man, and an older subject would have more body fat than a younger individual.

Various tables listing BMI stratified by height and weight are available for quick reference. In general, an adult with a BMI between 25 and 29.9 kg/m^2 is overweight, and one with a BMI of 30 kg/m^2 or higher is considered to be obese.[8,24] These numbers may not be appropriate for older subjects, especially those older than 60 years, where a BMI between 27 kg/m^2 and 30 kg/m^2 has not been associated with the same increased nutrition-related risks as seen in younger individuals.[25] BMI has also been used to assess undernutrition with a BMI less than 18.5 kg/m^2 indicating undernutrition (see Table 149–3).[8,24] Children 2 years of age and older are considered overweight if their BMI is at or above the 85th percentile on the age- and gender-specific NCHS BMI chart and obese if the BMI is at or above the 95th percentile.[5,6] Use of these charts helps to heighten parental and healthcare provider awareness of children whose BMI and family history put them at risk for adult obesity and its associated risks.

CLINICAL CONTROVERSY

Clinicians disagree whether an individual's nutrition status is best evaluated using IBW, ABW, adjusted IBW, or BMI. Frame size and muscle mass, as well as gender and height, can influence both IBW and BMI, leading to misclassification of nutrition status in some individuals. Use of adjusted IBW in obese individuals may lead to under- or overestimation of nutrition needs.

SKINFOLD THICKNESS AND MIDARM MUSCLE CIRCUMFERENCE

More than 50% of the body's fat is subcutaneous, thus changes in subcutaneous fat usually reflect changes in total body fat. Skinfold thickness measurement provides an estimate of subcutaneous fat, whereas midarm muscle circumference, which is calculated using the skinfold thickness, estimates skeletal muscle mass. Although simple and noninvasive, these anthropometric measurements are not used commonly in clinical practice but can be used for both population analysis and long-term monitoring of individuals. Triceps skinfold thickness is the most commonly used skinfold measurement, although reference standards also exist for subscapular and iliac sites. Careful technique in the use of pressure-regulated calipers is essential for reproducibility and reliability in measuring triceps skinfold thickness. Midarm muscle circumference is a calculated value based on the measurement of the midarm circumference and triceps skinfold thickness.

These measurements in individuals should be interpreted cautiously because standards do not account for individual variations in bone size, muscle mass, hydration status, or skin compressibility; reference standards do not account for obesity, ethnicity, illness, and increased age; and technique is critical (interobserver error can be significant). Furthermore, these parameters are slow to change in adults, often requiring weeks before significant alterations from baseline can be detected.

WAIST CIRCUMFERENCE

Waist circumference is a simple measurement used to assess abdominal (visceral) fat. Excess abdominal fat, rather than excess peripheral (subcutaneous) fat, is an independent predictor of risk for obesity-related complications, especially diabetes mellitus and cardiovascular disease.[26,27] Waist circumference is determined by measuring the distance around the smallest area below the rib cage and the top of the iliac crest. Interpretation varies with gender. Men are considered at increased risk (beyond the BMI-related risk) if the waist circumference is greater than 40 inches (102 cm); women are at increased risk if the waist circumference is greater than 35 inches (89 cm), and children are at risk if the waist circumference is at the 90th percentile or greater according to age- and gender-specific standards.

WAIST-TO-HIP AND WAIST-TO-HEIGHT RATIO

For most people, extra weight around the waist confers more of a health risk than extra weight around the hips and thighs. The waist-to-hip ratio is determined by dividing the waist circumference by the hip circumference (maximal posterior extension of the buttocks). In adults, a waist-to-hip ratio of greater than 0.9 in men and 0.85 in women is considered an independent risk factor for adverse health consequences.[26] Waist-to-height ratio (both measured in centimeters) has been used to evaluate children at risk for the metabolic syndrome because, unlike waist circumference, it is age and gender independent. A child with a waist-to-height ratio of 0.5 or less is generally not considered to be at metabolic risk.[28]

BIOELECTRICAL IMPEDANCE

BIA is a simple, noninvasive, and relatively inexpensive technique used to measure LBM.[29,30] The technology is based on the fact that lean tissue has a higher electrical conductivity (less resistance) than fat, which is a poor current conductor because of its lower water and electrolyte content. By applying a very small electric current to appendages (wrist and ankle or both feet), impedance (resistance) to flow can be measured. Assessment of LBM, TBW, and water's distribution into compartments can be determined with BIA. Increased TBW decreases impedance; therefore, it is important to evaluate fluid status along with BIA measurements. Other potential limitations of BIA include variability with electrolyte imbalance, interference by large fat masses (obesity), and the lack of reference standards that reflect variations in individual body size and clinical condition. Although BIA equations have high validity when used in the population in which they were developed (mostly young healthy adults), BIA calculations are subject to considerable errors if applied to other populations. BIA is not superior to BMI as a predictor of overall adiposity in the general population and is therefore used primarily as a research tool.

TABLE 149-5 Visceral Proteins Used for Assessment of Lean Body Mass

Serum Protein	Half-Life (Days)	Function	Factors Resulting in Increased Values	Factors Resulting in Decreased Values
Albumin	18–20	Maintains plasma oncotic pressure; transports small molecules	Dehydration, anabolic steroids, insulin, infection	Overhydration, edema, kidney dysfunction, nephrotic syndrome, poor dietary intake, impaired digestion, burns, congestive heart failure, cirrhosis, thyroid/adrenal/pituitary hormones, trauma, sepsis
Transferrin	8–9	Binds Fe in plasma; transports Fe to bone	Fe deficiency, pregnancy, hypoxia, chronic blood loss, estrogens	Chronic infection, cirrhosis, burns, enteropathies, nephrotic syndrome, cortisone, testosterone
Prealbumin (transthyretin)	2–3	Binds T_3 and to a lesser extent T_4; carrier for retinol-binding protein	Kidney dysfunction	Cirrhosis, hepatitis, stress, surgery, inflammation, hyperthyroidism, cystic fibrosis, burns, kidney dysfunction, zinc deficiency

Fe, iron; T_3, triiodothyronine; T_4, thyroxine.
Data from references 8, 10, and 31.

BIOCHEMICAL ASSESSMENT OF LBM

❻ LBM includes skeletal muscle, somatic protein, and functional proteins such as the circulating and visceral proteins. Biochemically, LBM can be assessed by measuring the serum visceral proteins, ALB, TFN, and prealbumin (thyroxine-binding prealbumin or transthyretin). Retinol-binding protein, fibronectin (an opsonic protein), and somatomedin-C (insulin-like growth factor-1), proteins with a very short half-life (less than 12 to 24 hours), have also been evaluated as indicators of nutrition status. However, the clinical availability of these alternative tests is limited, and their relevance to nutrition status and patient outcome has not been established. Creatinine-height index has historically been used to assess LBM but is seldom used today because of the lack of evidence to support its usefulness in assessing muscle mass.

Visceral Proteins

Measurement of serum concentrations of the transport proteins synthesized by hepatocytes can be used to assess the visceral protein compartment. It is assumed that a low serum protein concentration in states of undernutrition reflects the hepatic protein synthetic mass, and therefore indirectly reflects the functional protein mass of other organs such as the heart, lung, kidney, and intestines. The visceral proteins with the greatest relevance for nutrition assessment are serum ALB, TFN, and prealbumin. Many factors other than nutrition may affect the serum concentration of these proteins, including age, abnormal kidney (nephrotic syndrome), GI tract (protein-losing enteropathy), or skin (burns) losses, hydration status (dehydration results in hemoconcentration, overhydration in hemodilution), liver function (because this is the primary synthesis site), and metabolic stress (sepsis, trauma, surgery, and infection). Visceral protein concentrations must be interpreted relative to the individual's overall clinical condition (Table 149–5). Serum visceral proteins are of greatest value in assessing the presence of uncomplicated semi-starvation and recovery. During severe acute stress (trauma, burns, or sepsis), these proteins are relatively poor markers of nutrition status because their synthesis is downregulated as the liver increases the production of acute-phase reactants such as C-reactive protein, α_1-acid glycoprotein, and α_1-antitrypsin.[31]

Albumin is the most abundant plasma protein and is involved in maintenance of colloid oncotic pressure and binding and transport of numerous hormones, anions, drugs, and fatty acids. It is one of the most widely used biochemical markers of malnutrition in population studies and in individuals. It is, however, a relatively insensitive index of early protein malnutrition because there is a large amount normally found in the body (4–5 g/kg of body weight), it is highly distributed in the extravascular compartment (60%), and it has a long half-life (18–20 days). However, chronic protein deficiency in the setting of adequate nonprotein calorie intake leads to marked hypoalbuminemia because of a net ALB loss from the intravascular and extravascular compartments. Serum ALB concentrations also are affected by moderate-to-severe calorie deficiency and liver, kidney, and GI disease. Because it is a negative acute phase reactant, serum concentrations will decrease with infection, trauma, stress, and burns. A positive correlation between decreased serum ALB concentrations and poor clinical outcome has been demonstrated in most of the above mentioned settings. Additionally, serum ALB concentrations less than 2.5 g/dL (25 g/L) can be expected to exacerbate ascites and peripheral, pulmonary, and GI mucosal edema as a result of decreased colloid oncotic pressure, Hypoalbuminemia will also affect the interpretation of serum calcium concentrations as well as serum concentrations of highly protein bound drugs.[8,10,31]

TFN is a glycoprotein that binds and transports ferric iron to the liver and reticuloendothelial system for storage. As a surrogate marker of nutrition status, TFN will decrease in response to protein depletion before the serum ALB concentration decreases because it has a shorter half-life (8–9 days), and there is less of it in the body (less than 100 mg/kg of body weight). Serum TFN concentrations may be determined by direct measurement or can be estimated indirectly from measurement of total iron-binding capacity (in μg/dL), where TFN (in mg/dL) = (total iron binding capacity × 0.8) − 43. Critical illness, hydration status, and iron stores affect the serum TFN concentration. In iron deficiency, hepatic TFN synthesis is increased, resulting in increased serum TFN concentrations unrelated to protein status.[8,10]

Prealbumin is the transport protein for thyroxine and a carrier for retinol-binding protein. The body's content of prealbumin is low (10 mg/kg of body weight), and it has a very short half-life (2–3 days). The serum prealbumin concentration may be reduced in as few as 3 days after calorie and protein intake is significantly decreased or when hypercatabolism or severe metabolic stress (trauma or burns) is present. Because of its short half-life, it is most useful in monitoring the short-term, acute effects of nutrition support or deficits, as it responds very quickly in both situations. As with ALB and TFN, serum prealbumin concentrations are depressed in those with liver disease as a consequence of decreased synthesis. Increased serum prealbumin concentrations have been noted in patients with kidney disease as a result of impaired excretion.[8,10]

IMMUNE FUNCTION TESTS

The frequency of impaired immunocompetence and an increased incidence of infection in malnourished patients suggest that certain immune function tests can be used as nutrition status markers. Nutrition affects immune status either directly, affecting primarily the lymphoid system, or indirectly by affecting cellular metabolism or organ systems that are involved with immune system regulation. Immune function tests used in nutrition assessment are the total lymphocyte count and DCH reactions. Both tests are simple, readily available, and inexpensive.

Total lymphocyte count reflects the number of circulating T and B lymphocytes. Tissues that generate T cells are very sensitive to malnutrition and undergo involution resulting in decreased T cell production and eventually lymphocytopenia. Total lymphocyte count is calculated from a complete blood count with differential: total lymphocyte count = (% lymphocytes × total number of white blood cells). Values less than 1,500 cells/mm³ (1.5×10^9 cells/L) have been associated with nutrition depletion.[2] DCH is commonly assessed using antigens to which the patient was likely previously sensitized. The recall antigens used most frequently in nutrition assessment are mumps, *Candida albicans*, and *Trichophyton*. Anergy is associated with severe malnutrition, and immune response may be restored with nutrition repletion. Other more sophisticated immune function tests have been used to evaluate nutrition status in research settings, including lymphocyte surface antigens (CD4 and CD8 counts, CD4:CD8 ratio), T lymphocyte responsiveness, and serum interleukin concentrations.

Other factors besides nutrition can affect immune status. Nonnutrition factors that affect total lymphocyte count include infection (e.g., human immunodeficiency virus [HIV], viruses, and tuberculosis), immunosuppressive drugs (e.g., corticosteroids, cyclosporine, tacrolimus, sirolimus, chemotherapy, and anti-lymphocyte globulin), leukemia, and lymphoma. DCH can be affected by a number of factors, including fever, viral illness, recent live virus vaccination, critical illness, irradiation, immunosuppressive drugs, diabetes mellitus, HIV, cancer, and surgery. This lack of specificity currently limits the usefulness of these tests as nutrition status markers. Nutrients such as arginine, omega-3 fatty acids, and nucleic acids given in pharmacologic doses have been shown to improve immune function. Monitoring the efficacy of a nutrition care plan that includes these potentially immunomodulating nutrients may need to include immune function assessment with these or other immune function indicators.[32,33]

SPECIFIC NUTRIENT DEFICIENCIES AND TOXICITIES

7 A comprehensive nutrition assessment must include an evaluation for possible trace element, vitamin, and essential fatty acid deficiencies. Because of their key role in metabolic processes (as coenzymes and cofactors), a deficiency of any of these nutrients may result in altered metabolism and cell dysfunction and may interfere with metabolic processes necessary for nutritional repletion. The evaluation of a single nutrient deficiency or toxicity state includes an accurate history to identify symptoms and risk factors that may indicate deficiency or toxicity or a predisposition of the patient to developing a deficiency or toxicity state. A nutrition-focused physical examination for signs of deficiencies and biochemical assessment to confirm a suspected diagnosis should be done. Ideally, biochemical assessment would be based on the nutrient's function (e.g., metalloenzyme activity) rather than simply measuring the nutrient's serum concentration. Unfortunately, few practical methods to assess micronutrient function are available, and most assays measure the serum concentration of an individual nutrient.

TRACE ELEMENTS

Clinical syndromes are associated with deficiency states of the essential trace elements zinc, copper, manganese, selenium, chromium, iodine, fluoride, molybdenum, and iron in children and adults.[34–37] Each element is involved in a variety of biologic functions and is necessary for normal metabolism, serving as a coenzyme and/or playing a role in hormonal metabolism or erythropoiesis. Other essential trace elements for which deficiency states have not been recognized include tin, nickel, vanadium, cobalt, gallium,

aluminum, arsenic, boron, bromine, cadmium, germanium, and silicon. Toxicities can occur with excess intake of some trace elements. With the current public interest in alternative and complementary medicine, clinicians must ask patients about their use of dietary supplements and assess for signs and symptoms of toxicities (overdose) as well as deficiencies (Table 149–6).

Zinc is a component of many enzymes and proteins and is involved in the regulation of gene expression. Excess zinc intake is usually eliminated by the kidneys and GI tract. Zinc deficiency is characterized by several signs and symptoms, including a moist eczematous dermatitis that is most apparent in the nasolabial folds and around orifices (see Table 149–6). Recovery is rapid with oral zinc supplementation; severe dermatitis can remit in as little as 4 to 5 days.[37] Acrodermatitis enteropathica is an autosomal recessive genetic disorder of zinc metabolism, and zinc deficiency may also occur with abnormal GI losses, such as in Crohn's disease, malabsorptive states (e.g., cystic fibrosis, short bowel syndrome), and extensive ostomy or fistula losses, or from prolonged inadequate intake, such as with zinc-free or inadequately zinc-supplemented parenteral nutrition. Low zinc stores have also been reported in premature infants and in children with sickle cell disease. Zinc deficiency can be documented by the presence of low plasma zinc concentrations.[38] However, plasma zinc concentrations decrease during acute stress states, such as trauma, surgery, burns, or sepsis, and generally remain depressed until the stress resolves. Also, because zinc is a normal contaminant of most blood collection tubes, special zinc-free collection tubes must be used for plasma assays. Hair zinc analysis and urinary zinc excretion are also biomarkers of zinc status.[38]

Copper is a component of ceruloplasmin and key metalloenzymes involved in iron metabolism (ceruloplasmin), electron transport and energy metabolism (cytochrome oxidase), connective tissue and collagen cross-linking (lysyl oxidase, elastase, and monamine oxidase), and free radical scavenging (superoxide dismutase). Copper intake in excess of metabolic requirements is excreted through the bile. The signs and symptoms of copper deficiency include hypochromic anemia, neutropenia, neurologic dysfunction, skeletal demineralization, and hypercholesterolemia (see Table 149–6). In severe cases, such as in Menkes syndrome, copper deficiency is further manifested as hypothermia, hair and skin depigmentation, progressive mental deterioration, and growth retardation. Factors predisposing to copper deficiency include malabsorption states, protein-losing enteropathy, nephrotic syndrome, and copper-free parenteral nutrition.[39] The chronic ingestion of too much copper or inadequate elimination can result in cirrhosis as seen in Wilson disease, an autosomal-recessive genetic disorder. Copper deficiency is best assessed using serum copper concentrations which appear to reflect changes in copper status in both copper-depleted and copper-replete individuals.[40] As with zinc, serum copper concentrations may not accurately reflect total body copper status because serum concentrations may be altered by a variety of conditions (see Table 149–6). Copper function also may be assessed by measuring ceruloplasmin total protein; however this test appears to be more copper status dependent, reflecting copper status changes only in highly depleted individuals.[40]

Trivalent chromium is an important cofactor, along with insulin, in the maintenance of normal blood glucose concentrations. Recent data indicate that a low-molecular-weight chromium binding substance, sometimes referred to as the glucose tolerance factor, may enhance the response of the insulin receptor to insulin.[41] Chromium deficiency is characterized by glucose intolerance, impaired protein utilization, and increased insulin requirements. Patients with chromium deficiency also may have increased free fatty acid concentrations and a low respiratory quotient (RQ) (see Table 149–6). Chromium deficiency has only been identified in patients receiving long-term parenteral nutrition with inadequate chromium intake.

TABLE 149-6 Assessment of Trace Element Status

Trace Element	Signs of Deficiency	Signs of Toxicity	Factors Associated with Altered Plasma Concentrations
Chromium	Impaired glucose/protein utilization, peripheral neuropathy, low RQ, weight loss, increased LDL-C, increased free fatty acid concentrations	Industrial exposure: skin/nasal septum lesions, allergic dermatitis, increased incidence of lung cancer	Decreased: long-term inadequate intake Increased: kidney failure
Copper	Menkes syndrome, progressive mental deterioration, vomiting, diarrhea, protein-losing enteropathy, hypopigmentation, bone and hair changes Deficiency: neutropenia, hypochromic anemia, pallor, dermatitis, neurologic dysfunction	Wilson disease: cirrhosis, Kayser-Fleischer ring;[a] kidney dysfunction, neurologic/psychiatric symptoms (tremors, slow speech, inappropriate behavior, personality changes) Mild chronic toxicity: fatigue, anemia, thrombocytopenia Acute toxicity: nausea, vomiting, diarrhea	Decreased: high zinc, iron or vitamin C intake, corticosteroid use Increased: infection, rheumatoid arthritis, pregnancy, oral contraceptives, decreased biliary excretion
Iodine	Hypothyroid goiter, neuromuscular impairment, deaf-mutism, increased embryonic and postnatal mortality, cognitive impairment, impaired fertility, cretinism (severe cases)	Thyrotoxicosis: nodular goiter, weight loss, tachycardia, muscle weakness, warm skin	Decreased: long-term inadequate intake
Iron	Microcytic, hypochromic anemia (weakness, pallor, fatigue), glossitis, headache, dysphagia, nail changes, gastric atrophy, paresthesia, decreased cognitive function	Cirrhosis, cardiomyopathy, pancreatic damage, skin pigmentation changes	Increased: blood transfusion Decreased: blood loss
Manganese	Nausea, vomiting, dermatitis, hair color changes, hypocholesterolemia, growth retardation, defective carbohydrate, lipid, and protein metabolism	Parkinsonian-like symptoms, hyperirritability, hallucinations, libido disturbances, ataxia, mental confusion, lack of attention, memory loss	Increased: decreased biliary excretion, high iron or vitamin C intake
Molybdenum	Tachycardia, tachypnea, altered mental status, visual changes, headache, nausea, vomiting	Gout-like syndrome, increased urinary copper	Decreased: low birth weight, excessive GI losses
Selenium	Muscle weakness/pain, cardiomyopathy, skin and hair pigmentation changes	Nausea, vomiting, hair/nail loss, tooth decay, skin lesions, irritability, fatigue, peripheral neuropathy	Decreased: malignancy, liver failure, pregnancy Increased: reticuloendothelial neoplasia
Zinc	Dermatitis (scaly, hyperpigmented lesions of elbows/knees), altered taste and smell, alopecia, diarrhea, apathy, depression, growth retardation, impaired wound healing, anorexia, immunosuppression, delayed sexual maturation	Acute: diarrhea, vomiting, nausea, dizziness, garlic-smelling breath; death with large intravenous doses Chronic: immunosuppression, decreased HDL-C, copper deficiency	Decreased: infection, burns, stress, hypoalbuminemia, corticosteroids, pregnancy, inflammation Increased: tissue injury, hemolysis, contaminated collection tube

GI, gastrointestinal; HDL-C, high-density-lipoprotein cholesterol; LDL-C, low-density-lipoprotein cholesterol; RQ, respiratory quotient.
[a]Kayser-Fleischer rings are dark rings that appear to encircle the iris of the eye.
Data from references 8 and 34 to 37.

Plasma chromium concentrations do not accurately reflect total body chromium status, presumably because the biologically active form of chromium is the low-molecular-weight chromium binding substance. Toxicity from trivalent chromium is not a common clinical concern, and chromium toxicity has been reported only with contaminated drinking water or industrial exposure. Chromium supplementation as an adjunct for weight loss has not been proven effective.

Manganese is important in the function of many enzymes, including arginase (amino acid metabolism via the urea cycle), pyruvate carboxylase and phosphoenolpyruvate carboxykinase (carbohydrate and cholesterol metabolism), superoxide dismutase (mitochondrial antioxidant), glycosyltransferases (bone formation via proteoglycans), and prolidase (wound healing).[35,37,42] Excess manganese is eliminated via the bile. Manganese deficiency has only been reported in association with the ingestion of chemically defined manganese-deficient oral diets. Table 149-6 lists common symptoms associated with manganese deficiency. Manganese toxicity is more concerning and has been described in industrial exposures via inhaled manganese and in several patients receiving long-term parenteral nutrition supplemented with manganese (standard trace element preparation), especially in the setting of chronic cholestasis.[35,37,42-44] Manganese can accumulate in brain tissue and the newborn brain may be more susceptible to the effects of manganese toxicity.[37,43] Clinical toxicity is evidenced primarily by extrapyramidal symptoms mimicking Parkinson's disease, such as tremors, ataxia, and fascial muscle spasms. These symptoms may be preceded by psychiatric symptoms, including irritability, aggressiveness, and hallucinations. In most reported cases, discontinuation of manganese from the parenteral nutrition solution resulted in resolution of neurologic symptoms in 6 months with partial or total normalization of the magnetic resonance image after 1 to 2 years. Whole-blood manganese concentrations can be obtained to ascertain manganese status. Magnetic resonance imaging with intensity and T1 values in the globus pallidus may be useful for assessing manganese toxicity.[44,45]

Selenium is incorporated into at least 25 enzymes known as selenoproteins, about half of which have a defined metabolic function. Important selenoproteins include: five glutathione peroxidases (antioxidant activity), iodothyronine deiodinase (thyroid hormone regulation), thioredoxin reductase (vitamin C), selenoprotein P (antioxidant activity), selenoprotein V (spermatogenesis), and selenoprotein S (inflammation and immune response).[35,37] Prematurity, acute illness, chronic GI losses, and long-term selenium-free parenteral nutrition are associated with low serum selenium concentrations and decreased glutathione peroxidase activity.[35,37,46] The clinical significance of reduced serum selenium concentrations is unclear, but low selenium concentrations may make individuals more susceptible to physiologic stressors. Selenium deficiency has been described in patients receiving long-term selenium-free parenteral nutrition. Muscle pain, wasting, and weakness were the most frequently observed signs and symptoms (see Table 149-6), but severe biochemical deficiency is not always accompanied by these symptoms. Fatal cardiomyopathy has been reported in several cases. Selenium toxicity or selenosis generally only occurs in those with long-term exposure to foods grown in selenium-rich soil (e.g., Great Plains area of the United States) and may occur when intake exceeds 400 mcg/day for prolonged periods. Selenium toxicity results in hair and nail brittleness and loss, GI disturbance, skin rash, garlic breath odor, fatigue, irritability, and nervous system abnormalities. Plasma, erythrocyte, and whole-blood selenium, plasma selenoprotein P, and plasma, platelet, and whole-blood glutathione peroxidase activity respond to changes in selenium intake, but the response is heterogeneous.[47] Decreased plasma selenium concentrations may indicate selenium deficiency, but reductions have been observed in patients with malignancies, liver failure, and pregnancy.

Molybdenum is a cofactor for enzymes involved in catabolism of sulfur amino acids, purines, and pyrimidines (i.e., xanthine, aldehyde, and sulfite oxidases).[35,37] Molybdenum deficiency is rare, but an inborn error of metabolism resulting in molybdenum deficiency has been identified. One case of molybdenum deficiency has been reported in a patient receiving long-term parenteral nutrition who presented with symptoms that included tachycardia, tachypnea, headache, night blindness, nausea, vomiting, central scotomas, lethargy, disorientation, and ultimately coma (see Table 149–6). Symptoms were reversed when molybdenum was added to the parenteral nutrition solution.[48] Factors predisposing to molybdenum deficiency appear to be low birth weight,[49] excessive loss via the GI tract, and long-term inadequate intake, such as with molybdenum-free parenteral nutrition. Biochemical abnormalities expected in molybdenum deficiency include very low serum and urine uric acid concentrations (low xanthine oxidase activity) and low urine inorganic sulfate concentrations with high urine inorganic sulfite concentrations (low sulfate oxidase activity).[35,37] Molybdenum toxicity has not been described.

Deficiency of iodine, a component of thyroid hormones, may result in goiter formation (see Chap. 84). However, not everyone with an iodine-deficient diet will develop a goiter. Thyroxine (T_4) and triiodothyronine (T_3) can be used to assess iodine status (see Table 149–6). Intravenous iodine supplementation is not necessary except during long-term parenteral nutrition with minimal enteral intake. Iodine needs may be met by cutaneous absorption of iodine from germicides (e.g., povidone-iodine) used in catheter care or consumption of iodized salt.[35,37] Use of povidone-iodine as a topical antiseptic has decreased with the increased use of chlorhexidine for catheter care; thus the need for iodine supplementation must be individualized. Iodine excess is rarely a clinical concern when thyroid and kidney function are normal.

Iron is an important component of hemoglobin, myoglobin, and cytochrome enzymes; it is important in oxygen transport, muscle iron storage, and cellular energy production. Patients with iron-deficiency anemia generally present with fatigue, weakness, and pallor, but they may have other symptoms (see Chap. 109).[35,37] Inadequate iron intake, malabsorption, and blood loss are the principal causes of iron-deficiency anemia. Iron toxicity (overload) with possible organ damage can occur when chronic iron intake exceeds requirements, such as in patients receiving chronic blood transfusions. Iron deficiency or overload is confirmed by assessment of body iron stores, as reflected indirectly by measurement of hemoglobin, serum iron, total iron binding capacity, and serum ferritin, or directly by marrow staining and liver biopsy. Although the direct methods are the most accurate, they are invasive, and indirect measurements are used more commonly. Because indirect parameters may be altered by chronic illness independent of iron stores, concomitant illness must be considered in their interpretation.

VITAMINS

Vitamins act as both catalysts (cofactors) and substrates in essential metabolic reactions. A comprehensive nutrition-focused history and physical examination is the most valuable means of assessing patients for vitamin deficiency or toxicity (Table 149–7). A thorough review of all the complex interrelationships of vitamins and their effects on nutrition and metabolism is beyond the scope of this chapter.[34–36,50–52] Multiple vitamin deficiencies are most often associated with generalized malnutrition; however, single vitamin deficiencies may be noted. Thiamine deficiency results in lactic acidosis

and encephalopathy.[53] Pernicious anemia caused by vitamin B_{12} (cyanocobalamin) deficiency has been reported with increasing frequency, especially in the elderly, as a consequence of decreased gastric acidity.[54] The increasing prevalence of vitamin D deficiency is a growing concern, especially in children and the elderly.[55–57] Laboratory assessment may be useful to confirm the clinical suspicion of a deficiency or toxicity state. The first indication of a deficiency is usually a fall in circulating serum concentrations of the vitamin or its coenzyme. Subsequently, there is a decrease in urinary excretion of the vitamin, which is followed by diminished tissue concentrations. The most common measurements of vitamin status are assays of circulating amounts in plasma or serum. Assays of biochemical or metabolic function of the vitamin are more likely to reflect body stores than are serum concentrations. Most of these functional assays use erythrocyte or leukocyte extracts to determine apoenzyme activity, which is dependent on the vitamin coenzyme (Table 149–7).

Vitamin toxicity can occur, especially with the fat-soluble vitamins (A, D, E, and K), which are stored in the body. Excessive dietary intake of vitamin A (hypervitaminosis A) is linked to an increased risk of hip fractures in both men and women.[58,59] With the exception of cyanocobalamin, which is stored in the liver, water-soluble vitamins are not stored in the body; consequently, the risk of toxicity is considered minimal unless ingested in very high doses. Recent evidence, however, suggests that even water-soluble vitamins may be associated with adverse events when taken chronically in high doses. Although administration of folic acid is definitively associated with a reduction in neural tube defects, its ability to improve some cardiac outcomes (a result of its effect on homocysteine concentrations) is not established.[60] The administration of folic acid, vitamin B_6 (pyridoxine), and vitamin B_{12} after coronary artery stenting has been associated with an increase in the risk of in-stent restenosis.[61] With the current use of nutrition supplements by Americans, the clinician should be alert for the signs of hypervitaminosis (Table 149–7).

ESSENTIAL FATTY ACIDS

The human body can synthesize all fatty acids except linoleic acid (an omega-6 fatty acid) and α-linolenic acid (an omega-3 fatty acid). If approximately 5% of total calories are ingested as these fatty acids, development of a deficiency state can be prevented.[62] Essential fatty acid deficiency is rare in adults and children but can occur with prolonged use of lipid-free parenteral nutrition, with severe fat malabsorption, with very-low-fat enteral feeding formulations or diets, and with severe malnutrition, especially in stressed patients.[63,64] In critically ill adults and older children with increased metabolic demands, biochemical evidence of essential fatty acid deficiency can occur within 1 week of starting lipid-free parenteral nutrition.[63,64] Because newborns, especially those born prematurely, have limited fat stores, they may develop essential fatty acid deficiency more rapidly than adults. Biochemical essential fatty acid deficiency has been noted within 72 hours after birth in preterm infants receiving fat-free intravenous solutions.[65] Symptoms of essential fatty acid deficiency include dermatitis (dry, cracked, scaly skin), alopecia, impaired wound healing, growth failure, thrombocytopenia, and anemia.

Linoleic acid normally is converted to arachidonic acid (a tetraene fatty acid). If linoleic acid is unavailable, oleic acid will be substituted, which results in production of eicosatrienoic acid (a triene fatty acid) as the metabolic end product, enabling an essential fatty acid deficiency to be detected on the basis of decreased tetraene production and increased triene production. Normally, the ratio of trienes to tetraenes is less than 0.4; when this ratio becomes greater than 0.4, the diagnosis of essential fatty acid deficiency is established. However, because analysis of plasma fatty acids is

TABLE 149-7 Assessment of Vitamin Status

Vitamin	Signs of Deficiency	Laboratory Assay	Comments
Water-soluble vitamins			
Thiamine (B₁)	Early: anorexia, fatigue, depression, impaired memory/concentration Late: paresthesia, nystagmus, GI beriberi (nausea, vomiting, abdominal pain, lactic acidosis), beriberi (congestive heart failure, edema), Wernicke encephalopathy, Korsakoff's psychosis, peripheral neuropathy	Whole blood or erythrocyte transketolase activation test Blood thiamine pyrophosphate Erythrocyte glutathione reductase activity coefficient	Increased need with hemo- and peritoneal dialysis, alcoholism, malabsorption, hypermetabolism
Riboflavin (B₂)	Mucositis, dermatitis, cheilosis, glossitis, photophobia, corneal vascularization, lacrimation, decreased vision, impaired wound healing and growth, normocytic anemia	Urinary riboflavin	
Pantothenic acid	Fatigue, malaise, headache, insomnia, vomiting, abdominal cramps	Serum pantothenic acid	
Niacin	Pellagra: dermatitis, dementia, glossitis, diarrhea, memory loss, headaches	Urinary niacin and N₁-methylnicotinamide Erythrocyte NAD and NADP concentrations to determine "niacin number"	Flushing, nausea, and vomiting seen with hyperlipidemia treatment; increased need with hemo- and peritoneal dialysis
Pyridoxine (B₆)	Pellagra, dermatitis, glossitis, cheilosis, distal limb numbness/paresthesia, convulsions, microcytic anemia	Plasma pyridoxal 5-phosphate Urinary 4-pyridoxic acid	Sensory neuropathy and seizures with very high doses (more than 2 g/day)
Folic acid	Macrocytic anemia, diarrhea, glossitis, cheilosis, angular stomatitis, fatigue, difficulty concentrating, irritability, headache, palpitations, shortness of breath, heart failure, tachycardia, postural hypotension, lactic acidosis, neural tube defects, impaired cellular immunity, paranoid behavior	Serum or plasma folate (acute) Red blood cell folate (chronic) Serum homocysteine	Decreased with increased cellular/tissue turnover (pregnancy, malignancy, hemolytic anemia); masks diagnosis of vitamin B₁₂ deficiency; decreases risks of neural tube defects
Cyanocobalamin (B₁₂)	Pernicious anemia, glossitis, spinal cord degeneration, peripheral neuropathy	Serum cobalamin Plasma homocysteine Urinary methylmalonic acid	Decreased absorption in the elderly, distal ileal resection, loss of gastric intrinsic factor by gastrectomy or long-term gastric acid suppression
Biotin	Dermatitis, depression, lassitude, somnolence	Urinary biotin	
Ascorbic acid (C)	Enlargement/keratosis of hair follicles, impaired wound healing, anemia, lethargy, depression, bleeding, ecchymosis, scurvy	Plasma ascorbic acid Leukocyte ascorbate	GI disturbances, hyperoxaluria and kidney stones, excess iron absorption with excess intake; smokers need 35 mg/day more than nonsmokers; rebound scurvy with abrupt discontinuation after long-term high doses
Fat-soluble vitamins			
Vitamin A (includes retinol, retinal, retinoic acid, and retinyl esters)	Dermatitis, night blindness, xerophthalmia, Bitot spots,ᵃ pruritus, follicular hyperkeratosis, excessive deposition of periosteal bone, hair changes, poor growth and wound healing, impaired resistance to infection Irreversible: punctate keratopathy, keratomalacia, corneal perforation	Serum retinol Serum retinol-binding protein Serum retinyl esters (toxicity)	Teratogenic, liver toxicity with excessive intake; alcohol intake, liver disease, hyperlipidemia, and severe protein malnutrition increase susceptibility to adverse effects of high intake; β-carotene supplements recommended only for those at risk of deficiency (fat malabsorption); can reverse corticosteroid-induced poor wound healing
D	Rickets, osteomalacia and osteoporosis, muscle weakness, poor growth, hypocalcemia, immune dysfunction, cardiomyopathy	Serum 25-hydroxy vitamin D	Elevated intake causes hypercalcemia, nephrocalcinosis, azotemia, poor growth; decreased in uremia, elderly (especially in winter), fat malabsorption
α-Tocopherol (E)	Hemolysis	Serum α-tocopherol Ratios of serum α-tocopherol to total lipids	Excess intake: hemorrhagic toxicity; increased risk of bleeding with anticoagulants; impaired leukocyte function
K	Bleeding (ecchymosis, petechiae, hematomas)	Prothrombin time INR	Anticoagulant therapy can be affected by supplements or diet

GI, gastrointestinal; INR, international normalized ratio; NAD, nicotinamide adenine dinucleotide; NADP, nicotinamide adenine dinucleotide phosphate.
ᵃBitot spots are spots located superficially in the conjunctiva, which are oval, triangular, or irregular in shape.
Data from references 8, 34 to 36, 50, and 51.

expensive and not widely available, diagnosis is generally made based on clinical findings and risk assessment.

CARNITINE

Carnitine is a quaternary amine required for transport of long-chain fatty acids into the mitochondria for β-oxidation and energy produc-

tion. Carnitine also binds acyl residues and helps in their elimination (detoxification), thereby decreasing the number conjugated with coenzyme A and increasing the ratio of free to acetylated coenzyme A. Carnitine is available from a wide variety of dietary sources (especially meats) and can be synthesized by the liver and kidneys from lysine and methionine. Hepatic synthesis is decreased in premature infants, and low plasma carnitine concentrations and/or overt carnitine deficiency have been documented in premature infants receiving parenteral nutrition or carnitine-free diets, as well as in those with inborn errors of metabolism.[66,67] Other predisposing factors for carnitine deficiency include chronic kidney[68] or liver disease, chronic use of valproic acid and zidovudine,[69] and a vegetarian diet. The clinical presentation of carnitine deficiency includes generalized skeletal muscle weakness, fatty liver, and fasting hypoglycemia.[66,67]

In clinical practice, carnitine status is most often assessed by measurement of plasma total and free carnitine concentrations and acylcarnitine; although tissue concentrations, especially muscle, are higher than plasma concentrations.[66,67] Plasma and urine carnitine concentrations are most helpful in primary carnitine deficiency (an inborn error of metabolism); acylcarnitine concentrations are more helpful in secondary causes of carnitine deficiency. When only total and free concentrations are available, the free is subtracted from the total to give the acylcarnitine concentration.

MUSCLE FUNCTION TESTS

Diminished skeletal muscle function can be a useful indicator of malnutrition as muscle function is an end-organ response. Muscle function also recovers more rapidly in response to initiation of nutrition support than anthropometric measurements. Hand-grip strength (forearm muscle dynamometry), respiratory muscle strength, and muscle response to electrical stimulation have been used. Measuring hand-grip strength is a relatively simple, noninvasive, and inexpensive (most hand-grip dynamometers cost less than $400) procedure that correlates with patient outcome.[70-72] Ulnar nerve stimulation causes measurable muscle contraction and is currently used in the intensive care unit to monitor the adequacy of neuromuscular blockade. In the setting of malnutrition, increased fatigue and a slowed muscle relaxation rate have been noted; these indices return to normal after refeeding. Both these parameters have the advantage of being indicators of tissue function rather than composition. Their usefulness in clinical practice is currently hampered by a lack of appropriate reference standards and limited data confirming their sensitivity and specificity for nutrition assessment.

OTHER NUTRITION ASSESSMENT TOOLS

Various methods to determine body composition have been used in the research setting. These methods generally are complex, require expensive technology, and at present are limited to research centers. One of the most promising for routine clinical practice is dual-energy x-ray absorptiometry (DXA). DXA is best known for its use in measuring bone density for the evaluation of osteoporosis, but DXA can be used to quantify the mineral, fat, and LBM compartments of the body.[73-76] DXA is available in most hospitals and many outpatient clinics. Equipment for a central DXA scan requires a fair amount of space and is expensive; that is, $40,000 to $160,000 depending on complexity of the scanner. Portable (or peripheral) DXA devices that use ultrasound and infrared interactance can be used to measure bone density in peripheral bones, such as the wrist, fingers, or heel, and have also been used to assess subcutaneous fat. These portable DXA scanners are much less expensive ($10,000–$20,000 or less) and are amenable for use in community screenings in malls, health fairs, and pharmacies. Further research is needed to determine if DXA will be useful clinically in nutrition assessment.

Magnetic resonance imaging and computed tomography can measure subcutaneous, intraabdominal, and regional fat distribution. Neutron activation is a means of measuring body nitrogen, calcium, sodium, chloride, and phosphorus. These measurements can then be used to calculate total body fat, bone, and protein. Isotope dilution methods determine TBW, and underwater weighing determines density. In addition, these methods can be used to estimate LBM and body fat because fat tissue is less dense than muscle and bone. LBM also can be estimated using total body electrical conductivity and by measuring the naturally occurring isotope ^{40}K. These techniques are used primarily in research and seldom in clinical practice.

ASSESSMENT OF NUTRIENT REQUIREMENTS

8 Nutrition requirements depend on an individual's clinical condition and the need for continued maintenance of adequate nutrition or whether starvation or ongoing metabolic stress dictates a need for repletion. For obese patients, usual nutrition requirements may be altered because of the need for weight loss. In children, there is the added consideration of sustaining or reestablishing normal growth and development. Organ function (e.g., intestine, kidney, liver, and pancreas) may affect nutrient utilization.

Nutrient requirements vary with age, gender, size, disease state, clinical condition, nutrition status, and physical activity. An estimate of nutrient requirements must be made using guidelines interpreted in the context of these patient-specific factors. The Recommended Dietary Allowances (RDAs) were initially established in 1941. In the early 1990s, the Food and Nutrition Board began a significant revision of the RDAs and introduced a new family of nutrition reference values, the Dietary Reference Intakes (DRIs), in 1997.[77]

The four categories of the DRIs are Estimated Average Requirements (EARs), RDAs, Adequate Intakes (AIs), and Tolerable Upper Intake Levels (ULs). EARs can be used for planning nutrient intakes for groups, as they are defined as the amount of the nutrient that meets the needs of 50% of persons in a given group or population. The RDA is designated as the nutrient intake that meets the needs of almost all persons in the designated group. The RDA is approximately 2 standard deviations above the EAR for nutrients for which the requirement is well defined, and 1.2 times the EAR for other nutrients. To evaluate an individual's daily intake, the RDA is the most appropriate comparator. AIs are defined as the average intake for the designated group that appears to sustain a particular nutrition state, growth, or other functional indication of health. This category is reserved for nutrients for which no EAR or RDA has been determined. Finally, the UL is the maximum nutrient intake that is unlikely to pose adverse effects in almost all persons in a designated group.[77]

DRIs have been established for six of the seven established nutrient groups: calcium, phosphorus, magnesium, vitamin D, and fluoride; folate and other B vitamins; antioxidants (e.g., selenium and vitamins C and E); trace elements; macronutrients (e.g., protein, fat, carbohydrates, and fiber); and electrolytes and water.[77] Recommendations for group seven, which includes other food components (e.g., phytoestrogens), are still in development. Due to the increased prevalence of vitamin D deficiency, the calcium and vitamin D recommendations are being reassessed. The United States Department of Agriculture's Website includes an Interactive DRI for Healthcare Professionals which easily calculates a generally healthy individual's nutrition needs based on the DRIs.[78]

ENERGY

According to the DRIs, adults should consume 45% to 65% of their total calories as carbohydrates, 20% to 35% as fat, and 10% to 35% as protein.[62] The recommendations for children are similar: carbohydrate, 45% to 65%; fat, 30% to 40%; and, protein, 10% to 30%. Infants, especially premature infants, need a higher proportion of fat (approximately 40%–50% of total calories) in their diets to ensure normal neurologic development. The RDA for total daily carbohydrates for adults and children is 130 g.[62]

TABLE 149-8 Dietary Reference Intakes for Energy and Protein in Healthy Children

Age (Reference Age/Weight)	Estimated Energy Requirement (kcal/day)[a] Boy	Estimated Energy Requirement (kcal/day)[a] Girl	Protein RDA (g/kg/day)[b]
0–6 months (3 months/6 kg)	570	520	1.52[c]
7–12 months (9 months/9 kg)	743	676	1.5
1–2 years (24 months/12 kg)	1,046	992	
1–3 years (24 months/12 kg)			1.1
3–8 years (6 years/20 kg)	1,742	1,642	
4–8 years (6 years/20 kg)			0.95
9–13 years (11 years/M: 36 kg; W: 37 kg)	2,279	2,071	0.95
14–18 years (16 years/M: 61 kg; W: 54 kg)	3,152	2,368	0.85

M, men; RDA, recommended dietary allowance; W, women.

[a]One kcal/day is approximately 4.19 kJ/day.

[b]Protein requirements in metabolically stressed children increase by 50% or more.

[c]Adequate Intake (AI).

Data from reference 62.

Estimating Energy Expenditure

An individual's total daily energy expenditure depends on the basal energy expenditure (BEE), the energy used for substrate metabolism, and energy used for physical activity. More than 200 methods for determining an individual's total energy or calorie (kcal) requirement have been published. The most commonly used methods to determine energy requirements use population estimates of calories per kilogram of body weight (kcal/kg), equations that estimate an individual's energy expenditure, or indirect calorimetry. The corresponding SI unit is kilojoule per kilogram of body weight (kJ/kg) where 1 kcal/kg is equivalent to 4.186 kJ/kg. The simplest method to assess energy requirements is to use population estimates of calories required per kilogram of body weight. This method assumes standard values for the energy requirements associated with various disease states or clinical conditions, as well as the additional requirements for repletion of a malnourished individual. It does not take into consideration age- or gender-related differences in energy needs. Daily adult requirements determined by this method are accepted to be[2,79]:

Healthy/normal nutrition status/minimal illness severity: 20 to 25 kcal ABW/kg/day (84–105 kJ ABW/kg/day)

Illness, metabolic stress (BMI <30 kg/m²): 25 to 30 kcal ABW/kg/day (105–126 kJ ABW/kg/day)

Illness, metabolic stress (BMI ≥30 kg/m²): 11 to 14 kcal ABW/kg/day or 22 to 25 kcal IBW/kg/day (92–105 kJ ABW/kg/day)

Major burn injury (≥50% total body surface area) or repletion: ≥30 kcal ABW/kg/day (≥126 kJ ABW/kg/day)[80]

Table 149-8 shows suggested calorie intakes for maintenance and normal growth of healthy infants and children.[62] For children, these maintenance energy requirements are approximately 150% of basal metabolic rate, with the additional calories needed to support activity and growth. Caloric requirements increase with fever, sepsis, major surgery, trauma, burns, and long-term growth failure, and in the presence of chronic conditions such as bronchopulmonary dysplasia, congenital heart disease, and cystic fibrosis. Energy needs may decrease with obesity and neurologic disability (e.g., cerebral palsy).[20] Close monitoring and appropriate clinical decisions are essential to ensure that the desired nutrition therapy outcomes are attained.

Various equations are used to estimate energy needs of adults and children (see Table 149-9). The Harris-Benedict equations which were derived in 1919 based on a study of 239 individuals are still a

TABLE 149-9 Equations to Estimate Energy Expenditure in Adults and Children[a]

Adults

Harris-Benedict[b] (kcal/day)[c]

Men: BEE = 66 + [(13.7W(kg)] + [5H(cm)] − (6.8A)

Women: BEE = 655 + [(9.6W(kg)] + [1.8H(cm)] − (4.7A)

DRI equations (kcal/day)[c]

Men: EER = 662 − 9.53A + (PA × 15.91W) + 539.6H(m)

Women: EER = 354 − 6.91A + (PA × 9.36W) + 726H(m)

PA = 1 if sedentary; 1.12 if low active; 1.27 if active; and 1.45 if very active.

Children

FAO/WHO/UNU (kcal/day)[c]

0–3 years of age

  Boys: BMR = 60.9W − 54

  Girls: BMR = 61W − 51

4–10 years of age

  Boys: BMR = 22.7W + 495

  Girls: BMR = 22.5W + 499

11–18 years of age

  Boys: BMR = 17.5W + 651

  Girls: BMR = 12.2W + 746

DRI equations (kcal/day)

Birth through 2 years of age

  EER = (89W − 100) + GF

  GF = 175 kcal if 0–3 months; 56 kcal if 4–6 months; 22 kcal if 7–12 months; 20 kcal if 13–35 months

3–18 years of age

  Boys: EER = 88.5 - (61.9A) + PA [26.7W + 903H(m)] + GF

  Girls: EER = 135.3 - (30.8A) + PA [10W + 934H(m)] + GF

  GF = 20 kcal if 3–8 years; 25 kcal if 9–18 years.

  PA = 1 if sedentary; 1.13–1.16 if low activity; 1.26–1.31 if normal activity; and 1.42–1.56 if very active

A, age in years; BEE, basal energy expenditure; BMR, basal metabolic rate; DRI, Dietary Reference Intakes; EER, estimated energy requirement; FAO/WHO/UNU, Food and Agriculture Organization/World Health Organization/United Nations University; GF, growth factor, H, height in centimeters (cm) or meters (m), as indicated; PA, physical activity factor; W, weight in kilograms.

[a]No real consensus exists as to which formula is best in all situations. Many clinicians use more than one equation and calculate a range of acceptable intakes.

[b]The common practice of using an adjusted body weight for obesity in these calculations is not supported by the original data which used actual body weight in all cases up to a BMI of 56 kg/m² in men and 40 kg/m² in women.[64]

[c]One kcal/day is equivalent to 4.19 kJ/day.

Data from references 2, 62, 64, 79, and 81.

popular means for assessing energy requirements in adults. They have the advantage of taking into consideration the patient's age, height, weight, gender, and clinical condition. These equations were derived from oxygen (O_2) consumption measurements made on normally nourished healthy individuals who were in a fasting and resting state. Although these equations are commonly referred to as the "BEE equations," they actually estimate resting energy expenditure (REE), the amount of energy expended at rest by a fasting, awake individual in a temperature-controlled environment performing only basal functions such as breathing, circulation, and metabolic processes.

Because these equations approximate REE, their results must be modified by a factor that is most representative of the individual's clinical condition. For example, an individual who is confined to bed may require a calorie intake that is only 20% to 30% above the REE; whereas a person who is suffering from a severe burn injury may require 150% to 200% of the calculated REE. Some clinicians multiply the calculated REE by both a stress factor and an activity factor. Because validation studies in healthy subjects have shown that these equations overestimate REE by 6% to 15%, the calculated REE should be multiplied by either a stress factor or an activity factor to avoid further overestimation of the individual's energy needs.[2] It should also be noted that ABW (up to a BMI of 57 kg/m² in men and 40 kg/m² in women), not IBW or adjusted IBW, was

TABLE 149-10 Stress Factors for Use in Children and Adults

Condition	Factor
No stress	
Confined to bed	1.2
Out of bed: normal activity	1.3
Catch-up growth	1.5
Mild stress[a]	
Postoperative recovery: uncomplicated surgery	1–1.15
Trauma: mild (e.g., long-bone fracture)	1.2
Moderate stress[a]	
Sepsis (moderate)	1.2–1.4
Trauma: central nervous system (sedated)	1.3
Trauma: moderate to severe	Children: 1.5
	Adults: 1.3–1.4
Severe stress[a]	
Sepsis (severe)	Children: 1.6
	Adults: 1.3
Trauma: central nervous system (severe)	Children: up to 2.0
	Adults: up to 1.3
Burns (proportionate to burned area)[b]	Up to 2.0

[a]Implies decreased activity during period of stress.

[b]Formulas specifically for estimating energy needs in burned children and adults have been published and are likely more accurate. See reference 80.

Data from references 2 and 82

used to generate the original data with these equations.[64] The metabolic response to stress in children appears to be similar to that seen in critically ill adults, and the "stress factors" used in adults, shown in Table 149–10, can be used in children once the REE has been determined using one of the equations shown in Table 149–9. Controversy exists over the accuracy and reliability of predicting energy expenditure based on these equations because clinical judgments of stress or activity level will vary between clinicians and the variability of the Harris-Benedict equations in predicting BEE is well documented.[64,81]

CLINICAL CONTROVERSY

Numerous equations and "stress" factors have been published for estimating energy requirements, but none has been shown to be superior in all situations. Measuring energy expenditure with indirect calorimetry is more accurate, especially for the obese, stressed, and mechanically ventilated patient, but it is neither appropriate nor available for all patients. Regardless of the method chosen, recognition that it is only an estimate and careful monitoring of the response to nutrition intervention are imperative.

Measuring Energy Expenditure

The most accurate method to determine energy expenditure, especially in acutely ill or obese patients, is to measure it using indirect calorimetry, also referred to as metabolic gas monitoring. Indirect calorimetry methodology is based on the fact that when substrates (carbohydrates, fat, and protein) are oxidized, O_2 is consumed and carbon dioxide (CO_2) is produced in varying amounts depending on the substrate being oxidized. Indirect calorimetry is a noninvasive procedure where oxygen consumption (VO_2, mL/min) and carbon dioxide production (VCO_2, mL/min) are measured, and the measured resting energy expenditure (MREE; kcal/day) is calculated using the abbreviated Weir equation as MREE = [(3.94 VO_2 + 1.11 VCO_2) + (2.17 uN_2] × 1.44.[82–85] The urinary nitrogen component (uN_2) is often excluded when calculating energy expenditure because

it accounts for less than 4% of the energy expenditure in critically ill patients and thus results in only a 1% to 2% error in calculation. Excluding the nitrogen component obviates the need for a 24-hour urine collection which can be problematic in many patients.[82,83]

MREE represents the total energy expended by the patient during the time period over which the measurements were taken. It is often extrapolated to a 24-hour period to approximate daily energy requirements. MREE reflects alterations in energy requirements as a result of disease or clinical condition, but it does not include energy required for nutritional repletion of a malnourished individual or growth in a child. The energy intake required for these functions is accounted for by multiplying MREE by a metabolic or activity factor: mechanically ventilated, critically ill, 1; critically ill, no mechanical ventilation, 1 to 1.1; adult acute noncritically ill, 1.1 to 1.4, depending on activity; adult needing repletion or a child, 1.3 to 2; adult outpatient, 1.1 to 2, depending on activity; and adult depletion (weight loss), less than 1.[85]

The data obtained from indirect calorimetry also can be used to determine the RQ, which reflects substrate oxidation, characterizes substrate use, and is calculated as VCO_2/VO_2. RQ values for nutrient substrates are fat, 0.7; carbohydrate, 1; protein, 0.8; and mixed substrate (fat, carbohydrate, and protein), 0.85. RQ values of greater than 1 represent either lipogenesis or hyperventilation; less than 0.7 may indicate a ketogenic diet, fat gluconeogenesis, or ethanol oxidation. Values outside the physiologic range of 0.67 to 1.3 should raise doubts as to the test's validity. Clinically, the RQ is used to determine if a patient is being overfed, which is likely if the RQ value is greater than 1.

There are limitations to the use of indirect calorimetry.[64,82–85] Not all institutions have metabolic carts available or personnel trained to use them. Calibration errors are common, and indirect calorimetry overestimates REE for patients with hyperventilation, metabolic acidosis, overfeeding, and air leaks anywhere in the system. Underestimation of REE is likely with hypoventilation, metabolic alkalosis, underfeeding, and gluconeogenesis. Mechanically ventilated patients are technically easier to study because the indirect calorimeter circuit can be integrated into the ventilator circuit. The patient must be at complete rest for 1 hour, must not receive bolus feedings either by feeding tube or orally for 4 hours, should have no changes in substrate delivery for 12 hours, must be on a fraction of inspired O_2 of less than 0.6, and the positive end-expiratory pressure must be less than 5 cm H_2O to ensure a steady-state reading. Unfortunately, many of the patients in whom indirect calorimetry would be most useful will not meet these requirements. Indirect calorimetry should be considered in obese patients (BMI >30 kg/m²); patients who are metabolically stressed; patients receiving mechanical ventilation, continuous sedatives or paralytics, or dialysis; and patients with HIV infection.[79,83] In the outpatient setting, less expensive, portable devices have allowed an increase in the use of indirect calorimetry for weight management, including both weight loss and weight gain.[86]

CLINICAL CONTROVERSY

Clinicians continue to debate whether an individual's energy requirements should be expressed as total or nonprotein calories. Proponents of nonprotein calories argue that sufficient energy must be provided from nonprotein sources (dextrose and fat) to spare protein from conversion to energy to be used for wound healing and LBM maintenance. Supporters of total calories state that the nonprotein calorie approach overestimates energy needs because 15% of daily energy expenditure is derived from protein breakdown. Regardless of the method chosen, the practitioner should consistently document which method was used.

PROTEIN

Daily protein requirements are based on age, gender, nutrition status, disease state, and clinical condition. Table 149–8 lists the RDA for protein for children; for individuals older than 18 years of age, the RDA is 0.8 g/kg/day, which is significantly less than most Americans typically consume.[62] In adults older than 60 years of age, protein needs are increased to 1 to 1.5 g/kg/day to help reduce loss of LBM that occurs with aging, and 1.5 to 2 g/kg/day may be needed in states of metabolic stress, such as infection, trauma, and surgery, to prevent loss of LBM.[62,79,87] Protein requirements are also higher in pregnant and lactating women (1.1 g/kg/day or 6–10 g protein per day above the usual RDA).[62,88]

Protein metabolism depends on both kidney and liver function; thus protein requirements are altered with kidney or liver dysfunction (see Chap. 153). Critical illness (e.g., sepsis, burns, or trauma) results in a hypercatabolic state in which there is increased protein synthesis and degradation. Consequently, protein requirements are increased to 1.2 to 2 g/kg/day. For critically ill obese patients, protein needs are 2 g/kg IBW or more if the BMI is 30 to 40 kg/m^2 and 2.5 g/kg IBW or more if the BMI is greater than 40 kg/m^2.[79] In burned patients, protein requirements may be 2.5 to 3 g/kg/day or more or 20% to 25% of total calories in children.[80] Liver failure typically results in the need for protein restriction (0.5 g/kg/day) except if a hypercatabolic state is also present, in which case the requirement may be increased to 1.5 g/kg/day. Protein needs in kidney failure are variable and affected by the various kidney replacement therapies available. The application of these guidelines requires both clinical judgment and frequent monitoring of kidney and liver function, serum chemistries, clinical condition, and nutrition outcomes.

Nitrogen is found only in protein and at a relatively constant ratio of 1 g nitrogen per 6.25 g protein. This ratio may vary somewhat for enteral and parenteral feeding formulations, depending on the biologic value of the protein source. Adequacy of protein intake can be assessed clinically by a nitrogen balance study—measuring urinary nitrogen excretion and comparing it with nitrogen intake. Nitrogen balance indirectly reflects an individual's protein use or protein catabolic rate, which increases with hypercatabolism. As the stress level increases, a concomitant increase in protein catabolism results in an increase in urinary nitrogen excretion. Usually the amount of urea nitrogen is measured in a 24-hour urine urea collection. In healthy individuals, urine urea nitrogen accounts for 80% to 90% of the total urine nitrogen excreted. Nitrogen output (g/day) can be approximated as 24-hour urine urea nitrogen + 4, where 4 is a factor representing usual skin, fecal, and respiratory nitrogen losses. Alternatively, if available, total urine nitrogen can be measured and may be more accurate, especially in critically ill patients. If total urine nitrogen is used, then the best estimate of nitrogen output is total urine nitrogen × 1.05.[89] In patients with kidney failure, in which case neither urine urea nitrogen nor total urine nitrogen accurately represents net protein degradation, nitrogen balance can be approximated with equations based on urea nitrogen appearance.[90]

FAT

The daily adequate intake (AI) for men and women for α-linolenic acid is 1.6 and 1.1 g, respectively; for linoleic acid, it is 14 to 17 g/day for men and 11 to 12 g/day for women.[62] Overall, for adults, fat should represent no more than 10% to 35% of total calories, with the recommendation that saturated fatty acids, *trans* fatty acids, and dietary cholesterol intake be kept as low as possible while consuming a nutritionally adequate diet. Fat should constitute 30% to 40% of energy in children 1 to 3 years of age and 25% to 35% of energy in children 4 to 18 years of age. Fat intake in children younger than 3 years of age is critical for proper central nervous system growth and development; generally, fat-restricted diets (e.g., skim milk) should not be imposed until after the age of 2 to 3 years except under strict medical supervision. A lower limit of 15% of total energy intake has been suggested as the minimum fat intake in children, when fat restriction is warranted.[91]

FIBER

Maintenance of normal bowel habits, lower blood pressure, and lower serum cholesterol concentrations has been attributed to dietary fiber intake. Fiber intake may also have a role in the prevention of colon cancer and may promote weight control through its effect on satiety. Men and women 50 years of age and younger should ingest 38 g/day and 25 to 26 g/day, respectively, of total fiber. For men and women older than 50 years of age, the recommended intakes are 30 g/day and 21 g/day, respectively.[62,92] An adequate intake for fiber has not been set for children younger than 1 year of age. For other children, the recommended fiber intake is 19 g/day for children 1 to 3 years of age, 24 g/day for children 4 to 8 g/day, and 26 to 31 g/day for children 9 to 13 years of age.[62] Another method to determine fiber need in children is the "age + 5" rule. The recommended daily intake of fiber is calculated by adding 5 g to the child's age in years.[93] Using this rule, a 6-year-old child should ingest 11 g/day of dietary fiber.

FLUID

The daily fluid requirement for an adult depends on many factors but is generally estimated to be 30 to 35 mL/kg, 1 mL for each kcal (or per every 4.19 kJ) ingested, or 1,500 mL/m^2. Fluid requirements per kilogram of body weight are higher for children and even higher for preterm infants because of their higher percentage of TBW and basal energy needs. Additionally, premature neonates have increased fluid requirements because of greater insensible losses and the kidney's inefficiency in concentrating urine. The Holliday-Segar method is a commonly employed, quick, and simple method for estimating minimum daily fluid needs of children that also can be applied to adults. Children who weigh less than 10 kg should receive at least 100 mL/kg per day. An additional 50 mL/kg/day should be provided for each kilogram of body weight between 11 kg and 20 kg, and 20 mL/kg/day for each kilogram above 20 kg. Thus daily fluid needs for a child weighing 8 kg would be at least 800 mL/day, whereas at least 1,350 mL/day would be needed for a 17-kg child.

Table 149–11 lists factors that alter fluid needs for both adults and children. All sources of fluid intake should be assessed (e.g., fluid vehicles for intravenous medications and intravenous or feeding tube

TABLE 149-11 Factors That Alter Fluid Requirements	
Increased Requirements	**Decreased Requirements**
Fever	Fluid overload
Radiant warmers	Cardiac failure
Diuretics	Decreased urinary output
Vomiting	Heat shields
Nasogastric suction	Relatively high humidity
Ostomy/fistula drainage	Humidified air via endotracheal tube
Diarrhea	Kidney failure
Glycosuria	Hypoalbuminemia with starvation
Phototherapy	Syndrome of inappropriate secretion
Diabetes insipidus	of antidiuretic hormone (SIADH)
Increased ambient temperatures	
Hyperventilation	
Prematurity	
Excessive sweating	
Increased metabolism (e.g., hyperthyroidism)	

TABLE 149-12 Recommended Daily Electrolytes, Trace Elements, and Vitamins Intakes[a]

Nutrient	Adult (≥19 years of age)		Pediatric	
	Enteral	*Parenteral*	*Enteral*	*Parenteral*
Electrolytes and minerals				
Acetate[b]	—	—	—	—
Calcium	1,000–1,200 mg	0–15 mEq (0-7.5 mmol)	0–12 months: 210–270 mg 1–3 years: 500 mg 4–8 years: 800 mg 9–18 years: 1,300 mg	Premature: 2–4 mEq/kg (1–2 mmol/kg) Other: 1–2.5 mEq/kg (0.5–1.25 mmol/kg)
Chloride[b]		—	—	2–6 mEq/kg (1–3 mmol/kg)
Magnesium	M: 400–420 mg W: 310–320 mg	10–20 mEq (5–10 mmol)	0–6 months: 30 mg 7–12 months: 75 mg 1–3 years: 80 mg 4–8 years: 130 mg 9–18 years: 240–410 mg	0.25–1 mEq/kg (0.12–0.5 mmol/kg)
Phosphorus	700 mg	20–45 mmol	0–6 months: 100 mg 7–12 months: 275 mg 1–8 years: 460–500 mg 9–18 years: 1,250 mg	Premature: 1–2 mmol/kg Others: 0.5–1 mmol/kg
Potassium[cd]	4,700 mg	60–100 mEq (60-100 mmol) (1–2 mEq/kg [1-2 mmol/kg])	0–6 months: 400 mg 7–12 months: 700 mg 1–8 years: 3,000–3,800 mg 9–18 years: 4,500–4,700 mg	2–5 mEq/kg (2–5 mmol/kg)
Sodium[cd]	1,200–1,500 mg	60–100 mEq (60-100 mmol) (1–2 mEq/kg [1-2 mmol/kg])	0–6 months: 120 mg 7–12 months: 370 mg 1–8 years: 1,000–1,200 mg 9–18 years: 1,500 mg	2–6 mEq/kg (2–6 mmol/kg)
Trace elements				
Chromium[e] (mcg)	20–35	10–15	0–6 months: 0.2 7–12 months: 5.5 1–8 years: 11–15 9–18 years: 21–35	0.14–0.2 mcg/kg (max 5 mcg)
Copper[f] (mcg)	900	0.3–1.5	0–12 months: 200–220 1–8 years: 340–440 9–18 years: 700–890	20 mcg/kg (max 300 mcg)
Fluoride	3–4 mg	—	0–6 months: 0.01 mg 7–12 months: 0.5 mg 1–8 years: 0.7–1 mg 9–18 years: 2–3 mg	—
Iodine[g] (mcg)	150	70–140 (not well defined)	0–12 months: 110–130 1–8 years: 90 9–18 years: 120–150	1 mcg/kg
Iron (mg)	M: 8 W (≤50 years): 18 W (>50 years): 8	Varies	0–6 months: 0.27 7 months–8 years: 7–11 M (9–18 years): 8–11 F (9–13): 8 F (14–18): 15	Varies
Manganese[f] (mg)	1.8–2.3	0.15–1	0–6 months: 0.003 7–12 months: 0.6 1–8 years: 1.2–1.5 9–18 years: 1.6–2.2	1 mcg/kg (max 50 mcg)
Molybdenum (mcg)	45	100–200	0–12 months: 2–3 1–8 years: 17–22 9–18 years: 34–43	0.25 mcg/kg (max 5 mcg)
Selenium (mcg)	55	20–60	0–12 months: 15–20 1–8 years: 20–30 9–18 years: 40–55	1.5–3 mcg/kg (max 30 mcg)
Zinc[b] (mg)	8–11	2.5–5	0–12 months: 2–3 1–8 years: 3–5 9–18 years: 8–11	Premature: 300–400 mcg/kg Other: 50–250 mcg/kg
Vitamins				
Ascorbic acid (mg) (Vitamin C)	75–90	100	0–12 months: 40–50 1–8 years: 15–25 9–18 years: 45–75	80
Biotin (mcg)	30	60	0–12 months: 5–6 1–8 years: 8–12 9–18 years: 20–25	20

(continued)

TABLE 149-12 Recommended Daily Electrolytes, Trace Elements, and Vitamins Intakes[a] (continued)

	Adult (≥19 years of age)		Pediatric	
Nutrient	*Enteral*	*Parenteral*	*Enteral*	*Parenteral*
Cobalamin (mcg) (Vitamin B$_{12}$)	2.4	5	0–12 months: 0.4–0.5 1–8 years: 0.9–1.2 9–18 years: 1.8–2.4	1
Folic acid (mcg)	400	400	0–12 months: 65–80 1–8 years: 150–200 9–18 years: 300–400	140
Niacin (mg NE)	14–16	40	0–12 months: 2–4 1–8 years: 6–8 9–18 years: 12–16	17
Pantothenic acid (mg)	5	15	0–12 months: 1.7–1.8 1–8 years: 2–3 9–18 years: 4–5	5
Pyridoxine (mg) (Vitamin B$_6$)	1.3–1.7	4	0–12 months: 0.1–0.3 1–8 years: 0.5–0.6 9–18 years: 1–1.3	1
Riboflavin (mg)	1.1–1.3	3.6	0–12 months: 0.3–0.4 1–8 years: 0.5–0.6 9–18 years: 0.9–1.3	1.4
Thiamin (mg)	1.1–1.2	3	0–12 months: 0.2–0.3 1–8 years: 0.5–0.6 9–18 years: 0.9–1.2	1.2
Vitamin A (mcg RE) (Retinol)	700–900	600–1,000 (3,300–5,500 international units)	0–12 months: 400–500 1–8 years: 300–400 9–18 years: 600–900	700 (2,300 international units)
Vitamin D^i (mcg)	≤50 years: 5 (200 IU) 51–70 years: 10 (400 international units) >70 years: 15 (600 international units)	5 (200 international units)	All ages: 5 (200 international units)	5–10 (200–400 international units)
Vitamin E (mg TE) (α-tocopherol)	15 (15 international units)	10 (10 international units)	0–12 months: 4–5 (4–5 international units) 1–8 years: 6–7 9–18 years: 11–15	7 (7 international units)
Vitamin K (mcg)	90–120	0.7–2.5 mg	0–12 months: 2–2.5 1–8 years: 30–55 9–18 years: 60–75	200

M, men; NE, niacin equivalents; RE, retinol equivalents; TE, tocopherol equivalent; W, women.

[a]Data represent either the recommended dietary allowance (RDA) or the adequate intake (AI) for each nutrient where established.

[b]Not established; as needed to maintain acid–base balance.

[c]Newborns and low-birth-weight or very-low-birth-weight infants or with concomitant disease (e.g., necrotizing enterocolitis) may have higher requirements. Intake in nonhealthy children must be individualized.

[d]No recommended dietary allowance or adequate intake has been established.

[e]An additional 20 mcg/day is recommended in patients with significant intestinal losses.

[f]May accumulate in cholestasis

[g]Long-term parenteral nutrition only if no topical preparations containing iodide or iodized table salt are used.

[h]Additional intake needed with small bowel losses which can be 12.2 mg zinc/L or 17.1 mg zinc/kg of stool or ileostomy output; an additional 2 mg/day needed for acute catabolic stress.

[i]Data suggest that intakes should be higher; currently being reviewed.

Data from references 34, 35, 37, 50, 51, and 94.

flushes) when determining fluid requirements. Monitoring of urine output and specific gravity as well as serum electrolytes and weight changes can be used to assess fluid status. A urine output of at least 1 mL/kg/hour (in children) and approximately 40 to 50 mL/hour (in adults) is considered adequate to ensure tissue perfusion. Urine output should be higher if large fluid volumes or high renal solute loads (e.g., parenteral nutrition or concentrated enteral feeding formulations) are being administered. Urine specific gravity depends on the kidney's concentrating and diluting capabilities. Concomitant diuretic therapy, as a result of increased solute excretion, limits the usefulness of urine specific gravity as an index of fluid status.

MICRONUTRIENTS

Requirements for micronutrients (e.g., electrolytes, trace elements, and vitamins) vary with age, gender, and the route by which the nutrient is ingested (Table 149–12; see Chaps. 58 to 60).[34–37,50,51,94]

The variability between oral and parenteral requirements is a result of bioavailability considerations. Micronutrients poorly absorbed via the GI tract usually are required in greater doses enterally than parenterally. However, many water-soluble micronutrients are excreted more rapidly via the kidneys when administered intravenously. In these situations, the intravenous dose is greater than the oral dose. Other factors that affect micronutrient requirements include GI losses through diarrhea, vomiting, or high-output fistula; wound healing; and hyper-metabolism/catabolism. Cutaneous micronutrient losses (e.g., zinc, copper, and selenium) also may be significant after major burn injury. Sodium, potassium, magnesium, and phosphorus excretion are particularly dependent on kidney function, and in the setting of kidney failure, intake will likely need to be restricted. Calcium needs, on the other hand, may be increased in these patients. (See Chaps. 51 and 53.) Patients who are severely malnourished will have increased electrolyte requirements during early refeeding owing to preexisting deficiencies and/

or rapid intracellular uptake with anabolism. Failure to provide adequate electrolytes during refeeding has resulted in death from the refeeding syndrome.[95]

DRUG–NUTRIENT INTERACTIONS

9 Drug-induced nutrient deficiency, poor therapeutic response, enhanced drug toxicity, and failure to achieve desired nutrition outcomes can occur if either nutrition support or drug therapy is stopped as a consequence of adverse effects.[96-100] Patient outcomes may be enhanced when an effective screening method to identify significant drug–nutrient interactions is coupled with a patient-counseling program. An important part of the screening process is to recognize risk factors that influence drug–nutrient interactions. The potential for drug–nutrient interactions is greatest in pediatric and elderly individuals, those with poor nutrition status (obesity and marasmus), those receiving multiple drug therapies, and those receiving tube feedings.

Mineral and electrolyte serum concentrations may change because of drug therapy. For example, with loop diuretics, urine sodium, potassium, calcium, and magnesium wasting may occur, causing a reduction in their respective serum concentrations (see Chaps. 58 to 60). Alternatively, calcium excretion is reduced with thiazide diuretics. Serum electrolyte concentrations also may increase as a direct result of the drug's mechanism (e.g., potassium-sparing diuretics) or because of the drug's salt form. Corticosteroids and cyclosporine are known to cause hyperglycemia, whereas other drugs are prescribed to pharmacologically lower blood glucose concentrations, for example, insulin and oral hypoglycemics (see Chap. 83).

Vitamin status also may be affected by drugs (Table 149–13). For example, sulfasalazine therapy causes a decrease in folic acid, isoniazid therapy causes pyridoxine deficiency, and furosemide therapy may result in decreased thiamin concentrations. Drug therapy outcomes also may be affected by vitamin intake. The ingestion of high doses of folic acid may decrease methotrexate's therapeutic effect, whereas changes in an individual's usual vitamin K or vitamin E intake may cause variability in warfarin's anticoagulant effects.

Drug-delivery vehicles also may contain nutrients. Most intravenous therapies (maintenance intravenous fluids, drugs, and electrolyte replacements) are delivered using either dextrose (e.g., dextrose 5% or 10% in water) or sodium (e.g., 0.9% normal saline) in the admixture. Lipid emulsion (10%) is used as the vehicle for the anesthetic agent propofol and the intravenous calcium channel blocker clevidipine and will contribute fat calories when continuous infusions are used. In these instances, nutrition support regimens must be adjusted to accommodate the calories and other nutrients delivered through these therapies.

PRACTICAL GUIDELINES FOR NUTRITION ASSESSMENT

10 The value of any given marker used for nutrition assessment is only as great as its ability to accurately identify the patient with malnutrition and to correlate with malnutrition-associated complications. Most of the currently available markers of nutrition status were first used in epidemiologic studies to define large populations suffering from malnutrition caused by famine. The response of the various nutrition status markers to nutrition therapy and the correlation between improvement in these markers and decreased morbidity and mortality further support their validity. However, when applied to an individual, most of these markers lack specificity and sensitivity, which makes the development of a clinically useful,

TABLE 149-13 Drug and Vitamin Interactions

Drug	Effect
Antacids	Thiamin deficiency
Antibiotics	Vitamin K deficiency
Aspirin	Folic acid and deficiency; increased vitamin C excretion
Cathartics	Increased requirements for vitamins D, C, and B_6
Cathartics	Increased requirements for vitamins D, C, and B_6
Cholestyramine	Vitamins A, D, E, and K, β-carotene malabsorption
Colestipol	Vitamins A, D, E, and K, β-carotene malabsorption
Corticosteroids	Decreased vitamins A, D, and C
Diuretics (loop)	Thiamin deficiency
Histamine$_2$ antagonists	Vitamin B_{12} deficiency
Isoniazid	Vitamin B_6 and niacin deficiency
Isotretinoin	Vitamin A increases toxicity
Mercaptopurine	Niacin deficiency
Methotrexate	Folic acid inhibits effect
Orlistat	Vitamins A, D, E, and K malabsorption
Pentamidine	Folic acid deficiency
Phenobarbital	Vitamin D malabsorption; vitamin C affects protein binding
Phenytoin	Vitamin D malabsorption; altered vitamin C binding; effect reversed by folic acid
Primidone	Folic acid deficiency
Proton pump inhibitors	Vitamin B_{12} deficiency
Sulfasalazine	Folic acid malabsorption
Trimethoprim	Folic acid depletion
Warfarin	Vitamin K inhibits effect; vitamins A, C, and E may affect prothrombin time
Zidovudine	Folic acid and B_{12} deficiencies increase myelosuppression

cost-effective approach to individual patient nutrition assessment challenging.

The importance of the nutrition-focused history and physical examination in both nutrition screening and nutrition assessment cannot be overemphasized. The least amount of objective data that can further substantiate the clinical impression and provide a baseline for subsequent monitoring are those markers that show the best correlation with outcome: weight and serum albumin concentration. The cost-effectiveness of the addition of further biochemical parameters is yet to be determined. The assessment of other anthropometric measures is most useful in the setting of anticipated long-term nutrition support in which these measurements will serve as a longitudinal marker of an individual's response to the nutrition care plan.

Initially, nutrition requirements are determined on the basis of assumptions made about the patient's clinical condition and the nutrition needs associated with repletion or growth, if needed. Once a nutrition intervention has been initiated, periodic reassessment of nutrition status is critical to determine the accuracy of the initial estimate of nutrition requirements. Also, nutrition requirements are dynamic in the setting of acute or critical illness—as the patient's clinical status changes, so will protein and energy requirements, further emphasizing the need for continued reassessment.

Better markers of nutrition status and methods for determining patient-specific nutrition requirements are needed to allow further refinement of estimates of an individual's nutrition needs. Functional tests and simple, noninvasive tests for body composition analysis hold promise for the future. However, until better methods of assessment become available clinically and are demonstrated to be cost-effective, the currently available battery of tests will continue to be the mainstay of nutrition assessment.

Information in this chapter can be used to establish empiric goals for a nutrition care plan. However, as with other forms of therapy, continuous monitoring and reassessment are required to determine if these goals are appropriate for an individual patient.

ABBREVIATIONS

ABW: actual body weight

AI: Adequate Intake

ALB: albumin

BEE: basal energy expenditure

BIA: bioelectrical impedance analysis

BMI: body mass index

DCH: delayed cutaneous hypersensitivity

DRI: Dietary Reference Intake

DXA: dual-energy x-ray absorptiometry

EAR: Estimated Average Requirement

GI: gastrointestinal

HIV: human immunodeficiency virus

IBW: ideal body weight

LBM: lean body mass

MREE: measured resting energy expenditure

NCHS: National Center for Health Statistics

RDA: Recommended Dietary Allowance

REE: resting energy expenditure

RQ: respiratory quotient

TBW: total body water

TFN: transferrin

UBW: usual body weight

UL: Tolerable Upper Intake Level

VCO_2: carbon dioxide production

VO_2: oxygen consumption

REFERENCES

1. Kotler DP. Cachexia. Ann Intern Med 2000;133:622-634.
2. DeLegge MH, Drake LM. Nutritional assessment. Gastroenterol Clin North Am 2007;36:1-22.
3. Ogden CL, Carroll MD, Curtin LR, et al. Prevalence of overweight and obesity in the United States, 1999-2004. JAMA 2006;295:1549-1555.
4. Centers for Disease Control and Prevention. Overweight and obesity. U.S. Obesity Trends: Trends by State, 1985-2008; 2009. *http://www.cdc.gov/obesity/data/trends.html.*
5. Ogden CL, Caroll MD, Flegal KM. High body mass index for age among US children and adolescents, 2003-2006. JAMA 2008;299:2401-2405.
6. Centers for Disease Control and Prevention, National Center for Health Statistics. CDC growth charts; 2009. *http://www.cdc.gov/growthcharts/.*
7. Kondrup J, Allison SP, Elia M, et al. ESPEN guidelines for nutrition screening 2002. Clin Nutr 2003;22:415-421.
8. Russell MK, Mueller C. Nutrition screening and assessment. In: Gottschlich MM, ed. The A.S.P.E.N. Nutrition Support Core Curriculum: A Case-Based Approach—The Adult Patient. Silver Spring, MD: America Society for Parenteral and Enteral Nutrition; 2007: 163-186.
9. Soeters PB, Reijven PLM, van Bokhorst-de van der Schueren MAE, et al. A rational approach to nutritional assessment. Clin Nutr 2008;27:706-716.
10. ASPEN Board of Directors and the Clinical Guidelines Task Force. Guidelines for the use of parenteral and enteral nutrition in adult and pediatric patients. J Parenter Enteral Nutr 2002;26 (suppl 1):1SA-138SA.
11. Joint Commission on Accreditation of Healthcare Organizations. Comprehensive Accreditation Manual for Hospitals: The Official Handbook, 2010. Oakbrook Terrace, IL: Joint Commission Resources; 2009. *www.jointcommission.org.*
12. Charney P. Nutrition screening vs nutrition assessment: how do they differ? Nutr Clin Pract 2008;23:366-372.
13. Anthony PS. Nutrition screening tools for hospitalized patients. Nutr Clin Pract 2008;23:373-382.
14. Makhija S, Baker J. The subjective global assessment: a review of its use in clinical practice. Nutr Clin Pract 2008;23:405-409.
15. Keith J. Bedside nutrition assessment past, present, and future: a review of the subjective global assessment. Nutr Clin Pract 2008;23:410-416.
16. Bauer JM, Kaiser MJ, Anthony P, et al. The Mini Nutritional Assessment® - its history, today's practice, and future perspectives. Nutr Clin Pract 2008;23:388-396.
17. Hickson M, Frost G. A comparison of three methods for estimating height in the acutely ill elderly population. J Hum Nutr Diet 2003;16:13-20.
18. Bell KL, Davies PS. Prediction of height from knee height in children with cerebral palsy and non-disabled children. Ann Hum Biol 2006;33:493-499.
19. Chumlea WC, Guo SS, Steinbaugh ML. Prediction of stature from knee height for black and white adults and children with application to mobility-impaired or handicapped persons. J Am Diet Assoc 1994;94:1385-1388.
20. Marchand V, Motil KJ, and the NASPGHAN Committee on Nutrition. Nutrition support for neurologically impaired children: a clinical report of the North American Society for Pediatric Gastroenterology, Hepatology, and Nutrition. J Pediatr Gastroenterol Nutr 2006;43: 123-135.
21. Fenton TR. A new growth chart for preterm babies: Babson and Benda's chart updated with recent data and a new format. BMC Pediatrics 2003:3:13. *http://www.biomedcentral.com/1471-2431/3/13.*
22. Rao SC, Tompkins J, World Health Organization. Growth curves for preterm infants. Early Human Dev 2007;83:643-651.
23. Cronk C, Crocker AC, Pueschel SM, et al. Growth charts for children with Down syndrome: 1 month to 18 years of age. Pediatrics 1988;81:102-110.
24. Centers for Disease Control and Prevention. Body mass index; 2009. *http://www.cdc.gov/healthyweight/assessing/bmi.*
25. Cook Z, Kirk S, Lawrenson S, Sandford S. Use of BMI in the assessment of undernutrition in older subjects: reflecting on practice. Proc Nutr Soc 2005;64:313-317.
26. Ness-Abramof R, Apovian CM. Waist circumference measurement in clinical practice. Nutr Clin Pract 2008;23:397-404.
27. Klein S, Allison DB, Heymsfield SB, et al. Waist circumference and cardiometabolic risk: a consensus statement from Shaping America's Health: Association for Weight Management and Obesity Prevention; NAASO, The Obesity Society; the American Society for Nutrition; and the American Diabetes Association. Diabetes Care 2007;30: 1647-1652.
28. Maffeis C, Banzato C, Talamini G, on behalf of the Obesity Study Group of the Italian Society of Pediatric Endocrinology and Diabetology. Waist-to-height ratio, a useful index to identify high metabolic risk in overweight children. J Pediatr 2008;152:207-213.
29. Buchholz AC, Bartok C, Schoeller DA. The validity of bioelectrical impedance models in clinical populations. Nutr Clin Pract 2004;19: 433-446.
30. Willett K, Jiang R, Lenart E, et al. Comparison of bioelectrical impedance and BMI in predicting obesity-related medical conditions. Obesity (Silver Spring) 2006;14:480-490.
31. Crook MA. Hypoalbuminemia: the importance of correct interpretation. Nutrition 2009;25:1004-1005.
32. Grimble RF. Immunonutrition. Curr Opin Gastroenterol 2006;21: 216-222.
33. Kudsk KA. Immunonutrition in surgery and critical care. Annu Rev Nutr 2006;26:463-479.
34. Food and Nutrition Board, Institute of Medicine, National Academy of Sciences. Dietary Reference Intakes: Elements; 2009. *http://www.iom.edu/Home/Global/News%20Announcements/~/media/48FAAA2F D9E74D95BBDA2236E7387B49.ashx.*
35. Clark SF. Vitamins and trace elements. In: Gottschlich MM, ed. The A.S.P.E.N. Nutrition Support Core Curriculum: A Case-Based

Approach—The Adult Patient. Silver Spring, MD: America Society for Parenteral and Enteral Nutrition, 2007:129–159.

36. Sriram K, Lonchyna VA. Micronutrient supplementation in adult nutrition therapy: practical considerations. J Parenter Enteral Nutr 2009;33:548–562.

37. Kleinman RE, ed. Trace elements. In: Pediatric Nutrition Handbook, 6th ed. Elk Grove Village, IL: American Academy of Pediatrics, 2009: 423–451.

38. Lowe NM, Fekete K, Decsi T. Methods of assessment of zinc status in humans: a systematic review. Am J Clin Nutr 2009;89(suppl):2040S-2051S.

39. Hurwitz M, Garcia MG, Poole RL, Kerner JA. Copper deficiency during parenteral nutrition: a report of four pediatric cases. Nutr Clin Pract 2004;19:305–308.

40. Harvey LJ, Ashton K, Hooper L, et al. Methods of assessment of copper status in humans: a systematic review. Am J Clin Nutr 2009;89(suppl):2009S-2024S.

41. Vincent JB. Quest for the molecular mechanism of chromium action and its relationship to diabetes. Nutr Rev 2000;58:67–72.

42. Dickerson RN. Manganese intoxication and parenteral nutrition. Nutrition 2001;17:689–693.

43. Erikson KM, Thompson K, Aschner J, Aschner M. Manganese neurotoxicity: a focus on the neonate. Pharmacol Therapeut 2007;113:369–377.

44. Iinuma Y, Kubota M, Uchiyama M, et al. Whole-blood manganese levels and brain manganese accumulation in children receiving long-term home parenteral nutrition. Pediatr Surg Int 2003;19:268–272.

45. Takagi Y, Okada A, Sando K, et al. Evaluation of indexes of in vivo manganese status and the optimal intravenous dose for adult patients undergoing home parenteral nutrition. Am J Clin Nutr 2002;75:112–118.

46. Geoghegan M, McAuley D, Eaton S, Powell-Tuck J. Selenium in critical illness. Curr Opin Crit Care 2006;12:136–141.

47. Ashton K, Hooper L, Harvey LJ, et al. Methods of assessment of selenium status in humans: a systematic review. Am J Clin Nutr 2009;89(suppl):2025S-2039S.

48. Sardesai VM. Molybdenum: an essential trace element. Nutr Clin Pract 1993;8:277–281.

49. Friel JK, MacDonald AC, Mercer CN, et al. Molybdenum requirements in low-birth-weight infants receiving parenteral and enteral nutrition. J Parenter Enteral Nutr 1999;23:155–159.

50. Food and Nutrition Board, Institute of Medicine, National Academy of Sciences. Dietary Reference Intakes: Vitamins; 2009. http://www.iom.edu/Home/Global/News%20Announcements/~/media/48FAAA2FD9E74D95BBDA2236E7387B49.ashx.

51. Kleinman RE, ed. Vitamins. In: Pediatric Nutrition Handbook, 6th ed. Elk Grove Village, IL: American Academy of Pediatrics, 2009: 453–495.

52. Willett WC, Stampfer MJ. What vitamins should I be taking, doctor? N Engl J Med 2001;345:1819–1824.

53. Centers for Disease Control and Prevention. Lactic acidosis traced to thiamin deficiency related to nationwide shortage of multivitamins for total parenteral nutrition—United States, 1997. JAMA 1997;278: 109–111.

54. Allen LH. How common is vitamin B-12 deficiency? Am J Clin Nutr 2009;89(suppl):693S-696S.

55. Wagner CL, Greer FR, and the American Academy of Pediatrics Section on Breastfeeding and Committee on Nutrition. Prevention of rickets and vitamin D deficiency in infants, children, and adolescents. Pediatrics 2008;122:1142–1152.

56. Reis JR, von Mühlen D, Miller ER, et al. Vitamin D status and cardiometabolic risk factors in the United States adolescent population. Pediatrics 2009;124:e371-e379.

57. Holick MF. Vitamin D deficiency. N Engl J Med 2007;357:266–281.

58. Peskanich D, Singh V, Willett WC, Colditz GA. Vitamin A intake and hip fractures among postmenopausal women. JAMA 2002;287:47–54.

59. Michaëlsson K, Lithell H, Vessby B, Melhus H. Serum retinol levels and the risk of fracture. N Engl J Med 2003;348:287–294.

60. The Heart Outcomes Prevention Evaluation (HOPE) 2 Investigators. Homocysteine lowering with folic acid and B vitamins in vascular disease. N Engl J Med 2006;354:1567–1577.

61. Lange H, Suryapranata H, De Luca G, et al. Folate therapy and in-stent restenosis after coronary stenting. N Engl J Med 2004;350:2673–2681.

62. Food and Nutrition Board, Institute of Medicine, National Academy of Sciences. Dietary Reference Intakes for Energy, Carbohydrate, Fiber, Fat, Fatty Acids, Cholesterol, Protein, and Amino Acids; 2005. http://www.nap.edu/books/0309085373/html/R2.html.

63. Adolph M, Hailer S, Echart J. Serum phospholipid fatty acids in severely injured patients on total parenteral nutrition with medium chain/long chain triglyceride emulsions. Ann Nutr Metab 1995;39:251–260.

64. Wooley JA, Frankenfield D. Energy. In: Gottschlich MM, ed. The A.S.P.E.N. Nutrition Support Core Curriculum: A Case-Based Approach—The Adult Patient. Silver Spring, MD: American Society for Parenteral and Enteral Nutrition, 2007:19–32.

65. Foote KD, MacKinnon MJ, Innis SM. Effect of early introduction of formula versus fat-free parenteral nutrition on essential fatty acid status of preterm infants. Am J Clin Nutr 1991;54:93–97.

66. Crill CM, Helms RA. The use of carnitine in pediatric nutrition. Nutr Clin Prac 2007;22:204–213.

67. Scaglia F. Carnitine deficiencies. EMedicine.com, Inc. July 26, 2006, http://www.emedicine.com/ped/topic321.htm.

68. Schreiber B. Levocarnitine and dialysis: a review. Nutr Clin Prac 2005;20:218–243.

69. Scruggs ER, Dirks Naylor AJ. Mechanisms of zidovudine-induced mitochondrial toxicity and myopathy. Pharmacology 2008;82:83–88.

70. Schlüssel MM, dos Anjos LA, de Vasconcellos MTL, Kac G. Reference values of handgrip dynamometry of healthy adults: a population-based study. Clin Nutr 2008;27:601–607.

71. Budziareck MB, Duerte RRP, Barbosa-Silva MCG. Reference values and determinants for handgrip strength in healthy subjects. Clin Nutr 2008;27:357–362.

72. Kerr A, Syddall HE, Cooper C, et al. Does admission grip strength predict length of stay in hospitalized older patients? Age Ageing 2006;35:82–84.

73. Genton L, Hans D, Kyle UG, Pichard C. Dual-energy x-ray absorptiometry and body composition: difference between devices and comparison with reference models. Nutrition 2002;18:66–70.

74. King S, Wilson J, Kotsimbos T, et al. Body composition assessment in adults with cystic fibrosis: comparison of dual-energy x-ray absorptiometry with skinfolds and bioelectrical impedance analysis. Nutrition 2005;21:1087–1094.

75. Liu LF, Roberts R, Moyer-Mileur L, Samson-Fang L. Determination of body composition in children with cerebral palsy: bioelectrical impedance analysis and anthropometry vs dual-energy x-ray absorptiometry. J Am Diet Assoc 2005;105:794–797.

76. Steiner MC, Barton RL, Singh SJ, Morgan MDL. Bedside methods versus dual energy x-ray absorptiometry for body composition measurement in COPD. Eur Respir J 2002;19:626–631.

77. Food and Nutrition Board, Institute of Medicine, National Academy of Sciences. Dietary Reference Intakes (DRIs): The Development of DRIS 1994-2004: Lessons Learned and New Challenges; 2008. http://books.nap.edu/openbook.php?record_id=12086&page=R1.

78. United States Department of Agriculture web site. Interactive DRI for Healthcare Professionals; 2010. http://fnic.nal.usda.gov/interactiveDRI/.

79. McClave SA, Martindale RG, Vanek VW, et al. Guidelines for the provision and assessment of nutrition support therapy in the adult critically ill patient: Society of Critical Care Medicine (SCCM) and American Society for Parenteral and Enteral Nutrition (A.S.P.E.N.). J Parenter Enter Nutr 2009;33:277–316.

80. Chan MM, Chan GM. Nutrition therapy for burns in children and adults. Nutrition 2009;25:261–9.

81. Frankenfield DC, Coleman A, Alam S, Cooney RN. Analysis of estimation methods for resting metabolic rate in critically ill adults. J Parenter Enteral Nutr 2009;33:27–36.

82. Malone AM. Methods of assessing energy expenditure in the intensive care unit. Nutr Clin Pract 2002;17:21–28.

83. Haugen HA, Chan L-N, Li F. Indirect calorimetry: a practical guide for clinicians. Nutr Clin Pract 2007;22:377–388.

84. Moreira de Rocha EE, Alves VGF, da Fonseca RBV. Indirect calorimetry: methodology, instruments and clinical application. Curr Opin Clin Nutr Metab Care 2006;9:247–256.

85. Holdy KE. Monitoring energy metabolism with indirect calorimetry: instruments, interpretation, and clinical application. Nutr Clin Pract 2004;19:447–454.

86. Rubenbauer JR, Johannsen DL, Baier SM, et al. The use of a handheld calorimetry unit to estimate energy expenditure during different physiological conditions. J Parenter Enteral Nutr 2006;30:246–250.

87. Wolfe RR, Miller SL, Miller KB. Optimal protein intake in the elderly. Clin Nutr 2008;27:675–684.

88. Duggleby SL, Jackson AA. Protein, amino acid and nitrogen metabolism during pregnancy: how might the mother meet the needs of her fetus? Curr Opin Clin Nutr Metab Care 2002;5:503–509.

89. Velasco N, Long CL, Otto DA, et al. Comparison of three methods for the estimation of total nitrogen losses in hospitalized patients. J Parenter Enteral Nutr 1990;14:517–522.

90. Wolk R, Moore E, Foulks C. Renal disease. In: Gottschlich MM, ed. The A.S.P.E.N. Nutrition Support Core Curriculum: A Case-Based Approach—The Adult Patient. Silver Spring, MD: American Society for Parenteral and Enteral Nutrition, 2007:575–598.

91. Kleinman RE, ed. Fats and fatty acids. In: Pediatric Nutrition Handbook, 6th ed. Elk Grove Village, IL: American Academy of Pediatrics, 2009:357–386.

92. American Dietetic Association. Position of the American Dietetic Association: Health implications of dietary fiber. J Am Diet Assoc 2002;102:993–1000.

93. Dwyer JT. Dietary fiber for children: How much? Pediatr 1995;96:1019–1022.

94. Greene HL, Hambidge KM, Schanler R, Tsang RC. Guidelines for the use of vitamins, trace elements, calcium, magnesium, and phosphorus in infants and children receiving total parenteral nutrition: Report of the Subcommittee on Pediatric Parenteral Nutrient Requirements from the Committee on Clinical Practice Issues of the American Society for Clinical Nutrition. Am J Clin Nutr 1988;48:1324–1342.

95. Kraft MD, Btaiche IF, Sacks GS. Review of the refeeding syndrome. Nutr Clin Pract 2005;20:625–633.

96. Jefferson JW. Drug and diet interactions: Avoiding therapeutic paralysis. J Clin Psychiatry 1998;59:31–39.

97. Saito M, Hirata-Koizumi M, Matsumoto M, et al. Undesirable effects of citrus juice on the pharmacokinetics of drugs: focus on recent studies. Drug Saf 2005;28:677–694.

98. Santos CA, Boullata JI. An approach to evaluating drug-nutrient interactions. Pharmacotherapy 2005;25:1789–1800.

99. Singh BN. Effects of food on clinical pharmacokinetics. Clin Pharmacokinet 1999;37:213–255.

100. McCabe BJ. Prevention of food–drug interactions with special emphasis on older adults. Curr Opin Clin Nutr Metab Care 2004;7:21–26.

150

Medication Administration Considerations with Specialized Nutrition Support

ROLAND N. DICKERSON AND GORDON S. SACKS

KEY CONCEPTS

❶ Enteral feeding access site and tube characteristics influence which drug administration and enteral feeding techniques will be used to optimize pharmacotherapy.

❷ The drug formulation often guides the medication administration protocol for patients receiving enteral nutrition (EN).

❸ Potential physical incompatibilities of liquid, elixir, and suspension medication formulations with enteral feeding necessitate the use of alternative dosage forms, changes in the route of administration, changes in the medication administration protocol, or selection of a different medication.

❹ Many medication formulations, particularly delayed-release and enteric-coated products, should not be crushed.

❺ Gastrointestinal (GI) intolerance to liquid and suspended medication forms are usually related to either the hypertonicity or the sorbitol content of the drug product.

❻ It is important that the clinician closely evaluate every enterally administered medication for efficacy as well as toxicity for those patients receiving EN, given the particular characteristics of drug absorption, the location of the feeding tube within the GI tract, and the potential adsorption to the feeding.

❼ A critical part of evaluating parenteral nutrition (PN) medication admixtures is understanding the difference between stability and compatibility.

❽ It is important to determine if the PN is either a two-in-one or three-in-one admixture when considering adding a medication, as the presence of an intravenous (IV) lipid emulsion can markedly change the stability characteristics of the PN.

❾ IV Y-site administration of calcium, potassium phosphate, sodium phosphate, and magnesium with PN admixtures must be avoided.

The use of parenteral and enteral nutrition requires a high level of clinical expertise and careful attention to ensure that patient outcomes are optimized and that untoward events are minimized. This chapter provides a foundational framework for the identifica-

tion and management of drug–nutrient interactions associated with enteral nutrition (EN) and parenteral nutrition (PN). Issues related to EN include feeding tube access site factors, medication administration techniques, dosage form–associated physical incompatibilities, and prevention of enteral tube occlusions. The key factors associated with PN formulation and drug interactions include physiochemical issues affecting compatibility and stability, adverse events associated with trace element contamination, treatments for vascular access device occlusions, and IV lipid emulsion (IVLE)–associated risks and adverse events.

MEDICATION ADMINISTRATION CONSIDERATIONS WITH ENTERAL NUTRITION

It is usually preferable for patients who require EN that medications also be given via their feeding tube when possible. When administering medications via a feeding tube, only syringes manufactured and intended for oral or enteral use should be used to measure and administer medications. In addition, the tips of the oral syringes should be too wide to fit IV Luer ports in an effort to prevent inadvertent IV delivery of oral medications. The administration of oral medications for patients receiving continuous enteral tube feeding is problematic, as mixing enteral feeding with medications may lead to reduced drug bioavailability, tube clogging, or adverse GI effects, such as cramping and diarrhea. Parenteral administration of medications obviates the potentiality of any physical interaction with the enteral regimen; however, IV medications are usually more expensive and may be associated with venous access problems, such as infection. Alternative routes, such as buccal, sublingual, and transdermal, are available for only a limited number of medications and may not be practical for critically ill patients. Therefore, enteral administration of drugs is preferred.

ENTERAL FEEDING TUBE ACCESS SITE, TUBE CHARACTERISTICS, AND METHODS OF MEDICATION ADMINISTRATION

❶ The characteristics of the feeding tube may dictate the selection of the appropriate medication administration technique for the patient. Medications should not be administered via a needle catheter jejunostomy due to the small internal diameter and the high risk for tube clogging. Conversely, larger bore feeding tubes (e.g., 20 and 28 Fr), such as a gastrostomy or nasogastric tube, can be easily used for medication administration with minimal risk for tube clogging.

❷ Although some medications are available in ready-to-administer liquid forms, suspensions, or elixirs, the majority are not. It is necessary to consider the type of available dosage form (e.g., tablets,

TABLE 150-1 Medication Administration Guidelines for Patients Receiving Enteral Nutrition[1-5]

1. Oral administration is preferred.
2. Medications should not be added directly to the feeding formulation.
3. Immediate-release tablets should be crushed to a fine powder, or capsules should be opened and mixed with water to form a slurry.
4. Soft gelatin immediate-release capsules can be dissolved in 15 to 30 mL of warm water.
5. Flush the feeding tube with at least 15 mL of water before and after medication administration.
6. When multiple medications are to be administered at the same time, they should be given separately, with water flushes done between each medication.
7. A liquid/suspension/elixir should be diluted when administered directly into the small bowel if the medication is substantially hypertonic.
8. Sustained-release products should be replaced with a therapeutically equivalent lower dose and increased frequency of administration.
9. Alternative pharmacotherapy or a different dosage form should be considered for enteric-coated tablets.
10. When providing medications in which the absorption of the medication is significantly impaired in the presence of continuous enteral feeding, the feeding should be held for at least 1 to 2 hours before and after the dose.

capsules, suspensions, or liquids) when determining an appropriate method for medication delivery. When suitable formulations are not available, tablets may need to be crushed or pulverized to a fine powder, then mixed with water to make a slurry mixture, or powder-containing capsules must be opened and the contents administered in the same manner as with crushed tablets. Gelatinous liquid capsules may be cut in half or dissolved in warm water, then administered as a solution. Care should be taken not to administer the undissolved gelatin remnants, as they may clog the feeding tube. Suspensions tend to have a higher viscosity than solutions; some are granular and contain modified-release particles. The resistance to flow through the enteral feeding tube is greater for suspensions than liquids and may be reduced by dilution of the suspension. It is recommended that the feeding tube be irrigated with 15 to 30 mL of water before and after each medication is administered. General recommendations for administration of medications via an enteral feeding tube are given in Table 150–1.[1-5]

CONSIDERATION OF THE LOCATION OF THE TIP OF THE FEEDING TUBE FOR DRUG DELIVERY

Although the absorption of some drugs occurs throughout the GI tract, the location of the distal tip of the feeding tube may alter the bioavailability of drugs. Administration of a drug into the jejunum whose primary site of absorption is in the duodenum/early jejunum can result in a significant reduction in bioavailability (e.g., 27% to 67% decrease for ciprofloxacin[6]). Drugs that require an acidic environment for maximum absorption (e.g., ketoconazole[7] and itraconazole[8]) can have a reduced absorption when administered directly into the small bowel, bypassing the stomach. Some drugs, such as digoxin, undergo considerable metabolism within the GI tract.[9] Because postpyloric administration would avoid acid hydrolysis of digoxin, increased drug concentrations delivered to the small bowel result in improved absorption and likely explain why an increased dosage is not necessary for patients with short bowel syndrome, unlike other drugs, such as warfarin.[9-11] Finally, it would be inappropriate to administer a drug via the small bowel whose intended action is through direct administration into the stomach (e.g., antacids and sucralfate).

MEDICATION BINDING TO THE FEEDING TUBE

Some medications, such as phenytoin[12] and carbamazepine,[13] have been shown to adsorb to enteral feeding tubes in vitro, with a loss ranging from ~10% to 25% of the drug dose. Because the degree of adsorption is not linear, less drug loss would occur with higher doses. The potential effect of drug adsorption to the tubing is easily attenuated by the dilution of the liquid medication (with an equal part of water) and with adequate flushing of the tube after drug administration.[12,13]

PHYSICAL INCOMPATIBILITY OF LIQUID, ELIXIR, AND SUSPENSION MEDICATION FORMULATIONS WITH ENTERAL FEEDING

❸ Many liquid medications are physically incompatible with EN formulas, and their coadministration may lead to tube clogging.[1-5] The clogging of the enteral feeding tube is due in part to the viscosity of the medication carrier solution itself or the acidic pH of the syrup, which may result in the formation of viscous flocculent precipitates, gelatinous adhesive material, or particulate granulation. Elixirs, which contain varying amounts of alcohol, have been reported to cause tube clogging when coadministered with enteral feedings. The higher the alcohol content, the more likely the elixir is to cause precipitation of inorganic salts present in the EN product.[14] Common liquid forms of medications known to be incompatible with enteral feeding are brompheniramine elixir, calcium glubionate syrup, cimetidine oral solution, ferrous sulfate elixir, potassium chloride liquid and syrup, and pseudoephedrine syrup.[1-3] Ferrous sulfate elixir is the most frequent EN-incompatible medication encountered in clinical practice.[2] Because of the potential incompatibilities, enteral feedings and liquid medications, regardless of their formulation, should not be mixed together.[14]

CONSIDERATIONS FOR SUSTAINED-RELEASE, PH-ACTIVATED, AND ENTERIC-COATED PRODUCTS

❹ Most medications are initially marketed as immediate-release tablets; however, the number of medications that are formulated to enhance drug delivery or to improve patient compliance has increased in recent years. Some medications can be immediately identified by their suffix as pharmaceutically modified products. It is important to ascertain whether the medication is formulated as a sustained- or delayed-release, pH-activated, or enteric-coated product, as crushing destroys the properties of the medication. For sustained- and extended-release products, this can result in higher peak serum concentrations and potentially clinical toxicity as the result of the rapid release of a much larger dose. Thus, one should avoid the use of this type of formulation whenever possible in the EN patient. Switching from an extended-release product to an immediate-release (preferably liquid or suspension) formula requires that the clinician appropriately lower the dose and increase the frequency of dosing. Disregard for this pharmacotherapeutic intervention has resulted in significant adverse effects and even death.[15-17]

Enteric- and film-coated medications when crushed and administered into the stomach often yield decreased clinical effectiveness because of acid degradation. This approach has also been known to result in increased gastric mucosa irritation for some medications. Enteric- and film-coated medications in general do not crush well and tend to aggregate in clumps when wet, which increases the risk of tube clogging.[5] Results from a national survey indicated that drug-related feeding tube obstruction occurred in 11% and 16% of patients when enteric-coated or modified-release drug products, respectively, were routinely crushed.[18]

Some modified-release, microencapsulated drug products can be safely administered via large-bore feeding tubes (e.g., percutaneous endoscopic gastrostomy and nasogastric tubes). The pellets or "beads" in these formulations can be poured down the feeding tube provided that they are not crushed. Medications that have been given in this manner include diltiazem, ferrous gluconate, nizatidine, pancreatic enzymes, theophylline, and verapamil.[1] Antineoplastic drugs such as methotrexate and capecitabine should not be crushed because exposure to the dispersed aerosolized particles may be harmful to the healthcare professional.[1,19] Many medication formulations should not be crushed, and an up-to-date listing can be obtained from the Institute of Safe Medication Practices at *http://www.ismp.org/tools/donotcrush.pdf.*

PROBLEMS WITH THE USE OF LIQUID AND SUSPENDED MEDICATIONS

5 GI intolerance to liquid and suspended medication forms is usually related to either the hypertonicity or the sorbitol content of the drug product. The osmolality of GI tract secretions ranges from 280 to 360 mOsm/kg (280 to 360 mmol/kg).[2] One of the major functions of the colon is to reabsorb excess water prior to passage of the excrement from the body. When this process is impaired, diarrhea occurs. Osmotic diarrhea is the result of excessive unabsorbed substances in the GI that results in retention of water. An analytical method that may help ascertain whether diarrhea is being induced by the administration of osmotically active nonabsorbable substances from the medication is to measure and calculate the stool osmotic gap. This technique involves obtaining a liquid stool sample for sodium (Na) concentration, potassium (K) concentration, and osmolality. The stool osmotic gap is then calculated using the following formula:

$$\text{Osmotic gap (mOsm/kg or mmol/kg)} = \text{Stool osmolality} \\ \text{(mOsm/kg or mmol/kg)} - 2 \times \text{(stool Na [mEq/L or mmol/L]} + \\ \text{stool K [mEq/L or mmol/l])}$$

For patients with secretory diarrhea (intestinal secretion of fluid and electrolytes), the osmotic gap should be <50 mOsm/kg (50 mmol/kg), and measured stool osmolality should be roughly equivalent to serum osmolality. A larger gap (>100 mOsm/kg [>100 mmol/kg]) often indicates the presence of an unabsorbed osmotic substance in the stool.[20]

Administration of a hypertonic medication may cause GI intolerance depending on the drug solution itself, the method of administration, and/or the location of the enteral feeding tube.[21] If a hypertonic medication solution is enterally given to a patient, an influx of water is secreted into the GI lumen. Administration of these hypertonic medications are better tolerated when administered intragastrically, as one of the functions of the stomach is to act as a reservoir and dilute hypertonic substances with gastric secretions as it prepares nutrients to be transferred to the small bowel.[1-3] However, very rapid administration of a hyperosmolar solution into the stomach can lead to dumping of large volumes of hyperosmolar solutions into the small intestine, with resultant diarrhea. Additionally, gastric emptying may be slowed by hypertonic solutions because of the regulatory effects of osmoreceptors in the duodenum. This delayed gastric emptying may lead to bloating and nausea. Osmotic diarrhea can be more readily induced by administration of hyperosmolar medications, without dilution, directly into the small bowel, as the physiologic diluting function and the volume reservoir to accommodate additional luminal secretions of the stomach are averted.

When assessing whether the osmolality of a drug solution or suspension may be problematic, it is necessary that the volume of the drug solution and the total osmotic load of the medication be considered. For example, potassium chloride liquid (10%), with an osmolality of ~3,500 mOsm/kg (3,500 mmol/kg), often requires a volume (e.g., 30 mL) for the desired dose (e.g., 40 mEq [40 mmol]), which may cause adverse effects, particularly when given directly into the small bowel. Osmotic loads from common liquid medications are given in Table 150–2.

CLINICAL CONTROVERSY

Hypertonic medication solutions can also be diluted with water prior to administration; however, this practice is limited by the amount of volume that can be practically delivered, as large volumes can also cause GI intolerance. Large water bolus volumes (e.g., >300 mL) administered directly into the small bowel in an effort to reduce osmotic load is not recommended, as this technique has been associated with bowel necrosis[22] and is thus considered to be contraindicated for some patients.

TABLE 150-2	Maximum Reported Osmolalities of Common Drug Solutions and Suspensions[2]		
Medication	**Osmolality (mOsm/kg or mmol/kg)**	**Dosage Volume (mL)**	**Osmotic Load (mOsm or mmol)**
Acetaminophen elixir, 65 mg/mL solution, 60 mg/mL	5,400	10–15	54–81
Cimetidine	5,550	5	58
Digoxin elixir, 50 mcg/mL	4,420	5	28
Docusate sodium syrup, 3.3 mg/mL	4,700	30	147
Furosemide solution, 10 mg/mL	3,938	4–8	16–32
Haloperidol concentrate, 2 mg/mL	500	5	3
Hydroxyzine syrup, 2 mg/mL	4,450	25	111
Metoclopramide HCl syrup, 1 mg/mL	8,350	10–20	84–167
Multivitamin liquid	5,700	5	29
Phenobarbital elixir, 4 mg/mL	11,630	15	174
Potassium chloride liquid, 10%	3,500	30	105
Potassium iodide saturated solution, 1 g/mL	10,950	0.05–0.25	1–3
Promethazine HCl syrup, 1.25 mg/mL	3,500	20–40	70–140
Sodium citrate liquid, 0.5 g/mL	2,050	10–30	20–60
Theophylline solution, 5.33 mg/mL	4,980	30	147
Trimethoprim/sulfamethoxazole 40/200 per 5 mL	4,560	20	91

Some liquid and elixir medication formulations contain sorbitol as a sweetening or solubilizing agent. Sorbitol is an inert sweetening agent that can induce osmotic diarrhea.[23] The usual minimal laxative dosage for sorbitol is ~20 g; however, some patients may be sensitive to smaller doses, such as 10 g. The most common culprits of high sorbitol-containing liquid medication formulations are acetaminophen, ibuprofen, potassium gluconate, pseudoephedrine, and theophylline.[24,25] Unfortunately, some manufacturers do not list the sorbitol content of their preparations, whereas others change the sorbitol content without notification. It is recommended that the manufacturer be contacted for the sorbitol content for any medication solution in question if the patient is experiencing unexplained diarrhea or if the medication cannot be stopped or changed to an alternative dosage form. For enterally fed patients with diarrhea, consider an alternative dosage form, or substitute a therapeutically equivalent drug. For example, if frequent acetaminophen administration is required, tablets can be crushed to a fine powder and mixed with water to form a slurry mixture.

Lesser known nonabsorbable osmotically active ingredients in some drug solutions that can also induce osmotic diarrhea are polyethylene glycol and propylene glycol.[26] Lorazepam liquid (2 mg/mL) contains 60 g of polyethylene glycol per 100 mL of solution and has been reported to induce diarrhea in an adult patient receiving 240 mg/day of lorazepam (72 g/day of polyethylene glycol). The diarrhea resolved when the dosage form was changed from liquid to crushed tablets.[26]

RELEVANT DRUG–LIQUID ENTERAL NUTRITION INTERACTIONS

Changes in bioavailability of certain medications can result in an impaired or failed therapeutic response, as the drug may not be adequately absorbed into the systemic circulation. Some clinicians have advocated holding the EN for 1 or 2 hours prior to and after each dose of a medication whose absorption is impaired when taken with food. Because the majority of hospitalized patients receive continuous enteral feeding, the feeding rate will need to be increased to account for the time period when feeding is not being given. For a patient receiving drug therapy twice or three times daily, this could result in a significant increase in feeding rate for which the patient may not be able to tolerate the feeding due to adverse GI symptoms, such as abdominal distention, diarrhea, and emesis. In addition, because many critically ill patients are given insulin therapy for effective glycemic control, withholding the feedings for 2 to 4 hours could place the patient at significant risk of hypoglycemia. Therefore, it is extremely important that the clinical relevancy of the drug–nutrient interaction be rigorously scrutinized before withholding the feeding and that the pharmacotherapy be closely monitored to ensure the appropriate therapeutic response. Data regarding many potential drug–liquid EN interactions are limited and often require further study. For drugs with no such data, it is recommended that the package insert for the medication be consulted regarding its administration with food and that its recommendation be applied to the patient receiving continuous EN when possible.

❻ It is important that the clinician closely evaluate every enterally administered drug therapy for efficacy as well as toxicity for those patients receiving EN.

Amiodarone

Although the manufacturer's data indicate improved absorption when taken with meals,[4] it has been reported that a nearly threefold increase in amiodarone dosage was required to achieve therapeutic drug concentrations for 8 patients receiving the medication nasoduodenally compared with 85 patients given the medication by the oral route.[27] Unfortunately, details regarding the nutritional regimen and the method of medication administration relative to the enteral feeding were not noted in this study. It is unclear whether this interaction was partially due to the loss of the drug in the dosage process (tablet crushing, etc.), adherence to the enteral feeding formula, or the medication's delivery directly into the duodenum/jejunum. It is advised that amiodarone be given consistently with regard to timing of the enteral feeding and that the patient be monitored closely.

Atovaquone

The bioavailability of a single dose of atovaquone oral suspension is more than doubled when administered with meals compared with fasting.[28] Bioavailability of atovaquone is equivocal with an oral liquid supplement containing 28 g of fat compared with a meal containing 21 g of fat.[28] Atovaquone may be given to patients receiving concurrent EN.

Azole Antifungal Agents: Fluconazole

Three studies[29–31] compared the pharmacokinetics of IV administration to enterally administered fluconazole during continuous enteral feeding for critically ill intensive care units (ICU) patients with invasive mycoses. Doses ranged from 100 mg[29] to 400 mg[31] between studies. The mean bioavailability for the enteral fluconazole for each study was determined to be 80%,[29] 97%,[30] and 100%.[31] Fluconazole may be given intragastrically or via a duodenostomy to patients receiving concurrent EN.

Itraconazole

Itraconazole has been plagued by erratic bioavailability, which has been improved with the development of an oral solution that is given in the fasted state.[32] Steady-state nadir plasma concentrations of IV itraconazole were compared with equidosage enteral itraconazole solution in critically ill, tube-fed patients.[8] The oral solution was administered via the feeding tube with a minimum interval of 2 hours from the enteral feeding or oral food intake. Despite holding the enteral tube feeding, plasma concentrations of itraconazole observed during enteral administration were about two-thirds of plasma concentrations achieved after IV administration. Doubling the enteral dosage to 200 mg twice daily achieved similar plasma concentrations to 100 mg of IV itraconazole; however, increased GI adverse effects (diarrhea) occurred.[8] Itraconazole should not be administered with concurrent EN.

Posaconazole

Concomitant administration of the liquid nutritional supplement with posaconazole resulted in a marked increase in bioavailability compared with the fasted state in healthy volunteers.[33,34] Posaconazole bioavailability increased linearly with coadministration of increasing amounts of liquid supplementation from 35% with fasting, to 60% with 60 mL, to 77% with 120 mL when compared with the area under the curve plasma concentrations achieved with concurrent ingestion of 240 mL of liquid supplement.[33] Posaconazole may be given to patients receiving concurrent EN.

Voriconazole

One small case series in critically ill patients examined peak and nadir plasma concentrations of voriconazole after 3 days of nasogastric administration with concurrent EN.[35] The voriconazole tablets were crushed and suspended in water for medication delivery, and the enteral feeding was interrupted only for the dosage administration and resumed immediately afterward. The investigators concluded that administration of the voriconazole by nasogastric tube was associated with adequate plasma concentrations for seven of the eight studied patients. No clear explanation could be provided for the single patient without acceptable plasma concentrations, and the study's authors questioned whether this variability could be due to polymorphic expression of CYP2C19, the major isozyme implicated in the metabolism of voriconazole.[35] Voriconazole may be given to patients receiving concurrent EN; patients should be monitored closely.

Carbamazepine

It has been shown that carbamazepine can significantly adsorb to the enteral feeding tube.[13] This interaction was easily alleviated by dilution of the suspension with an equal part of water followed by a water flush after medication administration.[13] In a randomized, crossover design in normal volunteers, continuous nasogastric enteral feeding has been shown to reduce carbamazepine absorption only by ~10%.[36] Carbamazepine may be given to patients receiving concurrent EN; patients should be monitored closely.

Digoxin

Although the detrimental effect of a high-fiber diet on digoxin absorption is well established,[37] it is unknown to what extent fiber-containing enteral formulas affect digoxin absorption. It is advised that the medication be given consistently with regard to timing of the enteral feeding and the patient be monitored closely.

Fluoroquinolone Antibiotics

The concentration of fluoroquinolones (ciprofloxacin, levofloxacin, and oflaxacin) is markedly reduced when they are admixed with enteral feedings in vitro.[38] This loss was originally thought to be due to chelation of the antibiotic with cationic minerals,[39] but other evidence indicates that chelation by cations cannot fully explain the magnitude of this drug–nutrient interaction.[14,38] It is possible that protein content of the liquid formulation may also have a significant effect on fluoroquinolone availability[14] analogous to the warfarin–enteral feeding interaction.[40]

CLINICAL CONTROVERSY

The appropriate timing and dosage for changing from IV to enterally administered ciprofloxacin for a patient receiving continuous gastric feeding is controversial. Factors to consider are the severity and location of the infection, sensitivity of the infecting organism, and whether withholding of the feeding before and after medication administration is a viable, safe option.

Ciprofloxacin

Ciprofloxacin is the most widely studied fluoroquinolone for an enteral feeding interaction, and its absorption is detrimentally influenced, more than the other fluoroquinolones, by the presence of enteral feeding. Studies in hospitalized and critically ill patients indicate an overall 33% to 73% bioavailability of ciprofloxacin when coadministered with continuous enteral feeding compared with IV ciprofloxacin.[6,41,42] The bioavailability of ciprofloxacin is also improved by ~28% when administered intragastrically versus intrajejunostomy during continuous enteral feeding.[6] Despite decreased GI absorption of ciprofloxacin in critically ill, enterally fed patients, use of a higher dose (750 mg every 12 hours) given via a nasogastric tube resulted in plasma concentrations similar to IV administration of 400 mg every 12 hours and were well above the minimum inhibitory concen-

tration values for many pathogenic bacteria.[43] Ciprofloxacin may be given to patients receiving concurrent EN, with close clinical monitoring and dosage adjustment.

Levofloxacin

In vitro data demonstrate that levofloxacin binds to liquid nutrition formulas less than ciprofloxacin but more than moxifloxacin.[38] Unfortunately, in vivo data regarding coadministration with enteral feeding is lacking. Levofloxacin may be given to patients receiving concurrent EN, with close clinical monitoring and dosage adjustment.

Moxifloxacin

Because of its good absorption characteristics, moxifloxacin has the best bioavailability of the fluoroquinolones when coadministered with enteral feedings. In a crossover design, healthy volunteers were given equal doses of moxifloxacin as an intact tablet, a crushed tablet as a suspension through a nasogastric tube with 200 mL of water, or a crushed tablet as a suspension through a nasogastric tube with a polymeric enteral feeding solution at 100 mL/hour starting 30 minutes before moxifloxacin administration and continued for another 2 hours after drug administration.[44] The relative bioavailability for the latter two regimens compared with intact tablet control was 91%. These preliminary data indicate that moxifloxacin may be administered to patients receiving concurrent EN.

Ofloxacin

In healthy volunteers, the coadministration of a liquid enteral supplement reduced the relative bioavailability of ofloxacin to only 90% (in contrast to ciprofloxacin, at 72%).[45] These preliminary data indicate that ofloxacin may be given to patients receiving concurrent EN.

Histamine$_2$ Receptor Antagonists

In vitro evaluation of ranitidine and cimetidine binding to enteral feeding demonstrates >90% recovery when admixed with an array of EN formulations; however, in vivo bioavailability studies are lacking.[46,47] These medications likely can be given to patients receiving concurrent EN.

Levetiracetam

In a crossover study of 10 healthy subjects, the absorption of a single dose of levetiracetam was not significantly altered when administered as an intact tablet, crushed powder mixed in applesauce, or crushed powder mixed with 120 mL of liquid EN.[48] Levetiracetam may be given to patients receiving concurrent EN.

Levothyroxine

Bioavailability studies indicate that levothyroxine is better absorbed when ingested in the fasting state (~79% vs 64%, respectively). Additionally, coadministration of levothyroxine with calcium carbonate,[49] magnesium-containing antacids,[50] iron preparations,[51] soy protein,[52] and fiber supplements[53] resulted in significantly decreased absorption of levothyroxine. Some clinicians have suggested that enteral feedings should be held 1 to 2 hours prior to and after levothyroxine administration despite the lack of data on continuous enteral feedings. A recent study examined 15 patients who received levothyroxine therapy during continuous EN.[54] All patients were euthyrotic prior to the initiation of concurrent levothyroxine–enteral feeding. About half of the patients developed a significant increase in serum thyrotropin concentration reflective of subclinical or clinical hypothyroidism. In a small subpopulation, holding the feedings for 1 hour before and after levothyroxine administration was inadequate for restoring euthyroidism. A modest increase in levothyroxine dosage by 25 mcg/day appeared effective in restoring euthyroidism for those who developed hypothyroidism during continuous enteral feeding. When levothyroxine is administered to patients receiving concurrent EN, routine periodic monitoring of thyroid function tests and a dosage adjustment may be necessary.

Linezolid

In a single-dose, crossover study, 11 elderly hospitalized patients receiving enteral feeding were given equal doses of IV or intragastric linezolid.[55] The intragastrically administered linezolid was given as a suspension. A separate control group of six patients who did not receive continuous liquid enteral feeding were also given IV or an oral suspension of linezolid. The absolute bioavailability (85% to 90% of the IV dose) of linezolid was unaltered by the presence of enteral feeding. Linezolid may be given to patients receiving concurrent EN.

Phenytoin

One of the most well documented drug–enteral feeding interactions is with the antiepileptic drug phenytoin. Since the first report of this interaction in 1982, more than 30 studies, case series, case reports, and reviews have been published.[14,56] Despite this abundance of literature, controversy exists whether dramatic decreases in bioavailability occur when given to individuals receiving continuous EN. Part of the controversy stems from four prospective, randomized, controlled trials in normal volunteers that refute the existence of this interaction.[56] However, there are numerous case series and reports that demonstrate dramatic decreases in serum phenytoin concentrations requiring a dosage adjustment when the medication is coadministered with continuous intragastric enteral feeding with different types of formulas.[14,56] The exact mechanism underlying this interaction is still unknown; however, some in vitro studies demonstrate significant complexation of phenytoin to various liquid enteral formulations.[56] Significant improvement in serum phenytoin concentrations has been observed for patients when the intragastric feeding was held for either 1 or 2 hours before and after phenytoin suspension administration compared with continuous administration. A common clinical practice, in addition to withholding the EN before and after phenytoin administration, is to modify the phenytoin dosing interval to twice daily to minimize the time of interrupted feeding.[2,57] Another strategy is to open the contents of an extended-release capsule, mix with water to make a slurry, and administer via the feeding tube. This method involves giving the total daily dose once daily and holding the feedings for 2 hours before and after phenytoin administration.[57] Unfortunately, the latter method has not been studied and cannot be recommended until confirmatory research confirms its effectiveness. Close monitoring of serum phenytoin concentrations during concurrent phenytoin and enteral feeding is warranted. If a dose escalation is required during EN, a reduction in dosage may be necessary when the feeding is discontinued or if the mode of feeding (continuous vs. bolus) is changed.

Proton-Pump Inhibitors

Omeprazole, esomeprazole, lansoprazole, pantoprazole, and rabeprazole are all acid-labile medications, so they are especially formulated to maintain their integrity until delivery to the alkaline pH of the duodenum, where absorption occurs. The medication forms designated for oral use are manufactured as delayed-release enteric-coated tablets, delayed-release capsules containing enteric-coated granules, or powdered packets for reconstitution. Previously, it was necessary to open the capsules and mix the granules/beads into a solution, then administer via the enteral feeding tube. Depending on the location of the tip of the feeding tube, either an acidic solution for administering the medication into the stomach or an alkalemic solution when the drug was administered into the small bowel was used as the liquid vehicle of choice. However, recent studies have demonstrated the efficacy of using an alkalemic solution when the drug was administered into either the stomach or the small bowel, simplifying the process.[58,59] Some commercially available proton-pump inhibitors (e.g., esomeprazole, lansoprazole, and omeprazole) can be reconstituted with water from a powder packet to make a suspension and administered via an intragastric feeding tube. Pantoprazole is less desirable for administration via a feeding tube. The manufacturer recommends that pantoprazole powder be diluted with apple juice (not water) for administration via an intragastric feeding tube. However, acidic fluids, such as apple juice, can denature proteins, cause enteral formula clumping, and potentially clog the small-bore feeding tube. Care should be taken to flush the enteral feeding tube well when esomeprazole and omeprazole suspensions reconstituted from powders are used, as they contain xanthan gum. This inert ingredient causes the suspension to expand, increasing the suspension's viscosity and thus the potential for clogging the small-bore enteral feeding tube.[60] Immediate-release omeprazole/sodium bicarbonate powder for oral suspension can be given either intragastrically or intraduodenally because it is immediately activated by its mixture with bicarbonate in the suspension.

Sevelamer

The manufacturer recommends against administering sevelamer via a feeding tube because of its viscosity and risk of tube clogging. Sevelamer should be used cautiously in tube-fed patients. The capsule contents must be dissolved and diluted with water and the feeding tube flushed extremely well before and after administration to prevent tube clogging.

Sucralfate

It has been noted that sucralfate complexes with protein sources in the enteral formulation may lead to tube clogging[4] and should not be administered via a small-bore feeding tube. Rare reports of esophageal bezoar formation have also occurred due to the prosthetic device (nasogastric suction tube), allowing regurgitation of gastric contents, particularly in those with esophageal reflux or gastric motility disorders.[61] For high-risk patients, use of sucralfate administration via a large-bore feeding tube warrants vigilant adherence to prevent reflux and gastric pooling.

Tacrolimus

A crossover evaluation of tacrolimus absorption was performed in 10 transplant patients receiving continuous nasoduodenal feeding.[62] One treatment arm consisted of coadministration of tacrolimus with the enteral feeding; in the other treatment arm, the feeding was held for 1 hour prior to and 8 hours after drug administration. No significant differences were noted in pharmacokinetic parameters between administration techniques. Tacrolimus may be given to patients receiving concurrent EN.

CLINICAL CONTROVERSY

Some clinicians still consider warfarin resistance to be attributed to vitamin K content of the liquid enteral formulation. However, more recent data indicate that binding of the warfarin to the enteral feeding during continuous feeding may be a more significant contributor to warfarin resistance.

Warfarin

Warfarin resistance associated with continuous enteral tube feedings was first reported in the early 1980s. This resistance was attributable to the large amounts of vitamin K in the feedings at that time.[63] The nutritional industries subsequently responded to this adverse effect by significantly reducing the vitamin K content of liquid EN formulations. Most current liquid formulations now contain <80 mcg/L of vitamin K. A vitamin K intake of 150 mcg/day significantly decreases International Normalized Ratio (INR) by 0.4 during acenocoumarol anticoagulation.[64] With conservative caloric intakes to avoid overfeeding, it was uncommon for patients to receive more than 160 mcg of vitamin K daily from the liquid enteral formula, yet warfarin resistance was still being encountered in clinical practice. Warfarin, a highly protein-bound drug, has been shown to bind to EN formula in vitro, with 35% to 50% of the warfarin dose being bound to the EN formula.[63] Clinical evidence for this warfarin–enteral feeding binding phenomenon stems from a crossover study of six adult patients who required combined enteral tube feeding and warfarin therapy for at least 10 days.[40] Each patient had at least 3 consecutive days during which the feedings were withheld for 1 hour before and after warfarin administration and at least 3 days when the feedings were not withheld. A significant difference in INR response over each 3-day observation period was noted: a mean rise in INR by 0.74 when feedings were held versus a mean fall in INR by 0.13 when the feedings were given concurrently with the warfarin therapy. These divergent changes in INR occurred despite similar mean warfarin doses (5.6 vs. 5.7 mg/day) and clinically irrelevant differences in mean vitamin K intake (77 vs. 102 mcg/day).[40] It is recommended that enteral feedings be withheld for 1 hour before and after warfarin administration. Close monitoring of the INR is essential.

MEDICATION CONSIDERATIONS WITH PARENTERAL NUTRITION

PN formulations are complex admixtures containing as many as 40 base components (e.g., amino acids, dextrose, and lipid emulsions) and additives (e.g., water, lipids, electrolytes, vitamins, trace elements, and insulin). Two types of PN are used in clinical practice: two-in-one and three-in-one formulations. A two-in-one formulation is a combination of dextrose and amino acids without IVLE. It has a yellow appearance due to the presence of the multivitamins. A three-in-one formulation (also referred to as total nutrient admixture [TNA]) includes the IVLE in the same container with dextrose and amino acids, so it has a milky white appearance.

STABILITY AND COMPATIBILITY

7 A critical part in evaluating PN–medication admixtures is understanding the difference between stability and compatibility. Although often used interchangeably, a distinction exists between these two terms in reference to parenteral admixtures. The inability of PN additives, including medications, to maintain their chemical integrity and pharmacologic activity would suggest instability. Compatibility issues with PN formulations generally involve the formation of precipitates. These precipitates may be solid, such as crystalline matter, or liquid, such as phase separation of oil and water in a TNA. The distinction between stability and compatibility with IVLE can be difficult to discern, as all emulsions are inherently unstable systems that will return to their oils and water components over time, yet there are clearly compatibility issues that result in phase separation of the IVLE components. As a result, compatibility of medications in PN admixtures is often determined by the presence or absence of IVLE.

PARENTERAL NUTRITION AS A DRUG DELIVERY VEHICLE

Adding medications to PN admixtures has been reviewed in the literature.[65–67] The rationale for adding medications to the PN solution may be necessary (e.g., to restrict fluid intake), or due to a limitation of available access for medication administration, or for ease of medication administration, particularly for the home PN patient. Because of the potential for numerous physiochemical drug–PN component interactions, this method of drug delivery is usually not the preferred route.

8 The presence of IVLE in a three-in-one admixture can markedly change the stability characteristics of the PN. Stability of IVLE is maintained by the addition of an emulsifying agent, egg yolk phosphatide. The emulsifier is anionic and renders a negative charge to the surface, which creates repulsive forces between individual lipid droplets. Certain medications or high concentrations of divalent or trivalent cations, such as magnesium, calcium, and iron, can neutralize the negative surface charge and promote attraction among the lipid particles. Ultimately, lipid droplets begin to join or aggregate into large lipid globules (i.e., >1 micron in diameter), and the emulsion becomes destabilized. Animal studies have suggested adverse effects on lung and liver function when unstable lipid emulsions are infused.[68,69] Under those conditions when no other reasonable alternative exists, the following criteria should be used for determining whether PN can be used as a drug administration vehicle:[67]

- The stability and compatibility of the drug with the PN admixture and the PN admixture with the drug have been determined.
- The medication must be clinically effective during continuous infusion.
- The drug dosage is constant during the previous 24-hour period.
- The PN infusion rate is stable during the previous 24-hour period.

In addition, the clinician must be cognizant of when the drug therapy needs to be continued when the PN is discontinued. Given these constraints, there are only a limited number of drugs with which this therapy may be considered. Of these medications, only histamine$_2$ antagonists and regular human insulin (RHI) are considered safe and effective with both two-in-one and TNA solutions; however, other medications have been employed in two-in-one PN solutions. Medications that have been added to the PN formulation for a continuous infusion are given in the following sections.

Albumin

Albumin historically has been added to lipid-free PN solutions as a way to provide a continuous source of colloid for those patients with edema associated with severe hypoalbuminemia.[70] Indications for the use of albumin and the best method for its administration (continuous vs short-term infusion vs. bolus) are still subject to considerable debate among clinical practitioners. Recent data indicate that albumin, when exposed to high concentrations of dextrose, results in glycosylation of a portion of the albumin, which alters its physiologic properties.[70] When added to a two-in-one admixture at a concentration of 25 g/L, albumin has clogged 0.2 micron filters.[70] Addition of albumin to an IVLE-containing PN admixture results in creaming by 4 hours.[71] As a result of these detrimental effects, the addition of albumin to PN formulations is not recommended.

Heparin

Heparin has been added to PN solutions to prevent catheter thrombosis in lipid-free PN admixtures and is clinically effective at concentrations of 3,000 units/L.[67] When undiluted heparin solution (100 units/mL) was admixed in a 1:1 volume mixture with a lipid-containing PN formulation (final heparin concentration of 50,000 units/L), the IVLE portion of the PN was not stable.[72] This instability was believed to be due to heparin's ability to form a bridge between lipid particles, keeping them in close proximity and leading to lipid globule aggregation.[67] It is possible that this adverse effect on IVLE stability is dose-related, as a heparin concentration of 2,158 units/L does not adversely influence IVLE stability over a 24-hour observation period.[65] Therefore, low heparin concentrations used for catheter thrombosis prophylaxis can be added to lipid-containing PN admixtures. Although high concentrations (35,000 units/L) of heparin are stable in lipid-free PN solutions,[65] this approach is not recommended, as titration of the heparin rate to the targeted activated partial thromboplastin time warrants infusion rate adjustments that may cause PN-associated electrolyte and macronutrient metabolic disturbances.

Histamine₂ Receptor Antagonists

Stress ulcer prophylaxis with either histamine₂ antagonists or proton-pump inhibitors is routine therapy for most patients in ICUs. Also, patients with hypergastrinemia during the early course of their short bowel syndrome are often given histamine₂ antagonists for several months with their home PN regimen. Ranitidine, famotidine, and cimetidine are efficacious and stable when admixed with either two-in-one or three-in-one PN admixtures.[65,67,73]

Hydrochloric Acid and Sodium Bicarbonate

Disturbance in acid–base homeostasis due to various etiologies is prevalent among patients receiving PN. In addition to treatment of the primary etiology for the acid–base disorder, sometimes the provision of HCl or $NaHCO_3$ is warranted. The stability of HCl when added to a lipid-free PN solution at a final HCl concentration of 100 mEq/L (100 mmol/L; 0.1 N) has been documented.[65] With consideration of the addition of HCl to a TNA admixture, it is pertinent to note that an extremely low pH <5 can effectively overcome the negative surface charge imparted by the emulsifier and irreversibly destabilize or "crack" the emulsion. This leads to separation of oil from the water phase and appears as an amber oil layer at the top of the PN bag or as yellow-brown streaks of oil throughout the formulation (referred to as "marbling" or "oiling out"). As a result, HCl cannot be added to IVLE-containing PN. Sodium bicarbonate must not be admixed with lipid-free or lipid-containing PN. When added to a PN formulation, it combines with calcium included in the PN to form a calcium carbonate precipitate, also known as chalk.[67]

Iron

Iron dextran has been used safely when added to a two-in-one PN formulation at a concentration of 100 mg/L.[74] The addition of iron dextran at a concentration of 10 mg/L to lipid-free pediatric PN solutions was compatible when the final amino acid concentration was ≥2%.[74] However, the trivalent cation from iron (dextran) disrupts the IVLE component of the TNA when added to IVLE-containing PN, even when given in doses as little as 2 mg/L.[75] Therefore, the addition of iron dextran to IVLE-containing PN is not recommended. The compatibility and stability of sodium ferric gluconate or iron sucrose when added to PN have not been evaluated, and their addition to a two-in-one or TNA solution is not recommended.

Octreotide

Although octreotide is listed as physically compatible when admixed with PN formulations,[72] glycosylation of the octreotide results in formation of pharmacologically inactive metabolites (thus the lack of stability of the medication) due to the availability of dextrose in the PN.[76] Decreased clinical efficacy has also been noted.[76] Therefore, octreotide should not be added to lipid-containing or lipid-free PN admixtures.

Regular Human Insulin

The addition of RHI to two-in-one or three-in-one PN admixtures has been shown to be compatible and effective. Only RHI is compatible with PN formulations; all other insulin formulations, such as neutral protamine Hagedorn (NPH), insulin glargine, lispro, and aspart, are not compatible and should never be added to the PN.[66] It is recommended to add the RHI to the PN formulation to control hyperglycemia after patient stability is achieved or to control mild hyperglycemia. For critically ill patients, an RHI infusion or sliding scale insulin coverage with only modest amounts of RHI provided in the PN is recommended.

COMPATIBILITY OF MEDICATION WHEN COADMINISTERED WITH PARENTERAL NUTRITION FORMULATIONS

Another method of medication administration is by coinfusion through the same IV tubing as the PN. In general, this method should be avoided unless the physical and chemical compatibility of the medication with the PN formulation is assured.[66] Even with the use of double and triple lumen catheters, there are situations encountered in clinical practice in which there are insufficient ports/lumens to provide for the patient's complicated IV therapy, and various medications/PN may need to be coinfused.[77] This is done using a Y-site, where two IV tubes are joined as a single tube. As a result, the two separate infusions are briefly mixed together as one infusion prior to delivery to the patient.

Unfortunately, these data are limited as, typically, only physical compatibility has been evaluated in the majority of studies assessing additive and Y-site compatibility with PN formulations;[72,77] very few consider stability. Unstable substances should not be added to or coinfused with PN regardless of physical compatibility. Another limitation is that the majority of studies examine only a single concentration of the medication with the PN admixture. Morphine is one example; its concentration may affect PN stability. For a two-in-one PN solution, morphine is compatible at both 1 mg/mL and 15 mg/mL concentrations. However, in one study, only morphine 1 mg/mL was compatible with TNA solutions, and "oiling out" of the IVLE-containing PN occurred with the 15 mg/mL concentration.[72] The clinician should consult resources such as *Trissel's Handbook on Injectable Drugs*[78] and the *King Guide to Parenteral Admixtures*[79] for comprehensive current information concerning the compatibility and stability of PN solutions when admixed with medications prior to coadministration of any medication with PN. Common examples of medications known to be incompatible or not recommended to be given concurrently via a Y-site with either a two-in-one or a three-in-one PN formulation are acyclovir, amphotericin B, cyclosporine, doxorubicin, fluorouracil, ganciclovir, immune globulin, midazolam, phenytoin, and sodium bicarbonate. Common drugs known to be compatible with two-in-one PN solutions but not TNA formulations include dopamine, HCl, heparin, iron dextran, and pentobarbitol. Conversely, some chemotherapy agents, such as cisplatin, cytarabine, and methotrexate, are not compatible with two-in-one PN solutions, but they are compatible with IVLE-containing PN solutions because of the lipid solubility of these medications.[67]

❾ IV Y-site administration of calcium, potassium phosphate, sodium phosphate, or magnesium with PN admixtures must be avoided. Given the characteristics of the PN (e.g., pH, amino acid concentration, calcium and phosphorus concentrations, and lipid concentration), the formulation may already be near the point of approaching solubility or stability limits. PN admixtures generally contain a fourfold higher concentration of calcium and a 25-fold higher concentration of phosphorus compared with serum (45 to 56 mg/L vs. 200 mg/L of calcium, respectively; 40 mg/L vs. 1,000 mg/L of phosphorus, respectively). Hence, rapid increases in pH (from the acidic pH of the PN solution to a neutral pH) and the heating of the PN to body temperature (resulting in increased calcium ion availability for interacting with phosphorus) as the PN solution flows from the bag to the body might make a marginal difference between solubility and precipitation.[80] Use of the same catheter tubing or lumen as the PN formulation for the treatment of hypocalcemia or hypophosphatemia can easily overwhelm calcium phosphate concentrations that exceed solubility limits, resulting in formation of dibasic calcium phosphate precipitants. These precipitants, which are virtually insoluble in water, pose the greatest threat and are implicated in reports of significant morbidity and mortality among patients receiving incompatible PN mixtures.[81,82] Another consideration beyond calcium phosphate precipitation is lipid stability. Phase separation (e.g., "oiling out") can occur when an excess of cations is added to an IVLE-containing PN formulation.[66,72] The higher the cation valence, the greater the destabilizing effect. Therefore, a trivalent cation such as iron is the most disruptive, followed by the divalent cations calcium and magnesium. Monovalent cations such as sodium and potassium are the least disruptive to the emulsifier, yet when given in high concentrations, they may produce instability.[66]

CONCLUSION

There are numerous issues related to the concurrent delivery of EN, PN, and medications. Because of these difficulties, considerations for the safe and effective administration of medications with EN and PN have been compiled and summarized in this chapter. The issues and provided recommendations should address many of the medication administration situations encountered in clinical practice. As more data become available, recommendations are likely to change. For drugs with a narrow therapeutic index, changes in the patient's pharmacotherapy need to be reevaluated with clinical monitoring for therapeutic efficacy or adverse effects, including serum concentrations of the medication.

ABBREVIATIONS

APPT: Activated partial thromboplastin time

EN: Enteral nutrition

HCl : Hydrochloric acid

IVLE: Intravenous lipid emulsion

NaHCO$_3$: Sodium bicarbonate

NPH: Neutral protamine Hagedorn (insulin)

PN: Parenteral nutrition

RHI: Regular human insulin

TNA: Total nutrient admixture (three-in-one parenteral nutrition)

REFERENCES

1. Beckwith MC. A guide to drug therapy in patients with enteral feeding tubes: Dosage form selection and administration methods. Hosp Pharm 2004;39:225–237.
2. Dickerson RN. Medication administration considerations for patients receiving enteral tube feedings. Hosp Pharm 2004;39:84–95.
3. Williams NT. Medication administration through enteral feeding tubes. Am J Health Syst Pharm 2008;65:2347–2357.
4. Wohlt PD, Zheng L, Gunderson S, Balzar SA, Johnson BD, Fish JT. Recommendations for the use of medications with continuous enteral nutrition. Am J Health Syst Pharm 2009;66:1458–1467.
5. Bankhead R, Boullata J, Brantley S, et al. Enteral nutrition practice recommendations. JPEN J Parenter Enteral Nutr 2009;33:122–167.
6. Healy DP, Brodbeck MC, Clendening CE. Ciprofloxacin absorption is impaired in patients given enteral feedings orally and via gastrostomy and jejunostomy tubes. Antimicrob Agents Chemother 1996;40:6–10.
7. Lourenco R. Enteral feeding: Drug/nutrient interaction. Clin Nutr 2001;20:187–193.
8. Vandewoude K, Vogelaers D, Decruyenaere J, et al. Concentrations in plasma and safety of 7 days of intravenous itraconazole followed by 2 weeks of oral itraconazole solution in patients in intensive care units. Antimicrob Agents Chemother 1997;41:2714–2718.
9. Beermann B, Hellstrom K, Rosen A. The gastrointestinal absorption of digoxin in seven patients with gastric or small intestinal reconstructions. Acta Med Scand 1973;193:293–297.
10. Severijnen R, Bayat N, Bakker H, Tolboom J, Bongaerts G. Enteral drug absorption in patients with short small bowel: A review. Clin Pharmacokinet 2004;43:951–962.
11. Brophy DF, Ford SL, Crouch MA. Warfarin resistance in a patient with short bowel syndrome. Pharmacotherapy 1998;18:646–649.
12. Seifert CF, McGoodwin PL, Allen LV, Jr. Phenytoin recovery from percutaneous endoscopic gastrostomy Pezzer catheters after long-term in vitro administration. JPEN J Parenter Enteral Nutr 1993;17:370–374.
13. Clark-Schmidt AL, Garnett WR, Lowe DR, Karnes HT. Loss of carbamazepine suspension through nasogastric feeding tubes. Am J Hosp Pharm 1990;47:2034–2037.
14. Chan LN. Drug-nutrient interaction in clinical nutrition. Curr Opin Clin Nutr Metab Care 2002;5:327–332.
15. Dickerson RN, Tidwell AC, Brown RO. Adverse effects from inappropriate medication administration via a jejunostomy feeding tube. Nutr Clin Pract 2003;18:402–405.
16. Schier JG, Howland MA, Hoffman RS, Nelson LS. Fatality from administration of labetalol and crushed extended-release nifedipine. Ann Pharmacother 2003;37:1420–1423.
17. Lesar TS. Prescribing errors involving medication dosage forms. J Gen Intern Med 2002;17:579–587.
18. Seifert CF, Johnston BA. A nationwide survey of long-term care facilities to determine the characteristics of medication administration through enteral feeding catheters. Nutr Clin Pract 2005;20:354–362.
19. Magnuson BL, Clifford TM, Hoskins LA, Bernard AC. Enteral nutrition and drug administration, interactions, and complications. Nutr Clin Pract 2005;20:618–624.
20. Topazian M, Binder HJ. Brief report: Factitious diarrhea detected by measurement of stool osmolality. N Engl J Med 1994;330:1418–1419.
21. Dickerson RN, Melnik G. Osmolality of oral drug solutions and suspensions. Am J Hosp Pharm 1988;45:832–834.
22. Schloerb PR, Wood JG, Casillan AJ, Tawfik O, Udobi K. Bowel necrosis caused by water in jejunal feeding. JPEN J Parenter Enteral Nutr 2004;28:27–29.
23. Johnston KR, Govel LA, Andritz MH. Gastrointestinal effects of sorbitol as an additive in liquid medications. Am J Med 1994;97:185–191.
24. Lutomski DM, Gora ML, Wright SM, Martin JE. Sorbitol content of selected oral liquids. Ann Pharmacother 1993;27:269–274.
25. Miller SJ, Oliver AD. Sorbitol content of selected sugar-free liquid medications. Hosp Pharm 1993;28:741–744.
26. Shepherd MF, Felt-Gunderson PA. Diarrhea associated with lorazepam solution in a tube-fed patient. Nutr Clin Prac 1996;11:117–120.

27. Kotake T, Takada M, Goto T, Komamura K, Kamakura S, Morishita H. Serum amiodarone and desethylamiodarone concentrations following nasogastric versus oral administration. J Clin Pharm Ther 2006;31:237–243.

28. Freeman CD, Klutman NE, Lamp KC, Dall LH, Strayer AH. Relative bioavailability of atovaquone suspension when administered with an enteral nutrition supplement. Ann Pharmacother 1998;32:1004–1007.

29. Rosemurgy AS, Markowsky S, Goode SE, Plastino K, Kearney RE. Bioavailability of fluconazole in surgical intensive care unit patients: A study comparing routes of administration. J Trauma 1995;39:445–447.

30. Nicolau DP, Crowe H, Nightingale CH, Quintiliani R. Bioavailability of fluconazole administered via a feeding tube in intensive care unit patients. J Antimicrob Chemother 1995;36:395–401.

31. Buijk SL, Gyssens IC, Mouton JW, Verbrugh HA, Touw DJ, Bruining HA. Pharmacokinetics of sequential intravenous and enteral fluconazole in critically ill surgical patients with invasive mycoses and compromised gastro-intestinal function. Intensive Care Med 2001;27:115–121.

32. Barone JA, Moskovitz BL, Guarnieri J, et al. Food interaction and steady-state pharmacokinetics of itraconazole oral solution in healthy volunteers. Pharmacotherapy 1998;18:295–301.

33. Krishna G, Ma L, Vickery D, et al. Effect of varying amounts of a liquid nutritional supplement on the pharmacokinetics of posaconazole in healthy volunteers. Antimicrob Agents Chemother 2009;53:4749–4752.

34. Sansone-Parsons A, Krishna G, Calzetta A, et al. Effect of a nutritional supplement on posaconazole pharmacokinetics following oral administration to healthy volunteers. Antimicrob Agents Chemother 2006;50:1881–1883.

35. Mohammedi I, Piens MA, Padoin C, Robert D. Plasma levels of voriconazole administered via a nasogastric tube to critically ill patients. Eur J Clin Microbiol Infect Dis 2005;24:358–360.

36. Bass J, Miles MV, Tennison MB, Holcombe BJ, Thorn MD. Effects of enteral tube feeding on the absorption and pharmacokinetic profile of carbamazepine suspension. Epilepsia 1989;30:364–369.

37. Kasper H, Zilly W, Fassl H, Fehle F. The effect of dietary fiber on postprandial serum digoxin concentration in man. Am J Clin Nutr 1979;32:2436–2438.

38. Wright DH, Pietz SL, Konstantinides FN, Rotschafer JC. Decreased in vitro fluoroquinolone concentrations after admixture with an enteral feeding formulation. JPEN J Parenter Enteral Nutr 2000;24:42–48.

39. Deppermann KM, Lode H. Fluoroquinolones: Interaction profile during enteral absorption. Drugs 1993;45(3 Suppl):65–72.

40. Dickerson RN, Garmon WM, Kuhl DA, Minard G, Brown RO. Vitamin K-independent warfarin resistance after concurrent administration of warfarin and continuous enteral nutrition. Pharmacotherapy 2008;28:308–313.

41. de Marie S, VandenBergh MF, Buijk SL, et al. Bioavailability of ciprofloxacin after multiple enteral and intravenous doses in ICU patients with severe gram-negative intra-abdominal infections. Intensive Care Med 1998;24:343–346.

42. Mimoz O, Binter V, Jacolot A, et al. Pharmacokinetics and absolute bioavailability of ciprofloxacin administered through a nasogastric tube with continuous enteral feeding to critically ill patients. Intensive Care Med 1998;24:1047–1051.

43. Cohn SM, Sawyer MD, Burns GA, Tolomeo C, Milner KA. Enteric absorption of ciprofloxacin during tube feeding in the critically ill. J Antimicrob Chemother 1996;38:871–876.

44. Burkhardt O, Stass H, Thuss U, Borner K, Welte T. Effects of enteral feeding on the oral bioavailability of moxifloxacin in healthy volunteers. Clin Pharmacokinet 2005;44:969–976.

45. Mueller BA, Brierton DG, Abel SR, Bowman L. Effect of enteral feeding with ensure on oral bioavailabilities of ofloxacin and ciprofloxacin. Antimicrob Agents Chemother 1994;38:2101–2105.

46. Crowther RS, Bellanger R, Szauter KE. In vitro stability of ranitidine hydrochloride in enteral nutrient formulas. Ann Pharmacother 1995;29:859–862.

47. Rochard EB, Rogeron B, Barthes DM, Courtois PY. Stability of cimetidine hydrochloride in Sondalis Iso enteral nutrition formula. Am J Hosp Pharm 1991;48:1681–1682.

48. Fay MA, Sheth RD, Gidal BE. Oral absorption kinetics of levetiracetam: The effect of mixing with food or enteral nutrition formulas. Clin Ther 2005;27:594–598.

49. Singh N, Singh PN, Hershman JM. Effect of calcium carbonate on the absorption of levothyroxine. JAMA 2000;283:2822–2825.

50. Mersebach H, Rasmussen AK, Kirkegaard L, Feldt-Rasmussen U. Intestinal adsorption of levothyroxine by antacids and laxatives: Case stories and in vitro experiments. Pharmacol Toxicol 1999;84:107–109.

51. Campbell NR, Hasinoff BB, Stalts H, Rao B, Wong NC. Ferrous sulfate reduces thyroxine efficacy in patients with hypothyroidism. Ann Intern Med 1992;117:1010–1013.

52. Bell DS, Ovalle F. Use of soy protein supplement and resultant need for increased dose of levothyroxine. Endocr Pract 2001;7:193–194.

53. Chiu AC, Sherman SI. Effects of pharmacological fiber supplements on levothyroxine absorption. Thyroid 1998;8:667–671.

54. Dickerson RN, Maish GO, Minard G, Brown RO. Clinical relevancy of the levothyroxine-continuous enteral nutrition interaction. JPEN J Parenter Enteral Nutr 2010;34:194–195.

55. Beringer P, Nguyen M, Hoem N, et al. Absolute bioavailability and pharmacokinetics of linezolid in hospitalized patients given enteral feedings. Antimicrob Agents Chemother 2005;49:3676–3681.

56. Au Yeung SC, Ensom MH. Phenytoin and enteral feedings: Does evidence support an interaction? Ann Pharmacother 2000;34:896–905.

57. Gilbert S, Hatton J, Magnuson B. How to minimize interaction between phenytoin and enteral feedings: Two approaches. Nutr Clin Pract 1996;11:28–31.

58. Phillips JO, Olsen KM, Rebuck JA, Rangnekar NJ, Miedema BW, Metzler MH. A randomized, pharmacokinetic and pharmacodynamic, cross-over study of duodenal or jejunal administration compared to nasogastric administration of omeprazole suspension in patients at risk for stress ulcers. Am J Gastroenterol 2001;96:367–372.

59. Sharma VK, Vasudeva R, Howden CW. The effects on intragastric acidity of per-gastrostomy administration of an alkaline suspension of omeprazole. Aliment Pharmacol Ther 1999;13:1091–1095.

60. Sacks GS. Drug-nutrient considerations in patients receiving parenteral and enteral nutrition. Pract Gastro 2004;19:39–48.

61. Shueke M, Mihas AA. Esophageal bezoar due to sucralfate. Endoscopy 1991;23:305–306.

62. Murray M, Grogan TA, Lever J, Warty VS, Fung J, Venkataramanan R. Comparison of tacrolimus absorption in transplant patients receiving continuous versus interrupted enteral nutritional feeding. Ann Pharmacother 1998;32:633–636.

63. Dickerson RN. Warfarin resistance and enteral tube feeding: A vitamin K–independent interaction. Nutrition 2008;24:1048–1052.

64. Schurgers LJ, Shearer MJ, Hamulyak K, Stocklin E, Vermeer C. Effect of vitamin K intake on the stability of oral anticoagulant treatment: Dose-response relationships in healthy subjects. Blood 2004;104:2682–2689.

65. Driscoll DF, Baptista RJ, Mitrano FP, Mascioli EA, Blackburn GL, Bistrian BR. Parenteral nutrient admixtures as drug vehicles: Theory and practice in the critical care setting. DICP 1991;25:276–283.

66. Mirtallo J, Canada T, Johnson D, et al. Safe practices for parenteral nutrition. JPEN J Parenter Enteral Nutr 2004;28:S39-S70.

67. Mirtallo JM. Complications associated with drug and nutrient interactions. J Infus Nurs 2004;27:19–24.

68. Driscoll DF, Ling PR, Quist WC, Bistrian BR. Pathological consequences from the infusion of unstable lipid emulsion admixtures in guinea pigs. Clin Nutr 2005;24:105–113.

69. Driscoll DF, Ling PR, Andersson C, Bistrian BR. Hepatic indicators of oxidative stress and tissue damage accompanied by systemic inflammation in rats following a 24-hour infusion of an unstable lipid emulsion admixture. JPEN J Parenter Enteral Nutr 2009;33:327–335.

70. Lester LR, Crill CM, Hak EB. Should adding albumin to parenteral nutrient solutions be considered an unsafe practice? Am J Health Syst Pharm 2006;63:1656–1661.

71. Ambados F. Destabilization of fat emulsion in total nutrient admixtures by concentrated albumin 20% infusion. Aust J Hosp Pharm 1999;29:210–212.

72. Trissel LA, Gilbert DL, Martinez JF, Baker MB, Walter WV, Mirtallo JM. Compatibility of medications with 3-in-1 parenteral nutrition admixtures. JPEN J Parenter Enteral Nutr 1999;23:67–74.

73. Puzovic M, Hardy G. Stability and compatibility of histamine H2-receptor antagonists in parenteral nutrition mixtures. Curr Opin Clin Nutr Metab Care 2007;10:311–317.

74. Kumpf VJ. Update on parenteral iron therapy. Nutr Clin Pract 2003;18:318–326.

75. Driscoll DF, Bhargava HN, Li L, Zaim RH, Babayan VK, Bistrian BR. Physicochemical stability of total nutrient admixtures. Am J Health Syst Pharm 1995;52:623–634.

76. Trexler K. No, octreotide cannot be added to parenteral nutrition solutions. Nutr Clin Prac 1998;13:87–88.

77. Trissel LA, Gilbert DL, Martinez JF, Baker MB, Walter WV, Mirtallo JM. Compatibility of parenteral nutrient solutions with selected drugs during simulated Y-site administration. Am J Health Syst Pharm 1997;54:1295–1300.

78. Trissel LA, ed. Handbook on Injectable Drugs. 15th ed. Bethesda, MD: American Society for Health-System Pharmacists; 2009.

79. King JC, Catania PN, ed. King Guide to Parenteral Admixtures. Napa, CA: King Guide Publications; 2009.

80. Driscoll DF, Newton DW, Bistrian BR. Precipitation of calcium phosphate from parenteral nutrient fluids. Am J Hosp Pharm 1994;51:2834–2836.

81. Hill SE, Heldman LS, Goo ED, Whippo PE, Perkinson JC. Fatal microvascular pulmonary emboli from precipitation of a total nutrient admixture solution. JPEN J Parenter Enteral Nutr 1996;20:81–87.

82. Shay DK, Fann LM, Jarvis WR. Respiratory distress and sudden death associated with receipt of a peripheral parenteral nutrition admixture. Infect Control Hosp Epidemiol 1997;18:814–817.

151

Parenteral Nutrition

TODD W. MATTOX AND CATHERINE M. CRILL

KEY CONCEPTS

❶ Four steps to developing a successful nutrition plan include definition of nutrition goals, determination of nutrition requirements, determination of appropriate route of delivery of nutrients, and subsequent monitoring of the nutrition regimen to evaluate suitability of the regimen as a patient's clinical condition changes and to minimize or treat complications.

❷ The appropriate route of nutrition support depends on the functional condition of the patient's gastrointestinal (GI) tract, risk of aspiration, expected duration of nutrition therapy, and clinical condition.

❸ Identifying the patient who is most likely to benefit from parenteral nutrition (PN) therapy includes consideration of the patient's age, nutrition status, expected duration of GI dysfunction, and potential risks of initiating therapy.

❹ PN formulations include intravenous (IV) sources of protein, dextrose, fat, water, electrolytes, vitamins, trace elements, and other additives.

❺ PN solutions may be appropriately formulated for administration by peripheral or central venous access.

❻ PN solutions may be infused continuously or intermittently.

❼ Biochemical and clinical measurements considered necessary for effective monitoring of patients receiving PN include serum chemistries, vital signs, weight, total daily fluid intake and losses, and nutritional intake.

❽ Non–catheter-related complications of PN therapy are minimized with application of age-appropriate nutrient dosing guidelines, frequent monitoring, and rational adjustments to the PN regimen when metabolic abnormalities occur.

❾ Expenses associated with PN therapy may be minimized by using PN in appropriate patients, appropriate use of laboratory measurements associated with PN therapy, maximizing efficient purchasing practices for PN solutions and compounding supplies, implementing a standardized process for PN management, and minimizing PN waste.

Learning objectives, review questions, and other resources can be found at **www.pharmacotherapyonline.com**.

Maintenance of adequate nutrition status during illness has been recognized for more than 50 years as an integral part of the medical treatment plan for patients who are unable to use normal physiologic means of nourishment. Successful techniques for providing intravenous (IV) nutrition support were introduced to clinical practice in adults and subsequently, infants in the late 1960s.[1] Use of central venous access was investigated to reduce risk of metabolic complications associated with fluid overload and electrolyte imbalances. The use of larger vessels permitted infusion of concentrated formulas, which decreased the fluid volume required and avoided the phlebitis that commonly occurred when hypertonic infusions were given peripherally.

Further clinical experience and research fostered development of protocols that promoted better patient care and resulted in a decline in complications associated with parenteral nutrition (PN) therapy.[2] The scope of practice for nutrition support clinicians has broadened as a result of increasing knowledge regarding the metabolic consequences associated with acute injury and chronic disease states. The pharmacist's role in providing safe and effective nutrition-support care requires knowledge of the principles of patient selection, initial therapy design, preparation and dispensing of the nutritional formulations, and outcome monitoring. Other responsibilities of the nutrition support pharmacist may include development of policy and procedures as well as quality improvement activities for patient care and operational processes associated with providing parenteral and enteral nutrition.[3–5] However, the role of other healthcare professionals may be similar because of the evolving interdisciplinary approach to nutritional support.[6–8] This chapter reviews indications for PN, components of PN formulations, routes of IV administration, practical aspects of regimen design, solution admixture, outcome monitoring, and management of complications for both adult and pediatric (neonates, infants, and children) patients.

DESIRED OUTCOMES

❶ The primary objective of nutrition support therapy is to promote positive clinical outcomes of an illness and improve a patient's quality of life. Four fundamental steps are key to providing optimal care for patients who require nutrition support. They are definition of nutrition goals, determination of nutrient requirements for achievement of the nutrition goals, delivery of the required nutrients, and subsequent assessment of the nutrition regimen.[4,5]

A patient's nutrition goals can be established after a thorough nutritional assessment (see Chap. 149). Nutrient requirements and an appropriate route for delivery of the required nutrients can then be determined. Nutrition support goals include correction of the patient's caloric and nitrogen imbalances, and any fluid or electrolyte abnormalities, or known vitamin or trace element abnormalities. An additional goal is to lessen the metabolic response to injury by minimizing oxidant stress and favorably modulating immune response. These interventions should not cause or worsen other metabolic complications.

Specific caloric goals include (a) adequate energy intake to promote normal growth and development in neonates, infants, and children, (b) energy equilibrium and preservation of fat calorie stores in well-nourished adults, and (c) positive energy balance in malnourished patients with depleted endogenous fat stores. Overweight patients with >120% of ideal body weight or a body mass index >30 kg/m^2) may require less caloric support than non-obese patients with the same clinical condition.[9] Specific nitrogen goals are positive nitrogen balance or nitrogen equilibrium and improvement in the serum concentration of visceral protein markers such as transferrin or prealbumin.

❷ The gastrointestinal (GI) tract is the optimal route for providing nutrients unless obstruction, severe pancreatitis, or other GI complications are present (see Chap. 149).[10] Other considerations that may impact determination of an appropriate route for delivery of nutrition support include expected duration of nutrition therapy and risk of aspiration. Patients who have nonfunctional GI tracts or are otherwise not candidates for enteral nutrition may benefit from PN. Routine monitoring is necessary to ensure that the nutrition regimen is suitable for a given patient as the patient's clinical condition changes and to minimize or treat complications.

INDICATIONS FOR PARENTERAL NUTRITION SUPPORT

The association between malnutrition and development of complications and mortality is well documented for adult and pediatric patients.[11,12] Although improvement in nutrition status as defined by various clinical nutrition markers has been reported for patients who received PN, the impact on clinical outcome is difficult to demonstrate in many adult populations. Several investigations have reported a positive effect of PN on complications and mortality, whereas others have failed to demonstrate any difference.[11,13,14,15] Early studies have been criticized for defects in study design, such as small sample sizes, inappropriate randomization, and inconsistent baseline nutrition status among the study group, which hindered demonstration of the effectiveness of PN therapy. The impact of PN on clinical outcome has been more successfully demonstrated for critically ill infants and children, particularly those with acquired or congenital GI tract anomalies.[16] Consensus guidelines for PN use for adults (Table 151–1) and pediatric (Table 151–2) patients are based on clinical experience and investigations in specific patient populations.[13–19] Unfortunately, conflicting data have resulted in a lack of consistency in published guidelines from different sources, which complicates identification of the patient who is most likely to benefit from PN. However, these published reports may serve as resources for development of institution-specific standards.

❸ The decision to initiate PN is based on the assessment that the patient cannot meet his or her nutritional requirements through the GI tract. This assessment must include an evaluation of the patient's nutrition status, clinical status, age, and potential risks of initiating therapy, such as infection and other metabolic abnormalities. The appropriate length of time to wait prior to starting PN therapy is dependent on patient age and clinical status.[10–19]

Adult PN therapy is not an emergent intervention and should not be initiated until the patient is hemodynamically stable.[10] In general, adults who are not candidates for enteral nutrition should be considered candidates for PN after 7 to 14 days of suboptimal nutritional intake.[10] Guidelines for use in infants and children are primarily influenced by age. The most appropriate time to initiate therapy for infants and children varies with age and nutritional status. Early PN

TABLE 151–1 Indications for Adult Parenteral Nutrition

1. Inability to absorb nutrients via the GI tract because of one or more of the following:
   a. Massive small bowel resection: usually patients with <100 cm (39 in) of small bowel distal to the ligament of Treitz without a colon or <50 cm (20 in) of small bowel with an intact colon
   b. Intractable vomiting when adequate EN is not expected for 7–14 days.
   c. Severe diarrhea
   d. Bowel obstruction
   e. GI fistulae: PN is indicated for patients with prolonged inadequate nutritional intake longer than 5–7 days who are not candidates for EN.
2. Cancer: antineoplastic therapy, radiation therapy, or HSCT
   a. PN may be used for moderately to severely malnourished patients receiving active anticancer treatment who are not candidates for EN.
   b. PN is not routinely indicated for well-nourished or mildly malnourished patients undergoing surgery, chemotherapy, or radiation therapy.
   c. PN is unlikely to benefit patients with advanced cancer whose malignancy is unresponsive to treatment. However, use may be appropriate for carefully selected patients who have failed trials of less-invasive medical therapies and have good performance status, an estimated life expectancy of longer than 40–60 days, and strong social and financial support.
   d. PN is appropriate for patients undergoing HSCT who are malnourished and who are anticipated to be unable to ingest and/or absorb adequate nutrients for 7–14 days. PN should be discontinued as soon as toxicities have resolved after stem cell engraftment.
3. Pancreatitis: PN may be used for patients with severe pancreatitis with prolonged inadequate nutritional intake longer than 5–7 days who are not candidates for EN. PN should be used when EN exacerbates abdominal pain, ascites, or fistula output.
4. Critical care
   a. PN should be used for those patients in whom EN is contraindicated or is unlikely to provide adequate nutritional requirements within 5–10 days.
   b. Organ failure (liver, renal, or respiratory): PN should be used for patients with moderate to severe catabolism when EN is contraindicated.
   c. Burns: PN should be used for those patients in whom EN is contraindicated or is unlikely to provide adequate nutritional requirements within 4–5 days.
5. Perioperative PN
   a. Preoperative: for 7–14 days for patients with moderate to severe malnutrition who are undergoing major GI surgery, if the operation can be safely postponed.
   b. Postoperative: PN should be used for patients in whom EN is contraindicated or is unlikely to provide adequate nutritional requirements within 7–10 days.
6. Hyperemesis gravidarum: when EN is not tolerated
7. Eating disorders: PN should be considered for patients with anorexia nervosa and severe malnutrition who are unable or unwilling to ingest adequate nutrition.

EN, enteral nutrition; GI, gastrointestinal; HSCT, hematopoietic stem cell transplantation; PN, parenteral nutrition; SBS, short-bowel syndrome.
From references 10, 13, 14, and 18.

TABLE 151–2 Indications for Pediatric Parenteral Nutrition

1. When enteral nutrition is unlikely to provide adequate nutritional requirements
   a. Premature infant within 24–48 hours
   b. Other pediatric patients within 5–7 days
2. When the GI tract is not functional or cannot be assessed
   a. Massive small bowel resection resulting in short-bowel syndrome
   b. Neonatal necrotizing enterocolitis
   c. Severe inflammatory bowel disease
   d. Intractable diarrhea and/or vomiting
   e. Graft-versus-host disease
   f. Postchemotherapy
3. Infants and children requiring extracorporeal membrane oxygenation
4. Organ failure (liver, renal, pulmonary, pancreas) when enteral nutrition is contraindicated and child is catabolic

From references 16, 17, 19.

within the first 24 hours of life has been recommended for infants with a birth weight of 1,500 g.[20–22] Protein loss in extremely low-birth-weight infants can be twofold higher than in term infants, and frequently results in a negative nitrogen balance that cannot be corrected by glucose as a sole nutrient. Early aggressive PN in neonates can enhance protein accretion and somatic growth.[20,22,23] While there has been some concern regarding protein tolerance with early initiation of PN, most clinicians now support the practice. Withholding PN for 2 to 3 days after birth, coupled with a slow advancement of substrate, only appears to contribute to the acute semistarvation and growth failure seen for many neonates.[20,22,23] PN should be initiated within 5 to 7 days for other pediatric patients who are unable to meet their nutrient requirements with enteral nutrition.[16,21] Earlier intervention should be considered for term infants (within 2 to 3 days), critically ill children (within 3 to 5 days), and children with preexisting malnutrition. Guidelines for older children are similar to those for adults.

CLINICAL CONTROVERSY

The most appropriate time to initiate PN in adults differs among various consensus reports because few data specifically address this issue. Some recommend initiating PN for patients who are not candidates for enteral nutrition as early as after 7 days of inadequate oral intake, whereas others recommend waiting up to 14 days for previously well-nourished or moderately malnourished patients.

COMPONENTS OF PARENTERAL NUTRITION

❹ PN formulations include IV sources of protein, dextrose, fat, water, electrolytes, vitamins, trace elements, and other additives. PN solutions should provide the optimal combination of macro- and micronutrients to provide a patient's specific nutritional requirements. Macronutrients include water, protein, dextrose, and IV fat emulsion (IVFE) (Table 151-3). Micronutrients include vitamins, trace elements, and electrolytes. Both macronutrients and micronutrients are necessary for maintenance of normal metabolism. In general, macronutrients are used for energy (dextrose and fat) and as structural substrates (protein and fat). Micronutrients are required to support a variety of metabolic activities necessary for cellular homeostasis such as enzymatic reactions, fluid balance, and regulation of electrophysiologic processes. These components usually require individualized adjustments as the patient's clinical condition affects changes in metabolic stress, organ function, fluid and electrolyte balance, and acid–base status.

AMINO ACIDS

Protein in PN solutions is provided in the form of crystalline amino acids (CAAs), which are used primarily for protein synthesis. When oxidized for energy, 1 g of protein yields 4 cal (or ~17 J). However, including the caloric contribution from protein when calculating calories provided by the PN regimen is controversial.[24]

Commercially available CAA solutions may be categorized as standard amino acid solutions or modified amino acid solutions. Standard CAA solutions are designed for patients with "normal" organ function and nutritional requirements (see Table 151-3). Although standard CAA solutions differ in the proportion of specific amino acids, they contain a balanced profile of essential, semi-essential, and nonessential L-amino acids. Despite these differences, similar effects on markers of protein use have been reported.[25] The protein concentration, total nitrogen, and electrolyte content are also

TABLE 151-3 Macronutrient Components of PN Solutions

Nutritional Substrate	Intravenous Source	Description
Fluid	Sterile water for injection USP	
Nitrogen	Crystalline amino acids standard solutions	Contain a balanced profile of essential, semi-essential, and nonessential L-amino acids.
	Disease-specific solutions	
	Hepatic encephalopathy	Amino acid profile includes higher BCAA concentrations and lower AAA and methionine concentrations.
	Renal failure	Amino acid profile includes higher EAA and histidine concentrations.
	Metabolic stress/ trauma	Amino acid profile provides standard essential, semi-essential, and nonessential amino acids with higher BCAA concentrations.
	Pediatrics	Amino acid profile includes standard essential, semi-essential, and nonessential amino acids with lower methionine, phenylalanine, and glycine concentrations; these solutions also contain taurine, glutamate, and aspartate.
Energy		
Carbohydrate	Dextrose	
	Glycerol	Used in ProcalAmine (B. Braun Medical, Inc.)
Fat	Intravenous fat emulsion	Fatty acid source
	LCT emulsions	Soybean

	Alternative fat emulsions (investigational)	MCT-LCT
		Olive oil
		Fish oil
		Mixed fat emulsions:
		  SMOF (soybean oil, MCT, olive, and fish oils)
		  MSF (MCT, soybean, and fish oils)

AAA, aromatic amino acids (includes phenylalanine and tyrosine); BCAA, branched-chain amino acids (leucine, isoleucine, and valine); EAA, essential amino acids (leucine, isoleucine, valine, phenylalanine, tryptophan, methionine, threonine, and lysine); LCT, long-chain triglycerides; MCT, medium-chain triglycerides; PN, parenteral nutrition

different among products. Because the nitrogen concentration of dietary protein is approximately 16%, 6.25 (100 g protein/16 g nitrogen) is commonly accepted as the conversion figure for calculating the nitrogen amount provided by CAA protein. Differences in nitrogen content per gram of amino acids among CAA products may affect calculation of nitrogen amounts infused when determining nitrogen balance.[25,26] The clinical significance of these differences in determining nitrogen balance for routine clinical use is unknown.[26]

Electrolyte composition of standard CAA solutions varies from small, obligatory amounts to the provision of maintenance requirements of most electrolytes for an adult. Electrolytes provided by CAA solutions must be considered when determining a patient's individual requirements. CAAs are available in several different concentrations, which facilitates compounding of patient-specific PN regimens. Use of highly concentrated products (15% to 20%) is attractive for critically ill patients who typically require fluid restriction but have large protein needs. Modified amino acid solutions are designed for patients who have altered protein requirements, such as those with hepatic encephalopathy, renal failure, and metabolic stress or trauma, as well as for neonates and pediatric patients (see Table 151-3). These solutions tend to be more expensive than standard CAA solutions. The rationale for and clinical efficacy of modified amino acids in disease-specific PN regimens is controversial (see Chap. 153).

Several commercially available CAA solutions are designed to provide conditionally essential amino acids, which are considered nonessential during health because they are produced from other amino acids. However, under certain physiologic conditions, such as prematurity or sepsis, these amino acids cannot be synthesized in sufficient quantities.[25] CAA solutions specifically designed for neonates and pediatric patients contain increased amounts of taurine, aspartic acid, and glutamic acid. Other conditionally essential amino acids, such as cysteine, carnitine, and glutamine, are not available in commercial CAA solutions in pharmacologic amounts because they are relatively unstable or poorly soluble.[25]

Consequently, PN solutions may need to be modified to provide the desired amount of supplemental conditionally essential amino acids. For example, cysteine is a conditionally essential amino acid for preterm and term infants because of their enzymatic immaturity of the trans-sulfuration pathway. Cysteine may be added to PN solutions at the time of compounding as a supplement to CAA solutions and also to enhance calcium and phosphate solubility by decreasing solution pH.[27] Carnitine is a quaternary amine required for long-chain fatty acid transport into the mitochondria for β-oxidation and energy production. Newborns are at risk for carnitine deficiency because of their immature biosynthetic capacity. Decreased plasma carnitine concentrations have been reported for infants and children receiving PN without carnitine.[28] Supplemental carnitine may be added to the PN solution at the time of compounding. While the benefit of carnitine supplementation in PN has not been clearly identified, positive effects on nutritional markers, including improved fatty acid oxidation, weight gain, and nitrogen balance have been documented. In general, carnitine supplementation is reserved for neonates expected to receive PN support for 7 days or longer.[28]

Glutamine is the most abundant free amino acid in the body and is an important intermediate for many metabolic processes. Glutamine is reported to have an important role in maintaining intestinal integrity, immune function, and protein synthesis during conditions of metabolic stress.[25,29] Investigations in humans and animals have reported positive effects on nutritional markers such as nitrogen balance, whereas others have reported significant improvement in other outcome markers, such as decreased length of hospitalization, incidence of infections, and GI toxicities associated with chemotherapy or radiation.[29] However, the best adult candidate for response to glutamine therapy has not been clearly identified.[29] The clinical usefulness of glutamine in neonates is less clear.[30] Plasma glutamine concentrations increase with supplementation, but no beneficial effect on sepsis, enteral feeding tolerance, necrotizing enterocolitis, growth, or mortality has been reported.[30] The clinical use of glutamine is further complicated because there is no IV glutamine formulation commercially available in the United States. Currently available CAA solutions do not contain glutamine because of poor solubility and instability. Use of IV glutamine requires special manufacturing techniques not readily available in many institutional pharmacies.[31] Additional controlled trials are warranted to characterize the risks and costs associated with extemporaneous compounding before routine IV glutamine use can be recommended.[29,31] Dipeptide amino acids are a potential parenteral source for conditionally essential amino acids that may provide a solution to the instability and solubility limitations. Dipeptides are synthesized by combining two amino acids with a peptide bond. The resulting protein is more soluble and stable than the individual amino acids.[25] IV dipeptide formulations would be advantageous clinically because they incorporate higher concentrations of some specific amino acids as well as some low-solubility, low-stability

amino acids that are omitted or present in small quantities in current CAA solutions. In addition, dipeptide use would allow formulation of CAA solutions with higher nitrogen content. Further studies are needed to assess long-term safety and optimal combinations of amino acids in different disease states. Dipeptide CAA formulations are currently not available in the United States.

CLINICAL CONTROVERSY

Although sufficient energy substrate should be provided to support amino acid use for protein synthesis, amino acid oxidation for energy has been demonstrated in critically ill patients and is thought to occur because of altered metabolism associated with severe metabolic stress. Hence, some practice settings may express calories provided by PN as total calories (protein, carbohydrate, fat calories), whereas others may use nonprotein calories (carbohydrate and fat).

DEXTROSE

The primary energy source in PN solutions is carbohydrate, usually in the form of dextrose monohydrate, which is available in concentrations ranging from 5% to 70%. When oxidized, each gram of hydrated dextrose provides 3.4 kcal (14.2 kJ). The appropriate IV dextrose dose depends on the patient's age, estimated caloric requirements, and clinical condition. For example, minimum dextrose requirements for neonates are estimated to be approximately 6 to 10 mg/kg/min.[22,32] However, IV dextrose infusion rates should not exceed 10 to 14 mg/kg per minute for infants and 4 to 7 mg/kg per minute for adults.[32-34] The recommended dextrose dose for routine clinical care rarely exceeds 5 mg/kg per minute for older critically ill children (1 to 11 years old) and adults.[33,35] Maintaining an age-appropriate dextrose infusion rate is necessary to minimize risk of adverse effects. If the dextrose infusion rate exceeds the glucose oxidation rate, metabolically expensive pathways, such as glycogen repletion and lipid synthesis, are favored, resulting in increased energy expenditure, increased oxygen consumption, and increased carbon dioxide production. Excessive dextrose infusion rates also may contribute to the development of hyperglycemia, excess carbon dioxide production, and increased biochemical markers for liver function associated with fatty infiltration of the liver.[33-35]

Carbohydrate sources that are not insulin dependent have been investigated as an alternative to dextrose to improve glycemic control for patients with impaired insulin secretion or activity who require PN. Glycerol, a sugar alcohol that provides 4.3 kcal/g (18 kJ/g), is the only dextrose alternative commercially available for clinical use. It is available as an isotonic, 3% solution in combination with 3% amino acids and supplemental electrolytes (ProcalAmine, B. Braun Medical, Irvine, CA). Although the solution may be peripherally infused, a major disadvantage of this formula is the dilute amino acid and carbohydrate concentrations. Most adult patients require up to 3 to 4 L/day of ProcalAmine solution together with IVFE as a caloric source to provide minimum energy requirements.[36] IV glycerol use for catabolic adults is safe and effective, but similar data are not available for infants and children.[37]

INTRAVENOUS FAT EMULSION

IVFE is used as a concentrated source of calories and essential fatty acids. While commercially available IVFE products have traditionally contained soybean oil or a combination of soybean oil and safflower oil, IVFE products containing safflower oil are no longer manufactured. Soybean-oil-based IVFE products are available in various concentrations (10%, 20%, and 30%) and contain egg phospholipids as an emulsifying agent and glycerol to make the emulsion isotonic. Although the caloric contribution of fat is 9 kcal/g (38 kJ/g), the caloric content of IVFE is 1.1 kcal/mL (4.6 kJ/mL) for 10% emulsion, 2 kcal/mL (8.4 kJ/mL) for 20% emulsion, and 3 kcal/mL (12.6 kJ/mL) for 30% emulsion because of the caloric contribution of the egg phospholipid and glycerol.[38] The fatty acid composition of soybean-oil-based IVFEs is approximately 44% to 62% linoleic acid and 4% to 11% linolenic acid.[38] Linolenic acid, an omega-3 fatty acid, and linoleic acid, an omega-6 fatty acid, are both polyunsaturated long-chain triglycerides (LCTs).[39] IVFE products differ in phospholipid and triglyceride concentrations. Higher-concentrated IVFEs (20% and 30%) have a lower phospholipid-to-triglyceride ratio compared with 10% IVFE.[31,40] Because higher amounts of circulating phospholipids are associated with impaired triglyceride clearance in neonates and infants, 20% IVFE is the preferred product for this population.[31,40,41]

Soybean-oil-based IVFE is effective for treatment or prevention of essential fatty acid deficiency (EFAD). EFAD is the result of a biochemical deficiency of linoleic acid and arachidonic acid, which are considered essential for humans.[42] Linoleic and linolenic acids are important for a variety of functions such as cellular integrity, platelet function, postnatal brain development, and wound healing.[42] Normally, linoleic acid is converted to the tetraene arachidonic acid. When linoleic acid is not present in sufficient amounts, oleic acid is converted to the triene 5,8,11-eicosatrienoic acid, a fatty acid of lesser physiologic integrity, and EFAD occurs. EFAD may be prevented by providing 2% to 4% of total calories as linoleic acid and 0.25% to 0.5% of total calories as linolenic acid.[31] This may be achieved for most adult patients by giving approximately 100 g IVFE weekly.[31,33] Neonates and infants require a minimum of 0.5 to 1 g/kg daily.[40,41,43]

Plasma IVFE clearance is directly related to gestational age of infants and appears to be influenced by the infusion rate and the patient's clinical status.[40,41,43] The risk of developing hypertriglyceridemia decreases with longer infusion times.[31,40,43] Rapid IVFE infusions are reported to contribute to decreased oxygenation for neonates.[40,43] Adverse pulmonary effects are thought to be caused by polyunsaturated fatty acid (PUFA)-driven prostaglandin production, which results in altered vascular tone. Although the association between IVFE and pulmonary dysfunction is not clear, a black-box warning appears in the FDA labeling for soybean-oil-based IVFE that acknowledges deaths in preterm infants associated with pulmonary fat accumulation thought to be related to IVFE infusions.[40,43,44] In addition, data for animals and humans also suggest that rapid infusion of long-chain fatty acid formulations may have a negative impact on immunocompetence by saturating the reticuloendothelial system.[33,45]

As a caloric source, IVFE use may facilitate provision of adequate calories and minimize complications of nutrition therapy such as hyperglycemia, hepatotoxicity, or increased carbon dioxide production.[33] Although the frequency of acute adverse effects is reported to be <1% with current formulations, patients receiving their first IVFE dose should be monitored for dyspnea, chest tightness, palpitations, and chills. Headache, nausea, and fever also have been reported and might be associated with a rapid infusion rate. In general, IVFE use is contraindicated for patients with an impaired ability to clear fat emulsion, such as patients with pathologic hyperlipidemia, lipoid nephrosis, and hypertriglyceridemia associated with pancreatitis.[44] Finally, patients with a reported egg allergy should be evaluated carefully for the nature and severity of the reaction before deciding to initiate a fat-based PN regimen.

Commercially available 10% and 20% IVFE products may be administered by either the central or the peripheral route. They may be added directly to the PN solution as a total nutrient admixture (TNA), also referred to as a 3-in-1 system (lipids, protein, glucose, and additives), or they may be piggybacked with the CAA-dextrose solution, commonly referred to as a 2-in-1 solution.[31,38,44] The more concentrated 30% IVFE is only approved for use in the preparation of TNA and is not intended for direct IV administration.

Soybean-oil-based IVFEs have negative effects on immune function as the result of omega-6 PUFA influence on proinflammatory eicosanoid production. These negative effects on immune function have stimulated a search for alternative IVFE sources that provide adequate essential fatty acids but lower amounts of omega-6 FA.[39,45] Medium-chain triglycerides (MCTs) may offer several advantages, especially for critically ill patients. MCTs are hydrolyzed and cleared more rapidly than LCTs, and they do not accumulate in the liver. In addition, MCTs do not require carnitine for entrance into mitochondria for oxidation. However, MCTs are not a source of essential fatty acids. Subsequent studies of IV MCT-LCT mixtures in a number of patients demonstrate safety and efficacy comparable with standard LCT emulsions.[39,42,45] Several MCT-LCT products are available in Europe, although no IV MCT formulations are currently available commercially in the United States. Other IVFE that are available outside the United States include a fish oil-based emulsion, an olive-oil- and soybean-oil-based emulsion and mixed fat source emulsions including a soybean, MCT, olive oil, and fish oil combination and a soybean, MCT, and fish oil combination.[39,45] Fish-oil-based IVFE contain predominantly omega-3 PUFAs, which are metabolized to cytokine mediators that may be less inflammatory and immunosuppressive than those derived from omega-6 PUFAs. Olive-oil-based IVFEs provide essential fatty acids, are a rich source of vitamin E, and may have a neutral effect on immune function. The clinical effect of IVFE administration on immune function, as well as on patient morbidity and mortality, is not clear.[39,43,45] However, investigations of enteral solutions with a higher concentration of omega-3 PUFAs have reported decreased infections and improvement of in vitro immunologic indices in critically ill patients.[42,46] Recent evidence suggests that soybean-based IVFE, which contains phytosterols and predominantly omega-6 PUFAs, may play a greater role in the development of PN-associated liver disease (PNALD). Investigations of fish-oil-based IVFE have reported improved or reversal of PNALD.[47–49] Although IVFE products remain the most common source of parenteral fat, a number of drugs have been introduced that contain lipid either as a vehicle for delivery or as a portion of the drug molecular formulation. Propofol, an IV anesthetic, is delivered in a soybean-oil-in-water emulsion that has essentially the same composition and caloric concentration as 10% IVFE. This agent is used commonly for continuous sedation of ventilated patients and should be considered a potentially significant source of calories that may require adjustment of a patient's nutrition regimen.[31] The antifungal amphotericin B is available in several lipid-containing combinations such as liposomal and lipid complex formulations. The caloric contribution from these products when used in standard doses generally is small and is not relevant clinically.

VITAMINS

Maintenance guidelines for daily parenteral vitamin supplements were initially established by the Nutrition Advisory Group of the American Medical Association (NAG-AMA) for adults, children, and infants.[50] The NAG-AMA identified 13 essential vitamins that include 4 fat-soluble vitamins and 9 water-soluble vitamins based on requirements for healthy people. These original guidelines have been revised based on clinical experience and research for specific adult and pediatric patient groups who required PN. [21,43,51–53]

For example, the NAG-AMA guidelines for infants and children were later revised to primarily reflect changes for preterm infants requiring PN.[53] In addition, the U.S. Food and Drug Administration (FDA) mandated reformulation of adult parenteral multiple-vitamin product guidelines to include 150 mcg of vitamin K in addition to higher doses of vitamins B1, B6, and C compared with the original AMA-NAG recommendations.[54]

Vitamin K was not included in previous parenteral multiple-vitamin formulations to minimize the risk of a drug–nutrient interaction for patients receiving anticoagulants, which antagonize vitamin K–dependent coagulation factors. The NAG-AMA recommendation for vitamin K for adults is 2 to 4 mg weekly. Other practitioners recommend larger doses of 0.5 to 1 mg/day or 5 to 10 mg weekly.[31] An investigation of patients receiving long-term IVFE-containing PN with vitamin K–free parenteral multivitamins at home suggests that supplemental vitamin K may not be necessary to maintain normal prothrombin times and plasma vitamin K concentrations.[55] Soybean oil used in IVFEs is a natural source of phylloquinone (vitamin K1). However, the vitamin K concentration is dependent on the soybean oil concentration in the IVFE.[54-56] Mean concentrations of 30.9 and 67.5 mcg/100 mL were reported for 10% and 20% Intralipid (Baxter Healthcare Corporation, Deerfield, IL), a soybean-oil-based IVFE. The bioavailability of vitamin K1 from IVFEs is unknown. Although hospitalized patients who received no additional vitamin K supplementation during short-term PN that included a low vitamin K–containing IVFE experienced minimal effects on international normalized ratio, supplemental vitamin K may be given intramuscularly or subcutaneously or added to the PN solution if needed.[54] Current recommendations suggest supplemental vitamin K is unnecessary when a vitamin K–containing multiple-vitamin product is used.[31]

Adult parenteral multiple-vitamin products formulated to comply with the FDA-mandated changes to the NAG-AMA guidelines are available commercially. In addition, a parenteral multiple-vitamin formulation containing no vitamin K is commercially available for adult patients receiving home PN and warfarin anticoagulation. (MVI-12, multivitamin infusion without vitamin K, Hospira Inc. Lake Forest, IL.) Two parenteral multiple-vitamin products are commercially available for use for pediatric patients. MVI-Pediatric (Hospira Inc., Lake Forest, IL) and Infuvite Pediatric (Baxter Healthcare Corporation, Deerfield, IL) are formulated to meet the revised NAG-AMA guidelines for infants weighing <1 kg (2.2 lb) to children up to 11 years old. However, there are no commercially available IV multivitamin products designed to specifically meet the unique requirements of premature infants, including higher vitamin A and lower doses of vitamins B1, B2, B6, and B12 compared with recommendations for term infants and older children.

Vitamin requirements may be altered in malnutrition and other specific disease states or with certain drug therapies. Individual and combination products are available to provide additional or tailored supplementation, which may be necessary to prevent development of vitamin toxicities or deficiencies caused by altered metabolism or drug therapy.

TRACE ELEMENTS

Many trace elements are an important part of metalloenzymes and also function as cofactors in a variety of regulatory metabolic pathways.[51,53] Although 17 trace elements have demonstrated biologic importance, clear deficiency syndromes in humans have been described only for cobalt (as vitamin B12), copper, iodine, iron, and zinc.[53,57,58] The NAG-AMA recognized chromium, copper, and zinc as being essential for IV supplementation for patients receiving PN.[59] Although a clear deficiency syndrome for manganese has not been reported in humans, the NAG-AMA considered manganese essential based on case reports of patients receiving PN with metabolic complications that corrected after manganese supplementation. Reports of syndromes associated with selenium and molybdenum

deficiency suggest that they also may be essential.[53,57] Although iodine deficiency has not been reported for patients receiving short-term PN, it has been observed for patients receiving long-term PN and may be related to the use of chlorhexidine for central-line care instead of povidone–iodine.[60]

IV trace elements are available as single-trace element solutions and as multiple-trace element combinations. Most products for adults provide the daily requirements for the trace elements considered essential by the NAG-AMA (i.e., chromium, copper, manganese, selenium, and zinc). Currently available combination products for neonates and pediatric patients contain only chromium, copper, manganese, and zinc. Combination products containing iodide and molybdenum are no longer commercially available in the United States. Single entity IV products are available that allow for individualization of trace mineral supplementation of chromium, copper, iodine, manganese, selenium, and zinc.

Requirements for trace elements also change depending on the clinical condition of the patient. For example, higher doses of supplemental zinc likely are necessary for patients with high-output ostomies or diarrhea because the GI tract is the predominant excretion route for zinc. Manganese and copper are excreted through the biliary tract, whereas chromium, molybdenum, and selenium are excreted renally. Hence, these trace elements should be restricted or withheld from PN solutions for patients with cholestatic liver disease and renal failure, respectively.

ELECTROLYTES

Electrolytes such as sodium, potassium, calcium, magnesium, phosphorus, chloride, and acetate are necessary PN components for the maintenance of numerous cellular functions. Electrolytes may be given to maintain normal serum concentrations or to correct deficits. Patients who have "normal" organ function and relatively normal serum concentrations of any electrolyte should receive normal maintenance electrolyte doses when PN is initiated and daily thereafter. Specific electrolyte requirements vary according to the patient's age, disease state, organ function (see Chap. 153), previous and current drug therapy, nutrition status, and extrarenal losses. Electrolytes are available commercially as single- and multiple-nutrient solutions. Multiple-electrolyte solutions are useful for stable patients with normal organ function who are receiving PN. Concentrated multiple-electrolyte solutions designed for addition to PN solutions generally contain only sodium, potassium, calcium, and magnesium. Phosphorus must be added as a separate additive. Further information regarding metabolism and requirements of vitamins, trace elements, and electrolytes is given elsewhere.[31,61]

DESIGNING A PARENTERAL NUTRITION REGIMEN

❺ Several factors, including the patient's venous access, fluid status, and macronutrient and micronutrient requirements, are important considerations when designing the PN regimen. A patient's venous access and fluid status determines how concentrated the PN solution may be compounded and, hence, have an impact on the nutrient amount that may be provided. PN solutions may be administered by central or peripheral venous access. The patient's clinical condition determines which route is most appropriate (Fig. 151–1).

PN solutions may be provided as a 2-in-1 formulation that contains dextrose, CAA, and other necessary micronutrients or as a 3-in-1 formulation or TNA that contains dextrose, CAA, and IVFE, as well as other necessary micronutrients. Use of TNA solutions offers several potential advantages, including reduced inventory

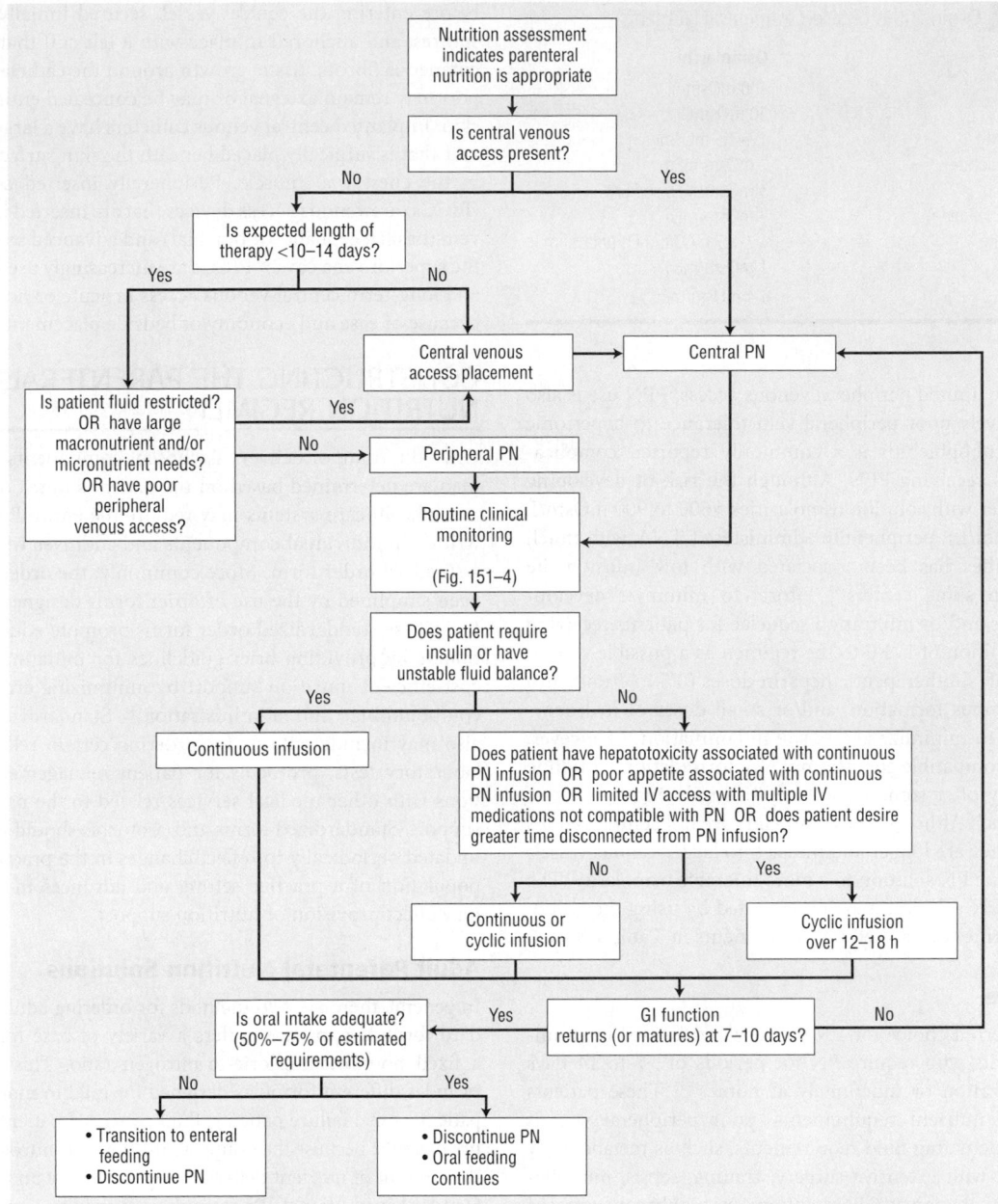

FIGURE 151-1. The route of parenteral nutrition (PN) and the infusion type depend on the patient's clinical status and the expected length of therapy.

(infusion pumps, tubing, and other related supplies), decreased time for compounding and administration, a potential decrease in manipulations of the infusion line (which should correspond with a decreased risk of catheter contamination), and ease of delivery and storage for patients receiving home PN.[62] Potential disadvantages include increased risk of infections and stability and compatibility concerns. For example, the stability of TNA solutions is less predictable than that of 2-in-1 solutions, which makes their use less desirable in specific patient populations such as neonates and infants.[31]

ROUTES OF PARENTERAL NUTRITION ADMINISTRATION

Peripheral Route

Peripheral parenteral nutrition (PPN) is an option for mild to moderately stressed patients for whom central access is unavailable

or undesirable and function of their GI tract is expected to return within 10 to 14 days.[63] Potential PPN candidates should not be fluid restricted or require large nutrient amounts. Lower concentrations of amino acid (3% to 5% final concentration), dextrose (5% to 10% final concentration), and micronutrients compared with central parenteral nutrition (CPN) are necessary for peripheral administration. Because PPN solutions are relatively dilute, larger volumes are usually necessary to provide nutrient requirements. Additionally, many patients who receive PPN likely will require the use of IVFE to increase caloric support to levels more consistent with CPN regimens. The primary advantages of PPN include a lower risk of infectious, metabolic, and technical complications.[63] However, several other factors may complicate PPN use in many patient populations. Patients who have received multiple courses of chemotherapy, malnourished patients, premature infants, elderly patients, and others with an illness of long duration who have already been subjected to multiple venous accesses for fluid and medication administration

TABLE 151-4 Osmolarities of Select Parenteral Nutrients

Nutrient	Osmolarity
Amino acid	100 mOsm/%
Dextrose	50 mOsm/%
Lipid emulsion (20%)	1.3–1.5 mOsm/g
Sodium (acetate, chloride)	2 mOsm/mEq
Sodium phosphate	3 mOsm/mEq sodium
Potassium (acetate, chloride)	2 mOsm/mEq
Potassium phosphate	1.7–2.7 mOsm/mEq potassium
Magnesium sulfate	1 mOsm/mEq
Calcium gluconate	1.4 mOsm/mEq

are likely to have limited peripheral venous access. PPN use is also limited by relatively poor peripheral vein tolerance to hypertonic solutions. Thrombophlebitis is a commonly reported complication for patients receiving PPN. Although the risk of developing phlebitis is greater with solution osmolarities >600 to 900 mOsm/L (600 to 900 mmol/L), peripherally administered TNA with much higher osmolarities has been associated with low infusion-site complications in some centers.[63] Efforts to minimize development of phlebitis and/or infiltration sequelae for patients receiving PPN include addition of IVFE to the regimen as a possible venous lumen protectant, subtherapeutic heparin doses (0.5 to 1 unit/mL) to prevent thrombus formation, and/or small doses of hydrocortisone (5 mg/L) to minimize access site inflammation.[63] However, heparin is not compatible for use in TNA formulations. Midline catheter use may offer some advantage with reducing the risk of thrombophlebitis.[64] Although these catheters are not central venous access devices, they are longer and infuse into larger venous vessels that may dilute the PN solution to a more tolerable osmolarity. The osmolarity of a PN solution may be estimated by using the guidelines for osmolarities of selected PN components in Table 151–4.

Central Route

CPN is the preferred choice for PN delivery and is used predominantly for patients who require PN for periods of >7 to 14 days during hospitalization or indefinitely at home.[31,65] These patients may have large nutrient requirements, poor peripheral venous access, and/or fluctuating fluid requirements, such as metabolically stressed patients with extensive surgery, trauma, sepsis, multiple-organ failure, or malignancy. CPN solutions are highly concentrated hypertonic solutions that must be administered through a large central vein. Unlike peripheral veins, central veins have a higher blood flow, which quickly dilutes the hypertonic solutions. Disadvantages of CPN include risks associated with catheter insertion, routine catheter use, and care of the access site. Relative to peripheral venous access, central venous catheter access is associated with a greater potential for infection. In addition, the risk of more serious catheter-induced trauma and related sequelae and other serious technical or mechanical problems is greater than that with peripheral access.

The choice of central venous access site depends on a number of factors, including the patient's age and anatomy. Central venous catheters vary in composition, lumen size, number of injection ports, and other special features that affect ease or convenience of care and maintenance. Central venous catheters for short-term use for adults are commonly inserted percutaneously into the subclavian vein and advanced so that the tip is at the superior vena cava.[64] If this approach is not possible, the internal jugular vein can be used. Frequently, short-term central venous access is obtained for critically ill neonates via a catheter placed in the umbilical vein. Other sites for central venous access in infants and older children are similar to those in adults. When therapy is expected to last longer than 4 weeks, the catheter usually is tunneled subcutaneously

before entering the central vessel, secured initially with retaining sutures, and anchored in place with a felt cuff that promotes subcutaneous fibrotic tissue growth around the catheter. The injection port may remain external or may be concealed entirely beneath the skin. Implanted central venous catheters have a larger port or reservoir that is surgically placed beneath the skin surface and anchored in the chest wall muscle. Peripherally inserted central catheters (PICCs) are venous access devices that are inserted into a peripheral vein (basilic, cephalic, or brachial) and advanced so that the tip is at the superior vena cava.[64] PICCs are increasingly used for both short- and long-term central venous access in acute or home care settings because of ease and economy of bedside placement.[31,65]

CONSTRUCTING THE PARENTERAL NUTRITION REGIMEN

Once the route of delivery is chosen, components of the PN regimen are determined based on the patient's nutritional assessment. Some healthcare systems may require the entire PN formula to be written in individual components and additives without the use of a standard order form. More commonly, the ordering process has been simplified by the use of order forms designed specifically for PN. These standardized order forms promote education of practitioners by providing brief guidelines for initiating PN and foster cost-efficient nutrition support by minimizing errors in ordering, compounding, and administration.[31] Standardized order forms also may include options for ordering certain related procedures, laboratory tests, protocols for patient management, or consultations with other medical services related to the patient's nutrition support. Standardized forms and protocols should be reviewed and updated periodically to reflect changes in the practices and patient population of a practice setting and advances in technology that may affect provision of nutrition support.

Adult Parenteral Nutrition Solutions

In general, there are two methods for ordering adult PN. The "standard formula approach" offers a variety of base formulations with a fixed nonprotein-calorie-to-nitrogen ratio. This method usually includes different formulas designed for mild to moderately stressed patients, renal failure patients, fluid-restricted patients, and liver failure patients. Because the nonprotein-calorie-to-nitrogen ratio is fixed, the amount of nutrient delivered depends solely on the infusion rate. Standard institutional PN formulations may be compounded; however, standardized commercial PN products or "premixed" solutions are available from manufacturers.[66] Use of a standard institutional formula may promote clinician prescribing of a complete, balanced formulation. Their use may also promote consistent provision of stable, compatible admixtures. However, efficiencies associated with use of the standard formula approach may be hindered if there is a frequent need to modify the PN formulation. Finally, standard PN formulations may be difficult to use in potentially complicated patients, such as neonatal or pediatric patients, or those with severe malnutrition, organ failure, glucose intolerance, large GI losses, or critical illness.[66]

The "individualized formula approach" permits compounding of patient-specific solutions. Compounding of the PN solution is limited only by the concentrations of stock solutions and stability of the additives. The nutrient amount delivered depends on the daily volume of the PN solution infused and the nutrient concentrations in the PN solution. The total daily amount of PN solution may be prepared in multiple bags or more cost-effectively in a single container.[31]

Traditionally, adult PN solutions have been ordered by expressing the final concentrations of each component in the solution. For example, CAA and dextrose are ordered commonly in final percentage, electrolytes in milliequivalents per liter, and other additives in amount (milliliters or units) per day. This inconsistency may promote confu-

Calculation of an Adult Parenteral Nutrition Regimen

Patient case: A patient's daily nutritional requirements have been estimated to be 100 g protein and 2,000 total kcal. The patient has central venous access and reports no history of hyperlipidemia or egg allergy. The patient is not fluid restricted. The PN solution will be compounded as an individualized regimen using a single-bag, 24-hour infusion of a 2-in-1 solution with intravenous fat emulsion (IVFE) piggybacked into the PN infusion line. Determine the total PN volume and administration rate by calculating the macronutrient stock solution volumes required to provide the desired daily nutrients. The stock solutions used to compound this regimen are 10% crystalline amino acids (CAA), 70% dextrose, and 20% IVFE.

1. Determine the daily IVFE calories and volume

   - 2,000 kcal/day × 30%–40% of total calories as fat = 600–800 kcal/day
     Choose IVFE 20% 250 mL/day × 2 kcal/mL = 500 kcal/day

2. Determine the 70% dextrose stock solution volume

   - Determine dextrose calories
     Dextrose calories = TOTAL − IVFE − Protein
     2,000 kcal − 500 kcal IVFE − (4 kcal/g × 100 g CAA) = 1,100 kcal

   - Calculate required dextrose (grams)
     1,100 kcal ÷ 3.4 kcal/g dextrose = 324 g dextrose

   - Determine 70% dextrose volume
     70 g/100 mL = 324 g/X mL 70% dextrose;   X = 463 mL 70% dextrose

3. Calculate the 10% CAA stock solution volume

   - 10 g/100 mL = 100 g/X mL 10% CAA;   X = 1,000 mL 10% CAA

4. Determine the 2-in-1 PN volume and administration rate

   - Calculate CAA/dextrose volume
     463 mL 70% dextrose + 1,000 mL 10% CAA = 1,463 mL CAA–dextrose

   - Add 100–200 mL for additives
     Total 2-in-1 volume = approximately 1,600–1,700 mL/day

   - Calculate the administration rate
     1,600–1,700 mL/day ÷ 24 hours = 67–71 mL/hour; round to 65–70 mL/hour

5. Choose final 2-in-1 PN regimen and determine provided nutrient amounts:

   - Final 2-in-1 regimen
     100 g CAA/324 gm dextrose in 1,680 mL/day to infuse at 70 mL/hour
     + 20% IVFE 250 mL to infuse at 2 mL/hour

   - Calculate macronutrient calories

20% IVFE calories:	250 mL × 2 kcal/mL =	500 kcal
Dextrose calories:	324 g × 3.4 kcal/g =	1,102 kcal
Protein calories:	100 g × 4 kcal/g =	400 kcal
Total kcal:		2,002 kcal
Nonprotein kcal:		1,602 kcal

FIGURE 151-2. Calculation of an adult parenteral nutrition (PN) regimen. To convert to energy units of kilojoules (kJ) multiply values with kilocalories as the numerator (kcal, kcal/mL, kcal/kg, kcal/g) by 4.18 to give the corresponding value in kilojoules (kJ, kJ/mL, kJ/kg, kJ/g).

sion and misinterpretation of PN solution contents that may result in harm, especially when patients are transferred between health system environments. To ensure that PN labels in all health system environments clearly and accurately reflect the PN solution contents, guidelines for standardized adult PN labeling have been recommended.[31] In addition to including a variety of other information on the label such as dosing weight and administration route, the guidelines recommend expressing PN ingredients in amounts per total volume, which minimizes the need for pharmaceutical calculations to determine the nutrient value of the admixture. Computer software for calculating PN solutions is widely available, and several programs have adapted the recommended labeling guidelines. Pharmaceutical calculations of a 2-in-1 PN regimen are briefly reviewed (see Fig. 151–2).

Several guidelines or clinical rules of thumb are available to help simplify calculation of a PN regimen after a patient's nutritional requirements have been decided. For example, adult patients receiving only PN therapy may need larger volumes of fluid to provide maintenance requirements and replace extrarenal losses. However, patients requiring other IV drug therapy may receive adequate fluid from an additional IV maintenance solution (e.g., 0.45% NaCl in 5% dextrose) and/or piggybacked medications. Depending on individual institutional practices, maximally concentrating the PN solution and using an inexpensive maintenance fluid to manage hydration may provide a cost-effective regimen that requires fewer adjustments. Another guideline that may be helpful in designing a PN regimen is to allow a volume of approximately 100 to 150 mL/L of base solution (approximately 200 to 300 mL per day) for electrolytes and other additives. PN regimens for patients who require very small amounts of additives, such as patients with renal failure, may be further concentrated.

Pediatric Parenteral Nutrition Solutions

Pediatric PN solutions are typically ordered using an individualized approach because clinical practice guidelines often recommend nutrient intakes based on the patient's weight. To simplify pediatric PN ordering many institutions use a pediatric-specific PN order form that expresses daily nutrient amount based on weight. For example, protein and fat are ordered as grams per kilogram per day, dextrose as milligrams per kilogram per minute, and electrolytes as milliequivalents per kilogram per day. However, some institutions may order macronutrients by expressing the final concentration of each component in the solution. Current safe practice guidelines suggest that the pediatric PN label identify components as an "amount per day" with a secondary expression of components as "amount per kilogram per day."[31] Auxiliary labels may be needed when the format between PN ordering and PN labeling is different. Calculations for determining a pediatric PN solution are reviewed to illustrate fundamental concepts for ordering pediatric PN solutions (Fig. 151–3). Additional features of the pediatric PN label include the dosing weight, administration date and time, expiration date, infusion rate, and duration of infusion. Because infants and children generally receive daily maintenance fluid from the PN regimen, supplemental IV solutions are rarely needed. Pediatric PN may be provided as a 2-in-1 or TNA formulation. However, the TNA system is not recommended for compounding neonatal and infant PN because of IVFE instability with the often needed higher calcium and phosphorus concentrations.[31] The IVFE labeling guidelines for pediatric PN are similar to adult IVFE labeling recommendations.

Administration Techniques

PN solutions should be administered with an infusion pump. The IV administration line for CAA-dextrose solutions should include a 0.22 μm inline filter to remove particulate matter, air, and any microorganisms that may be present in the solution. IVFEs administered separately from the CAA-dextrose solution must be infused into the PN line by utilizing a y-site port beyond the inline filter because the average size of IVFE particles is approximately 0.5 μm.[31] The FDA recommends use of a 1.2 μm filter with TNA solutions, which may be effective in preventing catheter occlusion caused by precipitates or lipid aggregates.[31] This filter size is also reported to remove *Candida albicans*.

INITIATING AND ADVANCING THE PARENTERAL NUTRITION INFUSION

ADULT PARENTERAL NUTRITION

The patient's nutrition status, current clinical status, history of glucose tolerance, and dextrose concentration in the formula will dictate the infusion rate at which the adult PN solution should be initiated. Stable patients with normal organ function and stable baseline serum glucose concentrations have demonstrated minimal effect on serum glucose concentrations when abruptly initiating or discontinuing PN therapy.[67,68] However, another approach is to begin the PN infusion and increase the rate gradually over 12 to 24 hours to the desired rate. The infusion rate is likewise reduced in a stepwise fashion, such as decreasing the rate by 50% for 1 hour prior to discontinuation, when the PN therapy ends.[67] This approach

should prevent development of hyperglycemia and rebound hypoglycemia, respectively. Alternatively, the PN regimen may be initiated at the goal infusion rate but with a hypocaloric dextrose dose. The dextrose dose can be increased daily to the goal based on patient response. Tapered initiation and cessation should be considered for patients receiving intermittent subcutaneous regular insulin, patients with severe renal or hepatic disease, and patients with other disease states that may increase the risk for development of hyperglycemia or hypoglycemia, such as severe diabetes or pancreatic malignancy.

Although the IVFE dose should not exceed 2.5 g/kg per day or 60% of total daily calories, lower doses of 1 g/kg per day not to exceed 30% of calories have been recommended to minimize negative effects associated with long-chain fatty acids.[31] Manufacturer's information recommends IVFE infusion over 4 to 8 hours for adults. However, infusion over 12 to 24 hours appears to be the best clinical strategy to promote IVFE clearance and minimize risk of negative effects on pulmonary and immune function.[31,40,43]

The manufacturer's guidelines recommend initiating IVFE for adults with a test dose of 0.5 to 1 mL/min for the first 15 to 30 minutes because of the potential for an immediate hypersensitivity reaction. For most patients, this is probably not necessary because of the relatively low incidence and benign nature of acute adverse reactions. In addition, infusion over 12 to 24 hours eliminates the need for a test dose because the infusion rate is within the range of the test dose rates recommended by the manufacturer. Appropriate electrolytes should be provided to patients with normal organ function based on standard nutrient ranges.[31] Adjustments may be necessary depending on the patient's clinical condition. Adults and children older than 11 years of age should receive daily amounts of trace elements and an adult vitamin formulation.

PEDIATRIC PARENTERAL NUTRITION

Pediatric PN solutions are typically initiated with a volume calculated to provide the patient's daily maintenance fluid requirements on the first day of therapy. Individual substrates are then advanced daily as tolerated with the goal PN regimen generally being achieved by day 3 of therapy. PN should be initiated with the goal protein dose. The initial dextrose dose for older infants and children is based on previous glucose tolerance. Although practices may vary, one approach is to start with 10% dextrose and advance the concentration in 5% increments daily as tolerated to a goal not to exceed 5 to 7 mg/kg per minute. Initial dextrose doses for premature infants should approximate fetal nutrient delivery rates of 5 to 6 mg/kg per minute. Frequently this mathematically translates into a final concentration range of 5% to 10% dextrose. The dextrose concentration for the neonatal PN should be advanced daily by 1% to 2.5% or by 2 to 4 mg/kg/min increments to a goal that does not exceed 12 to 14 mg/kg/min. IVFE is usually initiated at 0.5 g/kg/day for neonates and 0.5 to 1 g/kg/day for older children and increased daily by 0.5 to 1 g/kg/day. Incremental increases of IVFE dose allow daily serum triglyceride evaluation and early detection of those with impaired fat clearance. The IVFE dose should not exceed 60% of total daily calories for neonates and 30% of total calories for children, and the maximum IVFE dose should not exceed 3 g/kg/day (approximately 30 kcal/kg/day) for infants and children.[41] The best clinical strategy for minimizing the risk of adverse effects associated with rapid IVFE administration and promoting IVFE clearance is to infuse IVFE over 20 to 24 hours or at a rate of 0.15 g/kg/h.[40,41] This slow infusion also eliminates the need for a test dose because the infusion rate is less than the test-dose rate recommended by the manufacturer.

IV electrolytes, vitamins, and trace elements should be initiated on the first day of therapy and continued as a daily component of the PN solution.[31] Children younger than age 11 years should receive a vitamin

Calculation of a pediatric parenteral nutrition regimen

Patient case: A 30-week gestational age infant (weight 2 kg) with an estimated nutrition goal of 3 g/kg/day protein, 3 g/kg/day intravenous fat emulsion (IVFE), and 100 nonprotein kcal/kg/day. The infant has central venous access and no history of hyperlipidemia or egg allergy. The PN regimen will be compounded as an individualized regimen using a single-bag, 24-hour infusion of a 2-in-1 solution with 20% IVFE piggybacked into the PN infusion line. Determine the macronutrient calculations to deliver this infant's nutrition goals; 10% crystalline amino acids (CAA) and 70% dextrose stock solutions will be used to compound the solution.

1. Determine the goal daily IVFE amount, volume, and administration rate

   - 3 g/kg/day IVFE × 2 kg = 6 g/kg

   - Calculate 20% IVFE volume
     20 g/100 mL = 6 g/X mL   X = 30 mL/day of 20% IVFE

   - Calculate the IVFE administration rate
     30 mL 20% IVFE ÷ 24 hours = 1.25 mL/hour

2. Determine the goal 2-in-1 PN volume and administration rate

   - PN volume based on maintenance fluid requirements
     120 mL/kg/day × 2 kg = 240 mL/day

   - PN infusion rate is 240 mL/day ÷ 24 hours/day = 10 mL/hour

3. Determine the daily protein amount and the corresponding 10% CAA volume

   - Calculate the goal protein amount
     3 g/kg/day × 2 kg = 6 g/day

   - Calculate the 10% CAA stock solution volume
     10 g/100 mL = 6 g/X mL 10% CAA   X = 60 mL 10% CAA

4. Determine the daily dextrose amount, corresponding 70% dextrose volume, and final dextrose concentration in the 2-in-1 PN solution

   - Goal is to provide approximately 14 mg/kg/min dextrose
     14 g × 2 kg × 1440 minutes/day ÷ 1000 mg/g = 40.3 g dextrose

   - Calculate the 70% dextrose volume
     70 g/100 mL = 40.3 g/X mL 70% dextrose   X = 57.6 mL 70% dextrose

   - Calculate the final dextrose concentration of the PN solution
     40.3 g dextrose/240 mL = X g/100 mL   X = 16.8% dextrose

5. Determine available volume for additives

   - 240 mL − 60 mL (10% CAA) − 57.6 mL (70% dextrose) = ~122 mL
     Sterile water for injection may be necessary to QS to total volume of 240 mL

6. Determine the final PN regimen and provided nutrient amounts

   - Final PN regimen
     3 g/kg/day CAA and 16.8% dextrose to infuse at 10 mL/hour
     3 g/kg/day (or 30 mL) 20% IVFE to infuse at 1.25 mL/hour

   - Macronutrient calories

20% IVFE:	30 mL × 2 kcal/mL =	60 kcal
Dextrose:	40.3 g × 3.4 kcal/g =	137 kcal
Protein:	6 g × 4 kcal/g =	24 kcal
Total kcal (kcal/kg):		221 kcal (111 kcal/kg)
Nonprotein kcal (kcal/kg):		197 kcal/kg (99 kcal/kg)

To convert to energy units of kilojoules (kj) multiply values with kcal as the numerator (kcal, kcal/mL, kcal/kg, kcal/g) by 4.18 to give the corresponding value in kJ (kJ, kJ/mL, kJ/kg, kJ/g).

FIGURE 151-3. Calculation of a pediatric parenteral nutrition (PN) regimen.

product formulated for pediatric patients. Two multivitamin dosing schemas have been suggested for infants and children.[31] One method recommends 2 mL/kg/day for infants weighing <2.5 kg (5.5 lb) and 5 mL/day for infants and children weighing more than 2.5 kg (5.5 lb).

The other suggests 30% of a vial (1.5 mL/day) for infants weighing <1 kg (2.2 lb), 65% of a vial (3.25 mL/day) for infants weighing 1 to 3 kg (2.2 to 6.6 lb), and 100% of the vial (5 mL/day) for children weighing more than 3 kg (6.6 lb)(up to 11 years of age). Adult IV vitamin formulations should not be used for infants because of potential neurotoxicity from accumulation of polysorbate and propylene glycol preservatives. Weight-based dosage recommendations for pediatric multiple-trace-element formulations are 0.3 mL/kg for children weighing <3 kg (6.6 lb) and 0.2 mL/kg for children weighing more than 3 kg (6.6 lb) (maximum 5 mL/day). Children weighing more than 25 kg (55 lb) should receive an adult trace-element formulation. However, weight-based doses do not provide the recommended daily intake for all trace elements, so individual dosing with single entity products may be necessary. This approach also allows for dose adjustment based on serum trace element assessment, individual patient characteristics (e.g., cholestasis, stool losses, wounds), and the need to minimize administration of trace elements that accumulate in patients receiving chronic PN such as chromium and manganese. Pediatric patients receiving PN commonly transition from PN support to enteral nutrition by gradually, over a period of days to weeks, decreasing the PN infusion rate while increasing the enteral intake. The PN infusion rate should be reduced for 1 to 2 hours prior to stopping the infusion for neonates and infants because of their immature counterregulatory mechanisms that contribute to an increased risk for developing rebound hypoglycemia.[16] Blood glucose concentrations should be checked within 15 to 60 minutes after the PN infusion ends.

CLINICAL CONTROVERSY

Initiation of IVFE earlier than 4 to 7 days of life for infants with a birth weight <800 g remains controversial because of the potential increased risk of chronic lung disease and death. Some clinicians advocate initiating IVFE at 1 to 1.5 g/kg/day within the first week of life and advancing the dose after the second week of life.

CONTINUOUS VERSUS CYCLIC INFUSIONS

6 Use of continuous infusions is attractive for patients with unstable fluid balance or glucose control (see Fig. 151–1). The intermittent or cyclic infusion of PN over a period of time <24 hours, usually for 12 to 18 hours each day, is useful for hospitalized patients with limited venous access in whom administration of multiple other medications requires interruption of the PN infusion.[67] Cyclic PN also may prevent or treat hepatotoxicities associated with continuous PN therapy. In addition, this delivery mode allows patients receiving PN at home the ability to resume a relatively normal lifestyle.[67] Various protocols have been reported that suggest incremental increases to the maximum infusion rate for a desired period of time followed by a gradual taper to discontinue the solution.[16,67] However, metabolically stable adults and older children (older than age 2 years) receiving fat-based PN regimens are likely candidates for abrupt initiation and discontinuation of their intermittent PN regimen.[16,67] Cyclic PN is not optimal for all patients and should be used with caution for those with severe glucose intolerance or diabetes, or unstable fluid balance.

EVALUATION OF THERAPEUTIC OUTCOMES

7 Thorough and consistent monitoring of patients who are receiving PN is necessary to ensure that the desired nutritional outcomes are achieved and to prevent the occurrence of adverse effects or complications. Routine evaluation should include the assessment of the patient's clinical condition with a focus on nutritional and metabolic effects of the PN regimen. Serial documentation of a patient's response to a particular regimen is a helpful guide for determining appropriate adjustments in fluid, electrolyte, and nutrient therapies.

Several biochemical and clinical measurements are necessary for effective monitoring of patients receiving PN. Serum concentrations of electrolytes, hematologic indices, and biochemical markers for renal function, liver function, and nutrition status should be measured prior to PN initiation and periodically thereafter depending on the patient's age, nutrition status, and clinical condition. The frequency of blood laboratory measurements for neonates and infants tends to be more conservative because of their smaller circulating blood volumes and, in some cases, lack of central vascular access. Other important clinical measurements include vital signs, weight, total fluid intake and losses, and nutritional intakes. Weekly measurements of height/length and head circumference are helpful for monitoring nutritional changes in neonates. Monitoring parameters considered important for patients receiving PN and the suggested frequency of measurement for each are outlined in Figure 151–4. Appropriate assessment and evaluation of patient data can identify potential complications that may be avoided or treated early. Monitoring protocols should be developed and tailored for the patient population, medical practices, and resources of individual practice settings.

COMPOUNDING, STORAGE, AND INFECTION CONTROL

The United States Pharmacopeia (USP) Chap. 797 details the procedures and requirements for compounding sterile preparations including PN formulations.[69] These standards apply to all healthcare settings in which sterile preparations are compounded and are used by boards of pharmacy, the FDA, and accreditation organizations such as the Joint Commission. Compounded sterile preparations are defined by risk level (immediate use, low, low with 12-hour beyond use date, medium, and high) based on the probability of microbial, chemical, or physical contamination. PN solutions are classified as a medium-risk compounded sterile preparation. In general, PN solutions should be prepared using aseptic technique in a device or room that meets International Organization for Standardization (ISO) Class 5 standards that is located in an ISO Class 7 buffer area with an ISO Class 8 ante area.[69] Personnel must be trained adequately for personnel cleansing and garbing procedures and aseptic manipulations. Supervision by a pharmacist experienced in compounding IV solutions and knowledgeable about stability, compatibility, and storage of PN solutions is necessary. Quality assurance procedures should be developed to maintain safe and accurate admixture preparation. A standardized process for PN ordering, labeling, determining nutrient requirements, screening of the PN order, PN administration, and monitoring has been recommended to minimize risk of potentially life-threatening compounding errors.[31,66,70,71] The potential risk of infectious complications associated with PN solution contamination can be decreased greatly when pharmacy-based admixture programs follow specific guidelines developed to ensure proper compounding of PN solutions.[69]

In general, the type of solution being prepared dictates the methods of compounding, storage, and infusion. Currently, the two most commonly used types of PN solutions are 2-in-1 solutions with or without IVFE piggybacked into the PN line and TNAs. Methods for compounding PN solutions vary based on a healthcare system's patient population and medical practices and the number of PN solutions that need to be prepared. PN base solutions may be prepared by using gravity-driven transfer of CAA stock solutions to partially filled bags of concentrated dextrose stock solutions.[31,72] Other practice settings may use standardized

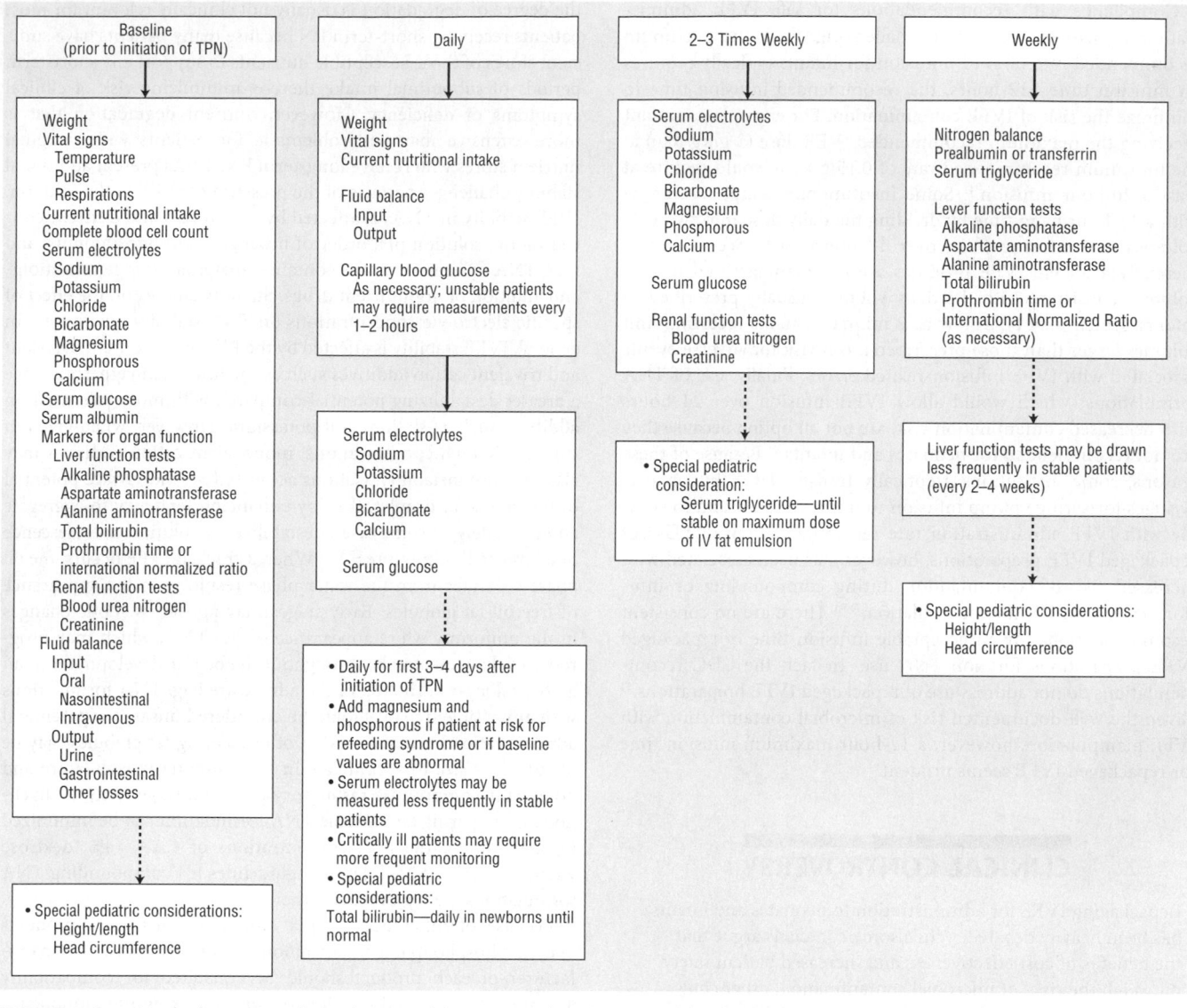

FIGURE 151-4. Monitoring strategy for patients receiving parenteral nutrition (PN).

commercial PN products with CAA and dextrose separated within a single bag that must be mixed prior to use.[31,66] Advances in compounding technology have facilitated use of automated compounders for preparing PN solutions. Automated compounders are computer-based systems that perform the calculations necessary to determine volumes of nutrient stock solutions for PN formulations. In addition, most automated compounder systems include software that communicates the determined calculations directly to a transfer pump device that delivers fluid from the source container to the final container by either a volumetric or gravimetric fluid pumping system.[72] Advantages associated with automated compounders include reduced personnel time and compounding materials and improved compounding accuracy. Disadvantages include the potential for equipment failure and power outages.

Assurance of solution sterility during compounding, storage, and administration is necessary to reduce the risk of infection and related complications. Because of their acidic pH and hypertonicity, 2-in-1 PN formulations are poor media for microbial growth.[31,73] However, several characteristics of IVFE such as iso-osmotic tonicity, near-neutral to alkaline pH, and glycerol content favor microbial growth, particularly at room temperature.[31]

When IVFEs are added to dextrose-CAA solutions to make TNAs, the growth potential is decreased, presumably due to the protective effects of the hypertonic dextrose-CAA solution and decreased pH.[64,74]

CAA-dextrose solutions generally are stable for 30 days if refrigerated at 4°C (39.2°F) and protected from light.[27] However, because of the risk for microbial contamination, manufacturers recommend storage of PN solutions for as little time as possible after preparation. The USP 797 standards recommend storage times of not more than 30 hours at controlled room temperature [20°C (68°F) to 25°C (77°F)] and not more than 9 days at cold temperatures [2°C (36°F) to 8°C(46°F)] for all medium-risk compounded sterile preparations, including PN solutions.[69]

Because IVFEs support growth of gram-positive and gram-negative bacteria as well as fungi, the Centers for Disease Control and Prevention (CDC) recommend that infusion time for IVFE administered as a separate infusion should not exceed 12 hours, unless volume considerations require more time, in which case the infusion should be completed within 24 hours.[64] The CDC guidelines also recommend use of administration sets for 2-in-1 PN for up to 72 hours, but those used for TNA solutions and IVFE should be changed every 24 hours.[64]

Compliance with recommendations for safe IVFE administration to pediatric patients is challenging. First, the maximum recommended rate of IVFE infusion for infants typically requires an infusion time >12 hours, the recommended infusion time to minimize the risk of IVFE contamination. For example, an infant receiving the maximum recommended IVFE dose (3 g/kg/day) at the maximum recommended rate of 0.15 g/kg/h would require at least a 20-hour infusion.[41] Some institutions attempt to comply with a 12-hour hang time by dividing the daily dose into two unit volumes and infusing them over 12 hours each. Second, commercially available IVFE products are not manufactured in unit volumes consistent with the daily volumes usually prescribed to infants, which may be as low as 2 mL/day. Infants receiving unit volumes larger than those prescribed are at risk for adverse events associated with IVFE infusion-related errors. Finally, use of TNA formulations, which would allow IVFE infusion over 24 hours with decreased contamination risk, are not an option because they are not recommended for neonates and infants.[31] Because of these reasons, some institutions aseptically transfer IVFE into plastic syringes for syringe pump infusion to improve safety and to comply with IVFE administration rate recommendations.[74–76] Use of repackaged IVFE preparations, however, has been associated with increased risk of contamination during compounding or infusion because of IV line manipulation.[74,76] There are no consistent recommendations for an acceptable infusion time of repackaged IVFE preparations for non-TNA use. In fact, the CDC recommendations do not address use of repackaged IVFE preparations.[64] Given the well-documented risk of microbial contamination with IVFE manipulation, however, a 12-hour maximum infusion time for repackaged IVFE seems prudent.

CLINICAL CONTROVERSY

Repackaging IVFE for administration to neonates and infants has been heavily debated. While some clinicians argue that the benefits of cost effectiveness and increased patient safety outweigh the risks of microbial contamination, other clinicians continue to advocate for the delivery of IVFE direct from the manufacturer's container to decrease infection risk. Other IVFE practices vary greatly from institution to institution, including the most appropriate IVFE infusion rate, hang times for repackaged and nonrepackaged IVFE, and the number of IVFE units prepared and administered per patient per day based on established IVFE hang times.

STABILITY AND COMPATIBILITY

Comprehensive current information regarding compatibility and stability of PN solutions can be found in several reference sources such as *Handbook on Injectable Drugs*[73] and *King Guide to Parenteral Admixtures*.[77] In many cases, the answer to a compatibility question may not be readily available, and a review of the primary literature may be necessary. When information is not available, clinical judgment and experience must be used carefully to resolve the situation.

The stability of a PN formulation is determined by the rate or degree of component degradation and any resulting changes in chemical integrity or pharmacologic activity that may render the formulation unsuitable for safe administration. In general, the sterile combination of PN components accelerates the rate of physicochemical destabilization of all of the components in the formulation; certain amino acids, vitamins, and IVFE are the most susceptible nutrients.[31] When compounded and stored appropriately, the degree of degradation is usually not clinically relevant for most patients receiving short-term PN because many patients have sufficient stores of those susceptible nutrients to support any short-term periods of suboptimal intake thereby minimizing risk of clinical symptoms of deficiency. However, nutrient degradation that is more extensive may be problematic for patients with marginal nutrient stores who receive long-term PN. TNAs present additional stability challenges because of the presence of IVFE in the solution. IVFE stability in TNAs is affected by amino acid and dextrose concentration, solution pH, order of mixing, electrolyte amounts, and final TNA volume as well as container material, storage conditions, and addition of nonnutrient drugs. Stability studies on the effect of specific electrolyte concentrations on TNA stability are limited. In general, IVFE stability is affected by the PN cation content. Divalent and trivalent cation additives such as calcium and magnesium have a greater destabilizing potential compared with monovalent cation additives such as sodium and potassium. However, when given in sufficiently high concentrations, monovalent cation additives may also produce instability. Cations act to reduce the surface potential of the emulsion droplet, thereby enhancing tendency to aggregate and ultimately, in some cases, destabilize the solution to coalescence or a "cracked" admixture.[27,31,78] When a cracked IVFE occurs, the oil phase separates from the water phase resulting in the appearance of free oil fat globules. Early stages may appear as subtle changes in the uniformly white appearance of the TNA, which may progress to yellow oil streaks throughout the bag or development of an amber oil layer at the top of the admixture bag. TNA formulations with any visible free oil should be considered unsafe for parenteral administration because infusion of circulating fat globules may be of sufficient size to accumulate in the pulmonary vasculature and potentially compromise respiratory function. In general, the likelihood of preparing an unstable TNA formulation can be minimized by maintaining the final concentrations of CAA >4%, dextrose >10%, and IVFE >2%.[78] Specific guidelines for compounding TNA formulations are reviewed elsewhere.[27]

Because of differences in pH among various CAA products and in phospholipid content among IVFE products, the manufacturer of each product should be consulted for compatibility and stability information prior to routine mixing of components. One approach to compounding TNA formulations manually is to first combine CAA, dextrose, and sterile water (if necessary). Add electrolytes, vitamins, and trace elements, and then visually inspect the solution for precipitate or other particulates. Finally, add IVFE and visually inspect the solution to ensure a uniform emulsion exists.[27,44] However, mixing components in this specific order and time sequence may not be possible with the use of automated compounders. Although CAA, dextrose, and IVFE may be simultaneously transferred to an admixture container, the compounder's manufacturer should be consulted for the optimal mixing sequence to ensure safe compounding of TNA solutions.

The precipitation of calcium and phosphorus is a common interaction that is potentially life-threatening.[27,31,79] Factors that enhance the risk of precipitate formation include high concentrations of calcium and phosphorus salts, use of the chloride salt of calcium, decreased amino acid and dextrose concentrations, increased solution temperature, increased solution pH, use of an improper sequence when mixing calcium and phosphorus salts, and the presence of other additives including IVFEs.[27,31,79] In general, steps to minimize risk of calcium and phosphate precipitation in PN formulations include use of calcium gluconate instead of calcium chloride because it is less reactive, adding phosphate salts early in the mixing sequence, adding calcium last or nearly last, and agitating the mixture throughout the admixture process to achieve homogeneity. PN formulations with a lower final pH should be used when clinically appropriate. Higher final concentrations of dextrose and CAA and lower final concentrations of IVFE favor a lower admixture pH. CAA product-specific solubility curves that are available from the manufacturer or primary literature should be used for determining solubility. Use of a calculation to derive a sum or product of calcium and phosphate concentrations should not be used as the sole criterion for determining solubility since products of calcium and phosphate concentrations vary inconsistently as calcium concentration decreases and phosphate concentration increases.[79]

Electrolyte stability in TNA solutions is difficult to assess because of poor visualization of a precipitate should one occur. PN solutions for neonates and infants tend to have larger calcium and phosphorus amounts, as well as other divalent cations, that limit the use of TNA formulations. Because of the relatively limited amount of published stability information, the use of a 2-in-1 formulation with separate administration of IVFEs is recommended for neonates and infants.[31] In general, alternative methods of delivering electrolytes or other medications should be pursued in any clinical situation in which compatibility information involving a TNA solution is lacking. Because the addition of bicarbonate to acidic PN solutions may result in the formation of carbon dioxide gas and insoluble calcium and magnesium carbonates, sodium bicarbonate use in PN solutions is not recommended.[31] Use of a bicarbonate precursor salt such as acetate usually is preferred.

Vitamins may be affected adversely by changes in solution pH, presence of other additives, storage time, solution temperature, and exposure to light.[27] Because of variable stabilities of individual vitamins, IV vitamin solutions should be added to the PN solution as near to the time of administration as is clinically feasible and should not be in the PN solution longer than 24 hours.

Increased peroxide concentrations have been reported in IVFE and dextrose-amino acid solutions after addition of IV multivitamins and/or exposure to air or light.[80] Multiple in vitro experiments have reported negative effects of peroxides and associated metabolites on organ and immune function. Peroxides are associated with neonatal hypoxic–ischemic encephalopathy, intraventricular hemorrhage, periventricular leukomalacia, chronic lung disease, retinopathy of prematurity, and necrotizing enterocolitis.[80] Neonates and infants are at increased risk for harmful effects of peroxides because they receive a higher daily peroxide load from PN solutions and they have lower endogenous antioxidant levels. Protecting PN and IVFE solutions from light is therefore recommended to minimize peroxide formation.[21,80]

Many patients receiving PN also receive other IV medications. The compatibility of these medications and other IV solutions is an important concern. Although some medications may be added directly to the PN solution and administered at the same rate as the PN infusion, most are administered as a separate admixture piggybacked in the PN line. Several criteria should be considered before medications are added directly to the PN solution because of the potential for ineffective drug therapy or other complications associated with physiochemical incompatibility and stability of the PN solution.[31] First, the drug should be stable for at least 24-hours and should have pharmacokinetic properties appropriate for continuous infusion. Second, there should be documented chemical and physical compatibility of the medication with PN mixture components and other medications that may be piggybacked concomitantly into the PN line. Advantages of using PN admixtures as drug vehicles include consolidation of dosage units, improved pharmacodynamics for certain drugs, conservation of fluid in volume-restricted patients, fewer venous catheter violations, and decreased compounding and administration times. However, a major disadvantage to the use of PN solutions as drug-delivery vehicles is the lack of compatibility and stability data for the PN solutions that are used commonly in clinical practice. Medications frequently added to PN solutions include regular insulin and histamine-2 receptor antagonists.[31,73,77]

COMPLICATIONS OF PARENTERAL NUTRITION

MECHANICAL OR TECHNICAL COMPLICATIONS

Mechanical or technical complications include malfunctions in the system used for IV delivery of the solution, such as infusion pump failure, problems with administration sets or tubing, and problems with the catheter. While problems associated with infusion pumps and administration sets can be decreased by appropriate equipment selection and routine care and monitoring, catheter-related complications are potentially life threatening. Pneumothorax, catheter misdirection or migration into the wrong vein or improperly positioned within the cardiac chambers, arterial puncture, bleeding, and hematoma formation may occur during surgical placement of the catheter. Many of these complications, in addition to venous thrombosis and air embolism, can occur after insertion. Catheters occasionally occlude or break during use. If these problems cannot be rectified easily, the catheter may need to be surgically replaced.

INFECTIOUS COMPLICATIONS

Infectious complications can be a major hazard for patients receiving CPN because of the increased risk associated with the presence of an indwelling central venous catheter (CVC). The source of a CVC infection may be skin organisms at the catheter insertion site, contamination of the catheter hub, or hematogenous seeding of the catheter from a distant site. In addition, patients receiving PN therapy are often predisposed to infection because of compromised immunity and/or concomitant infection. Frequent use of broad-spectrum antibiotic therapy and malnutrition are also predisposing factors for development of infection. The risk of catheter infection is increased for those who require multiple manipulations of the line used for PN administration. The risks for infection are also increased for those who experience failure of in-line bacterial filter, poor catheter placement technique, and poor CVC and insertion site care.[64]

Infection rarely develops secondary to solution contamination.[64,81] Strict adherence to protocols for preparation of PN solutions should minimize this occurrence.[31,69] Catheter-related bloodstream infection (CRBSI), defined as the presence of clinical manifestations of infection (e.g., fever, chills, and/or hypotension), associated with bacteremia or fungemia resulting from no apparent source other than the catheter is a common source of systemic infection.[81] Before this diagnosis can be made, there should be evidence of more than one positive blood culture obtained from the peripheral vein with growth of the same organism from a blood culture obtained from the catheter or catheter segment. When a CRBSI is suspected or confirmed, appropriate antimicrobial therapy is initiated. Retention or removal of the central catheter depends on the patient's severity of illness, the suspected or identified pathogen, and the type of catheter involved. The catheter may be removed and replaced in the same site; the catheter may be removed and replaced at a different anatomic location, or it may not be replaced.[81] Recently, the use of 70% ethanol lock therapy has shown promising results for the prevention and treatment of CRBSI for patients receiving long-term PN.[82,83] Specific guidelines for treatment of CRSBI have been recently reviewed.[81]

METABOLIC AND NUTRITIONAL COMPLICATIONS

❽ Metabolic and nutritional complications associated with PN therapy are numerous, frequently multifactorial in origin, and if left untreated, some are potentially fatal. Metabolic abnormalities

TABLE 151-5 Metabolic Abnormalities Associated with PN Macronutrients

Abnormality	Possible Etiologies
Hyperglycemia	Metabolic stress, infection, corticosteroids, pancreatitis, diabetes mellitus, peritoneal dialysis, excessive dextrose administration
Hypoglycemia	Abrupt dextrose withdrawal, excessive insulin
Excess carbon dioxide production	Excess dextrose administration
Hypertriglyceridemia	Metabolic stress, familial hyperlipidemia, pancreatitis, excess IVFE dose; rapid IVFE infusion rate
Abnormal liver function tests (elevated ALT, AST, Alk Phos, Bili)	Metabolic stress, infection, excess carbohydrate intake, excess caloric intake, EFAD; long-term PN therapy

ALT, alanine aminotransferase (SGPT); AST, aspartate aminotransferase (SGOT); Alk Phos, alkaline phosphatase; Bili, bilirubin; EFAD, essential fatty acid deficiency; EN, enteral nutrition; IVFE, intravenous fat emulsion; PN, parenteral nutrition.

related to substrate intolerance, fluid and electrolyte disorders, and acid–base disorders are summarized in Table 151–5 and multiple review articles.[31,33,42,43,61,67,84–94]

Parenteral Nutrition–Associated Liver Disease

PN-associated liver disease (PNALD) as evidenced by elevations in total bilirubin, aspartate aminotransferase, alanine aminotransferase, and alkaline phosphatase is well documented.[84,85] No single etiology has been identified, although several risk factors have been reported. Risk factors for children include degree of prematurity, sepsis, hypoxia, lack of enteral nutrition, small bowel bacterial overgrowth, GI conditions requiring surgical intervention, duration of PN therapy, and long-term administration of excessive calories.[43,84,85] PNALD in infants is characterized clinically by a serum direct bilirubin concentration >2 mg/dL (34.2 μmol/L).[84] Taurine deficiency has been proposed as an etiology of cholestasis for preterm infants and neonates.[84,85] Taurine is a conditionally essential amino acid that is not present in standard CAA solutions but is important for neonatal and infant bile metabolism. However, the effectiveness of PN regimens with CAA solutions containing supplemental taurine is unclear. Recent studies have focused on the potential relationship between IVFE and the development of PNALD.[47–49] Soybean-oil-based IVFEs contain large concentrations of plant sterols or phytosterols which are inefficiently metabolized to bile acids by the liver. Experimental data suggest parenteral phytosterols may impair bile flow. Improvement or reversal of PNALD has been reported for patients who received a fish-oil-based IVFE that is not currently commercially available in the United States.

Risk factors for PNALD in adults include preexisting liver diseases, sepsis, preexisting malnutrition, extensive bowel resection, prolonged duration of PN therapy, lack of enteral intake, nutrient deficiencies such as choline deficiency, and long-term administration of excessive calories.[84,85] PNALD in adults typically presents as steatosis and steatohepatitis on biopsy. Clinically, PNALD is characterized by mild elevations in serum liver enzymes, usually less than three times the upper limit of normal, with peak enzyme levels usually occurring between 1 and 4 weeks after initiating PN. In many cases, the liver abnormalities improve or resolve with manipulation of substrate intake or discontinuation of PN therapy. However, in severe cases, liver dysfunction may progress to overt failure and death despite use of traditional therapies such as using cyclic PN, ursodiol, and oral antibiotics for bacterial overgrowth; maximizing enteral feeding; and avoiding sepsis and parenteral overfeeding.[84,85] Intestinal transplant with or without liver transplantation has become a treatment option for those PN-dependent patients who have progressive PNALD.

Hypertriglyceridemia

Hypertriglyceridemia, defined as serum triglyceride concentrations >400 mg/dL (4.52 mmol/L) for adults and 150 mg/dL (1.70 mmol/L) to 200 mg/dL (2.26 mmol/L) for preterm infants, neonates, and older pediatric patients, may occur for patients receiving IVFE-based PN. Risk factors include preexisting liver or pancreatic dysfunction, sepsis, multiple-organ failure, degree of prematurity, IVFE infusion rate, and dose.[31,40,43]

IVFE-associated hypertriglyceridemia is generally thought to be caused by defective lipid clearance or an excessive rate of IVFE administration.[31,41] Premature infants and neonates have relatively slower lipid clearance than do adults because of immature metabolic pathways, including decreased lipoprotein lipase activity.[40,41,43] Reducing the IVFE infusion rate or dose or withholding IVFE therapy should be considered when patients present with hypertriglyceridemia or lipemic serum.[31,41] Use of low-dose heparin (1 unit/mL of 2-in-1 PN formulation) to stimulate lipoprotein lipase activity has been suggested as a potential therapeutic intervention to treat IVFE-associated hypertriglyceridemia in neonates.[16,41] However, others have suggested that the risk associated with heparin delivery via PN outweighs clinical benefits because of the potential for compounding errors associated with heparin and insulin confusion.[70] The role of carnitine for treatment of IVFE-associated hypertriglyceridemia is not clear.[16,41]

CLINICAL CONTROVERSY

Carnitine may be considered conditionally essential for neonates, particularly preterm neonates, due to lack of placental carnitine transfer in the third trimester and immature neonatal biosynthetic capacity. While some clinicians refrain from using carnitine beyond the neonatal period, others argue that a trial of carnitine supplementation for patients with hypertriglyceridemia receiving standard doses of IVFE is warranted.

Hyperglycemia

Hyperglycemia is one of the most common complications associated with PN administration and is associated with a history of diabetes, metabolic stress, adverse effects of medications such as glucocorticoids and excessive carbohydrate administration. In the pediatric population, additional risks for hyperglycemia include prematurity and surgery. The optimal blood glucose concentration for acutely ill hospitalized patients receiving PN is not known. A target range of 100 to 150 mg/dL (5.6 to 8.3 mmol/L) has been suggested, but a recent investigation of blood glucose control for critically ill adult medical and surgical patients reported decreased mortality when blood glucose was maintained in a target range of 144 to 180 mg/dL (8.0 to 10.0 mmol/L).[31,86] Clinical management of PN patients with hyperglycemia has not been well studied and is largely empiric. Blood glucose concentrations can be controlled with regular insulin, which may be given subcutaneously or added to the PN formulation. One approach for adult PN patients requiring insulin or oral hypoglycemic agents prior to starting PN therapy is to initiate PN with approximately 100 to 200 g of dextrose and add 0.05 to 0.1 units of regular insulin per gram of dextrose in the PN solution for those patients with mild hyperglycemia [130 to 150 mg/dL (7.2 to 8.3 mmol/L)]. The insulin dose may be increased to 0.15 to 0.2 units per gram of dextrose for patients with moderate hyperglycemia [151 to 200 mg/dL (8.4 to 11.1 mmol/L)].[31,87] Blood glucose concentrations should be monitored every 4 to 6 hours. Blood glucose measurements above the goal range should be treated with regular insulin administered subcutaneously according to an appropriate sliding scale. The insulin dose is modified daily by adding 60% to 100% of the sliding-scale insulin given over the previous 24 hours to the PN formulation daily until blood glucose concentrations are stable and within the target range. Once blood glucose measurements are stable, the dextrose dose may be advanced. The frequency of monitoring blood glucose concentrations may be decreased once blood glucose concentrations are stable within the target range at the goal dextrose dose. Use of a separate IV insulin infusion is most commonly used for pediatric patients, but it may also provide better and safer glycemic control for patients with very large insulin requirements or unstable marked fluctuations in their blood glucose concentrations.

Refeeding Syndrome

Severe and rapid declines in serum phosphate, potassium and magnesium concentrations, fluid retention, and other micronutrient deficiencies are common features of the refeeding syndrome.[88,89] Individuals at risk for refeeding syndrome include those who are severely malnourished with significant weight loss and who receive aggressive nutritional supplementation. Other examples of patients receiving PN therapy who may be at risk for developing refeeding syndrome abnormalities include those who are unfed for 7 to 10 days with evidence of stress or nutritional depletion; those with chronic diseases causing undernutrition such as cancer, cardiac cachexia, chronic obstructive pulmonary disease, or cirrhosis; and those individuals who were previously morbidly obese and have experienced massive weight loss.[88] The mechanism of the electrolyte abnormalities appears to be related to acute provision of macronutrient substrates that promote anabolism in an environment of depleted total body stores of phosphorus, potassium, and magnesium. Recommendations for initiating PN in adults at risk for refeeding syndrome include providing 25% to 50% of the calculated nonprotein caloric requirements initially. The dextrose dose should be initiated at approximately 100 to 200 g/day. Calories should be advanced over 3 to 4 days to the desired goal. Because the metabolic abnormalities described with refeeding syndrome appear to be related primarily to acute provision of large amounts of dextrose, the goal protein dose may be provided with the initial PN infusion. Pediatric PN regimens are usually advanced over several days as a general practice for all pediatric patients. Additional recommendations for minimizing the risk of refeeding syndrome for pediatric patients include provision of additional phosphorus and potassium above standard nutrient requirements at the time PN is initiated.[43]

Complications Associated with Long-Term PN

Other nutritional complications of PN therapy may develop over a prolonged course of therapy (weeks to months) as a result of inappropriate intake of a particular nutrient. Certain conditions, such as metabolic stress in a previously malnourished patient, may elicit symptoms of deficiency much earlier if a nutrient is not appropriately provided. For example, lactic acidosis and other life-threatening complications associated with severe thiamine deficiency have been reported for patients who received PN solutions without multivitamin supplementation.[90] Maintenance doses of vitamins, trace elements, and essential fatty acids should be provided to all patients with normal age-related organ function receiving PN.

Essential Fatty Acid Deficiency

Patients receiving PN regimens without IVFEs for extended periods (weeks to months) are at risk for development of EFAD. Clinical signs of EFAD include hair loss, desquamative dermatitis, thrombocytopenia, and malabsorption and diarrhea resulting from changes in intestinal mucosa.[31,42] EFAD also may be diagnosed by evaluating plasma fatty acid profiles. Although this assessment is not routinely available, it can be provided by several larger regional labs. A triene-to-tetraene ratio more than 0.4 is biochemical evidence for EFAD. Although the time in which EFAD may develop is dependent on the patient's nutrition status, disease state, and age, these manifestations may occur 2 to 4 weeks after initiation of fat-free PN in adults and within 48 hours in newborn infants[40,42] (see Chap. 149).

Metabolic Bone Disease

Metabolic bone disease has been reported for adults and children receiving long-term home PN.[84] This disorder in adults is characterized by osteomalacia with or without osteoporosis that may present without associated clinical, radiologic, or biochemical abnormalities. The diagnosis may not be made for premature infants until after the development of bone fractures or overt rickets. The etiology is poorly understood and likely multifactorial. Treatment options include pharmacologic intervention, calcium and vitamin D supplementation, and exercise. Since excessive vitamin D has also been implicated in the development of metabolic bone disease, others have recommended removal of vitamin D from the PN for patients with a normal 25-hydroxyvitamin D concentration and low serum parathyroid hormone and 1,25-hydroxyvitamin D concentrations.[16,84]

Trace Elements and Vitamin Complications

Clinical symptoms of trace element deficiencies, although rare, have been reported for patients receiving PN. More commonly, decreased serum trace element concentrations have been reported in a variety of patient populations. However, the clinical significance of decreased concentrations of many trace elements is not known because serum concentrations often do not correlate with total body stores.[57,58] Occasionally, patients may develop clinical toxicities from elevated vitamin or trace element intakes or decreased metabolism. These abnormalities are frequently associated with an underlying disease state such as severe renal or hepatic failure and may necessitate reduction in vitamin and trace element intake. (See Chap. 153.)

Many trace elements are present in PN components as contaminants.[50] Some investigations of patients with normal organ function who were receiving PN supplemented with commercially available parenteral multiple trace element solutions have reported concern with elevated serum concentrations of trace elements such as chromium and manganese.[91] Aluminum is a common contaminant of many sterile IV solutions, including those used for compounding PN. Calcium and phosphorus solutions are among those components with higher levels of aluminum contamination.[92,93] Aluminum accumulation may occur during long-term PN therapy, especially for patients with renal insufficiency, and is associated with abnormal neurologic and hematologic function and metabolic bone disease in adults and premature infants.[84,92,93] Preterm infants are at higher risk of aluminum toxicities because they receive larger doses (micrograms per kilogram) from PN solutions than adults.[92] Preterm infants are also more likely to retain aluminum because of immature renal function. Although the maximum safe level of IV aluminum intake is unknown, the FDA has reported that parenteral doses of 4 to 5 mcg/kg/day were associated with central nervous system and bone toxicity for patients with impaired renal function, including premature neonates.[94] Even smaller amounts may result in tissue accumulation but no documented toxicity.

Recent data suggest that the aluminum content of sterile solutions used for compounding PN has declined as a result of awareness of toxicity and improvements in industrial PN component preparation.[92] However, in 2004 the FDA implemented a restriction of aluminum content in large-volume PN stock solutions

(CAA, dextrose, sterile water for injection, IVFE) to a maximum of 25 mcg/L and a requirement for manufacturers to indicate the maximum aluminum concentration at expiration for both large and small volume parenteral products used for PN.[94] After the FDA standards were in effect, a study evaluating the amount of aluminum in parenteral products revealed that aluminum content varied considerably during the shelf life of the product and tended to increase with time due to leaching from glass containers. The amount of aluminum contamination delivered to patients receiving long-term parenteral therapy, such as chronic PN patients or dialysis patients, is substantially reduced if newer stock is used for their therapy.[93]

HOME PARENTERAL NUTRITION

Advances in technology for the delivery of IV solutions have allowed medically stable patients who require extended PN therapy to be maintained indefinitely on IV nutrition. An increasing concern for cost containment of healthcare services has fostered use of sophisticated infusion devices to provide PN at home. Numerous programs are now available outside the traditional healthcare setting to support patients with various long-term or permanent medical conditions. Standards have been developed to promote safe and effective care.[95] Home PN services may be coordinated and administered through a hospital or by a commercial home care company.

Many factors are considered in selecting candidates for home PN therapy. Significant benefit must be expected from the therapy. Examples of patients who have been maintained successfully with home PN include those with severe GI dysfunction secondary to Crohn disease, ischemic bowel disease, severe GI motility disorders, extensive intestinal obstruction, and congenital bowel dysfunction.[96] The patient and the patient's caregiver must be willing to complete training and assume numerous responsibilities for managing the new daily routine in the home. Other logistics such as funding, procurement of solutions and supplies, and clinical management and followup must be evaluated, resolved, and individualized for each patient in order to achieve the desired outcomes.[95]

Patients commonly receive PN solutions from the home care provider. IV vitamins or other additives may be added daily by the patient or caregiver, depending on the arrangement with the home care provider. The solution generally is administered through the night by infusion pump over 10 to 12 hours.[67] A cycled regimen allows the patient time away from the pump during daylight hours and provides many patients with the freedom to have a reasonably normal daily routine. Clinical management and followup are performed periodically according to the needs of the patient and the protocol of the home care provider or the managing healthcare team. A coordinated effort among several healthcare professionals, including physicians, pharmacists, nurses, social workers, and the patient and the patient's caregiver, as well as the suppliers, is paramount to providing safe and effective management. Home PN affords some patients the potential for an ambulatory lifestyle while maintaining an IV feeding regimen that was previously only available in the hospital setting. For others, home PN may contribute to a better quality of life in the comfort of their home.[96]

PHARMACOECONOMIC CONSIDERATIONS

❾ Because numerous variables have an impact on the provision of PN support and the response to therapy, determining the true cost of PN is difficult.[96–99] In general, PN is an expensive intervention, and cost varies depending on the underlying indication for treatment

and whether PN is provided at home or in an acute care setting.[96–99] Expenses associated with PN therapy may be categorized as direct and indirect costs.[100] Direct costs may be further categorized as fixed or variable costs. Fixed costs do not depend on the volume of patients receiving therapy. For example, an automatic compounder and the tubing sets required to transfer volumes of stock solutions to the administration bag would be considered fixed costs in many practice settings. These costs per patient tend to be highest in low-volume environments. Variable costs such as PN administration bags depend directly on the number of patients receiving PN. Other direct costs include ancillary services required by patients receiving PN and costs related to the management of nutritionally associated complications.

Benefits and other clinical effects of PN (i.e., length of stay and frequency of complications) in specific patient populations have been evaluated.[15,16,18,19] Few investigations have reported an economic assessment of the therapy. However, economic data from many of these reports would not necessarily reflect current costs. Indeed, the direct cost of PN solution components generally has declined over the past 10 to 15 years. Attempting to measure the cost or cost savings associated with reported benefits of PN therapy and other clinical effects based on results of controlled clinical trials is difficult.[97,98] Clinical outcomes measurements and hence economic outcomes are influenced by multiple factors, including experimental design, sample size, and specific health system practices. Several investigations used for determining costs and benefits of PN therapy have been criticized for such biases.[99]

Although the results of economic analyses of PN remain controversial, similarities among several reports provide a basis for minimizing the costs of PN therapy. These similarities include the following:

1. Use PN only for the most appropriate patients as described by institution-specific criteria based on current consensus statements.[101] The costs and complications associated with enteral nutrition are demonstrated to be less than those associated with PN.[102]

2. Reassess the need for routine laboratory measurements used for monitoring PN therapy. In general, the level of laboratory monitoring should decrease as a patient's clinical condition stabilizes.

3. Minimize the direct cost of PN by using efficient purchasing practices for PN solutions and compounding supplies through contract purchasing, streamlined compounding procedures, standardized administration times, and 24-hour hang times to reduce waste, single-bag PN solutions, and optimized monitoring plans.

CONCLUSIONS

Appropriate patient selection, assessment, and monitoring are key to successful PN therapy and the prevention of unnecessary complications. Because pharmacists are actively involved in the provision of PN at many levels, including direct patient care, education, and research, nutrition support is recognized as a pharmacy practice specialty.[103] In addition, as the interdisciplinary approach to specialized nutrition support has evolved, standards of practice have been defined for pharmacists as well as for other healthcare professionals who provide nutrition support care.[3,6–8] Standardized order forms and monitoring protocols are useful tools to ensure appropriate administration and monitoring of PN therapy. The future of PN therapy and the role of the nutrition-support clinician will be affected primarily by new insights from clinical research and economic challenges in the healthcare environment.

ABBREVIATIONS

AAP: American Academy of Pediatrics

CAA: crystalline amino acid

CDC: Centers for Disease Control and Prevention

CPN: central parenteral nutrition

CRBSI: catheter-related bloodstream infection

CVC: central venous catheter

EFAD: essential fatty acid deficiency

FDA: Food and Drug Administration

GI: gastrointestinal

IVFE: intravenous fat emulsion

IV: intravenous

LCT: long-chain triglyceride

MCT: medium-chain triglyceride

NAG-AMA: Nutrition Advisory Group of the American
Medical Association

PICC: peripherally inserted central catheter

PN: parenteral nutrition

PNALD: parenteral nutrition-associated liver disease

PPN: peripheral parenteral nutrition

PUFA: polyunsaturated fatty acid

TNA: total nutrient admixture

REFERENCES

1. Dudrick SJ. A three and one-half decade nutritional and metabolic iliad. J Am Coll Surg 2007;205(4 suppl):S59–S64.
2. Schneider PJ. Nutrition support teams: An evidence-based practice. Nutr Clin Pract 2006;21:62–67.
3. Rollins C, Durfee SM, Holcombe BJ, et al. Standards of practice for nutrition support pharmacists. Nutr Clin Pract 2008;23:189–194.
4. American Society for Parenteral and Enteral Nutrition Board of Directors and Task Force on Standards for Specialized Nutrition Support for Hospitalized Adult Patients. Standards for specialized nutrition support: Adult hospitalized patients. Nutr Clin Pract 2002;17:384–391.
5. American Society for Parenteral and Enteral Nutrition Board of Directors and Task Force on Standards for Specialized Nutrition Support for Hospitalized Pediatric Patients. Standards for specialized nutrition support: hospitalized pediatric patients. Nutr Clin Pract 2005;20:103–116.
6. Task Force of A.S.P.E.N; American Dietetic Association Dietitians in Nutrition Support Dietetic Practice Group, Russell M, Stieber M, et al. American Society for Parenteral and Enteral Nutrition (A.S.P.E.N.) and American Dietetic Association (ADA): standards of practice and standards of professional performance for registered dietitians (generalist, specialty, and advanced) in nutrition support. Nutr Clin Pract 2007;22:558–586.
7. American Society for Parenteral and Enteral Nutrition (A.S.P.E.N.) Board of Directors and Nurses Standards Revision Task Force, DiMaria-Ghalili RA, Bankhead R, Fisher AA, Kovacevich D, Resler R, Guenter PA. Standards of practice for nutrition support nurses. Nutr Clin Pract 2007;22:458–465.
8. Seashore JH, McMahon MM, Wolfson M, D'Angelo DW; American Society for Parenteral and Enteral Nutrition; Task Force on Standards for Nutrition Support Physicians. Standards of practice for nutrition support physicians. Nutr Clin Pract 2003;18:270–275.
9. Dickerson RN. Hypocaloric feeding of obese patients in the intensive care unit. Curr Opin Clin Nutr Metab Care 2005;8:189–196.
10. ASPEN Board of Directors and the Clinical Guidelines Taskforce. Administration of specialized nutrition support. JPEN J Parenter Enteral Nutr 2002;26:18SA–21SA.
11. ASPEN Board of Directors and the Clinical Guidelines Taskforce. Nutrition assessment—Adults. JPEN J Parenter Enteral Nutr 2002;26:9SA–12SA.
12. ASPEN Board of Directors and the Clinical Guidelines Taskforce. Nutrition Assessment-pediatrics. JPEN J Parenter Enteral Nutr 2002;26:13SA–18SA.
13. McClave SA, Martindale RG, Vanek VW, et al. Guidelines for the provision and assessment of nutrition support therapy in the adult critically ill patient: Society of Critical Care Medicine (SCCM) and American Society for Parenteral and Enteral Nutrition (A.S.P.E.N.). JPEN J Parenter Enteral Nutr 2009;33:277–316.
14. August DA, Huhmann MB; American Society for Parenteral and Enteral Nutrition (A.S.P.E.N.) Board of Directors. A.S.P.E.N. clinical guidelines: nutrition support therapy during adult anticancer treatment and in hematopoietic cell transplantation. JPEN J Parenter Enteral Nutr 2009;33:472–500.
15. Koretz RL, Lipman TO, Klein S. AGA technical review on parenteral nutrition. Gastroenterology 2001;121:970–1001.
16. ASPEN Board of Directors and the Clinical Guidelines Taskforce. Administration of specialized nutrition support—Issues unique to pediatrics. JPEN J Parenter Enteral Nutr 2002;26:97SA–110SA.
17. Mehta NM, Compher C, and A.S.P.E.N. Board of Directors. A.S.P.E.N. Clinical guidelines: nutrition support of the critically ill child. JPEN J Parenter Enteral Nutr 2009;33:260–276.
18. ASPEN Board of Directors and the Clinical Guidelines Taskforce. Specific guidelines for disease—Adults. JPEN J Parenter Enteral Nutr 2002;26:61SA–96SA.
19. ASPEN Board of Directors and the Clinical Guidelines Taskforce. Specific guidelines for disease—Pediatrics. JPEN J Parenter Enteral Nutr 2002;26:111SA–138SA.
20. Denne SC, Poindexter BB. Evidence supporting early nutritional support with parenteral amino acid infusion. Semin Perinatol 2007;31:56–60.
21. Koletzko B, Goulet O, Hunt J, et al. Guidelines on paediatric parenteral nutrition of the European Society of Paediatric Gastroenterology, Hepatology and Nutrition (ESPGHAN) and the European Society for Clinical Nutrition and Metabolism (ESPEN), supported by the European Society of Paediatric Research (ESPR). J Pediatr Gastroenterol Nutr 2005;41(suppl 2):S1–S87.
22. Hay WW Jr. Strategies for feeding the preterm infant. Neonatology 2008;94:245–254.
23. Poindexter BB, Langer JC, Dusick AM, Ehrenkranz RA; National Institute of Child Health and Human Development Neonatal Research Network. Early provision of parenteral amino acids in extremely low birth weight infants: Relation to growth and neurodevelopmental outcome. J Pediatr 2006;148:300–305.
24. Van Way CW. Editorial: total calories vs nonprotein calories. Nutr Clin Pract 2001;16:271–272.
25. Furst P, Stehle P. Are intravenous amino acid solutions unbalanced? New Horizons 1994;2:215–223.
26. Dickerson RN. Using nitrogen balance in clinical practice. Hosp Pharm 2005; 40:1081–1085.
27. Trissel LA. Amino acid injection In: Trissel LA, ed. Handbook on Injectable Drugs, 15th ed. Bethesda, MD: American Society of Health-System Pharmacists; 2009:49–95.
28. Crill CM, Helms RA. The use of carnitine in pediatric nutrition. Nutr Clin Pract 2007;22:204–213.
29. Alpers DH. Glutamine: do the data support the cause for glutamine supplementation in humans? Gastroenterology 2006;130:S106–S116.
30. Tubman TR, Thompson SW, McGuire W. Glutamine supplementation to prevent morbidity and mortality in preterm infants. Cochrane Database Syst Rev 2008;1:CD001457.
31. Task Force for the Revision of Safe Practices for Parenteral Nutrition. Safe Practices for Parenteral Nutrition. JPEN J Parenter Enteral Nutr 2004;28:539–570.
32. Hay WW. Early postnatal nutritional requirements of the very preterm infant based on a presentation at the NICHD-AAP workshop on research in neonatology. J Perinatol 2006,S13–S18.
33. Btaiche IF, Khalidi N. Metabolic complications of parenteral nutrition in adults, part 1. Am J Health Syst Pharm 2004;61:1938–1949.

34. A.S.P.E.N. Board of Directors and the Clinical Guidelines Taskforce. Normal requirements-pediatrics. JPEN J Parenter Enteral Nutr 2002; 26:25SA–32SA

35. Sheridan RL, Yu YM, Prelack K, et al. Maximal parenteral glucose oxidation in hypermetabolic young children: A stable isotope study. JPEN J Parenter Enteral Nutr 1998;22:212–216.

36. Waxman K, Day AT, Stellin GP, et al. Safety and efficacy of glycerol and amino acids in combination with lipid emulsion for peripheral parenteral nutrition support. JPEN J Parenter Enteral Nutr 1992;16:374–378.

37. ProcalAmine. Product information. Irvine, CA: B. Braun Medical; 2003.

38. Fat emulsion intravenous. Drug Facts and Comparisons. *http://online.factsandcomparisons.com*. 2010 by Wolters Kluwer Health, Inc. Accessed September 2010.

39. Waitzberg DL, Torrinhas RS, Jacintho TM. New parenteral lipid emulsions for clinical use. JPEN J Parenter Enteral Nutr 2006;30:351–366.

40. Kerner JA Jr, Poole RL. The use of IV fat in neonates. Nutr Clin Pract 2006;21:374–380.

41. Parenteral Nutrition. In: American Academy of Pediatrics Committee on Nutrition. Pediatric Nutrition Handbook, 6th edition. Kleinman RE, ed. Elk Grove, IL: American Academy of Pediatrics; 2009: 519–540.

42. Bistrian BR. Clinical aspects of essential fatty acid metabolism: Johnathon Rhoads Lecture. JPEN J Parenter Enteral Nutr 2003;27:168–175.

43. Shulman RJ, Phillips S. Parenteral nutrition in infants and children. J Pediatr Gastroenterol Nutr 2003;36:587–607.

44. Intralipid. Product information. Uppsala, Sweden: Fresnius Kabi, 2007.

45. Waitzberg DL, Torrinhas RS. Fish oil based lipid emulsions and immune response: what clinicians need to know. Nutr Clin Pract 2009;24:487–499.

46. Marik PE, Zaloga GP. Immunonutrition in critically ill patients: a systematic review and analysis of the literature. Intensive Care Med 2008;11:1980–1990.

47. Gura KM, Duggan CP, Collier SB, et al. Reversal of parenteral nutrition-associated liver disease in two infants with short bowel syndrome using parenteral fish oil: Implications for future management. Pediatrics 2006;118:e197–e201.

48. Gura KM, Lee S, Valim C, et al. Safety and efficacy of a fish-oil-based fat emulsion in the treatment of parenteral nutrition-associated liver disease. Pediatrics 2008;121:e678–86.

49. de Meijer VE, Gura KM, Le HD, Meisel JA, Puder M. Fish oil-based lipid emulsions prevent and reverse parenteral nutrition-associated liver disease: the Boston experience. JPEN J Parenter Enteral Nutr 2009;33:541–547.

50. American Medical Association Department of Foods and Nutrition. Multivitamin preparations for parenteral use: A statement by the nutritional advisory group. JPEN J Parenter Enteral Nutr 1979;3:258–262.

51. Demling RH, DeBiasse MA. Micronutrients in critical illness. Crit Care Clin 1995;11:651–673.

52. Greer FR. Vitamin metabolism and requirements in the micropremie. Clin Perinatol 2000;27:95–118.

53. Green HL, Hambidge KM, Schanler R, Tsang RC. Guidelines for the use of vitamins, trace elements, calcium, magnesium, and phosphorus in infants and children receiving total parenteral nutrition: Report of the Subcommittee on Pediatric Parenteral Nutrient Requirements from the Committee on Clinical Practice Issues of the American Society for Clinical Nutrition. Am J Clin Nutr 1988;48:1324–1342.

54. Helphingstine CJ, Bistrian BR. New food and drug administration requirements for inclusion of vitamin K in adult parenteral multivitamins. JPEN J Parenter Enteral Nutr 2003;27:220–224.

55. Chambrier C, Lellerq M, Saudin F, et al. Is vitamin K_1 supplementation necessary in long-term parenteral nutrition? JPEN J Parenter Enteral Nutr 1998;22:87–90.

56. Lennon C, Davidson KW, Sandowski JA, Mason JB. The vitamin K content of intravenous lipid emulsion. JPEN J Parenter Enteral Nutr 1993;17:142–144.

57. Misra S, Kirby DF. Micronutrient and trace element monitoring in adult nutrition support. Nutr Clin Pract 2000;15:120–126.

58. Aggett PJ. Trace elements of the micropremie. Clin Perinatol 2000;27:119–129.

59. American Medical Association. Guidelines for essential trace element preparations for parenteral use: A statement by the Nutrition Advisory Group. JPEN J Parenter Enteral Nutr 1979;3:263–267.

60. Zimmermann MB, Crill CM. Iodine in enteral and parenteral nutrition. Best Pract Res Clin Endocrinol Metab 2010;24:143–158.

61. Kraft MD, Btaiche IF, Sacks GS, Kudsk KA. Treatment of electrolyte disorders in adult patients in the intensive care unit. Am J Health Syst Pharm 2005;62:1663–1682.

62. Parenteral Nutrition Formulations. In: Canada T, Crill C, Guenter P, eds. A.S.P.E.N. Parenteral Nutrition Handbook. Silver Spring, MD: The American Society for Parenteral and Enteral Nutrition; 2009.

63. Anderson ADG, Palmer D, MacFie J. Peripheral parenteral nutrition. Br J Surg 2003;90:1048–1054.

64. O'Grady NP, Alexander M, Dellinger EP, et al. Guidelines for the prevention of intravascular catheter-related infections. MMWR Morb Mortal Wkly Rep 2002;51(RR10):1–26.

65. A.S.P.E.N. Board of Directors and The Clinical Guidelines Taskforce. Access for administration of nutrition support. JPEN J Parenter Enteral Nutr 2002;26:33SA–41SA.

66. A.S.P.E.N. Statement on Parenteral Nutrition Standardization. A.S.P.E.N. Board of Directors and Task Force on Parenteral Nutrition Standardization, Kochevar M, Guenter P, Holcombe B, Malone A, Mirtallo J. JPEN J Parenter Enteral Nutr 2007; 31; 441–448.

67. Speerhas R, Wang J, Seidner D, Steiger E. Maintaining normal blood glucose concentrations with total parenteral nutrition: Is it necessary to taper total parenteral nutrition? Nutr Clin Pract 2003;18:414–416.

68. Krzyda EA, Andris DA, Whipple JK, et al. Glucose response to abrupt initiation and discontinuation of total parenteral nutrition. JPEN J Parenter Enteral Nutr 1993;17:64–67.

69. USP <797> Guidebook to Pharmaceutical Compounding—Sterile Preparations. Rockville, MD: United States Pharmacopeia Convention; 2008.

70. ISMP Medication Safety Alert!®Acute Care. Action needed to prevent dangerous heparin-insulin confusion; May 3, 2007, *http://www.ismp.org/Newsletters/acutecare/articles/20070503.asp*.

71. ISMP Medication Safety Alert!®Acute Care. Fatal 1,000-fold overdoses can occur, particularly in neonates, by transposing mcg and mg; September 6, 2007, *http://www.ismp.org/Newsletters/acutecare/articles/20070906.asp*.

72. American Society for Health-System Pharmacists. ASHP guidelines on the safe use of automated compounding devices for the preparation of parenteral nutrition admixtures. Am J Health Syst Pharm 2000;57:1343–1348.

73. Trissel LA, ed. Handbook on Injectable Drugs. 15th ed. Bethesda, MD: American Society of Health-System Pharmacists; 2009.

74. Crill CM, Hak EB, Robinson LA, Helms RA. Evaluation of microbial contamination associated with different preparation methods for neonatal intravenous fat emulsion infusion. Am J Health-Syst Pharm 2010;67:914–918.

75. Hicks RW, Becker SC, Chuo J. A summary of NICU fat emulsion medication errors and nursing services. Data from MEDMARX. Adv Neonatal Care 2007;7:299–310.

76. Reiter PD, Robles J, Dowell EB. Effect of 24-hour intravenous tubing set change on the sterility of repackaged fat emulsion in neonates. Ann Pharmacother 2004;38:1603–1607.

77. King JC, Catania PN, ed. King Guide to Parenteral Admixtures, Napa, CA: King Guide Publications; 2009.

78. Driscoll DF. Lipid injectable emulsions: 2006. Nutr Clin Pract 2006;21:381–386.

79. Newton DW, Driscoll DF. Calcium and phosphate compatibility: revisited again. Am J Health-Syst Pharm 2008; 65:73–80.

80. Hoff DS, Michaelson AS. Effects of light exposure on total parenteral nutrition and its implications in the neonatal population. J Pediatr Pharmacol Ther 2009;14:132–143.

81. Mermel LA, Allon M, Bouza E, et al. Clinical Practice Guidelines for the Diagnosis and Management of Intravascular Catheter-Related Infection: 2009 Update by the Infectious Diseases Society of America. Clin Infect Dis 2009;49:1–45.

82. Mouw E, Chessman K, Lesher A, Tagge E. Use of ethanol lock to prevent catheter-related infections in children with short bowel syndrome. J Pediatr Surg 2008;43:1025–1029.

83. Opilla MT, Kirby DF, Edmond MB. Use of ethanol lock therapy to reduce the incidence of catheter-related bloodstream infections in home parenteral nutrition patients. J Parenter Enteral Nutr 2007;31:302–305.

84. Btaiche IF, Khalidi N. Metabolic complications of parenteral nutrition in adults, part 2. Am J Health Syst Pharm 2004;61:2050–2057.

85. Buchman AL, Iyore K, Fryer J. Parenteral nutrition-associated liver disease and the role for isolated intestine and intestine/liver transplantation. Hepatology 2006;43:9–19.

86. The NICE-SUGAR Study Investigators. Intensive versus conventional glucose control in critically ill patients. N Engl J Med 2009;360: 1283–1297.

87. Marie E., McDonnell ME, Apovian CM. Diabetes Mellitus In: The A.S.P.E.N. Nutrition Support Core Curriculum. A Case-Based Approach-The Adult Patient. Gottschlich MM, ed. Silver Spring, MD: American Society for Parenteral and Enteral Nutrition (A.S.P.E.N.); 2007;676–694.

88. Kraft MD, Btaiche IF, Sacks F. Review of the refeeding syndrome. Nutr Clin Pract 2005;20:625–633.

89. Mehanna HM, Moledina J, Travis J. Refeeding syndrome: What it is, and how to prevent and treat it. BMJ 2008;336;1495–1498.

90. Centers for Disease Control. Lactic acidosis traced to thiamine deficiency related to nationwide shortage of multivitamins for total parenteral nutrition—United States, 1997. MMWR Morb Mortal Wkly Rep 1997;46:523–528.

91. Krishnan Sriram K, Lonchyna VA. Micronutrient supplementation in adult nutrition therapy: practical considerations. JPEN J Parenter Enteral Nutr 2009;33:548.

92. Gura KM, Puder M. Recent developments in aluminum contamination of products used in parenteral nutrition. Curr Opin Clin Nutr Metab Care 2006;9:239–246.

93. Speerhas RA, Seidner DL. Measured versus estimated aluminum content of parenteral nutrient solutions. Am J Health Syst Pharm 2007;64:740–746.

94. Food and Drug Administration. Aluminum in large and small volume parenterals used in total parenteral nutrition. Fed Regist 2000;65:4103–4111.

95. American Society for Parenteral and Enteral Nutrition Board of Directors and the Standards for Specialized Nutrition Support Task Force. Standards for specialized nutrition support: home care patients. Nutr Clin Pract 2005;20:579–590.

96. Howard L. Home parenteral nutrition: Survival, cost, and quality of life. Gastroenterology 2006;130:S52–S59.

97. Lipman TO. The cost of TPN: Is the price right? JPEN J Parenter Enteral Nutr 1993;17:199–200.

98. Eisenberg JM, Glick HA, Buzby GP, et al. Does perioperative total parenteral nutrition reduce medical care costs? JPEN J Parenter Enteral Nutr 1993;17:201–209.

99. Twomey PL, Patching SC. Cost effectiveness of nutritional support. JPEN J Parenter Enteral Nutr 1985;9:3–10.

100. Eisenberg JM, Glick H, Hillman AL, et al. Measuring the economic impact of perioperative total parenteral nutrition: Principles and design. Am J Clin Nutr 1988;47:382–391.

101. Trujillo EB, Young LS, Chertow GM, et al. Metabolic and monetary costs of avoidable parenteral nutrition use. JPEN J Parenter Enteral Nutr 1999;23:109–113.

102. Zaloga GP. Parenteral nutrition in adult inpatients with functioning gastrointestinal tracts: Assessment of outcomes. Lancet 2006;367: 1101–1111.

103. Mirtallo JM. Advancement of nutrition support in clinical pharmacy. Ann Pharmacother 2007;41:869–872.

CHAPTER

152

Enteral Nutrition

VANESSA J. KUMPF AND KATHERINE HAMMOND CHESSMAN

KEY CONCEPTS

❶ The GI tract defends the host from toxins and antigens by both immunologic and nonimmunologic mechanisms, collectively referred to as the gut barrier function. Whenever possible, enteral nutrition (EN) is preferred over parenteral nutrition (PN) because it is as effective, may reduce metabolic and infectious complications, and is less expensive.

❷ Candidates for EN are those who cannot or will not eat, those who exhibit a sufficiently functioning GI tract to allow adequate nutrient absorption, and in whom enteral access can be safely obtained.

❸ The most common route for both short- and long-term EN access is directly into the stomach. The method of delivery may be either continuously via an infusion pump, intermittently via a pump or gravity drip, or by gravity or syringe bolus administration.

❹ Patients unable to tolerate feeding directly into the stomach because of impaired gastric motility and for those at high risk of aspiration, feeding tube tip placement into the duodenum or jejunum may be indicated. When feeding into the small bowel, the continuous method of delivery via an infusion pump is required to enhance tolerance.

❺ Selection of the enteral feeding formulation depends on nutritional requirements, the patient's primary disease state and related complications, and nutrient digestibility and absorption. A standard polymeric formulation will meet the needs of the majority of adult patients and children.

❻ Measurement of gastric residual volumes can be used to monitor GI tolerance in patients receiving gastric feeding. Although not always reliable, excessive residual volumes may be associated with nausea, abdominal distension, and increased risk for aspiration.

❼ Management of diarrhea in patients receiving EN should focus on identification and correction of the most likely cause(s). Tube feeding–related causes include too rapid delivery or advancement, intolerance to the formula composition, and occasionally formula contamination.

❽ Prior to administering medications through a feeding tube, the feeding tube tip location should be verified (stomach or small bowel) and the most suitable dosage form selected. Medications that should not be crushed and administered through a tube include enteric-coated or sustained-release capsules or tablets and sublingual or buccal tablets.

❾ The coadministration of medications with EN can result in alterations in bioavailability and/or changes in the desired pharmacologic effects of several medications, including phenytoin, warfarin, selected antibiotics, antacids, and proton-pump inhibitors.

Enteral nutrition (EN) is defined as the delivery of nutrients by tube or by mouth into the GI tract. This chapter focuses on nutrient delivery through a feeding tube rather than the oral ingestion of food. The terms *enteral nutrition* and *tube feeding* are thus used interchangeably in this context. The goal of EN is to provide calories, macronutrients, and micronutrients to those patients who are unable to achieve these requirements from an oral diet. Over the past 20 to 30 years, EN has replaced parenteral nutrition (PN) as the preferred method of specialized nutrition support in many patients who are at risk of malnutrition. Improvements in enteral access techniques and feeding formulations and the recognition of methods to prevent and manage complications have resulted in an increased use of EN across all healthcare settings.

In this chapter, principles and practices related to the successful use of EN support are described. Digestive and absorptive physiology is reviewed, and the beneficial effects of EN are presented. The indications for EN and descriptions of various enteral access and administration methods are also summarized. Characteristics of commercially available enteral feeding formulations are presented, as well as administration and monitoring guidelines. Strategies to prevent and manage complications are discussed, and clinical therapeutic controversies are highlighted. In addition, issues of drug compatibility, drug–nutrient interactions, and drug administration via feeding tubes are discussed. Finally, the effectiveness and pharmacoeconomics of EN in enhancing nutrition and disease outcome goals are reviewed.

GASTROINTESTINAL TRACT PHYSIOLOGY

DIGESTION AND ABSORPTION

Digestion and absorption are GI processes that generate the body's usable fuels.[1,2] Digestion consists of the stepwise conversion of a complex chemical and physical nutrient into a molecular form that is absorbable by the intestinal mucosa. Absorption from the

TABLE 152-1 Gastrointestinal Enzymes and Hormones

Enzyme/Hormone	Site of Secretion	Main Actions
Amylase	Salivary glands, pancreas	Converts carbohydrates, starch, and glycogen to simple disaccharides
Cholecystokinin	Duodenum, jejunum	Stimulates pancreatic enzyme secretion and gallbladder contraction
Chymotrypsinogen	Pancreas	Breaks down proteins into peptides
Enteroglucagon	Duodenum, small intestine	Inhibits pancreatic enzyme secretion and bowel motility
Gastric inhibitory peptide	Small intestine	Decreases gastric motility and stimulates insulin secretion
Gastrin	Stomach, duodenum	Stimulates gastric acid secretion and mucosal growth
Glucagon	Pancreas	Stimulates hepatic glycogenolysis and inhibits motility
Lipase	Pancreas	Hydrolyzes dietary fat to release fatty acids
Pancreatic polypeptide	Pancreas	Inhibits gallbladder contraction and pancreatic and biliary secretion
Pepsinogen	Stomach	Converts large proteins into polypeptides
Secretin	Small intestine	Stimulates hepatic and pancreatic water and bicarbonate release
Trypsinogen	Pancreas	Breaks down proteins into peptides
Vasoactive inhibitory peptide	Small intestine, pancreas	Vasodilator; stimulates water and bicarbonate secretion, release of insulin and glucagon, and production of small intestinal secretions

GI tract is a multistep process that includes the transfer of a nutrient across the intestinal cell membrane. The nutrient ultimately reaches the systemic circulation through the portal venous or splanchnic lymphatic systems, provided the GI or biliary tract does not excrete it. Ingested nutrients are primarily large polymers that cannot be absorbed by the intestinal cell membrane unless they are transformed into an absorbable molecular form. In addition, a coordinated interplay of GI motility and neurohormonal secretion is required to facilitate adequate digestion and absorption.

Nutrient digestion involves the complex coordination of multiple mechanical, enzymatic, and physiochemical processes.[1,2] Mechanical dissolution of food occurs by chewing, then mixing and grinding the stomach contents. Food stimulates the secretion of numerous hormones and enzymes from the salivary glands, stomach, liver and biliary system, pancreas, and intestines (Table 152–1). As food passes along the gut lumen, these hormones modulate GI motility and the secretions from subsequent organs of the digestive system. Nutrient digestion occurs within the gut lumen and is a specific function of the intestinal cell membrane, which is comprised of fingerlike projections called villi. Each individual villus is made up of epithelial cells called enterocytes. The enterocyte surface contains special luminal projections called microvilli, which provide an increased surface area that is referred to as the brush-border membrane.

Figure 152–1 illustrates the digestion and absorption of carbohydrate, fat, and protein within the small intestine. Carbohydrates are presented to the small intestine in either a digestible or a nondigestible form. Polysaccharides (starches) and oligosaccharides (sucrose and lactose) undergo enzymatic digestion within the small intestine to produce simple sugars. The simple sugars are absorbed via active and passive transport mechanisms and are eventually released into the portal vein. Polysaccharides, such as cellulose complexes and other fiber components, pass undigested to the colon, where they are digested by bacteria and enzymes to form short-chain fatty acids. Absorption of short-chain fatty acids by the colon stimulates sodium and water reabsorption, serves as an energy source, and provides nourishment to the colonic mucosa cells.

Fat is presented to the small intestine as long-chain triglycerides. Its digestion requires pancreatic enzyme release and formation of mixed bile salt micelles, which then facilitate absorption across the intestinal enterocyte. Within the enterocyte, triglycerides are reesterified and packaged into chylomicrons for release into the lymphatic system. Medium-chain triglycerides (MCTs) can be absorbed intact by the mucosal membrane and are acted on by intracellular lipase within the enterocyte to release free fatty acids that pass directly into the portal vein.[3]

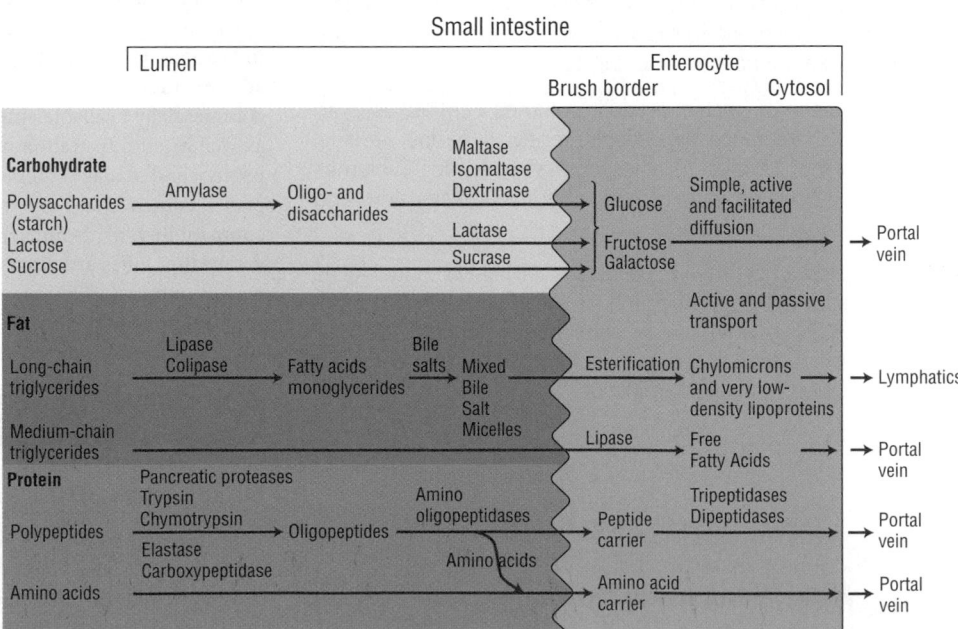

FIGURE 152-1. Schematic of carbohydrate, fat, and protein digestion.

Protein is presented to the small intestine primarily as large polypeptides and to a small extent as free amino acids because of the denaturation of protein within the stomach. Luminal polypeptide digestion generates oligopeptides, which are further hydrolyzed to dipeptides and tripeptides. Absorption of peptides occurs via a peptide transport system; free amino acids are carried via specific amino acid transport systems. The carriers for the peptides are very efficient, whereas absorption of free amino acids appears to be more limited and less efficient.[2]

Understanding the mechanisms of digestive and absorptive physiology can greatly enhance the rational use of EN during conditions of normal or altered GI anatomy and/or function. Several circumstances may alter the efficacy of nutrient digestion and absorption. For example, the functional immaturity of the neonatal gut may lead to clinical problems associated with inadequate digestion and absorption of EN. These factors, as they relate to successful EN practice, are discussed in detail throughout this chapter.

GUT HOST DEFENSE MECHANISMS

❶ Besides digesting and absorbing nutrients to maintain nutritional health, the GI tract is actively involved in defending the host from toxins and antigens by means of both immunologic and nonimmunologic mechanisms.[4] These gut host defense mechanisms are collectively referred to as the gut barrier function. The gut barrier acts to prevent the spread of intraluminal bacteria and endotoxins to systemic organs and tissues. Hydrochloric acid secreted by the stomach kills most of the bacteria ingested with food. Under normal circumstances, a mucus layer coats the intestinal epithelium and thereby alters the adherence of bacteria to the cells of the GI tract and provides a favorable environment for anaerobic bacteria. Anaerobic bacteria, which normally colonize the mucus layer, aid in preventing tissue colonization by potential pathogens. Small bowel peristalsis further prevents bacterial stasis and overgrowth. The gut barrier function is also maintained by the intestinal immune system, known as the gut-associated lymphoid tissue (GALT). GALT regulates the local immune response to antigens within the GI tract. Specific immunoglobulins are secreted to kill the remaining organisms and neutralize any toxins they produce. The liver Kupffer cells help to maintain gut barrier function by clearing the portal blood of gut-derived bacteria and endotoxins. The integrity of gut barrier function may be affected negatively by numerous pathogenic insults, such as physiologic stress and ischemia, and a variety of drugs, including chemotherapeutic agents. The administration of certain probiotics can modify intestinal flora and may have beneficial effects in various disease states and patient populations by positively affecting the maintenance of gut barrier function and intestinal immune function.[5,6]

INDICATIONS FOR ENTERAL NUTRITION

❷ The decision to initiate EN is based on a variety of factors. Suitable candidates are those who cannot or will not eat a sufficient amount to meet nutritional requirements, those who exhibit a sufficient functioning GI tract to allow the absorption of nutrients, and those in whom a method of enteral access can be safely obtained.[7-9] EN may be indicated in a variety of conditions or disease states (Table 152–2). For example, patients who have neurologic disorders, such as a cerebrovascular accident, and have difficulty swallowing often require EN. Patients unable to eat because of conditions such as facial or jaw injuries, lesions of the oral cavity or esophagus, esophageal stricture, or head and neck cancer may also be candidates for EN delivered distal to the affected site. Extreme prematurity necessitates tube feeding

TABLE 152-2 Potential Indications for Enteral Nutrition

Neoplastic disease	GI disease
Chemotherapy	Inflammatory bowel disease
Radiation therapy	Short bowel syndrome
Upper GI tumors	Esophageal motility disorder
Cancer cachexia	Pancreatitis
Organ dysfunction	Fistulas
Liver disease/failure	Gastroesophageal reflux disease (severe)
Kidney insufficiency/failure	Esophageal or intestinal atresia
Cardiac cachexia	**Neurologic impairment**
ARDS/ALI	Comatose state
Bronchopulmonary dysplasia	Cerebrovascular accident
Congenital heart disease	Demyelinating disease
Organ transplantation	Severe depression
Hypermetabolic states	Cerebral palsy
Closed head injury	**Other indications**
Burns	AIDS
Trauma	Anorexia nervosa
Postoperative major surgery	Complications during pregnancy
Sepsis	Failure to-thrive
	Geriatric patients with multiple chronic diseases
	Extreme prematurity
	Inborn errors of metabolism
	Cystic fibrosis

AIDS = acquired immune deficiency syndrome, ALI = acute lung injury, ARDS = acute respiratory distress syndrome.

because the suck–swallow mechanism has not yet developed sufficiently to allow safe oral intake.

Critically ill patients who are endotracheally intubated for mechanical ventilation represent a large percentage of patients requiring EN. Traditionally, EN in the critically ill population was regarded as supportive care designed to provide nutrients during the period of time the patient was unable to maintain oral dietary intake. Recently, the use of EN has been initiated to modulate the stress response to critical illness and improve patient outcomes. Nutrition guidelines support the initiation of EN in critically ill adults[10,11] and children[12] who are unable to maintain volitional intake. Some of these patients may have reduced gastric motility and emptying caused by sepsis, GI surgery, anesthetic agents, opioid analgesics, and underlying pathology, such as diabetic gastroparesis. However, successful EN can often be achieved by bypassing the stomach and placing the tip of the feeding tube beyond the pylorus into the duodenum, or preferably into the jejunum. Small bowel feeding may also be appropriate for patients with gastric outlet obstruction and those with pancreatitis.

The only absolute contraindications for EN are mechanical intestinal obstruction[13] and necrotizing enterocolitis.[14] However, conditions such as severe diarrhea, protracted vomiting, enteric fistulas, severe GI hemorrhage, and intestinal dysmotility may result in significant challenges to the successful use of EN.

BENEFITS OF ENTERAL NUTRITION

The importance of maintaining nutrient delivery through the GI tract in patients without a contraindication to its use is well supported. The beneficial effects of EN, specifically in the critically ill patient, are further enhanced if EN is initiated within 24 to 48 hours of admission to an intensive care unit (ICU).[10]

ENTERAL VERSUS PARENTERAL NUTRITION

Clinical studies comparing EN and PN in the critically ill patient demonstrate a decrease in infectious complications and thus improved outcomes with the use of EN.[15-19] Infectious complications are less common with EN in part because EN supports the functional integrity of the gut by stimulating bile flow and the release of endogenous trophic agents, such as cholecystokinin, gastrin, and bile salts. Provision of enteral nutrients appears to help maintain the villous height of the intestinal mucosa and support the mass of secretory immunoglobulin A (IgA)–producing immunocytes that comprise the GALT. In the setting of critical illness or injury, adverse changes in gut permeability and gut barrier function that result in increased risk for systemic infection and multiorgan dysfunction syndrome often have been noted. By supporting gut integrity, the enteral route of feeding is more likely than the parenteral route to lower the risk of infection and minimize organ failure.[10]

Critical reviews of available prospective randomized, controlled trials comparing EN with PN in the critically ill adult patient with an intact GI tract suggest a significant reduction in infectious complications associated with EN.[10,11,14] Decreased infectious complications have been documented in patients with abdominal trauma, burns, severe head injury, major surgery, and acute pancreatitis. The reduced infectious complications are primarily the result of a lower incidence of pneumonia and catheter-related bloodstream infections in most of these patient populations and a decrease in abdominal abscess in trauma patients. EN is thus preferred over PN for the feeding of critically ill adult patients requiring specialized nutrition support.[10,11] There are no randomized, controlled trials that compare the use of EN and PN in children.[12]

EN is more physiologic than PN in terms of nutrient utilization and therefore is generally associated with fewer metabolic complications, such as glucose intolerance and elevated insulin requirements.[20] Enteral formulations contain both complex and simple carbohydrates compared with the simple carbohydrate in the form of dextrose that is used in PN. This may account for better blood glucose control when carbohydrate is given via the enteral route. An additional physiologic benefit of enteral feeding is that it stimulates bile flow through the biliary tract and thus reduces the risk of developing cholestasis, gallbladder sludge, and gallstones, conditions that have been associated with long-term PN and bowel rest.[21] Also, EN avoids the potential infectious and technical complications associated with the placement and use of a central venous access device required for PN. Finally, EN is less costly than PN when all factors are considered.

EARLY VERSUS DELAYED INITIATION

The timing of initiation of EN in the critically ill patient is of clinical significance. Initiating EN in the first 24 to 72 hours following admission appears to attenuate the stress response and may reduce disease severity and infectious complications when compared with the initiation of feedings after 72 hours.[10,11] Early EN has also been associated with a decrease in the release of inflammatory cytokines and fewer alterations in gut permeability.[22] Clinical studies demonstrating a decrease in infectious complications with the use of EN compared with PN in the critically ill patient initiated feeding within 24 to 48 hours of hospital admission.[10,11,15,22,23] The benefits of decreased infectious complications are not apparent when the initiation of EN is delayed. A review of available studies comparing early versus delayed EN in critically ill patients showed a trend toward a reduction in infectious complications with early EN.[10,11] In addition, a trend toward reduction in mortality associated with early EN has been noted.[10,11,24]

In critically ill patients who are hemodynamically unstable, early EN may result in gut ischemia because of poor gut blood flow and increased oxygen demand. Consequently, it is recommended that initiation of EN be delayed until the patient is fluid resuscitated

and has an adequate perfusion pressure. Once this goal is achieved, often within 6 hours of hospitalization, the initiation of EN at a low administration rate is considered appropriate, along with clinical monitoring to ensure GI tolerance.[25,26] Therefore, early EN (within 24–48 hours after hospital admission) is recommended in critically ill adult patients.[10,11] Although no randomized, controlled trials have assessed early EN in critically ill children, initiation of EN within 48 to 72 hours of admission is common.[12] Early initiation of EN is not warranted for the mild to moderately stressed adult patient who is otherwise well nourished. It is reasonable to delay the initiation of EN in these patients until oral intake is inadequate for 7 to 14 days.[7] In the mild to moderately stressed adult patient with inadequate oral intake who is malnourished, it is unclear when to initiate EN, but most clinicians would not wait more than 7 days.

ENTERAL ACCESS

Advances in enteral access techniques have contributed to the expanded use of EN for conditions in which PN had previously been used. In particular, improved methods of achieving jejunal access for feeding have allowed for the use of EN during the early postoperative and postinjury period when gastric motility is typically impaired. As outlined in Table 152–3, various factors influence the selection of enteral access site and device, including anticipated duration of use (short- or long-term) and whether to feed into the stomach or small bowel. Figure 152–2 illustrates the predominant enteral access options.

SHORT-TERM ACCESS

❸ Short-term enteral access is easier to initiate, less invasive, and less costly than the establishment of long-term access.[27] The most frequently used routes for short-term enteral access are established by inserting a tube through the nose and passing the tip into the stomach (nasogastric [NG]), duodenum (nasoduodenal), or jejunum (nasojejunal). In general, these tubes are used in the hospitalized patient when the anticipated tube feeding duration is less than 4 to 6 weeks. The orogastric route is generally reserved for patients in whom the nasopharyngeal area is inaccessible or in young infants who are obligate nasal breathers. Because these routes do not require surgical intervention, they are the least invasive. The feeding tube is frequently held in place only by a piece of tape on the nose or face; therefore, it can be inadvertently pulled out relatively easily.

NG tubes vary in diameter size and stiffness. The large-bore (≥14F) rigid NG tubes are used primarily to decompress the stomach but can also be used for feeding. There is a low incidence of clogging with these tubes, and they provide a reliable way to measure gastric residual volumes. The major disadvantage associated with the use of these tubes is patient discomfort. Small-bore nasal tubes designed solely for feeding are available in varying lengths (16–60 inches [41–152 cm]) and diameter sizes (4F to 12F) to accommodate both pediatric (including neonates) and adult patients. The tip of the tube can be placed into the stomach, duodenum, or jejunum. These tubes consist of a lightweight, pliable silicone or polyurethane material that is more comfortable for the patient. A disadvantage of the small-bore tubes is that they may become easily occluded, often as a result of improper medication administration or tube-flushing technique.

❹ In general, the stomach is the least expensive and the least labor-intensive access site to use for enteral feeding; however, feeding into the stomach is not as well tolerated. Patients with impaired gastric motility may be predisposed to aspiration and pneumonia when feedings are delivered into the stomach. Many critically ill, injured, and postoperative patients exhibit delayed gastric emptying, limiting their ability to tolerate gastric feeding.

TABLE 152-3 Options and Considerations in the Selection of Enteral Access

Access	EN Duration/Patient Characteristics	Tube Placement Options	Advantages	Disadvantages
Nasogastric or orogastric	Short term Intact gag reflex Normal gastric emptying	Manually at bedside	Ease of placement Allows for all methods of administration Inexpensive Multiple commercially available tubes and sizes	Potential tube displacement Potential increased aspiration risk
Nasoduodenal or nasojejunal	Short term Impaired gastric motility or emptying High risk of GER or aspiration	Manually at bedside Fluoroscopically Endoscopically	Potential reduced aspiration risk Allows for early postinjury or postoperative feeding Multiple commercially available tubes and sizes	Manual transpyloric passage requires greater skill Potential tube displacement or clogging Bolus or intermittent feeding not tolerated
Gastrostomy	Long term Normal gastric emptying	Surgically Endoscopically Radiologically Laparoscopically	Allows for all methods of administration Low-profile buttons available Large-bore tubes less likely to clog Multiple commercially available tubes and sizes	Attendant risks associated with each type of procedure Potential increased aspiration risk Risk of stoma site complications
Jejunostomy	Long term Impaired gastric motility or gastric emptying High risk of GER or aspiration	Surgically Endoscopically Radiologically Laparoscopically	Allows for early postinjury or postoperative feeding Potential reduced aspiration risk Multiple commercially available tubes and sizes Low-profile buttons available	Attendant risks associated with each type of procedure Bolus or intermittent feeding not tolerated Risk of stoma site complications

EN = enteral nutrition, GER = gastroesophageal reflux.

In addition, patients with diabetic gastroparesis or patients with severe gastroesophageal reflux disease or intractable vomiting are at a higher risk for aspiration of gastric contents, resulting in pneumonia. In these patients, placing the tip of the tube into the duodenum or jejunum (also referred to as transpyloric placement) may be required to enable successful enteral feeding. However, studies have yet to prove definitively that transpyloric tube feedings actually do decrease the risk of aspiration and pneumonia. One meta-analysis of studies comparing gastric and transpyloric feeding in critically ill patients demonstrated no difference in the incidence of pneumonia;[28] another critical review of the same patient population suggested that small bowel feedings were associated with a reduction in gastroesophageal regurgitation and a lower rate of ventilator-associated pneumonia.[29] Thus, the true difference in aspiration and pneumonia risk associated with gastric and small bowel feeding remains unclear.

In general, small bowel feeding may be beneficial in patients who do not tolerate gastric feeding and offers an alternative to PN.[10–12] Nasoenteric feeding tubes can be inserted at the patient's bedside by trained medical personnel. However, greater skill is required to advance the tip of the feeding tube beyond the pylorus. Several techniques have been described in the literature to help facilitate bedside placement. Variable success rates have been reported with these techniques and are largely dependent on clinician experience. Electromagnetic tube placement devices that can be used at the bedside to guide tip position into the small bowel have been shown to be safe and cost-effective for small bowel feeding tube placement.[30] Alternatively, a variety of endoscopic and fluoroscopic techniques have been described to insert transpyloric tubes.[27] Radiographic confirmation of appropriate tip placement for feeding tubes inserted by bedside techniques should be obtained prior to use.[7,8]

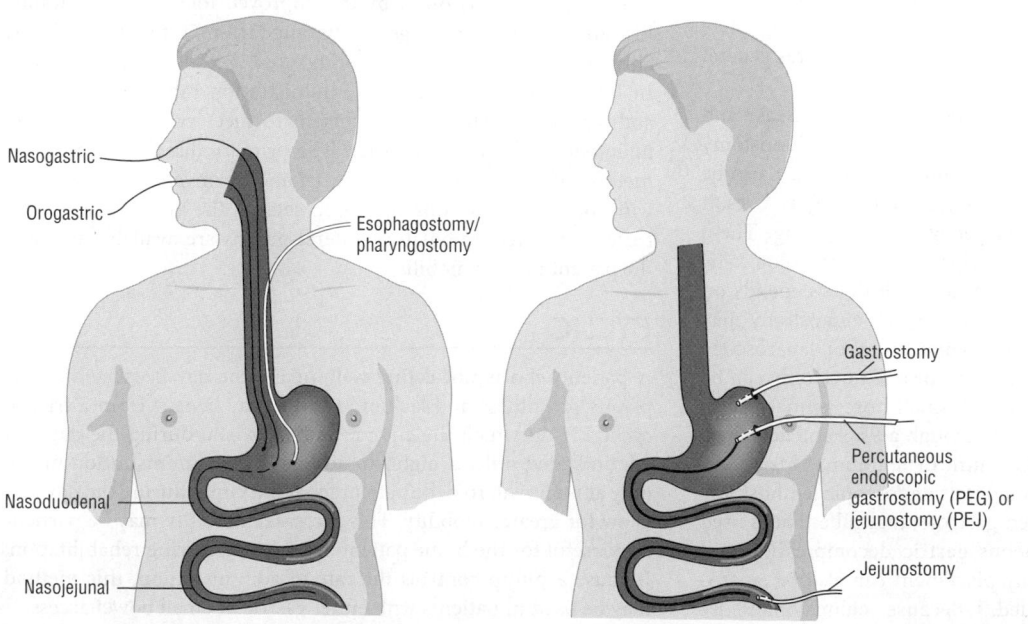

Nasogastric

Orogastric

Esophagostomy/ pharyngostomy

Nasoduodenal

Nasojejunal

Gastrostomy

Percutaneous endoscopic gastrostomy (PEG) or jejunostomy (PEJ)

Jejunostomy

FIGURE 152-2. Access sites for tube feeding.

LONG-TERM ACCESS

Feeding tubes used for short-term enteral access are usually not optimal for long-term use because of patient discomfort, long-term complications, and mechanical failures that develop over time. Long-term access should generally be considered when EN is anticipated for longer than 4 to 6 weeks. Many techniques can be used to establish long-term enteral access, including laparotomy, laparoscopy, endoscopy, and fluoroscopy. The ability to perform the various techniques will be somewhat dependent on the expertise and facilities available within each institution. Long-term enteral access options include gastrostomy and jejunostomy tubes.

A gastrostomy is the most common type of long-term enteral access. It eliminates the nasal irritation and discomfort associated with nasoenteric feeding tubes and inadvertent removal is uncommon. In addition, because feeding gastrostomies use large-bore tubes, clogging is less of a problem. Multiple techniques for insertion of a gastrostomy tube have been described, including surgical laparotomy, endoscopy, radiography, and laparoscopy. The most common technique is the percutaneous endoscopic gastrostomy (PEG). It is minimally invasive and can be performed safely and cost-effectively in an endoscopy suite or at the bedside using conscious sedation and local anesthesia. Young children, however, will usually require general anesthesia for the procedure. Numerous kits are available for PEG placement in both children and adults and vary in size (12F–28F; 1–4.5 cm shaft lengths), material used, internal and external bolsters, and insertion techniques. There are, however, ethical implications regarding determination of appropriate candidates for PEG placement.[31–33] Because of its relative ease of placement, the PEG tube is often placed inappropriately based on unrealistic expectations of what EN can accomplish in patients who are unable to eat. In adults, PEG placement is associated with an unexpectedly high 30-day mortality rate, which suggests that the procedure is being performed in patients who have multiple coexisting morbid conditions.[31] Evaluation by a multidisciplinary team is warranted for those patients near end of life to establish whether the benefit outweighs the risk of PEG placement.[8,31]

For patient convenience and comfort, a low-profile skin-level gastrostomy device may be placed in 2 to 3 months, once the gastrostomy tract has matured, if this type of device was not placed initially. This "gastric button" consists of a short, silicone, self-retaining conduit with either a mushroom tip or a balloon at the internal end and a one-way valve and small flange at the skin surface. Because this averts the external tube presence, it tends to be preferred in children or ambulatory adults who are receiving intermittent feedings. The exit site of all gastrostomies requires general stoma care to prevent inflammation and infection.

In patients at high risk of gastroesophageal reflux disease and aspiration who require long-term enteral access, a jejunostomy may be the most appropriate option.[34] Jejunostomies may also be indicated in patients unable to tolerate gastric feeding as a result of impaired gastric motility or delayed gastric emptying. These tubes can be inserted surgically, endoscopically, radiologically, or laparoscopically. The most appropriate technique depends on the expertise and facilities available. A surgical jejunostomy may be preferred if the patient requires a laparotomy or laparoscopy for other reasons. Endoscopic placement of a jejunostomy can be done by various methods. Typically, a small-bore jejunal extension tube (6F, 8F, or 10F) is inserted through a PEG and advanced through the pylorus into the duodenum or jejunum. This procedure has been referred to as percutaneous endoscopic jejunostomy (PEJ). A PEG/PEJ is a dual-lumen gastrojejunal tube that is used for patients who need simultaneous gastric decompression and small bowel feedings. Jejunostomy placement can also be laparoscopically or radiologically guided.[34] Because jejunostomies use

smaller-bore tubes, occlusion occurs more commonly than with gastrostomy tubes.

Pharyngostomies and esophagostomies are invasive because the tube is located in the neck and passes through the skin into the pharynx or esophagus, respectively. They have been used in patients with head and neck malignancies and in those with impaired swallowing caused by neuromuscular disorders. However, better long-term enteral access techniques have replaced the need for the pharyngostomy and esophagotomy routes. They are rarely performed today because of the high complication rate and extreme difficulty associated with their care.[31]

ADMINISTRATION METHODS

EN may be administered by continuous, cyclic (i.e., a continuous rate over a portion of the day), or bolus methods and may be accomplished by syringe, gravity, or pump-controlled techniques. The method of delivery depends on the location of the tip of the feeding tube, the clinical condition and intestinal function of the patient, the environment in which the patient resides, and the patient's tolerance to the tube feeding.

CONTINUOUS

In hospitalized patients, the continuous administration of EN is most commonly used for initiation and is generally the preferred method.[35,36] When initiating feeding into the stomach, the continuous method of delivery is usually better tolerated than the intermittent bolus method. Once tolerance is established, a conversion to intermittent bolus administration may be warranted. When EN is delivered into the small intestine, the continuous method is preferred because it is associated with enhanced tolerance. The rapid delivery of feeding into the small intestine, especially hyperosmotic formulations, may contribute to abdominal distension, cramps, hyperperistalsis, and diarrhea. Therefore, conversion to intermittent bolus administration is not recommended for those who have an access placed into the duodenum or jejunum.

The delivery system for continuous administration generally includes a feeding reservoir or bag attached to an extension set that is connected to a pump. The delivery system is then attached to the patient's enteral access tube. Continuous administration may increase nursing time because routine checks are needed, but this disadvantage is offset by the improved tolerance. For adults, EN administration rates generally range from 50 to 125 mL/hour, although higher rates have been used without complications. In infants and children, goal administration rates vary with age and weight and should be sufficient to meet caloric needs while maintaining good GI tolerance. The primary disadvantage to this method of administration is the cost and inconvenience associated with the pump and administration sets. In the home care setting, battery-operated ambulatory enteral pumps are available to allow the patient greater mobility.

CYCLIC

A patient who is not eating well during the day because of complaints of fullness and lack of appetite may benefit from a trial of cyclic EN, in which the enteral feeding is held during the day and administered only at night. In addition, the administration of EN only at night will free the patient from the pump during the day and allow for greater mobility. This increased mobility may be particularly useful for the home patient or patient requiring rehabilitation. Because a pump controls the rate of administration, this method may be used in patients with either gastric or small bowel access.

BOLUS

The bolus administration of EN is commonly used for patients in long-term care settings who have a gastrostomy. This administration technique involves the delivery of the enteral feeding formulation over 5 to 10 minutes. Essentially, the only equipment needed is a syringe to instill the feeding solution into the tube. Depending on the patient's nutritional requirements, an instillation volume of 240 to 500 mL is generally used and repeated four to six times daily. From a convenience standpoint, it is generally preferable to adjust the bolus volume in increments of the feeding formulation container size (usually 240–250 mL). Bolus volumes given to infants and children vary with age and weight (usually 30–240 mL) and should be sufficient to meet the calorie needs of most patients. In neonates, the bolus regimen is usually begun with an every 3-hour schedule; as the child grows, feedings may be given less frequently.[37] In patients with duodenal or jejunal access, bolus delivery may result in cramping, nausea, vomiting, aspiration, and diarrhea. Bolus administration also should be avoided in patients with delayed gastric emptying and in patients who are at high risk of aspiration.

INTERMITTENT

If a patient is experiencing intolerance to bolus administration over 5 to 10 minutes, it may be helpful to administer the prescribed volume over a longer time period, generally 20 to 60 minutes. For this method, the desired volume of feeding formulation is emptied into a reservoir bag or container and administered by an enteral pump or via gravity drip using a roller clamp. The bolus method of administration is more consistent physiologically with normal eating patterns than the continuous method. One study in infants demonstrated that normal gallbladder emptying did not occur with continuous feedings but was present in those infants receiving bolus feedings.[38] Thus, those patients who need long-term EN and PN, especially children, may benefit when this approach is used because it may minimize the development of cholestatic liver disease.

INITIATION AND ADVANCEMENT PROTOCOL

Guidelines for the initiation and advancement of enteral feeding formulations vary greatly, and scientific support for any of the guidelines is weak or nonexistent. The typical recommendation for continuous administration of EN for adults is to start at 20 to 50 mL/hour and advance by 10 to 25 mL/hour every 4 to 8 hours until the desired goal is achieved. For intermittent administration, the typical recommendation is to start with 120 mL every 4 hours and advance by 30 to 60 mL every 8 to 12 hours.[8,36] In children, the recommendation for continuous administration is initiation at a rate of 1 to 2 mL/kg per hour (25–30 mL/h) or 2 to 4 mL/kg per bolus (30–90 mL) with advancement by similar amounts every 4 to 24 hours. In premature infants, feedings may be initiated at lower rates usually 10 to 20 mL/kg per day and advanced by similar rates daily. Schedules for progression of tube feeding from initial to target rates are important and may influence tolerance. If the protocol is too conservative, it may take an excessively long period of time to reach nutrient goals. The practice of diluting enteral feeding formulations is not routinely recommended unless necessary to increase fluid intake.[8,36] The development of an EN protocol within an institution that outlines initiation and advancement criteria may be a useful strategy to optimize achievement of nutrient goals.[10,11] Such a protocol should allow nursing to advance the rate (i.e., 25 mL/hour every 4 hours until the goal rate is achieved) based on GI tolerance. Clinical signs of intolerance

include abdominal distension, abdominal cramping, high gastric residual volumes, aspiration, and diarrhea.

ENTERAL FEEDING FORMULATION SELECTION

Historically, enteral formulas were created to provide essential nutrients. Over the years, enhancements have been made to meet specific patient needs and improve tolerance. For example, nutrient composition has been enhanced by changing the content of the amino acids (e.g., glutamine and arginine), changing the omega-3 polyunsaturated fatty acid content, and adding ribonucleic acid to enhance immune function and improve therapeutic outcomes. These specific nutrients have been called nutraceuticals or pharmaconutrients because of the intent to use them to modify the disease process and improve clinical outcomes. Currently, enteral feeding formulations are categorized by the FDA as medical foods.[8] They are considered components of supportive care and are simply regulated to ensure sanitary manufacture. Unfortunately, they are not subject to rules governing health claims, and promotion of medical foods for therapeutic intent is currently not regulated by the FDA.[39,40]

The macronutrient content of enteral formulas (namely, protein, carbohydrate, and fat) varies in nutrient complexity (Table 152–4). Nutrient complexity refers to the amount of hydrolysis and digestion a substrate requires prior to intestinal absorption. Polymeric or intact substrates are of similar molecular form as the food we eat. Enteral formulas that contain partially hydrolyzed or elemental substrates are characterized as elemental or defined-formula diets. The caloric contribution of each of the macronutrients is as follows: carbohydrates, 4 kcal/g (17 kJ/g); protein, 4 kcal/g (17 kJ/g); and fat, 9 kcal/g (38 kJ/g). Micronutrients, including electrolytes, vitamins, trace elements, and water, do not contribute to caloric content.

PROTEIN COMPOSITION

The essential amino acid content of the protein source determines the quality of the protein, and most commercially available enteral feeding formulations contain proteins of high quality. The molecular form of the protein source in enteral formulas will determine the amount of digestion that is required for absorption within the

TABLE 152-4 Enteral Formula Nutrient Complexity

Nutrient	Polymeric or Intact	Partially Hydrolyzed or Elemental
Carbohydrate	Starches	Oligosaccharides
	Fruit, vegetable, cereal solids	Maltodextrins
	Glucose polymers	Disaccharides
	Corn syrup solids	Maltose, sucrose, lactose
	Polysaccharides	Monosaccharides
		Glucose
		Galactose
Fat	Long-chain triglycerides	Medium-chain triglycerides
	Polyunsaturated fatty acids	Coconut oil
	Corn oil	Palm kernel oil
	Safflower oil	Free fatty acids
	Soybean oil	Linoleic
	Canola oil	
	Marine oils	
Protein	Whole	Oligopeptides
	Egg, milk, wheat, whey	Dipeptides
	Isolates	Tripeptides
	Caseinate salts	L-amino acids
	Lactalbumin	

small bowel. Polymeric or intact protein sources require digestion to smaller peptides and free amino acids before absorption from the GI tract. Therefore, enteral formulation protein sources such as meat, milk, eggs, and caseinates require digestion by hydrochloric acid, specific protein enzymes, and pancreatic proteases. Enteral formulations may also contain protein sources that are partially hydrolyzed to peptides or L-amino acids. As the molecular form of protein is reduced in size, the osmotic load of the enteral formulation is increased. Many commercially available enteral feeding formulations contain combinations of intact and partially hydrolyzed protein sources.

CONDITIONALLY ESSENTIAL AMINO ACIDS

Glutamine and arginine are generally considered nonessential amino acids. However, during periods of high physiologic stress, the need for these nutrients may be increased beyond the body's synthetic ability; consequently, these amino acids are characterized as conditionally essential. Because they are usually present in low amounts in most enteral feeding formulations, those formulations targeted for the critically ill may be supplemented with glutamine and/or arginine.

Glutamine serves as a key fuel for rapidly dividing cells, including enterocytes, endothelial cells, lymphocytes, and fibroblasts. The primary site of glutamine production is skeletal muscle. During critical illness, the catabolism of skeletal muscle provides an increased supply of glutamine, but this may not be enough to meet the high rate of glutamine use by cells of the immune system and other cells involved in recovery and repair. Glutamine depletion may develop, particularly during prolonged periods of metabolic stress. Favorable outcomes have been documented in critically ill patients when enteral formulations have been supplemented with glutamine.[10,41,42]

Arginine has been added to some immune-modulating enteral formulations in concentrations that range from 4.5 to 14 g/L. However, arginine supplementation remains controversial, especially in patients with sepsis.[43,44] Many of the physiologic effects of arginine are mediated by its conversion to nitric oxide, which, in turn, modulates immune function, inflammation, and response to sepsis. Some of these effects may be potentially harmful in the patient with sepsis, especially when higher arginine intakes are used.[10,11]

CARBOHYDRATE COMPOSITION

The carbohydrate component of enteral feeding formulations usually provides the major source of calories. Polymeric or intact enteral formulations contain starches and numerous types of glucose polymers, which require digestion to monosaccharide moieties prior to intestinal absorption (see Fig. 152–1). As the hydrolysis of carbohydrate increases within an enteral formulation, the osmolality of the formulation increases. Elemental carbohydrates, such as glucose and galactose, contribute significantly to the osmolality of enteral formulations. Consequently, polymeric entities, rather than elemental sugars, are preferred in enteral formulas. Glucose polymers provide a useful carbohydrate source that is tolerated by most individuals (see Table 152–4). The polymers are large chains that provide minimal osmotic load, yet are absorbed easily in the intestine. The one shortcoming of glucose polymers and oligosaccharides is that they are not as sweet as simple glucose and thus may decrease the palatability of orally consumed products. Finally, almost all commercially available enteral feeding formulations used in adults and older children are lactose-free because disaccharidase production within the gut lumen is reduced during illness and periods of prolonged bowel rest. Additionally, there is a high incidence of lactose intolerance in those of certain ethnic decent: rates range from 5% in white northern Europeans, North Americans, and Australians to over 50% in people from South America, Africa, and Asia.[45] Infant formulas are available with or without lactose.[37]

FAT AND FATTY ACID COMPOSITION

Fat is an important constituent in the diet because it provides a concentrated calorie source and serves as a carrier for fat-soluble vitamins. Sufficient linoleic acid is required to prevent essential fatty acid deficiency and should approximate 1% to 3% of total daily calories. The most common sources of fat in enteral feeding formulations are vegetable oils (soy or corn) rich in polyunsaturated fatty acids. The concentration of fat varies between less than 2% to 45% of total calories. High fat content of the diet is associated with delayed gastric emptying. Enteral feeding formulations can also contain fat in the form of MCTs derived from palm kernel or coconut oils. Because MCTs do not contain linoleic acid, most enteral formulations that contain MCTs will also have a source of long-chain triglycerides to provide essential fatty acids. Potential advantages of MCTs compared as opposed to long-chain triglycerides are that they are more water soluble, undergo rapid hydrolysis, require little to no pancreatic lipase or bile salts for absorption, and do not require carnitine for transport into the mitochondria, where they are converted to energy. They also do not require chylomicron formation for small bowel enterocyte absorption.

The source of long-chain fat within some enteral formulations has been modified from omega-6 to omega-3 fatty acids in an effort to modulate the inflammatory response in patients with acute respiratory distress syndrome (ARDS), acute lung injury (ALI), and sepsis.[46] The omega-6 fatty acids serve as precursors to certain cytokines that are potent inflammatory mediators and also decrease cell-mediated immune response. The omega-6 fatty acids are high in linoleic acid and are derived from vegetable oil, whereas the omega-3 fatty acids, derived from coldwater fish oils, are high in linolenic acid. It has been proposed that if the dietary proportion of omega-3 fatty acids is increased and omega-6 fatty acids is decreased, less inflammation and immunosuppression may occur during metabolic stress.

Docosahexaenoic acid (DHA) and arachidonic acid (ARA) are two fatty acids abundant in human milk, but until recently, they were not contained in commercial infant formulas. Although the role of ARA supplementation is unclear, DHA is known to be important in both brain and eye development. In some studies, DHA and ARA supplementation provided benefits to a child's visual function and/or cognitive and behavioral development.[47] The FDA has classified plant-based fatty acid blends of DHA and ARA as generally recognized as safe (GRAS), and most infant formulas, as well as some products for pregnant and lactating women, are supplemented with these fatty acids.

FIBER CONTENT

Fiber, in the form of soy polysaccharides, has been added to several enteral feeding formulations intended for use in both children and adults in amounts ranging from 5.9 to 24 g/L. Infant formulas generally do not contain fiber; however, at least one formula intended for use in infants with diarrhea contains soy fiber. Fiber supplementation is common in clinical practice, primarily because fiber-free enteral formulations are implicated as a contributing factor to both diarrhea and constipation. Ingested fiber undergoes bacterial degradation within the colon to produce short-chain fatty acids. Potential benefits of fiber are the trophic effects on the colonic mucosa and the promotion of sodium and water absorption within the colon. Fiber supplementation may help regulate bowel function in both normal individuals and those with altered colonic motility. In addition, the resulting short-chain fatty acids are an excellent energy source. Although beneficial effects of fiber supplementation have not been clearly proven in clinical studies, there is experimental evidence that fiber may play an integral role in normal nutrition, and risk is generally minimal.[48] Fiber supplementation may be beneficial when long-term EN is required or in patients who experience diarrhea or constipation while receiving a fiber-free enteral formulation. Soluble fiber may also be beneficial in the critically ill patient who is hemodynamically stable and develops diarrhea while receiving EN.[10,49] Insoluble fiber should be avoided in all critically ill patients due to case reports of bowel obstruction.[10]

OSMOLALITY AND RENAL SOLUTE LOAD

Osmolality and renal solute load can affect tolerance to enteral feeding formulations. The osmolality of a given enteral formulation is a function of the size and quantity of ionic and molecular particles, primarily related to the protein, carbohydrate, electrolyte, and mineral content within a given volume. The unit of measure of osmolality is milliosmoles per kilogram (mOsm/kg) or millimoles per kilogram (mmol/kg). Iso-osmolar is considered to be ~300 mOsm/kg (300 mmol/kg). Enteral formulations with greater amounts of partially hydrolyzed or elemental substrates have a higher osmolality than formulations containing polymeric or intact substrate forms. Therefore, formulations that contain sucrose or glucose, dipeptides and tripeptides, and amino acids are generally hyperosmolar. Increased caloric density also increases the osmolality of an enteral formulation. In general, the osmolality of commercially available enteral feeding formulations ranges from 300 to 900 mOsm/kg (300–900 mmol/kg). The American Academy of Pediatrics recommends that enteral formulations for use in infants have an osmolality of 450 mOsm/kg (450 mmol/kg) or less.

Symptoms of gastric retention, diarrhea, abdominal distension, nausea, and vomiting have been attributed to enteral formulations having high osmolality based on the assumption that a higher osmolality will draw water into the gut lumen. However, clinical evidence to support the relationship between osmolality and GI tolerance is lacking. The practice of diluting hyperosmolar formulations has not been shown to enhance tolerance and should be discouraged unless dilution is done to increase fluid intake.[8,36] Factors such as concurrent antibiotic therapy, method of enteral feeding administration, and the formulation's composition are likely to play a greater role in GI tolerance than the osmolality.

The renal solute load is determined by the protein, sodium, potassium, and chloride content of the enteral formulation. Formulations that contain a greater solute load increase the obligatory water loss via the kidney. It is estimated that 40 to 60 mL of water is the minimal amount necessary to excrete 1 g of nitrogen. Those receiving high-protein enteral formulations unable to ingest more water, such as a geriatric patient and a patient with altered mental status, may be at risk for significant dehydration.

CLASSIFICATION OF ENTERAL FEEDING FORMULATIONS

⑤ Although most patients' needs can probably be met using three or four different formulations, certain disease states or clinical conditions may warrant the use of a specialty feeding formulation. Development of an effective formulary system should focus on clinically significant characteristics of available formulations, avoid duplicate feeding formulations, and use only those specialty formulations with evidence-based indications. Categorizing enteral feeding formulations according to therapeutic class is necessary in developing a formulary system for adults (Table 152–5) and children (Table 152–6).

TABLE 152-5 Adult Enteral Feeding Formulation Classification System

Category	Features	Indications
Standard polymeric	Isotonic 1–1.2 kcal/mL (4.2–kJ/mL) NPC:N 125:1 to 150:1 May contain fiber	Designed to meet the needs of the majority of patients Patients with functional GI tract Not suitable for oral use
High protein	NPC:N <125:1	Patients with protein requirements >1.5 g/kg/day, such as trauma patients and those with burns, pressure sores, or wounds
	May contain fiber	Patients receiving propofol
High caloric density	1.5–2 kcal/mL (6.3–8.4 kJ/mL) Lower electrolyte content per calorie Hypertonic	Patients requiring fluid and/or electrolyte restriction, such as kidney insufficiency
Elemental	High proportion of free amino acids Low in fat	Patients who require low fat Use has generally been replaced by peptide-based formulations
Peptide-based	Contains dipeptides and tripeptides Contains MCTs	Indications/benefits not clearly established Trial may be warranted in patients who do not tolerate intact protein due to malabsorption
Disease-specific		
Kidney	Caloric dense Protein content varies Low electrolyte content	Alternative to high caloric density formulations, but generally more expensive
Liver	Increased branched-chain and decreased aromatic amino acids	Patients with hepatic encephalopathy
Lung	High fat, low carbohydrate Antiinflammatory lipid profile and antioxidants	Patients with ARDS and severe ALI
Diabetes mellitus	High fat, low carbohydrate	Alternative to standard, fiber-containing formulation in patients with uncontrolled hyperglycemia.
Immune-modulating	Supplemented with glutamine, arginine, nucleotides, and/or omega-3 fatty acids	Patients undergoing major elective GI surgery, trauma, burns, head and neck cancer, and critically ill patients on mechanical ventilation Use with caution in patients with sepsis Select nutrients may be beneficial or harmful in subgroups of critically ill patients
Oral supplement	Sweetened for taste Hypertonic	Patients who require supplementation to an oral diet

ALI = acute lung injury, ARDS = acute respiratory distress syndrome, GI = gastrointestinal, MCT = medium-chain triglyceride, NPC:N = nonprotein calorie-to-nitrogen ratio.

TABLE 152-6 Pediatric Enteral Feeding Formulation Classification System

Formula Type	Features	Indications
Infants		
Cow's milk-based	Standard energy density for feeding: 20–24 kcal/oz (2.8–3.3 kJ/mL); also available in concentrate (40 kcal/oz [5.6 kJ/mL)) and powder forms Standard formulation contains lactose, but also available as lactose-free	Normal, healthy infant
Soy protein-based	Standard energy density for feeding: 20 kcal/oz (2.8 kJ/mL); also available in concentrate (40 kcal/oz [5.6 kJ/mL]) and powder forms Lactose free May contain added soy fiber	Lactase deficiency or intolerance, galactosemia, diarrhea (fiber added)
Prematurity	Standard energy density for feeding: 24 kcal/oz (3.3 kJ/mL); also available in 20 (2.8 kJ/mL) and 30 kcal/oz (4.2 kJ/mL) forms Provide increased protein, mineral, electrolytes, and vitamins compared with term infant formulations	Preterm infants weighing <2–3 kg (4.4–6.6 lb)
Transition	Standard energy density for feeding: 22 kcal/oz (3.1 kJ/mL) Provide higher calcium and phosphorus content compared with term infant formulas	Preterm infants weighing <3 kg (6.6 lb) and ready for discharge
Semielemental/elemental	Standard energy density for feeding: 20 kcal/oz (2.8 kJ/mL) Hydrolyzed protein and free amino acids May contain ARA and DHA Lactose free Typically contain MCTs ranging from 5% to 86% of fat content	Malabsorption, cow's milk protein allergy, chylothorax, cystic fibrosis, biliary atresia, short bowel syndrome, food allergies
Special diets	Low electrolyte/mineral content	Kidney disease
Children ages 1–10 years		
Standard	Standard energy density for feeding: 30 kcal/oz (1 kcal/mL [4.2 kJ/mL]) Intact protein; 30–38 g/L May contain added fiber	Functioning GI tract requiring tube feedings
Semielemental/elemental	Standard energy density for feeding: 20–30 kcal/oz (2.8–4.2 kJ/mL) Hydrolyzed protein and free amino acids Lactose-free MCTs range from 33% to 87% of fat content	Malabsorption, cow's milk protein allergy, chylothorax, cystic fibrosis, biliary atresia, short bowel syndrome, food allergies

ARA = arachidonic acid, DHA = docosahexaenoic acid, GI =gastrointestinal, MCT = medium-chain triglyceride.

STANDARD POLYMERIC

A large number of commercially available enteral feeding formulations fall within the category of a standard polymeric formulation. These formulations are approximately isotonic (300 mOsm/L [300 mmol/L]), provide about 1 kcal/mL (4.2 kJ/mL), and are composed of intact nutrients in a nutritionally balanced mix of carbohydrate, fat, and protein. They are provided with or without dietary fiber. The nonprotein calorie-to-nitrogen ratio of these products

is ~125:1 to 150:1. This ratio is a useful parameter for assessing protein density in relation to calories provided. Certain feeding formulations in this category may be promoted as high nitrogen but fall within standard protein amounts. To maintain their isotonicity, many products within this category are not sweetened, making them not very palatable and generally suited only for tube feeding and not oral supplementation; however, flavored products are available. The nutrient requirements of the majority of adult patients and children older than 1 year receiving EN can generally be met using feeding formulations in this category. Many infant formulas will also fall into this category because they provide 20 to 30 kcal/oz (2.8–4.2 kJ/mL).[37]

HIGH PROTEIN

Enteral feeding formulations with a nonprotein calorie-to-nitrogen ratio less than 125:1 can be categorized as high protein. The lower the ratio, the higher the protein density in relation to calories provided. In patients with high protein requirements, it is generally unacceptable to use a feeding formulation with standard protein amounts because the volume necessary to meet protein requirements will often result in excessive calorie intake. Patients who may be candidates for a high-protein feeding formulation are critically ill patients and those with pressure sores, surgical wounds, and high fistula output. In general, adult patients with estimated protein requirements exceeding 1.5 g/kg per day may benefit from a high-protein formulation. High-protein formulations may also be beneficial in mechanically ventilated patients who are receiving propofol for sedation. The vehicle for propofol is a soybean fat emulsion that contains 1.1 kcal/mL (4.6 kJ/mL). At therapeutic dosages, the use of propofol can significantly contribute to caloric intake, and a high protein formulation may be beneficial in allowing for the provision of protein requirements while minimizing the risk of overfeeding.

HIGH CALORIC DENSITY

High caloric density formulations are concentrated to provide less fluid and electrolyte intake in comparison to a standard polymeric formulation. They provide ~2 kcal/mL (8.4 kJ/mL) and will achieve similar calorie and protein intake as a standard polymeric formulation, using half the volume. High caloric density formulations are often necessary for patients who require fluid and/or electrolyte restriction, such as those with kidney insufficiency or congestive heart failure. Although specialty enteral formulations targeted for acute and chronic kidney failure are also available, many patients with kidney failure can be managed using a product in this category (see Chapter 153).

ELEMENTAL/PEPTIDE BASED

Formulations in this category contain protein and/or fat components that are hydrolyzed into smaller, predigested forms. Traditionally, enteral formulations in this category were referred to as elemental and contained a high proportion of protein in the form of free amino acids and a low amount of fat. Although still commercially available, the use of these formulations has been replaced in clinical practice with formulations containing a portion of the protein in the form of dipeptides and tripeptides and thus fewer free amino acids. These formulations are referred to as peptide based. This alteration in protein composition was made in an effort to optimize protein absorption in patients with impaired digestive or absorptive capacity. Results from human and animal intestinal perfusion studies indicate that the partially hydrolyzed sources of protein provide an absorptive advantage over formulas that contain only free amino acids.[50] Peptide-based formulations are generally higher in fat than the older, elemental formulations and use MCTs in varying proportions as the fat source.

Evidence to support the use of elemental or peptide-based formulations is limited, and their routine use is generally not recommended. Patients who do not tolerate standard, intact nutrient formulations as a result of malabsorption or short bowel syndrome might be candidates for a trial of a peptide-based formulation. In addition, elemental or peptide-based products that have higher percentages of MCTs and small amounts of long-chain triglycerides may be beneficial for patients with severe pancreatic insufficiency, such as chronic pancreatitis and cystic fibrosis; severe abnormalities of the intestinal mucosa, such as untreated celiac disease; biliary tract disease, such as biliary atresia or severe cholestasis; or chylothorax.

DISEASE SPECIFIC

Newer enteral feeding formulations have been designed to meet unique nutrient requirements and manage metabolic abnormalities associated with specific disease states. Conditions for which specialized enteral feeding formulations exist include kidney and liver failure, lung disease, including ARDS, diabetes mellitus, wound healing, and metabolic stress. Chapter 153 discusses specific nutrient concerns during organ failure. Specialized enteral formulations designed to modulate the inflammatory response in patients with severe metabolic stress have been referred to as immune-modulating formulations or immunonutrition. These specialized formulations are supplemented with nutrients such as glutamine, arginine, branched-chain amino acids, nucleotides, and omega-3 polyunsaturated fatty acids, as a result of their potential role in regulating immune function; guidelines for their use in critically ill patients have been published.[10,11,51] Positive results have been reported in patients undergoing major elective GI surgery and major cancer surgery of the head and neck, patients with severe trauma or burns, and critically ill patients on mechanical ventilation. Multiple meta-analyses have shown that the use of immune-modulating enteral formulations in these select patient populations is associated with significant reductions in infectious complications, hospital length of stay, and duration of mechanical ventilation.[52,53] However, use of immune-modulating formulations has been associated with increased mortality in patients with preexisting severe sepsis and should therefore not be used or used with caution in these patients and in those who become septic while receiving these products.[10] Because of the lack of evidence to support their use, immune-modulating formulations are not recommended for use in children.[12]

CLINICAL CONTROVERSY

Although there appears to be a role for immune-modulating enteral formulations in critically ill patients, the optimal pharmaconutrient composition and type of critically ill patient most likely to benefit are unclear. Available literature has been criticized for the heterogeneity of studies, including a wide range of patient populations and a variety of enteral formulations. The specific effects and optimal dose of individual nutrient components contained in immune-modulating enteral formulations also remain unclear. Caution is suggested in patients with severe sepsis due to arginine content, but available evidence is conflicting.

In patients with ARDS, improved outcomes from using a low carbohydrate formulation supplemented with specific fatty acids (eicosapentaenoic acid and γ-linolenic acid) and antioxidants have been documented.[44,56] When compared with a high fat for-

mulation, the specialized diet was associated with fewer days of ventilatory support, fewer ICU days, and fewer new organ failures. Consequently, it is recommended that this specialized formulation be used for patients with ARDS and severe ALI.[10,11,51]

There are no disease-specific enteral products currently marketed for use in infants or children from 1 to 10 years of age. The use of modular supplements is often necessary in children with special nutrition needs (see Modular Products below).

ORAL SUPPLEMENTS

In general, oral supplements are not intended for tube feeding but to enhance an oral diet. They are sweetened to improve taste and therefore are hypertonic (~450–700 mOsm/kg [450–700 mmol/kg]). Osmolality is generally not a problem in the patient with a functioning GI tract. However, in the tube-fed patient, a sweetened product is unnecessary and may contribute to GI intolerance, particularly diarrhea. Powder supplements that are mixed with milk should be avoided in lactose-intolerant patients. In addition to liquid supplements, puddings, gelatins, bars, and milkshake-like supplements are available.

MODULAR PRODUCTS

A module is a powder or liquid form of nutrients (e.g., protein, carbohydrate, or fat) that is used to supplement a commercially available enteral formulation. Addition of a modular product may be necessary, especially in children, to achieve a nutrient mix not supplied by a single commercially available product.[37,57] Alternatively, formulations available in powder or concentrate can be mixed with less water than needed for the standard dilution to deliver more nutrients in less volume. Infant formulas generally are concentrated beyond their standard concentration in this way. The mixing process required for modular components increases the potential for bacterial contamination and incorrect preparation. Contamination is a particular concern with the use of blenders and reconstitution of powders.[8,58] Human milk fortifiers are available for supplementation of human milk so that it meets the needs of a premature infant. Human milk fortifiers add calories, protein, and minerals and have been shown to improve nutritional outcomes in human milk–fed premature infants.[37,59–62]

REHYDRATION

Oral rehydration formulations are useful in maintaining hydration or treating dehydration in adult and pediatric patients with high GI output. Such formulations are available commercially in powder or liquid form or can be extemporaneously compounded. They can be administered orally or given via a feeding tube. The glucose content of oral rehydration solutions is important because it stimulates active transport systems, which, in turn, stimulate passive sodium and water uptake simultaneously with the glucose. Therefore, oral or enteral administration of rehydration solutions may decrease fecal water loss and generate a positive electrolyte balance.[63]

FORMULARY AND DELIVERY SYSTEM CONSIDERATIONS

The selection of a product for an individual should be based on the patient's nutritional requirements. In general, no more than one product is necessary per category of enteral feeding formulation, and it may be possible to omit certain categories based on the specific patient population within a given institution. Additional selection criteria include container size and type, liquid or powder form, shelf life, ease of use, and cost.

Most enteral products are available as ready-to-use, prepackaged liquids, and a few are available in the powdered state and require reconstitution prior to use. Advantages of ready-to-use liquid formulations are convenience and lower susceptibility to microbiologic contamination. One disadvantage is that more storage space is required. The ease or convenience of a ready-to-use liquid is especially important for self-care patients, the disabled, and those who have difficulty reading or following printed instructions. Ready-to-use liquid enteral formulations are generally available in rigid plastic containers, cans, or closed, ready-to-hang bags. Bolus administration of EN is usually achieved using formulas available in cans. However, when formula from a can is used for continuous or cyclic administration, it must first be poured into a bag or bottle to allow for administration via a pump. This "open system" differs from the closed, ready-to-hang containers from the standpoint of microbial contamination risk. The use of a powder formula is also considered an open system of delivery.

Contaminated enteral feeding formulations are a potential source of infectious complications.[8,63] The GI tract may serve as a portal of entry for bacteria into the systemic circulation, especially in patients who are receiving multiple antibiotics, have undergone a surgical procedure, are immunosuppressed, or have GI tract stasis from a variety of causes. The contamination of enteral feeding formulations is associated with a lack of attention to proper handling techniques, inability to disinfect preparation equipment, and nonsterile or contaminated tube-feeding additives. Unlike liquid formulations, powdered products are not guaranteed by the manufacturer to be sterile because of the inability to properly sterilize the powder without destruction of some of its components. Occasional contamination of milk powder and consequently powdered infant formulas with *Enterobacter sakazakii* (*Cronobacter* species) has been reported.[58] Contamination of one infant formula with *E. sakazakii* at the manufacturing site was implicated in the death of an infant in a neonatal ICU, prompting FDA warnings regarding the use of powdered formulations in premature neonates and other immunocompromised infants. Because powder formulations require reconstitution, often in a blender that is difficult to sterilize, they are also more susceptible to contamination at the time of preparation. Stringent handling procedures are recommended during all aspects of enteral feeding preparation and delivery to minimize contamination risk. The closed-system containers supply a ready-to-hang, prefilled, sterile supply of formula in volumes of 1 to 1.5 L. Numerous, but not all, enteral formulations intended for use in adults and some of the pediatric formulations are available in the closed-administration system. The closed-administration system also offers the advantage of not requiring refrigeration and allowing hang times beyond 24 to 36 hours, whereas the conventional open-delivery system necessitates hang times of generally 4 to 8 hours.

COMPLICATIONS AND MONITORING

The majority of complications associated with EN are metabolic, GI, and mechanical. The early detection and management of potential complications is necessary to allow for the successful use of EN. In addition, measures to avoid complications should be incorporated into the management of all patients receiving EN (Table 152–7).

METABOLIC COMPLICATIONS

Metabolic complications associated with EN are similar to those associated with PN, but the incidence tends to be lower. EN is associated with a lower incidence of hyperglycemia than PN.[64] Complications related to hydration and electrolyte imbalance and

TABLE 152-7	Suggested Monitoring for Patients on Enteral Nutrition	
Parameter	During Initiation of EN Therapy	During Stable EN Therapy
Vital signs	Every 4–6 hours	As needed with suspected change (i.e., fever)
Clinical assessment		
Weight	Daily	Weekly
Length/height (children)	Weekly–monthly	Monthly
Head circumference (<3 years of age)	Weekly–monthly	Monthly
Total intake/output	Daily	As needed with suspected change in intake/output
Tube-feeding intake	Daily	Daily
Enterostomy tube site assessment	Daily	Daily
GI tolerance		
Stool frequency/volume	Daily	Daily
Abdomen assessment	Daily	Daily
Nausea or vomiting	Daily	Daily
Gastric residual volumes	Every 4–8 hours (varies)	As needed when delayed gastric emptying suspected
Tube placement	Prior to starting, then ongoing	Ongoing
Laboratory		
Electrolytes, blood urea nitrogen/serum creatinine, glucose	Daily	Every 1–3 months
Calcium, magnesium, phosphorus	3–7 times/week	Every 1–3 months
Liver function tests	Weekly	Every 1–3 months
Trace elements, vitamins	If deficiency/toxicity suspected	If deficiency/toxicity suspected

EN = enteral nutrition, GI = gastrointestinal.

altered glucose control are observed more frequently in critically ill patients, especially those with underlying organ dysfunction. The micronutrient and water contents within enteral feeding formulations are in fixed amounts intended to meet recommended dietary allowances for the average patient. Consequently, the frequency of clinical and laboratory assessment to monitor hydration, electrolyte, organ function, and glucose control adequately for a patient who is critically ill is greater than for a stable patient residing in a rehabilitation unit or at home. Patients receiving long-term EN at home may require laboratory monitoring only every 2 to 3 months, depending on their clinical status. Besides macronutrient content, it is important to evaluate the actual content of water and micronutrients provided by the enteral formulation, especially in critically ill patients at high risk of metabolic complications. Supplemental fluid and electrolytes may be required in some patients. Conversely, for patients who have fluid retention or increased serum electrolytes, the enteral formulation may need to be changed to one that is more concentrated or provides less of a particular nutrient.

GASTROINTESTINAL COMPLICATIONS

❻ The GI complications associated with tube feeding include nausea, vomiting, abdominal distension, cramping, aspiration, diarrhea, and constipation. Gastric residual volume refers to the volume of contents in the stomach and is measured by using a syringe and aspirating from a large-bore NG or gastrostomy tube. For patients receiving tube feeding into the stomach, gastric residual volumes are widely used as an indicator of tolerance. It is believed, although not well documented, that patients with high gastric residual volumes are at higher risk of vomiting and/or aspiration. The frequency of measuring gastric residual volumes generally varies between 4 and 8 hours, and most institutions follow a protocol that directs the frequency of monitoring and when to hold feedings.[65]

CLINICAL CONTROVERSY

Clinicians disagree as to what constitutes excessive gastric residual volume. In adults, the definition of a high residual volume ranges from greater than 200 mL to 500 mL. In children, residual volumes greater than 2 to 3 times the bolus volume or twice the hourly infusion rate for continuous gastric feedings are considered excessive.

If high gastric residuals occur, the response is often to withhold the next scheduled bolus or stop or decrease the rate of a continuous feeding. However, frequent interruptions in the delivery of EN can adversely affect the attainment of nutrient goals. Because gastric residual volumes are unreliable, symptoms such as abdominal distension, fullness, bloating, and discomfort are generally more reliable indicators of EN intolerance and should be assessed frequently. A trend in elevated gastric residual volumes is generally more important than an isolated high measurement. If symptoms are present, and residual volumes are elevated, a decrease in tube-feeding rate may be warranted. In general, abruptly stopping tube feeding should be reserved for patients with overt regurgitation or aspiration.[66] Gastric residual volumes should generally be reinstilled through the tube to the patient unless they are excessive (greater than 500 mL in adults).[8,35,66] It may be beneficial to initiate a prokinetic agent such as metoclopramide or erythromycin to increase the gastric emptying rate and decrease residual volume, thereby enhancing tolerance.[35,67,68] If high gastric residual volumes persist, a transpyloric feeding tube may be considered for feeding into the small bowel. Other interventions may include a trial of a proton-pump inhibitor or histamine$_2$-receptor antagonist to decrease the volume of gastric secretions and minimizing the use of narcotics, sedatives, or other agents that may delay gastric emptying.[35,36]

Aspiration pneumonia is considered the most serious complication associated with tube feeding and is potentially life-threatening. Although aspiration is a fairly common event for critically ill patients receiving tube feeding, progression to aspiration pneumonia is difficult to predict. Risk factors for aspiration include a previous aspiration episode, decreased level of consciousness, neuromuscular disease, structural airway or GI tract abnormalities, endotracheal intubation, vomiting, persistently high gastric residual volumes, and prolonged supine positioning.[35] Identification of these risk factors, along with close monitoring of gastric residual volumes, is recommended for the management of critically ill patients receiving tube feeding. Historically, blue food coloring had been added to enteral formulations in an attempt to detect aspiration. However, because of its low sensitivity for detection and association with several serious adverse events, including death, the addition of blue food dye to enteral formulations is no longer advised.[10,35,69] There are currently no reliable methods available to detect aspiration in enterally fed patients.[10,70]

Strategies to decrease aspiration risk include keeping the patient's head of the bed elevated to a 30- to 45-degree angle during feeding and for 30 to 60 minutes after intermittent boluses, in addition to those mentioned above. This positioning makes it more difficult for the EN formulation to migrate up the esophagus against gravity. Changing from bolus or intermittent to continuous administration may also reduce the risk, although this has not been proven. Aspiration may occur with improper feeding tube placement or displacement; therefore, regular assessment of tube position is recommended.[8,35]

The reported incidence of diarrhea in patients receiving EN ranges from 20% to 70% because of the lack of a standard definition and the number of contributing factors.[36,71,72] When monitoring for diarrhea, stool frequency, consistency, and volume should be evaluated, and previous bowel habits should be considered. One commonly accepted definition of diarrhea is the occurrence of more than three to five liquid stools daily or a stool volume >250 to 500 mL/day (10 mL/kg per day in children) for at least 2 consecutive days.[71] Therefore, the occurrence of one or two loose stools does not constitute diarrhea or require intervention.

❼ Diarrhea in patients receiving tube feeding may be caused by a number of factors, and management should be directed at identifying and correcting the most likely cause(s). Tube feeding–related factors that may contribute to diarrhea include too rapid delivery or advancement of formula, intolerance to the formula composition, administration of large volumes of feeding into the small bowel, and formula contamination. Measures to prevent or manage the development of diarrhea related directly to the tube feeding should address these potential causes.[63,72] If diarrhea occurs when using a fiber-free formulation, consider switching to a fiber-containing formulation. If using a high-fat formulation, it may be beneficial to switch to a formulation lower in fat or having a proportion of the fat supplied as MCTs. Finally, it is important to assess the risk of bacterial contamination of the formula and take steps to minimize any potential risk factors. Once infectious etiologies have been excluded, pharmacologic intervention may be required to control severe diarrhea, including the use of opioids, diphenoxylate, and loperamide.

A common cause of diarrhea that is unrelated to tube feeding is drug therapy, particularly the use of broad-spectrum antibiotics. Another drug-related cause is the sorbitol contained in many liquid medication formulations. Sorbitol is used as a sweetening agent to enhance palatability, but it acts as an osmotic laxative. In addition, many drugs available in a liquid form are hyperosmolar, which may contribute to diarrhea. Because many patients receiving tube feeding also receive medications in a liquid form, all medications should be evaluated for their potential contribution. Infectious causes of diarrhea, such as antibiotic-induced bacterial overgrowth by *Clostridium difficile* or other intestinal flora, need to be considered when diarrhea develops. Diarrhea also may occur as a result of malabsorption, secondary to the underlying disease state or condition.

MECHANICAL COMPLICATIONS

Mechanical complications of EN are those associated with the feeding tube, including tube occlusion or malposition, and nasopulmonary intubation. Feeding tube occlusion is usually a result of the improper administration of medications and/or flushing technique. Kinking of the tube also may cause occlusion. The tube should be flushed with at least 30 mL of water before and after administering any medication. The recommended volume used in children is generally less than 30 mL and depends on the size of the tube. The frequency of flushing should be at least every 8 hours during continuous feeding and before and after each intermittent feeding. If tube occlusion occurs, an attempt to irrigate the tube with warm water should be made. Other fluids such as colas and cranberry juice have been used to irrigate occluded tubes but have not been shown to be any better than warm water. Some success in reestablishing patency has been shown with the use of pancreatic enzymes mixed in sodium bicarbonate.[73] Declogging devices that are specifically designed to unclog feeding tubes are available. They have been designed to either mechanically break through or remove the occlusion or provide an applicator and syringe prefilled with pancreatic enzymes and various powders targeted to restore patency.

CLINICAL CONTROVERSY

The source of water used to flush the feeding tube and maintain patient hydration via the feeding tube is controversial. Tap water is adequate for the otherwise healthy, immunocompetent patient. However, the acute or chronically ill patient receiving EN may be at higher risk from exposure to nonsterile tap water and may benefit from the use of purified water. Nosocomial infections from contaminated tap water sources have been reported in critically ill patients. The use of purified water for tube-feeding flushes in at-risk patients has been recommended by some clinicians.

Inadvertent tube removal or displacement has been reported in ~40% of patients receiving EN.[74] An agitated or confused patient may pull at the feeding tube and cause its removal or malposition. Measures to decrease agitation and confusion should be attempted. Various manipulations done to the patient throughout the day may also cause malposition. Securing the tube with tape may be helpful, as well as marking the tube with permanent ink at the exit site to assess for change in position. A recently developed nasal bridle that uses a magnetic retrieval system has proven to be a simple and effective method for securing nasoenteric feeding tubes and preventing accidental tube removal.[74]

When a feeding tube is inserted nasally or orally, there is a risk that the tube may inadvertently enter the tracheobronchial tree. The risk may be higher in patients who have an impaired cough or gag reflex and when a stylet is used for tube insertion. Proper positioning of the tube should always be confirmed by radiography prior to feeding initiation and routinely reassessed to avoid inadvertent administration of enteral formula into the lung.

OTHER COMPLICATIONS

Infectious complications of feeding tube placement include sinusitis (with nasoenteric placement), exit site-related infections (e.g., cellulitis, subcutaneous abscess, and necrotizing fasciitis), and intraabdominal infections (e.g., peritonitis and abscess). Leaking and bleeding around the exit site can also occur.[31,34] Formation of excessive granulation tissue around the exit site is often the cause of leaking and bleeding and can be managed by applying a line layer of silver nitrate.

A unique complication of tube feedings in children, especially in the first year of life, is the development of feeding disorders as a consequence of oral hypersensitivity, poor oral/motor skills, and food aversion. In these children, transitioning from tube to oral nutrition is often difficult and protracted. The involvement of an occupational or speech therapist, behavioral psychologist, or other trained individual, as well as perseverance by the family, often is necessary to improve oral intake. Avoidance of a strict nothing by mouth (NPO) status, if possible, and oral stimulation programs for those children who must remain NPO are recommended to avoid this complication.[75]

DRUG DELIVERY VIA FEEDING TUBE

Using enteral feeding tubes to deliver drugs is a common practice and offers an alternative for patients unable to take drugs by the oral route. However, in addition to complications of tube occlusion, effects on drug bioavailability and other potential interactions need to be considered when using this route. Medications have been given as a concomitant bolus administration via the feeding tube or admixed with the enteral feeding formulation.

CONCOMITANT DRUG ADMINISTRATION

❽ Concomitant administration of medications with enteral feedings requires awareness of certain limitations. Medications delivered directly into the stomach allow for the normal process of drug dissolution. Medications delivered into the small bowel may result in alterations of drug dissolution because the stomach is bypassed. In addition, therapeutic effect designed to occur within the stomach, such as with antacids and sucralfate, may be influenced by the feeding tube route. Because many drugs are best absorbed in the fasting state, they should be administered on an empty stomach whenever possible. Patients on bolus gastric feeding may receive medications appropriately spaced between the feedings, but patients on continuous feeding will require interruption for drug administration.

Selecting the proper medication dosage form for coadministration with the tube feeding is another important consideration. Medications in sublingual form, sustained-release capsules or tablets, and enteric-coated tablets should not be crushed and therefore should not be administered via enteral feeding tubes.[8,76] Solid dosage forms that are appropriate to crush should be prepared as a very fine powder and mixed with 15 to 30 mL of water or other appropriate solvent before administering through the tube. In addition, many capsules may be opened and the contents administered in the same manner. Pellets contained inside microencapsulated dosage forms should generally not be crushed. It may be acceptable to administer intact pellets through feeding tubes, provided that the pellets are small enough and drug absorption is not compromised.[76-79] To avoid the need to crush a solid dosage form and mix with water, liquid dosage preparations have been used for administration through feeding tubes. However, the risk of GI intolerance should be considered because of the hyperosmolality of many liquid formulations and possible sorbitol content.[76-78] Although the use of a liquid dosage preparation may be more convenient than a solid dosage form, it may not be the best choice if GI intolerance is an issue.

As previously mentioned, adherence to proper flushing technique is necessary to prevent occlusion when administering medication through a feeding tube. At least 15 mL of water should be given before and after medication administration to clear the drug through the tube and help get the drug into the stomach.[8] If more than one medication is scheduled for a given time, each should be administered separately, and the tube should be flushed with at least 15 mL of water between them.[8,76] Flush volume will be less for children but generally should be at least 5 mL to ensure adequate flushing of the tube.[8]

ADMIXTURE OF DRUGS WITH ENTERAL FEEDING

Mixing liquid medications with certain enteral feeding formulations is associated with several types of physical incompatibilities, including granulation, gel formation, separation, and precipitation.[76,77] Not only can these physical incompatibilities inhibit drug absorption, but gel formation potentially may clog small-bore feeding tubes. Physical incompatibility with medications is more common in formulations that contain intact protein than in those with hydrolyzed protein. Also, medication and enteral formula incompatibilities are more common with the use of acidic pharmaceutical syrups. The most prudent recommendation is to avoid the routine admixture whenever possible, especially for nonaqueous preparations and syrups. In the clinical setting, exceptions do exist, such as adding electrolyte injections of potassium or sodium to enteral formulas to assist in maintaining or repleting electrolytes.

TABLE 152-8 Medications with Special Considerations for Enteral Feeding Tube Administration

Drug	Interaction	Comments
Phenytoin	Reduced bioavailability in the presence of tube feedings Possible binding of phenytoin to calcium caseinates or protein hydrolysates in enteral feeding	To minimize interaction, holding tube feedings 1–2 hours before and after phenytoin has been suggested; this has no proven benefit Adjust tube-feeding rate to account for time held for phenytoin administration Monitor phenytoin serum concentration and clinical response closely Consider switching to IV phenytoin route if unable to reach therapeutic serum concentration
Fluoroquinolones Tetracyclines	Potential for reduced bioavailability because of complexation of drug with divalent and trivalent cations found in enteral feeding	Consider holding tube feeding 1 hour before and after administration Avoid jejunal administration of ciprofloxacin Monitor clinical response
Warfarin	Decreased absorption of warfarin because of enteral feeding; therapeutic effect antagonized by vitamin K in enteral formulations	Adjust warfarin dose based on INR Anticipate need to increase warfarin dose when enteral feedings are started and decrease dose when enteral feedings are stopped Consider holding tube feeding 1 hour before and after administration
Omeprazole Lansoprazole	Administration via feeding tube complicated by acid-labile medication within delayed-release, base-labile granules	Granules become sticky when moistened with water and may occlude small-bore tubes Suggested that granules be mixed with acidic liquid when given via a gastric feeding tube An oral liquid suspension can be extemporaneously prepared for administration via a feeding tube

INR= International Normalized Ratio, IV = intravenous(ly).

DRUG–NUTRIENT INTERACTIONS

❾ The most significant drug–nutrient interactions that can occur during continuous enteral feeding are those in which the bioavailability of the drug is reduced, and the desired pharmacologic effect is not achieved (Table 152–8). Unfortunately, limited clinical studies are available to document the extent of this problem with enteral feeding. Most of the observations are anecdotal case reports involving few patients. One of the most studied interactions has been the interaction between phenytoin and enteral feeding that results in decreased phenytoin bioavailability. The interaction was first reported in 1982,[80] yet the precise mechanism for the interaction remains unclear. Phenytoin serum concentrations may decrease by as much as 50% to 75% when phenytoin is given concomitantly with EN, possibly as a result of the binding of phenytoin to calcium caseinates or protein hydrolysates in the enteral formulation. Patients typically require higher than normal phenytoin doses while receiving EN.[76,77,81] The patient's clinical response and phenytoin serum concentrations should be monitored closely if phenytoin is given enterally during continuous enteral feeding and after its discontinuation.

Decreased bioavailability of certain antibiotics, particularly quinolones, has been documented when coadministered with enteral feeding.[76,77,82] Although the practice of holding tube feeding for 30 minutes before and 30 minutes after quinolone administration has been recommended, it has not been shown to improve drug absorption. There is evidence to suggest that ciprofloxacin absorption is significantly decreased when given via a jejunostomy tube, so this practice should be avoided.[82]

Warfarin resistance has been documented during enteral feeding, possibly as a consequence of decreased absorption or the antagonist effects of vitamin K. Before 1980, it was thought that the content of vitamin K (up to 1,330 mcg/1,000 kcal [or 317 mcg/1000 kJ] of enteral feeding formula) was contributing to the pharmacologic interaction with warfarin. Subsequently, the vitamin K content within formulas intended for use in adults was reformulated to less than 200 mcg/1,000 kcal (or 48 mcg/1000 kJ). However, warfarin resistance continues to be reported, and a warfarin dosage increase may be required in patients receiving EN.[76,77,83] The patient's International Normalized Ratio should be closely monitored in patients receiving both warfarin and enteral feedings. Conversely, when EN is discontinued, a reduction in warfarin dose may be required.

NUTRITION OUTCOME GOALS

Nutrition outcome goals of EN are to promote an adequate nutritional state in adults and promote growth and development of infants and children. Assessing the outcome of EN includes monitoring objective measures of body composition, protein and energy balance, and subjective outcome for physiologic muscle function and wound healing. Besides an improvement in nutrition outcome, a goal of EN is to reduce disease-related morbidity and mortality. Measures of disease-related morbidity include length of hospital stay, infectious complications, and the patient's sense of well-being. Such clinical outcome goals are extremely difficult to document with the use of EN, in part because other factors, such as age, underlying comorbidities, extent of injury, immunocompetence, and end-organ complications, also affect disease outcome. However, no disease process improves significantly with prolonged starvation. Ultimately, the successful use of EN can avoid the need for PN in patients unable to meet nutrient requirements with an oral diet.

PHARMACOECONOMIC CONSIDERATIONS

EN has consistently been shown to be less expensive than PN. The pharmacoeconomic comparison between EN and PN should include an evaluation of therapeutic outcome relative to the cumulative cost associated with providing the therapy. Therapy costs should include costs related to placement and maintenance of enteral or parenteral access; costs of nutrients and related supplies; time spent by professional staff in ordering, compounding, delivering, administering, and managing therapy; costs of laboratory monitoring; and costs of managing complications that result from therapy. However, it is very difficult to capture all of these costs and separate actual cost from charge-based estimates. None of the existing pharmacoeconomic analyses incorporate all costs related to EN and PN therapy, but selected cost comparisons derived from clinical research trials in institutional settings have been published.[84–86] The cost of EN has been reported to be ~25% to 50% that of PN. Incorporating the cost of managing complications related to therapy greatly increases the overall cost of PN compared with EN.[86] In situations in which improved outcome has not been demonstrated with PN, EN appears preferable on a cost basis.[7]

ABBREVIATIONS

ALI: Acute lung injury

ARA: Arachidonic acid

ARDS: Acute respiratory distress syndrome

DHA: Docosahexaenoic acid

EN: Enteral nutrition

IgA: Immunoglobulin A

MCT: Medium-chain triglyceride

NG: Nasogastric

NPO: Nothing by mouth

PEG: Percutaneous endoscopic gastrostomy

PEJ: Percutaneous endoscopic jejunostomy

PN: Parenteral nutrition

REFERENCES

1. Colaizzo-Anas T. Nutrient intake, digestion, absorption, and excretion. In: Gottschlich MM, ed. The A.S.P.E.N. Nutrition Support Core Curriculum: A Case-based Approach—The Adult Patient. Silver Spring, MD: American Society for Parenteral and Enteral Nutrition; 2007:3–18.

2. Farrell JJ. Digestion and absorption of nutrients and vitamins. In: Feldman M, Friedman LS, Brandt LJ, eds. Sleisenger & Fordtran's Gastrointestinal and Liver Disease: Pathophysiology/Diagnosis/Management. 8th ed. Philadelphia, PA: Saunders Elsevier; 2006:2147–2188.

3. Hise ME, Brown JC. Lipids. In: Gottschlich MM, ed. The A.S.P.E.N. Nutrition Support Core Curriculum: A Case-based Approach—The Adult Patient. Silver Spring, MD: American Society for Parenteral and Enteral Nutrition; 2007:48–70.

4. Jabbar A, Chang WK, Dryden GW, McClave S. Gut immunology and the differential response to feeding and starvation. Nutr Clin Pract 2003;18:461–482.

5. Minocha A. Probiotics for preventive health. Nutr Clin Prac 2009;24:227–241.

6. Wallace B. Clinical use of probiotics in the pediatric population. Nutr Clin Prac 2009;24:50–59.

7. A.S.P.E.N. Board of Directors and the Clinical Guidelines Task Force. Guidelines for the use of parenteral and enteral nutrition in adult and pediatric patients. JPEN J Parenter Enteral Nutr 2002;26(1 Suppl):1SA–138SA.

8. Bankhead R, Boullata J, Brantley S, et al. A.S.P.E.N. enteral nutrition practice recommendations. JPEN J Parenter Enteral Nutr 2009;33: 122–167.

9. Stroud M, Duncan H, Nightingale J. Guidelines for enteral feeding in adult hospital patients. Gut 2003;52(Suppl 7):1–12.

10. McClave SA, Martindale RG, Vanek VW, et al. Guidelines for the provision and assessment of nutrition support therapy in the adult critically ill patient: Society of Critical Care Medicine (SCCM) and American Society for Parenteral and Enteral Nutrition (A.S.P.E.N.). JPEN J Parenter Enteral Nutr 2009;33:277–316.

11. Heyland DK, Dhaliwal R, Drover JW, et al. Canadian clinical practice guidelines for nutrition support in mechanically ventilated, critically ill adult patients. JPEN J Parenter Enteral Nutr 2003;27:355–373.

12. Mehta NM, Compher C, A.S.P.E.N. Board of Directors. A.S.P.E.N. clinical guidelines: Nutrition support of the critically ill child. JPEN J Parenter Enteral Nutr 2009;33:260–276.

13. Kirby DF, DeLegge MH, Fleming CR. American Gastroenterological Association technical review on tube feeding for enteral nutrition. Gastroenterology 1995;108:1282–1301.

14. Thompson AM, Bizzarro MJ. Necrotizing enterocolitis in newborns: pathogenesis, prevention and management. Drugs 2008;68:1227–1238.

15. Dhaliwal R, Heyland DK. Nutrition and infection in the intensive care unit: What does the evidence show? Curr Opin Crit Care 2005;11: 461–467.

16. Braunschweig CL, Levy P, Sheean PM, Wang X. Enteral compared with parenteral nutrition: A meta-analysis. Am J Clin Nutr 2001;74:534–542.

17. Simpson F, Doig GS. Parenteral vs. enteral nutrition in the critically ill patient: A meta-analysis of trials using the intention to treat principle. Intensive Care Med 2005;31:12–23.

18. Gramlich L, Kichian K, Pinilla J, et al. Does enteral nutrition compared to parenteral nutrition result in better outcomes in critically ill adult patients? A systematic review of the literature. Nutrition 2004;20: 843–848.

19. Peter JV, Moran JL, Phillips-Hughes J. A meta-analysis of treatment outcomes of early enteral versus early parenteral nutrition in hospitalized patients. Crit Care Med 2005;33:213–220.

20. van den Berghe G, Wouters PJ, Bouillon R, et al. Outcome benefit of intensive insulin therapy in the critically ill: Insulin dose versus glycemic control. Crit Care Med 2003;31:359–366.

21. Kumpf VJ. Parenteral nutrition-associated liver disease in adult and pediatric patients. Nutr Clin Pract 2006;21:279–290.

22. McClave SA, Heyland DK. The physiologic response and associated clinical benefits from provision of early enteral nutrition. Nutr Clin Pract 2009;24:305–315.

23. Artinian V, Krayem H, DiGiovine B. Effects of early enteral feeding on the outcome of critically ill mechanically ventilated medical patients. Chest 2006;129:960–967.

24. Marik PE, Zaloga GP. Early enteral nutrition in acutely ill patients: A systemic review. Crit Care Med 2001;29:2264–2270.

25. McClave SA, Wei-Kuo Chang. Feeding the hypotensive patient: Does enteral feeding precipitate or protect against ischemic bowel? Nutr Clin Pract 2003;18:279–284.

26. Zaloga GP, Roberts PR, Marik P. Feeding the hemodynamically unstable patient: A critical evaluation of the evidence. Nutr Clin Pract 2003;18:285–293.

27. Vanek VW. Ins and outs of enteral access: 1. Short-term enteral access. Nutr Clin Pract 2002;17:275–283.

28. Marik PE, Zaloga GP. Gastric versus post-pyloric feeding: A systematic review. Crit Care 2003;7:46–51.

29. Heyland DK, Drover JW, Dkaliwal R, Greenwood J. Optimizing the benefits and minimizing the risks of enteral nutrition in the critically ill: Role of small bowel feeding. JPEN J Parenter Enteral Nutr 2002;26(6 Suppl):S51–S55.

30. Rivera RJ, Campana J, Seidner D, Hamilton C. Small bowel feeding tube placement using an electromagnetic tube placement device: accuracy of tip placement [Abstract]. JPEN J Parenter Enteral Nutr 2009;33:225.

31. Vanek VW. Ins and outs of enteral access: 2. Long-term access—Esophagostomy and gastrostomy. Nutr Clin Pract 2003;18:50–74.

32. Angus F, Burakoff R. The percutaneous endoscopic gastrostomy tube: Medical and ethical issues in placement. Am J Gastroenterol 2003;98:272–277.

33. Gauderer MW. Percutaneous endoscopic gastrostomy and the evolution of contemporary long-term enteral access. Clin Nutr 2002;21: 103–110.

34. Vanek VW. Ins and outs of enteral access: 3. Long-term access-jejunostomy. Nutr Clin Pract 2003;18:201–220.

35. McClave SA, DeMeo MT, DeLegge MH, et al. North American Summit on Aspiration in the Critically Ill Patient: Consensus statement. JPEN J Parenter Enteral Nutr 2002;26(6 Suppl):S80–S85.

36. Parrish CR. Enteral feeding: The art and the science. Nutr Clin Pract 2003;18:76–85.

37. Chessman KH. Infant nutrition and special nutritional needs of children. In: Berardi RR, Kroon LA, McDermott JH, et al, eds. Handbook of Nonprescription Drugs. 15th ed. Washington, DC: American Pharmacists Association; 2006:521–552.

38. Jawaheer G, Shaw NJ, Pierro A. Continuous enteral feeding impairs gallbladder emptying in infants. J Pediatr 2001;138:822–825.

39. Mueller C, Nestle M. Regulation of medical foods: Toward a rational policy. Nutr Clin Pract 1995;10:8–15.

40. Heymsfield SB. Enteral solutions: Is there a solution? Nutr Clin Pract 1995;10:4–7.

41. Hall JC, Dobb G, Hall J, et al. A prospective randomized trial of enteral glutamine in critical illness. Intensive Care Med 2003;29:1710–1716.

42. Garrel DR, Patenaude J, Nedelec B, et al. Decreased mortality and infectious morbidity in adult burn patients given enteral glutamine supplements: A prospective, controlled, randomized clinical trial. Crit Care Med 2003;31:2444–2449.

43. Heyland DK, Samis A. Does immunonutrition in patients with sepsis do more harm than good? Int Care Med 2003;29:669–671.

44. Zaloga GP, Siddiqui R, Terry C, Marik P. Arginine: Mediator or modulator of sepsis? Nutr Clin Pract 2004;19:201–215.

45. Lomer MCE, Parkes GC, Sanderson JD. Review article: Lactose intolerance in clinical practice—myths and realities. Aliment Pharmacol Ther 2009;27:93–103.

46. Singer P, Theilla M, Fisher H, et al. Benefit of an enteral diet enriched with eicosapentaenoic acid and gamma-linolenic acid in ventilated patients with acute lung injury. Crit Care Med 2006;34:1033–1038.

47. Koletzko B, Lien E, Agostoni C, et al. The roles of long-chain polyunsaturated fatty acids in pregnancy, lactation and infancy: Review of current knowledge and consensus recommendations. J Perinat Med 2008;36:5–14.

48. Roy CC, Kien L, Bouthillier L, Levy E. Short-chain fatty acids: Ready for prime time? Nutr Clin Pract 2006;21:351–366.

49. Rushdi TA, Pichard C, Khater YH. Control of diarrhea by fiber-enriched diet in ICU patients on enteral nutrition: A prospective randomized controlled trial. Clin Nutr 2004;23:1344–1352.

50. Silk DBA, Grimble GK. Relevance of physiology of nutrient absorption to formulation of enteral diets. Nutrition 1992;8:1–12.

51. Kreymann KG, Berger MM, Deutz NEP, et al. ESPEN guidelines on enteral nutrition: Intensive care. Clin Nutr 2006;25:210–223.

52. Waitzberg DL, Saito H, Plank LD, et al. Postsurgical infections are reduced with specialized nutrition support. World J Surg 2006;30:1592–1604.

53. Montejo JC, Zarazaga A, Lopez-Martinez J, et al. Immunonutrition in the intensive care unit: A systematic review and consensus statement. Clin Nutr 2003;22:221–233.

54. Beale RJ, Bryg DJ, Bihari DJ. Immunonutrition in the critically ill: A systematic review of clinical outcome. Crit Care Med 1999;27:2799–2805.

55. Heyland DK, Novak F, Drover JW, et al. Should immunonutrition become routine in critically ill patients? A systematic review of the evidence. JAMA 2001;286:944–953.

56. Gadek JE, DeMichele SJ, Karlstad MD, et al. Effect of enteral feeding with eicosapentaenoic acid, gamma-linolenic acid, and antioxidants in patients with acute respiratory distress syndrome. Crit Care Med 1999;27:1409–1420.

57. Davis A, Baker S. The use of modular nutrients in pediatrics. JPEN J Parenter Enteral Nutr 1996;20:228–236.

58. Chenu JW, Cox JM. Cronobacter (Enterobacter sakazakii): Current status and future prospects. Lett Appl Microbiol 2009;49:153–159.

59. Groh-Wargo S, Sapsford A. Enteral nutrition support of the preterm infant in the neonatal intensive care unit. Nutr Clin Prac 2009;24:363–376.

60. Berseth CL, Van Aerde JE, Gross S, et al. Growth, efficacy, and safety of feeding an iron-fortified human milk fortifier. Pediatrics 2004;114:e699–e706.

61. Porcelli P, Schanler R, Greer F, et al. Growth in human milk-fed very low birth weight infants receiving a new human milk fortifier. Ann Nutr Metab 2000;44:2–10.

62. Reis BB, Hall RT, Schanler RJ. Enhanced growth of preterm infants fed a new powdered human milk fortifier: A randomized controlled trial. Pediatrics 2000;106:581–588.

63. Corkins MR, Scolapio J. Diarrhea. In: Merritt R, ed. The A.S.P.E.N. Nutrition Support Practice Manual. 2nd ed. Silver Spring, MD: A.S.P.E.N.; 2005:203–210.

64. Zaloga GP. Parenteral nutrition in adult inpatients with functioning gastrointestinal tracts: Assessment of outcomes. Lancet 2006;367:1101–1111.

65. Williams TA, Leslie GD. A review of the nursing care of enteral feeding tubes in critically ill adults: Part 1. Intensive Crit Care Nurs 2004;20:330–343.

66. McClave SA, Lukan JK, Stefater JA, et al. Poor validity of residual volumes as a marker for risk of aspiration in critically ill patients. Crit Care Med 2005;33:324–330.

67. Nguyen NQ, Chapman MJ, Fraser RJ, Bryant LK, Holloway RH. Erythromycin in more effective than metoclopramide in the treatment of feed intolerance in critical illness. Crit Care Med 2007;35:483–489.

68. Booth CM, Heyland DK, Paterson WG. Gastrointestinal promotility drugs in the critical care setting: A systematic review of the evidence. Crit Care Med 2002;30:1429–1435.

69. Maloney JP, Ryan TA, Brasel KJ, et al. Food dye use in enteral feedings: A review and a call for a moratorium. Nutr Clin Pract 2002;17:168–181.

70. Maloney JP, Ryan TA. Detection of aspiration in enterally fed patients: A requiem for bedside monitors of aspiration. JPEN J Parenter Enteral Nutr 2002;26(6 Suppl):S34–S42.

71. Bliss DZ, Guenter PA, Settle RG. Defining and reporting diarrhea in tube-fed patients—What a mess! Am J Clin Nutr 1992;55:753–759.

72. Eisenberg PG. Causes of diarrhea in tube-fed patients: A comprehensive approach to diagnosis and management. Nutr Clin Pract 1993;8:119–123.

73. Frankel EH, Enow NB, Jackson KC, et al. Methods of restoring patency to occluded feeding tubes. Nutr Clin Pract 1998;13:129–131.

74. Gunn SR, Early BJ, Zenati MS, Ochoa JB. Use of a nasal bridle prevents accidental nasoenteral feeding tube removal. JPEN J Parenter Enteral Nutr 2009;33:50–54.

75. Rommel N, DeMeyer AM, Feenstra L, Veereman-Wauters G. The complexity of feeding problems in 700 infants and young children presenting to a tertiary care institution. J Pediatr Gastroenterol Nutr 2003;37:75–84.

76. Beckwith MC, Feddema SS, Barton RG, Graves C. A guide to drug therapy in patients with enteral feeding tubes: Dosage form selection and administration methods. Hosp Pharm 2004;39:225–237.

77. Wohlt PD, Zheng L, Gunderson S, et al. Recommendations for the use of medications with continuous enteral nutrition. Am J Health-Syst Pharm 2009;66:1458–1467.

78. Dickerson RN. Medication administration considerations for patients receiving enteral tube feedings. Hosp Pharm 2004;39:84–89.

79. Magnuson BL, Clifford TM, Hoskins LA, Bernard AC. Enteral nutrition and drug administration, interactions, and complications. Nutr Clin Pract 2005;20:618–624.

80. Bauer LA. Interference of oral phenytoin absorption by continuous nasogastric feedings. Neurology 1982;32:570–572.

81. Gilbert S, Hatton J, Magnuson B. How to minimize interaction between phenytoin and enteral feedings: Two approaches. Nutr Clin Pract 1996;11:28–31.

82. Nyffeler MS. Ciprofloxacin use in the enterally fed patient. Nutr Clin Pract 1999;14:73–77.

83. Dickerson RN, Garmon WM, Kuhl DA, Minard G, Brown RO. Vitamin K-independent warfarin resistance after concurrent administration of warfarin and continuous enteral nutrition. Pharmacotherapy 2008;28:308–313.

84. Senkel M, Mumme A, Eickhoff U, et al. Early postoperative enteral immunonutrition: Clinical outcome and cost-comparison analyses in surgical patients. Crit Care Med 1997;25:1489–1496.

85. McClave SA, Greene LM, Snider HL, et al. Comparison of the safety of early enteral vs parenteral nutrition in mild acute pancreatitis. JPEN J Parenter Enteral Nutr 1996;21:14–20.

86. Trice S, Melnik G, Page CP. Complications and costs of early postoperative parenteral versus enteral nutrition in trauma patients. Nutr Clin Pract 1997;12:114–119.

153

Nutritional Considerations in Major Organ Failure

BRIAN M. HODGES AND MARK DELEGGE

KEY CONCEPTS

❶ Carbohydrate calories absorbed and protein lost via renal replacement therapy must be accounted for when designing a parenteral (PN) or enteral nutrition (EN) regimen for patients with renal failure.

❷ Administration of renally excreted or regulated electrolytes, such as potassium, magnesium, and phosphorus, should be limited in patients with renal failure unless refeeding syndrome is present or continuous renal replacement therapies are used.

❸ Hyperglycemia is common in cirrhosis. Patients with fulminant hepatitis are prone instead to hypoglycemia.

❹ Folic acid and thiamine supplementation is important in patients with liver disease for the prevention of anemia and Wernicke encephalopathy, respectively.

❺ In short bowel syndrome, PN should be used to meet nutritional needs in the immediate postoperative period after intestinal resection.

❻ Increased fluid and electrolyte replacement is often necessary in patients with short bowel syndrome to replace GI losses. Patients may need increased calcium, magnesium, zinc, and other trace elements because of decreased absorption and/ or excessive GI losses.

❼ Patients with ileal resection commonly develop vitamin B_{12} deficiency, necessitating therapy with parenteral cyanocobalamin.

❽ As small bowel adaptation occurs, some patients with short bowel syndrome receiving PN can be transitioned successfully to EN. Early initiation of enteral intake affects adaptation because intraluminal nutrients are a stimulus for this process.

❾ Care should be taken to avoid overfeeding of patients with respiratory failure, as excessive carbon dioxide production may limit the patients' ability to have mechanical ventilation discontinued.

❿ Excessive fluid administration should be avoided in patients with pulmonary disease because it may worsen already compromised pulmonary function.

Learning objectives, review questions, and other resources can be found at **www.pharmacotherapyonline.com**.

Because organ failure may alter absorption, use, and excretion of nutrients, administration of standard nutrients to patients with organ dysfunction may be inappropriate. Individualization of a nutritional regimen for these patients often requires a planned, disease-specific approach. Different laboratory testing or more frequent monitoring of traditional markers may be necessary to ensure that the desired therapeutic goals are achieved. For example, it is impossible to collect a 24-hour urine specimen to measure urea nitrogen and nitrogen balance in an anuric patient. In this situation, an alternative method of calculating urea nitrogen appearance is required.

Patients with acute organ failure requiring nutrition support often are hospitalized in intensive care units (ICUs). With advances in treating chronic organ failure, increasing numbers of older, chronically ill patients will require nutritional support on a long-term basis. It therefore will become increasingly common for nutrition support to be provided in community and ambulatory settings. Regardless of the setting, the clinician needs a firm pathophysiologic foundation on which to build a pharmaceutical care plan to ensure appropriate outcomes for patients requiring nutritional support.

This chapter discusses the nutritional needs of patients with renal, hepatic, GI, and pulmonary failure. The predominant approaches to ensure delivery of safe and efficacious nutrients to patients with these disorders are critically reviewed.

RENAL FAILURE

Major differences exist between the metabolic, fluid, and electrolyte management of patients with acute kidney injury (AKI) versus those with stable chronic kidney disease (CKD) and those with an AKI episode that complicates preexisting CKD. For example, positive nitrogen balance is more difficult to achieve in patients with AKI because of the increased rate of protein catabolism. Additionally, patients with AKI are more likely to develop hyperglycemia during nutritional support and frequently are dialyzed by modalities that are not used commonly for those with end-stage kidney disease. Because of these differences, the nutritional management of patients with AKI is discussed separately.

ACUTE KIDNEY INJURY

Epidemiology

AKI, as defined in Chapter 51, is a decrease in glomerular filtration rate occurring over hours to weeks that is associated with an increase in the serum concentrations of waste products, such as urea and creatinine. AKI has been observed in as many as 5% of hospitalized patients and in up to 50% of patients receiving care in an ICU.[1] The mortality rate of AKI patients who require renal replacement therapy ranges from 40% to 70%. A study in Austria demonstrated that despite the recent advancements made in renal replacement therapies and ICU care, the mortality rate of patients was still 62.8%.[2] Severe malnutrition has been documented in 42% of patients with AKI and is an independent predictor of in-hospital mortality and increased morbidity from sepsis, shock, dysrhythmias, and acute respiratory failure.[3] Because malnutrition is an apparently independent contributor to mortality in patients with AKI, nutrition support remains a cornerstone in the treatment of these patients, despite a lack of evidence demonstrating improvement in patient survival.[1,4]

Pathophysiology

Energy Requirements AKI does not itself change patient energy requirements. Energy requirements in AKI are greatly influenced by comorbid critical illness and the types of renal replacement therapies used.[4,5] In this patient population, they ideally should be measured by indirect calorimetry (see Chapter 149) because energy expenditures of patients with AKI are highly variable. Energy expenditure is close to normal in patients with uncomplicated AKI, but resting energy expenditure (REE) increases of up to 30% have been reported in the presence of sepsis and AKI.[6] Typically, patients with AKI and without underlying hypermetabolic conditions should receive 20 to 30 kcal/kg (84–126 kJ/kg) per day. Those with underlying hypermetabolic conditions, such as thermal injury or head injury, usually need even greater caloric intake, up to 35 kcal/kg (147 kJ/kg) per day, unless indirect calorimetry indicates otherwise.[7,8] Patients with stage 4 or 5 CKD and acute metabolic illness or injury should receive similar energy provisions.[5] Increasing energy provision beyond this to 40 kcal/kg/day (167 kJ/kg/day) is not associated with better nutritional outcomes but has been associated with more frequent metabolic complications.[9]

Carbohydrates Hyperglycemia and peripheral insulin resistance are common in AKI. Patients usually have a superimposed illness that exacerbates glucose intolerance. The etiology of glucose intolerance in AKI is thought to be a result of increased levels of glucagon, growth hormone, and catecholamines—all known antagonists of insulin. Other proposed mechanisms are an elevated glucagon-to-insulin ratio secondary to impaired degradation of these hormones and elevated secretion of inflammatory cytokines.

Fat Intolerance to IV lipid emulsion (IVLE), evidenced by increased serum triglyceride concentrations, is common in AKI. Hypertriglyceridemia is thought to be caused by decreased catabolism of triglycerides and increased triglyceride synthesis from free fatty acids.[1] Hepatic triglyceride lipase and peripheral lipoprotein lipase activity may be reduced significantly in AKI patients.[6] Insulin resistance and metabolic acidosis may contribute to this process by inhibiting lipoprotein lipase.[9] Triglyceride concentrations therefore should be measured before administering IVLE to patients with AKI.

Protein AKI is associated with marked protein catabolism and urea accumulation. Most patients with AKI have a primary stressful illness that results in ureagenesis; thus, protein breakdown is accelerated. Protein catabolism in AKI may be stimulated as the result of insulin resistance, metabolic acidosis, circulating proteases and inflammatory mediators, and the effects of uremic toxins.[1] The mechanism may be direct, via modulation of protein synthesis, or indirect, by inhibiting the action of anabolic hormones. Unlike healthy patients or those with CKD, protein catabolism in the presence of AKI is not significantly attenuated by the administration of exogenous nutrition support.[4]

Significant amounts of protein and amino acids are also removed by dialysis. Amino acid losses of 5.2 g per conventional hemodialysis (HD) treatment, 7.3 g per high-flux HD session, and up to 13 to 16 g/day during continuous renal replacement therapy (CRRT) have been reported.[10,11] The clearance of histidine and tryptophan are enhanced, whereas the clearance of phenylalanine and valine is reduced in nondialyzed patients with AKI.[12] In patients undergoing CRRT, glutamine represents roughly one-third of all amino acid dialysate losses. Serum glutamine concentrations decrease significantly early during CRRT but may return to baseline subsequently, suggesting altered glutamine metabolism early in the course of CRRT.[13]

Fluid, Electrolyte, And Acid–Base Disorders The volume status of patients with AKI depends primarily on residual urine output and the type of dialysis received, if any. The patient with oliguric AKI will have impaired excretion of sodium and water. In nonoliguric AKI, considerable sodium may be lost in the urine, necessitating replacement to maintain sodium balance. This also applies to the patient who is losing considerable gastric fluids. Patients on CRRT will lose sodium via hemofiltration or dialysis and should be given sodium as part of their CRRT replacement fluid regimen. To maintain sodium balance, most replacement fluids contain between 140 and 154 mEq/L (140 and 154 mmol/L) of sodium. The rate of administration of these fluids varies based on the type of CRRT, the rate of ultrafiltration, and the patient's clinical condition.[14]

Hyperkalemia is observed frequently in AKI secondary to protein catabolism and intracellular potassium release, as discussed in Chapter 60. Hyperkalemia also results from the impaired secretion and excretion of potassium by the kidney and the endogenous release secondary to tissue breakdown. If this is severe, emergent dialysis may be indicated. Patients on CRRT, however, usually require potassium replacement to avoid hypokalemia as a consequence of the significant dialytic potassium losses.

Because phosphorus is excreted renally, hyperphosphatemia is commonly observed in patients with AKI. Like potassium, large amounts of phosphorus are released into the circulation secondary to tissue breakdown. Control of hyperphosphatemia is important because as the calcium–phosphorus product (serum calcium in milligrams per deciliter multiplied by serum phosphorus in milligrams per deciliter) exceeds 55, the risk of developing metastatic calcification increases (see Chapter 58). Conversely, with initiation of dialysis, particularly CRRT, patients must be monitored for hypophosphatemia due to the enhanced clearance by the CRRT procedure. Hypophosphatemia may also be observed in patients with AKI or CKD who continue to receive oral phosphate binders despite decreased oral phosphorus intake.

The net removal of calcium during the continuous dialysis modalities depends on the calcium concentration of the dialysate fluid. Severe hypocalcemia has been reported when regional citrate anticoagulation has been used for CRRT in AKI and hepatic failure patients.[14]

Hypermagnesemia is less common than other electrolyte abnormalities, but it has been noted in those with AKI as the result of impaired excretion and endogenous release from tissues. Both magnesium and calcium losses via CRRT have been quantified: average daily losses were 24 mmol and 70 mmol of magnesium and calcium, respectively.[11]

Patients with AKI usually have metabolic acidosis because of impaired excretion of organic acids. If potassium and sodium are needed in the parenteral nutrition (PN) regimen, they should be added as acetate salts, which are converted to bicarbonate in the liver. This increase in bicarbonate partially compensates the patient's metabolic acidosis. Intermittent and continuous dialytic therapies also may help improve the metabolic acidosis because they increase the removal of endogenously generated acids and serum bicarbonate levels as the result of diffusion of bicarbonate from the dialysate into the blood. Correction of acidosis may be best managed with the use of lactate buffers (lactate > bicarbonate > acetate).[15]

Trace Elements The requirements for trace elements during nutritional support of AKI patients are not well established because trace element accumulation or losses during AKI have not been characterized. Additionally, many of the trace element alterations in AKI may represent an "acute-phase reaction."[7] Zinc and chromium are excreted by the kidney and theoretically can accumulate because of reduced excretion and increased intake secondary to impurities in dialysate or IV fluids. In patients with AKI undergoing CRRT, zinc intake via nutrition support exceeds losses.[11] Selenium concentrations are reduced in AKI and may result in a decrease in thyroxine concentrations.[16,17] Because manganese and copper are excreted in bile, and zinc and copper are removed by peritoneal dialysis (PD) and HD, most patients receiving PN should also receive standard daily trace element supplementation; in addition, some experts recommend that selenium supplementation may be necessary.[4,17] Supplemental doses of 50 to 70 mcg/day may be necessary to maintain selenium balance.[7]

Vitamins The little available information available indicates that AKI-associated alterations in vitamin requirements are minimal; thus, there is no need to alter patient treatment.[18] Losses of vitamins via dialysis also must be considered. Traditional HD enhances the clearance of several water-soluble vitamins, such as folic acid, vitamins C and B_{12}, and pyridoxine, but not the highly protein-bound, fat-soluble vitamins A and D.[19] Significant reductions in the plasma concentrations of water-soluble vitamins have also been observed in patients receiving CRRT.[13,17] Currently, it seems prudent to administer vitamins at least daily in doses recommended by the Nutrition Advisory Group of the American Medical Association for patients receiving PN (see Chapter 149).[7] Administration of ascorbic acid should be restricted to 30 to 50 mg/day to offset losses caused by renal replacement therapies but to avoid secondary oxalosis, which may worsen renal function.[8,20] If the enteral route is used for nutritional support, vitamin administration should at least meet the recommended daily allowances.

TREATMENT

■ DESIRED OUTCOME

The maintenance of lean muscle mass and the prevention of disorders of macro- and micronutrient excess or deficiency are the primary goals in the nutritional management of the patient with AKI. Although it has yet to be proven that nutrition support is associated with a reduction in mortality, the secondary goals of nutrition therapy are to optimize immunocompetence and promote wound healing. Additionally, the attenuation of the inflammatory state, metabolic derangements, and alterations of the patient's antioxidant capacity should be considered in the design of specialized nutrition support for patients with AKI.[4]

■ GENERALIZED APPROACH TO TREATMENT

Enteral nutrition (EN) is the preferred route of nutrient delivery in patients with AKI.[4,5] Calorically dense, electrolyte-free or -reduced formulas are preferred.[21] These formulas are useful in patients with fluid overload, hyperkalemia, hypermagnesemia, and hyperphosphatemia. EN is well tolerated by many patients with AKI[22] and is associated with improved maintenance of GI tract function and survival in nonrandomized studies of patients with AKI.[2,23] It is recommended that EN be used for all patients to the degree tolerated, even if PN must be used as a supplement to meet the patient's nutritional needs. Unfortunately, because of the high incidence of GI complications, many patients may not tolerate EN to meet their nutritional goals and thus require PN support.[2]

■ PHARMACOLOGIC THERAPIES

Drug Treatments of First Choice

Patients with AKI and comorbid hypermetabolism typically require 20 to 30 kcal/kg (84–126 kJ/kg) per day.[8] Increasing energy provision beyond this does not improve nutritional outcomes and is associated with metabolic complications and a greater net fluid imbalance.[24] A relatively conservative initial estimate of patient energy needs is appropriate because the results of slightly underfeeding the patient are far less serious than those associated with overfeeding.[4,25]

❶ In the absence of dialysis, the nutritional formula should be concentrated in a small volume and contain minimal sodium (Table 153–1). In the oliguric patient who is receiving renal replacement therapy, these restrictions may be less rigorous, but the formula generally will need to be concentrated.[5] When using these high-dextrose-concentration formulas, careful monitoring of

TABLE 153-1 Empiric Parenteral Nutrition Formulas for Patients with Organ Failure					
	Acute Renal Failure	**Chronic Renal Failure**	**Hepatic Failure**	**Short Bowel**	**Pulmonary Failure**
Dextrose (%)[a]	40	30	25	20	20
Crystalline amino acids (%)[a]	Variable	4	5[b]	5	5
Lipids (%)[a]	1	2	2	2	3
NaCl (mEq/L)	0	0	0	80[c]	10
Na acetate (mEq/L)	0	30	0	0	0
Na phosphate (mEq/L)	0[d]	7.5	15	7.5	30
K acetate (mEq/L)	0[d]	0	50	60	20
K chloride (mEq/L)	0	10	0	0	20
Ca gluconate (mEq/L)	5[d]	5	5	10	5
Magnesium sulfate (mEq/L)	0[d]	6	16	10	5
Multivitamins (mL/day)	10	10	10	10	10
Zinc (mg/day)	3	3–6	8	10	3
Copper (mg/day)	1.2	1.2	<1.2	1.2	1.2
Manganese (mcg/day)	300	300	<300	≥300	300
Chromium (mcg/day)	12	12	<12	20	12
Selenium (mcg/day)	–	40	40	60	40

[a]Final concentrations after admixture.
[b]Hepatamine 4% when criteria for use are met.
[c]Does not include 0.45% Na chloride injection or lipid.
[d]The continuous renal replacement therapies frequently require variable additions of electrolytes and trace elements.

glucose homeostasis (every 6 hours) is important because the maintenance of glycemic control in a range of 110 to 150 mg/dL (6.1–8.3 mmol/L) has been associated with improved clinical outcomes of critically ill adults.[25,26] Additionally, CRRT, which is increasingly popular in the treatment of AKI (see Chapter 50), contributes significant calories to a nutritional regimen. This is a direct result of the absorption of glucose from the dialysate or ultrafiltrate replacement fluids: net uptakes of up to 355 g/day have been reported.[13] Total glucose intake should range from 3 to 7 g/kg/day.[5]

CLINICAL CONTROVERSY

There is debate as to the most appropriate protein provision for patients with ARF who are receiving CRRT. Although initial data has shown an association between higher protein intake (up to 2.5 g/kg/day) and improved survival, many express concern about the effectiveness and safety of this practice.

AKI is not a contraindication to IVLE use, despite the changes in lipid metabolism. When the serum triglyceride concentration is less than 300 mg/dL (3.39 mmol/L), IVLE is recommended to prevent essential fatty acid deficiency and to provide a balanced caloric intake. Current recommendations call for patients to receive between 0.8 and 1.2 g/kg/day, but no more than 1.5 g/kg/day.[5]

Although individual patient assessment for the presence of hypercatabolism and dialytic losses is necessary, it is not uncommon for patients to require 2.5 g/kg/day of protein or more to achieve a positive nitrogen balance.[27] Protein restriction, to reduce the urea nitrogen appearance rate from exogenous protein intake in an effort to avoid dialysis, should not be used unless the AKI is thought to be temporary (e.g., expected to resolve in 7 to 10 days), and hypercatabolism is not present.[5,7,28] Once dialysis therapy is instituted, protein intake should be liberalized to 1 to 1.5 g/kg/day for noncatabolic patients and at least 1.5 g/kg/day for hypercatabolic patients.[28] Patients undergoing CRRT with hypermetabolism may need to receive 1.5 to 2 g/kg/day[26] or more (up to 2.5 g/kg/day) to achieve positive nitrogen balance.[23] The safety and efficacy of this aggressive strategy remain to be confirmed before it can be routinely recommended.[8,26,29]

❷ Several electrolytes (i.e., phosphorus, magnesium, and potassium) warrant special attention in patients with AKI.[5] During early AKI, PN solutions should not contain potassium unless the patient is hypokalemic or undergoing CRRT. After several days, the serum potassium concentrations tend to decrease, often necessitating cautious addition of potassium to the PN solution. If the enteral route is used, formulas with minimal potassium may be needed. Serum potassium concentrations may decrease more rapidly in patients receiving CRRT. Potassium losses during CRRT are proportional to the potassium gradient between blood and dialysate. Therefore, cautious additions of potassium may be considered early in the course of AKI for those patients treated with CRRT. Serum magnesium concentrations do not decrease as quickly as potassium concentrations in patients receiving electrolyte-free nutrition regimens. As serum concentrations decrease toward normal and/or renal function returns, magnesium should be added to the PN solution in small amounts (4–6 mEq/L [2–3 mmol/L]).

Phosphorus can be omitted from the nutritional formula of AKI patients receiving PN until the phosphorus level approaches normal (<5 mg/dL [<1.62 mmol/L]). It is prudent to monitor phosphorus concentrations daily and to add phosphorus in small doses once the serum concentration is <4 mg/dL (1.29 mmol/L). Failure to do so can lead to severe hypophosphatemia (see Chapter 59), especially in patients treated with CRRT. Patients with persistently high serum phosphorus concentrations who have a functional GI tract can be prescribed phosphate-binding therapy (see Chapter 53) and enteral feedings low in phosphorus to minimize the absorption of exogenous phosphorus.

Alternative Drug Treatments

Standard mixed amino acids rather than essential amino acid solutions should be used.[5,28] Early studies assessing essential amino acid products were promising. Subsequently, several prospective, double-blind studies have indicated no significant reduction in mortality when the essential amino acid formulations were used.[1,5,28]

■ PHARMACOECONOMIC CONSIDERATIONS

Although analyses of total costs of AKI care have been published,[30] no specific research has yet been published assessing the cost-effectiveness of nutrition support in patients with AKI.

■ EVALUATION OF THERAPEUTIC OUTCOMES

Although the clinical and quality-of-life (QOL) outcomes for patients with AKI have been reported, data specifically analyzing the effects of nutrition support are limited.[30] To date, there is no clear consensus regarding the degree of benefit, if any, of nutrition support on the outcome parameters of renal recovery or mortality. Data suggest that malnourished AKI patients experience significantly higher mortality rates (odds ratio of in-hospital mortality of 7.21) than AKI patients without malnutrition.[3] In one retrospective analysis, EN was associated with a survival benefit, even when controlling for severity of illness.[2] No prospective studies to date show a survival benefit from aggressive nutritional support in patients with AKI. When nutrition support is used, the evaluation tools employed in monitoring patients with AKI are similar to those for other patients receiving PN and EN (see Chapters 151 and 152).

CHRONIC KIDNEY DISEASE

CKD is defined by either structural or functional damage to the kidneys that is present for at least 3 months (see Chapter 52). Malnutrition secondary to reduced oral nutrient intake frequently is evident when the glomerular filtration rate drops below 20 to 25 mL/min (0.33–0.42 mL/s). Stage 5 CKD has been associated with inflammatory and metabolic changes that increase the likelihood of malnutrition, and increased nutrient losses have been documented in those receiving hemodialysis and peritoneal dialysis. Because of its chronicity, malnutrition in these patients is treated most frequently in the ambulatory setting with oral nutritional supplements and EN.

Epidemiology

Protein-energy malnutrition is very common in patients with CKD and is a significant predictor of morbidity and mortality. Significant malnutrition, typically represented by deficiency of visceral proteins or being underweight, has been noted in 28% to 48% of predialysis patients, in 9% to 72% of patients undergoing HD, and in up to 45% of patients commencing PD.[31,32] In one of the larger studies to date (n = 1,397), mean dietary calorie and protein intake in those 50 years of age and older was 22 kcal/kg/day (92 kJ/kg/day) and 0.9 g/kg/day, respectively.[33] Both these values are lower than published recommendations for patients with CKD.[34] Protein-energy malnutrition and wasting at initiation of dialysis are significant predictors of morbidity and mortality in patients with stage 5 CKD.[31]

However, there appears to be a gender-confounding factor: women tend to have a higher prevalence of malnutrition[32] and poorer nutritional outcomes, yet a lower mortality rate.[35]

Pathophysiology

Carbohydrate In general, patients with stage 5 CKD are not as nutritionally stressed as those with AKI; however, more than half of patients with stage 5 CKD have insulin resistance and hyperglycemia. This is attributed to the increased glucagon-to-insulin ratio, resulting in protein breakdown and gluconeogenesis. In patients with normal peritoneal transport on PD, ~60% of glucose in the dialysate is absorbed. One method of estimating the quantity of glucose absorbed is as follows: glucose absorbed (g/day) = $0.89x$ (g/day) − 43, where x is the total amount of dialysate glucose instilled daily. This dialysate glucose absorption can worsen existing hyperglycemia and contribute significantly to the patient's energy intake, making kwashiorkor-type malnutrition common. Although glucose control is not problematic unless the patient is diabetic, infected, or subjected to operative stress, insulin can be added to chronic ambulatory PD bags to control hyperglycemia (see Chapter 54).

Fat Hypertriglyceridemia is common in patients with stage 5 CKD. This is mainly a result of decreased catabolism of triglycerides secondary to decreased hepatic lipoprotein lipase activity.[36] Most patients with stage 5 CKD receiving HD also receive heparin, which activates lipoprotein lipase and converts triglycerides to free fatty acids and glycerol. Carnitine, an amino acid necessary for the transport of long-chain fatty acids across mitochondria, is removed by HD and PD; therefore, serum carnitine concentrations typically are reduced in patients with stage 5 CKD.[37]

Current guidelines do not advocate carnitine administration for the treatment of hypertriglyceridemia.[38] Studies of carnitine for this indication have varied widely in duration and have used both oral and IV administration in varying doses (1–2 mg/kg/day IV to as much as 10 mg/kg/day to 3 g/day orally).

Leptin, which is produced and secreted by fat cells, regulates satiety and energy balance (see Chapter 154). Leptin concentrations often are elevated in patients with stage 5 CKD, particularly those undergoing PD probably as the result of decreased renal degradation of leptin and increased production as the result of chronic inflammation. Hyperleptinemia in CKD is associated with decreased protein intake and weight loss. Further study is required to better define the relationship between leptin concentrations and nutrition status in patients with CKD.[39,40]

Protein Secondary analysis of the Modification of Diet in Renal Disease Study indicated that in nondiabetics, a reduction of dietary protein intake may slow the rate of renal disease progression and ultimately delay the onset of dialysis (see Chapter 52).[41] The National Kidney Foundation Kidney Disease Outcomes Quality Initiative (NKF K/DOQI) guidelines for nutrition in patients with CKD recommend a diet providing 0.6 g/kg of protein per day for those with a glomerular filtration rate less than 25 mL/min (0.42 mL/s).[38] Although the safety of low-protein diets has been questioned, it has been suggested that for carefully selected and monitored patients, protein intakes of as low as 0.3 g/kg/day supplemented with essential amino acids can be used safely.[5,28]

Patients with stage 5 CKD receiving PD require special attention as a consequence of protein losses across the peritoneal membrane. Peritoneal protein losses typically range from 5 to 15 g/day for patients undergoing PD.[38] PD protein losses, however, do not predict the risk for malnutrition (as measured by serum albumin concentration) in all patients.[38] The American Society for Parenteral and Enteral Nutrition (ASPEN) and K/DOQI guidelines suggest that dietary protein intake of at least 1.2 to 1.3 g/kg/day (at least 50% of high biologic value) is needed to consistently achieve neutral

or positive nitrogen balance in nonacutely ill peritoneal dialysis patients and clinically stable HD patients.[38] Dialysate protein losses also must be considered for the patient with stage 5 CKD undergoing HD. The amount of protein lost via HD depends on the dialysis membrane used and whether the dialyzer is being reused. Typical losses are 10 to 12 g per dialysis session, but this may be increased by up to 50% with dialyzer reuse.[38]

Fluid and Electrolytes Hyponatremia, often due to overhydration, is common in patients with CKD (see Chapter 58). Regular dialysis is the principal means for control of body water and serum sodium concentration in the stage 5 CKD. Patients with CKD who develop hyperkalemia generally have ingested excessive potassium relative to the potassium-removing capacity of the failing kidney (and dialysis, in the case of stage 5 CKD). The undernourished CKD patient receiving PN, however, may require considerable potassium as new body cell mass is synthesized.

Patients with CKD often are treated for hyperphosphatemia with phosphorus-restricted diets and phosphate-binding agents (see Chapters 52 and 53). When these patients receive aggressive nutritional support, the combination of refeeding (cellular uptake of phosphorus for synthesis of body cell mass) and vigorous phosphate-binding therapy can result in hypophosphatemia.

Metabolic acidosis, a common complication of stage 5 CKD, is associated with increased protein degradation and decreased synthesis of albumin.[38] Correction of acidosis in patients with stage 5 CKD may be associated with increases in serum albumin, body weight, and midarm muscle circumference, along with fewer hospitalizations.[42] Stabilization of serum bicarbonate concentrations (>22 mEq/L [>22 mmol/L]) via alteration of the dialysate bicarbonate concentration or administration of oral bicarbonate salts is a prudent nutritional intervention in these patients (see Chapters 53 and 61).

Trace Elements There are considerable data regarding trace element requirements in patients with stage 5 CKD.[19] Decreased zinc concentrations have been linked to taste disturbances and sexual dysfunction. Zinc supplementation, however, does not universally reverse these anomalies. Although serum concentrations of this trace element are decreased, total body stores of zinc in stage 5 CKD often are increased. This suggests a redistribution of zinc or increased need to maintain normal enzymatic function in patients with stage 5 CKD.

Serum chromium concentrations are elevated in patients on chronic HD and PD, perhaps because the needles used during HD and the peritoneal and hemodialysate fluids are sources of chromium. Such patients have decreased selenium concentrations that can be increased with oral selenium supplements of 135 to 140 mcg/day.[43] It appears that for patients undergoing HD, significant selenium losses occur during dialysis.[19]

Vitamins Patients with CKD are prone to develop water-soluble vitamin deficiencies because of decreased dietary intake secondary to anorexia and restriction of many foods because of their protein, potassium, or phosphorus content. Additionally, vitamin losses due to hemodialysis are similar to those mentioned for AKI. The decrease in ascorbic acid serum levels observed in patients with CKD was recently associated with increased cardiovascular morbidity and mortality. Plasma ascorbic acid concentrations are usually normal in patients on PD. The highly protein-bound vitamins (A, D, and B_{12}) are not removed significantly by HD.[19] Vitamin D deficiency is correlated with decreased serum albumin concentrations, and supplementation of vitamin D has increased serum albumin concentrations significantly in deficient patients.[44] Vitamin A concentrations often are elevated in CKD and can lead to hypervitaminosis A and its cirrhosis-like syndrome. Conversely, vitamin E supplementation may have a distinct benefit to patients with stage 5 CKD. Increased oxidative stress in stage 5 CKD may contribute to the accelerated atherosclerosis. Vitamin E in doses of 800 international units (IU) per day decreases low-density lipoprotein oxidation in patients with stage 5 CKD, especially in those undergoing PD.[45] Thiamine concentrations decrease during dialysis; supplementation within the daily recommended intake norms is sufficient to keep concentrations in the normal range. Hyperhomocysteinemia is common in patients with stage 5 CKD. Folate doses from 2.5 mg three times weekly to 60 mg/day have lowered homocysteine concentrations in patients with stage 5 but have not completely reduced concentrations to normal. In patients with stage 3 or 4 CKD, elevated homocysteine concentrations are associated with increased cardiovascular risk. In those with stage 5 CKD, lower homocysteine concentrations are associated with an increased risk of cardiovascular events. It is thought that in these patients, ongoing malnutrition and inflammation suppress homocysteine concentrations while continuing to accelerate atherosclerosis.[46]

TREATMENT

■ DESIRED OUTCOMES

Goals of nutrition support in CKD are similar to those in other patient populations, with only a few additional considerations because of the metabolic derangements that are commonly observed. Prevention of undernutrition and maintenance of lean body mass are of primary importance. Other goals are correction and prevention of metabolic disorders, maintenance of electrolyte homeostasis, minimization of CKD progression, and preservation of optimal GI structure and function.[5] The ultimate goal of

nutritional interventions, considering the strong relationship between malnutrition and morbidity and mortality in CKD, is to optimize patient survival.[31]

■ GENERAL APPROACH TO TREATMENT

Nutrition support for patients with CKD can usually be managed with oral supplementation or EN. These patients rarely need PN because their GI tract is usually functional. Guidelines for nutrition support have been developed by NKF K/DOQI, ASPEN, and the European Society for Parenteral and Enteral Nutrition (ESPEN) (Fig. 153–1).[5,8,28,38] The calorically dense low-electrolyte (potassium, phosphorus, and magnesium) enteral formulas are particularly useful. For protein-restricted predialysis patients with CKD, Suplena and Renalcal, which have relatively low protein content, should be used. Even though patients with stage 5 CKD receive regular dialysis, many are anuric between dialysis sessions, so excess fluid intake is a potential problem. Nepro and Novasource Renal are marketed specifically (because of their high caloric density and low electrolyte content) for the dialysis-dependent patient with stage 5 CKD.[21] If there is superimposed illness that precludes EN, balanced amino acid products should be used as the protein component of PN formulations. There are no data supporting the use of essential amino acid parenteral formulations.

■ NONPHARMACOLOGIC THERAPIES

Nutritional interviews, diaries, and counseling are essential parts of the nutrition support plan for patients with CKD. The NKF K/DOQI guidelines stress the importance of renal dietetic interventions and recommend that patients maintain 3-day dietary diaries intermittently and discuss the results with their dietary

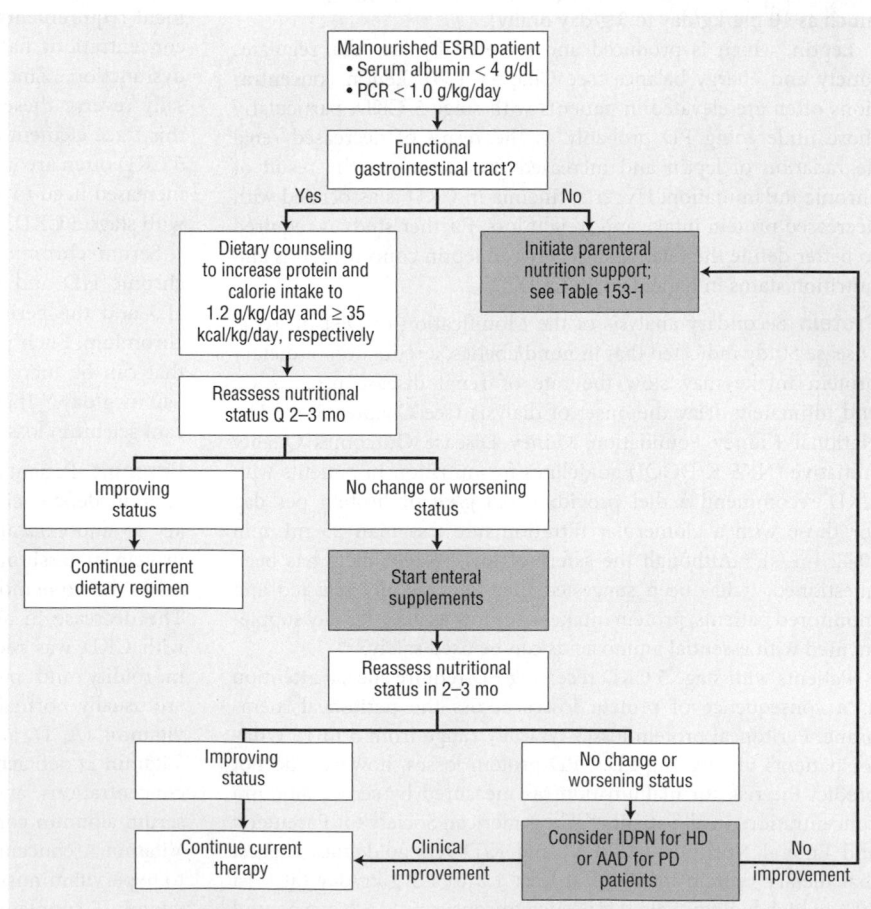

FIGURE 153-1. An algorithmic approach to nutritional support in the patient with end-stage renal disease. Serum albumin <4 g/dL is equivalent to <40 g/L. Energy intake ≥35 kcal/kg/day is equivalent to ≥147 kJ/kg/day. AAD, amino acid dialysate; CAPD, continuous ambulatory peritoneal dialysis; ESRD, end-stage renal disease; IDPN, intradialytic parenteral nutrition; HD, hemodialysis; PCR, protein catabolic rate.

care provider. These interventions are conducted to optimize the quantity and quality of patient energy and protein intake. In other populations, such interventions with frequent nutritional counseling have resulted in increased adherence to the recommended dietary intake.[38]

■ PHARMACOLOGIC THERAPIES

Drug Treatments of First Choice

Current recommendations from NKF K/DOQI that factor in concurrent illnesses and the likelihood of preexisting malnutrition advocate 35 kcal/kg/day (147 kJ/kg/day) and 1.2 g/kg/day of protein for patients on chronic HD who are younger than 65 years and 1.2 to 1.3 g/kg/day of protein for patients on chronic PD.[38] This is higher than the spontaneous dietary intake in most dialysis patients. This emphasizes the importance of dietary counseling to encourage compliance with current dietary recommendations, especially for patients with concurrent hypercatabolic illnesses.

For patients who cannot achieve recommended dietary intake goals, several studies have examined the effect of EN on nutritional outcomes. A systematic review of these studies across all stages of CKD reveals that EN is associated with significant increases in energy and protein intake and serum albumin concentration.[31] No significant increases in metabolic or electrolyte imbalances were noted. However, no significant differences in CKD patient morbidity or survival were noted.

Several electrolytes warrant special attention for patients with CKD. Generally, sodium should be administered only to replace losses to avoid overhydration. Examples of initial daily supplementation can be found in Tables 153-1 and 153-2, and supplementation may be adjusted based on the patient's serum sodium concentration and fluid balance. Although these patients also are predisposed to hyperkalemia, once anabolism is attained, potassium requirements may be as high as 40 to 80 mEq/day (40–80 mmol/L/day). This dose needs to be given carefully and requires serum potassium concentration monitoring. Clinically significant hypermagnesemia is less common in patients with CKD than those with AKI. It is usually added to the PN solution in reduced doses (4 mEq/L [4 mmol/L]).

Patients with end-stage renal disease (ESRD) or stage 5 CKD often are treated for hyperphosphatemia. With aggressive nutritional support, the combination of refeeding and compliance with phosphate-binding therapy can result in hypophosphatemia within a matter of days. Decreasing or temporarily discontinuing the phosphate-binding therapy is appropriate if this occurs. Thereafter conservative amounts of phosphorus may need to be administered.

Some practitioners advocate withholding trace elements from patients with CKD who are receiving PN. Others recommend the administration of standard dietary intake of trace elements, because in stage 5 CKD, serum concentrations of certain trace elements are normal (e.g., manganese), and others are decreased (e.g., zinc and selenium).[19] Additional zinc and selenium supplementation may be considered in documented cases of deficiency.[5]

During PN, avoidance of vitamin A is recommended. Dialytic losses of ascorbic acid, folic acid, and pyridoxine are common. Thus, patients with stage 5 CKD should receive ascorbic acid 50 to 100 mg/day, pyridoxine 5 to 10 mg/day, and at least 1 mg/day folic acid in addition to the other essential vitamins.[19] Typical PN and EN prescriptions for a patient with stage 5 CKD are presented in Tables 153-1 and 153-2, respectively.[34] Figure 153-1 is an algorithmic approach to improve nutritional status and ensure optimal outcomes integrating recommendations from NKF K/DOQI, ASPEN, and ESPEN.[5,8,28,38]

Alternative Drug Treatments

Poor nutritional intake due to anorexia and impaired GI motility have led to research assessing the impact of appetite stimulants and prokinetic agents on nutritional outcomes in patients with CKD. The use of the appetite stimulant megestrol acetate and prokinetic agent metoclopramide are associated with increases in serum albumin in patients with CKD.[42] Further research is needed to better define the effect and optimal dosing if their use is to be applied more widely for nutritional intervention in CKD. The association of poor nutritional status and increased morbidity and mortality in stage 5 CKD has led to the development of alternative nutritional delivery systems. One such approach is intradialytic parenteral nutrition (IDPN), or the provision of glucose–amino acid–lipid admixture during HD. IDPN typically allows for the infusion of 650 to 1,100 kcal (2,721–4,604 kJ) per session (250 mL of 50–70% dextrose and 250 mL of 10–20% lipids) and 50 to 90 g of protein (500 mL of 10–15% amino acids).[47] An evidence-based evaluation of 24 studies employing IDPN found that the use of IDPN was associated with decreased mortality, but only 3 of the 24 studies were randomized. Because of the limitations of presently available data, IDPN should be reserved for malnourished patients who have serum albumin <3.4 g/dL (<34 g/L), weight loss >10% of ideal body weight, dietary history of intake of <25 kcal/kg/day (<105 kJ/kg/day), and who failed attempts at oral supplements and enteral tube feedings or who are not appropriate for such attempts.[28,48]

Amino acid dialysate is the IDPN counterpart for the patient on PD. This technique entails using a 1.1% amino acid solution in place of one or two of the dextrose-containing PD exchanges per day. Improvements in serum transferrin and total protein concentrations have been observed in malnourished patients on PD; however, no beneficial effect has been noted on patient mortality. Adverse effects of this therapy have included exacerbations of uremic symptoms (because of increases in blood urea nitrogen) and metabolic acidosis. In the longest study to date, amino acid dialysate was associated with improved maintenance of albumin and cholesterol concentrations but no significant difference in morbidity or mortality.[49] In summary, amino acid dialysate may be useful in the treatment of malnourished patients on PD, but better-designed studies are needed.

Recombinant human growth hormone (rhGH) in doses of 0.2 IU/kg/day subcutaneously has been used experimentally in adults with stage 5 CKD to enhance anabolism; weight gain and increased transferrin concentrations have been reported after

TABLE 153-2	Initial Enteral Nutrition Prescription for Patients with End-Stage Renal Disease
Nutrient	**Recommendation**
Nonprotein calories	35 kcal/kg (147 kJ/kg) per day for HD
	35 kcal/kg (147 kJ/kg) per day PD (including calories from glucose absorption from dialysate)
Protein	1.2 g/kg IBW for HD
	1.2–1.3 g/kg IBW for PD
Sodium	2–3 g/day for HD[a]
	2 g/day for PD[a]
Potassium	2,000–2,500 mg/day[a]
Phosphorus	800–1,000 mg/day[a]
Calcium	<2,500 mg/day total intake[a]
Fluid	1,000 mL + daily urine output for HD
	To maintain appropriate fluid balance for PD

[a]Individualized based on patient's laboratory values.
CAPD = continuous ambulatory peritoneal dialysis HD = hemodialysis, IBW = ideal body weight, PD = peritoneal dialysis.
Data from references 5, 9, and 41.

TABLE 153-3 Routine Nutritional Monitoring in Patients with End-Stage Renal Disease

Parameter	Frequency
Predialysis serum albumin1	Monthly
Percentage of usual postdialysis or postdrain body weight	Monthly
Subjective global assessment	Every 6 months
Protein equivalent of total nitrogen appearance(PNA)^a	Monthly for HD, every 3–4 months for PD
Dietary interview and/or diary	Every 6 months
Predialysis prealbumin	As needed
Anthropometry	As needed
Dual-energy X-ray absorptiometry	As needed

^{a}Beginning of week PNA = $Co/[36.3 + (5.48)$ $(spKt/V) + (53.5/spKt/V)] = 0.168$, where Co is predialysis BUN, and $spKt/V$, the single-pool index of hemodialysis adequacy = $Ln(R - 0.08 \times t)$ $+ [4 - (3.5 \times R)] \times UF/W$, where R is postdialysis:predialysis BUN ratio, t is dialysis session in hours, UF is ultrafiltration in liters, and W is postdialysis weight in kilograms. (See Chapter 48.)
BUN = blood urea nitrogen, PD = peritoneal dialysis, HD = hemodialysis.
Reprinted from Am J Kidney Dis, Vol. 35 (6 Suppl 2), K/DOQI, National Kidney Foundation, Clinical practice guidelines for nutrition in chronic renal failure, pages S1–S140, Copyright © 2000, with permission from the National Kidney Foundation.

4 weeks.[50] Despite these gains, rhGH is associated with sodium and water retention, and the fact that its effects may be lessened by catabolic illness or decreased dietary intake limits its utility. In the future, there may be a role for rhGH or other anabolic agents in the treatment of patients with stage 5 CKD who have inadequate oral intake despite appropriate dietary counseling and oral supplements.[42]

■ PHARMACOECONOMIC CONSIDERATIONS

There are no data demonstrating the economic value of nutrition support in patients with CKD.

■ EVALUATION OF THERAPEUTIC OUTCOMES

The short- and long-term monitoring plan for patient with stage 5 CKD receiving PN or EN needs to be carefully tailored. This can be achieved via frequent (daily) monitoring of serum electrolyte concentrations (e.g., sodium, potassium, phosphorus, magnesium, and calcium) and fluid balance. Serum glucose concentrations should be followed frequently (four times daily) in those who develop persistent hyperglycemia.

Because protein-energy malnutrition is a significant predictor of morbidity and mortality in patients with stage 5 CKD, monitoring to ensure the effectiveness of the long-term nutritional plan becomes critical. Increased serum albumin concentrations are correlated with increased survival; thus, monitoring of serum albumin concentrations is recommended for all patients undergoing HD and PD (Table 153–3).

HEPATIC FAILURE

The liver is the primary organ involved in the digestion, metabolism, and storage of nutrients. When functional capacity is depressed, profound nutrient intolerance (hyper- or hypoglycemia, hypertriglyceridemia, and hepatic encephalopathy) may result. Other sequelae that accompany the failing liver are fluid and electrolyte imbalances, vitamin deficiencies, and malnutrition. It is estimated that 65% to 90% of patients with advanced liver disease and almost 100% of patients awaiting liver transplantation have some degree of malnutrition, which increases morbidity and mortality. Nutritional support is an important component of the overall care of the patient with liver disease that may decrease complications and extend survival.[51]

EPIDEMIOLOGY

It is estimated that 30% of cirrhotic patients have protein-energy malnutrition, 40% have protein malnutrition, and 10% have energy malnutrition.[52] Changes in body composition such as decreases in body cell mass may be seen in early phases of the disease and become more severe as cirrhosis progresses. In general, there is no significant difference in the incidence of malnutrition between those with cirrhosis caused by alcoholism and those with postviral cirrhosis. One study, however, found that abstinent patients with alcoholic cirrhosis had lower average measures of nutritional adequacy than those with cirrhosis caused by chronic hepatitis C.[53]

PATHOPHYSIOLOGY

Energy

A decrease in spontaneous oral intake is quite common in patients with cirrhosis and appears to be multifactorial in nature. Potential causes of decreased oral intake include altered taste, early satiety as a result of ascites and/or hyperleptinemia, impaired GI motility, bacterial overgrowth in the small intestine, malabsorption as a consequence of GI dysfunction and treatment with neomycin or lactulose, nausea, and chronic encephalopathy.[28,51]

Resting energy requirements in stable cirrhotics can appear to be normal, but approximately one-third are hypometabolic, and one-third are hypermetabolic when energy expenditure is corrected for alterations in lean body mass.[51] The Harris-Benedict equation for estimating caloric needs usually underestimates their needs by 15% to 20%.[54] The marked variability in energy expenditure underscores the need for patient-specific regimen design and monitoring and may suggest the need for indirect calorimetry measurement.[51] An initial energy provision of 35 to 40 kcal/kg/day (147–167 kJ/kg/day) is recommended by ESPEN for patients with alcoholic steatohepatitis and liver cirrhosis.[55]

Carbohydrates

❸ In healthy adults, ~60% of absorbed glucose is taken up by the liver and used for glycogen synthesis, triglyceride synthesis, and glycolysis. In general, glycogen synthesis and glycolysis are enhanced by insulin, whereas gluconeogenesis and glycogen breakdown are controlled by glucagon. Hyperglycemia is common in cirrhosis as a result of peripheral insulin resistance, which is mediated by a decreased binding to insulin receptors and defective postreceptor signal handling in peripheral tissues. Plasma concentrations of insulin are elevated with or without a glucose stimulus. This makes administration of large doses of glucose problematic because administration of insulin to control hyperglycemia may not improve its utilization substantially.

Patients with fulminant hepatitis are prone to hypoglycemia because hepatic glucose production is depressed secondary to decreased glycogen stores, diminished gluconeogenesis, and impaired degradation of insulin. A continuous IV infusion of 5% dextrose usually prevents hypoglycemia in acute hepatitis, but concentrations greater than 10% dextrose may be needed in more severe cases.

Fat

The liver is responsible for synthesis of cholesterol, high-density lipoproteins, and very low density lipoproteins. The enzymes lipoprotein lipase and lecithin-cholesterol acyltransferase are synthesized in the liver. Increased serum triglyceride and free fatty acid concentrations are thus encountered in patients with hepatic failure, primarily as a result of the increased lipolysis. The significant insulin resistance that can be seen in those with cirrhosis causes a shift to lipids as a primary fuel source.[51] Whereas only 35% of total calories are derived from fat in normal patients, this can increase to 75% in patients with cirrhosis.[54] Incorporation of late-evening snacks may correct abnormal substrate metabolism, increase carbohydrate metabolism, and decrease fat oxidation rates.[56,57]

Patients with severe liver failure may be at increased risk for essential fatty acid deficiency; the ratio of nonessential to essential fatty acids was found to be increased in patients with acute and chronic liver failure. Poor oral intake of fat and dietary fat malabsorption in patients with cirrhosis both contribute to essential fatty acid deficiency.[58] The concentrations of linoleic acid can be increased with administration of an average of 33 g/day of IVLE supplementation.[59] Despite concerns of impaired clearance of long-chain triglycerides in IVLE as a consequence of impaired synthesis of apoprotein CII in cirrhotic patents, IVLE solutions have been given safely to patients with fulminant hepatic failure.[60]

Diarrhea and steatorrhea are common in patients with hepatic cholestasis because of intestinal malabsorption (partly as a result of mucosal edema from hypoalbuminemia), inadequate bile acid delivery to the duodenum, and pancreatic dysfunction with decreased secretion of lipase.[54] Because the micelle formation is impeded, the long-chain fatty acids pass through the colon, resulting in a foul-smelling, soapy diarrhea.

Protein

Nitrogen requirements for the patient with liver failure are similar to those of normal subjects, but intolerance to protein may limit the achievement of this goal. Thus, some experts have advocated restriction of dietary protein intake. Recent research indicates, however, that protein restriction is not beneficial for patients with cirrhosis even in the midst of episodic hepatic encephalopathy.[61]

Because the liver metabolizes the aromatic amino acids (i.e., phenylalanine, tyrosine, and tryptophan), methionine, and glutamine, the plasma concentrations of these amino acids are elevated in cirrhotic patients. Plasma concentrations of the branched-chain amino acids (i.e., valine, leucine, and isoleucine) often are depressed because these amino acids are metabolized by skeletal muscle. This altered plasma aminogram most likely contributes to the development of hepatic encephalopathy.

Fluid and Electrolytes

Patients with severe cirrhosis often have ascites and peripheral edema. The excess of total body sodium in the presence of an even greater excess of total body water results in hyponatremia. Salt and fluid restrictions are required to avoid exacerbating this overhydrated state (see Chapter 58).

Hypokalemia is common in patients with liver failure who have normal renal function. Poor nutritional intake and vomiting may initiate this disorder. Severe vomiting may also lead to volume contraction metabolic alkalosis, with increased renal excretion of potassium (see Chapter 61). Secondary hyperaldosteronism, a common finding in patients with liver failure and intravascular volume depletion, also increases renal excretion of potassium. Loop diuretic therapy causes increased renal excretion of potassium, whereas diarrhea from lactulose therapy increases fecal excretion of potassium. All these conditions can lead to profound hypokalemia. Therefore, potassium requirements in patients with liver failure who are receiving specialized nutritional support may be substantially larger than those in otherwise healthy adults.

Poor nutritional intake secondary to alcohol abuse and increased excretion of magnesium secondary to diuretic therapy contribute to hypomagnesemia. Even in cirrhotic patients with normal serum magnesium concentrations, muscle magnesium is depleted; this has been independently associated with the development of hepatic encephalopathy.[62] During nutrition support, requirements for phosphorus are also substantially elevated because synthesis of body cell mass occurs, placing this population at risk for developing hypophosphatemia during refeeding.

Trace Elements

Zinc deficiency is seen in many patients with liver failure because of malabsorption, chronic diarrhea, or elevated cytokine concentrations. Thus, patients with chronic diarrhea should be suspected of having zinc deficiency; the measurement of serum concentrations, however, is rarely used to confirm such deficiencies. Tumor necrosis factor, interleukin-1, and interleukin-6 may stimulate metallothionein, an intestinal zinc-binding protein, thereby inhibiting zinc absorption. Finally, patients receiving a protein-restricted diet may be at additional risk because substantial amounts of zinc are found in red meat.

Because copper and manganese are excreted in the bile, it has been recommended that these two trace elements not be administered or be administered in reduced doses to patients with serious cholestasis. Direct measurements of manganese in the globus pallidus of cirrhotic patients who died in hepatic coma were two- to sevenfold higher than expected.[63] These findings suggest that reduced quantities of manganese should be provided in the nutritional formulation to avoid exacerbating encephalopathy in the patient with chronic liver disease. There are no prospective evaluations, however, demonstrating the benefits of low copper or manganese diets.

An association between alcoholism and low serum selenium concentrations has been reported.[64] Because selenium is important in maintaining the enzyme glutathione peroxidase, a deficiency of this trace element has been implicated as a cause of hepatic injury in the alcoholic patient. However, because human serum contains at least three fractions of selenium, the use of serum selenium concentrations as a marker for selenium deficiency is controversial. At this time, maintaining a daily selenium intake of 40 mcg is the most appropriate approach in patients with chronic liver disease.

Vitamins

❹ Folic acid deficiency may lead to megaloblastic anemia, whereas thiamine deficiency may result in Wernicke encephalopathy after rehydration with IV glucose. Depletion of hepatic stores of vitamin A, pyridoxine, folic acid, riboflavin, pantothenic acid, vitamin B_{12}, and thiamine has been reported in patients with hepatic failure. Poor intake and malabsorption are the principal causes of vitamin deficiencies in patients with chronic liver disease.

Because vitamin D is metabolized to 25-hydroxyvitamin D in the liver, low concentrations of this vitamin are seen in patients with biliary cirrhosis. Impaired absorption of dietary vitamin D as a consequence of decreased bile production may also contribute to these low serum concentrations and ultimately lead to the development of osteoporosis. The most appropriate approach at this time is to provide the daily recommended intake of these vitamins and consider additional supplementation when a deficiency is documented.

TREATMENT

■ DESIRED OUTCOMES

The primary objective of nutrition support in patients with cirrhosis is the provision of the recommended amounts of energy and protein. Adequate nutrition support may slow disease progression, prevent morbidity, enhance the structure and function of the GI tract, and decrease mortality.[51,55]

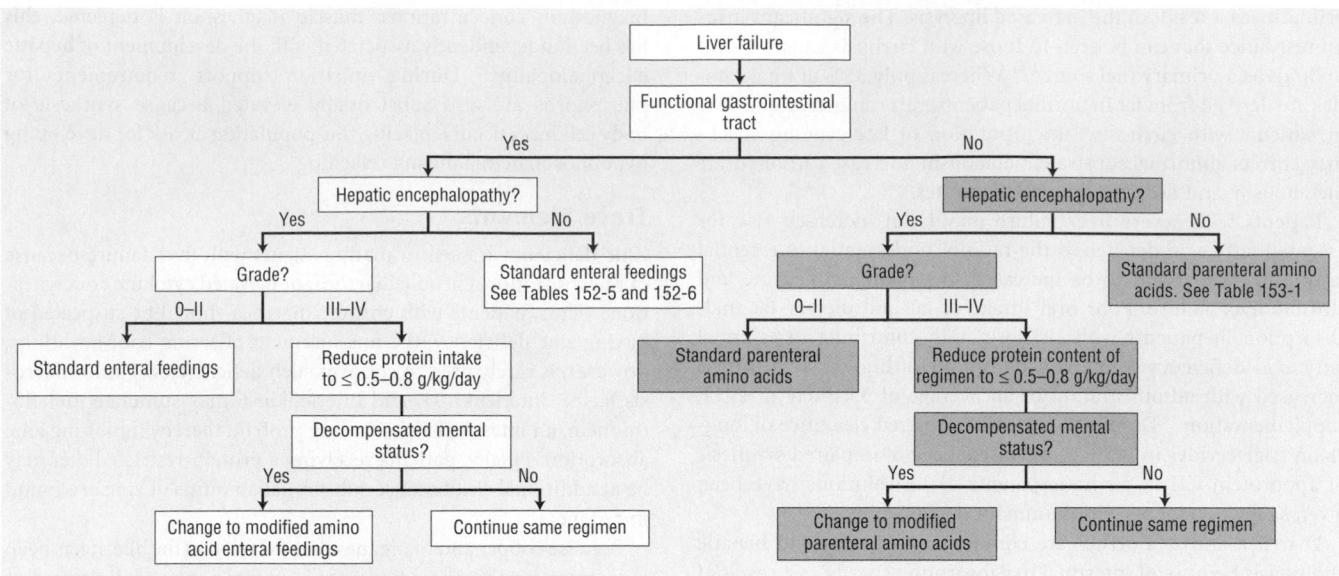

FIGURE 153-2. An algorithmic approach to nutritional support for the patient with hepatic failure. *Adapted from references 28 and 55.*

GENERAL APPROACH TO TREATMENT

Enteral nutrition is preferred in patients with cirrhosis when the GI tract is functional and accessible (Fig. 153–2).[28,55] The indications for PN in the patient with liver failure are similar to those for general hospitalized patients. Because EN can contribute to hyperammonemia in cirrhotic patients with transjugular intrahepatic portosystemic shunts,[65] the use of PN in such patients might be preferable. In most cases, PN in the patient with liver failure can be accomplished via the administration of standard mixed amino acids (Fig. 153–2).[66]

NONPHARMACOLOGIC THERAPIES

Dietary counseling makes patients aware of the risks that malnutrition poses for the progression of their disease and can provide strategies for patients to attain goal intakes, while being mindful of dietary restrictions. Many patients will have a higher likelihood of maintaining normal substrate utilization if they eat four or five small meals a day and a snack at bedtime. At least one study has found that intensive counseling is equivalent to providing oral nutritional supplements in increasing patient intake.[51] Cirrhotic patients may also derive up to a 26% increase in energy intake and a significant increase in lean body mass after the insertion of a transjugular intrahepatic portosystemic shunt.[67]

There is considerable interest in the use of vegetable-protein diets in the chronic management of patients with cirrhosis and hepatic encephalopathy. Enthusiasm for this therapy is based on the reduced amounts of aromatic amino acids and methionine in vegetable protein and a decrease in nitrogen absorption as the result of a decreased GI transit time and an increase in fecal nitrogen excretion by colonic bacterial flora. However, compliance is more difficult to achieve with vegetable-based than animal-based protein diets. ASPEN recommends that a diet with vegetable-based protein be considered for those patients who do not tolerate at least 1 g/kg/day of protein from their normal diet.[28]

PHARMACOLOGIC THERAPIES

Drug Treatments of First Choice

In patients with liver disease who are unable to meet their nutritional needs despite dietary counseling, ESPEN guidelines recommend that EN be initiated with a goal of providing 35 to 40 kcal/kg/day (147–167 kJ/kg/day) and protein intake of 1.2 to 1.5 g/kg/day.[55] Indirect calorimetry quantification may be preferred to empiric estimates of caloric requirements in this setting. Excessive calorie provision actually may promote liver dysfunction and increased production of carbon dioxide with an associated increased work of breathing. Standard whole-protein formulas are recommended, but more concentrated formulations are appropriate to avoid excessive fluid overload in patients with ascites.[55]

When dextrose-based PN is started in those who cannot tolerate EN, additional thiamine may be needed to prevent Wernicke encephalopathy. Standard mixed amino acids are appropriate for most patients. IVLE should be used in patients with liver failure only to prevent essential fatty acid deficiency when initial serum triglyceride concentrations exceed 300 mg/dL (3.39 mmol/L). If serum triglyceride concentrations are low or normal, IVLE may be used as a calorie source. Monitoring serum triglyceride concentration and free fatty acid oxidation (not available in all facilities) to ensure that lipid is both cleared and oxidized appropriately has been suggested. Oral medium-chain triglycerides have been used occasionally with success because they do not require pancreatic enzymes or micelle formation before absorption. However, these products do not provide essential fatty acids.

The electrolytes that warrant the most careful monitoring in those with liver disease are sodium, potassium, phosphorus, and magnesium. During fluid and salt restriction, patients (especially those receiving concurrent lactulose therapy for encephalopathy) should be observed for symptoms of volume depletion (e.g., increased pulse rate, decreased blood pressure, or dry mucous membranes). Magnesium concentrations as high as 24 mEq/L (12 mmol/L) in the PN solution, which is two to three times the standard daily dose, may be required to maintain plasma concentrations in the normal range.

Trace elements that warrant individual attention include zinc, copper, and manganese. For patients receiving PN, withholding copper from the solution until a copper serum concentration in the normal range is documented or the cholestasis resolves are appropriate. Patients who have chronic cholestasis may require copper in reduced doses (e.g., 0.6 mg/day); however, they should have serum copper concentrations checked regularly (once per month in the acute care setting and every 6 months in the ambulatory setting). Manganese restriction also may be required in these patients.

TABLE 153-4 Nutrition Recommendations for Patients with Liver Disease

Patient Type	Calorie Energy (kcal/kg/day)[b]	Protein (g/kg/day)	Comments
Compensated cirrhosis	25–35	1–1.2	Use a bedtime snack and frequent small meals
Decompensated cirrhosis[a]	25–35	0.5–1.5 for mild; 0.5 for severe	Use branched-chain amino acids for refractory cases of encephalopathy unresponsive to protein restriction
Decompenstated cirrhosis[a] with malnutrition	35–40	1.5	May have to temporarily decrease protein for encephalopathy worsening

[a]Decompensated cirrhosis: cirrhosis accompanied by significant ascites or encephalopathy.
[b]One kcal/kg/day is equivalent to 4.2 kJ/kg/day.
Adapted from reference 51 and 55.

Table 153–4 lists the nutritional requirements of patients with liver failure secondary to cirrhosis, and Table 153–1 presents an empiric PN formula for the patient with hepatic failure.[54,60,66]

Alternative Drug Treatments

The major controversy in nutritional support of the patient with liver failure has centered on the selection of the optimal protein product. Modified amino acid solutions for PN (e.g., HepatAmine) are marketed for patients with liver failure and hepatic encephalopathy. They are enriched with branched-chain amino acids and have reduced amounts of aromatic amino acids and methionine. These products are formulated on the basis of the false neurotransmitter hypothesis, which postulates that hepatic encephalopathy may be a result of increased aromatic amino acid concentrations in the central nervous system.

NutriHep, a supplement for patients with hepatic encephalopathy, usually provides adequate amounts of vitamins and minerals, contains a high percentage of medium-chain triglycerides, and is supplemented with carnitine. Clinical trials using this and other branched-chain amino acid products have yielded promising outcomes, including decreases in morbidity and mortality. These results, however, have not been consistent. Enteral products with branched-chain amino acids are associated with significant nonadherence because of poor taste.[51] This, coupled with the increased cost of these products, has led ASPEN and ESPEN to recommend reserving these products for patients with severe encephalopathy who decompensate on standard protein formulations despite continued lactulose–neomycin therapy.[28,55]

■ PHARMACOECONOMIC CONSIDERATIONS

Nutritional supplementation in patients with alcoholic cirrhosis reduces the frequency of hospitalizations.[68] Intuitively, this should be a cost-saving intervention, but without formal analysis, the degree of benefit cannot be quantified.

■ EVALUATION OF THERAPEUTIC OUTCOMES

Weight, albumin concentration, and prealbumin concentration are commonly used markers of nutrition status that may not be as reliable in patients with hepatic failure. Ascites, edema, and impaired hepatic protein synthesis make nutritional evaluation difficult in this patient population. Indeed, many of the commonly used markers of nutritional status correlate poorly with body cell mass in those with ESLD. Subjective global assessment, prognostic nutritional index, bioelectrical impedance, midarm muscle circumference, and hand grip strength have been tested as predictors of body cell mass.[51] Hand grip strength best correlates with malnutrition and is a better predictor of major complications in patients with cirrhosis.[69]

SHORT BOWEL SYNDROME

Short bowel syndrome (SBS) is generally a consequence of significant surgical resection of the small bowel that results in the malabsorption of nutrients and fluids. Morbidity and mortality caused by GI failure in SBS patients have been improved with the provision of PN and EN. The goal of nutritional support with EN and PN is to maintain nutritional status, prevent or correct nutritional deficiencies, and enhance quality of life.[70]

EPIDEMIOLOGY

There are at least 10,000 patients who have SBS in the United States.[71] The most common etiologies in adults are surgical resections because of Crohn disease, mesenteric vascular disease, and cancer. In infants, necrotizing enterocolitis, midgut volvulus, and intestinal atresia are the most common etiologies for resection leading to SBS.[71] SBS occurs more commonly in women than in men, most likely as a consequence of women having less small intestine length to begin with. This condition also may be functional as opposed to anatomic and occurs in individuals who have not had resections, but who have a decreased small bowel absorptive capacity as a result of radiation enteritis or severe inflammatory bowel disease.[70] Symptoms of SBS generally include diarrhea, dehydration, electrolyte disturbances, and progressive malnutrition.[71]

PATHOPHYSIOLOGY

The average length of the small intestine, where the majority of nutrients are absorbed, in adults is 400 to 600 cm (157–236 inches). The American Gastroenterological Association considers a patient to have SBS when the patient has 200 cm (79 inches) or less of functional small intestine.[72] Losing this absorptive capacity leads to deficiencies in multiple nutrients, requiring the initiation of interventional nutrition.

❺ PN must be used at least immediately following resection of the small intestine while the GI tract is healing and adapting. Enteral nutrition may be used later during the transition to oral feedings, as the GI tract is able to adapt with time, by increasing absorptive capacity, in ~50% of patients with SBS.[71] The length and type of nutritional support a patient may require are based on such factors as the length of remaining small intestine and the presence or absence of a functional colon. Adult patients have the highest likelihood of transitioning off PN if the residual jejunum–ileum length is greater than 100 cm (40 inches) for individuals without a colon, or greater than 60 cm (24 inches) if a portion of the colon is in continuity with the remaining small intestine.[73] Factors that are predictive of a poor outcome include older age, disease in the residual bowel, and removal of the ileocecal valve, the physiologic sphincter that controls the rate of passage of intestinal contents from the small to large bowel and prevents small bowel bacterial overgrowth.[74]

Intestinal Adaptation

The adaptation process of the residual small intestine to compensate for the loss of the resected area begins 24 to 48 hours after bowel resection and may continue to occur for 1 to 2 years.[75] Several factors act as stimuli for adaptation, including enteral nutrients, pancreatic biliary secretions, and intestinal hormones.[28] The ability of the remaining intestine to adjust after resection is also influenced by the area of bowel loss. The jejunum is the primary site for absorption of most nutrients, but if it is removed, the ileum usually can accommodate and take on the structural characteristics and functional roles. Even with this compensation, patients with less than 50 to 60 cm (<20–24 inches) of jejunum typically need indefinite PN. With ileal resection, the jejunum has a decreased capacity to adapt and perform the functions of the ileum.[75]

Energy Requirements

Caloric intake and energy needs of SBS patients are highly variable. Individuals who have lost >50% of their small intestine typically require 25 to 30 kcal/kg (105–126 kJ/kg) of ideal body weight when receiving PN, but they may need to ingest 50 to 60 kcal/kg (209–251 kJ/kg) of ideal body weight when receiving enteral feedings to compensate for malabsorption.[72,76] This condition is referred to as *adaptive hyperphagia*.[77]

Carbohydrates

Carbohydrate malabsorption plays a major role in diarrhea associated with SBS. Unabsorbed carbohydrates, especially simple carbohydrates, represent a substantial osmotic load in patients with SBS and are associated with an increased output. In patients with an intact colon, however, soluble fiber and complex carbohydrates are broken down by colonic bacteria to short-chain fatty acids, hydrogen, and methane. This fermentation causes flatulence; however, the colon is able to use the short-chain fatty acids as a source of energy. Thus, complex carbohydrates may provide a significant caloric source for patients with a massive resection and a preserved colon.[73]

Fat

Fat malabsorption also is common in SBS. The pathophysiology of this problem is complex and related to alterations in pancreatic enzyme secretion and bile salt absorption. The ileum is the major site of the latter process, and with its removal, bile salt malabsorption is common. Eventually, the total bile salt pool may be depleted, resulting in increased fat malabsorption and steatorrhea.[71] There has been much debate regarding the restriction of oral fats, which may decrease steatorrhea, number of stools, and stool weight in some patients. Fats have the highest number of kilocalories per gram and make the diet more palatable; thus, patients with SBS without a colon should not be restricted in the amount of fats they take in. For patients with SBS but with a healthy colon, a diet higher in complex carbohydrates and lower in fat may result in lower stool volume and electrolyte loss, so this type of diet may be more beneficial.[73] Medium-chain triglycerides have also been suggested for patients with SBS and an intact colon, as MCTs are better absorbed than long-chain triglycerides. MCTs may be especially useful in decreasing steatorrhea in patients with bile acid or pancreatic insufficiency. Care must be taken, however, because medium-chain triglycerides do not contain essential fatty acids.[71,73]

Protein

Protein typically is well tolerated as a caloric source in patients with SBS. The optimal form for the delivery of protein to patients with SBS is the subject of much study and debate.[73] In the past, EN was often initiated with elemental formulas that contain free amino acids as the protein source because the efficiency of protein uptake was perceived to be better. However, total protein absorption is faster and more complete with dipeptide and tripeptide formulations. Absorption of free amino acids by the enteral route is a saturable process, whereas the absorption of small peptides is not. These more complex protein sources also may stimulate intestinal adaptation.[75] The American Gastroenterological Association now recommends that standard enteral formulas be used preferentially in SBS.[72]

Fluid, Electrolyte, and Acid–Base Disorders

❻ After substantial resections of the small bowel, the postoperative course is complicated by fluid and electrolyte imbalances that typically last 1 to 3 months.[75] Patients may have high-volume gastric fluid loss from nasogastric tubes and small intestine fluid loss from ostomies. Sodium content usually is elevated in these secretions, with concentrations reaching 80 to 100 mEq/L (80–100 mmol/L).[71] Acute gastric hypersecretion may occur after massive resection and contribute significantly to these deficits.[75] Secretory diarrhea (see Chapter 43) also results in fluid and electrolyte losses that may be difficult to quantify.

Patients with end jejunostomies or proximal ileostomies (surgically created openings into the jejunum and ileum, respectively, that divert the intestinal contents externally through a stoma) can have recurrent dehydration and electrolyte deficiencies. A high jejunostomy can produce fluid output of 3 to 4 L/day, with sodium loss of 90 mEq/L (90 mmol/L). To overcome the net secretion of sodium and water into the jejunum, the sodium content of fluids ingested by the patient needs to be ~90 mEq/L (90 mmol/L). In patients who have a small intestine in continuity with the colon, the malabsorbed bile and fatty acids stimulate sodium and water excretion into the large bowel, but in general, these patients are at less risk for sodium and water depletion.[71]

Patients with a jejunostomy and individuals with long-term sodium depletion, magnesium deficiency, or excessive loss from diarrhea are at risk for hypokalemia.[70] Metabolic alkalosis, which may occur when a patient becomes dehydrated, accelerates the renal excretion of potassium, as all hydrogen ions are conserved in an attempt to correct the acid–base disorder. As bicarbonate ions are excreted renally, potassium is taken with them to maintain osmotic balance.

The unusually large amount of unabsorbed fatty acids within the remaining small intestine and colon of the patient with SBS will cause increased binding to calcium, resulting in a deficiency. This also may result in hyperoxaluria because dietary oxalate usually complexes with the intraluminal calcium and is excreted in the stool. As a result of decreased calcium available for binding, more oxalate is absorbed and available for renal excretion; thus, the risk of calcium oxalate renal stone formation is increased.[73] Because vitamin D deficiency results in insufficient calcium absorption, patients with SBS requiring long-term PN are at risk for metabolic bone disease. Magnesium deficiency is common in patients with large ostomy or diarrheal losses. This deficiency should be corrected aggressively because of the correlation between low magnesium and potassium concentrations with the development of calcium oxalate stones. Serum concentrations are commonly monitored, but urinary magnesium concentrations may decrease earlier with deficiency and be a better estimate of total body stores than serum levels. Oral supplementation may be difficult because it can contribute to increased diarrhea or ostomy output. However, repletion is necessary to prevent complications and to effectively correct potassium deficits.[70]

Patients with SBS can lose substantial amounts of chloride (60–140 mEq/L [60–140 mmol/L]) in addition to sodium from ostomy output. These individuals have a high risk of developing hypochloremic metabolic alkalosis. Patients who have SBS complicated by a pancreatic fistula and severe diarrhea lose considerable potassium and bicarbonate and may develop metabolic acidosis. Patients with severe diarrhea who have an intact colon will conserve sodium and chloride, resulting in considerable loss of potassium and bicarbonate and the development of metabolic acidosis. Quantifying fluid losses with particular attention to the sources of loss will aid in the acid–base management of these patients (see Chapter 61).

Lactic acidosis can occur in patients with SBS who have an intact colon and may result in symptoms of ataxia and delirium.[75] D-lactic acid is produced by the fermentation of malabsorbed carbohydrates by colonic bacteria, and increased concentrations are associated with small bowel bacterial overgrowth. The diagnosis of D-lactic acidosis should be considered in patients with a functional colon who have an unexplained metabolic acidosis and an elevated anion gap.[75]

Trace Elements

Patients with SBS are particularly prone to zinc deficiency as a result of excessive losses from stool, ostomy outputs, and fistula drainage. Although serum zinc concentrations are not always reflective of body zinc status, a low serum zinc concentration requires an adjustment in the replacement amount.[71] Significant bowel resection, GI losses, and impaired intestinal absorption also contribute to imbalances of other trace elements, such as copper, selenium, and manganese. Because trace element deficiencies are common, the need for supplementation of these micronutrients is essential for SBS patients, including those receiving PN, EN, or an adequate diet.[75]

Vitamins

❼ Patients with ileal resection commonly develop vitamin B$_{12}$ deficiency, necessitating therapy with parenteral or intranasal cyanocobalamin. Most other water-soluble vitamins are absorbed in the proximal jejunum, and deficits of these vitamins are less common. There are reports, however, of SBS patients with symptomatic thiamine, folate, and biotin deficiencies.[71] Small bowel bacterial overgrowth can contribute to diminished vitamin B$_{12}$ because bacteria may metabolize the nutrient within the intestine, decreasing its availability for absorption. Patients with SBS with fat malabsorption can acquire deficiencies in vitamins A, D, E, and K.[71]

TREATMENT

■ DESIRED OUTCOMES

The desired outcomes of the nutritional management of patients with SBS are to provide effective energy, protein, micronutrients, and fluids in amounts adequate to maintain patient health and normal growth, avoid complications of SBS or the nutrition support regimen, and optimize quality of life.[70] Finally, one wants to maximize the use of the GI tract for nutrient provision to maintain GI tract function.

■ GENERAL APPROACH TO TREATMENT

After intestinal resection, the clinical course and nutritional management of patients with SBS may be described in three stages (Fig. 152–3).[72,74] The first stage typically covers the initial postoperative week; however, it may continue for up to 3 months. It is complicated by major fluid and electrolyte losses (up to 5 L/day).

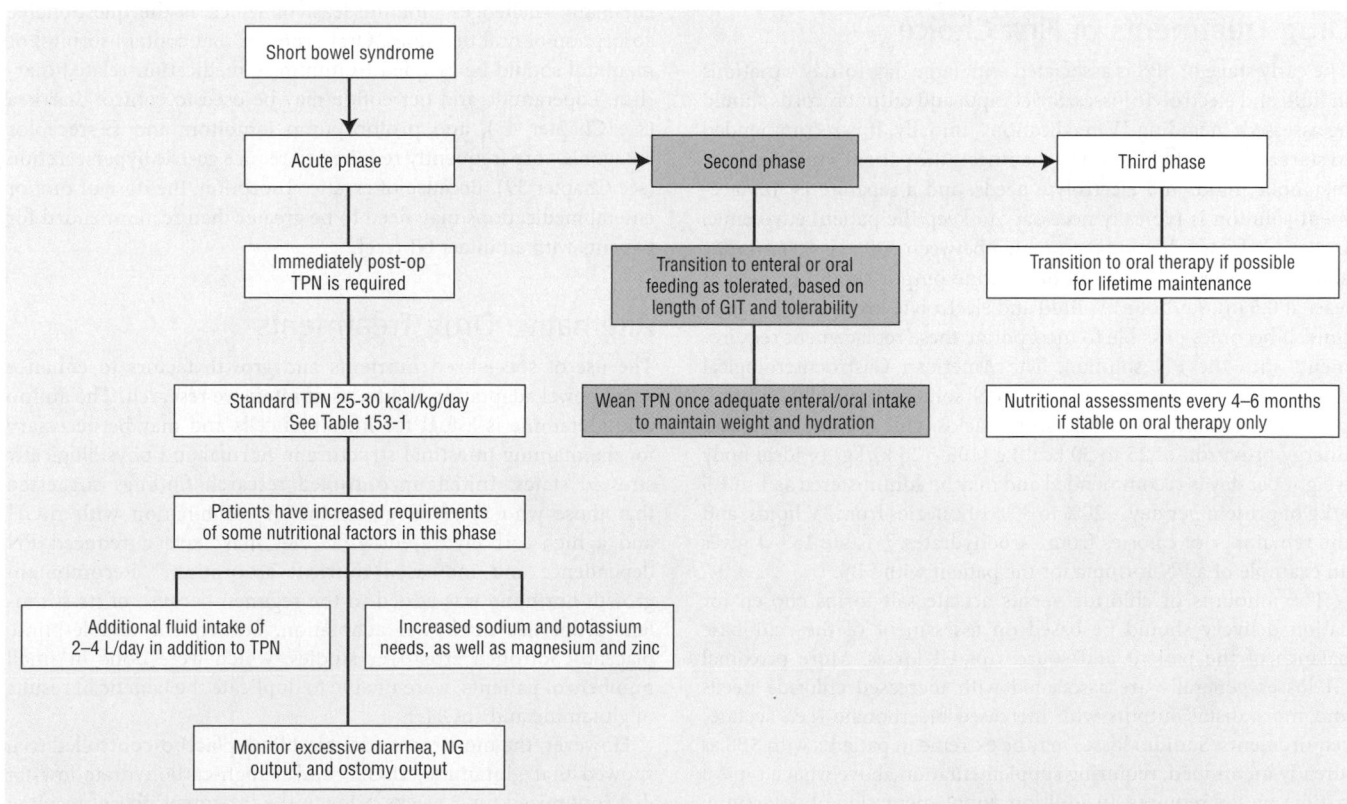

FIGURE 153-3. An algorithmic approach to nutritional support for the patient with short bowel syndrome. Energy intake of 25 to 30 kcal/kg/day is equivalent to 105 to 126 kJ/kg/day. GIT, gastrointestinal tract; NG, nasogastric; TPN, total parenteral nutrition. *Adapted from data in reference 70 and 72.*

The parenteral route should be used to supply nutritional needs during this stage of recovery.

❽ The second stage lasts from a few months to longer than a year, and institution of enteral or oral intake early during this stage is important because intraluminal nutrients are essential stimuli for intestinal adaptation. The amount of enteral/oral nutrition can be advanced as the patient tolerates; concomitantly, the duration and/or rate of PN may be decreased. If a PN regimen is to be reduced or discontinued, it should be done slowly; initially, 1 or 2 nights of PN may be eliminated each week. In the third and final stage, adaptation is maximized, and many patients can be maintained with oral nutrition alone. However, PN may not be required on a daily basis for some. Eventually, some patients may be able to tolerate administration on an every-other-night or every-third-night basis.[74,75]

■ NONPHARMACOLOGIC THERAPY

Initially, surgical management focuses on preserving as much GI tract as possible. Intestinal transplantation is a surgical treatment option for some patients with SBS, and ~1,200 such procedures have been performed worldwide as of 2006.[70] With refinement of patient selection and surgical techniques, the 1-year survival rate after small bowel transplantation is 88% to 92%, which is similar to that of those receiving home PN. Five-year survival, however, is still poorer than that reported in patients receiving home PN.[78] After transplantation, the majority of survivors are able to completely discontinue PN.[70] Small bowel transplantation is currently reserved for those patients with SBS who fail PN therapy because of recurrent line sepsis, loss of vascular access, PN-induced liver failure, or frequent severe dehydration.[72] As patient selection and immunosuppressive regimens continue to evolve, the indications for small bowel transplantation will likely expand.

■ PHARMACOLOGIC THERAPY

Drug Treatments of First Choice

The early stage of SBS is associated with large day-to-day variations in fluid and electrolyte losses. Strict input and output records should be assessed, including IV medications. Initially, it is recommended to start a standard PN solution that meets the patient's maintenance metabolic, fluid, and electrolyte needs, and a separate IV replacement solution is typically necessary to keep the patient euvolemic. Insensible losses should be estimated between 300 and 800 mL/day above measured output, and daily urine output should be kept at least at 0.5 mL/kg/hour. As fluid and electrolyte losses stabilize over time, it becomes possible to incorporate these replacement requirements into the PN solution. The American Gastroenterological Association recommends that the PN solution typically be composed of standard crystalline amino acids, glucose, and IV lipids. Energy provision of 25 to 30 kcal/kg (105–126 kJ/kg) of ideal body weight per day is recommended and may be administered as 1 to 1.5 g/kg of protein per day, ~20% to 30% of calories from IV lipids, and the remainder of calories from carbohydrates.[72] Table 153–1 gives an example of a PN formula for the patient with SBS.

The amounts of chloride versus acetate salt forms chosen for cation delivery should be based on assessment of the acid–base balance of the patient and sources of GI losses. More proximal GI losses generally are associated with increased chloride needs and more distal outputs with increased bicarbonate (i.e., acetate) requirements. Sodium losses may be extreme in patients with SBS as already mentioned, requiring supplementation above what a typical patient on PN requires. In addition, supplementation of potassium, calcium, magnesium, zinc, or other micronutrients over their maintenance amounts may be necessary to meet replacement needs.[75]

The transition from PN to enteral feedings is desirable because EN serves as a stimulus for intestinal adaptation. Thus, EN should be instituted as the patient progresses throughout the postoperative period.[71] Enteral nutrition, given as a continuous infusion through a nasogastric or gastric feeding tube, may be advantageous over bolus feedings because it can maximize absorptive capacity, decrease recovery time, and minimize diarrhea.[75] Although specialized and elemental formulas have been studied, standard EN formulations are preferred in SBS.[72] Avoiding lactose-containing foods and enteral formulations is also appropriate in patients who have extensive jejunal resection or who demonstrate lactose intolerance.[71]

Small volumes (600–1,000 mL/day) of oral electrolyte solutions, such as low-carbohydrate sports drinks and sugar- and caffeine-free beverages, are optimal for patients with a colon, and oral rehydration solutions (with ~90 mEq/L [90 mmol/L] of sodium) for those without a colon. Frequent, small amounts of solid food composed primarily of complex carbohydrates and proteins (600–1,000 kcal/day [2,511–4,186 kJ/day]) have been recommended, with avoidance of concentrated sweets and dairy products.[73] When a patient is able to maintain hydration and weight via EN and/or eating, PN may be tapered.[74] Many factors must be considered once a patient with SBS begins to transition off interventional nutrition when determining the content of a long-term oral diet. Factors such as the site and length of remaining intestine, tolerance, and patient acceptance must be considered. Fat generally is not restricted in patients without a colon. However, patients with a colon may experience more diarrhea with a high-fat diet and may benefit from oral intake that has more calories from carbohydrates and less fat content.[73] The oral diet for patients with remaining functional colon also must account for oxalate content, and patients should avoid foods with high amounts of oxalate (e.g., spinach, parsley, rhubarb, cocoa, and tea) to decrease formation of calcium oxalate renal stones.[73] Finally, oral diets in patients with SBS often need to be supplemented to maintain electrolyte, mineral, vitamin, and trace element balance.

The delivery of medications to patients with SBS may present many challenges, not the least of which is the questionable absorption of oral therapies. Oral products that contain sorbitol or mannitol should be avoided to minimize medication-related diarrhea. Loperamide and octreotide may be used to control diarrhea (see Chapter 43), and proton-pump inhibitors and H_2-receptor antagonists are frequently required to reduce gastric hypersecretion (see Chapter 39). Because of erratic absorption, the dose of oral or enteral medications may need to be greater than recommended for patients with an intact GI tract.

Alternative Drug Treatments

The use of specialized nutrients and growth factors to enhance small bowel adaptation is a focus of intensive research. The amino acid glutamine is a fuel for intestinal cells and may be necessary for maintaining intestinal structure in normal and physiologically stressed states. Initial uncontrolled research findings suggested that those who received glutamine in combination with rhGH and a high-carbohydrate/low-fat diet may have a reduced PN dependence and increased nutrient absorption.[79] Recombinant growth hormone was added to the regimen because of its stimulant properties on bowel adaptation. Subsequent double-blind, placebo-controlled crossover studies, which were done in small numbers of patients, were unable to duplicate the beneficial results of glutamine and rhGH.[80]

However, the most recent double-blind, placebo-controlled trial showed that glutamine, rhGH, and a high-carbohydrate/low-fat diet (optimized for 2 weeks prior to the treatment phase) resulted in a significant reduction in PN volume and caloric requirements.[76] Patients in the group receiving glutamine and rhGH were able to maintain their nutritional status while decreasing their average PN requirements from 5 to 6 days per week down to 2 days per week.[76] In the wake of this study, the FDA approved one form of rhGH for use in patients with SBS who are receiving specialized nutrition support.

A consensus panel convened by a manufacturer of rhGH recommended the FDA-labeled dose of 0.1 mg/kg subcutaneously daily for 4 weeks be considered a reasonable therapeutic intervention. The panel suggested that appropriate patients are PN-dependent patients who are nutritionally stable and on an optimized diet and medication regimen, and that treatment be given 6 to 24 months after bowel resection.[80] This treatment, however, is not recommended by the American Gastroenterological Association.[72] Other experts question the benefit of rhGH and suggested that before incorporating it into SBS treatment, it should be studied during the adaptive phase of SBS.[71] The safety of prolonged use of rhGH is also unknown.

CLINICAL CONTROVERSY

Although there are some data indicating that rhGH in combination with dietary optimization and glutamine may decrease PN dependence in patients with SBS, the role of these therapies is still not well defined. There are conflicting data as to whether this therapy enhances nutrient absorption. The timing of therapy and the identification of appropriate patient populations are also still areas of active research.

■ PHARMACOECONOMIC CONSIDERATIONS

Nutritional management of SBS is quite costly, especially in patients who require home PN. One year of home PN therapy is estimated to cost $100,000.[78] This figure does not include home nursing, equipment, and the costs of intermittent hospitalizations. Significant savings may be realized in patients who are able to transition from PN, but this is unlikely to occur in patients who are still PN dependent after 2 years. A study in pediatric patients found the average total cost of care for the first year following SBS was $505, 250 and over the first 5 years was $619,851.[81]

No analyses have yet been published that describe the economic consequences of the potential PN-reducing effect of rhGH.[80] It has been reported that intestinal transplantation is a cost-effective intervention relative to the cost of home parenteral nutrition in patients who survive for 2 years postoperatively.[82]

■ EVALUATION OF THERAPEUTIC OUTCOMES

Therapeutic monitoring of patients with SBS who are receiving PN for metabolic complications should follow the guidelines outlined in Chapter 151. This patient population differs in that serum electrolytes should be obtained daily until the patient has stabilized postoperatively. Special consideration should also be given to the fluid status of patients with SBS, especially in the period immediately following surgery, when fluid losses are extreme. Monitoring of stool output is such a large factor that it must be taken into consideration for all such patients. Because many patients with SBS remain on PN for extended periods of time, clinicians must be careful to monitor for elevations in liver enzymes, and cycling PN for 12 to 14 hours daily should be considered in those patients to minimize these complications. Obtaining a serum fatty acid profile may be judicious in those patients on long-term PN without oral intake to ensure they do not have essential fatty acid deficiency.[83]

The most comprehensive and thorough analysis of the clinical outcomes of patients receiving home PN or EN comes from Medicare and the North American Home Parenteral and Enteral Patient Registry.[84] It was estimated that 40,000 and 152,000 patients in the United States were receiving home PN and EN support, respectively as of 1995. Patients with GI failure, which included those with Crohn disease, ischemic bowel disease, motility disorders, and congenital bowel defects, had relatively good clinical outcomes, especially when compared with the groups with cancer or acquired immune deficiency syndrome. The patients with GI failure had an 87% annual survival rate and a 50% to 75% likelihood of complete rehabilitation. Sepsis, metabolic disorders, and mechanical problems with catheters resulted in one or two hospitalizations per year for all patients.[84]

■ QUALITY-OF-LIFE ISSUES

Initially, those patients on extended PN therapy have a significant gain in QOL when transitioning from the hospital to their home setting. This is often followed by the reality of restrictions in daily living, dehydration and malnutrition despite PN, and complications such as sepsis and liver dysfunction. Patients with SBS on home PN have reported that their QOL is significantly reduced in comparison to those with anatomic or functional SBS not on home PN.[80] There are currently no data assessing the effect of treatment with growth factors such as rhGH on QOL, although one might expect to see an improvement. Valid comparisons of home PN and intestinal transplantation are not available, as a consequence of the limited indications for transplantation.[82] Preparing patients and their caregivers for the possible stresses associated with this therapy (e.g., financial challenges, fatigue, depression, complications, and social or emotional problems) through education and referral to support groups, such as the Oley Foundation, may help to increase QOL.[85]

PULMONARY FAILURE

Nutrition support is an important aspect of preventing and treating both acute and chronic pulmonary failure. Malnourished patients are at increased risk of acute respiratory distress syndrome (ARDS), and malnutrition in patients with chronic obstructive pulmonary disease (COPD) is well documented. There is also a correlation between the outcomes of patients with alterations in nutritional status and concurrent pulmonary diseases.[86] Loss of lean muscle mass is detrimental because the depletion of diaphragm and intercostal muscles makes the effort of breathing harder, and progression of weight loss leads to muscle fatigue and respiratory failure. The ventilatory drive, as well as compensation to hypoxia, is depressed in patients with COPD who are malnourished, and nutritional support plays a key role in optimizing respiratory muscle function in patients with pulmonary disease.[87]

EPIDEMIOLOGY

More than 10% of the U.S. population over 45 years of age have COPD, resulting in significant cost to the healthcare system.[87] Weight loss and protein–calorie malnutrition may occur in up to half of these patients, and weight loss often coincides with disease progression.[28,87] In those with acute respiratory failure, nutritional abnormalities have been reported in up to 70%.[86] Engelen et al evaluated the body composition of patients with COPD, specifically those with emphysema and chronic bronchitis. They found a higher incidence of lean mass depletion in patients with emphysema than in those with chronic bronchitis. Body weight and body mass index (BMI) were also lower in the group with emphysema.[88] In a subsequent evaluation, the same investigators reported that skeletal muscle weakness was associated with wasting of extremity fat-free mass that was independent of COPD subtype.[89] Finally, malnutrition is associated with an increased mortality rate in patients with COPD with low BMI.[90]

PATHOPHYSIOLOGY

Energy Requirements

❾ Patients with COPD have highly variable REE, and commonly used predictive measures may underestimate their energy needs.[91] Those who are losing weight tend to have significantly higher REE adjusted for fat-free mass compared with weight-stable patients. Total daily energy expenditure also was found to be elevated in clinically stable COPD patients with both normal and increased REE. The cause of elevated total daily energy expenditure despite a normal REE is still unknown, although the oxygen cost of breathing, acute or chronic systemic inflammation, and medications may contribute.[86] Although the optimal approach to energy needs in COPD has not been identified, it is evident that there is no advantage to providing 1.7 × REE compared with 1.3 × REE.[92] Hypermetabolism likely contributes to the decreased body weight and fat-free mass, although it has been shown that in this patient population, intake may be suboptimal. During meals hypoxic patients tend to experience decreases in oxygen saturation and increased dyspnea. Gastric filling may also be impaired because of diaphragmatic expansion and a false feeling of fullness.[86] These problems, combined with increased daily requirements, may result in the negative energy balance seen in many patients with COPD. Several specialized equations have been developed to estimate energy requirements in this patient population, and indirect calorimetry may be used, but clinical benefit is questionable. Patients with acute respiratory failure also may have alterations in energy expenditure, but the situation is similar in that predictive formulas for energy needs exist, and indirect calorimetry may be used. Providing excess calories to the acutely ill patient in respiratory failure should be avoided because this may increase CO_2 production and the associated work of breathing.[28,87]

Carbohydrates

Malnutrition in patients with pulmonary disease has been consistently identified in the literature, and nutrition support should be considered as part of the overall treatment plan. However, increasing nutritional intake can be complicated because it may elevate the respiratory quotient, which may lead to a corresponding increase in the work of breathing and resulting hypercapnia. The respiratory quotient is the ratio of the amount of CO_2 produced divided by the amount of O_2 consumed. When a subject is overfed, the amount of CO_2 produced markedly exceeds the amount of O_2 consumed, which can result in increased ventilatory demand.[93] Ventilatory drive may be improved in some patients with moderate infusions of carbohydrates; however, administration of glucose formulas at a rate greater than 5 mg/kg/min has been shown to increase production of CO_2 and is associated with the inability to wean from mechanical ventilation.[87]

Fat

Fats have the lowest respiratory quotient, but administration of IV fat emulsions to mechanically ventilated patients has the potential to adversely affect pulmonary gas exchange in some clinical conditions.[94]

The administration of lipid emulsions to patients with ARDS may decrease oxygenation. A trial assessing both long-chain triglyceride and combination long-chain triglyceride/medium-chain triglyceride administration showed that there was no deleterious effect on oxygenation. Discrepancies in trial data may be a result of differing lipid infusion rates and duration, as well as preexisting lung status.[95] Rapid administration of IV lipids should be avoided; a rate of 3 mg/kg/min increases pulmonary vascular resistance in patients with ARDS.[95] A review of nutritional intervention in ambulatory patients with COPD revealed that diets high in fat placed a lower demand on the respiratory system in comparison to diets with a higher carbohydrate content. In addition to an improvement in forced expiratory volume, the number of breaths needed per minute decreased within 3 weeks in patients with COPD who switched to a high-fat/low-carbohydrate diet.[93] Although these effects are important, the most critical element in managing patients with pulmonary compromise is avoiding overfeeding.[28]

Protein

Undernourished patients demonstrate a blunted response to hypercapnia that improves after as little as 1 week of adequate nutritional support. This response is thought to result from protein administration, as evidenced by decreased partial CO_2 pressure, increased minute ventilation, and improved breathing patterns after the start of PN. Protein administration also may influence ventilatory demand by increasing ventilatory response to hypoxia and hypercapnia. This stimulation may be altered by the amino acid composition of the protein source, with increased amounts of branched-chain amino acids having a greater effect compared with standard amino acids. Although this protein effect is potentially beneficial in some patients, excessive protein administration could theoretically lead to increased work of breathing and fatigue.[87]

Fluid, Electrolyte, and Acid–Base Disorders

❿ In patients with ARDS or pulmonary edema, excessive fluid intake should be avoided, as fluid accumulation is associated with a poor outcome. Patients in the ICU often receive substantial fluid loads from medication administration... When possible, it is important to limit intake by concentrating these sources.[28,87]

Alteration of micronutrient requirements in respiratory failure is commonly focused on phosphorus replacement. Phosphorus has an essential role in the synthesis of adenosine triphosphate (ATP) and 2,3-diphosphoglycerate (2,3-DPG). Inadequate stores of ATP can lead to respiratory muscle weakness, and normal contractility of the diaphragm muscles is dependent on phosphate.[87] Finally, a significant percentage of critically ill patients experience hypophosphatemia from refeeding. Most patients with moderate to severe hypophosphatemia and respiratory failure should be treated with IV sodium or potassium phosphate (see Chapter 59). Correction of hypophosphatemia in patients in the ICU receiving nutritional support with a graduated weight-based dosing scheme of phosphorus replacement has been reported.[96]

Ventilator-dependent patients and those with stable COPD often have respiratory acidosis. A balanced mixture of chloride and acetate salts often is appropriate in these patients. The acid–base status of the patient in the ICU with pulmonary compromise should be monitored daily, whereas every 2 to 3 days may be adequate for the stable hospitalized patient with COPD.

Vitamins and Trace Elements

Patients with pulmonary disease usually do not have significant alterations in vitamin and trace element requirements, and they can receive standard doses of these micronutrients. There are some data that support the supplementation of vitamin C, vitamin E, and β-carotene because of a correlation with moderately improved pulmonary function. Patients with COPD may have an increased burden of oxidants from cigarette smoke or release of oxygen free radicals from inflammatory leukocytes in the lungs, and deficiencies of antioxidants may contribute to oxidant/antioxidant imbalances in these individuals.[97]

TREATMENT

■ DESIRED OUTCOMES

In patients with pulmonary failure, nutritional support should be given to meet energy and protein requirements and to limit wasting of respiratory muscles. In stable patients with COPD, this may be done in addition to exercise rehabilitation programs to optimize weight and fat-free body mass. To date, nutrition support has not been shown to affect long-term survival in these patients.[98]

■ GENERAL APPROACH TO TREATMENT

When oral feedings are inadequate, ASPEN recommends that EN be used in those who have a functional gut and can meet their needs through this route.[28] PN is recommended when the GI tract is not usable or as a supplement to EN if sufficient energy intake is otherwise not possible.[28,87]

Most general EN formulas contain an equal balance of nonprotein energy between carbohydrates and fat. Elemental or chemically defined products are the exception because they are intended to be high-carbohydrate, low-fat formulas to enhance absorption and digestion. In pulmonary patients, administration of a high-carbohydrate formula may result in a significant increase in minute ventilation, heat production, and CO_2 production when compared with a high-fat formula. Because most general formulas contain balanced nonprotein calories, moderate doses of these products may be appropriate in most patients with pulmonary disease.[26,90] Patients who are fluid restricted should be given a higher energy formulation so as to maintain an appropriate fluid balance.[28]

■ NONPHARMACOLOGIC THERAPY

Patient education and nutritional counseling are essential to maximizing the health of patients with COPD. Education about appropriate energy and caloric intake and the proper use of oral nutritional supplements may enhance patient adherence to these practices. Ambulatory patients with COPD may also benefit from a pulmonary rehabilitation program that integrates diet, supplements, and exercise.[90]

■ PHARMACOLOGIC THERAPY

Drug Treatment of First Choice

Moderate doses of carbohydrate, fat, and protein given enterally are appropriate in most conditions. Total calorie provision 30% above basal energy expenditure does not have any untoward effects on pulmonary status. However, patients who are overfed, that is, those who are receiving twice the basal energy expenditure, often produce excessive CO_2. Critically ill patients with respiratory failure can be fed 25 to 30 kcal/kg/day (105–126 kJ/kg/day) as they recover.[28,99] In patients with borderline ventilatory status, the nutritional regimen should be monitored closely to prevent excessive CO_2 production, and increasing the proportion of nonprotein calories as fat relative to the amount of carbohydrates may be beneficial.[87]

A concentrated enteral formula (Oxepa) has been marketed specifically for critically ill patients on mechanical ventilation and studied in patients with acute lung injury and ARDS. The macronutrient composition of Oxepa is similar to that of the other specialized pulmonary enteral formulas, with 55% of the nonprotein caloric content being from fat. However, the lipid blend in the formula was altered to decrease the production of proinflammatory cytokines by including eicosapentaenoic acid from fish oil and γ-linolenic acid from borage oil. Nutrients with antioxidant properties (i.e., vitamin C, vitamin E, and β-carotene) also are included in this product.[100,101] This formulation is associated with improved respiratory mechanics, decreased ventilatory dependence, and an attenuation of the inflammatory state in those with acute lung injury/ARDS. In one study of patients with a diagnosis of ARDS, as well as severe sepsis/septic shock, the use of this formulation resulted in a statistically significant decrease in 28-day mortality. These results have led ASPEN and the Society of Critical Care Medicine to recommend the preferential use of this product in critically ill patients with severe acute lung injury or ARDS.[28,26,99]

In general, patients with ARDS who need PN may receive nonprotein calories administered within the following ranges: 60% to 70% carbohydrate and 30% to 40% lipid. A reasonable protein dose is 1 to 1.5 g/kg/day for the patient with stable COPD. Patients who are mechanically ventilated with superimposed illness may require higher doses of protein (1.5–2.5 g/kg/day). Figure 153–4 illustrates an approach to the patient with acute respiratory failure requiring PN or EN support based on recommendations from ASPEN and ESPEN.[28,99] Table 153–1 includes an empirical PN formula for the patient with respiratory failure.

CLINICAL CONTROVERSY

There are conflicting data on the safety of administration of lipid emulsions to patients with ARDS. Discrepancies in trial data may be due to the use of differing lipid infusion rates and duration, as well as preexisting lung function.

Alternative Drug Therapies

Enteral formulas (e.g., Pulmocare) marketed for use specifically in patients with pulmonary disease are commercially available. These products contain a higher percentage of nonprotein calories as fat (>50%). Several studies evaluated the use of these high-fat/low-carbohydrate products in patients with COPD and acute respiratory failure, and generally the outcomes were favorable.[93] These specialized pulmonary EN products are calorically dense (1.5 kcal/mL [6.3 kJ/mL]), which may be helpful for patients with severe ARDS or pulmonary edema, as well as others who may require fluid restriction. There are no data, however, indicating that these formulas result in improved clinical outcomes in patients with pulmonary failure. Nonspecialty formulations and high-concentration formulations for those requiring fluid restriction are still preferred for routine use.[28,90]

Recombinant human growth hormone is known to induce general muscle growth, lipolysis, and protein anabolism. When used as adjunctive therapy to EN support, patients with COPD have shown improvements in lean body mass, maximal inspiratory pressure, and exercise capacity. The benefit of rhGH is debatable, with trials having differing results, but body mass and fat-free mass typically increase in patients after use of this product. The benefit in pulmonary patients as shown by improvements in respiratory muscle function and pulmonary function testing is questionable. The effects of anabolic steroids also have been evaluated for use in COPD as an adjunct to nutritional intervention. Patients on anabolic steroids tend to have larger increases in fat-free mass and

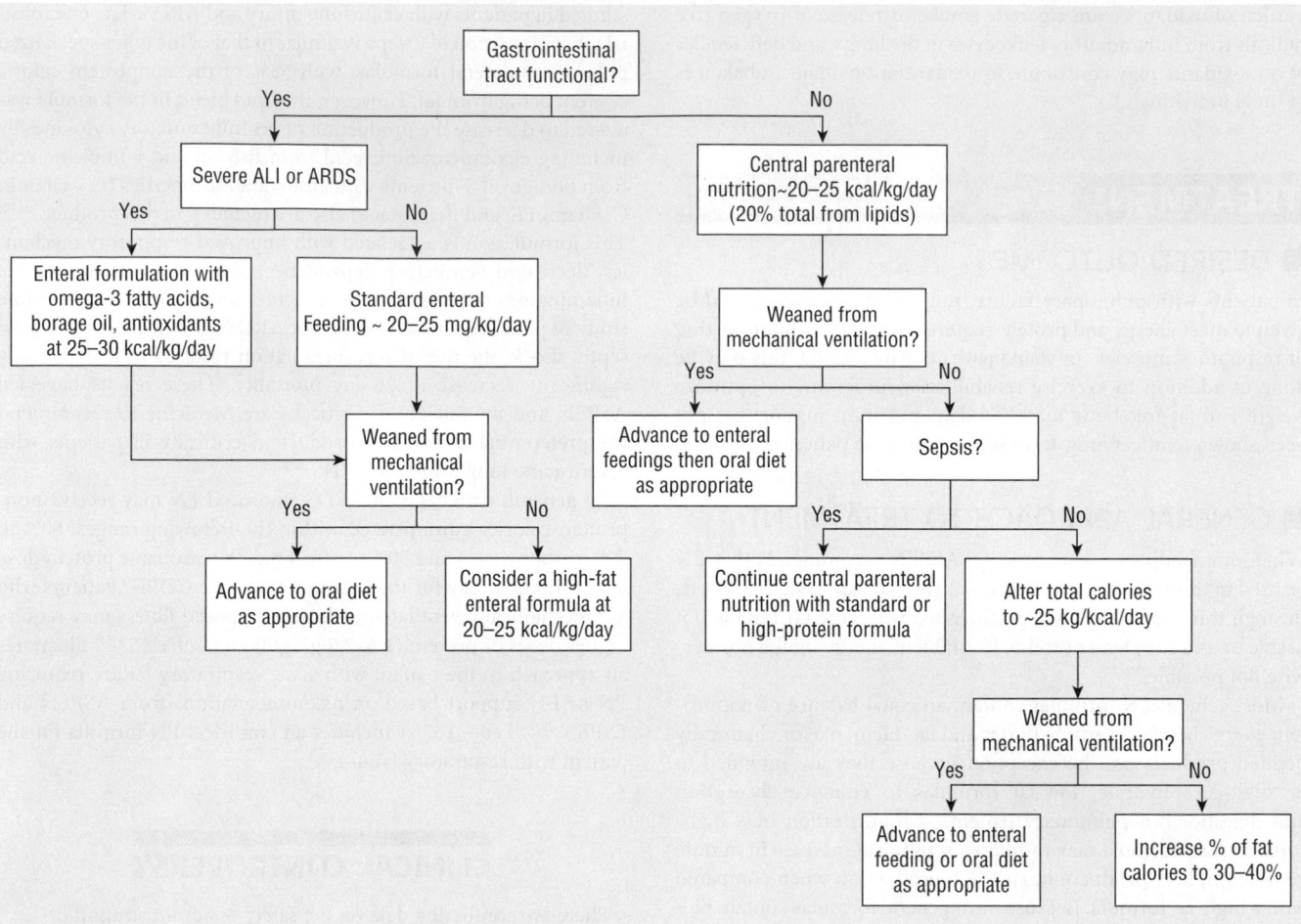

FIGURE 153-4. An algorithmic approach to nutritional support for the patient with acute respiratory failure. Energy intake of 20 to 25 kcal/kg/day is equivalent to 84 to 105 kJ/kg/day. Energy intake of 25 to 30 kcal/kg/day is equivalent to 105 to 126 kJ/kg/day.

more favorable distributions in weight gain in comparison to interventional nutrition alone.[102] More studies are needed to characterize the benefits of rhGH, as well as anabolic steroids, and to determine the risk-to-benefit ratio.

PHARMACOECONOMIC CONSIDERATIONS

There are no data available that establish the pharmacoeconomic value of nutrition support in patients with respiratory failure.

EVALUATION OF THERAPEUTIC OUTCOMES

Because pulmonary patients are at extreme risk of malnutrition, monitoring the progression of the patient on interventional nutrition is extremely important. Therapeutic monitoring of pulmonary patients on PN for metabolic complications should follow the guidelines presented in Chapter 151. Patients on EN should be monitored as described in Chapter 152. Pulmonary status must be assessed for any changes, especially with the initiation of higher carbohydrate formulas of PN or EN. Weights should be charted frequently, and it is important that prealbumin concentrations are assessed weekly for hospitalized patients. It is important to remember that patients with ARDS in critical care units are prone to fluid overload from medication administration, so careful monitoring of intake and output is necessary to avoid pulmonary edema. Nutritional status should be monitored every 4 to 6 months for those patients with stable pulmonary disease and COPD.

QUALITY-OF-LIFE ISSUES

Patients with COPD who have fat-free mass depletion experience decreased disease-specific QOL when compared with control patients.[103] Decreased activity and exercise capacity are associated with low fat-free mass, which appears to be related to decreasing patient satisfaction.[86] Dyspnea also has been shown to be correlated strongly with health-related QOL in patients with decreased fat-free mass and may be the strongest predictor of patient satisfaction. Nutrition support supplementation has not been shown to definitively improve QOL in COPD. In one study, however, patients who received a diet of 1.3 × REE stated that they had an improved feeling of control over their COPD, whereas those fed 1.7 × REE did not report any improvement in QOL.[92]

ABBREVIATIONS

AKI: Acute kidney injury

ARDS: Acute respiratory distress syndrome

ASPEN: American Society for Parenteral and Enteral Nutrition

ATP: Adenosine triphosphate

CKD: Chronic kidney disease

COPD: Chronic obstructive pulmonary disease

CRRT: Continuous renal replacement therapy

EN: Enteral nutrition

ESPEN: European Society for Clinical Nutrition and Metabolism

ESRD: End-stage renal disease

HD: Hemodialysis

ICU: Intensive care unit

IDPN: Intradialytic parenteral nutrition

IVLE: Intravenous lipid emulsion

NKF K/DOQI: National Kidney Foundation Kidney Disease Outcomes Quality Initiative

PD: Peritoneal dialysis

PN: Parenteral nutrition

QOL: Quality of life

REE: Resting energy expenditure

rhGH: Recombinant human growth hormone

SBS: Short bowel syndrome

REFERENCES

1. Strejc JM. Considerations in the nutritional management of patients with acute renal failure. Hemodial Int 2005;9(2):135–142.

2. Metnitz PG, Krenn CG, Steltzer H, et al. Effect of acute renal failure requiring renal replacement therapy on outcome in critically ill patients. Crit Care Med 2002;30(9):2051–2058.

3. Fiaccadori E, Lombardi M, Leonardi S, et al. Prevalence and clinical outcome associated with preexisting malnutrition in acute renal failure: A prospective cohort study. J Am Soc Nephrol 1999;10(3):581–593.

4. Druml W. Nutritional management of acute renal failure. J Ren Nutr 2005;15(1):63–70.

5. Cano N, Fiaccadori E, Tesinsky P, et al. ESPEN guidelines on enteral nutrition: Adult renal failure. Clin Nutr 2006;25(2):295–310.

6. Bozfakioglu S. Nutrition in patients with acute renal failure. Nephrol Dial Transplant 2001;16(Suppl 6):21–22.

7. Druml W. Nutritional management of acute renal failure. Am J Kidney Dis 2001;37(1, Suppl 2):S89–S94.

8. Cano NJ, Aparicio M, Brunori G, et al. ESPEN guidelines on parenteral nutrition: Adult renal failure. Clin Nutr 2009;28(4):401–414.

9. Fiaccadori E, Parenti E, Maggiore U. Nutritional support in acute kidney injury. J Nephrol 2008;21(5):645–656.

10. Maxvold NJ, Smoyer WE, Custer JR, Bunchman TE. Amino acid loss and nitrogen balance in critically ill children with acute renal failure: A prospective comparison between classic hemofiltration and hemofiltration with dialysis. Crit Care Med 2000;28(4):1161–1165.

11. Klein CJ, Moser-Veillon PB, Schweitzer A, et al. Magnesium, calcium, zinc, and nitrogen loss in trauma patients during continuous renal replacement therapy. JPEN J Parenter Enteral Nutr 2002;26(2):77–92, discussion 93.

12. Druml W, Fischer M, Liebisch B, et al. Elimination of amino acids in renal failure. Am J Clin Nutr 1994;60(3):418–423.

13. Marin A, Hardy G. Practical implications of nutritional support during continuous renal replacement therapy. Curr Opin Clin Nutr Metab Care 2001;4(3):219–225.

14. Mehta RL. Acid-base and electrolyte management in continuous renal replacement therapy. Blood Purif 2002;20(3):262–268.

15. Heering P, Ivens K, Thumer O, et al. The use of different buffers during continuous hemofiltration in critically ill patients with acute renal failure. Intensive Care Med 1999;25(11):1244–1251.

16. Metnitz GH, Fischer M, Bartens C, et al. Impact of acute renal failure on antioxidant status in multiple organ failure. Acta Anaesthesiol Scand 2000;44(3):236–240.

17. Berger MM, Shenkin A, Revelly JP, et al. Copper, selenium, zinc, and thiamine balances during continuous venovenous hemodiafiltration in critically ill patients. Am J Clin Nutr 2004;80(2):410–416.

18. Druml W, Schwarzenhofer M, Apsner R, Horl WH. Fat-soluble vitamins in patients with acute renal failure. Miner Electrolyte Metab 1998;24(4):220–226.

19. Kalantar-Zadeh K, Kopple JD. Trace elements and vitamins in maintenance dialysis patients. Adv Ren Replace Ther 2003;10(3):170–182.

20. Bellomo R, Ronco C. How to feed patients with renal dysfunction. Curr Opin Crit Care 2000;6(4):239–246.

21. Wickersham R, ed. Drug Facts and Comparisons. St. Louis, MO: Wolters Kluwer Health; 2006.

22. Fiaccadori E, Maggiore U, Giacosa R, et al. Enteral nutrition in patients with acute renal failure. Kidney Int 2004;65(3):999–1008.

23. Scheinkestel CD, Kar L, Marshall K, et al. Prospective randomized trial to assess caloric and protein needs of critically ill, anuric, ventilated patients requiring continuous renal replacement therapy. Nutrition 2003;19(11–12):909–916.

24. Fiaccadori E, Maggiore U, Rotelli C, et al. Effects of different energy intakes on nitrogen balance in patients with acute renal failure: A pilot study. Nephrol Dial Transplant 2005;20(9):1976–1980.

25. Van den Berghe G, Wouters PJ, Bouillon R, et al. Outcome benefit of intensive insulin therapy in the critically ill: Insulin dose versus glycemic control. Crit Care Med 2003;31(2):359–366.

26. McClave SA, Martindale RG, Vanek VW, et al. Guidelines for the provision and assessment of nutrition support therapy in the adult critically ill patient: Society of Critical Care Medicine (SCCM) and American Society for Parenteral and Enteral Nutrition (A.S.P.E.N.). JPEN J Parenter Enteral Nutr 2009;33(3):277–316.

27. Bellomo R, Tan HK, Bhonagiri S, et al. High protein intake during continuous hemodiafiltration: Impact on amino acids and nitrogen balance. Int J Artif Organs 2002;25(4):261–268.

28. Guidelines for the use of parenteral and enteral nutrition in adult and pediatric patients. JPEN J Parenter Enteral Nutr 2002;26 (1 Suppl):1SA–138SA.

29. Stein MY, Stein TP. High-protein feedings and the critically ill renal patient. Nutrition 2003;19(11–12):1030–1031.

30. Korkeila M, Ruokonen E, Takala J. Costs of care, long-term prognosis and quality of life in patients requiring renal replacement therapy during intensive care. Intensive Care Med. 2000 (Dec);26(12): 1824–1831.

31. Stratton RJ, Bircher G, Fouque D, et al. Multinutrient oral supplements and tube feeding in maintenance dialysis: A systematic review and meta-analysis. Am J Kidney Dis 2005;46(3):387–405.

32. Chung SH, Lindholm B, Lee HB. Influence of initial nutritional status on continuous ambulatory peritoneal dialysis patient survival. Perit Dial Int 2000;20(1):19–26.

33. Burrowes JD, Cockram DB, Dwyer JT, et al. Cross-sectional relationship between dietary protein and energy intake, nutritional status, functional status, and comorbidity in older versus younger hemodialysis patients. J Ren Nutr 2002;12(2):87–95.

34. Wiggins KL, Harvey KS. A review of guidelines for nutrition care of renal patients. J Ren Nutr 2002;12(3):190–196.

35. Sehgal AR. Outcomes of renal replacement therapy among blacks and women. Am J Kidney Dis 2000;35(4, Suppl 1):S148–S152.

36. Vaziri ND, Moradi H. Mechanisms of dyslipidemia of chronic renal failure. Hemodial Int 2006;10(1):1–7.

37. Evans AM, Faull R, Fornasini G, et al. Pharmacokinetics of L-carnitine in patients with end-stage renal disease undergoing long-term hemodialysis. Clin Pharmacol Ther 2000;68(3):238–249.

38. Clinical practice guidelines for nutrition in chronic renal failure. K/ DOQI, National Kidney Foundation. Am J Kidney Dis 2000;35(6, Suppl 2):S1–S140.

39. Mehrotra R, Kopple JD. Nutritional management of maintenance dialysis patients: Why aren't we doing better? Annu Rev Nutr 2001;21:343–379.

40. Mak RH, Cheung W, Cone RD, Marks DL. Leptin and inflammation-associated cachexia in chronic kidney disease. Kidney Int 2006;69(5):794–797.

41. Levey AS, Adler S, Caggiula AW, et al. Effects of dietary protein restriction on the progression of advanced renal disease in the Modification of Diet in Renal Disease Study. Am J Kidney Dis 1996;27(5): 652–663.

42. Mehrotra R, Kopple JD. Protein and energy nutrition among adult patients treated with chronic peritoneal dialysis. Adv Ren Replace Ther 2003;10(3):194–212.

43. Temple KA, Smith AM, Cockram DB. Selenate-supplemented nutritional formula increases plasma selenium in hemodialysis patients. J Ren Nutr 2000;10(1):16–23.

44. Yonemura K, Fujimoto T, Fujigaki Y, Hishida A. Vitamin D deficiency is implicated in reduced serum albumin concentrations in patients with end-stage renal disease. Am J Kidney Dis 2000;36(2):337–344.

45. Islam KN, O'Byrne D, Devaraj S, et al. Alpha-tocopherol supplementation decreases the oxidative susceptibility of LDL in renal failure patients on dialysis therapy. Atherosclerosis 2000;150(1):217–224.

46. Wrone EM, Hornberger JM, Zehnder JL, et al. Randomized trial of folic acid for prevention of cardiovascular events in end-stage renal disease. J Am Soc Nephrol 2004;15(2):420–426.

47. Serna-Thome MG, Padilla-Rosciano AE, Suchil-Bernal L. Practical aspects of intradialytic nutritional support. Curr Opin Clin Nutr Metab Care 2002;5(3):293–296.

48. How PP, Lau AH. Malnutrition in patients undergoing hemodialysis: Is intradialytic parenteral nutrition the answer? Pharmacotherapy 2004;24(12):1748–1758.

49. Li FK, Chan LY, Woo JC, et al. A 3-year, prospective, randomized, controlled study on amino acid dialysate in patients on CAPD. Am J Kidney Dis 2003;42(1):173–183.

50. Iglesias P, Diez JJ, Fernandez-Reyes MJ, et al. Recombinant human growth hormone therapy in malnourished dialysis patients: A randomized controlled study. Am J Kidney Dis 1998;32(3):454–463.

51. Henkel AS, Buchman AL. Nutritional support in patients with chronic liver disease. Nat Clin Pract Gastroenterol Hepatol 2006;3(4):202–209.

52. Moriwaki H, Tajika M, Miwa Y, et al. Nutritional pharmacotherapy of chronic liver disease: From support of liver failure to prevention of liver cancer. J Gastroenterol 2000;35(Suppl 12):13–17.

53. Caly WR, Strauss E, Carrilho FJ, Laudanna AA. Different degrees of malnutrition and immunological alterations according to the aetiology of cirrhosis: A prospective and sequential study. Nutr J 2003;2:10.

54. Dudrick SJ, Kavic SM. Hepatobiliary nutrition: History and future. J Hepatobiliary Pancreat Surg 2002;9(4):459–468.

55. Plauth M, Cabre E, Riggio O, et al. ESPEN guidelines on enteral nutrition: Liver disease. Clin Nutr 2006;25(2):285–294.

56. Okamoto M, Sakaida I, Tsuchiya M, et al. Effect of a late evening snack on the blood glucose level and energy metabolism in patients with liver cirrhosis. Hepatol Res 2003;27(1):45–50.

57. Miwa Y, Shiraki M, Kato M, et al. Improvement of fuel metabolism by nocturnal energy supplementation in patients with liver cirrhosis. Hepatol Res 2000;18(3):184–189.

58. Clemmesen JO, Hoy CE, Jeppesen PB, Ott P. Plasma phospholipid fatty acid pattern in severe liver disease. J Hepatol 2000;32(3):481–487.

59. Duerksen DR, Nehra V, Palombo JD, et al. Essential fatty acid deficiencies in patients with chronic liver disease are not reversed by short-term intravenous lipid supplementation. Dig Dis Sci 1999;44(7):1342–1348.

60. Matos C, Porayko MK, Francisco-Ziller N, DiCecco S. Nutrition and chronic liver disease. J Clin Gastroenterol 2002;35(5):391–397.

61. Cordoba J, Lopez-Hellin J, Planas M, et al. Normal protein diet for episodic hepatic encephalopathy: Results of a randomized study. J Hepatol 2004;41(1):38–43.

62. Chacko RT, Chacko A. Serum and muscle magnesium in Indians with cirrhosis of liver. Indian J Med Res 1997;106:469–474.

63. Layrargues GP, Rose C, Spahr L, et al. Role of manganese in the pathogenesis of portal-systemic encephalopathy. Metab Brain Dis. 1998 Dec;13(4):311–7.

64. Dworkin B, Rosenthal WS, Jankowski RH, et al. Low blood selenium levels in alcoholics with and without advanced liver disease. Correlations with clinical and nutritional status. Dig Dis Sci. 1985;30(9):838–44.

65. Plauth M, Roske AE, Romaniuk P, et al. Post-feeding hyperammonaemia in patients with transjugular intrahepatic portosystemic shunt and liver cirrhosis: Role of small intestinal ammonia release and route of nutrient administration. Gut 2000;46(6):849–855.

66. Plauth M, Cabre E, Campillo B, et al. ESPEN guidelines on parenteral nutrition: hepatology. Clin Nutr 2009;28(4):436–444.

67. Plauth M, Schutz T, Buckendahl DP, et al. Weight gain after transjugular intrahepatic portosystemic shunt is associated with improvement in body composition in malnourished patients with cirrhosis and hypermetabolism. J Hepatol 2004;40(2):228–233.

68. Hirsch S, Bunout D, de la Maza P, et al. Controlled trial on nutrition supplementation in outpatients with symptomatic alcoholic cirrhosis. JPEN J Parenter Enteral Nutr 1993;17(2):119–124.

69. Alvares-da-Silva MR, Reverbel da Silveira T. Comparison between handgrip strength, subjective global assessment, and prognostic nutritional index in assessing malnutrition and predicting clinical outcome in cirrhotic outpatients. Nutrition 2005;21(2):113–117.

70. Nightingale J, Woodward JM. Guidelines for management of patients with a short bowel. Gut 2006;55(Suppl 4):1–12.

71. Buchman AL. Etiology and initial management of short bowel syndrome. Gastroenterology 2006;130(2, Suppl 1):S5–S15.

72. American Gastroenterological Association medical position statement: Short bowel syndrome and intestinal transplantation. Gastroenterology 2003;124(4):1105–1110.

73. Matarese LE, Steiger E. Dietary and medical management of short bowel syndrome in adult patients. J Clin Gastroenterol 2006;40 (Suppl 2):S85–S93.

74. DiBaise JK, Matarese LE, Messing B, Steiger E. Strategies for parenteral nutrition weaning in adult patients with short bowel syndrome. J Clin Gastroenterol 2006;40(Suppl 2):S94–S98.

75. Sundaram A, Koutkia P, Apovian CM. Nutritional management of short bowel syndrome in adults. J Clin Gastroenterol 2002;34(3):207–220.

76. Byrne TA, Wilmore DW, Iyer K, et al. Growth hormone, glutamine, and an optimal diet reduces parenteral nutrition in patients with short bowel syndrome: A prospective, randomized, placebo-controlled, double-blind clinical trial. Ann Surg 2005;242(5):655–661.

77. Crenn P, Morin MC, Joly F, et al. Net digestive absorption and adaptive hyperphagia in adult short bowel patients. Gut 2004;53(9):1279–1286.

78. Sudan D. Cost and quality of life after intestinal transplantation. Gastroenterology 2006;130(2, Suppl 1):S158–S162.

79. Byrne TA, Persinger RL, Young LS, et al. A new treatment for patients with short-bowel syndrome: Growth hormone, glutamine, and a modified diet. Ann Surg 1995;222(3):243–254, discussion 254–255.

80. Steiger E, DiBaise JK, Messing B, et al. Indications and recommendations for the use of recombinant human growth hormone in adult short bowel syndrome patients dependent on parenteral nutrition. J Clin Gastroenterol 2006;40(Suppl 2):S99–S106.

81. Spencer AU, Kovacevich D, McKinney-Barnett M, et al. Pediatric short-bowel syndrome: The cost of comprehensive care. Am J Clin Nutr 2008;88(6):1552–1529.

82. Abu-Elmagd KM. Intestinal transplantation for short bowel syndrome and gastrointestinal failure: Current consensus, rewarding outcomes, and practical guidelines. Gastroenterology 2006;130(2 Suppl 1):S132–S137.

83. Lord LM, Schaffner R, DeCross AJ, Sax HC. Management of the patient with short bowel syndrome. AACN Clin Issues 2000;11(4):604–618.

84. Howard L, Ament M, Fleming CR, et al. Current use and clinical outcome of home parenteral and enteral nutrition therapies in the United States. Gastroenterology 1995;109(2):355–365.

85. The Oley Foundation. Available from: http://www.oley.org/.

86. Schols AM, Wouters EF. Nutritional abnormalities and supplementation in chronic obstructive pulmonary disease. Clin Chest Med 2000;21(4):753–762.

87. Berry JK, Baum CL. Malnutrition in chronic obstructive pulmonary disease: Adding insult to injury. AACN Clin Issues 2001;12(2):210–219.

88. Engelen MP, Schols AM, Lamers RJ, Wouters EF. Different patterns of chronic tissue wasting among patients with chronic obstructive pulmonary disease. Clin Nutr 1999;18(5):275–280.

89. Engelen MP, Schols AM, Does JD, Wouters EF. Skeletal muscle weakness is associated with wasting of extremity fat-free mass but not with airflow obstruction in patients with chronic obstructive pulmonary disease. Am J Clin Nutr 2000;71(3):733–738.

90. Anker SD, John M, Pedersen PU, et al. ESPEN guidelines on enteral nutrition: Cardiology and pulmonology. Clin Nutr 2006;25(2):311–318.

91. Slinde F, Ellegard L, Gronberg AM, et al. Total energy expenditure in underweight patients with severe chronic obstructive pulmonary disease living at home. Clin Nutr 2003;22(2):159–165.

92. Planas M, Alvarez J, Garcia-Peris PA, et al. Nutritional support and quality of life in stable chronic obstructive pulmonary disease (COPD) patients. Clin Nutr 2005;24(3):433–441.

93. Cai B, Zhu Y, Ma Y, et al. Effect of supplementing a high-fat, low-carbohydrate enteral formula in COPD patients. Nutrition 2003;19(3):229–232.

94. Hasselmann M, Reimund JM. Lipids in the nutritional support of the critically ill patients. Curr Opin Crit Care 2004;10(6):449–455.

95. Faucher M, Bregeon F, Gainnier M, et al. Cardiopulmonary effects of lipid emulsions in patients with ARDS. Chest 2003;124(1):285–291.

96. Clark CL, Sacks GS, Dickerson RN, et al. Treatment of hypophosphatemia in patients receiving specialized nutrition support using a graduated dosing scheme: Results from a prospective clinical trial. Crit Care Med 1995;23(9):1504–1511.

97. MacNee W. Oxidants/antioxidants and COPD. Chest 2000;117 (5 Suppl 1):303S–317S.

98. Ferreira IM, Brooks D, Lacasse Y, et al. Nutritional supplementation for stable chronic obstructive pulmonary disease. Cochrane Database Syst Rev 2005;2:CD000998.

99. Kreymann KG, Berger MM, Deutz NE, et al. ESPEN guidelines on enteral nutrition: Intensive care. Clin Nutr 2006;25(2):210–223.

100. Gadek JE, DeMichele SJ, Karlstad MD, et al. Effect of enteral feeding with eicosapentaenoic acid, gamma-linolenic acid, and antioxidants in patients with acute respiratory distress syndrome. Enteral Nutrition in ARDS Study Group. Crit Care Med 1999;27(8):1409–1420.

101. Singer P, Theilla M, Fisher H, et al. Benefit of an enteral diet enriched with eicosapentaenoic acid and gamma-linolenic acid in ventilated patients with acute lung injury. Crit Care Med 2006;34(4):1033–1038.

102. Schols AM. Nutrition in chronic obstructive pulmonary disease. Curr Opin Pulm Med 2000;6(2):110–115.

103. Katsura H, Yamada K, Kida K. Both generic and disease specific health-related quality of life are deteriorated in patients with underweight COPD. Respir Med 2005;99(5):624–630.

CHAPTER

154

Obesity

JUDY T. CHEN, AMY HECK SHEEHAN, JACK A. YANOVSKI,
AND KARIM ANTON CALIS

KEY CONCEPTS

❶ Two clinical measures of excess body fat, regardless of sex, are the body mass index (BMI) and the waist circumference (WC). BMI and WC provide a better assessment of total body fat than weight alone and are independent predictors of obesity-related disease risk.

❷ Excessive central adiposity increases risk for development of type 2 diabetes, hypertension, and dyslipidemia.

❸ Weight loss of as little as 5% of total body weight can significantly improve blood pressure, lipid levels, and glucose tolerance in overweight and obese patients. Sustained, large weight losses (i.e., after bariatric surgery) are associated with long-term improvements in many of the complications associated with obesity and a lower risk of both myocardial infarction and death.

❹ Pharmacotherapy may be considered in patients with a BMI ≥30 kg/m² and/or a WC ≥40 inches (≥ 102 cm) for men or 35 inches (89 cm) for women, or BMI of 27 to 30 kg/m² with concurrent risk factors if 6 months of diet, exercise, and behavioral modification fail to achieve weight loss.

❺ There is a high probability of weight regain when obesity pharmacotherapy is discontinued.

❻ The FDA does not regulate labeling of herbal and food supplement diet agents, and content is not guaranteed.

It is now estimated that more than 140 million or approximately two out of every three adults are overweight or obese in the United States.[1] Additionally, the number of children and adolescents who are overweight has been increasing at an alarming rate in the last 40 years,[2] with one out of every three adolescents currently considered overweight or obese.[3] Based on the national trend, this epidemic is projected to affect ~80% of the U.S. adults by 2020, and the prevalence of overweight among children is expected to double by 2030.[4] The presence of obesity and overweight is associated with

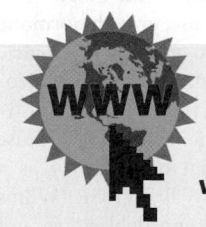

The complete chapter, learning objectives, and other resources can be found at **www.pharmacotherapyonline.com**.

a significantly increased risk for the development of many diseases (Table 154–1),[5–18] poorer outcomes of comorbid disease states, and increased healthcare costs. Prospective cohort studies show that overall mortality parallels increases in adiposity.[19,20] The evidence is strongest for middle-aged adults. In older individuals, excess body weight and adiposity increase the risk of death, but the degree of impact diminishes with age.[19,20] Annually, up to 35% of Americans have actively resolved to lose weight, spending between $30 billion and $50 billion on such attempts.[21] As of 2003, it was estimated that overweight and obesity account for 5% to 7% of total medical expenditures in the United States, and the sum of direct and indirect costs approaches $150 billion annually.[21] The inclusion of several aggressive Healthy People 2020 goals stimulated national initiatives to reverse the obesity epidemic through implementation of prevention strategies, consensus guidelines, and best practices.[22–26] This chapter reviews the epidemiology, pathophysiology, and therapeutic approaches for the management of obesity. Although nonpharmacologic treatment modalities are discussed, the pharmacotherapy of obesity is highlighted, and the role of pharmacotherapy relative to the other therapeutic options is critically reviewed.[27–30]

EPIDEMIOLOGY

Obesity is increasing in prevalence in the United States. The National Health and Nutrition Examination Survey (NHANES) II data (1976–1980) estimated the prevalence of obese adults in the United States at 15%.[2] During NHANES 1999–2000, the prevalence had increased twofold to 30.9%,[2] and by 2006, obesity affected 35.1% of the adult population,[1] making the prevention of obesity a public health priority.[23] This is further emphasized by the continued pursuit of safe and effective long-term therapies for obesity. Existing evidence consistently reports children who are overweight are at least twice as likely to remain overweight as adults when compared with normal-weight children.[31] In particular, obese adolescents have a higher risk of obesity that persists into adulthood that is associated with significant affects on psychological and physical health. Therefore, childhood and early adulthood are critical intervention periods for prevention of obesity in the future. The prevalence of obesity varies by sex among racial and ethnic minorities within the United States.[2] The highest prevalence is observed among non-Hispanic black women (52.9% obese and 13.7% with extreme obesity) compared with values of 37.2% and 5.9% of non-Hispanic black men, respectively.[32] This gender disparity is also associated with the level of parental education. Young black women from the lowest-educated families are at greater risk of obesity compared with young black men.[33] The prevalence of obesity also increases with age, reaching a maximum by the eighth decade.[2] After the age of 80, the prevalence falls progressively for both genders. Socioeconomic status clearly affects the prevalence

TABLE 154-1 Conditions More Prevalent in Obese Populations[5-18]

Cancer	**Genitourinary**
Breast cancer (postmenopausal)	Chronic kidney disease
Colorectal cancer	Increased serum urate
Gallbladder cancer	End-stage renal disease
Endometrial cancer	Obesity-related glomerulopathy
Esophageal carcinoma	Urinary stress incontinence
Hepatic cancer	**Metabolic**
Kidney cancer	Diabetes mellitus
Ovarian cancer	Hyperlipidemia
Pancreatic cancer	Hyperinsulinemia
Prostate cancer	Hypertriglyceridemia
Rectal cancer	Low high-density lipoprotein
Cardiovascular	Impaired glucose tolerance
Atrial fibrillation	Metabolic syndrome
Cerebral vascular accidents	**Musculoskeletal**
Congestive heart failure	Degenerative joint disease
Coronary artery disease	Diffuse idiopathic skeletal hyperostosis
Cor pulmonale	Disc disease
Hypertension	Gait disturbance
Left ventricular hypertrophy	Gout and hyperuricemia
Myocardial infarction	Fibromyalgia
Peripheral vascular disease	Immobility
Peripheral venous insufficiency	Low back pain/back strain
Pulmonary embolism	Osteoarthritis (knee, hips, ankles, feet)
Thrombophlebitis	Plantar fasciitis
Varicose veins	**Neurologic**
Dermatologic	Carpal tunnel syndrome
Acanthosis nigricans	Idiopathic intracranial hypertension
Cellulitis	Meralgia parethetica
Intertrigo, carbuncles	Pseudotumor cerebri
Lymphedema	Stroke
Skin tags	**Oral health**
Status pigmentation of legs	Dental caries
Striae distensae (stretch marks)	Loss of teeth
Psoriasis (women)	Periodontitis
Endocrine/reproductive	Xerostomia
Amenorrhea/menstrual	**Psychological**
disorders	Affective disorders
Congenital anomalies	Body image disturbance
Fetal abnormalities	Depression
Hirsutism	Eating disorders
Hypogonadism (male)	Low self-esteem
Infertility	Social stigmatization
Polycystic ovarian syndrome/	**Respiratory**
androgenicity	Asthma
Pregnancy complications	Chronic obstructive pulmonary
Sexual dysfunction	disease
Gastrointestinal	Dyspnea
Cholelithiasis	Hypoventilation syndrome
Gastroesophageal reflux	Obstructive sleep apnea
disease	Pickwickian syndrome
Hepatic cirrhosis	Pneumonia
Hernias	Pulmonary hypertension
Nonalcoholic fatty liver disease	Venous thromboembolism

of obesity among non-Hispanic white adults; a strong inverse association is observed among non-Hispanic white women from lower socioeconomic classes.[2] Educational achievement, which is linked to socioeconomic status, is also correlated with the fraction of people who are overweight; the prevalence of overweight is greatest in those with less than a high school education.

ETIOLOGY

Obesity occurs when there is an imbalance between energy intake and energy expenditure over time, resulting in increased energy storage. The specific etiology for this imbalance in the vast majority of

individuals is multifactorial, with genetic and environmental factors contributing to various degrees. In a small minority of individuals, excess weight may be attributed to an underlying medical condition or an unintended effect of a medication.

GENETIC INFLUENCES

Observational studies in humans and experimental studies in animal models have demonstrated the strong role of genetics in determining both obesity and distribution of body fat. In some individuals, genetic factors are the primary determinants of obesity, whereas in others, the obesity may be caused primarily by environmental factors. The genetic contribution to the actual variance in BMI and body fat distribution is estimated to be between 50% and 80%.[34] The increase in the prevalence of obesity that has taken place in the United States over the past 40 years is without doubt the result of alterations in our environment.

The role of genetic influences in the development of obesity is an area of extensive research. A number of single-gene mutations producing extreme obesity have been identified, but such mutations are rare and account for an extremely small number of the total cases of obesity.[35] Some common alleles, for instance, the rs9939609 obesity-risk allele in the *FTO* (fat mass and obesity associated) gene that is found in almost 70% of people, increases BMI by about 2 kg/m².[36] The total number and identity of contributing genes are still being determined, as is the means by which the many potential "obesity" genes interact with each other, and with the environment, to produce the obesity phenotype. The Human Obesity Gene Map Database provides a repository listing of candidate genes that may be associated with obesity.[37]

ENVIRONMENTAL FACTORS

Many of the societal changes associated with economic development over the past 30 years have been implicated as potential causes for the increase in the prevalence of obesity. The comforts of modern life in Western civilizations have ultimately resulted in reduced physical activity, in combination with an abundant food supply.[38] Advances in technology and automation have resulted in relatively sedentary lifestyles during both work and leisure time for most individuals. At the same time, there has been a significant increase in the availability and portion size of high-fat foods, which are aggressively marketed and are often more convenient and less expensive than healthier alternatives. This modern environment has been described by some as "obesogenic," as it is likely to result in a state of positive energy balance in many individuals (Fig. 154–1).[39] Obesity has also been reported more frequently among individuals within close social networks (e.g., siblings, spouses, and friends), with a person's risk of becoming obese increasing significantly if a friend in his or her social network is obese.[40] Finally, it should be noted that cultural factors, socioeconomic status, and religious beliefs may influence eating habits and body weights.

MEDICAL CONDITIONS

Occasionally, patients present with obesity secondary to an identifiable medical condition. Conditions associated with weight gain include iatrogenic and idiopathic Cushing disease, growth hormone deficiency, insulinoma, leptin deficiency, and various psychiatric disorders, such as depression, binge-eating disorder, and schizophrenia. Hypothyroidism is often included in this list, but it mostly causes fluid retention (myxedema) and is generally not a cause of significant obesity. Genetic syndromes that have obesity as a major component are extremely rare: Prader-Willi, WAGR (Wilms tumor, Aniridia, Genitourinary abnormalities or gonadoblastoma, and

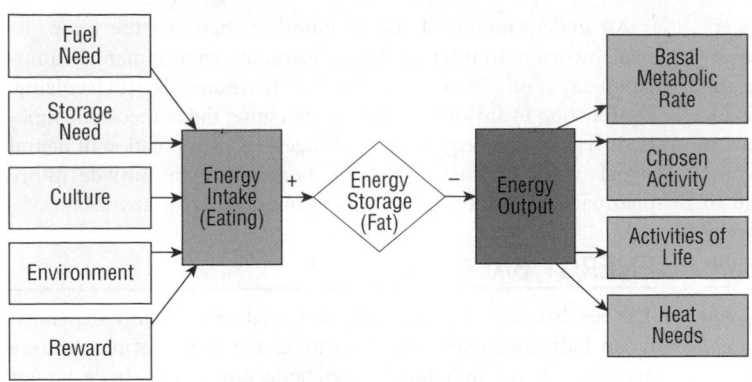

FIGURE 154-1. Net energy stores are determined by various inputs and outputs. Simply stated, obesity occurs when there is an imbalance between energy intake and expenditure.

mental Retardation), Simpson-Goabi-Behmel, Cohen, Bardet-Biedl, Carpenter, Börjeson, and Wilson-Turner. The clinician evaluating a patient for obesity needs to be aware of these potential conditions. The physical examination of obese patients always should include an assessment for secondary causes of obesity, including genetic syndromes.

MEDICATIONS

An increasing number of medications are associated with unintended weight gain.[41] These include several anticonvulsants (i.e., carbamazepine, gabapentin, pregabalin, and valproic acid), antidepressants (i.e., mirtazapine and tricyclic antidepressants), atypical antipsychotics (e.g., clozapine, olanzapine, quetiepine, and risperidone), conventional antipsychotics (e.g., haloperidol), and hormones (e.g., corticosteroids, insulin, and medroxyprogesterone). Although the pharmacologic mechanism responsible for weight gain is usually drug specific, in most cases the exact cause has not been determined.

PATHOPHYSIOLOGY

The pathophysiology of obesity involves numerous factors that regulate appetite, energy storage, and energy expenditure. Disturbance of these homeostatic functions results in an imbalance between energy intake and energy expenditure.

APPETITE

Human appetite is a complex process that is the net result of many inputs within a neural network involving principally the hypothalamus, limbic system, brainstem, hippocampus, and elements of the cortex.[42] Within this neural network, many neurotransmitters and neuropeptides have been identified that can stimulate or depress the brain's appetite network and thereby affect total caloric intake.

Biogenic Amines

The first receptor systems found to alter food intake in animals and humans were the biogenic amines. These neurotransmitters are the foundation from which the most robust pharmacologic interventions for obesity have been developed. Serotonin, also known as 5-hydroxytryptamine (5-HT), and cells known to respond to 5-HT are found throughout the central nervous system and the periphery. Currently, two major noradrenergic receptor subtypes are recognized (α and β), each with multiple subtypes. Histamine and dopamine also demonstrate multiple receptor subtypes, but their role in the regulation of human eating behaviors and food intake is less well documented. Direct stimulation of 5-HT$_{1A}$ and noradrenergic α_2-receptors will increase food intake, whereas the opposite occurs with 5-HT$_{2C}$ and noradrenergic α_1- or β_2-receptor

activation. Table 154-2 summarizes the major effects of direct receptor stimulation, inhibition, or changes in synaptic cleft amine concentrations on food intake.

Neuropeptides

Many neuropeptides that influence appetite exert their effects within the hypothalamus. Thus, in the last several years research has focused on the neural projection between parts of the hypothalamus and the arcuate nucleus sending signals to the paraventricular nucleus. The key peptides in this projection are currently thought to be neuropeptide Y and α-melanocyte–stimulating hormone, which engages melanocortin receptors in the paraventricular nucleus. Neuropeptide Y is the most potent known stimulator of eating, and α-melanocyte–stimulating hormone action at the melanocortin 3 and 4 receptors is one of the crucial inhibitors of eating.[42,43]

TABLE 154-2	Effects of Various Neurotransmitters, Receptors, and Peptides on Food Intake	
Anatomic Region	**Increased Eating**	**Decreased Eating**
Arcuate nucleus of hypothalamus	Ghrelin	Leptin Insulin Glucagon-like peptide-1 Peptide YY
Paraventricular nucleus of hypothalamus	Neuropeptide Y Agouti-related protein Opioids (especially mu) Galanin	Melanocyte stimulating hormone (melanocortin) Corticotropin-releasing hormone Cholecystokinin
Lateral hypothalamus	Orexin Melanocyte concentration hormone	
Hypothalamus	Norepinephrine α_2 Serotonin 5-HT$_{1A}$	Norepinephrine α_1 and β_2 Serotonin 5-HT$_{1B}$ and 5-HT$_{2C}$ Histamine H$_1$ and H$_3$
Nucleus accumbens	Dopamine	
Amygdala	Opioids (especially mu)	
Brainstem (Hindbrain)	Neuropeptide Y Agouti-related protein Opioids (especially mu)	Leptin Melanocyte stimulating hormone (melanocortin) Cholecystokinin (CCK)
Vagus nerve	Ghrelin	Leptin Cholecystokinin Glucagon-like peptide-1 Peptide YY
Various or undetermined	Cannabinoid CB$_1$	Dopamine D$_1$ and D$_2$

Adapted from Dhillo WS. Appetite regulation: An overview. Thyroid 2007;17(5):433–445; and Valassi E, Scacchi M, Cavagnini F. Neuroendocrine control of food intake. Nutr Metab Cardiovasc Dis 2008;18(2):158–168.

The lateral hypothalamus has been referred to as the "hunger" center within the brain. The most prominent of these lateral hypothalamic peptides, orexin, increases food intake stimuli within the lateral hypothalamus.[42] Another important neuropeptide stimulator of eating that principally originates in the lateral hypothalamus is melanocyte-concentrating hormone. Neurons in the lateral hypothalamus use orexin and melanocyte-concentrating hormone to communicate with other neurons throughout the brain and thereby affect a number of functions beyond appetite.[42,43] Table 154–2 summarizes the major effects of various neuropeptides on food intake. Although hunger and satiety functions are thought to be primarily regulated by the hypothalamus, humans eat in response to a broad set of stimuli, such as reward, pleasure, learning, and memory.

Peripheral Appetite–Related Signals to the Brain

Peripheral appetite signals also dramatically affect food intake. Leptin, a hormone that is secreted by adipose cells, acts on the arcuate nucleus of the hypothalamus and elsewhere in the brain to decrease appetite and increase energy expenditure.[44,45] Studies conducted in leptin-deficient mice and humans revealed that exogenous leptin administration produced significant weight loss. However, recombinant leptin replacement therapy in obese humans who are not leptin deficient has not proved successful, as obese humans appear to be leptin resistant. Figure 154–2 shows the peripheral link that leptin appears to provide in signaling the central nervous system about the status of fat cell mass. Leptin also has been found to regulate various functions outside the central nervous system, including insulin and glucocorticoid secretion, reproduction, and glucose transport within the small intestine.[44]

Other peripheral signals important to the brain's processing of appetite include several gut hormones, notably those released by the intestine in response to passage of digesting food such as glucagon-related peptide-1, oxyntomodulin, and peptide YY.[46] Each of these hormonal signals suppresses eating in animals and humans. Glucagon-related peptide-1 has other effects, most importantly as an incretin, which facilitates release of insulin by pancreatic β cells in response to meal-related glucose. Ghrelin, another important gut hormone that is released from the distal stomach and duodenum, stimulates appetite.

An understanding of the relationships between the brain, its many neurotransmitters and neuropeptides, environmental stimulation of brain activities, and other hormones is still evolving. Dysfunction in any of these factors can upset the homeostatic functions regulating energy balance. Exogenous manipulation of neural signals and associated peripheral hormones may provide future pharmacotherapeutic approaches to obesity management.

ENERGY BALANCE

The net balance of energy ingested relative to energy expended by an individual over time determines the degree of obesity (see Fig. 154–1). An individual's metabolic rate is the single largest determinant of energy expenditure. Resting energy expenditure (REE) is defined as the energy expended by a person at rest under conditions of thermal neutrality. Basal metabolic rate (BMR) is defined as the REE measured soon after awakening in the morning, at least 12 hours after the last meal. Metabolic rate increases after eating, based on the size and composition of the meal. It reaches a maximum approximately 1 hour after the meal is consumed and returns to basal levels 4 hours after the meal. This increase in metabolic rate is known as the *thermogenic effect of food*. The REE measures the energy costs of the wakeful state and may include the residual thermogenic effect of a previous meal; it is thus usually higher than metabolic rate measured during quiet sleep. Physical activity is the other major factor that affects total energy expenditure and is the most variable component.

PERIPHERAL STORAGE AND THERMOGENESIS

There are two major types of adipose tissue, white and brown. The primary function of white adipose tissue is lipid manufacture, storage, and release. Brown adipose tissue, once believed to be found only in infants, is now recognized to exist in most adults.[47] It is more commonly identified in lean than obese individuals, but its importance for human obesity remains unclear. Lipid storage occurs in response to insulin, whereas lipid release is seen during periods of calorie restriction. Brown adipose tissue is notable for its ability to dissipate energy via uncoupled mitochondrial respiration.[48]

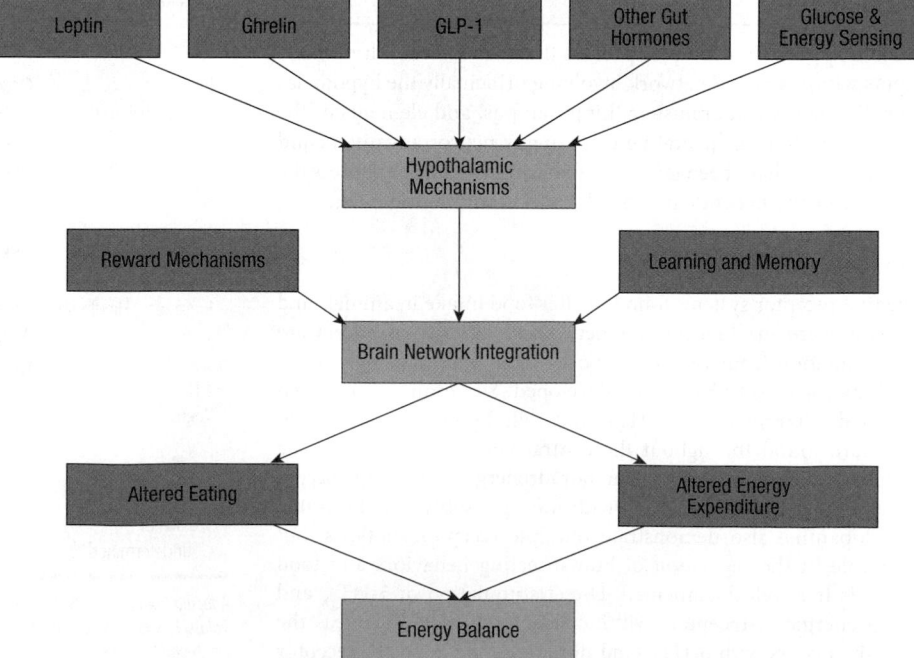

FIGURE 154-2. Intrinsic hypothalamic hunger and satiety mechanisms are modified by input from fat tissue via leptin, the gut via ghrelin, glucagon-like peptide-1 (GLP-1) and other hormones, and also by direct sensing of prevailing glucose and other energy signals. The hypothalamus generates signals that are integrated within brain networks, which are also receiving signals and food hedonics, learning and memory, and other motivations. The brain network effects change in energy balance by modifying food intake and energy expenditure.

Both white and brown adipose tissues are highly innervated by the sympathetic nervous system, and adrenergic stimulation via β-adrenergic receptors (β_1, β_2, and β_3) is known to activate lipolysis in fat cells as well as increase energy expenditure in adipose tissue and skeletal muscle. Genetic polymorphisms have been identified in both the β_2- and β_3-receptor systems that are associated with obesity or excess weight gain.[49] Thus, genetic susceptibility for excess weight status may in part be related to adrenergic dysfunction.

CLINICAL PRESENTATION

Although obesity is readily apparent, most obese patients seek healthcare only when obesity-associated comorbidities become problematic. A consistent and reproducible description of weight status is essential in the diagnosis and management of obesity. Evidence-based guidelines issued by many groups, notably the World Health Organization and the National Institutes of Health (NIH), have established a stratification of weight excess based on associated medical risks.[50] The first increment of excess weight is termed *overweight*, with the term *obesity* reserved for the higher levels of weight excess. These levels of excess weight are defined on the basis of body mass index (BMI), a measure of total body weight relative to height. Those with a BMI of 18.5 to 24.9 are considered to have "normal" weight; the terms *overweight, obese*, and *severely obese* are reserved for those with a BMI of 25 to 29.9, 30 to 39.9, and 40 and over, respectively. Using metric units, BMI (kg/m²) is defined as weight in kilograms divided by height in meters squared (kg/m²). Using pounds and inches, BMI (lb/inch²) is estimated as (weight [lb]/height [inches²]) × 703. Because BMI may overestimate the degree of excess body fat in some clinical situations (e.g., edematous states, extreme muscularity, muscle wasting, and short stature), the assessment of body composition in such cases often requires clinical judgment.

❶ BMI is an acceptable measure of obesity and is the practical method of defining obesity in the clinic and epidemiologic studies; however, it does not always correspond to excess fat. There are well-established differences in the relationship between BMI and obesity-related risks among disparate racial and ethnic groups. For examples, BMI overestimates adiposity among non-Hispanic blacks and underestimates risk among Asians.[51–54] Ideally, obesity refers to a state of excess body fat as determined by measures of adiposity. Direct ways to assess fat-free body mass include skinfold thickness, body density using underwater body weight, bioelectric impedance and conductivity, dual-energy radiographic absorptiometry, computed tomography (CT), and magnetic resonance imaging (MRI).[55] These measurement techniques that determine body fat directly are currently too expensive and time-consuming to be used routinely in the clinical setting. Furthermore, all fat is not equal in its danger to health. Superficial subcutaneous fat has a weak association with metabolic markers of insulin production, release, and resistance, whereas deep subcutaneous fat demonstrates a strong relationship with insulin resistance.[48] Central obesity reflects high levels of intraabdominal or visceral fat, and this pattern of obesity is associated with an increased propensity for the development of hypertension, dyslipidemia, type 2 diabetes, and cardiovascular disease (sometimes referred to as the "metabolic syndrome"). Thus, in addition to the absolute excess fat mass, the distribution of this fat regionally in the body has important clinical effects. Intraabdominal fat is best estimated by imaging techniques such as CT and MRI but can be estimated through measurement of the waist circumference (WC). Clinically, WC is the narrowest circumference measured in the area between the last rib and the top of the iliac crest.[56] The current definition for high-risk WC is greater than 40 inches (102 cm) in men and greater than 35 inches (89 cm) in women.[56] Notably,

TABLE 154-3 Classification of Overweight and Obesity by Body Mass Index (BMI), Waist Circumference, and Associated Disease Risk

| | BMI (kg/m²) | Obesity Class | Disease Risk[a] (Relative to Normal Weight and Waist Circumference) | |
			Men ≤ 40 inches / Women ≤ 35 inches	Men > 40 inches / Women > 35 inches
Underweight	<18.5		–	–
Normal weight[b]	18.5–24.9		–	High
Overweight	25.0–29.9		Increased	High
Obesity	30.0–34.9	I	High	Very high
	35.0–39.9	II	Very high	Very high
Extreme obesity	≥40	III	Extremely high	Extremely high

[a]Disease risk for type 2 diabetes, hypertension, and cardiovascular disease.
[b]Increased waist circumference can also be a marker for increased risk even in persons of normal weight.
Adapted from Preventing and Managing the Global Epidemic of Obesity. Report of the World Health Organization Consultation on Obesity. Geneva: World Health Organization, 1997. National Institutes of Health, National Heart, Lung and Blood Institute, http://www.nhlbi.nih.gov/guidelines/obesity/ob_home.htm.

epidemiologic studies demonstrate that WC adds little in terms of risk prediction once a patient's BMI reaches 35 kg/m². Thus, routine determination of WC should be implemented in those with BMIs between 25 and 34.9 kg/m².

❷ Although BMI and WC are related, each measure independently predicts disease risk. Both measurements should be assessed and monitored during therapy for obesity.[57] The risks for development of type 2 diabetes, hypertension, or cardiovascular disease at various stages of obesity based on BMI or WC are outlined in Table 154–3. Note that increased WC confers increased risk even in normal-weight individuals.

COMORBIDITIES

Although overall mortality is not increased among those classified as overweight, those who are obese have serious health risks and increased mortality,[57] particularly adults with BMI greater than 35 kg/m².[58] Substantial reductions in life expectancy have been predicted in adults with BMI greater than 35 kg/m².[58] Further reduction in life span has been observed in obese individuals who are current or former smokers.[58] Several disease states and/or conditions are more prevalent in obese patients (see Table 154–1).[5–18] Increased body fat, increased total body weight, and a central distribution of body fat all are associated with an increased incidence of mortality, primarily as a result of cardiovascular disease. Hypertension, hyperlipidemia, insulin resistance, and glucose intolerance are all known cardiac risk factors that tend to cluster in obese individuals. Therefore, the obese individual is exposed to multiple risk factors. Some of the earliest studies from Framingham have confirmed the relationship between obesity and increased risk of stroke and coronary heart disease in both men and women.[59] Blood pressure frequently is elevated in obese individuals and may in part explain the increased incidence of stroke and cardiovascular disease observed with obesity. Hypertension in lean individuals is associated with concentric cardiac hypertrophy as a consequence of an increased afterload, which increases the risk of cardiac ischemia. In contrast, eccentric dilation is observed in obesity, leading to an increased volume load. This dilated cardiomyopathy is associated with a reduction in ventricular ejection fraction and a high-output cardiac state.

The combination of obesity and hypertension is associated with thickening of the ventricular wall, ischemia, and increased heart volume. This leads more rapidly to heart failure, an association that has been recognized for more than 2 decades.[60,61] Alterations in pulmonary function are common in patients with obesity. Sleep apnea, which is more common in men, is a significant and costly condition that is associated with increased morbidity and mortality in the obese.[60,61] The exact mechanism by which obesity leads to sleep apnea is unknown, but weight loss often results in significant and sometimes dramatic improvements in the condition.

Diabetes mellitus and impaired glucose tolerance are associated with insulin resistance and obesity. As insulin response becomes impaired, the pancreatic β cells respond by increasing insulin production and release, resulting in a state of relative hyperinsulinemia. Although hyperinsulinemia is known to be associated with an increased risk of cardiovascular disease, it is not known whether the increased insulin levels contribute directly to cardiac disease, or if they are a marker for the underlying defect of insulin resistance and glucose intolerance. Insulin resistance, in turn, also frequently leads to impaired lipid metabolism (increased cholesterol, increased triglycerides, and low circulating high-density lipoprotein) and hypertension. As with cardiovascular disease, central obesity is an important factor in determining the risk of developing type 2 diabetes.

Osteoarthritis in weight-bearing joints, such as the knees, may be related directly to the mechanical effects of excess body weight and the resulting forces exerted on these joint surfaces. The increase of osteoarthritis in non-weight-bearing joints, however, suggests that obesity may lead to altered cartilage, collagen, and even bone metabolism.[8] Increasing evidence has suggested proinflammatory adipocytokines, such as tumor necrosis factor-α and leptin, may play an important role in the metabolic influence of overweight on osteoarthritis. Osteoarthritis and its symptoms, such as pain, are a significant barrier to physical activity and a key impediment to sustained weight loss.

Obesity affects the human reproductive system in a number of ways. Obesity is associated with earlier menarche in girls and hyperandrogenism, hirsutism, and anovulatory menstrual cycles in women. In some women, this disorder manifests as overt polycystic ovary syndrome, a condition in which insulin resistance is common.[62] Weight loss therapy with insulin-sensitizing drugs, such as the thiazolidinediones and biguanides, has been shown to restore normal ovulation in some women.[62] These observations suggest that insulin resistance plays a part in the causation of polycystic ovary syndrome associated with obesity.

TREATMENT

■ DESIRED OUTCOME

Weight management is commonly considered successful when a predefined amount of weight has been lost such that a final goal is achieved. However, desired outcomes are fully dependent on the clinical situation. Success may also include end points of decreasing the rate of weight gain or maintaining a weight-neutral status. A significant number of web-based resources for supporting both patient and practitioner weight management activities are available.[23,24,56]

■ GENERAL APPROACH TO TREATMENT

The success of obesity therapy has been measured most often as weight loss over a defined study period of up to 4 years in duration. Successful obesity treatment plans have incorporated an integrated dietary intervention, exercise, behavior modification (with or without pharmacologic therapy), and/or surgical intervention. Specific weight goals should be established that are consistent with medical needs and the patient's personal desire. For most obese patients, a weight loss goal of 5% to 10% of initial weight is reasonable. Patients should not be allowed to attain abnormally low body weight (i.e., less than their estimated ideal body weight).

Patients seeking help for obesity do so for many reasons, including improvement in their quality of life, a reduction in associated morbidity, and increased life expectancy. Unfortunately, numerous individuals seek therapy for obesity primarily for cosmetic purposes and often have unrealistic goals and expectations. Aggressive marketing of weight loss programs, therapies, and diets—parallel to the fashion industry's standards of desirable body profiles—has led many individuals to set impossible goals and expectations. In some cases, these persons will go to extreme measures to achieve weight loss. Consequently, clinicians must be careful to fully discuss the risks of therapies and to clearly define the achievable benefits and magnitude of weight loss. Obese patients should be redirected away from trying to achieve an "ideal weight" to the more reasonable goals of modest (e.g., loss of 5–10% of body weight) but sustained, medically relevant weight loss. In practice, the goal has to be set based on many factors, including initial body weight, patient motivation and desire, presence of comorbid conditions, and age. For example, in patients with diabetes, even modest weight loss can improve glucose control and may reduce mortality,[63–66] yet in individuals with osteoarthritis, significantly more weight reduction may be required to improve symptoms. Indeed, dietary modification and exercise have been shown to ameliorate hyperglycemia, hyperlipidemia, and hypertension with weight loss of less than 5% of initial body weight. These data emphasize the importance of defining end points and measures of success in any weight loss plan.

❸ Weight loss interventions must be founded on lifestyle changes, such as a modification in eating practices, complemented by drug therapy if indicated, and in some cases surgery (Fig. 154–3). Prior to recommending any therapy, the clinician must evaluate the patient for the presence of secondary causes of obesity. If a secondary cause is suspected, then a more complete diagnostic workup and the initiation of appropriate therapy may be warranted. The next step in patient evaluation is to determine the presence and severity of other medical conditions that are either directly associated with obesity (e.g., diabetes) or that have an impact on therapeutic decision making (e.g., history of liver disease or cardiac arrhythmia). Appropriate laboratory tests to exclude and/or quantify the degree of specific conditions such as diabetes, liver dysfunction, and nephropathy should be done as indicated by the history and physical examination. Based on the outcome of this medical evaluation, the patient should be counseled on treatment options, benefits, and risks. No matter what the treatment options are, they all require significant effort on the part of the patient to change lifestyle and comply with the management plan. If the patient is not yet ready to meet these expectations, then early counseling will reduce the chance of frustration for the patient, clinician, and in some cases other family members. Providing basic education can lead to a significant change in motivation and desire to lose weight and improved compliance.

The ultimate goals of treatment must be defined clearly. These goals may be absolute weight loss if obesity is present without other comorbid conditions. If improvement in blood glucose, blood cholesterol, and hypertension are primary goals, then these must be defined appropriately and may include setting target levels for low-density lipoprotein cholesterol, glycosylated hemoglobin, or blood pressure. Per current national guidelines, the recommended weight loss goal for adults is 10% of initial weight gradually over 6 months of therapy to achieve a reasonable rate of weight loss of ~1 to 2 lb (0.5–0.9 kg) per week.[6] All too often patients expect to lose

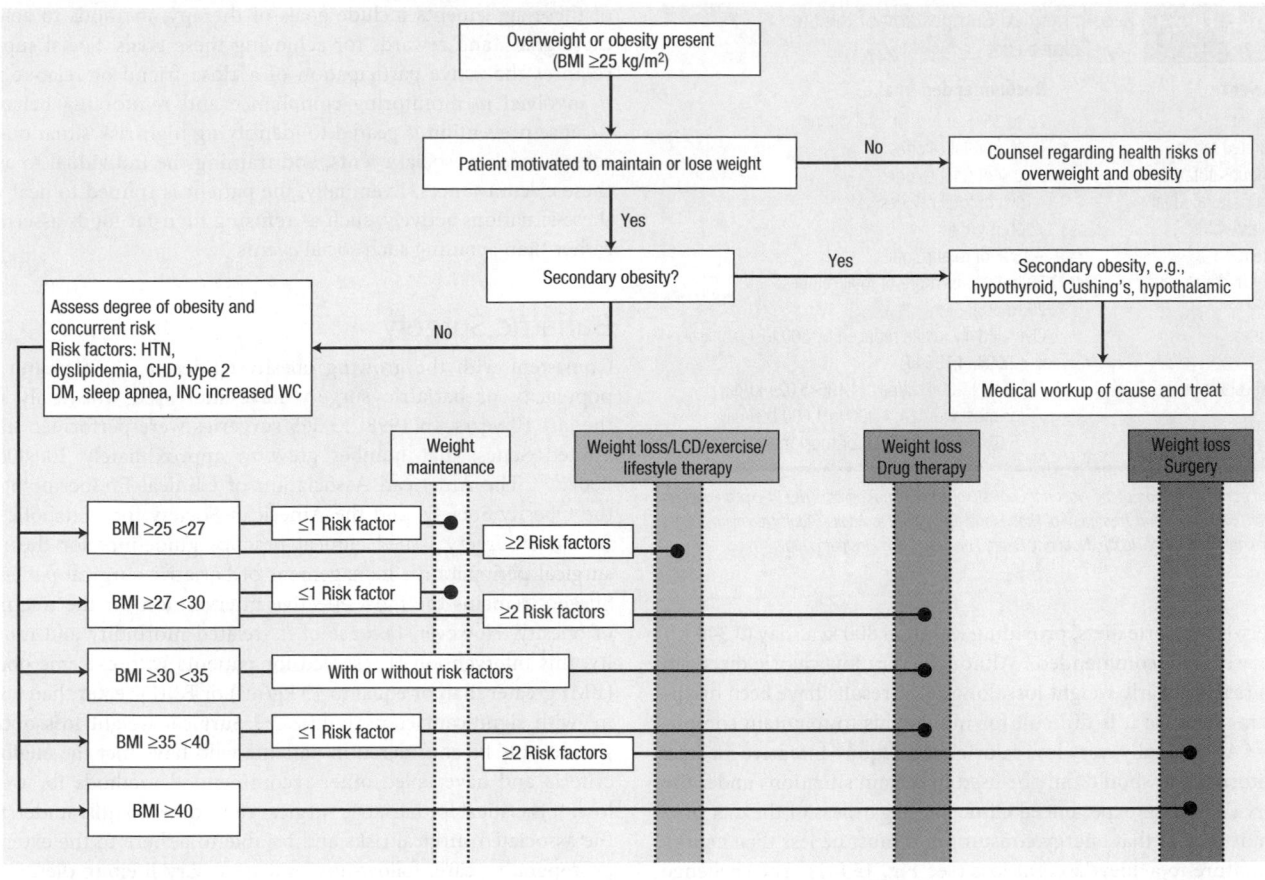

FIGURE 154-3. Pharmacotherapy treatment algorithm. Candidates for pharmacotherapy are selected on the basis of body mass index and waist circumference criteria, along with consideration of concurrent risk factors. Medication therapy is always used as an adjunct to a comprehensive weight-loss program that includes diet, exercise, and behavioral modification. CHD, coronary heart disease; DM, diabetes mellitus; HTN, hypertension; WC, waist circumference, ≥40 inches [≥102 cm] for men and ≥35 inches [≥89 cm] for women; LCD, low-calorie diet.

weight overnight, only to be disappointed. Thus, it is important to set a time course for the plan. Ultimately, lifelong therapeutic goals should consist of maintenance of reduced body weight and prevention of weight gain.

◾ NONPHARMACOLOGIC THERAPY

Nonpharmacologic therapy including reduced caloric intake, increased physical activity, and behavioral modification is the mainstay of obesity management. This combination is recommended as first-line therapy in current evidence-based clinical guidelines for the treatment of overweight and obesity in adults set forth by the NIH.[6]

Reduced Caloric Intake

CLINICAL CONTROVERSY

Because of the popularity of diets such as Atkins's New Diet Revolution (high fat, low carbohydrate, high protein), there is extensive coverage in the media and ongoing debate in academic circles regarding the risks, benefits, and outcomes related to diets that preferentially employ macronutrient extremes (i.e., high protein vs high carbohydrate vs low fat). However, recent information suggests that macronutrient composition of the diet may not be as important as consistent adherence to reduced energy consumption.

Current adult guidelines recommend reduced caloric intake through adherence to a low-calorie diet (LCD).[6] The LCD should provide a daily caloric deficit of 500 to 1,000 (kcal) (2,093–4,486 kJ), which generally correlates to a total intake of 800 to 1,200 kcal/day (3,349–5,024 kJ/day). Severely obese individuals will require more energy, at least at the start of dietary restriction. The composition of the LCD is outlined in the Step I Diet recommended by the third report of the Expert Panel on the Detection, Evaluation, and Treatment of High Blood Cholesterol in Adults (ATP III), as shown in Table 154-4.[67] Adherence to the LCD has been shown to result in an average weight loss of 8% after 6 months.[6]

Numerous diet and nutrition plans are available to aid patients in their pursuit of weight loss. Popular diets include moderate energy-deficient plans (e.g., Weight Watchers, LEARN [Lifestyle, Exercise, Attitude, Relationships, Nutrition], and Jenny Craig), vegetarian-based plans (e.g., Ornish), and low carbohydrate plans (e.g., Zone and Atkins).[68] Short-term weight loss is significant for almost all diet plans. However, long-term weight loss and maintenance of weight loss is less promising, primarily because of difficulty with adherence. Low-carbohydrate diets have been found to achieve better weight loss than low-fat diets for the first 6 months of treatment, but similar efficacy is generally seen after 1 year.[69,70] More recently, a long-term trial reported no significant difference in the amount of weight loss achieved with adherence to various types of reduced-calorie diets.[71] Therefore, macronutrient composition of the diet may not be as important as consistent adherence to reduced energy consumption.

TABLE 154-4 Recommended Composition of the Step I Low-Calorie Diet

Nutrient	Recommended Intake
Total fat	25 to 35% or less of total calories
Saturated fat	<7% of total calories
Monounsaturated fat	≤20% of total calories
Polyunsaturated fat	≤10% of total calories
Cholesterol	<200 mg/day
Protein	~15% of total calories
Carbohydrates	50 to 60% or more of total calories
Fiber	20 to 30 g
Calories	Overall daily intake reduced by 500 to 1,000 kcal (2,094–4,186 kJ)
Total caloric intake	1,000 to 1,200 kcal/day (4,186–5,024 kJ/day) for most women; 1,200 to 1,600 kcal/day (5,024–6,698 kJ/day) for most men

Adapted from Third report of the National Cholesterol Education Program (NCEP) Expert Panel on Detection, Evaluation, and Treatment of High Blood Cholesterol in Adults (Adult Treatment Panel III). National Institutes of Health, National, Heart, Lung and Blood Institute, 2002.

Very low calorie diets, providing less than 800 kcal/day (3,349 kJ/day), are not recommended.[6] Although, very low calorie diets can often result in early weight loss, long-term results have been disappointing because it is difficult for individuals to maintain compliance.[72] Additionally, very low calorie diets require intensive medical monitoring and should only be used in certain situations under the supervision of an experienced clinician. Regardless of the diet program, it is clear that energy consumption must be less than energy expenditure to achieve weight loss (see Fig. 154–1). The challenge is to develop a diet plan that leads to consistent adherence by the patient and therefore sustained weight loss and/or maintenance.

Increased Physical Activity

Increased physical activity is an important component in achieving the state of greater energy expenditure than energy intake that is necessary to lose weight and maintain weight loss. When increased physical activity is attempted as monotherapy, only modest weight loss has been reported.[73] However, when it is combined with reduced calorie intake and behavior modification, it can augment weight loss and improve obesity-related comorbidities and cardiovascular risk factors.[6,73] Current recommendations suggest at least 30 minutes of moderate physical activity on most days of the week. However, 1 hour of moderate physical activity per day may be required to augment weight loss.[74] Patients should be advised to start slowly and gradually increase intensity. All obese patients should receive a medical examination prior to embarking on a physical activity program.

Behavioral Modification

Behavior modification is common to almost all weight loss interventions. The primary aim is to help patients choose lifestyles that are conducive to safe and sustained weight loss. Behavioral therapy is based on principles of human learning and thus attempts to substitute desirable behaviors for learned undesirable habits using a combination of stimulus control and reinforcement. Most such programs use self-monitoring of diet and exercise both to increase patient awareness of behavior and as a tool for the clinician to determine patient compliance as well as patient motivation.[75,76] Behavior is reinforced by techniques including behavioral contracting, social support, relapse prevention, and in some cases booster treatments. Behavioral contracts are written agreements jointly developed by the patient and ther clinician. Components

of these agreements include goals of therapy, methods to achieve these goals, and rewards for achieving these goals. Social support requires the active participation of a close friend or relative who is involved in monitoring compliance and reinforcing behavior. Relapse prevention is geared to identifying high-risk situations for relapse, such as social events, and training the individual to avoid these circumstances. Eventually, the patient is trained to deal with these situations actively, such as refusing high-fat foods assertively rather than avoiding such social events.

Bariatric Surgery

Consistent with the growing obesity epidemic, the demand and popularity of bariatric surgery have increased drastically over the last 10 years. In 1998, 13,365 surgeries were performed in the United States; that number grew to approximately 200,000 in 2007.[77,78] The American Association of Clinical Endocrinologists, the Obesity Society, and the American Society for Metabolic and Bariatric Surgery issued clinical practice guidelines for the non-surgical perioperative management of bariatric surgical patients.[78] Surgery remains the most effective intervention for the treatment of obesity. However, because of its related morbidity and mortality, this intervention is reserved for patients with extreme obesity (BMI greater than or equal to 40 kg/m²) or BMI greater than 35 kg/m² with significant comorbidities.[6,78] Surgical weight loss options should only be considered in patients who have met the eligibility criteria and have failed other recommended methods for weight loss. It is critical for bariatric surgical candidates to fully understand the associated surgical risks and be able to adhere to the extensive postoperative care, follow-ups, and necessary lifelong dietary and lifestyle adjustments to ensure long-term success of the procedure. Careful patient selection and choice of procedure are critical to achieving a successful outcome. The input of an experienced surgeon working with a multidisciplinary team is invaluable in the care of these patients.

All bariatric surgical procedures achieve weight loss and maintenance through two principle mechanisms: 1) restriction or reduction of food intake by reducing stomach volume or 2) malabsorption by reducing the absorptive surface of the alimentary tract. Currently, the four major types of procedures are adjustable gastric banding, vertical banded gastroplasty, biliopancreatic diversion with duodenal switch, and conventional Roux-en-Y gastric bypass. Gastroplasty and adjustable gastric banding are designed to reduce the volume of the stomach and thus restrict the rate of nutrient intake. The biliopancreatic diversion with duodenal switch is primarily malabsorptive in nature, and the length of the diversion determines the extent of nutrient malabsorption. The conventional Roux-en-Y gastric bypass is the most common procedure currently performed in the United States. It combines a restrictive approach with a degree of malabsorption induced by excluding 90% to 95% of the stomach, the entire duodenum, and a portion of the proximal jejunum from the effective alimentary tract. Conventional Roux-en-Y gastric bypass yields greater and longer lasting weight loss than the other purely restrictive methods. Ultimately, reductions in excess body weight of ~48% to 85% can be achieved within the first 1 or 2 years, and weight loss maintenance of 25% to 68% of presurgery weight has been reported after 7 to 10 years with this procedure.[78]

Improvements in the peri- and postoperative care of gastric surgery patients have reduced morbidity and mortality associated with bariatric surgeries. The operative 30-day mortality rate is ~0.3% with conventional bypass or laparoscopic gastric banding[79] and 1.1% with malabsorptive procedures.[78] Some of the most common early complications of conventional gastric bypass are deep venous thrombosis, pulmonary emboli, anastomotic leaks, bleeding, and wound infections. Approximately one-third of patients who do not receive vitamin supplementation will develop significant vitamin B_{12} and iron deficiency, with a large proportion demonstrating microcytic anemia.[78] Empiric supplementation with one or two tablets of daily multivitamin, 1,200 to 2,000 mg/day of calcium citrate with 400 to 800 IU/day of vitamin D, 400 mcg/day of folic acid, 40 to 65 mg/day of elemental iron, and at least 350 mcg/day of oral vitamin B_{12} (or 500 mcg intranasally once weekly) is essential to prevent nutritional deficiencies in bariatric recipients.[78] Dumping syndrome, characterized by abdominal pain and cramping, nausea, diarrhea, and bloating, tachycardia, and syncope can occur in 70% to 76% of patients after Roux-en-Y gastric bypass procedure[78] and may complicate provision of drug therapy in some cases. Dietary changes such as eating small, frequent meals, avoiding refined sugars, and increasing intake of fiber, complex carbohydrates, and protein can help alleviate the symptoms associated with dumping syndrome.

Weight losses resulting from bariatric surgery are often accompanied by dramatic improvements, and sometimes complete resolution, of many obesity-related complications. With improved glycemic control and reduced insulin resistance, remission rates for type 2 diabetes mellitus have been as high as 83% to 92% after Roux-en-Y gastric bypass and ~50% after gastric banding.[78] Other clinical benefits are improvements in hypertension, hypertriglyceridemia, high-density lipoprotein cholesterol, cardiomyopathy, cardiac function, degenerative joint diseases, mobility, nonalcoholic fatty liver disease, respiratory functions, obstructive sleep apnea, obesity–hypoventilation syndrome, polycystic ovary syndrome, infertility, pregnancy complications, and positive psychosocial changes, as well as enhanced quality of life.[78] Reduced risk of cancer-related mortality has also been documented after bariatric surgery. Furthermore, data from the prospective controlled Swedish Obese Subjects study have demonstrated a significant 29% reduction in overall mortality for patients who underwent bariatric surgery compared with those who received conventional treatments (ranging from lifestyle or behavioral medications to no interventions) after an average follow-up duration of 10.9 years.[80]

After experiencing weight loss, many gastric surgery patients are able to discontinue pharmacotherapy for glucose lowering, dyslipidemia, and hypertension. Frequently, however, antihypertensive medications must be restarted postsurgery, despite the fact that the patient has not experienced marked weight regain. It is imperative for clinicians to recognize that bariatric interventions not only alter nutrient absorption but also may impede drug absorption.[81] Achlorhydria and reduced surface area for intestinal and gastric absorption after bariatric surgery can lead to altered dissolution of certain pH-dependent medications, such as ketoconazole, enalapril, simvastatin, tacrolimus, sirolimus, and mycophenolic acid.[81,82] Data regarding absorption challenges associated with bariatric surgery remain scarce; thus, close therapeutic monitoring of any orally administered medication after surgery is highly recommended as dosage form selection, dose conversion, or therapeutic interchange may be necessary to avoid or minimize absorption problems and ensure bariatric surgery success.

■ PHARMACOLOGIC THERAPY

❹ The debate regarding the appropriateness of obesity pharmacotherapy remains heated, fueled by the recognized national need to treat a growing epidemic and the medical and litigious fallout from the failed use of fenfluramine and dexfenfluramine (Redux).[83] Strategies for the pharmacologic management of obesity have historically focused on modulating central and/or peripheral sites that regulate energy balance. Figure 154–4 depicts the sites of action of these therapies within the energy intake, storage, and expenditure cycle. Short-term use of anorexic agents is difficult to justify because of the predictable weight regain that occurs with discontinuation of therapy. Long-term pharmacotherapy may have a place in the treatment of obesity for patients who have no obvious contraindications to approved drug therapy.[56,84] According to the NIH guidelines for treatment of overweight and obese patients, pharmacotherapy may be considered in adults with a BMI ≥30 kg/m² and/or a WC ≥40 inches (102 cm) for men or 35 inches (89 cm) for women, or

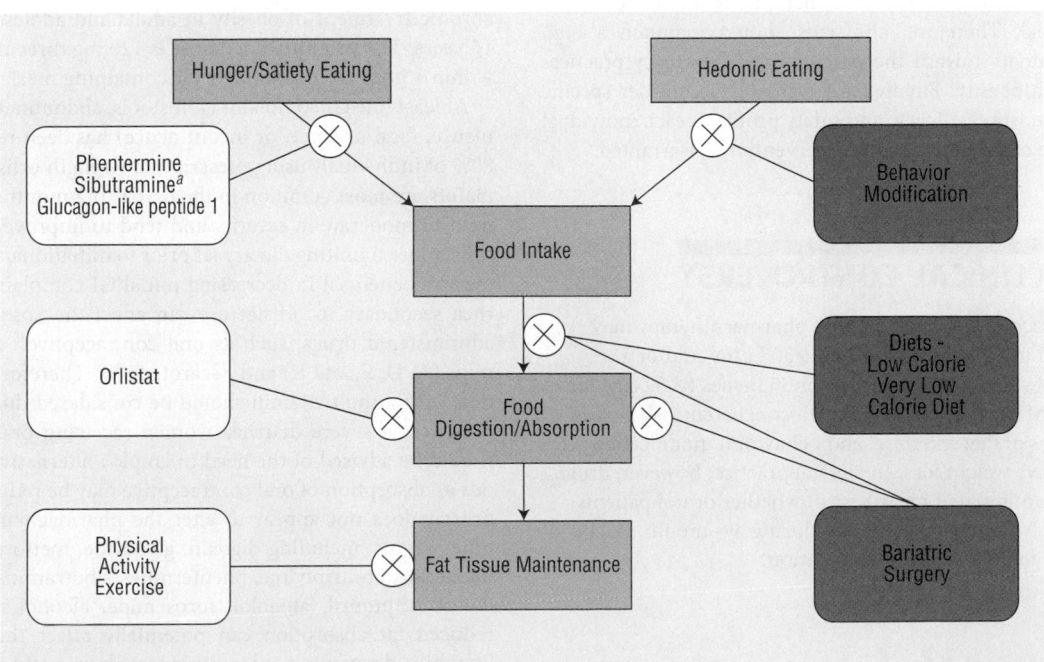

FIGURE 154-4. Sites of action for obesity treatments are represented by a circled X. Most appetite suppressants act on hunger and satiety mechanisms. Traditional diets and bariatric surgery act by limiting food intake. Orlistat interferes with fat absorption in the gut, whereas gastric bypass surgery interferes with absorption more generally. *aSibutramine was withdrawn from the U.S. market in October of 2010.*

TABLE 154-5 Pharmacotherapeutic Agents for Weight Loss

Class	Availability	Status	Daily Dosages (mg)
Gastrointestinal lipase inhibitor			
Orlistat (Xenical)	Rx	Long-term use	360 (3 divided doses)
Orlistat (Alli)	OTC	Long-term use	180 (3 divided doses)
Noradrenergic/serotonergic agent			
Sibutramine (Meridia, Reductil)[a]	Rx	Long-term use	5–15
Noradrenergic agents			
Phendimetrazine (Prelu-2, Bontril, Plegine, Obezine, Statobex, X-trozine)	Rx	Short-term use	70–105
Phentermine (Fastin, Adipex-P, Ionamin)	Rx	Short-term use	15–37.5
Diethylpropion (Tenuate, Tenuate Dospan)	Rx	Short-term use	75

[a]Sibutramine was withdrawn from the U.S. market in October of 2010.
OTC = over-the-counter, Rx = prescription

BMI of 27 to 30 kg/m^2 with at least two concurrent risk factors if 6 months of diet, exercise, and behavioral modification failed to achieve weight loss (Fig. 154–3).[6] Table 154–5 lists the status of the most common classes of agents currently available.

❺ A multidisciplinary team approach to the management of obesity is necessary to ensure long-term success. The U.S. Preventive Services Task Force published an exhaustive summary of evidence related to screening and interventions for adult obesity that incorporates a graded assessment of obesity pharmacotherapy randomized controlled trials.[75] The discovery of cardiac valve disease in relation to serotonergic appetite suppressant use and its resulting multibillion-dollar class action litigation affirms the task force's call for further study of available therapies.[83,85] It is common for patients to use a combination of nonprescription, prescription, and other complementary and alternative therapies to attain the desired weight loss goal. Therefore, clinicians should maintain a high degree of sensitivity toward the potential polypharmacy practices of patients with obesity. Finally, is it prudent to consider specific patient characteristics, efficacy, and safety profile of each individual agent when use of a pharmacologic intervention is warranted.

CLINICAL CONTROVERSY

Current practice guidelines state that pharmacotherapy may be considered in patients with a BMI ≥30 kg/m^2 and/or a WC ≥40 inches (≥ 102 cm) for men or 35 inches (≥ 89 cm) for women, or BMI of 27 to 30 kg/m^2 with concurrent risk factors after 6 months of diet, exercise, and behavioral modification failed to achieve weight loss. In clinical practice, however, drug therapy is often initiated regardless of whether or not patients have previously failed to lose weight during a 6-month trial of diet exercise, and behavioral modification.

Agents Approved for Long-Term Use
Lipase Inhibitors

Orlistat Excessive intake of dietary fat is one of the contributing factors in the development of obesity. Gastrointestinal (gastric,

pancreatic, and carboxyl ester) lipases are essential in the absorption of the long-chain triglycerides. Additionally, lipase is known to play a role in facilitating gastric emptying and secretion of other pancreaticobiliary substances. Orlistat (Xenical,) is a synthetic derivative of lipstatin, a natural lipase inhibitor produced by *Streptomyces toxytricini*. The drug is minimally absorbed and induces weight loss by persistent lowering of dietary fat absorption through selective inhibition of the gastrointestinal (GI) lipase. Furthermore, lower luminal free fatty acid concentrations result in malabsorption of cholesterol. Up to 30% reduction in fat absorption occurred with daily doses of 120 mg three times daily with meals.[86] A nonprescription formulation of orlistat (Alli) is approved in the United States at a reduced daily dose of 60 mg three times daily.[87] The drug must be taken within 1 hour of consuming foods that contain fat in order to exert its effect. If a meal is skipped or contains no fat, the dose of orlistat can be omitted.

Clinical studies employing orlistat as an adjunct to diet therapy demonstrate dose-dependent reductions in fat absorption. Overall, results from clinical trials demonstrate that orlistat effectively increases the amount of weight lost and decreases the amount of weight regained during medically supervised weight loss programs.[86,88] The longest trial that evaluated the safety and efficacy of orlistat is XENDOS (XENical in the prevention of Diabetes in Obese Subjects), a 4-year, double-blind, randomized, placebo-controlled prospective study.[89] Although weight regain was observed with continual therapy beyond the first year of orlistat therapy, results from this study show moderate weight loss sustained after 4 years of treatment compared with placebo, 12.8 lb (5.8 kg) and 6.6 lb (3.0 kg), respectively. Weight loss using orlistat also decreased the rate of development of type 2 diabetes by 37.3% in patients with impaired glucose tolerance. Improved glycemic control can be attained in patients with type 2 diabetes by inducing or increasing weight loss with orlistat in addition to diet management.[86,88] In some cases, dosages or the number of antidiabetic medications may be reduced or discontinued.[86] Significant improvements in lipid profile (reduction in total and low-density lipoprotein [LDL] cholesterol), glucose control, and other markers of metabolism are seen when using orlistat in addition to diet.[86,88] Orlistat is approved for the chronic treatment of obesity in adults and adolescents ages 12 to 16 years. The recommended dose is 120 mg three times daily taken within 1 hour of consuming a fat-containing meal.

At least one GI complaint (soft stools, abdominal pain/colic, flatulence, fecal urgency, or incontinence) has been reported in up to 80% of individuals using prescription strength orlistat. These complaints are most common in the first 1 to 2 months of therapy, are mild to moderate in severity and tend to improve with continued orlistat use. Limiting dietary fat prior to initiation of orlistat therapy may be beneficial in decreasing initial GI complaints. Severe diarrhea secondary to orlistat use can affect the absorption of orally administered drugs, such as oral contraceptives, fat-soluble vitamins (A, D, E, and K) and β–carotene.[86,89] Therefore, supplementation with a multivitamin should be considered during therapy. In presence of severe diarrhea women receiving oral contraceptives should be advised of the need to employ alternative backup methods as absorption of oral contraceptive may be reduced.[86] Although orlistat does not appear to alter the pharmacokinetic profiles of other agents, including digoxin, glyburide, metformin, phenytoin, fluoxetine, amitriptyline, phentermine, sibutramine, losartan, nifedipine, captopril, atenolol, furosemide, alcohol, or atorvastatin, reduced fat absorption can potentially affect the absorption of lipophilic drugs, such as lamotrigine, valporic acid, gabapentin, and amiodarone.[90] Decreased vitamin K absorption has also been noted and can alter the patients warfarin dosage needs.[90] Clinicians should also be aware that orlistat may directly interfere with the absorption of other narrow therapeutic range drugs, such as cyclosporine and levothyroxine.[90] In patients requiring concomitant therapies with orlistat, close monitoring is warranted to ensure an adequate therapeutic response. Separation of the administration times of the medications may minimize these potential drug interactions.

The Food and Drug Administration (FDA) is reviewing safety information for the possible risk of liver damage with the use of orlistat. Between 1999 and October 2008, there were 32 reports of serious liver injury, including 27 hospitalizations and 6 reports of liver failure, in patients using orlistat.[91] Causality has not been definitively linked to orlistat, and those taking prescription and nonprescription orlistat are advised to continue using the product as directed by their healthcare providers.

Noradrenergic–Serotonergic Agents

Sibutramine Until recently sibutramine was available in the U.S. for long-term use. This drug induces weight loss by decreasing appetite and maintaining or increasing thermogenesis via increasing the synaptic concentration of serotonin, norepinephrine (NE), and dopamine through reuptake inhibition. Reuptake inhibition appears to be greatest for NE, followed by serotonin, with dopamine the least inhibited. In humans, the degree to which these effects can be attributed to central versus peripheral activity is currently unknown.

In adults, the recommended starting dose is 10 mg daily, with a recommended dose range of 5 to 15 mg daily. A meta-analysis of available randomized trials suggests after 1 year of therapy sibutramine-treated patients on average lost 9.2 lb (4.2 kg) more weight than placebo-treated patients.[88] After 12 months of therapy, sibutramine-treated patients had a 32% higher chance of achieving a 5% reduction in total body weight and an 18% higher chance of achieving a 10% reduction in body weight compared to those taking placebo. As with other centrally active appetite suppressants, weight regain occurs with cessation of therapy; patients can regain up to 55% of weight lost 18 months after treatment is discontinued. STORM (Sibutramine Trial of Obesity Reduction and Maintenance) was the longest randomized, double-blind study to evaluate the effectiveness of sibutramine, lasting up to 2 years.[92] The group receiving sibutramine achieved more weight loss than the placebo group (22.4 lb [10.2 kg] vs 10.3 lb [4.7 kg]), respectively] and had more subjects who retained at least 80% of the weight loss (43% and 16%, respectively). Sibutramine-related weight loss was associated with a decline in triglycerides, very low-density lipoprotein cholesterol, insulin C-peptides, and uric acid concentrations. The 20% improvement in high-density lipoprotein (HDL) cholesterol is comparable to the average effects of the ingestion of fibric acid derivatives or statins.[67] Few studies have evaluated the safety and efficacy of sibutramine in children and adolescents.

Dry mouth, anorexia, insomnia, constipation, dizziness, and nausea were noted two- to threefold more frequently in sibutramine-treated subjects than in placebo-treated subjects. Statistically significant increases in blood pressure (1.7 mm Hg systolic and 2.8 mm Hg diastolic pressure) and pulse rate (4.5 beats/min) have been reported with sibutramine use.[88] Baseline blood pressure should be established prior to beginning therapy, and close monitoring is required when using this agent. Sibutramine's product labeling has indicated that the drug should not be used in patients with hypertension. Interestingly, however, some evidence suggests that the central α-adrenergic (clonidine-like) effect of sibutramine may predominate in patients with elevated sympathetic activity resulting in decreased blood pressure in hypertensive patients.[93] Nonetheless, use of sibutramine has been contraindicated in all patients with a history of cardiovascular disease, including coronary artery disease, stroke or transient ischemic attack, heart arrhythmias, uncontrolled hypertension, congestive heart failure, and peripheral arterial disease. The SCOUT (Sibutramine Cardiovascular OUTcomes)

study—a prospective trial that evaluated the potential benefits of sibutramine on cardiovascular outcomes in obese or overweight individuals with preexisting cardiovascular disease, type 2 diabetes mellitus, or both—failed to provide any reassurance regarding sibutramine's safety.[94] Although individuals taking sibutramine had modest weight loss, improvement in cardiovascular outcomes was not seen. Conversely, subjects with preexisting cardiovascular disease actually had an increased risk of nonfatal myocardial infarction and nonfatal stroke. Because of concerns that the effectiveness of sibutramine on weight loss is counterbalanced by increased rather than decreased cardiovascular risk, the drug was voluntarily withdrawn from the U.S. market in late 2010.[95]

Combination Therapy Theoretically, the combination of orlistat and sibutramine would produce a synergistic effect because they work through different mechanisms of action to induce weight loss. However, none of the few studies to look at this combination has shown that it would result in greater weight loss compared with sibutramine alone.[96–99] The concomitant use of these two drugs may lead to increased adverse effects without improved therapeutic outcomes. Therefore, the combination of orlistat and sibutramine is not recommended over the use of either product individually.

CLINICAL CONTROVERSY

Obesity is considered a chronic disease. Agents approved by the FDA for long-term management of obesity have limited long-term data regarding morbidity and mortality outcomes; therefore, the optimal duration of treatment beyond the studied treatment periods remains unknown. Although discontinuation of drug treatment tends to result in weight regain, continuation of an effective and well-tolerated drug regimen is the current practice until additional evidence is available.

Agents Approved for Short-Term Use

Noradrenergic Agents

Phentermine Phentermine is structurally similar to amphetamine, but it has less severe CNS stimulation and a lower abuse potential. Its mechanism of action centers on its ability to enhance NE and dopamine neurotransmission. Phentermine is available in both immediate-release and sustained-release formulations. However, the value of sustained-release formulations is questionable based on the reported phentermine plasma half-life of 12 to 24 hours.[100] Phentermine is an effective adjunct to diet, exercise, and behavior modification for producing weight loss in excess of that seen with placebo.[101] Intermittent phentermine therapy appears to elicit comparable weight loss as that seen with continuous use. However, most individuals experience weight regains during therapy and generally always after discontinuing use.[100] A single dose of 30 mg once daily in the morning provides effective appetite suppression throughout the day. Divided doses of 8 mg immediately before meals, however, are common. Doses >30 mg daily do not improve effectiveness.[101] Evening or nighttime dosing should be avoided because of insomnia. Significant increases in blood pressure, palpitations, and arrhythmias can occur with phentermine administration. Use is not advisable in hypertensive patients and those with underlying cardiac abnormalities.

The potential for hypertensive crisis with coadministration of phentermine and MAOIs is noted in the product labeling of each agent; therefore, patients should be off an MAOI for at least 14 days prior to use of any adrenergic agent to avoid excessive adrenergic stimulation syndromes.[102] Phentermine use is contraindicated in patients with hyperthyroidism or agitated states and in those who are abusers of substances such as cocaine, phencyclidine, and methamphetamine, again because of the potential for excessive adrenergic stimulation syndromes and abuse potential. Mydriasis from adrenergic stimulation can worsen glaucoma, and patients diagnosed with glaucoma should not receive phentermine. Diabetic patients may experience altered insulin or oral hypoglycemic dosage requirements soon after beginning therapy and prior to any substantial weight loss. Phentermine remains the most widely prescribed weight management medication by obesity specialists in spite of product labeling that indicates short-term (a few weeks), monotherapy use only.[103] This usage pattern deviates from the current national recommendations that promote only long-term drug intervention when obesity pharmacotherapy is appropriate.[56]

Diethylpropion Diethylpropion stimulates NE release from presynaptic storage granules. Increased adrenergic neurotransmitter concentrations activate hypothalamic centers, which results in decreased appetite and food intake. This drug undergoes extensive first-pass hepatic metabolism. Active metabolites are eliminated renally and account for ~70% of the administered dose. The elimination half-life of these metabolites is about 8 hours.[101] Less than 10% of the parent compound is recovered in urine. No specific dosing recommendations exist for use in patients with renal or hepatic insufficiency. Diethylpropion can be taken in divided daily doses, generally 25 mg three times daily before meals. An extended-release formulation is also employed by some clinicians, usually as 75 mg taken once daily in the morning or midmorning. Both dosing regimens are effective in achieving short-term weight loss in excess of placebo.[29] Complaints of insomnia increase if late afternoon dosing is used. Diethylpropion causes less stimulation of the central nervous system than mazindol and generally causes less insomnia than phentermine. Patients with severe hypertension or significant cardiovascular disease should not receive diethylpropion. Diabetic patients may experience decreased insulin or oral hypoglycemic dosage requirements soon after beginning therapy and prior to any substantial weight loss. More frequent blood glucose self-monitoring and medical follow-up are warranted when treating diabetic patients with diethylpropion.

Amphetamines Appetite suppressant effects of the amphetamines were well recognized in the 1930s. Amphetamines activate central noradrenergic receptor systems as well as dopaminergic pathways at higher doses by stimulating neurotransmitter release. Increases in blood pressure and mild bronchodilation are attributed to peripheral α- and β-receptor activation. Amphetamines are no longer widely used for the treatment of obesity due to their powerful stimulant effects and addictive potential.

Mazindol Chemically distinct from amphetamines and phentermine, mazindol's tricyclic structure results in amphetamine-like appetite suppression.[29] Despite demonstrated efficacy as a short-term therapy for weight reduction, mazindol is no longer available in the United States.[86]

Other Agents Used for Weight Management

Serotonergic Agents Serotonin is an important neurotransmitter involved in many human physiologic systems such as sleep–wake cycles, sensitivity to pain, blood pressure, mood, and eating behaviors. Increasing central serotonin levels disrupts the body's natural development of satiety by decreasing the amount of food consumed and prolongs the time between food intake.[104] Some serotonergic agents increase central serotonin concentrations via stimulating release of presynaptic stores and/or inhibition of reuptake into storage granules. Additionally, either the parent

compound or metabolites of these agents may stimulate postsynaptic 5-HT receptors directly. Peripheral serotonin effects that have an impact on appetite, such as slowing gastric motility, have been described. A major distinction between serotonergic and noradrenergic anorexiants is that serotonergic agents lack the central stimulant effects and thus the abuse potential seen with the noradrenergic compounds.[27,29] Conversely, decreased wakefulness, altered sleep patterns, and changes in affect can be seen.

Antidepressants: Selective Serotonin Reuptake Inhibitors Some of the serotonergic appetite-suppressing agents were first studied as antidepressants (see Chapter 77) and when weight loss was noted in some patients, they began to be used as weight management agents. These drugs are not approved by the FDA as weight management agents and currently not recommended for treatment of obesity. Nonetheless, some practitioners have prescribed these agents for the treatment of obesity "off-label" either alone or in combination with phentermine.

Fluoxetine is a serotonergic agent that has been prescribed as an appetite-suppressing agent. Higher doses of fluoxetine (60 mg) were generally employed for weight loss as opposed to the lower doses (20 mg) frequently used for the treatment of depression. A meta-analysis of six fluoxetine trials demonstrated a variable effect on weight loss, ranging from 14.5 kg (31.9 lb) lost to 0.4 kg (0.9 lb) gained, when compared with placebo over periods of up to 1 year.[29] Weight regain was noted to occur despite continued medication use.[105]

The safety and efficacy of phentermine–serotonin reuptake inhibitor combinations is limited. A case report of adverse experiences (e.g., impaired mentation, tremor, hyperreflexia, and GI symptoms) with unintentional concurrent use of phentermine and fluoxetine reinforces the need for caution by prescribers of this unapproved combination therapy.[106] Although cases of pulmonary hypertension have been reported in patients exposed to fluoxetine,[107] serious adverse effects such as cardiac valve abnormalities in excess of baseline prevalence have not been reported in relation to selective serotonin reuptake inhibitor use for obesity therapy.[108]

Endocannabinoid System Agents Over the past 20 years, arachidonic acid derivatives, known as endocannabinoids, were identified as endogenous substances that activate cannabinoid receptors.[109,110] A complex relationship exists between the endocannabinoid system, energy regulatory hormones, and neuropeptides.[110] The endocannabinoid system appears to be overactive in states of overweight and obesity. Additionally, the endocannabinoid system appears to be involved in the propagation of addictive behaviors related to ingestion of substances such as nicotine, alcohol, marijuana, opioid, and other psychostimulants.

Two distinct cannabinoid receptors are known and have been cloned, CB_1 and CB_2. The existence of a third, CB_3, has also been described.[111] These G-protein-coupled receptors have wide and differing tissue distribution. CB_1 receptors are found in high concentrations in brain and peripheral organs, including the liver, GI tract, adipocytes, and cardiac muscle.[109] Central and peripheral CB_1 receptors are involved in many aspects of energy balance, regulation of food intake, glucose and lipid metabolism, and body composition. CB_2 receptors are mainly expressed within immune system tissues and are not currently recognized as affecting energy balance.

Rimonabant Rimonabant (SR141716A), first described in 1994 as an inhibitor of brain CB_1 receptors, has potent central and peripheral effects on feeding, nutrient metabolism, and body composition.[27,109] However, the FDA's Endocrinologic and Metabolic Drugs Advisory Committee in 2007 unanimously agreed that rimonabant did not demonstrate a favorable risk-to-benefit profile to enable it to be approved for weight management.[112] The committee's concerns centered on increased risk of serious neurologic side effects—seizures, depression, anxiety, aggressiveness, and suicidal thoughts among patients randomized to rimonabant. Following a safety review from the European Medicines Agency's Committee for Medicinal Products for Human Use, marketing of rimonabant was withdrawn across the European Union in 2008 due to its serious psychiatric concerns.[113] Sanofi-Aventis subsequently decided to discontinue clinical development of rimonabant.[114] Similarly, the development of other CB[1] receptor antagonists has been suspended.[115]

■ COMPLEMENTARY AND ALTERNATIVE THERAPIES

6 Many complementary and alternative therapy products are currently promoted for weight loss. A survey of consumers revealed that ~18% of Americans reported use of "natural products" (i.e., dietary supplements other than vitamins and minerals) within the past year.[116] It is important for clinicians to be aware that the regulation of dietary supplements is less rigorous than that of prescription and over-the-counter drug products. As such, a manufacturer of a dietary supplement does not have to prove the safety or effectiveness of the product before it is marketed. Of concern, some herbal and food supplement diet agents contain pharmacologically active substances that should be used with caution or avoided in obese patients with conditions such as diabetes, hypertension, and significant cardiovascular disease. In addition, many marketed products have been reported to lack consistency in labeling versus actual product content. More recently, a number of dietary supplements have been found to contain undeclared prescription drugs.[117] Clinicians may access the FDA Dietary Supplement Alerts and Safety Information website to keep informed of these issues.[118] Table 154–6 lists some of the common herbal/natural products used for weight loss and the constituents found in many of these products.

Bitter Orange

Bitter orange (*Citrus aurantium*) contains m-synephrine, a sympathomimetic amine with structural similarities to ephedrine.[119] After FDA banned the sale of ephedra-containing dietary supplements in 2004, several manufacturers replaced the ephedra constituents within their products with bitter orange. Bitter orange–containing products are commonly promoted as "ephedra-free." Although bitter orange has been shown to effectively promote weight loss, it may also increase heart rate and blood pressure, potentially causing the same adverse cardiovascular effects that were observed with ephedra.[119]

| **TABLE 154-6** | Common Herbal/Natural Products and Food Supplements Used for Weight Loss[a] |

Herbal/Natural/Food Supplements	Active Component	Proposed Mechanism
Bitter orange	M-synephrine	Noradrenergic
Calcium pyruvate	Pyruvate	Unknown
Chromium picolinate	Chromium	Unknown
Chitosan	Cationic polysaccharide	Block fat absorption
Garcinia gambogia extract (citrin)	Hydroxycitric acid	Unknown
Guarana extract	Caffeine	Noradrenergic
Hoodia	P57	Unknown
Various tea extracts	Caffeine	Noradrenergic

[a]Safety and efficacy are not documented.

Chromium

Chromium is considered an essential nutrient and experimentally in animals is an insulin cofactor active in carbohydrate, protein, and lipid metabolism. In humans, insulin resistance has been reported in a few cases of apparent severe chromium deficiency during long-term total parenteral nutrition (see Chapter 151). Currently, there is no reliable means of assessing total body chromium status, making diagnosis of deficiency difficult. The tryptophan metabolite, picolinic acid, forms a complex with trivalent chromium, which improves bioavailability. Food sources with highly available chromium include brewer's yeast, calves' liver, American cheese, and wheat germ. Clinical trials assessing chromium picolinate as a supplement to aerobic exercise in the treatment of obesity have failed to demonstrate any effectiveness.[120,121]

Chitosan

Chitosan is a cationic polysaccharide, specifically a partially N-deacetylated form of chitin. This nonhydrolyzable fiber exhibits properties similar to those of cellulose. In vitro and preclinical data indicate that chitosan may be effective in blocking absorption of fat from the gut. It has been suggested that orally administered chitosan may be an effective weight reduction agent by blocking calories ingested as fat. Chitosan is a major constituent in several heavily advertised weight management food supplements and nonprescription preparations. However, a small number of randomized and blinded or open-label investigations have demonstrated that orally administered chitosan is not an effective inhibitor of fat absorption in humans.[122] Although further research may be warranted with respect to the appropriate dose in humans needed to impair fat absorption, current claims of chitosan effectiveness are unsubstantiated.

Ephedra Alkaloids

Based on the known effects of ephedrine, dietary supplements claiming weight management effects have employed plant sources of ephedra alkaloids. Various parts of the Ephedraceae, ma huang, *Sida cordifolia,* and *Pinellia ternata* plants are known to produce ephedra alkaloids, including L-ephedrine, D-pseudoephedrine, L-norephedrine, D-norpseudoephedrine, L-N-methylephedrine, and D-N-methylpseudoephedrine.[123] Common names routinely included in dietary supplement labeling for these alkaloid sources include joint fir, popotillo, country mallow, sea grape, and yellow horse. From 1994 through July 1997, the FDA received more than 800 reports of serious adverse events; including seizures, stroke, and death, coincident with ephedrine alkaloid-containing dietary supplement use. An in-depth review of 140 reports of adverse events related to ephedrine alkaloid-containing dietary supplements demonstrated that approximately half the reports involved cardiovascular symptoms.[124] In 2004, the FDA determined that all sources of ephedra alkaloids must be excluded from dietary supplements because they present an unreasonably high health risk.[125]

Guarana Extract and Various Tea Extracts

Guarana and tea are sources of caffeine that have inherent adrenergic properties and increase the effects of stimulant substances, such as ephedrine and ephedra alkaloids. Guarana and various tea extracts are commonly found in energy drinks and combination weight loss products that contain other substances with stimulant properties.[126,127]

Hoodia

Hoodia is a desert cactus of the Apocynaceae plant family. Natives indigenous to the Kalahari Desert are purported to consume the stems and roots of this plant for their appetite suppressant effects.[128] Other names appearing on product labels are Kalahari cactus, Hoodia cactus or extract, *Hoodia gordonii* cactus, and Kalahari diet. Hoodia extract, sometimes referred to as P57, is rumored to elicit weight loss; however, no peer-reviewed reports of effectiveness are currently available.

Pyruvate

Pyruvate is a commonly listed ingredient in many herbal weight management preparations. Multiple salt forms are used, including sodium, magnesium, potassium, and calcium. Other names are α-ketopropionic acid, 2-oxypropanoic acid, and acetylformic acid. Pyruvate is a three-carbon intermediate formed during normal glucose metabolism and/or during glycolysis. It is advertised in the lay press for its ability to "increase metabolism" and thus promote weight loss. Objective data documenting these effects are lacking.[129,130] Although most pyruvate nutritional weight management supplements contain less than 2 g per dose, large exposures (>20 g) are known to cause noticeable GI side effects, including bloating and diarrhea.

■ AGENTS UNDER INVESTIGATION

Several investigational pharmacologic agents are currently being evaluated for weight management. Lorcaserin, a selective serotonin (5-HT$_{2C}$) receptor agonist, is one such agent currently in phase III development. Activation of central 5-HT$_{2C}$ receptors results in appetite suppression. A clinical trial evaluating the efficacy and safety of lorcaserin in healthy obese men and women reported dose-dependent weight loss and a favorable safety profile.[131] Subjects who received 10 mg of lorcaserin twice daily for 12 weeks experienced an average weight loss of 3.6 kg (7.9 lb), compared with 0.3 kg (0.7 lb) in placebo-treated subjects. It is important to note that this trial did not include any modifications in dietary intake or physical activity. The most common adverse events reported in subjects receiving lorcaserin were headache, nausea, and dizziness.

Another agent in the final stages of testing for obesity treatment is cetilistat, a lipase inhibitor. A trial involving 371 obese subjects reported an average weight loss of 4.1 kg (9 lb) over 12 weeks in patients who received 240 mg of cetilistat three times daily in combination with a hypocaloric diet.[132] Cetilistat also improved total and LDL cholesterol. The safety profile of cetilistat is similar to that of orlistat and includes primarily GI adverse events. Other products currently being studied for weight management include the following drug combinations: bupropion and naltrexone (Contrave), phentermine and topiramate (Qnexa), and pramlintide and metreleptin.[133,134]

■ PHARMACOECONOMIC CONSIDERATIONS

The economic consequences of treating obesity and obesity-related comorbidities are significant. The annual cost of health care attributed to obesity was estimated to be at least $147 billion in 2008.[135] Weight reduction has been reported to reduce prescription costs. A study conducted by Collins and colleagues evaluated the savings in prescription costs following a 12-week weight reduction program in 40 type 2 diabetic patients. A cost analysis was completed on 32 of 40 patients who were taking antihypertensive and/or antidiabetic medications based on their out-of-pocket costs for these medications at the beginning of the study and after 1 year. The average cost

of these prescriptions at the beginning as compared with the 1-year follow-up was $63.30 versus $32.50 per month. The estimated annual average saving in prescription costs per patient was $443.[136] Another study evaluating the economic impact of weight change in patients with type 2 diabetes examined total healthcare cost and diabetes-related costs in 458 patients.[137] Patients were classified as either weight gainers (n = 224; average weight gain 3.9% in 6 months) or non–weight gainers (n = 234; average weight loss 3.3%). The overall pharmacy cost after 1 year was significantly less for the non–weight gainers than the weight gainers ($1,703 vs $2,225; P = 0.044). The cost of antidiabetic agents was also significantly less in the non–weight gainer group ($499 vs $769; P = 0.001). This evidence suggests that weight reduction can lead to decreased prescription medication costs. A systematic review of published economic evaluations of orlistat, sibutramine, and rimonabant reported incremental cost-effectiveness ratios (ICERs).[138] The authors reported a median ICER of $23,364 per quality-adjusted life-year (QALY). It was determined that most of the ICERs were within the appropriate range to be considered cost-effective. However, the authors concluded uncertainty regarding the utility gain associated with weight loss and weight regain. Of note, adverse events were not explicitly taken into account in any study.

Martin and colleagues compared the costs associated with medical and surgical treatment of obesity.[139] Medical therapy groups received diet therapy only (no medications), and cost included weekly clinic visits for behavioral modification. A successful outcome was defined as loss of at least one-third of excess body weight above ideal body weight. The authors monitored all patients for 2 years and some for as long as 7 years so that long-term weight control could be addressed. As expected, the costs of surgery were much higher than medical therapy over the first 2 years ($24,000 vs $3,000). However, when costs were extrapolated out to 6 years, the cost per pound lost for medical therapy exceeded surgical therapy (about $313 vs $261 per pound lost).

Finally, third-party payer and insurance reimbursement for provision of obesity treatment services continue to be inconsistent. For example, a recent questionnaire administered to 25 health plans in Pennsylvania reported that less than 50% of payers reimbursed for lifestyle modification (other than dietary counseling) or weight loss medication. All of the health plans that responded to the questionnaire provided some coverage for bariatric surgery.[140]

It is clear from the preceding data that weight loss can be expensive. Prospectively designed cost–benefit or cost-effectiveness analyses are needed to determine if costs of weight loss therapy or surgery are balanced by lower costs of hospitalizations for other medical problems associated with obesity or the additional life-years gained. Quality-of-life measures also need to be taken into consideration when evaluating these types of data.

■ EVALUATION OF THERAPEUTIC OUTCOMES

Monitoring the Pharmaceutical Care Plan

Assessment of patient progress should be documented once or twice monthly for 1 to 2 months and then monthly thereafter.[6] Each encounter should document weight, WC, BMI, blood pressure, medical history, and patient assessment of obesity medication tolerability.[6] Chronic use of obesity medications should be consistent with the approved product labeling, and medication therapy should be discontinued after 3 to 4 months if the patient has failed to demonstrate weight loss or maintenance of prior weight. To achieve optimal weight loss, patients should be instructed about the importance of adherence to prescribed medication and lifestyle changes. Numerous tools for both patient and practitioner are readily available through the Department of Human Services and NIH–National Heart Lung and Blood Institute (NHLBI) Obesity Education Initiative.[141] The Short Form 36 (SF-36) also has been used as a quality-of-life evaluation tool for obese patients undergoing programmatic weight loss. Quarterly assessments of well-being and quality of life using validated assessment tools can be helpful in objectively quantifying the effectiveness of therapy, as well as potential drug-induced side effects (e.g., depression).

Diabetic patients receiving weight loss medication require more intense medical monitoring and self-monitoring of blood glucose. Insulin therapy may need to be adjusted with the start of obesity medication therapy. Some diabetic patients may require daily telephone contact with a healthcare provider to assist in adjusting their hypoglycemic therapy. Weekly patient visits to a healthcare setting may be necessary for 1 to 2 months until the effects of diet, exercise, and weight loss medication become more predictable. As frequent as quarterly assessment of hemoglobin A_{1c} may be appropriate in type 2 diabetics who lose weight to aid in adjustment of hypoglycemic therapy. Lipid profiles can normalize or improve with weight loss. Lipid status should be assessed semiannually or annually in patients with hyperlipidemia to determine the need for continued hyperlipidemia therapies. Weight loss also can result in normalization of blood pressure in hypertensive obese patients. Assessment of appropriateness of antihypertensive therapy should occur with each follow-up visit.

The evaluation and management of a patient with obesity requires careful clinical, biochemical, and, if necessary, psychological evaluation. The evaluation must include an assessment of current medical conditions and medications the patient uses. Clearly, a multidisciplinary team including, but not limited to, a physician, nutritionist, psychologist, and pharmacist best achieves this.

CONCLUSION

Obesity is a chronic disease with a prevalence that has increased dramatically over the past 30 years. Increased body weight is a consequence of an imbalance between energy intake and energy expenditure over time, which is influenced by many factors, including genetic and environmental aspects. Nonpharmacologic therapy, including reduced caloric intake, increased physical activity, and behavioral modification, is currently the mainstay of obesity management. Drug therapy may be considered as an adjunct for those patients who fail to achieve adequate weight loss after 6 months of diet, exercise, and behavioral modification. Currently, only orlistat is available in the United States for the long-term treatment of overweight and obesity. Bariatric procedures have evidence for long-term efficacy for weight reduction, but they also introduce surgical comorbidities and, for the most efficacious procedures, may cause significant nutritional deficiencies. Treatment of obesity should be individualized, considering factors such as patient desires, age, degree and duration of obesity, and the presence or absence of medical conditions both directly related to obesity and those that may have an impact on the therapeutic decisions. Regardless of the chosen treatment plan, the management of obesity is a lifelong process requiring patient support and careful monitoring for safety and efficacy.

ABBREVIATIONS

ATP III: Third Report of the Expert Panel on the Detection, Evaluation, and Treatment of High Blood Cholesterol in Adults

5-HT: 5-hydroxytryptamine (serotonin)

BMI: Body mass index

BMR: Basal metabolic rate

CT: Computed tomography

HDL: High-density lipoprotein

ICER: Incremental cost-effectiveness ratio

LCD: Low-calorie diet

LDL: Low-density lipoprotein

Kcal: Kilocalories

MAOI: Monoamine oxidase inhibitor

MRI: Magnetic resonance imaging

NE: Norepinephrine

NHANES: National Health and Nutrition Examination Survey

NIH: National Institutes of Health

QALY: Quality-adjusted life-year

REE: Resting energy expenditure

WC: Waist circumference

REFERENCES

1. Centers for Disease Control and Prevention. NCHS Health and Statistics. Prevalence of overweight, obesity and extreme obesity among adults: United States, trends 1960–62 through 2005–2006, 2008. http://www.cdc.gov/nchs/data/hestat/overweight/overweight_adult.pdf. Last accessed, September 26, 2009.

2. Ogden CL, Yanovski SZ, Carroll MD, Flegal KM. The epidemiology of obesity. Gastroenterology 2007;132(6):2087–2102.

3. Ogden CL, Carroll MD, Flegal KM. High body mass index for age among US children and adolescents, 2003–2006. JAMA 2008;299(20):2401–2405.

4. Wang Y, Beydoun MA, Liang L, Caballero B, Kumanyika SK. Will all Americans become overweight or obese? Estimating the progression and cost of the US obesity epidemic. Obesity 2008;16(10):2323–2330.

5. Kushner RF. Assessment and management of adult obesity: A primer for physicians. Chicago, IL: American Medical Association, 2003. http://www.ama-assn.org/ama/pub/category/print/10931.html. Last accessed, October 2, 2009.

6. U.S. Department of Health and Human Services. National Heart Lung and Blood Institute: Obesity Initiative Expert Panel on the Identification, Evaluation, and Treatment of Overweight and Obesity in Adults. Washington, DC: U.S. Public Health Service; 1998.

7. Anand RG, Peters RW, Donahue TP. Obesity and dysrhythmias. J Cardiometab Syndr 2008;3(3):149–154.

8. Anandacoomarasamy A, Caterson I, Sambrook P, Fransen M, March L. The impact of obesity on the musculoskeletal system. Int J Obes 2008;32(2):211–222.

9. Buchwald H. Bariatric surgery for morbid obesity: Health implications for patients, health professionals, and third-party payers. J Am Coll Surg 2005;200(4):593–604.

10. Esposito K, Giugliano F, Ciotola M, De Sio M, D'Armiento M, Giugliano D. Obesity and sexual dysfunction, male and female. Int J Impot Res 2008;20(4):358–365.

11. Guh DP, Zhang W, Bansback N, Amarsi Z, Birmingham CL, Anis AH. The incidence of co-morbidities related to obesity and overweight: A systematic review and meta-analysis. BMC Public Health 2009;9:88. doi:10.1186/1471-2458-9-88.

12. Kushner RF, Roth JL. Assessment of the obese patient. Endocrinol Metab Clin North Am 2003;32(4):915–933.

13. Mathus-Vliegen EM, Nikkel D, Brand HS. Oral aspects of obesity. Int Dent J 2007;57(4):249–256.

14. Murugan AT, Sharma G. Obesity and respiratory diseases. Chron Respir Dis 2008;5(4):233–242.

15. Nguyen S, Hsu CY. Excess weight as a risk factor for kidney failure. Curr Opin Nephrol Hypertens 2007;16(2):71–76.

16. Pan SY, DesMeules M. Energy intake, physical activity, energy balance, and cancer: epidemiologic evidence. Methods Mol Biol 2009;472: 191–215.

17. Setty AR, Curhan G, Choi HK. Obesity, waist circumference, weight change, and the risk of psoriasis in women: Nurses' Health Study II. Arch Intern Med 2007;167(15):1670–1675.

18. Stothard KJ, Tennant PW, Bell R, Rankin J. Maternal overweight and obesity and the risk of congenital anomalies: A systematic review and meta-analysis. JAMA 2009;301(6):636–650.

19. Janssen I, Bacon E. Effect of current and midlife obesity status on mortality risk in the elderly. Obesity 2008;16(11):2504–2509.

20. Reis JP, Macera CA, Araneta MR, Lindsay SP, Marshall SJ, Wingard DL. Comparison of overall obesity and body fat distribution in predicting risk of mortality. Obesity 2009;17(6):1232–1239.

21. Finkelstein EA, Ruhm CJ, Kosa KM. Economic causes and consequences of obesity. Annu Rev Public Health 2005;26:239–257.

22. Office of the Surgeon General. Overweight and obesity. 2003. http://www.surgeongeneral.gov/topics/obesity/.

23. U.S. Department of Health and Human Services. Healthy People 2010. Objectives: List for public comment. http://www.healthypeople.gov/hp2020/objectives.htm.

24. U.S. Department of Health and Human Services, NIH-NHLBI. Obesity Education Initiative. 2003. http://www.nhlbi.nih.gov/about/oei/oei_pd.htm.

24. U.S. Preventative Services Task Force. Screening for obesity in adults: Recommendations and rationale. Ann Intern Med 2003;139(11): 930–932.

26. Institute of Medicine Committee on Prevention of Obesity in Children and Youth. Preventing Childhood Obesity: Health in the Balance. Washington, DC: National Academies Press; 2005.

27. Ioannides-Demos LL, Proietto J, McNeil JJ. Pharmacotherapy for obesity. Drugs 2005;65(10):1391–1418.

28. Lakka TA, Bouchard C. Physical activity, obesity and cardiovascular diseases. Handb Exp Pharmacol 2005(170):137–163.

29. Li Z, Maglione M, Tu W, et al. Meta-analysis: Pharmacologic treatment of obesity. Ann Intern Med 2005;142(7):532–546.

30. Wadden TA, Berkowitz RI, Womble LG, et al. Randomized trial of lifestyle modification and pharmacotherapy for obesity. N Engl J Med 2005;353(20):2111–2120.

31. Singh AS, Mulder C, Twisk JW, van Mechelen W, Chinapaw MJ. Tracking of childhood overweight into adulthood: A systematic review of the literature. Obes Rev 2008;9(5):474–488.

32. Ogden CL. Disparities in obesity prevalence in the United States: Black women at risk. Am J Clin Nutr 2009;89(4):1001–1002.

33. Robinson WR, Gordon-Larsen P, Kaufman JS, Suchindran CM, Stevens J. The female-male disparity in obesity prevalence among black American young adults: Contributions of sociodemographic characteristics of the childhood family. Am J Clin Nutr 2009;89(4): 1204–1212.

34. Lee YS. The role of genes in the current obesity epidemic. Ann Acad Med Singapore 2009;38(1):45–43.

35. Rankinen T, Zuberi A, Chagnon YC, et al. The human obesity gene map: The 2005 update. Obesity 2006;14(4):529–644.

36. Frayling TM, Timpson NJ, Weedon MN, et al. A common variant in the FTO gene is associated with body mass index and predisposes to childhood and adult obesity. Science 2007;316(5826):889–894.

37. Obesity Gene Map Database. Human Genomics Laboratory. http://obesitygene.pbrc.edu/. Last accessed, October 6, 2009.

38. French SA, Story M, Jeffery RW. Environmental influences on eating and physical activity. Annu Rev Public Health 2001;22:309–335.

39. Hill JO, Peters JC. Environmental contributions to the obesity epidemic. Science 1998;280(5368):1371–1374.

40. Christakis NA, Fowler JH. The spread of obesity in a large social network over 32 years. N Engl J Med 2007;357(4):370–379.

41. Sheehan AH. Weight gain. In: Tisdale JE, Miller DA, eds. Drug-Induced Diseases: Prevention, Detection and Management. 2nd ed. Bethesda, MD: American Society of Health-System Pharmacists; 2010.

42. Dhillo WS. Appetite regulation: An overview. Thyroid 2007;17(5): 433–445.

43. Valassi E, Scacchi M, Cavagnini F. Neuroendocrine control of food intake. Nutr Metab Cardiovasc Dis 2008;18(2):158–168.

44. Farooqi IS, O'Rahilly S. Leptin: A pivotal regulator of human energy homeostasis. Am J Clin Nutr 2009;89(3):980S–984S.

45. Friedman JM. Leptin at 14 years of age: An ongoing story. Am J Clin Nutr 2009;89(3):973S–979S.

46. Small CJ, Bloom SR. Gut hormones and the control of appetite. Trends Endocrinol Metab 2004;15(6):259–263.

47. Cypess AM, Lehman S, Williams G, et al. Identification and importance of brown adipose tissue in adult humans. N Engl J Med 2009;360(15):1509–1517.

48. Avram AS, Avram MM, James WD. Subcutaneous fat in normal and diseased states: 2. Anatomy and physiology of white and brown adipose tissue. J Am Acad Dermatol 2005;53(4):671–683.

49. Arner P, Hoffstedt J. Adrenoceptor genes in human obesity. J Intern Med 1999;245(6):667–672.

50. Clinical guidelines on the identification, evaluation, and treatment of overweight and obesity in adults: The Evidence Report. National Institutes of Health. Obes Res 1998;6(Suppl 2):51S–209S.

51. Carroll JF, Chiapa AL, Rodriquez M, et al. Visceral fat, waist circumference, and BMI: impact of race/ethnicity. Obesity 2008;16(3):600–607.

52. Cheng CY, Reich D, Coresh J, et al. Admixture mapping of obesity-related traits in African Americans: The Atherosclerosis Risk in Communities (ARIC) Study. Obesity 2010;18(3):563–572.

53. Cossrow N, Falkner B. Race/ethnic issues in obesity and obesity-related comorbidities. J Clin Endocrinol Metab 2004;89(6):2590–2594.

54. Rahman M, Temple JR, Breitkopf CR, Berenson AB. Racial differences in body fat distribution among reproductive-aged women. Metabolism 2009;58(9):1329–1337.

55. Lee SY, Gallagher D. Assessment methods in human body composition. Curr Opin Clin Nutr Metab Care 2008;11(5):566–572.

56. U.S. Department of Health and Human Services. National Heart Lung and Blood Institute: Clinical guidelines on the identification, evaluation, and treatment of overweight and obesity in adults–Practical guide. 2003. http://www.nhlbi.nih.gov/guidelines/obesity/ob_home.htm.

57. Pischon T, Boeing H, Hoffmann K, et al. General and abdominal adiposity and risk of death in Europe. N Engl J Med 2008;359(20):2105–2120.

58. Finkelstein EA, Brown DS, Wrage LA, Allaire BT, Hoerger TJ. Individual and aggregate years-of-life-lost associated with overweight and obesity. Obesity 2010;18(2):333–339.

59. Hubert HB, Feinleib M, McNamara PM, Castelli WP. Obesity as an independent risk factor for cardiovascular disease: A 26-year follow-up of participants in the Framingham Heart Study. Circulation 1983;67(5):968–977.

60. Poirier P, Giles TD, Bray GA, et al. Obesity and cardiovascular disease: Pathophysiology, evaluation, and effect of weight loss–An update of the 1997 American Heart Association Scientific Statement on Obesity and Heart Disease from the Obesity Committee of the Council on Nutrition, Physical Activity, and Metabolism. Circulation 2006;113(6):898–918.

61. Poirier P, Giles TD, Bray GA, et al. Obesity and cardiovascular disease: Pathophysiology, evaluation, and effect of weight loss. Arterioscler Thromb Vasc Biol 2006;26(5):968–976.

62. Escobar-Morreale HF. Polycystic ovary syndrome: Treatment strategies and management. Expert Opin Pharmacother 2008;9(17):2995–3008.

63. Gregg EW, Gerzoff RB, Thompson TJ, Williamson DF. Trying to lose weight, losing weight, and 9-year mortality in overweight U.S. adults with diabetes. Diabetes Care 2004;27(3):657–662.

64. Klein S, Sheard NF, Pi-Sunyer X, et al. Weight management through lifestyle modification for the prevention and management of type 2 diabetes: Rationale and strategies. A statement of the American Diabetes Association, the North American Association for the Study of Obesity, and the American Society for Clinical Nutrition. Diabetes Care 2004;27(8):2067–2073.

65. Norris SL, Zhang X, Avenell A, et al. Long-term non-pharmacologic weight loss interventions for adults with type 2 diabetes. Cochrane Database Syst Rev 2005(2):CD004095.

66. Williamson DF, Thompson TJ, Thun M, Flanders D, Pamuk E, Byers T. Intentional weight loss and mortality among overweight individuals with diabetes. Diabetes Care 2000;23(10):1499–1504.

67. Third report of the National Cholesterol Education Program (NCEP) Expert Panel on Detection, Evaluation, and Treatment of High Blood Cholesterol in Adults (Adult Treatment Panel III) final report. Circulation 2002;106(25):3143–3421.

68. Volpe SL. Popular weight reduction diets. J Cardiovasc Nurs 2006;21(1):34–39.

69. Gardner CD, Kiazand A, Alhassan S, et al. Comparison of the Atkins, Zone, Ornish, and LEARN diets for change in weight and related risk factors among overweight premenopausal women: The A TO Z Weight Loss Study–A randomized trial. JAMA 2007;297(9):969–977.

70. Nordmann AJ, Nordmann A, Briel M, et al. Effects of low-carbohydrate vs low-fat diets on weight loss and cardiovascular risk factors: A meta-analysis of randomized controlled trials. Arch Intern Med 2006;166(3):285–293.

71. Sacks FM, Bray GA, Carey VJ, et al. Comparison of weight-loss diets with different compositions of fat, protein, and carbohydrates. N Engl J Med 2009;360(9):859–873.

72. Franz MJ, VanWormer JJ, Crain AL, et al. Weight-loss outcomes: A systematic review and meta-analysis of weight-loss clinical trials with a minimum 1-year follow-up. J Am Diet Assoc 2007;107(10):1755–1767.

73. Shaw K, Gennat H, O'Rourke P, Del Mar C. Exercise for overweight or obesity. Cochrane Database Syst Rev 2006(4):CD003817.

74. Jakicic JM, Otto AD. Physical activity considerations for the treatment and prevention of obesity. Am J Clin Nutr 2005;82:226S–229S.

75. McTigue KM, Harris R, Hemphill B, et al. Screening and interventions for obesity in adults: Summary of the evidence for the U.S. Preventive Services Task Force. Ann Intern Med 2003;139(11):933–949.

76. Williamson DA, Perrin LA. Behavioral therapy for obesity. Endocrinol Metab Clin North Am 1996;25(4):943–954.

77. Santry HP, Gillen DL, Lauderdale DS. Trends in bariatric surgical procedures. JAMA 2005;294(15):1909–1917.

78. Mechanick JI, Kushner RF, Sugerman HJ, et al. American Association of Clinical Endocrinologists, the Obesity Society, and the American Society for Metabolic and Bariatric Surgery medical guidelines for clinical practice for the perioperative nutritional, metabolic, and nonsurgical support of the bariatric surgery patient. Surg Obes Relat Dis 2008;4(5 Suppl):S109–S184.

79. Flum DR, Belle SH, King WC, et al. Perioperative safety in the longitudinal assessment of bariatric surgery. N Engl J Med 2009;361(5):445–454.

80. Sjostrom L, Narbro K, Sjostrom CD, et al. Effects of bariatric surgery on mortality in Swedish obese subjects. N Engl J Med 2007;357(8):741–752.

81. Miller AD, Smith KM. Medication and nutrient administration considerations after bariatric surgery. Am J Health Syst Pharm 2006;63(19):1852–1857.

82. Rogers CC, Alloway RR, Alexander JW, Cardi M, Trofe J, Vinks AA. Pharmacokinetics of mycophenolic acid, tacrolimus and sirolimus after gastric bypass surgery in end-stage renal disease and transplant patients: A pilot study. Clin Transplant 2008;22(3):281–291.

83. AHP diet drug settlement, 1999. http://www.settlementdietdrugs.com/. Last accessed, October 10, 2009.

84. Yanovski SZ. Pharmacotherapy for obesity: Promise and uncertainty. N Engl J Med 2005;353(20):2187–2189.

85. Seghatol FF, Rigolin VH. Appetite suppressants and valvular heart disease. Curr Opin Cardiol 2002;17(5):486–492.

86. Henness S, Perry CM. Orlistat: A review of its use in the management of obesity. Drugs 2006;66(12):1625–1656.

87. Anderson JW. Orlistat for the management of overweight individuals and obesity: A review of potential for the 60-mg, over-the-counter dosage. Expert Opin Pharmacother 2007;8(11):1733–1742.

88. Rucker D, Padwal R, Li SK, Curioni C, Lau DC. Long term pharmacotherapy for obesity and overweight: Updated meta-analysis. BMJ 2007;335(7631):1194–1199.

89. Torgerson JS, Hauptman J, Boldrin MN, Sjostrom L. XENical in the prevention of diabetes in obese subjects (XENDOS) study: A randomized study of orlistat as an adjunct to lifestyle changes for the prevention of type 2 diabetes in obese patients. Diabetes Care 2004;27(1):155–161.

90. Filippatos TD, Derdemezis CS, Gazi IF, Nakou ES, Mikhailidis DP, Elisaf MS. Orlistat-associated adverse effects and drug interactions: A critical review. Drug Saf 2008;31(1):53–65.

91. Early communication about an ongoing safety review of orlistat (marketed as Alli and Xenical). August 2009. http://www.fda.gov/Drugs/DrugSafety/PostmarketDrugSafetyInformationforPatientsandProviders/DrugSafetyInformationforHeathcareProfessionals/ucm179166.htm.

92. James WP, Astrup A, Finer N, et al. Effect of sibutramine on weight maintenance after weight loss: A randomised trial. STORM Study Group. Sibutramine Trial of Obesity Reduction and Maintenance. Lancet 2000;356(9248):2119–2125.

93. Sharma AM. Does pharmacologically induced weight loss improve cardiovascular outcome? Sibutramine pharmacology and the cardiovascular system. Eur Heart J Suppl 2005;7:L39–L43.

94. James WPT, Caterson ID, Coutinho W, et al. Effect of sibutramine on cardiovascular outcomes in overweight and obese subjects. N Engl J Med 2010;363(10):905–917.

95. U.S. Food and Drug Administration. Drug safety information for healthcare professionals. Follow-up to the November 2009 early communication about an ongoing safety review of sibutramine, marketed as Meridia. http://www.fda.gov/Drugs/DrugSafety/PostmarketDrugSafetyInformationforPatientsandProviders/DrugSafetyInformationforHeathcareProfessionals/ucm198206.htm.

96. Wadden TA, Berkowitz RI, Womble LG, Sarwer DB, Arnold ME, Steinberg CM. Effects of sibutramine plus orlistat in obese women following 1 year of treatment by sibutramine alone: A placebo-controlled trial. Obes Res 2000;8(6):431–437.

97. Aydin N, Topsever P, Kaya A, Karasakal M, Duman C, Dagar A. Orlistat, sibutramine, or combination therapy: Which performs better on waist circumference in relation with body mass index in obese patients? Tohoku J Exp Med 2004;202(3):173–180.

98. Sari R, Balci MK, Cakir M, Altunbas H, Karayalcin U. Comparison of efficacy of sibutramine or orlistat versus their combination in obese women. Endocr Res 2004;30(2):159–167.

99. Kaya A, Aydin N, Topsever P, et al. Efficacy of sibutramine, orlistat and combination therapy on short-term weight management in obese patients. Biomed Pharmacother 2004;58(10):582–587.

100. Bray GA, Greenway FL. Current and potential drugs for treatment of obesity. Endocr Rev 1999;20(6):805–875.

101. Silverstone T. Appetite suppressants: A review. Drugs 1992;43(6):820–836.

102. Adipex-P (phentermine hydrochloride) product information. Sellersville, PA: Teva Pharmaceuticals; North Wales, PA 1 2005.

103. Hendricks EJ, Rothman RB, Greenway FL. How physician obesity specialists use drugs to treat obesity. Obesity 2009;17(9):1730–1735.

104. Halford JC, Harrold JA, Boyland EJ, Lawton CL, Blundell JE. Serotonergic drugs: Effects on appetite expression and use for the treatment of obesity. Drugs 2007;67(1):27–55.

105. Goldstein DJ, Rampey AH, Jr., Enas GG, Potvin JH, Fludzinski LA, Levine LR. Fluoxetine: A randomized clinical trial in the treatment of obesity. Int J Obes Relat Metab Disord 1994;18(3):129–135.

106. Bostwick JM, Brown TM. A toxic reaction from combining fluoxetine and phentermine. J Clin Psychopharmacol 1996;16(2):189–190.

107. Anchors M. Fluoxetine is a safer alternative to fenfluramine in the medical treatment of obesity. Arch Intern Med 1997;157(11):1270.

108. Whigham LD, Dhurandhar NV, Rahko PS, Atkinson RL. Comparison of combinations of drugs for treatment of obesity: Body weight and echocardiographic status. Int J Obes 2007;31(5):850–857.

109. Leite CE, Mocelin CA, Petersen GO, Leal MB, Thiesen FV. Rimonabant: An antagonist drug of the endocannabinoid system for the treatment of obesity. Pharmacol Rep 2009;61(2):217–224.

110. Wegener N, Koch M. Neurobiology and systems physiology of the endocannabinoid system. Pharmacopsychiatry 2009;42(Suppl 1):S79–S86.

111. Ryberg E, Larsson N, Sjogren S, et al. The orphan receptor GPR55 is a novel cannabinoid receptor. Br J Pharmacol 2007;152(7):1092–1101.

112. U.S. Food and Drug Administration. Endocrinologic and Metabolis Drugs Advisory Committee. FDA briefing document. NDA 21-888. Zimulti (rimonabant) tablets, 20 mg, Sanofi-Aventis. June 13, 2007. http://www.fda.gov/ohrms/dockets/ac/07/briefing/2007-4306b1-fda-backgrounder.pdf.

113. The European Medicines Agency recommends suspension of the marketing authorisation of Acomplia, 2008. http://www.emea.europa.eu/humandocs/PDFs/EPAR/acomplia/53777708en.pdf. Last accessed, October 8, 2009.

114. Sanofi-aventi to discontinue all clinical trials with rimonabant. 2008. http://en.sanofi-aventis.com/binaries/20081105_rimonabant_en_tcm28-22682.pdf. Last accessed, October 7, 2009.

115. Janero DR, Makriyannis A. Cannabinoid receptor antagonists: Pharmacological opportunities, clinical experience, and translational prognosis. Expert Opin Emerg Drugs 2009;14(1):43–65.

116. Blanck HM, Serdula MK, Gillespie C, et al. Use of nonprescription dietary supplements for weight loss is common among Americans. J Am Diet Assoc 2007;107(3):441–447.

117. Cohen PA. American roulette: Contaminated dietary supplements. N Engl J Med 2009;361(16):1523–1525.

118. United States Food and Drug Administration. Dietary supplement alerts and safety information, 2009. http://www.fda.gov/Food/DietarySupplements/Alerts/default.htm. Last accessed, October 9, 2009.

119. Haaz S, Fontaine KR, Cutter G, Limdi N, Perumean-Chaney S, Allison DB. Citrus aurantium and synephrine alkaloids in the treatment of overweight and obesity: An update. Obes Rev 2006;7(1):79–88.

120. Lukaski HC, Siders WA, Penland JG. Chromium picolinate supplementation in women: Effects on body weight, composition, and iron status. Nutrition 2007;23(3):187–195.

121. Trent LK, Thieding-Cancel D. Effects of chromium picolinate on body composition. J Sports Med Phys Fitness 1995;35(4):273–280.

122. Ni Mhurchu C, Dunshea-Mooij CA, Bennett D, Rodgers A. Chitosan for overweight or obesity. Cochrane Database Syst Rev 2005(3):CD003892.

123. Betz JM, Gay ML, Mossoba MM, Adams S, Portz BS. Chiral gas chromatographic determination of ephedrine-type alkaloids in dietary supplements containing Ma Huang. J AOAC Int 1997;80(2):303–315.

124. Haller CA, Benowitz NL. Adverse cardiovascular and central nervous system events associated with dietary supplements containing ephedra alkaloids. N Engl J Med 2000;343(25):1833–1838.

125. Department of Health and Human Services, Food and Drug Administration. Final rule declaring dietary supplements containing ephedrine alkaloids adulterated because they present an unreasonable risk. Fed Regist 2004;69(28):6787–6854.

126. Clauson KA, Shields KM, McQueen CE, Persad N. Safety issues associated with commercially available energy drinks. J Am Pharm Assoc 2008;48(3):e55–e63.

127. Morelli V, Zoorob RJ. Alternative therapies: Part I. Depression, diabetes, obesity. Am Fam Physician 2000;62(5):1051–1060.

128. Van Heerden FR. Hoodia gordonii: A natural appetite suppressant. J Ethnopharmacol 2008;119(3):434–437.

129. Koh-Banerjee PK, Ferreira MP, Greenwood M, et al. Effects of calcium pyruvate supplementation during training on body composition, exercise capacity, and metabolic responses to exercise. Nutrition 2005;21(3):312–319.

130. Pittler MH, Ernst E. Dietary supplements for body-weight reduction: A systematic review. Am J Clin Nutr 2004;79(4):529–536.

131. Smith SR, Prosser WA, Donahue DJ, Morgan ME, Anderson CM, Shanahan WR. Lorcaserin (APD356), a selective 5-HT(2C) agonist, reduces body weight in obese men and women. Obesity 2009;17(3):494–503.

132. Kopelman P, Bryson A, Hickling R, et al. Cetilistat (ATL-962), a novel lipase inhibitor: A 12-week randomized, placebo-controlled study of weight reduction in obese patients. Int J Obes 2007;31(3):494–499.

133. Klonoff DC, Greenway F. Drugs in the pipeline for the obesity market. J Diabetes Sci Technol 2008;2(5):913–918.

134. Padwal R. Contrave, a bupropion and naltrexone combination therapy for the potential treatment of obesity. Curr Opin Investig Drugs 2009;10(10):1117–1125.

135. Finkelstein EA, Trogdon JG, Cohen JW, Dietz W. Annual medical spending attributable to obesity: payer and service-specific estimates. Health Aff 2009;28(5):w822–w831.

136. Collins RW, Anderson JW. Medication cost savings associated with weight loss for obese non-insulin-dependent diabetic men and women. Prev Med 1995;24(4):369–374.

137. Yu AP, Wu EQ, Birnbaum HG, et al. Short-term economic impact of body weight change among patients with type 2 diabetes treated with antidiabetic agents: analysis using claims, laboratory, and medical record data. Curr Med Res Opin 2007;23(9):2157–2169.

138. Neovius M, Narbro K. Cost-effectiveness of pharmacological anti-obesity treatments: A systematic review. Int J Obes 2008;32(12):1752–1763.

139. Martin LF, Tan TL, Horn JR, et al. Comparison of the costs associated with medical and surgical treatment of obesity. Surgery 1995;118(4):599–606.

140. Tsai AG, Asch DA, Wadden TA. Insurance coverage for obesity treatment. J Am Diet Assoc 2006;106(10):1651–1655.

141. National Heart Lung and Blood Institute, 1991. Obesity education initiative. http://www.nhlbi.nih.gov/about/oei/. Last accessed, October 9, 2009.

GLOSSARY

2,3-Bisphosphoglycerate: An intermediate in the Rapoport-Luebering shunt, formed between 1,3-bisphosphoglycerate and 3-phospho-glycerate; an important regulator of the affinity of hemoglobin for oxygen.

5-α-reductase: Enzyme responsible for conversion of testosterone to its active metabolite dihydrotesterone. Two types of this enzyme exist. Type 2 is predominant in prostate cells.

α-Amino-3-hydroxy-5-methyl-4 isoxazolepropionate (AMPA)/ kainate receptors: Two of three types of ionotropic post-synaptic glutamate receptors. These receptors are similar and are often considered together. Upon binding glutamate, these receptors permit the influx of Na⁺ ions and results in brain excitation. These are one of the two primary receptors for excitatory neurotransmission in the brain.

α-Amino-3-hydroxy-5-methylisoxazole-4-propionate: See *AMPA*.

α-Hydroxy acids: Exfoliating products such as lactic, glycolic, malic, mandelic, and tartaric acid used in cosmetics.

β-Hydroxy acid: Salicylic acid.

γ-Aminobutyric acid (GABA): The major inhibitory neurotransmitter in the central nervous system.

γ-Aminobutyric acid (GABA$_A$) receptors: Postsynaptic ionotropic receptors that bind to GABA and result in Cl⁻ influx and neuronal hyperpolarization. GABA is the main inhibitory neurotransmitter in the brain and GABA$_A$ receptors mediate fast CNS inhibitory neurotransmission.

Abscess: A purulent collection of fluid separated from surrounding tissue by a wall comprised of inflammatory cells and adjacent organs. It usually contains necrotic debris, bacteria, and inflammatory cells.

Abstinence: Refraining from the indulgence in something, as sexual intercourse or substances, by one's own choice. The absence of genital contact that could permit a pregnancy (i.e., penile penetration into the vagina).

Acanthosis: Increased thickness of the prickle cell layer of the skin.

Acculturation: The process by which individuals from one cultural group adopt or change behaviors, attitudes and/or beliefs through contact with a different culture.

Acetabular: Relating to the acetabulum, the hollow, cuplike portion of the pelvis into which the head of the thigh bone (femur) fits.

Achalasia: Problem that occurs when a ring of muscle fibers, such as a sphincter of the esophagus, fail to relax.

Acne: Inflammatory eruption of the sebaceous gland.

Acnegenicity: Product effect that causes irritation of follicles resulting in papules and pustules.

Acquired resistance: See *Secondary resistance*.

Acromegaly: A pathologic condition characterized by excessive production of growth hormone.

Activities of daily living: Dressing, bathing, getting around inside the home, feeding, toileting, and grooming. See also *Instrumental activities of daily living*.

Acute bacterial pharyngitis: Acute bacterial infection of the oropharynx or nasopharynx.

Acute bacterial sinusitis: Acute bacterial infection of the paranasal sinuses lasting less than 30 days.

Acute coronary syndrome (ACS): Ischemic chest discomfort at rest most often accompanied by ST-segment elevation, ST-segment depression, or T-wave inversion on the 12-lead electrocardiogram and caused by plaque rupture and partial or complete occlusion of the coronary artery by thrombus. Acute coronary syndromes include infarction and unstable angina. Former terms used to describe types of ACS include *Q-wave myocardial infarction*, *non–Q-wave myocardial infarction*, and *unstable angina*.

Acute otitis media: Acute inflammation of the middle ear.

Acute pain: Can be a useful physiologic process warning individuals of disease states and potentially harmful situations. Severe, unremitting, undertreated, acute pain, when it outlives its biologic usefulness, can produce many deleterious effects (e.g., psychological problems). It usually subsides when the healing process decreases the pain-producing stimuli.

Acute pancreatitis: Acute inflammation of the pancreas that can be mild with minimal or no organ dysfunction or severe with organ failure and local complications.

Acute stress disorder: A disorder characterized by anxiety, dissociative, and other symptoms that occurs within 1 month after exposure to an extreme traumatic stressor.

Acute tubular necrosis: Acute renal failure as the result of renal tubular epithelial cell damage, which can be caused by either direct toxic or ischemic effects of drugs.

Adaptive functioning: Individual effectiveness coping with everyday stressors compared to a peer with similar background, and socioeconomic and psychosocial opportunities.

Adaptive inflammation: Inflammatory pain that promotes the shifting from prevention of tissue damage to promotion of healing.

Addiction: A primary, chronic, neurobiologic disease, with genetic, psychosocial, and environmental factors influencing its development and manifestations. It is characterized by behaviors that include one or more of the following five Cs: *c*hronicity, impaired *c*ontrol over drug use, *c*ompulsive use, *c*ontinued use despite harm, and *c*raving.

Adjuvant analgesics: Agents that are useful in the treatment of pain but are usually not classified as analgesics.

Administrative burden: The demands placed on those who administer an instrument.

Adolescents: Pediatric patients who are 12 to 16 years of age.

Adoptive immunotherapy: Administration of immune cells for the purpose of cancer treatment.

Adrenergic: Neuronal or neurologic activity caused by neurotransmitters such as epinephrine, norepinephrine, and dopamine.

Adrenocorticotropic hormone (ACTH): A polypeptide hormone secreted by the anterior pituitary that controls secretion of cortisol from the adrenal glands.

Adverse drug events: Injuries resulting from administration of a drug or other circumstances surrounding use of the drug but not necessarily caused by the drug itself. See also *Adverse drug reaction*.

Adverse drug reaction: Any noxious, unintended, and undesired effect of a drug that occurs at doses used in humans for prophylaxis, diagnosis, or therapy.

Affect: Pattern of behaviors that a clinician can observe that expresses a person's current state of emotion.

Afterload: The pressure or the "load" the heart must generate to eject blood into the systemic circulation. Although approximated by the systemic vascular resistance, it is a complex measure that includes blood viscosity, aortic impedance, and ventricular wall thickness. Along with preload, it is an important determinant of cardiac output.

Aganglionosis: The state of being without ganglia.

Agnosia: Cardinal symptom of Alzheimer's disease; inability to recognize or identify a familiar object in the absence of impaired sensory function.

Agoraphobia: Anxiety about, or avoidance of, places or situations from which escape might be difficult (or embarrassing) or in which help might not be available in the event of having a panic attack or panic-like symptoms.

Akathisia: The sensation of inner restlessness resulting in the need to make movements such as pacing or moving the legs. Akathisia has subjective and objective components.

Albumin: The major protein in plasma, with a molecular weight of 65 kDa.

Albuminuria: A condition where a large amount of albumin (>300 mg/day) is present in the urine, often indicating glomerular damage in the kidney.

Alcohol ablation: Alcohol ablation of the septum is a nonsurgical procedure to improve outflow tract obstruction. It is a percutaneous catheter-based method to decrease septal thickness by therapeutic myocardial infarction.

Alcoholism: A chronic, progressive, and potentially fatal biogenic and psychosocial disease characterized by tolerance and physical dependence and manifested by a total loss of control, as well as diverse personality changes and social consequences.

Algorithm (treatment algorithm): Identifies and specifies sequences for treatment alternatives, with specific options and tactics for care. Based on scientific data and on expert consensus in areas where there is little scientific data, algorithms are divided into stages so that the simplest, most efficacious, and best-tolerated treatments available are tried first. If results are not optimal, treatment advances to the next stage. Unless a patient's illness fails to improve sufficiently with early stage treatments, he or she is spared treatments that are more complex, that might be less well tolerated, or that have more potential for drug interactions or serious side effects. Algorithms recommend key decision points in treatment decision making.

Allergic interstitial nephritis: Inflammation of the interstitial region of the kidney often associated with acute onset of renal insufficiency.

Allergic salute: Constant upward rubbing of the nose as a result of allergies.

Allergic shiners: Dark circles under the eyes as a result of nasal congestion leading to venous pooling.

Allodynia: Painful response to normally non-noxious stimuli.

Allogeneic transplantation: Transfer of cells between different individuals.

Allograft: An organ or tissue transplant from one human to another.

Allokinesis: A phenomenon whereby pruritic skin affects the surrounding normally nonpruritic skin area, whether inflamed or noninflamed. The nonpruritic skin becomes very sensitive, reacts to light stimuli, and begins itching.

Alloimmunization: Rapid consumption of transfused platelets through an immune-mediated reaction.

Alternate forms: All modes of administration other than the mode for which the instrument was originally developed.

Amenorrhea: Lack of menstruation or the abnormal ending of the female menstrual cycle.

American Urological Association (AUA) Symptom Index: A validated questionnaire of seven questions that can be used by patients to assess the bothersomeness of their voiding symptoms. The total score range is 0 to 35. Higher scores are consistent with severely bothersome symptoms.

Amnesia: A pathologic impairment of memory.

AMPA/kainate receptors: Two of three types of ionotropic postsynaptic glutamate receptors. These receptors are similar and are often considered together. On binding glutamate, these receptors permit the influx of sodium ions (Na^+) and results in brain excitation. These are one of the two primary receptors for excitatory neurotransmission in the brain.

Amygdala: A small almond-shaped temporal lobe structure that plays a role in emotions and fear control.

Anaphylactoid: Anaphylaxis-like reactions that do not involve immunoglobulin E (IgE)-mediated mechanisms.

Anaphylaxis: Acute, life-threatening allergic reaction involving multiple organ systems.

Anastomosis: The surgical connection of two tubular structures, such as blood vessels, in a transplanted organ.

Andropause: Refers to a number of symptoms associated with decreased testosterone production by the testes in aging men. The symptoms include decreased libido, increased body fat, depressed mood, and osteoporosis. The symptoms of andropause generally worsen as the patient ages. Andropause in men parallels menopause in women.

Anemia of chronic disease: Mild to moderate anemia not associated with blood loss or hemolysis. Usually with normal cell size. Can be seen with chronic inflammation (e.g., rheumatoid arthritis, chronic infection) or malignancy.

Anemia of chronic kidney disease: A decrease in red blood cell production caused by a deficiency in the hormone erythropoietin normally produced by progenitor cells of the kidney. As kidney function declines, less erythropoietin is available to stimulate red blood cell production (erythropoiesis) in the bone marrow. Contributing factors include iron deficiency and a shortened, red-blood-cell life span.

Aneuploid: Deviation by a whole number in the total number of chromosomes in a cell compared to normal (46 in humans).

Angioedema: An allergic reaction characterized by edema of a tissue such as the lips, eyes, mouth, joints, or other structures because of leak of fluid from blood vessels.

Anhedonia: A lack of pleasure or interest in usual activities.

Anisocytosis: Considerable variation in the size of cells that are normally uniform, especially with reference to red blood cells.

Ankylosis: Bony fusion resulting from chronic joint inflammation.

Anomia: Cardinal symptom of Alzheimer's disease; inability to name objects or to recognize names.

Anorexia nervosa: A psychiatric disorder in which patients present with a fear of being obese. These patients often express a dislike or lack of interest in food; it is most common in young females and can disrupt normal menstrual cycles. It is associated with poor medication treatment response and can result in fatal medical complications.

Antenatal: Time between conception and birth; same as prenatal.

Anterograde amnesia: Inability to remember events or actions that occur after taking a sedative hypnotic medication.

Antibiogram: A summary of antimicrobial susceptibilities.

Anticipatory anxiety: The fear of having an anxiety attack, which is often a trigger by itself; "fear of fear."

Anticoagulant: Any substance that inhibits, suppresses, or delays the formation of blood clots. These substances occur naturally and regulate the clotting cascade. Several anticoagulants have been identified in a variety of animal tissues and have been commercially developed for medicinal use.

Antigenic drift: The creation of antigenic variants by point mutations in the surface antigens, hemagglutinin and/or neuraminidase, of a particular subtype of influenza.

Antigenic shift: Occurs when an influenza virus acquires a new hemagglutinin and/or neuraminidase.

Antimicrobial cycling: A predetermined change in an antimicrobial recommendation for empiric therapy of a specific infection at a predetermined time.

Antimycotic: Inhibiting fungal growth.

Antithrombotic: A pharmacologic agent that prevents thrombus/clot formation. This category includes both antiplatelet agents and anticoagulants.

Anuria: Production of less than 50 mL of urine/day.

Anxiety: A state of apprehension, uncertainty, and fear resulting from the anticipation of a realistic or fantasized threatening event or situation that often impairs physical and psychological functioning.

Aortic stenosis: Aortic stenosis is the obstruction of blood flow across the aortic valve. This disorder has several etiologies: congenital unicuspid or bicuspid valve, rheumatic fever, and degenerative calcific changes of the valve.

Aphasia: Cardinal symptom of Alzheimer's disease; inability to generate or comprehend spoken language.

Aphthous ulcer: A small superficial area of ulceration within the gastrointestinal mucosa, typically found in the oral cavity.

Apical pulse: Point at the apex (bottom portion) of the heart impacts the chest wall.

Apoptosis: Programmed cell death.

Appendageal: Referring to hair, sweat glands, and nails.

Apraxia: Cardinal symptom of Alzheimer's disease; inability to carry out a motor task in the absence of impaired motor function.

Arteriovenous (AV) fistula: In hemodialysis, a vascular access surgically created by connection of an artery directly to a vein, usually in the forearm.

Arteriovenous (AV) graft: In hemodialysis, a vascular access surgically created using a synthetic tube to connect an artery to a vein.

Arteriovenous malformations: A tangle of blood vessels, both arterial and venous, that can rupture and cause hemorrhage in the brain.

Arthrodesis: The surgical immobilization of a joint (i.e., joint fusion).

Arthropathy: Disease of the joints.

Ascites: Accumulation of serous fluid in the peritoneal cavity.

Asherman's syndrome: A cause for menstrual flow obstruction; often resulting from infection or surgery affecting the endometrium.

Asperger's disorder: A type of pervasive developmental disorder characterized by severe and sustained impairment in social interaction, restricted and repetitive patterns of behavioral/interested activities—similar to autism but without clinically significant delays in language and cognitive development or age-appropriate self-help skills.

Aspiration pneumonitis: The inflammation of lung tissue caused by the aspiration of fluids and gastric contents that often leads to dyspnea, pulmonary edema, secondary infections, and adult respiratory distress syndrome. Hydrocarbon pneumonitis is caused by the pulmonary aspiration of hydrocarbons such as kerosene and gasoline.

Assertive community treatment: A treatment program for the care of individuals with schizophrenia in which teams provide comprehensive wraparound services for the patient, including going to the home to provide support for daily living skills, housing, and supported employment. Team members are available 24 hours daily if needed to meet the patient's comprehensive care needs.

Asystole: The presence of a flat line on the electrocardiogram monitor.

Ataxia: Loss of the ability to coordinate muscular movement.

Atelectasis: Pulmonary parenchymal collapse caused by alveolar or bronchial obstruction.

Atopic dermatitis: Skin inflammation that causes itching, scales, and erythema.

Atopic pleat (Dennie–Morgan fold): An extra fold of skin that develops under the eye, characteristic of atopic dermatitis.

Atopy: An allergic syndrome characterized by asthma, hay fever, and urticaria or eczema.

Atrial fibrillation: Rapid beating of the atria that results in variable ventricular rates.

Atropinism: Symptoms of poisoning by atropine or belladonna.

Aura: Sensory or somatosensory alteration without loss of consciousness.

Augmentation: Addition of a medication not usually used as monotherapy for a disorder to a core medication for a disorder in an attempt to enhance the patient's clinical response.

Auscultation: Listening to the heart or other organs with a stethoscope.

Autism/Autistic disorder: A type of pervasive developmental disorder with a neurobiologic etiology, characterized by impaired reciprocal social interaction, impaired communication skills, and a limited range of activities and interests; frequently associated with mental retardation; sometimes referred to as early infantile autism, childhood autism, or Kanner autism.

Autologous transplantation: Readministration of the same person's cells that were previously collected.

Autosomal: Pertaining to a chromosome.

Axonal transaction: Destroying or severing the axon so that electrical impulses are impeded along the nerve sheath or across the nerve synapse. Axonal damage is not reversible and leads to long-term disability and the formation of black holes.

Azotemia: Term referring to elevated levels of urea in the serum or blood.

Azotorrhea: An excessive loss of protein in the feces.

Bacteremia: Presence of viable bacteria (fungi) in the bloodstream.

Bacterial prostatitis: An inflammation of the prostate gland and surrounding tissue as a result of infection.

Bacteriuria: The presence of bacteria in the urine.

Barrett esophagus: Inflammatory changes in the esophagus resulting in replacement of epithelial lining by columnar-type cells that can lead to stricture or adenocarcinoma.

Basal ganglia and striatum: Parts of the brain regulating movements.

Behavioral phenotype: The actions or reactions of a person to internal or external environmental influences.

Benign prostatic hyperplasia: Nonmalignant enlargement of the prostate gland in elderly men.

Bilateral salpingo-oophorectomy: Surgical excision (removal) of both ovaries.

Biliverdin: A green bile pigment formed from the oxidation of heme.

Binge eating: Excessive intake of calorie-laden food over a short period of time.

Bioavailability: The fraction of drug absorbed into the systemic circulation after extravascular administration.

Biochemical markers: Intracellular macromolecules released into the peripheral circulation from necrotic myocytes as a result of myocardial cell death (infarction). These laboratory tests are used in the diagnosis of myocardial infarction. Examples include troponin I, troponin T, creatinine kinase myocardial band (MB), and myoglobin.

Biofilm: A population or community of microorganisms adhering to a surface by a secreted coating. This coating also reduces microorganism vulnerability to antibiotics.

Biopsy: A procedure in which a tiny piece of a body part, such as the kidney or bladder, is removed for examination under a microscope.

Bioterrorism agents: Organisms or toxins that can cause disease and death in humans, animals, or plants for the purpose of eliciting terror.

Bipolar I disorder: Characterized by one or more manic or mixed episodes, and is usually accompanied by major depressive episodes.

Bipolar II disorder: Characterized by one or more major depressive episodes and accompanied by at least one hypomanic episode.

Bleeding diathesis: A condition in which there is an unusual susceptibility or predisposition to bleeding.

Blood urea nitrogen (BUN): A waste product in the blood that comes from the breakdown of food protein. The kidneys filter blood to remove urea and thus maintain homeostasis. As kidney function decreases, the BUN level increases.

Blood–brain barrier: The relative lack of permeability of large molecules (and those molecules lacking lipid solubility) into the central nervous system because of the nonfenestrated capillary beds of the cerebral vasculature.

Borborygmi: Rumbling or gurgling noises produced by movement of gas, fluid, or both in the alimentary canal and audible at a distance.

Brachytherapy: A procedure in which radioactive material sealed in needles, seeds, wires, or catheters is placed directly into or near a tumor. Also called internal radiation, implant radiation, or interstitial radiation therapy.

Bradykinesia: Delay or slowness in initiating and performing purposeful, voluntary movement as seen in Parkinsonism.

Breakthrough bleeding: The unpredictable and irregular bleeding associated with hormone therapy.

Bronchiectasis: Dilation of a bronchus or bronchi, usually related to excessive secretions.

Bronchioles: A subdivision of bronchi; smaller in diameter and without cartilage.

Bronchiolitis: Inflammation of the bronchioles.

Bronchoalveolar lavage: Instilling and then removing a lavage fluid to reveal the secretory and/or cellular contents from deep in the lung.

Bronchorrhea: Excessive bronchial secretions that can impair pulmonary ventilation.

Bruit: An abnormal and often harsh sound heard over a blood vessel, usually an artery, on examination with a stethoscope caused by turbulent blood flow.

B-type natriuretic peptide: B-type natriuretic peptide is a 32-amino-acid polypeptide secreted by the ventricles in response to excessive myocyte stretching. Elevated levels are typically seen in patients with left ventricular dysfunction and can correlate with both the heart failure severity and the prognosis.

Bulimia nervosa: A psychiatric disorder manifested by episodes of consuming a large caloric load over a short period of time (binge eating), with subsequent self-induced vomiting, use of cathartics or diuretics, fasting, or excessive exercise to prevent weight gain.

BUN (blood urea nitrogen): A waste product in the blood that comes from the breakdown of food protein. The kidneys filter blood to remove urea. As kidney function decreases, the BUN level increases.

Bursitis: Inflammation of the bursa, a fluid-filled soft tissue structure that usually results in pain and swelling.

Caffeinism: A clinical syndrome produced by acute or chronic overuse of caffeine characterized by anxiety, psychomotor alterations, sleep disturbances, mood changes, and psychophysiologic complaints.

Calcimimetic: A class of agents that stimulate calcium-sensing receptors on the parathyroid gland and *mimic* the effects of extracellular calcium. They suppress parathyroid hormone (PTH) release and increase the sensitivity of the receptor to extracellular calcium.

Calcium-sensing receptor: The calcium receptor on the chief cells of the parathyroid gland, activation of which leads to suppression of PTH release.

Candidiasis: Fungal infection involving *Candida* species.

Carbuncles: Broad, swollen, erythematous, deep, and painful, follicular masses commonly associated with fever, chills, and malaise.

Carcinoid: A carcinoid is a slow-growing tumor usually located in the gastrointestinal system and sometimes in the lungs or other sites. Carcinoids can spread to the liver and can secrete serotonin or prostaglandins.

Cardiac arrest: The cessation of cardiac mechanical activity as confirmed by the absence of signs of circulation.

Cardiac index: Cardiac output standardized for body surface area. Mathematically, cardiac index = cardiac output/body surface area.

Cardiac output: The volume of blood pumped by the heart per unit of time. Cardiac output is the product of heart rate and stroke volume.

Cardioembolic stroke: An ischemic stroke thought to be caused by an embolism arising from the heart. Cardioembolic stroke can be assumed in patients with significant cardiovascular disease including atrial fibrillation, dilated cardiomyopathy, prosthetic valves, recent myocardial infarction (MI), and patent foramen ovale.

Cardiopulmonary arrest: The abrupt cessation of spontaneous and effective ventilation and circulation following a cardiac or respiratory event.

Cardiopulmonary bypass: The use of extracorporeal devices to pump blood and oxygenate the blood while the heart or lungs are not functional. Extracorporeal membrane oxygenation (ECMO) is a form of long-term cardiopulmonary bypass that is typically used for days to weeks.

Cardiopulmonary resuscitation: The attempt to restore spontaneous circulation by performing chest compressions with or without ventilations.

Carotid Doppler: A technique that provides information about the presence and severity of atherosclerosis of the carotid artery using noninvasive sound wave technology.

Carotid endarterectomy: Removal of the atherosclerotic plaque from the inside of a stenotic carotid artery by a surgical technique. The vessel is surgically opened and sewn and/or patched after removal of the plaque.

Carpal tunnel syndrome: A medical condition in which the median nerve is compressed at the wrist, leading to parethesias, numbness, and muscle weakness in the hand.

Case-control study: An observational study of persons with the disease of interest (cases) and a suitable control group of persons without the disease to establish the extent of association between exposure(s) of interest and disease.

Cataplexy: A sudden loss of muscle control with retention of clear consciousness that follows a strong emotional stimulus (e.g., elation, surprise, or anger) and is a characteristic symptom of narcolepsy.

Cellulitis: An acute, infectious process that initially affects the epidermis and dermis and can subsequently spread within the superficial fascia.

Centrilobular: Affecting the central portion of the lobe.

Cerebral autoregulation: The process by which cerebral blood flow is maintained in a tight range over a wide range of peripheral blood pressures. It is accomplished by reactive dilation and constriction of cerebral arteries.

Cerebral blood flow (CBF): The volume of blood perfusing a given brain mass as a function of time.

Cerebral blood volume (CBV): The total volume of blood within the cerebral vasculature at a given point in time.

Cerebral microdialysis: A sampling method that allows continuous acquisition of a small volume of cerebral extracellular fluid specimens using a microdialysis probe inserted into the brain.

Cerebral oxygen consumption (CMRo$_2$): The cerebral metabolic rate for oxygen consumption calculated as the mean hemispheric CBF and the arteriovenous oxygen content difference (AVDo$_2$).

Cerebral oxygen delivery (CDo$_2$): The product of CBF and arterial oxygen content.

Cerebral perfusion pressure: A critical monitoring parameter in traumatic brain injury patients defined as the difference between the mean arterial pressure and the intracranial pressure.

Cerebrospinal fluid: The clear, colorless fluid that bathes and cushions the brain and spinal cord.

Cervical cap: A thimble-shaped latex rubber device that is held on the cervix by suction, thus acting as a barrier to reduce the risk of pregnancy.

Cervical effacement: During the first stage of labor, as the cervix is opening, it is also thinning. The thinning of the cervix is termed *effacement.*

Cervical ripening: Prior to inducing labor, the cervix must be favorable, approximately 2 cm dilated and 80% thinned out. If this is not the case, an agent must be used to induce histochemical changes to make the cervix more favorable.

Cervical stenosis: A cause for menstrual flow obstruction; often caused by surgical interventions for cervical dysplasia.

Cervicitis: Inflammation of the cervix.

Chancre: A sore or ulcer, the dermal lesion of primary syphilis.

Chancroid: A venereal dermal lesion caused by agents other than syphilis.

Cheilitis: Inflammation of the lips; can be related to retinoid use.

Children: Pediatric patients who are 1 to 11 years of age.

Cholelithiasis: A solid formation in the gallbladder or bile duct composed of cholesterol and bile salts. Also known as gallstone.

Cholestatic hepatitis: Rare form of hepatitis marked by stopped or suppressed flow of bile; characterized by pruritus, dark urine, light-colored stools, elevated alkaline phosphatase, and conjugated bilirubin.

Cholinesterase inhibitors: Class of medication that inhibits enzymatic activity of acetylcholinesterase, butyrylcholinesterase, or both to prevent the degradation of acetylcholine.

Chronic condition: An illness or impairment that cannot be cured.

Chronic kidney disease (CKD): Slow and progressive loss of kidney function that takes several years, often resulting in permanent kidney failure requiring dialysis or transplantation.

Chronic pain/persistent pain: Pain persisting for months to years.

Chronic pancreatitis: Chronic inflammation of the pancreas caused by the many sequelae of long-standing pancreatic injury leading to irreversible pancreatic damage.

Chvostek's sign: A facial twitch produced by tapping on the cheek over the branches of the facial nerve.

Circumstantial speech: Speech pattern whereby the expressed ideas are characterized by unnecessary detail. The speaker ultimately makes their point, but in a very roundabout manner.

Clearance: the volume of blood per unit of time (e.g. L/h, mL/min) completely cleared of a drug.

Clinical inertia: A clinical situation in which no therapeutic move was made to treat a medical condition in a patient that is not considered adequately treated, or at their treatment goal.

Clinical outcomes: Medical events that occur as a result of the condition or its treatment.

Clinical pharmacokinetics: The discipline that describes the absorption, distribution, metabolism, and elimination of drugs in patients.

Clinical proteinuria: Total protein in the urine in amounts greater than 300 mg/day.

Clinical resistance: Refers to failure of an antifungal agent in the treatment of a fungal infection that arises from factors other than microbial resistance, such as failure of the antifungal agent to reach the site of infection, or inability of a patient's immune system to eradicate a fungus whose growth is retarded by an antifungal agent.

Clinically isolated syndrome: The first attack of multiple sclerosis characterized by a neurologic syndrome such as optic neuritis and generally seen with silent or asymptomatic white matter lesions (seen on magnetic resonance imaging) suggestive of demyelination. Individuals that experience a clinically isolated syndrome are at high risk of developing definite multiple sclerosis.

Clotting cascade: A series of enzymatic reactions by clotting factors leading to the formation of a blood clot. The clotting cascade is initiated by several thrombogenic substances. Each reaction in the cascade is triggered by the preceding one, and the effect is amplified by positive feedback loops.

Clotting factor: Plasma proteins found in the blood that are essential to the formation of blood clots. Clotting factors circulate in inactive forms but are activated by their predecessor in the clotting cascade or a thrombogenic substance. Each clotting factor is designated by a Roman numeral (e.g., factor VII) and by the letter "a" when activated (e.g., factor VIIa).

Cluster headache: A primary headache disorder characterized by attacks of severe unilateral headache pain that occurs in series of weeks or months (cluster periods) separated by remission periods usually lasting months or years.

Cluster period: The time during which cluster-headache attacks occur regularly and at least once every other day.

Codon: A sequence of three consecutive nucleotides that specify an amino acid or amino acid chain termination.

Coelomic metaplasia: Transformation of normal cells into endometrial cells.

Cognitive behavioral therapy: A form of psychotherapy designed to replace distorted or inappropriate ways of thinking with healthy, more realistic thoughts to alter maladaptive moods and behavior. It is instructional in approach and is based on the theory that thoughts (not external influences such as people, situations, and events) cause feelings and behaviors. Patients learn to identify the thinking that causes the negative feelings and behaviors and then learn how to replace that thinking with thoughts that lead to more desirable feelings and behaviors.

Cogwheeling: A ratchet-like movement in the joints, characteristic of Parkinson disease.

Cohort study: Assembly of a group of persons without a disease(s) of interest at the onset of the study, determination of the exposure status of each person, and observation of the cohort over time to determine the development of disease in exposed and nonexposed persons.

Colectomy: Surgical removal of the colon.

Colonization resistance: Preservation of anaerobic flora by selective gut decontamination to prevent colonization by potentially pathogenic gram-negative organisms.

Colony-stimulating factors: Proteins that regulate the proliferation, maturation, and differentiation of stem cells to red blood cells, white blood cells, and platelets.

Coma: A state of unconsciousness whereby a patient is not opening his or her eyes, not obeying commands, and not uttering understandable words.

Comedo, comedones (pl.): Plug of sebum and keratinous material in a hair follicle; blackhead.

Comedogenicity: Product effect that causes follicular plugging resulting in comedones.

Comedolytic: Prevents shed keratinocytes from aggregating in follicle and clogging pores.

Communities: Organized groups of people with a shared identity or relationship that may be based on history, culture, context, or geography.

Comorbidity: A concomitant but unrelated pathologic or disease process.

Complementary and alternative medicine (CAM): Any practice for the prevention and treatment of disease that is not usual conventional medicine.

Complex partial seizure: A seizure beginning in one hemisphere of the brain. It is manifested by automatisms, periods of memory loss, or aberrations of behavior.

Compulsion: Repetitive ritualistic behavior such as ordering or hand washing or a mental act such as repeating words silently with the intent of preventing or reducing distress or some dreaded event or situation.

Conceptual model: The rationale for and description of the concepts that a measurement instrument is intended to assess and the interrelationships of those concepts.

Condom: A sheath, usually made of thin rubber, used to cover the penis during sexual intercourse to prevent conception or infection.

Confounding: A situation in which the effects of two processes are not separated. The distortion of the apparent effect of an exposure on risk brought about by the association of other factors that can influence the outcome.

Constrictive pericarditis: Constrictive pericarditis is a disorder caused by inflammation of the pericardium with subsequent thickening, scarring, and contracture of the pericardium. The pericardium cannot stretch during contraction, thereby preventing chamber filling.

Construct validity: The strength of the relationship between measures purporting to measure or reflect the same underlying theoretical construct.

Content validity: Refers to how adequately the questions/items capture the relevant aspects of the domain or concept being measured.

Continuation therapy: The second phase in drug therapy during which the goal is to eliminate any remaining symptoms and prevent a relapse.

Continuous-combined estrogen-progestogen therapy: Daily administration of both estrogen and a progestogen.

Continuous long-cycle estrogen-progestogen therapy: Estrogen is given daily and a progestogen is given six times a year (every other month for 12 to 14 days).

Convection: The movement of solutes, or metabolic waste products, by bulk flow in association with fluid removal. Convective clearance is not dependent on concentration gradients, and the magnitude of its contribution to total clearance is directly related to the ultrafiltration (fluid removal) rate.

Convulsion: Specific seizure type where the seizure is manifested by involuntary muscle contractions.

Cor pulmonale: Right-sided heart failure caused by lung disease.

Corneocytes: Flattened, dead, keratin-filled epidermal cells.

Coronary artery bypass graft surgery (CABGS): Thoracic surgery where parts of a saphenous vein from a leg or internal mammary artery from the arm are placed as conduits to restore blood flow between the aorta and one or more coronary arteries to *bypass* the coronary artery stenosis (occlusion).

Corpus cavernosum: Two chambers on the dorsal side of the penis. Chambers composed of sinusoidal tissue, which can fill with arterial blood to produce an erection.

Corpus luteum: The small yellow endocrine structure that develops within a ruptured ovarian follicle and secretes progesterone and estrogen.

Corpus spongiosum: One chamber on the ventral side of the penis. Chamber is composed of sinusoidal tissue, which can fill with arterial blood to produce an erection. The urethra passes through the corpus spongiosum.

Cortical necrosis: Acute renal failure secondary to ischemic necrosis of the renal cortex usually caused by significantly diminished renal arterial perfusion.

Corticotropin-releasing hormone (CRH): A trophic hormone released by the hypothalamus that stimulates release of adrenocorticotropic hormone (ACTH).

Cost-effectiveness ratio: The outcome of cost-effective analysis. The numerator of the ratio summarizes the costs and financial savings associated with the therapy, including the costs of the therapy itself, side effects, medical costs, and savings from avoided illness and disability. The denominator of the cost-effectiveness ratio reflects the health effect of the intervention. The year of life saved is probably the most commonly used measure of the health effect.

Cranial nerve palsy: Paralysis of one or more of the 12 cranial (brain) nerves.

Craniectomy (for stroke): Removal of part of the skull overlying an area of injury to relieve the pressure of cerebral edema.

C-reactive protein: An endogenous marker released by the body in response to inflammation.

Creatine kinase, creatine kinase MB: Creatine kinase (CK) enzymes are found in many isoforms, with varying concentrations depending on the type of tissue. Creatine kinase is a general term used to describe the nonspecific total release of all types of CK, including that found in skeletal muscle (MM), brain (BB), and heart (MB). Creatine kinase MB is released into the blood from necrotic myocytes in response to infarction and is a useful laboratory test for diagnosing myocardial infarction. If the total CK is elevated, then the relative index (RI), or fraction of the total that is composed of CK-MB, is calculated as follows:

$$RI = (CK\text{-}MB/CK\ total) \times 100$$

A RI greater than 2 is typically diagnostic of infarction.

Creatinine (serum): A protein metabolic by-product obtained from the diet or generated from muscles of the body. Creatinine is removed from blood by the kidneys; as kidney disease progresses, the level of creatinine in the blood increases.

Creatinine clearance: A test that measures how efficiently the kidneys filter creatinine and other waste products from the blood. Low creatinine clearance (<60 mL/min) usually indicates the presence of kidney damage.

Crepitus: A crinkly, crackling, or grating feeling or sound in the joints, skin, or lungs.

Cronbach α-coefficient: Commonly used statistical measure to quantify internal consistency reliability for multi-item scales or tests.

Crossmatch: A test to determine if a recipient has antibodies against donor antigens. A positive crossmatch indicates that the recipient has antibodies against the donor, and the two are incompatible. A negative crossmatch means the recipient does not have antibodies against the donor, and the two are considered compatible.

Crust: Dried exudate, secretion, or hemorrhage; scab.

Crypt abscess: Neutrophilic infiltration of the intestinal glands (Crypts of Lieberkuhn); a characteristic finding for patients with UC.

Cultural competency: The attitudes, knowledge, skills, and values that an individual and/or an organization acquires, develops, and uses to work effectively in a cross-cultural environment.

Culture: The acquired and shared attitudes, beliefs, knowledge, and values that individuals and/or groups use to influence their actions and behavior.

Culture negative endocarditis: Describes a patient in whom a clinical diagnosis of infective endocarditis is likely, but blood cultures do not yield a pathogen.

Cutaneous: Pertaining to the skin.

Cutis: Skin.

Cyanopsia: A condition when a patient sees a blue halo around objects, or objects appear to be blue-colored.

Cyanosis: Bluish tint to the skin or mucous membranes because of lack of oxygen.

Cyclic estrogen-progestogen therapy: Estrogen is taken continuously, with a progestogen added cyclically the last 10 to 14 days during each 28-day cycle.

Cyst: Sac or closed cavity containing fluid, semifluid, or solid material.

Cystitis: Inflammation of the bladder, usually caused by infection.

Cytokines: Protein molecules that are released by one cell (e.g., T-lymphocytes) that can have an influence on other cells. These proteins are important in numerous cell functions, such as regulating the immune response and cell-to-cell communication.

Dactylitis: Erythema and swollen hands, feet, fingers, and toes. Also known as *hand-and-foot syndrome*.

Deep vein thrombosis: A disorder of thrombus formation causing obstruction of a deep vein in the leg, pelvis, or abdomen.

Defibrillation: The therapeutic use of electric current in attempt to completely depolarize the myocardium and provide an opportunity for the natural pacemaker centers of the heart to resume normal activity.

Delayed cerebral ischemia: A worsening in neurologic function in a subarachnoid hemorrhage patient, occurring several days after the initial bleed, not due to another cause.

Delusion: Fixed, false beliefs that are not based in reality or consistent with the patient's religion or culture. Delusions can be classified as paranoid, somatic, or grandiose in nature. Delusions are often unshakable in spite of evidence to the contrary.

Dementia: A chronic progressive neurodegenerative syndrome characterized by a decline in memory and at least one other cognitive function.

Demyelination: Destruction of myelin in the spinal cord and brain leading to the formation of plaques that impair communication between neurons. Demyelination is classically found in the central nervous system of patients with multiple sclerosis and may be reversible.

Depersonalization: A change in an individual's self-awareness, during anxiety disorder, such that one feels detached from his or her own experiences, with the self, body, and mind seeming alien or distant. Persistent or recurrent experiences as if one is an outside observer of one's mental processes or body (e.g., feeling like one is in a dream).

Derealization: A feeling of estrangement or detachment from one's environment.

Dermatitis: Inflammation of the skin.

Dermatophyte: Fungal infection of the skin.

Dermis: The inner layer of skin between the epidermis and hypodermis.

Desensitization: Administration of increasing doses of drug to achieve patient tolerance and avoidance of hypersensitivity reactions.

Detoxification programs: A medically supervised treatment program for alcohol or drug addiction designed to purge the body of intoxicating or addictive substances. Such a program is used as a first step in overcoming physiologic or psychologic addiction.

Detumescence: Process by which an erect penis becomes flaccid.

Diagnostic overshadowing: Underestimating the significance of the emotional disturbances because of the presence of significant cognitive deficits.

Dialysate: The cleansing solution used in dialysis to remove excess fluids and waste products from the blood.

Dialysis: The process of removing toxic substances and fluid across a semipermeable membrane to maintain fluid, electrolyte, and acid–base balance.

Diaphragm: (1) A flexible ring covered with rubber or other plastic material, fitted over the cervix of the uterus to prevent pregnancy. (2) Muscular membrane separating the abdominal and thoracic cavities, used for respiration.

Diastolic blood pressure: The arterial BP that occurs after cardiac contraction when the cardiac chambers are filling.

Diastolic heart failure: A condition caused by increased resistance to the filling of one or both ventricles; this leads to symptoms of congestion from the inappropriate upward shift of the diastolic pressure-volume relation.

Diffuse idiopathic skeletal hyperostosis (DISH): A form of degenerative arthritis caused by calcification or a bony hardening of ligaments alongside the vertebrae of the spine. Also known as Forestier disease.

Diffuse idiopathic skeletal hyperostosis (DISH): Abnormal bone formation with calcifications and ossifications along the anterolateral aspect of vertebral bodies. A variant of Forestier disease.

Diffusion-weighted imaging: A type of magnetic resonance imaging (MRI) that can sensitively detect changes in water movement in tissue. It is particularly sensitive to the early changes seen during brain ischemia.

Digital clubbing: Rounded and swollen tip of finger usually associated with long-term pulmonary disease.

Dihydrotestosterone: The active androgen metabolite, which is formed inside various cells. In the case of benign prostatic hyperplasia (BPH), dihydrotestosterone is formed inside prostate cells by the action of 5-α-reductase, which converts testosterone to dihydrotestosterone. Dihydrotestosterone stimulates the glandular portion of the prostate to undergo hyperplasia.

Disinhibition: A physiologic effect that occurs during psychoactive substance use characterized by a loss of normal, executive functioning and normal behavior. An increase in behaviors with the propensity to harm the individual is common.

Dissociative amnesia: Inability to remember some important aspect of an event.

Diverticulitis: Inflammation of a diverticulum, especially of the small pockets in the wall of the colon that fill with stagnant fecal material and become inflamed; rarely, they can cause obstruction, perforation, or bleeding.

Dopamine: A monoamine neurotransmitter formed in the brain by the decarboxylation of dopa and essential to the normal functioning of the central nervous system.

Doppler imaging: With Doppler imaging, a probe generates sound waves typically at 2.5 MHz. When encountering an object, sound waves are scattered or reflected back toward the probe from the object's interface with adjacent structures; this is repeated in many times per second to build up a moving real-time image of the heart.

Drug abuse: A maladaptive pattern of substance use indicated by repeated adverse consequences related to the repeated use of the substance. Examples include failure to fulfill important obligations at work, school, or home; repeated use in situations in which it is physically dangerous, such as driving under the influence; legal problems; and social or interpersonal problems such as arguments and fights.

Drug addiction: A chronic disorder characterized by the compulsive use of a substance resulting in physical, psychologic, or social harm to the user and continued use despite that harm.

Dual diagnosis: A developmentally disabled person comorbid with a psychiatric disorder.

Dumping syndrome: A condition characterized by weakness, dizziness, flushing/warmth, nausea, and palpitation immediately or shortly after eating and produced by abnormally rapid emptying of the stomach, particularly in individuals who have had part of the stomach removed.

Dysentery: Diarrhea characterized by blood, mucus, and leukocytes in the stool with tenesmus and fever.

Dyskinesia: Choreiform abnormal involuntary movements involving usually the face, neck, trunk, and extremities.

Dysmenorrhea: Crampy pelvic pain occurring with or just prior to menses. *Primary* dysmenorrhea implies pain in the setting of normal pelvic anatomy, whereas *secondary* dysmenorrhea is secondary to underlying pelvic pathology.

Dyspareunia: Painful sexual intercourse.

Dyspepsia: Literally means "bad digestion" but refers to persistent or recurrent pain or discomfort centered in the upper abdomen. Symptoms may include epigastric pain, bloating, abdominal distention, postprandial fullness, early satiety, and nausea.

Dysphagia: Difficulty swallowing.

Dysphoria or dysphoric: A feeling of discomfort or an unpleasant mood, such as sadness, anxiety, or irritability.

Dyspnea: Dyspnea is referred to as shortness of breath or difficulty or distress in breathing.

Dystonia: Sustained muscular spasm or abnormal postures.

Early empirical therapy: The administration of systemic antifungal agents at the onset of fever and neutropenia.

Economic outcomes: The direct, indirect, and intangible costs compared with the consequences of a medical intervention.

Edema: Accumulation of fluid in tissues.

Effective renal plasma flow (ERPF): The flow of plasma through the kidneys; often measured by *p*-aminohippurate (PAH) clearance and expressed in volume per unit of time (mL/min). The ERPF is less than the true renal plasma flow (RPF) because plasma flow through renal connective and adipose tissue is not measured and the extraction of PAH, although high (>0.9), is not complete.

Ejaculatory dysfunction: This is a type of sexual dysfunction that can present as premature ejaculation (before orgasm has occurred), anejaculation (failure of emission), or retrograde ejaculation (when ejaculate moves backward into the bladder as opposed to forward and out of the body during orgasm). In some cases, ejaculatory dysfunction can decrease sexual enjoyment in the patient.

Ejection fraction: The ejection fraction is the percentage of blood ejected from the left ventricle with each heart beat.

Elation: An exaggerated feeling of well-being, euphoria, or elation.

Electroconvulsive therapy: A treatment for severe mental illness in which a precisely calculated electric stimulus is administered in a controlled medical setting to produce a generalized seizure.

Electroencephalograph (EEG): Used to evaluate brain electrical activity.

Electroencephalography: A test that measures electrical brain wave activity through the use of multiple scalp electrodes.

Electromyography: Test of muscle function because of either primary muscle disease or secondary to nerve injury.

Embolism: The sudden blockage of a vessel caused by a blood clot or foreign material that has been brought to the site by the flow of blood.

Embolization: The process by which a blood clot or foreign material dislodges from its site of origin, flows in the blood, and blocks a distant vessel.

Emergency contraception: Any method of contraception that acts after intercourse to prevent pregnancy.

Emesis: See *Vomiting*.

Empirical therapy: With systemic antifungal agents is administered to granulocytopenic patients with persistent or recurrent fever despite the administration of appropriate antimicrobial therapy.

Enanthem: Eruption on a mucous membrane (as the inside of the mouth) occurring as a symptom of a disease

Encephalitis: Inflammation of the brain tissue.

Encephalopathy: An altered brain state that may occur with altered brain structure. Many etiologies are associated with encephalopathy (toxins, cancer, metabolic disorders, CNS infections, increased cranial pressure, radiation, alcohol, psychotropic drugs, trauma, inadequate nutrition, decreased brain oxygen, and CNS injury). Consciousness is impaired with patients having a decreased/altered mental state and diffuse slowing of the EEG.

Endobronchitis: Inflammation of the epithelial lining of the bronchi.

Endocarditis: An infection of the endocardial surface of the heart, which can include one or more heart valves, the mural endocardium, or a septal defect.

Endometriosis: Presence of endometrial tissue outside the uterus.

Enkephalins: Pentapeptide endorphins, found in many parts of the brain, that bind to specific receptor sites, some of which can be pain-related opiate receptors.

Enteric fever: Intestinal inflammation and ulceration with high fever and abdominal complaints caused by infection.

Enterocolitis: Inflammation of the small intestine and colon.

Enterotoxin: A cholera-like disease that produces secretory diarrhea.

Enuresis: Urinary incontinence, especially at night.

Enzymuria: Presence of enzymes in the urine.

Epidermis: The outer layer of skin.

Epigenetic: A change in the genome that is heritable and potentially reversible that does not alter the nucleotide sequence of DNA.

Epilepsy: Two or more unprovoked seizures; symptoms of disturbed electrical activity in the brain.

Epilepsy syndrome: The combination of seizure type with other components of the patient history such as age of onset, intellectual development, findings on neurologic examination, and results of neuroimaging.

Episodic: Recurring and remitting in a regular or irregular pattern.

Epistaxis: Nose bleed.

Epithelial cells: Cells that make up epithelium.

Epithelial tissue of the prostate: Also known as glandular tissue. This portion of the prostate is responsible for producing prostatic secretions, and this comprises only approximately 25% of the total volume of the enlarged prostate gland in patients with benign prostatic hyperplasia. Epithelial tissue is androgen dependent.

Epithelium: Layer of avascular cells covering body surfaces.

Erectile dysfunction: Also known as *impotence*. This is a failure of the penis to become rigid enough to allow for vaginal penetration of the sexual partner.

Erysipelas: Infection of the more superficial layers of the skin and cutaneous lymphatics.

Erythema: Redness.

Erythema multiforme: Symmetrical patches of raised, red skin.

Erythema nodosum: Raised, red, tender nodules on the skin that vary in size from 1 cm.

Erythroderma: Generalized redness of the skin.

Erythropoiesis: The production of erythrocytes (red blood cells) within the bone marrow.

Erythropoietic agents: Agents developed with recombinant DNA technology that have the same biologic activity as endogenous erythropoietin to stimulate red blood cell production. Available agents in the United States include epoetin alfa and darbepoetin alfa.

Erythropoietin: A hormone made by the kidneys that is required for red blood cell formation in the bone marrow. Lack of this hormone leads to anemia.

Eschar: Black, painless skin ulcer characteristic of cutaneous anthrax.

Esophageal: Involving the esophagus.

Esophageal stricture: A narrowing of the esophageal lumen because of acid reflux into the lower esophagus.

Esophagitis: Inflammation of the esophagus.

Essential hypertension: Persistently elevated BP that results from unknown pathophysiological etiology.

Essential or primary hypertension: Persistently elevated blood pressure that results from unknown pathophysiological etiology.

Estrogen therapy: Unopposed estrogen regimens administered to postmenopausal women following hysterectomy.

Euphoria: A mood state characterized by an exaggerated, superficial sense of well-being, characterized extreme happiness, sometimes more than is reasonable in a particular situation.

Euthymia or euthymic: A mood in a *normal* range without depression or mood elevation.

Evidence-based medicine (EBM): Evidence-based medicine emphasizes the consideration of results from clinical research as the basis for clinical decision making. Under this practice approach, unless individual patient-specific factors dictate otherwise, treatment should generally be guided by those approaches that have the best research evidence for efficacy, tolerability, and patient acceptance.

Evoked potentials: EEG-based technique involving measurement of brain-wave activity in response to stimuli, usually visual or auditory.

Exanthema: An eruption on the skin occurring as a symptom of a disease.

External beam radiotherapy: Treatment by radiation emitted from a source located at a distance from the body; also called beam therapy and external beam therapy.

Extrapyramidal: Regarding involuntary motor movement.

Extrapyramidal system: Neurotransmitter tracts in the midbrain with dopamine as the primary ascending neurotransmitter, with cell bodies in the substantial nigra and axons terminating in the basal ganglia (e.g., caudate nucleus, putamen). The extrapyramidal system is largely involved in the control of fine motor movements, and with some degree of emotional expression as well.

Fasciculations: The localized contractions of muscle groups, often visible through the skin, because of excessive neuronal discharge.

Fear: A direct, focused response to a specific event or object of which an individual is consciously aware.

Felty syndrome: Rheumatoid arthritis associated with splenomegaly and neutropenia.

Fibrin: An insoluble protein that is one of the principle ingredients of a blood clot. Fibrin strands bind to one another to form a fibrin mesh. The fibrin mesh often traps platelets and other blood cells.

Fibromyalgia: A syndrome characterized by chronic widespread pain, multiple tender points, abnormal pain, sleep disturbances, fatigue, and psychological distress.

Fibrosis: Formation of fibrous tissue as a reparative or reactive process.

First-generation (typical or traditional) antipsychotic: An antipsychotic medication with a mechanism of action thought to be primarily caused by the blockade of dopamine-2 (D_2) receptors. D_2-blockade is associated with hyperprolactinemia and extrapyramidal side effects.

Fistula: A communicating tube-like passage from one organ to another or from an organ to an external surface; often seen in severe cases of Crohn's disease.

Flight of ideas: An accelerated flow of speech with thoughts that change rapidly from one topic to another.

Focal seizures: Partial seizures.

Follicle-stimulating hormone (FSH): A polypeptide hormone secreted by the anterior pituitary gland that promotes ovarian follicle development and stimulates estradiol and progesterone.

Fragile X syndrome: A genetic disorder commonly associated with mental retardation in which the tip of the long arms of the X chromosome separates from the rest of the genetic material; most males and 30% of females with fragile X syndrome have mental retardation; males develop enlarged testicles, enlarged ears, and a prominent jaw.

Freezing: Intermittent immobility lasting a few seconds, particularly in walking, seen in Parkinsonism.

Fulminant hepatitis: Acute hepatic failure; rare complication of viral hepatitis, it can also result from hepatotoxins, or drug sensitivity and causes massive necrosis of the liver; marked by a high fatality rate.

Functional analysis: Evaluation performed by a psychologist qualified in applied behavioral analysis to determine if a behavior is caused by some environmental factor.

Functional pain: Pain due to abnormal operation of the nervous system.

Functional psychiatric disorder: A mental disorder that is primarily defined by a constellation of symptoms and behaviors and for which the pathophysiologic etiology is still largely unknown.

Fungemia: The presence of fungi in the blood.

Gastroesophageal reflux disease (GERD): Symptomatic clinical condition or histologic alteration that results from episodes of gastroesophageal reflux.

Gene: Series of codons that specify a particular protein.

Generalized anxiety disorder (GAD): Excessive anxiety and worry occurring more days than not for a period of at least 6 months.

Generalized convulsive status epilepticus (GCSE): Most common and dangerous type of status epilepticus. It consists of bilateral (both brain hemispheres) electrical seizure activity that manifests as tonic and/or clonic motor activity. The convulsions and/or brain discharges can be symmetrical or asymmetrical (i.e., parts of body and brain mirroring or not mirroring each other in activity). Consciousness is not maintained during the seizures episodes. The duration is sufficient enough in length to meet the definition of status epilepticus.

Generalized seizures: Seizures occurring in both hemispheres of the brain. They can be primary or secondarily generalized.

Generic/general measures: Instruments designed to be applicable across a wide variety of conditions/diseases, medical interventions, and populations.

Genotype: The genetic constitution of an individual.

Genu valgum: A deformity marked by lateral angulation of the leg in relation to the thigh.

Genu varum: A deformity marked by medial angulation of the leg in relation to the thigh; an outward bowing of the legs.

Gestation: Time from fertilization of egg until birth.

Gigantism: Excess secretion of growth hormone prior to epiphyseal closure in children.

Glasgow coma scale: The most widely used system to grade the arousal and functional capacity of the cerebral cortex consisting of eye opening, motor responses, and verbal responses.

Glaucoma: Any of a group of ocular disorders that lead to an optic neuropathy characterized by changes in the optic nerve head (optic disk) that is associated with loss of visual sensitivity and field. Open angle and closed angle are the two major types of glaucoma.

Glomerular filtration rate (GFR): The primary index of overall kidney function; the volume of plasma that is filtered by the glomerulus per unit of time; often reported in mL/min or mL/min/1.73 m².

Glomerulonephritis: Glomerular lesions characterized by inflammation of the capillary loops in the glomerulus caused by immunologic, vascular, and other idiopathic diseases (may be diffuse or membranoproliferative).

Glomerulosclerosis: Fibrosis of the glomeruli.

Glomerulus: A coiled capillary bed in the kidney that is responsible for filtering water and small molecular weight substances from the blood.

Gonadotropin: A sex hormone that promotes gonadal growth and functioning in both males and females.

Gonadotropin-releasing hormone (GnRH): A trophic hormone released by the hypothalamus that stimulates release of follicle-stimulating hormone (FSH) and luteinizing hormone (LH).

Gout: A disease spectrum that includes hyperuricemia, recurrent attacks of acute arthritis associated with monosodium urate crystals in leukocytes found in synovial fluid, deposits of monosodium urate crystals in tissues (tophi), interstitial renal disease, and uric acid nephrolithiasis.

gp120: The glycoprotein structure on the surface of human immunodeficiency virus (HIV) that binds to CD4 on human cells.

Grandiosity: An inflated self-appraisal of one's status, power, or identity.

Granuloma inguinale: Granuloma lesions affecting the genital area.

Growth hormone (GH): A polypeptide hormone secreted by the anterior pituitary gland that stimulates insulinlike growth factor-1 (IGF-1) production and promotes growth of all body cells.

Growth hormone-releasing hormone (GHRH): A trophic hormone released by the hypothalamus that stimulates release of growth hormone.

Guillain-Barré's syndrome: A disorder characterized by progressive symmetrical paralysis and loss of reflexes, usually beginning in the legs. The paralysis typically involves more than one limb, is progressive, and usually proceeds from the end of an extremity toward the torso. Areflexia or hyporeflexia can occur in the limbs. It typically occurs after recovery from a viral infection.

Gumma: A granulomatous lesion found in organs or tissues as a result of syphilis.

Gynecomastia: Gynecomastia is the abnormal development of large breasts in men.

Half-life: The time required for serum concentrations to decrease by one-half after absorption and distribution are complete.

Hallucination: A sensory perception (e.g., auditory, gustatory, olfactory, somatic, tactile, visual) that occurs without external stimulation of the relevant sensory organ.

Haplotype: Set of polymorphisms that are inherited together.

Haptocorrin: A group of carrier proteins that bind with vitamin B_{12} in the blood and aid in its transport.

Haptoglobin: A group of α_2-globulins in human serum, so called because of their ability to combine with hemoglobin, preventing loss in the urine; levels are decreased in hemolytic disorders and increased in inflammatory conditions or with tissue damage.

Hay fever: See *Rhinitis.*

Health literacy: The degree to which individuals have the capacity to obtain, process, and understand basic health information and services needed to make appropriate health decisions (as defined by the Institute of Medicine).

Health outcomes: The consequences or ends results of a disease and/or its treatment.

Health profiles: Generic instruments that provide an array of scores representing individual dimensions or domains of health-related quality of life (HRQOL) or health status.

Health-related quality of life (HRQOL): A person's perception of how health impacts his or her physical, social, and psychologic functioning and well-being.

Health state preference: The perceived relative desirability of a health state measured on a scale where 1.0 equals full health, and 0.0 equals dead.

Heart failure: A clinical syndrome that can result from any disorder that impairs the ability of the heart to fill with or eject blood. Although heart failure may be caused by numerous cardiac disorders, the primary clinical signs and symptoms of dyspnea, fatigue, and volume overload are similar regardless of the initial cause.

Heinz bodies: Intracellular inclusions usually attached to the red cell membrane composed of denatured hemoglobin.

Hemagglutinin: The major antigenic determinant of the influenza virus; a surface antigen that allows the influenza virus to enter host cells by attaching to sialic acid receptors.

Hematemesis: Vomiting up blood that can be bright red or similar to coffee grounds in appearance.

Hematochezia: The presence of visible bright red blood in the stool.

Hematopoiesis: The formation and maturation of blood cells and their derivatives.

Hematopoietic growth factors: See *Colony-stimulating factors.*

Hematopoietic stem cell: An immature cell capable of self-renewal and subsequent differentiation into mature blood cells.

Hematuria: Presence of red blood cells in the urine.

Hemetemesis: Vomiting up blood that may be bright red or appear like coffee grounds. The digestive action of acid and enzymes may cause blood in the stomach to darken and appear like coffee grounds in the vomitus.

Hemochromatosis: Hemochromatosis is a disorder that interferes with iron metabolism, which results in excess iron deposition throughout the body.

Hemodialysis: A dialysis procedure during which blood is pumped outside the body through a dialyzer that acts like an artificial kidney; the dialyzer removes extra fluids and wastes from the blood and returns the clean blood to the body.

Hemolytic uremic syndrome: A condition characterized by the breakup of red blood cells (hemolysis) and kidney failure. Platelets clump together within the kidney's small blood vessels resulting in ischemia leading to kidney failure.

Hemosiderin: A golden yellow or yellow-brown insoluble protein produced by phagocytic digestion of hematin; found in most tissues, especially in the liver, spleen, and bone marrow, in the form of granules much larger than ferritin molecules (of which they are believed to be aggregates) but with a higher content, as much as 37%, of iron.

Hepatosplenic candidiasis: Clinical presentation often manifested only as fever while a patient remains neutropenic (<1,000 white blood cells/mm³). When the white blood cell (WBC) count increases to >1000 cells/mm³, imaging studies can detect the presence of abscess or microabscesses in the liver and spleen, often found with acute suppurative and granulomatous reactions. Infection can persist for months and ultimately cause the patient's death despite aggressive systemic therapy with antifungal agents.

Heterozygous: Presence of different (alleles) genes at one location.

Hippocampal sclerosis: A condition in which there is histopathological changes in the hippocampus that have been associated with patients with a history of prolonged status epilepticus. There is an association with hippocampal sclerosis and temporal lobe epilepsy.

Hippocampus: A sea horse–shaped structure located within the brain that is an important part of the limbic system. The hippocampus is involved in some aspects of memory, in the control of the autonomic functions, and in emotional expression.

Hirsutism: Heavy, abnormal growth of hair on the face or body; excess body hair appearing on the lower abdomen, around the nipples, around the chin and upper lip, between the breasts, and on the lower back.

HLA (human leukocyte antigen): See *Human leukocyte antigen.*

Hollenhorst plaque: Cholesterol emboli that usually dislodges from the carotid arteries, or calcific fragments from a stenosed aortic valve that can be visualized on a retinal exam.

Homocysteine: A homolog of cysteine, produced by the demethylation of methionine, and an intermediate in the biosynthesis of 1-cysteine from 1-methionine through 1-cystathionine. Elevated levels of homocysteine have been associated with certain forms of heart disease.

Homozygous: Presence of identical genes (alleles) at one location.

Hormone therapy: Either estrogen-only therapy or combined estrogen and progestogen therapy.

Hot flashes/flushes: A sensation of warmth, frequently accompanied by skin flushing and perspiration.

Human leukocyte antigen (HLA): The *self antigens* are the histocompatibility antigens found on human leukocytes and tissues that enable the body to differentiate *self* from *foreign* cells. The HLA antigens are used in histocompatibility testing to determine the suitability of an organ for transplant.

Humanistic outcomes: Patient-reported outcomes such as patient satisfaction and health-related quality of life.

Hydrocephalus: An uncharacteristic increase in the amount of cerebrospinal fluid within the skull, causing dangerous expansion of the cerebral ventricles.

Hyperalgesia: Exaggerated painful response to normally noxious stimuli.

Hyperarousal: A state of elevated or increased alertness, awareness, or wakefulness.

Hypercapnia: Elevation of carbon dioxide gas in the blood.

Hypercoagulable state: A disorder or state of excessive or frequent thrombus formation; also known as *thrombophilia*.

Hypereosinophilic syndrome: Hypereosinophilic syndrome is a group of leukoproliferative disorders characterized by an overproduction of eosinophils resulting in organ damage.

Hyperkalemia: Serum potassium concentration above 5.5 mEq/L.

Hyperlinear palms: Increased number of skin creases on the palms.

Hypermagnesemia: Serum magnesium concentration above 1.8 mEq/L or 2.3 mg/dL.

Hyperpigmentation: Excess pigment in skin causing an area of darker color than surrounding skin.

Hyperprolactinemia: A state of persistent serum prolactin elevation characterized by prolactin concentrations greater than 20 mcg/L observed on multiple occasions.

Hyperresponsiveness: In the airways, the characteristic of an exaggerated response to stimuli.

Hypertensive crises: Clinical situations where BP values are very elevated, typically greater than 180/120 mm Hg. They are categorized as either a hypertensive emergency or hypertensive urgency depending on the clinical presentation.

Hypertensive emergency: A clinical situation in which a patient has extremely high BP values, typically greater than 180/120 mm Hg that is also accompanied by the presence of acute and/or progressing target-organ damage. Immediate but gradual reduction in BP using intravenous antihypertensive agents is needed to prevent acute morbidity and/or mortality.

Hypertensive urgency: A clinical situation in which a patient has extremely high BP values, typically >180/120 mmHg, that is not accompanied by acuter or progressing target-organ injury. These situations require oral antihypertensive therapy to reduce BP to Stage 1 values over a period of several hours to several days.

Hypertrichosis: Abnormal hair growth on the body in areas where hair does not usually grow.

Hypertrophic cardiomyopathy: Hypertrophic cardiomyopathy is a genetic disorder characterized by disproportionate hypertrophy of the left ventricle, and occasionally of the right ventricle.

Hypervigilance: An enhanced state of sensory sensitivity accompanied by an exaggerated intensity of behaviors whose purpose it is to detect threats.

Hypnagogic hallucinations: Dreamlike experiences on the threshold of sleep that intrude into wakefulness.

Hypnopompic hallucinations: Dreamlike experiences on the threshold of awakening that intrude into wakefulness.

Hypochlorhydria: Presence of an abnormally small amount of hydrochloric acid in the stomach.

Hypogonadism: Little or no hormone production by the testes (in men) or ovaries (in women).

Hypokalemia: Serum potassium concentration below 3.5 mEq/L.

Hypomagnesemia: Serum magnesium concentration below 1.4 mEq/L or 1.7 mg/dL.

Hypomania: An abnormally and persistently elevated, expansive, or irritable mood that lasts at least 4 days but does not cause marked impairment in functioning.

Hypomimia: Decreased facial expression often associated with decreased blink rate.

Hypophonia: Decreased volume of speech.

Hypothalamus: A small region at the base of the brain that controls the release of hormones from the anterior and posterior regions of the pituitary gland and regulates limbic functions, fluid balance, body temperature, cardiovascular function, respiratory function, and diurnal rhythms.

Hysterectomy: Excision of the uterus.

Hysteresis: A situation in which concentration-effect curves do not always follow the same pattern when serum concentrations increase as they do when serum concentrations decrease. This can result from tolerance to a drug (clockwise hysteresis) or accumulation of active metabolites (counterclockwise hysteresis).

Iatrogenesis or iatrogenic disease: A disease produced as a consequence of medical or surgical treatment.

Ichthyosis: Dry, rectangular scales on the skin.

Ictal: The period during a seizure.

Icteric: Relating to or marked by jaundice.

Idiopathic: Unknown etiology of status epilepticus, often considered a genetic etiology for the prolonged seizure.

Ileitis: Inflammation of the ileus.

Illusions: Visual perceptions that are misinterpreted but have a real sensory stimulus.

Immunocompromised host: A patient with defects in host defenses that predisposes him or her to infection (risk factors can include neutropenia, immune system defects from disease or immunosuppressive drug therapy, compromise of natural host defenses, environmental contamination, and changes in normal flora of the host).

Immunoglobulin: Structurally related glycoproteins that function as antibodies and are divided into classes on the basis of structure/biologic activity.

Impaction: An immovable packing; a lodgment of something in a strait or passage of the body; as, impaction of the fetal head in the strait of the pelvis; impaction of food or feces in the intestines of man or beast.

Impedance-pH monitoring: New technique used to detect reflux by measuring changes in intraluminal resistance determined by the presence of liquid or gas inside the esophagus. When combined with pH monitoring, it can differentiate between acid and nonacid reflux.

Impending status epilepticus: Any seizure that does not stop automatically within 5 minutes has been termed impending status epilepticus. This is a fairly new term that was created to recognize the importance of early treatment of status epilepticus. Pharmacologic and nonpharmacologic treatment of status epilepticus should be initiated for those seizures that do not spontaneously terminate within 5 minutes.

Impetigo: A superficial skin infection that is seen most commonly in children.

Implantable cardioverter-defibrillator (ICD): The ICD is a surgically implanted electronic device that monitors, detects, and treats potentially life-threatening ventricular tachycardia with rate-responsive ventricular pacing.

Inanition: Severe weakness and wasting as occurs from lack of food, defect in assimilation, or neoplastic disease.

Incubation period: The time between exposure of a biologic (i.e., pathogen), chemical, or radiologic substance and when symptoms first start to appear (also known as latency).

Induction: Administration of a highly intense level of immunosuppression in the perioperative period or use of antibody therapy to provide enough immunosuppression to delay administration of nephrotoxic calcineurin inhibitors.

Infant mortality: Deaths occurring in those younger than the age of 1 year per 1,000 live births.

Infants: Pediatric patients who are 1 month to 1 year of age.

Infection: Inflammatory response to invasion of host tissue by microorganisms.

Information bias: A flaw in measuring exposure or outcome data that results in systematic differences in the quality of information gathered for study and comparison groups. See also *Selection bias.*

Instrumental activities of daily living: Housekeeping chores, shopping, going outside, medication management. See also *Activities of daily living.*

Insulin-like growth factor-1: An anabolic peptide that acts as a direct stimulator of cell proliferation and growth in all body cells.

Integumentary system: Skin, subcutaneous tissue, and skin appendages.

Interleukin: A type of cytokine, usually influencing a white blood cell.

Intermittent-combined estrogen-progestogen therapy: A regimen that combines a daily estrogen with a progestogen administered intermittently in cycles of 3 days on and 3 days off (which is then repeated without interruption).

International normalized ratio (INR): A measure of coagulation calculated from the patient's prothrombin time (PT) measurement compared to the laboratory's mean normal control measurement and takes into account the sensitivity of the thromboplastin used to perform the test.

Interpersonal psychotherapy: A psychologic intervention that focuses on interpersonal relationships and psychosocial functioning.

Interpretability: The degree to which one can assign qualitative meaning to an instrument's quantitative scores.

Intertriginous areas: Body fold areas (e.g., between buttocks, beneath breasts, between toes, under arms).

Intertrigo: An inflammatory condition of skinfolds induced or aggravated by heat, moisture, maceration, friction, and lack of air circulation.

Intoxication: The development of a substance-specific syndrome after recent ingestion and presence in the body of a substance; associated with maladaptive behavior during the waking state caused by the effect of the substance on the central nervous system.

Intracavernosal injection: Injection into the corpus spongiosum.

Intracranial hypertension: Excessive pressure (>20 mm Hg) within the nondistensible intracranial cavity (i.e., skull) that can develop following traumatic brain injury.

Intracranial pressure: The pressure of the cerebral spinal fluid that is essentially the same as the pressure within the brain tissue (i.e., intraparenchymal pressure).

Intraperitoneal: Within the peritoneal cavity.

Intrauterine device: A device inserted in the uterus to prevent pregnancy, either through spermicidal action (copper device) or thickening cervical mucus to inhibit sperm penetration and migration (progesterone device).

Intrinsic resistance: See *Primary resistance.*

Intussusception: Invagination of one portion of the intestine into an adjacent part of the intestines.

Inulin: A fructose polysaccharide that is filtered by the glomerulus; its clearance is often used as an index of GFR.

Iothalamate: A nonradiolabeled or radiolabeled iodinated contrast agent that is filtered by the glomerulus; its clearance is often used as an index of GFR.

Irritable: Easily annoyed and provoked to anger.

Irritative voiding symptoms: Urinary urgency and frequency. This results from detrusor muscle decompensation that results from long-standing bladder outlet obstruction.

Isolated systolic hypertension: Patients with DBP values that are less than or equal to 90 mm Hg and SBP values that are greater than or equal to 140 mm Hg.

Janeway lesion: These lesions appear as flat, painless, red to bluish-red spots on the palms and soles of patients with acute bacterial endocarditis.

Jarisch-Herxheimer reaction: An increase in symptoms of spirochetal disease caused by the initiation of treatment.

J-curve phenomenon (in hypertension): A theoretical situation where lowering BP provides a reduced risk of cardiovascular events, but when BP is lowered too much, can paradoxically increase the risk of cardiovascular events.

Jugular venous oxygen saturation (Sjvo$_2$): Oxygen hemoglobin saturation of blood in the jugular bulb, which is a key element in estimating CMRo$_2$.

Just Culture of Patient Safety: an approach to analysis and prevention of medication errors that relies on encouragement of internal risk transparency, coaching and consoling of employees, avoiding negative retribution for errors, and gathering then using information to prevent error recurrence.

K complexes: Electronegative waves followed by electropositive waves seen on the EEG during sleep.

Karyotyping: Chromosomal analysis.

Keratinization: Keratin formation.

Keratinized: Skin that has developed thicker areas of keratin in the stratum corneum.

Keratinocyte: Cell of the epidermis that produces keratin.

Keratoconjunctivitis sicca: Dry, itchy eyes that result from atrophy of the lacrimal ducts, which can be seen in inflammatory arthritis.

Keratolytic: Agent that solubilizes intracellular cement of keratin cells in the stratum corneum.

Keratosis pilaris: Small, rough bumps, generally on the face, upper arms, and thighs.

Ketogenic diet: A special antiseizure diet that is high in fat and low in carbohydrates and protein.

Kleptomania: An impulse control disorder characterized by frequent and repeated theft.

Köbner phenomenon: De novo lesion psoriasis appearing at the site of cutaneous trauma.

Kt/V: A measurement of how much urea is being removed from the blood during dialysis. The measurement takes into account the efficiency of the dialyzer (clearance, K), the treatment time (t), and the volume of distribution of urea (V).

Kussmaul sign: Kussmaul sign is a rise in jugular venous pressure on inspiration. Kussmaul sign is seen in conditions in which there is right ventricular filling.

Lactation: Production and secretion of breast milk.

Lactogenesis II: Copious milk production that begins between 24 and 102 hours postpartum resulting from decreased maternal progesterone serum concentration.

Lanugo: Fine body hair normally found on a fetus. The hair develops in patients with anorexia nervosa when they are very underweight and malnourished.

Laparoscopic: Abdominal exploration or surgery employing a type of endoscope called laparoscope.

Laparotomy: Surgical opening of the abdominal cavity.

Laryngospasm: The spasmodic closure of the larynx because of a variety of causes such as allergic reactions, response to irritants, and pharmacologic actions.

Lavage: Washing out.

Laxative: A medication or agent used to produce a bowel movement.

Left ventricular ejection fraction: Also known simply as the ejection fraction, it is the fraction or percentage of the end diastolic blood volume ejected by the left ventricle during systole. It is a measurement of cardiac systolic function with a normal ejection being >60%. It can be determined noninvasively by an echocardiogram.

Left ventricular end diastolic volume: Left ventricular end diastolic volume refers to the volume of blood found in the left ventricular at the end of heart relaxation or diastole.

Left ventricular hypertrophy: Enlargement of the left ventricle, which is seen in heart failure and can give rise to arrhythmias.

Lentigines, PUVA: Brown to black macules resulting from long-term use of psoralens plus ultraviolet A light.

Leptospirosis: A bacterial disease that affects humans and animals caused by the genus Leptospira.

Lewy bodies: Pink-staining spheres found inside neuronal cells of the substantia nigra and other brain regions, considered to be a histopathologic marker for Parkinson's disease.

Lichenification: Thick, leathery skin, usually the result of constant scratching and rubbing.

Linear pharmacokinetics: The situation when changes in long-term daily doses of drugs result in proportional changes in steady-state serum drug concentrations. Most drugs follow this pattern.

Linguistic competency: The ability of individuals and organizations to communicate effectively with people from diverse language backgrounds.

Linkage disequilibrium: Two or more polymorphisms that are inherited together more frequently than would be expected based on chance.

Lipid peroxidation: A pathophysiologic process involving the iron-catalyzed attack of lipid membranes by reactive oxygen species.

Liposomes: Spherical amphiphilic vesicles capable of sustained release of water-soluble substances.

Locus ceruleus: A small area in the brainstem containing norepinephrine neurons that is considered to be a key brain center for anxiety and fear.

Low-glycemic-load diet: A low-glycemic-load diet emphasizes consuming carbohydrates with a low glycemic index. To eat a low-glycemic-load diet, avoid foods such as white bread, refined cereal, cookies, and sugary drinks. Emphasize fruits, vegetables, legumes, and minimally processed grains.

Low glycemic index: The term low glycemic index refers to the quality of carbohydrates and how fast they are absorbed. Foods with a low glycemic index are absorbed more slowly, thus keeping insulin levels more stable.

Lumbar puncture: The procedure used to withdraw cerebrospinal fluid through a needle inserted in the lumbar region of the spinal column.

Luteinizing hormone (LH): A polypeptide hormone secreted by the anterior pituitary gland that stimulates ovulation and maintains the corpus luteum.

Luteolysis: Death of the corpus luteum.

Lymphangitis: An inflammation involving the subcutaneous lymphatic channels.

Lymphocytosis: Increased blood concentration of lymphocytes ($>4 \times 10^9$ cells/mm^3) commonly observed in mononucleosis, pertussis, measles, chickenpox, or lymphoid malignancies.

Lymphedema: A lymphatic obstruction of localized fluid retention and tissue swelling caused by compromised lymphatic system.

Lymphogranuloma venereum: Inflammation of the lymph nodes caused by *Chlamydia trachomatis* resulting in destruction and scarring of tissue.

Macule: Flat, nonpalpable, variable-colored lesion.

Maculopapular: Skin eruption containing both macules and papules.

Magnetic resonance angiography (MRA): A noninvasive method to evaluate the patency of blood vessels using magnetic resonance imaging.

Magnetic resonance imaging (MRI): An imaging technique based on the magnetic properties of the hydrogen atom. It provides an accurate, computer-processed image that can be more sensitive than computed tomography.

Major depression: A psychiatric disorder in which the patient can present with symptoms of depressed mood, a lack of interest in usual activities or inability to experience pleasure, changes in sleep and eating habits, guilt, reduced energy, thoughts of self-harm, and a sense of helplessness or hopelessness.

Major histocompatibility complex (MHC): A set of genes responsible for most of the proteins on the surface of cells in the body that are responsible for recognition of *self*.

Mania: An abnormally and persistently elevated, expansive, or irritable mood that lasts at least 1 week and causes marked impairment in functioning.

Masked hypertension: Patients that have elevated BP measurements based on home measurements but have normal BP measurements when measured in a clinical setting. These patients have chronic hypertension but either may not be diagnosed or may have a diagnosis of hypertension that is undertreated.

Mass effect: Distortion or displacement of the brain anatomy because of an implied or apparent mass (such as stroke or tumor).

Mastalgia or mastodynia: Pain in the breast.

Mean arterial pressure: The mean arterial pressure is the product of the cardiac output and systemic vascular resistance. Since the cardiac output is pulsatile, rather than continuous, and since two thirds of the normal cardiac cycle is spent in diastole, the mean arterial pressure is not the arithmetic mean of the systolic and diastolic blood pressures. Mean arterial pressure = diastolic blood pressure + (1/3)(systolic blood pressure – diastolic blood pressure).

Measurement model: An instrument's scale and subscale structure and the procedures followed to create scale and subscale scores.

Meconium ileus: Intestinal obstruction caused by meconium.

Medication error: Any preventable event that may cause or lead to inappropriate medication use or patient harm while the medication is in the control of the healthcare professional, patient, or consumer (per the National Coordinating Council for Medication Error Reporting and Prevention).

Megakaryocytes: Precursors of platelets.

Melanin: Dark pigment that is part of determining skin color.

Melena: Dark-colored stools resulting from upper gastrointestinal bleed.

Membrane stripping: When the cervix is dilated, a practitioner can use a hand to separate the amniotic membranes from the uterus. This technique has been shown to reduce the need for labor induction.

Menarche: The time of the first menstrual period or flow.

Meningitis: Inflammation, usually infectious, of the meninges, a covering of the brain.

Menopause: The permanent cessation of menses following the loss of ovarian follicular activity.

Menorrhagia: Menstrual blood loss of greater than 80 mL per cycle; a more practical definition is heavy menstrual flow associated with problems of containment of flow, unpredictably heavy flow days, or other associated symptoms.

Menses: Periodic bloody discharge from the uterus.

Mental status examination: An objective patient evaluation conducted through a direct patient interview and used to make a diagnosis, assess the course of illness, or determine treatment response.

Meralgia parethetica: A disorder characterized by tingling, numbness, and burning pain in the outer side of the thigh. The disorder is caused by compression of the lateral femoral cutaneous nerve, a sensory nerve to the skin, as it exits the pelvis.

Mesolimbic pathway: A dopaminergic pathway in the brain that connects the ventral tegmental area in the midbrain to the nucleus accumbens in the striatum and is involved in motivation and reward.

Metabolic syndrome: A constellation of metabolic and cardiovascular changes consisting of at least three of the following: obesity, low high-density lipoprotein (HDL), elevated triglycerides, hypertension, and elevated fasting blood glucose.

Metastasis: Movement or spread of disease from one organ or part to new location not directly connected.

Methemoglobin: A form of hemoglobin that occurs when its iron is oxidized to the +3 state, which decreases oxygen binding.

Methionine: The 1-isomer is a nutritionally essential amino acid and the most important natural source of *active methyl* groups in the body, hence usually involved in methylations in vivo.

Michaelis–Menten kinetics: the situation in which changes in steady-state serum drug concentrations of drugs are disproportional to changes in long-term daily doses due to alterations in drug metabolism.

Microalbuminuria: A condition in which a small amount of albumin (30–300 mg/day) is present in the urine; often indicates an early stage of chronic kidney disease (CKD).

Microcephalic: Abnormally small head.

Microcomedo: Microscopic lesion formed from the combination of sloughed, clumping keratinocytes reacting with sebum and fatty acids from the sebaceous gland.

Micrographia: Handwriting that is small, trails off in size, or very slow.

Midsystolic: Middle of systole.

Migraine aura: Early symptom of an attack of migraine with aura, which is the manifestation of focal cerebral dysfunction. The aura typically precedes the headache.

Mild cognitive impairment: A syndrome characterized by cognitive impairment that is not of sufficient severity to warrant a diagnosis of dementia.

Milia: Small, white cysts containing keratin.

Mixed states: Rapidly alternating mood states (mania and major depressive episodes) that last at least 1 week, and cause marked impairment in functioning.

Molds: Fungal organisms that grow as multicellular branching, thread-like filaments (hyphae) that are either *septate* (divided by transverse walls) or *coenocytic* (multinucleate without cross walls). On agar media, molds grow outward from the point of inoculation by extension of the tips of filaments, and then branch repeatedly, interweaving to form fuzzy, matted growths called *mycelium*. Germ tubes are the beginning of *hyphae*, which arise as perpendicular extensions from the yeast cell, with no constriction at their point of origin.

Molybdenum (Mo): A bioelement found in a number of proteins.

Monoamine neurotransmitters: Neurotransmitters that contain one amino group and are derived from amino acids such as tyrosine and tryptophan. Includes, among others, the catecholamines (dopamine and norepinephrine) and an indoleamine (serotonin).

Mood: A more pervasive and sustained emotional state that colors a person's perception of the world.

Morbilliform: Maculopapular lesions that become confluent on the face and body.

Mucolytic: The ability to break down mucus.

Mucositis: Inflammation of the mucosa.

Multiattribute health status classification systems: Preference-based HRQOL instruments for which health-state preferences have been derived from population studies. The instruments assess respondents' health status, and then population preferences are applied to produce the index score.

Multiparity: Condition of having given birth to multiple children.

Multiple-organ dysfunction syndrome (MODS): Presence of altered organ function requiring intervention to maintain homeostasis.

Multiple sclerosis (MS): A demyelinating disease, caused by inflammation, leading to neurologic deficits and often, disability.

Mutism: A state in which a person either has the inability or refuses to speak or vocalize sounds.

Mycotic: A fungal infection.

Myectomy: A surgical removal of the overgrown septal muscle to decrease the outflow tract obstruction.

Myocarditis: Inflammation of the cardiac muscle.

Myoclonic seizures: Brief shock-like muscular contractions of the face, trunk, and extremities. They usually begin in adolescence and are referred to as *juvenile myoclonic epilepsy* (JME).

Myoclonus: A sudden twitching of muscles or parts of muscles, without any rhythm or pattern.

Myositis: Inflammation of the muscle, characterized by pain, tenderness, and sometimes spasm in the affected area.

Narrowband UVB (NB-UVB): 311 nm ultraviolet B light.

National Kidney Foundation (NKF): A major voluntary health organization that seeks to prevent kidney and urinary tract diseases, improve the health and well-being of individuals and families affected by these diseases, and increase the availability of all organs for transplantation.

Nausea: An unpleasant sensation associated with an awareness of the urge to vomit.

Necrosis: Local death of cells or tissue.

Necrotizing fasciitis: A rare, but very severe infection of the subcutaneous tissue that can be caused by aerobic and/or anaerobic bacteria and results in progressive destruction of the superficial fascia and subcutaneous fat.

Negative symptoms: Those symptoms of schizophrenia that are largely associated with a deficit in psychosocial functioning, emotional expression, and interpersonal interactions. Examples include blunted affect, alogia, decreased interest and involvement in social and occupational activities, and decreased grooming and hygiene.

Neonatal: Within the first 4 weeks (28 days) of life.

Neonates: Newborns who are 1 day to 1 month of age.

Nephritis: Inflammation of the kidney.

Nephrolithiasis: Presence of one or more stones in the renal pelvis, collecting system, or ureters.

Nephron: The working unit of the kidney that is comprised of a glomerulus and tubule. Each kidney is made up of approximately 1 million nephrons, which collectively remove drugs, toxins, and fluid from the blood.

Nephropathy: Refers to a pathologic alteration of the kidney.

Nephrotic range proteinuria: Proteinuria >3 g/day associated with glomerular disease and nephrotic syndrome.

Nephrotoxicity: Toxic insult to the kidney.

Nerve conduction studies: Measurement of the speed of electrical conduction through a nerve.

Neuraminidase: The second major antigenic determinant of the influenza virus; a surface antigen that allows the release of new viral particles from host cells by catalyzing the cleavage of linkages to sialic acid.

Neuritic plaques: Hallmark pathologic marker of Alzheimer's disease comprised of β-amyloid protein and masses of broken neurites.

Neurofibrillary tangles: Hallmark pathologic marker of Alzheimer's disease derived from abnormal phosphorylation of τ-protein filaments.

Neuropathic pain: Pain due to nervous system damage.

Neutropenia: An abnormally reduced number of neutrophils circulating in peripheral blood; although exact definitions of neutropenia often vary, an absolute neutrophil count of <1000 cells/mm^3 indicates a reduction sufficient to predispose patients to infection.

New York Heart Association classification: The New York Heart Association classification provides a simple way of classifying the extent of heart failure. It places patients in one of four categories based on how much they are limited during physical activity.

***N*-methyl-D-aspartate antagonists:** Class of medications that decreases the activity of synaptic glutamate, thus decreasing the likelihood of cell death.

***N*-methyl-D-aspartate (NMDA) receptors:** One of three types of ionotropic postsynaptic glutamate receptors. Upon binding glutamate, these receptors permit the influx of Ca^{+2} ions and results in brain excitation. These are one of the two primary receptors for excitatory neurotransmission in the brain.

Nociceptive pain: Pain due to physiologic processes that involve stimulation, transmission, perception, and modulation.

Nocturia: Frequent nighttime urination (>2 micturitions per night).

Nodule: Elevated, palpable, solid, round or oval lesion more than 0.5 cm in diameter.

Nonalcoholic fatty liver disease (NAFLD): Refers to a wide spectrum of liver disease ranging from simple fatty liver (steatosis), to nonalcoholic steatohepatitis (NASH), to cirrhosis (irreversible, advanced scarring of the liver). All of the stages of NAFLD have in common the accumulation of fatty infiltration in the liver cells.

Nonarteritic, anterior, ischemic optic neuropathy: A disorder caused by an acute decrease of blood flow to the optic nerve, which results in sudden vision loss. If persistent, it can lead to permanent vision loss.

Nonconvulsive status epilepticus (NCSE): Believed to be less common and have a better prognosis than GCSE. The most common two types are absence status epilepticus and complex partial status epilepticus. Both are associated with an impairment in consciousness. For the more common of the two, absence status, the patient appears in a twilight state to lethargy, there is no return to consciousness as occurs in complex partial status epilepticus. For complex partial status epilepticus partial return to consciousness can occur. It may or may not be associated with motor activity or automatisms. The duration is sufficient enough in length to meet the definition of status epilepticus.

Nonoliguria: Production of >450 mL urine/day.

Nonpolyposis: Absence of polyps.

Nonulcer dyspepsia: Ulcer-like dyspepsia that has been investigated, but endoscopic findings yield no evidence of mucosal injury (ulcer).

Norepinephrine (NE): A hormone secreted by the adrenal medulla and also released at synapses.

Nosocomial infection: An infection acquired in a healthcare facility.

NSAID: Nonsteroidal antiinflammatory drug.

N-terminal proBNP: The biologically inactive fragment of B-type natriuretic peptide (BNP). Compared to BNP, N-terminal proBNP circulates at higher plasma concentrations and has a longer half-life.

Nulliparity: Condition of not having given birth to a child.

Obesity–hypoventilation syndrome: Also known as Pickwickian syndrome.

Oblique lie: The fetus is at an angle to the cervix. The head is not the presenting part, and often the patient will need to be delivered by cesarean section.

Obsession: Recurrent and persistent thoughts, images, or impulses experienced as intrusive and distressing.

Obsessive–compulsive disorder (OCD): An anxiety disorder characterized by obsessions and/or compulsions that are time-consuming and interfere significantly with normal routine, social or occupational functioning, or relationships.

Obstructive voiding symptoms: Decreased force of the urinary stream, hesitancy, incomplete bladder emptying, urinary dribbling. This results from bladder outlet obstruction as could be caused by benign prostatic hyperplasia.

Odynophagia: Painful swallowing.

Oligoanovulation: The condition of having few to no ovulatory menstrual cycles.

Oligomenorrhea: Reduced frequency of menses with a time interval between periods greater than 40 days but less than 6 months.

Oliguria: Diminished volume of urine output (volume <400 to 500 mL/day).

Omentumectomy: Excision of the double fold of peritoneum attached to the stomach and connecting it with abdominal viscera (omentum).

Onychomycosis: Fungal infection of the nail apparatus.

Open prostatectomy: In this surgical procedure, an enlarged prostate is removed in its entirety. Access to the prostate can be achieved by cutting through the bladder and reaching down to the prostate, or by cutting through the perineum (between the legs).

Ophthalmia neonatorum: Inflammation of the conjunctiva resulting from acquisition of gonococcal infection at birth.

Opioid addiction: A behavioral pattern manifesting as loss of control over opioid use, compulsive use, and continued use despite harm.

Opioid dependence: State that occurs subsequent to extended exposure to an opioid and manifests as withdrawal symptoms after abrupt dose reduction, discontinuation or after the administration of an opioid antagonist.

Opioid tolerance: Decreased effectiveness of opioid over time due to opioid exposure.

Opportunistic infection (OI): Infection with microorganism that occurs because of altered physiologic state of the patient.

Orchiectomy: The surgical removal of the testicles.

Organic erectile dysfunction: Term used to refer to erectile dysfunction that is caused by vascular, neurologic, and/or hormonal causes.

Orthopnea: Difficulty breathing after lying down.

Orthostatic hypotension: A significant drop in BP, defined as a SBP decrease of greater than 20 mm Hg or a DBP decrease of greater than 10 mm Hg, that occurs when changing from a supine to a standing position.

Osler nodes: Osler nodes are red, raised tender nodules usually 5 mm in diameter on the pulps of toes or fingers. Seen in patients with endocarditis, they are thought to be caused by the deposition of immune complexes.

Osteogenesis imperfecta: Genetic disorder characterized by low trabecular and cortical bone density.

Osteomalacia: Abnormal bone mineralization, referred to as rickets in children.

Osteomyelitis: Infection involving the bone.

Osteopenia: Low bone density, dual-energy x-ray absorptiometry (DXA) T-score of –1 to –2.5.

Osteophyte: A bony outgrowth or protuberance.

Osteoporosis: Very low bone density, DXA T-score less than –2.5, with or without a low trauma fracture. National Osteoporosis Foundation definition: "A chronic, progressive disease characterized by low bone mass, microarchitectural deterioration and decreased bone strength, bone fragility and a consequent increase in fracture risk."

Osteotomy: The surgical cutting of a bone.

Otitis media: Inflammation of the middle ear.

Ovulation: Periodic ripening and rupture of mature follicle and the discharge of ovum from the cortex of the ovary.

Oxytocin: A polypeptide hormone secreted by the posterior pituitary gland that stimulates uterine contraction.

Paget's disease: Disorder of bone remodeling in discrete sections of bone.

PAH: *p*-aminohippurate, a small molecule that is completely secreted from the tubules into urine, so that blood leaving the kidney is virtually free of PAH; a marker that is often used to measure renal plasma flow (RPF).

Pain: An unpleasant sensory and emotional experience associated with actual or potential tissue damage or described in terms of such damage.

Palpation: Touching the skin to feel the outline of an organ.

Pan- or holosystolic: Throughout the end time of systole.

Pancolitis: Inflammation that involves the majority of the colon for patients with inflammatory bowel disease.

Pancreatitis: An acute or chronic inflammation of the pancreas with variable involvement of local tissues and remote organs.

Panel reactive antibody (PRA): The percentage of cells from a panel of donors with which a potential recipient's bloodstream reacts. The more antibodies in the recipient's bloodstream, the higher the PRA. The higher the PRA, the higher the risk for a positive crossmatch.

Panhypopituitarism: A condition of complete or partial loss of anterior and posterior pituitary function resulting in a complex disorder characterized by multiple pituitary-hormone deficiencies.

Panic attack: A discrete period in which there is the sudden onset of intense apprehension, fearfulness, or terror, often associated with feelings of impending doom.

Panic disorder: The presence of recurrent, unexpected panic attacks followed by at least 1 month of persistent concern about having another panic attack, worry about the possible implications or consequences of the panic attacks, or a significant behavioral change related to the attacks.

Panlobular: Affecting the entire lobe.

Papillary: Upper layer of the dermis.

Papilledema: Swelling around the optic nerve, usually caused by pressure on the nerve by a tumor or stroke.

Papule: Solid, elevated, lesion more than 0.5 cm in diameter.

Papules: Small raised bumps that may open when scratched and become crusty and infected.

Papulosquamous: Raised plaque or papule with scaling.

***p*-Aminohippurate (PAH):** A small molecule that is completely secreted from the tubules into urine, so that blood leaving the kidney is virtually free of PAH; a marker that is often used to measure renal plasma flow (RPF).

Paranoia: Ideation involving suspiciousness or the belief that one is being harassed, persecuted, or unfairly treated.

Parenchyma: Specific cells or tissue of an organ.

Paresthesia: An abnormal sensation, such as of burning, pricking, tickling, or tingling.

Parkinsonism: A constellation of symptoms with atypical features such that a diagnosis of idiopathic Parkinson disease cannot be made.

Parous: Having borne one or more children.

Paroxysmal nocturnal dyspnea: Onset of difficulty breathing after lying down for several hours.

Partial agonist: A drug with high binding affinity to a receptor and that elicits a weaker response than the endogenous neurotransmitter. At least theoretically, this causes an agonist effect in states of decreased endogenous neurotransmitter tone and an antagonist effect in the endogenous state of heightened neurotransmitter activity.

Partial seizure: A seizure that begins in one hemisphere of the brain. It can be simple, complex, or secondarily generalized.

Patch: Large macule (more than 2 cm in diameter).

Patient-reported outcomes: The consequences of the disease and/or its treatment as perceived and reported by the patient.

Pelvic inflammatory disease (PID): Infection of the lining of the uterus, the fallopian tubes, or the ovaries.

Penumbra (ischemic): The area of brain tissue around the core of the infarct that has decreased function but remains viable. It is proposed that reperfusion of this tissue will allow survival of the affected neurons and other brain cells.

Peptic ulcer: Cellular distribution of the gastrointestinal mucosa, submucosa, and muscular layer. Chronic peptic ulcers usually occur as a "single hole" and are found most often in the stomach and duodenum.

Percussion: Tapping on a structure to elicit a sound.

Percussion and postural drainage: Tapping on the thorax to physically loosen pulmonary secretions and posturing the body to facilitate expectoration.

Percutaneous coronary intervention (PCI): A minimally invasive procedure whereby access to the coronary arteries is obtained through the femoral artery up the aorta to the coronary os. Contrast media is used to visualize the coronary artery stenosis using a coronary angiogram. A guidewire is used to cross the stenosis and small balloon is inflated and/or stent is deployed to break up atherosclerotic plaque and restore coronary artery blood flow. The stent is left in place to prevent restenosis of the coronary artery.

Pericarditis: Inflammation of the pericardium, which is the fibroserous sac enclosing the heart.

Perimenopause: The period immediately prior to the menopause and the first year after menopause. Reflects the transition to menopause (with irregular menstrual cycles) and includes the 3 to 5 years before and 1 year after the cessation of menstrual flow.

Perinatal: Time shortly before and after birth.

Periodontitis: A serious gum infection caused by inflammation and infection of the ligaments that support the teeth.

Perioral dermatitis: Rash around the mouth. In patients with anorexia nervosa or bulimia nervosa, the rash is secondary to repeated vomiting that creates skin irritation from exposure to the gastric contents.

Peripheral arterial disease (PAD): Atherosclerotic occlusive disease of the extremities, usually diagnosed by symptoms (claudication) or assessment of the blood flow to an extremity.

Peripheral blood progenitor cells: Immature blood cells, which are capable of producing white blood cells, platelets, and red blood cells.

Peritoneal dialysis (PD): A dialysis procedure performed in the peritoneal cavity in which the peritoneum acts as the semipermeable membrane.

Peritonitis: The acute, inflammatory response of the peritoneal lining to microorganisms, chemicals, irradiation, or foreign body injury.

Periungual pyogenic granulomas: Benign vascular lesion around the fingernails or toenails; can relate to acitretin use.

Perseveration: Persistent repetition of the same verbal or motor response despite differing stimuli.

Pervasive developmental disorder: A group of disorders characterized by severe and pervasive impairments in the development of socialization and communication skills, as well as behavioral repertoire, with a typical diagnosis younger than age 3 years; includes autistic disorder, Rett syndrome, pervasive development disorder not otherwise specified, childhood disintegrative disorder, and Asperger disorder.

Petechiae: Pinpoint, flat, round, red spots under the skin caused by intradermal hemorrhage.

Peyronie's disease: Disease of the penis associated with fibrous tissue scarring along the inside of the penile shaft resulting in significant and abnormal curvature of the erect penis. Associated with penile pain; deformity makes sexual intercourse difficult or impossible.

P-glycoprotein: An adenosine triphosphatase (ATPase)-dependent membrane transporter efflux pump coded for by the multidrug-resistance gene 1 (MDR1 or ABCB1 or PGY1) found in the human blood-brain barrier and intestine as well as other tissues; lipophilic molecules are good substrates for the ABCB1 efflux transport system at the blood–brain barrier.

Pharmacodynamics: The study of the relationship between the concentration of a drug and the response obtained in a patient.

Pharmacoepidemiology: The study of the use of and the effects of drugs in large numbers of people with the purpose of supporting safe and effective drug therapies. This type of observational research is useful when more rigorous, experimental designs are not feasible.

Pharmacogenetics: Genetic basis for interindividual differences in drug response.

Pharmacovigilance: The science and activities relating to the detection, assessment, understanding, and prevention of adverse effects or any other drug-related problems.

Pharyngitis: An acute infection of the oropharynx or nasopharynx.

Phase I reactions: Metabolic changes by the body that generally make the drug molecule more polar and water soluble so that it is prone to elimination by the kidney, such as oxidation, hydrolysis, and reduction.

Phase II reactions: Metabolic changes by the body that generally make the drug molecule more prone to elimination by the kidney, such as conjugation to form glucuronides, acetates, or sulfates.

Phenotype: Outward expression of the genotype.

Phenotypes: How a gene is expressed (e.g., eye color, height, drug metabolism capacity). The expression of genetic alleles (genotype) as an observable physical or biochemical trait.

Phobia: A persistent, abnormal, and irrational fear of a specific thing or situation that compels one to avoid it, despite the awareness and reassurance that it is not dangerous.

Phonophobia: Hypersensitivity to sound, usually causing avoidance.

Photic stimulation: Stimulation of the visual cortex through visual stimulation with bright and alternating light.

Photoallergy: Photosensitivity disorder of skin (light and photo-allergic agent).

Photophobia: Hypersensitivity to light, usually causing avoidance.

Phototoxicity: Photosensitivity disorder of skin (light and photo-toxic agent).

Physical dependence: A state of adaptation that is manifested by a drug class–specific withdrawal syndrome that can be produced by abrupt cessation, rapid dose reduction, decreasing blood level of the drug, and/or administration of an antagonist.

Pickwickian syndrome: Excess load of excess body fat on the chest tissues resulting in a constellation of syndromes that include excessive daytime sleepiness, shortness of breath due to elevated blood carbon dioxide pressure, disturbed sleep at night, and flushed face.

Pilonidal: Hair-containing cyst.

Pilosebaceous: Sebaceous gland and adjacent hair follicle.

Placenta accreta: Attachment of placental villi to the muscle of the uterine wall causing abnormally firm placental adherence. Complications include intractable postpartum hemorrhage.

Placenta previa: Placental implantation at or near the opening of the cervix. Severe maternal hemorrhage can occur because the placenta precedes the infant during birth.

Plantar fasciitis: A condition that causes heel and arch pain as a result of irritation and inflammation of the plantar fascia, the connective tissues that form the arch of the foot.

Plaque: Raised, flat lesion (more than 2 cm in diameter).

Pneumonitis: Inflammation of lung tissue.

Poikilocytosis: The presence of irregularly shaped red blood cells in the peripheral blood.

Poikilothermia: Inability to maintain normal body temperature.

Polyarteritis nodosa: A systemic necrotizing vasculitis of small and medium-sized arteries.

Polycystic ovarian syndrome: An endocrine disorder with a constellation of symptoms with excessive androgen activity, including irregular or no menstrual periods, acne, excessive hair growth, and infertility.

Polycythemia: An increase in the number of red cells present in the blood.

Polymorphism: Genetic variations occurring at a frequency of at least one percent in the human population.

Porphyria: A group of disorders involving heme biosynthesis, characterized by excessive excretion of porphyrins or their precursors; can be inherited or can be acquired, as from the effects of certain chemical agents.

Porphyrins: Pigments widely distributed throughout nature (e.g., heme, bile pigments, cytochromes) consisting of four pyrroles joined in a ring (porphin) structure.

Positive symptoms: Those symptoms of schizophrenia, largely based on perceptual and thought disturbances, that are typically associated with psychosis. Examples are suspiciousness, paranoia, delusions, hallucinations, and disorganized thought processes.

Positron emission tomography (PET): Specialized nuclear scanning technique that allows the measurement of regional blood flow and glucose metabolism. With radiolabeled ligands, also allows for the measurement of the binding of drugs to receptors.

Posterior fossa: The cavity in the back part of the skull that contains the cerebellum, brainstem, and cranial nerves 5–12.

Postexposure prophylaxis: Dispensing or administering a medication (including a vaccine) to start immediately after exposure to a disease or organism, to prevent the disease from developing or spreading.

Postictal: The recovery period after a seizure, when a patient can be lethargic or confused. Duration can be variable.

Posttraumatic seizures: Seizure event(s) that can occur following a traumatic brain injury within the first 7 days postinjury (early) or beyond 7 days postinjury (late).

Postrenal acute renal failure (ARF): Acute renal failure with an anatomical cause that is in the urinary tract.

Posttraumatic stress disorder: An anxiety disorder in which exposure to an exceptional mental or physical stressor is followed by persistent reexperiencing of the event, avoidance of reminders of the event, and arousal symptoms.

Postvoid residual urine volume: Urine left in the bladder after the patient has been asked to completely empty urine out of the bladder. Normally the postvoid residual urine volume should be zero. A high postvoid residual urine volume is associated with recurrent urinary tract infection.

PRA (panel reactive antibody): The percentage of cells from a panel of donors with which a potential recipient's bloodstream reacts. The more antibodies in the recipient's bloodstream, the higher the PRA. The higher the PRA, the higher the risk for a positive crossmatch.

Preexposure vaccination: Administration of a protective vaccine to the public, military troops, or high-risk individuals prior to the potential exposure to an infectious disease.

Preference-based measures: Measures that provide an overall HRQOL index score based on a scale anchored by 1.0 (full health) and 0.0 (dead).

Prefrontal cortex: Part of the brain that integrates thought, emotion, and motivation.

Preload: Along with afterload, it is an important determinant of cardiac output. It is the degree of stretch of the myocardial fibers (sarcomeres) at the end of diastole. As the sarcomeres are stretched, the force of contraction increases. Preload is approximated by the left ventricular end diastolic volume or pressure.

Premature infants: Those born before 37 weeks of gestational age.

Premature ovarian failure: Amenorrhea, sex-steroid deficiency, and infertility in women younger than 40 years of age.

Premenstrual dysphoric disorder (PMDD): Severe psychiatric mood disorder with marked affective symptoms causing significant interference in work or relationships temporally associated with the luteal phase and not caused by an underlying psychiatric disturbance; a severe form of premenstrual syndrome and is listed in the appendix of the *Diagnostic and Statistical Manual of Mental Disorders, Fourth Edition Revised*. The diagnostic criteria require prospective documentation of symptoms, a specific constellation of symptoms, and functional impairment.

Premenstrual molimina: Includes premenstrual symptoms such as breast tenderness, pelvic heaviness or bloating, and food cravings that are not distressing and do not interfere with daily functioning.

Premenstrual syndrome (PMS): A constellation of symptoms including mild mood disturbance and physical symptoms that occur prior to the menses and resolve with initiation of menses.

Premonitory migraine symptoms: Symptoms preceding and forewarning of a migraine attack by 2 to 48 hours, occurring before the aura in migraine with aura and before the onset of pain in migraine without aura.

Prerenal ARF: Acute renal failure caused by a reduction of renal blood flow. Often associated with volume depletion or poor cardiac function.

Presbycusis: Progressive bilateral loss of hearing that occurs in the aged.

Pressured speech: More and faster speech that is difficult or impossible to interrupt.

Preterm: Before 37 weeks of gestation.

Priapism: Painful prolonged erection.

Primary amenorrhea: Absence of menses by age 16 years in the presence of normal secondary sexual development or absence of menses by age 14 years in the absence of normal secondary sexual development.

Primary hypertension: Same as essential hypertension; persistently elevated BP that results from unknown pathophysiological etiology.

Primary hypogonadism: Failure of the testes to produce an adequate supply of testosterone to meet physiologic needs.

Primary lesion: Basic skin lesion that appears at the beginning of skin disorder.

Primary resistance: Refers to resistance recorded prior to drug exposure in vitro or in vivo, as determined by in-vitro susceptibility testing using standardized methodology.

Proctitis: Inflammation confined to the rectum for patients with inflammatory bowel disease.

Prodrome: Early symptom indicating that disease or further symptoms are imminent.

Progestogen: A term referring to progesterone and the synthetic progestational compounds (sometimes referred to as *progestins*).

Progressive multifocal leukoencephalopathy (PML): Rapidly progressive neuromuscular disease caused by opportunistic infection of brain cells by the JC virus.

Prolactin: A polypeptide hormone secreted by the anterior pituitary gland that stimulates lactation.

Proprioception: A sense or perception, usually at a subconscious level, of the movements and position of the body and especially its limbs, independent of vision; this sense is gained primarily from input from sensory nerve terminals in muscles and tendons and the fibrous capsule of joints combined with input from the vestibular apparatus.

Prostate-specific antigen (PSA): A clinical laboratory test; PSA is a tumor marker that is used to screen for, monitor response to treatment of, and determine degree of spread of prostate cancer. Normally, PSA blood levels should be low as PSA is passed out of the body in the ejaculate.

Prostatectomy: Removal of all or part of the prostate gland. There are two main types: (1) transurethral resection of the prostate (TURP)—removes part of the tissue surrounding the urethra that can be blocking the flow of urine; and (2) radical prostatectomy, which removes all of the prostate and the seminal vesicles.

Protease: An enzyme in HIV that cleaves large precursor polypeptides into functional proteins that are necessary to produce a complete virus.

Proteinuria: A condition in which the urine contains large amounts of protein (>150 mg/day); often a sign of glomerular or tubular damage in the kidney.

Proteolytic: The ability to break down protein.

Prothrombin: A clotting factor that is converted to thrombin; also known as factor II.

Prothrombin time (PT): A measure of coagulation representing the amount of time required to form a blood clot after the addition of thromboplastin to the blood sample; also known as Quick's test.

Pruritus: Itching.

Pseudoaddiction: A behavior pattern reflective of seeking relief of pain and resembling that of addictive behavior.

Pseudoallergic: Adverse reactions that appear like allergic reactions but do not have an immunologic mechanism.

Pseudocyst: Collection of pancreatic juice and tissue debris enclosed by a wall of fibrous or granulation tissue.

Pseudohypertension: A falsely elevated BP measurement that is usually because of rigid, calcified brachial arteries; this can be seen in patients who are elderly, have longstanding diabetes, or have chronic kidney disease.

Pseudomembranous colitis: Inflammation of the colon caused by the toxin of *Clostridium difficile* and resulting in bloody diarrhea.

Pseudopolyps: An area of hypertrophied gastrointestinal mucosa that resembles a polyp and contains nonmalignant cells.

Pseudotumor cerebri: Increased intracranial pressure caused by decreased venous drainage from the brain as a result of increased intraabdominal pressure. Symptoms usually include severe headache, bilateral pulsatile auditory tinnitus, and visual field cuts. Also known as idiopathic intracranial hypertension.

Pseudoxanthoma elasticum: Pseudoxanthoma elasticum is a chronic degenerative disease of connection tissues of the skin, eyes, and cardiovascular system resulting from fragmentation and calcification of elastic fibers.

Psoriasis: A chronic, noncontagious autoimmune disease that affects the skin in the form of thick, red, scaly patches.

Psychoeducation: Education geared toward patients becoming more informed about their mental illness and treatment. Additional goals include self-monitoring, efforts to improve treatment adherence, interactions between patient and clinicians, and empowerment.

Psychogenic erectile dysfunction: Erectile dysfunction because of failure of central nervous system to perceive or process sexually stimulating information.

Psychometrics: The measurement of psychologic constructs, such as quality of life.

Psychomotor: Movement or muscular activity related to mental processes.

Psychomotor retardation: A slowing or limitation of motor functioning or muscular movements.

Psychosocial functioning: A person's level of functioning on a daily basis that encompasses all the domains of life experience (e.g., interpersonal relationships, work, school, recreation).

Psychosocial rehabilitation programs: Care programs oriented toward improving patient's daily adaptive functioning. Includes such interventions as basic living skills, social skills training, basic education, work programs, and supported housing.

Psychosocial stressor: Any significant life event or change that can be associated with the onset, occurrence, or exacerbation of a mental disorder.

Psychotherapy: A general term used to describe a form of treatment based on talking with a therapist. Psychotherapy aims to relieve distress by discussing and expressing feelings, to help the patient to change attitudes, behavior, and habits and to develop better ways of coping.

Pulmonary artery occlusion pressure: It is usually determined by a balloon-tipped Swan-Ganz catheter that is advanced into a distal branch of the pulmonary artery. Inflation of the balloon at the catheter tip occludes the pulmonary artery and allows measurement of the left atrial pressure that reflects the left ventricular diastolic pressure. Therefore, it is a measure of the left ventricular preload.

Pulmonary aspiration: The inhalation of fluids and gastric contents into the lungs that can cause aspiration pneumonitis.

Pulmonary capillary wedge pressure: It is usually determined by a balloon-tipped Swan-Ganz catheter that is advanced into a distal branch of the pulmonary artery. Inflation of the balloon at the catheter tip occludes the pulmonary artery and allows measurement of the left atrial pressure, which reflects the left ventricular diastolic pressure. Therefore, it is a measure of the left ventricular preload.

Pulmonary embolism: A disorder of thrombus formation causing obstruction of a pulmonary artery or one of its branches and results in pulmonary infarction.

Pulsating: Throbbing or beating with a rhythm.

Pulseless electrical activity: The absence of a detectable pulse and the presence of some type of electrical activity other than VF or PVT.

Purgatives: An agent used for purging the bowels.

Purpura: Discoloration of skin because of a hemorrhagic spot more than 0.5 cm in diameter.

Pustule: Small, raised lesion containing pus or exudates.

Pyelonephritis: An infection involving the kidneys and representing upper tract infection.

Pyoderma: Purulent skin disease.

Pyoderma gangrenosum: Skin ulceration with necrotic edges.

Pyuria: Presence of pus or white blood cells in the urine.

Quality-adjusted life-years (QALY): A health outcome summary measure in which quantity of life is adjusted for its quality. A year in full health is equivalent to 1.0 QALY. A year in a health state considered worse than full health, such as 0.5, would equal 0.5 QALY, which is equivalent to living half a year in full health.

Radionuclide ventriculography: Radionuclide ventriculography, also known as contrast ventriculography, provides imaging of a ventricle of the heart after the injection of a radioactive contrast medium. The technique is less invasive than cardiac catheterization and is used to assess ventricular function.

Rales: The clicking, rattling, or crackling noises heard on auscultation of the lungs during inhalation.

Rating scales: Tools used to objectively describe, assess, and measure subjective findings common in psychiatric illnesses. Rating scales are also used to diagnose specific psychiatric conditions.

Rational polytherapy: The concurrent use of two or more drugs for patients not responding to monotherapy. The combination of drugs is based on a consideration of mechanism of action, clinical pharmacokinetics, adverse reactions, and drug interactions.

Rebound insomnia: Sleep that is worsened compared with patient's baseline sleep for a few days after discontinuation of a sedative hypnotic medication.

Rebound vasodilation or congestion: See *Rhinitis medicamentosa*.

Refractory status epilepticus: Status epilepticus is considered refractory when adequate doses of a benzodiazepine, hydantoin, or barbiturate have failed to terminate the seizures, that is, a patient must have failed two first line therapies to be considered refractory.

Rejection: The response of the immune system, usually involving T- or B-lymphocytes, to the recognition of foreign antigens in transplanted tissue, which destroys the cells in the transplanted organ and ultimately leads to organ failure, if not treated successfully.

Relapse: New or old multiple sclerosis symptoms lasting 24 hours or longer often associated with demyelination or inflammation in the brain or spinal cord. Relapses are also referred to as an attack, exacerbation, or flare-up of multiple sclerosis.

Relapsing-remitting multiple sclerosis: The most common form of multiple sclerosis at the time of diagnosis. It is characterized by attacks usually with full or partial recovery and no disease progression between attacks.

Relative risk reduction: The amount of risk reduced when compared to a control. When one sees a 5% event rate in the control group and a 4% event rate in the treatment group, the relative risk reduction is 20%. The absolute risk reduction is 1%.

Reliability: The extent to which measures give consistent or accurate results.

Remote symptomatic: When the cause of the status epilepticus is from a previous neurological injury or anatomical malformation, e.g., a patient with a prior stroke, head trauma or brain tumor.

Renal osteodystrophy (ROD): The condition resulting from sustained metabolic changes that occur with chronic kidney disease including secondary hyperparathyroidism, hyperphosphatemia, hypocalcemia, and vitamin D deficiency. The skeletal complications associated with ROD include osteitis fibrosa cystica (high bone turnover disease), osteomalacia (low bone turnover disease), adynamic bone disease, and mixed bone disorders.

Renal replacement therapy: Any form of dialysis or hemofiltration used to support patients without adequate kidney function. Goals of renal replacement therapy are to remove excess fluid; remove waste products and toxins; and control electrolyte concentrations.

Renal: General term referring to the kidneys.

Renin-angiotensin-aldosterone system: A complex endogenous humoral mediated system that is involved with most of the regulatory components involved with arterial BP.

Renovascular: Pertaining to blood vessels located within the kidney, such as the afferent and efferent arterioles, and renal arteries.

Resistant hypertension: Patients with hypertension that have not achieved their goal BP value despite treatment with three or more antihypertensive drugs.

Respiratory disturbance index: A summary measure that quantifies the number of apneas, hypopneas, and respiratory effort-related arousals per hour of sleep.

Respondent burden: The time, energy, and other demands placed on those to whom the instrument is administered.

Responsiveness: The ability or power of a measure to detect clinically important change when it occurs.

Resting tremor: Tremor that occurs or exacerbates when the affected body part is at rest; it decreases or disappears with active motions.

Restrictive cardiomyopathy: Restrictive cardiomyopathy is characterized by nondilated ventricles with impaired ventricular filling. Hypertrophy is typically absent, although the infiltrative and storage diseases can cause a left ventricular wall thickness elevation.

Retching: Contractions of the diaphragm, thoracic, and abdominal muscles without expulsion of gastric contents.

Retinitis: Inflammation of the retina, often caused by infection with cytomegalovirus.

Retinoid dermatitis: Erythematous scaly patches with superficial skin fissuring.

Retrograde pyelography: A procedure where radiocontrast dye is injected into the ureter to produce detailed radiographs of the ureter and kidneys.

Rett's syndrome: A type of pervasive developmental disorder typically associated with severe to profound mental retardation, seen in females only, with the development of significant multiple progressively worsening deficits following a period of normal development (microcephaly, loss of purposeful hand motor skills, and acquisition of stereotyped hand movements, diminished social interests, and appearance of poorly coordinated gait or trunk movements).

Reverse transcriptase: The enzyme in HIV that synthesizes a complementary strand of DNA.

Reversible posterior leukoencephalopathy syndrome (RPLS): Rare, life-threatening condition affecting the brain. Symptoms include headaches, seizures, confusion, and vision problems. Prognosis good with early identification and treatment.

Reye's syndrome: Acute encephalopathy characterized by fever, vomiting, fatty infiltration of the liver, disorientation, and coma, occurring mainly in children and usually following a viral infection, such as chicken pox or influenza.

Rhabdomyolysis: The breakdown of muscle tissue and release of myoglobin and intracellular electrolytes into the circulation because of a variety of causes such as crush injuries, drug-induced immobilization, and status epilepticus. It often leads to acute renal failure.

Rheumatoid arthritis: A systemic, symmetric autoimmune disease with swelling, pain, and inflammation of joints as a key finding.

Rhinitis: Inflammation of the nasal mucous membrane. Can be seasonal (*hay fever*) or perennial (increasingly called *intermittent* or *persistent*).

Rhinitis medicamentosa: Nasal congestion associated with tolerance to and resulting overuse of topical decongestants. Also known as *rebound vasodilation* or *rebound congestion*.

Rickets: See *Osteomalacia*.

Rigidity: Increased resistance detectable with the passive movement of a limb.

Roth spots: A hemorrhage in the retina with a white center. Roth spots are often associated with bacterial endocarditis.

Russell sign: Callus on dorsum of the hand secondary to self-induced vomiting.

S_4 gallop: An S_4 gallop is a presystolic atrial sound that immediately precedes the first heart sound (S_1). This finding on auscultation of the heart can be indicative of myocardial disease.

Salicylism: Poisoning by salicylic acid or any of its compounds.

Salpingo-oophorectomy: Surgical removal of the ovaries and fallopian tubes.

Sarcoidosis: Sarcoidosis is a multisystem granulomatous disorder of unknown etiology characterized histologically by noncaseating epithelioid granulomas involving various organs or tissues, with symptoms dependent on the site and degree of involvement.

Scale: Flake of stratum corneum.

Scar: Fibrous tissue formed during healing of injury to skin.

Schizophrenia: A chronic disorder of thought and affect encompassing different constellations of symptoms (i.e., positive symptoms, negative symptoms, cognitive dysfunction), with the individual having a significant disturbance in interpersonal relationships and ability to function in society on a daily basis.

Scleritis: Inflammation of the white portion of the eyeball, which can be superficial (episcleritis) or involve deeper layers of the eye.

Scleroderma: Scleroderma is a diffuse connective tissue disease characterized by changes in the skin, blood vessels, skeletal muscles, and internal organs.

Sebaceous gland: Gland that secretes sebum.

Sebosuppressive: Decreasing amount of sebum produced by the sebaceous gland.

Sebum: Oil produced by the sebaceous gland.

Second-generation antipsychotic (atypical antipsychotic): An antipsychotic medication that has pharmacodynamic and clinical properties different than the first generation (typical or traditional) antipsychotics that act primarily by having high levels of binding to dopamine-2 (D_2) receptors. Although definitions of atypicality vary, all second-generation antipsychotics share the property of causing a much lower incidence of extrapyramidal side effects.

Secondary amenorrhea: Cessation of menses in a woman previously menstruating for 6 months or more.

Secondary brain injury: A complex sequence of pathophysiologic events precipitated by the initial or primary brain injury that disrupts the normal central nervous system balance between oxygen supply and demand resulting in a worsened patient outcome.

Secondary hypertension: Persistently elevated BP that results from a known pathophysiological etiology or drug-induced cause.

Secondary hypogonadism: Failure of hypothalamus or pituitary gland to produce adequate amount of luteinizing hormone-releasing hormone (LHRH) or luteinizing hormone (LH). Thus, testicular production of testosterone is reduced.

Secondary prophylaxis (or suppressive therapy): Refers to administration of systemic antifungal agents (generally prior to and throughout the period of granulocytopenia) to prevent relapse of a documented invasive fungal infection that was treated during a previous episode of granulocytopenia.

Secondary resistance: Develops on exposure to an antifungal agent and can be either reversible, because of transient adaptation, or acquired as a result of one or more genetic alterations.

Secondary-progressive multiple sclerosis: Often follows relapsing-remitting multiple sclerosis whereby attacks become continuously progressive over time. It is sometimes accompanied by acute relapses.

Seizure: Paroxysmal disorder of central nervous system, characterized by abnormal neuronal discharges with or without loss of consciousness. They vary in cause, presentation, consequences, duration, and management.

Selection bias: Systematic differences in characteristics between those selected for study and those who are not. See also *Information bias*.

Sepsis: The systemic inflammatory response syndrome (SIRS) secondary to infection. See also *Systemic inflammatory response syndrome*.

Septic arthritis: Infection involving a joint.

Septic shock: Sepsis with persistent hypotension despite fluid resuscitation, along with the presence of perfusion abnormalities. Patients who are on inotropic or vasopressor agents might not be hypotensive at the time perfusion abnormalities are measured.

Serotonin (5-hydroxytryptamine [5-HT]): An inhibitory neurotransmitter present in the raphe nucleus of the brainstem, platelets, carcinoid tumors, and other tissues. It is a vasoconstrictor and neurochemical involved in mood and sleep.

Serum urea nitrogen (SUN): See *Blood urea nitrogen*.

Severe sepsis: Sepsis associated with organ dysfunction, hypoperfusion, or hypotension. Hypoperfusion and perfusion abnormalities can include, but are not limited to, lactic acidosis, oliguria, or acute alteration in mental status.

Short stature: A broad term describing a condition commonly defined by a physical height that is more than two standard deviations below the population mean and lower than the third percentile for height in a specific age group.

Sickle cell disease: A group of inherited red blood cell (RBC) disorder in which sickle cell hemoglobin (HbS) is present. Hemolytic anemia and painful vasoocclusion are the main features.

Simple partial seizure: A seizure beginning in one hemisphere of the brain. It is manifested by alterations in motor functions, sensory or somatosensory symptoms without loss of consciousness. It can progress to a complex partial seizure or to a secondarily generalized seizure with loss of consciousness.

Single-nephron GFR (SNGFR): The rate of filtration through a single glomerulus of a nephron; often reported in nL/min.

Sinus ostia: The pathways that drain the sinuses.

Sinusitis: An inflammation and/or infection of the paranasal sinus mucosa.

Sjögren's syndrome: An inflammatory process affecting the mucous membranes. Can cause dry mouth with difficulty swallowing. Can occur secondary to autoimmune diseases such as rheumatoid arthritis or systemic lupus erythematosus.

Sleep latency: The amount of time it takes to fall asleep.

Sleep spindles: Brief burst of electrical activity seen on the EEG, 12 to 14 Hz.

Slipped capital femoral epiphysis (SCFE): Increased width of the femoral plate observed during GH treatment resulting in hip or knee pain.

Social anxiety disorder (SAD): A disorder characterized by clinically significant anxiety provoked by exposure to certain types of social or performance situations, often leading to avoidance behavior.

Social phobia: See *Social anxiety disorder.*

Somatic pain: Pain arising from skin, bone, joint, muscle, or connective tissue.

Specific measures: Instruments intended to provide greater detail concerning particular outcomes, in terms of functioning and well-being, uniquely associated with a condition and/or its treatment.

Specific phobia: A phobia characterized by clinically significant anxiety provoked by exposure to a specific feared object or situation, often leading to avoidance behavior.

Spermicide: A substance (nonoxynol-9 in the United States) placed in the vagina to inhibit the activity of sperm, thus reducing the risk of pregnancy; available as vaginal creams, films, foams, gels, suppositories, sponges, and tablets.

Spirochete: The class of microorganism that is the agent of syphilis (*Treponema pallidum*).

Standard gamble: An approach to health-state preference elicitation in which the respondent is offered a choice between two alternatives: choice A—living in health state *i* (a health state between full health and death) with certainty, or choice B—taking a gamble on a new treatment for which the outcome is uncertain.

Status epilepticus: Defined as any recurrent or continuous seizure activity lasting longer than 30 minutes in which the patient does not regain baseline mental status. The two most common types are generalized convulsive status epilepticus and nonconvulsive status epilepticus.

Steatorrhea: Excessive fat in stool.

Stereotypy: Persistent repetition of senseless acts or words.

Stevens–Johnson syndrome: A serious dermatologic reaction characterized by blistering of the mucous membranes (mouth, eyes, vagina) with patchy rashes that can cover most of the body. Patients can also experience fever, headache, and cough.

Stress-related mucosal damage: Superficial gastritis-like lesions associated with critical illness in hospitalized patients.

Striae: Linear, atrophic, pink, purple, or white lesions of skin secondary to changes in connective tissue.

Stricture: An area of narrowing or constriction in the gastrointestinal tract due to buildup of fibrotic tissue; often a result of longstanding inflammation.

Stroke: A sudden onset, focal neurologic deficit, of presumed vascular origin, lasting longer than 24 hours.

Stroke volume: The volume of blood ejected from the heart during systole.

Stromal tissue of the prostate: This portion of the prostate is composed of smooth muscle tissue, which is embedded with α-adrenergic receptors. When stimulated, the muscle contracts around the urethra. This comprises approximately 75% of the total volume of the enlarged prostate gland in patients with benign prostatic hyperplasia.

Subarachnoid hemorrhage: Accumulation of blood in the space (subarachnoid space) surrounding the brain that usually contains the cerebrospinal fluid. It is usually caused by rupture of an intracranial aneurysm or trauma. It is a type of hemorrhagic stroke and can cause focal neurologic deficits.

Substance abuse: A maladaptive pattern of substance use indicated by repeated adverse consequences related to the repeated use of the substance. Examples include failure to fulfill important obligations at work, school, or home; repeated use in situations in which it is physically dangerous, such as driving under the influence; legal problems; and social or interpersonal problems such as arguments and fights.

Substance dependence: The continued use of the substance despite adverse substance-related problems. The criteria for substance dependence are the same for each of the drugs or drug classes, varying only to fit the unique pharmacologic properties of each drug.

Substantia nigra: Area of the brain (basal ganglia) where cells produce dopamine; characterized by neuromelanin deposits.

Subtle status epilepticus: For patients with prolonged refractory status epilepticus. The electrographical seizures persist; however, the motor manifestations of the seizures may not be apparent. In such cases the patient is considered in subtle status epilepticus.

Sudden death: Also known as sudden cardiac death; an unexpected death because of cardiac causes occurring in a short time period (generally within 1 hour of symptom onset) in a person with known or unknown cardiac disease in whom no previously diagnosed fatal condition is apparent. Most cases are related to cardiac arrhythmias, particularly ventricular fibrillation.

SUN (serum urea nitrogen): See *Blood urea nitrogen.*

Suppressive therapy: See *Secondary prophylaxis.*

Surge capacity: A term that refers to a healthcare system's ability to handle a large influx of patients in the event of an epidemic or disaster.

SV2A: A presynaptic vesicle protein found in the hippocampus as well as other areas of the brain believed to be important in the mechanism of action of levetiracetam.

Swan–Ganz catheter: A catheter (tube) inserted into the heart to measure pressure and cardiac output.

Symptomatic intracerebral hemorrhage: Collection of blood in the brain, usually after an ischemic stroke, that is associated with neurologic worsening.

Symptomatic status epilepticus: Status epilepticus occurring during the time of an acute neurological injury. This etiology is associated with a poorer prognosis.

Systemic vascular resistance: The resistance to blood flow that is primarily determined by the vascular tone of the arteriolar blood vessels.

Symptomatic: SE occurring during the time of an acute neurological injury. This etiology is associated with a poorer prognosis.

Syncope: Fainting.

Synechiae: A *creeping* angle closure that sometimes occurs in patients between attacks of closed-angle glaucoma.

Synergism: The combination of two drugs (such as antibiotics) that produces an effect greater than the sum of the two drugs if used alone.

Synesthesias: The overflow of one sensory modality to another. For example, colors are heard, sounds are seen.

Synovitis: Inflammation of the synovial lining of the joint.

Synovium: Synovial membrane, the inner of the two layers of the articular capsule of a synovial joint, composed of loose connective tissue and having a free smooth surface that lines the joint cavity. It secretes the synovial fluid.

Systemic inflammatory response syndrome (SIRS): Systemic inflammatory response to a variety of clinical insults, which can be of infectious or noninfectious etiology.

Systemic vascular resistance (SVR): The resistance to blood flow that is primarily determined by the vascular tone of the arteriolar blood vessels.

Systolic blood pressure: The arterial BP that occurs during cardiac contraction.

Systolic heart failure: Systolic heart failure is a condition characterized by a decrease in myocardial contractility, which results in a reduction in the cardiac output and left ventricular ejection fraction.

Tachy-brady syndrome: Tachy-brady syndrome, also known as sick sinus syndrome, is a condition in which the sinoatrial node is unable to perform as the pacemaker of the heart.

Tangential speech: Speech pattern whereby the connections between expressed ideas are unrelated or have little relationship to each other.

Taper: To gradually decrease the dosage of a drug over a period of time.

Tardive: A modifier used to describe movement disorders secondary to chronic antipsychotic treatment (duration of treatment must be greater than 3 months). The disorder must persist for greater than 4 weeks and exhibit masking and unmasking characteristics. Tardive dyskinesia, tardive chorea, tardive dystonia, and tardive akathisia are examples of tardive movement disorders.

Telangiectases: Spidery red skin lesions caused by dilated blood vessels.

Tendonitis: Inflammation of tendons.

Tenesmus: Difficulty with bowel evacuation despite the urgency to defecate.

Teratogenicity: Ability of an agent to cause a defect or malformation in a fetus.

TEWL (transepidermal water loss): The rate of water loss by evaporation from the skin.

Thalassemia: Any of a group of inherited disorders of hemoglobin metabolism in which there is impaired synthesis of one or more of the polypeptide chains of globin.

Third-spacing: The shift of fluid and protein into the peritoneal cavity and bowel wall lumen that occurs as a result of peritonitis.

Thought blocking: Interruption of a train of thought whereby the person stops speaking suddenly and without warning, even in the middle of a sentence. Person may report that the thoughts were taken out of his or her head.

Thought broadcasting: Belief that one's thoughts are audible to others.

Thrombin: The enzyme formed from prothrombin that converts fibrinogen to fibrin. It is the principle driving force in the clotting cascade.

Thrombogenesis: The process of forming a blood clot.

Thrombolysis: The process of enzymatically dissolving or breaking apart a blood clot.

Thrombolytic: An enzyme that dissolves or breaks apart blood clots.

Thromboplastin: A substance that triggers the coagulation cascade. Tissue factor is a naturally occurring thromboplastin and used in the prothrombin time (PT) test.

Thrombopoiesis: The process of platelet production from immature cells.

Thrombosis: The process of forming a thrombus.

Thrombotic thrombocytopenic purpura: A life-threatening disease involving embolism and thrombosis of the small blood vessels in the brain and kidney.

Thrombus: An aggregation of fibrin and platelets within a blood vessel. A thrombus often causes vessel obstruction, inflammation, and injury.

Thrush: Fungal infection of the oral mucosa.

Thyroid-stimulating hormone (TSH): A polypeptide hormone secreted by the anterior pituitary gland that stimulates iodine uptake and thyroid hormone synthesis.

Thyrotropin-releasing hormone (TRH): A trophic hormone released by the hypothalamus that stimulates release of thyroid-stimulating hormone (TSH).

Time trade-off: An approach to health-state preference elicitation in which the respondent is asked to trade off years of life in less than full health for a shorter number of years in full health.

Tinea barbae: Fungal infection of the hair follicles of the beard or mustache.

Tinea capitis: Fungal infection of the scalp, hair follicles, or adjacent skin.

Tinea corporis: Fungal infection of the glabrous skin of the trunk and extremities.

Tinea cruris: Fungal infection of the proximal thighs and buttocks.

Tinea manuum: Fungal infection of the palmar surface of the hands.

Tinea pedis: Fungal infection of the feet.

Tinnitus: A noise in the ears, as ringing, buzzing, roaring, clicking, etc. Such sounds can at times be heard by those other than the patient.

Tocolytic: Agent that stops labor contractions.

Tolerance: (1) A state of adaptation in which exposure to a drug induces changes that result in a diminution of one or more of the drug's effects over time. (2) The ability of the immune system to accept a transplanted allograft as part of *self*.

Tonic-clonic seizures: Sharp tonic contraction of muscles followed by a period of rigidity and clonic movement.

Tophi: Urate deposits.

Toxic epidermal necrolysis: A syndrome similar to Stevens-Johnson syndrome characterized by blistering of skin and mucous membranes in response to administration of a drug. Large areas of skin may peel off.

Toxic megacolon: A segmental or total colonic distension of >6 cm with acute colitis and signs of systemic toxicity.

Toxic shock syndrome: Sudden onset of fever, muscle ache, vomiting and diarrhea, accompanied by a peeling rash and followed by low body temperature and shock; caused by staphylococcal endotoxin, especially from infection of the vagina associated with tampon use.

Toxoplasmosis: Clinical infection with *Toxoplasma gondii*.

Transmural: Across the wall of an organ or structure; in the case of CD, inflammation may extend through all four layers of the intestinal wall.

Transurethral incision of the prostate: In this surgical procedure, the bladder neck opening is widened by making incisions at various locations around the bladder neck with a resectoscope, which is inserted into the penis. Excess prostate tissue is not removed.

Transurethral prostatectomy: In this surgical procedure, an enlarged prostate core is removed from the inside out. That is, a resectoscope is inserted into the penis. A cutting blade at the end shaves out excess prostate tissue.

Transverse lie: The fetus is perpendicular to the mother. Usually the shoulder is the presenting part. Fetuses in this position must be delivered by cesarean section.

Transverse myelitis: Inflammation of the full width of the spinal cord that disrupts communication to the muscles, resulting in pain, weakness, and muscle paralysis.

Traveler's diarrhea: Diarrhea caused by contaminated food or water and usually attributed to enterotoxigenic *Escherichia coli* (ETEC), *Shigella*, *Campylobacter*, *Salmonella* species, or viruses.

Troponin: A protein found predominately in cardiac, but not skeletal, muscle, which regulates calcium-mediated interaction of actin and myosin. Troponin I and T are released into the blood from the myocytes at the time of myocardial cell necrosis secondary to infarction. These biochemical markers become elevated and are used in the diagnosis of myocardial infarction. Troponin I and T are more sensitive and specific for infarction than creatinine kinase, which is found in both skeletal and myocardial cells. The exact value of troponin I or T, which is diagnostic of infarction, differs based on assay.

Trousseau's sign: A hand spasm produced by placing a blood pressure cuff over the forearm and inflating the pressure above the systolic pressure for 3 minutes.

Tubule: Section of the nephron that is responsible for secretion and reabsorption of water, electrolytes, and drugs.

Tumor: Elevated, solid lesion.

Tumor necrosis factor-α (TNF-α): A proinflammatory cytokine.

Type I reaction: An immediate, immunoglobulin E (IgE)-mediated allergic reaction.

Ulcer: Loss of epidermis and dermis caused by sloughing of necrotic tissue.

Ultradian sleep–wake rhythm: Is a cycle of sleep and wake that repeats in less than 24 hours. Babies have an ultradian sleep–wake rhythm with multiple sleep and wake periods in a 24-hour period.

Ultrafiltration: The process of removing water from the blood during dialysis.

Ultraviolet A light: 315–400 nm ultraviolet A light.

Ultraviolet A light 1: 340–400 nm ultraviolet A light.

Ultraviolet B light, broadband: 280–315 nm ultraviolet B light.

Ultraviolet B light, narrow band: 311 nm ultraviolet B light.

Umbilication: Slight, navel-like depression, or dimpling, of the center of a rounded body.

Unilateral: On either the right or left side, not crossing the midline. When used for defining sensory or motor disturbances of migraine aura, it includes complete or partial hemi-distribution.

Upper respiratory tract infection: Otitis media, sinusitis, pharyngitis, laryngitis (croup), rhinitis, or epiglottitis.

Urea: A waste product found in the blood and caused by the normal breakdown of protein in the body.

Uremia: An array of symptoms associated with accumulation of metabolic by-products and endogenous toxins in the blood due to impaired kidney function. Symptoms include nausea, vomiting, loss of appetite, weakness, and mental confusion.

Urethritis: Inflammation of the urethra.

Urinalysis: The diagnostic analysis of urine and its components; can be microscopic or macroscopic in nature.

Urinary incontinence: Involuntary leakage of urine; can result from urethral underactivity (stress urinary incontinence), urethral overactivity (overflow incontinence), or mixed pathophysiologic mechanisms.

Urine: Fluid waste resulting from filtration of blood by the kidneys; transferred to the bladder by ureters and expelled from the body through the urethra by the act of voiding or urinating.

Urticaria: Hives (red, raised bumps) that may occur after exposure to an allergen.

Vacuum erection device: Medical device used to manually induce an erection.

Vagal nerve stimulator (VNS): A medical device that is surgically implanted in patients with refractory epilepsy.

Validity: An estimation of the extent to which an instrument is measuring what it is purported to be measuring.

Valsalva maneuver: The Valsalva maneuver is the expiratory effort against a closed glottis, which increases thoracic cavity pressure, which impedes venous return to the heart. This maneuver results in blood pressure and heart rate changes and is used to diagnose treat various cardiac conditions.

Vasculitis: Inflammation of blood vessels.

Vasopressin: A posterior pituitary hormone that controls fluid balance by acting on the renal collecting ducts to prevent water loss.

Vector: Carrier (person, animal, or insect) of disease.

Vegetation: Bacterial growth on heart valves.

Ventricular remodeling: Alterations in myocardial cells and the extracellular matrix that result in changes in the size, shape, structure, and function of the heart. The remodeling process leads to reductions in myocardial systolic and/or diastolic function that, in turn, leads to further myocardial injury, perpetuating the remodeling process and the decline in ventricular dysfunction and progression of heart failure.

Vesicle: Clear blister (<0.5 cm in diameter) filled with fluid.

Visceral pain: Pain arising from internal organs such as the large intestine or pancreas.

Visual analog scale: A response scale that is a line with the end points well defined (e.g., 0 = worst imaginable health state, and 100 = best imaginable health state).

Volume of distribution: A proportionality constant that relates the amount of drug in the body to its serum concentration.

Vomiting: Contraction of the abdominal muscles, descent of the diaphragm, and opening of the gastric cardia resulting in expulsion of stomach contents from the mouth.

Vulgaris: Ordinary, common.

Wearing-off phenomena: Also known as end-of-dose wearing-off or motor fluctuations. The waning of the effects of a dose of levodopa prior to the scheduled time for the next dose, resulting in return of parkinsonian features, such as, tremor, slowness, and rigidity.

White coat hypertension: Patients have normal BP measurements based on home measurements but have elevated BP measurements when measured in a clinical setting.

Withdrawal: The development of a substance-specific syndrome after cessation of or reduction in intake of a substance that was used regularly by the individual to induce a state of intoxication. Withdrawal causes significant distress to the individual and is associated with impairment in social, occupational, or other areas of functioning. Withdrawal is usually associated with substance dependence. Withdrawal generally is also associated with a craving to readminister the drug to relieve the symptoms.

Withdrawal bleeding: The predictable bleeding that results from cessation of a progestogen.

Withdrawal syndrome: The onset of a predictable constellation of signs and symptoms involving alerted activity of the central nervous system after the abrupt discontinuation of, or rapid decrease in, dosage of a drug.

Xerosis: Dry skin.

Xerostomia: Dry mouth caused by decreased salivary production.

Yeasts: Oval or spherically shaped unicellular forms that generally produce pasty or mucoid colonies on agar media, similar to those observed with bacterial cultures. Yeasts have rigid cell walls that reproduce by budding, a process in which daughter cells arise from pinching off a portion of the parent cell.

Zeitgeber: Environmental cue.

Zollinger–Ellison syndrome: Gastric acid hypersecretory disease caused by a gastrin-secreting tumor and leading to multiple, severe duodenal ulcers.

INDEX

Page numbers followed by *f* or *t* indicate figures or tables, respectively.

Laboratory	Conventional Units	Conversion Factor	SI Units
Haptoglobin	60–270 mg/dL	0.01	0.6–2.7 g/L
HBeAg	Negative		
HbsAg	Negative		
HBV DNA	Negative		
Hematocrit			
Male	40.7–50.3%	0.01	0.407–0.503
Female	36.1–44.3%	0.01	0.361–0.443
Hemoglobin (blood)			
Male	13.8–17.2 g/dL	10	138–172 g/L
		Alternate SI: 0.62	8.56–10.67 mmol/L
Female	12.1–15.1 g/dL	10	121–151 g/L
		Alternate SI: 0.62	7.5–9.36 mmol/L
Hemoglobin A1c	4.0–6.0%	0.01	0.04–0.06
Heparin			
Via protamine titration method	0.2–0.4 mcg/mL		
Via anti-factor Xa assay	0.3–0.7 mcg/mL		
High-density lipoprotein (HDL) cholesterol	Greater than 35 mg/dL	0.0259	Greater than 0.91 mmol/L
Homocysteine	3.3–10.4 µmol/L		
Ibuprofen			
Therapeutic	10–50 mcg/mL	4.85	49–243 µmol/L
Toxic	100–700 mcg/mL or more	4.85	485–3395 µmol/L or more
Imipramine, therapeutic	100–300 ng/mL or mcg/L	3.57	357–1071 nmol/L
Immunoglobulin A (IgA)	85–385 mg/dL	0.01	0.85–3.85 g/L
Immunoglobulin G (IgG)	565–1765 mg/dL	0.01	5.65–17.65 g/L
Immunoglobulin M (IgM)	53–375 mg/dL	0.01	0.53–3.75 g/L
Insulin (fasting)	2–20 microunits/mL or milliunits/L	7.175	14.35–143.5 pmol/L
International normalized ratio (INR), therapeutic	2.0–3.0 (2.5–3.5 for some indications)		
Iron			
Male	45–160 mcg/dL	0.179	8.1–31.3 µmol/L
Female	30–160 mcg/dL	0.179	5.4–31.3 µmol/L
Iron binding capacity (total)	220–420 mcg/dL	0.179	39.4–75.2 µmol/L
Iron saturation	15–50%	0.01	0.15–0.50
Lactate (plasma)	0.7–2.1 mEq/L	1	0.7–2.1 mmol/L
	6.3–18.9 mg/dL	0.111	
Lactate dehydrogenase	100–250 IU/L	0.01667	1.67–4.17 µkat/L
Lead	Less than 25 mcg/dL	0.0483	Less than 1.21 µmol/L
Leukocyte count	3.8–9.8 × 10³/µL	10⁶	3.8–9.8 × 10⁹/L
Lidocaine, therapeutic	1.5–6.0 mcg/mL or mg/L	4.27	6.4–25.6 µmol/L
Lipase	Less than 100 IU/L	0.01667	1.7 µkat/L
Lithium, therapeutic	0.5–1.25 mEq/L	1	0.5–1.25 mmol/L
Low-density lipoprotein (LDL) cholesterol			
Desirable	Less than 130 mg/dL	0.0259	Less than 3.36 mmol/L
Borderline high risk	130–159 mg/dL	0.0259	3.36–4.11 mmol/L
High risk	Greater than or equal to 160 mg/dL	0.0259	Greater than or equal to 4.13 mmol/L
Luteinizing hormone (LH)			
Male	1–8 milliunits/mL	1	1–8 units/L
Female			
Follicular phase	1–12 milliunits/mL	1	1–12 units/L
Midcycle	16–104 milliunits/mL	1	16–104 units/L
Luteal phase	1–12 milliunits/mL	1	1–12 units/L
Postmenopausal	16–66 milliunits/mL	1	16–66 units/L
Lymphocyte count	1.2–3.3 × 10³/µL	10⁶	1.2–3.3 × 10⁹/L
Magnesium	1.3–2.2 mEq/L	0.5	0.65–1.10 mmol/L
	1.58–2.68 mg/dL	0.411	0.65–1.10 mmol/L
Mean corpuscular volume	80.0–97.6 µm³	1	80.0–97.6 fL
Mononuclear cell count	0.2–0.7 × 10³/µL	10⁶	0.2–0.7 × 10⁹/L
Nortriptyline, therapeutic	50–150 ng/mL or mcg/L	3.8	190–570 nmol/L
NT-ProBNP (see Pro-BNP)			
Osmolality (serum)	275–300 mOsm/kg	1	275–300 mmol/kg
Osmolality (urine)	250–900 mOsm/kg	1	250–900 mmol/kg
Parathyroid hormone (PTH), intact	10–60 pg/mL or ng/L	0.107	1.1–6.4 pmol/L
Parathyroid hormone (PTH), N-terminal	8–24 pg/mL or ng/L		
Parathyroid hormone (PTH), C-terminal	50–330 pg/mL or ng/L		
Phenobarbital, therapeutic	15–40 mcg/mL or mg/L	4.31	65–172 µmol/L
Phenytoin, therapeutic	10–20 mcg/mL or mg/L	3.96	40–79 µmol/L
Phosphate	2.5–4.5 mg/dL	0.323	0.81–1.45 mmol/L
Platelet count	140–440 × 10³/µL	10⁶	140–440 × 10⁹/L
Potassium (plasma)	3.3–4.9 mEq/L	1	3.3–4.9 mmol/L
Prealbumin (adult)	19.5–35.8 mg/dL	10	195–358 mg/dL
Primidone, therapeutic	5–12 mcg/mL or mg/L	4.58	23–55 µmol/L
ProBNP	Less than 125 pg/mL or ng/L	0.118	Less than 14.75 pmol/L
Procainamide, therapeutic	4–10 mcg/mL or mg/L	4.23	17–42 µmol/L
Progesterone			
Male	13–97 ng/dL	0.0318	0.4–3.1 nmol/L
Female			
Follicular phase	15–70 ng/dL		0.5–2.2 nmol/L
Luteal phase	200–2500 ng/dL		6.4–79.5 nmol/L
Prolactin	Less than 20 ng/mL	1	Less than 20 mcg/L
Prostate-specific antigen (PSA)	Less than 4 ng/mL	1	Less than 4 mcg/L
Protein, total	6.0–8.0 g/dL	10	60–80 g/L
Prothrombin time (PT)	10–12 seconds		
Quinidine, therapeutic	2–5 mcg/mL or mg/L	3.08	6.2–15.4 µmol/L
Radioactive iodine uptake (RAIU)	Less than 6% in 2 hours		
Red blood cell (RBC) count (blood)			
Male	4–6.2 × 10⁶/µL	10⁶	4–6.2 × 10¹²/L
Female	4–6.2 × 10⁶/µL	10⁶	4–6.2 × 10¹²/L
Pregnant			
Trimester 1	4–5 × 10⁶/µL	10⁶	4–5 × 10¹²/L
Trimester 2	3.2–4.5 × 10⁶/µL	10⁶	3.2–4.5 × 10¹²/L
Trimester 3	3–4.9 × 10⁶/µL	10⁶	3–4.9 × 10¹²/L
Post partum	3.2–5 × 10⁶/µL	10⁶	3.2–5 × 10⁶/L

(continued)